CANCER

Principles and Practice of Oncology

Edited by

Vincent T. DeVita, Jr., M.D.

DIRECTOR, NATIONAL CANCER INSTITUTE
CLINICAL DIRECTOR, NATIONAL CANCER INSTITUTE
BETHESDA, MARYLAND
PROFESSOR OF MEDICINE
GEORGE WASHINGTON UNIVERSITY SCHOOL OF MEDICINE AND HEALTH SCIENCES
WASHINGTON, D.C.

Samuel Hellman, M.D.

DIRECTOR, JOINT CENTER FOR RADIATION THERAPY
ALVAN T. AND VIOLA D. FULLER—
AMERICAN CANCER SOCIETY PROFESSOR AND CHAIRMAN
DEPARTMENT OF RADIATION THERAPY
HARVARD MEDICAL SCHOOL
BOSTON, MASSACHUSETTS

Steven A. Rosenberg, M.D., Ph.D.

CHIEF OF SURGERY
NATIONAL CANCER INSTITUTE
PROFESSOR OF SURGERY
UNIFORMED SERVICES UNIVERSITY OF THE HEALTH SCIENCES SCHOOL OF MEDICINE
BETHESDA, MARYLAND

104 Contributors

CANCER

Principles and Practice of Oncology

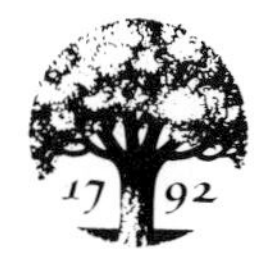

J. B. LIPPINCOTT COMPANY
Philadelphia · Toronto

The authors and publisher have exerted every effort to ensure that drug selection and dosage set forth in this text are in accord with current recommendations and practice at the time of publication. However, in view of ongoing research, changes in government regulations, and the constant flow of information relating to drug therapy and drug reactions, the reader is urged to check the package insert for each drug for any change in indications and dosage and for added warnings and precautions. This is particularly important when the recommended agent is a new or infrequently employed drug.

For information address J. B. Lippincott Company, East Washington Square, Philadelphia, Pennsylvania 19105.

5 6 4

Library of Congress Cataloging in Publication Data
Main entry under title:

Cancer, principles and practice of oncology.

Bibliography
Includes index.
1. Cancer. 2. Oncology. I. DeVita, Vincent T. II. Hellman, Samuel. III. Rosenberg, Steven A.
[DNLM: 1. Neoplasms. QZ 200 C21537]
RC261.C274 616.99'4 81-5974
ISBN 0-397-50440-3 AACR2

Printed in the United States of America

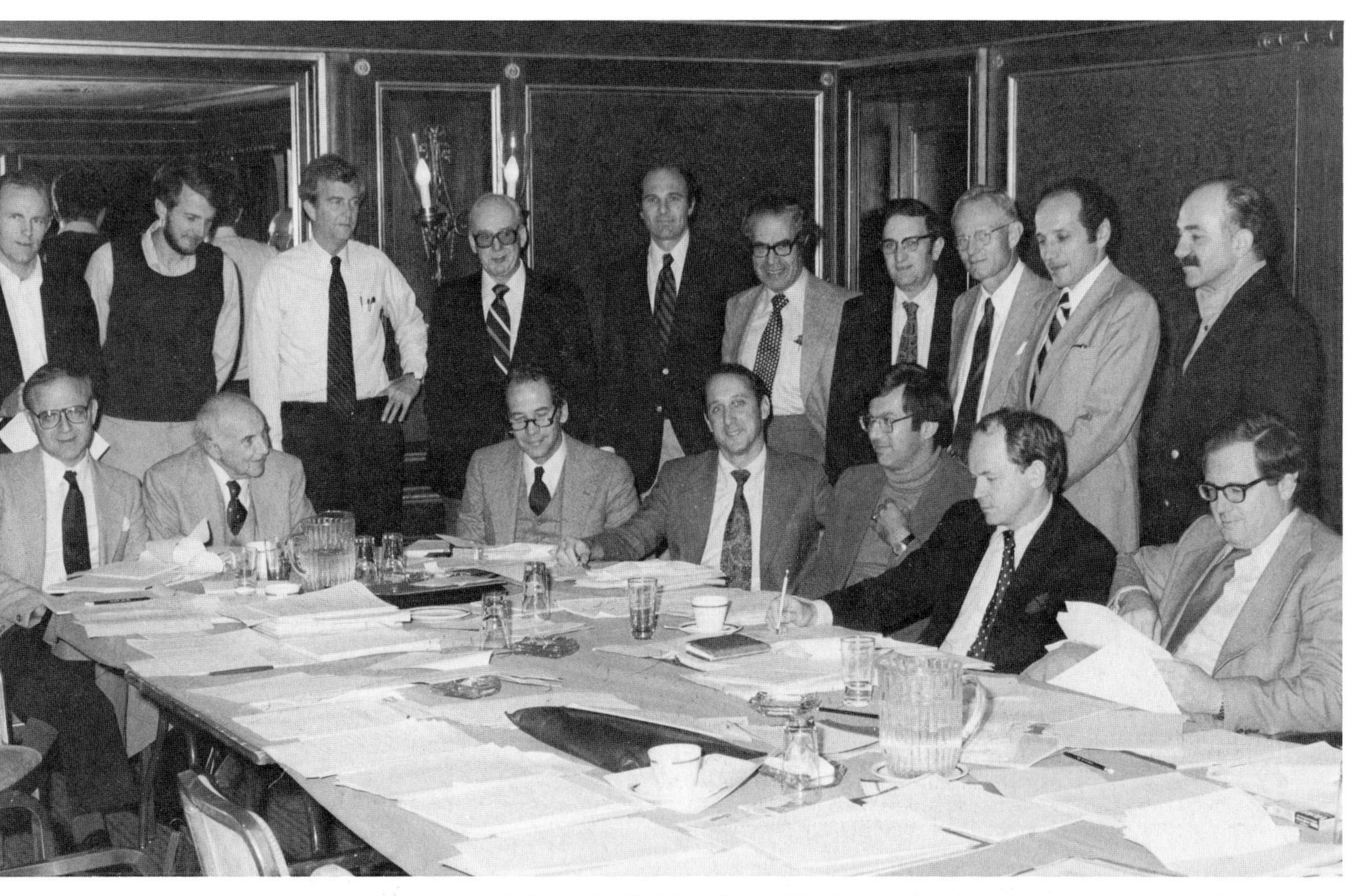

On November 7th, 8th, and 9th, 1979, fifteen prominent American oncologists met in Montreal with the three editors, Vincent T. DeVita, Jr., Samuel Hellman, and Steven A. Rosenberg, to plan a comprehensive book on cancer, emphasizing the integrated use of all available modalities for management of the cancer patient.

Seated, left to right: George P. Canellos, Martin B. Levene, Samuel Hellman, Steven A. Rosenberg, Vincent T. DeVita, Jr., Murray F. Brennan, Alan R. Baker.

Standing, left to right: John S. Macdonald, Paul H. Sugarbaker, David F. Paulson, Daniel E. Bergsagel, John D. Minna, John E. Ultmann, Paul L. Kornblith, Rodney R. Million, Jerry C. Rosenberg, Joseph V. Simone.

Dedicated to

Mary Kay
Rusty
Alice

Contents

PART TWO. Practice of Oncology

13 — 301

Cancer in the Head and Neck

RODNEY R. MILLION
NICHOLAS J. CASSISI
ROBERT E. WITTES

14 — 396

Cancer of the Lung

JOHN D. MINNA
GEORGE A. HIGGINS
ELI J. GLATSTEIN

15 — 475

Neoplasms of the Mediastinum

JERRY C. ROSENBERG

16 — 499

Cancer of the Esophagus

JERRY C. ROSENBERG
JAMES G. SCHWADE
VAINUTIS K. VAITKEVICIUS

21 — 643

Colorectal Cancer

PAUL H. SUGARBAKER
JOHN S. MACDONALD
LEONARD L. GUNDERSON

22 — 724

Cancer of the Anal Region

PAUL H. SUGARBAKER
LEONARD L. GUNDERSON
JOHN S. MACDONALD

23 — 732

Genito-Urinary Malignancies

DAVID F. PAULSON
CARLOS A. PEREZ
TOM ANDERSON

24 — 786

Cancer of the Testis

DAVID F. PAULSON
LAURENCE H. EINHORN
MICHAEL J. PECKHAM
STEPHEN D. WILLIAMS

25 — 823

Gynecologic Tumors

CARLOS A. PEREZ
ROBERT C. KNAPP
ROBERT C. YOUNG

26 — 884

Cancer of the Ovary

ROBERT C. YOUNG
ROBERT C. KNAPP
CARLOS A. PEREZ

27 — 914

Cancer of the Breast

SAMUEL HELLMAN
JAY R. HARRIS
GEORGE P. CANELLOS
BERNARD FISHER

28 — 971

Cancer of the Endocrine System

MURRAY F. BRENNAN

32 — 1171

Intraocular Melanomas

DANIEL M. ALBERT

33 — 1181

Neoplasms of the Central Nervous System

PAUL L. KORNBLITH
MICHAEL D. WALKER
J. ROBERT CASSADY

34 — 1254

Cancers of Childhood

JOSEPH V. SIMONE
J. ROBERT CASSADY
ROBERT M. FILLER

35 — 1331

Hodgkin's Disease and the Non-Hodgkin's Lymphomas

VINCENT T. DEVITA, JR.
SAMUEL HELLMAN

36 — 1402

Acute Leukemias of Adults

PETER H. WIERNIK

37 1427

Chronic Leukemias

GEORGE P. CANELLOS

38 1439

Plasma Cell Neoplasms

DANIEL E. BERGSAGEL
WALTER D. RIDER

39 1476

Paraneoplastic Syndromes

JOHN D. MINNA
PAUL A. BUNN, JR.

40 1518

Management of the Patient with Cancer of Unknown Primary Site

JOHN E. ULTMANN
THEODORE L. PHILLIPS

41 1534

Treatment of Metastatic Cancer

JOHN E. ULTMANN
THEODORE L. PHILLIPS

43 1628

Supportive Care of the Cancer Patient

44 1677

Management of Infections of the Cancer Patient

45 1703

Management of the Adverse Effects of Treatment

Associate Editors

Surgery

MURRAY F. BRENNAN, M.D.

Attending Surgeon
Memorial Sloan–Kettering Cancer Center
Professor of Surgery
Cornell University
New York, New York

BERNARD FISHER, M.D.

Professor of Surgery
Department of Surgery
University of Pittsburgh School of Medicine
Pittsburgh, Pennsylvania

PAUL H. SUGARBAKER, M.D.

Senior Investigator
Surgery Branch
National Cancer Institute
National Institutes of Health
Assistant Professor of Surgery
Uniformed Services University School of the Health Sciences
Bethesda, Maryland

Radiation Therapy

RODNEY R. MILLION, M.D.

American Cancer Society
Professor of Clinical Oncology
Professor and Chief
Division of Radiation Therapy
University of Florida
Gainesville, Florida

CARLOS A. PEREZ, M.D.

Professor of Radiology
Director
Division of Radiation Oncology
Mallinckrodt Institute of Radiology
Washington University School of Medicine
Saint Louis, Missouri

THEODORE L. PHILLIPS, M.D.

Professor of Radiation Oncology
Department of Radiation Oncology
University of California, San Francisco
San Francisco, California

Medical Oncology

DANIEL E. BERGSAGEL, M.D., D. Phil.

Professor of Medicine
University of Toronto
Chief of Medicine
Princess Margaret Hospital
Toronto, Ontario, Canada

GEORGE P. CANELLOS, M.D.

Chief of Medical Oncology
Sidney Farber Cancer Institute
Boston, Massachusetts

JOHN E. ULTMANN, M.D.

Professor of Medicine
Director
Cancer Research Center
Division of Biological Sciences
University of Chicago
Pritzker School of Medicine
Chicago, Illinois

Contributors

ROSS A. ABRAMS, M.D.
Assistant Professor of Medicine
Hematology/Oncology Section
Medical College of Wisconsin
Milwaukee County Medical Complex
Froedtert Memorial Lutheran Hospital
Milwaukee Children's Hospital
Blood Center of Southeastern Wisconsin
Milwaukee, Wisconsin

MARTIN A. ADSON, M.D.
Professor of Surgery
Mayo Medical School
Consultant
Department of Surgery
Mayo Clinic and Foundation
Rochester, Minnesota

DANIEL M. ALBERT, M.D.
Professor of Ophthalmology
Harvard Medical School
Associate Surgeon and Director
Eye Pathology Laboratory
Massachusetts Eye and Ear Infirmary
Boston, Massachusetts

TOM ANDERSON, M.D.
Chief, Section of Hematology/Oncology
The Medical College of Wisconsin
Milwaukee County Medical Complex
Milwaukee, Wisconsin

ALAN R. BAKER, M.D.
Senior Investigator
Surgery Branch
National Cancer Institute
Bethesda, Maryland

LAURENCE H. BAKER, D.O.
Professor and Associate Chairman
Department of Oncology
Wayne State University School of Medicine
Coordinator of Cancer Programs
Wayne State University
Deputy Director
Comprehensive Cancer Center of Metropolitan Detroit
Detroit, Michigan

WILLIAM D. BLOOMER, M.D.
Associate Professor of Radiation Therapy
Harvard Medical School
Boston, Massachusetts

W. BRYANT BOUTWELL, M.P.H.
Division of Cancer Prevention
The University of Texas System Cancer Center
M. D. Anderson Hospital and Tumor Institute
Houston, Texas

DONN G. BOYLE
Cancer Research Scientist
Division of Radiation Biology
Roswell Park Memorial Institute
Buffalo, New York

EVELYN S. BRANYON, M.P.H.
Division of Cancer Prevention
The University of Texas System Cancer Center
M. D. Anderson Hospital and Tumor Institute
Houston, Texas

PAUL A. BUNN, JR., M.D.
Senior Investigator
National Cancer Institute–Navy Medical Oncology Branch
Division of Cancer Treatment
National Cancer Institute
National Naval Medical Center
Bethesda, Maryland

CHARLES V. BURTON, M.D.
Director
Department of Neuroaugmentation
Sister Kenny Institute
Minneapolis, Minnesota

STEVEN C. CARABELL, M.D.
Associate Professor
Division of Radiation Oncology
Department of Radiology
George Washington University Medical Center
Washington, D.C.

J. ROBERT CASSADY, M.D.
Associate Professor of Radiation Therapy
Joint Center for Radiation Therapy
Harvard Medical School
Children's Hospital Medical Center
Boston, Massachusetts

NICHOLAS J. CASSISI, D.D.S., M.D.
Professor
Division of Otolaryngology
Department of Surgery
Chief
Division of Otolaryngology
Professor
Gainesville Veterans Administration Hospital
Gainesville, Florida

BRUCE A. CHABNER, M.D.
Associate Director
Clinical Oncology Program
Division of Cancer Treatment
National Cancer Institute
Bethesda, Maryland

VINCENT P. CHUANG, M.D.
Professor of Radiology
Head
Special Procedure Section
Department of Diagnostic Radiology
The University of Texas System Cancer Center
M. D. Anderson Hospital and Tumor Institute
Houston, Texas

ISIDORE COHN, JR., M.D., D.Sc.
Professor and Chairman
Department of Surgery
Louisiana State University School of Medicine
New Orleans, Louisiana

CAROL M. CRONIN, M.S.
Clinical Research Assistant and Consultant
Sidney Farber Cancer Institute
Boston, Massachusetts

ALBERT DEISSEROTH, M.D., Ph.D.
Head
Experimental Hematology Section
National Cancer Institute
Bethesda, Maryland

JOEL A. DELISA, M.D.
Associate Chief of Staff/Education
Veterans Administration Medical Center
Associate Professor
Department of Rehabilitation Medicine
University of Washington
Seattle, Washington

THOMAS J. DOUGHERTY, Ph.D.
Head
Division of Radiation Biology
Department of Radiation Medicine
Roswell Park Memorial Institute
Buffalo, New York

N. REED DUNNICK, M.D.
Associate Professor
Department of Radiology
Duke University Medical Center
Durham, North Carolina

LAURENCE H. EINHORN, M.D.
Professor of Medicine
Indiana University Medical Center
Indianapolis, Indiana

ISAIAH J. FIDLER, D.V.M., Ph.D.
Director
Cancer Metastasis and Treatment Laboratory
Frederick Cancer Research Center
Frederick, Maryland

ANTHONY L. A. FIELDS, M.D.
Assistant Professor
Division of Medical Oncology
Faculty of Medicine
University of Alberta
Physician
Cross Cancer Institute
Edmonton, Alberta, Canada

ROBERT M. FILLER, M.D.
Surgeon-in-Chief
The Hospital for Sick Children
Professor of Surgery
University of Toronto
Toronto, Ontario, Canada

M. WAYNE FLYE, M.D., Ph.D.
Associate Professor of General and Thoracic Surgery
Associate Professor of Microbiology (Immunology)
Director
Vascular Surgical Service
University of Texas Medical Branch
Galveston, Texas

JAMES H. FOSTER, M.D.
Professor and Chairman
Department of Surgery
University of Connecticut School of Medicine
Farmington, Connecticut

ELI J. GLATSTEIN, M.D.
Chief
Radiation Oncology Branch
Clinical Oncology Program
Division of Cancer Treatment
National Cancer Institute
Bethesda, Maryland

ALFRED L. GOLDSON, M.D.
Chairman
Department of Radiotherapy
Howard University Hospital and
Regional Cancer Research Center
Washington, D.C.

ROBERT M. GOLDWYN, M.D.
Clinical Professor of Surgery
Harvard Medical School
Surgeon
Brigham and Women's Hospital
Head
Division of Plastic Surgery
Beth Israel Hospital
Boston, Massachusetts

ROBERT L. GOODMAN, M.D.
Professor and Chairman
Department of Radiation Therapy
University of Pennsylvania School of Medicine
Fox Chase Cancer Center
Philadelphia, Pennsylvania

LEONARD L. GUNDERSON, M.D.
Consultant in Therapeutic Radiology
Mayo Clinic
Associate Professor in Oncology
Mayo Medical School
Rochester, Minnesota

GEORGE M. HAHN, Ph.D.
Associate Professor of Radiology
Stanford University
Palo Alto, California

JAY R. HARRIS, M.D.
Department of Radiation Therapy
Harvard Medical School
Joint Center for Radiation Therapy
Boston, Massachusetts

IAN R. HART, B.V.Sc., Ph.D.
Cancer Metastasis and Treatment Laboratory
Frederick Cancer Research Center
Frederick, Maryland

ANDREA S. HAY, M.S.S.A
Clinical Social Worker
Social Work Department
Clinical Center
National Institutes of Health
Lanham, Maryland

HARLEY A. HAYNES, M.D.
Director
Dermatology Division
Department of Medicine
Brigham and Women's Hospital
Associate Professor of Dermatology
Harvard Medical School
Boston, Massachusetts

JANE E. HENNEY, M.D.
Special Assistant for Clinical Affairs
Division of Cancer Treatment
National Cancer Institute
Bethesda, Maryland

STEPHEN P. HERSH, M.D.
Chairperson
Saint Jude Scientific Advisory Board
Saint Jude Children's Research Hospital
Memphis, Tennessee

GEORGE A. HIGGINS, M.D.
Veterans Administration Surgical Oncology Group
Professor of Surgery
Georgetown Medical School
Clinical Professor of Surgery
George Washington Medical School
Washington, D.C.

RICHARD J. HODES, M.D.
Chief
Immunological Therapy Section
Immunology Branch
National Cancer Institute
Bethesda, Maryland

SUSAN MOLLOY HUBBARD, B.S., R.N.
Chief
Scientific Information Branch
Division of Cancer Treatment
National Cancer Institute
Bethesda, Maryland

NASSER JAVADPOUR, M.D.
Senior Investigator and Staff Urologist
National Cancer Institute
Bethesda, Maryland

ROBERT G. JOSSE, M.B.
Assistant Professor of Medicine
University of Toronto
Staff Endocrinologist
Saint Michael's Hospital
Toronto, Ontario, Canada

HARRY R. KATZ, M.D.
Assistant Professor of Radiation Therapy
University of Pennsylvania School of Medicine
Associate Radiotherapist
Fox Chase Cancer Center
Philadelphia, Pennsylvania

ROBERT C. KNAPP, M.D.
Professor of Gynecology
Harvard Medical School
Director
Gynecologic Oncology and Gynecologic Surgery
Brigham and Women's Hospital
Boston, Massachusetts

PAUL L. KORNBLITH, M.D.
Chief
Surgical Neurology Branch
National Institute of Neurological and Communicative Disorders and Stroke
Bethesda, Maryland

MARTIN B. LEVENE, M.D. (deceased)
Deputy Director
Joint Center for Radiation Therapy
Associate Professor of Radiation Therapy
Harvard Medical School
Boston, Massachusetts

BRIAN J. LEWIS, M.D.
Associate Clinical Professor of Medicine
Cancer Research Institute
Department of Medicine
University of California, San Francisco
San Francisco, California

FREDERICK P. LI, M.D.
Clinical Studies Section
National Cancer Institute
Bethesda, Maryland
Division of Biostatistics and Epidemiology
Sidney Farber Cancer Institute
Boston, Massachusetts

JOHN S. MACDONALD, M.D.
Associate Director
Cancer Therapy Evaluation Program
Division of Cancer Treatment
National Cancer Institute
Bethesda, Maryland

MICHAEL J. MASTRANGELO, M.D.
Department of Medicine
Fox Chase Cancer Center
Temple University School of Medicine
Philadelphia, Pennsylvania

PETER M. MAUCH, M.D.
Assistant Professor
Harvard Joint Center for Radiation Therapy
Department of Radiation Therapy
Harvard Medical School
Boston, Massachusetts

ROSALIE RAPS MELNICK, Ph.D.
Coordinator
Rehabilitation Medicine Service
Veterans Administration Medical Center
Clinical Instructor
Department of Rehabilitation Medicine
University of Washington
Seattle, Washington

MARY ANN MIKULIC, M.N., R.N.
Rehabilitation Nurse Clinical Specialist
Veterans Administration Medical Center
Clinical Assistant Professor
Department of Physical Medicine and Rehabilitation
School of Medicine
Clinical Assistant Professor
Department of Physiological Nursing
School of Nursing
University of Washington
Seattle, Washington

ROBERT M. MILLER, Ph.D.
Speech Pathologist
Veterans Administration Medical Center
Clinical Assistant Professor
Department of Speech and Hearing Sciences
University of Washington
Seattle, Washington

JOHN D. MINNA, M.D.
Chief
National Cancer Institute–Navy Medical Oncology Branch
Division of Cancer Treatment
National Cancer Institute
National Naval Medical Center
Bethesda, Maryland

DEXTER L. MORRIS, Ph.D.
Division of Cancer Prevention
The University of Texas System Cancer Center
M. D. Anderson Hospital and Tumor Institute
Houston, Texas

CHARLES E. MYERS, M.D.
Chief
Clinical Pharmacology Branch
Attending Physician
Medicine Branch
Clinical Oncology Program
Division of Clinical Treatment
National Cancer Institute
Bethesda, Maryland

GUY R. NEWELL, M.D.
Division of Cancer Prevention
The University of Texas System Cancer Center
M. D. Anderson Hospital and Tumor Institute
Houston, Texas

ARTHUR B. PARDEE, Ph.D.
Sidney Farber Cancer Institute
Chief
Division of Cell Growth and Regulation
Professor of Pharmacology
Harvard Medical School
Boston, Massachusetts

DAVID F. PAULSON, M.D.
Professor and Chairman
Division of Urology
Duke University Medical Center
Durham, North Carolina

MICHAEL J. PECKHAM, M.D.
Professor of Radiotherapy
Institute of Cancer Research
The Royal Marsden Hospital
London, England

DAVID A. PISTENMAA, M.D.
Chief
Radiotherapy Development Branch
Cancer Therapy Evaluation Program
Division of Cancer Treatment
National Cancer Institute
Bethesda, Maryland

PHILIP A. PIZZO, M.D.
Head
Infectious Disease Section
Pediatric Oncology Branch
National Cancer Institute
Bethesda, Maryland

EUGENE A. QUINDLEN, M.D.
Attending Neurosurgeon
Clinical Center
Surgical Neurology Branch
National Institute of Neurological and Communicative Diso and Stroke
Bethesda, Maryland
Assistant Clinical Professor of Neurosurgery
George Washington University Hospital
Washington, D.C.

CHARLES D. RAY, M.D.
Senior Consulting Neurosurgeon
Sister Kenny Institute
Clinical Associate Professor
Department of Neurosurgery
University of Minnesota
Minneapolis, Minnesota

WALTER D. RIDER, M.B., Ch.B.
Head
Radiation Oncology
Princess Margaret Hospital
Professor of Radiology
Associate Professor of Medical Biophysics
University of Toronto
Toronto, Ontario, Canada

GERALD ROSEN, M.D.
Department of Pediatrics and Medicine
Memorial Sloan-Kettering Cancer Center
New York, New York

JERRY C. ROSENBERG, M.D., Ph.D.
Chief of Surgery
Hutzel Hospital
Professor of Surgery
Wayne State University
Detroit, Michigan

STEPHEN E. SALLAN, M.D.
Clinical Director
Pediatric Oncology
Sidney Farber Cancer Institute
Children's Hospital Medical Center
Assistant Professor of Pediatrics
Harvard Medical School
Boston, Massachusetts

WENDY S. SCHAIN, Ed.D.
Rehabilitation Department
Medical Care Consultant
Clinical Center
National Institutes of Health
Bethesda, Maryland

RICHARD L. SCHILSKY, M.D.
Medical Service
Harry S Truman Veterans Administration Hospital
Columbia, Missouri

JAMES G. SCHWADE, M.D.
Head
Radiobiology Section
Radiation Oncology Branch
Division of Cancer Treatment
National Cancer Institute
Bethesda, Maryland
Assistant Professor
Department of Radiation Oncology
University of California, San Francisco
San Francisco, California

CLAUDIA A. SEIPP, R.N.
Clinical Nurse Specialist for Surgical Oncology
Surgery Branch
National Cancer Institute
Clinical Center Nursing Department
National Institutes of Health
Bethesda, Maryland

RICHARD J. SHERINS, M.D.
Senior Investigator
Developmental Endocrinology Branch
National Institute of Child Health and Human Development
Bethesda, Maryland

RICHARD M. SIMON, Ph.D.
Chief
Biometric Research Branch
Division of Cancer Treatment
National Cancer Institute
Bethesda, Maryland

JOSEPH V. SIMONE, M.D.
Associate Director for Clinical Research
Saint Jude's Children's Research Hospital
University of Tennessee Center for the Health Sciences
Memphis, Tennessee

WILLIAM F. SINDELAR, M.D., Ph.D.
Surgery Branch
National Cancer Institute
Bethesda, Maryland

EVERETT V. SUGARBAKER, M.D.
Director
Surgical Oncology
Miami Cancer Institute
Miami, Florida

HERMAN D. SUIT, M.D., D. Phil.
Chief
Department of Radiation Medicine
Massachusetts General Hospital
Professor of Radiation Therapy
Harvard Medical School
Boston, Massachusetts

WILLIAM D. TERRY, M.D.
Chief
Immunology Branch
National Cancer Institute
Bethesda, Maryland

BARBARA C. TILLEY, Ph.D.
Division of Cancer Prevention
The University of Texas System Cancer Center
M. D. Anderson Hospital and Tumor Institute
Houston, Texas

ARTHUR C. UPTON, M.D.
Professor and Chairman
Department of Environmental Medicine
New York University Medical Center
New York, New York

VAINUTIS K. VAITKEVICIUS, M.D.
Professor and Chairman
Department of Oncology
Wayne State University School of Medicine
Detroit, Michigan

MICHAEL D. WALKER, M.D.
Director
Stroke and Trauma Program
National Institute of Neurological and Communicative Disorders and Stroke
Bethesda, Maryland

SIDNEY WALLACE, M.D.
Professor of Radiology
Deputy Head
Department of Diagnostic Radiology
The University of Texas System Cancer Center
Houston, Texas

KENNETH R. WEISHAUPT, M.D.
Cancer Research Scientist
Division of Radiation Biology
Roswell Park Memorial Institute
Buffalo, New York

PETER H. WIERNIK, M.D.
Professor of Medicine
University of Maryland School of Medicine
Director
Baltimore Cancer Research Program
National Cancer Institute
Baltimore, Maryland

STEPHEN D. WILLIAMS, M.D.
Assistant Professor of Medicine
Indiana University Medical Center
Indianapolis, Indiana

RICHARD E. WILSON, M.D.
Professor of Surgery
Chief
Surgical Oncology
Brigham and Women's Hospital
Sidney Farber Cancer Institute
Boston, Massachusetts

ROBERT E. WITTES, M.D.
Associate Attending Physician
Department of Medicine
Memorial Sloan-Kettering Cancer Center
New York, New York

ROBERT C. YOUNG, M.D.
Chief
Medicine Branch
National Cancer Institute
Bethesda, Maryland

Publisher's Foreword

The development of the manuscript on a fundamental subject in medicine remained the same for generations. An authority in a given field, acting as editor, would originate the concept for a new book. He would select contributors to write separate chapters. In the fullness of time—often a *long* time—the chapters would be written and delivered to the editor. Even though he might review and change the written text, the published book remained a collection of these separate chapters. That textbooks are too often "a sum of parts" rather than "a divisible, integrated whole" has plagued generations of medical students and practitioners.

Over two years ago, Drs. DeVita, Hellman, and Rosenberg proposed to the publisher that enlightened and effective oncologic therapy required a comprehensive text that would offer a true integration of what was known of the principal treatment modalities—surgery, radiotherapy, and chemotherapy. As they point out in the preface to this work, "treatment modalities have been refined to the point that all produce significant positive results by themselves," but that "the best treatment a cancer patient can receive is the balanced application of some of each. . . ."

To realize the editors' objective of integration, the book would have to be written as a divisible whole and not as a sum of parts. How could this be realized when the complexities of the subject required the collaboration of 104 specialists?

Before any text was written, the editors met with 19 contributors in Montreal, Quebec. During intensive sessions that lasted all day and into the night for three full days, each topic, and each subtopic in each chapter, was subjected to evaluation and criticism. The meeting was a learning experience for everyone. The concept for the book did not change in those three days, but the means of its implementation did. Only after this meeting was the final table of contents decided upon. Contributors were chosen. Each contributor received a copy of the entire table of contents. Chapters were drafted and redrafted. Prior to acceptance of the text and illustrations, the editors met with the editorial representatives of the publisher for one week. During that intensive week all chapters were critically reviewed by each editor. Only after subsequent revision was the manuscript delivered to the publisher.

Revision and correction continued during in-house redaction and production, with the result that the text before you contains today's most accurate and useful information.

The increasing complexities of medical teaching and practice have placed new burdens on authors and publishers alike. We hope that our publishing efforts will stand as a complement to the efforts of all 104 contributors, and that CANCER: PRINCIPLES AND PRACTICE OF ONCOLOGY is now an instrument that will benefit all cancer patients.

The Publisher

Preface

The management of cancer has changed dramatically during the past two decades. Treatment modalities have been refined to the point that all produce significant positive results by themselves. The most important advance, however, has come from the realization that often the best treatment a cancer patient can receive is the balanced application of some of each: surgery, radiation therapy, and chemotherapy. Thus the need has existed for a book that stresses the integrated management of the cancer patient.

In November 1979, the three editors met with 15 prominent oncologists to plan a book that considered the integrated multidisciplinary approach to cancer, which became the basis of this volume. Freshness of information has been a major concern, and unusually tight writing, editing, and publication deadlines were imposed to ensure up-to-date discussions of each subject. This book has been extensively referenced, and the bibliography after each chapter serves to validate and to amplify the information presented.

The book is divided into two major parts. The first section, Principles of Oncology, covers aspects of the cause and evolution of cancer as a biologic phenomenon and the essential principles that serve as the underpinning of modern cancer diagnosis and treatment. The second section, Practice of Oncology, deals with the management of the specific cancers themselves, the complications that cancers cause, and the complications of therapy. The unique feature of the book is that each disease-oriented chapter has been prepared by cancer specialists in each of the treatment modalities and tightly edited by the three editors to conform to the standards of accuracy and practicality we believe are essential elements of a comprehensive textbook on cancer.

A word about how to use the text: The emphasis in the practice section is on treatment planning, and in each of the major specialties a consistent format is followed.

Advances in surgical technique have led to the introduction of new or alternative therapies that have had increased effectiveness or diminished adverse impact on the quality of life. Chapter 6, Principles of Surgical Oncology, outlines the underlying principles of modern surgery as applied to the patient with cancer. The surgical approaches to each cancer have been carefully integrated into each of the disease-oriented chapters. Anatomical considerations are of major importance to overall treatment planning and an understanding of the natural spread of each type of cancer, and they should be familiar to all oncologists. In considering the treatment of each individual type of cancer, the anatomical bases that underlie the natural history of each cancer have been presented in simple diagrams. An attempt has been made to present, in sufficient detail, the major surgical procedures used to treat cancer so as to familiarize the nonsurgeon with the steps of the operative procedure and as a basis for understanding the advantages, limitations, possible complications, and ultimate morbidity of each major surgical operation. The operative diagrams presented are unique in a general oncologic textbook and will serve as an important guide to all oncologists. Surgical options available for the treatment of individual cancers are presented along with modifications of surgery required by the application of other treatment modalities. Operative risks and morbidity that weigh in the decision to use surgery in specific clinical situations are discussed. Surgical considerations have been woven throughout the book, and, where appropriate, the role of surgery in patient palliation and rehabilitation has been considered, along with other treatment options.

Because the major effects of radiotherapy are on the reproductive viability of the cells irradiated, the reader should be acquainted with the principles of cellular proliferation. In Chapter 4, Kinetics of Cellular Proliferation, and Chapter 7, Principles of Radiation Therapy, are described the basic physics and cell biology needed to understand the effects of radiation on tumors and normal tissues. In the practice section of the book are described the indications and uses of radiation therapy alone and in combination with other modalities for each major disease. Explanations of treatment technique, including the prescription, treatment plan, dose distribution, and portal films, are included in a form accessible to the radiation-therapist and nonradiation therapist. The use of radiation therapy in special or emergency circumstances is discussed in Chapters 40 through 42. Some of the newer methods of radiation are discussed as they are relevant to individual diseases, and a number have been separately highlighted in Chapter 48, Newer Methods of Cancer Treatment.

The chemotherapy data are organized into four distinct areas that should facilitate their understanding and use. The major principles guiding the development of chemotherapy as a discipline are covered in Chapter 8, Principles of Chemotherapy, and in Chapter 4, Kinetics of Cellular Proliferation, whereas the details of pharmacokinetics, metabolism, excretion, and mechanism of action of anticancer drugs are discussed in Chapter 9, Clinical Pharmacology of Cancer Chemotherapy. Physicians can identify specific drugs, or combinations of drugs, the indications for their use, and their therapeutic effects in the disease-oriented chapters. Detailed treatment plans indicating doses and schedules are arrayed in these chapters in tabular form. Practical points in the administration of these drugs are given in Chapter 47, Administration of Cancer Treatments: Practical Guide for Physicians and Oncology Nurses, along with the common side effects of chemotherapy and how to deal with them.

The emphasis throughout the practice section of the book is on how each type of therapy interacts and complements the others. The goal of this book is to present the broad scope of modern oncology in a cohesive fashion to help all physicians consider and select the best approach to the management of patients with cancer.

Vincent T. DeVita, Jr., M.D.
Samuel Hellman, M.D.
Steven A. Rosenberg, M.D., Ph.D.

Acknowledgments

The editors are grateful to several people whose excellent help contributed to this book.

Alice Rosenberg assumed responsibility for the overall compilation of the contributions to this volume and for many of the organizational details involved in assembling this book.

Sally Gwin, administrative assistant to Dr. Samuel Hellman, contributed to the editing and compilation of many of the manuscripts.

Susan Hubbard, Chief, Scientific Information Branch, National Cancer Institute, contributed important editorial assistance.

Stuart Freeman, Editor-in-Chief, Medical Books, and Lisa Biello, Editor, Medical Books, provided valuable help and worked closely with the editors from the book's inception to its completion.

CANCER

Principles and Practice of Oncology

PART ONE

PRINCIPLES OF ONCOLOGY

Guy R. Newell
W. Bryant Boutwell
Dexter L. Morris
Barbara C. Tilley
Evelyn S. Branyon

CHAPTER 1

Epidemiology of Cancer

Cancer epidemiology, an analytical discipline focusing on the patterns of distribution of neoplasia in humans, is primarily concerned with disease as it manifests itself in populations as opposed to individuals, and its primary goal is prevention rather than cure.

It has been stated recently that epidemiologic studies have contributed to knowledge of cancer in five ways.[1]

1. By demonstrating geographical and temporal variations in incidence.
2. By correlating incidence in different communities with the prevalence of social habits and environmental agents.
3. By comparing the experience of persons with and without cancer.
4. By intervening to remove suspected agents and observing the results.
5. By making quantitative observations that test the applicability to humans of models of the mechanism by which the disease is produced.

Historically, epidemiology has evolved in relation to the study of acute, infectious disease.[2] In industrialized countries, however, chronic, noninfectious diseases such as cancer and cardiovascular disease have increased in both relative and absolute importance, resulting in a shift of interest among many epidemiologists. As a result, we are witnessing today a trend toward specialization in epidemiology, with a growing emphasis in the area of chronic diseases.

On the surface, identifying the cause of a chronic disease appears to be a simple task. Unfortunately, cancer, like most other chronic diseases, rarely has a single cause. Rather, the cancer epidemiologist must address a number of confounding or intervening factors, including differences in age, sex, race, life-style, genetic background, patient's state of health, and exposure to one or more cancer-causing agents. In addition, cancer is by no means a single disease, but rather a group of more than 100 pathologically and epidemiologically distinct diseases.[3] Thus, cancer epidemiology calls for a strong combination of logical thought, medical knowledge, and biostatistics.

Generally, investigators use one of three rather different classes of epidemiologic studies in their work, some of which will be discussed in greater detail in other portions of this chapter.[4]

- Descriptive studies on the distribution and progression of disease in populations.
- Analytical studies of hypotheses suggested by the descriptive studies.
- Experimental or intervention studies of the effect on the population of manipulating environmental influences thought to be harmful, or by introducing in a controlled way preventive, curative, or ameliorative services.

This chapter focuses on the basic principles of cancer epidemiology. Our goal is to provide a working knowledge of selected epidemiologic principles as they relate to oncology. Included are sections on epidemiologic principles, study designs, statistical procedures, data sources, incidence and mortality, and screening. The contributions of epidemiology to environmental carcinogenesis have recently been reviewed.[5] The following chapter focuses on cancer etiology per se.

This chapter is not intended to substitute for entire epidemiology textbooks devoted to detailed treatment of methods and statistical testing. It does provide, however, a better understanding of epidemiology as it relates to cancer and a list of references for the reader who needs more detailed information on the subject.

HISTORICAL HIGHLIGHTS

The foundations of medicine and science were laid in 500 B.C. in Greece in the narrative descriptions and historical accounts of epidemics. There the practice of medicine became separated from religion and philosophy but kept an association in both. The scope of observational medicine was born based upon prognosis by the natural history of disease as described by the Hippocratic writings, which are filled with descriptions and accounts of various epidemics.[6]

The word "epidemiology" is derived from the Greek: "epi" means "on, above, over"; "demos" means "people"; "logos" means "study." Hence it is a science concerned with the understanding of all factors related to the occurrence of disease among groups of people. It involves the study of populations, both the sick and the well, and their relationships to each other and to the environmental facts of the population.

Fox has observed the following.[2]

> Epidemiology is not the proprietor of a well-defined and homogenous body of knowledge as is the case with a basic or pure science such as chemistry. Rather, epidemiology is a discipline which has evolved relatively specialized methods for investigating disease causation and bringing to bear, according to needs of the moment, specific knowledge and special skills from many other sciences. With some justice, epidemiology has been called a method rather than an independent science.

In the beginning, epidemiologic investigations were oriented solely to infectious diseases because of their importance. More recently, with the ever-growing importance of noninfectious diseases, investigations have been directed toward their control as well. Today, epidemiology embraces all illnesses, with a growing emphasis on chronic diseases such as cancer. Application of epidemiologic knowledge is directed primarily to the control and ultimate prevention of disease occurrence. Thus, it has become one of the basic principles for the practice of oncology.

It was Hippocrates (c. 460–c. 370) who first described cancer by the terms "carcinos" and "carcinoma" and defined its grave prognosis.[7] Using his observational approach to medicine, Hippocrates set the foundation of epidemiology inwards and first described the general concept of environmental influences on disease. The four elements—air, fire, earth, and water—were thought to have biologic counterparts that, in combinations, produced the qualities of heat, cold, wetness, and dryness. Black bile, a subtance thought to be produced by the spleen and the stomach, was thought to be the etiologic agent of cancer for several thousand years.[8] Galen, a physician–scientist who was the most prominent medical authority before the Renaissance, concurred with Hippocrates that cancer was caused by excess black bile and noted it should be left alone without treatment.

STATISTICS

Statistics of people were the subject of many treatises published late in the 16th and 17th centuries. In England, for example, statistical analysis of production and population began in the 17th century with the works of John Graunt and William Petty.[7] *The Bills of Mortality*, published weekly in London, began at the end of the 16th century. Eventually, these bills became a measure of morbidity and mortality but were not used statistically until John Graunt's treatise on vital statistics in 1772. Graunt studied the Bills to ascertain birth, death, morbidity rates, and therefore the health of the community. Graunt found a higher rate of male than female births, a high rate of infant and child mortality, and a higher rate of urban than rural deaths. Although Graunt appears to have grasped the significance of biostatistics, it was William Petty who used these data to urge the passage of laws and regulations to foster public health.

Not until Fanchou gathered statistical data around Paris between 1830 and 1840 and Rigoni-Stern collected data around Verona between 1760 and 1839 did cancer statistics emerge in the modern sense.[9,10] Rigoni-Stern's analysis of data by age, sex, occupation, and other features resembles modern demographic studies on cancer. He first noted that the incidence of cancer generally increases with age; the frequency of breast cancer is inversely related to the incidence of uterine cancer for different age groups; unmarried women have a greater chance of contracting cancer, especially breast cancer; married women contract uterine cancer more than do unmarried women; cancer is generally more frequent in cities than in suburbs; and cancer of different anatomic sites probably has different causes.[11]

The need for reliable cancer statistics became increasingly apparent during the first decade of the 20th century. In 1915 Hoffman, a statistician for the Prudential Insurance Company of America, published a monumental compilation of cancer statistics available thoughout the world.[12] Hoffman was instrumental in having the U.S. Census Bureau analyze cancer mortality in registration areas of the United States for 1914. This eventually led to field surveys of cancer incidence in 1937 by Harold Dorn.[13] Greenwood, a British epidemiologist and statistician, analyzed data on survival of untreated patients with cancer, and from this came the concept of 5-year cures.[14]

BREAST CANCER

Bernadino Ramazzini in 1713 first noted that breast cancer was found more frequently among nuns than among other women.[15] In 1913 Stevenson found that breast cancer mortality rates were higher for single than for married women after age 45.[16] The first case-control study of breast cancer was done in 1926 by Lane-Claypon, who demonstrated differences in marital and reproductive histories and evidence of familiality between English women with breast cancer and control subjects.[17] This stimulated many other studies of breast cancer. DeWaard first presented data supporting a different etiology for premenopausal and postmenopausal breast cancer, while Staszewski found a relationship between breast cancer and age at menarche.[18] That lower rates of breast cancer found in parous women were not related to the number of children but rather to the mother's age at first pregnancy was first noted in 1960 by MacMahon and associates.[19]

CERVICAL CANCER

In 1931 Smith conducted the first case-control study on the relation of cervical cancer and socioeconomic status and found that the highest rates for the disease were among the lower classes.[20] Logan in 1949 reported that the lowest rates of cervical cancer were among single women and the highest rates were among parous women and widowed women.[21] Other studies, suggesting that cultural or possibly genetic factors may be related to disease, reported a rarity of cervical cancer among Jewish women.[22] Evidence that a sexually released factor might be important in the etiology of cervical cancer was reported by Ganon and Røjel.[23,24] In the study conducted by Ganon no cases of cervical cancer were found over a 20-year period among nuns in Canadian convents. The importance of the role of sexual activity in cervical cancer etiology was suggested by Røjel, who reported a more significant proportion of prostitutes among cervical cancer patients than among control subjects.

All of these findings suggest that cancer of the cervix is a sexually transmitted disease that may have etiologic effects that could lead to an increased risk of cervical cancer.

NUTRITION

Differences in the constitution of food components may explain variations in some cancer rates. In 1849 Bennett suggested that overnutrition might play a role in carcinogenesis.[25] Williams in 1908 noted the infrequent occurrence of cancer in persons who were largely vegetarians; he thus made the association between cancer and civilization. In 1926 came the idea that rich food, particularly meat, contributed to cancer and that this might be related to intestinal stasis or use of preservatives.[26] Russell in 1912 studied nutrition and cancer among monks in Cistercian and Benedictine monasteries and found one death from cancer when at least 20 were expected.[27] This finding, however, was not duplicated subsequently.[28] The first case-control study found no consistent association between diet and cancer.[29] During the past 20 years there have been numerous studies suggesting that excess intake of total fat and reduced intake of fiber might play a role in cancer of the breast and colon. Recently Doll has stated, "Joint investigation of dietetic factors by epidemiologists and laboratory workers offers the brightest prospect of discovering new ways of preventing cancer in the near future."[1]

ENVIRONMENT

Schneiderman has grouped the major achievements of epidemiology and biostatistics in cancer research into three areas.[30]

TABLE 1-1. Some Work Leading to the General Recognition of Environmental Contributions to Cancer

- Association of lung cancer with cigarette smoking
- Evidence that, for cancer of the large bowel, migrants took on the cancer patterns of the country to which they migrated.
- The enormous differences in cancer incidence in different parts of the world*
- Gross associations between diet and some forms of cancer
- Discovery of industrial carcinogens†
- Elucidation of dose-response relations between ionizing radiation exposure and the later development of some forms of cancer in humans

(Adapted from Schneiderman MA: The numerate sciences—epidemiology and biometry. J Natl Cancer Inst 59:633–644, 1977)

* Knowledge of this difference came through the development of accurate cancer registries.

† Obviously these carcinogens directly affect small numbers of persons but possibly could involve very large populations through spillovers into the air and water of surrounding communities.

1. Work leading to the general recognition of environmental contributions to cancer. Some of these are shown in Table 1-1.
2. Recognition of the place of genetic-environment interactions and developmental anomalies in the origin of cancer. Schneiderman cites as examples genetic and environmental effects in childhood cancer, familial clustering, and specific markers, antigens, and cell or chromosome abnormalities that might be associated with cancer susceptibility.
3. Influence of the direction of cancer research through the epidemiologic testing of hypotheses. He cites as examples the viral hypothesis for cancer transmission, clustering of certain tumors in time and space, and the concept of immune surveillance.

Much of this work provides the first step in the ascertainment of risk factors associated with environmental carcinogens or the recognition of risk factors associated with specific sites of cancer.

EPIDEMIOLOGIC STUDIES

A major purpose of epidemiologic studies of cancer is to investigate the causes of cancer. Systematic investigations usually begin with a hypothesis associating a suspected etiologic factor to a specific type of cancer. Hypotheses can be generated from animal experimentations, clinical observations, observations of geographic differences, changes in cancer occurrence over time, international differences, or other astute observations or inductive reasoning. Special studies are usually undertaken to test an epidemiologic hypothesis. The question is whether a statistical association exists between the suspected etiologic factor and the cancer, and, if so, is this association causal in nature?

CAUSATION AND ASSOCIATION

When microbes were discovered and associated with disease, the precise cause of disease was thought to have been identified. Microorganisms meant disease; no microorganisms meant no disease. As medical knowledge progressed, however, it became apparent that even for infectious diseases, the process was not that simple. Although the microbiologic agent was necessary for the disease to occur, many other factors were related to its cause. From this knowledge, the concept of a web of causation evolved. Basically the web of causation is meant to represent the relation and inter-relation of factors contributing to the occurrence of a disease. This concept adapts particularly well to chronic diseases such as lung cancer. Smoking is a cause of lung cancer, but not all smokers develop lung cancer. The development of lung cancer may partially relate to the amount smoked or whether there has been exposure to asbestos or some other known carcinogen. Overlying this may be a genetic predisposition that makes one more likely to develop lung cancer or more likely to smoke. It has been suggested that a high vitamin A consumption may be associated with a reduced risk of lung cancer. People who consume more vitamin A may tend to live on farms, where there is less air pollution. Thus, one can envision an endless set of interconnecting relationships.

The web of causation is an important concept in cancer epidemiology. In attempts to narrow the scope of studies and examine only a few variables, often the larger picture is forgotten. The total picture is virtually never known. Relationships between the variables and the disease are not isolated, and in reality these interactions are very complex. To plan successful prevention measures, one must understand both the relation of the factor to the rest of the web and to the disease itself.

Two variables are said to be associated if the distribution of one is affected by knowledge of the value of the other.[31] For example, a proportion of those who develop lung cancer are smokers. If this proportion is larger than would be expected by chance based on the frequencies of smokers and lung cancer cases in the U.S. population, then it can be said that there is a statistical association between smoking and lung cancer. Associations can be broken down into noncausal, or secondary association and causal association.[32] Thus, the detection of a statistical association does not necessarily prove a causal association. In fact, most statistical associations can be shown to be secondary associations. Number of sexual partners, for example, has been shown to be associated with development of cervical cancer. However, evidence also exists that an agent transmitted through sexual intercourse might cause the cervical cancer, rather than the actual number of partners. In other words, the number of partners cannot be said to cause cervical cancer. Investigators should be cautious in presenting their results as causal when only secondary associations have been shown.

Given that the cause of a disease is not clear-cut, it is difficult to judge whether an association is causally related to a disease. The causal significance of an association is a matter of judgment that goes beyond any statement or statistical probability.[33] Several criteria have been developed as aides to determine whether a factor is causally related to a disease.[31] Five criteria are discussed below.

Strength of Association

The stronger the association, the more likely it is to be causal. The association between lung cancer and smoking, for example, produced an increased relative risk of tenfold,[34] whereas the association between leukemia and smoking was twofold or less.[35] Relative risks of three or greater are considered more than modest risks. Relative risks between one and three require careful interpretation. As the risk increases, an association is more likely to be causal.

Replication or Consistency

If the results of several studies are the same, the association is probably real rather than spurious. On the other hand, if several studies have different results, a causal association must be questioned. More than 10 studies examined the relationship between reserpine use and breast cancer in women. A review of these concluded that the association, if present, was weak.[36]

Biologic Plausibility

An association should have some grounding in biologic knowledge. It is more convincing if similar observations have been made in cellular or animal systems, even though these do not constitute absolute proof of causality. A plausible physiologic mechanism adds strength to a suspected causal association.

Temporal Sequence

Exposure to the suspected etiologic factor should precede the onset of disease. With cancer's relatively long latent period this concept becomes particularly important. Determination of the precise time of exposure or length of the latent period may be difficult or impossible. If, for example, one examines diet in patients with lung cancer and in their control subjects and finds a deficit of vitamin A in the diet of the former, it is difficult to know whether the deficit was a result of the cancer or if the deficiency was a pre-existing condition and contributed to the development of the disease. Differentiation between the two possibilities would affect one's judgment about the causality of the relationship.

Dose-Response

Most agents that cause cancer have a dose-response relation between exposure to the agent and development of the cancer. It is important in examining epidemiologic data to establish a dose-response relationship if one is present. The risk of developing leukemia from ionizing radiation from the atomic bomb blasts at Hiroshima and Nagasaki clearly showed such a relationship.[37] Coffee drinking has been associated with bladder cancer,[38] but its lack of a dose-response relation makes its role in the etiology of bladder cancer seem unlikely.

All of these criteria are important when evaluating causality, and they should be used as a scale with which to weigh the evidence. In the end, good epidemiologic judgment must prevail just as good clinical judgment must often be exercised.

CASE OBSERVATIONS

An important part of the practice of oncology is contributing to knowledge about the causes of cancer. The concept of the practicing oncologist making observations about the etiology of cancer has been termed "bedside etiology" or "clinical astuteness in etiology" and the oncologist himself, a "clinical etiologist" or "alert practitioner." This concept was first introduced by Miller.[39] Historically, much of what we know about the etiology of cancer was first brought to attention by a physician in practice who made astute clinical observations on a case or a group of cases.

The first such observation often cited is attributed to Sir Percivall Pott, who was not an epidemiologist by training but rather a surgeon. He related scrotal cancer in chimney sweeps to their exposure to soot.[7] Experimental studies produced similar tumors in mice and rabbits about 150 years after the carcinogen was first identified in humans.[39]

As a medical student at Washington University of St. Louis, Alton Ochsner was called to witness an autopsy of a patient with lung cancer because the pathologist said the condition was so rare he thought the students might never see another case. Seventeen years later as a young surgeon at Tulane, Dr. Ochsner witnessed his second case of this extremely rare condition. Although there was nothing particularly unusual about seeing one rare case in 17 years, 6 months later he realized that he had seen eight additional cases and that this was extremely unusual. In his words, "the sudden increase in incidence represented an epidemic, and there had to be some reason for it."[40] He further noted that all the patients were men who smoked cigarettes heavily and who had begun smoking during [illegible]d War I. This led to the first case-control study of lung [illegible] and cigarette smoking reported by Wynder and Gr[illegible] 1950.[41] Cigarette smoking has become the single mo[illegible]ant health hazard of our time.[34] Its relation to ma[illegible]f cancer, especially lung cancer, and other diseases [illegible]table.[42]

In 1971 a gynecologist observed a cluster of eight young women with clear-cell adenocarcinoma of the vagina, a rare tumor except in old age. This led to a case-comparison study that found a strong association with in utero exposure to diethylstilbesterol. Several hundred cases have since been found among an estimated 1 million daughters so exposed.[43]

These examples show the importance of clinical observations by physicians and oncologists. When rare forms of cancers are observed together or as a cluster, such as several cases of lung cancer before 1930 occurring over a short time, or clear-cell adenocarcinoma of the vagina occurring in young women, important clues to etiology can be uncovered. This is an important source for the generation of hypotheses, which can then be tested by more rigorous epidemiologic studies or laboratory investigations, or both.

Analysis of case series data is generally straightforward. Usually, case series consist of a few cases for which it is possible to publish a complete description. If the case series is large, however, the data can be reported using various descriptive statistics such as histograms, cross-tabulations, graphs, box and whisker plots, stem and leaf plots, means, medians, standard deviations, or standard errors. Details on how to calculate box and whiskers and stem and leaf plots are provided by Tukey.[44] If the data are exceptionally complex, multivariate statistical techniques may be used. However, the emphasis with these methods should be on description rather than on testing.

The advantages of case observations are that they can be done at minimal cost by anyone with access to the case material. The disadvantage is that they are rarely, if ever, conclusive and must be followed up by more rigorous studies that lend themselves to statistical and other kinds of interpretation. Case series studies can contribute information in several ways: by providing a description of disease status; by detecting patient characteristics related to prognosis; by being a source of special studies of changes in disease; or by providing patient characteristics over time given sufficient information. Thus, the importance of clinical observations by physicians and oncologists should not be underestimated.

CASE-COMPARISON STUDIES

Case-comparison studies, also referred to as case-control studies, case history studies, and retrospective studies, compose the largest part of active investigations in cancer epidemiology. If done properly, they allow a great deal of information to be learned in a time- and cost-efficient manner. In case-comparison studies, the frequency of a suspected etiologic factor is compared in a group of persons who have a cancer (cases) and a group who do not (compeers). If a greater frequency of the suspected etiologic factor is found among those with cancer than among those without, an association between the disease and the factor may be indicated. In this type of study the investigator starts with the disease and goes back in time to ascertain the suspected etiologic event—hence use of the term "retrospective." A classic example of a case-comparison study is the investigation of cigarette smoking histories among lung cancer patients and hospital control subjects first reported by Wynder and Graham in 1950.[41]

Selection of cases for inclusion in a case-comparison study is important. Ideally, criteria for inclusion should provide clear and reproducible disease entities. Criteria that reproduce more homogeneous groups of cases are usually desirable. Inclusion of variants of the cancer could dilute a possible association. Even though criteria must be specific to each investigation, histologic confirmation of cases is desirable.

Commonly, cases are taken from a hospital or a particular medical care facility or by ascertaining all persons with the cancer in a defined geographical area such as a city or county. Institutional data are more commonly used because they are relatively easier, inexpensive, and faster to obtain. Geographic data are more desirable because they avoid hospital selection bias and allow for calculation of rates of the disease related to the suspected etiologic factor.

The selection of a comparison group or groups is the most difficult problem in designing a case-comparison study. In choosing a case-comparison design the investigator gives up the chance of comparing all cases of cancer and noncancer in the community. Hopefully, however, almost as much can be learned about relationship of the cancer to other factors by studying a group of cases and the comparison group.

Ideally, compeers should be similar to cases in every way except for the factor being studied. Because this is virtually impossible, compromises must be made depending on financial considerations and availability of potential compeers. One of the most important considerations in selecting compeers involves the information to be collected on study variables or suspected etiologic factors. The availability and quality of this information should be identical in both cases and compeers.

Potential sources of bias must also be avoided when choosing a compeer group, as discussed later. Financial and statistical considerations are important as well. Compeers may come from hospital patients, relatives of cases, friends of cases, neighbors of cases, or from the community as a whole. Some different sources of cases and compeers are summarized in Table 1-2. The number of compeers should be at least as great as the number of cases. Often twice as many compeers are used in order to increase the statistical power to detect a difference between groups. More than two compeers per case are occasionally used, but the small increase in power is usually not cost-effective.[45] An alternative used by some investigators is to have two compeer groups, one from the hospital and one from the case's neighborhood. When the groups are combined the investigator has the advantage of increased power, but, more important, when examined separately, many sources of potential bias may be examined.

Once the source of compeers is identified they must be matched to cases to minimize difference between the groups.

TABLE 1-2. Different Sources of Cases and Controls in Case-Comparison Studies

CASES	CONTROLS
All cases diagnosed in the community (in hospitals and other medical facilities, including physicians' offices)	Sample* of the general population in a community
All cases diagnosed in a sample of the general population	Noncases in a sample of the general population, or subgroup of a sample of the general population
All cases diagnosed in all hospitals in the community	Sample of patients in all hospitals in the community, who do not have the disease or related diseases being studied
All cases diagnosed in a single hospital	Sample of patients in the same hospital where cases were selected
All cases diagnosed in one or more hospitals	Sample of persons who are residents in the same block or neighborhood of cases
Cases selected by any of the above methods	Spouses, siblings, or associates of cases; accident victims

(Adapted from Lilienfeld AM: Foundations of Epidemiology. New York, Oxford University Press, 1976)

* When the term "sample" is used, it means a probability sample.

Groups of compeers may be matched to groups of cases (stratification) or individual compeers to individual cases. Several possibilities exist on the degree of matching. The matching may range from very loose (age only) to very specific (age, race, sex, smoking habits, socioeconomic status, and so forth). Undermatching allows investigation of factors other than the one of primary interest but may result in significant differences between cases and compeers that might affect the distribution of the factor under study. Overmatching assures minimal confounding from known risk factors but may result in matching out the suspected association when, in fact, it does exist. An alternative to a high degree of matching is to stratify the important variables in the analysis. There is some debate as to whether it is more efficient to match or to stratify in the analysis.[46]

Advantages of case-comparison studies are that they usually can be conducted more quickly and less expensively than cohort or prospective studies. They are also more suited to study when the disease outcome is infrequent or rare. Limitations of case-comparison studies lie in their interpretation, which is related to problems of bias, confounding variables, indirect associations, and low level of risks. If an association is found, it may be direct or indirect, and if direct it may be causal. Case-comparison studies are usually the first step in deciding whether a suspect association exists. They are often followed by cohort studies. For example, as MacMahon and Pugh point out, there had been some 15 published case-comparison studies on the relation between smoking and lung cancer before the first cohort study in 1954.[32,47]

Analysis of case-comparison studies is usually done by estimating relative risks using the odds ratio or by other measures of association discussed later. A complete discussion of case-comparison studies is beyond the scope of this chapter, but there are several excellent resources.[32,48–50]

COHORT STUDIES

In a cohort study, also referred to as a prospective study, the investigator begins with a group of persons exposed to a suspect etiologic factor before onset of the resultant disease, then follows the group over time and measures the frequency of the disease. The control group constitutes a group of persons similar to the cohort group but without exposure to the suspected etiologic factor. A classic cohort study is the ascertainment of mortality among British physicians in relation to their cigarette smoking habits.[51] Occupation groups provide a rich source of cohorts with unusually heavy exposures to chemical, physical, or other agents, such as the study of bladder cancer among workers in the dyestuffs industry.[52] Certain groups offer special opportunities for follow-up, including persons in prepaid medical plans, insured populations, veterans, college alumni, or volunteer groups such as the large study group assembled by Hammond and Horn.[53] The availability of opportunities for conducting cohort studies is limited only by the imagination of the investigator and the resources available.

The term "prospective cohort" means that the group has been identified but the investigator must wait for the disease to occur.[51] If disease has already occurred among the cohort ("retrospective cohort"), then the investigator can retrospectively conduct the study without having to wait for time to lapse.[52]

The advantages of cohort studies are that they provide a direct estimate of the risk of developing the disease in the group exposed to the suspected etiologic factor. Usually the suspect etiologic factor can be measured more precisely than in case-comparison studies, thus decreasing the possibility of subjective bias, such as having to remember whether some event occurred. All persons with the disease can be related to the etiologic event, not just those who survive a certain time-interval as in a case-comparison study. Other diseases may be studied at little or no extra expense.

Cohort studies also have some severe limitations. They are difficult and expensive to conduct. They usually require large populations to be observed and followed up for long periods. It may be difficult to engage the whole cohort. Physical examinations may be desirable to detect early or unsuspected disease. Cohort studies are very inefficient for studying rare diseases, such as most individual types of cancer, because an extremely large number of subjects must be followed up to detect a sufficient number of cases for study.

Analysis of cohort studies and a discussion of bias and confounding factors as they relate to cohort studies are presented in later sections. For detailed methods of conducting cohort studies, refer to classic texts on the subject.[32,48,54] The advantages and disadvantages of case-comparison and cohort studies are summarized in Table 1-3.

CROSS-SECTIONAL STUDIES

In a cross-sectional study, measurements of cause and effect are made at the same time, in contrast to a longitudinal study where the observations relate to two different times. Most, but not all, case-comparison and cohort studies are longitudinal. In case-comparison studies, the suspect etiologic factor has occurred before onset of disease. In cohort studies, the disease is measured after the group with the suspect etiologic factor has been assembled. Cross-sectional studies require that suspected causes be permanent or long-lasting so that suspected relations to disease are still measurable at the same time the disease is measured. A case-comparison study of ABO blood groups and cancer, for example, can be considered cross-sectional.[55] In practice, distinctions among all types of epidemiologic studies are not clear, and flexibility should be maintained to allow maximum use of the investigator's imagination.

Cross-sectional studies include population surveys such as the U.S. National Health Survey and can be used to test hypotheses. However, the conclusion of association will often be less firm than that derived from case-comparison studies, generally because of the lack of control or lack of information on confounding factors. In these studies, the classification and definition of events depend on both the quality of the data collection mechanism and the availability of data. There is often little chance to standardize definitions. Illness surveys, for example, may rely on information from various physicians who have been recording information in their own way. Population surveys often place greater reliance on questionnaires than do other types of studies. Thus, it is essential that questionnaires be clear and use terms the respondent can understand.

For reasons of cost, population surveys generally involve studies of subsets of the population of interest. The validity and interpretability of results from a survey will be enhanced if the survey is a random sample from a well-defined population. This enables generalization to the population from

TABLE 1-3. Summary of Advantages and Disadvantages of Case-Comparison and Cohort Studies

	ADVANTAGES	DISADVANTAGES
CASE-COMPARISON STUDY	Relatively inexpensive	Incomplete information
	Smaller number of subjects	Biased recall
	Relatively quick results	Problems of selecting control group and matching variables
	Suitable for rare diseases	Estimation of relative risk
COHORT STUDY	Lack of bias in factor	Possible bias in ascertainment of disease
	Yielding of incidence rates as well as relative risk	Large numbers of subjects required
	Possible yielding of associations with additional disease as by-product	Long follow-up period
		Problem of attrition
		Changes over time in criteria and methods
		Very costly

(Adapted from Mausner JS, Bahn AK: Epidemiology: An Introductory Text, p 324. Philadelphia, WB Saunders, 1974)

which the sample was taken. Surveys that involve complete ascertainment of a population or that represent the entire population can be used to ascertain or estimate prevalence. However, because there may be shifts in the population from one survey to the next, it would be difficult in most instances to ascertain incidence using survey data.

In interpreting results of survey or other cross-sectional studies it is important to look carefully at the group studied. Depending on the method by which the group was selected, generalizations to a larger population may not be possible.

For analysis, standard statistical techniques may be used. However, if there is sampling and some subsets are sampled more heavily than others, a weighting scheme for most analysis will be needed.[56] When complicated sampling schemes are used, there may be difficulties in estimating variances, which may hamper interpretation of results.

SELECTED EPIDEMIOLOGIC AND STATISTICAL CONCEPTS

Fundamental to interpreting epidemiologic studies that relate suspected etiologic factors to cancer are some selected epidemiologic and statistical concepts. The concept of causation has been discussed previously. Causation is usually thought of in terms of associations, which may be independent of each other or not statistically related. If they are statistically related they may be noncausally related or causal. Associations can be misleading or even spurious because of biases and confounding variables. Measures of association are usually made in terms of different risks or by comparing rates or proportions. In addition to measures of association, this section discusses bias, confounding, ecologic fallacy, and cohort effect.

RISKS

Relative Risk

Relative risk of cancer is defined as the probability of cancer given the characteristic or exposure factor divided by probability of cancer given the person does not have the characteristic or exposure factor. It is calculated as follows.

$$\text{Relative risk} = \frac{\left(\dfrac{\text{number exposed population with cancer}}{\text{number exposed population}}\right)}{\left(\dfrac{\text{number unexposed population with cancer}}{\text{number unexposed population}}\right)}$$

If the relative risk is unity, the cancer and the exposure or characteristic are not associated. If the relative risk is greater than one, a person with the exposure or characteristic is more likely to contract cancer than a person without the characteristic. If the relative risk is less than one, a person with the exposure or characteristic is less likely to contract cancer than the person without the characteristic, implying the characteristic may be protective.[57] Instead of cancer, mortality or some other outcome event could be used and a relative risk computed. The relative risks for smokers compared to nonsmokers are computed in Table 1-4. The data, taken from the Doll and Hill study, show an increase in relative risk with an increase in the amount of tobacco, giving a dose-response relation.[58] The likelihood that an association between two variables is a secondary association decreases as the relative risk increases.

Relative Odds

If population data are not available, relative risk can still be estimated using a retrospective or case-comparison study if the following assumptions are made: [1] the comparison group represents the general population; [2] the cancer cases are representative of all cancer cases; and [3] the frequency of the disease in the general population is small.[54] When these assumptions are satisfied, the relative risk can then be estimated by the relative odds or odds ratio. The odds ratio is calculated from the frequencies presented in Table 1-5. An example is given in Table 1-6. The relative odds are 1.7 and are greater than unity. Methods for testing that the relative odds are not equal to unity are described by Lilienfeld.[59]

Attributable Risk

Attributable risk is defined as the proportion of cancer in exposed persons that can be attributed to exposure.

$$\text{Attributable risk} = \frac{\text{number exposed population with cancer}}{\text{number in exposed population}} - \frac{\text{number in unexposed population with cancer}}{\text{number in unexposed population}}.$$

Attributable risk can also be calculated from retrospective studies from the frequencies presented in Table 1-5.[60]

$$\text{Attributable risk} = \frac{\dfrac{a}{a+c} - \dfrac{b}{b+d}}{1 - \dfrac{b}{b+d}}$$

An example of the calculation of attributable risk from a case-comparison study is given in Table 1-6. The calculated value of 0.26 indicates a small risk attributable to being a user of tobacco. Walter has developed tests of significance and approximate confidence intervals for attributable risk.[61]

In cohort studies, the relative risk will give a better measure of the effect of a factor than attributable risk. For example, in Table 1-4 the attributable risk for a smoker of 1 to 14 g of tobacco daily would be 0.57 − 0.07 = 0.5. The size of the relative risk is also a better index than attributable risk of the likelihood that a causal relationship exists between suspect etiologic factors and the disease. If a causal relationship has been demonstrated, then attributable risk is a useful measure of the potential impact of a prevention program.

RATES AND PROPORTIONS

Rates and proportions are measures of disease frequency. For epidemiologic purposes, three items of information are needed: the number of persons affected (numerator), the

TABLE 1-4. Death Rates from Lung Cancer by Smoking Status*

SMOKING STATUS	ANNUAL RATE PER 1000	RELATIVE RISK	ATTRIBUTABLE RISK
Nonsmoker	0.07		0
Smoker (1–14 g daily)	0.57	(0.57/0.07) = 8.14	0.50
Smoker (15–24 g daily)	1.39	(1.39/0.07) = 19.86	1.32
Smoker (25 g or more daily)	2.27	(2.27/0.07) = 32.43	2.20

(Adapted from Doll R, Hill AB: Lung cancer and other causes of death in relation to smoking: A second report of the mortality of British doctors. Br Med J 2:1071–1081, 1956)
* British male physicians aged 35 and older, 1951–1956.

population from which the affected persons come (denominator), and a specified time-period. If the numerator is restricted to a certain age, sex, race, or other group, the denominator should have similar restrictions. The denominator is called the *reference population.* When the denominator is restricted solely to those persons capable of contracting the disease, it is a population *at risk.*[32]

Numbers of cases of a disease when expressed as a proportion of the total number of cases of all disease, or as a proportion of all cases seen at the same institution, are called *proportional rates.* Proportional rates do not reflect the risk of persons in the population acquiring or dying from the disease. Such proportions may be useful in comparing areas in which, or population subgroups in whom, differences may exist and may be worth investigating. Without computing rates against a population base, it is impossible to know whether observed differences are due to differences in the sizes of the numerators or of the denominators. Basing conclusions on numerator data alone can be misleading.[62]

Among the common rates and proportions used in cancer epidemiology are *prevalence*, a measure of existing disease at a designated point in time; *incidence*, the number of new cases diagnosed during a specified period; *mortality*, the number of deaths from a disease during a specified period; and *case-specific fatality*, the number of deaths of a disease divided by the number of persons with the disease during a specified period.

TABLE 1-5. Fourfold Table for Calculating Relative Odds*

SUSPECTED ETIOLOGIC FACTOR	CASES	CONTROLS	TOTAL
Exposed	a†	b	a+b
Not exposed	c	d	c+d
Total	a+c	b+d	N

* Relative odds $= \frac{ad}{bc}$.

† a, b, c, d = frequencies of individuals in each cell.

TABLE 1-6. Case-Control Study of Bladder Cancer and Smoking Habits

TOBACCO USE	CASES WITH BLADDER CANCER	CONTROL SUBJECTS
Any	192	156
Never	129	181

(Lilienfeld AM: Foundations of Epidemiology. New York: Oxford University Press, 1976)

$$\text{Relative odds} = \frac{192 \times 181}{129 \times 156} = 1.7$$

$$\text{Attributable risk} = \frac{\dfrac{192}{192 + 129} - \dfrac{156}{156 + 181}}{1 - \dfrac{156}{156 + 181}} = 0.26$$

Definitions

1. Cancer prevalence

$$= \frac{\text{number of persons with a cancer at a specified time}}{\text{total number in group at the specified time}}$$

This has sometimes been referred to as a prevalence rate but is actually a proportion.[63] For example, from the data in Table 1-7, prevalence of acute leukemia per million is computed as follows.

$$\text{prevalence} = \frac{17}{2{,}525{,}000} \times 1{,}000{,}000 = 6.7$$

2. Cancer incidence

$$= \frac{\text{number of new cases of cancer in a given period}}{\text{total number in population exposed to the risk of developing cancer during that period}}$$

If the period is 1 year, the midyear population would be used as a denominator. For example, from the data in Table 1-7, incidence of acute leukemia is computed as follows.

$$\text{incidence} = \frac{83}{2{,}525{,}000} \times 1{,}000{,}000 = 32.9$$

This gives an estimate of the risk of developing cancer during the specified period, in contrast to prevalence, which measures the number of cases present at a particular time.

3. Cancer mortality

$$= \frac{\text{number of persons dying of disease during the time period}}{\text{total number in population during that period}}$$

TABLE 1-7. White Patients with Leukemia, Brooklyn, New York, 1950*

TYPE OF LEUKEMIA	PATIENTS ALIVE AT THE BEGINNING OF THE YEAR	NEW CASES DIAGNOSED IN YEAR	DEATHS IN YEAR
Acute	17	83	73
Chronic	157	90	90

(Adapted from MacMahon B, Pugh TF: Epidemiology: Principles and Methods. Boston, Little, Brown & Co, 1979)

* 1950 white population = 2,525,000.

From Table 1-7, mortality for acute leukemia is computed as follows.

$$\text{mortality} = \frac{73}{2{,}525{,}000} \times 1{,}000{,}000 = 28.9$$

4. Case-specific fatality

$$= \frac{\text{number of persons dying of cancer during the time period}}{\text{total number of persons with cancer during that period}}$$

From Table 1-7, case-specific fatalities for acute and chronic leukemia are computed as follows.

$$\text{case fatality (acute leukemia)} = \frac{73}{17 + 83} = 0.73$$

$$\text{case fatality (chronic leukemia)} = \frac{90}{157 + 90} = 0.36$$

Table 1-8 gives a summary of prevalence, incidence, and mortality for the leukemia data. Although there are similarities in incidence, there are differences in prevalence. This is due to a difference in case fatality, as noted above.

When comparing rates and proportions across time or populations, some adjustment for differences in factors such as age and sex may be needed. Methods of adjustment are discussed in the Appendix to this chapter.

BIAS

Whether studies are case-comparison or cohort, it is possible to introduce errors. Some errors may be random and others nonrandom or systematic. It is the systematic error that is referred to as *bias*. In case-comparison studies various types of bias can occur. A fairly complete catalogue of bias in analytic research is presented by Sackett and Vessey.[64] One of the more well-known types of bias is Berkson's paradox.[65] This is a spurious association arising when there are differing rates of admission to the case or control group from the population with respect to the suspected etiologic factor. In hospital studies of lung cancer and cigarette smoking, for example, more hospital patients as a control group smoke than do control groups from the general population. This can lead to a minimizing or underestimating of the association between cigarette smoking and lung cancer. Thus, the admission bias must be carefully considered in any study with hospital control subjects.

TABLE 1-8. Measures of Frequency of Acute and Chronic Leukemia (Rates per Million Population)

MEASURE	ACUTE LEUKEMIA	CHRONIC LEUKEMIA
Prevalence	6.7	66.1
Incidence	32.5	29.0
Mortality per annum	31.3	30.4

(Adapted from MacMahon B, Pugh TF: Epidemiology: Principles and Methods. Boston, Little, Brown & Co, 1979)

Another type of bias is selection bias. This is demonstrated in an example by Cornfield and Haenszel.[57] In an autopsy study of cancer, the autopsied controls were found to have more tuberculosis than were the cancer cases. It was subsequently shown that those who died of tuberculosis were more likely to have had an autopsy, thus overestimating the amount of tuberculosis in the control group relative to the cancer group.

To guard against the two previous types of hospital bias, controls should be drawn where possible from a representative sample of hospital admissions or from the general population rather than the hospital. Also, patients questioned in the hospital may give different responses than patients questioned in their own homes. One possible solution would be to use both general populations and hospital controls as a further protection against bias.

Another type of bias is interviewer bias. If the interviewer knows the hypothesis under study, the interviewer may inadvertently obtain better information from one group than from the other. Doll and Hill in 1950 had a unique opportunity to test for interviewer bias.[66] A group of patients in their lung cancer study, after being interviewed, were found to have respiratory disease rather than lung cancer. They were able to compare the response of the patients with respiratory diseases with the response of the controls and found no difference. Thus, they were somewhat assured that the difference in smoking rates in the lung cancer group and in the control group was not due to interviewer bias. To avoid this type of bias, interviewers, if possible, should not know if they are interviewing a case or control. Blinding is not possible if the case is a hospitalized lung cancer patient and the control comes from the population. It may also be helpful if the case and control groups do not know the actual hypothesis being tested. However, this has become more difficult given the strict regulations on informed consent.

In cohort studies additional types of biases are possible, including that in the selection of participants for study. A graphic example is given by the DESAD Project, a study of young women exposed *in utero* to diethylstilbestrol (DES).[67] Some participants were chosen by reviewing all prenatal records in selected physicians' practices, identifying those women exposed to DES during pregnancy and their daughters. These daughters were then asked to participate. In addition, women who voluntarily presented themselves at study clinics with documentation of DES exposure and women referred to the clinics by their private physicians in the documentation of *in utero* DES exposure were enrolled. An earlier report by Stafl had indicated that young DES-exposed daughters were at high risk of squamous cancer of the cervix.[68] The DESAD data showed that depending on the method of selection the prevalence of cancer and dysplasia varied greatly across the three groups, with the referral group having the highest, the walk-in group the second highest, and no findings beyond moderate dysplasia in the record review group.[69] The data show that conclusions based on walk-in or referral populations alone may be erroneous.

Case-comparison and cohort studies can also be subject to nonresponse bias. Case-comparison studies, however, more often rely on recall and hospital records, while cohort studies generally rely on other records or require contact with participants, making it more likely that there will be problems with response bias. Cohort studies have an additional difficulty with bias created by dropouts or lost to follow-up. For example, if a group of smokers and nonsmokers are being followed over a long time, the nonsmokers may be more likely to drop out because they do not have incentive for continuing annual physical examinations, as the smokers do. This may lead to greater loss to follow-up among nonsmokers than smokers. If follow-up procedures are not carefully planned, those who died may be registered as lost to follow-up rather than recorded as deaths, and again bias may result.

It is not possible to present a complete catalogue of biases. In designing a study, however, appropriate types of biases should be considered and eliminated if possible.

CONFOUNDING

Confounding may exist between a suspected etiologic factor and a disease when a second factor (the confounder) is associated with both the disease and the first factor. As a hypothetical example, consider a study of the mortality experience of several occupational categories. Age-adjusted rates revealed that painters had a higher rate of lung cancer than did persons in other occupations included in the study. The suggestion was made that the excess lung cancer was due to the painters breathing potential carcinogens in the paint and fumes from the thinner. Because the study used death certificates, information on smoking habits was not available. Further investigation revealed that a higher percentage of painters were smokers. When persons were divided into smoker and nonsmoker groups, little variation was seen in lung cancer rates between occupational groups.

Often potential confounding variables are not as obvious or measurable. In any study the relationship between a factor and a disease may be the result of a confounding factor. It is important to think about possible confounding variables and investigate them where possible. Methods of adjustment for confounding variables are presented in the Appendix to this chapter.

ECOLOGIC FALLACY

Erroneous conclusions can also result from an ecologic fallacy. An ecologic fallacy can arise when the relationship between a factor and a disease is measured in groups of persons (cities, counties, countries, and so forth) as opposed to individuals. Suppose, for example, that examination of leukemia rates by cities in the United States showed higher rates among those having nuclear power plants. It could then be hypothesized that the excess rates of leukemia were due to radiation exposure of workers at the plants. However, cities with nuclear power plants might be more highly industrialized than other cities and therefore might contain industries whose workers may be exposed to leukemogenic compounds. If this exposure were responsible for the high rates of leukemia, rather than the nuclear power plant, the original conclusion would be wrong and considered an ecologic fallacy. Examination of individuals and their place of work would not have resulted in this erroneous conclusion.

COHORT EFFECT

A *cohort* is defined as those people within a geographic or otherwise delineated population who experience the same significant life event within a given time. For example, a birth cohort might include all persons born in a particular year. The cohort might also be defined by birth of the first child, retirement, or some other event of that nature. A cohort analysis of several groups may indicate variation because of a cohort effect or variations because of a period effect. Lung cancer in men older than age 70 provides an example of a cohort effect. The lung cancer rate for these men is low because they belong to a birth cohort with less exposure to cigarette smoking than cohorts of men born later. An example of a period effect would be the bombing of Hiroshima. Persons of all ages in the area at the time of the atomic explosion would be more likely to develop radiation-induced cancer than would persons living in the area before or after that time. Tables 1-9 and 1-10 give hypothetical examples where all variation is due to cohort effects and where all variation is due to period effects.[70] These cohort tables are the standard

TABLE 1-9. Cohort Table Showing Hypothetical Data (Percentages) in Which All Variation Is Due to Cohort Effects

	YEAR			
AGE	*1940*	*1950*	*1960*	*1970*
20–29	50	40	30	20
30–39	60	50	40	30
40–49	70	60	50	40
50–59	80	70	60	50
60–69	90	80	70	60
70–79	100	90	80	70
Age-adjusted total*	75	65	55	45

(Reprinted from Glenn ND: Cohort Analysis (Series on Quantitative Applications in the Social Sciences), pp 50–51. Beverly Hills, Sage Publications, 1977)

* Standardized to an age distribution with an equal number of persons at each age level.

TABLE 1-10. Cohort Table Showing Hypothetical Data (Percentages) in Which All Variation Is Due to Period Effects

	YEAR			
AGE	*1940*	*1950*	*1960*	*1970*
20–29	70	60	50	40
30–39	70	60	50	40
40–49	70	60	50	40
50–59	70	60	50	40
60–69	70	60	50	40
70–79	70	60	50	40
Age-adjusted total*	70	60	50	40

(Reprinted from Glenn ND: Cohort Analysis [Series on Quantitative Applications in the Social Sciences], pp 50–51. Beverly Hills, Sage Publications, 1977)

* Standardized to an age distribution with an equal number of persons at each age level. In this table, the age-adjusted total equals the unadjusted total.

method of cohort analysis. There are also complex statistical techniques, especially analysis of variance and covariance, that can be used to adjust for interactions that would otherwise distort the standard cohort table.

When analyzing cohort data, researchers should avoid the tendency to overinterpret small differences that could be due to random fluctuations over time. This could, of course, lead to incorrect conclusions. The investigator should also assure that observed changes over time do not reflect changes in the data collection instrument rather than actual changes. If a type of cancer is more easily diagnosed today than in the past, for example, it may look as though there is a rise in cancer in the cohort of people born in 1920 as compared to that in the cohort of people born in 1900, even though the difference is strictly due to the ability to diagnose the disease.

SOURCES OF EPIDEMIOLOGIC DATA

There are many sources of epidemiologic data for investigating cancer, ranging from a single case observation to basic laboratory investigation. Each source has its own limitations. Death certificate data are the most widely used because of their availability. Other organized sources of data in this country include collection of survival information, incidence surveys, and hospital-based registries. International data are available as well. The major sources of these data are summarized below and have been discussed in more detail.[30,71]

DEATH CERTIFICATES

Cause-specific death rates are the single most useful source of information on the distribution of many diseases. In the United States, state laws require the registration of deaths, births, marriages, and divorces. Copies are sent to the National Center for Health Statistics where tabulations of national statistics are made. In 1933 the death registration for the entire United States was completed. Because death registration varies from state to state and from time to time and classification systems have changed, data must be interpreted cautiously, especially in considering time trends from 1900.

Death rate is the result of the case fatality rate of the disease (number of persons who die from the disease divided by number of persons who get the disease), the incidence of the disease (number of new cases of the disease in a defined population for a given time), the responsiveness of the disease to treatment, and other factors in the natural history of the disease. Death rates are most reliable as indicators of disease occurrence when the interval between onset of the case and death is short and deaths from the disease are frequent, such as with lung cancer.

Some of the problems with the use of mortality data include ascertainment of the cause of death, adequacy of diagnostic work-up, assignment of a single cause of death from multiple disorders present at the time of death, and changes in classification systems over time. The physician completing the death certificate may not be the attending physician. Death certificates are completed before autopsy and are not amended to reflect autopsy findings. However, most cancers are recorded on a very high proportion of death certificates if they are present at death[32], thus, even considering the limitations, death certificates can serve as a valuable resource.

CANCER MORTALITY BY COUNTY IN THE UNITED STATES

Differences in occurrence of cancer by geographic distribution can be useful in developing etiologic hypotheses. In 1971, Burbank first published maps showing the distribution of age-adjusted death rates for the United States by state.[72] This volume provided new information on the geographic distribution of cancer and showed decreased cancer mortality among younger persons and a downturn in childhood leukemia. Most investigators wanted geographic distribution in more detail and for smaller areas.[30]

In 1975, tabulations of total number of cancer deaths and age-adjusted death rates by U.S. county, sex, and race (whites and nonwhites) for the 20-year period 1950 to 1969 were published.[73] The county, as a geographic unit of study, has advantages over larger areas in that counties have greater homogeneity of demographic and environmental characteristics. For most counties sufficient numbers were available to calculate meaningful values. For more uncommon sites, state economic-area boundaries were used. These are single counties or groups of counties that share similar economic and social characteristics. County tabulations of cancer deaths have been supplemented by an atlas of mortality maps for whites and nonwhites.[74,75] These maps identify counties or clusters of counties with high cancer rates that may provide etiologic clues to the causes of cancer. The maps also designate high-risk areas where special carcinogenic hazards may be detected or where control programs for prevention or early detection of cancer may be beneficial.

SURVIVAL OF CANCER PATIENTS

The "End Results Group," a system for reporting cancer patient survival, was developed by the National Cancer Institute. A series of survival reports has been published, the most recent in 1976.[76] This is the largest collection of survival data on cancer patients in the world, covering 450,000 patients contributed by two population-based registries (Connecticut and California) and two teaching hospitals (Charity Hospital in New Orleans and the University of Iowa Hospital). It is impossible to assess whether these data truly reflect cancer patient survival throughout the United States.

THIRD NATIONAL CANCER SURVEY (TNCS)

The Third National Cancer Survey (TNCS) was a sequel to earlier national surveys, commonly referred to as the Ten Cities Survey of 1937 and 1947 and the Iowa Study of 1950.[13,77,78] These surveys sought to collect incidence data, that is, all newly diagnosed cases of cancer (except nonmelanoma skin cancer) in a defined population using 1970 census data covering 3 years, 1969 to 1971.[79] In addition, information was collected on costs of cancer care.[80] In theory, incidence data should be more useful for the study of etiology than should mortality data. To date, however, the TNCS data have probably been used less than the mortality maps.[30]

SURVEILLANCE, EPIDEMIOLOGY, AND END RESULTS (SEER)

To monitor the occurrence of cancer continuously, the periodic survey represented by the TNCS was transformed into a continuous reporting system consisting, at this date, of 11 population-based registries.* This is called the Surveillance, Epidemiology, and End Results (SEER) program.[81] Through active surveillance, these registries attempt to ascertain all cancer cases occurring within a specified geographic area. In addition, follow-up of identified cases provides treatment and survival information. Although these registries are not representative of the population of the United States as a whole, they are very useful because as a group they provide incidence data for many ethnic groups, including American Indians, Japanese, Chinese, Polynesians, Mexican–Americans, and blacks.

The importance of these population-based registries is that they provide, for the most part, extremely accurate cancer incidence rates by site, age, and ethnicity. This allows the epidemiologist to monitor changes in incidence over time and to make comparisons between ethnic and geographic groups with the confidence that the data are accurate. The registries also serve as a reservoir from which cases can be drawn for case-comparison studies. For cases so selected, accurate information on tumor type and address of patient, for instance, is readily available, thus simplifying the study procedure. The population-based nature of the registry also facilitates the use of "neighborhood" controls if so desired.

Population-based tumor registries have two major drawbacks. First, because of the logistics involved, they are difficult to set up and manage. Continuous cooperation is needed on several levels to assure accurate and complete reporting of cases. As the completeness and accuracy of reporting drop, the value of registry similarly declines. Second, the expense of the endeavor is a drawback. The large populations and large geographical areas covered necessitate a rather large amount of resources. In times of limited resources it will be difficult deciding whether to continue these unquestionably valuable programs in light of their high dollar costs.

HOSPITAL-BASED CANCER REGISTRIES

Since 1956 cancer registries have been an integral part of the American College of Surgeons' effort to improve the quality care of cancer patients through hospital-based cancer programs. These registries should provide a stimulus and a resource for clinical investigations and epidemiologic research. They aid the physician in the mechanics of following patients and in providing continuity of patient care regardless of eventualities such as change of residence, retirement, or death of a physician. Additionally they serve as a resource for continuing education of physicians and paramedical personnel at clinical conferences, medical society meetings, seminars, and discussion groups. Tumor registries in hospitals can serve as the focus for the interdisciplinary approach to cancer management, including surgery, radiotherapy, chemotherapy, immunotherapy, and hormone therapy. Last, they can provide the hospital staffs, both medical and administrative, with statistical and analytic summary reports evaluating the cancer problem in the institution and in the community. These reports assist administrators with solving their operational problems and assist physicians with the development of comprehensive cancer care.

There are important limitations in the use and interpretation of hospital-based cancer registry data. The population of patients included are served usually by a single hospital that may have various criteria for admission eligibility. Thus, disease occurrence in these patients does not necessarily represent that of the general population, and extrapolation of findings to the general population is limited. Geographic variation in cancer occurrence is well known, whereas these groups of patients usually represent one geographic area. Just as important is the fact that large referral centers may have patients from all over the country or the world. Denominator data are usually impossible to derive; hence calculation of rates is usually not possible. When comparing observed numbers to expected numbers, the application of a single set of incidence rates may not provide an accurate estimate of

* Metropolitan Atlanta, Detroit, and New Orleans; San Francisco-Oakland Standard Metropolitan Statistical Area; the Seattle-Puget Sound (13 counties) area; the states of Connecticut, Hawaii, Iowa, New Mexico, and Utah; and the Commonwealth of Puerto Rico.

expected numbers. Patient entries may cover many years, during which some cancer incidence changes or treatment methods change. In some categories the numbers are small.

For epidemiologic purposes, hospital-based registries are most useful as sources of cases for case-comparison studies or as part of the surveillance system of a population-based registry.

INTERNATIONAL CANCER INCIDENCE

International differences in cancer occurrence have been of great interest and have contributed to the current notion that much of cancer is caused by environmental factors. A large number of cancer registries exist throughout the world. Data from several of them have been compiled under the auspices of the World Health Organization.[82] The latest volume, titled *Cancer Incidence in Five Continents* (volume III), reports data for 58 populations. Caution must be exercised in comparing international cancer incidence data because of variation in the way data are collected, assembled, and treated around the world.

CANCER INCIDENCE AND MORTALITY

Numerous geographic factors as well as individual characteristics of a population contribute to the computation and understanding of cancer incidence and mortality data. By identifying the distribution of the disease and its patterns of occurrence within a population, the epidemiologist puts together various clues to gain insight into the etiology of the disease.

In using cancer rates to suggest etiologic clues, one must continually be aware of the limitations of data and recognize that rates are only as good as the data from which they were computed. Incomplete ascertainment, poor coding, and misdiagnosis may all lead to errors in rate calculation and interpretation.

One must also understand the limitations of the type of rate one is working. For example, mortality rates reflect not only incidence but survival. Although this may not be a problem for cancers of the lung or pancreas where survival is generally poor, for carcinoma of the cervix or breast, incidence and mortality rates may be markedly different. Finally, as discussed earlier in this chapter, an association by no means always implies a cause.

DIFFERENCES BY AGE

Age has the greatest effect on cancer morbidity and mortality. In the United States, cancer incidence doubles, after age 25, with every 5-year increase in age.[83] This increase is probably due to an accumulation of premalignant changes occurring over a long period, so that cancer exists primarily in the aged.[84] There are several typical patterns by which cancer

FIG. 1-1. Incidence of prostate, colon, and stomach cancer among males, aged 20 to 80 years. (Third National Cancer Survey rates)

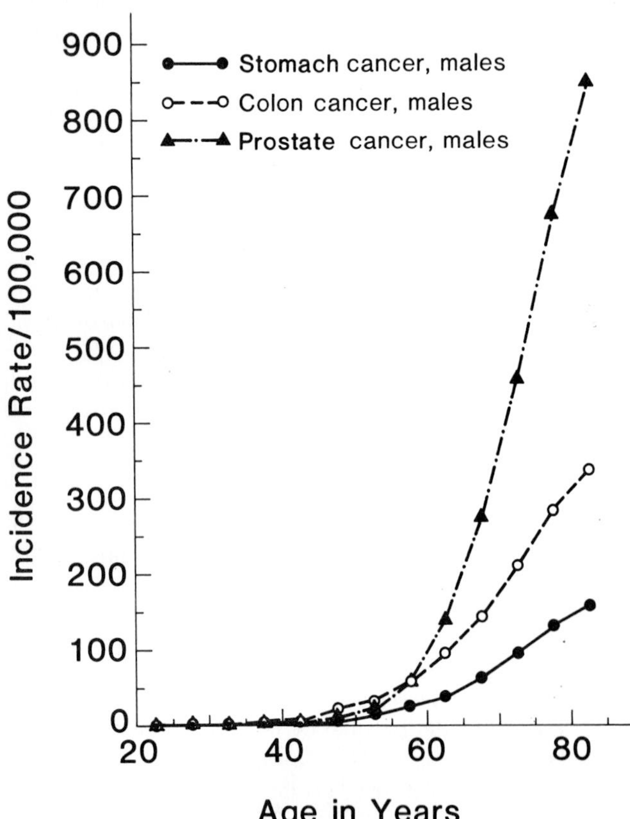

FIG. 1-2. Incidence of breast cancer among white and black females, aged 20 to 80 years. (Third National Cancer Survey rates)

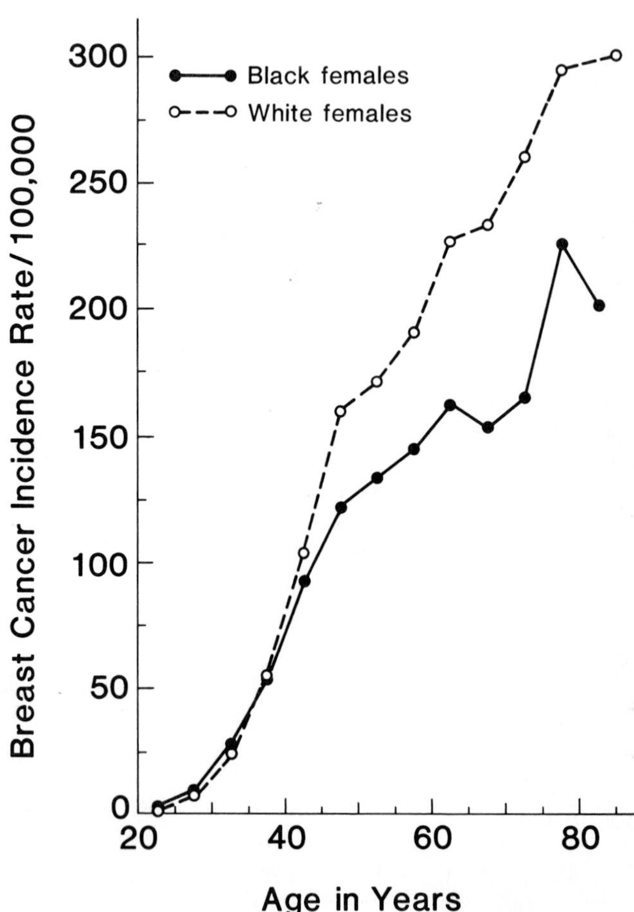

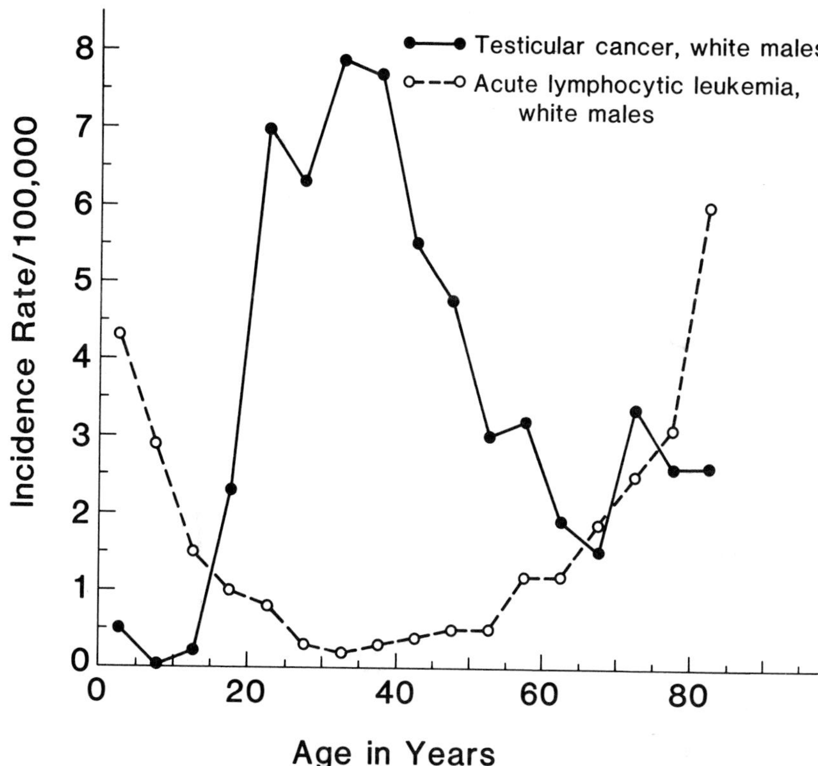

FIG. 1-3. Incidence of testicular cancer and acute lymphocytic leukemia among white males. (Third National Cancer Survey rates)

FIG. 1-4. Age-specific incidence rates of Hodgkin's disease in Brooklyn, New York, 1943–1952. (Adapted from MacMahon B, Pugh TF: Epidemiology: Principles and Methods. Boston, Little, Brown & Co., 1979)

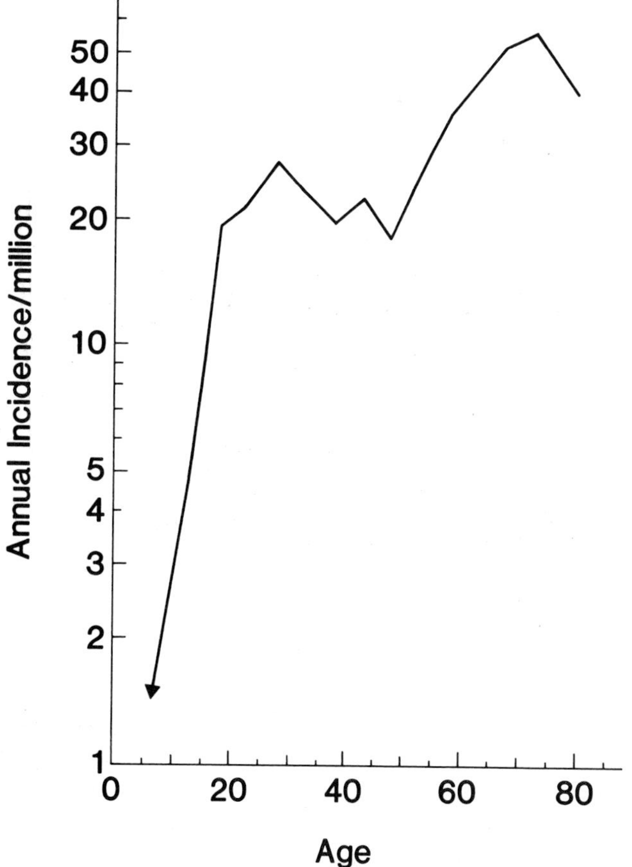

rates vary with age. Perhaps the most common pattern is a sharp, uninterrupted, and regular increase in magnitude that occurs from adulthood into the 80s. This is illustrated in Figure 1-1, which shows rates for prostate, colon, and stomach cancer in males. This type of pattern is generally associated with tumors of epithelial origin.

The incidence of carcinoma of the breast also increases with age but not in a regular manner. Breast cancer incidence rates for blacks and whites by age are shown in Figure 1-2, where the change in slope of the curves after age 45 is evident. This change is probably related to a change in hormonal status associated with menopause.[85] Not all cancers increase with age. Incidence rates for testicular cancer and acute lymphocytic leukemia in white males are shown in Figure 1-3. Testicular cancer has an almost trimodal distribution with a small peak in the first few years of life, a major peak at age 35, and a minor peak at age 75. Acute lymphocytic leukemia, on the other hand, has a clearly bimodal distribution with peaks occurring in infants and in the elderly, with very low rates in between. Hodgkin's disease also has a bimodal age distribution, as shown in Figure 1-4. Histologic differences between the two age groups have been shown.[86] These distributions may represent true changes in incidence by age, or each peak may represent different disease entities.

DIFFERENCES BY CHRONOLOGICAL TIME

Cancer rates vary not only by the age of the person but also by chronological time. Age-adjusted U.S. death rates for males and females from 1930 to 1979 are shown in Figures 1-5 and 1-6, where several marked changes in rates are evident. There are many reasons for changes in death rates not related to an actual change in occurrence of the disease. For example, a change in the survival rate or curability of a cancer may affect death rates. This is probably the case with uterine cancer, which has shown a steady decline since at least the 1930s. A change in the classification of disease may appear as an abrupt change in rates, while more subtle changes may occur with increasing or decreasing diagnostic capability.

Of course, changes in death rates do reflect actual changes in the incidence of a disease. Two prime examples in the United States are stomach cancer and lung cancer. Stomach cancer has been decreasing for many years in both men and women. In men the death rate has declined from about 30 of 100,000 in 1930 to 7 of 100,000 in the 1970s. Although no one factor can be singled out, it is suspected that the decrease in stomach cancer is related to changes in diet or food preservation occurring over this time.

The death rate for lung cancer has increased dramatically during the past 40 years. For men, the rates have increased by almost 20-fold, and the rates for women are following a similar trend, although the increase started at a later date. This increase in lung cancer rates, almost entirely attributed to cigarette smoking, is a well-worn but particularly frustrating example. It is a case in which an increase in rates has been definitely attributed to a clearly preventable factor, and yet relatively little progress has been made in reducing the rates.

GEOGRAPHIC DIFFERENCES—INTERNATIONAL

Data from cancer registries around the world show a range of diversity. The common cancer sites, with high and low international incidence areas and the range of this variation, are listed in Table 1-11. Some sites (breast and bladder) have a relatively small variance in rates, 6- or 7-fold, while other sites (skin, esophagus, and penis) have a variance greater than 200-fold. Comparisons of geographical areas with high and low rates may lead to important etiologic clues. As with death rates, however, one must be aware that the differences observed may be an artifact related more to differences in reporting or diagnosis rather than differences in actual occurrence of the cancer.

GEOGRAPHICAL DIFFERENCES—NATIONAL

Differences in cancer rates also exist on a national level. As described in a previous section, site-specific cancer mortality

FIG. 1-5. Age-adjusted cancer death rates for males from selected sites in the United States, 1930–1977. (American Cancer Society: Facts and Figures. New York, American Cancer Society, 1980)

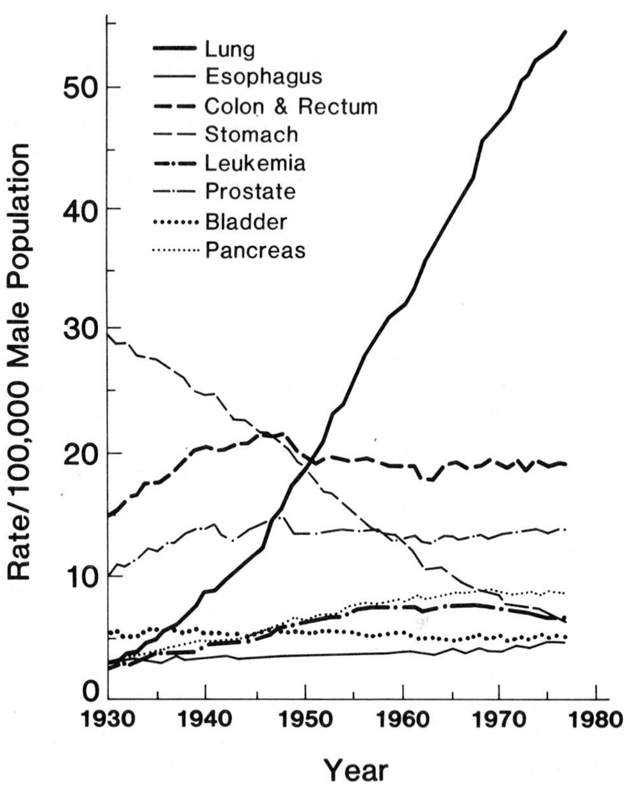

FIG. 1-6. Age-adjusted cancer death rates for females from selected sites in the United States, 1930–1977. (American Cancer Society: Facts and Figures. New York, American Cancer Society, 1980)

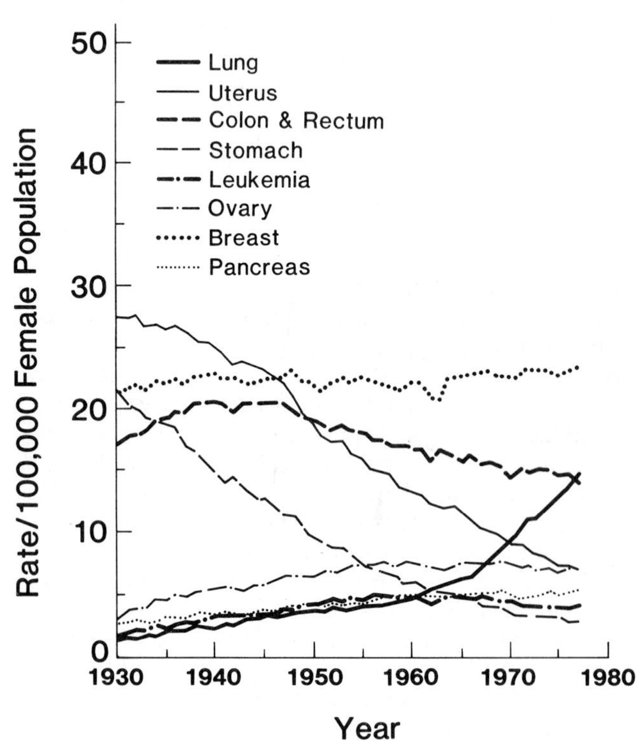

TABLE 1-11. Variation in the Incidence of Common Cancers

	HIGH INCIDENCE AREA	CUMULATIVE RISK	LOW INCIDENCE AREA	RANGE OF VARIATION
		%		
Skin	Australia (Queensland)	>20	India (Bombay)	>200*
Esophagus	Iran (Northeast)	20	Nigeria (Ibadan)	300
Bronchus	England	11	Nigeria (Ibadan)	35
Stomach	Japan (Okayama)	11	Uganda (Kampala)	25
Cervix uteri (F)†	Columbia (Cali)	10	Israel (Jewish persons)	15
Prostate	USA (black persons)	9	Japan (Miyagi)	40
Liver	Mozambique (Lower Marques)	8	England	100
Breast (F)	Canada (British Columbia)	7	Israel (non-Jewish persons)	7
Colon	USA (Connecticut)	3	Nigeria (Ibadan)	10
Corpus uteri (F)	USA (California, white persons)	3	Japan (Osaka)	30
Buccal cavity	India	>2	Denmark	>25
Rectum	Denmark	2	Nigeria (Ibadan)	6
Bladder	USA (Connecticut)	2	Japan (Miyagi)	6
Ovary	Denmark	2	Japan (Miyagi)	6
Nasopharynx	Singapore (Chinese)	2	England	40
Larynx	Brazil (Sao Paulo)	2	Japan (Miyagi)	10
Pharynx	India (Bombay)	2	Denmark	20
Pancreas	NZ (Maori)	1	India (Bombay)	8
Penis	Uganda (part)	1	Israel (Jewish persons)	300

(Reprinted from Doll R: The epidemiology of cancer. In Fortner JG, Rhoads JE (eds): Accomplishments in Cancer Research. Philadelphia, JB Lippincott, 1979)
* Rate, for example, 200-fold.
† F = female.

rates by U.S. counties have been computed and examined in the form of atlases indicating areas of high and low rates.[74,75] These maps are useful in defining problem areas from a health care viewpoint as well as areas in which epidemiologic investigations might be warranted. By comparison with the distribution of other factors, the maps may provide etiologic clues. Three examples follow.

The distribution of male lung cancer death rates is shown in Figure 1-7. Areas of high incidence are evident along the Gulf Coast and Eastern Seabord. Subsequent studies have indicated the high rates associated with the shipbuilding, fishing, and petroleum industries.[87,88]

Stomach cancer in white males, a much rarer entity, shows a striking pattern when rates are plotted by county. A cluster of counties with high rates is found in the north-central region, particularly in Minnesota, the Dakotas, Michigan, and Wisconsin, as seen in Figure 1-8. This area is known to have a large portion of foreign-born residents, particularly of Russian, Austrian, Scandinavian, and German origin. It is believed that the high rates in these areas are a result of the disposition this ethnic group has to develop the disease and is compatible with the high incidence of this tumor in the countries of origin. The smaller cluster in New Mexico and Colorado is suggestive of high stomach cancer among Spanish-surnamed persons in these areas.[89]

The distribution of cancer of the liver and billiary passage among nonwhite females is shown in Figure 1-9. Several areas with high rates are seen in the western states, with a small concentration in the north-central area as well. This corresponds well to the distribution of American Indians residing in this country. Previous studies have shown that gallbladder disease and gallbladder cancer occurs at an extremely high rate among American Indian women.[90] Thus, the distribution of Indians, to a large extent, explains the pattern seen on this particular map. Many other interesting patterns exist, some of which can be explained by current knowledge and some of which await further investigation.

MIGRANT STUDIES

Population migration represents a natural experiment and thus an opportunity to investigate host and environmental factors as determinants of cancer risk. When cancer rates assume the levels of the host country, the influencing factors are thought to be environmental rather than genetic. Studies of migrant groups lend themselves to several generalizations, as described by Haenszel.[91] For stomach cancer, migrants from high-risk areas show some reduction in rates but still retain some characteristic experience of the country of origin. Stomach cancer rates are high in Japan and low in the United States. These studies indicate that the level of stomach cancer risk is determined primarily by events in early life. Thus, primary prevention by environmental modification offers limited prospects. For large bowel cancer the Japanese migrants with high rates assume the low rates of the United States. The pattern is different than for stomach cancer in that changes of environment in adult life may have an effect on risk relatively soon.[92] This could have significant implications for primary prevention, especially as large bowel cancer is being related to diets high in fat and low in fiber.[93] The risk

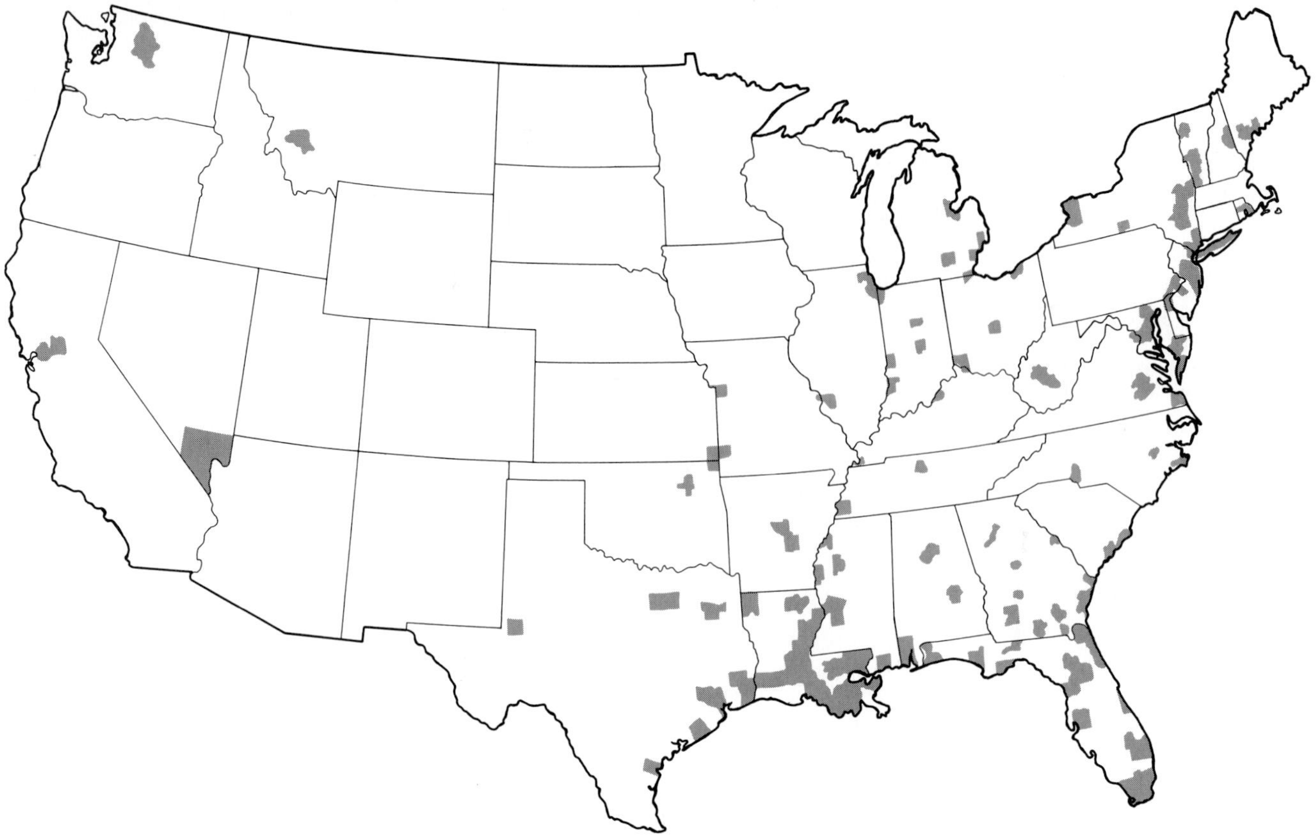

FIG. 1-7. Cancer mortality, 1950–1969, by U.S. county for cancer of the trachea, bronchus, and lung among white males. Denotes counties significantly higher than U.S. average. (Adapted from Mason TJ, McKay FW, Hoover, R, et al: Atlas of Cancer Mortality for U.S. Counties: 1950–1969. Washington DC, US Government Printing Office, 1975)

FIG. 1-8. Cancer mortality, 1950–1969, by county for cancer of the stomach among white males. Denotes counties significantly higher than the U.S. average. (Adapted from Mason TJ, McKay FW, Hoover R, et al: Atlas of Cancer Mortality for U.S. Counties: 1950–1969. Washington DC, US Government Printing Office, 1975)

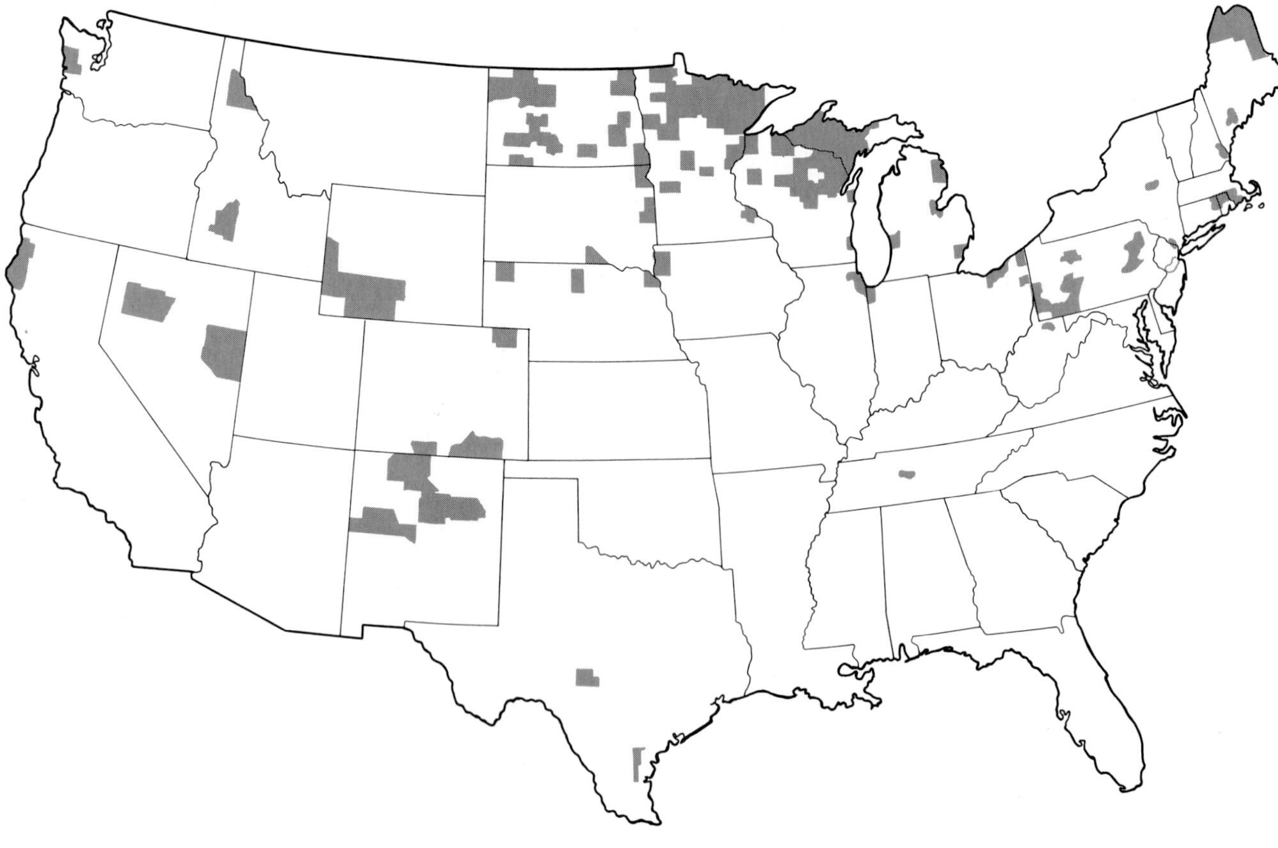

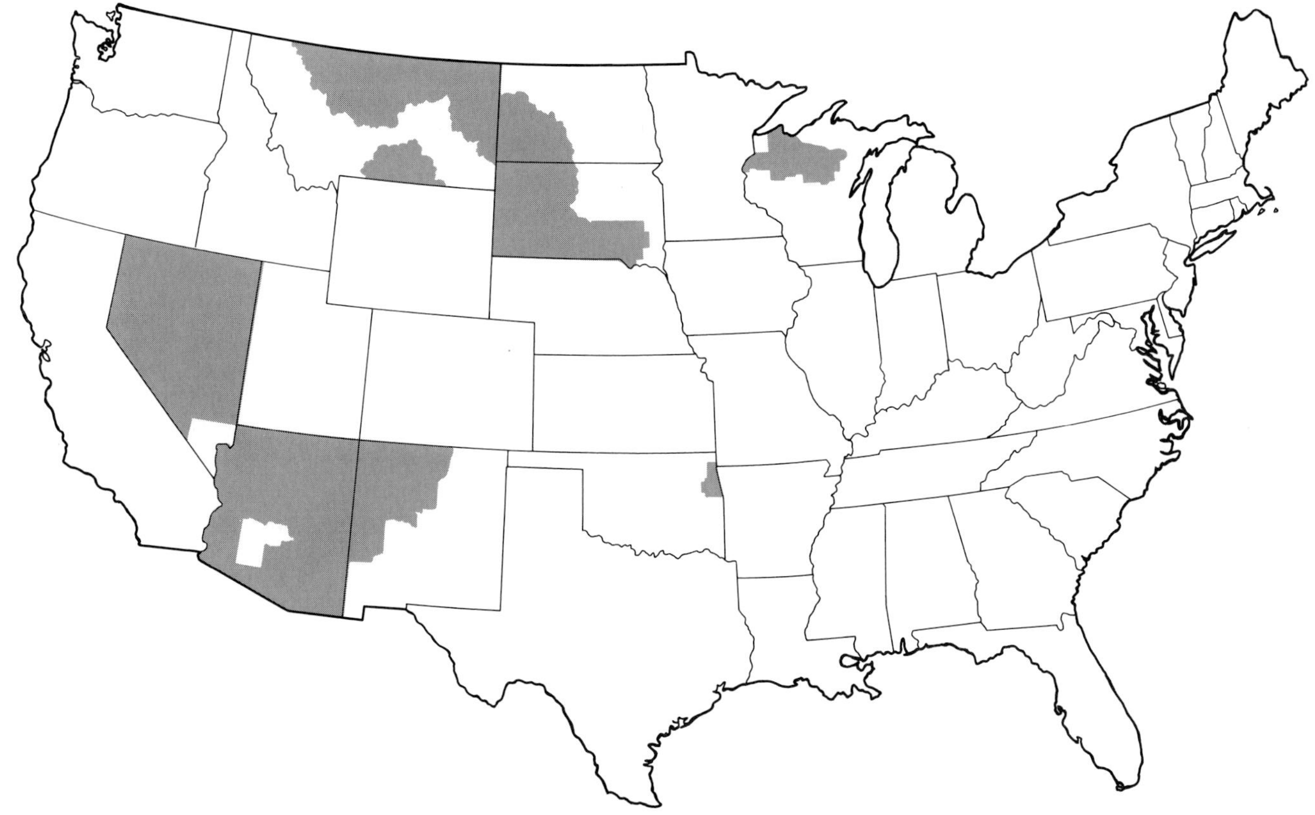

FIG. 1-9. Cancer mortality, 1950–1969, by state economic area for cancer of the biliary passages and liver among nonwhite females. Denotes state economic areas significantly higher than the U.S. average. (Adapted from Mason TJ, McKay FW, Hoover R, et al: Atlas of Cancer Mortality Among U.S. Nonwhites: 1950–1969. Washington DC, US Government Printing Office, 1976)

for developing breast cancer also assumes the rates of the host country, although it occurs over two generations. As with large bowel cancer, breast cancer changes have been associated with changes in dietary factors.[94] Japanese women have a low breast cancer risk in Japan and assume a high risk when they move to the United States.

ETHNIC GROUPS

Blacks

Cancer among black Americans has increased during the past 25 years. Although some of this increase may be due to underreporting and under numeration of census figures, most epidemiologists believe there has been a real increase.[95] Among black males there has been an overall 63% increase compared to a 24% increase in white males. Lung cancer has increased more than 400%. Colonic and rectal, prostatic, pancreatic, and esophageal cancers have also increased. Among black females, the overall rate has decreased by 4% compared to 9% for white females. Deaths from lung cancer among black females have increased, as they have among white females. Large bowel and breast cancers have also increased. There is a striking difference between cancer of the cervix and cancer of the corpus uterus. Cancer of the cervix is 120% higher among blacks than among whites, whereas cancer of the corpus uterus is 53% lower in black females. Differences in dietary, occupational, genetic, and other life-style factors may explain these differing rates eventually.

Asians, American Indians, and Hispanics

Thomas summarized the occurrence of cancer in the main racial groups residing in the four western states bordering the Pacific Ocean (Alaska, Washington, Oregon, and California).[96] These groups include blacks, Japanese, Chinese, Filipinos, American Indians, and Hispanics. Although cautioning about the use of such diversified data, Thomas makes some interesting generalizations. Cancers associated with cigarette smoke (lung, larynx, and bladder) tend to occur less frequently in migrants (and in their native lands) than in white Americans. Cancers etiologically related to reproductive and endocrine factors (prostate, ovary, corpus uteri, breast, and testis) tend to occur less frequently in minorities and in their countries of origin. Conversely, cancers related to diets rich in meat and animal protein (colon-rectum, kidney, and other endocrine-related cancers) develop more frequently among white Americans than among other groups. Cancers of the stomach and esophagus, which have a different relation to diet, tend to occur at higher rates among minorities. Neoplasms that have a suspected viral etiology (nasopharynx, cervix, and liver) occur more frequently in minorities (and in their homeland) than in white Americans. Hodgkin's disease tends to occur less frequently in minority populations (and their countries of origin) than in white Americans. This is consistent with the model suggested by Newell that, like paralytic polio, Hodgkin's disease is a rare manifestation of a common infection.[97] High rates of cancer of the gallbladder were seen in Indians and Spanish-surnamed groups. A more detailed review of cancer in Asian populations is available.[98] Further studies of these groups hold great promise.

MULTIPLE PRIMARIES

Study of multiple primary cancers can be helpful in the ascertainment of etiologies, in clinical management, and in improvement of treatment techniques. Etiologic mechanisms suggested by these studies include hormonal factors (acting alone or in combination with dietary factors), dietary and nutritional factors, chemicals in the environment, social factors (especially cigarette smoking), radiation, chemotherapeutic agents, and genetic determinants.[99]

Although there are many case reports in the literature of aggregate multiple primary cancers, few studies attempt to measure these occurrences. All of these studies have inherent and unavoidable biases. There is a need for additional large studies using population-based registries with long-term follow-up. Data from the Third National Cancer Survey and the Surveillance, Epidemiology, and End Results programs of the National Cancer Institute would be particularly useful resources for some of these studies.

The multiple occurrence of breast, corpus uterus, ovary, and colon cancer suggests a hormonal priming of breast tissue, perhaps leading to hyperplasia, followed by nutritional alterations (low-fiber diet) leading to greater increase in carcinogens acting on hormonally primed tissue.[100,101] This combination of hormonally dependent tissues exposed to dietary carcinogens could explain why multiple tumors in humans occur mainly in the sex organs and digestive tract.[102]

The multiple occurrences of cancer of the cervix, lung, oral cavity, bladder, and pancreas suggest a common relation to cigarette smoking. The lack of association between cancer of the cervix and breast and cancer of the colon suggests this cluster is not related to hormonal or nutritional influences.

Synchronous occurrence of primary cancers of the breast, colon, and stomach suggests multicentric origins for these cancers and possible etiologic relation to the interaction between hormonal and dietary factors. Significant excesses in multiple epidermoid carcinomas are shared by tissues of the oral cavity, pharynx, glottis, supraglottis, and esophagus and are largely preventable by abstinence from cigarette smoking. Similarly, multiple-occurring cancers of the lung, larynx, bladder, and pancreas are attributed to cigarette smoking and are thus preventable.

Multiple occurrence of cancers of the nervous system, in childhood cancers and in families, indicates genetic predisposition by some, either by gene damage or predisposing diseases. In children, previous radiotherapy can account for a large number of second cancers.

Differences among racial groups within the United States for multiple primary breast cancers have been shown. Spanish–Americans have the highest rate, whites are intermediate, and blacks have the lowest rate. This observation needs to be confirmed and should be followed up by studies on environmental or other etiologic factors. There were no increased risks for second cancers among American Indians, although the numbers were extremely small.[99]

The carcinogenic potential of cancer chemotherapeutic agents in humans is now well recognized.[103] Many, and probably all, of the alkylating agents, many of the antitumor antibiotics, and some of the antitumor antimetabolites are carcinogens in animals. Acute myelogenous leukemia has been reported after treatment for Hodgkin's disease, multiple myeloma, ovarian carcinoma, chronic leukemia, and various solid tumors. Because many of these descriptions are isolated, it is difficult to estimate the frequency with which a second tumor emerges after cancer chemotherapy.

CORRELATION STUDIES

The relationship of diet to breast cancer has been widely investigated using correlation studies.[104,105] In these studies, total fat consumption was highly correlated with incidence of the disease. In Japan, where fat consumption and breast cancer have been increasing, Hirayama reported that the highest correlation was with the amount of per capita pork intake.[94] Death rates were also closely associated with the daily amount of animal fat consumed. Carroll and coworkers found significant positive correlations for per capita calorie and fat intakes with age-adjusted death rates for breast cancer in their study of persons from 24 countries.[106] In addition to fat, intake of protein and sugar has also been correlated with breast cancer incidence and mortality, respectively.[104,107] Conversely, a negative association has been found with starch intake.[108]

Studies of this type must be interpreted with care, in that they compare gross patterns of food availability with overall incidence and mortality rates. No conclusions on individual consumption and disease experience can be drawn.

SCREENING FOR CANCER

There is an intuitive appeal that screening for cancer will be rewarding in detecting early cancers when they are more amenable to successful treatment. In recent years screening programs for the control of cancer have steadily increased in number. Screening is not a simple, straightforward approach to cancer control and is difficult in terms of establishing screening objectives, the mechanics of conducting large programs over time, measuring desired outcomes, and justifying cost-benefits. Principles of cancer screening have been reviewed by several sources.[109,110]

PRINCIPLES OF SCREENING

To justify screening for any disease, the disease must have certain characteristics and a suitable cost effective screening test must be available. Diseases that have serious consequences such as severe or prolonged morbidity or that are fatal, including nearly all cancers if not treated, are suitable

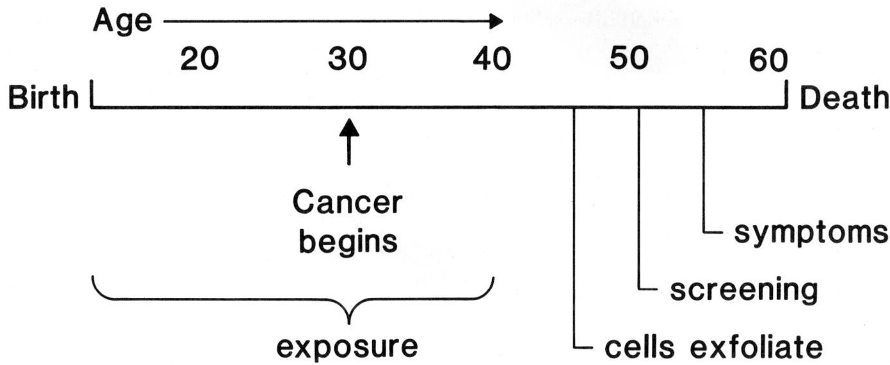

Interval	Age	Duration
1. Preclinical phase (Theoretical maximum lead time)	30 to 55	25 years
2. Detectable preclinical phase (Practical maximum lead time)	45 to 55	10
3. Observed lead time	(55–50)	5
4. Duration of survival from symptom diagnosis	(60–55)	5
5. Duration of survival from screen diagnosis	(60–50)	10

FIG. 1-10. Disease process relative to critical events for screening purposes. (Cole P, Morrison AS: Basic issues in population screening for cancer. J Natl Cancer Inst 64:1263–1272, 1980)

for screening. Treatment for the disease must be effective because there is no point in screening for a disease for which no effective treatment exists, such as most lung cancers. The amount of disease in the preclinical detectable form should be high among those screened, such as carcinoma-in-situ of the cervix among high-risk women. Most cancers do not meet this criteria. Figure 1-10 depicts the disease process relative to critical events for screening purposes.

The screening test should be inexpensive, easy to apply, and have a high consistent level of accurate interpretations. Ideally, it should be conveniently administered and painless. The test itself should not carry any untoward risk for the screened person. It is expected to separate persons with early disease as positive (reflection of sensitivity) and those without disease as negative (reflection of specificity). Usually if opting for high sensitivity, specificity must be sacrificed, and vice versa. Table 1-12 shows how sensitivity and specificity calculations are derived. The positive predictive value is the likelihood that a patient whose results are positive on a given test will prove to have cancer after diagnostic work-up. Calculations are shown in Table 1-13. Most important, remember that all screening tests have limitations and there is no ideal cancer screening test.

Galen and Gambino describe the relationships between sensitivity and specificity, and positive predictive value as follows.[111]

The highest sensitivity (preferably 100%) is desired in these situations.

- The disease is serious and should not be missed.
- The disease is treatable.
- False-positive results do not lead to serious psychologic or economic trauma to the patient.

Example: Cancer of the cervix can be fatal if missed but if diagnosed is nearly 100% curable. Other examples include

TABLE 1-12. Sensitivity* and Specificity† of a Screening Test

	EARLY DISEASE		
TEST OUTCOME	*Yes*	*No*	TOTAL
Positive‡	a	b	a + b
Negative	c	d	c + d
Total	(a + c)	(b + d)	N = a + b + c + d

* Sensitivity = a/(a + c).
† Specificity = d/(b + d).
‡ Positive predictive value = a/(a + b).

TABLE 1-13. Sample Screening Test

	EARLY DISEASE		
TEST OUTCOME	*Yes*	*No*	*Total*
Positive	400	995	1,395
Negative	100	98,505	98,605
Total	500	99,500	100,000

Disease prevalence = 5/1,000 (500/100,000); sensitivity = 80% (400/500); specificity = 99% (98,505/99,500); positive predictive value = 29% (400/1,395).

phenylketonuria, venereal disease, and other treatable infectious disease.

The highest specificity (preferably 100%) is desired in these situations.

- The disease is serious but is not treatable or curable.
- The knowledge that the disease is absent has psychologic or public health value.
- False-positive results can lead to serious phychologic or economic trauma to the patient.

Example: Cancer of the pancreas is serious but generally not treatable.

A high predictive value for a positive result is essential in this situation.

- Treatment of a false-positive might have serious consequences.

Example: For occult cancer of the lung, if a lobectomy is done or radiation given to a patient without the cancer, the consequences might be disastrous.

Consideration must also be given to the diagnostic work-up to which each person who screens positive will be subjected. This includes the psychic trauma to the person being screened, the cost of the diagnostic work-up (which can be considerable), and the morbidity of the diagnostic procedures. For example, the work-up of a positive sputum cytology is traumatic and costly and may include bronchoscopy and exploratory surgery.

CANCER SCREENING OF HEALTHY POPULATIONS

In mid-1980 the American Cancer Society (ACS) issued updated guidelines for screening for cancer.[112] It stressed that these recommendations pertain to the early detection of cancer in asymptomatic persons on an individual basis. These guidelines are summarized in Table 1-14. The ACS also stresses that these recommendations are intended to help individual physicians and patients select the best early detection protocol for their personal needs and recognizes that no single recommendation is best for everyone.

The new recommendations reflect very important findings. First, the ACS continues to find that the early detection of cancer is a very important health promotion activity. It continues to believe that early detection provides a very effective way to reduce the morbidity and mortality of several cancers to protect people's health. Second, the new recommendations provide essentially the same benefits at greatly reduced risk, costs, and inconvenience. Finally, the ACS states that it is important to interpret these recommendations as interim guidelines, based on the best information available at the time, to be reviewed as new tests and more information become available.

SCREENING FOR EARLY-STAGE CANCER

The value of organized and efficient screening programs as an active component of cancer prevention programs should not be underestimated.[113] Ideally, prevention of cancer is always preferable to detecting the disease in its various phases,

TABLE 1-14. Proposed American Cancer Society Recommendations for Screening Asymptomatic Patients (March 1980)

TEST OR PROCEDURE	SEX	POPULATION AGE	RISK	FREQUENCY	PREVIOUS RECOMMENDATION
Chest x-ray film	Not recommended for any population				High-risk persons annually*
Sputum cytology	Not recommended for any population				Not recommended
Sigmoidoscopy	M, F	Over 50	. . .	Every 3 years†	Persons over 40 annually
Stool guaiac slide test	M, F	Over 50	. . .	Every year	Persons over 40 annually
Digital rectal examination‡	M, F	Over 40	. . .	Every year	Same
Papanicolaou's (Pap) test	F	20–65§	. . .	Every 3 years‖	Annually
Pelvic examination	F	20–40	. . .	Every 3 years	Annually
		Over 40	. . .	Every year	Same
Endometrial tissue sample	F	At menopause	High#	At menopause	Same
Breast self-examination	F	Over 20	. . .	Every month	Same
Breast physical examination	F	20–40	. . .	Every 3 years	Annually
		Over 40	. . .	Every year	Same
Mammography	F	35–40	. . .	Base-line	No policy
		Under 50	. . .	Consult physician	Policy related only to BCDDP**
		Over 50	. . .	Every year	Policy related only to BCDDP
Health counseling and cancer check-	M, F	Over 20	. . .	Every 3 years	"Periodic"
up††	M, F	Over 40	. . .	Every year	

(Reprinted with permission of the American Cancer Society, New York)
* Persons over 40 who smoke or are exposed to other lung carcinogens.
† After two initial negative examinations a year apart.
‡ Includes single guaiac test.
§ Pap test should also be done on women under 20 who are sexually active.
‖ After two initial Pap tests done a year apart are negative; high-risk women should have more frequent Pap tests.
History of infertility, obesity, failure of ovulation, abnormal uterine bleeding, or estrogen therapy.
** BCDDP = Breast Cancer Detection Demonstration Project.
†† To include examination for cancers of the thyroid, testicles, prostate, ovaries, lymph nodes, oral region, and skin.

when aggressive and expensive treatments are often called for. Unfortunately, knowledge of how to prevent most cancers does not yet exist. Even if all cancers could now be prevented, millions of people already exposed to cancer-causing agents face diagnosis of the disease well into the 21st century. Thus, screening for early-stage cancer becomes a significant subject for all health professionals involved in primary care.[114]

Cervical Cancer

Cancer of the cervix is essentially preventable, and if detected during its early stages may be reversed. Occurrence has been related to socioeconomic and cultural conditions. Although in recent years incidence in black and white women in the United States has dropped, it is still more than double among blacks compared to whites. Risk factors associated with cancer of the cervix are coitus at an early age, multiple pregnancies, multiple sex partners, and a history of venereal disease.[115]

The screening test most often used for detecting cervical cancer is cytology. The clinician should obtain two specimens, one from the endocervical canal and one from the squamocolumnar junction. If the squamocolumnar junction is not visible, a scraping should be taken from the anatomic os. The test should be repeated at appropriate intervals to identify the malignancy at an early stage. The examination for asymptomatic women is an important screening procedure that should be encouraged by all providers of health care. As with any screening test, cytology should be available and affordable to everyone at risk for this type of cancer.

The annual Papanicolaou (Pap) smear has been reviewed by different authors as to its cost-benefit, and controversy exists among different groups. The new ACS recommendations advise Pap smears every 3 years for most women after two consecutive negative Pap smears. These new recommendations have raised some important questions. Many women have periodic examinations including Pap smear and examination of the breast, vulva, vagina, uterus, and ovaries. In short, they have come to accept the Pap test as their annual cancer test. If certain women are told they should have Pap smears every 3 to 5 years, will they, in the interim, continue to receive regular examinations of the breast and genital area? More recently, a National Institutes of Health consensus development conference panel has recommended rescreening "at regular intervals of one to three years." The panel was unable to agree precisely on how frequently asymptomatic women should undergo the Pap smear test.[116]

Breast Cancer

Screening for breast cancer appears to offer promise of reduced mortality from this disease, which remains the primary cause of cancer mortality among American women. It is known that when breast cancer is clinically localized before nodal involvement, the 5-year survival rate is 85%. The survival rate drops with nodal involvement, which unfortunately has occurred by the time most breast cancer is detected.

Because most breast cancers are not localized when first seen by the clinician, earlier detection of preclinical cancer in asymptomatic women should be considered an important goal.[117] This point has been emphasized by many breast cancer screening program studies, including that conducted by the Health Insurance Plan of Greater New York (HIP) on women 50 to 60 years of age. Combining physical examination and mammography, the 9-year HIP follow-up program demonstrated a 30% reduction in mortality for women with breast cancer over the control group.[118]

With improvement in mammographic techniques, the potential exists for even higher cure rates for breast cancer. Although mammography or any method used alone is not 100% accurate, a combination of methods, including breast self-examination, professional palpation, and mammography, increases the accuracy of earlier detection and, in turn, reduces mortality.

The importance of breast self-examination should not be underestimated. The health care provider, whether physician or nurse, must learn to teach breast self-examination and encourage patients to take advantage of this important early detection method.[119] Of particular importance is that the patient understand the rationale behind each step of the self-examination procedure, as well as being knowledgeable about subtle breast changes.

Colon and Rectal Cancer

Colon-rectal cancer is second only to lung cancer as a cause of death among American males and is the third highest cause of death among women. This cancer comprises the largest group of all the gastrointestinal tumors, of which most lesions are adenocarcinomas. Survival is dependent on the stage of disease at the time of diagnosis. Persons at higher risk for colon-rectal cancer are those with familial polyposis, Gardner's syndrome, ulcerative colitis, a history of the disease, or a change in bowel habits. In recent years, a growing awareness has been focused on the association between high-fat/low-fiber diets and the occurrence of colon-rectal cancer.[120,121]

Some cancers of the colon-rectum can be found by digital examination. This safe, cost-efficient examination should be used as a routine screening procedure during any physical examination. Other methods of detection include the Hemoccult test and sigmoidoscopy. Polyps associated with cancer of the colon-rectum can also be detected by the sigmoidoscope.

Hemoccult slide testing (examination of a stool specimen for occult blood) appears to be an inexpensive and simple procedure for screening in persons over 40 years of age. However, no long-term study data are available to ascertain the efficacy of the test in early detection of colon-rectal cancer.

The ability of the Hemoccult slide to predict cancer is highly dependent on the investigator following the proper procedure.[122] Although the accuracy of the test has been questioned, false-negatives can be reduced by correct procedures such as dietary preparation, three consecutive stool specimens, and prompt analysis. Patients with positive Hemoccult results under proper procedure should be referred for diagnostic work-up. Patients with higher risk may need special observation.

Studies supporting sigmoidoscopic examination were conducted by the Kaiser Medical Center Multiphasic Screening

Program and showed, in a controlled trial, that periodic check-ups, including digital rectal and sigmoidoscopic examination, can reduce colon-rectal cancer mortality.[123]

Some errors commonly encountered in colon-rectum screening include the assumption that blood in the stool is caused only by hemorrhoids and the failure to perform a digital examination because of discomfort to the patient. Patients with cancer in one site are at a higher risk for other primary tumors and should be followed-up for life for recurrence of colon-rectal cancer, as well as for second primary cancers.

Skin Cancer

Nonmelanoma skin cancer accounts for an estimated 400,000 new cases annually, most of which are highly curable basal or squamous cell cancers. The accessibility of the skin for screening simplifies early detection. With early detection and proper treatment, 90% to 95% of basal cell carcinomas of the skin can be cured; in lesions less than 1 cm in diameter, 99% cure is possible.[124]

Screening for skin cancer involves inspection and palpation of the skin. Any lesion that appears suspicious should be properly evaluated for early diagnosis and proper treatment. Basal and squamous cell skin cancers may appear on the skin either as pale, waxlike, pearly nodules that ulcerate and crust or as a red, scaly, sharply outlined patch. People should be educated to recognize unusual skin changes, changes in moles, or the presence of new lesions. Once treated for a skin cancer, the patient must recognize that new primary tumors are likely and a continued awareness of early warning signs is essential.

Oral Cancer

Oral cancer accounts for about 3% of all cancers occurring in the United States and is seen most frequently in men over 40 years of age. Although the exact cause of oral cancer is unknown, several well-known factors contribute. Oral cancers occur most frequently in persons who smoke and drink excessively, have poor oral hygiene, and have chronic irritation from jagged teeth or ill-fitting dentures. The smoking of pipes and cigars is thought to be the cause of mouth cancer because of the high heat that irritates the mouth tissue.

When inspecting the oral cavity, the professional should have a good light, a tongue blade, finger cots, and gauze. When the patient performs oral self-examination, he should be instructed to use whatever materials are available at home to visualize the mouth, such as a washcloth, spoon, flashlight, and mirror.

Lesions of the mucosal linings may appear as hyperkeratosis (white patches) or erythroplakia (red velvety patches), and as the lesion progresses it may appear as ulceration or exophytic growth. Any suspicious lesion should be evaluated for early diagnosis and proper treatment.

Lung Cancer

Several organized attempts at early tumor detection through large-scale screening of asymptomatic populations have been undertaken. Although results have been mixed, no strong evidence emerges from these studies that screening of asymptomatic populations improves lung cancer mortality. More recently, a study applicable to the primary care setting and lacking some of the shortcomings of previous studies has been initiated at the Mayo Clinic, Memorial Sloan-Kettering, and Johns Hopkins. The Mayo study involves asymptomatic, male, heavy cigarette smokers over age 45 screened with chest radiographs and sputum cytology examinations every 4 months and compared to a control group having only a chest x-ray film yearly.[125] Although it is too early to draw conclusions, unless these data prove otherwise, any decision to undertake lung cancer screening among the general population must be considered at best empiric and possibly ineffective. However, physicians may want to follow patients at high risk for lung cancer (heavy cigarette smokers over the age of 50) with chest x-ray films and cytologic tests of sputum for the detection of lung cancer in a nonsymptomatic stage when it is more amenable to curative surgery.

APPENDIX: SELECTED APPLICATIONS OF STATISTICAL TESTS

ADJUSTING FOR CONFOUNDING VARIABLES

Mantel–Haenszel Approach

When analyzing the results of case-comparison or cohort studies, one must sometimes take into account confounding variables (*see* section on confounders). For retrospective studies, a commonly used procedure was developed by Mantel and Haenszel.[126] To use the Mantel–Haenszel approach, the data are subdivided by the confounding factors such as age, sex, or residence. Relative risk estimates (relative odds) are calculated for each individual subtable and the values combined. Denote the frequencies in the 2 × 2 tables in the ith subdivision.

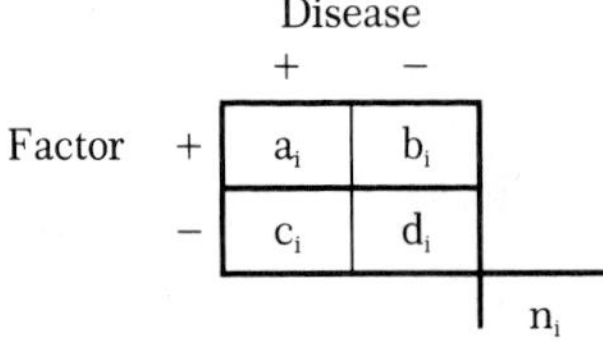

The pooled estimate of the relative risk is then $R = \sum_i \frac{a_i d_i / n_i}{b_i c_i / n_i}$

The Mantel–Haenszel statistic gives a reasonable estimate of the relative risk if the true relative risk is constant within each of the subtables. If the true relative risk is not constant, however, the Mantel–Haenszel procedure may fail to detect an association when one exists. To ascertain the constancy of the relative risk, visually inspect the relative odds computed for each of the subtables. If these appear quite different from each other, it is advisable to use another procedure such as GENCAT, a weighted least squares approach for categorical data analysis.[127]

Logistic Regression

Logistic regression has also been proposed as a means of adjusting for confounders when analyzing both case-comparison and cohort studies.[115] In a prospective study, the dependent or outcome variable is a (0, 1) indicator of whether the subject is a case or compeer (for example, 0 = compeer; 1 = case). The regression variables or independent variables represent both variables associated with risk and confounding factors, along with interaction terms. In case-comparison studies the outcome variable is a (0, 1) indicator of exposure to a particular risk factor (for example, 0 = no exposure; 1 = exposed). Here the regression variables or independent variables represent case or compeer status, other risk factors, confounding factors, and interaction terms involved with disease status. The logistic function is defined as follows.

$$\ln\left[\frac{P(\pi_1|x)}{1 - P(\pi_1|x)}\right] = \ln \exp(\alpha_0 + \beta_1 x_1 + \cdots \beta_k x_k).$$

The beta coefficients can be estimated using standard linear discriminant techniques, assuming that the distribution is multivariate normal with different means and the same variances and covariances.[129] The beta coefficients can also be estimated using more complicated methods such as maximum likelihood. For testing hypotheses, however, the linear discriminate function coefficients are satisfactory, even when the assumptions are somewhat violated.[130] The beta coefficients calculated for various risk factors and interaction terms can be tested individually to ascertain whether, given a fixed level of the remaining factors, the particular factor being tested significantly affects the outcome. Most computer programs that do a multiple logistics analysis will give these tests of coefficients. Also, $e^{\beta i}$ gives an estimate of the relative risk associated with the ith factor after fixing levels of the other factors. For example, if cancer was the outcome and the risk factors included estrogen exposure, smoking, and fibroid tumors, the value of e^{β} for fibroid tumors would be the increased risk of cancer given that a person had fibroid tumors.

The main caution in using the logistic approach relates to interactions. If testing of the coefficients indicates interactions are present in the model, then the estimates of the beta coefficients for the main effects cannot really be interpreted. When interactions are present, it is best to subdivide the data into strata indicated by the interactions and do a separate logistic analysis within each stratum. For example, if the investigator is studying a particular cancer and its association with exposure to estrogens in a drug manufacturing plant, he might find that males react in one way to the exposure and females in another. Thus, the best approach would be to do a logistics analysis for males and another one for females.

ADJUSTMENT OF RATES

Many etiologic clues can be found by comparing different populations for cancer incidence and mortality. However, an adjustment must often be made before comparing rates, because of differences in the structure of the populations being compared. For example, one might wish to compare cancer rates in a community before and after construction of a nuclear power plant. Before the plant is built, the community consists of a retired, elderly population. Construction of the plant attracts to the community a population of young, healthy workers and families. The age structure of the population of the community shifts from an elderly to a young industrial population. Comparison of cancer rates in the population of the community before and after construction of the nuclear power plant would then require adjustment for age.

Several methods are available to make comparisons of cancer mortality rates when there must be an adjustment for a related factor.[131] The first method is to compute specific rates for each population. Using age as an example, this would involve ascertaining the age distribution of each population and the age distribution of the cancer cases. The age-specific rate is then the number of persons with cancer in a particular group divided by the number of persons of that age in the population. Of course, specific rates can be calculated for factors other than age. Specific rates are advantageous because they give an accurate and detailed description of variation in cancer incidence or mortality among different strata, such as different age groups.

Direct and indirect standardization can provide a single summary index for each population. This summary index is more easily compared than the schedule of the specific rates for each population. Also, if some strata are quite small, the specific rates may not be precise or reliable. For some populations or groups of special interest, specific rates may not exist because only the total number of events such as cancer may be available, not the subdivision by such strata as age. Direct and indirect standardization have the disadvantage that standardization may mask differences across the various strata. Therefore, when a single summary index is desired, it is also important to look at specific rates as well as the summary index.

Indirect Standardization

When specific rates for a particular population are unreliable or do not exist, indirect standardization can be used. To do indirect standardization, it is necessary to know the crude cancer incidence or mortality rate (C) for the population being studied, that is, the number of persons with cancer in the population divided by the number of persons in the population. It is also necessary to know the distribution of the event being studied across strata, that is, the numbers of persons in each age group who have the cancer being studied (e_i). However, it is not necessary to know the number in the population who are in each age group. The data for the population being studied are then adjusted to a standard population for which specific rates (S_i), such as the age-specific rates for the cancer being studied, are available and the crude rate (R) for the standard population is also available.

The indirect rate is then calculated as follows.

$$C' = S_1e_1 + S_2e_2 + \cdots S_Ie_I = \sum_{i=1}^{I} S_ie_i$$

where I = total number of strata. The indirect adjusted rate is then

$$C_{indirect} = RC/C'.$$

If the specific rates are equal and the study population is indirectly adjusted, the adjusted rates may not be equal. This distortion, however, is not great. If the standard population is a composite of the populations being studied, this will not happen. Indirect standardization does not completely adjust for differences in the distribution of factors, such as age in the population studies.

Direct Standardization

A second method is called direct standardization. This may be applied only when the specific rates for the study populations (s_i) and the distribution across the various strata, such as age for the selected standard population (P_i), are available. For example, the age-specific rates for breast cancer for the study population and the proportion of women in each age group in the standard population would be needed. The direct adjusted rate is then

$$C_{direct} = s_1P_1 + s_2P_2 + \cdots s_IP_I = \sum_{i=1}^{I} s_iP_i$$

where I = total number of strata.

Direct adjusted rates have the property that if specific rates for two populations are equal, their directly adjusted rates will be equal no matter what population is used as a standard. The magnitude of the rate, however, depends strongly on the composition of the standard population.

For both direct and indirect adjusted rates, it is important to remember that the rate has meaning only when compared with a similarly adjusted rate. For example, Doll and Cook looked at total incidence of stomach cancer standardized (indirectly) for age.[132] Three different populations were used as standard populations to which all countries' age distributions were adjusted. These included Africa with a high proportion of young people, the world population (46 nations), and a European (predominantly Scandinavian) population with a high proportion of older people. Although the ranking changes little, the magnitude varies greatly depending on the population chosen as a standard.

OTHER STATISTICAL MEASURES FOR INFERENCE AND TESTING

The choice of statistical measures to be used in inference and testing depends on properties of data being collected. Data can be subdivided into discrete and continous measurements. Discrete data are those that take on distinct and separate values, usually including counts that must be whole numbers or a grading such as assessment of the healing of a bone. Continous data are those that assume a continuous uninterrupted range of values, including such variables as height, weight, age, and blood pressure.[31] Sometimes continuous data are categorized into discrete intervals such as age group (0–10 years, 11–20 years, and so forth). When continous data are categorized, they can be analyzed as discrete data.

The following is a brief summary of some available statistical measurements and an indication of when they should be used. For more complete discussions, *see* elementary statistical books such as those by Christensen and Colton.[133,134]

Discrete Data, Single Sample Compared to Standard

For discrete data where a single sample is being compared to a standard, the test statistic would be as follows.

p = observed proportion

π_0 = hypothesized value of the proportion (standard)

n = sample size

Then

$$Z = \frac{p - \pi_0}{(\pi_0(1 - \pi_0))/n}$$

Z is approximately distributed as a standard normal deviate if np is greater than 5 and $n(1 - p) > 5$. The probability of obtaining this observed value of Z can be obtained from statistical tables for the normal distribution. If np or $n(1 - p)$ is small, the probability for the binomial distribution should be calculated exactly. This can be done using binomial tables as found in the *CRC Handbook of Tables for Probability and Statistics.*[135]

Discrete Data, Paired Samples

When there are two samples to be compared, determine if the samples are paired or independent before proceeding with analysis. Examples of paired samples would be measures taken before and after treatment, observations on twins, and eye tests on the right and left eyes for a series of women. An example of independent samples would be measurement on a group of cancer cases and measurements on a group of compeers. For paired two sample test on a 2 × 2 table, McNemar's test would be used. It is computed as follows.

		Case Exposed	Not Exposed	
Control	Exposed	k	r	k + r
	Not Exposed	s	m	s + m
				N
		k + s	r + m	

$$Z = \frac{r - \left(\frac{r + s}{2}\right)}{(\sqrt{r + s})/2}$$

Z is distributed as a standard normal deviate if $(r + s)/2 > 5$, and thus the probability of obtaining the observed value of Z can be obtained from stastical tables for the normal distribution. If $(r + s)/2 \leq 5$, a nonparametric sign test should be used on r and s.

Discrete Data, Two Independent Samples

If there are two independent samples to be tested and a 2 × 2 table, the test statistic would be as follows.

$$\frac{r_1}{n_1} = p_1 = \text{observed proportion in sample 1}$$

$$\frac{r_2}{n_2} = p_2 = \text{observed proportion in sample 2}$$

$$p = \frac{r_1 + r_2}{n_1 + n_2}$$

$$n = n_1 + n_2$$

Then

$$Z = \frac{p_1 - p_2}{p\sqrt{\frac{1}{n_1} + \frac{1}{n_2}}}$$

Z is distributed approximately as a standard normal deviate if $np > 5$ and $n(1 - p) > 5$.

For smaller values of np and $n(1 - p)$, Fischer's exact test should be used. For the 2 × 2 table the Z test is equivalent to a chi-squre (χ^2) test. The advantage of using this test rather than the χ^2 test is that a confidence interval can be obtained and a two-sided test can be done. Using the χ^2 test, only a one-sided test can be done.

A χ^2 test for a 2 × 2 table is defined as follows.

$$\chi^2 = \sum_{i=1}^{4} \frac{(\text{observed ith cell value} - \text{expected ith cell value})^2}{(\text{expected ith cell value})}$$

Expected cell values are calculated for a 2 × 2 table (using letter notation from Table 1-5) as follows.

$$E(a) = \frac{(a + c)(a + b)}{N}$$

$$E(b) = \frac{(a + b)(b + d)}{N}$$

$$E(c) = \frac{(a + c)(c + d)}{N}$$

$$E(d) = \frac{(b + d)(c + d)}{N}$$

Note that the sums (a + b) and (c + d) are called the row marginals or sum of the rows. The sums (a + c) and (b + d) are the column marginals or column totals. If i refers to row and j to column, then

$$E(\text{cell}_{ij}) = \frac{(\text{row i total})(\text{column j total})}{N}$$

Thus for tables larger than 2 × 2 the χ^2 value can be calculated as above summing over all cells in the table. The probability of obtaining a χ^2 value as large as computed can be found in a statistical table for the χ^2 distribution under the appropriate degrees of freedom. Degrees of freedom = (number of rows − 1) × (number of columns − 1); for example, in a 2 × 2 table, degrees of freedom = (2 − 1) × (2 − 1) = 1. For χ^2 tests the entries in the cells in the tables must be counts or frequencies, not percentages.

Continuous Data, One Sample Compared Against Standard

For continuous data in the one sample case where the investigator is again testing against a standard, a t-statistic would be used where

n = sample size

$\bar{x}$ = observed mean value $\sum_{i=1}^{n} x_i/n$

μ_0 = hypothesized mean value (standard)

s = observed standard deviation = $\sqrt{\sum_{i=1}^{n} \frac{(x_i - \bar{x})^2}{n-1}}$

$$t = \frac{\bar{x} - \mu_0}{s/\sqrt{n}} \quad \text{degrees of freedom} = n - 1.$$

The probability of obtaining a t-value as computed can be obtained from a statistical table of the t-distribution for the appropriate degrees of freedom. The computation of t is based on the assumption that the distribution being tested is normal. If it suspected to be other than normally distributed, Kolmogorov-Smirnov or one-sample runs test should be used.

Continuous Data, Paired Samples

If in the two sample cases the samples are paired, then the t-statistic to be used would be as follows.

n = number of pairs

Sample 1 = $x_{11}, x_{12}, \cdots x_{1n}$

Sample 2 = $x_{21}, x_{22}, \cdots x_{2n}$

$$d_i = x_{1i} - x_{2i}$$

$$\bar{d} = \sum_{i=1}^{n} \frac{(x_{1i} - x_{2i})}{n}$$

$$s_d = \sqrt{\sum_{i=1}^{n} (di - \bar{d})^2/(n-1)}$$

$$t = \frac{\bar{d}}{s_d\sqrt{n}} \quad \text{degrees of freedom} = n - 1.$$

The probability of obtaining the observed value of t can be obtained as before from statistical tables of the t-distribution. If the distribution of the d_i is not normal, a sign test or Wilcoxon matched-pairs signed rank test can be used.

Continuous Data, Two Independent Samples

If in the two-sample case the samples are independent, then the following t-statistic would be used.

n_1 = sample size for sample 1

n_2 = sample size for sample 2

$\bar{x}_1 = \sum_{i=1}^{n_1} x_i/n$ = mean for sample 1

$\bar{x}_2 = \sum_{j=1}^{n_2} x_j/n$ = mean for sample 2

$s_1 = \sqrt{\sum_{i=1}^{n_1} \frac{(x_i - \bar{x}_1)^2}{(n_1 - 1)}}$ = standard deviation for sample 1

$s_2 = \sqrt{\sum_{j=1}^{n_2} \frac{(x_j - \bar{x}_2)^2}{(n_2 - 1)}}$ = standard deviation for sample 2

$$s_p = \sqrt{\frac{s_1^2(n_1 - 1) + s_2^2(n_2 - 1)}{n_1 + n_2 - 2}}$$

$$t = \frac{\bar{x}_1 - \bar{x}_2}{s_p\sqrt{\frac{1}{n_1} + \frac{1}{n_2}}} \quad \text{degrees of freedom} = n_1 + n_2 - 2$$

Again the statistical tables of the t-distribution can be used. If the distributions are not normal, various nonparametric procedures can be used.

More Than Two Samples

When there are more than two samples, other statistical tests are available. To test for equality of means, for example, among several populations that were subjected to different treatments and are of different sexes and ages, analysis of variance could be used. Again there is the underlying assumption of normality, and there are nonparametric methods for analysis of variance available in the situations where normality does not hold.

Regression

If building a mathematical model for the relationship between the variables studied, one may use regression analysis. This is similar to the multiple logistic approach discussed earlier. In this case, however, the purpose is to use the information from the variables to predict an outcome rather than to estimate a relative risk.

In epidemiologic studies relative risks and the logistic function are generally used rather than a standard regression analysis because the outcome variable, rather than being some measurement such as lung capacity, is a (0, 1) variable such as disease, no disease; alive, dead; or exposed, nonexposed. Also, the probability to be predicted is generally small and the variance not constant across groups.

Correlation

Correlation analysis measures the strength of the relationship and ranges from −1 to +1. A "−1" indicates a negative association. As one variable gets larger the other gets smaller. For example, if the number of colonic cancer cases increases as the amount of vitamin A consumed decreases, this would indicate a negative association. A "+1" indicates a positive association. Both variables move together. As one variable becomes larger the other becomes larger, or as one becomes smaller the other becomes smaller. For example, if the number of cancer cases increases as the amount of alcohol consumed increases, this would indicate a positive association. If the correlation coefficient is zero or near zero, this implies little or no relationship between the variables being studied. One may also calculate a multiple correlation among a group of variables and test that the correlation coefficient is equal to zero.

SAMPLE SIZE

Whether a study is retrospective or prospective, an investigator needs to make several decisions before the sample size can be ascertained. First, the investigator must ascertain the significance or alpha (α) level of the test. The α level is the probability of rejecting the hypothesis being tested when the hypothesis is actually true. It is desirable, of course, to make this probability as small as possible. However, the smaller the probability the larger the sample size needed to guarantee the probability. Commonly chosen α-levels are 0.05 and 0.01.

Second, the investigator must ascertain the power or the probability of rejecting the hypothesis when it actually should be rejected. Common values for power are 0.8, 0.85, and 0.9. The higher the power the larger the sample size required.

The investigator must also decide on a one-tailed or two-tailed test. For example, suppose the hypothesis being tested in a retrospective study is that smoking is positively associated with liver cancer, that is, smokers are more likely to have liver cancer. This would be a one-sided or one-tailed test. If the hypothesis was a negative association with liver cancer, that is, smokers are less likely to have liver cancer, this would also be a one-tailed test. However, if the investigator was testing any association, positive or negative, this would be a two-tailed or two-sided test. If the α level is 0.05 for a one-sided test, the rejection region would be 0.05. For a two-sided test with $\alpha = 0.05$, the rejection region would be 0.025 in each tail. A two-sided test at $\alpha = 0.05$ would require a larger sample than a one-sided test at $\alpha = 0.05$.

Another critical consideration in the ascertainment of sample size is the difference the investigator expects to detect. If the investigator wishes to detect very small differences in the groups being studied, then the sample size must be larger than if the investigator wishes to find very large differences in the two groups. In retrospective studies the difference could be measured by the size of the relative risk that the investigator wishes to detect.

The actual details of the sample size calculations appear in various statistical books and articles.[136–138] Depending on the type of study, information other than that already specified may also be required. In a retrospective study, for example, it is necessary to have an estimate of the prevalence of the risk factor in the general population before sample size can be ascertained.

REFERENCES

1. Doll R: The epidemiology of cancer. Cancer 45:2475–2485, 1980
2. Fox JP, Hall CE, Elveback LR: Epidemiology: Man and Disease, New York, Macmillan, 1970
3. Ackerman LV, del Regato JA: Cancer: Diagnosis, Treatment, and Prognosis, 4th ed, pp 1–13. St Louis, CV Mosby, 1970
4. Alderson M: An Introduction to Epidemiology, pp 1–6. London, Macmillan Press, 1976
5. Maclure KM, MacMahon B: An epidemiologic perspective of environmental carcinogenesis. Epidemiol Rev 2:19–48, 1980
6. Winslow C: The Conquest of Epidemic Disease; A Chapter in the History of Ideas. Princeton, Princeton University Press, 1943
7. Shimkin MB: Contrary to Nature: (US Department of Health, Education, and Welfare; National Institutes of Health (NIH) 76-720), Washington DC, US Government Printing Office, 1977
8. Adams F (trans): The Genuine Works of Hippocrates, 2 vols. London, Syndenham Society, 1849
9. Fanchou S: Recherches sur la frequence du cancer. Gaz Haspitaux 16, Ser 2,5:313, 1843
10. Rigoni-Stern D: Fatti statistici relativi alle mallatti cancerose che servirono di base alle poche case. G Progr Patol Terap 2:499–517, 1842
11. Scotto J, Bailor JC: Rigoni-Stern and medical statistics: A nineteenth-century approach to cancer research. J Hist Med 24:65–75, 1969
12. Hoffman FL: The Mortality From Cancer Throughout the World. Newark, NJ, Prudential Press, 1915
13. Dorn HF: Illness from cancer in the United States. Public Health Rep 59:33–48, 65–77, 97–115, 1944
14. Greenwood M: A Report on the Natural Duration of Cancer (Ministry of Health Reports on Public Health and Medical Subjects No. 33) London, His Majesty's Stationery Office, 1926
15. Ramazzini B: Diseases of Workers (The Latin text of 1713). Wright WC, (trans). New York, Hafner, 1964
16. Stevenson THC: Seventy-sixth Annual Report of the Registrar-General of Births, Deaths and Marriages in England and Wales. London, Great Britain General Registry Office, 1915
17. Lane-Claypon JE: A further report on cancer of the breast, with special reference to its associated antecedent conditions. (Ministry of Health Reports on Public Health and Medical Subjects No. 32) London, His Majesty's Stationery Office, 1926
18. DeWaard F, Baanders-van Halewijn EA, Huizinga J: The bimodal age distribution of patients with mammary carcinoma: Evidence for the existence of two types of human breast cancer. Cancer 17:141–151, 1963
19. MacMahon B, Cole P, Lin TM, et al: Age at first birth and breast cancer risk. Bull WHO 43:209–221, 1970
20. Smith FR: Etiologic factors in carcinoma of the cervix. Am J Obstet Gynecol 21:18–25, 1931
21. Logan WPD: Marriage and childbearing in relation to cancer of the breast and uterus. Lancet 264:1119–1202, 1953
22. Clemmesen J: Statistical studies in the aetiology of malignant neoplasms. Acta Pathol Microbiol Scand [Suppl] 174:1–319, 1965
23. Ganon F: Contribution to the etiology and prevention of cancer of the cervix of the uterus. Am J Obstet Gynecol. 60:516–522, 1950
24. Røjel J: The interrelation between uterine cancer and syphilis. Acta Pathol Microbiol Scand [Suppl] 97:1–82, 1953
25. Hoffman FL: Cancer and Diet. Baltimore, Williams & Wilkins, 1937
26. Williams WR: The Natural History of Cancer. New York, Wood, 1908
27. Russell R: Preventable Cancer: A Statistical Research. London, Longmans & Green, 1912
28. Copeman SM, Greenwood M: Diet and Cancer: With Special Reference to the Incidence of Cancer upon Members of Certain Religious Orders (Ministry of Health Reports on Public Health and Medical Subjects No. 36). London, His Majesty's Stationery Office, 1926
29. Stocks P, Korn MN: A cooperative study of the habits, home life, dietary and family histories of 450 cancer patients and of an equal number of control patients. Ann Eugen (Lond) 5:237–280, 1933
30. Schneiderman MA: The numerate sciences—epidemiology and biometry. J Natl Cancer Inst 59:633–644, 1977
31. Armitage P: Statistical Methods in Medical Research. Oxford, Blackwell Scientific Publications, 1971
32. MacMahon B, Pugh TF: Epidemiology: Principles and Methods. Boston, Little, Brown & Co, 1979
33. Stolley PD: The use of epidemiologic methods in the elucidation of the relationship between oral contraceptives and cardiovascular disease. In Colombo F, Shapiro S, Sloane D et al (eds), Epidemiological Evaluation of Drugs, p 85. Littleton, Massachusetts, PSG Publishing Co, 1977

34. Surgeon General's Advisory Committee on Smoking and Health: Smoking and Health: A Report of the Surgeon General (US Department of Health, Education, and Welfare; Public Health Service (PHS) 79-50066). Washington DC, US Government Printing Office, 1979
35. Hammond EC: Smoking in relation to the death rates of one million men and women. In Haenszel W (ed): Epidemiology of Cancer and Other Diseases, pp 127–204. Bethesda, National Cancer Institute, 1966
36. Labarthe DR: Methodologic variation in case-control studies of reserpine and breast cancer. J Chronic Dis 32:95–104, 1979
37. Beebe GW, Kato H, Land CE: Studies of the mortality of A-bomb survivors. Radiat Res 75:138–201, 1978
38. Cole P: Coffee drinking and cancer of the lower urinary tract. Lancet 1:1335–1337, 1971
39. Miller RW: The discovery of human teratogens, carcinogens, and mutagens: Lessons for the future. In Hollaender A, deSerres FJ (eds): Chemical Mutagens, pp 101–126. New York, Plenum Press, 1978
40. Ochsner A: My first recognition of the relationship of smoking and lung cancer. Prev Med 2:611–614, 1973
41. Wynder EL, Graham EA: Tobacco smoking as a possible etiologic factor in bronchogenic carcinoma: A study of six hundred and eighty-four proven cases. JAMA 143:329–333, 1950
42. Newell GR: Comments on epidemiology, etiology, and prevention of lung cancer. Cancer Bull 32:76–77, 1980
43. Herbst AL, Ulfelder H, Postkanzer DC: Adenocarcinoma of the vagina: Association of maternal stilbesterol therapy with tumor appearance in young women. N Engl J Med 284:878–881, 1971
44. Tukey JW: Exploratory Data Analysis, pp 1–8, 12, 23–24, 39. Reading, Addison-Wesley Publishing Co. 1977
45. Ury HK: Efficiency of case-control studies with multiple controls per case: Continuous or dichotomous data. Biometrics 31:643–649, 1975
46. Miettinen OS: Matching and design efficiency in retrospective studies. Am J Epidemiol 91:111, 1970
47. Doll R, Hill AB: Mortality of doctors in relation to their smoking habits: A preliminary report. Br Med J 1:1451–1455, 1954
48. Lilienfeld AM: Foundations of Epidemiology. New York, Oxford University Press, 1976
49. Ibrahim MA (ed): The case control study: consensus and controversy. J Chronic Dis 32:1–190, 1979
50. Breslow NE, Day NE: Statistical Methods in Cancer Research: I: The Analysis of Case-Control Studies. Lyons, IARC Press, 1980
51. Doll R, Hill AB: Mortality in relation to smoking: Ten years' observations of British doctors. Br Med J 1:1399–1410, 1460–1467, 1964
52. Caes RAM, Hosker ME, McDonald DB, et al: Tumours of the urinary bladder in workmen engaged in the manufacture and use of certain dyestuff intermediators in the British chemical industry. Br J Ind Med 11:75–104, 1954
53. Hammond EC, Horn D: Smoking and death rates—report on forty-four months of followup of 187,783 men. JAMA 166:1159–1172, 1294–1308, 1958
54. Mausner JS, Bahn AK: Epidemiology: An Introductory Text, p 324. Philadelphia, WB Saunders, 1974
55. Newell GR, Gordon JE, Monlezun AP et al: ABO blood groups and cancer. JNCI 52:1425–1430, 1974
56. Cochran WG: Sampling Techniques, 2nd ed. New York, John Wiley and Sons, 1963
57. Cornfield J, Haenszel W: Some aspects of retrospective studies. J Chronic Dis 11:523–534, 1960
58. Doll R, Hill AB: Lung cancer and other causes of death in relation to smoking: A second report of the mortality of British doctors. Br Med J 2:1071–1081, 1956
59. Lilienfeld DE: Foundations of Epidemiology, 2nd ed, pp 342–346. New York, Oxford University Press, 1980
60. Levin ML, Bertell R: Simple estimation of population attributable risk from case-control studies. Am J Epidemiol 108:78–79, 1978
61. Walter SD: The distribution of Levin's measure of attributable risk. Biometrika 62:371–374, 1975
62. Friedman GD: Primer of Epidemiology. New York, McGraw-Hill, 1974
63. Elandt-Johnson RC: Definition of rates: Some remarks on their use and misuse. Am J Epidemiol 102:267–71, 1975
64. Sackett DL, Vessey MP: Bias in analytic research. J Chronic Dis 32:51–68, 1979
65. Berkson J: Limitations of the application of four-fold table analysis to hospital data. Biometrics Bull 2:47–53, 1946
66. Doll R, Hill AB: A study of the aetiology of carcinoma of the lung. Br Med J 2:1271, 1952
67. Labarthe D, Adam E, Noller KL, et al: Design and preliminary observations of National Cooperative Diethylstilbestrol Adenosis (DESAD) Project. Obstet Gynecol 51:453–458, 1978
68. Stafl A, Mattingly RF: Vaginal adenosis: A precancerous lesion? Am J Obstet Gynecol 126:666, 1974
69. O'Brien PC, Noller KL, Robboy SJ et al: Vaginal epithelial changes in young women enrolled in the National Cooperative Diethylstilbestrol Adenosis (DESAD) Project. Obstet Gynecol 53:300–308, 1979
70. Glenn ND: Cohort Analysis (Series on Quantitative Applications in the Social Sciences), pp 50–51. Beverly Hills, Sage Publications, 1977
71. Cutler SJ: Cancer registries: opportunities and responsibilities. JNCI 57:741–742, 1976
72. Burbank F: Patterns in cancer mortality in the United States: 1950–1967. Natl Cancer Inst Monogr 3:1–594, 1971
73. Mason RJ, McKay FW: Cancer Mortality by County: 1950–1969 (US Department of Health, Education, and Welfare; National Institute of Health (NIH) 74-615). Washington DC, US Government Printing Office, 1973
74. Mason TJ, McKay FW, Hoover R et al: Atlas of Cancer Mortality for U.S. Counties: 1950–1969 (US Department of Health, Education and Welfare; National Institutes of Health (NIH) 75-780). Washington DC, US Government Printing Office, 1975
75. Mason TJ, McKay FW, Hoover R et al: Atlas of Cancer Mortality Among U.S. Nonwhites: 1950–1969 (US Department of Health, Education, and Welfare; National Institutes of Health (NIH) 76-1204). Washington DC, US Government Printing Office, 1976
76. Axtell LM, Asire AJ, Myers MH: Cancer Patient Survival: Report No. 5. (US Department of Health, Education, and Welfare; National Institutes of Health (NIH) 77-992). Washington DC, US Government Printing Office, 1976
77. Dorn HF, Cutler SJ: Morbidity from Cancer in the United States: Parts I and II (US Department of Health, Education, and Welfare; Public Health Monograph 56). Washington DC, US Government Printing Office, 1956
78. Haencel W, Marcus SC, Zimmer EG: Cancer Morbidity in Urban and Rural Iowa (US Department of Health, Education, and Welfare; Public Health Monograph 37). Washington DC, US Government Printing Office, 1956
79. Cutler SJ, Young JL: Third National Cancer Survey: incidence data (US Department of Health, Education, and Welfare; National Institutes of Health (NIH) 75-787). Natl Cancer Inst Monogr 41:1–454, 1975
80. Scotto J, Chiazze L: Third National Cancer Survey: Hospitalizations and Payments to Hospitals, Part A (US Department of Health, Education, and Welfare; National Institutes of Health (NIH) 76-1094). Washington DC, US Government Printing Office, 1976
81. Young JL, Asire AJ, Pollack ES: SEER Program: Cancer Incidence and Mortality in the U.S., 1973–1976 (US Department of Health, Education, and Welfare; National Institutes of Health (NIH) 78-1837). Washington DC, US Government Printing Office, 1976
82. Waterhouse J, Muir CS, Correa P et al (eds): Cancer Incidence in Five Continents, Vol III. Berlin, Springer-Verlag, 1976
83. Miller DG: On the nature of susceptibility to cancer. Cancer 46:1307–1318, 1980
84. Doll R: The age distribution of cancer: Implications for models of carcinogenesis. J R Stat Soc (A) 134–155, 1971

85. Kelsey JL: A review of the epidemiology of human breast cancer. Epidemiol Rev 1:74–109, 1979
86. Newell GR, Cole SR, Meittinen OS et al: Age differences in the histology of Hodgkin's disease. JNCI 45:311–317, 1970
87. Blot WJ, Harrington JM, Toledo A et al: Lung cancer after employment in shipyards during World War II. N Engl J Med 299:620–623, 1978
88. Gottlieb MS, Pickle LW, Blot WJ et al: Lung cancer in Louisiana: Death certificate analysis. JNCI 63:1131–1137, 1979
89. Hoover R, Mason TJ, McKay FW et al: Geographic patterns of cancer mortality in the United States. In Fraumeni JF (ed): Persons at High Risk of Cancer: An Approach to Cancer Etiology and Control, pp 343–359. New York, Academic Press, 1975
90. Morris DL, Buechley RW, Key CR et al: Gallbladder disease and gallbladder cancer among American Indians in tricultural New Mexico. Cancer 42:2474–2477, 1978
91. Haenszel W: Migrant studies. See Reference 89, pp 361–371
92. Bjelke E; Epidemiology of colorectal cancer with emphasis on diet. In Davis W, Harrap KR, Stathopoulos G (eds): Human Cancer: Its Characterization and Treatment. Proceedings of the Eighth International Symposium on the Biological Characterization of Human Tumors, pp 158–174. Amesterdam, Excerpta Media, 1980 (International Congress Series No. 484)
93. Ellison NM, Newell GR: Relationship between diet and cancer: A brief review for the practicing physician. Cancer Bull 32:157–160, 1980
94. Hirayama T: Epidemiology of breast cancer with special reference to the role of diet. Prev Med 7:173–195, 1978
95. Garfinkel L, Poindexter CE, Silverberg E: Cancer in black Americans. CA 30:39–44, 1980
96. Thomas DB: Epidemiologic studies of cancer in minority groups in the western United States (Second Symposium on Epidemiology and Cancer Registries in the Pacific Basin). Natl Cancer Inst Monogr 53:103–113, 1979
97. Newell GR: Etiology of multiple sclerosis and Hodgkin's disease. Am J Epidemiol 91:119–122, 1970
98. Henderson BE, Thompson DJ, Hirohata T (eds): Second Symposium on Epidemiology and Cancer Registries in the Pacific Basin. Natl Cancer Inst Monogr 53:1–212, 1979
99. Newell GR: Multiple primary cancers: Suggested etiologic implications. Cancer Bull 32:160–164, 1980
100. Lemon HM: Experimental basis for multiple primary carcinogenesis by sex hormones: A review. Cancer 40:1825–1832, 1977
101. Modan B: Role of diet in cancer etiology. Cancer 40:1887–1889, 1977
102. Schoental R: The role of nicotinamide and of certain other modifying factors in diethylnitrosamine carcinogenesis. Cancer 40:1833–1840, 1977
103. Adamson RH, Sieber SM: Carcinogenic potential of cancer chemotherapeutic agents in man. Cancer Bull 29:179–183, 1977
104. Drasar BS, Irving D: Environmental factors and cancers of the colon and breast. Br J Cancer 27:167–172, 1973
105. Lea AJ: Dietary factors associated with death rates from certain neoplasms in man. Lancet 2:332–333, 1966
106. Carroll KK, Gammal EB, Plunkett ER: Dietary fat and mammary cancer. Canadian Med Assoc J 98:590–594, 1968
107. Hems G, Stuart A: Breast cancer rates in populations of single women. Br J Cancer 31:118–123, 1975
108. Hems G: Epidemiological characteristics of breast cancer in middle and late age. Br J Cancer 24:226–234, 1970
109. Cole P, Morrison AS: Basic issues in population screening for cancer. JNCI 64:1263–1272, 1980
110. Hall DJ, Wood MD: Cancer Screening: When Is It Worthwhile? A Guide for Primary Care Physicians. Boston, Sidney Farber Cancer Institute, 1979
111. Galen RS, Gambino SR: Beyond Normality: The Predictive Value and Efficiency of Medical Diagnoses, p 50. New York, John Wiley and Sons, 1975
112. Guidelines for the cancer-related checkup: Recommendations and rationale. CA 30:194–240, 1980
113. White LN, Boutwell WB: Screening for early stage cancer. Cancer Bull 32:151–153, 1980
114. Breslow L: Review of future perspective of cancer screening. In Nieburgs HE (ed): Prevention and Detection of Cancer, Vol I, Part II, pp 1177–1210. New York, Marcel Dekker, 1976
115. Rotkin ID: A comparison review of key epidemiological studies in cervical cancer related to current searches for transmissible agents. Cancer Res 33:1353, 1973
116. Compromise reached on suggested intervals between Pap tests. JAMA 24:1411–1419, 1980
117. Strax P: Screening for breast cancer. Clin Obstet 20:781–801, 1977
118. Sadowsky NL: Radiologic detection of breast cancer, review and recommendations. N Engl J Med 294:370, 1976
119. Judkins AF: The art of teaching self-examination of the breast. Cancer Bull 31:149–152, 1979
120. Burkitt DP, Walker AR, Painter NS: Effect of dietary fibre on stools and transit-times, and its role in the causation of diseases. Lancet 2:1408–1412, 1972
121. Graham S, Sayal H, Swanson M et al: Diet in the epidemiology of cancer of the colon and rectum. JNCI 61:709–714, 1978
122. Smeltzer CV, Verba P: Hemoccult screening: Nurses' role. Cancer Nurs 2:475–479, 1979
123. Doles LG, Friedman GD, Collen MF: Evaluating periodic multiphasic health checkups: A controlled trial. J Chronic Dis 32:385–404, 1979
124. McCormack R, Rubin P: Skin cancer. In Rubin P (ed): Clinical Oncology: A Multidisciplinary Approach, 5th ed, pp 157–162. New York, American Cancer Society, 1978
125. Fontana RS: Editorial: Early diagnosis of lung cancer. Am Rev Respir Dis 116:399, 1977
126. Mantel N, Haenszel W: Statistical aspects of the analysis of data from retrospective studies of disease. JNCI 22:719–748, 1959
127. Landis JR, Stanish WM, Koch GG: A Computer Program in the Generalized Chi-Square Analysis of Categorical Data Using Weighted Least Squares to Compute Wald Statistics (GENCAT) (Biostatistics Technical Report No. 8). Ann Arbor, Department of Biostatistics, University of Michigan; and Chapel Hill, Department of Biostatistics, University of North Carolina, 1976
128. Truett J, Cornfield J, Kannel MD: A multivariate analysis of the risk of coronary heart disease in Framingham. J Chronic Dis 20:511–524, 1967
129. Prentice R: Use of the logistic model in retrospective studies. Biometrics 32:599–606, 1976
130. Breslow N, Powers W: Are there two logistic regressions for retrospective studies? Biometrics 34:100–105, 1978
131. Fleiss JL: Statistical Methods for Rates and Proportions, pp 155–172. New York, John Wiley and Sons, 1973
132. Doll R, Cook P: Summarizing indices for comparison of cancer incidence data. Int J Cancer 2:269–279, 1967
133. Christensen HB: Statistics Step by Step. Boston, Houghton Mifflin, 1977
134. Colton T: Statistics in Medicine. Boston, Little, Brown & Co, 1974
135. Beyer WH (ed): CRC Handbook of Tables for Probability and Statistics, 2nd ed, pp 182–205. Cleveland, The Chemical Rubber Co, 1968
136. Mace AE: Sample Size Determination. New York, Robert E Krieger, 1974
137. Cassagrande JT, Pike MC: An improved approximation formula for calculating sample sizes for comparing two binomial distributions, Biometrics 34:483–486, 1978
138. Schlesselman JJ: Sample size requirements in cohort and case-control studies of disease. Am J Epidemiol 99:381–384, 1974

CHAPTER 2 **Arthur C. Upton**

Principles of Cancer Biology: Etiology and Prevention of Cancer

GENERAL NATURE OF NEOPLASIA

The term neoplasia literally means "new growth." The mass of tissue comprising the new growth is known as a neoplasm. It is difficult to describe the properties of neoplasms concisely. Nevertheless, the following definition by Willis is useful: "A neoplasm is an abnormal mass of tissue, the growth of which exceeds and is uncoordinated with that of the normal tissues, and persists in the same excessive manner after cessation of the stimuli which evoked change."[1] Implicit in this definition is the propensity for a neoplasm to enlarge at the expense of its host, behaving as a parasite, competing for nutrients, usurping for itself some degree of autonomy, and ultimately threatening the host's survival.

While this definition provides a useful characterization of neoplastic growth in general, variations among neoplasms reflect a broad spectrum of abnormalities in growth and differentiation. To place these abnormalities in perspective, the process of neoplasia must be considered in relation to non-neoplastic patterns of proliferation.

TYPES OF PROLIFERATIVE GROWTH

HYPERPLASIA

Hyperplasia denotes an increase in cell number, in contrast to "hypertrophy," which denotes an increase in cell or organ size. Hyperplasia may be physiologic, as in the case of normal growth during prenatal development, childhood, and adolescence, or in the case of the mammary gland during pregnancy and lactation. It may also be compensatory, as in the regenerative and reparative proliferation of cells during wound healing.

Hyperplasia may be pathologic when it exceeds the level needed in degree and duration to maintain or restore normal tissue structure, size, and function. Pathologic hyperplasia of the endometrium, for example, may be encountered in the presence of excessive estrogen stimulation, being reversible when normal hormone levels are restored. Although reversibility is a hallmark of hyperplasia, sustained pathologic hyperplasia frequently precedes neoplasia, possibly because it favors the outgrowth of transformed cells.

METAPLASIA

Metaplasia denotes a reversible process in which one type of differentiated cell is substituted for another. For example, squamous metaplasia of ciliated columnar epithelium in the respiratory tract may occur in vitamin A deficiency. Such metaplastic transformation results from redirection of tissue stem cell differentiation into a new pathway.

While metaplasia usually gives rise to an orderly arrangement of cells, it may, at times, produce disorderly patterns (*i.e.*, cells varying in size, shape, orientation to one another) and staining properties. The resulting atypical metaplasia, which represents a step toward dysplasia, is occasionally encountered in chronic inflammation.

DYSPLASIA

Dysplasia consists of a loss in the regularity and normal arrangement of cells. Although it is a common feature of neoplastic growth, it can occur in the absence of neoplasia.

In non-neoplastic cells, where it is reversible, it is seen most often in the presence of a long-standing inflammation.

ANAPLASIA

The term anaplasia is used to denote lack of cellular differentiation and is seldom encountered, except in malignant neoplasms. In an anaplastic or undifferentiated neoplasm, the cells tend to be disorganized, poorly differentiated, pleomorphic, and tend to show increased nucleocytoplasmic ratio and staining intensity.

NEOPLASIA

As indicated by the above definition, neoplasia is broadly characterized by cellular proliferation that exceeds and is uncoordinated with normal growth, and that persists at the expense of the host. In general, the proliferative abnormality of neoplastic cells behaves as a stable and irreversible phenotypic change. Depending on the specific properties of neoplasms, they are classified into various subgroups.

Benign Neoplasia

Benign neoplasms are distinguished from malignant neoplasms on the basis of the differences summarized in Table 2-1. Most of the differences are relative, except for the propensity to invade and metastasize. Although, by definition, benign neoplasms do not invade or metastasize, some of them are neither encapsulated nor discretely demarcated (*e.g.*, certain fibromatous and vascular tumors of the dermis).

Malignant Neoplasia

Malignant neoplasia is synonomous with the term cancer. Cancers grow by invasion of surrounding structures, including blood vessels, lymphatics, and nerves. Cancers can also metastasize to distant sites by seeding body cavities, transportation via blood vessels and lymphatics, or direct surgical or mechanical transplantation. While these attributes are common to cancer cells in general, they vary in detail among different types of cancer and in the same cancer from one stage of development to another.

With time, neoplasms tend to become increasingly autonomous, or malignant—a process known as *tumor progression*. This phenomenon implies that cancer may evolve stepwise through a succession of stages, beginning as a relatively benign growth and culminating as a highly malignant one. Depending on the circumstances, this process may occupy a large fraction of the natural lifespan of the affected person. In humans, benign tumors have only been rarely observed to transform into cancers. Notable exceptions have occurred in papillomas of the colon and pigmented nevi of the skin. For most human cancers, the patterns of growth and metastasis are more or less predictable, although they vary from one type of cancer to another.[1]

TABLE 2-1. General Differences between Benign and Malignant Neoplasms

BENIGN	MALIGNANT
1. Frequently encapsulated	1. Nonencapsulated
2. Noninvasive	2. Invasive
3. Well differentiated	3. Poorly differentiated
4. Slowly growing	4. Rapidly growing
5. Low mitotic rate	5. High mitotic rate
6. Nonmetastasizing	6. Metastasizing

(Modified from Pitot HC: Fundamentals of Oncology. New York, Marcel Dekker, 1978)

PHYLOGENETIC DISTRIBUTION OF NEOPLASIA

Neoplasms have been reported in virtually all vertebrates, and some invertebrates, higher plants, and insects. It can be inferred, therefore, that the process may be essentially universal among complex, multicellular organisms.[3] The occurrence of neoplastic lesions in dinosaur bones and other fossils proves that neoplasia made its appearance early in the evolutionary scale. The observation of bone tumors in mummies and descriptions of cancer in early Egyption and Greek records attests to the disease in humans since the dawn of history.[4]

THEORIES OF CARCINOGENESIS

To explain the causation of cancer, many theories have been propounded, all of which have sought in various ways to account for the phenotypic changes that typify the cancer cell.[2,6–8] These changes include the following:

1. Tendency for relatively uncontrolled and unlimited proliferation, ultimately at the expense of the host
2. Transmissibility of the proliferative abnormality from one neoplastic cell to successive generations of daughter cells, as a relatively "stable" and "heritable" phenotype
3. Tendency for the proliferative abnormality to progress with time toward increasing malignancy, associated with increasingly marked alterations in cell morphology, karyotype, antigen specificity, metabolism, and other properties.[2,9]

Although many theories of carcinogenesis have failed to stand the test of time, and none by itself has successfully accounted for all of the observed aspects of neoplasia, several theories form the basis for contemporary concepts. These theories can be grouped under the four major mechanisms they invoke:

1. Somatic mutation
2. Aberrant differentiation
3. Virus activation and
4. Cell selection[2,8–10]

SOMATIC MUTATION THEORY

The somatic mutation theory attributes neoplasia to abnormalities in one or more of the genes regulating growth and differentiation. According to this theory, such genetic abnormalities can occur at any time during life. To the extent that one or more of the requisite mutations is inherited via the zygote, the affected person is made more susceptible to cancer, since fewer mutational steps remain necessary to complete the carcinogenic process in a somatic cell. The carcinogenic action of agents such as ionizing radiation and alkylating chemicals is ascribed to their mutagenic effects on exposed cells.

Evidence for the somatic mutation theory includes:

1. The influence of genetic constitution on susceptibility to cancer
2. The correlation between mutagenicity and carcinogenicity
3. The frequent occurrence of chromosomal aberrations in cancer cells

Influence of Genetic Background

CHROMOSOMAL DISORDERS. Since the classical observations of Boveri, the frequent presence of chromosomal abnormalities in cancer cells has prompted speculation that such abnormalities may bear a causal relationship to neoplasia.[11–13] With the development of modern cytogenetic techniques and their systematic clinical application, an accumulating body of evidence has disclosed that certain chromosomal disorders often precede, and hence predispose to, specific types of neoplasms.[13–17]

These chromosomal disorders include trisomies, such as Down's syndrome (trisomy 21), trisomy–D, and Klinefelter's syndrome (XXY), all of which predispose to leukemia.[14,15] Associated with these disorders, there is also an increased susceptibility of fibroblast transformation by SV_{40} *in vitro*.[18] Another trisomy, apparently predisposing to dysplasia and neoplasia, is trisomy–18, which has been followed by Wilm's tumor of the kidney in some instances and by multiple proliferative lesions resembling Wilm's tumor in others.[14,15]

The D–deletion syndrome, a disorder in which there is deletion of the long arm of chromosome 13 with multiple congenital anomalies, has been accompanied by retinoblastoma in a high proportion of cases, the tumors usually being bilateral.[14]

A number of syndromes characterized by chromosomal instability predispose to cancer. These include Bloom's syndrome, Fanconi's syndrome, ataxia–telangiectasia, xeroderma pigmentosum, porokeratosis of Mibelli, nevoid basal cell carcinoma syndrome, incontinentia pigmenti, and scleroderma.[17]

The presence of the Y chromosome in phenotypically female patients with gonadal dysgenesis may account for the high rate of gonadoblastoma in such patients (25–30%), even when the cells containing the Y chromosome in such patients are restricted to the gonadal line.[16] In this case, the carcinogenic effect of the Y chromosome may result from its presence in an abnormal environment; this occurs in heterotopic transplantation of embryo cells in mice, which causes neoplasia under certain conditions, as will be discussed below.

The Philadelphia chromosome (which involves translocation of the long arm of the chromosome 22 usually to chromosome 9) is present in the leukemic cells of up to 90% of patients with chronic myelocytic leukemia (CML).[12,16] The consistency and specificity of this association have suggested to many observers that the chromosomal abnormality may play a causal role in the pathogenesis of the leukemia, especially since it has been observed in nonleukemic carriers in whom the disease has later supervened.[13–15] The abnormality has been documented unequivocally only in cells of hemopoietic origin. In addition, several pairs of identical twins have been described who were discordant both for the Philadelphia chromosome and for CML. Hence, it is assumed to arise postzygotically.[14,19,20]

Other evidence that chromosomal imbalance can predispose to neoplasia is provided by the so-called Kostoff genetic tumors of plants.[21] These tumors arise regularly in mature interploid F_1 hybrids resulting from the crossbreeding of certain species within the genus Nicotiniana. For example, when N. glauca ($2n = 24$) is crossed with N. lagsdorffii ($2n = 18$), the resulting f_1 hybrid ($2n = 21$) develops a profusion of tumors after maturation. When cells from parental species are fused in culture, the resulting amphiploid cells ($2n = 42$) give rise to either well or poorly differentiated derivatives, depending on the environment in which they are grown.[21]

MENDELIAN RECESSIVE DISEASES. A number of recessive diseases are accompanied by heightened susceptibility to cancer. Xeroderma pigmentosum (XP) is one of the most noteworthy. In this disease, sensitivity to UV light is greatly increased, causing affected persons to develop solar keratoses and recurrent cutaneous cancers on exposed body parts early in life. This extreme photosensitivity is related to a defect in the repair of UV light-induced damage in DNA, which appears to be variable in kind and degree.[23,24] Although repair-deficient fibroblasts cultured from patients with XP have been found lacking in their ability to repair DNA damage induced by UV light and certain alkylating agents, their ability to repair damage induced by x-rays and other alkylating agents is not impaired.[24–26] Such fibroblasts do, however, give rise spontaneously to an increased frequency of pseudodiploid clones and exhibit an increased yield of chromosome aberrations on UV irradiation.[17]

Other recessive diseases predisposing to cancer include Fanconi's syndrome, Bloom's syndrome, and ataxia-telangiectasia, in which the increased risk of cancer is associated with chromosomal fragility, as noted above.[17] Cultured cells from affected persons are abnormally sensitive to the induction of chromosome abnormalities by x-rays and radiomimetic chemicals and to transformation by SV_{40} virus.[15,18] In ataxia-telangiectasia, clones of circulating lymphocytes with chromosome translocations have been noted, one such clone multiplying during a four-year observation period so as to outnumber the normal circulating lymphocytes. This occurred in a patient who died from pulmonary insufficiency at age 23.[16,27] The basis for the chromosomal fragility remains to be determined, but it has been suggested that it may result from a defect in DNA repair.[24,28] Another abnormality that may also contribute to the high risk of cancer in these diseases is the immunologic deficiency that is present.[15,29]

An additional category of primary immunodeficiency diseases in which there is a heightened risk of cancer, without detectable chromosomal fragility, includes Bruton's agammaglobulinemia, the Wiscott–Aldrich syndrome, and the Chediak–Higashi syndrome.[14,15] In these diseases, the cancer excess is attributable primarily to an increased frequency of leukemias and lymphoreticular tissue neoplasms.[29,30]

Werner's syndrome, a recessive form of progeria inherited as an autosomal recessive, also predisposes to cancer at an early age.[14] As in some other syndromes mentioned above, the basis for the increased susceptibility to neoplasia may conceivably be linked to a cellular defect associated with deficient repair of DNA damage.[31,32]

DOMINANT TUMOR SYNDROMES. Susceptibility to a number of specific types of neoplasms is inherited as a Mendelian dominant, in some instances with a high degree of penetrance. The development of a particular form of tumor at a given site may be the only manifestation of an inherited syndrome in some cases; in other cases, tumors may occur at different sites, with or without additional abnormalities.[14,22]

The phacomatoses comprise one group of disorders in this category, characterized by congenital defects and tumor syndromes of various types, neurofibromatosis being the most familiar.[14] The observation that the cells of neurofibromata comprise more than one G–6–PD phenotype, as do those of hereditary trichoepitheliomata, argues against a unicellular origin in these growths; in this respect, these tumors differ from most other neoplasms that have but one G–6–PD phenotype, implying a monoclonal nature.[14,19] Other rarer phacomatoses include the von Hippel–Lindau syndrome and tuberous sclerosis. Early onset and multiplicity are broadly characteristic of the tumors in this entire group.[14]

Embryonal tumors, notably retinoblastoma, Wilm's tumor of the kidney, and neuroblastoma, constitute another group of neoplasms showing a familial distribution consistent with a dominant Mendelian form of inheritance. In members of affected families, the tumors tend to occur earlier and are more frequently bilateral than in the general population. These differences have been interpreted as evidence that the tumors arise in each case as the consequence of two mutations, one of which may be inherited and the other acquired postzygotically through a somatic mutation.[14,15,33,34] Use of the model to estimate the relative frequency of hereditary, as opposed to non-hereditary, permits estimates that roughly 40% of all retinoblastomas, 38% of all Wilm's tumors, and 20–25% of all neuroblastomas are hereditary.[14] The model can also apply to other neoplastic diseases showing dominant inheritance, some of which characteristically occur during adult life. These include pheochromocytoma, multiple endocrine adenomatosis, basal cell nevus syndrome, malignant melanoma, polyposis of the colon, tylosis, and hereditary adenocarcinomatosis.[14]

COMMON CANCERS. The two-step mutational model has been inferred to apply, to a lesser extent, to many of the more common neoplasms, for which evidence of a polygenic component has emerged from family studies.[14,15,35] Prominent examples include:

1. Carcinoma of the breast, with the risk of early and bilateral tumors being far higher in women with relatives who have developed the premenopausal form of the disease than in the general population
2. Carcinoma of the endometrium, with the risk exceeding 30% in women with the dominantly inherited Stein–Levinthal syndrome
3. Carcinoma of the colon
4. Carcinoma of the stomach
5. Carcinoma of the prostate
6. Carcinoma of the bronchus
7. Leukemia [14]

The powerful influence of genetic determinants is strikingly manifest in twins. A child whose identical twin has already developed leukemia has a risk of about 1 in 5 of developing the same disease within a matter of weeks or months, whereas a child in the general population has a risk of roughly 1 in 2900 of developing the disease during the first decade of life.[36] A similar degree of concordance is seen in animals of highly inbred strains, which approach identical twins in the extent to which they are genetically uniform.[37]

In certain instances, the basis for genetic differences in susceptibility has been analyzed in detail, and the genes involved have been characterized. In the laboratory mouse, for example, a number of genetic loci affect susceptibility to leukemia, with effects at different levels, ranging from the assembly of leukemia virus on the one hand to the immunological resistance of the host on the other.[38,39] From such investigations, it is evident that many genes are involved in regulating susceptibility to neoplasia. With the exception of determinants like the major histocompatibility loci and the loci regulating mixed oxidase function enzyme activities, which affect overall resistance broadly, the influence of a given gene tends to be relatively specific for the pathogenesis of a particular type of neoplasm.[37]

Chromosomal Abnormalities in Cancer Cells

The cells of nearly all human malignant solid tumors contain chromosomal abnormalities, and the extent of abnormality tends to parallel the stage of progression of the tumor.[12,40,41] In the leukemias, the presence of chromosomal abnormalities is more variable, depending on the hematologic type and stage of the disease. For instance, in CML nearly all typical cases show the Philadelphia chromosome in every cell.[12] Similarly, the majority of Burkitt's lymphoma (BL) cells contain a characteristic 8:14 translocation.[41] The frequency and types of abnormalities in other human leukemias are more variable, although not random.[12,13]

Likewise, the cells of neoplasms in animals have been observed to contain chromosomal abnormalities, but not as frequently as their human counterparts. Nor has a particular form of aberration been observed as consistently in animal tumors of a given type as has the Philadelphia chromosome in human CML.[12,40,41]

Although microscopically visible chromosome abnormalities are not detectable in all cancer cells, the existing evidence amply justifies the generalization that the karyotype in neoplastic cells tends to be unstable and variable.[40] In a given neoplasm, however, the cells frequently exhibit the same chromosomal abnormality as would be consistent with their clonal origin from a single precursor, particularly in the case of the leukemias and lymphomas. With time, especially in animal tumors that are transplanted serially through successive transplant generations, clones of progressively greater abnormality tend to appear and to predominate successively. Ultimately, the karyotype may become stabilized in a highly aneuploid state, as in canine venereal sarcoma. Throughout the world, this sarcoma exhibits the same bizarre stemline.[12,32,40,42]

Although the Philadelphia chromosome in CML and the 8:14 translocation in BL are exceptional in the regularity of their occurrence compared with the aberrations associated with other cancers that are more variable from case to case, monosomy for chromosome 22 has been noted repeatedly in human meningiomas.[13,44-46]

There is evidence that the chromosomal abnormalities of cancer cells, though variable, are not random. In leukemias other than human CML and BL, specific types of cytogenetic abnormalities have been observed recurrently, both in human patients and in experimental animals.[12,47,48] Moreover, in solid tumors, the stemline has been observed to bear some relationship to the organ involved. In certain sites it tends toward the tetraploid range, while in others it remains closer to the diploid mode.[12]

Observations on golden hamster embryo cells transformed by SV_{40} or dimethylnitrosamine in culture have led to the hypothesis that specific chromosomal changes are correlated with transformation. The outcome depends on the balance between gain or loss of sites in the genome that is stimulating or restraining cell growth.[12,49,50]

Correlation Between Carcinogenicity and Mutagenicity

In keeping with the somatic mutation hypothesis, there is a general correlation between carcinogenicity and mutagenicity. This is exemplified by ionizing radiation, nitrogen mustard, certain polycyclic aromatic hydrocarbons, and other alkylating agents.[51-54] The correlation is now known to extend to many chemical carcinogens previously thought not to have mutagenic activity because they had been assayed in lower organisms lacking the metabolic capability for activating them.[55] With the recognition that many of the compounds causing cancer are not carcinogenic in their ambient form but are merely precursors of reactive metabolites, efforts to determine the mutagenicity of such agents have sought to provide for their appropriate metabolic activation by including mammalian activating enzymes in the assay system.[51,56,57] With such refined techniques, the vast majority of carcinogens tested to date have turned out showing mutagenicity.[53,54,56,57] In a number of chemicals, there appears to be a correlation between relative carcinogenic and relative mutagenic potency.[58]

It remains doubtful that the correlation between carcinogenicity and mutagenicity will ever prove to be absolute, in view of the likelihood that some types of carcinogens act through mechanisms other than somatic mutation. This difference would seem particularly applicable to the hormones as a class and will be discussed later.

Other evidence put forward in support of the somatic mutation theory is the propensity for chemical carcinogens to bind to DNA[9,51,59-61] As yet, the extent to which such effects of a carcinogen on DNA are related to its ultimate carcinogenicity remains to be determined, especially since the chemicals in question characteristically interact with other intracellular macromolecules and organellae.[9,52]

Additional evidence consistent with the somatic mutation hypothesis is the single-hit character of the dose-response relation for chemical-induced cellular neoplastic transformation *in vitro*. This is despite the requirement for successive cell divisions after exposure to the chemical in order for its effects to become "fixed."[50,62]

The extent to which "misrepair" of carcinogen-induced damage to DNA may contribute to the induction of cancer remains to be evaluated.[9,24,63-65]

ABERRANT DIFFERENTIATION THEORY

In contrast to the somatic mutation hypothesis, which attributes carcinogenesis to abnormalities of genes or chromosomes, the aberrant differentiation theory supposes that such changes need not occur. Instead, it postulates that disturbances in gene regulation, through faulty repression or depression, may cause a derangement of growth and differentiation expressed in the form of cancer. Since the defect merely involves changes in the regulation of genes and not changes in their structure, it can be considered epigenetic rather than genetic.[10]

Since stable patterns of gene expression are known to occur during differentiation (and since plausible theoretical mechanisms exist showing that carcinogens may cause stable changes in gene expression through epigenetic means alone) without necessarily altering the genetic material itself, the distinction between the aberrant differentiation mechanism and the mutational mechanism calls for special kinds of evidence.[66,67] Some of the cogent evidence is reviewed below.

Totipotentiality of Cancer Cell Genome

To determine whether the cancer cell arises through mutation, one ingenious approach has involved the transplantation of diploid mouse teratocarcinoma cells (derived from an ascites tumor in about the 200th transplant generation) into the blastocysts of normal recipient mouse embryos. In such blastocysts, the tumors cells have been observed to lose their neoplastic phenotype and to give rise to normal differentiated tissue derivatives, including fertile sperm.[67,68]

A similar experiment has involved the transplantation of nuclei from Lucke frog renal carcinoma cells into enucleate frog eggs, which have been observed to give rise to normal embryos and ultimately normal-appearing tadpoles.[69]

Although the aforementioned experiments were not performed with cloned cells, their methodology strongly argues against the possibility that the donor cells used for transplantation were non-neoplastic contaminants. Therefore, the results constitute persuasive evidence that the genes responsible for normal differentiation and cell regulation are intact in at least some tumor cells, in which they are capable of being expressed if given the appropriate stimulus. The neoplastic phenotype may merely reflect a reversible derangement in gene regulation and not necessarily a mutation-like alteration, at least in the experimental neoplasms in question.

Reversibility of the Neoplastic Phenotype in Vitro

In keeping with the results described above are observations indicating that the neoplastic behavior of cells transformed *in vitro* may be reversibly modulated in many instances. Notable examples include cases in which varying degrees of phenotypic reversion have been induced by cyclic AMP, testosterone, bromodeoxyuridine, or dimethyl sulfoxide.[9,62]

Other noteworthy examples include temperature-sensitive mutants, in which the neoplastic phenotype can be switched off and on at will by varying the culture temperature.[10,62] In some instances, the mutants have been derived from cells transformed by chemical carcinogens.[10] In others, the mutants have been derived from cells transformed by temperature-sensitive oncogenic viruses.[70,71]

Another class of cells in which modulation and reversion of the neoplastic phenotype have been observed to be readily inducible includes various plant tumors.[72]

Although the above observations do not suggest that phenotypic reversion is possible in all cancer cells, they indicate that many of the properties of neoplastic cells are capable of modulation under appropriate conditions. The data are consistent with the interpretation that the fundamental lesion in cancer cells need not reside at the genetic level in the form of mutational changes, but may instead reside at the epigenetic level.

Differentiation of Cancer Cells in Vivo

It is common knowledge that neoplasms differ in the extent to which they show "dedifferentiation," and that it is only the occasional cancer that can be called "undifferentiated." The formation of differentiated structures (*e.g.*, keratohyaline pearls) or products (*e.g.*, hormones) by neoplastic cells attests to their capacity for some degree of differentiation under appropriate conditions. It is the exceedingly rare tumor in which differentiation becomes so marked and pervasive that it causes the growth to regress. Perhaps the best evidence for this type of regression exists when malignant neuroblastomas have been found to evolve into benign ganglioneuromas, presumably through the differentiation of neuroblastoma cells into ganglion cells.[73] The regression of neuroblastomatous nodules in the fetal adrenal gland would appear to be more common than has generally been recognized, as is the regression of disseminated neuroblastomas in infancy.[74,75]

Cancer Associated with Developmental Disturbances

As previously mentioned, the risk of cancer is frequently increased in association with certain disturbances of growth and development.[76] This association, coupled with the occurrence of neoplastic growth in dermoid cysts, hamartomas, and teratomas, accounts for one of the oldest theories of carcinogenesis, often known as Cohnheim's theory. This theory ascribes cancer to embryonic rests.[8] Although it is no longer considered a unifying hypotheses by experimental oncologists, concern with the role of morphogenetic interactions in carcinogenesis remains at the forefront, along with inquiry into the nature and action of morphogenetic inducers and other regulatory influences.

One of the most intriguing experimental models illustrating the oncogenic action of disturbed morphogenetic interactions is the murine teratocarcinoma that results from heterotopic transplantation of the mouse embryo beneath the testis capsule. In this location, the tissues of the embryo become disorganized, give rise to teratomas, and ultimately produce metastasizing malignant teratocarcinomas.[77,78]

Another experimental situation in which carcinogenesis may conceivably result from derangement in the morphogenetic interactions necessary for normal homeostasis is that involving tumor induction by inert plastic films subcutaneously imbedded in the rat.[79] In this case, tumor induction is prevented if the films are sufficiently perforated to allow broad contact between cells on opposite sides of the membrane. It has been tentatively inferred that the carcinogenic stimulus may result in interference with some yet undisclosed form of cell–cell interaction.[80]

It is thus tempting to speculate that the transplacental carcinogenic action of diethylstilbestrol on the human vagina, which first involves interference with the normal structural development of the organ, constitutes another example in which oncogenesis supervenes on a derangement of tissue homeostasis.[81]

High Rate of Transformation in Vitro

In some experimental systems, the frequency of transformation of cells in response to a given stimulus has exceeded the maximum frequency consistent with known mutation rates at any given locus. This difference has been interpreted as additional evidence for an epigenetic, as opposed to genetic, mechanism of neoplastic transformation. Examples of this phenomenon include the activation of a cell division-promoting factor in cultured plant cells. This factor is involved in the process of "habituation" that leads to tumor-like growth, and which occurs with a frequency two to three orders of magnitude higher than spontaneous randomly occurring mutations at any given gene locus.[72,82] Another example is the high rate of transformation (100%) exhibited in clones derived from cultured cells of a mouse prostate line exposed to a single pulse dose of methylcholanthrene *in vitro*.[50,62]

VIRAL THEORY

Experimental Tumor Viruses

Since the discovery of the myeloblastosis virus in chickens by Ellerman and Bang in 1908, many other oncogenic viruses have been identified.[83,84] The lengthening list of such agents now encompasses viruses and viral tumors of virtually every type, with examples in nearly all of the commonly studied species of animals. Viewed historically, the evolution of viral oncology can be divided into four major phases:

The first period, from 1910 to about 1935, was dominated by studies on avian tumor viruses and efforts to establish etiologic relationships in terms of Koch's postulates. These efforts were often frustrated by expectations now known not to be strictly applicable to oncogenic viruses; namely, that the virus should cause rapid onset of the disease and remain present at the height of the disease. At that time, however, the failure to fulfill Koch's postulates consistently, especially in any mammalian tumors, prevented the viral hypothesis from gaining wide credence.

The second period, from about 1935 to 1960, saw the discovery of a growing number of mammalian tumor viruses and the important realization that such viruses might not necessarily act alone, that they might require the interaction of specific genetic, physiologic, or environmental cofactors. It was also recognized during this period that the induced neoplasms might develop only after a long latency, appear in but few of the infected animals, and be non-infectious themselves. Because of these restrictions, viruses continued to be viewed as having little importance in the etiology of cancer.

During the third era, the early 1960's, it became apparent that tumorigenesis by DNA viruses was characteristically accompanied by integration of viral genes into the genome of the host cell. After this, the viral genes were transmitted vertically and could be expressed without production of infectious virus. These observations reconciled the puzzling lack of correlation between patterns of cancer incidence and epidemiological evidence for an infectious causative agent. The observations also suggested the possibility that any DNA virus might conceivably exert carcinogenic effects under appropriate circumstances, thus stimulating the search for oncogenic activity among common viruses. This has since led to demonstration of tumorigenesis by adenoviruses and also to implication of herpes simplex virus in the pathogenesis of certain types of cancer.

The fourth phase of viral oncology has seen the emergence of the revolutionary concept that RNA tumor viruses (oncornaviruses), like their DNA counterparts, contribute genetic information that becomes part of the genome of the affected host cell. With this latest development in viral oncology, tumor viruses have come to be considered more endogenous than exogenous to the host, thus, requiring for their elucidation, approaches used in research on molecular genetics and cell regulation.[39]

Viruses as Cofactors in Human Neoplasms

With the exception of the wart virus, viral agents have yet to be implicated conclusively in the pathogenesis of neoplastic lesions in humans. However, the susceptibility of human cells to virus-induced "neoplastic" transformation *in vitro* is amply documented. Indirect evidence implicating viruses in human neoplasia is also mounting; for example, the frequent occurrence of characteristic virus particles in the cells of certain malignancies; the association of group-specific, possibly viral or virus-mediated, antigens with the cells of some neoplasms; the presence of reverse transcriptase of oncornavirus-type in certain cancer cells; and the presence in certain cancer cell nuclei of DNA base sequences complementary to the base sequences of known or suspected tumor viruses.[85–88] These and other findings, which are analogous to those associated with virus-induced neoplasms in animals, strongly suggest the involvement of viruses as cofactors in the etiology of certain human cancers (see Table 2-2).[85,86]

Mechanism of Viral Transformation

Prevailing evidence favors the view that the virus exerts its oncogenic effects through integration of genetic information encoded in its nucleic acid into the genome of the infected host cell. In the case of DNA viruses, the integration and subsequent transcription of viral nucleic acid may be analogous to processes that have been best characterized in lysogenic bacteriophages.[88] On the other hand, in the case of the RNA virsus, the process of integration is thought to involve a DNA intermediate, synthesized from viral RNA through the action of a virus-specified, RNA-directed, DNA polymerase, or "reverse transcriptase."[84,89]

The viral information integrated into the genome of the host cell is viewed in each of the two currently prevailing hypotheses as constituting part of the normal inheritance of the cell, the virus-derived genes being subject to regulation

TABLE 2-2. Evidence of Association between Viruses and Certain Human Tumors

	LEUKEMIAS, SARCOMAS	BREAST CANCER	CERVICAL CARCINOMA	BURKITT'S LYMPHOMA	NASOPHA-RYNGEAL CARCINOMA	HEPATOCEL-LULAR CARCINOMA
Epidemiologic charcteristics favoring viral etiology	±	±	+ +	+	+	+
Candidate virus	–	–	HSV-2, CMV, papilloma	EBV	EBV	Hepatitis B
Viral markers in tumor cells	+	+	–	+ +	+ +	+
Patient's immune response to viral products	–	–	±	+ +	+ +	+
In vitro transforming activity of virus	N.A.	N.A.	+	+	+	N.A.
In vivo oncogenic potential at the same site in experimental animals	N.A.	N.A.	±	+	–	N.A.
Prospective studies	N.A.	N.A.	+	+	–	Planned
Intervention trials	N.A.	N.A.	–	Planned	–	Planned

(Adapted from material in de The G: Viruses as causes of some human tumors? Results and perspectives of the epidemiologic approach. *In* Hiatt HH, Watson JD, Winsten JA (eds): Origins of Human Cancer, pp 1113–1131. New York, Cold Spring Harbor, 1977, and from material in Szmuness W: Hepatocellular carcinoma and the hepatitis B virus: evidence for a causal association. Prog Med Virol 24:40–69, 1978)

N.A. = Not Applicable; + = positive; – = negative.

by mechanisms of repression and derepression similar to those controlling normal genes. These hypotheses are known as the "oncogene" hypothesis and the "protovirus" hypothesis.[90,91] Viewed in this context, the viral theory of carcinogenesis and the genetic theory of carcinogenesis become merged into a single unifying framework.

The "oncogene" hypothesis postulates that the genomes of C-type RNA viruses consist of "virogenes," which code for replication of the virus, and "oncogenes," which code for neoplastic transformation of the host cell. Such viral genomes are widespread, if not universal, in vertebrates, being transmitted vertically in the germ line and playing a functional role in normal cellular growth and differentiation by coding for alloantigens, or differentiation antigens, on the cell surface. According to this hypothesis, cancer is envisioned to result from de-repression of viral oncogenes, either through the action of external carcinogens or through spontaneously occurring mutational events. De-repression of virogenes, leading to virus production, is not considered necessary for the induction of neoplasia.[88,92,93]

The "protovirus" hypothesis postulates that genetic information can be transmitted within or among somatic cells from the DNA in "protovirus" regions of the genome into RNA intermediates. Then, via reverse transcriptase, it is transmitted back into DNA sequences reinserted into the genome. Through this mechanism, existing genes are thought to be amplified and new DNA sequences evolved in differentiation without affecting the stability of the germ line. "Misevolution" of protoviruses, either by mutation of their base sequences or their faulty integration into the wrong sites in the genome, is postulated to result in neoplastic transformation of the affected cell.[84,89]

Knowledge of the genetic composition of the oncogenic viruses and of the mechanisms regulating its expression is still meager. However, it is clear that viral mutants exist that differ to varying degrees in their ability to transform host cells and their host cell range, ability to replicate, and specification of virus-associated cell surface antigens. Depending on the nature of the mutation, the affected form of the virus may be said to be "defective" for the property in question. The occurrence of genetic interactions between defective and nondefective viruses, and between defective mutants and host cell genomes, is indicated by "marker rescue" phenomena. However, at present, genetic mapping of the viruses and characterization of their genetic interactions are in a rudimentary state.

The genetic complexity and heterogeneity of tumor viruses are paralleled by heterogeneity of host cells in susceptibility to transformation by a given virus. This further reflects the complexity of interactions between viral gene sequences and host cell genomes. In avian cells, as well as in mouse cells, several genetic loci influence the control of spontaneous and induced virus activation, expression of viral antigen, susceptibility to spreading of viral infection, and the host's ability to respond immunologically to virus-induced antigens in the transformed cells.[88] These observations demonstrate unequivocally that the expression and host range of endogenous viruses can be controlled in different ways and at more than one level in the viral life cycle; however, the extent to which the mechanisms are comparable in different tumor viruses and different host species, including man, remains to be determined.

The failure of transformation to result from infection alone or to persist without the continued expression of critical viral "oncogenes" has been clearly demonstrated in studies with temperature-sensitive mutant RNA and DNA viruses.[71,94] In Burkitt's lymphoma, the Epstein–Barr virus is postulated merely to initiate the process of carcinogenesis. Its completion is thought to require two additional steps, the final one being an 8:14 chromosomal translocation.[95] The crucial challenge in viral carcinogenesis, therefore, is to identify the viral "oncogenes" and their active products, and to elucidate their modes of action and regulation.

The mapping of tumor virus genomes, the identification of their transforming genetic sequences, or "oncogenes," and, the isolation and characterization of the transforming gene products have been the most successful to date in the case of the avian sarcoma virus. The ability of this virus to transform chick fibroblasts has been linked to a viral gene *src*.[96] The active product of src has been identified as a protein kinase associated with a phosphoprotein.[97,98]

CELL SELECTION THEORY

In certain situations, stimuli that increase the probability of cancer are thought to do so by favoring the proliferation of transformed cells which might not otherwise express their neoplastic proclivities. Although this mechanism is principally invoked to account for the effects of agents that are not carcinogenic by themselves, but which enhance the efficacy of carcinogens, it has been proposed as one of the modes of carcinogenic action.[8,9] The rationale is partially derived from evidence that under some conditions, carcinogenesis can be demonstrated to be a multistage process. Early stages may be reversed or arrested in the absence of a further tumor-inciting stimulus. The stimulus required to promote further evolution frequently involves cytotoxic effects that tend to select for cells that have already passed through the initial stages of neoplastic transformation. In this context, the progression of the tumor toward malignancy is viewed as the sequential appearance and selective outgrowth of progressively more autonomous subpopulations of cells, evolving through stepwise mutation-like changes, and proliferating under the influence of sustained selection pressure.[8,9]

In experimental carcinogenesis, the aforementioned process is well exemplified in the tumor-inciting action of phorbol esters and certain other "promoting" agents, as well as in the tumorigenic effects of hormonal imbalance on endocrine target organs.[8,99–102] These effects are discussed in the next section, in relation to the multistage pathogenesis of the cancer process.

Another situation favoring selection of dormant tumor cells occurs in immunodeficiency states. In animals and humans, spontaneous or induced immunodeficiency often increases susceptibility to neoplasia.[29,30] However, the results show more variability than can be explained simply by impairment of immunologic surveillance.[30] In humans, the excess is largely due to an increase in the frequency of leukemias, lymphoreticular neoplasms, cutaneous cancers, and gastric carcinomas, except in those immunodeficiency states associated with chromosomal fragility, such as ataxia-telangiectasia.[29,103,104] The situation is further complicated by evidence that a weak immunologic reaction against tumor cells may even enhance their survival and growth under certain conditions.[30,106,107]

In an attempt to explain the long latency of neoplasia in terms of a step-wise evolution and expression of the neoplastic phenotype, other possible explanations must not be overlooked. One of these is the puzzling phenomenon of tumor cell dormancy. The long interval occasionally intervening between the treatment of a neoplasm and its subsequent recurrence (this may amount to more than a decade) far exceeds the time that would be required merely for the regrowth of the tumor from residual tumor cells. That tumor cells can remain dormant indefinitely *in vivo,* under certain conditions, has been demonstrated repeatedly in experimental animals. One of the most striking examples is the experiment by Fisher and Fisher in which injected carcinoma cells that had remained dormant in rats for weeks were dislodged.[107] They were caused to form rapidly growing metastases in the lungs merely by mechanical manipulation of the liver. Clearly, the factors within the internal environment that account for such behavior of tumor cells cannot be adequately characterized at present. The many factors presumably involved include those which are concerned with the regulation of normal growth and differentiation, such as chalones, morphogenetic inducers, and other growth-regulating substances.[108-110]

CHEMICALS AS ETIOLOGIC AGENTS

CLASSES OF AGENTS (COMPLETE CARCINOGENS, INITIATING AGENTS, PROMOTING AGENTS)

Following the observation by Sir Percival Pott that cancer of the scrotum was relatively common among chimney sweeps, nearly 150 years elapsed before systematic efforts were made to identify the chemicals causing cancer in this occupational group and in other populations.[111,112] During recent years, the number of chemicals known or suspected to be carcinogenic has grown rapidly. Of a total of 368 chemicals (or industrial processes) evaluated between 1971 and 1977 by the International Agency for Research on Cancer, 26 were judged to be carcinogenic in humans (see Table 2-3) and 221 showed some evidence of carcinogenicity in animals.[113,114] A breakdown of these chemicals according to the circumstances in which they are usually encountered is shown in Table 2-4.[113]

Since there are millions of compounds in nature, efforts to evaluate them for carcinogenicity and then to proceed with effective interim measures to minimize exposure, if carcinogenic, must rest on some theoretical knowledge of the relation between molecular structure and biological activity, and on some understanding of the mechanisms of chemical carcinogenesis. One of the earliest insights into differences in modes of action came from observations more than 20 years ago by Rous, Berenblum, and others. They claimed that the process of carcinogenesis can be divided into at least two steps—initiation and promotion.[115] The changes produced by initiating agents are essentially permanent and irreversible, while those produced by promoting agents are transitory and elicit neoplasia only if preceded by appropriate initiating effects (see Fig. 2-1).[116] While the distinction between initiation and promotion is based on the operational differences illustrated in Fig. 2-1, many compounds that appear capable of merely initiating carcinogenesis at low doses may behave as complete carcinogens at higher doses or in animals of appropriate susceptibility. Similarly, chemicals that behave as promoting agents under some experimental conditions, failing to cause neoplasia unless preceded by an initiating agent, may, under other conditions, elicit neoplasia by themselves, possibly because the process of carcinogenesis has been initiated "spontaneously."

The nature and mechanisms of the changes responsible for initiation and promotion in cocarcinogenesis have yet to be established; however, initiation is generally postulated to involve some permanent, mutation-like alteration in DNA, while promotion is suspected to involve reversible alterations in epigenetic regulation (see Table 2-5).[112] This is possibly mediated through effects on the cell membrane.[60,112,117,118] Mutagens, as a class, tend to behave as initiators, while hormones and other growth stimulating factors behave as promoters. Both types of agents appear to be important in the causation of cancer in humans. The fact that the risk of lung cancer stops rising relatively soon after cessation of cigarette smoking is attributable to its ability to promote late stages in the process of carcinogenesis (see Fig. 2-2).[119]

METABOLIC ACTIVATION AND INACTIVATION

Most environmental carcinogens are not directly active in their ambient form. They require metabolic activation in the body in order to become carcinogenic (Fig. 2-3).[52,60] As yet, in few instances do we know the precise metabolic sequence through which derivatives of a parent compound are converted into more active "proximate" carcinogens and finally into the "ultimate" form, or forms, which react with cellular macromolecular targets to initiate carcinogenesis.[60] Based on present evidence, the ultimate carcinogens as a class are strongly electrophilic.[52,60]

The enzymatic machinery involved in the metabolic activation process resides in multicomponent, microsomal, mixed-function oxidase systems, notably the cytochrome P–450 mono-oxygenases. The concentration of carcinogenic derivatives formed during metabolism of a chemical by these enzyme systems depends on the inducibility and levels of activation, as opposed to inactivation, pathways. These vary markedly under the influence of environmental and genetic factors.[120-123] This helps to explain age-, species-, and strain-dependent differences in susceptibility to the carcinogenic effects of a given chemical.

MUTAGENICITY

As previously indicated, most carcinogens tested under conditions enabling their activation have been found to be mutagens. However, the correlation is better for certain classes of chemicals than for others, perhaps in part because of inadequacies in existing test methodology.[54] False negatives

(*Text continues on p. 44*)

TABLE 2-3. Chemicals or Industrial Processes Associated with Cancer Induction in Humans: Comparison of Target Organs and Main Routes of Exposure in Animals and Humans

	HUMANS			ANIMALS		
Chemical or industrial process	*Main type of exposure**	*Target organ*	*Main route of exposure†*	*Animal*	*Target organ*	*Route of exposure*
1. Aflatoxins	Environmental, occupational‡	Liver	PO, inhalation‡	Rat	Liver, stomach, colon, kidney	PO
				Fish, duck, marmoset, tree shrew, monkey	Liver	PO
				Rat	Liver, trachea	IT
					Liver	IP
				Mouse, rat	Local	SC injection
				Mouse	Lung	IP
2. 4-Aminobiphenyl	Occupational	Bladder	Inhalation, skin, PO	Mouse, rabbit, dog	Bladder	PO
				Newborn mouse	Liver	SC injection
				Rat	Mammary gland, intestine	SC injection
3. Arsenic compounds	Occupational, medicinal, and environmental	Skin, lung, liver‡	Inhalation, PO, skin	Mouse, rat, dog	Inadequate, negative	PO
				Mouse	Inadequate, negative	Topical, IV
4. Asbestos	Occupational	Lung, pleural cavity, gastrointestinal tract	Inhalation, PO	Mouse, rat, hamster, rabbit	Lung, pleura	Inhalation or IT
				Rat, hamster	Local	Intrapleural
				Rat	Local	IP, SC injection
						PO
5. Auramine (manufacture of)	Occupational	Bladder	Inhalation, skin, PO	Mouse, rat	Liver	PO
				Rabbit, dog	Rat	PO
				Rat	Negative	SC injection
					Local, liver, intestine	
6. Benzene	Occupational	Hemopoietic system	Inhalation, skin	Mouse	Inadequate	Topical, SC injection
7. Benzidine	Occupational	Bladder	Inhalation, skin, PO	Mouse	Liver	SC injection
				Rat	Liver	PO
					Zymbal gland, liver, colon	SC injection
				Hamster	Liver	PO
				Dog	Bladder	PO
8. Bis(chloromethyl) ether	Occupational	Lung	Inhalation	Mouse, rat	Lung, nasal cavity	Inhalation
				Mouse	Skin	Topical
					Local, lung	SC injection
				Rat	Local	SC injection
9. Cadmium-using industries (possibly cadmium oxide)	Occupational	Prostate, lung‡	Inhalation, PO	Rat	Local, testis	SC or IM injection
10. Chloramphenicol	Medicinal	Hemopoietic system	PO, injection		No adequate tests	
11. Chloromethyl methyl ether (possibly associated with bis(chloro-methyl)ether)	Occupational	Lung	Inhalation	Mouse	Initiator	Skin
					Lung‡	Inhalation
				Rat	Local, lung‡	SC injection
						SC injection
12. Chromium (chromate-producing industries)	Occupational	Lung, nasal cavities‡	Inhalation	Mouse, rat	Local	SC, IM injection
				Rat	Lung	Intrabronchial implantation

TABLE 2-3. (Continued)

	HUMANS			ANIMALS		
Chemical or industrial process	*Main type of exposure**	*Target organ*	*Main route of exposure†*	*Animal*	*Target organ*	*Route of exposure*
13. Cyclophosphamide	Medicinal	Bladder	PO, injection	Mouse	Hemopoietic system, lung	IP, SC injection
					Various sites	PO
				Rat	Bladder‡	IP
					Mammary gland	IP
					Various sites	IV
14. Diethylstilbestrol (DES)	Medicinal	Uterus, vagina	PO	Mouse	Mammary	PO
				Mouse	Mammary, lymphoreticular, testis	SC injection, SC implantation
					vagina	Local
				Rat	Mammary, hypophysis‡ bladder	SC implantation
				Hamster	Kidney	SC injection, SC implantation
				Squirrel monkey	Uterine serosa	SC implantation
15. Hematite mining (? radon)	Occupational	Lung	Inhalation	Mouse, hamster, guinea pig	Negative	Inhalation, IT
				Rat	Negative	SC injection
16. Isopropyl oils	Occupational	Nasal cavity, larynx	Inhalation		No adequate tests	
17. Melphalan	Medicinal	Hemopoietic system	PO, injection	Mouse	Initiator	Skin
					Lung, lymphosarcomas	IP
				Rat	Local	IP
18. Mustard gas	Occupational	Lung, larynx	Inhalation	Mouse	Lung	Inhalation, IV
					Local, mammary	SC injection
19. 2-Naphthylamine	Occupational	Bladder	Inhalation, skin, PO	Hamster, dog, monkey	Bladder	PO
				Mouse	Liver, lung	SC injection
				Rat, rabbit	Inadequate	PO
20. Nickel (nickel refining)	Occupational	Nasal cavity, lung	Inhalation	Rat	Lung	Inhalation
				Mouse, rat, hamster	Local	SC, IM injection
				Mouse, rat	Local	IM implantation
21. *N,N*-Bis(2-chloroethyl)-2-naphthylamine	Medicinal	Bladder	PO	Mouse	Lung	IP
				Rat	Local	SC injection
22. Oxymetholone	Medicinal	Liver	PO		No adequate tests	
23. Phenacetin	Medicinal	Kidney	PO		No adequate tests§	
24. Phenytoin	Medicinal	Lymphoreticular tissues	PO, injection	Mouse	Lymphoreticular tissues	PO, IP
25. Soot, tars, and oils	Occupational, environmental	Lung, skin (scrotum)	Inhalation, skin	Mouse, rabbit	Skin	Topical
26. Vinyl chloride	Occupational	Liver, brain,‡ lung‡	Inhalation, skin	Mouse, rat	Lung, liver, blood vessels, mammary, Zymbal gland, kidney	Inhalation

(Tomatis L, Agtha C, Bartsch H, et al: Evaluation of the carcinogenicity of chemicals: a review of the monograph program of the International Agency for Research on Cancer. Cancer Res 38:877–881, 1978. Reproduced with the permission of the American Association for Cancer Research, 1978)

* The main types of exposures mentioned are those by which association has been demonstrated; exposures other than those mentioned may also occur

† The main routes of exposure given may not be the only ones by which such effects could occur

‡ Indicative evidence

§ The induction of tumors of the nasal cavities in rats given phenacetin has recently been reported (S. Odashima, personal communication, 1977)

TABLE 2-4. Major Use Exposure Categories for the Chemicals or Industrial Processes Evaluated in Volumes 1 to 16 of the International Agency for Research on Cancer Monographs

MAJOR USE OR EXPOSURE	NUMBER OF CHEMICALS
Industrial chemicals	173
Drugs	84
Pesticides	34
Naturally occurring substances	32
Food additives or cosmetics	31
Miscellaneous chemicals and analogs	7
Industrial processes	5
Industrial by-products	2
TOTAL	368

(Tomatis L, Agtha C, Bartsch H, et al: Evaluation of the carcinogenicity of chemicals: a review of the monograph program of the International Agency for Research on Cancer. Cancer Res 38:877–881, 1978.)

FIG. 2-1. Outline of the so-called two-stage process of carcinogenesis, involving initiation and promotion components. Each horizontal line represents an experimental condition in which there may or may not be a single application of initiating agent and multiple applications of a promoting agent. The time span may extend to 50 weeks in carcinogenesis in mouse skin, depending on dosages of the initiator and promoter. The term "tumors" refers to papillomas, or to carcinomas provided the experiment is extended for a sufficiently long time. Time = →, Initiator = ┬, Promoter = ┬. (Boutwell) RK: Biochemical Mechanism of Tumor Promotion. In Slaga TJ, Sivak A, Boutwell RK (eds): Carcinogenesis, vol 2, Mechanisms of Tumor Promotion and Carcinogenesis, pp. 49–58. New York, Raven Press, 1978)

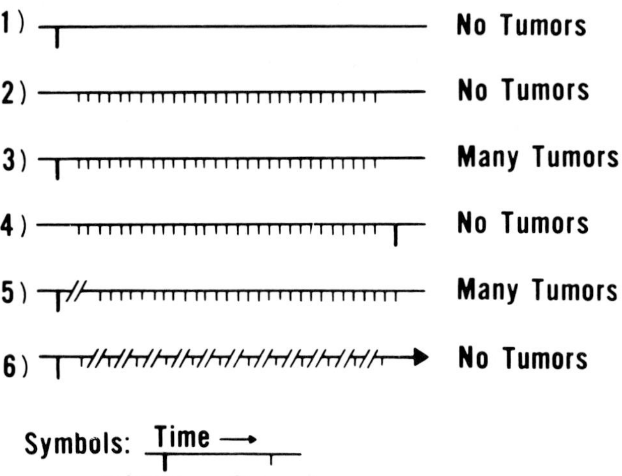

in a microbial assay system, which may conceivably result from inadequate activation *in vitro* or from inability of the system to detect the entire spectrum of mutational events that might lead to cancer, do not necessarily exclude possible damage to DNA *in vivo*. At the same time, there is no reason to implicate mutagenesis as the only mechanism of carcinogenesis, and hence to postulate that all carcinogens should be mutagens.

TABLE 2-5. Biological Properties of Initiating Agents as Compared with Promoting Agents

INITIATING AGENTS	PROMOTING AGENTS
1. Carcinogenic by themselves—"solitary carcinogens"	1. Not carcinogenic alone; must be given after the initiating agent
2. Single exposure is sufficient	2. Require prolonged exposure
3. Action is "irreversible" and additive	3. Action is reversible (at early stage) and not additive
4. No apparent threshold	4. Probable threshold
5. Yield electrophiles—bind covalently to cell macromolecules	5. No evidence of covalent binding
6. Mutagenic	6. Not mutagenic

(Weinstein IB: Current concepts of mechanisms of chemical carcinogenesis. Bull NY Acad Med 54:366–383, 1978)

FIG. 2-2. Relationship between the incidence of bronchial carcinoma and time since cigarette smoking was stopped, compared with the relationship in continuing smokers and nonsmokers. (Doll R: Cancer and Aging: The Epidemiologic Evidence. In Clark RL, Cumley RW, McKay JE et al (eds): The Harold Dorn Memorial Lecture. Oncology 1970, Vol. V, pp. 1–28. Chicago, Year Book Medical Publishers, 1971)

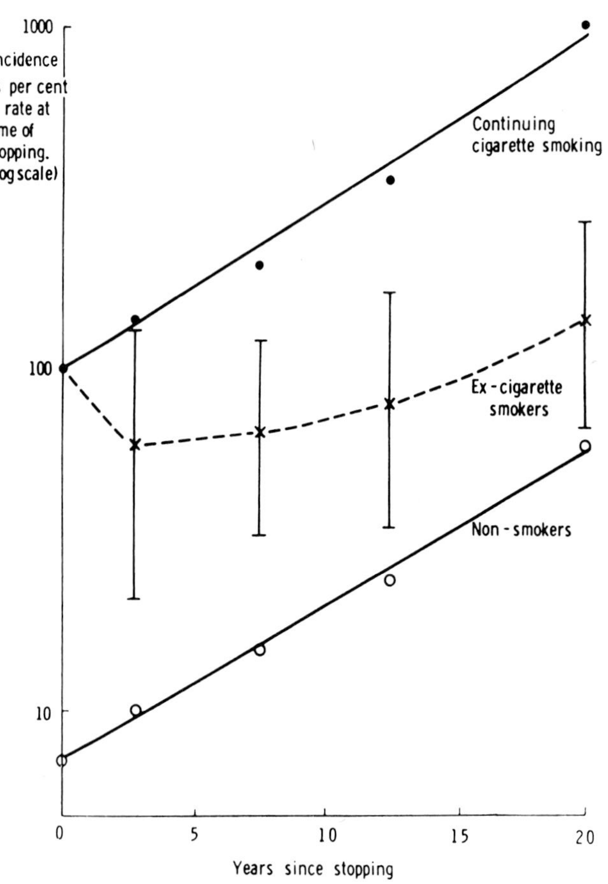

SCREENING METHODS

The identification of chemicals with carcinogenic activity calls for epidemiologic as well as laboratory approaches. Since the epidemiologic approaches were discussed in Chapter 1,

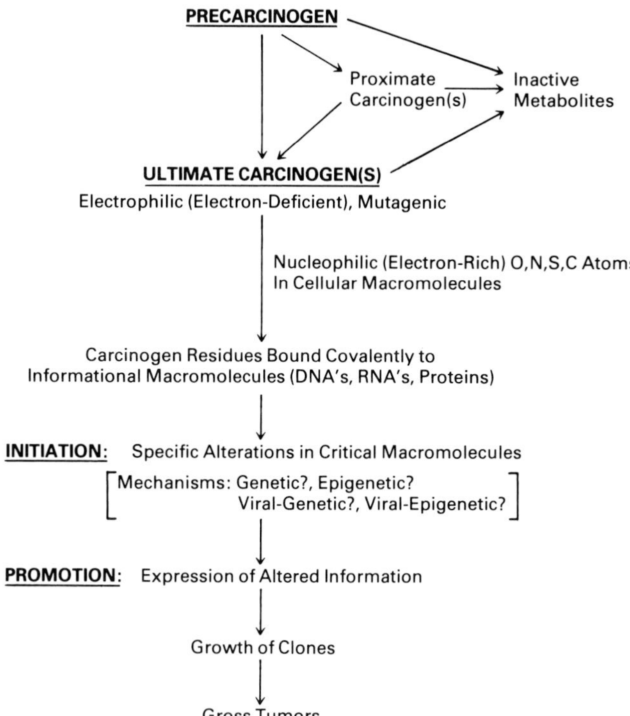

FIG. 2-3. The processes involved in carcinogenesis by chemical carcinogens. (Miller JA: Concluding Remarks on Chemicals and Chemical Carcinogenesis. In Griffin AC, Shaw CR (eds): Carcinogens: Identification and Mechanisms of Action, pp. 455–464. New York, Raven Press, 1979)

only the laboratory approaches will be treated here. These include assays in laboratory animals and short-term tests in microorganisms, Drosophila, cultured cells, and other systems.

In Vivo *Assays*

Because chemicals known to cause cancer in humans also generally show carcinogenecity in animals (see Table 2-3), and because the carcinogenicity of a chemical in laboratory animals is generally not species-specific, chemicals shown to cause neoplasms in animals are ordinarily classified as *presumptive* carcinogens for humans.[111,113,124–128] Evidence for the chemical carcinogenicity in laboratory animals has preceded the observation of human carcinogenicity in the case of diethylstilbestrol (DES), 4-aminobiphenyl, vinyl chloride, bis(chloromethyl)ether, acetylaminofluorene, and others. In some of these instances, had the predictive warning given by the laboratory evidence been more fully heeded, and human exposure curtailed accordingly, a number of cancers could have been prevented.[113]

Methods for evaluating the carcinogenicity of chemicals in laboratory animals are now based on criteria recommended by several national and international groups of experts.[124,127] These criteria are embodied in the carcinogen bioassay program conducted by the U.S. National Cancer Institute. The standard test protocol in this program involves the life-long dietary administration of suspect chemicals at high dose levels to rats and mice of both sexes.[130,120] When a chemical is found to be carcinogenic in such tests, assessment of its potential risks to humans who are likely to be exposed at much lower dose levels involves two kinds of extrapolation. One extrapolation is across species and the other across differences in dose and conditions of exposure. These extrapolations are fraught with great uncertainty because of gaps in our knowledge about species differences in susceptibility and dose-response relations. Further uncertainty results from the fact that exposure of human populations is almost never limited to one chemical alone, but involves untold myriads of chemicals, which may interact with one another in additive, synergistic, or mutally inhibitory ways, depending on the chemicals and circumstances in question.

Because each of the standard feeding tests described above costs several hundred thousand dollars and takes 4 to 5 years to complete, only a few of the many thousands of chemicals to be tested can be investigated with the limited resources available. To increase the testing capacity, more economical and rapid assay systems are called for. Hence, *in vitro* tests of the sort described below are now under active exploration.

In Vitro *Assays*

Short-term tests under study include mutagenicity tests in various assay systems, morphologic transformation of cells in culture, binding of chemicals to DNA, DNA damage and repair, induction of latent virus, and other endpoints.[131] To date, the most widely used assays have been the Salmonella mutagenicity test and the *in vitro* cell transformation test.[56,57,132–134] In the Salmonella test, (known after its developer as the Ames test) one of a number of histidine-requiring mutant strains of *S. typhimurium* is plated on culture medium containing the chemical to be tested and a rat liver enzyme fraction that is capable of converting carcinogen and mutagen precursors into active metabolites. Because the bacteria cannot grow on the medium in question until the mutation for histidine-dependence is reverted by a back-mutation, the assay scores for colonies of revertants, the frequency of which reflects the mutagenicity of metabolites of the chemical under testing.

As indicated in Table 2-6, the predictive value of the Salmonella test varies, depending on the type of carcinogenic chemical in question. The cell transformation assay, while used less widely thus far, appears to give fewer false–negative and false–positive results.[134] While a combination of *in vitro* tests may collectively provide greater predictability than any one test alone, the limitations of these tests have not yet been investigated sufficiently to indicate their ultimate usefulness.

At present, although the *in vitro* tests are not able to replace *in vivo* tests as an approach for identifying carcinogens, their rapidity, economy, and sensitivity make them valuable for prescreening suspect compounds. Also enhancing their usefulness is their applicability to crude mixtures of various kinds, including specimens of urine, blood, feces, and tissue fluid. The mutagenicity assays have the additional virtue of indicating whether a carcinogen possesses mutagenic activity, thus contributing to the evaluation of its mechanism of action.

TABLE 2-6. Summary of Relative Mutagenic Activities of 465 Known or Suspected Carinogens in Relation to their Chemical Structure

ACTIVITY*	CATEGORY	CHEMICALS	TESTED IN SALMONELLA	POSITIVE IN SALMONELLA
NOT EVALUABLE	Cyanamide	1	0/1	0/0
	Substituted diphenylethane	1	1/1	0/1
	Stilbenediol	3	1/3	0/1
	Dioxane	1	0/1	0/0
	Anhydride	2	1/2	0/1
	Pyrazolinone	1	1/1	0/1
	Pyrrolizidine	5	0/5	0/0
	Haloalkyl ether	3	1/3	1/1
	Sulfanilamide	2	0/2	0/0
	Polysaccharide	4	1/4	0/1
	Polymer	3	1/3	0/1
	Metal complex	5	0/5	0/0
	Miscellaneous	7	5/7	0/5
SUBTOTAL	13 categories† (33)‡·§	38 (8)§	12/38 (32)	1/12 (8)
HIGH	Triazene	3	2/3	2/2
	Diazo	4	3/4	3/3
	Azoxy	5	4/5	3/4
	Nitroso	53	39/53	39/39
	Diaryl alkynyl carbamate	3	3/3	3/3
	Aromatic amine	67	43/67	36/43
	Nitroaromatic	38	32/38	32/32
	Polyaromatic	50	18/50	18/18
	Aziridine	16	6/16	6/6
	Oxirane, thirane	11	6/11	6/6
	Heteroaromatic	20	13/20	12/13
	Halomethane, haloethane	15	13/15	11/13
	N-, S-, or O-mustard	17	10/17	10/10
	Sulfate, sulfonate, sultone	9	6/9	6/6
	Phosphate	1	1/1	1/1
SUBTOTAL	15 categories (38)§	312 (67)§	199/312 (64)	188/199 (94)
MEDIUM	Hydrazine	12	8/12	5/8
	Lactone	8	4/8	2/4
	Chloroethylene	6	6/6	4/6
	Inorganic	8	5/8	2/5
SUBTOTAL	4 categories (10)§	34 (7)§	23/34 (68)	13/23 (57)
LOW	Azo	11	6/11	2/6
	Carbamyl, thiocarbamyl	21	9/21	3/9
	Phenyl	8	5/8	0/5
	Benzodioxole	8	4/8	1/4
	Polychlorinated cyclic	9	8/9	1/8
	Steroid	15	2/15	0/2
	Antimetabolite	9	3/9	1/3
SUBTOTAL	7 categories (18)§	81 (17)§	37/81 (46)	8/37 (22)
TOTAL	39 categories†	465	271/465 (58)	210/271 (77)

(Rinkus SJ, Legator MS: Chemical characterization of 465 known or suspected carcinogens and their correlation with mutagenic activity in the salmonella typhimurium system. Cancer Res 39:3289–3318, 1979)

* Relative ability of the Salmonella S-9 system to detect carcinogens in the given categories. "Not evaluable" indicates either a small number of chemicals in the category or a lack of testing; "high", "medium", and "low" indicate that individual category correlations are in the upper, middle, and lower 33rd percentiles, respectively

† Includes a miscellaneous category

‡ Numbers in parentheses, percentages

§ Percentages of respective total

INHIBITORS OF CARCINOGENESIS

In view of the multistage nature of the cancer process, strategies for preventing carcinogenesis should include, in addition to the identification of cancer-causing agents and their removal from the environment:

1. Interference with the formation of carcinogens *in vivo*
2. Strengthening of defenses that prevent carcinogens from reaching or reacting with critical target sites
3. Blocking or reversing tumor progression at early stages[135,136]

A number of substances have been experimentally observed to inhibit the formation of carcinogens *in vivo*.[135,136] These include ascorbic acid, which inhibits the formation of nitroso compounds in the stomach and decreases the content of mutagens in human feces. Other agents may inhibit carcinogen formation by modifying microsomal mixed function oxidase activity in ways that decrease the activation or increase the detoxification of carcinogens; examples include butylated hydroxyanisole, disulfuram, certain flavones, and various other enzyme inducers and inhibitors. The use of nucleophilic trapping agents to bind competitively with electrophilic carcinogens and thus protect critical target sites is another approach deserving of study.[135,136]

Under certain conditions, various agents have been observed to inhibit the promotion and progression of neoplasia in experimental animals; for example, retinoids, protease inhibitors, and anti-inflammatory steroids.[137,139] As yet, the range of neoplasms against which these agents protect and the ultimate value of this approach for cancer prevention in humans remain to be determined.

The rationale for use of retinoids derives from their essentiality for the maintenance of normal differentiation. Without them, normal epithelial differentiation does not occur in the respiratory tract, urinary bladder, breast, gastrointestinal tract, and other organs. Instead, the epithelium gives rise to squamous metaplastic lesions that are readily reversible by administering appropriate retinoids. Retinoids also are capable of reversing, to some extent, epithelial lesions induced experimentally by chemical carcinogens. However, the natural retinoids, including vitamin A, are relatively ineffective in preventing cancer in experimental animals because of toxicity at the high dose levels required. More promising are synthetic retinoids, such as 13-cis-retinoic acid, which inhibits carcinogenesis in the rat bladder and breast. Further advances in our knowledge of structure–function relationships may ultimately enable the synthesis of retinoids that are sufficiently non-toxic to be of practical use in preventing human cancer.[137] In the meantime, toxicity remains a limiting problem.

PHYSICAL AGENTS AS CARCINOGENS

IONIZING RADIATION

More than 75 years have elapsed since the carcinogenic effects of ionizing radiation were first recognized. In the interim, these effects have been studied extensively in human populations and laboratory animals. Ionizing radiations of all forms possess carcinogenic activity, although potency varies. Furthermore, depending on the conditions of irradiation and the susceptibility of irradiated tissue, radiation-induced neoplasms of virtually all types have been observed.[140–142]

Because the dose of radiation to a given organ can be measured relatively precisely, considerable effort has gone into analysis of the dose-incidence relation for radiation carcinogenesis. The existing data indicate that with radiations of high linear energy transfer (LET)—alpha particles, protons, and neutrons—the incidence of neoplasms generally increases as a linear function of the dose to tumor-forming cells, irrespective of the duration of irradiation, at least in the low-to-intermediate dose range (see Fig. 2-4). In contrast, the dose-incidence curve for low-LET radiations tends to increase in slope with increasing dose and dose rate.[142–144] Above a certain dose, the curves for high dose rate irradiation tend to saturate, pass through a maximum, and decrease with further increase in the dose (see Fig. 2-4).[145]

The above dose-incidence relationships can be described by the following expression:

$$I_D = I_o + (aD + bD^2)e^{-(pD+qD^2)}$$

where I_D is the control incidence and a, b, p, and q are constants. In the case of high-LET radiations, the linear term characteristically predominates at high doses as well as at low doses, whereas in the case of low-LET radiations, it characteristically predominates only in the low-to-intermediate dose region.[146] It is noteworthy that these dose-effect curves are consistent with the curves for such radiation-induced changes at the cellular level as mutations, chromosome abberations, cell transformation *in vitro*, and cell killing.[146]

Although the mechanisms of radiation carcinogenesis are unknown, one can postulate that the dose-incidence curves for carcinogenic effects at low-to-intermediate doses predominantly reflect the neoplastic transformation of cells, while at high doses, the curves saturate because of damage that interferes with transformation expression. The decline of the dose-incidence curve for radiation-induced leukemia at high doses (see Fig. 2-4), which can be described by the negative exponential term in the above equation, is attributable to excessive killing of hematopoietic stem cells.[142–147]

While excessive killing of cells may interfere with carcinogenesis at high radiation doses, there are circumstances under which cell killing has been observed to play an important role in promoting neoplasia. These include the induction of thymic lymphoma in the mouse, in which extensive destruction of hemopoietic cells in the marrow and other sites is essential to maximal tumorigenesis; the induction of osteosarcomas by internally deposited radium-226 in humans and dogs, in which the outgrowth of transformed osteoblasts is presumed to be promoted by the killing of other osteoblasts; and the induction of hair follicle tumors in rats, in which sufficient killing of cells to damage follicles irreparably is required for maximal yields of tumors.[148–150]

Additional variables affecting the induction of neoplasms by radiation include species, strain, sex, age at irradiation, immunologic reactivity, hormonal balance, and other physiological factors, as well as the possible interactive effects of

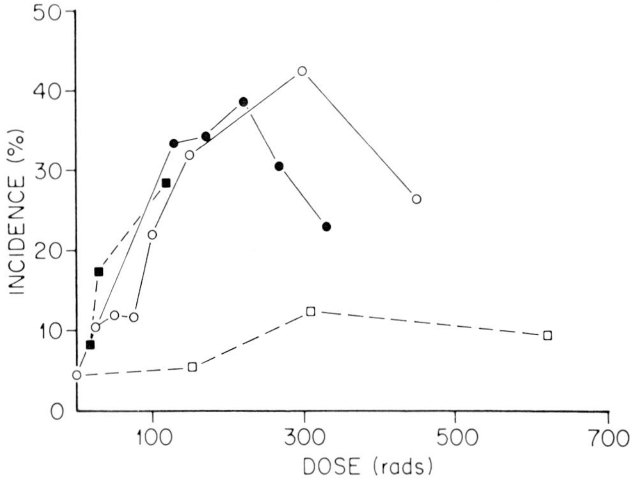

FIG. 2-4. Myeloid leukemia in male mice. ○ single exposure; □ daily exposures. (Open symbols denote results with gamma rays and x rays; solid symbols, neutrons.)

other physical or chemical agents.[142,143] The effects of hormonal and immunologic modifiers are consistent in general with their growth-promoting and growth-inhibiting actions.[142]

Study of the mechanisms of radiation carcinogenesis has been materially advanced by the development of techniques to investigate the neoplastic transformation of cells in culture. Analysis of the transformation of Syrian hamster embryo cells by x-rays and fast neutrons has revealed dose-response relations (see Fig. 2-5) consistent with those for mutations, chromosome aberrations, and cell killing.[145,146] Paradoxically, however, at doses below 300 rads, fractionation of low-LET radiation into two exposures separated by an interval of five hours has been observed to induce a higher rate of transformation than the same dose delivered in a single exposure.[152] This fractionation effect, which remains to be explained, may conceivably indicate that repair processes induced by the first exposure can affect the susceptibility of DNA to damage by an appropriately timed second exposure.

FIG. 2-5. Incidence of hamster embryo cell transformation following exposure to neutrons. For doses at which more than one experiment was performed the data were pooled. The mean value together with the standard deviation is plotted in the figure. (Borek C: In vitro cell transformation by low doses of x-irradiation and neutrons. In Yuhas JM, Tennant RW, Regan JD (eds): Biology of Radiation Carcinogenesis, pp. 309–326. New York, Raven Press, 1976)

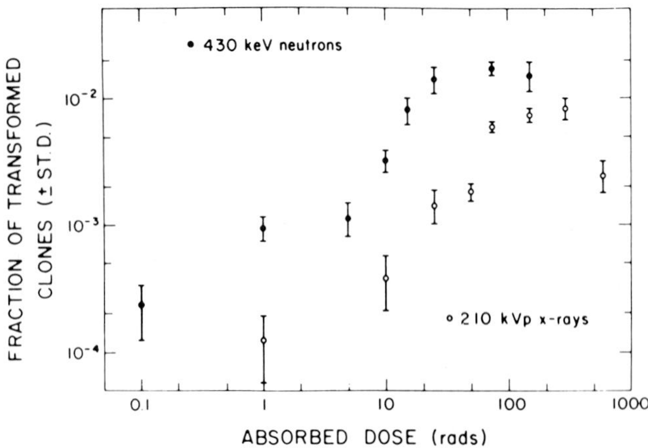

Attempts to estimate the carcinogenic risks associated with low-level radiation have generally utilized the linear nonthreshold extrapolation model as a prudently conservative working hypothesis, although the possibility of a threshold cannot be excluded.[142,153] It has more recently been suggested that a linear-quadratic model, such as is represented by the above equation, may provide more realistic risk estimates for some of the carcinogenic effects of low-LET radiation.[146,154] Based on the use of a linear nonthreshold extrapolation model, it has been estimated that exposure of the population to natural background radiation, which corresponds to an average dose of about 0.1 rem per year, may account for roughly 1% to 2% of the total cancer incidence (see Table 2-7).[155]

ULTRAVIOLET RADIATION

An association between skin cancer and exposure to sunlight was recognized more than a century ago.[156] In the interim, the carcinogenic action of UV radiation of the skin has been documented extensively by several lines of evidence:

1. Skin cancer occurs most frequently on exposed parts (head, neck, arms, hands)
2. There is an inverse correlation between pigmentation of the skin, which filters out UV, and the incidence of cutaneous cancer—skin cancer is most common in fair-skinned people, such as Celts, and relatively rare in dark-skinned races
3. Increased incidence of skin cancer among those who are occupationally exposed to sunlight, such as farmers, sailors, fishermen
4. The incidence of skin cancer in whites living in various parts of the world is correlated with the intensity of the sunlight to which they are exposed, being highest in those closest to the equator
5. Susceptibility to skin cancer is greatly increased in xeroderma pigmentosum, an inherited disease characterized by defective repair of UV-induced damage to DNA

TABLE 2-7. Estimate of Annual Contribution of Radiation Exposure to Lifetime Burden of Fatal Cancer in the U.S. Population
(Total Cancer Mortality in 1975: 365,000)

SOURCE	LIFETIME CANCER MORTALITY COMMITMENT (Number of deaths)
Natural Background	5,000
Technologically Enhanced Natural Radiation	250
Healing Arts	4,250
Nuclear Weapons Fallout	250–450
Nuclear Energy	9
Consumer Products	1.5
TOTAL = 2.7 percent of cancer mortality	10,000

(Jablon S, Bailar JA: The contribution of ionizing radiation to cancer mortality in the United States. Prev Med 9:212–226, 1980)

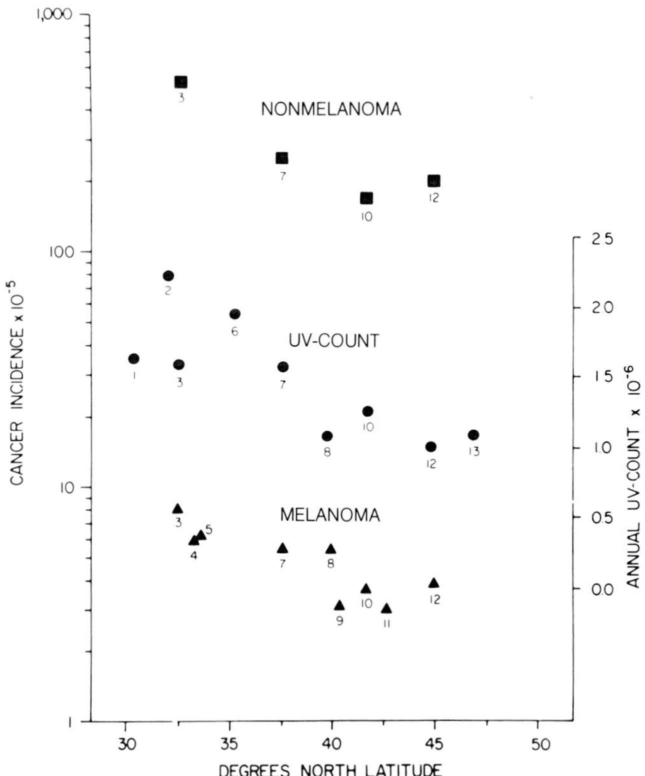

FIG. 2-6. Variation with latitude in UV radiation levels and age-adjusted skin cancer rates for white mice in various U. S. cities and states, 1970. ((*1*) Tallahassee, FL; (2) El Paso, TX; (*3*) Fort Worth, TX; (*4*) Birmingham, AL; (*5*) Atlanta, GA; (*6*) Albuquerque, NM; (*7*) Oakland, CA; (*8*) Colorado; (*9*) Pittsburgh, PA; (*10*) Des Moines, IA; (*11*) Detroit, MI; (*12*) Minneapolis, MN; (*13*) Bismarck, ND. (Hiatt HH, Watson JD, Winsten JA (eds): Origins of Human Cancer, pp. 2–61. Cold Spring Harbor Laboratory, Cold Spring Harbor, New York, 1977)

6. Skin cancer can be readily induced in experimental animals by repeated exposure to UV, but not to visible light alone[157–161]

Melanomatous, as well as non-melanomatous, skin cancers are increased in frequency by UV.[141]

The mode of UV action is not known precisely, but evidence suggests that the induction of pyrimidine dimers in the DNA of skin cells may be the critical molecular lesion in UV-induced skin carcinogenesis.[159] In addition, there is evidence in the mouse that UV irradiation causes immunologic changes that contribute to cutaneous carcinogenesis, possibly through the production of suppressor T-lymphocytes.[162,163]

In mice exposed daily to UV radiation, the incidence of skin cancer has been observed to vary with the logarithm of the square of the number of days of exposure.[156,164]

FOREIGN BODIES

Asbestos

The inhalation of asbestos fibers has been associated with an increase in the incidence of bronchial, gastrointestinal, and mesothelial cancers in human populations.[165] In cigarette smokers, the combined effects of smoking and asbestos on the incidence of bronchial cancer are synergistic, being equivalent to the product of the increments in risk attributable to each agent alone rather than merely to the sum of the two.[166,167] An asbestos worker who smokes cigarettes has eight times the risk compared to smokers of the same age who do not work with asbestos and 92 times the risk of men who neither smoke nor work with asbestos.[165]

In animals, the introduction of asbestos fibers into the pleural space can induce mesotheliomas, thus reproducing the human disease.[168] Analysis of the carcinogenicity of asbestos fibers in relation to their size and shape has disclosed that long, slender fibers are significantly more carcinogenic than short, thick ones, indicating that crocidolite is a more hazardous form of asbestos than amosite.[168] The carcinogenic effect of intrapleurally-injected asbestos fibers can be duplicated by glass fibers, the carcinogenicity of which is also more marked in the case of long, slender fibers than in the case of short, thick ones.[168] These data indicate that it is the physical properties of the fibers rather than their chemical composition that account for their carcinogenic activity; however, the precise nature of the physiologic stimulus through which they act remains obscure.

Films and Planar Surfaces

Implantation of plastic films into various body sites has been observed to induce fibrosarcomas in rats, mice, Syrian hamsters, and dogs.[80] The carcinogenicity of the implants is dependent on their size, surface area, and porosity. For example, Millipore filters of about 150 μm in width with pore sizes larger than 0.22 μm fail to induce tumors in rats, in contrast to those of finer porosity. The dependency of the carcinogenic activity of implanted films on their physical properties points to a physical, or mechanical, mechanism of carcinogenesis, the nature of which remains to be disclosed. However, it is noteworthy that development of film-induced tumors is characteristically preceded by exuberant foreign body reactions.[80]

Sarcomas have sporadically been reported in association with foreign body reactions in humans, with latencies of up to 40 years.[80] In comparison with the rodent, however, man appears much less susceptible to such tumors, since their occurrence after implantation of prostheses has been extremely rare.[80]

Schistosomiasis

Squamous cell carcinoma of the urinary bladder in association with infestation of the urinary tract by the parasite *Schistosomia hematobium* is unusually common in inhabitants of the Nile river valley, Mozambique, and Rhodesia.[6,169] Cancer development is characteristically preceded by long-standing inflammation and fibrosis of the bladder mucosa, with squamous metaplasia of its transitional epithleium.[169] In experimental animals, *S. hematobium* infestation has been observed to enhance susceptibility of the bladder mucosa to the carcinogenic effects of 2-AAF and methylnitrosourea.[170,171]

The mechanism of carcinogenesis in *S. hematobium* infestation is obscure, but the presence of chronic inflammation

TABLE 2-8. Some Factors Related to the Occurrence of Neoplasia

	CAUSATIVE OR PREDISPOSING FACTORS		
Site	*Exogenous*	*Endogenous*	*"Premalignant" states or lesions*
Mouth and pharynx	Tobacco	Plummer–Vinson syndrome (sideropenia)	Leukoplakia
	Alcohol		—
	Nutritional deficiency		—
Esophagus	Alcohol	Sideropenia	?Dysplasia
	Tobacco	Tylosis	—
	Nutritional deficiency		—
	Stricture (lye)		—
Stomach	?	Achlorhydria	Atrophic gastritis
		Pernicious anemia	Polyp
Colorectum	Diet	Familial (multiple polyposis)	—
		Ulcerative colitis	—
		Gardner's syndrone	—
Liver	Alcohol	Hemochromatosis	?
	?Nutritional deficiency	Cirrhosis	—
	?Aflatoxin		—
Larynx	Tobacco	?	Leukoplakia
	Alcohol		—
Lung	Tobacco	Family history	Cytologic atypia
	Air pollution		Bronchial adenoma
	Occupational inhalation of chromate, asbestos, nickel, uranium, etc.		—
Urinary bladder	Tobacco	?Tryptophan metabolism abnormality	Leukoplakia
	Schistosoma hematobium		Papilloma
	Occupational: aniline dye products		—
Skin (including genitalia)	Actinic radiation	Fair complexion	Senile keratosis
	Ionizing radiation	Xeroderma pigmentosum	Arsenical keratosis
	Arsenic		Leukoplakia
	Petroleum, tar products		—
	Burn scars		—
Leukemia (myelocytic)	Ionizing radiation	Mongolism	Myeloproliferative states (preleukemia)
	?Phenylbutazone	Bloom syndrome	
	?Benzol	Fanconi syndrome	
	?Alkylating agents		—
Lymphoma	Immunosuppression	Agammaglobulinemia	?
		Wiskott–Aldrich syndrome	—
Thyroid	Ionizing radiation	Family history	?Adenoma
	Iodine deficiency		—
Bone	Ionizing radiation (radium)	Paget's disease	—
		Fibrous dysplasia	—
		Osteochondroma	—
Testis	?Mumps orchitis	Cryptorchidism	?
Uterine cervix	Early sexual intercourse	?	Leukoplakia
	Promiscuity		Cytologic dysplasia
	?Uncircumcised partner		—
Endometrium	?Diet	Endocrine: obesity, infertility, diabetes	Cytologic atypia ?Hyperplasia
		?Ovarian hyperfunction	—
Breast	Ionizing radiation	Nulliparity	Intraductile papilloma
	?Diet	Family history	
		Endocrine: obesity, diabetes	Chronic cystic disease

(Shimkin MB: Preventive oncology. Prev Med 4:106–114, 1975. Reproduced with the permission of Academic Press, Inc., New York, 1975)

incited, along with leukoplakia, has led some observers to compare this carcinogen process with the induction of the foreign body sarcomas mentioned above. However, at the same time, the possible role of bacterial infection, with nitrosamine formation, disturbances in tryptophan metabolism, and other biochemical abnormalities, must also be considered.[171]

Mineral Oil

Intraperitoneal injections of mineral oil into BALB/c mice incite granulomatous inflammation of the peritoneum, followed several months later by the development of plasma cell tumors in discrete peritoneal nodules.[172] The tumor cells have been observed to contain type-A, virus-like particles, but the

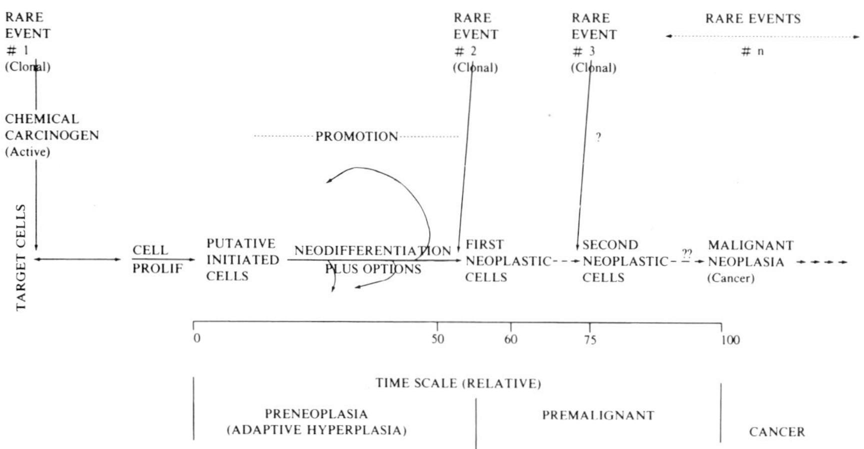

FIG. 2-7. Diagrammatic representation of our current concept of the steps in the development of liver cancer with chemicals. The rare events occur in a very small number of cells in a much larger population and therefore are analogous to a mutation-like phenomenon. In contrast, the steps between the rare events involve essentially the whole of the bulk of that population. As indicated, the rare events are probably clonal in origin. (Farber EE, Camera RG, Laishes B et al: Cellular and molecular markers of the carcinogenic process. 313–335. In Griffin AC, Shaw CR (eds): Carcinogens: Identification and Mechanisms of Action, 313–335. New York, Raven Press, 1979)

role of such particles in the pathogenesis of the disease is unknown.[172]

The origin of these tumors in a peritoneal granuloma suggests that their pathogenesis may have features in common with the other foreign body-induced neoplasms described above.

NATURAL HISTORY OF CANCER *IN VIVO*

PRECANCEROUS LESIONS

A number of lesions are known to predispose to cancer. A few of the more common examples are listed in Table 2-8.[173] The frequency and rapidity with which such precancerous lesions give rise to invasive cancer is variable, depending on the type of lesion, the organ affected, and other factors.

Women with dysplasia of the epithelium of the uterine cervix are estimated to have a 1600 times greater-than-normal chance of developing carcinoma of the cervix *in situ*.[174] However, the course of progression is predictable only for histologic classes of lesions and not for the lesion in any given person.[175] Similarly, with carcinoma of the skin *in situ* and with lobular carcinoma of the breast *in situ*, it is difficult to distinguish lesions that will progress from lesions that will remain stationary or regress.[175] The course of carcinoma of the urinary bladder, stomach, and bronchus (all *in situ*) tends to be more predictable.[175].

The study of experimentally-induced carcinogenesis in laboratory animals has also disclosed a variety of preneoplastic lesions. These have been investigated most extensively in the liver (see Fig. 2-7), where the appearance of altered clones is detectable by foci of phenotypically modified cells. These tend to remain stationary unless stimulated to further proliferation or change.[176,177] Analogous preneoplastic changes have been observed in the development of adenomas of the mouse pituitary gland.[102]

PROGRESSION

The progression of a neoplasm from a relatively benign pattern of growth to one of increasing malignancy has been observed repeatedly in experimental animals and human patients.[8] It is characteristically accompanied by step-wise changes in the morphology, mitotic activity, biochemical properties, and karyotype of the neoplastic cells. The process is interpreted to reflect the successive emergence of progressively more autonomous clones, each in turn outgrowing its predecessors.[8,9,40]

TUMOR–HOST RELATION

Hormones

Neoplastic cells retain their responsiveness to normal growth-regulating factors to varying degrees. This is particularly evident in tumors of endocrine target tissues, where cell growth may be dependent on appropriate endocrine stimulation, enabling hormonal control of such neoplasms.[102] By the same token, derangement of endocrine balance, leading to excessive and sustained horomonal stimulation, may elicit the development of neoplasia in overstimulated target cells.[102] The evolution of malignancy in such cells has been observed to occur step-wise in the mouse, passing through successive stages, characterized first by hyperplasia, followed by hormone-dependent growth, and culminating in complete autonomy.[178]

Immune Response

Neoplasms induced in experimental animals by chemicals and viruses generally possess neoantigens that distinguish them from their normal tissue counterparts.[30,179,180] While such antigens have not been consistently detected in spontaneously-occurring animal neoplasms, evidence for them has

EVOLUTION OF CANCERS

Sequence of changes	Basic change	Responsiveness to hormones
↓ **NORMAL** cell hyperplasia **DEPENDENT T**	In host	Correction can be complete
↓ **AUTONOMOUS T** highly responsive ↓ less and less responsive ↘ reversely responsive	In cell	Growth can be retarded but not arrested
↓ full autonomy		None

FIG. 2-8. Scheme of the sequence of changes induced by derangement of physiologic forces regulating cell growth, which can result in evolution of cancer cells from normal cells. (Furth J: Hormones as etiological agents in neoplasia. In Becker FF (ed): Cancer: A Comprehensive Treatise, Vol. 1, pp. 75–120. New York and London, Plenum Press, 1975)

been observed in human cancers of various types. They have often been accompanied by blocking factors that protect them against the cytotoxic action of sensitized immunocytes.[30]

The evidence that neoplasms may develop in spite of their antigenicity to the host led to the "immunologic surveillance" hypothesis, which postulates that antigenic differences between normal and neoplastic cells constitute an important homeostatic mechanism through which the body normally rids itself of transformed cells.[181] A corollary of this hypothesis is that immunosuppression should enhance susceptibility to carcinogenesis.

While immunosuppression has indeed been observed to increase the susceptibility of laboratory animals to chemical and viral carcinogenesis, it has not increased their susceptibility to spontaneous carcinogenesis.[30] In humans with immunodeficiency states, susceptibility to some, but not all, forms of cancer is increased, depending on whether the immunodeficiency is complicated by chromosomal instability and other abnormalities.[30] Also, in patients whose immunity has been suppressed therapeutically for organ transplantation, certain types of cancer, especially cutaneous and lymphoproliferative neoplasms, are generally increased in frequency.[104]

Nonspecific stimulation of immunity, by BCG or other agents, has been observed to inhibit the experimental induction of neoplasia under some conditions. The possibility that suppressor cells may also be stimulated by bacillus Calmette-Guérin may partially account for the fact that inhibition of tumorigenesis has been obtained only inconsistently with this approach.[182]

Diet

Dietary and nutritional factors have been observed to influence the occurrence of cancer in experimental animals through a number of mechanisms (see Table 2-9).[183] The extent to which these factors may affect the incidence of cancer in humans largely remains to be determined, but the overall influence of diet is considered to be appreciable.[184] Among the most dramatic effects in experimental animals is the influence of caloric restriction, which postpones the onset and reduces the overall incidence of spontaneous and induced neoplasms, at the same time extending the life span.[185,186] Much less striking are the effects of variations in individual constituents of the normal diet, although carcinogenesis can be enhanced under certain conditions by increasing fat intake.[177] The levels of protein, fiber, vitamins, and trace minerals have also been observed to influence susceptibility through various mechanisms.[187] Of the carcinogens identified in foodstuffs thus far, the mycotoxins are the most potent, microgram quantities causing hepatocellular carcinomas in animals.[188] The recent finding that mutagenic protein pyrolysis products are formed in food when it is cooked at high temperature, as in broiling or frying, points to the possibility that such materials may also constitute a carcinogenic risk, but their potency in animals and their practical significance for humans remain to be determined.[189]

TABLE 2-9. Ways in Which Diet may Affect the Occurrence of Cancer

BY PROVIDING A SOURCE OF CARCINOGENS OR PRECARCINOGENS
Natural components of plants
Products of chemical, bacterial, or fungal action during processing or storage
Products of cooking
Food additives
Contaminants (products of fuel combustion, agricultural chemicals, pesticide residues)
BY AFFECTING FORMATION OF CARCINOGENS
Provision of nitrosamine precursors
Inhibition of nitrosamine formation, as in stomach (vitamin C)
Alteration of excretion of bile salts and cholesterol (fat)
Alteration of bacterial flora of gut (fiber? meat?)
Alteration of metabolism of carcinogens (enzyme induction by meat, fat, indoles in vegetables, antioxidants)
Alteration of enzyme formation (trace elements)
Effect on hormone levels (fats, total calories)
BY MODIFYING EFFECTS OF CARCINOGENS
Through transport (alcohol, fiber)
Through effect on concentration in bowel (fiber)
Inhibition of promotion (vitamin A, B-carotene)

(Doll R: The epidemiology of cancer. In Fortner JG, Rhoads JE (eds): Accomplishments in Cancer Research, 1979 Prize Year, General Motors Cancer Research Foundation, pp 103–121. Philadelphia, JB Lippincott, 1980)

STRATEGIES FOR CANCER PREVENTION

DETECTION OF CARCINOGENS

Epidemiological Approaches

Evidence suggesting that the bulk of cancer arises at least in part through nonhereditary influences calls for a concerted effort to identify the risk factors in question and to develop means to eliminate or counteract them.[190–192] For this purpose, study of variations in cancer rates among different human populations provides one of the most effective approaches.[192,193] This is especially true when it comes to the quantitative assessment of a given risk factor, since, as mentioned previously, the magnitude of carcinogenic effects in humans cannot be confidently predicted by extrapolation from effects in animals.

Bioassay Methods

Because there is a high correlation between the carcinogenicity of a given chemical in one species and its carcinogenicity in others, chemicals are tested in animals as a means of determining their potential carcinogenicity for humans.[127] Chemicals found to cause neoplasia in animals, through appropriately conducted tests, are generally classified as presumptive carcinogens for humans and treated accordingly.[127] By heeding the warnings of animal test results, precautionary measures can be instituted to minimize human exposure long before there may be direct evidence of carcinogenic effects in humans themselves, owing to the long induction period for cancer formation in man. Thus, bioassay of suspect chemicals for carcinogenic activity constitutes an essential part of the cancer prevention strategy, especially as a means for preventing exposure of the human population to newly synthesized compounds for which no previous experience is available.

Because of the relatively high cost and slowness of animal bioassays, efforts to develop more rapid and economical short-term tests deserve high priority. Although the reliability of these tests is yet to be determined, they are widely used in prescreening compounds for further study, and their inclusion in a multitier assay system (see Fig. 2-9) or battery of *in vitro* tests is an approach that has been widely recommended.[134]

Multagenicity Test(s)
↓
Cell Transformation Test(s)
↓
Carcinogenicity Test(s) in Animals

FIG. 2-9. Framework of test procedures in a multitier carcinogenicity assay system.

DETECTION OF HIGH RISK INDIVIDUALS

Precancerous Lesions

A variety of lesions are known to predispose to cancer development (see Table 2-7).[193] For example, in women with dysplasia of the uterine cervix the risk of developing carcinoma of the cervix *in situ* is estimated to be 1600 times higher than it is in normal women, and the systematic excision of carcinoma *in situ* has been observed to prevent invasive carcinoma of the cervix.[174,175]

Because detection and treatment of precancerous lesions may reduce the risk of cancer in affected persons, efforts to identify and treat such lesions should be part of any strategy for cancer prevention.

Heightened Susceptibility States

A number of inherited conditions are associated with increased susceptibility to cancer, as indicated above. One of the most striking conditions is xeroderma pigmentosum, an autosomal recessive disease characterized by defective repair of DNA, markedly exaggerated sensitivity to sunlight, and greatly increased risk to skin cancer early in life.[23] Another category of inherited diseases associated wih high susceptibility to cancer comprises the so-called dominant tumor syndromes.[14] These diseases are characterized by familial occurrence of specific types of tumors that often develop early in life and may be multiple. One theory postulates that these diseases arise through a multistage mutation process in which there are a minimum of two steps. The first step involves an inherited mutation that is present in every cell of the body. The second step involves a mutation that is acquired during or after embryonal development.[34] Persons who have inherited the first step of the process are assumed to be at high risk to cancer induction by mutagenic agents capable of effecting the second step.[14,34]

Also affecting susceptibility to cancer is enzyme system activity responsible for converting carcinogen precursors into their ultimate reactive forms. The inducibility and activity of such enzymes appear to be under genetic control with the result that susceptibility to carcinogens can be expected to vary.[121–123]

To the extent that persons with inherited susceptibility states can be identified, measures to minimize their exposure to carcinogens and to monitor them for preneoplastic lesions are called for.

SURVEILLANCE

To identify persons at high risk, to monitor them for preneoplastic or neoplastic changes, and to treat them with indicated countermeasures requires the systematic surveillance of population groups. Presently, however, above and beyond sound principles of clinical diagnosis, the methodology for screening asymptomatic persons to detect early stages of neoplasia is limited. Among the accepted techniques for this purpose, two are noteworthy. These are the Papanicoloau smear technique, used in examining the uterine cervix, and x-ray mammography, used in screening for early detection of breast cancer. These procedures are discussed in detail later in the book.

EDUCATION

Because of the widespread occurrence of carcinogenic risk factors and the importance of detecting cancer at early stages of development, education of the public, as well as of the health professions, is essential to cancer prevention. It is tragic that it has taken our society so long to react to the evidence incriminating cigarette smoking as a major cause of cancer. This situation reflects not only a persistent lack of awareness, but also conflicts between value systems, involving various philosophical, political, psychological, and socio-economic ramifications.

Similar problems are likely to recur in the future as other risk factors are identified, since it is probable that the cancer burden will be found to result predominantly from long-term exposure to many weak carcinogens, acting together, rather than from exposure to a few potent carcinogens one at a time. Moreover, because the evidence incriminating new risk factors will almost invariably be inconclusive when first introduced, especially if based solely on animal studies, adequate public understanding of the problem will be crucial to an effective societal response.

REGULATION

Risk avoidance is best assured through the development of sound safety standards and codes of practice. Society customarily relies on such standards to protect itself against the hazardous actions of persons or subgroups. Standards for the protection of workers, consumers, and other members of the population against carcinogens are now an integral part of many federal, state and municipal laws. It must be acknowledged, however, that the development of such standards has frequently lagged behind the demonstration of carcinogenicity, and also that compliance with standards has not always been faithful, or adequately enforced.[194]

Clearly, the problem has been complicated in the past by uncertainty and controversy concerning the criteria for determining carcinogenicity of a given agent and about assessment of the magnitude of any risk it might pose for human populations. These problems remain to be resolved, but workable interim approaches are prospected.[127,128]

REFERENCES

1. Willis RA: The Spread of Tumors in the Human Body. London, Butterworth & Co, 1952
2. Pitot HC: Fundamentals of Oncology. New York, Marcel Dekker, 1978
3. Dawe C: Comparative neoplasia. In Holland JF, Frei E (eds): Cancer Medicine, Lea & Febiger, Philadelphia, 1973 pp. 193–240.
4. Bett WR: Historical aspects of cancer. In Raven WR (ed): Cancer, Vol 1, p 1. London, Butterworth & Co, 1957
5. Ewing J: Neoplastic Diseases, 3rd ed. Philadelphia, WB Saunders, 1928
6. Nicholson GW: Studies on Tumor Formation. London, Butterworth & Co, 1950
7. Huxley J: Biological Aspects of Cancer. London, George Allen & Unwin, 1958
8. Foulds L: Neoplastic Development. London and New York, Academic Press, Vol I, 1959, Vol II, 1975
9. Farber EE: Carcinogenesis—cellular evolution as a unifying thread: Presidential Address. Cancer Res 33:2537–2550, 1973
10. Weinstein IB, Yamaguchi N, Gebert R: Use of epithelial cell cultures for studies on the mechanism of transformation by chemical carcinogens. In Vitro 11:130–141, 1975
11. Boveri T: ZurFrage der Enstehung maligner Tumoren. Jena, Gustav Fischer, 1914
12. Nowell PC: Cytogenetics. In Becker FF (ed): Cancer: A Comprehensive Treatise, Vol 1, pp 3–31, New York and London, Plenum Press, 1975
13. Harnden DG: Cytogenetics of human neoplasia. In Mulvihill JJ, Miller RW, Fraumeni JF Jr (eds): Progress in Cancer Research and Therapy, Vol 3, Genetics of Human Cancer, pp 87–104. New York, Raven Press, 1977
14. Knudson AG: Mutation and cancer. Adv Cancer Res 17:317–352, 1973
15. Knudson AG: Genetic influences in human tumors. In Becker FF (ed): Cancer: A Comprehensive Treatise, Vol 1, pp 59–74. New York, Plenum Press, 1975
16. Mulvihill JJ: Congenital and genetic diseases. In Fraumeni JF Jr (ed): Persons at High Risk of Cancer, pp 3–35. New York, Academic Press, 1975
17. Hecht F, McCaw BK: Chromosome instability syndrome. In Mulvihill JJ, Miller RW, Fraumeni JF Jr (eds): Progress in Cancer Research and Therapy, Vol 3, Genetics of Human Cancer, pp 105–123. New York, Raven Press, 1977
18. Miller RW, Todaro GJ: Viral transformation of cells from persons at high risk of cancer. Lancet 1:81–82, 1969
19. Fialkow PJ: Clonal origin and stem cell evolution of human tumors. In Mulvihill JJ, Miller RW, Fraumeni JF Jr (eds): Progress in Cancer Research and Therapy, Vol 3, Genetics of Human Cancer, pp 439–452. New York, Raven Press, 1977
20. Nance WE: Relevance of twin studies in cancer research. In Mulvihill JJ, Miller RW, Fraumeni JF Jr (eds): Progress in Cancer Research and Therapy, Vol 3, Genetics of Human Cancer, pp 27–38. New York, Raven Press, 1977
21. Braun AC: Plant tumors. In Becker FF (ed): Cancer: A Comprehensive Treatise, Vol 4, pp 411–427. New York and London, Plenum Press, 1975
22. Mulvihill JJ: Genetic repertory of human cancer. In Mulvihill JJ, Miller RW, Fraumeni JF Jr (eds): Progress in Cancer Research and Therapy, Vol 3, Genetics of Human Cancer, pp 137–143. New York, Raven Press, 1977
23. Cleaver JE: Human diseases with *in vitro* manifestations of altered repair and replication of DNA. In Mulvihill JJ, Miller RW, Fraumeni JF Jr (eds): Progress in Cancer Research and Therapy, Vol 3, Genetics of Human Cancer, pp 355–363. New York, Raven Press, 1977
24. Patterson MC: Environmental carcinogenesis and imperfect repair of damaged DNA in Homo sapiens: causal relation revealed by rare hereditary disorders. In Griffin AC, Shaw CR (eds): Carcinogens: Identification and Mechanisms of Action, pp 251–276. New York, Raven Press, 1979
25. Cook K, Friedberg EC, Cleaver JE: Excision of thymine dimers from specifically incised DNA by extracts of xeroderma pigmentosum cells. Nature 256:235–236, 1975
26. Lehman AR, Kirk–Bell S, Arlett CF et al: Xeroderma pigmentosum cells with normal levels of excision repair have a defect in DNA synthesis after UV irradiation. Proc Natl Acad Sci USA 72:219–223, 1975
27. Hecht F, McCaw BK: Chromosomally marked lymphocyte clones in ataxiatelangiectasia. Lancet 1:563–564, 1975
28. Poon PK, O'Brien RL, Parker JW: Defective DNA repair in Fanconi's anemia. Nature 250:223–225, 1974
29. Kersey JH, Spector BD: Immune deficiency diseases. In Fraumeni JF Jr (ed): Persons at High Risk of Cancer, pp 55–66. New York, Academic Press, 1975
30. Melief CJM, Schwartz RS: Immunocompetence and malignancy. In Becker FF (ed): Cancer: A Comprehensive Treatise, Vol 1, pp 121–160. New York and London, Plenum Press, 1975
31. Holliday R, Porterfield JS, Gibbs DD: Premature aging and occurrence of altered enzyme in Werner's syndrome fibroblasts. Nature 248:762–763, 1974
32. Epstein J, Williams JR, Little JB: Deficient DNA repair in human progerioid cells. Proc Natl Acad Sci USA 70:977–981, 1973
33. Knudson AG, Strong LC: Mutation and cancer: a model for Wilm's tumor of the kidney. JNCI 48:313–324, 1972
34. Knudson AG: Genetic and environmental interactions in the origin of human cancer. In Mulvihill JJ, Miller RW, Fraumeni JF Jr (eds): Progress in Cancer Research and Therapy, Vol 3, Genetics of Human Cancer, pp 391–397. New York, Raven Press, 1977
35. Anderson DE: Familial susceptibility. In Fraumeni JF Jr (ed): Persons at High Risk of Cancer, pp 39–53. New York, Academic Press, 1975
36. Miller RW: Persons with exceptionally high risk of leukemia. Cancer Res 27:2420–2423, 1967
37. Heston WE: Genetics: animal tumors. In Becker FF (ed): Cancer: A Comprehensive Treatise, Vol 1, pp 33–57. New York and London, Plenum Press, 1975

38. Lilly F, Pinars T: Genetic control of murine viral leukemogenesis. Adv Cancer Res 17:231–277, 1973
39. Rowe WP: Genetic factors in the natural history of murine leukemia virus infection: G.H.A. Clowes Memorial Lecture. Cancer Res 33:3061–3068, 1973
40. Nowell PC: The clonal evolution of tumor cell populations. Science 194:23–28, 1976
41. Sandberg AA: The Chromosomes in Human Cancer and Leukemia. New York, Elsevier Publishing Co, 1980
42. Makino S: Some epidemiological aspects of venereal tumors of dogs as revealed by chromosome and DNA studies. Ann NY Acad Sci 108:1106–1122, 1963
43. Weber WT, Nowell PC, Hare WCD: Chromosome studies of a transplanted and a primary canine venereal sarcoma. JNCI 35:537–547, 1965
44. Benedict WF, Porter IH, Brown CD et al: Cytogenetic diagnosis of malignancy in recurrent meningioma. Lancet 1:971–973, 1970
45. Mark J, Levan G, Mitelman F: Identification by fluorescence of the G chromosome lost in human meningiomas. Hereditas 71:163–171, 1972
46. Zankl H, Weiss AF, Zang KD: Cytological and cytogenetical studies on brain tumors: VI. No evidence for a translocation in 22-monosomic meningiomas. HumGenet 30, No. 4: 343–348, 1975
47. Rowley JD: Are nonrandom karyotypic changes related to etiologic agents? In Mulvihill JJ, Miller RW, Fraumeni JF Jr (eds): Progress in Cancer Research and Therapy, Vol 3, Genetics of Human Cancer, pp 125–134. New York, Raven Press, 1977
48. Wiener F, Spira J, Ohno S et al: Chromosome changes (trisomy 15) in murine T-cell leukemia induced by 7,12-dimethylbenz(a) anthracine (DMBA). Int J Cancer 22:447–453, 1978
49. Sachs SL: Regulation of membrane changes, differentiation, and malignancy in carcinogenesis. Harvey Lect 68:1–35, 1974
50. Heidelberger C: Chemical carcinogenesis. Annu Rev Biochem 44:79–121, 1975
51. Miller EC, Miller JA: The mutagenicity of chemical carcinogens: correlations, problems, and interpretations. In Hollaender A (ed): Chemical Mutagens: Principles and Methods for Detection, Vol 1, pp 83–119. New York, Plenum Press, 1971
52. Miller JA, Miller EC: Ultimate chemical carcinogens as reactive mutagenic electrophiles. In Hiatt HH, Watson JD, Winsten JA (eds): Origins of Human Cancer, pp 605–627. New York, Cold Spring Harbor Laboratory, 1977
53. Magee PN: The relationship between mutagenesis, carcinogenesis, and teratogenesis. In Scott D, Bridges BA, Sobels F (eds): Progress in Genetic Toxicology, Vol 2, pp 15–27. North Holland Biomedical Press, Amsterdam, Elsevier, 1977
54. Rinkus SJ, Legator MS: Chemical characterization of 465 known or suspected carcinogens and their correlation with mutagenic activity in the Salmonella typhimurium system. Cancer Res 39:3289–3318, 1979
55. Sugimura T, Sato S, Nagao M et al: Overlapping of carcinogens and mutagens. In Magee PN et al (eds): Fundamentals in Cancer Prevention, pp 191–215. University of Tokyo Press, Tokyo/University Park Press, Baltimore, 1976
56. Ames BN, Durston WE, Yamasaki E et al: Carcinogens are mutagens: a simple test system combining liver homogenates for activation and bacteria for detection. Proc Natl Acad Sci 70:2281–2285, 1973
57. Ames BN, McCann J, Yamasaki E: Methods for detecting carcinogens and mutagens with the Salmonella/mammalian-microsome mutagenicity test. Mutat Res 31:347–363, 1975
58. Meselson M, Russell K: Comparisons of carcinogenic and mutagenic potency. In Hiatt HH, Watson JD, Winsten JA (eds): Origins of Human Cancer, pp 1473–1481. New York, Cold Spring Harbor Laboratory, 1977
59. Miller JA: Carcinogenesis by chemical: an overview: G.H.A. Clowes Memorial Lecture. Cancer Res 30:559–576, 1970
60. Miller JA: Concluding remarks on chemicals and chemical carcinogenesis. In Griffin AC, Shaw CR (eds): Carcinogens: Identification and Mechanisms of Action, pp 455–469. New York, Raven Press, 1979
61. Stich HF, Kieser D, Laishes BA et al: The use of DNA repair in the identification of carcinogens, precarcinogens, and target tissue. In Scholefield PG (ed): Proceedings of the Tenth Canadian Cancer Conference, Vol 10, pp 83–110. Toronto, University of Toronto Press, 1973
62. Heidelberger C: Chemical carcinogenesis in culture. Adv Cancer Res 18:317–366, 1973
63. Zajdela F, Latarjet R: Effect inhibiteur de la cafeine sur l'induction de cancers cutanes par les rayons ultraviolets chez la souris. C R Acad Sci (Paris) 277, Ser D:1073–1076, 1973
64. Terzaghi M, Little JB: Repair of potentially lethal radiation damage in mammalian cells is associated with enhancement of malignant transformation. Nature 253:548–549, 1975
65. vanBekkum DW: Mechanisms of radiation carcinogenesis. In Nygaard OF, Adler HI, Sinclair WK (eds): Radiation Research: Biomedical, Chemical, and Physical Perspectives, pp 886–894. New York, Academic Press, 1975
66. Pitot HC, Heidelberger C: Metabolic regulatory circuits and carcinogenesis. Cancer Res 23:1694–1700, 1963
67. Mintz B: Genetic mosaicism and *in vivo* analyses of neoplasia and differentiation. In Saunders GF (ed): Cell Differentiation and Neoplasia, pp 27–53. New York, Raven Press, 1978
68. Mintz B, Illmensee K: Normal genetically mosaic mice produced from malignant teratocarcinoma cells. Proc Natl Acad Sci USA 72:3585–3589, 1975
69. McKinnell RG, Deggins BA, Labat DD: Transplantation of pluripotent nuclei from triploid frog tumors. Science 165:394–396, 1969
70. Stephenson JR, Reynolds RK, Aaronson SA: Characterization of morphologic revertants of murine and avian sarcoma virus-transformed cells. J Virol 11:218–222, 1973
71. Khoury G, Salzman NP: Replication and transformation by papovaviruses. In Becker FF (ed): Cancer: A Comprehensive Treatise, Vol 2, pp 343–427. New York and London, Plenum Press, 1975
72. Braun AC: Differentiation and dedifferentiation. In Becker FF (ed): Cancer: A Comprehensive Treatise, Vol 3, pp 3–20. New York and London, Plenum Press, 1975
73. Everson TC, Cole WH: Spontaneous Regression of Cancer. Philadelphia, WB Saunders, 1966
74. Turkel SB, Itabashi HH: The natural history of neuroblastic cells in the fetal adrenal gland. Am J Pathol 76:225–244, 1974
75. Schwartz AD, Dadash-Zadek M, Lee H et al: Spontaneous regression of disseminated neuroblastoma. J Pediatr 85: 760–763, 1974
76. Miller RW: Relation between cancer and congenital defects: an epidemiological evaluation. JNCI 40:1079–1085, 1968
77. Stevens LC: The development of transplantable teratocarcinomas from intratesticular grafts of pre- and post-implantation mouse embryos. Dev Biol 21:364–382, 1970
78. Pierce GB, Cox WF: Neoplasms as caricatures of tissue renewal. In Saunders GF (ed): Cell Differentiation and Neoplasia, pp 57–66. New York, Raven Press, 1978
79. Oppenheimer BS, Oppenheimer ET, Stout AP et al: Malignant tumors resulting from embedding plastics in rodents. Science 118:305–306, 1953
80. Brand KG: Foreign body induced sarcomas. In Becker FF (ed): Cancer: A Comprehensive Treatise, Vol 7, pp 485–511. New York, Plenum Press, 1975
81. Herbst AI, Ulfelder U, Poskanzer DC: Adenocarcinoma of the vagina. N Engl J Med 284:878–881, 1971
82. Binns A, Meins F Jr: Habituation of tobacco pith cells for factors promoting cell division is heritable and potentially reversible. Proc Natl Acad Sci USA 70:2620–2662, 1973
83. Rauscher FJ, O'Connor TE: Virology. In Holland JF, Frei E III (eds): Cancer Medicine, pp 15–44. Philadelphia, Lea & Febiger, 1973
84. Baltimore D: Tumor viruses. 1974 Cold Spring Harbor Symposium on Quantitative Biology 39:1187–1200, 1975
85. de The G: Viruses as causes of some human tumors? Results

and perspectives of the epidemiologic approach. In Hiatt HH, Watson JD, Winsten JA (eds): Origins of Human Cancer, pp 1113–1131. New York, Cold Spring Harbor Laboratory, 1977

86. Szmuness W: Hepatocellular carcinoma and the hepatitis B virus: evidence for a causal association. Prog Med Virol 24:40–69, 1978
87. Tooze J (ed): DNA Tumor Viruses. New York, Cold Spring Harbor Laboratory, 1980
88. Tooze J (ed): The Molecular Biology of Tumor Viruses. New York, Cold Spring Harbor Laboratory, 1973
89. Temin HM: On the origin of RNA tumor viruses. Harvey Lect 69:173–196, 1975
90. Huebner RJ, Todaro GJ: Oncogenes of RNA tumor viruses as determinants of cancer. Proc Natl Acad Sci USA 64:1087–1094, 1969
91. Temin HM, Baltimore D: RNA-directed DNA synthesis and RNA tumor viruses. Adv Virus Res 17:129–186, 1972
92. Huebner RJ, Kelloff GJ, Sarma PS et al: Group-specific antigen expression during embryogenesis of the genome of the C-type RNA tumor virus: implications for ontogenesis and oncogenesis. Proc Natl Acad Sci USA 67:366–373, 1970
93. Todaro GJ: RNA tumor virus genes (virogenes) and the transforming genes (oncogenes): genetic transmission, infectious spread, and modes of expression. In Hiatt HH, Watson JD, Winsten JA (eds): Origins of Human Cancer, pp 1169–1196. New York, Cold Spring Harbor Laboratory, 1977
94. Varmus HE, Guntaka RV, Deng CT et al: Synthesis, structure, and function of avian sarcoma virus-specific DNA in permissive and non-permissive cells. Cold Spring Harbor Symposium on Quantitative Biology 39:987–994, 1975
95. Klein F: Cancer, viruses, and environmental factors. In Kurstak E, Maramorosch K (eds): Third International Conference on Comparative Virology, pp 1–12. New York, Academic Press, 1978
96. Vogt PK: The genetics of RNA tumor viruses. In Fraenkel-Conrat H, Wagner R (eds): Comprehensive Virology, pp 341–455. New York, Plenum Press, 1977
97. Brugge JS, Erikson RL: Identification of a transformation-specific antigen induced by an avian sarcoma virus. Nature 269:346–347, 1977
98. Levinson AD, Oppermann H, Levintow L et al: Evidence that the transforming gene of avian sarcoma virus encodes a protein kinase associated with a phospho-protein. Cell 15:561–572, 1978
99. Van Duuren BL: Tumor-promoting agents in two-stage carcinogenesis. Prog Exp Tumor Res 11:31–68, 1969
100. Berenblum I: Sequential aspects of chemical carcinogenesis: skin. In Becker FF (ed): Cancer: A Comprehensive Treatise, Vol 1, pp 323–344. New York and London, Plenum Press, 1975
101. Clifton KH, Sridharan BN: Endocrine factors and tumor growth. In Becker FF (ed): Cancer: A Comprehensive Treatise, Vol 3, pp 249–287. New York and London, Plenum Press, 1975
102. Furth J: Hormones as etiological agents in neoplasia. In Becker FF (ed): Cancer: A Comprehensive Treatise, Vol 1, pp 75–120. New York and London, Plenum Press, 1975
103. Spector BD: Immunodeficiency—Cancer Registry: 1975 update. In Mulvihill, JJ, Miller RW, Fraumeni JF Jr (eds): Progress in Cancer Research and Therapy, Vol 3, Genetics of Human Cancer, pp 339–342. New York, Raven Press, 1977
104. Penn I: Tumors arising in organ transplant recipients. Adv Cancer Res 28:31–62, 1978
105. Prehn RT: The immune reaction as stimulator of tumor growth. Science 176:170–171, 1972
106. Prehn RT: Tumor progression and homeostasis. Adv Cancer Res 23:203–206, 1976
107. Fisher B, Fisher ER: Experimental evidence in support of the dormant tumor cell. Science 130:918–919, 1959
108. Folkman J: Tumor angiogenesis. In Becker FF (ed): Cancer: A Comprehensive Treatise, pp 355–388. New York, Plenum Press, 1975
109. Houck JC, Attallah AM: Chalones (specific and endogenous mitotic inhibitors) and cancer. In Becker FF (ed): Cancer: A Comprehensive Treatise, Vol 3, pp 287–326. New York, Plenum Press, 1975
110. LoBue J, Potmesil M: Stimulation. In Becker FF (ed): Cancer: A Comprehensive Treatise, Vol 3, pp 217–224. New York, Plenum Press, 1975
111. Weisburger JH: Chemical carcinogenesis. In Holland JS, Frei E (eds): Cancer Medicine, pp. 45–90. Philadelphia, Lea & Febiger, 1973
112. Weinstein IB: Current concepts of mechanisms of chemical carcinogenesis. Bull NY Acad Med 54:366–383, 1978
113. Tomatis L, Agtha C, Bartsch H et al: Evaluation of the carcinogenicity of chemicals: a review of the monograph program of the International Agency for Research on Cancer. Cancer Res 38:877–885, 1978
114. Althouse R, Huff J, Tomatis L et al: An evaluation of chemicals and industrial processes associated with cancer in humans based on human and animal data: IARC monographs, volumes 1 to 20. Report of an IARC working group. Cancer Res 40:1–12, 1980
115. Berenblum I: Theoretical and practical aspects of the two-stage mechanism of carcinogenesis. In Griffin AC, Shaw CR (eds): Carcinogens: Identification and Mechanisms of Action, pp 25–36. New York, Raven Press, 1979
116. Boutwell RK: Biochemical mechanism of tumor promotion. In Slaga TJ, Sivak A, Boutwell RK (eds): Carcinogenesis, Vol 2, Mechanisms of Tumor Promotion and Cocarcinogenesis, pp 49–58. New York, Raven Press, 1978
117. Van Duuren BL, Witz F, Goldschmidt BM: Structure-activity relationship of tumor promoters and co-carcinogens and interaction of phorbol myristate acetate and related esters with plasma membranes. In Slaga TJ, Sivak A, Boutwell RK (eds): Mechanisms of Tumor Promotion and Cocarcinogenesis, Vol 2, pp 491–507. New York, Raven Press, 1978
118. Benner CE, Moroney J, Porter CW: Early membrane effects of phorbol esters in 3T3 cells. In Slaga TJ, Sivak A, Boutwell RK (eds): Mechanisms of Tumor Promotion and Cocarcinogenesis, pp 363–387. New York, Raven Press, 1978
119. Doll R: Cancer and aging: the epidemiological evidence. In Clark RL, Cumley RW, McKay JE et al (eds): Proceedings of the 10th International Cancer Congress, Vol 5, pp 1–28. Chicago, Year Book Medical Publishers, 1971
120. Kouri RE, Nebert DW: Genetic regulation of susceptibility to polycyclic-hydrocarbon-induced tumors in the mouse. In Hiatt HH, Watson JD, Winsten JA (eds): Origins of Human Cancer, pp 811–835. New York, Cold Spring Harbor Laboratory, 1977
121. Nebert DW, Atlas SA: The Ah locus: aromatic hydrocarbon responsiveness . . . of mice and men. Hum Genet (Suppl) 1:149–160, 1978
122. Kellerman G, Luyteon-Kellerman M, Jett JR et al: Aryl hydrocarbon hydroxylase in man and lung cancer. Hum Genet (Suppl) 1:161–168, 1978
123. Arnott MS, Yamauchi T, Johnson DA: Aryl hydrocarbon hydroxylase in normal and cancer populations. In Griffin AC, Shaw CR, (eds): Carcinogens: Identification and Mechanisms of Action, pp 145–156. New York, Raven Press, 1979
124. Saffiotti U: Identifying and defining chemical carcinogens. In Hiatt HH, Watson JD, Winsten JA (eds): Origins of Human Cancer, pp 1311–1326. New York, Cold Spring Harbor Laboratory, 1977
125. Saffiotti U: Experimental identification of chemical carcinogens, risk evaluation, and animal-to-human correlations. Environ Health Perspect 22:107–113, 1978
126. Shubik P: Identification of environmental carcinogens: animal test models. In Griffin AC, Shaw CR (eds): Carcinogens: Identification and Mechanisms of Action, pp 39–47. New York, Raven Press, 1979
127. Interagency Regulatory Liaison Group: Scientific bases for identification of potential carcinogens and estimation of risks. JNCI 63:241–268, 1979
128. Calkins DR, Dixon RL, Gerber CR et al: Identification, characterization, and control of potential human carcinogens: a framework for federal decision-making. JNCI 64:169–176, 1980

129. Page NP: Concepts of bioassay program in environmental carcinogenesis. In Mehlman M, Kraybill H (eds): Environmental Cancer. Adv Mod Toxicol 3:87–171, 1977
130. Sontag JM: Aspects in carcinogen bioassay. In Hiatt HH, Watson JD, Winsten JA (eds): Origins of Human Cancer, pp 1327–1338. New York, Cold Spring Harbor Laboratory, 1977
131. Montesano R, Bartsch H, Tomatis L (eds): Screening Tests in Chemical Carcinogenesis, No. 12. Lyon, France, International Agency for Research on Cancer, 1976
132. McCann J, Ames BN: The Salmonella/microsome mutagenicity test: predictive value for animal carcinogenecity. In Hiatt HH, Watson JD, Winsten JA (eds): Origins of Human Cancer, pp 1431–1450. New York, Cold Spring Harbor Laboratory, 1977
133. Heidleberger C, Mondal S: *In vitro* chemical carcinogenesis. In Griffin AC, Shaw CR, (eds): Carcinogens: Identification and Mechanisms of Action, pp 85–92. New York, Raven Press, 1979
134. Pienta RJ: A hamster embryo cell model system for identifying carcinogens. In Griffin AC, Shaw CR (eds): Carcinogens: Identification and Mechanisms of Action, pp 123–141. New York, Raven Press, 1979
135. Wattenburg LW: Inhibitors of chemical carcinogenesis. Adv Cancer Res 23:203–236, 1978
136. Wattenberg LW: Inhibitors of carcinogenesis. In Griffin AC, Shaw CR (eds): Carcinogens: Identification and Mechanisms of Action, pp 299–316. New York, Raven Press, 1979
137. Sporn MB, Newton DL, Smith JM et al: Retinoids and cancer prevention: the importance of the terminal group of the retinoid molecule in modifying activity and toxicity. In Griffin AC, Shaw CR, (eds): Carcinogens: Identification and Mechanisms of Action, pp 441–452. New York, Raven Press, 1979
138. Troll W, Meyn S, Rossman TG: Mechanisms of protease action in carcinogenesis. In Slaga TJ, Sivak A, Boutwell RK (eds): Carcinogenesis: A Comprehensive Survey, Vol 2, Mechanisms of Tumor Promotion and Cocarcinogenesis, pp 301–312. New York, Raven Press, 1978
139. Slaga TJ, Fischer SM, Viaje A et al: Inhibition of tumor promotion by antiinflammatory agents: an approach to the biological mechanism of promotion. In Slaga TJ, Sivak A, Boutwell RK (eds): Carcinogenesis: A Comprehensive Survey, Vol 2, Mechanisms of Tumor Promotion and Cocarcinogenesis, pp 173–195. New York, Raven Press, 1978
140. Upton AC: Physical carcinogenesis: radiation—history and sources. In Becker FF (ed): Cancer: A Comprehensive Treatise, Vol 1, pp 387–403. New York, Plenum Press, 1975
141. Upton AC: Radiation effects. In Hiatt HH, Watson JD, Winsten JA (eds): Origins of Human Cancer, pp 477–500. New York, Cold Spring Harbor Laboratory, 1977
142. United Nations Scientific Committee on the Effects of Atomic Radiation: Sources and Effects of Ionizing Radiation. Report to the General Assembly. New York, United Nations, 1977
143. Storer JB: Radiation carcinogenesis. In Becker FF (ed): Cancer: A Comprehensive Treatise, Vol 1, pp 453–483. New York, Plenum Press, 1975
144. Brown JM: The shape of the dose-response curve for radiation carcinogenesis: extrapolation to low doses. Radiat Res 71:34–50, 1977
145. Upton AC, Randolph ML, Conklin JW: Late effects of fast neutrons and gamma-rays in mice as influenced by the dose rate of irradiation: induction of neoplasia. Radiat Res 41:467–491, 1970
146. Upton AC: Radiobiological effects of low doses: implications for radiological protection. Radiat Res 71:51–74, 1977
147. Barendsen GW: RBE-LET relations for induction of reproductive death and chromosome aberrations in mammalian cells. In Booz J, Ebert HG (eds): Proceedings of the Sixth Symposium on Microdosimetry, Brussels. London, Harwood Academic Publishers, 1978
148. Kaplan HS: On the natural history of the murine leukemias: Presidential Address. Cancer Res 27:1325–1340, 1967
149. Marshall JH, Groer PG: A theory of the induction of bone cancer by alpha radiation. Radiat Res 71:149–192 1977
150. Albert RE, Burns FJ, Bennett P: Radiation induced hair follicle damage and tumor formation in mouse and rat skin. JNCI 49:1131–1137, 1972
151. Borek C: *In vitro* cell transformation by low doses of x-irradiation and neutrons. In Yuhas JM, Tennant RW, Regan JD (eds): Biology of Radiation Carcinogenesis, pp 309–326. New York, Raven Press, 1976
152. Miller R, Hall EJ: X-ray dose fractionation and oncogenic transformation in cultured mouse embryo cells. Nature 272: 58–60, 1978
153. Advisory Committee on the Biological Effects of Ionizing Radiation: Effects on populations of exposure to low levels of ionizing radiation. Washington, DC, National Academy of Sciences, 1972
154. Advisory Committee on the Biological Effects of Ionizing Radiation: The effects on populations of exposure to low levels of ionizing radiation. Washington, DC, National Academy of Sciences, 1980
155. Jablon S, Bailar JA: The contribution of ionizing radiation to cancer mortality in the United States. Prev Med 9:212–226, 1980
156. Thiersch K: Der Epithelialkrebs. Leipzig, Germany, Namentlieh der Ausseren Haut., 1875
157. Blum HF: Ultraviolet radiation and skin cancer in mice and men: accumulation of effect and uncertainty of prediction. Natl Cancer Inst Monogr 50:11–12, 1978
158. Urbach F: Ultraviolet radiation: interaction with biological molecules. In Becker FF (ed): Cancer: A Comprehensive Treatise, pp 441–451. New York, Plenum Press, 1975
159. Scott EL:, Straf ML: Ultraviolet radiation as a cause of cancer. In Hiatt HH, Watson JD, Winsten JA (eds): Origins of Human Cancer, pp 529–546. New York, Cold Spring Harbor Laboratory, 1977
160. Setlow RB, Ahmed FE, Grist E: Xeroderma pigmentosum: damage to DNA is involved in carcinogenesis. In Hiatt HH, Watson JD, Winsten JA (eds): Origins of Human Cancer, pp 889–902. New York, Cold Spring Harbor Laboratory, 1977
161. Epstein JH: Photocarcinogenesis: a review. Natl Cancer Inst Monogr 50:13–25, 1978
162. Kripke ML, Fisher MS: Immunologic aspects of tumor induction by ultraviolet radiation. Natl Cancer Inst Monogr 50:179–183, 1978
163. Fisher MS: A systemic effect of ultraviolet irradiation and its relationship to tumor immunity. Natl Cancer Inst Monogr 50:185–188, 1978
164. Blum HF: Carcinogenesis by Ultraviolet Light. Princeton, Princeton University Press, 1959
165. Selikoff IJ: Cancer risk of asbestos exposure. In Hiatt HH, Watson JD, Winsten JA (eds): Origins of Human Cancer, pp 1765–1784. New York, Cold Spring Harbor Laboratory, 1977
166. Doll R: An epidemiological perspective of the biology of cancer. Cancer Res 38:3573–3583, 1978
167. Surgeon General: Smoking and Health. (PHS) 79-50066, Washington, DC, Department of Health, Education and Welfare, 1979
168. Stanton MF, Wrench C: Mechanisms of mesothelioma induction with asbestos and fibrous glass. JNC 48:797–821, 1972
169. Mustacchi P: Parasites. In Holland JS, Frei E III (eds): Cancer Medicine, pp 106–112. Philadelphia, Lea & Febiger, 1973
170. Hashem M, Boutros K: The influence of bilharzial infection on the carcinogenesis of the mouse bladder: an experimental study. J Egypt Med Assoc 44:598, 1961
171. Hicks RM, James C, Webbe G et al: Schistosoma haematobium and bladder cancer. Trans R Soc Trop Med Hyg 71:288, 1977
172. Potter M, Cancro M: Plasmacytomagenesis and the differentiation of immunoglobulin-producing cells. In Saunders GF (ed): Cell Differentiation and Neoplasia, pp 145–161. New York, Raven Press, 1978
173. Shimkin MB: Preventive oncology. Prev Med 4:106–114, 1975
174. Stern E, Neely PM: Dysplasia of the uterine cervix: incidence of regression, recurrence and cancer. Cancer 17:508–512, 1964

175. Koss LG: Precancerous lesions. In Fraumeni JF Jr (ed): Persons at High Risk of Cancer, pp 85–101. New York, Academic Press, 1975
176. Farber EE, Cameron RG, Laishes B et al: Cellular and molecular markers of the carcinogenic process. In Griffin AC, Shaw CR (eds): Carcinogens: Identification and Mechanisms of Action, pp 319–335. New York, Raven Press, 1979
177. Pitot HC, Barsness L, Kitagawa T: Stages in the process of hepatocarcinogenesis in rat liver. In Slaga TJ, Sivak A, Boutwell RK (eds): Carcinogenesis: A Comprehensive Survey, Vol 2, Mechanisms of Tumor Promotion and Cocarcinogenesis, pp 433–442. New York, Raven Press, 1978
178. Furth J: Hormones as etiological agents in neoplasia. In Becker FF (ed): Cancer: A Comprehensive Treatise, Vol 1, pp 75–120. New York and London, Plenum Press, 1975
179. Klein G: The Epstein-Barr virus and neoplasia. N Engl J Med 293:1353–1357, 1975
180. Baldwin RW, Embleton MJ, Pimm MV: Neoantigens in chemical carcinogenesis. In Griffin AC, Shaw CR (eds): Carcinogens: Identification and Mechanisms of Action, pp 365–379. New York, Raven Press 1979
181. Thomas L: Discussion. In Lawrence HS (ed): Cellular and Humoral Aspects of the Hypersensitive States, pp 529–532. New York, Hoeber-Harper, 1959
182. Naor D: Suppressor cells: permitters and promoters of malignancy? Adv Cancer Res 29:45–126, 1979
183. Doll R: The epidemiology of cancer. In Fortner JG, Rhoads JE (eds): Accomplishments in Cancer Research, 1979 Prize Year, General Motors Cancer Research Foundation, pp 103–121. Philadelphia, JB Lippincott, 1980
184. Berg JW: Diet. In Fraumeni JF Jr (ed): Persons at High Risk of Cancer, pp 201–224. New York, Academic Press, 1975
185. Tannenbaum A, Silverstone H: Nutrition in relation to cancer. Adv Cancer Res 1:452–501, 1953
186. Sacher GA: Life table modification and life prolongation. In Finch CE, Hayflick L (eds): Handbook of the Biology of Aging, pp 582–638. New York, Reinhold, 1977
187. Clayson DB: Nutrition and experimental carcinogenesis: a review. Cancer Res 35:3292–3300, 1975
188. Goldblatt LA (ed): Aflatoxin: Scientific Background, Control, and Implication. New York, Acadmic Press, 1969
189. Sugimura T, Nagao M, Kawachi T et al: Mutagen-carcinogens in food, with special reference to highly mutagenic pyrolytic products in broiled foods. In Hiatt HH, Watson JD, Winsten JA (eds): Origins of Human Cancer, pp 1561–1577. New York, Cold Spring Harbor Laboratory, 1977
190. Doll R: Strategy for the detection of cancer hazards to man. Nature 265:589–596, 1977
191. Upton AC: Progress in the prevention of cancer. Prev Med 7:476–485, 1978
192. Higginson J, Muir CS: Environmental carcinogenesis: misconceptions and limitations to cancer control. JNCI 63:1291–1298, 1979
193. Fraumeni JF Jr: Epidemiologic studies in cancer. In Griffin AC, Shaw CR (eds): Carcinogens: Identification and Mechanisms of Action, pp 53–63. New York, Raven Press, 1979
194. Wolfe SM: Standards for carcinogens: science affronted by politics. In Hiatt HH, Watson JD, Winsten JA (eds): Origins of Human Cancer, pp 1735–1747. New York, Cold Spring Harbor Laboratory, 1977

CHAPTER 3

Arthur B. Pardee

Principles of Cancer Biology: Cell Biology and Biochemistry of Cancer

IDEAS BASIC TO THE STUDY OF NEOPLASIA

SPONTANEOUS TUMORS

Spontaneous human tumors are the ultimate objects of applied or basic cancer research. Fundamental studies of malignancy at all levels thus rest on studies of spontaneous cancers, and the ultimate value of any result or theory is its influence or utility in preventing or eradicating neoplasms. Cancer *in vivo* is thus the subject of almost all the rest of this treatise, and of other comprehensive works. But investigations *in vivo*, in spite of enormous efforts, have not provided a clear insight into how cancer comes about, what it is basically, or how to cure it. This is largely because the problem is extremely difficult. But also, incisive experiments with rigorous controls and varied protocols can hardly be performed on patients with differing, poorly defined, and irreproducible diseases. Some of these problems persist, even when transplanted tumors are studied in whole animals.

The purpose of this section is to provide an overview of current ideas and research on the fundamental nature of cancer. What advantages are there to pursuing these problems from the animal into cellular and subcellular levels? Simplifications and controllability are obtained. However, experiments *in vitro* have their costs. They must not abstract so far from reality that relevance to the ultimate goals of being better able to prevent the disease or improve treatment are lost, remembering that relevance of a result may not initially be evident.

A principal justification for studying cancer abstracted from the entire organism is that a neoplasm is conceived of as arising from a single, altered cell (see Chapter 2). That the essential elements of uncontrolled growth *in vivo* lie within a cell is supported by at least two sorts of evidence. First, only one cell from a preexisting tumor injected into an animal host can produce a tumor.[1] Second, many tumors have been shown to be clonal;[2] every cell of a spontaneous tumor can carry the same biochemical marker, one that is present in some cells of the host but not in others. This mosaicism is determined by the activity in each cell of one but not the other of two different X chromosomes in females (see Chapter 2). Also, chromosome patterns in a tumor are clonal.

The conclusion that isolated cells are suitable objects for cancer research does not require that the entire process occur in one single cell. Indeed, as the cells of a cancer grow and divide there are generally progressive stages, from pre-neoplasia to malignancy.[3] To study cancer we must investigate cells in these different stages; and also study normal cells since disease can be illuminated by its contrast to the normal. Spontaneous or induced mutants have aided studies of other diseases and of metabolic processes. And effects of the *in vivo* environment on the properties of cells cannot be underestimated and must eventually be explored.

As a prologue, an investigator needs to ascertain major properties that are to be the rational basis of investigation *in vitro*, from the vast literature on *in vivo* cancer. This subsection will be devoted to pointing out briefly some of these properties.

Definitions are designed to summarize the most relevant features of cancer. They all emphasize the property of neoplasia. From his many observations on cancer in humans Ewing says, "A neoplasm is a relatively autonomous growth of tissue".[4] Ponten proposes, "For descriptive purposes the functional abnormalities of neoplastic cells may be divided into those which concern the control of position, proliferation, or differentiation".[5] The definition of Willis, cited by Upton (see Chapter 2), also stresses excessive, uncoordinated growth autonomous from normal regulatory stimuli. These views of cancer focus on tissues, composed of cells that have become independent to some degree of the normal growth controlling forces of the host. A normal cell's characteristics, including growth patterns, are determined genetically and by surroundings, previous and present. Neoplastic cells have changed so as to become "asocial;" their environment, including neighboring cells, affects them less stringently. Thus the basic nature of neoplasia is a major question, whether partial or complete loss of normal, externally imposed growth controls.

A second major property of cancer cells *in vivo* is *anaplasia*, which is the loss to various degrees of the normal differentiated properties of cells. Anaplastic changes include the tendency of cells to metastasize—lose positional control (see Chapter 5); the altered morphologies in tumor tissues that are basic to identification by pathologists; changes from the constant chromosome structures characteristic of normal cells (Chapter 2); and altered biochemical properties. The last usually are manifest as loss of cell specific differentiated properties and reversion to more embryonic patterns. But tumor cells can also gain new properties, such as altered enzyme patterns in pheochromocytes that overproduce catecholamines, or oat cell carcinomas that produce a variety of hormones. Understanding anaplasia, therefore, is closely dependent on and connected to understanding normal differentiation and cellular biochemistry.

Cancers differ greatly one from another in numerous properties. Many kinds of observations of spontaneous neoplasms lead to this conclusion. Thus, cancers arise from initially dissimilar differentiated tissues and cells; and widely different agents are causative—chemicals, mutagens, and both RNA- and DNA-containing viruses (see Chapter 2). Preexisting mutations also can contribute; *e.g.*, as in familial polyposis of the colon.[6] Successive stages provide further diversity. Tumor progession from preneoplastic lesions to metastatic disease,[3] the multi-step nature of cancer that is deduced from genetic evidence[7,8] and from increasing incidence of cancer with age,[9] and the two-step generation of malignancies under the influences of initiating and promoting chemicals[10] or virus and environment[11] all point to variety of tumors (Chapter 2). The differences between neoplasms are indeed only too clearly demonstrated by their varied responses to chemotherapy. The ability of a neoplasm to change is illustrated by rapidly developing drug resistance. Furthermore a single cancer mass can differ within itself in important ways, including resistance to antineoplastic drugs.[12]

From the observations made *in vivo* we expect and find a diversity of properties of tumors and tumor cells in culture. Only the general properties of neoplasia and anaplasia appear evidently universal. Even these are only quantitative; neoplastic growth can be fast or slow. Tumors can take weeks to develop at one extreme, and years at the other. Tissue pathologies are minimal and difficult to detect as different from the normal in some cancers but are obvious in others. Common special properties of anaplasia appear to be concealed in the profusion of forms that cancer takes. Discovery of some basic anaplastic property, common to even a subclass of neoplastic cells, would seem to require more guided insight or more sophisticated methods than we possess at present.

Growth of a cell *in vivo* into a clinical neoplasm is an exceedingly rare event, even though frequency of cancer in the human population is high. An adult has more than 10^{14} cells, and in a lifetime produces perhaps 10^{16} cells. Yet, the chance of one of these cells growing into a lethal neoplasm in 70 years is less than 50%. Immune surveillance mechanisms may prevent the overt appearance of neoplasias. But, beyond such possible protective mechanisms, the initial event of cell transformation must be very uncommon. For comparison, dominant mutations appear spontaneously at frequencies of around 10^{-7} per newly formed cell, and recessive mutations theoretically are expressed at 10^{-14} per cell. Carcinogens can increase the frequency of mutations by an order of magnitude or more (see Chapter 2). The several step sequence of tumor production requires that two or more rather rare stimuli be applied in the proper order; carcinogenesis is, therefore, much less likely to occur than is any single mutationally induced event. The initial carcinogenic event should also be rare in cultures of normal cells.

Clinical chemotherapy has provided basic information, although the main conclusion is a negative one. Namely, although responses of individual tumors to drugs differ, all cancer cells are sufficiently similar to some normal cells that the drug effects are extremely difficult to exploit for effective treatment. Both biochemical and immunological properties of most spontaneous tumors are so like those of normal cells that in spite of enormous efforts only a few drugs have been found capable of eliminating a few types of tumor cells without killing the host.[13] Most effective antineoplastic drugs take advantage of the neoplastic property—the larger growth fraction of cells in tumors relative to their tissues of origin (see Chapter 4). This empirical finding once again stresses the importance of neoplasia as a fundamental characteristic for basic investigation. We are unlikely to discover in tumors some fundamental biochemical difference of the magnitude that has made chemotherapy of infectious diseases successful.

In vivo studies have not provided firm evidence regarding the biochemical basis of neoplastic or anaplastic changes. The diversity of agents that cause cancer does not provide much of a clue. As discussed in Chapter 2, competing theories of the origin of cancer assume: (1) effects of a mutational nature, (2) differentiation-like effects, and (3) viruses. Analysis is especially difficult because normal growth control and differentiation are not at all well understood. The multistage nature of malignancy[14] provides further obstacles. The great ability of chromosomes in cancer cells to be rearranged, as contrasted to normal cells which have extremely stable chromosome patterns, is a most striking characteristic. This mechanism may only appear as a later event in the progression of neoplasia.

TRANSPLANTED TUMORS

Spontaneous human neoplasms help define the problem but they have drawbacks for gaining a deeper understanding of cancer. Clinical material is not reproducible, tumors varying from one patient to another, and the variations are so numerous that sorting out which are important is almost impossible. Control experiments are not readily performed. Thus, it is little wonder that for many years the three main subjects of cancer research—origins of cancer through the actions of various agents, growth kinetics, and treatment—often have been investigated using tumors that can be repetitively transplanted into animals. Lessons learned with these *in vivo* tumors provide a further basis for valid studies with cells and subcellular systems.

The whole problem of cancer and growth control is intimately bound up with agents acting from outside the cell and with the responses of cells to them. Cancer cells continue to grow in environments that stop normal cells. Some tumors, as in the breast, are at least initially dependent on steroid hormones; they can progress to become hormone-independent. Normal stem cells are susceptible to a variety of positively and negatively acting growth factors[15] which provide a growth-regulatory feedback network.[16,17]

Growth of a tumor is limited by availability of substances, hormones, growth factors, and nutrients that are provided by blood. Large tumors can have necrotic centers owing to inadequate blood supply to their interiors. Small metastatic nodules are more likely to be sensitive to antineoplastic drugs than are large tumors,[18] since a greater fraction of metastases is composed of cells in a growing state, being better supplied with growth factors and nutrients.

A striking example of growth limitation by blood supply is seen after a few tumor cells are implanted into the vitreous humor of the eye.[19] These cells grow into spheres with a maximum diameter of a millimeter of so. But if they come into contact with the internal surface of the eye or attract capillaries they rapidly become vascularized and then proliferate explosively under the influence of the factors and nutrients provided by blood.

The observation that transplanted tumors from a great range of species can grow in immunodeficient athymic (nude) mice, and that normal tissues cannot,[20] strongly suggests that the growth regulatory mechanisms and growth factors are species non-specific. (Failure of some tumors to grow probably can be attributed to residual immune defenses in these animals.) This is an important conclusion in regard to species universality of a basic defect of neoplasia, and a further justification for work with non-human tumors.

Carcinogenesis has often been studied with transplanted tumors and cells. The development of teratoma cells and teratocarcinomas from mouse embryo cells that have been implanted into the testes underscores the importance of local environment *in vivo*.[21] There is evidence from this system also for the reversibility of tumor growth,[21,22] a result consistent with the differentiation hypothesis of the origin of cancer and hard to reconcile with the equally well supported mutational hypotheses (see Chapter 3A). A most striking result is that incorporation of a teratocarcinoma cell into a very early embryo (blastocyst) permits growth to maturity of a mouse that contains apparently normal cells derived from these teratocarcinoma cells.[21]

Differentiation may be due to a pattern of expression of unique sets of genes among many present, others being silent. Differentiation includes regulation of cell proliferation as one of its traits. Differentiation patterns are genetically determined, and hence they can be modified by alterations of the genetic material, either by mutations and chromosome rearrangements or by (poorly understood) phenotypic DNA modifications that are the basis of differentiation. The possibilities are not exclusive, and indeed viruses cause neoplastic changes by introducing new genetic material. The multistep process of neoplasia could be initiated in any of these ways, and be followed by chromosomal rearrangements, to further modify the classes of genes that are expressed. Some so modified cells would later be selected, owing to their rapid growth, and they could progress into neoplasms.[11]

Identification of the chromosomes on which determinants of neoplasia are located has been attempted using transplantable tumors and techniques of somatic cell genetics.[23] Normal and tumor cells are fused into a hybrid that contains both sets of chromosomes. Surprisingly, these hybrids are not neoplastic when injected into a suitable host.[24] This result indicates that neoplasia is recessive, and perhaps is permitted by absence of a normal cellular element. After a few of the normal chromosomes are spontaneously lost from some cells in hybrid populations, these cells become neoplastic.[25] Attempts to correlate neoplasia with a specific chromosome loss have not been successful. Nonetheless, these *in vivo* expriments point to critical alterations of DNA as important subjects for *in vitro* investigation.

The great experimental advantage of using transplanted tumors is that one has a ready source of reproducible material; but a long recognized problem with any tissue or cell specimen that is passed from animal to animal (or from culture to culture) for many generations is that properties of the material change. Also, human cells become senescent and lose their proliferative potential *in vitro* and in transplantation.[26] There is selection for the most rapidly growing cells in a transplanted tumor during successive passages; consequently, the tumors which finally emerge contain these rapidly growing cells. Many old, established lines such as Ehrlich ascites and HeLa are stripped-down versions that bear little resemblance to original tumors.[27]

Results obtained by treating tumor lines with antineoplastic drugs may have limited applicability to chemotherapy of spontaneous, early stage human tumors. The transplantable tumors have a large proportion of growing cells (growth fraction) that are susceptible to cycle-specific antineoplastic drugs, in contrast to natural, slowly growing tumors with a small growth ratio.[28] It is not surprising that the main successes of drugs selected using transplantable tumors have been against rapidly growing neoplasias such as leukemias.

NORMAL AND NEOPLASTIC CELLS IN CULTURE

Transplantable tumors can be caricatures of spontaneously occurring neoplasms and yet have value as experimental material. One can carry abstractions a step farther from reality and study normal and tumor cells in culture. The primary defect of neoplasia lies within a cell, so we are justified in investigating properties of cultured cells and their relationships to their environment. The rest of this chapter will be on *in vitro* studies, divided between investigations of cells in culture and of truly *in vitro* subcellular, biochemical systems.

TISSUE CULTURE

Neoplasia, considered as a cell's relaxed growth responses to its environment, can be studied most incisively in tissue culture. Homogeneous populations of cells can thereby be placed into defined environments and their responses and properties measured precisely. Only in about the past 20 years have conditions been developed for relatively rapidly and conveniently growing and experimenting on non-tumor and tumor-derived fibroblastic cells in culture.[29,30] Numerous conditions have to be optimized for obtaining good growth, including: (1) a suitable substratum for those cells that need to grow on a surface; (2) a variety of inorganic ions, CO_2, and controlled pH; (3) small organic molecules, such as essential amino acids and vitamins; (4) additional organic molecules, such as pyruvate, fatty acids, purines, polyamines, and so forth, which aid growth of more fastidious cells; (5) antibiotics such as penicillin and streptomycin to help maintain sterility; (6) and, beyond these simpler essentials, various growth factors, which are generally supplied by ten-fold diluted bovine serum. Mammalian cells grow best at 37°C, and can tolerate a temperature ranging from about 31 to 39°C for adequate growth. The cells can divide about every 12 hours as a maximum, but usually divide more slowly.

Primary cells that are taken directly from an animal are often not readily started in culture. Conditions have to be optimized for growth of each kind of cell, as for example human breast cells,[31] including empirical modifications of the medium such as using fetal calf serum and providing additional nutrients. The substratum can be of great importance, and a layer of "feeder cells," preplated on the plastic tissue culture surface permits growth of some fastidious cells, such as epidermal cells.[32] Most cultured cells have a fibroblastic appearance though they may not actually be fibroblasts. The recent successes in culturing epithelial cells[31,33] is a development of great interest since most neoplasms are of epithelial origin. The fibroblasts in tissue specimens take over cultures because they grow relatively readily on plastic surfaces. Techniques have been developed to remove them[32] or limit their growth in order to allow other cells to be grown.

Cells from tumors often are as difficult to culture as are normal cells.[34] This problem is an important one for devising "clonogenic assays" of resistance to antineoplastic drugs, in which the ability of cells to grow in the presence of each drug is determined.[35] Cells neoplastically transformed in culture require nearly the same growth conditions as do untransformed cells. However, transformed cells in general require lower concentrations of serum and growth factors than do untransformed cells, and their requirements for adhesion to a surface are not so stringent (see below). It is an irony and a measure of our ignorance that we do not know how to grow most carcinoma cells in culture, and that, on the other hand, we cannot stop their growth *in vivo*.

After cells are in culture and cloned to isolate a single cell type, a cell line is obtained, the properties of which depend on the conditions of cultivation. A classic study of this kind showed that the different lines eventually emerge from the same initial culture, depending on durations of culture time between cell transfers to new dishes and on the initial densities of cells at the times of transfer.[36] The 3T3 line of mouse cells was obtained after transferring Swiss mouse cells at three-fold dilutions every three days (initial density 3×10^5 cells/21 cm^3 plate). This cell line shows a highly regulated growth mode (see below). But, when three-fold dilutions were made at initial densities of 6 or 12×10^5/plate the 3T6 and 3T12 lines were obtained. These lines show progressively less growth control, and form tumors in nude mice. In general, cells in culture can in time lose their tissue-specific properties and spontaneously become tumorigenic.

Normal cells may be able to continue proliferation in culture only for a limited number of generations. For example, chick cells can be cultured for only a very few cell generations, and human cells can no longer grow after about 50 generations.[26,37] Rodent cells exhibit decreased growth rates with generation number, and after about 30 generations mouse cells come to a crisis; cultures nearly stop growing. From these cultures altered cells emerge which grow rapidly.[36] They are aneuploid and can be grown indefinitely in culture. This property of "immortalization" is a common characteristic of neoplastic cells,[5] although not all tumor-forming cells are immortal. Also a few "immortalized" cell lines are not tumor-forming.

TRANSFORMED CELLS

Normal cells, which cannot form tumors in an appropriate animal, generally also are limited in their growth in culture. Their most evident characteristic is density dependent inhibition of growth: there is virtual cessation of increase in cell number and DNA synthesis when a culture covers the surface of the vessel.[38] Also, the cells do not migrate across one another, and they line up in a monolayer of parallel cells, owing to density dependent inhibition of motility.[39] Non-tumor-forming fibroblasts must be able to attach and spread on a substratum, such as glass or the plastic suitable for tissue culture. These cells also require several percent serum in their medium in order to grow, and they often have other properties different from tumor forming cells, which have frequently been summarized and some of which will be referred to later.[5,38,40,41]

In non-tumorigenic populations, rare cells can arise that continue to grow into piled-up cell foci in confluent cultures. These cells have undergone a spontaneous transformation. They can be isolated (cloned) and then are found to differ from the original cells in various "transformed" properties. They often can form tumors *in vivo* (tumorigenic transformation). They continue to grow at confluence, showing losses of density dependent inhibition of growth and motility. The cells disregard one another, and are seen as dense colonies in which cells cross over one another. These neoplastically transformed cells often can grow in suspension, not needing the surface attachment required by the original cells. Their surface adhesion or anchorage requirement is changed, as can be shown quantitatively by the degree to which cells grow on a graded set of surfaces covered with increasing quantities of the plastic Hydron.[42] Also, they generally can grow in media containing less serum than is required by untransformed cells.[43] As mentioned earlier, neoplastically transformed lines are more likely to be immortalized in culture.

Cells in culture can be transformed by various agents including carcinogenic chemicals,[44] ultraviolet light or roentgen rays and some viruses (see Chapter 2). Cells transformed by the small RNA retroviruses and by DNA tumor viruses, particularly SV40, polyoma, and adenoviruses,[45] have been investigated very extensively in culture. Cells transformed by the DNA viruses can show the most marked neoplastic alterations; but even their transformed properties are quite diverse in independently isolated lines.[46]

SV40 virus can transform human cells in culture, although these cells do not readily form tumors in the nude mouse.[47] A few human tumors are related to DNA virus infection, such as Burkitt's lymphoma to a Herpes virus,[11] and hepatomas to hepatitis B virus.[48] RNA viruses have not been shown to cause cancers in humans, in spite of exhaustive experimentation. In contrast, rodent tumor production *in vivo* and transformation of rodent cells in culture are readily accomplished by RNA viruses, as well as by chemical and other physical agents. Chemical transformation of human cells in culture is very difficult, although tumors in humans are thought to be mainly produced by chemical carcinogens.[9] There are only a few reports of success, requiring months of culture.[49,50] This difficulty may relate to our inability to mimic well in culture the growth conditions on which epithelial tumor cells (carcinomas) thrive *in vivo,* also perhaps because several stages are required.

Transformed cells show a spectrum of properties, ranging from barely changed to completely altered from the normal. These properties are often possessed by spontaneously, chemically, or virally transformed cells; but all of them do not occur in all transformed cells.[46,51] Some properties are related; thus density-dependent inhibition of growth can be overcome by increasing serum in the medium, final density being proportional to serum concentration.[52] Confluent cultures have been theorized to stop growing because they may simply have run out of a localized supply of growth factors for normal cells, or of nutrients for transformed cells.[53] Transformation changes might lie in a progressive series, more or less in the sequence of loss of high serum requirement, altered morphology, decreased anchorage requirement, and tumorigenicity. No one property in culture assures that a cell is capable of forming a tumor *in vivo;*[54] but cells which have several of these properties, particularly loss of the anchorage requirement, are quite likely to be tumorigenic.[55] Tumor-forming ability was lost and yet transformed properties were retained in cells formed by fusing HeLa cells and normal human fibroblasts;[56] thus, even these two properties are separable.

Quiescent (Resting) Cells

Most cells *in vivo* are in a quiescent state; some brain cells remain quiescent for a lifetime. Such cells are in a special state named G0, which is different from any state of growing cells.[57] Other cells have a finite lifetime before they are eliminated; lymphocytes are a well-known example. To replace lost, dead cells, quiescent stem cells are activated to grow and divide. One of the daughter cells replaces the original stem cell and the other replaces a lost cell; a finely tuned regulatory mechanism evidently is involved in maintaining this balance.[17,26] In cases of hyperplasia or increase in number of a given type of cell, such as when fibroblasts proliferate after wounding, or the increased numbers of erythrocytes arising under lower O_2 pressure at higher elevations, or specific production of lymphocytes following stimulation of the immune system, there is only a transient shift to restore equilibrium. The balance remains upset in a neoplasm, so that proliferation exceeds cell loss. Nevertheless, many cells in tumors are temporarily quiescent.[28,57] The total cell number increases only slowly when new cell production only slightly exceeds cell death; and tumors thus can require many years to develop.

The rate of a tissue's growth mainly depends on the fraction of total cells which are going through the cell cycle and are not resting (quiescent) minus the fraction dying.[16,28] The actual rate of progress through the cycle of these non-resting cells is relatively constant and has only a minor effect on growth rate. Control is applied at cycle initiation and termination events, the shifts between quiescence and growth.

The regulation of cell numbers as a result of stimulation and inhibition by external factors is a complex subject, under active investigation with a variety of cell types including fibroblasts, lymphocytes, endothelial, epidermal, and smooth muscle cells.[58] As an example, the platelet derived growth factor (PDGF) is required by fibroblasts to initiate their escape from high-density induced G0 arrest.[59] Stem cell proliferation has until recently been difficult to study in culture; evidently stem cell activation is a subject of great importance to cancer chemotherapy: neoplastic stem cells in a G0 state present a major obstacle to any chemotherapy based on selectively killing only growing, cycling cells.[16]

In tissue cultures, as *in vivo,* viable cells can either be quiescent or cycling (Fig. 3-1). The quiescent (G0) cells differ in many ways from cycling cells;[40] they only resemble G1 phase cells in having the same DNA content. The main emphasis in tissue culture initially is to get cells to grow, and so a major emphasis is on finding conditions that move quiescent cells into cycle and keep them there. Conversely, untransformed cells can be moved from the cycle into G0 if suboptimal conditions of various sorts are provided—if they are starved for a nutrient such as an essential amino acid, or are deprived of serum or a growth factor such as insulin, or after they become confluent, or are put into suspension.[60] Some drugs also put cells in culture into the G0 state.[51] As cells shift between growth and quiescence they exhibit a set of biochemical changes named "the pleiotypic response."[61] In terms of growth control mechanisms, it is equally important to consider transition out of G0 as transition from the cycle into quiescence. The conditions that determine these tran-

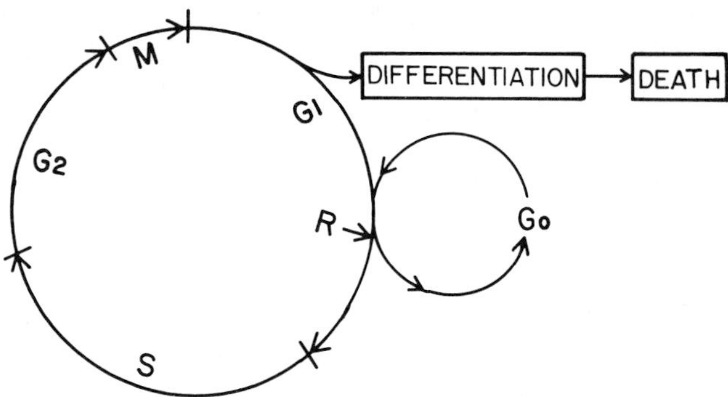

FIG. 3-1. A cell cycle diagram. The larger circle represents the cell cycle. After division, (at the top of the circle) cells spend several hours in the G1 phase and pass the control event (restriction point R). After G1, during S phase, they synthesize DNA. Then there is the second "gap", G2, followed by chromosomal rearrangements in mitosis, and another division. The smaller circle indicates that if a cell cannot pass R it is shunted into the resting state G0, from which it can re-enter G1 after an indeterminate time, if conditions become favorable. Finally, the branch at the top indicates that one cell in stem cell systems can take a different path, to become differentiated, and possibly to eventually die.

sitions and hence growth are different for fibroblasts and epithelial cells.[62]

Transformed and tumor derived cells in culture are not arrested in G0 as readily as are non-tumor cells.[40,41] The difference is usually quantitative, and for most neoplastic cells arrest of growth takes place if sufficiently stringent conditions are applied.[51] In the extreme—cells transformed by the DNA virus SV40—adverse conditions merely slow their rate of cycle traverse; the cells are incapable of entering the G0 state[43] and die in a few days.[63] The effects of transformation on differentiation in culture (anaplasia) have so far been little investigated, compared to effects on neoplasia.

Cell Cycle Kinetics

The cell cycle is classically divided into four stages (Fig. 3-1). After cells divide they pass through G1, S (DNA synthesis), G2, and M (mitosis). G1 is the "gap" between division and S, and G2 is between S and M. The times of transit for a typical cycle in culture (e.g., 3T3 cells) are G1:S:G2:M = 6:8:3:0.7 hr. Quiescent fibroblasts in culture enter the cell cycle and duplicate when placed at low cell density into fresh medium. The interval before their DNA synthesis commences is usually longer than the G1 period of cycling cells.[40] This time (lag) suggests that extra events must occur for cells to get back into the cycle from G0. The lengths of the S, G2, and M phases that follow are the same as for cells previously in cycle.

The G1 phase is most important for cell growth control. It is primarily in G1 that external conditions determine whether cycling cells will continue in the proliferative cycle or be switched into G0. These conditions affect the other parts of the cycle less; cells usually transit the cycle and enter into G0 (quiescence) in suboptimal conditions, stopping only following division and prior to DNA synthesis.[40,41,64] The "place" in G1 at which the decision is made between proliferation and quiescence has been named the restriction point.[65]

A remarkable feature of the cycle is that its duration is highly variable from one cell to another in the same culture. Most of this variability lies in G1, and the more adverse the growth conditions (*e.g.*, the lower the serum concentration) the greater becomes this variability and the average G1 lengthens.[66] These and other results suggest that an event in G1 is particularly sensitive to environmental conditions, and the abilities of individual cells to progress past this event differ. Transit of G1 can be delayed for long periods under adverse conditions without the cells entering S or G0.[59] This variability of entry into S phase probably is a barrier to chemotherapy by cycle phase–specific drugs; some tumor cells will not have time to leave G1 during the period that a drug can be safely applied, and therefore these cells will survive treatment.

These results and others have led to the idea of a special event (restriction point[65] or transition[67]) at which an event in G1 must be accomplished before a cell can initiate DNA synthesis. This is the event mainly sensitive to the external influences that determine whether or not a cell will cycle, and thus how fast a population will grow. Additional regulatory points have been proposed.[59,64,67] In neoplastic cells the restriction point event in G1 is less dependent than in non-tumor cells on external signals such as growth factors, nearby cells, or substratum;[68,51] transformed cells continue to pass this point under the physiological conditions that arrest growth of non-transformed cells.[63,69,70] The regulatory events are of prime interest for understanding normal and abnormal growth.

Relatively little is known about the biochemistry of the restriction event. Indeed, very little is known about the biochemistry of the entire G1 part of the cycle. Synthesis of proteins is necessary for transit of G1, as is RNA synthesis, as shown by studies with inhibitors.[40] The restriction point appears to be located 2 or 3 hours prior to the actual initiation of S phase.[71] It is highly dependent on rapid protein synthesis; and many of the factors that control cell growth also influence rates of net protein accumulation, affecting rates of protein synthesis or degradation. The critical event for growth may be the growth factor–dependent accumulation of a rather unstable protein (half life of a few hours) during G1.[72,73,74] Very recent data suggest that transformed cells can more readily accumulate this protein, need less of it, or (most likely) degrade it slowly;[75] a shift in the balance from quiescence toward proliferation results in any case. Both transformation[76] and high serum concentration[77] increase proliferation and also decrease overall protein turnover.

BIOCHEMISTRY OF NEOPLASTIC CELLS

The cell biology just summarized needs eventually to be understood at a subcellular, biochemical level. Numerous biochemical changes have been reported relating to growth, regulation, and neoplasia. Difficulties in their interpretation arise from the complexity of cell growth, with its multitude of biochemical reactions that are connected into a great metabolic network, the modification of which in any part creates changes throughout, and from the variety and progression of properties of tumor cells. Tumor progression creates alterations of many sorts, many of which must be secondary to the presumed primary events of neoplasia. Some current biochemical information contrasting normal and tumor cells will be summarized in the following sections, in the order from extracellular to nuclear processes.

EXTRACELLULAR MOLECULES

As discussed above, normal cell growth and differentiation *in vivo* and in culture both depend heavily on external factors.[58,78] A striking example of *in vivo* environment on differentiation is the conversion of normal cells into multipotential teratocarcinoma cells after early embryos are implanted under the testes capsule.[21]

Growth of cells in culture depends on serum to provide growth factors, in an extremely complicated mixture with other substances. Most of the factors are not yet known. Attempts to isolate factors by fractionating whole serum have not been very successful. Incomplete sera may not support growth unless a missing factor is added. Thus fibroblasts in culture require somatomedin C, as shown by inability of serum from hypophysectomized animals (thereby lacking somatomedin C) to support growth unless somatomedin C is also provided.[79] Media that contain combinations of known factors in place of serum allow cell growth.[80,81] These factors include proteins and peptides such as transferrin, insulin, epidermal growth factor (EGF), and fibroblast growth factor (FGF). These and other factors permit excellent growth of various normal and transformed cells in culture, though other cells require still unknown factors (present in serum). Specially designed media can decrease or eliminate factor requirements.[82] Additional factors are being found, such as one from platelets that is released when serum is formed during blood clotting. It stimulates G0 fibroblasts' growth at a step prior to the other factors which are provided by plasma,[59] and it also is needed to prevent growth arrest in G1.[83]

Transformed cells generally grow well in media containing less serum than is needed by non-transformed cells, indicating that some factors are dispensible or are required in smaller amounts.[40,41] Transformation of fibroblasts has been particularly correlated with a diminished requirement for EGF, using a defined medium.[81] Tumor cells can in some instances supply their own factors.[84] A line of mouse cells transformed by Moloney sarcoma (RNA) virus produces a peptide that replaces EGF for cell growth,[85] one of several examples of the ability of tumor cells to overproduce growth factors and hormones, as known also to occur *in vivo*. Other transformed cells could have a decreased requirement for extracellular supply of growth factors because of intracellular changes in their regulatory mechanism.

Most studies with defined growth factors suggest that cell growth is under positive control, i.e., growth factors must be available for growth. But cells have been proposed to produce inhibitory substances, called chalones, which limit their growth.[85] Tumor cells could be less sensitive to extracellular chalones or might underproduce them. This attractive hypothesis is unfortunately not supported by hard data. No chalone has been isolated to date, as contrasted to isolation of a number of positive growth factors. The cellular experiments on growth inhibition by chalones are generally interpretable in other ways. Furthermore, toxic factors such as spermidine are produced by cells, and their ability at high concentrations to inhibit growth can be confused with physiologically relevant inhibitions. On the other hand, the proliferation of stem cells *in vivo,* in contrast to fibroblastic cells in culture, may well be subject to negative feedback regulation.[15,17]

Numerous externally supplied compounds, such as metabolic inhibitors, arrest cell growth. In a few cases they appear to affect the physiological (G1) control event.[63,74] A fascinating recent example is arrest of fibroblasts by compactin, an inhibitor of the pathway leading to cholesterol and other isoprenoid compounds.[87,88] In a few instances unusual compounds are growth stimulatory, as for example, the tumor promoter TPA.[89]

THE CELL SURFACE

The external factors that determine a cell's pattern of growth, *e.g.*, substratum, adjacent cells, and growth stimulating compounds, must first impinge on the cell surface. They therefore either change this surface or pass through it to have effects inside the cell. The cell surface has three components: extracellular matrix, cytoplasmic or plasma membrane, and an intracellular matrix that passes into the cytoplasm from the membrane's internal surface. Each of these components may be involved in growth regulation, and each can be altered in transformed cells. Ability to metastasize also depends on properties of the cell surface. Indeed, it was proposed many years ago that a fundamental defect of tumor cells could reside in the cell membrane.[90]

Literally thousands of papers have been written comparing normal and cancer cell's surface chemistry.[91,92,93,94] Differences have been reported in nearly every surface component. Transformed and non-transformed cells' proteins, antigens,[95] glycoproteins,[96] glycolipids, phospholipids, cholesterol, and so forth all differ. But a function has not been found for any of these, nor more than a correlation with neoplastic growth.[97]

The extracellular matrix is secreted as a complex of proteins and other components which adheres to the cell exterior and also coats the dish's surface. It appears to be important as a substratum for permitting growth. A plastic surface that has been covered with residues of other, detergent-extracted cells or with proteins extracted from other cells, permits readier cell growth and more regular colony morphology than does plastic alone.[98] What is actually supplied by these complex coatings that aids growth is unknown; they may well contain absorbed growth factors. There are indications that these preparations have tissue specificity; but little is yet known regarding requirements for them by tumor cells versus normal cells.

A great deal of work has been done on a large extracellular protein called fibronectin. It is absent from some neoplastic cells, possibly because it is removed by a proteolytic system, plasminogen activator, that is secreted by these cells.[99] It does not seem to be related to neoplasia, although it is possibly related to metastatic activity.[100]

The plasma membrane holds cells together; it presents a

barrier between extra- and intra-cellular molecules. Two of its main activities are, therefore, selective transport of molecules into and out of the cell, and the binding of growth factors and other proteins to its exterior surface.

Nearly all small molecules, such as ions, sugars, and amino acids, are brought across the membrane by specific transport mechanisms, and are often actively concentrated within the cell. Some of these transport mechanisms (*e.g.*, those for amino acids and sugars) increase several-fold in activity after cells are transformed.[101] Changes of some transport activities occur within minutes after cells are shifted between quiescence and growth.[102] Growing (transformed or non-transformed) chick fibroblasts transport glucose about ten times as rapidly as do quiescent and non-transformed cells.[101] Although rates of nutrient or ion[103] transport could actually determine growth rates, by limiting the supply of an essential nutrient or element, evidence in support of this idea is not conclusive for any nutrient.[104] The membrane's functional properties more likely are changed upon transformation as adaptations to altered metabolic rates.

Proteins in solution can be taken into cells by endocytosis. A protein is first bound to a membrane receptor site, and then invagination of part of the membrane which contains the bound protein forms a vesicle within the cell. This vesicle fuses with a lysosome, the enzymes of which digest the endocytotic vesicle's contents and release them to the cytoplasm. Little or nothing is known about differences in this mechanism between tumor and non-tumor cells, although differences have been reported in mobilities of molecules in membranes and in membrane fluidity.[93,94]

Proteins may not have to enter a cell in order to function, but may act on the surface. Some growth factors can function from outside when they are attached to large beads that prevent their entry into cells.[105] Interaction of growth factors with the cell surface currently provides a very active area of research on growth regulation.[97] A cell can have 100,000 or more specific membrane receptors for a growth factor such as insulin. Variations in the number of these receptors have been noted after transformation. These changes could in some cases arise from competition for binding sites between the radioactively labelled factor used as a probe and a non-radioactive, similar factor produced by the transformed cell.[85] Various receptor sites are being isolated and purified.

Research has been particularly active on the epidermal growth factor, a small protein. After EGF binds to the surface membrane it is quite rapidly internalized and digested.[107] Thus, its action in stimulating cell growth might be due to these internal fragments of EGF or receptor. But EGF also phosphorylates a membrane protein,[108] and new, functionally active proteins appear inside the cells as well.[109] Thus, there are at least three possibilities as to the next step in its action.

The cell surface can specifically bind other proteins. One class comprises lectins, proteins usually of plant origins that have affinities for specific carbohydrate residues on surface glycoproteins.[91] Lectins can stimulate cell growth, the best known being the stimulation of lymphocytes by phytohemagglutinin. Although the amounts of lectins bound to neoplastic and non-neoplastic cells are not very different, some lectins more readily agglutinate the former than the latter. The basis for this difference may reside in surface compositions, or receptor site distribution and their mobilities within the membrane.[94] Specific antigens are located on the membrane of cells transformed by various agents,[95] and of tumor cells.

The subcellular matrix consists of filamentous structures[110] composed of several proteins, mainly actin and tubulin and also the proteins of intermediate filaments.[111] Filaments are associated with the interior side of the membrane, and extend through the cell, as can be seen with the aid of fluorescent antibodies or with the electron microscope. Their functions relate to cell shape, spreading, and division, and possibly to transmission of signals from the membrane into the cell. Microfilaments and microtubules are often found to have more organized structures in untransformed cells than in transformed cells,[112] although these findings have been disputed.[113] Microtubules are disrupted by colchicine, an agent that either inhibits or stimulates growth, depending on the cell type and its state of growth.[114]

Microtubules are associated with the centrioles, and they are condensed into a cilium when cells are in G0 or mid-G1. The exact duplication of centrioles during the cell cycle and the cycle-dependent changes they undergo have suggested a centriole cycle.[115]

THE CYTOPLASM

Second Messengers

Externally available growth factors initially must impinge on the membrane to activate growth; somehow they pass a signal through the cytoplasm in order to activate nuclear, DNA-related functions. Factors can pass into the cell; a clear example is seen with steroid hormones.[116] Estrogen enters the cytoplasm of uterine cells, where it binds to and changes the properties of a specific receptor protein. This protein moves into the nucleus where it binds to DNA, and enhanced macromolecular synthesis and cell proliferation follow.

Whether protein growth factors function after they enter the cell is not yet clear. Epidermal growth factor (EGF) and its receptor protein form a complex on the cell surface which is internalized, degraded, and released into the cytoplasm,[107] but it is not at all clear that these pieces of internalized receptor and growth factor are functional. The balance of data currently suggests that protein growth factors probably function by acting on the membrane to produce and release a "second messenger" into the cytoplasm. Proteins appear in the cytoplasm of cells treated with EGF which activate DNA synthesis when added to nuclei of frog cells.[109]

The nature of putative second messengers is obscure. A few years ago a great deal of work attempted to relate cyclic nucleotides, cAMP and cGMP, to regulation of cell growth.[117] Thus, if the amount of intercellular cAMP was increased by adding dibutyryl-cAMP, prostaglandin-E1, or cholera toxin in the medium, growth of non-transformed fibroblasts generally was inhibited and the cells accumulated in G0 or G1. Also, some transformed cultures became morphologically untransformed cultures. The effects of cGMP were thought generally to be opposite of those of cAMP. There is now no agreement regarding a simple role of cAMP or cGMP in growth control, owing to conflicting data.[118] For example, concentrations of cAMP actually increase when growth of epithelial and lymphoid cells is stimulated.

The main function of cyclic nucleotides is to activate protein kinases, enzymes that phosphorylate a variety of proteins and thereby either increase or decrease their activities.[119] Indications that cAMP-dependent protein kinases are involved in growth control are, first, that a mutant cell that lacks a protein kinase cannot be arrested in the G1 phase of the cell cycle;[120] second, that two cAMP-dependent protein kinases are synthesized at specific stages of the cell cycle, in a fashion that correlates with cell growth events.[121]

Other candidates for second messengers are metal ions, such as Ca^{2+}, Mg^{2+}, Na^{+}, and K^{+}. Intracellular concentrations of these ions depend on transport systems,[101,104] and uptake is stimulated by serum and growth factors.[82] Ions activate various enzymes and metabolic processes, including protein kinases and ATPase, stimulating both protein synthesis and the energy producing glycolytic system.[101] Functions of Ca^{2+} are mediated by calmodulin, a specific binding protein for this ion.[122,123] Ca^{2+} and cAMP are interrelated in their effects on various important processes such as protein kinase activities and microtubule formation.[124]

Protein and Enzymes

In an overall way, neoplastic cells become traps for nitrogen compounds in the body, rapidly taking up amino acids and metabolizing them into new proteins via highly active anabolic pathways.[4] Neoplastic cells also have active key enzymes for assimilating precursors into nucleic acids.[125] Protein synthesis takes place mainly on cytoplasmic ribosomes which are connected into polyribosomes in actively synthesizing cells. This metabolic machinery does not seem to be qualitatively altered by neoplastic transformation. But active protein synthesis requires growth factors, on which normal cells are more dependent than are transformed cells. Protein synthesis rates are similar in growing cells, whether neoplastic or non-neoplastic; quiescent cells synthesize proteins more slowly. Thus, neoplastic cells on the average synthesize proteins more rapidly than do non-neoplastic cells because the former have a greater growth fraction. This typical kind of correlation, between growth and protein synthesis, does not tell us whether it is growth or protein synthesis that is primary. Protein synthesis, activated by external factors, could be permitting growth, since protein synthesis is essential to growth in all parts of the cycle,[40,44] and particularly in the G1 phase (see above).

Protein degradation, in contrast to protein synthesis, has been reported to be decreased in transformed cells.[76] Detailed studies on specific proteinases and their activities in various neoplastic cells have not been pursued extensively. Cells shifted to low serum degrade their proteins relatively rapidly,[77] possibly confusing the comparisons of neoplastic and non-neoplastic cells. These data are in general consistent with a scheme outlined earlier here, that growth may be controlled by a labile protein, the accumulation of which depends on a balance between synthesis and degradation.[74]

The cytoplasm also contains most of the enzymes that catalyze all of biosynthetic and degradative metabolism. Attempts to find distinctive differences between enzymes in tumor and non-tumor cells were made by Greenstein and his associates in the 1940's.[126] Various differences were found. But one now knows that the state of growth must be taken into account. For example, ornithine decarboxylase is much more active in growing cells. Progression of neoplastic cells also at least quantitatively changes enzymes, as metabolism shifts to enzyme patterns presumably permitting more rapid growth.[27]

Weber and his colleagues[125] more recently have made detailed studies of enzyme patterns in hepatic cells and hepatomas. Some slow growing tumors show minimal deviations in their enzymes' patterns, and resemble neonatal cells in general. If the tumors are faster growing, both their enzyme and their chromosome patterns change. Although no enzyme change is typical of all neoplasia, a few alterations have utility in therapy, such as inability of some neoplasms to synthesize asparagine. The enzyme asparaginase injected into the blood restricts growth of these tumors by depriving them of a source of asparagine (see Chapter 8).

Pitot[4] has performed a remarkable series of investigations on hepatomas and normal hepatocytes to show that, whereas the production of some enzymes in normal cells is inducible—flexibility dependent on environmental stimuli—each hepatoma has a fixed level of each of these enzymes that differs from one neoplasm to the other. It is as if for each enzyme a control system were frozen at some arbitrary setting. These controls thus appear to be much more affected than are the enzymes' catalytic properties or actual amounts. This result could be based on the poorer communication of tumor cells with their environments, and with neighboring cells.[127] These cells' growth oriented, independent behavior appears to correlate with anaplastic metabolism.

Novel proteins appear in cells transformed by tumorigenic viruses.[128] The sarc protein is produced in cells transformed by Rous Sarcoma (RNA) virus.[129] This protein is present in very small amounts in non-transformed cells. It has protein kinase activity that phosphorylates tyrosine residues.[130] Cells transformed by SV40 or polyoma (DNA) viruses produce new proteins named T antigens, which also are reported to have protein ATPase and kinase activity.[131] Transformation by Rous, SV40 or polyoma in each case depends on only a single viral gene. These results reinforce the idea (*e.g.*, from studies with EGF and cyclic AMP) that protein kinases are important in growth control.

Organelles and Energy Metabolism

The first biochemical hypothesis of cancer was proposed by Warburg in 1925: that all tumors have higher rates of glycolysis under aerobic conditions than do non-tumor cells.[132] Subsequent work has not supported the universality of this hypothesis, which probably was based on this property existing in transplanted, progressing, and rapidly growing tumors.[27] Some of these neoplasms have high rates of glucose utilization and lactic acid production in the presence of oxygen. Their regulation of glucose utilization has been studied intensively for many years.[133] It is not clear at this time whether some tumors use glucose more rapidly because the sugar is transported into the cell faster[134] or because the regulation of glycolysis by various factors—ATP and K^{+} among others—is relaxed so that the pathway goes faster.[138] Each may be correct for some tumor cells, since good data support both possibilities.

Aerobic energy production occurs in mitochondria, which are semi-autonomous organelles. They contain a small amount of DNA which codes for a few proteins and are sensitive to inhibitors (such as chloramphenicol) different from ones that affect cytoplasmic ribosomes. Some transformed cells are more sensitive to chloramphenicol and to inhibitors of oxidative phosphorylation than are untransformed cells, suggesting that their mitochondrial ribosomes have altered structures and functions.[136] These differences could diminish oxidative energy producing abilities of tumor cells, and could be responsible for the smaller effects of aerobic (mitochondrial) energy metabolism or glycolysis in tumor cells, as proposed by Warburg.

THE NUCLEUS

Nuclear Composition

The nucleus is the site of all this hereditary information, aside from the important but relatively small amount of DNA in organelles.

The nucleus is the focus of two major questions in cancer research. First, nuclear DNA is assumed to be the site of the hereditary changes produced by carcinogens (see Chapter 2). All possible normal and neoplastic properties of a cell ultimately are limited by the available functioning genes. Cancer thus results from gene expression patterns that are altered from normal ones. Modifications of genetic structure—by localized mutation and rearrangements, or modifications of expression (aberrant differentiations), or introduction of new genes by DNA[128] or RNA[137] viruses, or as free DNA from transformed cells[138,139]—could be responsible for neoplasia (see Chapter 2). From this viewpoint of neoplasia, gene modifications are the primary objects of study. Methods are now being developed that should allow detection of fine-structure DNA changes relevant to cancer, as contrasted to the gross chromosomal rearrangements.

A second goal of basic cancer research is the one mainly discussed in this chapter, to understand control of cell growth by modifications of the system that activates DNA replication. DNA is the target of agents that control cell growth by their ultimate interactions with available genes and are all of interest in terms of the regulation of cell growth and differentiation.

Nuclei of neoplastic tumor cells appear to have distorted morphologies, found to be the most obvious characteristic of breast cancer cells.[140] But tumor and non-tumor cells are not evidently different within the nucleus, with the exception of frequent chromosomal rearrangements. The structure of chromatin—DNA wrapped around nucleosomes composed of histones, and the other proteins associated with DNA—does not seem to be different according to present methods.

DNA Replication

A major measurable event in the cell cycle is initiation of S phase. The rapid incorporation of ^{3}H-thymidine into DNA is generally taken as the initial point of S phase, although a small incorporation can be detected, by autoradiography, to commence a couple of hours earlier. DNA synthesis starts bulk DNA replication and later mitosis and cell division follow without much overall control from external agents.

Synthesis of DNA in all parts of chromosomes does not commence at the beginning of S phase.[141] Rather, chromosomes are divided into replicons, units of DNA replication, of which there are tens of thousands having lengths from a few μm up to several hundred. They replicate at different times during S phase, proceeding in both directions from an origin. There thus must be sequential signals for initiations of groups of replicons. What these signals are and whether they are altered in any way in neoplastic cells is unknown. The duration of S phase does not appear to be shorter in neoplastic cells.

There are several DNA polymerases of which α appears to be the major one.[142] The enzymes of DNA precursor production and of DNA synthesis do not seem to be different in activities or regulation in normal vs. neoplastic cells. But in simpler organisms, such as *Escherichia coli,* at least a dozen proteins are required for DNA elongation; and numerous genes are involved; as yet, comparable information is not available for animal cells. DNA is associated with a matrix associated with the nuclear membrane of mammalian cells.[143] In *E. coli,*[144] and as very recently found in mammalian cells,[145] DNA replication (like protein synthesis) is performed by a multiprotein complex, rather than being catalyzed by free enzymes. Formation of the multienzyme complex for DNA replication may be a major event of cell cycle control that is modified by transformation.[145]

Various proteins are associated with DNA in chromatin. These proteins change during cell growth, and the morphology of chromatin changes as well. Histones are modified by acetylation and phosphorylation, particularly histone H-1 at the onset of S phase.[146] The synthesis of some nuclear acidic proteins increases within 30 minutes after serum stimulation of quiescent human fibroblasts, long before DNA synthesis commences.[147] The relation of these early nuclear changes to the long progression of events in G1 is obscure,[40] though it may indicate initiations of RNA transcription.

Nuclear division is affected differently by cytochalasin B in transformed cells as compared to untransformed cells.[148] The former show limited nuclear division by producing only binucleate cells. The transformed cells showed uncontrolled nuclear division; the drug creates cells with many nuclei.

DNA Damage and Repair

Many antineoplastic drugs kill only cells that are in S phase. They are incorporated into replicating DNA or stop its synthesis, which is lethal for S phase cells. Other mutagens and carcinogens damage non-replicating DNA. Cells contain enzymic mechanisms that repair these lesions; for a recent review see Hanawalt, Cooper, Ganesan, et al.[149] Their importance is illustrated in individuals with the genetic disease xeroderma pigmentosum by the high incidence of skin cancer, after exposure to DNA-damaging ultraviolet rays (UV) in sunlight. Xeroderma cells cannot effectively repair lesions created by UV. Relatively little is known about DNA repair mechanisms in higher organisms, not even how many major repair mechanisms are in human cells. The mechanism mainly responsible for repairing UV lesions appears to be almost error-free, but other repair mechanisms are proposed to make errors relatively frequently; these defective repairs can be mutagenic and possibly lead to carcinogenesis. There are relatively few studies of error repair in normal versus tumor cells, although a few differences have been noted.[150]

DNA Function: Transcription

In a mammal all normal cells possess the same genes. Differentiation and development are thought to depend on biochemical processes that activate some of these genes but not others. What these activating factors and their mechanisms are is not known. Some current models for gene activation in eucaryotic cells are based on enzyme induction and repression mechanisms in bacteria.[151]

Genes are expressed through RNA that is copied from them. Before the RNA can be used, *e.g.*, as templates for protein synthesis (mRNA) or as structural and functional components (tRNA and rRNA), it has to be processed and exported from the nucleus into the cytoplasm.

Processing of RNA, a subject of very active investigation, is a set of biochemical changes and includes altering bases, terminally adding adenylic acids, and removing long sequences with splicing of the remaining sequences.[152]

The production and processing of RNA do not as yet seem to be very different in normal and neoplastic cells. Changes in methylation of tRNAs of tumor cells have been reported.[153] Quiescent cells produce RNA less rapidly than do growing cells, and after quiescent cells are activated to grow their transport of RNA precursors and RNA synthesis rise within a few hours.[40] Strong inhibition of RNA synthesis blocks entry of these stimulated cells into S phase,[40] though some recent data indicate that new ribosomal RNA is not essential.

PROSPECTS AND QUESTIONS

An attempt has been made here to summarize briefly, with emphasis on growth control, major concepts under investigation regarding cell biology and biochemistry of neoplastic and non-neoplastic cells. Though an outline is now possible, much remains to be learned and understood. Questions that are somewhat more specific than those asked before have emerged from recent studies; we are entering a period when we should be able to provide biochemical answers to observations of cell biology, using improved technologies of tissue culture, cell biology, biochemistry and genetics.

Some questions currently raised are:

1. What growth factors are required by normal and by neoplastic cells?
2. What biochemical mechanisms determine cell number increase or non-growth?
3. How many "cancer" genes are there and where are they located on chromosomes?
4. What mechanism is responsible for the rapid appearance of chromosomal changes in cancer cells? What roles have these changes?
5. What is the basis of anaplastic morphological and biochemical differentiation in cancer cells?
6. What surface, membrane, and cytoplasmic structural changes are relevant to neoplasia?
7. What role does error-prone DNA repair have in causing malignancy and in creating drug resistance?

The ultimate practical aims of cancer research are to prevent the appearance of cancer cells, and to differentially kill them or at least limit their growth if they do appear. Extensive theoretical and empirical studies have not revealed any differences between tumor and non-tumor cells which serve as a basis for a universally effective therapy. A few empirically discovered drugs inhibit a limited group of tumors, particularly childhood leukemias. The main rationale in current cancer chemotherapy is to try to selectively kill cancer cells by virtue of their greater growth fraction. Perhaps the difference between tumor forming and non-tumor forming cells in the early stages of tumor progression is small and qualitative. Research should tell us what these differences are, and help us to take advantage of them in therapy and prevention.

REFERENCES

1. Skipper HE: In The Proliferation and Spread of Neoplastic Cells, pp 213–233. Baltimore, Williams & Wilkins, 1968
2. Fialkow PJ: Clonal origin and stem cell evolution of human tumors. In Mulvihill JJ, Miller RW, Fraumeni JF Jr (eds): Genetics of Human Cancer, pp 439–452. New York, Raven Press, 1977
3. Foulds L: Neoplastic Development. New York, Academic Press, 1975
4. Pitot HC: Fundamentals of Oncology. New York, Marcel Dekker, 1978
5. Ponten J: The relationship between *in vitro* transformation and tumor formation *in vivo*. Biochim Biophys Acta 458:397–422, 1976
6. Kopelovich L, Bias NE, Helson L: Tumor promoter alone induces neoplastic transformation of fibroblasts from humans genetically predisposed to cancer. Nature 282:619–621, 1979
7. Cohen AJ, Li FP, Berg S et al: Hereditary renal-cell carcinoma associated with a chromosomal translocation. N Engl J Med 301:592–595, 1979
8. Knudson AG Jr, Meadows AT: Regression of neuroblastoma IV-S: a genetic hypothesis. N Engl J Med 302:1254–1256, 1980
9. Cairns J: Cancer: Science and Society. San Francisco, WH Freeman, 1978
10. Diamond L, O'Brien TG, Bard WM: Tumor promoters and the mechanism of tumor promotion. Adv Cancer Res 32:1–74, 1980
11. Klein G: Lymphoma development in mice and humans: diversity of initiation is followed by convergent cytogenetic evolution. Proc Natl Acad Sci USA 76:2442–2446, 1979
12. Heppner GH, Dexter DL, DeNucci T et al: Heterogeneity in drug sensitivity among tumor cell subpopulations of a single mammary tumor. Cancer Res 38:3758–3763, 1978
13. Pratt WB, Ruddon RW: The Anticancer Drugs. Fairlawn, NJ, Oxford Press, 1979
14. Peto R: Epidemiology, multistage models, and short term mutagenicity tests. In Hiatt HH, Watson JD, Winsten JA (eds): Origins of Human Cancer, pp 1403–1428. New York, Cold Spring Harbor Laboratory, 1977
15. Waksman BH, Namba Y: On soluble mediators of immunologic regulation. Cell Immunol 21:161–176, 1976

16. Hill BT: Cancer chemotherapy: the relevance of certain concepts of cell cycle kinetics. Biochim Biophys Acta 516:389–417, 1978
17. McCulloch EA: Granulopoiesis in cultures of human haemopoietic cells. Clin Haematol 4:509–533, 1975
18. Simpson-Herren L, Springer TA, Sanford AH et al: Kinetics of metastases in human tumors. In Day SB (ed): Cancer Invasion and Metastasis: Biologic Mechanisms and Therapy, pp 117–133. New York, Raven Press, 1977
19. Folkman J, Cotran R: Relation of vascular proliferation to tumor growth. Int Rev Exp Pathol 16:207–248, 1976
20. Stiles CD, Kawahara AA: The growth behavior of virus-transformed cells in nude mice. In Fogh J, Giovanella B (eds): The Nude Mouse in Experimental and Clinical Research, pp 385–409. New York, Academic Press, 1978
21. Mintz B: Gene expression in neoplasia and differentiation. Harvey Lect 71:193–246, 1978
22. Pierce GB, Shikes R, Fink LM: Cancer: A Problem of Developmental Biology. Englewood Cliffs, Prentice-Hall, 1978
23. Ringertz NR, Savage RE (eds): Cell Hybrids. New York, Academic Press, 1976
24. Harris H: Some thoughts about genetics, differentiation and malignancy. Somatic Cell Genet 5:923–930, 1979
25. Sager R, Kovac PE: Genetic analysis of tumorigenesis, I. Expression of tumor-forming ability in hamster hybrid cell lines. Somatic Cell Genet 4:375–392, 1978
26. Hellman S, Botnick LE, Hannon EC et al: Proliferative capacity of murine hematopoietic stem cells. Proc Natl Acad Sci USA 75:490–494, 1978
27. Potter VR: Mechanisms of carcinogenesis in relation to studies on minimal deviation hepatomas. In Exploitable Molecular Mechanisms and Neoplasia, pp 587–610. Austin, University of Texas Press, 1968
28. Steele G: Growth Kinetics of Tumors. Oxford, Clarendon Press, 1977
29. Clarkson B, Baserga R (eds): Control of Proliferation in Animal Cells. New York, Cold Spring Harbor Laboratory, 1976
30. Jakoby WB, Pastan IH (eds): Methods in Enzymology 58: Cell Culture. New York, Academic Press, 1979
31. Owens R, Smith H, Nelson-Rees W et al: Epithelial cell cultures from normal and cancerous human tissues. JNCI 56:843–849, 1976
32. Rheinwald JG, Green H: Serial cultivation of strains of human epidermal keratinocytes: the formation of keratinizing colonies from single cells. Cell 6:331–344, 1975
33. Kirkland WL, Yang NS, Jorgensen T et al: Growth of normal and malignant human mammary epithelial cells in culture. JNCI 63:29–41, 1979
34. Giard DJ, Aaronson SA, Todaro GJ et al: *In vitro* cultivation of human tumors: establishment of cell lines derived from a series of solid tumors. JNCI 51:1417–1423, 1973
35. Salmon SE, Hamburger AW, Soehnlen B et al: Quantitation of differential sensitivity of human-tumor stem cells to anticancer drugs. N Engl J Med 298:1321–1327, 1978
36. Todaro GJ, Green H: Quantitative studies of the growth of mouse embryo cells in culture and their development into established lines. J Cell Biol 17:299–313, 1963
37. Good PI: Aging in mammalian cell populations: a review. Mech Ageing Dev 4:339–348, 1975
38. Smets LA: Cell transformation as a model for tumor induction and neoplastic growth. Biochim Biophys Acta 605:93–111, 1980
39. Abercrombie M: Contact inhibition and malignancy. Nature 281:259–262, 1979
40. Baserga R: Multiplication and Division in Mammalian Cells. New York, Marcel Dekker, 1976
41. Prescott DM: The cell cycle and the control of cellular reproduction. Adv Genet 18:99–177, 1976
42. Folkman J, Moscona A: Role of cell shape in growth control. Nature 273:345–349, 1978
43. Bartholomew JC, Yokoto H, Ross P: Effect of serum on the growth of Balb 3T3 A31 mouse fibroblasts and an SV40-transformed derivative. J Cell Physiol 88:277–286, 1976
44. Barrett JC, Ts'o PO: Relationship between somatic mutation and neoplastic transformation. Proc Natl Acad Sci USA 75:3297–3301, 1978
45. Tooze J (ed): The Molecular Biology of Tumor Viruses. New York, Cold Spring Harbor Laboratory, 1980
46. Risser R, Pollack R: A non-selective analysis of SV40 transformation of mouse 3T3 cells. Virology 59:477–489, 1974
47. Stiles CD, Desmond W, Sato G et al: Failure of human cells transformed by SV40 virus to form tumors in athymic nude mice. Proc Natl Acad Sci USA 72:4971–4975, 1975
48. Blumberg BS, Larouzé B, London WT et al: Primary hepatic carcinoma and hepatitis B infection: a summary of recent work. In Nieburgs HE (ed): Prevention and Detection of Cancer, Vol 2, Cancer Detection in Specific Sites, pp 2151–2162. New York, Marcel Dekker, 1980
49. Kakunaga T: Neoplastic transformation of human diploid fibroblast cells by chemical carcinogens. Proc Natl Acad Sci USA 75:1334–1338, 1978
50. Milo GE, DiPaolo JA: Neoplastic transformation of human diploid cells *in vitro* after chemical carcinogen treatment. Nature 275:130–132, 1978
51. Dubrow R, Riddle VGH, Pardee AB: Different responses to drugs and serum of cells transformed by various means. Cancer Res 39:2718–2726, 1979
52. Holley RW, Kiernan JA: "Contact inhibition" of cell division in 3T3 cells. Proc Natl Acad Sci USA 60:300–304, 1968
53. Stoker MGP: Role of diffusion boundary layer in contact inhibition of growth. Nature 246:200–203, 1973
54. Eagle H, Foley GE, Koprowski H et al: Growth characteristics of virus-transformed cells. J Exp Med 131:863–879, 1970
55. Barrett JC, Ts'o PO: Evidence for the progressive nature of neoplastic transformation *in vitro*. Proc Natl Acad Sci USA 75:3761–3765, 1978
56. Stanbridge EJ, Wilkinson J: Analysis of malignancy in human cells: malignant and transformed phenotypes are under separate genetic control. Proc Natl Acad Sci USA 75:1466–1469, 1978
57. Epifanova OI: Mechanisms underlying the differential sensitivity of proliferating and resting cells to external factors. In International Review of Cytology, Supplement F, pp 303–335. New York, Academic Press, 1977
58. Sato GH, Ross R: Hormones and Cell Culture: A and B. New York, Cold Spring Harbor Laboratory, 1979
59. Pledger WJ, Stiles CD, Antoniades HN et al: An ordered sequence of events is required before BALB/c-3T3 cells become committed to DNA synthesis. Proc Natl Acad Sci USA 75:2839–2843, 1978
60. Benecke B, Ben-Ze'ev A, Penman S: The control of mRNA production, translation and turnover in suspended and reattached anchorage-dependent fibroblasts. Cell 14:931–939, 1978
61. Hershko A, Mamont P, Shields R et al: Pleiotypic response. Nature [New Biol] 232:206–211, 1971
62. Holley RH: Control of growth of kidney epithelial cells in culture. In Sato GH, Ross R (eds): Hormones and Cell Culture, pp 455–459. New York, Cold Spring Harbor Laboratory, 1979
63. Pardee AB, James LJ: Selective killing of transformed baby hamster kidney (BHK) cells. Proc Natl Acad Sci USA 72:4994–4998, 1975
64. Gelfant S: A new concept of tissue and tumor cell proliferation. Cancer Res 37:3845–3862, 1977
65. Pardee AB: A restriction point for control of normal animal cell proliferation. Proc Natl Acad Sci USA 71:1286–1290, 1974
66. Brooks RF: The kinetics of serum-induced initiation of DNA synthesis in BHK 21/C13 cells, and the influence of exogenous adenosine. J Cell Physiol 86:369–377, 1975
67. Brooks RF, Bennett DC, Smith JA: Mammalian cell cycles need two random transitions. Cell 19:493–504, 1980
68. Holley RW, Baldwin JH, Kiernan JA et al: Control of growth of benzo(a)pyrene-transformed 3T3 cells. Proc Natl Acad Sci USA 73:3229–3232, 1976
69. O'Neill FJ: Differential *in vitro* growth properties of cells transformed by DNA and RNA tumor viruses. Exp Cell Res 117:393–401, 1978
70. Moses HL, Wells DJ, Swartzendruber DE et al: Comparison of

RNA metabolism in G1-arrested and stimulated nontransformed and chemically transformed mouse embryo cells in culture. Cancer Res 39:4516–4524, 1979
71. Yen A, Pardee AB: Exponential 3T3 cells escape in mid-G1 from their high serum requirement. Exp Cell Res 116:103–113, 1978
72. Schneiderman MH, Dewey WC, Highfield DP: Inhibition of DNA synthesis in synchronized Chinese hamster cells treated in G1 with cycloheximide. Exp Cell Res 67:147–155, 1971
73. Brooks RF: Continuous protein synthesis is required to maintain the probability of entry into S phase. Cell 12:311–317, 1977
74. Rossow PW, Riddle VGH, Pardee AB: Synthesis of labile, serum-dependent protein in early G1 controls animal cell growth. Proc Natl Acad Sci USA 76:4446–4450, 1979
75. Medrano EE, Pardee AB: A prevalent deficiency in tumor cells of cycle arrest by cycloheximide. Proc Natl Acad Sci USA 77:4123–4126, 1980
76. Gunn JM, Clark MG, Knowles SE et al: Reduced rates of proteolysis in transformed cells. Nature 266:58–60, 1977
77. Warburton MJ, Poole B: Effect of medium composition on protein degradation and DNA synthesis in rat embryo fibroblasts. Proc Natl Acad Sci USA 74:2427–2431, 1977
78. Gospodarowicz D, Greenburg G, Bialecki H et al: Factors involved in the modulation of cell proliferation *in vivo* and *in vitro*: the role of fibroblast and epidermal growth factors in the proliferative response of mammalian cells. In Vitro 14:85–118, 1978
79. Stiles CD, Capone GT, Scher CD et al: Dual control of cell growth by somatomedins and platelet-derived growth factor. Proc Natl Acad Sci USA 76:1279–1283, 1979
80. Murakami H, Masui H: Hormonal control of human colon carcinoma cell growth in serum-free medium. Proc Natl Acad Sci USA 77:3464–3468, 1980
81. Cherington PV, Smith BL, Pardee AB: Loss of epidermal growth factor requirement and malignant transformation. Proc Natl Acad Sci USA 76:3937–3941, 1979
82. McKeehan WL, McKeehan KA: Serum factors modify the cellular requirement for Ca^{2+}, K^{+}, Mg^{2+}, phosphate ions, and 2-oxocarboxylic acids for multiplication of normal human fibroblasts. Proc Natl Acad Sci USA 77:3417–3421, 1980
83. Scher CD, Stone ME, Stiles CD: Platelet-derived growth factor prevents G0 arrest. Nature 281:390–392, 1979
84. Shields R: Growth factors for tumors. Nature 272:670–671, 1978
85. DeLarco JE, Reynolds R, Carlberg K et al: Sarcoma growth factor from mouse sarcoma virus-transformed cells. J Biol Chem 255:3685–3690, 1980
86. Houck JC (ed): Chalones. Amsterdam, North-Holland, 1976
87. Habenicht AJR, Glomset JA, Ross R: Relation of cholesterol and mevalonic acid to the cell cycle in smooth muscle and Swiss 3T3 cells stimulated to divide by platelet-derived growth factor. J Biol Chem 255:5134–5140, 1980
88. Brown MS, Goldstein JL: Multivalent feedback regulation of HMG CoA reductase, a control mechanism coordinating isoprenoid synthesis and cell growth. J Lipid Res 21:505–517, 1980
89. Frantz CN, Stiles CD, Scher CD: The tumor promoter 12-0-tetradecanoyl-phorbol-13-acetate enhances the proliferative response of Balb/c-3T3 cells to hormonal growth factors. J Cell Physiol 100:413–424, 1979
90. Pardee AB: Cell division and a hypothesis of cancer. JNCI 14:7–20, 1964
91. Burger MM: Cell surfaces in neoplastic transformation. In Horecker BL, Stadtman ER (eds): Current Topics in Cellular Regulation, Vol 3, pp 135–193. New York, Academic Press, 1971
92. Emmelot P: Biochemical properties of normal and neoplastic cell surfaces: a review. Eur J Cancer 9:319–333, 1973
93. Nicolson GL, Poste G: The cancer cell: dynamic aspects and modifications in cell-surface organization. N Engl J Med 295:197–203, 1976
94. Nicolson GL: Transmembrane control of the receptors on normal and tumor cells. Biochim Biophys Acta 458:1–72, 1976
95. DeLeo AB, Jay G, Appella E et al: Detection of a transformation-related antigen in chemically induced sarcomas and other transformed cells of the mouse. Proc Natl Acad Sci USA 76:2420–2424, 1979
96. Bramwell ME, Harris H: Some further information about the abnormal membrane glycoprotein associated with malignancy. Proc R Soc Lond (B) 203:93–99, 1978
97. Hynes RO, Fox CF (eds): Tumor Cell Surfaces and Malignancy. New York, Alan R Liss, 1980
98. Gospodarowicz D, Ill CR: Do plasma and serum have different abilities to promote cell growth? Proc Natl Acad Sci USA 77:2726–2730, 1980
99. Reich E, Rifkin D, Shaw E (eds): Proteases and Biological Control. New York, Cold Spring Harbor Laboratory, 1975
100. Chen LB, Summerhayes I, Hsieh P et al: Possible role of fibronectin in malignancy. J Supramol Struct 12:139–150, 1979
101. Hatanaka M: Transport of sugars in tumor cell membranes. Biochim Biophys Acta 355:77–104, 1974
102. Rozengurt E: Early events in growth stimulation. In Hynes RO (ed): Surfaces of Normal and Malignant Cells, pp 323–353. New York, John Wiley & Sons, 1979
103. Leffert HL (ed): Growth Regulation by Ion Fluxes. Ann NY Acad Sci 339: 1980
104. Naiditch WP, Cunningham DD: Hexose uptake and control of fibroblast proliferation. J Cell Physiol 92:319–332, 1977
105. Carney DH, Cunningham DD: Cell surface action of thrombin is sufficient to initiate division of chick cells. Cell 14:811–823, 1978
106. Gorden P, Carpentier J, Cohen S et al: Epidermal growth factor: morphological demonstration of binding, internalization, and lysosomal association in human fibroblasts. Proc Natl Acad Sci USA 75:5025–5029, 1978
107. Das M, Fox CF: Molecular mechanism of mitogen action: processing of receptor induced by epidermal growth factor. Proc Natl Acad Sci USA 75:2644–2648, 1978
108. Carpenter G, King L, Cohen S: Rapid enhancement of protein phosphorylation in A-431 cell membrane preparations by epidermal growth factor. J Biol Chem 254:4884–4891, 1979
109. Das M: Mitogenic hormone-induced intracellular message: assay and partial characterization of an activator of DNA replication induced by epidermal growth factor. Proc Natl Acad Sci USA 77:112–116, 1980
110. Singer SJ, Ash JF, Bourguignon LYW et al: Transmembrane interactions and the mechanisms of transport of proteins across membranes. J Supramol Struct 9:373–389, 1978
111. Lazarides E: Intermediate filaments as mechanical integrators of cellular space. Nature 283:249–256, 1980
112. Hynes RO: Cell surface proteins and malignant transformation. Biochim Biophys Acta 458:73–107, 1976
113. Tucker RW, Sanford KK, Frankel FR: Tubulin and actin in paired nonneoplastic and spontaneously transformed neoplastic cell lines *in vitro*: fluorescent antibody studies. Cell 13:629–642, 1978
114. McClain DA, Edelman GM: Density-dependent stimulation and inhibition of cell growth by agents that disrupt microtubules. Proc Natl Acad Sci USA 77:2748–2752, 1980
115. Tucker RW, Pardee AB, Fujiwara K: Centriole ciliation is related to quiescence and DNA synthesis in 3T3 cells. Cell 17:527–535, 1979
116. Yamamoto KR, Alberts BM: Steroid receptors: elements for modulation of eukaryotic transcription. Annual Rev Biochem 45:721–746, 1976
117. Pastan I, Johnson GS: Cyclic AMP and the transformation of fibroblasts. Adv Cancer Res 19:303–329, 1974
118. Rebhun LI: Cyclic nucleotides, calcium, and cell division. Int Rev Cytol 49:1–54, 1977
119. Greengard P: Phosphorylated proteins as physiological effectors. Science 199:146–152, 1978
120. Coffino P, Bourne HR, Friedrich U et al: Molecular mechanisms of cyclic AMP action: a genetic approach. Recent Prog Horm Res 32:669–684, 1976
121. Haddox MK, Magun BE, Russell DH: Differential expression

of type I and type II cyclic AMP-dependent protein kinases during cell cycle and cyclic AMP-induced growth arrest. Proc Natl Acad Sci USA 77:3445–3449, 1980

122. Cheung WY: Calmodulin plays a pivotal role in cellular regulation. Science 207:19–27, 1980
123. Means AR, Dedman JR: Calmodulin: an intracellular calcium receptor. Nature 285:73–77, 1980
124. Whitfield JF, Boynton AL, MacManus JP et al: The roles of calcium and cyclic AMP in cell proliferation. Ann NY Acad Sci 339:216–240, 1980
125. Weber G: Enzymology of cancer cells. N Engl J Med 296:486, 1977; 296:551, 1977
126. Greenstein JP: Biochemistry of Cancer, 2nd ed. New York, Academic Press, 1954
127. Loewenstein WR: Junctional intercellular communication and the control of growth. Biochim Biophys Acta 560:1–65, 1979
128. Weil R: Viral 'tumor antigens': a novel type of mammalian regulator protein. Biochim Biophys Acta 516:301–388, 1978
129. Collett MS, Erickson RL: Protein kinase activity associated with the avian sarcoma virus *src* gene product. Proc Natl Acad Sci USA 75:2021–2024, 1978
130. Hunter T, Sefton BM: Transforming gene product of Rous sarcoma virus phosphorylates tyrosine. Proc Natl Acad Sci USA 77:1311–1315, 1980
131. Rigby P: The transforming genes of SV40 and polyoma. Nature 282:781–784, 1979
132. Warburg O: On the origin of cancer cells. Science 123:309–315, 1956
133. Weinhouse S: Metabolism and isozyme alterations in experimental hepatomas. Fed Proc 32:2162–2167, 1973
134. Bissell MJ: Transport as a rate limiting step in glucose metabolism in virus-transformed cells. J Cell Physiol 89:701–710, 1976
135. Racker E: Why do tumor cells have a high aerobic glycolysis? J Cell Physiol 89:697–700, 1976
136. Howell N, Sager R: Differential effects of mitochondrial inhibitors on normal and tumorigenic mouse cells. Fed Proc 36:356, 1977
137. Taylor JM: DNA intermediates of avian RNA tumor viruses. Curr Top Microbiol Immunol 87:23–41, 1979
138. Shih C, Shilo B, Goldfarb MP et al: Passage of phenotypes of chemically transformed cells via transfection of DNA and chromatin. Proc Natl Acad Sci USA 76:5714–5718, 1979
139. Cooper GM, Okenquist S, Silverman L: Transforming activity of DNA of chemically transformed and normal cells. Nature 284:418–421, 1980
140. Smith HS, Springer EL, Hackett AJ: Nuclear ultrastructure of epithelial cell lines derived from human carcinomas and nonmalignant tissues. Cancer Res 39:332–344, 1979
141. Hamlin JL, Pardee AB: Control of DNA synthesis in tissue culture cells. In Vitro 14:119–127, 1978
142. Kornberg A: DNA Replication. San Francisco, WH Freeman, 1979
143. Pardoll DM, Vogelstein B, Coffey DS: A fixed site of DNA replication in eucaryotic cells. Cell 19:527–536, 1980
144. Mathews CK, North TW, Reddy GPV: Multienzyme complexes in DNA precursor biosynthesis. Adv Enzyme Regul 17:133–156, 1979
145. Reddy GPV, Pardee AB: Multienzyme complex for metabolic channeling in mammalian DNA replication. Proc Natl Acad Sci USA 77:3312–3316, 1980
146. Rattle HWE, Kneale GG, Baldwin JP et al: Histone complexes, nucleosomes, chromatin and cell-cycle dependent modification of histones. In Nicolini CA (ed): Chromatin Structure and Function, pp 451–513. New York, Plenum Press, 1978
147. Tsuboi A, Baserga R: Synthesis of nuclear acidic proteins in density-inhibited fibroblasts stimulated to proliferate. J Cell Physiol 80:107–117, 1972
148. O'Neill FJ: Control of nuclear division and chromosomal abnormalities in cytochalasin B-treated normal and transformed cells. In Tanenbaum SW (ed): Cytochalasins: Biochemical and Cell Biological Aspects, pp 217–255. Amsterdam, North-Holland–Elsevier, 1978
149. Hanawalt PC, Cooper PK, Ganesan AK et al: DNA repair in bacteria and mammalian cells. Annu Rev Biochem 48:783–836, 1979
150. Day RS, Ziolkowski CHJ: Human brain tumour cell strains with deficient host-cell reactivation of *N*-methyl-*N'*-nitro-*N*-nitrosoguanidine-damaged adenovirus 5. Nature 279:797–799, 1979
151. Miller JH, Reznikoff WS (ed): The Operon. New York, Cold Spring Harbor Laboratory, 1978
152. Abelson J: RNA process and the intervening sequence problem. Annu Rev Biochem 48:1035–1069, 1979
153. Kuchino Y, Borek E: Tumour-specific phenylalanine tRNA contains two supernumerary methylated bases. Nature 271:126–129, 1978

CHAPTER 4

Samuel Hellman
Vincent T. DeVita, Jr.

Principles of Cancer Biology: Kinetics of Cellular Proliferation

An understanding of the kinetics of cellular proliferation and of the cell replication cycle is a prerequisite to studies of the growth and maturation of normal tissues, response of normal tissues to cytotoxic agents, growth of malignant tissue, and treatment strategies of malignant disease. A malignant tumor may be characterized as a cell population that continually increases. This increase may not be regular, rapid, or efficient, but it occurs until the host's death. In contrast, cells of many normal tissues proliferate to achieve and to maintain a population size that is useful physiologically. In both tumors and these normal tissues there will be cell birth and cell death. However, in normal tissue during the steady state, cell birth equals death. As tumors grow, cell birth must exceed cell death. The control of the normal tissues in the steady state is not well understood but such control may be: positive (stimulatory) or negative (inhibitory); humoral and effective at great distances (hormones); substances released locally (chalones); or contact-related (contact inhibition by like cells or stimulation by matrix produced by cells).

CELL REPLICATION CYCLE

The cell replication cycle was first described by Howard and Pelc in 1951, using ^{32}P as as a cell marker synthesizing DNA.[1] Tritiated thymidine has replaced this. As shown in Figure 4-1, the cell replication cycle can be divided into discrete phases.[2] Beginning at the completion of mitosis, cells may spend a variable period of time in a presynthetic phase, (G1). Following this, the cells enter the DNA synthetic phase (S); then the cells cease DNA synthesis and enter the G2 phase before mitosis (M). The mitotic phase can be identified under the light microscope while the synthetic phase (S) can be determined by incorporating tritiated thymidine, as described below. G1 and G2 are the gaps between these two identifiable events. The durations of S, G2, and M are fairly constant; however, the variation is very great for G1. The term G0 has been introduced for cells not in cycle but able to be recruited into cycle, entering in the G1 period.[3] Some believe that G1 is not so variable, but measurements of it include both G1 and a variable number of cells in G0. In mammalian cells, M appears to be consistently short (30–90 minutes), S usually 8–30 hours in both normal and malignant tissues, G2 is less accurately determined, but is quite short (probably an hour or so). The great variability is in G1.[4]

The basic technique for determining the length of the cell cycle and duration of the four separate phases is the *percent labeled mitosis curve* (PLM), derived from autoradiographs prepared after the injection of tritiated thymidine.[5] Following a single injection of tritiated thymidine, samples of the tumor are taken and autoradiographs prepared. Cells in S at injection or their progeny will be labeled (silver grains over the nucleus) due to decay of the radioactive tritium exposing the photographic emulsion overlayed on the cells (see Fig. 4-2). In tissues sampled shortly after injection, all labeled cells are still in S. However, if a longer period of time were allowed then the labeled cells would have moved through G2 and into the next cell cycle. An idealized plot of the percent of mitoses labeled as a function of time after the injection of tritiated thymidine is illustrated in Fig. 4-3. Immediately following injection no mitoses are labeled since the only labeled cells are in S. Therefore, the minimum time before the beginning

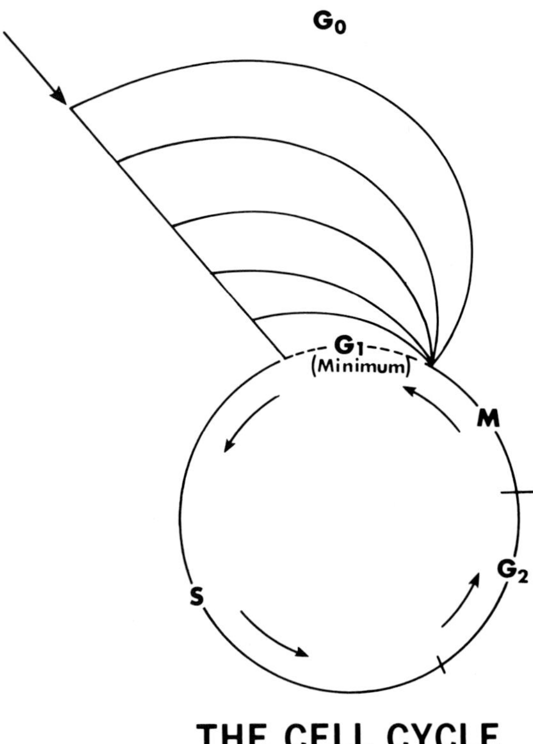

FIG. 4-1. The cell cycle.

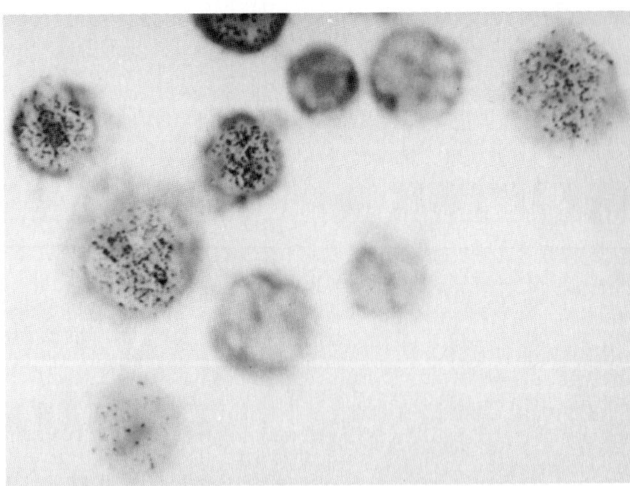

FIG. 4-2. An example of cells labeled with tritiated thymidine. The black silver grains that have formed due to exposure of the photographic emulsion are restricted to the nucleus indicating that the labeled cell was synthesizing DNA at the time of sampling.

of labeled mitoses is an estimate of the time it took cells in late S to traverse G2 and enter mitosis. The percent of labeled mitotic figures increases rapidly as all those cells in S pass through M. Then it begins to fall. An estimate of the duration of S is then this large plateau of labeled mitoses with a second wave of labeled mitoses occurring with the next cell cycle. From any point in the first wave to that in the second gives an estimate of the cycle time. This is the basic technique for determining cell cycle characteristics. The rise in the second peak is a measure of the extent of variation of cell cycle times. If it is equal in height to the first peak, the cells all have the same cycle time. Alternatively, if it cannot be discerned, the cells have a very varied cycle time. The latter is the case in human tumors (see Fig. 4-4).[6] Computer programs have been described to make some estimate of the range of cell cycle time using this parameter.[7,8]

Another technique using tritiated thymidine requiring only a single sample of the tumor is the *labeling index*. This measures the proportion of cells that are labelled as compared to the total population of cells. If all cells are in the cell cycle, the labeling index will be proportional to the duration of S. Since this is usually not the case, the labeling index is used as a general measure of proliferative activity.

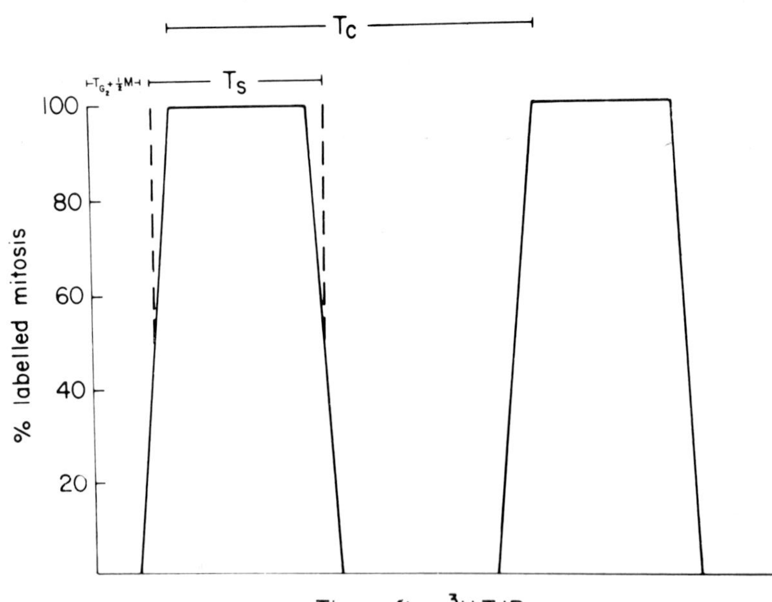

FIG. 4-3. An idealized percent labelled mitosis curve.

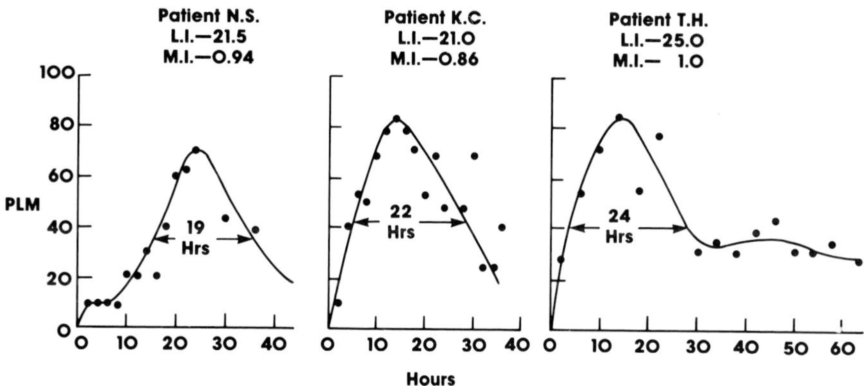

FIG. 4-4. Actual labelled mitosis curves for human breast cancer. L.I. = labelling index; M.I. = mitotic index.

NORMAL TISSUES

From a kinetic standpoint, normal tissues may be divided into four categories.

CELL RENEWAL TISSUES

In these, proliferation occurs to replace cells of limited life span. There is both extensive cell birth and cell death. Examples of such tissues include the mucosa of the gastrointestinal system, bladder, vagina, and the skin. A variation of these are the exocrine glands whose pattern of proliferation is in response to stimulation, either locally or systemically. An example of the latter is the breast.

NON-PROLIFERATING TISSUES

Examples of these include neuronal cells and striated muscle.

CELLS EXHIBITING LITTLE IF ANY PROLIFERATIVE ACTIVITY DURING THE STEADY STATE

Examples include smooth muscle, connective tissue, capillary endothelium, and hepatic parenchyma.

CELL PROLIFERATION IN RESPONSE TO PHYSIOLOGIC NEEDS

Periosteal cells after a fracture and the liver after hepatectomy are two examples of cell proliferation in response to physiologic needs.

The renewing cell populations are most important to the oncologist. It is their continued proliferation that is most susceptible to cytotoxic agents These tissues are thought to have the compartments described in Fig. 4-5, with the stem cells as the progenitors of the compartment. In the steady state, they are usually proliferatively inactive and serve as reserve cells. Their active proliferation is seen only when the pool size is markedly reduced or during the expansion of fetal life. The committed stem cell population tends to be active with extensive proliferation. These cells give rise to the proliferative compartment when great expansion as well as maturation occurs. Finally, the cells are no longer capable of cell division and continue maturation until the adult functioning cell is produced. This has a finite life span that is usually short. As long as entrance into the maturation compartment exactly equals cell death, the pool of cells will not expand regardless of the proliferative rate of the compartment. There is some evidence that stem cells have a limitation on their proliferative capacity, which may be the cause of many

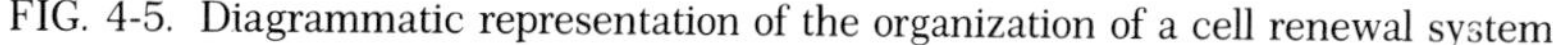
FIG. 4-5. Diagrammatic representation of the organization of a cell renewal system.

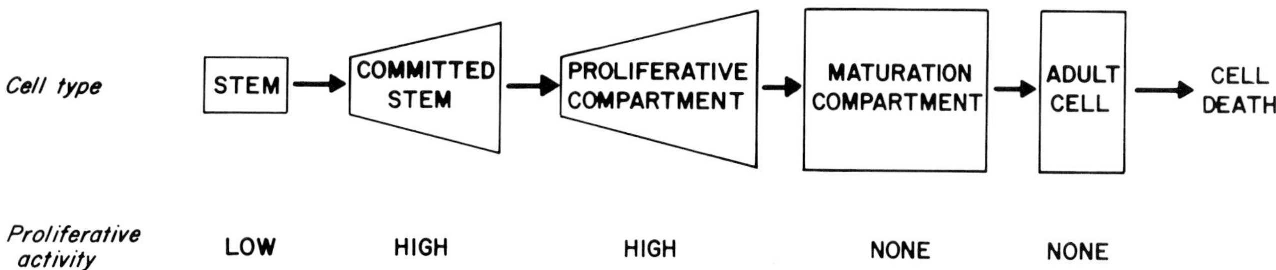

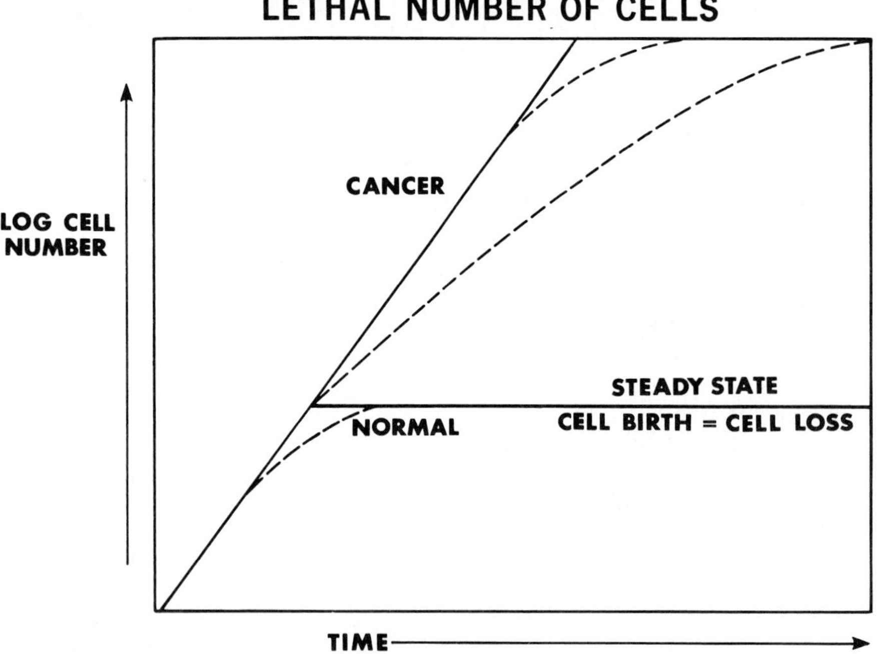

FIG. 4-6. A comparison of normal and malignant growth.

of the late effects seen following certain cytotoxic agents.[9,10] This is discussed in greater detail in Chapter 7.

A comparison of normal and malignant growth, emphasizing that both may be kinetically quite active, is depicted in Fig. 4-6. Tumors too may have stem cells and mature cells as well as significant cell death.[11] Whatever the organization, cell birth must exceed cell death in order for the tumor to expand. Since not all cells in a tumor may be participating in active proliferation, Mendelsohn defined the term *growth fraction* (GF) to describe that portion of the population involved in proliferation.[12] The remaining cells may or may not be able to be stimulated to divide. Some may not because they have matured and thus are really committed end cells. Examples of these include the keratinized cells frequently seen in squamous carcinoma of the skin. Others may be capable of extensive proliferation but are deprived of nutrients due to geographic separation from the capillary caused by the tumor growth. Finally, these non-proliferating cells may be quiescent in response to some unknown inhibitor.

Tumors may also have significant *cell loss*. This is difficult to determine directly. Steel related cell loss to the difference between the actual doubling time measured and the potential doubling time possible based on all the kinetic parameters of tumor growth.[13] The causes of cell loss in a tumor might include maturation of the cells and eventual death. The latter might merely be exfoliation of mature cells from the surface of differentiating cancer, such as those of the skin and oral mucosa. Cell death due to inadequate nutrition may also be a cause. Tumors appear to have areas of necrosis at distances of 150 μ or so from the nutrient capillaries.[13] Cell loss may also be due to failed mitosis. Observation of tumors often shows bizarre mitotic figures. These unsuccessful mitoses may be related to the aneuploid nature of tumors. Host defenses may also destroy some tumor cells causing some cell loss. Finally, it is conceivable that shedding of cells in the formation of metastases accounts for some of the cell loss seen.

A diagram of an experimental murine mammary carcinoma with some of the kinetic parameters enumerated is shown in Fig. 4-7. Cells closest to the capillary have the highest growth fraction.[15] As the distance from the capillary increases, the GF decreases. However, the cell cycle time remains the same.

Much research has been concerned with cell population kinetics following administration of radiation or chemotherapy. Following radiation, tumors can be shown to decrease or increase their intermitotic time.[16–19] Extrapolation of tumor regrowth after chemotherapy or radiation suggests decrease in the doubling time. It has been suggested that the effect of treatment may not only be to reduce cell number, but also to return the tumor to the rapid growth seen in smaller tumors.[20]

STUDIES OF HUMAN TUMORS

The first quantitative study of the human tumor growth rate was made by Collins and coworkers in 1956 using serial radiographs of pulmonary metastases.[21] This work has been greatly expanded by a number of authors and reviewed by Tubiana and Malaise.[22] Tumors appear to grow exponentially. However, with experimental tumors the doubling time increases as the tumor grows. That is to say that the exponent of growth reduces as a function of tumor size. This relationship is described mathematically as a Gompertzian function.[23] Whether this also occurs in humans is difficult to determine since the range of tumor growth available to be studied is quite limited in ethically justifiable clinical circumstances. It appears highly likely, however, that human tumors as well as experimental tumors have Gompertzian growth kinetics. This is important when the physician attempts to extrapolate from

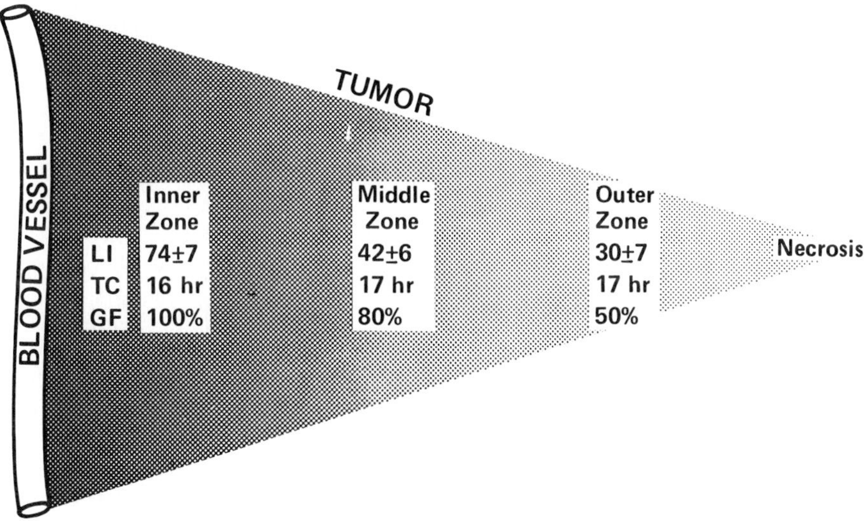

FIG. 4-7. Cell kinetic parameters of a mouse mammary carcinoma. (Tannock LF: The relation between cell proliferation and the vascular system in a transplanted mouse mammary tumour. Br J Cancer 22:258–273, 1968)

doubling times in the clinic to preclinical circumstances in order to estimate the time the tumor growth started. Such extrapolations are almost certainly erroneous and tend to overestimate the tumor lifespan in the preclinical period. In the extreme case, it may be determined that tumors begin before conception. Salmon, using data obtained from the immunoglobulin produced in multiple myeloma, suggests that the growth of this human tumor is indeed Gompertzian.[24]

Despite these considerations, the doubling times of clinical tumors have been determined. They may vary widely but some useful general statements can be made about them. Metastases in the same patient tend to grow at approximately the same rate while the same histologic tumor type arising in different patients may differ widely. The doubling times for various histologic types are shown in Table 4-1.[22,25,26] Also, while there is a general order of doubling times the distribution bution within each histologic group is very wide and therefore the doubling times greatly overlap each other. There is a crude relationship between the doubling time of human tumors and survival time. This effect, however, is quite muted.

Metastases tend to grow more rapidly than the primary tumor as demonstrated in Table 4-2. A number of reasons have been suggested for this:

1. The selection of the more malignant clone by the metastatic process
2. Tumor progression
3. These are usually measured in the lung or on the skin and these sites may be especially conducive to more rapid growth.

A number of human tumor cell cycle times have been measured by a number of authors. These are illustrated in Table 4-3.[22,27–37] Ninety percent of the values of the cell cycle time vary between 15 and 120 hours with a modal value of approximately 48 hours. S seems to be less variable with 90% of the values falling between 9½ and 24 hours with a modal value of approximately 16. Using the techniques previously described (doubling times; labeling index; GF; cell loss factor; and daily tumor turnover, another measurement of cell loss), were measured and are shown in Table 4-1. Cell loss from

TABLE 4-1. Kinetic parameters of some human tumors

TYPE	DOUBLING TIME (DAYS)	LABELING INDEX (%)	GROWTH FRACTION (%)	CELL LOSS (%)	DAILY TURNOVER RATE (%)
Embryomal Tumors	27 (76)	30 (30)	90	93	49
Lymphomas	29 (41)	29 (15)	90	93	47
Sarcomas	41 (87)	4 (32)	11	68	5.5
Squamous Carcinomas	58 (51)	8 (68)	25	89	10
Adenocarcinomas	83 (134)	2 (121)	6	71	2

(Adapted from Tubiana M: Malaise EP: Growth rate and cell kinetics in human tumours: some prognostic and therapeutic implications. In Symington T, Carter RL (eds). Scientific Foundations of Oncology, pp 126–136. Chicago, Year Book, 1976)

TABLE 4-2. Doubling time (measured in days) of primary tumors and their pulmonary metastases

TYPE	PRIMARY	METASTASES
Squamous Carcinomas	82 (97)	58 (51)
Adenocarinomas	166 (34)	83 (134)

(Adapted from Charbit A, Malaise E, Tubiana M: Relation between the pathological nature and the growth rate of human tumours. Europ J Cancer 7:307–315, 1971)

TABLE 4-3. Some cell cycle measurements (measured in hours) of human solid tumors

AUTHORS	CELL CYCLE TIME
Frindel and coworkers	97, 51, 28, 48, 50
Bennington	16, 15
Young and DeVita	42, 82, 74
Shirakawa and coworkers	120, 144
Weinstein and Frost	217
Terz and coworkers	45, 31, 14, 26, 26, 42
Peckham and Steel	59
Estevez and coworkers	37, 30, 48, 30, 38, 96, 48
Terz and Curutchet	18, 19, 19, 120
Malaise and coworkers	24, 33, 48, 42
Muggia and coworkers	64
Bresciani and coworkers	82, 50, 67, 53, 58

(Tubiana M, Malaise EP: Growth rate and cell kinetics in human tumours: some prognostic and therapeutic implications. *In* Symington T, Carter RL (eds), Scientific Foundations of Oncology, pp 126–136. Chicago, Year Book, 1976)

solid tumors is sometimes considerable, possibly explaining why the doubling time may be 30 to 90 times longer than the duration of the cell cycle. It cannot, however, be invoked to account for the differences between the mean duration of doubling time for the various histologic groups. The latter appears to be more closely related to the GF. Use of the PLM curve for human tumors in general shows a very poorly defined second peak.[6] This suggests that the cells have almost completely lost synchrony by the second division, indicating that the spread of intermitotic times must be very large.

Ascites tumors and leukemias have also been studied and compared to solid tumors.[38–41] Clarkson and coworkers have shown that ascites tumors appear to have a longer duration of S and G1 than do the corresponding solid tumor. In experimental animals, it appears as though the GF of ascites tumors is unified but that cell cycle length can be variable.[42,43] As ascites tumors and leukemia decelerate growth, the cell cycle lengthens and there is also some decrease in GF. Solid tumors usually decrease growth rate by decreasing GF and increasing cell loss without significant change in cell cycle time. In the leukemias there appear to be two types of cells—large and small. The large cells tend to be stimulated to reenter mitosis.[39] The rapidly proliferating L-1210 leukemia of mice has been used to develop strategies of chemotherapy and will be described separately in Chapter 8.

NEW METHODS OF CELL KINETICS

The data described have largely been obtained by the use of the autoradiography techniques that are difficult to use on humans. They are also very slow and time consuming and thus cannot be used to influence the therapy of an individual patient. The possibility of using cell kinetics data on a routine basis to plan treatment may now be possible because of the development of flow cytometry. This technique uses suspensions of tumor cells and fluorescent stains that label DNA. The amount of fluorescence is proportional to the DNA content. Presynthetic cells have two n DNA, postsynthetic cells have four n DNA and those in S vary between 2n and 4n. Using this information, a great deal of cell kinetic information can be determined. Gray and colleagues have used a cell sorter to separate cells in a narrow intermediate range of DNA content using fluorescent labeling.[44] They then inject tritiated thymidine and study its rise and fall through this narrow window of intermediary DNA. This technique can be likened to the PLMs. However, it requires no autoradiography, can be done promptly, and its results can be related to therapy. Time will tell whether these or other techniques will have an important role in the planning of therapy.

REFERENCES

1. Howard P, Pelc SR: Nuclear incorporation of ^{32}P as demonstrated by autoradiographs. Exp Cell Res 2:178–187, 1951
2. DeVita VT: Cell kinetics and the chemotherapy of cancer. Cancer Treat Rep 2:23–33, 1971
3. Baserga R: Multiplication and Division in Mammalian Cells, pp 53–77. New York, Marcel Dekker, 1976.
4. Baserga R: The relationship of the cell cycle to tumor growth and control of cell division: a review. Cancer Res 25:581–595, 1965
5. Quastler H, Sherman FG: Cell population kinetics in the intestinal epithelium of the mouse. Exp Cell Res 17:428–438, 1959.
6. Steel GG: Growth Kinetics of Tumors, pp 204–205. Oxford, Clarendon Press, 1977
7. Barrett JC: A mathematical model of the mitotic cycle and its application to the interpretation of percent labelled mitosis data J. Nat Cancer Inst 37:443–450, 1966
8. Steel GG, Hanes S: The technique of labelled mitosis: analysis by automatic curve fitting. Cell Tissue Kinet 4:93–105, 1971
9. Botnick LE, Hannon E, Hellman S: Limited proliferation of stem cells surviving alkylating agents. Nature 262:68–70, 1976
10. Botnick LE, Hannon EL, Hellman S: Multisystem stem cell failure following apparent recovery from alkylating agents. Cancer Res 38:1942–1947, 1978
11. Steel GG: Growth kinetics of tumours, pp 176–177. Oxford, Clarendon Press, 1977
12. Mendelsohn ML: The growth fraction: a new concept applied to tumors. Science 132:1496, 1960
13. Steel GG: Cell loss as a factor in the growth rate of human tumours. Eur J Cancer 3:381–387, 1967
14. Thomlinson RH, Gray LH: The histological structure of some human lung cancers and the possible implications for radiotherapy. Br J Cancer 9:539–549, 1955
15. Tannock IF: The relation between cell proliferation and the vascular system in a transplanted mouse mammary tumour. Br J Cancer 22:258–273, 1968
16. Hermens AF, Barendson GW: Changes in cell proliferation characteristics in a rat before and after x-irradiation. Eur J Cancer 5:173–189, 1969

17. Brown JM, Berrz RJ: Effect of x-irradiation on the cell population kinetics in a model tumour and normal tissue system: implications for the treatment of human malignancies Br J Radiol 42:372–377, 1969
18. Brown JM: The effect of acute x-irradiation on the cell proliferation kinetics of induced carcinomas and their normal counterpart. Radiat Res 43:627–653, 1970
19. Frindel E, Vassort F, Tubiana M: Effects of irradiation on the cell cycle of an experimental ascites tumour of the mouse. Int J Radiat Biol 17:329–337, 1970
20. Steel GG: Growth Kinetics of Tumours pp 286–287. Oxford, Clarendon Press, 1977
21. Collins VP, Loeffler RK, Twey H: Observation on growth rates of human tumours. Am J Roentgen 76:988–1000, 1956
22. Tubiana M, Malaise EP: Growth rate and cell kinetics in human tumours: some prognostic and therapeutic implications. In Symington T, Carter RL (eds), Scientific Foundations of Oncology, pp 126–136 Chicago, Year Book, 1976
23. Lird AK: The dynamics of tumour growth. Br J Cancer 28:490–502, 1966
24. Salmon SE, Smith BA: Immunoglobulin synthesis and total body tumor cell number in igG multiple myeloma. J Clin Invest 49:1114–1121, 1970
25. Charbit A, Malaise E, Tubiana M: Relation between the pathological nature and the growth rate of human tumours. Europ J Cancer 7:307–315, 1971
26. Malaise E, Chavaudra N, Tubiana M: The relationship between growth rate, labelling index and histological type of tumours. Europ J Cancer 9:305–312, 1973
27. Frindel E, Malaise E, Tubiana M: Cell proliferation kinetics in five solid tumours. Cancer 22:611–620, 1968
28. Bennington JL: Cellular kinetics of invasive squamous carcinoma of the human cervix. Cancer Res 29:1082–1087, 1969
29. Young RC, DeVita VT: Cell cycle characteristics of human solid tumors in vivo. Cell Tissue Kinet 3:285–290, 1970
30. Shirakawa S, Luce JK, Tammock IF et al: Cell proliferation in human melanoma. J. Clin Invest 49:1188–1199, 1970
31. Weinstein GD, Frost P: Cell proliferation in human basal cell carcinoma. Cancer Res 30:724–728, 1970
32. Terz JJ, Curutchet HP, Lawrence, W: Analysis of the cell cycle kinetics of human solid tumors. Cancer 28:1100–1110, 1971
33. Peckham MJ, Steel GG: Cell kinetics in reticulum cell sarcoma. Cancer 29:1724–1728, 1972
34. Estevez RA, Chacon RD, Cardiello C: Parameters cineticos de tumores humanos in vivo. Rev Lat Am Radioth Anti-neopl 5:116, 1972
35. Terz JJ, Curutchet HP: Cell cycle kinetics of human solid tumors following continuous infusion of 3H-TDR. In The Cell Cycle in Malignancy and Immunity. Proceedings of the 13th Annual Handford Biology Symposium, Richland, Washington, 1973, pp 323–329. US Energy Research and Development Administration, Technical Information Center, 1975
36. Muggia FM, Oster SK, Hanon HH: Cell kinetics studies in small cell carcinoma of the lung. Proc Am Assoc Cancer Res 13:16, 1972
37. Bresciano F, Paoluzi R, Benassi M et al: Cell kinetics and growth of squamous cell carcinoma in man. Cancer Res 34:2405–2415, 1974
38. Clarkson B, Ota K, Olkita T et al: Kinetics of proliferation of cancer cells in neoplastic effusions in man. Cancer 18:1189–1213, 1965
39. Clarkson BD, Fried J: Studies of cellular proliferation in adult leukemia III: Behavior of leukemia cells in three adults with acute leukemia given continuous infusions of ^{3}H-thymidine for 9 or 10 days. Cancer 25:1237, 1970
40. Gavosto F: Granulopoiesis and cell kinetics in chronic myeloid leukemia. Cell Tissue Kinet 7:151–163, 1974
41. Killmann S-A: Kinetics of Leukaemia Blast Cells in Man. Clin Haematol 1:95–113, 1972
42. Lula PK, Patt HM: Cytokinetic analysis of tumor growth. Proc Natl Acad Sci 56:1735–1742, 1966
43. Tannock IF: A comparison of cell proliferation parameters in solid and ascites Ehrlich tumours. Cancer Res 29:1527–1534, 1969
44. Gray JW, Carva JH, George YS et al: Rapid cell cycle analysis by measurement of the radioactivity per cell in a marrow window in 5 phases (RCSi). Cell Tissue Kinet 10:97–104, 1977

CHAPTER 5

Isaiah J. Fidler
Ian R. Hart

Principles of Cancer Biology: Biology of Cancer Metastasis

Most neoplasms can be conveniently divided into three major categories: benign tumors that are noninvasive and nonmetastatic; invasive tumors that are nonmetastatic (*e.g.*, carcinoma *in situ*, basal cell carcinoma); and metastatic tumors. Benign tumors are characterized by a structure that is often typical of the tissue of origin; they are well-differentiated and grow slowly. Mitotic figures are infrequent, and those present are usually normal. In contrast, malignant tumors are usually undifferentiated and consist of a large percentage of dividing cells. These dividing cells can have many abnormal chromosomes and can exhibit varying degrees of anaplasia.[1]

Metastasis can be defined as "the transfer of disease from one organ, or part, to another not directly connected with it. It may be due either to the transfer of pathogenic organisms, or to transfer of cells as in malignant tumors."[2] Indeed, this ability to invade and metastasize is the only characteristic unique to malignant neoplasms and is responsible for most therapeutic failures in clinical oncology.[3,4] Metastasis involves the release of cells from the primary tumor, dissemination to distant sites, arrest in the microcirculation of organs, extravasation and infiltration into the stroma of those organs, and survival and growth into new tumor colonies. The outcome of the process depends on host factors and tumor cell properties. These may vary among tumor systems. Much remains to be discovered about the pathogenesis of metastasis, but recent research has shed considerable light on some of the processes involved. In this chapter, a broad overview of cancer metastasis will be given, with particular emphasis on recent findings that have implications for therapy. (For more detailed discussion on the biology of cancer invasion and metastasis, the reader is referred to recently published reviews.[5,6])

THE PATHOGENESIS OF METASTASIS (MECHANISMS)

INVASION

Tumor cell dispersion can take place by direct spread or migration through coelomic cavities.[7] However, such routes of dissemination are generally secondary to those involving hematogenous or lymphatic spread. Invasion and infiltration into host tissues surrounding the primary tumor lead to penetration of blood, lymph vessels, or both, and provide the opportunity for widespread dissemination. Little is known about the mechanisms responsible for invasion of local host tissues. Mechanical pressure produced by the rapid proliferation of neoplasms may force finger-like cords of tumor cells along lines of least resistance.[8] Not all invasive tumors are rapidly growing; in fact, many highly invasive tumors have very slow growth rates.[1,4] Moreover, tumor cells added to the surface of organ explants maintained *in vitro* are capable of infiltrating these tissues without any pressure factors.[9,10]

Individual cell motility may play a role in tumor cell invasion though at present, evidence for such a mechanism is circumstantial.[11,12] The rates of migration of tumor cells and homologous normal cells have been assayed by *in vitro* techniques. Several investigators have demonstrated an association between increased cell motility and tumorigenic potential.[13–15] Conversely, investigations of variant murine tumor lines of differing invasive behavior have failed to reveal a correlation between *in vitro* motility and malignant capacity *in vivo*.[16–18] Interpretation of these results is difficult since movement of cells on a two-dimensional, serum-coated plastic petri dish may not be analogous with behavior within host tissue. Normal cells grown in monolayer culture are contact-inhibited with regard to directional locomotion.[19] If such a lack of constraint were displayed within three-dimensional structures, it might be supposed that invasive cells would demonstrate considerable mobility. Unfortunately, there is poor correlation between the contact inhibition of tumor cells growing as monolayer cultures and their invasive behavior when implanted in the three-dimensional developing chick wing bud.[20] Certainly, tumor cells possess the organelles necessary for active locomotion and can form cellular cytoplasmic processes, presumably indicative of motility, during the invasive process.[23–25] The inhibition of cell motility can prevent invasion in some, but not all, *in vitro* systems.[9,26] Pretreatment of tumor cells with cytoskeleton-disrupting agents, prior to their injection into experimental animals, had produced altered metastatic patterns that have been ascribed to the prevention of cell movement. However, such agents may affect a variety of processes in the metastatic sequence other than motility *per se*.[28] At this time, it appears that the role of cell motility in tumor invasion needs further clarification. Invasion by leukemic cells, without individual cell motility, is almost inconceivable but the situation with regard to solid tumors is far from clear.[29]

Similar uncertainty surrounds the involvement of tissue-destructive enzymes in tumor invasion, such as lysosomal hydrolases and collagenases. Destruction of host tissue by these enzymes, aided by pressure atrophy and the occlusion of blood and lymph vessels mediated by an expanding tumor mass, could facilitate infiltration of neoplastic tissue. Histological examination of tissues obtained from sites of tumor invasion shows considerable variation in the degree of tissue damage.[1,23] Many human and animal malignancies possess higher levels of lytic enzymes than benign tumors or corresponding normal tissues.[30–33] Though direct sampling may cause tissue damage itself and an elevation of enzyme activity, evidence for the involvement of tissue-degradative enzymes in neoplastic invasion is compelling.[34] Lysosomal catheptic enzymes have shown elevated levels of activity within some tumor tissues.[32,35] Recently, Poole and coworkers have demonstrated an increased production of cathepsin B in breast carcinomas as compared to that of normal or benign tissue.[36,37] This suggests a role for this enzyme in the expression of the aggressive malignant phenotype.

Enhanced production and secretion of the serine protease, plasminogen activator, has been associated with the neoplastic transformation of a variety of cell types.[38,39] Considerable interest has centered on the possible role of this enzyme in invasion and metastasis.[40] However, many normal cells are known to produce high levels of plasminogen activator and examination of variant murine melanoma cell lines with different invasive capacities has failed to reveal a consistent correlation between malignant behavior *in vivo* and plasminogen activator production or secretion.[16,39,41,42] It may be that the relative importance of different enzymes rather than one enzyme being responsible for all tumor invasion, may vary from one tumor system to another or, within the same tumor system, from one anatomical site to another.

The penetration of blood vessels, both during invasion and extravasation, is of pivotal importance in metastasis. Therefore, it is of interest that a strong correlation between the ability of tumor cells to produce spontaneous metastasis and possession of high levels of collagenase IV has been demonstrated.[143] Type IV collagen is a major structural protein of basement membranes that exist between parenchymal cells and the connective tissue on which such cells rest. Tumor cells that invade blood vessels or egress from the capillaries of distant organs in which they have been lodged must penetrate the basement membrane. Dissolution of the basement membrane, suggestive of enzymatic action, has been observed in areas adjacent to arrested tumor cells.[44] Collagen IV is chemically and genetically distinct from cartilage collagen type II and stromal collagen types I and III. The collagenase prepared from metastatic murine tumor cells exhibits preferential digestion of this basement membrane collagen.[49] Cells recovered from the venous effluent of a murine fibrosarcoma, presumptively the invasive population, solubilized basement membrane collagen to a significantly greater extent than cells from the parent population.[46] It appears that metastatic tumor cells exhibit a preferential attachment to type IV collagen substrates.[47] Since tumor cells can lodge selectively in areas of endothelial damage, the possession of high levels of collagenase type IV could be of fundamental importance in invasion and metastasis.[48,49]

DIRECT SPREAD

Tumors that grow in or penetrate body cavities may shed cells or emboli that travel in the cavity to seed on serosal surfaces of other organs. Lung or mediastinal tumors entering the pleural cavity can shed cells into the pleural fluid, which can result in multiple parietal or visceral metastases. Ovarian tumors, primary or metastatic in origin, frequently shed cells into the peritoneal cavity that grow to cover the peritoneal surface of abdominal organs. Though cells shed from primary ovarian tumors adhere to the surfaces of the viscera, they rarely infiltrate and grow within the organ parenchyma. It appears that the ability of tumor cells to adhere may be distinct from their ability to invade, or it could be that this tumor type invades tissue by mechanical pressure.

Primary tumors of the CNS rarely develop metastases outside the CNS in spite of their highly invasive capacity. Spread appears to occur by the cerebrospinal fluid or by direct extension. Tumors such as medulloblastomas and ependymomas can invade the cerebral ventricles and have cells transported to the leptomeninges of the spinal canal by the cerebrospinal fluid. Attachment to the leptomeninges is followed by growth and the development of secondary tumor deposits.

LYMPHATIC–HEMATOGENOUS SPREAD

Clinically, it is often stated that carcinomas spread by the lymphatic route and mesenchymal tumors spread by means of the bloodstream. However, lymphatic and vascular systems have numerous connections.[50] Experimentally, it has been shown that disseminating tumor cells may pass from one system to another.[51,52] Therefore, the two systems are inseparable, and the division into lymphatic spread and hematogenous spread is an arbitrary one used for the sake of clarity.

Lymphatic Spread

During tumor cell invasion, the process of infiltration and expansion into host tissue results in the penetration of small lymphatic vessels. The release of tumor cell emboli into these vessels is responsible for lymphatic metastases. Tumor emboli may be trapped in the first lymph node encountered on their route; they may traverse lymph nodes or even bypass them to form distant nodal metastases (the "skip" metastasis). Though this phenomenon was recognized in the late 1800's, its implications for treatment were frequently ignored in the development of surgical approaches.[4,53,54]

Apart from connections at the venular angles in the neck, there are numerous lymphatic–venous communications.[50,55] There is considerable evidence to suggest that tumor cells are capable of passing freely between blood vessels and lymphatics.[51,52] The view that tumors of mesenchymal origin tend to spread by way of the bloodstream, and carcinomas spread predominantly by way of the lymphatics appears to be an oversimplification of the process. What appears to be of prime importance is the role that the lymphatic system, in general, and lymph nodes, in particular, may play in the control or regulation of metastatic spread.

The Regional Lymph Node in Neoplasia

Lymph nodes in the area of a primary neoplasm may be enlarged and clinically palpable. Histologically, the enlargement could be due to either hyperplasia of lymph node follicles accompanied by proliferation of reticulum cells and sinus endothelium or active growth of tumor cells. A hyperplastic response could indicate reactivity to autochthonous tumors, which may be of benefit to the host. In a study of breast cancer patients, Berg and others found that the presence of an enlarged, nontumorous, apical lymph node was associated with a more favorable prognosis than if the node was small or absent. A more favorable prognosis has also been described for patients demonstrating lymphocytic infiltration into the tumor; such infiltrations were seen more frequently in patients who lived at least ten years after surgical tumor removal than in those from patients who were not cured by surgery.[57] Although the use of morphologic criteria for assessing prognoses based on lymph node appearance is debatable, it has been generally accepted that inactive lymphocyte-depleted lymph nodes are indicative of a less favorable prognosis than those demonstrating reactive patterns.[56,58,59]

Lymph nodes are immunologically reactive in patients with neoplasms. Tumor presence may stimulate the production and release of immunocompetent cells in the lymphoreticular system.[60] The reaction commences in the regional lymph nodes (RLN), but later extends to distant nodes and the spleen. Proliferative changes in the RLNs can therefore precede the spread and subsequent growth of tumor emboli in them. Initial entrapment and growth of lymphatic-borne tumor emboli usually occur in the subcapsular sinus of the lymph node. Additional emboli may be released from there, or the tumor may grow toward the hilar region and the efferent channels.

The Barrier Effect of Lymph Nodes

Whether lymph nodes can serve as a temporary "filter" for metastatic tumor cells is not clear.[4] The lymph nodes (of normal animals) can be an effective but temporary barrier to tumor spread. Zeidman and Buss injected Brown–Pearce or VX2 carcinoma cells into the afferent popliteal lymphatics of rabbits and removed the lymph nodes 1–42 days after injection.[52] Only two of 30 animals developed distant metastases. This was taken as evidence for the effectiveness of the lymph node as a temporary barrier to tumor spread. However, other studies indicate that most tumor cells that reach the lymph node rapidly enter the efferent lymphatics and then the bloodstream.[51] If, indeed, tumor cells can pass from lymphatic to blood vessels and back again with great ease, then the question may not actually be of clinical importance. In most of the experimental animal systems used to investigate this question, normal nodes have been subjected to an influx of a large number of tumor cells, a situation that may not be at all analagous to the RLN in the early stages of cancer spread in a human patient.

Several mechanisms can alter the filtration capacity of lymph nodes. Tumor growth, or even acute or chronic inflammatory reactions, may reduce the efficiency of filtration, as can fibrosis resulting from local irradiation. However, it could be that the properties of tumor cells *per se* rather than the filtration capacity of the lymph node determine whether neoplastic cells are trapped.

The role of the RLN in neoplasia, in general, and in metastasis, in particular, is as important as it is controversial. Unquestionably, the RLN may be involved immunologically in the host response to neoplasms. The importance of the RLN to the initiation of systemic immunity has been established in various systems. Mitchison first reported adoptive transfer of tumor allograft immunity by the IP administration of RLN cells of tumor-bearing animals to normal animals.[61] Billingham and others showed that skin allografts lacking lymphatic connections were tolerated only until restoration of the lymphatic system occurred.[62] Construction of skin pedicles in guinea pigs lacking afferent lymphatics led to indefinite retention of skin allografts.[63] Using a similar system, Futrell and Myers found that tumor allografts were rejected, although skin allografts remained viable.[64]

In 1965, Crile challenged the classical concept of "en bloc" resection of primary breast tumor and its regional lymphatics.[65] He advocated simple mastectomy, which preserved the RLN, basing the choice on experiments in which depressed immunity to tumor challenge after excision of the RLN was observed. The retention of the RLN free of metastatic cells was hypothesized to be important in maintaining a high level of systemic tumor immunity, which, theoretically, could aid in growth prevention of disseminated micrometastases. Indeed, the results of the early clinical survival data of patients with breast cancer who underwent simple mastectomy seemed to confirm the hypothesis stating that the RLN should be preserved.[65,66]

Additional animal experiments complicated the interpretation of RLN's role in controlling tumor spread. It appears from the work of Fisher and Fisher, who have done the most detailed work on this problem, that the RLN could be important for the initiation of immunity against a transplantable syngeneic tumor in mice.[67] The effect, however, is dependent on the antigenicity of the tumor. When the tumor was weakly antigenic, the RLN were important in the initiation of systemic immunity. Such was not the case when strongly antigenic tumors were used.[68]

Clinical trials comparing simple and radical mastectomy have not confirmed Crile's original observations since no significant differences in survival times have been observed.[69] Nonetheless, an increase in axillary nodal metastases has been observed in breast cancer patients treated with simple mastectomy as compared to those treated with mastectomy and regional radiotherapy.[70] The role of RLN in the control of metastatic spread remains uncertain. Determining the exact nature of this role is important since the decision to surgically remove the RLN must be based upon the degree of involvement in the metastatic process.

Hematogenous Spread

As mentioned above, widespread tumor cell dissemination is a consequence of the penetration of blood vessels, lymphatics, or both. Cells of malignant neoplasms frequently penetrate thin-walled capillaries, but rarely manage to invade artery or arteriole walls rich in elastin fibers.[55] This resistance to invasion is not necessarily mediated by mechanical strength alone. Connective tissues have been shown to possess protease inhibitors, which may block the enzyme-dependent process of invasion.[71-73] Malignant tumors do not produce their own blood vessels but induce the ingrowth of new capillaries from host tissue by releasing tumor angiogenesis factor.[74] The penetration of these vascular channels can be aided by the defective endothelium and increased permeability of such vessels.

Once tumor cells have penetrated blood vessels, they can passively be carried away or develop and grow at the penetration site and only subsequently release tumor emboli into the circulation. The appearance of tumor emboli correlates with the development of tumor vascularization.[75] The rate of tumor cell release from an implanted murine fibrosarcoma rose with post-implantation time and could be related mathematically to the development of pulmonary metastases.[76] The mere presence of tumor cells in the circulation does not in itself constitute a metastasis.[77] Most cells released into the bloodstream are eliminated rapidly.[78,79] Although most tumor cells are destroyed within the bloodstream, it appears that the greater the number of cells released by a primary tumor, the greater the probability that some cells will survive to form metastases. The number of tumor emboli in the circulation appears to correlate well with the size and clinical duration of the primary tumor.[4] The development of necrotic and hemorrhagic areas within large tumors facilitates this process by providing tumor cells with easy access to the circulation.[80]

The rapid demise of most circulating tumor cells is probably due to the traumatic nature of blood turbulence, but the isolated nature of the emboli allows for interaction with a variety of blood components. Tumor cells can aggregate with each other (homotypic aggregation) or with host cells (heterotypic aggregation), such as platelets and lymphocytes.[5] Formation of such multicellular emboli can assist tumors in establishing secondary growths. The number of pulmonary metastases formed after IV injection of tumor cells has been related to the size of tumor emboli.[81-83] Although such an effect is presumably related to an enhanced trapping of larger emboli in the microcirculation, it can also be due to the protective effect of an outer layer of cells. Metastases can result from undamaged "central" cells protected from the hostile circulatory environment by peripheal tumor or host cells in the embolus.

Tumor cell entrapment in the capillary bed of distant organs is a necessary prelude to secondary tumor growth. Although the morphologic aspects of tumor cell arrests have been studied extensively, relatively little is known about the dynamics of the process.[49] Exposure of the capillary basement membrane is a result of the normal and continuous physiologic process of endothelial cell-shedding and may allow adhesion of tumor emboli.[49] Platelet adherence to damaged areas (naked basement membrane) followed by degranulation can cause further retraction of endothelial cells and the further attachment of tumor emboli or platelet/tumor cell emboli.[49,84-86] Fibrin deposits around an arrested tumor embolus have frequently been observed, but not invariably.[86-90] The role of fibrin in tumor cell arrest and metastasis is uncertain. Theoretically, a protective coat of fibrin around the tumor embolus can shield the neoplastic cells from the attack of host immunocytes or blood turbulence. Increased coagulability is commonly observed in patients with cancer and could be related to the high levels of thromboplastin found in certain tumors.[91,92] Recently, it has been demonstrated that some neoplasms have the capability of producing high levels of procoagulant-A activity, which can directly activate factor X in the clotting process.[93,94] A reduced rate of blood flow could lead to increased trapping of circulating tumor cells and the increased survival of already trapped cells. The use of anticoagulants, in the treatment or control of metastasis, is based on the consideration of such factors.[95]

Extravasation of arrested tumor cells is thought to occur by mechanisms comparable to those that affect invasion. Tumor cells can grow and destroy the arresting vessel as a prelude to attaining an extravasuclar position or can migrate in the wake of white blood cells.[86,87,96]

PATTERNS OF METASTASIS

There is a tendency for primary tumors of defined histologic classification to metastasize to and grow in specific, distant organs.[3-5] These selective patterns of metastases have also been demonstrated in experimental animal systems.[5] Two hypotheses have been proposed to explain this non-random pattern of tumor spread. Ewing has suggested that metastases are influenced purely by mechanical considerations, such as anatomic and hemodynamic factors in the vasculature.[97] Paget has theorized that host and tumor cell properties were both important in determining metastasic growth.[53] Experimental studies tend to support the "seed and soil" hypothesis of Paget and to suggest that sites of secondary tumor growth are determined by both host and tumor factors. Distribution studies of radiolabeled tumor cells in experimental animals have revealed that the initial arrest of viable cells in a particular organ does not always correlate with subsequent tumor development.[76,98] Hemodynamic considerations alone do not explain why organs such as the spleen or skeletal muscle are infrequent sites of metastatic development.

Certainly, vascularity of organs may contribute to the frequency with which metastatic deposits are formed. For example, the lung may be a common site of metastatic development simply because it is the first capillary bed encountered by tumor cells entering the venous circulation. Other effects of host tissues on tumor development are less well-established. Differences in local immune defenses could regulate the observed preferential growth, whereas some tissues could release diffusible inhibitors of tumor development.[99,100] The dramatic nature of the specificity of host–organ control of metastastic patterns has been demonstrated by using organ grafts maintained in ectopic sites.[101–103] Grafts of tissue were implanted into the thighs of syngeneic mice, which were subsequently inoculated, either IV or intraarterially (IA), with tumor cell suspensions. Tumors developed only in those grafts derived from the organ tissues that normally supported tumor growth in the intact animal.

More work has been performed on the role of tumor cell properties in determining the outcome of metastatic development. The selection of organ-specific variant tumor lines from heterogeneous parent tumor populations has been reported extensively, and the modification of many tumor cell properties can alter tumor dissemination patterns.[27,28,104–108] Selective entrapment and arrest of circulating tumor cells can be determined by the specificity of cell-to-cell recognition, control of which may reside at the cell surface. Tumor cells showing preferential "homing" to specific organs have exhibited increased aggregation or adherence to cells derived from that organ.[109–111] The ability of melanoma cells of low metastatic potential to be arrested and form metastases in the lungs of recipient mice was recently enhanced by fusing these cells with plasma membrane vesicles derived from highly metastatic cells. The results suggest that differences in the localization of cells with low and high metastatic potential are determined by surface properties.[108]

IMMUNITY AND METASTASIS

Experimental animal tumors, induced by the administration of carcinogens, frequently express cell surface, tumor-specific transplantation antigens (TSTA).[112] Although the situation in man is less certain, it appears likely that at least some human tumors can possess specific antigens on their cell surface.[113] The exact role that the immune response plays in regulating the development and growth of spontaneous tumors is unclear. Nonetheless, it could be that the process of metastasis, with the detachment of cells from the primary tumor mass and circulation as single cells or small groups of cells, is particularly susceptible to modification by the immune system.

CELL-MEDIATED IMMUNITY AND METASTASIS

Evidence that the immune response can be important in determining metastatic spread has been obtained from a number of studies.[113] Arrest patterns of tumor cells, and their subsequent development into metastatic foci following IV injection can be modified by the immune manipulation of recipient animals.[98,114] However, the nature of the immune system's effect on tumor metastasis varies from tumor to tumor. Depression of immunologic reactivity has, on occasion, increased the incidence of both spontaneous and experimental metastasis whereas in other tumor systems, the same manipulation has produced the opposite effect or no effect at all.[98,112–121] Such conflicting data are difficult to analyze since they have not only been obtained in different laboratories, but they are the result of studies utilizing vastly different tumor systems.

Recently, Fidler and Hart have attempted to study, in a more systematic way, the role of tumor cell antigenicity in the formation of experimental and spontaneous metastasis.[122] Three C3H mouse fibrosarcomas of differing immunogenicities were tested for metastatic behavior in normal, sham-suppressed, immuno-suppressed, and immunologically reconstituted syngeneic mice. Immunosuppression affected experimental metastasis of the three tumors in various ways. The highly immunogenic fibrosarcoma formed more pulmonary tumor colonies in immunosuppressed mice than in normal, sham-suppressed or reconstituted animals. A fibrosarcoma of intermediate immunogenicity also formed more pulmonary metastases in immunosuppressed recipients, but this increase could not be reversed by immune reconstitution. In contrast, the least immunogenic tumor formed fewer pulmonary tumor colonies in immunosuppressed mice than in normal, sham-suppressed or reconstituted mice. Therefore, it appears that generalizations about the nature of metastatic spread and the immune response cannot be made; there is no simple correlation between the outcome of experimental metastasis and the immune status of the recipient animal from tumor to tumor.

Such results lend credence to Prehn's suggestion that the response of the immune system to tumors is of a dual nature.[123,124] During the initial stages of neoplasia or in cases in which the tumors are weakly antigenic, the response was suggested to be stimulatory; in contrast, a strong immune response or a strongly antigenic tumor was thought to produce inhibition of cancer growth by the immune system.

As Prehn has suggested, these stimulatory effects may result from a direct effect of lymphoid cells or their product on tumor growth.[123,124] For example, lymphocyte aggregation with circulating tumor cells can aid embolic lodgement and lymphocytes can be the source of angiogenic factors.[119,120,125] In other systems, enhanced tumor growth *in vivo* can result from an excess of regulatory T-lymphocytes that suppress an antitumor immune response.[126,127]

Obviously, experimental observations such as these can be meaningful to the clinical oncologist. If some human tumors are spontaneous and are weakly immunogenic, then the stimulation of the T-lymphocyte system as a mode of immunotheapy could be fraught with hidden dangers. Many of these difficulties will be discussed in greater detail in the tumor heterogeneity and therapy section.

The concept of immune surveillance arose out of the need to justify teleologically the host-versus-graft reaction.[128] Refined and expanded by Burnet, this hypothesis was accepted widely in the early 1970's, questioned and revised in the mid 1970's, and is now generally believed to exist in a somewhat modified form from that which was proposed originally.[129,130] Although the immune surveillance mechanism and its relevance to tumor development can be questioned, it remains an attractive hypothesis that such a phenomenon could operate in the control of metastatic disease.

One of the strongest objections to the immune surveillance theory of neoplasm regulation was that, if the hypotheses were correct, immunodeficient animals should show an increased frequency of tumor development.[131] The nude mouse, lacking T-cell function and unable to reject foreign grafts, could be expected to develop a high incidence of spontaneous tumors of different types. This does not appear to be the case.[132,133] It has, therefore, been of considerable interest that a subpopulation of lymphocytes, termed natural killer (NK) cells, responsible for natural cell-mediated cytotoxicity is present at a high level in nude and neonatally thymectomized mice.[134]

The possible significance of this subpopulation of cells, in the control of tumor development, has been reviewed elsewhere.[134,135] Measurements of the *in vivo* growth of IV injected tumor cells have shown a strong correlation between high NK activity and inhibition of tumor development.[135,137]

In spite of the widespread use of nude mice in experimental tumor biology, there are very few reported cases of allogeneic or xenogeneic tumors metastasizing in nude mice.[138–140] It is becoming apparent that one of the factors that may be operative in this restriction of metastasis is the high level of NK cell activity found in these animals.[140,141] Most studies, involving nude mice as tumor bearers, have utilized animals six weeks of age or older. By this time, the level of NK cell activity has risen from previously low levels.[140] If specific-pathogen-free (SPF), healthy three-week-old animals are used, either for IV injection followed by pulmonary nodule quantitation, or for SC or IM implantation with assessment of subsequent spontaneous metastasis, then both allogeneic and xenogeneic tumors of different types can metastasize.[142] The age-related reduction in metastasis is due to the maturation of the NK cell system. This has been shown by artificial stimulation of NK cell activity in three-week-old nude mice, using such agents as interferon, and the decrease in experimental metastasis that accompanies this stimulation.[140–142]

HUMORAL IMMUNITY

The role of the humoral response in the control of metastatic disease awaits clarification. It seems likely that if a tumor is capable of provoking a humoral immune response, then the exposure of single cells, or small clumps of cells, to the circulatory environment during metastasis could allow humoral immunity to profoundly influence the course of disseminated disease. Antibodies directed against tumor antigens have been detected using a variety of techniques in many experimental and a few human tumors.[143,144] The clinical relevance of these antibodies is uncertain, but in malignant melanoma (perhaps the best characterized human tumor by serological analysis) there is good evidence that the presence of circulating antibody correlates with localization of the disease.[145] It could be that the presence of both complement and antibody allows lysis of disseminating cells; alternatively, a coating of antibody could prevent adherence to the endothelium and thus prevent tumor cell lodgement.[146]

A somewhat negative role for humoral responses in the control of metastasis was suggested by the studies of Hellstrom and Hellstrom.[147] Serum from tumor-bearing patients was capable of abrogating lymphocyte-mediated cytotoxicity *in vitro*.[148,149] From this finding the concept arose that this serum contained a blocking antibody that bound to tumor cell surfaces and masked these sites from circulating cytotoxic lymphocytes. Further experiments have shown that such "blocking factors" need not be antibodies but can be antigen, immune complexes, autoantibody, or an unidentified repressor protein.[150]

What is the clinical relevance of such a phenomenon? If this mechanism were to operate *in vivo* it could be that the masking of tumor antigen sites provided by blocking factors could allow the escape of metastatic cells from host immune defenses. However, most data on so-called blocking factors have been obtained from *in vitro* studies, and little information is available on the role that such substances could play *in vivo*. Serum from tumor-bearing animals administered to other tumor-bearing animals has brought about both the facilitation and regression of tumor growth.[151,152] Serum obtained from animals bearing tumor lung nodules has enhanced the metastatic ability of an immunologically related tumor in a second group of animals.[153] If data acquired from experimental animal systems could be extrapolated to the clinic, it could be assumed that the presence of excess, free tumor antigen in a tumor-bearing host is a negative factor in host immune resistance such that the use of immunoadsorption techniques to remove circulating tumor antigen could be beneficial.[154,155] Unfortunately, the contradictory nature of much of the data suggests that more than variation in technique could be responsible for observed differences and, as with so much of metastasis biology, generalizations are unwarranted.

THE HETEROGENEOUS NATURE OF METASTATIC NEOPLASMS

METASTASIS AS A SELECTIVE PROCESS

The development of metastases appears to be dependent on an interplay between host factors and intrinsic characteristics of the tumor cells. To establish metastases, tumor cells must complete all of the steps involved in the metastatic process. Therefore, enhanced performance of a cell in one step of the process does not compensate for an inability to complete a subsequent step. Metastatic cells are analogous to a decathlon athlete who must perform well in every event to succeed.[3,4,156] The failure to produce metastases by most tumor cells cannot be attributed to a single common factor. For example, only a small proportion of cells in a primary neoplasm can enter the circulation. Only as few as 0.1% of circulating tumor cells can survive the trauma of dissemination and arrest in the capillary bed of an organ.[76] This tremendous loss of cells in the circulation is probably due to mechanical destruction and host-mediated destruction by NK cells.[5,6,78,139,140] Not all cells arresting in the capillary bed can undergo extravasation. The ability of extravasated cells to proliferate into clinical metastases could depend on the availability of appropriate nutrients and escape from destruction by host defense mechanism(s), such as the reticuloendothelial (RE) system.

The fact that only a few circulating tumor cells survive to form metastases is not surprising. However, it raises the important question of whether their survival is random or nonrandom. The possibility that cells with high metastatic potential can be isolated from a heterogeneous parental tumor by selection procedures was first suggested by Koch's experiments, who demonstrated that a highly metastatic subline of the Ehrlich carcinoma tumor could be isolated by serially transplanting lymph node metastases.[157] Klein demonstrated that the gradual conversion of some solid murine neoplasms into ascites variants is due to the selective overgrowth of a small number of cells that differ from the parental population in their ability to proliferate in the peritoneal cavity and metastasize to the lungs. Since the change was stable and heritable, it was concluded that the gradual transformation of a solid tumor into ascites form was due to mutation selection and not adaptation.[158] Further evidence of heterogeneity in the metastatic potential of tumor cells has come from experiments in a large number of tumor systems that show that harvesting of cells from metastases during successive *in vivo* selections yields cell populations with a greater metastatic potential than cells from the original cell population. In this type of *in vivo* selection, the enhanced metastatic potential detected in the population is due to enrichment of highly metastatic cells in the population with each successive passage *in vivo*.[104-108,159-165]

Metastatic and nonmetastatic tumor cell variants have also been isolated from the same parent tumor cell population using *in vitro* selection methods. Cell populations were selected for expression (or failure to express), a property considered to be important in one step of the metastatic process. The metastatic behavior of such isolated cells is then assayed *in vivo* to determine whether the particular selection has enriched the population for cells with increased or decreased metastatic phenotype. *In vitro* selection for detachment from a monolayer culture, resistance to lysis by lymphocytes, resistance to lectin-mediated toxicity, attachment to collagen, degradation of collagen type IV, and ability to invade various tissues maintained in organ culture have all been used successfully to isolate tumor cell lines with increased or decreased metastatic capabilities.[16,43,46,47,163-166]

TUMOR HETEROGENEITY FOR INVASION AND METASTASIS

The first direct experimental evidence that malignant neoplasms do indeed contain subpopulations of cells with differing metastatic capabilities was demonstrated in 1977 by Fidler and Kripke using the B16 melanoma syngeneic to the C57BL/6 mouse.[167] To investigate whether the tumor contained cells of differing or uniform metastatic potential, they performed an experiment similar in design to the classical fluctuation test devised by Luria and Delbruck to distinguish between selection and adaptation in the origin of bacterial mutants.[168] A cell suspension of the B16 melanoma parent line was divided into two parts. One portion was injected IV into syngeneic C57BL/6 mice. The other portion was used to produce clones, which were then injected IV into groups of C57BL/6 mice. If the tumor had been populated by cells of uniform metastatic potential, then the cloned sublines would have each produced the same number of metastases in different animals. However, the cloned sublines differed markedly in their metastatic potential. There was also considerable variation among the clones in the number and sites of extrapulmonary metastases. Control subcloning experiments demonstrated that the variability among the clones was not generated during the cloning procedure. These experiments concluded that the parent tumor is heterogeneous and that highly metastatic tumor cell variants preexisted in the parental population.[168]

To exclude the possibility that the metastatic heterogeneity found in the B16 melanoma might have been introduced as a result of the lengthy *in vivo* and *in vitro* cultivation, the same experiment was performed with two newly induced primary mouse tumors. The metastatic potential of cells isolated from the UV-induced fibrosarcoma and a C3H melanoma after only five passages *in vitro* was demonstrated.[169,170] The results obtained with these tumors were strikingly similar to those obtained with the B16 melanoma. Moreover, the cloned cell lines isolated from these tumors varied greatly in their ability to grow at SC sites and to produce spontaneous metastases in distant organs. In these tumor systems, the ability of cells to produce spontaneous metastases originating from a SC tumor strongly correlated with production of artificial metastases following introduction into the circulation.

Similar heterogeneity in metastatic potential has now been demonstrated with murine mammary tumors, MCA-induced fibrosarcoma, sarcoma virus-transformed fibrosarcoma, mouse lymphosarcoma, and rat transformed epithelioid cell line of liver.[171-175] More recently, Fidler and Hart have shown that whereas clones with widely differing metastatic potential can be isolated from the primary tumor, cloned sublines isolated from metastases exhibit a much more uniform metastatic potential. This suggests that metastases, in contrast to a primary tumor, are populated by a more homogeneous population of cells with similar metastatic capabilities.[6,170]

THE ORIGIN OF CELLULAR DIVERSITY IN MALIGNANT NEOPLASMS

Whether or not neoplasms are unicellular or multicellular in origin, most can be heterogeneous and contain many subpopulations of cells with differing biological behavior by the time of diagnosis. Tumors can arise as the result of a rare event such as a somatic mutation, and thus their origin can be expected to be unicellular. Indeed, there is strong evidence (from studies using a marker immunoglobulin or glucose 6-

phosphate dehydrogenase [G6PD] in human females with X-chromosome inactivation mosaicism) that chronic myelogeneous leukemia, Burkitt's lymphoma (BL), and multiple myeloma arise from a single cell.[176,177] Other human tumors, such as hereditary trichoepithelioma and colon carcinoma, are suspected to arise from multicellular origin.[178] In this regard, it is interesting to note that chemically-induced murine fibrosarcomas have also recently been shown to have a multicellular origin.[179]

It is easy to understand the source of cellular diversity in neoplasms that are multicellular in their origin. Such tumors are probably populated by the progenies of several transformed cells. Thus, cells obtained from different parts of chemically-induced sarcomas, known to be multicellular in origin, differed in their growth rate, susceptibility to cytotoxic drugs, and antigenicity.[179-182] It is more difficult to perceive the source of heterogeneity in neoplasms that are unicellular in origin. In this regard, Nowell has recently hypothesized that neoplasms can arise from a single cell of origin and that tumor progression results from an acquired genetic variability within developing clones of cells.[183] Variant cells can arise within the progressing neoplasm and be subjected to selection pressure by the host. Such forces can allow for the emergence of new sublines with increased potential for survival, which we clinically define as *malignant potential*. Therefore, regardless of whether neoplasms are monoclonal or multiclonal in origin, most can be heterogeneous at diagnosis and contain subpopulations of cells with a broad range of characteristics.

Collectively, a large body of experimental data indicates that malignant tumors are not populated by cells of equal metastatic potential. Rather, primary tumors are populated by subpopulations of cells of widely differing metastatic potential. The heterogeneous nature of neoplasms with regard to many characteristics is well-recognized. Cells populating both human and animal neoplasms are known to differ with respect to their immunogenicity, antigenic properties, growth rate, metabolic characteristics, hormone receptors, pigment production, karyotypes, radiosensitivity, and susceptibility to cytotoxic drugs.[5,160,180-182,184-199]

HETEROGENEITY OF HUMAN NEOPLASMS

Clinical and histopathologic studies of cancer in humans have suggested that neoplasms may undergo changes during the course of disease. For example, a growth that originally appeared to be a benign tumor, and behaved as such, seemed to transform or progress in one area or another over a period of months or sometimes even years into a malignant, metastatic, and lethal tumor.[200-203] Tumor progression need not be an all or none process. Not all cells within a tumor progress at the same rate or time. This may indeed contribute to the development of heterogeneity. The heterogeneous nature of human neoplasms is now being recognized. Differences in the cell karyotype populating a primary human uterine adenocarcinoma and its metastases have been described.[195] Heterogeneity in response to cytotoxic agents has been found in human adenocarcinoma of the colon and stomach, in advanced ovarian carcinoma and in non-Hodgkins lymphoma.[193,199,204-206] Several other examples of tumor cell heterogeneity in human neoplasms other than morphologic features have now been described. For example, the content of estrogen receptors in breast carcinoma can vary within or among lesions from a patient.[191-193] Variations in cell content of enzymes and small polypeptide hormones have also been observed between primary and metastatic foci.[191,207,208]

The problem that extensive cellular diversity inherent in some neoplasms can present for therapy is illustrated by Baylin and coworkers.[207] Elevation of serum levels of histaminase, L-dopa decarboxylase and calcitonin had been used as clinical markers for the presence of growing small-cell lung cancer. However, simultaneous sampling of primary and metastatic lesions of small-cell lung cancer found significant differences in the content of these markers. All primary lesions produced high levels of these markers. In contrast, either low or no levels of the three products could be detected in four of seven metastases isolated from livers of several patients. Subsequent immunohistochemical studies for histaminase indicated that even cells within the primary tumor were heterogeneous for this enzyme. Since Baylin and coworkers found that some metastases were populated with cells that did not produce or release any of the biomarkers, the usefulness of such markers in correlating systemic tumor burden is obviously doubtful.[207,208]

IMPLICATIONS FOR THERAPY

The existence of specialized subpopulations of cells within primary neoplasms that have high metastatic potential has far reaching consequences for testing potential agents for treating metastatic disease. Differences in the response of primary and metastatic lesions to therapeutic agents have been documented in clinical practice, and metastatic cells showing increased resistance to chemotherapeutic agents have been selected in experimental tumor systems.[6,191,193,198,199]

Schabel and coworkers pointed out that most of the methods presently used to define the drug sensitivity of experimental animal tumors could be misleading since they are based on the assumption that transplantable tumors are homogeneous, and syngeneic recipients respond uniformly to growing tumors or drug treatments.[209] Partial regression of a transplantable tumor could be an inadequate assay for screening agents for their antimetastatic activity. Assays in which a drug or combination of drugs limits tumor growth (injected at a "primary site", *i.e.*, SC or IM) to 50% of that in untreated controls does not necessarily offer any insight into the pharmacologic susceptibility of the tumor cell subpopulations that will give rise to metastases. Moreover, the response of tumor cells to cytotoxic agents can be influenced by the site of growth. Indeed, it is not uncommon to clinically observe the regression of some metastases in one organ, whereas other metastases (in the same patient) in another organ grow progressively.

Immunologic heterogeneity among tumor cells within a "primary neoplasm" and between primary neoplasms and their metastases could pose serious problems in treatment of metastases by specific immunotherapy.[5,6,113,185] For example, analysis of a number of AKR mouse lymphomas of recent origin has shown that these tumors are immunologically polyclonal, and consist of a dominant major subpopulation and several minor subpopulations that could comprise less than 3% of the total tumor. Immunization of tumor-bearing animals with unfractionated tumor cells was unsuccessful since only the dominant clone was rejected, and the minor subclones in the vaccine did not offer a sufficient immunologic mass to stimulate the immune response. Thus, rejection of the major clone permitted the other subpopulations to proliferate and become dominant.[210] This situation is similar to the well-recognized problem of drug-resistance in cancer chemotherapy. Drug-resistant variants may preexist within the parental tumor population, and following the destruction of the original dominant drug-sensitive populations, they proliferate unchecked. Many clinical examples for the emergence of drug-resistant phenotype exist. For example, the small-cell carcinoma of the lung is usually sensitive to initial chemotherapy with or without radiotherapy. Recurrence is a common feature of this neoplasm and most recurring tumors are resistant to continued treatment regardless of the initial responsiveness to therapy.[191,211,212] Recognition that primary malignant tumors are not populated by cells of equal metastatic potential, but contain subpopulations of cells with widely differing metastatic capabilities thus calls for reappraisal of the adequacy of many of the experimental systems presently used to study "malignancy" and to identify potential therapeutic agents for treating metastatic disease.

CONCLUSIONS

The development of metastasis is a complex and highly selective process that is dependent upon the interplay of host and tumor cell properties. Characteristics of tumor cells, such as their cell surface properties, adhesive capacities, cell motility, and enzyme secretion, appear to be of paramount importance in determining the eventual outcome of metastasis. To establish metastases, tumor cells must complete all steps involved in the metastatic process. Enhanced performance by a cell in one step of the process does not compensate for an inability to complete a subsequent step. Interruption of the sequence at any stage can prevent the production of clinical, visible metastasis. The recognition that primary malignant tumors are not composed of uniform cells with regard to metastatic behavior, but contain subpopulations of cells with differing biologic behavior calls for critical reappraisal of the adequacy of many of the tumor systems now used to study the process of metastasis and for testing new approaches or agents for treating metastatic disease.

REFERENCES

1. Franks LM: Structure and biological malignancy of tumors. In Garattini S, Franchi G (eds): Chemotherapy of Cancer Dissemination and Metastasis, pp 71–78. New York, Raven Press, 1973
2. Dorland WA: Dorland's Illustrated Medical Dictionary, 24th ed. Philadelphia, WB Saunders, 1965
3. Sugarbaker EV, Ketcham AS: Mechanisms and prevention of cancer dissemination: an overview. Semin Oncol 4:19–32, 1977
4. Sugarbaker EV: Cancer metastasis: a product of tumor-host interactions. Curr Probl Cancer 7:1–59, 1979
5. Fidler IJ, Gersten DM, Hart IR: The biology of cancer invasion and metastasis. Adv Cancer Res 28:149–250, 1978
6. Poste G, Fidler IJ: The pathogenesis of cancer metastasis. Nature 283:139–146, 1979
7. Willis RA: The Spread of Tumors in the Human Body. London, Butterworth & Co, 1972
8. Eaves G: The invasive growth of malignant tumors as a purely mechanical process. J Pathol 109:233–237, 1973
9. Easty DM, Easty GC: Measurement of the ability of cells to infiltrate normal tissues *in vitro*. Br J Cancer 19:36–49, 1974
10. Noguchi PD, Johnson JB, O'Donnell R et al: Chick embryonic skin as a rapid organ culture assay for cellular neoplasia. Science 199:980–983, 1978
11. Easty GC, Easty DM: Mechanisms of tumor invasion. In Symington T, Carter RL (eds): Scientific Foundations of Oncology, pp 167–172. London, William Heinemann, 1976
12. Strauli P, Weiss L: Cell locomotion and tumour penetration. Eur J Cancer 13:1–12, 1977
13. Gail MH, Boone CW: Density inhibition of motility in 3T3 fibroblasts and their SV40 transformants. Exp Cell Res 64:156–162, 1971
14. Gershman H, Drumm J, Rosen JJ: Dibuturyl cyclic AMP treatment of 3T3 and SV40 virus-transformed 3T3 cells in aggregates. J Cell Biol 72:424–440, 1977
15. Gershman H, Katzin W, Cook RT: Mobility of cells from solid tumors. Int J Cancer 21:309–316, 1978
16. Hart IR: Selection and characterization of an invasive variant of the B16 melanoma. Am J Pathol 97:587–600, 1979
17. Varani J, Orr W, Ward PA: Comparison of subpopulations of tumor cells with altered migratory activity, attachment characteristics enzyme levels and *in vivo* behavior. Eur J Cancer 15:585–591, 1979
18. Varani J, Orr W, Ward PA: Hydrolytic enzyme activities, migratory activity and *in vivo* growth and metastatic potential of recent tumor isolates. Cancer Res 39:2376–2380, 1979
19. Abercrombie M, Heaysman JEM: Social behavior of cells in tissue culture, II. "Monolayering" of fibroblasts. Exp Cell Res 6:293–306, 1954
20. Tickle A, Crawley A, Goodman M: Cell movement and the mechanism of invasiveness: a survey of the developing chick wing bud. J Cell Sci 31:293–322, 1978
21. Franks LM, Riddle PN, Seal P: Actin-like filaments and cell movement in human ascites tumour cells: an ultrastructural and cinemicrographic study. Exp Cell Res 54:157–162, 1969
22. Malech HL, Lenz TL: Microfilaments in epidermal cancer cells. J Cell Biol 60:473–482, 1974
23. Babai F, Tremblay A: Ultrastructural study of liver invasion by Novikoff hepatoma. Cancer Res 32:2765–2770, 1972
24. Dingemans KP: Invasion of liver tissue by blood-borne mammary carcinoma cells. JNCI 53:1813–1824, 1974
25. Roos E, Dingemans KP, van de Pavert IV, et al: Invasion of lymphosarcoma cells into the perfused mouse liver. JNCI 58:399–407, 1977
26. Ambrose EJ, Easty DM: Time-lapse filming of cellular interactions within living tissues, II. The role of cell shape. Differentiation 6:61–70, 1976
27. Hagmar B, Ryd W: Tumor cell locomotion: a factor in metastasis formation: influence of cytochalasin B on a tumor dissemination pattern. Int J Cancer 19:576–580, 1977
28. Hart IR, Raz A, Fidler IJ: Effect of cytoskeleton-disrupting agents on the metastatic behavior of melanoma cells. JNCI 64:891–900, 1980
29. Strauli P: Remarks on locomotion of normal and neoplastic white blood cells in the organism. Blood Cells 2:467–471, 1976
30. Dresden MH, Heilman SA, Schmidt JD: Collagenolytic enzymes in human neoplasms. Cancer Res 32:993–996, 1972
31. Strauch L: The role of collagenases in tumor invasion. In Tarin D (ed): Tissue Interactions in Carcinogenesis, pp 399–407. London, Academic Press, 1972
32. Sylven B: Lysosomal enzyme activity in the interstitial fluid of solid mouse tumour transplants. Eur J Cancer 4:463–474, 1968
33. Yamanishi T, Maeyens E, Dabbous MK et al: Collagenolytic activity in malignant melanoma: physichochemical studies. Cancer Res 33:2507–2512, 1973

34. Sylven B: Biochemical and enzymatic factors involved in cellular detachment. In Garattini S, Franchi G (eds): Chemotherapy of Cancer Dissemination and Metastasis, pp 129–138. New York, Raven Press, 1973
35. Bosmann HB, Hall TC: Enzyme activity in invasive tumors of human breast and colon. Proc Natl Acad Sci USA 71:1833–1837, 1974
36. Poole AR, Tiltman KJ, Recklies AD et al: Differences in secretion of the proteinase cathepsin B at the edges of human breast carcinomas and fibroadenomas. Nature 273:545–547, 1978
37. Recklies AD, Tiltman KJ, Stoker TAM et al: Secretion of proteinases from malignant and nonmalignant human breast tissue. Cancer Res 40:550–556, 1980
38. Roblin RO, Chou IN, Black PH: Proteolytic enzymes, cell surface changes and viral transformation. Adv Cancer Res 22:203–259, 1975
39. Roblin RO: Plasminogen activator production as a possible biological marker for human neoplasia: some fundamental questions. In Ruddon R (ed): Biological Markers of Neoplasia: Basic and Applied Aspects, pp 421–432. New York, Elsevier Publishing Co, 1978
40. Reich E: Tumor-associated fibrinolysis: abstracted comments. Fed Proc 32:2174–2175, 1973
41. Nicolson GL, Birdwell CR, Brunson KW et al: Cell interactions in the metastatic process: some cell surface properties associated with successful blood-borne tumor spread. In Burger MM, Lash J (eds): Cell and Tissue Interactions, pp 225–241. New York, Raven Press, 1977
42. Wang BS, McLoughlin GA, Richie JP et al: Correlation of the production of plasminogen activator with tumor metastasis in B16 mouse melanoma cell lines. Cancer Res 40:288–292, 1980
43. Liotta LA, Tryggvason K, Garbisa S et al: Metastatic potential correlates with enzymatic degradation of basement membrane collagen. Nature 284:67–68, 1980
44. Babai F: Etude ultrastructurale sur la pathogenie de l'invasion du muscle strie par des tumeurs transplantables. J Ultrastruct Res 56:287–303, 1976
45. Liotta LA, Abe S, Robey PG et al: Preferential digestion of basement membrane collagen by an enzyme derived from a metastatic murine tumor. Proc Natl Acad Sci USA 76:2268–2272, 1979
46. Liotta LA, Kleinerman J, Catanzaro P et al: Degradation of basement membrane by murine tumor cells. JNCI 58:1427–1431, 1977
47. Murray JC, Liotta L, Rennard SI et al: Adhesion characteristics of murine metastatic and nonmetastatic tumor cells *in vitro*. Cancer Res 40:347–351, 1980
48. Warren BA: Environment of the blood-borne tumor embolus adherent to vessel wall. J Med 4:150–177, 1973
49. Warren BA, Chaurin WJ, Philips J: Blood-borne tumor emboli and their adherence to vessel walls. In Day SB (ed): Cancer Invasion and Metastasis: Biologic Mechanisms and Therapy, pp 185–197. New York, Raven Press, 1977
50. del Regato JA: Pathways of metastatic spread of malignant tumors. Semin Oncol 4:33–38, 1977
51. Fisher B, Fisher ER: The interrelationship of hematogenous and lymphatic tumor cell dissemination. Surg Gynecol Obstet 122:791–798, 1966
52. Zeidman I, Buss JM: Experimental studies on the spread of cancer in the lymphatic system, I. Effectiveness of the lymph node as a barrier to the passage of embolic tumor cells. Cancer Res 14:403–410, 1954
53. Paget S: The distribution of secondary growths in cancer of the breast. Lancet i:571–573, 1889
54. Fisher ER, Fisher B: Recent observations on the concept of metastasis. Arch Pathol 83:321–324, 1967
55. del Regato JA: Physiopathology of metastasis. In Weiss L, Gilbert HA (eds): Pulmonary Metastasis, pp 104–113. Boston, GK Hall, 1978
56. Berg JW, Huvos AG, Axtell LM et al: A new sign of favorable prognosis in mammary cancer: hyperplastic reactive lymph nodes in the apex of the axilla. Ann Surg 177:8–16, 1973
57. Lane M, Goksel H, Salerno RA et al: Clinicopathologic analysis of the surgical curability of breast cancers: a minimum ten-year study of a personal series. Ann Surg 153:483–504, 1961
58. Black MM, Freeman C, Mork T et al: Prognostic significance of microscopic structure of gastic carcinomas and their regional lymph nodes. Cancer 27:703–710, 1971
59. Carter RL: Recurrent and metastatic malignant disease: immunological considerations. Proc R Soc Med 67:852–854, 1974
60. Alexander P: Metastatic spread and "escape" from the immune defenses of the host. Natl Cancer Inst Monogr 44:125–129, 1976
61. Mitchinson NA: Passive transfer of transplantation immunity. Proc R Soc Lond Ser B 142:72–87, 1954
62. Billingham RE, Brent L, Medawar PB: Quantitative studies on tissue transplantation immunity. Philos Trans R Soc Lond Ser B 239:357–366, 1956
63. Barker CF, Billingham RE: The role of afferent lymphatics in the rejection of skin homografts. J Exp Med 128:197–222, 1968
64. Futrell JW, Myers GH: Role of regional lymphatics in tumor allograft rejection. Transplantation 13:551–557, 1972
65. Crile G: Rationale of simple mastectomy without radiation for clinical stage 1 cancer of the breast. Surg Gynecol Obstet 120:975–982, 1965
66. Crile G: Possible role of uninvolved regional nodes in preventing metastasis from breast cancer. Cancer 24:1283–1289, 1969
67. Fisher B, Wolmark N, Coyle J et al: Studies concerning the regional lymph node in cancer, VIII. Effect of two asynchronous tumor foci on lymph node cell cytotoxicity. Cancer 36: 521–527, 1975
68. Fisher B, Saffer EA, Fisher ER: Studies concerning the regional lymph node in cancer, IV. Tumor inhibition by regional lymph node cells. Cancer 33:631–636, 1972
69. Fisher B, Wolmark N: New concepts in the management of primary breast cancer. Cancer 36:627–632, 1975
70. Editorial: Management of early cancer of the breast: report on an international multicentre trial supported by the Cancer Research Campaign. Br Med J 1:1035–1038, 1976
71. Brem H, Foldman J: Inhibition of tumor angiogenesis mediated by cartilage. J Exp Med 141:427–439, 1975
72. Sorgente N, Kuettner KE, Soble LW et al: The resistance of certain tissues to invasion, II. Evidence for extractable factors in cartilage which inhibit invasion by vascularized mesenchyme. Lab Invest 32:217–222, 1975
73. Eisenstein R, Kuettner KE, Neopolitan C et al: The resistance of certain tissues to invasion, III. Cartilage extracts inhibit the growth of fibroblasts and endothelial cells in culture. Am J Pathol 81:337–347, 1975
74. Folkman J: Tumor angiogenesis. Adv Cancer Res 19:331–358, 1974
75. Liotta LA, Kleinerman J, Saidel GM: Quantitative relationships of intravascular tumor cells, tumor vessels and pulmonary metastases following tumor implantation. Cancer Res 34:997–1004, 1974
76. Liotta LA, Saidel G, Kleinerman J: Stochastic model of metastases formation. Biometrics 32:535–550, 1976
77. Salsbury AJ: The significance of the circulating cancer cell. Cancer Treat Rev 2:55–72, 1975
78. Fidler IJ: Metastasis: quantitative analysis of distribution and fate of tumor emboli labeled with ^{125}I-5-iodo-2′-deoxyuridine. JNCI 45:773–782, 1970
79. Butler T, Gullino P: Quantitation of cell-shedding into efferent blood of mammary adenocarcinoma. Cancer Res 35:512–517, 1975
80. Weiss L: Some mechanisms involved in cancer cell detachment by necrotic material. Int J Cancer 22:196–203, 1978
81. Fidler IJ: The relationship of embolic homogeneity, number, size and viability to the incidence of experimental metastasis. Eur J Cancer 9:223–227, 1973
82. Liotta LA, Kleinerman J, Saidel G: The significance of hematogenous tumor cell clumps in the metastatic process. Cancer Res 36:889–894, 1976
83. Ryd W, Hagmar B: Effect of cell aggregation on intravenous

tumor transplantation. Acta Pathol Microbiol Scand 85:405–412, 1977
84. Mason RG, Saba HI: Normal and abnormal hemostasis: an integrated view. Am J Pathol 92:775–811, 1978
85. Gasic GJ, Gasic TB, Galanti N et al: Platelet-tumor cell interaction in mice: the role of platelets in the spread of malignant disease. Int J Cancer 11:704–718, 1973
86. Chew EC, Josephson RL, Wallace AC: Morphological aspects of the arrest of circulating cancer cells. In Weiss L (ed): Fundamental Aspects of Metastasis, pp 121–150. Amsterdam, North Holland Biomedical Press, 1976
87. Wood S Jr: Experimental studies of the intravascular dissemination of ascitic V2 carcinoma cells in the rabbit with special reference to fibinogen and fibrinolytic agents. Bull Schweiz Akad Med Wiss 20:92–121, 1964
88. Cliffton EE, Agostino D: The effects of fibrin formation and alterations in the clotting mechanism on the development of metastases. Vasc Dis 2:43–52, 1965
89. Cotmore SF, Carter RL: Mechanism of enhanced intrahepatic metastases in surfactant-treated hamsters: an electron microscopy study. Int J Cancer 11:725–738, 1973
90. Sindelar WF, Tralka TS, Ketcham AS: Electron microscope observations on formation of pulmonary metastases. J Surg Res 18:137–161, 1975
91. Cliffton EE, Grossi CE: The rationale of anticoagulants in the treatment of cancer. J Med 5:107–116, 1974
92. Svanberg L: Thromboplastic activity of human ovarian tumours. Thromb Res 6:307–311, 1975
93. Gordon SG, Franks JJ, Lewis B: Cancer procoagulant A: a factor X activating procoagulant from malignant tissue. Thromb Res 6:127–133, 1975
94. Curatolo L et al: Evidence that cells from experimental tumours can activate coagulation factor X. Br J Cancer 40:228–233, 1979
95. Hoover HC, Ketcham AS, Millar RC, et al: Osteosarcoma: improved survival with anticoagulation and amputation. Cancer 41:2475–2480, 1978
96. Baserga R, Saffioti U: Experimental studies on histogenesis of blood-borne metastases. Arch Pathol 59:26–34, 1955
97. Ewing J: Neoplastic Diseases, 3rd ed. Philadelphia, WB Saunders, 1928
98. Fidler IJ, Gersten DM, Riggs CW: Relationship of host immune status to tumor cell arrest, distribution and survival in experimental metastasis. Cancer 40:23–30, 1977
99. Reif A: Evidence for organ specificity of defenses against tumors. In Waters H (ed): The Handbook of Cancer Immunology, Vol 1, pp 174–240. New York, Garland STPM Press, 1978
100. Klein K, Coetzee ML, Madhav R et al: Inhibition of tritiated thymidine incorporation in cultured cells by rat kidney extract. JNCI 62:1557–1564, 1979
101. Kinsey DL: An experimental study of preferential metastasis. Cancer 13:674–676, 1960
102. Sugarbaker EV, Cohen AM, Ketcham AS: Do metastases metastasize? Ann Surg 174:161–166, 1971
103. Hart IR, Fidler IJ: The role of organ selectivity in the determination of metastatic patterns of the B16 melanoma. Cancer Res (in press)
104. Brunson KW, Beattie G, Nicolson GL: Selection and altered tumour cell properties of brain-colonizing metastatic melanoma. Nature 272:543–545, 1978
105. Brunson KW, Nicolson GL: Selection of malignant melanoma variant cell lines for ovary colonization. J Supramol Struct 11:517–528, 1979
106. Tao T, Matter A, Vogel K et al: Liver colonizing melanoma cells selected from B16 melanoma. Int J Cancer 23:854–857, 1979
107. Raz A, Hart IR: Murine melanoma: a model for intracranial metastasis. Br J Cancer (in press)
108. Poste G, Nicolson GL: Modification of the arrest of poorly metastatic tumor cells in the microcirculation after treatment with plasma membrane vesicles from highly metastatic cells. Proc Natl Acad Sci USA 77:399–403, 1980
109. Winkelhake JL, Nicolson GL: Determination of adhesive properties of variant metastatic melanoma cells to BALB/3T3 cells and their virus-transformed derivatives by a monolayer attachment assay. JNCI 56:285–291, 1976
110. Kahan B: Ovarian localization by embryonal teratocarcinoma cells derived from female germ cells. Somatic Cell Genet 5:763–780, 1979
111. Schirrmacher V, Cheingson-Popov R, Arnheiter H: Hepatocyte-tumor cell interaction *in vitro*, I. Conditions for rosette formation and inhibition by anti-H-2 antibody. J Exp Med 151:984–989, 1980
112. Baldwin RW: Role of immunosurveillance against chemically induced rat tumors. Transplant Rev 28:62–69, 1976
113. Fidler IJ, Kripke ML: Tumor cell antigenicity, host immunity and cancer metastasis. Cancer Immunol Immunother 7:201–205, 1980
114. Weiss L, Glaves D, Waite D: The influence of host immunity on the arrest of circulating cancer cells in tumor-bearing mice. Int J Cancer 18:850–862, 1974
115. Alexander P: Dormant metastases which manifest on immunosuppression and the role of macrophages in tumors. In Weiss L (ed): Fundamental Aspects of Metastasis, pp 227–239. Amsterdam, North Holland Biomedical Press, 1976
116. Fisher ER, Soliman O, Fisher B: Effect of anti-lymphocyte serum on parameters of growth of MCA-induced tumors. Nature 221:287–288, 1969
117. Kim U, Baumler A, Carruthers C et al: Immunological escape mechanism in spontaneously metastasizing mammary tumors. Proc Natl Acad Sci USA 72:1012–1016, 1975
118. Sadler TE, Castro JE: Abrogation of the anti-metastatic activity of *Corynebacterium parvum* by antilymphocyte serum. Br J Cancer 34:291–295, 1976
119. Fidler IJ: Immune stimulation-inhibition of experimental cancer metastasis. Cancer Res 34:491–498, 1974
120. Vaage J: A survey of the growth characteristics of and the host reactions to one hundred C3H/HeN mammary carcinomas. Cancer Res 38:331–338, 1978
121. Hewitt HB, Blake ER, Walder AS: A critique of the evidence for active host defense against cancer based on personal studies of 27 murine tumors of spontaneous origin. Br J Cancer 33:241–249, 1976
122. Fidler IJ, Gersten DM, Kripke ML: Influence of immune status on the metastasis of three murine fibrosarcomas of different immunogenicities. Cancer Res 39:3816–3821, 1979
123. Prehn RT: The immune reaction as a stimulator of tumor growth. Science 176:170–171, 1972
124. Prehn RT: Immunostimulation of the lymphodependent phase of neoplastic growth. JNCI 59:1043–1049, 1977
125. Auerbach T, Kubai L, Sidky Y: Angiogenesis induction by tumors, embryonic tissues and lymphocytes. Cancer Res 36:3435–3440, 1976
126. Fisher MS, Kripke ML: Systemic alteration induced in mice by ultraviolet light irradiation and its relationship to ultraviolet carcinogenesis. Proc Natl Acad Sci USA 74:1688–1693, 1977
127. Fisher MS, Kripke ML: Further studies on the tumor-specific suppressor cells induced by ultraviolet radiation. J Immunol 121:1139–1144, 1978
128. Thomas L: Discussion. In Lawrence HS (ed): Cellular and Humoral Aspects of the Hypersensitive States, pp 529–532. New York, Paul B Hoeber, 1959
129. Burnet FM: Self and Not-Self, pp 286–308. London, Cambridge University Press, 1969
130. Allison AC: Immunological surveillance of tumors. Cancer Immunol Immunother 2:151–155, 1977
131. Stutman O: Immunodepression and malignancy. Adv Cancer Res 22:261–422, 1975
132. Rygaard J, Povlsen O: The nude mouse in the hypothesis of immunological surveillance. Transplant Rev 28:43–61, 1976
133. Outzen HC, Custer RP, Eaton GJ: Spontaneous and induced tumor incidence in germ-free nude mice. J Reticuloendothel Soc 17:1–9, 1975
134. Herberman RB, Holden HT: Natural cell-mediated immunity. Adv Cancer Res 27:305–351, 1978

135. Herberman RB et al: Natural killer cells: characteristics and regulation of activity. Immunol Rev 44:43–70, 1979
136. Campanile F, Crino L, Bonmassar E et al: Radio-resistant inhibition of lymphoma growth in congenitally athymic (nude) mice. Cancer Res 37:394–399, 1977
137. Iorio A, Campanile F, Neri M et al: Inhibition of lymphoma growth in the spleen and liver of lethally irradiated mice. J Immunol 120:1679–1686, 1978
138. Fidler IJ, Caines S, Dolan Z: Survival of hematogenously disseminated allogeneic tumor cells in athymic nude mice. Transplantation 22: 208–212, 1976
139. Hanna N, Fidler IJ: Expression of metastatic potential of allogeneic and xenogeneic neoplasms in young nude mice. Cancer Res (in press)
140. Hanna N, Fidler IJ: The role of natural killer cells in the destruction of circulating tumor emboli. JNCI (in press)
141. Talmadge JE, Meyers KM, Prieur DJ et al: Role of NK cells in tumour growth and metastasis in beige mice. Nature 284:622–624, 1980
142. Sordat B, Merenda C, Carrel S: Invasive growth and dissemination of human solid tumors and malignant cell lines grafted subcutaneously to newborn nude mice. In Nomura T, Ohsawa N, Tamaoki N et al (eds): Proceedings of the Second International Workshop on Nude Mice, pp 313–326. Tokyo, University of Tokyo Press, 1977
143. Baldwin RW, Barker CR: Demonstration of tumour-specific humoral antibody against aminoazo dye-induced rat hepatoma. Br J Cancer 21:793–801, 1967
144. Morton DL, Malmgren RA, Holmes EC et al: Demonstration of antibodies against human malignant melanoma by immunofluorescence. Surgery 64:233–270, 1968
145. Lewis MG et al: Tumour-specific antibodies in human malignant melanoma and their relationship to the extent of the disease. Br Med J 3:547–552, 1969
146. Lewis MG, Phillips TM, Cook KB et al: Possible explanation of loss of detectable antibody in patients with disseminated melanoma. Nature 232:52–54, 1971
147. Hellstrom KE, Hellstrom I: Lymphocyte-mediated cytotoxicity and blocking serum activity to tumor antigens. Adv Immunol 18:209–277, 1974
148. Hellstrom I, Hellstrom KE: Studies on cellular immunity and its serum-mediated inhibition in Moloney virus-induced mouse sarcomas. Int J Cancer 4:587–593, 1969
149. Hellstrom I, Hellstrom KE: Colony inhibition studies on blocking and non-blocking serum effects on cellular immunity to Moloney sarcomas. Int J Cancer 5:195–201, 1970
150. Price MR, Robins RA: Circulating factors modifying cell-mediated immunity in experimental neoplasia. In Castro JE (ed): Immunological Aspects of Cancer, pp 155–181. Lancaster, MTP Press, 1978
151. Bansal SC, Hargreaves R, Sjogren HO: Facilitation of polyoma tumor growth in rats by blocking sera and tumor eluate. Int J Cancer 9:97–102, 1972
152. Bansal SC, Sjogren HO: Counteraction of the blocking of cell-mediated tumor immunity by inoculation of unblocking sera and splenectomy: immunotherapeutic effects on primary tumors in rats. Int J Cancer 9:490–496, 1972
153. Starkey JR, Talmadge JE, Ristow SS et al: Modification of tumor growth and metastasis by tumor-induced humoral factors or by the presence of a second tumor mass. Fed Proc 39:776, 1980
154. Alexander P: Escape from immune destruction by the host through shedding of surface antigens: is this a characteristic shared by malignant and embryonic cells? Cancer Res 34:2077–2082, 1974
155. Langvad E, Hyden H, Wolf H et al: Extracorporeal immunoadsorption of circulating specific serum factors in cancer patients. Br J Cancer 32:680–686, 1975
156. Fidler IJ, Cifone MA: Properties of metastatic and nonmetastatic cloned subpopulations of an ultraviolet-light-induced murine fibrosarcoma of recent origin. Am J Pathol 97:633–638, 1979
157. Koch FE: Zur frege be metastas-enbildung bei inpftumoren. Krebsforsch 48:495–507, 1939
158. Klein E: Gradual transformation of solid into ascites tumors: evidence favoring the mutation-selection theory. Exp Cell Res 8: 188–212, 1955
159. Fidler IJ: Selection of successive tumor lines for metastasis. Nature (New Biol) 242:148–149, 1973
160. Fidler IJ: Tumor heterogeneity and the biology of cancer invasion and metastasis. Cancer Res 38:2651–2660, 1978
161. Suzuki N, Withers HR, Koehler MW: Heterogeneity and variability of artificial lung colony-forming ability among clones from mouse fibrosarcoma. Cancer Res 38:3349–3351, 1978
162. Brunson KW, Nicolson GL: Selection and biologic properties of malignant variants of a murine lymphosarcoma. JNCI 61:1499–1503, 1978
163. Briles EB, Kornfeld S: Isolation and metastatic properties of detachment variants of B16 melanoma cells. JNCI 60:1217–1222, 1978
164. Fidler IJ, Gersten DM, Budmen MB: Characterization *in vivo* and *in vitro* of tumor cells selected for resistance to syngeneic lymphocyte-mediated cytotoxicity. Cancer Res 36:3160–3165, 1976
165. Tao TW, Burger MM: Nonmetastasizing variants selected from metastasizing melanoma cells. Nature 270:437–438, 1977
166. Reading CL, Brunson KW, Torrianni M et al: Malignancies of murine lymphosarcoma cells correlate with decreased cell surface display of RNA-tumor virus envelope glycoprotein gp70. Proc Natl Acad Sci USA (in press)
167. Fidler IJ, Kripke ML: Metastasis results from pre-existing variant cells within a malignant tumor. Science 197:893–895, 1977
168. Luria SE, Delbruck M: Mutations of bacteria from virus sensitivity to virus resistance. Genetics 28:491–511, 1943
169. Kripke ML, Gruys E, Fidler IJ: Metastatic heterogeneity of cells from an ultraviolet light-induced murine fibrosarcoma of recent origin. Cancer Res 38:2962–2967, 1978
170. Fidler IJ, Kripke ML: Metastatic heterogeneity of cells from the K-1735 melanoma. In Grundmann E (ed): Metastatic Tumor Growths. Stuttgart and New York, Gustav Fischer Verlag, 1980
171. Dexter LD, Kowalski HM, Blazar BA et al: Heterogeneity of tumor cells from a single mouse mammary tumor. Cancer Res 38:3179–3186, 1978
172. Suzuki N, Withers HR: Isolation from murine fibrosarcoma of cell lines with enhanced plating efficiency *in vitro*. JNCI 60:179–183, 1978
173. Nicolson GL, Brunson KW, Fidler IJ: Specificity of arrest, survival, and growth of selected metastatic variant cell lines. Cancer Res 38:4105–4111, 1978
174. Brunson KW, Nicolson GL: Selection and biologic properties of malignant variants of a murine lymphosarcoma. JNCI 61:1499–1503, 1978
175. Talmadge JE, Starkey JR, Davis WC et al: Introduction of metastatic heterogeneity by short term *in vivo* passage of a cloned transformed cell line. J Supramol Struct 12:227–243, 1979
176. Fialkow PJ: Genetic marker studies in neoplasia. In Genetic Concepts and Neoplasia, pp 112–130. Baltimore, Williams & Wilkins, 1970
177. Fialkow PJ: Clonal origin of human tumors. Biochim Biophys Acta 458:283–291, 1976
178. Ohno S: Genetic implication of karyological instability of malignant somatic cells. Physiol Rev 51:496–526, 1971
179. Reddy AL, Fialkow PJ: Multicellular origin of fibrosarcomas in mice induced by the chemical carcinogen 3-methylcholanthrene. J Exp Med 150:878–887, 1979
180. Hakansson L, Trope C: On the presence within tumors of clones that differ in sensitivity to cytostatic drugs. Acta Pathol Microbiol Scand 82:35–40, 1974
181. Hakansson L, Trope C: An *in vitro* study of the effect of cytostatic drugs on the DNA synthesis in methylcholanthrene induced mouse sarcomas and in rat Walker 256 tumours. Acta Pathol Microbiol Scand (A) 81:552–558, 1973
182. Prehn RT: Analysis of antigenic heterogeneity within individual 3-methylcholanthrene-induced mouse sarcomas. JNCI 45:1039–1045, 1970

183. Nowell PC: The clonal evolution of tumor cell populations. Science 194:23–28, 1976
184. Killion JJ, Kollmorgen GM: Isolation of immunogenic tumor cells by cell-affinity chromatography. Nature 259:674–676, 1976
185. Kerbel RS: Implications of immunological heterogeneity of tumours. Nature 280:358–360, 1979
186. Fugi H, Mihich E: Selection for high immunogenicity in drug resistant sublines of murine lymphomas demonstrated by plaque assay. Cancer Res 35:946–952, 1975
187. Fogel M, Gorelik E, Segal S et al: Differences in cell surface antigens of tumor metastases and those of the local tumor. JNCI 62:585–588, 1979
188. Schabel FM Jr: Concepts for systemic treatment of micrometastases. Cancer 35:15–24, 1975
189. Kirccuta I, Mustea I, Rogozaw I et al: Relations between tumor and metastases, I. Aspects of the crabtree effect. Cancer 18:978–984, 1965
190. Sluyser M, VanNie R: Estrogen receptor content and hormone-responsive growth of mouse mammary tumors. Cancer Res 34:3253–3257, 1974
191. Baylin SB: Clonal selection and heterogeneity of human solid neoplasms. In Fidler IJ, White RJ (eds): Design of Models for Testing Cancer Therapeutic Agents. New York, Van Nostrand (in press)
192. Gray JM, Pierce GB: Relationship between growth rate and differentiation of melanoma *in vivo*. JNCI 32:1201–1211, 1964
193. Trope C: Different susceptibilities of tumor cell subpopulations to cytotoxic agents. In Fidler IJ, White RJ (ed): Design of Models for Testing Cancer Therapeutic Agents. New York, Van Nostrand (in press)
194. Ito E, Moore GE: Characteristic differences in clones isolated from an S37 ascites tumor *in vitro*. Exp Cell Res 48:440–447, 1967
195. Mitelman F: The chromosomes of fifty primary Rous rat sarcomas. Hereditas 69:155–186, 1971
196. Barranco SC, Ho DHW, Drewinko B et al: Differential sensitivities of human melanoma cells grown *in vitro* to Arabinosylcytosine. Cancer Res 32:2733–2736, 1972
197. Heppner GH, Dexter DL, De Nucci T et al: Heterogeneity in drug sensitivity among tumor cell subpopulations of a single mammary tumor. Cancer Res 38:3758–3763, 1978
198. Trope C: Different sensitivity to cytostatic drugs of primary tumor and metastasis of the Lewis carcinoma. Neoplasma 22:171–180, 1975
199. Siracky J: An approach to the problem of heterogeneity of human tumour-cell populations. Br J Cancer 39:570–577, 1979
200. Foulds L: Neoplastic Development, Vol 1. London, Academic Press, 1969
201. Foulds L: Neoplastic Development, Vol 2. London, Academic Press, 1975
202. Prehn RT: Tumor progression and homeostasis. Adv Cancer Res 23: 203–236, 1976
203. Dunn T: Morphology of mammary tumors in mice. In Homburger F (ed): Physiopathology of Cancer, pp 38–84. New York, Paul B Hoeber, 1959
204. Trope C, Hakansson L, Dencker H: Heterogeneity of human adenocarcinomas of the colon and the stomach as regards sensitivity to cytostatic drugs. Neoplasma 22:423–430, 1975
205. Trope C, Aspegren K, Kullander S et al: Heterogeneous response of disseminated human ovarian cancers to cytostatis *in vitro*. Acta Obstet Gynecol Scand (in press)
206. Biorklund A, Hakansson L, Stenstam B et al: Heterogeneity of non-Hodgkin's lymphomas as regards sensitivity to cytostatic drugs: an *in vitro* study. Eur J Cancer (in press)
207. Baylin SD, Weissberger WR, Eggleston JC et al: Variable content of histaminase, L-dopa decarboxylase and calcitonin in small-cell carcinoma of the lung: biologic and clinical implications. N Engl J Med 229:105–110, 1978
208. Baylin SD, Abeloff, MD, Goodwin G et al: Activities of L-dopa decarboxylase and diamine oxidase (histaminase) in human lung cancers: the decarboxylase as a marker for small (oat) cell cancer in tissue culture. Cancer Res (in press)
209. Schabel FM Jr, Griswold DP Jr, Corbett RB et al: Testing therapeutic hypotheses in mice and man: observations on the therapeutic activity against advanced solid tumors of mice treated with anticancer drugs that have demonstrated or have potential clinical utility for treatment of advanced solid tumors of man. In Busch H, DeVita VT (eds): Cancer Drug Development, Part B. Methods in Cancer Research, Vol 17, pp 3–40. New York, Academic Press, 1979
210. Olsson L, Ebbesen P: Natural polyclonality of spontaneous AKR leukemia and its consequence for so-called specific immunotherapy. JNCI 62:623–627, 1979
211. Abeloff MD, Ettinger DS, Khouri NF et al: Intensive induction therapy for small cell carcinoma of the lung. Cancer Treat Rep 63:519–524, 1979
212. Livinston RB: Treatment of small cell carcinoma: evolution and future directions. Semin Oncol 5:299–308, 1979

CHAPTER 6

Steven A. Rosenberg

Principles of Surgical Oncology

Surgery is the oldest treatment for cancer and until recently was the only treatment modality capable of curing patients with cancer. The surgical treatment of cancer has changed dramatically in the last several decades. Advances in surgical technique and an increased understanding of the patterns of spread of individual cancers have provided surgeons with the tools and knowledge necessary to allow an extension of surgical resections to an increased number of patients. At the same time, the development of alternate treatment strategies that are capable of controlling microscopic disease has led the surgeon to a careful reassessment of the magnitude of surgery necessary in conjunction with other treatment modalities. These available alternative treatments increase the consideration of the quality of life that results from treatment interventions.

Consideration of these issues requires the surgeon treating cancer to be familiar with the natural history of individual cancers, the principles and potentialities of surgery, radiation therapy, chemotherapy, immunotherapy, and the other new treatment modalities developing.

The surgeon has a central role in the prevention, diagnosis, definitive treatment, palliation, and rehabilitation of the cancer patient. The principles underlying each of these roles of the surgical oncologist will be discussed in this chapter.

HISTORICAL PERSPECTIVES

Though the earliest discussions of the surgical treatment of tumors are found in the Edwin Smith Papyrus from the Egyptian Middle Kingdom (approximately 1600 B.C.), the modern era of elective surgery for visceral tumors began in frontier America in 1809.[1,2] Ephraim MacDowell removed a 22 pound ovarian tumor from a patient, Mrs. Jane Todd Crawford, who survived for 30 years after the operation. This procedure, the first of 13 ovarian resections performed by MacDowell, was the first elective abdominal operation and provided a great stimulus to the development of elective surgery.

However, the development of surgery for the treatment of most tumors was dependent on two developments in surgery. The first of these was the introduction of general anesthesia by two dentists, Dr. William Morton and Dr. Crawford Long. The first major operation under general ether anesthesia was an excision of the submaxillary gland and part of the tongue, performed by Dr. John Collins Warren on October 16, 1846, at the Massachusetts General Hospital. The second major development stimulating the widespread application of surgery resulted from the introduction of the principles of antisepsis by Joseph Lister in 1867. Based on the concepts of Pasteur, Lister introduced carbolic acid in 1867 and described the principles of antisepsis in an article in the Lancet in that same year.

These two developments freed surgery from both pain and sepsis and led to a flourishing of the use of surgery for the treatment of tumors. In the decade prior to the introduction of ether only 385 operations were performed at the Massachusetts General Hospital. By the last decade of the 19th century, over 20,000 operations per year were performed at that same hospital.[3]

Table 6-1 lists some selected historical landmarks in the development of surgical oncology. While this does not include

TABLE 6-1. Selected Historical Landmarks in Surgical Oncology

YEAR	SURGEON	EVENT
1809	Ephraim McDowell	Elective abdominal surgery (excised ovarian tumor)
1846	John Collins Warren	Use of ether anesthesia (excised submaxillary gland)
1867	Joseph Lister	Introduction of antisepsis
1850–1880	Albert Theodore Billroth	First gastrectomy, laryngectomy, and esophagectomy
1878	Richard von Volkmann	Excision of cancerous rectum
1880's	Theodore Kocher	Development of thyroid surgery
1890	William Stewart Halsted	Radical mastectomy
1896	G. T. Beatson	Oophorectomy for breast cancer
1904	Hugh H. Young	Radical prostatectomy
1906	Ernest Wertheim	Radical hysterectomy
1908	W. Ernest Miles	Abdomenoperineal resection for cancer of the rectum
1912	E. Martin	Cordotomy for the treatment of pain
1910–1930	Harvey Cushing	Development of surgery for brain tumors
1913	Franz Torek	Successful resection of cancer of the thoracic esophagus
1927	G. Divis	Successful resection of pulmonary metastases
1933	Evarts Graham	Pneumonectomy
1935	A. O. Whipple	Pancreaticoduodenectomy
1945	Charles B. Huggins	Adrenalectomy for prostate cancer

all of the important developments, it does provide the tempo of the application of surgery to cancer treatment.[4] Major figures in the evolution of surgical oncology included Albert Theodore Billroth who, in addition to the development of meticulous surgical technique, performed the first gastrectomy, laryngectomy, and esophagectomy. In the 1890's William Stewart Halsted elucidated the principles of en bloc resections for cancer as exemplified by his development of the radical mastectomy. Examples of radical resections for cancers of individual organs include the development of the radical prostatectomy by Hugh Young in 1904, the radical hysterectomy by Ernest Wertheim in 1906, the abdominoperineal resection for cancer of the rectum by Dr. W. Ernest Miles in 1908, and the first successful pneumonectomy performed for cancer by Evarts Graham in 1933. Developments in technical surgery continue at a rapid pace and modern technical innovations are continuing to significantly extend the surgeon's reach into a variety of areas. Examples of developments in the last several decades that have had profound impact on surgery include the development of microsurgical techniques that enable the performance of free grafts for reconstruction, automatic stapling devices, sophisticated endoscopic equipment that allow for a wide variety of "incisionless" surgery, and major improvements in postoperative management and critical care of patients that have extended the safety of major surgical therapy.

Many critics of modern surgery who feel that the application of surgery has reached a plateau beyond which it will not progress should remember the words of a famous British surgeon, Sir John Erichsen, who in his introductory address to the medical institutions at University College on October 4, 1873, said:

> ". . . there must be a final limit to the development of manipulative surgery, the knife cannot always have fresh fields for conquest and although methods of practice may be modified and varied and even improved to some extent, it must be within a certain limit. That this limit has nearly, if not quite, been reached will appear evident if we reflect on the great achievements of modern operative surgery. Very little remains for the boldest to devise or the most dextrous to perform."

These comments published in Lancet in 1873 by this prominent academic surgeon preceded the majority of important developments in modern surgical oncology.

THE OPERATION

ANESTHESIA

Modern anesthetic techniques have greatly increased the safety of major oncologic surgery. Regional and general anesthesia play an important role in a wide variety of diagnostic techniques and local therapeutic maneuvers, as well as in major surgery, and these should be understood by all oncologists.

Anesthetic techniques may be divided into *regional* and *general* anesthesia. *Regional* anesthesia implies a reversible blockade of pain perception by the application of local anesthetic drugs. These agents generally work by preventing the activation of pain receptors or blocking the transmission of nerve conduction. A variety of agents commonly used for regional anesthesia are shown in Table 6-2.[5] *Topical* anesthesia refers to the application of local anesthetics to the skin or mucous membranes. Good surface anesthesia of the conjunctiva and cornea, the oral- and nasopharynx, esophagus, larynx, trachea, urethra, and anus can result from the application of these agents.

Local anesthesia refers to the injection of anesthetic agents directly into the operative field. Field block refers to injection of local anesthetic by circumscribing the operative field with

TABLE 6-2. Regional Anesthetic Agents

TECHNIQUE	LOCAL ANESTHETIC	CONCENTRATION RANGE	DURATION OF ACTION	MAXIMAL SAFE DOSE
Topical anesthesia (mucous membranes)	Lidocaine	2–4%	15 minutes	100 mg
	Cocaine	4–10%	30 minutes	100–200 mg
	Tetracaine	1–2%	45 minutes	40 mg
	Benzocaine	2–10%	Several hours	
Local infiltration	Procaine	0.5%	¼–½ hour	1000 mg
	Lidocaine	0.5–1%	½–1 hour	500 mg
	Mepivacaine	0.5–1%	½–1 hour	500 mg
	Tetracaine	0.025–0.1%	2–3 hours	75 mg
Major nerve block	Lidocaine	1–2%	1–2 hours	500 mg
	Mepivacaine	1–2%	1–2 hours	500 mg
	Tetracaine	0.1–0.25%	2–3 hours	75 mg

(Adapted from Brunner EA, Eckenhoff JE: Anesthesia. *In* Sabiston DC Jr. (ed): Textbook of Surgery. Phila., W.B. Saunders, 1977)

a continuous wall of anesthetic agent. Lidocaine (Xylocaine) in concentrations from 0.5 to 1% is the most common anesthetic agent used for this purpose. Peripheral nerve block refers to the deposition of a local anesthetic surrounding major nerve trunks. It can provide local anesthesia to entire anatomic areas.

Major surgical procedures to the lower portion of the body can be performed under either epidural or spinal anesthesia. Epidural anesthesia results from the deposition of a local anesthetic agent into the extradural space within the vertebral canal. Catheters can be left in place in the epidural space, thus allowing the intermittent injection of local anesthetics for prolonged operations. The major advantage of epidural over spinal anesthesia is that it does not involve puncturing the dura and thus the injection of foreign substances directly into the cerebrospinal fluid.

Spinal anesthesia involves the direct injection of local anesthetic into the cerebrospinal fluid. Puncture of the dural sac is generally performed between the L2 and L4 vertebra. Spinal anesthesia provides excellent anesthesia for intraabdominal operations, operations on the pelvis, or the lower extremities. There is little systemic toxicity of spinal anesthesia and the safety of administration has led to widespread use of this technique.

General anesthesia refers to the reversible state of loss of consciousness produced by a variety of chemical agents that act directly on the brain. General anesthesia is commonly used for major surgical oncologic procedures. Many general anesthetic agents exist and are currently in clinical use, the most popular being nitrous oxide, generally in combination with narcotics and muscle relaxants. This technique provides a safe form of general anesthesia with the use of nonexplosive agents. Two other agents in current widespread use are the fluorinated hydrocarbons, halothane (Fluothane) and enflurane (Ethrane). Though in general use, the fluorinated hydrocarbons have a variety of side effects. Halothane is associated with significant hepatotoxicity. In addition, virtually all general anesthetics have effects on biochemical mechanisms including depression of bone marrow, alteration of the phagocytic activity of macrophages, and various immunosuppressive properties. General anesthetic agents such as cyclopropane and diethyl ether are rarely used in current practice because of their explosive potential.

OPERATIVE MORTALITY

As with any treatment, the potential benefits of surgical intervention in cancer patients must be weighed against the risks of surgery. The incidence of operative mortality is of major interest in formulating therapeutic decisions and varies greatly in different patient situations (see Table 6-3). The incidence of operative mortality is a complex function of the basic disease process that requires surgery, anesthetic technique, operative complications (related to the complexity of the surgical procedure being performed), and, most importantly, the general health status of the patient and his ability to withstand operative trauma.

In formulating estimates of operative mortality, the general health status of the patient is of primary importance. In an attempt to classify the physical status of patients and their surgical risks, the American Society of Anesthesiologists has formulated a General Classification of Physical Status that appears to correlate well with operative mortality.[6] Patients are classified into five groups depending on their general health status:

Class 1. The patient has no organic, physiologic, biochemical, or psychiatric disturbance. The pathologic process for which operation is to be performed is localized and does not entail a systemic disturbance. (Examples: A fit patient with a lipoma or an otherwise healthy woman with a fibroid uterus.)

Class 2. Mild to moderate systemic disturbance caused by either the condition to be surgically treated or by other pathophysiologic processes. The extremes of age are included here, either the neonate or the octogenarian, even though no discernible systemic disease is present. Extreme obesity and chronic bronchitis are also included in this category. (Examples: Nonlimiting or only slightly limiting organic heart disease, mild diabetes, essential hypertension, or anemia.)

TABLE 6-3. Determinants of Operative Risk

General health status
Severity of underlying illness
Degree to which surgery disrupts normal physiologic functions
Technical complexity of the procedure (related to incidence of complications)
Type of anesthesia required
Experience of personnel

Class 3. Severe systemic disturbance or disease from whatever cause, even though it may not be possible to firmly define the degree of disability. (Examples: severely limiting organic heart disease, severe diabetes with vascular complications, moderate to severe degrees of pulmonary insufficiency, angina pectoris, or healed myocardial infarction.)

Class 4. Indicative of the patient with severe systemic disorders that are already life-threatening and not always correctable by operation. (Examples: the severely cachectic patient with metastatic cancer; patients with organic heart disease showing marked signs of cardiac insufficiency, persistent anginal syndrome, or active myocarditis; advanced degrees of pulmonary, hepatic, renal, or endocrine insufficiency; severe neutropenia or thrombocytopenia in cancer patients.)

Class 5. The moribund patient who has little chance of survival but submitted to operation in desperation. Most of these patients require operation as a resuscitative measure with little, if any, anesthesia. (Examples: The burst abdominal aneurysm with profound shock, major cerebral trauma with rapidly increasing intracranial pressure, massive pulmonary embolus.)

Emergency Operation (E). Any patient in one of the classes listed previously who is operated upon as an emergency is considered to be in poorer physical condition. The letter *E* is placed beside the numerical classification. (Examples: patients with perforation of a viscus, major hemorrhage from a gastrointestinal mass, or hitherto uncomplicated hernia now incarcerated and associated with nausea and vomiting.)

Operative mortality is usually defined as mortality within 30 days of a major operative procedure. In oncologic patients, the basic disease process will be a major determinant of operative mortality. Patients undergoing palliative surgery for widely metastatic disease have a high operative mortality even if the surgical procedure can alleviate the emergent problem. Examples of these situations include surgery for intestinal obstruction in patients with widespread ovarian cancer and surgery for gastric outlet obstruction in patients with cancer of the head of the pancreas. Even these simple palliative procedures are associated with mortalities of 20–30% in most series because of the debilitated state of the patient, in addition to the rapidity of progression of the basic disease, which is not in itself being treated by the surgical procedure.

Mortality due to anesthetic administration alone is directly related to the physical status of the patient. In a review of 32,223 operations conducted by Dripps and coworkers, the mortality thought to be related to anesthetic administration alone is presented (see Table 6-4).[7] It is extremely difficult to differentiate the mortality due to anesthesia from that due to other contributors to operative mortality. However, this analysis indicates that operative mortality due to anesthesia in physical status Class 1 patients is extremely low. In this study, Class 1 patients had an anesthetic mortality of less than one in every 16,000 operations. The anesthetic mortality increased with increasing physical status. Most cancer patients undergoing elective cancer surgery fall somewhere between physical status 2 and 3. An anesthetic mortality in the range of approximately 0.1% is a realistic estimate.

In an attempt to dissect the operative mortality due to anesthesia alone, similar estimates to that found by Dripps and coworkers have been obtained. For example, Moir found the fatality rate for women undergoing caesarian sections in Great Britain to be one in 1250–2000 deliveries.[8] The mortality thought to be due to anesthesia alone was one patient in every 6000–7500 deliveries. A similar estimate was obtained by Collins and coworkers who estimated that the mortality due to general anesthesia alone was approximately one in 3000–5000 in otherwise healthy patients.[9]

The impact of general health status on operative mortality is also seen when analyzing operative mortality as a function of age. Palmberg and coworkers studied the postoperative mortality of 17,199 patients undergoing general surgical procedures.[10] The overall mortality rate of patients under 70 years old was 0.25% compared to 9.2% for patients over 70 years of age. In these elderly patients, the operative mortality for emergency operations was 36.8% compared to 7.8% for elective surgical procedures. The four leading causes of operative mortality in this age group that accounted for approximately 75% of all postoperative deaths were pulmonary embolism, pneumonia, cardiovascular collapse, and the primary illness itself.

Reports of most surgical series include an account of operative mortality and operative complications. These results, combined with a consideration of the general health status of the patient, should allow a reasonable estimate of the operative mortality for any given surgical intervention in the treatment of cancer.

THE ROLE OF SURGERY IN THE PREVENTION OF CANCER

The surgeon's role as a primary giver of medical care implies a responsibility for the education of patients about known

TABLE 6-4. Anesthetic Mortality Related to Physical Status

PHYSICAL STATUS	NUMBER OF PATIENTS	NUMBER OF DEATHS	ANESTHETIC MORTALITY (%)
Class I	16,192	0	<.006
Class II	12,154	7	0.058
Class III	4,070	11	0.27
Class IV	720	17	2.4
Class V	87	4	4.6
TOTAL	33,223	39	0.12

(Adapted from Dripps RD, Lamont A, Eckenhoff JE: The role of anesthesia in surgical mortality. JAMA, 178:261, 1961)

TABLE, 6-5. Surgery to Prevent Cancer

UNDERLYING CONDITION	ASSOCIATED CANCER	PROPHYLACTIC SURGERY
Cryptorchidism	Testicular	Orchiopexy
Polyposis coli	Colon	Colectomy
Familial colon cancer	Colon	Colectomy
Ulcerative colitis	Colon	Colectomy
Familial medullary carcinoma of the thyroid (MEN/II)	Medullary cancer of the thyroid	Thyroidectomy
Familial breast cancer	Breast	Mastectomy
Familial ovarian cancer	Ovary	Oophorectomy

(Adapted from Mulvihill JJ: Cancer control through genetics. *In* Avighi FE, Rao PN, Stubblefield E (eds): Genes, Chromosomes, and Neoplasia. New York, Raven Press, 1980)

carcinogenic hazards. In addition, there is a definite role for the surgeon concerning direct surgical intervention for the prevention of cancer. All surgical oncologists should be aware of those high risk situations that call for surgery to prevent subsequent malignant disease.

A variety of underlying conditions, or congenital or genetic traits are associated with an extremely high incidence of subsequent cancer. When these cancers are likely to occur in non-vital organs, there is a definite role for prophylactic removal of the offending organ to prevent subsequent malignancy.[11] Examples of diseases associated with a high incidence of cancer that can be prevented by prophylactic surgery are presented in Table 6-5. An excellent example is presented by patients with the genetic trait for multiple polyposis of the colon. If colectomy is not performed in these patients, approximately half will develop colon cancer by the age of 40. By the age of 70, virtually all patients with multiple polyposis will develop colon cancer.[11] It is therefore advisable for all patients containing the mutant gene for multiple polyposis to undergo prophylactic colectomy prior to the age of 20 in order to prevent these cancers.

In this situation, as for many of the other familial conditions associated with a high incidence of cancer, the surgeon has a responsibility for alerting the family to the hereditary nature of this disorder and its possible occurrence in other family members. Another disease associated with a high incidence of cancer of the colon is ulcerative colitis. Approximatley 40% of patients with total colonic involvement of ulcerative colitis will ultimately die of colon cancer if they survive the ulcerative colitis.[12] Three percent of children with ulcerative colitis will develop cancer of the colon by the age of 10 and 20% will develop cancer during each ensuing decade.[13] Colectomy is indicated for patients with cancer of the colon when the chronicity of this disease is well established.

Other disorders requiring early treatment in order to prevent subsequent cancers include cryptorchidism and multiple endocrine neoplasia. Cryptorchidism is associated with a high incidence of testicular cancer that can probably be prevented by early prophylactic surgery. Patients with multiple endocrine neoplasia (Type II) should be screened for the presence of C-cell hyperplasia using pentagastrin stimulation tests. If thyrocalcitonin levels are increased following this provocative test, thyroidectomy should be performed to prevent the subsequent occurrence of medullary cancer of the thyroid gland.

A more complex example of the role of surgery in cancer prevention involves women at high risk for breast cancer. Because the risk of breast cancer is some women is substantially increased over the normal risk (but does not yet approach 100%), counseling is required. Women in this situation must carefully balance the benefits and risks of prophylactic mastectomy. A careful understanding of the factors involved in increased breast cancer incidence is essential for the surgical oncologist to provide sound advice in this area. Statistical techniques can provide approximations of the risk for patients depending on the magnitude of disease in the family history, the age at the first pregnancy, and the presence of fibrocystic disease. For example, the woman with a family history of breast cancer in a sister or mother who has fibrocystic disease and is either nulliparous or who had a first pregnancy at a late age has an approximately 18% probability of developing breast cancer over a five year period.[11] These estimates can be of value in helping to advise women about prophylactic mastectomy.

THE ROLE OF SURGERY IN THE DIAGNOSIS OF CANCER

The major role of surgery in the diagnosis of cancer lies in the acquisition of tissue for exact histologic diagnosis. The principles underlying the biopsy of malignant lesions vary depending on the natural history of the tumor under consideration. A variety of techniques exists for obtaining tissues suspected of malignancy. These techniques include aspiration biopsy, needle biopsy, incisional biopsy, and excisional biopsy.

Aspiration biopsy involves the aspiration of cells and tissue fragments through a needle that has been guided into the suspect tissue. Cytologic analysis of this material can provide a tentative diagnosis of the presence of malignant tissue. In general, however, major surgical resections should not be undertaken solely on the basis of the evidence of aspiration biopsy. Even the most experienced cytologist can mistake inflammatory or benign repairative changes for malignant cells. This error is inherent in the uncertainties of individual cell analysis and, even in the best of hands, provides an error rate substantially higher than that of standard histologic diagnosis.

Needle biopsy refers to obtaining a core of tissue through a specially designed needle introduced into the suspect tissue.

The core of tissue provided by needle biopsies is sufficient for the diagnosis of most, but not all, tumor types. Soft tissue and bony sarcomas often present major difficulties in differentiating benign and repairative lesions from malignancies and often cannot be diagnosed with assurance. When these latter lesions are considered in the diagnosis, attempts should be made to obtain greater amounts of tissue than are possible from a needle biopsy.

Incisional biopsy refers to removal of a small wedge of tissue from a larger tumor mass. Incisional biopsies are often necessary for the diagnosis of large masses that would require major surgical procedures for even local excision. Incisional biopsies are the preferred method of diagnosis for soft tissue and bony sarcomas because of the magnitude of the surgical procedures necessary to definitively extirpate these lesions. The treatment of many visceral cancers cannot be undertaken without an incisional biopsy. For example, needle or incisional biopsies of masses in the head of the pancreas are essential before proceeding with the major operations necessary to cure these lesions. In addition, one must be aware of opening new tissue planes contaminated with tumor by performing excisional biopsies for large lesions. An inappropriately performed excisional biopsy can compromise subsequent surgical excision. When this is a possibility, incisional biopsies should be performed.

Excisional biopsy refers to an excision of the entire suspected tumor tissue with little or no margin of surrounding normal tissue. Excisional biopsies are the procedure of choice for most tumors when they can be performed without contaminating new tissue planes or further compromising the ultimate surgical procedure.

There is little evidence that differences exist between incisional and excisional biopsies with respect to tumor spread. Several studies comparing incisional and excisional biopsies of suspected melanoma lesions found no differences in ultimate outcome in these patients.[14,15] In general, however, the surgeon should avoid cutting directly into suspected tumor if it is not necessary to do so.

The following principles guide the performance of all surgical biopsies:

1. Needle tract or scars should be carefully placed so that they can be conveniently removed as part of the subsequent definitive surgical procedure. Placement of biopsy incisions is extremely important and can often compromise subsequent care. Incisions on the extremity should generally be placed in a longitudinal fashion so as to make the removal of underlying tissue and subsequent closure easier.
2. Care should be taken not to contaminate new tissue planes during the biopsy. Large hematomas following biopsy can lead to tumor spread and must be scrupulously avoided by securing excellent hemostasis during the biopsy. For biopsies on extremities, the use of a tourniquet may sometimes be helpful in controlling bleeding. Instruments used in a biopsy procedure are another potential source of contamination of new tissue planes. It is not uncommon to biopsy several suspected lesions at one time. Care should be taken not to use instruments that may have come in contact with tumor when obtaining tissue from a potentially noncontaminated area.
3. Choice of biopsy technique should be carefully selected in order to obtain sufficient tissue for the needs of the pathologist. For the diagnosis of selected tumors, electron microscopy, tissue culture, or other techniques may be necessary. Sufficient tissue must be obtained for these purposes if diagnostic difficulties are anticipated.
4. Handling of the biopsy tissue is also of importance to the pathologist. When orientation of the biopsy specimen is important for subsequent treatment, the surgeon should carefully mark distinctive areas of the tumor so as to facilitate subsequent orientation of the specimen by the pathologist. Different fixatives are best for different types or sizes of tissue. If all biopsies are immediately put in formalin, the opportunity to perform valuable diagnostic tests may be lost. The handling of excised tissue is a responsibility of the surgeon. Biopsy tissue obtained from breast cancer lesions, for example, should be saved for estrogen receptor studies and carefully placed in cold storage until ready for processing.

Surgery also has a role in the diagnosis of pathologic states in cancer patients that do not directly involve the diagnosis of cancer. That is, cancer patients are often immunosuppressed either by their disease or treatment and are subject to a variety of opportunistic infections not commonly seen in most general surgical patients. The use of open lung or liver biopsies is often important to adequately diagnose these lesions and to plan suitable therapy.

Oncologists are becoming increasingly aware of the need for precise staging of patients when planning treatment. Lack of proper staging information can lead to poor treatment planning and compromise the ability to cure patients with a variety of malignancies. Staging laparotomies have a role in determining the exact extent of spread of lymphomas. (This is considered in more detail in the chapter dealing with the treatment of these lesions.) The development of ovarian cancer treatment provides an excellent example of the need for adequate surgical staging prior to embarking on routine therapy. In performing accurate surgical staging, the surgeon must be familiar with the natural history of the diseases under consideration. The tendency of ovarian cancer to metastasize to the undersurface of the diaphragm represents an example of the need to biopsy an anatomic site based on the knowledge of the natural history of this disease that would not normally be considered by most surgeons. Extensive surgical staging may be required prior to undertaking other major surgical procedures with curative intent. For example, biopsy of the celiac and para-aortic lymph nodes in patients with cancer of the esophagus is often important so that unnecessary esophageal resections can be avoided.

Placement of radio-opaque clips during biopsy and staging procedures is important in order to delineate areas of known tumor and as a guide to the subsequent delivery of radiation therapy to these areas.

THE ROLE OF SURGERY IN THE TREATMENT OF CANCER

Surgery can be a simple and safe method for the cure of patients with solid tumors when the tumor is confined to the anatomic site of origin. Unfortunately, when patients with solid tumors present to the physician for the first time, approximately 70% will already have micrometastases beyond the primary site. The extension of the surgical resection, to include areas of regional spread, can cure some of these patients though regional spread is often an indication of undetectable distant micrometastases.

The emergence of effective nonsurgical therapies has had profound impact on the treatment of cancer patients and on the role and responsibilities of the surgeon treating the cancer patient. John Hunter, a brilliant 18th century surgeon, characterized surgery:

> "like an armed savage who attempts to get that by force which a civilized man would get by strategem".

While surgery continues to play the main role in the treatment of most patients presenting with solid tumors, modern clinical research in oncology has been devoted to applying other adjuvant "strategems" to improve the cure rates of those 70% who will ultimately fail surgical therapy alone.

The role of surgery in the treatment of cancer patients can be divided into six separate areas (see Table 6-6). In each area, interactions with other treatment modalities can be essential for a successful outcome.

TABLE 6-6. Surgeon's Role in the Treatment of Cancer Patients

1. Definitive surgical treatment for primary cancer
   - Selection of appropriate local therapy
   - Integration of surgery with other adjuvant modalities
2. Surgery to reduce the bulk of residual disease (Examples: Burkitt's lymphoma, ovarian cancer)
3. Surgical resection of metastatic disease with curative intent (Examples: pulmonary metastases in sarcoma patients, hepatic metastases from colorectal cancer)
4. Surgery for the treatment of oncologic emergencies
5. Surgery for palliation
6. Surgery for reconstruction and rehabilitation

DEFINITIVE SURGICAL TREATMENT FOR PRIMARY CANCER

The major challenges confronting the surgical oncologist in the definitive treatment of solid tumors may be summarized as:

1. Accurate identification of those patients who can be cured by local treatment alone
2. Development and selection of those local treatments that provide the best balance between local cure and the impact of treatment morbidity on the quality of life
3. Development and application of those adjuvant treatments that can improve the control of both local and distant invasive and metastatic disease.

The selection of the local therapy to be used in cancer treatment varies with the individual cancer type and the site of involvement. In many instances, definitive surgical therapy that encompasses a sufficient margin of normal tissue is sufficient local therapy. (The treatment of many solid tumors fall in this category.) Examples include the wide excision of primary melanomas in the skin that can be cured locally by surgery alone in approximately 90% of cases. The resection of colon cancers with a 5 cm margin from the tumor results in anastamotic recurrences in less than 5% of cases.

In other instances, surgery is used to obtain histologic confirmation of diagnosis but primary local therapy is achieved predominantly through the use of a nonsurgical modality such as radiation therapy. Examples of this include the treatment of Ewing's sarcoma in long bones and the treatment of selected primary malignancies in the head and neck. In each instance, selection of the definitive local treatment involves a careful consideration of the likelihood of cure balanced against the morbidity of the treatment modality.

The magnitude of surgical resection is modified in the treatment of many cancers by the use of adjuvant treatment modalities. Rationally integrating surgery with other treatment modalities requires a careful consideration of all effective treatment options. The surgical oncologist must be thoroughly familiar with adjuncts and alternatives to surgical treatment. It is a knowledge of this rapidly changing field that separates the surgical oncologist from the general surgeon most distinctly.

In some instances, the extension of local surgical procedures has provided marked improvement in cure rates. In the early 1970's, for example, retroperitoneal lymph node dissection for patients with Stage I and II nonseminomatous testicular tumors was introduced. In other instances, effective adjuvant modalities have led to a decrease in the magnitude of surgery. The evolution of childhood rhabdomyosarcoma treatment provides a striking example of the successful integration of adjuvant modalities with surgery in the treatment of cancer (see Table 6-7).[16,17]

Childhood rhabdomyosarcoma is the most common soft tissue sarcoma in infants and children. Prior to 1970, surgery alone was used almost exclusively and five year survivals of from 10–20% were commonly reported. Local surgery alone failed in patients with rhabdomyosarcomas of the prostate and

TABLE 6-7. Treatment of Childhood Rhabdomyosarcoma

TREATMENT	FIVE-YEAR SURVIVAL
Surgery alone	10–20%
Surgery + Radiotherapy	40–50%
Surgery + Radiotherapy + Chemotherapy	80—90%

(Adapted from Kilman JW, Clatworthy HW Jr, Newton WA, et al: Reasonable surgery for rhabdomyosarcoma: A study of 67 cases. Ann Surg 3:346, 1973; and from Heyn RM, Holland R, Newton WA, et al: The role of combined chemotherapy in the treatment of rhabdomyosarcoma in children. Cancer 34:2128–2142, 1974)

extremities, both because of extensive invasion of surrounding tissues and the early development of metastatic disease. The failure of surgery alone to control local disease in patients with childhood rhabdomyosarcoma led to the introduction of adjuvant radiation therapy. This resulted in a marked improvement in local control rates that was further improved dramatically by the introduction of combination chemotherapy with vincristine, actinomycin D, and cyclophosphamide. Long-term cure rates are now in the range of 80%. Treatment of childhood rhabdomyosarcoma represents a prime example of the need to modify surgical practice based on the availability of adjuvant modalities. Surgery alone was used for the treatment of rhabdomyosarcomas of the extremities and amputation was often necessary. With the introduction of adjuvant radiation therapy in these cases, local control rates of 90% can be accomplished. Local surgical excisions removing all gross tumor followed by aggressive radiation is the common mode of therapy. In one series, almost 90% of patients had positive microscopic margins at the time of gross tumor resection for rhabdomyosarcoma.[16] However, successful local control was achieved in virtually all of these patients by the addition of radiation therapy.

Current investigations are exploring the use of preoperative radiation therapy to see if the magnitude of surgery can be further reduced or perhaps even eliminated by using radiation and chemotherapy as primary treatment modalities with surgery reserved for elimination of residual disease. This latter approach has been successful in the treatment of Ewing's sarcoma and has largely replaced surgery. Many other examples of the integration of surgery with other treatment modalities appear throughout the text.

SURGERY TO REDUCE THE BULK OF RESIDUAL DISEASE

The concept of cytoreductive surgery has received wide attention in recent years. In some instances, the extensive local spread of cancer precludes the removal of even all gross disease by surgery. The surgical resection of bulk disease in the treatment of selected cancers may well lead to improvements in the ability to control residual gross disease that has not been resected. Studies will be discussed that suggest the merit of this approach in the sections on Burkitt's lymphoma and ovarian cancer.

Enthusiasm for cytoreductive surgery has led to the inappropriate use of surgery for reducing the bulk of tumor in some instances. Clearly, cytoreductive surgery will only be of benefit when other effective treatment modalities are available to control the residual disease that is unresectable. Except in a palliative setting, there is no role for cytoreductive surgery in patients where little other effective therapy currently exists.

SURGICAL RESECTION OF METASTATIC DISEASE WITH CURATIVE INTENT

The role of surgery in the cure of patients with metastatic disease tends to be overlooked. As a general principle (for which there are exceptions) patients with a single site of metastatic disease that can be resected without major morbidity should undergo resection of that metastatic cancer. Many patients with small numbers of metastases to lung or liver or brain can be cured by surgical resection (see Chapter 41). This approach is especially true for those cancers that tend not to be highly responsive to systemic chemotherapy. The resection of pulmonary metastases in patients with soft tissue and bony sarcomas can cure up to 30% of patients. As effective systemic chemotherapy is developed for the treatment of these diseases these cure rates may become higher. Recent studies have shown that adenocarcinomas will show similar cure rates when resected metastatic disease to the lung is the sole clinical site of metastases. Small numbers of pulmonary metastases are often the only clinically apparent metastatic disease in patients with sarcomas. However, this is rare in the natural history of most adenocarcinomas. When solitary metastases to the lung do occur in patients with carcinoma of the colon or other adenocarcinomas, then surgical resection is indicated.

Similarly, there is increasing enthusiasm for the resection of hepatic metastases, especially from colorectal cancer, in patients in which the liver is the only site of known metastatic disease. In patients with solitary hepatic metastases from colorectal cancer, resection can lead to long-term cure in approximately 25% of patients. This far exceeds the cure rates of any other currently available treatment approach.

The resection for cure of solitary brain metastases should also be considered when the brain is the only site of known metastatic disease. The exact location and functional sequellae of resection should be considered in making this treatment decision.

SURGERY FOR THE TREATMENT OF ONCOLOGIC EMERGENCIES

As in the treatment of all patients, emergent situations arise in oncologic patients that require surgical intervention. In oncologic patients, these emergencies generally involve the treatment of exsanguinating hemorrhage, perforation, drainage of abscesses, or impending destruction of vital organs. Each category of surgical emergency is unique and requires an individual approach. These are considered in detail later in this book (see chapter 42).

The oncologic patient is often neutropenic, thrombocytopenic, and presents an unusual threat of hemorrhage or sepsis. Perforations of an abdominal viscus can result from direct tumor invasion or from tumor lysis resulting from effective systemic treatments. Perforation of the gastrointestinal tract following effective treatment for lymphoma involving the intestine is not an uncommon occurrence. The ability to identify patients at high risk for perforation may lead to the use of surgery to prevent this problem. Surgery to decompress cancer invading the CNS represents another surgical emergency that can lead to preservation of function.

SURGERY FOR PALLIATION

Surgical resection is often required for the relief of pain or functional abnormalities. The appropriate use of surgery in these settings can improve the quality of life of cancer patients. Palliative surgery may include the relief of mechanical problems such as intestinal obstruction or the removal of masses that are causing severe pain or disfigurement.

SURGERY FOR RECONSTRUCTION AND REHABILITATION

Surgical techniques are being increasingly developed that aid in the reconstruction and rehabilitation of cancer patients following definitive therapy. For example, reconstruction has long been an important part of cancer treatment for surgical resections of the head and neck. The ability to reconstruct anatomic defects can substantially improve both function and cosmetic appearance. The recent development of free flaps using microvascular techniques is having a profound impact on the ability to bring fresh tissue to resected or heavily irradiated areas. Loss of function (especially of extremities) can often be rehabilitated by surgical approaches. This includes lysis of contractures or muscle transposition to bring back muscular function that has been damaged by prior surgery or radiation therapy.

THE SURGICAL ONCOLOGIST

Several factors have led to a recent increase in the development of surgical oncology and to the organization of separate sections of surgical oncology in large hospitals and university departments of surgery. A major reason for this enthusiasm involves the recognition that modern oncologic management requires levels of expertise in cancer surgery, chemotherapy, and radiation therapy that are not common to most general surgeons, as well as a desire to effectively utilize the resources being committed to cancer care and research by hospitals, private foundations, and the federal government. These factors have been accorded a sense of urgency due to the perception among some surgical leaders that the surgeon is experiencing a declining intellectual role in modern cancer treatment and research and that steps must be taken to reassert the surgeon's importance in modern oncology.

The development of surgical oncology as a speciality area of surgery depends upon a clear delineation of its role. There are six major areas in which the modern surgical oncologist can play a valuable role in the care of cancer patients at major treatment centers (see Table 6-8).

TABLE 6-8. Role of the Surgical Oncologist

1. Organize surgical oncology teaching programs for staff, residents, and students
2. Provide expert consultation for unusual or difficult oncologic patient problems
3. Provide unique surgical expertise in surgical cases unfamiliar to general surgeons (*e.g.*, major soft tissue resections, exenterations, head and neck resections, isolation-perfusions)
4. Organize clinical research protocols for surgical oncology patients
5. Coordinate surgical oncology efforts with medical and radiation oncologists
6. Conduct experimental research programs in oncology where possible

The rapid development of new information in surgery, chemotherapy, and medical oncology, in addition to newer disciplines of immunotherapy, hyperthermia, phototherapy, etc., requires the continuing education of all surgical staff. Surgical oncologists maintain close contact with all of these areas and should take responsibility for teaching programs for general surgical staff, residents, and students in these different areas.

Because of the unique training and exposure to oncologic problems, the surgical oncologist has unique expertise in dealing with unusual or difficult oncologic patient problems and can thus provide expert consultation in these areas. The surgical oncologist is also trained to perform many types of surgical procedures not commonly performed by most general surgeons. Examples of these procedures include major soft tissue resections, pelvic exenterations, extensive head and neck resections, and isolation–perfusions of extremities. While most surgeons are able to perform many of the standard cancer resections, some operations are infrequently performed by general surgeons and can be better performed by a specialist in surgical oncology.

In most hospital settings, a variety of general surgeons operate on cancer patients. It is often essential, however, that patients receiving care for a variety of cancers enter clinical protocols that will help answer important questions related to the treatment of that cancer. The surgical oncologist can help organize clinical research protocols for surgical oncology patients treated by all surgeons at that institution. A large surgical group should have a surgical specialist capable of coordinating efforts with medical and radiation oncologists. Successful coordination with these nonsurgical specialists requires expertise in medical oncology and radiation therapy that is not common among most general surgeons.

The surgical oncologist can also play a major role in administering and defining the need for a variety of adjuvant treatments. Adjuvant chemotherapy is commonly administered by surgeons when the chemotherapy regimens utilize well-known single or combination agent chemotherapy. The future development of immunotherapies and other new adjuvant treatments can be logically administered by the surgical oncologist to his patient following recovery from the surgical procedure.

Finally, the surgical oncologist, when the situation permits, is in a position to perform experimental research in oncology that will hopefully lead to the introduction of new diagnostic and treatment regimens in clinical care. Laboratory research programs that contribute to basic knowledge of cancer biology also provide an important source of stimulation to residents and students in the clinical area.

The emergence of a subspeciality of surgical oncology within general surgery requires that special attention be paid to the training of surgeons interested in pursuing this area of clinical care. While it is generally agreed that all surgical oncologists should be well-trained general surgeons, attempts have been made to define additional areas of expertise that must be studied. In September 1978 a meeting of surgical oncologists met under the sponsorship of the Society of Surgical Oncology and the Division of Cancer Research, Resources, and Centers of the National Cancer Institute to develop guidelines for the training of surgical oncologists.

The guidelines adopted by this meeting included a variety of suggestions for such training.[18] These include:

1. A two-year program of training on a surgical oncology service following completion of eligibility for general surgical certification by the American Board of Surgery or other surgical speciality board
2. Training at an institution whose cancer program is approved by the Commission on Cancer of the American College of Surgeons and whose clinical resources provide a sufficient variety and volume of clinical material to assure exposure to a broad variety of clinical cancer problems
3. Training at a center with sufficient basic science resources to provide education in these areas with exposure to both basic and clinical research
4. Training at an institution that will provide adequate operative experience including standard curative and palliative procedures with broad exposure to those surgical procedures unique to the oncologic patient
5. A full-time assignment during the training period to both radiation oncology and medical oncology services to permit the trainee to gain confidence and knowledge in these nonsurgical disciplines

These training recommendations are designed to provide general surgeons with the expertise in oncology and nonsurgical disciplines necessary to bring the best aspects of all disciplines of modern oncology to the care of the cancer patient.

REFERENCES

1. Brested JH: The Edwin Smith Surgical Papyrus. Chicago, University of Chicago Press, 1930
2. Thorwald J: Science and the Secrets of Early Medicine. New York, Hancourt, Borace, and World, 1962
3. Wangensteen OH: Has medical history importance for surgeons? Surg Gynec Obstet 140:434, 1975
4. Hill GJ: Historic milestones in cancer surgery. Semin Oncol 6:409–427, 1979
5. Brunner EA, Eckenhoff JE: Anesthesia. *In* Sabiston DC, Jr (ed): Textbook of Surgery. Phila., WB Saunders, 1977
6. Dripps RD, Eckenhoff JE, Vandam LD: Introduction to Anesthesia. Phila., WB Saunders, 1977
7. Dripps RD, Lamont A, Eckenhoff JE: The role of anesthesia in surgical mortality. JAMA 178:261, 1961
8. Moir DD: Maternal mortality and anesthesia. Br J Anaesth 52:1–3, 1980
9. Collins VJ: Principles of Anesthesiology. Phila., Lea and Febiger, 1976
10. Palmberg S, Hirsjarvi E: Mortality in geriatric surgery. Gerontology 25:103–112, 1979
11. Mulvihill JJ: Cancer control through genetics. *In* Avighi FE, Rao PN, Stubblefield E (eds): Genes, Chromosomes, and Neoplasia. New York, Raven Press, 1980
12. MacDougall IPM: The cancer risk in ulcerative colitis. Lancet 2:655, 1964
13. Devroede GJ, Taylor WF, Sauer WG: Cancer risk and life expectancy of children with ulcerative colitis. N Engl J Med 285:17, 1971
14. Epstein E, Bragg K, Linden GJ: Biopsy and prognosis of malignant melanoma. JAMA 208:1369, 1969
15. Knutson CO, Hori JM, Spratt JS Jr: Melanoma. Curr Probl Surg, Dec 1971
16. Kilman JW, Clatworthy HW Jr, Newton WA, et al: Reasonable surgery for rhabdomyosarcoma: A study of 67 cases. Ann Surg 3:346, 1973
17. Heyn RM, Holland R, Newton WA, et al: The role of combined chemotherapy in the treatment of rhabdomyosarcoma in children. Cancer 34:2128–2142, 1974
18. Leffall LD Jr: Presidential address. Surgical oncology—expectations for the future. Cancer 42:2925–2928, 1980

CHAPTER 7

Samuel Hellman

Principles of Radiation Therapy

To understand the practice of radiation therapy one must seek its roots in principles derived from three separate areas. The first is practical radiation physics. This must be understood much as the surgeon understands the use of the equipment available in the operating room and the internist understands the pharmacologic basis of therapeutics. The rudimentary physics concepts necessary to consider radiation therapy in the upcoming disease-related chapters will be introduced in this chapter.

The second important discipline to be understood is that of cell tissue and tumor biology. The basic principles of radiation biology and cell kinetics will be described in this chapter (cell kinetics as it relates to both chemotherapy and radiation therapy will be discussed in a separate chapter). These two discussions should give the rudiments of cell biology necessary to understand the uses of radiation.

Finally, a large clinical experience in radiation use has evolved from which certain principles of treatment have emerged, proven in the clinic. These will be discussed separately and will be related to the physical and biologic concepts which may underlie their success.

PHYSICAL CONSIDERATIONS

The physics of ionizing radiation cannot be discussed adequately in this chapter; only a very brief explanation of the most important concepts will be described. If more detailed information is needed, a standard textbook of radiation physics is a more appropriate source of information.[1]

Ionizing radiation is that radiation which, during absorption, causes the ejection of an orbital electron. A large amount of energy is associated with ionization. Such ionizing radiations may be electromagnetic or particulate. In fact, electromagnetic radiation can be considered both as a wave and as a packet of energy (a photon). This is important since it is the particulate nature of electromagnetic radiation that explains much of its biologic action. The packet of energy is large enough to cause ionizations and these are distributed unevenly through tissue. Examples of particulate radiations are the subatomic particles, electrons, protons, alpha particles, neutrons, negative pimesons, and atomic nuclei. All of these have been considered or are being used in radiation therapy, at least experimentally.

ELECTROMAGNETIC RADIATION

Electromagnetic radiation is divided into two types: roentgen and gamma radiation. Their only difference is the way in which they are produced. Gamma rays are produced intranuclearly while roentgen rays are produced extranuclearly. In practice, this means that gamma rays used in radiation therapy are produced by the decay of radioactive isotopes and that almost all the roentgen rays produced in radiation therapy are those made by electrical machines. An exception to this are the roentgen rays produced by orbital electron rearrangements in the decay of ^{125}I. The latter, while a radioactive isotope, produces photons by extranuclear processes. Thus, these are roentgen rays. ^{125}I also emits a small number of gamma rays from the nucleus.

The intensity of electromagnetic radiation dissipates as the inverse square of the distance from the source. Thus, the dose of radiation two centimeters from a point source is 25% of the dose at one centimeter. The dominant absorption mechanisms of electromagnetic radiation are of three types. The relative prevalence depends on the energy of the radiation. The first is known as photoelectric absorption. This predominates at the lower energies. In this circumstance, the photon interaction results in the ejection of a tightly bound orbital electron. The vacancy left in the atomic shell is then filled by another electron falling from an outer shell of the same atom or from outside the atom. All or most of the photon energy is lost in this process. Important in the photoelectric effect is that photoelectric absorbtion varies with the cube of the atomic number (Z^3). This has important practical implications since it is why materials with a high atomic number such as lead are such effective shielding materials. It also means that bones will absorb significantly more radiation than soft tissues at lower photon energies, the basis for conventional diagnostic radiology.

The second type of radiation absorption is of the Compton type. In this process, the interaction is with a distant orbital electron having a very low binding energy. In this absorptive process the photon does not give all its energy up to a single electron. An appreciable portion reappears as a secondary photon, created in the interaction. In contrast to the photoelectric effect, the probability of Compton absorption does not depend much on atomic number, but rather on electron density. The final type of absorption is the pair production process. This type of absorption requires an incident photon energy of greater than 1.02 MeV. In this process, a positive and negative electron are produced at the same time.

The fundamental quantity necessary to describe the interaction of radiation with matter is the amount of energy absorbed per unit mass. This quantity is called absorbed dose and the *Rad* is the most commonly used unit. In currently recommended nomenclature absorbed dose is measured in joules per kilogram. A special name for 1 joule/Kg is the Gray (1 Gray = 100 Rad). The Roentgen (R) is a unit of x-(roentgen) or gamma rays based on the ability of radiation to ionize air. At the energies used in radiation therapy, IR of roentgen ray or gamma ray results in a dose of somewhat less than 1 rad (0.01 Gy) in soft tissue.

The different ranges of electromagnetic radiations used in clinical practice are *superficial radiation,* or roentgen rays from approximately 10–125KeV, *orthovoltage* radiation, electromagnetic radiation between 125 and 400KeV, and *supervoltage* radiation or megavoltage for those energies above this. The important differences between these classes are as follows: 1. as energy increases, the penetration of the roentgen rays increases as shown in Fig. 7-1; and 2. at supervoltage energies, the bone is not higher than that in surrounding soft tissues (as is the case with lower energies). This is because at supervoltage energies Compton absorbtion predominates. Another difference between orthovoltage and supervoltage is that supervoltage radiation is "skin sparing." This means that the maximum dose is not reached in the skin but rather occurs some depth below the surface. The electrons created in the interaction travel some distance and do not reach full intensity until some depth. Clinically, this is important as it results in a reduced dose to the skin. With orthovoltage radiation the skin was frequently the dose-limiting normal tissue.

RADIATION TECHNIQUES

There are two general types of radiation techniques used—*brachytherapy* and *teletherapy*. In brachytherapy, the radiation device is placed either within or close to the target volume. Examples of this are the interstitial and intracavitary radiation used in the treatment of many gynecologic and oral tumors. Teletherapy uses a device quite removed from the patient, as is the case in most orthovoltage or supervoltage machines. Since the radiation source is quite close to the target volume with brachytherapy (in fact, it is usually within the target volume), then dose is largely determined by inverse square considerations. This means that the geometry of the implant is a very important detail. Spatial arrangements have been determined for different types of applications based on the particular anatomic considerations of the tumor and important tissues. An example of isotope distribution around a radium application for carcinoma of the cervix is shown in Fig. 7-2. Note how rapidly the dose decreases with distance from the applicator. This emphasizes the importance of proper

FIG. 7-1. Relative dose at different depths for various types of ionizing radiation.

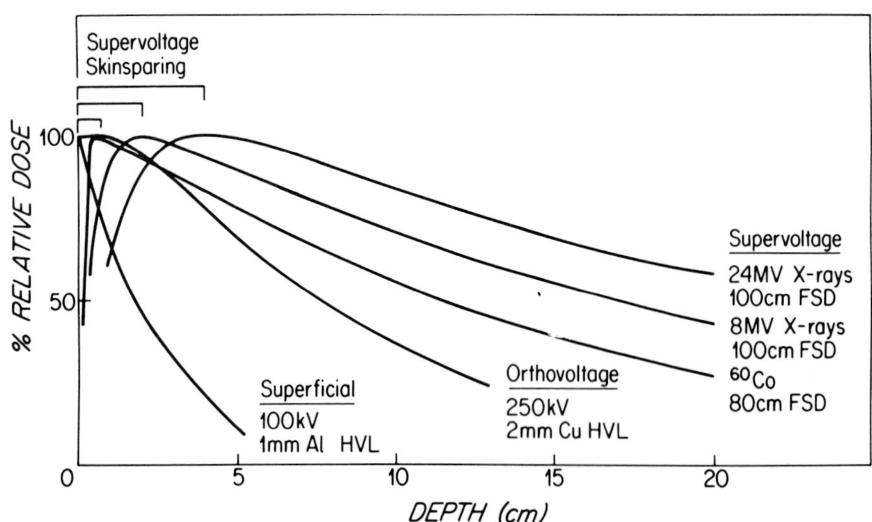

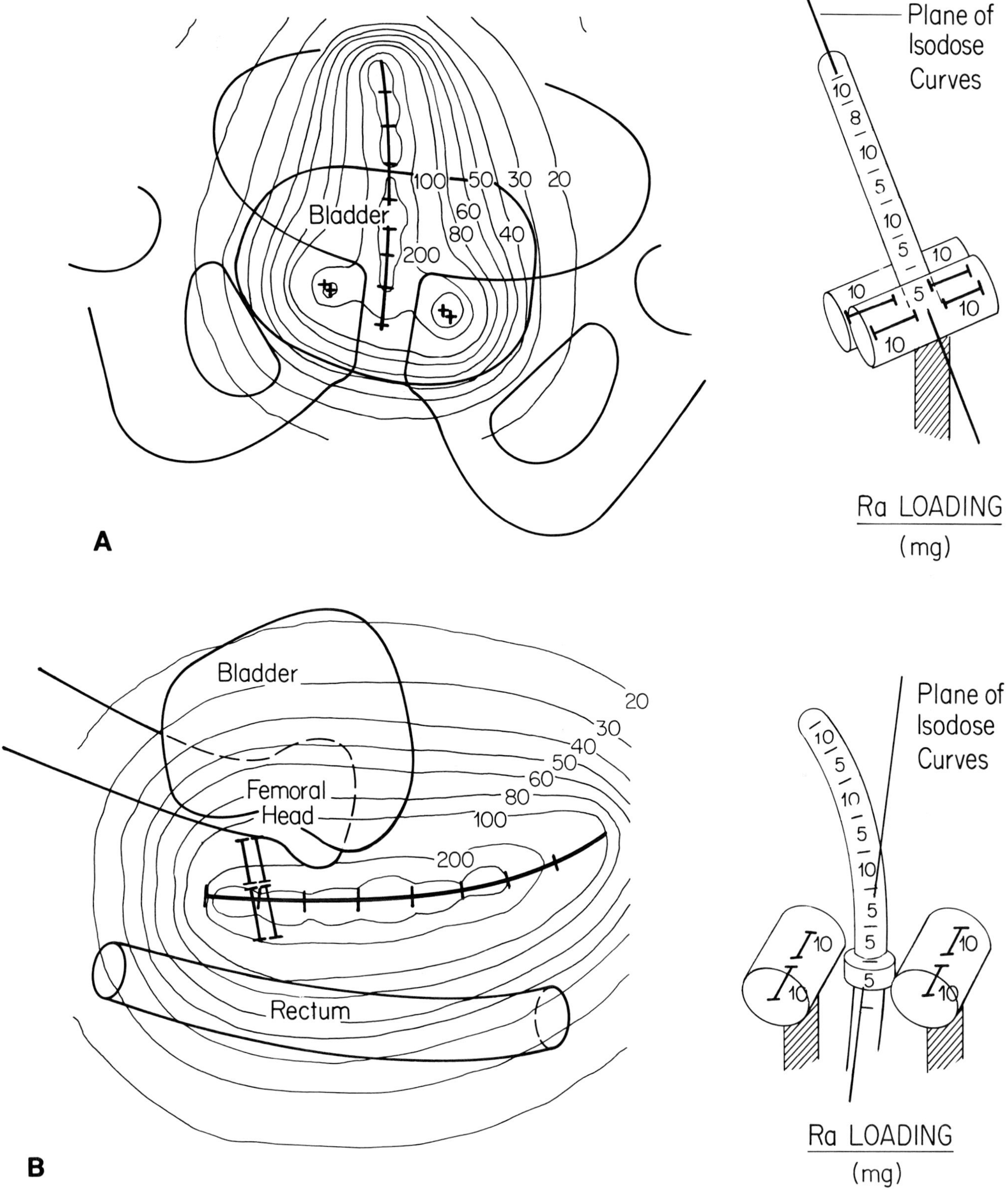

FIG. 7-2. *A*, AP view of isodose distribution around an intrauterine radium applicator. *B*, Lateral view.

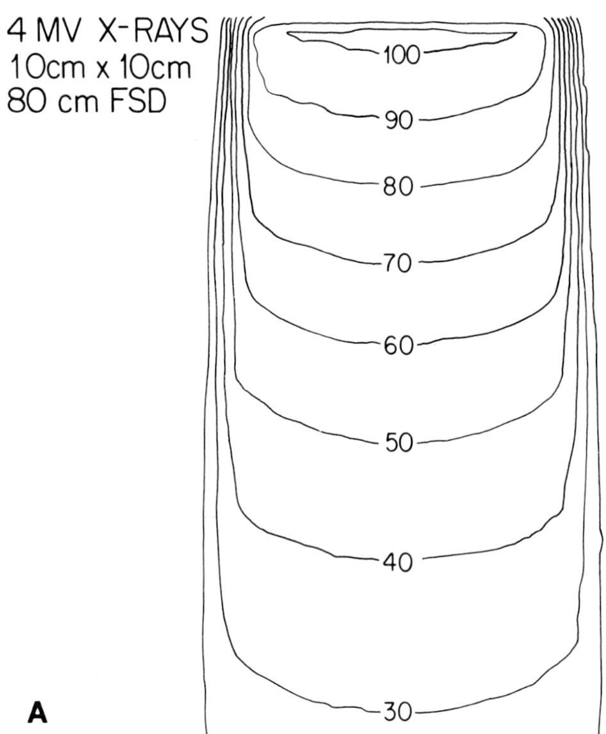

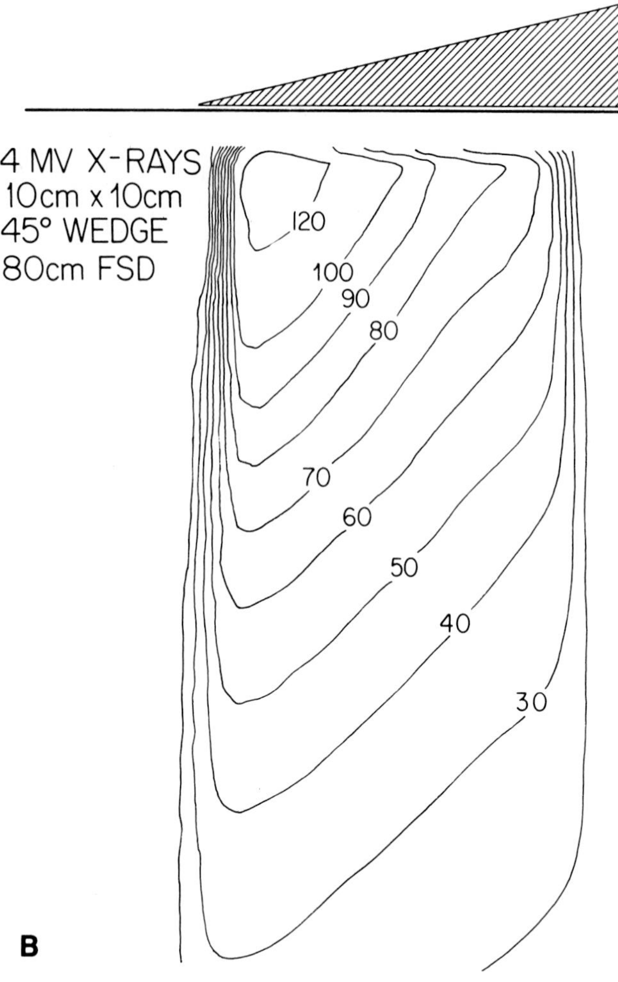

FIG. 7-3. Isodose distributions for *A*, 4MeV without a wedge filter and *B*, 4MeV with a wedge filter.

placement. This applicator attempts to treat the cervix, uterus, and important paracervical tissues while limiting excessive irradiation of the bladder and rectum in front of and behind the tumor.

Typical teletherapy isotope distributions are shown in Fig. 7-3. The dose depends both on inverse square considerations and tissue absorbtion. The distribution of radiation depends on characteristics of the machine and the patient. Thus, the isodose curve depends on the energy of radiation, the distance from the source of radiation, and the density and atomic number of the absorbing material. The beam of radiation produced in typical radiation treatment may be modified by devices to make isotope distributions best conform to the specific target volume. Individually designed shields are used to protect vital, normal tissues. Fig. 7-4 shows some radiation treatment plans in which the target volumes are shown. This volume contains the tumor and those normal tissues intimately involved with the tumor. The diagram also contains the transited normal tissues or *transit volume*. The purpose of the treatment plan is to maximize the dose to the target volume while minimizing that to the transit volume. *It is quite important that the tumor dose is relatively homogenous since the maximum dose in the target volume is often the cause of complications and the minimum dose in the target volume determines the likelihood of tumor recurrence.*

Beam Modifying Devices

In modern radiation therapy, teletherapy is given almost exclusively with supervoltage equipment. These radiations are produced by the decay of radioactive cobalt or with the production of roentgen rays in the 2–35 MeV range (the most common being 4–8 MeV roentgen rays). Higher energy photons and electrons can be made by various electrical machines of which the most common are linear accelerators and betatrons.

Regardless of the radiation source, the beam must be modified for clinical use. With electrical machines, the beam tends to have a much greater intensity in the center than on the sides. This must be modified to give a uniform dose of radiation across the beam and it is done with the *flattening filter*. (This is not necessary in cobalt units.) In order for the beam to be limited to the size designated there are collimators placed in the head of the machine. These are usually made of materials with a high atomic number Z and can be varied to conform to the exact rectangular beam dimensions desired for an individual case.

It is sometimes desirable that the beam not be flat but rather be more intense on one side than the other. This is especially important when fields at angles to each other are to be employed. In order to modify the beam in this fashion wedges are used (see Fig. 7-3b). These are literally wedge-shaped pieces of metal that absorb the beam differentially, depending on the thickness that allows the angled isodose curves desired. Depending on the anatomic volume being

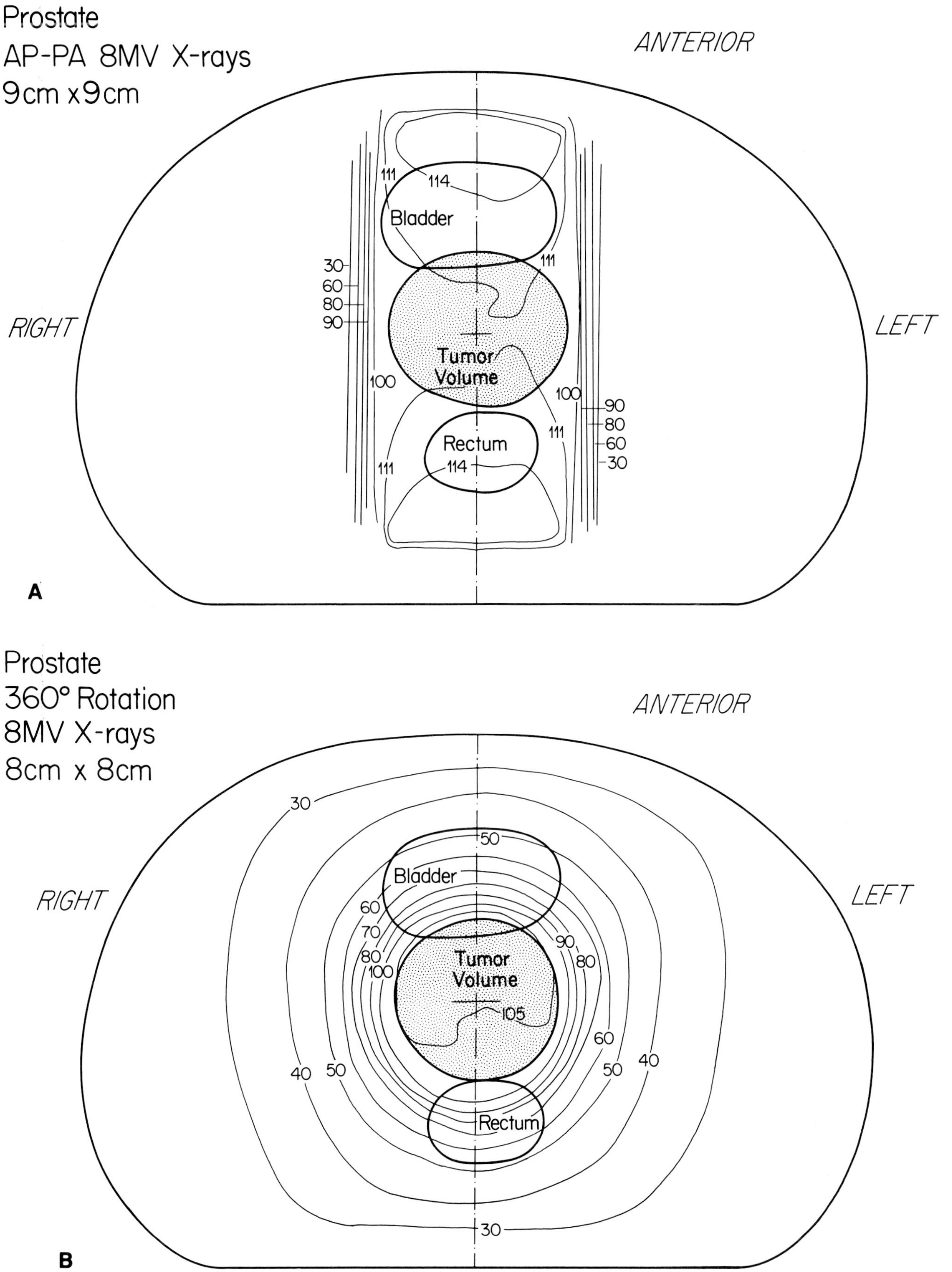

Prostate
AP-PA 8MV X-rays
9cm x9cm

ANTERIOR
RIGHT
LEFT
Bladder
Tumor Volume
Rectum
111
114
111
30
60
80
90
100
100
90
80
60
30
111
111
114

A

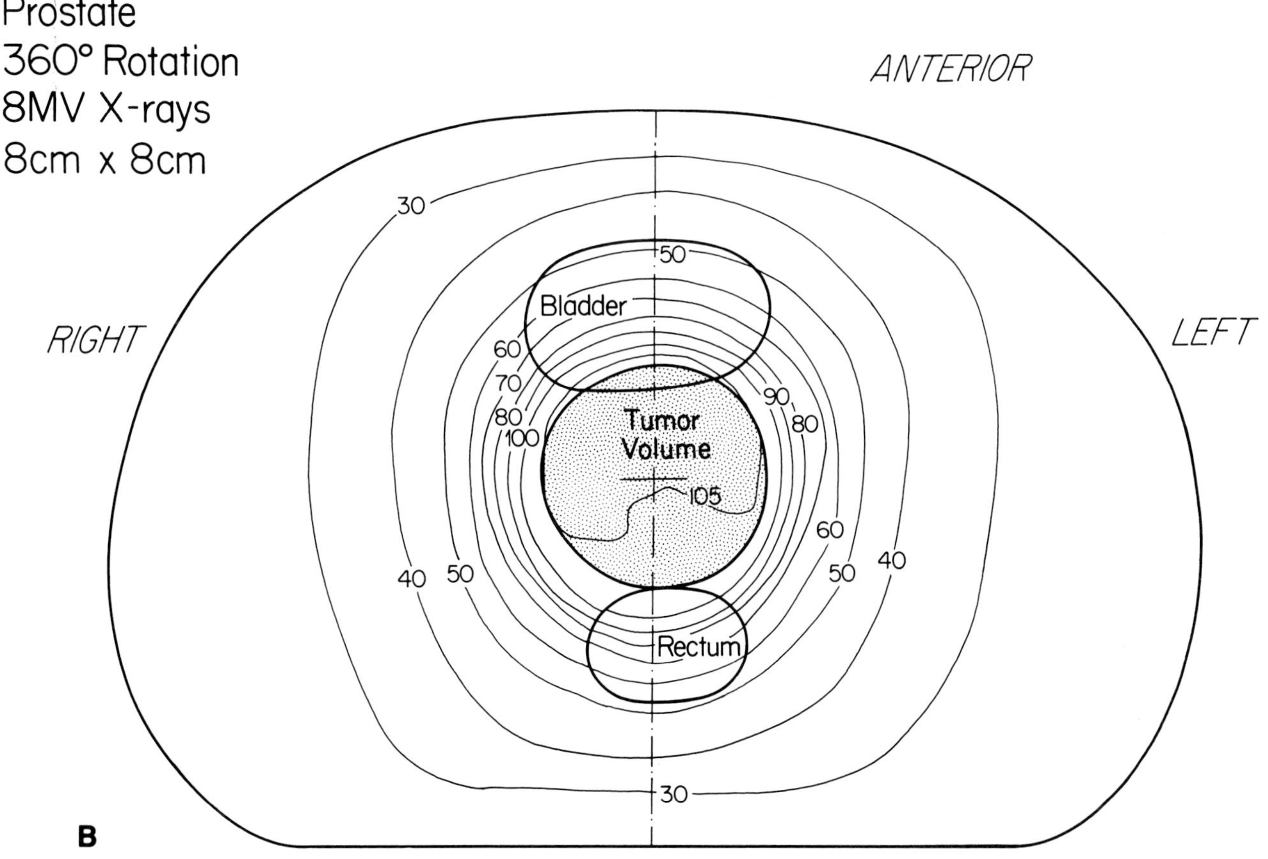

FIG. 7-4. Typical supervoltage treatment plans for opposing fields (*A*), rotation (*B*). (*Fig. 7-4 continues on p. 108.*)

Esophagus
3-Field Plan 8MV X-rays
Equal Scale
8cm x 8cm
ANTERIOR
RIGHT
LEFT
84
74
95
84
100
Tumor
Volume
105
42
53
63
63
53
42
74
63
32
74
74
C

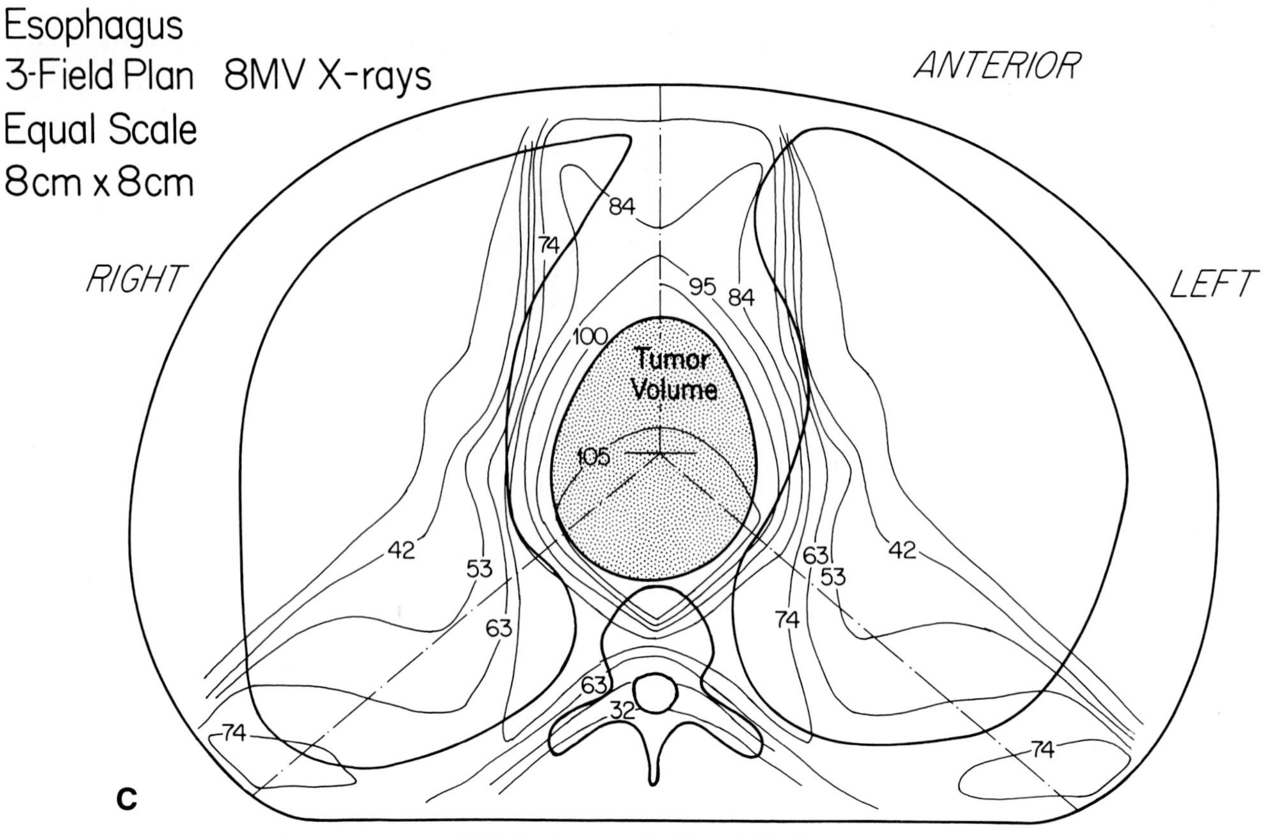

FIG. 7-4 (*continued*). Three field (*C*).

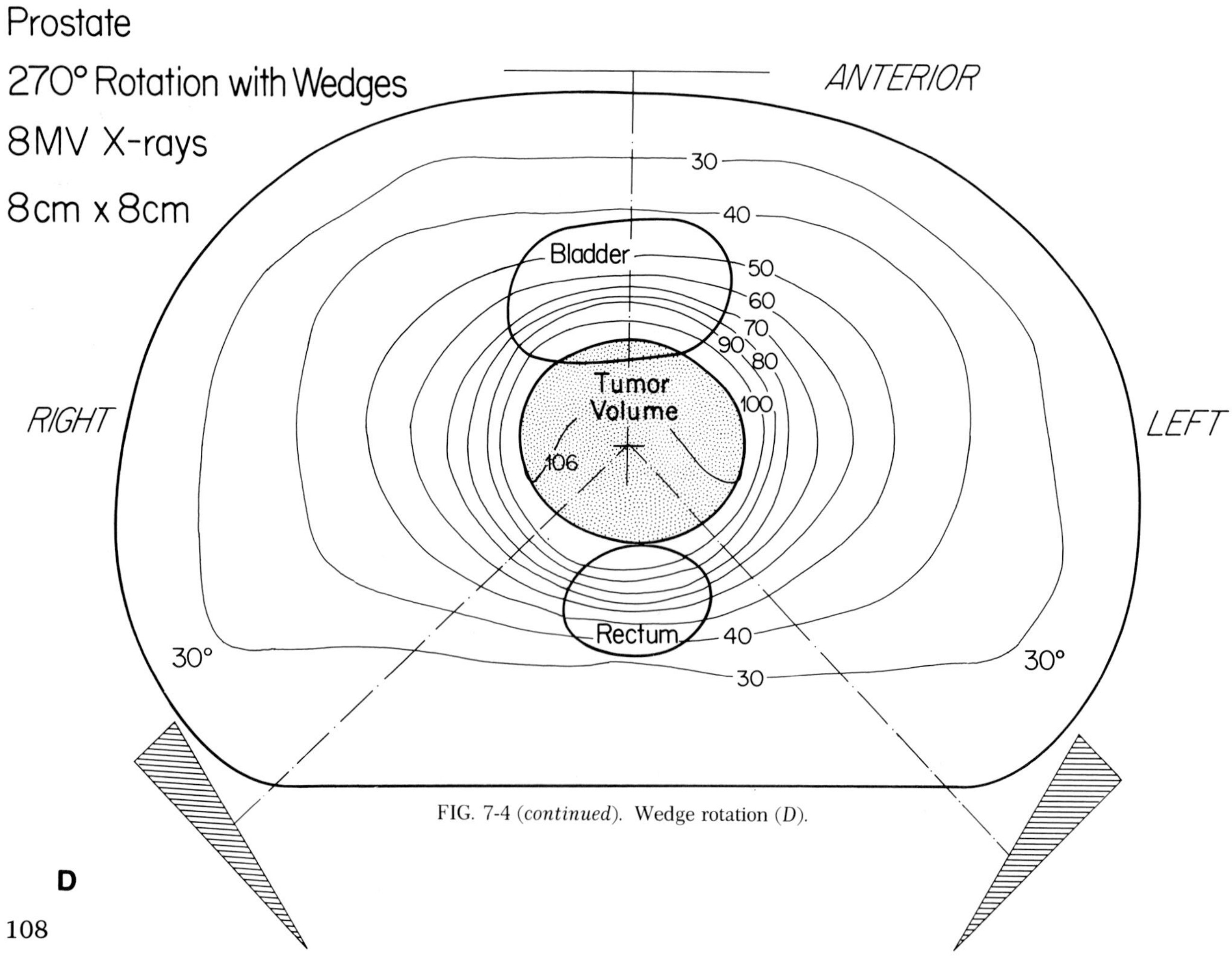

Prostate
270° Rotation with Wedges
8MV X-rays
8cm x 8cm
ANTERIOR
30
40
Bladder
50
60
70
90
80
Tumor
Volume
100
RIGHT
LEFT
106
Rectum
40
30°
30°
30
D

FIG. 7-4 (*continued*). Wedge rotation (*D*).

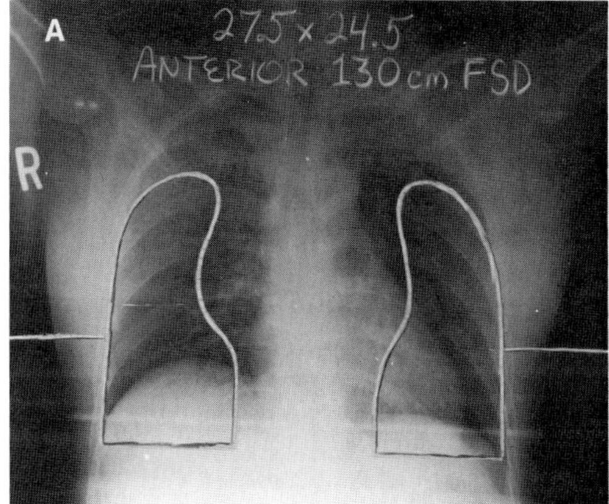

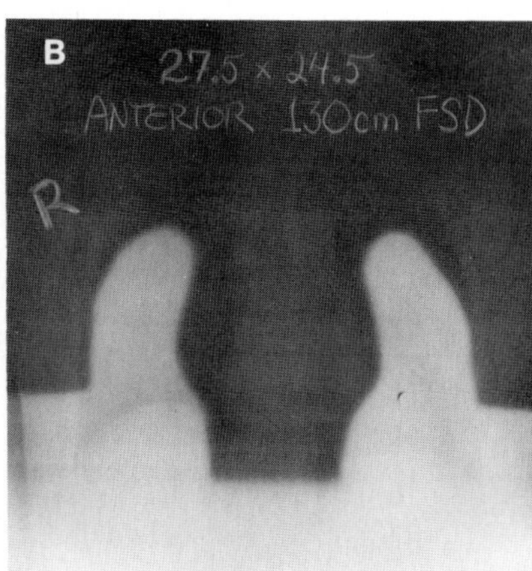

FIG. 7-5. *A*. A film made on a therapy simulator on which outlines for shielding blocks are drawn. *B*. Supervoltage portal film with blocks in place. *C*. Technique for checking accuracy of the blocks with simulator films.

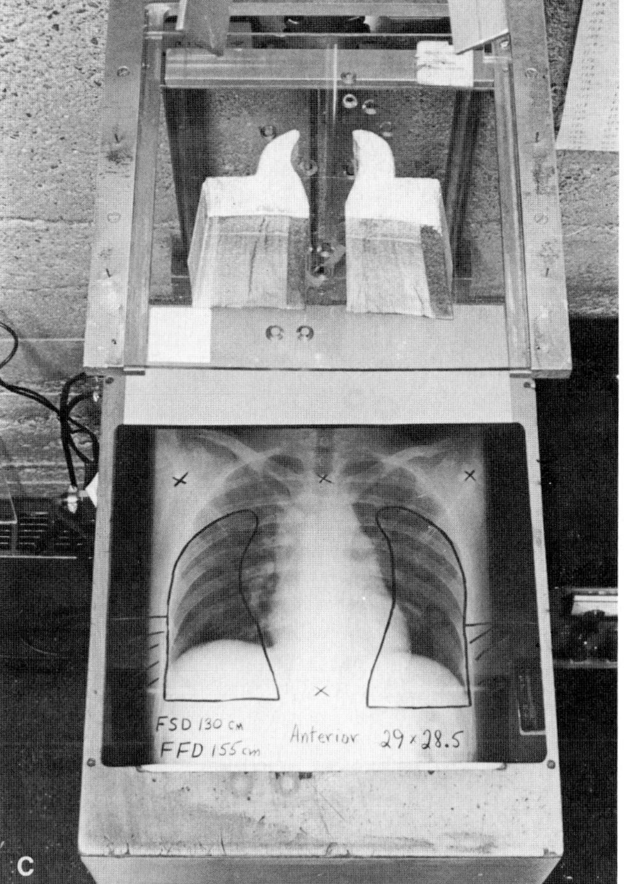

treated, it is often desirable to outline the beam in a fashion different than can be constructed by the rectangular collimators. On these certain areas within the beam should be shielded. In order to do this individually fashioned blocks are made. These are usually made to conform to the individual distributions desired for each patient and each beam. They are made out of high Z material, such as lead or the commercial product Libowitz metal, comprised of bismuth, lead, tin, and cadmium.

RADIATION TREATMENT

Once the decision has been made to treat a patient with radiation a number of pretreatment procedures must be undertaken. First, there must be accurate target volume localization as well as the dose-limiting, transited normal tissues. This localization requires physical examination, in addition to the use of radiographs, ultrasound, and other diagnostic procedures. Prior to this, the clinician must understand the natural history of the disease and its patterns of spread. Computerized tomography has greatly changed the process of tumor localization by allowing much greater accuracy in determining normal tissue location as well as tumor location. Once localization has been completed, the treatment planning process begins. Here alternative techniques of treatment are considered. The selection of the appropriate treatment plan is made by the clinician consulting with the radiologic physicist and dosimetrist. This team effort must consider the best beam distribution, homogeneity within the target volume, and appropriate minimizing of dose distribution in the transit volume. Once the appropriate treatment plan has been accepted, the technique is simulated using the radiation simulator. This device can mimic the treatment machine but produces superficial radiation that can be used for direct imaging, with an image intensifier for the production of radiographs that delineate exactly the beam location. Often treatment simulation causes modifications to be made in the treatment plan, allowing further sparing of the normal tissues. Examples of simulator films are shown in Fig. 7-5. These must be compared to the check or portal films on the supervoltage machine that confirm the treatment plan (also shown in Fig. 7-5). These are of much poorer image quality since they only distinguish bone from soft tissue. This is because supervoltage radiation is primarily absorbed by the Compton process that does not depend upon Z. In contrast, the simulator films are made with radiations of 80–110 KeV, well in the photoelectric range therefore depending on Z^3. In order for the treatment to be applied as designed on the radiation simulator, proper immobilization and marking techniques must be used. These also insure that daily treatments are given at the same volume. Markings on the patient's skin may be temporary or permanent. Usually temporary marks are used to supplement the permanent small dots or "tattoos." These insure that the treatment will be given at the same volume each day. In addition, should the patient require further therapy at later date, these markings will accurately indicate the location of previous treatment portals. Within the

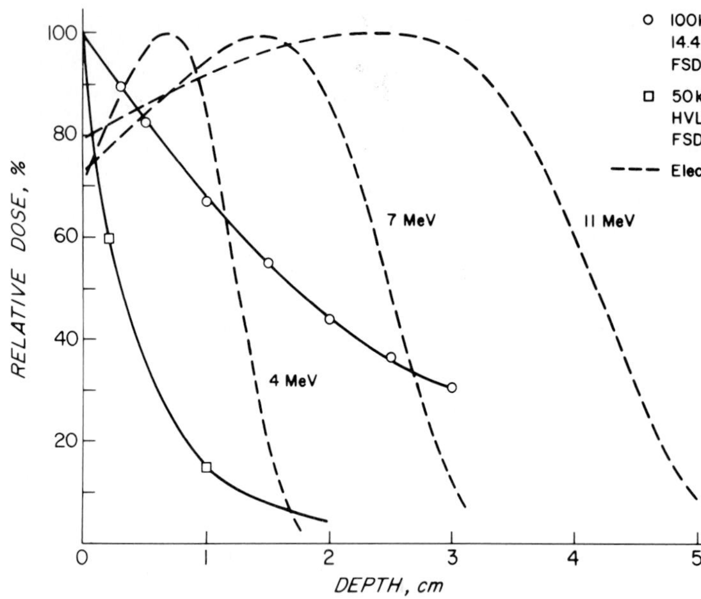

FIG. 7-6. Electron and superficial roentgen ray depth dose curves.

treatment room, light localizes the outline of the field and small laser dots are used to check that the patient is in the correct position. Immobilization of the patient is usually achieved by devices made of foam, plastic, and a variety of other materials, which can be made to conform to individual patient anatomy. Most important in this is that the patient is put in a position that is comfortable and easily reproduced from day to day.

Electron Therapy

With the development of betatrons and high energy accelerators, electron beam therapy has become available for teletherapy. Electrons differ greatly in their characteristic depth dose distributions (Fig. 7-6 shows the depth dose distributions for a few sample electron energies). As one can see there is little skin sparing. The maximum dose is reached and a very prompt fall follows. Obviously it is most useful to use this radiation in the treatment of superficial tumors since the deeper tissues will be spared by the prompt fall in the radiation. The higher the electron energy the greater the penetration and the less steep the fall in depth dose. A major problem with electrons is that this absorption can be greatly modified by bone or air-containing tissues. Bone will cause the depth dose to be greatly reduced as it will absorb much more of the radiation, while the contrary is true for air-containing spaces. Primarily, electron beams are used as a "boost" or supplementary treatment after photon therapy.

BIOLOGIC CONSIDERATIONS

RADIATION INTERACTION WITH BIOLOGICAL MATERIALS

Since mammalian cells may be considered dilute aqueous solutions, there are two possible mechanisms of interaction with biologically important molecules—the direct effect of radiation on the important target molecule or the indirect effect by way of intermediary radiation products. For most events, the important target molecule is thought to be the DNA. When considering the maintenance of reproductive integrity it is useful to assume DNA to be the target. Whatever the critical target, it can be directly affected by the ionizing radiation that causes a change in the molecular structure of the biologically important molecule. This direct effect is most common for high linear energy transfer (LET) radiation. Alternatively, the photon may interact with water, the predominant molecule in such a dilute solution, to produce free radicals. All of these forms are relatively short-lived; they can interact with biologically important material causing a detrimental effect; or, conversely, can react innocently to revert to their former state. The likelihood of interaction versus reversion can be modified by reaction with molecular oxygen, which would favor prolonging the life of a reactive species, or by reaction with sulfhydryl compounds, which will reduce the free radical lifespan by combining with them to return to innocuous substances.

CELL SURVIVAL CONSIDERATIONS

Radiation effects, whether direct or indirect, are random. This randomness is important in the general nature of cell killing. The major biologically important effects of radiation when considering radiation therapy are those concerned with reproductive integrity. It is usual to assume that DNA is the critical target for this radiation effect. While this is highly likely, it has not been proven with certainty. Surely other biologically important effects of radiation (*i.e.*, edema) are far more likely to be due to membrane effects of radiation. A cell damaged by radiation that loses its reproductive integrity may divide once or more often before all the progeny are rendered reproductively sterile. This is an important consequence of radiation; it means that an irradiated cell will not appear damaged until it faces at least the first division. At the time of reproduction, there are a number of possible paths for this cell:

1. It may die while trying to divide
2. It may produce unusual forms due to aberrant attempts at division

3. It may stay as it is, unable to divide, but physiologically functional for a very long period of time (such functional but sterile cells will not appear different from fertile cells)
4. It may divide, giving rise to one or more generations of daughter cells before some or all the progeny become sterile (those colonies in which some reproductively viable progeny emerge may then regrow)
5. The cell may suffer none or only minor alterations in the divisional process

Usually there is some division delay produced even in cells not lethally damaged. An example of cellular pedigrees photographed *in vitro* are shown in Fig. 7-7.[2]

Survival Curves

Plot the fraction of cells surviving radiation against the dose given (where survival is determined by the ability to form a macroscopic colony). The simplest relationship can be seen for bacteria in which survival is a constant exponential function of dose. The importance of this exponential relationship is that for a given dose increment a constant proportion rather than a given number of cells are killed. Because of the random deposition of radiation damage if one has, on average, one lethal lesion per cell, some cells will have the one lesion, some more than one, some less than one. The proportion of cells that have less than one, that is, no lethal events, under such circumstances, is e^{-1} or a survival fraction of 0.37. The dose required to reduce the survival fraction to this 37% on the exponential curve is known as the D_o. This term, therefore, is related to the slope of the exponential survival curve. The smaller the dose required to reduce the survival fraction to 37%, the more sensitive the cells are to radiation.

Survival curves of most mammalian cells differ from those of bacterial cells by having a "shoulder" in the low dose region and the exponential relationship described above at higher doses. This shoulder indicates a reduced efficiency of cell killing. Such an idealized curve is shown in Fig. 7-8. The remaining other important shorthand terminology used to describe survival curves is shown in this figure. The terminal exponential portion is described by the D_o while the initial shoulder region can be described by the extrapolation number n, or the D_q, the quasi-threshold dose. The latter is the dose at which the straight portion of the survival curve extrapolated backward intersects the line where the survival fraction is united. Knowing any two of these will allow one to calculate the third and describe the survival curve as follows: $\log e^n = D_q/D_o$.

FIG. 7-7. Two cell pedigrees indicating cell cycle times and the outcome of cells irradiated *in vitro*. *PYK* = pyknosis. (Thompson LH, Suit HD: Proliferation kinetics of x-irradiated mouse L cells studied with time lapse photography-II. Int J Radiat Biol 15:347–362, 1969) (*Fig. 7-7 continued on p. 112.*)

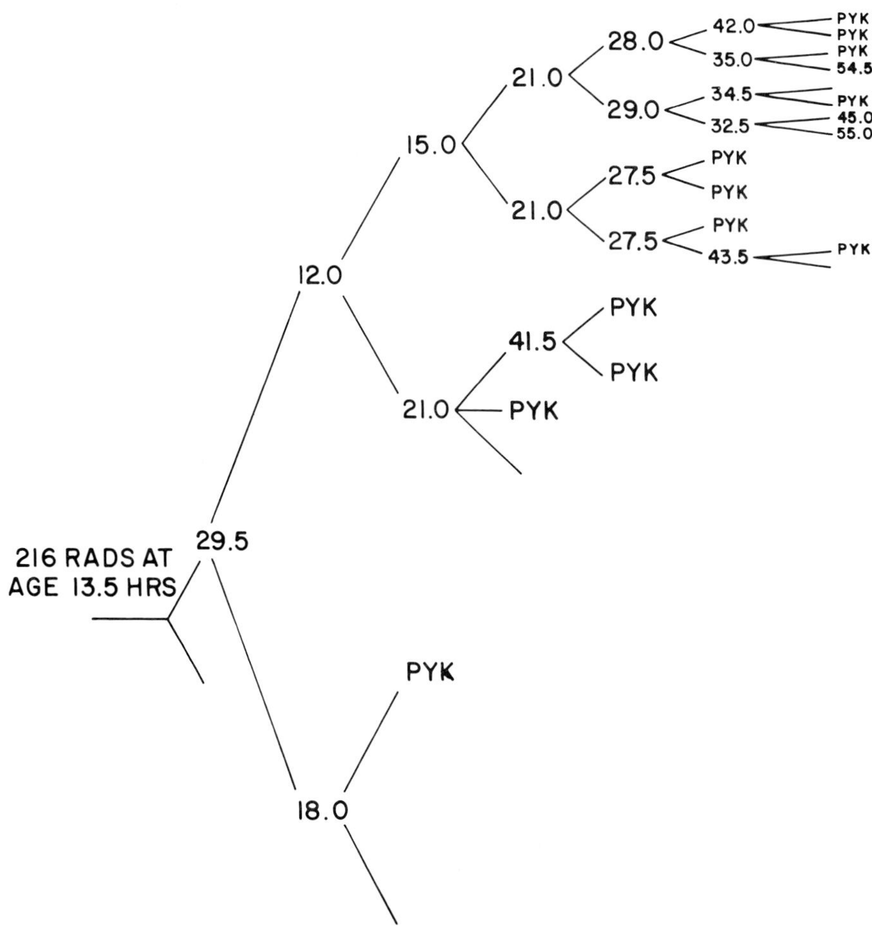

FIG. 7-7. (*Continued*).

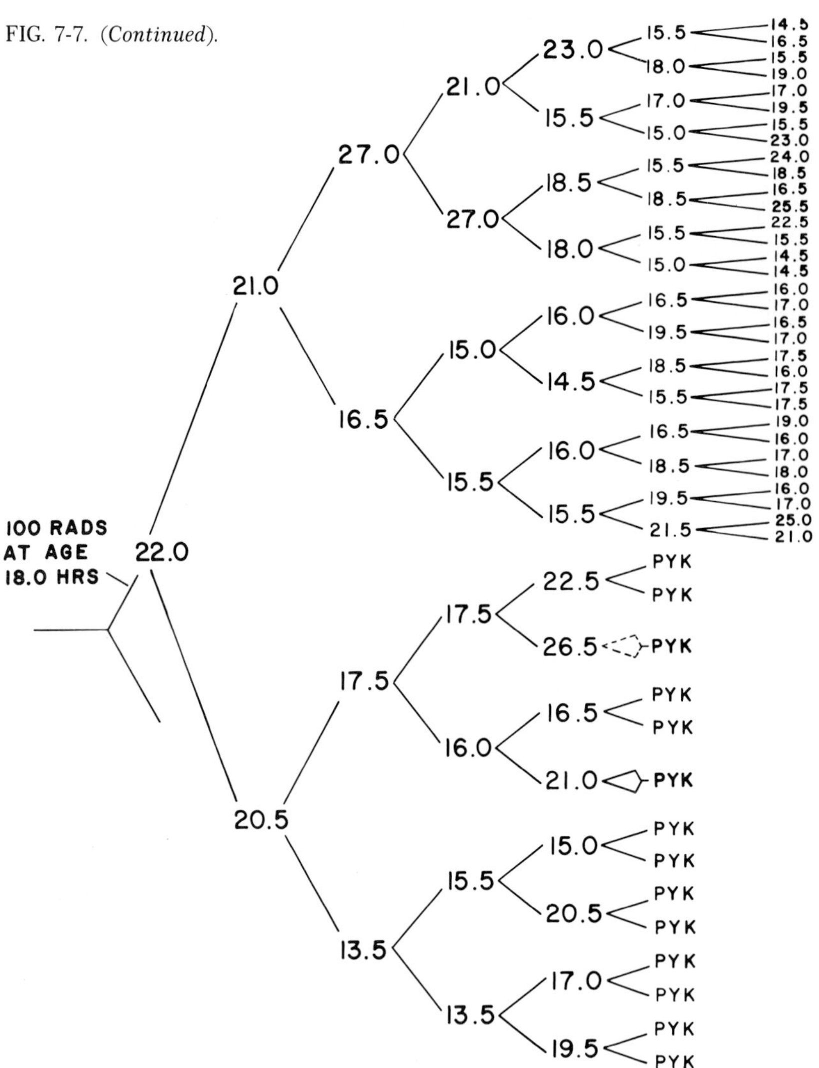

Survival curves have been determined for a variety of mammalian cells in culture of benign or neoplastic origin. There are no general characteristics of tumor cells that make them different from normal cells in culture. The survival curves for various human tumors thought to be both sensitive and resistant to radiation have been studied by Weichselbaum and coworkers,[3] and there are little, if any, survival curve characteristics that allow one to separate these two. Therefore, it is generally felt that the differences in clinical response cannot be explained by simple acute survival curve differences.

Normal tissues have also been studied using clonogenic survival as an end point with survival curves determined. The simplest clonal system as originally described by Till and McCullough is that used for murine bone marrow stem cells.[4] When bone marrow cells are injected into lethally irradiated recipient animals colonies are formed in the animals' spleen. These can be used to assess the reproductive integrity of the injected cells. Small intestinal clonogenic mucosal cell viability can be determined by looking at sections of the small intestine at various times following irradiation for the appearance of colonies derived from cells surviving this radiation.[5] Using these and other techniques, the general characteristics of survival curves of both normal and tumor cells are shown (see Table 7-1). There are no characteristic survival curve differences between normal tissues and tumors. In general, tumors tend to resemble their normal tissue of origin.

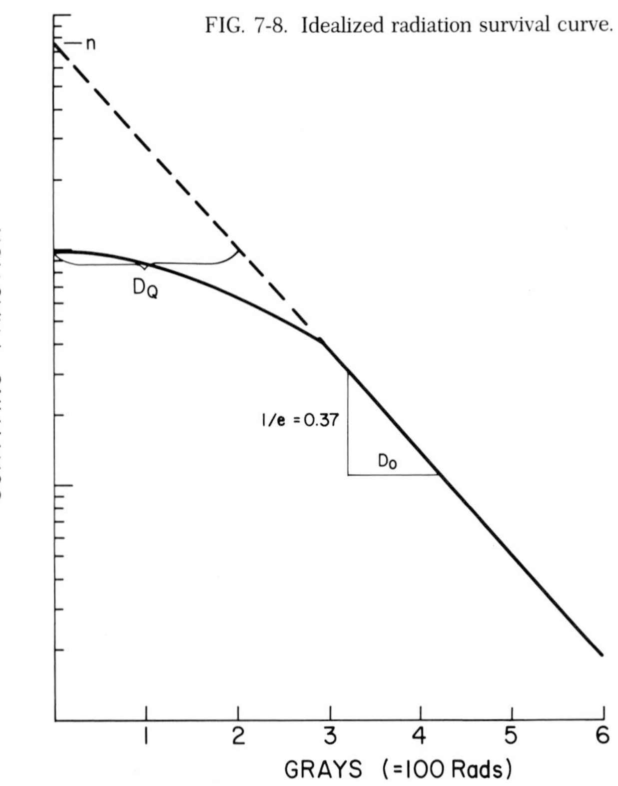

FIG. 7-8. Idealized radiation survival curve.

TABLE 7-1. Survival Curve Parameters for Some Mammalian Cells *In Vivo* or *In Vitro*

CELL TYPE	HOW DETER-MINED	Do	n	Dq
HAMSTER V-79 FIBROBLAST	*in vitro*	~160	~7	250–300
CHANG LIVER	*in vitro*	150	2	150
HE LA	*in vitro*	130	4	180
P 388 LEUKEMIA	*in vivo*	130	8.5	280
MOUSE BONE MARROW	*in vivo*	90–100	1.5–2.0	~60
MOUSE SMALL INTESTINE	*in vivo*	100	50	390
MOUSE CHONDROBLAST	*in vivo*	160	9	350
RAT ENDOTHELIUM	*in vivo*	170	7	340

Repair of Radiation Damage

When cells are irradiated, lethal damage can occur or the damage may be modified and not lead irrevocably to cell death. Such modification or amelioration of this damage is generally referred to as repair. This repair can be divided into *potentially lethal damage repair* and *sublethal damage repair.*

Potentially lethal damage is that which, under certain circumstances, will lead to cell death. However, if the post-irradiation conditions are modified to allow repair, cells which would have died can be salvaged. In general, those post-irradiation conditions that suppress cell division are most favorable to potentially lethal damage repair. The simplest example of this was first shown in bacteria for both UV- and X-radiation.[6] A similar effect was shown in mammalian cells and persists into the first few post-irradiation generations.[7–9] Potentially lethal damage repair may be most important in relating the cell culture studies of human tumors to their clinical response. Weichselbaum and coworkers[10] have shown that a tumor characteristically thought to be quite resistant to radiation (osteogenic sarcoma) has a great capacity for such potentially lethal damage repair, compared to tumors thought to be much more responsive to radiation. Following irradiation in the clinical circumstance the tumor cell may not be faced with the necessity of rapid cell division. Thus it may be allowed the opportunity for potentially lethal damage repair.

An explanation usually given for the shoulder of the radiation survival curve is that the cell is able to repair some of the radiation damage. This includes a great proportion of the damage incurred with low doses of radiation and is called *sublethal damage*. Elkind and colleagues have studied the shoulder and its return by using divided doses of radiation.[11] They have shown that if one divides the dose of radiation into two fractions allowing a few hours between radiation doses the shoulder will return. Therefore, two doses of radiation separated in time are less effective than the same dose given as a single dose. The difference between these two doses is the D_q when the two doses are sufficiently large enough to cause cell survival loss to extend to the exponential portion of the survival curve (see Fig. 7-9). The D_q can be considered to be a measure of sublethal damage repair. Table 7-2 shows the D_q for bone marrow, skin, lung, and gastrointestinal mucosa. The contrast is striking. Bone marrow stem cells

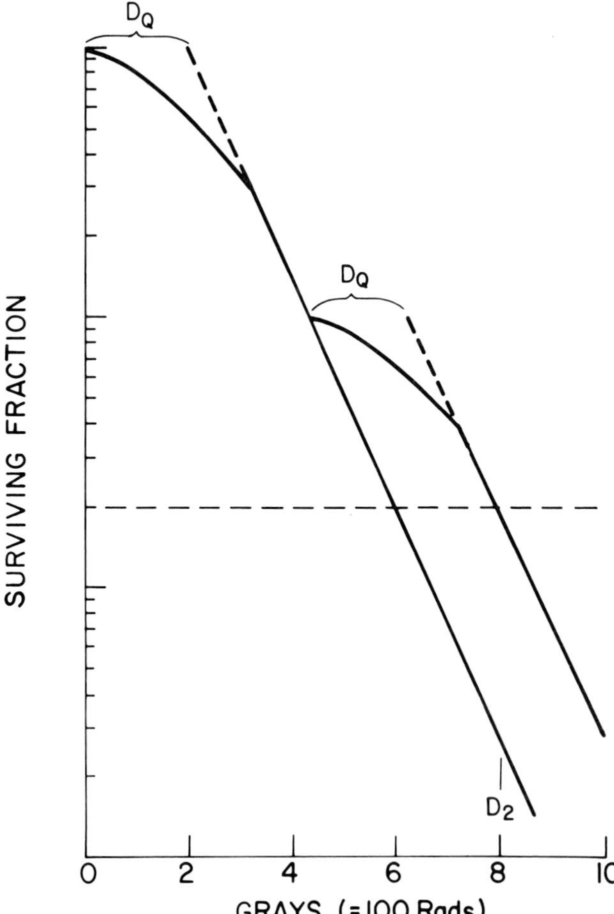

FIG. 7-9. Two dose radiation survival curves demonstrating return of the shoulder.

have a very small D_q while the others have considerable sublethal damage repair capacity. This suggests the great advantage of multiple small radiation fractions to preserve these tissues, but not bone marrow. When considering differences in radiation fractionation schemes, whether or not the fraction size is sufficient to be off the shoulder must be known. If all of the variations are on the shoulder there will be little difference in cell kill by varying the fractionations. With such small fractions essentially all the damage that can be repaired is already being repaired and fractionation becomes much less important. However, if the fractions are large enough to include a portion of the steeper part of the survival curve then differences in fraction size are very important since the proportion of shoulder-to-steep exponential portion varies for different fraction sizes.

TABLE 7-2. Dq Determination for Some Normal Tissues

NORMAL TISSUE	Dq (AVERAGE FROM LITERATURE) (GRAY)
Mouse skin	~4
Mouse intestine	3.50–4
Mouse lung	~3.75
Mouse bone marrow	~0.60

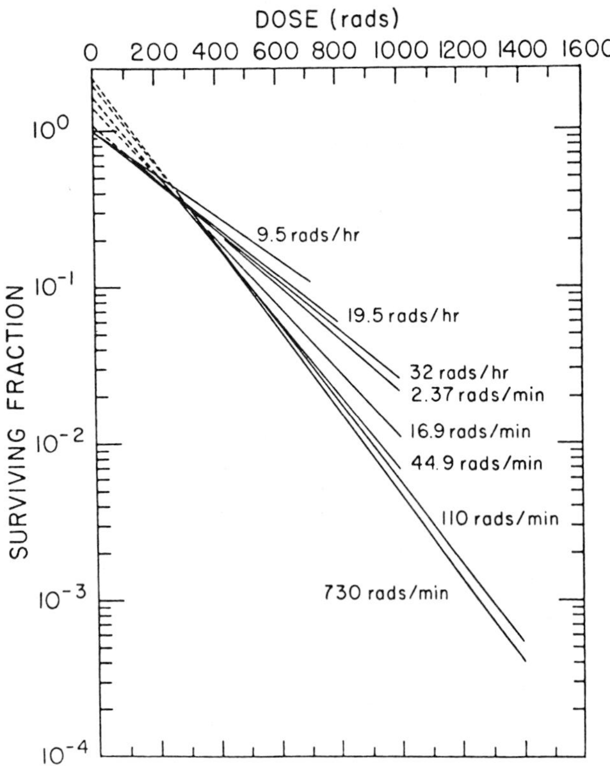

FIG. 7-10. *In vitro* survival curves for cells irradiated at different dose rates. (Hall EJ: Radiation dose-rate: a factor of importance in radiobiology and radiotherapy. Br J Radiol 45:81–97, 1972)

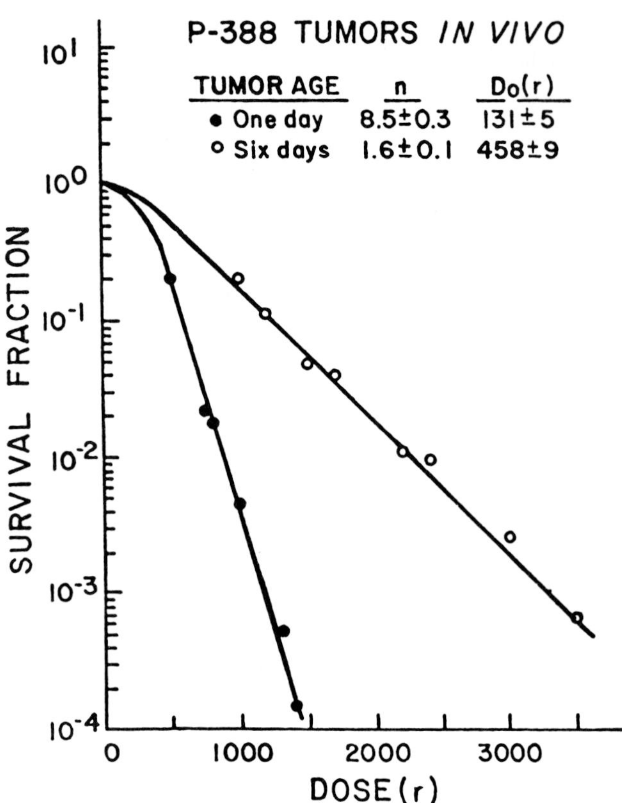

FIG. 7-11. *In vivo* survival curves for oxic and hypoxic tumor cells. (Belli JA, Discus GJ, Bonte FJ: Radiation response of mammalian tumor cells. 1. Repair of sublethal damage *in vivo*. Journal of the National Cancer Institute 38:673–682, 1967)

Varying the dose rate of radiation may be considered a form of radiation fractionation. When the dose rate is made quite low, such as during interstitial or intra-cavitary irradiation, this can be considered a large number of small doses on the shoulder of the survival curve.[11] Therefore, differences between the dose limiting normal tissues, the tumor in shoulder characteristics, and the break point between shoulder and steep exponential will have great clinical implications for such continuous radiation. A example of this for cells in culture is shown in Fig. 7-10.

The Importance of Oxygen

The most important modifier of the biologic effect of ionizing irradiation is molecular oxygen. This was noted in the 1920s but not understood or its importance realized until Mottram and colleagues studied this systematically.[13–15] The general scientific community became aware of this with the publications by Read and Gray in the early 1950s.[14,15] Figure 7-11 shows a survival curve for cells under aerobic and hypoxic conditions.[16] For every level of survival, greater doses are required under hypoxic conditions as compared to oxic conditions. There is some disagreement in the literature as to whether the dose ratio is the same throughout the survival curve. Some data suggest a smaller difference when low doses are used. A shorthand term, the oxygen enhancement ratio (OER), is often used. OER is the ratio of dose required for equivalent cell killing in the absence as compared to the presence of oxygen. This term has most relevance on the exponential portion of the curve. Some investigators report a reduced shoulder on a survival curve of cells under hypoxic conditions.[16] As shown in Fig. 7-12, tumor cells, when allowed to grow into physiologic hypoxia, have reduced capacity to repair sublethal damage.

The OER range for different cells studied varies from about 2.5 to 3.5. This means that for a *given survival level* three times as much radiation is required under hypoxic conditions than under oxic conditions. Since the curves are exponential, for a *given dose of radiation* the ratio of survival fraction may be much greater and will increase with dose. For example, in Fig. 7-11, at 1000 rads the ratio of survival is 30. Study of the phenomenon reveals that oxygen must be present during irradiation. Figure 7-13 shows the relative radiosensitivity of cells as a function of the oxygen tension at the time of irradiation. A very low oxygen tension must be reached before there is a protective effect of hypoxia. The exact mechanism of the oxygen effect has not been definitely determined. It is felt that oxygen affects the initial chemical products of radiation interaction with biologic material. The important free radicals have a short half-life. A useful way to think about them is that they may either return to an innocuous state or remain highly reactive molecules. Oxygen appears to favor the latter while the presence of high levels of sulfhydryl compounds favors the former. Thomlinson and Gray recognized the importance of the oxygen effect to clinical radiotherapy in a classic paper in which they showed that human

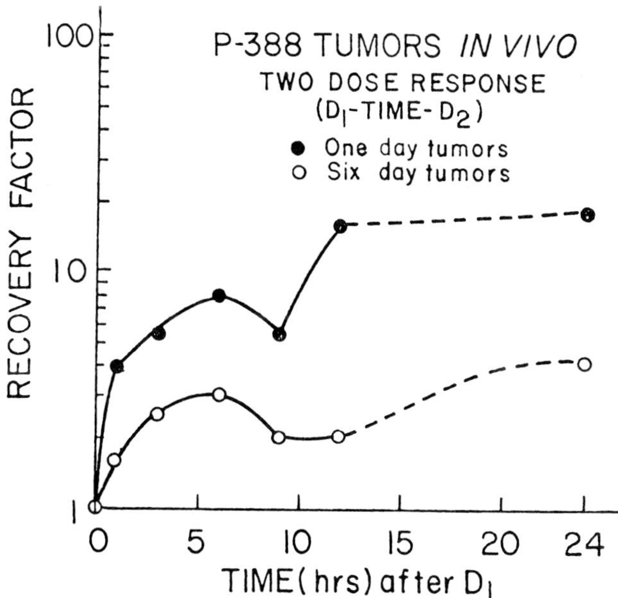

FIG. 7-12. *In vivo* curves comparing two dose survival to single dose survival for oxic and hypoxic tumor cells. (Belli JA, Discus GJ, Bonte FJ: Radiation response of mammalian tumor cells. 1. Repair of sublethal damage *in vivo*. Journal of the National Cancer Institute 38:673–682, 1967)

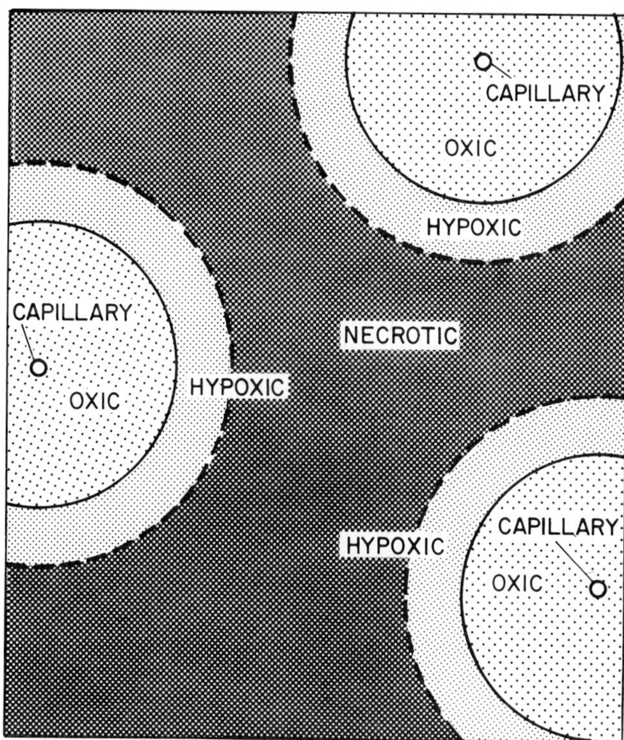

FIG. 7-14. Diagramatic representation of a tumor.

tumors frequently had anoxic regions.[18] Calculations of oxygen diffusion from capillaries and metabolism predicted that the oxygen tension would decrease to zero at about 150 microns. They measured the width of tumor cords and showed that tumors could be thought to be modeled as shown in Fig. 7-14. Those cells within 100 microns or so of the capillary are well oxygenated; those beyond 150 microns are anoxic and necrotic; those between 100 and 150 are hypoxic at an oxygen tension that might confer on such cells protection from radiation. This model has had a profound influence on radiobiologic and radiotherapeutic thinking. If all tumors look this way and such hypoxic regions contain cells that could

FIG. 7-13. Radiation sensitivity as a function of ambient oxygen pressure. (Modified from Deschner EE, Gray LH: Influence of oxygen tension on x-ray induced chromosomal damage in Ehrlich ascites tumor cells irradiated *in vitro* and *in vivo*. Radiat Res 11:115–146, 1959)

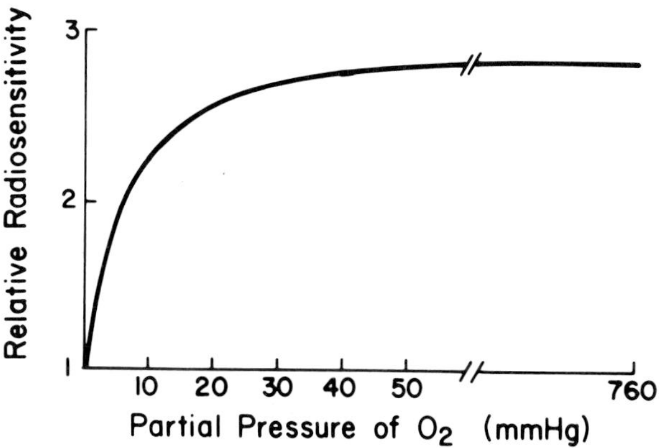

ultimately cause tumor regrowth then no clinically apparent tumor would be cured by radiation therapy. Since this is obviously not the case, one must explain this paradox. Laboratory experiments have indicated that immediately after a single dose of radiation the surviving tumor cells are largely the originally hypoxic ones. However, after a period of time the proportion of hypoxic cells returns to the preradiation level. This has been called *reoxygenation*.[19] The term can be confusing since these are very indirect experiments and do not record the fate of individual cells. These experiments can be explained by suggesting that tumor cells do reoxygenate because of:

1. Reduced total tumor cell population relative to the surface area of tumor blood vessels
2. Reduced separation of hypoxic cells from the blood vessels resulting from cell kill
3. Increased oxygen diffusion
4. Decreased intratumoral pressure allowing opening of blood vessels, in addition to a variety of other reasons.

Alternatively, a large number of these hypoxic cells might in fact be doomed since with proliferation in the oxic regions they will be pushed outward, ultimately forced to reside in the anoxic regions, and therefore die. Thus they may have only a limited clinical importance in determining tumor curability. It is likely that different mechanisms pertain under different circumstances, both in the laboratory and in the clinic. The obvious clinical importance of the oxygen effect has led to a number of clinical and laboratory experiments, including the use of high pressure oxygen with radiation therapy in order to improve results. These studies have indicated that with small number of fractions such hyperbaric

TABLE 7-3. Results of a Randomized Prospective Trial of Hyperbaric Oxygen in the Radiation Treatment of Head and Neck Cancer

	LOCAL CONTROL	SURVIVAL AT 4 YEARS
HP O_2	61%	56%
Conventional treatment	40%	27%

(Henk J, Kindler PB, Smith CW: Radiotherapy and head and neck cancer: Final report on the first clinical trial. Lancet 2:101–103, 1977)

TABLE 7-4. Effect of Anemia on Pelvic Recurrence in Stage IIB–III Cervical Cancer[27]

	CONTROL		TRANSFUSED
Hgb (gm%)	<12	>12	>12
Pelvic recurrence	50% (10/20)	23% (11/48)	16% (11/67)

(Bush RS, Jenkin RP, Allt WE et al: Definitive evidence for hypoxic cells influencing cure in cancer therapy. Br J Cancer 37:302–306, 1978)

oxygen will increase curability. However, when normal fractionation schemes are used, such hyperbaric oxygen has often failed to show an advantage. There are, however, some recent reports with tumors of the head, neck, and uterine cervix indicating that hyperbaric oxygen with 10 fractions of radiation results in greater cure than conventional daily fractionation.[20-22] Table 7-3 depicts the head and neck results. Despite these promising studies the technique is thought to be cumbersome, difficult for the patient, prohibiting the use of the careful beam definition and beam modification so important in radiation therapy. Thus the technique has been abandoned in most radiotherapy centers.

A more attractive alternative has been the development of *hypoxic cell sensitizers*. In the 1960s, Adams and colleagues began searching for compounds that would mimic oxygen in its effect.[23,24] Importantly, however, these agents should not be rapidly metabolized so that they can reach all portions of the tumor. This is an important distinction because high pressure oxygen increases diffusion only slightly, while such slowly metabolized sensitizers might reach all areas of the tumor.* While newer methods were based on replacing molecular oxygen there are apparently other effects of the nitro-imidazoles, the most well-studied class of these agents. They appear to be quite cytotoxic to hypoxic cells and may sensitize cells to chemotherapeutic agents.[25,26] How important these last two points are in their use remains to be seen. However, this general class of agents offers a whole new approach to the chemical treatment of tumors based on a known tumor–normal tissue difference (*i.e.*, the presence of hypoxic cells in tumors).

A practical clinical concern is whether the presence of anemia affects tumor response to radiation. Historic review and a recent prospective study from the Princess Margaret Hospital (see Table 7-4) appear to indicate that anemia results in an adverse effect on tumor curability by radiation, presumably because it increases the hypoxic component of tumor cells.

Variation of the Radiation Response During the Division Cycle

As described in Chapter 4 on cell kinetics the cell cycle can be divided into four phases: G1, S, G2, and M. Terasima, Tolmach, and Sinclair studied relatively synchronized populations to determine whether there is a difference in response to radiation as a function of the cell's position in the division cycle.[28,29] They found that in general the mitotic phase (M) is most sensitive with G2 almost as sensitive. G1 is relatively sensitive in cells with a short G1. Cells gradually increase in resistance as they proceed through late G1 and S phase, reaching a maximum of resistance in the late S. In those cells with a long G1 there appears to be a peak of resistance early in G1. These findings *in vitro* seem to be true *in vivo* as well for both normal cells and tumor tissues.[30,31] The changes are due to both changes in the shoulder as well as changes in the terminal slope. These differences can be quite large. The difference between the most resistant and the most sensitive can show slope ratios equal to that of the oxygen effect. The clinical consequence of a dose of 200 rad is shown for two different radiation fractionation schemes, one used in Hodgkin's disease (20 fractions) and one used in epithelial cancer (32 fractions) (see Table 7-5).[32] Note how small differences in survival fractions following a single dose may change the final survival level achieved. All of these fractional survivals are within the range seen for cells in different parts of the cell cycle. A second consequence of such differential cell killing as well as the mitotic delay induced by radiation is a tendency to partially synchronize the cells. Thus, the timing of the second dose of a fractionated scheme might be quite critical. However, this synchronization is short-lived as cells desynchronize rapidly and redistribute themselves according to the original cell age distribution. This phenomenon, which might have posed a clinical problem or a clinical advantage, does not seem to be important unless there is incomplete *redistribution* between fractions.

CELL PROLIFERATION. During a course of fractionated radiation the ultimate response of the tumor and normal tissue will depend on whether there has been cell proliferation between the fractions, thereby increasing the number of cells exposed to radiation. This may be due to cell proliferation

* These agents and their importance are described in Chapter 19 concerned with newer methods of treatment.

TABLE 7-5. Calculated Cumulative Survival Fraction*

SURVIVAL FRACTION	X^{32} X =	X^{20} X =
10^{-11}	0.45	0.28
10^{-10}	0.49	0.32
10^{-9}	0.52	0.35
10^{-8}	0.56	0.40
10^{-7}	0.60	0.45
10^{-6}	0.65	0.50
10^{-5}	0.70	0.56

* Calculated cumulative survival fraction for either 32 or 20 equal fractions when the fractional survival is varied.[32]

within the volume irradiated (*i.e.*, within the tumor or normal cell renewal tissue) or due to cells that migrate in from unirradiated adjacent areas. The latter is noted in the skin, oral, and gastrointestinal mucosa or from great distances as noted with bone marrow and lymph node repopulation. The balance between radiation-induced cell killing and repopulation is responsible for much of the clinical findings seen during fractionated radiotherapy treatment (discussed later in this chapter). In addition to this spontaneous repopulation there may be an induced cell proliferation or *recruitment* of cells.[33,34] Physiologically many tissues of the body respond to trauma by being recruited into rapid proliferation (*i.e.*, following a wound in the skin, a break of the bone, or a partial hepatectomy). The reparative process requires proliferation of the undamaged cells. Similarly, when the oral mucosa is irradiated there is good evidence that the cell cycle time is decreased and net cell proliferation increases. This may also occur in some tumors but appears to be of less magnitude than that in the normal tissues.[35] Part of the differential effect of fractionated radiation may lie in differential recruitment of normal versus tumor cells.

Pharmacologic Modification of Radiation Effects

There are a number of pharmacologic agents that can modify those basic parameters of radiation response discussed. Fig. 7-15 shows a radiation survival curve for cells that have semiconservatively incorporated the halogenated pyrimidine BUDR into their DNA. Under such circumstances these cells are more sensitive to radiation having both the slope and the shoulder modified.[36] This only occurs when the halogenated pyrimidines BUDR or IUDR are incorporated into the DNA; their being present at the time of radiation is not sufficient (see Fig. 7-15). Sublethal damage repair is also markedly inhibited under these circumstances. A second class of agents are those that primarily affect the shoulder and only slightly affect the slope. The two most important agents here are actinomycin D and adriamycin. Sublethal damage is apparently inhibited by actinomycin D but not by adriamycin.[37,41–43] The mechanisms by which these drugs affect the radiation response are quite complicated. From a clinical standpoint, however, there appears to be strong evidence that these drugs can and do modify radiation effects when given simultaneously. Furthermore, when given after radiation therapy they can "recall" the irradiated volumes by erythema on the skin or by producing pulmonary reactions.[38,41,44,45] Whether this is due to interaction of the damage done by radiation and drug or whether it only represents additivity of the effects is uncertain. Chemicals may also interact with radiation by preferentially killing cells more resistant to radiation. For example, agents that preferentially destroy cells in the most resistant phase of the cell cycle (S) together with radiation will increase the cell kill; an example of this is hydroxyurea.[46] The hypoxic sensitizers also kill hypoxic cells and therefore would act similarly in destroying a population of cells resistant to radiation. Radioprotective agents such as sulfhydryl-containing compounds act in the reverse fashion and tend to make cells more resistant.[47]

When considering the whole animal, agents with different dose-limiting normal tissue toxicities than radiation may be

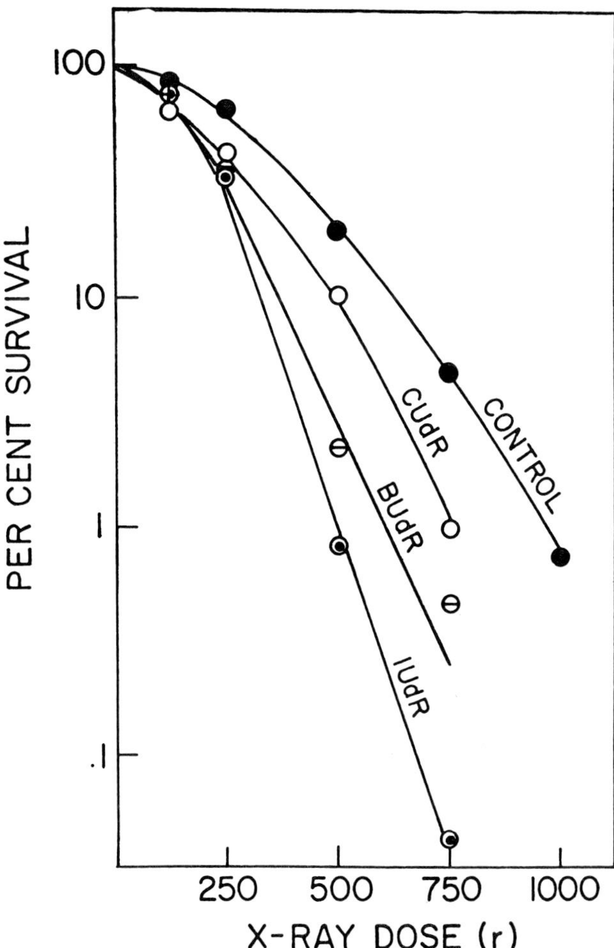

FIG. 7-15. Radiation survival curve for cells incorporating halogenated pyrimidines. (Szybalski W: X-ray sensitization by halopyrimidines. Cancer Chemotherapy Rep 58:539–557, 1974)

used very effectively with radiation. This applies one of the basic principles of multiple drug chemotherapy—to add agents with non-overlapping toxicities. This also works well with radiation.

The combined effects of drugs and radiation, or of two drugs, can be divided into the following types:

1. Independent—the agents act independently, their mechanisms of action are independent and their damage is independent.
2. Additivity—the agents act on the same loci and therefore both their sublethal damage as well as their lethal damage are additive. Because of additive sublethal damage the lethality of the two together may be greater than the lethality of each alone
3. Synergism—when the two agents have a result that is more effective than pure additivity
4. Antagonism—where the cell killing is less than independent action

The most important parameter for the clinician is the therapeutic index. The sigmoid curve of tumor cure and that of dose-limiting toxicity are portrayed in Fig. 7-16. If both curves are moved but their relative place (one to the other)

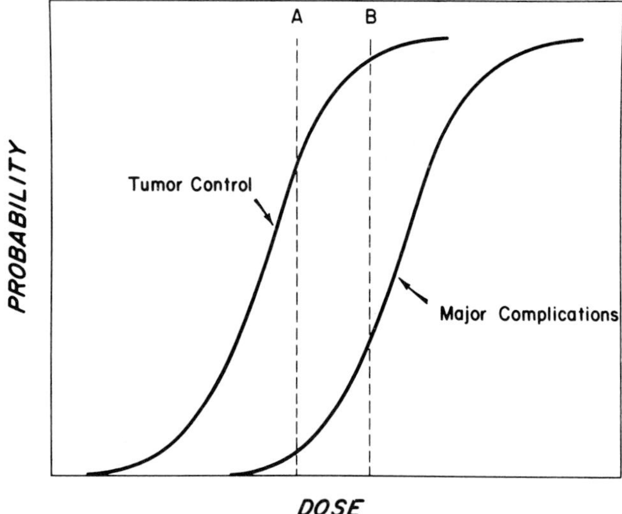

FIG. 7-16. Sigmoid curves of tumor control and complications. *A*, Dose for tumor control with minimum complications. *B*, Maximum tumor dose with significant complications.

is not changed then the proportion cured for a given level of toxicity is unchanged. Drug–roentgen ray interaction is only useful when the curves are separated and not merely displaced.

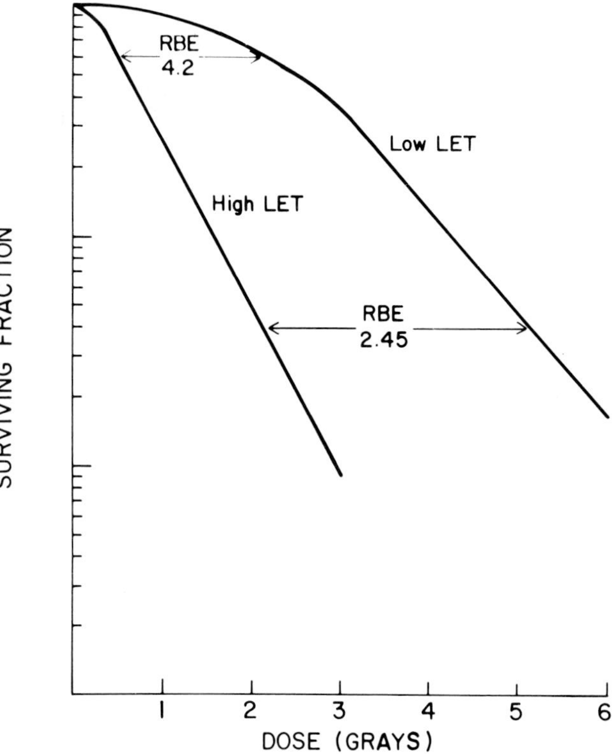

FIG. 7-17. Survival fractions for high and low *LET* radiations.

HIGH LET RADIATION

Most of the previous discussion has been concerned with sparsely ionizing radiation such as that produced by photons or high energy electrons. More densely ionizing radiation is produced by larger atomic particles. The biologic actions of these two types of radiation are quite different and relate to the density of ionization. *LET or linear energy transfer* is the rate of energy loss along the path of the particle (de/dl). High LET radiations are very densely ionizing, de/dl being very high. In general the density of ionization is dependent on z^2/v^2 where z equals the atomic number and v the particle velocity. Photons and electrons are characterized as having high energy and very low mass. Therefore, the density of ionization will be low until the secondary electrons come to rest at the very end of their path. Particulate radiation ionizes directly. Alpha particles and stripped nuclei have a high LET; neutrons have an intermediate LET due to recoil protons. The z^2 is quite large for large particles, intermediate for protons, and low for photons.

RELATIVE BIOLOGIC EFFECTIVENESS (RBE)

RBE is commonly used in radiation biology. It is the dose ratio of different average LET beams required to produce the same biologic effect. This term is generally a descriptive one but its numerical value is fraught with many difficulties since it varies with the biologic end point used. High LET radiation differs from low LET radiation in affecting both the shoulder and slope of the radiation survival curves (see Fig. 7-17). If the biologic endpoint of interest is one associated with a high survival fraction then the RBE will be large as it considers shoulder differences as well as those of the terminal slope. However, if it has to do with a very low survival fraction, the RBE will be less as it primarily considers slope differences. In general then, RBE increases as the dose decreases. Not only is the shoulder reduced but other measures of sublethal damage repair or potentially lethal damage repair are markedly reduced with high LET radiation. A general explanation for this is ionization is so dense that when a cell is hit the damage is so great that it is not possible to be repaired. It is also true that the oxygen effect decreases as the LET increases. With very high LET radiation there is no oxygen effect. Fig. 7-18 plots both RBE and OER as a function of LET.[48] With very high LET radiation there is a fall in RBE. This is because these very densely ionizing radiations deposit more than one lethal event per cell. Thus, some of the absorbed dose is redundant and becomes less efficient.

While this obvious advantage in RBE and OER would suggest the possible therapeutic use of these radiations a cautionary note should be made. Increasing RBE in itself does not afford a therapeutic advantage. What is important is the therapeutic gain factor—the RBE of the tumor versus the RBE of the normal tissue. This is quite complicated and very much depends on the specific tumor and the dose-limiting normal tissue being considered.[49] (These forms of radiation will be discussed further in Chapter 48.)

TUMOR RADIOBIOLOGY

A great deal of experimental work has been done using a variety of animal tumors. In general, these tumors are either spontaneous tumors occurring with reasonably high fre-

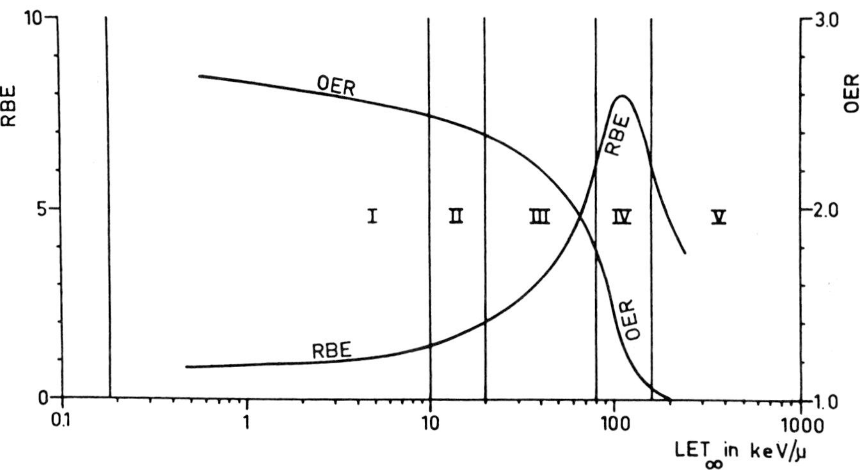

FIG. 7-18. Oxygen enhancement ratio (*OER*) and relative biological effectiveness as a function of linear energy transfer *OER*. Five regions of *LET* are suggested. *I*, Corresponds to shouldered survival curves; affected greatly by fraction size and dose rate. *II*, Transition region. *III*, Exponential survival curve, independent of fractionization and dose rate. *RBE* changes considerably with *LET* as does *OER*. *IV*, Transition region. *V*, *LET* in excess of 160 *KeV/u* independent of fractionization and dose rate. *RBE* decreases as *LET* increases since any cell damaged is so extensively damaged by high density of interactions that some interactions are "wasted."

quency in certain strains of mice (*i.e.*, the mammary carcinoma in the C3H mice) or tumors induced by carcinogens. Such primary tumors of animals are difficult to use because their production is time-consuming and numbers of tumors of the same size and location are limited, restricting some experimental designs. The use of transplanted tumors is much more common. These are tumors that may have occurred spontaneously or due to the application of a carcinogen but have now been transplanted from animal to animal. They grow with predictable and known kinetics. While this is a great advantage in experimental work, it does increase the likelihood that the application of the results may be somewhat limited. Since these tumors are selected for rapid growth and for the ability to serially transplant they may not represent tumors occurring spontaneously in the host animal.

Tumors can be used in radiobiologic experiments and assayed in a number of ways. The simplest is to study the likelihood for cure. One implants a tumor into animals, allows it to grow to palpable size, treats with a specific regimen, and then determines how many tumors of this type in various host animals are cured. If the dose of radiation is plotted against the likelihood for cure a sigmoid curve is generated as seen in Fig. 7-19. There is insufficient cell kill to cause tumor cure at very low doses. However, as the dose is raised (close to about one lethal event per cell) then the statistics of random cell kill become important. Then there are occasions when tumors will have zero viable cells and are cured. Cure likelihood rises rapidly with dose at this portion of the curve; it starts to plateau when the maximum effect of the particular technique is reached. The dose required to increase a 10% to a 90% likelihood of tumor control is about three times the D_0 dose. This sigmoid relationship is very important as it is not only true for tumors in experimental animals but for clinical situations as well.

The shape and steepness of the sigmoid dose response relationship for tumors can be affected by many factors. If the radiation survival curve is quite shallow for individual tumor cells (*i.e.*, the D_0 is large), then the dose response curve will be shallow also. It will also be affected by host defense mechanisms. This curve is quite steep with non-immunogenic tumors or when the immune response is abrogated but significantly more shallow in immunogenic tumors.[51] The shallowness means that there will be occasional cures at low doses and occasional failures at very high doses. A similar sigmoid relationship is also seen when plotting the likelihood for complications against tumor control. Figure 7-16 shows the two sigmoid curves, one for cure and one for complications. This is presented optimistically (*i.e.*, the important complication curve is placed to the right of the tumor

FIG. 7-19. Sigmoid curve of tumor control.

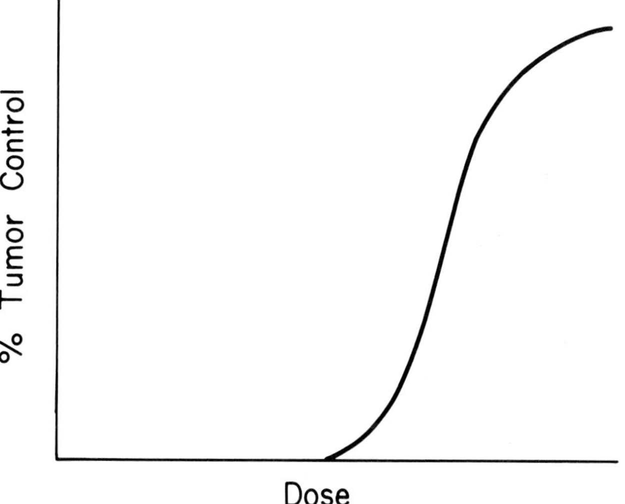

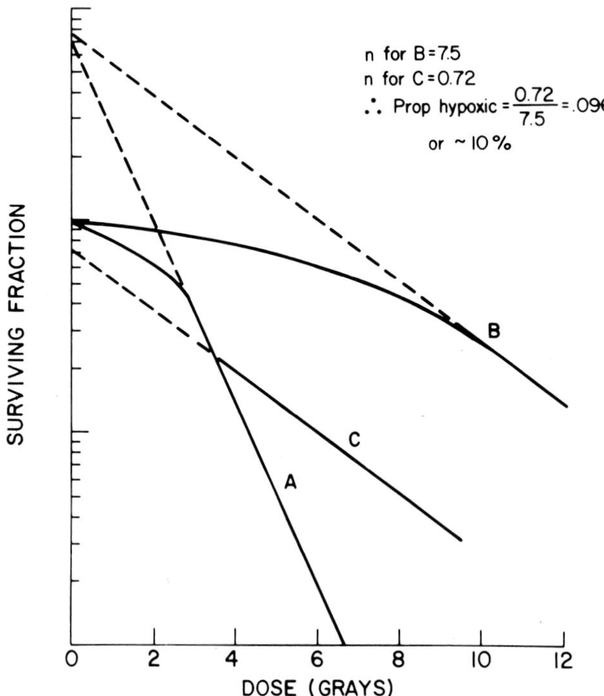

FIG. 7-20. Idealized survival curves for *A*, Oxic tumor cells; *B*, Hypoxic tumor cells; *C*, A tumor containing both oxic and hypoxic tumor cells.

cure curve). The difference between these curves is therefore a measure of therapeutic gain. Much of clinical medicine and research in cancer treatment is concerned with separating these curves.[49] Once the curves are separated then, for a given level of complications, the likelihood for cure can be increased. Or, for a high likelihood for cure, the likelihood for complications can be decreased.

Another method of measuring tumor response to treatment is to determine the growth delay of tumors following treatment. The longer the time for regrowth, the more effective was the treatment. If it is assumed that tumors grow and regrow with the same kinetics when they are at similar sizes then the separation between the original curve and the regrowth curve is a direct measure of cell kill.[52] A direct measure of tumor cell kill is to remove the tumor after treatment, separate the cells, and score the surviving colony-forming cells either *in vivo* or *in vitro*. Assay techniques include transplantation and measurement of recipient animal death, tumor growth, or the number of colonies in the lung, liver, or brain. *In vitro* techniques require tumors to adapt to grow both *in vivo* and *in vitro*.

It is important to realize that tumors, like normal tissues, have certain physiologic characteristics. Some of these we associate with the definition of malignancy (*i.e.*, continued growth and extension into surrounding tissues as well as, in most cases, the ability to metastasize). In addition, if tumors are to grow they must induce a blood supply to meet their increasing metabolic needs. The production of these blood vessels appears to be a consequence of the release of a substance described by Folkman and colleagues as "tumor angiogenesis factor." This may have very important clinical implications. If tumors can be prevented from producing such substances then they should not grow beyond that tumor size supported by diffusion alone.[53,54] From the radiobiologic point of view it also means that when irradiating a tumor both the radiobiology of the tumor and the vascular endothelial cells are of concern. Complete destruction of the ability of the tumor blood vessels to proliferate will effectively limit tumor growth. As tumors grow they appear to exceed their blood supply and develop areas of necrosis and hypoxia (see Fig. 7-14). The proportion of hypoxic cells in a tumor can be determined by study of the radiation survival curves (see Fig. 7-20). In this figure, curve A is that found with a well-oxygenated cell population, curve B for hypoxic cells, and curve C for a mixture of oxic and hypoxic cells (as in a tumor). Extrapolation of the curves to the ordinate will give the proportion of hypoxic cells within a tumor as first described by Powers and Tolmach.[55] In most experimental tumors studied the percent of hypoxic cells is 10–20%. Calculation of the likelihood to cure tumors based on the D_0, N, repopulation, repair, and hypoxia indicates that since each fraction of radiation should increase the proportion of hypoxic cells the current clinically used treatment regimens should not be effective. Since radiotherapy cures a large number of tumors of a sufficient size to have hypoxic components and, in fact, show necrosis on pathologic examination, then this conclusion must be erroneous. After multiple fractions of radiation a marked increase in the proportion of the more resistant hypoxic cells would be expected. In fact, the proportion remained constant when observed 72 hours after the last of five radiation fractions. Kallman has called this *reoxygenation*.[19] It may well be that hypoxic cells are not at all important in those tumors cured but may be important in some of those tumors that are not cured. Clinical evidence that this is important is the benefit of correcting anemia, hyperbaric oxygen, and the hypoxic sensitizers. All appear to beneficially influence tumor curability in certain clinical circumstances.

NORMAL TISSUE RADIATION BIOLOGY

To understand this, an appreciation of cell kinetics of the cell renewal tissues is vital (see Chapter 4 on cell kinetics). The effects on organ function very much depend on the reproductive requirements of the irradiated cells. Those tissues whose functional activity does not require cell renewal (*i.e.*, muscle and neurologic tissue) are quite "resistant" to radiation. Both of these also have important vasculo–connective tissue stroma that support them.[56] These stromal cells may be required to divide, therefore determining the organ response to radiation. The radiation response of endothelial cells demonstrates a D_q = 340 rads, N = 7, and a D_o = 170 rads, values similar to those of epithelial cells.[57] There are, of course, many tissues of the body that require continued cellular proliferation for their function. These cell renewal tissues include the skin and its appendages, the gastrointestinal mucosa, bone marrow, reproductive tissues, and many exocrine glands. Since continued reproduction is essential in these systems they promptly demonstrate the effects of radiation. Clonogenic survival curves for bone marrow stem cells, gastrointestinal epithelial cells, and skin are all available. There are also more slowly proliferating tissues (*i.e.*, lung) where the effects of radiation are seen significantly later but it is an effect dependent on radiation damage to proliferating cells.

Tissues such as the liver and bone require little or no proliferation during the steady state. However, both of these respond to injury with rapid cell renewal. In these tissues normal function can be maintained despite large doses of radiation. Should trauma (fracture or partial hepatectomy) occur then the cells will die when they attempt repair. Irradiation of the liver appears to have little consequence in moderate doses. Should this be followed by a partial hepatectomy then hepatic failure can occur. This has been of clinical importance in the pre-operative irradiation of right-sided Wilm's tumors attached to the liver in which a significant amount of liver must be removed. When this is done liver failure may occur post-operatively, as the hepatocytes attempt to repopulate and die.[58] Under such circumstances it is far better to operate, allow the liver to regenerate, and then irradiate.

Patients who have received large amounts of radiation to the bone do perfectly well unless the bone is fractured. Such damaged bones will either fail to be reconstituted or will heal in a very delayed fashion, causing a significant deformity and disability to the patient. These examples are included to make the point that it is not the different cells that have such great differences in radiation response, but rather, that the differing proliferative requirements of different tissues largely determine the radiation effects. When the proliferative requirements are low, the organ will be considered relatively resistant to radiation. When the proliferative requirements are high, it will be considered quite "radiosensitive." There may be some common limitations on all systems based on the radiosensitivity of the vascular connective tissue and endothelial cells.[56]

There are many other effects of radiation that do not depend on reproductive viability. These may have clear clinical relevance. For example, radiation is quite damaging to the cell membrane and will change membrane transport. One obvious clinical consequence of this is radiation-induced edema seen with quite moderate doses of radiation. These non-reproductive effects of radiation are far less well-understood but may be quite important in understanding the effects of radiation on non-dividing tissue—most importantly the central nervous system.

When given to the whole animal there are some general effects of radiation. Large doses of whole body irradiation have obvious clinical consequences. These effects are, in general, not relevant to conventional radiation therapy. However, since whole body irradiation has been used in the treatment of the lymphomas in low doses, and high doses in the treatment of metastatic carcinoma this will be mentioned briefly. Following large doses of radiation, there is the prodromal syndrome of nausea, vomiting, diarrhea, cramps, fatigue, sweating, fever, and headache. Following this, three distinct modes of death may occur. The first, with very high doses of radiation (in excess of 10,000 rad), is seen in a matter of hours and appears to result from neurologic and cardiovascular damage. Since this occurs so quickly, it is probably due to a failure of a proliferating cell system to extranuclear events within these organs. At intermediate doses of radiation of the order of 500–1000 rads, death occurs in a matter of days. It is associated with extensive gastrointestinal mucosal damage, resulting in prolonged severe bloody diarrhea, dehydration, and secondary infection occurring as the gastrointestinal mucosa is denuded. At lower doses of radiation (around the LD_{50}), death is due to hematopoietic failure. This has a latency period as the formed blood elements are non-dividing and bone marrow failure does not occur until the progeny of the proliferating cells are required to maintain the patient. Lymphocytes fall promptly as some of these cells die without dividing. The granulocyte level will fall on about day 5–6 and finally, thrombocytopenia will occur. In general, anemia does not occur directly due to failure of red cell production because of the long life of the red cell. However, anemia may occur due to hemorrhage.

There appears to be significant antitumor activity of whole body radiation which exceeds that seen when the same dose is given to the tumor alone.[59,60] Very low doses of whole body radiation in man (10–15 rads, 2–3 times per week for 6–10 fractions) may be quite effective treatment for lymphomas and may cause marked depression of the formed blood elements. The mechanism of action of this type of treatment is not understood. The effects on both tumor and normal tissue are greater than one can explain by considering the typical survival curve.

ADVERSE EFFECTS OF RADIATION

There are some biologic considerations of localized radiation that may conceivably decrease the likelihood for tumor control. First and most discussed is the effect of radiation on the *immune response*. High dose, whole body radiation has a well-known and profound effect on the immune response. However, this generalized treatment is rarely used in clinical radiation therapy except as preparation for bone marrow transplantation.

Shortly after the discovery of roentgen rays whole body irradiation prior to antigen administration was found to suppress antibody production. Following whole body radiation there is a prompt fall in the lymphatic count. The lymphocytes appear to have two types of radiation response. About 80% die a prompt intermitotic death while some lymphocytes survive this radiation. When assayed on the basis of reproductive capacity by either exposure to mitogens after radiation or other functional endpoints, their radiation survival curves looked similar to hematopoietic cells with a D_o of about 70–80 rad and an N of about one.[61] Response depends on the classes of lymphocytes involved in the response, the extent of cell proliferation required, cell traffic, and the balance between inhibiting (suppressor) and stimulatory (helper) systems involved. In general, the following conclusions concerning the effect of radiation on the immune response can be made:[61]

1. B-lymphocytes are quite radiosensitive and undergo both interphase and mitotic death following irradiation
2. All functional T-cell subpopulations have sensitive precursor cells (suppressor T-cell precursors may undergo interphase death)
3. The homing potential of cells is affected by radiation
4. Resting cells are more sensitive to interphase death than the same cells when stimulated to divide before

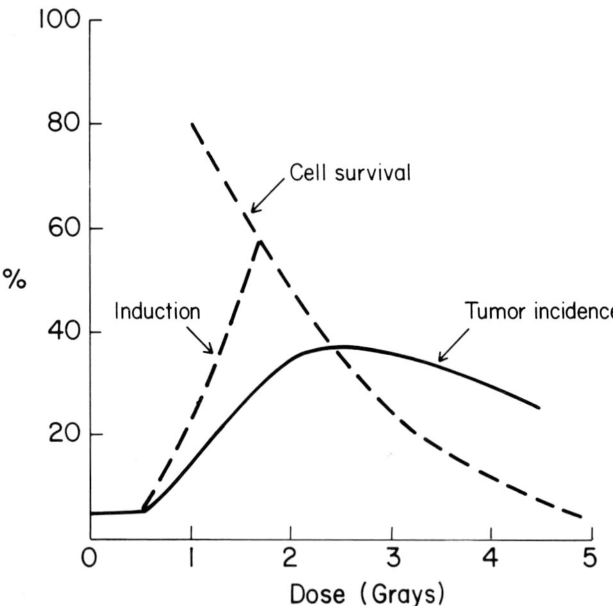

FIG. 7-21. Biphase curve of tumor incidence. (Redrawn from Gray LH: Radiation biology and cancer. In Cellular Radiation Biology, p. 7–25. M. D. Anderson Hospital and Tumor Institute 18th Symposium on Fundamental Cancer Research. Baltimore, Williams and Wilkins, 1975; and Upton AC, Randolph ML, Conklin JW: Late effects of fast neutrons and gamma rays in mice as influenced by the dose rate of irradiation: induction of neoplasia. Radiat Res 41:467–491, 1970)

irradiation (in the latter case they have an n and D_0 similar to hematopoietic stem cells)

5. The effects of whole body radiation are qualitatively and quantitatively different than those due to localized or regional radiation

Whole body radiation is more effective in preventing response to new antigens than in modifying response to an antigen to which the subject has been previously exposed. Survival of second set skin grafts are affected much less than the initial grafts. Localized radiation, as used in radiation therapy, affects the immune response by decreasing the number of circulating lymphocytes by presumably irradiating and destroying them as they pass through the irradiated volume. The consequences of this irradiation appear to be small if the tumor has been in place for a significant period of time before the irradiation and if the irradiated volume is relatively small. If the animal is irradiated at the time the tumor is implanted, then the immune response will be inhibited. However, this is rarely the clinical situation. There have been reports suggesting the deleterious effects on the immune response of localized radiation, but this does not appear to be the case in either the original series studied or in subsequent studies.[62–64] It is clear that localized radiation, despite producing a chronic lymphopenia of both T- and B-cells, does not affect the immune response to bacterial or viral agents since treated patients do not seem to be more susceptible. This is the case with the immune suppression produced by whole body radiation or systemic chemotherapy. Clearly, regional irradiation of the lymph nodes adjacent to tumors has been associated with increased curability in head and neck tumors without adverse effects.[65]

There may also be adverse effects of radiation on the patient other than those on host defense mechanisms. Radiation induced *mutagenesis* is of concern for both germ line as well as somatic cells. Obviously, if the gonads are not irradiated there is no increase in germ line mutations. If the gonads are irradiated then there is an increased likelihood of mutation with increasing doses without any evidence of threshold dose or of an ameliorating effect of fractionation. At higher doses, however, there is significant cell killing and the dose response curve is no longer linear, presumably because those cells mutated receive sufficient radiation to become sterile. Abnormal live births are surprisingly uncommon following gonadal irradiation. This is because most radiation-induced mutations are recessive. Further, dominant mutations, when they occur, are usually lethal. There is some evidence in the mouse that the risk of mutation decreases with time after ovarian irradiation. Whether this is true in humans, in addition to the mechanism by which it occurs in animals, is not known. This does not appear true for irradiation of the testes. The mutagenic effects of radiation are very dependent on the type of irradiation. The RBE for high LET radiation can be extremely high for mutations. It is very difficult to quantify the risk since the experiments on mice indicate a large difference in the mutation rate for different loci with a factor of as much as 1000-fold variation in the mutarate.[66] In general, the prudent figure used is that the mutation rate doubles for approximately every 50 rads.

Perhaps of even greater concern are somatic mutations, especially those that might lead to tumors. There is a great deal of evidence available that indicates that low doses of radiation increase tumor incidence after significant latent periods. This information comes largely from whole body exposures secondary to the atomic bomb and patients irradiated for a variety of benign diseases.[67-69] In general, there appears to be a linear increase in tumor incidence with dose until high doses are reached when the incidence plateaus or even falls.[70,71] Presumably, this is true again due to cell killing. Fig. 7-21 is an example of this biphasic dose response curve. Such tumor induction is associated with a latent period of three to five years of leukemia but is much longer for solid tumors. There are different ages at which tumor induction is most likely and ages when the organ at risk does not appear significantly at risk. For example, breast cancer induction by radiation appears primarily for exposure in the first and second decades of life and decreases with radiation later in life.[72] Except for irradiation of children, it is very difficult to demonstrate a significant increased incidence of tumors in patients receiving therapeutic radiation for malignant disease. This may be an example of the biphasic nature of the tumor induction curve. For example, long-term studies of patients with carcinoma of the cervix do not show increased incidence of pelvic cancer.[72,73] In contrast, when patients are irradiated to the same volume for benign diseases with much lower doses of radiation an increased tumor incidence can be seen.[68] Thus there appears to be a difference in tumorigenicity of doses of radiation used for benign disease, (between 200 and 1000 rads) than that seen when therapeutic doses of radiation are used.

Radiation is clearly a teratogen when a woman is exposed during the rapidly proliferating period of embryogenesis (somewhere between weeks 2 and 16).

CLINICAL CONSIDERATIONS

It is often suggested that the goal of treatment is the greatest probability of uncomplicated cure. While this is desirable, the circumstances may actually dictate a different policy. Consider Fig. 7-16 where the curve for complications is to the right of the sigmoid curve for tumor control. The ideal dose would be that dose that gives as many cures before the steep portion of the complication curve as shown by line A. This, however, may not be the optimal dose. It depends very much on the consequences of both tumor failure and the nature of the complications. If tumor failure can be salvaged by subsequent surgery but complications are severe, long-lived, and difficult to manage then line A is indeed the optimal line.[49] An example of this would be the treatment of T2 and T3 glottic cancer. On the other hand, if the complications are either not severe or remediable, but cancer failure is fatal then a line closer to line B would be appropriate. This is the case in Stages II and III carcinoma of the uterine cervix. Therefore, there is no simple answer. Often the worst complication of treatment is tumor recurrence.

There are many clinical examples of sigmoid dose response curves. An example for tumors of the head and neck is shown in Fig. 7-22 and for Hodgkin's disease in Fig. 7-23.[74,75] Even these are simple since they do not consider time-dose relations or tumor volume. A quite instructive clinical experience is described by Stewart and Jackson in which a consistent ~10% change in dose was used.[76] Fig 7-24 shows the results in both control and complications seen. The small dose increase markedly improved the curability of the larger tumors, presumably because this dose is on the steep portion of the sigmoid dose response curve. It did not change the cure of small tumors very much since, presumably, the dose was already large enough to be on the top of the dose response curve where changes in dose do not affect cure very much. Similarly, complications were not increased very much, presumably because the complication curve was to the right and still on the shallow portion of this curve. This is a good example of separation of response between tumor and normal tissues. It also shows displacement of the curve for cure as a function of tumor size.

FIG. 7-22. Tumor control versus dose for supraglottic carcinoma. (Shukovsky LJ: Dose, time, volume relationships in squamous cell carcinoma of the supraglottic larynx. Am J Roentgenol Rad Ther Nucl Med 108:27–29, 1970)

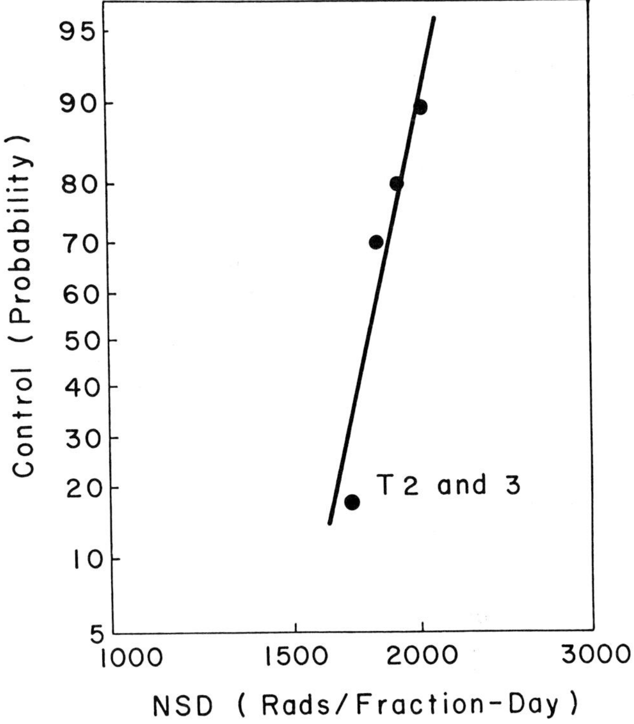

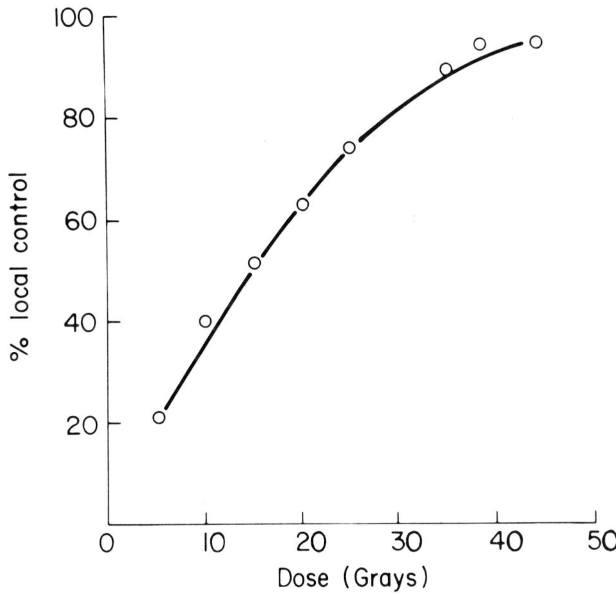

FIG. 7-23. Tumor control versus dose. (Kaplan HS: Evidence for a tumorcidal dose level in the radiotherapy of Hodgkin's disease. Cancer Res 26:1221–1224, 1966)

Early in this century, as the practice of radiation therapy evolved, the virtues of dividing the radiation into small fractions was noted. The reasons given were often incorrect but the clear observation was that such fractionation of the dose allowed more effective tumor cure without excessive complications. The fashioning of a plan for fractionated radiation therapy for carcinoma of the larynx by Coutard based on the principles of Regaud laid the basis for the development of radiation therapy.[77,78] The principles of such treatment were:

1. Fractionation is important
2. Relationship between the acute reaction of the skin and oropharyngeal mucosa to both cure and to late effects.

It was felt that one had to have complete epidermititis and mucositis with confluent reactions with primary healing from without in order to have a dose sufficient to cure the tumor. The fractionation schemes recommended resulted in tolerable late effects.

The association between acute and late effects has sometimes led radiotherapists astray. This relationship very much depends on the fractionation scheme, the energy of radiation used, in addition to other factors. In general, acute effects are

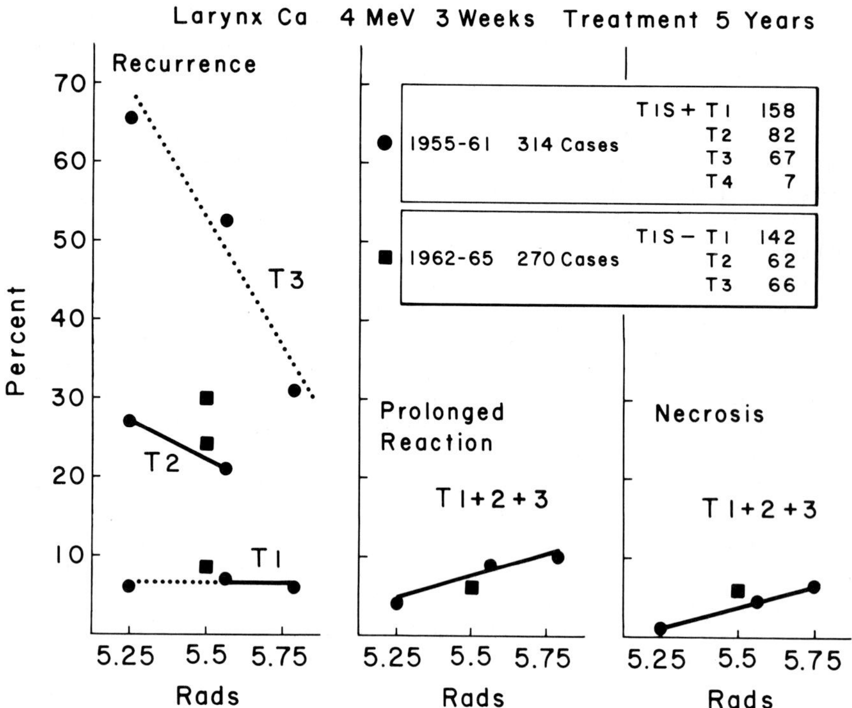

FIG. 7-24. Tumor control versus dose for cancer of the larynx. (From Stewart JG, Jackson AW: The steepness of the dose response curve both for tumor and normal tissue injury. Laryngoscope 85:1107–1111, 1975)

very dependent on the time factor while late effects are much less dependent on time. They are primarily influenced by total dose and fraction size.

Another important technique of radiation therapy that evolved in the early part of the century was the use of continuous radiation by interstitial or intracavitary application.[79] If the dose rate was too high or the volume too large then unacceptable complications occurred. Rules for treatment were developed resulting in the cure of certain tumors without unacceptable complications. These required that the dose rate be kept moderate (less than 100 rad/hour) and an attempt at a good implant geometry be made to avoid unnecessary hot spots and cold spots as much as possible. The whole question of homogeneity of dose is much more difficult in intracavitary and interstitial radiation than with external beam. To a great extent the clinical development of the use of radioactive isotopes, especially by the implantation techniques proceeded separately from that of external beam. There are those physicians who practiced only the latter, rarely, if ever, using the former and vice versa. In more recent years, both external beam and interstitial treatment have been used together to take advantage of the virtues of both treatment modalities. Some good examples of this combined treatment are described in the chapters dealing with tumors of the head, neck, uterine cervix.

ACUTE AND LATE NORMAL TISSUE EFFECTS

Acute radiation effects are largely on the cell renewal tissues—skin, oropharyngeal mucosa, small intestine, rectum, bladder mucosa, and vaginal mucosa. These cell renewal tissues are rapidly proliferating and as they are confronted with fractionated radiation, the processes of repair, repopulation, and recruitment all obtain. Some terms need definition here to add clarity to understanding of radiation treatment programs. *Fractionation* is the size and number of radiation increments. *Protraction* is the time over which the radiation is given. Since the effect on such rapid cell renewal tissues will be dependent on the balance between cell birth and cell death it will be crucially affected by the time allowed for repopulation, therefore very dependent on protraction. It will also be dependent on the cell kill per fraction. Therefore, fraction size will be important. The radiotherapist frequently observing the oral mucosa and seeing an excessive reaction knows that a small decrease in fraction size or a small treatment break may allow rapid resolution of the problem since these changes will permit reconstitution of the normal tissue.

Late effects are really the dose-limiting effect in radiation therapy. These include necrosis, fibrosis, fistula formation, non-healing ulceration, and damage to specific organs, such as spinal cord transection, blindness, etc. While the mechanisms of these phenomena are not clear they do not appear to primarily depend upon the rapid proliferation of a cell renewal tissue. Clinically they appear much less dependent upon protraction and much more dependent upon the total dose of radiation and the size of the radiation fraction. Thus, only if the same fractionation scheme is used with the same normal tissue endpoint, the same volume irradiated and the same treatment technique can acute and late effects be correlated. If any of these parameters are varied the acute reactions to radiation may be dissociated from eventual late effects. Rather than serve as a guide, these acute reactions will be misleading. There are a number of examples in radiation therapy where the total dose has been increased, the fraction size increased or kept the same, but the time has been protracted to minimize acute effects. Such techniques have resulted in unacceptable late complications.

Two hypotheses for late effects are worth some discussion. One theory holds that all late effects are due to damage to vasculo–connective tissue stroma. Since this is common throughout the body this would employ a common mechanism for the late effects in any organ.[56] A variation on this hypothesis is that it is damage to the endothelial cells, ubiquitous throughout the body, that determines late effects.[58] An alternate hypothesis suggests that both the acute and the late effects of radiation and cytotoxic chemotherapy are due to cell depletion of the major target cell renewal tissues. Acute effects depend on the balance between cell killing and compensatory cellular replication of both the stem and proliferative compartments. The development of late effects requires that stem cells have only a limited proliferative capacity.[80,81] Compensation for extensive or repeated cell killing may exhaust this capacity, resulting in eventual tissue failure.

Altering the Therapeutic Index

Goodman and Gilman define the therapeutic index as the relationship between desired and undesired effects of therapy.[82] Clearly for the oncologist, separation of the sigmoid curve of complications from that of local control (see Fig. 7-16) is the graphic representation of the manipulation of the therapeutic index. Some techniques of time-dose relationships used by the radiotherapist to take advantage of this are: fractionation, protraction, split course technique, the use of interstitial treatment, and manipulation of the target volume. Though fractionation has been discussed, use of multiple small fractions two, three, or more times a day has been described as *hyperfractionation* and is just beginning to be explored with some good results. The experiments that stimulated the recent interest administered two fractions of radiation separated by six hours, and this was compared to a single fraction as the method of giving daily radiation. The six hours is felt to be sufficiently long enough to allow complete sublethal damage repair and not long enough for significant proliferation. Since both are daily treatments this should allow separation of repair from repopulation and recruitment. The general results of the experiments were presented as the recovered radiation, that being the dose difference seen when giving the radiation as two divided doses separated by six hours, as compared to giving it in one fraction. When the single fraction was 200 rads or less there was little recovered dose. This recovered dose increased rapidly between 200 and 800 rads; then, with very large fractions the recovered dose tended to level off. Clinically this means when dividing the usually used radiation sizes of about 200 rads into two smaller fractions only little more should be given as a recovered dose is small. This has been confirmed in a number of clinics.[84] The use of this "hyperfractionation" is being tried for a number of tumors; however, it is too early to determine whether this will be useful.

In general, most radiotherapists administer the conventional radiation in fractions of between 180 and 250 rads a day. This is consistent with tumor control without excessive acute or late effects. The fraction size tolerated in terms of acute effects is dependent on the volume irradiated (the larger the volume the smaller the fraction size), the amount and type of dose-limiting normal tissue, the age of the patient, and other clinical factors. Small changes in fraction size will make a big difference in tolerance. Patients are often given small breaks during the treatment. Those rest periods most regularly used are those caused by the weekend interruptions of daily fractionation. This protraction of the treatment allows for repopulation and recruitment. These days of rest also allow amelioration of many acute effects. They may also allow time for tumor regression resulting in reoxygenation. An attempt to formalize and extend treatment breaks is the so-called *split course technique*.[85,86,87] Two to three weeks are allowed in the middle of treatment for recovery of the acute effects as well as to permit tumor regression. When the dose of radiation is not increased there is some evidence that this treatment (while it is clearly better tolerated) may be associated with less tumor control.[88] When the split course is administered with an increase in total dose the results seem to be comparable to conventional fractionation but perhaps with greater late effects.

Interstitial radiation, as used in radium needle implants, gold and radon seed implants, iridium wire implants, and a variety of other techniques of either permanently or temporary placing radioactive material into tissues, require both biological and physical considerations. Clearly there is great inhomogeneity in even the most geometrically perfect implant (this has been discussed earlier in the physics section). Not only is there large inhomogeneity of dose but similar variation in dose rate; the dose rate of radiation being greater in those areas of high dose. In general, with temporary implants attempts at administering a calculated dose of between 30 and 100 rads per hour to the minimum tumor location are made. This is impossible with permanent implants since isotopes decrease their radiation intensity as they decay. The most commonly used of these isotopes are radon and ^{198}Au. More recently, ^{125}I has been used creating unusual new problems. The half life of ^{125}I is quite long (60 days), resulting in a significant amount of the dose given quite slowly, so long that there may be significant cell division occurring in both the tumor and some normal cells. Therefore, the important dose may not be the total dose, but rather, the dose per cell cycle, different for each cell type and different as the isotope decays. Secondly, ^{125}I irradiates primarily by the emission of very low energy photons, some of which are absorbed by the seeds themselves leading to even further inhomogeneity.[88]

Generally, when implants can be done alone or in a combination with external irradiation the results tend to be better in terms of the therapeutic index than with external beam alone. The high local dose, continuous radiation, and even inhomogeneity allowing normal tissue regrowth all may contribute to better cosmetic and functional results along with tumor cure. Examples of these are tumors of the tongue and other head and neck sites.[90]

Tumor volume is also quite important to consider in clinical radiotherapy. While the gross tumor extent can be determined, most clinicians recognize that a characteristic of tumors is to

TABLE 7-6. Control (%) of Subclinical Disease[65]

DOSE (GRAY)	ADENOCARCINOMA OF THE BREAST	CARCINOMA OF UPPER AERO-DIGESTIVE TRACT
30–35	60–70%	60–70%
40	80–90%	>90%
50	>90%	>90%

(Fletcher GH: Clinical dose-response curves of human malignant epithelial tumours. Br J Radiol 46:1–12, 1973)

extend far beyond those macroscopically identifiable borders. Determination of the target volume must include this consideration but the larger the volume required to irradiate, the smaller the dose that is tolerated. Conversely, the larger the volume of tumor the more dose is required. This dilemma limited the success of early radiotherapy of certain tumors by either reducing the target volume, resulting in recurrences at the treatment margins or in significant complications in the treatment of large target volumes. Today distinctions are made between gross tumor and the subclinical extensions into apparently normal tissues. Subclinical disease means small numbers of cells, perhaps in physiologic circumstances favorable to irradiation (well-oxygenated), which can be controlled with modest doses of radiation (see Table 7-6). The large number of cells present in the clinically evidenced tumor requires higher doses, as noted in the sigmoid curves shown in Fig. 7-22 and 7-23. This difference has led to a variety of techniques developed to administer different doses to microscopic tumor extensions as compared to the gross tumor. These include shrinking field techniques, boost treatments, and certain of the strategies of combined surgery and radiotherapy to be described later in this chapter.

Shrinking field technique simply means giving the largest potential tumor bed a moderate dose of radiation, then reducing the target volume to the tumor and its immediate confines, raising the dose. This can be done by simply reducing the fields by changing the treatment technique and target volume, or by using a treatment technique that gives, at the same time, the desired moderate dose to the larger volume and a higher dose to the smaller volume. It can also be done by combining the moderate dose external beam radiation with an interstitial implant to a smaller volume. A modification of this is the *boost technique* where maximum tolerated dose is given to a volume and then very localized radiation is used to raise the dose to the tumor bed. An implant or an electron boost can be used for this technique. A number of attempts have been made to consider fractionation, protraction, and even implantation with external beam in some form of some mathematical formulae. All of these tend to even simplify more complex clinical circumstances and can be very misleading.

The normal tissues that limit the dose of radiation given may be so closely applied to the tumor that any target volume which includes a tumor must include these normal tissues. These are to be distinguished from those normal tissues transited by the radiation but not in the target volume. Both may contribute to the production of complications and thus be dose limiting. Fig. 7-25 shows the difference between the target volume and transit volume. Radiotherapy with detailed treatment planning, CT scanning, and a variety of techniques (perhaps the ultimate of which is computer controlled radiation therapy) may reduce the dose to the transit volume, possibly changing the therapeutic index.[90] However, it is unlikely that there will be significant physical techniques of reducing the dose to the normal tissues in the target volume. This can only be done by some biologic mechanism that distinguishes tumor from normal tissues.

RADIOSENSITIVITY

The term radiosensitivity is used in a number of different ways in the literature and can mean what we define as *radiosensitivity*, *radioresponsiveness*, or *radiocurability*. Each are somewhat different concepts. *Radiosensitivity* means the innate sensitivity of the cells to radiation. For cells that die a reproductive death it is related to the slope of the survival curve or the D^o. *Radioresponsiveness* means the clinical appearance of tumor regression promptly following moderate doses of radiation. This may be a function of the cell's radiosensitivity but it also may be a function of the active cell kinetics of a tumor. Bergonie and Tribondeau first established an association between the rate of proliferation and the response of normal tissues although they considered this equal with radiosensitivity.[91] A similar relationship was presumed to apply to tumors. Since cells will not die until they face mitosis, some tumors that rapidly proliferate will regress rapidly but also regrow rapidly. This is frequently confused with radiosensitivity. An excellent example of this is the adenoidcystic tumor of the salivary gland or cylindroma. Such tumors are quite radioresponsive; however, they require very large doses to be cured.

Radiocurability means that the tumor–normal tissue relationships are such that curative doses of radiation can be regularly applied without excessive damage to the normal tissues. Such radiocurable tumors are carcinomas of the cervix, larynx, breast, prostate, in addition to Hodgkin's disease, seminomas, etc. Some of these are quite radioresponsive, some are radiosensitive, some are neither.

COMBINATIONS OF RADIATION AND SURGERY

Radiation and surgery can be combined in many different ways. The general rationale for combining surgery and radiation is that the mechanism of failure for the two techniques is quite different. Radiation rarely fails at the periphery of tumors where cells are small in number and well-vascularized. When radiation fails it usually does so in the center of the tumor where there are large volumes of tumor cells often under hypoxic conditions. Surgery, in contrast, is often limited by the required preservation of vital normal tissues adjacent to the tumor. In resectable cancers the gross tumor can be removed but it is these vital normal tissues that limit the anatomic extent of the dissection. When surgery fails under these circumstances it is usually because microscopic tumor cells are left behind because of these limitations. Thus, the mechanism of tumor recurrence may be quite different for surgery as compared to radiation therapy. It seems logical, therefore, to consider combining the two techniques. Radia-

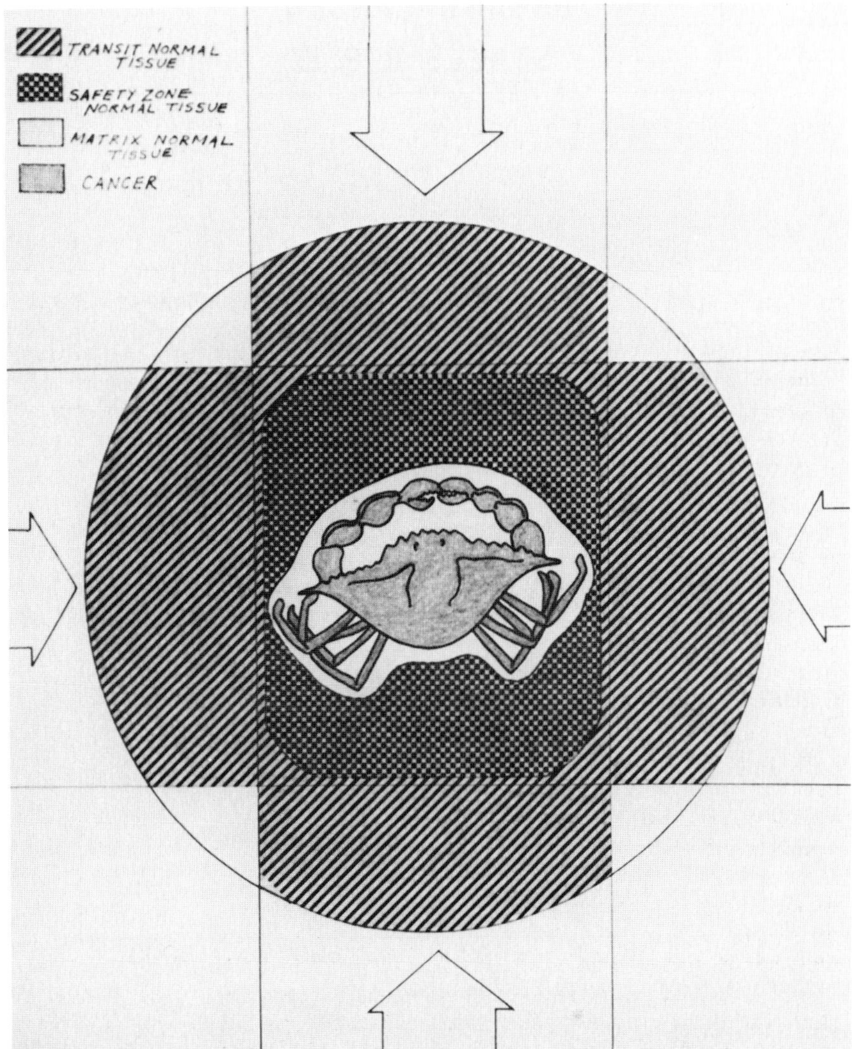

FIG. 7-25. Schematic representation of normal tissues in radiotherapy planning. (Kramer S: The biomedical problem in radiation therapy. In Particle Accelerators in Radiation Therapy, pp 6–10. Los Alamos, Los Alamos Scientific Laboratory, LA 5180–C, 1973)

tion can be given before or after surgery. Preoperative radiation has the advantages of sterilizing cells at the edges of the resection, sterilizing cells that would perhaps be dislodged and seeded at the time of surgery, and in the special circumstance of unresectable tumors, reducing the tumor volume sufficiently to allow resection. It is not clear how often this really ends up effecting a cure as it may only change gross tumor to microscopic tumor and still result in tumor recurrence. It does seem to be of benefit in certain selected cases of large unresectable cancers.[92]

There are disadvantages in the use of preoperative irradiation. The pathology reports are not evaluable since if sufficent time is allowed between the radiation and the surgery, by causing much tumor destruction the preoperative radiation will prevent ascertainment of the initial anatomic tumor extent. In contrast, if the tumor is slow-growing or if the surgery is done shortly after the radiation, the radiation consequences will not be represented in the pathologic evaluation of the material since sufficient time was not allowed for tumor destruction and regression. Another disadvantage is that the patient is irradiated before the careful staging available at surgical exploration and so some patients who would not benefit from the preoperative radiation are given this treatment (*e.g.,* preoperative radiation to a colorectal carcinoma in a patient with occult liver metastases). These metastases may be found only at the time of surgery. If recognized previously, the preoperative radiation would not have been given. Another disadvantage often quoted is the delay before surgical resection. This may not be a disadvantage since as long as the patient is having treatment to the tumor the order of treatments should make no difference. The radiation dose is usually moderate (4,000–5,000 rads) in conventional 200 rad fractions five days a week, or smaller total doses given more quickly in larger fractions. If the total dose of radiation is kept quite small (2000 rad or less) then there need not be much delay between radiation and surgery.

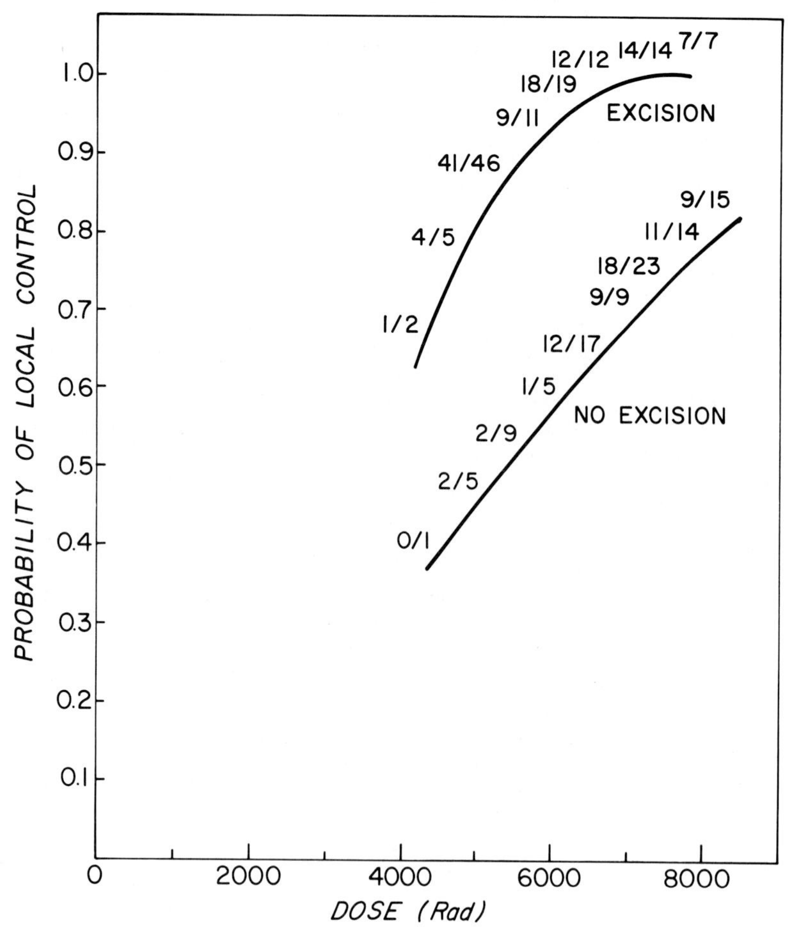

FIG. 7-26. Tumor control versus dose for breast cancer. (Hellman S: Improving the therapeutic index in breast cancer treatment. Cancer Res 40:4335–4342, 1980)

When the dose reaches approximately 4000 rads, some delay to allow the tissues to recover from the radiation is of value (usually 4–6 weeks). If the total dose is greater than 5000 rads, then the surgery will often be more difficult. However, with moderate doses of radiation and some time allowed between radiation and surgery the resection can proceed without undue difficulty. The use of smaller doses of radiation over very short periods of time without delay allows many advantages and is becoming the preferred treatment technique. With this technique the pathology is less destorted, tumor reduction does not occur significantly, and the surgeon is not lulled into doing too small an operation. If the major value of the preoperative radiation is to prevent seeding then large doses of radiation are not necessary. For example, preoperative use of intrauterine radium before the surgical treatment of carcinoma of the endometrium is an effective way of preventing seeding. This can be done immediately before surgery.

Postoperative radiation has a number of advantages as well. The subgroup of patients who might be helped by radiation can be very accurately defined as a consequence of the surgical exploration and pathologic review. Unnecessary irradiation to patients not likely to benefit can be avoided and the target volumes can be tailored based on what is found at surgery. Time can be allowed for wound healing so that the radiation will not interfere with this process. A disadvantage of such treatment is that it has no effect on seeding at the time of surgery when the seeded cells extend outside the target volume. It may also alter the physiology of the tumor left behind because of reduction of the vascular supply. Cells which were well-oxygenated (had they been irradiated before surgery) may be rendered physiologically hypoxic and thus more resistant to radiation. Another disadvantage in the peritoneal cavity is that the surgery will cause loops of bowel to be fixed in specific positions and thus will increase the likelihood of small intestinal damage by radiation.

In general, there is some uncertainty as to which technique is better under which clinical circumstance. Both preoperative and postoperative radiation appear to have value and the choice of the method, the dose of radiation, and the time between radiation and surgery should be considered in terms of the goals planned.

An additional technique in combining surgery with radiation that deserves some specific discussion is the limited surgical removal of the gross tumor. Since it is this gross tumor that limits the radiotherapeutic treatment new interest has been raised in using surgery as the "boost" technique. Full courses of radiation are given combined with tumorectomy. This surgery can be done either before or after the irradiation. An example of this is the "lumpectomy" used in the treatment of breast masses before definitive radiation (see chapter 27).[93,94] In the latter there appears to be evidence that the gross tumor removal both displaces the sigmoid curve of cure to lower radiation doses and makes it change more steeply with dose (see Fig. 7-26).

CLINICAL COMBINATIONS OF RADIATION AND CHEMOTHERAPY

The principles of combination radiation and chemotherapy were discussed earlier and emphasized that the purpose of such combined treatment is not to decrease the dose of radiation to gain the same effect, but rather to increase the therapeutic index. This may be achieved by a number of techniques that take advantage of the different mechanisms of action of systemic chemotherapy and regional irradiation. Chemotherapeutic agents may be used, which directly modify the radiation survival curve. Perhaps a good example of this is the use of actinomycin D in the treatment of childhood rhabdomyosarcoma or Wilm's tumor. A second way to increase the therapeutic index is by using drugs that specifically affect tumor response to radiation; the most exciting of these are the hypoxic sensitizers, since these affect hypoxic cells that are usually restricted to tumors. A third mechanism is the combination of drugs and roentgen ray with either independent action or additivity (but which do not have overlapping toxicity with radiation). This is just beginning to be explored but appears to be of value in the increased local control seen in recent studies of head and neck cancer when chemotherapy is given before radiation.[97] It is also seen in the enhanced local control when radiotherapy is followed or administered concomitantly with adjuvant chemotherapy in locally advanced breast cancer.[98] Finally, since the major advantage of chemotherapy is that it is distributed widely throughout the body the combination of radiation and chemotherapy may improve the therapeutic index because, like the combination of surgery and irradiation, the target volumes are different. Adjuvant chemotherapy with radiation for breast cancer or with surgery and radiation for colon cancer may improve survival because the chemotherapy is effective on occult micro-metastases outside the radiation field. Similarly, radiation may be of value in the treatment of leukemia by chemotherapy since the radiation can be applied to specific sanctuary sites, such as the central nervous system. (This is discussed further in Chapter 34 on pediatric tumors.)

REFERENCES

1. Johns HE, Cunningham JR: The Physics of Radiology. Springfield, ILL, Charles C Thomas, 1977
2. Thompson LH, Suit HD: Proliferation kinetics of x-irradiated mouse L cells studied with timelapse photography-II. Int J Radiat Biol 15: 347–362, 1969
3. Weichselbaum RR, Nove J, Little JB: X-ray sensitivity of human tumor cells *in vitro*. Int J Radiat Onc Biol Phys 6:437–440, 1980
4. Till JE, McCulloch EA: A direct measurement of the radiation sensitivity of normal mouse bone marrow cells. Radiat Res 14:213–222, 1961
5. Withers HR, Elkind MM: Microcolony survival assay for cells of mouse intestinal mucosa exposed to radiation. Int J Radiat Biol 17:261–267, 1970
6. Alper T, Gillies NE: Restoration of *Escherichia coli* Strain B irradiation: its dependence on suboptimal growth conditions. J Gen Microbiol 18:461–472, 1958
7. Phillips RA, Tolmach LJ: Repair of potentially lethal damage in x-irradiated HeLa cells. Radiat Res 29:413–432, 1966
8. Little JB, Hahn GM, Frindel E et al: Repair of potentially lethal radiation damage *in vitro* and *in vivo*. Radiology, 106:689–694, 1973
9. Belli JA, Shelton M: Potentially lethal radiation damage: repair of mammalian cells in culture. Science 165:490–492, 1969
10. Weichselbaum R, Little JB, Nove J: Response of human osteosarcoma *in vitro* to irradiation: evidence for unusual cellular repair activity. Int J Radiat Biol 31:295–299, 1977
11. Elkind MM, Sutton H: Radiation response of mammalian cells grown in culture. 1. Repair of x-ray damage in surviving Chinese hamster cells. Radiat Res 13:556–593,1960
12. Hall EJ: Radiation dose–rate: a factor of importance in radiobiology and radiotherapy. Br J Radiol 45:81–97, 1972
13. Mottram JC: Factors of importance in radiosensitivity of tumors. Br J Radiol 9:606–614, 1936
14. Read J: The effect of ionizing radiation on the broad beam root: the dependence of the x-ray sensitivity on dissolved oxygen. Br J Radiol 25:89–99, 1952
15. Gray LH, Coger AD, Ebert M et al: The concentration of oxygen dissolved in tissues at the time of irradiation as a factor in radiotherapy. Br J Radiol 26:638–648, 1953
16. Belli JA, Dicus GJ, Bonte FJ: Radiation response of mammalian tumor cells. 1. Repair of sublethal damage *in vivo*. JNCI 38:673–682, 1967
17. Deschner EE, Gray LH: Influence of oxygen tension on x-ray induced chromosomal damage in Ehrlich ascites tumor cells irradiated *in vitro* and *in vivo*. Radiat Res 11:115–146, 1959
18. Thomlinson RH, Gray LH: The histological structure of some human lung cancers and possible implications for radiotherapy. Br J Cancer 9:539–549, 1955
19. Kallman RF: The phenomenon of reoxygenation and its implications for fractionated radiotherapy. Radiology 105:135–142, 1972
20. Henk JM, Kindler PB, Smith CW: Radiotherapy and head and neck cancer: final report of the first clinical trial. Lancet 2:101–103, 1977
21. Henk J, Smith CW: Radiotherapy and head and neck cancer: interim report of second clinical trial. Lancet 2:104–105, 1977
22. Watson ER, Halman KE, Dische S et al: Hyperbaric oxygen and radiotherapy: A Medical Research Council trial in carcinoma of the cervix. Br J Radiol 51:879–887, 1978
23. Adams GE, Dewez DL: Hydrated electrons and radiobiological sensitization. Biochem Biophys Res Common 12:473–477, 1963
24. Adams GE, Ahmed L, Fielden EM et al: The development of some mitromidazoles as hypoxic cell sensitizers. Cancer Clin Trials 3:37–42, 1980
25. Stratford LJ, Adams GE: Effect of hyperthermia on differential cytotoxicity of a hypoxic cell radiosensitizer RO–07–0582 on mammalian cells *in vitro*. Br J Cancer 35:307–313, 1977
26. Rose CM, Millar JL, Peacock JH et al: Differential enhancement of toxicity in tumors and normal tissues by misonidizole. Proceedings of the Key Biscayne Conference on Hypoxic Cell Sensitizers and Radioprotectors. New York, Masson, 1980
27. Bush RS, Jenkin RP, Allt WE et al: Definitive evidence for hypoxic cells influencing cure in cancer therapy. Br J Cancer 37:302–306, 1978
28. Terasima R, Tolmach LJ: X-ray sensitivity and DNA synthesis in synchronous populations of HeLa cells. Science 140:490–492, 1963
29. Sinclair WK, Morton RA: X-ray sensitivity during the cell generation cycle of cultured Chinese hamster cells. Radiat Res 29:450–474, 1966
30. Chaffey JT, Hellman S: Differing responses to radiation of murine

bone marrow stem cells in relation to the cell cycle. Cancer Res 31:1613–1615, 1971

31. Madoc-Jones H, Mauro F: Age responses to x-rays vinca alkaloids and hydroxyurea of murine lymphoma cells synchronized *in vivo*. JNCI 45:1131–1143, 1970
32. Hellman S: Cell kinetics, models and cancer treatment: some principles for the radiation oncologist. Radiology 114:219–223, 1975
33. Chaffey JT, Hellman S: Radiation fractionation as applied to murine colony-forming units in differing proliferative states. Radiology 93:1167–1172, 1969
34. Chaffey JT, Hellman S: Studies on dose fractionation as measured by endogenous spleen colonies in the mouse. Radiology 90:363–365, 1968
35. Hermens AF, Barendson GW: Changes in cell proliferation characteristics in a rat rhabdomyosarcoma before and after x-irradiation. Eur J Cancer 5:173–189, 1969
36. Szybalski W: X-ray sensitization by halopyrimidines. Cancer Chemother Rep 58:539–557, 1974
37. Piro AJ, Taylor CC, Belli JA: Interaction between radiation and drug damage in mammalian cells. 1. Delayed expression of actinomycin D/x-ray effects in exponential and plateau phase cells. Radiat Res 63:346–362, 1975
38. D'Angio GJ, Farber S, Maddock CL: Potentiation of x-ray effects by actinomycin D. Radiology 73:175–177, 1959
39. Bases RE: Modification of the radiation response determined by single-cell techniques: actinomycin D. Cancer Res 19:1223–1229, 1959
40. Elkind MM, Whitmore GF, Alescio T: Actinomycin D: Suppression of recovery in x-irradiated mammalian cells. Science 143:1454–1456, 1964
41. Pinkel D: Actinomycin D in childhood cancer: a preliminary report. Pediatrics 23:342–347, 1959
42. Hellman S, Hannon E: Effects of Adriamycin on the radiation response of murine hematopoietic stem cells. Radiat Res 67:162–167, 1976
43. Belli JA, Piro AJ: The interaction between radiation and adriamycin damage in mammalian cells. Canc Res 37:1624–1630, 1977
44. Cassady JR, Richter MP, Piro AJ et al: Radiation–adriamycin interactions: Preliminary clinical observations. Cancer 36:946–949, 1975
45. Donaldson SC, Glick JM, Wilbur JR: Adriamycin activating a recall phenomenon after radiation therapy. Ann Intern Med 81:407–408, 1974
46. Sinclair WK: Hydroxyurea: effects on Chinese hamster cells grown in culture. Cancer Res 27:297–308, 1967
47. Yuhas JM, Yurconic M, Kligerman MM et al: Combined use of radioprotective and radiosensitizing drugs in experimental radiotherapy. Radiat Res 70:433–443, 1977
48. Barendsen GW: Response of cultured cells, tumours, and normal tissues to radiations of different linear energy transfer. Curr Top Radiat Res 4:293–356, 1968
49. Bloomer WD, Hellman S: Normal tissue responses to radiation therapy. N Engl J Med 293:80–83, 1975
50. Holthusen H: Erfahrungen uber die Vertaglichkeitsgrenze fur Rontgenstrahler und deren Nutzanwendung zur Verhutung von Schaden. Strahlentherapie 57:254–269, 1936
51. Suit HD, Goitein M: Rationale for use of charged particle and fast neutron beams in radiation therapy. Radiation Biology in Cancer Research. Meyn RE, Withers HR (eds). New York, Raven Press, 1980
52. Thomlinson RH: An experimental method for comparing treatments of intact tumors in animals and its application to the use of oxygen in radiotherapy. Brit J Can 14:555–576, 1960
53. Folkman J, Tyler K: Tumor angiogenesis: its possible role in metastasis and invasion. In Day B, Myers WP, Stans Garattini S et al (eds): Cancer Invasion and Metastasis: Mechanisms and Therapy, pp 95–103. Vol. 5 in Progress in Cancer Research and Therapy. New York, Raven Press, 1977
54. Folkman J: Tumor angiogensis: a possible control point in tumor growth. Ann Intern Med 82:96–100, 1975
55. Powers WE, Tolmach LV: A multicomponent x-ray survival curve for mouse lymphosarcoma cells irradiated *in vitro*. Nature 197:710–711, 1963
56. Rubin P, Casarett GW: Clinical Radiation Pathology. Philadelphia, WB Saunders, 1968
57. Filler RM, Tefft M, Vawter GF et al: Hepatic lobectomy in childhood: effects of x-ray and chemotherapy. J Pediatr Surg 4:31–41, 1969
58. Reinhold HS, Buisman GH: Radiosensitivity of capillary endothelium. Br J Radiol 46:54–57, 1973
59. Medinger FG, Craver LF: Total body irradiation. Am J Roentgenol Radium Ther Nucl Med 48:651–671, 1942
60. Hellman S, Chaffey JT, Rosenthal DS et al: Place of radiation therapy in the treatment of non-Hodgkin's lymphomas. Cancer 39:843–851, 1977
61. Anderson RE, Warner NL: Ionizing radiation and the immune response. Adv Immunol 24:215–335, 1976
62. Stjernsward J: Decreased survival related to irradiation postoperatively in early operable breast cancer. Lancet ii: 11:1285–1286, 1974
63. Levitt SH, McHugh RB: Early breast cancer and postoperative irradiation. Lancet 2:1258–1259, 1975
64. Cancer Research Campaign (Kings/Cambridge) Trial for Early Breast Cancer. Lancet 2:55–60, 1980
65. Fletcher GH: Clinical dose-response curves of human malignant epithelial tumours. Br J Radiol 46:1–12, 1973
66. Kohn HI,Melvold RW: Divergent x-ray induced mutation rates in the mouse for Hand "7 locus" groups of loci. Nature 259:209–210, 1976
67. Folley JH, Borges W, Yamawaki T: Incidence of leukemia in survivors of the atomic bomb in Hiroshima and Nagasaki, Japan. Am J Med 13:311–321, 1952
68. Smith PG, Doll R: Late effects of x-irradiation in patients healed for metropathia hemorrhagica. Br J Radiol 49:224–232, 1976
69. Court Brown WM, Doll R: Mortality from cancer and other causes after radiotherapy for ankylosing spondylitis. Br Med J z: 1327–1332, 1965
70. Gray LH: Radiation biology and cancer. *In* Cellular Radiation Biology p 7–25 M.D. Anderson Hospital and Tumor Institute 18th Symposium on Fundamental Cancer Research. Baltimore, Williams and Wilkins, 1965
71. Upton AC, Randolph ML, Conklin JW: Late effects of fast neutrons and gamma rays in mice as influenced by the dose rate of irradiation: induction of neoplasia. Radiat Res 41:467–491, 1970
72. Boice JD, Hutchinson GB: Leukemia in women following radiotherapy for cervical cancer: ten year follow up of an international study. JNCI 65:115–129, 1980
73. Zippen C, Bailar JC III, Kohn HI et al: Radiation therapy and cervical cancer: late effects on life span and leukemia incidence. Cancer 28:937–942, 1971
74. Shukovsky LJ: Dose, time, volume relationships in squamous cell carcinoma of the supraglottic larynx. Am J Roentgenol Radium Ther Nucl Med 108:27–29, 1970
75. Kaplan HS: Evidence for a tumorcidal dose level in the radiotherapy of Hodgkin's disease. Cancer Res 26:1221–1224, 1966
76. Stewart JG, Jackson AW: The steepness of the dose response curve for tumor and normal tissue injury. Laryngoscope 85:1107–1111, 1975
77. Coutard H: Roentgen therapy of epitheliomas of the tonsillar region, hypopharynx and larynx from 1920 to 1926. Am J Roentgenol 28:313–331, 1932.
78. Regaud C, Ferroux R: Discordance des effets des rayons X, d'une part dans la peau, d'autre part dans le testicule par le fractionement de la dose: diminution de l'efficacite dans le peau, maintien de l'efficacite dans le testicule. Compt Rend Soc Biol 97:431–434, 15 July, 1927
79. Finzi NS: Inoperable recurrent carcinoma of the breast under treatment by radium. Proc R Soc Med 2: clin sec 226–227, 1909
80. Botnick L, Hannon EC, Hellman S: Multisystem stem cell failure after apparent recovery from alkylating agents. Canc Res 38:1942–1947, 1978

81. Hellman S, Botnick LE: Stem cell depletion: an explanation of the late effects of cytotoxins. Int J Radiat Oncol Biol Phys z: 181–184, 1977
82. Goodman LS, Gilman A: The Pharmacological Basis of Therapeutics, p 21. London, Macmillan, 1970
83. Dutreix J,Wambersie A, Bounik C: Cellular recovery in human skin reactions: application to dose, fraction number, overall time relationship in radiotherapy. Eur J Cancer 9:159–167, 1973
84. Marks RD, Witherspoon BJ, Davis LW et al: Hyperfractionation—where do we stand: a preliminary report. Int J Radiat Oncol Biol Phys 4(suppl): 139–140, 1978
85. Scanlon P: Split-dose radiotherapy: the original premise. Int J Radiat Oncol Biol Phys 6:527–528, 1980
86. Sambrook DK: Split-course radiation therapy in malignant tumors. Am J Roentgenol 91:37–45, 1964
87. Parson JT, Thar TL, Bova FJ et al: An Evaluation of split-course irradiation for pelvic malignancies. Int J Radiat Oncol Biol Phys 6:175–181, 1980
88. Parsons JT, Bova FJ, Million RR: A re-evaluation of the University of Florida split-course technique for squamous carcinoma of the head and neck. Int J Radiat Oncol Biol Phys (in press) 6:1645–1652, 1980
89. Ling CC, Anderson LL, Shipley WU: Dose in homogeneity in interstitial implants using ^{125}I seeds. Int J Radiat Oncol Biol Phys 5:419–425, 1979
90. Kramer S: The biomedical problem in radiation therapy. In Particle Accelerators in Radiation Therapy, pp 6–10. Los Alamos, Los Alamos Scientific Laboratory, LA 5180-C, 1973
91. Pierquin B, Chassagne D, Baillet F et al: Clinical observations on the time factor in interstitital radiotherapy using Iridium-192. Clin Radiol 24:506–509, 1973
92. Levene MB, Kijewski PK, Chin LM et al: Computer controlled radiation therapy. Radiology 129:769–775, 1978
93. Bergonie J, Tribondeau L: Interpretation of some results of radiotherapy and an attempt at determining a logical technique of treatment. Radiat Res 11:587–588, 1959
94. Kligerman MM: Radiotherapy and rectal cancer. Cancer 39:896–900, 1977
95. Hellman S, Harris JR, Levene MB: Radiation therapy of early carcinoma of the breast without mastectomy. Cancer 46:988–994, 1980
96. Hellman S: Improving the therapeutic index in breast cancer treatment. Cancer Res 40:4335–4342, 1980
97. Miller D, Ervin T: Improved survival for patients with advanced carcinoma of the head and neck treated with methotrexate-leukovorin prior to definitive radiotherapy or surgery. Proc Am Assoc Cancer Res 21:562, 1980
98. Bruckman JE, Harris JR, Levene MB et al: Results of treating Stage III carcinoma of the breast by primary radiation therapy. Cancer 43:985–993, 1979

CHAPTER 8

Vincent T. DeVita, Jr.

Principles of Chemotherapy

CHEMOTHERAPY OF INFECTIOUS DISEASES AND CANCER

HISTORICAL PERSPECTIVES

The chemotherapy of cancer is the treatment of metastases. Current data support a clonal origin of most cancers since most tumors arise from a single cell as a result of a spontaneous mutation, or after exposure to an oncogenic virus or chemical carcinogen, and expand to the detectable level while continually shedding viable cells.[1,2] The ability to cure the cancer then depends on numerous variables, the most important being the presence of viable metastases. The need for chemotherapy arose out of the appreciation that cancer is uncommonly a localized process, not amenable to control by purely local means.

The idea that chemicals might be useful in treating cancer received great impetus from the successful use of synthetic chemicals and natural products used to cure parasitic, common bacterial infections and tuberculosis in rodents and man. In each case, the possible success of drug therapy was greeted with great pessimism, but none more so than the possibility that chemotherapy could cure cancer.

At the turn of the 20th century, Paul Erhlich, an optimist by all other accounts and considered the father of chemotherapy, was paid to work on the problem of cancer. This time he was not at all optimistic about the possible outcome. The part of the laboratory at that time that was devoted to cancer research is reported to have had a sign over it stating "Abandon all hope all ye who enter here."[3] In 1898, Erhlich discovered the first alkylating agent and it was nearly 50 years before this observation was applied to the treatment of neoplastic diseases in humans.

There are two types of drugs used for treatment of any disease—those that suppress symptoms but do nothing to remove the cause of disease and those that cure. Curative drug therapy, as we know it, began with the use of antimalarials. The use of cinchona bark (containing quinine) and ipecac (containing emetine) for the treatment of malaria can probably be considered the first successful chemotherapeutic agents. These remedies, discovered accidentally, date back to the seventeenth century. Introduced into Europe from South America by the Jesuits, they were used without knowledge of the causes of the diseases, the identity of the chemicals, or the mode of action of the drugs. Nevertheless, they worked.

Paul Erhlich coined the word "chemotherapy" for the use of a chemical of known composition that treated parasites. Between 1903 and 1915, Erhlich devoted most of his attention to the development of chemotherapeutic agents, much in the fashion used to identify anticancer drugs today.[3] He stressed the value of models using diseased animals to study the effects of drugs. Around 1900, such models existed for infectious diseases. For example, mice could be infected with the tubercle bacillus and pneumococci, mice and rats with trypanosomes, and rabbits with syphilis. With the help of an organic chemist and the support of the pharmaceutical industry, Erhlich synthesized a long series of organic arsenic compounds and tested them on these test animals. The 606th derivative was found highly effective, not only against trypanosome infections, but also (much to his surprise) against rabbit syphilis. Erhlich called the drug *salvarsan* (the savior of mankind). This was the first man-made chemical found to be effective in human parasitic disease. This work was completed by 1910.

By the 1930s, the first easy-to-use successful chemotherapeutic agents against bacterial infections were discovered. Sulfanilamide was found to be curative for some highly fatal human infections, such as streptococcus and meningococcal meningitis. The discovery, isolation, purification, and demonstration of the effectiveness of penicillin radically altered the approach to infectious diseases after that. Penicillin was effective against gram-positive organisms and it was correctly assumed that drugs could also be found effective against gram-negative organisms as well. This occurred when streptomycin was discovered.[4] However, the effectiveness of streptomycin against gram-negative bacteria was overshadowed by an unexpected surprise—it was effective against the bacillus of tuberculosis—a finding just as accidental as the efficacy of penicillin against syphilis.

The parallels in the development of anticancer drugs and anti-infectious agents are striking. Erhlich's introduction of arsphenamine in 1910 is a paradigm of the cancer chemotherapy work of the 1960s. Erhlich's work was an important milestone because it proved infectious diseases, especially syphilis, could be cured in rodents and humans and that the rodent model predicted for human effectiveness. This has now been shown to be true for anticancer drugs as well. The treatment of syphilis with arsphenamine took 18 long months of injections. Erhlich's discovery was not followed by any further significant advance until the discovery of (1926) and the clinical use of penicillin (1939–1943) despite the expenditure of much effort on the synthesis of numerous organic compounds. Now the treatment of syphilis with penicillin can be accomplished in a single injection.

Resistance of bacteria to antibiotics was soon identified as a major obstacle to successful treatment, as it now is for the chemotherapy of cancer. In the case of tuberculosis, resistance developed to streptomycin when it was used alone. When other drugs with antituberculous activity were found, it was quickly demonstrated that two drugs were better than one, and three better than two. It is now appreciated that combination chemotherapy of tuberculosis is effective because of the delay in the development of resistance and because they provide broad coverage of the heterogeneic population of organisms with different *de novo* sensitivity to antibiotics. Today, the dose and dose rate (schedule) of antituberculous agents is known to be important. Similar studies are underway with anticancer agents, as a greater appreciation of the differences between bacterial and cancer cells has emerged.[5]

Cancer treatment research began in earnest at the turn of the century with three major pieces of work.[6–8] The first was the development of the principles of cancer surgery leading Halsted, in 1894, to propose *en-bloc* resection as part of a cancer operation, particularly the radical mastectomy. At about the same time, Roentgen discovered x-rays, or roentgen rays, and gave physicians a second means of treating localized cancer. The third advance had its roots in the work of Paul Erhlich. Erhlich's use of rodent models for infectious diseases led George Clowes, of Roswell Park Memorial Institute in Buffalo, to develop in the early 1900's inbred rodent lines that could carry transplanted rodent tumors. These models and others have since served as the testing ground for potential cancer chemotherapeutic agents. Alkylating agents were developed in the secret gas warfare program in both world wars. An explosion in Naples harbor and the exposure of seamen to these agents in World War II led to the observation that these particular agents caused marrow and lymphoid hypoplasia, and led to the use of these chemicals in the lymphomas. They were first tested in humans with Hodgkin's disease in 1943 at Yale University but, because of the secret nature of the gas warfare program, the work was not published until 1946.[6–8] The demonstration of remissions in chemically treated human cancers caused much excitement, which led to accelerated testing and later disappointment when all tumors grew back. The results are detailed in the chapter on lymphomas.

After Farber's observation on the effects of folic acid on leukemic cell growth in children with lymphoblastic leukemia and the development of the antifols as cancer drugs, the chemotherapy of cancer began in earnest.

BIOLOGIC PRINCIPLES

In the early 1960s, Skipper and colleagues laid down the guiding principles of chemotherapy using the rodent leukemia L1210 as a model. (These are detailed in Table 8-1.)[9–11] Applying these principles to the drug treatment of human cancers required an understanding of the differences between growth characteristics of rodent leukemia and those of human cancers, and the differences in growth rates of normal target tissue in mice and men. The growth characteristics of L1210 are illustrated in Chapter 4 and other sources as well.[12]

L1210 leukemia resembles no human tumor with the possible exception of Burkitt's lymphoma. Because L1210 leukemia is a rapidly growing tumor with a high percentage of cells actively synthesizing DNA at any given moment (60%) and because it has a growth fraction of one hundred percent, its life cycle is consistent and predictable. On the other hand, the cell cycles of human tumors are heterogeneous and prolonged.[1,13–16] The number of cells synthesizing DNA or actively in cycle (the growth fraction) is small, many cells contributing to tumor masses are not clonogenic, and many cannot form metastases. While these differences between the kinetics of mouse and human cancer are striking, the contrast between the kinetics of cell division (*i.e.*, cancer cell and bacterial cell division) are on a different order of magnitude. The doubling time of bacteria is on the order of 2 hours. Qualitative differences between human and bacterial cells can be identified as targets for drug therapy. Thus, the implied assumption that treatment of cancer could be as simple as that of bacterial infections misled investigators during the 1950s.

Little attention was paid to integrating treatment schedules with growth characteristics of cancer cells. Because of the tedious methodology required to gather it, information on the growth characteristics of human tumors and normal tissue only became available in the early 1960s.[1,13–16] An example of the contrast between growth patterns of a normal tissue of mouse and those of a human is shown in Fig. 8-1.[17,18] There is a substantial difference between the peak egress of leukocytes in the blood of mouse and that of man, and also of the life cycle of mouse and human myeloblasts, as measured by

TABLE 8-1. Some Models, Concepts, or Theories That Have Been Useful in the Theory and/or Practice of Cancer Treatment

BRIEF DESCRIPTION OF THE CONCEPT(s)	QUALITATIVE OR QUANTITATIVE IMPLICATIONS	COMMENTS
1. Reasons why surgery or radiation often cure localized cancers, but fail to cure widespread neoplasia.	One or a few surviving neoplastic cells may result in relapse (documented many times in experimental cancers).	This knowledge was the basis of the beginning research on cancer chemotherapy immediately after World War II.
2. a. First-order rates of bacterial cell kill by certain chemicals and drugs (the theory of Arrhenius developed in the early 1900's) was based on knowledge of chemical reaction rates and the shape of dose-response and time-action curves observed when growing bacterial cells were exposed to certain chemicals. b. Logarithmic order of neoplastic cell kill by anticancer drugs, before the limitations due to cell population heterogeneity comes into play.	a. Reaction (death) of a constant percentage of a comparably exposed cell population *regardless* of its size. b. Reaction (death) of an equal percentage of the surviving cells in *equal units of time* when the total population is exposed to a constant concentration of certain chemicals or drugs. A given dose of a given drug will kill the same percentage, not the same number, of widely different sized cancer cell populations *so long as they are similarly exposed and both the growth fraction and the ratio of the sensitive to permanently drug-resistant cancer cells are the same.*	The objections to this fundamental concept raised repeatedly over the first half of the 20th century have been resolved by new knowledge gained during the past two decades. Cell population heterogeneity of two types limits the range over which first-order rates of cell killing are observed, but this does not negate the validity of the theory of Arrhenius. This often-confirmed theory is similar to and compatible with (a) and the same limitations obtain. The major limitations are underlined.
3. The *invariable* inverse relationship between the tumor cell burden at the initiation of chemotherapy and "curability."	As in 2(b), this relationship stems from two other well documented relationships. a. the higher the tumor cell burden, the lower the growth fraction; and b. the higher the tumor cell burden, the higher the probability of drug-resistant sublines.	This concept underlies the importance and the usefulness of combination chemotherapy and modality treatment.
4. The influence of growth fraction and cell death on the rates, and the changing rates, of tumor growth. (See Chapter 4)	Growth fraction: the fraction of cells that are replicating their DNA in preparation for division at a particular time. Growth rates of tumors are related to their growth fraction and the rate of cell death, lysis, and resorption at a particular time in their growth history. Deviation from exponential growth (asymptotic phase) results from a decreasing growth fraction, increasing cell death, or both.	Differing growth rates and labeling indices of primary tumors and micrometastases in the lungs of the same animals have been demonstrated. The micrometastases are easier to eradicate with chemotherapy for several reasons.
5. a. Resting cells are temporarily resistant to a variety of agents. b. The direct relationship between growth fraction and cell kill (neoplastic and normal) by a given exposure to a drug or drugs.	a. Resting bacterial cells are refractory to penicillin and certain other antibiotics. b. Resting mammalian cells are markedly refractory to antimetabolites and are refractory to other classes of anticancer drugs if such resting cells do not attempt DNA replication prior to "repair." c. Resting cells again become sensitive to drugs when they resume DNA replication. d. The cell kill resulting from a given exposure to an anticancer drug is directly related to the growth fractions of (1) neoplastic cells and (2) the stem cells in normal cell renewal systems. e. The minimum cytotoxic concentration of a variety of drugs is essentially the same for a variety of neoplastic and normal cells (of animal or human origin) *when their growth fractions are similar.* f. The responsiveness to chemotherapy of animal and human cancers is generally related to their growth fractions when exposed to drugs.	a. The selective toxicity of ionizing radiation and almost all anticancer drugs is directed toward stem cells of cell renewal systems. The limiting toxicity usually is reflected in stem cells of intestinal epithelium (high growth fraction) and/or hematopoietic stem cells (high growth fraction) after damage by radiation or cytotoxic drugs. b. There can be little doubt that rapidly growing neoplasms in animals and man (high labeling index, short median cell cycle time, and relatively high growth fraction) are more responsive to chemotherapy than large tumor masses with low growth fractions. c. Micrometastases usually have a higher growth fraction than larger tumor masses and are easier to eradicate with chemotherapy. (Micrometastases also are much less apt to contain permanently drug-resistant neoplastic cells.)

TABLE 8-1. (Continued)

BRIEF DESCRIPTION OF THE CONCEPT(S)	QUALITATIVE OR QUANTITATIVE IMPLICATIONS	COMMENTS
6. Animal "screening models," when properly employed, are useful in selecting drugs and combinations of drugs that will be useful in treating human cancers (alone or in an adjuvant setting).	a. No single animal tumor is a perfect model for any single human cancer, much less for all human cancers. In the same context, no single human cancer is a good model for all animal cancer nor is any single human cancer a good model for all human cancer. b. On the more positive side, chemotherapeutic results obtained in animal models have gone a long way toward identifying the criteria for cure of any disseminated cancer.	a. Animal models have selected many drugs and combinations of drugs (and schedule patterns) now widely used in treating many human cancers. b. Animal models have selected "false positives." This usually has occurred when the endpoints used in the experimental system were *unrealistic* in the context of what would be considered a useful therapeutic response in man.
7. Combination modality treatment (surgery + chemotherapy and radiation + chemotherapy).	The major tumor cell burden often is contained in primary tumor mass(es). When the primary is removed by surgery or largely destroyed by radiation, chemotherapy has a much greater chance of producing cure because micrometastases may be expected to have a higher growth fraction and to contain smaller numbers of specifically drug-resistant neoplastic cells (zero if the residual burden after local treatment is small).	a. The value of surgery + chemotherapy has been documented in a variety of metastatic animal cancers. b. The value of surgery + chemotherapy and radiation + chemotherapy has been documented in certain human cancers, so long as the metastatic burden is not too large after local treatment.

(Modified from Skipper HE: Southern Research Booklet #9, 1980, Personal Communication)

the appearance of tritiated thymidine-labeled leukocytes in the peripheral blood.[1] A treatment devised to be given at intervals to avoid lethal bone marrow suppression in the mouse can easily be expected to prove too toxic for human bone marrow. On the other hand, arbitrarily prolonging the interval between treatments to adjust for the differences in the kinetics of mouse and human bone marrow may allow tumor regrowth.

Skipper quantitated the effects of chemotherapy on cancer cells. He clarified the influence of the burden of cancer cells on the body on the outcome of treatment. Skipper showed that the survival of CDF_1 mice, bearing transplanted L1210, is inversely related to the number of tumor cells inoculated or surviving after treatment.[9] For example:

1. Injection of a single malignant clonogenic cell can ultimately lead to the death of the host animal
2. The larger the number of cells inoculated into an animal the shorter its survival
3. The interval between the injection of cells and death in the mouse can be predicted by a knowledge of the number of cells injected and the doubling time of the tumor population

These relationships are shown in Fig. 8-2. The time to death of animals bearing L1210 leukemia is the interval required to achieve a population size of about one billion cells (10^9). With a growth fraction of 100% and a doubling time of 12 hours, 10^9 cells will accumulate 19 days after the injection of a single cell, 10 days after the injection of 10^5 cells, and 5 days after the administration of 10^8 cells. Skipper further postulated that the increase in host life-span after cytotoxic chemotherapy of L1210 leukemia is largely due to the cytocidal effect of treatment on the tumor cell population. In these early elegant mouse experiments he could calculate the residual number of cells after treatment by extrapolating back from the duration of prolongation of life after a single treatment. An increase in life-span of 2 days would be equivalent to a 90% cell kill, or a reduction of cell numbers from 10^6 to 10^5 (1 log kill). A 99.999% cell kill, a figure that seems enormous to most clinicians, represents only a five log kill and will not cure these animals unless the initial inoculum of cells is small, say 10^4 cells or less. If multiple treatments are given,

FIG. 8-1. Peripheral blood granulocytes labeled with a pulse or tritiated thymidine in CDF_1 mice and normal humans. The difference in peak radioactivity represents, in part, shorter generation time of cells of stem cell pool in mice.

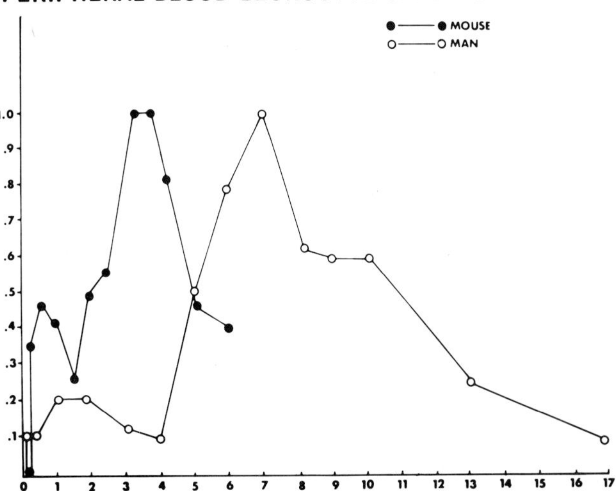

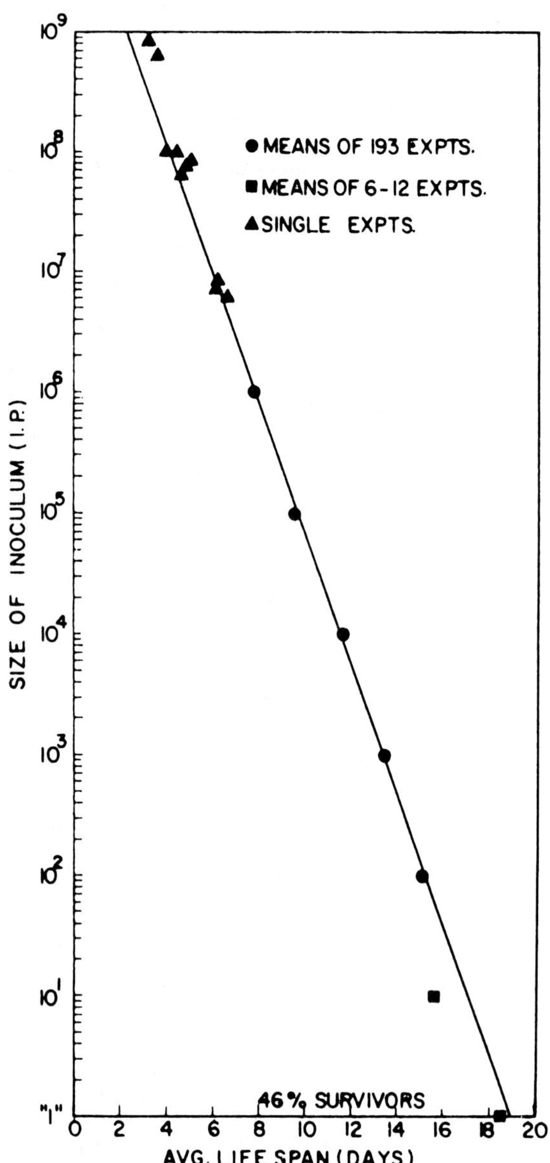

FIG. 8-2. Relationship between size of tumor cell inoculation and time to death of the host in L1210 leukemia in CDF_1 mice.

the net tumor cell kill per treatment is the sum of the surviving cells plus the regrowth of the tumor cell population before the next treatment.

Skipper showed that anticancer drugs killed cancer cells by first order kinetics, that is, a given dose of drug will kill a constant fraction of a population of cells regardless of its size. (Zero order kinetics had been assumed prior to this time.) In zero order kinetics a dose of drug would kill a fixed number of cells regardless of body burden. With a first order reaction, a dose of drug that reduces a population of 100,000 cells to one cell will leave 1,000 residual cells if a billion cells were present at the start of treatment (assuming the population had equivalent growth fraction and an equal number of sensitive and resistant cell lines). Thus, the chance of eradicating a cancer is *greater* when the population size is *small*. This is particularly true since cell kinetic data in animal models indicate that the growth fraction increases with decreasing tumor size.[19,20] Or, conversely, as the tumor mass increases, growth slows by a reduction in growth fraction. Exponential growth in large tumors is then matched by exponential retardation of growth (Gompertzian growth curve). Recently, Goldie and Coldman have reemphasized that resistance of bacteria to phage and of tuberculosis organisms to antituberculosis drugs arises *de novo* without prior exposure to the agent in question.[21] They propose that in genetically unstable exponentially growing human cancer cells, spontaneous development of phenotypic resistance to anticancer drugs is likely. Using the original work of Luria and Delbruck that describes the fluctuation of bacterial resistance to phage (see Table 8-2 for details), the chance of drug resistant cells lines being present was calculated to be related to the inherent mutation rate in a tumor cell population.[22] By their model, this varies directly with tumor mass. Thus, the chance of having multiple drug resistant lines and the percentage of resistant cells increases directly with tumor size.[21]

These observations have important implications when applied to the treatment of human tumors. They provide a basis for the effectiveness of combination chemotherapy over single agents against tumor cell populations with constant growth fractions. In other words, according to the model of Goldie and Coldman, for the first time a basis is provided for the invariable inverse relationship between drug curability and cell number independent of tumor growth kinetics. Since the number and fraction of resistant cells will vary with mass of tumor, it is easy to appreciate that the possibility of multiple resistant lines is high when patients present with widespread metastases. Furthermore, the Goldie and Coldman formula indicates that such resistance can develop over only two logs of growth (about six doublings). Thus, delays in starting treatment may assume considerable importance.

The presence of a small fraction of resistant tumor cells in a large mass may not influence the initial response to chemotherapy but can explain why patients who have complete remissions are not always cured. On the other hand, slow regression of killed tumor cells may create the impression of lack of responsiveness since repopulation by the resistant line may outstrip lysis. Figure 8-4 illustrates this problem. For each increment of tumor cell death indicated by the arrows there is lysis of tumors (line C) and regrowth of the residual surviving cells (line B). Since lysis can be a slow process, the actual reduction of tumor mass (line D) may not reflect the magnitude of tumor destruction. In fact, for a 90% cell kill the tumor mass shown in this hypothetical case may not shrink below the limits of palpation.

Contrary to popular opinion among physicians, the killing effect of cancer chemotherapeutic agents has a definite selectivity for cancer cells over the normal host cells. Although individual cancer cells do not divide faster than their normal tissue counterpart, the population of cancer cells generally has a higher growth fraction.[20] Also, the stem cell fraction of normal renewing tissues (bone marrow, gastrointestinal mucosa), the chief normal target tissue, remains partially in a resting phase unless perturbed by chemotherapy. This selectivity is illustrated by the work of Bruce and coworkers in Table 8-2.[23] These workers quantitated the survival of murine lymphoma cells and normal murine bone marrow cells after *in vivo* exposure to a variety of chemotherapeutic agents. The

TABLE 8-2. Some Pharmacological Concepts or Theories That Have Been Useful in the Theory or Practice of Cancer Chemotherapy

BRIEF DESCRIPTION OF THE CONCEPTS(s)	QUALITATIVE OR QUANTITATIVE IMPLICATIONS	COMMENTS
1. Mechanisms of action of various anticancer agents at the molecular level.	Almost all available anticancer drugs kill neoplastic or normal cells by affecting DNA synthesis or function. These drugs usually do not kill cells that are "resting" (not making new DNA) during exposure and some period afterwards.	This information has been and continues to be a focal point for integration of knowledge across disciplines.
2. The correlation of data on the toxicity of anticancer drugs across species including man: the mg/m^2 relationship.	Dosage on mg/kg basis relates to the maximum drug concentration achieved in body fluids, but does not carry across species in a direct manner with respect to sublethal or lethal toxicity. A reasonably good direct correlation with respect to toxicity across species is observed on a mg/m^2 dosage basis.	The mg/m^2 correlation relates to cardiac output in different species and, in turn, to the rates drugs are delivered to the kidneys and liver—the chief routes responsible for loss of drugs from the blood. In confirmation, we note that the serum half-life of drugs is usually longer (*e.g.*, 10×) in man than in the mouse.
3. Haber's toxicologic principles (C × t = k).	a. Over a considerable range of drug concentrations (C) and times of exposure (t), the same degree of toxicity (or cytotoxicity) results from the same C × t (μg/mi-minutes). b. The limitations to this principle are most apparent for antimetabolites, which kill cells only as rapidly as they intiate DNA replication during exposure. Alkylating agents and DNA binders will kill cells that are exposed in a resting state if they attempt division prior to repair.	a. This principle was widely employed in interpreting the lethal and sublethal toxicity of certain chemical warfare agents during World Wars I and II (*e.g.*, alkylating agents). b. This concept is compatible with first-order rates and cell kill and the same limitations obtained.
4. The relative pharmacokinetic behavior of anticancer agents in animals and man in relation to anticipated usefulness of different doses of a single drug or each drug in combination.	a. The dose levels required to achieve *minimum* cytotoxic serum levels and any possible therapeutic benefit. b. The quite different C, t, and C × t achievable by maximally tolerated doses of different drugs when administered in the same manner to both animals and man.	a. With knowledge of the minimum cytotoxic concentrations of different drugs for dividing neoplastic cells and pharmacokinetic information it is possible to anticipate whether or not each drug in a proposed combination (as delivered) is likely to be contributory. b. Also see (2) above regarding the serum half-life differences between small animals and man.
5. a. Bacterial cells mutate spontaneously to a state of specific resistance to phage and to drugs. b. Neoplastic cells mutate spontaneously to a state of specific resistance to a wide variety of anticancer drugs.	a. Specific and permanent drug-resistant bacterial and neoplastic cells arise spontaneously and with a definite frequency, independent of the selecting agent. b. *Depending upon the tumor burden* chemotherapy "cures" or fails to "cure" a variety of animal cancers. When tumor cell populations regress and then relapse during continued undiminished treatment, the surviving tumor cells are now specifically resistant to the drug(s) employed. This has been documented repeatedly by passage and retesting with the same drug(s).	The classical studies of Luria and Delbruck showed that when independent lines of bacterial cells were grown from a few cells to 10^8 and 10^9 and tested for the ratio of cells resistant to phage, the variation was great.[34] But when multiple samples from a single subline were tested, the variation was small (the "fluctuation test"). This implies that mutation to resistance was random and could occur at different times in the growth process. This principle was later obtained with respect to bacterial cells with resistance to drugs and leukemia cells resistant to methotrexate.
6. a. Essentially all classes of anticancer drugs select and allow overgrowth of specifically drug-resistant neoplastic cells. b. The rate of selection of a drug-resistant subline of cancer cells is directly related to the rate of eradication of the drug-sensitive cells and is influenced by the tumor cell burden and the intensity and duration of treatment. c. Clinical resistance is observed when selection has reached the point where 1–50% of the surviving cells are resistant to the selecting agent(s).	a. When a neoplastic cell population is large, the chances of it containing a small fraction of cells (*e.g.*, 0.01–0.0001%) that are specifically resistant to a given drug are high. b. After selection to the point of, say, 50% cells that are resistant to maximally tolerated doses of a given drug, that drug cannot achieve a second remission.	a. Selection and overgrowth of drug-resistant neoplastic cell populations is a major cause of chemotherapeutic failure in animal cancers and probably in human cancers as well. b. Switching drugs at or near the nadir achievable with a remission-inducing combination is a rational approach to minimizing treatment failures—if such a median nadir can be deduced from the remission duration in past treatment failures.

TABLE 8-2. (Continued)

BRIEF DESCRIPTION OF THE CONCEPT(s)	QUALITATIVE OR QUANTITATIVE IMPLICATIONS	COMMENTS
d. If the tumor cell population is large, combination chemotherapy may select sublines that are resistant to two or more drugs. The rate of mutation to a state of resistance to two different classes of drugs is *not* proportional to the product of the rate of mutation to resistance to each drug; it is much higher. Experimental data suggest that the origin of doubly resistant neoplastic cells is as follows: Drug A-resistant cells grow to some number and then begin mutating to a state of resistance to Drug B, Drug C, etc., and retain their resistance to Drug A. e. Combination chemotherapy (simultaneous, cyclic, or sequential) will often prevent or delay failures due to overgrowth of drug-resistant sublines of neoplastic cells. The doses and schedules employed are usually of greater importance than the variable of simultaneous, cyclic, or sequential delivery of combinations. f. When a neoplastic cell population shows resistance to maximally tolerated doses of a combination, it will also show resistance to maximally tolerated doses of some (but perhaps not all) of the individual drugs in the combination.		
7. The numbers of anticancer drugs that show little or no cross-resistance is larger than some realize.	a. Generally, drug-resistant neoplastic cells that have been selected by antimetabolites or alkylating agents or DNA binders never show cross-resistance across these broad drug classifications. b. Cells selected by methotrexate are not cross-resistant to purine and pyrimidine antagonists. c. Cells selected by different purine analogs are not cross-resistant to all purine analogs. d. Cells selected by different pyrimidine analogs are not cross-resistant to all pyrimidine analogs. e. Cells selected by different alkylating agents are not cross-resistant to all alkylating agents.	a. To date, neoplastic cells resistant to a given purine or pyrimidine antagonist have shown cross-resistance only to others that require the *same enzyme* for activation (conversion to respective nucleotides). b. A variety of alkylating agents that do not show cross-resistance have been shown to provide therapeutic potentiation when used in combination (animal tumor systems).

(Modified from Skipper HE, Southern Research Booklet #9, 1980, Personal Communication)

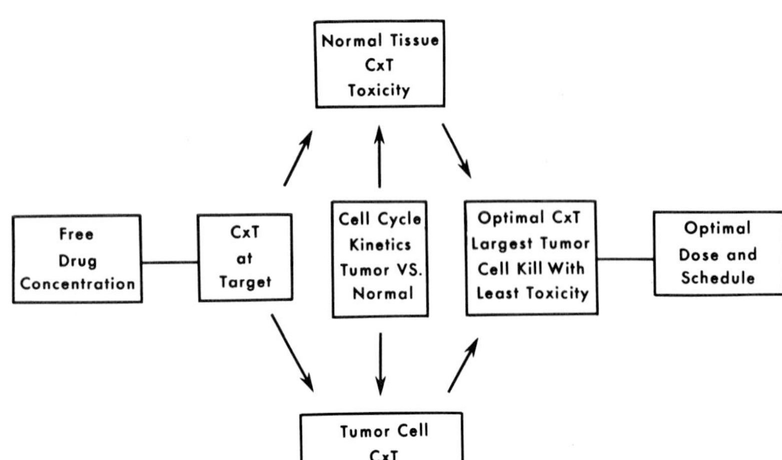

FIG. 8-3. Drug-cell interaction. Plasma concentration versus time of exposure to target ($C \times T$).

killing effect of different types of antitumor agents varied considerably depending on whether they acted during a specific phase of the cell cycle (cell cycle specific), or affected cells in the resting phase as well (cell cycle nonspecific) (Table 8-3). Some agents achieve as much as a 10,000 times greater cell kill of lymphoma cells over marrow cells. In the clinic this difference is quite visible when a nonlethal treatment produces severe but reversible leukopenia and thrombocytopenia, eradicating the tumor permanently (as seen in many cases of Hodgkin's disease, childhood leukemia, and diffuse hystiocytic lymphoma). (See Chapters 34 and 35 in this book.)

PHARMACOLOGIC PRINCIPLES

The cancer cell presents a variable and moving target to drugs. The interrelationship of anticancer drug pharmacokinetics and cell kinetics is the mainstay of clinical cancer chemotherapy. The major pharmacologic concepts important to cancer treatment and their implications are given in Table 8-2. Almost all anticancer drugs share two common properties: they work by affecting DNA synthesis and they usually do not kill resting cells unless such cells are destined to divide soon after exposure to the drug. The therapeutic and the toxic effects of chemotherapeutic agents are related to the time the active principal is exposed in an effective concentration to its target. This relationship is shown in Figure 8-3. The same degree of cytotoxicity can be achieved on different schedules

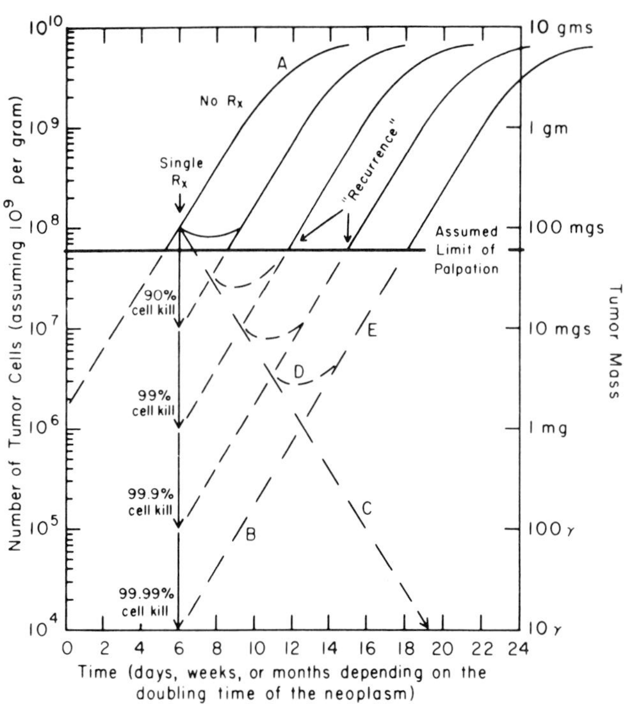

FIG. 8-4. A hypothetical depiction of the relationship between fractional tumor reduction, tumor regrowth, and tumor mass. Line *A* is the unperturbed tumor. Line *B* is the regrowth rate of the surviving fraction. Line *C* repesents slow lysis of tumor cells. Line *D* represents the net effect of lysis and regrowth.

TABLE 8-3. Classification of Chemotherapeutic Agents According to Dose-Survival Curves for Lymphoma and Marrow-Colony Forming Cells

CLASS	AGENTS ASSIGNED	SURVIVAL CURVES OBTAINED	DIFFERENTIAL SENSITIVITY BETWEEN MARROW AND LYMPHOMA CELLS	SUGGESTED ACTION AT CELLULAR LEVEL
I	Gamma radiation Nitrogen mustard BCNU	Exponential	None	Agents kill in all phases of cell cycle; not too dependent on proliferative capacity of cells.
II	3H–thymidine Vinblastine Amethopterin Azaserine	Decrease to constant saturation point at high doses	500–fold greater cell kill of lymphoma colony-forming cells	Agents kill in only one portion of the cycle; cells not entering this portion during treatment survive.
III	Cyclophosphamide Actinomycin D 5-Fluorouracil	Exponential	10,000–fold greater cell kill of lymphoma colony-forming cells	Agents kill in all phases of the cell cycle, but sensitivity strongly depends on fraction in proliferative state.

Bruce WR, Meeker BE, Valeriote FA: Comparison of the sensitivity of normal hematopoietic and transplanted lymphoma colony-forming cells to chemotherapeutic agents administered *in vivo.* Journal of the National Cancer Institute 37:233–245, 1966

from the same concentration of drug multiplied by the time of exposure (C × T). This relationship generally pertains across species barriers provided that the drugs are both metabolized and excreted in a similar fashion. This principle has made it possible to translate doses of drugs devised in animals to humans for early clinical testing.[9–11,24] Doses expressed allow for more accurate cross species comparisons in mg/sq m of body surface area for some agents. This is because body surface area is more closely related to cardiac output and cardiac output to the blood flow to the liver and the kidney (the principal organs of excretion and detoxification).[25] A given C × T will be equally cytotoxic only in populations of cells with equivalent growth characteristics.

The most important reason for treatment failure is drug resistance. Resistance to drugs occurs in cell populations either because some cells are resistant *de novo* to the agent or the agents used, or, because resistant cell lines develop under the pressure of exposure to the drug.[21,25–32] The situation is quite different for radiotherapy. *De novo* resistance is rare. It is relative to the sensitivity of normal surrounding tissue. Radiotherapy resistant lines do not appear with treatment. The presence and overgrowth of drug resistant cell lines is not, of course, the only reason for treatment failure. The tendency of large masses of tumor cells to consist of noncycling cancer cells, and the presence of pharmacologic sanctuaries also play important roles. Nonetheless, since a single viable cancer cell can lead to the death of the host, the appearance of a cell from a sanctuary or the presence or selection of a resistant mutant line is the major cause of chemotherapeutic failure in the clinics.[9,10,33,34] The mathematical analysis of Goldie and Coldman, relating drug sensitivity to spontaneous mutation rate and to drug resistance, indicates that the probability of resistant clones increases, as tumor size increases.[21] The likelihood of there being at least one resistant cell present in a population can change from the condition of low to high probability over a relatively short interval of growth. The higher the mutation rate, the earlier in the growth of the tumor this transition is likely to occur.[21,35–39] The striking implication of this statement is emphasized by the fact that to reach a size of one billion cancer cells (10^9), which is the lower limit of palpability or visability of a tumor mass on x-ray, a cancer cell must go through 27 to 30 doublings.[27] Ten additional doublings will yield 10^{12} cells, usually the lethal tumor body burden for humans. It may, therefore, be safely assumed that in most clinical situations when metastases are visible some cells have spontaneously mutated to resistance to current drugs by the time the patient presents to the doctor. Also, under the pressure of exposure to chemotherapeutic agents, phenotypically resistant cell lines very likely appear and grow at an increasing rate. A clinical example of fluctuating resistance affecting response to treatment can be found in the treatment of Hodgkin's disease with the four drug combination MOPP. Patients who achieve a complete remission and do not relapse for more than a year after treatment is stopped usually respond again to the same treatment while those who relapse early (12 months) do not.[40] This suggests that treatment failure in the first case was due to early discontinuation of treatment while the population of cancer cells was still sensitive to drugs. In the latter case, the data suggest resistance had already developed during treatment and regrowth occurred quickly, and would have occurred even if treatment were continued.[40] As previously emphasized, all evidence listed in Tables 8-1 and 8-2 point to an advantage to initiating treatment early when the population size is small, growth fraction is high, and the likelihood of *de novo* cell lines resistant to treatment is less. These principles form the basis for the use of postoperative chemotherapy.[42–45]

TABLE 8-4. Mechanisms of Resistance to Anticancer Drugs

MECHANISM	EXAMPLE
Insufficient drug uptake by the neoplastic cell	Methotrexate Daunomycin
Insufficient activation of drug	6-Mercaptopurine 5-Fluorouracil
Increased inactivation	Arabinosyl cytosine
Increased concentration of a target enzyme; gene amplification	Methotrexate
Decreased requirement for a specific metabolic product	L-Asparaginase
Increased utilization of an alternative biochemical pathway (salvage)	Antimetabolites
Rapid repair of a drug-induced lesion	Alkylating agents

General mechanisms of resistance to anticancer drugs are shown in Table 8-4, and discussed in more detail in the chapter on clinical pharmacology, in addition to other sources.[45,46] It should be emphasized, however, that resistance to an agent of one class does not necessarily imply resistance to all agents in the same class. Alkylating agents, for example, differ in modes of transport into cells, in activation by cellular enzymes, and in reactive alkylating moieties. This has important clinical implications since a patient initially responsive to an alkylating agent but now resistant may get a useful clinical response to a second alkylating agent of different structure.[25,29]

In contrast, it has been observed in rodent leukemia that resistance to drugs like adriamycin often confers resistance to other large complex molecules such as actinomycin D and vincristine. This may reflect a general alteration in cell membranes and altered cell transport of these agents. This phenomenon appears to carry over with these latter drugs in the clinic. On the other hand, the development of resistance to one drug sometimes results in increased sensitivity to another that acts by a different mechanism. This phenomenon has been called *collateral sensitivity*.[30] In experimental animals, resistance to methotrexate, or 6-mercaptopurine, can lead to increased sensitivity to the other drug. Resistance to arabinosyl cytosine has led to sensitivity to the experimental drug PALA, (phosphonacetyl-L-aspartate). The usefulness of the combination of methotrexate and 6-mercaptopurine in the treatment of acute lymphocytic leukemia of childhood may owe some of its effect to this collateral sensitivity.[47]

The Importance of Dose and Schedule

In applying the principles of chemotherapy, nothing is of greater importance to the clinician than proper dosing.[48] Since anticancer drugs are quite toxic, it is very appealing to find reason to reduce dosage with the hope of achieving an effect equal to that seen at higher doses. All the principles espoused earlier in the chapter argue strongly against this approach. The dose response curve for almost all known antitumor agents is steep for both toxic and therapeutic effects. For example, in high growth rate experimental animal tumors there is a linear-log relationship between dose and tumor cell kill. A twofold increase in dose will often increase tumor cell kill by one log (a 10-fold increase). Small changes in dose can effect large changes in response rate as well. Numerous studies in experimental animals show that if doses achieving a high complete response rate are reduced even by a small amount (20%) a large reduction of therapeutic effectiveness occurs and may even result in the disappearance of any response at all.[24,48] There are now several clinical examples of the same effect. In lymphomas, a twofold difference in dose of alkylating agent and the antimetabolite methotrexate resulted in a three- to fivefold greater antitumor effect.[49,50] In the oat cell carcinoma of the lung, the triple drug combination (cyclophosphamide, CCNU, and methotrexate) used in a regimen that doubled the doses of two of the three agents, doubled the overall response rate compared to the standard regimen and increased the complete response rate from 0 to 30%.[51] Similar effects have been noted in the treatment of childhood leukemia.[52] These dose response effects are only expressed clinically in treatment of tumors known to be at least partially responsive to the drugs used. Marginally chemosensitive tumors do not display a dose response curve, as measured by regression of large metastases, at least within the range of two- to threefold differences in dose. Increasing doses of ineffective drugs alone, or in combination, usually only produces in increased toxicity rather than therapeutic effect.

Dose rate is equally important. Faced with severe marrow hypoplasia from a cycle of chemotherapy, the physician is often tempted to prolong the interval between cycles without considering the potential for tumor regrowth during the increased interval. In a study of the treatment of acute myelocytic leukemia by the Southwest Oncology Group, a major variation in response rate was noted among these institutions.[53] An explanation was found in the dose rate between two types of institutions. Those with supportive care facilities and greater experience in the management of acute myelocytic leukemia gave the second cycle of treatment as prescribed by protocol. This usually meant initiating treatment in the face of marrow hypoplasia. Those institutions with less experience and less access to supportive care tended to prolong the interval between the first and the second cycle to 3 weeks. This reduction in dose rate by 50% made a greater than twofold difference in the complete remission rate and decreased it from 53% to 25%. A similar result has been noted for chemotherapy used in the postoperative period for breast cancer. Bonadonna and Valagussa have reported that relapse-free survival was significantly higher in patients receiving greater than 75% of the drug combination cyclophosphamide, methotrexate, and 5-flourouracil (CMF), as compared to those receiving less than 75% of the protocol dose. A substantially larger proportion of postmenopausal patients received less than 75% of the prescribed dose since it was unfortunately assumed that older women would tolerate the drugs less well. In this study, the initial lack of effectiveness of chemotherapy in the postmenopausal women with positive lymph nodes can largely be attributed to this modest reduction in dose and dose rate.

The questions of dose and dose rate impact on the use of maintenance chemotherapy. In all cases, maintenance treatment implies a reduction in the dose of individual drugs or deletion of drugs used in the induction treatment, or widening of the intervals between cycles (reduction in dose rate). There is, at present, no evidence from any study that drug maintenance treatment improves the cure rate of any chemotherapeutic regimen. This is again perhaps best illustrated using the treatment of Hodgkin's disease with the MOPP program as an example.[55-58] Several groups initiated studies to explore the prevention of relapse after remission induction with the MOPP combination (see Chapter 35) by supplying continued treatment in the form of maintenance therapy with MOPP or other drugs. All studies invariably used treatments of lower dose or dose rate. Ultimately, all studies have shown that there is no impact of these treatments on relapse-free survival; however, temporary prolongation of remission was noted in one study.[58] All evidence points strongly toward the position that the program that initially produces maximal cytocidal effect should be continued for an optimum duration of time rather than reducing the dose in favor of a maintenance program.

The entire philosophy of maintenance chemotherapy in drug responsive tumors needs to be reexamined. A serious area of clinical research involves the establishment of clinical trials to determine the proper duration for the administration of induction programs in drug responsive tumors. Most present data point to a duration of no less than 6 months and probably a year. Studies are also under way to explore increasing the intensity of treatment by escalating the doses and dose rate in the early treatment period while reducing the duration of the induction period.

PRINCIPLES OF COMBINATION CHEMOTHERAPY

The use of drugs in combination largely evolved out of the clinics because (with the two exceptions of choriocarcinoma and Burkitt's lymphoma), treatment with single agents, unlike the treatment of bacterial infections, was unable to produce either significant remissions or to cure patients with cancer.[45,59] Early attempts to design drug combinations based on biochemical principles were largely ineffective.[60-63] It seems this failure was due to the selection of individual drugs ineffective against the tumors studied. To combine effective drugs, a variety were obviously required. The availability of multiple clinically useful drugs for leukemia and lymphomas fortunately coincided with the principles of chemotherapy outlined previously by Skipper.

The era of effective combination chemotherapy began with the treatment of leukemias and lymphomas and has now extended to the treatment of more common malignancies described throughout this text.[27,40,41,45,64-72] It now seems likely that drug combinations are effective because they accomplish three important feats not possible with single agent treatment.

1. They provide maximal cell kill within the range of toxicity tolerated by the host for each drug.
2. They provide a broader range of coverage of *de novo* resistant cell lines in the heterogeneous tumor population.
3. They prevent, or slow, the development of new resistant lines.

Failure of combination chemotherapy to work in marginally sensitive tumors seems related to the absence of a dose response curve for cytoreduction within the range of doses tolerable to the host.

Several principles that have characterized the selection of drugs in the most effective drug combination treatment programs guide the development of new programs.[41] They include:

1. Only drugs known to be partially effective when used alone should be selected for use in combination. If available, drugs that produce some fraction of complete remission should be preferred to those that produce only partial responses.
2. When several drugs of a class are available, a drug should be selected for toxicity that does not overlap with other drugs used in the combination. While such selection leads to a wider range of side effects and greater discomfort to the patient, it minimizes the risk of a lethal effect.
3. Drugs should be used in their optimal dose and schedule. (The previous comments on dose response and dose rate effects are pertinent here).
4. Drug combinations should be given at consistent intervals. The interval selected between cycles should be the narrowest possible to allow for recovery of the most sensitive normal target tissue. In most cases, this is bone marrow, but on occasion, it can be gastrointestinal tract.

The physician should keep in mind that bone marrow has a storage compartment that can supply mature cells to the peripheral blood for 8 to 10 days after the stem cell pool has ceased to function. Thus, events measured in the peripheral blood are usually a week behind the events in the bone marrow. In previously untreated patients, leukemia and thrombocytopenia are discernible on the 9th or 10th day after initial dosing. The nadir of these blood counts is reached by the 14th to 18th day, with recovery apparent by the 21st and usually complete by the 28th day. Prior treatment with drugs or x-ray may alter the sequence by shortening the time to the appearance of leukopenia and thrombocytopenia and prolonging the recovery time. Curiously, the habit of giving the second half of the drug combination in the clinic 1 week later (day 8), just preceding the usual onset of leukopenia and thrombocytopenia, has proven safe even though peripheral blood count suppression will appear even if the second dose is omitted. The cytotoxic dose response effect is usually the nadir white cell and platelet count, not the duration of cytopenia. This is fortunate since the most dangerous depression of blood counts (a granulocyte count of less than $500/ml^3$ and a platelet count less than $20{,}000/ml^3$) lasts only 4 to 7 days and is tolerated by most patients even without supplemental support. Increasing doses of most anticancer drugs beyond the level that produces such severe granulocytopenia and thrombocytopenia usually does not ablate the marrow or even prolong the duration to recovery. This is due to the resting state of the stem cells of normal bone marrow which protects them from damage.

However, scheduling is critical. Repeated dosing at early recovery (days 16–21) of the marrow may cause more severe toxicity for the second treatment cycle in patients whose marrow is not the source of, or involved with, tumor. These sequences do not apply to the treatment of leukemia. These data have led to the familiar 2-week interval between cycles (new cycle begins on day 28 after first dose) of the most effective drug combinations that accommodate the recovery time of human bone marrow. While this schedule is useful for the individual tumors whose regrowth characteristics permit marrow to return to normal before the tumor mass returns to pretreatment levels, the interval is excessively long for some rapidly growing tumors (e.g., diffuse histiocytic lymphoma and Burkitt's lymphoma). To circumvent this, investigators have resorted to several approaches. The simplest approach is the use of non-marrow toxic chemotherapeutic agents (bleomycin, asparaginase, or high-dose methotrexate with citrovorum factor rescue) between cycles of treatment with marrow toxic agents to permit the bone marrow to recover in face of continued treatment.[6] This approach is limited by the sensitivity of the tumor in question to available non-marrow toxic agents. Other attempts to match the treatment schedule to the individual tumor growth rate have used autologous bone marrow transfusions to facilitate recovery (see Chapter 43) in addition to alternating cycles of drug combinations (consisting of non-cross resistant drugs).[69b-72] The latter approach is attractive but requires available and effective drugs. This approach also theoretically prevents the development of multiple resistant cell lines. Thus far it has only been effectively applied in the treatment of Hodgkin's disease (see Chapter 35).

In reality, no rigid schedule can accommodate all the clinical variables in the practice of medical oncology. Physicians must often adjust doses and intervals to administer drugs safely. The surety that the therapeutic effect of a drug or combination of drugs might be lost if the dose or schedule is adjusted should temper these judgments. Both physician and patient must consider the risk of dying from the cancer along with the more obvious, but transient, benefits of reducing the acute side effects of the treatment. Adhering to a standard sliding scale of dose adjustment usually published with most new treatments is quite useful. In addition to providing guidelines for dose reduction, these sliding scales provide consistency by preserving both the intervals between cycles and the integrity of the drug combination. Alteration of a drug combination by omitting a drug is also likely to alter its effect. Every attempt should be made to administer at least a partial dose of each drug in combination unless a clinical study has indicated that changes can be made without altering the therapeutic effect.

Selection of Drugs for Postoperative Treatment

Drugs should be used in the postoperative period if clinical studies indicate that they provide benefit. In most studies the selection is made based on two criteria: if the risk of developing recurrent tumor is great (in spite of apparently effective local treatment), and, if the drugs used are known to be effective against the same type of tumor in those patients with visible metastases.

Risk of recurrence is relative to the toxicity of the regimen used. An easy to use nontoxic regimen might be used with acceptable risk, even if the chance of recurrence is less than 50%. The limiting factor in all adjuvant studies is that patients who would not recur must be exposed to cytotoxic drugs to extend the benefit to those who will recur.

It is also difficult to define the level of effectiveness that warrants the selection of a treatment for adjuvant chemotherapy. Clearly, the most effective, least toxic regimen is the best. But what if a clearly superior treatment is not available? Those treatments that produce complete remissions in patients with high volume metastatic disease are more cytocidal than those that only produce partial responses; those treatments should be the selection of choice. Høwever, L-phenylaline mustard (L-PAM) is useful as an adjuvant to surgery in some patients with breast cancer while producing only a 20% partial response rate (with rare complete remissions) in patients with metastatic breast cancer. Therefore, the success of postoperative chemotherapy is undoubtedly conditioned by the population kinetics of small tumor masses previously described, and the decreased likelihood that multiple resistant cell lines are present at the time of diagnosis when compared to massive, visible tumor. The suggestion that drugs ineffective against metastatic disease of the same type might be useful in the postoperative chemotherapy has not been tested clinically. There is some evidence that this is true in rodents. The tenets of Goldie and Coldman provide a theoretical basis for such an approach as well.[21] Given the steep dose response curves of most anticancer drugs, one factor appears certain: there is no evidence of benefit, and much to fear, from a reduction in dose or dose rate of treatment programs used in the postoperative period. Physicians are advised to adhere closely to the use of chemotherapeutic agents in full doses and schedules unless reductions have been proven to be effective in a clinical trial.

Selection of Individual Drugs for Treatment

An assay of clonogenic cancer cells has been described by Hamburger and Salmon whereby a sample of fresh tissue is plated with growth factors on soft agar leading tumor colonies to form.[73-75] Using this test individual patient sensitivity to cancer drugs can be assayed. Although the slowness of this procedure obviates its use for the initial treatment, it can identify potentially useful drugs for future treatment, avoiding exposure of the patient to ineffective toxic drugs. Thus far, the clinical correlation with the *in vitro* results has been quite good. Nonetheless, the technique has limited value today in clinical cancer chemotherapy. This is because most tumors cannot yet be consistently grown in soft agar. In others, the plating efficiency is too low to provide a reliable assessment of sensitivity to a panel of drugs. In addition, there is no assurance that the assay is selecting a population of stem cells or even an adequate sample of the heterogenous cell population. The most important drawback, however, is that the pool of active drugs available today is not sufficient to make this assay routinely useful. It is highly unlikely that a tumor type thought to be resistant to all available chemotherapy will be found sensitive by virtue of *in vitro* assay results. The value of this system will undoubtably increase in a fashion similar to sensitivity assays for antibiotics when a wider array of excellent anticancer drugs is available. Until then, selection of drugs for treatment is best done by using data from large Phase II clinical trials.

SPECIAL USES OF CHEMOTHERAPY

Special uses of chemotherapy include the instillation of drugs into the spinal fluid either directly through a lumbar puncture needle or into an implanted Ommaya reservoir to treat CNS leukemia and lymphoma; the instillation of drugs into the pleural or pericardial space to control effusions; splenic infusion to control spleen size; hepatic artery infusions to selectively treat hepatic metastases; and carotid artery infusions to treat head and neck cancers. These are discussed throughout the text. In all cases, the rationale for local use is based on achieving a greater C × T against the target tumor tissue and sparing the normal tissue. The technology for infusion and the appreciation of the pharmacokinetics of available antitumor agents have not been sufficient to fully evaluate many of these approaches, although the place of intracerebrospinal fluid and intrapleural treatment is established. Further experimental studies are now indicated since the capacity to measure active principles of anticancer drugs and their target has improved enormously with the availability of techniques such as high-pressure liquid chromatography, gas chromatographic mass spectroscopy, and radioimmune assays.

Two recent approaches warrant an additional comment. Drugs can be encompassed in lipid bilayer droplets called liposomes.[76,77] The surface characteristics of these liposomes can be altered to direct their delivery to specific organ sites or into resistant cell lines. Labile liposomes that dissolve at temperatures of 41°C or greater have also recently been developed.[77] In experimental animals, drugs can be deposited selectively in preheated areas.

Another regional use of chemotherapy is the intraperitoneal administration of drugs to treat ovarian cancer, a disease which kills almost exclusively by local effects in the abdomen (see Chapter 26).[78-80]

Older data indicating the failure of intraperitoneal treatment to exceed results with systemic treatment was flawed by a failure both to appreciate the varying transport characteristics of antitumor agents across the peritoneal membrane and to appreciate the need for high volume fluid administration to assure adequate drug distribution. A series of preclinical experiments established the pharmocokinetics of peritoneal transport of common antitumor agents in rodents.[78] Human studies were facilitated by the development and use of peritoneal dialysis techniques, for example, the Tenkhoff catheter (see Chapter 47). Table 8-5 shows data derived from such early human studies. The concentration of drug achievable in the peritoneal cavity using this "belly bath" technique for the three drugs shown far exceeds the plasma level, thus achieving a favorable C × T for the tumor over normal tissue. The effect is particularly marked for 5-fluorouracil (which has a metabolic clearance in the liver as well as a renal clearance) and adriamycin (which, because of its molecular size, diffuses

TABLE 8-5. Intraperitoneal Drug Therapy

	RATIO OF MEAN CONCENTRATION PERITONEAL FLUID TO PLASMA	MAXIMUM PLASMA CONCENTRATION
Methotrexate	23	2–3 × 10^{-7} M
5 Fluorouracil	298	1.67 × 10^{-5} M
Adriamycin	343	1.1 × 10^{-7} M

slowly across the peritoneal membrane). The difference is less with methotrexate which is cleared exclusively by the kidney. Nonetheless, even for methotrexate, renal clearance significantly exceeds peritoneal clearance. Clinical trials exploiting this technique in the treatment of ovarian cancer, and, as a potential postoperative treatment of the peritoneal cavity and liver for Dukes C colorectal cancer are in progress at the National Cancer Institute.

CANCER DRUG DEVELOPMENT

The steps in development of anticancer agents are shown in Fig. 8-5. The most important step in the drug selection process is screening, the mechanism used for narrowing the number of chemicals that are potential treatments for human cancer to a manageable number of high priority drugs. This is accomplished by testing the drugs in rodents bearing transplantable tumors of uniform and predictable behavior.[84–86] The quality of drugs selected by the screening program is dependent on the procedures used for the acquisition of materials.

In the early days of screening, acquisition of agents was purely random. Random screening faced two major problems—both repetition and screening of analogues of drugs known to be active. With the refinement of knowledge of cell biology, chemistry, pharmacology, and biochemistry, more predesigned agents are entering all screening programs. As new, effective agents are discovered, there is also a tendency to synthesize and screen analogues of these active compounds. While this approach is useful in the search for less toxic versions of existing anticancer drugs, it will not yield the new, potentially more active structures that are sorely required.

FIG. 8-5. Steps in cancer drug development.

ACQUISITION
↓
SCREENING
↓
PRODUCTION AND FORMULATION
↓
TOXICOLOGY
↓
PHASE I CLINICAL TRIALS
↓
PHASE II CLINICAL TRIALS
↓
PHASE III—IV CLINICAL TRIALS
↓
GENERAL MEDICAL PRACTICE

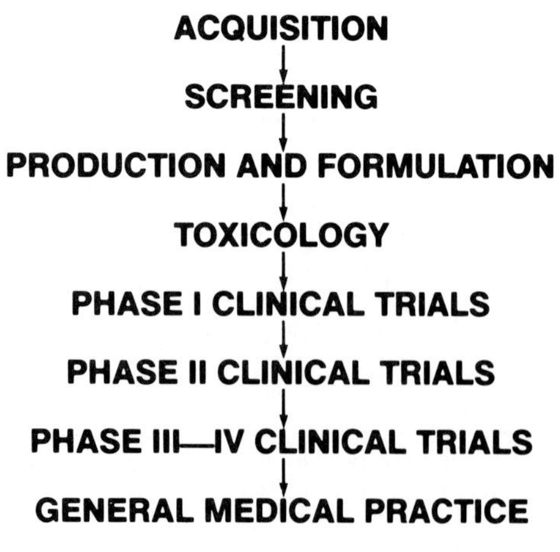

From its inception in 1955 until 1975, the mainstay of the National Cancer Institute's screening program was murine L1210 leukemia. Drugs found to be active in L1210 leukemia were evaluated further in other rodent tumors for schedule dependency but entrance in the clinic was usually based on antitumor effect in L1210. The input to the screening program reached its maximum number of 40,000 compounds per year in 1975; a major shift in emphasis was made in the NCI screening program because of the availability of a plethora of rodent models then. More rational selection of compounds was coupled with testing in a broader panel of rodent tumors before selection was made for clinical use. The elements of the new screening program are shown in Figure 8-6. Input to the screen has been decreased from 40,000 to approximately 15,000 compounds per year. Now, prescreening is performed in the sensitive rodent P388 mouse leukemia. An agent shown to have an antitumor effect in this system passes to a tumor panel. The decision to initiate clinical trials is made only upon demonstration of antitumor effect against one of the tumors in the tumor panel. The panel is made up of rodent tumors equivalent to common human tumors as well as xenographs of human tumors grown in "nude" (immune-deprived or hairless) mice.[86] A bypass was built into the early stages of the system to allow for chemicals not active in the P388 prescreen. However, these chemicals must have biologic activity in other systems, to bypass the P388 screen and to proceed to the panel.

The panel poses several questions of the screening procedure itself. For example, could the use of models of slower growing (low growth fraction) tumors select a different type of anticancer drug that would be more effective against the low growth fraction common visceral malignancies of humans? And of special interest would be drugs selected by activity against human tumors grown in immune deprived mice. Also, the pairing of a human tumor in nude mice with a rodent tumor of the same organ system questions the potential of rodent screens for agent selection with organ specificity against human cancer *in vivo*. Since rodent tumors such as leukemia L1210 are tested in parallel with human tumors in nude mice in the panel, the question of whether the older screening systems are as good as new approaches is also addressed. The latter question has assumed some importance since the expense of the older systems is far less than that of the newer screens. Since human tumors grown in soft agar have been useful in predicting antitumor effect of existing drugs *in vivo*, these *in vitro* systems have also been introduced in parallel with the *in vivo* systems to test their capacity to select new structures for human use.[73–75]

Inherent in all screening systems is the tenet that biological activity in some preclinical system must be demonstrated before human testing is performed. To date, no currently marketed useful anticancer agent is devoid of such preclinical activity. It should be kept in mind, however, that all have been selected for clinical testing using these systems. Thus, the basic question has never been adequately tested. Given the need to use some selection criteria to narrow the drug choice for clinical trials, screening systems are likely to remain the mainstay for decision-making for some time. Ultimately,

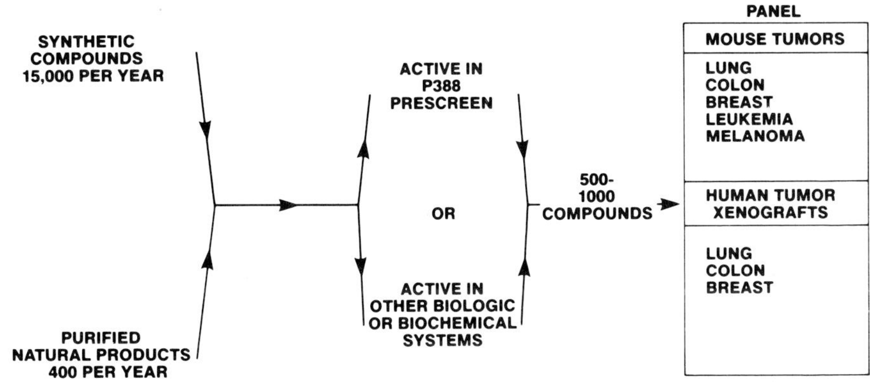

FIG. 8-6. Organization of the cancer drug screening program of the National Cancer Institute.

sophisticated *in vitro* systems offer the best hope of using human tumors to select for clinical use.

Workers in cancer drug development often face enthusiasts for various anticancer agents who by reason of theory or personal interest feel their material shows great promise as a human cancer treatment. Without activity in one of the many rodent systems in use, the decision is usually not to initiate clinical testing of these materials. Nowhere is this point better dramatized than in the issue of the clinical testing of Laetrile (amygdalin), which is discussed in Chapter 48.

Formulation and production of anticancer drugs often present formidable obstacles for chemists. Anticancer agents with great activity in rodents have been discarded for lack of an adequate formulation for human use. This is particularly true of the more complicated products extracted from plants. Once these formulation problems have been solved, preclinical testing for toxicity is required. Then, the Food and Drug Administration will approve an Investigational New Drug application (IND), which permits clinical testing. Toxicology testing has evolved over the last decade from complicated testing in rodents, dogs, and monkeys to a less expensive system that relies on toxicity testing in mice. Data accumulated since 1955 on the clinical testing of numerous anticancer drugs in humans have allowed for comparisons across species. These data have shown there is no real safety advantage in using larger animal species instead of rodents.[87] In the current system, implemented in 1980, a dose response curve of a new drug is developed in mice. The lethal dose (LD) in 10%, 50%, and 90% of animals is determined and the reproducible dose that is lethal in 10% of tested animals (LD_{10}) is hence used to establish an initial dose for clinical trials. This dose is further tested for toxicity in dogs prior to its use in humans. To maximize safety when administering an unknown compound in humans, 10% of the LD_{10} dose in rodents is selected for the initial human dose.

While correlation of toxic effects on rapidly dividing normal tissue (marrow and gastrointestinal tract) between rodents, dogs, monkeys, and man is good, correlation of other toxic effects is not as consistent. Therefore, routine pathologic examination of rodent tissues is not performed prior to clinical testing.

A note about dosing: the practive of dosing without reference to either weight or body surface area is archaic and should be abandoned. The preferable reference point is body surface area since better cross-species comparisons can be made. Also, the use of body surface area as a reference point allows dosing between adults and children without adjustment. The assumptions leading to the dose conversion factors have been described in detail by Freireich and coworkers, and are shown in Tables 8-6 and 8-7.[26]

Early Clinical Trials of Antitumor Agents

Antitumor agents go through four phases of clinical testing (see Fig. 8-5) before they are accepted for general medical practice and marketed or discarded.[82,88-90] The average time

TABLE 8-6. Representative Surface Area to Weight Ratios (km) For Various Species*

SPECIES	BODY WEIGHT (kg)	SURFACE AREA	SURFACE AREA TO WEIGHT RATIO (km)
Mouse	0.02	0.0066	3.0
Rat	0.15	0.025	5.9
Monkey	3	0.24	12
Dog	8	0.40	20
Human: Child	20	0.80	25
Adult	60	1.6	37

* To express a mg/kg in any given species as the equivalent mg/Sq.M dose, multiply the dose by the appropriate *km*. In the adult human, for example, 100 mg/kg is equivalent to 100 mg/kg × 37 kg/Sq.M = 3700 mg/Sq.M.

TABLE 8-7. Equivalent Surface Area Dosage Conversion Factors*

FROM	MOUSE 20 g	RAT 150 g	MONKEY 3.0 kg	DOG 8 kg	MAN 60 kg
Mouse	1	1/2	1/4	1/6	1/12
Rat	2	1	1/2	1/4	1/7
Monkey	4	2	1	3/5	1/3
Dog	6	4	5/3	1	1/2
Man	12	7	3	2	1

* This table gives approximate factors for converting doses expressed in terms of mg/kg from one species to an equivalent *surface area* dose expressed in the same terms mg/kg in the other species. For example, given a dose of 50 mg/kg in the mouse, what is the appropriate dose in man assuming equivalency on the basis of mg/m^2?

$$50 \text{ mg/kg} \times 1/12 = 4.1 \text{ mg/kg}$$

from the discovery of an effective antitumor agent to the marketing of that agent is unfortunately long, (somewhere in the range of 10–12 years). Fortunately, however, anticancer drugs with known efficacy against one or more human tumors in a premarketing phase are now made available to physicians by the National Cancer Institute (see Tables 8-8 and 8-9). Table 8-10 details the phases of clinical testing and the main purpose of each step. Phase I trials are done on small groups of patients, usually no more than 15–30 per study. Although the main purpose of Phase I trials is to identify a maximally tolerated dose in one or several schedules suggested by preclinical data, therapeutic effects should not be overlooked. When discussing participating in Phase I trials with patients, it is appropriate to emphasize that the patient has few other options. The Phase I trial usually offers the best hope available. For the most effective older anticancer drugs, therapeutic effects were often first seen in the Phase I trial. However, physicians should avoid drawing therapeutic conclusions from results of Phase I trials, especially if clinical responses are not noted. Since a limited number of patients with a variety of diseases are treated in Phase I trials, and doses may be below the ultimate therapeutic range, the absence of any positive clinical effect is never a reason to discontinue further studies. The only reason not to proceed to a Phase II study is prohibitive toxicity. Escalation of doses in Phase I trials is usually done by a modified Fibonacci system.[88] At first doses are doubled, and then increased in fractions of 66, 50, and 33% in succeeding groups of patients (usually three patients at a time) until toxicity is noted. In general, the practice of escalating doses in the same patient, if no toxic effect is seen with the first or several doses, is to be discouraged since delayed toxic effects of the first dose can appear to be early toxic effects of subsequent doses and can also be irreversible.

Once a decision is made to proceed with Phase II testing, trials are begun in a panel of clinical tumors matching those in the preclinical tumor panel. The panel used by the National Cancer Institute is illustrated in Fig. 8-7. The main difficulty with Phase II trials is testing agents in a uniform way and in

TABLE 8-8. The National Cancer Institute Classification of New Anticancer Drugs in Clinical Testing.

GROUP A DRUGS
This group includes drugs in Phase I clinical trials and Phase II clinical trials in specified tumors. Protocol acceptance and drug distribution are limited to clinical investigators.

GROUP B DRUGS
This group includes drugs already tested in initial Phase II studies and of clinical interest. Protocol acceptance and drug distribution are extended to include clinical cooperative groups, NCI contractors, and cancer centers.

GROUP C DRUGS
Group C includes drugs that demonstrate efficacy within a tumor type in more than one study, that alter the pattern of care of the disease in question, and that are safely administered by properly trained physicians without requiring specialized supportive care facilities. This group includes:

1. Streptozotocin (NSC 85998)—for islet cell carcinoma of the pancreas and carcinoid tumors
2. Methylcyclohexyl Nitrosourea (MeCCNU, NSC 95441)—for carcinoma of the colon and stomach, melanoma
3. Azacytidine (NSC 102816)—for refractory acute myelogenous leukemia
4. Ervinia Asparaginase (NSC 106977)—for acute lymphatic leukemia in patients sensitive to *E. coli* L-asparaginase
5. Hexamethylmelamine (NSC 13875)—for ovarian carcinoma
6. VP 16-213 (NSC 141540)—for small cell carcinoma of the lung
7. Tetrahydrocannabinol (THC) (NSC 134454)—for patients who have nausea and vomiting due to chemotherapy that is refractory to marketed antiemetics. (See Table 8-9.)

Drugs in Group C are available for use by physicians for specific indications. (See text and Table 8-10 as well.)

TABLE 8-9. The Procedure to be Followed to Obtain Drugs in Group C of the National Cancer Institute Classification of New Anticancer Drugs in Clinical Testing*

1. A physician must be registered with the National Cancer Institute as an investigator by having completed an FDA-Form 1573.
2. A written request for the drug, indicating the disease to be treated, must be submitted.
3. The use of the drugs shall be limited to indications outlined in the guidelines that will be provided to the physician.
4. All adverse reactions must be reported to the Investigational Drug Branch, DCT, NCI.
5. In contrast to the usual procedures for obtaining Group C drugs, THC will be distributed by hospital pharmacies registered with NCI as designated distribution facilities. At this time, more than 300 pharmacies are registered with NCI to participate in the program. Physicians requiring information on particular pharmacies in their local areas should contact the Office of the Chief, Investigational Drug Branch, CTEP, DCT, National Cancer Institute, Building 37, Room 6E20, Bethesda, Maryland 20205.†

* See Table 8-8.
† CTEP = Cancer Therapy Evaluation Program.

TABLE 8-10. Stages in the Clinical Testing of New Anticancer Agents

STAGE OF DRUG TESTING	OBJECTIVES	PATIENT POPULATION STUDIED
Phase I	*Determine Tolerance* 1. Maximally tolerable dose (MTD) 2. Limiting toxicity 3. Reversibility of toxicity 4. Properly scheduling administration *Pharmacology* 1. Bioavailability 2. Plasma clearance 3. Biotransformation 4. Excretion *Therapeutic Effect* Secondary	Histologically confirmed advanced malignancy. No longer amenable to conventional therapy. Physiologically well compensated. A variety of tumor types per study permissible.
Phase II	*Therapeutic Effect* 1. Types of tumor that respond 2. Dose response relationships *Non-therapeutic Effects* Extent of toxicity in relationship to therapeutic effect	Histologically confirmed advanced malignancy. Measurable tumor masses. No longer amenable to conventional therapy. A variety of tumor types in groups of 15 to 30. Physiologically well compensated.
Phase III	*Therapeutic Effectiveness* Compare experimental therapy to existing standard therapy *Non-therapeutic Effect* Are toxic effects tolerable in the context of observed therapeutic effect and in comparison to standard therapy?	Histologically confirmed malignancy. Patient sample must be of adequate size and uniformity. Usually untreated previously. Controls are usually randomly selected but historical controls are used on occasion.
Phase IV	*Therapeutic Effectiveness* 1. Integration of drug therapy into primary treatment in combination with surgery or radiation therapy (*e.g.*, postoperative drug treatment in breast cancer) 2. Compared to standard program without drugs added *Non-therapeutic Effects* 1. Are toxic effects minimal enough to risk giving drug to patients whose tumor will not necessarily recur? 2. Long-term toxic effects require monitoring (second tumors, sterility, marrow aplasia)	Histologically confirmed malignancy. Patient sample must be of adequate size and uniformity. Controls usually randomized.

a uniform population of patients. Under the best of circumstances, a drug that produces no antitumor effect in 14 patients of the same tumor type has a greater than 95% chance of being ineffective against that tumor and could reasonably be dropped from further studies against that specific cancer. One or two responses, on the other hand, increase the chance of efficacy sufficiently to dictate an expansion of the trial to 30 or more patients so as not to miss a drug with a response rate in the 20% range. Such studies will determine the actual response rate for a given dose and schedule. In general, partial response rates in excess of 20% place the agent in a category of potential clinical usefulness. Response rates in the range of 5%–10% are consistent with observer variation in Phase II trials. Response rates below 20% can be meaningful if the quality of the responses is good. A few complete remissions, even if the overall frequence of response is low, should lead to a decision to proceed with further testing in that disease. Since multiple doses and schedules may be tested, a Phase II trial for each dose, schedule, and tumor type is required before a drug can be disqualified from further clinical testing. Such decisions are complicated by the heterogeneity of the clinical presentation of most human tumors. For example, a Phase II trial of a new drug in breast cancer can result in different conclusions if the first 14 patients tested have primarily soft tissue involvement (usually quite responsive to chemotherapy), visceral involvement (usually more resistant to drugs), or varying

FIG. 8-7. Strategy for clinical testing of potential new anticancer drugs.

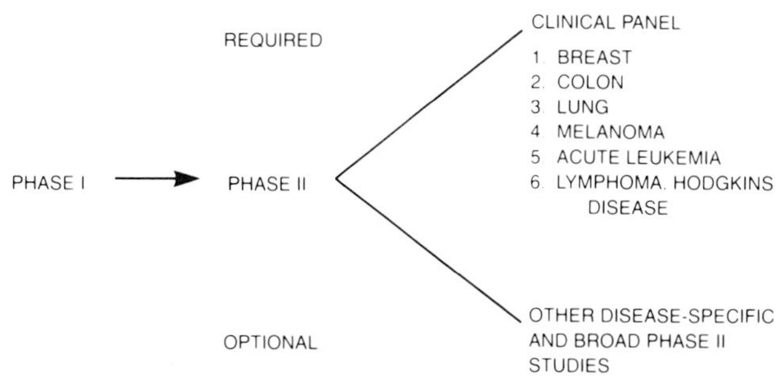

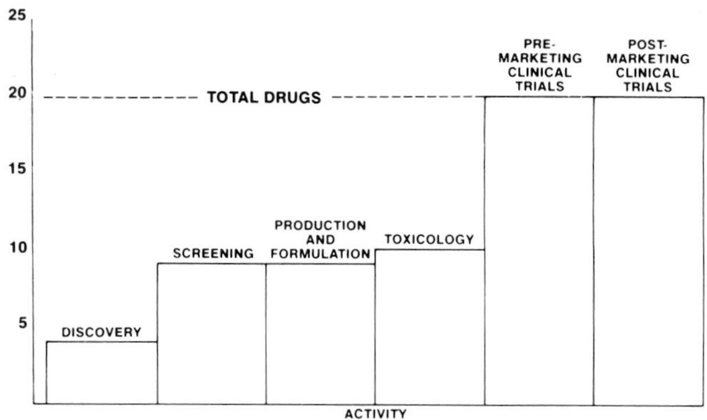

FIG. 8-8. The role that the National Cancer Institute's drug development program has played in development of marketed anticancer drugs since its inception in 1955 (excludes pre-National Cancer Institute drugs).

mixtures of both. The type of previous treatment these patients received, their age, and physical status also will affect the antitumor effect. Given these confounding variables, as a general rule, Phase II studies should be conducted on groups of 30 or more previously untreated patients (if ethically permissible) who have uniform clinical presentations and measurable disease. Using these criteria, a complete Phase II trial can require 600 patients or more.

At the completion of a Phase II trial, a decision is made to proceed or discard the agent. This decision is based on lack of efficacy, excessive, or intolerable toxicity, given the observed therapeutic effect. Since it is not possible to test each new agent against every tumor type, the potential for discarding agents that might be useful in rare tumors is significant.[91] This point is well-illustrated with the drug streptozotocin, which is primarily effective against the rare islet cell carcinoma of the pancreas.[92,93] Its antitumor effect in the rodent screens was minimal and it would have been dropped; however, its diabetogenic effect was noted quite incidentally.[93] In broad Phase II studies, it also has had minimal effectiveness in other tumors. But for its effect in islet cell tumors, dictated by its diabetogenic effect in rodents, it would have been discarded.

If a drug is found effective in Phase II trials, Phase III and IV testing establishes its place in the therapeutic armamentarium. These clinical trials usually require large numbers of patients and are logistically difficult to perform. The issue of randomized vs. historic controls in Phase III and IV tumors is an important one and is discussed in detail in Chapter 10.

Cost–benefit ratio of the development of anticancer drugs approximates that of other drugs developed by industry. For example, for each 4,000 compounds screened in rodents, approximately one is deemed effective and safe enough to reach clinical testing in a Phase I trial. However, only one of about 40,000 compounds screened is eventually found to be useful in the clinics. Preclinical development costs for synthetic products, fermentation products, and plant products averaged \$215,000, \$450,000, and \$400,00 respectively in 1980. Clinical testing through Phase II trials adds an average cost of 1 million dollars to the preclinical costs for each drug, thus, the development of a useful anticancer agent through Phase II testing costs approximately 1.5 million dollars. The cost of running a drug development program is markedly increased, however, by the cost of all the compounds

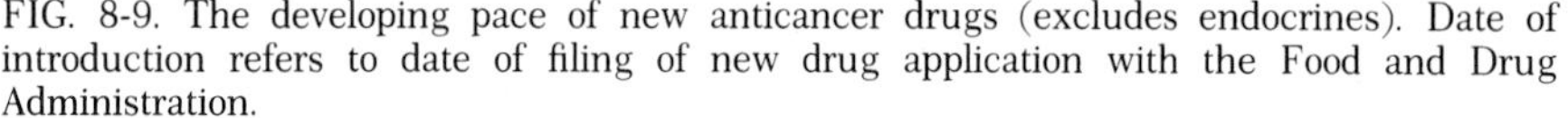
FIG. 8-9. The developing pace of new anticancer drugs (excludes endocrines). Date of introduction refers to date of filing of new drug application with the Food and Drug Administration.

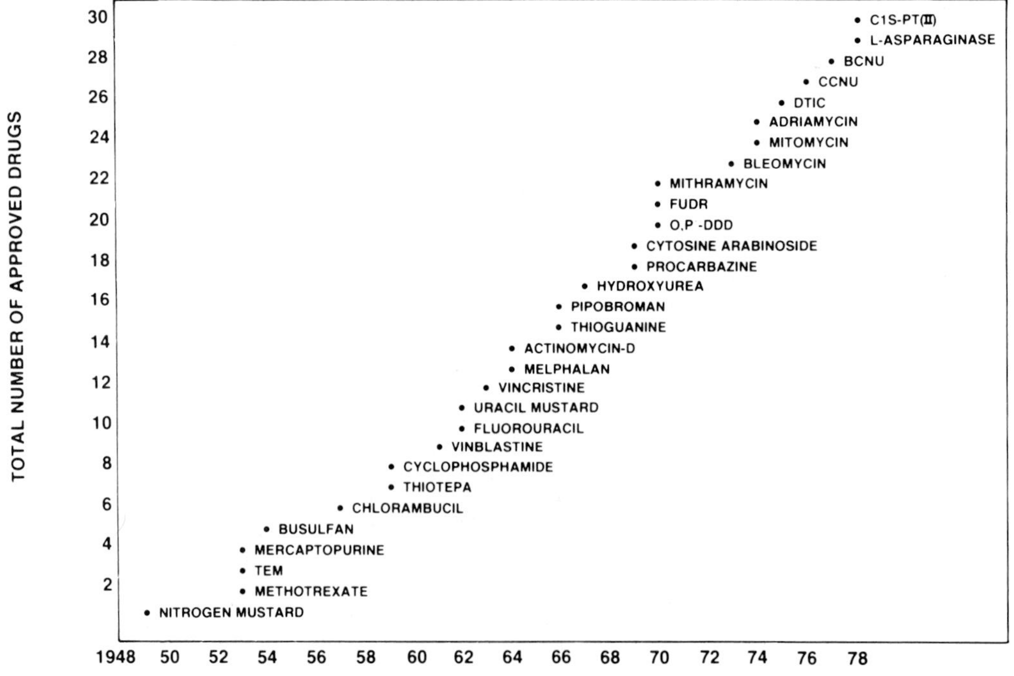

discarded because of toxicity, difficulty in formulation, or lack of human effectiveness as discussed earlier in this chapter.

To date, approximately 30 antitumor drugs are commercially available. Another 70 are in some stage of clinical development. The role played by National Cancer Institute's drug development program in bringing drugs to the market is illustrated in Fig. 8-8. Ten marketed drugs, mostly closely related alkylating agents and antimetabolites, were available prior to the organization of the program. Of the 20 remaining drugs, the program has been involved in premarketing and postmarketing testing of all (and of most in other stages of development) regardless of their origin. This close collaboration with the pharmaceutical industry has been a model of government–industry cooperation. Fig. 8-9 illustrates the pace of the introduction of the new anticancer drugs from 1948 to 1978.

Cancer drugs and their congeners also often have useful effects in noncancerous illness. These are illustrated in Table 8-11.[94]

TABLE 8-11. Antitumor Drugs with Clinical Effectiveness in Non-Neoplastic Diseases

Drug	Use
Vidarabine	Antiviral agent
Allopurinol	Uricosuric agent
Fluorocytosine	Antifungal agent
Azathioprine (Imuran)	Immunosuppressive agent for organ transplantation
Iododeoxyuridine	Antiviral agent
Pyrimethamine	Antimalarial agent
Trifluoromethyl thymidine	Antiviral agent

Clinical Application of Cancer Chemotherapy

The clinical setting for most cancer patients is illustrated in Fig. 8-10. On the left ordinate of the figure, the three separate scales indicate the relationship of size, weight, and cell number of a tumor mass. The line indicating the lethal cell number intersects with 10^{12} cells, approximately 1000 grams (1 kg) of tumor, of large but indeterminant size (the sum total of multiple metastases). The lower level of detectability of a mass occurs when it reaches about 1cm^3 in size, weighs approximately 1 g, and contains 10^9 or 1 billion cancer cells. One cancer cell and its progeny must go through nearly 30 doublings to reach that size; in ten more doublings the cell number will reach the lethal number of 10^{12} cells.[25] Thus, even small cancers at the limits of detection are far advanced in their life cycle. It is also important to realize that each undetectable micrometastasis may contain from 10^1 to 10^8 cells. The total tumor burden will be the sum of all micrometastases. Keep in mind that a patient with one clinically detectable (1 cm) mass may actually have a tumor burden well in excess of 1 billion cells.

As shown by the solid line originating in the left lower corner of Fig. 8-10, a tumor may grow and spontaneously regress due to host influences that are at present unclear, or continue to grow to a detectable level, as shown in the shaded gray area. If a patient presents with a solitary mass that is resected or treated with surgery or x-irradiation, the tumor burden is reduced abruptly below the level of host control and cure may result. If viable micrometastases are present outside the treatment field, recurrence may occur leading to the reappearance of the tumor at point C. If visible metastases were present at point A, drug therapy may result in reduction of visible tumor to levels below clinical detectability, that is, a complete clinical remission. For those tumors very responsive to chemotherapy, continued treatment may lead to cure. But more often, after variable periods of time, regrowth occurs as indicated by the arrow at point E. In this case, the interval between points B and E in Fig. 8-10 represent the duration of complete remission. For cancers that are systemic at the outset (leukemias, multiple myeloma, and others) this interval may be relatively long and the prolongation of life equals the duration of remission. For most visceral malignancies that

FIG. 8-10. Relationship of size, weight, and cell number to the clinical course of patient with cancer over time.

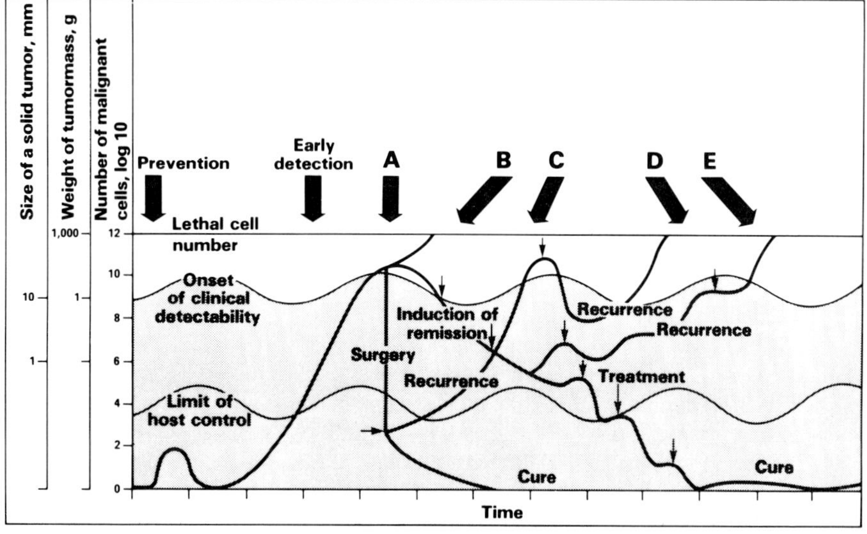

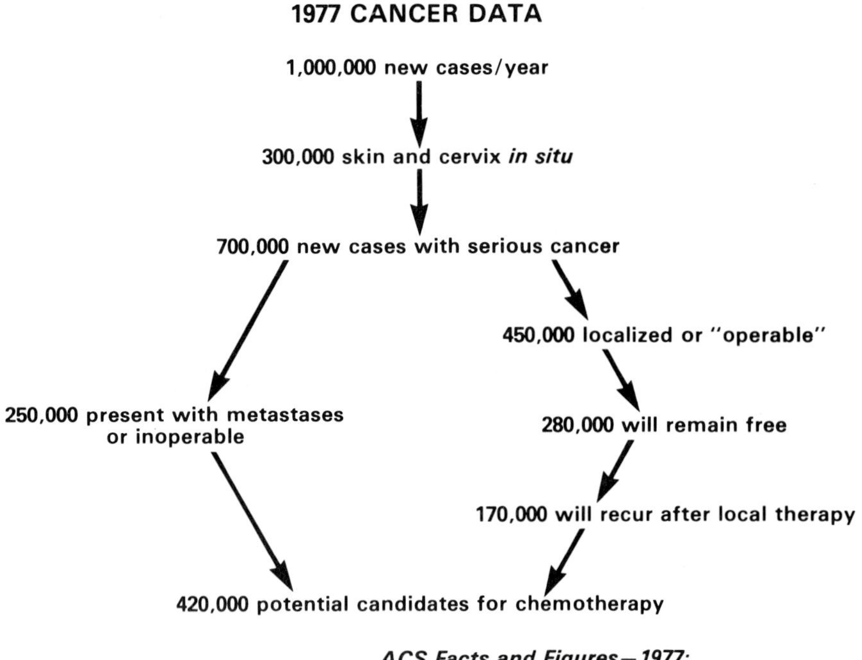

FIG. 8-11. Subdivision of one million cases of cancer in 1977 according to presentation and eligibility for chemotherapy.

recur after surgery (at point C) reduction of tumor mass by currently available chemotherapy may be less and the interval of remission may be shorter (between points C and D). Thus, patients present to their doctor in one of four different ways (as illustrated in Fig. 8-10): 1) with a solitary mass (point A) that either lends itself to resection or treatment with radiotherapy; 2) with a cancer that presents as a systemic disease (point B); 3) with recurrent cancer after local treatment with surgery or radiation therapy (point C); or 4) with recurrent cancer after systemic treatment (points D and E).

The majority of newly diagnosed cancer patients present at point A, and are managed for cure by surgeons or radiotherapist (with or without the help of a chemotherapist). Those that present at points B, C, D, and E are usually seen by medical oncologists since the correct treatment is chemotherapy, or by radiotherapists and surgeons for palliative treatment. One notable exception are those patients who present at point C. Recent data suggest that resection of metastases to the lung in patients with osteosarcoma may be most effectively managed by resection with or without chemotherapy (see Chapter 29).

The use of chemotherapy has expanded widely.[8] If the year 1977, when a convenient figure of 1 million new cases of cancer diagnosed in the United States is taken as a reference point, the application of chemotherapy can be easily illustrated (see Fig. 8-11).[95] Of the 1 million new cases, approximately 300,000 had easily curable skin cancer or *in situ* carcinoma of the cervix. When these 300,000 patients are excluded from consideration because they are easily cured, 700,000 patients with "more serious" cancers remain. To estimate the fraction of these 700,000 patients who presented to their physicians with apparently localized cancer and those curable with local treatment, several pieces of information can be used. To obtain the fraction potentially cured by local treatment in 1977, look at the relative survival rate reported in the Public Health Service Report #5 published in 1976 (41%).[96] This figure of 41% is reduced by 1% to remove patients who are cured *exclusively* by chemotherapy (see below). Multiply this by 700,000, yielding 280,000 patients. To estimate the number of patients who presented with localized or operable cancers (shown in Fig. 8-11), some 450,000, data from standard textbooks on operating rates were used. This corresponds to the patients who present at point A in Fig. 8-10. When those who survive 5 years (some 280,000) are subtracted from the number of patients with localized disease (450,000), 170,000 patients remain who, although operable, will develop recurrent tumor and are therefore potential candidates for adjuvant chemotherapy (point C, Fig. 8-10). The difference between 700,000 (total serious cancers) and 450,000 (localized or operable cases) also provides an estimate of the number of patients (250,000) who initially present with inoperable tumors or with evidence of distant metastases (point B, Fig. 8-10.) The addition of the 250,000 patients who present with inoperable or metastic disease to the 170,000 patients who recur after local therapy provides a total of 420,000 patients who were potential candidates for chemotherapy in 1977 (points B and C, Fig. 8-10).

The group of patients who presented with metastatic disease (250,000) has always been the first to receive new forms of chemotherapy. They can now be divided into two important subunits—those who experience demonstrable benefit from chemotherapy and those who do not (see Fig. 8-12). Benefit in this case is defined as evidence that the prolongation of survival occurs in patients who respond to chemotherapy

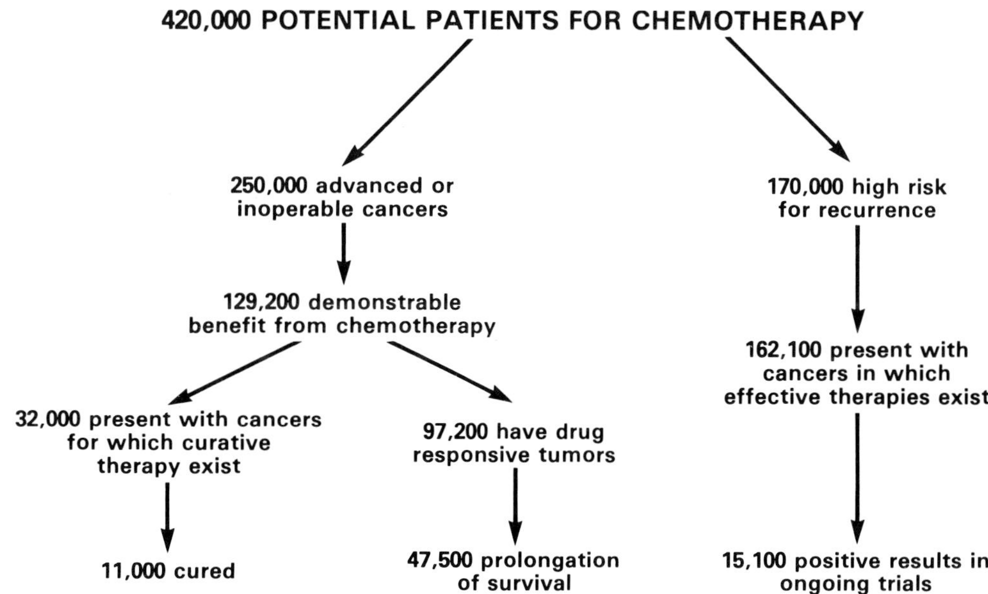

FIG. 8-12. Subdivision of patients who might be candidates for chemotherapy. Groups established according to response to treatment.[8] Incidence figures are from 1977 American Cancer Society data.[85]

compared to those who do not. A minimal response rate of 20% is used here to define drug-responsive tumors. While it is certainly apparent that a partial response rate of 20% is of minimal clinical benefit, clinical investigators have always used such data as the starting point for future, more effective treatment programs.

Using these criteria, nearly 129,000 of the 250,000 patients are estimated to derive benefit from chemotherapy. Patients who experience benefit from chemotherapy can also be divided into two sharply distinctive groups—those patients with advanced cancer potentially curable using chemotherapy alone (32,000 in 1977), and, those who have drug-responsive tumors but cannot be considered curable with existing chemotherapy (97,000 in 1977). These two groups are depicted in Tables 8-12 and 8-13.

In Table 8-12, 12 cancers are listed in which a fraction of patients with advanced cancer can now be considered curable with chemotherapy alone. Approximately 44,500 new cases of these 12 cancers were diagnosed in 1977. Of these, 32,000 patients had advanced cancer at the time of presentation. By applying the results of the best available treatment programs described in this text and extrapolating these results to nationwide application, the fraction who remain free of disease beyond 5 years can be estimated. Those calculations result in the identification of approximately 11,000 of the 32,000 patients as potentially curable with drug programs current in 1977. It should be noted that this group represented less than 10% of all cancers in 1977 and less than 10% of all cancer deaths. Thus, the greatest successes of chemotherapy have occurred in the least common cancers. It is important to note, however, that the successful use of chemotherapy in combination with other modalities extends beyond the groups with metastatic cancer. Some 12,500 of these patients had localized disease (44,500 new cases minus 32,000 with advanced disease) and are potentially curable using the combination of surgery, or x-ray, or both and chemotherapy.

TABLE 8-12. Twelve Cancers in Which a Fraction of Patients with Advanced Disease can be Cured with Chemotherapy*

Choriocarcinoma	Ovarian carcinoma
Acute lymphocytic leukemia in children	Acute myelogenous leukemia
Hodgkin's disease	Wilms' tumor
Diffuse histiocytic lymphoma	Burkitt's lymphoma
Nodular mixed lymphoma	Embryonal rhabdomyosarcoma
Testicular carcinoma	Ewing's sarcoma

* These 12 cancers accounted for about 44,550 new cases in 1977. About 11,000 of these patients were cured with current therapy. These 12 cancers account for less than 10% of all cancers per year and less than 10% of all cancer deaths per year.

TABLE 8-13. Advanced Cancers in which a Fraction of Patients Respond to Chemotherapy and Improved Survival is Demonstrable*

Breast carcinoma	Gastric carcinoma
Chronic myelogenous leukemia	Malignant insulinoma
Chronic lymphocytic leukemia	Endometrial carcinoma
Nodular poorly differentiated lymphocytic lymphoma	Adrenal cortical carcinoma
Multiple myeloma	Medulloblastoma
Small cell carcinoma of the lung	Neuroblastoma
Soft tissue sarcomas	Polycythemia vera
	Prostatic carcinoma
	Glioblastoma

* The cancers listed above account for about 40% of all new cancers per year and about 30% of all cancer deaths.

These 12,500 patients appear as part of the 280,000 patients curable in 1977 (see Fig. 8-11).

Of considerable interest are the 97,200 patients shown in Table 8-13 who have drug-responsive but not drug curable advanced tumors. In this group, responding patients do demonstrate survival benefit, however brief. Complete remissions occur in 20% to 68% of treated patients (*e.g.*, breast cancer–20%, nodular poorly differentiated lymphocytic lymphoma–68%, small cell carcinoma of the lung to 50%, and so on). Using the best response rates in the current literature for each of the tumors listed in Table 8-13, 47,500 of these 97,200 patients (49%) can respond sufficiently to have some prolongation of life. Since the average prolongation of life is approximately one year, the use of chemotherapy may result in the addition of 47,500 person-years of life annually. The issue of the quality of this prolonged life is debatable for many of these patients. It depends largely on the type of chemotherapy, the stage of the disease, the motivation and age of the patients, and often the attitude of the physician. Of greater importance, however, is the fact that chemotherapy, partially effective in advanced disease, is identified. This therapy may have its greatest potential for success in the immediate postoperative period for reasons previously discussed. This has certainly been true in breast cancer. The tumors listed in Table 8-13 are among the most common cancers and comprise nearly 40% of all new cancers and approximately 30% of all cancer deaths in 1977.

TABLE 8-14. Some Advanced Cancers in which a Fraction of Patients Respond but no Improvement in Survival has yet been Demonstrated*

Adenocarcinoma of lung	Malignant carcinoid tumors
Bladder carcinoma	Malignant melanoma
Carcinoma of cervix	Thyroid carcinoma
Colon carcinoma	Rectal carcinoma
Head and neck carcinoma	Hepatocellular carcinoma
Hypernephroma	Carcinoma of the penis

* The cancers listed above account for about 35% of all new cancers per year and 30% of all cancer deaths.

TABLE 8-15. Patients Potentially Benefiting from Adjuvant Therapy

	PATIENTS WITH LOCAL DISEASE	NUMBERS BENEFITTED
Breast carcinoma	35,600	7,120
Rectal carcinoma	14,600	2,920
Colon carcinoma	29,400	2,940
Gastric carcinoma	4,400	880
Melanoma	6,800	680
Soft tissue sarcoma	1,400	560
Lung carcinoma	17,600	—
Testicular carcinoma	2,000	1,800
Ovarian carcinoma	4,800	—
Bladder carcinoma	24.200	—
Cervical carcinoma	9,800	—
Head and neck carcinoma	11,500	—
TOTALS	162,100	16,900

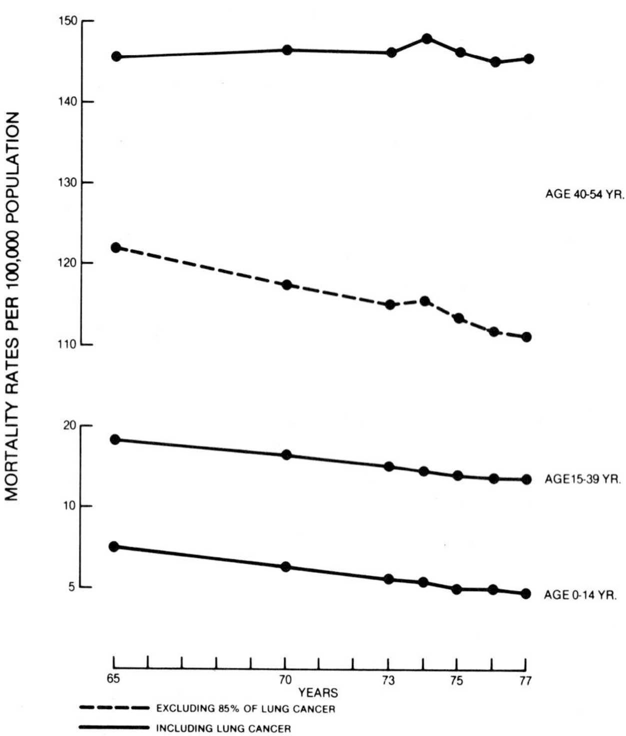

FIG. 8-13. Age-specific cancer mortality rates: all sites, all races, both sexes—1965–1977. A significant decrease in mortality from cancer is noted for the 40–54 age group when 85% of lung cancers are excluded.

Table 8-14 shows the remaining group of 121,000 patients who may show evidence of a partial response to drug treatment, but usually experience no demonstrable survival benefit. Patients in this group represent one-third of all cancers diagnosed in 1977 and nearly 30% of all cancer deaths. While partial responses in these patients have not led to survival benefit, the use of some of the therapies developed in patients with advanced disease has resulted in demonstrable clinical benefit in adjuvant chemotherapy programs as has been noted in rectal cancer (see Chapter 22).

Estimates of Those Who May Benefit from Postoperative Chemotherapy

In 1977, the estimate of patients who develop tumor recurrences following primary treatment was 170,000 (see Figs. 8-11 and 8-12). The number of patients in this group for whom there is a testable drug regimen (using the criteria previously described) is calculated to be 162,100 (see Table 8-15). The number of patients in each category of disease who will develop recurrences after local treatment is estimated in the left column of this table. The column on the right is the estimated number of patients that could benefit if the drug therapy available today were applied, on a nationwide basis, in 1977.

Summary of the Numerical Impact of Chemotherapy

Using the 1977 data and assuming widespread use of chemotherapy, long-term useful benefit (disease-free survival off therapy) can be expected in the following 38,600 patients:

1. the 11,000 patients with advanced cancers that are now curable by chemotherapy alone (Table 8-12)
2. The 12,500 patients with localized presentations of these same tumors that are effectively treated with combinations of local treatment and chemotherapy and
3. the 15,100 patients who may be deriving benefit from widespread application of current adjuvant chemotherapy programs (Table 8-15).

It is difficult to accurately predict the actual degree of the use of chemotherapy. It is likely that between 200,000 and 400,000 patients a year are receiving it while only about 40,000 are cured by it. National mortality data suggest the application is wide-spread. For example, the tumors shown in Table 8-12 occur at younger ages. Age-specific mortality data show sharp reduction in national mortality in patients with cancer under the age of 45 (see Fig. 8-13).[97]

REFERENCES

1. DeVita VT: Cell kinetics and the chemotherapy of cancer. Cancer Chemother Rep. 2:23–33, part 3, 1971
2. Steel GG: Cell loss from experimental tumors. Cell Tissue Kinet 1:193–207, 1968
3. Marshall EK Jr: Historical perspectives in chemotherapy. *In* Goldin A and Hawking IF (eds): Advances in Chemotherapy, vol. 1, pp. 1–8. New York, Academic Press, 1964
4. Waksman SA (ed): Streptomycin, Nature and Practical Applications. Baltimore, Williams & Wilkins, 1949
5. Glassroth J, Robins AG, Snider DE Jr: Tuberculosis in the 1980's. N Engl J Med 302:1441–1450, 1980
6. DeVita VT: Human models of human diseases: breast cancer and the lymphomas. Int J Radiat Oncol Biol Phys 5:1855–1867, 1979
7. DeVita VT: The evolution of therapeutic research in cancer. N Engl J Med 298:907–910, 1978
8. DeVita VT, Henney JE, Hubbard SM: Estimation of the numerical and economic impact of chemotherapy in the treatment of cancer. In Burchenal JH and Oettgen HS (eds): Cancer Achievements, Challenges, and Prospects for the 1980's, pp 857–880. New York, Grune and Stratton, 1981
9. Skipper HE, Schabel FM Jr, Wilcox WS: Experimental evaluation of potential anticancer agents. XII. On the criteria and kinetics associated with "curability" of experimental leukemia. Cancer Chemother Rep. 35:1–111, 1964
10. Skipper HE: Reasons for success and failure in treatment of murine leukemias with the drugs now employed in treating human leukemias. Cancer Chemotherapy, vol. 1. pp 1–166. Ann Arbor, MI, University Microfilms International, 1978
11. Skipper HE, Schabel FM Jr, Mellet LB et al: Implications of biochemical, cytokinetic, pharmacologic, and toxicologic relationships in the design of optimal therapeutic schedules. Cancer Chemother Rep. 54:431–450, 1950
12. Yankee RA, DeVita VT, Perry S: The cell cycle of leukemia L1210 cells *in vivo*. Cancer Res 27:2381–2385, 1967
13. Young RC, DeVita VT: Cell cycle characteristics of human solid tumors *in vivo*. Cell Tissue Kinet 3:285–295, 1970
14. Clarkson B, Ohkita T, Ota K et al: Studies of the cellular proliferation in human leukemia. I. Estimation of growth rates of leukemic and normal hematopoietic cells in two adults with acute leukemia given single injections of tritiated thymidine. J Clin Invest 46:506–529, 1967
15. Whang-Peng J, Perry S, Knutsen TA et al: Cell cycle characteristics, maturation and phagocytosis *in vitro* in blast cells from patients with chronic myelocytic leukemia. Blood 38:153–161, 1971
16. Tannock I: Cell kinetics and chemotherapy: A critical review. Cancer Treat Rep 62:1117–1133, 1978
17. Perry S, Moxley JH, Weiss GH et al: Studies of leukocyte function by liquid scintillation counting in normal individuals and in patients with chronic myelocytic leukemia. J Clin Invest 45:1388–1399, 1966
18. DeVita VT, Denham C, Perry S: Relationship of normal CDFl mouse leukocyte kinetics to growth characteristics of leukemia L1210. Cancer Res 29:1067–1071, 1969
19. Simpson-Herren L, Sanford AH, Holmquist JP: Cell population kinetics of transplanted Lewis lung carcinoma. Cell Tissue Kinet 7:349–361, 1974
20. Mendelsohn ML: The growth fraction: A new concept applied to tumors. Science 132:1496, 1960
21. Goldie JH, Coldman AJ: A mathematic model for relating the drug sensitivity of tumors to the spontaneous mutation rate. Cancer Treat Rep 63:1727–1733, 1979
22. Luria SE, Delbruck M: Mutations of bacteria from virus sensitivity to virus resistance. Genetics 28: 491–511, 1943
23. Bruce WR, Meeker BE, Valeriote FA: Comparison of the sensitivity of normal hematopoietic and transplanted lymphoma colony-forming cells to chemotherapeutic agents administered *in vivo*. JNCI 37:233–245, 1966
24. Schabel FM Jr, Simpson-Herren L: Some variables in experimental tumor systems which complicate interpretation of data from *in vivo* kinetic and pharmacologic studies with anticancer drugs. Antibiotics Chemotherapy 23:113–127, 1978
25. Brockman RW: Circumvention of resistance. Pharmacologic basis of cancer chemotherapy. 27th Annual Symposium on Fundamental Research, University of Texas, M.D. Anderson Hospital and Tumor Institute, pp. 691–711. Baltimore, Williams & Wilkins, 1975
26. Freireich EJ et al: Quantitative comparison of toxicity of anticancer agents in mouse, rat, dog, monkey and man. Cancer Chemother Rep. 50:219–244, 1966
27. DeVita VT Jr, Young RC, Canellos GP: Combination versus single-agent chemotherapy: review of the basis of selection of drug treatment of cancer. Cancer 35:98, 1975
28. Hutchison DJ, Schmid FA: Cross-resistance and collateral sensitivity. Drug-Resistance and Selectivity: Biochemical and Cellular Basis, pp. 73–126. New York, Academic Press, 1973
29. Brockman RW: Resistance to therapeutic agents. In Burchenal JH and Oettgen HS (eds): Cancer Achievements, Challenges, and Prospects for the 1980's. New York, Grune and Stratton, (in press)
30. Hutchison DJ: Cross-resistance and collateral sensitivity studies in cancer chemotherapy. In Haddow A, Weinhouse S (eds): Advances in Cancer Research, Vol 7, pp. 235–350. New York, Academic Press, Inc., 1963
31. Klein M: A mechanism for the development of resistance to streptomycin and penicillin. J Bacteriol 53:463–467, 1947
32. Shannon JA, Earle DP, Brodie BB et al: The pharmacologic basis for the rational use of atabrene in the treatment of malaria. J Pharmacol Exp Therap 81:307–330, 1944
33. Furth J, Kahn MC: The transmission of leukemia of mice with a single cell. Am J Cancer 31:276–282, 1937
34. Goldin A, Venditti JM, Humphries SR et al: Influences of the concentration of leukemic inoculum on the effectiveness of treatment. Science 123:840, 1956
35. Law LW: Origin of the resistance of leukemic cells to folic acid antagonists. Nature 169:628–629, 1952
36. Luria SE, Delbruck M: Mutations of bacteria from virus sensitivity to virus resistance. Genetics 28:491–511, 1943
37. Siminovitch L: On the nature of heritable variation in cultured somatic cells. Cell 7:1–11, 1976
38. Skipper HE: Concurrent comparisons of some 2-, 3-, and 4-drug

combinations delivered simultaneously and sequentially (L1210 and P388 leukemia systems). Cancer Chemotherapy, Vol 9, pp 1–76. Ann Arbor, MI, University Microfilms International, 1980
39. Skipper HE, Hutchison DJ, Schabel FM Jr et al: A quick reference chart on cross-resistance between anticancer agents. Cancer Treat Rep 56:493–498, 1972
40. Fisher RI, DeVita VT, Hubbard SP et al: Prolonged disease-free survival in Hodgkin's disease with MOPP reinduction after first relapse. Ann Intern Med 90:761–763, 1979
41. DeVita VT: The consequences of the chemotherapy of Hodgkin's disease: The 10th annual David A. Karnofsky lecture. Cancer 47:1–13, 1981
42. Schabel FM: Concepts from systemic treatment of micrometastases. Cancer 35:15–24, 1975
43. Schabel FM: Rationale for adjuvant chemotherapy. Cancer 39:2875–2882, 1977
44. Schabel FM Jr: Concepts for treatment of micrometastases developed in murine systems. Am J Roentgenol Radium Ther Nucl Med 127:500–511, 1976
45. DeVita VT, Schein PS: The use of drugs in combination for the treatment of cancer: rationale and results. N Engl J Med 288:998–1006, 1973
46. Schimke RT, Kaufman RJ, Alt FW et al: Gene amplification and drug resistance in cultured mammalian cell. Science 202:1051–1055, 1978
47. Frei E III, Freireich EJ, Gehan E et al: Studies of sequential and combination antimetabolite therapy in acute leukemia: 6-mercaptopurine and methotrexate: from the acute leukemia group. Blood 18:431–454, 1961
48. Frei E III, Canellos GP: Dose: A critical factor in cancer chemotherapy. Amer J Med (in press)
49. Brindley CO et al: Further comparative trial of thio-phosphoroamide and mechlorethamine in patients with melanoma and Hodgkin's disease. J Chronic Dis 17:19, 1964
50. Frei E III, Spurr CL, Brindley CO et al: Clinical studies of dichloromethotrexate (NSC 29630). Clin Pharmacol Ther 6:160–171, 1965
51. Cullen MH, Creaven PJ, Fossieck JR et al: Intensive chemotherapy of small cell bronchogenic carcinoma. Cancer Treat Rep 61:349–353, 1977
52. Pinkel D, Hernandez K, Borella L et al: Drug dose and remission duration in childhood lymphocytic leukemia. Cancer 27:247–256, 1971
53. Gehan E, Coltman C: Southwest Oncology Group, unpublished observations, 1980
54. Bonadonna G, Valagussa P: Dose-response effect of CMF in breast cancer. Proc Am Soc Clin Oncol 21:413, 1980
55. DeVita VT, Serpick AA, Carbone PP: Combination chemotherapy in the treatment of advanced Hodgkin's disease. Ann Intern Med 73:881–895, 1970
56. Young RC, Canellos GP, Chabner BA et al: Maintenance chemotherapy for advanced Hodgkin's disease in remission. Lancet 1:1339, 1973
57. Frei E III, Luce JK, Gamble JF et al: Combination chemotherapy in advanced Hodgkin's disease—induction and maintenance of remission. Ann Intern Med 79:376–382, 1973
58. Lewis BJ, DeVita VT: Combination chemotherapy of the lymphomas. Semin Hematol 15:431–462, 1978
59. Li MC, Hertz R, Spencer DB: The effect of methotrexate upon choriocarcinoma and chorioadenoma. Proc Soc Exp Biol Med 93:361–366, 1956
60. Nathanson L, Hall TC, Schilling AC et al: Concurrent combination chemotherapy of human solid tumors: Experience with three-drug regimen and review of the literature. Cancer Res 29:419–425, 1969
61. Potter VR: Sequential blocking of metabolic pathways *in vivo*. Proc Soc Exp Biol Med 76:41–46, 1951
62. Elion GB, Singer S, Hitchings GH: Antagonists of nucleic acid derivatives. VIII. Synergism in combinations of biochemically related antimetabolites. J Biol Chem 208:477–488, 1954
63. Sartorelli AC: Approaches to the combination chemotherapy of transplantable neoplasms. Prog Exp Tumor Res 6:228–288, 1965
64. Freireich EJ, Karon M, Frei E III: Quadruple combination therapy (VAMP) for acute lymphocytic leukemia of childhood. Proc Am Assoc Cancer Res 5:20, 1974
65. Einhorn LH, Donohue JP: Combination chemotherapy in disseminated testicular cancer: The Indiana University experience. Semin Oncol 6:87–93, 1979
66. DeVita VT, Canellos GP, Chabner BA et al: Advanced diffuse histiocytic lymphoma, a potentially curable disease. Lancet 1:248–254, 1975
67. Santoro A, Bonadonna G, Bonfante V et al: Non-cross-resistant regimens (MOPP–ABVD) versus Mopp alone in Stage IV Hodgkin's disease. Proc Am Soc Clin Oncol 21:470, 1980
68. Canellos GP, DeVita VT, Gold CL et al: Cyclical combination chemotherapy in the treatment of advanced breast cancer. Br Med J 1:218–220, 1974
69. Spitzer G, Dicke KA, Valdivieso KB et al: High-dose combination chemotherapy with autologous marrow transplantation in adult solid tumors. Proc Am Soc Clin Oncol 20:406, 1979
70. Phillips GL, Fay JW, Hertzig GP et al: Intensive BCNU autologous bone marrow transplantation therapy of refractory cancer. Exp Hematol 7 (suppl 5):372–384, 1979
71. McIlwain TJ, Healy DW, Gordon MY et al: High-dose melphalan and non-cryopreserved autologous bone marrow treatment of malignant melanoma and neuroblastoma. Exp Hematol 7 (suppl 5):360–372, 1979
72. Takvorian R, Parker IN, Hochberg FH et al: High-dose BCNU with autologous bone marrow rescue for glioblastomas. Proc 11th Internatl Cong Chemother, Abstract 538, 1979
73. Hamburger AW, Salmon SE: Primary bioassay of human tumor stem cells. Science 197:461–463, 1977
74. Salmon SE, Hamburger AW, Soehnlen BJ et al: Quantitation of differential sensitivity of human tumor stem cells to anticancer drugs. N Engl J Med 298:1321–1327, 1978
75. Salmon SE: Application of the human tumor stem cell assay in the development of anticancer therapy. In Burchenal JH and Oettgen HS (eds): Cancer Achievements, Challenges, and Prospects for the 1980's. New York, Grune and Stratton, (in press)
76. Papahadjopoulos D, Poste G, Vail WJ et al: Use of lipid vesicles as carriers to introduce actinomycin D into resistant tumor cells. Cancer Res 36:2988–3012, 1976
77. Weinstein JM, Magin RL, Cysyk RL et al: Treatment of solid L1210 murine tumors with local hyperthermia and temperature-sensitive liposomes containing methotrexate. Cancer Res 40:1388–1396, 1980
78. Dedrick RL, Myers CE, Bungay PM et al: Pharmacokinetic rationale for peritoneal drug administration in treatment of ovarian cancer. Cancer Treat Rep 62:1–11, 1978
79. Jones RB, Myers CE, Guarino AM et al: High volume intraperitoneal chemotherapy ("belly bath") for ovarian cancer: Pharmacologic basis and early results. Cancer Chemother Pharmacol 1:161–166, 1978
80. Jones RB, Collins JM, Myers CE et al: High volume intraperitoneal chemotherapy with methotrexate in patients with cancer. Cancer Res (in press)
81. Goldin A, Schepartz SA, Venditti JM et al: Historical development and current strategy of the National Cancer Institute Drug Development Program. In DeVita VT and Busch H (eds): Methods of Cancer Research, Vol XVI, Cancer Drug Development, Part A, pp. 165–247. New York, Academic Press, 1979
82. DeVita, VT Oliverio VT, Muggia FM et al: The Drug Development Program and Clinical Trials Programs of the Division of Cancer Treatment, National Cancer Institute. Cancer Clin Trials 2:195–216, 1979
83. Zubrod CG, Schepartz S, Leiter J et al: The Chemotherapy Program of the National Cancer Institute: history, analysis, and plans. Cancer Chemother Rep 50:349–540, 1966
84. Hirschberg E: Patterns of response of animal tumors to anticancer agents. Cancer Res (suppl) 23:(no 5, part 2) 521–980, 1963
85. Johnson RK, Goldin A: The clinical impact of screening and other experimental tumor studies. Cancer Treat Rev 2:1–31, 1975
86. Mihich E, Laurence DJR, Laurence DM et al: UICC Workshop on New Animal Models for Chemotherapy of Human Solid Tumors. UICC Technical Report Series 15:1–50, 1974

87. Rosencweig M, Von Hoff DD, Staquet MJ et al: Animal toxicity for early clinical trials with anticancer agents. Cancer Clin Trials (in press)
88. Muggia FM, Rozencweig M, Chiuten DF et al: Phase II trials: Use of a clinical tumor panel and overview of current resources and studies. Cancer Treat Rep 64:1–9, 1980
89. Wooley PV, Schein PS: Clinical pharmacology and phase I trial design. In DeVita VT and Busch H (eds): Methods in Cancer Research. XVII. Cancer Drug Development, part B, pp. 177–199, 1979
90. Muggia FM, McGuire WP, Rosencweig M: Rationale, design and methodology of phase II clinical trials. In DeVita VT and Busch H (eds): Methods in Cancer Research. XVII. Cancer Drug Development, part B, pp. 199–215, 1979
91. Van Hoff DD, Rozencweig M, Soper WT et al: Commentary: Whatever happened to NSC——? An analysis of clinical results of discontinued anticancer agents. Cancer Treat Rep 61:759–768, 1977
92. Arlson RN, Ciaccio EI, Glitzer MS et al: Light and electron microscopy of lesions in rats rendered diabetic with streptozotocin. Diabetes 16:51–56, 1967
93. Schein PS, O'Connell NJ, Blom J et al: Clinical antitumor activity and toxicity of streptozotocin (NSC 85998). Cancer 34:993–1000, 1974
94. Steinberg AD, Plotz PH, Wolff SM et al: Cytotoxic drugs in treatment of non-malignant disease. Ann Intern Med 76:619–642, 1972
95. American Cancer Society: Cancer Facts and Figures. New York, American Cancer Society, 1977
96. Axtell LM, Asire AJ, Myers MH (eds): Cancer Patient Survival, Report No. 5, Cancer Surveillance, Epidemiology, and End Results (SEER) Program. National Cancer Institute, NIH, US-DHEW Publ. No. (NIH)77-992, 1976
97. DeVita VT, Henney JE, Stonehill E: Cancer mortality: The good news. In Jones SE and Salmon SE (eds): Adjuvant Therapy of Cancer II, pp. xv–xx. New York, Grune and Stratton, 1979

Bruce A. Chabner
Charles E. Myers

CHAPTER 9

Clinical Pharmacology of Cancer Chemotherapy

The primary goal of clinical pharmacology is to develop a rational basis for the treatment of disease. Unfortunately, the required information often comes many years after the empirical discovery of active pharmacologic agents, and only in hindsight are the mechanisms of toxicity and therapeutic action illuminated. In dealing with highly toxic agents that possess a narrow therapeutic index, such information is all the more important. It can safely be said that the effective use of cancer chemotherapeutic agents requires a level of pharmacologic understanding unique to the practice of internal medical specialties. The objective of this chapter is to provide the fundamental information on drug action, metabolism, disposition, and toxicity in man that will allow optimal clinical use of the anticancer drugs. This discussion assumes a basic understanding of cell constituents, the general scheme of synthesis of DNA, RNA, and protein, and the fundamental principles of drug transport, metabolism, and excretion. The syntheses of DNA and its precursors is summarized in Figure 9-1. For a further review of these latter topics, the reader is referred to primary texts in biochemistry and pharmacology.[1,2]

Before becoming absorbed in the intricacies of drug action, the reader should be reminded that the essential aspects of safe usage require a few elementary steps:

1. Determination of safe dosage range
2. Choice of an appropriate route of administration
3. Awareness of the incidence and time course of potentially life-threatening toxicity
4. Routes of drug elimination and adjustment of dose to accommodate organ dysfunction
5. Reduction of dose to accommodate overlapping drug toxicities

A few basic tables are provided to allow a rapid confirmation of these essential drug characteristics. Dose, toxicity, and pharmacokinetics of the most important agents are summarized in Table 9-1. Table 9-2 provides dose adjustment guidelines for agents affected by organ dysfunction. Table 9-3 provides a summary of indications for drug level monitoring of anticancer agents. The reader is referred to Chapter 47 for a practical guide to the administration of chemotherapy, its complications, and further information on drug side-effects. The reader should also consult the text for specific discussion and for references to "Methods" papers.

Not all agents listed or discussed in this text are commercially available. For further information on noncommercial drugs, the interested reader should contact the Investigational Drug Branch of the National Cancer Institute, Bethesda, Maryland 20205.

ANTIMETABOLITES

ANTIFOLATES

Antimetabolites are agents that, by virtue of structural similarity with physiologic intermediates, are accepted as fraudulent substrates for vital biochemical reactions and thus interfere with a required cell process. The first agent in the antifolate class of antimetabolites to find clinical application was aminopterin, a 4-NH_2 analog of folic acid (Fig. 9-2). Aminopterin has since been replaced in common usage by the 4-NH_2,N^{10}-methyl analog amethopterin, or methotrexate. The latter, although a less potent antifolate, has more predictable clinical toxicity and at least equal clinical activity.

In the past 20 years, several new antifolate compounds, such as the diaminopyrimidines and quinazolines, have entered clinical trial (see Fig. 9-2); however, none of these compounds has shown clinical activity superior to that of methotrexate.

Mechanism of Action

Methotrexate exerts its cytotoxic effects through inhibition of the enzyme dihydrofolate reductase (Fig. 9-3).[3] This enzyme is responsible for maintaining the intracellular pool of folates in a reduced state; the tetrahydrofolates in turn function as carriers of one-carbon groups required for synthesis of the purine nucleotides and of thymidylate. In the thymidylate synthesis reaction (catalyzed by thymidylate synthestase), N^{5-10} methylene tetrahydrofolate is simultaneously relieved of its one-carbon methylene group and is oxidized to dihydrofolate, an inactive form of folic acid. Thus, in the presence of ongoing thymidylate synthesis, an intact dihydrofolate reductase pathway is needed to recycle oxidized folates to their active tetrahydrofolate form.

Methotrexate, through inhibition of reductase, causes an accumulation of cellular folates in the inactive oxidized form, and a cessation first of thymidylate and then of purine nucleotide synthesis.[4] Thymidylate synthesis inhibition appears to be more sensitive to reduced folate depletion and occurs at free extracellular methotrexate concentrations of 1×10^{-8} M, whereas inhibition of purine synthesis takes place at somewhat higher free drug concentrations (above 1×10^{-7} M). Cell killing proceeds somewhat more efficiently at higher drug levels, presumably because of the greater lethality of the antipurine effects.[5]

The requirement for an excess of free (unbound) drug to produce inhibition of nucleotide biosynthesis is thought to result from the reversible nature of methotrexate binding to dihydrofolate reductase. Although methotrexate is extremely tightly bound in its complex with reductase, a measurable off-rate of inhibitor from enzyme is found in living cells. In the presence of excess dihydrofolate, which builds up "behind" the inhibited reaction, an excess of free drug is required to compete for unoccupied binding sites.

The biomedical effects of methotrexate can be reversed by administration of a reduced folate. The most commonly used rescue agent, leucovorin, or D,L-N^5-formyl-tetrahydrofolic acid, effectively prevents methotrexate toxicity to bone marrow and gastrointestinal epithelium if administered in sufficient doses following 6- to 36-hour infusions of high doses of methotrexate. Longer durations of methotrexate exposure lead to clinically significant toxicity.

The dose of leucovorin required to reverse methotrexate toxicity is dependent upon the antifolate concentration at the time of antidote administration.[6] The reason for this competitive relationship is unclear but may relate to the common use of the reduced folate transport systems by both methotrexate and leucovorin. Other rescue measures employed clinically include administration of thymidine, which restores intracellular pools of thymidine triphosphate (TTP) and of carboxypeptidase G_1, an enzyme that hydrolyzes and inactivates methotrexate. These latter measures are not available for general use.

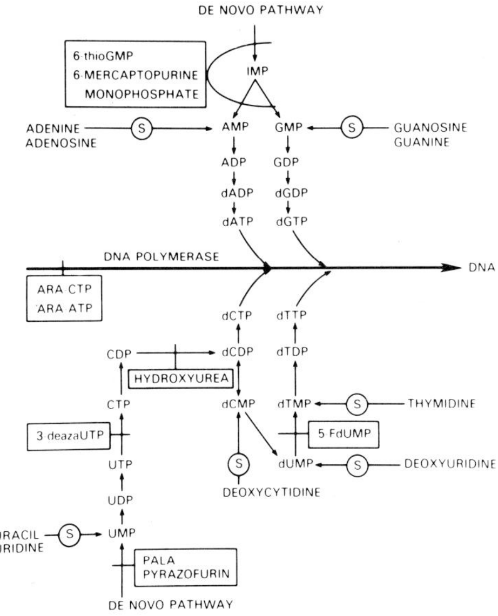

FIG. 9-1. Pathways for synthesis of triphosphate precursors of DNA, and site of action of antimetabolites. Salvage pathways of nucleotide biosynthesis are indicated by —Ⓢ→. Agents, or their metabolites, that inhibit specific synthetic reactions are enclosed in box: □. The inhibited pathway is indicated by ⫱. d = deoxyribose; MP = monophosphate; DP = diphosphate; TP = triphosphate.

U = uracil

G = guanine

T = thymine

A = adenine

C = cytosine

I = inosine

Methotrexate enters cells by a carrier-mediated, active transport mechanism shared by the physiologic reduced folates and reaches equilibrium concentrations in most cells in less than 30 minutes. The affinity constant of the transport system lies in the range of 1 to 10 μM for most mammalian cells; there is some evidence for a second low-affinity transport mechanism that would become important at high drug concentrations, when the high-affinity system is saturated.[7] An active efflux carrier is also found in mammalian cells and is

(Text continues on p. 160.)

TABLE 9-1. Dose, Toxicity, and Pharmacokinetics of Major Antineoplastic Agents

CLASS	DOSE (mg/m²)	ROUTE*	SCHEDULE	ACUTE TOXICITY *WBC*	ACUTE TOXICITY *Platelets*	ACUTE TOXICITY *Nausea/ Vomiting*	OTHER TOXICITY	ELIMINATION (R = renal, M = metabolic)	PLASMA HALF-LIFE (hr)
PLANT ALKALOIDS									
1. Vincristine	1.0	IV	q.w.	Mild	Mild	Mild	Distal neuropathy, inappropriate ADH	M	2.6
2. Vinblastine	4.0	IV	q.d. × 5, or q.w.	Marked	Marked	Mild	Mucositis	M	3.1
3. VP-16	86	IV	2 days q.w.	Moderate	Mild	Mild	Distal neuropathy	M & R	0.5/4/26
	200	PO	2 days q.w.	Moderate	Mild	Moderate			
4. VM-26	67	IV	q.w.	Moderate	Mild	Mild	Distal neuropathy	M & R	3/15
ANTIBIOTICS									
1. Actinomycin D	0.6	IV	q.d. × 5	Marked	Marked	Moderate	Alopecia, mucositis	M & R	?
2. Doxorubicin	75	IV	q.3.w	Marked	Marked	Moderate	Alopecia, cardiomyopathy	M	3/25
3. Daunorubicin	30	IV	q.d. × 3 q.3.w.	Marked	Marked	Moderate	Alopecia, cardiomyopathy	M	?
4. Mithramycin	1.75	IV	q.o.d. to toxicity	Mild	Marked	Severe	Renal, hepatic, neurologic, fever, rash	M	?
For high Ca^{2+}	0.75	IV	q.d. × 3–4 d.	Mild	Mild	Mild			
5. Mitomycin C	2.0	IV	q.d. × 3, q.3.w.	Marked	Marked	Moderate	Renal, pulmonary	M	?
6. Bleomycin	10–15	IV, SC, or IM	q.w.	Rare	Rare	Mild	Skin, pulmonary fibrosis, fever, allergic reactions	R	0.4/2
ANTIMETABOLITES									
1. Methotrexate	25	IM, IV, PO	2 d.q.w.	Moderate–marked	Moderate–marked	Mild	Mucositis, hepatic fibrosis, pneumonitis	R	2/8
	1500 and higher with rescue	IV	6–42 hr infusion q.1–3 w.	Mild	Mild	Moderate	Mucositis, renal failure, rash, anaphylaxis	R	2/8
	12	IT	q.4–7 d.	Mild	Mild	None	Seizures, coma, arachnoiditis	R	12 (CSF)
2. 5-Fluorouracil	500	IV	q.d. × 5 or q.w.	Moderate–marked	Moderate–marked	Moderate	Diarrhea, conjunctivitis, mucositis	M	0.3
	500	IA	q.d. × 10	Mild	Mild	Mild	Catheter-related	M	0.3
	500	IV	infusion × 5 d.	Mild	Mild	Mild	Mucositis, diarrhea	M	0.3
3. 6-Mercaptopurine	100	PO	q.d. × 5	Moderate–marked	Moderate–marked	Mild	Cholestasis	M	0.3–0.6
4. 6-Thioguanine	100	IV	q.d. × 5	Moderate–marked	Moderate–marked	Mild	Cholestasis	M	1.5
5. Cytosine arabinoside	100	IV infusion or bolus	q.12 h × 5–10 d	Marked	Marked	Moderate	Cholestasis, mucositis	M	0.15
				Marked	Marked	Severe	Neurotoxicity, mucositis	M	rapid
				Marked	Marked	Mild	Gastritis	R & M	1.7
6. 5-Azacytidine	200	IV	q.5 d						
7. Hydroxyurea	1000	PO, IV	q.d.						

MISCELLANEOUS									
1. DTIC	250	IV	q.d. × 5	Moderate	Moderate	Marked	Flulike syndrome	M	3
2. Procarbazine	100	PO	q.d. × 10–14 d	Moderate	Moderate	Moderate	Rash, pneumonitis, MAO inhibition	M	3
3. Hexamethylmelamine	150–300	PO	q.d. × 10–14 d.	Mild	Mild	Moderate–marked	Peripheral and central neurotoxicity	M	5–10
4. L-asparaginase	1000–2000 units	IV	q.d. × 10–20 d.	Rare	Rare	Moderate	Pancreatitis, clotting abnormalities, hyperglycemia (see Table 5)	M	14
5. o,p′-DDD	5000	PO	q.d.	None	None	Marked	Diarrhea, skin, depression	M	?
ALKYLATING AGENTS									
1. Cyclophosphamide	400	IV	q.d. × 5	Marked	Mild	Moderate	Cystitis, water retention, alopecia	M	6–12
	100	PO	q.d. × 14	Moderate	Mild	Mild			
2. Melphalan	4	PO	q.d.	Moderate	Moderate	Mild		M	2
	8	IV	q.d. × 5	Marked	Marked	Moderate			
3. Busulfan	2–6	PO	q.d.	Marked	Marked	Mild	Pulmonary fibrosis	M	?
4. BCNU	225	IV	q.6 w.	Marked	Marked	Marked	Alopecia, pulmonary fibrosis, renal failure	M	?
5. CCNU	100–150	PO	q.6 w.	Marked	Marked	Moderate	Alopecia	M	?
6. MeCCNU	150–200	PO	q.6 w.	Marked	Marked	Moderate	Alopecia, pulmonary fibrosis, renal failure	M	?
7. Streptozotocin	500	IV	q.d. × 5 q.3–4 w.	Mild	Mild	Moderate–marked	Renal failure, hyperglycemia, hepatic enzyme elevation	R	0.25
8. cis-diamminedichloroplatinum	50–125	IV	q.4 w.	Moderate	Moderate	Severe	Renal failure, Mg^{2+} wasting, peripheral neuropathy	R & M	0.3/72 +

* IV = intravenously.
PO = per os.
SC = subcutaneously.
IM = intramuscularly.
IT = intrathecally.
IA = intra-abdominally.

TABLE 9-2. Drugs Requiring Dose Modification for Organ Dysfunction

AGENT	ORGAN DYSFUNCTION	SUGGESTED DOSE MODIFICATION
Methotrexate	Renal failure or ↓ creatinine clearance	In proportion to ↓ creatinine clearance (normal 60 ml/min/m^2)
cis-Platinum	Renal failure	In proportion to creatinine clearance
Cyclophosphamide	Renal failure (creatinine clearance below 25 ml/min)	50% decrease
Bleomycin	Renal failure (creatinine clearance below 25 ml/min)	50–75% decrease
Streptozotocin	Renal failure (creatinine clearance below 25 ml/min)	50–75% decrease
Doxorubicin Daunorubicin Vincristine Vinblastine VP-16 VM-26	Hepatic dysfunction	1. Only approximate guidelines can be offered and are probably inaccurate. 2. For bilirubin of >1.5 mg/100 ml, reduce dose by 50%. 3. For bilirubin of >3.0 mg/100 ml, reduce dose by 75%.

readily blocked by the antitumor alkaloid, vincristine. This inhibition has led to the use of vincristine prior to methotrexate in clinical protocols, although there is no evidence that this combination produces enhanced intracellular methotrexate concentrations or augmented therapeutic activity. It is likely that the vincristine concentrations present after clinical use are too low to affect methotrexate transport.

Methotrexate undergoes transformation to polyglutamate forms by a process analogous to the polyglutamation of physiologic folates.[8] The methotrexate polyglutamates, consisting of the parent molecule plus from one to four additional glutamates in γ-peptide linkage, are slowly formed in hepatic and tumor cells and in skin fibroblasts, and over a matter of hours gradually become the predominant form of drug found intracellularly. The polyglutamates bind with equal or greater avidity to dihydrofolate reductase, as compared to the binding of the parent drug, and after removal of free drug, persist intracellularly for a longer period than the parent compound. Thus, polyglutamate formation may constitute an important determinant of the duration of drug action in both normal and malignant cells.

The kinetic aspects of methotrexate cytotoxicity are important considerations in clinical chemotherapy. For bone marrow granulocyte precursors and for experimental tumors, cell kill is proportional to the duration of exposure to methotrexate. Greater cell kill is also seen with increases in drug concentration above the threshold required for inhibition of DNA synthesis, but in this relationship cell kill is approximately

TABLE 9-3. Drug Monitoring in Cancer Therapy*

AGENT	ASSAY (see text)	USES
Methotrexate	Competitive binding to enzyme or to antibody	1. Early detection of patients at high risk of toxicity in high-dose therapy. Drug level $>5 \times 10^{-7}$ M at 48 hr alerts to need for increased and prolonged leucovorin. In toxic patients, tailor leucovorin dosage to plasma methotrexate level. 2. Aid in differential diagnosis of neurotoxicity. High drug level in cerebrospinal fluid favors drug reaction. 3. Predict drug clearance in patients with altered renal function. Allow choice of safe dose.
5-Fluorouracil	HPLC	Design intra-arterial and intraperitoneal chemotherapy regimens with acceptable systemic toxicity. Detect inappropriately elevated ($>10^{-5}$ M) venous blood levels.
Hexamethylmelamine L-Phenylalanine mustard	HPLC HPLC	Determine plasma levels after oral therapy to assure adequate bioavailability.
Adriamycin	HPLC	Determine plasma pharmacokinetics in patients with hepatic dysfunction.

* See text for references to specific drug assays.

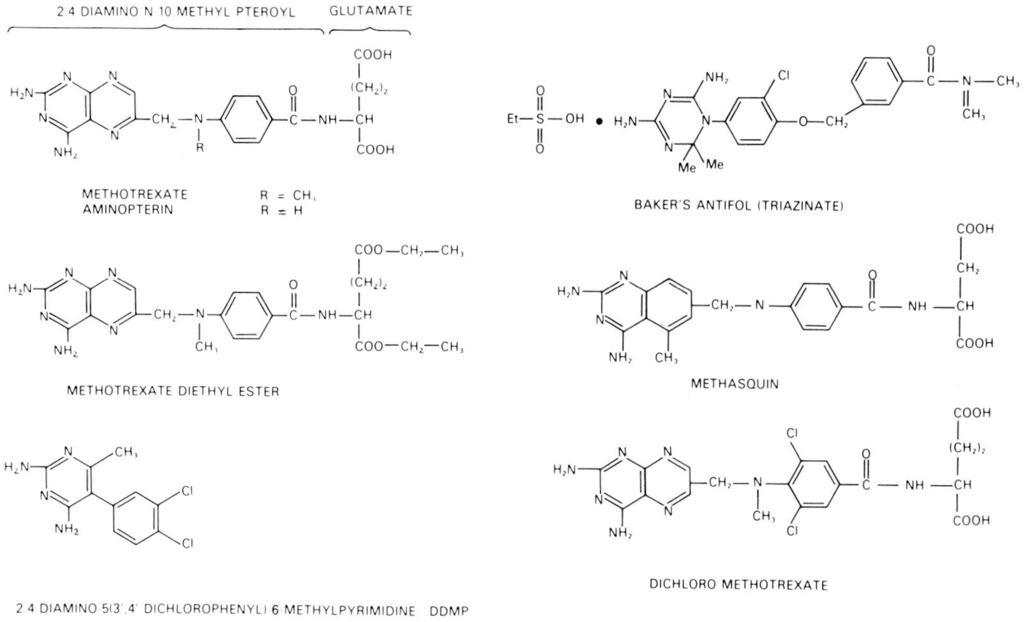

2,4 DIAMINO N 10 METHYL PTEROYL
GLUTAMATE
METHOTREXATE R = CH3
AMINOPTERIN R = H
BAKER'S ANTIFOL (TRIAZINATE)
METHOTREXATE DIETHYL ESTER
METHASQUIN
DICHLORO METHOTREXATE
2,4 DIAMINO-5(3',4' DICHLOROPHENYL)-6-METHYLPYRIMIDINE (DDMP)

FIG. 9-2. Structure of antifolates.

correlated with the log of drug concentration. The dependence on duration of exposure can best be explained by the S-phase specifically of cell kill by antifolates; nonproliferating cells are extremely resistant to this class of compounds.

Resistance of tumor cells to antifolates is conferred by several different biochemical mechanisms. It is unclear which of these mechanisms accounts for the development of resistance in the clinical setting. The best understood of these mechanisms are the deletion of the reduced folate transport system and an increase in the concentration of dihydrofolate reductase. The increase in enzyme concentration occurs as the result of amplification of the gene coding for this enzyme and can readily be induced by exposure of cells to graded increases in drug concentration in cell culture systems.[9] The appearance of increased enzyme levels is correlated with new bits of chromosomal material called double minutes, which become integrated into chromosomes and appear as broad new bands of homogeneously staining genetic material. This integrated genetic material is then heritable and becomes a stable characteristic of the resistant cell lines. It is not known whether gene amplification accounts for the increased enzyme levels in resistant human tumor cells, although this seems to be a probable mechanism of resistance to methotrexate and other metabolic inhibitors.

Clinical Pharmacology and Pharmacokinetics

Because of the common use of methotrexate in high-dose regimens and the well-understood relationship between extracellular drug concentration and inhibition of DNA synthesis, monitoring of methotrexate concentrations in plasma has assumed importance as a tool for guiding drug dosage, detecting patients at high risk of toxicity, and allowing institution of rescue measures in high-risk situations. At least four methods are available for methotrexate assay,[10] all providing rapid and sensitive analysis; these include an enzyme inhibition assay using dihydrofolate reductase (the most cumbersome of the group); a competitive protein binding assay that uses reductase as the binding protein[11]; a radioimmunoassay that utilizes an antibody to the methotrexate–albumin complex[11]; and an enzyme-linked immunoassay. The competitive protein binding assay is specific for ligands that bind tightly to the enzyme active site, whereas the immunoassays show degrees of cross-reactivity

FIG. 9-3. Sites of action of methotrexate (*MTX*) and 5-fluorodeoxyuridylate (*5-FdUMP*). Methotrexate block of dihydrofolate reductase (*DHFR*) and 5-FdUMP inhibition of thymidylate synthetase (*T.S.*) are shown. Folate abbreviations: FH_2 = dihydrofolate; FH_4 = tetrahydrofolate. (Donehower RC, Myers CE, Chabner BA: New developments on the mechanism of action of antineoplastic drugs. Life Sci 25:1–14, 1979)

N5 Formyl FH4 (Leucovorin)
MTX
dTMP
FH2
DHFR
FH4
N10 Formyl FH4
Purine Nucleotides
5-FdUMP
T.S.
N5,10 Methenyl FH4
dUMP
N5,10 Methylene FH4

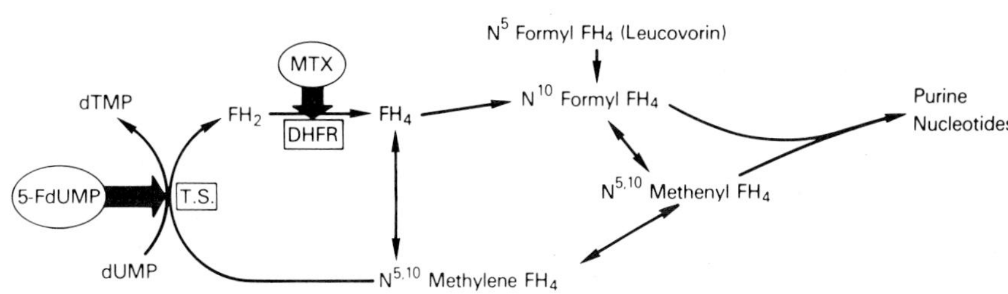

with a methotrexate metabolite, 2,4-diamino-N^{10} methylpteroic acid (DAMPA). This metabolite is found in increasing concentrations in later time samples and thus produces spuriously high assay results. High-pressure liquid chromatographic assay systems can be used to produce clean separation of methotrexate from contaminants and metabolites, with quantitation of the various peaks by spectral or other assay methods, but are not practical for routine clinical monitoring.

Methotrexate is well absorbed orally in doses less than 25 mg per m^2, but bioavailability becomes erratic for larger doses. Thus, the drug is usually administered intravenously. The plasma pharmacokinetics after intravenous administration vary from patient to patient, but over the clinical dose range of 25 to 1500 mg/m^2 generally follow a three-phase disappearance pattern. A brief distributional phase is followed by a primary elimination half-life of 2 to 3 hours, and a final phase of elimination with a half-life of 8 to 10 hours. Drug excretion occurs primarily through renal elimination. Methotrexate is filtered by the glomerulus, reabsorbed in the proximal tubule (a process blocked by probenecid), and secreted by the distal tubule. Its clearance equals or exceeds creatinine clearance but is not entirely predictable on the basis of clinical measures of renal function. Thus, in patients with compromised renal function or in those receiving potentially lethal doses (above 1000 mg/m^2), monitoring of plasma concentration is recommended to avoid serious toxicity. In high-dose therapy, small test doses may be used to establish pharmacokinetic characteristics in an individual patient, thus allowing calculation of a safe dose.[13]

Methotrexate distributes slowly into third-space accumulations of fluid, such as ascites or pleural effusions, but exits slowly from these spaces as well. The reentry of drug into the systemic circulation from these spaces has been associated with a prolongation of the terminal phase of plasma drug disappearance and with unexpected toxicity. It is advisable to evacuate such effusions or to monitor drug levels in patients with ascites or massive pleural effusions.

Methotrexate also enters the cerebrospinal fluid slowly, producing concentrations that are (during continuous intravenous infusion) approximately one-thirtieth the concentration found simultaneously in plasma. Cytotoxic drug concentrations can be achieved in the spinal fluid by administration of a high dose of methotrexate; peak levels approach 1×10^{-5} M in regimens employing 500 to 1500 mg/m^2. However, these peak concentrations and the concentration × time product are considerably lower than those achieved by direct installation of small doses of methotrexate into the intrathecal space, and the efficacy of systemic high-dose regimens in preventing or treating meningeal leukemia or carcinomatosis is not confirmed.

Dose Adjustment

Special emphasis must be given to the rationale, methods, and results of monitoring drug levels during therapy with high doses of methotrexate. These are summarized in Table 9-4. Methotrexate infusions of 6 to 36 hours duration, in total dosages of 1000 mg/m^2 or greater, can be given without toxic consequences if preceded by intensive hydration and urinary alkalinization and if followed by a series of leucovorin doses. Because of the competitive relationship between leucovorin and methotrexate, the actual dose of leucovorin required to provide rescue is dependent on the plasma concentration of antifolate at the time of rescue. Doses of leucovorin in the range of 15 to 25 mg/m^2 usually provide plasma levels of 1×10^{-6} M and are adequate to prevent toxicity of similar concentrations of antifolate. However, in patients with altered renal function, either induced by methotrexate (*vida infra*) or antedating this treatment, methotrexate excretion is delayed, plasma concentrations are higher than anticipated, and conventional doses of leucovorin are inadequate to rescue. The occurrence of severe myelosuppression and mucositis in patients receiving high dosages of methotrexate has been directly correlated with delayed drug elimination and elevated drug levels in plasma.[14] An appreciation of this relationship has allowed the establishment of critical guidelines for leucovorin administration based on drug-level monitoring at specific time points following infusion and has allowed adjustment of leucovorin dosage to compensate for elevations of plasma methotrexate levels. For the commonly used Jaffe regimen (Table 9-4) (50 to 250 mg/kg methotrexate given

TABLE 9-4. High-Dose Methotrexate Therapy

1. *Prehydration*
   In 12 hr prior to treatment establish diuresis with 1.5 liters/m^2 with 100 mEq HCO_3^- and 20 mEq KCl per liter. Test urine *p*H to assure neutrality (*p*H 7 or >) at time of drug infusion.
2. *Drug Infusion*
   a. Jaffe regimen: 50 to 250 mg/kg methotrexate (MTX) over 6-hr infusion. Continue hydration for 24 hr. Begin leucovorin 2 hr after end of infusion, 15 mg/m^2 1 M q6h × 7 doses.
   b. Alternative: bolus administration of 50 mg/m^2 MTX intravenously followed by infusion of MTX over 36-hr period at dose of 1.5 g/m^2. At 36 hr, begin leucovorin infusion 200 mg/m^2 for 12 hr. At 48 hr, give leucovorin 25 mg/m^2 q6h × 6 doses 1 M.
3. *Monitor Points*
   For Jaffe regimen and for 36-hr infusion, drug levels above 5×10^{-7} M at 48 hr require additional leucovorin rescue.

Drug Level	*Dose Leucovorin*
5×10^{-7} M	15 mg/m^2 q6h × 8 doses
1×10^{-6} M	100 mg/m^2 q6h × 8 doses
2×10^{-6} M	200 mg/m^2 q6h × 8 doses

Drug levels should be repeated every 48 hr and leucovorin dose adjusted until drug concentration is less than 5×10^{-8} M.

over a 6-hour period,[14] followed by 8 doses of leucovorin, 15 mg/m² q6h), a plasma methotrexate level above 9×10^{-7} M at 48 hours is associated with a high risk of severe myelosuppression. Increased leucovorin dosage (100 mg/m² for levels of 10^{-6} M, with proportional increases for higher antifolate concentrations) is effective in preventing myelosuppression.

Alternate high-dose regimens have been employed. Infusions of equivalent doses of methotrexate (1.5 to 7.5 g/m²) over an infusion period prolonged for more than 6 hours produces lower plateau concentrations of drug in the range of 10 to 100 μM, but for longer periods of time. A typical 36-hour regimen used for preoperative chemotherapy of head and neck carcinoma is given in Table 9-4. In this regimen, extreme precautions were taken to assure the adequacy of hydration, alkalinization of the urine, and the adequacy of leucovorin rescue in treating a high-risk patient population. A comparison of the pharmacokinetics of high-dose methotrexate given as a 6-hour infusion and 36-hour infusion is shown in Figure 9-4.

There are no known effective means for removing methotrexate from body fluids in the absence of normal renal function. Hemodialysis produces clearances rates of only 35 to 40 ml/min. Circulating drug can be effectively hydrolized and inactivated by a bacterial enzyme, carboxypeptidase G_1, [15] but this enzyme is not available for general clinical use.

Only a small fraction of administered drug is metabolized to inactive products. However, two metabolites, DAMPA and 7-OH methotrexate, the latter a product of hepatic aldehyde oxidase, tend to accumulate in plasma at later time points in patients receiving high doses of methotrexate.[14] Neither has potent antifolate activity, but both are less soluble than the parent compound and may contribute to the renal precipitation of methotrexate-derived material observed in high-dose therapy.

The pharmacokinetics of methotrexate in the cerebrospinal fluid have an important bearing on both therapeutic and toxic effects. Drug injected in the lumbar intrathecal space distributes poorly into the ventricular spinal fluid, a factor that may contribute to the frequency of relapse of meningeal leukemia.[16] Thus, for patients with known meningeal leukemia, direct intraventricular injection through an indwelling reservoir is recommended. Peak drug concentrations of approximately 10^{-3} M are achieved in the cerebrospinal fluid by injection of 12-mg doses; the major half-life in patients without active meningeal disease is approximately 12 hours but may be considerably prolonged in patients with active leukemic meningitis. Delayed methotrexate elimination from the spinal fluid is associated with methotrexate neurotoxicity.[17] In preliminary studies, a lower incidence of such toxicity was found in patients who received small (1-mg) doses every 12 hours in an effort to provide more constant spinal fluid concentrations without the high peaks associated with the larger doses.

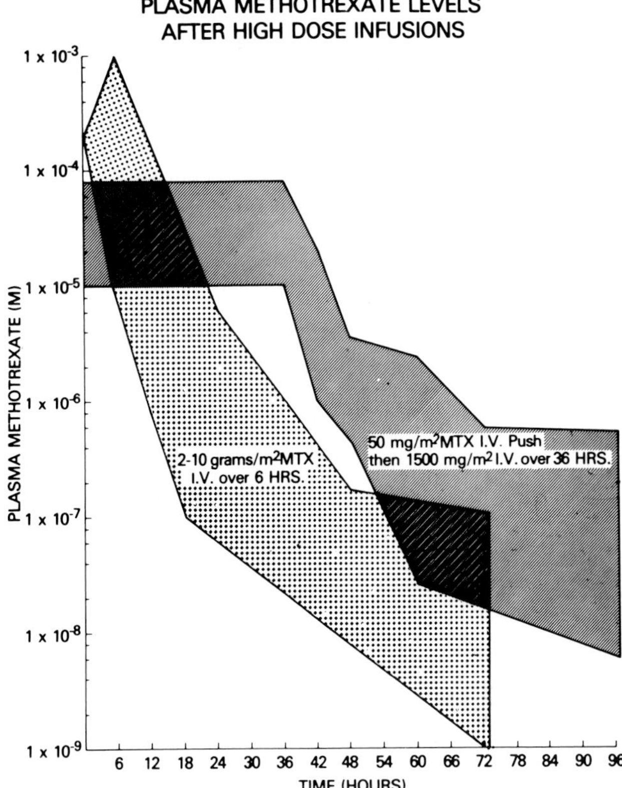

FIG. 9-4. A comparison of methotrexate pharmacokinetics in two high-dose regimens, the first a 6-hr infusion of 50 to 250 mg/kg, the second a bolus dose of 50 mg/m² followed by a 36-hr infusion of 1500 mg/m².

Toxicity

The toxicities observed in man as a consequence of methotrexate therapy fall into two categories: those related to the drug's action on rapidly proliferating tissues (bone marrow and intestinal and oral epithelium) and those manifested by nondividing tissues and less predictable in their incidence. Myelosuppression and mucositis reach their maximum 5 to 14 days following a bolus dose or short-term infusion, and recovery is usually rapid thereafter. More prolonged and severe toxicity has been observed in patients receiving high doses of methotrexate and seems to be related to the long duration of exposure (greater than 48 hours) of these sensitive tissues to circulating drug. These toxicities are preventable by administration of adequate doses of leucovorin or of thymidine, although the latter form of rescue is less reliable and less predictable than is rescue with leucovorin. It should be remembered that in the presence of renal dysfunction even small doses of methotrexate may cause serious, or fatal, myelosuppression.

Conventional doses of methotrexate rarely cause renal injury, but high-dose therapy, in the absence of adequate hydration and urine alkalinization, is associated with at least a 10% incidence of acute renal injury, as indicated by an acute rise in BUN and serum creatinine levels and a decrease in urine volume. In most cases, the mechanism of renal toxicity is believed to be renal precipitation of methotrexate or of methotrexate-derived material;[18] however, the possibility of other mechanisms of renal damage is suggested by the finding that 30-fold lower doses of aminopterin, a more potent antifolate, cause similar deterioration in renal function.[19] These adverse effects can largely be prevented by vigorous pretreatment hydration (3 liters of fluid per m² for 24 hours), by urinary alkalinization (pH 7 or greater), and proportional dose reduction in patients with underlying renal disease (see Tables 9-3 and 9-4).

Both acute and chronic hepatotoxicity are caused by methotrexate. Acute rises in levels of hepatic enzymes are often observed during high-dose therapy, but the levels return to normal within one week. Hyperbilirubinemia is rarely observed in high-dose treatment. Long-term administration of oral methotrexate, as employed in leukemia maintenance therapy and for treatment of psoriasis, is associated with evidence of hepatic fibrosis in up to 30% of patients and with a smaller but definite occurrence of cirrhosis. The etiology of this lesion is unknown; the results of animal experiments suggest impairment of choline synthesis and consequent inhibition of lipid mobilization, and this postulate is borne out by the finding of fatty infiltration in biopsy material of patients who exhibit acute hepatotoxicity.[20]

Acute pneumonitis is infrequently observed in patients receiving methotrexate.[21] When biopsied, the lung often shows granuloma formation and eosinophilia, suggesting a hypersensitivity reaction. However, retreatment of such patients has not been reported to cause a recurrence of this syndrome. Lung biopsy is usually required to rule out the possibility of infection or tumor as the cause of the pulmonary infiltrate.

Rare episodes of acute hypersensitivity with wheezing, urticaria, and hypotension have been reported, including two patients who were receiving immunotherapy with the antifolate. Anaphylaxis has not been documented following conventional doses of methotrexate.

Various manifestations of neurotoxicity are observed in up to 30% of patients receiving intrathecal methotrexate.[22] Symptoms include motor dysfunction of the extremities or cranial nerve palsies, coma, or seizures. This syndrome is distinct from the acute arachonoiditis often seen in the 48 hours following drug injection. Neurotoxicity usually occurs after the third or fourth course of intrathecal injection and is most frequent in adult patients and in those with active meningeal leukemia. Symptoms may be accompanied by an increase in spinal fluid pressure and protein concentration and a reactive pleocytosis. When the syndrome is recognized, a change in therapy to cytarabine (Cytosine Arabinoside) or thiotepa is indicated, because continued treatment may have fatal consequences. Chronic brain injury is believed to occur in the many children treated prophylactically with the standard combination of intrathecal methotrexate and cranial irradiation. In these children, computed tomography reveals intracerebral calcification, thinning of the cerebral cortex, and ventricular dilatation. An effective alternative to intrathecal methotrexate for prophylaxis of meningeal leukemia has not yet been established in comparative clinical trials.

FLUOROPYRIMIDINES

Few of the active antitumor agents now in clinical use have resulted from rational design; rather, most are the product of serendipitous observations or random screening procedures. 5-Fluorouracil (5-FU), which was conceived and synthesized by Dr. Charles Heidelberger at the University of Wisconsin, represents a notable exception (Fig. 9-5).[23] Heidelberger observed that certain malignant cells utilized the base uracil more efficiently than did rat intestinal mucosa and designed a series of uracil analogs with fluorine substitutions at the 5 position. This substitution, after suitable intracellular transformation of the derivative, yields a nucleotide, 5-fluorodeoxyuridylate (5-FdUMP), which is highly inhibitory for the thymidylate synthetase reaction and thus for DNA synthesis.

5-FU has antitumor activity against many types of solid tumors, including breast, colon, and ovarian carcinoma. In these tumors, the response rates vary from 10 to 40%, but complete remissions are unusual. The drug is now commonly used in combination therapy and has interesting biochemical interactions with methotrexate, physiologic nucleosides and bases, and allopurinol, all of which have prompted new clinical trials. The important pharmacologic actions of 5-FU, as well as the biochemical basis of its interactions with other agents, are discussed in this chapter.

Mechanism of Action

5-FU has at least two biochemical actions that may account for its cytotoxicity. It is converted by one of several possible pathways (Fig. 9-6) to the nucleotide fluorouridine monophosphate (FUMP); from this point, two "active" nucleotides may be formed: Fluorouridine triphosphate (FUTP), which is incorporated into RNA and inhibits RNA processing and function, and 5-FdUMP, which binds tightly to thymidylate synthetase and inhibits the eventual formation of deoxythym-

FIG. 9-5. Structures of clinically useful 5-fluoropyrimidines.

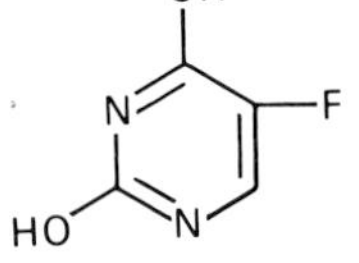

FU

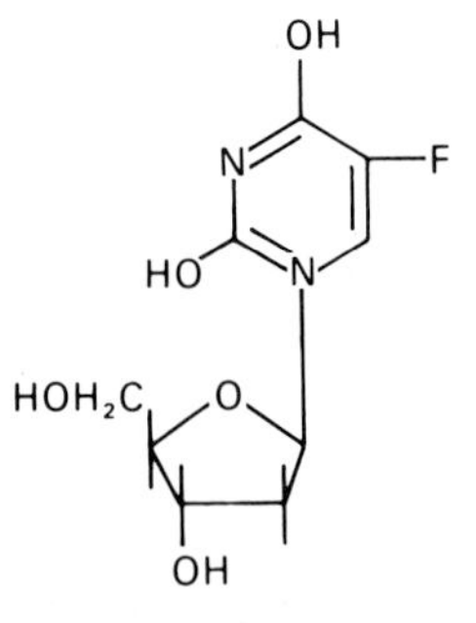

FUdR

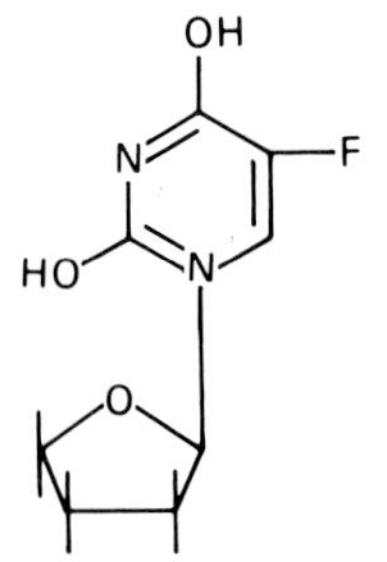

FTORAFUR

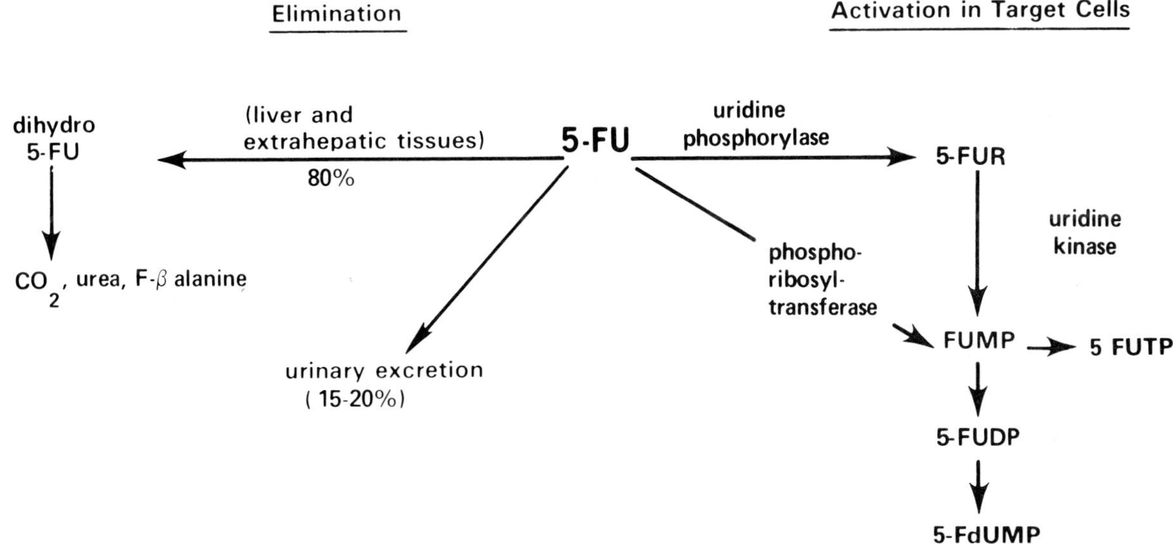

FIG. 9-6. Pathways of 5-fluorouracil elimination and activation.

idine triphosphate (dTTP), one the four necessary precursors of DNA. Although the greater research interest was focused on 5-FdUMP action, evidence from both tissue culture and *in vivo* experiments suggests that the toxicity of 5-FU cannot be completely reversed by thymidine, a direct precursor of dTMP. Secondly, manipulations that increase 5-FU incorporation into RNA also produce increased cytotoxicity.[24]

It is unclear how 5-FU incorporation into RNA produces cytotoxicity; its incorporation into RNA inhibits conversion of high-molecular-weight RNA precursors to the lower molecular weight forms normally found in ribosomes. At somewhat higher concentrations, 5-FU also inhibits the polyadenylation of messenger RNA and thus might affect the stability of this species of RNA. However, these effects have not been correlated with disordered protein synthesis in mammalian cells or in cell-free systems.

The interaction of FU with thymidylate synthetase is more clearly understood in murine tumor systems. Both the peak concentration of 5-FdUMP and the persistence of 5-FdUMP in cells correlate with sensitivity to 5-FU[25]; however, a third factor, the concentration of dUMP (the physiologic substrate), may also determine the duration of inhibition of thymidylate synthetase. This inhibition may be reversed by accumulation of dUMP behind the blocked reaction. dUMP is known to compete with 5-FdUMP for binding to the enzyme and for slowing the rate of enzyme inactivation. The complex formed between 5-FdUMP–thymidylate synthetase–N^{5-10} methylene tetrahydrofolate is extremely stable, but slowly dissociable with a half-life of 6 hours in intact cells. A folate cofactor is an absolute requirement for complex formation; severe depletion of intracellular reduced folates may compromise complex formation in tissue culture experiments, but pretreatment of cells with methotrexate does not affect 5-FU toxicity, perhaps because methotrexate itself can participate in the complex in place of the folate.

Because the active forms of 5-FU are nucleotides, it is logical that resistance to 5-FU develops through deletion of one of the key enzymes required for its activation. In murine tumors, resistance has been associated with deletion of uridine kinase, nucleoside phosphorylase, or orotic acid phosphoribosyl transferase. In addition, an increase in thymidylate synthetase has been found in resistant cells. It is not known which of these changes is responsible for resistance in human tumors.

In an effort to enhance 5-FU activation and overcome resistance, various antitumor agents and nucleosides have been used in combination with the fluoropyrimidine. Methotrexate given prior to 5-FU increases 5-FU nucleotide formation by increasing the intracellular content of phosphoribosylpyrophosphate (PRPP), a required substrate in the orotic acid phosphoribosyltransferase reaction.[26] A nucleotide metabolite of allopurinol inhibits this enzyme, which appears to be the preferred pathway for 5-FU activation in normal tissues but not in all the tumors and thus improves the therapeutic index of 5-FU against some experimental tumors. The combination of 5-FU and allopurinal has antitumor activity in man.[27] Thymidine and other nucleosides enhance 5-FU incorporation into RNA by unknown mechanisms; in addition, thymidine delays 5-FU breakdown by the hepatic enzyme dihydrouracil dehydrogenase and thus prolongs 5-FU plasma half-life and increases its toxicity for both normal and malignant cells.[28] None of these combinations has received thorough phase II testing in clinical trials at this writing.

Clinical Pharmacology and Pharmacokinetics

A variety of methods may be used to measure 5-FU levels in biologic specimens. The most rapid and most sensitive of these methods are those utilizing high-pressure liquid chromatography, either with anion enchange resins or with reverse-phase columns.[29] The sensitivity of this method, with appropriate sample clean-up, is less than 0.1 μM, or less than the threshold for bone marrow toxicity (probably 1 μM). Gas chromatographic–mass spectrophotometric methods, which are equally sensitive and specific, require derivatization and longer processing time.

An understanding of 5-FU pharmacokinetics is required for an informed choice of route, schedule, and dose of administration. The alternative routes of administration (oral, intravenous, intra-arterial, and even intraperitoneal) each have unique advantages and disadvantages that determine their usefulness in clinical chemotherapy. The clinical effectiveness and pattern of toxicity seen with each of these routes can largely be explained by pharmacokinetic considerations.

5-FU is usually administered intravenously. Plasma levels vary considerably after oral administration, probably because of erratic absorption and variable first-pass metabolism in the liver from the gastrointestinal tract.[30] Clinical results reflect the variation in bioavailability by this route. After intravenous dosage, the drug penetrates well into the cerebrospinal fluid and extracellular "third space" fluids, such as ascites or pleural fluid. Following conventional single doses of 10 to 15 mg per kg, peak plasma concentrations reach 0.1 mM to 1 mM, but rapid metabolic breakdown to dihydrofluorouracil in the liver and other tissues leads to an abrupt fall in plasma concentrations. The primary plasma half-life of about 10 minutes varies considerably from patient to patient, but is not clearly correlated with clinical tests of hepatic function. Within 6 hours of injection, plasma concentrations of 5-FU fall below 1 μM, the approximate threshold for exerting cytotoxic effects in tissue culture, and thereafter decline more slowly.

Because of its metabolism by the liver, 5-FU can be infused into the hepatic artery or portal vein for treatment of hepatic metastases, and only limited amounts of drug reach the systemic circulation. Preliminary data indicate that infusion of 30 mg per kg per day produces plasma levels of 0.13 to 0.35 μM, although these figures are likely to be dependent on catheter position and hepatic function.[31] At this infusion rate, greater than 50% of the infused drug is cleared in its first pass through the liver.[32]

5-FU has also been administered by peritoneal instillation for treatment of ovarian cancer.[33] This route attempts to exploit the high local concentration of drug tolerated by this route (4 mM), the primary absorption of drug into the portal circulation and its metabolism in the liver, and the limited direct absorption into the systemic circulation. Minimal systemic toxicity occurs if drug concentrations are maintained at or below 4 mM in the peritoneal cavity, because a 100:1 to 1000:1 gradient in drug concentration is established between the peritoneal fluid and plasma. The therapeutic effects of this type of regimen have not been conclusively evaluated.

Greater than 80% of administered 5-FU (by intravenous or intra-arterial route) is eliminated by metabolic conversion to dihydrofluorouracil, the remainder being excreted intact in the urine. The primary metabolite, dihydro-5-FU, is then further cleaved to yield α-fluoro-β-ureidoproprionic acid and CO_2. The liver and gastrointestinal mucosa are primary sites of this conversion; it is not known whether neoplastic cells also degrade 5-FU. Doses do not have to be modified in the presence of hepatic dysfunction, because metabolism occurs in extrahepatic tissues.

The active intracellular nucleotides, 5-FdUMP and FUTP, have prolonged half-lives intracellularly; their decay rates vary among tissues, and their persistence is thought to be an important determinant of the duration and, ultimately, of the magnitude of drug effect.

Clinical Toxicity

The primary clinical toxicity of 5-FU results from its effects on rapidly dividing tissues, specifically intestinal and oral mucosa and bone marrow. After bolus intravenous administration, using either a 5-day course or single weekly doses, suppression of the white cell count and platelet count occurs in 4 to 7 days with full recovery within 2 weeks after the last dose. Stomatitis and diarrhea are also frequent toxicities, particularly in patients receiving a 5-day course of treatment.

An alternative regimen employing continuous intravenous infusion of 5-FU at doses of 30 mg per kg per day for 5 days gives equivalent therapeutic results, but a different pattern of toxicity. Myelosuppression is usually mild, whereas gastrointestinal symptoms are the predominant toxicities (again, stomatitis and diarrhea). Continuous intrahepatic infusion of 5-FU is also a useful alternative to intravenous therapy in patients with metastases to the liver. In patients with colonic carcinoma with hepatic metastases, response rates of 50% have been achieved by this mode of therapy. Because at least 50% of the drug is cleared in its first pass through the liver, systemic toxicity is mild, consisting primarily of mucositis and, less frequently, myelosuppression. The primary complications are related to catheter slippage into the gastroduodenal artery, with resultant necrosis of the intestinal epithelium, hemorrhage, or perforation. The physician must be alert to sudden onset of epigastric pain or ileus as an early sign of catheter displacement into a feeding artery of the stomach or the small bowel. Thrombosis of the extremity artery used for insertion of the cannula can also be anticipated if the catheter is inserted into a brachial artery. Hepatic portal perfusion is a less favorable form of local therapy because most large hepatic metastases derive their blood supply from the arterial rather than the portal circulation.

Other less common toxicities of 5-FU include acute neurologic symptoms (somnolence, ataxia, and upper motoneuron signs) seen primarily in patients receiving intracarotid infusions; this syndrome is thought to be caused by a neurotoxic metabolite, 5-fluorocitrate. A syndrome of chest pain, serum enzyme elevations consistent with myocardial necrosis, and electrocardiographic findings consistent with myocardial ischemia, have been described in patients undergoing 5-FU infusion. Whether these episodes represent incidental myocardial infarction or are related to 5-FU is unclear.

5-FU causes acute and chronic conjunctivitis that may lead to tear-duct stenosis and ectropion. The acute inflammatory response is reversible with discontinuation of the drug, but surgical correction of tear-duct stenosis may be required.

Other Fluoropyrimidines

Two other fluoropyrimidines (see Fig. 9-5), 5-fluoro-2-deoxyuridine (FUdR) and ftorafur (1-2-tetrahydrofuranyl)-5-fluorouracil, have had extensive clinical trial but have not replaced 5-FU in general clinical use. FUdR is converted by a nucleoside kinase to 5-FdUMP and functions primarily as an inhibitor of thymidylate synthetase, with lesser effects than 5-FU on RNA. The deoxyribose group is readily removed by the ubiquitous enzyme thymidine phosphorylase, and the resulting 5-FU undergoes metabolic degradation as outlined previously. More than 90% of FUdR is removed in its first pass through the liver.[32] Its pattern of toxicity and the advantages of its use in hepatic perfusion closely parallel the characteristics of 5-FU.

Ftorafur acts as a depot form of 5-FU, producing little myelosuppression. However, significant diarrhea, nausea, and vomiting and neurotoxicity in the form of altered mental status and ataxia are the usual dose-limiting complaints.[34] It is administered intravenously in doses of 1.5 g per m^2 per day for 5 days and is reliably absorbed orally. The parent compound, ftorafur, has a prolonged plasma half-life of 6 to 16 hours and is eliminated by conversion to hydroxylated metabolites. The circulating concentrations of 5-FU produced are low (less than 0.1 mg/ml), suggesting that conversion to 5-FU may occur predominantly with tumor cells and the liver and that the circulating level of 5-FU may not adequately reflect the extent of this conversion.[35]

CYTOSINE ARABINOSIDE

Cytosine arabinoside (ara-C) is one of several arabinose nucleosides first isolated from the sponge, *Cryptothethya crypta,* differing from its physiologic counterpart, deoxycytidine, in the presence of an OH group in the β configuration at the 2′ position (see Fig. 9-6). Since this initial discovery, many arabinose nucleosides have been synthesized or isolated from bacterial broths, and a few have been tested as antitumor agents, the most prominent of those being ara-adenine, a purine analog. However, none of these compounds has as potent clinical activity against human acute myeloblastic leukemia as does ara-C. As a single agent, ara-C induces remission in almost 50% of patients with acute myeloblastic leukemia (AML) and is the standard agent in combination with anthracyclines for treatment of this disease. It has definite but lesser activity against other human tumors, including the blastic crisis of chronic granulocytic leukemia and acute lymphoblastic leukemia, but its selective activity against rapidly growing tumors and its pharmacokinetic features have rendered this agent less useful in treating most solid malignancies.

Structure and Mechanism of Action

Because of the absence of a 2′-OH group in the α position, ara-C is recognized enzymatically as an analog of 2′-deoxycytidine and is metabolized by salvage pathway enzymes to its active form, ara-CTP (Fig. 9-7). This nucleotide acts as an inhibitor of DNA polymerase in competition with deoxycytidine triphosphate (dCTP) with a K_i of approximately 0.1 μM.[36] Repair synthesis of DNA seems less effectively inhibited than does replicative synthesis. Ara-C is also incorporated into DNA, leading to a defect in ligation of fragments of newly synthesized DNA.[37] There is also evidence that cells exposed to ara-C during their S, or DNA synthetic, phase of the cell cycle re-initiate DNA synthesis upon removal of ara-C, causing an abnormal duplication of early portions of the DNA strand.[38]

Ara-C penetrates cells by a carrier-mediated process that allows the achievement of equilibrium of extra- and intracellular drug concentrations within seconds. There is no evidence that transport limits the response of normal or resistant cells. Intracellular metabolism of ara-C by three sequential phosphorylation reactions, mediated by deoxycytidine kinase, deoxycytidine monophosphate (dCMP) kinase, and nucleoside diphosphate kinase, leads to formation of aracytidine triphosphate (CTP). Two inactivating enzymes, cytidine deaminase and dCMP deaminase, may also act on ara-C or ara-CMP, respectively.[39] These deaminating enzymes are found in high concentration relative to the activating enzymes and are thought to exert an important negative influence on drug action (see Fig. 9-7).

The enzymatic changes responsible for resistance to ara-C have not been clearly pinpointed in man, although a deletion of deoxycitidine kinase is often observed in resistant murine leukemia cells and has been implicated by at least one study in AML.[40] A second mechanism of resistance, documented only in preclinical studies, is an increased intracellular pool

FIG. 9-7. Structures of cytosine arabinoside, 5-azacytidine, and related physiologic nucleosides.

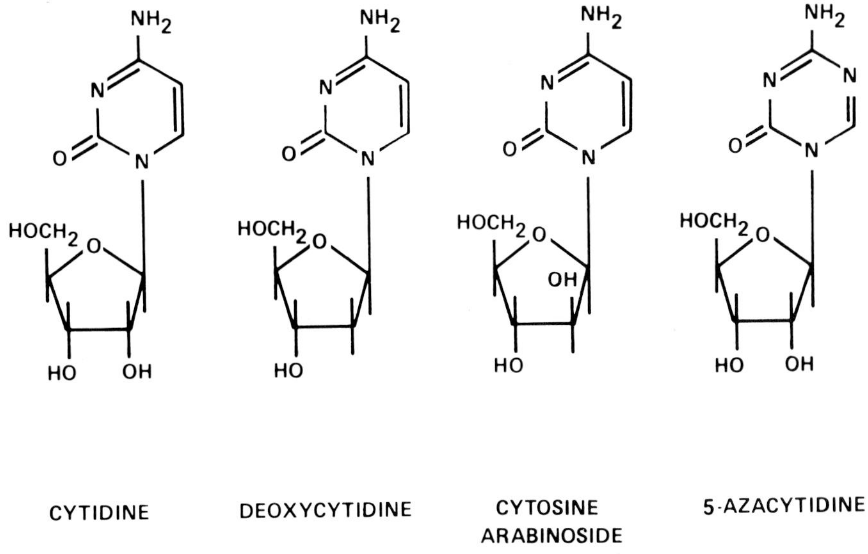

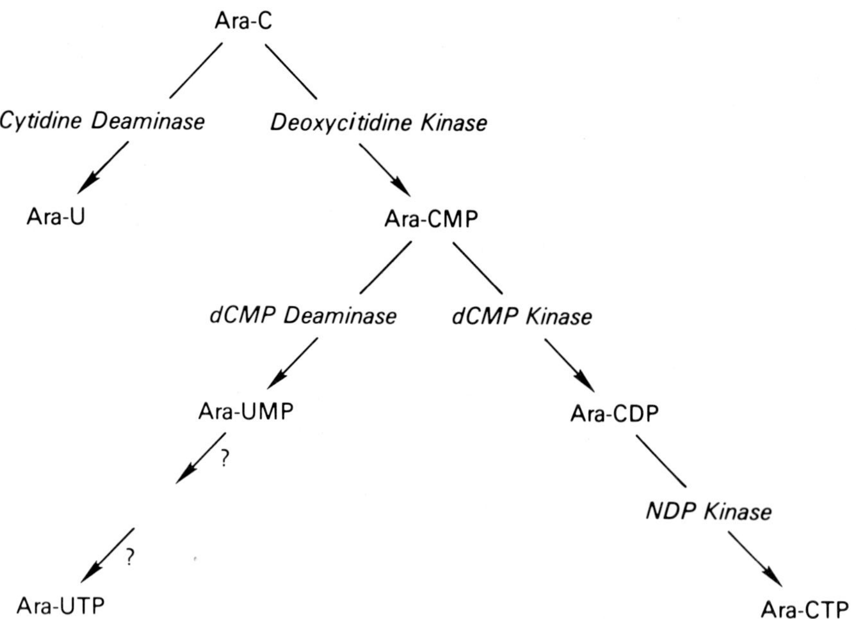

FIG. 9-8. Metabolism of cytosine arabinoside by tumor cells. The names of important enzymes are in italics. The conversion of ara-UMP to a triphosphate has not been demonstrated in mammalian cells. d = deoxyribose; MP = monophosphate; DP = diphosphate; TP = triphosphate.

of dCTP (the nucleotide that competes with ara-CTP). Increased activity of cytidine deaminase has been correlated with resistance in a single study in AML,[41] but has not been confirmed subsequently. It is possible to predict clinical response to ara-C by a test incubation of leukemic cells with the drug *in vitro;* the ability of cells to form and to retain ara-CTP after exposure to ara-C can be used to predict the duration of a subsequent remission (Fig. 9-8).[42] These studies require the separation and quantitation of ara-C nucleotides by high-pressure liquid chromatography and are not easily adapted to routine clinical use.

As an inhibitor of DNA synthesis, ara-C kills cells selectively during the S phase of the cell cycle, although exposure of cells during other phases may lead to chromatid deletions and to a failure to repair strand breaks induced by x-rays or other agents. The cytotoxicity of ara-C is not only cell-cycle specific, but also dependent on the rate of DNA synthesis. Cytotoxic effects are greatest if cells are exposed to ara-C during periods of rapid DNA synthesis, as for example in the recovery phase after treatment with an initial dose of ara-C or another S-phase-specific drug. Thus, the timing of second doses of ara-C may have critical impact on the therapeutic outcome.

Clinical Pharmacology

The measurement of ara-C in biologic fluids presents significant problems. Because of its close structural similarity to physiologic nucleosides (deoxycytidine, cytidine), it is difficult to separate from these endogenous compounds. Further, ara-C is subject to deamination by cytidine deaminase, an enzyme found in plasma and in granulocytes; thus, one must include a deaminase inhibitor, such as tetrahydrouridine, in samples at the time of their collection. Various chemical and microbiologic assays for ara-C have been developed and applied to clinical pharmacokinetic studies; the best of these employs high-pressure liquid chromatography, with a cation-exchange column, and cleanly separates ara-C from its primary metabolite ara-U.[43] The sensitivity of this method approaches 0.1 μM in plasma. A simpler and more rapid method is the radioimmunoassay based on a sheep antibody to an ara-C: albumin conjugate.[44] This assay is highly specific for ara-C (and its nucleotides, which are not found in plasma), takes less than 3 hours to complete, and is thus applicable to routine pharmacokinetic monitoring and other clinical uses.

Because of the presence of cytidine deaminase in gastrointestinal epithelium and its first-pass elimination in the liver, the drug is not given orally. When administered by the intravenous route, it distributes rapidly into total body water; concentrations in the cerebrospinal fluid reach 50% of simultaneous plasma levels after 2 hours of continuous intravenous administration. Peak plasma concentrations reach 1×10^{-4} M after a 100-mg dose and thereafter fall with a primary half-life of 7 to 20 min.[45] A second half-life of 0.5 to 2.6 hours has been detected by the more sensitive assay precedures, but is probably of little clinical significance. Over 70% of a clinical dose is excreted in the urine, primarily in the form of the inactive metabolite ara-U. Within minutes of injection, ara-U becomes the predominant drug form found in plasma, its formation taking place in liver, plasma, peripheral granulocytes, and other sites.

Plasma concentrations are not consistently predictable on the basis of dose or infusion rate. An average plasma concentration of about 3×10^{-7} M can be expected in patients receiving 5 to 10 mg per hour by constant infusion; a loading dose of 3 times the hourly infusion rate should be given prior to infusion to allow rapid achievement of the steady-state level.

There is some evidence that a correlation exists between remission induction and the plasma half-life of ara-C in individual patients; in one study of 14 patients with AML, those with more prolonged plasma half-life had the best chance of achieving a complete remission.[46] These preliminary findings require confirmation.

Ara-C may also be administered intrathecally for treatment of meningeal leukemia or carcinomatosis. Because deamination is much slower in the cerebrospinal fluid, doses of 50 mg per m^2 yield peak levels of 1 mM, which decline slowly with a half-life of approximately 2 hours, and cytotoxic concentrations of greater than 0.1 μM are maintained for 24 hours.

Because of the rapid inactivation of ara-C by cytidine deaminase and its phase-dependent killing, the drug is usually administered as a continuous infusion or in bolus doses of 50 to 100 mg every 8 to 12 hours for 5 to 10 days. Single bolus doses of 4 g per m^2 produce minimal toxicity because of rapid drug inactivation, whereas the continuous infusion of 1 g per m^2 over a 48-hour period produces severe myelosuppression.

The primary toxic side-effects of ara-C are myelosuppression and gastrointestinal epithelial injury. With conventional doses of 100 mg/m^2/day, leukopenia and thrombocytopenia reach their maximum in 7 to 14 days. The duration of myelosuppression depends on the rate of achievement of remission, the nature of concomitant therapy, and prior treatment experience. There is little acute effect on the circulating lymphocyte count, but a depression of cell-mediated immunity is found during therapy.

Gastrointestinal toxicity is prominent in patients receiving ara-C. The most frequent complaints include nausea, vomiting, and diarrhea; a spectrum of pathologic changes is observed in the intestinal mucosa, from superficial ulceration to intramural hematoma formation and perforation. Patients receiving ara-C frequently develop elevated levels of serum enzymes consistent with mild hepatocellular damage, but hepatotoxicity necessitates discontinuation of treatment in less than 25% of patients.

Ara-C is often used intrathecally as a substitute for methotrexate in patients experiencing antifolate neurotoxicity; however, ara-C may also cause neurotoxic side-effects, including seizures and alteration in mental status.[47]

Drug Interactions

Ara-C has shown synergistic interaction with many other antitumor agents including alkylating agents, thiopurines, uridine analogs, and antifolates. Each of these interactions has been explained on a biochemical or cellular kinetic basis, although the application of these interactions to the design of clinical trials is not straightforward, in view of differences in the biochemical and kinetic characteristics of the experimental and clinical treatment situation. The enhancement of cyclophosphamide and bischloroethylnitrosourea (BCNU) activity by ara-C can be ascribed to ara-C inhibition of the repair of strand breaks caused by the alkylating agents. 3-Deazauridine inhibits dCTP formation and blocks deamination of ara-C and ara-CMP[48]; these actions lead to increased ara-CTP formation in some but not all experimental tumors. This combination has not yet been tested clinically. Likewise, methotrexate given prior to ara-C enhances ara-CTP formation in experimental tumors, perhaps through expansion of the dUMP pool and consequent inhibition of dCMP deaminase.[49] Thymidine also enhances ara-C cytotoxicity in some cell lines by inhibiting formation of dCDP through its effects on ribonucleotide reductase.[50] However, this latter interaction has not been observed in experiments with human AML cells.

Potent enhancement of ara-C cytotoxicity is observed when patients are pretreated with a cytidine deaminase inhibitor, tetrahydrouridine (THU). This compound markedly prolongs the plasma half-life of ara-C and reduces the tolerable dose 30-fold.[51] It is not known whether the THU:ara-C combination will have selective toxic effects on human tumor cells, although, on the basis of experimental work, this combination would be expected to have synergistic activity only against cells with high deaminase levels, as found in a fraction of patients with acute myeloblastic leukemia.

Alternative Anticytidine Therapy

Because of the rapid metabolism of ara-C, attempts have been made to develop alternate therapies that would be resistant to deamination. Ara-C enclosed in lipid vesicles, or liposomes, has increased potency,[52] probably because of the prolonged half-life of the vesicles in plasma, but this increased potency has not been translated into improved therapeutic efficacy, as compared to optimal use of free ara-C. Various conjugates of ara-C, including N^4-acyl analogs, ara-C or ara-CMP esters, and the anhydro compound cyclocytidine have all shown antitumor activity and are not subject to deamination, but, again, do not have a superior therapeutic index. Most of these derivatives owe their activity to ara-CTP and thus have the same mechanism of action as ara-C.

Analogs with distinctly different mechanisms of action have been developed, and two, 5-azacytidine (5-azaC) (Fig. 9-6) and 3-deazauridine (3-deazaU) (Fig. 9-9) have entered clinical trial. 5-AzaC has significant activity in the treatment of leukemia. Like ara-C, it is subject to deamination in plasma and liver, as well as in tumor cells, but its activation proceeds by a separate pathway. It is phosphorylated by uridine-cytidine kinase and then follows the same pathways as ara-CMP to reach its active form, 5-azaCTP. The latter is a substrate for RNA polymerase, and when it is incorporated into RNA it causes defective protein synthesis and polyribosomal degradation.[53] Resistance to 5-azaC in murine leukemia cells develops through deletion of uridine-cytidine kinase.

The 5-azaC ring system is unstable in solution; this instability may contribute to its lethal effects after incorporation into RNA.

The rapid decomposition of 5-azaC in alkaline or neutral solution necessitates either fresh mixing prior to administration or formulation at a slightly acid *p*H in Ringer's lactate (*p*H 6.2), in which it has a half-life of 65 hours at 25°C.

The pharmacokinetics of 5-azaC are poorly understood, although it is clear that the drug undergoes rapid removal from the plasma, either through metabolism or chemical decomposition. Less than 2% of an administered dose remains in plasma as parent compound 30 minutes after administra-

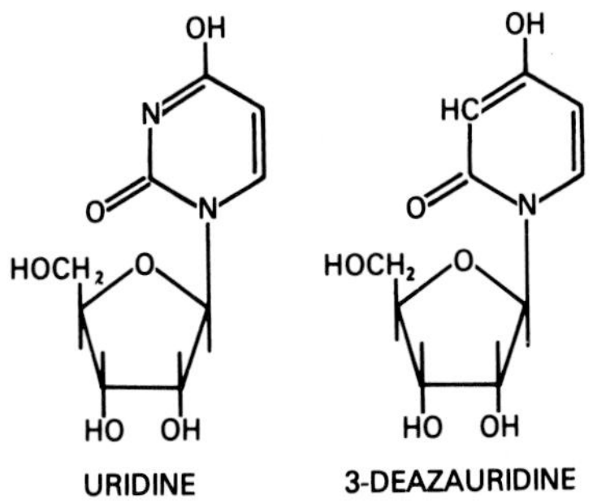

URIDINE 3-DEAZAURIDINE

FIG. 9-9. Structure of 3-deazauridine and its physiologic counterpart, uridine.

tion. The compound is a substrate for cytidine deaminase, but the product, 5-azauridine, is chemically unstable and has not been identified in human urine or plasma.

The primary toxicities of 5-azaC are myelosuppression and severe and prolonged nausea and vomiting. The latter symptoms are ameliorated if the drug is administered by a prolonged or continuous infusion, and there is no apparent change in its therapeutic efficacy or myelosuppressive effects by this alternate schedule. Patients may infrequently develop abnormal liver function tests, myalgias, transient temperature elevation, or rash following 5-azaC therapy.

A new antipyrimidine, 3-deazauridine (3-deazaU) (see Fig. 9-9), acts by a completely different mechanism. 3-DeazaU inhibits CTP synthetase and thus depletes cells of CTP and dCTP, although salvage of circulating nucleosides presents an alternative route for making these triphosphates. In selected experimental tumors, 3-deazaU enhances the cytotoxicity of cytidine analogs, including ara-C, 5-azaC, and 5-aza-2′deoxy-C.

Little is known of the disposition and elimination of 3-deazaU in man. Less than 10% of the drug is recovered in urine intact. Its likely metabolic pathway involves removal of the ribose group by uridine phosphorylase and further catabolism of 3-deazaU. The plasma half-life of the parent compound is 4.4 hours.[54]

PURINE ANALOGS

The development of purine analogs for treatment of cancer has been one of the most fruitful endeavors in rational synthesis undertaken by the pharmaceutical industry. Not only have effective antileukemic agents, such as 6-mercaptopurine (6-MP) and 6-thioguanine (6-TG), resulted from these efforts, but potent immunosuppressive agents, such as azathioprine, the xanthine oxidase inhibitor, allopurinol, and the antiviral compound ara-adenine, have found significant clinical application in nononcologic fields.[55] A new area of great potential has been opened by the discovery of adenosine deaminase inhibitors such as deoxycoformycin, which have selective action against T lymphocytes and promise useful application in cancer treatment and immunologic disorders. This chapter deals with established as well as potentially important new antipurine agents in cancer chemotherapy.

Structure and Mechanism of Action of 6-Thiopurines

6-MP and 6-TG are commonly used in treating acute lymphocytic leukemia of childhood and acute myelogenous leukemia, respectively, but have no appreciable activity against human solid malignancies. Because of the similarities in the mechanisms of action, pharmacokinetic properties, and patterns of clinical toxicity of these two agents, they are considered jointly in the following section. The newer purine analogs are dealt with in a subsequent section of this chapter.

The 6-thiopurine analogs have the single substitution of a thiol group in place of the 6-hydroxyl group found in guanine or in the basic purine nucleus (Fig. 9-10). Both 6-MP and 6-TG are inactive compounds in their native state and require further activation to the nucleotide level by the enzyme hypoxanthine-guanine phosphoribosyl transferase (HGPRT'ase). As monophosphate nucleotides, these analogs inhibit *de novo* purine biosynthesis at its first step (phosphoribosylpyrophosphate amidotransferase) and also block the conversion of inosinic acid to adenylic acid or to guanylic acid. The triphosphate nucleotides of 6-TG and 6MP are incorporated into DNA and produce toxicity that is manifested in a delayed manner after drug exposure.[56] The specific consequences of this incorporation into DNA are poorly understood.

Biochemical resistance to these agents has been ascribed to the absence of the activating enzyme (HGPRT'ase) in experimental tumors, but in human leukemic cells, resistance is more commonly associated with increased concentrations of a degrading enzyme, a membrane-bound alkaline phosphatase.[57] This phosphatase has specific properties, such as greater heat lability and a higher *p*H maximum, which distinguish it from phosphatases found in sensitive tumor cells.

The purine analogs penetrate cells readily. Their intracellular metabolism proceeds in several phases, as defined by studies using ^{35}S-6-MP (Fig. 9-9).[58] Substantial quantities are converted first to the inactive product, 6-thiouric acid; then to the monophosphate nucleotides of 6-thioxanthine and 6-thioguanosine, which inhibit *de novo* purine synthesis; and finally to the triphosphate nucleotides, which are incorporated over time into DNA. It is believed that the initial inhibition

FIG. 9-10. Purine analogs and their physiologic counterparts, hypoxanthine and guanine.

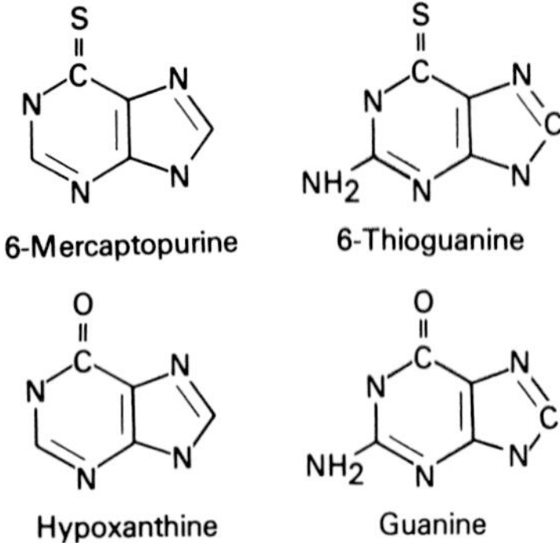

of purine synthesis allows a build-up of PRPP pools and thus allows conversion of 6-MP to its various nucleotides.

Clinical Pharmacology and Pharmacokinetics

Although initial information on 6-MP pharmacokinetics came from the use of radiolabeled drug, this approach is impractical for routine monitoring or for repetitive studies in a single patient. Improved analytic techniques using high-pressure liquid chromatography have been described, but none has been applied as yet in a systematic examination of 6-thiopurine pharmacokinetics. The most sensitive of these new methods employs derivatization of the thiopurines to phenyl mercury derivatives,[59] or oxidation to sulfonates with alkaline permanganate, followed by column separation and fluorometric detection.[60] The level of sensitivity of these procedures is approximately 0.1 μM.

6-MP is well absorbed orally; approximately 50% of a dose reaches the systemic circulation. 6-TG is erratically absorbed and is thus administered by intravenous infusion. The plasma half-lives vary from 80 to 90 minutes for 6-TG to 20 to 45 minutes for 6-MP. The major determinants of drug elimination are metabolic alteration by several pathways (Fig. 9-11). 6-MP is oxidized to 6-thiouric acid by xanthine oxidase, a reaction sequence inhibited by allopurinol. In the presence of allopurinol, 6-thioxanthine, an intermediate oxidation product, becomes the predominant elimination product. There is clinical evidence of increased 6-MP toxicity in patients receiving concomitant allopurinol, but a detailed pharmacokinetic examination of this interaction has not been undertaken; nonetheless, a dose reduction of 75% is recommended in the presence of the xanthine oxidase inhibitor. 6-MP also undergoes S-methylation to yield 6-methylmercaptopurine, which, upon phosphorylation, becomes an active antipurine in its own right. Finally, methylated 6-MP derivatives may undergo oxidation to sulfonic acid products, with ultimate liberation of inorganic sulfate.

The catabolism of 6-TG is somewhat different. Methylation of the sulfur substituent plays a prominent role, leading ultimately to oxidation and elimination of the sulfur molecule. 6-TG also is converted to 6-thioxanthine in a reaction catalyzed by the enzyme guanase. This intermediate is further oxidized to 6-thiouric acid by xanthine oxidase, but because the substrate for this reaction, 6-thioxanthine, is inactive, no reduction in 6-TG dosage is required for patients who are also receiving allopurinol.

Dose, Schedule, and Toxicity

6-MP, given by the oral route, and 6-TG, given intravenously, are well tolerated in doses of approximately 100 mg per m^2. These doses are usually given for at least 5 days in leukemic induction therapy or, in the case of 6-MP, for longer courses at slightly reduced doses for maintenance of remission. As mentioned previously, a 6-MP dosage reduction of 75% is indicated for patients also receiving allopurinol. Extremely high doses of 6-MP have been employed (up to 1000 mg/m^2/day for 5 days by intravenous infusion) without effectively increasing antitumor activity.[61]

Because both 6-MP and 6-TG produce cytotoxicity by virtue of their incorporation into DNA, it follows that their primary toxicity would be exerted against the rapidly dividing precursor cells of the bone marrow and intestinal epithelium. Myelosuppression is maximal within 7 days of drug administration; the time to recovery is dose dependent, but is usually complete in 14 days. Reversible hepatoxicity is occasionally observed after treatment with either thiopurine, although most frequently after 6-MP. Serum alkaline phosphatase, direct bilirubin, and transaminase levels are elevated during this acute toxicity, in a pattern consistent with cholestatic jaundice. Mucositis, esophagitis, and gastrointestinal complaints are usually mild and not a significant hindrance to antipurine therapy.

The 6-thiopurines and the related compound azathioprine, which releases 6-mercaptopurine through hepatic metabolism following oral administration, are potent suppressors of cell-mediated immunity and are used for suppression of rejection of transplanted organs or for treatment of autoimmune diseases such as Crohn's disease, ulcerative colitis, or rheumatoid arthritis.[62] Therapeutic immunosuppression can be realized at doses of 100 mg per day (1.5 mg per m^2), which

FIG. 9-11. Pathways for degradation of 6-mercaptopurine (*6-MP*).

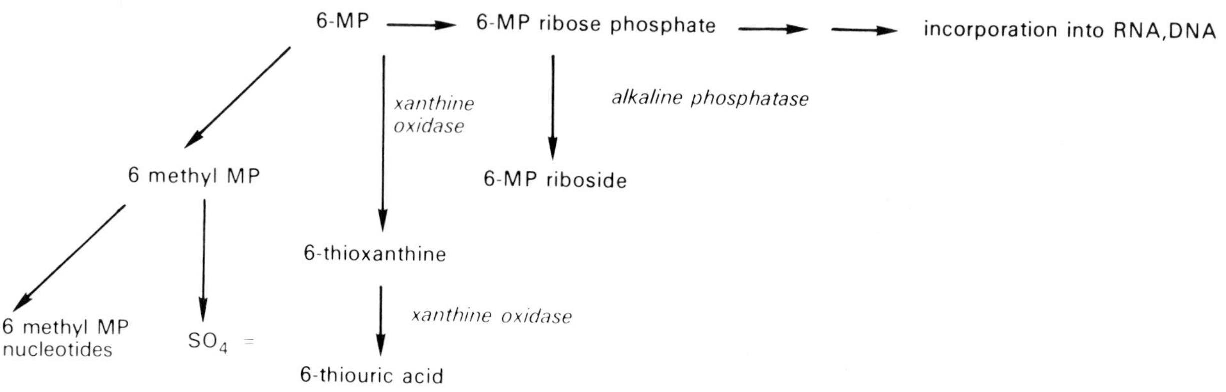

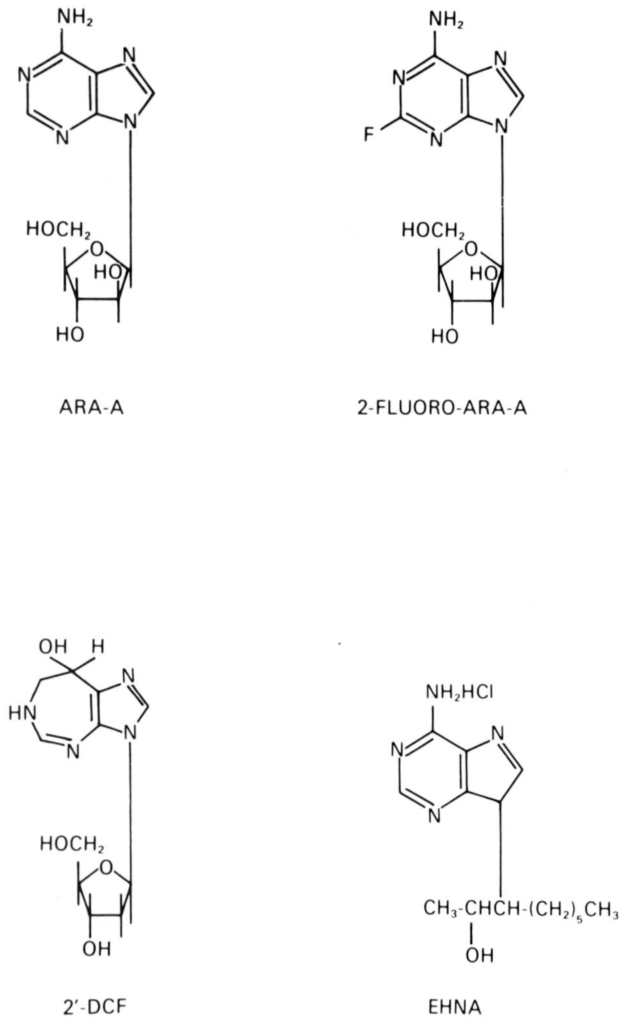

FIG. 9-12. Adenine arabinoside (*ARA-A*), 2-fluoro-ara-A, 2′-deoxycoformycin (*2′-DCF*), and EHNA.

produce little decrease in the white blood cell count. Long-term immunosuppressive therapy with azathioprine has been associated with an increased risk of squamous carcinomas of skin and histiocytic lymphoma; these complications have not been reported secondary to chronic 6-MP therapy. Other complications related to chronic 6-thiopurine treatment include a predisposition to bacterial and opportunistic infection.

ADENOSINE ANALOGS

In addition to the 6-thiopurines, which act as guanine analogs, a number of analogs of adenosine have been synthesized or isolated from fermentation broths. The most prominent among these is 9-β-D-arabinofuranosyladenine (ara-A) (Fig. 9-12), which, as a triphosphate, inhibits DNA polymerase. This compound has antiviral activity against DNA viruses, particularly those of the herpes group.[63] Although ara-A has shown potent antitumor activity in animal tumors, its clinical utility has been hampered by its limited aqueous solubility and its rapid deamination by adenosine deaminase, which have prevented achievement of clinically toxic dose levels. The nucleotide ara-AMP, a more soluble compound that is not susceptible to hydrolysis by adenosine deaminase but is slowly cleaved to ara-A by plasma phosphatase activity, is expected to enter clinical trial.

The susceptibility of adenosine analogs to hydrolysis by adenosine deaminase and the high activity of the latter enzyme in certain human tumors (particularly T-cell lymphoblastic leukemia and selected cases of acute myelocytic leukemia) have prompted interest in the combination of these analogs with inhibitors of the deaminase (Fig. 9-12). Two potent inhibitors of adenosine deaminase, 2′-deoxycoformycin and erythro-9-(2-hydroxy-3-nanyl)adenine(EHNA), enhance antitumor potency of ara-A and other adenosine analogs such as tubercidin, xylosyl adenine, and 3′-deoxyadenosine.[64] These combinations are curative against the L1210 leukemia, which is highly resistant to ara-A alone because of high deaminase levels. The increase in intracellular ara-ATP concentrations produced by deoxycoformycin is greatest in tumor cells that contain adenosine deaminase, whereas there is less increase in bone marrow or gastrointestinal epithelium. Thus, it is likely that the combination of ara-A or ara-AMP with the deaminase inhibitor will have selective effects only against tumors with high enzyme levels. These combinations can be expected to have potent immunosuppressive effects, because T lymphocytes have extremely active enzyme systems for activating adenosine, deoxyadenosine, and their analogs, and are protected against toxicity of these compounds only by the presence of high concentrations of adenosine deaminase.[65]

An alternative to the combination of an adenosine analog with 2′-deoxycoformycin is the new compound 2-fluoro-ara-A (Fig. 9-12), which is resistant to deamination by adenosine deaminase[66] and thus is active as a single agent against various ara-A-resistant tumors.

ALKYLATING AGENTS

Two primary classes of cytotoxic compounds have proved useful in the treatment of cancer: those that interfere with the synthesis of precursors of DNA and those that chemically interact with DNA itself. Most prominent among the latter compounds are drugs known as alkylating agents on the basis of their ability to form covalent bonds with nucleic acid. The alkyl groups that become attached to DNA in this reaction interfere with the integrity or function of DNA in poorly understood ways, but the process of alkylation is known to have significant cytotoxic, mutagenic, and carcinogenic effects.

The biochemical process of alkylation is depicted in Fig. 9-13. Most alkylating agents posses the characteristic of forming positively charged carbonium ions in aqueous solution. In the cases of the chloroethyl alkylating groups, a preliminary cyclization to form an unstable imonium ion takes place, with spontaneous opening of the three-member ring to yield the alkylating intermediate, $R—CH_2—CH_2+$. This charged group then attacks nucleophilic (electron-rich) sites on nucleic acids, protein, and, in addition, small molecules such as sulfhydrils (glutathione) and amino acids. It is likely that the primary cytotoxic and mutagenic effects of alkylating agents are the result of their interactions with DNA.[67] The

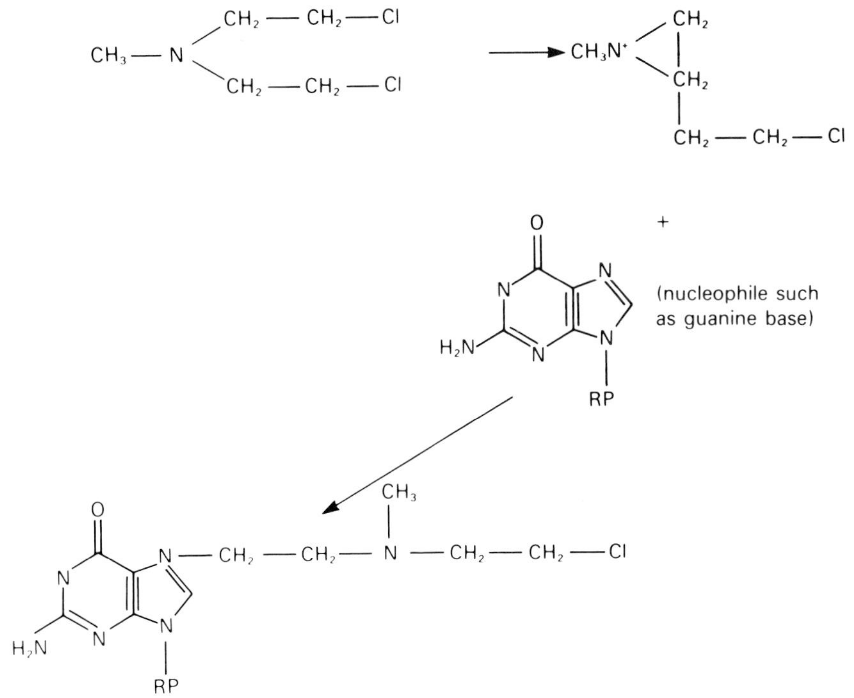

(nucleophile such as guanine base)

FIG. 9-13. Spontaneous activation of nitrogen mustard to an imonium ion that forms a covalent bond with nucleophilic sites such as the N-7 position of guanine. The remaining free chloroethyl arm of nitrogen mustard can repeat the same sequence of reactions to form DNA crosslinks.

favored sites of DNA attack are the N^7 position of guanine, which accounts for about 90% of alkylated sites, the 1 position of guanine, the 1, 3, and 7 positions of adenine, and the N^3 position of cytosine. It is not clear which of these sites of attack is most crucial in producing the pharmacologic action of this class of compounds; alkylation of the N^7 position of guanine has a lesser effect on misreading the DNA template than does alteration of the N^3 position of cytidine or the 0^6 position of guanine, both of which interfere with accurate base pairing.

The consequences of base alkylation include not only misreading of the DNA code but also single-strand breakage and cross-linking of DNA. Further effects include an inhibition of DNA, RNA, and protein synthesis is rapidly dividing tissues. Single-strand breakage occurs primarily as a consequence of the enzymatic processes of repair; the alkylated base is excised by endonuclease enzymes that specifically open the DNA strand at sites of base alkylation or in sequences lacking a purine base. The resulting gap can be repaired by a ligase enzyme, if such an enzyme is present in the affected cell.

Cross-linkage of DNA occurs when so-called bifunctional alkylating agents are employed. For example, the prototype drug nitrogen mustard possesses two chloroethyl groups, each of which is capable of forming a carbonium ion. The establishment of cross-strand covalent binding correlates closely with the lethality of exposure to alkylating agents and to nitrosourea derivatives.[68]

Alkylating agents as a class exert cytotoxic effects on cells throughout the cell cycle, but have quantitatively greater activity against rapidly dividing cells, possibly because these cells have less time to repair damage before entering the vulnerable DNA-synthetic phase of the cycle.

Although the alkylating agents as a class share a common molecular mechanism of action and possess cytotoxic, mutagenic, and carcinogenic potential, they differ greatly in their pharmacokinetic features, lipid solubility, chemical reactivity, and membrane transport properties and thus do not uniformly share cross-resistance in experimental or clinical chemotherapy. [69] Thus, the nitrosoureas and cyclophosphamide are not cross-resistant clinically in the treatment of lymphomas, nor does multiple myeloma necessarily show cross-resistance to cyclophosphamide and melphalan. Thus, a consideration of the individual agents is necessary in order to understand their unique properties and optimal clinical usage. The structures of commonly used alkylating agents are shown in Figure 9-14.

NITROGEN MUSTARD

Nitrogen mustard, or mechlorethamine, was the first alkylating agent to receive clinical trial and was found to produce responses in patients with lymphoma. This agent is highly reactive in aqueous solution and must be administered by intravenous injection. It is also effective as a topical solution for treatment of mycosis fungoides, but produces hypersensitivity to its chloroethyl side chain when used in this way. Nitrogen mustard penetrates cells through an active transport mechanism shared with the physiologic amine choline.[70] Resistance to the agent is poorly understood; it is believed to

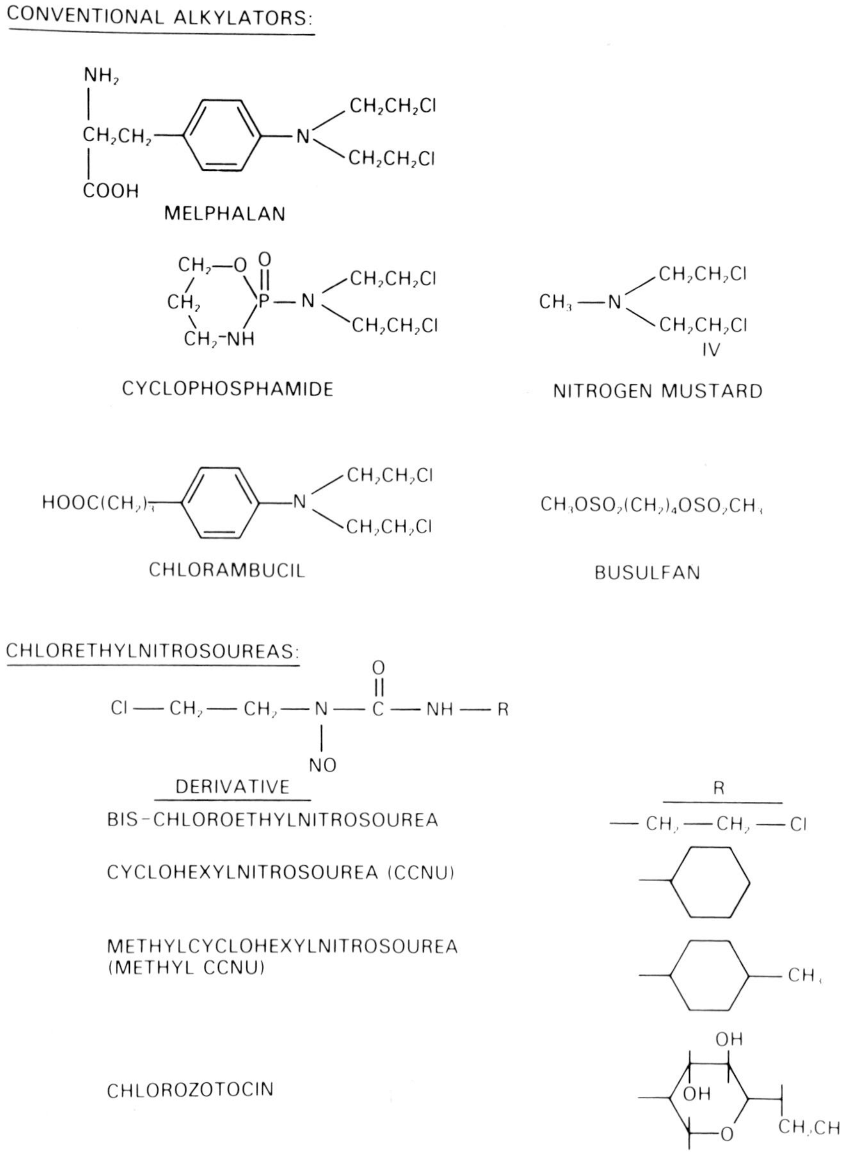

CONVENTIONAL ALKYLATORS:

MELPHALAN

CYCLOPHOSPHAMIDE

NITROGEN MUSTARD

$CH_3OSO_2(CH_2)_4OSO_2CH_3$

CHLORAMBUCIL

BUSULFAN

CHLORETHYLNITROSOUREAS:

$Cl—CH_2—CH_2—N(NO)—C(=O)—NH—R$

DERIVATIVE	R
BIS-CHLOROETHYLNITROSOUREA	$—CH_2—CH_2—Cl$
CYCLOHEXYLNITROSOUREA (CCNU)	
METHYLCYCLOHEXYLNITROSOUREA (METHYL CCNU)	CH_3
CHLOROZOTOCIN	OH, OH, O, CH_2CH

FIG. 9-14. Structures of commonly used alkylating agents and chloroethylnitrosoureas.

result from enhanced ability to repair DNA alkylation,[71] but other mechanisms—such as defective transport or increased inactivation of the carbonium ion by enzymatic conjugation with intracellular sulfhydril groups—have not been examined.

The primary clinical toxicities of nitrogen mustard are shown in Table 9-1 and consist of myelosuppression and gastrointestinal symptoms (nausea and vomiting). Minor cholinergic side-effects are noted at high doses and include lacrimation, diarrhea, and diaphoresis. Because of the high chemical reactivity of this compound, it is a potent vesicant and causes severe local tissue injury when infiltrated into the skin. It is thus useful for ablating the pleural space in patients with chronic pleural effusion due to malignant disease. Nitrogen mustard has been largely replaced in clinical use by more stable agents, as described below.

CYCLOPHOSPHAMIDE

In an attempt to improve the selectivity of alkylating agents, cyclophosphamide was designed based on the rationale that tumor cells possess a high concentration of enzyme activity capable of cleaving the P—N bond, liberating the potent phosphoramide mustard. In fact, the drug is activated in a multistep process. The first metabolite, hydroxycyclophosphamide, is produced by hepatic microsomal metabolism (Fig. 9-15).[72] This latter compound undergoes spontaneous tautomerization to aldophosphamide, which is hydrolysed within target cells to yield the final active compound, phosphoramide mustard, and a side product, acrolein. (Acrolein, a weakly cytotoxic compound, may be responsible for the common side-effect, hemorrhagic cystitis.) The intermediates in this

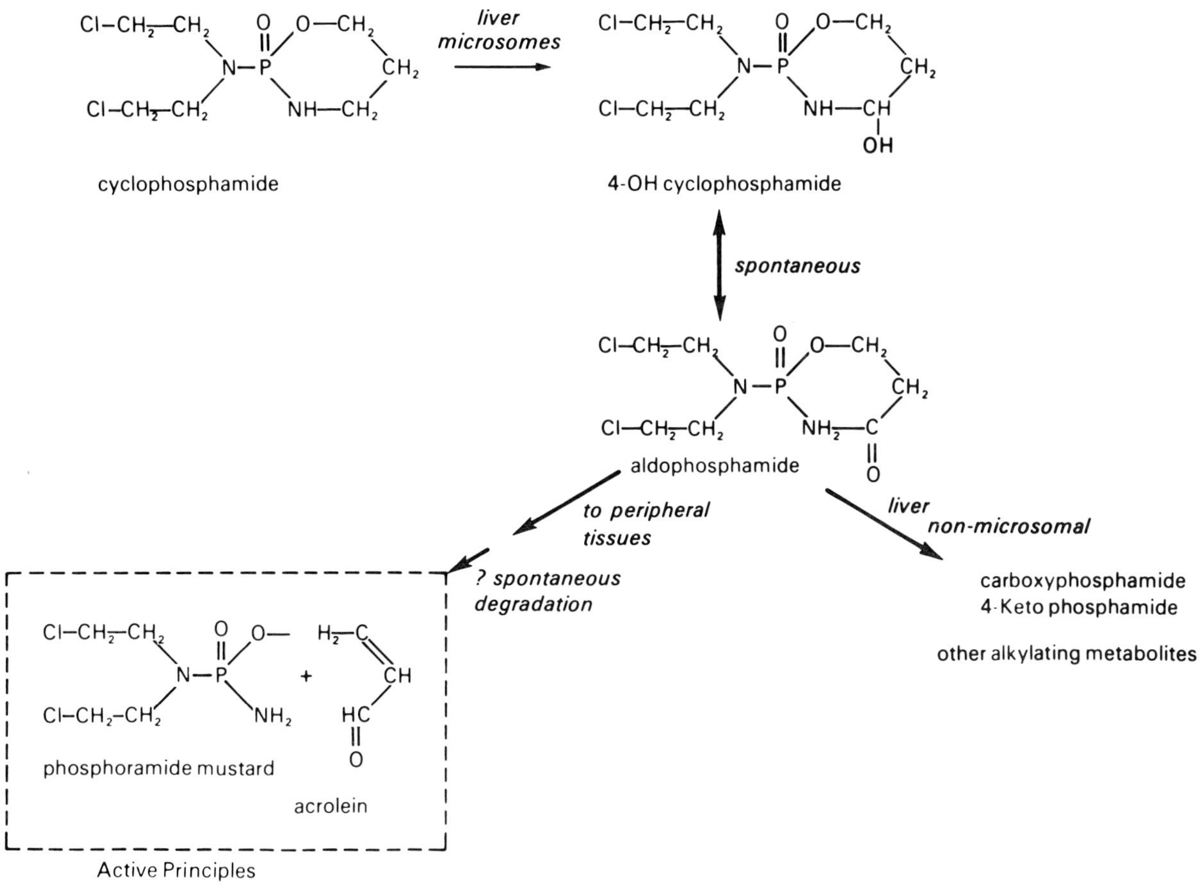

cyclophosphamide

liver microsomes

4-OH cyclophosphamide

spontaneous

aldophosphamide

to peripheral tissues

liver non-microsomal

carboxyphosphamide
4-Keto phosphamide

other alkylating metabolites

? spontaneous degradation

phosphoramide mustard

acrolein

Active Principles

FIG. 9-15. Metabolism of cyclophosphamide by hepatic mixed-function oxidase, and transformation into active intermediates.

reaction sequence have been identified in plasma, but the pharmacokinetics of cyclophosphamide have not been thoroughly studied.

The toxicities produced by cyclophosphamide differ from those of nitrogen mustard. Cyclophosphamide is stable as the parent compound, is well absorbed orally, and does not cause local irritation if infiltrated during attempted intravenous infusion. It produces only mild thrombocytopenia in comparison to leukopenia. Nausea, vomiting, and alopecia are common side-effects with high-dose intravenous therapy. In addition, active products excreted in the urine produce two unusual toxicities: (1) hemorrhagic cystitis and (2) inappropriate retention of water by the distal nephron. Cystitis is particularly common in high-dose chemotherapy regimens or with prolonged periods of oral therapy and may lead to significant blood loss, necessitating discontinuation of the drug. Because cystitis is caused by local irritation from drug products in the urine (possibly acrolein), it has been suggested that instillation of agents such as thiol compounds into the bladder or systemic administration of N-acetyl cysteine might prevent this toxicity; the effectiveness of these measures has not been proved clinically, and the major preventive maneuver is simply to reduce alkylating metabolite concentration by diuresis.[73] Hydration of such patients carries some risk, however, because in high-dose infusion regimens cyclophosphamide causes a syndrome of inappropriate water retention because of direct effects on the renal tubule. Hyponatremia, seizures, and death have been reported as a consequence of water retention.

Other toxicities include potent suppression of both humoral and delayed hypersensitivity[74]; carcinogenicity in animals and leukemogenesis in man; sterility that is probably irreversible in male and possibly reversible in female patients; and, rarely, interstitial pulmonary fibrosis.[75] Acute myocardial necrosis has also been observed in patients receiving extremely large doses (greater than 100 mg per kg) of cyclophosphamide prior to bone marrow transplantation.

MELPHALAN

A second, rationally designed alkylating agent, melphalan, was conceived as a compound that would localize preferentially in tumors actively utilizing phenylalanine or tyrosine, such as melanin-producing malignancies. The resulting compound has a broad spectrum of antitumor activity similar to that of cyclophosphamide (lymphomas, breast and ovarian cancer, multiple myeloma) but has the additional advantage of not causing hemorrhagic cystitis.

The drug shows variable bioavailability when given orally,[76] and thus doses must be adjusted by this route according to bone marrow tolerance. Melphalan enters cells by active transport, utilizing a high affinity carrier—the "L" amino acid transport system—that also transports the amino acids leucine and glutamine. In some tumor cells, a second transport system (that also carries alanine, cysteine, and serine) promotes melphalan uptake but is less effective than the L system at high drug concentrations.[77] High concentrations of leucine and glutamine can reduce melphalan toxicity both to bone marrow colony-forming units *in vitro* and to tumor cells.[78] It is not known whether the amino acid concentration of the plasma or ascitic fluid influences the uptake and cytotoxicity of melphalan, or whether hyperalimentation with an intravenous amino acid mixture might alter melphalan transport.

Melphalan is variably absorbed after oral adminsitration. Between 20 and 50% of oral drug is excreted in the stool. After intravenous administration, the parent compound disappears from plasma with a half-life of approximately 2 hours, a rate consistent with the rate of hydrolysis of the chloride groups in plasma. Mono- and dihydroxy metabolites as well as alkylated proteins are found in plasma soon after intravenous drug administration. Less than 15% of the drug is excreted in the urine intact.[79]

Melphalan causes equal suppression of granulocyte and platelet production, with reversal of these effects in 10 to 14 days. Alopecia is also common during extended courses of treatment.

CHLORAMBUCIL

This close structural congener of melphalan has similar stability in aqueous solution because of the electron-withdrawing properties of its unsaturated ring. Chlorambucil is given orally and thus is a convenient alkylating agent for treatment of malignancies such as chronic lymphocytic leukemia, nodular lymphomas, or multiple myeloma, which require long-term management. It has predictable myelosuppressive effects on both granulocytes and platelets, but few other side-effects. Like other alkylating agents, chlorambucil has been implicated in late occurrences of acute myeloblastic leukemia[80] and in a single case of pulmonary fibrosis.[81] Its pharmacokinetics are poorly understood, but it appears to be eliminated by metabolic transformation.

BUSULFAN

Busulfan consists of two labile methane-sulfonate groups attached at opposite ends of a four-carbon alkyl chain. This compound is sufficiently stable to allow oral administration, but it rapidly forms carbonium ions after systemic absorption through release of the methane-sulfonate group, leading to alkylation of DNA.[82] Although the potential for interstrand cross-linkage exists in the bifunctional structure of busulfan, such cross-linkage has not been demonstrated.

This agent is primarily used in schedules of daily oral administration for the treatment of chronic granulocytic leukemia, where its strongly myelosuppressive action provides smooth, long-term regulation of the white blood cell count. However, myelosuppression produced by busulfan is not quickly reversible; bone marrow "burn out" may last indefinitely if excessive doses are used. Thus, close monitoring of blood counts is essential. The relationship between drug concentration in plasma and myelotoxicity is not known.

In addition to myelosuppression, busulfan causes two unusual side effects: diffuse pulmonary fibrosis and an Addisonian-like state characterized by cutaneous hyperpigmentation and weakness, but without abnormalities of adrenal function.

NITROSOUREA

The chloroethylnitrosoureas are highly lipid-soluble and chemically reactive compounds that have clinical activity against the lymphomas, malignant melanoma, brain neoplasms, and gastrointestinal carcinomas. Many derivatives incorporating this basic structure, but differing in their lipid solubility, side-group substitution, and aqueous stability, have been synthesized in an effort to improve their therapeutic index[83]; the most recent of these, chlorozotocin, a glycosylated nitrosourea, has a spectrum of activity similar to that of the established agents, but lesser bone marrow toxicity, and it is currently undergoing trials in various tumor types.

Chemical decomposition of these agents in aqueous solution yields two reactive intermediates, a chloroethyldiazohydroxide and an isocyanate group (Fig. 9-16). The former decomposes further to yield a reactive chloroethyl carbonium ion that alkylates DNA in the same manner as the classic mustards, producing strand breaks and crosslinks. Crosslinks are produced both by the monofunctional and bifunctional nitrosoureas[84]; the monofunctional cyclohexylnitrosoureas (CCNU and methylCCNU) probably crosslink by an initial formation of the chloroethyl adduct to DNA, followed by loss of the chloride substituent and formation of a second reactive carbonium ion. This second reactive site then attacks the opposite DNA strand.

In distinction to the classic alkylating agents, decomposition of nitrosoureas also yields isocyanates that react with amine groups such as the epsilon amino group of lysine, in a carbamoylation reaction. The isocyanates are believed to inhibit DNA repair and to alter maturation of RNA. However, although carbamoylation may contribute to the overall effects of the nitrosoureas, compounds such as chlorozotocin, which lack significant carbamoylating activity, still preserve significant antitumor activity. Thus, alkylation seems to be a more important feature of nitrosourea action.[85]

The reduced bone marrow toxicity of glycosylated nitrosoureas (streptozotocin and chlorozotocin) is believed to result from the reduced alkylation of bone marrow DNA, possibly because of altered transport properties of these compounds. The high antitumor potency of chlorozotocin has been attributed to its preferential binding to transcriptionally active portions of chromatin.[86]

Because of the extreme clinical reactivity of these compounds in aqueous solution, they disappear rapidly from the blood after absorption or intravenous infusion. Intact parent compounds (BCNU, CCNU or methylCCNU) have not been detected in plasma in man. It is likely that the cyclohexylnitrosoureas undergo ring hydroxylation by hepatic micro-

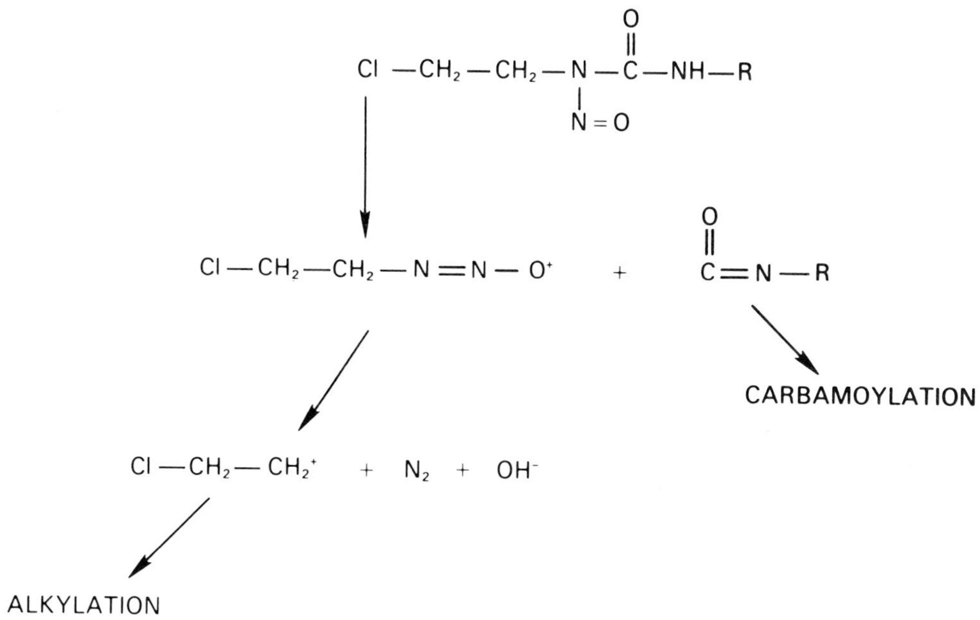

$$Cl-CH_2-CH_2-N(N{=}O)-C(=O)-NH-R$$

$$\downarrow$$

$$Cl-CH_2-CH_2-N{=}N-O^{+} \quad + \quad O{=}C{=}N-R \rightarrow \text{CARBAMOYLATION}$$

$$\downarrow$$

$$Cl-CH_2-CH_2^{+} \quad + \quad N_2 \quad + \quad OH^{-}$$

$$\downarrow$$

ALKYLATION

FIG. 9-16. Decomposition of chloroethylnitrosoureas to form chloroethyl carbonium ion and a carbamoylating isocyanate group.

somes, resulting in decreased carbamoylating potential but increased alkylating activity.[87] The high lipid solubility of the nitrosoureas may account for their excellent activity against experimental and clinical intracranial tumors; the chloroethyl portion of CCNU crosses readily into the central nervous system reaching concentrations 30% of those found simultaneously in plasma.

The toxicities of the clinically useful nitrosoureas are listed in Table 9-1. The most notable and consistent toxicity is delayed myelosuppression, which reaches a nadir 4 to 6 weeks after treatment and prevents the repetition of cyclic therapy at intervals shorter than 6 to 8 weeks. Severe and protracted leukopenia and thromocytopenia may occur in patients receiving conventional doses of BCNU, CCNU, or methyl-CCNU, particularly in patients who have received extensive prior chemotherapy. Prolonged use of these drugs leads to cumulative bone marrow toxicity and, in occasional patients, to an aplastic bone marrow. Acute myelocytic leukemia has been reported following long-term CCNU treatment, and these agents are known to be highly carcinogenic and mutagenic in animals and in *in vitro* tests.

Prolonged courses of treatment with BCNU and with methylCCNU have been associated with pulmonary fibrosis. The total dose of BCNU was 1000 mg/m^2 or greater in all cases reported and was 2733 mg/m^2 for the one reported case of pulmonary fibrosis induced by methylCCNU.[88] Chronic renal failure has been reported in children receiving methylCCNU for brain tumor treatment.[89] Azotemia or elevated serum creatinine levels developed after the cessation of treatment in 5 of 6 patients who received more than 1500 mg/m^2 methylCCNU, and a decrease in kidney size was observed in all 6 patients. This toxicity in man bears out the consistent finding of renal toxicity of methylCCNU in preclinical toxicologic studies. Renal toxicity has also been observed in patients receiving more than 1200 mg/m^2 of BCNU and appears to be a common, but late-developing, complication of prolonged nitrosourea treatment.

CIS-PLATINUM

Cis (II) platinum diamminedichloride (*cis*-DDP) is the only heavy metal compound in common use as a cancer chemotherapeutic agent, and as such has a mechanism of action and a spectrum of biologic effects unique to this group of drugs. The biologic activity of platinum coordinate compounds was first recognized in 1965, when Rosenberg and colleagues observed inhibition of bacterial growth in a medium subjected to an electric current transmitted by platinum electrodes. Of the several forms of platinum found in the solution, the *cis*-DDP compound had both antibacterial and antitumor action.[90,91] This compound subsequently entered clinical trials in 1971 and since has become established as a highly effective drug for treating testicular tumors, ovarian carcinoma, and head and neck cancer.

The antitumor activity of *cis*-DDP is best understood in terms of its chemistry in aqueous solution (Fig. 9-17). The divalent heavy metal platinum (Pt) binds two potential leaving groups, the chloride ions; in transposition, to the chlorides are bound two NH_3 groups in a firm covalent linkage. Only the *cis*-dichloro structure is an active antitumor agent; the *trans*-DDP isomer lacks cytotoxic activity, possibly because of its inability to form intrastrand DNA crosslinks.[92] Both chloride ions undergo a slow displacement by water, a process thought to occur at an accelerated rate in an environment of low chloride concentration (*e.g.*, inside the cell), generating a positively charged, aquated complex. This activated complex can then interact with a nucleophilic site on DNA, RNA, or protein to form bifunctional covalent links analogous to

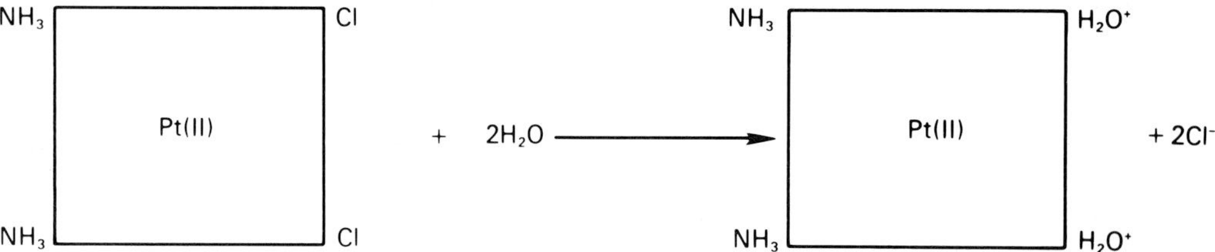

FIG. 9-17. Cis-diamminedichloroplatinum: generation of a reactive complex in aqueous solution.

alkylating reactions. Favored sites of attack are the N^7 position of guanine and the N^3 position of cytosine.[93] A variety of bifunctional and monofunctional covalent bonds are possible, including intrastrand crosslinks, interstrand links, and DNA–protein complexes.[94] There is preliminary evidence that the formation of intrastrand crosslinks may be a crucial feature of *cis*-DDP action, because this type of bond is not formed by the inactive *trans*-DDP complex.

The consequences of *cis*-DDP attack on DNA include changes in DNA conformation and inhibition of DNA synthesis.[95] The formation of crosslinks is a slow process that continues for hours after drug exposure and is opposed by enzymatic repair processes that excise and rebuild damaged segments of DNA.[96] DNA crosslinks may also be prevented by preincubation of the drug with thiourea,[97] which combines readily with the aquated platinum binding sites; thiourea can also reverse interstrand crosslinks in isolated DNA, but the concentrations of thiol required for this reversal are not achievable within intact cells.

The cell-cycle dependence of *cis*-DDP is poorly understood; it appears that some cells are most sensitive to *cis*-DDP if exposed during the G_1 (intermitotic) phase of the cycle, possibly because of the delay in crosslink formation, which would then be maximal during the following S phase.[98] A delay in transit through S phase and the succeeding cell cycle is induced by drug treatment.

Little is known about mechanisms of resistance to *cis*-DDP. It is likely that the ability to prevent (through sulfhydril reaction) or repair DNA crosslinks plays an important role in determining sensitivity to this drug.

Clinical Pharmacology

Cis-platinum is readily measured in biologic fluids by flameless atomic absorption spectroscopy,[99] a technique that has high sensitivity (about 0.3 μg/ml) and specificity but is not routinely available in pharmacology laboratories. A high-pressure liquid chromatographic technique has also been described[100]; it has comparable or greater sensitivity and the added advantage of separating the parent drug from the aquated species. Because of the high degree of covalent binding to protein, plasma samples must undergo ultrafiltration to separate the active unbound drug from the inactive protein-bound complex.

The clearance of total platinum from plasma proceeds rapidly during the first four hours after injection,[101] but thereafter levels decline very slowly because of covalent binding of the drug to serum proteins.[102] Unbound platinum, presumably the parent drug or the aquated derivative, falls with a half-life of 20 minutes to 1 hour, depending upon the rate of drug infusion. Maximum drug concentrations reach approximately 2.5×10^{-5} M for doses of 100 mg per m^2. Twenty to 75% of administered drug is excreted in the urine in the 24 hours after administration, the remainder representing drug bound to tissues or plasma protein.[103] *Cis*-DDP penetrates poorly into the central nervous system.[104] In monkeys, the ratio of drug concentration in plasma to cerebrospinal fluid was 25:1 or greater.

Cis-DDP is excreted in the urine as the result of glomerular filtration of unbound platinum coordinate complexes such as *cis*-DDP itself or other small-molecular-weight derivatives. In addition, there is evidence for tubular secretion of *cis*-DDP in animals.[105]

Clinical Administration and Toxicity

The mode of clinical administration of *cis*-DDP is largely determined by its primary toxicities. Because of its nephrotoxic potential, *cis*-DDP is usually administered after a 4- to 6-hour period of hydration with 1 liter fluid and 25 to 50 g mannitol.[106] The total dose administered is usually between 40 and 120 mg per m^2, depending on the frequency of administration and individual patient tolerance. An alternative schedule is the use of 20 mg per m^2 per day for 5 days, a regimen that causes lesser nephrotoxicity and nausea.

In the absence of hydration, the incidence of nephrotoxicity reaches 30% in patients treated with 50 to 75 mg per m^2 per course.[107] Although in animals both the proximal and distal tubules are pathologically affected, in man the primary finding is coagulative necrosis of the distal tubular epithelium and collecting ducts.[108] A reduction in renal blood flow and glomerular filtration rate also occurs in patients with platinum nephrotoxicity,[107] as well as a series of changes in tubular function, including magnesium wasting[109] and the excretion of various high-molecular-weight proteins.[110] Asymptomatic hypomagnesemia is a common finding in patients treated with *cis*-DDP, but magnesium loss may lead to symptomatic tetany.

Other experimental approaches to the prevention of *cis*-DDP toxicity have been considered and include development of new analogs and the testing of various thiol compounds that might inactivate *cis*-DDP in the urine. Thus far, none of the various analogs has been adequately tested in man. A promising thiol compound, diethyldithiocarbamate, is able to prevent renal toxicity in rats if given simultaneously with *cis*-DDP.[111] It remains to be established that this compound does not affect the antitumor action of *cis*-DDP.

Nausea and vomiting are quite frequent and persistent in patients taking *cis*-DDP and are poorly relieved by standard antiemetics. The severity of these symptoms is reduced by dividing the dose into smaller doses given once daily for 5 days. Myelosuppression is only moderate at usual clinical doses but becomes clinically significant in patients who have received prior myelosuppressive treatment or in patients receiving combination chemotherapy. Both leukopenia and thrombocytopenia are observed; significant anemia may develop after extended periods of treatment.

Other toxicities include a distal, sensory neuropathy that develops after prolonged treatment; hypersensitivity reactions such as urticaria, wheezing, and hypotension, which can be controlled in subsequent doses by pretreatment with antihistamines and corticosteroids[112]; and a progressive loss of high-frequency hearing, a toxicity that is most often seen in older patients. *Cis*-DDP is mutagenic to mammalian cells and is carcinogenic in whole animals.

ANTITUMOR ANTIBIOTICS

BLEOMYCIN

One of the most unusual structures with antitumor activity is bleomycin, a mixture of small-molecular-weight (1500 daltons) peptides isolated from the fungus *Streptomyces verticullus*. Bleomycin is one of a family of antibiotic peptides that possess both antitumor and antimicrobial activity. The bleomycin mixture contains predominantly the A_2 peptide, the unique pharmacologic properties of which have been extensively characterized.

The structure of the A_2 compound is shown in Figure 9-18; it consists of a DNA binding fragment, the "S" peptide, and an iron-binding portion located at the opposite end of the molecule. The primary action of bleomycin is to produce single- and double-strand breaks in DNA, an action that can be reproduced in cell-free mixtures of the A_2 peptide and DNA.[113] The sequence of events leading to DNA breakage begins with the binding of the S peptide to DNA in a ratio of 1 molecule of bleomycin to 4 to 5 base pairs of DNA. This binding occurs preferentially to guanine bases in DNA. Ferrous ion (Fe^{2+}), which is intimately bound to the imidazole, pyrimidine, and other nitrogen-containing groups of bleomycin, undergoes spontaneous oxidation to the Fe^{3+} state. The electron liberated in this reaction is accepted by oxygen to form active oxygen intermediates such as the superoxide or hydroxyl radicals. These radicals in turn attack the phosphodiester bonds between guanine and either thymine or cytosine. Free bases, particularly the pyrimidines, are released from DNA, leading to strand breaks. The action of bleomycin is specific for DNA and is not exerted against RNA.

There appears to be some cytokinetic specificity to bleomycin cell kill.[114] Cells in synchronized culture systems seem most susceptible during the premitotic, or G_2 phase, or in the mitotic phase of the cell cycle. However, cells exposed during G_1 are also killed, and there is no consensus as to whether rapid cell division predisposes to cytotoxicity. The possibility of increasing cell kill by exposing cells during the G_2 phase

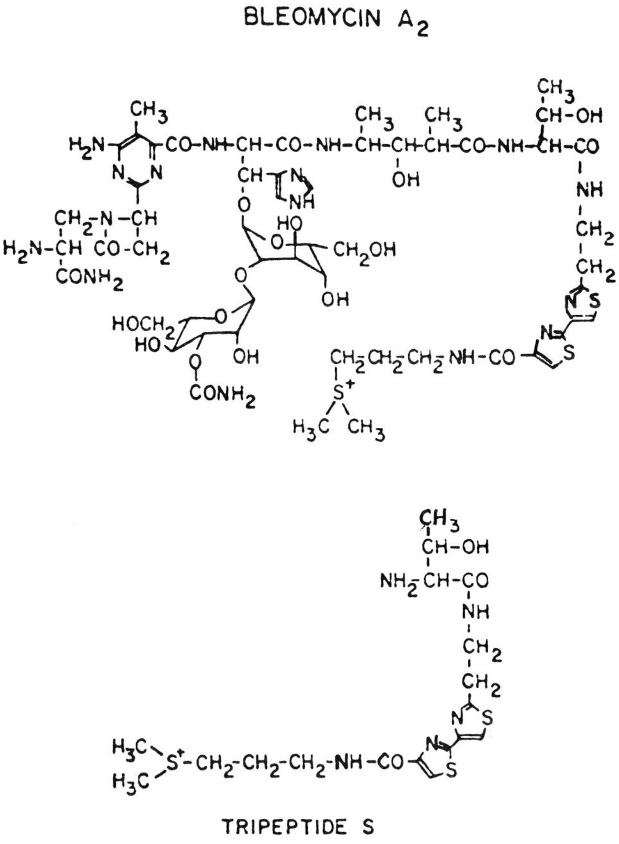

BLEOMYCIN A_2

TRIPEPTIDE S

FIG. 9-18. Structure of bleomycin A_2. The terminal S-tripeptide, which binds to DNA, is also shown.

has prompted bleomycin administration by continuous infusion.

The DNA lesions produced by bleomycin are visible as chromosomal breaks and deletions. It is likely that repair processes play an important role in determining the lethality of these lesions, because repair of potentially lethal damage has been demonstrated in cultured cells exposed to this agent.[115] There is indirect evidence that the same processes required to repair ionizing radiation damage are operative in bleomycin repair.

Little is known about the determinants of bleomycin response in tumor cells. The drug appears to penetrate cells slowly, requiring several hours to reach maximal uptake. A bleomycin-inactivating enzyme has been detected in both normal and malignant cells and is particularly prominent in liver.[116] The enzyme is not found in lung or skin, two normal tissues sensitive to bleomycin action. Increased degradative activity has been found in resistant experimental tumors.

Clinical Pharmacology

The most sensitive and reliable technique for assay of bleomycin is radioimmunoassay.[117] ^{125}I- or ^{57}Co-labeled bleomycin is used in this assay. The predominant peptides in the clinical mixture, the A_2 and B_2 compounds, give 75 to 100% reactivity when compared with the clinically used mixture of peptides.

Bleomycin is administered by parenteral injection, either

subcutaneously, intramuscularly, or intravenously. There are no obvious differences in clinical response rates associated with the different routes, although the continuous intravenous infusion has been widely used in the curative treatment of testicular cancer (see Chapter 24). Bleomycin exhibits a two-phased plasma disappearance curve with half-lives of 24 minutes and 2 to 4 hours. Peak plasma concentrations reach 1 to 10 m units per ml following intravenous bolus doses of 15 units/m^2. The postinfusion half-life is approximately 3 hours, a value similar to the β-half-life following bolus administration. Most bleomycin is excreted unchanged in the urine in patients with normal renal function.[118] As mentioned previously, a bleomycin-degrading aminopeptidase has been isolated from liver, but this enzyme plays no apparent important role in drug elimination in patients with normal renal function.

Preliminary evidence suggests that bleomycin pharmacokinetics are markedly altered in patients with abnormal renal function.[119] A half-life of 21 hours has been observed in a patient with a creatinine clearance of 11 ml/min. It would thus appear to be wise to decrease dosage of bleomycin by 50 to 75% in patients with severely compromised renal function.

In addition to conventional routes of administration, bleomycin may be injected into the pleural or peritoneal space to control malignant effusions.[119] Intracavitary doses of 60 mg/m^2 provide high-effusion concentrations of up to 50 m units/ml, or approximately tenfold higher levels than in plasma. About 50% of an intracavitary dose enters the systemic circulation; the remaining fraction is either metabolized in the pleural or peritoneal cavity or eliminated in its first pass through the portal circulation.

Clinical Toxicity

In contrast to most antitumor agents, bleomycin has little myelosuppressive toxicity. Only at high doses (above 25 mg/m^2) or in patients with severely compromised bone marrow is a fall in white count or platelet count observed. The primary toxicity of bleomycin is a subacute or chronic pneumonitis that progresses to interstitial fibrosis and may be fatal. The first manifestations of this toxicity are usually cough, dyspnea, and bibasilar pulmonary infiltrates on chest roentgenograms. The diffusion capacity of the lung is progressively decreased with increased total doses of the drug; total doses above 250 mg are associated with a more rapid decrease in diffusion capacity, and the incidence of clinically significant pulmonary toxicity reaches 10% at total doses of 450 mg or greater.[120] Toxicity is most frequent in older patients (over 70 years of age), in those with underlying lung disease such as emphysema, and in those previously treated with pulmonary or mediastinal irradiation. Although there appears to be a close relationship between total dose and risk of toxicity, well-documented cases have been observed at total doses below 100 mg.

The pulmonary lesion induced by bleomycin, as indicated by animal models of this toxicity, begins as an acute inflammatory intra-alveolar process with edema and proliferation of type II alveolar macrophages. Interstitial fibrosis, the hallmark of the mature lesion, becomes apparent in later stages, and leads to the decrease in diffusion capacity. There is no evidence at present that this fibrosis can be prevented by anti-inflammatory agents such as corticosteroid nor is it known whether the fibrosis is reversible upon withdrawal of the drug.

The clinical symptoms and x-ray findings of bleomycin pulmonary toxicity are not easily distinguished from other syndromes commonly observed in cancer patients, including progressive metastatic tumor (especially lymphangitic tumor), infectious processes such as *Pneumocystis carinii* or cytomegalovirus, or radiation injury. Open lung biopsy is often required, and reveals an acute inflammatory infiltrate, interstitial and intra-alveolar edema, pulmonary hyaline membrane formation, and intra-alveolar and interstitial fibrosis. In addition, squamous metaplasia of the alveolar lining cells is a common finding.

Bleomycin frequently produces an unusual cutaneous toxicity. Almost 50% of patients develop erythma, induration, thickening, and eventual peeling of skin over the fingers, palms, and extremity joints. In addition, most patients develop hyperpigmentation of skin creases and a general darkening of the skin. Occasional patients may develop Reynaud's phenomenon during bleomycin therapy.

Other, less frequent, toxicities include acute hypertension, primarily in patients receiving doses greater than 25 mg per day, and hyperbilirubinemia. Fever is often observed in the first 48 hours after drug administration, and occasional hypersensitivity reactions, with urticaria and bronchospasm, have been observed. These reactions usually do not necessitate discontinuation of the drug, but pretreatment with antihistamines and corticosteroids is advisable in patients with a history of allergic reactions to bleomycin.

In addition to its conventional use systemically, bleomycin has been administered by intra-arterial infusion[121] and by direct instillation into the urinary bladder.[122] The latter route causes a predictable and at times severe cystitis. Neither of these routes has been established as beneficial in cancer treatment.

ANTHRACYCLINES

The first anthracyclines in clinical use, daunomycin and doxorubicin, are antibiotics produced by *Streptomyces* species. These antibiotics are, in fact, part of a large group of usually highly colored *Streptomyces* products known as the rhodomycins. The reader is referred to the available exhaustive reviews of the structure and properties of the rhodomycins.[123,124] In general, these compounds share with daunomycin and doxorubicin a planar anthroquinone nucleus attached to an amino sugar (Fig. 9-19). Within this group or closely related to it are compounds with a wide range of biologic activity, which include antibacterial as well as antitumor agents.

As antitumor agents, anthracyclines are matched only by alkylating agents in terms of their clinical utility. Daunorubicin is one of the most effective agents in the treatment of acute lymphocytic and myelocytic leukemia. Doxorubicin, on the other hand, has a significant role in the treatment of solid tumors such as carcinoma of breast, lung, thyroid, and ovary, as well as soft tissue sarcomas. As a result of this clinical activity, a large number of analogs (over 500) have been synthesized or isolated from *Streptomyces*. It is likely that this activity will provide the clinician with a steady stream of new anthracyclines with different therapeutic spectra or altered toxicity. For this reason, we will place some emphasis in this section on pertinent structure–activity relationships.

Mechanism of Action

There is no single clearly defined mechanism of action. Anthraquinones, of which the anthracyclines are a subset, exhibit a wide range of biologic, biochemical, and chemical properties.[125] They are known to chelate divalent cations, especially calcium and, as a result, can alter bone metabolism and dissolve kidney stones. Other anthraquinones exhibit laxative effects. Because of the quinone-hydroquinone functionalities characteristic of the anthraquinones, these compounds can participate in oxidation–reduction reactions. Finally, because of the size and planar nature of the anthraquinones, many agents in this group intercalate between strands of the DNA double helix.

Thus, it is not surprising that doxorubicin and daunorubicin are known to intercalate DNA, chelate divalent cations, and engage in oxidation–reduction reactions.[126,127] In addition, these agents have been shown to react directly with cell membranes at low concentrations with resultant alterations in membrane function.[128,129]

Of these actions, we know most about the interaction with DNA. Both doxorubicin and daunorubicin act as intercalators with the planar anthracycline ring structure lying perpendicular to the long axis of the DNA double helix. The B and C rings appear to be buried within the helix with the A and D rings projecting out on either side. The amino sugar appears to confer added stability to the binding through its interaction with the sugar-phosphate backbone of DNA. Most available evidence suggests that this DNA binding is central to the antitumor activity of these compounds. The intercalation has been shown to result in the blockade of DNA, RNA, and protein synthesis, actions that can readily be understood to affect rapidly growing tumor cells. There is also an excellent correlation between DNA binding affinity and relative antitumor activity of a wide range of anthracycline analogs. Recently, the consequences of DNA binding have been described in more detail.

DNA-dependent DNA synthesis appears to be most affected through replicon initiation rather than through elongation of the nascent DNA chain. RNA synthesis is also not evenly affected; preribosomal RNA synthesis is more sensitive than is messenger or transfer RNA synthesis. In addition, there are significant differences among anthracyclines as to whether they exert their effects predominantly on DNA-dependent DNA synthesis or RNA synthesis. The major structural determinant here is the presence of multiple rather than single sugars; those with multiple sugars tend to be RNA selective.[130]

Many of the anthracyclines are also mutagenic, carcinogenic, and teratogenic. There is now abundant evidence that both these agents cause single-stranded DNA breaks and impair DNA repair. The mechanism of this DNA damage remains a point of some controversy. One school of thought holds that intercalation leads to changes in the topography of the double helix that trigger "nicking" of the DNA by some as yet to be specified repair enzyme. In support of this hypothesis, its proponents cite the appearance of DNA protein crosslinks adjacent to the single-stranded breaks. The alternate school proposes that anthracyclines are activated to free radicals in the nuclear membrane and that this leads to oxygen radical-mediated DNA damage. Workers in this school have confirmed the existence of a nuclear membrane P-450 reductase with capacity to convert doxorubicin to a free radical. Results of *in vitro* studies have, in turn, shown that doxorubicin radicals participate in oxygen-mediated DNA cleavage.[131] Thus, in part, it may be difficult to separate the effect of an anthracycline on DNA from its ability to act as a free radical.

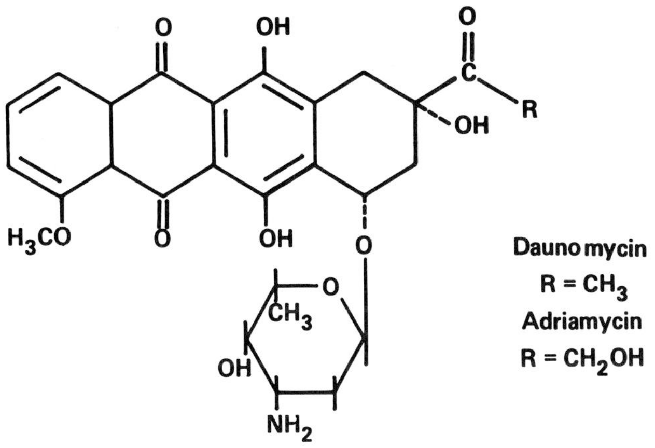

Daunomycin
$R = CH_3$
Adriamycin
$R = CH_2OH$

FIG. 9-19. Structure of anthracyclines.

The activation of doxorubicin into a free radical intermediate has been the subject of intense research interest over the past few years, since its initial description by Handa and Sato.[126] Yet, the picture here is far less complete than it is for DNA intercalation. We now know that a wide range of flavin-dependent oxidoreductases appear capable of reducing doxorubicin to a semiquinone radical. In turn, it has been shown that this semiquinone radical rapidly donates its electron to molecular oxygen to create the superoxide radical. Finally, tocopherol, a known free radical scavenger, has been shown to lessen doxorubicin-mediated oxygen radical generation *in vitro*. Superoxide radical production is the common final pathway of injury in radiation damage, phagocytic killing, and, as discussed later, DNA damage by mitomycin C and bleomycin. The reader is referred to several excellent reviews of the chemistry and biology of superoxide for further details of its action.[132,133]

The major difficulty with the free radical hypothesis occurs when one tries to use it to explain tumor response or toxicity of a specific tissue. It has been proposed that the cardiac toxicity of these agents is on a free radical basis whereas tumor response is secondary to DNA binding. In support of this hypothesis, it was shown that tocopherol, a radical scavenger, lessens cardiac toxicity without affecting tumor response. Although the differential effect of tocopherol on cardiac toxicity versus tumor effect has been amply confirmed, it soon became evident that these effects were not due to the presence in cardiac tissue of uniquely high levels of the enzymes that convert doxorubicin to a free radical. In fact, such enzymatic machinery seems to be ubiquitous and has been shown to be present in red blood cells and platelets, for example. This problem has recently been partially resolved by the discovery that cardiac tissue not only lacks the enzyme catalase but loses glutathione peroxidase after doxorubicin administration.[134] Thus, cardiac tissue, after doxorubicin, is without any known mechanism for disposing of hydrogen peroxide at the same time that doxorubicin is catalyzing the production of superoxide and hydrogen peroxide.

Finally, anthracyclines react directly with cell membranes to alter membrane function in a number of ways.[128,129] Specific binding has been shown to two membrane sites, the phospholipid cardiolipin and the protein spectrin. The latter is critical for membrane structure, the former is found in particularly high concentrations in cardiac mitochondria and in the membranes of malignant cells. This interaction with cardiolipin has led one worker to propose that binding to this cardiolipin explains both cardiac toxicity and tumor-cell kill.[129] Much work needs to be done to validate this interesting hypothesis.

Clinical Pharmacology and Pharmacokinetics

The clinical pharmacology of the anthracyclines is in its infancy. It is only within the last two years that adequate assay methodology has become available. For many years, thin-layer chromatography was used as a method of separating parent drug from metabolite. It is now apparent that many anthracyclines, doxorubicin for example, are unstable on thin-layer chromatographic plates and that significant artifacts were created by this process. Currently, the only valid assay methodology is via high-pressure liquid chromatography, which allows rapid resolution of doxorubicin and its metabolites.[135,136] The major doxorubicin metabolite is doxorubicinol, the product of reduction via the aldo-keto reductase. This compound does exhibit antitumor effect, although less than the parent drug. Parent drug and this metabolite also predominate in bile and urine. Another metabolite of interest, deoxyadriamycin aglycone, is one of the by-products of semiquinone radical formation and is thus a marker for this process *in vivo*. Other minor metabolites have been described whose importance is obscure at present.[137] Although the pharmacokinetics of this drug are undoubtedly complex, its disappearance curves can be fit to a three-compartment model with half-lives of 11 minutes, 3 hours, and 25 to 28 hours.[138] Clearance of doxorubicinol appears often but not always to parallel that of the parent drug.

The effect of renal and liver failure on doxorubicin and daunomycin clearance is of great interest to the clinician because this information can then provide a basis for rational modification of drug dosage in the face of malfunction of these organs. Renal clearance of doxorubicin is minor in magnitude, and there is thus no need to modify drug dosages in the face of renal failure. The liver is a site of significant metabolism of both doxorubicin and daunorubicin. As a result, drug dosages are often modified based on abnormal liver function, especially elevated bilirubin. Precise guidelines based on a sound pharmacokinetic basis are, however, completely lacking, and this subject warrants more careful study.

Toxicity

Doxorubicin and daunorubicin both cause bone marrow suppression and mucositis, which represent the dose-limiting acute toxicity of these agents. Alopecia is a common, nearly universal, toxicity that although not life-threatening, often causes patients significant distress. Extravasation of these agents leads to severe local reaction. Typically, erythema and pain develop within 24 hours and can progress over weeks, eventuating in deep ulceration that can reach tendon and bone. These lesions heal very slowly and are difficult to skin graft. Multiple local measures used to manage this compromise include ice packs and local injections of steroid, bicarbonate, or saline solution. Nevertheless, the best approach is clearly to take all possible precautions to avoid extravasation.

Perhaps the most perplexing toxicity these agents exhibit is cardiac toxicity. Clinically, there are two aspects to this toxicity. There is an acute syndrome that can be seen from hours to days after a dose of doxorubicin or daunorubicin; it is unrelated to cumulative dose and can manifest as either disturbances in conduction and rhythm or pump failure. Electrocardiographic (ECG) studies have revealed supraventricular arrythmias, heart block, and ventricular tachycardia. In addition, ECG-gated pool scans have shown major drops in ejection fraction that reach a nadir within 24 to 48 hours after drug administration. In certain patients, this is sufficient to cause congestive heart failure. Some of these patients develop pericardial effusions, and this whole complex has been termed the myocarditis–pericarditis syndrome. It can be severe enough to lead to the sudden demise of the patient.

The other aspect to this toxicity is a cumulative, dose-dependent cardiomyopathy that can lead to congestive heart failure in 1 to 10% of the patients who receive a total dose of 550 mg/m^2 of doxorubicin. The pathology of this lesion is unique and can readily be quantitated by endocardial biopsy. This technique is of value both in diagnosing the cause of congestive heart failure in patients who may have received doxorubicin and in detecting subclinical cardiac damage, which contraindicates further doxorubicin treatment. ECG-gated pool scan measurement of ejection fraction has also proved of value in detecting heart damage. This modality may be more practical for widespread clinical use than is endocardial biopsy.

The mechanism of this cardiac toxicity was discussed in part earlier. Here it is important to note that two independent lines of investigation suggest that this toxicity may be dissociable from the antitumor activity of these agents. First, antidotal agents such as tocopherol have been shown in animals to lessen cardiac toxicity without affecting tumor response. Second, new anthracyclines have been developed that in animals possess significantly less cardiac toxicity while preserving antitumor activity.[139,140]

MITOMYCIN C

Mitomycin C is an antibiotic whose antitumor activity has been known for over 20 years. Its clinical use has been restricted because it causes severe marrow aplasia. Interest in this agent has increased because of its activity in carcinoma of the stomach and ovary. Also, it has been discovered that high-dose intermittent therapy preserves antitumor effect and reduces the myelosuppression to manageable proportions. The reader is referred to several reviews for more detail of the clinical activity and pharmacologic aspects of this agent.[141,142]

Structure and Mechanism of Action

Mitomycin has three groups capable of damaging tissue: a quinone that can participate in free radical reactions in a fashion analogous to that of the anthracyclines;[143] an azuridinal group that can clearly function as an alkylator; and a urethane functionality that might act as an alkylator.

With this background, it is not surprising that activation of mitomycin C proceeds by means of reduction of the quinone and loss of the methoxy group.[144] This is followed by alkylation of DNA with intrastrand and interstrand crosslinks that results in inhibition of DNA synthesis and cell death.

Clinical Pharmacology

Limited information is available on the pharmacokinetics of this agent. The drug may be measured in patient samples by high-pressure liquid chromatography, mass spectrophotometry, or microbiologic assay. The first two methods provide greater inherent specificity, but the latter is, at present, more sensitive.

After bolus intravenous administration of 22.5 mg/m^2 to 45 mg/m^2, plasma levels peak at an average of 0.4 μg/ml. The drug appears to have a volume of distribution that approaches that of total body water.

Metabolic activation by reduction appears to occur in all tissues. It does not, therefore, explain the selectivity of this agent for tumor tissue. As a result of this ubiquitous metabolism, clearance of the drug is rapid. As with the anthracyclines, renal clearance is minor, and the role of the liver is so poorly defined that no guidelines can be given for dose modification in the presence of liver disease.

Toxicity

As mentioned, the major dose-limiting toxicity of mitomycin C is myelosuppression. This myelosuppression is delayed and cumulative in a fashion analogous to that of the nitrosoureas. After a single bolus dose, leukocyte and platelet counts usually reach a nadir between the fourth and sixth weeks. Typically, by the third course of treatment, doses have to be modified, usually to 50% or less of the initial dose.

Less commonly, this drug has also been associated with interstitial pneumonitis, nephrotoxicity, and cardiomyopathy. The pneumonitis is uncommon, not dose-related, and exhibits pathology similar to that of busulfan lung.[145] The nephrotoxicity is at present rare and poorly described. The cardiomyopathy has been reported in patients receiving doxorubicin and mitomycin C in combination and manifests itself as accelerated appearance of cardiac toxicity at doses of doxorubicin that are not, by themselves, associated with significant damage. This phenomenon is not unexpected because both doxorubicin and mitomycin C can be activated to radicals by reduction and,[143] in the former case, this radical production has been proposed as the mechanism of the cardiac toxicity.[134]

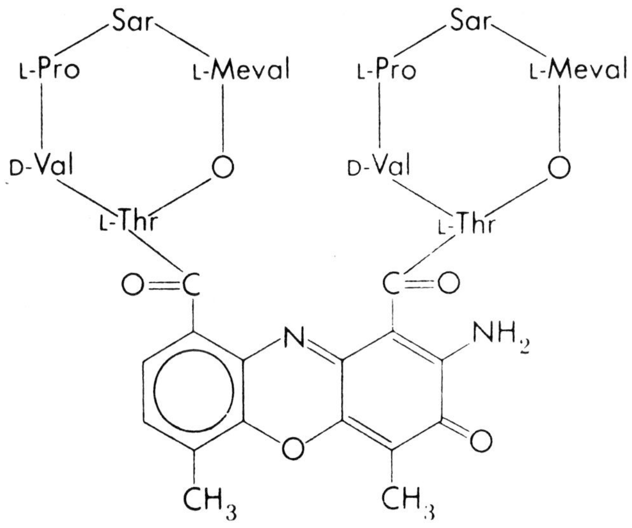

FIG. 9-20. Actinomycin D.

ACTINOMYCIN D

This antibiotic is a member of a large class of similar drugs either isolated from *Streptomyces* or synthesized chemically.[146] It is the only member of the class to achieve significant clinical use. This drug has a fairly well-defined clinical role in the treatment of a limited group of malignancies. It is clearly effective in the treatment of Wilms' tumor, Ewing's sarcoma, embryonal rhabdomyosarcoma, and gestational choriocarcinoma.[147] Responses are also seen in testicular cancer, Kaposi's sarcoma, and lymphoma.

Structure and Mechanism of Action

This drug has an interesting structure in that it is composed of a phenoxazone ring chromophore that confers a red color to the drug and to which are bound two identical cyclic polypeptides (Fig. 9-20). This antibiotic binds to DNA by intercalation with the phenoxazone ring inserted perpendicularly to the long axis of the DNA double helix and the polypeptide chains extending into the minor groove. This intercalation depends on a specific interaction between the polypeptide chains and deoxyguanosine.[148] The result of this intercalation is a block in the ability of DNA to act as a template for both RNA and DNA synthesis. At low drug concentrations, inhibition of RNA synthesis predominates, whereas at higher cocentrations both RNA and DNA synthesis are affected.[149]

In addition to these effects, actinomycin D also causes single-stranded DNA breaks in a fashion similar to that of doxorubicin.[150] As with doxorubicin, there are several possible explanations for this observation. Actinomycin D can be reduced via P-450 reductase to a radical intermediate, and this has been postulated to be the cause of the single-strand breaking. The alternate hypothesis is that intercalation results in sufficient strain on the three-dimensional topography of the double helix to trigger enzymatic nicking and strand breakage. This picture is complicated by the fact that of the many actinomycin D analogs that have been examined, there is no correlation between their affinity for DNA, the occurrence of single-stranded breaks, and cytotoxicity.

Clinical Pharmacology

Metabolism does not play a significant role in the clearance of actinomycin D, and most of the drug is excreted unchanged in bile and urine. Clearance of the drug from plasma is rapid initially and is dominated by tissue uptake and DNA binding.[151] The slow phase (half-life of 36 hours) of the drug disappearance curve is dominated by slow release of drug from tissue pools with excretion into bile and urine.[152] Because human pharmacologic data are so fragmentary, no firm guidelines can be given for dose modification in the face of liver or renal failure.

Toxicity

The dose-limiting toxicity of this agent is most commonly myelosuppression but may occasionally be gastrointestinal toxicity. The latter can manifest as ulceration of oral mucosa and gastrointestinal tract with pain and diarrhea. Alopecia occurs and skin toxicity can also be severe on occasion.

One of the most interesting and perplexing toxicities associated with actinomycin D is its interaction with x-irradiation. Combined treatment with these two modalities leads to accelerated skin and gastrointestinal toxicity. In addition, late radiation damage to lung and liver appears to be increased. This effect has been postulated to result from the ability of actinomycin D to block repair of radiation-mediated DNA damage. This explanation cannot, however, explain the recall effect observed in patients who are treated with actinomycin D after x-irradiation. This recall reaction can be observed even after an interval of several months between radiation and drug treatment.

MITHRAMYCIN

Mithramycin is an antibiotic isolated from *Streptomyces plicatus* that has antitumor activity against testicular carcinoma, but in addition has a specific hypocalcemic effect that has value in the treatment of malignant hypercalcemia.

Mithramycin is an inhibitor of DNA-directed RNA synthesis by virtue of its binding to guanine bases of DNA. Mg^{2+} is required for this binding, and the resulting complex is only slowly reversible.

Mithramycin is administered intravenously. Little is known about its pharmacokinetics and disposition in man. There are no suitable assays for this drug at the present time. This agent has a number of unusual side effects in addition to its antitumor activity. It causes acute nausea and vomiting and, occasionally, diarrhea and stomatitis. More importantly, a hemorrhagic diathesis is associated with daily treatment and is manifested as a fall in platelet count, a lengthening of the prothrombin time, and a depression of clotting factors II, V, VII, and X. Deaths due to uncontrolled gastrointestinal hemorrhage have been reported with this schedule of administration. In addition, mithramycin has serious renal and hepatic toxicity, the mechanisms of which are again unclear. An alternate day regimen of 50 μg/kg/day appears to cause more predictable and tolerable toxicity and is associated with a nearly 50% response rate in testicular carcinoma. This schedule is maintained on an alternate day basis until signs of hepatic (LDH greater than 2000 units/100 ml), renal (azotemia), or clotting (prothrombin time greater than 15 seconds, platelet count below 100,000 cells per mm^3) dysfunction appear.

Other toxicities include fever, myalgias, headache, and uncommonly, vascular thrombosis. Because of its many serious toxic side-effects, mithramycin at present is indicated only for treatment of testicular neoplasms. However, in lower doses and for brief courses of treatment (15–25 μg/kg/day for 3 days), mithramycin effectively lowers serum calcium concentration in patients with hypercalcemia of malignant and nonmalignant origin. Its effects are mediated through decreased bone resorption and last for 7 to 21 days. In most instances, specific therapy directed against the neoplasm in question is required to produce permanent and effective control of the serum calcium.

PLANT ALKALOIDS

The search for new anticancer drugs through chemical synthesis of antimetabolites and through the isolation of fungal fermentation products has paid considerable dividends. An equally intensive screening of plant extracts has yielded many unusual and cytotoxic compounds, as reviewed by Creasey,[154] but few of these products have had a significant impact on clinical chemotherapy. The exceptions to this generality are the vinca alkaloids vincristine and vinblastine, derived from the ornamental shrub *Vinca rosea,* and the epipodophyllotoxins VM-26 and VP-16, derived by modification of a product of the mandrake plant.

The vinca alkaloids are closely related structures composed of two paired multiringed systems linked by a carbon–carbon bridge. A single modification on the catharanthine ring, as shown in Figure 9-21, constitutes the sole difference in structure, but the two compounds have significant differences in their spectrum of clinical action and toxicity. A third analog, vindesine (deacetylvinblastine), which is also a metabolic product of vinblastine in man, has entered clinical trial and has activity against the blastic phase of chronic granulocytic leukemia, the lymphomas, and various hematologic malignancies.[155]

The vinca alkaloids possess cytotoxic activity by virtue of their binding to tubulin. The latter is a dimeric protein found in the soluble fraction of the cytoplasm of all cells; it exists in equilibrium with a polymerized form, the microtubular apparatus, which forms the spindle along which chromosomes migrate during mitosis. In addition, microtubules play a vital role in maintaining cell structure, providing a conduit for cellular secretions and for neurotransmitter transit along axons. The vinca alkaloids, through their binding to tubulin, inhibit the process of assembly of microtubules and lead to the dissolution of the mitotic spindle.[156] A separate site for binding on tubulin is shared by two other spindle poisons, colchicine and podophyllotoxin.[157]

The primary manifestation of vinca action is an arrest of cells in the metaphase of mitosis. However, cells in culture appear to be most sensitive to the cytotoxic effects of these compounds during the late S phase of the cell cycle; this sensitivity may be related to the synthesis of a vital microtubular structure at this point, but is not clearly reconcilable with the hypothesis that the primary effect is on the synthesis of the mitotic spindle.[158]

The vinca alkaloids traverse the cell membrane by an active uptake process that has an affinity constant of approximately 10 μM.[159] This concentration is not achieved during clinical use of either vincristine or vinblastine; thus, the transport system is operating well below maximal velocity under treatment circumstances. However, only minute concentrations (in the range of 1×10^{-8} M) of either drug are required to kill murine leukemia cells in culture or to inhibit the proliferation of human lymphoblastic leukemia cells.[160]

Mechanisms of resistance to the vinca alkaloids have not been characterized. Patterns of cross resistance with other drugs such as anthracyclines and actinomycin D suggest that these agents share a common transport pathway, the absence of which might lead to resistance.[161,162] However, the biochemical lesion in resistant cells has not been adequately defined.

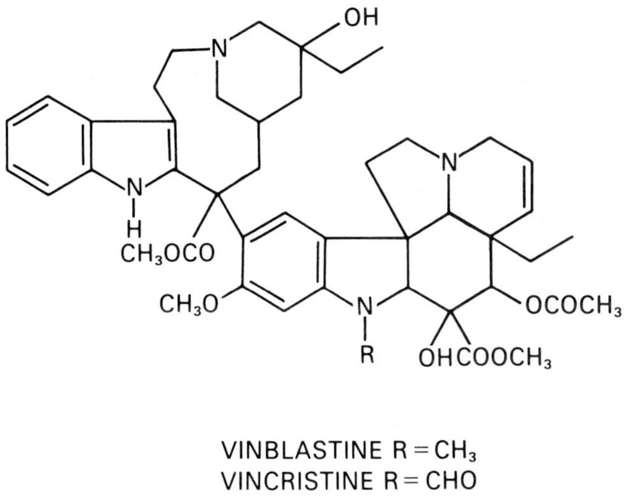

CLINICAL PHARMACOLOGY

The development of a comprehensive understanding of vinca alkaloid pharmacokinetics has been hampered by the lack of sufficiently sensitive and specific methods for drug assay. Most information has been obtained using radiolabeled drug, supplemented with chromatographic separation of parent drug from metabolites.[163] Radioimmunoassays for vincristine and vinblastine have been described, although their specificity is unproven.[164]

The primary pharmacokinetic characteristics of vincristine and vinblastine are given in Table 9-5. The main features of drug disposition are similar for the two agents and include the achievement of peak plasma concentrations of approximately 0.4 μM, followed by a multiphasic plasma disappearance with half-lives of 7.4 and 164 minutes for vincristine and 4.5 and 190 minutes for vinblastine.[163,164] A terminal velban half-life of 20 hours has been observed using the

OH
N
N
H
CH_3OCO
N
CH_3O
N
R
$OCOCH_3$
$OHCOOCH_3$

VINBLASTINE $R = CH_3$
VINCRISTINE $R = CHO$

FIG. 9-21. Structure of vinblastine and vincristine.

radioimmunoassay. A minimal amount of either drug is excreted in the urine. Almost 70% of a vincristine dose is excreted in the feces, primarily as metabolites resulting from hepatic metabolism and biliary excretion.[165,166] The fecal excretion of vinblastine is only 10%, as measured by radioimmunoassay, although drug metabolites may not be measured by this technique.[167]

Both vincristine and vinblastine are administred by intravenous bolus in doses of 1 to 1.4 mg per m^2 for the former and 0.1 mg per kg for the latter. Vincristine doses may be repeated at weekly intervals or at longer time intervals. Total doses in excess of 2 mg are often associated with a progressive and disabling neurotoxicity, particularly in older patients and in those receiving weekly treatment. The first signs of neuropathy are a decrease in deep tendon reflexes and paresthesias of the fingers and lower extremities. More advanced neurotoxicity may lead to cranial nerve palsies and profound weakness of the dorsiflexors of the foot and extensors of the wrist. At higher doses of vincristine, above 3 mg total dose, constipation, obstipation, and paralytic ileus may occur because of autonomic neuropathy. Rarely, alterations in mental status accompany signs and symptoms of peripheral neuropathy.[168] Although the sensory changes and reflex changes may improve with discontinuation of vincristine, motor deficits show little improvement and may be permanent.

Vincristine causes little myelosuppression. As the result of

TABLE 9-5. Pharmacokinetics of the Vinca Alkaloids

	VINCRISTINE	VINBLASTINE	VINDESINE
PEAK BLOOD LEVEL	0.4 μM	0.4 μM	0.4 μM
PRIMARY ELIMINATION ROUTE	Hepatic metabolism	Metabolism	?
PLASMA HALF-LIFE—ALPHA	0.85 min	4.5 min	3.2 min
—BETA	7.4 min	53 min	99 min
—GAMMA	164 min	20 hr	20 hr
URINARY EXCRETION (% DOSE)	12	14 (ring-label) 19–23 (acetyl-label)	13
FECAL EXCRETION (% DOSE)	70	10 (ring-label) 25–41 (acetyl-label)	?

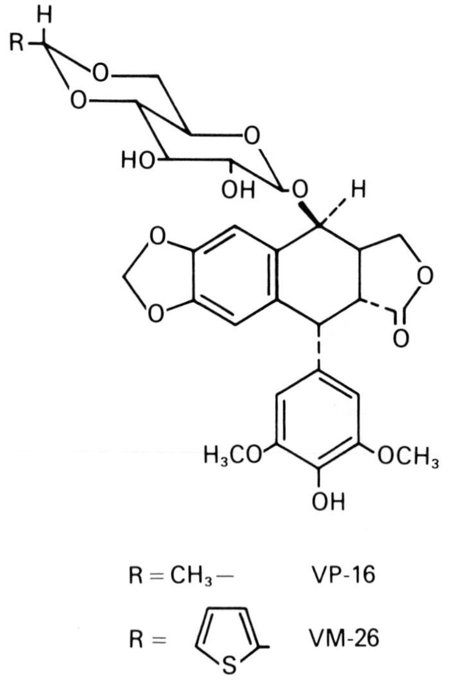

R = CH_3— VP-16

R = (thienyl) VM-26

FIG. 9-22. Structure of VP-16 and VM-26.

inhibition of mitosis, megakaryocytes undergo endoreduplication and, at low doses of vincristine, the platelet count may actually rise during treatment. In contrast, the primary toxicity of vinblastine is borne by the bone marrow. Leukopenia is usually dose limiting. Mucositis is also a frequent side-effect, and neurotoxicity is rarely observed at conventional doses. Vindesine, a new vinca alkaloid, causes both myelosuppression and mild, but consistent, neurotoxicity similar to that of vincristine.[155,169]

In addition to the more common toxicities, vincristine promotes release of antidiuretic hormone and in rare instances may lead to symptomatic dilutional hyponatremia.[170] This syndrome is self-limited and, if recognized early, treatable with simple fluid restriction. Vigorous hydration should be used with caution in patients receiving high doses of vincristine (above 2 mg total dose).

Although specific pharmacokinetic information is not available as the basis for dose modification, it is advisable to reduce the dose of either vincristine or vinblastine in patients with hepatic failure. A reduction of 50% is recommended in patients with bilirubin above 3 mg per 100 ml. No modification is recommended for patients with impaired renal function.

The only well-documented drug interaction of note is the enhancement of total methotrexate uptake by vincristine and vinblastine. This effect is the result of an inhibition of the efflux of methotrexate by the vinca alkaloids. However, this enhancement requires relatively high concentrations of the vinca alkaloids (0.1 μM or above) and the combination of methotrexate following vincristine has not been shown to improve treatment results in experiments with murine leukemia.[171]

TABLE 9-6. Pharmacokinetics of VP-16 and VM-26

	VM-26	VP-16
MEAN PEAK BLOOD LEVELS	14 μg/ml	30 μg/ml
PLASMA HALF-LIFE—ALPHA	0.49 hr	2.8 hr
—BETA	3.85 hr	15.1 hr
—GAMMA	26.3 hr	
URINARY EXCRETION (% DOSE)	45	45
% EXCRETED AS METABOLITE	79	33

THE EPIPODOPHYLLOTOXINS

Podophyllotoxin, an extract of the mandrake plant, has a prominent place in folk medicine as a remedy for poisoning, parasites, and warts. Like vincristine and vinblastine, it binds to tubulin and inhibits microtubular assembly but failed initial clinical trials because of prohibitive toxicity. Two glycosidic derivatives, VP-16 and VM-26, have been synthesized and have important clinical activity in the treatment of lymphomas, small-cell carcinoma of the lung, and testicular cancer. These derivatives differ only in their substitution on the 4,6-acetal carbon (Fig. 9-22) and have basic similarities in their pharmacokinetics, toxicity, and spectrum of clinical action.[172]

The mechanism of action of these synthetic derivatives remains in doubt. They have no discernible effect on microtubular assembly and arrest cells in G_2 rather than in mitosis.[173] VP-16 and VM-26 have the unusual property of inhibiting nucleoside transport into HeLa cells in tissue culture, but this observation is of uncertain relevance to their cytotoxicity.[174]

The primary features of epipodophyllotoxin disposition in man are given in Table 9-6.[175] VP-16 is administered either in the form of a drinking ampule or by intravenous infusion, whereas VM-26 is given only intravenously. VP-16 has a more rapid renal clearance, shorter terminal half-life, and undergoes less metabolism than VM-26. Both drugs penetrate poorly into the cerebrospinal fluid despite their high lipid solubility. The primary route of elimination for VM-26 is metabolic, although the products have not been identified; at least 30% of VP-16 is excreted unchanged.

VP-16 has been used in a variety of schedules and by both oral and intravenous routes of administration. At least a twofold increase in dose is required if the drug is given orally, in order to compensate for only 50% bioavailability by this route. Maximum tolerated doses intravenously are 45 mg per m^2 per day for 7 days, 86 mg per m^2 per day for twice-weekly doses, and 290 mg per m^2 once weekly. VM-26 is usually given in weekly doses of 67 mg per m^2.

The dose-limiting toxicity for both drugs is leukopenia. Thrombocytopenia occurs in less than 25% of patients. Mild gastrointestinal complaints such as nausea and vomiting are reported by less than 20% of patients receiving intravenous VP-16 or VM-26, but increase to a 55% incidence in those receiving oral VP-16. A mild peripheral neuropathy, usually paresthesias or tendon reflex depression, is observed in less than half the patients receiving these drugs.

OTHER AGENTS

HEXAMETHYLMELAMINE

Hexamethylmelamine (HMM) and pentamethylmelamine (PMM) belong to a unique class of antitumor agents that have an uncertain mechanism of action, but significant antineoplastic activity against ovarian cancer, breast cancer, the lymphomas, and small cell carcinoma of the lung. Despite partial elucidation of the complex metabolism of HMM, the active intermediate has not been identified, and the drug has no clear relationship to conventional classes of chemotherapeutic agents such as antimetabolites or alkylating agents. Its relatively mild myelosuppressive effects render this agent a useful candidate for combination therapy.

HMM consists of a symmetric 6-member triazene ring, to which are attached three dimethylamine groups (Fig. 9-23). PMM, a more water-soluble analog, has one less methyl side group. These methyl substitutions are readily removed by microsomal metabolism to yield various possible methylmelamine derivatives[176] plus corresponding quantities of formaldehyde, which is itself a weakly cytotoxic compound.[177] None of these melamine metabolites is cytotoxic *in vitro* in the absence of microsomes. HMM and several of its demethyl metabolites can be converted by enzymatic hydroxylation to methylol (R–CH_2OH) analogs, which are cytotoxic in tissue culture. However, these compounds have not been identified *in vivo* at this writing, and their role in HMM or PMM cytotoxicity remains unproved.

Experimental studies with HMM labeled in either the triazene ring or in the methyl groups have demonstrated covalent binding of both types of labeled compound to acid-insoluble material in both tumor cells and normal tissues, indicating possible alkylating action.[178] However, HMM is not consistently cross-resistant with classic alkylating agents in rodent tumors or in human cancer treatment.

As in rodents, both HMM and PMM undergo extensive and rapid N-demethylation in man. The S-triazene ring is excreted intact, whereas the methyl groups appear as respiratory CO_2, undergo metabolic reutilization by the intermediate formaldehyde, or remain attached to the ring system of partially demethylating metabolites.

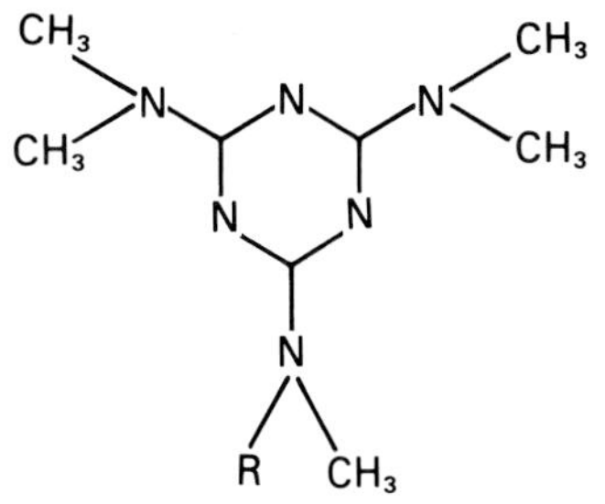

Clinical Pharmacology and Pharmacokinetics

HMM, PMM, and other polymethylated metabolites are readily extracted from plasma or urine by heptane or toluene[179] or, alternatively, may be concentrated from these fluids by cation exchange chromatography in acid solution.[180] Following these concentration steps, PMM and HMM are best measured by gas chromatography with a nitrogen detector[179] or by gas chromatography–mass spectrometry[180]; both of these methods can detect as little as 0.1 μM of either compound in plasma.

Because of its limited aqueous solubility, HMM can only be given by the oral route. Usual doses of 4 to 12 mg per kg per day are given for courses of 14 to 21 days. The bioavailability of HMM by this route is highly variable, yielding peak blood levels of 0.2 to 0.8 μg per ml.[181] This variability may be due either to variable absorption or variable first-pass metabolism in the liver. The parent compound has a half-life of 4.7 to 10.2 hours in plasma. PMM, which is given intravenously, has half-lives of 27 and 133 minutes and thus is eliminated somewhat faster than HMM.

R = CH_3 FOR HEXAMETHYLMELAMINE
R = H FOR PENTAMETHYLMELAMINE

FIG. 9-23. Structure of melamine derivatives.

Both HMM and PMM produce nausea and vomiting as their dose-limiting toxicity. These symptoms, produced by bolus administration of PMM, are particularly severe and have led to use of more protracted infusion of PMM, which causes less emesis. Oral administration of HMM leads to a gradual increase in these symptoms over a period of days, limiting the duration of therapy to 2 to 3 weeks. Higher daily doses of HMM (above 12 mg per kg per day) are tolerated for shorter periods of time. No standard schedule of PMM dosage has been established in preliminary clinical trials, although single doses of 1500 mg per m^2 repeated every week produce dose-limiting gastrointestinal symptoms in most patients.

Both PMM and HMM also produce neurotoxic symptoms. HMM treatment may lead to mood alterations, hallucinations, and peripheral neuropathy; these effects appear gradually during a protracted course of treatment and disappear upon drug withdrawal. PMM has caused convulsive death in preclinical trials and acute coma after rapid intravenous injection in man.

DACARBAZINE

Dacarbazine (DTIC) [5-methyl-(3,3-dimethyl-1-trizeno)-imidazole-4-carboxamidel] is the product of a fortuitous misadventure in drug design. This compound was the outgrowth of efforts to synthesize analogs of 5-amino-imidazole-4-carboxamide, an intermediate in purine biosynthesis, but in actuality DTIC functions as an alkylating agent. DTIC is active against a broad spectrum of murine solid and ascitic tumors, but its clinical effectiveness is limited to Hodgkin's disease, malignant melanoma, and soft tissue sarcomas.

The probable pathway of metabolic activation of this agent is shown in Figure 9-24 and consists of microsomal-mediated demethylation, followed by spontaneous rearrangement of the product, leading to elimination of a methyl diazonium cation ($+N = NCH_3$). This cation further yields an active methyl cation (CH_3+) and N_2. Methylation of nucleic acids has been observed in both experimental systems and in urinary excre-

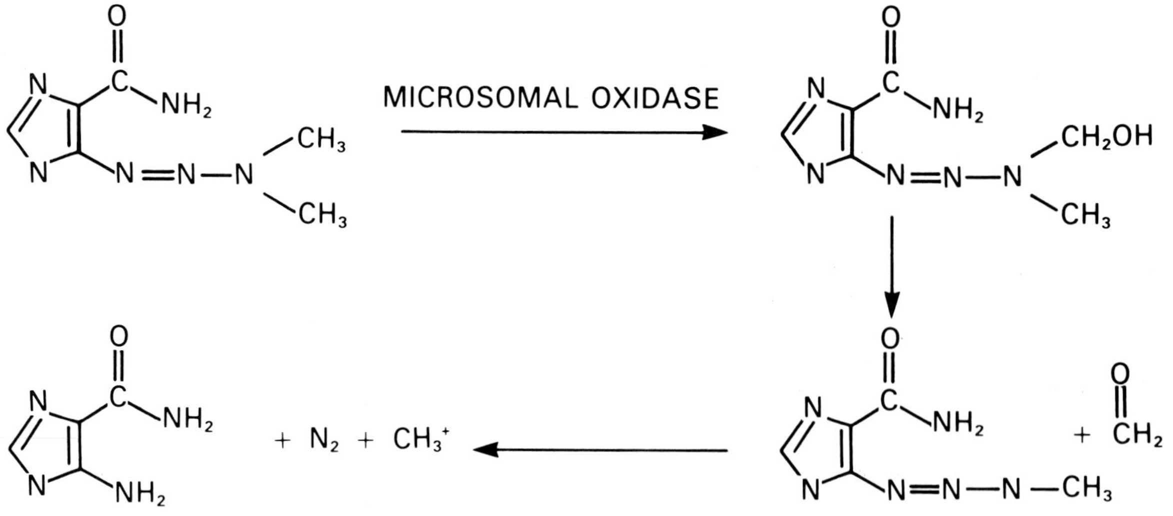

FIG. 9-24. Metabolic activation of dacarbazine (DTIC). The initial step is enzymatically mediated, but the mechanism of subsequent reactions has not been clarified.

tion products in man, but the active species of drug and the route of its generation are still in doubt.[182]

In addition to its microsomal metabolism, DTIC undergoes spontaneous decomposition when exposed to light, yielding diazoimidazole carboxamide and azahypoxanthine, an active antimetabolite in its own right. This light-activation pathway may account for the antitumor effects of DTIC in tissue culture in the absence of microsomes, but there is little evidence to support any relevance of this reaction sequence to *in vivo* toxicity.

The effects of DTIC on cell cycle progression, and its cycle specificity, are uncertain. It appears to kill cells in all phases of the cell cycle and shows little schedule dependency in experimental studies.

Clinical Pharmacology

There is no routine method for measurement of DTIC or any of its metabolites. Preliminary information has been forthcoming from studies employing a method in which the parent compound is decomposed by photolysis, followed by coupling of the decomposition products with the Bratton-Marshall reagent and ultraviolet spectroscopic detection,[183] but this approach is not specific for the parent compound. A less sensitive high-pressure liquid chematography method has been described, and it does provide separation of the parent compound from its monomethyl derivative and aminoimidazole carboxamide, but it has not been applied in a comprehensive study as yet and lacks requisite sensitivity for pharmacokinetic purposes.[184]

The preliminary information indicates that the drug is adequately absorbed orally, but, as expected, a comparable dose given intravenously yields fivefold higher peak blood levels. Its disappearance half-life from plasma is about 3 hours. Little is known concerning its route(s) of elimination. An ultimate breakdown product, aminoimidazolecarboxamide, has been detected in man.[185] The primary half-life is prolonged by concurrent *C. parvum* administration, but this effect is reversed by addition of actinomycin D.[184] The basis for these interactions is not understood.

A variety of schedules of administration are used in man. Intravenous doses vary from 150 to 300 mg/m^2 per day for 5 to 10 days, depending on prior treatment history, concurrent therapy, and patient tolerance. The drug has also been given by intra-arterial infusion, but this route lacks rationale in view of the likely requirement for hepatic microsomal activation. The most significant toxicity is usually nausea and vomiting, which is most severe during the first days of treatment and which may be lessened by reducing the initial dose and gradually increasing the dose during the course of treatment. Moderate myelosuppression may occur during the 2 to 3 weeks following treatment but is usually not dose-limiting. Other toxicities include a flulike syndrome and a possible enhancement of adriamycin cardiac toxicity.[186]

PROCARBAZINE

Procarbazine [N-isopropyl-a-(2-methylhydrazino)-p-toluamide hydrochloride] was discovered during a search for new inhibitors of monoamine oxidase; in addition to preserving that capability, it was found to have antitumor activity and has since become an important agent in the treatment of Hodgkin's disease, brain tumors, and lung cancer.

The mechanism of action and metabolism of procarbazine are incompletely understood; it is certain, however, that the drug requires metabolic activation, and the likely end product is an alkylating agent, probably a methyldiazonium ion. A proposed pathway for this activation is given in Figure 9-25. Microsomal oxidation of the diazene side group leads to formation of the azo metabolite, which has been identified in hepatic perfusion experiments or with isolated microsomes.[187] This reaction is inducible with phenobarbital. Further oxidation produces two azoxy isomers, depending on which side chain nitrogen undergoes oxidation. Through further oxidation of the alkyl group, a chemically unstable intermediate is produced that then yields the active alkylating species, prob-

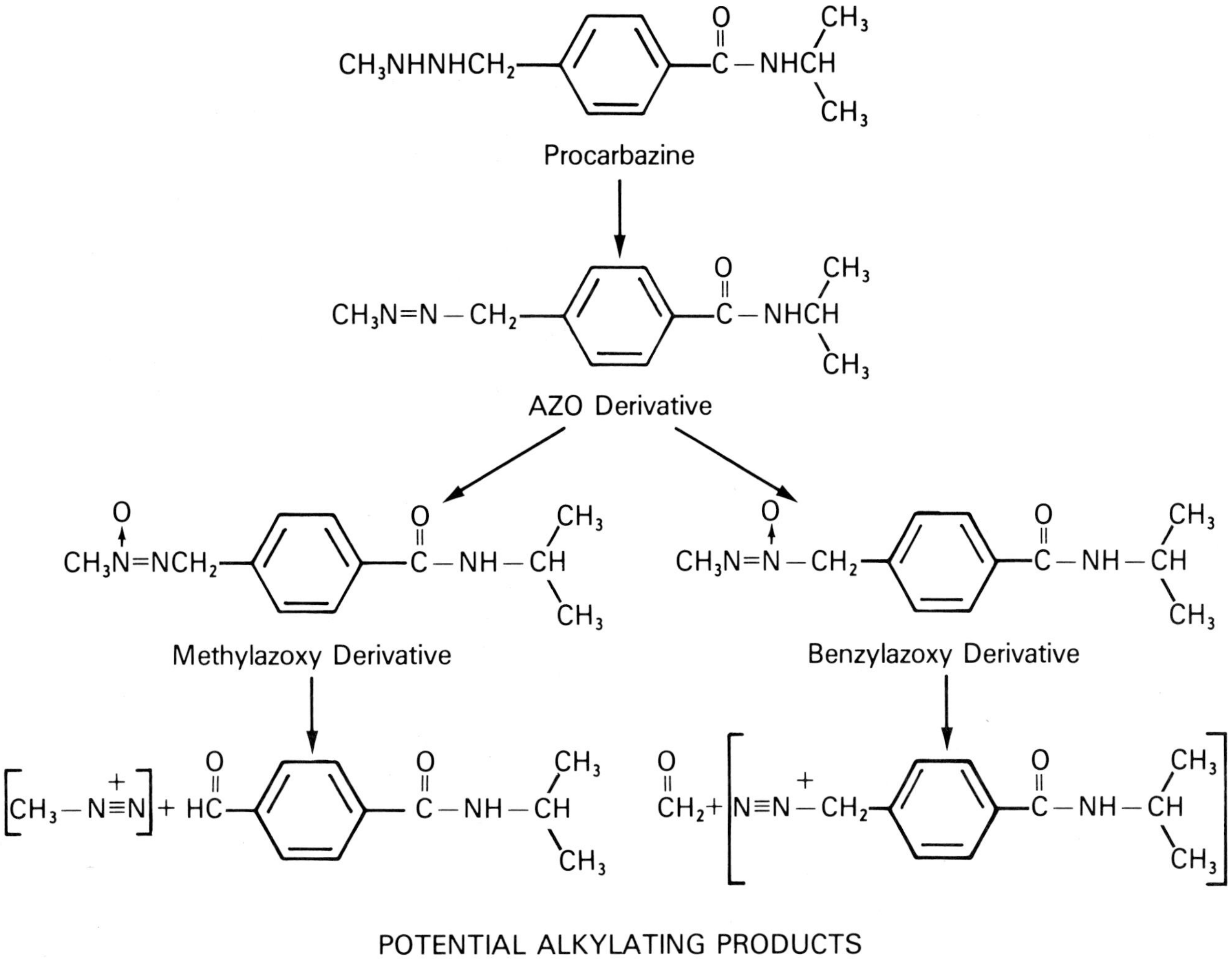

Procarbazine

AZO Derivative

Methylazoxy Derivative

Benzylazoxy Derivative

POTENTIAL ALKYLATING PRODUCTS

FIG. 9-25. Activation of procarbazine by liver microsomes to yield alkylating species (in brackets).

ably a methyldiazonium ion or a benzyl diazonium ion. Only the azo and azoxy intermediates have been identified in mammalian plasma. N-methyl-labeled procarbazine does become bound to nucleic acids, phospholipids, and protein, indicating that alkylation does occur *in vivo*.[188]

A second pathway of procarbazine metabolism leads to the generation of free radical intermediates, but its primary side product, N-isoprophyl-p-toluamide, is formed in extremely small quantities in rats.[189]

There is no reliable information regarding mechanisms of cellular resistance to procarbazine.

Clinical Pharmacology and Pharmacokinetics

The pharmacokinetics of procarbazine in man have been incompletely characterized. The parent drug disappears rapidly from plasma with a half-life of 7 minutes following intravenous administration. The primary excretion product is N-isopropylterephthalamic acid. Procarbazine-derived radioactivity in the cerebrospinal fluid reaches equilibrium with plasma within 15 minutes of injection; the highly lipophilic azoxy metabolites have also been found in rat brain 10 to 30 minutes after intravenous administration.

The antitumor activity and the rate of microsomal metabolism of procarbazine are increased by pretreatment of rodents with phenobarbital, a microsomal enzyme inducer.[190] However, procarbazine itself inhibits microsomal biotransformation of pentobarbital and aminopyrene, indicating that it may have important interactions with antitumor drugs that undergo microsomal metabolism in man, such as DTIC and cyclophosphamide.

Procarbazine is usually administered orally in daily doses of 100 mg per m^2 per day for 10 to 14 days. Given orally, procarbazine causes moderate nausea and decreased appetite, mild to moderate leukopenia and thrombocytopenia, and, less frequently, neurotoxicity, which is manifested by paresthesias of the extremities, drowsiness, or depression. These changes in mental status may be related to its inhibition of monoamine oxidase. Patients receiving procarbazine should be warned to avoid foods that contain significant quantities of tyramine, such as wine, bananas, yogurt, and ripe cheese, because these may provoke a hypertensive crisis. Other monoamine oxidase inhibitors such as tricyclic antidepressants and sympathomimetic drugs should not be used concurrently with procarbazine. Neither should potent hypnotics be used, because procarbazine has mild hypnotic effects in its own right

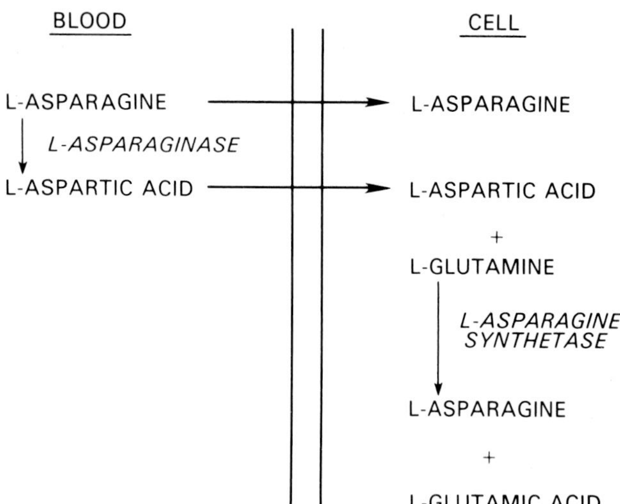

FIG. 9-26. Pathways for synthesis of L-asparagine intracellularly, and on circulating L-asparagine.

and is known to depress the microsomal inactivation of other agents.

The neurotoxicity of procarbazine becomes the most prominent and disabling side-effect when the drug is given intravenously.[191] Total doses of 2 g per m^2 by this route produce confusion or coma but little myelosuppression, and uncertain clinical benefit.

Procarbazine has an Antabuse-like action that may lead to an unpleasant syndrome of sweating, flushing, and headache upon ingestion of alcohol by patients receiving procarbazine. Hypersensitivity reactions have also been observed and include most prominently a maculopapular rash and pulmonary infiltrates. In the author's experience, the development of a rash is not an indication for discontinuation of procarbazine. This rash usually abates with concurrent use of corticosteroids, and continued treatment with procarbazine plus corticosteroids does not lead to progressive cutaneous reaction or anaphylaxis.

Procarbazine is a potent immunosuppressant in rodents; it prolongs the survival of first or second set skin grafts across major histocompatibility barriers.[192] It has been used as an immunosuppressant in patients with lupus erythematosus and for suppression of graft-versus-host disease in bone marrow transplantation. Procarbazine is also a highly teratogenic and carcinogenic agent in rodents.[193] Fetal rats acquire a variety of skeletal and nervous system abnormalities when exposed to the drug *in utero.* The compound is highly mutagenic in the Ames assay and produces both adenocarcinomas and acute myelocytic leukemia in rodents and monkeys. An increased incidence of both sarcomas and acute leukemias has been observed in patients receiving MOPP combination chemotherapy with irradiation for Hodgkin's disease (see Chap. 35), and procarbazine is suspected of being the responsible carcinogen. Thus, its use in treating nonneoplastic diseases should be carefully weighed with these late toxicities in mind.

L-ASPARAGINASE

The growth of malignant as well as normal cells depends on the availability of specific nutrients used in the synthesis of protein, nucleic acids, and lipids. Some of these nutrients can be synthesized within the cell, but others are required from external sources such as another organ (liver) or from food sources (essential amino acids). Nutritional therapy of cancer has been directed at identifying differences between the host and malignant cells that might be exploited in treatment; these attempts have largely been unsuccessful because of difficulties in producing a deficiency state by dietary means and a lack of clear differences between the rapidly proliferating host cells and the tumor. The only exception has been the use of L-asparaginase in the treatment of childhood acute leukemia.

L-asparagine is a nonessential amino acid that is synthesized by transamination of L-aspartic acid (Fig. 9-26). The amine group in this reaction is donated by glutamine, and the reaction is catalyzed by the enzyme L-asparagine synthetase. This enzyme is constitutive in many tissues, thus accounting for the lack of toxicity of asparagine depletion, but is present in low concentrations in certain human malignancies, particularly those of T-lymphocyte derivation. In tumor cells lacking L-asparagine synthetase, the amino acid can be obtained only from the circulating pool of amino acids.

In 1953, Kidd observed that guinea pig serum had antileukemic effects when administered to mice.[194] Ten years later, Broome and co-workers demonstrated that the responsible factor co-purified with the enzyme L-asparaginase.[195] Subsequently, highly purified preparations of enzyme from *E. coli* and *Erwinia carotovora* have shown significant activity against childhood acute lymphocytic leukemia and have become standard components of induction regimens in this disease. Their antitumor effects result from the rapid and complete depletion of circulating pools of L-asparagine, whereas resistance to this treatment arises through an increase in L-asparagine synthetase activity in tumor cells. This increase occurs either by a process of mutation or by enzyme induction in response to the fall in intracellular asparagine levels.

Purified L-asparaginase enzyme has a molecular weight of 133,000 daltons and is composed of four subunits, each having one active catalytic site.[196] Preparations of enzyme from different bacterial strains and by different purification methods have slight differences in specific activity, isoelectric point, and substrate specificity and affinity. Of greater importance clinically is the fact that enzyme prepared from *Erwinia* does not cross-react immunologically with *E. coli* preparations and therefore may be used in patients who are hypersensitive to the *E. coli* L-asparaginase.[197] The clinical preparations have an affinity constant for L-asparagine of approximately 1×10^{-5} M, a figure tenfold higher than the minimum L-asparagine concentration at which the growth of sensitive tumors is retarded *in vitro.*[198] Thus, considerable excess of enzyme is required to degrade L-asparagine to sufficiently low concentrations.

The cellular effects of L-asparaginase result from inhibition of protein synthesis and correlate well with the effects of the enzyme on the incorporation of an amino acid such as ^{3}H-valine into protein. Inhibition of nucleic acid synthesis is also observed in sensitive cells but is believed to be secondary to the block in protein synthesis. Cells insensitive to asparagine depletion from growth medium *in vitro* are also insensitive to L-asparaginase and show little inhibition of RNA or protein synthesis in the presence of the enzyme. As might be expected, these resistant cells have high endogenous activity of asparagine synthetase.

Most bacterial L-asparaginase preparations contain significant L-glutaminase activity, which is 3 to 5% of the L-asparaginase activity. The enzyme from mammalian sources and from certain bacterial sources (*V. succinogenes*) lacks L-glutaminase activity, but has lesser affinity for L-asparaginase.[199] There is some evidence to suggest that the immunosuppressive properties of *E. coli* L-asparaginase may result from L-glutamine depletion[200] and that cerebral dysfunction observed clinically may be the result of degradation of L-glutamine.

TABLE 9-7. Toxicity of L-Asparaginase

Immediate Reactions	(70%)
Nausea, vomiting, fever, chills	
Hypersensitivity Reactions	(<10%)
Urticaria	
Bronchospasm	
Hypotension	
Decreased Protein Synthesis	(100%)
Albumin	
Insulin	
Clotting factors II, V, VII, VIII, IX, X	
Serum lipoproteins	
Cerebral Dysfunction	(33%)
Disorientation	
Coma	
Seizures	
Organ Toxicities	
Pancreatitis	(15%)
Liver function test abnormalities	(100%)
Azotemia (? increased nitrogen load)	(78%)

(Ohnuma T, Holland JF, Sinks LF: Biochemical and pharmacological studies with L-asparaginase in man. Cancer Res. 30:2297–2305, 1970)

Clinical Pharmacology

L-asparaginase is easily measured in biologic fluids by assays that detect ammonia release[201] or by a coupled enzymic assay.[202] The drug is given intravenously or by intramuscular administration; the latter route produces peak blood levels that are 50% lower than the former. The usual doses are 6000 International Units (IU) per m^2 every other day for 3 to 4 weeks, or daily doses of 1000 to 2000 IU/m^2 for 10 to 20 days. Although blood levels of L-asparaginase are detectable for 1 to 3 weeks after these doses, widely spaced schedules of administration are infrequently used because of the increased risk of anaphylaxis.[203] Blood concentrations of L-asparagine fall below 1 μM within minutes of enzyme injection and remain unmeasurable for 7 to 10 days after completion of therapy.[204]

L-asparaginase concentration in plasma is proportional to dose for doses up to 200,000 IU per m^2 and falls with a primary half-life of 14 to 22 hours. (The Merck & Co. preparation of L-asparaginase has a somewhat longer half-life than the Bayer preparation.) In patients who develop hypersensitivity to the enzyme, plasma clearance is greatly accelerated and enzyme activity may be undetectable in plasma as soon as 4 hours after administration.[205] The enzyme distributes primarily within the intravascular space. However, the cerebrospinal fluid concentration of asparagine falls rapidly, and an antileukemic effect is exerted in this sanctuary, despite the poor penetration of enzyme into the cerebrospinal fluid. The drug can be given directly into the cerebrospinal fluid but exits rapidly from this site and there appears to be no clear therapeutic advantage for this route.

The primary toxicities of L-asparaginase, listed in Table 9-7,[204] fall into two main groups—those related to immunologic sensitization to the foreign protein and those resulting from decreased protein synthesis. Positive skin tests to L-asparaginase are rarely observed prior to drug administration, but anaphylaxis may occur with the initial dose of drug. More commonly, hypersensitivity phenomena, such as urticaria, laryngeal edema, bronchospasm, or hypotension, occur following multiple courses of the enzyme. Passive hemagglutinating antibodies are observed in patients who subsequently develop anaphylaxis, and complement-fixing antibodies are found in serum after an anaphylactic episode.[205] The reason for the low incidence of hypersensitivity reactions (less than 10%) in patients receiving L-asparaginase is unknown but may be related to the immunosuppressive properties of the drug itself (which inhibits delayed hypersensitivity) or may be due to the concomitant administration of other immunosuppressive agents.

Other toxic effects relate to the inhibition of protein synthesis and include hypoalbuminemia; decrease in serum fibrinogen, prothrombin, and other clotting factors; decreased serum insulin with hyperglycemia; decreased serum lipoproteins; and, in 25% of patients, cerebral dysfunction with confusion, stupor, or frank coma.[204] The latter syndrome resembles ammonia toxicity but is not clearly correlated with serum ammonia levels and may be the result of low concentrations of either L-asparagine or L-glutamine in the brain. Probable or definite improvement in cerebral dysfunction has been observed in three patients treated with infusions of L-asparagine, 1 to 2 mmol per kg per day for up to 44 days.[204]

Other toxicities are not as easily explained by the mode of action of the drug; the most important of these is acute pancreatitis, which occurs in less than 15% of patients, but which may progress to severe hemorrhagic pancreatitis. L-asparaginase is frequently the cause of abnormal liver function tests, including increased serum bilirubin, SGOT, and alkaline phosphatase. Histologic examination reveals fatty metamorphosis, probably due to decreased mobilization of lipids.

Approximately two-thirds of patients receiving L-asparaginase experience nausea, vomiting, and chills as an immediate reaction, but these side-effects can be mitigated by antiemetics, antihistamines, or, in extreme cases, corticosteroids.

L-asparaginase has no known toxicity for gastrointestinal mucosa or bone marrow and is thus a favorable agent for use

TABLE 9-8. Amino Acid-Directed Antitumor Therapy

AMINO ACID-DEGRADING ENZYMES WITH ANTITUMOR ACTIVITY			
Enzyme	*Substrate*	*Comment*	*Ref.*
L-glutaminase	L-glutamine L-asparagine	Antitumor activity in man	207,208
L-threonine deaminase	L-threonine	Active vs. murine leukemia	209
L-methionase	L-methionine	Active vs. cultured human lymphoblasts	210
L-tyrosine phenol-lyase	L-tyrosine L-phenylalanine	Active vs. murine B16 melanoma	211
L-phenylalanine ammonia-lyase	L-phenylalanine	Active vs. murine leukemia	212
L-tryptophan hydroxylase	L-tryptophan	Active vs. murine leukemia	213

AMINO ACID ANALOGS			
	Compound	*Mechanism of Action*	*Antitumor Activity in Man*
L-glutamine analogs (214)	1. 6-diazo-5-oxonorleucine (DON)	Inhibits glutamine-dependent transaminases	Breast, lung, choriocarcinoma
	2. Azaserine	Inhibits glutamine-dependent transaminases	Childhood acute leukemia, Hodgkin's disease
	3. Azotomycin	Precursor of DON	Colorectal carcinomas, soft tissue sarcoma
L-aspartate analogs (215, 216)	1. L-alanosine	Inhibits purine biosynthesis	Unknown
	2. N-phosphonacetyl-L-aspartic acid (PALA)	Inhibits *de novo* pyrimidine synthesis	Breast, colon carcinoma; soft tissue sarcoma

(Uren R, Handschumacher RE: Enzyme therapy. *In* Cancer: A Comprehensive Treatise, Becker, FF (ed.), Plenum Press, New York, 1977, pp. 457–487)

in combination chemotherapy. The only well-established drug interaction is its ability to terminate methotrexate action.[206] The antagonism between L-asparaginase with methotrexate is probably the result of L-asparginase inhibition of protein synthesis, with consequent prevention of cellular entry into the vulnerable phase of the cell cycle. When the enzyme is given after methotrexate, the action of the antifolate is abbreviated at that point. Large doses of the antifolate are thus well tolerated if followed by L-asparaginase rescue because of the limited time exposure of the bone marrow and gastrointestinal mucosa. The combination of methotrexate and L-asparaginase has been employed, with promising results, in acute leukemia refractory to conventional methotrexate doses (8 of 10 patients achieved remissions).

OTHER FORMS OF ENZYME THERAPY AND AMINO ACID ANTAGONISTS

A number of other enzymes, primarily of bacterial origin, have antitumor activity in animal systems and may undergo clinical trial in the future. The most prominent of these are listed in Table 9-8. L-glutaminase–L-asparaginase from *Acinetobacter glutaminasificans*,[207] and a succinylated derivative that has a longer plasma half-life, have received preliminary trials in acute leukemia.[208] With the nonsuccinylated enzyme, doses in excess of 10,000 IU/m^2 per day are required to produce continuous depletion of serum L-glutamine and L-asparagine. The succinylated enzyme used in doses of less than 2000 IU/m^2 per day produces rapid depletion of L-glutamine lasting for at least 24 hours. A lowering of peripheral lymphoblast count was reported in patients resistant to L-asparaginase, but severe neurotoxicity with coma was observed in 4 patients and marked elevation of plasma ammonia levels occurred in all patients tested. The more common toxicities associated with L-asparaginase are also seen in patients treated with L-glutaminase, including decreases in various serum proteins and hyperglycemia.

L-glutamine analogs (see Table 9-8) have also received limited clinical trial, but with little success. The strong activity of 6-diazo-5-oxonorleucine (DON) against human xenografts in nude mice has prompted a reexamination of this drug. Inhibitors of the L-asparagine synthetase reaction have also been described and may have use in combination with L-asparaginase.

REFERENCES

1. Chabner BA (ed): Pharmacologic Basis of Cancer Treatment, Philadelphia, WB Saunders, 1981, in press
2. Pratt WB, Ruddon RW: The Anticancer Drugs. New York, Oxford Press, 1979
3. Werkheiser WC: The biochemical, cellular, and pharmacological action and effects of the folic acid antagonists. Cancer Res 23:1277–1285, 1963
4. Zaharko DS, Fung W-P, Yang F-H: Relative biochemical aspects of low and high doses of methotrexate in mice. Cancer Res 37:1602–1607, 1977
5. Pinedo HM, Zaharko DS, Bull JM et al: The relative contribution of drug concentration and duration of exposure to mouse bone marrow toxicity during continuous methotrexate infusion. Cancer Res 37:445–450, 1977
6. Goldin A, Mantel N, Greenhouse SW et al: Effect of delayed administration of citrovorum factor on antileukemic effectiveness of aminopterin in mice. Cancer Res 14:43–48, 1954
7. Warren RD, Nichols AP, Bender RA: Membrane transport of methotrexate in human lymphoblastoid cells. Cancer Res 38:668–671, 1978
8. Schilsky RL, Bailey BD, Chabner BA: Methotrexate polyglutamate synthesis by cultured human breast cancer cells. Proc Natl Acad Sci USA 77:2919–2922, 1980

9. Alt FW, Kellems RE, Schimke RT: Synthesis and degradation of folate reductase in sensitive and resistant lines of S-180 cells. J Biol Chem 251:3063–3074, 1976
10. Bertino JR, Isacoff WH: Methods of measuring methotrexate in body fluids. In Pinedo HM (ed): Clinical Pharmacology of Antineoplastic Drugs, pp. 3–11. Amsterdam, Elsevier/North Holland, 1978
11. Myers CE, Lippman M, Eliot HM et al: Competitive protein binding assay for methotrexate. Proc Natl Acad Sci USA 72:3683–3686, 1975
12. Donehower RC, Hande KR, Drake JC et al: Presence of 2,4-diamino-N^{10}-methyl pteroic acid after high-dose methotrexate. Clin Pharmacol Ther 26:63–72, 1979
13. Monjanel S, Rigault JP, Cano JP et al: High-dose methotrexate: Preliminary evaluation of a pharmacokinetic approach. Cancer Chemother Pharmacol 3:189–196, 1979
14. Stoller RG, Hande KR, Jacobs SA et al: Use of plasma pharmacokinetics to predict and prevent methotrexate toxicity. N Engl J Med 297:630–634, 1977
15. Abelson HT, Ensminger W, Rosowsky A et al: Competitive effects of citrovorum factor and carboxypeptidase G_1 on cerebrospinal fluid methotrexate pharmacokinetics. Cancer Treat Rep 62:1549–1552, 1978.
16. Shapiro WR, Young DG, Mehta BM: Methotrexate distribution in cerebrospinal fluid after intravenous, verticular, and lumbar injection. N Engl J Med 293:161–166, 1975
17. Bleyer WA: The clinical pharmacology of methotrexate. Cancer 41:36–51, 1978
18. Jacobs SA, Stoller RG, Chabner BA et al: 7-Hydroxymethotrexate as a urinary metabolite in human subjects and Rhesus monkeys receiving high-dose methotrexate. J Clin Invest 57:534–538, 1976
19. Glode LM, Pitman SW, Ensminger WD et al: A phase I study of high-dose aminopterin with leucovorin rescue in patients with advanced metastatic tumor. Cancer Res 39:3707–3714, 1979
20. Dahl MGC, Gregory MM, Scheuer PJ: Liver damage due to methotrexate in patients with psoriasis. Br Med J 1:625–630, 1971
21. Sostman HD, Matthay RA, Putman C et al: Methotrexate-induced pneumonitis. Medicine 55:371–388, 1976
22. Bleyer WA, Drake JC, Chabner BA: Neurotoxicity and elevated cerebrospinal-fluid methotrexate concentration in meningeal leukemia. N Engl J Med 289:770–773, 1973
23. Heidelberger C, Chandhari NK, Dannenberg et al: Fluorinated pyrimidines; a new class of tumor inhibitory compounds. Nature 179:663–666, 1957
24. Mandel HG: Incorporation of 5-fluorouracil into RNA and its molecular consequences. Prog Mol Subcell Biol 1:82–135, 1969
25. Myers CE, Young RC, Chabner BA: Biochemical determinants of 5-fluorouracil response *in vivo:* the role of deoxyuridylate pool expansion. J Clin Invest 56:1231–1238, 1975
26. Cadman EC, Heimer R, Davis L: Enhanced 5-fluorouracil nucleotide formation following methotrexate: Biochemical explanation for drug synergism. Science 205:1135–1137, 1979
27. Schwartz PM, Handschumacher RE: Selective antagonism of 5-fluorouracil cytotoxicity by 4-hydroxypyrazolopyrimidine (Allopurinol) *in vitro*. Cancer Res 39:3095–3101, 1979
28. Vogel SJ, Presant CA, Ratkin GA et al: Phase I study of thymidine plus 5-fluorouracil infusions in advanced colorectal carcinoma. Cancer Treat Rep 63:1–5, 1979
29. Buckpitt AR, Boyd MR: A sensitive method for determination of 5-fluorouracil and 5-fluorodeoxyuridine in human plasma by high-pressure liquid chromatography. Anal Biochem, in press
30. Christophidis N, Vajda FJE, Lucas I et al: Fluorouracil therapy in patients with carcinoma of the large bowel: A pharmacokinetic comparison of various rates and routes of administration. Clin Pharmacokinet 3:330–336, 1978
31. Jones RB, Buckpitt AR, Londer H et al: Potential clinical application of a new method for quantitation of plasma levels of 5-fluoruracil and 5-fluorodeoxyuridine. Bull Cancer (Paris) 66:75–78, 1979
32. Ensminger WD, Rosowsky A, Raso V: A clinical pharmacological evaluation of hepatic arterial infusion of 5-fluoro 2'-dexoyuridine and 5-fluorouracil. Cancer Res 38:3784–3792, 1978
33. Speyer JL, Collins JM, Dedrick RL et al: Phase I and pharmacologic studies of intraperitoneal 5-fluorouracil. Cancer Res 40:567–572, 1980
34. Valdivieso M, Body GP, Gottlieb JA et al: Clinical evaluation of ftorafur (pyrimidine-deoxyribose N,-2′-furanidyl-5-fluorouracil). Cancer Res 36:1821–1824, 1976
35. Au JL, Wu AT, Friedman MA et al: Pharmacokinetics and metabolism of ftorafur in man. Cancer Treat Rep 63:343–350, 1979
36. Cohen SS: The lethality of ara nucleotides. Med Biol 54:299–326, 1976
37. Fridland A: Inhibition of DNA chain initiation by 1-β-D-arabinofuranosylcytosine (ara-C) in human lymphoblasts. J Supramol Struct 771:331, 1978
38. Woodcock DM, Fox RM, Cooper IA: Evidence for a new mechanism of cytotoxicity of 1-β-D-arabinofuranosyl cytosine. Cancer Res 39:1418–1424, 1979
39. Chabner BA, Hande KR, Drake JC: Ara-C metabolism: Implications for drug resistance and drug interactions. Bull Cancer 66:89–92, 1979
40. Tattersall MNH, Ganeshagura K, Hoffbrand AV: Mechanisms of resistance of human acute leukaemia cells to cytosine arabinoside. Br J Haematol 27:39–46, 1974
41. Steuart CD, Burke PJ: Cytidine deaminase and the development of resistance to arabinosyl cytosine. Nature (New Biol) 233:109–110, 1971
42. Rustum YM, Preisler HD: Correlation between leukemic cell retention of 1-β-D-arabinofuranosyl cytosine 5′-tri-phosphate and response to therapy. Cancer Res 39:42–49, 1979
43. Wan SH, Huffman DH, Azarnoff DL et al: Pharmacokinetics of 1-β-D-arabinofuranosylcytosine in humans. Cancer Res 34:392–397, 1974
44. Piall EM, Aherne GW, Marks VM: A radioimmunoassay for cytosine arabinoside. Br J Cancer 40:548–556, 1979.
45. Ho DHW, Frei E III: Clinical pharmacology of 1-β-D-arabinofuranosylcytosine. Clin Pharmacol Ther 12:944–954, 1971
46. van Prooijen R, vander Kleijn E, Hagnen C: Pharmacokinetics of cytosine arabinoside in acute leukemia. Clin Pharmacol Ther 21:744–750, 1977
47. Aden OB, Goldie W, Wood T et al: seizures following intrathecal cytosine arabinoside in young children with acute lymphoblastic leukemia. Cancer 42:53–58, 1978
48. Drake JC, Hande KR, Fuller RW et al: Cytidine and deoxycytidylate deaminase inhibition by uridine analogs. Biochem Pharmacol 29:807–811, 1980
49. Cadman E, Eiferman F: Mechanism of synergistic cell killing when methotrexate precedes cytosine arabinoside. Study of L1210 and human leukemic cell. J Clin Invest 64:788–797, 1979
50. Harris AW, Reynolds EC, Finch LR: Effect of thymidine on the sensitivity of cultured mouse tumor cells to 1-B-D-arabinofuranosylcytosine. Cancer Res 39:538–541, 1979
51. Kreis W, Wokcock TM, Gordon CS, Krakoff IH: Tetrahydrouridine physiologic disposition and effect upon deamination of cytosine arabinoside in man. Cancer Treat Rep 61:1347–1353, 1977
52. Rustum YM, Dave C, Mayhew E et al: Role of liposome type and route of administration in the antitumor activity of liposome-entrapped 1-β-D-arabinofuranosylcytosine against mouse L1210 leukemia. Cancer Res 39:1390–1395, 1979
53. Lu LJW, Randerath K: Effects of 5-azacytidine on transfer RNA methyltransferases. Cancer Res 39:940–948, 1979
54. Benvenuto JA, Hall SW, Farquhar D et al: Pharmacokinetics and disposition of 3-deazauridine in humans. Cancer Res 39:349–352, 1979
55. Elion GB: Biochemistry and pharmacology of purine analogs. Fed Proc 26:898–904, 1967
56. Tidd DM, Paterson ARP: Distinction between inhibition of purine nucleotide synthesis and the delayed cytotoxic reaction of 6-mercaptopurine. Cancer Res 34:733–737, 1974
57. Lee MH, Huang Y-M, Sartorelli AC: Alkaline phosphatase

activities of 6-thiopurine-sensitive and -resistant sublines of sarcoma 180. Cancer Res 38:2413–2418, 1978

58. Breter HJ, Zahn RK: Quantitation of intracellular metabolites of [^{35}]-6-mercaptopurine in L5178Y cells grown in time-course incubates. Cancer Res 39:3744–3748, 1979
59. Ding TL, Benet LZ: Determination of 6-mercaptopurine and azathioprine in plasma by high-performance liquid chromatography. J Chromatog 163:281–288, 1979
60. Tidd DM, Dedhar S: Specific and sensitive combined high performance liquid chromatographic-flow fluorometric assay for intracellular 6-thioguanine metabolites of 6-mercaptopurine and 6-thioguanine. J Chromatog 145:237–246, 1978
61. Esterhay RJ, Aisner J, Levi JA et al: High-dose 6-mercaptopurine in advanced refractory cancer. Cancer Treat Rep 62:1229–1231, 1978
62. Present DH, Korelitz BI, Wisch N et al: Treatment of Crohn's disease with 6-mercaptopurine. N Engl J Med 302:981–986, 1980
63. Pavan-Langston D, Buchanan RA, Alford CA Jr (eds): Adenine Arabinoside: An Antiviral Agent. New York, Raven Press, 1979
64. Plunkett W, Alexander L, Chubb S et al: Biochemical basis of the increased activity of 9-beta-D-arabinofuranosyladenine in the presence of inhibitors of adenosine deaminase. Cancer Res 39:3655–3660, 1979
65. Smyth JF, Poplack DG, Holiman BJ et al: Correlation of adenosine deaminase activity with cell surface markers in acute lymphoblastic leukemia. J Clin Invest 901:710–712, 1978
66. Brockman RW, Schabel FM, Montgomery JH: Biologic activity of 9-β-D-arabinofuranosyl-2-fluoro adenine, a metabolically stable analog of 9-β-D-arabinofuranosyladenine. Biochem Pharmacol 26:2193–2196, 1977
67. Ludlum DB: Alkylating agents and the nitrosoureas. In Becker FF (ed): Cancer: A Comprehensive Treatise, Vol. 5, pp. 285–307. New York, Plenum Press, 1977
68. Kohn KW: Interstrand cross-linking of DNA by 1,3-bis(2-chlorethyl)-1-nitrosourea and other 1-(2-haloethyl)-1-nitrosoureas. Cancer Res 37:1450–1454, 1977
69. Bergsagel DE: Treatment of plasma cell myeloma with cytotoxic agents. Arch Intern Med 135:172–176, 1975
70. Lyons RM, Goldenberg GJ: Active transport of nitrogen mustard and choline by normal and leukemic human lymphoid cells. Cancer Res 32:1679–1685, 1972
71. Lawley PD, Brookes P: Molecular mechanisms of the cytotoxic action of difunctil alkylating agents and of resistance to this action. Nature 206:480–483, 1965
72. Colvin M: A review of the pharmacology and clinical use of cyclophosphamide. In Pinedo HM (ed): Clinical Pharmacology of Antineoplastic Drugs, pp. 245–261. Amsterdam, Elsevier/North Holland, 1978
73. Cox PJ: Cyclophosphamide cystitis. Identification of acrolein as the causative agent. Biochem Pharmacol 28:2045–2049, 1979
74. Connors TA: Alkylating drugs, nitrosourea and dialkyl triazenes. In Pinedo HM (ed): Cancer Chemotherapy 1979, pp. 25–55. Amsterdam, Elsevier/North Holland, 1979
75. Alvarado CS, Boat TF, Newman AJ: Late onset pulmonary fibrosis and chest deformity in two children treated with cyclophosphamide. J Pediatr 92:443–446, 1978
76. Tattersall MN, Jarman M, Newlands ES et al: Pharmacokinetics of melphalan following oral or intravenous administration in patients with malignant disease. Eur J Cancer 14:507–514, 1978
77. Vistica DT, Toal JN, Rabinovitz M: Amino acid-conferred protection against melphalan. Biochem Pharmacol 27:2865–2870, 1978
78. Vistica DT, Toal JN, Rabinovitz M: Amino acid-conferred protection against melphalan: Interference with leucine protection of melphalan cytotoxicity by the basic amino acids in cultured murine L1210 leukemic cells. Mol Pharmacol 14:1136–1142, 1978
79. Alberts DS, Chang SY, Chen HSG et al: Kinetics of intravenous melphalan. Clin Pharmacol Ther 26:73–80, 1979
80. Cole SR, Myers TJ, Klatsky AU: Pulmonary disease with chlorambucil therapy. Cancer 41:455–459, 1978
81. Fiere D, Felman P, Vivian H et al: Acute myeloid leukemia following the administration of chlorambucil. Two cases. Nouv Presse Med 7:756, 1978
82. Nadkarni MV, Trams EG, Smith PK: Preliminary studies on the distribution and fate of TEM, TEPA, and myleran in the human. Cancer Res 19:713–718, 1959
83. Heal JM, Franza BR, Schein PS: Pharmacology of nitrosourea antitumor agents. *In* Pinedo HM (ed): Clinical Pharmacology of Anti-Neoplastic Drugs, pp. 263–275. Amsterdam, Elsevier/North Holland, 1978
84. Ewig RAG, Kohn KW: DNA damage and repair in mouse leukemia L1210 cells treated with nitrogen mustard, 1,3-bis(2-chloroethyl)-1-nitrosourea, and other nitrosoureas. Cancer Res 37:2114–2122, 1977
85. Kann HE Jr: Comparison of biochemical and biological effects of four nitrosoureas with differing carbamoylating activities. Cancer Res 38:2363–2366, 1978
86. Tew KD, Sudhakar S, Schein PS et al: Binding of chlorozotocin and 1-(2-chlorethyl)-3-cyclohexyl-1-nitrosourea to chromatin and nucleosomal fractions of HeLa cells. Cancer Res 38:3371–3378, 1978
87. Reed DJ, May HE: Cytochrome P-450 interactions with the 2-chloroethylnitrosoureas and procarbazine. Biochimie 60:989–995, 1978
88. Hundley R, Lukens JN: Nitrosourea-associated pulmonary fibrosis. Cancer Treat Rep 63:2128–2130, 1979
89. Harmon WE, Cohen HJ, Schneeberger EE et al: Chronic renal failure in children treated with methyl CCNU. N Engl J Med 300:1200–1203, 1979
90. Rosenberg B, Van Camp L, Krigas T: Inhibition of cell division in *Escherichia coli* by electrolysis products from a platinum electrode. Nature 205:698–699, 1965
91. Rosenberg B, Van Camp L, Trosko JE et al: Platinum compounds: A new class of potent antitumor agents. Nature 222:385–386, 1969
92. Filipski J, Kohn KW, Bonner WM: The nature of inactivating lesions produced by platinum(II) complexes produced by platinum(II) complexes in phage DNA. Chem-Biol Interact, submitted for publication
93. Scovell WM, O'Connor T: Interaction of aquated *cis*-[$(NH_3)_2$PtII] with nucleic acid constituents. 1. Ribonucleosides. J Am Chem Soc 99:120–126, 1977
94. Zwelling LA, Kohn KW: Mechanism of action of *cis*-dichlorodiammineplatinum(II). Cancer Treat Rep 63:1439–1444, 1979
95. Cohen GL, Bauer WR, Barton JK et al: Binding of *cis*- and *trans*-dichlorodiammineplatinum(II) to DNA: Evidence for unwinding and shortening of the double helix. Science 203:1014–1016, 1979
96. Roberts JJ, Thomson AJ: The mechanism of action of antitumor platinum compounds. Prog Nucleic Acid Res Mol Biol 22:71–133, 1979
97. Burchenal JH, Kalaher K, Dew K et al: Studies of cross-resistance, synergistic combination and blocking activity of platinum derivatives. Biochimie 60:961–965, 1978
98. Fraval HNA, Roberts JJ: G_1 phase Chinese hamster V79-379A cells are inherently more sensitive to platinum bound to their DNA than mid S phase or asynchronously treated cells. Biochem Pharmacol 28:1575–1580, 1979
99. LeRoy AF, Wehling ML, Sponseller HL et al: Analysis of platinum in biological materials by flameless atomic absorption spectrophotometry. Biochem Med 18:184–191, 1977
100. Bannister SJ, Sternson LA, Repta AJ: Urine analysis of platinum species derived from *cis*-dichlorodiammineplatinum(II) by high-performance liquid chromatography following derivitization with sodium diethyldithiocarbomate. J Chromatog 173:333–342, 1979
101. Litterst CL, LeRoy AF, Guarino AM: The disposition and distribution of platinum following parenteral administration to animals of *cis*-dichlorodiammineplatinum(II). Cancer Treat Rep 63:1485–1492, 1979
102. LeRoy AF, Lutz RJ, Dedrick RL et al: Pharmacokinetic study of *cis*-dichlorodiammineplatinum in the beagle dog: Thermo-

dynamic and kinetic behavior of DDP in a biological milieu. Cancer Treat Rep 63:59–71, 1979
103. Patton TF, Himmelstein KJ, Belt R et al: Plasma levels and urinary excretion of filterable platinum species following bolus injection and i.v. infusion of *cis*-dichlorodiammineplatinum(II) in man. Cancer Treat Rep 63:1359–1361, 1979
104. Gormley P, Poplack D, Pizzo P: The cerebrospinal fluid pharmacokinetics of *cis*-diamminedichloroplatinum(II) and several platinum analogues. Proc Am Assoc Cancer Res 20:279, 1979
105. Jacobs C, Kalman SM, Tretton M et al: Renal handling of *cis*-diamminedichloroplatinum. Submitted for publication
106. Chary KK, Higby DJ, Henderson ES et al: Phase I study of high-dose *cis*-dichlorodiammineplatinum(II) with forced diuresis. Cancer Treat Rep 61:367–370, 1977
107. Madias NE and Harrington JT: Platinum nephrotoxicity. Am J Med 65:307–314, 1978
108. Gonzalez-Vitale JC, Hayes DM, Cvitkovic E et al: The renal pathology in clinical trials of *cis*-platinum (II) diamminedichloride. Cancer 39:1362–1371, 1977
109. Schilsky RL, Anderson T: Hypomagnesemia and renal magnesium wasting in patients receiving *cis*-platin. Ann Intern Med 90:929–931, 1979
110. Jones B, Mladek J, Bhalla R et al: Enzymuria and $beta_2$ microglobulinuria as a sensitive index of *cis*-platinum nephrotoxicity. Proc Am Soc Clin Oncol 20:336, 1979
111. Borch RF, Pleasants ME: Inhibition of *cis*-platinum nephrotoxicity by diethyldithiocarbamate rescue in a rat model. Proc Natl Acad Sci USA 76:6611–6614, 1979
112. Wiesenfeld M, Reinders E, Corder M et al: Successful retreatment with *cis*-DDP after apparent allergic reactions. Cancer Treat Rep 63:219–221, 1979
113. Takeshita M, Grollman AP, Ohtsubo E et al: Interaction of bleomycin with DNA. Proc Natl Acad Sci USA 75:5983–5987, 1978
114. Barranco SC, Humphrey RM: The effects of bleomycin on survival and cell progression in Chinese hamster cells *in vitro*. Cancer Res 31:1218–1223, 1971
115. Barranco SC, Novak JK, Humphrey RM: Studies on recovery from chemically induced damage in mammalian cells. Cancer Res 35:1194–1204, 1975
116. Umezawa H, Hori S, Sawa T et al: A bleomycin-inactivating enzyme in mouse liver. J Antibiotics 27:419–424, 1974
117. Broughton A, Strong JE: Radioimmunoassay of bleomycin. Cancer Res 36:1418–1421, 1976
118. Alberts DS, Chen HSG, Liu R et al: Bleomycin pharmacokinetics in man. I. Intravenous administration. Cancer Chemother Pharmacol 1:177–181, 1978
119. Alberts DS, Chen HSG, Mayersohn M et al: Bleomycin pharmacokinetics in man. II. Intracavitary administration. Cancer Chemother Pharmacol 2:127–132, 1979
120. Blum RH, Carter SK, Agre K: A clinical review of bleomycin—a new antineoplastic agent. Cancer 31:903–914, 1973
121. Morrow CP, DiSaia PJ, Mangan CF: Continuous pelvic arterial infusion with bleomycin for squamous carcinoma of the cervix recurrent after irradiation therapy. Cancer Treat Rep 61:1403–1405, 1977
122. Bracken RB, Johnson DE, Rodriquez L et al: Treatment of multiple superficial tumors of bladder with intravesical bleomycin. Urology 9:161–163, 1977
123. Thompson RH: Naturally Occurring Quinones, pp. 536–575. London, Academic Press, 1971
124. DiMarco A, Galtani M, Orezzi PO: Daunomycin, a new antibiotic of the rhodomycin group. Nature 201:706–707, 1964
125. Friedmann CA: Structure–activity relationships of anthraquinones in some pathological conditions. Pharmacology 20:113–122, 1980
126. Handa K, Sato S: Generation of free radicals of quinone group containing anticancer chemicals in NADPH-microsome system as evidenced by initiation of sulfite oxidation. Gann 66:43–47, 1975
127. Pigram WJ, Fuller W, Amilton LDH: Stereochemistry of intercalation: Interaction of daunomycin with DNA. Nature (New Biol) 235:17–19, 1972
128. Murphree SA, Cunningham LS, Hwang KM et al: Effects of adriamycin on surface properties of sarcoma 180 ascites cells. Biochem Pharmacol 25:1227–1231, 1976
129. Mikkelsen RB, Lin PS, Wallach DF: Interaction of adriamycin with human red blood cells: A biochemical and morphologic study. J Mol Med 2:33–40, 1977
130. Crooke ST, DuVernay VH, Galvan L et al: Structure–activity relationships of anthracyclines relative to effects on macromolecular synthesis. Mol Pharmacol 14:290–298, 1978
131. Lown JM, Sim S, Majumdar KC et al: Strand scission of DNA by bound adriamycin and daunomycin in the presence of reducing agents. Biochem Biophys Res Commun 79:705–710, 1977
132. Fridovich J: The biology of oxygen radicals. Science 201:875–880, 1978
133. Chance B, Boveris A, Nakase Y et al: Hydroperoxide metabolism: An overview. *In* Sies H, Wendel A (eds): Functions of Glutathione in Liver and Kidney, pp. 95–147. New York, Springer-Verlag, 1978
134. Doroshow JH, Locker GY, Myers CE: Enzymatic defenses of the mouse heart against reactive oxygen: Alterations produced by doxorubicin. J Clin Invest 65:128–135, 1980
135. Israel M, Pegg WJ, Wilkinson PM et al: Liquid chromatographic analysis of adriamycin and metabolites in biological fluids. J Liquid Chromatogr 1:795–809, 1978
136. Eksborg S: Reversed-phase liquid chromatography of adriamycin and daunorubicin and their hydroxyl metabolites, adriamycinol, and daunorubicinol. J Chromatogr 149:225–232, 1978
137. Takanashi S, Bachur NR: Adriamycin metabolism in man: Evidence from urinary metabolites. Drug Metab Disp 4:79–87, 1976
138. Benjamin RS: Pharmacokinetics of adriamycin in patients with sarcomas. Cancer Chemother Rep 58:271–273, 1974
139. Dantchev D, Slioussantchouk V, Paintrand M et al: Electron microscopic studies of the heart and light microscopic studies of golden hamsters with adriamycin, doxorubicin, AD 32, and aclacinomycin. Cancer Treat Rep 63:875–888, 1979
140. Tong GL, Wu HY, Smith TH et al: Adriamycin analogues. 3. Synthesis of N-alkylated anthracyclines with enhanced efficacy and reduced cardiotoxicity. J Med Chem 22:912–918, 1979
141. Crooke ST, Bradner WT: Mitomycin C: A review. Cancer Treat Rev 3:121–139, 1976
142. Reich SD: Clinical pharmacology of mitomycin C. *In* Carter SK, Crooke ST (eds): Mitomycin C: Current Status and New Developments, p 243. New York, Academic Press, 1979
143. Bachur NR, Gordon SL, Gee RV: A general mechanism for microsomal activation of quinone anticancer agents to free radicals. Cancer Res 38:1745–1750, 1978
144. Iyer V, Szybalski W: Mitomycins and porfiromycin: Chemical mechanisms of activation and crosslinking of DNA. Science 145:55–58, 1964
145. Oswoll ES, Kiessling PJ, Patterson JR: Interstitial pneumonia from mitomycin. Ann Intern Med 89:352–355, 1978
146. Selman Waksman Conference on actinomycins: Their potential for cancer chemotherapy. Cancer Chemother Rep 58:1–123, 1974
147. Frei E: The clinical use of actinomycin. Cancer Chemother Rep 58:49–54, 1974
148. Sobell HM, Jain SC, Sakere TD et al: Stereochemistry of actinomycin-DNA binding. Nature (New Biol) 231:200–205, 1971
149. Reich E, Franklin RM, Shatkin AJ et al: Action of actinomycin D on animal cells and viruses. Proc Natl Acad Sci USA 48:1238–1245, 1962
150. Ross WE, Glaubiger DL, Kohn KW: Quantitative and qualitative aspects of intercalator-induced DNA damage. Biochim Biophys Acta 562:41–50, 1979
151. Galbraith WM, Mellett LB: Tissue disposition of ^{3}H-actinomycin D in rat, monkey and dog. Cancer Chemother Rep 59:1061–1069, 1975
152. Tattersall MHN, Sodergren JE, Segupta SK et al: Pharmacokinetics of actinomycin D in patients with malignant melanoma. Clin Pharmacol Ther 17:701–708, 1975

153. Kennedy BJ: Mithramycin therapy in testicular cancer. J Urol 107:429–433, 1972
154. Creasey WA: Plant Alkaloids. *In* Becker FA (ed): Cancer: A Comprehensive Treatise, Vol. 5, pp. 379–425. New York, Plenum Press, 1977
155. Mathe G, Misset JL, de Vassal F et al: Phase II clinical trial with vindesine for remission induction in acute leukemia, blastic crisis of chronic myeloid leukemia, lymphosarcoma, and Hodgkin's disease: Absence of cross-resistance with vincristine. Cancer Treat Rep 62:805–809, 1978
156. Owellen RJ, Hartke CA, Dickerson RM et al: Inhibition of tubulin-microtubule polymerization by drugs of the vinca alkaloid class. Cancer Res. 36:1499–1502, 1976
157. Owellen RJ, Owens AH, Donigian DW: The binding of vincristine, vinblastine and colchicine to tubulin. Biochem Biophys Res Commun 47:685–691, 1972
158. Madoc-Jones H, Mauro F: Interphase action of vinblastine and vincristine: Differences in their lethal action through the mitotic cycle of cultured mammalian cells. J Cell Physiol 72:185–196, 1968
159. Bleyer WA, Frisby SA, Oliverio VT: Uptake and binding of vincristine by murine leukemia cells. Biochem Pharmacol 24:633–639, 1975
160. Jackson DV, Bender RA: Cytotoxic thresholds of vincristine in L1210 murine leukemia and a human lymphoblastic cell line *in vitro.* Cancer Res 39:4346–4349, 1979
161. Dan K: Development of resistance to daunomycin (NSC 83151) in Ehrlich ascites tumor. Cancer Chemother Rep 55:133–141, 1971
162. Beidler JL, Riehm H: Cellular resistance to actinomycin D in Chinese hamster cells *in vitro:* Cross resistance, radioautographic, and cytogenetic studies. Cancer Res 30:1174–1184, 1970
163. Bender RA, Castle MC, Margileth DA et al: The pharmacokinetics of ^{3}H-vincristine in man. Clin Pharmacol Therap 22:430–438, 1977
164. Owellen RJ, Root MA, Hains FO: Pharmacokinetics of vindesine and vincristine in humans. Cancer Res 37:2603–2607, 1977
165. Castle MC, Margileth DA, Oliverio VT: Distribution and excretion of ^{3}H-vincristine in the rat and the dog. Cancer Res 36:3684–3689, 1976
166. Jackson DV, Castle MC, Bender RA: Biliary excretion of vincristine. Clin Pharmacol Ther 24:101–107, 1978
167. Owellen RJ, Hartke CA, Hains FO: Pharmacokinetics and metabolism of vinblastine in humans. Cancer Res 37:2567–2602, 1977
168. Weiss HD, Walker MD, Wiernik PH: Neurotoxicity of commonly used antineoplastic agents. N Engl J Med 291:127–133, 1974
169. Dyke RW, Nelson RL: Phase I anticancer agents. Vindesine (desacetyl vinblastine amide sulfate). Cancer Treat Rep 4:135–142, 1977
170. Robertson GL, Bhoopalam N, Zelkowitz LJ: Vincristine neurotoxicity and abnormal secretion of antidiuretic hormone. Arch Intern Med 132:717–720, 1973
171. Bender RA, Nichols AP, Norton L et al: Lack of therapeutic synergism of vincristine and methotrexate in L1210 murine leukemia *in vivo.* Cancer Treat Rep 62:997–1003, 1978
172. Radice PA, Bunn PA, Ihde DC: Therapeutic trials with VP-16-213 and VM-26: Active single agents in small cell lung cancer, non-Hodgkin's lymphoma, and other malignancies. Cancer Treat Rep 63:1231–1239, 1979
173. Drewinko B, Barlogie B: Survival and cycle-progression delay of human lymphoma cells *in vitro* exposed to VP-16-213. Cancer Treat Rep 60:1295–1306, 1976
174. Loike JD, Horwitz SB: Effects of podophyllotoxin and VP-16-213 on microtubule assembly *in vitro* and nucleoside transport in HeLa cells. Biochemistry 15:5435–5442, 1976
175. Allen LM, Creaven PJ: Comparison of the human pharmacokinetics of VM-26 and VP-16, two antineoplastic epipodophyllotoxin glucopyranoside derivatives. Eur J Cancer 11:697–707, 1975
176. Worzalla JF, Kaima BD, Johnson BM et al: N-demethylation of the antineoplastic agent hexamethylmelamine by rats and man. Cancer Res 33:2810–2815, 1972
177. Lake LM, Gruden EE, Johnson BM: Toxicity and antitumor activity of hexamethylmelamine and its N-demethylated metabolites in mice with transplantable tumors. Cancer Res 35:2858–2863, 1975
178. Rutty CJ, Connors TA, Nguyen-Hoang-Nam et al: *In vivo* studies with hexamethylmelamine. Eur J Cancer 14:713–720, 1978
179. Ames MM, Powis G: Determination of pentamethylmelamine and hexamethylmelamine in plasma and urine by nitrogen-phosphorous gas-liquid chromatography. J Chromatogr 174: 245–249, 1979
180. Dutcher JS, Jones RB, Boyd MR: A sensitive and specific assay for pentamethylmelamine in plasma: Applicability to clinical studies. Cancer Treat Rep 64:99–104, 1980
181. D'Incalci M, Bolis G, Mangioni C et al: Variable oral absorption of hexamethylmelamine in man. Cancer Treat Rep 62:2117–2119, 1978
182. Montgomery JA: Experimental studies at Southern Research Institute with DTIC (NSC-45388). Cancer Treat Rep 60: 125–134, 1976
183. Skibba JL, Ramirez G, Beal DD et al: Preliminary clinical trial and the physiologic disposition of 4(5)-(3,3-dimethyl-1-triazeno)imidazole-5(4)-carboxamide in man. Cancer Res 29: 1944–1951, 1969
184. Benvenuto JA, Hall SW, Farquhar D et al: High-pressure liquid chromatography in pharmacological studies of anticancer drugs. Chromatogr Sci 10:377–395, 1979
185. Householder GE, Loo TL: Elevated urinary excretion of 4-aminoimidazole-5-carboxamide in patients after intravenous injection of 4-(3,3-dimethyl-1-triazeno)imidazole-5-5 carboxamide. Life Sci 8:533–536, 1969
186. Smith PJ, Ekert H, Waters KD et al: High incidence of cardiomyopathy in children treated with adriamycin and DTIC in combination chemotherapy. Cancer Treat Rep 61:1736–1738, 1977
187. Weinkam RJ, Shiba DA: Metabolic activation of procarbazine. Life Sci 22:937–945, 1978
188. Kreis W, Yen Y: An antineoplastic C^{14}-labeled methyl hydrazine derivative in P815 mouse leukemia. A metabolic study. Experentia 21:284–285, 1965
189. Dost F, Reed D: Methane formation *in vivo* from N-isopropyl-alpha-(2-methylhydrazino)-p-toluamide hydrochloride, a tumor-inhibiting methyl hydrazine derivative. Biochem Pharmacol 16:1741–1746, 1967
190. Shiba DA, Weinkam RJ: Metabolic activation of procarbazine: Activity of the intermediates and the effects of pretreatment. Proc Am Assoc Cancer Res 20:139, 1979
191. Chabner BA, Sponzo R, Hubbard S et al: High-dose intermittent intravenous infusion of procarbazine. Cancer Chemother Rep 57:361–363, 1973
192. Liske R: A comparative study of the activity of cyclophosphamide and procarbazine on the antibody production in mice. Clin Exp Immunol 15:271–280, 1973
193. Le IP, Dixon RL: Mutagenicity, carcinogenicity, and teratogenicity of procarbazine. Mutat Res 55:1–14, 1978
194. Kidd JG: Regression of transplanted lymphomas induced *in vivo* by means of normal guinea pig serum. I. Course of transplanted cancers of various kinds in mice and rats given guinea pig serum, horse serum, or rabbit serum. J Exp Med 98:565–582, 1953
195. Broome JD: Evidence that the L-asparaginase of guinea pig serum is responsible for its antilymphoma effects. I. Properties of the L-asparaginase of guinea pig serum in relation to those of the antilymphoma substance. J Exp Med 118:99–120, 1963
196. Jackson RC, Handschumacher RE: *Escherichia coli* L-asparaginase. Catalytic activity and subunit nature. Biochemistry 9:3585–3590, 1970
197. Ohnama T, Holland JF, Meyer P: *Erwinia carotovora* asparaginase in patients with prior anaphylaxis to asparaginase from *E. coli.* Cancer 30:376–381, 1972

198. Haley EE, Fischer GA, Welsch AD: The requirement for L-asparagine of mouse leukemia cells L5178Y in culture. Cancer Res 21:532–536, 1961
199. Distasio JA, Neederman RA, Kafkewitz D et al: Purification and characterization of L-asparaginase with antilymphoma activity from *Vibrio succinogenes*. J Biol Chem 251:6929–6933, 1976
200. Haw T, Ohnuma T: L-asparaginase: *In vitro* inhibition of blastogenesis by enzyme from *Erwinia carotovora*. Nature (New Biol) 239:50–51, 1972
201. Meister A, Levintow L, Greenfield RE et al: Hydrolysis and transfer reactions catalyzed by amidase preparations. J Biol Chem 215:441–460, 1955
202. Cooney DA, Capizzi RL, Handschumacher RE: Evaluation of L-asparagine metabolism in animals and man. Cancer Res 30:929–935, 1970
203. Nesbitt M, Chard R, Evans A et al: Intermittent L-asparaginase therapy for acute childhood leukemia. Proc 10th Int Cancer Cong, p 447, 1970
204. Ohnuma T, Holland JF, Sinks LF: Biochemical and pharmacological studies with L-asparaginase in man. Cancer Res 30:2297–2305, 1970
205. Peterson RC, Handschumacher RF, Mitchell MS: Immunological responses to L-asparaginase. J Clin Invest 50:1080–1090, 1971
206. Capizzi R: Improvement in the therapeutic index of L-asparaginase by methotrexate. Cancer Chemother Rep, Pt. 3, 6:37–41, 1975
207. Spiers ASD, Wade HE: *Achromobacter* L-glutaminase-L-asparaginase: Human pharmacology, toxicology, and activity in acute leukemia. Cancer Treat Rep 63:1019–1024, 1979
208. Holcenberg JS, Camitta BM, Borella LD et al: Phase I study of succinylated *Acinetobacter* L-glutaminase-L-asparaginase. Cancer Treat Rep 63:1025–1030, 1979
209. Wellner D, Greenfield RS: L-threonine deaminase as a possible antitumor agent. Cancer Treat Rep 1089–1094, 1979
210. Kreis W: Tumor therapy by deprivation of L-methionine: Rationale and results. Cancer Treat Rep 63:1069–1072, 1979
211. Elmer GW, Linden C, Meadows GG: Influence of L-tyrosine phenol-lyase on the growth and metabolism of B^{16} melanoma. Cancer Treat Rep 63:1055–1062, 1979
212. Abell CW, Smith WJ, Hodgkins DS: An *in vivo* evaluation of the chemotherapeutic potency of phenylalanine ammonia-lyase. Cancer Res 33:2529–2532, 1973
213. Schmer G, Roberts J: Molecular engineering of the L-tryptophan-depleting enzyme indolyl-3 alkane alpha-hydroxylase. Cancer Treat Rep 63:1123–1126, 1979
214. Catane, R, Von Hoff DD, Glaubiger DL et al: Azaserine, DON, and azotomycin: Three diazo analogs of L-glutamine with clinical antitumor activity. Cancer Treat Rep 63:1033–1038, 1979
215. Jayaram HN, Cooney DA: Analogs of L-aspartic acid in chemotherapy for cancer. Cancer Treat Rep 63:1095–1108, 1979
216. Erlichman E, Strong JM, Wiernik PH et al: Phase I trial of N-(phosphonacetyl)-L-aspartate. Cancer Res 39:3992–3995, 1979
217. For a detailed discussion of therapies directed at amino acid depletion or analog development, see Uren R, Handschumacher RE: Enzyme therapy. *In* Becker FF (ed): Cancer: A Comprehensive Treatise, pp 457–487. New York, Plenum Press, 1977

CHAPTER 10 **Richard M. Simon**

Design and Conduct of Clinical Trials

The purpose of this chapter is to highlight principles for the design and conduct of valuable therapeutic clinical trials in oncology. Many such studies are one of the following types.

1. *Phase I Studies*. Determine the relationship between toxicity and dose-schedule of treatment.
2. *Phase II Studies*. Identify tumor types for which the treatment appears promising.
3. *Phase III Studies*.
   a. Determine the effects of a treatment relative to the natural history of the disease;
   b. Determine whether a new treatment is more effective than a standard therapy;
   c. Determine whether a new treatment is as effective as a standard therapy but is associated with less morbidity.

These classes of studies include evaluation of surgical procedures, radiotherapeutic treatments, chemotherapeutic drugs, immunostimulants, biological response modifiers, antibiotics, antiemetics and pain control agents. Each of the objectives stated above is meaningful, however, only within the context of a clearly defined patient population.

The experimental approach plays an important role in clinical oncology today. By the experimental approach, I refer roughly to two components. First, that clinical results, rather than deductive reasoning, are required for the evaluation of a treatment.[1] We try to avoid reasoning of the type that deduces that since disease is caused by evil spirits, and since bleeding purges evil spirits, bleeding must be good treatment. Second, the experimental approach requires that pre-planned therapeutic interventions be administered to specified types of patients under conditions that are controlled to enable well defined medical questions to be directly answered. Comparing the survivals of breast cancer patients treated with mastectomy to survivals of those receiving mastectomy plus post-operative radiotherapy based upon regional tumor registry data is an example of a non-experimental survey. In such surveys the investigator is a passive observer and abstracts records that he hopes will provide information about the phenomena he wishes to study. Treatment assignments, diagnostic tests and follow-up procedures are determined by the patients and physicians independently of the investigator. The statistical associations resulting from such studies are in themselves a weak basis for causal inferences concerning the relationship between treatment administered and results observed. Treatments are usually selected based upon subjective assessment of prognosis for the patient, capabilities of the physician, and variable diagnostic evaluations. It is generally impossible to identify and eliminate all the biases inherent in survey data.

Surveys are sometimes called "observational studies", though this is inaccurate since all knowledge is based upon observations. Surveys are generally the only feasible mechanisms for epidemiologic assessment of disease etiology and, when performed by highly trained and critical investigators, can contribute greatly to public welfare.[2,3] Acute observations in poorly structured therapeutic settings can also lead to immensely valuable ideas to be pursued and tested in the laboratory and planned clinical trials. Surveys are however sometimes proposed as an easy alternative to planned clinical trials for the evaluation of treatments.[4,5] For this purpose the survey is distinctly inferior with regard to inherent reliability of conclusions concerning therapeutic effects. MacMahon and Pugh point out:

> Only a minority of statistical associations are causal. . . . Once a statistical association has been demonstrated, how can it be determined whether or not it is causal. . . . The most satisfactory procedure is direct experiment. . . . The evaluation of the causal nature of a relationship, in the absence of direct experiment, is neither easy nor objective. . . . The field of cancer therapy is replete with examples of new modalities that were taken up with enthusiasm and proved worthless only after they had resulted in many years of futile cost and suffering.[3]

The difficult problems in analysis of survey data are discussed elsewhere.[6-8] Improvements in computer technology have increased the ease of conducting medical surveys, but have not had a major role in solving the basic weaknesses of this approach.

This chapter will address principles for the design and conduct of therapeutic clinical trials in oncology. Such studies can be direct and easily interpretable mechanisms for answering important medical questions. In order to achieve this objective, however, certain principles must be followed in planning the study. The following sections will address certain key aspects of this planning process.

The first result of the planning process is a written protocol. Typical subject headings for the protocol are shown in Table 10-1. This document should be self-contained, consistent and carefully prepared. It should define uniform treatment and evaluation policies for a well defined set of patients, and should not leave important decisions up to the discretion of the physician or the study chairperson. The protocol should clearly define the questions to be answered by the study and should directly justify that the number of patients and nature of controls are adequate to definitively answer these questions. It is very easy to embark on a futile or trivial study, and to write the protocol merely as a guideline for clinical management supplemented by lofty objectives of no scientific meaning. Rushing the protocol development process, and not being sufficiently critical of what is written or omitted, contributes to this tendency. From the presentaion of scientific background through the definition of data forms, the protocol should evidence clear, precise, and practical thinking.

TABLE 10-1. Subject Headings for a Protocol

1. Introduction and scientific background
2. Objectives
3. Selection of patients
4. Design of study (including schematic diagram)
5. Treatment programs
6. Procedures in event of toxicity
7. Required clinical and laboratory data
8. Criteria for evaluating the effect of treatment
9. Statistical considerations
10. Informed consent
11. Data forms
12. References
13. Study chairperson, collaborating participants, addresses, and telephone numbers

STUDY OBJECTIVES

It is important to describe the study objectives quite specifically in the protocol. This helps orient the protocol to represent a clearly thought-out research plan, rather than merely a guide for clinical management. Clearly stated objectives are also necessary to ensure that size of the study, nature of controls, and plans for patient management are adequate and unbiased with regard to the questions posed.

There are many studies in the social sciences that are fishing expeditions, that include numerous batteries of tests, resulting in exhaustive analyses. Such unstructured investigations are likely to result in some erroneous conclusions due to the multiplicity of the questions addressed.[9] Therapeutic studies in oncology generally have a more specific natural focus. Nevertheless, it is useful to describe the objectives in terms of specific questions to be answered by the study. Some protocols state that the objective is to "improve treatment" and some list numerous objectives that are not feasible within the size of study planned or for which there are inadequate controls. These characteristics are often an indication that insufficient critical thinking has been done in the planning stage to permit clear interpretation of the results that will be obtained.

The realities of numbers of patients required dictate that most studies should be restricted to one major question. It is best when either positive or negative results are informative for patient management and developing better treatments. Two examples of such studies are: (a) comparison of mastectomy to tumor resection for patients with stage I breast cancer; and (b) comparison of high dose versus conventional dose therapy with an effective drug. Many current studies provide no leads to build on when the results are negative.

Many current studies also fail to address the most important medical questions. The most important studies are often the most difficult to initiate. They may involve withholding a treatment established by tradition, potential transfer of patient management responsibility across specialties, standardization of procedures among individuals who believe their way is best, and sharing recognition with a large group of collaborators.

PATIENT ELIGIBILITY

The two main principles guiding the specification of eligibility criteria are (a) generalizability of conclusions to patients other than those actually involved in the study, and (b) identification of patients most likely to benefit from a new therapy. For phase I and phase II studies, these principles are secondary because an established therapy that prolongs life cannot be withheld in favor of a new treatment with undemonstrated therapeutic benefit. Phase I studies are therefore generally conducted with previously treated patients. The organ systems that are the expected targets of toxicity, however, should be competent in patients selected for the study. Otherwise, the relationships between dose schedule and toxicity found in the study will not be relevant to the treatment of less debilitated patients.

Whereas phase I studies need not be performed separately by histologic tumor type, this is not the case for phase II studies. In phase II studies the biologic response of major interest is that of the tumor itself. Because cytosensitivities vary among histologic types, it is important to have enough patients studied so that evaluation of tumor response can be made separately by type.

There are some kinds of advanced cancer for which there is no known therapy that prolongs survival (e.g., melanoma, esophogeal, pancreatic). For such sites, phase II studies should primarily include non-previously-treated patients. The chance of tumor response generally decreases with prior treatment. Consequently, including previously treated patients in phase II studies of diseases where treatment does not prolong survival constitutes a decrease in the potential sensitivity of the study.

For phase III studies, determination of eligibility criteria involves a trade-off between broad applicability of conclusions and addressing the study to those patients most likely to benefit from the new treatment. In a study with broad eligibility requirements, a conclusion of no difference between the treatments may result from a positive effect in one subset being cancelled by a negative effect in another. More frequently, a positive effect in one subset may be hidden in the overall comparison by the variability introduced by including patients less likely to benefit. For most studies, the basic analysis should include all patients, thus broad eligibility requirements may entail a loss of sensitivity.

Some statisticians advise that the eligibility criteria be very broad, because subset analyses can always be performed later.[10,11] This approach has the following deficiencies: (a) considerable effort and resources may be expended studying patients who may not be expected to benefit from or tolerate a new therapy; (b) misleading conclusions may result from multiple subset analyses; and (c) one must be careful to plan the study so that adequate numbers of patients within each major subset are available for separate analysis.

Studies with relatively narrow eligibility criteria may not yield results which are generalizable to patients of the types excluded. Such studies have been criticized for this. But if the narrow eligibility criteria provide improved homogeneity of prognosis, then such studies can yield more clearcut answers to therapeutic questions with reasonable numbers of patients of a well defined type.

In general, clearcut evidence of benefit for a well defined class of patients is likely to be more valuable than a finding of no effect for a mixed population. Though it is often not obvious which patients are most likely to benefit, some studies of intensive treatment include debilitated patients for whom reduced doses are planned from the outset. Generally, their inclusion is detrimental to the study. The added numbers they represent is more than compensated for by the increase in variability of response, and uncertainty of to whom the conclusions apply. Sir Bradford Hill made this point in discussing a clinical trial of streptomycin for respiratory tuberculosis[12]:

> . . . for it was realized that no two patients have an identical form of the disease and it was desired to eliminate as many of the obvious variations as possible. This planning . . . is a fundamental feature of the successful trial. To start out upon a trial with all and sundry included, and with the hope that the results can be sorted out statistically in the end is to court disaster.

ENDPOINT

The term endpoint refers to the criterion by which patient benefit is measured. A meaningful and reliable endpoint is essential for a worthwhile study. In some of the social sciences, lack of an adequate endpoint is a major impediment to progress. For clinical oncology this is not generally a severe problem. Nevertheless, explicit definition of the endpoint(s) is important for determining the size and duration of the trial, for ensuring that the proper measurements are taken and that follow-up evaluations are performed without bias.

Survival is generally the most meaningful measure of benefit for phase III studies. For several reasons, other endpoints are also used. Survival sometimes takes a long time to observe and one may wish to plan a new study before survivals are analyzable. Survival can also be influenced by treatments administered subsequently and by a variety of extraneous factors. When historical controls are used, survival may not be an adequate endpoint. For example, the recent aggressive use of thoracotomy for patients with osteosarcoma appears to have considerably prolonged survival making it impossible to use this endpoint in evaluating chemotherapeutic adjuvants to primary surgery with historical controls.

The endpoints commonly used instead of or in addition to survival are degree of tumor shrinkage, and duration of tumor disappearance. These are basically subjective measures. Whether or not a patient has a partial response depends upon who is doing the measuring.[13-17] Most patients who eventually "relapse" really had no disease-free period. Rather, the disease was below the level of detection with the procedures used. The more closely one looks, the fewer complete remissions are obtained and the more rapidly will recurrent disease be detected. Consequently, it is important that follow-up procedures be standardized in the protocol to ensure that the study is not jeopardized by biased evaluation of response. It is equally important to avoid excessive inadvertant bias resulting from having detailed diagnostic procedures during follow-up applied at the discretion of the participants. In some studies evaluating prolonged chemotherapy as a surgical adjuvant, the chemotherapy patients are followed by medical oncologists and the surgery-alone patients are followed by surgeons. This is a poor procedure, for their differing views about follow-up procedures may confound the comparison of the treatments.

Complete elimination of the prerogative of participating physicians to perform more detailed follow-up procedures that are based upon suspected tumor recurrence is impossible and undesirable. It is very important, however, to build into the study adequate follow-up procedures to be performed at specified intervals uniformly for all patients (*e.g.*, chest roentgens every three months). The procedures should be both reasonably complete and practical. The protocol should also specify in as great a detail as is possible the conditions under which more detailed unscheduled diagnostic procedures should be performed.

In some studies, time till tumor progression cannot be used as an unbiased endpoint. For example, in studies comparing surgical to nonsurgical treatments of a visceral malignancy, tumor dissemination will be detected earlier in the surgical group.

A great number of conflicting literature reports are due in

part to subjectivity in quantitating tumor response.[13-17] The concept of partial response is certainly useful in phase II studies, and to some extent in phase III studies as one guide for how to combine agents or modalities. In some cases, however, improving partial response rates are not an index to improving therapy. In metastatic breast cancer for example, though partial response rates may approach 75 percent, only about 15 to 20 percent of patients obtain complete responses and few if any are cured of their disease. As more and more drugs are introduced into a combination regimen, the partial response rate may increase via a spectrum coverage effect, though individual patients may not benefit compared to their response to the correct single agent (if it could be identified). This was certainly not the case for diseases like acute lymphoblastic leukemia or Hodgkin's disease, but it may be the case in settings where the complete response rate, and duration of complete responses do not improve as treatment becomes more complex. For such diseases, complete response rate, duration of complete responses, and survival should probably be the primary study endpoints. This has definite implications for the size and duration of such studies.

TREATMENT ALLOCATION

PHASE I STUDIES

The simplest phase I studies involve estimation of the relationship between dose and toxicity for a single schedule and mode of administration. Such studies are usually performed by starting with a low dose not expected to produce serious toxicity in any patients and increasing the dose for subsequent patients according to a series of pre-planned steps. Several patients are treated at each dosage level, often three patients per step when no toxicity is encountered and six patients per step thereafter.[18-20] The initial dose selection is generally based upon animal toxicology data. A starting dose of one-third the lowest toxic dose expressed as milligrams per square meter of body surface area in the most sensitive animal species (usually the dog or the monkey) is widely employed.[21-25]

Dose escalation for subsequent patients occurs only after sufficient time has passed to observe acute toxic effects for patients treated at lower doses. Insufficient attention has been given to quantitative methods of determining dose steps. One commonly employed is based upon a modified Fibonacci series.[26,27] The second step is twice the starting dose, the third step is 67 percent greater than the second, the fourth step is 50 percent greater than the third, the fifth step is 40 percent greater than the fourth, and each subsequent step is 33 percent greater than that preceding it. In some cases this procedure may result in an insufficiently rapid escalation.[28] Some workers believe that it is safe to continue to double the dose as long as no toxicity is seen,[19] however this requires better substantiation with past data. Other methods of dose escalation have also been proposed.[29,30]

Escalating doses for subsequent courses of the same patient is generally to be discouraged because it may mask the presence of cumulative toxicity and invalidly reduce the apparent inter-patient variability in maximum tolerable dose. An escalated second dose for a patient may be toxic because it is a higher dose or because it is a second dose. Many phase I studies which escalate doses within patients are not analyzed in a way that distinguishes patients from courses of therapy.

Some phase I studies evaluate several schedules or modes of administration. If study of the second schedule is begun after evaluation of the first is complete or well under way, then the accumulated information can be used to establish a starting dose. Otherwise it may be useful to randomly allocate the schedules to newly eligible patients. This is not crucial, but serves to eliminate bias in selecting patients for one schedule or other based upon their condition. Such randomization is not for the purpose of directly comparing the schedules, but to better ensure that the maximum tolerable dose determined for one schedule is not misleadingly high or low due to patient selection. Random assignment of doses to patients has been proposed even for phase I studies of one schedule[31,32] though it is not widely used today.

For any phase I study, and particularly for studies of combinations, criteria for dose reductions should be clearly specified in the protocol and closely monitored.

PHASE II STUDIES

Most phase II studies are performed by treating all accepted patients with the regimen being evaluated.[33,34] The results of such a study can be misleading in two ways. First, little antitumor effect may be seen but the patients may be so debilitated or extensively pre-treated that the results do not reflect true potential usefulness of the agent. Second, because of patient selection or inadequately rigorous response criteria, more favorable results are obtained than will be substantiated by further trials. The first type of result is generally viewed as more serious than the second, because it may cause the abandonment of a useful agent. The second result is quite undesirable, however, because it may be the basis of costly and futile phase III studies. If the misleading results are sufficiently favorable, investigators may find it unethical to withhold the agent from their patients in phase III studies resulting in extensive controversy, false research directions, and possibly adoption of an ineffective drug.

To deal with these potential problems it has been suggested that phase II studies involve a randomization between the experimental agent and a treatment known to have antitumor value.[11,35,36] The purpose of randomization would not be for determining which treatment was better, but for having a baseline response rate of similar patients treated with a known therapy. The known therapy would not be a "standard therapy" in the sense of being the treatment of choice. Peto has suggested that two-thirds of the patients should be randomized to the new treatment.[11] For phase II studies of previously treated patients it is not always possible to identify an active control treatment. When it is possible, this design can effectively deal with the false positivity problem. Adequate standardization or response criteria would usually be just as effective, however. The randomized design appears to have less value for dealing with the false negativity problem. The control therapy will generally have a low response rate for such patients and it will not serve as a sensitive control. A better safeguard against false negative results is to use non-previously treated patients in phase II studies when it is ethically possible.

For cooperative groups with sufficient patients to simultaneously conduct several phase II studies in a disease, randomization among the new agents is desirable. There is no question that patient selection can influence results.[37] Such selection can lead to bias in the ranking of new agents. Differences among institutions in evaluation of response can make the problem even more severe. The conduct of one master phase II study with randomized treatment assignment helps alleviate these problems. Some current trials of the Eastern Cooperative Oncology Group are performed in this manner and are adaptively weighted so that the new agents doing best receive more allocated patients.

Phase II trials may be designed with crossover to a specified treatment (either another experimental agent or an established drug) when the patient fails the initial therapy. This aspect of the design usually supplies little information because so few patients make it through the secondary treatment, because there are so few responses, and because the condition of the patient has changed.

PHASE III STUDIES

Controls

The interpretation of most phase III studies involves some type of comparison of results. In some cases the basis of comparison will be the natural history of the disease, and in others it will be another treatment. We shall use the term "control" to represent the basis against which a treatment is to be evaluated. Rarely if ever do we just want to know if a treatment is better or worse than the control. We want to estimate the degree of difference. All measurement is ultimately comparative, however, and the categorization of a treatment as "good" or "bad" involves an implicit comparison to the natural history of the disease.

To determine whether a new treatment cures any patients with a disease that is uniformly and rapidly fatal, history is a satisfactory control. In this situation the patient population is completely homogeneous with regard to cure in the absence of the new therapy. If 20 percent of patients are cured by conventional therapy and we can identify them by patient and tumor characteristics measured at diagnosis, then we can restrict a study to the remaining 80 percent and have complete homogeneity. Once we leave the setting of complete homogeneity with regard to the chosen endpoint, the definition of an adequate non-randomized control becomes problematical.

In many studies the controls are either numbers determined from publications or patients treated in non-experimental settings in which the information is abstracted from tumor registries, data banks, or medical records. The meaningfulness of such controls is questionable. Often diagnostic and staging procedures, supportive care, secondary treatments, and methods of evaluation and follow-up are different for the controls and the current treatment group. There is generally differential bias in the selection of patients to be treated resulting from judgments by the physicians, self-selection by the patients and differences in referral patterns. There may be bias in treatment ineligibility rates.[38] Current patients are sometimes excluded from analysis because of not meeting eligibility criteria, not receiving "adequate" treatment, refusing treatment, or a major protocol violation. The controls, on the other hand, generally contain all the patients. There may be differences in the distribution of known and unknown prognostic factors between the controls and the current treatment group. Often there is inadequate information to determine whether such differences are present, and current known prognostic factors may not have been measured or recorded for the controls. It is generally difficult to tell whether the controls would have been eligible for the current study and in what way they represent a selection of all eligible patients.

In the best of circumstances historical controls will be patients treated within the previous few years at the same institution or institutions performing the new study. The controls would be treated on a protocol having exactly the same eligibility requirements, work-up, follow-up, and response evaluation procedures as the current study, referral patterns and accrual rates would be static, no patients in either group would be excluded from analysis because of ineligibility or nonevaluability, and an exhaustive demonstration of similarity in distribution of all suspected prognostic factors would be presented. These circumstances are rarely encountered in practice. Pocock[39] has reported 19 unselected instances under circumstances approaching these where a collaborative group carried one treatment over for two successive studies. Even here, for four of the 19 pairs of trials the differences in outcome were statistically significant at the $P < 0.02$ level.

Formation of the control group by random assignment of treatment as an integral part of the planned study can avoid most of the systematic biases mentioned above.[40-43] The random assignment should not be performed till the patient is found eligible, and then a truly random or non-decipherable mechanism should be used. Alternation, day of the week, or other predictable procedures are not adequate because they permit bias in the decision of whether to enter a patient into a study based upon knowledge beforehand of what treatment the patient will receive. Randomization does not ensure that the study will include a representative sample of all patients with the disease, but it does help ensure an unbiased evaluation of the relative merits of the two treatments for the types of patients entered.

Some of the advantages of randomization are subtle and not widely understood. For example, it is sometimes said that randomization is unnecessary because matched historical or concurrent controls can be selected. But one can only match with regard to known prognostic factors, and these generally explain only a minor portion of the heterogeneity in prognosis among patients. Matching with regard to known factors gives no assurance that the distributions of unknown factors are similar between the treatment groups. It is also sometimes said that randomization is not effective in ensuring that the treatment groups are similar with regard to unknown prognostic factors unless the number of patients is large. This is true but reflects a misunderstanding of randomization. Randomization does not ensure that the groups are medically equivalent, but it distributes the unknown biasing factors according to a known random distribution so that their effects can be rigorously allowed for in significance tests and confidence intervals.[44] This is true regardless of the study size. A significance level represents the probability that differences in outcome are due to random fluctuations. Without randomized treatment allocation, a "statistically significant difference" may be due to a non-random difference in the distribution of unknown prognostic factors.

Randomization (or stratified randomization, to be discussed later) is inherently the method of treatment assignment that results in the most reliable basis for inference.[45,46] This is not to say that all randomized studies are good or that all non-randomized studies are bad, but that everything else being equal, randomization adds considerably to the ease of interpretability of the study since one need not worry about conscious or inadvertent systematic biases in patient selection or treatment assignment. Gehan and Freireich[47] and Pocock[48] have listed conditions under which non-randomized studies can be considered reliable. The majority of non-randomized studies do not meet these conditions. The oncology literature is filled with reports of non-randomized studies in which scant attention is paid to comparability with regard to known prognostic factors. At this point the major advantages of randomization are not the subtle aspects mentioned, but avoidance of the major biases of the majority of poorly done, non-randomized studies. If non-randomized studies were scrupulously conducted and critically reported under the conditions described above for consecutive trials, then the subtle advantages that randomization will always have might be less decisive. "Modern" alternative approaches based upon non-experimental data bases and tumor registries[4] having "concurrent" non-randomized controls are a poor alternative to either method.

Are randomized trials necessary for identifying major advances in treatment? No. There are many examples of therapeutic breakthroughs that were recognized without randomized trials. For the most part, however, these occurred in diseases where the prognosis was 100 percent predictable before the advent of the new therapy and hence there was no possibility of bias with regard to patient selection. False innovations are much more numerous than real breakthroughs, however, and it is difficult to distinguish one from the other.[49] There certainly is a role for innovative non-randomized studies, in diseases with uniformly bleak prognosis.

Some physicians are uncomfortable with the notion of randomization feeling that they have an obligation to develop an opinion about the relative merits of alternative possible treatments and to recommend a therapy to their patients accordingly.[50] This position is understandable but must be tempered by the following considerations: (a) different competent physicians often hold widely divergent opinions about the relative merits of alternative treatments for the same patient;[51] (b) the little research done indicates that experienced, well-educated adults are likely to overrate the correctness of their opinions and hunches;[52] and (c) the experimental treatment is generally neither much better nor much worse than the control, and we have little real basis for selecting between the treatments prior to the trial. Gilbert, McPeek and Mosteller point out:[52]

> Much of current popular discussion of the ethical issue takes the position that physicians should use their best judgment in prescribing for a patient. To what extent the physician is responsible for the quality of the judgment is not much discussed, except to say that he must keep abreast of the times. Some physicians will feel an obligation to find out that goes beyond the mere holding of an opinion. Such physicians will feel a responsibility to contribute to the research. In similar fashion, some current patients may feel a responsibility to contribute to the better care of future patients. The current model of the passive patient and the active outgoing physician is not the most effective one for a society that not only wants cures rather than sympathy, but insists on them—a society that has been willing to pay both in patient cooperation and material resources for the necessary research.

If randomization is employed, it should generally take place as late as possible before effecting treatment of the patient.[10] For example, in evaluating a chemotherapeutic regimen as a post-surgical adjuvant treatment, randomization should take place after the surgery is complete and the patient has sufficiently recovered to begin receiving chemotherapy. This approach serves to reduce bias in the surgery administered, and possible bias in disqualifications of randomized patients due to surgical findings, morbidity, or mortality.

Stratified Randomization

When there are known major prognostic factors for patients in randomized study, it is often advisable to stratify the randomization to assure equal distribution of these factors.[53] This is usually accomplished by preparing a separate randomization list (or set of cards in sealed envelopes) for each distinct subset of patients (stratum). Each list must be balanced so that after each block of four to ten patients within the stratum, the treatment groups contain equal numbers of patients. Within the blocks, the sequence of treatment assignments is random. The stratification factors must, of course, be known for each patient at the time of randomization.

For example, as shown in Figure 10-1, in a comparison of treatments for testicular cancer the factors may be histology and stage. These two stratification factors determine six patient strata. For a comparison of two treatments, designated A and B, the sequence of treatment assignments for a stratum can be determined in the following manner. We shall assume that it has been decided that the sequence for each stratum will be balanced in blocks of six patients. One obtains a table of two-digit random numbers and starts reading the table down an arbitrarily selected column. Random numbers in the range 00–49 will indicate treatment A and random numbers in the range 50–99 will indicate treatment B. If no more than 30 patients are anticipated in the stratum, then the tentative treatment assignments are determined by the first 30 random numbers read. This determines a sequence of a total of 30 A's and B's. This list must be modified in the following way to ensure balance after each block of six patients in the stratum. If the random sequence is

ABAAAABBABABBBBAAAABBAABBAAABB

then it is modified to

ABAABB AABBAB ABBBAA BAAABB ABBAAB.

Histology	*Stage* II	III
Teratocarcinoma with or without seminoma		
Embryonal carcinoma with or without seminoma		
Either of above with elements of choriocarcinoma		

FIG. 10-1. Example of stratification for a randomized clinical trial.

If three A's occur in a block before three B's, then the remainder of the block is automatically filled in with B's before the random sequence is continued. Similarly, if three B's occur in a block before three A's, then the remainder of the block is automatically filled in with A's. This procedure is performed separately for each stratum. The sequence of treatment assignments for each stratum is then transferred to a randomization list or to sealed and numbered randomization envelopes. The randomization sequences should be prepared by someone who will not be entering patients into the study. Generally, the blocksize should not be known to the participants and they should not be permitted to examine the partially used randomization sequences. These procedures are easily generalized to more than two treatments or to blocksizes other than six. For unstratified randomizations, the sequence of treatment assignments can be prepared in exactly the same way except that the blocksize is often larger.

The number of strata increases multiplicatively with the number of stratification factors, because the patient subsets are defined by combinations of these factors. Though limited stratification is often desirable, overstratification is detrimental to the trial. If there is extensive stratification, numerous strata will contain very few patients. Consequently, balance with regard to the most important factor or factors may be seriously impaired by the inclusion of factors of secondary importance. Even the total numbers of patients assigned each of the treatments may be very unequal. Extensive overstratification becomes equivalent to randomization with no stratification at all.[54]

It is generally best to limit stratification to those factors definitely known to have important independent effects on response. If two factors are closely correlated, one, at most, should be included in the stratification. Peto and others[10] feel that stratification is an unnecessary complication because adjustment for imbalances of known factors can be made in the analysis. For small studies, however, such adjustments should not be relied upon. Stratification may obviate the chance of gross imbalances that cannot be adjusted for, and ensures that the treatment comparisons are not totally dependent upon statistical adjustment methods.[55,56] Simon[57] has reviewed the various stratification methods available, and Zelen[58] has described a method particularly suited to multi-institution studies.

Crossover Designs

Crossover designs have been discussed in the context of phase II studies, but they are also used in other settings, such as the comparative evaluation of anti-emetics and anti-pain treatments. For example, patients might be randomized to receive either an anti-emetic during the first course of chemotherapy and a placebo during the second, or the alternate sequence. This design is motivated by the desire to increase the sensitivity of a study by using each patient as his own control, and to thereby reduce the number of patients required. The usefulness of this approach is limited by the fact that the condition of the patient changes with time, and the effect of a treatment may be influenced by previous treatments or conditioned by previous responses.

Crossover designs in which there are more than two treatment episodes per patient are almost always difficult or impossible to clearly interpret. Frequently such studies are analyzed and reported in a manner that fails to distinguish distinct patients from multiple treatment episodes of the same patient.

Useful methods for the analysis of a two-period crossover design are described by Hills and Armitage[59] and by Koch.[60] Use of the crossover design is controversial, and has been discouraged by the Biometric and Epidemiologic Advisory Committee of the Food and Drug Administration.[61] If the relative efficacy of the treatments in the second period differs from that in the first period or is conditioned by first period response, then it is not possible to use each patient as his own control. In order to determine whether such an interaction exists requires as many patients as a non-crossover design, and one should seriously weigh these considerations before adopting the crossover design.[62]

It is always best to administer a treatment in a clinical trial the way that it would be recommended for administration in general medical practice. The crossover design is artificial in this regard. Less structured designs that repeatedly re-randomize the same patients are subject to this criticism and suffer from the introduction of additional correlations that are generally impossible to properly account for in the analysis.

Common Control Designs

In randomized multi-institution studies it is sometimes difficult to obtain agreement among all participants concerning the treatments to be used. A compromise design sometimes suggested is to permit each institution to select between doing a randomized study of treatments A and C or doing a randomized study of treatments B and C. These two studies are conducted simultaneously, but at different institutions. It is usually recognized that this design is inferior to a simple randomization among all treatments A, B, and C within each institution, but it is hoped that it is better than a totally non-randomized design. Schoenfeld and Gelber[63] have shown that unless one can assume that there are no differences among institutions in response to treatment, this design is very inefficient. With three treatments (one being the common control), this design requires twice as many patients as a straightforward three-way randomized design. Makuch and Simon[64] have pointed out that similar results for the common control treatment between the sets of institutions selecting the two options does not ensure that the other two treatments can be validly compared. Systematic differences among the institutions may only be manifested in intensively treated patients. Consequently, the common control design is not a good alternative unless the experimental treatments are minor variants of each other. In general, it is best to rigorously standardize the treatments in order to eliminate extraneous causes of variability and bias.

Factorial Designs

In a 2 × 2 factorial design there are actually four treatments under study. The first factor represents two alternative treatment interventions, such as amputation or resection. The second factor represents two other alternative interventions superimposed upon the first factor, such as adjuvant chemotherapy or no further treatment. Though there are actually four treatment groups (amputation alone, resection alone, amputation plus chemotherapy, resection plus chemotherapy), proponents of such designs[11,46] suggest that the effect of each treatment factor can be addressed using all of the patients and pooling with regard to the other factor (or with the influence of the other factor accounted for in the analysis, but not separate analysis for each level of the other factor). The validity of such an analysis depends upon the following types of assumptions: if adjuvant chemotherapy is beneficial for amputees then it is also beneficial for resected patients, and the difference in efficacy of the two surgical procedures is either concurrently positive, negative, or zero, both for patients receiving adjuvant chemotherapy and for those not receiving further treatment. If these assumptions are not satisfied then the study must be analyzed by the simultaneous comparison of all four treatment groups. The risk in planning such a study is that the number of patients established will be sufficient only for pooled two-group comparisons, yet the data may suggest that such an analysis is not adequate. Also, the number of patients required to determine whether such an interaction is present is greater than the number required to perform two group comparisons. Thus, the factorial design offers the possibility of increased efficiency, but with a definite risk of difficulty in interpretation.

Combining Randomized and Historical Controls

Randomized studies are sometimes conducted weighted 2/1 in favor of the new treatment with the intent of incorporating historical controls in the analysis if their outcomes are similar to those of the randomized controls.[10] This design rarely provides enough randomized controls for an adequate comparison with results for the historical control group.[65] Pocock[48] has investigated other methods for combining controls from two successive studies but he assumes that the expected difference between outcomes from the control groups is zero. As discussed in the next section, a 2/1 randomization is often reasonable, but not for the purpose of including historical controls.

SIZE AND DURATION OF THE STUDY

PHASE I AND PHASE II TRIALS

The size of phase I studies cannot be completely determined in advanced. Guidelines that exist for planning the size of such studies have been presented in a previous section.

Gehan[66] presented the following useful two-stage patient accrual plan for phase II trials. The plan is applied separately to each subset of patients for whom inferences are to be made (*e.g.*, non-previously treated advanced colon cancer patients). If no partial responses in 14 such patients are obtained, then the trial is terminated for such patients and the drug is considered inactive for that subset. The basis for this conclusion is that a drug with a 20 percent response rate in an infinite number of such patients has a 95 percent chance of causing at least one response in 14 patients. Thus, if we "reject" the drug for this subset when no responses are seen in the first 14 patients, the rejection error is 5 percent for a true effectiveness of 20 percent. Table 10-2 shows the number of patients to be treated in the first stage as a function of the rejection error and true effectiveness proportion. If no responses are seen in the tabulated number of patients, then the drug is "rejected" for this subset.

For a rejection error of 5 percent and a true effectiveness proportion of 20 percent, if at least one response is obtained in the first 14 such patients, then a second stage of the trial is conducted in order to better estimate the response rate of the drug. Table 10-3 indicates the size of the second stage as a function of the precision desired for the estimate. For a standard error of 10 percent in the estimate of response rate, about ten additional patients in the subset should be treated.

This plan is frequently misapplied by having too heterogeneous a set of patients in the first stage. If no responses are

TABLE 10-2. Sample Size (n_1) Required for Preliminary Trial of a New Agent for Given Levels of Therapeutic Effectiveness and Rejection Error

REJECTION ERROR (β)	THERAPEUTIC EFFECTIVENESS (%)									
	5	10	15	20	25	30	35	40	45	50
5%	59	29	19	14	11	9	7	6	6	5
10%	45	22	15	11	9	7	6	5	4	4

TABLE 10-3. Number of Additional Patients (n_2) Required in a Follow-Up Trial to Estimate the Therapeutic Effectiveness of an Agent With Specified Precision (Standard Error)

REJECTION ERROR OF PRELIMINARY TRIAL	REQUIRED STANDARD ERROR	NO. OF TREATMENT SUCCESSES IN PRELIMINARY TRIAL	THERAPEUTIC EFFECTIVENESS (%) 5	10	15	20	25	30
	NO OF PATIENTS IN PRELIMINARY TRIAL		59	29	19	14	11	9
5%	5%	1	0	4	30	45	60	70
		2	0	17	45	63	78	87
		3	0	28	58	76	87	91
		4	0	38	67	83	89	91
		5	0	46	75	86	89	91
	10%	1	0	0	0	1	7	11
		2	0	0	0	6	12	15
		3	0	0	1	9	14	16
		4	0	0	3	11	14	16
		5	0	0	5	11	14	16
	NO. OF PATIENTS IN PRELIMINARY TRIAL		45	22	15	11	9	7
10%	5%	1	0	21	42	60	70	83
		2	0	35	60	78	87	93
		3	0	47	72	87	91	93
		4	4	57	81	89	91	93
		5	9	65	85	89	91	93
	10%	1	0	0	0	7	11	16
		2	0	0	4	12	15	18
		3	0	0	7	14	16	18
		4	0	0	9	14	16	18
		5	0	0	10	14	16	18

observed among 14 patients of diverse tumor types or previous treatment experiences, no conclusion can be reached for any single well defined class of patients. Homogeneity can be carried beyond the point of practicality, because even tumors of the same histologic type differ in sites of metastasis and in other ways. One should usually strive for separate evaluation of results by tumor histology and by whether or not the patient has previously received chemotherapy. It is important to describe the sites of metastatic disease of the patients treated and how the response rate observed varied among sites. It will not generally be practical however, to treat at least 14 patients with each histology, prior treatment experience, and metastatic site combination.

Gehan's plan is also frequently misapplied by failure to conduct the second stage for strata that exhibit at least one response in the first 14 patients. The second stage is important because a modest or moderate response rate in the first stage is consistent with both a very poor and a very good drug. This two-stage design is often simplified by specifying at the outset that 25 patients will be treated for each relevant subset. Other patient accrual plans for phase II trials have also been described.[67–70]

PHASE III TRIALS

The protocol for a phase III study should specify the number of patients and duration of follow-up planned. These plans should be based upon the specific study objectives and endpoints used. In many cases the same protocol will include plans for treating very distinct subsets of patients (*e.g.*, stage I and stage II breast cancer patients). In such instances, plans should be made for accruing sufficient numbers of patients of each type for separate analyses, because the relative merits of the treatments may vary substantially. Because of unforeseen complications or larger than expected treatment differences, patient accrual may have to be terminated prematurely. Nevertheless, target sample sizes are essential in order to ensure that the study is feasible and in order to know when to stop in the absence of premature termination. If too few patients are studied, the results may be ambiguous or erroneous and this commonly happens.[71–72] It is equally undesirable to have more patients studied than is necessary to reliably answer the questions posed by the study.

The usual statistical methods of sample-size determination in comparative trials are oversimplified as rigid models of the complete analysis, but have been found useful for planning purposes. These methods are based upon the assumption that at the conclusion of the trial, a statistical significance test will be performed comparing the treatment groups with regard to the major endpoint(s). A statistical significance level of 0.05 resulting from a treatment comparison has the following meaning: if there is no true difference in treatment efficacy, the probability of obtaining a difference in outcomes as extreme as that observed in the data is 0.05. The significance level does not represent the probability that the null hypothesis is true, it represents a probability of an observed difference, *assuming* that the null hypothesis is true. Conventional statistical theory ascribes no probabilities to hypotheses, only to data.

With few patients in each of the treatment groups being compared, the difference in observed outcomes must be very extreme in order for the significance level to be as small as 0.05. As the sample size increases, smaller differences in response will be statistically significant at the 0.05 level. In comparing proportions, 10/10 compared to 7/10 (a difference of 30 percent) is not statistically significant at the 0.05 level, whereas 40/40 compared to 35/40 (a difference of 12 percent) is.

For comparing two proportions, the usual method of sample size determination is as follows. It is assumed that after n patients have been observed on treatment A and n patients have been observed on treatment B, a statistical significance test will be performed. One wishes to determine n to be just large enough so that if the true response rate for A is p_A percent (*i.e.*, the response rate that would be observed in an infinite number of patients receiving A) and the true response rate for B is p_B percent, then 80 percent of the time the significance level will be no greater than 0.05. The 80 percent figure is called the power of the test.

If we think of a study resulting in a significance level of less than 0.05 for the major comparison as a positive study, then the power represents the probability of getting a true positive result when the actual response rates are p_A and p_B. The power is a design parameter which is usually specified between 80 percent and 95 percent. Whereas performing a significance test does not require knowledge of the unknown p_A and p_B, these parameters are an integral part of determining n to achieve a pre-planned power. If treatment A is a standard treatment, p_A is estimated from past data. The absolute magnitude $| p_B - p_A |$ is viewed as a difference that we wish to have a power of 80 percent (say) for detecting.

For comparing two proportions, Tables 10-4 and 10-5 can be used to determine the number of patients to be assigned each of two treatments in order to achieve a specified power as a function of the true response rates. Table 10-4 is for obtaining one-sided significance levels less than 0.05, and Table 10-5 is for two-sided significance levels of less than 0.05. A two-sided significance level represents the probability by chance alone of obtaining a difference in either direction as large as the one actually observed. A one-sided significance level represents the probability by chance alone of obtaining a difference as large as and in the same direction as that actually observed. Controversy exists over the appropriateness of one-sided or two-sided significance levels. This will be discussed later in this chapter. A conservative approach is to use two-sided significance levels. Suppose that based upon past data we estimate the response rate for treatment A to be

TABLE 10-4. Number of Patients in Each of Two Treatment Groups (One-Sided Test)

SMALLER SUCCESS RATE	LARGER MINUS SMALLER SUCCESS RATE									
	.05	.10	.15	.20	.25	.30	.35	.40	.45	.50
.05	512* 381†	172 129	94 72	62 48	45 35	35 27	28 22	23 18	19 15	16 13
.10	786 579	236 176	121 91	76 58	54 41	40 31	31 24	25 20	21 16	17 14
.15	1026 752	292 216	144 108	88 66	60 46	44 34	34 26	27 21	22 17	18 14
.20	1231 900	339 250	163 121	98 73	66 50	48 37	36 28	29 22	23 18	19 15
.25	1402 1024	377 278	178 132	105 79	70 53	50 38	38 29	29 23	23 18	19 15
.30	1539 1122	407 300	189 141	111 83	73 55	52 39	38 30	30 23	23 18	19 15
.35	1642 1196	429 315	197 146	114 85	74 56	52 40	38 30	29 23	23 18	18 14
.40	1711 1246	441 324	201 149	115 86	74 56	52 39	38 29	29 22	22 17	17 14
.45	1745 1271	446 327	201 149	114 85	73 55	50 38	36 28	27 21	21 16	16 13
.50	1745 1271	441 324	197 146	111 83	70 53	48 37	34 26	25 20	19 15	15 12

* Upper figure: significance level 0.05, power 0.90.
† Lower figure: significance level 0.05, power 0.80.

TABLE 10-5. Number of Patients in Each of Two Treatment Groups (Two-Sided Test)

SMALLER SUCCESS RATE	LARGER MINUS SMALLER SUCCESS RATE									
	.05	.10	.15	.20	.25	.30	.35	.40	.45	.50
.05	620*	206	113	74	54	42	33	27	23	19
	473†	159	88	58	43	33	27	22	18	16
.10	956	285	146	92	64	48	38	30	25	21
	724	218	112	71	50	38	30	24	20	17
.15	1250	354	174	106	73	53	41	33	26	22
	944	269	133	82	57	42	32	26	21	18
.20	1502	411	197	118	79	57	44	34	27	22
	1132	313	151	91	62	45	34	27	22	18
.25	1712	459	216	127	84	60	45	35	28	23
	1289	348	165	98	65	47	36	28	22	18
.30	1880	495	230	134	88	62	46	36	28	22
	1414	375	175	103	68	48	36	28	22	18
.35	2006	522	239	138	89	63	46	35	27	22
	1509	395	182	106	69	49	36	28	22	18
.40	2090	537	244	139	89	62	45	34	26	21
	1571	407	186	107	69	48	36	27	21	17
.45	2132	543	244	138	88	60	44	33	25	19
	1603	411	186	106	68	47	34	26	20	16
.50	2132	537	239	134	84	57	41	30	23	17
	1603	407	182	103	65	45	32	24	18	14

* Upper figure: significance level 0.05, power 0.90.
† Lower figure: significance level 0.05, power 0.80.

30 percent, and that we wish to have 80 percent power for detecting a true response rate of treatment B of 55 percent. For a two-sided statistical significance test, we find from Table 10-5 that 68 patients for each of the two treatments are required (136 patients total). If we wish power of 80 percent for detecting a true response rate of treatment B of 50 percent, then 103 patients per treatment are required. The required number of patients increases rapidly as size of the difference to be detected decreases. Planning a study not large enough to reliably detect a difference of 25 percent in success rate is usually unrealistic. The "not significantly different" results of smaller comparative studies are often mistakenly interpreted as saying something about the treatments, whereas they may be just a consequence of the inadequate numbers of patients.[71,72]

Tables 10-4 and 10-5 presented here were constructed according to the methods of Casagrande, Pike, and Smith,[73] and are considered more accurate than tables previously published based upon other approximations.[74-77] When the smaller response rate is thought to exceed 50 percent, the tables given here should be used with regard to comparing failure rates (100 percent minus response rate).

When an unbalanced $K/1$ randomization is contemplated for comparing two treatments, the total sample size obtained from Tables 10-4 and 10-5 should be multiplied by $(K + 1)^2/4K$. For example, a 2/1 randomization requires 12.5 percent more total patients than an equally weighted design of the same power. Weightings more extreme than 2/1 are rarely desirable.

For comparative trials of proportions using historical controls, appropriate tables are given by Makuch and Simon,[78] and are reproduced here as Tables 10-6 through 10-8. These tables are more bulky because the number of patients to be given the experimental treatment depends upon the size of the historical control group. Tables 10-6 through 10-8 are for achieving 80 percent power with a one sided significance level of 0.05. If our historical control group of 50 patients showed a response rate of 30 percent and we want 80 percent power for detecting a true response rate of 50 percent for the new treatment, then Table 10-6 indicates that 69 new patients should be treated with the new experimental therapy. If there were 100 appropriate historical controls, then Table 10-7 indicates that 48 new patients should be treated with the experimental therapy. Tables 10-6 through 10-8 assume that all new patients will be given the experimental therapy. Mixtures of historical and concurrent controls have not been studied in this way.

These tables for comparing proportions are useful when the endpoint can be dichotomized as success or failure. This can be done for response rate or complete response rate. The tables can also be used when survival or continuous disease-free survival is to be compared. In such cases the table is used with regard to the proportion of patients who survive (or remain without evidence of disease) for some meaningful

TABLE 10-6. Number of patients needed in an experimental group for a given probability of obtaining a significant result (one-sided test) with significance level α = 0.05 and power $(1 - \beta) = 0.80$. When N_c = 20, 30, 40, and 50 historical controls are used for comparison

PROPORTION OF SUCCESS (π_e) FOR EXPERIMENTAL PATIENTS	PROPORTION OF SUCCESS (π_c) FOR HISTORICAL-CONTROL PATIENTS							
	0.1	0.2	0.3	0.4	0.5	0.6	0.7	0.8
0.2	*†							
	*‡							
	>40,000§							
	944‖							
0.3	116	*						
	53	*						
	40	*						
	35	*						
0.4	22	385	*					
	17	98	*					
	15	67	*					
	14	55	*					
0.5	11	31	882	*				
	9	23	137	*				
	9	21	87	*				
	8	19	69	*				
0.6	7	13	37	913	*			
	6	12	27	147	*			
	6	11	24	92	*			
	6	10	22	74	*			
0.7	5	8	14	36	455	*		
	4	7	13	27	122	*		
	4	7	12	24	83	*		
	4	7	11	22	68	*		
0.8	4	5	8	14	30	179	*	
	3	5	8	12	24	83	*	
	3	5	7	12	22	63	*	
	3	5	7	11	20	55	*	
0.9	3	4	5	8	12	22	68	*
	3	4	5	7	11	19	47	>40,000
	3	4	5	7	10	17	40	745
	3	4	5	7	10	17	37	355

*No solution.
†Sample size for N_c = 20 historical controls.
‡Sample size for N_c = 30 historical controls.
§Sample size for N_c = 40 historical controls.
‖Sample size for N_c = 50 historical controls.

time period (*e.g.*, five years). The number of patients required must then be observed for this time period. The final analysis of such studies will generally consist of a comparison of the entire survival curves, rather than just the proportions surviving five years. It is not possible, however, to produce general tables of required number of patients for comparing survival curves because the results depend upon the form of the survival distributions. For example, fewer patients are required to detect a 50 percent increase in median survival when the variability in survival time among similarly treated patients is small than would be required to detect the same 50 percent increase when variability is large.

George and Desu[79] have produced tables for determining the required number of patients when the survival distributions have an exponential form. Exponential survival corresponds to a constant force of mortality. That is, a constant percentage of the remaining patients die each month. For exponential survivals, the number of deaths required to achieve a specified power depends only upon the ratio of median survivals to be detected, not upon the actual median values. In using the tables of George and Desu one must be careful to remember that the number of deaths (or recurrences) are given, not the number of patients. Similarly, for using the tables presented here to plan survival studies, it must be remembered that the tabulated entry represents the number of patients per group followed for the specified period of time.

When survival or remission data are available from previous studies of the same type of patients, one can check whether the survival distribution is approximately exponential. If $S(t)$ denotes the probability of surviving at least t months, then the graph of log $S(t)$ versus t is linear for exponential survival. For diseases where a proportion of the patients are cured, however, the exponential distribution will not be appropriate.

TABLE 10-7. Number of patients needed in an experimental group for a given probability on obtaining a significant result (one-sided test) with significance level α = 0.05 and power $(1 - \beta)$ = 0.80. When N_c = 75, 100, 125, and 150 historical controls are used for comparison

PROPORTION OF SUCCESS (π_e) FOR EXPERIMENTAL PATIENTS	PROPORTION OF SUCCESS (π_e) FOR HISTORICAL-CONTROL PATIENTS							
	0.1	0.2	0.3	0.4	0.5	0.6	0.7	0.8
0.2	232*							
	156†							
	129‡							
	115§							
0.3	29	907						
	27	383						
	26	271						
	25	223						
0.4	13	44	3373					
	13	40	702					
	12	38	424					
	12	36	327					
0.5	8	18	54	8392				
	8	17	48	949				
	8	16	46	525				
	8	16	44	390				
0.6	5	10	20	58	6016			
	5	10	19	52	893			
	5	10	19	49	511			
	5	9	18	47	385			
0.7	4	7	11	21	55	1944		
	4	6	11	20	50	609		
	4	6	10	19	47	398		
	4	6	10	19	45	316		
0.8	3	5	7	11	19	46	596	
	3	5	7	11	18	42	331	
	3	5	7	10	18	40	253	
	3	5	7	10	18	39	217	
0.9	3	4	5	7	10	16	33	187
	3	4	5	7	10	15	31	146
	3	4	5	6	9	15	30	129
	3	4	5	6	9	15	30	119

*Sample size for N_c = 75 historical controls.
†Sample size for N_c = 100 historical controls.
‡Sample size for N_c = 125 historical controls.
§Sample size for N_c = 150 historical controls.

Unfortunately, tables such as those in George and Desu have not been prepared for other types of distributions with censored survival data. Consequently, the tables for comparing proportions are commonly used for planning the size of survival studies.

The kinds of methods described are useful for ensuring that sufficient numbers of patients are treated so that an improvement in response is not erroneously missed due to the random fluctuations of small numbers. For studies comparing a standard treatment to a more conservative or less invasive therapy, it is particularly important that the sample size be large for the following reason. With few patients, it is unlikely that the difference in outcomes will be statistically significant at a level as small as 0.05 even though the conservative treatment may be truly inferior. In the usual statistical formulation, the null hypothesis specifies that the two treatments are equivalent. Acceptance of the null hypothesis may result in erroneous adoption of a new, more conservative therapy. The burden of proof for studies of this type should be on showing that results are similar, not on demonstrating that they are dissimilar. Consequently, accepting the null hypothesis based upon a significance test of low power is very inappropriate. Large numbers of patients are required to ensure that important differences can be ruled out in the analysis by calculating confidence intervals for the true difference in efficacy. The confidence interval provides a much clearer picture of what differences in efficacy are consistent with the data than does a significance test. Makuch and Simon[65] discuss this approach for planning the size and duration of studies evaluating a conservative therapy.

INTERIM ANALYSES OF PHASE III TRIALS

The methods described above for determining the required number of patients assume that statistical analysis will be performed only at the conclusion of the trial. If statistical

TABLE 10-8. Number of patients needed in an experimental group for a given probability of obtaining a significant result (one-sided test) with significant level $\alpha = 0.05$ and power $(1 - \beta = 0.80$. When $N_c = 200$, 250, 300, and 500 historical controls are used for comparison

PROPORTION OF SUCCESS (π_e) FOR EXPERIMENTAL PATIENTS	PROPORTION OF SUCCESS (π_e) FOR HISTORICAL-CONTROL PATIENTS							
	0.1	0.2	0.3	0.4	0.5	0.6	0.7	0.8
0.2	101*							
	94†							
	90‡							
	82§							
0.3	24	181						
	24	162						
	23	151						
	23	133						
0.4	12	35	250					
	12	34	217					
	12	33	199					
	12	32	170					
0.5	7	16	42	289				
	7	16	41	248				
	7	16	40	226				
	7	15	38	190				
0.6	5	9	18	44	288			
	5	9	18	43	248			
	5	9	18	42	226			
	5	9	17	41	191			
0.7	4	6	10	19	43	248		
	4	6	10	18	42	218		
	4	6	10	18	41	201		
	4	6	10	18	40	174		
0.8	3	5	7	10	17	38	182	
	3	5	7	10	17	37	166	
	3	5	7	10	17	36	156	
	3	5	7	10	17	35	139	
0.9	3	4	5	6	9	15	29	108
	3	3	5	6	9	15	28	102
	3	3	5	6	9	15	28	99
	3	3	5	6	9	14	28	92

*Sample size for $N_c = 200$ historical controls.
†Sample size for $N_c = 250$ historical controls.
‡Sample size for $N_c = 300$ historical controls.
§Sample size for $N_c = 350$ historical controls.

significance tests are performed repeatedly throughout the trial then the probability that the difference in outcomes will be statistically significant at the 0.05 level at some point is greater than 5 percent by chance alone.[80,81] This probability is called the type 1 error of the design. Peto and others[10] state that the type 1 error is approximately 15 percent if you perform a significance test every six months of a three-year trial comparing two identical treatments. If the times of the analyses are determined by visual trends in the accumulating data, this error may be even greater. If we think of a study that reports a significance level of less than 0.05 for the major comparison as a positive study, then the type 1 error represents the probability of getting a false positive result.

Interim analyses can be misleading because they may be dominated by differences in treatment efficacy for minor subsets of patients of poorer prognosis, and by transient differences in the distribution of prognostic factors.[71] Interim analyses may also influence the types and numbers of patients subsequently entered and even cause undesirable changes in patient management and evaluation of response. For these reasons, it is common in fields other than oncology to review interim results only by a monitoring board rather than by the participating physicians.

The decision to stop a study and the conclusions drawn from a study are two distinct entities, though they are often confused.[82,83] Similarly, the significance level of a statistical test and the type 1 error of a monitoring plan are distinct. The significance level depends only upon the data, the test statistic, the probability distributions, and the definition of "more extreme" difference. The type 1 error depends upon how often we looked at the data, what the decision to stop was based upon, and what decisions we would have made previously if the data had looked differently than it did. If the monitoring plan consists of performing repeated significance tests and stopping as soon as a level less than 0.05 is achieved, then one must accept that the type 1 error will exceed 0.05.

Armitage[84] has pioneered continuous monitoring plans which limit the type 1 error to a specified level, say 0.05. These methods have been successfully utilized and extended for application to survival data[85] and for interim analyses at discrete points rather than continuously.[86,87] With these approaches, the decision to stop and the specification of which treatment is preferred are given by the same decision rule. For complex clinical trials involving several endpoints, complications, patient heterogeneity, and delays in reporting outcomes, these designs may represent too great an oversimplication.[88] If there is no difference between the treatments or if the difference is modest, sequential monitoring plans generally require increased numbers of patients, since the chance of falsely terminating the trial at each interim point is allowed for. Consequently, it may be desirable to use these methods with only a few (2 or 3) interim decision points.[9]

Peto and others[11] have suggested a reasonable alternative to the problem of monitoring results. They suggest that interim statistical comparisons be performed at fixed times, and premature termination occur when the significance level for a major comparison achieves a very small value (such as $p < .001$). This provides protection against extreme unanticipated differences. If the interim differences are not significant at this level, then the trial is terminated at its originally intended size. The final statistical analysis is performed without regard to the interim analyses, and the type 1 error is affected little by the monitoring. They claim that with such an approach the objectives of interim monitoring are achieved in a manner that affects the final statistical analysis in a very minor way, if causes for early termination do not materialize.

The effect of interim analyses on type 1 error should be recognized, but the two concepts should not be confused. Suppose that in a simple trial comparing complete response rates for two treatments the following early termination rule is used. Interim significance tests are performed once each year for a four-year study, and accrual is terminated if the difference in complete response rate is statistically significant at the 0.01 level. In the absence of early termination, a difference significant at the 0.05 level in the final analysis would be associated with a type 1 error of no greater than 0.08 for the monitoring plan.

Generally the protocol should specify a single target number of patients to be accrued, a minimum duration of follow-up for each patient, and the estimated time necessary for accrual and follow-up. Though the rationale for early termination decisions are often more complex than those encompassed in mathematical plans,[83,89] the effect of repeated significance tests should be recognized and such tests limited as much as possible.

THE EPIDEMIOLOGY OF CLINICAL TRIALS

Some critics argue against small or moderate size trials on the following basis. Of the many small trials performed, at least 5 percent will by chance alone yield differences significant at the 0.05 level when there is no true difference in treatment efficacy. Journal publication policies are biased toward accepting positive results. These individuals believe that there are few true treatment differences of sufficient magnitude to be detected in small clinical trials. Hence they claim that the literature of positive results from small trials is dominated by false positive claims. For example, Peto states:[11]

> My interpretation is that, having done what resections we can, almost all past claims or hopes of great therapeutic improvements have been mistaken, and so, despite appearances, almost all current therapeutic suggestions will likewise eventually be found to yield either small or no benefits . . . Because the need is to distinguish between small benefits and no benefits, historically controlled comparisons will not suffice, nor will small randomized trials suffice . . .

This point of view seems to be gaining in popularity.[90] It is true that preferential publication of positive studies may result in a disproportionate number of false positive claims from small clinical trials. But the solution offered, elimination of small and moderate sized clinical trials, would make this nihilistic viewpoint a self-fulfilling prophecy. Williams and Whitehouse point out that though there have been major advances in cancer treatment:[91]

> It is difficult to find a single instance where dramatic improvements in the management of a cancer have come from a large scale multicentre study . . . Improved management of cancer will not come from the large-scale application of standard therapies—which we already know fail. New treatments are needed and these cannot be developed in large multicentre trials.

Though large multi-institution clinical trials can be very valuable, they also frequently have limitations. Decisions about regimens are made by committee. These decisions are often conservative and commitment to a radically new approach is difficult to achieve. Chemotherapy is often watered down and trials often fail to have a no-treatment arm because some of the participants deem it unethical.[92] It is difficult to standardize the application of surgery, radiotherapy, or chemotherapy in multi-institution trials, it is difficult to uniformly utilize the most sensitive diagnostic procedures, and it is difficult to study complex treatments such as bone marrow transplantation. Ensuring data quality is also a difficult task for such studies.

The elimination of moderate sized innovative clinical trials conducted by one or a few cooperating major research centers would eliminate much of the possibility of real breakthrough as well as the false positive claims. Such studies generally need substantiation, however, on a larger scale. There are so few effective therapies, that failure to examine promising intensive treatments may be more troublesome than false positives. Staquet[91] and others are correct in pointing out that the proportion of false positive claims in the literature is probably much greater than 5 percent. But for developing improved treatments, it is probably better to encourage innovative clinical research with cautious reporting of results and requiring confirmation of apparently positive findings in large studies. For many studies it is clear at the outset that a large number of patients is necessary. Single institutions with inadequate accrual do a disservice by initiating such trials, for misleading results are likely.

DATA MANAGEMENT

Data management is a very important part of the conduct of a clinical trial, particularly for multi-institution studies. Obtaining reliable data requires the same planning and professional expertise as the other aspects of the study. Some general guidelines for data management follow, though these are not applicable to all situations.

1. Data forms should be as simple and unambiguous as possible.
2. Collect relatively extensive initial information about patients, but severely limit follow-up information to the major endpoints and acute complications.
3. Details of treatment administration should continuously go to the study chairman or modality coordinator so that errors and misinterpretations can be quickly corrected for future patients. This detailed data should generally not be computerized.
4. Forms should be filled out only by fully qualified individuals. Uniformity of subjective evaluations should be ensured.
5. Epidemiologic, psycho-social, and optional laboratory data should not be included for addressing peripherally related questions. These should be viewed as independent studies to be critically reviewed and requiring additional resource allocation.
6. Whenever possible use an existing computerized data management system rather than hiring programmers to start from scratch.
7. Treat data management seriously and resolve problems quickly.

Generally, physicians are tempted to design more elaborate data collection than is really useful. This results in unnecessary complexity in the conduct of the study, increased effort on the part of all involved in data collection, and reduced reliability of the most important data elements. For multi-

FIG. 10-2. Osteosarcoma study registration form (for all new osteosarcoma patients admitted).

Patient Name ______________________________ Institution |__| Hospital Number |__|__|__|__|__|__|__|__|

1. Sex ....(M/F) .... |__| 2. Age at diagnosis .... |__|__|
3. Date of first symptoms .... (MM-YY) .... |__|__|—|__|__|
4. Date of diagnostic biopsy .... (MM-DD-YY) .... |__|__|—|__|__|—|__|__|
5. Primary site .... (see code list) .... |__|__|
6. Primary size by x-ray .... (cm X cm) .... |__|__|__| X |__|__|__|
7. Date of surgery for primary .... (MM-DD-YY) .... |__|__|—|__|__|—|__|__|
   Type of surgery .... (see code list) .... |__|__|
   Margins .... (0= Negative 1= Positive) .... |__|
   Place of surgery .... (1= Referral institution 2= Before referral) .... |__|
8. Date first admitted .... (MM-DD-YY) .... |__|__|—|__|__|—|__|__|
9. Extra-surgical treatment prior to admission? .... (Y/N) .... |__|
10. Metastatic work-up at admission .... (0= Negative 1= Positive) .... |__|
   If postitive:
   Chest x-ray .... (0= Negative 1= Positive 2= Not done) .... |__|
   Lung tomograms .... (0= Negative 1= Positive 2= Not done) .... |__|
   CT scan .... (0= Negative 1= Positive 2= Not done) .... |__|
11. Is patient eligible for this study? .... (Y/N) .... |__|
   If NO, specify ______________________________

   ____
12. If eligible, is patient entered on this study? .... (Y/N) .... |__|
   If NO, describe: ______________________________

   ____

Patient Name ______________________________ Institution |__| Hospital Number |__|__|__|__|__|__|__|__|__|

If patient has not recurred, skip to Item 4.

1. Date of local recurrence .... (MM-DD-YY) .... |__|__|—|__|__|—|__|__|

2. Date metastases first diagnosed .... (MM-DD-YY) .... |__|__|—|__|__|—|__|__|

   Pulmonary metastases .... (Y/N) .... |__|

   Other metastases (specify ____________________) (Y/N) .... |__|

   For pulmonary metastases:

   Current chest x-rays* .... |__|

   Current lung tomograms* .... |__|

   Current CT scan* .... |__|

   *Codes: 0= Negative

   1= Unilateral single nodule

   2= Unilateral multiple nodules

   3= Unilateral, otherwise unknown

   4= Bilateral

   Was a thoracotomy performed? .... (Y/N) .... |__|

   If YES:

   Date .... (MM-DD-YY) .... |__|__|—|__|__|—|__|__|

   Number of lesions found .... (R) |__|__| .... (L) |__|__|

   Were all apparent lesions removed? .... (Y/N) .... |__|

3. Treatment of first recurrence:

   Describe treatment ____

   ____

   Date treatment began .... (MM-YY) .... |__|__|—|__|__|

   Response .... (1= CR 2= PR 3= No response) .... |__|

   If CR:

   Has patient recurred? .... (Y/N) .... |__|

   Date recurrence or

   last known NED .... (MM-YY) .... |__|__|—|__|__|

If patient has recurred, skip to Item 6.

4. If no recurrence or metastasis, date last known

   to be continuously NED .... (MM-DD-YY) .... |__|__|—|__|__|—|__|__|

5. Worst toxicity before recurrence: (see code list)

WBC .... |__|	Skin rash .... |__|
Platelets .... |__|	Cardiac .... |__|
Nausea/vomiting .... |__|	Renal .... |__|
Stomatitis .... |__|	Mucositis .... |__|
Sepsis .... |__|	Other .... |__|
If present, describe:	If present, describe:
______________________________	______________________________
______________________________	______________________________

6. Patient status .... |__|

1= Alive, NED	3= Alive, tumor status unknown
2= Alive, with tumor	4= Dead

7. Date of death or date last known alive .... (MM-YY) .... |__|__|—|__|__|

If dead:

Tumor status at death .... |__|

1= NED with autopsy	3= Macroscopic tumor present
2= NED, no autopsy	4= Only microscopic tumor present

Primary cause of death .... |__|

1= Osteosarcoma	3= Infection
2= Treatment (describe) ________________	4= Other
______________________________)	5= Unknown

FIG. 10-3. Osteosarcoma study follow-up information (for all patients entered into study).

institution studies data management can be very complex, expensive, and time consuming. The development of good forms and procedures should occupy a prominent role in the planning process. If it is not treated with due respect by the trial organizers or adequately supported, the consequences are severe. Wright and Haybittle[93] have described specific considerations for the design of data forms.

Figures 10-2 through 10-4 show an example of data collection forms for a multi-institution clinical trial of primary osteosarcoma. These forms are supplemented by a code sheet, the operative report, flow sheets, and pathology slides. The registration form is filled in at the participating institution and sent to the statistical center. The information is computer-stored there and the computer prints a mirror image copy of the completed form to be returned to the institution in case later corrections must be made. The pathology reference center form is routed from the institution to the reference center with slides and then to the statistical center. The follow-up form is updated every six months by the participating institution and sent to the statistical center. The statistical center updates their computer files and returns a mirror image of the form for the next six-month update. The surgical coordinator receives operative reports, and the study chairman receives flow sheets from the participating institutions.

ETHICS

INFORMED CONSENT

The basic principle of a clinical trial is to give patients the best known treatment in a pre-planned manner that permits reliable conclusions to be drawn that can benefit future patients. Medical experiments have been performed by the Nazis and others that were clearly not in the interest of the human subjects. The United States and some other countries

Patient Name ________________________________ Institution |__| Hospital Number |__|__|__|__|__|__|__|__|

1. Date of biopsy .... (MM-DD-YY) .... |__|__|—|__|__|—|__|__|
2. Site of biopsy .... (see code list) .... |__|
3. Age at biopsy .... |__|__|
4. Date slides sent .... (MM-DD-YY) .... |__|__|—|__|__|—|__|__|
5. Histologic diagnosis .... |__|

   1= Osteosarcoma   2= Other   3= Indeterminate

   If not osteosarcoma, specify: ________________________________

6. Primary subtype .... |__|

   1= Osteoblastic   3= Fibroblastic   5= Anaplastic

   2= Chondroblastic   4= Telangiectatic   6= Well differentiated

   7= Not classifiable

7. Grade .... (1/2/3/4) .... |__|

TO BE COMPLETED BY STATISTICAL CENTER:

8. Randomized treatment .... (1= Surgery alone 2= Surgery+ chemo 9= None) ..... |__|
9. Date of randomization .... (MM-DD-YY) .... |__|__|—|__|__|—|__|__|

FIG. 10-4. Osteosarcoma study pathology reference center report.

have adopted the view that treating a patient as part of a clinical trial implies that the physician may have an interest in conflict with offering the best available therapy. Regulations and laws have dealt with this potential conflict of interest by requiring that the patient be told that he or she is part of a research study, that the patient be informed of all reasonable possible treatments and their potential side effects, and that the patient agree in writing to be treated according to the study protocol.

Informed consent is required today in the United States for clinical trials. Some physicians feel that the process may be detrimental to the mental health of patients who do not want to know all of the potential, though perhaps unlikely, complications of therapy. For randomized studies informed consent is generally sought before the randomization is performed. Consequently, the patient must agree to accept any of the treatments being compared. This makes clear to the patient that the physician does not reliably know which treatment is best. This may be embarrassing to the physician and unsettling to the patient. However, for best reliability of conclusions drawn from a randomized study, the randomization should occur after the patient agrees to receive any of the treatments; otherwise the informed consent process may serve to unconsciously select patients for one treatment or another based on his or her prognosis. For example, some relatively poor prognosis patients may refuse to participate in a surgical adjuvant study unless they know ahead of time that they will be in the chemotherapy group.

Zelen[94] proposed a design in which patients are randomly assigned either the standard or experimental treatment before consent is sought. Then, only patients in the experimental group are informed that they have been randomly selected and their consent sought for participation in the study to receive the experimental treatment. Those who refuse and ask for the standard therapy are so treated, but for purposes of statistical analysis are still included as part of the experimental treatment group. By analyzing the patients based on their randomized treatment assignment, this design avoids the selection bias mentioned above. If many patients randomized to the experimental therapy refuse that treatment, the design is obviously not effective. The fact that those patients randomized to receive the standard treatment are not told that they have been so randomized or that they are participants in a clinical trial has been controversial.[95,96]

Some clinical trials use pre-randomization, but then seek informed consent of all patients regardless of the results of the randomization. Though it is generally felt that the fact that randomization was employed should be described to the patient, the patient is consenting to receive a specific therapy, not one of several possibilities. If potential bias is to be avoided, all patients should be analyzed as part of the group to which they were randomized, regardless of whether they refused to consent to that treatment. Again, if there are many refusals, then the design is ineffective and the study compromised.

Some groups have found the second type of pre-randomization described above very beneficial. For many physicians, however, the conventional method of seeking informed consent, before randomization, does not pose a problem. Even for comparisons of treatments as different as amputation versus local resection, many physicians have found that patients can accept the honest presentation of lack of knowledge on the part of their physician.

It has been pointed out by many people that "informed consent" is not really informed because most patients have neither the educational background nor the psychological composure to be truly informed. Research is being conducted on ways of more effectively informing patients. Some individuals, however, believe that the process of informed consent is "a legalistic trick to devolve what should properly be the doctor's responsibility onto the patient."[11] It is likely that most abuses of good medical treatment today occur outside of clinical trials.

ACCUMULATING INFORMATION

Many individuals have struggled with the following question: Though it may be ethical to initiate a randomized clinical trial, doesn't the accumulation of interim results favoring one treatment make it unethical for a physician to continue entering patients? If the rate of patient entry is rapid compared to the time required to observe the major endpoints (*e.g.*, survival or duration of remission), then this problem does not arise. A strong impetus for the development of sequential analysis methods has been to enable a reliable conclusion to be reached as early as possible for trials with slower accrual. Statistical methods of sequential analysis are not in themselves, however, substitutes for the human monitoring of interim results. Chalmers and others[97] have suggested that the decision of when a trial should stop should be in the hands of a small monitoring committee, containing individuals who are not themselves entering patients into the study. The physicians entering patients would not see interim results and hence, in a multi-institution study, their opinions about the relative value of the treatments would remain essentially unchanged. Though the concept of "ethical behavior" inherent in this plan seems controversial, it is likely that the patients in general would in fact benefit. Clinical trials would not be prematurely terminated or accrual reduced when results remain questionable causing ambiguity to persist or new trials of the same treatments to be required. This approach is widely used in fields other than oncology.

The focus on ethical problems of accumulating information in randomized clinical trials derives to some extent from an oversimplified view of such studies. Most major trials are complex, requiring long term follow-up for evaluation of survival and complications and warranting subset analyses to determine which treatment is best for which patients. It is often difficult to thoroughly evaluate the treatments after adequate follow-up and to interpret the results in the context of other studies. This type of reliable evaluation is usually impossible during accrual with limited follow-up on limited numbers of patients. In addition, few randomized studies result in treatments that differ so greatly in efficacy and with such slow accrual as to require early termination.

ANALYSIS

There are good treatises on the technical aspects of statistical analysis,[10,98–104] and in the Appendix to this chapter some of the most commonly used methods are described. In this section we shall address several general aspects of analysis which are important for interpreting your own results and those of others.

SIGNIFICANCE LEVELS AND HYPOTHESIS TESTS

Medical decision making is complicated, and clinicians frequently misinterpret statistical significance tests in search of clearcut answers from ambiguous data. A statistical significance test for comparing outcomes of two treatment groups is performed in the following way. We define a test statistic, say difference in response rates, and then calculate the probability of getting a difference as large as that actually obtained if the treatments are actually of equal efficacy and differences occur merely by chance. That probability is called the significance level. If we calculate the probability of getting a difference in either direction as large in absolute value as the one we actually obtained, then the significance level is called two-sided. If the probability is calculated only for differences in the same direction as that actually obtained, then the significance level is called one-sided. Generally the two-sided significance level is twice the one-sided level.

After significance tests were used for many years, J. Neyman and E. S. Pearson[105] formalized a mathematical theory of "hypothesis testing." In this theory, before conducting the study you rigidly specify a null statistical hypothesis, an alternative statistical hypothesis, and a decision rule for accepting one hypothesis and rejecting the other, based upon the data obtained. The fraction of the time that the null hypothesis will be rejected in hypothetical repetitions of the experiment when it is in fact true is called the type 1 error. Similarly, the type 2 error is the fraction of the time that the alternative hypothesis would be rejected when it is true. The study involves collecting the data, applying the decision rule, and announcing whether you accept or reject the null hypothesis. This theory had great appeal to mathematical statisticians, because its tight structure opened up fields of statistical research devoted to finding decision rules having minimum type 2 errors for a given type 1 error and specified probability distribution.

This hypothesis testing framework has dominated introductory statistical courses, in large part because academic statisticians liked its mathematical niceties. The theory also appealed to clinicians because it simplified complex medical decision-making by providing yes or no answers; either the difference is "statistically significant" or it is not, period. With this theory the value of 0.05 for type 1 error has become very special. The distinction between one-sided and two-sided decision rules becomes crucial because a one-sided $p = 0.05$ is simply "non-significant" if a type 1 error of 0.05 based upon a two-sided decision rule is pre-specified (the two-sided $p = 0.10$). Within this theory the interpretation of results depends critically upon what was written in the experimental plan, because the specific statistical hypotheses, type 1 and 2 errors, monitoring plan, and decision rules must be pre-specified. Consideration of hypotheses suggested by the data is strictly forbidden in this framework.

It is ironic that so many physicians accept the theory of hypothesis testing as the ultimate model of a "scientific" study while it has been questioned by so many prominent statisticians as a basis for inference in research.[82,89,106–111] Sir Ronald Fisher, a pioneer of modern statistics, dismissed this approach as being applicable only to routine assembly line testing.

> Neyman, thinking that he was correcting and improving my own early work on tests of significance, as a means to the "improvement of natural knowledge," in fact reinterpreted them . . . as an acceptance procedure . . . I am casting no contempt on acceptance procedures . . . but the logical differences between such an operation and the work of scientific discovery . . . seem to me so wide that the analogy between them is not helpful, and the identification of the two sorts of operations is decidedly misleading . . . the conclusions drawn by a scientific worker from a test of significance are provisional and involve an intelligent attempt to understand the experimental situation . . . We have the duty of formulating, of summarising, and of communicating our conclusions, in intelligible form, in recognition of the right of other free minds to utilize them in making their own decisions.[106]

Other prominent statisticians have expressed similar views. Anscombe says of this approach:

> The concept of error probabilities of the first and second kinds . . . has no direct relevance to experimentation. The formation of opinions, decisions concerning further experimentation and other required actions, are not dictated in a simple prearranged way by the formal analysis of the experiment, but call for judgment and imagination . . . Sequential rules are simultaneously two things, stopping rules and decision rules . . . When the experiment has been completed, the number of observations taken is an unalterable fact. The verdict, on the other hand, is no better than an opinion of the experimenter, and if anyone considers it to be a mistaken opinion he can form a different opinion of his own . . . the primary aim of the statistical analysis of the experiment should be to present as clearly and accurately as possible the evidence concerning relative effectiveness . . .[108]

Cox and Hinkley comment:

> An approach to the analysis of data that confines us to questions and a model laid down in advance would be seriously inhibiting . . . The relation of the decision problem with significance testing is no more than a crude resemblance.[111]

Greenhouse comments:

> . . . the classical precepts of the specification of the two possible types of error and their relationship to the determination of sample size should serve as a guide . . . in the planning stage of the study . . . But, it should not bind the investigator or the statistician in the analysis of the data . . .[89]

It is not the intention here to imply that one should adopt an "anything goes" attitude in the analysis of data. But the hypothesis testing framework is not entirely satisfactory and should not be viewed as a rigid prescription for good science. Significance levels play a prominent role in the reporting of clinical trial results, but they often cannot be interpreted as type 1 errors. Determination of type 1 error is virtually impossible unless a rigid decision rule is used for monitoring interim results. Significance levels can serve as useful aids to interpretation of results, but quibbling about whether a one-sided $p = .04$ is "significant" makes little sense. Significance levels are influenced by sample sizes and failure to "reject the null hypothesis" does not mean that the outcomes are not different. In many cases the calculation of confidence intervals is more informative than significance levels. There is no simple index of truth for interpreting results. Many physicians attempt to use the notion of "statistical significance" in this way, but the attempt has an unsound basis. Thorough presentation, skeptical evaluation, and cautious interpretation of results are always required.

EXCLUSIONS

Excluding patients from analysis because of treatment deviations, early death, or patient withdrawal for other reasons may seriously bias the results.[10,11,19] Often, excluded patients have poorer outcomes than those not excluded. One can rationalize that patients not receiving treatment as specified in the protocol did worse because of that fact. But this is just a rationalization, which may be erroneous. The poor prognosis of these patients may have led directly or indirectly to their exclusion. There may be more potential exclusions in one treatment group or the reasons for potential exclusion may differ among treatments. Excluding patients (or "analyzing them separately," which is equivalent to excluding them) for reasons other than that they did not satisfy the eligibility criteria of the study is a major problem in interpreting many studies. If the conclusions of a study depend upon exclusions, then these conclusions are suspect. Eligibility criteria for both patients and collaborators should be established in such a way that there will be few protocol deviations. Generally the treatment plan should be viewed as a policy to be evaluated. This policy cannot be applied completely to all patients, but all patients should generally be evaluable in phase III studies.

PROGNOSTIC FACTORS AND MULTIPLE ANALYSES

The results of a clinical trial are often multifaceted and require analysis with regard to several endpoints. If there are major prognostic factors known beforehand, then it will frequently be desirable to incorporate these factors into the analysis either to correct for imbalances or to improve the precision of the estimates of treatment differences. Ignoring major prognostic factors in the analysis unnecessarily increases background patient variability, and obscures comparisons between the treatments.[112] The identification and careful utilization of major prognostic factors can considerably increase the sensitivity of clinical trials. For some major patient or tumor characteristics it may be desirable to evaluate the treatments separately by the determined subsets.

Multiple analyses can be carried too far, however, and result in erroneous conclusions caused by ransacking the data. The subsets and adjusting variables should preferably represent characteristics known to be of major prognostic importance before the analysis is begun. It is not necessary that these factors be included as stratification variables in randomized studies, but they should represent characteristics measurable at the time of patient entry to the protocol. It is generally not valid to subset or adjust the analysis by characteristics measured subsequent to the start of treatment (*e.g.*, treatment compliance). Analyses not restricted to the widely recognized endpoints and the few major prognostic factors known at the outset should be interpreted very cautiously.

As mentioned previously, it is often important to perform interim monitoring of results, even though interim results may be misleading and adversely affect the subsequent conduct of the study. In reporting the results of a study it is desirable to specify whether, when, and on what basis interim analyses were performed, to describe the nature of the interim analyses, and to specify how it was decided to terminate the trial. To some statisticians and clinicians, interpretation of results will be independent of these factors and based solely upon the data which should be clearly and thoroughly summarized. Some readers, however, may wish to revise their assessment of the results based upon such information, and adequate information should be presented to permit them to do this. For either type of reader, your conclusions and significance levels are no substitute for extensive data presentations and descriptions of the conduct of the trial.

APPENDIX: STATISTICAL METHODS

The proper analysis of clinical data often requires a greater degree of statistical knowledge than is recognized. It makes little sense to decrease the interpretability of an important study by using deficient methods of analysis. One should generally plan to have a statistical collaborator for the design and analysis of phase III studies. Nevertheless, many clinical studies are analyzed and reported without statistical collaboration. Consequently, some useful methods of analysis are presented in this appendix. These methods are applicable to common relatively simple situations, but more complex problems should not be forced into this framework.

ESTIMATION OF SURVIVAL FUNCTIONS

Representation of the distribution of survivals for a group of patients is a commonly encountered problem. The problem of representing the distribution of remission duration or time till disease progression is mathematically identical, though we will refer to survivals here. The usual elementary methods of plotting histograms or calculating means and medians are generally not applicable, because some patients will not have died at the time of analysis. Thus the data contains "censored" observations, in the sense that survivals are known only to be at least as great as the observed values for the living patients.

The most satisfactory way of representing such data is to estimate the survival function $S(t)$. This function represents the probability of surviving for at least t time units. Time t is measured from diagnosis, start of treatment or some other meaningful time point. For randomized studies it is best to measure time from the date of randomization. There are numerous *ad hoc* and deficient ways of estimating $S(t)$, but a generally satisfactory method of estimation for samples of small to moderate size will now be described.[113] This procedure is called the "product-limit" method of Kaplan and Meier.

Let $t_1, t_2, \ldots, t_n$ denote the distinct times of death in increasing order. Let $d_1, d_2, \ldots, d_n$ denote the number of deaths at each of these times. If survival is measured in days, then it is likely that no two patients die at the exact same time and so one will usually have all of the d's equal to 1. It is sometimes convenient, however, to measure survival in integral weeks or months, in which case there may be multiple patients with the same survival. Let a_1 denote the number of living patients with censored survivals less than t_1. Let a_2 denote the number of living patients with censored survivals at least as great as t_1 but less than t_2. In general, let a_i denote the number of living patients with censored survivals at least as great as t_{i-1}, but less than t_i. Let a_{n+1} denote the number of alive patients with censored survivals at least as great as t_n.

The non-parametric maximum likelihood estimator of $S(t_i)$ is calculated as follows:

$$\hat{S}(t_1) = (R_1 - d_i)/R_1$$
$$\hat{S}(t_i) = [(R_i - d_i)/R_i]\hat{S}(t_{i-1}), \qquad \text{for } i = 2, 3, \ldots, n$$

where

$$R_1 = N - a_1$$
$$R_i = R_{i-1} - d_{i-1} - a_i, \qquad \text{for } i = 2, 3, \ldots, n.$$

In these equations, R_i represents the number of patients at risk just before time t_i. The number at risk at the first time of death t_1 equals the total number of patients N minus the number of patients a_1 not yet followed for t_1. The number R_i at risk at any t_i equals the number R_{i-1} at risk just before the previous time of death (t_{i-1}), minus the number d_{i-1} that expired then minus the number a_i censored after t_{i-1} but before t_i. The estimated probability of surviving past t_1 equals the proportion of patients at risk just before t_1 who survive past that time. The estimated probability of surviving past any t_i ($i = 2, 3, \ldots, n$) equals the product of two factors. One factor is the estimated probability of surviving past t_{i-1} [$\hat{S}(t_{i-1})$]. The other factor is the proportion of patients at risk just before t_i who survive beyond that time.

Once $\hat{S}(t_1), \hat{S}(t_2), \ldots, \hat{S}(t_n)$ have been calculated, they may be graphed with time on the horizontal axis and the vertical axis taking values between 0 and 1. Unless $t_1 = 0$, the point $\hat{S}(0) = 1$ is included. The points $[t_i, \hat{S}(t_i)]$ should be joined by a step function in which the value at $\hat{S}(t_{i-1})$ is drawn horizontally to t_i where it drops to $\hat{S}(t_i)$.

As a numerical example, assume that the data consists of survivals 3, 3, 3^+, 5, 6, 8^+, 8^+, 10, 10, 12^+ where censored survivals are suffixed with a plus. In the previous notation, $N = 10$; $n = 4$; $t_1 = 3$, $t_2 = 5$, $t_3 = 6$, $t_4 = 10$; $d_1 = 2$, $d_2 = 1$, $d_3 = 1$, $d_4 = 2$; $a_1 = 0$, $a_2 = 1$, $a_3 = 0$, $a_4 = 2$, $a_5 = 1$. Using the equations given, one obtains $R_1 = 10$, $R_2 = 7$, $R_3 = 6$, $R_4 = 3$; $\hat{S}(3) = (10 - 2)/10 = 0.80$, $\hat{S}(5) = (7 - 1)(.80)/7 = 0.69$, $\hat{S}(6) = (6 - 1)(.69)/6 = 0.57$, $\hat{S}(10) = (3 - 2)(.57)/3 = 0.19$. The median survival is the value of t for which $S(t) = 0.50$. The plotted curve does have a point for which $\hat{S}(t) = 0.50$, but the median is often estimated by linear interpolation. Interpolating between 6 months and 10 months, the estimated median equals $6^+(.57 - .50)(10 - 6)/(.57 - 19) = 6.74$ months. Tic marks are placed on the graphed step function at 3, 8, and 12 months to represent the follow-up times of living patients. The step function is extended horizontally from $t_4 = 10$ months out to 12 months to represent follow-up of the last patient. The estimator

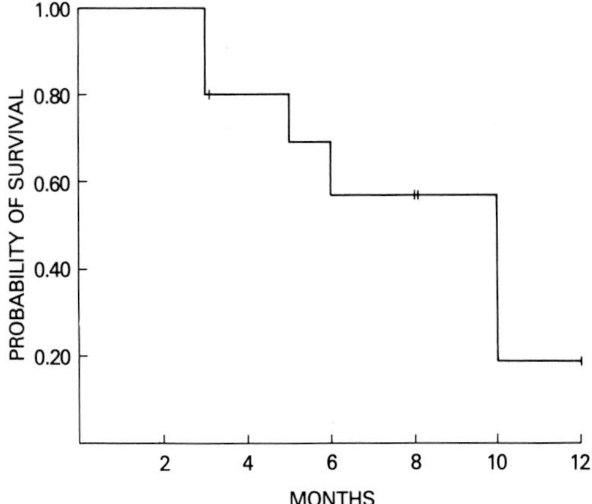

FIG. 10-5. Example of estimated survival distribution.

of the survival distribution is not determined beyond the largest observation. Figure 10-5 shows the estimated survival distribution.

For any time t, $\hat{S}(t)$ is an estimator of the true unknown value $S(t)$. This estimator is approximately normally distributed in large samples. If m patients remain alive at time t, then the standard error of $\hat{S}(t)$ can be conservatively estimated as $\hat{S}(t)\sqrt{[(1 - \hat{S}(t)]/m)}$.[10] Another commonly used estimator of the standard error is[113]

$$\hat{S}(t)\sqrt{\Sigma\, d_i/R_i(R_i - d_i)}$$

where the summation is taken over all times of death no later than t.

The life-table method described above can also be used for representing the distribution of remission duration or time till progression. As for survival analyses, censored observations result from the limited period of observation at the time of analysis or because patients are lost to follow-up when still in remission.

With censored survival data there are really only two valid general methods for estimating the probability of surviving beyond a specified time, say five years. One method is that described above. This can be modified for large samples by grouping deaths into, say, six month intervals, but the idea is the same. The second method is to disregard results for all patients who have not had a potential follow-up of five years. Their results are disregarded regardless of whether they are dead or alive. Of the remaining patients, the proportion who have survived five years is the absolute or crude estimate. This method is adequate for very large samples, but it does not give as precise estimates for smaller samples, as does the product-limit method described. In reporting a product-limit estimate of five-year survival derived from 100 patients, it is not accurate to say that "X percent of 100 patients survived five years." It is better to say "the estimated probability of surviving at least five years is X percent."

COMPARISON OF TWO SURVIVAL FUNCTIONS

A number of statistical significance tests have been developed for comparing sets of patients with regard to survival or remission duration with censored observations. As with all statistical significance tests, a finding of "no significant difference" with small sample sizes may contribute only confusion to the interpretation of the data, because of limited power of the test. This error is made both in therapeutic studies of small size, and in studies large enough to evaluate treatments, but too small to support the evaluation of prognostic factors.

For simplicity we will present here one method for comparing the survivals of two sets of patients. The method is the Mantel-Haenszel test.[102] Let $t_1, t_2, \ldots, t_n$ denote the distinct times of death for patients in both of the two groups being compared. Let r_{1i} and r_{2i} denote the number of living patients in the first and second groups respectively just before time t_i. The r's represent numbers of patients at risk. Let d_{1i} and d_{2i} denote the numbers of deaths in the two groups at t_i. The total number of observed deaths in the first group is thus

$$D = \sum_{i=1}^{n} d_{1i}. \quad (1)$$

If the survival distributions for the groups are the same, then the expected value of D is

$$E = \sum_{i=1}^{n} r_{1i}(d_{1i} + d_{2i})/(r_{1i} + r_{2i}). \quad (2)$$

Each term of this summation is the product of the total number of deaths $(d_{1i} + d_{2i})$ at t_i times the proportion of the patients at risk who are in the first group. Under the null hypothesis of no difference in the survival distributions, the variance of D is

$$V = \sum_{i=1}^{n} (d_{1i} + d_{2i})(r_{1i} + r_{2i} - d_{1i} - d_{2i})r_{1i}r_{2i}/[(r_{1i} + r_{2i})^2(r_{1i} + r_{2i} - 1)]. \quad (3)$$

A significance test can be performed by calculating $z = |D - E|/\sqrt{V}$ and referring to tables of the standard normal distribution. If z is greater than 1.96, then the difference is significant at a two-sided level of less than 0.05.

This test is easily modified to account for an important prognostic factor. One may wish to do this because of an imbalance in the groups being compared with regard to this factor. It is important to recognize that the fact that an imbalance is not "statistically significant" does not mean it is not distorting the survival comparison; lack of "statistical significance" merely means that the imbalance may have arisen by chance. One may also wish to incorporate into the analysis an important prognostic factor for which there is no imbalance. One sometimes obtains a more powerful survival comparison by accounting in this way for known sources of variability. To incorporate such information one subdivides each of the two treatment groups into distinct strata determined by the prognostic factors. Considering each stratum *entirely separately* one calculates D_j, E_j, and V_j for group one, in which the subscript j is used here to denote stratum. One then calculates $D = \Sigma D_j$, $E = \Sigma E_j$, $V = \Sigma V_j$, summing over the strata, and performs the test $z = |D - E|/\sqrt{V}$ as before.[104] Only a few strata can be accommodated in this type of analysis unless there are many patients. The resulting test is an overall comparison of the two groups adjusted for the influences of the prognostic factors.

There are a number of ways in which significance tests described here are commonly misused. If there are more than two groups to be compared, an overall test comparing all groups simultaneously should be employed before contrasting all pairs. It is also not valid to compare various subsets of one treatment group to another without first demonstrating that the relative treatment efficacy varies among the subsets. These more complex analyses require more sophisticated methods.[114]

To illustrate the use of the Mantel-Haenszel test, consider the following survival data in months.

	Treatment 1	Treatment 2
Grade 1–2	12,13,14,15,16$^+$	9,10,11,12,13$^+$
Grade 3–4	6,8,9,10,11$^+$	1,3,4,7,8$^+$

Table 10-9 illustrates the calculations for performing the Mantel-Haenszel test to compare survivals between the two treatment groups pooled over grade. The columns labeled $E(d_{1i})$ and $V(d_{1i})$ represent the terms of the summations in equations (2) and (3) respectively. For treatment 1, $D = 8$, $E = 10.731$, and $V = 3.047$. This results in $z = |8 - 10.731|/\sqrt{3.047} = 1.564$, corresponding to a two-sided significance level of 0.12. Table 10-10 shows the calculations for grade 1 to 2 patients alone. For treatment 1, $D = 4$, $E = 5.909$, and $V = 1.231$. This results in $z = 1.720$, corresponding to a two-sided significance level of 0.085. If the calculations are performed for grade 3 to 4 patients alone, one again obtains for treatment group 1 $D = 4$, $E = 5.909$, and $V = 1.231$. Hence the Mantel-Haenszel test comparing treatments adjusted for grade gives $D = 8$, $E = 11.818$, $V = 2.462$, and $z = 2.433$, corresponding to a two-sided significance level of 0.015. For this example, even though there is no imbalance between the treatments with regard to grade, the adjusted test is much more powerful than the pooled test. Pooling implies ignoring an important known source of variability and considering it due to unknown causes. Adjustment for an unimportant variable, however, can result in a test of decreased power. Adjustment should never be made with regard to variables observed after the start of treatment such as dose received, toxicity experienced, or protocol violations. Such characteristics should be viewed as part of the outcome rather than a cause of the outcome.

COMPARISON OF PROPORTIONS

Many investigators are familiar with the contingency chi-square test for comparing two proportions; where one treatment group has d_1 responses in r_1 patients and the other has d_2 responses in r_2 patients. The test is based on the null hypothesis that the number of responses in the first group can be viewed as a random selection of r_1 items from an urn containing $r_1 + r_2$ items in which $d_1 + d_2$ are labeled response. If the numbers are adequately large, then $X^2 = (|d_1 - E| - 0.5)^2/V$ is well approximated by the chi-square distribution with one degree of freedom in which

$$E = r_1(d_1 + d_2)/(r_1 + r_2)$$

$$V = r_1r_2(d_1 + d_2)(r_1 + r_2 - d_1 - d_2)/(r_1 + r_2)^2(r_1 + r_2 - 1).$$

The usual chi-square test has $(r_1 + r_2)^3$ in the denominator of V instead of $(r_1 + r_2)^2(r_1 + r_2 - 1)$. The results will generally be similar. An exact test of the null hypothesis which does not use the chi-square approximation is called the Fisher-Irwin exact test. When r_1 and r_2 are both less than 50, tables for the exact one-sided significance levels are available.[115] It is difficult to give general guidelines for how large the sample sizes must be for the chi-square approximation to be adequate. If $r_iA \geqq 5$ and $m_i(1 - A) \geqq 5$ for each treatment $i = 1$ and 2, where $A = (d_1 + d_2)/(r_1 + r_2)$, then there should be no problem. Use of the exact Fisher-Irwin test, doubling the tabulated significance values if two-sided levels are desired, is always the safest procedure. The 0.5 term in the above expression for X^2 is called the continuity correction. Statisticians are divided on when it would be used. This author believes that it would always be included in the chi-square test for comparing two proportions unadjusted for other variables.

An implicit assumption of these tests is that all observations are independent. That is, if the same patient is represented multiple times in the sample then the tests are not appropriate. As an extreme

TABLE 10-9. Calculations for Pooled Survival Comparison

	TREATMENT 1		TREATMENT 2			
t_i	r_{1i}	d_{1i}	r_{2i}	d_{2i}	$E(d_{1i})$	$V(d_{1i})$
1	10	0	10	1	10/20	$10^2/20^2$
3	10	0	9	1	10/19	$10\times 9/19^2$
4	10	0	8	1	10/18	$10\times 8/18^2$
6	10	1	7	0	10/17	$10\times 7/17^2$
7	9	0	7	1	9/16	$9\times 7/16^2$
8	9	1	6	0	9/15	$9\times 6/15^2$
9	8	1	5	1	$(8/13)\times 2$	$2\times 11\times 8\times 5/13^2\times 12$
10	7	1	4	1	$(7/11)\times 2$	$2\times 9\times 7\times 4/11^2\times 10$
11	6	0	3	1	6/9	$6\times 3/9^2$
12	5	1	2	1	$(5/7)\times 2$	$2\times 5\times 5\times 2/7^2\times 6$
13	4	1	1	0	(4/5)	$4\times 1/5^2$
14	3	1	0	0	3/3	0
15	2	1	0	0	2/2	0
		D = 8			E = 10.731	V = 3.047

TABLE 10-10. Calculations for Survival Comparison of Grade 1–2 Patients

	TREATMENT 1		TREATMENT 2			
t_i	r_{1i}	d_{1i}	r_{2i}	d_{2i}	$E(d_{1i})$	$V(d_{1i})$
9	5	0	5	1	5/10	$5\times 5/10^2$
10	5	0	4	1	5/9	$5\times 4/9^2$
11	5	0	3	1	5/8	$5\times 3/8^2$
12	5	1	2	1	$(5/7)\times 2$	$(2)(5)(5)(2)/7^2\times 6$
13	4	1	1	0	4/5	$4\times 1/5^2$
14	3	1	0	0	3/3	0
15	2	1	0	0	2/2	0
		D = 4			E = 5.909	V = 1.231

hypothetical example, consider the case where one patient experiences leukopenia on each of six cycles of drug A where a second patient experiences no leukopenia on each of six cycles of drug B. Based on only this data we cannot derive any conclusions about drug A versus drug B (even though 6/6 versus 0/6 is a "statistically significant" difference) because our sample size for estimating the proportion of patients who experience leukopenia is only one for each drug.

As for comparing survival curves, it may be of interest to compare the response rates of two groups after adjusting for other factors. The Mantel-Haenszel test can be used for this. Let d_{1i} and d_{2i} denote the number of responders for the two groups in stratum i, and let r_{1i} and r_{2i} denote the number of patients for the two groups in stratum i. Then equations (1), (2), and (3) are used to calculate D, E, and V and the overall adjusted test is $z = |D - E|/\sqrt{V}$, which has a standard normal distribution under the null hypothesis. Comparisons among more than two groups, tests that the relative response rates between groups differ among subsets, and comparisons with paired data require other methods.[100,116]

Paired data with binary outcomes may arise in several ways. For example, by selecting one historical control paired to each new patient in which matching is done with regard to characteristics of potential importance. The simple chi-square test or Fisher-Irwin test ignores pairing and is not truly appropriate to the data. An exact analysis can be performed in the following way. Let u denote the number of pairs in which exactly one patient responds, and let u_1 denote the number of those u pairs in which the responder received treatment 1. Then, under the null hypothesis of no difference in efficacy between the two treatments, u_1 has a binomial distribution with parameters 0.5 and u. Exact binomial tables (see Beyer, p. 195[117]) can be used to determine the significance level. For large u, u_1 is approximately normally distributed with mean $u/2$ and variance $u/4$. Thus $z = (\left|u_1 - \mu/2\right| - 0.5)/\sqrt{u/4}$ can be looked up in standard normal distribution tables to determine the approximate significance level. This normal approximation is (except for continuity correction) equivalent to using the Mantel-Haenszel test as described above in which each pair constitutes a stratum. As for all adjustment procedures, pairing is only beneficial to power if the pairing variables have important effects on prognosis. Pairing does ensure, however, that the treatment groups are "comparable" with regard to the pairing variables.

Paired data can also arise from crossover trials in which each patient receives both treatments under study. Such experiments require special methods of analysis, however, because there may be time effects and order effects.

COMPARISON OF TWO DISTRIBUTIONS OF ORDERED RESPONSE

The final topic to be considered is the comparison of two groups of patients with regard to some uncensored quantitative or semi-quantitative outcome. For example, the outcome may be nadir platelet count which is fully numerical. Alternatively, the outcome may be objective tumor response, in which the values complete response, partial response, no change, and progressive disease are only ordered. The significance tests presented here are rank tests. In some cases, tests based upon normal distributions, such as Student's t test, could be used, but such methods are often inappropriately applied. The validity of the t test depends upon assumptions such as equality of variance and either normal distributions or large sample sizes, assumptions which users often fail to examine. The rank tests are valid in broader circumstances, and generally are of almost equivalent power.

Applying some of the formulae given here with an outcome such as objective tumor response requires one to assign numerical scores to the degrees of response; such as progressive disease = 0, no change = 1, partial response = 2, and complete response = 3. The tests are, however, independent of these numerical values and depend only on the ordering of the response levels. Assume that group 1 consists of m observations from a distribution F and that group 2 consists of n observations from a distribution G. The assumptions are that the observations are independent (*e.g.*, no patients are represented more than once in the total sample of $m + n$). The null hypothesis is that $F = G$.

The test is performed in the following way. Rank the combined data in ascending order from 1 to $m + n$, ignoring which observation came from which group. If two or more observations are tied, assign them each the average of the ranks involved (called the midrank). For example, if two observations are tied for sixth and seventh smallest, assign them each rank 6.5 and give the next largest observation rank 8. If three observations are tied for sixth, seventh and eighth smallest, assign them each rank 7 and give the next largest observation rank 9. After doing this combined ranking, calculate T, the sum of the ranks of the group with fewer observations (group 1 if m is less than or equal to n). The calculated value T, together with the sample sizes m and n are then referred to published tables for the Wilcoxon two-sample rank sum test (Beyer, p. 409[117]). From such tables one can determine whether the total T is outside of the range of variation expected, say 95 percent of the time, with samples of size m and n. These exact tables are accurate if there are not many ties. This will be the case for a fully quantitative variable.

If the sample sizes are large (at least 20 in each group), then the calculations can be simplified even if there are many ties. Let T denote the sum of the ranks (or midranks) for group 1 consisting of m observations. The second group consists of n observations. For the normal approximation it does not matter whether m or n is larger. The distribution of T can be approximated by a normal distribution with mean $E = m(N + 1)/2$ and variance

$$V = mn(N + 1)/12 - mn \sum (d_i^3 - d_i)/12N(N - 1).$$

In this formula for the variance, $N = m + n$, and d_i represents the number of observations tied for the ith smallest distinct value. For example, if no observations are tied for the smallest value, $d_1 = 1$; if four observations are tied for the third smallest distinct value, $d_3 = 4$. In determining the number of ties, observations in both groups are included. The summation is taken over all distinct values. The significance level of the difference between the two groups can be assessed by calculating $z = (|T - E| - 0.5)/\sqrt{V}$ and referring to tables for the standard normal distribution. For example, values of z greater than 1.96 imply a two-sided significance level of less than 0.05.

To illustrate this method consider the following data which might represent the numbers of days per patient with leukopenia less than 1000 cells/cc for two treatment regimens.

Treatment 1: 0, 0, 0, 0   1 2 4 5 6
Treatment 2: 0   4   6, 6   12   13, 13   14, 14   20

This data is written in a way that permits easy visual ranking. There are nine observations on treatment 1 and ten observations on treatment 2. Thus, $m = 9$, $n = 10$, $N = 19$. The ranks for treatment 1 are 3, 3, 3, 3, 6, 7, 8.5, 10, 12. Thus $T = 55.5$. Table X.5 of Beyer[117] indicates that the approximate two-sided significance level is less than 0.01. For the normal approximation, $E = 9 \times 20/2 = 90$. $d_1 = 5$, $d_4 = 2$, $d_6 = 3$ and all other $d_i = 1$. Thus

$$V = 9 \times 10 \times 20/12 - (9 \times 10/12 \times 19 \times 18)(120 + 6 + 24) = 146.71$$

and $z = (|55.5 - 90| - 0.5)/\sqrt{146.71} = 2.81$. Using the standard normal distribution tables, this corresponds to an approximate two-sided significance level of 0.005.

Though the rank test given here is valid for testing whether the underlying distributions F and G are equal, regardless of their form, the test is most powerful for detecting alternatives where one distribution is a displacement of the other. The test does not assume that the variability in the two groups are equal, as does Student's t test, but does assume that within each group all observations are measured with the same precision. If a data value is the average of k_i observations for patient i, and the k's vary considerably, then this assumption is violated. For such situations, for situations in which more than two groups are being compared, or where the data is paired, other methods are required. A good reference for such problems is Lehmann.[101]

If the sample sizes are adequate, the Wilcoxon rank-sum test described here is easily generalized for comparing two treatments adjusted for prognostic factors. Suppose that we have several distinct strata determined by prognostic variables. Analyze each stratum entirely separately, that is, ignore patients from other strata in calculating T_i, E_i and V_i as described above for each stratum i. T_i should represent the sum of the ranks for treatment group 1 among patients in stratum i. Do not renumber the treatments in going from stratum to stratum. Then one accepted adjusted test is performed by calculating[101]

$$T = \Sigma\, T_i/(N_i + 1)$$

$$E = \Sigma\, E_i/(N_i + 1)$$

$$V = \Sigma\, V_i/(N_i + 1)^2$$

where N_i is the total number of patients in stratum i. One then calculates $z = |T - E|/\sqrt{V}$ and obtains the approximate significance level from tables of the standard normal distribution.

REFERENCES

1. Bull JP: The historical development of clinical therapeutic trials. J Chron Dis 10:218–248, 1959
2. Doll R, Hill AE: A study of the aetiology of carcinoma of the lung. Brit Med J 2:1271–1286, 1952
3. MacMahon B, Pugh TF: Epidemiology: Principles and Methods. Boston, Little, Brown & Co, 1970
4. Starmer CF, Rosati RA, McNeer JF: Data bank use in the management of chronic disease. Comput Biomed Res 7:111–116, 1974
5. McShane DJ, Porta J, Fries JF: Comparison of therapy in severe systemic lupus erythematosus employing stratification techniques. J Rheumatol 5:51–58, 1978
6. Cochran WG: The planning of observational studies of human populations. JR Stat Soc A 128:234–250, 1965
7. Byar DP: Why data bases should not replace randomized clinical trials. Biometrics 36:337–342, 1980
8. Dambrosia JM, Ellenberg JH: Statistical considerations for a medical data base. Biometrics 36:323–332, 1980
9. Tukey JW: Some thoughts on clinical trials, especially problems of multiplicity. Science 198:679–684, 1977
10. Peto R, Pike MC, Armitage P et al: Design and analysis of randomized clinical trials requiring prolonged observation of each patient. 1. Introduction and Design. Br J Cancer 34:585–612, 1976; 2. Analysis and Examples. Br J Cancer 35:1–39, 1977
11. Peto R: Clinical trial methodology. Biomedicine 28: 24–36, 1978
12. Hill AB: The clinical trial. Br Med Bull 7:278–282, 1951
13. Moertel CG, and Reitmeier RG: Advanced Gastrointestinal Cancer: Clinical Management and Chemotherapy. New York, Harper & Row, 1969
14. Schneiderman M: Non-objective art and objective evaluation in cancer chemotherapy. In Brodsky I, Kahn SB, Moyer JH (eds): Cancer Chemotherapy pp 67–76. New York, Grune & Stratton, 1969
15. Schneiderman MA: The clinical excursion into 5-flurouracil. Cancer Chemother Rep 16:107–118, 1962
16. Moertel CG, Hanley JA: The effect of measuring error on the results of therapeutic trials in advanced cancer. Cancer 38:388–394, 1976
17. Gurland J, Johnson RO: How reliable are tumor measurements? J Am Med Assoc 29:973–978, 1965
18. Carter SK, Selawry O, Slavik M: Phase I clinical trials. In Saunders JP, and Carter SK (eds): Methods of Development of New Anticancer Drugs, pp 75–80. Natl Cancer Inst Monogr 45, US Dept Health, Educ, Welfare, Bethesda, 1977
19. Williams DJ, Carter SK: Management of trials in the development of cancer chemotherapy. Br J Cancer 37:434–447, 1978
20. Woolley PV, Schein PS: Clinical pharmacology and phase I trial design. In DeVita VT, Jr, Busch H (eds): Methods in Cancer Research, vol. XVII, Cancer Drug Development Part B, pp 177–198. New York, Academic Press, 1979
21. Freireich EJ, Gehan EA, Rall DP et al: Quantitative comparison of toxicity of anticancer agents in mouse, rat, hamster, dog, monkey, and man. Cancer Chemother Rep 50:219–244, 1966
22. Shein PS, David RD, Carter S et al: The evaluation of anticancer drugs in dogs and monkeys for the prediction of qualitative toxicities in man. Clin Pharmacol Ther 11:3–40, 1970
23. Homan ER: Quantitative relationships between toxic doses of antitumor chemotherapeutic agents in animals and man. Cancer Chemother Rep. 3:13–19, 1972
24. Shein PS: The prediction of clinical toxicities of anticancer drugs. In the Pharmacologic Basis of Cancer Chemotherapy, pp 383–399. Baltimore, Williams & Wilkins, 1975
25. Guarino AM: Pharmacologic and toxicologic studies of anticancer drugs: of sharks, mice, and men (and dogs and monkeys). In DeVita VT, Jr, Busch H (eds): Methods in Cancer Research, vol. XVII, Cancer Drug Development Part B, pp 91–174. New York, Academic Press, 1979
26. Schneiderman MA: Mouse to man: statistical problems in bringing a drug to clinical trial. In Proc Fifth Berkeley Symp Math Statis Prob, Univ. of California 4:855–866. Berkeley, University of California Press, 1967
27. Hansen H, Selawry OS, Muggia FM et al: Clinical studies with 1-(2-chloroethyl)-3-cyclohexyl-1-nitrosourea (NSC 79037). Cancer Res 31:223–227, 1971
28. Goldsmith MA, Slavik M, Carter SK: Quantitative prediction of drug toxicity in humans from toxicity in small and large animals. Cancer Res 35:1354–1364, 1975
29. Louis J: Coordinated phase I studies for cooperative chemotherapy groups. Cancer Chemother Rep. 16: 99–105, 1962
30. Gottlieb JA: Phase I and II clinical trials: a critical reappraisal. In The Pharmacological Basis of Cancer Chemotherapy, pp 485–498. Baltimore, Williams and Wilkins, 1974
31. Carbone PP, Krant MJ, Miller SP, et al. The feasibility of using randomization schemes early in the clinical trials of new chemotherapeutic agents: Hydroxyurea. Clin Pharmacol Ther 6:17–24, 1965
32. DeVita VT, Carbone PP, Owens AH et al: Clinical trials with 1,3-bis(2-chloroethyl)-1-nitrosourea. Cancer Res 25:1876–1881, 1965
33. Carter SK, Selawry O: Phase II clinical trials. In Saunders JP, Carter SK, (eds): Methods of Development of New Anticancer Drugs, pp 81–92. Natl Cancer Inst Monogr 45, US Dept Health Educ Welfare, Bethesda, 1977
34. Muggia FM, McGuire WP, Rozencweig M: Rationale, design and methodology of phase II clinical trials. In DeVita VT, Jr, Busch H (eds): Methods in Cancer Research, vol. XVII, Cancer Drug Development Part B, pp 199–214. New York, Academic Press, 1979
35. Chalmers TC: Randomization of the first patient. Med Clin N. Amer 59:1035–1038, 1975
36. Lee YJ, and Wesley RA: Statistical considerations to phase II trials in cancer: Interpretation, analysis and design. Semin Onco 8:403–416, 1981
37. Moertel CG, Schutt AJ, Hahan RG et al: Effects of patient selection on results of phase II chemotherapy trials in gastrointestinal cancer. Cancer Chemother Rep 59:257, 1974
38. Zelen M: Statistical options in clinical trials. Semin Onco 4:441–446, 1977.

39. Pocock SJ: Randomized clinical trials (letter). Br Med J 1:1161, 1977
40. Lasagna L: The controlled clinical trial: Theory and practice. J Chron Dis 1:353–367, 1955
41. Ingelfinger FJ: The randomized clinical trial. New Engl J Med 287:100–101, 1972
42. Chalmers TC, Block JB, Lee S: Controlled studies in clinical cancer research. New Engl J Med 287:75–78, 1972
43. Schneiderman MA: Looking backward: is it worth the crick in the neck? Or: Pitfalls in using retrospective data. Am J Roentgen Rad Ther. Nucl Med 96:230–235, 1966
44. Wendel HA: Randomization in clinical trials. Science 199:368, 1979
45. Byar DP, Simon RM, Friedewald WT et al: Randomized clinical trials: perspectives on some recent ideas. New Engl J Med 295:74–80, 1976
46. Pocock SJ: Allocation of patients to treatment in clinical trials. Biometrics 35:183–197, 1979
47. Gehan EA, Freireich EJ: Non-randomized controls in cancer clinical trials. New Engl J Med 290:198–203, 1974
48. Pocock SJ: The combination of randomized and historical controls in clinical trials. J Chron Dis 29:175–188, 1976
49. Silverman WA: The lesson of retrolental fibroplasia. Sci Am 236,6:100–107, 1977
50. Hellman S: Editorial: Randomized clinical trials and the doctor-patient relationship. Cancer Clin Trials 2:189–193, 1979
51. Shapiro AR: The evaluation of clinical predictions. N Engl J Med 296:1509–1514, 1977
52. Gilbert JP, McPeek B, and Mosteller F: Statistics and ethics in surgery and anesthesia. Science 198:684–689, 1977
53. Zelen M: Aspects of the planning and analysis of clinical trials in cancer. In Srivastava JN (ed): A Survey of Statistical Design and Linear Models, pp 629–645. New York, North-Holland Publ Co, 1975
54. Pocock SJ, Simon R: Sequential treatment assignment with balancing for prognostic factors in the controlled clinical trial. Biometrics 31:103–115, 1975
55. Brown BW, Jr: Statistical controversies in the design of clinical trials. Controlled Clinical Trials 1:13–27, 1980
56. Simon R: Heterogeneity and standardization in clinical trials. In Tagnon HJ, Staquet MJ (eds): Controversies in Cancer, Design of Trials and Treatment, pp 37–49. New York, Masson Publishing, 1978
57. Simon R: Restricted randomization designs in clinical trials. Biometrics 35:503–512, 1979
58. Zelen M: The randomization and stratification of patients to clinical trials. J Chron Dis 27:365–375, 1974
59. Hills M, and Armitage P: The two period cross-over clinical trial. Br J Clin Pharm 8:7–20, 1979
60. Koch GG: The use of non-parametric methods in the statistical analysis of the two-period change-over design. Biometrics 28:577–584, 1972
61. Brown BW, Jr: The crossover experiment for clinical trials. Biometrics 36:69–79, 1980
62. Meier P, Free SM, Jr, Jackson GL: Reconsideration of methodology in studies of pain relief. Biometrics 14:330–342, 1958
63. Schoenfeld DA, Gelber RD: Designing and analyzing clinical trials which allow institutions to randomize patients to a subset of the treatments under study. Biometrics 35:825–830, 1979
64. Makuch RW, Simon R: A note on the design of multi-institution three-treatment studies. Cancer Clin Trials 1:301–303, 1978
65. Makuch R, Simon R: Sample size requirements for evaluating a conservative therapy. Cancer Treatment Rep 62:1037–1040, 1978
66. Gehan EA: The determination of the number of patients required in a preliminary and follow-up trial of a new chemotherapeutic agent. J Chron Dis 13:346–353, 1961
67. Sylvester RJ, Staquet M: An application of decision theory to phase II clinical trials in cancer. In Tagnon HJ, Staquet MJ (eds): Recent Advances in Cancer Treatment, pp 1–11. New York, Raven Press, 1977
68. Staquet M, Sylvester R: A decision theory approach to phase II clinical trials. Biomedicine 26:262–264, 1977
69. Lee YJ, Staquet JJ, Simon R et al: Two-stage plans for patient-accrual in phase II cancer clinical trials. Cancer Treatment Rep. 63–1721–1726, 1979
70. Herson J: Predictive probability early termination plans for phase II clinical trials. Biometrics 35:775–784, 1979
71. Pocock SJ: Size of cancer clinical trials and stopping rules. Br J Cancer 38:757–766, 1978
72. Freiman JA, Chalmers TC, Smith H, Jr., et al: The importance of beta, the type II error and sample size in the design and interpretation of the randomized control trial: Survey of 71 "negative" trials. New Engl J Med 299:690–694, 1978
73. Casagrande JT, Pike MC, Smith PG: An improved formula for calculating sample sizes for comparing two binomial distributions. Biometrics 34:483–486, 1978
74. Cochran WG, Cox GM: Experimental Designs. New York, John Wiley & Sons, 1957
75. Kramer M, Greenhouse SW: Determination of sample size and selection of cases. In Cole JO, Gerard RW (eds): Psychopharmacology: Problems in Evaluation, pp 356–371. Natl Acad Sci, Natl Research Council, Washington, D.C., Publication 583, 1959
76. Burdette WJ, Gehan EA: Planning and Analysis of Clinical Studies. Springfield, Charles C. Thomas, 1970.
77. Gehan EA, Schneiderman MD: Experimental design of clinical trials. In Holland JF, Frei E (eds): Cancer Medicine, Philadelphia, Lea & Febiger, 1973.
78. Makuch RW, Simon R: Sample size considerations for non-randomized comparative studies. J Chron Dis 33:175–171, 1980.
79. George SL, Desu MM: Planning the size and duration of a clinical trial studying the time to some critical event. J Chron Dis 27:15–24, 1974
80. Armitage P, McPherson CK, Rowe BC: Repeated significance tests on accumulating data. J R Stat Soc A 132:235–244, 1969
81. McPherson K: Statistics: The problem of examining accumulating data more than once. New Engl J Med 290:501–502, 1974
82. Tukey JW: Conclusions versus decisions. Technometrics 2:423–434, 1960
83. Meier P: Statistics and medical experimentation. Biometrics 31:511–529, 1975
84. Armitage P: Sequential Medical Trials, 2nd ed. New York, John Wiley & Sons, 1975
85. Jones D, Whitehead J: Sequential forms of the log rank and modified Wilcoxon tests for censored data. Biometrika 66:105–113, 1979
86. Elfring GL, Schultz JR: Group sequential designs for clinical trials. Biometrics 29:471–477, 1973
87. Pocock SJ: Group sequential methods in the design and analysis of clinical trials. Biometrika 64:191–199, 1977
88. Pocock SJ: Can sequential methods be used for the analysis of cancer clinical trials? In Tagnon HJ, and Staquet MJ (eds): Controversies in Cancer—Design of Trials and Treatment, pp 63–74. New York, Masson Publishing, 1978
89. Cutler SJ, Greenhouse SW, Cornfield J et al: The role of hypothesis testing in clinical trials. J Chron Dis 19:857–882, 1966
90. Staquet MJ, Rozencweig M, Von Hoff DD et al: The delta and epsilon errors in the assessment of cancer clinical trials. Cancer Treatment Rep 63:1917–1921, 1979
91. Williams CJ, Whitehouse JMA: Cancer trials. Lancet 2:909, 1979
92. Sikora K: Multicentre cancer trials. Lancet 8184:41–42, 1980
93. Wright P, Haybittle J: Design of forms for clinical trials. Brit Med J 2:529–530, 590–592, 650–651, 1979
94. Zelen M: A new design for randomized clinical trials. N Engl J Med 300:1242–1245, 1979
95. Frost N: Consent as a barrier to research. N Engl J Med 300:1272–1273, 1979
96. Curran WJ: Reasonableness and randomization in clinical trials: Fundamental law and government regulation. N Engl J Med 300:1273–1275, 1979
97. Chalmers TC, Block JB, Lee S: Controlled studies in clinical cancer research. N Engl J Med 287:75–78, 1972

98. Armitage P: Statistical Methods In Medical Research. Oxford, Blackwell, 1971
99. Brown BW, Jr, Hollander M: Statistics—A Biomedical Introduction. New York, John Wiley & Sons, 1977
100. Fleiss JL: Statistical Methods for Rates and Proportions. New York, John Wiley & Sons, 1973
101. Lehmann EL: Nonparametrics—Statistical Methods Based on Ranks. San Francisco, Holden-Day, 1975
102. Mantel N: Evaluation of survival data and two new rank order statistics arising in its consideration. Cancer Chemother Rep 50:163–170, 1966
103. Gehan EA: Statistical methods for survival time studies. In Staquet MJ (ed): Cancer Therapy: Prognostic Factors and Criteria of Response, pp 7–35. New York, Raven Press, 1975
104. Hankey BF, Myers MH: Evaluating differences in survival between two groups of patients. J Chron Dis 24:523–531, 1971
105. Neyman J, Pearson ES: On the use and interpretation of certain test criteria. Biometrika 20A:175–240, 263–294, 1928
106. Fisher RA: Statistical methods and scientific induction. J R Stat Soc B 17:69–78, 1955
107. Cox DR: Some problems connected with statistical inference. Ann Math Stat 29:357–372, 1958
108. Anscombe F: Sequential medical trials. J Am Stat Assoc 58:365–382, 1963
109. Gibbons JD, Pratt JW: P-values : Interpretation and methodology. Am Statistician 29:20–25, 1975
110. Kempthorne O: Of what use are tests of significance and tests of hypothesis? Commun Stat Theor Meth 8:763–777, 1976
111. Cox DR, Hinkley DV: Theoretical Statistics. New York, Halsted Press, 1974
112. Zelen M: Importance of prognostic factors in planning therapeutic trials. In Staquet MJ (ed): Cancer Therapy: Prognostic Factors and Criteria of Response, New York, Raven Press, 1975
113. Kaplan EL, Meier P: Nonparametric estimation from incomplete observations. J Am Stat Assoc 53:457–481, 1958
114. Cox DR: Regression models and life tables. J R Stat Soc B 34:187–220, 1972
115. Finney DJ, Latscha R, Bennet BM et al: Tables for Testing Significance in a 2 × 2 Contingency Table. Cambridge, Massachusetts, Cambridge University Press, 1966
116. Cox DR: Analysis of Binary Data. New York, Methuen Co, 1970
117. Beyer WH: CRC Handbook of Tables for Probability and Statistics. Chemical Rubber, Cleveland, 1968

Paul H. Sugarbaker
N. Reed Dunnick
Everett V. Sugarbaker

CHAPTER 11

Diagnosis and Staging

Accurate diagnosis and staging of malignant tumors commonly depends upon a series of diagnostic tests rather than one individual study. Unfortunately, often no single test is a precise reflection of the disease state. Some tests, such as a surgical biopsy with histologic evaluation, are definitive studies with no superior examination; other tests, such as the serum sedimentation rate, are extremely nonspecific and their significance can only be appreciated in the context of numerous other clinical data.

Whenever a diagnostic examination is performed, the result must be interpreted in the context of how accurately it reflects the presence or absence of disease. The fundamentals of decision analysis as reviewed by McNeil and Adelstein have made possible a clearer understanding of the use of diagnostic tests.[1] The two methods commonly used to convey this information are the decision matrix and the receiver operating characteristic (ROC) curve. If a test is asked to predict the presence or absence of disease (binary outcome) a decision matrix is used. In this system a series of ratios is calculated:

1. True positive ratio—the fraction of patients with disease who had a positive test result;
2. False positive ratio—the fraction of patients who do not have disease but have a positive test result;
3. True negative ratio—the fraction of patients without disease who have a negative test result;
4. False negative ratio—the fraction of patients with disease who have a negative test result.

Often the term sensitivity is used for the true positive ratio and specificity for the true negative or false-positive ratio. The overall accuracy may be defined as the number of correct tests over the total number of tests.

When tests have a range of results and any given level may be selected to separate normal from abnormal, the ratios of the decision matrix will vary with the level of the cutoff point. The ROC curve is a graphical representation of changes in the probability of disease being present as the level of the cutoff point is varied.

DIAGNOSIS OF HEPATIC METASTASES BY LABORATORY TESTS

The use of decision analysis in test interpretation is especially valuable in the detection of liver metastases by laboratory tests, for no single procedure consistently gives evidence of a nodular or infiltrative process in the liver. The laboratory tests in current use for detection of hepatic metastases include measurements of serum alkaline phosphatase, 5′-nucleotidase, leucine aminopeptidase, gamma-glutamyl transpeptidase (GGT), lactic dehydrogenase (LDH), glutamic oxaloacetic transaminase (GOT), glutamic pyruvic transaminase (GPT), and bilirubin. Also, carcinoembryonic antigen (CEA) is a tumor marker that, when yielding abnormal findings, may assist in the diagnosis of hepatic metastatic disease.

In a large proportion of patients with extensive hepatic metastatic disease, the alkaline phosphatase values are elevated. Schaefer and Schiff found 92 percent of jaundiced patients and 72 percent of patients without jaundice but with hepatic metastases confirmed by closed liver biopsy to have increased alkaline phosphatase.[2] However, abnormal laboratory tests in patients with physical signs of hepatic involvement by tumor are of little or no value clinically. Ranson, Adams, and Localio determined the clinically more relevant evaluation of alkaline phosphatase in patients with occult metastases appreciated at the time of surgery, but not causing hepatomegaly by physical examination preoperatively.[3] Only 1 of 16 (6 percent true positive ratio) patients had abnormal alkaline phosphatase giving this test very low sensitivity in this group of patients. Sixty-seven percent of patients with physical signs of hepatic metastases had elevated alkaline phosphatase in the study.

Just as the sensitivity of alkaline phosphatase determinations is low, so is its specificity. As discussed by Combes and Schenker, alkaline phosphatase elevation may result from excessive production by liver, bone, or placenta.[4] Hepatic metastases result in elevations in liver alkaline phosphatase and not the bone or placental coenzymes. Good separation of the protein bands with alkaline phosphatase activity by electrophoresis has been reported, but the techniques are complicated and not yet suitable for clinical use. A second approach to the specificity problem is based on the differential sensitivity of the 3 isoenzymes to heat inactivation. Placental alkaline phosphatase is fully heat stable, hepatobiliary alkaline phosphatase activity is moderately stable, and bone alkaline phosphatase most heat labile.[5] However, use of heat inactivation is not accurate enough to be diagnostically useful in unselected patients.[6] The best approach to the problem of specificity with alkaline phosphatase is to use enzymes elevated only with liver defects. Most studies indicate that 5′-nucleotidase is just as sensitive as liver alkaline phosphatase to space-occupying lesions in the liver, but only becomes abnormal with hepatic dysfunction.[7] Leucine amino peptidase should be used, as 5′-nucleotidase, to improve the specificity of abnormal alkaline phosphatase determinations. Some consider leucine aminopeptase more sensitive than alkaline phosphatase or 5′-nucleotidase in the detection of metastatic disease.[8] GGT determinants are used in a similar manner, as is 5′-nucleotidase and leucine aminopeptidase. In addition to detecting metastatic lesions in the liver, recent studies would indicate that these serum enzymes from liver may be useful tumor markers for hepatoma.[9]

Ranson and colleagues found serum LDH to be the most sensitive laboratory test for the presence of hepatic metastases.[3] With occult metastases, 13 of 16 patients (81 percent) had abnormal determinations and, with palpable metastases, 4 of 5 patients (80 percent). GOT was elevated in 38 and 83 percent of the two groups and GPT in 13 and 50 percent.

Wanebo and coworkers found CEA assays to be a very sensitive test for the presence of recurrent colorectal cancer metastases in the liver; 48 of 52 patients (92 percent true positive ratio) had CEA elevations greater than 5.0 ng/ml if recurrence in the liver was confirmed.[10]

In summary, several laboratory tests are available to assist in a search for evidence of hepatic metastases. However, all the laboratory and radiologic tests currently in use for detection of liver metastases have significant numbers of false negative and false positive determinations. Only histologic examination of tissue provides reliable proof of the presence of hepatic metastases; such tissue diagnosis may be obtained by blind liver biopsy or directed biopsy under peritoneoscopic, ultrasound, or CT control. False positive tests may present an even more difficult clinical problem, requiring exploratory laparotomy to rule out the presence of hepatic metastases.

DIAGNOSIS OF METASTASES USING RADIOLOGIC TECHNIQUES

During the past decade diagnostic radiology has experienced a technological explosion which has resulted in significant improvement in the ability to diagnose and follow tumor metastases. The most dramatic example of this has been computed tomography (CT) which is rapidly becoming a most accurate method of detecting metastases in a wide variety of locations. Rapid technical change has also resulted in vastly improved diagnostic ultrasound and radionuclide imaging. Continued improvement in gray scale equipment with digital-based scan conversion and real-time imaging has brought marked changes in ultrasound. In addition to improved scanning equipment and refinement in radionuclide carriers, computerized data manipulation has added flow measurements to nuclear medicine. While diagnostic images are increasingly accurate, the introduction of fine-needle percutaneous aspiration biopsy techniques has enabled radiologists to obtain specimens to prove suspected lesions or to clarify equivocal findings.

Although further studies are needed to define the role of these various diagnostic modalities, the application of certain principles may help to gain most efficiently the desired information in any given patient. CT, ultrasound, and radionuclide imaging measure different parameters of morphology and physiology. CT detects differences in radiodensity. Not only does it display this information in a cross-sectional format, but it also has a far greater capability to show minor density differences than plain film radiographs. In the retroperitoneal space, low density fat provides the contrast by which higher density tumor masses can be identified. Since CT scans have longer exposure times than routine radiographs, the ability to suspend respiration is important for high quality images of the chest and upper abdomen. In general, patients who are unable to suspend respiration or who have a paucity of retroperitoneal fat will be poor subjects for CT examination.

Diagnostic ultrasound displays reflections from sound waves which may be obtained at any degree of angulation or obliquity. This aspect of ultrasound may be crucial in determining the precise anatomic location of a given image. Real-time image units scan at such a speed that physiologic motion may be observed. This is particularly useful in examining the abdomen where motion may allow discrimination of vascular or enteric structures from mass lesions. Gas transmits sound poorly, and adipose tissue is sufficiently echogenic that diagnostic information regarding deeper structures is degraded. Thus, patients with overlying bowel gas and obese patients are difficult to examine. Currently, ultrasound tissue signatures are being developed to allow the identification of the type of tissue based upon its pattern of sound reflection.[11]

Radionuclide imaging combines physiology and morphology. Rapid sequence scanning provides information on vascular supply while delayed scanning demonstrates a more precise anatomic image. By attaching a radionuclide to carriers with varying physiologic properties, information can be gained about different functional systems within the same organ.

Percutaneous aspiration has become more useful since the introduction of fine-needle techniques. In the abdomen, 22 or 23 gauge needles may be passed into a variety of targets without significant complications. Percutaneous needle aspirations have been successfully incorporated into the routine evaluation of potential tumor masses, particularly when they are of renal or pancreatic origin. Percutaneous liver biopsies performed at the bedside are a blind sampling of hepatic parenchyma. Under radiographic guidance, usually CT or ultrasound, the lesion may be entered and a biopsy obtained from the abnormal area of the liver. Following bipedal lymphography the aspirating needle can be guided fluoroscopically, not merely into an abnormal node but into the most abnormal portion of the lymph node. Pulmonary parenchymal lesions are readily accessible to fine-needle aspiration if they are large enough to be visualized under fluoroscopy. When pulmonary lesions are subpleural or pleural based, CT may be the most effective imaging modality for needle placement. Fine needles may even be used in bone lesions if they have a significant soft tissue component or if the cortex has been destroyed. However, if the cortex is intact, a larger needle will be required to penetrate the lesion.

The complication rate of percutaneous needle aspiration varies with the size and location of the target and the gauge needle used. In the abdomen, where 22 gauge needles are used, the complication rate is extremely low. No significant complications have yet been reported with lymph node aspirations. One case of needle tract seeding after biopsy of a pancreatic carcinoma has been reported.[12] As many as 30 percent of pulmonary aspirations will result in pneumothorax, the majority of which resolve spontaneously.[13] Higher complication rates are expected in patients with obstructive lung disease, when larger needles are used or when more centrally located nodules are aspirated. When one considers that thoracotomy is often required for diagnosis if aspiration is unsuccessful, even higher complication rates may be acceptable.

DIAGNOSIS OF PULMONARY METASTASES

The pulmonary interstitium is the most common site of metastases for a wide variety of tumors, and the chest radiograph is a simple method of screening for such metastases. As demonstrated by Figure 11-1, whole lung tomography (WLT) has been shown to detect lesions in 3 to 18 percent of patients with normal chest radiographs and multiple pulmonary nodules are seen in 20 to 36 percent of patients when only solitary lesions are identified on plain chest films.[14–16] Data from Chang and coworkers (Table 11-1) demonstrated CT to be more sensitive, but less specific than whole lung tomography in detecting metastases.[17] As experience grows, the specificity of CT appears to be improving. In a recent report by Muhm and colleagues, CT demonstrated more pulmonary nodules than WLT in 35 percent of patients. In 5 patients, no pulmonary nodules were seen by WLT but were present by CT. In 13 patients, bilateral nodules were identified by CT when only unilateral nodules were present on WLT.[18] Contrary to other reports in which most of the additional nodules identified by CT were benign lesions, the lesions in 27 of the 31 patients in whom these additional nodules were resected were proven metastases (Fig. 11-2).

More recent work by Siegelman and co-workers has demonstrated that density differentials provided by CT can detect calcium within pulmonary nodules in smaller amounts than can be detected by WLT.[19] This has been quite helpful in assessing the probability of malignancy of a pulmonary nodule. Unless the primary tumor is an osteogenic sarcoma, even small amounts of calcium in a pulmonary nodule make the lesion more likely benign. Computed tomography may become the standard for detection of pulmonary metastases; however, due to limitations in its availability, it is still reserved for a relatively small group of high-risk patients and plain chest radiographs supplemented by WLT are more commonly used.

When multiple pulmonary nodules appear in a patient with an underlying malignancy, pulmonary metastases are most likely present. However, since inflammatory processes may have the same appearance, tissue proof may be desired. Of greater uncertainty is the development of a single pulmonary nodule by a cancer patient. Almost two-thirds of such patients who underwent thoracotomy at the Sloan-Kettering Cancer Center were found to have primary cancer of the lung as the etiology of the solitary nodule.[20] Less than 25 percent of these patients had solitary metastases from their underlying primary malignancy. Thus, tissue proof is required for proper management.

Fine-needle percutaneous aspiration biopsy has become a routine radiologic procedure for pulmonary lesions large enough to be localized under fluoroscopy (Fig. 11-3). A variety of needles have been used, from 16-gauge cutting needles to 23-gauge thin walled aspiration needles. Twenty- to 23-gauge aspiration needles are more popular since the complications are fewer than with the large cutting needles.[21] Larger (>2 cm) and more central lesions are also amenable to evaluation by bronchoscopy with brush cytology or forceps biopsy.[22] The complication rate, particularly when the nylon brush is used for tissue sampling, is lower than for percutaneous biopsy. Percutaneous aspiration is preferred for peripheral lesions, as it is more likely to be diagnostic.[23]

The accuracy of percutaneous pulmonary aspiration is approximately 90 percent with virtually all errors due to false negative results. False positive diagnoses are rare (24–26). Complication rates are low enough that this procedure may be performed on an outpatient basis. If the patient has normal platelets and clotting factors and a 22- or 23-gauge aspiration needle is used; pulmonary hemorrhage or hemoptysis is unlikely. Pneumothorax will still occur in 5 to 30 percent of patients, but most are small and will revolve spontaneously.

DIAGNOSIS OF HEPATIC METASTASES

In many medical centers, evidence of hepatic metastases is most readily obtained by radionuclide scanning with ^{99m}Tc-labeled sulfur colloid. This is a rapid, relatively inexpensive method of imaging the reticuloendothelial system of the liver and spleen. Metastatic deposits appear as areas of decreased radionuclide uptake (Fig. 11-4). The resolution is sufficient to detect lesions as small as 1 cm in diameter, but varies with the location of the lesion. Lesions near the camera or in the "thin" portion of the liver are more easily detected than those deep within the organ or located near the porta hepatis.

Using radionuclide scanning, an overall accuracy of approximately 80 percent in detecting metastases may be

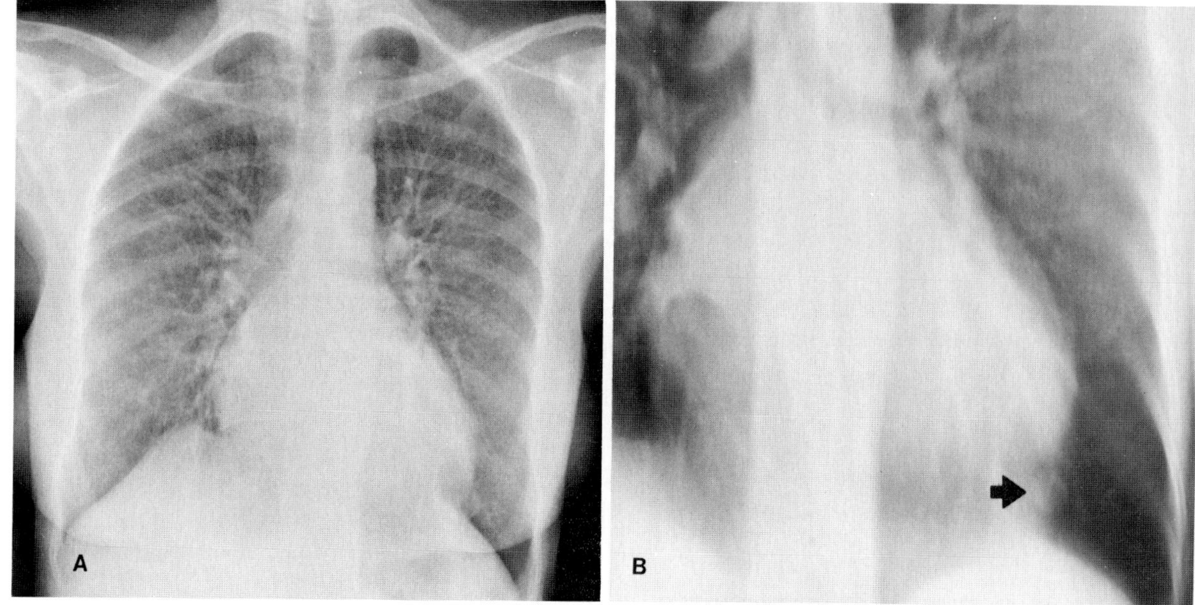

FIG. 11-1. Forty-four-year-old woman with adenocarcinoma of the colon and a pulmonary metastasis. **(A)** Plain chest radiograph fails to show the pulmonary nodule as it overlies the cardiac silhouette. **(B)** The nodule is readily seen on linear tomography (*arrow*).

expected, although significant variation exists depending upon the underlying malignancy.[27,28] In general, the sensitivity is quite good, but significant false positive determinations reduce the specificity.

Diagnostic ultrasound with gray scale imaging has an accuracy similar to radionuclide scanning.[29] Although generally not as sensitive, it does not suffer from the relatively high number of false positive interpretations seen with radionuclide scans. Ultrasound is useful in confirming a positive radionuclide scan and in differentiating metastatic lesions from benign cysts or normal anatomic variants. It may be used to clarify an equivocal radionuclide scan and has the added virtue of permitting the examination of the biliary tree and porta hepatis.[30]

TABLE 11-1. Detection of S3 Pulmonary Metastases in 27 Patients by Chest Radiography, Conventional Tomography and Computed Tomography

	CHEST RADIOG-RAPHY	WHOLE LUNG TOMOG-RAPHY	COMPU-TERIZED TOMOG-RAPHY
Nodules visualized	21	38	69
Nodules identified as metastases at operation	19	25	31
Number of metastases confirmed pathologically	53	53	53
True-positive ratio (sensitivity)	19/53 (36%)	25/53 (47%)	31/53 (58%)

(From Chang AE, Schaner EG, Conkle DM, Flye MW, Doppman JL, Rosenberg SA: Evaluation of computed tomography in the detection of pulmonary metastases. Cancer 43:913–916, 1979)

A variety of ultrasound appearances are seen with hepatic metastases and occasionally more than one pattern may be seen in the same patient.[31,32] The most frequent appearance is localized areas of increased echogenicity. This is commonly seen when metastases from adenocarcinoma are present. Areas of decreased attenuation or "bull's-eye" lesions are other ultrasound manifestations (Fig. 11-5). Some of these reflect central necrosis.[33] Occasionally, hepatic metastases appear only as a diffuse alteration in the normal pattern of hepatic parenchyma. Although the ultrasonographic appearance is suggestive, it is not sufficiently specific to indicate the tissue of origin of hepatic metastases.[34]

Most hepatic metastases are identified on CT as areas of decreased attenuation coefficient.[35,36] The degree of contrast

FIG. 11-2. Thirteen-year-old girl with osteosarcoma. A subpleural metastasis is seen on computed tomography (*arrow*) that was not appreciated by plain chest radiography or linear tomography.

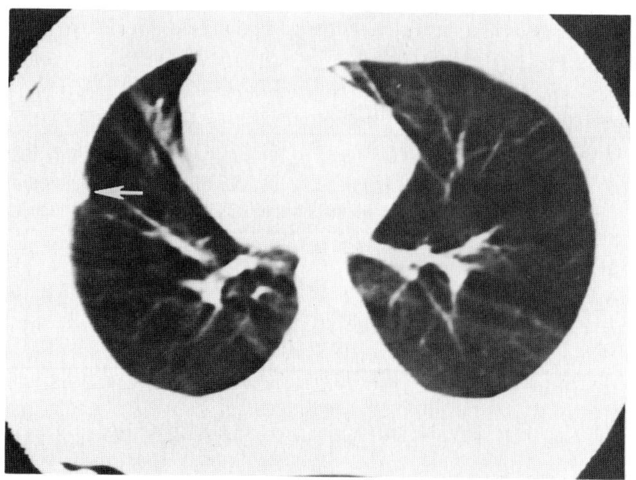

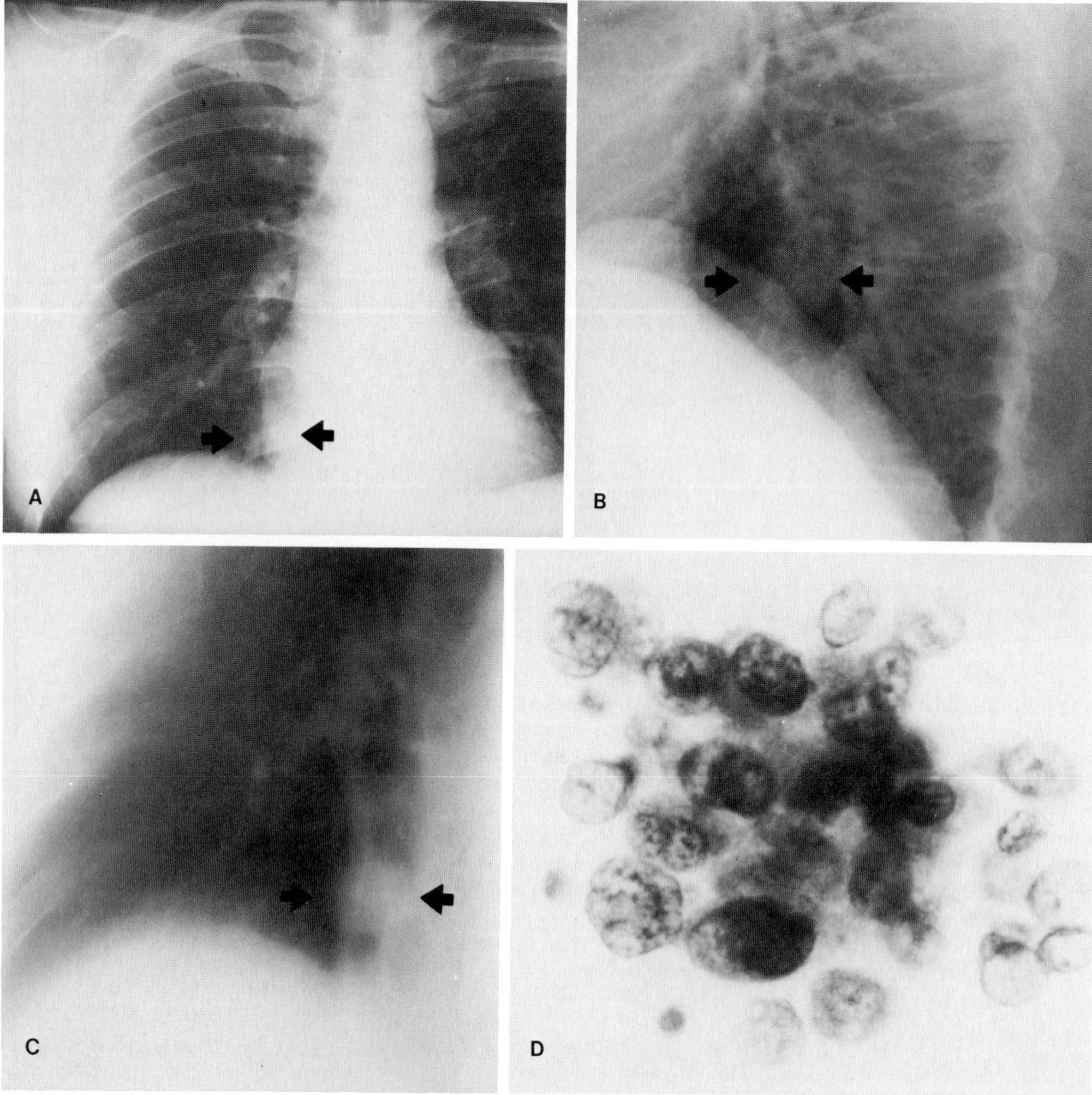

FIG. 11-3. Forty-seven-year-old man with malignant melanoma. A pulmonary nodule is seen **(A)** poorly on the posterior-anterior film (*arrow*) and **(B)** better on the lateral radiograph (*arrow*). **(C)** Linear tomagraph defines the nodule (*arrow*) more clearly. **(D)** Percutaneous pulmonary aspiration with a 22-gauge fine needle reveals metastatic melanoma.

TABLE 11-2. Liver Imaging

	SENSITIVITY (+ tests/abnormal livers)	SPECIFICITY (− tests/normal livers)	ACCURACY (corrrect tests/total Pts.)
Liver scan	13/20 65%	17/21 81%	30/41 73%
	____P = .1		
Ultrasound	9/20 45%	19/21 90%	28/41 68%
	____P .05		____P<.1
CT	14/20 70%	19/21 90%	33/41 83%

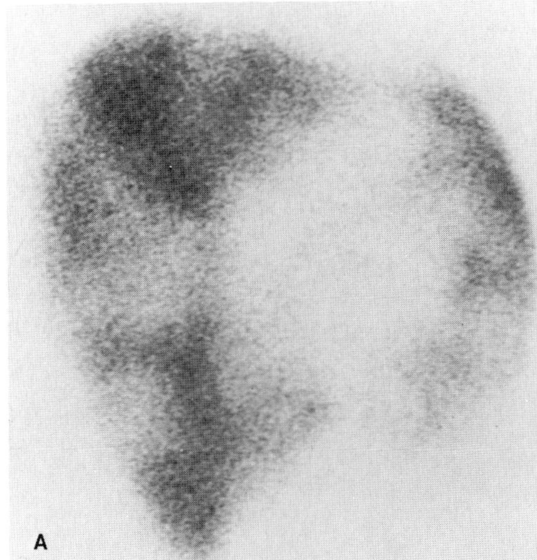

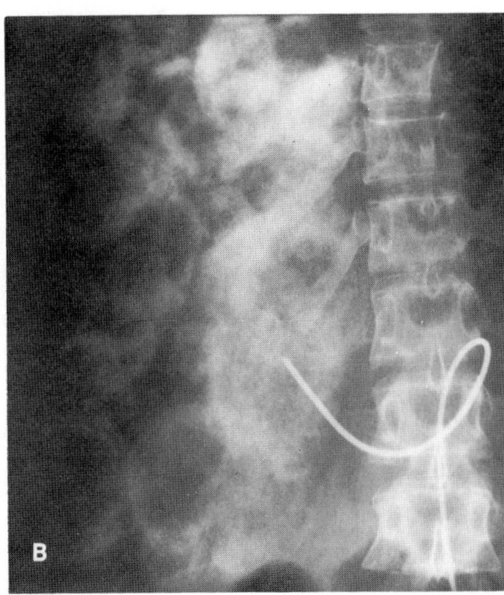

FIG. 11-4. Fifty-five-year-old woman with carcinoma of the breast metastatic to the liver. **(A)** Radionuclide liver-spleen scan reveals an enlarged liver, with multiple focal areas of decreased radionuclide activity. **(B)** A hepatic arteriogram shows multiple vascular metastases.

enhancement after intravenous administration of iodinated dye is variable and metastases may become either more or less apparent. While overall accuracy in detecting metastases with CT has been generally comparable to radionuclide scanning and ultrasound, a recent study from the M.D. Anderson Hospital found CT superior to either of these methods.[37] Smith and coworkers at the NIH prospectively compared radionuclide scans, ultrasound, and CT in the evaluation of patients with suspect liver metastases.[38] The standard for evaluation of these tests was the objective findings at surgery or autopsy within one month of liver imaging studies (Table 11-2). CT proved to be the most accurate study. Figure 11-6 shows a new contrast agent currently being evaluated to further improve the ability of CT to detect metastatic lesions.[39] Vermess and colleagues have developed a lipid soluble contrast agent that is preferentially (80 percent) taken up by the liver. This contrast agent reliably increases the density of the liver, but has no effect on tumor density. Early studies show a low incidence of toxicity and an increased accuracy of CT studies.

The success of these noninvasive methods in detecting hepatic metastases has relegated angiography to a secondary role. When solitary lesions are present or when surgery is contemplated for unilobar disease, angiography is indicated to search for further metastases and define the vascular anatomy of the liver. Most hepatic metastases are sufficiently vascular to allow differentiation from the normal liver parenchyma, but pharmacoangiography with epinephrine or priscoline may be needed to confirm the diagnosis.[40] When assessing resectability, subselective injection of right and left main hepatic artery branches is quite helpful. Angiographic differentiation of suspected metastases from vascular lesions is particularly helpful in view of the similarity of their CT appearance.

DIAGNOSIS OF CNS METASTASES

Radionuclide brain scans have been replaced by CT as the most sensitive method of detecting CNS metastases.[41-43]

FIG. 11-5. Twenty-seven-year-old woman with malignant melanoma. **(A)** The ultrasonographic pattern of the liver **(L)** is disrupted by an area of decreased echogenicity **(T)**, indicating a metastasis. The right kidney **(K)** is posteromedial to the liver in this transverse scan. **(B)** A contrast-enhanced computed tomography scan shows two low-density areas (*arrow*), confirming the presence of metastasis.

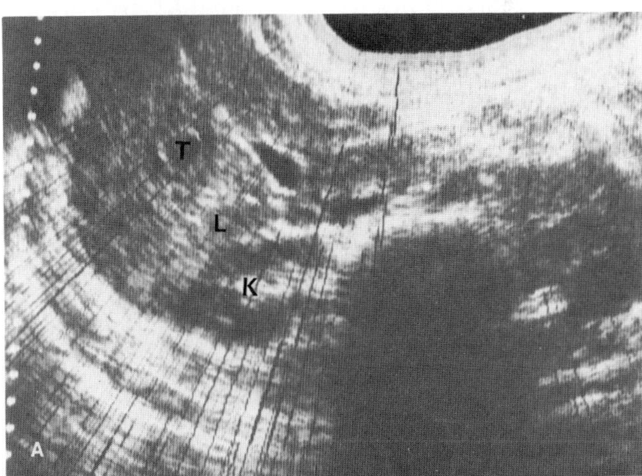

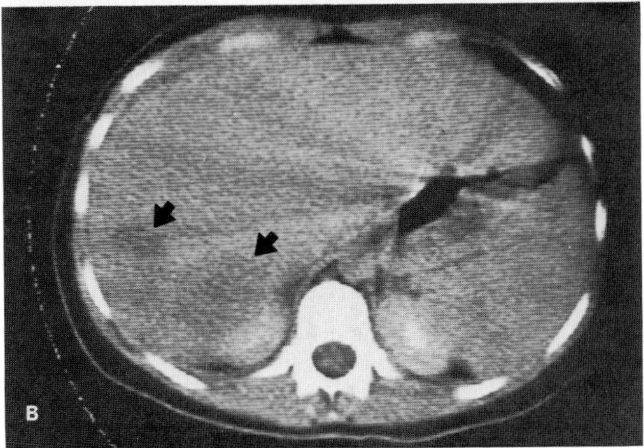

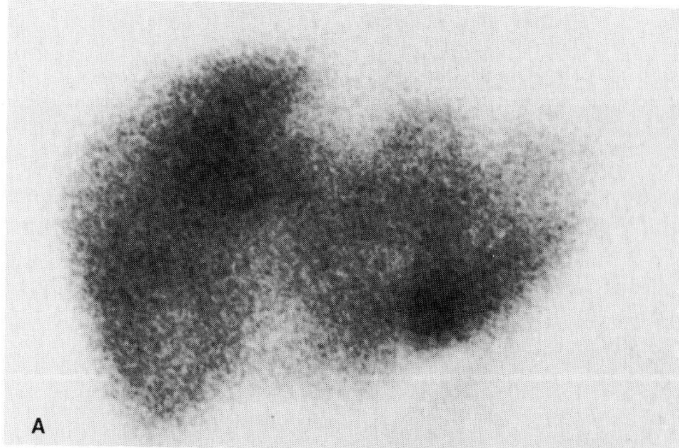

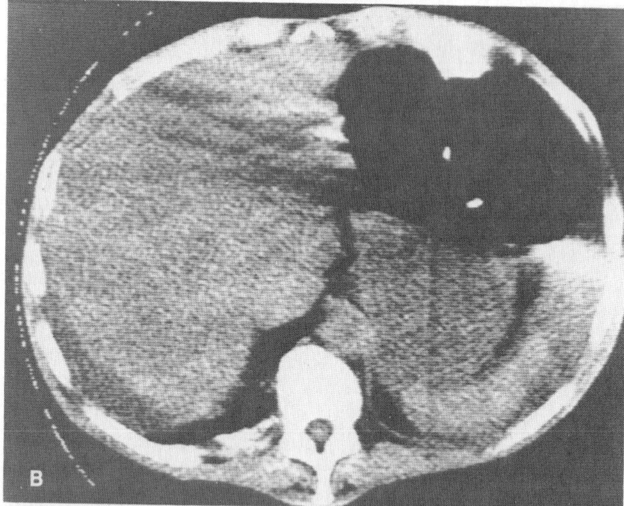

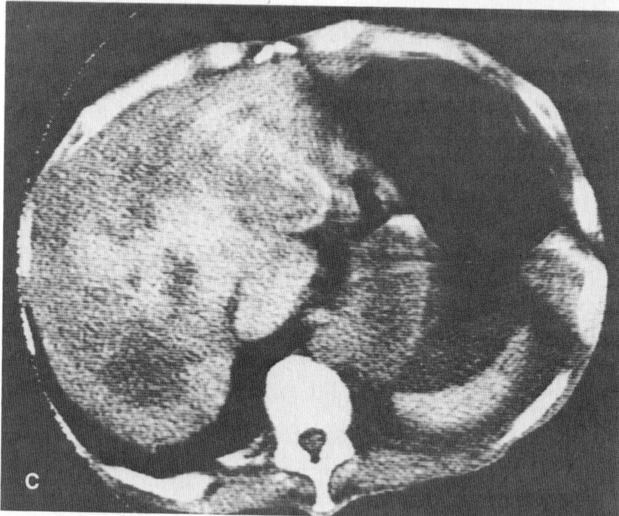

FIG. 11-6. Fifty-year-old man with carcinoma of the rectum. **(A)** Radionuclide scan appearance of multiple areas of decreased activity indicates hepatic metastases. **(B)** Computed tomography scan shows only mild inhomogeneity of the liver, suggesting the presence of metastatic disease. **(C)** After intravenous injection of an experimental contrast material of ethiodized oil in emulsion, the extent of hepatic metastases becomes apparent. (The case is courtesy of Dr. Michael Vermess, National Institutes of Health.)

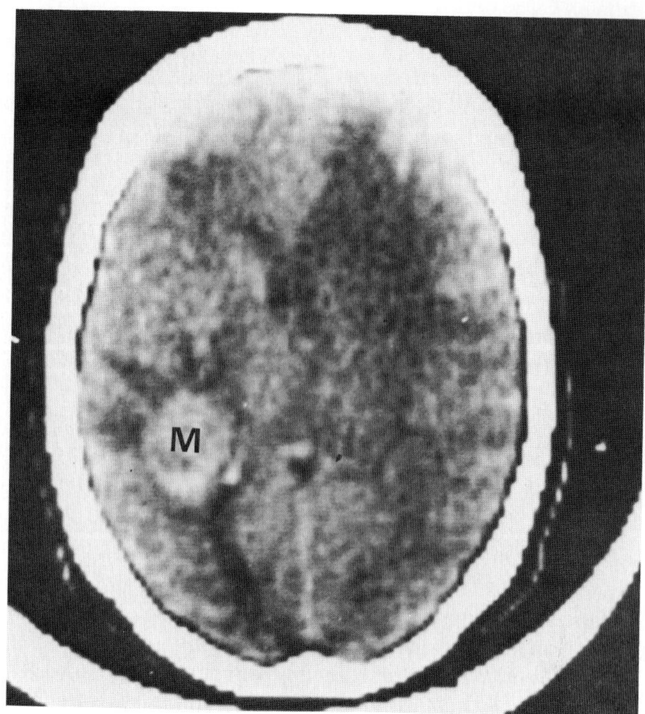

FIG. 11-7. Fifty-four-year-old woman with malignant melanoma. A contrast-enhanced computed tomography scan shows the typical appearance of a metastatic lesion **(M)** with surrounding edema in the left parietal lobe. The low-density area on the right side with leftward shift of the midline structures indicates the mass effect from a larger metastasis seen on lower sections.

Although both of these noninvasive imaging modalities provide good sensitivity for cerebral hemispheric lesions, CT has proven superior in the more troublesome infratentorial region. In addition to the demonstration of cerebral metastases, CT provides invaluable information regarding the size of the tumor and the presence of mass effect, cerebral herniation, or the development of obstructive hydrocephalus.

Most cerebral metastases will be detected on pre-contrast scans as areas of decreased attenuation coefficient. If there has been hemorrhage within the tumor, which is not infrequently seen in metastases from malignant melanoma or choriocarcinoma, there will be an area of increased attenuation coefficient representing the fresh blood. Following the injection of intravenous contrast material, metastatic lesions usually show contrast enhancement. Densely enhancing lesions with surrounding edema are most commonly seen with metastases from adenocarcinoma. Peripheral rim enhancement with a lucent center is more typical of epidermoid or squamous cell tumors. The contrast enhancement shown by metastatic lesions is usually striking, and whenever possible, intravenous contrast should be used to examine for metastatic disease (Fig. 11-7).

In approximately two-thirds of cases of CNS metastases, multiple lesions will be demonstrated. In a recent series of 190 patients with intracranial metastases reported by Weisberg, 120 had multiple lesions.[44] In 52 cases only a solitary lesion was seen prior to contrast enhancement but multiple lesions were identified after injection of intravenous contrast material.

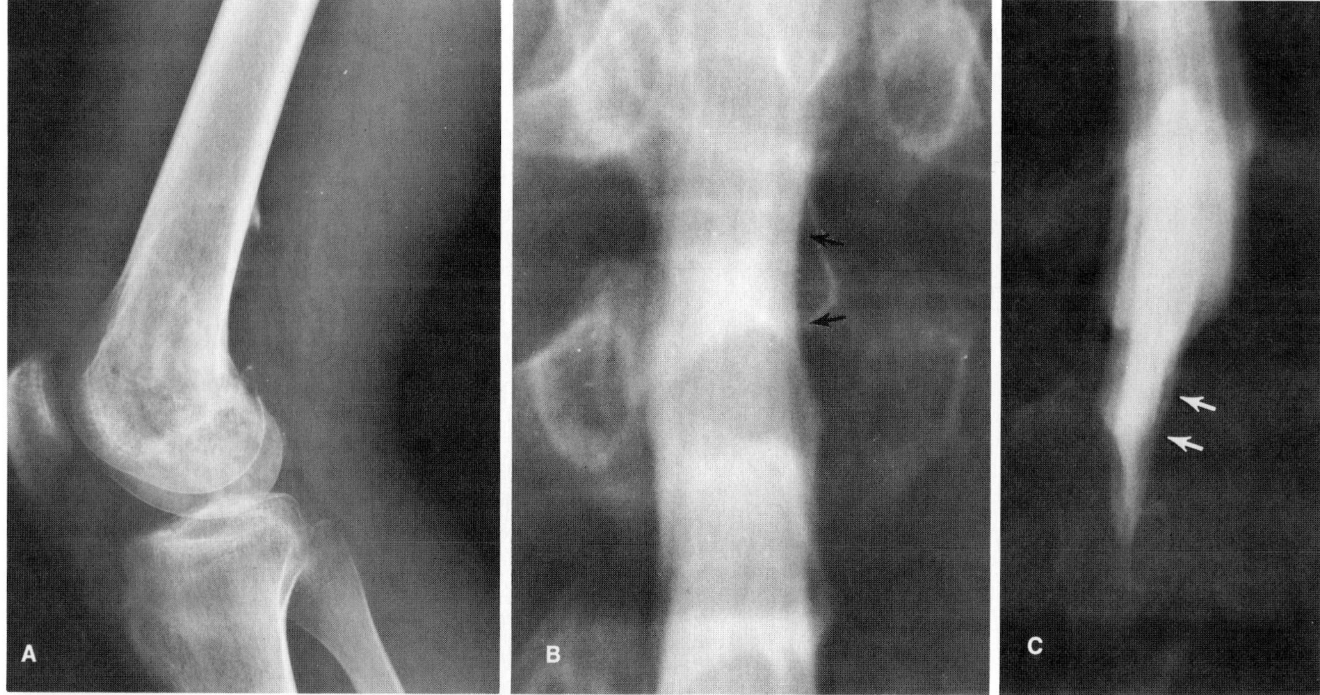

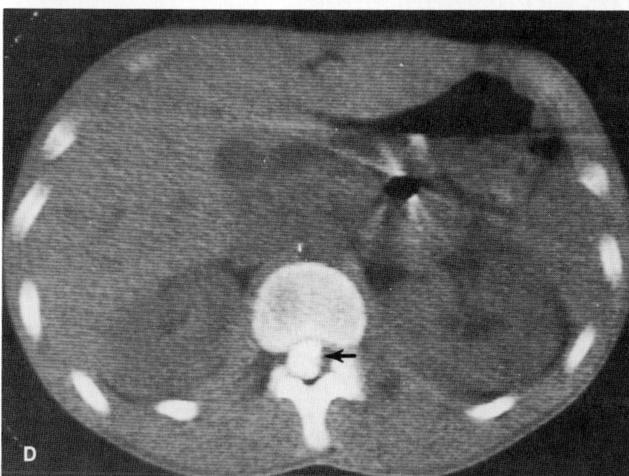

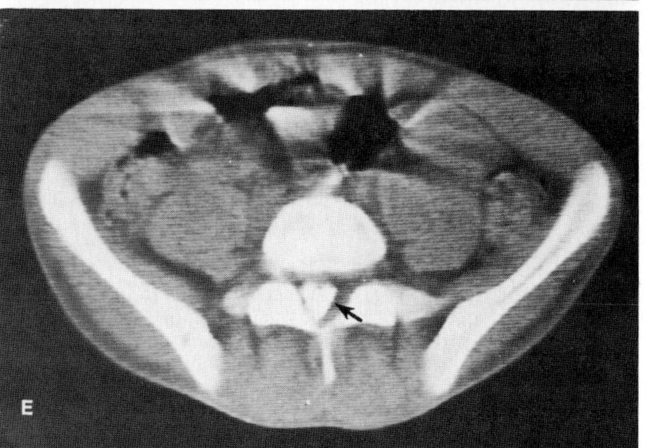

FIG. 11-8. Seventeen-year-old boy with Ewing's sarcoma of the distal femur. **(A)** Metrizamide myelogram reveals extrinsic compression defects at L_{1-2} **(B)** (*arrows*) and at the sacral level **(C)** (*arrows*). Computed tomography scans done immediately after the myelogram shows the shift of the dense contrast material by water density tumor **(D,E)** (*arrows*).

Impairment of the spinal cord function by compression from epidural metastases has a profound effect upon patient comfort and function.[45] Most commonly, this results from bone metastases to the vertebral column that produce a mass effect and cause extrinsic compression of the spinal cord. Thus, a radionuclide bone scan is a simple screening examination when spinal cord compression is suspected. However, as shown in Figure 11-8, bone involvement is not a necessary component, as metastases to the epidural space may occur and cause similar cord compression without involving the bones.[46] Whenever pain, a change in the neurologic examination, or an abnormal radionuclide bone scan suggests spinal cord compression, a myelogram should be performed. Precise anatomic localization of the defect allows proper placement of radiation ports or surgical decompression. When possible, the myelogram should examine the entire spine to detect other mass lesions which have not yet caused clinical symptoms. Although technically more difficult, the thoracic area should be carefully studied, as this is the most common location of compression upon the spinal cord by metastatic lesions.[46,47]

DIAGNOSIS OF SKELETAL METASTASES

As shown in Table 11-3, the superiority of radionuclide bone scanning over plain film radiographs for the detection of bone metastases has been amply proven.[48-52] In a review of 200 patients with a variety of tumors, Pistenma and colleagues found that scanning with technetium-99^{m}-labeled diphos-

TABLE 11-3. Comparison of Radiographs and Radionuclide Bone Scans in Detecting Bone Metastases

	RADIOGRAPH (+)	RADIOGRAPH (−)
Radionuclide (+) scan	100	63
Radionuclide (−) scan	2	189

NOTE: This table assumes that all lesions detected were caused by a neoplastic lesion, however, no histopathologic confirmation was made in all patients. In only 2 of 102 patients was radiograph positive when bone scan was negative. In 63 of 189 patients radiograph was negative in patients with positive bone scans and a strong clinical suspicion of bony metastases.

(From Citrin DL, Bessent RG, Grieg WR: A comparison of the sensitivity and accuracy of the ^{99m}Tc phosphate bone scan and skeletal radiograph in the diagnosis of bone metastases. Clin Radiol 28:107–117, 1977)

phonate detected almost three times as many metastases as plain radiographs.[48] Technetium-99^{m}-labeled phosphate compounds are currently used, but work continues to determine if other agents are superior.

The avid radionuclide uptake of the metaphyses and the tendency for symmetric metastases from neuroblastoma may make bone scan interpretation more difficult in children. Gilday, however, examined 159 children with an underlying malignancy and detected bone metastases in 44.[53] In 30 patients, lesions were seen on the radionuclide scan, but not the plain film radiograph; 14 were present on both scan and radiograph. There were no false negative radionuclide scans.

Skeletal uptake of the technetium-labeled phosphates is dependent upon blood flow and new bone formation. Most metastatic deposits elicit sufficient hyperemia and osteoblastic activity to be imaged as areas of increased uptake (Figure 11-9). If there is either impairment of blood flow or a primarily destructive lesion with little reparative bone formation, the concentration of radionuclide may be equal to or less than

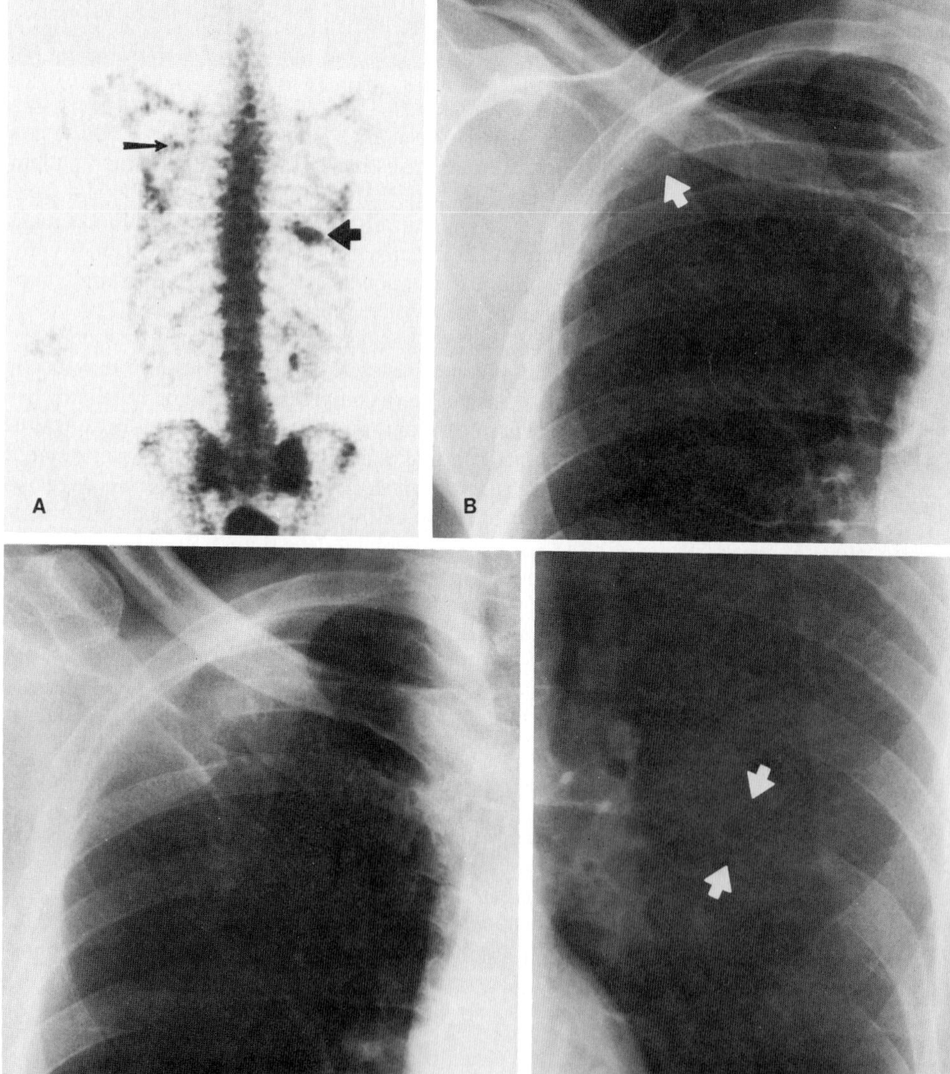

FIG. 11-9. Sixty-three-year-old man with esophageal carcinoma. **(A)** Radionuclide bone scan reveals increased uptake in the left eighth (*large arrow*) and right fourth (*small arrow*) ribs posteriorly. **(B)** Plain radiographs confirm destruction of the right fourth rib (*arrow*), which developed a large soft tissue component 2 months later **(C)**. **(D)** The involvement of the left eighth rib is difficult to see (*arrows*), even in coned views.

that of adjacent bone. In such a case the bone scan may appear normal or a metastatic lesion could actually present as a "cold lesion" or area of diminished radionuclide uptake.[54] Decreased uptake in metastatic lesions on radionuclide bone scans is seen in multiple myeloma and has been reported with malignant lymphoma and carcinomas of the lung, breast, and nasopharynx. If the concentration of radionuclide within the lesion is equal to that in the adjacent bone, the scan will appear normal. This presumably accounts for the few false negative examinations in which metastatic lesions are detected by other methods.

Areas of increased radionuclide uptake do not necessarily indicate metastatic disease. Trauma, surgery, infection, arthritis, and benign bone neoplasms are common nonmalignant causes of increased radionuclide concentration. In the majority of patients, metastases will appear as multiple asymmetric foci; however, even when solitary lesions appear, approximately two-thirds represent malignant disease.[55]

Radionuclide bone scans should be obtained as the screening examination for bone metastases. Areas of abnormal radionuclide uptake should be examined radiographically to exclude a benign etiology such as previous trauma, as even remote trauma may cause increased radionuclide concentration.

Even when the radiograph is compatible with metastatic disease, tissue characterization may be desired before a pivotal therapeutic choice is made. If there has been extensive bone destruction and the cortex is gone, the lesion is amenable to thin-needle biopsy with a 22-gauge needle. Adler and Rosenberger reported 26 such biopsies on 24 patients with no complications.[56] Positive cytologic diagnoses were obtained in 21 patients (88 percent). Similar results were reported using a larger cutting needle by Collins and associates.[57]

DIAGNOSIS OF LYMPH NODE METASTASES

Among the earliest metastases are those that travel along the lymphatics and involve the draining lymph nodes. Depending on the site of the tumor, these lymph nodes may be palpable or amenable to radiographic imaging. Bipedal lymphography opacifies retroperitoneal lymph nodes in the iliac and paraaortic chains. While this is a valuable contribution, metastases to other abdominal node regions, such as mesenteric, splenic or renal hilar, and porta hepatis, can not be examined by this method. The injection of lymphatics in the arm or neck has been used to visualize axillary and cervical lymph nodes. Occasionally, indirect injection of the organ involved, such as testis, prostate, or breast, has been used to provide radiographic evaluation of the specific draining nodes. However, these lymphographic techniques have not gained favor and bipedal lymphography is currently the only form in routine use for the evaluation of metastatic disease.

Improved resolution of ultrasound equipment now allows this noninvasive modality to be used to supplement lymphography as ultrasound permits visualization of areas not demonstrated by lymphography. Enlarged lymph nodes are imaged as areas of decreased echogenicity adjacent to the aorta or inferior vena cava.[58] Although sometimes limited by the presence of overlying bowel gas, ultrasound can examine the renal and splenic hilar areas, as well as the region of the porta hepatis. When significant adenopathy exists, ultrasound may detect tumor metastases in the mesenteric or hypogastric regions as well.

Figure 11-10 demonstrates why CT was quickly embraced as a valuable method of evaluating patients for lymph node metastases in the abdomen.[59] It shares with ultrasound the ability to examine areas outside the region of lymphographic opacification. While not limited by overlying bowel gas, the absence of significant retroperitoneal fat makes interpretation more difficult.

Although specific protocols vary with institutions, bipedal lymphography is routinely used in the pretreatment evaluation of patients with malignant lymphomas, and tumors of the genitourinary system.[60–66] The accuracy of bipedal lymphography in detecting metastases to the opacified lymph nodes depends in part upon the specific tumor examined, but is approximately 80 to 90 percent.[66] More significant to the clinician, however, is the sensitivity and specificity such that this information can be incorporated into the treatment protocol (Table 11-4). If more rigid criteria for the diagnosis of metastatic disease are employed, there will be fewer false positive, but more false negative, interpretations. Conversely, rigid criteria for negative studies will result in few false negative, but more false positive, interpretations.[67]

Following lymphography, routine surveillance abdominal radiographs are used to assess response to therapy and early detection of recurrent disease. After approximately 12 to 18 months, residual contrast remaining in retroperitoneal lymph nodes will be insufficient for evaluation and a reopacification lymphangiogram may be performed. The value of repeat lymphograms has been demonstrated for Hodgkin's disease as well as other malignant lymphomas.[68,69]

Figure 11-11 illustrates that percutaneous fine-needle aspiration of opacified lymph nodes may be performed under fluoroscopic guidance to confirm the presence of tumor in suspicious areas.[70–73] This is helpful in equivocal or atypical lymphograms and is particularly useful in following the response to therapy. Residual scarring in a previously involved site cannot always be distinguished from residual tumor on surveillance, abdominal radiographs, or even repeat lymphography, but fine needle aspiration is quite useful for this purpose.[74] The technique is remarkably free of complications and can be performed on outpatients.[75]

ENDOSCOPY

Endoscopy is one of the few medical technological advances that has resulted in simultaneous decrease in patient morbidity and mortality as well as cost. These advances have been made possible by the delivery of high-intensity cold light and high-resolution images through fiberoptic light bundles. Direct visual inspection of many internal organs and structures is now possible, permitting tissue diagnosis, assessment of operability, and endoscopic surgery without requiring major exploratory procedures. Photography, biopsy, and excision of many pathologic processes is now possible. In this section we explore the indications and results, techniques and complications of endoscopic procedures often useful to oncologists. Throughout the discussion we will emphasize proper tech-

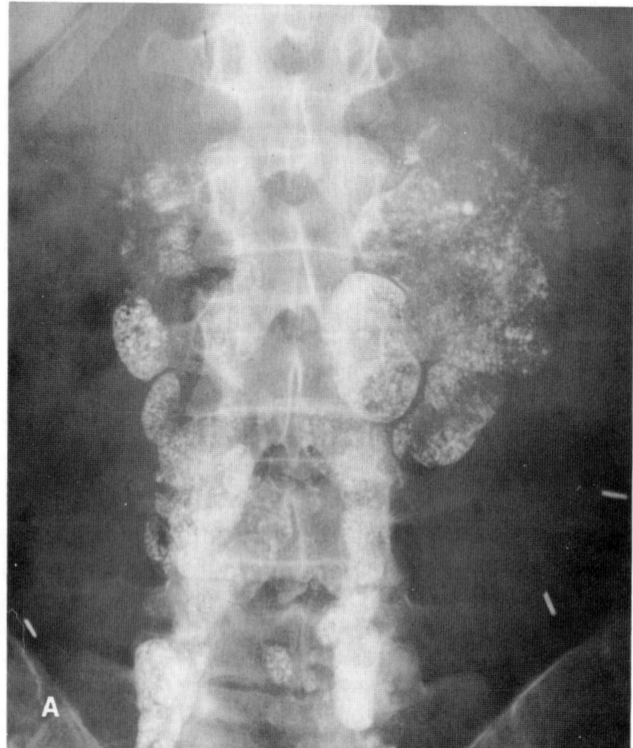

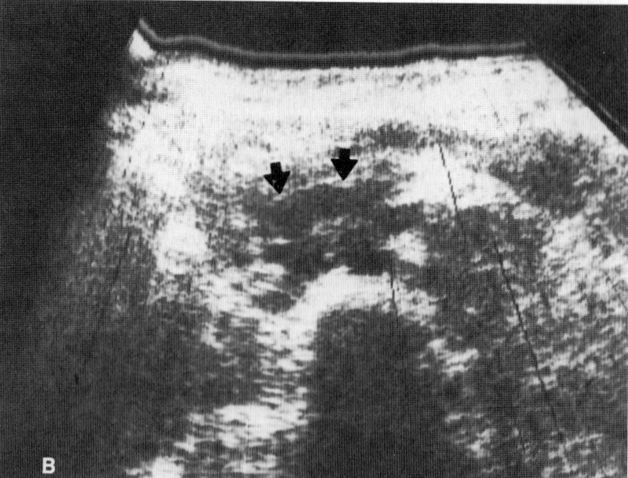

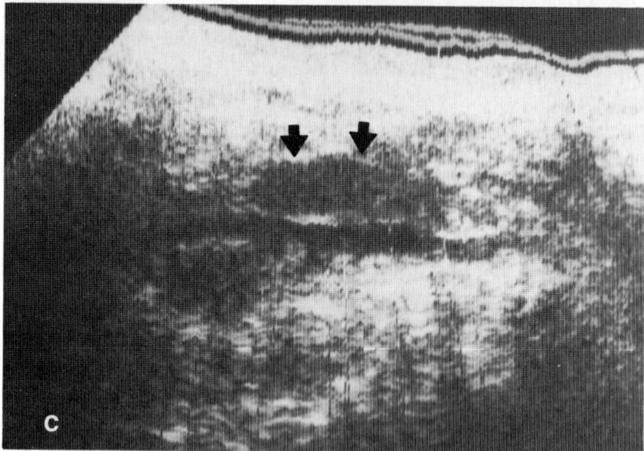

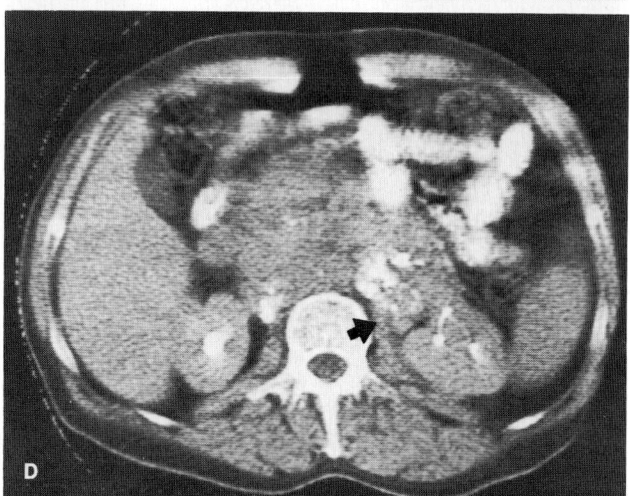

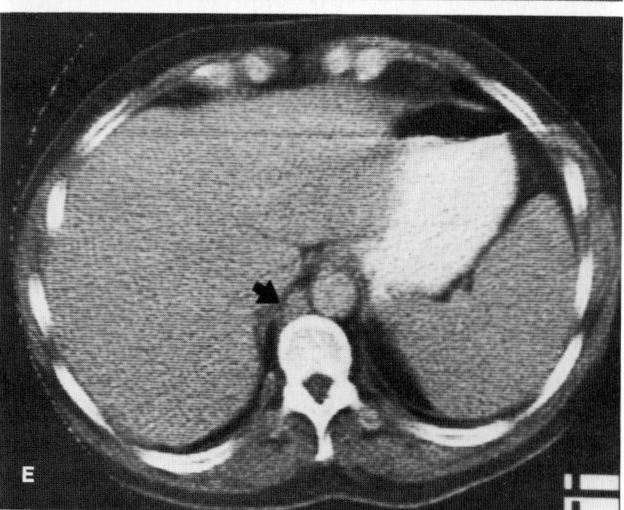

FIG. 11-10. Fifty-three-year-old man with non-Hodgkin's lymphoma. **(A)** Lymphogram is grossly abnormal, with enlarged foamy nodes throughout but most markedly in the left para-aortic region. Ultrasound in transverse **(B)** longitudinal **(C)** projections demonstrates relatively echolucent areas adjacent to the great vessels (*arrows*) confirming the adenopathy. **(D)** Computed tomography reveals not only para-aortic disease but also tumor extending into the left renal hilum (*arrow*). **(E)** At a higher level retrocrural adenopathy can also be appreciated (*arrow*).

TABLE 11-4. Lymphographic Accuracy in 240 Patients with Malignant Lymphoma

		LYMPHOGRAPHIC DIAGNOSIS	
		Negative	*Positive*
HISTOLOGY	Benign	147	18
	Tumor	3	72
	TOTAL	150	90

Sensitivity 72/75 = 96%
Specificity 147/165 = 89%
Accuracy 219/240 = 91%

(From: Castellino RA, Billingham M, Doffman FR: Lymphographic accuracy in Hodgkin's disease and malignant lymphoma with a note on the "Reactive" lymph node as a cause of most false-positive lymphograms. Invest Radiol 9:115–165, 1974)

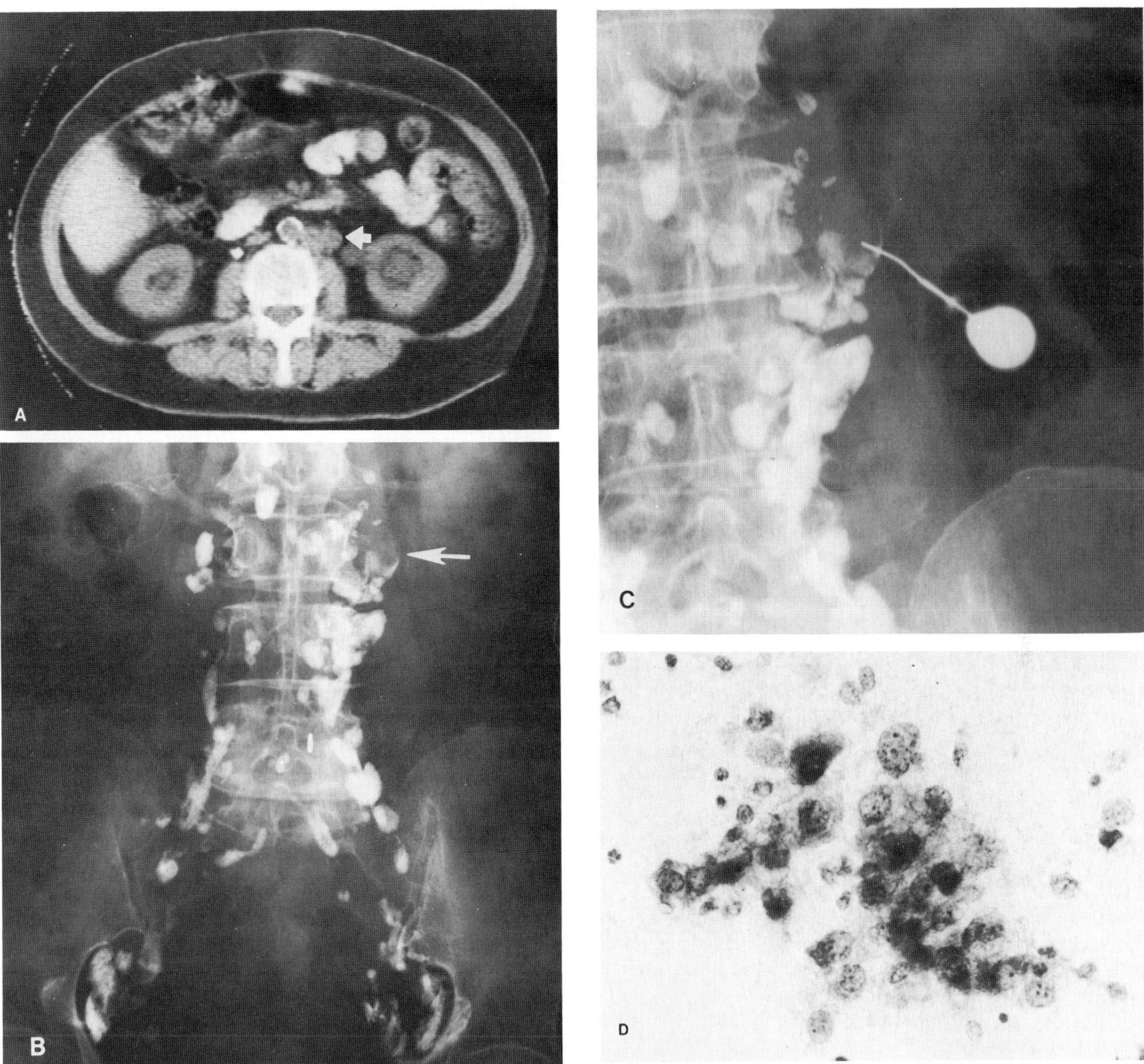

FIG. 11-11. Forty-seven-year-old woman with ovarian carcinoma **(A)** Computed tomography shows a left para-aortic mass (*arrow*). **(B)** Lymphography confirms this impression. The peripheral filling defect (*arrow*) is typical for metastatic carcinoma. **(C)** Percutaneous needle aspiration, done with a 22-gauge fine needle, reveals metastatic ovarian **(D)**.

niques, for only with meticulous attention to technical detail can these procedures be repeatedly employed without appreciable morbidity or mortality.

PERITONEOSCOPY (CELIOSCOPY, LAPAROSCOPY)

Indications and Results

ASSESS OPERABILITY IN PATIENTS WITH CANCER. Peritoneoscopy frequently provides information traditionally obtained only by exploratory laparotomy. It enables the physician to *assess operability* without making an abdominal incision; consequently, many patients can be spared exploratory surgery. Liver metastases, plus peritoneal and pelvic tumor implants, can be visualized and biopsied to determine the stage of intra-abdominal malignant neoplasms. Perhaps, in order to establish operability, all patients who have advanced primary cancer with statistically low cure rates should undergo peritoneoscopy before proceeding with potentially curative surgical therapy.[76] For example, 11 percent of 140 patients undergoing what was considered a curative resection for lung cancer had, at autopsy, within one month of surgery metastatic spread to the liver.[77] Patients in this category might include those with pulmonary, gastric, and pancreatic cancers. Advanced endometrial and rectal cancer patients would also be included. Patients with primary colonic

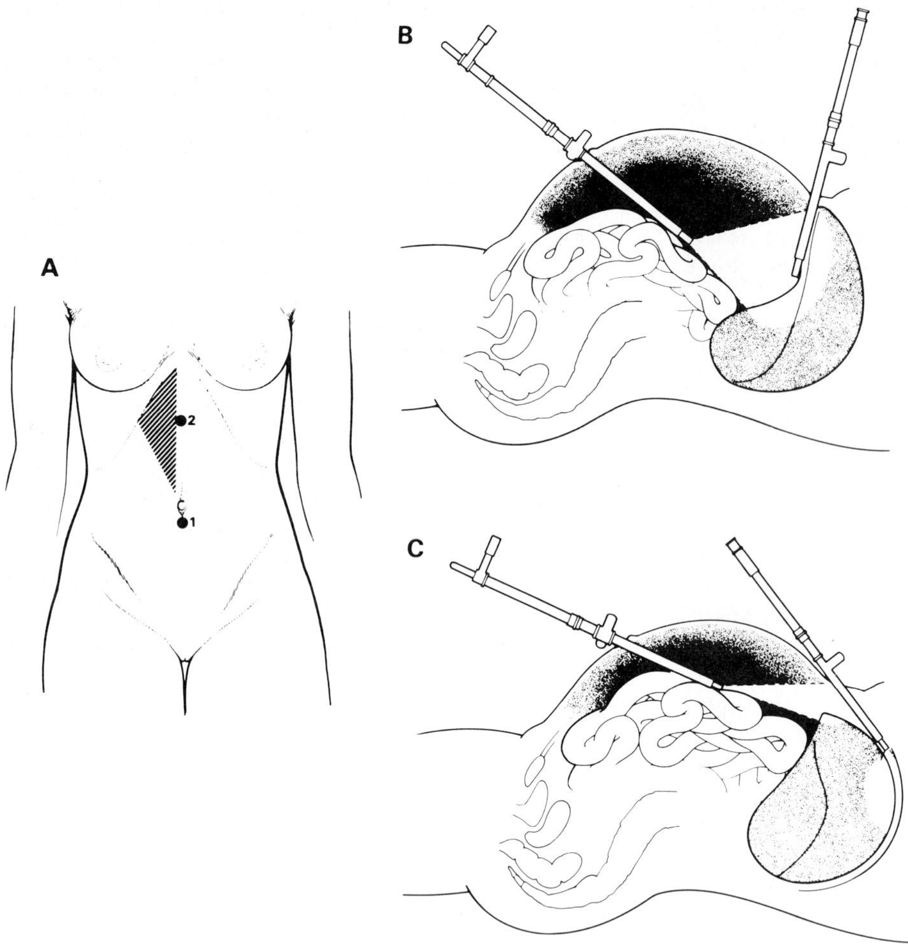

FIG. 11-12. Double puncture peritoneoscopy. **(A)** An end-viewing peritoneoscope is inserted through the abdominal wall, and under direct vision a second oblique viewing telescope is inserted in the epigastrium. **(B)** The first telescope is used to visualize the lower surface of the liver while the second telescope elevates the liver edge. **(C)** The second telescope also visualizes the entire upper surface of the liver.

or ovarian cancer do not require preoperative peritoneoscopy, for colonic cancer (and occasionally, gastric cancer) requires resection to prevent intestinal obstruction and bleeding. If possible, ovarian cancer requires an attempt at resection of bulk disease to improve local control and perhaps augment response to subsequent chemotherapy.

DETECTION OF LIVER METASTASES. Few pieces of clinical information change patient management more than the presence or absence of hepatic metastases. The tests used to detect hepatic disease are multiple; however, all the noninvasive techniques can only provide clues to the presence or absence of liver metastases. From a theoretical point of view, one would suspect that direct visualization of the liver surface would give an accurate assessment of the presence or absence of hepatic metastases. In an autopsy study Ozarda and Pickren determined that if liver metastases were present, at least one would be visible on the surface of the liver in 89 percent of patients.[78] Hogg and Pack found that if metastases were absent from the liver surface at the time of liver exploration, they were absent at autopsy in 95 percent of patients.[79] Obviously the greater the amount of liver surface seen by peritoneoscopy, the higher the true positive and true negative ratios will be. The false positive ratio for peritoneoscopic detection of hepatic metastases should be extremely low, for biospy confirmation of the presence or absence of disease should be possible in most patients. As emphasized by Bleiberg and colleagues adequate biopsy may often require general anesthesia.[80]

As emphasized in the section on laboratory tests for the detection of hepatic metastases, only histologic examination of liver biopsy specimens provides reliable proof of hepatic metastases. Blind percutaneous liver biopsy can sometimes provide this information, but biopsies taken under peritoneoscopic control detect hepatic neoplastic disease nearly twice as frequently.[81-83] As illustrated in Figure 11-12, double puncture peritoneoscopy under general anesthesia should maximize the accuracy of detection of metastases.[84] This technique should also markedly reduce the reported false-negative rate of 36 percent.[80]

STAGING OF LYMPHOMA. DeVita and coworkers performed peritoneoscopy on 38 previously untreated patients with Hodgkins disease.[85] In six patients (16 percent), positive liver biopsies for Hodgkins lymphoma were obtained at the time of peritoneoscopy. These researchers suggest that such patients may be spared staging laparotomy if visceral involvement can be determined by peritoneoscopic biopsy. These findings were confirmed by Coleman and colleagues and Hoffken and Schmidt.[86,87] False negative examinations were uncommon, but all three groups of investigators urge that a negative peritoneoscopy should not be used to rule out visceral involvement; patients whose peritoneoscopy is unrevealing should move to staging laparotomy.

STAGING AND FOLLOW UP OF OVARIAN CANCER. Ozols and coworkers recently reviewed their experience with 159 peritoneoscopic examinations in the management of 99 patients with ovarian cancer.[88] In these patients, all of whom had undergone prior abdominal surgical procedures, peritoneoscopy was reported to be safe and feasible. It could not be technically performed in only six percent of patients. Peritoneoscopy-documented sites of cancer spread undetected by conventional radiologic and nuclear medicine studies in 64 percent of examinations and provided the only evidence of followable disease in 38 percent of patients. Twenty-one percent of patients referred with Stage I or II disease were upstaged to Stage III on the basis of diaphragmatic disease detected at peritoneoscopy. In 66 restaging examinations, residual intra-abdominal disease was found in 33 patients (50 percent) and peritoneoscopic findings were the only evidence of disease in 24 patients (36 percent). Twenty-two patients with negative restaging peritoneoscopy went on to exploratory laparotomy; in 12 (55 percent), residual ovarian cancer was found. Ozols and coworkers urged that a negative peritoneoscopy must be followed by a laparotomy before a patient with ovarian cancer can be considered disease-free. However, a majority of patients in whom recurrent or persistent intra-abdominal disease was present were spared by peritoneoscopy an exploratory laparotomy.

Techniques

All examinations are done in the operating room. In women patients with the uterus and cervix present, the legs should be in stirrups with the buttocks 5 cm off the end of the table. If local anesthesia is planned, intravenous administration of diazepam (Valium), 5 mg, and morphine sulfate, 5 mg is given through an indwelling intravenous catheter. An umbilical block of lidocaine (Xylocaine) hydrochloride is used; local anesthetic is also injected just above the peritoneum, inferior to the umbilicus. A second puncture site lateral to the course of the deep epigastric artery may be infiltrated at this time. However, we have found general anesthesia to be more satisfactory when double-puncture technique is being used. If general anesthesia is used, a nasogastric tube should be passed into the stomach to allow escape of air that is often introduced during induction. This will prevent possible gastric perforation as the trocar is introduced. In women, a Cohen-Eder cannula is placed in the uterus and secured with a tenaculum to allow elevation of the uterus out of the pelvis.

A 2 to 3 cm incision is made through the skin only at the lower edge of the umbilicus; the subcutaneous tissue is spread with a large hemostat until the fascia is clearly seen. If a patient has had a midline abdominal incision with possible diffuse fibrous adhesions, the puncture site is made just lateral to the rectus muscle, or the peritoneum is surgically exposed and the Verres needle is introduced under direct vision. After the peritoneum is punctured two liters of nitrous oxide are introduced into the abdominal cavity under manometric control. As the gas is insufflated, the air pressure noted on the gauge should be below 15 cm of water. It is difficult and usually impossible to determine if an endoscope is within the abdominal cavity before gas infusion allows visualization. Insufflation of subcutaneous tissue in the space of Retzius gives a pressure of 20 to 30 cm of water; pressure within the bowel is about the same. Patients who strain while intubated under general anesthesia may cause much higher pressures to develop. The patient must be relaxed so insufflation pressures are low; when this is so, one is sure that gas is going into the free peritoneal cavity. Pressure within venules of the anterior abdominal wall is 16 to 22 cm of water in supine normovolemic persons, and just a few centimeters of water higher within the portal system. Uncontrolled insufflation of gas by syringe or hand pump should not be performed because it exposes patients to a needless risk of air embolism.

The trocar in the sleeve is introduced at an angle of 45 degrees to the abdominal wall. It is passed through the abdominal incision and toward the pouch of Douglas. During penetration, the anterior abdominal wall is stabilized by grasping a fold of skin midway between the umbilicus and the os pubis and pulling upward. If the patient is under local anesthesia, the abdominal wall is tensed by asking the patient to raise her head off of the operating table. As the trocar is removed from its sleeve, a rush of air from the abdominal cavity is noted. The operating peritoneoscope is advanced through the sleeve; a second puncture can now be made in other parts of the abdomen under direct vision.

When the peritoneal cavity is entered, it is visualized by a standard routine starting at the pelvis and proceeding clockwise around the abdominal cavity. A complete exploration is not performed in all patients, especially if local anesthesia is used. A percutaneous needle biopsy of most intra-abdominal organs can be performed under direct vision. Biopsy examinations of less stationary lesions or organs are performed using forceps through the peritoneoscope. Irrigation and aspiration for recovery of cytologic specimens is frequently indicated.

We have found it useful to tilt the table to examine different abdominal quadrants; reverse Trendelenburg position is used to look into the upper part of the abdomen and Trendelenburg position to look into the pelvis. The spleen is only seen in sharp reverse Trendelenburg position with the patient's right side downward. In women, the entire pelvis is visualized if the uterus is moved inward and upward. Rotation and elevation of the uterus using the tenaculum to the opposite side of the abdomen allows improved visualization of a fallopian tube. All gas should be evacuated from the abdomen at the end of the procedure. The skin incision is closed with absorbable subcuticular sutures.

Complications

In the study by Ozols and associates, severe complications included bleeding, wound infection, hypotension, and pneumothorax; these complications occurred in only three percent of examinations and none required surgical corrections. There were no deaths or viscus perforations in this group of 159 examinations, although they are known to occasionally occur in this clinical setting.[88] Bleeding most frequently occurs from a biopsy site. If bleeding develops after a needle biopsy of the liver, hemorrhage into the free peritoneal cavity or into the bile (hemobilia) may occur. This blood loss can sometimes be controlled by hepatic angiography and clot embolization. Bleeding from other more accessible biopsy sites is usually easily controlled by electrocoagulation through the peritoneoscope. Bleeding that occurs from the anterior abdominal wall as a result of the trocar puncture can be controlled without surgery. A large Foley catheter is inserted into the abdominal cavity through the bleeding puncture wound; the Foley balloon is inflated and traction exerted until bleeding stops.

Bowel perforation rarely occurs as the trocar is being introduced into the abdominal cavity. A more common cause of perforation is full thickness heat necrosis occurring inadvertently as a biopsy using electrocautery is being performed. Perforations almost always involve small bowel; they are difficult to diagnose, for free air is introduced into the peritoneal cavity by peritoneoscopy and symptoms may be delayed in their onset. Surgical repair of a perforation immediately after diagnosis is indicated.

COLONOSCOPY

Indications and Results

COLONOSCOPIC POLYPECTOMY. Colonoscopy has had its greatest impact by reducing the morbidity, mortality, and cost of medical care by allowing colonic polypectomy without laparotomy.[89,90] All but the largest and most sessile benign lesions can be removed *in toto*.

DIFFERENTIAL DIAGNOSIS OF DIVERTICULITIS AND CANCER. Not infrequently diverticulitis and colon cancer produce similar clinical and radiologic findings. Colonoscopy has been found useful in making this differential.[91–93] Cancer can be ruled out if the colonoscope can be passed through the entire segment of colon in question and no neoplasm is seen. A diagnosis of cancer is made if biopsy or cytologic brushing reveals malignancy.[92]

DETERMINATION OF THE EXTENT, SEVERITY AND DIFFERENTIAL DIAGNOSIS OF INFLAMMATORY BOWEL DISEASE. Not infrequently, patients who have abdominal pain, blood per rectum and leukocytosis may have inflammatory bowel disease with an entirely normal barium enema.[92,94–96] In these patients, colonoscopy with biopsy of each segment of the colon has revealed inflammatory changes in the mucosa. Also, serial colonoscopic examination with biopsy has been useful to follow the response to therapy in patients with colitis and assist in making a differential diagnosis of ulcerative colitis and Crohn's disease of the colon.[97,98]

DETECTION OF DYSPLASIA IN PATIENTS WITH ULCERATIVE COLITIS. Ulcerative colitis, *in situ* carcinoma (dysplasia) is thought to precede the development of colon cancer. Several authors have suggested that sampling the colonic mucosa in multiple areas at frequent intervals may enable the clinician to predict when a colitic colon is undergoing malignant degeneration. Prophylactic colectomy may no longer be necessary, for selection of patients for surgery may be based on a histopathologic study of biopsy specimens obtained at colonoscopy.[99,100]

EVALUATION OF SUTURE LINES. Following resection and anastomosis for colon cancer, tumor cells may implant on the suture line and result in recurrent disease (see chapter 21, section on natural history of colon cancer). These mucosal recurrences are difficult to diagnose by barium enema and are often too far from the anus to visualize by sigmoidoscopy. Colonoscopy and suture line biopsy may lead to a diagnosis of local recurrence and result in a curative repeat resection.

CLARIFICATION OF CONFUSING FINDINGS SEEN ON BARIUM ENEMA. The ileocecal valve and midsigmoid areas often are not clearly defined even with the most meticulous radiologic techniques. Colonoscopy may often complement barium enema, especially if the radiologic findings are confusing.[101–104] Barium enema is the indicated procedure after a careful history, physical examination, rectal examination, and stool test for occult blood are made. The endoscopist should not perform colonoscopy prior to obtaining a barium enema for several reasons: (1) Colonoscopy with biopsy delays barium enema examination by at least 10 days, to allow healing of mucosal and submucosal damage produced by biopsy. This prevents submucosal dissection of barium or perforation at the time of barium enema. (2) The barium enema tells if diverticuli are present; if they are, special precautions need to be taken so the colonoscope is not moved into a diverticulum and then through the colon wall, causing perforation. (3) The barium enema in identifying pathology gives the endoscopist a definite area within the colon to reach and then to inspect and photograph. A narrowed or obstructing lesion presents a serious risk for perforation if not recognized prior to examination. Sometimes the segment of colon in question by barium enema may look entirely normal by colonoscopy. Success rates in reaching lesions known to exist are much better than success rates in reaching undefined lesions. (4) A barium enema defines the anatomy of the colon so that the endoscopist knows the length and configuration of the bowel. (5) Patients whose barium enema suggests inflammatory bowel disease should have multiple biopsies performed.

IDENTIFICATION OF A LESION IN PATIENTS WITH OCCULT BLOOD PER RECTUM. In patients with occult blood in the stool and a negative sigmoidoscopy and barium enema, colonoscopy may find a lesion in about 50 percent of patients.[105]

Techniques

ADVANCEMENT OF THE COLONOSCOPE TIP. The most difficult aspect of colonoscopy is the most fundamental maneuver—advancement of the colonoscope tip up into the colon. Experience indicates that a definite sequence of maneuvers repreated in every patient allows most rapid advancement.[106] A barium enema is displayed and is used as a road map. The well lubricated tip of the colonoscope is introduced into the anus on the index finger, as in performing a rectal examination. Upon insufflation of air, the rectal ampulla

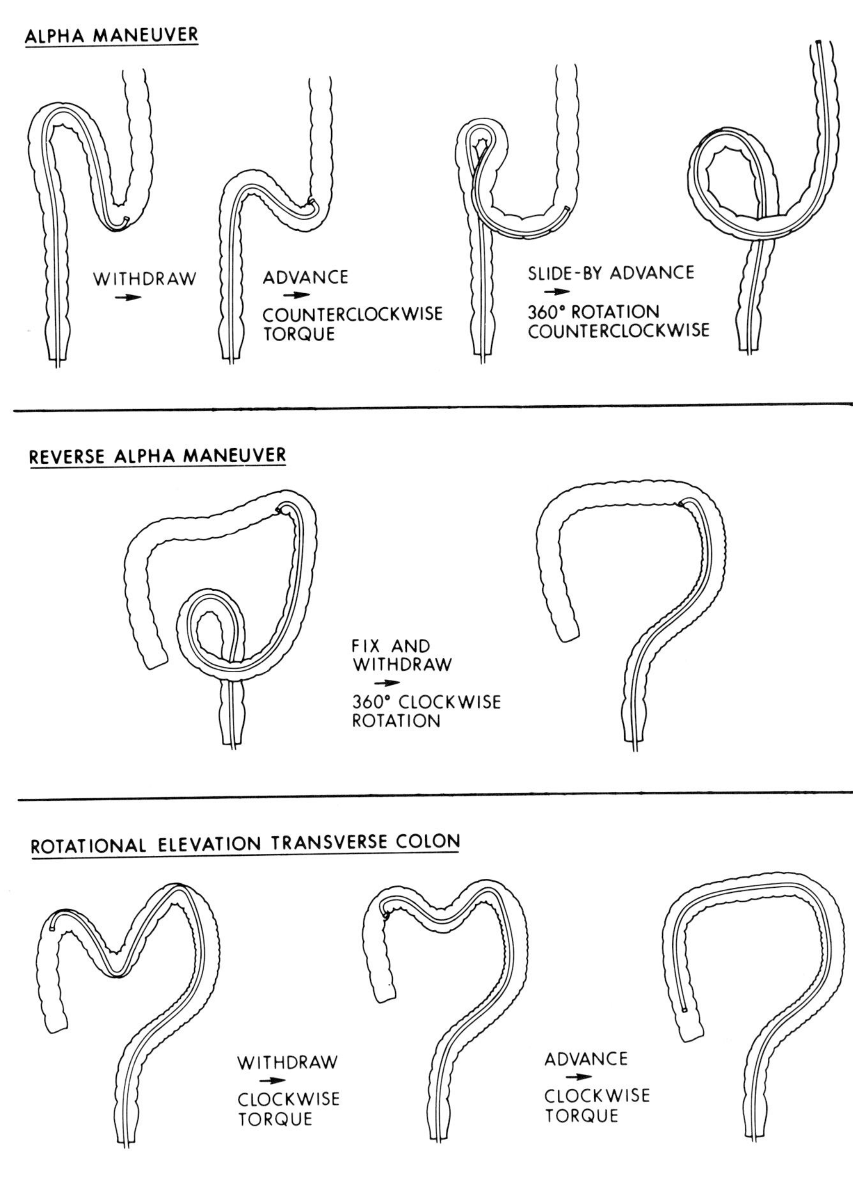

FIG. 11-13. Maneuvers for colonoscopic advancement. (Sugarbaker PH, Vineyard GC, Peterson LM, et al: Anatomic localization and stepwise advancement of the fiberoptic endoscope. Surg Gynecol Obstet 143:451-462, 1976)

appears as a large cavern; its exit can be located using moderate flexion and then rotation of the tip. The sigmoid colon is usually navigable under direct vision until the acute angle at the junction of the sigmoid and descending colon is encountered. Often, despite an open lumen ahead, insertion does not advance the tip but merely increases the sigmoid inverted U-loop. As shown at the top of Figure 11-13, 2 to 3 inches of retraction are used to relax, but not completely reduce, the loop of the sigmoid; 360 degrees of counterclockwise rotation modify the loop into an alpha configuration, markedly decreasing the acute angle the colon makes with itself at the junction of the sigmoid and descending colon. If the loop of the sigmoid is completely reduced, the colonoscope may merely turn within the lumen of the colon rather than change its configuration. Advancement through an alpha loop causes the tip to slide by into the descending colon. During a slide-by maneuver, insertion should be discontinued if the mucosa blanches or the patient experiences pain. Because the descending colon is fixed to the retroperitoneum, navigation straight to the splenic flexure is usually uncomplicated. The middle of Figure 11-13 shows how, after entering the splenic flexure, the tip of the colonoscope is gently fixed in a mucosal fold, and the reverse alpha maneuver is performed by retraction and 360 degrees of clockwise rotation. This straightens the sigmoid colon on the colonoscope and lowers the splenic flexure. If complete straightening has occurred, motion of the instrument at the anus is transmitted one to one to the colonoscope tip.

The transverse colon usually becomes quite ptotic as the tip of the colonoscope reaches the hepatic flexure. More insertion only evaluates splenic and hepatic flexures while depressing further the middle portion of the transverse colon. The lower portion of Figure 11-13 illustrates how rotational elevation of a ptotic transverse colon is accomplished by partial reduction of the U-loop and clockwise rotation. This maneuver slides the colon onto the undersurface of the diaphragm, relieves the ptosis and pushes the tip of the colonoscope down into the ascending colon. Slight, continued clockwise torque upon further insertion moves the tip into the cecum.

Localization of the colonoscope tip can be accomplished with fluoroscopy; however, colonoscopy without fluoroscopy acquires increased versatility, for examinations can then be performed in the operating room, at the patient's bedside, or in the physician's office, replacing the use of the rigid sigmoidoscope. Guidance for locating the tip of the colonoscope is available from the light transmitted through the abdominal wall, the internal appearance of the colon, and certain gross anatomic landmarks.

EXTERNAL LOCALIZATION FROM TRANSMITTED LIGHT. As the colonoscope is passed from the anus to ileocecal valve, the transilluminated intracolonic light on the abdominal wall can be located at key check points in a darkened room in most patients. The patient is initially positioned in the right lateral decubitus position. As the colonoscope is passed up into the midportion of the sigmoid colon, transmitted light first appears in the left lower quadrant; then the light disappears as the junction of the sigmoid and descending colon is tranversed. As the tip of the colonoscope moves up the descending colon, transmitted light appears in the left flank at the level of the splenic flexure; at this point the patient is turned onto the back. Light travels across the abdomen at the level of the umbilicus during navigation of the transverse colon and then disappears behind the liver to reappear at McBurney's point when the cecum is entered.

LOCALIZATION USING INTERNAL APPEARANCE OF COLON. Often, the internal appearance is sufficient to localize the tip of the colonoscope but over-insufflation of air may distort characteristic anatomic features. The rectum is a smooth-walled cavity partially divided by transverse rectal folds, the valves of Houston. The inferior fold lies left and posterior in the patient; the middle fold lies right and anterior; the superior fold lies left and posterior. The sigmoid colon is characterized by low profile, irregular mucosal folds, tubular lumen and, if the colonoscopic examination is prolonged, forceful peristaltic waves. Acute angulations from pelvic adhesions or from over-distention with air may occur upon insertion, for the mesentery allows great mobility of the sigmoid colon within the abdominal cavity. The transverse colon is characterized by a triangular lumen with prominent, repetitive, drapery-like mucosal folds, the interhaustral septa. Deep pockets, the haustra, separate triangular interhaustral septa at regular intervals. In the ascending colon and cecum, the lumen is capacious and circular in outline; the folds between irregular haustra are widely separated and deep. Small mucosal lesions may be especially difficult to locate. The appendicular orifice may be patulous, a mere dimple if the lumen of the appendix is scarred shut, or a shallow diverticulum if a previous appendectomy was done. When viewed from the ascending colon, the ileocecal valve appears merely as a mound of mucosa projecting from an interhaustral fold. It is often recognized by a fleck of ileal contents within it. In the terminal ileum, the delicate mucosa is arranged in closely spaced folds around the oval lumen. Peristalsis is continuous and makes further advancement of the colonoscope difficult.

LOCALIZATION USING GROSS ANATOMIC LANDMARKS. A major landmark may be the obstruction to easy advance encountered at the junction of sigmoid and descending colon, which may be navigated using the alpha maneuver. At the splenic flexure, respiratory excursions are seen. Beneath the right hemidiaphragm, motion imparted by cardiac contractions is first noted. A darkened indentation caused by the spleen is frequently seen at the splenic flexure, and a similar darkened area is produced by the liver at the hepatic flexure. Both cardiac and respiratory movements disappear as the instrument enters the hepatic flexure. The cecum is usually close enough to the anterior abdominal wall so that the application of localized pressure at McBurney's point can be seen from within this part of the colon.

Once the navigation from anus to cecum is complete, the colonoscope is slowly withdrawn to visualize, biopsy, or remove pathologic findings. Usually, location of the lesion seen on barium enema is not difficult; however, certain portions of the colon just beyond acute angulations should be considered blind spots and require special effort to visualize (junction of sigmoid and descending colon, splenic flexure, hepatic flexure).

Biopsy is seldom difficult; problems in passing the biopsy forceps through the biopsy channel do occur unless this channel is kept well cleaned and lubricated. If difficulty arises during a procedure, 10 to 20 cc of mineral oil injected down the biopsy channel will facilitate passing the biopsy forceps.

TECHNIQUE OF COLONOSCOPIC POLYPECTOMY. Few recent technical advances have impacted on the standard of medical practice as has colonoscopic polypectomy. Doctors William Wolff and Hiromi Shinya must be congratulated for developing and popularizing the technique in the United States. The technique is basically a simple one.[107,108] A wire loop is passed over the head of a polyp and secured loosely around the stalk. The loop is pulled into its catheter as electrocautery is applied. However, no two polyps are the same and multiple technical details must be practiced to keep complications at a minimum (Fig. 11-14). For some very small lesions, excision should not be attempted, for "hot biopsy" can be used to sample and destroy the lesion simultaneously.[109]

Complications

Complications resulting from diagnostic colonoscopy have been few (0.3 percent) and usually occur in patients with

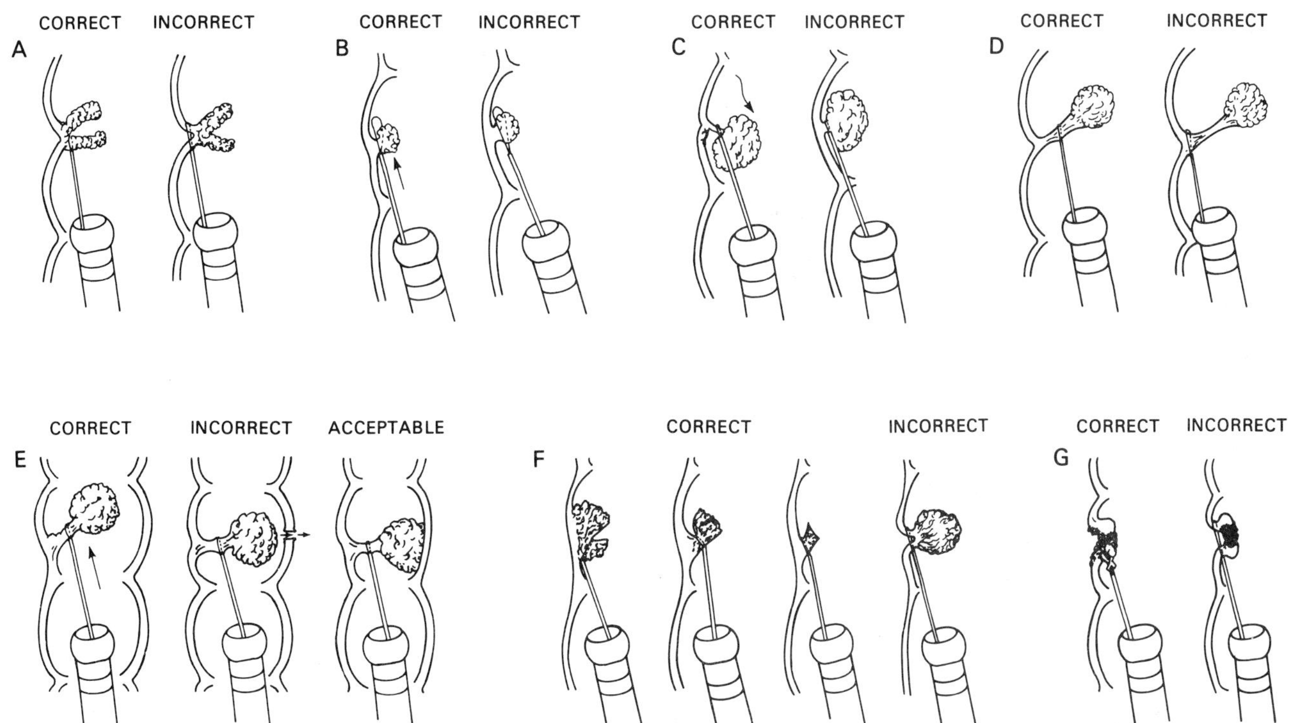

FIG. 11-14. Techniques of colonoscopic polypectomy.
(A) Sessile multilobed polyps. Sessile multilobed polyps should be excised piecemeal. En bloc excision may include bowel wall in the specimen especially if the polyp occurs on an interhaustral fold. **(B)** Excision of small polyps. In excising small sessile or small pedunculated polyps the catheter should be advanced to the base of the polyp before beginning to even up on the snare wires. If this is not done, the polyp will slip out of the snare as the wires are manipulated to secure the polyp (Shinya maneuver). **(C)** Minimally pedunculated polyps. Many polyps that do not appear pedunculated grossly will on microscopic examination be shown to be completely excised. Small sessile polyps can be gently lifted away from the colon wall by tenting up the mucosa. **(D)** Polyps with long stalks. Excision of polyps with long stalks at their base incurs unnecessary risk of full thickness heat necrosis of the colon wall. Division of the stalk at its midpoint should always be attempted. **(E)** Minimizing sparking. Sparking to the bowel wall has caused perforation and should be avoided. The profile of a polyp may be lowered by pushing out on the tightened snare. Or sparking may be avoided if a large portion of opposite colon wall is in contact with the polyp head. **(F)** Piecemeal excision of sessile polyps. Sessile polyps if they are to be removed by colonoscopic polypectomy, should be excised piecemeal. Snare excision of a large tissue mass allows the colon wall to be included in the specimen. If the snare wire is slowly tightened while (not before) electrocautery is applied, hemostasis will be better and the colon wall less likely to be puckered into the resected specimen. **(G)** Carcinoma in sessile polyps. Because of distortion and retraction of tissue surrounding invasive cancer, perforation or bleeding has occurred frequently with excision of carcinomatous polyps. A suspicious sessile lesion should be biopsied before excision attempted.

underlying colorectal pathology that weakens the colon wall.[110] Diverticular disease causes problems in that increased intracolonic air pressure can result in a "blow-out." Also, the orifice of a large diverticulum can be mistaken for the colon lumen and the colonoscope passed into the free peritoneal cavity. These problems are greatly magnified in the patient with diverticular disease on corticosteroid medication. Active ulcerative colitis results in a weak colon wall, making examination and biopsy more hazardous. Active granulomatous colitis does not usually weaken the bowel wall, but patients experience severe pain if traction is placed on the involved segment of bowel. A narrowed segment of bowel caused by adenocarcinoma may be extremely friable and minimal pressure from the colonoscope tip may result in free perforation.

The management of colonoscopic complications only rarely requires laparotomy. Bleeding occurs at the time of polypectomy, in approximately two percent of patients; it can usually be controlled with the "hot biopsy" forceps. This is most easily accomplished if a double-channel colonoscope is available. Good exposure of the bleeding point is maintained by sucking blood through the large channel and passing the hot-biopsy forceps through the small channel. Not infrequently, bleeding may start three to five days after polypectomy. Early or late after polypectomy, persistent bleeding usually is controlled by blood replacement and peripheral venous vasopressin infusion, if necessary. If unsuccessful, arteriography should be used to identify the bleeding point and Gelfoam or blood clot then used to occlude the bleeding vessel.

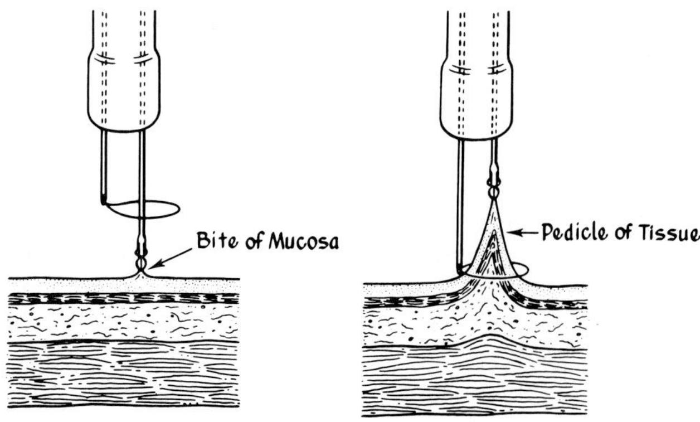

FIG. 11-15. "Macrobiopsy" of gastric mucosa (Martin TR, Onstad GR, Silvis SE, et al: Lift and cut biopsy technique for submucosal sampling. Gastrointest Endosc 23:29-30, 1976)

Perforations occur in approximately 1.0 percent of polypectomies; this is a more serious problem and requires good surgical judgement to prevent a life-endangering situation from occurring. Perforations through a segment of diseased bowel or those caused by the colonoscope being pushed through the colon wall are unlikely to close on their own; the danger of bacterial contamination of the peritoneal cavity by bowel flora is great and laparotomy to close the leak is indicated. If the patient has suspect carcinoma, biopsy confirmation on an emergency basis should be obtained, and definitive surgery undertaken. In other situations, where a small perforation has occurred through a segment of healthy colon, expectant management is indicated. This can only be recommended if the bowel preparation at the time of endoscopy was excellent.

UPPER GASTROINTESTINAL (UGI) ENDOSCOPY

Indications and Results

Upper gastrointestinal endoscopy is a clinical skill shared by the surgeon and gastroenterologist. However, the nature of the disease process usually indicates who should manage a particular patient. The gastroenterologist is asked to consult on those patients whose problems require medical management. On the other hand, cancer patients who are likely to need surgical intervention in the near future are usually directed to the surgeon.

Upper gastrointestinal endoscopy is of great use in a preoperative setting. Visualization and biopsy of pathologic lesions allow the surgeon to better define the type of operation to be performed and its extent. Endoscopy preoperatively will supply more accurate histopathological diagnosis and allow the pathophysiology of the lesion to be better defined.

ESOPHAGEAL STRICTURES. Differentiation of esophageal strictures as benign or malignant by biopsy and brush cytology is possible nearly 100 percent of the time.[111-113] Care should be taken to measure the distance of the esophageal lesion from the teeth and its extent for this is important in determining an operative approach. Benign strictures can be related to reflux (acid or alkaline) infection (monilia) or scar (from ingestion of corrosives). In patients with hiatus hernia, esophageal cancer can be ruled out, the presence of reflux and extent of associated esophagitis evaluated, and the type of mucosa (squamous or columnar as seen with Barrett's ulcer) determined by biopsy.

GASTRIC ULCER. Gastric ulcers can be visualized and their appearance evaluated as suggesting a benign (mucosal folds radiating into a flat "punched-out" ulcer) or malignant (mucosal folds terminating before they reach a "shaggy" ulcer with raised edges) process. However, no matter what the gross appearance of the ulcer, multiple biopsies from each quadrant of the ulcer must be taken, followed by brushings from the ulcer crater. If the gross appearance and histopathological examination suggest a benign process, a second endoscopic study after three weeks of conservative management should be performed. If again, malignancy is not suggested, cancer is highly unlikely, for the accuracy of diagnosis approaches 100 percent using this plan of management.

A not uncommon problem in differential diagnosis occurs in patients seen to have remarkably thickened gastric mucosal folds by UGI radiologic examination. These patients may have hypertrophic gastritis, Menetrier's disease, gastric lymphoma, or superficial spreading carcinoma of the stomach. As shown in Figure 11-15, endoscopy with "macrobiopsy" is the procedure of choice to definitively differentiate these entities.[114]

UPPER GASTROINTESTINAL BLEEDING. In patients with acute upper gastrointestinal bleeding, endoscopic study of esophagus, stomach, and duodenum will afford a correct diagnosis about 90 percent of the time, if the endoscopy is performed soon after the onset of the bleeding episode.[115] Knowledge of the patient's history is helpful but must not be relied on for diagnosis. In about half the patients with esophageal varices, the actual bleeding site is erosive gastritis or peptic ulcer. A Mallory-Weiss tear at the esophagogastric junction occurs usually without prior symptomatology, but may cause as many as 25 percent of UGI bleeding episodes.

SURGICAL FOLLOW-UP. UGI endoscopy is useful for follow-up. Gastric cancer may often first recur at a previous suture line; anastomoses are traditionally difficult to evaluate radiologically because of postoperative changes distorting the normal anatomy. The size and shape of an anastomotic channel, marginal ulceration, and inflammatory changes can be readily evaluated. One must be cautioned, however, that although endoscopy is sensitive to detect the presence of recurrent cancer intrinsic to the gut wall, recurrent disease extrinsic to intestinal lumen is difficult or impossible to evaluate. Radiologic examination is more accurate than endoscopic examination in assessing progressive extrinsic distortion of a hollow viscus.

ENDOSCOPIC RETROGRADE CHOLANGIOPANCREATOGRAPHY (ERCP). A final UGI endoscopy technique, seldom performed by surgeons, but occasionally useful to them in clinical decision-making, is ERCP. This procedure may be indicated in patients with jaundice in whom a definite diagnosis cannot be established. Percutaneous transhepatic cholangiography with the Chiba needle may also be helpful in this clinical situation (see Chapter 18 on pancreatic cancer).

Techniques

UGI endoscopy is probably the least technically demanding of the procedures discussed so far. The sedated patient is asked to gargle a local anesthetic agent while seated. Then with the patient in the right lateral decubitus position, the endoscope tip is passed on the forefinger into the pharynx. The patient is asked to swallow to open the cricopharyngeal sphincter and the endoscope passes into the esophagus. The cardioesophageal sphincter is visualized from above and then from below by retroflexing the endoscope. If the endoscope tip just below the cardioesophageal sphincter is flexed 45 degrees to the left of the plane of the esophagus, the greater curvature comes into view. Rotation of the endoscope clockwise scans the anterior surface of the stomach; rotation counterclockwise scans the posterior surface of the stomach. If the endoscope tip is repositioned just below the cardioesophageal sphincter and extended 45 degrees to the right of the esophagus, the lesser curvature is visualized. The lesser curvature is followed to the antrum and then through the pylorus into duodenum. Persistent advancement will move the tip to the ligament of Treitz and even beyond.

It should be mentioned that the techniques involved in UGI endoscopy and colonoscopy are quite different. The esophagus, stomach, and duodenum are structures whose position within the abdominal cavity is fixed; therefore, as the hollow viscus is inflated with air, the endoscope is moved readily ahead under direct vision. Not so with the colon. The sigmoid, transverse, and often ascending colon are free to move nearly anywhere within the abdominal cavity; therefore, maneuvers to reduce bowel loops by accumulating collapsed colon on the endoscope are required.

Complications

The number one rule for the UGI endoscopist is "dont't push." Perforations are rare, but they do occur, often through a cancer. If this occurs, surgery needs to be performed immediately and the pathologic lesion resected. If a perforation occurs through normal stomach or through a benign duodenal ulcer, nasogastric suctioning, intravenous antibiotics, and careful observation are usually enough. Perforation of the normal esophagus should be rare, but does occur. If the diagnosis is suspected (substernal pain, subcutaneous emphysema in the neck, elevated temperature) pharyngeal suctioning, antibiotics, and careful observation are indicated. Patients may often need surgical drainage; this is done through the neck if the perforation is in the upper mediastinum or through the left chest if it is in the middle or lower third of the esophagus.

BRONCHOSCOPY

Indications and Results

Bronchoscopy is indicated for diagnosis and staging of most pulmonary, esophageal and mediastinal lesions. Using fiberoptic instruments, lesions that distort or invade primary, secondary, or even tertiary bronchi should be readily appreciated (see Chapter 14 on lung cancer).

Techniques

Flexible fiberoptic instruments are safer, less traumatic, and better tolerated by patients; they should be used unless there are special indications for rigid instruments. Usually under general anesthesia (often prior to mediastinoscopy or other endoscopic procedure), with the patient on the back, an orotracheal tube is inserted just below the vocal cords. Through this the fiberoptic bronchoscope is inserted with the patient ventilated through a side arm on the orotracheal tube. Cytological specimens are recovered from the right and left mainstem bronchi. Biopsy and brushings for cytology are taken from suspect lesions. The pharynx is carefully inspected as the orotracheal tube is slowly pulled back.

Complications

Problems with bronchoscopy are few and are generally related to inadequate oxygenation of the patient during the procedure.

MEDIASTINOSCOPY

Mediastinoscopy as practiced today was devised by Carlens, with results reported in 1959. The midline approach through a small, low cervical incision made biopsy of lymph nodes on both sides of the superior mediastinum possible. Through this technique, visualization and biopsy of nearly all paratracheal and hilar lymph nodes in the middle and lower portions of the superior mediastinum were possible. However, Pearson has pointed out that the surgeon is anatomically limited in sampling anterior mediastinal, subaortic, and subcarinal nodes posterior to the trachea.[116] The subcarinal nodes anterior to the tracheal bifurcation are important nodes for visualization and sampling at the lowermost extent of the endoscopic dissection.

Two important anatomical features of the lymphatic drainage of the lung should be made. First, lymphatic crossover from a lung on one side of the mediastinum to lymph nodes on the opposite side is not unusual. Goldberg, Shapiro, and Glicksman reported that 28 of 46 patients (60 percent) with positive mediastinal nodes from lung carcinoma in the right upper lobe had bilateral spread of disease within the mediastinum.[117] One patient (3 percent) had only contralateral spread detected. Similarly, five of 20 patients (25 percent) with positive mediastinal nodes from left upper lobe cancer had bilateral mediastinal nodal spread and six (30 percent) had only contralateral spread detected. Bilateral spread in patients with mediastinal involvement from lower lobe lesions was 37 percent on the right and 25 percent on the left.

Borrie documented a second important anatomic fact.[118] Cancer in the upper lobe of the left lung, in addition to its previously recognized tracheo-bronchial lymphatic drainage, has alternate anterior mediastinal pathways of lymphatic spread. Carcinoma of the left upper lobe can spread directly to anterior mediastinal lymph nodes. These nodes are not available to study by cervical mediastinoscopy. However, as shown by Bowen and colleagues and Jolly and Anderson, anterior mediastinoscopy revealed lymphatic metastasis in nearly one-third of patients having previously negative cervical mediastinoscopy.[119,120] Anterior medastinoscopy was performed by inserting the mediastinoscope through the left second intercostal space so that anterior mediastinal lymph nodes could be evaluated.

Indications and Results

ASSESSMENT OF MEDIASTINAL SPREAD OF LUNG CARCINOMA. Perhaps the most widespread use of mediastinoscopy is to prevent patients unlikely from profiting from thoracotomy from undergoing this exploratory procedure. Most surgeons agree that patients with lung cancer spread to mediastinal lymph nodes carry a prolonged survival rate of less than ten percent. The definitive study of Gibbons showed that thoracotomy and an attempt to curatively resect tumors in patients with positive mediastinal biopsy is rarely, if ever, possible. In 28 patients with positive mediastinal biopsies, thoracotomy with resection was attempted; none of these 28 survived longer than two and one-half years and, at one year, only three of those with positive biopsy were alive.[121] It can be concluded that surgery alone is not proper therapy for patients with positive mediastinal nodes. Therefore, mediastinoscopy should keep patients with positive nodes from needless thoracotomy and direct them to irradiation and chemotherapy, possibly followed at a later date by pulmonary resection.

Some authors have presented data to suggest that not all lung cancer patients need mediastinoscopy prior to thoracotomy; size, location (peripheral versus central) and cell type of the primary tumor influence the incidence of positive mediastinal nodes. Hutchinson and Mills found a high incidence of mediastinal metastases associated with central tumors (63 to 100 percent) of all cell types and with peripheral lesions (63 percent) of undifferentiated cell types. However, only 8.6 percent of peripheral carcinomas of adeno- or squamous type with a radiographically normal mediastinum were found to have mediastinal metastases.[122] Baker and coworkers found only three of 40 patients with T_1 lesions (3 cm in size or less) to have mediastinal node metastases detected by mediastinoscopy. All three patients had large-cell undifferentiated tumors.[123] Therefore, in patients with small, peripherally located tumors of well-differentiated histology and a normal mediastinum by radiologic examination, mediastinoscopy need not precede thoracotomy. In this group of patients the slight risk of mediastinoscopy can be avoided.

Smith suggested that some patients may profit from thoracotomy with extensive pulmonary resection even if mediastinal nodes are positive for malignancy.[124] If patients with low grade tumor in ipsilateral mediastinal nodes are selected to proceed to resection, some five year survivors and good palliation of other patients may be achieved; irradiation as primary therapy must also be considered in this group of patients.[125]

The beneficial results of mediastinoscopy in the evaluation of patients with lung cancer has been reviewed by Baker, Stibb, and Summer.[126] Mediastinoscopy has become such a standard of practice that Goldberg, Shapiro, and Glickman have suggested that the findings at mediastinoscopy be included in the preoperative TNM staging system for lung cancer[117] (see Chapter 14 on lung cancer).

DIAGNOSIS OF MEDIASTINAL HODGKIN'S DISEASE. Vaeth, Moskowitz, and Green reviewed a group of patients with Hodgkin's disease limited to the mediastinum at the time of initial presentation. From their experience, they suggested that if bone marrow biopsy was negative, a tissue diagnosis was best established by mediastinoscopy rather than thoracotomy.[127] An attempt to resect mediastinal Hodgkin's disease is not indicated. Redding, Anagnostopoulos, and Ultman found that routine use of mediastinoscopy as a staging procedure in all patients with Hodgkin's disease similar to staging laparotomy was not indicated.[128]

ASSESSMENT OF OPERABILITY OF ESOPHAGEAL CARCINOMA. Murray, Wilcox, and Starek used combined mediastinoscopy and laparotomy to assess operability of patients with esophageal cancer.[129] Evidence of extra-esophageal mediastinal spread was detected and the proportion of patients undergoing curative resection was increased to 70 percent by the combined staging procedure. Further clinical studies utilizing this approach seem indicated.

Techniques

The patient is placed on his back with the neck hyperextended by a cushion beneath the scapulae (Figure 11-16). Under general anesthesia a 4 cm incision is made in the suprasternal notch about 2 cm above the manubrium. The strap muscles are separated in the midline so that the loose alveolar tissue anterior to the trachea can be bluntly and bloodlessly dissected using the index finger. The exploring finger moves along the anterior surface of the trachea beneath the innominate vein, innominate artery, and aortic arch to the level of the tracheal bifurcation. During this dissection the surgeon should note the position of pathologic feeling nodes for possible later biopsy.[130]

After a tunnel is prepared the mediastinoscope is introduced and advanced, keeping the anterior tracheal wall in view. Further dissection through the endoscope using a blunt suction apparatus and gauze pledgets is accomplished. In a complete exploration, which may not be necessary in every patient, both main bronchi, the azygos vein, paratracheal and parabronchial lymph nodes, the right pulmonary artery, the undersurface of the aortic arch, and the left recurrent nerve are visualized.

Biopsy sampling or removal of suspicious lymph nodes is performed; needle aspiration of structures to be removed may prevent subsequent hemorrhage from damage to vascular channels. Metal clips are useful for hemostasis and to mark biopsy sites. Preparation for emergency thoracotomy should always be made prior to beginning mediastinoscopy to deal with complications.

Complications

Foster, Murro, and Dobell reviewed 14 mediastinoscopy series published between 1968 and 1970; three (0.08 percent) deaths and 60 (1.6 percent) complications among 3742 examinations were reported. Postoperative respiratory insuf-

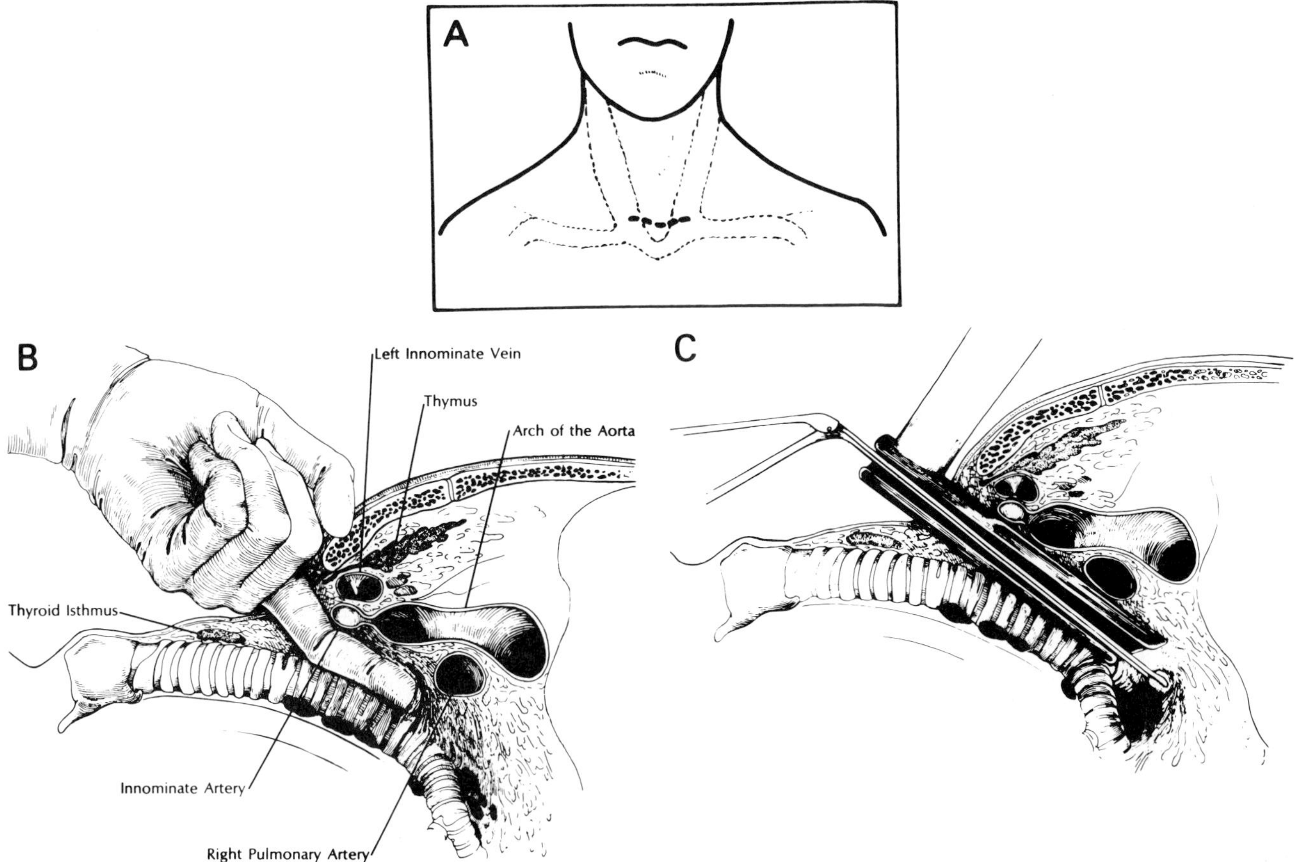

FIG. 11-16. Technique of mediastinoscopy. (Modified from Kirschner PA: Transcervical approach to the superior mediastinum. Hosp Pract, June 1970)

ficiency in two patients and cardiac arrest in one accounted for the three deaths.[131] Despite the large number of major vascular structures immediately associated with the dissection, hemorrhage is an unusual problem. Should it occur, tamponade of the operative channel with gauze seems to prevent prolonged blood loss. Other complications occasionally encountered include left recurrent nerve paresis, pneumothorax, and elevation of the right hemidiaphragm from phrenic nerve irritation.[132,133]

THORACOSCOPY

Indications and Results

Bloomberg has recently reviewed thoracoscopy from a historical and clinical perspective.[134] This procedure was originally developed to lyse pleural adhesions that prevented complete pneumothorax for the treatment of tuberculosis. Presently, rigid fiberoptic instruments and double-puncture techniques under general or local anesthesia in select patients allow safe examination and a high yield of valuable diagnostic information.

THORACOSCOPY IN THE DIAGNOSIS OF PLEURAL EFFUSIONS. Not infrequently, patients present with pleural effusions, and diagnosis is unobtainable by all the usual diagnostic modalities. These include bronchoscopy, scalene node biopsy, mediastinoscopy, thoracentesis, and closed pleural biopsy. Thoracoscopy in these settings can usually provide a definitive diagnosis and often spare the patient a thoracotomy. Pepper studied 39 patients with pleural effusion by thoracoscopy. In 31 patients a definitive diagnosis was provided by thoracic endoscopy and in 22 of those the cause of the pleural effusion was malignancy.[135] Lewis and coworkers recently reported similarly good results in this group of patients.[136]

PREOPERATIVE SCREENING OF PATIENTS WITH BRONCHIAL CARCINOMA. LeRoux found seven percent of patients with bronchial carcinoma to present with pleural fluid. Because pulmonary resection is likely to always fail in the presence of pleural metastases, LeRoux recommended preoperative thoracoscopy for patients with pleural fluid prior to lung surgery. In 82 of 139 patients pleural metastases were found, and a needless thoracotomy averted.[137]

Techniques

Oldenberg and Newhouse describe the preferred method for performing thoracoscopy.[138] The procedure is performed under local anesthesia in the operating room with adequate premedication. Patients are placed in the lateral decubitus position, the skin prepared, local anesthesia administered, and a 1.5 cm incision made in the mid-axillary line of the sixth to eighth intercostal space. The pleural space is entered bluntly and after assuring an adequate cavity the trocar and sleeve are inserted. A rigid 11 cm diameter thorascope (Stortz) is used for visualization; biopsy, cytological brushing, and photography is possible of pleural and some parenchymal lesions. Except where adhesions interfere, the parietal pleura, visceral pleura, mediastinum, and diaphragm are well visualized. Areas difficult to examine are the hilar area and the peripheral pleura at the point of insertion of the thorascope. The degree of pneumothorax is controlled by applying suction or by opening the suction channel to atmospheric pressure. At the completion of the procedure, the thorascope is removed, a rubber catheter inserted into the chest through the trocar, and then the trocar removed around the catheter. The chest tube is connected to underwater drainage until air leak, if present, has sealed.

Complications

Few complications have resulted from thoracoscopy; bleeding and persistent air leak from generous parenchymal biopsy may be the most common problems. Care must be taken not to compromise the patient's oxygenation seriously during the procedure. Patients with respiratory compromise prior to examination should probably undergo general anesthesia using a Carlen's endotracheal tube. This allows controlled collapse of one lung while maintaining optimal ventilation of the opposite one.

INTRAOPERATIVE ENDOSCOPY

Espiner and coworkers and Bombeck have related their experiences with intraoperative endoscopy.[139,140] Intraoperative colonoscopy above an obstructing cancer is indicated if the bowel can be properly prepared; such a practice will prevent concomitant polyps and cancers from being missed. With proper preparation all portions of the bowel can be seen from within the lumen by telescoping bowel over the endoscope. This may be of great help in patients with gastrointestinal bleeding of unknown source. A possible complication of this procedure is contamination of the operative site by bowel contents and resultant infection.

TUMOR MARKERS

A large number of "biologic markers" for cancer have been described and these and new markers are the focus of much ongoing research. These markers may be classified as tumor-associated oncofetal antigens, ectopic hormones (most of these are discussed in the section on paraneoplastic syndromes), enzymes, and products of tumor or host metabolism. Unfortunately, the specificity for tumor of nearly all of the tumor markers described to date is quite poor, for the metabolic and immunologic properties of tumor cells closely resemble those of normal cells. There are a large number of individuals in a population with abnormal tests for a tumor marker caused by nonmalignant conditions. Also, the sensitivity of these tests to the presence of malignancy is often lacking. The small volume of tumor present at the time an early diagnosis is made and inconsistent production of markers by the same tumor type in different individuals result in a large proportion of false negative tests. Frequent false positive and false negative tests result in a very limited use of tumor markers as a screening test for malignancy. However, use of tumor markers in a population of patients known to have cancer has impacted favorably on the management of patients with several types of tumors. Tumor markers have been used as definitive tests through which a clinician can monitor the response of a tumor to therapy and to determining disease recurrence. Decisions to start, continue or withhold treatment are frequently influenced by serial determinations of the level of a tumor marker.

In the discussion of tumor markers in this chapter, only markers currently in clinical use will be discussed. Often, specific clinical indications for use of individual tumor markers will be discussed in greater detail in the appropriate treatment chapter.

ONCOFETAL PROTEINS

Two oncofetal proteins used as biologic markers of human malignancy have evolved into valuable clinical tools for use in management of selected patients. Carcinoembryonic antigen (CEA) and alpha-fetoprotein (AFP) circulate at high levels during fetal life, but are detectable in only minute amounts in the serum or plasma of normal adults. However, in the neoplastic cell, synthesis of oncofetal proteins may begin again. Tumor cells derived from gut epithelium, a prominent CEA producer in fetal life, may regain their ability to produce CEA in large quantities. Also, tumor cells derived from liver or yolk sac tissue may begin AFP production again. This phenomenon may be consistent with the numerous theories that attribute the carcinogenic process to dedifferentration or regression of cellular processes.

Carcinoembryonic Antigen

CHARACTERIZATION OF THE CEA MOLECULE. The original studies by Gold and Freedman were thought to suggest that the CEA antigen was produced only by colon cancer cells and was of uniform molecular structure.[141] Molecular weight was estimated at 200,000 and the structure was that of a complex glycoprotein. Further studies by the group in Montreal and others showed CEA production by multiple different tissues; also, the substances that have CEA immunoreactivity consisted of a family of related glycoprotein molecules. The heterogeneity of CEA's molecular structure rests in its carbohydrate portion, which may vary from 50 to 75 percent of its composition.[142,143] The terminal carbohydrate structures are also quite variable, particularly with respect to sialic acid.[142–144] Also, several different forms are separable by differences in net charge, using ion exchange chromatography or isoelectric focusing.[143–145]

The antigenic determinants of CEA were originally thought to reside in the carbohydrate portion of the molecule. However, Vrba and coworkers at the Massachusetts General Hospital were unable to competitively inhibit CEA immunoreactivity with a wide variety of simple carbohydrates or carbohydrate chains.[146] As opposed to the variable carbohydrate structure, the protein structure of the molecule seems quite uniform. Terry and coworkers showed a constant sequence of the 24 N-terminal amino acids in several different CEA preparations.[143] Arnon and colleagues synthesized the amino terminal peptide of CEA and showed it to have CEA immunoreactivity.[147] These data strongly suggest that the internal protein structure of the molecule contains at least part of the antigenic determinants critical for immunoreactivity.

CEA PRODUCTION AND METABOLISM. The biologic function of the CEA molecule remains a mystery. Its inconstant presence in a whole host of epithelial tumors, plus the fact that its production may cease and the malignant process continue makes its production unlikely as an essential step in the malignant process. CEA, like other embryonic antigens and ectopic hormones, is an epigenetic process not essential to the neoplastic event.[148] The degree to which the neoplastic cell machinery reverts to CEA production over and above that produced by normal tissues may be a random, and therefore inconsistent, event.

Only occasionally is CEA found by immunofluorescent or immunoperoxidase studies to be within cancer cells; usually it is seen accumulating at the cell surface as a glycocalyx.[149] CEA at this extracellular site enters the extracellular space, then diffuses into lymphatics and blood capillaries to reach the systemic circulation.

It is well established that CEA is present in many normal as well as malignant tissues; also, alterations in nonmalignant tissue can result in elevated plasma CEA. CEA is present in feces of normal individuals, in normal colonic tissue, in normal liver and in bile.[150–154] The common denominator for increased plasma levels of CEA in the absence of malignancy may be a breakdown in the anatomic barrier between an epithelial surface and its underlying tissues. The structure that must be disrupted to give CEA elevations is probably the epithelial basement membrane. This structure is disrupted in conditions associated with nontumor CEA elevations such as in inflammatory bowel disease, pancreatitis, gastritis, and the bronchitis that accompanies heavy smoking.

Tumors also disrupt the epithelial basement membrane; after invasion, the tumor must release substances it produces in normal or increased amounts into the interstitial fluids and hence into lymphatics and blood. Many colonic tumors have no more CEA in their tissue than does normal colonic epithelium.[152,153,155] However, normal colonic epithelium excretes CEA into the gut; an invasive adenocarcinoma of the colon lacks this capability.

The other pathophysiologic cause for nontumor CEA elevation is decreased metabolism by the liver. There is strong evidence that CEA degradation and excretion takes place almost exclusively in the liver.[154,156–160] Direct evidence for a prominent role for the liver in CEA metabolism comes from the clinical studies of Lurie and colleagues.[161] Patients with elevated CEA levels and biliary tract obstruction from stones were studied pre- and postoperatively. CEA levels returned to normal in patients who had successful relief of biliary obstruction. Recent studies by Lowenstein and coworkers, showed that cirrhotic livers excreted less CEA into the duodenal juice, even when plasma CEA levels were elevated.[162] From these studies it was clear that decreased excretion of CEA from biliary obstruction or cirrhosis can result in elevated plasma CEA levels.

NONTUMOR CEA ELEVATIONS. Zamcheck and collaborators at the Boston City Hospital established through clinical studies that CEA elevations could result from many nontumor disease processes. Alcoholic patients often had CEA levels greater than 2.5 ng/ml but less than 10 ng/ml. Forty-five percent of 88 patients with alcoholic liver disease had positive CEA tests, whereas none of 14 patients with nonalcoholic liver disease had positive CEA assays.[153,163,164]

Numerous other nontumor causes of CEA elevation have been reported: pancreatitis, recent blood transfusion, ulcerative colitis, heavy cigarette smoking, gastritis following partial gastrectomy, and colonic polpys.[165–182]

The multiple nontumor causes for elevated CEA may cause a clinician considerable difficulty as he or she seeks to utilize the CEA test in patient management decisions. The following suggestions can be made to assist in differentiating tumor from nontumor CEA elevations. First, the magnitude of the elevation is important. CEA elevations in the 2.5 ng/ml to 10 ng/ml range may be from tumor or nontumor. However, nontumor CEA elevations greater than 10 ng/ml are very unlikely without jaundice and other obvious signs of biliary tract obstruction. Therefore, only patients with moderate CEA elevations (2.5–10 ng/ml range) are those likely to create clinical dilemmas. In these patients the clinician must make a search for possible nontumor causes of CEA elevations. Hepatic cirrhosis and hepatitis, heavy smoking, and gastrointestinal inflammatory states are the most common causes of these nontumor elevations. Most commonly, as emphasized by Gardner and coworkers, these conditions are usually in an active state when associated with plasma CEA elevations.[176] If present in a state of complete remission, it is not safe to assume they are responsible for an elevated CEA. These clinical entities can usually be identified by a careful medical history and routine laboratory and radiologic tests. Liver function tests including tests for hepatitis antigens are needed. Sugarbaker suggested that liver biopsy as a routine in all patients undergoing surgery for colorectal cancer should be performed to assist in interpreting postoperative serial CEA assays.[183]

Second, to differentiate tumor from nontumor CEA elevation, several sequential CEA assays as opposed to individual determinations may be required. If the titer is progressively rising, cancer is the most likely cause; if the serial titers are erratic, with both elevated and normal values, nontumor causes are more common.

The first successful efforts to distinguish tumor CEA from nontumor CEA elevation on a laboratory basis were recently reported by Lowenstein and colleagues.[162] Duodenal juice was collected through a double lumen gastroduodenal (Dreiling) tube and CEA outputs determined for 100 minutes. Normal patients had duodenal CEA outputs of less than 150 ng/min. Six of seven patients with CEA associated cancers had duodenal outputs of greater than 150 ng/min. Seven of nine patients with benign liver disease or extrahepatic biliary obstruction had normal duodenal CEA outputs. Lowenstein and coworkers suggested that determinations of duodenal juice CEA may assist the oncologist in two ways: (1) It may detect increased CEA production even prior to the occurrence of elevated circulating levels. This may provide a more sensitive CEA assay system than currently available using plasma sampling. (2) Determinations of duodenal juice CEA may assist in distinguishing between increased plasma CEA due to increased production (by cancer or inflammatory diseases) and that due to impaired metabolism and excretion due to liver disease.

A second approach to the specificity problem was that taken by Nakamura, Plow, and Edgington.[184] They devised a radioimmunoassay for CEA-S which may yield fewer false positive results than CEA.

CEA IN THE DIAGNOSIS OF PRIMARY AND RECURRENT CANCER. McNeil and Adelstein in their studies on the interpretation of laboratory tests show how a laboratory test is "only as good as the patient population in whom it is employed."[1] This explains how CEA can be of little or no value in mass screening for cancer, but of great value for detection of recurrence in a high risk population such as postoperative colorectal cancer patients.[185–187] Data obtained from screening asymptomatic populations can be summarized as *"too little information too late."*[188–190] Unfortunately, the patients with advanced primary tumors in whom a low cure rate is expected generally have CEA levels greater than 2.5 ng/ml and good prognosis cancers are missed because CEA levels are normal.

Ona and coworkers showed that CEA may be of value when used in a population of patients suspect of having pancreatic cancer.[191] They reported 23 of 27 patients (85 percent) with pancreatic cancer had elevated CEA assays. The CEA assay was more frequently positive in patients with cancer of the pancreas than were any other diagnostic tests used, including upper gastrointestinal series, hypotonic duodenography, celial arteriography, and percutaneous transhepatic cholangiography. Also, if CEA levels greater than 10 ng/ml were assumed to indicate liver disease, CEA detected liver metastasis in more patients than did the liver scan.

Sugarbaker, Beard, and Drum combined the liver scan and CEA as a composite in patients with suspect hepatic recurrence of breast cancer.[192] In this study the composite test was positive if both tests were positive, negative if both tests were negative and equivocal (further studies indicated) if the results disagreed. The number of false positive scans was markedly reduced by the composite. The false positive rate for the liver scan was 14 percent and for the CEA assay 25 percent; however, there were no false positive composite tests. Similar studies have been reported by McCartney and Hoffer for composites of liver scan plus CEA and of barium enema plus CEA.[193,194]

An interesting use for anti-CEA antibody has recently been developed by Goldenberg and coworkers at the University of Kentucky.[195] This group took anti-CEA antibody made in goats, coupled it to radioactive iodine and, after injecting this into cancer patients, performed total body isotope scans. Tumor location could be demonstrated at 48 hours after injection in almost all patients studied. Circulating antigen levels up to 350 μg/ml did not prevent successful tumor imaging.

Perhaps the most important current use of CEA is as an indicator of early recurrent colorectal cancer and guide to selected second-look surgery. Many studies suggested that progressively rising serial CEA assays were in many patients the first signal of recurrent cancer.[183,196–200] Martin and colleagues at Ohio State University performed second-look surgery on 60 patients because of rising CEA levels. In 59, recurrent tumor was found at re-exploration, or occurred later. In 60.5 percent of patients studied prospectively, repeat excision for cure was reported. Results of long-term survival in this group of patients will be of great interest.[201]

The high percentage of early elevations of CEA in patients with hepatic metastases, plus the development of resection techniques to remove liver metastases but preserve liver parenchyma, suggests that salvage of patients with early hepatic metastatic disease may be possible.[202,203] Successful resection of metastatic colorectal cancer in the liver, similar to the resection of osteosarcoma in the lungs, may be possible.[204,205]

Rittgers and colleagues interjected a timely precautionary note regarding transient CEA elevations occasionally seen following resection of colorectal cancer.[206] Nine of 25 patients showed transient elevations without cancer recurrence upon follow-up and close clinical investigation. Trends in serial CEA titers rather than isolated CEA values must be used, along with all other clinical and laboratory data available, in making the decision to perform second-look surgery.

CEA IN ASSESSING PROGNOSIS IN PATIENTS WITH KNOWN MALIGNANCY. Perhaps the most crucial clinical assessment of a patient with cancer is the initial one made immediately after the diagnosis is established and prior to any definitive therapy. Laurence and coworkers and Booth and colleagues suggested that CEA tests done at the time of initial patient evaluation were of prognostic value.[189,207] This was determined retrospectively by correlating preoperative CEA levels with Dukes Classification in patients with colorectal cancer. Wanebo and coworkers at the Memorial-Sloan Kettering Cancer Center showed conclusively that recurrence rates were higher in patients with Dukes B and Dukes C lesions who had preoperative levels higher than 5 ng/ml. Also, as the preoperative CEA level increased, the mean time to recurrence decreased as a linear inverse correlation.[202]

Although preoperative CEA blood tests are prognostic indicators, nevertheless some patients with very large Dukes C, Dukes D, or even metastatic tumors may have normal CEA assays. This is likely due to decreased production or decreased release of CEA by the tumor. Poorly differentiated tumors, even though often or large mass, often are associated with normal circulating CEA values.[152,183,189,208] Shamberg showed definitively that preoperative plasma CEA levels were statistically significantly related to the degree of tumor differentiation.* The consistency of this observation is not always appreciated clinically, for primary tumor size also correlates with circulating CEA levels, and poorly differentiated tumors

* Shamberg JF: Personal communication

with lesser CEA production tend to be of larger size and to invade more deeply. Consequently, in poorly differentiated tumors, the variables of tumor differentiation and tumor size conflict and tend, therefore, to nullify each other.

CEA has been identified as a prognosticator in several other tumors besides colorectal cancer. Kalser and coworkers found tha pancreatic cancer patients with locally unresectable or metastatic carcinoma had a significantly longer survival if CEA was normal at the time of diagnosis.[209] Wang and coworkers showed a relationship between plasma CEA and prognosis in women with breast cancer.[210] Patients after mastectomy with CEA levels above 2.5 ng/ml had a significantly ($P < 0.001$) more rapid recurrence rate than similar patients with CEA levels below this level. At two years after mastectomy the disease had recurred in 65 percent of the patients with CEA greater than 2.5 ng/ml compared to 20 percent of those with CEA less than 2.5 ng/ml. Haagensen and others, and Meyers and coworkers both also showed a poor prognosis in patients with elevated postmastectomy CEA levels.[211,212] Haagensen and colleagues also showed an increased incidence of tumor recurrence with preoperative CEA levels greater than 3 ng/ml. Tormey and Waalkes noted that patients with metastatic breast cancer with CEA greater than 5 ng/ml prior to treatment had lower response rates and a shorter time to treatment failure than did patients with CEA equal to or less than 5 ng/ml.[213]

Dent and coworkers reported from Hamilton, Ontario on the prognostic significance of pretreatment CEA values in patients with bronchogenic carcinoma.[214] The use of the CEA assay for diagnostic purposes was somewhat limited, for heavy smokers frequently have elevated CEA levels in the absence of cancer. In groups of nonsmokers, smokers, patients with limited bronchogenic cancer, patients with inoperable cancer, and patients with metastatic cancer there were different and progressively higher mean CEA values. Concannon and colleagues made the interesting observation that all epidermoid and adenocarcinoma patients in a series of 147 who had pretreatment CEA levels greater than 6 μg/ml died in less than three years.[215]

SERIAL CEA IN MONITORING CANCER THERAPY. Serial CEA titers during a period of intensive therapy may also be used as a monitor of the effectiveness of a treatment regimen. After surgical excision of a colorectal cancer, elevated preoperative CEA levels usually fall into the normal range of 2.5 ng/ml or less. Several groups have noted that failure of postoperative CEA values to fall into the normal range is associated with poor prognosis.[196,216–220] In the careful report from the Royal Victoria Hospital, Montreal, colorectal cancer patients were divided into three groups according to their preoperative and postoperative CEA levels.[220] Thirty-six patients (Group 1) had preoperative and postoperative CEA values less than 2.5 ng/ml. Eleven patients (Group 2) had a preoperative CEA greater than 2.5 ng/ml but the postoperative value failed to decline below 2.5 mg/ml. In Group 1, 14 percent of patients had recurred by 19 months postoperatively, in Group 2, 18 percent of patients had recurred, while in Group 3, 73 percent of patients had recurred (Fig. 11-17).

Vider and colleagues, Sugarbaker and colleagues, and

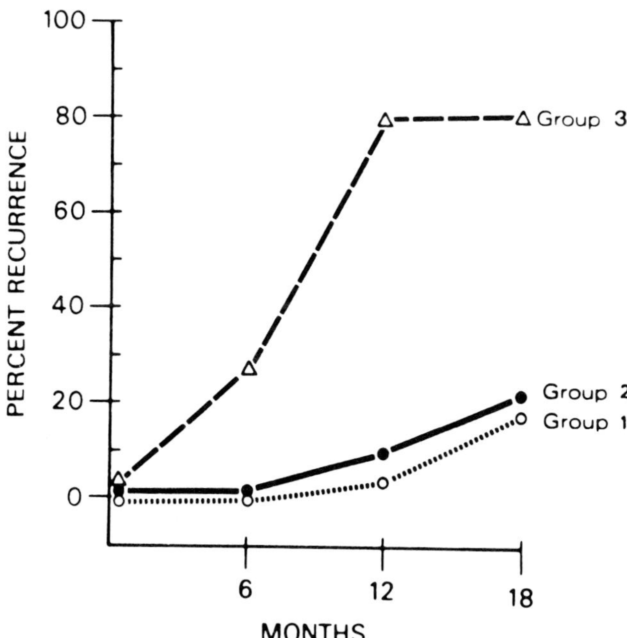

FIG. 11-17. Recurrence rates of colonic cancer after curative surgery. Group 1 preoperative and postoperative CEA values < 2.5 μg/ml; Group 2 preoperative value > 2.5 μg/ml. Postoperative value < 2.5 μg/ml; Group 3 preoperative and postoperative values > 2.5 μg/ml. (Oh JH, MacLean LD: Prognostic use of preoperative and immediate postoperative carcinoembryonic antigen determinations in colonic cancer. Can J Surg 20:64-67, 1977)

Donaldson and coworkers reported a correlation of CEA levels and the clinical response to radiation therapy.[221–224] Mulcare and LoGerfo noted good correlations between the pattern of change of serial CEA assays and the patients response to systemic chemotherapy.[225] They and other groups emphasize that the CEA test was useful in those cancer patients with elevated CEA in the plasma, but was of no help if the titer was not increased.[226–228]

Herrera and coworkers offer an important *caveat* in interpreting serial CEA values in patients treated with nitrosourea compounds.[226] In these patients they report a tendency to lower CEA levels regardless of the patient's tumor response to the drug. This could be due to the nitrosoureas producing a diffuse block of cellular activity, including glycoprotein production both at the nucleolus and in the cytoplasm.

In summary, serial CEA assays in patients whose tumors produce CEA elevations in the blood can be a valuable monitor of treatment. The adequacy of surgical resection, the likelihood of disease control by radiation therapy, and the response to systemic chemotherapy can be assessed in many patients. Of course, whenever possible, a correlation of serial CEA levels with other clinical assessments should be made.

Alphafetoprotein (AFP)

AFP is a serum protein similar in size, structure, and amino acid composition to serum albumin; it is present in only minute amounts in the serum of humans one week after

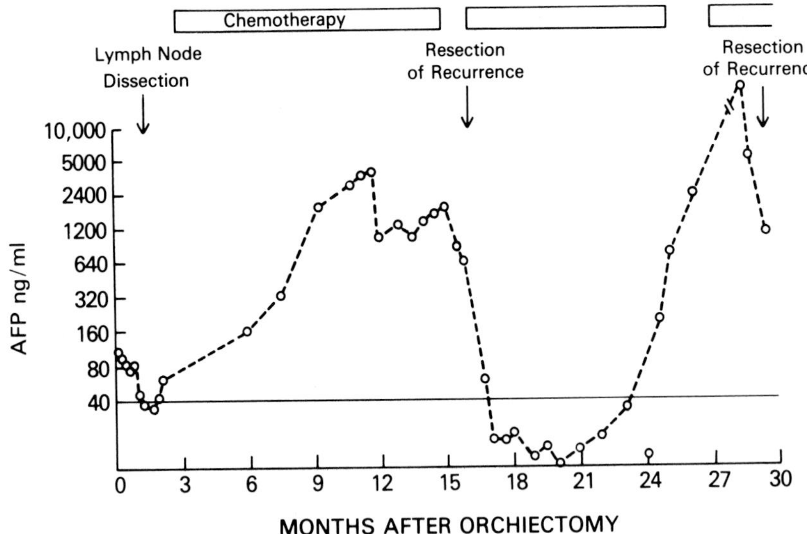

FIG. 11-18. Use of alphafetoprotein in the management of a patient with embryonal carcinoma of the testicle with an element of choriocarcinoma. Surgical resection of tumor mass resulted in marked reductions in AFP levels. Chemotherapy did not prevent regrowth of tumor in this patient. (Modified from Javadpour N, McIntire R, Waldmann TA, et al: The role of radioimmunoassay of serum alphafetoprotein and human chorionic gonadotropin in the intensive chemotherapy and surgery of metastatic testicular tumors. J Urol 119:759-762, 1978)

birth, but is present in high concentration prenatally. This oncofetal protein was identified in cord blood of human infants by electrophoresis in 1957 by Bergstrand and Czar and designated as X component.[229] In 1963 Abelev and coworkers associated an alpha migrating protein, normally detected only in pregnancy, as identical to a protein found in mice-bearing transplanted hepatocellular carcinomas.[230] Shortly thereafter, Tatarinov reported the presence of a fetal protein in patients with hepatocellular carcinoma.[231] Development of sensitive radioimmunoassays allowed precise quantitation of AFP levels.[232-234] Extensive clinical investigation has determined the tumor and nontumor processes associated with AFP elevation and led the way to useful application of this tumor marker in oncology.

NONTUMOR AFP ELEVATIONS. During prenatal development, AFP reaches its peak at 15 weeks of gestation in the fetus; maternal levels of AFP are also elevated, but more transiently. Some conditions such as anencephaly, esophageal artresia, intrauterine fetal distress, and congenital nephrosis may result in prolonged high concentrations of AFP. These conditions probably result in decreased turnover by AFP by the fetus.

Rapid generation of liver tissue, normally present in the fetus, may be caused by a variety of conditions in the adult and result in AFP elevations. Partial hepatectomy, chemically induced liver necrosis, viral hepatitis all result in liver damage, then hepatocyte proliferation.[235,236]

Exposure to chemical hepatocarcinogens is associated with AFP elevations in animals followed by a decline toward normal levels. If an adequate dose of carcinogen is continued long enough to result in malignant change, the decline in AFP is followed by a progressive rise that reflects an accumulation of hepatic tumor mass.[237]

AFP IN THE DIAGNOSIS AND MONITORING OF HEPATIC, YOLK SAC, AND SOME GASTROINTESTINAL TUMORS. Sell and Becker refer to a report from within the Peoples Republic of China in which AFP was successfully used to screen populations for primary liver cancer. More than 490,000 persons were screened, with 75 asymptomatic patients with liver cancer being detected and only seven false positive tests recorded.[238]

The widespread clinical use of AFP is to follow tumor growth and the effects of therapy. Nearly 80 percent of Africans with hepatoma have elevated AFP tests. However, American and English patients show AFP elevation in only about 30 percent of patients.[239] Some have speculated that differences in seropositivity may vary with the etiologic factors responsible for the appearance of the hepatoma.

Teratocarcinomas that contain elements of yolk sac tumor almost invariably result in AFP elevations unless tumor mass is minute. Nonseminomatous testicular tumors and teratocarcinoma of the ovary constitute the tumors in this group. The clinical use of AFP in the management of patients with embryonal carcinoma of the testis has been reviewed by Javadpour and Bergman and an example of the clinical use of AFP in patient management is shown in Figure 11-18.[240,241]

AFP is also found in smaller quantities in the fetal gut. It may not be surprising, therefore, that some patients with gastrointestinal cancer show AFP elevations. Waldmann and McIntire in a sensitive double antibody radioimmunoassay for AFP found 23 percent of 44 patients with pancreatic carcinoma, 18 percent of 91 patients with gastric carcinoma and five to seven percent with colonic and bronchogenic carcinoma having AFP elevations.

Pancreatic Oncofetal Antigen (POA)

Banwo, Versey, and Hobbs in 1974 described a new oncofetal antigen which was utilized for the detection of pancreatic cancer.[242] Wood and Moosa used an assay for POA, CEA, and AFP to prospectively evaluate 136 patients with intra-abdominal disease, 38 were subsequently shown to have pancreatic cancer. The true positive rate (sensitivity) of POA was 60 percent, of CEA, 48 percent, and of AFP, 33 percent. The true negative rate (specificity) for POA was 94 percent, for CEA 75 percent, and for AFP, 71 percent.[243] The conclusions from this study should be that if POA is positive, pancreatic cancer is the likely diagnosis; if the test is negative, a further search for pancreatic cancer must proceed. A full 40 percent of negative tests are false negatives.

ECTOPIC HORMONES—HUMAN CHORIONIC GONADOTROPIN

Only a few tumors consistently produce an ectopic hormone that can be used as a circulating marker in all patients. Those tumors that *consistently* produce a hormone are generally of neuroendocrine origin, so are by definition not "ectopic" hormone producers. Hormone production and the clinical manifestations of endocrine tumors are discussed in Chapter 28 on endocrine tumors; ectopic hormone production by tumors and the associated clinical findings are discussed in the chapter on paraneoplastic syndromes. Here we focus on an ectopic hormone that, although produced in large amounts, has few if any clinical signs or symptoms. In this section the use of human chorionic gonadotropin (hCG) as a tumor marker is discussed. Accurate measurement of low levels of hCG activity was not possible before 1972 because of the inherent biologic and immunologic cross reaction between luteinizing hormone (hLH) and hCG. Therefore, these two hormones were indistinguishable in a precipitive reaction or radiommunoassay utilizing antibody against the intact molecule. Normal levels of endogenous pituitary hLH in a conventional radioimmunoassay for hCG was measured as hCG, so that a cut-off point had to be established to rule out false positive results. Therefore, low levels of circulating hCG went undetected. However, Vaitukaitis and her coworkers developed a radioimmunoassay to measure hCG in the presence of hLH by utilizing an antibody which is specific for the beta subunit chain of hCG.[244] The clinical use of this subunit radioimmunoassay was the culmination of much biochemical effort directed toward elucidating the structure of several glycoprotein hormones normally produced by the pituitary. In fact, the alpha subunits of hCG, hLH, human follicle-stimulating hormone, and human thyroid-stimulating hormone have been found to be interchangeable; the immunological specificity of each hormone appears to be determined by its beta subunit.[245]

Human chorionic gonadotropin is normally produced only by the placenta and is the basis for most tests for pregnancy. Indeed, the presence of elevated levels of beta hCG can be detected within seven to ten days following implantation of the fertilized egg in the uterus.[246] The most common use of beta hCG in oncology comes in the detection, monitoring of therapy and follow-up of placental and testicular tumors.[247,248] The beta hCG assay has been shown to reflect the mass of choriocarcinoma and to accurately assess any recurrence of tumor (Fig. 11-19). Also, Braunstein and coworkers and Vaitukaitis found elevated hCG in the sera of patients with liver, breast, stomach and ovarian tumors.[249,250] Javadpour and Bergman have recently summarized the important contribution the use of beta hCG has made to the management of nonseminomatous testicular cancer.[240]

Surprisingly, in spite of the very high levels of circulating hCG with some tumors, no clinical manifestations are consistently present. Gynecomastia in men with testicular tumor and precocious puberty in boys with teratomas are the most common findings. Frequently, the clinical syndrome may precede localization of the tumor.

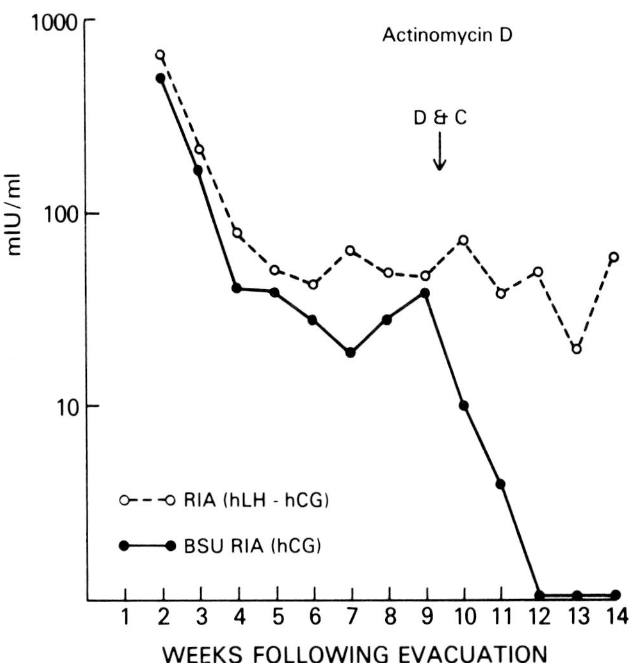

FIG. 11-19. Use of beta hCG assay in the management of a patient with hydatidiform mole. Following uterine evacuation of a molar pregnancy beta hCG activity remained elevated; levels returned to normal after D&C plus actinomycin administration. (Modified from Goldstein DP, Kozasa TS, Skariñ AT: The clinical application of a specific radioimmunoassay for human chorionic gonadotropin in trophoblastic and nontrophoblastic tumors. Surg Gynecol Obstet 138:747-751, 1974)

SERUM ENZYMES AS TUMOR MARKERS

As a tumor progresses, many alterations in host metabolism may be found. One change which may be found by serum or plasma assay is in enzyme activity. Because of uncontrolled metabolic activities, some tumors release increased amounts of various enzymes. The activity of a circulating enzyme may then be used to detect the presence or absence of tumors or to estimate its increasing or decreasing mass. Because these enzymes are not consistently produced by most tumor types, they must be considered of only occasional utility in clinical management.

The tumor enzymes currently in clinical use will be discussed in this section; the alterations in serum enzyme levels that result from tumor impairing the function of surrounding tissue (usually liver) is discussed in the section on laboratory diagnosis of hepatic metastases.

Placental Alkaline Phosphatase (Regan Isoenzyme)

Stalbach and coworkers described the ectopic synthesis of placental alkaline phosphatase by a variety of tumors.[251] This enzyme was biochemically and immunologically indistinguishable from that normally produced within the placenta. Changes in serum levels were shown to correlate with a clinical assessment of tumor response to chemotherapy followed by subsequent tumor progression. In 27 patients with elevated placental alkaline phosphatase, only about half had elevated total serum alkaline phosphatase; starch gel electrophoresis without and with antiserum to placental alkaline phosphatase was necessary to reliably detect increased quantities of this enzyme in serum. Placental alkaline phosphatase was found to be elevated in 40 percent of patients with seminoma.[252]

Bone Alkaline Phosphatase

Thorpe and coworkers reported that elevated preoperative alkaline phosphatase levels in patients with osteogenic sarcoma indicated a poor prognosis. Twelve of 17 patients with elevated preoperative enzyme levels recurred ($P < .05$). Unfortunately, postoperative alkaline phosphatase levels were found to have no relationship to recurrence. It may be that the bulk of tumor that is clinically detectable (usually in the lungs) is not sufficient to result in serum enzyme elevations over and above that normally produced.[253]

Levine and Rosenberg found that elevated tissue alkaline phosphatase levels were present in 17 patients, 16 of whom developed pulmonary metastases. It may be that an aggressive biologic behavior of a primary osteosarcoma is reflected by its production of alkaline phosphatase.[254]

Acid Phosphatase and Prostatic Acid Phosphatase

The enzyme acid phosphatase is abundant in the human prostate gland following puberty. When prostatic carcinoma develops the serum acid phosphatase level may become markedly increased, especially if bony metastases are present. However, enzymes with acid phosphatase activity are present in erythrocytes, leucocytes, platelets, liver, spleen, kidney, and other tissue. Hemolysis of blood and cytolysis within a large number of organs will result in serum elevations of acid phosphatase; these conditions will, therefore, result in a false positive test for prostatic cancer. Romas, Rose, and Tannenbaum called attention to the large number of nonprostatic disorders that may result in elevation of this enzyme.[255]

Several groups have successfully separated prostatic acid phosphatase as a purified protein. This was then used to prepare antiprostatic acid phosphatase serums in rabbits. Human acid phosphatase from liver, lung pancreas, and human cell cultures did not cross react. The use of specific antisera has led to the development of a radioimmunoassay by several laboratories. Foti found that use of the radioimmunoassay may allow detection of over half the cases of intracapsular prostatic carcinoma. The enzyme method detected only 10 to 20 percent of these tumors.[256] Also, several groups have reported favorable results with the use of the immunoassay on bone marrow fluid to detect prostatic cancer spread to the marrow cavity.[257] However, false positive results appear to preclude use of prostatic acid phosphatase radioimmunoassay for use as a screening test for asymptomatic carcinoma of the prostate.[258]

ACUTE PHASE PROTEINS

Cancer patients frequently show altered levels of normally occurring serum proteins. In multiple studies, acute phase proteins normally synthesized in the liver (haptoglobin, alpha 1-acid glycoprotein, and alpha 1-antitrypsis) were increased. Some normally occurring proteins (alpha 2HS-glycoprotein, prealbumin, and albumin) were often depressed in cancer patients. The immunosuppressive nature of some serum glycoproteins has been proposed as a mechanism whereby host immune responses to tumor growth may be diminished. Recently, Israel and Edelstein have reviewed data which would support this mechanism of immunosuppression and have suggested plasmaphoresis as a treatment for patients with disseminated cancer.[259] Baskies and Chretien and coworkers correlated serum levels of acute phase proteins with tumor extent and the immune status of patients as assessed by lymphocyte reactivity to PHA and delayed type hypersensitivity to skin testing with DNCB. Serum proteins were more closely related to the immune status of the patient than to tumor extent. These authors suggest that further attempts to improve the immune status of cancer patients by alterations in serum glycoprotein levels should be made in hopes of impacting favorably on the host–tumor relationship.[260]

COMBINED DETERMINATIONS OF TUMOR MARKERS

Because of the unpredictable occurrence of an elevation of a single tumor marker in a particular individual, some researchers have suggested that multiple markers be evaluated in each tumor patient. Ravry and coworkers reported on the combined use of CEA and AFP in 37 gastric cancer patients with distant metastases. Nine (24 percent) had abnormal CEA and 12 (32 percent) had abnormal AFP. Only 1 patient had both elevated CEA and AFP, so that the combined assays were positive in 20 of 37 patients (54 percent).[261] Similarly, Tormey and colleagues used CEA, N2, N2-dimethyl-guanosine, and hCG in patients with breast cancer. The performance of all three tests in each patient revealed one or more abnormalities in 97 percent of 60 patients with distant metastases and 67 percent of 15 patients with positive nodes.[262] The work by Munjal and colleagues with breast cancer should also be noted.[263] Javadpour and Millan have studied the combined use of placental alkaline phosphatase, gamma glutamyl transferase, and beta hCG in patients with testicular cancer; over 90 percent of patients with seminoma have elevated serum levels of at least one of these markers.[252]

STAGING

The objective of this section is to assemble a constellation of tumor and host characteristics that will provide an accurate prognosis. The *prognosis* is the outcome of a disease. This section will outline the general principles of cancer staging, and relate these principles to the currently employed TNM cancer staging system. Also, some of the problems and inadequacies with the current "state of the art" as relates to cancer staging will be pointed out. For the purposes of this discussion of staging, it is assumed that optimal treatments are being rendered, and yet treatment failure remains a significant problem.

IMPORTANCE OF CANCER STAGING

The prognosis as determined by cancer staging is of paramount importance to *patient, physician, and clinical researcher*. The patient asks his physician "What is my prognosis (forecast)?" "Will I live or die?" "If I am to die—when?" Patients need to prepare in a timely fashion multiple social, education, and administrative aspects of their life in accord with the prognosis for cure. An accurate prognosis allows the physician to meaningfully *counsel* the patient in this regard.

The physician must also use the prognosis as his guide for *planning treatment*. If the prognosis is good, radical treatment can be a major contribution to patient care. On the other hand, if the outlook is hopeless, the physician must refrain from inflicting unnecessary morbidity. The risk–gain judgments often faced daily in cancer management would be greatly facilitated by accurate and exacting cancer staging which could reliably be translated into a definitive prognosis.

Additionally, *clinical trials* of new treatment modalities require that homogenous groups of patients be available for comparison. If prognosis cannot be accurately determined, spurious conclusions are possible, since undefined and therefore nonstratifiable variables, rather than the treatments under comparison, determine the outcome of a study. The need for accurate prognosis is of greater importance when projected new therapies hold promise for only a minor incremental improvement over the existing therapy.

CANCER STAGING EQUIVALENT TO A DETERMINATION OF METASTATIC POTENTIAL

For most common adult malignancies, a development of systemic metastases is equivalent to death from the disease. Thus, we find that for each stage of a given malignancy—other than that of widespread dissemination—the objective of cancer staging is to assess the eventual risk for systemic metastasis. Accurate assessment of this property of *metastatic potential* of a given tumor or class of tumors is therefore the essential objective of cancer staging and the key determinant of prognosis.

TUMOR CHARACTERISTICS AFFECTING PROGNOSIS

Table 11–5 lists the characteristics of a primary neoplasm which are known to affect prognosis and therefore can enter into a cancer staging system. First, the *organ of origin* is important. As an obvious example, by virtue of strategic location, a benign brain tumor can be rapidly lethal, while an equal tumor mass in the viscera, breast, or skin proves relatively harmless. The interrelationship of satisfactory treatment and cancer staging, in this comparison, is of obvious importance. Furthermore, the propensity for metastasis seems regulated in an unexplained way by the organ of origin. For example, squamous cell carcinoma of the skin is more than 95 percent curable, while a histologically identical squamous cell carcinoma of the lung or esophagus is about 95 percent lethal. Mucosal melanoma is highly lethal, while cutaneous melanoma carries a reasonable cure rate. Therefore, the organ of origin is a basic tumor characteristic which greatly affects prognosis and, therefore, cancer staging.

TABLE 11-5. Tumor Characteristics of Prognostic Importance

1. Organ of origin.
2. Histologic (histogenetic) classification
3. Age of patient
4. Extent of established dissemination
   Primary
   Regional nodes
   Distant metastases
5. Metastatic potential of tumors without distant metastases

The histological type of neoplasm, along with the organ of origin, likewise affects prognosis. The prognosis for malignancies of different histogenetic types, even within the same organ system, can vary greatly. A comparison of cutaneous melanoma and cutaneous basal cell carcinoma or a comparison of small cell carcinoma of the lung with squamous cell carcinoma of the lung emphasizes the importance of histologic classification as a major factor in cancer staging and, therefore, prognosis.

It should be emphasized that for some malignancies, these two characteristics alone (organ of origin and histologic type) are sufficient to establish the prognosis and therefore provide accurate cancer staging. Diagnoses characterized as small cell carcinoma of the lung, undifferentiated carcinoma of the thyroid, acute myeloid leukemia, and so forth designate a nearly uniformly fatal prognosis and unfortunately designate a timeframe for patient demise.

However, for the majority of the common malignancies—colon, lung, breast, prostate, head and neck carcinoma, and so forth—these two characteristics are not sufficient to establish prognosis for a given patient. For instance, approximately 50 percent of women with adenocarcinoma of the breast are cured. Forty-five percent of adults with adenocarcinoma of the colon and 40 to 60 percent of women with carcinoma of the cervix are cured. Therefore, it has long been recognized that other tumor characteristics must be found which would better predict outcome and effectively stage these lesions.

Extent of Established Dissemination

Observations of the clinical progression of human malignancy from the growth at the primary site, in a delayed fashion through regional lymphatics and lymph nodes, and subsequently to distant organ sites, were extensively recorded in the literature of the late 19th and early 20th century. These clinical and pathologic observations on human cancer growth and metastasis were therapeutically translated into cancer operations designed to remove the primary tumor *en bloc* with regional lymph nodes, unless systemic metastasis was apparent. The radical mastectomy, abdominoperineal resection, and neck and jaw resection are all examples of such procedures. Analyses of the surgical specimens resected were correlated with the eventual patient prognosis, and it became established that *the extent of established tumor dissemination was the most significant factor in determining prognosis.* The staging systems published by Dukes for carcinoma of the colon and by Haagensen for carcinoma of the breast, emphasized the dominant effect which established tumor dissemination had on patient prognosis.[264,265] Clinical and histologic assessment of the extent of regional dissemination became the most important variables integrated into these two published staging systems, and have greatly influenced the design of subsequent staging systems, including the TNM staging system devised by the American Joint Committee on Cancer Staging and End Result Reporting.[266]

In these early published staging systems, an objective was to predict from the examination of a surgical specimen whether the subsequent phase of the cascade of dissemination from primary site to regional lymph nodes to systemic sites would be reached. Or, was surgical intervention in a particular patient likely to interrupt the natural history of the cancer? Thus, one of the central objectives of assembling the characteristics of a given stage of malignancy became to predict whether the next stage of the cascade of neoplastic progression would be reached.

It was apparent from these studies that once the primary tumor had reached the regional lymph nodes, the involvement and characterization of involvement of regional lymph nodes was a more important prognostic determinant than the characteristics of the primary tumor. Therefore, for a primary malignancy the most important part of staging is to assemble a set of characteristics which predict whether or not regional lymph nodes are occultly involved, or will subsequently become involved with time. Additionally, one seeks descriptors for eventual systemic spread.

CHARACTERISTICS OF PRIMARY TUMORS PREDICTIVE OF REGIONAL NODE OR DISTANT METASTASIS

If a given malignancy is localized by clinical and diagnostic criteria to the primary site at the organ of origin, cancer staging attempts to predict its metastatic potential to clinically uninvolved regional lymph nodes and also the metastatic potential for eventual distant metastasis. The secondary objective with significant surgical and radiotherapeutic implications for many "localized" primary malignancies is to determine the risk for occult regional nodal metastasis. Table 11-6 lists the major primary tumor characteristics which have been shown to correlate with regional node systemic metastasis. There are three types of partially interrelated primary tumor characteristics affecting metastatic potential. First, and most objectively measured for clinically accessible cancers, is the measured *tumor size.* Tumor size correlates well with the statistical probability for regional metastasis in adenocarcinoma of the breast with survival in carcinoma of the lung. This readily measured and also reproducible tumor characteristic has been integrated extensively into the T (primary) stage of assessment of many clinical cancers, as published in the Manual for Staging Cancer.

The relative inadequacy of size alone in predicting metastatic potential, however, is obvious. Some very large tumors fail to metastasize, while some small (even clinically occult) carcinomas of the breast metastasize early.

TABLE 11-6. Primary Tumor Characteristics Predictive of Regional and/or Systemic Metastasis

1. Size (diameter, volume).
2. Extent of local invasion:
   a. Clinical:
      Skin retraction, ulceration, edema
      Fixation to bone or muscle
      Obstruction, perforation of bowel, ureters, etc.
      Adjacent visceral organ invasion
      Nerve paralyses
   b. Histopathologic:
      Depth of organ, cutaneous invasion
      Venous, lymphatic, perineural invasion
3. Biologic:
   a. Histologic grade, i.e., degree of retention of characteristics or function of cell or origin.
   b. Historical growth note
   c. Tumor cell kinetics:
      Growth fraction
      Cell cycle time
      Proliferation index
   d. Growth pattern:
      Circumscribed versus stellate
      Lateral spreading versus nodular
      Virgin versus recurrent

A related, but clearly not coincident, primary tumor characteristic is the extent of *local tumor invasion,* assessed clinically or histopathologically. Physically large tumors of many organ systems may be only minimally invasive regionally and carry a good prognosis, while physically small tumors can deeply penetrate the layers of the organ of origin (colon, skin, mucosa of upper airway, or bladder). As a tumor becomes even more deeply invasive than the confines of its organ of origin, many descriptive clinical terms are used to indicate this tumor characteristic, such as "fixation," "skin retraction," "ulceration," and so forth, as listed in Table 11-6. These clinical characteristics for assessment of extensive regional invasion about a primary tumor site have been variably employed in tumor staging systems, as is indicated in the staging of head and neck squamous cell carcinoma, and also carcinoma of the breast. The details of these staging systems are presented in other chapters. Histopathologically, the extent of local invasion has also been suggested as an important parameter for the assessment of metastatic potential beyond the primary site. Blood vessel, lymphatic, or perineural invasion have been used to assess metastatic potential microscopically. The problem with these findings has always been the possible sampling error. For this reason, these histopathological features have generally not been employed in comprehensive staging systems, although logically are a very important addition to complete understanding of the metastatic potential of an individual patient's lesion.

The third and least well-defined (or standardized) set of primary tumor characteristics can be termed *"biological characteristics."* A rapidly growing lung carcinoma (with a short tumor doubling time) carries an ominous prognosis, as is true for other malignancies. However, these observations can only be made retrospectively in very selected circumstances, since it is not ethical to observe a tumor's growth rate prior to employing definitive therapy as soon as satisfactory diagnostic work has been accomplished. However, quantitation of the growth rate may be possible by employing newer techniques in tumor cell kinetics, and this kinetic prognostic variable may well become sufficiently refined to have a major impact in the staging of a primary tumor. It is obvious that most of the primary tumors become available after surgical resection, and indeed, if the primary tumor holds the answer to its future metastatic potential, the appropriate analysis of this specimen indeed should provide an improved amplification of current tumor staging. The "grade" of a malignancy reflects the degree of its retention of the characteristics of the tissue of its origin, that is, well differentiated versus poorly differentiated. This degree of differentiation is also thought to correlate with the rate of cell division, and also with the "nuclear grade," reflecting changes in tumor ploidy. The assessment of tumor ploidy, using flow cytometry, holds promise for quantitating this nuclear characteristic with precision not available previously in histopathologic analysis. It is possible that DNA histogram analysis will also greatly amplify the ability to determine metastatic potential of a given primary lesion.[267]

TMN STAGING SYSTEM

Primary Tumor Staging (T)

Since, as has been discussed, the physical size of a given primary cancer, the extent of regional invasion assessed either clinically or histopathologically, and other biological characteristics of the primary tumor, all affect prognosis, the characterization of the primary stage (designated as the "T" stage) has involved controversy and compromises in the TNM system. For example, in squamous carcinoma of the head and neck area, the T stage is determined "almost" exclusively by the measured primary tumor size, actually, the surface dimension. For other malignancies, including carcinoma of the stomach, colon, bladder, and malignant melanoma, it is the extent of local invasion that is formulated into the T stage. In carcinoma of the lung and esophagus, a very complex formula involving both the size and the degree of invasion and involvement of regional structures, has been utilized. For soft tissue sarcomas, the histologic grading of primary tumor—a biologic characteristic—is thought to be the major determinant of prognosis in Stage I to III. The T stage for soft tissue sarcomas has little weight, unless there is extensive invasion of bone, nerve, or regional structures that causes escalation of the stage to Stage IV. Although the TNM system proposed by various organ site committees of the American Joint Committee for Cancer Staging and End Result Reporting have attempted to define the T characteristics of prognostic importance, one can see significant variation in the way various T characteristics are assembled in the various TNM staging systems. The fact that prognosis from a T2N0M0 (Duke's B) carcinoma of the colon (which is 50 percent five-year outlook) is equally well-determined by the flip of a coin as by the actual T staging is further evidence for the imperfection of the state of the art in primary tumor staging. It would seem, therefore, that the most important test of predicting outcome before the tumor has shown evidence for dissemination has been the variable that to date is least satisfactorily identified. In most common adult neoplasia, accurate primary staging would seem to await more precise biologic parameters for assessment of metastatic potential. As is discussed in another chapter of this volume for carcinoma of the breast, such a biologic characteristic is at least partially available. An estrogen receptor positive T1N0M0 carcinoma of the breast establishes a significantly better prognosis than that of a T1N0M0 estrogen receptor negative lesion.

Regional Lymph Nodes Staging (N)

Correlations of the results of analysis of surgical specimens with eventual patient prognosis has also indicated a number of characteristics of regional lymph nodes that are predictive of the development of systemic metastases. These characteristics are listed in Table 11-7 and include the size of the involved lymph nodes. For lymph nodes that are microscopic only in extent and not detectable grossly, the prognosis is consistently better in carcinoma of the breast, and also in malignant melanoma, as well as other lesions. The location of the lymph node in relationship to the primary tumor likewise has been shown to be of prognostic importance, and is integrated into the staging of squamous cell carcinomas of the head and neck and other lesions. The extent of nodal invasion assessed by clinical or histopathological criteria likewise has been shown to be of importance for eventual prognosis. Other biologic parameters, such as historical growth rate and whether the metastasis is synchronous or metachronous with the primary, have also been shown to influence prognosis.

The actual growth potential of some micrometastatic foci has been questioned by studies which show that occult foci statistically present in comparison with resected specimens show virtually no growth potential with long-term followup. Better assessment of the true meaning of "occult foci of metastatic disease" in relation to prognosis needs to be accomplished.

TABLE 11-7. Regional Lymph Node Characteristics Predictive of Systemic Metastasis

1. Size (occult versus gross).
2. Number and location
   a. "Sentinel" versus secondary level
   b. Ipsilateral versus bilateral
3. Extent of nodal invasion:
   a. Clinical
      Mobility versus "fixed", edema
   b. Histopathologic
      Pericapsular sinus versus replacement
      Extracapsular invasion
      Vascular, lymphatic, neural, soft tissue invasion
4. Biologic:
   a. Historical growth rate
   b. Synchronous versus metachronous with primary
   c. "Growth potential" of occult metastases

TABLE 11-8. Characteristics of Distant Organ Metastasis Predictive of Prognosis

1. Organ site(s) involved
   Skin/distant nodes
   Bone
   Lung
   Liver
   Brain
2. Solitary versus multiple
3. First capillary network versus systemic spread
4. Doubling time
5. Synchronous versus metachronous with primary

Staging of Distant Organ Metastasis (M)

Even when disease has reached to distant organ sites, certain features of involvement have been shown to be very important in predicting outcome (Table 11-8). Involvement of skin or distant lymph nodes for essentially all metastatic malignancies shows a better prognosis than involvement of visceral organs. It is also clear that a solitary metastasis carries a better prognosis than do multiple metastases. Metastases in the first capillary network beyond a tumor may be resectable for cure whereas systemic metastases are not. The more rapidly the metastatic focus is growing, the shorter the prognosis, so that measured tumor doubling time is important in the staging of systemic metastatic disease.

HOST FACTORS AND PROGNOSIS

A number of characteristics of the human host have also been found to influence prognosis, particularly in patients who have systemic metastatic disease (Table 11-9).

The staging of malignant disease is imperfect and at this time, accurate prognoses are not available for the individual patient with a given malignant disease process. Rather, a statistical probability for eventual metastasis or death is the best that can be offered. The TNM staging system has assembled both clinical and pathological morphologic characteristics of primary tumors, regional metastases, and systemic metastases, and has provided a major contribution to standardizing the morphological classification of neoplastic diseases. However, for most malignancies, this system is insufficient for helping with the accurate prognosis for the individual patient. Such accurate individualized prognostication would seem to await development of biological characteristics that will more accurately determine the prognosis of a patient. It is possible that multivariant analyses that will combine multiple aspects of a given tumor will amplify the currently available staging systems.

TABLE 11-9. Host Characteristics Predictive of Prognosis

1. Nutritional status
2. Performance status
3. Immunologic skin reactivity
4. Concomitant nonmalignant conditions curtailing treatment(s)
5. Other undefined

REFERENCES

1. McNeil BJ, Adelstein: Determining the value of diagnostic and screening tests. J Nucl Med 17:349–448, 1976
2. Schaefer J, Schiff L: Liver function tests in metastatic tumor of the liver: Study of 100 cases. Gastroenterol 49:360–363, 1965
3. Ranson JHC, Adams PX, Localio SA: Preoperative assessment for hepatic metastases in carcinoma of the colon and rectum. Surg Gynecol Obstet 137:435–438, 1973
4. Combes B, Schenker S: Laboratory test. In Schiff L (ed). Disease of the Liver, 4th ed. Philadelphia, JB Lippincott, 1975
5. Posen S, Neale FC, Clubb JS: Heat inactivation in the study of human alkaline phosphatase. Ann Intern Med 62:1234–1243, 1965
6. Winkelman J, Nadler S, Demetriou J et al: The clinical usefulness of alkaline phosphatase isoenzyme determinations. Am J Clin Pathol 57:625–634, 1972
7. Kowlessar OD, Haeffner IJ, Riley EM et al: Comparative study of serum leucine aminopeptidase, 5′-nucleotidase and nonspecific alkaline phosphatase in diseases affecting the pancreas, hepatobiliary tree and bone. Am J Med 31:231–237, 1961
8. Rutenburg AM, Banks BM, Pineda EP et al: A comparison of serum amino–peptidase and alkaline phosphatase in the detection of hepatobiliary disease in anicteric patients. Ann Intern Med 61:50–55, 1964
9. Tsou KC, Lo KW: Serum 5′-nucleotide phosphodiesterase isozyme-V test for human liver cancer. Cancer 45:209–213, 1980
10. Wanebo HJ, Bhaskar R, Pinsky CM et al: Preoperative carcinoembryonic antigen level as a prognostic indicator on colorectal cancer. NEJM 299:448–451, 1978
11. Rosenfield AT, Taylor JKW, Jaffe CC: Clinical applications of ultrasound tissue characterization. Radiol Clin North Am 18:31–58, 1980
12. Ferrucci JT, Jr, Witttenberg J, Margolies MN et al: Malignant seeding of the tract after thin needle aspiration biopsy. Radiology 130:345–346, 1979
13. Sanders DE, Thompson DW, Pudden BJ: Percutaneous aspiration lung biopsy. Can Med Assoc J 104:139, 1971
14. Polga JP, Watnick M: Whole lung tomography in metastatic disease. Clin Radiol 27:53–56, 1976
15. Sindelar WF, Bagley DH, Felix EL et al: Lung tomography in cancer patients. Full lung tomograms in screening for pulmonary metastases. JAMA 240:2060–2063, 1978
16. Neifeld JP, Michaelis LL, Doppman JL: Suspected pulmonary metastases. Correlation of chest x-ray, whole lung tomograms and operative findings. Cancer 39:383–387, 1977
17. Chang AE, Schaner EG, Conkle DM et al: Evaluation of computed tomography in the detection of pulmonary metastases. Cancer 43:913–916, 1979
18. Muhm JR, Brown LR, Crowe JK: Use of computed tomography in the detection of pulmonary nodules. Mayo Clin Proc 52:345–348, 1977
19. Siegelman SS, Zerhouni E, Leo F et al: Computed tomography of a solitary pulmonary nodule. Am J Roentgenol 135:1–13, 1980
20. Cahan WG, Shah JP, Castro EB: Benign solitary lung lesions in patients with cancer. Ann Surg 187:241–244, 1978
21. Sinner WM: Complications of percutaneous transthoracic needle aspiration biopsy. Acta Radio (Diagn) 17:813, 1976
22. Radke JR, Conway WA, Eyler WR et al: Diagnostic accuracy in peripheral lung lesions. Factors predicting success with flexible fiberoptic bronchoscopy. Chest 76:176–179, 1979
23. Mark JBD, Marglin SI, Castellino RA: The role of bronchoscopy and aspiration in the diagnosis of peripheral lung masses. J Thorac Cardiovasc Surg 76:266–268, 1978
24. Kline TS, Neal HS: Needle aspiration biopsy: A critical appraisal eight years and 3267 specimens later. JAMA 239:36–39, 1978
25. Sagel SS, Ferguson TB, Forrest JV et al: Percutaneous transthoracic aspiration needle biopsy. Ann Thorac Surg 26:399–404, 1978
26. Tao LC, Pearson FG, Delarue NC et al: Percutaneous fine

needle aspiration biopsy. I. Its value to clinical practice. Cancer 45:1480–1485, 1980

27. Lunia S, Parthasarathy KL, Bakshi S et al: An evaluation of ^{99m}Tc-sulfur colloid liver scintiscans and their usefulness in metastatic workup: A review of 1,424 studies. J Nucl Med 16:62–65, 1975
28. Drum DE: Optimizing the clinical value of hepatic scintiphotography. Semin Nucl Med 8:346–357, 1978
29. Vicary FR, Shirley I: Ultrasound and hepatic metastases. Brit J Radiol 51:596–598, 1978
30. Taylor KJW, Sullivan D, Rosenfield T et al: Gray scale ultrasound and isotope scanning: Complementary techniques for imaging the liver. Am J Roentgenol 128:277–281, 1977
31. Scheible W, Gosink BB, Leopold GR: Gray scale echographic patterns of hepatic metastatic disease. Am J Roentgenol 129:983–987, 1977
32. Green B, Bree RL, Goldstein HM et al: Gray scale ultrasound evaluation of hepatic neoplasms: Patterns and correlations. Radiology 124:203–208, 1977
33. Wooten WB, Green B, Goldstein HM: Ultrasonography of necrotic hepatic metastases. Radiology 128:447–450, 1978
34. Hillman BJ, Smith EH, Gammelgaard J et al: Ultrasonographic–pathologic correlation of malignant hepatic masses. Gastrointest Radiol 4:361–365, 1979
35. Scherer U, Rothe R, Eisenburg J et al: Diagnostic accuracy of CT in circumscript liver disease. Am J Roentgenol 130:711–714, 1978
36. Dunnick NR, Ihde DC, Johnston-Early A: Abdominal CT in the evaluation of small cell carcinoma of the lung. Am J Roentgenol 133:1085–1088, 1979
37. Snow JH, Jr, Goldstein HM, Wallace S: Comparison of scintigraphy, sonography and computed tomography in the evaluation of hepatic neoplasms. Am J Roentgenol 132:915–918, 1979
38. Smith TJ, Jones E, Shawker T et al: The current status of liver imaging in the detection of metastases. (in press)
39. Vermess M, Chatterji DC, Doppman JL et al: Development and experimental evaluation of a contrast medium for computed tomographic examination of the liver and spleen. J Comput Asst Tomogr 3:25–31, 1979
40. Coldstein HM, Thaggard A, Wallace S et al: Priscoline-augmented hepatic angiography. Radiology 119:275–279, 1976
41. Deck MDF, Messina AV, Sackett JF: Computed tomography in metastatic disease of the brain. Radiol 119:115–120, 1976
42. Bardfeld PA, Passalaqua AM, Braunstein P et al: A comparison of radionuclide scanning and computed tomography in metastatic lesions of the brain. J Comput Asst Tomogr 1:315–318, 1977
43. Buell V, Niendorf HP, Kazner E et al: Computerized transaxial tomography and cerebral serial scintigraphy in intracranial tumors—Rates of detection and tumor-type identfication: Concise communication. J Nucl Med 19:476–479, 1978
44. Weisberg LA: Computerized tomography in intracranial metastases. Arch Neurol 36:630–634, 1979
45. Gilbert H, Apuzzo M, Marshall L et al: Neoplastic epidural spinal cord compression: A current preospective. JAMA 240:2271–2773, 1978
46. Hatam A, Hindmarsh T, Greitz T: Myelography in metastatic lesions. Acta Radiol 16:321–330, 1976
47. Livingston KE, Perrin RG: The neurosurgical management of spnal metastases causing cord and cauda equina compression. J Neurosurg 49:839–843, 1978
48. Pistenma DA, McDougall IR, Kriss JP: Screening for bone metastases. JAMA 231:46–50, 1975
49. Citrin DL, Bessent RG, Grieg WR: A comparison of the sensitivity and accuracy of the $^{99}{}_{m}$Tc phosphate bone scan and skeletal radiograph in the diagnosis of bone metastases. Clin Radiol 28:107–117, 1977
50. Parthasarathy KL, Landsberg R, Bakshi SP et al: Detection of bone metastases in urogenital malignancies utilizing Tc^{99m}-labeled phospate compounds. Urology 11:99–102, 1978
51. Donato AT, Ammerman EG, Sullesta O: Bone scanning in the evaluation of patients with lung cancer. Ann Thorac Surg 27:300–304, 1979
52. Brady LW, Croll MN: The role of bone scanning in the cancer patient. Skeletal Radiol 3:217–222, 1979
53. Gilday DL, Ash JM, Reilly BJ: Radionuclide skeletal survey for pediatric neoplasms. Radiology 123:399–406, 1977
54. Kim EE, DeLano FH, Maruyama Y: Decreased uptake in bone scans ("Cold Lesions") in metastatic carcinoma. Two case reports. J Bone Joint Surg 60A:844–846, 1978
55. McNeil BJ: Rationale for the use of bone scans in selected metastatic and primary bone tumors. Semin Nucl Med 8:336–345, 1978
56. Adler O, Rosenberger A: Fine needle aspiration biopsy of osteolytic metastatic lesions. Am J Roentgenol 133:15–18, 1979
57. Collins JD, Bassett L, Main GD et al: Percutaneous biopsy following positive bone scans. Radiology 132:439–442, 1979
58. Brascho DJ, Durant JR, Green LE: The accuracy of retroperitoneal ultrasonography in Hodgkin's disease and nonHodgkin's lymphoma. Radiology 125:485–487, 1977
59. Lee JKT, Stanley RJ, Sagel SS et al: Accuracy of computed tomography in detecting intra-abdominal and pelvic adenopathy in lymphoma. Am J Roentgenol 131:311–315, 1978
60. Castellino RA, Blank N, Cassady JR et al: Roentgenologic aspects of Hodgkin's disease. II. Role of routine radiographs in detecting initial relapse. Cancer 31:316–323, 1973
61. Castellino RA, Billingham M, Dorfman FR: Lymphographic accuracy in Hodgkin's disease and malignant lymphoma with a note on the "Reactive" lymph node as a cause of most false-positive lymphograms. Invest Radiol 9:115–165, 1974
62. Parker BR, Castellino RA, Fuks Z et al: The role lymphography in patients with ovarian cancer. Cancer 34:100–105, 1974
63. Athey PA, Wallace S, Jing BS et al: Lymphangiography in ovarian cancer. Am J Roentgenol 123:106–113, 1975
64. Musumeci R, Banfi A, Bolis G et al: Lymphangiography in patients with ovarian epithelial cancer. An evaluation of 289 consecutive cases. Cancer 1444–1449, 1977
65. Spellman MC, Castellino RA, Ray GR et al: An evaluation of lymphography in localized carcinoma of the prostate. Radiology 125:637–644, 1977
66. Watson RC: Lymphography of testicular carcinoma. Semin Oncol 6:31–35, 1979
67. Dunnick NR, Javadpour N: The value of CT and lymphography in detecting retroperitoneal metastases from nonseminomatous testicular tumors. (in press)
68. Castellino RA, Fuks Z, Blank N et al: Roentgenologic aspects of Hodgkin's disease; Repeat lymphangiography. Radiology 109:53–58, 1973
69. Dunnick NR, Fuks Z, Castellino RA: Repeat lymphography in non-Hodgkin's lymphoma. Radiology 115:349–354, 1975
70. Gothlin JH: Postlymphographic percutaneous fine needle biopsy of lymph nodes guided by fluoroscopy. Radiology 120:205–207, 1976
71. Zornoza J, Jonsson K, Wallace S et al: Fine needle aspiration biopsy of retroperitoneal lymph nodes and abdominal masses: An updated report. Radiology 125:87–88, 1977
72. Prando A, Wallace S, VonEschenbach AC et al: Lymphangiography in staging carcinoma of the prostate. The potential value of percutaneous lymph node biopsy. Radiology 131:641–645, 1979
73. MacIntosh PK, Thompson KR, Barbaric ZL: Percutaneous transperitoneal lymph node biopsy as a means of improving lymphographic diagnosis. Radiology 131:647–649, 1979
74. Dunnick NR, Fisher RI, Chu EW et al: Percutaneous aspiration of retroperitoneal lymph nodes in patients with ovarian carcinoma. Am J Roentgenol 135:109–113, 1980
75. Gothlin JH, MacIntosh PK: Interventional radiology in the assessment of retroperitoneal lymph nodes. Radiol Clin North Am 17:461–473, 1979
76. Sugarbaker PH, Wilson RE: Using celioscopy to determine stages of intraabdominal malignant neoplasms. Arch Surg 111:41–44, 1976
77. Matthews MJ, Kanhouwa S, Pickren J et al: Frequency of residual and metastatic tumor in patients undergoing curative surgical resection for lung cancer. Cancer Chemotherapy Reports 4:63–67, 1973

78. Ozarda A, Pickren J: The topographic distribution of liver metastases—its relation to surgical and isotope diagnosis. J Nucl Med 3:149–152, 1962
79. Hogg L, Pack GT: Diagnostic accuracy of hepatic metastases at laparotomy. Ann Surg 72:251–252, 1966
80. Bleiberg H, Rozencweig M, Mathieu M et al: The use of peritoneoscopy in the detection of liver metastases. Cancer 41:863–867, 1978
81. Jori GP, Peshle C: Combined peritoneoscopy and liver biopsy in the diagnosis of hepatic neoplasm. Gastroenterol 63:1016–1019, 1972
82. Czaja AJ, Steinberg AS, Saldana M et al: Peritoneoscopy: its value in the diagnosis of liver disease. Gastrointest Endosc 20:23–25, 1973
83. McCallum RW, Berci G: Laparoscopy in hepatic disease. Gastrointest Endosc 23:20–24, 1976
84. Sugarbaker PH: Double puncture peritoneoscopy. Surg Gynecol Obstet (in press)
85. DeVita VT, Bagley CM, Goodell B et al: Peritoneoscopy in the staging of Hodgkin's disease. Cancer Res 31:1746–1750, 1971
86. Coleman M, Lightdale CJ, Vinciguerra VP et al: Peritoneoscopy in Hodgkin's disease. Confirmation of results by laparotomy. JAMA 236:2634–2636, 1976
87. Hoffken K, Schmidt CG: Laparoscopy bei Morbus Hodgkin. Dtsch Med Wschr 101:814–818, 1976
88. Ozols RF, Fisher RI, Anderson T et al: Peritoneoscopy in the management of ovarian cancer. (Submitted for publication)
89. Goldhaber Z, Bloom BS, Sugarbaker PH et al: Effects of the fiberoptic laparoscope and colonoscope on morbidity and cost. Ann Surg 179:160–162, 1974
90. Knutson CO, Schrock LG, Polk HC: Polypoid lesions of the proximal colon: Comparison of experiences with removal at laparotomy and by colonoscopy. Ann Surg 179:657–662, 1974
91. Dean ACB, Newell JP: colonoscopy in the differential diagnosis of carcinoma from diverticulitis of the sigmoid colon. Br J Surg 60:633–635, 1973
92. Sugarbaker PH, Vineyard GC, Lewicki AM et al: Colonoscopy in the management of diseases of the colon and rectum. Surg Gynecol Obstet 139:341–349, 1974
93. Glerum J, Agenant D, Tytgat GN: Value of coloscopy in the detection of sigmoid malignancy in patients with diverticular disease. Endoscopy 9:228–230, 1977
94. Warwick RRG, Sumerling MD, Gilmour HM et al: Colonoscopy and double contrast barium enema examination in chronic ulcerative colitis. Am J Roentgenol 117:292–296, 1973
95. Schmitt MG, Wu WC, Geenen JE et al: Diagnostic colonoscopy. An assessment of the clinical indications. Gastroenterology 69:765–769, 1975
96. Tawile NT, Priest RJ, Schuman BM: Colonoscopy in inflammatory bowel disease. Gastrointest Endosc 22:11–13, 1975
97. Waye JD: The role of colonoscopy in the differential diagnosis of inflammatory bowel disease. Gastrointest Endosc 23:150–154, 1977
98. Banche M, Rossini FP, Ferrari A et al: The role of coloscopy in the differential diagnosis between idiopathic ulcerative colitis and Crohn's disease of the colon. Am J Gastroenterol 65:539–545, 1976
99. Dobbins WO, Stock M, Ginsberg AL: Early detection and prevention of carcinoma of the colon in patients with ulcerative colitis. Cancer 40:2542–2548, 1977
100. Riddel RH: Dysplasia in inflammatory bowel disease. Clin Gastroenterol 9:439–458, 1980
101. Wolff WI, Shinya H, Geffen A et al: Comparison of colonoscopy and barium enema in five hundred patients with colorectal disease. Am J Surg 129:181–186, 1975
102. Leinicke JL, Dodds WJ, Hogan WJ et al: A comparison of colonoscopy and roentgenography for detecting polypoid lesions of the colon. Gastrointest Radiol 2:125–128, 1977
103. Amberg JR, Berk RN, Burhenne J et al: Colonic polyp detection: Role of roentgenography and colonoscopy. Radiology 125:255–257, 1977
104. Thoeni RF, Menuck L: Comparison of barium enema and colonscopy in the detection of small colonic polyps. Radiology 124:631–635, 1977
105. Teague RH, Salmon PR, Read AE: Fiberoptic examination of the colon: A review of 255 cases. Gut 14:139–142, 1973
106. Sugarbaker PH, Vineyard GC, Peterson LM: Anatomic localization and step by step advancement of the fiberoptic colonoscopic. Surg Gynecol Obstet 143:457–462, 1976
107. Shinya H, Wolff WI: Colonoscopic polypectomy: Technique and safety. Hospital Practice 10:71–78, 1975
108. Sugarbaker PH, Vineyard GC: Snare polypectomy with the fiberoptic colonoscope. Surg Gynecol Obstet 138:581–583, 1974
109. Williams CB: Diathermy-biopsy—a technique for the endoscopic management of small polyps. Endoscopy 5:215–218, 1973
110. Shamir M, Schuman BM: Complications of fiberoptic endoscopy. Gastrointest Endosc 26:86–91, 1980
111. Kobayashi S, Yoshii Y, Kasugai T: Selective use of brushing cytology in gastrointestinal strictures. Gastrointest Endosc 2:76–77, 1972
112. Winawer S, Posner G, Belladonna J et al: Application of panendoscopic directed brush cytology to the diagnosis of esophageal cancer. Gastrointest Endosc 21:188, 1974
113. Hanson LT, Thoreson C, Morrissey JF: Brush cytology in the diagnosis of upper gastrointestinal malignancy. Gastrointest Endosc 26:33–35, 1980
114. Martin TR, Onstad GR, Silvis SE et al: Lift and cut biopsy technique for submucosal sampling. Gastrointest Endosc 23:29–30, 1976
115. Sherlock P, Winawer SJ: Differential diagnosis of upper gastrointestinal bleeding and cancer. Cancer J Clinicians 28:7–16, 1978
116. Pearson FG: An evaluation of mediastinoscopy in the management of presumably operable bronchial carcinoma. J Thorac Cardiovasc Surg 55:617–625, 1968
117. Goldberg EM, Shapiro CM, Glicksman AS: Mediastinoscopy for assessing mediastinal spread in clinical staging of lung carcinoma. Semin Oncol 1:205–215, 1974
118. Borrie J: Lung Cancer Surgery and Survival. New York, Appleton-Century-Crofts, 1965
119. Bowen TE, Zajtchuk R, Green DC et al: Value of anterior mediastinotomy in bronchogenic carcinoma of the left upper lobe. J Thorac Cardiovasc Surg 79:269–271, 1978
120. Jolly PC, Li W, Anderson RP: Anterior and cervical mediastinoscopy for determining operability and predicting resectability in lung cancer. J Thorac Cardiovasc Surg 79:366–371, 1980
121. Gibbons JRP: The value of mediastinoscopy in assessing operability in carcinoma of the lung. Br J Dis Chest 66:162–166, 1972
122. Hutchinson CM, Mills NL: The selection of patients with bronchogenic carcinoma for mediastinoscopy. J Thorac Cardiovasc Surg 71:768–733, 1976
123. Baker RR, Lillemoe KD, Tockman MS: The indications for transcervical mediastinoscopy in patients with small peripheral bronchial carcinoma. Surg Gynecol Obstet 148:860–862, 1979
124. Smith R: The importance of mediastinal lymph node invasion by pulmonary carcinoma in selection of patients for resection. Ann Thorac Surg 25:5–11, 1978
125. Paulson DL, Urschel HC: Selectivity in the surgical treatment of bronchogenic carcinoma. J Thorac Cardiovasc Surg 62:554–567, 1971
126. Baker BR, Stibb FP, Summer W: Bronchogenic carcinoma. Current Probl Surg 74:1–48, 1974
127. Vaeth JM, Moskowitz SA, Green JP: Mediastinal Hodgkin's disease. Am J Roentgenol 126:123–126, 1976
128. Redding ME, Anagnostopoulos CE, Ultmann JE: The possible value of mediastinoscopy in staging Hodgkin's disease. Cancer Res 31:1741–1745, 1971
129. Murray GF, Wilcox BR, Starek PJK: The assessment of operability of esophageal carcinoma. Ann Thorac Surg 23:393–399, 1977
130. Kirschner PA: Transcervical approach to the superior mediastinum. Hosp Prac, June 1970
131. Foster ED, Munro DD, Dobell ARC: Mediastinoscopy. A review of anatomical relationships and complications. Ann Thorac Surg 13:273–286, 1972
132. Bacsa S, Czaro Z, Vezendi S: The complications of mediastinoscopy. Pan Med 74:402–406, 1974

133. Kliems G, Savic B: Complications of mediastinoscopy. Endoscopy 1:9–12, 1979
134. Bloomberg AE: Thoracoscopy in perspective. Surg Gynecol Obstet 147:433–443, 1978
135. Pepper JR: Thoracoscopy in the diagnosis of pleural effusions and tumours. Br J Dis Chest 72:74–75, 1978
136. Lewis RJ, Kunderman PJ, Sisler GE et al: Direct diagnostic thoracoscopy. Ann Thorac Surg 21:536–539, 1976
137. Le Roux BT: Bronchial Carcinoma, p 127. London, E and S Livingston Ltd., 1968
138. Oldenburg FA, Newhouse MT: Thoracoscopy. A safe, accurate diagnostic procedure using the rigid thoracoscope and local anesthesia. Chest 75:45–50, 1979
139. Espiner HJ, Salmon PR, Teague RH et al: Operative colonoscopy. Br Med J 1:453–454, 1973
140. Bombeck CT: Intraoperative esophagoscopy, gastroscopy, colonoscopy and endoscopy of the small bowel. Surg Clin N Am 55:135–142, 1975
141. Gold P, Freedman SO: Demonstration of tumor-specific antigens in human colonic carcinomata by immunologic tolerance and absorption techniques. J Exp Med 122:467–481, 1965
142. Banjo C, Shuster J, Gold P: Intermolecular heterogeneity of the carcinoembryonic antigen. Cancer Res 34:2114–2121, 1974
143. Terry WD, Henkart PA, Coligan JE et al: Structural studies of the major glycoprotein in preparations with carcinoembryonic antigen activity. J Exp Med 136:100–129, 1972
144. Coligan JE, Henkart PA, Todd CW et al: Heterogeneity of the carcinoembryonic antigen. Immunochemistry 10:591–599, 1973
145. Eveleigh JW: Heterogeneity of carcinoembryonic antigen. Cancer Res 34:2122–2124, 1974
146. Vrba R, Alpert E, Isselbacher KJ: Carcinoembryonic antigen: Evidence for multiple antigenic determinants and isoantigens. Proc Natl Acad Sci USA 72:4602–4606, 1975
147. Arnon R, Bustin M, Calef E et al: Immunologic cross-reactivity of antibodies to a synthetic undecapeptide analogous to the aminoterminal segment of the carcinoembryonic antigen, with the intact protein and with human sera. Proc Natl Acad Sci USA 73:2123–2127, 1976
148. Sherbet GV: Epigenetic processes and their relevance to the study of neoplasia. Advances in Cancer Res 97–167, 1970
149. Burton P, von Kleist S, Sabine MC et al: Immunohistological localization of carcinoembryonic antigen and nonspecific cross-reacting antigen in gastrointestinal normal and tumor tissues. Cancer Res 33:3299–3302, 1973
150. Freed DJL, Taylor G: Carcinoembryonic antigen in feces. Br Med J 1:85–87, 1972
151. Elias EG, Holyoke ED, Chu TM: Carcinoembryonic antigen in feces and plasma of normal subjects and patients with colorectal cancer. Dis Colon Rectum 1:38–41, 1974
152. Martin F, Martin MS: Radioimmunoassay of carcinoembryonic antigen in extracts of human colon and stomach. Int J Cancer 9:641–647, 1972
153. Khoo SK, Warner NL, Lie JT et al: Carcinoembryonic antigenic activity of tissue extracts: A quantitative study of malignant and benign neoplasms, cirrhotic liver, normal adult and fetal organs. Int J Cancer 11:681–687, 1973
154. Molnar IG, Vandevoorde JP, Gitnick GL: CEA levels in fluids bathing gastrointestinal tumors. Gastroenterology 70:513–515, 1976
155. Dyce BJ, Haverback BJ: Free and bound carcinoembryonic antigen in neoplasms and in normal adult and fetal tissue. Immunochemistry 11:423–430, 1974
156. Schuster J, Silverman M, Gold P: Metabolism of human carcinoembryonic antigen in xenogeneic animals. Cancer Res 33:65–68, 1973
157. Primus FJ, Goldenberg DM, Hansen HJ: Metabolism of carcinoembryonic antigen (CEA) in a human tumor-hamster model (abstr). Fed Proc 32:834, 1973
158. Thomas P, Heims PA: The hepatic clearance of circulating carcinoembryonic antigen by the mouse. Biochem Soc Trans 5:312–313, 1977
159. Holyoke ED, Reynoso G, Chu T: Carcinoembryonic antigen in patients with carcinoma of the digestive tract. In Proceedings of second conference on embryonic and fetal antigens in cancer, p 215. National Technical Information Service, Springfield, Va., US Department of Commerce, 1972
160. Go VLW, Ammon HV, Holtermuller KH et al: Quantitation of carcinoembryonic antigen-like activities in normal human gastrointestinal secretions. Cancer 36:2346–2350, 1975
161. Lurie BB, Lowenstein MS, Zamcheck N: Elevated circulating CEA levels in benign extrahepatic biliary tract obstruction and inflammation. JAMA 233:326–330, 1975
162. Lowenstein MS, Rau P, Rittgers RA et al: CEA in duodenal aspirates of patients with benign and malignant disease; preliminary observations. JNCI (in press)
163. Moore T, Dhar P, Zamcheck N et al: Carcinoembryonic antigen(s) in liver disease. I. Clinical and Morphologic studies. Gastroenterology 63:88–94, 1972
164. Kupchik JZ, Zamcheck N: Carcinoembryonic antigen(s) in liver disease. II. Isolation from human cirrhotic liver and serum and from normal liver. Gastroenterology 63:95–101, 1972
165. Delwiche R, Zamcheck N, Marcon N: Carcinoembryonic antigen in pancreatitis Cancer 31:328–330, 1973
166. Sharma MP, Gregg JA, Lowenstein MS, Ona FV, Zamcheck N, Dhar P: CEA in the diagnosis of pancreatic cancer. Cancer 31:324–327, 1973
167. Gitnick GL, Molnar IG: Carcinoembryonic antigen transmission by blood products. Cancer 42:1568–1573, 1978
168. LoGerfo P, Krupey J, Hansen HJ: Demonstration of an antigen common to several varieties of neoplasia. Assay using zirconyl phosphate gel. NEJM 285:138–141, 1971
169. Wight DGD, Gazet J-C: Carcinoembryonic antigen levels in inflammatory disease of the large bowel. Proc Royl Soc Med 65:967–968, 1972
170. Moore TL, Kantrowitz PA, Zamcheck N: Carcinoembryonic antigen (CEA) in inflammatory bowel disease. JAMA 222:944–947, 1972
171. Rule AH, Straus E, Vandevoorde J et al: Tumor associated (CEA reacting) antigen in patients with inflammatory bowel disease. NEJM 287:24–26, 1972
172. Dilawari JB, Lennard-Jones JE, MacKay AM et al: Estimation of carcinoembryonic antigen in ulcerative colitis with special reference to malignant change. Gut 16:255–260, 1975
173. Morson BC, Pang LSC: Rectal biopsy as an aid to cancer control in ulcerative colitis. Gut 8:423–434, 1967
174. Yardley JH, Keren DF: "Precancer" lesions in ulcerative colitis. A retrospective study of rectal biopsy and colectomy specimens. Cancer 34:835–844, 1974
175. Cook MG, Path MRC, Golighan JC: Carcinoma and epithelial dysplasia complicating ulcerative colitis. Gastroenterology 68:1127–1136, 1975
176. Gardner RC, Feinerman AE, Kantrowitz PA et al: Serial carcinoembryonic antigen (CEA) levels in patients with ulcerative colitis. Am J Dig Dis 23:129–133, 1978
177. Stevens DP, MacKay IR: Increased carcinoembryonic antigen in heavy cigarette smokers. Lancet 1:1238–1239, 1973
178. Alexander JC, Silverman NA, Chretien PG: Effect of age and cigarette smoking on carcinoembryonic antigen levels. J Am Med Assoc 235:1975–1979, 1976
179. Pulimood BM, Knudsen A, Coghill NF: Gastric mucosa after partial gastrectomy. Gut 17:463–470, 1976
180. Doos WG, Wolff WI, Shinya H et al: CEA levels in patients with colorectal polyps. Cancer 36:1996–2003, 1975
181. Alm T, Wahren B: Carcinoembryonic antigen in hereditary adenomatosis of the colon and rectum. Scan J Gastroenterol 10:875–879, 1975
182. Guirgis HA, Lynch HT, Harris RE et al: Carcinoembryonic antigen (CEA) in the cancer family syndrome. Cancer 42:1574–1578, 1978
183. Sugarbaker P, Zamcheck N, Moore FDK: Assessment of serial carcinoembryonic antigen (CEA) in postoperative management of colon and rectal cancer. Cancer 38:2310–2315, 1976
184. Nakamura RM, Plow EF, Edgington TS: Current status of carcinoembryonic antigen (CEA) and CEA-S assays in the evaluation of neoplasm of the gastrointestinal tract. Ann Clin Lab Sci 8:4–10, 1978
185. Joint National Cancer Institute of Canada/American Cancer

Society Investigation, a collaborative study of a test for carcinoembryonic antigen (CEA) in the sera of patients with carcinoma of the colon and rectum. Can Med Assoc J 107:25–33, 1972
186. Hansen JG, Snyder BS, Miller E et al: Carcinoembryonic antigen (CEA) assay, a laboratory adjunct in the diagnosis and management of cancer. Hum Pathol 5:139–147, 1974
187. Chu TM, Holyoke ED: Can CEA assay be used as a screening test for cancer? Proc XI Int Cancer Congress, Florence, Italy 1:351, 1974
188. Dykes PW, King J: Progress report: Carcinoembryonic antigen. Gut 13:1000–1013, 1972
189. Laurence JJR, Stevens U, Bettelheim R et al: Evaluation of the role of plasma carcinoembryonic antigen (CEA) in the diagnosis of gastrointestinal, mammary and bronchial carcinoma. Br Med J 3:605–609, 1972
190. Concannon JP, Dalbow MH, Frich JC: Carcinoembryonic antigen (CEA) plasma levels in untreated cancer patients and patients with metastatic disease. Radiology 108:191–193, 1973
191. Ona F, Zamcheck N, Dhar P et al: Carcinoembryonic antigen (CEA) in the diagnosis of pancreatic cancer. Cancer 31:324–327, 1973
192. Sugarbaker PH, Beard JO, Drum DE: Detection of hepatic metastases from cancer of the breast. Am J Surg 133:531–535, 1977
193. McCartney WH, Hoffer PB: Carcinoembryonic antigen assay: An adjunct to liver scanning in hepatic metastases detection. Cancer 42:1457–1462, 1978
194. McCartney WH, Hoffer PB: The value of carcinoembryonic antigen as an adjunct to the radiological colon examination in the diagnosis of malignancy. Radiology 110:325–328, 1974
195. Goldenberg DM, Deland F, Kim E et al: Use of radiolabeled antibodies to carcinoembryonic antigen for the detection and localization of diverse cancers by external photoscanning. NEJM 298:1384–1388, 1978
196. Mach JP, Jaeger PH, Bertholet MM et al: Detection of recurrence of large bowel carcinoma by radioimmunoassay of circulating carcinoembryonic antigen (CEA). Lancet 2:535–540, 1974
197. MacKay AM, Patel S, Carter S et al: Role of serial plasma CEA assays in detection of recurrent and metastatic colorectal carcinoma. Br Med J 4:382–385, 1974
98. Herrera MA, Chu TM, Holyoke ED: Carcinoembryonic antigen (CEA) as a prognostic and monitoring test in clinically complete resection of colorectal carcinoma. Ann Surg 183:5–9, 1976
199. Martin EW, James KK, Hurtubise PE et al: The use of CEA as an early indicator for gastrointestinal tumor recurrence and second-look procedures. Cancer 39:440–446, 1977
200. Ratcliffe JG, Wood CB, Burt RW et al: Patterns of change in carcinoembryonic antigen (CEA) levels in patients developing recurrent colorectal cancer. Sixth Meeting of the International Research Group for Carcinoembryonic Proteins held in Marburg/Lahn, W. Germany 17–21 Sept, 1978
201. Martin EW, Cooperman M, Carey LC et al: Sixty second look procedures indicated primarily by rise in serial CEA. Abstract presented at Thirteenth Annual Meeting Association for Academic Surgery, November 1979
202. Wanebo HJ, Rao B, Pinsky CM et al: Preoperative carcinoembryonic antigen level as a prognostic indicator in colorectal cancer. NEJM 299:448–457, 1978
203. Foster JH, Berman MM: Solid Liver Tumors, p 225. Philadelphia, WB Saunders, 1977
204. Martini N, Huvos AG, Mike V: Multiple pulmonary resection in the treatment of osteogenic sarcoma. Ann Thorac Surg 12:271–280, 1971
205. Rosenberg SA, Flye MW, Conkle D et al: The treatment of osteogenic sarcoma. II Aggressive resection of pulmonary metastases. Cancer Treatment Reports 63:753–756, 1979
206. Rittgers RA, Steele G, Zamcheck N et al: Transient carcinoembryonic antigen (CEA) elevations following resection for colorectal cancer: A limitation in the use of serial CEA levels as an indicator for second look surgery. Cancer Institute 61:315–318, 1978
207. Booth SN, Jamison GG, King JPG et al: Carcinoembryonic antigen in the management of colorectal carcinoma. Br Med J 4:183–187, 1974
208. Denk H, Tappeiner G, Eckerstorfer R et al: Carcinoembryonic antigen (CEA) in gastrointestinal and extragastrointestinal tumors and its relationship to tumor cell differentiation. Int J Cancer 10:262–272, 1972
209. Kalser MH, Barkin JS, Redlhammer D et al: Circulating carcinoembryonic antigen in pancreatic carcinoma. Cancer 42:1468–1471, 1978
210. Wang DY, Bulbrook RD, Hayward JC et al: Relationship between plasma carcinoembryonic antigen and prognosis in women with breast cancer. Eur J Cancer 11:615–618, 1975
211. Haagensen DE, Kister SJ, Vandervoord JP et al: Evaluation of carcinoembryonic antigen as a plasma monitor for human breast carcinoma. Cancer 42:1512–1519, 1978
212. Myers RE, Sutherland DJ, Meakin JW et al: Carcinoembryonic antigen in breast cancer. Cancer 42:1520–1526, 1978
213. Tormey DC, Waalkes TP: Clinical correlation between CEA and breast cancer. Cancer 42:1507–1511, 1978
214. Dent PG, McCulloch PB, Wesley-James O et al: Measurement of carcinoembryonic antigen in patients with bronchogenic carcinoma. Cancer 42:1484–1491, 1978
215. Concannon JP, Dalbow MH, Hodgson SE et al: Prognostic value of preoperative carcinoembryonic antigen (CEA) plasma levels in patients with bronchogenic carcinoma. Cancer 42:1477–1483, 1978
216. Dhar P, Moore T, Zamcheck N et al: Carcinoembryonic antigen (CEA) in colonic cancer. Use in preoperative and postoperative diagnosis and prognosis. J Am Med Assoc 221:31–35, 1972
217. LoGerfo P, Herter F, Hansen JG: Tumor-associated antigen in patients with carcinoma of the colon. Am J Surg 123:127–131, 1972
218. Livingstone AS, Hampson LG, Schuster J et al: Carcinoembryonic antigen in the diagnosis and management of colorectal carcinoma. Arch Surg 109:259–264, 1974
219. Sorokin JJ, Sugarbaker PH, Zamcheck PM et al: Serial carcinoembryonic antigen assays. Use in detection of cancer recurrence. J Am Med Assoc 228:49–53, 1974
220. Oh JH, MacLean LD: Prognostic use of preoperative and immediate postoperative carcinoembryonic antigen determinations in colonic cancer. Can J Surg 20:64–67, 1977
221. Vider M, Kashmiri R, Hunter L et al: Carcinoembryonic antigen (CEA) monitoring in the management of radiotherapeutic patients. Oncology 30:257–272, 1974
222. Vider M. Kashmiri R, Meeker WR et al: Carcinoembryonic antigen (CEA) monitoring in the management of radiotherapeutic and chemotherapeutic patients. Am J Roentgenol 124:630–635, 1975
223. Sugarbaker PH, Bloomer WD, Corbett ED et al: Carcinoembryonic antigen (CEA) monitoring of radiation therapy for colorectal cancer. Am J Roentgenol 127:641–644, 1976
224. Donaldson E, Van Nagell JR, Wood EG et al: Carcinoembryonic antigen in patients treated with radiation therapy for invasive squamous cell carcinoma of the cervix. Ann J Roentgenol 127:829–831, 1976
225. Mulcare R, LoGerfo P: Tumor associated antigen in chemotherapy of solid tumors. J Surg Oncol 4:407–417, 1972
226. Herrea MA, Chu TM, Holyoke ED et al: CEA monitoring of palliative treatment for colorectal carcinoma. Ann Surg 185:23–30, 1977
227. Young VL, Kashmiri R, Hazen R et al: Usefulness of serial carcinoembryonic antigen (CEA) determinations in monitoring chemotherapy. South Med J 69:1274–1276, 1976
228. Mayer RJ, Garnick MB, Steele GD et al: Carcinoembryonic antigen (CEA) as a monitor of chemotherapy in disseminated colorectal cancer. Cancer 42:1428–1433, 1978
229. Bergstrand CG, Czar B: Demonstration of a new protein fraction in serum from the human fetus. Scan J Clin Lab Invest 8:174–179, 1956
230. Abelev GI, Perova SD, Khramkova NI: Production of embryonal alphaglobulin by transplantable mouse hepatomas. Transplantation 1:174–180, 1963
231. Tatarinoy Y: Detection of embryospecific alphaglobulin in the

blood sera of patients with primary liver tumors. Vopr Med Khim 10:90–91, 1972
232. Oakes DD, Schuster J, Gold P: Radioimmunoassay for alpha-1-fetoprotein in serum of rats. Cancer Res 32:2753–2760, 1972
233. Sell S, Gord D: Rat alpha-1-fetoprotein. III. Refinement of radioimmunoassay for detection of 1 ng rat alpha-1-F. Immunochemistry 10:439–442, 1973
234. Waldmann TA, McIntire KR: The use of a radioimmunoassay of alphafetoprotein in the diagnosis of malignancy. Cancer 34:1510–1515, 1974
235. Silver HKB, Deneault J, Gold P: The detection of alpha-1-fetoprotein in patients with viral hepatitis. Cancer Res 34:244–247, 1974
236. Silver HKB, Gold P, Shuster J et al: Alpha-1-fetoprotein in chronic liver disease. NEJM 291:506–508, 1974
237. Becker FF, Horland AA, Shurgin A: A study of alpha-1-fetoprotein levels during exposure to 3′-methyl-4-dimethylaminocyobenzene and its analogs. Cancer Res 35:1510–1513, 1975
238. Sell S, Becker FF: Alphafetoprotein. JNCI 60:19–26, 1978
239. LoGerfo P, Barker HG: Immunologic tests for the detection of gastrointestinal cancers. Surg Clin N Am 52:829–837, 1972
240. Javadpour N, Bergman S: Recent advances in testicular cancer. Curr Probl Surg 15:1–64, 1978
241. Javadpour N, McIntire R, Waldmann TA et al: The role of radioimmunoassay of serum alphafetoprotein and human chorionic gonadotropin in the intensive chemotherapy and surgery of metastatic testicular tumors. J Urol 119:759–762, 1978
242. Banwo O, Versey J, Hobbs JR: New oncofetal antigen for human pancreas. Lancet 1:643–645, 1974
243. Wood RAB, Moosa AR: The prospective evaluation of tumour-associated antigens for the early diagnosis of pancreatic cancer. Br J Surg 64:718–720, 1977
244. Vaitukaitis JL, Braunstein GD, Ross GT: A radioimmunoassay which specifically measures human chorionic gonadotropin in the presence of human luteinizing hormone. Am J Obstet Gynecol 113:751–758, 1972
245. Amir SM: Dissociation of glycoprotein hormones. Acta Endocrinol 70:21–34, 1972
246. Goldstein DP, Kosasa TS: The subunit radioimmunoassay for hCG—clinical application. Progress in Gynecol 6:145–184, 1975
247. Hertz R, Lewis J, Lipsett MB: Five years' experience with the chemotherapy of metastatic choriocarcinoma and related trophoblastic tumor in women. Am J Obstet Gynecol 82:631–640, 1961
248. Goldstein DP, Kosasa TS, Skarim AT: The clinical application of a specific radioimmunoassay for human chorionic gonadotropin in trophoblastic and nontrophoblastic tumors. Surg Gynecol Obstet 138:747–751, 1974
249. Braunstein GD, Vaitukaitis JL, Carbone PP et al: Ectopic production of human chorionic gonadotropin by neoplasms. Ann Intern Med 78:39–45, 1973
250. Vaitukaitis JL: Tumors and human chorionic gonadotropin, In Ruddon RW (ed): Biological markers of neoplasia: Basic and applied aspects. New York, Elesevier, 1978
251. Stolback LL, Krant MJ, Fishman WH: Ectopic production of an alkaline phosphatase isoenzyme in patients with cancer. NEJM 281:757–762, 1969
252. Javadpour N, Millan HL: Multiple biochemical tumor markers in testicular seminoma (Submitted for publication)
253. Thorpe WP, Reilly JJ, Rosenberg SA: Prognostic significance of alkaline phosphatase measurements in patients with osteogenic sarcoma receiving chemotherapy. Cancer 43:2178–2181, 1979
254. Levine AM, Rosenberg SA: Alkaline phosphatase levels in osteosarcoma tissue are related to prognosis. Cancer 44:2291–2293, 1979
255. Romas NA, Rose NR, Tannenbaum M: Acid phosphatase: New developments. Hum Pathol 10:501–512, 1979
256. Foti AG, Cooper JF, Herschman H et al: Detection of prostatic cancer by solid phase radioimmunoassay of serum prostatic acid phosphatase. NEJM 297:1357–1361, 1977
257. Cooper JF, Foti A, Herschman H: Combined serum and bone marrow radioimmunoassays for prostatic acid phosphatase. J Urol 122:498–502, 1979
258. Watson RA, Tang DB: The predictive value of prostatic acid phosphatase as a screening test for prostatic cancer. N Engl J Med 303:497–499, 1980
259. Israel L, Edelstein R: In vivo and in vitro studies on nonspecific blocking factors of host origin in cancer patients. Role of plasma exchange as an immunotherapeutic modality. Israel J Med Sc 14:105–130, 1978
260. Baskies AM, Chretien PB, Weiss JF et al: Serum glycoproteins in cancer patients: First report of correlations with in vitro and in vivo parameters of cellular immunity. Cancer 45:3050–3060, 1980
261. Ravry M, McIntire KR, Moertell CG et al: Brief communication: Carcinoembryonic antigen and alphafetoprotein in the diagnosis of gastric and colonic cancer: A comparative clinical evaluation. JNCI 52:1019–1021, 1974
262. Tormey SC, Waalkes TP, Ahman D et al: Biological markers in breast carcinoma. 1. Incidence of abnormalities of CEA, hCG, three polyamines and three minor nucleotides. Cancer 35:1095–1100, 1975
263. Munjal D, Chawla PL, Lokich JJ et al: Carcinoembryonic antigen and phosphohexose isomerase, gammaglutamyltranspeptidase and lactate dehydrogenase levels on patients with and without liver metastases. Cancer 37:1800–1907, 1976
264. Dukes CE: The classification of cancer of the rectum. J Pathol Bacteriol 35:323–332, 1932
265. Haagensen CD, Stout AP: Carcinoma of the breast. Ann Surg 118:1–32, 1943
266. Manual for staging of cancer, 1978. American Joint Committee for Cancer Staging and End Result Reporting, Chicago, 1978
267. Sugarbaker EV: Cancer metastases, a product of tumor host interactions. Curr Probl Cancer 3:1–59, 1979

CHAPTER 12

Psychosocial Aspects of Patients with Cancer

Section 1

Stephen P. Hersh

Psychologic Aspects of Patients with Cancer

The medical community still categorizes concerns about the psychological and social functioning of patients as "supportive care." This approach continues despite accumulated insights of behavioral science research over the past fifty years.

Research documents the reality of the exciting, complex interactions among physiologic, psychologic, and the social state in man. Current information forces us to recognize that only through informed attention to the psychologic and social dimensions of a patient can the physician practice completely responsible care. When the patient suffers from a chronic disease, the importance of this reality is further magnified.

CANCER: A GROUP OF DISEASES AND AN ALLEGORY

Most of the diseases called cancer fall into the category of chronic illness. Informed attention, by the treating physician to psychosocial issues is now as basic to proper care as is expert knowledge of surgery, chemotherapy, and radiation therapy. There exists for this dimension of cancer treatment a complicating factor—the allegory of the *disease* called cancer—those feelings and meanings that our society has attributed to it, and, indeed, the folklore surrounding it. An awareness of this dimension becomes a necessary part of the physician's general sophistication.

The widespread fear that the word, no less the diagnosis of cancer, generates in people is well-recognized.[1–6] Hersh has written that the psychologic dimensions of cancer are strongly colored by society's fears projecting onto the disease. These fears consist of loss of control and of mortality:

> It presents one's own body destroying one's self. Appearing to come from nowhere, it strikes without warning . . . (showing) itself anywhere within the patient at any time. . . . Cancer represents *the* abnormal condition of physical self that symbolizes both our tenuous hold on life and the fragile reality of our own control.[7]

Cancer conjures up images of loneliness, abandonment, and helplessness. To ignore its allegorical/symbolic nature makes the practitioner more of a technician than a physician.

At different times in human history various diseases have represented for the populace the reality of everyone's mortality and, most particularly, the limitations that exist to our control over life's events. The various diseases (*i.e.*, leprosy, bubonic plague, blackwater fever, tuberculosis) that have served as such symbols have, in addition, been considered mysteries in their time themselves. Even the "wise men" and healers of the time were ignorant of etiology. Obviously, they were relatively helpless in modifying the course and person-to-person spread of these illnesses. Such mystery always encourages persons to formulate reasons that explain their misfortune.

In our culture, assisted by the Judeo–Christian reference contained in the story of Job, mysteries resulting in personal suffering tend to be associated with punishment for known or unknown transgressions (sins).[8] This provides an identifiable cause, a reason. It also, given the association to sin, forms one of the bases for stigma—a special marking of the person—a marking associated with disgrace, reproach, and infamy.

Despite the educational efforts of the American Cancer Society, its local affiliates, the National Cancer Institute, and various self-help organizations such as "Make Today Count," the diseases called cancer continue to stigmatize people in their families, their friendships, groups, neighborhoods, and workplaces. This stigmatization finds expression today in numerous ways. For example, it is expressed through the morbid curiosity displayed by persons not previously interested in the person who has now become a cancer patient; through the distancing behavior of others who previously related well to that individual (the distancing is often based on secret fears of contagion); through occasional cruel behaviors by employers who fire or will not hire when aware of the diagnosis; through neighborhoods that attempt to block the purchasing of a new home by a family whose child has cancer.

Thus, in considering the psychologic aspects of cancer in the cancer patient the physician must be aware of the social mark the individual bears and the potential effects it has on relationships, work lives, and on the patient's sense of himself. When stigma becomes the active social process called stigmatization, the stress placed on the patient can be unbearable, enough to cause depression, loss of appetite, withdrawal, and poor tolerance of and even poor response to treatments. Moreover, stigma combined with the fears generated by the loss of control implied in the diagnosis produces many ostensibly puzzling behaviors. Among these is "delay behavior," the reluctance or inability of a person with symptoms to follow through with a diagnostic visit to a physician.[9,10]

Complicating the mythology of cancer are the many hypotheses and insights concerning its possible causes that receive such widespread coverage in the lay and scientific press. Examples include such items as the delineation of chemical agents, including alcohol, that can produce cancers; the discovery that a certain transmissable chromosomal difference dramatically increases the probability of persons in certain genetic lines having cancer; the possible relationships of slow-virus infections in humans to certain cancers; and the hypotheses that chronic, stress-induced emotional states can predispose at least certain human beings to have some form of cancer.[11-17] The result appears to be greatly heightened by anxiety, vigilence, and fear in the lay public about this "disease." Cancer in the U.S. today is associated with everything from punishment for sins, to problems with closeness to parents, to bad luck, evil eyes, bad thoughts, bad genes, and bad people who irresponsibly manage the environment.[18] It seems to be everywhere and to be caused by everything. It is no wonder that some people began to joke not too long ago, making such statements as, "Did you know that leisure suits cause cancer in men!"

THE WAYS PEOPLE ARE AFFECTED BY CANCER

General Perspectives

Consider stress as an altered state of the organism.[19] Many things influence a person's capacity for dealing (or coping) with that altered state. These variables include:

- genetic makeup
- intactness and functioning of the nervous system
- growth and development experiences
- general health
- sex
- age
- culture
- psychological processes and self-image
- the specific "outside-of-self" resources (family, work, school, community)
- stress-producing life events (death, divorce, job change, moving, promotion, etc.)

Stress reactions to cancer are universal. The kind of cancer, the ability to locate it, where it is located, or the inability to locate it, all affect or influence the patient's psychological response, that of the family, and sometimes even that of the physicians. Specifically, the initial reaction, if the cancer is in a site easily visible and away from the internal organs, tends to be one of lesser fear and greater hope, based on a fantasy (sometimes a knowledge) that control and cure are possible. This applies to the reactions to cancers that involve both the extremities and the skin. Often cancers that physicians recognize as having great malignant potential, such as the melanomas and sarcomas, the patient will react to with more hope. The victim will immediately hone in on the apparent reality of the tumor being localized, away from head and vital organs, and therefore something that can be cut out with a resulting cure. Tumors associated with vital organs produce more fear and greater challenges to hopefulness. Tumors associated with the sexual organs have the additional emotion-laden dimensions of the intactness of one's maleness or femaleness. Most challenging of all, in a psychologic sense, are those cancers that require the patient to accept the reality of the disease based on their own feelings of "unwellness," the physician's statements, and laboratory test results. These particular cancers, referred to in this book as the *hematologic malignancies*, are the most frightening. To the lay mind they are simultaneously everywhere and nowhere. The patient does not feel well, may have some gross symptoms or signs, but relies very heavily on another person for an explanation. The physician tells the patient that according to tests, the "unwellness" is due to a malignant disease that cannot be localized to a single site for control or excision.

Other factors known to influence a person's reactions to cancer include the disease's visability to the patient and disfigurement and loss of functional capacity caused by treatment. Changes in contour of part of the body, changes in pigmentation, an unchanging sore throat, a bloody discharge, and chronic loss of weight are all examples of the ways various forms of cancer make themselves visible. Disfigurement and loss of function can include a greatly swollen neck, a grossly enlarged testicle, a hoarse voice, or diminished energy levels and strength. Treatment, of course, often produces the disfigurement of amputations, hair loss, and mouth ulcerations as well as physical weakness, lability of mood, and reduction in libido.

Although extensive studies of women with breast cancer reveal that most cope quite well with their disease and its treatments, very real difficulties do exist.[20,21] Examples of documented responses include suicidal ideation, increased anxiety, transient mood and behavioral changes, and transient increases in the use of alcohol and tranquilizers.[20] All patients experience increased anxiety with mood and behavioral change. These range from stoic silence, to withdrawal and depression, to restless agitation. These changes most often are transient. Psychological and social equilibrium is usually regained through the use of personal strengths that most persons have within the context of their belief systems, family, and other support systems (see the Essential Approaches and Intervention section of this chapter for further discussion). Those who have acute, severe problems in dealing with the stress of their disease and its treatments, or more chronic difficulties, usually have premorbid conditions that considerably enhance their vulnerability.[22] Problems in coping are not a matter of accident. Not only should the disease and its treatments be considered but the patient's personality structure, support network, and the treating physician's conduct and statements, especially when stress reactions are greater in intensity or duration than expected.[23]

The coping problems of Hodgkin's disease patients have not been studied as well as those of breast cancer patients. Optimism about the medical community's ability to treat the disease clearly influences patients and their families. Today, this optimism is rather high for Hodgkin's disease patients. Yet the reality for Hodgkin's disease patients is that chemotherapy-induced changes in sexual functioning and loss of fertility have produced severe adjustment reactions. These reactions can be dealt with successfully by early recognition of the emotional problem and subsequent professional intervention. Such intervention helps the patient successfully modify his self-image and reduce the number of resultant problems, such as disruptions in friendship and family relationships.[24,25]

Cancers of the external genitalia present direct, special challenges to an individual's body image and sexual functioning. Penile or vulvar lesions are often dealt with by radical surgical treatments with resultant disfigurements and functional disabilities.[25] With such cancers the risks of delay behavior are understandably high. Private, silent, emotional suffering is so likely that responsible management requires open, ongoing attention for each patient. Individual and group counseling have reduced the levels of psychologic and physical dysfunction in these patients.[26,27]

Cancer of the larynx presents a series of challenges beyond the physical changes of post-neck dissection and laryngectomy. Loss of those capacities and functions that most of us take for granted generates great concern in the patients over their control of various functions including speech, chewing, salivating, and swallowing. Depression is so likely to be a more-than-transient phenomenon in total laryngectomy patients that planned pre-operative and post-operative preparation of the patient should be part of routine care.[28,29] Such preparation is best accomplished by a multidisciplinary approach including surgeon, speech pathologist, and social worker. Access to a psychiatric consultant is also highly desirable. In addition, work should be done with both the patient and the patient's family, rehearsing expected changes and reviewing ways of regaining both control and function.

AGE. A cancer patient's age has a great deal to do with how the patient and family cope. Many problems as well as strengths can be predicted on this basis as long as the physician recognizes that chronological age and developmental stage do *not* always coincide. No matter what a patient's age, the diagnosis and initial treatments experienced by patient and family are shattering to the continuity of the life cycle, at some level. This produces regressive behavior in people and family systems including withdrawal from social interactions, increased dependency on family members for assistance in everyday activities and decisions, and "acting-out" rather than direct recognition and expression of feelings.* Such behaviors usually are self-limited and quite amenable to direct guidance by the physician.

Very young children cope by adapting so well to their experience that it becomes truly their "norm." An example of this kind of adaptation is a mother's recounting this statement by her six-year-old, a child diagnosed as having acute lymphocytic leukemia at age three years: Mother and daughter are in their kitchen and the afflicted daughter asks, "Mommy, when you were a little girl and had leukemia, did you also have trouble finding friends?"

As children age, they gradually develop the same cognitive capacities and "vocabulary" of psychological defenses as adults. They can rationalize, intellectualize, repress, sublimate, etc. In addition, they incorporate cultural reference points and belief systems as well as myths that help them and their families provide explanations for current experiences.[19] Child, adolescent, and adult cancer patients can become victims of the anxiety, intrusiveness, and defensiveness of others. Those "others" may be family members or medical care staff.

HOSPITALIZATION. Hospitalization itself is an experience that generates anxiety and predisposes the person to depression and withdrawal. This is especially so in the younger child.[30] For this reason, as much care as possible should be delivered through outpatient visits. In young children, a widely-noted coping style involves intense identification with doctors, nurses, and other members of the medical team. As part of such identification, these children assume the nonverbal behaviors and vocabulary of the medical adults who

* The phrase "acting-out" is commonly used psychiatric jargon. It refers to a person expressing feelings through specific behaviors. Conscious awareness of such feelings is often absent or partial. Examples of "acting-out" are repeated sarcasm directed at others when the underlying feelings may be bitterness and anger at being ill; dramatic disregard for previously respected limits such as curfews, drinking, reckless driving, in a teenager whose underlying feelings are anger and fear bordering on panic as a reaction to receiving the diagnosis of cancer.

surround them. The children absorb as much information about the disease and treatments as they can, becoming quite glib in recounting details of their illness, its progress, and its treatments. Hersh labels this coping style as a "pseudo-sophistication." The physician must often make an effort with such children to realize what they are encountering, that underneath the veneer is a child with all the bewilderments and needs appropriate for the age group.

ADOLESCENTS. Some of the most poignant age-related struggles in cancer patients are seen with adolescents. The necessary involvement with the treatment process, the compliance, the surrendering of much control, all force the adolescent to suspend the important struggles for autonomy and independence from the family.

THE AGED. Adjustment to the loss of function or limitations on function is not necessarily easier in the aged. Their continuity of life experiences is interrupted just as is that of the younger patient. The knowledge that developing a form of cancer is more likely in someone their age does not make the reality of cancer more acceptable for the person. He may clearly remember past physical functioning, energy levels, and abilities to fulfill needs and expectations. Thus, an apparent easy adjustment in an elderly person to an important loss of function may be deceptive. Similarly, the development of apparent dementia in an elderly person may not be a function of the disease, or of age, but an expression of severe depression and anxiety bordering on panic.[31] Appropriate treatment of such pseudodementia begins with something that is unfortunately not-so-obvious: the physician must consider pseudodementia in the differential diagnosis when confronted with marked deterioration in the psychosocial functioning of an elderly patient.[32]

SPECIFIC AREAS OF FUNCTIONING AFFECTED BY THE CANCERS

Self-Image and General Psychological State

How a person thinks and feels about himself defines "self-image." Self-image influences each person's level of comfort with themselves and with other people. Self-image is derived from developmental experiences from infancy within the context of particular physical and intellectual resources. The major components include physical self, psychological self, and social self.

Any of the cancers and their treatments produce changes—some transient, some permanent—in all three areas. When these changes occur, they are based on both the immediate reality as well as the anticipation of possible further changes. For example, amputation, impotency, and inability to work, may all be immediate changes with which a person must deal. Simultaneously, further disfigurement, future ability to be a sexual partner, and the actual loss of employment are of major concern. The required adjustments to change are significant and sometimes dramatic.[33] However, as stated earlier, psychological decompensation of sufficient degree to result in a clinical problem is rarely seen.[34] Challenges to a person's self-image, despite alterations in energy level, strength, agility, and mood, should be understood by the physician to be dramatic but manageable.[35] The techniques physicians can use to assist patients in these areas are discussed later in the chapter.

As background information, the physician must recall that the human armamentarium for dealing with challenges to self-image and alterations in moods and vegetative functions, as well as other forms of stress, relies heavily on psychological defense mechanisms. These are protective and usually unconscious mental processes used to shield the patient from feeling excessive anxiety. At the same time, they help the person deal with whatever external or internal stresses are producing the anxiety. The 19 traditionally identified defense mechanisms are illustrated in several psychiatric references.[36] These include

> displacement, denial, projection, condensation, conversion, dissociation, idealization, identification, incorporation, intellectualization, introjection, undoing, rationalization, reaction formation, regression, repression, sublimation, substitution, and symbolization.

In our culture, the most frequently mobilized defense mechanisms used by cancer patients are denial, intellectualization, and rationalization. Denial may be understood as the psychological rejection of feelings associated with certain events or thoughts. Or, it may be more generalized to total experiences or realities. It is one of the most important, adaptive, and effective defense mechanisms. Generally, the physician should avoid challenging it unless denial is interfering with either the treatment process or the patient's handling of essential family responsibilities (*i.e.*, finances, wills, etc.). Intellectualization and rationalization are closely related. The former refers to the use of intellectual processes to control or avoid the experience and expression of feelings. The latter refers to the use of intellectual processes to hide from oneself and others instinctual motives for particular behavior. For example, when a situation is perceived as dangerous an instinctual response would be to escape from the situation. However, what is presented to self and others may be the sudden need for a vacation.

Sex and Sexuality

Sexuality is a "pattern of learned human conduct, a set of skills and feelings . . ." that relate to both gender identity (sense of maleness or femaleness) and sexual behavior.[38] Given our common birth and early nurturent (bonding) experiences, sexuality includes those behaviors and feelings associated with touching, holding, and cuddling, as well as with genital sex acts.[7,38] Sexual demands and expectations placed on people vary through the life cycle.[39]

Thoughtful physician attention to the complex subject of sex and sexuality is needed more than ever. This is because of the tendency of patients and families to totally hand themselves over to the medical community when cancer is diagnosed. The medical community's attention to this issue is recent. Until now, society has tended to be symptom-oriented, focusing mostly on such issues as libido and performance capabilities in the cardiac or hemodialysis patient. An educational approach for cancer patients is needed on this subject. Such an approach relates to the particular stresses generated by the disease and its treatments. In addition, for persons with a chronic disability or disease, their "level of knowledge and skills" concerning their capacities becomes a significant factor influencing autonomy, control, and sense of responsibility for self.[40]

Cancers and their treatments can effect any aspect of body image and physiology that relates to sexual identity. For the prepubertal patient, delays or permanent changes in development can occur.[41] For the postpubertal patient, functional capacities and sexual interest (libido) changes vary in significance, depending on age, stage of development, personality, expectations, and social role (spouse, parent, lover). Such changes may be primarily physical (*i.e.*, amputation, resection, etc.).[26,42–45] Changes may also be physiological, although both produce emotional distress. Physical changes include altered secondary sexual characteristics, most commonly breast and hair loss. These have been studied for a long time.[20,46,47] Other important physical changes not as well studied include altered sensory abilities, such as hypersensitivity of the skin and other paresthesias. Physiologic changes secondary to therapeutic castration have major effects on the person. Vasomotor instability, headaches, nervousness and depression can also be observed in the same person.[48]

A person's sense of intactness as a sexual being significantly influences their sense of wholeness, strength, and health. This is further colored by the expectations made upon that person by others, and also by messages concerning what is whole and healthy from the culture.

Today, the physician who treats oncologic diseases should no longer join the collusion of silence about sexuality any more than he should join the collusion of silence about death. Sexuality is part of life and hence, a part of cancer patients and their families.

Family

Given the many forms the family assumes in society, it is best when the physician thinks of it in the broadest terms. Therefore, family is defined as any group of persons with a legal or biological relationship. The kind of family structure within which the cancer patient lives, as well as the dynamics within that structure, obviously determine many of the specific issues concerning how the family and family system are affected by cancer in one of its members.

Families are systems that exist within larger systems—neighborhoods, communities, cultures—and these larger systems influence the family. Cultural mythologies about cancer and the community's integration of those mythologies have been discussed earlier as important influencing factors. They color the assistance given as well as stigmatization suffered by the family.

Families differ in their structural and behavioral characteristics. Some families are closed systems with clear boundaries. They have very selective "transport" of ideas, influencing people into or out of them. This quality makes them less sensitive to the larger systems and, obviously, less dependent on them. Other families have less clearly defined boundaries. Often such families include non-related individuals (friends), bonded to the unit as closely or more so than the traditional biologically-related members. More vulnerable to outside systems, such families also have greater degrees of flexibility than the "closed boundary" family.

Many other characteristics also need to be considered. For example,

Is it a single or two parent family?
How career-oriented are its members?
What are the relationships of adults and children?
Is the major breadwinner the patient?
Is it a family in which information is easily shared?
Are feelings shared, and in what way?
What are the family members' styles of communication with one another?

This type of awareness about the patient's family provides insight into the nature of the support system available to the patient.

Families have their own stages of development. These stages are associated with changing values, changing perceptions of their members, and changing behaviors. Usually, families coalesce at moments of crisis. Their attention focuses on the member who becomes ill. Simultaneously, the family's networks of relations, friends, and acquaintances is set in motion with the news and prepared for potential support. Support may range from providing interest and sympathy to donations of blood, blood fractions, or bone marrow. A hierarchy in the intensity of initial response to the cancer diagnosis does seem to exist based either upon the age or roles of the ill member—children, adolescents, young adults, and principle breadwinners receive the strongest supportive reactions. (Such reactions are equally intense for older people if the family holds them in great affection.) Once the first moment of crisis has passed, family members tend to shift back to their previous rhythms, interests, and activities. However, the network, maintained by the nuclear family (whatever form it takes), remains especially tuned in to new crises.

When the diagnosis leads rapidly to treatment followed by cure, the stress on the family remains almost always within its tolerance capacities. This is similarly true when diagnosis leads rapidly to treatment and, despite all treatments, to death. The situations that sorely test family systems, demanding all of their supportive capabilities and those of their supportive networks, are situations where the course from diagnosis to either cure or death is a prolonged one. In such circumstances, attentions and energies wax and wane; relationships (intimate and distant) are stressed and shift; and people change because of their experiences and exposure to new ideas and to new people.[49] Today, these chronic situations are the most common reality for cancer patients and their families. As a result, major alterations of the pre-morbid family system occur because that system has both engrafted onto it and intruded into it the medical care system and other parts of the human service system such as social services.[7,50]

Although families respond quite well over time to calls for special attention, frequent cycling of crises causes fatigue. Indeed, a family can become desensitized, with partial extinction of empathetic responses. An extreme form of this is seen with the Lazarus syndrome, which develops guilt-generating, barely conscious anger and hostility.*[51] Wishes that

* And he that was dead came forth. (John 11:44)

the ill person will die surface in response to the stress of the unpredictable, painful, disruptive process. Healthy family members, particularly adolescents, may act out in various ways (*i.e.*, sexual promiscuity, drug abuse, running away).[52]

However, many families adapt very well despite all the challenges and pain. Indeed, there is reason to question the belief that parents of children with cancer suffer higher separation and divorce rates.[53] Successful adaptation has its price, too. For some it is paid when the ill family member dies and the entire family equilibrium, as well as the members within it, must painfully shift their life styles to adapt to the new post-death reality. For others, when cure becomes a probability, the adjustment can often prove equally as challenging.[54]

Families function in terms of group dynamics, with forming, fragmenting, and then reforming alliances. Psychological defenses are also employed by family members, but most families provide tremendous resources to their members. Some families do find themselves to be more vulnerable than others to problems in coping with cancer. Such families containing a cancer victim almost always have pre-existing problems that weakened them, such as marital conflict, economic difficulties, alcohol or drug abuse, or frank psychopathology (*e.g.*, schizophrenia, severe depressive disorders). Extra demands such as frequent moves, moves to different cultures, or dramatic career involvements, may also heighten a family's vulnerability. Common supports to family systems include their values, traditions, religion, and role in the community. All of these can be used in times of stress.

Work, School, and the Community

Work, school, and the community are tremendously important to cancer patients. Schools of any level, from nursery to university, are just as defined as places of employment—these are special environments where people find themselves interacting closely with others. All members of these environments react to and affect one another. When one member is diagnosed as having cancer, and that diagnosis becomes known, the behaviors within the school or workplace will change. Both are influenced not only by the people within them, but also by the values of the culture. Hence, they become sites for positive and negative behavior, for support and stigmatization. Helpful coalescing of members can occur; so can hurtful, but innocent, misunderstandings. Kind assistance can be found, as can frank, cruel rejection.

Information concerning what is actually happening in the school or workplace must be specifically gathered by the physician, nurse, or social worker. Other sources of information beyond the patient include family members, and (if permission is obtained) teachers or supervisors. Interventions are possible for any problems that arise in these sites. The basic guiding principle for the physician is to keep the cancer patient as involved as possible for as long as possible in the school, work, and the community.

Community refers to the immediate neighborhood, place of religious worship and involvement, and the social and civic organizations to which a person belongs. For the cancer patient, community offers tremendous potentials for economic, social, and emotional support. The physician's primary responsibility toward a community on behalf of the cancer patient is accurate information-sharing while simultaneously respecting privacy. This can be done through public education about cancer and its treatments geared toward reducing misunderstandings based on misinformation or prejudice.

THE CHALLENGE OF TREATING CANCER PATIENTS

Whether the physician is an oncologist, hematologist, surgeon, or primary care physician, treating cancer patients proves to be a personal as well as a professional challenge. Combine cancer's symbolic meanings in this society (as described at the beginning of this chapter) with the limitations and nature of available treatments, our culture's intolerance of disability, fear of death, and obsession with control. Together, these elements form the bases for the challenge caring for cancer patients presents. Of course, the extent of this challenge varies with the particular role the physician has (*i.e.*, consultant, primary care, terminal care). It also depends on the psychological structure and available support system. Cancer care is an issue of much greater complexity for the physician than implied in the traditional laments about the poor quality or missing elements of a physician's training.[55,56] Those laments seem to be based on sound realities. Yet, cancer care makes special demands on the people involved in its delivery. The many stories of physicians who withdraw from treating cancer patients, who become chronically gruff and distant, who become depressed or suicidal, are based on true occurrences.

Physicians should educate themselves with a continuing awareness of at least three dimensions of their work in oncology—the demands and effects of those demands made upon us as human beings; our own physical and psychological reactions to those demands; the psychological and behavioral defenses we mobilize to deal with the resultant stress.[57]

The demands made upon the physician are numerous. They include control and care of the disease process. Less articulated demands are for these goals to be achieved with as little discomfort, inconvenience, and expense to the patient and family as possible. Physicians face such demands from those they treat, knowing in reality that treatments frequently trade-off one kind of morbidity for another (*e.g.*, removal of a painful sarcomatous limb with the resultant disability of an amputation) and even one kind of mortality for another (*e.g.*, death secondary to chemotherapy-induced cardiotoxicity instead of death secondary to metastases-induced asphyxiation). Unarticulated, but constant and intense are the expectations for physicians to provide assistance and support to the psychological as well as social functioning of their patients. These expectations provide the "vehicles" through which the physician is used as the primary person with whom the patient and family can share their anxieties, fears, anger, helplessness, and hopelessness.

All of us react consciously and unconsciously to these demands. Physicians may find their own desires for control and personal rescue fantasies vibrate and mix with those of patients, their families, even with other members of the medical team. The physician's anxieties, fears, and mood swings become colored by the situation as well as by the parallel psychological states of the patient. Fatigue that the physician feels is often related not only to long working hours, but also to the somatic tension and other physiologic changes experienced in response to the above-described reactions. Such fatigue and tension are probably heightened by the fact that by training, inclination, and opportunity the physician condemns himself to isolation within himself. The physician, like the patient, has no primary trusted person with whom he pours out his anxieties, fears, anger, helplessness, and hopelessness.

The physician automatically and unconsciously mobilizes various psychological and behavioral defenses. The defenses the physician is trained to employ are those of intellectualization and sublimation. These are used heavily and appropriately much of the time. A familiar example is the on-going struggle to have an intellectual grasp of what is known about the disease and its treatments. Another example is found with many clinicians being involved with various forms of research and problem-solving. Other defenses include displacement, projection, repression, and rationalization. Medical "humor," doctors' jokes, exaggerated medical lunchtime, OR dressing room, or postrounds camaraderie all derive from these defenses.

Isolation and distancing of self are defenses all too commonly used. These defenses are often behind the behavior of the physician who cannot allow the patient or family to ask questions, or who cannot differentiate between covert ("I'm frightened!") and overt ("Go over again in detail the new treatment regimen and all its side effects") messages in those questions allowed to the patient. Using these defenses, the physician often distances himself from patients by overwhelming them (the rationalization used is informed consent) with information.[58]

Of course, behavioral defenses cannot truly be separated from psychological defenses. However, such behaviors are certainly easier to recognize in others and sometimes even in yourself. Common behaviors include: outbursts of impatience or anger, no matter whom they are directed at (hospital "system," family, patient, nurses, other medical staff, consultants, etc.), in immediate response to minor or not even identifiable challenges; quiet sadness and withdrawal; and tremendous aggressiveness in relaxation activity (*i.e.,* golf, tennis, squash, etc.). Behavioral defenses may also include buying sprees for material goods; eating binges; rage reactions at home; and various forms of self-destructive behavior ranging from minor self-mutilation (severe nail biting, hair pulling/trichotillomania) to reckless driving, to substance abuse, to suicide.

The more successfully physicians cope, the better they serve the patients and families they care for. The physician's pleasure and pride in work parallels such coping. A necessary first step in coping is the physician's acceptance of himself as a human being with human responses to the stresses of work with oncology patients.

OTHER MEMBERS OF THE TREATMENT TEAM: THE PERSONAL CHALLENGES THEY FACE

Important issues for physicians apply in varying degrees to other members of the medical staff who have patient contact. The realm of such people is broad—medical consultants, clergy, dieticians, the various nursing personnel, the special therapies (*e.g.,* O.T., R.T., hearing and speech, etc.), psychiatrists, psychologists, social workers, and technicians (blood bank, radiology/radiotherapy, etc.). Some work closely with patients, while others have only fleeting contact. Most function in the usual outpatient or inpatient environments, dealing with the various day-to-day demands. Some work with patients in special protected environments, such as laminar air flow rooms that impose very special demands on everyone. For all disciplines the challenges and the success in meeting those challenges depends on several factors: basic training; the quality of the orientation received to work with oncology patients and to special work situations (*e.g.,* protected environments, bone marrow transplants, radical surgical procedures); the existence or non-existence of support systems; and the basic personality structure of each individual.

With the exception of physicians in consultant roles, these members of the medical team, while facing similar issues, have less authority, less potential for control, and fewer obvious resources at their disposal than the oncologist, hematologist, surgeon or primary care physician. Thus, one may wonder whether they are more vulnerable to the stress-induced reactive behaviors and states which Hersh has observed in oncology service staff members (*e.g.,* shopping sprees, sexual promiscuity, depression, confusion of work life and private life, extreme forms of compartmentalizing feelings from behaviors, withdrawal, fleeing from work, accident proneness, and suicide).

Various disciplines are now involved in intensely exploring these issues with the goals of creating greater understanding of and greater effectiveness in staff work with cancer patients.[59–62] As the multidisciplinary-treatment-team approach becomes more of a reality in cancer treatment, such exploration must be further encouraged by physicians. Greater understanding can provide a basis for better training, and improved training will definitely help reduce common problems. These may include nurses being overinvolved in surrogate–parent or surrogate family member roles; adversary-like, territorial battles between disciplines over the patient or patient care; and poor communication of physician specialists with primary care physicians.[63]

THE POWER, GLORY, AND MAGIC OF THE CANCER TREATMENT CENTER

The question of the effects that cancer treatment centers have on the psychosocial functioning of cancer patients and their families needs some thoughtful exploration. Dr. Hersh suggests that such centers have assumed an intrusive role. They are technological equivalents of Delphi and Lourdes. As such, the offerings medical centers demand are greater than the offerings demanded in historic places of pilgrimage for cure. Beyond the demand for goods (payment), medical centers demand a degree of compliance with care that has the patient and family yielding much autonomy. In many ways, family dynamics are altered; physicians and nurses, even for adult patients, become surrogate parent figures. Self-care is discouraged except where specifically designed into systems. For inpatients normal physical reassurance through holding, hugging, and touching is in many ways covertly discouraged. Personal and family rhythms become altered in the direction of the demands of the medical center's various schedules. Hersh presents the hypothesis that sensitive attention to these realities in working with families to maintain, as much as possible, their active involvement with the patient, and working with patients to maintain, as much as possible, their autonomy and control, will have salutary effects on the *quality of life* experienced by all concerned. Further hypothesized is that such an approach will minimize at least certain morbidities of cancer treatment, such as reactive depression or the degree of incapacity experienced by radiation and chemotherapy side-effects (reactions to hair loss, anorexia, nausea, vomiting, and fatigue). These hypotheses, stated in various ways, are being tested by others. At this time, support is developing for the quality of life hypothesis.[64–66] As the chronicity of cancer care continues to develop, these questions will grow in importance.

INFORMED CONSENT

The knowledgeable participation of patients in their medical care and in those decisions related to that care summarizes the goals of informed consent. Throughout the U.S., belief in informed consent is institutionalized by way of the widely-distributed, 12 article, American Hospital Association's *Patient's Bill of Rights*. Everything from hospital-based public defender services to hospital employed ombudsmen and patient advocates is found here. The Patient's Bill of Rights is a sincere effort to assure knowledgeable use of the rights of patients. The practical as well as the legal and ethical dimensions of informed consent generate ongoing debate.

Findings from some recent studies are worthy of note. Some 75% of 200 cancer patients recently studied believed that informed consent forms were necessary as well as important to help decide their treatment. Of these 200 patients, 28% believed that they had to sign consent forms if such forms were given to them. Some 25% indicated they would do what their doctor said anyway.[67] The same study agreed with earlier findings that many patients failed to recall major portions of the information contained on the forms. Those who had the best recall believed most in the importance of the consent forms, were younger, Caucasian, and more educated (high school or greater). Bed-ridden patients recalled information less well than healthier patients.

Another study of five surgical consent forms showed that those forms were dramatically poor vehicles for conveying information. This was based on their "readability" equivalent to that for college or higher educational level readers.[68] Earlier studies revealed that only 7% of consent forms were written in language as simple as that of Time magazine; 77% are written at the senior year of high school or above language competency level![69]

In this country, our value system is to inform patients and their families. Studies indicate that patients want to hear "straightforward, even harsh statements."[69] Some, such as the Simontons of Fort Worth, Texas, carry the value of informed consent even further. They strongly believe that active participation in medical treatment is essential to getting well again."* [65]

* A husband-wife team (he, a radiation oncologist, she, a lay psychotherapist) who founded the Cancer Counseling and Research Center of Fort Worth. The Center focuses on psychological aspects of cancer treatment and cancer etiology.

Whatever the stand on this spectrum of opinion, objective evidence indicates that the practice of informed consent needs to be brought closer to the value system. The majority of written consent forms tend to "obfuscate, intimidate, and alienate" while oral explanations often leave much to be desired in the eyes of patients, families, and physicians.[69]

Hersh strongly recommends that informed consent should be made an ongoing, basic issue and principle of physician practice. Current aides, such as the *Patient's Bill of Rights* should be used. Copies should be available in physician offices and in hospitals. Furthermore, physicians should periodically review with colleagues the oral explanations and written consent forms used. Finally, the physician must always remember that people require repetition over time *combined with* both listening and encouragement to ask questions.

ESSENTIAL APPROACHES AND INTERVENTIONS

The first section of this chapter elaborated on the necessity that the physician treating cancer patients must always consider the whole person—not only the maintenance of that person's physical integrity but their psychological and social integrity as well. This section reviews essential approaches to successfully fulfilling this complex role. These essential approaches can be subsumed under five general headings:

1. The physician as a healer—beliefs and personality
2. Presenting the diagnosis of cancer to the patient, to important others
3. Assisting the patient to live with cancer
4. Working with the dying patient
5. Helping the patient live with cure

THE PHYSICIAN AS HEALER: BELIEFS AND PERSONALITY

Throughout recorded history, the healer's belief in his remedies has always appeared essential to the relationship with those who seek help.[70] Conviction in the effectiveness of the remedies combined with confidence in the healer's ability to use those remedies provides the setting in which a physician/healer generates trust and hope. Lack of conviction and lack of confidence are quickly noted by patients. They may respond with anger, disappointment, and withdrawal. However, when patients experience the physician in control, they respond with a high degree of cooperation and compliance. In addition, both cooperation and compliance are severely undermined—no matter what the physician's levels of technical knowledge and skill—by uncertainty on the physician's part.

Coloring the patient's responses is the image, the persona, projected by the physician. Aloof efficiency combined with impatience, compared to outgoing warmth, empathy, and calm attentiveness, produces very different reactions in patients, families, and medical staff. Physicians with the former persona find that their patients are guarded in their presence. At best, their patients will allow themselves to be approached in terms of the overt physical dimensions of this illness. They will tend not to volunteer information about new symptoms, subtle reactions to therapies, or directly express psychological stress. Indeed, stress does tend to build up and be expressed in the form of physical complaints and exaggerated morbidity to prescribed treatments (*i.e.*, more nausea and vomiting, more mood changes, and more weakness, than expected). Compliance with treatments, if adequate, will be out of fear rather than out of a sense of participation with the physician.

The physician with warmth, calm attentiveness, and confidence, facilitates the adjustment of patient and family to their new reality. With such physicians, patients tend to openly express their various concerns and to recount or inquire about subtle symptoms that concern them. Their compliance with treatment and motivation to follow through with treatments (even in difficult times) are greater out of a sense of partnership with the physician. Even morbidities from the various forms of treatment present a greater potential for being successfully handled.

This latter approach is obviously recommended to all physicians without reservations. Time constraints, a possible source of reluctance in accepting this recommendation, need not be an issue. A sincerely nurturant approach to patients does not necessarily require more time than an efficient, brusque, technical approach. The key is for the physician to focus attention on the patient while allowing non-verbal (body language*) behaviors to be consistent with verbal expressions of empathy, interest, and concern. For example, talking with a patient while standing at the bedside for five minutes, eyes furtively glancing from patient's face to your watch, leaves the patient dissatisfied with the visit and with any information shared. The same five minutes spent while sitting at the bedside, leaning toward or touching the patient, looking into the patient's eyes, leaves a patient convinced that the visit was long, attentive, and full of clear and helpful information.

Presenting the Diagnosis

Clinical experience generally supports the observation that informed patients are more receptive to prescribed treatment.[71] Moreover, attitudes acquired at the time the diagnosis is presented often seem to influence the future handling of the illness by patient and family. As noted in the discussion on informed consent, patients do want to know about the procedures that they will undergo.[69] The specific question of whether or not patients want to be given their diagnosis is now being researched.[73] Early studies with potentially fatal illnesses other than cancer showed that selective denial by patients seemed to be correlated with improved survival.[74-77] More recent studies find that not only do patients vary in the degree of benefit obtained from the awareness of their illness but also both individuals and family groups vary in terms of their ability to use any information.[78,79]

With all of the above considered, how should the physician present the diagnosis of cancer to the patient? What should the physician do or not do?

1. The physician's objectives are to help the patient maintain physical and psychological integrity.
2. The physician should present the diagnosis to the patient and family, having as thorough a knowledge of the family as possible (*i.e.*, the information that can be obtained through the traditional history and review of systems).
3. The physician should plan for more than one meeting on the diagnosis because very little of what is shared during the first meeting is retained.[65,66,71]
4. Using information concerning the patient's age, personality, and family (availability, proximity, belief systems, style of communicating), the physician should decide in advance whether or not to inform the patient alone or together with his family. In general, the family's presence is preferred.[71,72] Such meetings should be designed with the goal of facilitating the family's functioning as a support system for the patient.
5. The presentation should be tailored to the patient's age, language, and cultural background, and even with highly educated patients, the physician should use basic English, not medical jargon.
6. The patients and family should be asked to repeat what they have heard and understood. (This can be done gently by the physician.) Such inquiry helps to identify for the physician as early as possible selective hearing and retention by patients and family. It is often wise for the physician to simply note such distortions rather than attempt to immediately correct them.
7. The physician should observe, as well as listen to, the patient and family during the interviews, using this information to guide both immediate and future interactions with them.
8. The patient will *not* tell the physician all his major concerns and fears. Concerns, fears, and questions should be expressed over time. Lists of issues and questions that come to mind after patient-physician meetings should be made by the patient and brought to future meetings.[66]
9. Patients should be allowed to adapt to the diagnosis and treatments in their own way, but the physician should examine carefully and consult with a colleague about adaptations that make him uncomfortable before taking action. There is a broad range of reasonable human behaviors. Often, the physician's feelings of discomfort may be based on different values, or a projection of his own feelings onto the situation, or on a control struggle of some kind that he is having with the patient. Problems usually arise around various dimensions of denial. Remember that for the patient, "Illness is one aspect of reality . . . (struggling with) the concept of denial of illness ignores the important values that make surviving the illness worthwhile to the individual."[79]
10. The above recommendation does not eliminate the fact that maladaptive reactions to the diagnosis and illness do occur. When the physician has identified such reactions, his responsibility is to intervene using one or more of the techniques outlined in the next section.

* Information given by somatic musculature of a person, for example, facial muscles, direction of gaze, posturing of limbs, and position of trunk.

Assisting the Patient to Live with Cancer

Information concerning the basic principles and general techniques for assisting patients to live with cancer is presented at great length by Rosenbaum and Kelly.[66,71] Based on Hersh's experience as well as the literature (including that by Rosenbaum and Kelly), an outline of key points follows:

1. The process for assisting the patient to live with cancer begins with informing him of the diagnosis.
2. Physicians must be concerned with the patient's autonomy. This involves participation in self-care, medical treatments, and maintaining self in the roles held prior to illness (student, parent, spouse, lover, bread-winner).
3. Problems in psychological and social adjustment should be identified and attended to as soon as possible.
4. Maintain your awareness of the tremendous potential, and frightening reality, cancer patients have for feeling lonely and isolated from others.
5. Monitor the status of each patient's support systems: family, friends; work/school; community; religious involvement.
6. Encourage the use of support systems, including appropriate and available self-help groups as well as telephone networking of patients.
7. Use speciality consultation and special resources when they can improve the patient's quality of life.

An extensive array of special resources and techniques exists for assisting patients to live with cancer. To employ them properly, the physician must maintain his awareness of the exquisite, ongoing interactions in humans among the physical, psychological, and social dimensions of existence. Everything influences and affects everything else. Renal, hepatic, pulmonary, and pancreatic functions (to name a few) affect brain function. Electrolyte imbalance and steroid levels affect brain function. All of the above are altered in various ways by the introduction of analgesics, other chemotherapeutic agents, surgery, and radiation. All can be altered, including the responses to chemotherapy, radiation, and surgery, by brain function as captured in the phrase "psychological states." To add to this marvelous complexity are variations influenced by age, genetic background, pre-morbid functioning and experiences, intelligence, and belief systems.

Obviously special resources and techniques must be employed in creative, individualized ways in order to deal with specific problems ranging from depression to sexual dysfunction and sleep disorders. Many special resources and techniques are familiar to the physician and employed to various degrees as part of the ongoing, usual treatment of patients.

COUNSELING AND COGNITIVE REHEARSAL refer to techniques employed by all health professionals. Counseling involves interacting with the patient, to share feelings and reactions. The process helps the patient to consciously identify concerns and fears. It sanctions expression of anxieties, concerns, fears, worries—a process called ventilation. Given the presence of another person, advice can be given and conscious attempts made by the counselor to correct misperceptions. Counseling can give the patient an ally in problem-solving.

Through counseling, patients can be helped to develop for themselves a technique called cognitive rehearsal. This technique assists the patient in order to anticipate stressful events and situations (*e.g.*, a procedure, sharing of painful information such as impotency or the need for disfiguring surgery, toxicity from chemotherapy or radiation, surgery, or a relapse) in such a way that through rehearsing events before they occur, the person's psychological defenses and other resources are mobilized. When properly used, both counseling and the special self-help technique called cognitive rehearsal give the patient a greater sense of control over his life. Although all health professionals can use these techniques, misuse is frequent without special training or active supervision by trained personnel (a psychiatrist, clinical psychologist, specially trained social worker, or cleric). Counseling can be done individually, with spouses, family systems, or in groups. The appropriate approach must be tailored to each situation and each individual.

INDIVIDUAL PSYCHOTHERAPY is usually employed for situations where psychological symptoms and associated behaviors appear to be dramatic in intensity, have not been responsive to counseling, and are not based primarily on cerebral dysfunction from the many possible toxic/metabolic causes of such dysfunction. It can be useful when dealing with chronic anxiety, depression, feelings of helplessness, self-destructive preoccupations, social withdrawal, the sudden development of compliance-with-treatment difficulties, or sexual dysfunction. Relevant communication should be ongoing between the psychotherapist and the physicians treating the cancer patient. Psychotherapists do not have to be medically trained (*i.e.*, psychiatrists), although for working with cancer patients this is a strong prejudice of Hersh's.

BEHAVIOR THERAPY and biofeedback involve the employment of very particular techniques to alter a person's responses to particular situations or stimuli. It proves useful in modifying certain compliance problems with young patients, phobic reactions, psychogenic nausea and emesis, certain forms of sexual dysfunction, and certain forms of sleep and eating disorders. Behavior therapists need not have a medical background; however, they must have special, supervised training in its use. Training in relaxation techniques (awareness of somatic muscle tension and relaxation, temperature control of hands and feet, breathing exercises, alpha and theta EEG rhythm control) has become a basic part of behavior therapy. The majority of accomplished behavior therapists are psychologists.

HYPNOSIS AND GUIDED IMAGERY are techniques related to a special focusing of the person's attention. Today, their uses in medicine and psychiatry are almost always combined with training the patient in somatic muscle relaxation. Both techniques are extremely useful in children and adults for problems of anxiety, nausea, and pain. Guided imagery, a term less familiar than hypnosis to most physicians, involves training the patient to create for himself a state of relaxation during which the patient creates in his mind a desired place, or goal. In this state the patient is experiencing, as intensely as his mind will allow, the conjured-up place or goal. The Simontons and their followers claim great improvement in the morbidity and even mortality of cancer patients using this technique.[65] Hypnosis, guided imagery, meditation with relaxation, are all being aggressively explored now as important adjuncts to the care of the seriously ill.* The popularity of these techniques increases the probability of outright charlatans as well as simply poorly trained practitioners. The techniques are legitimate, but are not learned overnight. Practitioners should have had supervised training in this area.

SELF-HELP GROUPS AND PATIENT/FAMILY ACQUAINTANCE NETWORKS are a powerful and highly recommended resource. They are a natural person-to-person support, an extension of the healthy family, in which mutuality and reciprocity predominate. They provide situations in which peers help each other, allowing for the crossing of normal social, economic, and cultural boundaries based on some common interest, experience, or stress. They involve themselves with important immediate needs of people and hence are ideal for cancer patients and their families. More than any form of therapy self-help groups and patient/family networks allow for information sharing, ventilation, and a reduction of feelings of isolation. Problem-solving in such situations often has greater legitimacy for those involved than in any other situation. Examples of such formally established groups include the Candlelighters, Make Today Count, Inc., Reach to Recovery, Ostomy Rehabilitation Program (American Cancer Society), and the International Association of Laryngectomies (American Cancer Society). Their current addresses and phone numbers can be found in the appendix to Kelly's, *Until Tomorrow Comes* and in the chapter on community resources.[66] As a spin-off of these groups, telephone networking of patients has developed providing a reduction in isolation, especially for the bed-ridden and those living in rural areas. Groups and networks also exist for survivors.[66]

THE USE OF PSYCHOPHARMACOLOGIC AGENTS (PSYCHOACTIVE DRUGS) must be governed by caution and respect. They encompass a broad range of chemical substances. The problems for which they are prescribed are complex. These agents include the analgesics, anti-anxiety agents (minor tranquilizers), antidepressants, hypnotics, major tranquilizers (neuroleptics), and the stimulants (*e.g.*, amphetamines, methylphenidate, etc.).

All psychoactive drugs should be considered as adjuncts to medical, psychologic, and social interventions. Used by themselves *none* provide lasting improvement in anxiety, depression, hyperactivity, mania, pain, psychosis, or sleeplessness. Used appropriately, they are powerful tools for the physician. They can provide significant reduction or elimination of symptoms, rendering patients more responsive to additional needed interventions designed to improve physical, psychological, and social functioning. One rather recent example of this is the discovery during the mid-1970's that tricyclic antidepressants significantly raise the pain threshold of animals and human subjects.

Some 15% of the U.S. population is estimated to need mental health care.[80] In that context, the findings that 20% of cancer patients develop problems needing psychiatric intervention are not so overwhelming.[81] In cancer patients, a great variety of symptoms associated with the CNS may be noted. The patient may show anxiety, mood swings, or irritability, and may demonstrate impaired concentration, confusion, and even hallucinations. Whatever the symptoms, the physician's first responsibility is, obviously, to consider what physiologic changes secondary to the disease, cancer treatments administered, infection, or unrelated metabolic problems (*i.e.*, diabetes, thyroid dysfunction, etc.), might be producing these symptoms. Responses to the treatments received—chemotherapy, radiation therapy, surgery—can all involve behavioral, mood, and perceptual changes. Of particular concern are the CNS effects of chemotherapy. All such agents (alkylating agents, antimetabolites, vinca alkaloids, the special antibiotics such as actinomycin D or daunorubicin, L-asparaginase, cis-platinum) produce symptoms expressive of CNS changes.[82] These symptoms can range from classic toxic encephalopathies to akathisia, depressions, mania, mood swings, or schizophrenic behavior.

Medical etiologies for behavioral and mood changes do not rule out use of psychoactive drugs. Clearly such causes do render these agents adjuncts to other treatments. All psychoactive drugs produce side effects. Thus, so as not to totally confuse a clinical situation or create more distress, these drugs must be carefully administered. People show such great variation in how they absorb and metabolize psychopharmacologic agents that prescription calls for upward titration of doses, starting with the recommended minimum effective levels. (Children under age 13 years should be prescribed to in a similar fashion but using mg/kg doses.) Package inserts or books such as the *AMA Drug Evaluations* can serve as responsible, prescribing information sources.

The metabolism and clinical effects of psychoactive drugs vary with changes in physiologic states, including fatigue, dehydration, electrolyte imbalance, and infection, to name just a few. Among these substances, serum levels are now tracked for lithium, tricyclic antidepressants, and phenothiazines. The tricyclics are well known for their ability to produce cardiac conduction problems with arrhythmia and even heart failure. Phenothiazines should not be administered when a patient has an infection. All psychoactive drugs can produce undesired CNS effects that will find behavioral, mood, and intellectual expression. Tricyclics can produce confused states in people over 40. Furthermore, they should be given carefully to high suicide potential patients. Protein binding in plasma is usually greater than 90% and tricyclics are soluble in lipids.[83] Tricyclics and the phenothiazine thioridazine have powerful anticholinergic effects that produce symptoms such as delayed ejaculation, which is found to be most distressing and bewildering by patients who have not been warned of this dose-related effect.

When employing psychoactive drugs, the physician's basic goal is to return a sense of comfort and control to the patient. Problems for which they can be employed and some recommended drugs follow.

* Physiologically, these techniques have been shown to relate to the release of β-endorphins in the CNS.

Anxiety. Antianxiety drugs should not be used to treat anxiety in children. However, these drugs can be helpful in adolescents and adults. Use should be *short-term*, remembering that gradual withdrawal is best. (Metabolites can remain in the system after long-term use for up to three weeks.) The major categories include the propanediols (meprobamate and tybamate); benzodiazepines (chlordiazepoxide, diazepam, oxazepam and flurazepam); and the diphenylmethane derivatives (hydroxyzine). Benzodiazepines are the most useful with cancer patients. Chlordiazepoxide is best avoided because of its unpredictable ability to produce paradoxical irritability and hostility; in some persons, it can also produce nighttime hallucinations.

Pain. As part of the pain treatment armamentarium, the physician should familiarize himself with the muscle relaxants, the tricyclic anti-depressants, and the phenothiazines. Somatic tension and spasm are an important component of pain. Low to moderate doses of diazepam are most effective in combination with analgesics. Of the tricyclics, imipramine, amitryptaline, and clomipramine have been found to effectively raise the pain threshold in moderate doses (for example with amitryptaline doses of 50-100 mg per day).[84] Phenothiazines, such as chlorpromazine, have long been used as adjuncts to the treatment of chronic, severe pain. Recent reports indicate that they can be quite effective in combination with a tricyclic.[85]

Depression. Depression should never be treated with a stimulant drug. In cancer patients, the origins of depression are usually multifactorial. When an endogenous depression (hallmarks include sleep disorder combined with eating, bowel, and mood disorder) has been diagnosed, the tricyclic drugs are the most readily and commonly employed. Their peripheral and central anticholinergic effects can considerably cloud the picture of patients on chemotherapy and can be downright dangerous. Physician consultation on depressed patients with a psychiatrist familiar with not only tricyclics but lithium carbonate and monamine oxidase inhibitors is recommended.

Psychotic episodes. Of the many antipsychotic drugs (neuroleptics) for example, it is wisest to stay with the best known groups—the phenothiazines (for example, chlorpromazine, trifluoperazine, fluphenazine, and thioridazine) and the butyrophenones (haloperidol). Powerful, affecting blood chemistries and producing extrapyramidal CNS symptoms, these drugs should be prescribed *only when titrated against specifically selected target symptoms* that the clinician wants to reduce or eliminate. Such symptoms include combativeness hyperactivity, tension, hostility, hallucinations, extreme negativism, and poor self-care and sociability. They should be used cautiously in the elderly where postural hypotension induced by antipsychotic drugs can be severe enough to create arrhythmias. Note that in prepubertal children, the first drug of choice for treating a psychotic episode is the well-known, extremely safe drug diphenydramine.[86] Only if there is no therapeutic response in the psychotic child should the clinician move on to the phenothiazines.

In assisting the patient to live with cancer, the clinician must mobilize all resources possible and the most basic resources to mobilize lie within each patient and that patient's family. Emphasis should be given to identifying areas of function that are significantly modified. For example, with all individuals, self-image and psychologic state ride in tandem with physiologic changes. It is very important to track those changes that interfere in any way with the neurological/sensorimotor intactness of the patient. Such changes can alter the patient's ability to organize internal and external stimuli. Confusion in sorting such stimuli out produces high levels of anxiety and tension. Besides difficulties from loss of function or changes in levels of motor control and proprioception, the signal called pain, in its chronic forms, very clearly influences self-image and the person's sense of wholeness.[37] It has psychologic representations as well as the physical ones (chronic skeletal muscle tension and increased lactic acid production). Therefore, appropriate treatment of chronic pain must involve more than the dulling of a patient's conscious perceptions of pain. The physician should help the patient to review changes in function as well as control during rehabilitation and changes during healing and remissions. Techniques that patients can use themselves should be favored. The control that cognitive rehearsal, guided imagery, and hyponosis place in the patient's grasp is a significant factor in the usefulness of these techniques.[87,88]

Sexual dysfunctions become major challenges to those living with cancer. In approaching this problem, the physician should encourage communication about the patient's sexual concerns, should warn the patient of changes, and work in collaboration with the patient toward obtaining as much sense of wholeness, integrity, and continued participation with others as possible.[89] Assisting the patient with sexual problems need not be difficult. The physician should learn the patient's previous habits and elicit the current problems and needs. Whether the patient craves holding and caressing, the pleasure of stimulating the partner or being stimulated, or both, these needs can usually be accommodated. Not trying is the major problem.

Working with the Dying Patient

Over the past 5 years, the hospice movement has burgeoned in this country. As a concept for bringing together in space and time medical, spiritual, psychologic, and social support, the hospice is excellent. However, true hospices need special physical environments and well-trained staff. A certain danger does exist in the hospice movement. It is that of becoming a fad and that of hospices developing as mere euphemisms for low-cost nursing homes.[91] Recently the home hospice movement has been receiving increasing attention, including by third-party health-insurance programs. This movement, based on the use of multidisciplinary teams that assist patients and their families in their homes, provides a healthy further development of the more classic hospice.

Patients who recognize they are dying should talk about that recognition while sharing their associated feelings and thoughts (*e.g.*, fears of aloneness, concern for those left behind, and relief). Physicians should do their best to assure that patients do not die with a sense of being isolated. Thus, encourage family involvement. Contact the family after the patient's death to assist them with their mourning and their sense of continuity in life. This post-death contact can be made by the physician in person or by letter.

The general subject of working with the dying patient has been written about extensively, particularly by Kübler–Ross.[90] As a basic source for all clinicians treating cancer patients, Hersh strongly recommends that they read Kelly's chapter "Facing Death When there is No Choice" in his book *Until Tomorrow Comes.*[66] That chapter briefly reviews the personal, philosophical, and family issues, while discussing practical issues such as the "living will" and burial arrangements.

Future Considerations

Rapid generation of ideas and information will occur over the next five years in several areas. The first of these involves the cancer patient as a handicapped person in the context of this country's changing values concerning the handicapped. Legal changes have already been made at the national level that promote the return to school and the return to work of the handicapped. Overt school and job discrimination will therefore decrease for the cancer patient.

The second of these areas involves the increasing numbers of former patients—persons who have survived cancer and its dramatic treatments. These people survive with physical, psychological, and social impairments. How extensive are these impairments? How much can they be ameliorated? Both questions need to be examined much more extensively than they have been thus far. Self-image has changed; areas of functioning have been altered; dependency relationships have shifted; future options are often narrowed; reference points have changed. How can the medical community assist cancer patients to live with such success?

Third, sex and sexuality as important issues for hospitalized and non-hospitalized chronically ill patients will "come out of the closet." Efforts will be made to clarify the effects of fatigue, disfigurement, parasthesias, pain, neurologic impairment, and mood changes on the cancer patient as a total human (hence, sexual) being. It will become acceptable for the physician to review this subject with cancer patients while working with them to develop strategies for meeting needs that are blocked by circumstances (*i.e.*, hospital rituals) or by physical/functional changes. Attention to this area will improve the quality of life for all concerned.

REFERENCES

1. Miller EL, Anderson EJ: Cancer education from school personnel. J Sch Health 49, No. 7:383, 1979
2. Clark RL: Psychologic reactions of patients and health professionals to cancer. In Cullen JW, Fox BH, Isom RN (eds): Cancer: The Behavioral Dimensions, p 1. New York, Raven Press, 1976
3. Rosenbaum EH: The human side of cancer. In Proceedings of the American Cancer Society Second National Conference on Human Values and Cancer, p 5, Chicago, 1977. New York, American Cancer Society, 1978
4. Wallace JH: Psychosocial adjustment of the cancer patient. In Proceedings of the American Cancer Society Second National Conference on Human Values and Cancer, p 112. New York, American Cancer Society, 1978
5. Burdick D: Living with cancer. In Proceedings of the American Cancer Society Second National Conference on Human Values and Cancer, p 136. New York, American Cancer Society, 1978
6. Hamilton PK: Counseling the patient with cancer. In Proceedings of the American Cancer Society Second National Conference on Human Values and Cancer, p 156. New York, American Cancer Society, 1978
7. Hersh SP: Views on the psychosocial dimensions of cancer and cancer treatment. In Ahmed P, Coelho G (eds): Toward A New Definition of Health, pp 175–190. New York, Plenum Press, 1979
8. The Book of Job: Old Testament
9. Rimer II: The impact of mass media on cancer control programs. In Cullen JW, Fox BH, Isom RN (eds): Cancer: The Behavioral Dimensions, p 183. New York, Raven Press, 1976
10. Greenwald HP, Becker SW, Nevitt MC: Delay and noncompliance in cancer detection: a behavioral perspective for health planners. Milbank Mem Fund Q 56, No. 2:212–230, 1978
11. Room R: Measurements of drinking patterns in the general population and possible application in studies of the role of alcohol in cancer. Cancer Res 39, No. 7:2830–2833, 1979
12. Knudson AG: Persons at high risk of cancer. N Engl J Med 301, No. 11:606, 1979
13. Gross L: Cancer and slow virus diseases: some common features. N Engl J Med 301, No. 8:432–433, 1979
14. Scurry MT, Levin EM: Psychosocial factors related to the incidence of cancer. Int J Psychiatry Med 9, No. 2:159–177, 1979
15. Sklar LS, Anisman H: Stress and coping factors influence tumor growth. Science 205:513, 1979
16. Holden C: Cancer and the mind: how are they connected? Science 200:1363–1369, 1978
17. Thomas CB, Duszynski KR, Shaffer JW: Family attitudes reported in youth as potential predictors of cancer. Psychosom Med 41, No. 4:287–302, 1979
18. Thomas CB, Duszynski KR, Shaffer JW: Family attitudes reported in youth as potential predictors of cancer. Psychosom Med 41, No. 4:287–302, 1979
19. Warheit GJ: Life events, coping, stress, and depressive symptomatology. Am J Psychiatry 136, No. 4:502–507, 1979
20. Jamison KR, Wallisch DK, Pasman RO: Psychosocial aspects of mastectomy, I. The women's perspective. Am J Psychiatry 135, No. 4:432–436, 1978
21. Silberfarb PM, Maurer LH, Crouthamel CS: Psychosocial aspects of neoplastic disease, I. Functional status of breast cancer patients during different treatment regimens. Am J Psychiatry 137, No. 4:450–455, 1980
22. Morris T, Greer HS, White P: Psychological and social adjustment to mastectomy: a two-year follow-up study. Cancer 40, No. 5:2381–2387, 1977
23. Lewis FM, Bloom JR: Psychosocial adjustment to breast cancer: a review of selected literature. Int J Psychiatry Med 9, No. 1:1–17, 1979
24. Chapman RM, Sutcliffe SB, Malpas JA: Cytotoxic-induced ovarian failure in Hodgkin's disease, II. Effects on sexual function. JAMA 242, No. 17:1882–1884, 1976
25. Sutcliffe SB: Cytotoxic chemotherapy and gonadal function in patients with Hodgkin's disease: facts and thoughts. JAMA 242, No. 17:1898–1899, 1976
26. Mathews D, Robinson S, Mazur T et al: Counseling after resection of the penis. Am Fam Physician 19, No. 4:127–128, 1979
27. Capone MA, Good RF, Westie KS et al: Psychosocial rehabilitation of gynecologic oncology patients. Arch Phys Med Rehabil 61:128–132, 1980
28. Minear D, Lucente FE: Current attitudes of laryngectomy patients. Laryngoscope 89, No. 7:1061–1065, 1979
29. Olson ML, Shedd DP: Disability and rehabilitation in head and neck cancer patients after treatment. Head Neck Surg 1, No. 1:52–58, 1978
30. Pawazek M, Groff JR, Schyving J et al: Emotional reactions of children to isolation in a cancer hospital. J Pediatr 92, No. 5:834–837, 1978
31. Salzman C, Shader RI: Depression in the elderly, I. Relationship between depression, psychologic defense mechanisms and physical illness. J Am Geriatr Soc 26, No. 6:253–260, 1978
32. Neurgarten BL: Time, age, and the life cycle. Am J Psychiatry 136, No. 7:887–894, 1979
33. Vettese JM: Problems of the patient confronting the diagnosis of cancer. In Cullen JW, Fox BH, Isom RN (eds): Cancer: The

Behavioral Dimensions, pp 275–282. New York, Raven Press, 1976

34. Wallace HJ, Forti LA: Psychosocial adjustment of the cancer patient. In Proceedings of the American Cancer Society Second National Conference on Human Values and Cancer, pp 112–117, Chicago, 1977. New York, American Cancer Society, 1978
35. Peck A: Emotional reactions to having cancer. Am J Roentgenol 114:571–599, 1972
36. Freedman AM, Kaplan HI, Sadock BJ: Comprehensive Textbook of Psychiatry, Vol III. Baltimore, Williams & Wilkins, 1980
37. Gagnon JH: Human Sexuality, p 2. Glenview, Scott, Foresman & Co, 1977
38. Blos P, Finch SM: Sexuality and the handicapped adolescent. In Downey JA, Low NL (eds): The Child With Disabling Illness: Principles of Rehabilitation, pp 537–538. Philadelphia, WB Saunders, 1974
39. Gagnon JH: Human Sexuality, p 383. Glenview, Scott, Foresman & Co, 1977
40. Gagnon JH: Human Sexuality, p 384. Glenview, Scott, Foresman & Co, 1977
41. Siris ES, Leventhal BG, Vaitukaitis JL: Effects of childhood leukemia and chemotherapy on puberty and reproductive function in girls. N Engl J Med 294:1143–1146, 1976
42. Herr HW: Preservation of sexual potency in prostatic cancer patients after 125 I implantation. J Am Geriatr Soc 27, No. 1:17–19, 1979
43. Herr HW: Preservation of sexual potency in prostatic cancer patients after pelvic lymphadenectomy and retropubic 125 I implantation. J Urol 121, No. 5:621–623, 1979
44. Bergman B, Nilsson S, Peterson I: The effect on erection and orgasm of cystectomy, prostatectomy and vesiculectomy for cancer of the bladder. Br J Urol 51, No. 2:114–120, 1979
45. Jamison KR, Wellisch DK, Pasman RO: Psychosocial aspects of mastectomy, I. The women's perspective. Am J Psychiatry 135, No. 4:432–436, 1978
46. Chodoff P, Friedman SB, Hamburg DA: Stress, defenses and coping behavior: observations in parents of children with malignant disease. Am J Psychiatry 120:743–749, 1964
47. Binger CM, Ablin AR, Fuerstein RC et al: Childhood leukemia: emotional impact on patient and family. N Engl J Med 280:414–418, 1969
48. Greenblatt RB, Nezhat C, Roesel RA et al: Update on the male and female climacteric. J Am Geriatr Soc 27, No. 11:481–490, 1979
49. Cohen MM, Wellisch DK: Living in limbo: psychosocial intervention in families with a cancer patient. Am J Psychother 32, No. 4:561–571, 1978
50. Levanthal BG, Hersh SP: Modern treatment of childhood leukemia: the patient and his family. Child Today 3, No. 3:2–6, 36, 1974
51. Easson WM: The Dying Child, p 80. Springfield, Ill, Charles C Thomas, 1970
52. Wellisch DK: Adolescent acting out when a parent has cancer. International Journal of Family Therapy 1, No. 3:230–243, 1979
53. Lansky SB, Cairns NU, Hassanein R et al: Childhood cancer: parental discord and divorce. Pediatrics 62, No. 2:184–188, 1978
54. O'Malley JE, Koocher G, Foster D et al: Psychiatric sequelae of surviving childhood cancer. Am J Orthopsychiatry 49, No. 4:608–616, 1979
55. Cullen JW, Fox BH, Isom RN: Cancer: The Behavioral Dimensions, p 286–287. New York, Raven Press, 1976
56. Heinemann HO: Incurable illness and the hospital in the twentieth century. Man and Medicine 1, No. 4:281–285, 1976
57. Levine AS: The doctor's dilemma: "I-It" or "I-Thou"? In Proceedings of the American Cancer Society Second National Conference on Human Values and Cancer, pp 29–35, 1977. New York, American Cancer Society, 1978
58. Hersh SP: How much should patients know? Washington Post, Letters to the Editor, Sunday, August 6, 1978
59. Pilsecker C: Terminal cancer: a challenge for social work. Soc Work Health Care 4, No. 4:369–379, 1979
60. MacMillan-Brett K: The IV nurse and the chemotherapy patient: a vital emotional support. Cancer Nurse 75, No. 6:28–30, 1979
61. McKegney FP, Visco G, Yates J et al: An exploration of cancer staff attitudes and values. Med Pediatr Oncol 6, No. 4:325–337, 1979
62. Anderson JL: A practical approach to teaching about communication with terminal cancer patients. J Med Educ 54, No. 10:823–8824, 1979
63. Kellerman J, Rigler D, Siegel S et al: Psychological evaluation and management of pediatric oncology patients in protected environments. Med Pediatr Oncol 2:353–360, 1976
64. Carey RG, Posavac EJ: Holistic care in a cancer care center. Nurs Res 28, No. 4:213–216, 1979
65. Simonton OC, Matthews-Simonton S, Creighton J: Getting Well Again. Los Angeles, JP Tarcher, 1978
66. Kelly OE: Until Tomorrow Comes. New York, Everest House, 1979
67. Cassileth BR, Zupkis RV, Sutton-Smith K et al: Informed consent: why are its goals imperfectly realized? N Engl J Med 302, No. 16:896–900, 1980
68. Grundner TM: On the readability of surgical consent forms. N Engl J Med 302, No. 16:900–903, 1980
69. Rennie D: Informed consent by "well-nigh abject" adults. N Engl J Med 302, No. 16:917–918, 1980
70. Frank JD: Persuasion and Healing: A Comparative Study of Psychotherapy 2nd rev ed. Baltimore, Johns Hopkins University Press, 1973
71. Rosenbaum EH: Living with Cancer. New York, Praeger, 1975
72. Holland J: Interview: understanding the cancer patient. CA 30, No. 2:104–106, 1980
73. Hartwich P: The question of disclosing the diagnosis to terminally ill patients. Arch Psychiatr Nervenkr 227, No. 1:23–32, 1979
74. Hackett TP, Cassem NH, Wishnie HA: The coronary care unit: an appraisal of its psychological hazards. N Engl J Med 279:1365–1370, 1968
75. Hackett TP et al: Detection and treatment of anxiety in the coronary care unit. Am Heart J 78:727–730, 1969
76. Hackett TP, Cassem NH: Psychological reaction to life-threatening stress: a study of acute myocardial infarction. In Abram HS (ed): Psychological Aspects of Stress. Springfield, Ill, Charles C Thomas, 1970
77. Cassem NH, Hackett TP: Psychiatric consultation in a coronary care unit. Ann Intern Med 75:9–14, 1971
78. Gottheil E, McGurn RM, Pollack O: Awareness and disengagement in cancer patients. Am J Psychiatry 136, No. 5:632–636, 1979
79. Beisser AR: Denial and affirmation in illness and health. Am J Psychiatry 136, No. 8:1026–1030, 1979
80. Report to the President from The President's Commission on Mental Health, Vol I, p 8. Washington, DC, United States Government Printing Office, 1978
81. Holland J: Understanding the cancer patient. CA 30, No. 2:103–112, 1980
82. Peterson LG, Poplin MK: Neuropsychiatric effects of chemotherapeutic agents for cancer. Psychosomatics 21, No. 2:141–153, 1980
83. Hollister LE: Tricyclic antidepressants. N Engl J Med 299, No. 20:1106–1109, 1978
84. Lee R, Spencer PS: Antidepressants and pain: a review. J Int Med Res (Suppl) 5 146–156, 1977
85. Duthie AM: The use of phenothiazines and tricyclic antidepressants in the treatment of intractable pain. S Afr Med J 51, No. 8:246–247, 1977
86. Campbell M: Psychopharmacology. In Noshpitz JD (ed): Basic Handbook of Child Psychiatry, Vol II. New York, Basic Books, 1979
87. Barber J, Gitelson J: Cancer pain: psychologic management using hypnosis. CA 30, No. 3:130–136, 1980
88. Weisman AD, Sobel HJ: Coping with cancer through self-instruction: a hypothesis. J Human Stress, 6:3–8, March 1980
89. Lieber L, Plumb MM, Gerstenzang ML et al: The communication of affection between cancer patients and their spouses. Psychosom Med 38:379–389, 1976
90. Kübler-Ross E: On Death and Dying. New York, MacMillan, 1969
91. Potter JF: A challenge for the hospice movement. N Engl J Med 302, No. 1:53–56, 1980

Section 2

Wendy S. Schain

Sexual Problems of Patients with Cancer

For decades, scientific energy has been focused on causes and cures of the many forms of malignant diseases. Only recently have the advances in technology extended longevity to the point that quality of life has become a major theme in oncology and captured the interest of scientists from multiple disciplines. *Quality of life* is an abstract concept with many different meanings but may be viewed as encompassing ". . . those problems, the problems of living that are sometimes called psychological and social, that are common to us all, and its inevitability, the fear of disability and deformity, and the loss of self-sufficiency; as well as the loss of ways to maintain self-esteem, and the ability to sustain and fulfill our social roles."[1] One additional element of the "human condition" is missing from this description—the importance of viewing one's self as a sexual person. A cancer diagnosis imposes a threat to the image of self-esteem and to the prospects of giving and receiving physical love.

SEXUAL HEALTH

It is just in the last decade or so that the issue of sexual health has gained prominence as a subject worthy of scientific inquiry and one respectable enough to be admitted to the major considerations of health care. Behavioral scientists have entered the field of oncology and have added both a holistic approach to patient management as well as the concept of psychosocial rehabilitation as integral to comprehensive cancer medicine.[2] Groups of researchers from psychology, sociology, and public health have begun to explore specific aspects of the psychological "plight" of the cancer patient and various family members. Attention has become focused on how the patient and family cope with the diagnosis of this disease and the vicissitudes associated with various treatments intended to control the cancer.[3] This increased interest in quality of life issues has stimulated research into examining a host of psychological sequelae of the cancer experience that includes descriptions of the impact which cancer has on a person's vocational productivity, interpersonal relations, functional adaptation, self-esteem, relationships with health care providers, and lastly, sexual functioning.[4,5,6,7]

The area of human sexuality in medical practice has often received a low priority compared to other psychological factors, especially as it applies to those persons who are disabled, chronically ill, or over age 60.[8,9] Moreover, oncologists have generally left this problem to random attention or casual conversation because they have not taken the time or been comfortable enough to attend to the fact that a significant proportion of distress experienced by the cancer patient is due to the absence of sexual gratification as well as a diminution of affectionate responses.

The acknowledgment that sexual concerns have been largely neglected in the care of the cancer patient is a recent revelation. Remedial efforts are just beginning to emerge in the professional community's educational programs. One example of this expanded awareness was a national conference sponsored by the West Coast Cancer Foundation in March, 1979. This conference resulted in a compendium entitled, "Body Image, Self-Esteem, and Sexuality in Cancer Patients."[10] Both the conference and the publication of papers presented concerned themselves solely with the needs, problems, professional resistances, and the possible resources that exist in the area of sexual functioning in cancer patients. Body Image, Self-Esteem, and Sexuality in Cancer Patients is the first text devoted entirely to this underemphasized area of health care. (It is an excellent resource for community physicians to use as an overview of sexual problems concommitant to cancer therapy.)

Cancer may be viewed as a *biosocial* disease since it affects a person's psychological, social, and sexual responses as well as the major anatomical organs. Lack of sufficient attention to this area has caused damage to patients and their loved ones because the emotional morbidity and frustration associated with sexual dysfunctions often goes undiagnosed, undiscussed, and untreated. Therefore, an attempt to remedy this problem is done by:

1. Identifying the major sexual dysfunctions experienced by cancer patients
2. Providing practical information about intervention strategies that can be employed by most health professionals working in the field of oncology

HISTORICAL PERSPECTIVE

While sex has always been of intense interest to every human being of no matter what age, gender, culture, or century, it has usually been considered an underground topic for social gatherings, and especially medical conferences. To understand why sexuality has been so much of a taboo subject, it is necessary to describe several of the cultural factors. These factors have:

1. Shaped contemporary reactions to the subject of human sexual functioning in general
2. Influenced its role in current medical training
3. Stimulated the recent impetus to address sexual dysfunctions as a topic worthy of medical attention and amenable to study by the scientific method[11]

Part of the resistance to the subject of sex is because of the intimate and special relationship it shares with religion. This factor colors attitudes about sexual behaviors with fears and fantasies of "eternal damnation" or punitive consequences of "over-indulgence" or excessive self-stimulation. Puritanism, extreme religious convictions, and censorship have been society's weapons to try to control the sexual attitudes and practices of its members. Even the medical profession has been concerned with reported ailments assumed to result from zealous masturbation or acknowledged sexual promiscuity. Out of this curious but repressive atmosphere there arose serious efforts to inhibit depraved behavior and to limit sexual activities solely for the purpose of procreation. For centuries the literal interpretation of biblical sex allowed only for this narrow view of intercourse. The concept of physical pleasuring or recreational sex, as aspects of healthful pursuits, did not gain popular acceptance in the public domain (much less the medical world) until past the middle of the 20th century.

A major factor that inclined physicians to a puritanical view of human sexuality was Krafft–Ebing's book, *Psychopathia Sexualis*, which stated that the only normal sexual pattern was occasional intercourse, for the purpose of begetting, with only the husband experiencing orgasm.[12] Any other behavior was identified as "perversion." More sophisticated contemporary attitudes, however, were shaped by academicians who documented a significant relationship between sexual urges, the socialization of the human animal, and the adaptive or maladaptive forms of the adult personality.[13,14] In addition, Ellis stipulated that a large number of negative reactions that people had to sexual issues could be eliminated if they could grow up in a climate of knowledge, acceptance, and wisdom about sexuality.[15] This view piques the interest and concern of sex educators today who see a significant need to revise the curricular offerings in medical school training to include specialized courses in the area of human sexuality. Our young physicians and mental health professionals need to acquire knowledge, comfort, and flexible attitudes regarding the nature of sexual functioning, the role this plays in health and illness, and the various types of people and behaviors that people select to provide gratification of this primary urge.[16]

Around the 1960's the so-called "Sexual Revolution" (which was almost entirely a woman's political campaign) changed the basic stereotypic image of females to view them as active, pleasure-seeking persons, interested in their own orgasms and possibly initiating sexual relations for the pure "sport" of it.[17,18,19] Prior to that time, women were regarded as passive creatures who were not sexual animals but merely receptacles for men's pleasures, and not capable of independent lustful yearnings.[20] This change in sex roles was part of the sexual enlightenment, which carried with it a view of sexual functioning as a topic worthy of scientific inquiry. Considerable credit should be attributed to William Masters and Virginia Johnson for spear-heading sexology as a science and for bringing sexual behaviors into the laboratory for investigation. Reports of their years of research have culminated in several major texts. Two of their books, *Human Sexual Rsponse* and *Human Sexual Inadequacy* described the various types and sources of sexual dysfunctions and proposed a "treatment package" with prescriptions for sexual homework assignments intended to remedy the identified problem.[21,22] While these works put the issue of human sexual functioning into the realm of treatable medical care concerns, recent adverse criticism is challenging the scientific validity of the claims reported. They state that the noted sex therapy experts did not define their criteria for success in clearly measurable or operational terms, making replication of findings difficult or impossible. The most vocal antagonists were Zilbergeld and Evans who claimed ". . . Masters and Johnson's research is so flawed by methodological errors and slipshod reporting that it fails to meet customary standards and their own—for evaluation research."[23] Additional investigations are necessary to determine the veracity of the criticism and the reliability of the original claims regarding the efficacy of the therapeutic interventions that have been so widely acclaimed.

A few other notable leaders in this field have contributed to the "rites of passage" of human sexuality in clinical medicine. These persons have established pragmatic remedies for various dysfunctions and have proposed an array of theoretical and sociocultural assumptions that provide the foundation for "the new sex therapy".[24,25]

Because "sexology" as a separate medical discipline is so new and not standardized with the same guidelines as subspecialties like cardiology or oncology, regulation of training and research publications is still somewhat loosely defined. Two excellent journals in the field are *Journal of Sex Education and Therapy*, and *Medical Aspects of Human Sexuality*.[26,27] In addition to the validity of printed information, which is somewhat regulated by peer review and an organization known as SIECUS (Sex Information and Education Council of the United States), there is also an association that provides quality control of training courses for health professionals who want to become certified as sex educators, counselors, or therapists. AASECT (American Association for Sex Education, Counsellors and Therapists) is a membership group that stipulates basic criteria for certification at these three levels and issues licensure to participants who complete specified training courses at various programs or institutes set up across the country over the course of the academic year. The text, *Sex Education for the Health Professional: A Curriculum Guide*, is a major resource describing the country's programs in human sexuality and the various strategies employed to increase the physician's sensitivities, comfort, and skills in working in the field of sexuality in clinical medicine.[28]

San Francisco's program in human sexuality at The University of California is an excellent example of a response to expressed needs to provide medical students with a course in human sexual functioning.[29] In addition, this particular program is comprised of several areas based upon principal functions including a "Sex and Disability Unit," which provides direct services as well as opportunities for research in this field. Other programs provide a combination of didactic education, direct services to patients, and small group discussions for professionals involved in this type of training. More and more medical schools are beginning to include at least an elective course on this topic.

In addition to finding reputable reading material in this field and locating accredited courses for acquiring skills and facts about human sexuality in medical care, there is also the need to be aware of various psychological tests and instruments that can be used to diagnose patient problems or to research issues relevant to the field of human sexual dysfunction. A partial list of validated measures of psychosexual functioning currently available for diagnosis or evaluation by Derogatis is shown in Table 12-1.[30]

Table 12-1 is just a sample list of tests with relevant descriptive information and is intended as an initial aid for potential selection and use of psychosexual assessment measures.

TABLE 12-1. A Partial List of Validated Measures of Psychosexual Functioning Currently Available

INSTRUMENT	AUTHOR	NATURE OF MEASURE	UNIT OF MEASUREMENT	PSYCHOMETRIC CHARACTERISTICS
Sex-Role Inventory (SRI)	S. L. Bern, Stanford University	A 60-item measure of Gender Role Definition, generating scores on masculinity, femininity, and androgeny	Individual subject	Systematic series of studies in the literature addressing almost all aspects of reliability and validity
Derogatis Sexual Functioning Inventory (DSFI)	L. R. Derogatis, Johns Hopkins University School of Medicine	A 225-item measure of current sexual functioning scored in terms of ten sub-tests and two global measures	Individual subject	Systematic series of monographs and papers in the literature
Sexual Knowledge and Attitude Test (SKAT)	H. I. Lief & D. M. Reed, University of Pennsylvania School of Medicine	A 149-item test measuring sexual attitudes, knowledge, demography, and experiences	Individual subject	Reliability and validity data available, most completely compiled in the technical manual of the test
Sexual Interaction Inventory (SII)	J. LoPiccolo & J. C. Steger, SUNY at Stony Brook	A measure of sexual adjustment and satisfaction in couples requiring 102 responses and deriving comparable 11 scale profiles for the members of the couple	Individual subject	Systematic series of studies addressed to reliability and discriminative validity of the scale
Mosher Forced-Choice Guilt Inventory (FCGI)	D. L. Mosher, University of Connecticut	A measure of sex-guilt involving 78 forced-choice items, resulting in scores of three dimensions of sex-related guilt	Individual subject	Related series of reports in the literature addressing various aspects of reliability and validity
Dyadic Adjustment Scale	G. B. Spanier, Pennsylvania State University	A 32-item scale designed to assess the quality of a marital or other dyad, in terms of four primary sub-scale scores	Couple	Instrument is relatively new; however, data on reliability and validity are available in several reports

* A more thorough compendium of psychosexual assessment measures may be found in Schiavi RC et al: J Sex Marital Ther 5:169–224, 1979

DEVELOPMENTAL SEQUENCE, SEXUALITY, AND CANCER CARE

It is naive and even untenable to attempt an overview of sexual functioning in cancer patients without providing the reader with the broader frame of reference described in the section Psychosocial Stages of Development in this chapter. Stage-related hierarchies are a fundamental concept in behavioral science. They are guidelines that help the clinician grasp the unfolding nature of the human animal and the various issues that influence personality dynamics and psychosocial adaptation. At every stage on this developmental ladder there is a struggle to resolve certain issues in order to move on to and master subsequent tasks. If basic conflicts are resolved and handled adequately, the patient travels along this hierarchy with little trauma. If impeded by disease, psychological stresses, or environmental obstacles, the person may become fixated, may regress to an earlier stage, or become flagrantly dysfunctional. For most persons, the developmental process is arduous, somewhat conflicted, but progressive. However, for the cancer patient, the "passages" may be delayed, traumatized, or even threatened of being permanently arrested. Therefore, it is essential to bear in mind what the major psychosocial and sexual tasks are that the person is trying to master at various stages of life and how the disease known as cancer and its related treatments complicate these issues (or exacerbate the developmental conflicts).

Table 12-2 shows a life stage description of developmental tasks, psychosocial behaviors, and associated sexual concerns. Understanding the intricate interaction between these occurrences can help health care providers as well as family members identify certain risk factors likely to occur within specific age groups and, in addition, what some of the demands that are internally experienced by the patient (unrelated, but perhaps complicated the disease) are. In addition to identifying the developmental stage of the cancer patient, it is critical to determine what the patient's ego mechanisms or coping strategies are. This gives important information about how the patient is likely to try to resolve some of the

TABLE 12-2. Basic Psychosocial vs. Sexual Tasks at Different Stages of Development[31]

STAGE	BASIC PSYCHOSOCIAL TASK	SEXUAL TASKS
Infancy (0–2 years)	Acquiring basic trust, learning to walk, talk	Gender identity
Childhood (2–12 years)	Acquiring a sense of autonomy vs. shame and doubt; entering and adjusting to school	Pleasure-pain associated with sexual organs and eliminative functions; masturbation takes place with resulting shame and acceptance; secondary sex characteristics become evident
Adolescence (13–20 years)	Acquiring sense of identify vs. role confusion	Mastery over impulse control, acceptance of conflict between moral proscription and sexual urges, handling new physiologic functions (menses for girls and ejaculate for boys)
Young Adulthood (20–45 years)	Acquiring a sense of intimacy vs. isolation; vocational effectiveness; interpersonal security, "sexual adequacy"	Sexual adequacy and performance plus fertility concerns and questions related to parenting
Middle Adulthood (50–70 years)	Acquiring a sense of self-esteem vs. despair; adjusting to diminuation of one's energy and competence; 'Empty nest syndrome' plus care of aging parents or their death; adjusting to change in physique and evidence of aging	For the female, menopause and resulting vasomotor changes, atrophy of breasts, clitoral size, and vaginal lubrication; for the male, delay on attaining an erection, a reduced compulsion to ejaculate, episodic impotence, possible prostatitis
Old age	Adjusting to loss of friends, family, confrontations with old age and dying, painful joint conditions, reduced hearing and visual acuity; adjustment to social stigmatization of being 'old'	Reduced vitality, fear of incompetence or injury (coital coronary); fear of being viewed as "dirty old person"; unavailability of a partner (widowhood); limited physical capacity and reduced options

burdens of a particular stage in life or ramifications of the disease state. Knowledge about the basic tasks inherent in developmental stages, combined with an understanding of the patient's major coping strategy (*i.e.*, whether the patient is a denier, tackler, intellectualizer) can provide important clues to finding out *"Who"* is at high risk for emotional distress, *"Why"* the stress is experienced so acutely at this stage (*i.e.*, oophorectomy in 22-year-old nulliparous woman), and *"How"* to intervene with these patients to minimize their morbidity and maximize their adaptation. Effective coping skills can be identified and improved through specialized training. Patients can be taught to strengthen or modify problem solving behaviors so that they are less self-defeating and more self-fulfilling, especially in conjunction with issues related to their cancer treatment.[32]

SEXUAL FUNCTIONING IN THE GENERAL POPULATION

Most people think of sexual functioning as a combination of neurologic, vascular, muscular, and hormonal reactions that involve vasocongestion causing the genitals to become engorged with blood, and aroused or excited; and myotonic reactions that cause the muscular contractions experienced as the pleasurable end-point release known as orgasm. While these components do indeed comprise the human sexual response, the actual experience or gratification associated with sexual interactions depends much more on the person's response to "friction and fantasy," rather than the actual anatomic or physiologic sensations. Multiple determinants interact to influence sexual responsiveness and may be affected not only by organic or psychogenic factors but also by the person's drive, experience, and basic knowledge about sexual functioning.[33] In light of the multiplicity of factors that influence the human sexual response cycle, it is important to review specific physiologic stages in order to know the natural sequence of events to occur, what does or does not transpire as a result of certain organic processes, and the events or feelings that might be interfering with the execution of that response. Accurate assessment of sexual dysfunctions will be contingent on an understanding of "normal" cyclical occurrences as well as personalized information about anatomy and psychology of the individual's sexual behavior. The four major stages in the human sexual response cycle are:

1. Excitement (biological tension)
2. Plateau (bioelectric charge)
3. Orgasm (bioelectric discharge)
4. Resolution (mechanical relaxation)

1. *Excitement* (biologic tension)—which is characterized by the onset of erotic feelings and the attainment of erection in men and vaginal lubrication in women. Another dominant factor of this stage is the feeling of sexual tension.

2. *Plateau* (bioelectric charge)—a more advanced stage of excitement where the sex glands are engorged to capacity and undergo positional changes (viz., in men, the testicles retracted up against perineum and, in women, the uterus ballooned out and pulled away from the pelvic floor). There are also a number of extragenital conditions involving color change, respiration shifts, and generalized increased arousal.

3. *Orgasm* (bioelectric discharge)—is experienced as the most significant intense and pleasurable aspect of the sexual response. For men, this phase is noted by contractions of the

internal organs with accompanying sensation of "ejaculatory inevitability," and then by semen spurting out of the erect penis in rhythmic contractions at about .8 second intervals. For women, irrespective of the source of her stimulation, orgasm is experienced by rhythmic contractions of the circumvaginal and perineal muscles and of the swollen tissues of the "orgasmic platform" at about the same contraction interval as men.

4. *Resolution* (mechanical relaxation)—during this phase, local sex-specific reactions abate and the body and internal functions return to the base line. The penis detumesces and the testicles descend to their usual "cool" position. The penis returns to its flaccid urinary state. (There are some notable changes in duration of the refractory phase for men at different stages in the life cycle.) While there are some corresponding reactions in the female which reinstate her resting phase of sexual response, the women is never physically refractory to orgasm and if she wishes, can be stimulated over and over to climax.[34]

Complementary to learning the nature of the human sexual response is the realization of the number of internal and external factors which can interfere with any or all of the above-described reactions. For purpose of clarity, one can think of three major areas in which dysfunctions can occur, irrespective of the reason for the disturbance. These three areas are:

1. Desire (interest);
2. Arousal (excitement);
3. Orgasm (tension release).

Planning for relief from the problems of sexual dysfunctions involves very careful assessment of the problems: accurate identification of the stage in which the problem originates, the probable causative factors, and the patient's motivation to have the situation remedied. For all intents and purposes, the major decision in sex therapy is to determine the cause of the problem (psychogenic, organic, iatrogenic) and then to decide whether the primary treatment should be:

1. Psychological (uncovering interpersonal or intrapsychic conflicts);
2. Behavioral (involving recommended sexual tasks);
3. Surgical (*i.e.*, penile prosthesis to correct impotence resulting from radical prostatectomy).

Most often a combination of intervention strategies will be necessary and primary physicians ought to be prepared to diagnose the problem and initiate inquiry about the patient's sexual functioning prior to and especially following cancer treatment.

While there is considerable variation in the sexual reactions of people and in response to cancer treatment, some general trends can be identified to help health professions ferret out what aspects of a patient's sexual dysfunction is a general consequence of cancer therapy and what components are affected by the individual's interpretation of the disease. There is often a unique interfacing of factors which shape the patient's psychological as well as sexual response to the disease, and an understanding of the individual's personality dynamics combined with the interpretation given to the specific site in which the cancer occurs must be ascertained in order to plan appropriate interventions.

GENERAL CONSIDERATIONS OF SEXUAL FUNCTIONING IN NEOPLASTIC DISEASE

It is essential to have some understanding of the general biological progression of cancer and the psychosocial sequelae often associated with neoplastic disease. A diagnosis of cancer often elicits fears of (1) death, (2) morbidity associated with the treatments, (3) recurrence, (4) abandonment, and (5) losses (loss of functional ability, social value, attractiveness, self-esteem, economic independence, role behaviors, and sexual responsiveness). Practical statements about these global quality-of-life concerns often involve questions from patients who inquire as to what their body will look like, how it will function, whether they will be able to give and receive pleasure, and whether their masculinity or femininity will be irreparably impaired. Men are often primarily worried about whether or not they can function as they did before. Women are often more concerned with the possibility of rejection from a partner because of perceived damage or decreased value resulting from radical surgery and what they experience as mutilating consequences.

There is an intimate association between body image, sexuality, and cancer care which gets reflected in an individual's verbalized responses as well as in his or her overt behavioral reactions. Health professions must learn to listen and "read between the lines." For example, when a young woman who has lost her breast says that she feels defeminized, she is referring to the fact that she is experiencing herself as defective and not as worthwhile as before (especially because of the way our society prizes "beautiful," firm breasts). A middle-aged man who is left impotent after colorectal surgery may casually comment that he thinks his wife is having an affair with her doctor. This accusation may reflect feelings of his sexual inadequacy and a projected view that he fears someone else will satisfy his partner because he feels he cannot. The health professional must be able to ferret out superficial or obvious concerns from those which are imbedded in more obscure communications. There is a great deal of anguish associated with impaired sexual functioning related to cancer treatment, but patients and their doctors may still be too embarrassed to discuss these problems and thereby miss opportunities for exploration and resolution.

SELF-ESTEEM AND IMPACT ON SEXUAL FUNCTIONING

A cornerstone concept in evaluating the degree to which sexual functioning is likely to be affected by cancer is to assess the patient's self-esteem and determine to what extent body image and sexual activity contribute to the individual's overall sense of adequacy and well-being. In essence, self-esteem is the sum total of all of our feelings about ourselves or as one researcher cogently described ". . . it is the reputation we share of ourselves with ourself."[35]

This author has attempted to develop a fairly concrete but useful conceptual model to be used by health professionals to diagnose a patient's self-esteem and to begin to plan intervention strategies to assist that person to regain emotional equilibrium following cancer treatment. This particular model is compartmentalized into four major components with subfactors contained in two of the four.[36]

1. The body self—which has a functional (what I can do) and an aesthetic (what do I look like) part;
2. The interpersonal self—which is comprised of both social and acquaintance relations as well as intimate sexual interactions;
3. The achieving self—which contains elements of work or competitive efforts such as career or school behaviors;
4. The identification self—which is made up of those attitudes and behaviors that are related to spiritual, ethical or ethnic concerns.

These four component parts work in conjunction with one another to form the experience felt as self-esteem or self worth. At different times and due to different circumstances, a person may experience a sense of loss, insult, or depreciation in any one of these areas or psychic compartments. For example, the severance of a long-term relationship may be viewed as rejection (an insult to interpersonal self) and the person may see herself as devalued. She may begin to compensate by borrowing "good feelings" or psychological stroking from the body image component of her self-esteem system. This would be seen by her working hard to developing a beautiful figure and for getting rewarded for physical attractiveness. On the other hand, a child who was not regarded as attractive or reinforced for being personable may begin to work very seriously in school to become number one and to get good feelings from achieving. The hard-working schoolgirl manages to improve her scholastic standing in order to compensate for her not feeling adequate or worthwhile in the body image area of self-esteem.

It is often useful to assess an individual's self-esteem at the time of first diagnosis or preoperative evaluation and then at several different "critical" episodes after that. One method for making this assessment is to think of the self-esteem model described above as a commercial banking system with the patient having access to four or six areas of potential revenue (or loss). This economic paradigm permits analogies which view patients as capable of establishing assets, recording debits, and negotiating for profits in their own psychological balance sheet.

The crisis of cancer diagnosis and subsequent treatments can almost always be viewed as a threat to self-esteem and a major withdrawal from the sense of body integrity (whether resulting from the loss or alteration of a major body part or the change in one's sense of being a healthy person). It is therefore essential to discover, with the help of the patient, what the proposed surgery and treatments are likely to do to his or her feelings of value and competence. How much invested is this person in the organ, limb, or body system which is involved and threatened (*e.g.*, sarcoma in the dominant arm of a professional basketball player)? What kind of reserves does the person have at this time (a woman with her spouse living and supportive compared to a lonely widow with no relatives within 500 miles)? Professional intervention may be necessary to help the patient and staff identify the patient's resources and the methods necessary to mobilize such psychological reserves to counteract the loss that is anticipated.

Preoperative assessment and planning of problem solving activities may act both as a prophylaxis for certain anticipated crises as well as rehearsal for coping more effectively with expected problems (such as what to tell the children about coming to the hospital for chemotherapy treatment one weekend a month for two years). Self-esteem assessment can be conducted at repeated intervals in a patient's treatment experience and can be gleaned in an informal discussion with the patient under a number of different conditions. Such information will be a useful aid to the health care team in identifying and remedying other problems that may arise in the patient's psychosocial adaptation and may include bona fide fatigue, physical effects from radiation or chemotherapy, and complications of surgery which may predispose patients to low level interest in sexual relations or actual hardships in executing the act (such as leverage problems associated with a hemipelvectomy).

SITE SPECIFIC CONSIDERATIONS OF SEXUAL FUNCTIONING IN NEOPLASTIC DISEASE

In addition to the universal problems and threats that cancer presents, each individual will experience a unique configuration of problems associated with his or her disease. While it is essential to understand the existential impact of cancer, it is equally important to learn about the specific reactions experienced and the interpretation the patient has given to the fact that he or she has contracted cancer in a specific organ. Some individuals will indeed view a cancer diagnosis as a punishment for promiscuity (genital cancer) or evidence of hostile impulses which need to be cut off (limb amputation). This is especially true when the cancer diagnosis affects a sex organ (testis) or a sex-related organ (lips, legs). Various researchers who have discussed case reports in this area bear testimony to the fact that patients may interpret both the incidence and reactions to neoplastic disease as related to sexual thoughts or activities.[37]

Sexual functioning is a multi-faceted behavior and may reflect an individual's coping strategies as well as his/her desire for recreation or procreation. It is important therefore, to know that people use sex in many different ways and the same behavior may reflect different motives at different times in an individual's experience. For example, an expressed interest in sexual intercourse may indicate one or more of the following motives:

1. a desire for closeness;
2. a wish to conceive;
3. an attempt to control or manipulate one's partner;
4. a non-verbal expression of affection;
5. a defense against depression or anxiety;
6. a bid for attention;
7. a confirmation of worth;
8. a defense against intimacy.

These precipitating factors may be operating in a given individual prior to the onset of disease but the strength or frequency of motives for sexual acts may change as a result of a cancer diagnosis. Recognition of the multiplicity of causes for sexual behaviors can be a clue both to the source of sexual dysfunction as well as a key to personality dynamics and/or possible psychopathology.

The most logical starting point for a discussion of specific types of sexual problems associated with malignant disease is a discussion of those areas of the anatomy that are either genital organs themselves or are organs likely to have a disruptive effect on sexual functioning as a result of cancer management. In the 1980 edition of *Cancer Facts and Figures*,[38] the estimated number of people who will develop a malignancy in their genitals, urinary tract, breast, colon, or rectum is projected at nearly one-half million (480,000). The numbers of people affected certainly warrants attention to the problems of sexual dysfunction in cancer patients, as well as the concerted effort necessary to remedy the problems in procreational or recreational sex that are a consequence of cancer diagnosis and related treatments.

PSYCHOSEXUAL ISSUES IN SITE-SPECIFIC CANCERS*

BREAST CANCER

Breast cancer affects over one hundred thousand women each year and is the leading cause of cancer deaths in women.[39] Numerous reports to date have documented the psychosocial distress associated with this type of cancer and the need for specialized intervention programs to lessen the symptoms of depression, anxiety, and compromised sexual attractiveness.[40,41,42] In addition, specific investigators have identified various sexual difficulties encountered by women who have had a breast amputated to control their cancer.[43,44,45] Specialized assistance is often required for both the identified patient and her partner to help them make a satisfactory adjustment to the loss of one or both breasts. Witkin makes specific recommendations to the couple about viewing the women's operative site in front of a mirror, having both partners observe themselves naked and comment on various feelings this elicits.[46] Not all patients will be able to carry out this exercise and often couples will need permission to handle the first confrontation with the woman's changed body in a manner which is compatible with their coping strategies. One suggestion is to conjure up some interesting underwear or nightgown apparel to feel attractive in and camouflage the mastectomy site until the woman is ready to disrobe or let her partner touch the wound area. Some couples move gradually into viewing the loss as a result of shared responsibility in caring for the wound and it can be helpful for the woman's partner to assist her to change dressings and irrigate problem areas from the time of surgery. Some partners can make the transition from the caretaking aspects of treating the wound to the role of lover; others cannot and should only be encouraged to assist with wound problems if no one else is available. Other pragmatic suggestions are to have the couple experiment with positions which are comfortable for the woman and to use the man on top ("male superior") position whenever possible, since this minimizes the most direct view of the woman's missing organ and her partner is more likely to look into her face than at her amputated breast region (when she is on the top for coitus). *The Joy of Sex*[47] is an excellent resource text for positions which the couple may use to try to increase sexual pleasure and minimize discomfort, physically and psychologically.

Major factors which will interfere with the woman's sexual responsiveness are her feelings about her femininity, sense of worth, her investment in her breasts as critical to her overall value, her physical discomfort, and trust in her partner's caring response to her. In addition to acknowledging contributions made by these conditions, the health professional working with a mastectomee (or other type of breast surgery patient) should ascertain the woman's premorbid sexual responsiveness and inquire how frequently and satisfying her sexual relations were before her operation. The health professional must assume responsibility for inquiring about the patient's sex life and must be willing to ask leading questions about specific acts, resistance, and sensations. To inquire, "How are things in the bedroom?" is too vague and banal and does not really convey permission that talking about explicit sexual issues is acceptable. Inquiry about the patient's sexual attitudes and responses must follow the medical model. This involves asking specific questions as to onset, precipitating events, current efforts to improve the situation, and information dissemination about alternative behaviors (such as making love by candlelight to lessen impact of change in body contour). Specific questions to ask include:

1. "Tell me a little about your sexual relations before surgery—How often did you have intercourse? How satisfying would you say that was (not very, somewhat, extremely)?"
2. "Have you been in the habit of undressing in front of your partner? Has this changed since your surgery?"
3. "How important would you say your breasts are in your overall sexual arousal, orgasm?"
4. "Has the type of activities or the actual amount of time you are accustomed to spending in "foreplay" (pleasuring) changed since surgery?"

If the patient describes a moderate amount of change in sexual reactions or resistance to resuming sexual relations, recommendations for sex counseling might be appropriate. Suggestions about readings that describe the various strategies called "sensate focus" which involve concentrating on certain sexual tasks to lessen anxiety, reduce performance concerns, and refocus interest in other parts of one's anatomy may be helpful. Specific books which explain or illustrate various sexual behaviors quite explicitly along with the rationale for obtaining pleasure in this way are *The New Sex Therapy*,[48] *What You Still Don't Know About Male Sexuality*,[49] and *The Joy of Sex*.[50] In addition, certain self-help groups across the country such as "Y Me" in Chicago, "Women to Women" in Los Angeles, and various local chapters of The American Cancer Society's "Reach to Recovery" program may have women who are both willing and able to talk about this problem and who feel they have acquired some success in

* Although this article works under the assumption that patients with partners are heterosexual, the author acknowledges that this premise is made only for expediency and explicitly acknowledges that all health professionals must never assume (1) that all patients have, or even wish to have, a partner, or (2) that all partners are of the opposite sex. Obtaining accurate information about this issue is essential to appropriate sex counseling.

managing this part of their adjustment to radical breast surgery.

Psychotherapy, sex therapy, support groups, and above all a loving and concerned partner are therapeutic agents in the rehabilitation process following breast cancer diagnosis. In addition to these psychosocial aids is the recent addition of surgical intervention in the form of reconstructive mammoplasty. Sexual consequences subsequent to breast reconstruction are not yet reported in the literature but anecdotal accounts reflect the view that for some women, a portion of their motivation to seek breast rebuilding is to improve their sexual identity and sense of "being whole again."[51] The field of breast reconstruction may have a potentially therapeutic effect on the woman's self-esteem and sense of body integrity, which if improved by the surgical outcome, may have a corresponding embellishing impact on her feelings about her sexual attractiveness.[52,53] Well-planned, prospective research into the physical and psychosexual aspects of breast reconstruction will provide some guidelines about the impact of this operation on a woman's survival, psychological response to mastectomy, and sexual functioning.

PELVIC GENITAL CANCER

The field of pelvic genital cancer is very broad and can encompass a number of different diagnoses, surgeries and aggressive therapies. For the sake of parsimony, this chapter will refer to the psychological and sexual ramifications associated with radical hysterectomies for cancer, radical vulvectomies, and total pelvic exenterations. Literature reports discuss the varying degrees of emotional distress and dysfunction associated with primary surgical intevention and subsequent radiotherapy.[54,55,56] Reactions are often strongly dependent on the life stage of the woman, the extensiveness and satisfaction of her significant relationship and the adequacy and appropriateness of her ego defenses. Women facing this type of cancer treatment are often preoccupied with intense fears of what their life will be like after surgery. They may not be able to verbalize their concerns, but often their fantasies include worrying about what their external region will look like and whether they will be able to have intercourse and if so, how painful it is likely to be. Critical psychosocial and sexual issues for this population of cancer patients include worrying about the threat to life (which is omnipresent in cancer), diminished feelings of femininity, loss of fertility, vitality, orgasmic potential, and feelings of nurturance and tenderness. Women are frightened about hormonal shifts and the resulting disability allegedly associated with the loss of estrogen. Concerns subsequent to this condition include physical aging, diminished libido, loss of lubrication, and dyspareunia (associated with vaginal stenosis). Reports in the literature reveal that some women with no vulva (after radical surgery) report experiences of full satisfying orgasmic release.[57] This one particular report also discusses patients' interest and motivation for vaginoplasty following radical pelvic surgery. While reconstructive vaginoplasty is still quite a new procedure, pioneer efforts in this area do suggest a correlation between pelvic repair and improved sexual functioning. It may be useful in counseling patients about reconstructive vaginoplasty to present pictures of what pre- and post-operative results look like. This type of "psychological rehearsal" has been found to be helpful to patients considering reconstructive breast surgery so that they can begin to develop realistic expectations about the outcome of their operation and to discuss with their partner (or children who may wish to see the pictures) how the partner will feel about this additional change in body image and sexual organ appearance.[58]

Counseling of the gynecological cancer patient is recommended early to abate her withdrawal and possible sexual dysfunction due to ignorance about the changes in her body and the possible alternative behaviors which may be available to her for giving and receiving pleasure. One particularly helpful treatment tactic as described by Goode and Capone is intended to facilitate women's psychological adaptation and resumption of sexual relations following radical surgeries for pelvic cancers.[59] This particular type of directive therapy includes disspelling myths, shaping expectations, reinforcing self-interest, and disseminating detailed information (about lubricating creams, mechanical vibrators, and new sexual behaviors) intended to minimize morbidity associated with this type of cancer therapy.[60]

Because so few professionals are familiar with these psychotherapies or sexual treatment tactics, in-service education programs (sponsored jointly by surgery and psychiatry) may be useful adjuncts to teach health professionals specific skills of sex counseling. For example, it is often helpful to recommend to a patient to set a specific goal in a measurable time frame ("By two weeks after discharge, I will buy new sexy underwear to put on to come to bed in.") This type of behavior can be both a stimulus to one's partner as well as a reinforcement of the patient's own feelings of worth and sense of attractiveness. Frequent inquiry and reinforcement for behaviors intended to increase sexual interest or performance are necessary. The physician or nurse should dedicate a portion of the office visit time to discussing sexual reactions, problems, or concerns as they relate to the cancer treatments. This acknowledgment of the possibility of a problem sets the stage for communication of these issues and establishes the precedent that attention to sexual concerns and disorders is part of comprehensive management.

In addition, the attending physician, oncology nurse, and sex therapist can encourage self-examination for the gynecological cancer patient to learn about her original or altered anatomy. Showing a patient her external genitalia with a mirror and encouraging her to explore her vulva, medial thigh region, and introitus helps her be able to identify pleasurable and painful areas. Recommending the use of mechanical vibrators may liberate a patient to experiment with sexual responsiveness and to discover new ways to obtain satisfaction that can be retained as autoerotic behavior or incorporated into sexual activities with a partner.

COLO-RECTAL CANCER AND THE STOMA PATIENT

Approximately 40,000 colostomies and ileal conduits are performed in North America annually.[61] These men and women can be expected to suffer moderate emotional distress and moderate to severe sexual dysfunctions.[62] Such a change in basic anatomy and function has a profound effect on body image and sexual responsiveness. The psychosocial sequelae following this type of surgery often result from both the physical changes which take place as well as the societal taboos which center around eliminative functions.

The critical concerns and conflicts of the anal stage of development may consciously or unconsciously get unleashed by this crisis. Issues may arise which have to do with cleanliness, control over one's impulses, struggles to maintain self-direction, ambivalence over active or passive behavior and the resurrection of negative feelings of shame and doubt (refer back to developmental table). Emotional or physical regression may also be a consequence to this type of surgery because it is often a significant trauma. A study by Drusset revealed that two-thirds of their patients reported unpleasant reactions to their stoma.[63] Subjects in a study by Orback and Tallent disclosed that some men reacted to their operation as if it represented castration or demasculinization.[64] Other male patients reported reacting to the early post-surgical bleeding of the stoma as if it were a menstrual flow and therefore felt feminized or asexual. Women, on the other hand, viewed this dramatic change in their body similar to a rape experience or to feelings of having been violated. A few reported sexualizing the cleaning of the stoma and revealed embarrassing feelings similar to masturbation in handling this particular opening in their body. In addition to the psychological problems associated with a stoma, patients report distress at having no "vacation" from the maintenance of their appliance. This awareness often results in feeling compelled to compromise leisure activities, avoid highway travel, and seek seclusion where one is able to achieve privacy for the necessary toilet activities required for proper ostomy care.

In addition to the neurological or iatrogenic causes of sexual dysfunction in the colo-rectal patient, there is an array of psychological and social concerns which contribute to the ostomate feeling undesirable or sexually inadequate. Furthermore, the ostomy patient may also have to deal with the effects of adjuvant radiation treatments or chemotherapy or with the debilitating effects of advancing disease, thereby increasing physical pain, diminishing psychic reserves and exacerbating malaise and depression.

For this subgroup of cancer patients, very careful sexual history-taking and counseling is necessary to identify what problems are experienced as most severe and how to facilitate adaptation to the demands of such a drastic change in body image, social roles, and effective use of time and energy. Men especially seem to feel particularly vulnerable and inadequate in terms of their sexual prowess, at least in regard to penetration efforts associated with coitus. Helpful intervention should include clearly defined instructions to the patient about preparation of the pouch prior to sex, specific suggestions about deodorizing the appliance, permission for testing out comfortable positions (such as lateral scissors embrace) and suggestions for wearing attractive camouflage or covers for the appliance. For women, there are some underpants which have openings up the center and conveniently cover the pouch but permit stimulation or intercourse through the opening directly to the clitoris and introitus. In addition to practical information from professionals, there are a number of paraprofessional resources such as the Ostomy Association with its publications and outreach activities which may prove of invaluable assistance in the area of sexual behavior and ostomy care.[65]

Table 12-3 shows the specific sexual behaviors which may be affected by various cancer surgeries or treatments. Iatrogenic dysfunctions of arousal or orgasm are fairly predictable, but subtle psychological reactions may interfere with biolog-

TABLE 12-3. Major Cancer Surgeries Expected to Affect Sexual Function

	MEN				
	Drive (Desire)	*Erection*	*Ejaculation*	*Experiential Orgasm*	*Fertility*
ABDOMINOPERINEAL RESECTION	?	–	+	+	+
RADICAL PROSTATECTOMY	+	–	+	+	–
RETROPERITONEAL LYMPHADENECTOMY	+	+	–	+	–

	WOMEN			
	Drive	*Lubrication*	*Orgasm*	*Fertility*
ABDOMINO PERINEAL RESECTION	?	+	+	?
HYSTERECTOMY	?	–	+	–
TOTAL PELVIC EXENTERATION	?	–	?	–
PELVIC RADIATION	?	–	+	–

+ = presence
– = absence
? = uncertainty

ical responses and sexual drive in any one of the major cancer conditions. Discussion about possible remediation of erectile incompetence by implantation of a penile prosthesis will be discussed in the next section, since planning for the implant surgery will be the same no matter what the genesis of the patient's sexual disorder.

CANCER OF THE PROSTATE, TESTIS, OR PENIS

Cancer of the male urological organs often results not only in a threat to life but, most often, in a threat to sexual competence. The various surgical procedures for cancer in these regions often involve disturbance in (1) erection, (2) emission and (3) ejaculation.[66] The location of the tumor, the type of therapy (and possible resulting injury to the involved neural fibers) as well as the attendant psychological response determine the magnitude and duration of the degree of sexual dysfunction. Since this type of cancer affects an estimated 64,000 men annually, serious attention must be paid both to the concerns about preservation of sexual performance and the re-establishment of primary satisfaction. Education in this area should address:

1. Helping patients and partners develop changes in attitudes which might be necessary to learn alternative responses to the notion that intercourse (with an erect penis in the vagina) is the point at which all sexual encounters should be finalized.
2. The possible risks and benefits of the penile prosthesis surgery for restoring erection and return of function desired for gratifying penetration.

Following radical prostatectomy, approximately 85 to 90 percent of patients experience erectile dysfunction.[67] Orgasmic and ejaculatory functions mediated through the intact pudendal nerve are not affected. However, emission of semen may be reduced because the prostate, seminal vesicles, and ampullae of the vasa deferentia have been excised. On the other hand, less dysfunction may be associated with definitive radiotherapy since encouraging reports have noted that external megavoltage irradiation is less destructive than radical surgery to the erectile functions in the treatment of prostate cancer.[68,69] More research that involves assessment of physical and psychosexual consequences of these two different treatments is necessary for more definitive guidelines to be established.

Another major concern for prostate cancer patients is that endocrine therapy is the principal treatment for those individuals with metastatic disease. In these men, sexual dysfunctions often occur because the treatments administered produce loss of libido, erectile incompetence, gynecomastia, and, sometimes, phallic atrophy. In addition, the psychological aspects of surgical castration combined with feminizing hormones play a significant role in altered sexual appetites as well as performance of middle-aged men.[70]

While cancer of the testis accounts for 2 percent of all male neoplastic disease, it is the second most common malignancy of men between the ages of 20 and 34. The diagnosis and primary treatment of testicular cancer is achieved by a radical inguinal orchiectomy: removing the testis epididymis and spermatic cord. Although orchiectomy may result in psychological trauma, no impairment of fertility or endocrine function is anticipated in the presence of a normal contralateral testis.[71] In addition to orchiectomy, retroperitoneal lymph node dissection is often employed when the primary tumor contains elements other than seminona. Because of the interruption of nerve fibers most patients report an absence of emission after retroperitoneal lymphadenectomy.[72] Patients often need some preoperative instruction (along with schematic drawings) to explain the nature of their altered sexual response and specific information about the cause and sensations associated with retrograde ejaculation. Carefully controlled psychosexual assessment studies of patients with prostatectomy, orchiectomy, and retroperitoneal lymphadenectomy are essential to discover to what extent the sensations and absence of overt emission influence the sexual responses of these men and their partners. The issues of reduced volume of ejaculate and impaired fertility also need to be explored to determine what types of psychological and behavioral distress are associated with these alterations in "normal" sexual responses. Any operation or sustained treatment (radiotherapy) performed directly on or around the external genitalia may be perceived as a castration threat and unresolved psychological responses may arise in an effort to compensate for the imagined (or real) danger to the genitals. The issue of the possibility for paternity as well as sexual adequacy need to be addressed for patients treated by these specific procedures.

Three major topics must be explored with the male patient who has severe sexual dysfunction associated with his cancer treatments. They include:

1. Careful assessment of causative factors related to the specific dysfunction. This may involve a detailed "Sexual Problem History" to ascertain the onset of the problem, the description of the problem and attempts to remedy it.
2. Recommendations for non-demand pleasuring and encouragement for manual or oral genital stimulation without expectations of coitus.
3. Inquiry about interest and motivation for internal implant prosthesis.

Health professionals treating oncology patients need to be aware of the new techniques for and types of prostheses used to restore erectile competence. The two major types of devices currently used are shown in Figures 12-1 and 12-2. It has been recommended that patients considering this type of surgery be evaluated for physical and urological disease, personality disturbance, and nocturnal penile tumescense reactions. At the present time, there is little substantive data about what types of personality characteristics would render a patient ineligible for implant surgery.[76] Currently, it would seem prudent to caution physicians and mental health professionals to conduct a rather intense interview with the patient and any partner to ascertain his motivation for this type of surgery, his expectations subsequent to the implant, and his understanding of the risks and benefits of the actual surgical procedure. Careful research studies should be undertaken to learn about the reasons, reactions, and possible resistances to restoring erectile competence in this manner. Many men and their partners do wish to regain the experience of penile erection and vaginal penetration and apparently this is achiev-

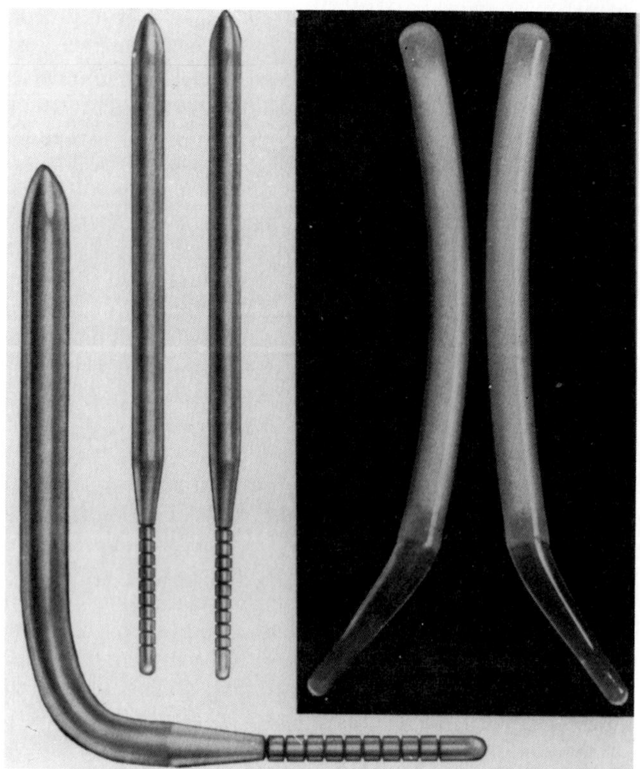

FIG. 12-1. Implantable penile prosthesis.

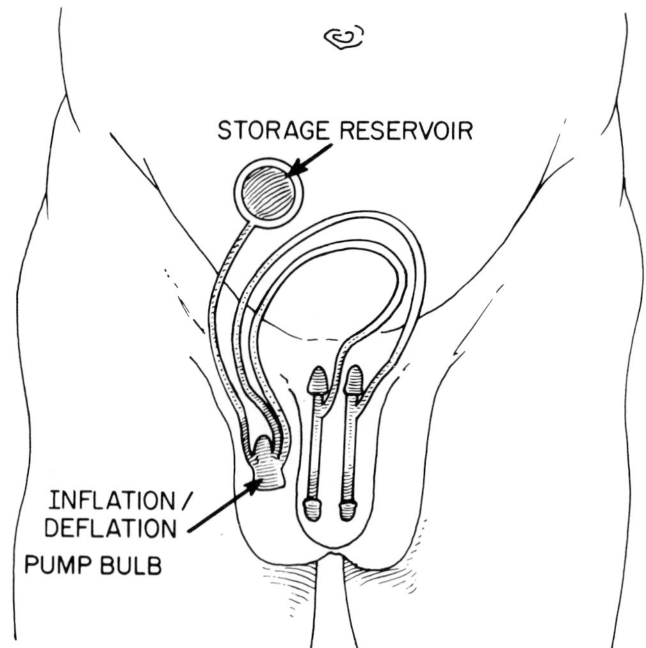

FIG. 12-2. Inflatable penile prosthesis.

able through a surgical technique even if it is not feasible through natural resources.

Table 12-3 shows the major cancer surgeries which can be expected negatively to affect sexual function. Again it is crucial to state that variations do occur. Function may be preserved when it is anticipated to be lost, and the contrary condition exists when there does not seem to be an organic reason for severe dysfunction but either erection, orgasm or desire is reported to be "subnormal" or not existing.[77]

NON-GENITAL CANCERS

Space does not permit a detailed description of psychosexual complications associated with other types of cancer diagnosis and treatments (such as limb amputation, head and neck surgeries, and hematological malignancies). However, it must be remembered that there is an intricate blending of psychological, physical, and iatrogenic factors which influence response or lack of response to affectional and sexual stimuli. Sometimes even when sexual interest is diminished, patients feel an increased desire for closeness and affection and even this behavior may be rebuffed, ignored, or blatantly denied because of the stigma, body mutilation or actual physical obstacles to the act of loving which certain cancers produce (such as radical neck surgery). A worthwhile overview of some of the psychosexual ramifications to these particular malignancies is contained in the text published by Karger entitled *Body Image, Self-Esteem, and Sexuality in Cancer Patients*.

What is most important to communicate here is that sensitive interviewing and acknowledgment of possible difficulties in this area may give patients permission to discuss these concerns and problems. Special attention must be given to radical head and neck surgery patients who often feel so grossly unattractive and have such difficulties in basic needs such as talking and eating that little or no attention is paid to their needs for closeness, touching, and genital sexual encounters.

THERAPEUTIC INTERVENTION: WHO? HOW?

WHO SHOULD INTERVENE

The most efficacious way to intervene in this manner and the best person for this function has not yet been established. There is no single course of events or sole source of care to take place except to make openness and communication of sexual concerns a serious issue in the care of cancer patients. There is a growing interest both in having primary physicians develop increased skills in sex counseling and also to develop interdisciplinary teams which include a certified sex therapist as an integral part of the treatment group. When the sex therapist is integrated into the oncology treatment team, this therapist has access to patients both pre- and post-surgery and is in pivotal position to (1) assess the possibility for dysfunction, (2) rehearse with patients and partners some preventive behaviors, and (3) evaluate candidacy for reconstructive or implant surgeries which might improve sexual functioning and self-esteem.

HOW TO INTERVENE

While there are several different strategies and techniques for intervention, one particularly useful approach is a specific hierarchical model known as the "P-LI-SS-IT" model. This theoretical framework allows the therapist to both diagnose and counsel patients and to move gradually (according to the therapist's skill and the treatment setting in which he or she works) from simple permission giving for thoughts, fantasies, or behaviors to providing specific information or recommendations which are uniquely relevant to the problem which is presented. One of the major values in using this particular model is that subsequent levels of involvement require the attending professional to use increasing degrees of knowledge, training, and skill. This stage-related sequence of activities therefore demands that the health professional adapt the approach to his or her level of competence and comfort or to refer elsewhere to someone who is specially trained in sex therapy.[81]

The following will be a brief discussion of the different stages employed in the "P-LI-SS-IT" model for a patient with erectile dysfunction (impotence) following radical prostatectomy. The patient is 61 yers old, lost his wife two years previously, but is keeping "regular" company with a 57-year-old widow who lives in his apartment house. These are the following steps to be taken:

1. *Permission*—the clinician needs to give permission to have or not to have certain thoughts, feelings, or behaviors. It is useful to acknowledge with this man that sexual desires and behaviors do not have to stop with his age or the fact that he cannot get an erection. Suggested readings such as "Sexual Life After Sixty" may be halpful.[82]

2. *Limited information*—refers to the need for very special information of a factual nature which will help the patient either feel better about his condition or recognize the "universality" of his problem. This would involve telling him about the percent of patients who are impotent after this type of surgery, explaining to him (perhaps before surgery) what causes the loss of erection or volume of seminal fluid. In addition, it may be helpful to mention to him that there is a surgical procedure which can restore erectile competence. If he is interested, detailed information about the inflatable and semi-rigid prosthesis could be provided.

3. *Specific suggestions—this stage involves the clinician actually giving specific recommendations intended to change or add new behaviors to the existing repetoire*. However, it is crucial to know that before embarking on any specific plans with the patient, one should have all the relevant background information about the presenting problem. (It would be destructive to suggest medication or hormone shots to bring on erectile competence in this patient, especially if nocturnal penile tumescence studies revealed physiological impotence.) Instead, it might be helpful to suggest some new behaviors such as oral-genital stimulation or attempting to "stuff" the penis into the vagina by forcing the flaccid organ into the introitus. Another recommendation which may be helpful (depending on the sophistication and openness of the patient) is to suggest mutual manual stimulation with his partner including the use of a mechanical vibrator to fulfill the woman's desire for vaginal containment.

It is important to bear in mind with this stage of intervention that the clinician should attempt to use the language which is familiar to the patient so that he (the doctor) does not appear condescending. Medical terminology is appropriate for the initial conversations, but incorporating the patient's terms for certain responses increases the usefulness of the communication. If a term is used that is absolutely unfamiliar, ask the patient to explain what he means. Also, always check with the patient that the term used (erection) has exactly the same meaning to both of you (some people confuse erection and ejaculation).

4. *Intensive therapy*—this stage is used when the attending physician or health professional does not feel that he or she has the time, expertise, or interest to delve into this issue in the manner which may be required for improvement or resolution of the problem. This then necessitates that the health professional recommend the patient to another individual for more appropriate intervention which may involve (1) more complex dynamic psychotherapy or (2) perhaps a surgical procedure for restoration of erectile competence. Specific recommendations to the appropriate health professional and plans for follow-up and feedback are important for closure to both patient and physician. This may be accomplished in either a formal office visit or an informal phone call assessment. It does, however, allow for some type of resolution to the initial relationship.

The issue of training health professionals who want to work in this field of sexual counseling is a matter of burgeoning concern. The decisions about who will specialize in sexuality is predicated on the needs of the patient population which one sees, the resources which can be made available and the responsibilities which the involved professional wishes to undertake. There are excellent resources today for the health professional who is interested in acquiring specialized training in sex therapy. The text *Sex Education for the Health Professional: A Curriculum Guide* has several chapters devoted to sample programs which are currently accredited in all areas of the country.[82]

In addition, there are a number of organizations which specialize in written, visual, and mechanical aids which may be used in teaching patients how to embellish their sexual satisfaction and to support their learning more about their range of sexual responsiveness (after cancer treatment). These aids to increase awareness and responsiveness to sexual stimuli are also described in the Pearsall and Rosenzweig text and are mentioned in Table 12-4 along with companies which provide mechanical aids and erotica for training health professionals, or to be used in therapy with patients.[82]

Oncology must expand its treatment efforts to go beyond survivorship, and this demands that professional attention be directed at identifying and remedying the sexual dysfunctions associated with cancer care. The negative and destructive impact that cancer has on one's body, personal resources, and options for healthful pursuits extends to the area of sexual intimacy and gratification. These cannot be ignored.

Helping patients to feel loved, experience being lovable,

TABLE 12-4. Suppliers of Audio-Visual Materials

COMPANY	ADDRESS
Carousel Films, Inc.	1501 Broadway Suite 1503 New York, New York 10036
Contemporary Films	McGraw-Hill, Inc. 330 W. 42nd Street New York, New York 10036
EdCoa Productions	310 Cedar Lane Teaneck, New Jersey 07666
Focus International, Inc.	505 West End Avenue New York, New York 10024
Multi-Media Resource Center	1525 Franklin Street San Francisco, California 94109
Perennial Education, Inc.	P.O. Box 236 1825 Willow Road Northfield, Illinois 60093
Sensory Research Corp.	
Texture Films, Inc.	1600 Broadway New York, New York 10019

(Adapted from Rosenzweig N, Pearsall FP (eds): Sex Education for the Health Professional: A Curriculum Guide. New York, Grune & Stratton, 1978)

and to be able to give and receive love should be a high priority item in comprehensive cancer management. Sexuality is a driving force of life, and as long as life exists, attention to that aspect of the human condition must be acknowledged, encouraged, and treated.

REFERENCES

1. Enelow A: Psychosocial rehabilitation for cancer patients. In Frontiers of Radiation Therapy and Oncology, Vol 10, pp 178–182. Basel, S Karger, AG, 1975
2. Cullen J, Fox B, Isom R (eds): Cancer: The Behavioral Dimensions. New York, Power Press, 1976
3. Weisman AD: Early diagnosis of vulnerability in cancer patients. Am J Med Sci 271, No. 2:187–196, 1976
4. Holland J: Psychologic aspects of cancer. In Holland J, Frei E (eds): Cancer Medicine. Philadelphia, Lea & Febiger, 1973
5. Schmale A: Recurrences, metastases, disseminated disease, psychological reactions. Radiat Oncol Biol Physics, 1:515–520, 1976
6. Garfield CA (ed): Stress and Survival: Emotional Realities of Life-Threatening Illness. St Louis, CV Mosby, 1979
7. Cassileth BR: The Cancer Patient: Social and Medical Aspects of Care. Philadelphia, Lea & Febiger, 1979
8. Hellerstein HK, Friedman EH: Sexual activity and the post-coronary patient. Arch Intern Med 125:987, 1970
9. Wise TN: Sexuality in chronic illness. Primary Care 4, No. 1:20, 1977
10. Vaeth JM, Blomberg RC, Adler L (eds): Body image, self-esteem, and sexuality in cancer patients. Frontiers of Radiation Therapy and Oncology, Vol 14. Basel, S Karger, AG, 1980
11. Calderone MS: Historical perspectives on the human sexuality movement: hindsights, insights, foresights. In Rosenzweig N, Pearsall FP (eds): Sex Education for the Health Professional: A Curriculum Guide. New York, Grune & Stratton, 1978
12. Brecher E, Sussman N: History of human sexual research and study. In Saddock BJ, Kaplan HI, Freedman AM (eds): The Sexual Experience, p 71. Baltimore, Williams & Wilkins, 1976
13. Freud S: An Outline of Psychoanalysis. New York, Norton, 1949
14. Kohlberg L: Moral stages and sex education. In Calderone MS (ed): Sexuality and Human Values, p 111. Chicago, Associated Press/Follet, 1975
15. Calderone MS: Historical perspectives on the human sexuality movement: hindsight, insights, foresights. In Rosenzweig H, Pearsall FP (eds): Sex Education for the Health Professional: A Curriculum Guide, p 11. New York, Grune & Stratton, 1978
16. Stayton WR: The core curriculum: what can be taught and what must be taught. In Rosenzweig N, Pearsall FP (eds): Sex Education for the Health Professional: A Curriculum Guide, pp 51–63. New York, Grune & Stratton, 1978
17. Mitchell J: Psychoanalysis and Women. New York, Vintage Books, 1974
18. Morgan R (ed): Sisterhood is Powerful: An Anthology of Writings from the Women's Liberation Movement. New York, Vintage Books, 1970
19. Millet K: Sexual Politics. New York, Avon Books, 1969
20. Kinsey AC, Pomeroy WB, Martin CE et al: Sexual Behavior in the Human Female. Philadelphia, WB Saunders, 1953
21. Masters WH, Johnson V: Human Sexual Response. Boston, Little, Brown & Co, 1965
22. Masters WH, Johnson V: Human Sexual Inadequacy. Boston, Little, Brown & Co, 1970
23. Zilbergeld B, Evans M: The inadequacy of Masters aand Johnson. Psychology Today August:29–42, 1980
24. Kaplan HS: The New Sex Therapy. New York, Brunner/Mazel, 1974
25. McCarthy B: What You Still Don't Know about Male Sexuality. New York, T. Crowell, 1977
26. Journal of Sex Education and Therapy. Chicago, American Association of Sex Educators, Counselors & Therapists
27. Medical Aspects of Human Sexuality. New York, Hospital Publications
28. Rosenzweig N, Pearsall FP (eds): Sex Education for the Health Professional: A Curriculum Guide, Part V, pp 201–303. New York, Gruen & Stratton, 1978
29. Wallace D: The University of California: San Francisco Program. In Rosenzweig N, Pearsall FP (eds): Sex Education for the Health Professional: A Curriculum Guide, Part V, pp 251–263. New York, Grune & Stratton, 1978
30. Derogatis LR: Psychological assessment of psychosexual functioning. Psychiatric Clinics of North America 3, No. 1:113–131, 1980
31. Schain WS: Sexual functioning, self-esteem, and cancer care. In Vaeth JM, Blomberg RC, Adler L (eds): Frontiers of Radiation Therapy and Oncology, Vol 14, pp 12–19. Basel, S Karger, AG, 1980
32. Weisman AD, Worden JW, Sobel HJ: Psychosocial Screening and Intervention with Cancer Patients. Boston, Project Omega, NCI Grant No. CA 19797, 1977–1980.
33. Derogatis LD, Melisaratos N: The DSFI: a multi-dimensional measure of sexual functioning. Sex and Marital Ther 5, No. 3:244–280, 1979
34. Kaplan HS: The New Sex Therapy, p 12. New York, Brunner/Mazel, 1974
35. Cantor RC: Self-esteem, sexuality and cancer-related stress. In Vaeth JM, Blomberg RC, Adler L (eds): Frontiers of Radiation Therapy and Oncology, Vol 14, p 52. Basel, S Karger, AG, 1980
36. Schain WS: Sexual functioning, self-esteem and cancer care. In Vaeth JM, Blomberg RC, Adler L (eds): Frontiers of Radiation Therapy and Oncology, Vol 14, p 15. Basel, S Karger, AG, 1980
37. Wise TN: Sexual functioning in neoplastic disease. Medical Aspects of Human Sexuality 12:16–31, 1978
38. American Cancer Society: Cancer Facts and Figures. New York, American Cancer Society, 1980
39. Cole P: Major aspects of the epidemiology of breast cancer. Cancer 46:865–867, 1980
40. Kusher R: Why Me: What Every Woman Should Know about Breast Cancer To Save Her Life. New York, Signet, 1977
41. Thomas SG: Breast cancer: the psychosocial issues. Cancer Nursing 1:1153–1160, 1978
42. Morris T: Psychological adjustment of mastectomy. Cancer Treatment 6:41–61, 1979

43. Schain WS: Guidelines for psychological management of breast cancer: a stage-related approach. In Gallagher HS, Leis HP, Snyderman RK et al: The Breast, pp 465–475. St Louis, C.V. Mosby, 1978
44. Abt V, McGurrin MC, Heintz AA: The impact of mastectomy on sexual self-image and behavior. Journal of Sex Education and Therapy 4, No. 2:45–46, 1978
45. Frank D, Dornbush R, Webster S et al: Mastectomy and sexual behavior: a pilot study. Sexuality Disability Vol 1: 1978
46. Witkin MH: Sex therapy and mastectomy. J Sex Marital Ther 1:290–304, 1975
47. Comfort A: The Joy of Sex: A Gourmet Guide to Love Making. New York, Simon & Schuster, 1972
48. Kaplan HS: The New Sex Therapy. New York, Brunner/Mazel, 1974
49. McCarthy B: What You Still Don't Know about Male Sexuality, pp 75–83. New York, T. Crowell, 1977
50. Kaplan HS: The Illustrated Manual of Sex Therapy. New York, Quadrangel, 1975
51. Zalon: I Am Whole Again: The Case for Breast Reconstruction. New York, Random House, 1978
52. Clifford E: The reconstruction experience: the search for restitution. In Georgiade N (ed): Breast Reconstruction following Mastectomy, pp 22–34. St Louis, C.V. Mosby, 1979
53. Schain WS: Reconstructive Mammoplasty: Reversibility of a Trauma. Paper presented at the American Psychological Association Annual Conference, San Francisco, August 1977
54. Abitol MM, Davenport JH: Sexual dysfunction after therapy for cervical carcinoma. Am J Obstet Gynecol 2:181–189, 1974
55. Fischer SG: Psychosexual adjustment following total pelvic exenteration. Cancer Nursing June, 2:218–225, 1979
56. Cobliner WG: Psychosocial factors in gynecological or breast malignancy. Hospital Physician 10:38–40, 1977
57. Morley GW, Lindenauer SM, Youngs D: Vaginal reconstruction following pelvic exenteration: surgical and psychological considerations. Am J Obstet Gynecol 117, No. 7:996–1002, 1973
58. NIH Study: The Treatment of Clinical Stage I and II Carcinoma and the Breast with Mastectomy and Axillary Dissection Versus Excisional Biopsy, Axillary Dissection and Definitive Radiation. Protocol No. 79-C-111
59. Vincent CE: Some marital sexual concomitants of the cervix. South Med J 68:552–558, 1975
60. Capone MA, Westie KS, Good RS: Sexual rehabilitation of the gynecological cancer patient: an effective counseling model. In Vaeth JM, Blomberg RC, Adler L (eds): Frontiers of Radiation Therapy and Oncology, Vol 14, pp 123–130. Basel, S Karger, AG, 1980
61. Kirkpatrick JR: The stoma patient and his return to society. In Vaeth JM, Blomberg RC, Adler L (eds): Frontiers of Radiation Therapy and Oncology, Vol 14, p 21. Basel, S Karger, AG, 1980
62. Bernstein W: Sexual dysfunction following radical surgery for cancer of the rectum and sigmoid colon. Medical Aspects of Human Sexuality 6:156–163, 1972
63. Druss R et al: Psychological response to colectomy II. Arch Gen Psychiatry 20:419–427, 1969
64. Orbach CE, Tallent N: Modification of perceived body and of body concepts. Arch Gen Psychiatry 12:126–135, 1965
65. Lyons AS, Brockmeir M: Sex after ileostomy and colostomy. Medical Aspects of Human Sexuality Jan, 1:107–108, 1975
66. Von Eschenbach AC: Sexual dysfunction following therapy for cancer of the prostate, testis, and penis. In Vaeth JM, Blomberg RC, Adler L (eds): Frontiers of Radiation Therapy and Oncology, Vol 14, pp 40–48. Basel, S Karger, AG, 1980
67. Jewett HJ: The present status of radical prostatectomy for stages A and B prostatic cancer. Urol Clin North Am 2:105–124 1975
68. Ray GR, Bashaw MA: The role of radiation therapy in the treatment of adenocarcinoma of the prostate. Annu Rev Med 26:567–588, 1975
69. Herr HW: Preservation of sexual potency in prostate cancer patients after iodine I-25 implantation. J Am Geriatr Soc 27:17–19, 1979
70. Ellis WJ, Grayhack JT: Sexual function in aging males after orchiectomy and estrogen therapy. J Urol 89:895–899, 1963
71. Von Eschenbach AC: Sexual dysfunction following therapy for cancer of the prostate, testis and penis. In Vaeth JM, Blomberg RC, Adler L (eds): Frontiers of Radiation Therapy and Oncology, Vol 14, p 45. Basel, S Karger, AG, 1980
72. Kedia KR, Markland C, Fraley EE: Sexual functioning following high retroperitoneal lymphadenectomy. Urol Clin North Am 4:523–527, 1977
73. Stoklosa JM, Bullard DG: Talking about sex suggestions for the health professional. In Vaeth JM, Blomberg RC, Adler L (eds): Frontiers of Radiation Therapy and Oncology, Vol 14, pp 79–82. Basel, S Karger, AG, 1980
74. Furlow WL: Prostate disease: prosthesis for surgical problems. Patient Care May, 2:1–12, 1978
75. Small MP: The Small-Carion prosthesis: surgical implant for the management of impotence. Sexuality and Disability 1, No. 4:282–291, 1978
76. Furlow WL: Sexual consequences of male genitourinary cancer: the role of sex prosthesis. In Vaeth JM, Blomberg RC, Adler L (eds): Frontiers of Radiation Therapy and Oncology, Vol 14, p 105. Basel, S Karger, AG, 1980
77. Personal communication from Nasser Javadpour
78. Leiber L, Plumb MM, Gerstenzang ML et al: The communication of affection between cancer patients and their spouses. Psychosom Med 38:379–389, 1976
79. Vaeth JM, Blomberg RC, Adler L (eds): Frontiers of Radiation Therapy and Oncology, Vol 14. Basel, S Karger, AG, 1980
80. Schain WS: The role of the sex therapist in oncology. In Frontiers of Radiation Therapy and Oncology, Vol 15. 1981 (in press)
81. Annon JS: The Behavioral Treatment of Sexual Problems, Vol 1. Honolulu, Mercantile Printing, 1974
82. Rosenzweig N, Pearsall FP (eds): Sex Education for the Health Professional: A Curriculum Guide, pp 201–315. New York, Grune & Stratton, 1978

Section 3

Andrea S. Hay

Community Resources for Patients with Cancer

Once an individual is diagnosed as having cancer and begins the treatment process, his life and that of his family change in many ways. Basic components of the individual's and family's life style which had previously been taken for granted, such as income, family relationships, and activities of daily living, must be re-assessed, and new ways must be found to meet new needs in new circumstances. In essence, the task for the patient and family is to develop a new equilibrium which allows them to function effectively, integrating the diagnosis of cancer and its implications. Fortunately, there are a variety of resources available to support the patient and family as they struggle to find solutions, either through societal institutions and agencies or health care providers or self help groups composed of people in similar situations grappling with similar issues.

INCOME MAINTENANCE

It is well recognized that the financial impact of a cancer diagnosis can be devastating. One of the first concerns expressed by adult patients and their families is maintaining an on-going source of income if they exhaust paid leave benefits from their place of employment. For the individual who has contributed to Social Security, submitting an application for Social Security disability benefits is the place to begin. Eligibility for benefits is based on the existence of the disease and on having accumulated sufficient quarters of Social Security coverage within the recent past. The availability of other financial assets is not considered in determining eligibility. In terms of eligibility relating to the disease state, the requirements are that the disease has been in existence for six months and is expected to last for at least one year, and the effect of the disease is such that the individual is unable to perform any "substantial gainful activity." In practice, "substantial gainful activity" means any type of employment whereby the individual earns more than $290.00 per month. The disability application should be initiated soon after a treatment plan is formulated. The requirement that the disease exist for six months is often met while the application is being processed. The stipulation that the disease must be expected to last for a year includes the period of active treatment whether in the presence of disease or not. Specifically, an individual undergoing an 18-month course of chemotherapy in the absence of disease would probably be eligible for benefits while a patient undergoing six weeks of radiation treatment only, also in the absence of disease probably would not be eligible. Should the initial application be rejected on medical grounds, there is an appeals process of several stages which may be undertaken. Application forms and detailed information can be obtained from the individual's local Social Security office.

Most people apply for Supplemental Security Income (SSI) at the same time as they apply for disability benefits. The process is identical. The purpose of this program is to provide income to the elderly and disabled who have very limited income and few assets. The amount of income or assets allowable in order to be eligible for benefits under this program varies from state to state. SSI may provide the cancer patient and his family with a source of income while the Social Security disability determination is being made. In most instances, once Social Security disability benefits begin, the SSI benefits cease, because the individual's income is now greater than the amount allowed for continuing SSI benefits. Children who have cancer may also be eligible for SSI using the same criteria. Parental financial resources will be considered in making the eligibility determination.

A few states, most notably New York, have state disability programs administered through the individual's place of employment. In New York, benefits begin after the worker has been absent for one week. The employer is the contact point for programs of this type.

Within each state, the Welfare Department provides financial assistance of various kinds. The financial eligibility requirements differ from jurisdiction to jurisdiction, making it impossible to delineate anything but the broadest outline of possible services. Again, income and assets must be extremely limited in order to be eligible. Some examples of the situations in which the Welfare Department would be an appropriate resource are: Aid for Dependent Children (AFDC) payments to support a child or children whose parent(s) has been determined to be disabled; General Relief payments to provide income, usually on a short term emergency basis, in situations where the disability determination has not yet been made or the adult has been found to not be disabled; Food Stamps to augment a family's food (only) budget. Applications for these services should be made at the local welfare or social services office.

The Veterans Administration (VA) provides a pension to veterans with non-service connected illnesses who meet very stringent financial requirements. The veteran must possess an honorable discharge following service during wartime. Vietnam veterans are included in this provision. He must also be totally and permanently disabled as certified by a VA Rating Board. The amount of the pension is determined by the amount of income available to the veteran, including income of a spouse, the number of his dependents, and the amount of his non-reimbursable medical bills.

INSURANCE

Inasmuch as medical insurance coverage is usually obtained through one's place of employment, choices in this area must also be explored. Once an employee is on leave without pay, most companies will not continue to pay their share of the medical insurance. Despite the financial hardship involved, the employee/patient should assume the full cost of this coverage as it will be difficult or impossible for him to obtain such coverage at a later date when he is once again financially secure. The same general rationale applies to all insurance of whatever type owned at the time a cancer diagnosis is made. Even after an individual has been disease-free for more than five years, he will likely have difficulty obtaining new or additional coverage.

It is always advisable to read carefully all of one's current insurance policies to determine if they offer particular benefits to the policyholder in the event of hospitalization or disability. Some policies pay a per diem rate to the patient while he is hospitalized. Others contain a clause waiving premiums while the policyholder is disabled. In addition, many people unknowingly carry insurance on loan agreements and/or mortgages which waives payment either completely or partially while the individual is disabled. One's insurance agent or the holder of the mortgage or loan agreement can answer questions about these options and assist with the necessary verification.

The Medicaid program, funded jointly by the federal and state governments, is designed to pay the medical expenses, primarily hospital, physician, and nursing home bills, of individuals found to be disabled according to the Social Security definition. In most states, an individual who is considered disabled, but whose income is greater than the SSI financial eligibility standards, will still be eligible for Medicaid benefits, especially if he owes large medical bills not covered by other insurance. Applications are made at the local welfare or social services office.

Medicare coverage is extended automatically to all individuals who are over 65 years of age or who have been receiving

Social Security disability benefits for two years. This program covers costs for hospitalizations, physicians' services, some home health care and limited days of nursing home placement.

FINANCIAL ASSISTANCE FOR TREATMENT EXPENDITURES

The dollar cost of treatment is high. In addition to the direct expenses of drugs, hospitalizations, and physicians' fees, there are the indirect expenses of transportation to and from the treatment center, lost wages of the patient and other family members, and often the expense of food and room near the treatment center for some member of the family while similar expenses continue at home. Payment of the direct medical expenses is usually at least partly covered through one's medical insurance. But problems may arise if there is a dollar limit on expenditures per diagnosis, per beneficiary, or within a specified time frame. The end result is that many families must absorb a major portion of all costs themselves, often going into debt, sometimes even being forced into bankruptcy.

The American Cancer Society, Inc., (ACS) provides some practical assistance in this area. Local chapters, which are usually county based, will provide transportation to and from the treatment center, either by car and volunteer driver or by the purchase of bus, train, or airplane tickets. ACS can also help pay for the cancer treatment itself as well as for a small portion of the cost of home health care personnel. These services are available to cancer patients regardless of diagnosis, but are based on need. Obviously, all financial needs of all patients cannot be met, as resources are limited. Contact the local ACS chapter for information about available assistance.

The Leukemia Society of America, Inc., provides similar kinds of financial assistance to a target population diagnosed with any of the leukemias, lymphomas, or Hodgkin's disease. They will reimburse the patient or family for the cost of some specific drugs and for other kinds of treatment, usually radiation, in specific medical situations. They will also help with transportation costs by reimbursing for mileage to and from the treatment center. There is a dollar limit on the amount of assistance provided to a family on a yearly basis. The Leukemia Society is organized on a national level with chapters in each state. Requests for assistance should be initiated through the state chapter.

Title V of the Social Security Act allocates funds through the Department of Health and Human Services to each state to locate and treat children who are crippled or who are suffering from crippling diseases. Under this title, a crippled child is defined as an individual less than 21 years of age suffering from an organic disease, defect, or condition which hinders the achievement of normal growth and development. While the federal definition is a broad one, individual states establish their own plans, which include eligibility standards according to diagnosis and family financial situation. The financial requirements are usually more generous than under the income maintenance programs. If the diagnosis of cancer is included in the state plan, the state Crippled Children's agency, usually a division of the State Health Department, will pay for some treatment costs, such as hospitalizations, surgeries, and appliances, provided the care is delivered by a physician who is a state-approved consultant.

EDUCATION/VOCATION

In some instances the prescribed cancer treatment is such that even upon its completion the patient is unable to resume his usual employment. The example of the coal miner who undergoes an above-knee amputation comes readily to mind. In such a situation the Bureau of Vocational Rehabilitation (BVR) is the desirable resource. This federal agency, part of the U.S. Department of Education, allocates monies to individual states. In turn, the states establish a plan which offers access to a variety of education and rehabilitation programs. The basic requirement to obtain assistance is inability to return to one's former employment because of a physical impairment. For students not previously in the labor force, there must be a need for education to ensure their successful competition in the job market. In most situations the agency will underwrite at least part of the cost of the education, whether it be technical training or a college program. Interested individuals must initiate their own applications.

Under Section 503 of the Rehabilitation Act of 1973, discrimination against physically handicapped individuals by companies holding contracts with the federal government is prohibited. Complaints in this area should be filed with the Office of Civil Rights at the Regional Office of the U.S. Department of Labor. Under Section 504 of the same act, discrimination is prohibited in federally assisted programs whether they be services, benefits, or employment. Complaints should be filed with the Office of Civil Rights at the Regional Office of the U.S. Department of Health and Human Services.

Interruption of schooling, the primary task or work of the child and adolescent, is a frequent consequence of cancer and its treatment. However, academic performance does not have to be sacrificed. Most comprehensive care hospitals offer an accredited school program, staffed by teachers provided by the local Board of Education. This service is usually available to inpatients and outpatients who do not live in the immediate area, but are remaining there for treatment. Close consultation with the child's own school program is standard procedure. Homebound tutoring, provided by the pupil's own school district, is available to those who are too ill to attend school, but are not hospitalized. Verification by a physician of the need for this service is usually required. Specific arrangements are made through the Office of Pupil Personnel, an administrative component of the local school system. In most systems, all schooling must be obtained either through homebound tutoring or the usual classroom program. In other words, a pupil cannot receive homebound instruction during the week immediately following chemotherapy when he is feeling particularly ill and then return to his classroom for a few weeks until his next treatment.

HEALTH CARE SERVICES

Currently, increased numbers of cancer treatment programs include an outpatient component where much of the therapy is administered. When hospitalizations do occur, they are usually brief. As a result, families must assume new responsibilities for their loved one's physical well being. Most families are initially unprepared to meet these responsibilities, but are quite willing to learn. Ideally, the family should have support from the community in this endeavor so that some of their time and energy remains to meet their own and the patient's emotional needs.

When nursing supervision is required for such tasks as dressing changes or evaluation of wound healing, a home health or public health nurse is invaluable. The services of these registered nurses can be obtained either through the local county or city Department of Health or the Visiting Nurse Association (VNA), a private, nonprofit agency. When contacting the health department, ask for the Home Health Section. The fee for this service through either source is usually based on a sliding scale, depending on the family's ability to pay. In some areas, the health department does not charge for its services. Depending on the individual's policy, the fee may be covered by medical insurance. Some health departments and VNA's employ additional staff usually referred to as Homemakers or Home Health Aides whose skills are oriented toward maintenance of routine activities. For instance, a Home Health Aide might come into the home on a daily basis to assist with morning care, such as bathing and getting the patient dressed for the day. A Homemaker might come daily to prepare a meal or weekly to do grocery shopping or laundry. The health department is listed under the local government heading in the white pages of the telephone directory. The VNA is also listed in the white pages, usually with the name of the place in which it is located. All of these services can also be purchased through proprietary agencies which are listed in the yellow pages of the telephone directory under Home Health Services.

Increasingly, community hospitals are developing home care programs as a distinct operating component separate from other departments of the hospital. These programs are usually quite comprehensive, offering services through one source to meet the majority of the physical and emotional needs of the patient and family. One does not always have to be a patient of the particular hospital in order to qualify for the service, as the service area may be defined by geographical location. To ascertain the availability of this kind of program, inquire of the hospital directly or ask other patients or health care providers.

Often the primary need is the provision of meals when other family members are at work or at school. Most communities have the Meals on Wheels program where, for a nominal fee, a well-balanced, nutritious meal is brought to the patient's home daily.

If specialized equipment or supplies are needed in order to keep the patient comfortable and safe at home, the local pharmacy or surgical supplies company can meet that need. Either source will have equipment such as wheelchairs, hospital beds, or bath seats to rent or buy. They will also have ostomy supplies, specific kinds of dressing and catheters which may be required. Some civic groups or chapters of the ACS operate loan closets from which one can borrow major pieces of equipment. ACS also provides the most common-sized dressings.

For those patients needing oxygen, surgical supply companies can supply the equipment and often the oxygen itself. In addition, in some areas there are companies which specialize in therapeutic, as opposed to industrial, oxygen services. They install and service the equipment on a 24-hour-per-day basis.

Occasionally, a very sick patient may need to be transported over a great distance and may be unable to travel by the usual commercial means or by automobile. There are private firms available which specialize in meeting this need, usually by air ambulance. They will coordinate the move from bedside to bedside, including the provision of all staff and equipment. Such firms can often be identified through contact with local privately operated ambulance companies.

In the United States, hospice care is a relatively new approach to the care of the dying patient. Although the term originally referred to a place to care for dying people and is still used somewhat in that sense in England, in this country it has come to reflect a philosophy of care. Thus, a hospice program might consist of a specific residence attached to or separate from a hospital, or a home care program designed to support the patient and family so that the patient can die at home if that is his wish. Indeed, many hospices offer a program containing both components. The basic goal of the hospice movement is to meet the physical, emotional, and spiritual needs of dying people and those important to them. The outstanding characteristics of a hospice program are compassionate concern for the patient and family as well as effective management of the severe pain often associated with a terminal cancer prognosis. The National Hospice Organization is an excellent source of information about all aspects of hospice care in the United States, including specific locations and contact people. The organization can be reached at 1311A Dolley Madison Boulevard, McLean, Virginia 22101.

In a few areas, private social service agencies have been funded to meet and coordinate the needs of individuals in the advanced stages of cancer and their families. Services include practical assistance to meet tangible needs, as well as family and bereavement counseling. An example of this type of agency is Cancer Care, Inc., a part of the National Cancer Foundation, which provides service to New York City and the surrounding area within a 50-mile radius. Nursing or social work staff of the hospital providing cancer treatment would be aware of the availability of a resource of this type.

EMOTIONAL SUPPORT RESOURCES

For many people, once the questions relating to tangible needs are answered, attention turns toward the emotional aspects of coping. Such needs can be met through a variety of resources, primarily self-help groups with varying degrees of professional support or supervision, veteran/peer counseling programs and traditional professional counseling. The underlying theme in both the self-help and veteran/peer approach is the sharing of needs, experiences, and feelings in order to help master the emotional impact of the cancer diagnosis. This kind of sharing generates a feeling of hope, the realization of not being alone in one's fears, and constructive suggestions for problem solving. A patient and/or family member affected directly by cancer can offer a kind of empathy and support to another patient or family member which cannot be found elsewhere. Professional counseling can help the patient and family deal with the overwhelming changes in their lives brought about by the cancer diagnosis or by the implications of the particular stage of the disease. It is also an appropriate resource for those individuals trying to manage multiple life stresses, many of which pre-date the cancer diagnosis. Self-help groups and professional counseling are not mutually exclusive. Various combinations may be helpful at different stages of the coping process.

The American Cancer Society (ACS) has long sponsored groups and peer support programs based on site-specific diagnoses. The Reach to Recovery program focuses on rehabilitative support to women who have undergone mastectomy. Upon referral from the woman's physician, a trained volunteer, who herself has had a mastectomy, visits the woman who has recently undergone the same surgery and provides her with appropriate exercises and a temporary prosthesis. The volunteer is an extremely effective role model, demonstrating that successful adaptation to mastectomy is possible. The Reach to Recovery volunteers can be contacted through the local ACS chapter.

The International Association of Laryngectomees is also sponsored by ACS and functions under the same principle of physician referral and early contact with a patient who is about to have his larynx removed or who has recently undergone such surgery. Members of the association also offer support to family members and provide information about alternative methods of communication, such as esophageal speech. If this organization is not listed separately in the telephone directory, the local ACS chapter can provide the necessary information to contact them.

For those individuals who have had ostomy surgery, the local chapter of the United Ostomy Association, Inc., is a very useful resource. The members offer each other emotional support, as well as practical information about various supplies and methods of caring for the ostomy. In addition to patient-to-patient visitation, chapter meetings are held on a regular basis. These meetings may be devoted to educational presentations or problem solving. Some chapters also sponsor groups for adolescents who have had ostomy surgery. If there is no listing in the white pages of the telephone directory for this group, the enterostomal therapist at the nearest comprehensive care hospital or the local chapter of ACS should have the necessary information. Contact can also be initiated through the organization's national headquarters, located at 2001 West Beverly Boulevard, Los Angeles, California 90057.

Make Today Count is an organization of cancer patients, their families and other members of the community, including, but not limited to, health professionals, who meet regularly for purposes of discussion and problem resolution. The primary focus of the organization is emotional self-help. To locate the nearest chapter or for information on starting a chapter, contact the national office at P.O. Box 303, Burlington, Iowa 52601.

Candlelighters is a nationwide association of local chapters focusing on the parents of the child with cancer. The goal of this organization is to provide emotional support to parents through the sharing of common concerns and information, to improve the quality of information available to parents, and to promote legislative action at all levels to benefit childhood cancer patients and their families. Local chapters can be located through ACS or by contacting the Candlelighters Foundation at 123 C Street S.E., Washington, D.C. 20003.

In addition to these national organizations, there are many excellent support programs available on a regional level. Most of these programs are affiliated with a local hospital, are available to all patients regardless of cancer site, and employ a veteran/peer counseling approach. Typically, a trained volunteer, a cancer veteran, visits a patient who is just beginning treatment, often while that individual is hospitalized. The goal of the linkage between the veteran and the new patient is to facilitate emotional coping. Ideally, a supportive relationship will be established which will continue throughout the treatment process. Examples of these kinds of programs include CanSurmount, based in Denver, Colorado; TOUCH, based at the Comprehensive Cancer Center at the University of Alabama in Birmingham; the SHANTI project in Berkeley, California; and the I Can Cope project in Minneapolis, Minnesota.

Professional counseling can take many forms, be located in many places and be provided by a variety of personnel trained in different fields. For many people, the first professional counselors they encounter are members of the hospital staff who are part of the team caring for the cancer patient. These counselors may be social workers, psychologists, chaplains, oncology or psychiatric nurses, or psychiatrists. Their services may be available routinely or by specific request from patient, family, staff nurse, or physician. The focus of their intervention is to help the patient and family deal with their reaction to the illness and its impact as well as their adaptation to the treatment regimen. In addition, they can provide emotional and spiritual support and information about resources.

For those desiring long-term counseling, the local community mental health clinic, again staffed by a variety of counselors with different professional training, is another appropriate resource. Most clinic staff members specialize in treating issues of family relationships, depression, and communication. Treatment can involve the cancer patient only, the spouse or children only, or the entire family. There is a fee for the counseling service which may be adjusted according to the individual's or family's ability to pay. Or the fee may be reimbursed through medical insurance coverage. The assistance of a member of the hospital care team can be invaluable in locating such counseling services.

An alternative to the community mental health clinic is the Family Service Association (FSAA), a private social work agency which offers similar counseling services. This agency, funded by the local United Fund charity campaign, also charges a fee based on ability to pay.

In some areas, the American Cancer Society employs a staff member specifically to counsel patients and families. In other situations, a counselor who is in private practice might be the desirable resource. Again, the counseling staff at the hospital providing cancer treatment or at the local community hospital can often provide the names of several counselors. It is perfectly reasonable for an individual to have an interview with a potential counselor prior to beginning treatment to

Listing of Resources and Services

INCOME MAINTENANCE	
Social Security Disability	Monthly payments to those unable to work because of disease or treatment.
Supplemental Security Income	Monthly payment to disabled individuals with very limited income and assets.
Aid for Dependent Children	Monthly support to children of disabled parents.
General Relief	Emergency, short term cash assistance.
Food Stamps	Coupons to purchase food items only.
Veterans Administration	Pension to veterans with non-service connected illness.
INSURANCE	
Medicaid	Payment of some medical expenses of disabled individuals.
Medicare	Payment of some medical expenses of individuals over 65 years of age or those who have received S.S. disability for two years.
FINANCIAL ASSISTANCE FOR TREATMENT	
American Cancer Society	Payment of some costs—transportation, treatment, home care, dressings.
Leukemia Society of America	Payment of some costs for leukemia patients—transportation, some drugs, radiation in specific instances.
Crippled Children's Program	Payment of approved hospitalizations, surgeries and appliances.
EDUCATION/VOCATION	
Bureau of Vocational Rehabilitation	Technical or academic education to ensure competition in job market.
Local School System	Homebound tutoring.
NON-ACUTE INPATIENT CARE	
Veterans Administration Hospital	Residential placement of veterans.
Nursing Home	Residential placement of those who cannot be cared for in own home.
Hospice	Care, in own home or residential for terminally ill patient and family.
HOME HEALTH CARE SERVICES	
Local Health Department	Personnel to assist with maintaining physical well-being of patient in home.
Visiting Nurse Association	Personnel to assist with maintaining physical well-being of patient in home.
Private Firms	Personnel to assist with maintaining physical well-being of patient in home.
Meals on Wheels	Meals delivered to patient in home.
Surgical Supply Companies	Specialized equipment for home.
Pharmacy	Specialized equipment for home.
Hospice	Comprehensive home care for terminally ill patient.
American Cancer Society	Payment of some home health care fees and provision of dressings.
TRANSPORTATION	
American Cancer Society	Some transportation or money for such between home and treatment center.
Leukemia Society of America	Reimbursement of mileage between home and treatment center.
Private Firms	Bedside to bedside transfer of patients usually by air-ambulance.
SELF-HELP GROUPS	
Reach to Recovery	Emotional support, exercises, and temporary prosthesis for women undergoing mastectomy.
International Assoc. of Laryngectomees	Emotional support and information to patients having larynx removed.
United Ostomy Association	Emotional support and practical information to those who have had ostomy surgery.
Make Today Count	Group discussion and problem solving relating to emotional coping with cancer.
Candlelighters	Emotional support and information to parents of children with cancer.
PROFESSIONAL COUNSELING	
Community Mental Health Clinics	Emotional support and therapy.
Family Service Association	Emotional support and therapy.
Private Practitioners	Emotional support and therapy.
INFORMATON SOURCES	
Hospital Staff	Emotional support and information about available resources of all types. Contact social worker, nurse or discharge planning coordinator.
Local County or City	Information and referral by telephone. Staff at health or social services department. All can provide information about available resources.
American Cancer Society	Information about local resources and educational material.
Leukemia Society of America	Information about local resources.
Cancer Information Service	Information about treatment resources, practical needs, emotional support groups, and the disease itself.

determine whether the trust and rapport essential to a productive relationship can be developed. It is equally important to discuss basic issues of the counselor's education and experience in the particular problem area, as well as fees and time commitment.

LOCAL INFORMATION SOURCES

Inasmuch as specific community resources vary from place to place and time to time, it is helpful to know of the services or people who are likely to be well informed about the current availability of such resources. Within the hospital setting, the staff of the social work department or the nursing department would be able to supply such information. If the questions are related to practical matters, such as obtaining health care services in the home, the person designated as the hospital's discharge planning coordinator could be helpful.

Many counties throughout the country offer telephone information and referral services which a consumer can call to present his problem and to receive information on local agencies which should be able to meet his need. County public health nurses and social service workers are also valuable sources of information. Again, the nurse can be reached through the Department of Health and the social service worker through the Welfare Department, Division of Social Services. Both agencies would be under the county government listings in the white pages of the telephone directory.

Local chapters of the American Cancer Society and the Leukemia Society of America possess much information about resources in their local area as well as educational material.

The Cancer Information Service (CIS) offers support and access to information on resources on a nationwide basis to the public and to health professionals. The CIS, affiliated with Comprehensive Cancer Centers and the American Cancer Society, can answer questions relating to treatment resources, financial assistance, counseling services, and home care programs. All requests for information are confidential. CIS can be contacted through the following toll-free telephone numbers:

Alabama: 1-800-292-6201
California: Area Codes 213, 714, and 805: 1-800-252-9066
 Rest of California: 213-226-2374
Colorado: 1-800-332-1850
Connecticut: 1-800-922-0824
Delaware: 1-800-523-3586
District of Columbia, including suburban Maryland and northern Virginia: 202-636-5700
Florida: Dade County: English: 305-547-6920 Spanish: 305-547-6960
 Rest of Florida: English: 1-800-432-5953 Spanish: 1-800-432-5955
Georgia: 1-800-327-7332
Hawaii: 536-0111
 Neighbor islands: Ask operator for Enterprise 6702
Illinois: Chicago: 312-226-2371
 Rest of Illinois: 800-972-0586
Kentucky: 800-432-9321
 Out of state regarding resources in Kentucky: 606-233-6333
Maine: 1-800-225-7034
Maryland: 800-492-1444
Massachusetts: 1-800-952-7420
Minnesota: 1-800-582-5262
New Hampshire: 1-800-225-7034
New Jersey: Southern: 800-523-3586
 Northern: 800-223-1000
New York: New York City: 212-794-7982
 Rest of New York: 1-800-462-7255
North Carolina: Durham County: 919-684-2230
 Rest of North Carolina: 800-672-0943
North Dakota: 1-800-328-5188
Ohio: 800-282-6522
Pennsylvania: 1-800-822-3963
South Dakota: 1-800-328-5188
Texas: Houston: 713-792-3245
 Rest of Texas: 1-800-392-2040
Vermont: 1-800-225-7034
Washington: 1-800-552-7212
Wisconsin: 800-362-8038

People living in areas not listed above should use the national line which is 800-638-6694.

CONCLUSION

While resources do exist which offer practical and emotional support to cancer patients and their families, they are by no means comprehensive enough to meet all the needs of those whose lives are so dramatically affected by the disease. Thus, cancer patients and all those who care about their well-being must continue to make known the many valid but as yet unmet needs which they face. Only in this way can change be generated in existing programs and new resources developed.

PART TWO

PRACTICE OF ONCOLOGY

Rodney R. Million
Nicholas J. Cassisi
Robert E. Wittes

CHAPTER 13

Cancer in the Head and Neck

EPIDEMIOLOGY OF HEAD AND NECK CANCER

The estimated number of new head and neck cancer cases (excluding skin cancer) for 1981 in the United States is approximately 37,000; this represents about 5% of the total new cancer cases. The ratio of male to female is approximately 3–4:1. The usual time for diagnosis is past the age of 40, except for salivary gland and nasopharyngeal tumors, which may occur in younger age groups. There has been no major change in the incidence of head and neck cancer over the past three decades in either the male or female population, which is a bit surprising since a common etiologic factor (namely, cigarette smoking) has resulted in a large increase in lung cancer. Cigarette smokers have an increased risk for not one, but multiple head and neck primaries as well as lung cancer. Alcohol has also been implicated as a causative factor for certain head and neck cancers, and the effects of alcohol and tobacco seem to be additive. Patients with pharyngeal cancer have an increased risk to develop esophageal cancer, and patients with major salivary gland tumors have an increased risk for breast cancer.

ANATOMY

The regional anatomy is described separately under specific sites.

LYMPHATIC SYSTEM

There are no capillary lymphatics in the epithelium. Tumor must penetrate the lamina propria before lymphatic invasion can occur. One may predict the richness of the capillary network in any given head and neck site by the relative incidence of lymph node metastases at presentation. The density of the capillary lymphatic network generally corresponds to the density of the vascular capillary system, but there are exceptions. The nasopharynx and pyriform sinus have the most profuse networks of capillary lymphatics. The paranasal sinuses, middle ear, and vocal cords have few or no capillary lymphatics, based on their low rate of lymph node metastases when tumor is confined to these sites. Muscle and fat contain few capillary lymphatics. Bone and cartilage are thought to have a few capillary lymphatics in the periosteum or perichondrium. There are no capillary lymphatics in the eye and few in the orbit. The capillary lymphatic system tends to undergo atrophy with age, particularly in the larynx and trachea.

There are an estimated 150–350 lymph nodes above the clavicle, nearly one-third of the total lymph nodes in the body. The lymphatic system probably originates embryonically from the venous system. Therefore, the lymph nodes and lymphatic trunks are associated with veins. Fig. 13-1 shows the arrangement of the important lymph nodes in the head and neck region.

The internal jugular vein nodes are an important group of lymph nodes in intimate relation with the internal jugular vein from the base of skull to the termination of its lymphatic trunks at the base of the neck. The highest group of nodes lies at the base of skull in the poststyloid portion of the lateral pharyngeal space and is referred to as the parapharyngeal nodes. They lie deep to the sternocleidomastoid muscle, the posterior belly of the digastric, and the tail of the parotid and are difficult to palpate (see Fig. 13-1).

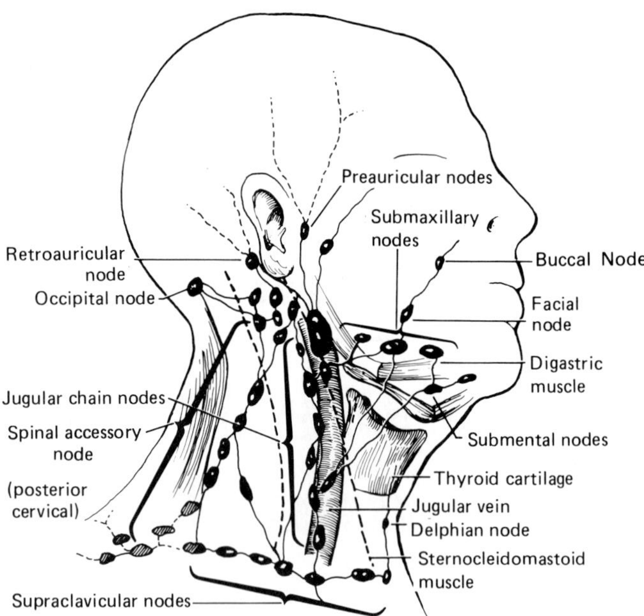

FIG. 13-1. The cervical lymphatics.

The remainder of the jugular chain nodes are divided, for practical purposes, into upper, middle, and lower. The upper group, frequently referred to as the subdigastric lymph nodes, is the most important, as virtually all head and neck malignancies spread to this area, either primarily or secondarily. The nodes lie anterior or lateral to the internal jugular vein and may be palpated in front of the sternocleidomastoid muscle, deep to it, or less commonly behind it. The midjugular nodes lie deep to the sternocleidomastoid. The low jugular nodes assume a more anterior and medial relationship to the internal jugular vein and lie quite close to the trachea.

The lymph nodes of the spinal accessory chain (posterior cervical chain) are distributed along the general course of the 11th cranial nerve. The superior nodes of the spinal accessory chain blend with the upper jugular chain nodes. The middle and lower spinal accessory chain nodes diverge posteriorly. They are covered only by the skin and thin platysma muscle and thus are quite superficial.

The supraclavicular lymph nodes (transverse cervical chain) lie in the lower neck along the upper margin of the clavicle. They communicate with the spinal accessory chain and flow toward the termination in the root of the neck with the internal jugular vein lymph nodes. They are actually a continuation of part of the axillary chain, and join other efferent trunks from the axilla before ending in the venous angle. They receive lymph from the head and neck, ipsilateral upper extremity, the breast, thorax, and abdomen.

The submaxillary lymph nodes, 3–6 in number, are related to the submaxillary gland, the undersurface of the mandible, and the anterior facial vein (see Fig. 13–1). These nodes drain the lips, floor of mouth, buccal mucosa, upper and lower gums, nasal vestibule, and skin of the anterior face.

The submental lymph nodes lie in the midline between the anterior belly of the digastric muscle and anterior to the hyoid. They are external to the mylohyoid muscle. They receive lymph from the lip, chin, cheeks, and, to a lesser extent, the floor of mouth, anterior lower gingiva, and tip of the tongue. The efferent vessels drain to the submaxillary or subdigastric lymph nodes.

PATHOLOGY

The vast majority of head and neck malignant neoplasms arise from the surface epithelium and are therefore squamous cell carcinoma or one of its many variants, including lymphoepithelioma, spindle cell carcinoma, verrucous carcinoma, and undifferentiated carcinoma.

Lymphoepithelioma is a carcinoma with a lymphoid stroma. The lymphoid stroma may or may not be present in regional lymph node or distant metastases. Lymphoepithelioma occurs at anatomic sites with lymphoid aggregates in the submucosa, namely, the nasopharynx, tonsil, and base of tongue. This histology has a higher rate of cure by radiation therapy than squamous cell carcinoma.

The spindle cell variant is a squamous cell carcinoma with a non-neoplastic spindle cell background. This variation has not been reported to change the prognosis or response to radiation.

Verrucous carcinoma is a grade one-half squamous cell carcinoma most often found in the oral cavity, particularly on the gingiva and buccal mucosa. It usually has an indolent growth pattern and is often associated with the chronic use of snuff or chewing tobacco. Verrucous tumors resemble a wart: white or pink, exophytic, with distinct margins and multiple filiform processes that produce a roughened, cobblestone surface. The lesion may be soft or firm to palpation depending on the degree of keratinization and associated inflammation. The patient with verrucous carcinoma very often has multiple biopsies of an obvious lesion, but the pathologist returns a diagnosis of hyperkeratosis or pseudoepitheliomatous hyperplasia. Eventually one may recommend cancer therapy based only on the appearance of the lesion and observation of its continued growth. If the pathologist can readily make a diagnosis of invasive carcinoma from histologic examination, the diagnosis of verrucous carcinoma is suspect.

Undifferentiated lymphomas and undifferentiated carcinomas may appear similar under the microscope. Unless the clinical picture and histologic reading are definitely lymphoma, it is better to treat the patient as if he has carcinoma.

The differentiation between tumor recurrence and radiation necrosis following irradiation is not always an easy histologic diagnosis. Since recurrence usually implies major ablation, the clinical picture must fit the diagnosis. Several examples of misdiagnosis of recurrent cancer have been seen in which the patient had either a laryngectomy, base of tongue resection, jaw-tongue-neck, or other major cancer operation, only to find that in fact the patient had a radiation necrosis that might have healed with conservative therapy. The opinion of a highly qualified pathologist is invaluable in these situations.

NATURAL HISTORY

PATTERNS OF SPREAD

Primary Lesion

Most epidermoid carcinomas begin as surface lesions, but occasionally may arise from ducts of minor salivary glands and therefore originate below the surface of the visible mucosa; this latter phenomenon is more likely to occur in the floor of mouth, base of tongue, and nasopharynx. The very early surface lesions may show only erythema and a slightly elevated, slightly roughened mucosa. These are the so-called "red lesions" and always deserve consideration for biopsy. Spread is dictated by local anatomy, and each anatomic site has its own peculiar spread patterns.

Muscle invasion is a common feature, and tumor may spread along muscle or fascial planes for a surprising distance from the palpable or visible lesion. Tumor may attach to periosteum or perichondrium quite early, but actual bone or cartilage invasion is usually a late event.

Bone and cartilage generally act as a barrier to spread, and these structures are generally spared until the neoplasm has explored easier avenues of growth. Tumor that encounters cartilage or bone on its path will usually be diverted and spread along a path of less resistance. Slow-growing neoplasms of the gingiva may produce a pressure defect or saucerization of the underlying bone without actual bone invasion.

Entrance of tumor into the parapharyngeal space allows superior or inferior spread from the base of the skull to the root of the neck.

Spread inside the lumen of the sublingual, submaxillary, and parotid gland ducts is not a prevalent pattern. The nasolacrimal duct, however, is frequently invaded in ethmoid sinus and nasal carcinoma.

Perineural spread is an important pathway for tumor spread; no site or histology is immune to this growth pattern. Squamous cell carcinoma and its variants and minor salivary gland tumors, especially adenoid cystic carcinoma, may show this pattern. Local recurrence increases the likelihood of perineural involvement, and tumors may track along a nerve to the base of the skull. Peripheral perineural spread, *i.e.*, growth away from the CNS, has been seen. Patients with perineural invasion will often develop neurologic symptoms. Some nerve palsies are secondary to compression or entrapment rather than actual nerve invasion.

Lymphatic Spread

The risk of lymph node metastasis may be predicted by the differentiation of the tumor (the more poorly differentiated, the greater the risk), by the size of the primary lesion, and by the availability of capillary lymphatics. Recurrent lesions likewise have an increased risk.

There is no exclusion of a particular histology from lymphatic spread; mere access to the capillary lymphatics determines the opportunity. In other words, minor salivary gland tumors and sarcomas assume a risk of lymphatic metastasis commensurate with the particular mucosal site.

It is common for a patient to present with a metastatic lymph node and, despite an extensive workup, have the site of origin remain undetermined. If only the neck is treated, a primary lesion may appear at a later date, but many never show a primary site. This strongly suggests permanent regression of the initial lesion.

The risk of subclinical disease in the patient with a clinically negative neck may be obtained either by studying the incidence of positive nodes found in elective neck dissection specimens or by counting the number of necks initially normal which become positive when the neck is not treated.

Table 13-1 outlines the relative risk for cervical metastatic disease for squamous cell carcinomas. Table 13-2 shows the

TABLE 13-1. Incidence of Lymph Node Metastasis by Site of Primary in Head and Neck Squamous Cell Carcinoma

SITE	PERCENTAGE N+ AT PRESENTATION (references)	PERCENTAGE NO CLINICALLY, N+ PATHOLOGICALLY (references)	PERCENTAGE NO → N+ WITH NO NECK TREATMENT (references)
Floor of mouth	30–59 (1–3)	40–50 (4, 5)	20–35 (6–8)
Gingiva	18–52 (1, 9–11)	19 (9)	17 (6, 9)
Hard palate	13–24 (11–13)		22 (6)
Buccal mucosa	9–31 (1, 3)		16 (6)
Oral tongue	34–65 (1–3, 14)	25–54 (5, 10, 15–17)	38–52 (8, 14, 16, 18)
Nasopharynx	86–90 (19–21)		19*–50 (22, 23)
Anterior tonsillar pillar/ retromolar trigone	39–56 (24–26)		10–15 (27)
Soft palate/uvula	37–56 (24–26)		16–25 (26)
Tonsillar fossa	58–76 (2, 19–21, 25)		22† (28)
Base of tongue	50–83 (21, 25, 27, 29)	22 (29)	
Pharyngeal walls	50–71 (21, 25, 27, 29)	66 (29)	
Supraglottic larynx	31–54 (2, 27)	16–26 (29, 30)	33 (30, 31)
Hypopharynx	52–72 (10, 27, 29)	38 (29)	

(Mendenhall WM, Million RR, Cassisi NJ: Elective neck irradiation in squamous cell carcinoma of the head and neck. Head Neck Surg 3:15–20, 1980)

* T1NO patients only.

† Patients received preoperative radiation.

TABLE 13-2. Percent of Clinically Detected Nodal Metastasis on Admission by T Stage—2044 Patients (M. D. Anderson Hospital, 1948–1965)

PRIMARY SITE	T STAGE	N0	N1	N2–3
Oral tongue*	T1	86	10	4
	T2	70	19	11
	T3	52	16	31
	T4	24	10	66
Floor of mouth*	T1	89	9	2
	T2	71	18	10
	T3	56	20	24
	T4	46	10	43
Retromolar trigone-anterior tonsillar pillar†	T1	88	2	9
	T2	62	18	20
	T3	46	21	33
	T4	32	18	50
Soft palate†	T1	92	0	8
	T2	64	12	24
	T3	35	26	39
	T4	33	11	56
Tonsillar fossa†	T1	30	41	30
	T2	32	14	54
	T3	30	18	52
	T4	10	13	76
Base of tongue†	T1	30	15	55
	T2	29	14	56
	T3	26	23	52
	T4	16	8	76
Oropharyngeal walls†	T1	75	0	25
	T2	70	10	20
	T3	33	22	44
	T4	24	24	52
Supraglottic larynx‡	T1	61	10	29
	T2	58	16	26
	T3	36	25	40
	T4	41	18	41
Hypopharynx§	T1	37	21	42
	T2	30	20	49
	T3	21	26	54
	T4	26	15	58
Nasopharynx‖	T1	8	11	82
	T2	16	12	72
	T3	12	9	80
	T4	17	6	78

(Lindberg R: Distribution of cervical lymph node metastases from squamous cell carcinoma of the upper respiratory and digestive tracts. Cancer 29:1446–1449, 1972)

* T stage defined in reference 32.

† T stage defined in reference 33.

‡ T stage defined in reference 34.

§ T stage defined in reference 35.

‖ T stage defined in reference 36.

relative incidence of clinically positive lymph nodes by anatomic site and T stage.

Well-lateralized lesions spread to ipsilateral neck lymph nodes. Lesions on or near the midline, and lateralized tongue and nasopharyngeal lesions, may spread to both sides, but tend to spread to the side occupied by the bulk of the lesion. Patients with clinically positive lymph nodes in the ipsilateral neck are at risk for contralateral disease, especially if the nodes are large or multiple. Obstruction of the lymphatic pathways by surgery or radiation therapy will also shunt the lymphatic flow to the opposite neck. This shunting is mainly through anastomotic channels by way of the submaxillary and submental shuttle.[37]

When contralateral metastases occur from well-lateralized lesions, the subdigastric node is the most commonly involved, but the subdigastric may be bypassed with the midjugular or low jugular next affected. When unusual lymph node metastases appear, a careful search must be made for a second primary.

Although there is usually an orderly progression of lymph node involvement, there are numerous examples of skips and random involvement. Eventually the lymphatic collecting trunks empty into the venous system at the root of the neck. Occasionally one will see retrograde lymph node metastases in the ipsilateral axilla associated with involvement of the lower neck nodes.

Distant Spread

The incidence of distant metastases reported by Merino and coworkers is about 10–12% for squamous cell carcinoma of all head and neck sites.[38] Table 13-3 shows incidence by site. There is no difference whether the patient is treated by radiation therapy or surgery. As expected, the risk of distant metastasis increases with T stage and especially N stage and total stage. Lung is the most common site, accounting for 52% of the first recognized sites. Mediastinal metastases are uncommon, occurring in only 3%. Almost one-half of the metastases are recognized by 9 months, 80% by 2 years, and 90% by 3 years. The risk of distant metastasis doubled in patients developing a recurrence above the clavicle: 16.7% for those having a recurrence, even if salvaged, and 7.9% for those never developing a recurrence. Only the nasopharynx and hypopharynx have a rate of distant metastasis of such proportions that successful adjuvant chemotherapy might significantly affect the cure rate.

TABLE 13-3. Incidence of Distant Metastasis by Site: Head and Neck Squamous Cell Carcinoma (5019 Cases)*

PRIMARY SITE	INCIDENCE OF DISTANT METASTASIS
Oral cavity	7.5%
Faucial arch	6.7%
Oropharynx	15.3%
Nasopharynx	28.1%
Paranasal sinuses and nasal cavity	9.1%
Supraglottic larynx	15.0%
Vocal cord	3.1%
Hypopharynx	23.6%
Total	10.9%†

(Merino OR, Lindberg RD, Fletcher GH: An analysis of distant metastases from squamous cell carcinoma of the upper respiratory and digestive tracts. Cancer 40:145–151, 1977)

* Minimum 2-year followup.

† Excludes 41 patients in whom distant metastasis was found only at autopsy.

METHODS OF DIAGNOSIS AND STAGING

PHYSICAL EXAMINATION

The routine techniques for head and neck examination are found in standard textbooks. Only special points will be added here.

Indirect laryngoscopy gives a better panorama of the lesion and more information regarding mobility than direct laryngoscopy under general anesthesia. However, direct laryngoscopy allows examination of areas invisible to the mirror, such as the ventricle, subglottic space, apex of the pyriform sinus, and postcricoid pharynx.

The fiberoptic laryngoscopes, both rigid and flexible, have added an important tool to outpatient laryngeal examination. The advantage of the fiberoptic laryngoscope compared to mirror examination is improved ability to view the laryngeal surface of the epiglottis and anterior commissure. It also allows laryngeal examination in those patients with an abnormal epiglottis (*e.g.*, horseshoe epiglottis), which virtually prevents good mirror examination. The fiberoptic laryngoscope is a great aid in examination of the nasopharynx and is the method of choice. The panorama obtained with the fiberoptic laryngoscope is equal to that of a small mirror, and certainly the light that enters the nasopharynx is considerably greater than can be obtained with the mirror. A small diameter (3 mm) fiberoptic nasoscope improves examination of the nasal cavity. In a small percentage of patients, especially children, the only satisfactory examination of the nasopharynx, nose, and larynx will be under general anesthesia.

Examination of the Neck

Clinically positive lymph nodes from cancer rarely produce symptoms until they are quite large. Therefore, the clinician must depend on physical examination to detect involved nodes. This technique will be described in detail since it is not generally taught in medical school or in standard physical diagnosis texts.

It takes at least 2–3 minutes to do a careful neck examination. It is important to repeat the examination at every opportunity, and even more important, to compare findings among several examiners. Detailed drawings complement the written report and are an essential part of the medical record.

The preferred position is with the patient sitting and the examiner standing behind. Since many examination chairs have a headrest or cannot be lowered sufficiently, it is often necessary to move the patient to a regular chair or stool so that the patient's neck is opposite the examiner's belt buckle.

When the clinician starts to examine the jugular chain and grasps the neck, the patient instinctively extends the neck, thereby tensing the sternocleidomastoid muscle. Since the nodes lie deep to the sternocleidomastoid, it is essential to have the neck muscles relaxed. Therefore, one hand is placed on the occiput to flex the patient's head forward and slightly to the side being examined. If the patient is quite tense, gentle rocking of the head along with gentle massage of the neck will often obtain the relaxation necessary.

The authors prefer to start at the sternal notch and work upward. First explore the suprasternal notch and the space that extends into the upper mediastinum with the index finger. Normally one should feel nothing except the anterior wall of the trachea. Clinically positive nodes are frequently found in this area, but only the top of the node may be felt. Metastatic lymph nodes from lung and breast cancers as well as metastatic nodes from cancers arising below the diaphragm are frequently felt. This is one of the most commonly missed physical findings. Since the discovery of a metastatic node in this position is so meaningful, it should be carefully sought before major operative or radiation procedures are enlisted. The differential diagnosis of a hard, discrete mass in this area includes thyroid, aneurysm of a major vessel, and mediastinal mass.

The jugular chain nodes are examined next. They lie deep to the sternocleidomastoid muscle in the lower neck; in the upper neck some of the nodes lie at the anterior border of the sternocleidomastoid. The thumb and index finger form a "C" around the sternocleidomastoid muscle. The tips of the examining fingers nearly meet on thin patients. As one proceeds up the jugular chain, the thumb and index finger are in constant motion, using a wiggle-waggle maneuver. Positive lymph nodes in the lower jugular area are often small, mobile, and deep; only slow, careful, gentle, repeated examinations will find them. Most clinically positive lymph nodes will be found in the upper jugular chain. Since the nodes are related to the jugular vein, they lie superficial to the carotid artery. The carotid artery is identified by the pulsation in the vessel. The carotid bulb represents a dilation of the internal carotid at its origin. The pressoreceptors in the carotid bulb respond to external pressure as well as internal vascular pressure. Stimulation will produce a drop in blood pressure and slowing of the pulse. The response is more sensitive in older patients. Patients may develop slight faintness or sudden syncope and collapse. Needless to say, palpation of this site must be gentle and *must not be done simultaneously on both sides*. Palpation of the carotid artery may rarely cause an atheromatous plaque to be splintered from the artery. In one such instance, the patient noted a sudden change in vision in the ipsilateral eye during neck examination. Eye examination confirmed that a branch of a retinal vessel had been occluded, presumably from a small thrombotic plaque entering the ophthalmic artery.

The subdigastric ("tonsillar node") is the largest normal node in the neck and can be identified in many persons. The most superior jugular nodes are difficult to palpate, particularly in men, because the sternocleidomastoid is attached to the mastoid tip and restricts the examining fingers.

There are a number of normal structures that may be confused with a lymph node. The lateral tip of the transverse process of C1 and C2 may feel like a deep lymph node. The transverse process is especially conspicuous in patients with long, skinny necks. The tail of the parotid gland becomes globular in older, obese patients, especially men, and resembles a node. This mass lies just below the ear lobe, between the horizontal ramus of the mandible and the tip of the mastoid. The parotid tails are usually symmetrical, which gives a clue to their identity; clinically positive nodes in the tail of the parotid are unusual except in parotid malignancies, skin cancers, or occasionally lymphomas or leukemias. The superior horn of the thyroid cartilage is not likely to be confused with a lymph node. The carotid bifurcation (carotid bulb) may be quite prominent in older persons and feel like a subdigastric lymph node. Gentle palpation to determine pulsation of the vessel helps to distinguish the vessel from the node. The differential diagnosis is especially difficult when a 1.5–2 cm node is closely approximated to the carotid bifurcation. Localized atheromatous plaques along the carotid may be confused with a small lymph node.

The neck examination is continued by examining along the horizontal ramus of the mandible. The submaxillary gland may be small and firm and tucked up behind the mandible, especially in younger persons. More frequently the gland lies below the mandible in the neck. If the submaxillary duct is obstructed by tumor, the gland may be enlarged, quite firm, and immobile. Several lymph nodes lie in juxtaposition to the submaxillary gland (see Fig. 13-1).

The submental lymph nodes lie in the midline between the digastric muscles. Both the submaxillary and submental nodes are examined bimanually with one index finger in the floor of the mouth. Examination of the spinal accessory and supraclavicular nodes requires only light, gentle palpation of the neck. Preauricular node examination is often overlooked. The ones involved by tumor lie just anterior to the tragus and may be quite small.

BIOPSY TECHNIQUES

Incisional biopsies are performed with knife or scissors; a piece of the lesion is removed. It is often wise to include an area of normal tissue for comparison, but this is not always necessary.

FIG. 13-2. American Joint Committee cancer staging grouping. (American Joint Committee for Cancer Staging and End-Results Reporting (AJC): Manual for Staging of Cancer 1978, pp. 27–52. Chicago, AJC, 1978)

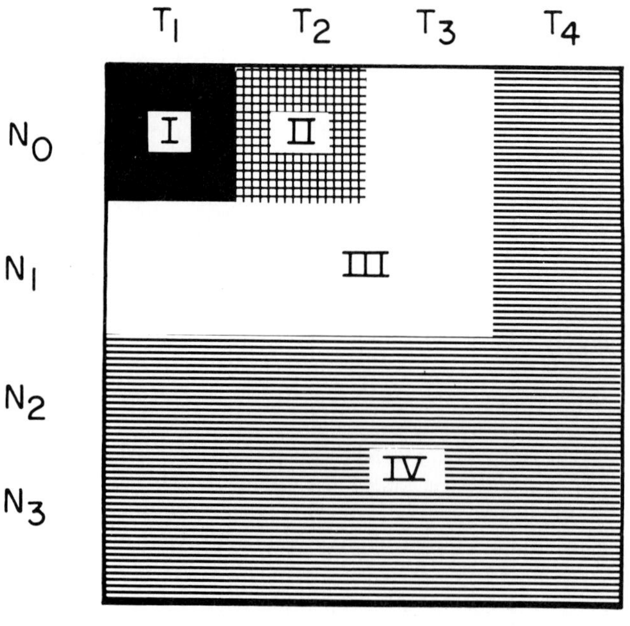

Excisional biopsies are performed not only for diagnosis, but for cure as well. This technique should be reserved for small lesions, or cases where a large amount of tissue may assist the pathologist. The lesion and an adequate margin should be included in the specimen.

A biopsy punch forceps is used for larger mucosal lesions where tumor is readily available or where use of a knife is impractical.

Needle biopsies are used mainly for neck masses and have the advantage of being simple outpatient procedures. Also, one may avoid incisional procedures that distort the lesion and perhaps spread tumor by way of a hematoma. Fine needle aspiration is done with a thin-gauge needle inserted into the mass. The mass is aspirated and the aspirate placed on a slide and stained. A biopsy needle is a large-bore needle that cuts a core of tissue that is studied like any tissue specimen. Two drawbacks to needle biopsy are that not all pathologists are willing to make a diagnosis from small amounts of tissue, and false negative results may occur because of sample size. A negative needle biopsy is followed by open biopsy.

Management of Biopsy Specimens

Frozen sections of specimens should be done for two reasons: first, to make sure that adequate material was obtained to make a diagnosis, and second, to determine the adequacy of margins of excisional biopsies. Aerobic and anaerobic, fungus, and acid-fast cultures of tissue should be requested if infection is suspected. Electron microscopy and special stains should be employed if the diagnosis is in question on routine permanent preparations. Special precautions should be exercised by the surgeon in the case of a patient who has been previously irradiated, because often what appears to be recurrence is in reality an area of necrosis. Close cooperation between the surgeon and the radiotherapist is necessary as to timing of the biopsy. Once the decision to biopsy has been made, deep biopsies may be necessary, often under general anesthesia; the highest yield is obtained by doing a second biopsy in the same site after the superficial tissue has been removed.

STAGING

The American Joint Committee staging system has been adopted for this chapter.[39] Like all staging systems it has numerous deficiencies. The staging for the primary lesions (T) is given in the appropriate section. The neck staging (N) is common to all head and neck sites and is listed under Principles of Treatment. Fig. 13-2 shows the format for combining T and N stages into a total stage represented by a Roman numeral. Evidence of distant metastasis automatically places the patient into stage IV.

Stage IV represents a wide spectrum of disease. A patient may have a T1 or T2 lesion with treatable N2 or N3 neck disease and represent a reasonable candidate for curative therapy, while another may have either a far-advanced primary or far-advanced neck disease, which is virtually a hopeless situation.

PRINCIPLES OF TREATMENT

GENERAL PRINCIPLES FOR SELECTION OF TREATMENT

Surgery and radiation therapy are the only curative treatments for carcinoma arising in the head and neck. Chemotherapy must be considered investigational at present; used alone, it is not curative, and its role as an adjunct to surgery, radiation therapy, or both is in a state of flux.

For most early-stage head and neck squamous cell carcinomas that can be cured by an operation, irradiation can be shown to produce comparable cure rates. The decision then rests on such factors as functional and cosmetic result, general state of the patient's health, and preference of the patient and family. Some patients prefer to join in the selection of treatment, but most prefer to be presented with the options and told which is the best treatment for them. Prior favorable or unfavorable experience with an operation or radiation therapy by a close friend or relative is frequently a major factor.

The advantages of an operation compared to radiation therapy, assuming comparable cure rates, *may* include the following:

1. A limited amount of tissue is exposed to treatment
2. Treatment time is shorter
3. The risk of immediate and late radiation sequelae is avoided
4. Irradiation is reserved for a subsequent head and neck primary which may not be as suitable for an operation
5. Pathologic examination of tissues permits identification of patients with more extensive disease than originally determined, in whom immediate postoperative irradiation can be added.

The advantages of irradiation *may* include:

1. The avoidance of the threat of a major operation. An operative mortality of only 1–2% may seem high to the patient compared to no immediate threat from radiation therapy.
2. The removal of no tissues. Resection of even a relatively small lesion may produce a functional or cosmetic defect. This risk must be weighed against the risk of a radiation necrosis.
3. Elective irradiation of the lymph nodes can be included with little added morbidity, whereas the surgeon must either adopt an attitude of "watch and wait" or proceed with elective neck dissection. This is important for lesions with a high rate of spread to the lymph nodes, especially so where there is a high opportunity for bilateral spread (*i.e.*, floor of mouth, base of tongue, soft palate, hypopharyngeal, and some supraglottic larynx lesions).
4. The surgical salvage of irradiation failures is more likely than the salvage of a surgical failure by either operation, irradiation, or both. When a primary lesion fails after irradiation, the recurrence is almost always in the center of the original lesion; marginal failures are uncommon. A rescue operation can often be done that would be similar in scope to the initial operation, albeit with a greater risk for a serious complication. In some cases, the rescue operation may entail a much more severe functional or cosmetic loss than if the operation had been performed initially. For example, if an epiglottic lesion suitable for supraglottic laryngectomy is treated by radiation therapy and fails, then the rescue procedure is usually a total laryngectomy.

Rescue of a surgical failure may be attempted by either operation, radiation therapy, or both. Surgical recurrences usually develop at the margins of the resection, in or near the suture line. It is difficult to distinguish the normal surgical scar from recurrent disease, and diagnosis of recurrence is often delayed. Tumor response to radiation therapy under these circumstances is poor. Small mucosal recurrences, however, can often be salvaged by an operation, radiation therapy, or both.

Management of the Primary Site

Patients with early-stage lesions (T1 NO-1, T2 NO-1) usually have a favorable prognosis when managed by either surgery or radiation therapy; combined treatment should be avoided as it only increases the morbidity with little or no benefit. The few failures are often salvaged by a second procedure.

Patients with moderately advanced lesions may benefit from combined therapy in some instances, but if either radiation therapy or surgery is reasonably successful by itself, then one modality may be held in reserve for treatment failure. When combined therapy is selected, it should be aggressive, since one rarely has a chance at salvage after combined approaches.

The most difficult decision is whether or not to offer a curative attempt to patients with advanced lesions but no distant metastases. There are anecdotal cases in which patients with advanced stage IV disease have been cured. However, the cure rate for some advanced lesions may be estimated at 1–2% at best. The question then becomes, is it rational to put 100 patients through major therapy with a treatment-related mortality rate of 5–10% and a high morbidity rate to cure one or two patients? Many of these patients with advanced lesions are in very poor general medical condition, and radical surgery or radiation therapy or both is simply unrealistic. However, if the patient is in relatively good condition, especially if in a young age group, then a curative approach may be considered. The patient and family must be presented the facts and assist in the decision. Frequently the patient will select a palliative course, usually radiation therapy, when faced with a low-yield major ablative procedure. Palliative surgery is used in selected cases (usually in cases in which radiation therapy has already been tried) to relieve major symptoms or reduce nursing care (*e.g.*, tumor fungating into skin). There are patients with very advanced disease for whom even a short course of palliative radiation therapy is considered inadvisable if symptoms can be controlled by simple means. Experimental chemotherapy may be advised for advanced lesions, often with spectacular, if temporary, tumor regression. The best treatment may be only observation;

about 5% of patients seen in our clinic receive no cancer therapy.

Management of the Neck

Management of the neck is closely tied to management of the primary site, but certain general principles can be outlined. Death due only to failure to control the neck with the primary tumor controlled should be an uncommon event if surgery and radiation therapy are used to their maximum advantage. The American Joint Committee cervical node classification system is used for all head and neck sites.[39]

- NX Nodes cannot be assessed
- NO No clinically positive node
- N1 Single clinically positive homolateral node 3 cm or less in diameter
- N2 Single clinically positive homolateral node more than 3 but not more than 6 cm in diameter or multiple clinically positive homolateral nodes, none more than 6 cm in diameter
- N2A Single clinically positive homolateral node more than 3 cm but not more than 6 cm in diameter
- N2B Multiple clinically positive homolateral nodes, none more than 6 cm in diameter
- N3 Massive homolateral node(s), bilateral nodes, or contralateral node(s)
- N3A Clinically positive homolateral node(s), one more than 6 cm in diameter
- N3B Bilateral clinically positive nodes (in this situation, each side of the neck should be staged separately; that is, N3B: right, N2A; left, N1)
- N3C Contralateral clinically positive node(s) only

CLINICALLY NEGATIVE NECK. Table 13-1 shows the incidence of subclinical disease in the regional lymphatics when the neck is clinically negative. The risk for any single primary lesion may be estimated by the size of the primary lesion and the differentiation of the neoplasm. A policy of "wait and see" may be adopted for the NO neck to avoid unnecessary treatment, and the neck may be successfully treated if nodes appear. However, even though the neck treatment may be successful, these patients are at an increased risk to develop distant metastasis and have a poorer prognosis. Elective neck treatment is indicated, therefore, where the associated morbidity is low. Elective neck treatment has the added advantage of giving complete treatment at the initial treatment and simplifying the followup neck examinations because of its high success rate.

There is a large volume of data supporting the success of irradiation in eradicating subclinical disease in regional lymphatics.[31]

Table 13-4 shows the results for elective neck irradiation at the University of Florida when the primary lesion is controlled.[41] Assuming a 25% overall risk for subclinical disease in the regional lymph nodes, the calculated efficiency is at least 90% for doses of 4500–6000 rads. If the primary lesion recurs, however, there is a renewed chance for lymphatic spread and the neck is at considerable risk even if elective neck irradiation has been given. If the primary lesion is to be treated with external beam irradiation, then elective neck irradiation incurs no added cost and, if properly done, little added morbidity.

Surgeons have argued for many years over the relative merits of elective neck dissection as compared to observation. It is a difficult decision to recommend a full radical neck dissection with the cosmetic and functional losses and possible shoulder discomfort unless the potential benefit is considerable. However, recent operative modifications reduce this morbidity. The so-called "functional neck dissection" popularized by Bocca preserves the 11th nerve, the jugular vein, and the sternocleidomastoid muscle and works as well as radical neck dissection for subclinical (NO) disease.[42]

The functional neck dissection is a more difficult and longer procedure than the standard radical neck dissection. For oral cavity lesions, an elective supraomohyoid neck dissection on one or both sides may be used as a staging procedure. If the nodes are negative, no further treatment is given. If the nodes are positive, the neck dissection is completed or postoperative radiation therapy is used. These two forms of neck dissection are at least 90% effective and create relatively few side effects. Partial neck dissection is not sufficient treatment, however, for lesions of the oropharynx, larynx, or hypopharynx (see Table 13-5).

TABLE 13-4. Efficacy of Elective Neck Irradiation (ENI) with Primary Tumor Controlled (126 Patients; University of Florida, 10/64–6/76; Minimum 2-Yr Followup)

PRIMARY STAGE	NO. OF PATIENTS WITH NECK CONTROLLED/NO. OF PATIENTS WITH PRIMARY CONTROLLED		
	No ENI	*Partial ENI*	*Whole ENI*
T1	11/12	17/18	9/10
T2	6/8	17/17	22/22
T3	0/1	10/10	18/18
T4	1/1	5/5	3/3
Total	18/22 (82%)*	49/50 (98%)*	52/53 (98%)*

(Mendenhall WM, Million Rr, Cassisi NJ: Elective neck irradiation in squamous cell carcinoma of the head and neck. Head Neck Surg 3:15–20, 1980)
* Significance level = 0.01, using exact test procedures.[40]

CLINICALLY POSITIVE NECK LYMPH NODES. Table 13-5 shows the rate of neck failure by N stage and therapeutic category reported from M. D. Anderson Hospital.[43] The irradiation precedes the operation if the primary site is to be treated by radiation therapy or if the node is fixed. The operation precedes the irradiation if the primary site is to be treated surgically.

Radical neck dissection is sufficient treatment for the ipsilateral neck for patients with N1 or N2A disease. Radiation therapy is added for other N stages or for control of contralateral subclinical disease (see Table 13-6). Invasion through the capsule of the node or the finding of multiple positive nodes in the specimen is an indication to add postoperative radiation therapy.

Radiation therapy alone is sufficient for patients with N1

TABLE 13-5. Failure of Initial Ipsilateral Neck Treatment (596 Patients with Carcinoma of the Tonsillar Fossa, Base of Tongue, Supraglottic Larynx, or Hypopharynx, M. D. Anderson Hospital, 1948–1967)

	STAGE							
	N0							
TREATMENT	NO TREATMENT	PARTIAL	COMPLETE	N1	N2A	N2B	N3A	N3B
Radiation	. . .	15%	2%	15%	27%	27%	38%	34%
Surgery	55% (16/29)	35%	7%	11%	8%	23%	42%	41%
Combined	. . .	1/5	0/6	0	0	0	23%	25%

(Barkley HT Jr, Fletcher GH, Jesse RH et al: Management of cervical lymph node metastases in squamous cell carcinoma of the tonsillar fossa, base of tongue, supraglottic larynx, and hypopharynx. Am J Surg 124:462–467, 1972)

(0–2 cm) disease, but should be combined with a neck dissection for N1 (3 cm), N2A, or N3A disease. The decision to add radical neck dissection for N2B and N3B disease is individualized, based on the diameter of the largest node or the multiplicity of palpable nodes. For example, a patient may be staged N2B based on a 2 cm subdigastric node and two 1 cm nodes in the middle and low jugular chain. This neck may be treated with radiation therapy alone. However, another patient staged N2B may have a 3–4 cm neck node and several other small nodes, and neck dissection should be added if possible. If the enlarged nodes disappear completely during the course of the radiation therapy, the likelihood of control by radiation therapy alone is improved, and neck dissection may be withheld. However, it is always safer to add the neck dissection immediately after radiation therapy since the detection of neck node recurrence after high-dose radiation therapy is difficult because of fibrosis and salvage is generally unsatisfactory. Large, fixed nodes (over 5 cm) require 6000–7500 rads prior to neck dissection; some of the specimens will show "no viable tumor" and quite a few patients will have the disease controlled in the neck.

GENERAL PRINCIPLES OF SURGERY

In general, many patients who present with head and neck malignancies are older patients who use alcohol and tobacco to excess and are in a poor nutritional state. Medical problems such as diabetes, pulmonary disease, and cardiovascular disease are often present. All of the factors must be considered and corrected prior to offering surgery to these patients. There are relatively few absolute contraindications to surgery, but if the medical problems are so severe that the risk of anesthesia is high, then surgery is contraindicated unless there is no feasible alternative and the patient strongly urges that the operation be done. A myocardial infarction within the previous 3 months is a contraindication to surgery. A relative contraindication to surgery is simultaneous double primaries that cannot be encompassed in a single operative procedure; individualization is required for these cases.

Surgery as the therapeutic modality of choice must be considered if the cure rate is at least as great as with radiation therapy and if the functional and cosmetic deformities are acceptable to the patient, or the anticipated complications from irradiation are severe enough to ultimately require surgery. The skills of the surgeon are another consideration; for instance, it would be better to treat an infrahyoid epiglottic lesion with radiation therapy rather than a total laryngectomy if the supraglottic laryngectomy is not in the surgeon's armamentarium, since a total laryngectomy is always an option for salvage.

There are also certain anatomic sites that lend themselves well to surgery, such as small lesions of the lip, retromolar trigone, tip of the tongue, gingiva, and epiglottis.

Advances in the treatment of the neck have been dramatic over the past few years. The concept of elective neck irradiation has changed the surgeon's options in neck dissection. Surgeons, motivated by the above concept, began to depart from the traditional standard radical neck dissection in which the sternocleidomastoid muscle, the internal and external jugular veins, and the spinal accessory nerve along with the submaxillary gland were removed as a single unit. The supra-

TABLE 13-6. Cervical Metastasis Appearing in the Contralateral Neck (596 Patients with Carcinoma of the Tonsillar Fossa, Base of Tongue, Supraglottic Larynx, or Hypopharynx, M. D. Anderson Hospital, 1948–1967)

TREATMENT	N0	N1	N2A	N2B	N3A
Radiation	2/50	1/52	2/22	2/27	0/21
Surgery	7/28	8/47	3/13	13/30	4/12
Combined	0/6	0/21	0/17	3/28	0/13

(Barkley HT Jr, Fletcher GH, Jesse RH et al: Management of cervical lymph node metastases in squamous cell carcinoma of the tonsillar fossa, base of tongue, supraglottic larynx, and hypopharynx. Am J Surg 124:462–467, 1972) omohyoid neck dissection was resurrected, and the functional neck dissection proved that the sternocleidomastoid muscle, internal jugular vein, and spinal accessory nerve could be preserved without any loss in survival when used in patients with a clinically negative neck.

As the options increase, the type of neck dissection may be individualized. The functional neck dissection should be done if there are no clinically positive nodes in the neck, the incidence of occult metastases is expected to be 15–20% or greater, and the primary site is to be treated surgically. The standard radical neck dissection preserving the spinal accessory nerve should be done in persons who, for occupational reasons, require use of the trapezius muscle. In general, this is carried out in patients undergoing a salvage operation who have no clinically palpable nodes, yet have a high risk of occult metastasis in the neck. The supraomohyoid neck dissection may be used when a primary lesion of the oral cavity is to be excised and the neck is clinically negative; in this case, only the first order of nodes is removed. If the nodes are found positive at the time of the operation, the dissection is extended to a full radical neck dissection. Another indication for the supraomohyoid neck dissection occurs for cases in which the primary lesion is to be treated with radiation therapy and the patient has a single large upper neck node. Irradiation is given to the primary and the entire neck on one or both sides. After irradiation, there is a residual mass in the upper neck, while the primary lesion appears to be controlled. It has been the author's experience that although the node may still be palpable, the pathologic specimen often fails to show residual tumor.

In a standard radical neck dissection, the superficial and deep cervical fascia with its enclosed lymph nodes is removed in continuity with the sternocleidomastoid muscle, the omohyoid muscle, the internal and external jugular veins, the spinal accessory nerve and the submaxillary gland. The incisions used by the surgeon will, to a large extent, be governed by the primary lesion. The indications for this procedure include disease high in the neck, along the spinal accessory nerve, and low in the neck. The functional deformity that occurs with sacrifice of the 11th cranial nerve, although sometimes significant, appears justified when the disease is this extensive. The functional loss and discomfort may be somewhat minimized with proper physical therapy.

The standard radical neck dissection sparing the 11th nerve is performed in clinically negative necks where surgery is the only modality of therapy to be used and in clinically positive necks that become clinically negative after radiation therapy.

The functional neck dissection as popularized by Bocca removes only the superficial and deep cervical fascia along with its enclosed nodes, leaving intact the sternocleidomastoid and omohyoid muscles, the internal jugular vein, and the spinal accessory nodes. Bocca reports no higher incidence of neck failure even in clinically positive necks than with a standard radical neck dissection.[42] The advantages are a lack of cosmetic or functional deformity. It is a technique not familiar to all surgeons, and, in general, takes longer to perform than the standard neck dissection.

The supraomohyoid neck dissection removes the superficial and deep cervical fascia above the omohyoid muscle as well as the submaxillary gland with its pre- and postvascular nodes. It is used for oral cavity lesions where the first echelon nodes are clinically negative, but are at risk, and in situations where the primary has been controlled with radiation therapy and the residual mass in the neck cannot be determined to be fibrosis or residual disease. The supraomohyoid neck dissection may be converted to a standard radical neck dissection if positive disease is found at the operation. Bilateral neck dissections may be done in patients with bilateral neck disease. They can be done simultaneously if one internal jugular vein can be preserved, usually on the less involved side. Fewer complications occur if the second neck dissection is carried out 4–6 weeks after the initial neck dissection.

Complications after radical neck dissection include hematoma, seroma, lymphedema, wound infections and dehiscence, damage to cranial nerves VII, X, and XII, carotid exposure, and carotid rupture. The latter can be minimized by covering the carotid wall with a dermal graft at the time of surgery.

GENERAL PRINCIPLES OF RADIATION THERAPY

SELECTION OF PATIENTS SUITABLE FOR RADIATION THERAPY

Prior high-dose irradiation to the head and neck area, even if given years previously, is nearly an absolute contraindication to radiation therapy unless the new cancer is clearly out of the prior radiation portals. There are a few exceptions to this rule (*e.g.*, recurrent lymphoepithelioma of the nasopharynx), but curative re-irradiation is rarely successful and the risk of major necrosis is high. An operation should be the treatment of choice with reirradiation used only in desperate or special circumstances.

A history of low-dose irradiation (*e.g.*, as used for acne) is a relative contraindication. The history of prior irradiation may be missed, since the irradiation was often given years ago. Irradiated skin has a characteristic appearance, and persistent questioning will frequently confirm the suspicion. Since radiation therapy records are usually not available, one must depend on the appearance of the skin and mucosa to guess the possible radiation dose.

The majority of patients with squamous cell carcinoma of the oral cavity, oropharynx, hypoharynx, and larynx either are or were confirmed tobacco or alcohol users. These patients are at a slightly greater risk to develop a radiation necrosis or edema if they continue their unsavory habits with zeal. However, if they moderate or stop smoking, drinking, or both, the risk of a complication is similar to that for other patients. The history of tobacco or alcohol use is not usually a decisive factor in treatment selection. The alcoholic is likely to refuse a major operation, but is also rather intolerant of the acute side effects of irradiation once treatment is started. About 50% of the patients who smoke will stop immediately when advised to do so, about 25% will decrease their tobacco use, and the remaining 25% do not change.

One of the common reasons for selecting radiation therapy instead of an operation is a concomitant medical condition. Radiation therapy has essentially a zero acute mortality rate, and it makes no sense to offer the patient an operation if the risk of an operative death is significant.

Young patients are best treated by an operation, all other factors being equal, since the risk of a radiation complication is ever present. Elderly or frail patients are frequently referred for radiation therapy even though they have a lesion preferably treated by an operation. A long, drawn-out, 7–8 week course of irradiation may be more wearing than an operation, which may entail only 7–14 days of hospitalization.

Adult patients with head and neck squamous cell carcinoma treated by high-dose radiation therapy have no greater chance of a second head and neck cancer than those treated by an operation.[44] Radiation-induced sarcomas are almost never seen when radiation is given to adults; there is a tiny risk for patients treated under the age of 20, especially in the very young.

A few patients have a fear of radiation therapy. If this fear is not easily reconciled, one should not force the issue.

SHRINKING FIELDS

The principle of shrinking fields is used to minimize the effects of a large treatment volume. The outer 1–3 cm perimeter of the treatment volume usually includes only tissues having the possibility of containing subclinical disease. If these tissues have not been surgically disturbed, 4500–5000 rads should be sufficient to sterilize minimal amounts of squamous cell carcinoma and the first reduction may occur at 4500–5000 rad. (Note: "Subclinical disease" refers to disease statistically known to be present in some cases, but that cannot be seen or palpated in areas accessible to physical examination nor seen on highly efficient roentgenographic studies.) Additional reductions are usually made at 6000 and 7000 rad. An interstitial implant to residual disease is considered a shrinking field technique. The final treatment portals are often quite small and are referred to as "boosts" or "booster treatments" to the center of the resolving mass. The final small fields are often used, however, to raise the dose in an undertreated zone to the same level as the remainder of the treatment volume. This situation occurs when there is a low dose due to lack of homogeneity of a treatment field and the actual dose is less than the specified tumor dose. This may occur because of tumor near the edge or corner of the field or due to partial shielding of the beam by bone. This maneuver is simply referred to as "make-up treatment". With the use of computers, CT scans, in-vivo dosimetry, irregular field computations, and special water phantom measurements, low-dose areas can be estimated and the dose adjusted.

REGIONAL NODE IRRADIATION

The regional nodes are included in the treatment planning for the primary lesion.

For almost all head and neck primaries, the subdigastric node area (*i.e.*, sentinal node, tonsillar node) is the major drainage site. For oral cavity lesions, the submaxillary nodes are also at high risk. For lesions of the nasopharynx, soft palate, and posterior tonsillar pillar, the high jugular and spinal accessory lymph nodes are also commonly involved. There is usually an orderly progression of lymphatic spread along the jugular chain. Patients with clinically positive neck nodes are at some risk for contralateral neck disease, even if the primary lesion is small and well-lateralized. When lymphatic obstruction develops from tumor or lymph node biopsy, the lymph flow is diverted. One common shunt is the submental pathway to the contralateral subdigastric and midjugular nodes.[37]

When the nodes are clinically negative and the risk of subclinical disease is around 15–20% or greater, the nodes are included and receive a minimum dose of 4500–5000 rads. In the treatment portals used for cancers of the oropharynx, supraglottic larynx, and hypopharynx, most of the high-risk upper neck nodes are automatically included with the primary lesion. For oral cavity, nasopharynx, large glottic, nasal cavity, and paranasal sinus lesions, the fields must be extended to include the nodes. Innovative treatment techniques must be devised to include the nodes, but keep mucosal irradiation to a minimum. The criteria for elective lymph node irradiation depend on several features:

1. Primary site and overall risk of subclinical disease
2. Risk for bilateral subclinical disease
3. Histologic grade
4. Size of primary (T stage)
5. Difficulty of neck examination
6. Relative morbidity for extending the lymph node coverage related to the risk of subclinical disease
7. Likelihood that patient will return for frequent followup examinations
8. Suitability of the patient for a radical neck dissection should tumor appear in the neck

Elective neck irradiation for oral cavity primary lesions includes the submaxillary and subdigastric lymph nodes and occasionally the midjugular nodes. For primary lesions of the oropharynx, nasopharynx, supraglottic larynx, and hypopharynx, the lower neck nodes are routinely included, although the risk for subclinical disease in some cases is admittedly quite small when the upper neck is negative. The well-tailored *en face* lower neck field adds little morbidity and assures neck control.

The justification for elective irradiation of the lower jugular and supraclavicular nodes is emphasized by Sagerman and coworkers, who reviewed 72 patients given 5000 rads/5 weeks preoperative irradiation for stage III and IV glottic, supraglottic, and pyriform sinus cancers.[45] Some 31 patients were treated with only lateral opposing portals that did not include the lower neck; 41 had similar portals but also an added 5000 rads through a separate lower neck portal. Ten of 31 (32%) treated with the two-field technique died with a local recurrence, while only four of 41 (10%) developed a local recurrence when the lower neck field was added. The complication rate was no different in the two groups.

Clinically positive nodes are included in the radiation portals. If radical neck dissection is to follow radiation therapy, the dose to the nodes varies with size, location, and response to irradiation. A preoperative dose of 5000–6000 rads is sufficient for nodes 3–5 cm in size, but larger, 6–8 cm masses require 7000–7500 rad to have a good chance at complete removal. If the node mass lies behind the plane of the spinal

TABLE 13-7. Guide to Dose for Neck Lymph Nodes

	SQUAMOUS CELL CARCINOMA	
	MINIMUM TUMOR DOSE (rad)	BOOST TO RESIDUAL (rad)*
No palpable nodes	5000	Not applicable
Small nodes, 1–2 cm	6000	500–1000
Nodes 3–5 cm	6000	1500–2000
Massive fixed nodes	6000	2000–3500

* Boost to residual: Boost dose added through portal just covering palpable residual disease.

cord, electrons are almost essential to obtain the required dose. Large nodes may not show much regression during the course of the radiation treatments, but will often show major change by the time the patient returns in 4–6 weeks for neck dissection. The node mass frequently has a thick capsule at this time which facilitates removal.

If neck dissection is undesirable from a medical standpoint, radiation therapy alone will cure a significant number of patients with positive neck nodes. The control of the lymph nodes seems to parallel the response and control of the primary lesion. The final dose to the lymph nodes is gauged by their original size (see Table 13-7). Interstitial implant may be used in selected cases for the boost dose. The dose for lymphoepithelioma nodes may be 500–1000 rads less if they show rapid, early regression.

Patients with bilateral neck disease require individualized planning with the surgeon. If the neck disease is minimal on one side, then irradiation is used for control on that side and neck dissection is used only on the side that has the major disease (N2A, N2B, N3A).

If there is major bilateral neck disease, then bilateral neck dissection follows the radiation therapy. The neck dissections may be one-stage or two-stage. Major lymphedema may be anticipated, but will gradually subside in 1–2 years. A few patients are salvaged in this manner.

Metastatic disease to the lower neck nodes is still compatible with cure. There is some indirect evidence that when comparing N stages (N2B, N3A, N3B) with or without lower neck nodes, the risk of distant metastasis is similar.[20]

DOSE/TIME/FRACTIONATION

Conventional head and neck external beam treatments employ a single daily treatment, 5 days/week, with a daily tumor dose that usually varies from 180 to 225 rads. The larger daily tumor doses (200–225 rads) shorten the overall treatment time and decrease the total dose, but also increase the acute sequelae and possibly the late complications. Smaller daily doses to the tumor (170–190 rads) require more treatment days and a slightly increased total dose to accomplish the same control rate, but produce fewer acute and late radiation effects on normal tissue. *Small differences in total dose* (300–500 rads) *may greatly affect the chance of local and regional control.* The specified tumor dose is based on the *volume of tumor* (size, diameter, T stage) and, to a lesser degree, the *site of origin*. The regression rate during treatment reflects the mitotic rate of the tumor, but does not accurately

TABLE 13-8. Guidelines to Dose-Time Schedules for Various Head and Neck Squamous Cell Carcinomas (5 Fractions per Week)

STAGE	LOCAL CONTROL	OROPHARYNX* (UF)† (46)	TONSIL (MDAH)‡ (47)	ANT. TONSILLAR PILLAR/RETROMOLAR TRIGONE (MDAH) (24)	GLOSSOTONSILLAR SULCUS (MDAH) (48)
	%			*rad/wk*	
T1	99		6300/6–6700/7	7000/7	
	95	6000/6–6500/7			
	85				
T2	99		6600/6–7000/7	7200/7	
	95	6000/6–6500/7			
	90				
	85				
T3	99		6800/6–7200/7	7500/7	
	80				
	65	6400/7–6800/8			
T2+T3	99			7000/6–7500/7	
	90				6750/6–7000/7
	85				
	80				
T4	50			7500/7.5	
T3+T4	≅90		6800/6–7200/7		
	≅50				
	≅25				

* Includes tonsillar region, base of tongue, and soft palate: 221 cases.
† UF = University of Florida data.
‡ MDAH = M. D. Anderson Hospital data.

predict the control rate, and is not used to select the dose. Persistent abnormality on physical examination at the completion of treatment predicts a higher rate of recurrence.

Tumor doses have been derived empirically from retrospective analysis. Table 13-8 summarizes the dose-response data by anatomic site and T stage from reports of the University of Florida and M. D. Anderson Hospital. Because of vagaries in specification of tumor dose, staging of lesions, and portal design, these time/dose schemes will not necessarily produce the same results in other departments, but they do serve as a guideline. Formulas (*e.g.*, NSD) are not recommended for use in adjusting dose schemes, since extrapolation beyond known empirical treatment schemes cannot be accurately predicted.

Other fractionation schemes have been tried, but they generally fail to improve local control or reduce the complication rate. Split-course schemes, which insert a rest period halfway through the treatment course, have been in vogue during the last decade, but no one has produced evidence that local control is as good as with conventional treatment plans. The advantage of a split-course is touted as allowing the severe mucosal reactions to heal part way through treatment, thereby reducing patient suffering. Table 13-9 shows a comparison of continuous-course and split-course schemes for each T stage, reported by Parsons and coworkers.[46] The local control and survival rates were poorer with split-course and the complication rates were not reduced.

A number of fractionation schemes have been tried in which treatments are given only one, two, three, or four times per week instead of five times per week. In these schemes the daily dose is higher. When these schemes are compared to five fractions per week, the local control is better with five treatments per week and the complication rates are less.[54]

RADIATION-INDUCED DENTAL DISEASE

The pathologic changes that occur in the teeth after irradiation are mainly due to the indirect effect of changes of salivary flow and, to a lesser degree, to the direct effect on the teeth and the surrounding bone and soft tissues. With the onset of irradiation of the salivary gland(s), the saliva is reduced in quantity and becomes increasingly acid. The saliva eventually becomes quite thick; it may be either white or discolored to a brown or black appearance. Simultaneously there is an increase in the organic nitrogen content of the saliva. As the saliva diminishes, the patient also begins to get a sore throat. He stops eating a normal, rough diet and changes to a soft, high-carbohydrate, sticky diet that does not have the cleansing value of an ordinary diet and favors a growth of cariogenic organisms and plaque. The patient stops routine dental care because the tissues are tender and it becomes uncomfortable to brush, floss, and maintain good oral hygiene. So the total result is an increased amount of organic material that sticks to the teeth, forming plaque; this plaque rapidly leads to caries.

The dentist must become involved prior to the initiation of irradiation to evaluate the requirements for each patient. The workup involves visual inspection and full-mouth roentgenograms. Inasmuch as the patient will receive high doses of radiation, the tiny doses from dental roentgenograms are not of any consequence, either at this point or during ensuing years.

BASE OF TONGUE (MDAH) (50)	PHARYNGEAL WALL (MDAH (50)	PYRIFORM SINUS (UF) (51)	SUPRAGLOTTIC LARYNX (UF) (52)	SUPRAGLOTTIC LARYNX (MDAH) (53)
		rad/wk		
6600/6–7000/7		6000/7–6500/8	6000/6–6250/7	
6300/6				
	7000/6			6000/6
6750/6–7250/7				
6900/6–7300/7				
			6700/7.5–7000/8	6250/6–7000/7.5
		6500/7–7000/8		
6750/6–7250/7				
	6600/6–7250/7			
	7000/6			
	6000/6			

TABLE 13-9. Comparison by Tumor Site of Continuous Course vs. Split Course External Beam Irradiation (University of Florida, 9/64–8/76; analysis 8/78) No. of patients with local control/no. treated

	STAGE T1–2*		STAGE T3		STAGE T4	
DISEASE SITE	SPLIT COURSE (6200 rad)†	CONTINUOUS (6100 rad)†	SPLIT COURSE (6600 rad)†	CONTINUOUS (6600 rad)†	SPLIT COURSE (6600 rad)†	CONTINUOUS (6600 rad)†
Oral cavity‡	4/8	2/5	2/5	1/3	No data	No data
Oropharynx‡	17/24	39/45	9/22	8/15	1/18	2/7
Nasopharynx	4/4	3/3	5/6	3/3	2/6	6/10
Hypopharynx	2/4	10/17	2/11	5/7	1/8	0/6
Supraglottic larynx	4/6	11/12	4/4	4/7	1/2	0/2
Total	31/46 (67%)	65/82 (79%)	22/48 (46%)	21/35 (60%)	5/34 (15%)	8/25 (32%)

(Parsons JT, Bova FJ, Million RR: A re-evaluation of split-course technique for squamous cell carcinoma of the head and neck. Int J Radiat Oncol Biol Phys 6:10645–10652, 1980)

* Forty percent of the split-course patients had T1 lesions vs. 35% of the continuous-course patients.

† Median dose of external irradiation.

‡ Patients with oral cavity and oropharynx primaries who received interstitial irradiation were excluded.

The edentulous patient requires the least amount of workup and study as there obviously is no risk for dental caries. The major risk is for a soft tissue necrosis or bone exposure due to irradiation effects. A few patients will have unerupted teeth in the molar area. If they are well-covered, they usually remain so in the postirradiation period. The authors have seen one patient who had an unerupted third molar who received irradiation and then returned several months later with a bone exposure and ulceration over the tooth. In addition, infected retained root tips may require removal.

The authors normally allow patients to wear their dentures during the course of irradiation as long as they can be tolerated. The gingiva tends to shrink, both during the treatment and for the first several months after the completion of irradiation, so the dentures may not fit snugly. They should be relined or, in some cases, new dentures should be made. The usual rule is to wait a full 6 months before old dentures are replaced with new ones, since there is remodeling and shrinkage of the gingiva during that period. The authors also encourage patients to use their dentures following completion of therapy.

It was a common practice in past years to remove all the normal teeth prior to irradiation. There are still a few physicians and dentists who hold this belief and will refer the patient to the radiotherapist, having already removed a very nice set of teeth prior to irradiation. In this situation, dentures should be made for use during the course of radiation treatment.

Soft silicone liners have been tried, but they actually caused more abrasion to the gingiva than the hard liners. It has even been reported that one can place dentures over bone exposures if the bone exposure is on the crest of the gingiva. The denture is simply relieved over the area of the exposed bone and the patient is watched very closely to make sure that the exposed bone is not increasing in size.

The management of dentulous patients requires several general considerations. First of all, the maxilla tolerates postirradiation surgery when it is required better than the mandible. Therefore, it is not as essential that the maxillary teeth be extracted prior to irradiation.

The patient with rapidly growing tumor and the patient with advanced cancer are best started immediately on therapy and their dental care patched up later.

Another consideration in the dental plan is whether or not that patient will comply with the dental recommendations the physician makes. A patient with poor teeth who may be an alcoholic or from a lower socioeconomic group will have neither the motivation nor the finances to save his teeth. In these patients, extractions prior to irradiation may be necessary; whereas, a patient who seems to be motivated and has the financial wherewithal will have his teeth saved.

When the dentulous patient is first seen, he is appraised by both the radiotherapist and the dentist to determine the appropriate treatment. Mobile and unrepairable teeth are extracted. Periodontal deficiencies indicate that the teeth will be very difficult to maintain and that the patient will be more susceptible to caries and infection than a patient with normal periodontal tissue. Exposure of the neck of the molars, a process called furcation, is an indication for extraction prior to irradiation. Periodontal bone loss, periapical abscesses, and caries with pulp exposure are relative indications for extraction.

Mandibular teeth within the radiation portal should receive special scrutiny as postirradiation extraction from an irradiated mandible is undesirable and may result in osteoradionecrosis. Teeth outside the irradiated zone may be extracted at a later date upon the completion of irradiation with very little risk. Extraction of teeth prior to irradiation does not prevent osteoradionecrosis—it only prevents dental caries.

If preirradiation extraction is indicated, a thorough alveolectomy is performed with a tight, sound closure of the gingiva. If this procedure is not done, then following recession of the gingival tissues at the completion of irradiation, spicules of bone will protrude through the mucosa. Hence, the underlying mandible will be irregular, making it difficult to place dentures.

The patient is examined at weekly intervals following the extractions, watching for complete healing and also trying to make sure that the tumor is not progressing. Healing generally occurs in about 11–14 days and treatment can then be started.

If radiotherapy is started before healing is complete, the suture line may dehisce.

Patients who require more extensive and traumatic extractions may require 3–6 weeks before complete healing. This may be disquieting to the patient; therefore, frequent examinations are needed to reassure both the patient and the physician.

Besides the recontouring of the alveolar bone after extraction, any other bony prominences such as a prominent or sharp mylohyoid ridge or tori in the anterior floor of the mouth should be recontoured. These are the favorite sites of bone exposure following irradiation. The gingiva is closely applied over these bony protuberances, and they are the most likely sites to break down at a later date. The remaining teeth should be put in order, which means cleaning, scaling, fluoride application, repair of carious teeth, and elimination of infection. At this point plastic dental carriers are made. A dental impression is taken and individualized vinyl carriers made for each patient.

The patient is then provided with a sodium fluoride gel, which he uses for 5 minutes per day, starting during the course of irradiation. Some patients complain of discomfort associated with the use of the fluoride gel and discontinue its use until the mucosa has healed. The patient is instructed to brush his teeth carefully and then apply the gel. Six to eight drops are placed in the carrier and the carrier applied to the teeth for about 5 minutes each day at bedtime. The gel can then be either swallowed or expectorated at the end of the application. Other self-applied fluorides are available.

Some dentists will tell patients that they can discontinue their fluoride treatments if their teeth seem to be in a healthy condition (dentists normally make fluoride applications once every 6 months). However, for prevention of radiation caries it is presently recommended that these treatments be continued for the lifetime of the patient. If there is a return of saliva, the number of fluoride applications may be reduced to 2–3 times a week.

In addition to the use of fluoride, patients are started on a salt-and-soda mouthwash or gargle that is to be used during the course of irradiation and during the followup period until healing of the mucosa. One teaspoon of table salt and one teaspoon of baking soda are added to a quart of water and used to rinse the mouth as often as necessary. This refreshes the mouth, decreases the pain from mucositis, and helps eliminate the thick, tenacious saliva that accumulates.

Patients may use a commercial preparation resembling saliva called Xero-lube. Glycerine may be used at bedtime to lubricate the surface of the mouth and has longer staying power than plain water. A soft brush with rounded tufts is recommended for routine dental care. Brushing must be done after every meal and at bedtime. The patient should use a disclosing solution such as Red–cote to show plaque to give it a little extra brushing attention. Unwaxed dental floss is used every day and a Water Pik at low pressure will assist in dental care.

The patient must see his dentist at regular intervals to keep his teeth clean, receive fluoride applications, have early repair of caries, and have any other dental care that will help preserve his teeth. The authors suggest that the patient see the dentist every 2 months following the completion of treatment for the first couple of years. If the teeth seem to be doing quite well, then the visits may be less frequent. The patient must have constant, repeated surveillance to maintain dentition, because once radiation caries start, they may take a very rampant course.

GENERAL PRINCIPLES OF CHEMOTHERAPY

The role of chemotherapy for squamous cell carcinoma of the head and neck is in the midst of intensive exploration and re-evaluation. The search for new agents, the development of potentially useful drug combinations, and the incorporation of chemotherapy into complex multimodal treatment plans along with surgery and radiotherapy are areas of current study.

In whatever setting chemotherapy is employed, however, certain general observations apply. Patients with advanced head and neck cancer are frequently symptomatic from their disease. Pain, local infection, odor, intermittent bleeding, and obstruction may all be significant problems. Since many of these epidermoid carcinomas are associated with alcohol and tobacco abuse and occur in the older age groups, patients may also suffer from various coincidental liver, renal, pulmonary, or cardiac disorders. Thus, patients about to embark on a course of chemotherapy may be in rather tenuous medical condition at the start of treatment. Clearly, all efforts should be directed toward reversing any potentially remediable abnormalities prior to institution of cytotoxic drug treatment. Specifically, dehydration, protein/calorie malnutrition, and specific vitamin deficiencies should be dealt with aggressively. Patients who are anorectic from analgesics, chemotherapy, or perhaps the cancer itself are a difficult group in which to secure adequate alimentation. Such patients may be nauseated by the sight or smell of food and may react similarly to synthetic diets. Although the use of an intact, functioning GI tract is preferable whenever possible, parenteral alimentation may sometimes be the better choice, particularly when small-diameter feeding tubes cannot be passed easily or when the patient objects to a gastrostomy. Parenteral hyperalimentation, however, is not universally available, is expensive, and usually requires a prolonged hospital stay.

SINGLE AGENTS

Table 13-10 shows the individual drugs that are generally regarded as active in the treatment of epidermoid cancer of the head and neck. These drugs come from the several major classes of antineoplastic compounds, including bifunctional alkylating agents, antimetabolites, antibiotics, plant alkaloids, and heavy metal coordination complexes. The response rates shown in this table are generally derived from pooled data taken from a large number of individual trials using various criteria for patient entry, variable doses and schedules of the individual drugs, and often discrepant criteria of response. In addition, some of the response rates are determined on a very small number of patients (hydroxyurea) or are unconfirmed reports from a single study (*e.g.*, vinblastine).[63] For these

TABLE 13-10. Drugs with Activity in Head and Neck Cancer[55-63]

DRUG	EVALUABLE CASES	RESPONSE RATE (%)
Methotrexate (weekly or twice a week)	100	50
Methotrexate (monthly loading courses)	107	29
Cis-platinum	108	33
Bleomycin	298	18
Hydroxyurea	18	39
Cyclophosphamide	77	36
Vinblastine	35	29
Doxorubicin (adriamycin)	34	23
5-Fluorouracil	118	15

reasons, most of these response rates should be regarded as approximations.

Methotrexate was the first antitumor agent to be regarded as truly useful in the treatment of epidermoid cancer of the head and neck. As can be seen in Table 13-11, methotrexate has been given in a large variety of doses and schedules.[64-69] Weekly or twice-weekly administration appears somewhat more effective than either loading courses once every 3–4 weeks or daily administration of small doses.[56,57] Over the dose range shown in Table 13-11, no obvious dose-response relationship exists. The relative efficacy of so-called "high-dose methotrexate with leucovorin rescue" compared to more conventional doses of methotrexate is difficult to assess. In a multi-institutional trial, Levitt and coworkers were unable to show a significant increase in response rate with moderate doses of methotrexate and leucovorin over that of methotrexate alone, but toxicity did appear to be somewhat less in the leucovorin group (see Table 13-12).[68] DeConti has found no significant difference in response rates among three regimens tested.[69] Woods and coworkers have compared three dose variations of a single methotrexate schedule over a 100-fold dosage range; a very preliminary analysis of their data suggests no obvious differences in response rates.[70] The early results of a trial in which high weekly doses of methotrexate with leucovorin were compared with much lower doses given twice a week with single injections of leucovorin after each dose suggest no differences in efficacy, and the low-dose biweekly regimen seemed somewhat less toxic.[71]

In summary, for head and neck cancer, no persuasive evidence has yet emerged that high doses of methotrexate with leucovorin are superior to conventional doses, with or without leucovorin, and the median response durations of low-dose methotrexate are not significantly increased as the dose of methotrexate is raised. Therefore, when using methotrexate in the palliation of advanced, incurable disease, it seems reasonable to begin with weekly IV administration at a dose of 40–50 mg/m^2 and to escalate the dose in small weekly increments until either mild toxicity or a therapeutic response is achieved. Before start of therapy, one must verify that renal function is normal, since methotrexate is excreted almost entirely by the kidneys. (*See* Chapter 43 in regard to precautions in the use of methotrexate.)

Initial studies with cis-platinum suggested that this agent had significant antitumor activity roughly equivalent to that of methotrexate, with respect to both remission rate and duration of remission.[72]

Bleomycin has also been recognized as an active agent, but the response rates from trials in the U.S. have been consistently lower than the Japanese results.[73] This drug has been employed in combination regimens because of its lack of significant myelosuppression.

In summary, at least three agents (methotrexate, cis-platinum, and bleomycin) show consistent antitumor effects in epidermoid carcinoma of the head and neck, and five other agents have shown suggestive signals of activity. Response duration with any of the active agents used singly is very short.

COMBINATION CHEMOTHERAPY OF ADVANCED DISEASE

Over the past few years, numerous clinical investigators have explored the effect of various combinations of drugs in advanced head and neck cancer. For the most part, the various combinations of drugs have been composed of agents from Table 13-10, although other compounds such as vincristine and the nitrosoureas have also been employed. All the available drugs in Table 13-10 cause either myelosuppression or mucositis or both. In addition, both cis-platinum and methotrexate are potentially nephrotoxic. These facts, coupled with the somewhat fragile nature of many patients with head and neck cancer, have frequently resulted in drug combina-

TABLE 13-11. Methotrexate (Weekly or Twice Weekly) in Head and Neck Cancer

INVESTIGATOR	SCHEDULE	NO. OF PATIENTS	RESPONSE (>50%)	RESPONSE RATE (%)
Papac et al[64]	0.8 mg/kg every four days IV	15	8	53
Lane et al[65]	25–50 mg every four to seven days IV	27	14	52
Leone et al[66]	60 mg/m^2 wk IV or 40 mg/m^2 biweekly IV	35	20	57
DePalo et al[67]	40 or 60 mg/m^2/wk IV	23	8	35
Levitt et al[68]	80 mg/m^2 for 30 hrs every two weeks with escalation to toxicity	16	7	44
DeConti[69]	40 mg/m^2 IV every week	Not available		24

TABLE 13-12. Methotrexate in Head and Neck Cancer: Randomized Trials Comparing High- and Low-Dose Schedules

AUTHOR	TREATMENT PLAN*	NO. OF PATIENTS	RESPONSE RATE (%)	MEDIAN DURATION OF RESPONSE (months)
Levitt et al[68]	1. M 80 mg/m² ×30 hr every two weeks with escalation to toxicity	16	44	3
	2. M 240–360 mg/m² ×36–42 h with escalation to 1080 mg/m² with L 40 mg/m² IV bolus; 25 mg/m² PO every six hours ×4 doses	25	60	3
DeConti[69]	1. M 40 mg/m² IV every week	Overall response rate 24%; median duration of response, 50 days; no significant differences among the three arms		
	2. M 240 mg/m² IV with L 25 mg every six hours ×8 doses every two weeks			
	3. M and L as in (2) plus C 500 mg/m² IV and Ara-C 300 mg/m² IV every two weeks			
Woods et al[70]	1. M 50 mg/m² bolus and L 15 mg PO every six hours ×12 doses	11	45	
	2. M 500 mg/m² bolus and L as in 1.	16	31	2
	3. M 5000 mg/m² bolus and L as in 1.	12	50	
Kirkwood et al[71]	1. M 40–200 mg/m² biweekly and L 50 mg/m² IV single dose	18	61	3
	2. M 1–7.5 g/m² ×24 h every week and L 10 mg/m² IV PO every six hours ×12 doses	16	50	3

* M—methotrexate; L—leucovorin; C—cyclophosphamide; Ara-C—cystosine arabinoside.

tions that produce formidable toxicity and no obvious therapeutic gain over the optimal use of either cis-platinum or methotrexate. The literature certainly contains reports of various drug combinations that appear very active in nonrandomized Phase II trials; such combinations, however, have almost never been subjected to direct randomized comparative trials against best single agent treatment, and it is therefore difficult to evaluate the clinical significance of many promising combinations.

From the available data, a few generalizations seem possible. Cis-platinum and methotrexate have been combined by at least three groups in a variety of dose and schedule variations.[74–76] Toxicity generally appears to be greater than with either drug used alone, except in the study of Tejada and coworkers, in which small individual doses of each agent are employed.[76] No persuasive evidence currently exists that any of these two-drug combinations is more active than either drug alone, perhaps only because the pertinent comparative studies have not yet been performed. Methotrexate and bleomycin have been given together in several small studies; mucositis is usually dose-limiting, and there is no evidence that the combination has a greater therapeutic index than methotrexate alone.[77–79] Cis-platinum and bleomycin would seem ideal for combination chemotherapy since the toxicities of these two agents do not overlap. In fact, it has been proven possible to give both drugs at full single-agent doses with acceptable toxicity.[80,81] Results in previously untreated patients suggest that this two-drug combination may be more active than cis-platinum alone, but there are no directly comparative data.[82] Reduction in dose of both drugs appears to compromise the response rate somewhat, but may also result in a parallel reduction in toxicity.[83,84] The addition of methotrexate to cis-platinum and bleomycin has frequently resulted in a substantial increase in toxicity without obvious therapeutic gain, although one such regimen appears surprisingly active.[82,85–87] A variety of combinations employing alkylating agents, nitrosoureas, or doxorubicin (adriamycin) appear no more effective than best single-agent treatment and generally have exhibited substantial toxicity.[88–92] Table 13-13 lists five promising combinations that have recently been described in which the response rate is about double the single-agent response rate. Since most of these combinations are either incompletely studied or have not yet been reported in final form, a full assessment is presently impossible.

GENERAL PRINCIPLES OF COMBINING MODALITIES

SURGERY PLUS RADIATION THERAPY

Either preoperative or postoperative radiation therapy may be used; there are advocates of each. Analysis of available data suggests that there is no difference in local-regional control or survival comparing the two sequences; the major difference is the increased operative morbidity associated with operations performed after radiation therapy.

Combined modality therapy should be avoided for lesions with a high cure rate (70% or greater) by either surgery or radiation therapy alone. The increased morbidity from combined treatment does not increase the control rate significantly, and many patients with local or regional failure can be salvaged by secondary procedures.

The advantages of postoperative compared to preoperative radiation therapy include less operative morbidity, more meaningful margin checks at the time of the operation, a knowledge of tumor spread for radiation treatment planning, safe use of a higher radiation dose, and no chance that the patient will refuse surgery.

TABLE 13-13. Promising Combinations of Drugs

AUTHOR	DRUGS	NUMBER OF PATIENTS	RESPONSE RATE (%)
Randolph et al[80]	Cis-platinum, bleomycin	12 (previously treated)	33
		21 (previously untreated)	71
Kaplan et al[87]	Bleomycin, methotrexate, cis-platinum	46	63
Price et al[93]	Vincristine, bleomycin, methotrexate, 5-fluorouracil, hydrocortisone, with and without doxorubicin	117 (total)	67
		58 (no previous radiotherapy)	72
Cortes et al[94]	Bleomycin, cyclophosphamide, methotrexate, 5-fluorouracil	26	58
Holoye et al[95]	Bleomycin, cyclophosphamide, methotrexate, 5-fluorouracil	22	59

The disadvantages of postoperative radiation therapy include the larger treatment volume necessary to cover surgical dissections and scars, a delay to the start of radiation therapy with possible growth of tumor (especially contralateral neck nodes), and the higher dose required to accomplish the same rate of local-regional control.

Preoperative Radiation Therapy

Preoperative radiation therapy is recommended for the following situations:

1. A trial of radiation therapy (5000 rads) is given to judge the response of the primary lesion. The patient is re-evaluated with the surgeon and a decision is made to continue for cure by radiation therapy or to stop the irradiation and proceed in 4–6 weeks to an operation. This philosophy is selected for moderately advanced lesions that have a reasonable chance to respond favorably to radiation therapy, thereby avoiding a major ablative procedure. The pyriform sinus and larynx are common primary sites for use of this strategy. There is no proof that one can select patients on this basis, but the concept is used by many groups and seems to work. In our practice, about four out of five patients selected for a trial will complete a full course of radiation therapy. On the other hand, a few patients initially selected for a full course of radiation therapy are re-evaluated at 5000 rads and the response is so poor that irradiation is stopped and an operation recommended.
2. Solitary neck nodes that are on the borderline of resectability are a reason to give radiation therapy before surgery. The preoperative dose to the primary lesion is 5000 rads, but treatment of the major neck mass is continued to a dose of 6000–7500 rads through a reduced portal. Most large nodes will become resectable, and in approximately 50% of the specimens no tumor is seen.
3. If the reconstruction and rehabilitation will delay the start of postoperative radiation therapy by more than 6 weeks, then preference should be given to preoperative radiation therapy.

The dose for preoperative radiation therapy is usually 5000 rads 5–6 weeks. Short treatment schemes using a few large fractions followed immediately by surgery have shown little or no advantage in comparison to surgery alone.[96–99] Moderate-dose schemes, 3000–4000 rad, have not shown any great increase in control rates. A dose of 5000 rad will control a large percentage of subclinical disease in lymph nodes and also reduce the recurrence rates for the primary site. A few venturesome groups have tried higher doses, 6000 rad, but the morbidity may exceed the gain in cures.

Postoperative Radiation Therapy

Postoperative radiation therapy is considered when the risk of recurrence above the clavicle exceeds 20%. The operative procedure should be one-stage and of such magnitude that irradiation is started no later than 6 weeks and preferably by 4 weeks. The operation should be undertaken only if it is believed to be highly likely that all gross disease will be removed and margins will be negative. It is fashionable to talk about "debulking" operations prior to radiation therapy. This term has no precise meaning and should be avoided, since it may imply partial removal of gross disease ("cut-through"), a maneuver that probably reduces the chance of control by radiation therapy rather than enhancing it.

The radiotherapist is frequently called upon to decide regarding further treatment based on the pathologist's report following a cancer operation. Positive margins or close margins are an indication for radiation therapy. Looser and coworkers compared the clinical significance of negative and positive margins for 1775 previously untreated squamous cell carcinomas of the head and neck (excluding glottic and skin).[100] Only 3.5% were scored as positive margins. The incidence of recurrence at the primary site was 31.7% for patients with negative margins and 71% for those with positive margins. There was no difference whether the positive margin was due to carcinoma *in situ,* invasive tumor, or close margin (within 5 mm). Other indications for postoperative irradiation may be cartilage or bone invasion, perineural spread, and high-grade histology.

The findings in the neck dissection are frequently the indication for postoperative radiation therapy. Multiple positive nodes, invasion through the capsule, and high-grade histology predict a high risk of recurrence in both the dissected neck and the contralateral neck.

TABLE 13-14. Number of Patients with Failure within the Primary Treatment Field According to Dose and Reason for Adding Postoperative Irradiation

	PRIMARY REASON FOR ADDING POSTOPERATIVE IRRADIATION (failures within field/total patients)							Total	
Dose (rad)	*Positive or Questionable Margins*	*Perinodal Extension*	*Perineural Involvement*	*Thyroid Cartilage Invasion*	*Mandible Involvement*	*Multiple Nodes*	*Misc.**	*No.*	*(%)*
<5000–5499	3/5	0/1	0	2/5	0	1/1	0/1	6/13	(46)
5500–6499	5/11	1/4	1/2	0/4	2/2	2/8	0/8	11/39	(28)
⩾6500	0/8	0/1	0/1	0/2	0/1	0	0	0/13	(0)
Total	8/24 (33%)	1/6 (17%)	1/3 (33%)	2/11 (18%)	2/3 (67%)	3/9 (33%)	0/9 (0%)	17/65 (26%)	

(Marcus RB Jr, Million RR, Cassisi NJ: Postoperative irradiation for squamous cell carcinomas of the head and neck: Analysis of time-dose factors related to control above the clavicles. Int J Radiat Oncol Biol Phys 5:1943–1949, 1979)
* Treated for reasons not clear in chart.

Marcus and coworkers analyzed the time-dose factors related to control above the clavicle for 71 patients with squamous cell carcinoma of the head and neck treated by operation and postoperative radiation therapy.[101] Table 13-14 analyzes the results according to the indication for treatment and the dose of radiation. The recurrence rate was increased by use of split-course schemes. There was no obvious difference in control between T3 and T4 lesions, and N stage did not predict success or failure. Oral cavity and oropharynx lesions tended to have a higher recurrence rate with combined treatment than larynx or pyriform sinus lesions. Fig. 13-3 shows a time-dose plot for control above the clavicle for a variety of head and neck sites. A dose of 6000 rads/6 weeks provides a control rate of approximately 90%, but for those patients requiring longer treatment times (7–8 weeks) or high-risk patients, a dose of 6500 rads/7 weeks is preferred. Serious late complications occurred in approximately 8% of the patients treated by postoperative irradiation. The main complication was pharyngeal stenosis in patients having laryngopharyngectomy (the complication rate was not dose dependent). Fig. 13-4 shows actuarial survival of the 65 patients evaluable for local control analysis. The higher local

FIG. 13-3. Failures within the primary fields for the 65 patients evaluable for local control after postoperative radiation therapy. Dose to the primary field (in rads) is shown on the ordinate and total treatment *time* (*days*) on the abscissa. Two patients received doses that would not fit on the scattergram: one received 3770 rad over 25 days and was controlled; the other received 4090 rad in 41 days and failed within the primary field. (Marcus RB Jr, Million RR, Cassisi NJ: Postoperative irradiation for squamous cell carcinomas of the head and neck: Analysis of time-dose factors related to control above the clavicles. Int J Radiat Oncol Biol Phys 5:1943–1949, 1979)

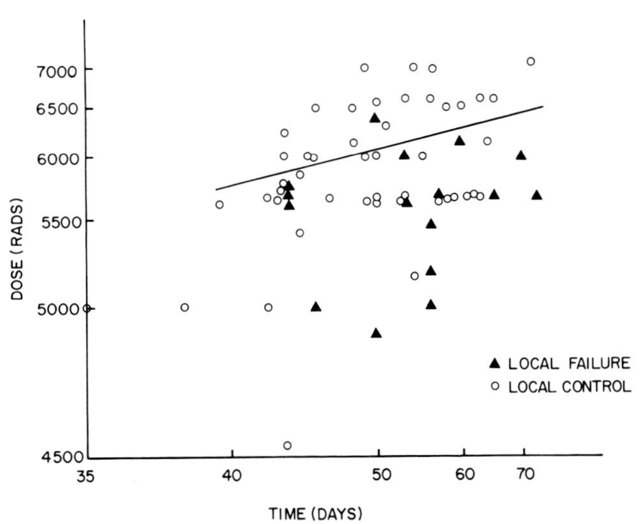

FIG. 13-4. Actuarial survival of the 65 patients evaluable for local control. The *p* value of the difference between the two curves was 0.10 by the Gehan method.[102,103] (Marcus RB Jr, Million RR, Cassisi NJ: Postoperative irradiation for squamous cell carcinomas of the head and neck: Analysis of time-dose factors related to control above the clavicles. Int J Radiat Oncol Biol Phys 5:1943–1949, 1979)

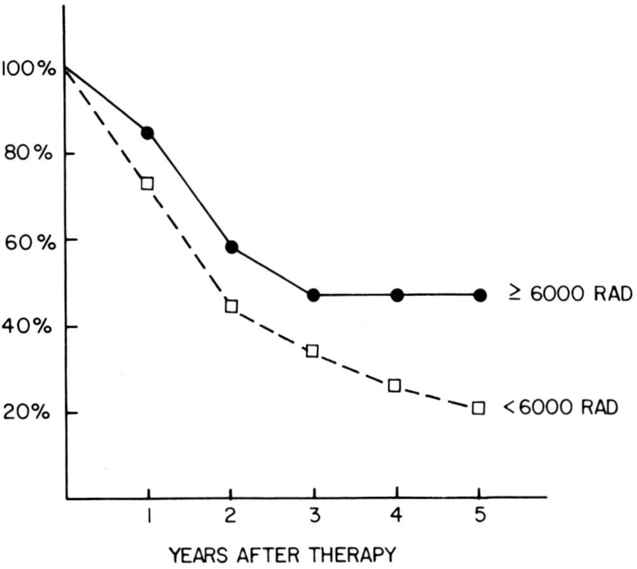

control rate of patients who received at least 6000 rads is reflected in a higher survival rate. The 5-year survival of these patients was 47%, while for those who received less than 6000 rads, the 5-year survival was only 22% ($p = 0.10$ by the Gehan method).[103]

CHEMOTHERAPY AND SURGERY OR RADIATION THERAPY

The intensive study of chemotherapy as an adjuvant to radiation or surgery for head and neck cancer has begun much more recently than similar efforts with other solid neoplasms, such as the carcinomas of breast, lung, and large bowel. The reason for this lag in interest has been the lack of effective regimens for the treatment of squamous cell carcinoma. In contrast to other solid tumors, in head and neck cancer the recent emphasis has been on the use of chemotherapy as initial treatment prior to irradiation or surgery. Although this use of chemotherapy is not new, the approach has gained recent impetus from several trials showing most impressive degrees of tumor necrosis by high-dose methotrexate cis-platinum-containing combinations and other regimens.[80–82,85,93,104–108] Since the achievement of local and regional control remains such a formidable problem in advanced disease, and since chemotherapy may produce dramatic tumor regression when given as initial treatment, it seems reasonable to expect benefit from effective chemotherapy in enhancing rates of local and regional control.

At present, nearly all the completed trials are small pilot studies. Valid conclusions at this time are that the use of chemotherapy prior to surgery or radiation therapy is feasible and that such treatment frequently results in regression of measurable tumor masses. The operative specimens following such treatment frequently show impressive histologic evidence of necrosis, although viable tumor cells are very much in evidence. Since all the completed studies have been uncontrolled, no firm statement about the effect of treatment on local control rates, duration of disease-free interval, or survival can be made. To study these questions definitively, a multi-institutional cooperative trial is currently in progress at several centers in the U.S.[84]

CHEMOTHERAPY AND RADIATION THERAPY

For a long time, clinical investigators have recognized that the simultaneous combination of chemotherapy and radiotherapy might offer therapeutic advantages over the use of either modality alone. Ample evidence exists from *in vitro* systems that the simultaneous administration of various drugs can potentiate the killing effect of ionizing radiation.[109] Obviously, however, extrapolation of cell culture results directly to the clinic is impossible. Since potentiation of radiation with drugs may have disastrous effects upon normal tissues, the question is whether the therapeutic effects of radiotherapy can be enhanced by simultaneous drug administration at tolerable levels of host toxicity.

Many exploratory trials have been performed in which various single agents have been given simultaneously with radiation.[56,57,110,111] The results of the controlled studies have been contradictory, with some suggesting benefit and others, little or none (see Table 13-15). Solid information concerning the effects of combinations of drugs administered simultaneously with radiotherapy is even more meager. Patient tolerance to this approach has been poor, with profound enhancement of the local effects of radiation in most studies.[125–128] On the other hand, Clifford's results with a vincristine-methotrexate-bleomycin regimen inserted into short interruptions in radiotherapy suggest a possible improvement in results over a group of historical controls treated with radiotherapy alone.[125,129] Despite the obvious problems of this general approach, there appear to be enough positive results to warrant further investigation.

REGIONAL CHEMOTHERAPY

The intraarterial administration of cytoxic agents has received extensive testing in head and neck cancer since 1959. The potential appeal of this approach lies in the possibility of maximizing drug concentration in the tumor and minimizing drug delivery to sensitive normal tissues elsewhere. Theoretical limits of the technique are its restriction to patients with disease localized to the distribution of the perfused vessel; in particular, cervical lymph nodes are difficult to perfuse.

Results with intraarterial chemotherapy have been reviewed by Carter who has concluded that, at least for methotrexate, the slight possible increment in response rate over systemic drug administration is nullified by the substantial rate of catheter-induced complications, which have included bleeding, infection, and vessel occlusion with stroke.[56,57] Intraarterial administration has been used in association with radiotherapy for treatment of carcinoma of the maxillary sinus and has shown some promise.[57,130] It is certainly possible that advances in catheter technology will allow for safer application of this type of drug administration and expanded trials in selected situations.

ORAL CAVITY

The oral cavity consists of the lip, floor of mouth, oral tongue (*i.e.*, the anterior two-thirds of the tongue), buccal mucosa, upper and lower gingiva, hard palate, and retromolar trigone. Squamous cell carcinomas of the oral cavity mostly occur after the age of 45 and are associated with the use of tobacco and alcohol.

The American Joint Committee staging system for all primary tumors of the oral cavity is:[39]

- TX No available information on primary tumor
- TO No evidence of primary tumor
- TIS Carcinoma *in situ*
- TI Greatest diameter of primary tumor 2 cm or less
- T2 Greatest diameter of primary tumor more than 2 cm but not more than 4 cm
- T3 Greatest diameter of primary tumor more than 4 cm
- T4 Massive tumor more than 4 cm in diameter with deep invasion to involve antrum, pterygoid muscles, base of tongue, or skin of neck

TABLE 13-15. Summary of Randomized Trials Comparing the Simultaneous Use of Single Agents and Radiation with Radiation Alone

AUTHOR	PRIMARY SITE	NO. OF PATIENTS	DRUG *	RADIATION THERAPY	SUMMARY OF RESULTS †
Kramer[112]	Oral cavity, oropharynx, supraglottic larynx, hypopharynx; advanced stages	631	M 25 mg IV every three days five times; then radiotherapy	5000–8000 rad in 5–10 wks	No survival difference
Knowlton et al[113]	Unresectable, stages III, IV	96	M 0.2 mg/kg/day IV five times (56 patients); then increased to 240 mg/m^2 IV days 1,5,9, with leucovorin (20 patients) each followed by radiotherapy	4500–5000 rad with boost to primary to total 6000–6600 rads in 6–7 wks, with or without implant	No significant differences in local control, distant metastases, or survival
Condit[114]	All sites, advanced stages	40	M 1–4 mg/kg every two weeks simultaneous with radiotherapy	1800–2500 rads in 3 days; repeat after 4 wk rest	No significant differences in local control rates or durations, but numbers very small
Bagshaw and Doggett[115]	All sites, T3–4	41	M 25 mg IA every day with leucovorin simutaneous with radiotherapy	6300 rads in 5.5 wks	No differences in local control; marked increase in local toxicity with simultaneous treatment
Steffani et al[116]	All sites, stages III, IV	110	HU 80 mg/kg PO bi-weekly simultaneous with radiotherapy	6000–10,000 rads in 8–12 wks with boost in selected cases (orthovoltage)	No differences in disease-free survival; borderline difference in total survival favoring radiotherapy alone
Richards and Chambers[117]	All sites	40	HU 80 mg/kg PO every third day during radiotherapy	5000–9000 rads in 6–12 wks	No significant differences, but numbers small
Gollin et al[118]	All sites, advanced stages	155	FU 10 mg/kg/day IV three times, then 5 mg/kg/day four times, then 5 mg/kg twice a week during radiotherapy	6000–7000 rads in 6–7 wks; stop at 5000 rads for surgery in selected cases	Significant superiority to combined treatment for oral cavity lesions
Ansfield et al[119]	All sites, advanced	134	FU 10 mg/kg/day IV three times, then 5 mg/kg/day four times, then 5 mg/kg twice a week during radiotherapy	6500 rads in 6 wks	Superior 5-yr survival in oral cavity and tonsil groups
Shigematsu et al[120]	Antrum	63	FU 5–10 mg/kg/day IA simultaneous with radiotherapy	8000 rads in 8 wks	No significant differences in survival at 2 yr; borderline difference in disease-free survival at 1 yr favoring combined treatment
Cachin et al[121]	Oropharynx, stages III, IV	186	B 5 mg IM or IV bi-weekly 2 hrs before radiotherapy	7000 rads in 7–9 wks	No significant differences in therapeutic effect; enhanced local toxicity in combined group
Shanta and Sundaram[122]	Tongue, buccal; stages III, IV	137	B 10–15 mg IV or IA twice weekly	5500–6500 rads in 6–7 wks	Striking improvement in CR rate with combined treatment (77% vs. 17%); disease-free survival at 2 yr: 66% combined vs. 11% radiotherapy alone
Abe et al[123]	Oral cavity, stages II, III, IV	67	B 15 mg IV bi-weekly	3000 rads in 3 wks, then additional therapy (surgery or radiotherapy)	After additional therapy, the combined treatment group had a higher incidence of CR (44%) than the group treated with radiotherapy alone (15%)
Kapstad et al[124]	All sites, stages III, IV	29	B 15 mg IM twice a week, 1 hr before radiotherapy	3000 rads in 5 wks with 1-wk rest after 1500 rads; then surgery	Higher CR rate with combined treatment (27%) than with radiotherapy alone (7%)

* M—methotrexate; HU—hydroxyurea; FU—fluorouracil; B—bleomycin. † CR—completed remission.

LIP

The ratio between men and women in cases of cancer of the lip is 50:1. Persons with light-colored skin or with prolonged exposure to sunlight are most prone to develop lip carcinoma; tobacco has not been definitely implicated as a causative agent.

Anatomy

The lips are composed of the orbicular muscle with skin on the external surface and mucous membrane on the internal surface. The transition from skin to mucous membrane of the oral cavity is the lip vermilion, where the muscle is covered by a very thin layer of squamous epithelium that allows the underlying vasculature to show, thus giving the lips their reddish color. The blood supply is by way of the labial artery, a branch of the facial artery. The motor nerves are branches of the seventh cranial nerve.

Pathology

The most common neoplasms are squamous cell carcinomas. Basal cell carcinoma usually starts on the skin of the lip and may invade the vermilion, but rarely arises from the vermilion. Benign lesions such as hemangiomas, fibromas, and cysts may involve the lips.

Leukoplakia is a common problem on the lower lip and may precede the appearance of carcinoma by many years. Primary lesions arising from the moist mucosa of the lip are considered under the section on the buccal mucosa.

Patterns of Spread

Squamous cell carcinoma starts on the vermilion of the lower lip and invades adjacent skin and the orbicular muscle. Advanced lesions invade the adjacent commissures of the lip and buccal mucosa, the skin and wet mucosa of the lip, the adjacent mandible, and eventually the mental nerve. Perineural invasion occurred in 2% of the cases reported by Byers and coworkers and was related to recurrent lesions, large tumor size, mandibular invasion, and poorly differentiated histology.[131] Lymphatic spread is to the submental, submaxillary, and subdigastric lymph nodes and occurs in 5–10% on admission, but in 19% for commissure lesions.[132] The risk of lymphatic involvement is increased by high-grade histology, large lesions, spread to involve the wet mucosa of the lip and buccal mucosa, and especially for patients with recurrent disease.

Clinical Picture

Carcinoma of the lip may present as an enlarging exophytic lesion that is non-tender unless it ulcerates and becomes infected. There will be occasional minor bleeding. These lesions are easily diagnosed by their appearance. However, some lesions develop very slowly on a background of leukoplakia and present as superficially ulcerated lesions with little or no bulk and a history of repeated episodes of scab formation without complete healing. These lesions are not so easy to diagnose clinically, and only excisional biopsy provides the answer.

Erythema of the adjacent skin suggests dermal lymphatic invasion. Palpation of the lip will reveal the extent of induration. Anesthesia of the skin of the lip indicates nerve invasion.

The diagnosis is readily established by biopsy, or if the lesion is not discrete, a lip shave may be done. Mandible films are requested when bone or mental nerve involvement is suspected.

The American Joint Committee staging for oral cavity cancer includes only those lesions arising from the vermilion.

Treatment

SELECTION OF TREATMENT MODALITY. Early lesions may be cured equally well with surgery or radiation. The length of the lower lip is 4–5 cm, but tends to be shorter in edentulous patients and in those who have received prior irradiation or surgery. Surgical excision is preferred for the majority of lower lip lesions up to 1–1.5 cm in diameter that do not involve the commissure; the treatment is simple and the cosmetic result quite satisfactory. Removal of more than 2 cm (40%) of the lip with simple closure usually results in a poor cosmetic and functional result and therefore requires an extensive plastic repair. Irradiation is usually preferred for lesions involving the commissure, for lesions over 1.5 cm in length, and for most upper lip carcinomas since complex reconstruction is required and radiation therapy avoids this problem. Advanced lesions with bone, nerve, or node involvement frequently require a combined approach. Surgery is preferred for the younger patient who will have years of climatic exposure and for previously irradiated patients.

SURIGICAL TREATMENT. Surgical treatment for early lesions (0.50–1.5 cm) involves a "W" or "U" excision (see Fig. 13-5). "V" excisions may be used for very small lesions, but do not give as good a margin with the larger tumors. Larger lesions (over 1.5 cm) may be closed with an Abbe flap from the upper lip to reconstruct the lower lip defect. If the vermilion is diffusely involved with little or no involvement of the muscle, then a lip shave may be done and the mucosa from the oral cavity advanced to cover the defect. If the commissure must be sacrificed, it must be reconstructed to prevent microstomia and to allow the patient to continue to wear dentures.

IRRADIATION TECHNIQUE. Lip cancer may be successfully treated by external beam, interstitial implants, or a combination of both.

Interstitial implants may be accomplished with removable sources such as radium needles or Iridium-192. Gold seeds may be permanently implanted under local anesthesia as an outpatient procedure and the patient sent home the same day.

External beam techniques use orthovoltage or electrons with lead shields behind the lip to limit exit irradiation. The dose schemes are similar to those used for skin cancer. Fractionation schemes of 4–6 weeks are preferred over the shorter regimens to decrease the normal tissue effects.

The regional lymphatics are not electively treated for early cases. Advanced lesions and especially recurrent lesions

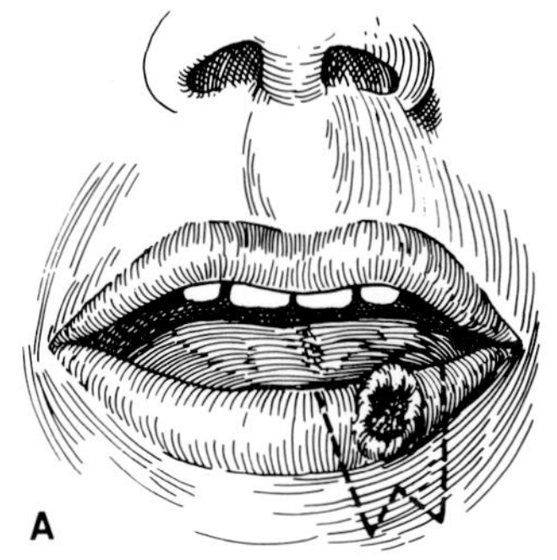

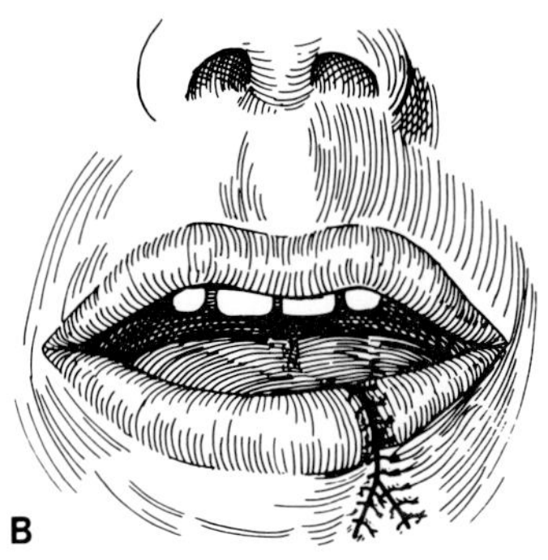

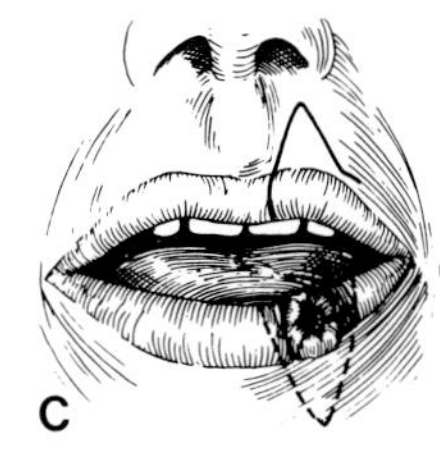

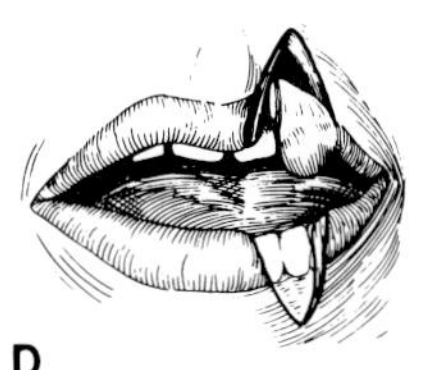

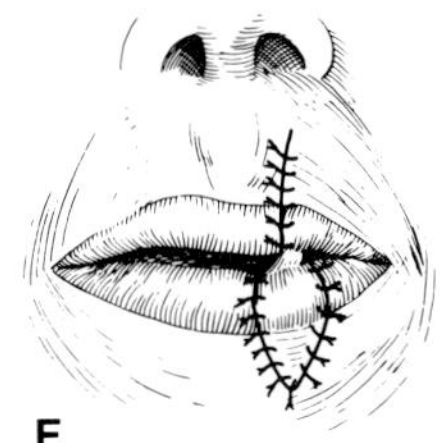

FIG. 13-5. Small lip lesions that do not involve the oral commissure can be removed using a "W" excision (*A*) and can be closed primarily (*B*). Larger lesions of the lip may be removed in a "V" fashion (*C*) and the defect can be closed using an Abbe flap from the upper lip (*D*). A second procedure to release the flap can also be performed two weeks later (*E*).

should have either elective neck irradiation or elective neck dissection, depending on the treatment selected for the primary lesion. Clinically positive nodes are managed according to policies outlined in "Principles of Treatment".

Results of Treatment

MacKay and Sellers reviewed 2854 patients with all stages of lip cancer, of whom 92% were managed initially by radiation therapy.[132] The primary lesion was controlled by the initial treatment in 84% of cases, and an additional 8% were saved by later treatment, for an overall local control rate of 92%. Fifty-eight percent of those who presented with clinically involved nodes had control of disease, but only 35% when neck nodes appeared later. The determinate 5-year survival rate was 89%; the absolute 5-year survival rate was 65%. Death due to intercurrent disease occurred in 17%.

Table 13-16 shows the M. D. Anderson Hospital local control rates for 444 previously untreated patients.[133] The 3- and 5-year determinate survival rate was 94%. With proper treatment and followup, very few patients should succumb to lip cancer.

Complications of Treatment

Microstomia and drooling secondary to oral incompetence may occur when a large flap reconstruction is necessary. If the oral opening is too small, the patient may not be able to insert a denture. Speech is not often affected.

There will be some atrophy of the irradiated tissues; this progresses with time. Continued exposure to the elements may result in a soft tissue necrosis; this problem is reduced by treatment schemes that prolong the treatment. The irradiated lip must be carefully protected from sun exposure by

TABLE 13-16. Cancer of the Lip—Previously Untreated Patients (M. D. Anderson Hospital)

SIZE OF LESION	TREATMENT*	NO. OF PATIENTS	NO. WITH LOCAL RECURRENCE	NO. SALVAGED
0–1 cm	RT	30	0	–
	S	239	6	6
1–2 cm	RT	36	2	1
	S	116	3	1
>2 cm	RT	7	0	–
	S	7	3	0
Massive	RT	1	0	–
	S	8	1	0

(MacComb WS, Fletcher GH, Healey JE Jr: Intra-oral cavity. In MacComb WS, Fletcher GH (ed): Cancer of the Head and Neck, pp 89–151. Baltimore, Williams & Wilkins, 1967)
* RT: Radiotherapy; S: Surgery

use of hats and UV protectants. Fishermen must wear a surgical face mask while on the water, as the various UV protectants are insufficient.

The anterior teeth are protected by lead shields when treatment is given by external beam.

FLOOR OF MOUTH

Anatomy

The floor of mouth is a U-shaped area bounded by the lower gum and the oral tongue; it terminates posteriorly at the insertion of the anterior tonsillar pillar into the tongue. The paired sublingual glands lie immediately below the mucous membrane. They are separated by the paired genioglossus and geniohyoid muscles. Bony protuberances, the genial tubercles, occur at the point of insertion of these two muscle groups at the symphysis. They may be quite prominent in some patients and interfere with the placement of interstitial sources. The mylohyoid muscle arises from the mylohyoid ridge of the mandible and is the muscular floor for the oral cavity. The mylohyoid muscle ends posteriorly at about the level of the third molars. The normal submaxillary gland is about the size of a walnut. Most of the gland rests on the external surface of the mylohyoid muscle in the niche between the mandible and the insertion of the mylohyoid. A tongue-like process wraps around the posterior border of the mylohyoid muscle and extends forward on the internal surface of the mylohyoid. This process is absent in about 10–20% of cases. The submaxillary duct (Wharton's duct) is about 5 cm long. It courses between the sublingual gland and the genioglossus muscle and exits in the anterior floor of mouth near the midline. Fig. 13-6 shows the relationships of the lingual nerve, hypoglossal nerve, and submaxillary duct.

Pathology

The majority of neoplasms are squamous cell carcinoma, usually of moderate grade. Adenoid cystic and mucoepidermoid carcinomas account for about 5% of malignant tumors in this area.

Patterns of Spread

PRIMARY. Approximately 90% of neoplasms originate within 2 cm of the anterior midline floor of mouth. They penetrate quite early beneath the mucosa into the sublingual gland and eventually into the midline genioglossus and geniohyoid muscles. The mylohyoid muscle acts as an effective barrier until the lesion becomes very advanced. Extension toward the gingiva and periosteum of the mandible occurs early and frequently. Even small lesions become attached to the periosteum. The periosteum is an effective barrier to mandibular invasion; when tumor reaches the periosteum, the tumor usually spreads along the periosteum rather than through it. Mandible invasion is usually a late manifestation. Tumor will sometimes grow over the alveolar ridge before it grossly invades bone. The skin of the lower lip may be involved in advanced cases. Posterior extension occurs into the muscles of the root of the tongue; this pattern of extension is usually associated with ulceration of the floor of mouth and undersurface of the tongue.

One or both submaxillary ducts are frequently obstructed by tumor or after biopsy. An enlarged duct may be palpated through the floor of mouth in some cases, and it may be difficult to distinguish between tumor extension and low-grade infection in an obstructed duct. Tumor rarely grows inside the duct, but may grow along the path of the duct. The submaxillary gland will frequently enlarge and become quite firm and occasionally painful when the duct is obstructed. It is difficult to distinguish between tumor directly invading the gland and chronic infection related to obstruction.

Tumors arising in the lateral floor of mouth are less common, but have the same general spread patterns. Extensive lesions may escape the oral cavity by following the anatomic plane of the mylohyoid muscle to its posterior extremity, emerging in the submaxillary space of the neck.

LYMPHATIC. Approximately 30% of patients will have clinically positive nodes on admission; 4% will have bilateral nodes. Southwick and coworkers report 50% pathologically positive nodes after elective neck dissection.[5] The reported incidence of conversion from NO to N^+ with no neck treatment varies from 20% to 35%.[6–8]

The first nodes involved are the submaxillary and the subdigastric nodes. The submental nodes are bypassed; Lindberg reports 2% clinically positive submental nodes in 258 cases.[32] Since most lesions either approach or cross the midline, the risk for bilateral spread is fairly high. Fletcher reports that 47% of patients (nine of 19) with ipsilateral positive necks (N1 or N2) developed contralateral neck disease if no elective neck treatment was given.[31] This rate was reduced to 10% (three of 28) after 3000–4000 rad to the upper neck.

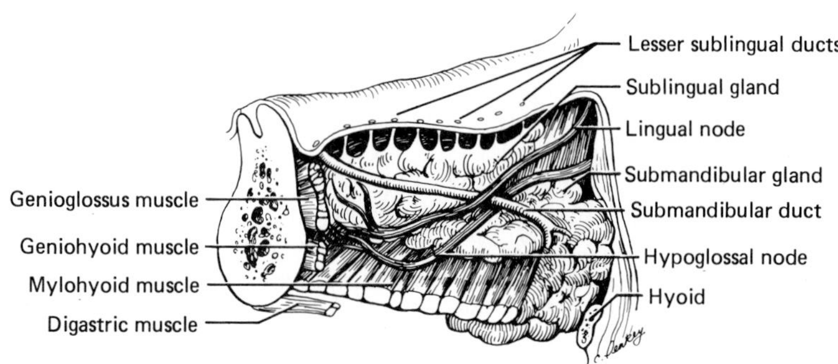

FIG. 13-6. The anatomical relationships of the floor of the oral cavity.

Clinical Picture

Early carcinomas are asymptomatic, red, slightly elevated mucosal lesions with ill-defined borders. A background of leukoplakia may be present. White lesions (leukoplakic) are less likely to be malignant, but 10% eventually become cancer. These lesions are usually diagnosed by the dentist or physician on routine oral examination.

T1–2 tumors are first noticed when the patient feels a lump in the floor of mouth with the tip of his tongue. There is mild soreness when eating or drinking that is usually thought by the patient (and sometimes the physician) to be due to a canker or denture sore. Advanced lesions produce increased pain, bleeding, foul breath, loose teeth, change in speech due to fixation of the root of the tongue, and a submaxillary mass that is often painful.

The earliest lesions appear as a red area, slightly elevated with ill-defined borders and very little induration. As the lesion enlarges, the edges of the tumor become distinct, elevated, and "rolled" with a central ulceration and induration.

Some lesions start with a background of leukoplakia. If the leukoplakia is extensive, it is difficult to know where or when to biopsy.

Bimanual palpation will determine the extent of the induration and the degree of fixation to the periosteum. Large lesions bulge into the submental space and rarely grow through the mylohyoid muscle into the soft tissues of the neck and even the skin.

The submaxillary duct and gland are evaluated by bimanual palpation. Small (5 mm) discrete lesions may be exised. Larger lesions have an incisional or punch forceps biopsy.

STAGING PROCEDURES. The occlusal view (dental film) of the arch or ramus of the mandible is the best technique for determining early invasion. Oblique mandible views and a Panorex view are not useful for determining early bone invasion, but may be obtained to evaluate the teeth and to determine the extent of invasion if extensive bony destruction is obviously present. These views also assist the surgeon in evaluating whether enough mandible exists in edentulous patients for a rim resection.

Submaxillary gland sialograms are not useful in determining the presence or absence of cancer in the gland.

The American Joint Committee staging was developed for all oral cavity lesions. No consideration is given to fixation to the periosteum of the mandible, and even small lesions may invade the periosteum. Extension to the gingivolabial sulcus, fixation of the tongue, growth through the mylohyoid muscle to the skin in the submental area, or bone invasion qualifies for T4.

Treatment

SELECTION OF TREATMENT MODALITY. *Leukoplakia.* Patches of thin leukoplakia are usually observed. Biopsy is done if the area becomes symptomatic or if the appearance changes and malignancy is suspected. Localized areas of leukoplakia may be exised, but many patients have extensive or scattered areas, which precludes excision. Cryotherapy may be tried in these cases.

Radiation therapy is not recommended for treatment of leukoplakia. However, when leukoplakia is inadvertantly irradiated along with an adjacent carcinoma, the leukoplakia may disappear. However, in most cases it will reappear at a later time.

Early Lesions. Operation and radiation therapy are equally effective treatments by themselves for many T1 and early T2 lesions; therefore treatment decisions are based on rather subtle differences in functional result and on the management of the neck.

A few patients are seen after excisional biopsy of a tiny lesion, and the only finding is a surgical scar with varying degrees of induration or nodularity under the scar (TX). The margins are stated to be free, close, or positive. If the excisional biopsy is judged to be inadequate, these patients are usually treated with an interstitial implant alone, since the surgeon has difficulty knowing where to start and stop the reexcision. The use of margin checks is essentially useless under these conditions since there are very few tumor cells present and the pathologist is "looking for a needle in a haystack." Additionally, a few tumor cells may be spread at some distance from the excision site by way of the hematoma. The radiotherapist can be generous with the treatment volume and cover potential spread without functional loss. The neck is usually observed. A review of six patients treated in this manner at M. D. Anderson Hospital revealed a 100% local control rate, similar patients treated at the University of Florida had a 100% local control rate.[134] None of the patients developed neck nodes. If the margins of the excisional biopsy are free and there is little or no induration or nodularity, 5500 rad are delivered. If the margins are positive or if there is slight induration or nodularity, the dose is raised to 6500 rad. In cases where gross cut-through is suspected, one may wish to use external beam, 5000 rad, to include regional nodes prior to the interstitial implant.

Small lesions, less than 1 cm in size, may be excised transorally if there is a margin between the lesion and the gingiva. If the submaxillary duct is surgically obstructed, then the submaxillary gland must also be removed. A common presentation is an anterior midline lesion, 1–3 cm in diameter, with a clinically negative neck; there is a risk for subclinical disease in one or both sides of the neck in 20–30% of cases. The authors recommend radiation therapy since it has the advantage of electively treating the nodes as well as the primary. If the nodes are clearly positive on one side, elective neck irradiation also sterilizes the subclinical disease on the opposite side and a neck dissection to the clinically positive neck follows the radiation therapy. Anterior midline lesions, 1–3 cm in size, may also be managed by a rim resection and bilateral supraomohyoid neck dissections. Well-lateralized floor of mouth lesions may be treated either with radiation therapy or by an operation with an incontinuity ipsilateral neck dissection. Lesions that lie against the mandible require a rim resection.

Moderately Advanced Lesions. An operation for moderately advanced floor of mouth cancers can produce major cosmetic and functional disability, especially if the arch of the mandible is removed. Rim resection, which preserves continuity of the mandible, produces a good cure rate with acceptable speech and swallowing. Success with irradiation

TABLE 13-17. Floor of Mouth Cancer: Local Control with Primary Radiation Therapy

		STAGE T1		STAGE T2		STAGE T3		
		RT ALONE*	ULTIMATE CONTROL	RT ALONE	ULTIMATE CONTROL	RT ALONE	SURGICAL SALVAGE	ULTIMATE CONTROL
M.D.A.H.†[135]	Mixed‡	48/49 (98%)	100%	68/77 (88%)	93%	46/60 (73%)	11/14	95%
U.F.§[136]	Mixed	14/16 (88%)	88%	13/17 (76%)	94%	12/25 (48%)	5/9	68%
U.C.(S.F.)‖[137]	External beam	29/38 (76%)	≃90%	21/39 (54%)	≃70%	8/32 (25%)	3	41%

* RT: Radiotherapy
† M.D.A.H.—M. D. Anderson Hospital.
‡ Mixed—external beam irradiation + interstitial implant.
§ U.F.—University of Florida.
‖ U.C.(S.F.)—University of California, San Francisco.

varies widely, but the highest local control occurs when interstitial irradiation is used either alone or as part of the treatment. Table 13-17 compares the local control rate by T stage for three different series.[135-137] The local control rates increase with increasing doses and a greater proportion of treatment given by interstitial implant; these high control rates are accompanied by a progressively higher risk of a complication.

The undesirable aspect of radical irradiation is simply the risk of soft tissue and bone necrosis with the doses required for a high rate of control. The complication rate has decreased over the past 10 years at the University of Florida due to changes in management of the teeth and improved interstitial technique[138]

Extension of tumor to the periosteum or gingiva does not exclude the use of radiation therapy. Table 13-18 shows the results of treatment according to the degree of gingival/periosteal involvement for 25 T2–3 lesions. The control rate is reasonably good, but the incidence of major complications in the patients with large, fixed lesions is quite high; if the alternative for the large, fixed lesion is a resection of the mandibular arch, floor of mouth, and anterior tongue, which produces major disability, then radiation therapy is frequently chosen as the initial treatment. However, if rim resection can be done, that is the preferred plan of management with irradiation added postoperatively.

Advanced Lesions. Patients who have stage T4 lesions only because of bone invasion have a small chance of cure with combined surgery and radiation therapy. Only palliation can be offered those who have tongue fixation, extension to submental skin, or massive neck disease.

SURGICAL TREATMENT. *Wide Local Excision.* Small lesions, 5 mm or less in size, may be excised transorally with a 1-cm margin and primary closure. If the duct is involved, the submaxillary gland and duct are removed in continuity.

Rim Resection. Rim resection of the mandible in continuity with excision of the primary lesion preserves the arch and usually gives an adequate surgical margin; the procedure may be combined with postoperative radiation therapy (see Figs. 13-7 and 13-8). Invasion of the periosteum is often an indication for this procedure. Even very early bone invasion (negative roentgenograms) may be treated in this fashion. Patients who have been edentulous for a long time may have a thin, atrophic mandible and are not suitable for rim resection since the mandible is likely to fracture.

Guillamondegui and Jesse report 20 patients treated by rim resection.[139] All patients had invasion of the periosteum and seven had early bone invasion on examination of the specimen. With 1-year minimum followup, there was only one local recurrence. Four patients, however, failed in the neck, and for this reason the authors recommend postoperative radiation therapy.

Mandibulectomy ("Jaw-Neck"). Lateral floor of mouth: A radical neck dissection is performed and the specimen remains attached to the mandible. Partial mandibulectomy with resection of the floor of mouth is done through a lip-splitting incision. A cheek flap is elevated to the level of the mandibular condyle to provide exposure. The mandible is separated at the mental foramen anteriorly and the neck of the condyle posteriorly. The primary lesion and neck specimen are then removed in continuity. Primary closure

TABLE 13-18. Floor of Mouth Cancer: Local Control (Radiation Therapy Alone) Related to Gingival Extension (Stage T2–3)—University of Florida, 10/64–12/77; analysis 12/79

EXTENT OF DISEASE	LOCAL CONTROL	SURGICAL SALVAGE	ULTIMATE LOCAL CONTROL	COMPLICATIONS REQUIRING SURGERY
Minimal gingival/periosteal extension	4/8	3/4	7/8	1
Tethered to gingiva/periosteum	4/6	1/2	5/6	0
Fixed to gingiva	6/11	1/2	7/11	4
Total			19/25 (76%)	

Mendenhall WH: unpublished data.

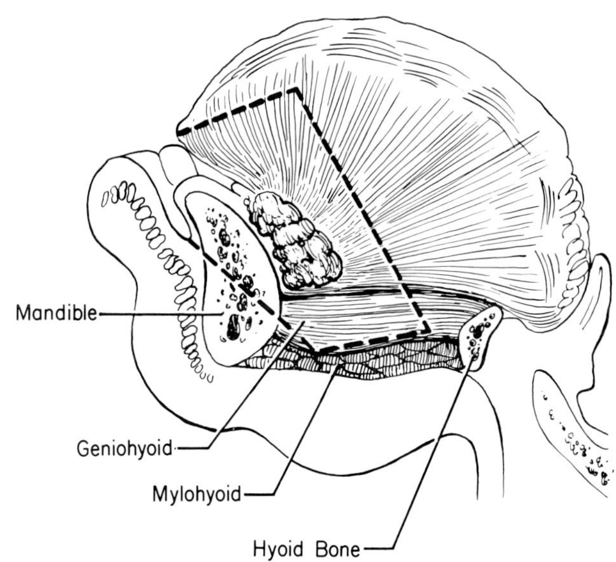

FIG. 13-7. Borders of rim resection for early carcinoma of the floor of mouth.

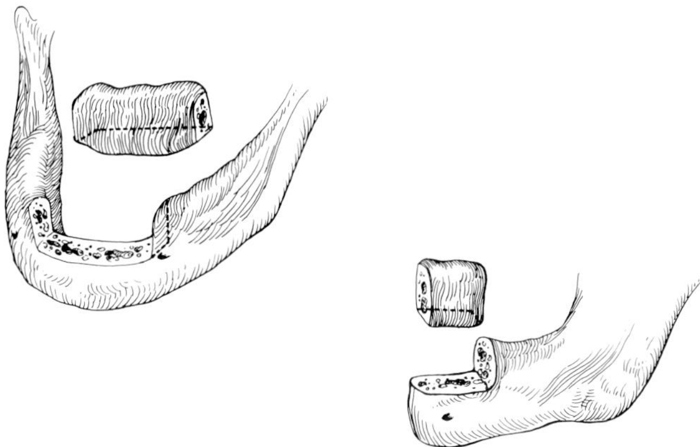

FIG. 13-8. Schematic for rim resection of the arch of the mandible. *A*, Anterior view; *B*, lateral view.

is usually feasible, unless a sizable portion of the oral tongue must be removed, in which case a myocutaneous flap is necessary to repair the defect.

The cosmetic and functional result is acceptable to patients, and very few request mandibular reconstruction. The mandible shifts to the opposite side, and if the patient has teeth, chewing may be impaired, but can be corrected with a glide plane. Edentulous patients cannot wear a lower denture.

Anterior floor of mouth: Lesions requiring full-thickness resection of the anterior mandible (arch) usually require removal from mental foramen to mental foramen. A spacer, such as a K wire or a cobalt-chromium alloy (Vitallium) tray, is necessary to maintain separation of the remaining mandible. This operation results in major cosmetic and functional loss and is usually reserved for advanced lesions with bone invasion or for irradiation failures.

IRRADIATION TECHNIQUE. Table 13-19 shows the dose schemes currently prescribed at the University of Florida. Doses are actually based on volume of tumor rather than diameter or T stage. A lesion may be 5 cm in total length and be very superficial and easily cured, while a 2–3 cm lesion may be 2–3 cm thick and invade the tongue and periosteum, requiring higher doses.

External Beam Irradiation. External beam portals for anterior floor of mouth carcinoma are opposed lateral portals. The entire width of the mandibular arch is included in the portal. The superior border is shaped to spare part of the parotid and minor salivary glands. The submaxillary and subdigastric nodes are included to the level of the thyroid notch if the neck is clinically negative. If the neck is clinically positive, the portals are enlarged to include all of the upper neck nodes, and an *en face* lower neck field is added.

Interstitial Irradiation. The availability of interstitial therapy is essential if maximum local control rates are to be obtained. External beam alone gives inferior local control results even for T1N0 lesions.[135,137]

Implantation of small lesions confined to the floor of mouth with minimal extension to the mucosa of the tongue or minimal extension to the gingiva or periosteum can be accomplished with either radium needles or iridium ("hairpins" or ribbons).

A preloaded custom-designed implant device for radium needles has been in use at the University of Florida since 1976.[138] It holds the radium needles in a fixed position. It is used only for T1–2 lesions. The arrangement of the needles for early lesions is usually a modified, curved, teardrop-shaped, two-plane implant with a single needle crossing the top of the implant. Fig. 13-9 shows the arrangement of needles for an

TABLE 13-19. Floor of Mouth Cancer: Dose Scheme Currently Prescribed at the University of Florida

	INTERSTITIAL ONLY (rads)	EXTERNAL BEAM + INTERSTITIAL (rads)
TX—No visible or palpable tumor	5500	Not recommended
TX—Palpable induration or nodularity	6500	Not recommended
TX—Tumor at margins, gross residual	Not recommended	5000 + 2500
Early (<1 cm)	6500	6000–6500 (ext. only)
Early (1–3 cm)	7000	5000 + 2500
Moderately advanced (3–5 cm)	Not recommended	5000 + 3000
Advanced	" "	6000–7000 ± implant
Postoperative radiation therapy	" "	6500/7 weeks
Preoperative radiation therapy	" "	5000/6 weeks

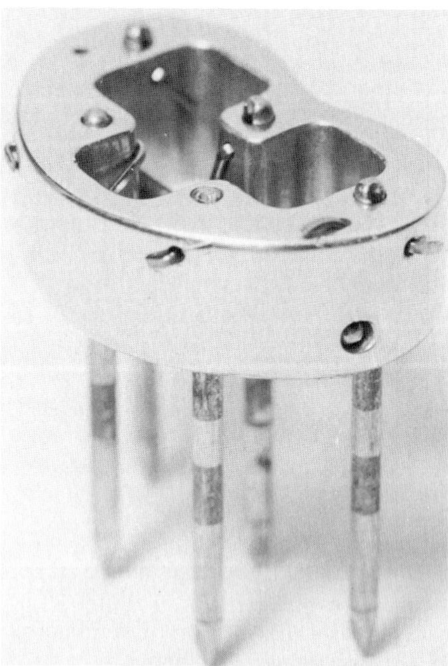

FIG. 13-9. Custom-made implant device for Stage T1-2 carcinoma of the floor of mouth. (Marcus RB Jr, Million RR, Mitchell TP: A preloaded, custom-designed implantation device for Stage T1-T2 carcinoma of the floor of mouth. Int J Radiat Oncol Biol Phys 6:111–113, 1980)

early T2 lesion; Fig. 13-10 shows the needles on a roentgenogram.

Implants for late T2 and T3 lesions are usually modified volume or multiplane arrangements. Needles or wires are inserted through the tongue. Sources at least 3.5–4.5 cm in active length are required.

Intraoral Cone Irradiation. An intraoral cone can be used for small anterior superficial lesions in the edentulous patient with a low alveolar ridge. Lesions that extend to involve the tongue are not suitable since the tongue is too mobile. Lesions more than 1 cm thick are not suitable for intraoral cone therapy because of the rapid fall-off in depth dose. The orthovoltage cones in use at the University of Florida are 2–6 cm in diameter; they are poured from lead and can be individually trimmed to adapt the cone to the anatomy. Electron beam cones can be individually fabricated as described by Tapley.[140] Intraoral cone therapy requires careful daily positioning by the physician.

Doses vary from 5000 rad 15 fractions/3 weeks to 5500 rad/20 fractions/4 weeks, depending on the size of the lesion.

Intraoral cone therapy may also be considered as a reduced field treatment in which only 1000–2000 rads is given in conjunction with external beam portals. It is preferable to use the intraoral cone before the external beam, because the mouth becomes sore and the lesion disappears.

Management of the Neck (Primary Treated by Irradiation Alone). N0: Small lesions, 1 cm or less in diameter, are treated by interstitial irradiation alone; the neck is not treated unless the histology is poorly differentiated, in which case the neck and the primary lesion are treated to 5000 rad by way of external beam followed by interstitial implant. Patients with lesions over 1 cm in size receive radiation therapy to the primary and the upper neck on both sides, 4500–5000 rad, to include the submaxillary and subdigastric nodes to the level of the thyroid notch; treatment of the primary lesion is completed by an interstitial implant.

N+: All patients receive bilateral whole neck irradiation, 5000 rad minimum. If a neck mass is large and fixed, the dose to the mass is increased to 6000–7000 rad through reduced fields and the floor of mouth is implanted. An appropriate neck dissection is added 4–6 weeks later. If the patient cannot have a neck dissection, the dose to the clinically positive node(s) is boosted.

COMBINED TREATMENT POLICIES. The results of combined surgery and irradiation may be better than those for

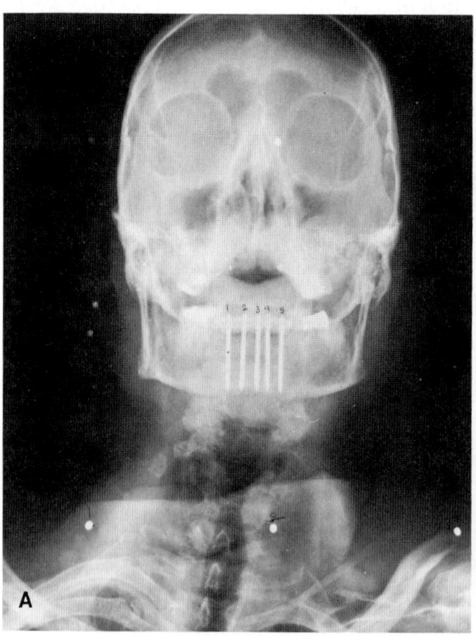

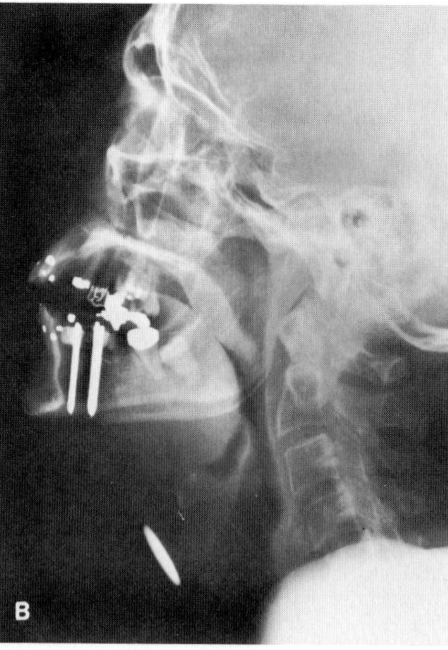

FIG. 13-10. Roentgenograms of an implant in place in the floor of mouth. *A*, AP and *B*, lateral views. (Marcus RB Jr, Million RR, Mitchell TP: A preloaded, custom-designed implantation device for Stage T1-T2 carcinoma of the floor of mouth. Int J Radiat Oncol Biol Phys 6:111–113, 1980)

TABLE 13-20. Floor of Mouth Carcinoma: Survival for Patients Treated Initially by Irradiation ± Radical Neck Dissection with Surgery for Salvage (University of Florida, 10/64–12/77; analysis 12/79)

STAGE	ABSOLUTE SURVIVAL		DETERMINE SURVIVAL*	
	2 YEARS	5 YEARS	2 YEARS	5 YEARS
I	14/17 (82%)	6/8 (75%)	14/14 (100%)	6/6 (100%)
II	11/14 (78.5%)	4/7 (57%)	11/13 (85%)	4/4 (100%)
III	20/28 (71%)	11/27 (41%)	20/24 (83%)	11/19 (58%)
IV	4/14 (28.5%)	0/7	4/11 (36%)	0/6
Total	49/73 (67%)	21/49 (43%)	49/62 (79%)	21/35 (60%)

(Mendenhall WM, Vancise WS, Bova FJ et al: Analysis of time-dose factors in squamous cell carcinoma of the oral tongue and floor of mouth treated with radiation therapy alone. Int J Radiat Oncol Biol Phys (in press))

* Excludes patients dead of intercurrent disease.

sequential therapy in the large, infiltrative, ulcerative lesions. Preoperative irradiation may be used if the patient has a large fixed node (5 cm or larger in size) or if a trial of radiation therapy is desired to evaluate response before the final decision on an operation. If rim resection is possible, postoperative irradiation is preferred, since the risk of bone complications and fistulae is higher with preoperative irradiation. Surgical clearance is most difficult in the tongue, and preoperative irradiation obscures the extent of disease. Postoperative irradiation portals usually include the entire oral tongue and floor of mouth. The daily dose is 180 rad and the tumor dose is 6500 rad. If the tongue margins were close or positive, the dose should be 7000 rad.

MANAGEMENT OF RECURRENCE. Radiation failures are treated by an operation. The salvage rate is quite high for patients with early lesions and moderately good for the more advanced lesions (see Table 13-18). Rim resection may be used for selected radiation therapy failures.

Surgical failures may be treated by a repeat operation, radiation therapy, or both on an individual basis. Radiation therapy is not likely to succeed except with limited lesions, which can be implanted as all or part of their treatment.

Results of Treatment

Table 13-20 shows survival rates at 2 and 5 years for patients initially treated with radiation.[136] Table 13-21 shows the local control rates for patients with stage III–IV disease treated by combined surgery and radiation therapy.[136,137,141]

Followup Policy

Patients are seen at 4–6 week intervals for the first 2 years. There are two major difficulties in followup after irradiation: soft tissue ulcer and enlarged submaxillary gland. An ulcer in the floor of mouth within 2 years of treatment can be either recurrence or necrosis. If the lesion appears to be soft tissue necrosis, a trial of conservative therapy and observation at close intervals is adequate. The soft tissue necroses are notoriously slow to heal. Failure to stabilize or show some indication of healing is an indication for biopsy. A negative biopsy does not rule out recurrence, and if the lesion remains suspicious, repeat deep biopsies are in order.

An enlarged submaxillary gland(s) is a common sequel to obstruction of the submaxillary duct. The gland may be enlarged on initial examination or it may enlarge during or after treatment. Since it is difficult to distinguish between an enlarged submaxillary gland and tumor in a lymph node, only removal will clarify the situation.

Complications of Treatment

A small soft-tissue necrosis may develop in the floor of mouth, usually in the site of the original lesion where the dose is highest. These ulcers are moderately painful and respond to local anesthesia, antibiotics, and tincture of time.

If the ulceration develops on the adjacent gingiva, then the underlying mandible is exposed. These areas are mildly painful. They are managed by discontinuing dentures, local anesthesia, antibiotics, and smoothing of the bone by filing if needed. These small bone exposures do not often progress to full-blown osteonecrosis. They either sequestrate a small piece of bone or are simply re-covered by mucous membrane. Healing is slow, and the patient requires constant reassurance that the discomfort and ulcer are not due to cancer.

Surgical complications include bone exposure and orocutaneous fistula. Salvage procedures after radiation therapy are associated with an increased risk of mandible complications.

ORAL TONGUE

Anatomy

Fig. 13-11 shows the muscular anatomy of the tongue. The circumvallate papillae locate the division between oral tongue

TABLE 13-21. Floor of Mouth Cancer: Stage III–IV, Local Control with Primary Combined Treatment (Surgery Plus Radiation Therapy)

	LOCAL CONTROL	ULTIMATE CONTROL
Louisville *[141]	13/15	13/15 (87%)
U.C. (S.F.) †[137]	9/10	9/10 (90%)
U.F. ‡[136]	5/11	5/11 (46%)

* Louisville—University of Louisville. † U.C. (S.F.)—University of California, San Francisco.

‡ U.F.—University of Florida.

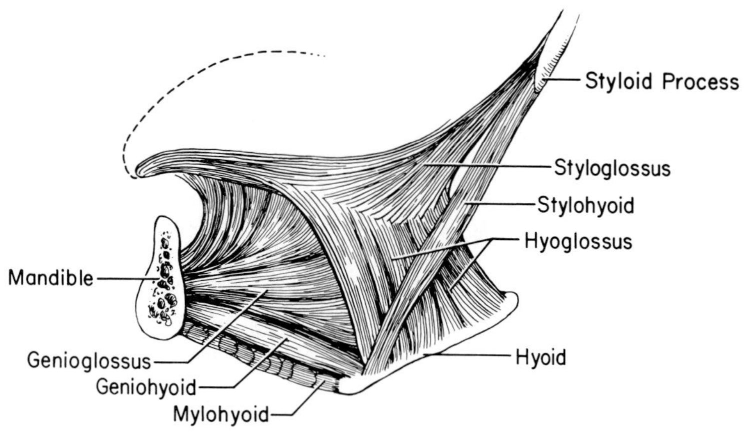

FIG. 13-11. Musculature of tongue and floor of oral cavity.

and base of tongue. The papillae foliatae may be recognized as 2–4 mm, slightly elevated, irregular areas on the dorsum at the junction with the anterior tonsillar pillar.

The arterial supply is mainly by way of paired lingual arteries, which are branches of the external carotid. One lingual artery may be sacrificed without danger of necrosis, but sacrifice of both lingual arteries results in an increased risk for loss of the oral tongue and almost certain loss of the base of tongue.

The sensory pathway is by way of the lingual nerve to the gasserian ganglion (see Fig. 13-12).

Fig. 13-13 shows the lymphatic pathways of the tongue.

Pathology

More than 95% of oral tongue lesions are squamous cell carcinomas. Coexisting leukoplakia is common. Verrucous carcinoma and minor salivary gland tumors are quite uncom-

FIG. 13-12. Pathways for referred pain to the ear. The *auricular nerve* is sensory to both the skin of the back of the pinna and the posterior wall of the external auditory canal. The *auriculotemporal nerve* supplies the skin covering the front of the helix and tragus, the skin of the anterior wall of the external auditory canal, the tympanic membrane, and the skin of the temple. The *tympanic nerve* (*Jacobson*) supplies the tympanic cavity and produces a constant, deep-seated earache.

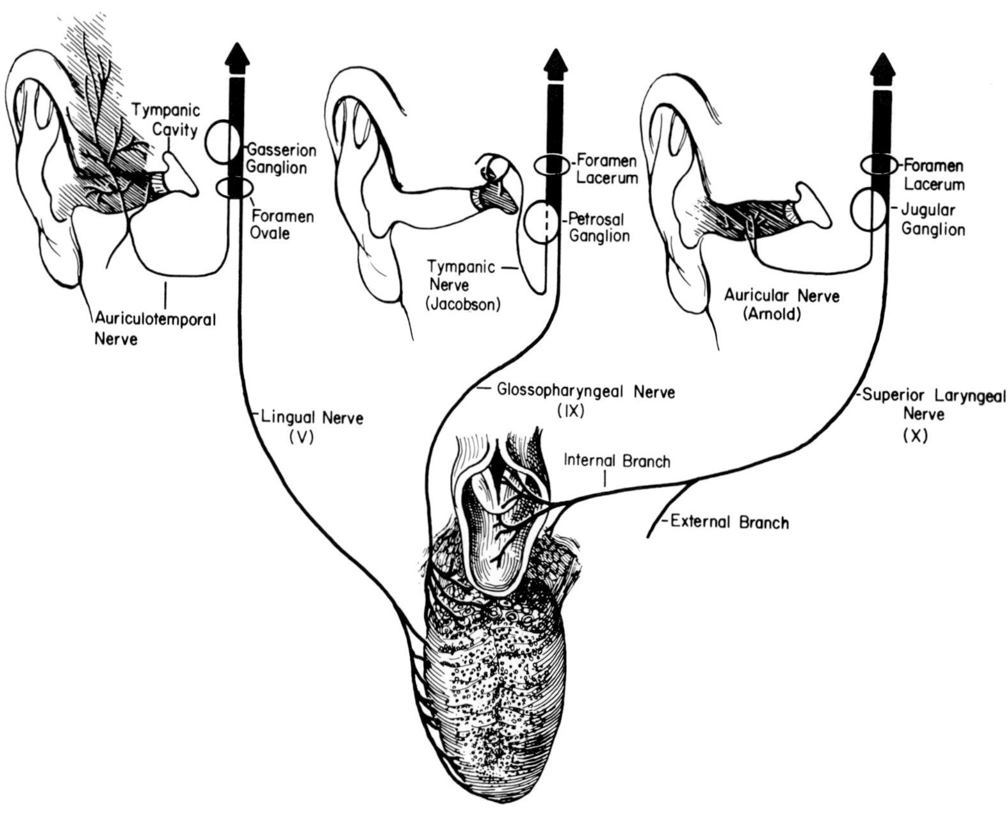

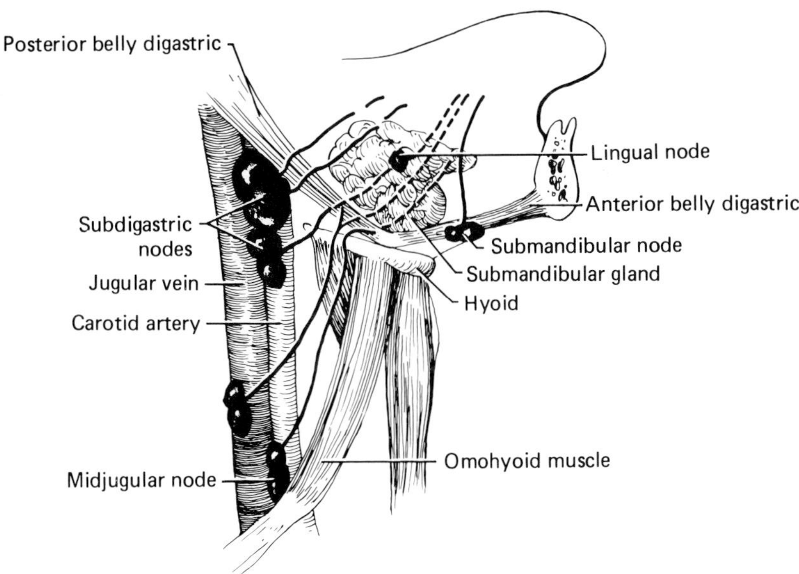

FIG. 13-13. Lymphatics and anatomical diagram of the tongue.

mon. Granular cell myoblastoma is a benign tumor of uncertain origin that commonly occurs on the dorsum of the tongue and may be confused histologically with carcinoma because of the associated pseudoepitheliomatous hyperplasia.

Patterns of Spread

PRIMARY. Nearly all oral tongue squamous cell carcinomas occur on the lateral and undersurfaces of the tongue. Rarelv, lesions appear on the dorsum, usually in the posterior midline. Most of the lateral border lesions occur on the middle and posterior thirds with a few on the anterior third. Oral tongue carcinomas tend to remain in the tongue until quite large.

Anterior third (tip) lesions are usually diagnosed early. Advanced lesions invade the floor of mouth and root of tongue, producing ulceration and fixation.

Middle third lesions invade the musculature of the tongue and later invade the lateral floor of mouth.

Posterior third lesions grow into the musculature of the tongue, the floor of mouth, anterior tonsillar pillar, base of tongue, and glossotonsillar sulcus. Posterior third lesions behave more like base of tongue cancer with a higher incidence of lymph node metastasis.

LYMPHATICS. The first echelon nodes are the subdigastric and submaxillary nodes. The submental and spinal accessory lymph nodes are seldom involved. Rouviere describes lymphatic trunks that bypass the subdigastric and submaxillary nodes and terminate in the midjugular lymph nodes (see Fig. 13-13). One seldom sees this pattern clinically. The lymphatic vessels of the tongue anastomose freely, allowing contralateral lymph flow, usually under conditions of partial obstruction by tumor or operation. Thirty-five percent of patients with oral tongue cancer have clinically positive nodes on admission; 5% are bilateral. The incidence of occult disease is approximately 30% (see Table 13-1). The incidence of positive nodes increases with T stage.[32]

Patients with N1–2 ipsilateral nodes have a 27% risk of developing node metastasis in the opposite neck.

Clinical Picture

PRESENTING SYMPTOMS. Mild irritation of the tongue is the most frequent complaint. The patient frequently presents because he thinks he has bitten his tongue. The pain may occur only during eating or drinking. As ulceration develops, the pain becomes progressively worse. The patient may present with pain referred to the external ear canal (see Fig. 13-12). Extensive infiltration of the muscles of the tongue affects speech and deglutition. Patients with advanced lesions have a foul odor.

The extent of disease is easily determined by visual examination and palpation. The tongue protrudes incompletely and toward the side of the lesion as fixation develops. Posterior oral tongue lesions may grow inferiorly, behind the mylohyoid, and present as a mass in the neck at the angle of the mandible; the mass may be confused with an enlarged lymph node. Invasion of the hypoglossal nerve is rare and may cause atrophy. Posterolateral lesions may be difficult to evaluate because of pain; examination under anesthesia is often required.

Method of Diagnosis and Staging

The differential diagnosis includes granular cell myoblastomas, which are usually slow-growing, non-tender masses, 0.5–2.0 cm in size. The lesions are well-circumscribed, firm, and slightly raised; they may be multiple. Malignant behavior is either nonexistent or rare, and wide local excision is the treatment of choice.

Treatment

SELECTION OF TREATMENT MODALITY. Both glossectomy and irradiation are curative for oral tongue cancer, and the reported cure rates are similar for similar stages. However, for irradiation to produce satisfactory control rates, the availability of interstitial therapy is essential. Since hemiglossectomy frequently produces some degree of speech impediment and difficulty in swallowing, irradiation is often selected as the initial treatment with glossectomy reserved for recurrence. Surgical salvage of irradiation failures is fairly successful for early lesions, but drops to a 50% success rate for larger lesions. For this reason, glossectomy and radiation therapy are often advised as initial therapy for the more advanced lesions, although many patients refuse glossectomy because of the anticipated morbidity.

Excisional Biopsy (TX). Excisional biopsy of a small lesion may show inadequate margins. An interstitial implant, 5500–6000 rad, will produce a high rate of control and is favored over re-excision.[134]

Early Lesions (T1–2). Operation and irradiation produce similar local control rates, and treatment decisions must be based on functional and cosmetic loss and patient preference.

Glossectomy implies possible speech impediment and difficulty in swallowing. It is difficult to predict which patients will have trouble. The surgeon has difficulty determining the extent of tumor invasion into the tongue at the time of the operation; for this reason, preoperative irradiation should be avoided, as it only obscures the margins and compounds the problem.

Glossectomy is the treatment of choice for small, well-circumscribed lesions that can be excised transorally, small lesions on the tip of the tongue, and the rare lesion on the dorsum of the tongue. Irradiation is usually selected for larger T1 and the T2 lesions to preserve speech and swallowing.

Moderately Advanced Lesions (T2–3). Lesions that have a large surface involvement, but minimal infiltration, are favorable lesions and can be cured with radiation therapy alone. Those lesions that are deeply infiltrative (more than 2 cm in depth) will have a higher control rate with combined surgery and radiation therapy, but the patient must be willing to accept glossectomy and possibly mandibulectomy.

FIG. 13-14. Small lesions on the anterior free margin of the tongue or in the midline of the tongue can be excised (*A*) and the defect closed primarily (*B*).

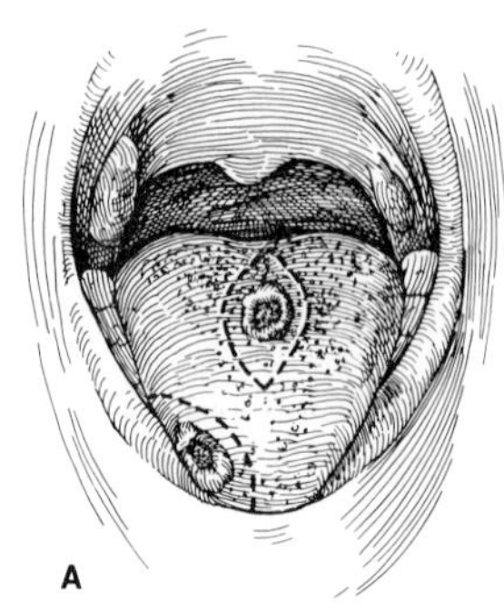

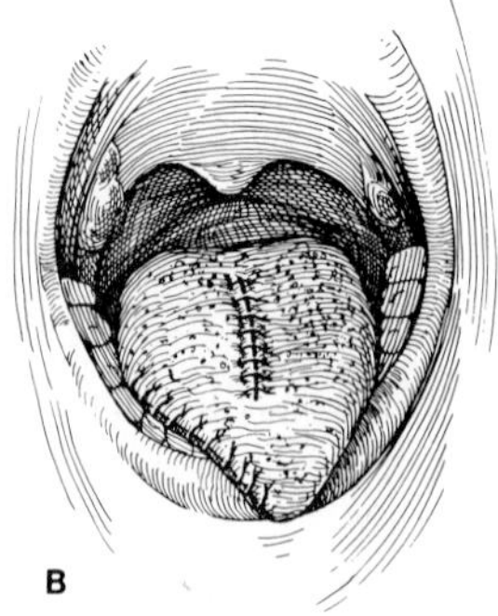

Advanced Lesions (T4). Combined treatment with surgery and radiation therapy will cure a few patients, especially those with minimal neck disease. Most patients in this category will receive palliative irradiation.

SURGICAL TREATMENT. *Early Lesions.* Fig. 13-14 shows examples of two lesions and the amount of tongue to be removed. Speech impediment and difficulty swallowing would be unlikely in these cases. Glossectomy offers the advantage of a short treatment time. Primary closure is generally done, although with large resections a flap may be necessary.

Moderately Advanced Lesions (T2–3). Deeply infiltrative lesions not suitable for irradiation alone are managed by glossectomy followed by postoperative radiation therapy. It is difficult when cutting the tongue to judge projections of tumor, and the likelihood of cutting across tumor is greater than for other head and neck sites. It is an advantage to the surgeon to be able to feel the tumor mass so that he can get a wide margin. This is not as easy if radiation therapy has preceded the glossectomy. Finally, if the mandible has to be sacrificed after high-dose radiation therapy, the likelihood of exposed bone, nonunion, and radionecrosis is increased.

Advanced Lesions (T4). Advanced lesions would require a total glossectomy and laryngectomy combined with postoperative radiation therapy. This procedure would only be offered to patients in good general condition and with minimal neck disease.

IRRADIATION TECHNIQUE. Table 13-22 gives the dose schemes currently prescribed at the University of Florida.

The ability to control the primary lesion is enhanced by giving all or part of the treatment by interstitial radiation therapy.[14,135,136,142,143] Table 13-23 shows the local control rate by T stage at the University of Florida and the rate of salvage by operation.[136] Treatment of the neck is an integral part of the treatment plan and is outlined in the section on principles of treatment. The authors favor elective neck irradiation for all lesions over 1 cm in size.

COMBINED TREATMENT POLICIES. When glossectomy is selected for large lesions, the operation is performed first. Even without previous irradiation, the surgeon has a difficult time estimating tumor extent in the tongue. The major indication for preoperative irradiation is a large node, in which case it is hoped that the irradiation will reduce the size and allow surgical clearance. Interstitial implant may be used to deliver a portion of the dose to the tongue if radiation therapy is given before an operation. Postoperative irradiation should begin within 4–6 weeks. Since most of the oral cavity is irradiated, the dose per fraction is 180 rad/day, with a total dose of 6500 rad. Interstititial implants are not usually employed in postoperative radiation therapy because recurrences may appear at any point along the surgical dissection. If the margins in the tongue are close or positive, 7000 rad is preferred because of the difficulty of eradicating even small amounts of tumor in the tongue.

MANAGEMENT OF RECURRENCE. Most recurrences appear in the first 2 years. Local recurrence after radiation

TABLE 13-22. Irradiation Policies for Oral Tongue Cancer at the University of Florida

	INTERSTITIAL ALONE (rads)	EXTERNAL BEAM + INTERSTITIAL (rads)
TX No visible or palpable tumor	6000	Not recommended
TX Palpable induration or nodularity	7000	" "
TX Tumor at margins; gross residual	7500	5000 + 3000
Early (<1 cm)	6500	Not recommended
Early (1–3 cm)	Not recommended	3000/2 weeks + 3500
Moderately advanced (3–5 cm)	" "	3000/2 weeks + 4000
Advanced	" "	5000 ± 3500
Postoperative radiation therapy	" "	6500–7000/7–8 weeks
Preoperative radiation therapy (fixed nodes)	" "	5000/6 weeks

therapy or surgery is heralded by ulceration, pain, or increased induration. A trial of antibiotics such as tetracycline will often reduce the pain of either radiation necrosis or recurrent tumor. Recurrences have a slightly elevated or rolled border, while necroses do not. The induration associated with necrosis is usually less than with recurrence. Biopsy should be done as soon as ulceration appears, if the ulcer is within the original cancer site and if no increased morbidity is likely from the biopsy. Ulcers that appear on adjacent normal tissues (*e.g.*, the gingiva) are due to radiation effect and not cancer. Outpatient biopsies under local anesthesia may miss the tumor. If suspicion remains high for local recurrence after a negative biopsy, generous biopsies under general anesthesia are required, and even this maneuver will occasionally miss persistent tumor.

Radiation failure is managed by glossectomy. Surgical failure is occasionally salvaged by radiation therapy or an operation, if the recurrence is limited to the mucosa. Recurrence in soft tissues of the neck is rarely eradicated by any procedure.

Nodes appearing in a previously untreated neck are managed by neck dissection with or without postoperative radiation therapy.

Results of Treatment

Table 13-23 shows the local control rates for a series of 57 patients treated initially by irradiation with or without radical neck dissection. Table 13-24 shows the absolute and determinate 2- and 5-year survival rates for the University of

TABLE 13-23. Oral Tongue Carcinoma—Local Control (University of Florida, 10/64–12/77; analysis 12/79)

	NO. OF PATIENTS WITH LOCAL CONTROL/NO. TREATED					
STAGE	RADIUM OR RADIUM + <3000 RAD	RADIUM + ≥3000 RAD	EXTERNAL BEAM	RT ALONE* (TOTAL)	NO. SALVAGED/ NO. ATTEMPTS	NO. ULTIMATELY CONTROLLED/ NO. TREATED
T1	5/5	2/2	0/1	7/8	1/1	8/8
T2	†10/11	7/15	1/1	18/27	4/7	22/27
T3	0/2	7/20	0	7/22	5/10	12/22
Total	15/18	16/37	1/2	32/57	10/18	42/57

(Mendenhall WM, VanCise WS, Bova FJ et al: Analysis of time-dose factors in squamous cell carcinoma of the oral tongue and floor of mouth treated with radiation therapy alone. Int J Radiat Oncol Biol Phys (in press))

* RT: Radiotherapy

† Significance level = 0.02, Fisher's exact test.[144]

TABLE 13-24. Oral Tongue Carcinoma: Survival for Patients Treated Initially by Irradiation ± Radical Neck Dissection with Surgery Reserved for Salvage (University of Florida, 10/64–12/77; analysis 12/79)

	ABSOLUTE		DETERMINATE*	
STAGE	2 YEARS	5 YEARS	2 YEARS	5 YEARS
I	7/12 (58%)	5/11 (45%)	7/7 (100%)	5/5 (100%)
II	16/22 (73%)	10/17 (59%)	16/18 (89%)	10/14 (71%)
III	17/24 (71%)	6/20 (30%)	17/24 (71%)	6/17 (35%)
IV	9/16 (56%)	1/12 (8%)	9/10 (90%)	1/2
Total	49/74 (66%)	22/60 (37%)	49/59 (83%)	22/38 (58%)

(Mendenhall WM, VanCise WS, Bova FJ et al: Analysis of time-dose factors in squamous cell carcinoma of the oral tongue and floor of the mouth treated with radiation therapy alone. Int J Radiat Oncol Biol Phys (in press))

* Excludes patients dead of intercurrent disease.

Florida radiation therapy series.[136] Approximately 20% will die of intercurrent disease; 10% will die of distant metastases.

Complications of Treatment

SURGICAL. Orocutaneous fistula, flap necrosis, and dysphagia are the three most common complications of surgery of the tongue. Damage to the lingual nerve or the hypoglossal nerve during the course of surgery, although rare, increases the difficulty in swallowing and in speaking.

Fistula and flap necrosis must be handled judiciously since the danger of carotid artery hemorrhage increases with either of these complications.

Enunciation difficulties occur whenever the tongue is bound down by scarring; it is often difficult to predict ahead of time which patients will have difficulty. The incidence of complications increases for surgical salvage attempts after radiation failure; the patient must be willing to accept these risks and must be informed that multiple procedures may be necessary.

RADIATION THERAPY. Many patients will compain of a sensitive tongue for many months after completion of treatment, even when the mucosa is quite well healed. This is hardly surprising since the tongue has been "burned" and, like any other burned area, remains extra sensitive for a period of time. This effect usually disappears with time.

Taste will reappear from one week to several months after treatment. Taste may return to normal, but more frequently it is "not quite as keen" as before. The dryness of the mouth may contribute to the poorer sense of taste.

Return of saliva is variable, depending on the treatment volume and the dose to the salivary glands. Patients treated with interstitial therapy alone will eventually have nearly normal saliva. Patients treated with 4500 rad external beam therapy plus interstitial therapy will eventually have 25–50% return of saliva if one parotid receives 3000 rad or less.

Soft Tissue Necrosis. Soft tissue necrosis is fairly common, although frequently of minor degree. Once recurrence has been ruled out, considerable patience is required for healing. The patient associates pain with recurrence of his cancer, since the original lesion frequently caused a similar pain. He needs to be constantly reassured that the ulcer will heal slowly and that there is no evidence of recurrence. Patients who develop a true necrosis rarely get a recurrence, so in a sense, there is some good news associated with the pain.

There is no good, simple treatment for soft tissue necrosis. The treatment plan is mainly to rule out recurrent cancer, provide local and general analgesia, and reduce local infection. If the ulcerated lesion has all the earmarks of necrosis, a conservative treatment trial is instituted. The patient is placed on a biweekly or monthly examination schedule, photographs are taken, and precise drawings are made. Broad-spectrum antibiotics (*e.g.*, tetracycline, 1 gm/day), local anesthesia to be applied by a cotton-tipped applicator, and analgesics as needed are prescribed. Chewable aspirin such as Aspergum will give good analgesia if the patient can chew gum. Frequently, pain will be reduced dramatically in 1–3 days after starting antibiotics, but sometimes the response is nil. Lidocaine (Xylocaine Viscous) can be applied to the ulcer with a cotton swab for local analgesia. The authors have had little success with alcohol nerve blocks. Hyperbaric oxygen treatment may be tried in difficult cases. The authors have tried local fulguration with silver nitrate to attempt pain relief, but with little success; they also have a variable experience with cryotherapy.

When all else fails and necrosis is persistent and pain uncontrollable, the necrosis must be resected. A myocutaneous flap may be needed to fill in the void.

The key word for management of radiation necroses is *patience*.

Radiation-Induced Bone Disease. The horizontal ramus above and behind the retromolar trigone is rarely the site of radiation-induced bone disease because it is covered and protected by muscle. Anterior to the retromolar trigone, the mandible is vulnerable. The edentulous person is less likely to develop serious radiation-induced disease of the mandible than one with teeth. There are several ways in which the mandible may be affected.

The most frequent problem involving the mandible is termed "bone exposure." The gingiva disappears, exposing the underlying bone. The exposed area or areas vary from 2 mm to 2 cm in diameter. There is either very little pain or modest discomfort. In fact, if the exposed area is small, the patient is often unaware of the problem. The bone appears intact. Biopsy is not needed unless there was tumor at that point on the gingiva prior to treatment. If the patient has dentures, they should be discontinued or, in certain cases, altered by the dentist to relieve the denture over the exposed bone. If sharp bony edges appear, they are filed to a smooth contour and the bone edge lowered to speed healing. The bone exposure may become more or less stationary at this point. Healing may require months to even years. Healing occurs when the gingiva regrows over the exposed area; a small, superficial piece of bone may sequestrate first and then the gingiva regrows to cover the exposed area. Again, *patience* is the major requirement.

In some instances, the bone exposure may progress so that a large area of bone is exposed. Pain is usually intermittent and mild to moderate, and occasionally severe. Antibiotics will usually reduce pain when it does occur. Local care is similar to that used for early bone exposures. It is amazing that rampant osteomyelitis rarely develops in the exposed, relatively avascular bone.

In some cases, the bone becomes frankly osteonecrotic with intermittent sequestration. Hyperbaric oxygen treatment has been used with some success. It is a matter of individualization as to when surgical intervention should be instituted. Conservative measures should be given a fair trial, but if pain becomes a problem, an operative procedure must be considered. The dead bone is removed and replaced with tissue such as myocutaneous flap, carrying its own blood supply.

BUCCAL MUCOSA

Anatomy

The buccal mucosa is the mucous membrane covering the inner surface of the cheeks and lips. It ends above and below with a transition to the gingiva. It ends posteriorly at the retromolar trigone. The parotid duct opens into the buccal mucosa opposite the second upper molar. The blood supply is a branch of the facial artery. The long buccal nerve, a branch of the mandibular (V), is sensory to the buccal mucosa and the skin of the cheek which covers the buccinator muscle.

Pathology

The majority of malignant tumors are low-grade squamous cell carcinoma, and they frequently appear on a background of leukoplakia. Verrucous carcinoma occurs and may be particularly difficult to diagnose histologically because of associated inflammatory changes.

Patterns of Spread

Almost all of the squamous cell carcinomas originate on the lateral walls. Early lesions are usually discrete, elevated tumors, often exophytic. As they enlarge, they penetrate the underlying muscles and eventually penetrate to the skin. Peripheral growth occurs into the gingivobuccal gutters and eventually onto the gingiva and underlying bone.

Squamous cell carcinomas arising from the moist mucosa of the lips are quite uncommon. The three cases observed were all in the midline of the lower lip near the gingivolabial sulcus in the precise area where snuff was held (see the section covering minor salivary gland tumors in this chapter).

The lymphatic spread is first to the submaxillary and subdigastric nodes. The incidence of positive nodes on admission is 9–31% and the risk of occult disease is 16% (see Tables 13-1 and 13-2).

Clinical Picture

Early, asymptomatic lesions may be discovered by the dentist or physician. A background of leukoplakia is common and sometimes quite extensive. Small lesions produce the sensation of a lump that is felt with the tongue. Pain is minimal even when the lesion becomes large, unless there is posterior extension to involve the lingual and dental nerves. Pain may be referred to the ear. Obstruction of Stensen's duct will produce parotid enlargement. Extension posteriorly behind the pterygomandibular raphe or into the buccinator and masseter muscles will eventually cause trismus. Intermittent bleeding occurs when the lesion is irritated by chewing or is ulcerated by growing against the teeth.

The differential diagnosis includes lues and tuberculosis, both of which are quite uncommon. If the first biopsy report is chronic inflammation or pseudoepitheliomatous hyperplasia and there is an obvious neoplasm present, repeat biopsy is in order. Sometimes multiple repeat biopsies are required to establish the diagnosis and the physician must be persistent.

Roentgenograms of the mandible and maxilla are requested when tumor has spread onto these areas and for posterior extension.

Treatment

SELECTION OF TREATMENT MODALITY. Small lesions (less than 1 cm) may simply be excised with primary closure; small lesions that involve the anterior commissure are best treated by radiation therapy. Lesions 1–3 cm in size are usually treated by radiation therapy. These lesions can be excised and grafted, but the graft tends to shrink and become firm; this makes detection of recurrence difficult, and the cheek feels tight and uncomfortable to the patient. Larger lesions are treated by either radical surgical excision, radiation therapy, or a combination of both on an individualized basis. Preference is given to radiation therapy when the tumor invades near the commissure. Preference is given to an operation when there is invasion of the mandible or maxilla.

SURGICAL TREATMENT. Lesions that invade the mandible or maxilla require that an appropriate amount of bone be resected along with the soft tissues. Repair may require a maxillary prosthesis. Full-thickness removal of the cheek is repaired by a myocutaneous flap.

IRRADIATION TECHNIQUE. These buccal mucosa lesions are suited for treatment with electrons, intraoral cone, and interstitial techniques to spare the contralateral normal tissues. When tumor extends into one of the gingivobuccal gutters or onto bone, treatment must be entirely by external beam. A lead block placed in the mouth will help decrease radiation to the opposite side. There are no data on the dose required for control.

Results of Treatment

Ash reports 35% absolute 5-year survival for 374 patients with carcinoma of the buccal mucosa for all stages.[6] The primary lesion was initially controlled in 53% of patients with early lesions and 25% with advanced lesions; salvage raised the ultimate control rates to 69% and 34%. The initial treatment to the primary lesion was radiation therapy in 97% of the patients.

Complications of Treatment

The buccal mucosa is quite tolerant of high-dose radiation therapy and complications are uncommon. Bone exposure may appear on the mandible or maxilla. Trismus may develop if the muscles of mastication receive high doses.

Surgical injury of Stensen's duct may cause obstruction and parotitis. The parotid gland will eventually atrophy.

GINGIVA AND HARD PALATE (INCLUDING RETROMOLAR TRIGONE)

Carcinomas arising from the upper and lower gingiva have a similar clinical picture and require a similar approach to diagnosis. Primary squamous cell carcinoma of the hard palate is quite unusual, the majority of hard palate neoplasms being minor salivary gland tumors (see section on minor salivary glands). Some authors include the retromolar trigone with the anterior tonsillar pillar, but in their natural history and management, these lesions are more similar to lesions of the lower gingiva.

Anatomy

The lower gingiva includes the mucosa covering the mandible from the gingivobuccal gutter to the origin of the mobile mucosa on the floor of the mouth. Behind the third molar is a small triangular surface covering the ascending ramus that is called the retromolar trigone; it is continuous above with the maxillary tuberosity.

Beneath the mucosa of the retromolar trigone is the tendinous pterygomandibular raphe, which is attached to the pterygoid hamulus and the posterior mylohyoid ridge of the mandible and serves as the insertion of the buccinator, orbicular oris, and superior constrictor muscles. Just behind the pterygomandibular raphe and between the medial pterygoid and the ascending ramus is the pterygomandibular space, which contains the lingual and dental nerves. The pterygomandibular space is related posteriorly to the deep lobe of the parotid and the contents of the parapharyngeal space.

There are no minor salivary glands in the mucous membrane over the alveolar ridges.

Pathology

The majority of neoplasms are squamous cell carcinoma. Verrucous lesions occur, usually on the lower gingiva. Melanoma is reported. Metastatic lesions to the underlying bone may be confused with primary tumors.

Epidermoid carcinoma may arise within the body of the mandible or maxilla (intraalveolar epidermoid carcinoma) either from odontogenic epithelium or from epithelium trapped during embryonic development. It is more frequent in the mandible than the maxilla, and is most common in the molar regions. It must be distinguished from metastatic squamous cell carcinoma and ameloblastoma.

Ameloblastoma is a rare tumor with an incidence of about 1% of all tumors of the maxilla and mandible. Most patients are in the age range of 20–50 years. Some 80% occur in the mandible with the molar-ramus region most commonly involved. No appreciable differences are found by sex or race.[145]

Histologically, the ameloblastoma is an epithelial tumor. The epithelium forms sheets or islands, and the peripheral layer is formed by atypical columnar cells.[146] The lesion may appear histologically benign, but is expansive and tends to recur locally.[147] Ameloblastoma is histologically similar to basal cell carcinoma.

Patterns of Spread

LOWER GUMS. Squamous cell carcinomas invade the periosteum and adjacent buccal mucosa and floor of mouth. Slow-growing, low-grade lesions tend to produce atrophy of adjacent bone and produce a smooth, saucerized defect before invading the mandible. Moderate- to high-grade lesions invade the bone directly or through recently opened dental sockets.

Lymphatic spread is to the submaxillary and subdigastric nodes. Eighteen to 52% have clinically positive nodes on admission; occult disease occurs in 17–19% (see Tables 13-1 and 13-2).

Ameloblastoma is a rather indolent tumor that destroys bone and slowly extends to adjacent areas by contiguous growth. Regional and even distant metastasis may occur in a few cases, but even when present, is compatible with a long natural course.

Metastatic disease is usually reported in the lungs, but bone and liver metastases have been reported.[148]

UPPER GUM AND HARD PALATE. Most of the carcinomas originate on the gingiva and spread secondarily to the hard palate, sofe palate, buccal mucosa, and underlying bone; the maxillary antrum is invaded quite late unless there are recent extractions that provide an open pathway. Primary carcinoma of the lower maxillary antrum must be excluded since it frequently presents in the upper gum and hard palate. The risk for positive lymph nodes is 13–24% on admission, and the incidence of occult disease is 22% (see Tables 13-1 and 13-2).

RETROMOLAR TRIGONE. The retromolar trigone is a small area, and spread to adjacent buccal mucosa, anterior tonsillar pillar, and maxilla occurs quite early. Posterior spread occurs early into the pterygomandibular space and the medial pterygoid muscle. Posterolateral spread occurs into the buccinator muscle and fat pad.

The submaxillary and subdigastric lymph nodes are the first relay.

The incidence of clinically positive nodes on presentation is about 40%, and the risk for occult disease about 25%.

Clinical Picture

The patient with squamous cell carcinoma may present first to the dentist with either ill-fitting dentures, dental pain, loose teeth, or a sore that will not heal. A history of inappropriate dental extractions or root canal therapy is common. Intermittent bleeding and mild pain occur when the lesion is traumatized. Invasion into the mandible may involve the inferior dental nerve and produce paresthesias or anesthesia of the lower lip. A background of leukoplakia is frequently present.

Retromolar trigone lesions, which involve the lingual and inferior dental nerve, cause local pain and pain referred to the external auditory canal and pre-auricular area. Invasion of the pterygoid muscle produces trismus, usually accompanied by severe pain.

Intra-alveolar epidermoid carcinoma presents with a submucosal mass and dental symptoms. Roentgenograms show a lytic lesion in the mandible.

Ameloblastoma is a slow-growing neoplasm with few symptoms in the early stages. Patients may notice a gradually increasing facial deformity or loosening of teeth in the area of tumor.[149]

On roentgenograms, a radiolucent area is seen with some of the following features: expansion of the overlying cortical plate, a scalloped margin, a multilocular appearance, or resorption of the roots of adjacent teeth.[150]

Methods of Diagnosis and Staging

The differential diagnosis includes dental disease and underlying bony cysts or tumors, including metastatic tumors.

Roentgenograms, including tomograms when needed, are required for almost all lesions. Dental roentgenograms should be used where fine detail is needed to look for early invasion.

It may be difficult to exclude early bone invasion when recent extractions have been done.

The American Joint Committee staging system for oral cavity lesions is difficult to apply to gum lesions. In fact, the possibility of mandible invasion is not even considered. Evidence of lytic bone invasion should qualify for T4. Since even small lesions (less than 2 cm) may invade bone, there will be a wide prognostic range for T4 tumors. Swearingen and coworkers report a 56% incidence of mandible involvement for gum lesions and 10% for retromolar trigone lesions.[151]

Treatment

SELECTION OF TREATMENT MODALITY. *Lower Gum.* The majority of lesions are managed by operation. Small lesions may be remedied by simple excision or a rim resection with split-thickness skin graft. When bone invasion is present, removal of a section of mandible is required. A neck dissection is included with mandibulectomy since the neck is entered in any event. Large lesions require hemimandibulectomy. Irradiation may be used for small lesions or those with only a pressure defect in the bone with good curative results, but the functional results are generally better after operation.

Ameloblastoma. The initial treatment of ameloblastoma is an operation, but local recurrence is a problem. Sehdev and coworkers report that curettage was followed by local recurrence in 90% of mandibular and all maxillary ameloblastomas.[148] Subsequent resection controlled 80% of the mandibular, but only 40% of the maxillary tumors. The initial use of segmental mandibular resection controlled 78% (18/23) with subsequent resection controlling those that failed. The use of partial maxillectomy as the first treatment controlled 100% (7/7) of maxillary ameloblastomas as opposed to only 40% when partial maxillectomy was performed for recurrence. Hemimandibulectomy controlled 100% of curettage failures in one series.[152]

The lesions respond quite readily to irradiation. However, since radiation therapy has generally been applied to patients only after multiple operative failures and in cases of advanced disease, the curative ability is not clear.

Retromolar Trigone. Small retromolar trigone lesions may appear innocuous and easily cured, but are often more extensive than they seem; early bone invasion not detected on roentgenograms is common. For early lesions without detectable bone invasion, a rim resection may be done to preserve continuity of the mandible. Evidence of bone invasion requires partial mandibulectomy. Preference is given to surgical treatment unless the cosmetic and functional result would be unacceptable to the patient, in which case operation is reserved for radiation therapy failure. Moderately advanced lesions are usually managed by resection followed by postoperative radiation therapy.

Upper Gum and Hard Palate. Surgical resection is the usual treatment for most lesions of the upper gum. Postoperative radiation therapy is added as needed. Squamous cell carcinoma on the hard palate is rare. If the lesion is superficial and extensively involves the hard palate or involves a significant portion of the soft palate, then radiation therapy should be used. If the lesion is small and discrete and there is no bone involvement, the resection includes the periosteum or occasionally some underlying bone. Bone invasion requires a partial maxillectomy. The defect is filled with a prosthesis.

SURGICAL TREATMENT. *Segmental Mandibulectomy.* For small lesions with minimal bone invasion, a short section of mandible is removed in continuity with the tumor (*e.g.*, removal of the mandible from the angle to the mental foramen).

Partial Mandibulectomy. The mandible and tumor are resected from the mental foramen anteriorly to include the coronoid process posteriorly, usually leaving the head of the condyle. The remaining mandible is stabilized by a K wire or a cobalt-chromium alloy (Vitallium) mesh spacer if there are teeth; if there are no teeth, no spacer is used. In certain cases, the mandible may be reconstructed at a later date, but few patients actually request the procedure since the cosmetic and functional loss is acceptable.

Hemimandibulectomy. Extensive lesions may require removal of the mandible from symphysis to condyle on one side. Massive anterior lesions require removal of the mandible from angle to angle. This produces a major cosmetic and functional loss and is reconstructed with flaps and metal trays.

IRRADIATION TECHNIQUE. Small lesions of the lower gum and retromolar trigone may be treated by intraoral cone for all or part of their therapy. Well-lateralized lesions are treated by ipsilateral mixed beam techniques with a lead intraoral stent. Anterior lesions are treated by parallel opposed portals.

The dose for retromolar trigone lesions is 7000 rad/7 weeks for T1-2; 7500 rad/7 weeks for T3 (See Table 13-8). The dose for gum lesions is similar. Local control by radiation therapy alone for lesions with early bone invasion is approximately 50% and for extensive invasion about 25% (Fayos JV: Personal communication, 1973).[153]

MANAGEMENT OF RECURRENCE. Radiation therapy failures may be salvaged by operation. Surgical failures may be salvaged by surgery, radiation therapy, or a combination of both (see Tables 13-25, 13-26, and 13-27).

Results of Treatment

Tables 13-25, 13-26, and 13-27 show the analysis of local control for lower gum, retromolar trigone, and upper gum lesions.[154] The high rate of local failure with radiation therapy alone for true retromolar trigone lesions is not explained by low dose or marginal failure. Thus, the authors' preference is to operate on these lesions. The absolute survival for 43 patients was 56% at 2 years and 34% at 5 years.

Cady and Catlin report an absolute 5-year survival rate of 43% for patients with lower gum lesions and 40% for upper gum lesions treated by surgery.[9]

Complications of Treatment

Surgical complications include orocutaneous fistula, bone exposure with sequestration, and loss of graft or flap.

TABLE 13-25. Carcinoma of the Lower Gum: Local control—19 Patients (University of Florida, 11/64–12/74; analysis 4/77)

STAGE	TREATMENT—NO. OF PATIENTS	PRIMARY RECURRENCE	SALVAGE* S/S	SALVAGE* RT/S	ULTIMATE LOCAL CONTROL
T1–2	Surgery—3	2	0/0	0/1	1/3
	Radiation—7	4	2/2	0/0	5/7
T3–4	Surgery—4	3	0/1	1/1	2/4
	Radiation—1	0	0/0	0/0	1/1
	Surgery + radiation—4	2	0/1	0/0	2/4

(Gefter JW: Carcinoma of the gums and retromolar trigone. 7th Annual Radiation Therapy Clinical Research Seminar, April 21–23, 1977, pp 191–210. Gainesville, Florida, Radiation Therapy Division, University of Florida, 1978)
* S/S—surgical salvage (no. salvaged/no. attempted); RT/S—radiation therapy salvage (no. salvaged/no. attempted).

TABLE 13-26. Carcinoma of the Retromolar Tongue: Local Control—15 Patients (University of Florida, 11/64–12/74; analysis 4/77)

STAGE	TREATMENT—NO. OF PATIENTS	PRIMARY RECURRENCE	SALVAGE* S/S	SALVAGE* RT/S	ULTIMATE LOCAL CONTROL
T1–2	Radiation—5	3	0/1	0/0	2/5
	Surgery + radiation—1	1	0/1	0/0	0/1
T3–4	Surgery—1	0	0/0	0/0	1/1
	Radiation—2	2	0/0	0/0	0/2
	Surgery + radiation—6	2	0/0	0/0	4/6

(Gefter JW: Carcinoma of the gums and retromolar trigone. 7th Annual Radiation Therapy Clinical Research Seminar, April 21–23, 1977, pp 191–210. Gainesville, Florida, Radiation Therapy Division, University of Florida, 1978)
* S/S—surgical salvage (no. salvaged/no. attempted); RT/S—radiation therapy salvage (no. salvaged/no. attempted)

TABLE 13-27. Carcinoma of the Upper Gum: Local Control—5 Patients (University of Florida, 11/64–12/74; analysis 4/77)

STAGE	TREATMENT—NO. OF PATIENTS	PRIMARY RECURRENCE	SALVAGE* S/S	SALVAGE* RT/S	ULTIMATE LOCAL CONTROL
T1–2	Radiation—3	3	2/2	0/1	2/3
T3–4	Surgery + radiation—2	2	0/0	1/1	1/2

(Gefter JW: Carcinoma of the gums and retromolar trigone. 7th Annual Radiation Therapy Clinical Research Seminar, April 21–23, 1977, pp 191–210. Gainesville, Florida, Radiation Therapy Division, University of Florida, 1978)
* S/S—surgical salvage (no. salvaged/no. attempted); RT/S—radiation therapy salvage (no. salvaged/no. attempted)

The complications of radiation therapy include soft tissue necrosis with bone exposure and subsequent osteoradionecrosis. The risk is greatest for patients with advanced lesions of the lower gum and retromolar trigone.

Eight patients in the University of Florida series had attempted surgical salvage, which was successful in four. Complications included fistula, wound infection requiring removal of bone graft, and chronic aspiration requiring a gastric tube. Four patients had attempted salvage by radiation therapy, which was successful in two. There were no complications.

OROPHARYNX

The oropharynx includes four areas: the base of tongue, the tonsillar region (tonsillar fossa and tonsillar pillars), the soft palate, and that portion of the pharyngeal wall between the pharyngoepiglottic fold and the nasopharynx. The pharyngeal walls will be considered in the section on the hypopharynx.

ANATOMY

The base of tongue is bounded anteriorly by the circumvallate papillae, laterally by the glossotonsillar sulci, and posteriorly by the epiglottis. The vallecula is a 1 cm, smooth strip of mucosa that is the transition from the base of tongue to the epiglottis; it is considered as part of the base of tongue. The surface of the base of tongue appears irregular and "bumpy" due to scattered submucosal lymphoid follicles; the mucous membrane itself is actually smooth compared to the dorsum of the oral tongue. The surface of the base of tongue lies in a nearly vertical position with the tongue at rest.

The musculature of the base of tongue is continuous with that of the oral tongue. Fig. 13-15 is a midsagittal section through the oropharynx which shows important relationships with neighboring sites. Fig. 13-16 is a cross-section through the oropharynx, showing relationships to the lateral pharyngeal space.

The tonsillar area is a triangular region bounded anteriorly by the anterior tonsillar pillar (palatoglossal muscle), posteriorly by the posterior tonsillar pillar (palatopharyngeal muscle), and inferiorly by the glossotonsillar sulcus and pharyngoepiglottic fold. The palatine tonsil lies within the triangle. The tonsillar region is bounded laterally by the pharyngeal constrictor muscle and its fascia, the mandible, and the lateral pharyngeal space.

The tonsillar area is separated from the base of tongue by the glossotonsillar sulcus. The narrow sulcus lies in a vertical plane between the anterior tonsillar pillar and the pharyngoepiglottic fold. Beneath the mucous membrane of the sulcus are the styloglossal muscle and the stylohyoid ligament.

The soft palate is a thin, mobile muscle complex that separates the nasopharynx from the oral cavity and oropharynx. The epithelium of the oral surface of the soft palate is squamous and the epithelium of the nasopharyngeal surface is respiratory. The soft palate is continuous laterally with the tonsillar pillars.

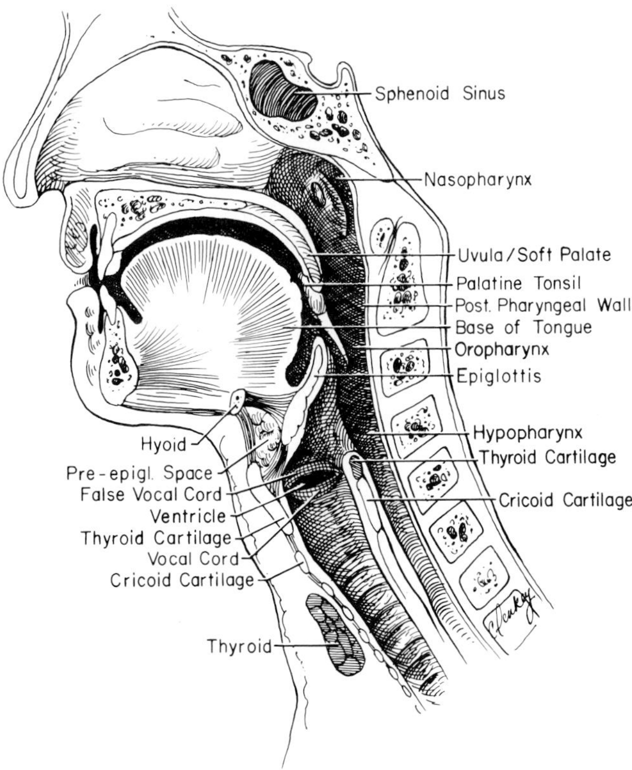

FIG. 13-15. Sagittal section of the upper aerodigestive tract.

PATHOLOGY

Squamous cell carcinoma or one of its variants accounts for 95% of malignant lesions. Lymphoepitheliomas occur in the tonsil and base of tongue. Verrucous carcinomas occur rarely. Malignant lymphomas account for approximately 5% of tonsillar and 1–2% of base of tongue malignancies. Minor salivary gland malignancies, plasmacytomas, and other rare tumors make up the remainder.

PATTERNS OF SPREAD

Base of Tongue

PRIMARY. Squamous cell carcinoma of the base of tongue tends to early, silent, deep infiltration. The tumor tends to

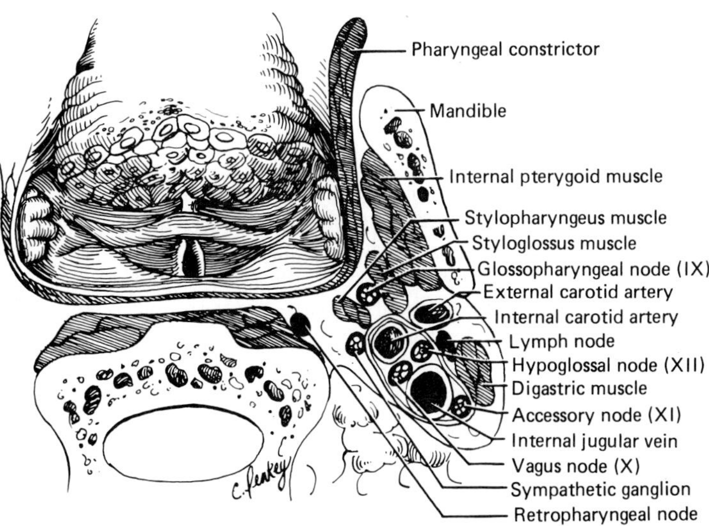

FIG. 13-16. Section at the level of the mid-oropharynx, depicting relationships in the parapharyngeal area.

remain in the base of tongue unless it begins at the very peripheral margin. Vallecular lesions spread along the mucosa to the lingual surface of the epiglottis, laterally along the pharyngoepiglottic fold, and then to the lateral pharyngeal wall and anterior wall of the pyriform sinus. They frequently penetrate through the thin mucous membrane of the vallecula; tumor spread is contained for a while by the hyoepiglottic ligament, but this thin, often incomplete structure is eventually breached and cancer enters the pre-epiglottic space.

Lesions that begin on the lateral base of tongue may invade the glossotonsillar sulcus. Deep penetration in the glossotonsillar sulcus allows tumor to escape into the neck, since there is no effective muscular barrier at this point. The mylohyoid muscle is an effective barrier for oral tongue lesions, but the mylohyoid terminates near the angle of the mandible. A tumor mass may be palpable below the angle of the mandible and be confused with an involved lymph node.

Advanced lesions tend to spread toward the larynx or oral tongue; spread into the parapharyngeal space is a late event.

LYMPHATICS. The first-echelon nodes are the subdigastric; the path of spread is then along the jugular chain to the midjugular and lower jugular nodes. The submaxillary nodes may become involved if tumor extends anteriorly into the oral tongue or if massive upper neck disease is present. Submental spread is rare. The posterior cervical nodes are involved often enough to be included in treatment plans.

Approximately 75% of patients with base of tongue cancer will have clinically positive neck nodes on admission; 30% will have bilateral nodes. The incidence of occult disease in clinically negative necks is reported at 22% but this figure is undoubtedly low, considering the selection of these patients for operation and the use of preoperative irradiation.[29]

Tonsillar Area

The tonsillar area includes the anterior and posterior tonsillar pillars and the tonsillar fossa. Some authors group the retromolar trigone lesions with those of the anterior tonsillar pillar. However, the retromolar trigone lesions are more appropriately considered as oral cavity lesions and grouped with the gingival (gum) lesions.

There are subtle differences in the spread patterns, clinical findings, treatment, and prognosis within the tonsillar area. When the lesions are early, the site of origin may be determined, but the more advanced lesions usually involve most, if not all, of the tonsillar area.

ANTERIOR TONSILLAR PILLAR. Almost all malignant tumors arising on the anterior tonsillar pillar are squamous cell carcinomas. The lesions tend to be early when diagnosed and have relatively little bulk or infiltration and therefore a good prognosis. Asymptomatic lesions are common and may be red lesions, white lesions, or a mixture of both. Their borders are usually indistinct. As the lesions progress they may develop a central ulcer with a rolled margin and infiltrate the palatoglossus. Superior medial spread occurs onto the soft palate, the most posterior hard palate, and the maxillary gingiva. Anterolateral spread to the retromolar trigone is frequent with later spread to the posterior gingivobuccal sulcus and buccal mucosa. Once tumor gains access to the buccal mucosa there is a threat for considerable anterior occult extension in the buccal pouch as exemplified by the occasional example of an anterior marginal failure in patients treated by irradiation or operation.

Invasion of the tongue is frequent; careful palpation may be necessary to distinguish the early submucosal nodule at the junction of the anterior tonsillar pillar and tongue.

As these lesions advance, they adhere to the mandible and eventually invade the bone. Extension toward the base of the skull and nasopharynx is a late phenomenon usually associated with infiltration of the medial pterygoid muscle and possible erosion of the medial pterygoid plate; such lesions produce trismus and marked temporal pain.

TONSILLAR FOSSA. Tonsillar fossa lesions arise either from the remnants of the palatine tonsil or from the mucous membrane within the triangle. There are a few differences in the development and spread patterns for squamous cell carcinoma of the tonsillar fossa compared to anterior tonsillar pillar lesions. Leukoplakia rarely occurs within the fossa, and asymptomatic red mucosal lesions are infrequently seen. The initial lesions tend to be exophytic with central ulceration plus an infiltrative component. Extension to the posterior tonsillar pillar and the oropharyngeal wall occurs early. Invasion into the glossotonsillar sulcus and base of tongue occurs in approximately 25% of cases. As the lesions advance, they penetrate to the parapharyngeal space and gain access to the base of the skull superiorly. Cranial nerve involvement, however, is uncommon. Advanced lesions invade the mandible, nasopharynx, and base of tongue and may extend below the pharyngoepiglottic fold into the pyriform sinus.

POSTERIOR TONSILLAR PILLAR. Early lesions arising from the posterior tonsillar pillar are uncommon and for some unknown reason have an evil reputation. The only two lesions the authors have seen were 1.0–1.5 cm discrete lesions with a raised border and central ulceration. Both were cured by radiation therapy. There are two major differences in their potential spread patterns. They may spread inferiorly along the palatopharyngeal muscle to its insertions into the middle pharyngeal constrictor, the pharyngo-epiglottic fold, and the posterior border of the thyroid cartilage. Second, the lymphatic trunks of the posterior tonsillar pillar are theoretically more likely to spread to the spinal accessory nodes and the high jugular chain node (*i.e.*, the nasopharyngeal node).

Soft Palate

Nearly all soft palate squamous cell carcinomas occur on the oral side of the palate. The nasopharyngeal side seems nearly immune to tumor production. Even large tumors of the nasopharynx avoid secondary invasion of the soft palate.

The earliest tumors are red lesions with ill-defined borders. White lesions are common on the soft palate and may be leukoplakia, carcinoma *in situ*, or early invasive carcinoma. Multiple sites of involvement with normal-appearing intervening mucosa are a common finding, dramatically demonstrated during the first week of radiation therapy when a tumoritis "lights up" the tumor sites, some of which are unsuspected.

The majority of soft palate carcinomas are diagnosed while still confined to the soft palate and adjacent pillars. The diameter of the lesions may qualify as T2 (2–4 cm) or T3 (>4 cm), but the lesions may be rather thin with a relatively small tumor volume compared to a T2 or T3 lesion of the base of tongue or tonsillar fossa. Spread from the soft palate occurs first to the tonsillar pillars and hard palate. Lateral spread may eventually penetrate the superior constrictor muscle with subsequent invasion of the medial pterygoid muscle and base of skull, and occasionally compression or invasion of cranial nerves in the parapharyngeal space. Involvement of the lateral wall(s) of the nasopharynx is common in advanced lesions, which may cause perforation or ulcerative destruction of part of the soft palate.

LYMPHATIC. The spread pattern is first to the subdigastric node and then along the jugular chain. The submaxillary, submental, and spinal accessory nodes are less commonly involved.

Approximately 56% of patients will have clinically positive nodes on admission; 16% will have bilateral nodes. The incidence of occult disease is not well-established since the first-echelon nodes are usually irradiated in all but the earliest lesions. Lindberg and coworkers noted an approximately 20% incidence of occult disease following either no or partial neck irradiation with the primary controlled.[26] The incidence of clinically positive nodes increases with T stage: 8% positive for T1, 36% for T2, and about 66% for T3 and T4.

CLINICAL PICTURE

Base of Tongue

PRESENTING SYMPTOMS. Asymptomatic lesions are rarely diagnosed since the base of tongue is visualized only by indirect mirror examination.

The earliest symptom is often a mild sore throat. The patient may sense a lump in the back of the tongue, and actually feel it by digital palpation; the patient is not amused by the physician who cannot see the lesion with a tongue depressor and fails to palpate the base of tongue. Since many of the early lesions are relatively silent, a subdigastric neck mass, often quite large, is often the first sign. The patient may insist that a 5 cm or larger neck mass "came about overnight." In a sense, the patient is correct. Small clinically positive lymph nodes 1–4 cm in diameter are almost always asymptomatic. Sudden enlargement occurs due to necrosis or internal bleeding with rapid increase in size and mild tenderness. Difficulty swallowing, a nasal voice quality, and deep-seated ear pain occur as the lesion enlarges (See Fig. 13-12). The earache is different from that produced by oral cavity and hypopharyngeal lesions.

Far-advanced lesions fix the tongue. Deep ulceration and necrosis result in foul breath.

Indirect mirror examination, digital palpation, and a high level of suspicion are the ingredients for diagnosis of early lesions of the base of tongue. Since early lesions are often submucosal and relatively soft and since the base of tongue is irregular, diagnosis is often a challenge. The rigid fiberoptic telescope will allow examination in some patients not easily visualized by indirect mirror examination, and the flexible fiberoptic laryngoscope allows outpatient examination by way of the nose. A small lesion originating in the glossotonsillar sulcus area may ulcerate and produce symptoms quite early; it may be overlooked unless the area is critically examined.

Lymphomas are usually large, entirely submucosal masses, suspected by their appearance. Minor salivary gland tumors are also usually submucosal, but more discrete and firm than lymphomas.

Tonsillar Area

ANTERIOR TONSILLAR PILLAR. Asymptomatic lesions are frequently found on routine examination by both dentists and physicians. Early symptoms include sore throat, usually aggravated by food or drink. Pain is referred to the ear as soon as ulceration takes place. If the lesion involves the hard palate or posterior upper gum, dentures may fit improperly or cause irritation. Advanced lesions invade the pterygoid or buccinator muscle and produce trismus and temporal pain. Invasion of the tongue will eventually limit tongue mobility and, when accompanied by ulceration at the junction of the anterior tonsillar pillar and oral tongue, causes a great deal of pain.

TONSILLAR FOSSA. Signs and symptoms are similar to those for anterior tonsillar pillar lesions except that the lesions tend to be larger before symptoms develop. Ipsilateral sore throat is the hallmark of these lesions. Detection by visual examination with a tongue depressor is sufficient for most lesions of the tonsillar fossa; however, a few cancers arise near the glossotonsillar sulcus or lower pole of the tonsillar area and are only visible by indirect examination. A few patients will present with a node in the neck. Lymphomas of the tonsil tend to be large submucosal masses, but may ulcerate and appear similar to carcinomas.

Soft Palate

The earliest symptom is usually mild sore throat, often aggravated by food or drink. The sore throat is not well localized; discomfort may improve temporarily if antibiotics are given. Advanced lesions interfere with swallowing and may cause a voice change. Regurgitation of food and liquid into the nasopharynx and nose occurs with destruction, perforation, or fixation of the soft palate. Lateral and superior spread to the nasopharynx and parapharyngeal space is associated with trismus, otitis media, temporal headache, and, occasionally, cranial nerve involvement.

Early lesions appear as red, white, or mixed changes in the mucosa; the mucosa may appear roughened. The margins are ill-defined. Multiple foci on the soft palate and anterior tonsillar pillars are common. Moderately advanced lesions have rolled edges with central ulceration, or they may be mainly exophytic, particularly around the uvula. The nasopharynx should be inspected and palpated for submucosal extension along the lateral wall; extension along the nasopharyngeal surface of the soft palate is uncommon until quite late. Extension to the posterior nasal cavity is seen only in advanced lesions that erode the posterior hard palate.

METHODS OF DIAGNOSIS AND STAGING

Most lesions of the oropharynx can be biopsied by incisional or punch forceps biopsy under local anesthesia in the outpatient clinic. Base of tongue lesions may require general anesthesia. Frozen section control is helpful in base of tongue lesions since it is sometimes difficult to obtain representative tissue. Special handling of tissue is required if lymphoma is suspected.

Early lesions are staged by physical examination; direct laryngoscopy under general anesthesia may be required for base of tongue/vallecula lesions. Mandible films and tomograms of the base of skull are obtained when involvement is suspected.

Staging

All oropharyngeal sites are included in one T stage system:[39]

TIS	Carcinoma *in situ*
T1	Tumor 2 cm or less in greatest diameter
T2	Tumor more than 2 cm, but not more than 4 cm in greatest diameter
T3	Tumor more than 4 cm in greatest diameter
T4	Massive tumor more than 4 cm in diameter with invasion of bone, soft tissues of neck, or root (deep musculature) of tongue

T1 and T2 are simply measurements of size and easy to apply. There is a tendency to overestimate the size of lesions in the oropharynx; insertion of a measuring device will help judge the maximum diameter. The difference between T3 and T4 is not so easily determined. Bone involvement is uncommon, but must be seen on roentgenograms to qualify. Invasion of soft tissues of the neck requires some judgment. Tumors of the tonsillar area or base of tongue that penetrate the glossotonsillar sulcus can frequently be palpated as a deep mass just under the angle of the jaw and qualify as T4 if the primary is larger than 4 cm in diameter. Invasion of the root or deep musculature of the tongue is easy to diagnose if the tongue is partially fixed. If a base of tongue cancer can be palpated easily through the lateral floor of mouth or in the submentum, then invasion of deep muscle has probably occurred. Tonsillar lesions that produce trismus or cranial nerve palsy or invade the nasopharynx should be classified as T4.

TREATMENT: BASE OF TONGUE

Selection of Treatment Modality

Although a few surgically-oriented centers continue to recommend glossectomy as the treatment of choice, irradiation is the more commonly prescribed treatment. Operation and irradiation produce similar cure rates for early base of tongue lesions, but since excision of the base of tongue generally causes greater disability, radiation therapy is the treatment of choice for the majority of lesions, with operation reserved for salvage of radiation therapy failures. Radiation therapy automatically encompasses the neck nodes on both sides of the neck. Extended supraglottic laryngectomy may be used for limited lateralized base of tongue lesions, but there are definite criteria that must be satisfied, and this selection limits its usefulness. The following conditions must be met: no gross involvement of the pharyngo-epiglottic fold; preservation of one lingual artery; resection of less than 80% of the base of tongue; pulmonary function suitable for supraglottic laryngectomy; and medical condition suitable for a major operation. At least an ipsilateral neck dissection is indicated, but with the high risk of bilateral neck disease even in the NO patient, this represents incomplete treatment. Finally, the surgeon has difficulty determining tumor extent in the tongue at the time of excision. Postoperative irradiation may have to be administered in any event for close margins or for fear of neck failure. Therefore, radiation therapy is usually the treatment of choice for the primary lesion with neck dissection added as needed (see section on the principles of treatment).

Surgical Treatment

The surgical approach for small neoplasms of the base of the tongue is either by splitting the lip, mandible, and tongue in the midline to reach the base of tongue, or to divide the mandible near the angle and approach the base of tongue in that fashion. After the tumor has been removed, the mandible is wired together. Only one lingual artery may be sacrificed. A radical neck dissection is done in continuity with excision of the base of tongue lesion. Removal of large base of tongue tumors requires simultaneous removal of part or all of the larynx.

Irradiation Technique

The irradiation of base of tongue cancer is basically accomplished by parallel opposed external beam portals that also encompass the regional nodes on both sides. Interstitial implants may be used for part of the treatment if the lesion is small, discrete, and located in the anterolateral base of tongue. Implants of posterior lesions are technically difficult; these implants are usually accomplished with a flexible source (*e.g.*, Iridium-192 ribbons), which allow through-and-through implantation from the base of tongue to the skin. There is no proven advantage in local control for interstitial as opposed to external beam treatment alone. (For oral tongue cancer, there is no doubt that interstitial treatment improves local control compared to external beam therapy alone.) Base of tongue lesions have a fairly good local control rate with external beam therapy alone. The base of tongue has quite a good vascular supply and tolerates rather high doses of radiation without soft tissue necrosis; most necroses appear in the glossotonsillar sulcus.

A boost of 1000–1500 rad may be delivered to the base of tongue by way of the submental route without traversing the mandible. The submental boost may be given with high-energy electrons or a photon beam with a superior angle to avoid the previously irradiated spinal cord. The submental boost has proven rather successful, partly because of the high dose achieved and the relatively small volume irradiated. It is selected for those base of tongue lesions that are central and posterior. Lateral lesions that involve the glossotonsillar sulcus lie immediately adjacent to the mandible; the tumor would be on the edge of the submental boost portal and would be underdosed. Large lesions that extend into the oral tongue near the junction with the anterior tonsillar pillar area are not suited for submental boost since the distance from the skin to the tongue surface is several centimeters and the portal is inefficient; an interstitial boost or reduced lateral portals are used for the final dose in these cases.

The doses usually prescribed are outlined in Table 13-8. Split-course techniques resulted in poorer local control and are not used. The usual dose per fraction is 180–200 rad; after 5000 rad, the treatment volume is reduced and the daily fraction is increased to 200–225 rad if patient tolerance is satisfactory.

One of the common errors in planning external beam portals is failure to recognize anterior growth of neoplasm as measured by palpation through the lateral floor of mouth.

The inferior border of the lateral portals is usually the thyroid notch unless tumor has extended into the upper pyriform sinus, lateral pharyngeal wall, or pre-epiglottic space. Extension of the lateral borders below the thyroid notch greatly increases mucosal and spinal cord irradiation.

The skin and subcutaneous fat in the submental area should be shielded, if possible, since high-dose radiation therapy to this area produces considerable fibrosis. It may not be possible to shield this area if the patient is quite thin or if tumor is bulging into the mylohyoid muscle.

Management of the lymphatics is critical. One of the major advantages of radiation therapy is the ease of irradiating all the nodes at risk. Even small, well-lateralized base of tongue lesions will spread to the opposite neck, and both sides are always treated. The primary portals include the upper jugular and submaxillary node(s). The superior border is approximately 2 cm above the tip of the mastoid even with clinically negative nodes to ensure coverage of the nodes near the base of skull.

The lower neck nodes on both sides are always treated. If the upper neck is clinically negative, the lower neck portals are carefully tailored to exclude as much normal tissue as possible; the midjugular nodes are the major risk area in this situation. If the upper neck is clinically positive, the lower neck portals become more generous.

Combined Treatment Policies

Combined treatment is seldom selected since an operation for moderately advanced lesions usually implies major functional loss, and few patients are willing to accept the morbidity and possible immediate mortality. The most common indication for offering glossectomy and laryngectomy is a lesion that is simply failing to respond to irradiation after 5000 rad. However, if the patient is offered and accepts a glossectomy-laryngectomy, the authors would prefer an immediate operation followed by postoperative radiation therapy.

Management of Recurrence

A painful ulcer must be biopsied to distinguish between recurrence and radiation necrosis; general anesthesia is usually necessary to obtain representative tissue. Radiation failures are treated surgically, but salvage is infrequent except for T1 lesions. At the University of Florida there have been 36 patients with local failure; 11 had a salvage operation, but only two were salvaged. Fletcher reports surgical salvage of radiation failure in two of nine patients with T1 disease, one of 13 T3, and two of 15 T4.[155]

Surgical failures are rarely salvaged by either an operation or radiation therapy, except for the early lesion with a discrete local recurrence in the base of tongue.

Recurrence of a small, discrete primary may be managed by a wide local excision. The remaining recurrences require either a jaw-tongue-neck resection or glossectomy/laryngectomy.

RESULTS OF TREATMENT: BASE OF TONGUE

Surgical Results

Whicker and coworkers of the Mayo Clinic report 102 patients selected for curative attempts by operation; 23 received pre- or postoperative radiation therapy.[156] Eleven were irradiation failures. Some 23% required partial or total laryngectomy; 56% had positive nodes in the specimen. The operative mortality was 4% with a 27% local recurrence rate and 10% neck failure rate. The 5-year survival was 37%.

Irradiation Results

Table 13-28 shows the local control and salvage rates for 69 patients treated for cure by irradiation.[157] Fig. 13-17 gives

TABLE 13-28. Base of Tongue Carcinoma—Local Control (69 Patients*, University of Florida, 9/64–9/77; analysis 9/79)

T STAGE (NO. PATIENTS)	LOCAL CONTROL BY RADIATION THERAPY ALONE	NO. SALVAGED/ NO. OF OPERATIONS ATTEMPTED	ULTIMATE CONTROL
T1 (8)	6 (75%)	0/2	6 (75%)
T2 (15)	10 (67%)	1/3	11 (73%)
T3 (22)	14 (64%)	0/1	14 (64%)
T4 (24)	3 (13%)	1/5	4 (17%)

(Parsons JT, Million RR, Cassisi NJ: Carcinoma of the base of tongue: Results of radical irradiation with surgery reserved for irradiation failure. (In preparation))

* 20 patients excluded from local control analysis due to death from intermittent disease.

the actuarial survival by stage. Only 10% had stage I or II disease, 19% stage III, and 71% stage IV. The 5-year absolute survival was 32%.

FOLLOWUP POLICY: BASE OF TONGUE

Surgical or radiation therapy or both will occasionally salvage the failure of an early lesion. Radiation failures may present as an ulcer and must be distinguished from radiation necrosis.

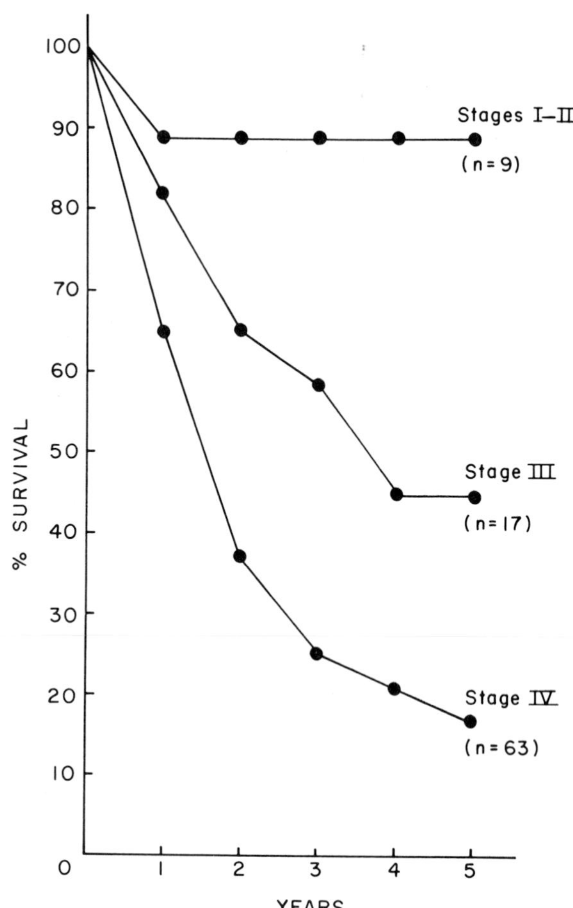

FIG. 13-17. Actuarial survival for patients with squamous cell carcinoma of the base of the tongue.[102] (Parsons JT, Million RR, Cassisi NJ: Carcinoma of the base of tongue: Results of radical irradiation with surgery reserved for irradiation failure. In press, 1981)

Most radiation ulcers will appear in the vallecula or glossotonsillar sulcus, not on the base of tongue proper. Biopsies will usually be done under general anesthesia to obtain adequate tissue and control of bleeding.

COMPLICATIONS OF TREATMENT: BASE OF TONGUE

Surgical Complications

The complications of surgery include an operative mortality of about 5%; fistula, mandibular necrosis, dysphagia, hoarseness, trismus, and carotid rupture are non-fatal complications.

Complications of Irradiation

Table 13-29 shows the risk of radiation therapy complications by boost technique.[157] Bone exposure and osteoradionecrosis are uncommon. Soft tissue necrosis is the major problem and occurs in approximately 6–10% of patients treated solely by external beam irradiation. Treatment of necrosis requires patience and reassurance to the patient, who assumes the pain is due to cancer. Antibiotics will often reduce pain. The patient will lose weight due to dysphagia and will require nutritional support. Many necroses persist several months. Serious hemorrhage is uncommon.

Hypoglossal nerve palsy occurred in two patients and is reported in other series. It is usually associated with an ulcer in the posterior glossotonsillar sulcus. Unilateral hypoglossal nerve palsy does not produce serious morbidity since the opposite side compensates very nicely.

An occasional patient cured of advanced base of tongue cancer by radiation therapy may have difficulty swallowing solid foods. The action of the base of tongue is to force the bolus of food into the hypopharynx, and loss of full motion impedes swallowing. This is probably a result of some fibrosis of the base of tongue compounded by a dry mouth. The addition of a radical neck dissection to radiation therapy increases the risk of this problem. Aspiration is unusual, however, even if the tip of the epiglottis has been amputated by tumor.

Complications of Combined Treatment

Preoperative irradiation will increase the risk of fistula, delayed healing, and carotid exposure. Postoperative irradiation in-

TABLE 13-29. Base of Tongue Carcinoma: Soft Tissue Necrosis and Bone Exposure by Boost Technique (University of Florida, 9/64–9/77; analysis 9/79)

BOOST TECHNIQUE (No. of patients)	NO. WITH SOFT TISSUE NECROSIS			NO. WITH BONE EXPOSURE		
	1+*	2+	3+	1+	2+	3+
Submental (47)	2 (4%)	3 (6%)	0	0 (0%)	†1 (2%)	0
Lateral (17)	0 (0%)	1 (6%)	0	0 (0%)	0 (0%)	0
Radium (25)	4 (16%)	2 (8%)	0	2 (8%)	3 (12%)	0

(Parsons JT, Million RR, Cassisi NJ: Carcinoma of the base of tongue: Results of radical irradiation with surgery reserved for irradiation failure. (in preparation))

* 1+ Healed with conservative management within 6 months; 2+ Healed with conservative management greater than 6 months; 3+ Required surgical treatment.

† Dental extractions 2 months after radiation therapy.

creases the amount of fibrosis in the neck. Radiation necrosis of the soft tissues or bone is uncommon. The added effect of xerostomia further worsens the swallowing defect produced by glossectomy.

TREATMENT: TONSILLAR AREA

Selection of Treatment Modality

EARLY (T1–T2). Early lesions are generally treated by irradiation with a high rate of success and relatively low morbidity; a neck dissection is added after radiation therapy as outlined in the section on principles of treatment. An occasional small lesion is cured by wide local excision or tonsillectomy, but surgical excision is usually prescribed only under unusual circumstances. A surgical attack usually implies removal of the mandible, the tonsillar area including both pillars and part of the soft palate, and perhaps a small amount of the tongue; additionally, an ipsilateral neck dissection is performed even with a clinically negative neck. The functional loss from this operation is not justified in view of the high success rate with irradiation, which leaves the patient intact; even a dry mouth may be avoided when well-lateralized lesions are treated by techniques that allow at least partial salivary recovery. An operation will often salvage the few radiation treatment failures. Table 13-30 shows the local control, surgical salvage, and ultimate control rates by T stage for tonsillar area lesions treated by radiation therapy.[158] These results are suboptimal due to inclusion of split-course cases and the use of lower doses in early years. Tonsillar fossa lesions have a slightly lower recurrence rate than those arising from the anterior tonsillar pillar area.

MODERATELY ADVANCED (T2–T3). The local failure rate with radiation therapy is approximately 30% when adequate doses are prescribed. Preoperative irradiation followed by an operation has not shown any improvement in the cure rate compared to radical radiation therapy with surgical salvage.[159-161] Surgical salvage is better for anterior tonsillar pillar failures than for those of the tonsillar fossa. The major indication for combined treatment is a lesion that is failing to regress after 5000 rad; these patients are offered an operation.

ADVANCED (T3–T4). If the lesion is assigned to stage T4 only because of mandible invasion, then an operation followed by radiation therapy should be considered. However, mandible invasion is usually associated with extensions that contraindicate surgical removal.

Radical irradiation will control a remarkable number of these advanced lesions if large doses are applied.

Surgical Treatment

Surgical treatment for very early cancers of the tonsillar area (less than 1 cm in size) consists of a wide local excision through a transoral approach. Larger lesions require removal of the adjacent mandible as well as a portion of the tongue and soft palate. Depending on the size of the defect, a tongue, deltopectoral, or myocutaneous flap may be required to close the defect. Flaps are usually necessary for extensive lesions or after radiation therapy failure. Deglutition is not generally a problem, but some patients remain on liquid diets. Chewing is difficult since a portion of the mandible has been removed and the patient will be unable to wear dentures. Speech may be impaired if a portion of the tongue or palate has been removed.

Irradiation Technique

The basic portal arrangement depends to a large degree on the extent of the local lesion and presence or absence of positive lymph nodes. The risk for contralateral lymph node metastases is very small unless there is tongue invasion, invasion of the soft palate within 1–2 cm of the midline, or clinically positive nodes in the ipsilateral neck. If these risk features are absent, mixed beam techniques that spare the contralateral mucosa and salivary glands may be used. If the medial extent of the primary lesion is no more than 4.5 cm from the ipsilateral skin surface, then mixed beam techniques can be used if high-energy photons (8–20 MV) and high-energy electrons (17–20 MeV) are available. The major advantage of these techniques is not a greater cure rate, but a lower incidence of xerostomia secondary to partial preservation of minor and major salivary gland function on the contralateral side. An intraoral lead block may also be added that further protects the minor salivary glands and a portion of the parotid. Since the lesions lie behind the mandible, an extra 1–1.5 cm is added to the depth dose calculations for the electron portion of the treatment.

Lesions with a medial extent greater than 4.5 cm are at risk for bilateral neck disease and are treated with parallel opposed photon portal, usually weighted 2:1 or 3:2, to the involved side; if there are positive contralateral nodes or extension across the midline, the portals are usually equally weighted. Table 13-8 shows the doses for local control.

The dose prescribed for tonsillar area lesions is critical if a high rate of control is to be achieved. Table 13-30 analyzes the rate of local control by T stage.[158]

Combined Treatment Policies

Patients selected for combined treatment preferably have resection first, followed by postoperative irradiation. A large, fixed node is the most common indication for preoperative irradiation.

Patients whose lesions show a poor response to radiation therapy are often re-evaluated at 5000 rad and offered an operation.

Management of Recurrence

An operation will salvage a good proportion of T1–2 radiation therapy failures, but only an occasional advanced lesion is salvaged. Table 13-31 shows the experience with surgical salvage at the University of Florida.[158]

A neck recurrence after radiation therapy only can occasionally be salvaged.

TABLE 13-30. Carcinoma of the Tonsillar Region—Local Control (University of Florida, 10/64–1/78, analysis 1/80; 24 month to unlimited followup)

STAGE	NO. PATIENTS EXCLUDED*	LOCAL CONTROL	NO. SALVAGED/ NO. OF OPERATIONS ATTEMPTED	ULTIMATE CONTROL
T1	4	15/18 (83%)	2/3	17/18 (94%)
T2	9	23/32 (72%)	†5/8	28/32 (88%)
T3	5	11/25 (44%)	1/6	12/25 (48%)
T4	4	4/18 (22%)	0/2	4/18 (22%)
Total		53/93 (57%)		61/93 (66%)

(Wickstrum DL: Carcinoma of the tonsillar region. 10th Annual Radiation Therapy Clinical Research Seminar, April 24–26, 1980, pp 249–270. Gainesville, Florida, Radiation Therapy Division, University of Florida, 1981)

* Dead of intercurrent disease less than 2 years after start of treatment and free of disease.

† One patient salvaged after third salvage attempt.

RESULTS OF TREATMENT: TONSILLAR AREA

Table 13-30 shows the local control, Table 13-32 the neck control, and Table 13-33 the survival rates by stage for 133 patients treated at the University of Florida.[158]

Fourteen patients were selected for combined treatment. Eight were treated with preoperative radiation therapy; only one has no evidence of disease over 2 years from treatment. Six were treated by resection and postoperative radiation therapy, and four have no evidence of disease over 2 years.

COMPLICATIONS OF TREATMENT: TONSILLAR AREA

Table 13-34 outlines the risk of bone and soft tissue complications for 115 patients treated by irradiation.[158] Five patients required an operative procedure. Improved management of the teeth has reduced the incidence of serious complications.

TREATMENT: SOFT PALATE

Selection of Treatment Modality

Very small (2–5 mm), well-defined lesions may be excised, but the multifocal nature of soft palate lesions predicts marginal recurrence after limited treatment unless patients are very carefully selected. Tiny lesions confined to the uvula may be treated by surgical excision with little morbidity. Irradiation is the modality most often selected for early and advanced soft palate carcinomas; neck dissection is added as needed. The success rate with irradiation is quite high, and it leaves the patient functionally intact without the need for a prosthesis or elaborate reconstruction. Fletcher reports a very high rate of success for patients treated by radiation therapy alone.[162] The control rates were: T1, 100%; T2, 88%; T3, 77%; and T4, 83%.

Surgical Treatment

Surgical excision for early lesions (less than 5 mm in size) of the soft palate can achieve a high cure rate with little or no functional loss if the full thickness of the palate does not have to be resected. However, if full-thickness resection is required, then a prosthesis is generally required to restore velopharyngeal competence. Surgical salvage of radiation recurrence should generally include full-thickness removal of the soft palate.

Irradiation Technique

The basic irradiation technique for early and advanced lesions involves parallel opposed external beam portals, which include the primary lesion and the first relay of upper neck nodes on both sides, since even very tiny lesions are at some risk for occult lymph node disease. If the primary lesion is discrete, a portion of the treatment may be given by way of intra-oral

TABLE 13-31. Carcinoma of the Tonsillar Region: Surgical Salvage at the Primary Site (University of Florida, 10/64–1/78; analysis 1/80)

PROCEDURE	NO. OF PATIENTS	POSITIVE MARGINS	LOCAL CONTROL	MAJOR COMPLICATIONS	NO EVIDENCE OF DISEASE
Local resection	4	0	2	0	2
Radical tonsillectomy ± radical neck dissection	15	6	7*	6†	7

(Wickstrum DL: Carcinoma of the tonsillar region. 10th Annual Radiation Therapy Clinical Research Seminar, April 24–26, 1980, pp 249–270. Gainesville, Florida, Radiation Therapy Division, University of Florida, 1981)

* One patient salvaged after third salvage attempt.

† One fatal complication: endocarditis after jaw-neck dissection.

TABLE 13-32. Carcinoma of the Tonsillar Region: Neck Control Analysis (University of Florida, 70 patients, 10/64–1/78; analysis 1/80)

STAGE	INITIAL TREATMENT*	NO. WITH NECK CONTROL/ NO. TREATED	SURGICAL SALVAGE	NO. WITH ULTIMATE CONTROL/ NO. TREATED
N0	RT	34/34	—	34/34
N1	RT	10/11 (1)†	—	10/11
	Exc + RT	1/1	—	1/1
	RT + RND	3/3	—	3/3
	Total			14/15
N2	RT	3/6 (1)	0/0	3/6
	RT + RND	3/4 (1)	—	3/4
	Total			6/10
N3	RT	1/6 (1)	0/1	1/6
	RT + RND	2/4	‡1/1	3/4
	RT + PND	1/1	—	1/1
	Total			5/11

(Wickstrum DL: Carcinoma of the tonsillar region. 10th Annual Radiation Therapy Clinical Research Seminar, April 24–26, 1980. Gainesville, Florida, Radiation Therapy Division, University of Florida, 1981)

* RT—radiation therapy; Exc—excision; RND—radical neck dissection; PND—partial neck dissection.

† ( )—Indicates patients with uncontrolled neck disease and failure at the primary site.

‡ Simple excision of recurrence after radical neck dissection.

cone or a single-plane seed implant. If intra-oral cone therapy is to be used, it should be given prior to external beam when the lesion is clearly visible and the mouth is not yet sore from the radiation reaction. Intra-oral cone therapy requires meticulous care to avoid geographic miss.

A small single-plane radioactive seed implant is an effective reduced-field technique. The seeds (radon or gold) are placed on a 1-cm grid to include the gross lesion with a small margin. The implant may be done prior to external beam if the lesion is flat or after external beam if the clinician wishes to flatten the lesion prior to implant.

The major advantage of the seed boost is a reduction of external beam dose by 1500–2500 rad with fewer late radiation side effects, increased moisture in the mouth, and hopefully a better local control rate due to the higher biologic dose.

The external beam technique is usually equally weighted, parallel opposed portals. The minimum treatment volume for early lesions includes the entire soft palate and the adjacent tonsillar areas. If the neck is clinically negative, high-energy photons (18–22 MeV) will produce an ideal isodose distribution allowing a tumor dose at the soft palate of 6500–7000 rad while maintaining the lymph node dose at 5000 rad. If the lymph nodes are clinically positive, then Cobalt-60 or 4–6 MeV is preferred on the involved side(s).

There is little information on dose for control of soft palate lesions, but schedules similar to those for the anterior tonsillar pillar are used.

TABLE 13-33. Carcinoma of the Tonsillar Region: Survival by Stage (University of Florida, 133 patients, 10/64–1/78; analysis 1/80)

STAGE	2 YEARS	5 YEARS
I	77%	51%
II	74%	50%
III	73%	46%
IV	37%	14%

(Wickstrum DL: Carcinoma of the tonsillar region. 10th Annual Radiation Therapy Clinical Research Seminar, April 24–26, 1980. Gainesville, Florida, Radiation Therapy Division, University of Florida, 1981)

Combined Treatment Policies

Combined therapy is rarely planned because of the success rate with radiation therapy and the morbidity associated with resection of the soft palate.

TABLE 13-34. Carcinoma of the Tonsillar Region: Complications of Radiation Therapy Alone (University of Florida, 10/64–1/78; analysis 1/80)

STAGE	NO. OF PATIENTS AT RISK	SOFT TISSUE COMPLICATIONS 1+*	2+	3+	BONE COMPLICATIONS 1+	2+	3+
T1–2	63	3	2	1	7	0	1
T3–4	52	1	1	1	6†	2	2

(Wickstrum DL: Carcinoma of the tonsillar region. 10th Annual Radiation Therapy Clinical Research Seminar, April 24–26, 1980. Gainesville, Florida, Radiation Therapy Division, University of Florida, 1981)

*1+ —Minor complications with minimal dysfunction and no functional loss; 2+ —Complications lasting more than 6 months or causing considerable pain or functional loss; 3+ —Complications requiring surgery.

† Three patients also had soft tissue complications.

Management of Recurrence

Soft tissue necrosis is uncommon after radiation therapy, so a persistent ulcer is the hallmark of recurrent disease following irradiation. Recurrence following irradiation is treated by surgical removal when feasible, and a few patients are salvaged.

RESULTS OF TREATMENT: SOFT PALATE

Surgical Results

Ratzer and coworkers report the Memorial Sloan-Kettering results for 299 patients with squamous cell carcinoma of the soft palate.[163] Some 112 were treated by surgery, 139 by radiation therapy, and 22 by combined treatment. The 5-year absolute survival rate was 21%, and the determinate survival rate was 30%. The determinate survival rate for just the group treated by surgery was 38%. The main cause of failure was recurrence at the primary site.

Irradiation Results

Weller and coworkers report a local failure rate of 50% in 30 patients with soft palate lesions.[164] Only five of the patients had T1 lesions.

Seydel and Scholl reviewed the results of 41 patients with previously untreated soft palate malignancies including four nonsquamous carcinomas.[165] Thirty-one patients were treated with doses between 6000 and 7000 rad, and 10 (32%) developed local recurrence.

Parsons analyzed the University of Florida data for 25 patients.* Local control was achieved in all of four patients with T1 lesions, eight of ten T2, two of seven T3, and one of four T4. A time-dose relationship could not be observed.

Lindberg and Fletcher report a high rate of control for soft palate lesions (T1, 100% T2, 88%; T3, 77% and T4, 83%).[166] A few failures were salvaged by operation.

COMPLICATIONS OF TREATMENT: SOFT PALATE

Surgical Complications

Nasal speech and regurgitation of food into the nasopharynx are sequelae of full-thickness resection of the soft palate. A prosthesis is only partially successful in correcting the functional defect.

Complications of Irradiation

Complications are few. Soft tissue necrosis of the soft palate is quite uncommon, and an ulcer must be considered to be a possible recurrence. The soft palate may become retracted following successful treatment of advanced lesions; this may result in regurgitation into the nasopharynx and slight alteration in speech. Small perforations may persist after successful treatment at sites where tumor has grown through the soft palate. These usually occur far laterally and do not interfere with function.

* JT Parsons, unpublished data, 1979.

LARYNX

Cancer of the larynx represents about 2% of the total cancer risk. The number of new cases in 1978 in the U.S. is estimated at 9200–8100 in men and 1100 in women, with an estimated 3300 deaths due to laryngeal cancer. Localized cases are estimated at 59%, those with regional spread around 31%, and those with distant metastasis at the time of first diagnosis at 10%.

A study of trends in cancer incidence in the U.S. from 1935 to 1970 shows that cancer of the larynx has increased by 33% in white males, but is 3½ times increased in nonwhite males. The incidence in females has shown only a very minimal increase in spite of the fact that lung cancer in women has quadrupled in the same period.

Cancer of the larynx seems to be primarily related to cigarette smoking. The risk of tobacco-related cancers of the upper alimentary and respiratory tract declines among ex-smokers after 5 years and is said to approach the risk of nonsmokers after 10 years of abstention.[167]

A 12-year American Cancer Society study has shown that low-tar and low-nicotine cigarettes (less than 15 mg of tar and less than 1 mg of nicotine) result in slightly lower death rates from lung cancer, but whether or not they affect the risk of laryngeal cancer is unknown.

The importance of alcohol in the etiology of laryngeal cancer remains unclear, but it is probably less important than in other head and neck sites, in which alcohol can be shown to be an associated factor that is synergistic to tobacco.[168]

The geographic distribution for laryngeal cancer in the U.S. shows excess occurrence in the Northeast, particularly in northern New Jersey, New York City, and along the Hudson River. The rates are also high along the southeastern Atlantic Coast and the Gulf Coast. This distribution closely resembles the high-risk areas for lung cancer.[169]

ANATOMY

The larynx is composed of several cartilages connected by ligaments and muscles. Anatomically it is divided into the supraglottic, glottic, and subglottic regions. The supraglottic larynx consists of the epiglottis, the false vocal cords, the ventricles, the aryepiglottic folds, and the arytenoids; the arytenoids are cartilages that articulate on the cricoid (see Figs. 13-18 and 13-19). The glottis includes the true vocal cords and the anterior commissure. The subglottic area is located below the vocal cords to the level of the first tracheal ring.

The pre-epiglottic space is an important anatomic region because the lymphatic trunks from the glottic and supraglottic region traverse this space; it is also an area where direct extension of tumor may occur.

Anatomically, the pre-epiglottic space is bounded by the epiglottis and thryoid cartilage posteriorly, the hyo-epiglottic ligament and central portion of the epiglottis superiorly, and the thyrohyoid membrane anteriorly and laterally. It can be seen as a low-density area on CT scan.

The supraglottic structures have a rich capillary lymphatic plexus, especially the false cords, ventricles, and suprahyoid epiglottis. The lymphatic trunks pass through the pre-epiglottic space and the thyrohyoid membrane to the subdigastric nodes. A few trunks drain directly to the middle or lower jugular chain.

There are essentially no capillary lymphatics of the true vocal cords; as a result, lymphatic spread from glottic cancer rarely occurs unless tumor extends to supraglottic or subglottic areas.

The infraglottic area has relatively few capillary lymphatics. The lymphatic trunks pass through the thyrocricoid membrane to the pretracheal (Delphian) node(s) in the region of the thyroid isthmus, or the trunks may carry the tumor to the lower jugular nodes. The pretracheal nodes are midline in position and even when clinically positive are small (1–5 mm to rarely over 1–2 cm). The subglottic area also drains posteriorly through the cricotracheal membrane with some trunks going to the paratracheal nodes while others pass to the inferior jugular chain.

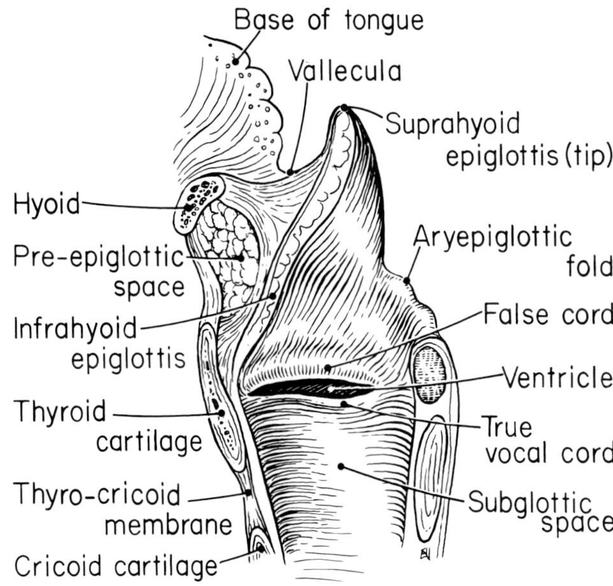

FIG. 13-18. Diagrammatic sagittal section of the larynx. (Million RR, Cassisi NJ: The management of local and regional laryngeal cancer. In Carter SK, Glatstein E, Livingston RB: Principles of Cancer Treatment. New York, McGraw-Hill, 1981)

PATHOLOGY

The laryngeal surfaces of the epiglottis and vocal cords are lined with stratified squamous epithelium and the remainder of the larynx with pseudostratified ciliated columnar epithelium. Nearly all malignant tumors of the larynx arise from the surface epithelium and therefore are squamous cell carcinoma or one of its variants.

Minor salivary gland tumors arise from the mucous glands, but are rare; even more rare is the appearance of fibrosarcoma, rhabdomyosarcoma, malignant lymphoma, or plasmacytoma. Benign chondromas and osteochondromas are reported, but their malignant counterparts are almost never seen.

Carcinoma *in situ* is rather common on the vocal cords. Distinction between dysplasia, carcinoma *in situ*, squamous cell carcinoma with microinvasion, and true invasive carcinoma is a problem frequently confronting the pathologist and the clinician. In patients with minimal lesions, the cord is biopsied by stripping the mucosa; the specimen tends to curl or fold, creating difficulty in orientation of the basement membrane. However, the precise distinction between carcinoma *in situ*, microinvasion, and invasive carcinoma is a bit academic. The authors recommend treatment, usually irradiation, in most patients. The local recurrence rate after irradiation for carcinoma *in situ* or microinvasive or invasive carcinoma is, surprisingly, about the same within the "T1" category; the recurrences are almost always invasive carcinoma.

Most of the vocal cord carcinomas are either well-differentiated or moderately well-differentiated. In a few cases there is an apparent carcinoma and sarcoma occurring together, but most of these are, in reality, an anaplastic carcinoma with pseudosarcomatous stromal reaction. It may be impossible for the pathologist to distinguish between a stromal reaction that mimics sarcoma in the presence of a carcinoma and a bona fide coexisting sarcoma and carcinoma. Only the course of the disease (*i.e.*, metastasis) may settle the argument. The term "pseudosarcoma" is applied to a rare laryngeal lesion, which is usually polypoid or pedunculated with a string-like umbilical cord. It has a favorable prognosis.

Verrucous carcinoma occurs on the vocal cords in about 1–2% of patients with carcinoma. The histologic diagnosis is difficult and must correlate with the gross appearance of the lesion.

Supraglottic carcinomas are less differentiated than those of the vocal cord; verrucous lesions are rare. Carcinoma *in situ* is rarely diagnosed as a distinct entity in the supraglottic larynx, although a zone of carcinoma *in situ* is seen at the margin between invasive tumor and normal mucosa.

FIG. 13-19. Photograph of the larynx (anterior view). *A*, posterior pharyngeal wall; *B*, arytenoid; *C*, aryepiglottic fold; *D*, false vocal cord; *E*, true vocal cord; *F*, infrahyoid epiglottis; *G*, suprahyoid epiglottis; *H*, pyriform sinus. (Million RR, Cassisi NJ: The management of local and regional laryngeal cancer. In Carter SK, Glatstein E, Livingston RB: Principles of Cancer Treatment. New York, McGraw-Hill, 1981)

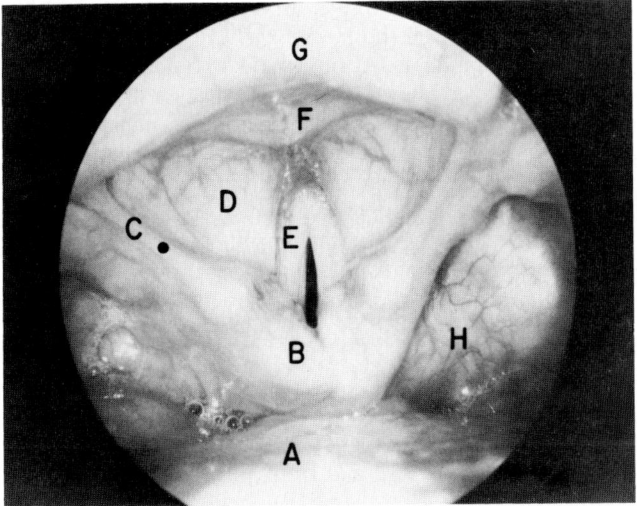

PATTERNS OF SPREAD

Supraglottic Larynx

The majority of lesions are epiglottic in origin. It is difficult to assign a site of origin for advanced lesions.

SUPRAHYOID EPIGLOTTIS. Lesions of the suprahyoid epiglottis may grow like a mushroom, producing a huge exophytic mass with little tendency to destruction of cartilage or spread to adjacent structures. Others may infiltrate the tip and produce destruction of cartilage and eventual amputation of the tip. The latter lesions tend to invade the vallecula and pre-epiglottic space, the lateral pharyngeal walls, and the remainder of the supraglottic larynx.

INFRAHYOID EPIGLOTTIS. Lesions of the infrahyoid epiglottis tend to produce irregular outgrowths of tumor nodules with simultaneous invasion through the porous epiglottic cartilage into the pre-epiglottic space and base of tongue. These lesions grow circumferentially to involve the false cords, aryepiglottic folds, and eventually, the medial wall of the pyriform sinus and the pharyngo-epiglottic fold. Invasion of the anterior commissure and cords is usually a late phenomenon, and subglottic extension occurs only in advanced lesions. Infrahyoid epiglottic lesions that extend onto or below the vocal cords are at high risk for cartilage invasion, even if the cords are mobile.[170] Tumor may burrow through the epiglottic cartilage and pre-epiglottic fat space, and present in the vallecula and base of tongue without involving the suprahyoid epiglottis. This anterior and superior extension is difficult to appreciate clinically; CT scan may be of assistance in outlining this spread pattern.

FALSE CORD. False cord carcinomas are usually infiltrative, ulcerative, and difficult to delineate accurately; they are therefore often understaged. They extend to the thyroid cartilage quite early. Extension to the infrahyoid epiglottis is common. Vocal cord involvement occurs late and is usually associated with thyroid cartilage invasion. Subglottic extension is uncommon until the lesion is advanced.

ARYEPIGLOTTIC FOLD/ARYTENOID. Early lesions are usually exophytic growths. It is often difficult to decide whether they start on the medial wall of the pyriform sinus or the aryepiglottic fold. As the lesions advance, they extend to adjacent sites and eventually cause fixation of the larynx. In some instances, the fixation may be secondary to mere bulk of tumor. However, involvement of the cricoarytenoid muscle and ligament and arytenoid cartilage also produces fixation. It is usually impossible to distinguish the cause of fixation at the time therapeutic decisions are made. Advanced lesions may invade the thyroid, epiglottic, or cricoid cartilage and eventually invade the base of tongue and pharyngeal wall.

Vocal Cord

The majority of lesions begin on the free margin and upper surface of the vocal cord and are easily visible. When diagnosed, about two-thirds are confined to usually one cord. The anterior portion of the cord is the most common site, and extension to the anterior commissure is frequent. Anterior commissure involvement is said to occur when no tumor-free cord can be seen anteriorly; when the lesion crosses over to the opposite cord, anterior commissure invasion is almost certain. Small lesions isolated to the anterior commissure account for only 1–2% of all cases.

As vocal cord lesions enlarge, they extend to the ventricle/false cord, vocal process of the arytenoid, and subglottic region. Infiltrative lesions invade the vocal ligament and and thyro-arytenoid muscles, eventually reaching the thyroid cartilage. As cancers reach the cartilage, they tend to grow up or down along the interface rather than attacking the cartilage. The conus elasticus acts as a barrier to subglottic penetration. Advanced glottic lesions eventually penetrate through the thyroid cartilage or thyrocricoid membrane to enter the neck and often invade the thyroid gland.

A fixed cord with less than 1 cm of subglottic extension and no false cord involvement does not ordinarily indicate invasion of the thyroid cartilage.[171] If the false cord is also involved, cartilage invasion is likely.

Subglottic Larynx

The boundaries of the subglottic area are ill-defined. The epithelium changes from squamous to respiratory about 5 mm below the free margin of the cord, and this is considered the beginning of the subglottic area; the inferior border is the inferior border of the cricoid cartilage.

Subglottic cancers are quite uncommon. It is difficult to define whether a tumor started on the undersurface of the vocal cord or in the true subglottic larynx with extension to the cord. These lesions involve the cricoid cartilage quite early, as there is no intervening muscle layer. Involvement of the undersurface of the vocal cord is usually present, and fixation of a cord is the rule.

Lymphatic Spread

SUPRAGLOTTIC. The incidence of clinically positive nodes is 55% at the time of diagnosis; 16% are bilateral.[32] Elective neck dissection will show pathologically positive nodes in 16–26% of cases; observation of the neck will be followed by the appearance of positive nodes in 33% of cases (see Table 13-1). Extralaryngeal spread to the pyriform sinus and vallecula/base of tongue increases the risk of node metastases. The infrahyoid epiglottis has a lower risk of lymph node involvement than the other portions of the supraglottic larynx.

GLOTTIC. The incidence of clinically positive nodes at diagnosis approaches zero for lesions confined to the cords (T1) and is 2–5% for T2 lesions and early, small-volume T3 lesions. The incidence of neck metastases increases to 20–30% for large T3 and T4 lesions. Supraglottic spread is associated with metastasis to the jugulodigastric nodes. Anterior commissure and anterior subglottic invasion is associated with midline pretracheal node involvement (Delphian node).

CLINICAL PICTURE

Presenting Symptoms

VOCAL CORD. Carcinoma arising on the true vocal cords produces hoarseness at a very early stage. Pain or sore throat is a symptom of advanced lesions. Airway obstruction producing respiratory distress is a feature of advanced lesions and is rarely seen even with bulky early-stage lesions.

SUPRAGLOTTIC LARYNX. Hoarseness is not a prominent symptom for cancer of the supraglottic larynx until the lesion becomes quite extensive. Changes in voice quality are often described as a "hot potato" quality, the voice quality associated with unexpectedly swallowing a bite of very hot food. Pain on swallowing, usually mild, is the most frequent initial symptom. The pain is often described as a mild, persistent irritation or sore throat, and often the patient can point to the area with one finger. Mild difficulty in swallowing is frequent; some patients report a sensation of a "lump in the throat." Cancer of the epiglottis may be quite large before symptoms are produced. Pain is referred to the ear by way of the vagus nerve and auricular nerve of Arnold (see Fig. 13-12). A mass in the neck may be the first sign of a supraglottic cancer. Late symptoms include weight loss, foul breath, dysphagia, and aspiration.

Physical Examination

In addition to the simple, inexpensive laryngeal mirror, there are rigid and flexible fiberoptic illuminated endoscopes that are now routinely used as a complement to the laryngeal mirror examination. The Hopkins rod with a right-angle lens gives excellent visualization of the infrahyoid epiglottis and anterior commissure, areas which may be difficult, if not impossible, to visualize with a laryngeal mirror. The mirror gives a larger image of the larynx/hypopharynx than that obtained by direct laryngoscopy or by fiberoptic endoscopes. The flexible fiberoptic laryngoscope is inserted through the nose and is useful in the more difficult cases.

A horseshoe-shaped epiglottis or other laryngeal abnormality may prohibit adequate laryngeal examination for even the most skilled examiner. The tip of the epiglottis may be amputated with a biopsy forceps to facilitate indirect examination of the larynx. This is performed at the time of direct laryngoscopy. Loss of the tip of the epiglottis does not result in functional problems.

Determination of the mobility of the larynx frequently requires multiple examinations as the subtle distinctions between mobile, partially fixed, and fixed cords are often difficult and in fact seem to change from examination to examination. A cord that appeared mobile to the surgeon prior to direct laryngoscopy, may show sluggish motion or even fixation after biopsy.

Invasion of the pre-epiglottic space occurs more frequently than one can diagnose clinically. Invasion of the pre-epiglottic space can be diagnosed clinically or radiographically only when tumor invasion is rather extensive. Ulceration of the infrahyoid epiglottis or fullness of the vallecula is an indirect sign of pre-epiglottic space invasion. Palpation of diffuse, firm fullness above the thyroid notch with widening of the space between the hyoid and thyroid cartilages signifies invasion of the pre-epiglottic space. Lateral soft tissue radiographs of the neck may show the presence of irregular air cavities inferior to the vallecula in patients with lesions of the suprahyoid epiglottis invading into the pre-epiglottic space by way of the vallecula.

Postcricoid extension may be suspected when the laryngeal "crackle" or "click" disappears on physical examination. The diagnosis is confirmed by direct laryngoscopy, by barium study of the hypopharynx, and by laryngogram.

Invasion of the thyroid cartilage is another difficult clinical diagnosis. Localized pain or tenderness to palpation over one ala of the thyroid cartilage is suggestive. Tumor may actually penetrate through the thyroid ala and be felt as a small bulge on the thyroid ala. Cartilage invasion may be diagnosed by roentgenographic examination, but the cartilage must be calcified to show destructive changes.[172] CT scan of the larynx may be of help in the future for staging, particularly to detect spread to the pre-epiglottic space.[173]

METHOD OF DIAGNOSIS AND STAGING

The differential diagnosis of laryngeal lesions includes papillomas, polyps, vocal nodules, fibromas, and granulomas. Papillomas can involve the epiglottis or false or true cords and can extend subglottically. They may be confused with verrucous carcinoma, generally occurring in children and young adults, possibly persisting into adulthood. Vocal polyps and nodules occur at the junction of the middle and anterior one-third of the true vocal cords. There is usually a history of voice abuse followed by hoarseness.

Granulomas of the larynx usually occur as a result of intubation and are located on the posterior one-third of the vocal cords, near the posterior commissure. Endoscopic removal is the definitive treatment.

Tuberculosis of the larynx, although rare, still occurs. Generally, the lesion is destructive in nature and occurs at the posterior commissure of the glottis, but the epiglottis and false cords may be involved. The appearance mimics cancer and pulmonary tuberculosis is usually present.

Direct laryngoscopy for biopsy with frozen section is usually performed under general anesthesia. A generous biopsy, taken from the bulk of the lesion, will help the pathologist make the diagnosis. Biopsies should be obtained from suspicious areas as well as areas grossly involved for staging purposes.

Staging

The American Joint Commission staging system for laryngeal primary cancer is:[39]

Supraglottis

TIS Carcinoma *in situ*
T1 Tumor confined to region of origin with normal mobility
T2 Tumor involves adjacent supraglottic site(s) or glottis without fixation
T3 Tumor limited to the larynx with fixation or exten-

sion to involve postcricoid area, medial wall of pyriform sinus, or pre-epiglottic space

T4 Massive tumor extending beyond the larynx to involve oropharynx, soft tissues of neck, or destruction of thyroid cartilage

Glottis

TIS Carcinoma *in situ*

T1 Tumor confined to vocal cord(s) with normal mobility (includes involvement of anterior or posterior commissures)

T2 Supraglottic or subglottic extension of tumor with normal or impaired cord mobility

T3 Tumor confined to the larynx with cord fixation

T4 Massive tumor with thyroid cartilage destruction or extension beyond the confines of the larynx

For lesions arising in the supraglottis, the sites of origin include the false cords, aryepiglottic folds, suprahyoid (tip) epiglottis, and infrahyoid epiglottis. Only in the early T stages can one identify the specific site of origin with certainty. As the lesions enlarge, the site of origin is an educated guess based on the location of the greatest bulk of tumor.

Therapeutic decisions should not be based on T staging as a single parameter; tumor volume and location are better for gauging prognosis. Fixation, for instance, is not a likely event for a lesion arising on the tip of the epiglottis. A small lesion arising from the aryepiglottic fold may invade the medial wall of the pyriform sinus quite early and qualify as a T3, and yet have a prognosis similar to a T1 or early T2.

Staging Procedures

Staging procedures for laryngeal cancer include:

- Indirect laryngoscopy (with photography)
- Direct laryngoscopy with multiple biopsies
- Tomograms
- Contrast laryngography
- CT scan
- Chest roentgenogram

Direct laryngoscopy with multiple biopsies is required to assess extent of tumor and confirm the diagnosis. The ventricles, subglottic area, apex of the pyriform sinus, and postcricoid area must be carefully examined, as these areas are not consistently seen by any other method.

Indirect laryngoscopy actually gives a better panorama and allows better evaluation of function than can be obtained at direct laryngoscopy.

Although a lot is written about roentgenographic examination of the larynx, it plays a very minor role in decision making.

Frontal tomograms are used by the radiotherapist to check the subglottic space and confirm the direct laryngoscopy findings, especially for the larger lesions.

Contrast laryngogram (lateral views) is sometimes useful in delineating tumor extent at the anterior commissure.

CT scan may show thyroid cartilage invasion, invasion of the pre-epiglottic fat pad, and soft tissue extension into the neck. The reliablity of the CT scan is not yet confirmed by large numbers of serially sectioned specimens; treatment should not yet be significantly modified based on this one test.

TREATMENT

Vocal Cord Carcinoma

SELECTION OF TREATMENT MODALITY. The goal is cure with the best functional result and the least risk of a serious complication. External beam irradiation and operation are the only curative modalities available. For purposes of treatment planning, patients may be considered to be in either an early group (T1, T2, early T3 lesions) or a late group (late T3, T4 lesions). The early group may be initially treated by irradiation or partial laryngectomy; the neck nodes are uncommonly involved and do not often figure in therapeutic decisions in this group. The late group almost always requires a total laryngectomy, and treatment of the lymph nodes is considered.

Early Vocal Cord Lesions (T1, T2, or Early T3). In most centers, irradiation is the initial treatment prescribed for early lesions with operation reserved for salvage of irradiation failures. While hemilaryngectomy will produce comparable cure rates for selected T1–T2 vocal cord lesions, irradiation is generally the preferred initial therapy. The major advantage of irradiation compared to hemilaryngectomy is that the quality of the voice is likely to be better. The voice after hemilaryngectomy remains hoarse; most physicians tell the patient that his voice will be as hoarse as it is now or even worse. The voice, after successful irradiation, is usually better than before therapy, but occasional cases are seen in which there is no improvement or, uncommonly, a worsening. Hemilaryngectomy finds its major use as a salvage operation in suitable cases after irradiation failure. Even if the patient has a local recurrence after a salvage hemilaryngectomy, there is a third chance with total laryngectomy, which may still be successful.[174]

Complete stripping of the mucosa of the cord is sometimes curative for lesions variously classified as leukoplakia, dysplasia, or carcinoma *in situ*. Careful observation is essential, as regrowth of the lesions is most often the rule. While repeated stripping may seem a satisfactory plan of management, the cords become thickened and the voice becomes harsh, and it becomes increasingly difficult to tell whether or not tumor is present. Through the years, the authors have come to recommend irradiation much earlier in these patients, realizing that most would eventually come to this treatment and that earlier use of irradiation means a better chance of preserving a good voice. Additionally, the difficulties in differentiating carcinoma *in situ* from microinvasion tend to push the decision toward irradiation (see the section on pathology).

Verrucous lesions have the reputation of being unresponsive to irradiation and, in some instances, losing their verrucous nature to convert into invasive, often anaplastic, metastasizing lesions after unsuccessful irradiation. The authors, however, have observed typical verrucous lesions that have disappeared with radiation therapy and not recurred. Burns and coworkers have also made this observation.[175] The authors do favor hemilaryngectomy for early verrucous carcinoma of the glottis, but do not hesitate to use radiation therapy if the alternative is total laryngectomy.

Hemilaryngectomy is also used in patients who have had prior head and neck irradiation that prohibits further irradiation and for the patient who cannot afford 6 weeks away from home or job for the irradiation series.

Fixed cord lesions (T3) treated by irradiation fall into two groups. One group consists of patients with fixed, bulky, advanced lesions who either refuse laryngectomy or are medically inoperable. Irradiation of these lesions is seldom successful; about 10% are cured. The second group includes patients with a fixed cord, but minimal total tumor bulk. They usually have subglottic extension and minor supraglottic extension confined to one side of the larynx. An attempt at irradiation in this group is worthwhile. The patient must be willing to return for followup every month for the first 2 years and understand that total laryngectomy may be recommended purely on clinical grounds without biopsy-proven recurrence. The reported local control rate for fixed cord lesions (T3NO) varies from 30% to 60%.[176]

The major difficulty in the use of irradiation for late T2 and early T3 lesions is in distinguishing between radiation edema and local recurrence during followup examinations. Persistent edema, increased hoarseness, and immobility of a formerly mobile cord are all signs of recurrence. The detection of recurrence is difficult because the surface epithelium may be intact with tumor growing submucosally. Deep biopsies are necessary, but may aggravate the radiation damage if no tumor is found. The patient must be apprised that total laryngectomy may be recommended if suspicion of recurrence is very high, even without proof of recurrence.

Advanced Vocal Cord Lesions (T3, T4). The mainstay of treatment is total laryngectomy with or without postoperative irradiation. The most frequent sites of local failure after total laryngectomy are around the tracheal stoma, in the base of tongue, and in the neck nodes. If the neck is clinically negative prior to operation and if postoperative irradiation is planned, no neck dissection is done and irradiation is used to treat both sides of the neck. If nodes are clinically positive, a radical neck dissection is done with total laryngectomy. Postoperative irradiation may be used to control subclinical disease in the opposite neck as well as to help prevent recurrence in the dissected neck.

Radical irradiation is prescribed for the patient who refuses total laryngectomy or is medically unsuitable for a major operation. A few patients in this category will be cured.

SURGICAL TREATMENT. Stripping of the cord implies transoral removal of the mucosa of the edge of the cord. The operating microscope assists the surgeon in total stripping of the mucosa.

Cordectomy is an excision of the vocal cord. Its use is confined to small lesions of the middle one-third of the cord. Cordectomy is generally reserved for the uncommon situation where there is a postirradiation recurrence limited to the middle one-third of the cord with normal mobility. Following cordectomy a pseudocord is formed, and the patient has a useful, if somewhat harsh, voice. A portion of the adjacent thyroid cartilage may be removed with the cord.

Hemilaryngectomy is a partial, "vertical" laryngectomy that allows removal of limited cord lesions with voice preservation. There are definite restrictions with this operation. One entire cord plus 5 mm of the opposite cord is the maximum cordal involvement suitable for the operation in men; generally the operation is reserved for lesions involving one cord. Partial fixation of one cord is not a contraindication to hemilaryngectomy, but only a few surgeons have attempted hemilaryngectomy for fixed cord lesions. The maximum subglottic extension allowable is 8–9 mm anteriorly and 5 mm posteriorly, since the cricoid must be preserved. Minor extension to the epiglottis, false cord, or arytenoid is a contraindication to hemilaryngectomy. If one arytenoid is sacrificed, postoperative aspiration is a possibility, and therefore the patient must have a satisfactory pulmonary status.

The last surgical alternative is total laryngectomy with or without radical neck dissection. Total laryngectomy is used as a salvage procedure for radiation failure in the early lesions that are not suited for conservative operations. It is the operation of choice for advanced lesions. The entire larynx is removed, the pharynx reconstituted, and a permanent tracheostomy is required.

Artificial speech is created by a number of techniques. Electronic devices may be used immediately after the operation, but are far from satisfactory. Esophageal speech is accomplished by belching swallowed air that is used to produce phonation. Only 10% of the patients develop satisfactory esophageal speech.

There have been numerous attempts to recreate the larynx after total laryngectomy, with very few producing predictable results. There have been attempts to surgically create a fistula between the trachea and esophagus to shunt air to the pharynx. The problem has been one of aspiration in a large number of cases. Recently, a plastic "duckbill" prosthesis has been developed for insertion into a tracheo-esophageal fistula; the prosthesis allows the patient to speak without the problem of aspiration. Air is shunted from the trachea to the pharynx by placing a finger over an opening in the "duckbill." This simple innovation has made the impact of total laryngectomy less devastating. Most patients can learn to speak quite quickly this way since it does not require the training and motivation needed for esophageal speech.

IRRADIATION TECHNIQUE. Irradiation for early vocal cord cancer is delivered by small portals covering only the primary lesion. The incidence of lymph node involvement is so small (0–1%) that elective irradiation of nodes is recommended only for late T2 or T3 lesions or poorly differentiated histology; only the subdigastric and midjugular nodes would be electively treated. Radiation portals extend from the thyroid notch superiorly to the inferior border of the cricoid; the posterior limits depend on posterior extension of the tumor. The field size ranges from 4 × 4 cm to 5 × 5 cm. Portals larger than this increase the risk of edema without increasing the cure rate. Since the portals are small and the skin of the neck is mobile, it is the authors' practice to have the physician check the portal on the treatment table each day by palpation of the anatomic landmarks. Table 13-35 shows the dose scheme used at the University of Florida.

TABLE 13-35. Radiation Treatment Plan for Vocal Cord Cancer at the University of Florida

STAGE	DESCRIPTION	EXTERNAL BEAM IRRADIATION
T1	Early, no visible tumor	5625 rad tumor dose/ 25 fractions/5 wk
T1	Moderate size	6300 rad tumor dose/ 28 fractions/5.5 wk
T1	Bulky	6550 rad tumor dose/ 29 fractions/6 wk
T2	Early, normal motion	6300 rad tumor dose/ 28 fractions/5.5 wk
T2	Moderate size, reduced motion	6775 rad tumor dose/ 30 fractions/6 wk
T3	Fixed cord	7000 rad tumor dose/ 31 fractions/6 wk

MANAGEMENT OF RECURRENCE. Most recurrences appear within 18 months, but late recurrences may appear after 5 years.[177] Additionally, these patients are prone to develop second primaries in the head and neck area, and 5–10% develop lung cancer; for this reason the authors recommend a chest roentgenogram every 6 months, although it is debatable if this will help in early detection.

With careful followup, recurrence is often detected before the patient notices return of hoarseness. Edema of the larynx, particularly the false cords and arytenoids, suggests recurrence. Fixation of the cord usually implies local recurrence; the authors have observed two patients who developed a fixed cord with an otherwise normal-appearing larynx and have not shown evidence of recurrence. A paralyzed left vocal cord should also suggest the possibility of lung cancer.

Irradiation failures are almost always salvaged by cordectomy, hemilaryngectomy, or total laryngectomy (see Table 13-36). Only 2–3% of patients will die of their cancer unless they refuse operation.

Salvage by radiation therapy for recurrences or new tumors that appear after hemilaryngectomy is about 50%. Lee and coworkers report seven successes in 12 patients; one lesion was subsequently controlled by total laryngectomy.[178]

Radiation therapy will occasionally cure a patient with recurrence in the neck or stoma after total laryngectomy.

Supraglottic Larynx Carcinoma

SELECTION OF TREATMENT MODALITY. External beam irradiation and operation are the only curative modalities available. For purposes of treatment planning, patients may be considered to be in either an early group (T1, T2, early T3 lesions) or a late group (late T3, T4 lesions). The early group may be treated by either irradiation or supraglottic laryngectomy with voice preservation. Neck nodes are commonly involved and influence the overall treatment plan.

The late group most often requires a total laryngectomy combined with either pre- or postoperative irradiation, although irradiation is selectively prescribed for favorable lesions with total laryngectomy reserved for irradiation failure. The authors prefer postoperative irradiation for technically resectable lesions since the operative morbidity is less. Preoperative irradiation is prescribed for lesions of borderline resectability, usually due to large or fixed nodes, or in patients where a trial of irradiation is used before deciding on laryngectomy.

Early Supraglottic Lesions (T1, T2, or Early T3).

Treatment of the primary lesion for the early group is either full-dose irradiation or supraglottic laryngectomy. Total laryngectomy would rarely be indicated today for this group of patients.

Supraglottic laryngectomy is a voice-sparing operation that can be tailored to the individual supraglottic lesion. Since the patient has an increased tendency to aspirate, it is essential that adequate pulmonary reserve be present as determined by blood gases, pulmonary function tests, chest roentgenogram, and a work test (walking the patient up two flights of stirs to determine tolerance to pulmonary stress). The voice quality is generally quite good following supraglottic laryngectomy. All patients have some difficulty swallowing in the immediate postoperative period, but most learn to swallow in a short time; motivation is a key factor in learning to swallow.

Supraglottic laryngectomy can be used successfully for lesions involving the epiglottis, a single arytenoid, the aryepiglottic fold, and false vocal cords. Extension of the tumor to the true vocal cords, to the anterior commissure, or to both arytenoids, or fixation, excludes supraglottic laryngectomy. The supraglottic laryngectomy may be extended to include the base of tongue to the level of circumvallate papillae as long as one lingual artery is preserved. A radical neck dissection on one or both sides may be added as part of the supraglottic laryngectomy; about 35% of patients will have histologically positive nodes even when the neck is negative to clinical appraisal. For small midline infrahyoid epiglottic lesions, which may spread to either side, neck dissection is usually reserved for the appearance of nodes since the risk of subclinical disease is less for this site compared to the rest of the supraglottic larynx.

Some centers use preoperative irradiation ranging from 2500 to 5000 rad prior to supraglottic laryngectomy; some have reported success with postoperative irradiation.

Irradiation is also highly successful in the early lesions and preserves both speech and normal swallowing.

How does one select supraglottic laryngectomy or irradiation when each produces a high degree of success? As a result of fact, this has not been a problem in the authors' practices. At least one-half of the patients technically suitable for a supraglottic laryngectomy are not suitable for medical reasons (*e.g.*, inadequate pulmonary status or major medical problems) or because they lack motivation to learn again how to swallow. The latter is particularly true in older patients. For some of the larger lesions, the surgeon calculates a 30–50% risk of converting to a total laryngectomy at the time of operation; radiation therapy may be preferred in these cases.

Medium-sized lesions of the infrahyoid epiglottis or false cords are preferably treated by supraglottic laryngectomy since they are frequently understaged and success in properly selected patients having supraglottic laryngectomy is quite high. Lesions of the suprahyoid epiglottis or aryepiglottic folds are preferably treated by irradiation. The status of the neck often determines the treatment of the primary.

When a patient presents with an early-stage primary lesion, but advanced neck disease (N2 or N3), combined treatment

TABLE 13-36. Results* of Radiation Plus Salvage for Vocal Cord Carcinoma in 155 Patients

STAGE	NO. OF PTS†	SITE OF FAILURE		SALVAGE			CAUSE OF DEATH	
		PRIMARY	NECK	HEMILARYNGECTOMY	TOTAL LARYNGECTOMY	RADIATION SALVAGE	LARYNX CANCER	INTERCURRENT DISEASE
T1	96	7**	0	1/3‡	4/4	0	1	14
T2	50	16§	1	2/2	11/12	1/1‖	4§	6
T3	10	7**	1	0	3/6	1/1	3	4

* University of Florida results: patients treated 10/64–12/77; analysis 12/80.

† Patients dead of intercurrent disease less than 2 years after treatment with primary controlled at the time of death are excluded from the analysis (7 with stage T1, 2 with stage T2).

‡ Two patients with failure had total laryngectomy; one died of neck node and distant metastases, one died due to intercurrent disease.

§ Two refused total laryngectomy and died of larynx cancer.

‖ Second failure.

** One patient refused attempted salvage and died of larynx cancer.

is frequently necessary. High-dose preoperative or postoperative irradiation is not recommended to the patient having a supraglottic laryngectomy because the incidence of lymphedema of the larynx increases rapidly. In this case, the primary is usually treated for cure by irradiation with surgery added to the involved neck. If the patient has resectable neck disease and surgery is elected for the primary site, postoperative irradiation may be added because of the risk of neck failure; patients treated by combined therapy are at greater risk to develop lymphedema of the larynx.

In selected cases, the patient is advised that the alternatives of either supraglottic laryngectomy or radiation therapy seem to be about equal.

Late Supraglottic Lesions (Late T3, T4). Selected T3 lesions of the upper supraglottic larynx that are mainly exophytic should be treated by irradiation, as the control rate is fairly high. A few T4 lesions may also be cured by irradiation. Borderline lesions are given a trial of irradiation to 4500–5000 rad and if response is good, irradiation is continued for cure. If response is unsatisfactory, irradiation is stopped and total laryngectomy is done 4–6 weeks later. There is no proof that one may select patients by this therapeutic trial, but many of the T3–4 successes were culled out in this fashion.

Lesions unsuitable for irradiation are managed by total laryngectomy. If the neck disease is resectable, then operation is the initial treatment, and postoperative irradiation is added if needed. If the neck disease is unresectable or borderline, preoperative irradiation is used.

SURGICAL TREATMENT. *Supraglottic Laryngectomy.* Supraglottic laryngectomy often entails a radical neck dissection in continuity with resection of the primary lesion. The structures removed include the entire epiglottis, both false vocal cords, the pre-epiglottic space, and in some instances, a single arytenoid. The incision is usually a modified Schobinger or a half H incision. If the likelihood of a total laryngectomy is high, then an apron flap is used. The neck dissection is completed and left attached to the thyrohyoid membrane. The perichondrium of the larynx is then elevated in continuity with the strap muscles. This is very important because it will be used to close the surgical defect. Saw cuts are made through the thyroid cartilage and the hyoid bone so that the pre-epiglottic space is included in the specimen. The pharynx is entered above the hyoid through the vallecula. The specimen is removed, leaving only the arytenoids and true vocal cords. If one arytenoid has to be sacrificed, the cord must be fixed in the midline to prevent aspiration. The defect is closed by suturing the previously saved perichondrium and muscle into the base of the tongue. Ten to 14 days later, the tracheostomy is removed and the patient is retrained in the act of swallowing. The patient is then discharged when he can swallow 2000 cc or more without significant coughing.

The complications are aspiration, fistula formation, wound breakdown, flap necrosis, and carotid exposure and rupture.

Total Laryngectomy. The entire larynx and pre-epiglottic space are resected *en bloc* and a permanent tracheostomy is fashioned. The pharynx is sutured to the base of tongue and a portion of the thyroid gland is usually included with the specimen.

IRRADIATION TECHNIQUE. The primary lesion and both sides of the neck are included with opposed lateral portals. The dose for T1 lesions is 6000–6500 rad and for T2-T3 lesions, 7000 rad, occasionally 7500. The lower neck nodes are irradiated through a separate anterior portal. A submental "boost" portal may be used for the last 1000 rad for suprahyoid epiglottic lesions that invade the vallecula (see the section on the base of the tongue).

Patients develop a sore throat, loss of taste, and moderate dryness during irradiation. Edema of the arytenoids may occur and give a lump-like sensation in the throat. Tracheostomy is seldom necessary even for bulky lesions; 180 rad treatment is favored for these lesions to avoid severe mucositis and edema.

Edema of the larynx may persist for several months to a year. Radical neck dissection increases the degree of lymphedema on the side of the operation. The lymphedema of the larynx and submental space resolves together. Patients who continue to smoke and drink heighten the side effects of dryness, dysphagia, and hoarseness.

COMBINED TREATMENT POLICIES. Either surgery or irradiation alone is preferred for the early primary lesions.

If total laryngectomy is required and the lesion is resectable, postoperative irradiation is preferred, since there is no evidence that preoperative irradiation produces any better local/regional control or improved survival. Radiation therapy is added for close or positive margins, invasion of soft tissues of the neck, cartilage invasion, and N2 or N3 neck disease. The high-risk areas are usually the base of tongue and neck; the stomal area is also at risk when subglottic extension is present. Complications related to postoperative irradiation are relatively uncommon in this group.

Irradiation is used prior to total laryngectomy for patients with technically unresectable neck nodes, as a trial of radiation therapy prior to deciding on radiation therapy alone or total laryngectomy, or when scheduling problems require a long delay to operation.

A number of patients either refuse laryngectomy or are medically unsuitable for the operation; hence, irradiation is the treatment by default. However, quite a few of these patients can be cured, and one should not take a hopeless attitude.[177]

MANAGEMENT OF RECURRENCE. Failures after supraglottic laryngectomy or irradiation can frequently be salvaged by further treatment; recognition of recurrence should be vigorously pursued.

Salvage of recurrences that develop after total laryngectomy and postoperative radiation therapy is quite uncommon.

RESULTS OF TREATMENT

Vocal Cord Cancer

SURGICAL RESULTS. Ogura and coworkers report a 3-year determinate survival without disease of 86% for patients treated by hemilaryngectomy.[179] The local and regional recurrence rate was 6%.

The 3-year determinate survival without disease for patients treated by total laryngectomy with or without radical neck dissection was 70%. The local and regional recurrence rate was 22%.

RADIATION THERAPY RESULTS. Table 13-36 shows the results of irradiation for 156 patients with squamous cell carcinoma of the vocal cord treated by irradiation. One of the T1 and four of the T2 patients died of cancer. The five deaths were due to recurrence of the vocal cord cancer in two patients who refused total laryngectomy, neck recurrence in two patients, and distant metastases in one. The high failure rate in the T3 lesions is partially explained by inclusion of patients who refused laryngectomy as initial therapy.

A few local failures continue to appear after 5 years of followup. Some of these late failures occur on the opposite cord and undoubtedly represent new cancers. The same pattern of late recurrence is also seen after hemilaryngectomy.

Anterior commissure extension does not affect success with irradiation unless it is associated with bulky disease, especially in the subglottic area. Lesions confined to the posterior half of the cord have a higher failure rate than lesions of a similar size in the anterior half; the reason is not known.

Within the T1 and T2 categories is a wide range of disease distribution and volume of tumor. Dickens and coworkers selected 84 patients (74 T1 and 12 T2) anatomically suitable for hemilaryngectomy.[180] The control rate by radiation therapy alone was 94%. All five patients with recurrence were saved by subsequent operations, four by total laryngectomy and one by hemilaryngectomy.

Dickens also selected 70 patients with T1 lesions confined to one cord that would have been anatomically suitable for cordectomy. The control rate by radiation therapy alone was 97%. The two patients with recurrence were salvaged by operations, one by total laryngectomy and one by hemilaryngectomy.

Supraglottic Larynx Cancer

The 3-year survival rate in a large series of patients with supraglottic larynx carcinoma treated by supraglottic laryngectomy was 82.5% for stage T1N0 and 79% for stage T2N0.[181] Overall, the salvage rate using surgery or radiation for recurrence after supraglottic laryngectomy was 47%. For patients with advanced lesions treated with preoperative radiation therapy followed by total laryngectomy and radical neck dissection, the 3- and 5-year survival rates are 70% and 67%, respectively. The 3-year survival rate for patients with clinically positive neck nodes is influenced by the size and fixation of the nodes. Survival rates range from 57.5% to 66% with Stage N1 having the best results.

The success with irradiation is outlined in Table 13-37. There is a very high local control rate with doses of 6000–6500 rad for T1 and 7000 rad for T2–T3 lesions.[53,177] Failures after supraglottic laryngectomy or irradiation can usually be salvaged by either total laryngectomy or irradiation in about one-half of the patients. Table 13-38 shows the local control rates obtained with combined operation and radiation therapy.

COMPLICATIONS OF TREATMENT

Surgical

Repeated stripping of the cord may result in a thickened cord and hoarse voice. Neel and coworkers reported a 26% incidence of nonfatal complications for cordectomy.[182] Immediate postoperative complications include atelectasis and pneumonia, severe subcutaneous emphysema in the neck, bleeding from the tracheotomy site or larynx, wound complications, and airway obstruction requiring tracheotomy. Late complications included removal of granulation tissue by direct laryngoscopy to exclude recurrence, extrusion of cartilage, laryngeal stenosis, and obstructing laryngeal web.

The postoperative complications of hemilaryngectomy include aspiration, chondritis, wound slough, inadequate glottic closure, and anterior commissure webs.

The postoperative complications of total laryngectomy may include operative death, hemorrhage, fistula, wound slough, carotid rupture, and dysphagia.

The complication rate following supraglottic laryngectomy is roughly 10%, including fistula formation, aspiration, chondritis, dysphagia, dyspnea, and carotid rupture.

Radiation Therapy

After irradiation, the quality and volume of the voice tend to diminish at the end of the day. Many patients report changes in voice with change in weather, with upper respiratory

TABLE 13-37. Local Control by T Stage in Carcinoma of the Supraglottic Larynx Treated by Radiation Therapy Alone (University of Florida, 10/64–11/77; analysis 11/79)

STAGE	INITIAL RADIATION THERAPY (No. Controlled/ No. Treated)	SURGICAL SALVAGE (No. Salvaged/ No. Attempted)	ULTIMATE CONTROL (No. Controlled/ No. Treated)
T1	12/13	1/1	13/13 (100%)
T2	8/13	1/4	9/13 (69%)
T3	7/9	0/0	7/9 (78%)
T4	2/8	3/4	5/8 (62%)
Total	29/43 (67%)	5/9 (55%)	34/43 (79%)

(Golder SL: Carcinoma of the supraglottic larynx. 10th Annual Radiation Therapy Clinical Research Seminar, April 24–26, 1980, pp 237–247. Gainesville, Florida, Radiation Therapy Division, University of Florida, 1981)

TABLE 13-38. Control of Primary Disease with Combined Treatment in Carcinoma of the Supraglottic Larynx (University of Florida, 10/64–11/77; analysis 11/79)

	SURGERY	
RADIATION THERAPY	TOTAL LARYNGECTOMY (No. controlled/ no. treated)	SUPRAGLOTTIC LARYNGECTOMY (No. controlled/ no. treated)
Preoperative	7/10 (70%)	2/2 (100%)
Postoperative	9/9 (100%)	2/3 (67%)

(Golder SL: Carcinoma of the supraglottic larynx. 10th Annual Radiation Therapy Clinical Research Seminar, April 24–26, 1980, pp 237–247. Gainesville, Florida, Radiation Therapy Division, University of Florida, 1981)

infections, and the like. Edema of the larynx is the most common sequela following irradiation for glottic or supraglottic lesions. The rate of clearance of the edema is related to dose of radiation, volume of tissue irradiated, addition of a neck dissection, continued use of alcohol and tobacco, and the size and extent of the original lesion. For instance, glottic lesions involving the posterior cord(s) require a higher dose to the arytenoids than small anterior glottic lesions; therefore, the posterior lesions have a higher incidence of edema. Edema is accentuated by a radical neck dissection; it may require 6 months to as long as 2 years for the lymphedema to disappear.

Soft tissue necrosis leading to chondritis occurs in about 1% of patients, usually in the person who continues to smoke and drink alcohol. Soft tissue and cartilage necroses mimic recurrence with hoarseness, pain, and edema; a laryngectomy may be recommended in desperation for fear of recurrent cancer, even though biopsies show only necrosis.

Steroids (*e.g.*, Decadron) have been used to reduce edema secondary to radiation effect after recurrence has been ruled out by biopsy. If ulceration and pain occur, antibiotics such as tetracycline may help.

Combined Treatment

Most surgeons agree that preoperative irradiation is generally associated with an increased risk of an operative complication and slightly prolonged hospitalization. The increased risk is not prohibitive by any means, but if the same goal can be accomplished by postoperative irradiation, the overall complication rates are reduced. The major late effects of combined treatment are an increased fibrosis of soft tissues.

HYPOPHARYNX: PHARYNGEAL WALLS, PYRIFORM SINUS, AND POSTCRICOID PHARYNX

Both the oropharyngeal and hypopharyngeal walls will be considered together as there is no distinct difference in the presentation, treatment, or prognosis. The great majority of hypopharyngeal lesions originate in the pyriform sinus. Postcricoid carcinomas are fortunately quite uncommon in the U.S.

ANATOMY

The epithelium of the pharyngeal mucous membrane is squamous. It is continuous with the mucous membrane of the nasopharynx; there is no visible point or line of transition. The dividing point between the nasopharynx and posterior pharyngeal wall is actually Passavant's ridge, a muscular ring that contracts to close the nasopharynx during swallowing. The posterior and lateral walls are surrounded by the thin constrictor muscles. Between the constrictor muscle and the prevertebral fascia that covers the longitudinal spine muscles (longus colli and longus capitis) is a thin layer of loose areolar tissue, the retropharyngeal space. The entire thickness of the posterior pharyngeal wall from the mucous membrane to the anterior vertebral body is no more than 1 cm in the midline. Lateral to the pharyngeal wall are the vessels, nerves, and muscles of the parapharyngeal space (see Fig. 13-16). The constrictor muscles are relatively thin, especially the superior constrictor, and do not present much of an obstacle to tumor penetration. There is a variable weak spot in the lateral pharyngeal wall just below the hyoid where the middle and the inferior constrictor muscles fail to overlap. The lateral wall in this area is composed of the fibrous thyrohyoid membrane, which is penetrated by the vessels, nerves, and lymphatics of the laryngopharynx.

The pharyngeal walls are continuous with the cervical esophagus below. The hypopharyngeal walls are visible by indirect mirror examination; the transition to cervical esophagus is below the arytenoids (C4) and invisible to mirror examination. The transition zone, 3–4 cm in length, is referred to as the postcricoid pharynx and will be dealt with separately, since tumors of this area present a special clinical picture.

The lateral pharyngeal wall is a rather narrow, ill-defined strip of mucosa. It lies behind the posterior tonsillar pillar in the oropharynx, is partially interrupted by the pharyngoepiglottic fold, and then continues into the hypopharynx, where it becomes the lateral wall of the pyriform sinus. The lateral pharyngeal wall has a maximum width of no more than 2 cm. The posterior cornu of the hyoid bone will occasionally protrude into the lateral pharyngeal wall on one or both sides, producing a submucosal bulge.

The posterior pharyngeal wall is about 4–5 cm wide and about 6–7 cm in height. Submucosal bulges may be seen due to osteophytes on the anterior lips of the cervical vertebrae and may be mistaken for submucosal tumor.

The pyriform sinus is created by the intrusion of the larynx into the anterior aspect of the pharynx. This creates pharyngeal grooves lateral to the larynx. The superior margin of the pyriform sinus is the pharyngo-epiglottic fold and the free margin of the aryepiglottic fold. The superolateral margin of the pyriform sinus is considered to be an oblique line along the lateral pharyngeal wall just opposite the aryepiglottic fold. The pyriform sinus therefore is made up of three walls: the anterior, lateral, and medial; there is no posterior wall. The pyriform sinus tapers inferiorly to the apex and usually terminates at the level of the cricoid cartilage. The superior limit of the pyriform sinus is opposite the hyoid. The thyrohyoid membrane is lateral to the upper portion of the pyriform sinus (membranous pyriform sinus), and the thyroid cartilage, cricothyroid membrane, and cricoid cartilage are lateral to the lower portion (cartilaginous pyriform sinus). The internal branch of the superior laryngeal nerve, a branch of the vagus, may produce a fold in the mucous membrane on the anterolateral wall of the pyriform sinus. Fig. 13-12 shows the pathway for referred pain to the external auditory canal by way of the auricular branch of the vagus. The auricular branch is sensory to the skin of the back of the pinna and the posterior wall of the external auditory canal.

Patients with pain associated with an oral cavity primary will point to the skin of the temple as well as the ear canal. Patients with referred pain from the larynx or hypopharynx will often point behind the ear and generally are more vague about the location of the earache.

The postcricoid pharynx is funnel-shaped to direct food into the gullet. There is no discrete superior margin, but it may be considered to begin just below the arytenoids. The anterior wall lies behind the cricoid cartilage and is the posterior wall of the lower larynx; this wall is often referred to as the "party wall." The posterior wall is merely a continuation of the hypopharyngeal walls. The recurrent laryngeal nerve lies between the lateral wall and the deep surface of the thyroid gland.

PATHOLOGY

Over 95% of malignant tumors are squamous cell carcinoma or one of its variants. Carcinoma *in situ* is commonly seen in surgical specimens at the edge of neoplasms of the pharyngeal wall, and multifocal skip areas of carcinoma *in situ* may make it difficult to obtain clear margins if excision is done. Minor salivary gland tumors are quite rare.

PATTERNS OF SPREAD

Posterior Pharyngeal Wall

Carcinomas of the posterior pharyngeal wall have a strong tendency to remain on the posterior wall, grow up or down the wall, and infiltrate posteriorly; they seldom spread circumferentially to the lateral walls, even when quite advanced. Early lesions are red lesions, sometimes with white areas sprinkled over the involved area. As the lesion progresses, the tumor bulges into the pharyngeal cavity and a ragged, midline, linear ulceration appears. The posterior tonsillar pillars may become involved, with spread up the pillars eventually reaching the palate. Advanced lesions tend to terminate inferiorly at the level of the arytenoids without growing into the postcricoid region. Superiorly they may extend into the nasopharynx. Direct invasion of the cervical vertebrae or base of skull is uncommon.

Lateral Pharyngeal Wall

Early tumors may be well-defined exophytic lesions. As they advance, they have a tendency to lateral penetration through the constrictor muscle, thus entering the lateral pharyngeal space or the soft tissues of the neck. A mass may become palpable in the neck just below the hyoid and be confused with a lymph node.

The muscles of the pharynx originate from the base of skull, eustachian tube, styloid process, pterygomandibular raphe, and hyoid bone; tumor may spread along muscle and fascial planes to all muscular points of origin.[183] Tumor also courses along cranial nerves IX and X and the sympathetic chain. The thyroid gland is adjacent to the lower walls and is often invaded. Tumor secondarily invades the pharyngoepiglottic fold, the vallecula, and the anterior and lateral walls of the pyriform sinus.

Pyriform Sinus

Early lesions are usually discrete and exophytic, particularly those high on the medial wall. Medial wall lesions may grow superficially along the aryepiglottic fold and arytenoids or invade directly into the false cord and aryepiglottic fold. They also extend posteriorly to the postcricoid region. Extensive submucosal spread is a characteristic feature.

Large bulky lesions arising in the upper medial wall may cause reduced motion that quickly returns to normal when gross tumor recedes during irradiation. The vocal cord becomes fixed due to infiltration of the intrinsic muscles of the larynx, the cricoaryntenoid joint, or less commonly the recurrent laryngeal nerve. These lesions grow posteriorly to involve the postcricoid pharynx and cricoid cartilage and may extend to the opposite pyriform sinus. Spread into the cervical esophagus is unusual.

Lesions arising on the lateral wall tend toward early invasion of the posterior thyroid cartilage and the posterior superior cricoid cartilage. The ipsilateral superior lobe of the thyroid gland may be invaded after tumor penetrates the cartilage, but thyroid invasion can occur in cases with no cartilage invasion when tumor penetrates behind the thyroid cartilage or through the cricothyroid membrane. Kirchner reports that thyroid cartilage invasion is associated with involvement of the apex of the pyriform sinus and the extent of invasion cannot be predicted on based visible disease.[184]

Lesions of the lateral walls tend to spread submucosally onto the posterior pharyngeal wall. It is often difficult to estimate the extent of posterior pharyngeal wall or postcricoid invasion except at direct laryngoscopy, since these areas are often impossible to visualize indirectly. Even with direct endoscopy, invasion may be underestimated.

Advanced lesions of the pyriform sinus invade all three walls, fix the larynx, involve the ipsilateral posterior pharyngeal wall, invade the thyroid cartilage and thyroid gland, and often escape into the soft tissues of the neck. The preepiglottic space is often not involved. Perineural invasion of the recurrent laryngeal nerve may be seen in whole organ sections.

Postcricoid Pharynx

Early lesions of the postcricoid area are rarely diagnosed. Lesions arising from the posterior wall tend to remain on the posterior wall. Lesions arising from the anterior wall tend to invade the posterior cricoarytenoid muscle and the cricoid and arytenoid cartilages. Advanced tumors eventually encircle the lumen. Since the apex of the pyriform sinus terminates in the postcricoid area, some lesions secondarily invade the apex of the pyriform sinus very early.

Lymphatics

PHARYNGEAL WALLS. The lymphatics of the pharyngeal walls terminate primarily in the jugular chain with a secondary avenue by way of the spinal accessory chain. The jugulodigastric node is the most commonly involved node.

Lindberg reports 59% clinically positive nodes on admission; 17% were bilateral.[32] Wang reports 55% positive nodes for lesions of the posterior pharyngeal wall, of which 10% were bilateral.[185] At the University of Florida, the incidence of clinically positive nodes for posterior pharyngeal wall lesions was 65%.

HYPOPHARYNX. The capillary lymphatics of the hypopharynx, especially the pyriform sinus, are quite profuse. The distribution of lymph node metastases is mainly to the jugular chain with a relatively small proportion to the spinal accessory chain. The subdigastric node is the most commonly involved, but midjugular involvement occurs without subdigastric node enlargement.

Seventy-five percent of patients have clinically positive nodes on admission and at least 10% are bilateral.

CLINICAL PICTURE

Tumors that are lateralized to the lateral pharyngeal wall or pyriform sinus produce a unilateral sore throat, a symptom rather specific for cancer since infectious sore throat is bilateral. The patient with cancer can point to the painful site with one finger, while the patient with inflammatory sore throat cannot. Dysphagia, sensation of foreign body, ear pain, blood-streaked saliva, and voice change occur later. A neck mass may be the presenting complaint.

Lesions of the posterior pharyngeal wall are often overlooked even by competent physicians because of failure to examine the posterior pharyngeal wall routinely during indirect laryngoscopy.

Small lesions of the pyriform sinus are easily missed unless very careful examinations are done. Many of these patients have active gag reflexes, and complete topical anesthesia coupled with patience is required by the examiner.

Lesions of the apex of the pyriform sinus or postcricoid area produce indirect findings that are clues to tumor not visible by indirect laryngoscopy. Pooling of secretions in the pyriform sinus and arytenoid area indicates obstruction of the upper gullet. Edema of the arytenoids and inability to see into the apex of the pyriform sinus are clues to postcricoid or low-lying pyriform sinus tumors. Invasion of the palatopharyngeus at its insertion into the inferior constrictor may cause shortening of the muscle and asymmetry of the posterior tonsillar pillars. As postcricoid tumor enlarges it pushes the larynx anteriorly. This produces a full, expanded neck appearance. The thyroid click or crackle is produced by the superior thyroid horns hitting against the spine while rocking the thyroid cartilage back and forth. This is lost when the larynx and thyroid cartilage protrude anteriorly.

METHODS OF DIAGNOSIS AND STAGING

Lesions of the oropharyngeal wall can often be biopsied in the outpatient clinic with topical anesthesia. Hypopharyngeal lesions usually require general anesthesia and biopsy under direct visualization.

Direct laryngoscopy and esophagoscopy are needed to map the extent of low pharyngeal wall, pyriform sinus, and postcricoid lesions.

Lateral soft tissue roentgenograms and xerograms are helpful to determine and confirm the extent of posterior pharyngeal wall involvement, particularly in the postcricoid area.

Anteroposterior tomograms of the larynx and hypopharynx are useful for pyriform sinus lesions to determine the degree of larynx invasion.

Laryngograms are useful for small to medium-sized pyriform sinus and postcricoid lesions to determine the extent of larynx invasion and invasion of the apex of the pyriform sinus. The "puffed cheek" view expands the pyriform sinus with air and contrast medium to demonstrate wall mobility. A lack of mobility suggests deep infiltration.

CT scans are useful in demonstrating invasion of the pre-epiglottic space and thyroid cartilage.

Staging

The American Joint Committee staging for the hypopharynx is satisfactory for the pyriform sinus, but unsatisfactory for the pharyngeal wall:[39]

- TX Tumor that cannot be assessed by the rules as listed
- TO No evidence of primary tumor
- TIS Carcinoma *in situ*
- T1 Tumor confined to the site of origin
- T2 Extension of tumor to adjacent region or site without fixation of hemilarynx
- T3 Extension of tumor to adjacent region or site with fixation of hemilarynx
- T4 Massive tumor invading bone or soft tissues of neck

If there is definite decrease in mobility, the lesion should be assigned to T3.

Lesions of the posterior pharyngeal wall tend to stay on the posterior pharyngeal wall rather than invade the larynx or lateral walls; therefore, fixation does not enter into staging. Posterior pharyngeal wall lesions would be more appropriately staged by tumor diameter.

TREATMENT

Selection of Treatment Modality

POSTERIOR PHARYNGEAL WALL. The majority of lesions on the posterior pharyngeal wall are treated by radiation therapy, although the results are far from outstanding. Attempts have been made to combine surgery and radiation therapy for selected, moderately-advanced lesions with limited success.

All aspects considered, high-dose radiotherapy will produce cure rates similar to those produced by either surgery alone or combined surgery plus radiation therapy, and with lesser morbidity. A few selected patients who fail to respond to radiation therapy or whose lesions recur after irradiation will be salvaged by pharyngectomy.

LATERAL PHARYNGEAL WALL. There is very little information specifically related to the lateral walls. Small (T1–2) lesions are usually exophytic and respond readily to irradiation. Larger lesions tend to be deeply infiltrative, and control by irradiation or surgery is only modest at best. An operation for a large lesion usually implies a laryngectomy in combination with pharyngectomy.

PYRIFORM SINUS. The pyriform sinus is the most common primary site in the hypopharynx. Lesions confined to the pyriform sinus with normal mobility (T1) are locally controlled in 85–90% of cases by irradiation or partial laryngopharyngectomy.[51] Irradiation is the preferred choice of the authors since it leaves the patient with nearly normal swallowing and speech while permitting wider coverage of the regional lymphatics. Irradiation is more generally applicable while there are certain restraints on use of partial laryngopharyngectomy.

Lesions that extend outside the pyriform sinus with normal or reduced mobility (T2–3) represent the group of cases where treatment selection is more complex.

Invasion of the pyriform sinus apex is a contraindication to partial laryngopharyngectomy, but these same patients do poorly with radiation therapy also; these patients are selected for total laryngopharyngectomy plus postoperative radiation therapy. Fixation is a relative indication for total laryngopharyngectomy and postoperative radiation therapy. If the lesion is mainly exophytic and in the upper pyriform sinus, a trial of radiation therapy is offered as an alternative to total laryngopharyngectomy. If the disease disappears at 4500–5000 rad and mobility is returning, radical irradiation is a reasonable choice with total laryngopharyngectomy reserved for failure. Partial laryngopharyngectomy is generally not attempted after 4500–5000 rad because of complications, so if the patient was suitable for partial laryngopharyngectomy at the initiation of radiation treatment, that option may be lost with a trial of radiation therapy. A select group of T2 lesions with minimal extension beyond the pyriform sinus and a normal apex are also suitable for partial laryngopharyngectomy. However, these are the very patients that do well with radiation therapy only. The local control rate by radiation therapy for selected T2–3 lesions is approximately 50–60% at the University of Florida. Radiation therapy failures may be salvaged by total laryngopharyngectomy, although the mortality and morbidity are considerable after high-dose irradiation.

The more advanced, infiltrative lesions are best treated with immediate total laryngopharyngectomy, radical neck dissection, and postoperative radiation therapy. While the control rate above the clavicles is reasonably good with combined treatment of unfavorable stage III and IV, the 5-year results average 10–15% due to deaths from distant metastasis, intercurrent disease, complications of treatment, or second primary cancers.

Surgical Treatment

POSTERIOR PHARYNGEAL WALL. Surgery for posterior pharyngeal wall tumors is usually reserved for radiation therapy failures. If the lesion is high on the posterior wall, then a transoral approach can be used; however, for lower lesions the midline mandibulolabial glossotomy approach may be used. Alternatives are the transhyoid approach or a lateral pharyngotomy approach. The lesion is removed down to the prevertebral fascia, and no skin graft is placed.

PYRIFORM SINUS. Conservation surgery offers an alternative mode of treatment in very early lesions of the pyriform sinus. A partial laryngopharyngectomy removes the false cords, epiglottis, and pyriform sinus on the involved side. Since the pyriform sinus extends beyond the inferior extent of the thyroid cartilage, the apex of the pyriform cannot be involved by tumor since the cricoid must be preserved. Also, the cord cannot be fixed; however, the arytenoid can be involved with tumor. Pulmonary function must be good since some degree of aspiration generally occurs for some time after the procedure.

If the lesion of the pyriform sinus extends to the apex or if the cord is fixed, then a total laryngopharyngectomy must be performed, often followed by postoperative radiation therapy. Complications include aspiration, fistula formation, wound breakdown, and occasionally carotid blowout. The morbidity is significantly higher after preoperative radiation therapy.

POSTCRICOID PHARYNX. Postcricoid carcinoma generally requires a total laryngopharyngectomy with immediate reconstruction, generally using a pectoralis major myocutaneous flap. Prior to undertaking the surgery, however, the patient must undergo direct laryngoscopy and esophagoscopy to determine the extent of the lesion. If the lesion extends into the cervical esophagus, then reconstruction becomes more difficult and often bowel or stomach will have to be used.

Irradiation Technique

POSTERIOR PHARYNGEAL WALL. The irradiation technique for lesions of the posterior pharyngeal wall is opposed lateral fields to include the primary lesion and the regional nodes. Since these lesions tend to have skip areas, the entire posterior pharyngeal wall is included initially. If the lesion extends near the arytenoids, the postcricoid pharynx, pyriform sinus, and upper cervical esophagus are included. The parapharyngeal and retropharyngeal nodes will automatically be included with these fields. The upper spinal accessory nodes are included even if the neck nodes are negative.

The critical portion of the treatment occurs when the field is reduced at 4500–5000 rad to avoid the spinal cord. The posterior border of the portal bisects the cervical vertebral bodies, which places tumor very near the edge of the portal.

Daily imaging films and precision setups are required. Table 13-8 shows the doses required for control.

External beam may be supplemented by either radon or gold seed single-plane implants. If implants are planned, it is probably wise to reduce the spinal cord dose from external beam to 3000–4000 rad and complete the lymph node treatment with either electrons or neck dissection.

PYRIFORM SINUS. Parallel opposed lateral portals are used to encompass the primary lesion and regional nodes on both sides. The superior border is placed 2–3 cm above the tip of the mastoid to cover lymph nodes in the parapharyngeal space. The posterior border encompasses the spinal accessory nodes. The spinal cord is shielded from the treatment field at 4500–5000 rad. Clinically positive nodes behind the plane of the spinal cord require the addition of a neck dissection or electron boosts. The anterior border is usually placed about 1 cm behind the anterior skin edge. When the anterior border is shielded, the radiotherapist checks the setup daily as the margin for error is rather slim. However, protection of this narrow anterior segment reduces irradiation of the anterior arch of the thyroid and cricoid cartilages, anterior commissure of the glottis, and anterior midline skin. The inferior border is 2 cm below the inferior border of the cricoid. The inferior recess or apex of the pyriform sinus varies, but generally terminates at the upper to middle cricoid. The remaining lower neck lymph nodes are treated through an *en face* portal.

Dosimetry is individualized using wedges, compensators, and unequal loadings as needed. Table 13-8 shows the doses prescribed.

Combined Treatment Policies

POSTERIOR PHARYNGEAL WALL. Operation should usually precede radiation therapy when a combination is selected. There is a high incidence of operative mortality and complications with a preoperative dose of 2500–3000 rad.[186] When postoperative irradiation is used, a dose of 6000–6500 rad is used.

PYRIFORM SINUS. Irradiation is given prior to total laryngopharyngectomy in those borderline T2–3 patients for whom a trial of radiation therapy is planned; the patients are re-evaluated at 4500 rads with the surgeon. Irradiation is also used prior to operation for patients with a large fixed node to reduce the size of the mass and help obtain surgical margins. The preoperative dose to the node may be 6000–7500 rad, although the dose to the primary will be only 4000–5000 rad.

Following total laryngopharyngectomy with or without radical neck dissection, radiation therapy is recommended if there are close or positive margins, multiple or large positive nodes, extension of nodal disease through the capsule, or cartilage invasion. In short, almost all patients receive postoperative radiation therapy. There is an increased risk of pharyngeal stenosis, especially if the pharyngeal closure is tight.

Management of Recurrence

POSTERIOR PHARYNGEAL WALL. Recurrence after radiation therapy may be limited to the posterior pharyngeal wall and suitable for surgical excision with occasional salvage. Meoz-Mendez and coworkers report 11 irradiation failures salvaged by an operation out of a total of 68 local failures.[50] Irradiation salvage of a surgical failure would be unusual.

There is frequently a persistent ulcer at the completion of radiation therapy for the more advanced lesions. If the ulcer does not heal in short order, it should be considered evidence of persistent disease. Excision of the ulcer and coverage of the defect with a split-thickness skin graft is a reasonable procedure. Random biopsies of the ulcer are difficult, but the persistent ulcer usually heralds future recurrence and early excision will salvage some patients. Surgical excision is limited posteriorly by the prevertebral fascia.

PYRIFORM SINUS. The hallmark of local recurrence after radical irradiation is persistent major edema and inability to visualize the pyriform sinus, pain on swallowing, and fixation of laryngeal structures. Direct laryngoscopy is required, but biopsy may be negative and misleading. Eventually a decision may be made to recommend total laryngopharyngectomy for salvage without a positive biopsy.

Recurrence after total laryngopharyngectomy is usually in the soft tissues of the neck, the untreated opposite neck, the base of tongue, or stoma.

Surgical failures after partial laryngopharyngectomy for early lesions may be salvaged by total laryngopharyngectomy. Surgical failures after total laryngopharyngectomy are rarely salvaged.

Radiation failure may occasionally be salvaged by total laryngopharyngectomy with or without radical neck dissection. The risk of an operative mortality or major morbidity is high.

RESULTS OF TREATMENT

Posterior Pharyngeal Wall

The treatment policy at the University of Florida has primarily been radical irradiation. The absolute 2-year survival rate was 25%

Wang reports a 25% 3-year survival without recurrence for 36 patients with carcinoma of the posterior pharyngeal wall treated by radiation therapy alone; the 3-year survival was 47% for patients with clinically negative nodes.[185] Sixteen (66%) of 24 patients with T1–2 lesions had their disease controlled by radiation therapy, as did three of 13 patients with T3 lesions.

Meoz-Mendez and coworkers reported the results of radiation therapy alone for 164 patients with lesions arising from the pharyngeal walls, both posterior and lateral.[50] Table 13-39 shows the local control by T stage and the salvage of radiation therapy failures. The cause of death was local failure in 38%, neck recurrence in 6%, distant metastases in 10%, and second primary cancer in 16%.

Marks and coworkers compared low-dose preoperative radiation therapy (2500–3000 rads) followed by operation to radiation therapy alone (see Table 13-40).[186] The local control was slightly better for the combined group, but the 3-year actuarial survival was 17%, and the 3-year absolute survival was 14%. An operative mortality of 14% and a high risk of major surgical complications offset any gain in local control.

TABLE 13-39. Squamous Cell Carcinoma of the Pharyngeal Walls: Local Control (164 Patients—M. D. Anderson Hospital, 1954–1974)

STAGE	LOCAL CONTROL WITH RT* ALONE (No. controlled/ no. treated)	SURGICAL SALVAGE (No. salvaged)	ULTIMATE LOCAL CONTROL (No. controlled/ no. treated)
T1 (0–2 cm)	10/11 (91%)	1	11/11 (100%)
T2 (2–4 cm)	33/45 (73%)	2	35/45 (78%)
T3 (>4 cm)	38/62 (61%)	6	44/62 (71%)
T4 (massive)	15/46 (37%)	2	17/46 (41%)

(Meoz-Mendez RT, Fletcher GH, Guillamondegui OM et al: Analysis of the results of irradiation in the treatment of squamous cell carcinomas of the pharyngeal walls. Int J Radiat Oncol Biol Phys 4:579–585, 1978)

* RT: Radiation therapy.

M. D. Anderson Hospital reports a group of 25 patients (five stage T2, 20 Stage T3–4) treated by combined surgery and radiation therapy.[50] Nineteen patients received postoperative radiation therapy, 7 had positive margins, and 3 had close margins. Fifteen patients were dead at 5 years; six died of local recurrence or neck recurrence, five of distant metastasis, one of intercurrent disease, and three of uncertain causes. The 5-year absolute survival was 4/19(21%).

TABLE 13-40. Local Control in Carcinoma of the Posterior Pharyngeal Wall (Washington University, St. Louis)

TREATMENT	LOCAL CONTROL T1	T2	T3	T4
Surgery (*31 patients)	6/8	7/12	4/12	0/1
Radiation therapy alone	1/1	3/6	0/5	1/1

(Marks JE, Freeman RB, Lee F et al: Pharyngeal wall cancer: An analysis of treatment results complications and patterns of failure. Int J Radiat Oncol Biol Phys 4:587–593, 1978)

* 29 patients had preoperative radiation therapy; 2 patients had postoperative radiation therapy.

Pyriform Sinus

Most reports paint a rather dismal outlook for pyriform sinus tumors treated by radiation therapy alone.[187,188] Kirchner and Owen report only two 3-year survivors of 55 patients treated by radiation therapy alone; all but four patients had advanced disease.[187]

Table 13-41 shows the 3-year absolute and determinate survival by stage for 181 patients treated at M. D. Anderson Hospital by surgery with or without radiation therapy or radiation therapy alone.[35] Combined surgery and radiation therapy did not seem to improve the results over surgery alone, but the factors of selection played an enormous role in who did or did not receive postoperative radiation therapy, which makes interpretation of the data somewhat difficult.

Table 13-42 gives the results of the treatment for 80 patients with carcinoma of the pyriform sinus treated at Washington University, St. Louis, by preoperative radiation therapy followed by partial laryngopharyngectomy.[189] Seventy patients had the equivalent of AJC T1 lesions (disease limited to the pyriform sinus) and 10 patients had disease extending beyond the pyriform sinus. None had invasion of the apex of the pyriform sinus, as determined prior to surgery. The cause of death was cancer in 26%, complications of treatment in 14%, and intercurrent disease in 20%. The 2-year absolute survival (38%) (Marks JE: Personal communication, 1979).

Table 13-42 shows the results of treatment for 57 patients from the same institution who were treated by preoperative radiation therapy followed by total laryngectomy and partial

TABLE 13-41. Carcinoma of the Pyriform Sinus: Absolute and Determinate Survival Without Evidence of Disease in 181 Patients Treated for Cure (M. D. Anderson Hospital)

	3-YEAR SURVIVAL STAGE II ABS	STAGE II DET	STAGE III ABS	STAGE III DET	STAGE IV ABS	STAGE IV DET
Radiation (51 Patients) (12% I.D.*)	3/7	3/6	1/7	1/6	3/37	3/33
Surgery† (130 Patients) (21% I.D.)	7/32	7/19	10/30	10/23	14/68	14/30

(MacComb WS, Healey JE Jr, McGraw JP et al: Hypopharynx and cervical esophagus. In MacComb WS, Fletcher GH (eds): Cancer of the Head and Neck, pp 213–240. Baltimore, © Williams & Wilkins, 1967)

* I.D.—death due to intercurrent disease, no evidence of recurrent cancer.

† 69 Patients had either pre- or postoperative radiation therapy.

TABLE 13-42. Carcinoma of the Pyriform Sinus: Results of Treatment by Low-Dose Radiation Therapy Plus Partial Laryngopharyngectomy (PLP) or Low-Dose Radiation Therapy Plus Total Laryngectomy and Partial Pharyngectomy (TLP) (Washington University, St. Louis, 1964–74)

RESULT	PLP (80 patients*)	TLP (57 patients†)
Local recurrence ± neck recurrence	14%‡	14%
Neck recurrence ± distant metastases (primary controlled)	9%	23%
Distant metastases alone	11%	21%
5-year actuarial survival (no evidence of disease)	40%	22%

(Marks JE, Kumick B, Powers WE et al: Carcinoma of the pyriform sinus: An analysis of treatment results and patterns of failure. Cancer 41: 1008–1015, 1978)
* T1, 70 patients; T2–4, 10 patients (AJC staging).
† T1, 35 patients; T2–4, 22 patients (AJC staging).
‡ Four patients salvaged.

TABLE 13-43. Local Control for Carcinoma of the Pyriform Sinus Treated by Radiation Therapy (University of Florida, 10/64–4/78; 24 months to unlimited followup)

PRIMARY STAGE	EXCLUDED*	LOCAL CONTROL (No. Controlled/ No. Treated)	SURGICAL SALVAGE† (No. Salvaged/ No. Attempted)	ULTIMATE CONTROL (No. Controlled/ No. Treated)
T1	1	11/14 (79%)	0/1‡	11/14 (79%)
T2	1	6/10	3/4	9/10
T3	3	3/6	0/0	3/6
T4	0	1/7	0/0	1/7

(Million RR, Cassisi NJ: Radical irradiation for carcinoma of the pyriform sinus. Laryngoscope 91:439–450, 1981)
* Dead of intercurrent disease less than 24 months after treatment with primary controlled.
† Successfully salvaged patients living 4, 4, and 5½ years.
‡ Patient refused operation for one year after recurrence was diagnosed.

pharyngectomy.[189] Thirty-five patients had lesions confined to the pyriform sinus (AJC T1) and the remainder had extension beyond the pyriform sinus (AJC T2–4). The cause of death was cancer in 56%, complications of treatment in 11%, and intercurrent disease in 18%.

Tables 13-43, 13-44, and 13-45 show the results of radiation therapy for carcinoma of the pyriform sinus with radical neck dissection added as outlined in the section on principles of treatment.[51] Most patients with T1–2 lesions were selected for radiation therapy; T3 lesions were irradiated if they were exophytic and in the upper pyriform sinus or because the patient refused operation. All T4 lesions were irradiated by default.

TABLE 13-44. Carcinoma of the Pyriform Sinus: Control of Neck Node Disease (University of Florida, 10/64–4/78; analysis 4/80)

NECK STAGE	TREATMENT*	NECK CONTROL (No. controlled/ no. treated)
N0	RT	8/8
N1	RT	4/4
	Excision + RT	1/1
	RT + RND	1/1
N2	RT	4/5†
	RT + PND	1/1
N3	RT	0/5
	RT + RND	3/4
	RT + PND	1/1

(Million RR, Cassisi NJ: Radical irradiation for carcinoma of the pyriform sinus. Laryngoscope 91:439–450, 1981)
* RT—radiation therapy; RND—radical neck dissection: PND—partial neck dissection.
† One patient refused RND.

COMPLICATIONS OF TREATMENT

Posterior Pharyngeal Wall

SURGICAL COMPLICATIONS. Cunningham and Catlin report an operative mortality of 9% and a complication rate of 57% for patients operated on during the period of 1951–1961.[190] Mucocutaneous fistula was the most common problem.

Marks and coworkers report a 14% operative mortality plus major complications including pharyngocutaneous fistula (31%) and carotid rupture (14%) for patients treated with preoperative radiation therapy, 2500–3000 rad.[186]

RADIATION THERAPY COMPLICATIONS. Meoz-Mendez and coworkers analyzed the complications for 164 patients with carcinoma of the pharyngeal wall treated by radiation therapy alone.[50] There was a 5% incidence of fatal complications. In seven patients the fatality was secondary to carotid rupture, associated with attempts at surgical salvage. Only

TABLE 13-45. Carcinoma of the Pyriform Sinus: Survival Free of Disease (University of Florida, 10/64–4/78; analysis 4/80)

STAGE	ABSOLUTE 2-YEAR	ABSOLUTE 5-YEAR	DETERMINATE 2-YEAR	DETERMINATE 5-YEAR
I & II	5/6	2/3	5/6	2/3
III	8/13 (62%)	3/8	8/11 (73%)	3/7
IV	12/23 (52%)	1/10 (10%)	12/22 (55%)	1/9
Total	25/42 (60%)	6/21 (29%)	25/39 (64%)	6/19 (32%)

(Million RR, Cassisi NJ: Radical irradiation for carcinoma of the pyriform sinus. Laryngoscope 91:439–450, 1981)

two patients developed severe laryngeal edema. Radiation myelitis was documented in two patients. The overall incidence of radiation therapy-related complications was 12%; the complication rate increased with rising T stage.

Pyriform Sinus

SURGICAL COMPLICATIONS. The complications of partial laryngopharyngectomy include a 12% operative mortality, fistula, aspiration, and dysphagia.[189]

The complications of total laryngopharyngectomy include a treatment-related mortality of 11%, fistula, and pharyngeal stenosis.[189]

The complication rate is increased by the addition of radiation therapy.

RADIATION THERAPY COMPLICATIONS. The major radiation therapy complication is laryngeal necrosis. Arytenoid edema occurs temporarily in most cases and is increased by radical neck dissection.

COMPLICATIONS OF COMBINED TREATMENT. Attempted surgical salvage of radiation therapy failures has a significant operative morbidity and mortality in the best of hands, but few cures are produced.

NASOPHARYNX

Malignant tumors of the nasopharynx are uncommon in the U.S. The Chinese have a high frequency; American-born second-generation Chinese maintain the risk of nasopharynx cancer. It is undecided whether or not the risk is reduced by moving away from the Orient. Nasopharynx cancer has also been shown to have an association with elevated titers of Epstein-Barr virus; this finding is independent of geography.[22]

There is a 3:1 ratio of predominance in males. The age distribution for carcinoma is much younger than for other head and neck sites. About 15–20% are less than 30 years of age.

ANATOMY

The nasopharynx is roughly cuboidal in shape. It is in direct continuity with the nasal cavity, inferiorly with the oropharynx, and laterally with the middle ears by way of the eustachian tubes.

The mucosa of the roof and posterior wall is often irregular due to the pharyngeal bursa, pharyngeal tonsil (adenoids), and the pharyngeal hypophysis. The mucosa tends to become smooth with age, but many folds may remain in the later years of life to add to the examiner's confusion as to whether tumor is present. Adenoids may persist well past puberty and may even be present in elderly people. Following successful irradiation, these irregularities are usually replaced by a smooth, atrophic appearance.

The lateral walls include the eustachian openings with the fossa of Rosenmuller (pharyngeal recess) located behind the torus tubarius. The superolateral muscular wall of the nasopharynx is incomplete and provides a meager barrier to tumor spread. Once tumor has penetrated the lateral wall, it enters the lateral pharyngeal space and its contents. The floor of the nasopharynx is incomplete and consists of the upper surface of the soft palate, which is rarely the origin of nasopharyngeal tumors and is uncommonly invaded, even with extensive local disease.

Lymphatics

There is an extensive submucosal lymphatic capillary plexus, attested to by the high incidence of neck metastases. Tumor cells spread mainly along two different lymph node pathways: the jugular chain and the spinal accessory chain.

A third avenue, the retropharyngeal nodes, is a possible route of spread, but is relatively unimportant. The lateral retropharyngeal nodes lie in the retropharyngeal space near the lateral border of the posterior pharyngeal wall and medial to the carotid artery. Directly behind the nodes are the lateral masses of the atlas. The clinical appreciation of enlarged retropharyngeal nodes usually requires peroral palpation of the high posterolateral pharyngeal wall. Marked nodal enlargement, such as that which occurs in lymphoma, may distort the posterior tonsillar pillar, shifting it medially and anteriorly.

The majority of lymphatic channels empty directly into either the jugulodigastric or the upper lateral jugular nodes. Inconstant lymphatic vessels are described as draining directly to the nodes below the bifurcation of the carotid (midjugular nodes) and to the spinal accessory nodes.[191]

PATHOLOGY

Most histologic varieties of malignant tumor have been reported to arise from the nasopharynx and its immediate supporting structures. Carcinomas comprise about 85% and lymphomas about 10% of the malignant lesions. Lymphoepithelioma and transitional cell carcinoma are considered variants within the epithelial group; the incidence of lymphoepithelioma varies from about 30%–50% in various series. A miscellaneous group of malignant tumors includes melanoma, plasmacytoma, adenocarcinoma, juvenile angiofibroma, carcinosarcoma, sarcomas, nonchromaffin paragangliomas, and unclassified malignancies.

SPREAD PATTERNS

Primary

Table 13-46 shows the recognized spread to contiguous structures on admission prior to treatment in 99 patients with epithelial lesions.[192]

Inferior extension along the lateral pharyngeal walls and tonsillar pillars is recognized in almost one-third of patients. Extension into the posterior nasal cavity is difficult to determine by indirect mirror examination since the nasopharyngeal mass frequently occludes the view. Similarly, it is difficult to examine the posterior nares by direct examination through the anterior nares. Thorough shrinking of the nasal mucosa and examination with a small-diameter fiberoptic nasoscope is the best method for detecting nasal extension. Tomography and CT scan are helpful to determine soft tissue extension into the nasal cavity, but inflammatory exudates or coagulated blood may give a false impression.

Invasion of the posterior ethmoids, the maxillary antrum, and the orbit occurs fairly often and is important to recognize since it dictates a modification of treatment techniques.

Invasion into or through the base of the skull is recognized roentgenographically or clinically in at least 25% of patients prior to treatment.[36,192] Early, unrecognized invasion presumably occurs in a far greater number of patients, since the base of the skull, brain, and cranial nerves are frequent sites of local recurrence. The sphenoid sinus is frequently invaded. Tumor may erode through the foramen ovale, the foramen lacerum, and the foramen spinosum. Tumor eventually reaches the cavernous sinus area and has access to cranial nerves (CN) II–VI.

The lateral muscular wall of the nasopharynx is incomplete superiorly. This defect, referred to as the sinus of Morgagni, is traversed by the cartilaginous portion of the eustachian tube and the levator palatine muscle, providing an avenue of egress for the nasopharynx cancer to the lateral pharyngeal space and base of skull.

TABLE 13-46. Malignant Tumors of the Nasopharynx—Incidence of Spread to Contiguous Structures on Admission (M. D. Anderson Hospital, August 1948 to December 1960)

SITE OF SPREAD*	NO. OF CASES
Oropharyngeal wall	29
Base of skull (sphenoid sinus—11)	25
Tonsillar bed	15
Cranial nerves	12
Pterygoid fossa	9
Nasal cavity	5
Maxillary antrum	4
Orbit	3
Soft palate	3
Hard palate	2
Ethmoids	2
Hypopharynx	1

(Fletcher GH, Million RR: Malignant tumors of the nasopharynx. AJR 93:44–55, 1965. © 1965, American Roentgen Ray Society)

* In several patients, more than one structure was involved.

Lymphatics

There is an 80–90% incidence of metastatic neck node disease on presentation; approximately 50% have bilateral lymph node metastases.

Low-grade squamous carcinomas produce fewer metastases (73%) compared to high-grade carcinomas (92%).

Metastases to submental and occipital nodes may appear when there is blockage of the common lymphatic pathways either by massive neck disease or by an untimely neck dissection.

CLINICAL PICTURE

The most common presenting complaint is a painless upper neck mass or masses, which may be quite large when first discovered. The neck mass may enlarge quite rapidly due to necrosis or hemorrhage. A rare patient will report exquisite tenderness of the nodes and will be unable to tolerate palpation of the masses.

Nasal obstruction, epistaxis, and otitis media are caused by local tumor effect.

Sore throat occurs in about 15% of patients and is related to spread into the oropharyngeal wall. Facial pain may be referred from any of the three divisions of the trigeminal nerve, usually the mandibular division. Occipital or temporal headache is frequently seen. Pain in the scalp over the left mastoid area is related to involvement of a high jugular lymph node that has become fixed to the skull and spine.

Pain in lifting the head and extending the neck is related to posterior infiltration of the prevertebral muscles. Proptosis occurs with posterior orbital invasion and usually displaces the eyeball straight forward. Trismus is related to the invasion of the pterygoid region.

Neurologic symptoms and signs occur in about 25% of patients. Involvement of CN II–VI indicates intracranial extension into the cavernous sinus and pituitary region. CN IX–XII and the sympathetic chain are involved in the lateral pharyngeal space.

Examination of the nasopharynx will show a lesion on the lateral wall or roof; the nasopharyngeal surface of the soft palate is almost never the site of origin and not often invaded secondarily, even by advanced lesions. In early lesions, the findings may be quite subtle—only slight fullness in the fossa of Rosenmuller or a small submucosal bulge in the roof. Lymphomas tend to remain submucosal until quite large.

Nasoscopy may show tumor growing into the posterior and superior nasal cavity.

Tumor may be seen infiltrating submucosally along the posterior tonsillar pillars, but uncommonly grows very far down the posterior pharyngeal wall. The posterior tonsillar pillars may bulge into the oropharynx if an enlarged node develops in the lateral pharyngeal space.

The cranial nerves should carefully be evaluated; the sixth nerve is the one most commonly involved. The eyes should be measured for proptosis. Ear examination may show findings of otitis media.

METHODS OF DIAGNOSIS AND STAGING

Adults with large, easily visible masses may have a biopsy performed in the outpatient clinic under local anesthesia. A straight biopsy forceps is placed through the nose and the procedure visualized indirectly from the nasopharynx, or a curved biopsy forceps may be inserted behind the retracted soft palate. Biopsy of a small lesion or random biopsies for suspected lesions require general anesthesia. The palate is retracted with a Yonkers speculum, providing direct visualization of the nasopharynx. Since some of these lesions tend to grow submucosally, random biopsies must be deep to detect an invisible lesion. A mucosal sample is taken and then the biopsy forceps is placed back into the biopsy site and a deeper sample is obtained. If a juvenile angiofibroma is suspected, workup, including angiogram, should precede diagnosis and treatment.

Staging

The American Joint Committee staging system for nasopharyngeal primary tumors is:[39]

- TIS Carcinoma *in situ*
- T1 Tumor confined to one site of nasopharynx or no tumor visible (positive biopsy only)
- T2 Tumor involving two sites (both posterosuperior and lateral walls)
- T3 Extension of tumor into nasal cavity or oropharynx
- T4 Tumor invasion of skull, cranial nerve involvement, or both

Tomography and CT scan of the nasopharynx, nasal cavity, paranasal sinuses, and base of skull are routinely obtained.

TREATMENT

Factors in the Selection of Treatment

The treatment of almost all malignancies of the nasopharynx is by radiation therapy since surgical resection is not feasible. A small adenocarcinoma or sarcoma may be excised. Juvenile angiofibromas are preferably excised because of the young age of the patient, although the tumors are quite successfully cured by radiation therapy when surgical excision is impossible or dangerous. Neck dissection is used less often in the management of neck disease in nasopharyngeal cancer because of the high success rate with radiation therapy alone. Neck dissection should be used for persistence or recurrence after irradiation.

Irradiation Technique

The anatomic planning is the same for the various grades of squamous cell carcinoma, transitional cell carcinoma, and lymphoepithelioma. The pathologist often has difficulty discerning between histiocytic lymphoma and a poorly differentiated carcinoma; the carcinoma dose should be prescribed for these patients. (See the section on lymphoma for further details.)

There is no place for small-volume irradiation even for an early epithelial tumor of the nasopharynx. If after complete clinical and roentgenographic workup the tumor is thought to be limited to the nasopharynx (T1 or T2) or to have minimal soft tissue extension (early T3), the following areas are included in the treatment volume:

1. Nasopharynx proper
2. Posterior 2 cm of the nasal cavity
3. Posterior ethmoid sinuses
4. Entire sphenoid sinus and basioccipital bone
5. Cavernous sinus
6. Base of skull (7–8 cm width encompassing the foramen ovale, carotid canal, and foramen spinosum laterally
7. Pterygoid fossae
8. Posterior one-third of orbit
9. Posterior one-third of maxillary sinus
10. Lateral and posterior oropharyngeal wall to the level of the midtonsillar fossa
11. Retropharyngeal nodes
12. Neck nodes on both sides

Extension to the base of skull or involvement of CN II–VI requires that the superior border be raised to include all of the pituitary, the base of the brain in the suprasellar area, the adjacent middle cranial fossa, and the posterior portion of the anterior cranial fossa. These patients are managed with a two- or four-field arrangement, depending on the experience of the radiation therapist.

When a four-field arrangement is used, the lateral fields deliver about two-thirds and the facial fields about one-third of the tumor dose.[193] The use of opposed lateral fields for the entire treatment course delivers a 5–10% higher dose to the temporomandibular joints, ear, and subcutaneous tissues as compared to the midline tumor, unless high-energy photons are available. Patients with anterior invasion into the orbit, ethmoids, or maxillary sinus require a three-field arrangement to produce a satisfactory volume distribution. Table 13-47 outlines the dose specified for the primary lesion.

NECK NODES. A comprehensive *en bloc* plan must be developed to irradiate the neck to the level of the clavicles for both the epithelial lesions and the lymphomas. Even patients with no palpable disease in the neck should probably have full neck irradiation.[19]

The retropharyngeal nodes are included in the treatment of the local lesion. The upper neck nodes are included in the lateral primary fields to the level of the thyroid notch. With no palpable nodes, the posterior margin is placed about 1 cm behind the posterior border of the sternocleidomastoid to encompass the high spinal accessory nodes and upper lateral internal jugular nodes. The portals are extended anteriorly into the submental area only if there is disease in the submaxillary triangle or if the patient had a neck dissection prior to irradiation.

The lower neck is treated through an anterior portal with

TABLE 13-47. Guide to Dosage for Primary Nasopharynx Tumors*

	SQUAMOUS CELL CARCINOMA (rad)	LYMPHO-EPITHELIOMA (rad)	LYMPHOCYTIC LYMPHOMA† (rad)	HISTIOCYTIC LYMPHOMA† (rad)
T1, T2, early T3	6500	6000	3000	5000
Late T3, T4	7000	6500	3500	6000

(Fletcher GH, Million RR: Nasopharynx. In Fletcher GH (ed): Textbook of Radiotherapy, 3rd ed, pp 364–383. Philadelphia, Lea & Febiger, 1980)
* 850–900 rad/week.
† See lymphoma chapter for additional information.

a shield over the larynx. The midjugular nodes lie immediately adjacent to the lateral wings of the thyroid cartilage, so the lateral margin of the larynx block should be located 1 cm medial to the lateral border of the cartilage. The lower border of the tapered larynx shield is drawn 1–2 cm below the inferior border of the cricoid cartilage. The inferior jugular nodes move to a medial position in relation to the jugular vein in the low neck, and since the vein also assumes a paratracheal position in the lower neck, it is not advisable to block the midline more than 2 cm below the cricoid cartilage.

Table 13-7 gives guidelines for selecting the dose. Large neck nodes from a lymphoepithelioma may show amazing regression after a few treatments or they may still be palpable after 5000 rad in 5 weeks. The reason for the unpredictable response rate is that the lymphoepithelioma pattern may be continued into the lymph nodes, or the lymph nodes may contain only squamous cell carcinoma.

ACUTE SEQUELAE. The large volume of mucosa irradiated produces unpleasant side effects during treatment. Sore throat begins at the end of the second week of therapy and persists for 3–4 weeks after the completion of treatment. Dryness is always present and may be quite severe. Loss of taste and appetite is often quite profound, but they return 1–6 months following completion of treatment.

The auditory tube is in the high-dose area, and obstruction may occur with secondary otitis media and hearing loss. This condition can be corrected by polyethelene tubes inserted through the eardrums to drain the middle ears. The obstruction often improves or clears completely following mucosal healing of the nasopharynx. Politzerization of the eustachian tubes may reopen the canal.

Although mild nausea may occur, severe nausea and vomiting are uncommon. The overall effect of the treatment is quite wearing on the patient, and a period of several months is required for successfully irradiated patients to regain their sense of well-being.

Management of Recurrence

The majority of recurrent squamous cell carcinomas are diagnosed within 2 years, but the lymphoepithelioma may reappear many years after initial therapy. Recurrence in the base of skull or middle cranial fossa may be difficult to diagnose even with CT scan. Headache and cranial nerve palsies usually indicate recurrence.

Retreatment for recurrence may be rewarding, particularly in the lymphoepitheliomas. Patients have been kept free of local disease for various lengths of time by irradiation to a limited portal with a high-energy beam or with brachytherapy sources inserted into the nasopharynx by mold technique.

RESULTS OF TREATMENT

The 5-year survival rate has improved considerably over the past 30 years. Survival rates of 10–30% were reported prior to the use of supervoltage techniques. Recent reports give an encouraging 44–59% 5-year survival rate (see Table 13-48).[23,194–196] The gains have not come from earlier diagnosis, but from better staging of the primary lesion with tomography, use of a larger treatment volume, higher doses, and comprehensive irradiation of the neck. Tables 13-49 and 13-50 give the local and regional control rates reported for the University of Florida.[195]

The 5-year survival rate for lymphoepithelioma is usually 20–30 % higher than for squamous cell carcinoma. The high

TABLE 13-48. Nasopharynx Cancer: Results of Radiation Therapy

INSTITUTION (Dates of Treatment)	NO. OF PATIENTS	5-YEAR SURVIVAL	PERCENTAGE T4 LESIONS	PERCENTAGE OF LYMPHOEPITHELIOMA
M. D. Anderson Hospital[194] (1954–77)	251	52% (actuarial)	30%	45%
University of Florida[195] (1964–78)	47	44% (absolute)	53%	24%
Stanford[196] (1956–73)	74	59% (absolute)	11%	36%
University of California[23] (1940–68)	146	37% (absolute)	Not available	25%

TABLE 13-49. Carcinoma of the Nasopharynx: Local Control at the Primary Site (University of Florida, 10/64–4/78; analysis 4/80)

STAGE	NO. CONTROLLED/ NO. TREATED
T1	4/4 (100%)
T2	4/5 (80%)
T3	9/10 (90%)
T4	10/20 (50%)
All stages*	27/39 (69%)

(Gefter JW: Carcinoma of the nasopharynx. 10th Annual Radiation Therapy Clinical Research Seminar, April 24–26, 1980. Gainesville, Florida, Radiation Therapy Division, University of Florida, 1981)

* Excludes 8 patients who died of other causes less than 1 yr after treatment, or in whom the cause of death was uncertain.

TABLE 13-50. Carcinoma of the Nasopharynx: Control of Neck Node Disease (University of Florida, 10/64–4/78; Analysis 4/80)

STAGE	NO. CONTROLLED/ NO. TREATED
N0–N3A	21/21 (100%)
N3B	11/18 (61%)
All stages*	32/39 (82%)

(Gefter JW: Carcinoma of the nasopharynx. 10th Annual Radiation Therapy Clinical Research Seminar, April 24–26, 1980. Gainesville, Florida, Radiation Therapy Division, University of Florida, 1981)

* Excludes 8 patients who died of other causes less than 1 yr after treatment or in whom the cause of death was uncertain.

rate of local and regional control in the lymphoepithelioma is offset by a high rate of distant metastasis.

Operative results for juvenile angiofibroma have improved in recent years with the use of arteriography to localize the tumor extent and preoperative arterial occlusion to reduce intraoperative blood loss. Billar and coworkers reported a 93% cure rate with modern techniques.[197]

Briant and coworkers reported the results for irradiation of 45 patients with juvenile angiofibroma treated at the Princess Margaret Hospital.[198] The disease was eventually controlled in all cases. Some 80% of the lesions were controlled by the initial treatment of 3000–3500 rad. Seven patients had their tumors controlled with a second course of radiation therapy and three by operation. No radiation-induced neoplasms have been observed with a followup of 2–20 years.

FOLLOWUP POLICY

Followup includes careful observation and laboratory testing for possible endocrine hypofunction of the thyroid and pituitary.

Dental care must be closely monitored because of the severe xerostomia.

The neck should be carefully followed because a patient with isolated neck recurrence may be salvaged by neck dissection. Documentation of local recurrence is important, but salvage is rarely possible if high-dose, large-volume treatment has been given initially. Localized recurrence of a lymphoepithelioma may be retreated for palliation, especially if the initial doses were low.

COMPLICATIONS OF TREATMENT

The unavoidable irradiation of part of the brain including the hypothalamus, temporal lobes, and pituitary to doses between 6000 and 7000 rad has not produced a single example of brain necrosis. Primary or secondary hypopituitarism due to a hypothalamic lesion has been reported. Hypothyroidism may result from either a direct effect on the thyroid gland or an indirect effect on the pituitary.[199] Delayed bone age and growth failure may be seen in young patients. A transitory CNS syndrome may appear about 2–3 months after irradiation.[200] The greater the volume of CNS irradiated, the longer it takes the patient to recover his sense of well-being; some patients require 6 months to a year to regain their general strength. General weakness and extreme fatigue may be symptoms of low serum cortisol levels. Radiation myelitis of the cervical cord or brain stem is the most severe CNS complication.

Trismus occurs to varying degrees due to fibrosis and contracture of the pterygoid muscles rather than temporomandibular joint fibrosis. This complication is more likely in those treated with two opposing portals for the entire course.

Palsy of CN IX–XII may occur several years following treatment. This is a problem related to entrapment in the lateral pharyngeal space.

Eye complications such as retrobulbar optic neuritis may develop due to irradiation of the optic nerve.

Irradiation of the posterior eyeball to high doses may produce a radiation retinopathy with decreased vision or even total loss of one eye.

NASAL VESTIBULE, NASAL CAVITY, AND PARANASAL SINUSES

Tumors of the nasal vestibule, the anterior entrance to the nasal cavity, are considered separately from nasal cavity tumors because they are essentially skin cancers and have a different natural history.

Primary tumors arising from the nasal cavity and paranasal sinuses are considered together because the lesions are frequently advanced when first seen and it is not always possible to determine the site of origin with certainty. Primary lesions of the lower half of the maxillary sinus can usually be identified as such.

Cancer of the nasal cavity or paranasal sinuses is a relatively rare problem with a yearly risk factor estimated at approximately one case for every 100,000 people. These cancers occur more often in males (2:1) and usually appear after the age of 40 except for an occasional tumor of minor salivary gland origin or esthesioneuroblastoma, which may appear even before the age of 20.

Nasal cavity and ethmoid sinus adenocarcinomas have been linked to occupations associated with wood dust: the furniture industry, sawmill work, and carpentry.[201–204]

Other dusty occupations such as boot- and shoemaking,

baking, and the flooring industry have also been implicated as a cause of adenocarcinomas.

Thorotrast, containing the radioactive metal thorium, is a known etiologic agent in maxillary sinus carcinomas. Thorotrast was used in past years as a contrast medium for roentgenographic study of the maxillary sinuses. The Thorotrast was retained in the sinus and responsible for tumor induction.

Primary carcinomas of the sphenoid sinuses are said to be rare. They mimic nasopharyngeal carcinoma and are most often diagnosed only after they penetrate the nasopharynx and are thought to be advanced nasopharyngeal cancer.

Frontal sinus neoplasms are rare.

ANATOMY

The nasal vestibule is the entrance to the nasal cavity. It is lined by skin in which there are numerous hair follicles and sebaceous glands. The vestibule is a three-sided, pear-shaped cavity about 1.5 cm in diameter that ends posteriorly at the limen nasi. The anterolateral wall is formed by the alar cartilages (see Fig. 13-20). The medial wall is the mobile columella, formed by the medial wing of the alar cartilage and the anterior portion of the cartilaginous septum. The floor is the superior surface of the hard palate (maxilla).

The nasal cavity begins at the limen nasi and ends at the posterior nares, where it communicates directly with the nasopharynx. Fig. 13-20 shows the composition of the midline septum and the bones and cartilages that compose the roof and sides of the external nose. Each lateral wall is composed of thin bony folds that project into the nasal cavity. These are the inferior, medial, and superior nasal turbinates. The nasolacrimal duct enters the nasal cavity beneath the inferior turbinate. The frontal sinus and ethmoid bullae connect to the nasal cavity with openings that lie under the middle turbinate. The sphenoid sinus communicates with the nasal cavity by an opening on the anterior wall of the sphenoid sinus. The olfactory nerves enter the nasal cavity through the cribriform plate and distribute nerve fibers over the upper one-third of the septum and superior nasal turbinate, which

FIG. 13-20. The bones and cartilages of the nose.

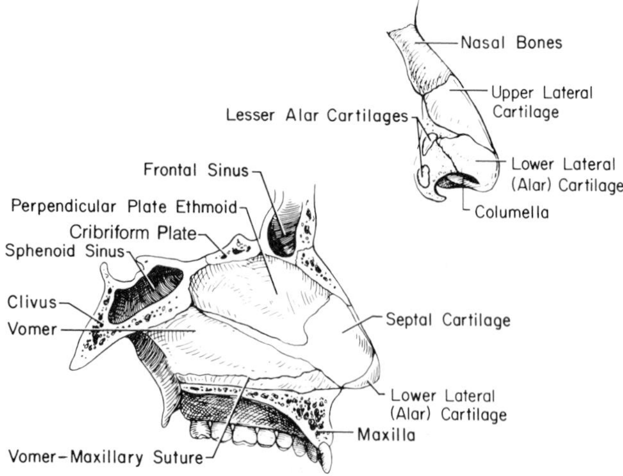

causes the mucous membrane of the olfactory portion to be tinted yellow. Approximately 20 branches of the olfactory nerve penetrate the cribriform plate, and these perforations provide an avenue of tumor spread to the floor of the anterior cranial fossa. The epithelium is nonciliated columnar. The lower half of the nasal cavity is the respiratory portion, and the epithelium is ciliated columnar. There are numerous collections of lymphoid tissue and mucous glands beneath the epithelium.

The maxillary sinuses are single pyramidal cavities with average measurements of approximately 3.7 cm in height by 2.5 cm in transverse diameter by 3 cm anteroposteriorly, and a volume of approximately 15 cc in adults. The medial wall is the lateral wall of the nasal cavity and has one or two openings that communicate with the middle meatus under the medial turbinate.

The inferior wall or floor is the hard palate. The roots of the teeth may penetrate into the cavity. The posterolateral wall is in relation to the zygomatic process and the pterygomaxillary space. The superior wall or roof separates the orbit from the sinus. All walls may be invaded and destroyed by cancer. The medial wall is easily breached by tumor because it is thin with one or two large natural perforations, and the inferolateral wall may be easily traversed when the roots of the teeth provide partial bone disruption.

The frontal sinuses are two irregular, asymmetrical air cavities separated by a thin bony septum. They connect to the middle meatus of the nasal cavity by the frontonasal duct. Frontal sinus cells may extend far laterally in the orbital process of the frontal bone. They are separated from the anterior ethmoid cells by thin bony walls. The posterior wall separating the frontal sinus from the anterior cranial fossa is quite thick in most patients.

The ethmoid sinuses consist of a number of air cells lying between the medial walls of the orbits and the lateral wall of the nasal cavity. The lateral border is the lamina papyracea, a very thin, porous bone, easily penetrated by tumor. Medially, the ethmoid air cells bulge into the lateral wall of the nasal cavity and form the superior and medial turbinates. The ethmoid cells communicate with the nasal cavity in the middle meatus. These bony walls are thin and easily traversed by tumor. The ethmoid air cells extend quite far anteriorly, and for this reason ethmoid lesions may present as a subcutaneous mass at the inner canthus. The anterior cells are actually covered laterally by the lacrimal bone. The ethmoid bone is porous and presents little resistance to tumor spread. The right and left ethmoid cells are anatomically separated, but the thinness of the walls and the narrow separation created by the midline perpendicular plate of the ethmoid indicate that extensive involvement of the ethmoid cells on one side should be considered as bilateral involvement, even if tomograms and CT scans are negative. The posterior ethmoids are particularly close together. There is no anatomic distinction or barrier between the anterior, middle, and posterior ethmoids.

The sphenoid sinus is a midline structure in the body of the sphenoid bone. The pituitary lies above, the cavernous sinuses laterally, the nasal cavity and ethmoid sinuses in front, and the nasopharynx beneath. The clivus and brain stem are posterior. The pneumatization varies widely and can extend into all portions of the sphenoid bone. The right and left sinuses are said to be separated by a septum, but are considered as one in treatment planning as the septum is said to be incomplete and easily penetrated. The sphenoid sinus connects anteriorly with the nasal cavity in the sphenoethmoidal recess.

Lymphatics

NASAL VESTIBULE. The lymphatic trunks run to the submaxillary nodes. There is a small risk for involvement of an intercalated facial node just behind the commissure of the lip along the course of the lymphatic trunk. In addition, preauricular nodes are occasionally involved, especially when tumor invades the lip or skin of the ala nasi.

NASAL CAVITY AND PARANASAL SINUSES. The lymphatics of the nasal cavity are separated into the olfactory group and the respiratory group. According to Rouvière, they do not communicate with each other.[191] There is a connection between the lymphatic network of the olfactory region and the subarachnoid spaces, which allows some absorption of cerebrospinal fluid by the lymphatics.

The lymphatics of the olfactory region of the nasal cavity run posteriorly to terminate in lymph nodes alongside the jugular vein at the base of the skull in the lateral pharyngeal space. The lymphatics of the respiratory nasal cavity also run posteriorly to terminate a bit lower, either in a lateral pharyngeal node or the subdigastric node. The capillary lymphatic plexus of the nasal mucosa must not be very profuse, as judged by the relatively small incidence of metastatic nodes even with advanced disease.

Metastases from carcinoma of the paranasal sinuses are uncommon, even though lesions are frequently quite advanced. It is literally unheard of for a paranasal sinus tumor to present with cervical lymphadenopathy and an asymptomatic primary lesion. Metastases probably only occur once tumor has extended beyond the paranasal sinuses to areas containing a rich supply of capillary lymphatics, such as the nasopharynx, buccal mucosa, nasal cavity, and skin.

PATHOLOGY

Benign Tumors

Many so-called benign lesions destroy bone and soft tissues and, if uncorrected, cause death. The management of some of these problems is not unlike cancer treatment.

Inflammatory polyps, giant cell reparative granuloma, benign mixed tumors of minor salivary gland origin, benign odontogenic tumors, and necrotizing sialometaplasia are some of the benign lesions appearing in this area.[205]

Malignant Tumors

Squamous cell carcinoma or one of its variants is the most common neoplasm. Minor salivary gland tumors account for about 10–15% of neoplasms in this region. Malignant melanoma accounts for less than 1% of all neoplasms of the nasal cavity and paranasal sinuses. Malignant lymphoma, usually histiocytic, occurs in about 5% of cases. It is frequently a locally destructive lesion because it more often arises in bone than in soft tissue (see Chapter 35 for more information on lymphomas).

Esthesioneuroblastoma (olfactory neuroblastoma) is a malignant tumor that originates from the olfactory nerves and has a histologic picture resembling adrenal neuroblastoma or retinoblastoma. Histologically, it may be confused with undifferentiated carcinoma or undifferentiated lymphoma. Esthesioneuroblastoma occurs at all ages with cases commonly seen in the second and third decades. Kadish and coworkers reported a 3-year-old boy with an advanced lesion; the authors have treated a 12-year-old boy.[206]

A wide range of soft tissue and bone sarcomas is reported for the nasal cavity and paranasal sinus region, including chondrosarcoma, osteosarcoma, Ewing's sarcoma, and most of the soft tissue sarcomas. (See pertinent chapters for a discussion of these neoplasms.)

Inverting papilloma is a confusing condition often referred to as benign, but for practical reasons, it is best classified under malignant since it may have a rather aggressive clinical picture that requires cancer-type management. It is best approached as a grade 1/2 neoplasm rather than as a benign polyp. The histologic picture is that of a papilloma which is growing into the stroma rather than growing outward. The lesion occurs predominantly in males 40–70 years of age. Any of the paranasal sinuses may be involved, as well as the nasal cavity. Squamous cell or transitional cell carcinoma is reported in association with inverting papilloma and may represent conversion of the papilloma to a more malignant tumor.

Midline lethal granuloma is a rather mysterious, progressively destructive condition that involves the nose, paranasal sinuses, and hard palate and produces secondary erosion of contiguous structures. Unchecked, the disease is fatal, usually after an extended illness. Death results from extension to the CNS, hemorrhage, sepsis, or inanition. Etiology is debatable. Midline lethal granuloma may be distinguished from Wegener's granulomatosis, which also produces inflammatory and destructive changes in the paranasal sinuses and nasal cavity. Wegener's granulomatosis also involves lung and kidney with a necrotizing vasculitis. Kassel and coworkers subdivide midline lethal granuloma into three different histologic entities: midline malignant reticulosis, malignant lymphoma (usually histiocytic lymphoma), and Wegener's granulomatosis.[207]

PATTERNS OF SPREAD

Nasal Vestibule

These lesions invade the alar and septal cartilages and occasionally will grow through to the skin surface of the nose. The upper lip is frequently invaded. Posterior growth into the nasal cavity occurs late or after recurrence. Early lesions originating on the anterior septum are often superficial lesions that ulcerate and produce a crust or scab and often present with perforation of the anterior septum.

LYMPHATICS. Lymph node spread is usually to a solitary ipsilateral submaxillary node, but may be bilateral. The facial, preauricular, and submental nodes are at small risk.

Goepfert and coworkers report only one of 26 patients with clinically positive lymph nodes on admission, but seven patients later developed positive lymph nodes, with four patients eventually showing bilateral disease.[208] Lymph node involvement is more likely in patients with recurrent local diseases, extension to the floor of the vestibule, base of the columella, or upper lip.

Nasal Cavity and Paranasal Sinuses

NASAL CAVITY. The routes of spread are essentially the same for the various histologies with the exception of minor salivary gland tumors. These have a greater propensity for perineural spread, although squamous carcinomas and esthesioneuroblastomas may also follow nerve pathways.

Lesions arising in the olfactory region invade into the ethmoids, the orbit, and through the seive-like cribriform plate to the anterior cranial fossa. These lesions also tend to destroy the septum and may invade through nasal bone to the skin. Lesions arising on the lateral wall of the respiratory portion of the nasal cavity invade the medial wall of the maxillary sinus, the ethmoids, and the orbit.

The nasopharynx and the sphenoid sinus are secondarily invaded in advanced lesions. Tumor may follow the numerous nasal nerves posteriorly and then superiorly toward the sphenopalatine ganglion near the base of the skull (pterygopalatine fossa) or along the maxillary branch of the trigeminal nerve.

MAXILLARY SINUS. All walls of the sinus may be penetrated by tumor. The pattern of spread and bone destruction is largely dependent on site of origin within the sinus. Lesions arising in the anterolateral infrastructure tend to invade through the lateral inferior wall or grow through dental sockets. Cancer presents in the oral cavity when tumor erodes through the maxillary gingiva or into the gingival-buccal sulcus. When tumor erupts through into the oral cavity, the tumor is at first submucosal, causing elevation of the mucosa, loosening of teeth, or improper seating of a denture. Ulceration follows, with the development of an oral-antral fistula.

Lesions arising on the medial infrastructure readily develop extension to the nasal cavity due to the thin, porous nature of the medial wall.

Posterior infrastructural lesions erode through the posterolateral wall. The diagnosis usually depends on sinus tomography and CT scan for definition. Recognition of this route of spread is important, since tumor escaping posteriorly has immediate access to the base of the skull and may defeat an operative attempt. Extension of lesions to the orbit occurs either directly through the roof of the maxillary sinus or by a circuitous route through the ethmoids and lamina papyracea.

Tumors arising in the upper half (suprastructure) of the antrum have two general patterns of development. One group develops laterally, invades the malar bone, and produces a mass just below the lateral floor of the orbit. The soft tissue mass may become quite large and eventually ulcerate through to the skin, producing an antrocutaneous fistula. The orbit is invaded laterally and displaces the eye inward and upward. The temporal fossa is often involved, as is the zygomatic bone in very advanced lesions.

The suprastructural cancers that develop medially invade the nasal cavity, ethmoids, and frontal sinus, lacrimal apparatus, and medial inferior orbit. It is often impossible to determine whether the origin is maxillary antrum, nasal cavity, or ethmoid.

ETHMOID SINUSES. Lesions of the ethmoid sinuses have many options for local spread due to their location and thin, porous bony walls, none of which offers particular resistance to tumor penetration. Invasion through the lamina papyracea into the medial orbit is common and must be considered to have occurred even when physical examination and roentgenograms of the orbit are normal. The lamina papyracea is normally indistinct on roentgenographic examination, and this makes interpretation of early destruction nearly impossible. The lamina papyracea is the lateral wall for the middle and posterior ethmoid air cells; the anterior ethmoid cells are covered laterally by the small, thin lacrimal bone and the frontal process of the maxilla. Thus, the ethmoid air cells extend quite far anteriorly, within a centimeter of the inner canthus.

The proximity of the maxillary antrum, the nasal cavity, and the ethmoids provides ready access for tumor spread among these three areas, a route often used, as judged by spread patterns. The medial surfaces of the ethmoid labyrinth are actually the middle and superior nasal conchae, which are formed by a thin, convoluted bone, easily traversed by tumor.

SPHENOID SINUS. There is little information regarding spread patterns for tumors arising in the sphenoid sinus. It is probable that some of the advanced nasopharyngeal lesions are, in reality, primary sphenoid sinus lesions. The fact that a disproportionate number of advanced nasopharynx lesions have no neck metastases is suggestive of their origin in the sphenoid sinus, a site with sparse, if any, capillary lymphatics, rather than from the nasopharynx with its copious capillary lymphatics.

The sphenoid sinus is in close relationship with the cranial nerves in the cavernous sinus: CN III, IV, and VI, and the ophthalmic and maxillary branches of the trigeminal nerve (see Fig. 13-21). Cranial nerve palsies and headache are frequently the first clinical evidence of a sphenoid sinus tumor. Diagnosis is usually made, however, when tumor eventually breaks through into the nasopharynx or nasal cavity where it can be seen and biopsied.

LYMPHATICS. The incidence of lymphatic metastases on admission is 10–15% for nasal cavity and ethmoid sinus tumors and probably even lower for antral and sphenoid tumors. The risk of lymphatic metastases is related to extension of tumor outside the sinus to areas with capillary lymphatics. Maxillary sinus tumors that invade the oral cavity and involve the buccal mucosa or the maxillary gingiva/hard palate may spread to the submaxillary and jugulodigastric nodes. Lesions that invade the nasal cavity or nasopharynx spread posteriorly to the parapharyngeal nodes and then to the jugulodigastric area. Esthesioneuroblastoma, minor salivary gland tumors, melanoma, and sarcomas may all demonstrate lymph node metastases.

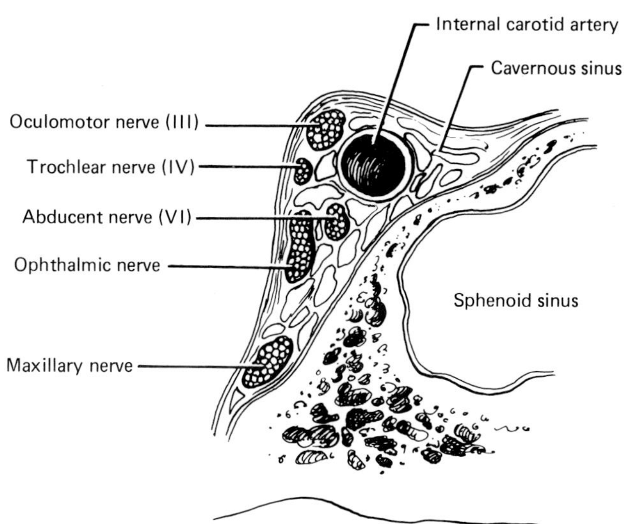

FIG. 13-21. Coronal section of the cavernous sinus.

CLINICAL PICTURE

Nasal Vestibule

These lesions present with few symptoms other than a mass growing in the entrance to the nose with crusting, scabbing, and occasional minor bleeding. Pain, if it occurs, is usually modest, even with destruction of cartilage or involvement of the lip. Secondary infection may occur, in which case the nose is painful with manipulation. The lesion may be localized to one district area of the nasal vestibule, but frequently fills the nasal vestibule so that the site of origin cannot be determined.

Nasal Cavity and Paranasal Sinuses

NASAL CAVITY. The earliest symptoms of nasal cavity neoplasm are a low-grade chronic infection with discharge, obstruction, and minor, intermittent bleeding. The symptoms mimic those associated with nasal polyps; since many of the patients with nasal neoplasms have a prior history of nasal operations for polyps, cancer is often missed in an early stage. The patient often complains of "sinus trouble" and intermittent anterior headache. Subsequent symptoms depend on pattern of growth. Lesions arising in the olfactory region may cause unilateral or bilateral nasal expansion of the bridge of the nose and a submucosal mass may appear near the inner canthus and eventually ulcerate. Obstruction of the nasolacrimal system may be a presenting complaint, with the patient treated by incision and drainage for a dacryocystitis. Extension through the cribriform plate or into the ethmoid sinuses is accompanied by frontal headache. Aberration of smell is rare.

Invasion of the medial orbit produces proptosis and diplopia; a mass may be palpated in the orbit. Indirect examination of the nasopharynx may show early submucosal invasion through the posterior nares.

MAXILLARY SINUS. These cancers develop silently as long as they are confined to the sinus and produce symptoms on extension outside the walls. If the tumor invades toward the oral cavity, the presenting symptoms relate to pain associated with the upper teeth; there may be loosening and eventually loss of teeth. The dentist is often the first one consulted, and the patient may have dental extraction without pain relief. Tumor may penetrate into the gingivobuccal sulcus or upper gum and eventually progress to an oral-antral fistula. If the patient wears upper dentures, the first symptom will be an ill-fitting denture. Palpation and observation of the face may show a mass. Early invasion of the floor of the orbit may be appreciated by feeling both orbits simultaneously with the tips of the index finger inserted between the bony rim and eyeball. Posterior invasion of the orbit will produce proptosis, diplopia, and edema of the conjunctiva. Invasion of the inferior orbital nerve or its branches in the floor of the orbit may cause paresthesias or anesthesia of the skin of the lower eyelid, upper lid, side of the nose, and the anterior premaxillary skin. Nasal obstruction and bleeding are common complaints, along with "sinus pain" or "fullness" over the involved antrum. Trismus and headache are associated with invasion posteriorly into the pterygomaxillary space with invasion of the pterygoid muscles and base of skull.

Cancers developing in the medial suprastructure of the antrum present with nasal symptoms of discharge or bleeding, mild infraorbital pain, infected lacrimal sac, and displacement of the eye upward and laterally with proptosis, diplopia, and conjunctival edema.

Cancer developing in the lateral suprastructure produces a mass below the lateral canthus with associated pain. The eye may be deviated medially and upward when orbital invasion occurs. There is edema of the conjunctiva, narrowing of the palpebral opening, diplopia, and proptosis. Tumor may extend to the temporal fossa, producing a diffuse fullness.

ETHMOID SINUS. Mild to moderate sinus ache or pain referred to the frontal/nasal area is an early symptom. A painless mass may present near the inner canthus. The mass may become infected and be interpreted as a boil or dacryocystitis, at which time an inappropriate incision and drainage procedure is done. Diplopia develops with invasion of the medial orbit. Proptosis is often present, and a mass can be felt by deep digital palpation of the orbit. Nasal discharge, epistaxis, and obstruction are frequent presenting complaints. Paresthesias may occur over the distribution of sensory nerves.

Physical examination includes anterior and posterior rhinoscopy after thorough shrinking of the nasal mucosa. A fiberoptic nasoscope is a great aid in visualizing the posterior and superior nasal cavity and the nasopharynx. Early invasion of the nasal cavity may produce only submucosal bulging into the superior or middle meatus, which is easily confused with allergic rhinitis, polyps, or inflammatory changes. Pus may be seen coming from beneath the superior, middle, or inferior turbinate.

Eye examination includes palpation of the orbit for masses. Palpation should be carried out simultaneously in both orbits, since the changes in the involved orbit are frequently subtle. Extraocular movements are examined and proptosis is measured with a ruler; there may be only 1–2 mm difference with early proptosis.

Invasion into the nasopharynx is usually submucosal and

appears on the roof and lateral wall. Advanced lesions may obstruct the eustachian canal.

METHODS OF DIAGNOSIS AND STAGING

Biopsy Technique

Tumor in the nasal cavity is biopsied with a punch forceps. Biopsy of tumor in the maxillary antrum is usually approached through a Caldwell-Luc procedure, which is an incision through the gingivobuccal sulcus opposite the premolars. This approach allows adequate visualization of the entire antrum.

Biopsy of ethmoid tumors is usually taken from the extension to the nasal cavity or inner canthus area. Tumor confined to the ethmoids may be found unexpectedly at the time of a lateral rhinotomy planned for diagnosis or treatment of benign disease.

An undiagnosed orbital mass may occasionally be the site of biopsy due to incomplete examination of other areas.

Sphenoid sinus tumors are biopsied by way of the transnasal route for the rare localized disease, but biopsy is usually made of an extension to the nasopharynx or nasal cavity.

Frontal sinus tumors are approached by supraorbital incision and osteotomy.

Staging

NASAL VESTIBULE. The staging used for skin cancer is appropriate for this area. Tomography and computerized axial tomography are useful for advanced or recurrent lesions.

NASAL CAVITY AND PARANASAL SINUSES. Physical examination alone is inadequate for staging these tumors. Tomograms in the coronal, sagittal, and occasionally the submental vertical views are necessary. CT scan is a valuable addition, particularly for detection of spread to the orbit and pterygomaxillary space. The primary tumor is staged as follows (maxillary sinus only)[39]:

- TX Tumor that cannot be assessed
- TO No evidence of primary tumor
- T1 Tumor confined to the antral mucosa of the infrastructure with no bone erosion or destruction
- T2 Tumor confined to the suprastructure mucosa without bone destruction, or to the infrastructure with destruction of medial or inferior bony walls only
- T3 More extensive tumor invading skin of cheek, orbit, anterior ethmoid sinuses, or pterygoid muscle
- T4 Massive tumor with invasion of cribriform plate, posterior ethmoids, sphenoid, nasopharynx, pterygoid plates, or base of skull

TREATMENT

Nasal Vestibule

SELECTION OF TREATMENT MODALITY. Both surgical resection and radiation therapy produce a high degree of success in experienced hands.[208–210] Radiation therapy is usually the preferred treatment because of the deformity produced by excision. Excision is preferred for very small lesions, the removal of which will not produce cosmetic deformity nor require reconstruction; few lesions fit this description. Radiation therapy is selected for the remainder with surgery reserved for radiation failure. Radiation therapy has been quite successful in salvaging surgical failures, but the nasal deformity has already been produced and the value of irradiation lost.

SURGICAL TREATMENT. Excision of lesions in the nasal vestibule usually involves removal of cartilage as well as skin. Depending on the site of the lesion, either the columella or the alar cartilages will have to be removed with a resulting cosmetic deformity, which may be difficult to reconstruct, particularly if the surgery is for radiation therapy failure. If the alar cartilage has been sacrificed, either a composite graft consisting of skin and cartilage from the ear or a nasolabial flap can be used to repair the defect. If the entire external nose is resected, a prosthesis is used to cover the defect.

IRRADIATION TECHNIQUE. Irradiation techniques are not standardized, but success is quite high with the several methods available. Selection of technique will depend on the extent of the disease and the experience of the radiation therapist.

External Beam. High energy (*e.g.*, Cobalt-60 or 4 MeV) is theoretically preferable to orthovoltage to reduce the dose in cartilage and adjacent bone. However, orthovoltage therapy fractionated over 4–6 weeks has produced quite excellent results; shorter courses with higher daily fractions will cure the cancer, but the cosmetic result after a couple of years is poor and the risk of a necrosis is increased.

There are two basic external beam treatment plans: opposed lateral portals and a single anterior portal. When the tumor volume can be encompassed by lateral portals, there is an advantage in avoiding unnecessary exit irradiation to the nasal cavity, nasopharynx, and CNS. This technique confines irradiation to the anterior nasal area, but has the disadvantage of full skin reaction, since a wax bolus nose block is made to ensure homogeneous irradiation. The portals may be angled posteriorly to ensure sufficient posterior coverage; wedges are added to compensate for the angle (see Fig. 13-22). Fractionation schemes are those used for orthovoltage since the bolus produces skin reactions comparable to orthovoltage therapy.

FIG. 13-22. Treatment plan for external beam irradiation of a nasal vestibule carcinoma.

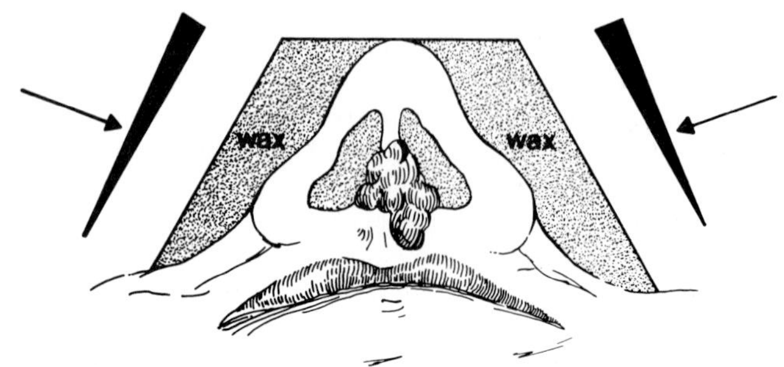

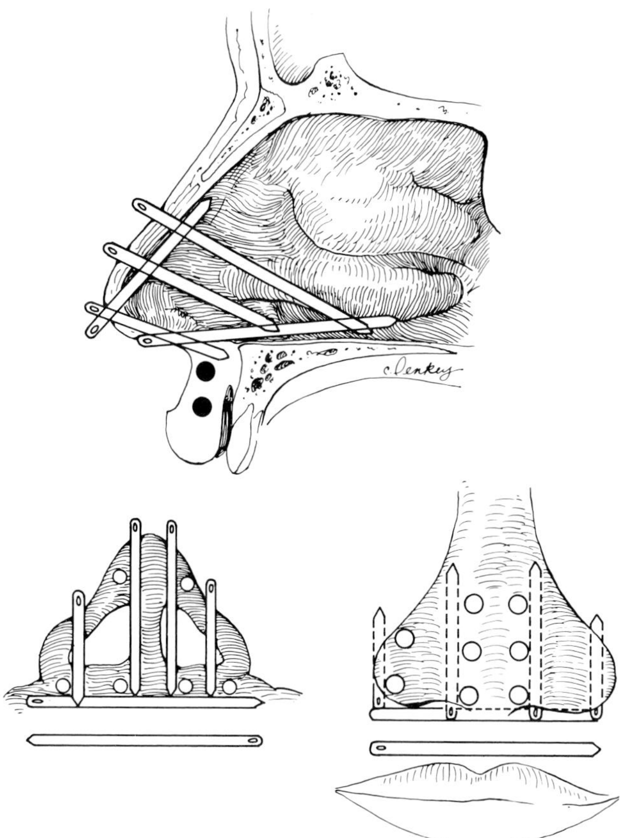

FIG. 13-23. Diagram of interstitial implant for carcinoma of the nasal vestibule.

Interstitial. Interstitial implants of the nasal vestibule and nasal cavity are highly individualized. The basic implant is usually composed of two, three, or four planes of needles inserted through the skin surface of the external nose. Fig. 13-23 shows the basic arrangement to cover the entire nasal vestibule and upper lip. Needles may be subtracted for smaller lesions or added for superior coverage toward the nasal cavity. The dose has varied from 5500–7500 rad, depending on the size of the lesion.

Nasal Cavity

SELECTION OF TREATMENT MODALITY. The histology, extent, and location of the malignant tumor in the nasal cavity are all considered when making treatment decisions.

Inverting papilloma is treated initially by surgical excision. The local recurrence rate is fairly high, and subsequent excisions may be required. When the lesion begins to act aggressively with rapid recurrences and invasion of the sinuses and cribriform plate, it should be considered a low-grade cancer and treated appropriately by more radical removal or irradiation.

Squamous cell carcinoma and adenocarcinoma of the nasal cavity may be treated either with surgery, irradiation, or both. Most analyses of nasal cavity carcinomas are included with paranasal sinus cancer series. Since standardized staging is not applied, it is difficult to compare the results of various therapies. Since regional and distant metastases are relatively uncommon, local control is tantamount to cure.

Either surgery or radiation therapy is used for discrete early lesions. Operative management is usually indicated for early lesions of the septum where good surgical margins may be expected without cosmetic or functional loss. Excision is also the treatment of choice for melanomas and sarcomas.

Radiation therapy is used for lateral wall and superior wall lesions, where resection implies cosmetic loss.

Midline lethal granuloma is treated by radiation therapy to the nasal cavity and all of the paranasal sinuses.

SURGICAL TREATMENT. Surgery for lesions of the nasal cavity is best carried out using a lateral rhinotomy approach to the nose, which allows the best access to the lesion. Generally reconstruction is not necessary unless the entire cartilaginous septum has been removed, in which case there will be a saddle deformity of the nose. The lateral wall of the nose may also be removed by this approach.

IRRADIATION TECHNIQUE. *External Beam.* The majority of cases are treated by external beam irradiation, which emphasizes an anterior portal with one or two lateral portals. Since satisfactory examination of the nasal cavity is difficult with cancer present, it is better to err on the side of a large treatment volume rather than rely too greatly on roentgenographic and physical examination findings. This means that contiguous structures such as the medial portion of the maxillary sinus, ethmoid sinus, medial orbit, nasopharynx, base of skull, and sphenoid sinus are generally included in the initial treatment volume, even though the lesion is thought to be rather localized. These lesions frequently invade the anterior cranial fossa and spread between bone and dura. Eventually they penetrate the dura and invade the frontal lobes. The treatment volume is reduced after 5000 rad to include the original gross disease with a margin.

Advanced lesions require inclusion of an entire orbit if tumor grossly invades the medial orbit; in these cases, loss of vision may occur, but an operation would require visual loss in any case. Fig. 13-24 shows a three-field distribution for advanced nasal cavity lesions.

FIG. 13-24. Isodose distribution for carcinoma of the ethmoid sinus with invasion of the orbit.

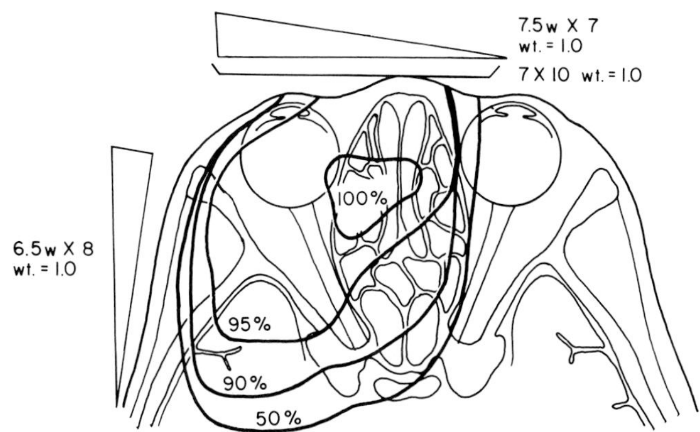

Treatment planning for midline lethal granuloma includes the nasal cavity and all of the paranasal sinuses. The dose is 4000 rad to normal areas and 5000 rad to areas of gross disease.

COMBINED TREATMENT POLICIES. If combined treatment is planned, the authors prefer to use the operation first to avoid obscuring the extent of tumor. Irradiation is started 4–6 weeks afterward. The dose is usually 6500 rad/6.5–7.5 weeks.

MANAGEMENT OF RECURRENCE. Diagnosis of recurrent lesions is important since salvage may be possible. Once the patient has had an operation or irradiation, it is difficult to determine the extent of recurrent disease by roentgenograms because of changes from the previous therapy. The most common situation for salvage is a radiation or surgical failure that can be treated successfully by a craniofacial resection. Tumor extension to the sphenopalatine fossa with definite destruction of a pterygoid plate is a contraindication to a craniofacial procedure, as is cranial nerve involvement, invasion posteriorly near the optic chiasm, or sphenoid sinus invasion. It is often impossible to roentgenographically distinguish between tumor and inflammatory changes in the sphenoid sinus unless there is obvious bone destruction; surgical exploration may be necessary for final diagnosis. The anterior wall of the sinus may be removed, but the sinus itself cannot be resected.[211] Postoperative irradiation should be considered whether or not margins are positive. About 25% of patients may be saved by this approach. Fig. 13-25 shows the limits of a craniofacial resection.

FIG. 13-25. Schematic diagram showing lines of resection for craniofacial resection of advanced paranasal sinus tumor with intracranial extension.

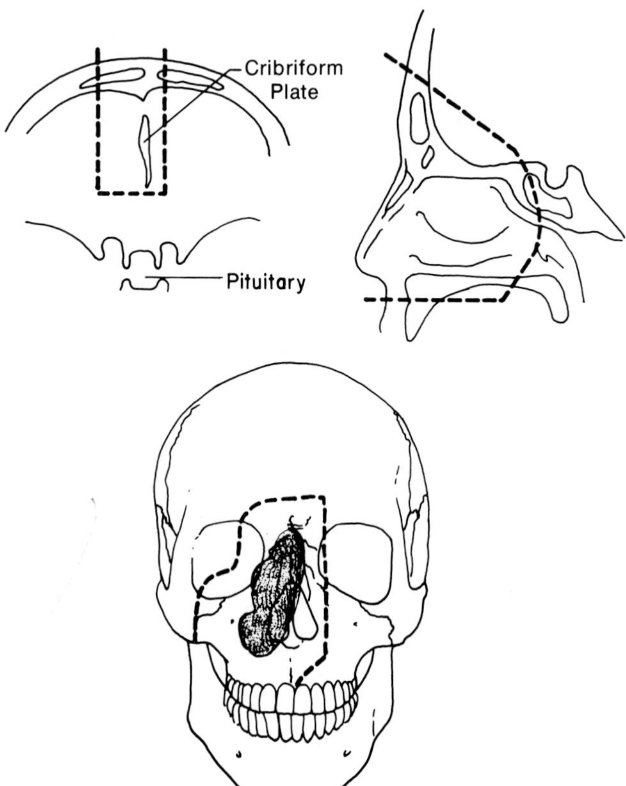

Maxillary Sinus

SELECTION OF TREATMENT MODALITY. Surgical resection gives the best results. Early infrastructural lesions may be excised and cured by surgery alone, but for most cases, irradiation is given postoperatively even if margins are negative. Extension of cancer to the base of skull and nasopharynx contraindicates surgical excision.

SURGICAL TREATMENT. Surgery for carcinoma of the maxillary sinus depends on which walls are involved. If the roof of the orbit is free of disease, then the eye and the orbital rim may be left undisturbed. If, however, there is involvement of the roof of the sinus, then a maxillectomy and orbital exenteration must be performed. If the posterior wall or the pterygoid plates are involved, they too must be included in the resection. A split-thickness skin graft is used to line the cavity, and a dental prosthesis is then used to fill the resulting deformity in the palate. It is preferable to construct the prosthesis prior to the surgery so it can be placed at the time of surgery and act as a stent.

IRRADIATION TECHNIQUE. Irradiation treatment planning includes the entire maxilla, the adjacent nasal cavity, ethmoid sinus, nasopharynx, and pterygopalatine fossa. The entire orbit is included in patients with extension into or near the orbital fossa; failure to include the orbital contents is one of the most common causes of failure. The prescribed dose is 6500–7000 rad.

COMBINED TREATMENT POLICIES. Except for the early infrastructural lesion, surgical resection is followed in 4 weeks by high-dose external beam radiation therapy. The dose should be 6500–7000 rad, as the recurrence rate at lower doses is substantial.

If radiation therapy alone is planned, localized drainage procedures may be done either before, during, or after radiation therapy.

Ethmoid Sinus

SELECTION OF TREATMENT MODALITY. Ethmoid sinus lesions are usually extensive when first diagnosed. Radiation therapy alone produces better results than surgery alone and is the preferred single treatment.[212] If resection is feasible with acceptable functional and cosmetic results, then the operation is carried out, followed by postoperative radiation therapy even if margins are clear.

SURGICAL TREATMENT. Localized lesions require resection of the ethmoids and the ipsilateral maxilla and orbit. Extensive lesions are removed by a craniofacial procedure.

IRRADIATION TECHNIQUE. Radiation treatment is entirely by external beam, emphasizing treatment through an anterior field combined with one or two lateral fields. A reduced anterior open field is often incorporated into the treatment plan to concentrate the dose to the major bulk of disease. This field arrangement, weighted 2:1 or 3:1 in favor of the anterior field, provides adequate treatment of the tumor volume while avoiding excessive irradiation of the contralateral eye. Wedges are added to achieve a satisfactory dose distribution.

MANAGEMENT OF RECURRENCE. Recurrent disease is heralded by recurrent pain and cranial nerve palsies. Exploration of the sinuses is necessary for diagnosis.

Localized recurrence after surgery only may be managed by radiation therapy alone or craniofacial resection and postoperative radiation therapy. Radiation therapy failures may be treated by craniofacial resection.

Sphenoid Sinus

The treatment is similar to that for advanced carcinoma of the nasopharynx.

RESULTS OF TREATMENT

Nasal Vestibule

Goepfert and coworkers reviewed the M. D. Anderson Hospital experience of 26 patients with squamous cell carcinoma of the nasal vestibule.[208] The absolute 5-year survival was 78%. Ten patients were treated initially by surgery; one developed a local recurrence and was salvaged by radiation therapy. Sixteen patients were treated by radiation therapy; three developed local recurrence and two were salvaged by an operation.

Nasal Cavity

Frazell and Lewis reported a 56% 5-year cure rate for 68 nasal cavity neoplasms treated surgically.[213]

Ellingwood and Million reported 15 patients with nasal cavity neoplasms.[212] Local control was achieved in eight of eight stage I and six of seven stage III lesions (see Table 13-51).

Elkon and coworkers, reviewed the world literature on esthesioneuroblastoma and presented results of 97 cases.[214] They conclude that either radiation therapy or surgery was sufficient treatment for early-stage disease, but that combined treatment might be advantageous for late-stage presentations. The 5-year absolute survival was: stage A, 75%; stage B, 60%; and stage C, 41%. The local recurrence rate after radiation therapy in this review is partially explained by the rather modest doses prescribed for most of the cases (see Table 13-52).

Fauci and coworkers reported the results of 10 patients with midline lethal granuloma treated by high-dose irradiation.[215] Long-term remissions occurred in seven patients. Four patients developed malignancies at other sites.

Maxillary Sinus

Jesse reviewed 87 patients with squamous cell carcinoma of the maxillary antrum.[216] The 3-year survival was about 30% for all cases, including 15 treated for palliation only and nine which were too advanced for any treatment. Sixty-three were treated for cure with a 3-year survival of 44%. Three-year survival after surgery alone for selected lesions was nine of 20 patients. Patients selected for combined treatment had either pre- or postoperative irradiation; the results were similar for both techniques. The local recurrence rate with combined treatment was 38%. Infrastructural lesions and superolateral lesions had a 3-year survival rate of 13/19 (68%), while superomedial or superoposterior lesions had a survival rate of only 29%.

Ethmoid Sinus

Table 13-51 gives the local control and absolute 2- and 5-year survival rates for 17 patients with cancer of the ethmoid sinus (included is one patient with sphenoid sinus cancer) treated by radiation therapy alone or for salvage of surgical cut-through.[212] Patients with relatively localized presentations had local control in seven of nine patients, while those with extension to the nasopharynx, base of skull, or middle cranial fossa had only two of eight controlled. The minor salivary gland tumors have good initial response and control, but may regrow locally many years later. Patients with carcinoma or esthesioneuroblastoma develop very few recurrences after 2 years.

COMPLICATIONS OF TREATMENT

Complications of radiation therapy for maxillary sinus cancer include osteonecrosis, radiation-induced CNS disease, loss of vision, nasal obstruction, and otitis media. Complications of

TABLE 13-51. Carcinoma of the Nasal Cavity and Ethmoid/Sphenoid Sinuses: Local Control and Survival by Primary Site (University of Florida; analysis 9/77)

	LOCAL CONTROL		ABSOLUTE SURVIVAL NED*	
SITE	MINIMUM 2-YR FOLLOWUP	MINIMUM 5-YR FOLLOWUP	MINIMUM 2-YR FOLLOWUP	MINIMUM 5-YR FOLLOWUP
Nasal cavity	14/15 (95%)	8/8 (100%)	14/15 (95%)	7/13 (54%)
Ethmoid/sphenoid	12/17 (71%)	5/9 (56%)	13/17 (77%)	6/13 (46%)
Total	26/32 (81%)	13/17 (76%)	27/32 (85%)	13/26 (50%)

(Ellingwood KE, Million RR: Cancer of the nasal cavity and ethmoid/sphenoid sinuses. Cancer 43:1517–1526, 1979)
* NED—no evidence of disease.

TABLE 13-52. Esthesioneuroblastoma: Results of Treatment by Modality and Stage (78 Patients; 6 mo–32 yr followup)

MODALITY	STAGE A			STAGE B			STAGE C		
	INITIAL TREAT-MENT	FOR RECURRENCE	TOTAL CONTROL RATE	INITIAL TREAT-MENT	FOR RECURRENCE	TOTAL CONTROL RATE	INITIAL TREAT-MENT	FOR RECURRENCE	TOTAL CONTROL RATE
Radiotherapy alone	2/5	5/5	70%	4/7	3/4	64%	1/5	1/1	33%
Surgery alone	5/9	4/4	69%	3/6	1/2	50%	1/1	0/0	—
Radiotherapy and surgery	7/10	0/0	70%	12/20	0/1	57%	7/15	0/0	47%

(Elkon D, Hightower SI, Lim ML et al: Esthesioneuroblastoma. Cancer 44:1087–1094, 1979)

maxillectomy include failure of the split-thickness skin graft to heal, trismus, cerebrospinal fluid leak, and hemorrhage.

Complications of ethmoid sinus surgery include hemorrhage, meningitis, cerebrospinal fluid leak, cellulitis and pansinusitis, brain abscess, and stroke. Complications of the craniofacial procedure are reported by Ketcham and coworkers.[211] About one-third of the patients had a life-threatening complication requiring intensive care and prolonged hospitalization. Operative mortality was 4%. Complications included meningitis, subdural abscess, cerebrospinal fluid leak, diplopia, and hemorrhage. Most of these patients had recurrent or far-advanced disease prior to surgery.

Eye complications are the most frequent and bothersome of the complications of radiation therapy.[217] When only a portion of the ipsilateral eyeball is irradiated (medial one-third), it is possible to preserve vision in the majority of patients. However, when there is gross disease in the orbit, the entire eyeball is irradiated to a high dose with almost certain loss of vision; however, these same patients would require orbital exenteration if treated by surgery.

An estimated 20% of patients will develop a transitory CNS syndrome that includes vertigo, headaches, decreased cerebration, and lethargy. This syndrome usually appears 2–3 months after completion of treatment, but has been seen as late as 12–15 months after completion of radiation therapy. The early-appearing CNS syndromes usually last 1–2 months, but the late-appearing syndromes last 6–12 months before slowly resolving. The mechanism of this condition is poorly understood, but is similar to the condition termed lymphogenous encephalopathy reported by Földi.[218] He reports that the symptoms and signs resolved with large doses of pantothenic acid and pyridoxine given every day.

Aseptic meningitis, chronic sinusitis, or serous otitis media may occur. High-dose irradiation of the nasal cavity may cause narrowing and synechiae of the nasal cavity. Douching with salt water and daily self-dilations with petrolatum jelly-coated cotton swabs will reduce this problem.

Septal perforations occur when tumor has destroyed part of the septum. These do not usually require treatment and may heal spontaneously.

Destruction of the nasal bone and septum by tumor may result in cosmetic deformity. Two patients had successful reconstructive rhinoplasties after 7000 rads.

Maxillary necrosis may develop if dental extraction is undertaken, but this can usually be successfully managed as the blood supply is much better than in the mandible.

CHEMODECTOMAS (GLOMUS BODY TUMORS)

Chemodectomas are a fascinating, but uncommon group of neoplasms that may originate anywhere glomus bodies are found. The lesions are uncommon before the age of 20, there is a female predominance in some series, and the lesions may occur in multiple sites in about 10–20% of cases, especially in families with a history of this tumor. Carotid body tumors are associated with conditions producing chronic hypoxia, such as high altitude habitation, and chronic hypoxemia (as occurs in cyanotic heart disease).

ANATOMY

The normal glomus bodies in the head and neck vary from 0.1–0.5 mm in diameter. An autopsy study showed a correlation between carotid body size and increased right ventricular weight secondary to emphysema.[219] Because of their small size, their total distribution in the head and neck remains speculative. Tumors arising from glomus bodies (*i.e.*, chemodectomas or nonchromaffin paragangliomas) occur most often from the carotid and temporal bone glomus bodies with rare reports of tumors arising from the orbit, nasopharynx, larynx, nasal cavity, paranasal sinuses, tongue, and jaw.

The glomus bodies arising in relation to the temporal bone require special mention in regard to their distribution, since the site of origin of the tumor explains the different clinical pictures. Guild reports an average of 2.82 glomera per ear with a range of 0–12.[220]

The temporal bone glomus bodies are not consistently found in any location, but vary from person to person. At least one-half of the glomus bodies are found in the general region of the jugular fossa and are located in the adventitia of the superior bulb of the internal jugular vein. The remainder are distributed along the course of the nerve of Jacobson (a branch of CN IX) and the nerve of Arnold (a branch of CN X). Approximately 20% of all temporal bone glomus bodies lie in the tympanic canaliculus and approximately 10% in relation to the cochlear promontory. A few glomus bodies are located in the descending part of the facial canal.

The carotid bodies are located in relation to the bifurcation of the common carotid, orbit bodies are in relation to the ciliary nerve.

PATHOLOGY

Chemodectomas are histologically benign tumors that resemble the parent tissue and consist of nests of epithelioid cells within stroma-containing thin-walled blood vessels and nonmyelinated nerve fibers. The tumor mass is well-circumscribed, but a true capsule is not seen. Dense fibrous bands occur in some tumors and account for the firmness of some masses. The histologic appearance varies, depending upon the relative amounts of epithelioid and vascular tissue present. The criterion of malignancy is based on the clinical progress of the disease rather than the histologic picture. Chemodectomas without cellular atypia may metastasize to regional nodes or to distant organ sites by way of hematogenous spread, although metastases are quite infrequent, probably in less than 5% of cases.

PATTERNS OF SPREAD

These lesions usually grow slowly; it is usual to have a history of symptoms for a few years and occasionally for 20 years.

Carotid Body Tumors

Carotid body tumors are usually located at the bifurcation of the common carotid and, as they expand, tend to displace and encircle the internal and external carotid vessels. The tumor begins in the adventitia of the artery and initially derives its blood supply from the vaso vasorum. An accessory blood supply may come from branches of the vertebral artery and the ascending cervical artery.[221] The tumor is usually closely adherent to the wall of the carotid adjacent to the vascular pedicle, and there may be thinning of the arterial wall due to pressure by the mass. Large masses extend toward the cervical spine, base of skull, angle of the mandible, and the lateral pharyngeal space and its contents.

Temporal Bone Tumors

Glomus tympanicum lesions tend to be small when diagnosed because they produce symptoms quite early in their course. Tumor may involve the ossicles, tympanic membrane, mastoid, external auditory canal, semicircular canal, and the facial, Jacobson's, and Arnold's nerves.

Glomus jugulare tumors invade the base of skull, petrous apex, jugular vein, middle ear, and middle and posterior cranial fossae. CN V–VII may be involved.

Lymphatic Spread

Lymphatic metastases are very uncommon. An upper neck mass may be an inferior extension of tumor rather than a lymph node metastasis. Capillary lymphatics have been described that drain the dura around the jugular foramen and could be the site of origin for lymph node metastasis.[218]

Distant metastases have been reported, but considering the frequency of jugular vein invasion, the risk of distant spread is quite small.

CLINICAL PICTURE

Symptoms may be present from a few months to many years prior to diagnosis; the average is 3–4 years. Tumors are reported in children.

Carotid Body Tumors

The most common presenting symptom is an asymptomatic, slow-growing mass in the upper neck near the bifurcation of the carotid. Large masses may encroach on the parapharyngeal space and produce dysphagia, pain, and cranial nerve palsies. A carotid sinus syndrome may occur because of the pressure of the mass.

On examination, the mass usually lies deep to the sternocleidomastoid muscle and is tethered to surrounding structures. Fixation occurs only in large tumors that extend to the spine and base of skull. A submucosal bulge may be seen in the tonsillar area. A bruit may be heard. Steady compression of the mass may reduce its size, which recovers when the pressure is released.

Temporal Bone Tumors

Since there is a range in the distribution of glomus bodies, the initial symptoms and signs depend on the site of origin.

Tumor arising in or near the middle ear presents with an insidious conductive hearing loss, pulsatile tinnitus, vertigo, and headache.

Patients with lesions developing in or around the jugular fossa develop headache, often pulsatile in nature, referred to the orbit or temple. CN V–XII and the sympathetics become affected.

Lesions developing in the facial canal present with facial nerve symptoms. Otorrhea and hemorrhage may occur when tumor breaks through into the external auditory canal.

A characteristic blue-red mass may be seen bulging the tympanic membrane or actually occupying the external auditory canal. A mass may be seen or felt in the upper neck between the mandible and mastoid and, at times, may be quite large.

CN V–XII and sympathetic nerves show varying neurologic loss.

METHODS OF DIAGNOSIS AND STAGING

When the diagnosis of glomus tumor is suspected, arteriography is the major step in establishing the diagnosis and, at the same time, outlining the extent of the tumor. Tomograms of the temporal bone and base of skull are helpful for showing bone involvement or destruction. CT scan may assist in outlining a soft tissue mass, but at present does not replace the other studies. A jugular venogram is added if the vein is not seen well on the outflow phase of the arteriogram.

TREATMENT

Selection of Treatment Modality

Although chemodectomas have a low potential for metastatic spread and a slow growth pattern, they may cause major disability and eventually death if unchecked. It may be appropriate to recommend no active treatment in selected cases, but the great majority should be treated.

Surgical excision is satisfactory for small lesions that can be removed without risk of operative death or damage to normal structures.

There remains a great deal of confusion regarding radiation treatment of chemodectomas. Since the histologic appearance of the tumors in the various locations is the same, there is no reason why radiation therapy will not work as well for lesions of the carotid body as for those of the temporal bone.

A recent review by Kim and coworkers of over 200 patients shows that the recurrence rate after adequate radiation therapy for temporal bone chemodectomas is 2% with doses of 4000 rad or greater.[222] In some cases, examination of the temporal bone after radiation therapy has shown either no definable tumor or a few microscopic residuals. However, in the majority of patients the tumor mass regresses, but stable remnants may be seen for years. Success in these patients is equated with the lack of tumor regrowth and permanent improvement in signs and symptoms. It seems poor judgment to risk any operative resection that carries an operative mortality or morbidity when irradiation has been so successful.

Early lesions of the tympanic cavity are successfully managed by excision without loss of hearing or vestibular function. The remainder of the lesions are best managed by irradiation, with a very high success rate and minimal morbidity with modern-day techniques. Partial removal of tumor prior to irradiation does not improve the results, but only increases the overall morbidity and puts the patient at risk for a fatal complication.

Surgical Treatment

TEMPORAL BONE TUMORS. *Glomus Tympanicum Tumors.* Small lesions are approached through the drum or mastoid and removed. Hearing loss may occur from the operation, but if there is conductive hearing loss from the tumor, hearing may improve.

Glomus Jugulare Tumors. The results with irradiation are very successful; attempted resection of these lesions is considered only for the now quite rare radiation failure.

CAROTID BODY TUMORS. Small lesions (1–5 cm) may be successfully removed with little risk to the patient. However, if ligation or replacement of the carotid vessels is anticipated, radiation therapy is the preferred treatment. These lesions are identical to temporal bone chemodectomas, and there is every indication that the response to radiation is similar. Scattered reports showed some patients with regression of the mass, while other reports declared little or no immediate response. There are numerous cases in which patients lived many years after radiation therapy with no progression or recurrence. The doses in some cases were well below the currently accepted level of 4000–5000 rad, and the lack of immediate regression is not necessarily tantamount to a therapeutic failure.[223]

Irradiation Techniques

The current treatment plan is 4500 rad/5 weeks, 180 rad/fraction, to the tumor volume. This dose is well below the tolerance of all normal tissues included, even if the brain stem and cord must be included for a large lesion.

Tumor-related symptoms may begin to improve during the first week of treatment, and the tumor mass, if visible, may show a decrease in size almost at once, which indicates a rather radiosensitive tumor.

Acute sequelae of treatment should be almost nil at 180 rad/fraction. The patient will have temporary hair loss in the entrance and exit areas beginning about the third week. Mild nausea may occur.

Late sequelae are few. The hair should regrow over a period of 2–4 months, but may show a slightly different texture or color. The patient may develop an otitis media, especially if the middle ear is involved with tumor.

Management of Recurrence

The diagnosis of recurrence is often delayed because of the inaccessibility to examination. Therefore, base-line roentgenograms should be obtained for reference.

Recurrence after irradiation is so uncommon that the diagnosis must be made only after complete re-evaluation and evidence of progression of symptoms or an enlarging mass. Pulsatile tinnitus may persist after irradiation because of incomplete regression of the vascular component of the tumor.[224,225]

Documented recurrence after operation is usually treated by irradiation; the complication rate in this group is higher than for those treated initially by irradiation. Recurrence after irradiation should be treated by operation if feasible; if operation is not possible, re-irradiation may be considered. Although there are no reports of re-irradiation for this tumor, there is experience with re-irradiation of nasopharynx and brain tumors. The potential for a complication would be significant, but in the face of advancing neoplasm, the risk would probably be acceptable.

RESULTS OF TREATMENT

Table 13-53 lists the local control rate for five irradiation series of chemodectomas in which adequate doses (3500 rad or more) were prescribed and the treatment volumes adequate.[226–230] No patients had documented evidence of disease progression in 71 patients treated. Table 13-54 lists the local control for operation for five series.[231–235]

FOLLOWUP POLICY

Repeat angiograms and other roentgenograms are only ordered for suspected recurrence. It is not unusual to have a persistent blue-red mass behind the eardrum after irradiation, even though the patient is clinically improved and there is no evidence of progression. About 5–10% of patients will develop a second chemodectoma (often in the head and neck area), either a carotid body tumor, or a contralateral temporal bone tumor.

TABLE 13-53. Local Control of Chemodectomas with Irradiation

INSTITUTION	TUMOR DOSE (rads)	LOCAL CONTROL*	FOLLOWUP
M. D. Anderson Hospital[226]	4250–5000	17/17	4–18 yr
University of Florida[227]	3750–5640	14/14	3–11 yr
Baylor Medical Center[228]	4000–5000	9/9	1–7 yr
Geisinger Medical Center[229]	4000–5000	11/11	1–12 yr
Princess Margaret Hospital[230]	3500	20/20	2–20 yr

(Dickens WJ, Million RR, Cassisi NJ et al: Chemodectomas arising in temporal bone structures. (in preparation))

* Local control: Regression and absence of disease progression.

TABLE 13-54. Local Control of Chemodectomas with Surgery

AUTHOR	YEAR	NO. OF PATIENTS	NO. WITH RECURRENCE
Newman et al[231]	1973	14	11
Grubb and Lampe[232]	1965	9	5
Hatfield et al[233]	1972	16	8
Rosenwasser[234]	1967	8	3
Spector et al[235]	1975	11 (GT)*	1
		45 (GJ)†	10

(Tidwell TJ, Montague ED: Chemodectomas involving the temporal bone. Radiology 116:147–149, 1975)

* GT—glomus tympanicum.

† GJ—glomus jugulare.

COMPLICATIONS OF TREATMENT

Surgical

Fatalities have been reported from biopsy and resection. The major risk during operation is hemorrhage and injury to cranial nerves. Other complications include hemiparesis, spinal fluid leak, and hearing loss.[236]

Irradiation

There have been isolated reports of brain necrosis; these cases were associated with high doses, high daily fractions, or repeat courses of irradiation. This complication should not occur at a dose of 4500 rad or less given at 180 rad/day, 5 days/week. Other complications include cholesteatoma and sequestrum of the mastoid and otitis media. Detectable damage to the hearing mechanism and vestibular apparatus does not occur at 4000–4500 rad to the normal temporal bone. Cranial nerves may regain complete or partial function, especially if the deficit is of recent onset; five of eight patients with cranial nerve deficits showed improvement in the University of Florida series.[227] However, the seventh nerve never improved. Cranial nerve palsy due to irradiation should not occur at 4500 rad. The complication rate is greater when both operation and irradiation are used.

MAJOR SALIVARY GLANDS

Tumors of the major salivary glands account for 3–4% of all head and neck neoplasms, with no known cause. The average age of patients with malignant neoplasms is approximately 55 years; for benign tumors, about 40 years. Approximately one-fourth of parotid tumors and one-half of submaxillary tumors are malignant.

ANATOMY

The parotid gland is a relatively simple structure with rather complex anatomic relationships. It is indented and formed by the muscles, bones, vessels, and nerves that come in contact with the gland. The major bulk of the parotid gland is superficial, extending superiorly to the zygomatic arch and anterior aspect of the external auditory canal. The anterior border is variable, but does not continue beyond the opening of the parotid duct into the oral cavity opposite the second molar. Inferiorly, the gland fills the gap between the mastoid and the angle of the mandible below the external auditory canal. A deep lobe extends into the parapharyngeal area, where it is in relationship to the lateral process of C1, the styloid process, and the contents of the parapharyngeal space.

The parotid gland is encompassed by fascia that are sufficient to contain most parotid infections, in addition to benign and low-grade malignant tumors. However, the fascia between the parotid gland and the conchal and tragal cartilages is quite thin; this is a weak spot that tumor quickly traverses. The fascia separating the deep lobe from the parapharyngeal space (stylomandibular fascial membrane) may be sufficiently thin to allow tumor or infection easy access to the parapharyngeal space and pharynx.

The sensory nerve supply to the parotid area and part of the pinna is by way of the greater auricular nerve (C2–3). This nerve is severed in removal of the parotid gland with permanent loss of sensation. The facial nerve penetrates the parotid gland almost immediately upon leaving the stylomastoid canal. The seventh nerve forms an extensive anastomotic network within the gland and gives off branches to the muscles of expression.

The parotid gland is richly supplied from several arteries that freely anastomose and create arteriovenous bleeding during parotidectomy. The external carotid, internal maxillary, and superficial temporal arteries and the posterior facial vein lie deep to the seventh nerve; if these vessels require attention during an operation, the seventh nerve may be damaged.

Fig. 13-26 shows the lymphatics associated with the parotid gland. The superficial preauricular nodes, usually one or two in number, lie outside the fascia of the parotid gland and immediately in front of the tragus. These nodes are quite important since they drain the skin of the anterior ear, temple, and upper face, including the eye and nose. They are most frequently involved by metastatic skin cancer (carcinoma and melanoma) and lymphoma, but not usually from parotid neoplasms.

The preauricular nodes then empty into the superficial cervical nodes along the external jugular vein as it crosses the sternocleidomastoid muscle or the vein may communicate with the jugular chain of nodes.

There are two groups of nodes within the fascia of the parotid gland. Within the substance of the parotid gland are numerous lymph follicles and 4–10 small lymph nodes scat-

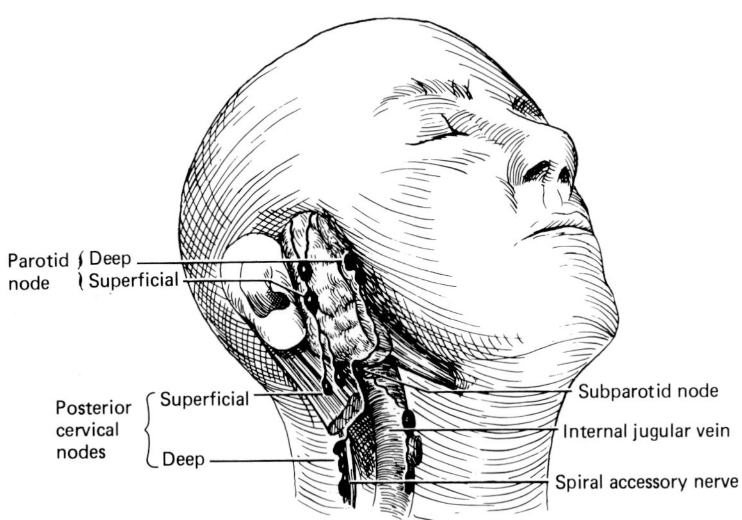

FIG. 13-26. Parotid gland lymphatic drainage system.

tered along the posterior facial and external jugular veins. Thus, they may lie deep to the seventh nerve. Outside the gland, but within the fascia, are one or two nodes that lie in front of the tragus and one or two nodes that lie between the inferior aspect of the tail of the parotid and the anterior border of the sternocleidomastoid muscle. These are referred to as the subparotid node(s). When enlarged, the subparotid node(s) are difficult to distinguish from a mass in the tail of the parotid gland.

For the anatomy of the submaxillary gland and lingual gland, see the section on the oral cavity.

PATHOLOGY

There is a large variety of benign and malignant neoplasms that occur in the major salivary glands. It is not at all unusual to have the diagnosis changed from that given at frozen section; the patient must be made aware of this risk.

Benign Tumors

BENIGN MIXED TUMORS. These slow-growing neoplasms are surrounded by an imperfect pseudocapsule that is traversed by fingers of tumor. Enucleation or removal of a narrow cuff of normal tissue usually results in recurrence. The histologic distinction between benign and malignant mixed tumor is often difficult. The age of appearance begins in the early 20's with a mean age of 40.

PAPILLARY CYSTADENOMA LYMPHOMATOSUM. This benign tumor, also called Warthin's tumor, probably arises from lymphoid elements. It is encased by a thin, but complete capsule occurring predominantly in older men. It is bilateral in approximately 10% of cases and may be multiple on one or both sides.

BENIGN LYMPHEPITHELIAL LESIONS. Benign lymphepithelial lesions (Godwin's tumor) account for about 5% of benign lesions. The tumor may be bilateral and is more common in women. Excision may be followed by recurrence.

ONCOCYTOMA. Oncocytoma is a benign, slow-growing tumor found mostly in the older age group. The encapsulated tumor has a dark appearance reminiscent of melanoma.

BASAL CELL ADENOMA. The basal cell adenoma is an uncommon benign lesion appearing in older people. It is histologically and clinically benign and is cured by simple excision. It must be distinguished from basal cell carcinoma of the skin metastatic to parotid lymph nodes.

Malignant Tumors

LOW-GRADE MALIGNANCY. *Acinic Cell Tumors.* Acinic cell tumors are typically slow-growing, low-grade neoplasms that appear in all age groups and are more common in women. They will recur after inadequate removal, sometimes as long as 25–30 years after initial treatment. Metastases occur in a small percentage of cases, but cannot be predicted by the histologic picture.

Mucoepidermoid Carcinoma, Low Grade. The majority of mucoepidermoid carcinomas are low-grade lesions readily cured by adequate excision and may appear in any age group. They grow slowly; there is little or no capsule, although they are well-circumscribed, but may widely infiltrate the normal gland or become fixed to skin. The mucin produced by the neoplasm may incite inflammatory changes about the edge of the mass.

HIGH-GRADE MALIGNANCY. *Mucoepidermoid Carcinoma, High Grade.* A few of the mucoepidermoid carcinomas behave in a very aggressive fashion and widely infiltrate the salivary gland and produce lymph node and distant metastases. They may be difficult to distinguish from high-grade epidermoid carcinoma.

Adenocarcinoma; Poorly Differentiated Carcinoma; Anaplastic Carcinoma; Squamous Cell Carcinoma. These histologies tend to appear late in life and have an aggressive behavior. True squamous cell carcinomas can arise from the salivary glands, but care must be taken to exclude metastases to the gland or to the lymph nodes contiguous to the gland. The great majority of so-called squamous cell carcinomas of the parotid are actually metastatic from skin cancer, especially of the temple area.[237]

Malignant Mixed Tumors. A small percentage of benign mixed tumors may develop into frank malignancy and have a very aggressive behavior.

Adenoid Cystic Carcinoma. This neoplasm is uncommon in the major salivary glands, varying in growth rate from slow to fast. Metastases to regional lymph nodes and distant sites occur; perineural involvement is characteristic; and recurrences may appear many years after initial treatment in the slow-growing lesions.

PATTERNS OF SPREAD

Benign Mixed Tumors

Benign mixed tumors of the parotid gland grow by expansion and local infiltration. Because of their slow growth they do not cause seventh nerve palsy, although the nerve may be severely stretched by large masses. When incompletely excised, multiple tumor nodules develop within the gland. Skin invasion may occur in recurrent lesions; bone invasion does not occur, but a mass may cause pressure defects of adjacent bone.

Malignant Tumors

The malignant neoplasms infiltrate the parotid gland, invade the seventh nerve, and spread along nerve sheaths for some distance. Tumor may invade the adjacent skin, muscles, and bone, depending on the site of origin. Lymph node metastases may occur from all of the histologies. Malignant tumors of the submaxillary gland invade the gland, fix the tumor to the adjacent mandible, and invade the mylohyoid muscle and eventually the tongue, hypoglossal nerve, and oral cavity or oropharynx. Skin invasion occurs in advanced cases.

CLINICAL PICTURE

The great majority of patients with either benign or malignant parotid tumors present with a mass that is easily seen and felt. Mild, intermittent pain is associated with a few of the masses, but does not distinguish between benign and malignant. Facial nerve palsy is an infrequent presenting complaint and indicates malignancy, as untreated benign tumors do not cause seventh nerve palsy. Tumors of the deep lobe may produce dysphagia.

The mobility of the mass depends on its size and location. Fixation or reduced mobility may occur in both benign and malignant neoplasms and does not distinguish the two. Tumors presenting in the deep lobe may cause bulging of the palate and tonsillar area.

Advanced malignant lesions may affect CN VII, and, more rarely, CN IX–XII and the sympathetic chain if the parapharyngeal space is invaded. The mandibular branch of CN V may be involved when tumor tracks along the auriculotemporal nerve to the base of the skull; pain is an associated finding. Nerve palsy is rarely seen with submaxillary gland tumors. These lesions may infiltrate the skin in advanced lesions. The tumor mass is usually partially fixed to the mandible unless quite small. Loss of mobility occurs with both benign and malignant lesions.

METHODS OF DIAGNOSIS AND STAGING

Biopsy Technique

Lesions lying in the superficial lobe of the parotid are usually biopsied by performing a superficial parotidectomy. Needle biopsy is often misleading and may delay diagnosis of submaxillary masses. If a careful search of the head and neck area fails to reveal a primary mucosal lesion, the submaxillary triangle is dissected as the biopsy procedure.

Staging Procedures

The proposed American Joint Committee staging for salivary gland tumors is[39]:

- TX Tumor that cannot be assessed by rules
- TO No evidence of primary tumor
- T1 Tumor 2 cm or less in diameter, solitary, freely mobile, facial nerve intact*
- T2 Tumor more than 2 cm but not more than 4 cm in diameter, solitary, freely mobile or reduced mobility or skin fixation, and facial nerve intact*
- T3 Tumor more than 4 cm but not more than 6 cm in diameter, or multiple nodes, skin ulceration, deep fixation, or facial nerve dysfunction*
- T4 Tumor more than 6 cm in diameter or involving mandible and adjacent bones

Benign tumors rarely invade bone, and routine roentgenograms are not necessary. Malignant tumors may invade the mandible or adjacent areas of skull such as the mastoid, styloid process, and base of skull, and appropriate roentgenograms are requested. Routine sialograms are not recommended to distinguish between malignant and benign neoplasms. However, a CT sialogram may show the distribution of the tumor mass prior to operation.[238] Sialograms are useful to distinguish a tumor mass from a stone, stricture, or sialectasis.

Nonneoplastic conditions that may be confused with a parotid tumor include:

- Acute or chronic parotitis
- Boeck's sarcoid
- Stone in duct
- Cysts (branchial cleft, dermoid)
- Hypertrophy associated with diabetes
- Hypertrophy of masseter muscle
- Neoplasms of the mandible
- Prominent transverse process of C1 (Atlas)
- Penetrating foreign bodies

TREATMENT

Selection of treatment modality

The initial treatment of resectable parotid lesions is exploration and *en bloc* superficial lobectomy for diagnosis and treatment.

* Applicable to parotid tumors only.

Involved skin is removed with the specimen. The tumor can usually be dissected free of the facial nerve. If the tumor involves the deep portion of the gland, the nerve is gently retracted and the deep portion excised. If the tumor grossly involves the facial nerve, one or more branches may have to be sacrificed. However, if tumor is merely adjacent to the nerve, it may be carefully dissected and spared; postoperative irradiation is essential in this situation.

Low-grade malignant neoplasms and small, favorable high-grade lesions may be treated by operation only. Radiation therapy is given postoperatively for most high-grade lesions, for low-grade lesions with positive margins or recurrence, and for selected benign mixed tumors when there is residual disease after operation for recurrence.

Inoperable tumors are treated by radiation therapy with an occasional success reported.

Submaxillary triangle dissection is used to make the diagnosis of lesions in this location. If frozen section diagnosis shows a malignant lesion and there is no involvement of nerves, mandible, or soft tissues, the operation is concluded, and postoperative irradiation is given to the submaxillary bed and ipsilateral neck.

If there is perineural invasion, bone invasion, a clinically positive node, or extension to contiguous soft tissues, then the resection is enlarged to encompass the necessary areas. This may include the mandible, mylohyoid muscle, digastric muscle, adjacent floor of mouth or tongue, and involved nerves. Postoperative radiation therapy is added based on the surgical findings.

The site of local recurrence includes the submaxillary triangle, adjacent oral cavity, pterygomaxillary fossa, base of skull, parotid gland, and neck. The irradiation portals must be tailored to cover the high-risk areas.

Surgical Treatment

SUPERFICIAL PAROTIDECTOMY. The parotid gland is really a unilobular gland, but is artificially divided into superficial and deep portions by the seventh nerve. A mass in the parotid gland is best approached by a superficial parotidectomy and frozen section diagnosis, since this affords the best method of diagnosis and often is the definitive treatment. The facial nerve is generally not sacrificed unless it is grossly involved with disease.

The incision is made in the preauricular crease and then curves under the earlobe posteriorly and then into the neck. The facial nerve must be identified in all superficial and total parotidectomies. Once this is accomplished, the dissection is carried out between the mass and the facial nerve. A margin of at least 1 cm around the mass is necessary if a benign tumor is suspected, and a larger margin if the mass is malignant. The adequacy of treatment is determined by frozen sections.

TOTAL PAROTIDECTOMY. Total parotidectomy is recommended for tumors in the deep lobe of the parotid gland, or for tumors that arise in the superficial lobe and extend into the deep lobe. A superficial parotidectomy is generally performed; then the nerve is dissected free from the underlying deep lobe and the deep lobe and tumor are removed. Occasionally, the mandible must be divided to gain access to the retromandibular portion of the deep lobe of the parotid gland. A partial mandibulectomy is required when the mandible is invaded by tumor. When pain is present, the auriculotemporal nerve should be explored to the base of the skull.

The paraparotid nodes are removed with the primary lesion. If the nodes are positive, a radical neck dissection is added. Radical neck dissection is always included for clinically positive nodes. Elective neck dissection is not done for low-grade lesions.

Generally, if a branch of the facial nerve or the entire nerve has to be sacrificed, a nerve graft or a crossover procedure is not performed immediately particularly if postoperative radiation therapy is to be used because the chances of success of the nerve graft or crossover are diminished. Attempts at nerve grafts and crossovers are delayed until local recurrence is thought to be unlikely.

Irradiation Technique

Radiation therapy plays its major role as an adjunct to surgery and is usually given postoperatively, although preoperative treatment may be considered in special situations. Postoperative irradiation is indicated for most high-grade lesions, for close or positive margins, for tumors of the deep lobe, for recurrent tumors, and for multiple regional node metastases.

The minimum treatment volume for parotid lesions includes the parotid bed and upper neck nodes. Perineural involvement indicates enlargement of the portals to cover the nerve pathways. The entire neck is included for high-grade lesions or for clinically positive nodes in the radical neck dissection specimen. The tumor dose to the primary area is 6000–6500 rad if there is no gross residual. Higher doses including interstitial implants are used for gross disease. There are no good data to show a difference in dose required for the various histologies, although the failure rate for malignant mixed tumors may be greater.[239–240]

Submaxillary tumor external beam portals are tailored to the extent of disease found in the surgical dissection. The entire ipsilateral neck is included. The postoperative dose is 6500–7000 rad as the rate of recurrences after combined treatment is substantial.

RESULTS OF TREATMENT

Benign Mixed Tumors

Enucleation or excision with a narrow rim of normal tissue will eventually result in a local recurrence rate of approximately 20% after 10–15 years of followup.

Rafla reported only a 2.7% recurrence rate when enucleation or excision was followed by postoperative radiation therapy.[241] Superficial parotidectomy (or excision for selected small lesions) will result in a recurrence rate of less than 5%.

The surgical success rate for recurrent lesions depends on the number of previous operations and the size and extent of the recurrence. It may be necessary to sacrifice one or several branches of the seventh nerve and repair the defect with a nerve graft. Postoperative irradiation of 6000–6500 rad is added in selected cases where there is residual disease, tumor dissected close to the seventh nerve, or a subsequent recurrence which would be almost impossible to manage surgically.

Death due to benign mixed tumor would be a rare event.

Malignant Tumors

Treatment results for paratoid tumors have been analyzed by histology, but tumors have not been staged by size or extent.

Table 13-55 shows the 5-year absolute survival rate by histology.[240]

The surgical results for low-grade malignant lesions are quite good, and radiation therapy is not often required. The local recurrence rate for operation alone is at least 30% for high-grade tumors. This recurrence rate was reduced to 14% by postoperative irradiation to a selected group in which half of the patients had gross residual tumor.[240]

Byers and coworkers report the results of treatment for 22 malignant tumors of the submaxillary gland with no prior therapy.[242] Treatment was resection followed selectively by postoperative irradiation. The local control was 64% and the survival 50%.

COMPLICATIONS OF TREATMENT

Surgical Treatment

Temporary facial nerve palsy may occur due to manipulation of the nerve during operation, and function will gradually return over a few months' time. Persistent weakness of the lower lip may occur, even though the remainder of the nerve recovers. Tarsorrhaphy may be required to protect the eye until function returns. Spontaneous return of facial movement has been reported to occur after surgical division of the seventh nerve. Facial nerve palsy may be repaired by a nerve graft. If grafting is not possible, a nerve crossover technique may be used, which connects the ipsilateral hypoglossal nerve to branches of the seventh nerve.

Gustatory sweating (Frey's syndrome) occurs in about 10% of patients after parotidectomy. This problem rarely requires treatment.

Persistent salivary fistula is a rare complication.

Radiation Therapy

Xerostomia is avoided by techniques which spare the contralateral salivary tissues.

TABLE 13-55. Parotid Cancer: Absolute 5-Year Survival (M. D. Anderson Hospital, 1944–65, 120 patients)

HISTOLOGY	NO. OF PATIENTS	5-YR SURVIVAL (Percentage)
Acinic cell	12	92
Mucoepidermoid (low grade)	28	76
Adenocarcinoma	12	66
Malignant mixed	27	50
Adenoid cystic	10	50
Squamous cell	6	50
Mucoepidermoid (high grade)	13	46
Undifferentiated	12	33

(Guillamondegui OM, Byers RM, Luna MA et al: Aggressive surgery in treatment for parotid cancer: The role of adjunctive postoperative radiotherapy. AJR 123:49–54, 1975 © 1975, American Roentgen Ray Society)

There may be trismus due to fibrosis of the masseter and pterygoid muscles with the temporomandibular joint. It should be possible to exclude the temporomandibular joint from high doses in most situations.

Otitis media may occur if the ear is irradiated and localized hair loss may occur with some techniques.

MINOR SALIVARY GLANDS

Tumors of minor salivary gland origin are uncommon, accounting for about 2–3% of all malignant neoplasms of the upper aerodigestive tract. They may appear at any age, but are uncommon before 20 and rare under 10. There is no known causative agent except for the adenocarcinomas of the nose (see the section on the nasal cavity.) They tend to occur most often in the hard palate, nasal cavity, and paranasal sinuses, areas infrequently involved by squamous carcinomas. Thus, the site of origin is related more to the population density of the minor salivary glands in a particular tissue than to any environmental factor.

ANATOMY

Minor salivary glands are ubiquitous in the mucosa of the upper aerodigestive tract with the exception of the gingivae and the anterior portion of the hard palate, which are free of minor salivary glands. They are distributed on the undersurface of the anterior and lateral oral tongue and the base of the tongue. Aberrant salivary tissue is sometimes seen in lymph nodes, in the body of the mandible just behind the third molar teeth, in the vestigial remnant of the nasopalatine canal in the anterior maxilla, the middle ear, lower neck, sternoclavicular joint, thyroglossal duct, and other sites.

PATHOLOGY

Approximately one-half of minor salivary gland tumors are malignant. The histologic varieties of malignant tumors include adenoid cystic carcinoma, mucoepidermoid carcinoma, adenocarcinoma, malignant mixed, acinic cell, and oncocytic carcinomas. About two-thirds are adenoid cystic. The mucoepidermoid carcinoma and adenocarcinoma arise predominantly in the oral cavity (see Table 13-56).[243]

The benign tumors are benign mixed (pleomorphic adenoma) in the great majority of cases with a sprinkling of intraductal papillomas, papillary cystadenomas, basal cell adenomas, and benign oncocytomas.[244]

PATTERNS OF SPREAD

Table 13-56 lists the site of origin for minor salivary gland tumors in 118 patients.[243] Tongue lesions usually originate from the base of tongue. There are no minor salivary glands in the anterior one-half or the midline of the hard palate, so tumors arise on the posterolateral hard palate and all of the soft palate. Almost all of the minor salivary gland tumors arising from lip mucosa occur on the upper lip. The site of origin for floor of mouth salivary gland tumors is moot—either the sublingual gland or a minor salivary gland.

TABLE 13-56. Site of Presentation and Histology for 118 Malignant Minor Salivary Gland Tumors (M. D. Anderson Hospital, January 1970–February 1978)

SITE	NO.	ADENOID CYSTIC	MUCO-EPIDERMOID (high grade)	MUCO-EPIDERMOID (low grade)	ADENO-CARCINOMA	MALIGNANT MIXED	ACINIC CELL
Lip	2	1	0	0	1	0	0
Buccal mucosa	16	9	1	3	3	0	0
Tongue	17	10	2	1	4	0	0
Floor of mouth	22	10	4	3	4	0	1
Gingivae	13	3	5	1	4	0	0
Palate	23	15	1	3	4	0	0
Paranasal sinuses and nasal cavity	20	16	1	1	2	0	0
Nasopharynx and pharynx	3	1	0	1	0	1	0
Trachea	1	1	0	0	0	0	0
Larynx	1	1	0	0	0	0	0
Total	118	67	14	13	22	1	1

(Schell S, Barkley HT Jr, Chiminazzo H Jr: Treatment of malignant minor salivary gland tumors. Unpublished data, 1980)

These tumors grow by extensive local infiltration with eventual invasion of muscle, bone, and cartilage. Perineural spread is a common feature, particularly for adenoid cystic carcinoma. Tumor may track both centrally and peripherally along nerves, but the central spread is the more common event since most lesions arise near the terminations of the nerves. Extension along nerves eventually may traverse the base of skull and surface intracranially, although this spread pattern may not become manifest for several years after the original treatment. Tumor growth along a nerve may be characterized by skipped areas, so that a normal nerve segment is no assurance of free margins. Adenoid cystic carcinoma may grow along the Haversian systems of bone without showing bone destruction.[245]

The risk of positive lymph nodes is related to the site of origin and the histology. Lymph node metastases are most likely from sites with a dense capillary lymphatic network, similar to patterns for squamous carcinoma. Adenoid cystic carcinoma, low-grade mucoepidermoid carcinoma, and acinic cell carcinoma are at low risk to spread to lymph nodes; about 20% of adenoid cystic carcinomas spread to lymph nodes, but this finding is partly related to their frequent site of origin in the hard palate and paranasal sinuses, areas that infrequently produce lymph node metastases. The high-grade tumors (high-grade mucoepidermoid carcinoma, adenocarcinoma, and malignant mixed tumor) have a 30% incidence of lymph node involvement on admission, and eventually 51% showed lymph node metastases. Schell and coworkers report a 17% incidence of positive nodes on admission for all histologies and grades and subsequent appearance in 11%.[243] Most were staged N1 or N2A and were usually associated with lesions of the tongue or floor of mouth. At least 25% of patients will develop distant metastasis. The lung is the site first recognized, but no site is exempt.

CLINICAL PICTURE

The clinical picture obviously depends on the site of origin. The signs and symptoms differ somewhat from those of squamous cell carcinoma arising in the same area. Many of the lesions are indolent, and the history may go back many months or even years; about 25% will give a history of a mass being present over 10 years. Since the lesions develop under the epithelium, the initial lesion is a submucosal mass that is often painless until ulceration develops. Perineural involvement is expressed as pain or paresthesias. Otherwise, the clinical picture resembles that for squamous cell carcinomas for a given size and site. Lymph node metastases surface at predictable sites. The clinically positive nodes are usually small and mobile, but neck dissection on such a patient may show numerous small, clinically undetectable positive nodes, particularly in the case of adenoid cystic carcinomas.

The differential diagnosis includes lesions that produce an enlarging submucosal mass, such as an abscess, a stone in a duct, a cyst of soft tissue or bone, sarcoma, or lymphoma.

Biopsy is required prior to treatment. Because of the infrequency of these lesions, faulty histologic interpretation is not unusual and often leads to inappropriate therapy.

The same staging systems applied to squamous cell carcinomas may be used, although very few reported series bother to correlate size and extent of tumor with results by various treatment modalities. Roentgenographic studies are similar to those used for squamous cell carcinomas for a specific site.

TREATMENT TECHNIQUES

There is little disagreement about the value of surgery but there remains considerable disagreement regarding the results of irradiation. Most series reporting poor results from radiation therapy mention neither the selection of patients for irradiation nor the doses and volumes used. Since radiation therapy has often been used as a last-ditch effort for high-grade, advanced lesions after multiple surgical procedures, it is hardly surprising that results in some reports have been poor. Those series using radiation therapy alone for early lesions or as an immediate postoperative adjunct to surgical removal have had a favorable experience. After all, the histologies of the minor salivary gland tumors are the same as those of parotid tumors, and it is generally accepted that routine postoperative irradiation will decrease the local recurrence rate in high-grade parotid lesions and that irradiation alone will even control a few locally recurrent or inoperable tumors.[239] Fig. 13-27 shows a typical response for primary adenoid cystic carcinoma of the palate treated by radiation therapy alone. The response of malignant minor salivary gland tumors to irradiation is similar to that of a squamous cell carcinoma of the same size and same anatomic site, and the doses used are quite similar.

The low-grade lesions (low-grade mucoepidermoid carcinoma, acinic cell carcinoma, and benign mixed tumors) are treated initially by an operation when feasible, but irradiation is sometimes used as the primary treatment for inaccessible lesions or where the functional loss would be considerable. Postoperative irradiation is added for close margins or for those lesions which have recurred more than once. If the patient presents after excisional biopsy of a small lesion, irradiation is an alternative to re-excision, particularly if the procedure would produce significant cosmetic or functional loss.

The treatment of high-grade lesions varies immensely, depending on the site of origin, stage of disease, and willingness of the patient to accept a major cosmetic or functional change subsequent to an operation. Since the philosophy at the University of Florida is to accept radiation therapy as a curative therapy, the authors essentially approach most lesions as they would a squamous cell carcinoma of similar stage and similar anatomic site.

When combined treatment is indicated, the operation should precede radiation therapy to facilitate healing and gain knowledge of tumor extent for radiation treatment planning.

An alternative to radical surgery is radical irradiation with operation reserved for persistence or recurrence. This concept has some merit in that recurrent tumors may be encompassed by the same operation, while if the radiation therapy is successful, the patient avoids the surgical morbidity.

The benign mixed tumors also respond to radiation therapy, although complete regression is unusual. Long-term cure by radiation therapy alone has been reported. Surgery, however, remains the treatment of choice, and the major use of radiation therapy has been an adjunct to operation in cases at significant risk for recurrence. The benign mixed tumors of minor salivary gland origin are reputed to be more radiosensitive than those arising in the parotid, but this may be a function of tumor volume rather than inherent differences in response.

Chemotherapy

Because of the rarity of these neoplasms, information about chemotherapy is almost entirely anecdotal. Some evidence of antitumor effects has been seen with 5-FU, hydroxyurea, methotrexate, and cis-platinum with bleomycin, but the magnitudes of responses are often difficult to evaluate in the context of broad Phase II studies or retrospective reviews of medical records.[246–249] Using a combination of methyl-CCNU,

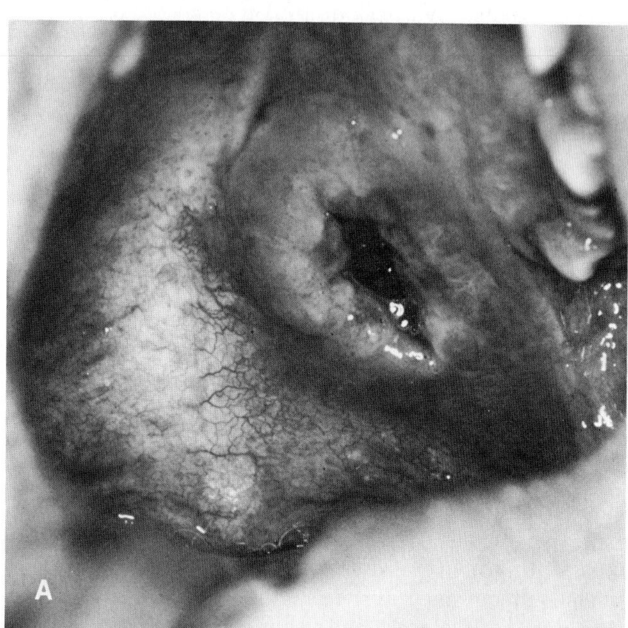

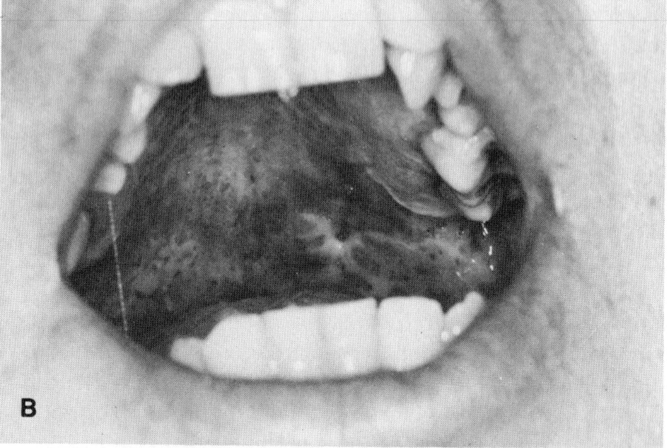

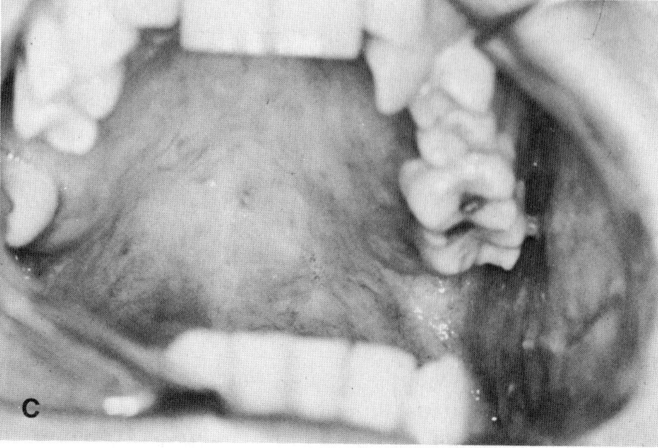

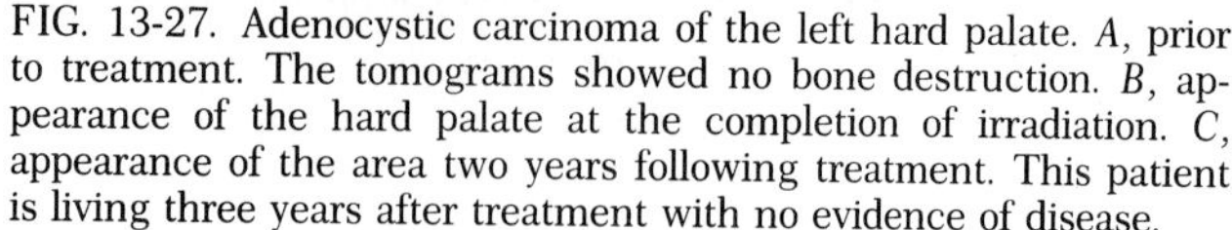
FIG. 13-27. Adenocystic carcinoma of the left hard palate. *A*, prior to treatment. The tomograms showed no bone destruction. *B*, appearance of the hard palate at the completion of irradiation. *C*, appearance of the area two years following treatment. This patient is living three years after treatment with no evidence of disease.

doxorubicin and vincristine, Hayes and coworkers have seen significant responses in adenoid cystic carcinoma.[250]

Surgical Treatment

Benign tumors are removed by wide local excision, which includes a cuff of normal tissue. Local excision or enucleation is insufficient treatment due to the high recurrence rate associated with limited procedures.

For malignant lesions, the surgical approach must allow for the propensity for perineural spread. Small low-grade lesions with a long history of slow growth may be treated with a wide local excision including a shell of normal tissue. Large low-grade lesions and high-grade lesions require a more radical resection. It is not possible, of course, to remove all the nerves potentially involved, but the nerves that are involved should be sacrificed wherever reasonable to do so. As an alternative, postoperative irradiation may be used to cover the perineural routes of spread. Since unsuccessfully treated patients often live many years before they eventually die of their disease, careful planning must go into reconstruction and rehabilitation.

Irradiation Technique

The irradiation techniques are similar to those for squamous cell carcinomas of the same anatomic site and similar tumor size, with the exception that nerve pathways must be covered, especially for high-grade lesions. Subclinical perineural spread is especially common for adenoid cystic carcinomas and must be considered to be present even though not seen on the biopsy or surgical sections. Recurrences are frequently manifested in and about the base of skull at the termination of the cranial nerves.

Dose and fractionation schedules are similar to those used for squamous cell carcinomas.

The regression rate of adenoid cystic carcinoma during treatment is similar to that of squamous cell carcinoma. Successfully treated adenocarcinomas or low-grade mucoepidermoid carcinomas may require several weeks or months to disappear after completion of treatment. The regional lymphatics are electively irradiated depending on the site of origin and grade of the lesion.

The response of benign mixed tumors is predictably slow and often incomplete.

TABLE 13-57. Results of Surgical Treatment of Minor Salivary Gland Tumors (Memorial Hospital, 1939–1963, 267 Patients*)

	NO. OF PATIENTS	LOCAL CONTROL
Oral cavity/oropharynx	198	68%
Sinus/nasal/nasopharynx	58	28%
Larynx	11	55%

(Spiro RH, Koss LG, Hajdu SI et al: Tumors of minor salivary origin: A clinicopathologic study of 492 cases. Cancer 31:117–129, 1973)

* 60%—no prior treatment; 14%—clinically positive nodes on admission; 90%—treated surgically; 5 yr. followup.

RESULTS OF TREATMENT

Spiro and coworkers report the Memorial Sloan-Kettering results for 434 malignant minor salivary gland tumors, of which 90% were treated surgically.[251] The determinate 5-, 10-, and 15-year cure rates were 44%, 32%, and 21%; 51% died of the original cancer. Patients with adenoid cystic carcinoma had the poorest prognosis, about 20% surviving without recurrence. Those with adenocarcinoma had an intermediate outlook, about 35% surviving without recurrence, and mucoepidermoid carcinomas had the best control rate with about 70% long-term cures. Local control differed considerably by site (see Table 13-57), but this difference is partly explained by the higher incidence of advanced adenoid cystic carcinoma in the sinuses. Local control was also better for small lesions and those without bone or lymph node involvement. Previous treatment had little effect on cure rate.

Bardwil and coworkers reported a similar series from M. D. Anderson Hospital with shorter followup (3–20 years) in which surgery was the sole treatment in 88% of cases (see Table 13-58).[252] Local control was reported to be 75%, but 47% died of their original cancer, a percentage similar to the Memorial Sloan-Kettering series.

Schell and coworkers recently have reported a group of 118 malignant salivary gland tumors of which only 10% were treated by operation alone, 58% by surgery plus radiation therapy, and 32% by radiation therapy alone (see Table 13-58).[243] The group treated by radiation therapy alone included 15 early and 23 advanced lesions; followup was 2–10 years. The initial local control rate for the entire group was 79%; 11

TABLE 13-58. Results of Treatment of Malignant Minor Salivary Gland Tumors (M. D. Anderson Hospital)

	NO. OF PATIENTS	NO PRIOR TREATMENT	FOLLOWUP	LOCAL CONTROL	DISTANT METASTASES	DOD OR LWD*	METHOD OF TREATMENT†	
1945–1962 Bardwil et al[252]	87	56%	3–20 yr	75%	30%	47%	S	71
							S + RT	10
							RT	6
1970–1978 Schell et al[243]	118	42%	2–10 yr	79%‡	25%	36%	S	11
							S + RT	69
							RT	38

* DOD or LWD—dead of disease or living with disease.
† S—surgery; RT—radiation therapy.
‡ 11 patients salvaged by repeat operations for ultimate control rate of 88%.

patients were saved by subsequent operation for an ultimate control of 88%.

There is a suggestion that overall local control may be improved by more frequent use of radiation therapy, but the eventual survival may be only slightly enhanced. Table 13-59 shows the risk of local recurrence by treatment category and histology.[243] The low incidence of recurrence with radiation therapy alone for adenoid cystic carcinoma indicates that this histology responds quite consistently to radiation. There are too few cases in the other categories to reach any conclusions except that surgery plus radiation therapy seems to provide better control than surgery alone for high-grade lesions. (Note: Adenoid cystic carcinoma is considered "high grade" because of its tendency to wide invasion, a high rate of local recurrence, and distant metastasis even though the growth rate may be indolent.)

Benign mixed tumors of minor salivary gland origin have a good prognosis. Enucleation, however, is followed by recurrence, and a cuff of normal tissue is required.

Bardwil and coworkers reported 13 patients with benign mixed tumors, all of whom were cured, 12 by operation and one by radiation therapy alone.[252]

Rafla-Demetrious reports the Royal Marsden experience of 44 cases of benign mixed tumor (see Table 13-60).[253] Eleven patients were treated by radiation therapy alone, and none of the tumors regrew, although not all had complete regression. Several excellent photographs demonstrate the response to radiation therapy. Local recurrence of benign mixed tumor may appear after many, many years and an occasional patient may eventually die from uncontrolled disease.

REFERENCES

1. Fletcher GH, MacComb WS, Braun EJ: Analysis of sites and causes of treatment failures in squamous cell carcinomas of the oral cavity. AJR 83:405–411, 1960
2. Goffinet DR, Gilbert EH, Weller SA et al: Irradiation of clinically uninvolved cervical lymph nodes. Can J Otolaryngol 4:927–933, 1975
3. Jesse RH, Barkley HT, Lindberg RD et al: Cancer of the oral cavity: Is elective neck dissection beneficial? Am J Surg 120:505–508, 1970
4. Hardingham M, Dalley VM, Shaw HJ: Cancer of the floor of the mouth: Clinical features and results of treatment. *Clin Oncol* 3:227–246, 1977
5. Southwick HW, Slaughter DP, Trevino ET: Elective neck dissection for intraoral cancer. Arch Surg 80:905–909, 1960
6. Ash CL: Oral Cancer: A twenty-five year study. AJR 87:417–430, 1962
7. Campos JL, Lampe I, Fayos JV: Radiotherapy of carcinoma of the floor of the mouth. Radiology 99:677–682, 1971

TABLE 13-59. Malignant Minor Salivary Gland Tumors: Primary Recurrence Related to Treatment Modality (No. of Patients with Recurrence after Initial Treatment at M. D. Anderson Hospital/Total Patients Treated)

HISTOLOGY	SURGERY ONLY	SURGERY + RADIATION THERAPY	RADIATION THERAPY ONLY	TOTAL
High grade				
Adenoid cystic	3/4	9/40	0/23	12/67
Mucoepidermoid	0/1	0/6	4/7	4/14
Adenocarcinoma	3/4	3/14	1/4	7/22
Malignant mixed	0/0	0/1	0/0	0/1
Low grade				
Mucoepidermoid	1/2	0/7	1/4	2/13
Acinic cell	0/0	0/1	0/0	0/1
Total	*7/11	†12/69	6/38	25/118

(Schell S, Barkley HT Jr, Chiminazzo H Jr: Treatment of malignant minor salivary gland tumors. Unpublished data, 1980)

* Five patients salvaged by repeated surgical resection(s).

† Six patients salvaged by surgery.

TABLE 13-60. Incidence of Recurrence of Pleomorphic Adenoma of Minor Salivary Glands in the Royal Marsden Series Distributed According to the Method of Treatment

METHOD OF TREATMENT	NO. OF PATIENTS	NO. WITH RECURRENCE	LENGTH OF FOLLOWUP
Radiation alone	11	0	5 for 5+ yr
Preoperative radiation and surgery	14	2	9 for 5+ yr
Surgery and postoperative radiation	18	0	14 for 5+ yr 9 for 10+ yr
Surgery alone	1	0	5 yr
Total	44	2	29 for 5+ yr

(Rafla-Demetrious SF: Mucous and Salivary Gland Tumours, p 118. Springfield, Illinois: Charles C Thomas, 1970)

8. Million RR: Elective neck irradiation for T_XN_O squamous carcinoma of the oral tongue and floor of mouth. Cancer 34:149–155, 1974
9. Cady B, Catlin D: Epidermoid carcinoma of the gum: A 20-year survey. Cancer 23:551–569, 1969
10. del Regato JA, Spjut HJ: Ackerman and del Regato's Cancer: Diagnosis, Treatment, and Prognosis, 5th ed pp 264, 281, 341–342, 345. St. Louis, CV Mosby, 1977
11. Martin CL, Craffey EJ: Cancer of the gums. AJR 67:420–427, 1952
12. Chung CK, Rahman SM, Lim ML et al: Squamous cell carcinoma of the hard palate. Int J Radiat Oncol Biol Phys 5:191–196, 1979
13. Eneroth CM, Hjertman L, Moberger G: Squamous cell carcinomas of the palate. Acta Otolaryngol (Stockh) 73:418–427, 1972
14. Horiuchi J, Adachi T: Some considerations on radiation therapy of tongue cancer. Cancer 28:335–339, 1971
15. Beahrs OH, Devine KD, Henson SW Jr: Treatment of carcinoma of the tongue: End-results in one hundred sixty-eight cases. Arch Surg 79:399–403, 1959
16. Frazell EL, Lucas JC Jr: Cancer of the tongue: Report of the management of 1554 patients. Cancer 15:1085–1099, 1962
17. Kremen AJ: Results of surgical treatment of cancer of the tongue. Surgery 39:49–53, 1956
18. Spiro RH, Strong EW: Discontinuous partial glossectomy and radical neck dissection in selected patients with epidermoid carcinoma of the mobile tongue. Am J Surg 126:544–546, 1973
19. Berger DS, Fletcher GH, Lindberg RD et al: Elective irradiation of the neck lymphatics for squamous cell carcinomas of the nasopharynx and oropharynx. AJR 111:66–72, 1971
20. Lindberg RD, Jesse RH: Treatment of cervical lymph node metastases from primary lesions of the oropharynx, supraglottic larynx, and hypopharynx. AJR 102:132–137, 1968
21. Million RR, Fletcher GH, Jesse RH Jr: Evaluation of elective irradiation of the neck for squamous cell carcinoma of the nasopharynx, tonsillar fossa, and base of tongue. Radiology 80:973–988, 1963
22. Ho JHC: An epidemiologic and clinical study of nasopharyngeal carcinoma. Int J Radiat Oncol Biol Phys 4:183–198, 1978
23. Moench HC, Phillips TL: Carcinoma of the nasopharynx: Review of 146 patients with emphasis on radiation dose and time factors. Am J Surg 124:515–518, 1972
24. Barker JL, Fletcher GH: Time, dose, and tumor volume relationships in megavoltage irradiation of squamous cell carcinomas of the retromolar trigone and anterior tonsillar pillar. Int J Radiat Oncol Biol Phys 2:407–414, 1977
25. Jesse RH, Fletcher GH: Metastases in cervical lymph nodes from oropharyngeal carcinoma: Treatment and results. AJR 90:990–996, 1963
26. Lindberg RD, Barkley HT Jr, Jesse RH et al: Evolution of the clinically negative neck in patients with squamous cell carcinoma of the facial arch. AJR 111:60–65, 1971
27. Southwick HW: Elective neck dissection for intraoral cancer. JAMA 217:454–455, 1971
28. Rolander TL, Everts EC, Shumrick DA: Carcinoma of the tonsil: A planned combined therapy approach. Laryngoscope 81:1199–1207, 1971
29. Ogura JH, Biller HF, Wette R: Elective neck dissection for pharyngeal and laryngeal cancers: An evaluation. Ann Otol Rhinol Laryngol 80:646–651, 1971
30. Putney FJ: Elective versus delayed neck dissection in cancer of the larynx. Surg Gynecol Obstet 112:736–742, 1961
31. Fletcher GH: Elective irradiation of subclinical disease in cancers of the head and neck. Cancer 29:1450–1454, 1972
32. Lindberg RD: Distribution of cervical lymph node metastases from squamous cell carcinoma of the upper respiratory and digestive tracts. Cancer 29:1446–1449, 1972
33. Fletcher GH, Jesse RH, Healey JE Jr, et al: Oropharynx. In MacComb WS, Fletcher GH (eds): Cancer of the Head and Neck pp 179–212. Baltimore, Williams & Wilkins, 1967
34. Fletcher GH, Jesse RH, Lindberg RD et al: The place of radiotherapy in the management of the squamous cell carcinomas of the supraglottic larynx. AJR 108:19–26, 1970
35. MacComb WS, Healey JE Jr, McGraw JP et al: Hypopharynx and cervical esophagus. In MacComb WS, Fletcher GH (eds): Cancer of the Head and Neck pp 213–240. Baltimore, Williams & Wilkins, 1967
36. Chen KY, Fletcher GH: Malignant tumors of the nasopharynx. Radiology 99:165–171, 1971
37. Fisch U: Lymphography of the Cervical Lymphatic System. Philadelphia, WB Saunders, 1968
38. Merino OR, Lindberg RD, Fletcher GH: An analysis of distant metastases from squamous cell carcinoma of the upper respiratory and digestive tracts. Cancer 40:145–151, 1977
39. American Joint Committee for Cancer Staging and End-Results Reporting (AJC): Manual for Staging of Cancer 1978 pp 27–52. Chicago, AJC, 1978
40. Agresti A, Wackerly D: Some exact conditional tests of independence for TxC cross-classification tables. Psychometrika 42:111–125, 1977
41. Mendenhall WM, Million RR, Cassisi NJ: Elective neck irradiation in squamous-cell carcinoma of the head and neck. Head Neck Surg 3:15–20, 1980
42. Bocca E, Pignataro O: A conservative technique in radical neck dissection. Ann Otol Rhinol Laryngol 76:975–987, 1967
43. Barkley HT Jr, Fletcher GH, Jesse RH et al: Management of cervical lymph node metastases in squamous cell carcinoma of the tonsillar fossa, base of tongue, supraglottic larynx, and hypopharynx. Am J Surg 124:462–467, 1972
44. Kogelnik HD, Fletcher GH, Jesse RH: Clinical course of patients with squamous cell carcinoma of the upper respiratory and digestive tracts with no evidence of disease 5 years after initial treatment. Radiology 115:423–427, 1975
45. Sagerman RH, Chung CT, King GA et al: High dose preoperative irradiation of the lower neck and supraclavicular fossae. AJR 132:357–359, 1979
46. Parsons JT, Bova FJ, Million RR: A re-evaluation of split-course technique for squamous cell carcinoma of the head and neck. Int J Radiat Oncol Biol Phys 46:1645–1652, 1980
47. Shukovsky LJ, Fletcher GH: Time-dose and tumor volume relationships in the irradiation of squamous cell carcinoma of the tonsillar fossa. Radiology 107:621–626, 1973
48. Shukovsky LJ, Baeza MR, Fletcher GH: Results of irradiation in squamous cell carcinomas of the glossopalatine sulcus. Radiology 120:405–408 1976
49. Spanos WJ Jr, Shukovsky LJ, Fletcher GH: Time, dose, and tumor volume relationships in irradiation of squamous cell carcinomas of the base of the tongue. Cancer 37:2591–2599, 1976
50. Meoz-Mendez RT, Fletcher GH, Guillamondegui OM et al: Analysis of the results of irradiation in the treatment of squamous cell carcinomas of the pharyngeal walls. Int J Radiat Oncol Biol Phys 4:579–585, 1978
51. Million RR, Cassisi NJ: Radical irradiation for carcinoma of the pyriform sinus. Laryngoscope 91:439–450, 1981
52. Golder SL: Carcinoma of the supraglottic larynx. Presented at the 10th Annual Radiation Therapy Clinical Research Seminar, April 26–26, 1980, pp 237–247. Gainesville, Florida, University of Florida, Radiation Therapy Division, 1981
53. Shukovsky LJ: Dose, time, volume relationships in squamous cell carcinoma of the supraglottic larynx. AJR 108:27–29, 1970
54. Cox JD, Byhardt RW, Komaki R et al: Reduced fractionation and the potential of hypoxic cell sensitizers in irradiation of malignant epithelial tumors. Int J Radiat Oncol Biol Phys 6:37–40, 1980
55. Bertino JR, Mosher MB, DeConti RC: Chemotherapy of cancer of the head and neck. Cancer 31:1141–1149, 1973
56. Carter SK: The chemotherapy of head and neck cancer. Semin Oncol 4:413–424, 1977
57. Goldsmith MA, Carter SK: The integration of chemotherapy into a combined modality approach to cancer therapy. V. Squamous cell cancer of the head and neck. Cancer Treat Rev. 2:137–158, 1975

58. Wittes RE, Cvitkovic E, Shah J et al: Cis-dichlorodiammineplatinum (II) in the treatment of epidermoid carcinoma of the head and neck. Cancer Treat Rep 61:359–366, 1977
59. Panettiere FJ, Lane M, Lehane D: Effectiveness of a new outpatient program utilizing CACP in the chemotherapy of advanced epidermoid head and neck tumors. A SWOG study. Proc Am Assoc Cancer Res 19:410, 1978
60. Jacobs C, Bertino J, Goffinet DR et al: 24-hour infusion of cis-platinum in head and neck cancers. Cancer 42:2135–2140, 1978
61. Sako K, Razack MS, Kalnins I: Chemotherapy for advanced and recurrent squamous cell carcinoma of the head and neck with high and low dose cis-diamminedichloroplatinum. Am J Surg 136:529–533, 1978
62. Randolph VL, Wittes RE: Weekly administration of cis-diamminedichloroplatinum (II) without hydration or osmotic diuresis. Eur J Cancer 14:753–756, 1978
63. Smart CR, Rochlin DB, Nahun AM et al: Clinical experience with vinblastine sulfate (NSC-49842) in squamous cell carcinoma and other malignancies. Cancer Chemother Rep 34:31–45, 1964
64. Papac R, Lefkowitz E, Bertino JR: Methotrexate (NSC-740) in squamous cell carcinoma of the head and neck. II. Intermittent intravenous therapy. Cancer Chemother Rep 51:69–72, 1967
65. Lane M, Moore JE, Levin H et al: Methotrexate therapy for squamous cell carcinoma of the head and neck. Intermittent intravenous dose program. JAMA 204:561–564, 1968
66. Leone LA, Albala MM, Rege VB: Treatment of carcinoma of the head and neck with intravenous methotrexate. Cancer 21:828–837, 1968
67. DePalo GM, DeLena M, Molinari R et al: Clinical evaluation of high weekly intravenous doses of methotrexate in advanced oropharyngeal carcinoma. Tumori 56:259–268, 1970
68. Levitt M, Mosher MB, DeConti RC et al: Improved therapeutic index of methotrexate with "leucovorin rescue." Cancer Res 33:1729–1734, 1973
69. DeConti RC: Phase III comparison of methotrexate with leucovorin versus methotrexate alone versus a combination of methotrexate plus leucovorin, cyclophosphamide, and cytosine arabinoside in head and neck cancer. Proc Am Assoc Cancer Res 17:248, 1976
70. Woods RL, Tattersall MHN, Sullivan J: A randomised study of three doses of methotrexate (MTX) in patients with advanced squamous cell cancer of the head and neck. Proc Am Assoc Cancer Res 20:262, 1979
71. Kirkwood JM, Ervin T, Pitman S et al: Twice-weekly low-dose methotrexate-leucovorin (MTX-LV) versus weekly high-dose methotrexate-leucovorin (MTX-LV) for advanced squamous carcinoma of the head and neck. Proc Am Assoc Cancer Res 20:314, 1979
72. Lippman AJ, Helson C, Helson L et al: Clinical trials of cis-diamminedichloroplatinum (NSC-119875). Cancer Chemother Rep 57:191–200, 1973
73. Turrisi AT III, Rosencweig M. VonHoff D et al: The role of bleomycin in the treatment of advanced head and neck cancer. In Carter SK, Crooke ST, Umezava H (eds): *Bleomycin: Current Status and New Developments,* pp 151–163. New York, Academic Press, 1978
74. Pitman SW, Minor DR, Papac R et al: Sequential methotrexate-leucovorin (MTX-LV) and cis-platinum (CDDP) in head and neck cancer. Proc Am Assoc Cancer Res 20:419, 1979
75. Jacobs C, Fee WE, Goffinet DR: Cis-platinum vs. high-dose methotrexate + cis-platinum in the treatment of recurrent head and neck cancer. Recent Results Cancer Res (in press)
76. Tejada F, Chandler JR, Salem E, et al: Preoperative time sequential chemotherapy for Stage III and IV head and neck cancer. Proc Am Assoc Cancer Res 21:478, 1980
77. Mosher MB, DeConti RC, Bertino JR: Bleomycin therapy in advanced Hodgkin's disease and epidermoid cancers. Cancer 30:56–60, 1972
78. Lokich JJ, Frei E III: Phase II study of concurrent methotrexate and bleomycin chemotherapy. Cancer Res 34:2240–2242, 1974
79. Yagoda A, Lippman AJ, Winn RJ et al: Combination chemotherapy with belomycin (BLM) and methotrexate (MTX) in patients with advanced epidermoid carcinomas. Proc Am Assoc Cancer Res 16:247, 1975
80. Randolph VL, Vallejo A, Spiro RH et al: Combination therapy of advanced head and neck cancer: Induction of remissions with diamminedichloroplatinum (II), bleomycin, and radiation therapy. Cancer 41:460–467, 1978
81. Hong WK, Shapshay SM, Bhutani R et al: Induction chemotherapy in advanced squamous head and neck carcinoma with high-dose cis-platinum and bleomycin infusion. Cancer 44:19–25, 1979
82. Wittes R, Heller K, Randolph V et al: cis-Dichlorodiammine-platinum (II)-based chemotherapy as initial treatment in advanced head and neck cancer. Cancer Treat Rep 63:1533–1538, 1979
83. Glick JH, Marcial V, Velez-Garcia E: The adjuvant treatment of inoperable Stage III and IV epidermoid carcinoma of the head and neck with platinum and bleomycin infusions prior to definitive radiotherapy: A RTOG pilot study. Proc Am Assoc Cancer Res 21:473, 1980
84. Wolf GT, Makuch RW: Preoperative cis-platinum (DDP) and bleomycin (BLM) in patients with head and neck squamous carcinoma (HNSCC): Toxicity and tumor response. Proc Am Assoc Cancer Res 21:400, 1980
85. Elias EG, Chretien PB, Monnard E et al: Chemotherapy prior to local therapy in advanced squamous cell carcinoma of the head and neck: Preliminary assessment of an intensive drug regimen. Cancer 43:1025–1031, 1979
86. Caradonna R, Paladine W, Goldstein J et al: Combination chemotherapy with high-dose cis-diamminedichloroplatinum (II) (CDDP), methotrexate (MTX), and bleomycin (Bleo) for epidermoid carcinoma of the head and neck. Proc Am Assoc Cancer Res 19:401, 1978
87. Kaplan BH, Vogl SE, Chiuten D et al: Chemotherapy of advanced cancer of the head and neck (HNCa) with methotrexate (M), bleomycin (B), and cis-diamminedichloroplatinum (D) in combination. Proc Am Assoc Cancer Res 20:384, 1979
88. Wittes RE, Spiro RH, Shah J et al: Chemotherapy of head and neck cancer: Combination treatment with cyclophosphamide, Adriamycin, methotrexate, and bleomycin. Med Pediatr Oncol 3:301–309, 1977
89. Livingston RB, Einhorn LH, Bodey GP et al: COMB (cyclophosphamide, Oncovin, methyl-CCNU, and bleomycin): A four-drug combination in solid tumors. Cancer 36:327–332, 1975
90. Livingston RB, Einhorn LH, Burgess MA et al: Sequential combination chemotherapy for advanced recurrent squamous carcinoma of the head and neck. Cancer Treat Rep 60:103–105, 1976
91. Richman SP, Livingston RB, Gutterman JU et al: Chemotherapy vs. chemoimmunotherapy of head and neck cancer. Report of a randomized study. Cancer Treat Rep 60:535–539, 1976
92. Presant CA, Ratkin G, Klahr C: Adriamycin (A), BCNU (B), plus cyclophosphamide (C) in head and neck carcinoma. Proc Am Assoc Cancer Res 18:281, 1977
93. Price LA, Hill BT, Calvert AH et al: Improved results in combination chemotherapy of head and neck cancer using a kinetically-based approach: A randomized study with and without adriamycin. Oncology 35:26–28, 1978
94. Cortes EP, Amin VC, Attie J et al: Combination of low-dose bleomycin (Bleo) followed by cyclophosphamide (C), methotrexate (M), and 5-fluorouracil (F) for advanced head and neck cancer. Proc Am Assoc Cancer Res 20:259, 1979
95. Holoye PY, Byers RM, Gard DA et al: Combination chemotherapy of head and neck cancer. Cancer 42:1661–1669, 1978
96. Ketcham AS, Hoye RC, Chretien PB et al: Irradiation twenty-four hours preoperatively. Am J Surg 118:691–697, 1969
97. Lawrence WL, Terz JJ, Rogers C et al: Preoperative irradiation for head and neck cancer: A prospective study. Cancer 33:318–323, 1974
98. Strong EW: Preoperative radiation and radical neck dissection. Surg Clin North Am 49:271–276, 1969

99. Fletcher GH: Basic principles of the combination of irradiation and surgery. Int J Radiat Oncol Biol Phys 5:2091–2096, 1979
100. Looser KG, Shah JP, Strong EW: The significance of "positive" margins in surgically resected epidermoid carcinomas. Head Neck Surg 1:107–111, 1978
101. Marcus RB Jr, Million RR, Cassisi NJ: Postoperative irradiation for squamous cell carcinomas of the head and neck: Analysis of time-dose factors related to control above the clavicles. Int J Radiat Oncol Biol Phys 5:1943–1949, 1979
102. Cutler SJ, Ederer F: Maximum utilization of the life table method in analyzing survival. J Chronic Dis 8:699–712, 1958
103. Gehan EA: A generalized Wilcoxon test for comparing arbitrarily single-censored samples. Biometrika 52:203–223, 1965
104. Kligerman MM, Hellman S, vonEssen CF et al: Sequential chemotherapy and radiotherapy. Preliminary results of clinical trial with methotrexate in head and neck cancer. Radiology 86:247–250, 1966
105. Kramer S: Radiation therapy and chemotherapy combination. JAMA 217:946–947, 1971
106. Helman P, Sealy R, Malherbe E et al: Intraarterial cytotoxic therapy and x-ray therapy for cancer of the head and neck. Lancet 1:128–130, 1965
107. Tarpley JL, Chretien PB, Alexander JC Jr et al: High-dose methotrexate as a preoperative adjuvant in the treatment of epidermoid carcinoma of the head and neck: A feasibility study and clinical trial. Am J Surg 130:481–486, 1975
108. Kirkwood J, Miller D, Pitman S et al: Initial high-dose methotrexate-leucovorin (MTX-LV) in advanced squamous cell carcinoma of the head and neck. Proc Am Assoc Cancer Res 19:398, 1978
109. Goffinet DR, Bagshaw MA: Clinical use of radiation sensitizing agents. Cancer Treat Rev 1:15–26, 1974
110. Borgelt BB, Davis LW: Combination chemotherapy and irradiation for head and neck cancer: A review. Cancer Clin Trials 1:49–59, 1978
111. Muggia FM, Cortes-Funes H, Wasserman TH: Radiotherapy and chemotherapy in combined clinical trials: Problems and promise. Int J Radiat Oncol Biol Phys 4:161–171, 1978
112. Kramer S: Methotrexate and radiation therapy in the treatment of advanced squamous cell carcinoma of the oral cavity, oropharynx, supraglottic larynx, and hypopharynx. (Preliminary report of a controlled clinical trial of the Radiation Therapy Oncology Group.) Can J Otolaryngol 4:213–218, 1975
113. Knowlton AH, Percarpio B, Bobrow S et al: Methotrexate and radiation therapy in the treatment of advanced head and neck tumors. Radiology 116:709–712, 1975
114. Condit PT: Treatment of carcinoma with radiation therapy and methotrexate. Missouri Med 65:832–835, 1968
115. Bagshaw MA, Doggett RLS: A clinical study of chemical radiosensitization. In Korger S, Vaeth JM (ed.): Frontiers of Radiation Therapy and Oncology, pp 164–173. Baltimore, University Park Press, 1969
116. Stefani S, Eells RW, Abbate J: Hydroxyurea and radiotherapy in head and neck cancer: Results of prospective controlled study in 126 patients. Radiology 101:391–396, 1971
117. Richards GJ Jr, Chambers RG: Hydroxyurea: A radiosensitizer in the treatment of neoplasms of the head and neck. AJR 105:555–565, 1969
118. Gollin FF, Ansfield FJ, Brandenburg JH et al: Combined therapy in advanced head and neck cancer: A randomized study. AJR 114:83–88, 1972
119. Ansfield FJ, Ramirez G, Davis HL Jr. et al: Treatment of advanced cancer of the head and neck. Cancer 25:78–82, 1970
120. Shigematsu Y, Sakai S, Fuchihata H: Recent trials in the treatment of maxillary sinus carcinoma, with special reference to the chemical potentiation of radiation therapy. Acta Otolaryngol (Stockh) 71:63–70, 1971
121. Cachin Y, Jortay A, Sancho H et al: Preliminary results of a randomized E.O.R.T.C. study comparing radiotherapy and concomitant bleomycin to radiotherapy alone in epidermoid carcinomas of the oropharynx. Eur J Cancer 13:1389–1395, 1977
122. Shanta V, Sundaram K: The combined therapy of oral cancer. GANN Monogr Cancer Res 19:159–170, 1976
123. Abe M, Shigematsu Y, Kimura S: Combined use of bleomycin with radiation in the treatment of cancer. Recent Results Cancer Res 63:169–178, 1978
124. Kapstad B, Bang G, Rennaes S et al: Combined preoperative treatment with cobalt and bleomycin in patients with head and neck carcinoma: A controlled clinical study. Int J Radiat Oncol Biol Phys 4:85–89, 1978
125. Clifford P, O'Connor AD, Durden-Smith J et al: Synchronous multiple drug chemotherapy and radiotherapy for advanced (Stage III and IV) squamous carcinoma of the head and neck. Antibiot Chemother 24:60–72, 1978
126. Seagren S, Byfield J, Nahum A et al: Concurrent cyclophosphamide (CY), bleomycin (BL), and ionizing radiation (XRT) in advanced squamous carcinoma of the head and neck (H&N). Proc Am Assoc Cancer Res 20:324, 1979
127. Fu KF, Silverberg IJ, Phillips TL et al: Combined radiotherapy and multi-drug chemotherapy for advanced head and neck cancer: Results of a Radiation Therapy Oncology Group pilot study. Cancer Treat Rep 63:351–357, 1979
128. Glick JH, Fazekas JT, Davis LW et al: Combination chemotherapy-radiotherapy for advanced inoperable head and neck cancer: A RTOG pilot study. Cancer Clin Trials 2:129–136, 1979
129. Clifford P: Synchronous multiple drug chemotherapy and radiotherapy in the treatment of advanced (Stage III and IV) squamous carcinoma of the head and neck. Proc Am Assoc Cancer Res 20:83, 1979
130. Sato Y, Morita M, Takahashi HO et al: Combined surgery, radiotherapy, and regional chemotherapy in carcinoma of the paranasal sinuses. Cancer 25:571–579, 1970
131. Byers RM, O'Brien J, Waxler J: The therapeutic and prognostic implications of nerve invasion in cancer of the lower lip. Int J Radiat Oncol Biol Phys 4:215–217, 1978
132. Mackay EN, Sellers AH: A statistical review of carcinoma of the lip. Can Med Assn J 90:670–672, 1964
133. MacComb WS, Fletcher GH, Healey JE Jr: Intra-oral cavity. In MacComb WS, Fletcher GH (eds): Cancer of the Head and Neck, pp 89–151. Baltimore, Williams & Wilkins, 1967
134. Ange DW, Lindberg RD, Guillamondegui OM: Management of squamous cell carcinoma of the oral tongue and floor of mouth after excisional biopsy. Radiology 116:143–146, 1975
135. Chu A, Fletcher GH: Incidence and causes of failures to control by irradiation the primary lesions in squamous cell carcinomas of the anterior two-thirds of the tongue and floor of mouth. AJR 117:502–508, 1973
136. Mendenhall WM, VanCise WS, Bova FJ et al: Analysis of time-dose factors in squamous cell carcinoma of the oral tongue and floor of mouth treated with radiation therapy alone. Int J Radiat Oncol Biol Phys (in press)
137. Fu KK, Lichter A, Galante M: Carcinoma of the floor of mouth: An analysis of treatment results and the sites and causes of failures. Int J Radiat Oncol Biol Phys 1:829–837, 1976
138. Marcus RB Jr, Million RR, Mitchell TP: A preloaded, custom-designed implantation device for Stage T1–T2 carcinoma of the floor of mouth. Int J Radiat Oncol Biol Phys 6:111–113, 1980
139. Guillamondegui OM, Jesse RH: Surgical treatment of advanced carcinoma of the floor of the mouth. AJR 126:1256–1259, 1976
140. Tapley N: Clinical Applications of the Electron Beam, pp 125–129. New York, John Wiley & Sons, 1976
141. Flynn MB, Mullins FX, Moore C: Selection of treatment in squamous carcinoma of the floor of the mouth. Am J Surg 126:477–481, 1973
142. Fu KK, Ray JW, Chan EK et al: External and interstitial radiation therapy of carcinoma of the oral tongue: A review of 32 years experience. AJR 126:107–115, 1976
143. Lees AW: The treatment of carcinoma of the anterior two-thirds of the tongue by radiotherapy. Int J Radiat Oncol Biol Phys 1:849–858, 1976
144. Mendenhall W: Introduction to Probability and Statistics (4th ed), pp. 284–286. North Scituate, Massachusetts, Doxbury Press, 1975

145. Small IA, Waldron CA: Ameloblastomas of the jaws. Oral Surg 8:281–297, 1955
146. Sinclair NA: Cysts and ameloblastomas: A relationship. Aust Dent J 22:27–30, 1977
147. Pandya NJ, Stuteville OH: Treatment of ameloblastoma. Plast Reconstr Surg 50:242–248, 1972
148. Sehdev MK, Huvos AG, Strong EW et al: Proceedings: Ameloblastoma of maxilla and mandible. Cancer 33:324–333, 1974
149. Goldberg SJ, Friedman JM: Ameloblastoma: Review of the literature and report of case. J Am Dent Assoc 90:432–438, 1975
150. McIvor J: The radiological features of ameloblastoma. Clin Radiol 25:237–242, 1974
151. Swearingen AG, McGraw JP, Palumbo VD: Roentgenographic pathologic correlation of carcinoma of the gingiva involving the mandible. AJR 96:15–18, 1966
152. Rankow RM, Hickey MJ: Adamantinoma of the mandible: Analysis of surgical treatment. Surgery 36:713–719, 1954
153. Fayos JV: Carcinoma of the mandible: Result of radiation therapy. Acta Radiol 12:378–386, 1973
154. Gefter JW: Carcinoma of the gums and retromolar trigone. 7th Annual Radiation Therapy Clinical Research Seminar, April 21–23, 1977, pp 191–210. Gainesville, Florida, Radiation Therapy Division, University of Florida, 1978
155. Fletcher GH: Oral cavity and oropharynx. In Fletcher GH (ed.): Textbook of Radiotherapy, 2nd ed, pp 212–254. Philadelphia, Lea & Febiger, 1973
156. Whicker JH, DeSanto LW, Devine KD: Surgical treatment of squamous cell carcinoma of the base of the tongue. Laryngoscope 82:1853–1860, 1972
157. Parsons JT, Million RR, Cassisi NJ: Carcinoma of the base of tongue: Results of radical irradiation with surgery reserved for irradiation failure. (in prep)
158. Wickstrum DL: Carcinoma of the tonsillar region. 10th Annual Radiation Therapy Clinical Research Seminar, April 24–26, 1980, pp 249–270. Gainesville, Florida, Radiation Therapy Division, University of Florida, 1981
159. Weichert KA, Aron BS, Maltz R et al: Carcinoma of the tonsil: Treatment by a planned combination of radiation and surgery. Int J Radiat Oncol Biol Phys 1:505–508, 1976
160. Perez CA, Lee FA, Ackerman LV et al: Non-randomized comparison of preoperative irradiation and surgery versus irradiation alone in the management of carcinoma of the tonsil. AJR 126:248–260, 1976
161. Strong MS, Vaughan, CW, Kayne HL et al: A randomized trial of preoperative radiotherapy in cancer of the oropharynx and hypopharynx. Am J Surg 136:494–500, 1978
162. Fletcher GH: The Third Annual Lectureship of the Juan A. del Regato Foundation: Squamous cell carcinomas of the oropharynx. Int J Radiat Oncol Biol Phys 5;2073–2090, 1979
163. Ratzer ER, Schweitzer RJ, Frazell EL: Epidermoid carcinoma of the palate. Am J Surg 119:294–297, 1970
164. Weller SA, Goffinet DR, Goode RL et al: Carcinoma of the oropharynx: Results of megavoltage radiation therapy in 305 patients. AJR 126:236–247, 1976
165. Seydel HG, Scholl H: Carcinoma of the soft palate and uvula. AJR 120:603–607, 1974
166. Lindberg RD, Fletcher GH: The role of irradiation in the management of head and neck cancer: Analysis of results and causes of failure. Tumori 64:313–325, 1978
167. Wynder EL: The epidemiology of cancer of the upper alimentary and upper respiratory tracts. Laryngoscope (Supp 8) 88:50–51, 1978
168. Vincent RG, Marchetta F: The relationship of the use of tobacco and alcohol to cancer of the oral cavity, pharynx or larynx. Am J Surg 105:501–505, 1963
169. Fraumeni JF Jr: Geographic distribution of head and neck cancers in the United States. Laryngoscope (Supp 8) 88:40–44, 1978
170. Pillsbury HRC, Kirchner JA: Clinical vs histopathologic staging in laryngeal cancer. Arch Otolaryngol 105:157–159, 1979
171. Kirchner JA: Staging as seen in serial sections. Laryngoscope 85:1816–1821, 1975
172. Fletcher GH, Jing B-S: The Head and Neck, p 168. Chicago, Year Book Medical Publishers, 1968
173. Mancuso AA, Hanafee WN, Juillard GJF et al: The role of computed tomography in the management of cancer of the larynx. Radiology 124:243–244, 1977
174. Biller HF, Barnhill FR Jr, Ogura JH et al: Hemilaryngectomy following radiation failure for carcinoma of the vocal cords. Laryngoscope 80:249–253, 1970
175. Burns HP, vanNostrand AWP, Bryce DP: Verrucous carcinoma of the larynx: Management by radiotherapy and surgery. Ann Otol Rhinol Laryngol 85:538–543, 1976
176. Harwood AR, Beale FA, Cummings BJ et al: T3 glottic cancer: An analysis of dose time-volume factors. Int J Radiat Oncol Biol Phys 6:675–680, 1980
177. Fletcher GH, Lindberg RD, Hamberger A et al: Reasons for irradiation failure in squamous cell carcinoma of the larynx. Laryngoscope 85:987–1003, 1975
178. Lee F, Perlmutter S, Ogura JH: Laryngeal radiation after hemilaryngectomy. Laryngoscope 90:1534–1539, 1980
179. Ogura JH, Sessions DG, Spector GJ: Analysis of surgical therapy for epidermoid carcinoma of the laryngeal glottis. Laryngoscope 85:1522–1530, 1975
180. Dickens WJ, Cassisi NJ, Million RR et al: Treatment of early vocal cord carcinoma: A comparison of apples and apples. Laryngoscope (in press)
181. Ogura JH, Sessions DG, Gershon JS: Conservation surgery for epidermoid carcinoma of the supraglottic larynx. Laryngoscope 85:1808–1815, 1975
182. Neel H III, Devine KD, Desanto LW: Laryngofissure and cordectomy for early cordal carcinoma: Outcome in 182 patients. Otolaryngol Head Neck Surg 88:79–84, 1980
183. Ballantyne AJ: Principles of surgical management of cancer of the pharyngeal walls. Cancer 20:663–667, 1965
184. Kirchner JA: Pyriform sinus cancer: A clinical and laboratory study. Ann Otol Rhinol Laryngol 84:793–803, 1975
185. Wang CC: Radiotherapeutic management of carcinoma of the posterior pharyngeal wall. Cancer 27:894–896, 1971
186. Marks JE, Freeman RB, Lee F et al: Pharyngeal wall cancer: An analysis of treatment results complications and patterns of failure. Int J Radiat Oncol Biol Phys 4:587–593, 1978
187. Kirchner JA, Owen JR: Five hundred cancers of the larynx and pyriform sinus: Results of treatment by radiation and surgery. Laryngoscope 87:1288–1303, 1977
188. Razack MS, Sako K, Marchetta FC et al: Carcinoma of the hypopharynx: Success and failure. Am J Surg 134:489–491, 1977
189. Marks JE, Kurnik B, Powers WE et al: Carcinoma of the pyriform sinus: An analysis of treatment results and patterns of failure. Cancer 41:1008–1015, 1978
190. Cunningham MP, Catlin D: Cancer of the pharyngeal wall. Cancer 20:1859–1866, 1965
191. Rouvière H: Anatomy of the Human Lymphatic System, p 53. Ann Arbor, Michigan, Edwards Brothers, 1938
192. Fletcher GH, Million RR: Malignant tumors of the nasopharynx. AJR 93:44–55, 1965
193. Fletcher GH, Million RR: Nasopharynx. In Fletcher GH (ed): *Textbook of Radiotherapy,* 3rd ed, pp 364–383. Philadelphia, Lea & Febiger, 1980
194. Mesic JB, Fletcher GH, Goepfert H: Megavoltage irradiation of epithelial tumors of the nasopharynx. Int J Radiat Oncol Biol Phys (in press)
195. Gefter JW: Carcinoma of the nasopharynx. 10th Annual Radiation Therapy Clinical Research Seminar, April 24–26, 1980, pp 229–235. Gainesville, Florida, Division of Radiation Therapy, University of Florida, 1981
196. Hoppe RT. Goffinet DR, Bagshaw MA: Carcinoma of the nasopharynx: Eighteen years' experience with megavoltage radiation therapy. Cancer 37:2605–2612, 1976
197. Biller HF, Sessions DG, Ogura JH: Angiofibroma: A treatment approach. Laryngoscope 84:695–706, 1974
198. Briant TDR, Fitzpatrick PJ, Berman J: Nasopharynx angiofibroma: A twenty year study. Laryngoscope 88:1247–1251, 1978
199. Samaan NA, Bakdash MM, Caderao JB et al: Hypopituitarism

after external irradiation: Evidence for both hypothalamic and pituitary origin. Ann Intern Med 83:771–777, 1975
200. Boldrey E, Sheline G: Delayed transitory clinical manifestations after radiation treatment of intracranial tumors. Acta Radiol Ther 5:5–10, 1966
201. Acheson ED, Cowdell RH, Hadfield EH et al: Nasal cancer in woodworkers in the furniture industry. Br Med J 2:587–596, 1968
202. Acheson ED, Cowdell RH, Jolles B: Nasal cancer in the Northamptonshire boot and shoe industry. Br Med J 1:385–393, 1970
203. Acheson ED, Hadfield EH, Macbeth RG: Carcinoma of the nasal cavity and accessory sinuses in woodworkers. Lancet 1:311–312, 1967
204. Ironside P, Matthews J: Adenocarcinoma of the nose and paranasal sinuses in woodworkers in the state of Victoria, Australia. Cancer 36:1115–1121, 1975
205. Maisel RH, Johnston WH, Anderson HA et al: Necrotizing sialometaplasia involving the nasal cavity. Laryngoscope 87:429–434, 1977
206. Kadish S, Goodman M, Wang CC: Olfactory neuroblastoma: A Clinical analysis of 17 cases. Cancer 37:1571–1576, 1976
207. Kassel SH, Echevarria RA, Guzzo FP: Midline malignant reticulosis (so-called lethal midline granuloma). Cancer 23:920–935, 1969
208. Goepfert H, Guillamondegui OM, Jesse RH et al: Squamous cell carcinoma of nasal vestibule. Arch Otolaryngol 100:8–10, 1974
209. Haynes WD, Tapley N: Radiation treatment of carcinoma of the nasal vestibule. AJR 120:595–602, 1974
210. Dickens WJ: Tumors of the nasal vestibule. Ninth Annual Radiation Therapy Clinical Research Seminar, April 26–28, 1979, pp 209–214. Gainesville, Florida, Radiation Therapy Division, University of Florida, 1980
211. Ketcham AS, Chretien PB, VanBuren JM et al: The ethmoid sinuses: A re-evaluation of surgical resection. Am J Surg 126:469–476, 1973
212. Ellingwood KE, Million RR: Cancer of the nasal cavity and ethmoid/sphenoid sinuses. Cancer 43:1517–1526, 1979
213. Frazell EL, Lewis JS: Cancer of the nasal cavity and accessory sinuses: A report of the management of 416 patients. Cancer 16:1293–1301, 1963
214. Elkon D, Hightower SI, Lim ML et al: Esthesioneuroblastoma. Cancer 44:1087–1094, 1979
215. Fauci AS, Johnson RE, Wolff SM: Radiation therapy of midline granuloma. Ann Intern Med 84:140–147, 1976
216. Jesse RH: Preoperative versus postoperative radiation in the treatment of squamous carcinoma of the paranasal sinuses. Am J Surg 110:552–556, 1965
217. Shukovsky LJ, Fletcher GH: Retinal and optic nerve complications in a high dose irradiation technique of ethmoid sinus and nasal cavity. Radiology 104:629–634, 1972
218. Földi M: Lymphogenous encephalopathy. In Mayerson HS (ed): Lymph and the Lymphatic System, pp 169–198. Springfield, Illinois, Charles C Thomas, 1968
219. Edwards C, Heath D, Harris P: The carotid body in emphysema and left ventricular hypertrophy. J Pathol 104:1–13, 1971
220. Guild SR: The glomus jugulare, a nonchromaffin paraganglion, in man. Ann Otol Rhinol Laryngol 62:1045–1071, 1953
221. Ward PH, Jenkins HA, Hanafee WN: Diagnosis and treatment of carotid body tumors. Ann Otol Rhinol Laryngol 87:614–621, 1978
222. Kim J-A, Elkon D, Lim M-L et al: Optimum dose of radiotherapy for chemodectomas of the middle ear. Int J Radiat Oncol Biol Phys 6:815–819, 1980
223. Warren KW: Symposium on surgical lesions of neck and upper mediastinum: Tumors of the carotid body: Recognition and treatment. Surg Clin North Am 53:677–693, 1953
224. Maruyama Y, Gold LHA, Kieffer SA: Clinical and angiographic evaluation of radiotherapeutic response of glomus jugulare tumors. Radiology 101:397–399, 1971
225. Myers EN, Newman J, Kaseff L et al: Glomus jugulare tumor: A radiographic-histologic correlation. Laryngoscope 81:1838–1851, 1971
226. Tidwell TJ, Montague ED: Chemodectomas involving the temporal bone. Radiology 116:147–149, 1975
227. Dickens WJ, Million RR, Cassisi NJ et al: Chemodectomas arising in temporal bone structures. (in prep)
228. Hudgins PT: Radiotherapy for extensive glomus jugulare tumors. Radiology 103:427–429, 1972
229. Cole JM: Glomus jugulare tumor. Laryngoscope 87:1244–1258, 1977
230. Smith PE: Management of chemodectomas (glomus jugulare). Laryngoscope 80:207–216, 1970
231. Newman H, Rowe JF Jr, Phillips TL: Radiation therapy of the glomus jugulare tumor. AJR 118:663–669, 1973
232. Grubb WB Jr, Lampe I: The role of radiation therapy in the treatment of chemodectomas of the glomus jugulare. Laryngoscope 75:1861–1871, 1965
233. Hatfield PM, James AE, Schulz MD: Chemodectomas of the glomus jugulare. Cancer 30:1164–1168, 1972
234. Rosenwasser H: Current management: Glomus jugulare tumors. Ann Otol Rhinol Laryngol 76:603–610, 1967
235. Spector GH, Fierstein J, Ogura JH: A comparison of therapeutic modalities of glomus tumors in the temporal bone. Laryngoscope 86:690–696, 1976
236. Glasscock ME III, Harris PF, Newsome G: Glomus tumors: Diagnosis and treatment. Laryngoscope 84:2006–2032, 1974
237. Cassisi NJ, Dickerson DR, Million RR: Squamous cell carcinoma of the skin metastatic to parotid nodes. Arch Otolaryngol 104:336–339, 1978
238. Som PM, Biller HF: The combined CT-sialogram. Radiology 135:387–390, 1980
239. King JJ, Fletcher GH: Malignant tumors of the major salivary glands. Radiology 100:381–384, 1971
240. Guillamondegui OM, Byers RM, Luna MA et al: Aggressive surgery in treatment for parotid cancer: The role of adjunctive postoperative radiotherapy. AJR 123:49–54, 1975
241. Rafla S: Submaxillary gland tumors. Cancer 26:821–826, 1970
242. Byers RM, Jesse RH, Guillamondegui OM et al: Malignant tumors of the submaxillary gland. Am J Surg 126:458–463, 1973
243. Schell S, Barkley HT Jr, Chiminazzo H Jr: Treatment of malignant minor salivary gland tumors. Submitted for publication, 1980
244. Thawley SE, Ward SP, Ogura JH: Basal cell adenoma of the salivary glands. Laryngoscope 84:1756–1766, 1974
245. Ranger D, Thackray AC, Lucas RB: Mucous gland tumors. Br J Cancer 10:1–16, 1956
246. Rentschler R, Burgess MA, Byers R: Chemotherapy of malignant major salivary gland neoplasms: A 25-year review of M. D. Anderson Hospital experience. Cancer 40:619–624, 1977
247. Vermeer RJ, Pinedo HM: Partial remission of advanced adenoid cystic carcinoma obtained with Adriamycin: A case report with a review of the literature. Cancer 43:1604–1606, 1979
248. Moore GE, Bross IDJ, Ausman R et al: Effects of chlorambucil (NSC-3088) in 374 patients with advanced cancer. Eastern Clinical Drug Evaluation Program. Cancer Chemother Rep (Part I) 52:661–666, 1968
249. Wittes RE, Brescia F, Young CW et al: Combination chemotherapy with cis-diamminedichloroplatinum (II) and bleomycin in tumors of the head and neck. Oncology 32:202–207, 1975
250. Hayes DM, Magill GB, Golbey RB et al: Methyl CCNU, Adriamycin, and vincristine (MAV) chemotherapy of adenoid cystic carcinoma. Proc Soc Surg Oncol, p 35, 1976
251. Spiro RH, Koss LG, Hajdu SI et al: Tumors of minor salivary origin: A clinicopathologic study of 492 cases. Cancer 31:117–129, 1973
252. Bardwil JM, Reynolds CT, Ibanez ML et al: Report of one hundred tumors of the minor salivary glands. Am J Surg 112:493–497, 1966
253. Rafla-Demetrious S: Mucous and Salivary Gland Tumours, p 118. Springfield, Illinois, Charles C Thomas, 1970

John D. Minna
George A. Higgins
Eli J. Glatstein

CHAPTER 14

Cancer of the Lung

LUNG CANCER: MAGNITUDE OF THE PROBLEM

Lung cancer is estimated to have developed in some 85,000 males and 32,000 females in the United States in 1980. Many of these victims died in the same year (see Table 14-1). The age-adjusted cancer death rates for both males and females are doubling approximately every 15 years (see Fig. 14-1). Lung cancer is the leading cause of cancer death in males from age 35 on, and the second leading cause of cancer deaths in females age 35–74.[1] In 1980, lung cancer caused some 22% of all male and 8% of all female cancers, yet caused 34% of all male and 14% of all female cancer deaths.[1] The majority of cases for both sexes are seen in the age range of 35–75 years, with a peak at age 55–65 years for each sex. At the time of diagnosis, in 70% of patients the disease has spread to regional nodes or distant sites (see Table 14-2). However, even in those patients with supposedly localized disease, five-year survival is the exception rather than the rule. In general, females have a better five-year survival than males for as yet unknown reasons.

Lung cancer is a major health problem. The epidemiology and etiology are discussed throughout the text, while several recent general references, in addition to some historical aspects, are cited in references at the end of this chapter.[3-19]

ANATOMIC CONSIDERATIONS

Because the lungs are paired organs with a large pulmonary reserve capacity, one lung may be sacrificed with little resultant disability in an otherwise healthy person. Graham, when performing the first pneumonectomy, was greatly concerned over the possible consequences of sudden occlusion of the left main pulmonary artery, having in mind the devastating consequences of pulmonary embolism.[17] However, sudden occlusion of one pulmonary artery with diversion of one-half the output from the right ventricle to the opposite lung produces almost imperceptible changes in the patient undergoing the operation.

Although the anatomy of the pulmonary hilus was well-known and the concept of the bronchopulmonary segment being the basic anatomic unit was first advanced by Ewart in 1889, early pulmonary resections were accomplished by mass ligature of these structures.[20] Clarification of the lobar and segmental anatomy greatly simplifies excisional pulmonary procedures.

The right lung is composed of three lobes—the upper, middle, and lower—and comprises approximately 55% of the ventilatory capacity. The left lung consists of only two lobes—the lingular portion of the upper lobe corresponding to the middle lobe on the right. The lobes are separated by fissures that can be identified on roentgenograms, particularly the lateral views. On the right side, there are usually two fissures present, the oblique or major fissure separating the lower lobe from the upper and middle lobes, and the horizontal or minor fissure separating the upper and middle lobes. On the left, the single fissure separates the upper and lower lobes, running obliquely from the level of the third rib posteriorly and forward, ending in the region of the sixth or seventh costochondral junction.

Ewart's original description of the bronchopulmonary segment as the basic anatomic unit was followed by a number of other anatomic studies. In 1942, Jackson and Huber published their own observations, along with those of others, outlining the most common segmental anatomy of the lungs with a system of nomenclature generally accepted in the United States.[21] In 1955, Boyden applied numerical designations to these various segments (see Fig. 14-2 and Table 14-3).[22]

TABLE 14-1. Lung Cancer: Magnitude of the Problem

		MALE	FEMALE
Estimated new cases in the U.S., 1980		85,000	32,000
Estimated deaths in the U.S., 1980		74,800	26,000
Deaths, 1977:	All Ages	68,481	22,029
Ages:	35–54	10,110	4,528
	55–74	44,112	13,045
	75+	14,060	4,341

(Silverberg E: Cancer Statistics, 1980. CA 30:2338, 1980)

Although the anatomic relationships of the pulmonary hilar structures as well as the arrangement of the bronchopulmonary segments are relatively constant, variations may be encountered with some frequency. Therefore, the thoracic surgeon must be on the alert for these anomalies. The main structures of the primary pulmonary hilus are the main bronchus, the pulmonary artery, and both the superior and inferior pulmonary veins (see Fig. 14-2). The relationships of these structures vary considerably on the two sides. On the left, the pulmonary artery curves around the upper lobe bronchus, while on the right side, it remains anterior and below the upper lobe bronchus. The segmental arteries follow the segmental bronchi; the veins occupy an intersegmental position converging to form segmental veins. These empty into the superior and inferior pulmonary veins. On the right side, the middle lobe vein empties into the superior pulmonary vein. Variations are common; in general, they occur in the veins, arteries, and bronchi (in that order of frequency). The pulmonary arterial tree is a low pressure system, compared with the peripheral arteries, and these vessels are thin-walled and fragile by comparison. While most centers report only on whether the lymph nodes are negative or positive for tumor, in addition to information on the general location of the nodes,

TABLE 14-2. Overall Extent of Disease at Time of Presentation and Overall 5-Year Survival for Lung Cancer

STAGE OF DISEASE (Cases Diagnosed 1970–73)		5-YEAR SURVIVAL (Cases Diagnosed 1965–1969)	
		Male	*Female*
	%	%	
Local	17	28	51
Regional spread	22	10	15
Distant metastases	48	(<0.1)†	(<0.1)†
All stages*		8	13

(Cancer Patient Survival, Report Number 5, DHEW Publ. No. (NIH) 77-912, 1977)

*Not all patients classified according to stage.

†Not stated, but estimated from data on survival of all stages to be less than 0.1%.

the American Joint Commission (AJC) feels there is inadequate information on the implication of nodal involvement as it relates to treatment. The AJC has thus developed a lymph node classification system (see Fig. 14-3).[24] Martini, of the Sloan Kettering Cancer Center in New York, along with colleagues at the National Cancer Center of Tokyo, are studying the importance of a lymph node mapping system and suggest recording the location number and extent of positive lymph nodes (see Fig. 14-3).[23]

PATHOLOGY OF LUNG CANCER

HISTOLOGIC TYPES

There are many different types of malignant pulmonary neoplasms. However, the histologic classfication of lung

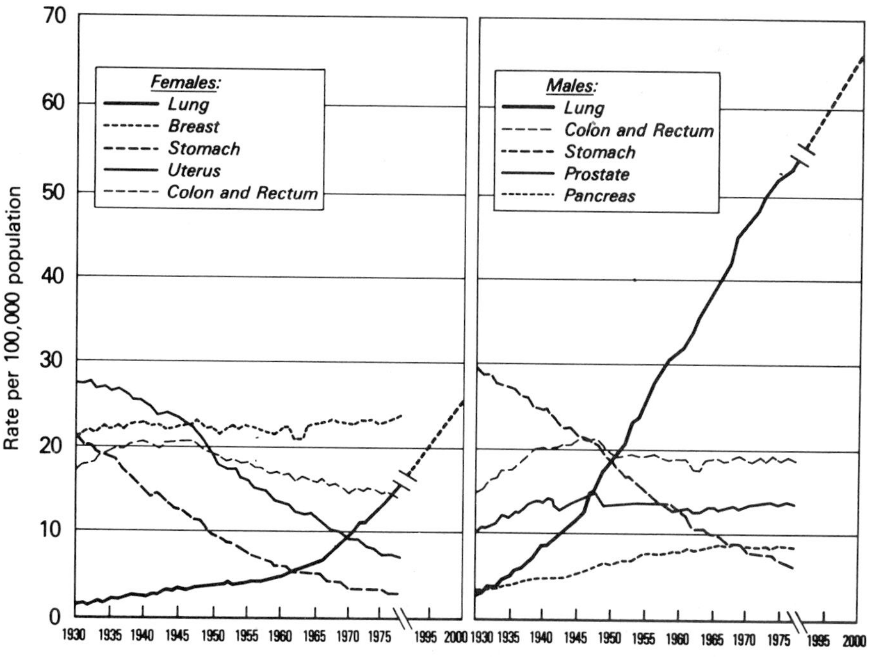

FIG. 14-1. Age-adjusted cancer death rates in the U.S. for lung cancer and other selected sites with theoretical projections for lung cancer mortality in the year 2,000. (The Cancer Bulletin 32 (3) 1980; Ca-A Cancer Journal for Clinicians 30 (1) 1980. Sources of data cited are the U.S. National Center for Health Statistics and the U.S. Bureau of the Census)

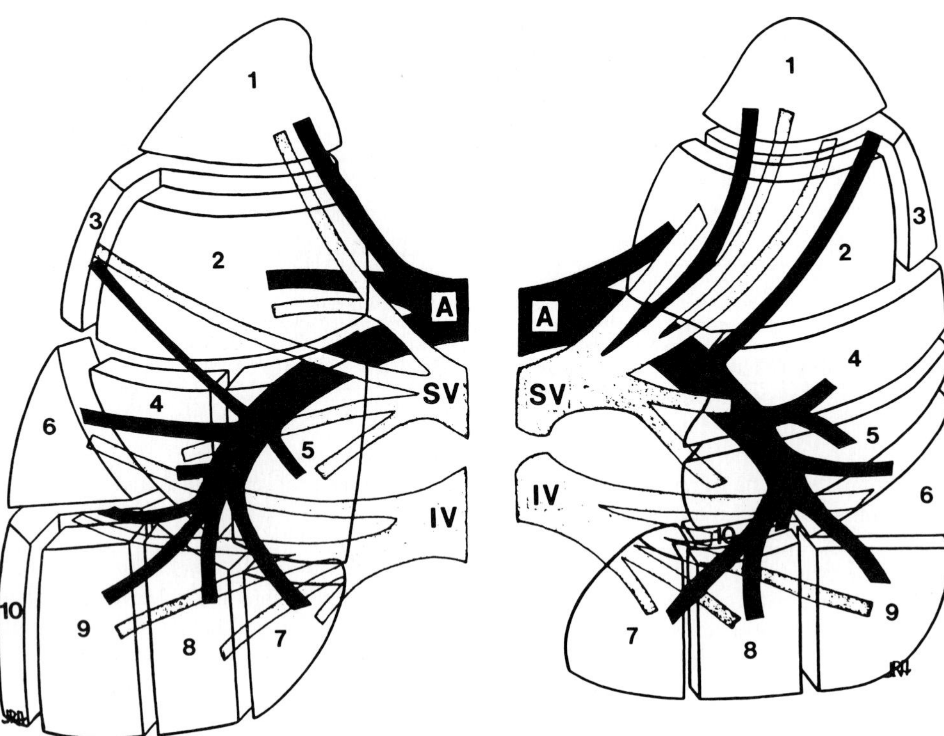

FIG. 14-2. Schematic diagram of the segmental and vascular anatomy of the lung. The anatomic distribution of the bronchopulmonary segments is numbered according to the Boyden scheme. (See text and Table 14-3 for description of bronchopulmonary segments.) *A*, pulmonary artery; *SV*, superior pulmonary veins; *IV*, inferior pulmonary veins. (Redrawn from Sweet RH: Surgical anatomy of the thorax. In Thoracic Surgery. Philadelphia, W B Saunders, 1950)

cancer recommended by the World Health Organization (WHO) in 1977 should be accepted as the definitive classification of this tumor for at least another decade (see Table 14-4).[25] Carcinomas arising from the bronchial or bronchioloalveolar surface epithelium and from the bronchial mucous glands make up 90–95% of lung cancers.[28] The four major cell types include squamous cell (or epidermoid) carcinoma, small cell (also called oat cell) carcinoma, adenocarcinoma, and large cell (also called large cell anaplastic) carcinoma (see Figs. 14-4 through 14-8). Approximately 2–4% of these tumors will be composed of a combination of squamous and glandular elements; thus, they are called adenosquamous cell carcinoma. These various cell types have different natural histories and responses to therapy. Therefore, correct histologic identification of the lung cancer cell type is a cornerstone of treatment planning. This is best accomplished by obtaining adequate amounts of tumor material for both tissue and cytologic evaluation. If discrepancies occur, it is important to

TABLE 14-3. Bronchopulmonary Segments

RIGHT LUNG		LEFT LUNG	
		Upper Lobe	
Jackson-Huber	Boyden	Jackson-Huber	Boyden
Apical	1	Apical-posterior	1–3
Anterior	2	Anterior	2
Posterior	3		
		Superior lingular	4
		Inferior lingular	5
		Middle Lobe	
Lateral	4		
Medial	5		
		Lower Lobe	
Superior	6	Superior	6
Medial basal	7	Anteriomedial	7–8
Anterior basal	8	Lateral basal	9
Lateral basal	9	Posterior basal	10
Posterior basal	10		

(Jackson CL, Huber JF: Correlated applied anatomy of bronchial tree and lungs with system nomenclature. Dis Chest 9:319–326, 1943; Boyden EA: Segmental anatomy of the lungs. New York, McGraw-Hill, 1955)

have the material reviewed by a pathologist experienced in the histologic typing of lung cancer.

Incidence of Types

Estimates of the incidence of the four major cell types depend on the source of pathologic materials reviewed (*e.g.*, by biopsy, cytology, surgical resection, or autopsy) (Table 14-5). For example, epidermoid carcinomas are more frequently identified in surgical resections while small cell carcinomas are more frequently identified in biopsy and cytologic materials. There appears to be a shift in incidence of the histologic types over the past 20 years, with a fall in the fraction of cases of epidermoid cancer and a rise in the percentage of adenocarcinomas.[28,34] This is partially because of the rise in the incidence of lung cancer in women who have more adenocarcinomas than epidermoid cancers.[3] However, an increase in adenocarcinomas is also seen in men.[34]

EMBRYOLOGY AND PATHOGENESIS

Embryologically, the laryngotracheobronchial tree is a ventral endodermal foregut derivative lined with five or more types of epithelial cells forming a pseudostratified mucosal sheath resting on a basement membrane.[35] Seen under electron microscopy are mucus-secreting goblet cells, ciliated cells, brush border cells, short basal, or reserve, cells, and granular basal cells which rest on the basement membrane, giving the mucosa a pseudostratified appearance. The granular basal cells are called Kulchitsky or K-type cells. They have "neurosecretory granules" with the capability of synthesizing polypeptide hormones or biogenic amines. Thus they are presumed to be the cell of origin of small cell carcinomas.[36]

As the embryonic lung diverticulum branches to form bronchopulmonary buds, splanchnic mesenchyme surrounds these structures and gives rise to the fibroelastic, vascular, muscular, and cartilaginous components of the lung, which form the visceral pleura. The parietal pleura is derived from the corresponding somatic mesenchyme.

TABLE 14-4. World Health Organization (WHO) Classification of Malignant Pleuro-Pulmonary Neoplasms

I. Epidermoid carcinoma
II. Small cell carcinoma
  1. Fusiform
  2. Polygonal
  3. Lymphocyte-like
  4. Others
III. Adenocarcinoma
  1. Bronchogenic (with or without mucin formation)
    a. Acinar
    b. Papillary
  2. Bronchioloalveolar
IV. Large cell carcinoma
  1. Solid tumor with mucin
  2. Solid tumor without mucin
  3. Giant cell
  4. Clear cell
V. Combined epidermoid and adenocarcinomas
VI. Carcinoid tumors
VII. Bronchial gland tumors
  1. Cylindromas
  2. Muco-epidermoid tumors
VIII. Papillary tumors of the surface epithelium
IX. "Mixed" tumors and carcinosarcomas
X. Sarcomas
XI. Unclassified
XII. Melanoma

(Kreyberg L: Histologic typing of lung tumors. In Kreyberg L (ed): International Histologic Classification of Tumors, No. 1, pp. 19–26. Geneva, World Health Organization, 1967)

(The Veterans Administration Lung Cancer Chemotherapy Study Group (VALG) and the Working Party for Therapy of Lung Cancer (WP-L) have developed similar schemes for the classification of malignant pleuro-pulmonary neoplasms but the authors' current recommendation is for use of the WHO scheme.[26,27])

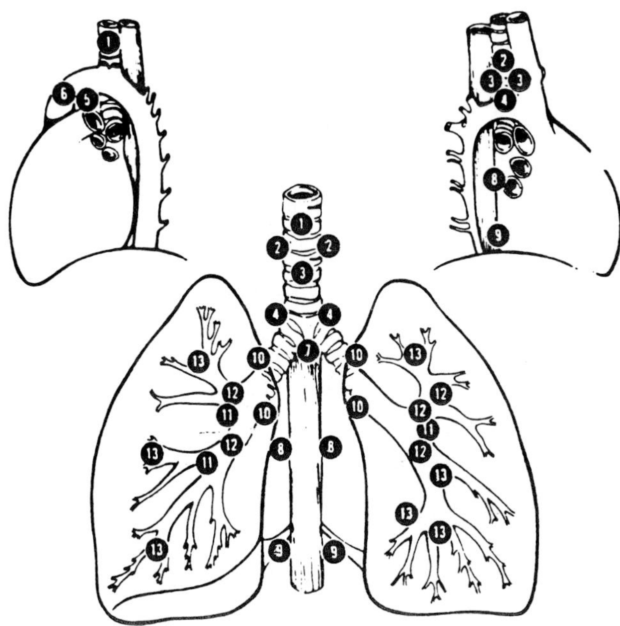

FIG. 14-3. Diagram of the regional lymph nodes of the lung and mediastinum. The lymph node nomenclature system has been adopted by the American Joint Committee (AJC) for Cancer Staging. Note that all single digit nodes are mediastinal. Nodal groups 1–4 = superior mediastinal nodes; 5–6 = aortic nodes; 7–9 = inferior mediastinal nodes. If involved with tumor, the nodes are scored *N2*. All double digit nodes (nodal groups 10–13) are hilar, peribronchial, or intrapulmonary; if these are involved with tumor, they are scored as *N1* by the AJC staging system. (Staging of Lung Cancer, 1979 Manual of the AJC for Cancer Staging and End-Results Reporting Task Force on Lung. Courtesy of N. Martini)

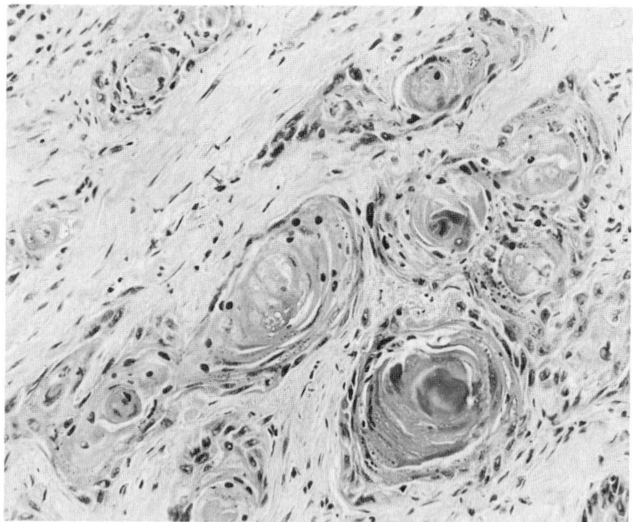

FIG. 14-4. Epidermoid (squamous) carcinoma of the lung. The key features illustrated here are cellular stratification and extracellular keratinization. Other features include intercellular bridges (desmosomes), which give the "prickle" appearance; intracellular keratinization, and atypical mitoses. In well-differentiated tumors (as illustrated here), nuclei are often pyknotic; in poorly differentiated tumors nuclei tend to be pleomorphic and enlarged. Original magnification × 95. (Courtesy of M. Matthews and A. Gazdar)

Lung cancer most commonly arises in segmental and subsegmental bronchi in response to repetitive injury and chronic inflammation.[28] At segmental bronchial bifurcations, bronchial epithelium is particularly susceptible to injury, and carcinogens may be deposited in these areas.[37] Initially, basal cells respond to injury by proliferating to generate mucin-secreting goblet cells. With added injury, the columnar cells are replaced by orderly, arranged, metaplastic, stratified squamous epithelium. Finally, the epithelium becomes disorganized and nuclear atypia and mitoses are seen in the basal half of the mucosa (findings which are called atypical metaplasia or dysplasia). When this process occurs throughout the full thickness of the mucosa, a diagnosis of carcinoma *in situ* (intraepithelial carcinoma) is made. Finally, the basement membrane is violated by the neoplastic cells; frank infiltration of neoplastic cells into the underlying stroma follows.[38–40] This process may take 10–20 years and represents the first

FIG. 14-5. Adenocarcinoma of the lung. The key histologic features of adenocarcinomas include the arrangement of cells in glands or acini, production of mucin, and enlarged cells with vesicular nuclei, prominent nucleoli, and abundant cytoplasm. Tumors that produce a significant amount of mucin but that do not form acini are accepted as poorly differentiated adenocarcinomas according to the 1977 WHO Lung Cancer Classification.[25] Original magnification × 300 (Courtesy of M. Matthews and A. Gazdar)

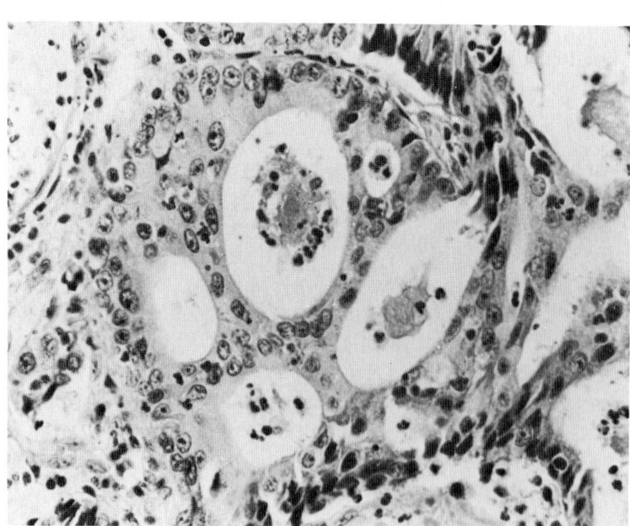

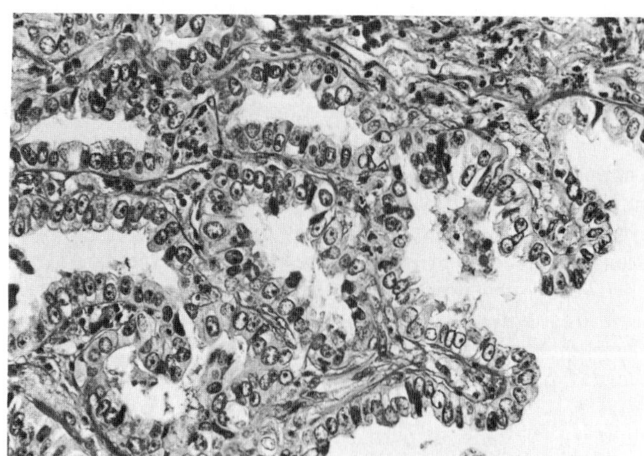

FIG. 14-6. Bronchioloalveolar cell carcinoma. The key histologic features of bronchioloalveolar carcinoma include alveolar septa lined by neoplastic columnar epithelial cells which invaginate to form intra–alveolar papillary processes supported by a fibrovascular stroma, in addition to rare mitoses and psammoma bodies in 5–15% of cases.[28] Original magnification × 120. (Courtesy of M. Matthews and A. Gazdar)

FIG. 14-7. Large cell carcinoma of the lung. The key histologic features here include large polygonal, spindle, or oval cells with abundant cytoplasm; large irregular pleomorphic nuclei with prominent nucleoli; and cells arranged in sheets, nests, or clusters. No evidence of maturation such as keratinization, 'prickle' cells, extracellular mucin, or acinar or gland formation is present. However, multinucleated giant cells, intracellular hyalin droplets, glycogen, and acidophilic nuclear inclusions may be present. A marked host response is present in the tumor shown here. Plasma cells and lymphocytes surround a sheet of tumor cells. Original magnification × 300 (Courtesy M. Matthews and A. Gazdar)

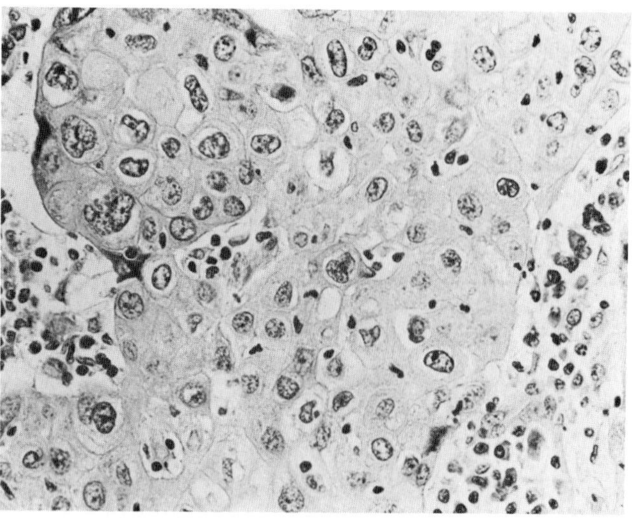

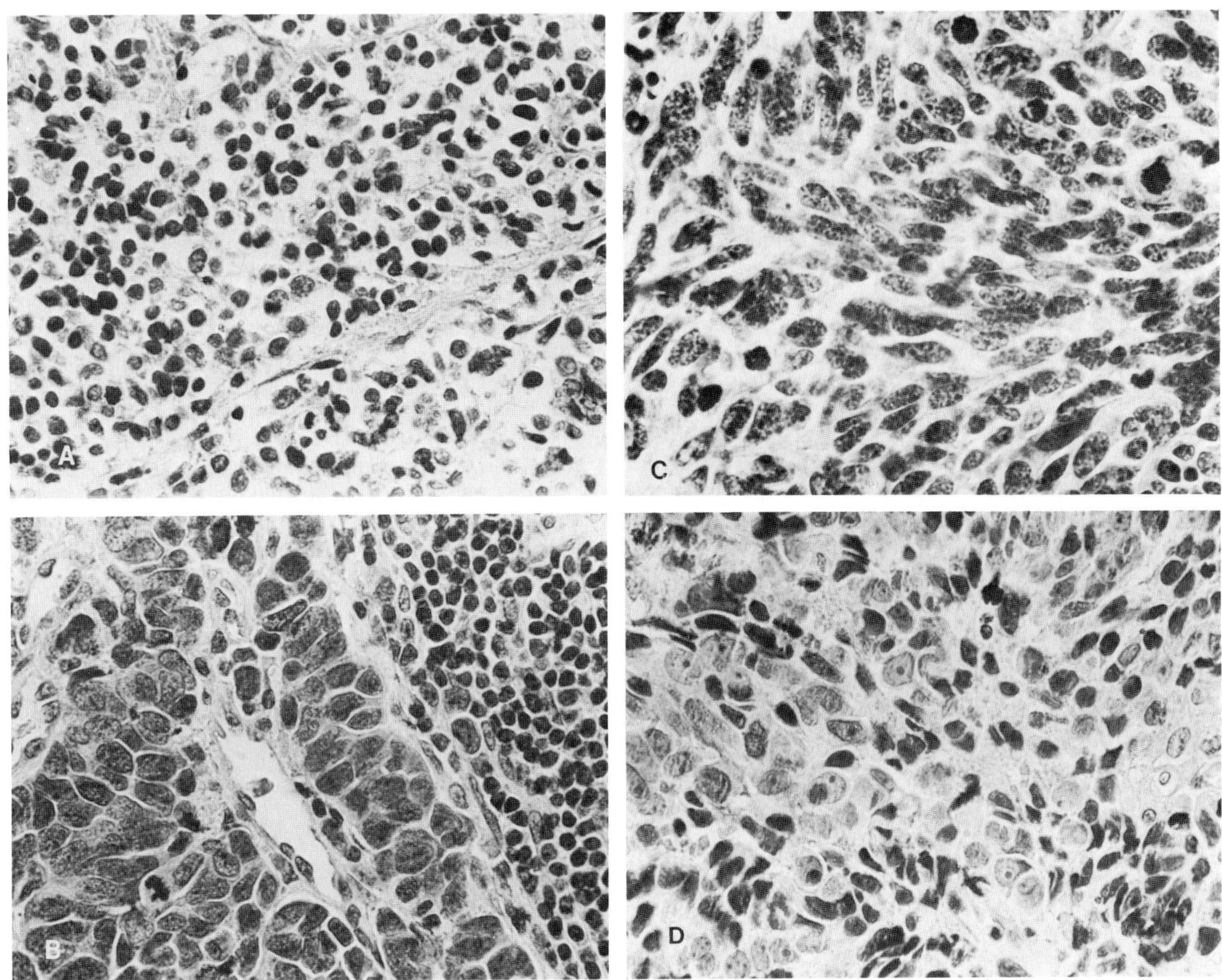

FIG. 14-8. Small cell carcinoma of the lung. *A*, lymphocyte-like type; *B*, polygonal type; *C*, fusiform type; *D*, mixed small-large cell carcinoma. In *A*, the nuclei are small and hyperchromatic, with little detail visible, and the cytoplasm is scant or not visible. In the intermediate types (*B* and *C*), the nuclei are larger, with characteristic salt and pepper distribution of the chromatin; the cytoplasm is also apparent. The key histologic features of all small cell carcinomas of the lung include the small cell being about two or three times the size of lymphocytes (see tumor cells in *B* compared to the surrounding lymphocytes), nuclear molding, necrotic areas, crush artifact, and depositions of basophilic granular DNA material on elastic fibrils. Cells are arranged in clusters, ribbons, trabeculae, or small nests with a thin vascular matrix. Host response in the form of inflammatory cells and desmoplastic reaction are seldom prominent. In *D*, cells having the characteristic features of small cell carcinoma are intermixed with larger, paler cells having large nuclei, prominent nucleoli, and distinct cytoplasmic borders. Original magnification × 300. (Courtesy M. Matthews and A. Gazdar)

TABLE 14-5. Incidence of the Major Histologic Types of Lung Cancer

HISTOLOGIC TYPE (*Number of Patients*)	BIOPSY-CYTOLOGY (*4,107*)	SURGICAL SPECIMENS (*1,206*)	AUTOPSY (*1,080*)	PRESENTING AT MAYO CLINIC (*2,926*)	JOHNS HOPKINS (1964–73) (*435*)
	% of Cases				
Epidermoid carcinoma	45	64	33	34	39
Adenocarcinoma	22	16	25	26	19
Large cell carcinoma	11	9	16	16	20
Small cell carcinoma	19	19	25	22	19
Other (*e.g.*, bronchoalveolar or mixed)	3	2	1	2	2
References	(26, 28–30)	(28, 31)	(28, 32)	(3)	(33)

phases of the natural history of lung cancer. The carcinogens implicated in this process include the constituents of tobacco smoke, radioisotopes, asbestos, polycyclic aromatic hydrocarbons, haloethers, nickel, chromium, inorganic arsenic, iron ore, printing inks, and other possible occupational and atmospheric pollutants.[41]

The above process appears to particularly relate to epidermoid carcinoma. A similar chain of events is seen in uranium miners who smoke. Here, a transition of the granular basal cells (K-type cells) to small cell carcinomas is evident.[42] The site of origin of small cell cancer is usually difficult to identify. These tumors infiltrate the submucosa while squamous metaplasia or dysplasia is seen in the overlying bronchial mucosa.

In most cases, it is also difficult to identify the site of origin of adenocarcinomas or large cell carcinomas in bronchial surface epithelium or underlying mucous glands. In contrast to epidermoid and small cell carcinomas, adenocarcinomas and large cell tumors are often peripheral in origin, associated with pulmonary conditions that cause lung destruction, fibrosis, reconstruction of the pulmonary airways into nonfunctional spaces, and hyperplasia of pneumocytes. Chronic interstitial lung diseases (*i.e.*, scleroderma, rheumatoid lung disease, sarcoidosis, interstitial pneumonitis, pulmonary scars and fibrosis from pulmonary infarcts, tuberculosis, chronic lung abscesses and other necrotizing pulmonary diseases) have been noted as predisposing factors.[43–47] With progressive pulmonary fibrosis, avascularity, local tissue anoxia, and proliferation of the bronchioloalveolar epithelium are stimulated, resulting in adenomatous foci that frequently become metaplastic and mucus-producing.[28] Exogenous agents involved in these processes include asbestos, cadmium, beryllium, chemical gases, mineral oils, viruses, mycobacteria, and pneumoconiotic dusts.[41]

Epidermoid Carcinoma

Epidermoid tumors (Fig. 14-4) grow centrally toward the main stem bronchus, and locally invade underlying bronchial cartilage, adjoining lung parenchyma, and lymph nodes. The bronchial mucosa usually shows evidence of squamous metaplasia, dysplasia, or frank intra-epithelial neoplasia, processes that provide evidence for the primary nature of the tumor in the lung.[28]

Adenocarcinoma

The majority of adenocarcinomas (Fig. 14-5) are peripheral in location, unrelated to bronchi, except by contiguous growth or lymph node metastases. The tumors provoke a desmoplastic response, present as firm, localized, subpleural masses, and tend to invade the overlying pleura. Tumors arising from the bronchial epithelium present as thick, firm, gray-white, pipe-stemmed structures with narrowed lumina. It may be difficult to distinguish the tumors in the lung from cancer of the pancreas, kidney, breast, or colon that metastasize to bronchi.[28] Adenocarcinomas arising from bronchial mucous glands form lobules of neoplastic glands that may be mucin-producing or exhibit a cribriform pattern.

Bronchioloalveolar Carcinoma

Bronchioloalveolar carcinoma (Fig. 14-6) presents either as single nodules or in a multinodular pattern. The multinodular presentation has led to the suspicion of multiple primaries.[48–52] Papillary configurations may be seen in adenocarcinomas arising from bronchial surface epithelium, those tumors associated with scars, as well the classic bronchioloalveolar carcinoma. Psammoma bodies are noted in 5–15% of papillary tumors. Bronchioloalveolar cancer in the lung may be indistinguishable from metastases to the lung from other adenocarcinomas such as the kidney, ovary, thyroid, uterus, or colon. Ultrastructural studies suggest that the cell of origin is the bronchiolar lining cell, with subcellular features of the Clara and ciliated epithelial cells.[53] Some of these tumors have osmiophilic lamellar bodies and demonstrate surfactant production, relating it to the type II pneumocyte. The tumor is similar to the viral-induced Jaagsiekte disease of sheep.[48] Mice, horses, and guinea pigs have similar disease as well.

Bronchioloalveolar carcinoma is usually reported to be associated with prior lung disease leading to fibrosis, including repeated pneumonias, idiopathic pulmonary fibrosis, granulomatas, inflammation, asbestosis, fibrosing alveolitis, scleroderma, and Hodgkin's disease.[50,54–56] However, in isolated reports no antecedent lung damage has been found. It is also found in families with other tumors, and has been seen in identical twins.[57,58] Interestingly, bronchioloalveolar carcinoma is not correlated with smoking.[52] Because of its association with fibrosing lung disease, any new roentgenographic mass or persistent infiltrate in such patients should be suspect for bronchioloalveolar carcinoma.[51]

Large Cell Carcinoma

Large cell carcinomas (Fig. 14-7) grossly present as peripheral, subpleural, large lesions with necrotic or cavitary surfaces. These tumors are also usually unrelated to bronchi except by contiguous growth, and they have a tendency to invade pulmonary parenchyma and the overlying pleura. In small foci, recognizable attempts at differentiation, usually glandular, may be identified, but the predominant anaplastic nature of the tumor is overwhelming. Microscopically, they are a composite of all the anaplastic features of poorly differentiated squamous and adenocarcinomas. A subtype of large cell carcinoma, giant cell carcinoma, is composed of bizarre cells with giant nuclei and very large quantities of cytoplasm, which often show phagocytic activity or contain mucin vacuoles. Approximately 30% of lung cancers (105 out of 348) have areas of clear cell changes. Over two-thirds of large cell carcinomas may show these changes and almost a third of adenocarcinomas and epidermoid carcinomas will also show these features.[59] The clear cells stain strongly for glycogen but weakly for mucin. However, it is very rare to find a tumor composed solely of clear cells. The prognosis of tumors containing large areas of clear cells is not different from the reported results for the other common lung cancer histologic types, however; the importance of recognizing the clear cell type of primary lung cancer is to differentiate it from metastatic renal carcinoma.[59]

Small Cell Carcinoma

Small cell carcinoma (Fig. 14-8) appears as submucosal infiltrates in the early phase of the disease. The mucosa may be normal or be slightly lifted by a plaque that obliterates normal bronchial markings. In advanced stages, bronchial lumina may be obstructed by extrinsic compression or endobronchial tumor.[28,60] Silver stains are negative, and neurosecretory granules are usually found in electron micrographic studies.[28] The classic oat cell or lymphocyte-type tumor is composed of cells with small, round, oval, or spindled, darkly staining nuclei and scant indistinct cytoplasm. The intermediate subtype of small cell carcinoma has cells with more fusiform or polygonal nuclei and the cytoplasm is often more distinct. Numerous atypical mitoses may be identified. Some tumors form distinct tubules as well as rosettes. Mixtures of lymphocyte-like and intermediate subtypes of small cell cancer are frequently seen in a single tumor. In some small cell tumors, prominent clusters of anaplastic large cells may be seen; in others, nests of squamous cells may be seen. Presently, it is unclear whether there are any clinical differences between the different subtypes of small cell carcinoma. However, the histologic distinction between small cell and non-small cell cancers is of great clinical importance. For example, the fusiform variety of small cell cancer may be confused with poorly differentiated epidermoid carcinoma; the polygonal form, with large cell cancer; while the rosette or tubular pattern may be confused with adenocarcinoma, particularly in metastatic sites.

Despite their submucosal location, small cell carcinomas often have malignant cells exfoliated into sputa and cytologic washings. Bronchoscopy yields malignant cytology in over 90% of clinically apparent disease.[60] Cytologic diagnosis appears as accurate as tissue diagnosis.[26] Other features of clinico-pathologic interest in small cell cancer include the presence of marked osteoblastic activity in 25% of patients with bony metastases, with new bone formation similar to prostate and breast cancer bony metastases; pancreatic involvement from peripancreatic nodal disease, associated focal acute pancreatitis, and possibly severe fat necrosis; and a significant number of metastases to endocrine organs (i.e., thyroid in 8%, pituitary in 15%, testes in 7%, and parathyroid in 1%).[4,28,41–43,60–62]

CLINICOPATHOLOGIC CORRELATION WITH HISTOLOGIC TYPE

Differences in long-term survival dependent on the histologic type of lung cancer have been analyzed in a large number of patients (see Table 14-6). In most instances, these patients have been treated with local modalities of therapy (*i.e.*, surgery and radiotherapy). (The figures for small cell lung cancer will probably be changing with the advent of intensive combination chemotherapy.) At present, epidermoid cancers have the best survival, followed by adenocarcinoma and large cell carcinoma. Until recently, small cell carcinoma has had only rare patients surviving for 5 years.

Epidermoid cancer is more common in males; adenocarcinoma is more common in females. An equal sex distribution exists for the other cell types (see Table 14-7). On the whole, females have a better survival than males independent of the stage of cancer.[64] Epidermoid and small cell cancers have a much higher incidence in smokers compared to non-smokers, while adenocarcinoma is the predominant type in non-smokers (see Table 14-7). This may be accounted for in part by the inclusion of adenocarcinomas of "unknown primary" with metastases to the lung in the non-smoker group. In any event,

TABLE 14-6. Overall 5-Year Survival Percentage for the Major Histologic Types of Lung Cancer

HISTOLOGIC TYPE	ALL CASES (N = 2,155)	RESECTED (N = 835)	
	5-Year Survival Percentage		Percentage Resectable
Epidermoid carcinoma	25	37	60
Adenocarcinoma	12	27	38*
Large cell carcinoma	13	27	38*
Small cell carcinoma	1	0	11

(Matthews MJ, Gordon PR: Morphology of pulmonary and pleural malignancies. In Straus MJ (ed): Lung Cancer Clinical Diagnosis and Treatment. New York, Grune and Stratton, 1977; Mountain CF, Carr DT, Martini N et al: Staging of lung cancer 1979. American Joint Committee for Cancer Staging and End Results Reporting. Chicago, Task Force on Lung Cancer, 1980)
*Combined in AJC report.

TABLE 14-7. Incidence by Sex and Smoking Status of Major Histologic Types of Lung Cancer at the Mayo Clinic

HISTOLOGIC TYPE (*Numbers of Patients*)	MALE (*2,411*)	FEMALE (*515*)	SMOKERS (*2,708*)	NEVER SMOKED (*218*)
	% of Cases			
Epidermoid carcinoma	37	18	36	9
Adenocarcinoma	22	44	23	64
Large cell carcinoma	17	12	16	14
Small cell carcinoma	22	20	23	3
Bronchioloalveolar	2	6	2	9

(Rosenow EC III, Carr DT: Bronchogenic carcinoma. CA 29:233–246, 1979)

it is clearly important in women with a lung adenocarcinoma to rule out a primary breast or gynecologic tumor that would need different therapy than a primary lung cancer. The location of the primary tumors (see Table 14-8) will determine the presenting signs and symptoms and dictate the methods for obtaining a histologic diagnosis in symptomatic patients and screening studies. Proximal tumors usually have histologic material obtained by bronchoscopy or sputum cytology, while distal lesions are usually detected on screening chest films and are thus diagnosed by transbronchial, percutaneous needle, open biopsy, or at time of resection.

In surgically resected specimens, small cell cancer involves lymph nodes in the great majority of cases, while the non-small cell cancers have lymph nodes involved in approximately 40% of cases (see Table 14-8). Epidermoid carcinomas (28%) and large cell carcinomas (22%) cavitate more frequently than adenocarcinoma (12%) or small cell carcinoma (8%).[65] In contrast, adenocarcinomas and large cell carcinomas show visceral pleural invasion more frequently than other types of surgically resected tumors because of their peripheral location.

The clinicopathologic correlation of therapeutic importance for bronchioloalveolar carcinoma relates to the number of nodules and the degree of differentiation. Lymph node metastases occur in 23% of patients with solitary nodules, but in more than 77% of patients with multicentric lesions.[66] A majority of patients with solitary nodules (84%) have well-differentiated tumors. In contrast, only 45% of multicentric tumors are scored as well-differentiated. Some 80% of poorly differentiated tumors have lymph node metastases, while only 20–30% of the more highly differentiated tumors show this spread.[66]

ACCURACY OF HISTOLOGIC DIAGNOSIS

The first principle of treatment is a correct histologic diagnosis. Central to a good histologic diagnosis are the quality and quantity of the histologic samples. Common problems for the clinical pathologist are crush artifact, poor fixation, overstaining, or inadequate amounts of material. A diagnosis of malignancy may also be based on a cytologic sample, and differentiated malignancies and small cell carcinomas may be diagnosed as readily and as accurately in cytologic specimens as in small biopsies.[67,68] However, a histologic (tissue block) diagnosis is preferred. A major problem in the use of histologic criteria when determining prognosis and types of treatment is the degree of inter- and intra-observer variability in reading the same specimens. In addition, there is heterogeneity within the tumor itself in both the primary and metastatic sites.[26,31,65,69,70] Tumors will often show features of several histologic subtypes, suggesting a morphologic continuum. This is a particular problem with small cell carcinoma.[71,72] Some series have reported imperfect correlations between cytologic and subsequent histologic cell type, and misleading results may be obtained from biopsy of cavitation lesions and necrotic tumors.[73] The distinction between small cell carcinoma and the non-small cell types is consistent in 80%–90% of cases when material is reviewed by well-trained observers experienced in lung cancer pathology.[65] The assignment of tumors to each of the other major types also appears to be correct in some 90% of cases.[65] In contrast, attempts to subdivide the major types are presently subject to a large degree of inter-observer variation.[70,74] This problem is particularly marked in the diagnosis of specimens with combinations of small cell carcinoma mixed with the other major histologic types, especially large cell carcinoma.[70] It may be necessary to get the opinion of several pathologists until biochemical or immunologic markers of small cell cancer are available. If several pathologists agree that a definite small cell component exists, the patient should probably be considered to have small cell carcinoma. At present, the authors feel the only treatment-related decisions that should be based on histologic type are between small cell cancer and the other "non-small cell" types, and possibly identification of well-differentiated epidermoid lesions (which often appear amenable to aggressive local therapy).

THE DEGREE OF TUMOR DIFFERENTIATION OR SUBTYPE

Despite scoring reliability problems, the role of the degree of histologic differentiation of the primary tumor on tumor survival and biology is being investigated. Small cell carcinoma

TABLE 14-8. Anatomic Location of Primary Tumors Related to Histologic Type of Lung Cancer and Frequency of Early Regional Spread of Disease

HISTOLOGIC TYPE	PROXIMAL LOCATION		RESECTED SURGICAL SPECIMEN: LYMPH NODE INVOLVEMENT		RESECTED SURGICAL SPECIMEN: VISCERAL PLEURAL INVOLVEMENT	
	*(N)**	%	*(N)*	%	*(N)*	%
Epidermoid Carcinoma	(275)	81	(158)	42	(109)	33
Adenocarcinoma	(140)	29	(109)	41	(59)	59
Large Cell Carcinoma	(113)	49	(65)	42	(27)	52
Small Cell Carcinoma	(96)	83	(29)	72	(13)	15
Overall	(641)	63	(631)	48	(211)	41

(Vincent RG, Pickren JW, Lane WW et al: The changing histopathology of lung cancer: A review of 1682 cases. Cancer 39:1647–1655, 1977; Rilke F, Carbone A, Clemente C et al: Surgical pathology of resectable lung cancer. Prog Cancer Ther Res Ther 11:129–142, 1979)

*Numbers (*N*) of patients in each group noted in parentheses.

(often called "small cell anaplastic" carcinoma) and large cell carcinoma (often called large cell "undifferentiated" carcinoma) have traditionally been regarded as "undifferentiated" tumors, although as more is learned about the cellular biology of lung cancer these concepts may change. Epidermoid and adenocarcinoma have been subdivided into groups exhibiting different degrees of histologic differentiation in the WHO classification. Squamous tumors present with about equal frequency as well, moderately, or poorly differentiated lesions while adenocarcinomas more frequently present as poorly differentiated lesions.[65] At present, there appears to be a 5-year survival advantage for well and moderately differentiated epidermoid carcinomas (20–39%) compared to poorly differentiated lesions. There is no difference between well and moderately differentiated (23%) and poorly differentiated (26%) adenocarcinomas.[33,74] This may be explained in part by the more frequent occurrence of lymph node metastases and increased tumor stage for the more poorly differentiated epidermoid lesions.[76]

In early studies of small cell carcinoma subtyping, conflicting results were obtained suggesting that one type or another may have a different prognosis. However, in three recent studies, large numbers of patients were extensively evaluated before therapy, then treated with intensive combination chemotherapy (or chemotherapy and radiotherapy) and no difference was seen between subtypes with respect to stage of disease, sites of metastases, response to therapy or number of complete responses, response duration, or survival.[71,72,77] When histologic subtypes in the primary biopsy were compared with the subtype of other pathologic specimens in the same patient, concordance of the subtypes was present in only 71% while two or three histologic subtypes were present in the remaining 29%.[77] Whether there are biochemical or antigenic correlates of small cell carcinoma histologic subtypes remains to be determined. At present, there appears to be no reason to base treatment decisions, or protocol stratification, on histologic subtype with one possible exception. The one histologic subtype of small cell lung cancer with a different prognosis is the mixed small cell-large cell carcinoma variant that occurs in approximately 6% of small cell lung cancer cases.[78] This type has a lower overall response to combination chemotherapy, a lower complete response rate, and a shorter median survival[78] compared to small cell carcinoma without large cell components. Cell biologic and autopsy studies indicate that a transition can occur between small cell carcinoma and large cell carcinoma accompanied by a switch in the expression of differentiated functions by the cells.[79,80,81] The cells with small cell carcinoma histology express the amine precursor uptake and decarboxylation (APUD) properties of high levels of dopa decarboxylase (L-aromatic amino-decarboxylase), formaldehyde-induced fluorescence after exposure to 5-hydroxytryptophan, and neurosecretory granules, while the large cell variants do not.[81] Autopsy studies at Johns Hopkins and the National Cancer Institute (NCI) conducted on 131 small cell carcinoma patients after intensive chemotherapy (or chemoradiotherapy) showed 27% of the patients had small cell carcinoma mixed with a giant cell, squamous cell, tubular, or carcinoid component; 4% had pure squamous cell carcinoma without small cell; 3% had pure large cell; and 1% had pure adenocarcinoma.[79,80] Thus, in a very large percentage of cases, other histologic types of lung cancer are found at autopsy. While some cases probably reflect separate primaries, the possible transition from one type of lung cancer to another must also be considered, a feature that must be resolved by chromosomal analysis.

NEWER METHODS OF PATHOLOGIC DIAGNOSIS

New approaches to the identification of malignant cells, particularly in sputum and bronchial washings, as part of screening studies are being explored. One approach is to develop antibodies reactive for lung cancer but not for normal respiratory epithelium, or, antibodies reactive for products produced by lung cancer cells, but not normally introduced into bronchial washings. Antisera against lung cancer antigens that react with antigens of apparent endodermal and neural crest derivation have been described.[82] Recently, monoclonal antibodies with specificity for lung cancer cells have been prepared.[75] Another approach involves identifying cells with increased DNA content, a condition frequently seen in malignant cells.[83] There appears to be a progressive increase in the amount of DNA per cell in squamous metaplastic cells or neoplastic cells exhibiting progressive amounts of atypia.[84] Combining DNA staining with new cell sorting instruments will allow for the screening of large numbers of cells ($10^{5/8}$–$10^{3/4}$) by flow cytometry in individual sputum samples.[85] Using flow cytometry, 90% of small cell and 100% of non-small cell cancer samples were aneuploid; DNA contents in primary and metastatic sites were similar.[85]

NATURAL HISTORY OF LUNG CANCER

Understanding the natural history of lung cancer is important for prevention, early detection (especially of patients with small tumor burdens), rationally planned initial curative and palliative therapy, anticipation of possible complications, and the institution of therapy at the time of relapse. The natural history of lung cancer begins with the exposure of a susceptible host to carcinogens, which eventually lead to the cytologic changes of cellular atypia seen in cells exfoliated into the sputum. These changes progress to carcinoma *in situ*, then to frank invasion. Accurate definition of these early events is important when planning preventive therapy in future trials, and for instituting surgery, radiotherapy, or chemotherapy in the asymptomatic patient with clinically occult disease. Information on early natural history will mostly come from the mass screening program data described later in this chapter.

SIGNS AND SYMPTOMS OF LUNG CANCER

With the onset of local tumor growth and invasion, lung cancer can give rise to signs and symptoms as well as chest radiograph or sputum cytology abnormalities (see Table 14-9). Findings may rise from local tumor growth, invasion of adjacent structures, regional growth (from metastasis to peribronchial, hilar, mediastinal, and supraclavicular nodes) by way of lymphatic spread, growth in distant metastatic sites from hematogenous dissemination, or result from a remote

TABLE 14-9. Common Signs and Symptoms of Lung Cancer

SYMPTOMS SECONDARY TO CENTRAL OR ENDOBRONCHIAL GROWTH OF THE PRIMARY TUMOR
- Cough
- Hemoptysis
- Wheeze and stridor
- Dyspnea from obstruction
- Pneumonitis from obstruction (fever, productive cough)

SYMPTOMS SECONDARY TO PERIPHERAL GROWTH OF THE PRIMARY TUMOR
- Pain from pleural or chest wall involvement
- Cough
- Dyspnea on a restrictive basis
- Lung abscess syndrome from tumor cavitation

SYMPTOMS RELATED TO REGIONAL SPREAD OF THE TUMOR IN THE THORAX BY CONTIGUITY OR BY METASTASIS TO REGIONAL LYMPH NODES
- Tracheal obstruction
- Esophageal compression with dysphagia
- Recurrent laryngeal nerve paralysis with hoarseness
- Phrenic nerve paralysis with hemidiaphragm elevation and dyspnea
- Sympathetic nerve paralysis with Horner's syndrome
- Eighth cervical and first thoracic nerves with ulnar pain and Pancoast's syndrome
- Superior vena cava syndrome from vascular obstruction
- Pericardial and cardiac extension with resultant tamponade, arrhythmia, or cardiac failure
- Lymphatic obstruction with pleural effusion
- Lymphangitic spread through lungs with hypoxemia and dyspnea

(Cohen MH: Signs and Symptoms of Bronchogenic Carcinoma. In Straus MJ (ed): Lung Cancer Clinical Diagnosis and Treatment, pp. 85–94. New York, Grune and Stratton, 1977)

effect of the tumor (paraneoplastic syndromes). Unfortunately, by the time a sign, symptom, or visible nodule appears on a chest roentgenograph, dissemination to regional or distant lymph nodes or distant metastatic sites has occurred in most patients. This is expressly seen at autopsy when the patient died shortly after a supposedly curative resection for lung cancer for reasons other than tumor (see Table 14-10). All histologic types of lung cancer in the autopsies examined had examples of microscopic residual disease; frequently these sites were outside the areas where postoperative chest radiotherapy would have been directed. Small cell carcinoma in particular has a high frequency of extra-thoracic metastases, followed by adenocarcinoma, and then the other non-small cell types. Often, these metastases were intra-abdominal.[88] Other data demonstrating the early metastatic nature of lung cancer come from analysis of surgical resection specimens. In non-small cell carcinoma, the approximate frequency of lymph node involvement in such specimens is 40%, invasion of veins occurs in 19%, invasion of arteries in 18%, and invasion of visceral pleura in 44% (see Table 14-8).[65]

Excluding the mass screening programs, most patients present with symptomatic disease. Feinstein found in 678 Yale New Haven Hospital and Yale Veterans Administration patients that 6% were asymptomatic, 27% had symptoms related to the primary tumor, 32% had symptoms of metastatic disease, and 34% had systemic symptoms suggesting tumor, such as anorexia, weight loss, and fatigue.[5] There was a significant difference in 5-year survival rate with 18% of asymptomatic, 12% of primary symptomatic, 6% of systemic symptomatic, and 0% of patients with metastatic symptoms surviving 5 years.[5] Patients with a long history of symptoms related to their primary tumor had a better 5-year survival (16%) compared to those with a short duration of symptoms (9%), suggesting that some tumors may have an inherently more indolent course and, in turn, this may be related to their rate of growth. Of great interest was the correlation of symptomatic stage with anatomic stage. Here there was an effect of symptoms independent of anatomic stage. Thus, the accurate determination of signs and symptoms can be of prognostic value as well and should be correlated with clinical and surgical–pathologic evidence of disease in planning treatment and determining prognosis for individual patients.

The frequency of the various presenting signs and symptoms will vary, depending on whether the series examined represents all patients presenting with lung cancer or the subpopulations selected for more limited disease, advanced disease, or those selected from mass screening series. Recently, a large series of patients undergoing radical radiotherapy for cure contained a high incidence of asymptomatic patients discovered on routine chest films and a lower percentage of patients with symptoms of regional spread, or systemic symptoms, compared to the Yale study (see Table 14-11).[89]

Signs, symptoms, and radiographic findings in the chest are related to the central or peripheral location of the primary

TABLE 14-10. Incidence at Autopsy of Persistent Tumor After "Curative" Surgical Therapy for Lung Cancer in Patients Dying of Other Causes Within a 30-Day Postoperative Period

		PERCENTAGE WITH PERSISTENT TUMOR		
CELL TYPE	NUMBER OF PATIENTS	TOTAL	LOCAL DISEASE ONLY	DISTANT METASTASES
Epidermoid carcinoma	131	34	17	17
Adenocarcinoma	30	43	3	40
Large cell carcinoma	22	14	0	14
Small cell carcinoma	19	69	6	63

(Matthews MJ, Kanhouwa S, Pickner J et al: Frequency of residual and metastatic tumors in patients undergoing curative surgical resection of lung cancer. Cancer Chemother Rep 3:63–67, 1973)

tumor, in addition to whether or not regional spread has occurred, both of which are related to the histologic type (see Table 14-12 and Figs. 14-9–14-14). In general, epidermoid cancers have a central location, atelectasis, pneumonitis (from bronchial obstruction), hilar adenopathy, and a tendency to cavitate; adenocarcinomas have a defined nodule in a peripheral location with pleural and chest wall involvement; large cell carcinomas have a large mass in a peripheral location with pneumonitis and hilar adenopathy; and small cell carcinomas present as a central lesion with atelectasis-pneumonitis, and hilar and mediastinal adenopathy.

Symptoms of centrally located tumors are cough, wheezing, stridor, deep chest pain, hemoptysis, and dyspnea due to obstruction, with or without postobstructive pneumonitis. Peripheral lesions present with pain and cough from pleural or chest wall involvement, or pleural effusion, and dyspnea on a restrictive basis.[86] Occasionally, large tumor masses, usually of epidermoid or large cell histology, will cavitate and present as lung abscesses.

When a tumor (usually epidermoid carcinoma) presents in the apex of the lung and grows by local extension to involve the eighth cervical and first thoracic nerves, the *Pancoast or superior sulcus tumor syndrome* results.[90–93] The syndrome characteristically has shoulder pain, which radiates in the ulnar nerve distribution of the arm. With sympathetic nerve involvement from paravertebral tumor extension, a Horner's syndrome of enophthalmus, ptosis, meiosis, and ipsilateral loss of ability to sweat develops. It is important to realize that with early involvement, mydriasis (pupillary dilation of the affected side) may result. Radiologic destruction of the first and second rib is often seen as well.

TABLE 14-11. Manner of Presentation of Lung Cancer Patients Referred for Treatment with Radical Radiotherapy

SYMPTOM OR FINDING	PERCENTAGE OF PATIENTS (N = 170)
Routine Chest Radiograph (Asymptomatic)	16
PRIMARY TUMOR (TOTAL)	81
Hemoptysis	30
Cough	25
Dyspnea	11
Pneumonitis	8
Pain	6
Wheeze	2
REGIONAL SPREAD (TOTAL)	2
Dysphagia	1
Hoarseness	0.5
SYSTEMIC SYMPTOMS	
Weight loss	0.5

(Coy P, Kennelly GM: The role of curative radiotherapy in the treatment of lung cancer. Cancer 45:698–702, 1980)

Intrathoracic spread of lung cancer, either by direct extension or by lymphatic metastases, produces regional disease symptoms in the thorax. Nerve entrapment can lead to recurrent laryngeal nerve paralysis and hoarseness. Because of the longer intrathoracic course, it is more common to have hoarseness from involvement of the left than the right recurrent laryngeal nerve. Involvement of the phrenic nerve can lead to paralysis and elevation of the hemidiaphragm with resulting dyspnea. Compression of the esophagus by the

TABLE 14-12. Presenting Chest Roentgenologic Findings in Lung Cancer by T, N, and M Factor

ROENTGEN RAY FINDING	PERCENTAGE OF PATIENTS WITH FINDING			
	EPIDERMOID CARCINOMA	SMALL CELL CARCINOMA	ADENO-CARCINOMA	LARGE CELL CARCINOMA
(Number of patients)	(N = 338–585)	(N = 114–252)	(N = 135–301)	(N = 97)
TUMOR (T) FACTOR				
Nodule less than 4 cm	14	21	46	18
Nodule greater than 4 cm	18	8	26	41
Peripheral location	29	26	65	61
Central location	64	74	5	42
Atelectasis	23	31	2	14
Pneumonitis	13	21	14	24
Cavitation	5	0	3	4
Pleural or chest wall	3	5	14	2
LYMPH NODE (N) FACTOR				
Hilar adenopathy	38	61	19	32
Mediastinal adenopathy	5	14	9	10

(Cohen MH: Signs and Symptoms of Bronchogenic Carcinoma. In Straus MJ (ed): Lung Cancer Clinical Diagnosis and Treatment, pp. 85–94. New York, Grune and Stratton, 1977; Byrd RB, Carr DT, Miller WE et al: Radiographic abnormalities in carcinoma of the lung as related to histologic cell type. Thorax 24:573–575, 1969; Green N, Kurohara SS, George FW III et al: The biologic behavior of lung cancer according to histologic type. Radiol Clin Biol 41:160–170, 1972)

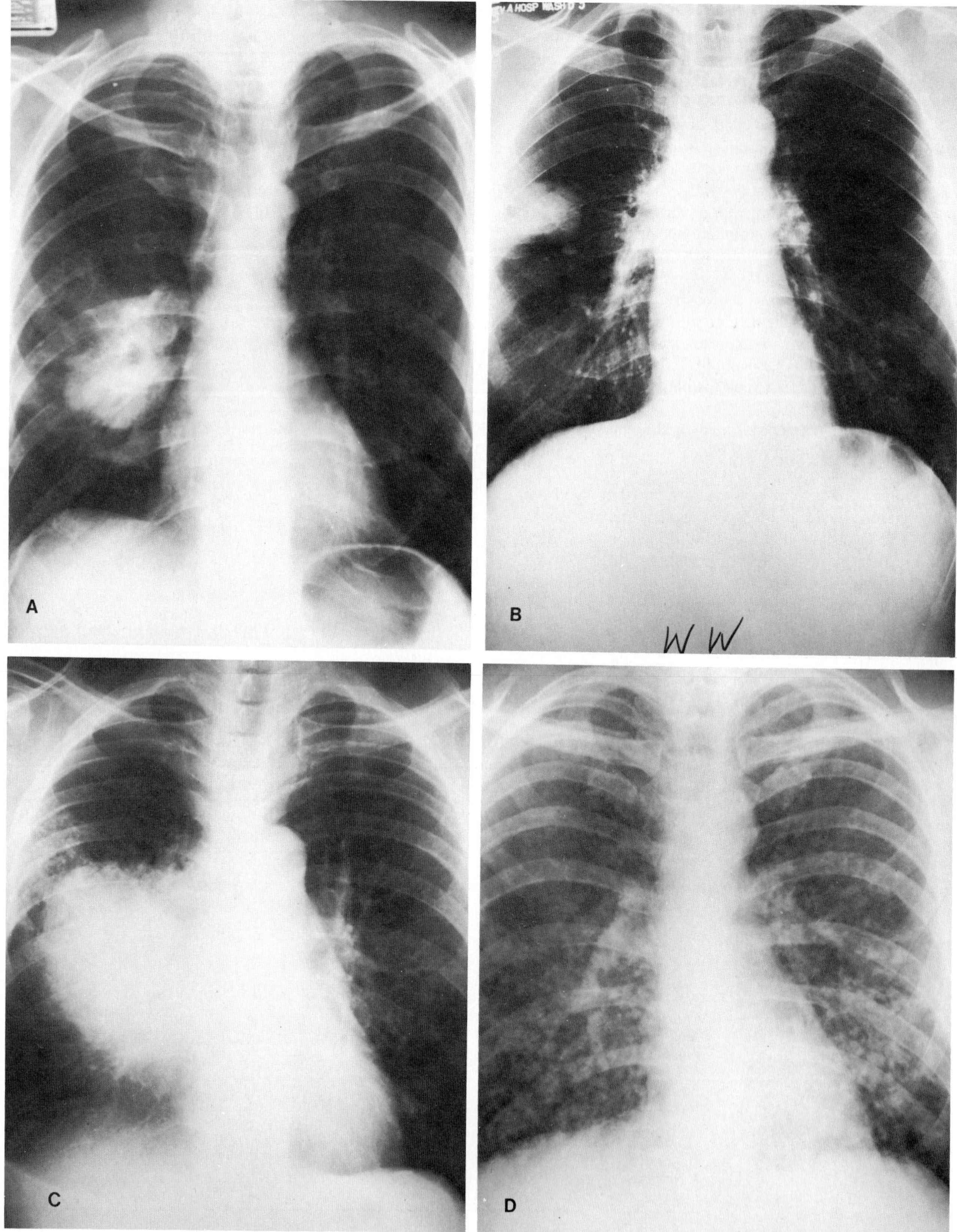
A
B
C
D

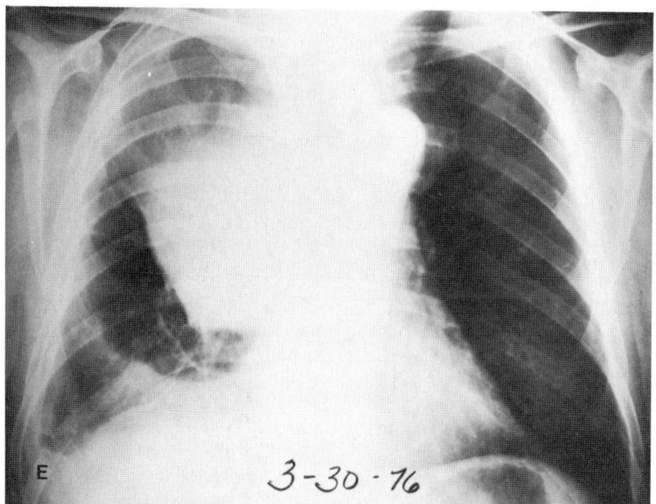

FIG. 14-9. Chest radiographs of patients with different histologic types of lung cancer. *A*, patient with epidermoid lung cancer where the tumor mass is centrally located, with beginning pneumonitis from bronchial obstruction, slight volume loss, and central cavitation. *B*, patient with adenocarcinoma of the lung. The tumor denotes a peripherally located nodule with early pleural thickening suggesting involvement. *C*, patient with large cell lung cancer, containing a large mass with some peripheral pneumonitis. *D*, patient with bronchioloalvelolar carcinoma with multiple bilateral pulmonary nodules present for over a year. *E*, patient with small cell lung cancer, which involves a large, bulky central mass with hilar and mediastinal adenopathy and obstruction of the right upper lobe.

tumor can lead to dysphagia. Also, with recurrent laryngeal nerve paralysis, dysphagia for both solids and liquids (and aspiration) may result since this nerve innervates part of the cricoid musculature and proximal esophagus.[94]

Frequently, a right-sided lung cancer or tumor in right mediastinal lymph nodes will compress the thin-walled, low pressure system of the superior vena cava; hence, an obstructive vascular syndrome, superior vena cava (SVC) syndrome, will result.[86,95,96] The type of SVC syndrome depends on the level of the obstruction and the rapidity of its development. In epidermoid carcinoma, the obstruction usually develops gradually and the patient presents with a well-developed collateral venous system visible on physical examination. With small cell carcinoma, the onset is more rapid and often collaterals will not have developed. If the obstruction is above the junction of the SVC and azygous veins, distention of the arm and neck veins, edema of the face, neck, arms, and suffusion of the mucous membranes, with dilated, tortuous collaterals on the upper chest and back result. If the obstruction is proximal to the entrance of the azygous vein, a more severe clinical syndrome results; collaterals are noted on the anterior and posterior abdominal walls (with downward blood flow) since blood must enter the heart by way of the inferior vena cava.[96]

Diagnosis of the SVC syndrome is usually obvious from physical examination and review of chest films. Because of

FIG. 14-10. Survival of lung cancer patients by clinical diagnostic stage as a function of histologic type using the AJC system. (Staging of Lung Cancer, 1979 Manual of the AJC on Cancer Staging and End-Results Reporting Task Force on Lung)

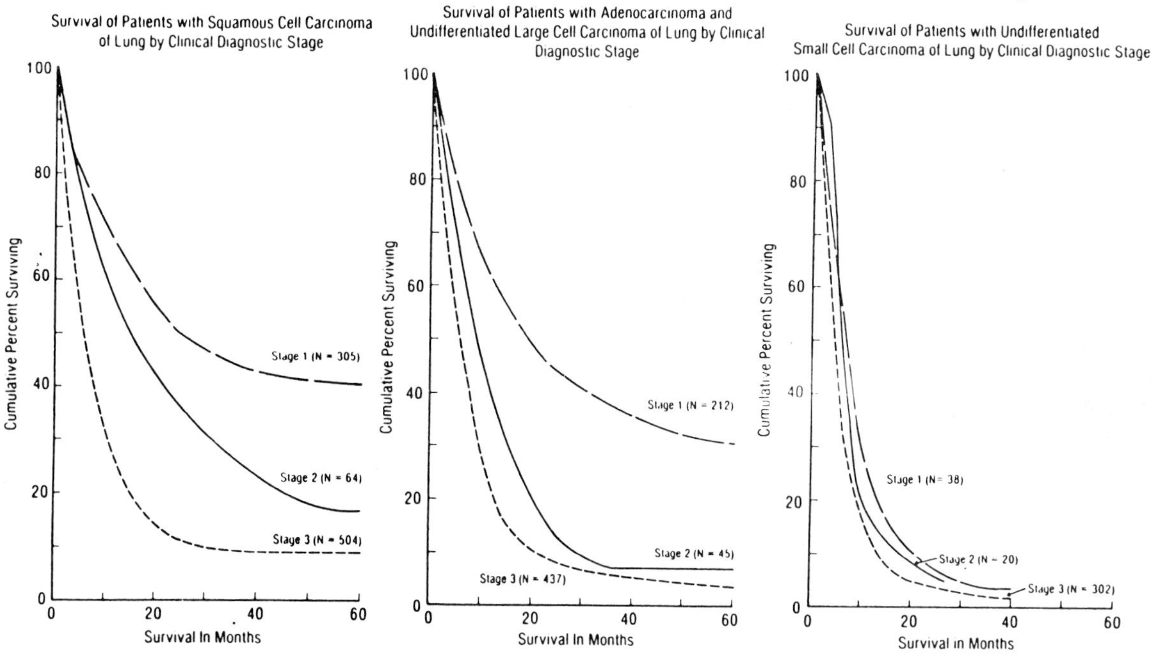

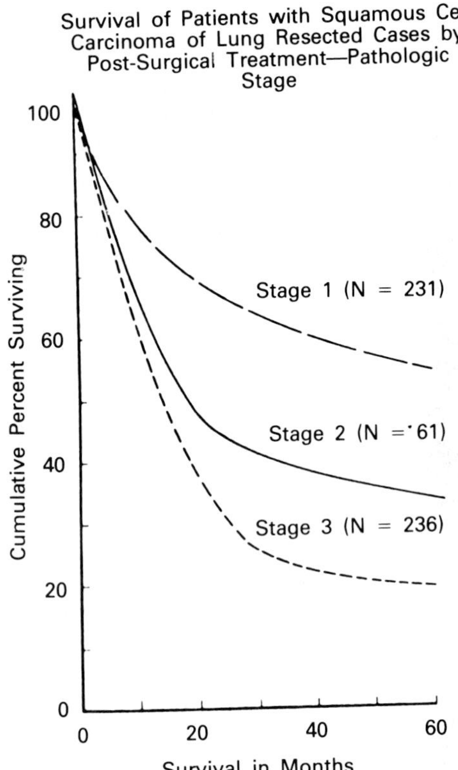

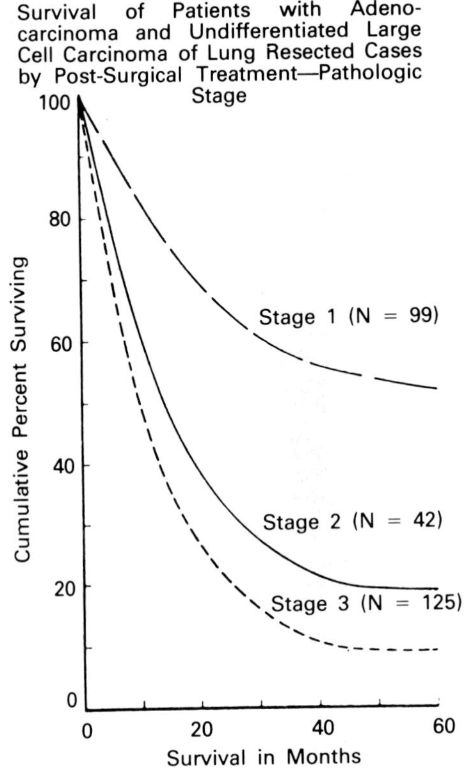

FIG. 14-11. Survival of lung cancer patients by post-surgical treatment pathologic stage as a function of histologic type using the AJC system. (Staging of Lung Cancer, 1979 Manual of the AJC on Cancer Staging and End-Results Reporting Task Force on Lung)

blood flow stasis, thrombosis occurs as a secondary phenomenon. For this reason, angiographic studies are not useful; while one can measure pressure in an arm and leg vein to demonstrate increased arm venous pressure, this is seldom necessary. It is important to be aware of the association of SVC syndrome with spinal cord compression from tumor extension and possibly vascular congestion.[97] A careful neurologic examination and review of x-ray films for bony abnormalities in this area are helpful as myelographic studies can be extremely difficult to perform in these patients. Another association is the co-existence of SVC syndrome with tumor extension into the pericardium with resultant tamponade. It is probably useful to perform an echocardiogram in all patients with SVC obstruction as well as in those suspected of having pericardial tamponade. The treatment of SVC obstruction is covered in Chapter 42 (Oncologic Emergencies).

Cardiac metastases occur in 15–35% of lung cancer patients.[98] Tumor extension into the pericardium and heart can result in pericardial tamponade, arrhythmias, and congestive heart failure. The exact frequency of these symptoms caused by lung cancer metastases is unknown at present, largely because cardiac metastases have only recently been sought antemortem. One retrospective review showed that only 4% of patients who were pathologically proved to have cardiac metastases had no clinical signs or symptoms related to the heart in addition to a normal electrocardiogram.[98] Thus, the development of cardiac signs or symptoms in lung cancer patients should prompt consideration in the differential diagnosis of heart involvement by tumor. At autopsy, the pericardium is more frequently involved (88% of heart metastases) than the myocardium (45% of metastases, often by extension) for all cell types.[98] (Diagnosis and management of pericardial tamponade is discussed in Chapter 42.) This is a common problem in lung cancer and its early detection requires recognition that the development of arrhythmias, enlarging cardiac silhouette, increasing venous pressure, or development of congestive failure can all precede tamponade. The diagnosis is readily confirmed by echocardiography. The absence of classic signs of tamponade (paradoxical pulse, grossly elevated venous pressure, distant heart sounds, friction rub, Kussmaul's sign, or low voltage on the electocardiogram) should not stop the physician from obtaining an echocardiogram if there is any clinical reason to suspect cardiac involvement by tumor. The treatment and definitive diagnosis are usually accomplished together in the cardiac catheterization laboratory with pericardiocentesis and decompression, followed by cytologic analysis of the pericardial fluid.[99]

Bronchioloalveolar carcinoma can present on x-ray films as a solitary nodule, multiple nodules, persistent infiltrate, lobar consolidation, or a cavitary lesion.[51] Some 60% of cases present as solitary nodules, 40% as multicentric disease.[58] However, what appears radiographically to be a single nodule in some 30% of cases is multifocal disease. On chest films, 50% of these cancers have a "rabbit" ear or "tail" sign with one or more fibrotic strands extending from the edge of a nodule toward the pleural surface.[51,100] Patients presenting with a persistent, unresolving, soft, fluffy infiltrate on chest films present a diagnostic problem as to whether this is inflammatory or neoplastic disease. Because the fluffy infiltrate represents alveolar involvement, an air bronchogram is seen on the film and there is no airway obstruction or atelectasis.[51] True cavitation is rare and what appears as cavities usually represents alveolar spaces not involved by tumor.[51] While a true solitary nodule is surgically curable, diffuse multinodular lesions represent an advanced stage of the disease, with survival less than 1–2 years.[49,66] While bronchioloalveolar carcinoma can have signs and symptoms similar to the other types of lung cancer (particularly adenocarcinoma), some findings are particularly suggestive of this cell type. Oxygen transfer across capillary membranes may be impaired by the tumor cells growing along alveolar surfaces; hence, respiratory insufficiency with dyspnea and hypoxemia becomes prominent. These patients sometimes produce large amounts of sputa (3–4 quarts daily), which accentuates the dyspnea and hypoxemia, induces electrolyte disturbances and hypovolemia, and predisposes to pneumonia.[51,101] In contrast to adenocarcinoma, pleura and chest wall invasion are not usually seen.[51]

FIG. 14-12. Standard position of patient for thoracotomy. *A*, lateral position (most frequently used); *B*, prone position; *C*, supine position. (Higgins GA:Thorax and respiratory system. In Operations in General Surgery, pp 190–254. Philadelphia, W B Saunders, 1968)

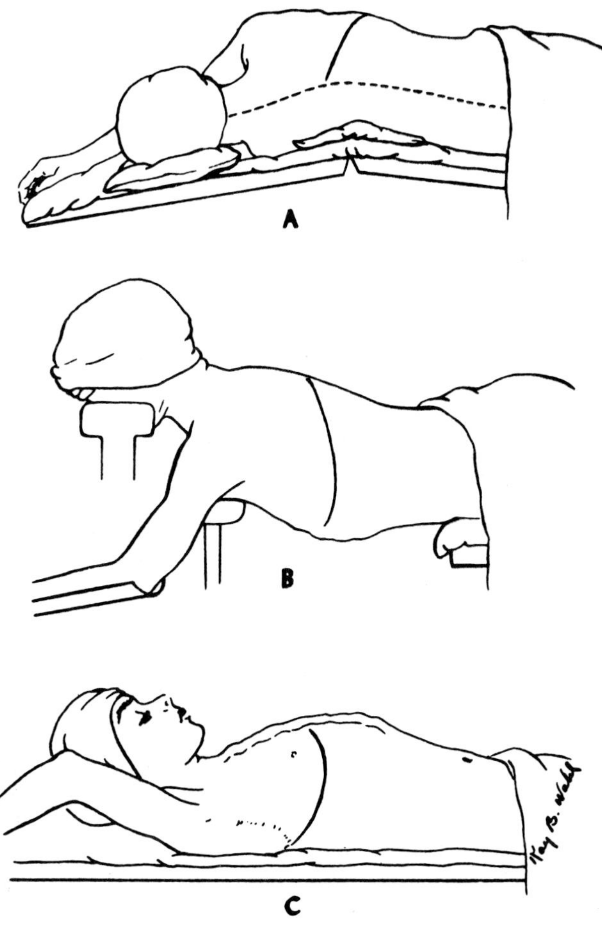

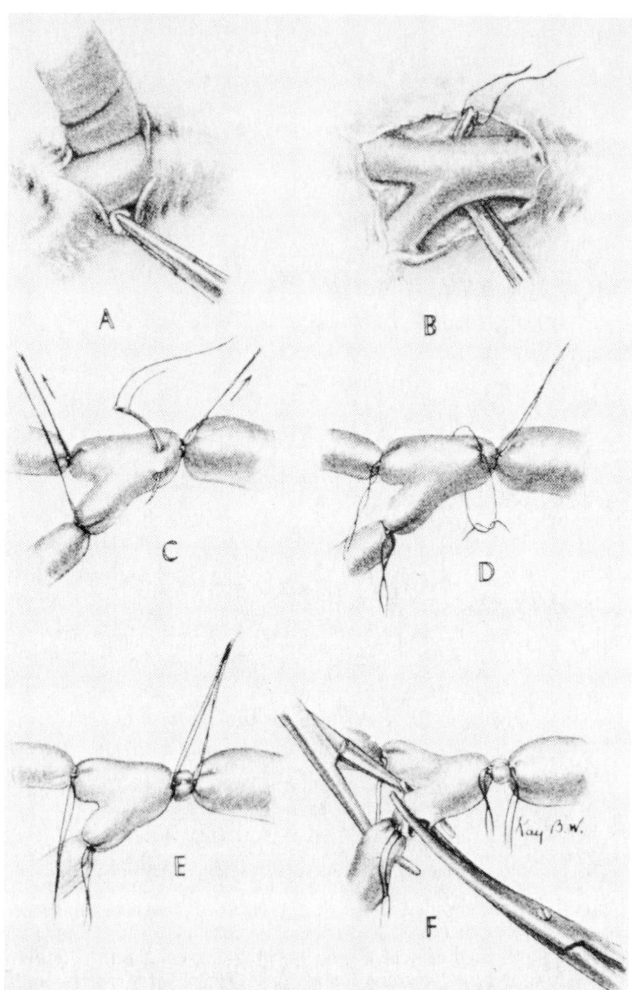

FIG. 14-13. Steps most commonly used in dissection and ligation of pulmonary vessels. *A*, Dissection and exposure of pulmonary vessel. *B*, Placement of free ligature. *C*. Placement of suture ligature. *D*. Encirclement of vessel by suture ligature. *E*. Completed ligation. *F*. Division of vessels. (See text also.) (Higgins GA: Thorax and respiratory system. In Operations in General Surgery, pp 190–254. Philadelphia, W B Saunders, 1968)

Extrathoracic Metastatic Disease

Autopsy studies have found lung cancer metastases in nearly every organ system of the body (see Table 14-13). Again, there are differences in the frequency of metastasis to different sites for each of the histologic types. At autopsy, the frequency of extrathoracic metastases are: epidermoid 25–54%; adenocarcinoma 50–82%; large cell carcinoma 48–86%; and small cell carcinoma 74–96%.[28,102] Common clinical problems related to distant metastatic disease of lung cancer include brain metastases with neurologic deficits, bone metastases with pain and pathologic fractures, and liver metastases that can cause liver dysfunction and pain. Lymph node metastases usually occur in the supraclavicular region, but occasionally axillary and groin node lesions can be painful and break down and ulcerate if not treated. Aside from the relatively small group of patients cured by primary treatment, the majority of lung cancer patients come to need therapy to palliate metastatic disease.

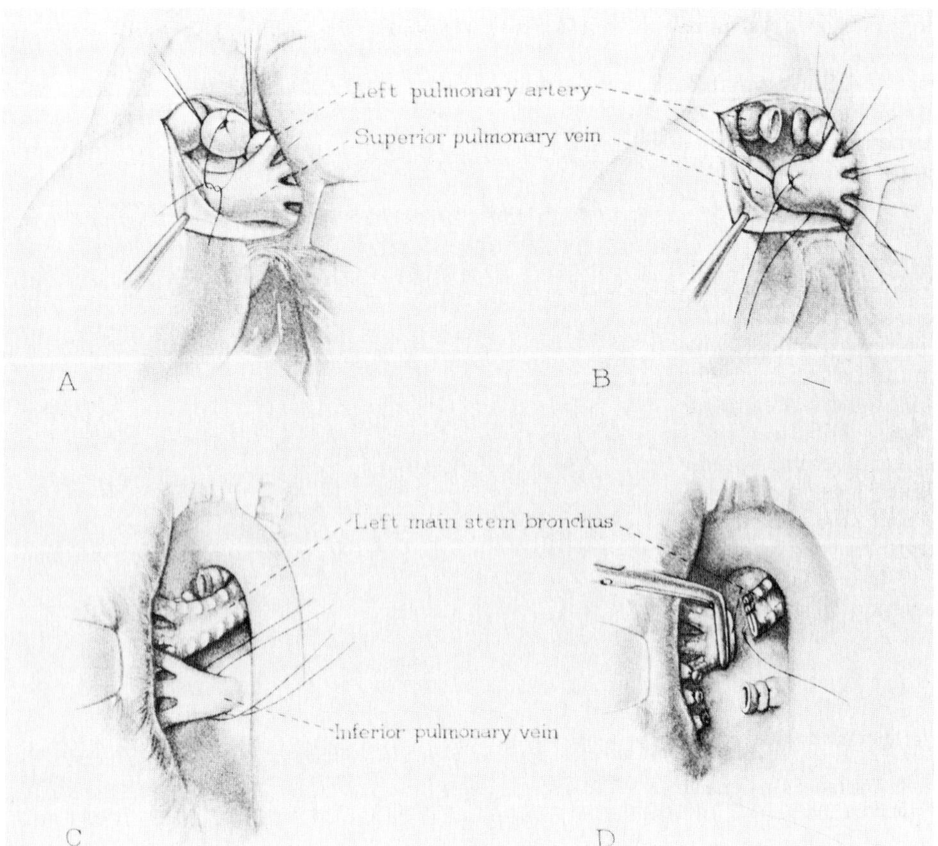

FIG. 14-14. Steps in hilar dissection for a left pneumonectomy. As indicated in *A*, the hilar pleura has been elevated and the lung retracted posteriorly and downward. The left pulmonary artery has been dissected and is being secured. In *B*, the pulmonary artery has been divided and the superior pulmonary vein has been dissected and is being secured with ligatures. In *C*, the lung has been retracted anteriorly and the inferior pulmonary vein has been freed from surrounding tissue prior to ligation and division. In *D*, the inferior pulmonary vein has been ligated and the left main stem bronchus has been cleared, clamped, and is presently being divided and sutured. (Higgins GA: Thorax and respiratory system. Operations in General Surgery, 4th ed, pp 190–254. Philadelphia, W B Saunders, 1968)

Paraneoplastic Syndromes

The diagnosis, management, and pathophysiology of paraneoplastic syndromes are covered in Chapter 39. However, they are frequently encountered in the clinical management of lung cancer patients.[103–108] Table 14-14 lists the types and approximate frequencies of paraneoplastic syndromes which are syndromes containing the effects of the tumor, seen in lung cancer patients.[103–113] In some cases, the paraneoplastic syndrome is associated with a particular histologic type of lung cancer. Examples of reversal of the clinical syndromes associated with successful treatment of the tumor exist in many cases. The paraneoplastic syndromes are frequently the first indication of tumor presence, thus prompting a search for an underlying tumor. In addition, many of the paraneoplastic syndromes may mimic metastatic disease and, unless detected, can lead to inappropriate palliative rather than curative treatment. For example, arterial emboli from marantic endocarditis can simulate brain metastases, as can cerebellar or cortical degeneration. Hypertrophic pulmonary osteoarthropathy with periostitis, in addition to clubbing, can give pain, tenderness, and swelling over the affected bones and can cause a positive bone scan, appearing as bone metastases.

Other Medical Problems in Lung Cancer Patients

Patients with lung cancer frequently have other medical problems. These are most commonly chronic obstructive pulmonary diseases related to smoking, chronic bronchitis and emphysema, cardiac problems related to coronary artery disease, and pulmonary disease. In addition, it is not uncommon to see lung cancer patients in whom the disease is associated with ethanol abuse and related liver damage. All of these, and the other medical problems commonly seen in the peak age range of lung cancer (55–65) have to be considered in planning and executing treatment. Often the treatment (*e.g.*, surgery, radiotherapy, or chemotherapy) can exacerbate these underlying medical problems. In addition, while lung cancer can metastasize and cause symptoms in many sites, new symptoms are frequently related to these non-malignant medical problems. The challenge to the physician caring for such patients is to sort these etiologies out and institute the proper treatment.

TABLE 14-13. Metastatic Patterns Found at Autopsy in Patients with Lung Cancer

	PERCENTAGE OF PATIENTS WITH METASTASIS			
SITE OF METASTASIS	EPIDERMOID CARCINOMA	ADENO-CARCINOMA	LARGE CELL CARCINOMA	SMALL CELL CARCINOMA
Number of patients studied	(N = 126)	(N = 110)	(N = 80)	(N = 102)
Hilar, mediastinal lymph nodes	77	80	84	96
Pleura	34	60	67	34
Chest wall	20	20	20	13
Diaphragm	9	11	15	14
Alternate lung	21	60	34	34
Cardiovascular system (total)	21	26	33	21
Pericardium	20	25	25	18
Myocardium	8	11	20	14
Limited to thorax	46	18	14	4
Liver	25	41	48	74
Adrenals	23	50	59	55
Bone	20	36	30	37
Kidney	21	23	28	22
CNS	18	37	25	29
Meninges	0	10	9	3
Dura	0	5	9	1
GI tract	12	5	20	14
Esophagus	13	8	3	14
Pancreas	4	12	22	41
Thyroid	4	2	6	18
Spleen	3	6	13	10
Parathyroid	1	0	0	1
Pituitary	1.6	4.5	3	15
Abdominal lymph nodes	10	24	30	52
Testes	0	0	0	7
Skin	0	0	6	0

(Matthews MJ: Problems in morphology and behavior of bronchopulmonary malignant disease. In Israel L, Chahanian P (eds): Lung Cancer: Natural History, Prognosis, and Therapy, pp 23–62. New York, Academic Press, 1976)

Multiple cancers are not infrequently seen in lung cancer patients.[114-116] These can either be synchronous or metachronous with the lung cancer. Common sites of secondary primary tumors include other lung cancers, head and neck cancer, esophageal cancer, bladder cancer, and pancreatic cancer.[115] These secondary neoplasms may have common etiologies with lung cancer in smoking and possible ethanol abuse.[117] Because the development of a new primary cancer in a patient previously treated for lung cancer may simulate metastatic disease, it is usually important to document (*i.e.*, biopsy) such a lesion, particularly if the patient could otherwise be cured of the first lung cancer.

Conversely, a solitary lung shadow may appear either at the same time or before or after a primary extrathoracic cancer. This single x-ray film abnormality should not automatically be assumed to be a metastasis from the extrathoracic cancer, since it can frequently be a primary lung cancer.[114] Because the natural history of lung cancer has a worse prognosis than most other primary tumors it is wise to approach a single pulmonary nodule (particularly in patients over 35 years who smoke) as though it were a primary lung cancer. Cahan, at the Memorial Sloan-Kettering Cancer Center, has studied this problem extensively and collected a large series of patients with multiple primaries, one of which was lung (see Table 14–15).[114] Because of these data, the authors recommend vigorous evaluation for surgical resection of the lung nodule in patients with a single pulmonary nodule in addition to an extrathoracic primary neoplasm. This will establish a firm histologic diagnosis, potentially curing the patients of either the lung cancer or the other neoplasm. For example, after surgical treatment in patients with colon cancer and a single pulmonary nodule, the total 5-year survival, free of cancer of either type (colon or primary lung), was 22%; the total fraction of patients alive or dead with no evidence of cancer was 31%. Of interest was the fact that all of the primary group who survived went on to develop a third primary tumor.[114]

SCREENING STUDIES FOR THE EARLY DIAGNOSIS OF LUNG CANCER

While the overall incidence and mortality rates of lung cancer have been rising in parallel, the percent of localized disease and overall resectability has remained approximately 20% for the past 30 years.[118] Local curative modalities (surgery and radiotherapy) have maintained an overall 5-year survival rate of 8–10% during the same period.[118] Staging studies have

TABLE 14-14. Some Clinically Manifest Paraneoplastic Syndromes in Lung Cancer Patients (Histologic type of lung cancer predominantly associated with the syndrome)[3,104–114]

SYSTEMIC SYMPTOMS

Anorexia-cachexia (31%)
Fever (21%)
Suppressed immunity

ENDOCRINE (12%)

Ectopic parathyroid hormone: hypercalcemia (epidermoid)
Inappropriate secretion of antidiuretic hormone: hyponatremia (small cell)
Ectopic secretion of ACTH: Cushing's syndrome (small cell)

SKELETAL

Clubbing (29%)
Hypertrophic pulmonary osteoarthropathy: periostitis (adenocarcinoma) (1–10%)

NEUROLOGIC-MYOPATHIC (1%)

Myasthenic syndrome: Eaton-Lambert syndrome (small cell)
Peripheral neuropathy
Subacute cerebellar degeneration
Cortical degeneration
Polymyositis

COAGULATION-THROMBOTIC (1–4%)

Migratory thrombophlebitis, Trousseau's syndrome: venous thrombosis
Nonbacterial thrombotic (marantic) endocarditis: arterial emboli
Disseminated intravascular coagulation: hemorrhage

CUTANEOUS (1%)

Dermatomyositis
Acanthosis nigricans

HEMATOLOGIC (8%)

Anemia
Granulocytosis
Leukoerythroblastosis

RENAL (<1%)

Nephrotic syndrome
Glomerulonephritis

(See Chapter 39 for a detailed discussion.)

suggested that in the earlier stage of disease more patients are likely to be cured of lung cancer. This has led to the hope that screening studies designed to detect early lung cancer would lead to earlier treatment and increased rates of cure. However, the actual survival benefits must be proven in prospective, controlled clinical trials.[119]

The highest incidence of lung cancer is seen in males over 40 who have smoked 40 or more cigarettes a day for a long period.[117] Several mass roentgenographic screenings of such patients have been done at 4–6 month intervals. Early studies suggest that cases discovered by x-ray screening have a 5-year survival of 15–18%, while control unscreened persons developing lung cancer had a 5-year survival of less than 10%.[120,121] The Philadelphia Pulmonary Neoplasm Research Project found lung cancer in 1.5% of the high-risk group they screened.[122] However, only 37% of the 94 lung cancers discovered were resectable; the 5-year survival for the resected group was 18% (7% for the entire group of cancers). Chest films and sputum cytologies complement one another in early lung cancer diagnosis; cytologies and radiographs pick up central tumors, while x-ray films alone pick up peripheral lesions.[123] Following this lead, Johns Hopkins, the Mayo Foundation, Memorial Sloan-Kettering Cancer Center (MSKCC), and the University of Cincinnati have undertaken prospective randomized trials using chest films and sputum cytologies when screening men over 45 years who smoke one pack/day or more of cigarettes, but who initially do not have signs or symptoms of lung cancer.[119]

The Mayo Foundation first screened asymptomatic persons entering the trial with chest films and sputum cytologies and detected prevalence cases (*i.e.*, cancer already present). They then randomized patients to an intensively screened group (chest films and sputum cytologies every 4 months) versus "unscreened" persons, meaning those who were only advised to have a yearly chest film and sputum test.[119] The MSKCC group initially screened for signs and symptoms of lung cancer and then randomized patients to annual chest films and sputum cytologies every 4 months, or annual radiographs alone.[124] At the start of the study, the Mayo group found a prevalence rate of 8.4/1,000 persons; MSKCC found a rate of 4–7/1,000. At Mayo, 62% of the prevalence cases were detected by radiographs, 18% by cytology, and 20% by both. For all prevalence cases, the overall curative resection rate was 57% and 5-year survival rate was 40%.[119] At MSKCC in the group screened by radiographs and cytology tests, 60% were detected by radiographs, 33% by cytology tests, and 7% by both. The overall curative resection rate was 69%; however, survival data were not presented.[124]

After the prevalence cases were removed, the Mayo group screening studies have identified lung cancer in 1.6% of the persons followed.[119] In the intensively screened group, 72% had lesions detected radiographically, 20% had cytologic detection, while 6% were detected by both procedures (see Table 14-16). In the screened group, fewer patients had symptoms at the time of detection than in the control group while the frequencies of lung cancer cell types were comparable in the two groups. More people in the screened group were resectable, more had postsurgical AJC Stage I cancer, and there is greater actuarial 5-year survival. In addition, sputum cytology has the added benefit of detecting upper airway cancers as well. In fact, by early 1978, in the screened group, 18 persons had an upper airway (head and neck) cancer detected. Of these, 44% were first detected by cytology.[125] Thus, screening a high risk population by chest films and sputum cytology detects lung cancer at an earlier and more resectable stage. However, the total death rate from lung cancer is not significantly lower yet in the screened group. For this reason, there is no justification at present for large scale population screening. However, the authors feel the data are suggestive enough for physicians to test their own high-risk patients similarly to the methods the Mayo, MSKCC, or Johns Hopkins groups until the trials are completed.[126]

BIOCHEMICAL MARKERS FOR EARLY DETECTION

At present no biochemical markers should be routinely used to screen for lung cancer. However, some markers, such as polypeptide hormones (*e.g.*, ACTH, calcitonin) have potential for clinical use. Of 74 patients with lung cancer, 72% had

TABLE 14-15. Probable Nature of a Solitary Lung Shadow with Known Cancer Elsewhere

SITE OF OTHER PRIMARY CANCER	NUMBER OF CASES	RATIO OF NEW LUNG PRIMARY: SOLITARY METASTASIS
Head and neck (excluding skin)	168	15.8
Trachea and lung (all types)	51	11.8
Prostate	26	All new lung primaries
Urinary bladder	22	6.3
Stomach	7	All new lung primary
Breast	63	1.7
Colo-rectal	52	1.4
Kidney	20	1.2
Testicle	18	0.5
Bone sarcoma	23	0.13
Melanoma	36	0.24
Soft tissue sarcoma	37	0.06

(Memorial Sloan-Kettering Cancer Center 1933–1972)
(Cahan WG: Multiple primary cancers of the lung, esophagus, and other sites. Cancer 40:1954–1960, 1977)

TABLE 14-16. Early Results of the Mayo Foundation Randomized Controlled Trial to Detect Early Lung Cancer

	PREVALENCE CASES	INCIDENCE CASES	
		RANDOMIZED GROUP (N = 9,223)	
		Screened	*Control*
Number of Patients with Lung Cancer	87	87	57
		% of Cases	
CELL TYPE			
Epidermoid	47	32	32
Adenocarcinoma	25	21	23
Large cell carcinoma	16	20	12
Small cell carcinoma	11	28	33
Symptoms at detection	?None	11	67
Resectability	57%	62	28
AJC post surgical stage			
Occult	10	Not stated	Not stated
I	39	53	21
II	6	Not stated	Not stated
III	45	37	68
Probability of 5-year survival	40	45	19
Rate/1,000 person/year incidence	Not applicable	4.4	3.0
Deaths from lung cancer		1.8	2.1

(11,001 patients initially screened)
(Fontana RS: Early diagnosis of lung cancer. Am Rev Respir Dis 116:399–402, 1977)

increased ACTH immunoreactivity.[127] In contrast, 0% of 24 patients with benign chest film abnormalities, and 20% of patients with chronic obstructive pulmonary disease (COPD), had elevated levels; 10% of patients with granulomatous lung disease had elevated ACTH levels during an acute exacerbation of their disease, which returned to normal with recovery. Some 25% of COPD patients with elevated ACTH levels and only 2% with normal ACTH levels developed lung cancer within two years.[127]

Carcinoembryonic antigen (CEA) is not a sensitive indicator to screen for lung cancer since 60% of 130 patients who underwent surgical resection of histologically proven lung cancer had normal levels (*i.e.*, values less than 2.5 ng/ml).[128] However, it may have prognostic value. A CEA level greater than 15 ng/ml reduced the possibility of a successful resection. In addition, patients who in follow-up appeared to be cured by surgery had significantly fewer elevated CEAs postoperatively than did patients who relapsed. Thus, a rising or persistently elevated CEA appears to predict for relapse or a second primary tumor.[128]

LOCALIZATION OF OCCULT (STAGE O) LUNG CANCER

The institution of sputum cytology screening studies has identified patients with cancer diagnosed cytologically who have normal chest radiographs (discussed later as Tx tumor stage). For treatment involving surgery or radiotherapy to be instituted, the lesion(s) must be localized. Conversely, lesions detected by chest radiographs are localized, but appropriate treatment requires a histologic diagnosis.[129] While chemotherapy is the primary treatment in small cell lung cancer, there are as yet no data on giving such systemic therapy to persons who only have malignant sputum cytology suggestive of small cell cancer but no radiographic, bronchoscopic, or metastatic lesions visible.

The groups at Johns Hopkins, Mayo Foundation, and MSKCC have investigated patients with positive sputum cytologies and normal chest radiographs in order to localize their tumors (see Table 14-17).[129–131] The method has been pioneered by Marsch at Johns Hopkins.[130,131] Smoking is discontinued before the procedure. In addition, bronchitis is treated because inflammatory cells can interfere with cytologic interpretation. First, the patient has a complete examination of the upper aerodigestive tract, particularly the nasopharynx, the base of tongue, larynx, and hypopharynx to detect an asymptomatic tumor by indirect and direct nasopharyngoscopy and laryngoscopy. Then, a detailed fiberoptic bronchoscopic examination under general anesthesia lasting up to two hours is performed with meticulous examination of the bronchial tree out to the fifth generation of bronchi. Suspicious areas, bronchial bifurcations (spurs), and prospective surgical margins are biopsied, and a series of differential brushings is collected. These biopsies are predictive that surgical margins will be clear or involved with *in situ* cancer.[129]

TABLE 14-17. Findings and Management of Patients with Positive Sputum Cytology and No Chest Film Lesions Localizing the Lung Cancer (Radiographically Occult Lung Cancer)—Follow-up of Three Years or More From Johns Hopkins and the Mayo Foundation

Number of patients	62
Age range	30–79 years (all males)
Upper aerodigestive cancer causing positive cytology	11%
IN REMAINING 55 PATIENTS:	
Fiberoptic bronchoscopic (FOB) localized the lesion	89% (49/55)
Squamous cancer found	98%
FOB visible gross lesion	48%
Carcinoma *in situ* found	43% (JH data only)
Multicentric *in situ* lesions or multiple tumors found	22% (6/27 patients with data)
OF THOSE LESIONS LOCALIZED	
Overall patients operated on	78% (38/49)
Patients resected	98%
AJC Stage I	85%
AJC Stage III	15%
Lymph nodes positive	5%
Pneumonectomy required	24% (9/38)
Radiation therapy required instead of surgery for technical or medical reasons	11% (Mayo data only)
No treatment given for medical or technical reasons	13% (Mayo data only)

(Baker RR, Ball WC Jr, Carter D et al: Identification and treatment of clinically occult cancer of the lung. Prog Cancer Res Ther II: 243–249, 1979; Sanderson DR, Fontana RS, Woolner LB et al: Bronchoscopic localization of radiographically occult lung cancer. Chest 65:608–612, 1974; Fontana RS: Editorial: The needle in the haystack. Mayo Clin Proc 53:616–617, 1978; Sanderson DR, Fontana RS: Early lung cancer detection and localization. Ann Otol Rhinol Laryngol 84:583–589, 1975)

Additional endobronchial tumor markers are needed for the 10% of tumors that cannot be localized bronchoscopically in order to assist in the initial localization and to detect multicentric lesions in those patients with a lesion localized by radiograph or bronchoscopy. The Johns Hopkins group has used tantalum powder bronchography (an experimental procedure).[129] Tantalum is instilled with a controlled catheter, bronchography is performed followed by a cine examination, and films are taken at 24 and 48 hours to detect delayed clearance of tantalum. The tantalum bronchogram localized lesions in over 90% of cases and thus can direct the fiberoptic bronchoscopic examination.

The Mayo group has pioneered the use of a derivative of hematoporphyrin (an experimental procedure) involving a photodynamically active dye that concentrates in cancer cells. It then exhibits a salmon-red fluorescence on excitation by UV light detected photoelectrically and connected to generate an audio signal for the fiberoptic bronchoscopist.[132–134] Early results show the concentration of dye in areas where no mucosal abnormalities are seen through the fiberoptic scope; however, biopsy reveals carcinoma *in situ*.[134] This method could greatly simplify bronchoscopic localization of tumor in patients with occult cancer.

MANAGEMENT AND TREATMENT DECISIONS IN PATIENTS WITH RADIOLOGICALLY OCCULT LUNG CANCER

Once localization of the radiologically occult lung cancer has taken place, treatment decisions can be formulated. These are complicated because of the multicentric nature of the lesions, the tendency for multiple primary lung cancers to develop, and reports of following patients with *in situ* lesions for several years without the development of invasive cancer.[129–131,132,135,136] Pathologically, the Johns Hopkins group found *in situ* carcinoma only in 43% of resected specimens but noted extensive glandular involvement in these cases.[129]

The Johns Hopkins and Mayo experiences in managing patients with radiographically occult lung cancer are similar. They are combined in Table 14-17.[129,130,132,136] Of the 55 patients in the combined group with lung cancer, nearly all had squamous carcinoma; 11% could not be localized. A large fraction had carcinoma *in situ* (including carcinoma *in situ* at the bronchial margins), or were multicentric, and new lung primaries have already started to appear in follow-up or resected cases. Thus, current recommendations are for the most conservative surgical resection permitted to remove the cancer and to conserve lung parenchyma, even if the bronchial margins are positive for carcinoma *in situ*.[129,131,135,136] Because of the multicentric nature, there is a need for a local ablative procedure to deal with the multiple foci of cancer. Fontana estimates the projected 5-year survival rate of these occult cancers detected by sputum cytology to be approximately 60% or greater, although follow-up is still short.[129,132,136] Screening studies continue, however, and the overall results suggest that 40% of patients with an early lung cancer detected will not be able to undergo surgery, will have metastatic disease, or will develop a new primary.

ESTABLISHING A TISSUE DIAGNOSIS OF LUNG CANCER

Once the signs and symptoms of lung cancer have developed or an abnormality on chest film or sputum cytology has been detected in a screening study, it is necessary to establish a histologic diagnosis of malignancy, determine lung cancer cell type, and stage the patient for appropriate treatment. The procedures employed depend on the individual clinical situation. In some cases (*i.e.*, a solitary, asymptomatic, pulmonary nodule), the tissue diagnosis will be made at the time of definitive surgical resection, while in others it will be made at the time of bronchial biopsy or biopsy of a distant metastatic focus. In all cases, it is mandatory that a histologic diagnosis of malignancy be made and the lung cancer cell type established.

A reasonable approach in the patient suspected of having lung cancer is first to review patient history and physical examination, specifically looking for signs or symptoms to direct a search for a tissue diagnosis. This involves careful review of supraclavicular lymph node areas for palpable masses, the skin for subcutaneous nodules, and the chest exam for signs and symptoms of endobronchial tumor. If an obvious tumor-bearing lymph node or skin nodule is found, it should be biopsied. If a pleural effusion is present, this should be sampled and cytology performed on a cytocentrifuge-prepared specimen. Also, needle biopsy of the pleura in such patients with effusion is an effective and simple method of obtaining a diagnosis with a moderate incidence of positive yield. If the liver is grossly enlarged or if it has nodular lesions on physical exam or radionuclide scan, a liver biopsy may be done. In an unexplained anemia, a bone marrow biopsy may be performed. Occasionally, lytic or blastic bone lesions on radiograph, or localized bone scan abnormalities in sites accessible to needle biopsy by an orthopedic surgeon, may be investigated when no other tumor tissue is available. If there are no obvious distant lesions, it is best to proceed to a flexible fiberoptic bronchoscopic study, examining washings, brushing, and biopsy of suspicious lesions.

FLEXIBLE FIBEROPTIC BRONCHOSCOPY

Flexible fiberoptic bronchoscopy, introduced in 1968, has revolutionized the evaluation of patients with lung cancer and has largely replaced rigid bronchoscopy for endoscopic examination of the tracheobronchial tree.[60,138–142] A far greater area of the tracheobronchial tree can be directly visualized during fiberoptic endoscopy than during rigid instrument examination. For example, in several series, 13–39% of lesions not seen by the rigid instrument were seen by the fiberoptic scope.[138] Bronchoscopy can be used to evaluate hemoptysis as well. Bronchogenic cancer is found in 23–33% of patients presenting with hemoptysis.[138] However, when massive hemoptysis is present, the rigid instrument is usually required to visualize the lesions. In large series of lung cancer patients, 59–74% of the lesions were visible through the fiberoptic scope; biopsy and brushings gave a true positive yield in 86–96% of these.[139,143] The combination of bronchial brushings and biopsy gave the optimum overall accuracy of 79% including 66–78% of peripheral lesions brushed under fluoroscopic control and 86% of central lesions.[139,143] The false positive rate is very low (0.8%) and is usually found in inflammatory lesions where squamous metaplasia masquerades as cancer.[139] Thus, it is important to perform washings, brushing, and biopsy during fiberoptic examination since additional positive samples are picked up with each.[140] In peripheral lesions not visualized endoscopically, brush biopsy under fluoroscopy of the suspected segment gave a positive (cancer cells found) diagnosis in 63–92% of lung cancers.[141,143,144] The fluoroscopic control is important in diagnosing the peripheral lesions.[140] In addition, when using a flexible fiberoptic scope, transbronchial forceps biopsy of peripheral lung lesions under fluoroscopic control made positive diagnoses in 70–75% of cases.[138,145] This method is good for peripheral lesions 2 cm in diameter or greater, but it had only a 28% yield in lesions under 2 cm (other diagnostic procedures should be used in these cases).[141] In addition, when suspicious cytology is seen in brushings or washings, 80% of the time this ultimately proves to be lung cancer from both peripheral and central lesions.[140] In patients presenting with a middle or anterior mediastinal mass or paratracheal mass on chest radiography, fiberoptic bronchoscopy gives an overall tissue diagnostic yield of 45%; if there is extrinsic compression of the trachea or mainstem bronchi, the yield is 72%.[142] In patients with radiographic findings of lung abscess subsequently proven to have lung cancer, 88% had a cytologic diagnosis of cancer made by fiberoptic bronchoscopy.[146]

TRANSTHORACIC FINE NEEDLE ASPIRATION BIOPSY

Until 5 years ago, cytologic or histologic diagnosis of lung cancer was made at the time of surgical exploration, bronchoscopy (including fiberoptic), sputum cytology, mediastinoscopy, or biopsy of some suspicious lesion. Recently, there has been rapid development of percutaneous, transthoracic fine needle aspiration biopsy under fluoroscopic guidance. Many intrapulmonary masses suspected of being malignant, including solitary pulmonary nodules, have been identified by this method.[147] Sinner reported on 5,300 transthoracic needle biopsies in 2,726 patients; Sagel and coworkers reported on 1,211 patients.[148–150]. The majority of biopsies were done in people 50–80-years-old. Final diagnosis was established in 91% of these patients, with 46–71% having cytologic evidence of a malignancy (approximately 85% of which were primary lung cancers).[149,150] There were 2.4% false positive and 0.23% false negative diagnoses. One aspiration provided malignant cells in 87% of patients subsequently proven to have malignant disease; this rose to 96% after two procedures.[150] Complications included pneumothorax in 27% (only 14% of which required chest tubes), hemoptysis in 2–5%, local bleeding around the lesion seen by chest films in 4–11% (requiring observation only), and only one instance of implantation metastasis in the 2,160 patients with lung cancer studied by the two groups. There was one case of air embolism and no immediate mortality reported. Contraindications to the procedure included unconscious or uncooperative patients, hemorrhagic diathesis, severe respiratory distress, or high fever and uncontrollable cough. When these acute symptoms recede, the procedure can be carried out. In cases of primary tumors 2 cm in diameter or less (verified cytologically by needle biopsy to be lung cancer) 5-year survival was 42%, comparing favorably to series where no needle biopsy was performed.[148] The procedure is relatively simple, rapid (15 minutes), generally causes little patient discomfort, and can be performed in most hospitals. However, it does require close cooperation between the cytopathologist and the physicians performing the needle biopsy.

While the authors foresee the widespread use of this technique in the future, several indications for aspiration needle biopsy in the lung cancer patient can currently be identified:

1. Pulmonary masses in the patient unsuitable for curative thoracotomy who needs a definitive tissue diagnosis
2. A localized or worsening pneumonic infiltrate in a immunocompromised patient despite standard therapy when a causative agent is not known
3. A patient with another malignancy allowing the differentiation between a new primary, a metastatic lesion, or an inflammatory process.

An area of controversy is the patient with a solitary pulmonary nodule and no contraindications to thoracotomy. Only 40% of peripheral pulmonary nodules surgically treated prove to be malignant; postoperative mortality and morbidity can be avoided in these patients.[151] However, in the patient at high risk of having lung cancer (*e.g.*, a 50-year-old male smoker with an irregular, expanding lesion), even needle biopsy advocates would proceed straight to thoracotomy.[150]

Fine needle aspiration cytology is reliable enough to permit a cytologic diagnosis of small cell carcinoma.[149] However, fiberoptic bronchoscopy usually provides cytologic or biopsy material for definitive diagnosis in a high percentage of proven small cell cancer cases.[60] In addition, adjuvant chemotherapy results for resected small cell carcinoma pulmonary nodules are good enough (see later in this chapter) to recommend resection for a single peripheral nodule without mediastinal adenopathy, even if small cell lung cancer was proven. Thus, aspiration biopsy in the patient with small cell lung cancer is primarily useful only in those occasional patients with a negative bronchoscopic examination.

Miscellaneous Techniques

Steel has described a *trefine needle biopsy* technique using a high speed air trefine drill to obtain a substantial core of pulmonary tissue for histopathologic study.[151] This method is valuable when diagnosing diffuse pulmonary infiltrative disease. It also has limited application in peripheral localized lesions suspected of being malignant.

Exploratory thoracotomy is the ultimate method when other diagnostic procedures fail. A more aggressive policy in recommending exploratory thoracotomy for the small indeterminate lesion found mainly in heavy smokers (in the cancer age group) has substantially improved postoperative survival percentages. Conversely, exploratory thoracotomy for diagnosis in elderly and poor-risk patients with limited functional pulmonary reserve should be approached with caution since thoracotomy alone carries a substantial mortality and morbidity in such patients.

STAGING OF PATIENTS WITH LUNG CANCER

Efficient and appropriate staging of the patient takes place once the tissue diagnosis of lung cancer is obtained. The purpose of staging is to aid in selection of treatment, estimate the probability of cure and survival, facilitate proper communication about a patient's status, and to compare results from different clinical treatment series. For non-small cell lung cancer, only surgery or, to a lesser degree, radiotherapy currently offers the opportunity for long-term survival to a significant number of patients. Selection of patients for a curative attempt by either of these modalities is determined by the anatomic stage of disease and the technical (determining "resectability" or "radiocurability") and physiologic considerations concerning the patient's ability to tolerate the treatment and be functional post therapy (this is referred to as "operability"). While there are biologic differences between epidermoid, adeno, and large cell carcinoma, these differences, at present, should probably not be used in ruling out curative local therapy. However, there are great biologic differences between these non-small cell cancers and small cell carcinoma of the lung. While anatomic considerations are also important in small cell cancer patients, the total tumor bulk and physiologic ability of the patient to tolerate chemotherapy with or without radiotherapy appear, at present, to be more important.

ANATOMIC STAGING

The task force on carcinoma of the lung of the American Joint Committee (AJC) for Staging and End Results Reporting has evaluated 2,155 cases of lung cancer. From this analysis they have established a TNM staging system with prognostic accuracy.[24,153-156] This system is based on the primary tumor size and extent (*T* factor), regional lymph node involvement (*N* factor), and presence or absence of distant metastases (*M* factor). While the AJC system can be applied to all histologic types of lung cancer, it currently has applicability only regarding treatment decisions the non-small cell group of tumors. A different staging system (discussed later in this chapter) is used for patients with proven small cell lung cancer. The TNM definitions and rules for stage groupings are given in Tables 14-18 and 14-19.

The AJC system identifies different types of evidence available for classifying the extent of disease at different sites and at different times in the course of disease and patient evaluation. These include clinical diagnostic staging (*i.e.*, all pretreatment information including that from endoscopy,

TABLE 14-18. American Joint Committee (AJC) for Cancer Staging and End Results Reporting—Definitions of TNM Categories*

PRIMARY TUMOR (T)	
TO	No evidence of primary tumor
TX	Tumor proven by the presence of malignant cells in bronchopulmonary secretions but not visualized roentgenographically or bronchoscopically, or any tumor that cannot be assessed (*i.e.*, a retreatment staging)
TIS	Carcinoma *in situ*
T1	Tumor that is 3 cm or less in greatest diameter, surrounded by lung or visceral pleura, and without evidence of invasion proximal to a lobar bronchus at bronchoscopy
T2	Tumor more than 3 cm in greatest diameter, or a tumor of any size that either invades visceral pleura or has associated atelectasis or obstructive pneumonitis extending to the hilar region. At bronchoscopy, the proximal extent of demonstrable tumor must be within a lobar bronchus or at least 2 cm distal to the carina. Any associated atelectasis or obstructive pneumonitis must involve less than an entire lung, and there must be no pleural effusion
T3	Tumor of any size with direct extension into an adjacent structure such as the perietal pleura or chest wall, the diaphragm, or the mediastinum and its contents, or a tumor demonstrable bronchoscopically to involve a main bronchus less than 2 cm distal to the carina, or any tumor associated with atelectasis or obstructive pneumonitis of an entire lung or pleural effusion (whether or not malignant cells are found)
REGIONAL LYMPH NODES (N)	
NO	No demonstrable metastasis to regional lymph nodes
N1	Metastasis to lymph nodes in the peribronchial or the ipsilateral hilar region, or both, including direct extension
N2	Metastasis to lymph nodes in the mediastinum†
DISTANT METASTASIS(M)	
MX	Not assessed
MO	No known distant metastasis
M1	Distant metastasis present with site specified (*i.e.*, scalene, cervical, or contralateral hilar lymph nodes; or metastasis to brain, bone, liver, soft tissue, or contralateral lung, etc.)

(Mountain CF (chairman): Staging of lung cancer, 1979. American Joint Committee for Cancer Staging and End-Results Reporting. Task Force on Lung Cancer)

* In all cases, the designation of the T, N, or M category should be for the greatest extent of disease providing the evidence of this extent is reasonable.

† Vocal cord paralysis, superior vena cava obstruction, and compression of the trachea or esophagus are scored as N2.

mediastinoscopy, or other biopsies), surgical–evaluative staging (*i.e.,* surgeon's findings at exploratory thoracotomy), postsurgical treatment pathologic staging (*i.e.,* surgical pathology report), retreatment staging (*i.e.,* staging at relapse), and finally, autopsy staging. Of most importance to the patient are the clinical diagnostic staging used to select the mode of primary treatment and the posttherapy staging (identified in the AJC system only as the postsurgical treatment pathologic stage, but technically applicable to patients after all forms of therapy). This method is used as an early indicator of the potential success of therapy and the need for additional treatment.

The TNM system can be applied with a consistency of greater than 90% in lung cancer patients by physicians trained in its use.[24] In all cases, the designation of the greatest extent of disease (for which there is reasonable evidence) should be used.[24] Multiple synchronous tumors of different histologic types should be considered as separate primary lung cancer and each one staged separately. If they are of the same histologic type, distinction between two primaries or a metastasis is made pathologically (*e.g.,* a primary is scored if the typical transition from normal bronchial epithelium to carcinoma *in situ* to invasive carcinoma is seen).

The accuracy of clinical TNM staging has been compared with results of surgicopathologic TNM determinations in 1,224 patients in Japan. There was agreement in only 46% of the patients; the disagreements were primarily in determination of the N stage.[157,158] In peripheral, non-small cell lesions the 5-year survival for clinical stage I was 50%; it was 72% for pathologic stage I.[158] Thus, the accuracy of nodal staging is very important in predicting outcome and is dependent on surgical assessment.

Hilar masses, particularly those near the mediastinum, can be difficult to classify by clinical–diagnostic staging as to whether they are the primary tumor or metastatic disease in hilar or mediastinal nodes. Vocal cord paralysis, superior vena cava obstruction, and compression of the trachea or esophagus are scored as N2 lesions since they usually are related to mediastinal node metastases. Those grouped within stage III at present are patients with disease confined to the chest (stage III MO and some stage III M1) as well as patients with extrathoracic metastatic disease (stage III M1). Some of

TABLE 14-19. American Joint Committee (AJC) for Cancer Staging and End Results Reporting—Stage Grouping for Lung Cancer

OCCULT CARCINOMA	
TX NO MO	An occult carcinoma with bronchopulmonary secretions containing malignant cells but without other evidence of the primary tumor or evidence of metastasis to the regional lymph nodes or distant metastasis
STAGE I*	
TIS NO MO	Carcinoma *in situ*
T1 NO MO T1 N1 MO T2 NO MO	Tumor that can be classified T1 without any metastasis or with metastasis to the lymph nodes in the peribronchial or ipsilateral hilar region only, or a tumor that can be classified T2 without any metastasis to nodes or distant metastasis.*
STAGE II	
T2 N1 MO	A tumor classified as T2 with metastasis to the lymph nodes in the peribronchial or ipsilateral hilar region only
STAGE III	
T3 with any N or M N2 with any T or M M1 with any T or N	Any tumor more extensive than T2, or any tumor with metastasis to the lymph nodes in the mediastinum, or any tumor with distant metastasis

(Mountain CF (chairman): Staging of Lung Cancer, 1979. American Joint Committee for Cancer Staging and End-Results Reporting. Task Force on Lung Cancer)

* TX N1 MO and TO N1 MO are also theoretically possible, but such a clinical diagnosis would be difficult, if not impossible, to make.

the intrathoracic stage III (stage III M0) patients and even those with contralateral hilar nodes (one type of stage III M1) could be treated with a tolerable radiotherapy port and thus are potentially curable. In contrast, patients with extrathoracic metastatic disease (another class of stage III M1) have essentially no probability of cure and thus these patients should be separately grouped.

The survival cures for the different histologic types of lung cancer by clinical–diagnostic stage grouping is shown in Fig. 14-10 and postsurgical treatment pathologic stage in Fig. 14-11. The percentage of resected cases in each postsurgical stage is similar for epidermoid, adeno, and large cell carcinoma (see Table 14-20).[24,155] Adenocarcinoma and large cell cancer have equivalent survival in the AJC study and thus are grouped together by stage. In all cases, there is a progressive loss of patients over the first 20–30 months and then plateaus in the survival curves appear that reflect the normal survival curves for this segment of the population. While patients will die from other causes than cancer in the first 30 months, the large majority die from recurrent tumor. Thus, disease-free survival after 30 months is another predictor of potential cure.

The prognostic value of the AJC postsurgical treatment pathologic stage grouping is identified in Fig. 14-10. For stage I, the rates are similar for epidermoid, adeno, and large cell carcinoma. For stages II and III, the rates are consistently better for epidermoid cancer (see Fig. 14-11 and Table 14-21). The T and N factors considered alone also predict survival (see Table 14-21). While the different stage groupings (*i.e.*, stage I, II, III M0, III M1) have prognostic value there are also significant differences in survival in the various TNM subsets that make up the stage groupings of patients resected for cure. Thus, it is reasonable to report data or make individual patient decisions based on the specific TNM subset.[160] However, for the non-small cell lung cancer patients with sufficiently limited disease permitting surgical resection, the overwhelming prognostic factor is whether or not the cancer has remained localized to the lung, has spread by local extension, or metastasized to the regional lymph nodes as determined by postsurgical treatment pathologic staging. For the average resectable lesion, cell type and size of the primary lesion do not exert independent influence over long-term survival.[162] When involved lymph nodes are present, long-term survival prospects are reduced by approximately 50%, compared to patients with disease confined to the lung. The ominous portent of lymph node involvement increases from peribronchial to hilar to mediastinal nodes.[160]

TABLE 14-20. Postsurgical Pathologic Treatment Stage of Non-Small Cell Carcinoma After Resection by Histologic Type

	PERCENTAGE OF PATIENTS IN EACH STAGE AFTER RESECTION	
	EPIDERMOID CARCINOMA	ADENOCARCINOMA-LARGE CELL CARCINOMA
Number of patients	(528)	(266)
AJC POSTSURGICAL PATH TREATMENT STAGE		
I	44	37
II	12	16
III	45	47

(Mountain CF, Hermes KE: Management implications of surgical staging studies. Prog Cancer Res Ther 11:233–242, 1979)

TABLE 14-21. Prognostic Value of AJC Postsurgical Treatment Staging in Non-Small Cell Lung Cancer Following Definitive Surgery for the Different T and N Variables

POSTSURGICAL TREATMENT STAGE		CUMULATIVE PERCENTAGE SURVIVING 5 YEARS
ALL PATIENTS RESECTED	N	(N = 794)
I	330	53
II	103	29
III	361	16
BY TUMOR STAGE		
T1		40
T2		20
T3		6
BY NODAL STAGE		
N0		46
N1 (Hilar nodes involved only)		33
N2 (Mediastinal nodes involved only)		8

(Mountain DC, Carr DT, Anderson WA: A system for the clinical staging of lung cancer. Am J Roentgenol Radium Ther Nucl Med 120:130–138, 1974; Mountain CF: Biologic, physiologic, and technical determinants in surgical therapy for lung cancer. In Straus MJ (ed): Lung Cancer: Clinical Diagnosis and Treatment, pp 185–198. New York, Grune and Stratton, 1977; Mountain CF: Surgery of lung cancer including adjunctive therapy. In Hansen HH, Rorth M (eds): Lung Cancer 1980, pp 71–92. Amsterdam, Excerpta Medica, 1980.)

It is clear that by initial clinical–diagnostic stage and postsurgical anatomic stage, the chances of a patient's being cured by resection can be determined and compared to operative mortality and postoperative functional status. However, in clinical practice, this question is usually posed: "Is there a finite chance of cure?" What most clinicians mean is whether the chance of cure is within the general range of operative mortality (*i.e.*, between 1 and 10%). Similar questions are posed in discussions advocating "curative" radiotherapy, although in this case the long-term complications of radiotherapy are often overlooked. In this case, the question is: "Has a patient with this stage of disease ever been cured by radiotherapy?" A group of patients exists who the majority of surgeons and radiotherapists feel are essentially not "curable" by current local modalities alone (see Table 14-22). When a patient has these findings the therapeutic approach is directed at "palliating" the patient.

A number of important implications can be drawn from the various studies done to relate staging to survival. Because of the greater than 50% long-term survival prospects in patients with stage I disease, adjuvant trials made up only of these patients must encompass large numbers to produce meaningful results. Conversely, the 70–90% failure rate for patients with resectable stage II and stage III disease demands an aggressive approach justifying increased risks of morbidity and mortality. However, the necessity for effective systemic

TABLE 14-22. Anatomic-Biologic Aspects of Tumor Involvement Which Are Major Contraindications to Curative Attempts by Surgery or Radiotherapy Alone by Standard Treatment Methods

Extrathoracic distant metastases
Superior vena cava syndrome
Vocal cord paralysis
Malignant pleural effusion
Cardiac tamponade with pericardial involvement
Tumor within 2 cm of the carina*
Metastasis to the contralateral lung
Bilateral endobronchial tumor*
Metastasis to the supraclavicular lymph nodes
Lymph node metastasis in the contralateral mediastinum*
Involvement of main stem pulmonary artery
Histologic diagnosis of small cell carcinoma†

* Depending on tumor location and physiologic factors, such tumors may be encompassed in a tolerable radiotherapy port and treated for cure.

† When an asymptomatic pulmonary nodule is resected and found to be small cell carcinoma, adjuvant chemotherapy is recommended.

adjuvant therapy even in stage I disease is obvious if long-term results are to be improved.

STAGING PROCEDURES

Pretreatment staging procedures to be carried out on patients with lung cancer of unknown histology or with non-small cell lung cancer are presented in Table 14-23, while those appropriate for patients with documented small cell cancer are given in Table 14-24.

All patients should have a complete history and physical examination with emphasis on eliciting signs and symptoms of the primary tumor, regional spread, distant metastases, and paraneoplastic syndromes. The staging procedures are directed at these same features as well as determining other medical problems that could complicate the treatment or course of the lung cancer. It is important to be systematic in this staging. On the one hand, a patient may present with what appears to be a solitary pulmonary nodule, but a careful history, physical examination, and brain scan would reveal a brain metastasis. On the other, a patient may present with an obvious liver metastasis but an impending lobar collapse from an endobronchial tumor may be missed and appropriate treatment delayed. In addition, paraneoplastic syndromes can either mimic metastatic disease or debilitate the patient so that what appears to be far advanced malignancy may be curable with local therapy modalities. As a general principle, paraneoplastic syndromes do not make the patient incurable.

Primary Tumor (T Factor)

The primary tumor (T factor) is evaluated by *chest roentgenogram and fiberoptic bronchoscopy.*[163,164] It is obviously important to have high quality roentgenograms to provide the radiologist with the pertinent clinical information and staging questions, and, if possible, to have old chest films available for comparison.[163] The major questions asked of the chest film include what is the size and location of the primary tumor;

TABLE 14-23. Pretreatment Staging Procedures for Lung Cancer Patients

ALL PATIENTS

Complete history, physical examination, and evaluation of all medical problems, including determination of performance status and weight loss
Ear, nose, and throat examination of the upper aerodigestive system
Chest posterior-anterior and lateral roentgenogram
Complete blood count with platelet determination
Routine complete blood chemistries including electrolytes, blood sugar, calcium, phosphorus, renal, and liver function tests
Electrocardiogram (EKG)
Pulmonary function studies and arterial blood gases if signs or symptoms of even minimal respiratory insufficiency are present
Skin tests for tuberculosis
Radionuclide scans of brain, liver, or bone if any of the above studies suggest presence of tumor in these organs; radiographs of any suspicious bony lesions by scan or symptom
Barium swallow radiographic examination if esophageal symptoms are present followed by esophagoscopy if abnormalities are found
Biopsy of any accessible lesions suspicious for cancer if a histologic diagnosis is not yet made or if treatment or staging decisions would be based on whether or not the lesion contained cancer
Routine medical evaluation of any abnormalities detected in the first part of the screen not related to cancer

PATIENTS PRESENTING WITH A SOLITARY PULMONARY NODULE

All of the above plus
Fiberoptic bronchoscopy with washings, brushings, and biopsy of suspicious areas; biopsy of the main carina
Pulmonary function tests, arterial blood gases
Coagulation tests
Transthoracic fine needle aspiration biopsy or transbronchial forceps biopsy of peripheral lesions if material from routine fiberoptic bronchoscopy is negative and patient is a poor surgical candidate

PATIENTS PRESENTING WITH A MASS LESION IN THE CHEST AND NO OBVIOUS CONTRAINDICATION TO A CURATIVE LOCAL APPROACH (SURGERY OR RADIOTHERAPY)

All of above plus
Radionuclide scans of brain, liver, and bone if signs, symptoms, or laboratory abnormalities are detected in these systems
CT scans of areas where regular radionuclide scans are nondiagnostic
Mediastinoscopy or lateral mediastinotomy in individual patients (see text for discussion)

PATIENTS PRESENTING WITH DISEASE THAT IS CONFINED TO THE CHEST BUT NOT RESECTABLE (CANDIDATE FOR CURATIVE RADIOTHERAPY)

All of above (except mediastinoscopy) plus
Transthoracic fine needle aspiration biopsy or transbronchial forceps biopsy of peripheral lesion if material from routine fiberoptic bronchoscopy is negative

PATIENTS PRESENTING WITH DISEASE THAT IS NOT CURABLE BY EITHER SURGERY OR RADIOTHERAPY, ALONE OR TOGETHER*

All under first entry plus
Biopsy of accessible lesions suspicious for tumor to obtain histologic diagnosis; or if therapy would be altered by findings of tumor
Fiberoptic bronchoscopy if indicated by hemoptysis, obstruction, pneumonitis, or no histologic diagnosis of cancer
Tap and cytologic examination of pleural effusion
Transthoracic fine needle aspiration biopsy or transbronchial forceps biopsy of peripheral lesions if material from routine fiberoptic bronchoscopy is negative and no other material exists to make a histologic diagnosis

* Extrathoracic metastatic disease or malignant pleural effusion.

TABLE 14-24. Pretreatment Staging Recommendations for Patients With Histologically Documented Small Cell Carcinoma of the Lung

Complete history and physical examination with performance status determination
Chest posterior-anterior and lateral roentgenograms
Abdominal plain film roentgenogram
Complete blood count including platelet determination
Routine complete blood chemistries including electrolytes, blood sugar, renal and liver function tests, prothrombin time, and partial thromboplastin time
Electrocardiogram (EKG)
Pulmonary function tests and arterial blood gases
Skin tests for tuberculosis
Fiberoptic bronchoscopic examination with washings and biopsies to determine disease extent
Bone marrow biopsy and aspiration
Radionuclide scan of liver, brain, and bone
Roentgenograms of suspicious areas on bone scan
Percutaneous liver biopsy if physical exam or liver function tests are abnormal; if no abnormalities are detected or if percutaneous biopsy is negative, perform peritoneoscopy with multiple liver biopsies if treatment would be altered by liver metastases
Radionuclide brain scan or CT scan if neurologic signs or symptoms present
Cerebrospinal fluid cytology if physical exam or scans indicate CNS tumor involvement
Myelogram if signs or symptoms of spinal cord compression are present
Routine evaluation and correction of any medical problems found on above-mentioned studies

is atelectasis or pneumonitis present and if so, does it involve the entire lung; is a pleural effusion present; is the primary tumor surrounded by lung; and is there evidence of hilar or mediastinal adenopathy, tracheal compression, rib or other bony invasion, contralateral lung or pericardial involvement, or a paralyzed diaphragm?

Pleural effusions can be caused by growth of malignant obtain a positive histologic diagnosis; if positive, this may tumor metastases in mediastinal nodes. The visceral pleura excretes and absorbs fluid by way of pulmonary lymphatics passing into the hilum. The parietal pleura drains through the inferior mediastinal lymphatics. Lymph from both areas goes through the superior mediastinum by way of the thoracic duct, emptying into the venous system. With nodal metastases, the resulting obstruction causes decreased absorption and accumulation of pleural fluid. Thus, any pleural effusion (unless it is caused by obvious congestive heart failure) makes the primary tumor a T3 lesion.[24]

Fiberoptic bronchoscopy defines the most proximal extension of the tumor and excludes bilateral endobronchial disease. A T1 lesion should not have proximal extension beyond the lobar bronchus. To be technically resectable a tumor must not be 2 cm or closer to the carina. Bronchoscopy will establish whether the chest film abnormality is a tumor, or atelectasis and pneumonitis secondary to bronchial obstruction. Biopsy of the carina has yielded evidence of tumor (and thus indicating unresectability) in 10% of patients without gross neoplastic involvement of this area.[165]

Lymphatic Spread (N Factor)

MEDIASTINOSCOPY. The most unfavorable anatomic prognostic factor in lung cancer is primary tumor spread beyond the lung. The first point of tumor cell lodgement is most often the lymph nodes of the hilum, mediastinum, or supraclavicular areas. Biopsy of these nodes may be used to obtain a positive histologic diagnosis; if positive, this may avoid an unnecessary thoracotomy.

At one time, excision biopsy of the prescalene fat pad was extensively used in patients being considered for thoracotomy. When palpable positive lymph nodes are present, biopsy is of course indicated. However, the yield of positive findings in routine study of the prescalene area has been so small that the procedure is generally reserved for particular situations such as patients with advanced roentgenologic findings or those who are poor-risk for major surgical procedures when a histologic diagnosis has not been established by other methods.[166,167] In 1954, Harken and associates extended this procedure deeper into the mediastinum by means of a lighted laryngoscope for exposure and biopsy of mediastinal lymph nodes.[168] Exposure of the pretracheal mediastinum was greatly facilitated by the introduction of a special modified instrument, the mediastinoscope. Mediastinoscopy, done through a small suprasternal incision, is now used extensively.[169] Nevertheless, considerable controversy remains concerning this procedure.[170–171] Some physicians use it almost routinely in all apparent resectable lesions; others believe that it is seldom useful and reserve it to establish the diagnosis in poor-risk patients, or for patients with a hilar mass or mediastinal lymph node enlargement demonstrated on either standard roentgenogram or tomogram. This procedure determines the presence or absence of metastatic tumor in the mediastinal lymph nodes. There is general agreement that involvement of the mediastinal nodes contraindicates surgery except in individual situations discussed later.

In 1966, McNeill and Chamberland described a different approach to the mediastinum using a limited parasternal thoracotomy through the second intercostal space.[172] This procedure, called mediastinotomy, provides a more direct approach to the mediastinal nodes that can be visualized either directly or by use of the mediastinoscope. In addition, when node biopsies are negative and the patient is not a candidate for thoracotomy, primary lung tumors may be biopsied by incising the mediastinal pleura and applying traction to the lung.[172] Mediastinotomy has been more readily accepted when evaluating the left mediastinum since the subaortic and anterior hilar nodes cannot be evaluated through the suprasternal approach. If these procedures are used extensively or routinely, both resectability and survival in those patients undergoing thoracotomy will be greatly increased. However, it must be pointed out that rigid adherence to this practice may well deny a chance of cure to a small percentage of patients. The prudent course followed by most surgeons at this time is selective use of these procedures based on clinical and roentgenologic findings in the individual patient rather than on the routine of the surgeon. None of these procedures visualize the subaortic nodes fully; the posterior subcarinal nodes are not visualized at all. When such involvement is suspected on bronchoscopic examination, transbronchial needle biopsy may be diagnostic.[173]

Standard mediastinoscopy cannot assess tumor involvement in the pericardium, heart, great vessels, posterior subcarinal nodes, anterior mediastinal nodes, and subaortic nodes, which includes locations inaccessible to the mediastinoscope.[174,177]

(Review mediastinal lymph node location in Fig. 14-3.) False negative standard mediastinoscopies are more frequent when the major tumor mass is in the left upper lobe or left hilum. In these cases, mediastinotomy can be performed through a left parasternal approach.[174,177] Mediastinoscopy is usually carried out under general endotracheal anesthesia. The mortality rate from large series is low (less than 0.2–0.04%), and the morbidity rate is less than 1.2–2%.[174,178,179] The specific complications include bleeding; vocal cord paralysis; esophageal perforation; infection in the mediastinum, incision, or lung; bradycardia; tumor seeding in the suture line; myocardial infarction; stroke; and air embolism.[174]

Large series of staging mediastinoscopies for potentially resectable patients have been reviewed and show tumor in the lymph nodes in 27% of epidermoid cancer, 47% of adenocarcinoma, 42% of large cell carcinoma, and 71% of small cell carcinoma for an overall positive rate of 39%.[4,177] In two series totaling 582 patients undergoing mediastinoscopy for potentially resectable disease, positive lymph nodes were found in 30% and 33% of cases. In the lymph node negative cases, the resectability rate was 85% and 90%.[178,179] In many other similar series, the resectability rates following a negative mediastinoscopy range from 83–97%.[174] In addition, no metastases were found in the resected specimens of 49% of 235 resected cases with a previously negative mediastinoscopy while another 29% had surgical–pathologic stage N1 nodes only.[179,180] The type of lymph node involvement found at mediastinosopy has prognostic value. For example, if the lymph node involvement at the time of mediastinoscopy or thoracotomy was intranodal only (a histologic diagnosis), the survival following resection was over 50%; it was less than 5% for resected patients with perinodal involvement.[179] Overall, peripheral tumors had 29% lymph node involvement while central tumors had a 33% involvement, not strikingly different.[179] Even in peripheral adenocarcinomas, 38% of cases had node involvement diagnosed by mediastinoscopy.[179] However, small peripheral lesions 3 cm in diameter or less, without obvious hilar or mediastinal lymph node enlargement on radiograph, had only an 8% positive mediastinoscopy rate. There was no survival difference between 40 patients with these lesions who had mediastinoscopy and 40 who did not.[181] Thus, for small peripheral lesions, patients can go straight to thoracotomy without a mediastinoscopy.

^{67}GALLIUM CITRATE SCANNING. ^{67}Gallium citrate is frequently concentrated in lung cancer. Scanning with this agent has been used to stage lung cancer patients.[6,182,183] Gallium uptake occurs in 80–96% of primary lung cancers.[180,183] If the primary chest tumor is gallium positive, and the mediastinum or contralateral hilar area is gallium positive, there is a 90–100% probability that the nodes contain tumor. If the primary tumor is gallium positive, and the mediastinum or contralateral hilar areas are negative, there is a 67–71% chance that the nodes do not contain tumor.[6,183] Likewise, if the primary tumor is positive there is a 90% probability that any extrathoracic uptake of gallium represents a metastatic lesion; 30% of these extrathoracic lesions will be clinically occult.[6] These results have led Golomb and DeMeester to propose a sequential staging program for lung cancer where gallium scanning is applied after the initial clinical evaluation.[6,180]

COMPUTED TOMOGRAPHY. Computed tomography (CT) of the thorax is being investigated as a staging procedure. Early results would indicate that it gives information on mediastinal or pleural extension of tumor.[184,185] It appears that CT scans, if positive, predict mediastinal node involvement in a large fraction of cases. However, a negative study does not exclude mediastinal involvement. When CT scanning was prospectively compared to mediastinoscopy or surgical pathologic results in 44 patients (57% of whom had proven nodal disease) there were 25–36% false negatives and 2% false positives found.[185,186] When comparing CT scans with regular tomography, conventional tomograms are more sensitive for determining the presence of mediastinal involvement. Pleural nodules, effusions, and masses are better delineated by a CT scan.[185] Until more data are available that prospectively compare CT scans with surgical–pathologic findings, CT scans for staging purposes should be used with caution and are not yet a routinely recommended part of preoperative staging.

OTHER INDIRECT TESTS OF MEDIASTINAL-HILAR NODAL INVOLVEMENT WITH TUMOR. A variety of indirect tests including mediastinal tomograms, esophagrams, pulmonary angiograms, and azygograms have been used to determine mediastinal lymph node involvement or involvement of great vessels.[187,188] Unfortunately, there is poor correlation between findings of the indirect tests and findings at mediastinoscopy.[178] This is particularly true for mediastinal tomograms where the false positive and false negative rates are both 30–40%.[178] At present, without mediastinoscopy, biopsy, or other histologic proof of nonresectability it is unwise to reject a patient for curative treatment based on tomograms, angiograms, or venograms alone.

Perfusion lung scans with macroaggregated albumin have shown that a perfusion defect larger than the mass lesion on radiograph has an 84% chance of having tumor in hilar nodes and a 58% chance of having tumor in mediastinal nodes, while those without such a large defect have only 23% chance of regional and 6% chance of mediastinal node involvement.[189] B mode gray scale echography (sonography) is useful in determining whether a large area of radiographic opacification such as an opaque hemithorax is due to fluid, tumor, or intrinsic pulmonary disease such as obstruction or consolidation.[190]

Staging Procedure for Distant Metastases (M Factor)

The value of ^{67}gallium scanning for detecting metastases discussed above appears to be useful. Routine radionuclide scans of brain, liver, and bone, or skeletal roentgen surveys and bone marrow biopsies (with the exception of small cell carcinoma) are only positive in 5–10% of patients without signs or symptoms referable to these organ systems.[191–195] If these scans are used to evaluate patients with potentially resectable non-small cell lung cancer not suspected of having metastases after initial clinical evaluation, the rate falls to less than 1% for brain, liver, and bone scans.[196] In addition, there is a significant false positive rate when the scan lesions are investigated by other clinical means.[196] Thus, current recommendations made by the authors are to perform radionuclide brain, liver, and bone scans, or skeletal surveys, only if there is other clinical evidence to suggest the possibility of metastases. A careful history and physical examination remain the best screening tools for detecting distant metastases.

Biopsy of the bone marrow and liver in patients with non-small cell carcinomas and no other clinical evidence pointing to metastases is positive in 10–15% or less of cases.[197–199] Therefore, the authors do not recommend routine biopsy of these sites unless some other clinical evidence points to the possibility of metastases.

PHYSIOLOGIC STAGING OF THE PATIENT

Assessment of the patient's physiologic and performance status is critical in order to determine the patient's ability to tolerate thoracotomy and pulmonary resection, aggressive radiotherapy, or intensive chemotherapy. Patients with lung cancer often present with cardiopulmonary problems related to chronic pulmonary disease or their age. Many studies have been performed to assess the ability to tolerate general anesthesia and pulmonary surgery, including whether pneumonectomy or lobectomy can be undertaken. The essence of this preoperative physiologic evaluation is to determine which patients can survive the surgery with reasonable operative mortality and still be functional post resection.[156,161,200] However, it is not always possible to predict whether a lobectomy or a pneumonectomy will be required until the time of surgery. The conservative approach tends to restrict resectional surgery to patients who could potentially tolerate a pneumonectomy. As yet, there are no similar data for physiologic staging of patients before curative radiotherapy–high dose combination chemotherapy, or combined chemoradiotherapy, but as these regimens become more intense similar guidelines to those for surgery must be applied.

PERFORMANCE STATUS, AGE, AND SEX

Performance status (PS) is an important prognostic factor. Patients who are fully ambulatory and either asymptomatic (PS = 0) or symptomatic (PS = 1) tolerate surgery or aggressive chemoradiotherapy better than those who are not fully ambulatory but out of bed more than 50% of the time (PS = 2). These patients do better than those who are ambulatory less than 50% of the time (PS = 3) and those patients who are bedridden (PS = 4). When other medical problems are identified and corrected (including nutritional status, anemia, electrolyte disorders, dehydration and infection), the performance status will also improve.[156,161,201]

The combination of a serious reduction in the patient's pulmonary reserve and significant cardiovascular, hepatic, or renal disease or poor performance status is a major contraindication to resectional pulmonary surgery.[156,201] While by definition patients who are candidates for resection will appear to have disease limited to the chest, many of them will have the symptoms and the presence of reduced performance status, weight loss, systemic symptoms, or anorexia, which suggest a poor prognosis. Stanley analyzed 77 prognostic factors in over 5000 patients with "inoperable" lung cancer entered onto Veteran's Administration Lung Group (VALG) protocols between 1968 and 1978.[202] The most important prognostic factors, in order of importance, were initial performance status, extent of disease, weight loss greater than 10 pounds in the previous 6 months, and the presence of any systemic symptoms (see Tables 14-25 and 14-26). The contribution of other factors (*i.e.*, tumor size and histologic type) were minor after correction for the major prognostic features, particularly performance status. Interestingly enough, age had no prognostic impact. While operative mortality is greater for older patients, the operative mortality in selected cases for patients over 70-years-old is not greater than the expected mortality for younger patients.[202a] Thus, it is of importance to assess the patient's physiologic rather than chronologic age when making borderline decisions.

In the U.S., female patients with lung cancer tend to have better survival rates than males (see Table 14-27). This is not explained by age, resectability, operative mortality, histopathology, location of the tumor, or differences in tumor stage between the sexes.[203–205] The difference is particularly marked

TABLE 14-25. Influence of Pretreatment Performance Status on Patients with Inoperable Lung Cancer*

PERFORMANCE STATUS SCALE				
ECOG† (Zubrod)	KARNOFSKY	DEFINITIONS	MEDIAN SURVIVAL (Weeks)	PERCENTAGE OF PATIENTS IN GROUP
0	100	Asymptomatic	34	2
1	80–90	Symptomatic, fully ambulatory	24–27	32
2	60–70	Symptomatic, in bed less than 50% of day	14–21	40
3	40–50	Symptomatic, in bed more than 50% of the day, but not bedridden	7–9	22
4	20–30	Bedridden	3–5	5

(Stanley KE: Prognostic factors for survival in patients with inoperable lung cancer. J Natl Cancer Inst 65:25–32, 1980)

* N = 5,022 males with "inoperable" lung cancer of all histologic types entered onto VALG protocols from 1968–1978.

† Eastern Cooperative Oncology Group (ECOG) or Zubrod performance status score.

TABLE 14-26. Influence of Various Pretreatment Variables on the Survival of Patients with Inoperable Lung Cancer*

VARIABLE	MEDIAN SURVIVAL (Weeks)	PERCENTAGE OF PATIENTS WITH VARIABLE
STAGE OF DISEASE		
Limited disease	28	21
Extensive disease	13	79
WEIGHT LOSS		
Less than 10 lb	22	52
More than 10 lb	11	48
PRESENCE OF SYSTEMIC SYMPTOMS		
No	28	49
Yes	15	51
REDUCED APPETITE		
No	27	53
Yes	15	47
INITIAL LYMPHOCYTE COUNT		
Over 2,000 per μl	16	42
Less than 1,000 per μl	8	19
ANY METASTATIC DISEASE SYMPTOMS		
No	22	64
Yes	15	36
SCALENE OR SUPRACLAVICULAR NODE INVOLVEMENT		
No	22	83
Yes	14	17

(Stanley KE: Prognostic factors for survival in patients with inoperable lung cancer. J Natl Cancer Inst 65:25–32, 1980)

* Limited stage disease is defined by VALG criteria as disease confined to one hemithorax with or without scalene or supraclavicular node involvement, while extensive stage disease is all disease beyond one hemithorax and the ipsilateral supraclavicular nodes.

in female patients with localized disease who undergo surgical resection (see Table 14-27). For unknown reasons, the prognosis for women is worse than that for men in Wales and England, and possibly worse in France, even after surgical resection of localized disease.[206]

CARDIAC STATUS

The signs or symptoms of a myocardial infarction in a patient with lung cancer in the past 6 months should be sought by the physician and serial EKGs reviewed. The presence of an infarct in this period would be a contraindication to surgery, and a documented infarct within the past 3 months is an absolute contraindication to thoracic surgery. Over 20% of such patients will die of a complication related to reinfarction alone.[156,207] About 10–15% of all patients evaluated for lung cancer surgery will have definitive EKG abnormalities. All cardiac arrhythmias should be identified and, if possible, corrected; serum potassium deficits and calcium excess should be identified and corrected as well, since these can potentiate digitalis toxicity and anesthetic hazard.[165,201] Uncontrolled major arrhythmias, such as multifocal premature ventricular contractions, carry a high-risk factor and will usually contraindicate surgery. Bundle branch block is not a contraindication to surgery. However, in estimating risk, a right bundle branch block or a left anterior fascicular block has less risk for the patient than a left posterior fascicular block, while combination and bifascicular blocks put the patient at greatest risk.[156] A history of angina by itself is not necessarily a contraindication to pulmonary resection. In patients with lung cancers that are otherwise favorable for resection, particularly by a conservative procedure, coronary arteriography can be done. In some cases where the coronary disease is deemed surgically correctable, simultaneous tumor resection and coronary bypass may be considered.[156]

PULMONARY FUNCTION STATUS

The assessment of pulmonary function status is of greatest importance in deciding whether or not the patient can tolerate pulmonary resection and how great a resection may be carried out. If possible, it is important to get the prospective patient to stop smoking, in order to treat any acute or chronic bronchitis or other pulmonary conditions and to start pulmonary physiotherapy, all of which may partially increase pulmonary function. Pulmonary function tests are important predictors of the patient's ability to withstand surgery. Measures of maximum air flow are the most reliable and significant index of the ability to tolerate pulmonary surgery.[156,208] Patients with maximum breathing capacities (MBC) of less than 40% predicted prior to pulmonary resection will have a near 100% fatal cardiopulmonary impairment postoperatively, while 90% of patients with an MBC greater than 40% will survive.[208] If

TABLE 14-27. Comparison of Survival Rates of Men and Women with Lung Cancer*

STAGE OF DISEASE	TIME PERIOD	5-YEAR SURVIVAL PERCENTAGE		REFERENCES
		MALE	FEMALE	
NCI SURVEILLANCE, EPIDEMIOLOGY, AND END RESULTS PROGRAM				(1, 2)
All stages	1965–1969	8	13	
Localized		28	51	
Regional spread		10	15	
LOCALIZED DISEASE, POSTSURGICAL RESECTION				
	1949–1962	29	49	(203)
	1950–1959	35	68	(204, 205)

* The number of patients in each group is over 1000.

the FEV_1 (forced expiratory volume in 1 sec) is 2.5 liters or more, the patient can tolerate pneumonectomy; if the FEV_1 is less than 1 liter, the patient cannot tolerate any loss of functional lung tissue; and, if the FEV_1 falls between 1.1 and 2.4 liters of flow, the risk of any resection and the maximum tolerable resection are judgmental and require further study.[156] Pulmonary resection is usually possible if the FEV_1 is greater than 50% of the total forced vital capacity (or greater than 2 liters); if the maximum voluntary ventilation (MVV) is greater than 50% of the predicted capacity and if the $PaCO_2$ is normal.[209,210] Patients with preoperative CO_2 retention cannot probably tolerate any loss of functioning pulmonary tissue.[156] Thus, abnormalities of $PaCO_2$ are more significant than abnormalities of PaO_2, since the former can result only from alveolar hypoventilation while the latter may result from an admixture of venous and arterial blood in the tumor area.[211] Many patients who appear marginal surgical risks may readily tolerate even extended resection if the burden of the ventilatory defect is in the tumor-bearing lung. If major shunting occurs on the affected side, these patients may have their pulmonary function and arterial blood gases improve after resection.[156] In patients with borderline pulmonary status or questionable pulmonary hypertension, split pulmonary function testing by bronchospirometry and right heart catheterization study with temporary unilateral pulmonary artery occlusion can define physiologic resectability.[210,212] Criteria of operability in these patients would be a mean pulmonary artery pressure after occlusion and exercise of less than 24 mm Hg, a systemic PaO_2 under similar conditions of greater than 45 mm Hg, and a predicted postpneumonectomy FEV_1 greater than 0.8 liters (where the predicted FEV_1 = the preoperative FEV_1 $\times$ the fraction of total perfusion to the contralateral lung).[210]

Radiospirometry using ^{132}Xe gas also allows regional pulmonary function studies so that ratios of perfusion and ventilation of unit volumes can be determined.[156,213] Pneumonectomy is functionally tolerable if the percentage of ventilation to the non-tumor-bearing lung when multiplied by the FEV_1 equals one liter or more of flow.[156] In contrast, if the volume of the normal lung exceeds its ventilation by more than 5%, there is a great chance of postpneumonectomy ventilatory failure.[156]

Influence of Other Factors on Survival

A comparison of the percentage of localized disease and survival rates as a function of race, socioeconomic status, and Veteran's Administration status has been made in male patients treated between 1955–1964.[213a] There was no significant difference between VA status, whites, blacks, indigent vs. nonindigent income status, or private vs. non-private patient status in the percentage of localized disease or survival. Thus, the biology of the disease appears to be more important than differences in natural history, detection, or treatment imposed by race or socioeconomic status.

An interesting association of increased one-year survival in non-small cell lung cancer correlated with the presence of HLA antigens of the AW19 and B5 complexes has also been reported.[213b]

STAGING OF PATIENTS WITH SMALL-CELL LUNG CANCER

In patients who have histologic or cytologic evidence indicating small-cell lung cancer, a different staging system and approach to staging procedures are used (see (Table 14-24). This is because the primary treatment modality will be chemotherapy with or without radiotherapy. In the uncommon case of a resected pulmonary nodule that turns out to be small-cell carcinoma, these staging procedures should also be employed.

Mountain, in review of 268 small-cell lung cancer patients for the AJC staging system, found no difference in survival for small-cell lung cancer for over 40 characteristics including sex; age; peripheral, central, or apical location; radiographic appearance; size of the lesion (including tumors less than 3 cm in diameter); presence, absence, or degree of atelectasis; pneumonitis; pleural effusion; mediastinal invasion; regional lymph node involvement; or presence or absence of distant metastases (see Table 14-28). There was no significant difference in 41 resected patients by postsurgical groups I, II, or III in survival; none were cured.[214] Because the TNM factors did not appear to be prognostic for survival in small-cell cancer patients treated predominantly with surgery or radiotherapy, the AJC initially recommended applying their system to small-cell cancer only for purposes of later reference. Because of the current advances in chemotherapy with or without radiotherapy, the AJC now recommends the general application of its system.[24] However, nearly all investigators

TABLE 14-28. Frequency of TNM Findings at Diagnosis in the AJC Group of Small Cell Lung Cancer Patients

	PERCENTAGE OF PATIENTS (N = 368)
Asymptomatic at diagnosis	6
Tumor location	
Hilar	68
Peripheral	12
Apical	2
Mainstem bronchus	17
Tumor size	
Less than 3 cm	20
Greater than 3 cm	80
Atelectasis/pneumonitis	
None	35
Segmental	43
Lobar	18
Entire lung	4
Pleural effusion	15
Clinical evidence of	
Mediastinal invasion	30
Metastases outside the hemithorax of origin and the mediastinum (M1)	48
Scalene or supraclavicular node involvement	30
Regional lymph node involvement clinically by radiograph	
N0	27
N1 (hilar)	26
N2 (mediastinal)	47

(Mountain CF: Clinical biology of small cell carcinoma: Relationship to surgical therapy. Semin Oncol 5:272–279, 1978)

studying the treatment of small-cell lung cancer have adopted the simple two-stage system of the VALG.[215]

In the two-stage system, *limited stage disease* is defined as disease confined to one hemithorax and to the regional lymph nodes (including mediastinal and contralateral hilar, and usually ipsilateral supraclavicular), while *extensive stage disease* is defined as disease beyond this (including distant lymph nodes, brain, liver, bone, bone marrow, and intra-abdominal and soft tissue metastases). The definition of stage relates to whether the known tumor can be encompassed within a tolerable radiation therapy port. Thus, ipsilateral pleural effusion, recurrent laryngeal nerve involvement, and superior vena caval obstruction can all still be considered limited stage disease. However, cardiac tamponade and bilateral pulmonary parenchymal involvement are generally scored as extensive stage disease because of the size of the radiation therapy port required to encompass all known disease, particularly if given with cytotoxic agents such as adriamycin.

Limited stage patients have both higher response rates and longer survival than extensive stage patients given identical or similar therapy.[216–223] In trials of combination chemotherapy with or without radiotherapy, patients classified as limited stage had a 86% total objective tumor regression rate, a 60% rate of complete clinical regression of tumor (complete response), and a median survival of 51 weeks. In contrast, patients scored as extensive stage had a 77% total response rate, a 25% complete response rate, and 33 weeks median survival.[216] Occasionally, similar response rates have been observed for both stages with stage predicting only survival differences.[224–226] The durability of the response is probably unaffected by stage. However, long-term survival in complete responders usually is reported to be superior in limited stage disease.[221,223]

While higher complete response rates are reported in limited versus extensive stage disease there are subsets of extensive stage patients who do as well as limited stage patients. In a review of 106 patients entered on NCI trials, extensive disease stage patients with only a single site of metastasis (outside of those included in the definition of limited stage disease) had indistinguishable survival from limited stage patients.[217] This group represents 33% of all patients and is thus clinically significant. In addition, in limited stage patients, neither ipsilateral nor contralateral supraclavicular lymph nodes influenced survival.[217,223] However, involvement of either the liver or central nervous system (CNS) presages an especially unfavorable outcome.[217] It is debatable whether the presence of a pleural effusion affects survival.[217,227]

Initial performance status strongly influences survival both in untreated patients and in patients receiving combination chemotherapy with or without radiotherapy.[215–217,222,228,229] While more favorable performance status occurs more frequently in limited stage patients, within either stage, performance status is the most important variable.[217,221,222,223] Also, in extensive stage patients a strong correlation exists between worsening performance status and the number of sites of metastatic disease, suggesting that the prognostic effect of performance status may largely be accounted for by its association with overall tumor burden.[217] In contrast, in patients treated with intensive combination chemotherapy there is no significant influence on survival of age, sex, previous pulmonary resection, or pretreatment total lymphocyte count.[217,222,225,228,230]

Patients may or may not be symptomatic from small-cell carcinoma metastatic sites. CNS metastases are symptomatic and clinically important in over 90% of instances. While bone metastases may be painful, they are not in the majority of patients, and pathologic fractures are rare. Liver metastases cause (usually mild) dysfunction of laboratory tests in 50–60% of cases with liver involvement but in only a few of these cases is liver function seriously impaired. Usually the liver involvement causes problems by its mass and overall contribution to tumor bulk and decreased performance status. Anemia, leukopenia, or thrombocytopenia related to bone marrow involvement is uncommon and hemoglobin and white cell levels are not indicative of marrow involvement.[62,230] During intensive induction chemotherapy, patients with positive bone marrows have more severe infections and require more red blood cell transfusions than patients without tumor in the marrow. However, leukopenia, thrombocytopenia, and the need for platelet transfusions during induction therapy do not appear to correlate with marrow involvement.[62]

The procedures the authors recommend for staging patients with small-cell lung cancer are listed in Table 14-24. The frequency of positive studies is listed in Table 14-29. The purpose of the studies is to document sites of disease before treatment and their response to therapy, and to assist in follow-up as recurrence appears to be primarily in sites of bulk disease.[236] The initial therapy (combination chemotherapy with or without radiotherapy) these patients will be

TABLE 14-29. Results of Pretreatment Staging Procedures in Small Cell Lung Cancer

FINAL STAGE	PERCENTAGE OF PATIENTS WITH FINDING	REFERENCES
Limited stage	31	(217)
Extensive stage	69	
CHEST STAGING		
Chest film mass	90	(60)
Fiberoptic bronchoscopy		(60)
Visual endobronchial tumor	83	
Washings/biopsy histocytologically positive	87	
Pleural effusion	9	(217)
Ipsilateral supraclavicular node	6	(217)
Contralateral lung	7	(217)
Bilateral endobronchial tumor	5	(217)
Bone (bone scan)	38	(217)
Liver (histologically proven by biopsy)	22–28	(217,231)
Bone marrow	17–23	(62,217,232,233)
(Ratio of positivity—aspiration: biopsy = 3:1; bilateral: unilateral biopsy = 2.2:1)		
Central nervous system	8–14	(217,230,234)
Brain	10	
Spinal	5	
Leptomeningeal	2	
Retroperitoneal metastases (CT scan)	16	(235)
Soft tissue, biopsy proven	24	(217)

Between 100 and 600 patients for each category

undergoing is, in many respects, as demanding as thoracotomy and pulmonary resection. Thus, physiologic as well as anatomic staging is required. The intensity of the initial therapy and the combined use of chemotherapy and aggressive radiotherapy produce induction mortality rates of 5% or more in many recent series. The most important factor appears to be the initial performance status. Although there are only few data from recent trials it would appear prudent to submit to aggressive induction therapy only those patients who are ambulatory more than 50% of the time and who have adequate cardiopulmonary, renal, and hepatic function. This is particularly true because drug metabolism may be altered by impaired renal or liver function, because most of the patients develop leukopenia and fever during induction therapy, and because moderate to severe cardiac and pulmonary toxicity is increasingly common with aggressive regimens.

The primary tumor and regional nodal spread are evaluated by chest posterior–anterior and lateral roentgenograms. In addition, fiberoptic bronchoscopy with bronchial washings and biopsy are essential to document the extent of disease, in addition to determining the degree and maintenance of tumor response during follow-up. Prior to treatment, fiberoptic bronchoscopy will reveal evidence of cancer in over 90% of cases including approximately 8–10% in whom the tumor is not evaluable on the chest film.[61] In follow-up patients with evidence of tumor, by restaging the bronchoscopy after initial therapy they have a much higher relapse rate in the chest within a 6 month period than patients with normal bronchoscopy at this time.[61]

The common sites of extrathoracic metastatic disease detected during pretreatment staging are bone in 38%, liver in 22–28%, bone marrow in 17–23%, and the CNS in 8–14%.[217,230] Bone metastases are best found with bone scans, while radiographic bone surveys have a low yield if the patient is asymptomatic.[230] If a bone scan abnormality is the sole site of metastatic disease and if the presence of this site would alter therapy, further evaluation of the site should be made with routine radiographs, obtaining a history of trauma, and (in selected cases) a needle biopsy of the site. After treatment, osteoblastic changes can sometimes be seen on bone radiographs. They probably represent regeneration of bone and not new metastases.[230] Thus, unless some other evidence of tumor progression exists, such changes should alone not be an indication for changing therapy. Bone marrow involvement is found with bone marrow aspiration and biopsy; often, the two procedures are complementary such that aspiration will be positive when the biopsy is not and vice versa.[230] Approximately 10% additional patients (30% of all positive marrows) will have bone marrow involvement if bilateral biopsies are done.[230] If the liver by physical exam appears grossly involved or if liver function tests are abnormal, a percutaneous needle biopsy is indicated. However, while liver function tests are abnormal in 93% of patients whose livers are histologically positive for tumor, they are also abnormal in 41% of patients with histologically negative livers.[230] Both false positive and false negative liver radionuclide scans are seen in small-cell cancer. Currently, the best way to detect all patients with liver metastases is with multiple biopsies at peritoneoscopy.[230,231,236a] If an initial percutaneous biopsy is negative and therapy would be altered by liver metastasis, the authors currently recommend proceeding to peritoneoscopy and multiple liver biopsies. Contraindications to obtaining liver biopsy confirmation are bleeding disorders, a patient unable to cooperate, massive pleural effusion, or respiratory decompensation so that the procedure cannot be tolerated.

CNS metastases are best documented by history and physical examination, followed by radionuclide brain or CT scans.[234,237] Routine radionuclide brain scans are only positive in 4% of asymptomatic patients; the value of CT scanning in asymptomatic patients is still being investigated.[234,236a] However, CT scans appear to detect a few lesions in symptomatic patients that conventional scans miss.[234] At present, in truly asymptomatic patients, after careful neurologic examination, the only indication for a radionuclide scan would be just prior to administration of prophylactic cranial irradiation. If asymptomatic lesions were discovered, a higher dose of radiotherapy would be delivered.[234,237]

CNS metastases can be intracranial, spinal epidural with spinal cord compression, or leptomeningeal with carcinomatous meningitis.[234,237] Screening asymptomatic patients with cerebrospinal fluid (CSF) cytologies is unrewarding.[234,237] However, it is important to know that once one site of CNS metastatic disease is discovered, the probability of finding metastatic disease at other CNS sites is greatly increased. Clinically apparent multiple sites are discovered in 20% of patients with CNS metastases and in 73% of such patients at autopsy.[237] Patients suspected of having spinal cord compression should promptly undergo a myelogram. Likewise, patients with signs and symptoms of leptomeningeal involvement should have CSF cytologies performed. However, both of these groups, as well as the patients with documented intracranial metastases, should have brain scans and CSF cytologies. Any indication of back pain, vertebral body bone scan, radiograph or minimal neurologic abnormalities suggesting an epidural lesion in the presence of an intracranial metastasis or carcinomatous leptomeningitis should be an indication for a myelogram.

Because of the high frequency of intra-abdominal metastases found at autopsy in the adrenals, pancreas, kidneys and lymph nodes, pretreatment staging of these areas would be useful (see Table 14-13).[28] In the future, abdominal CT scanning may be useful for such staging, but its general use in screening is not currently recommended. Upper abdominal CT scans performed prospectively reveal evidence of metastases in 36% of patients.[235] The most common site is the liver, while retroperitoneal metastases are found in 16%. The CT scan has a sensitivity of approximately 88% and a specificity of 94% compared with biopsy results.[235]

TREATMENT OF PATIENTS WITH LUNG CANCER BY SURGERY OR RADIOTHERAPY ADMINISTERED WITH CURATIVE INTENT

SURGICAL TREATMENT

Although a number of partial pulmonary resections for malignant lung disease had been recorded earlier, the first successful total pneumonectomy for bronchogenic carcinoma was performed by Graham in 1933.[17,18] The patient, a 48-year-old physician, not only survived the operation but continued in his medical practice for many years. Gradually, the development of modern technical methods brought pulmonary resection to its present level of safety. Preoperative assessment of both cardiopulmonary status and extent of disease of the lung cancer patient has improved greatly over recent years and enables most patients to avoid unnecessary thoracotomy and to withstand the operation with minimal risk. Performance of lobectomies rather than pneumonectomies has also reduced mortality. The modern anesthetic techniques of controlled respiration using a cuffed intratracheal tube, which today seems such a simple matter, evolved slowly. Simultaneously, the development of antimicrobial drugs, the ready availability of adequate blood replacement, along with immeasurably better support of the patient during the postoperative period, have contributed greatly to the safety of thoracic surgical procedures. At the time of the first successful pulmonary resection, the incidence of lung cancer was small compared with other major malignancies. Unfortunately, technical developments in the field of pulmonary surgery were paralleled by the alarming worldwide increase in incidence and mortality from lung cancer.

Selection of Patients For Surgical Treatment

Although careful assessment of the patient makes it possible to avoid unnecessary thoracotomy on the patient whose disease has progressed beyond the point of a possible cure, it must be strongly emphasized that surgical resection currently offers the best hope of cure in non-small cell lung cancer (NSCLC). This possible chance must not be denied unless there be unquestioned evidence to the contrary. Certain absolute contraindications to operation are generally accepted (see Table 14-22). However, under some circumstances, the palliative removal of a primary tumor may be justifiable to accomplish symptomatic relief of distressing complications such as bleeding, infection, or severe cough. Relative contraindications to thoracotomy are the presence of phrenic nerve involvement, as evidenced by paralysis of the diaphragm, and the presence of proven metastatic tumor in the ipsilateral mediastinal lymph nodes. Involvement of the chest wall or the presence of a Pancoast (superior sulcus) syndrome, while generally indicative of incurability, is not an absolute contraindication for operation. The combination of preoperative radiotherapy and resection for superior sulcus tumors as well as en bloc resection when other peripheral tumors have invaded the chest wall have resulted in sufficient numbers of long-term cures to justify operative intervention in selected patients.[238,248] As discussed earlier, patients with severe cardiac disease, recent myocardial infarction, or those with severe impairment of ventilatory function may not be candidates for operation if it can be determined that they will not tolerate the procedure. However, it is rare that advanced age alone or the presence of concurrent systemic disease is absolute contraindication to surgical exploration. Thus, the common major contraindications involve the anatomic extent of tumor and the histologic type.

Considerable discussion continues regarding the advisability of operation for patients with ipsilateral mediastinal lymph nodes.[23] Certainly the enlargement of these nodes on roentgenogram is not sufficient to preclude operation. Reports of 5-year survivals following resection and postoperative radiotherapy (discussed later in this chapter) when there is involvement of mediastinal nodes are sufficient, indicating that clinical judgement must be used in determining resectability even when such nodes are involved with cancer.

Patients with small-cell (oat cell) carcinoma have a very poor prognosis after resection alone. When this diagnosis is established the patient is, for the most part, not a candidate for surgical treatment. Yet, there may still be a selected role for surgery. When histologic proof is not obtained prior to thoracotomy in a peripheral lesion, certainly the appropriate resection should be carried out. In a large group of such patients with asymptomatic solitary pulmonary nodules, 5-year survival in patients with small-cell carcinoma was essentially the same as for the other cell types. A series (over 100 patients) of long-term small cell cancer survivors collected by Matthews in the NCI registry gives ample evidence that surgery can be effective in a highly selected segment of patients with this cell type who present atypically with a peripheral node.[239]

Any patient in the lung cancer age group with a non-determinant lung lesion, however small, which is undiagnosed by other methods should have thoracotomy, especially if there is a history of smoking. Following this approach and avoiding undue delay has resulted in increasing numbers of lung cancers less than 1 cm in diameter being resected with a higher prospect of cure. The Veterans Administration and Armed Services Hospitals conducted a combined study of asymptomatic solitary pulmonary nodules less than 6 cm in diameter.[240] Considering all ages, 35% of the nodules proved to be malignant; 86% of these were primary bronchogenic carcinomas. In patients over 50 years of age, 56% of the nodules were malignant. However, a significant number of lung cancer nodules had widespread disease at operation, and the observed five-year survival rate in patients with primary cancer was only 38%, emphasizing a tendency to early systemic involvement even in this apparently favorable group of patients with lung cancer. As a result of this study and others corroborating these findings, a more aggressive attitude toward the small indeterminate lung lesion has been pursued by many centers with consequently greater numbers of small lesions being resected.

TECHNICAL CONSIDERATIONS

The selection of the appropriate surgical procedure in resectable patients is determined by the size of the tumor, its anatomic extent, and the physiologic status of the patient. The actual extent of resection remains a matter of surgical judgement based on the findings at exploration. The surgeon should follow a procedure that will include all known disease and allow for the maximum conservation of lung tissue.[156] When conservative resection is technically feasible and encompasses all known tumor, the disease-free interval is equal to that obtained with more extensive procedures in patients of equivalent disease status.[156]

For many years, it was widely held that total pneumonectomy with dissection of the hilar nodes should always be carried out, even when the lesion was a small peripheral nodule. However, this concept was questioned as long ago as 1950 by Churchill and associates, who pointed out that not only does pneumonectomy (particularly on the right side) involve a higher short-term risk of morbidity and mortality, but there is a higher long-term risk of cardiopulmonary problems than when a smaller resection is performed.[241] When lesions are confined to one lobe and there are no demonstrable lymph nodes present, lobectomy is now considered the operation of choice by most surgeons.[242] In a large series of patients followed by the Veterans Administration Surgical Oncology Group (VASOG), long-term survival was essentially the same following lobectomy as for pneumonectomy.[243] However, it must be pointed out that the merits of the two procedures cannot be determined based on survival rates. The anatomic features of lesions suitable for a less radical operation introduce a selective factor that screens out patients with far advanced lesions. Each patient should be judged individually as to the extent and type of lesion, the operative risk, and pulmonary reserve. Thus, when there is an option, lobectomy is preferred over pneumonectomy.

Wedge resections and segmentectomies are usually reserved for patients with poor pulmonary reserve and small peripheral (3 cm or less) lesions.[156] The VASOG reported a small number of patients with lung cancer who had been treated by segmental or wedge resection.[243] This study and studies by Jensik and others have indicated that minimal resections may be selectively used in the treatment of bronchial carcinoma in patients with small peripheral tumors without lymph node involvement.[243,244]

In all cases, the decision to resect for cure should provide that no residual disease is anticipated. Exceptions to this rule would include patients in investigational studies with adjuvant therapy. Candidates for curative resection are thus all patients with clinical AJC stage I and stage II disease. Lobectomy is indicated for lesions totally confined within a lobe, so as to permit 1 cm or more of normal lobar bronchus proximally. In addition, there should be no gross evidence of lymph node involvement central to the origin of the lobar bronchus. Careful attention should be paid to en bloc dissection of the regional lymph nodes. In addition, frozen-section studies must be available during the course of surgery to guide an adequate resection. Pneumonectomy is indicated if more extensive involvement is found.[156]

For patients who are stage III M0 (no distant metastases) preoperatively (clinical stage), or if this stage becomes apparent during the surgical exploration, individual decisions must be made. One reasonable approach is to proceed with a curative resection in those physiologically able to tolerate the surgery in whom both the primary tumor is deemed technically resectable and the extent of nodal involvement is limited to the ipsilateral tracheobronchial angle or subcarinal space.[161] Resection may be attempted if there is more cephalad extension of tumor in ipsilateral peritracheal nodes; however, the outcome will depend on whether the nodal capsules are intact and whether the most peripheral nodes are microscopically free of metastatic disease.[161] In such cases, most radiotherapists believe postoperative irradiation would be indicated.

Although pulmonary resection can be carried out with the patient in either the face down or face up position using posterior or anterior thoracotomy, the most frequent procedure by far is to place the patient on his side with the lesion uppermost (see Fig. 14-12). There should always be current chest films available in the OR to be reviewed by the surgeon prior to beginning the procedure. The standard posterolateral thoracotomy incision begins just below the nipple in front, curving posteriorly below the tip of the scapula and extending slightly cephalad almost to the vertebral column behind. Following division of the intervening muscles, the thoracic cavity can be entered either by resecting a long portion of rib, usually the 5th, or by an intercostal incision (in which case a rib above and below may be transected to permit wider exposure). Assessment of the lesion can then be made, along with careful examination for any hilar or mediastinal lymph nodes. If frozen section diagnosis is to be done, small lesions can be resected *in toto* by wedge resection. The mechanical stapling device is an effective and quick method of accomplishing this type of excision.

Dissection, Ligation, and Division of Pulmonary Vessels

Whether segmental resection, lobectomy, or pneumonectomy is to be carried out, individual isolation, ligation, and division of the pulmonary vessels are indicated. In accomplishing this dissection, it must be kept in mind that these vessels are short and cannot be delivered into the wound as in other areas of the body. Because of their size, length, location, and fragility, injury during dissection may cause massive hemorrhage, which is extremely difficult to control; tears into these vessels will tend to extend. For these reasons, extreme care must be used in dissection and special methods of ligation are indicated. Fortunately, these vessels are enclosed by a layer of perivascular adventitial tissue in most instances, which separates readily from the vessel wall; this cleavage plan can be developed to secure an adequate length of vessel for ligation (see Fig. 14-13). It is customary to secure the pulmonary vessels by both ligature and suture ligature to prevent roll-off of the ties. Many surgeons prefer to secure the vessel with a non-crushing vascular clamp and oversew the ends of these sizable vessels. In certain instances when dissection of the pulmonary vessels in the pleural cavity is difficult or impossible because of extensive inflammatory reaction or encroachment by the tumor, the pericardium can be divided and the pulmonary vessels can be dissected, ligated, and divided inside the pericardial sac. Some surgeons prefer to secure these vessels with non-crushing vascular clamps and oversew the divided end of the vessel rather than depend on a circular ligature. The mechanical stapling device has been used for this purpose and has received considerable popularity for closure of the bronchus.

Detailed technical aspects of pulmonary excisional surgery are not indicated in a presentation of this type. However, steps in hilar dissection for accomplishing left pneumonectomy are shown in Fig. 14-14. When the thorax has been opened and the decision to proceed with pneumonectomy is made, the first step is incision and reflection of the perihilar pleura. The order in which the pulmonary artery, bronchus, and veins are handled varies somewhat with the anatomy, the nature of the underlying disease, and the position of the patient on the table. As indicated in Fig. 14-14, the usual order in which the hilar structures are approached are the main pulmonary artery, superior pulmonary vein, inferior pulmonary vein, and the bronchus, in that order. Following removal of the lung, it is common to rotate a piece of pleura over the bronchial stump, following which the pleural cavity is flushed out with saline solution. The chest is closed without drainage and when the patient has been turned to the supine position, the intrapleural pressure on the operated side is adjusted to normal or a negative value. This may be done by inserting a needle into the cavity through the second anterior intercostal space and withdrawing air until a slightly negative pressure is obtained. Postoperatively, the position of the mediastinum as well as the degree of inflation of the remaining lung are checked by portable chest film. For the procedures of lobectomy and segmental resection, the technique follows a similar pattern although at the completion of operation, tubes are inserted anteriorly and posteriorly into the pleural space and placed beneath a water seal to ensure expansion of the remaining lung as well as to remove any pleural fluid or air that accumulates.

Special Operative Procedures

Bronchoplastic or sleeve resections that conserve pulmonary tissue have been advocated under special circumstances by Naef, Jensik, and others.[245,246] This procedure, in which only a segment of the bronchus and lung containing the tumor is resected and the distal bronchial tree re-anastomosed to the proximal, is more applicable to the treatment of small bronchial adenomas, although it has been used in selected patients for carcinoma. Likewise, in selected instances when peripheral tumors have invaded the chest wall, a sizable portion of invaded wall (including the rib cage) can be resected along with the involved lobe and the defect covered with the intervening muscles or with a Marlex prosthesis. This aggressive approach by Beattie and colleagues at the Memorial Sloan-Kettering Cancer Center has resulted in a number of long-term survivals in selected patients. As previously noted, pulmonary resection is generally not indicated when the lesion has spread distally or to the mediastinum. However, the concept of cytoreductive surgery in experimental protocols for stage III M0 disease is being studied. The bulk of the tumor mass may be removed on the assumption that additional therapy (*i.e.*, radiotherapy, immunotherapy, or chemotherapy) will more likely be effective when applied to a lower tumor burden. However, presently this concept is only experimental.

Complications of Surgery

The more common complications following pulmonary resectional surgery are hemorrhage, cardiac dysrhythmias, pulmonary insufficiency, persistent air leakage, and bronchopleural fistula, atelectasis of any remaining lung, and empyema. Probably the most common complication following pulmonary resection is cardiac dysrhythmia. This is most often asymptomatic and, in most instances, responds to treatment with appropriate cardiac medications.

When postoperative bleeding does occur, it is most often from chest wall or mediastinal sites that carry the systemic pressure. Following partial pulmonary resection, tubes are placed in the pleural space. Excessive bleeding can thus be identified readily. Following pneumonectomy when no tubes are used, this must be detected by clinical signs of blood loss and accumulation of blood in the pleural space, as detected clinically and by radiograph. Occasionally, delayed bleeding from pulmonary vascular stumps may occur but is usually secondary to infection.

Since many patients undergoing pulmonary resection for carcinoma are in the older age group and have a history of heavy smoking, there is a susbstantial incidence of respiratory insufficiency or failure in which ventilation, respiration, or both are sufficiently altered to prevent the patients' meeting their basic respiratory needs. This may be apparent in the obviously dyspneic and hypoxic patient; however, frequently, agitation and mental confusion will precede these other more obvious manifestations. Careful monitoring of blood gases to detect low arterial oxygen tension with or without the accumulation of carbon dioxide can be monitored to anticipate respiratory insufficiency. Careful evaluation of patients prior to operation can provide a reasonably good indication of the patient's ability to withstand a pulmonary procedure and indeed may be an important factor in determining the extent of resection to be performed. When respiratory difficulties do arise, a multiplicity of factors may be involved including excessive resection of pulmonary tissue or unsuspected preexisting pulmonary disease in the remaining lung. Left ventricular failure or pulmonary hypertension may be contributing factors and, of course, fluid overload may greatly exaggerate these problems. Mechanical airway obstruction with resultant atelectasis of remaining pulmonary tissue is a serious hazard; therefore, diligent aspiration of the tracheobronchial tree combined with encouragement for the patient to cough are essential. In the postoperative period, these patients can be given excellent ventilatory support with mechanical volume respirators. However, care must be taken to ensure that secretions do not accumulate in the tracheobronchial tree. This can be accomplished by frequent tracheal suction and occasional bronchoscopy to remove encrusted plugs of mucus.

Persistent air leakage following partial pulmonary resection should be minimal. This is readily controlled by the placement of intrapleural tubes under water seal drainage. When air leakage is prolonged, one must suspect bronchopleural fistula with leakage through the bronchial closure. In general, this will be apparent since fluid accumulating in the pleural space will leak into the tracheobronchial tree and the patient will cough up the serosanguineous fluid. If the leak is small in the lobar or segmental bronchus, spontaneous closure and expansion of the remaining lung to fill the pleural space may occur. A bronchial stump leak following pneumonectomy, however, is a serious matter requiring early attention. The patient must be turned onto the operated side to prevent aspiration of the accumulated pleural fluid followed by adequate drainage of the pleural space. Contamination of the pleural space results in empyema. This may be handled adequately by tube drainage and antibiotics following partial pulmonary resection; however, in the post-pneumonectomy patient, the space remaining in the empty hemithorax must be closed by an obliterative thoracoplasty procedure. Most surgeons prefer to delay this for at least one year to assess the patient for recurrent or metastatic carcinoma prior to thoracoplasty.

Results of Surgical Treatment

Approximately 43% of all lung cancer patients will undergo thoracotomy, 33% will have a definitive resection, 5–8% will be explored for diagnosis or evaluation of disease extent, and 5% will have a palliative procedure (known residual disease will be left behind).[156] The end-results of the individual surgeon will be determined mainly by the preoperative assessment of physiologic operability, and the proportion of patients that fall into each histologic type and anatomic stage that is encountered. Despite improved diagnostic measures and technical advances that improve the safety of thoracotomy, 5-year survival of all patients with lung cancer remains discouragingly low—approximately 10% according to latest Cancer Patient Survival Report.[1,2] Numerous variables determine survival (both 30-day and 5-year) and all of these must be taken into account when comparing results. In extensive survival studies of large numbers of patients entered into various protocols by the VASOG, observed survival rates varied between 52% and 14%, depending on the presence or absence of various determinant factors.[247] For example, in the AJC study, patients with small primary tumors and no nodal involvement ($T_1N_0M_0$) had a 59% 5-year survival.[155] The phenomenon of improved postoperative survival rates related to more limited stage disease can readily be seen in Fig. 14-15, showing 5-year survival rates in older studies of the VASOG compared with the current trial.[248] This is entirely accounted for by a higher proportion of more favorable TNM subsets in the current trial.

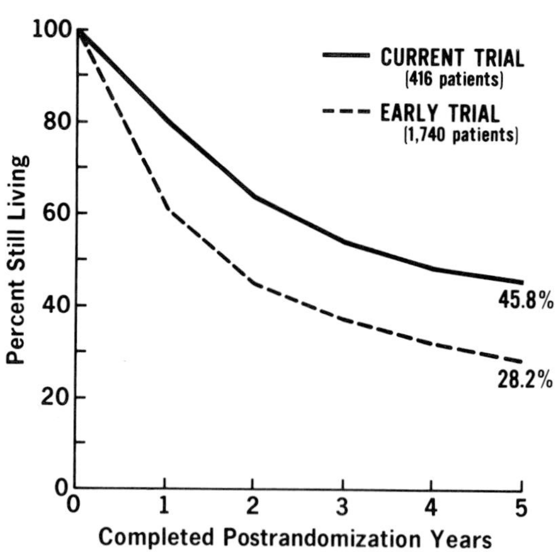

FIG. 14-15. Comparison of five-year survival curves in non-small cell lung cancer in VA surgical adjuvant trials conducted between 1965 and 1976 (*Early Trial*), and a trial conducted from 1976 on (*Current Trial*). The significant improvement in survival between the two curves can be accounted for by more careful selection of patients for thoracotomy. There was no difference between placebo and chemotherapy treated patients for any of the trials.

The fraction of long-term survivors following definitive surgical therapy is remarkably consistent throughout major centers performing lung cancer surgery in the U.S. (see Table 14-30).[161,249–253] Approximately 30% of all patients resected for cure survive five years. The 10-year survival is also remarkably constant at about 15% (795 of 5,164 resected patients pooled from ten series) and does not vary between epidermoid and adenocarcinoma, but is lower for large cell carcinoma.[249–252]

The 30-day hospital mortality following pulmonary resection at major centers with a large experience is also very constant, ranging from 4–9% for lobectomy and 9–11% for pneumonectomy.[249–252]

The causes of death during the immediate postoperative period include pulmonary thromboembolism (20%); myocardial infarction (24%); pneumonia-empyema (18%); bleeding (11%); respiratory insufficiency (20%); arterial embolism (4%); and tumor embolus (2%).[250,252] A detailed study of factors affecting 30-day postoperative mortality rates by the VASOG found the four most vital to be the age of the patient, the extent of the procedure, right pneumonectomy as opposed to left pneumonectomy, and the presence of significant nonpulmonary disease.[162] Cigarette smoking was also found

TABLE 14-30. Survival After Surgical Resection of Lung Cancer

HISTOLOGIC TYPE*	5- AND 10-YEAR SURVIVAL PERCENTAGE				
	5-Year	*(range)*	N	*10-Year*	N
Epidermoid Carcinoma	33	(26–43)	1,643	17	1,115
Adenocarcinoma	26	(20–34)	535	16	352
Large cell carcinoma	28	(6–36)	278	8	278
Bronchioloalveolar	51	(48–61)	76	24	76
Small cell carcinoma	1	(0–20)	125	<0.5	125
Totals	30	(26–36)	2,790	15	1,946

(Mountain CF: Assessment of the role of surgery for control of lung cancer. Ann Thor Surg 24:365–373, 1977; Paulson DL, Reisch JS: Long-term survival after resection for bronchogenic carcinoma. Ann Surg 184:324–332, 1976; Wilkins WE Jr, Scannell JG, Crauer JG: Four decades of experience with resection for bronchogenic carcinoma at the Massachusetts General Hospital. J Thorac Cardiovasc Surg 76:364–368, 1978; Ashor GL, Kem WH, Meyer BW et al: Long term survival in bronchogenic carcinoma. J Thorac Cardiovasc Surg 70:581–589, 1975; Kirsch MM, Rotman H, Argenta L et al: Carcinoma of the lung: results of treatment over ten years. Ann Thorac Surg 21:371–377, 1976)

* Miscellaneous histologic types (e.g., adenosquamous) had a 10 year survival of 14% for 87 patients.

TABLE 14-31. Five-year Survival Following Surgical Resection of Lung Cancer by Postsurgical Stage*

	CUMULATIVE 5-YEAR SURVIVAL PERCENTAGE			
	STAGE I	STAGE II	STAGE III (MO)§	STAGE III-N2
Epidermoid	54 (231)†	35 (61)	19 (236)	13 (62)
Adenocarcinoma and large cell carcinoma	51 (99)	18 (42)	10 (165)	2‡ (45)
Small cell carcinoma (N = 41)	0	0	0	0

* AJC data from reference 161
† Figures in parentheses refer to numbers of patients.
‡ The large cell cancer group had only a few patients but had an 11% five-year survival.
§ The fraction of these patients receiving postoperative radiotherapy is not reported.

to be an important factor, the postoperative mortality rate being five times greater in patients with a smoking history of over 20 years.

The AJC data provide a useful baseline for comparing the postsurgical staging results of the different histologic types by each of the anatomic stages (see Table 14-31, Figs. 14-10, 14-15, 14-16).[161] In NSCLC resected for cure, the postsurgical treatment pathologic stage I patients do consistently better than the stage II patients, who in turn do better than the stage III MO patients. It is important to emphasize that stage I patients have one year survival of 80–90% and a 3-year survival of approximately 60–75%.[161,253] Thus, the large majority of these patients do well in the first years after surgery. Small-cell carcinoma does consistently worse than the non-small cell types and there are only very rare long-term survivors following surgical resection alone. At 5 years in stage II and III patients, squamous cell carcinoma consistently does better than adenocarcinoma or large cell carcinoma; in stage I disease, however, there is no difference between the non-small cell lung cancer types in survival.

The single most important factor in postsurgical staging results in patients undergoing a "curative resection" is the presence or absence of nodal involvement. In patients with no clinical evidence of disseminated disease, and without consideration of other variables affecting prognosis, the cumulative 5-year survival rate is 46% without lymph node involvement, 33% if peribronchial or hilar lymph nodes are involved, and 8% with mediastinal lymph node metastases.[156] The 10-year survival is 33% without nodal involvement, 13% with hilar node involvement, and 3% with mediastinal node involvement.[249] Overall, the 5-year survival for resected NSCL with stage III disease, but negative mediastinal nodes and no

FIG. 14-16. Five-year cumulative survival patterns of patients with resected lung cancer, stratified by cell type and postsurgical treatment stage of disease. (Mountain CF: Assessment of the role of surgery for control of lung cancer. Ann Thorac Surg 24:365–373, 1977)

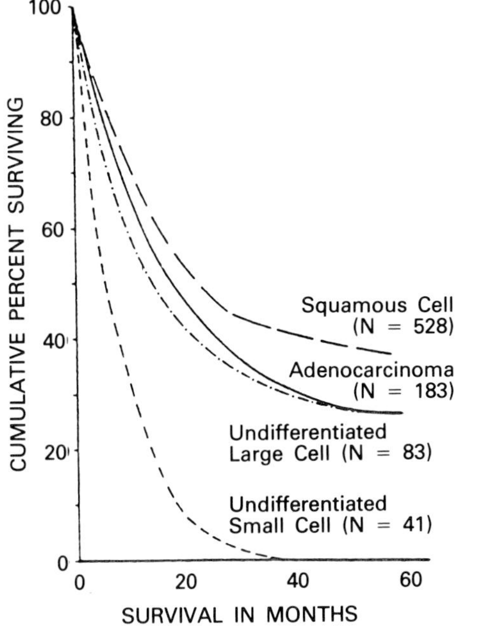

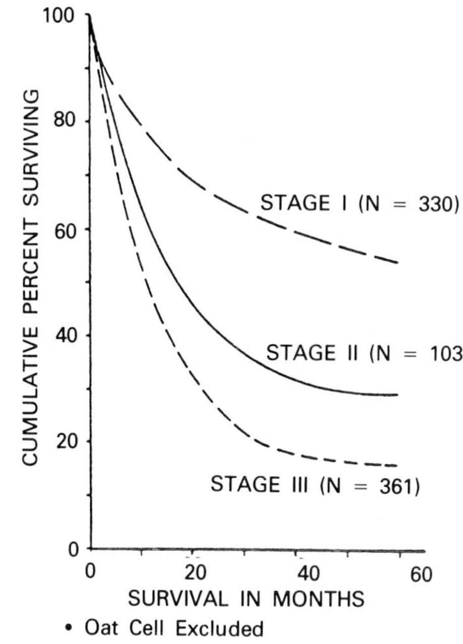

distant metastases, was 27% in the AJC series vs. 8% if the mediastinal nodes were positive. However, the fraction of stage III patients receiving postoperative radiotherapy is not reported and so the role of this treatment stage III N2 disease is not known. Because of better survival in N2 epidermoid than N2 adenocarcinoma, some would recommend proceeding with resection in stage III N2 patients only with squamous (and possibly large cell) histology.[156] The presence of a positive inlet node, contralateral peritracheal lymph node involvement, pleural effusion, and extension outside the hemithorax of primary tumor, or the findings of adenocarcinoma histology are contraindications as the survival does not equal the operative mortality rate.

While the surgeon's intent is curative in the resected cases, 16% have microscopic residual disease.[155] Even if no residual disease is suspected by the surgeon or pathologist, about one-half of the patients surviving the operation die within 2 years of recurrence or metastatic disease (see Figs. 14-15 and 14-16). This increases with increasing stage and is always worse for adenocarcinoma compared to epidermoid cancer on a stage-for-stage basis, especially when positive mediastinal nodes are present (see Table 14-32). In contrast, the size of the primary tumor does not influence survival when the mediastinal nodes are positive.[155] Thus, it appears that evidence of lymph node spread is extremely important in predicting survival but that distant metastases without regional nodal involvement may still be the most common pattern of failure in "early" disease.[155] Approximately 9–13% in each group die from causes unrelated to the primary tumor, and 2% die who were known to be tumor-free.

The analysis of the cause of death in patients surviving five or more years from their pulmonary resection is also interesting. In a group of 170 such patients reported from three institutions, 62% died without evidence of lung cancer, 25% died with lung cancer (recurrence or a new primary), 12% died of a new primary cancer, and 12% died of unknown causes.[249–252] Thus, cancer, whether it be recurrent disease or a new primary, is still a major threat to these patients long after definitive surgical treatment.

RESIDUAL TUMOR IN THE BRONCHIAL MARGIN AFTER RESECTION. A special postsurgical staging problem exists when microscopic residual tumor is found in the cut margin of the resected specimen. This occurs in approximately 15% of resected patients.[254] Bronchopleural fistulas will develop in approximately 10–12% of these patients and their perioperative mortality rate is higher (16–19%) in larger part because of these fistulas.[254,255] The overall 5-year survival rate is 22% (30/136 patients from three series) and the vast majority of the survivors all had epidermoid cancer histology.[254–256] The residual tumor group can be subdivided into those patients with direct extension of tumor (53%), lymphatic permeation (22%), clumps of cancer cells in the peribronchial tissue (9%), and the presence of carcinoma *in situ* (16%).[254] There were no 3-year survivors in the group with lymphatic permeation; these patients had nodal metastases as well.[254] The importance of these findings is that a short bronchial stump (distance from tumor to cut margin) does not preclude long-term survival. The inability to resect a 2-cm distance of apparently normal bronchus from the tumor should not be a contraindication to resection or an indication to convert a lobectomy to a pneumonectomy in a patient who might not tolerate the larger procedure.[254] The role of adjuvant radiotherapy in these patients remains to be determined.

RADIOTHERAPEUTIC TREATMENT

DETERMINATION OF THE ABILITY TO UNDERGO RADICAL RADIATION THERAPY FOR CURE

Patients with lung cancer represent a major problem in terms of selection of optimal treatment, precisely because their underlying pulmonary status often limits their ability to undergo a radical surgical procedure. The issue of resectability must also be put into perspective, inasmuch as mediastinal node involvement connotes a very poor prognosis with surgery alone.[252] Many of the same considerations hold for radical radiotherapy. Consideration for aggressive radiation therapy in the patient who has lung cancer is usually based on the extent of disease and the volume of the chest that requires irradiation. Whenever there is massive mediastinal involvement, the ability to restrict the volume of irradiation to mediastinum and nodes declines. A significant portion of the pulmonary parenchyma may lie anterior or posterior to the actual tumor mass and thus be incorporated in the irradiated tumor volume. As in presurgical evaluation, pulmonary function tests are useful as a baseline for future comparison, but no specific values preclude radiation therapy. There are times when part of the patient's pulmonary symptoms is actually

TABLE 14-32. Clinical Evidence for Residual Tumor After Surgical and Pathologic Exam Reveals No Tumor in "Curative Resections" for Non-Small Cell Lung Cancer

	PERCENTAGE OF PATIENTS DYING OF TUMOR RECURRENCE OR METASTASIS WITHIN 2 YEARS OF A "CURATIVE" RESECTION		
POSTSURGICAL TREATMENT STAGE	EPIDERMOID CARCINOMA	ADENO-CARCINOMA	LARGE CELL CARCINOMA
I	18	24	20
II	36	50	Not given
III	48	70	Not given

(Mountain CF, Hermes KE: Management implications of surgical staging studies. Prog Cancer Res Ther 11: 233–242, 1979)

due to bronchial obstruction. In such a patient, radiation therapy applied to the area of interest can in fact improve breathing, blood gases, and pulmonary symptoms. Midplane tomography and bronchoscopy can frequently be useful in identifying such endobronchial obstruction. Unfortunately, the typical patient referred for radiation therapy has fairly extensive disease that requires more than attention to relieve bronchial obstruction.

TREATMENT OF LUNG CANCER PATIENTS WITH RADIOTHERAPY ADMINISTERED WITH CURATIVE INTENT

For patients who have NSCLC, which after extensive evaluation appears to be stage I in its extent, surgery is unequivocally the treatment of choice (if the patient's underlying pulmonary status and other medical considerations suggest that they can tolerate a radical surgical procedure). Such surgery should also be considered the treatment of choice for the otherwise well patient who has stage II disease. Unfortunately, stage I and stage II represent only the minority of all patients with carcinoma of the lung. In addition, many patients who clinically appear to be stage I or II turn out to have microscopic involvement of lymph nodes in the mediastinum at surgery. Radiation therapy is considered an alternative treatment to surgery for patients who either decline thoracotomy with its attendant risks or for patients whose underlying pulmonary and other medical problems make surgery excessively risky.[257] There are only limited data concerning primary radiotherapy in lieu of surgery in resectable and operable patients with lung cancer. The reported series from England, in which relatively low (4000–5000 rads) doses were used, suggest that modern high dose radiotherapy is probably a reasonable approach for patients who decline surgery. Hilton and Smart reported over 20% of patients surviving over 5 years after radical radiotherapy for otherwise operable lung cancer.[258,259]

The vast majority of patients with lung cancer of the non-small cell varieties present with stage III disease that is unresectable. Stage III patients who have clinically evident mediastinal adenopathy can be considered for curative radiotherapy, with or without surgery, although the long-term survival figures remain poor. Patients with distant metastases and patients with positive supraclavicular nodes are not generally considered for curative radiation treatment. The median survival for unresectable patients undergoing primary radiotherapy is less than one year; however, the 5-year survival data show about 6% of patients alive and well with radiotherapy alone (see Table 14-33). This should not be compared to surgical results because patient selection in radiation series is less favorable than in surgical series.

TABLE 14-33. Five-Year Survival Data Following "Curative" Radiotherapy for Patients with Inoperable or Unresectable Lung Cancer

SERIES	REFERENCE	NUMBER OF PATIENTS	5-YEAR SURVIVAL
Stanford	(260)	284	6%
Columbia	(261,262)	253	5%
Hammersmith	(263)	513	6%

Radiation Therapy Treatment Planning

When curative treatment is planned with radiation therapy, the intention is to take the known tumor volume to midplane doses of 5500–6000 rad. If the tumor location is relatively small or favorable, one may consider boosting a small volume to an even higher dose. The major concern is the amount of lung parenchyma that will be included within the treatment plan. Organs that limit the amount of irradiation that can be applied to the thorax include lung parenchyma, spinal cord, and heart. The esophagus, although frequently symptomatic from acute desquamation during the course of treatment, is usually not considered a dose-limiting organ in terms of long-term complications. For patients who have no major degree of chronic obstructive lung disease, treatment plans may consist of opposing anterior and posterior fields, usually with a 2-cm margin around the entire tumor mass, for approximately 3000 rad, prior to switching to a second treatment plan, which usually consists of an anterior field in conjunction with a posteriorly obliqued field to keep the spinal cord dose well within tolerance levels (see Fig. 14-17). In most cases, the entire upper mediastinum is included while the inferior margin typically extends about 6–7 cm below the carina in the treatment position. Such treatment plans (which ideally require isocentric treatment planning) have considerably helped improve dosimetry in irradiating these patients (see Fig. 14-18). When such tools are available to assist in treatment planning, it is essential not only that the plan be documented at the tumor level, but that a second treatment plan be obtained at the level of the thoracic inlet, where the thickness of the chest is comparatively narrow compared to that at a lower level of the tumor itself. This discrepancy in anterior-posterior chest thickness means that the spinal cord dose at the upper level of the treatment volume may be higher than the actual dose being delivered at the tumor level, since there is less tissue at the upper level to attenuate the radiation than at the tumor level. Knowledge of the exact dose being applied at the upper portion of the chest to the spinal cord will allow appropriate decisions to be made to minimize the dose to the spinal cord at the upper thoracic level. Such consideration and meticulous execution of the dosimetric treatment plan should eliminate any concern about radiation myelitis.

For the patient who has a major degree of restrictive pulmonary disease, the treatment plan is usually confined to opposing anterior-posterior fields with a spinal cord block inserted posteriorly somewhere between 3000 and 4000 rad tumor dose to keep the total spinal cord dose below 4500 rad. Such a treatment plan is considered a major compromise from optimal tumor treatment since the block may attenuate tumor dose as well. If possible, it is preferable to reduce the tumor volume at the time of shifting to the obliqued field but this cannot always be done. Supraclavicular nodes are not usually included within the treatment volume in such patients, in contrast to the more typical unresectable patient in whom an anterior neck field is ordinarily used to treat the supraclavicular nodes routinely, regardless of their clinical status.

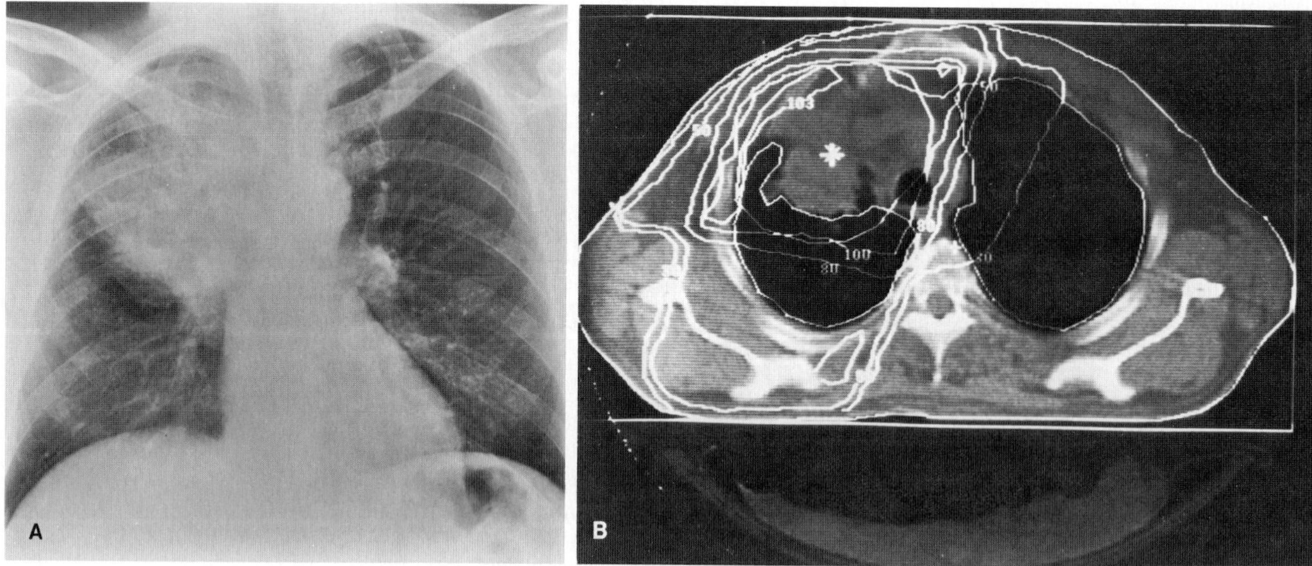

FIG. 14-17. *A*, prethoracotomy chest film of a 38-year-old male with locally unresectable large cell carcinoma of the lung. Only a biopsy was performed.

B, isodose distribution of the radiotherapy treatment plan superimposed upon the CT scan of the patient in question. An anterior field and a right lateral field are to be used with wedges to compensate for the obliquities of the patient's surface. The advantage of this treatment plan is that the dose distribution to the spinal cord will be well within patient tolerance and a portion of the posterior right upper lobe will be spared. A 100% isodose line will be carried to 5500 rad as part of the treatment plan for this patient. If there are no metastases, a further boost may be delivered to a coned down volume representing the residual tumor mass. In this particular patient, metastatic disease was present.

TIME, DOSE, AND FRACTIONATION. Concerning time, dose, and fractionation schemes, the question of split course treatment vs. continuous therapy has been raised. No major superiority has been achieved by split course treatment compared to continuous fractionation in terms of survival. The case for split course treatment (approximately 2500 to 3000 rad over two weeks time followed by 2–3 weeks off treatment before a final 2500–3000 rad in 2–3 weeks is delivered) is predicated upon better tolerance, a simplicity for integration into combined modality approaches, and an opportunity to reevaluate patients prior to their second half of treatment for new manifestations of metastatic disease that might have occurred.[260,264,265] It should be understood that if a tumor mass receives the same number of rad over a longer period of time with the same size of daily exposure, biological differences exist between those two fractionation schemes. In the simplest concept, to achieve the same effect from split course treatment, a higher total dose of radiation would be required to offset the tumor repopulation that may have occurred during the gap off treatment. Since the long-term success achieved with radiation therapy alone (predominantly in unresectable stage III patients or poor operative risks) remains relatively poor, no major superiority of split course treatment over continuous fractionation or vice versa has been determined.

The poor survival generally achieved in patients with lung cancer treated with irradiation may have led to unwarranted conclusions concerning local control with radiation therapy. In addition, it is often difficult to define accurately the pretreatment tumor volume because of atelectasis and collapse. Local tumor control in the chest remains difficult to determine because of problems distinguishing subtle differences between radiation changes and tumor on chest films. Inasmuch as metastatic disease has dominated the clinical course of these patients, it has been thought that local recurrence is not a major problem.[265] This remains to be seen, since local recurrence can be slow to manifest itself and certainly would predispose to further metastatic disease.[266]

Generally, most of the cardiac silhouette is outside the high dose radiation portal for treatment of lung cancer patients (unless the lesion in question is located in the lower thorax, well below the mainstem bronchi, or is associated with pericardial involvement). Thus, typically most of the pericardium of a patient with lung cancer has not been included in the high dose portion of the treatment plan. As a consequence, any interaction between radiotherapy and possible use of adriamycin should not be of major concern in most patients.[267]

CLINICAL CARE OF PATIENTS DURING RADIOTHERAPY. Most patients will tolerate daily doses of 200–300 rad midplane without major problems during treatment. Approximately 3 weeks after their treatment has started, dysphagia due to acute desquamation of the esophageal mucosa is noted. This will usually persist (and can be severe in some patients, necessitating an unplanned break) for approximately 2–3 weeks after the completion of radiation therapy. Bronchial secretions will become altered by radiation therapy and become noticeably more tenacious. A nonproductive cough is commonly seen during and after radiation therapy; it may be

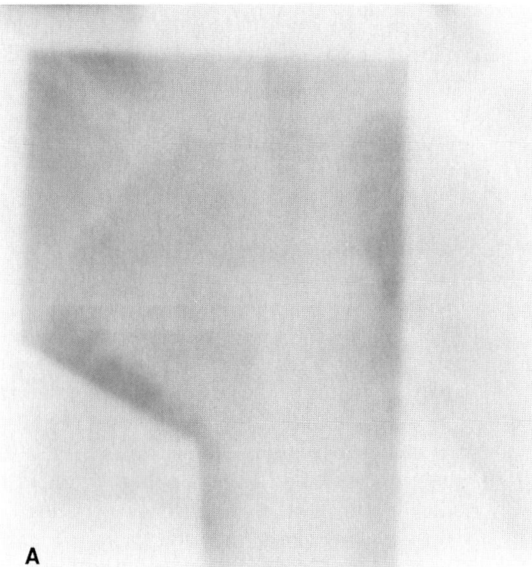

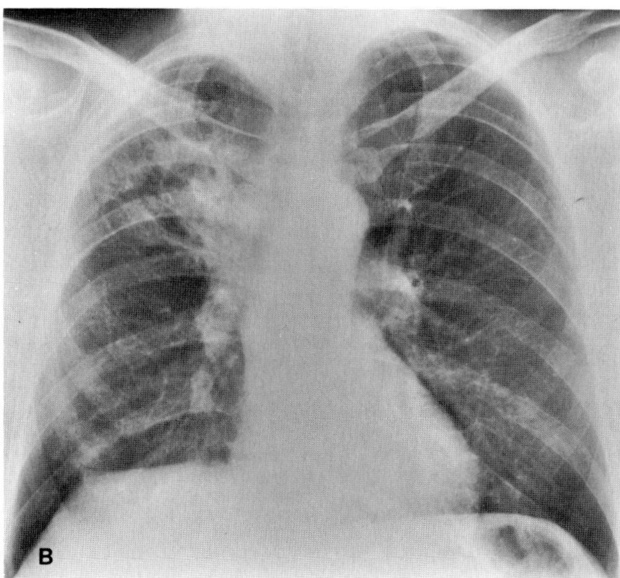

FIG. 14-18. *A*, anterior port used in the treatment. *B*, response to treatment after 5500 rad. Considerable tumor shrinkage has been achieved with good palliative results in terms of symptoms.

persistent for the rest of the patient's life. Frank radiation pneumonitis does not occur during treatment; it is more likely to be seen in the first 1–3 months after completion of radiation therapy. Care should be taken to evaluate the patients thoroughly prior to treatment to be sure that incipient obstructive pneumonia is not present. Such a problem may require antibiotics and delay treatment until cleared, particularly if intensive chemotherapy is planned as a portion of the treatment.

LONG-TERM FOLLOW-UP AND COMPLICATIONS. Problems with radiation pneumonitis will depend on the dose and volume of lung incorporated within the radiation field.[265] Pulmonary fibrosis may take months to years to develop; it can be disabling or even fatal. However, such lethal complications are relatively rare. The pathologic physiology appears to represent both vascular and parenchymal cell injury. The diffusion capacity is markedly reduced, and interstitial fibrosis of pulmonary septa occurs. Whenever pulmonary fibrosis occurs, marked decrease in pulmonary compliance and lung volume follows.[268] The optimal appoach to radiation pneumonitis and pulmonary fibrosis is to avoid them by means of sophisticated treatment planning and careful delineation of radiation portals. Often, patients will be asymptomatic while radiographic manifestations occur and coincide with the radiation treatment volume. Typically, such patients will have the manifestations decrease or disappear completely without symptoms or treatment. When shortness of breath or fever accompanies these radiologic changes, corticosteroids have been advocated. Roughly half the patients will claim marked symptomatic improvement.[268a] If radiation fibrosis has been well established, there is no value in the use of corticosteroids. In severe cases it may be necessary to use oxygen. There is no indication for antibiotics unless there is an associated secondary infecton. Prophylactic administration of corticosteroids to patients receiving large field lung irradiation has not prevented long-term radiation changes.

Radiation-induced cardiac disease has been seen following radiation therapy for lung cancer patients. It still remains relatively rare, probably because of the relatively short survival seen in patients who have this disease. Again, elimination of most of the cardiac silhouette from the high dose radiation volume obviates this problem for most patients. If the cancer is located close to the heart, this problem may be seen and can be difficult to distinguish from recurrent tumor. Paradoxical pulse may be present if pericardial constriction is present. Echocardiogram, cardiac catheterization, and pericardiocentesis may be necessary to perform for diagnostic and therapeutic purposes. Pericardial fluid must be evaluated cytologically to rule out a malignant pericardial effusion.

Acute radiation esophagitis usually occurs during treatment but proves self-limited in its duration once the mucosa has repopulated. During the acute esophagitis, viscous xylocaine is often helpful. Long-term esophageal problems are relatively rare, although esophageal stenosis has occasionally been reported. This is usually seen when relatively large daily fractions have been used (250–300 rad per day). For most patients who develop this uncommon problem, simple esophageal dilatation will be adequate.

Spinal cord injury should be avoided by careful treatment planning. As noted above, careful delineation of dose distribution within the patient, not only at the level of the tumor, but also at the upper thorax should allow the therapist to avoid this problem. When the patient receives a posterior oblique field, care must be taken to ensure that the spinal cord is still not included within the portal; if the location of the tumor makes the angle of the obliquity such that the spinal cord is included at the upper portion of the portal, an additional block must be inserted to reduce the exposure of the spinal cord to irradiation.

INTEGRATION OF SURGERY, RADIOTHERAPY, AND CHEMOTHERAPY IN THE PRIMARY TREATMENT OF NON-SMALL CELL LUNG CANCER WITH CURATIVE INTENT

Because of the frequent occurrence in non-small cell lung cancer (NSCLC) of metastatic disease outside the resected specimen, many groups have tried to combine radiotherapy and surgery. The radiotherapy has been given both pre- and postoperatively. For patients who have cancer in mediastinal nodes, this combined modality treatment appears appropriate.

PREOPERATIVE RADIOTHERAPY

The routine use of preoperative irradiation, pioneered by Bloedorn and associates, resulted in two large prospective studies that found no survival benefit from preoperative irradiation.[269–271] These studies did demonstrate that about a third of the specimens were free of tumor after irradiation. However, there was no survival benefit even in this supposedly favorable subgroup. It should be pointed out that in these two studies, many aspects were far from optimal; all stages and histologies were included but not stratified, pneumonectomy was the procedure of choice, and the quality of radiation therapy employed was suboptimal. Treatment planning by simulators and megavoltage equipment were often not employed in either study. Complications of routine prepneumonectomy irradiation were high, especially bronchopleural fistula. Thus, the prospective studies that have been reported have failed to answer questions definitively concerning preoperative irradiation. Moreover, Sherman and coworkers recently reported excellent results with preoperative radiation therapy in a subgroup of patients with "marginally resectable" disease.[272] Most of these patients received 3000 rad in ten fractions over 2 weeks and were then subjected to thoracotomy within 2 weeks of completion of the radiation. The vast majority of the patients (83%) proved to be resectable including those who had positive mediastinal nodes prior to treatment. The long-term results (18% 5-year survival) with preoperative irradiation in this group of selected stage III patients compares favorably to selected series in which surgery alone was used.[161] The results were best in epidermoid cancer. It also appears that a dramatic response to the preoperative radiotherapy (with only microscopic residual disease or no tumor found in the resected specimen) was associated with better survival than were lesser responses to the radiotherapy.[272] Thus, further study of a short course of preoperative irradiation in selected stage III patients appears indicated.

Patients should not routinely receive preoperative radiotherapy. However, there appear to be selected cases that may benefit from preoperative radiotherapy though it has not been proven. Such patients would include those in good physiologic shape with stage III epidermoid carcinoma in mediastinal nodes who otherwise would not be offered surgical resection. Such patients could be treated with 3000 rad in ten fractions over 2 weeks. If their visible tumor on chest film, by bronchoscopy, and at exploratory thoracotomy, underwent a major clinical regression, they could undergo an attempt at a curative resection. The lower dose of radiotherapy would probably not produce the postoperative complications seen with the higher doses. Whether this subgroup of patients would have done just as well with high dose radiotherapy alone or with a surgical debulking followed by postoperative radiotherapy is not known at this time.

POSTOPERATIVE RADIOTHERAPY

Postoperative irradiation has not been well studied. Uncontrolled studies suggest some advantage employing postoperative radiation therapy (approximately 5000 rad in 5 weeks) in patients who are proved by resection to have involved hilar or mediastinal nodes.[252,273,274] This is especially true in patients who had squamous cell histology.[252] These uncontrolled results suggest that 25–30% of patients with positive mediastinal nodes found at the time of surgery can be salvaged by postoperative irradiation to the chest, compared to a less than 8% long-term survival rate in similar patients treated with surgery alone.[161,252,273]

Another approach for patients who have non-metastatic lung cancer is conservative resection of the lesion coupled with mediastinal node resection and interstitial irradiation applied at thoracotomy utilizing ^{127}I seeds or ^{192}Ir implanted directly into the surgical bed.[253,275] This technique has not been routinely used, but is strongly advocated by some, often in conjunction with modest dose preoperative or postoperative external irradiation. It obviously requires close interaction between radiotherapists and surgeons both preoperatively and intraoperatively. The long-term results of this approach look promising for selected cases.

CURRENT RECOMMENDATIONS FOR THE USE OF COMBINED SURGERY AND RADIOTHERAPY

Patients who appear to have disease confined to stage I or stage II are probably best managed with surgery alone if they have suitable pulmonary function. If they turn out to have microscopic nodal involvement, postoperative irradiation (approximately 5000 rad) to the mediastinum is a common practice and appears appropriate, especially if the surgical procedure was suboptimal for any reason. The value of such therapy will be confirmed or denied in current randomized trials. For patients who have overt clinical involvement in mediastinal nodes, both resectability and prognosis appear poor. In such patients who do not have extrathoracic metastases, preoperative radiation therapy followed by resection may have value in selected patients, although this is not yet established. Whether the preoperative therapy should be 3000 rad in a short course as advocated by Sherman and coworkers or a more protracted course of 4000–5000 rad over 4–5 weeks remains to be seen. The determining factor will probably be the experience of the surgeon involved. For patients who do not have distant metastases but who are obviously clinically unresectable or who represent poor surgical risks, radical radiation therapy alone will continue to be the treatment standard with a small, but definite, cure rate (see Table 14-33).

Diagnosis and Management of Carcinomas in the Superior Pulmonary Sulcus

Carcinomas in the superior pulmonary sulcus produce a characteristic clinical pattern known as *Pancoast's syndrome.*[276–280] The tumor occurs in the sulcus or groove made by the subclavian artery in the cupola of the pleura and apices of the upper lobes of the lungs. It produces pain in the distribution of the eighth cervical and first and second thoracic nerve distribution, and a Horner's syndrome. A shadow is seen on chest films at the extreme apex of the lung; in 40% of patients, it appears only as an apical cap or thickening.[278,280] The pain is steady, severe, and unrelenting. It is first localized in the shoulder and vertebral border of the scapula and later extends down the ulnar distribution of the arm to the elbow (T1 distribution) and finally to the ulnar surface of the forearm and fourth and fifth fingers of the hand (C8 dermatome).[278] The first or second rib or vertebrae and the related intercostal nerves may also be involved, increasing the pain and, in some cases, leading to spinal cord compression. With involvement of the sympathetic chain and stellate ganglion by direct extension, Horner's syndrome and anhidrosis develop on the same side of the face and arm. However, rib destruction and Horner's syndrome do not have to be present to diagnose a superior sulcus tumor.

Paulson has pioneered an aggressive approach to these patients including preoperative irradiation followed by extended resection.[278,279] This was prompted by the observation that these tumors usually grow slowly and metastasize late. Patients should have the usual staging procedures done for any potentially resectable lung cancer lesion. However, there should be special emphasis on bone scans, bone and cervical spine roentgenograms, and CT scan of the area to determine tumor extent, as well as neurologic examination with electromyography to document the neurologic findings. Mediastinoscopy is usually recommended because of the poor survival of superior sulcus tumors even after radical procedures when these nodes are involved.[222] However, scalene node biopsy is only done when palpable nodes are present or the patient is of borderline operability.[278,280]

In contrast to other situations, a histologic diagnosis is often not made prior to radiation and surgery because of the inaccessibility of the lesions, even to needle biopsy, and a desire not to violate tissue planes.[278–280] If the precise definition of a tumor mass in the extreme apex of the chest, with pain down the ulnar distribution of the arm in T1 and C8 distribution, is strictly followed, the diagnostic accuracy for cancer is better than 90%.[278,279] With inoperable or doubtful cases, open biopsy of the cupola of the pleura may be made for histologic proof through a supraclavicular scalenotomy incision.[278]

Preoperative irradiation to a dose of 3000 rad in ten treatments over 12 days is given to the apex of the lung, upper ribs, upper mediastinum, ipsilateral hilum, and lower cervical spine.[279,280] This allows resection 3–6 weeks after completion of radiation therapy. Standard higher doses have not been routinely used preoperatively because of worry of increased radiotherapeutic and operative morbidity.[278] If surgery is not to be performed because of spread or underlying pulmonary risks, the dose to the spinal cord must be carefully limited. In these patients, shrinking field techniques are used to achieve tumor doses of approximately 6000 rad. Pancoast tumors can usually be treated to high dose, precisely because they are peripherally located away from the midline.

An extended en bloc resection of the chest wall is then carried out. This usually involves an extended radical lobectomy or segmental resection. The posterior portions of the first three ribs, portions of the upper thoracic vertebrae (including the transverse processes), the intercostal nerves, the lower trunk of the brachial plexus, the stellate ganglion, and a portion of the dorsal sympathetic chain are resected along with the involved lung.[278] Long-term complications include permanent ulnar nerve neurologic defects and Horner's syndrome, which do not appear to bother patients.[278] Immediate complications are respiratory in nature and include instability of the chest wall. They require endotracheal tube ventilatory support for the first three postoperative days, bronchoscopy for removal of secretions in the immediate postoperative period, and Velpeau dressing to stabilize the chest wall.[280] There is debate about the number of patients achieving pain relief, but at least two-thirds (and probably most long-term survivors) appear to do so.[278,280]

Contraindications to resection include extensive invasion of the brachial plexus, subclavian artery, vertebral bodies, esophagus, mediastinum, and distant metastases.[279,280] Patients with hilar, mediastinal, or scalene node involvement have such a poor prognosis following the procedure that these metastatic sites should probably also be considered as contraindications.[279,280] Only 50% of superior sulcus tumors are epidermoid, 30% are large cell or giant cell, and 15% are adenocarcinomas. While the fraction of 3-year survivors was 42% for the epidermoid cancers and 21% for the large cell and adenocarcinomas, histology alone should not determine resectability.[278]

ADJUVANT CHEMOTHERAPY WITH SURGERY

When the cancer chemotherapy era began two decades ago, great interest and anticipation spread throughout the surgical community concerning the administration of cytotoxic agents to patients undergoing standard surgical resection of cancer. It has been noted that the peripheral blood of patients with cancer contained cells which closely resembled the neoplastic cells found in the primary tumor and that the number of these cells increased greatly during operative manipulation of the tumor. Even greater numbers of cancer cells as well as clumps of cells were found in the venous blood draining the tumor area. It was hoped chemotherapy given as an adjuvant could kill these cells. Unfortunately, benefits from adjuvant chemotherapy in NSCLC have not been seen in prospective randomized clinical trials.

The results of randomized adjuvant chemotherapy trials in NSCLC are summarized in Tables 14-34 and 14-35. Two large cooperative groups, one composed of Veterans Administration Hospitals and the second of University Hospitals, began prospective randomized controlled trials in which

TABLE 14-34. Results of Adjuvant Chemotherapy in VA Surgical Oncology Group Trials

CELL TYPE	ADJUVANT TREATMENT RECEIVED		
	% Alive at 4 Years		
Cyclophosphamide Trial	*Cyclophosphamide*		*Control*
Total patients	33 (412)*		33 (430)
Squamous carcinoma	34		37
Adenocarcinoma	34		30
Other non-small cell types (Large cell carcinoma)	35		31
Small cell carcinoma (N = 58)	16		4
	% Alive at 3 Years		
Cyclophosphamide + Methotrexate Trial	*Cyclophosphamide*	*Cyclophosphamide + Methotrexate*	*Control*
Total patients	33 (132)	36 (142)	36 (143)
Squamous carcinoma	37	42	42
Adenocarcinoma	30	33	27
Other non-small cell types (Large cell carcinoma)	27	24	32
Small cell carcinoma (N = 18)	17	33	0

* Numbers of patients are given in parentheses.
(Higgins GA, Shields TW: Experience of the Veterans Administration Surgical Adjuvant Group. Prog Cancer Res Ther 11:433–422, 1979)

TABLE 14-35. Randomized Trials of Adjuvant Chemotherapy Versus Placebo in Non-Small Cell Lung Cancer

DRUG(S)	NUMBER OF PATIENTS RANDOMIZED	CONCLUSIONS	REFER-ENCES
Nitrogen mustard	1,136	No significant difference	(281)
Nitrogen mustard	1,192	No significant difference	(282)
Cyclophosphamide	661	No significant difference	(281)
Cyclophosphamide	189	More cancer recurrences in chemotherapy group	(283)
Cyclophosphamide or thiotepa	301	Possible benefit for squamous	(284)
Cyclophosphamide	234	No significant difference	(285)
Tetramethylene dimethanesul-phonate (busulphan)	243	No significant difference	(285)
Placebo	249		
Vinblastine	167	No significant difference	(286)
CCNU	72	More complications in chemotherapy group, no difference in survival	(287)
Cyclophosphamide + methotrexate	417	No significant difference	(281)
CCNU + hydroxyurea	471	No significant difference	(281)
Cyclophosphamide + methotrexate + vinblastine + 5-FU	82	Possible benefit in stage I	(288)
Cyclophosphamide + methotrexate + CCNU ± BCG immunotherapy ± chest radiotherapy	168	No significant difference	(289)

nitrogen mustard (HN_2) was administered IV and IP at the end of operation, and intravenously in the immediate post-operative period.[282,290] There were no demonstrable survival benefits in these trials and the University Cooperative Group did not continue with other chemotherapy adjuvant trials. The Veterans Administration Group continued adjuvant studies in lung cancer and has now entered approximately 4000 patients in a series of protocols.[281,291] For its second trial, the group used cyclophosphamide (CTX) as the cytotoxic agent, and in addition to administering the drug during and immediately following the operative procedure, a second course of drug was administered approximately 5 weeks into the postoperative period (see Table 14-34). Long-term follow-up of these patients again demonstrated no difference in survival in patients treated by surgery alone from those receiving adjuvant chemotherapy.

However, in a group of 58 patients classified as small-cell lung carcinoma (SCLC), there was a subtantially better survival in those who received chemotherapy (see Table 14-34).

In the third trial, the group developed a three-arm protocol comparing CTX alone with alternate courses of CTX and methotrexate (MTX) (the third arm being surgery alone). For this trial, chemotherapy was begun in patients randomized approximately 10–14 days following operation. The course of drug therapy was administered at 5-week intervals for a period of 18 months. Long-term survival data in this trial showed identical survival in all three arms. Again, there were 18 patients classified as having SCLC, 4 of these patients were long-term survivors, and all had received adjuvant chemotherapy, while there were no survivors in the control group (see Table 14-34).[281] For the fourth trial, a combination of CCNU and hydroxyurea, both administered by the oral route, were compared to placebo. Hydroxyurea was given twice weekly on a continuing basis, and CCNU was given at 6-week intervals, drug therapy being carried out for a 1-year period. These patients are currently in follow-up but again there is no demonstrable benefit from drug therapy.[281]

During this period, a number of reports were published in non- or partially randomized trials suggesting improved survival with adjuvant chemotherapy. Wingfield, from England, used IV CTX; Pirogov, from the Soviet Union, administered thiotepa as the adjuvant.[284,292] From Austria, Karrer and associates reported possible beneficial results for stage I patients using a combination of CTX, MTX, vinblastine and 5-fluorouracil (5-FU) intermittently for a period of three years in a partially randomized trial, while Katsuki and associates from Japan also reported beneficial results from a combination of chromomycin and mitomycin C in intermittent courses for a 3-year period.[293] However, all of these trials reporting beneficial survival figures were uncontrolled, involved small numbers of patients, or used an unacceptable selection of patients. There were also a number of other trials reported from outside the U.S.A. during this period, all indicating no benefit from adjuvant chemotherapy.[283,285,286,294,295] Of particular interest is the study of Brunner and associates who administered CTX chemotherapy for a 2-year period following surgical resection.[283] In this controlled trial in which 189 patients having resection were randomized after a nine-year follow-up, the authors found that the rate of recurrence and death from lung cancer was significantly higher in the group receiving long-term CTX therapy. This raises the question that CTX, a drug with strong immunosuppressive effects, may impair unspecified defense mechanisms against tumor cells.

The British Medical Research Council conducted a large randomized trial of busulphan vs. CTX vs. placebo and found no significant difference in survival at five years. However, the survival rates of 28%, 27%, and 34%, respectively, again suggested a possible slight detriment to the chemotherapy-treated groups.[285] A cooperative group effort studied adjuvant CCNU therapy to postsurgical stage I and II non-small cell cancer patients.[287] More pronounced and life-threatening complications were found in the CCNU-treated arm and, if anything, the cancer relapse rate was higher but not significantly so in the chemotherapy arm.

CURRENT RECOMMENDATIONS FOR SURGICAL ADJUVANT CHEMOTHERAPY

At present, the authors feel there is no good evidence suggesting the use of adjuvant chemotherapy after surgical resection for NSCLC. In contrast, there is good evidence that adjuvant chemotherapy for small-cell lung cancer (SCLC) is beneficial. Thus, the authors recommend that in the unusual circumstance when a lung cancer is resected and found to contain SCLC, that the patient be given adjuvant chemotherapy. Any of the standard treatment regimens discussed in the section on SCLC treatment are appropriate. While there has been much discussion and criticism of trial design, stratification, or chemotherapy dose or schedule in the NSCLS adjuvant trials, the positive results with SCLC, a chemotherapy sensitive tumor, underscore the major problem as lack of drug activity against squamous, adenocarcinoma, or large cell carcinoma of the lung. Current randomized trials by the Lung Cancer Study Group are testing some of the more active regimens in an adjuvant fashion, such as the combination of cyclophosphamide, adriamycin, and platinum.[159]

COMBINED MODALITY TREATMENT WITH RADIATION AND CHEMOTHERAPY IN NON-SMALL CELL LUNG CANCER WITH CURATIVE INTENT

The addition of chemotherapy to high-dose radiation therapy given with curative intent could, in theory, kill tumor cells outside the treatment field and also act as a possible radiation sensitizer. However, at present there is no convincing evidence that chemotherapy added to appropriately delivered high-dose radiation therapy has reproducibly and significantly increased the median survival or fraction of long-term, disease-free survivors.[296]

The following single agents plus radiotherapy have been compared to radiotherapy alone, given in doses over 4000 rad, and not found to benefit survival in controlled randomized trials: CTX, 5-FU, HN2, and vinblastine.[297–304,306] Isolated trials have reported statistically significant, but clinically slight positive results for CTX, 5-FU, and procarbazine.[307–309] However, the multiple negative trials indicate these are not reproducible findings. In a few cases, there appears to be a decrease in survival associated with the combined modality use of procarbazine, chromomycin, 5-FU, and actinomycin-D.[301,305,308] Combination chemotherapy + radiation has also not been shown to increase survival compared to high-dose radiation therapy alone in controlled randomized trials. In some cases, the radiotherapy alone appeared statistically better.[296] The combinations tested include 5-FU + actinomycin-D; CCNU and hydroxyurea; CTX or HN2 and MTX; and CTX + MTX + CCNU (for adeno and large cell carcinoma only).[296,301,310] With the combination chemotherapy added to the high-dose radiation therapy, more pronounced, life-threatening, and treatment-related complications were seen compared to radiotherapy alone.[296]

In some randomized trials, all patients have received high-dose radiation therapy and have been randomized to receive different types of chemotherapy. In this way, the regimen of CTX + adriamycin (ADRIA) + cis-platinum (CDDP) (CAP regimen) has significantly improved survival (in adeno and large cell carcinoma; 503 vs. 217 days), compared to patients who received CTX + ADRIA + DTIC.[311] In small numbers of patients, the combination of ADRIA + MTX + CTX + vincristine (VCR) and 5-FU was superior in median survival to CTX alone or the regimen minus ADRIA.[312] The major problem is, of course, whether the inferior chemotherapy was actually detrimental to survival rather than being similar to an untreated control.

There have been several reports of unrandomized trials that added combination chemotherapy to high-dose radiation therapy. Some of these claim to have improved either median or long-term survival compared to their own historical controls treated with radiotherapy alone. They include chemotherapy with CTX + MTX + actinomycin-D + VCR; bleomycin + MTX + VCR; CTX + ADRIA + MTX + procarbazine (CAMP); CTX + MTX + CCNU + ADRIA; CTX + ADRIA + VCR; CCNU + ADRIA + vinblastine.[313–319] These promising trials all use chemotherapy combinations with known objective response rates of 30–40% (see later section in this chapter on chemotherapy of NSCLC). This contrasts with the regimens tested in randomized trials (response rates of 10%). However, these new combinations must be compared in controlled randomized trials to the use of the best radiation therapy alone.

COMBINED MODALITY SURGERY, RADIOTHERAPY, AND CHEMOTHERAPY

There have been preliminary attempts to combine all three modalities in the treatment of NSCLS. Takita and coworkers from Roswell Park Memorial Institute have reported on 24 patients with inoperable NSCLS who were first treated with various combination chemotherapy regimens all of which contained CDDP followed by lung resection, irradiation, immunotherapy, and more chemotherapy.[320] Four patients died with no evidence of tumor and the remaining 20 patients were alive for periods of up to 27 months. DeMeester and colleagues from the University of Chicago have reported on 37 patients with resectable lesions confined to the chest who were treated with 3000 rads of radiation, in addition to resection of the primary tumor and 12–15 cycles of CAMP chemotherapy.[321] This group had a 47% survival at 42 months compared to 0% for nine historical control patients treated similarly but without the chemotherapy. In all such trials, there appears to be a cadre of long-term, potentially cured survivors. However, the major question remains: Does the combined modality approach (radiation + chemotherapy or radiation + surgery + chemotherapy) in these patients with disease confined to the chest represent an increase over the cures achieved by either radiation or surgery along? Because of the various possibilities of patient selection in comparisons to historical controls the question remains open. Therefore, the authors' current recommendation is only to treat stage III MO NSCLC patients with such combined modality therapy on approved clinical trials.

Prophylactic Cranial Irradiation in Non-Small Cell Lung Cancer

The role of prophylactic cranial irradiation in NSCLC is not yet defined. The frequency of brain metastases is less in this group compared to small-cell carcinoma of lung both initially and during follow-up. However, patients with stage III MO adenocarcinoma of the lung receiving combined modality therapy have been reported to have a very high rate (38%) of CNS metastases at the first site of relapse.[317] The VALG conducted a prospectively randomized trial of prophylactic cranial irradiation (PCI) in all types of lung cancer and found a significant reduction in the frequency of clinically detectable brain metastases in the NSCLC patients (13% in unirradiated and 6% in the irradiated group).[322] While there was, in effect, no survival of the PCI for these groups as a whole, patients exhibiting brain metastases had significantly shorter survival than those who did not. Thus, for the 7% of patients randomized to receive PCI who did not develop brain metastases a survival advantage probably exists. However, because of the present low incidence of brain metastases in NSCLC patients, the authors feel there is currently no routine role for PCI, particularly as an adjuvant to surgical resection despite the fact that PCI appears to work in the small fraction of patients at risk. In the uncommon adenocarcinoma patient with stage III disease and a dramatic ("complete" response) to chemotherapy or radiotherapy, PCI could be given with much the same rationale as the treatment of SCLC with PCI.

APPROACH TO PATIENTS WITH DISSEMINATED NON-SMALL CELL LUNG CANCER

The patient with histologically documented, unresectable, or inoperable NSCLC (*i.e.*, epidermoid, adenocarcinoma, large cell, or bronchoalveolar carcinoma) should first be evaluated for radiotherapy. If it is felt the disease is sufficiently limited (VALG limited stage; AJC stage III MO) so that it can be encompassed within a tolerable radiotherapy port (and thus treated "for cure"), or, if there are pressing symptomatic needs for palliation (*e.g.*, complete bronchial obstruction, hemcptysis, upper airway, or superior vena caval [SVC] obstruction), the initial treatment should be with radiotherapy (with or without chemotherapy or surgery, if part of an experimental protocol). If the patient has more disseminated disease (*i.e.*, VALG extensive stage or the TNM system stage III M_1 disease) and there is no pressing need for radiotherapy, the approach can involve supportive therapy alone if the patient is reliable for follow-up or consideration of the use of chemotherapy.[215,323]

THE USE OF RADIOTHERAPY IN THE PALLIATION OF LUNG CANCER

Patients who have AJC stage III lung cancer clearly have a poor prognosis; yet, there is a small but definite salvage rate with surgery or radiotherapy in patients whose disease has not spread beyond mediastinal nodes. In contrast, it is clear that NSCLC patients who have extrathoracic hematogenous metastatic disease are not curable by present therapeutic maneuvers.

When NSCLC patients present with these poor prognostic features, the question of whether or not their primary disease should be irradiated for palliation often arises. Since the patients have a poor prognosis, should they be subjected to therapy with the possibility of radiation pneumonitis and almost certainly esophagitis (short-term) if they have no symptoms? This has been elegantly addressed by others; the absence of symptoms along with the poor prognosis remains the major argument against immediate treatment.[324,325] It should be stressed, however, that the argument is not so much to avoid treatment as to defer it to a time at which the patient becomes symptomatic. The case for palliative treatment of the asymptomatic patient is to prevent major symptoms from occurring within the thorax. The case for delaying treatment really rests upon the reliability of the patient. If the patient can be followed closely, then deferring treatment until the development of symptoms may very well be appropriate. However, patients with a diagnosis of lung cancer are often followed at infrequent intervals. Thus, after diagnosis, these patients may present after a long follow-up interval with extreme symptoms (*e.g.*, superior vena caval obstruction, obstructive pneumonia, or lobar or lung collapse) all of which represent potentially life-threatening problems to the patient who has COPD in addition to lung cancer. When obstructive pneumonia complicates the patient's disease, the patient's treatment must often be started with larger fields than would have been used at presentation and under emergent conditions. In addition, sometimes treatment must be delayed until sepsis can be controlled.

When a patient with NSCLC relapses in the chest after primary surgical therapy, there may well be an indication for radiation therapy to the primary lesion. If prior radiation has been used, and the recurrence appears to be within the mediastinum, a course of low dose, palliative radiation (3000 rad in 2 weeks or slightly higher) is often employed to the mediastinum. The purpose of such treatment is to prevent progressive disease from obstructing the superior vena cava or airway, or from predisposing to pneumonia or sepsis. If the NSCLC patient has a local relapse after surgery, careful restaging reveals no distant metastases, and the patient is physiologically in good shape, a course of high-dose radiotherapy can be attempted. However, there are no data from controlled trials demonstrating benefit in these cases. A retreatment with irradiation after prior palliative radiation may also be considered, depending on the volume and dose previously exposed, the time-course of symptoms after the first course, the progression of disease at other sites, and alternative treatment plans. The decision should be made by the radiotherapist in conjunction with other physicians actively taking care of the patient.

COMMON PROBLEMS IN THE MANAGEMENT OF LUNG CANCER

The general principles of diagnosis and management of metastatic disease, oncologic emergencies, and paraneoplastic syndromes (all common problems in lung cancer patients) are discussed in Chapters 39, 41, and 42. However, when lung cancer of any cell type presents with a localized problem that manifests symptoms, radiation therapy is frequently used (see Table 14-36). Other approaches to the primary therapy of SCLC are discussed later. Such a problem as superior vena caval (SVC) obstruction can usually be relieved with a course of 3000–4000 rad over a 2–4 week period with most patients achieving a response.[95,96,326,328] Cardiac tamponade can also be alleviated in many patients with pericardiocentesis and radiation therapy to the entire cardiac silhouette.[99] Such treatment is usually fractionated more slowly than standard treatment because of concerns over later cardiac toxicity, interactions with adriamycin and other chemotherapeutic agents, and the typically large volume of lung that has to be incorporated into the treatment volume behind the enlarged heart silhouette. Malignant pleural effusion usually does not respond well to radiation, because the dose to the entire pleura is limited to about 2000 rad to spare the adjacent lung tissue. Hemoptysis as a symptom of tumor is usually successfully relieved with radiation therapy.

When an entire lobe or lung has been collapsed by bronchial obstruction, radiation therapy is frequently employed, but only with modest success. In general, a lobe or lung has the greatest probability of being re-expanded if collapsed only a short time (hours to few days). The longer the tissue has been collapsed, the less likely it appears that radiation therapy can induce re-expansion. This is far less true for SCLC than other types.

Symptomatic brain metastases and bone metastases usually respond to palliative doses of radiation therapy (approximately 3000 rad in 2 weeks). Occasionally, such lesions will clear completely with treatment, but usually careful evaluation of the site in question will still show persistent neoplasm that is asymptomatic. If such a metastasis is the only site of distant spread, physicians may occasionally decide to treat the metastasis and primary with curative doses, hoping that the known sites of involvement can be controlled and that no other involvement exists.

Spinal cord compression should be suspected in the lung cancer patient complaining of back pain, with or without lower extremity weakness. In general, patients with spinal cord compression represent an emergency in which the best neurologic results are achieved by continuous vigil of the physician. Early diagnosis when symptoms are modest is the

TABLE 14-36. Local Symptomatic Relief Achieved by Radiation Therapy in Patients with Bronchogenic Carcinoma (all cell types combined)

SYMPTOM	% RELIEF OF SYMPTOM	REFERENCES
Hemoptysis	84	(326,327)
Pain	66	(326,327)
Atelectasis	23	(326)
Superior vena caval obstruction	70–86	(326,328)
Dyspnea	60	(326,327)
Vocal cord paralysis	6	(326)
Cough	60	(326)

keystone of management. Radiation therapy will usually be the treatment of choice unless symptoms are very rapidly progressive. Paralysis of the lower legs, with or without a radicular component of pain, and with or without bowel or bladder dysfunction, makes the diagnosis obvious. When a spinal cord compression syndrome is suspected, a myelogram is essential to delineate the extent of the problem. Palliative irradiation is usually successful at alleviating the symptoms if major neurologic compromise has not already occurred. Since lung cancer is the most common neoplastic cause of spinal cord compression, a low threshold for the diagnosis is the most important variable in achieving a good functional result.[329–331] The more extensive the neurologic deficit at the time of diagnosis, the more difficult it is to achieve neurologic normality following radiation therapy.

Spinal cord compression can occur from either extension into the spinal canal from a vertebral metastasis or extension from a paravertebral mass through the intervertebral foramina. Because the compression may be occurring anywhere along the circumference of the spinal cord, decompressive laminectomy is usually reserved for: patients whose symptomatology is progressing so rapidly that there does not appear to be time for a response to irradiation; for those with recurrent cord compression in whom further irradiation cannot safely be delivered; and for those in whom a tissue diagnosis is not at hand. The more extensive the compression, the more difficult it is to return to normal neurologic function. Moreover, the more extensive the laminectomy, the greater is the instability of the spine that results. Since removal of the laminae only exposes the posterior aspect of the spinal cord, postoperative irradiation is still indicated in these patients, since metastatic disease is rarely confined solely to the posterior aspect of the cord. With or without surgery, doses of 3000–4000 rad over 2–4 weeks are necessary for palliation, often starting with 300–400 rad fractions. Concomitantly with radiotherapy, dexamethasone 25–100 mg/day divided into four doses is given initially and rapidly tapered to the lowest dosage that relieves the symptoms.[465] Again, the more extensive the neurologic deficit prior to treatment, the less recovery is expected. If the patient has had prior radiation therapy to the mediastinum and supraclavicular fossa, it can be difficult to distinguish between a brachial plexus syndrome caused by tumor and possible radiation injury. Typically, pain is more likely to be manifestation of tumor than a radiation injury.[332] The presence of a supraclavicular mass is certainly suggestive of tumor. If the patient had therapy more than 6 months prior to the development of the brachial plexus syndrome, does not manifest pain, and has induration throughout the supraclavicular fossa without a discrete mass, then the chance of radiation injury is high. Correlation with careful dosimetric reconstruction is necessary and a clinical diagnosis will often have to be made. When doubt exists and the patient is otherwise in good shape, surgical biopsy of the area may be necessary to plan treatment rationally.

USE OF CHEMOTHERAPY IN NON-SMALL CELL LUNG CANCER

A crucial question remains: Does chemotherapy benefit NSCLC patients in terms of either quality or quantity of survival? The answer is not straightforward and involves an individual assessment of each patient for prognostic variables.[333] Objective tumor shrinkage from chemotherapy is associated with prolonged survival compared to patients with tumor progression.[334–342] However, in most studies a significant survival difference has not been found between responders and patients with stable disease.[341,343,344] Complete tumor regressions are rare and the bulk of the tumor responses occur in patients with good performance status and with less total tumor bulk.[334,336,345] Thus, it is hard to separate out survival advantage resulting from chemotherapy-induced tumor shrinkage from the more favorable prognostic factors these same patients have initially.

The important prognostic factors governing the decision about the use of chemotherapy are stage of disease, performance status, weight loss, and age.[333,346] The initial history, physical examination, routine chest film, and laboratory tests will identify these factors. Nearly all current chemotherapy trials in NSCLC have performance status and stage of disease as stratification factors and all treatment comparisons should take these factors into account.[333] While pretreatment weight loss, in addition to sex, age, and immunologic tests have each been correlated with survival time in individual studies, none have consistently predicted survival as have performance status and extent of disease. For nonprotocol clinical care, all subsequent staging studies should be done only to investigate specific symptoms or signs.

SELECTION OF PATIENTS FOR CHEMOTHERAPY

Currently, there are no data demonstrating that single agent or combination chemotherapy affects survival of NSCLC patient treatment groups as a whole, independent of the prognostic variables discussed above. As a general principle, the bulk of chemotherapy responses occur in patients with good prognostic variables, particularly good performance status, and no prior chemotherapy.[334,338,339,341,343] Thus, the authors feel that nonprotocol chemotherapy should be reserved for those patients with good performance status (PS 0, 1, 2), under 70 years of age, weight loss less than 12%, and no prior chemotherapy. The results of chemotherapy even in this most favorable group are still relatively poor, and they become even more dismal in patients with poor prognostic factors.

CRITERIA OF TUMOR RESPONSE

Because objective tumor response is associated with prolonged survival, it is important to have standard criteria for determining such responses. However, these criteria can often be difficult to apply. The Eastern Cooperative Oncology Group (ECOG) objective tumor response criteria for NSCLC can be summarized as follows: a complete response (CR) is defined as disappearance of all lesions for at least one month; a partial response (PR) is defined as a 50% decrease in the product of the greatest perpendicular diameters of one or more measurable lesions. This must last at least one month and not be accompanied by increasing lesions elsewhere; neither should it be accompanied by declining performance status. Progressive disease is defined as the development of new lesions, a significantly enlarging old lesion, a significant drop in weight of 10% or more, or drop in PS of 2 scores (*e.g.*, PS 1 to PS 3). No change or stable disease represents patients with no significant increase or decrease in tumor size. Stable disease is an interim category as these patients, if followed sufficiently, will ultimately go on to either show tumor shrinkage or tumor progression.[335] "Minimal tumor responses" should be dealt with as no change or stable disease as they probably reflect difficulty in evaluating tumor responses.

A major problem in determining tumor responses in lung cancer is that the most visible tumor is usually apparent only on chest film and often does not have clearly defined, easily measurable borders. Frequently, these borders abut normal intrathoracic structures; while there usually is an easily measurable border this does not represent the largest perpendicular diameter. The Mayo Clinic has evaluated 191 NSCLC patients in their chemotherapy trials and found 54% had "measurable" lesions (tumor masses with clearly defined perpendicular diameters that were easily measured), while 43% had "evaluable" disease (tumor that was apparent but without clearly measurable borders).[335] The standard response criteria for CR and PR were applied to measurable tumors, for scoring a CR in evaluable disease. In evaluable disease, an objective tumor response (regression, R) was defined as a definite decrease in tumor size, agreed upon by two investigators with no new lesion(s).[335] For evaluable lesions, stable disease required no new lesions or definite progression, while to score progressive disease required a definite increase relative to the smallest measurement which again had to be agreed upon by two investigators. When these criteria were applied, the Mayo group could not detect significant differences in regression rates, times to regression, duration of regression or survival between the two categories. Of all patients treated, 31% (most with combination chemotherapy) had an objective tumor response of either a measurable or evaluable lesion. While there was no difference in survival between patients with measurable and evaluable lesions, there was a significant difference in the median survival of responders (13 months) vs. the non-responders (6 months).[335] Thus, either the definition of objective tumor response in measurable disease ("partial response") or a definite "regression" of evaluable tumor mass may be used. Both are associated with prolonged survival.

RESPONSES TO SINGLE AGENT CHEMOTHERAPY IN NON-SMALL CELL LUNG CANCER

No single agent chemotherapy has yet significantly increased overall survival in NSCLC. The duration of the objective tumor responses that occur is short, lasting 2–4 months; complete responses are rarely seen.[336,347] Response rates are almost uniformly higher in patients not having received prior chemotherapy of any type.[336,347] Using the relatively strict criteria outlined above, partial objective tumor responses are seen, but only in 10% or less of NSCLC patients treated with single agent alkalating agents (*e.g.*, NH2, CTX), nitrosoureas, MTX, and bleomycin.[336,347] In addition, 5-FU and VCR may have a similar level of activity but only in adenocarcinoma of the lung.[348,349] In contrast, vindesine, ADRIA, mitomycin-C (MMC), and VP-16-213 have all given objective tumor responses in approximately 15–20% of NSCLC patients treated; each has been tested in 40 or more patients (see Table 14-37). Recently, the EORTC Lung Cancer Working Party found a 26% response rate in 62 NSCLC patients treated with high-dose CDDP (120 mg/M every three weeks with a mannitol-induced diuresis). Thus, this agent may also have major activity (see Table 14-37). While many other agents have been tested, they have rarely shown activity.[347] Recently, Ifosfamide, an alkalating agent related to CTX, showed remarkable activity in epidermoid and large cell lung cancer (a 39% response including 7% complete responses).[360]

RESPONSES TO COMBINATION CHEMOTHERAPY IN NON-SMALL CELL LUNG CANCER

The evidence that combination chemotherapy is better than the most active of the single agents in NSCLC is just beginning to appear. Thus, a conservative approach is necessary.[336] The results of several large cooperative group randomized trials failed to find significant benefit between single agent chemotherapy and combinations of drugs that are now considered relatively inactive.[336,361] In these trials, the following comparisons showed no benefit of drug combinations: CTX vs. CTX + CCNU + HN2 vs. HN2 + CCNU; CTX vs. CTX + VCR + MeCCNU + bleomycin (BLEO); CCNU vs. BLEO vs. CCNU + BLEO; MECCNU vs. MeCCNU + VCR vs. MeCCNU + VCR + MTX; and ICRF-159 vs VCR + BLEO

TABLE 14-37. Response Rates of the Most Active Single Agents in the Chemotherapy of Non-Small Cell Lung Cancer.*

DRUG	NUMBER OF PATIENTS	OBJECTIVE RESPONSE PERCENTAGE	REFERENCES
Vindesine	73	23	(350,351)
Mitomycin-C	55	27	(352,353)
Cis-platinum			
120 mg/m^2 given every 3 weeks†	62	26	(354)
50 mg/m^2 given days 1, 8 every 4 weeks	54	17	(355)
75 mg/m^2 given weekly for 3 doses, then every 3 weeks	17	14	(356)
Adriamycin	154	18	(357,358)
VP-16-123	44	18	(359)

* In the vast majority of cases, no prior chemotherapy has been given.
† With mannitol diuresis.

+ ADRIA.[361] In all cases, there was no significant increase in response rate, median survival, or complete response rate; no long-term survivors appeared. In some cases, single agent CTX actually yielded increased survival compared to the combination therapy (*e.g.*, CTX + VCR + MeCCNU + BLEO or "COMB" regimen).[362] The VALG randomized 762 NSCLC patients to treatment with CTX alone, CTX + CCNU, CTX + ADRIA, or to CCNU + ADRIA.[337] There was no significant difference in the response rates (all low at 4–5%) for the different regimens. Also 20–25% of the patients treated with the drug combinations had severe and life-threatening side effects of the chemotherapy. However, there was a survival advantage for CTX + ADRIA compared to CTX in the subgroup of epidermoid carcinoma but not for adeno or large cell carcinoma.

Other combinations tested in large numbers of patients include: CTX + VCR + MTX + 5-FU + prednisone (206 patients, 14% responses, 3 months median survival); and "BACON" (BLEO + ADRIA + CCNU + VCR + HN2) in 50 patients with 43% response rate and 5 months overall median survival.[363,364] However, when BACON was compared to NAC (NH2 + ADRIA + CCNU), there was no significant benefit in terms of response rate (21%), response duration (4 months), or survival (median of 4 months).[365] Overall, there was a 4% treatment related mortality rate and an additional 10% had life-threatening therapy toxicities. This randomized cooperative group study was extremely important because it came at a time in the early 1970's when combination chemotherapy was being widely applied to a variety of unresponsive solid tumors including NSCLC. This study and many of the pilot phase II trials suggested a more conservative view. However, the trials did confirm the benefit of an objective tumor response on survival, and the importance of an initial good performance status on achieving such a response.

Beginning in 1975, the ECOG began a prospectively randomized trial of more than 16 different combination chemotherapies or single agents in over 680 patients with no prior chemotherapy of PS 0, 1, 2, 3.[334] Standard ECOG response criteria were used and randomized, comparisons were made to the "standard therapy" of 1975, CTX + CCNU. It is extremely sobering to consider the results of this trial for it represents a conservative estimate of the benefits of combination chemotherapy (see Table 14-38). The overall objective response rate for patients treated with combination chemotherapy was 14% (59/434 patients); only 0.9% complete response was seen. There was a general correlation between the objective response rate and the median survival. Thus, analysis of other factors correlating with response rate is important. The toxicity of the combination chemotherapy portions of the trial were not trivial as 19% had severe toxicity, 9% had life-threatening, and 3% had drug-related deaths. Thus, the fraction of patients with objective tumor responses was balanced by the number of patients with severe toxicity. This indicates the need for careful patient selection and close monitoring of combination chemotherapy in NSCLC. Regimens with significantly greater response rates than CTX + CCNU included: hexamethylmelamine (HMM) + ADRIA + MTX (HAM) regimen; CTX + CDDP + BLEO; ADRIA + 5-FU + CDDP; and mitomycin-C (MMC). Other combinations, including the MTX + ADRIA + CTX + CCNU (MACC) regimen, were not more active than CTX + CCNU. The need for confirmatory evidence of activity of new combinations is amply demonstrated by the MACC example. Previously, the MACC regimen had given an objective response rate of 44% in 68 patients in the initial phase II trial with a median survival for all NSCLC patients of 29–35 weeks, and for responders, 40–48 weeks.[366] However, the ECOG trial found only a 12% response rate in 43 patients

TABLE 14-38. Results of Combination Chemotherapy vs. Single Agents in the Eastern Cooperative Oncology Group Randomized Trials in Unresectable (Limited and Extensive Stage) Non-Small Cell Lung Cancer (N = 680 patients)

DRUG THERAPY*	NUMBER OF PATIENTS	OBJECTIVE RESPONSE PERCENTAGE	MEDIAN SURVIVAL WEEKS
HXM + ADRIA + MTX	41	27	34
ADRIA + 5-FU + CDDP	45	24	27
CTX + CDDP + BLEO	26	23	18
CTX + MTX	61	13	23
5-FU + procarbazine	19	11	16
VCR + BLEO + MTX	20	10	13
CTX + CCNU ("standard therapy")	140	9	16
MTX + ADRIA + CTX + CCNU	43	12	14
Dibromodulcitol + ADRIA	39	8	20
Seven single agents†	246	8 (overall)	12,12,13, 13,15,16,20

(Ruckdeschel J, Metha C, Creech R: Chemotherapy of advanced non-oat cell bronchogenic carcinoma: The Eastern Cooperative Oncology Group Experience. In Hansen HH, Dombernowsky P (eds): Abstracts II World Conference on Lung Cancer, p 237. Copenhagen, Amsterdam-Oxford-Princeton, Excerpta Medica, 1980)

* Hexamethylmelamine, HXM; doxorubicin, Adria; methotrexate, MTX; 5-flourouracil, 5-FU; cis-platinum, CDDP; bleomycin, Bleo; vincristine,VCR. CTX + CCNU was a common arm as "standard therapy" for several of the trials.

† Mitomycin-C, Baker's antifol, piperazinedione, actinomycin-D, Ftorafur, melphalan, galactitol.

TABLE 14-39. Results of Treating Non-Small Cell Lung Cancer Patients With Combination Chemotherapy with Cyclophosphamide + Adriamycin + Cis-platinum (CAP) (N = 268 patients)

	NUMBER OF PATIENTS TREATED	OBJECTIVE RESPONSE PERCENTAGE
All patients	268*	34 (1.4 % complete response)
Epidermoid	70	36
Adenocarcinoma	128	35
Large cell carcinoma	58	34
Fully ambulatory (PS 0, 1)	144	37
Less ambulatory (PS 2,3)	63	14
	Median Survival in Weeks for Each Study	
All patients treated	18, 24, 25, 29, 30, 37†	
Patients with objective tumor response	28, 32, 49+, 52,†, 56, 64	
Non-responders	10, 12, 16, 17, 18, 35†	
	Median Duration in Weeks	
Patients with objective tumor response	10+, 14, 28, 32	

(Eagan RT, Ingle JN, Frytak S et al: Platinum based polychemotherapy versus dianhydrogolactitol in advanced non-small cell cancer. Cancer Treat Rep 61:1339–1345, 1977; Galla RJ, Cvitkovic E, Golby RB: Cis-dichlorodiammine-platinum (II) in non-small cell carcinoma of the lung. Cancer Treat Rep 63:1585–1588, 1979; Evans, WK, Feld R, Deboer G et al: Cyclophosphamide, adriamycin, and cis-platinum in the treatment of non-small cell lung cancer. Proc AACR-ASCO 21:447, 1980; Britell JC, Eagan RT, Ingle JN et al: *cis*-Dichlorodiammineplatinum (II) alone followed by adriamycin plus cyclophosphamide at progression versus *cis*-dichlorodiammine platinum (II), adriamycin, and cyclophosphamide in combination for adenocarcinoma of the lung. Cancer Treat Rep 62:1207–1210, 1978.

* Data for each histologic type, performance status, and response category not always specified.

† Limited stage patients only.

with a median survival for all patients of 14 weeks, 25 weeks for the responders.[367]

Several other factors are demonstrated in the statistical analysis of this large ECOG trial that are similar to many other smaller series reported in the literature. There was no difference in response rates based on histologic type of NSCLC. However, initial performance status was correlated with response with significantly more responders in patients with PS 0, 1 than PS 2, 3.[334] Poor performance status, extensive stage disease, weight loss, and prior radiation therapy were all negative prognostic factors for survival, while prior surgery was a positive prognostic factor. This latter result probably relates to selection of patients with relatively limited stage disease, able to tolerate surgery, and who have had an early postsurgical recurrence. The median survival of responders to any of the regimens was 32–41 weeks, significantly better than the nonresponders who had a median survival of 16 weeks. However, because an objective response was highly correlated with good initial performance status, when all the prognostic variables are statistically accounted for, none of the treatments except the HAM regimen in limited stage disease appeared to prolong survival consistently and significantly.[334]

The most conclusive evidence for the benefits of combination chemotherapy comes in a series of randomized trials conducted by the Mayo Clinic.[338,368] They compared the combination of CTX + ADRIA + CDDP (CAP regimen) to some of the more active single agents and found that CAP had higher response rate (41%) compared to either dianhydrogalactitol (an alkalating agent), VP-16, or CDDP all given as single agents (11% response rate overall). In addition, upon failure on the single agent, 33% of patients responded to the CAP combination and these responders had median survivals of 56–88 weeks. While there was no significant difference in overall survival between single agent and combination chemotherapy (related in part to crossing patients over to combination chemotherapy from the single agents), the responders to both combination chemotherapy and single agent chemotherapy lived significantly longer (median survival of 56+ and 49+ weeks, respectively) than the nonresponders (17 and 12 weeks, respectively). Thus, over three times as many patients in the group treated with combination therapy had objective tumor responses and corresponding survival advantage compared to patients receiving only single agent chemotherapy.

Following the description by the Mayo Clinic of the CAP regimen, several other groups have confirmed the activity of this combination (see Table 14-39). The overall objective tumor response rate is 34% but the complete response rate remains very low. There is no difference in response by cell type but the bulk of the responders occur in fully ambulatory patients. Because some limited stage patients in these series also received chest radiotherapy, it is difficult to relate stage to response. However, there is no dramatic difference between limited and extensive stage. The median survival for all patients treated is about 6–7 months, while it is one year for the responders and 4 months for the nonresponders. The responses last about 7 months and most occur within the first two cycles of chemotherapy (although this has not always been reported). Various modifications of the CAP regimen have been made including increasing the dose of CDDP to 60 mg/m², or 120 mg/m², and adding VP-16-213, vindesine, or CCNU + VCR; there is no evidence reported from more than one institution of any response rate or survival benefit resulting from these changes.[339,340,369,372] Early results from a randomized trial comparing CAP to CTX + VCR + CDDP show no difference between the regimens.[370]

Other drug combinations tested in over 50 patients and having significant activity at more that one institution include the CAMP regimen (CTX + ADRIA + MTX + procarbazine: 31% responses); the combination of vindesine and CDDP (43% responses); and the FOMi combination (5-FU + VCR + mitomycin-C: 36% responses).[343,373–377] In all of these, the responders have significantly improved survival compared to the nonresponders although they do not have significant survival advantage when compared to those patients with stable disease. Whether the stable disease is related to response to drug therapy or is a function of tumor biology is as yet unknown. All of these regimens have similar median survivals to the CAP program for all patients treated (approximately 7 months depending on prognostic factors). Thus, at present there is no basis to select between them other than the relatively different toxicities contributed by CDDP (GI, renal), ADRIA (cardiac), vindesine (neurologic), and mitomycin-C (cumulative bone marrow or pulmonary). The doses of the drugs in these various programs are listed in Table 14-40 and the response rates of these and other recently reported combination chemotherapy regimens with reasonable numbers of patients and follow-up are presented in Tables 14-39 and 14-41. Consistent findings in all of these trials are overall objective response rates of 25–40%, complete response rates of 5–10%, overall median survivals of 5–10 months, and median survival of responders of about 12 months. In most cases, 1–5% of treatment related mortalities are seen. While overall this is discouraging, the consistent finding of complete responders five-fold over the rate seen in prior combination chemotherapy programs suggests that some progress is being made.[336] However, none of the regimens consistently gives tumor responses in over 90% of patients or complete responses in 50% of patients treated, which is the current status in

TABLE 14-40. Sample Drug Regimens Used in the Treatment of Non-Small Cell Lung Cancer

CAP[338,340,341,368]

Cyclophosphamide	400 mg/m² IV	All given day 1 and repeated every 4 weeks.
Adriamycin	40 mg/m² IV	
Cis-platinum	40 mg/m² IV	

1. Patients must have normal cardiac and renal status (creatinine less than 1.5 mg/dl).
2. Doses are given by rapid IV infusion with 1 liter of 5% glucose in half normal saline over 1–2 hours; no special diuresis program is routinely employed.
3. Doses are modified to obtain WBC nadirs of 1,500–2,500/μl or platelet nadirs of 75,000–100,000/μl measured at day 14. Prior to each subsequent treatment, WBC should be > 4,000/μl and platelets > 100,000/μl.
4. Stop cis-platinum permanently if creatinine rises above 2.0 mg/dl, or hearing loss develops.
5. Stop adriamycin at a maximum cumulative dose of 450 mg/m² or if signs of congestive heart failure or arrythmias develop.

CAMP[343,373,374]

Cyclophosphamide	300 mg/m²	days 1, 8 IV Repeat combination on day 29.
Adriamycin	20 mg/m²	days 1, 8 IV
Methotrexate	15 mg/m²	days 1, 8 IV
Procarbazine	100 mg/m²	days 1 through 10 orally

1. Patients must have normal cardiac status.
2. Doses are modified according to blood counts before next cycle or if nadir count (days 17–21) is unacceptably low. On day 1, 75% of dose if WBC less than 4,000/μ1, 50% if WBC is less than 3,000/μ1 or platelets less than 100,000; no drugs given when WBC less than 2,000 or platelets less than 75,000/μl.
3. Stop adriamycin at maximum cumulative dose of 450 mg/m² or if signs of congestive heart failure or arrythmias develop.
4. Reduce or omit dose of procarbazine for severe nausea and vomiting.

FOMI-[376,377]

5-fluorouracil	300 mg/m² IV days 1, 2, 3, 4	Repeat combination every 3 weeks for 3 courses then every 6 weeks.
Vincristine	2 mg total dose IV day 1	
Mitomycin-C	10 mg/m² IV day 1	

1. Appropriate drug reductions for hematologic toxicity, neurotoxicity, and mucositis.

VINDESINE + PLATINUM[375]

Vindesine	3 mg/m² IV	weekly for 7 doses then every 2 weeks
Cis-platinum	120 mg/m² IV	with mannitol diuresis days 1, 29 then every 6 weeks

1. Patients must have normal renal function, and no significant neurologic defect.
2. All patients will have nausea, vomiting, alopecia, and paraesthesias. Three percent of patients have had severe neuropathy and vindesine must be stopped if severe neuropathy develops.
3. Appropriate dose modifications for hematologic and renal toxicity. Omit cis-platinum if creatinine is 2 mg/dl or higher until creatinine returns to less than 1.5 mg/dl.

TABLE 14-41. Recent Results of Combination Chemotherapy in Non-Small Cell Lung Cancer*

DRUGS†	NUMBER OF PATIENTS TREATED	PR + CR‡	CR	CELL TYPE§	MEDIAN SURVIVAL (Months) ALL PATIENTS/ RESPONDERS	REFERENCES
		%	%			
CTX + ADRIA + MTX + PCZ ("CAMP")	131	31	7.5	All NSCLC	8/13	(343,373,374)
DVA + CDDP (120 mg/m²)‖	83	43	NS#	NS	NS/14+	(375)
5-FU+ VCR + MITO-C ("FOMi")	80	36	5	AC, LC	6/8	(376,377)
CDDP + ADRIA + CTX + CCNU + VCR	51	31	10	All NSCLC	5–12/20**	(371,372)
Ftorafur + ADRIA + CDDP	45	42	7	AC, LC	6/NS	(378)
VP-16 + CDDP	42	43	7	All NSCLC	NS	(379,380)
CTX + ADRIA + CDDP + VP-16		35		AC	6/	(369)
CTX + VP-16	24	63	8	All NSCLC	10/NS	(381)
CTX + ADRIA + VP-16	15	13	0	All NSCLC	6/NS	(382)
HMM + CDDP	51	16	0	All NSCLC	NS/8	(383)
MITO-C + VBL + CDDP	30	53	7	NS	NS	(345)
MITO-C + ADRIA + CTX	33	21	0	AC, LC	6/10	(384)
5-FU + ADRIA + MITO-C	25	36	8	AC	7/9+	(344)
5-FU + CTX + CCNU	31	22	3	AC	9/21	(385)
CTX + ADRIA + MTX††	34	29	9	AC	7/11	(386)
CCNU + ADRIA	23	35	9	All NSCLC	7/10	(387)
CCNU + MTX + ADRIA	53	19	4	EP	5/7	(342)
CTX + MTX + CCNU	28	25	0	AC	5/12	(342)
5-FU + ADRIA	26	15	0	AC	4/12	(342)

* Only results of no prior chemotherapy patients used. Median survivals rounded to nearest month.

† CTX, cyclophosphamide; ADRIA, doxorubicin, adriamycin; MTX, methotrexate; PCZ, procarbazine; DVA, vindesine; CDDP, cis-dichlorodiammineplatinum (II), cis-platinum; 5-FU, 5-fluorouracil; VCR, vincristine; MITO-C, mitomycin-C; HMM, hexamethylmelamine; VBL, vinblastine; VP-16, VP-16-213; CCNU, chloroethyl–cyclohexyl nitrosourea.

‡ PR, partial objective tumor response and "objective regressions" for patients with evaluable but not measurable disease; CR, complete tumor regression. PR + CR = all patients with an objective tumor response.

§ All NSCLC = epidermoid, adenocarcinoma, large cell, bronchioloalveolar, and other variants; AC, adenocarcinoma; LC, large cell carcinoma; EP, epidermoid carcinoma.

‖ High dose CDDP given with hydration, mannitol diuresis, furosemide.

\# NS (not stated).

** Long survival of responders reported in one study only.

†† Intermediate dose methotrexate with citrovorum factor rescue.

small cell carcinoma. In addition, the more optimistic of the regimens need to have their activities confirmed in more patients, at other institutions, and in cooperative group trials.

SUMMARY OF RECOMMENDATIONS FOR CHEMOTHERAPY OF NON-SMALL CELL LUNG CANCER

Only rarely have combination chemotherapy programs been reported to yield long-term (30-month plus) disease-free survivors in NSCLC without radiotherapy in unresectable disease.[388–390] In addition, it is possible in these rare cases that a mistake in histologic diagnosis was made and the tumor treatment was actually SCLC. Similarly, combination chemotherapy has not been shown to increase the number of long-term disease-free survivors when added to high-dose radiotherapy. While there is mention of improved quality of life and relief of symptoms in responding patients, these have not been clearly documented. This is in contrast to SCLC where the dramatic shrinkage of tumor masses usually gives relief of symptoms, in addition to improvement in performance status. For these reasons, and because of the importance of the prognostic factors mentioned above, the authors make the following recommendations for employing non-protocol chemotherapy in unresectable NSCLC (if the patient is a candidate for curative radiotherapy this should be given alone except as part of a clinical trial): Chemotherapy should be reserved until the time of disease progression. If a patient has a local symptom requiring palliation, it should be irradiated and the decision about chemotherapy reviewed later. To be eligible for non-protocol chemotherapy, patients should be fully ambulatory (PS 0, 1) with life expectancy of several months; less ambulatory patients (PS 2, 3, 4) should not be treated unless their PS improves to make them fully ambulatory. Patients should have had no prior chemotherapy and certainly no prior combination chemotherapy. They should have measurable or evaluable disease to assess tumor response and no medical contraindications (*e.g.*, heart or renal) to chemotherapy. Patients with 10% or more weight loss and some other negative prognostic feature, such as prior chemotherapy or radiotherapy, should probably not be given more chemotherapy. Finally, patients should be able to understand and accept the potential toxicities and the limited nature of the potential benefits involved.

One of the standard combination chemotherapy regimens with demonstrable activity shown in a large number of patients by several institutions should be used (*e.g.*, CAP, CAMP, FOMi, vindesine + CDDP). The dose schedules and modifications should be followed carefully. Patients should be treated for 2–3 months and then have their tumor status reassessed. Any patient with documented progressive disease at this time or in the future should immediately have the combination chemotherapy stopped. Patients with stable disease or an objective tumor response after 3–4 cycles should be continued on therapy. If there is significant toxicity at any time in stable disease patients, it is reasonable to discontinue chemotherapy as there is no evidence that chemotherapy benefits these patients. At the time of objective disease progression, decrease in PS by 2 scores, or loss of 10% or more of the true body weight chemotherapy should be stopped. Following these guidelines should allow patient selection with the greatest likelihood of benefit and the least chance of serious toxicities.

There are no data to determine the length of maintenance chemotherapy in the occasional NSCLC patient who achieves a complete clinical remission. At present, the authors recommend following the same principles laid down for the treatment of SCLC. Namely, to treat for approximately one year, restage the patient, and if they are still in a complete response to discontinue therapy. Alternatively, treatment could be maintained for up to 2 years depending on patient tolerance. The fact that at least some patients can achieve complete responses to combination chemotherapy in NSCLC is hopeful. What has to be discovered is whether these rare patients represent biologically different tumors (perhaps more closely related to SCLC), or whether their numbers can be increased by developing new chemotherapeutic agents, doses, or schedules, or rationally selecting already available agents through *in vitro* testing.

CLINICAL MANAGEMENT OF PATIENTS DURING PRIMARY TREATMENT OF SMALL CELL CARCINOMA OF THE LUNG (SCLC)

As discussed earlier, the stage of disease (limited versus extensive), the performance status, and prior therapy are important prognostic factors in SCLC. In addition, the degree of tumor response to initial chemotherapy (see Figure 14-19), radiotherapy, or chemoradiotherapy dramatically influences both median and long-term survival. In virtually all series, patients with complete clinical regression of tumor survive longer than patients with objective but only partial regression, who in turn survive longer than patients with no response.[216,218–229,236,330,391–393] Not only the median survival of the complete responders is increased compared to the other response groups, but the vast majority of the long-term survivors (*i.e.*, 2.5 years or greater) come from the complete response (CR) group. Thus, evaluation of benefits of various treatment plans for SCLC should focus on CR rate, number of long-term survivors, and median survival. Knowledge of the initial sites of disease is important in restaging patients after the initial course of treatment. The series with the most carefully documented complete responses after restaging appear to have the most durable tumor regressions and longer survivals when compared to series where the complete response status is less carefully ascertained.

As a background to current treatment plans, it is useful to stress that untreated SCLC patients have median survivals of only 6–17 weeks, and less than 0.5% of all patients are alive 5 years following surgical treatment alone.[214,215,394] In a randomized trial, radiotherapy alone was shown to be superior to surgery alone for patients with limited stage disease; however, the mean survival for these limited stage patients was short (10 months); less than 1–5% of such patients were alive at 5 years.[394] With the advent of systemic chemotherapy there was a dramatic impact on survival. Several reviews of single agent and combination chemotherapy exist for SCLC.[215,236,391–393,395,396] As already discussed, a significant survival advantage was seen in those SCLC patients who had pulmonary nodules resected and then were treated with cyclophosphamide, or cyclosphosphamide + methotrexate compared to patients treated with placebo. When data on SCLC from all of the prospectively randomized surgical adjuvant trials are pooled (because of the relatively small number of patients presenting with resectable lesions), the long-term survival advantage becomes apparent despite the less-than-optimal chemotherapy given (see Table 14-42). Small groups of long-term survivors are being reported from nonrandomized trials who had resectional surgery followed by high-dose combination chemotherapy. A large randomized chemotherapy trial in SCLC found superior survival in patients who had previously undergone pulmonary surgery.[225,399,400] Thus, while the preoperative diagnosis of SCLC is considered a contraindication to thoracotomy currently, the development of active combination chemotherapy will allow a selective re-exploration of the combined role of surgery and chemotherapy in this histologic type.

When chemotherapy and radiotherapy were both found to be active modalities in the treatment of SCLC, three randomized trials compared radiotherapy alone vs. chemotherapy alone.[299,401,402] Despite the inferior nature of the chemotherapy, in two of the three trials chemotherapy alone yielded better median survival compared to radiotherapy, while in the third trial, radiotherapy alone was superior. These trials revealed that metastatic dissemination was the most frequent cause of failure of radiation therapy even in patients with limited stage disease. Six randomized trials, all in limited stage disease, compared radiation therapy alone to radiation therapy plus systemic chemotherapy (which in many cases was not optimal).[298,307,309,403,405] The pooled data from all the trials show median survivals of 5–6 months for the patients treated with radiotherapy alone compared to 9–10 months for the patients treated with radiotherapy plus chemotherapy. In the trials employing the best combination chemotherapy (*e.g.*, using CTX + MTX + CCNU, or CTX + MTX + ADRIA) combined with radiotherapy, the results favored combined modality treatment. This was manifested by increases in 1- or 2-year survival and a decrease at 1 year in the percentage of patients with clinically evident metastases in the group receiving the combined modality therapy.[404,405] These trials demonstrate the superiority of combined chemoradiotherapy compared to radiotherapy alone.

SINGLE AGENT CHEMOTHERAPY

In 1969, Green and coworkers, in a randomized trial, demonstrated a doubling of lifespan in extensive stage SCLC

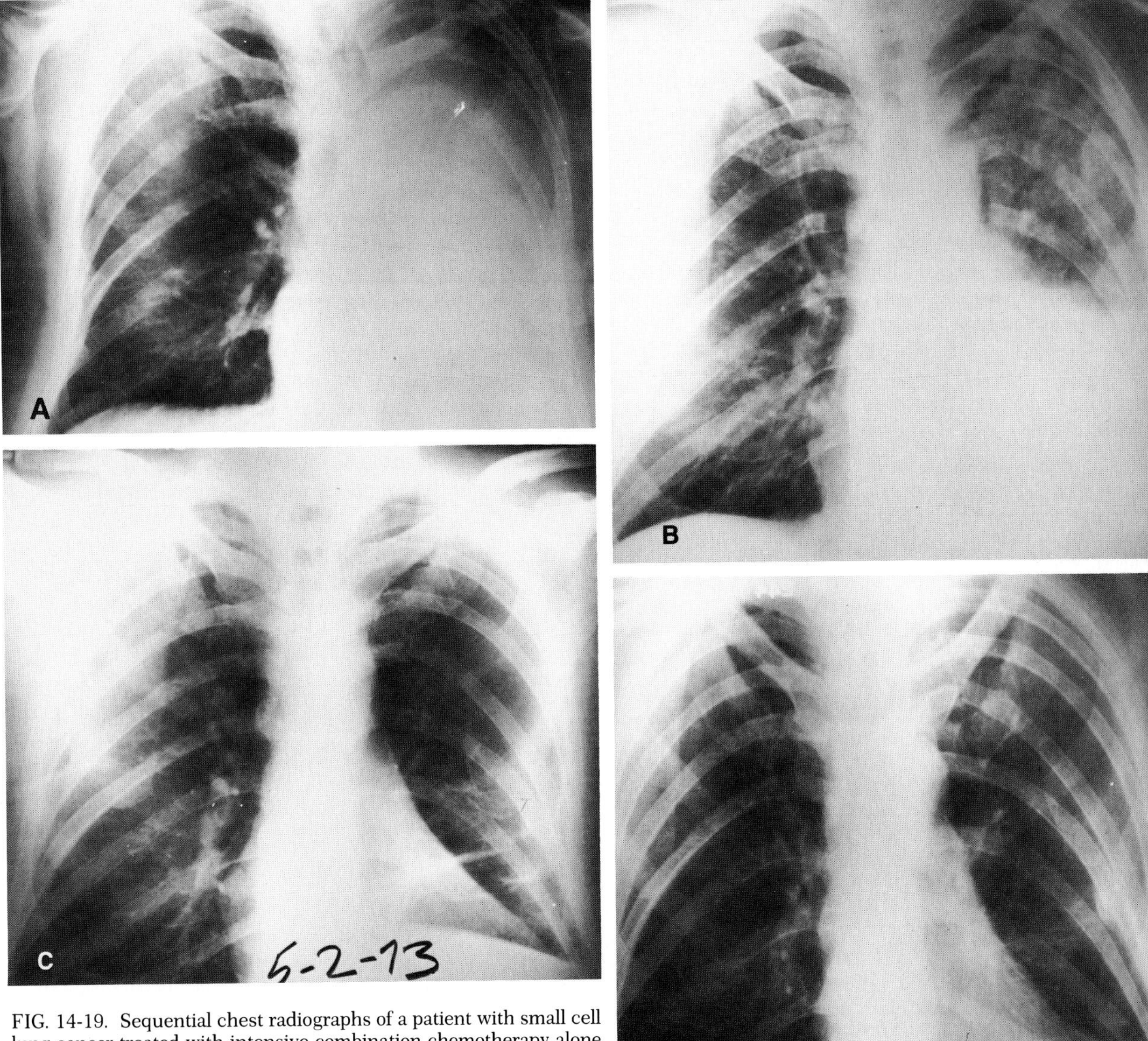

FIG. 14-19. Sequential chest radiographs of a patient with small cell lung cancer treated with intensive combination chemotherapy alone (cyclophosphamide + methotrexate + CCNU regimen). *A*, pretreatment showing large mass in left chest, with obstruction, collapse of left lower lobe, loss of volume, and tracheal deviation. *B*, one week after the start of therapy showing response of tumor, and revealing remaining bulk of tumor in pulmonary parenchyma, hilar, and mediastinal nodes. *C*, three weeks after the start of therapy. Almost complete resolution of tumor; however, there is still some residual stranding and possible mediastinal adenopathy. *D*, five weeks after the start of treatment; no tumor visible by chest radiograph. Fiberoptic bronchoscopy with washings and biopsy at six weeks revealed no evidence of tumor.

patients treated with three courses of CTX compared to patients receiving placebo.[405a] This led to the documentation of activity of a variety of single agents (see Table 14-43).[395] While single agent chemotherapy produced objective tumor responses it rarely produces complete regression of tumors in SCLC, even in previously untreated patients. In contrast, combination chemotherapy yields complete response rates of 25–50% (see Table 14-44). In comparing the results from the

TABLE 14-42. Pooled Results from Randomized Surgical Adjuvant Studies in Small-Cell Lung Cancer[281,291,397,398]

ADJUVANT THERAPY	NUMBER OF PATIENTS	PERCENTAGE OF 2-YEAR SURVIVORS
Chemotherapy	62	34
Placebo	61	8

TABLE 14-43. Chemotherapy Agents with Significant Activity Against Small-Cell Lung Cancer[392,393,395,417,418]

GROUP 1*
Cyclophosphamide
Nitrogen mustard
Adriamycin
Methotrexate
Hexamethylmelamine
VP-16-213
Vincristine

GROUP 2†
Procarbazine
(CCNU) 1–(2–chloroethyl)–3–cyclohexyl–1–nitrosourea
(BCNU) 1,3–bis(2-chloroethyl)–1–nitrosourea
(MeCCNU) methyl-CCNU

GROUP 3‡
Ifosphamide
Cis-platinum
Vindesine
High dose methotrexate with leucovorin rescue
Dibromodulcitol

*Evaluated in 40 or more patients with an overall response rate of 15% or more, including at least two studies with 10 or more patients which demonstrated at least a 20% objective response.
†Active in at least two or more trials.
‡Activity reported in one trial or for which conflicting data exist.

TABLE 14-44. Objective Tumor Responses to Single Agent or Combination Chemotherapy in Small-Cell Lung Cancer from Literature Review (No radiation therapy given; previously untreated patients)

	RESPONSES PERCENTAGE		
DRUG TREATMENT	NUMBER OF PATIENTS	ALL OBJECTIVE†	COMPLETE
Single agent*	753	15–20	2.5
Combination chemotherapy	1,236	70	31

(Bunn PA Jr, Ihde DC: Small cell bronchogenic carcinoma: a review of therapeutic results. In Livingston RB (ed): Lung Cancer: Advances in Research and Treatment. The Hague, Martinus Nijhosf (in press) 1981).
*Only includes data on, CTX, HN2, ADRIA, MTX, VP-16-213, hexamethylmelamine, VCR.
†Objective tumor responses include partial and complete responses. Complete responses rate data only available on 572 patients.

literature of median survivals of patients treated with either single agent or combination chemotherapy, the patients receiving combination chemotherapy survived longer.[392,393] A series of randomized trials have compared single agent to combination chemotherapy given with or without chest radiation.[223,225,226,406] As a whole, these randomized trials demonstrate a slight benefit from combination chemotherapy (in objective tumor response, in addition to a slight increase in the median survival). In contrast, the pooled results of many hundreds of patients from the literature show the complete response rate increased 10-fold over that screen with single agents. This is, in part, because some of the patients entering the trials had received prior radiation therapy and because many of the patients initially treated with single agent chemotherapy were subsequently treated with other drugs and drug combinations so that most trials were actually comparing initial vs. delayed combination chemotherapy. One randomized study compared giving the drugs CTX + MTX + VCR + procarbazine either sequentially or in combination. An increase was found in the response rate with the drugs given simultaneously.[407] Currently, all investigators studying SCLC use the simultaneous combination chemotherapy treatment method.

COMBINATION CHEMOTHERAPY

Related to the question of single agent vs. combination chemotherapy is determining the number of drugs to use in combination. In limited stage disease patients treated with combination chemotherapy without radiotherapy, nearly all trials have used three or more drugs. There is no significant difference in the complete response rate or long-term disease-free survival for using more than three drugs (see Table 14-45).[219,224–226,229,366,406,411,413,414,428,430,431,435,450,458] In extensive stage disease there is a definite increase in the complete response rate going from two to three or more drugs; the first long-term survivors appear with the use of three or more drugs. Whether adding more than three drugs helps is still in question, although there is a suggestion of benefit in extensive stage disease. Table 14-45 also demonstrates that patients initially scored as limited stage disease have a significantly higher initial complete response rate that later translates into more long-term disease-free survivors compared to patients scored as extensive stage disease. Thus, in addition to combination chemotherapy using known active agents, the use of at least three drugs in the combination is recommended.

Intensity of Chemotherapy

Most of the combination chemotherapy regimens currently in use produce substantial myelosuppression. The therapeutic results seem superior when compared to less aggressive single agent for combination chemotherapy given 5–10 years ago. However, only one prospective randomized trial has addressed the question of the value of moderate dose initial chemotherapy (chemotherapy given to outpatients with drug dose adjusted to keep the white blood counts [WBC] and platelet counts within safe ranges) vs. intensive combination chemotherapy where drug doses are given irrespective of the hematologic toxicity employed.[408] After the initial 6 weeks of treatment with either intensive or moderate doses, all patients were treated with the moderate dose regimen as outpatients. The results from this trial and pooled data from the literature using the same chemotherapy regimens in either the moderate- or the high-dose form demonstrate that initial high-dose therapy is better in terms of complete response rate and median survival (see Table 14-46). In addition, the only long-term disease-free survivors (when chemotherapy is used alone) have come from patients treated with the high-dose regimens (see Table 14-46). A series of other trials, particularly in extensive stage disease where the complete response rate remains around 30%, has further tested increasing the intensity of the initial chemotherapy. This has been done either

TABLE 14-45. Role of Number of Drugs in Combination Chemotherapy of Small-Cell Lung Cancer from Literature Review (No radiation therapy given)[219,224–226,229,366,406–411,413,414,428,430,431,435,450–458]

# DRUGS IN COMBINATION AND STAGE OF DISEASE	NUMBER OF PATIENTS	COMPLETE RESPONSE PERCENTAGE	2-YEAR DISEASE-FREE SURVIVAL PERCENTAGE
LIMITED STAGE			
3	88	44	6
4 or more	158	54	7
EXTENSIVE STAGE			
2	193	21	0
3	364	27	1
4 or more	433	30	3

(Bunn PA, Ihde DC: Small cell bronchogenic carcinoma: a review of therapeutic results. In Livingston RB (ed): Lung Cancer, vol 1: Advances in Research and Treatment, pp. 169–208. The Hague, Martinus Nijhoff, 1981; Ihde DC, Bunn PA: Chemotherapy of small cell bronchogenic carcinoma. In Whitehouse JMA, Williams CJ (eds): Recent Advances in Clinical Oncology, vol. 1. Edinburgh, Churchill Livingston, 1981)

by increasing the intensity of one of the drugs such as CTX or by increasing the number of cycles of induction chemotherapy given in the first 6–8 weeks of treatment. However, increasing the total dose of CTX delivered in the first 6–8 weeks from 2000 mg/M^2 to 6000 mg/M^2 resulted in the best complete response rates achieved with a total of 3000 mg/M^2 (usually, two 1500 mg/M^2 doses given three weeks apart) and only increased toxicity at the higher doses.[229,408,410,411] Similarly, increasing the number of induction cycles from three to six did not increase the complete response rate; it only resulted in increasing toxicity and death related to therapy.[412] Therefore, increasing the intensity of the induction therapy over that achieved with one of the standard regimens (to be described later) except as part of clinical trials is not recommended.

USE OF NON-CROSS RESISTANT DRUG COMBINATIONS

Several groups have tried to increase the complete response rate and improve survival by introducing non-cross resistant drug combinations. A list of various combinations that have given objective tumor responses after progression on an initial regimen are listed in Table 14-47. It appears that patients who have not yet entered a complete response with one combination may be induced to do so with the addition of a second non-cross resistant combination.[229] However, the durations of the complete responses occurring after the second combination are not as great as those occurring only after the first combination.[229] A series of randomized trials has tested the value of the early addition of alternative non-cross resistant combinations vs. the use of the non-cross resistant combination at tumor progression.[226,229,413,416] With the exception of one trial, which found a significant survival advantage in extensive stage disease patients, none of the randomized trials have demonstrated a survival benefit or increase in the number of long-term disease-free surviviors treated with the alternating combinations.[416] However, most of the trials indicate the second combination is doing something. This is represented by prolonged time to disease progression or improved response duration. Despite the suggestive results in some trials, most tumor regressions in SCLC due to chemotherapy occur quickly, usually within the first 3 to 6 weeks, and many series observe the maximum response to chemotherapy occurs within 5–8 weeks.[219,224,225,408,410,411,435] In several instances, the addition of a non-cross resistant combination after this period has failed to achieve a further tumor response.[410,411,435] The role of non-cross resistant combinations is being defined but does not appear to make a dramatic impact on treatment results.

TABLE 14-46. Effect of Intensity of Induction Combination Chemotherapy in Small-Cell Lung Cancer When No Chest Radiotherapy is Given (Randomized and non-randomized trial data)[229,418,419]

INDUCTION DOSE OF CHEMO-THERAPY*	NUMBER OF PATIENTS	COMPLETE RESPONSE PER-CENTAGE†	2-YEAR DISEASE-FREE SURVIVAL PERCENTAGE
Moderate dose	61	0	0
High dose	84	29	8

*The chemotherapy (CMC) used was CTX (500 mg/M^2 in moderate dose and 1000–1500 mg/M^2 every 3 weeks in high dose) + MTX (10 mg/M^2 in moderate dose and 15 mg/M^2 twice weekly in high dose) + CCNU (50 mg/M^2 in moderate dose and 100 mg/M^2 on day 1 in high dose regimens) for a 6-week induction cycle. After the initial six weeks of high dose induction therapy, all patients received the moderate dose therapy in 6 week cycles.

†The complete response rates were not always reported, but are taken from staging data six weeks after the start of therapy with the CMC combination. Some patients in both groups received subsequent therapy with VCR + ADRIA + procarbazine (VAP), and in some cases VP-16 or Ifosphamide. in the high dose group, some patients received this before tumor progression. However, only complete response at six weeks occurring after CMC alone are listed and nearly all long-term survivors came from this complete responder group.

TABLE 14-47. Non-Cross Resistant Drug Combinations and Single Agents in Small-Cell Lung Cancer[226,229,413–416]

PRIMARY COMBINATION CHEMOTHERAPY	SECONDARY CHEMOTHERAPY WITH ACTIVITY
Cyclophosphamide + methotrexate + CCNU (CMC)	Vincristine + adriamycin + Procarbazine (VAP); VP-16-213
Vincristine + adriamycin + cyclophosphamide (VAC)	VP-16-213; methotrexate; CCNU; procarbazine
Cyclosphosphamide + adriamycin + VP-16-213 (CAVP-16)	Vincristine + methotrexate + CCNU + procarbazine
VP-16-213 + methotrexate + adriamycin (VAM)	Cyclophosphamide + vincristine + procarbazine + CCNU (POCC)

COMBINED MODALITY RADIATION AND CHEMOTHERAPY

Radiation therapy can induce dramatic tumor regression in over 80% of SCLC patients. A dose response effect exists such that tumor regression and local control rise from 60% at 3000 rad to 79% with 4000 rad, to 88% with 4800 rad.[437–439] In patients treated with chemotherapy alone, relapse in the chest sites of bulk disease is common, occurring in over 60% of cases.[229,236] In patients entering a complete remission, 71% of relapses in limited and 56% of relapses in extensive disease were solely in the chest.[229] Thus, the rationale for combined modality therapy is for radiotherapy and chemotherapy together to deal with bulk disease in the chest primary site and for chemotherapy to take care of systemic metastases. The value of combination as opposed to single agent chemotherapy is also seen when chest radiotherapy is given (see Table 14-48). It appears the maximum benefit in combined modality therapy occurs when combination chemotherapy is used as well.

At present there is still considerable controversy concerning the role of radiotherapy. Table 14-49 summarizes the results of combined modality therapy (radiation + chemotherapy) vs. combination chemotherapy alone in the primary treatment of SCLC from a large number of non-randomized studies. Only studies that used three or more of the known active agents are included so as to provide for the best chemotherapy possible. Again, in both the combined modality group and the groups treated with chemotherapy alone, patients scored initially as having limited stage disease have a higher complete response rate, a higher median survival rate, and a greater number of long-term survivors. In limited stage disease there is no difference in the objective tumor response rate, complete response rate, or median survival range. There is, however, a 2.5-fold increase in the number of long-term disease-free survivors treated with combined modality therapy. In extensive stage disease, there is a higher objective tumor response rate, no difference in the complete response rate, and more long-term survivors in the patients treated with chemotherapy alone.

A series of randomized trials has been initiated to compare the value of adding radiotherapy to the best combination chemotherapy. Preliminary reports on four of them are available, although final long-term disease-free survival data are not yet available. The first three deal with limited stage disease.

In the University of Indiana trial, the combination of CTX + ADRIA + VCR was used with and without split course radiotherapy (3500 rad) sandwiched in between chemotherapy.[450] There was no difference in the median survival or long-term disease-free survival but a higher objective and complete response rate was seen for combined modality therapy. In the

TABLE 14-48. Role of Number of Drugs in Combination Chemotherapy Given With Chest Radiotherapy (Non-randomized trials)[218–223,228,400,419,420,422–433,440–449]

STAGE AND NUMBER OF DRUGS	NUMBER OF PATIENTS TREATED	COMPLETE RESPONSE PERCENTAGE	2-YEAR DISEASE-FREE SURVIVAL PERCENTAGE*
LIMITED STAGE			
NUMBER OF DRUGS			
1	26	27	0 (0/11)
2	89	42	19 (9/48)
3	304	58	20 (24/122)
4 or more	73	34	10 (4/40)
EXTENSIVE STAGE			
NUMBER OF DRUGS			
1	24	8	0 (0/12)
2	57	12	0 (0/17)
3	476	21	1 (3/411)
4 or more	120	31	4 (2/48)

(Bunn PA, Ihde DC: Small cell bronchogenic carcinoma: a review of therapeutic results. In Livingston RB (ed): Lung Cancer: Advances in Research and Treatment. pp. 169–208. The Hague, Martinus Nijhoff, 1981; Ihde DC, Bunn PA: Chemotherapy of small cell bronchogenic carcinoma. In Whitehouse JMA, Williams CJ (eds): Recent Advances in Clinical Oncology, vol. 1. Edinburgh, Churchill Livingston, 1981.

*Two year disease-free survival was not always reported. Number of patients reported given in parentheses.

Finsen Institute trial, the combination of CTX + VCR + CCNU + MTX was used with or without 4000 rad in the split course sandwich technique. While there was no difference in response rates, the chemotherapy alone group had a 3 month greater median survival; long-term survivals have not yet been reported.[457]

The National Cancer Institute trial employed CTX + MTX + CCNU (CMC) alternating with the combination of VCR + ARDIA + procarbazine (VAP regimen) with or without 4000 rad to the chest given concurrently with the chemotherapy beginning on day 1.[434] The complete response rate was higher in the combined modality arm (77% vs. 46% in the chemotherapy alone group) and there was a trend toward increased disease-free and overall survival in the combined modality group in this on-going study.

In extensive stage disease, the Stanford trial utilizing CTX + VCR + CCNU + procarbazine (POCC) with or without 3000 rad to the chest given between chemotherapy by the continuous technique and 1,500–2,500 rad to extrathoracic metastatic sites found no benefit for combined modality therapy and no long-term disease-free survivors.[457a] The University of Indiana trial is not yet complete but preliminary analysis shows no benefit for combined modality therapy in extensive stage disease.[450] At present there is no conclusive evidence of benefit of combined radiotherapy and chemotherapy together over chemotherapy alone. This appears to be particularly true in extensive stage disease. In limited stage disease, the comparison of non-randomized trials suggests a benefit for combined modality therapy. However, the final results of the randomized trials must be evaluated.

TABLE 14-49. Role of Combined Modality (Radiotherapy + Chemotherapy) versus Combination Chemotherapy Alone in the Primary Treatment of Small-Cell Lung Cancer*[219–223,400,419–434]

	RADIO-THERAPY + CHEMO-THERAPY	CHEMO-THERAPY
LIMITED STAGE DISEASE (3 OR MORE DRUGS)		
Number of patients	377	246
Number of studies	13	8
CR + PR (Objective tumor response rates) (%)	78	81
Complete response rate (%)	53	52
Median survival (months)	6 ± 18.5	5 ± 14
2-year disease-free survivors (%)	17	7
EXTENSIVE STAGE DISEASE		
Number of patients	1,232	797
Number of studies	17	24
CR + PR (Objective tumor response rate) (%)	57	71
Complete response rate (%)	21	29
Median survival (months)	3–10.5	4–11
2-year disease-free survivors (%)	0.9	2

*Studies include randomized and nonrandomized trials using combination chemotherapy with three or more of the known active drugs.

(Bunn PA, Ihde DC: Small cell bronchogenic carcinoma: a review of therapeutic results. In Livingston RB (ed): Lung Cancer, vol 1: Advances in Research and Treatment, pp 169–208. The Hague, Martinus Nijhoff, 1981; Ihde DC, Bunn PA: Chemotherapy of small cell bronchogenic carcinoma. In Whitehouse JMA, Williams CJ (eds): Recent Advances in Clinical Oncology, vol. 1. Edinburgh, Churchill Livingston, 1981.)

Dose, Schedule, and Timing of Radiotherapy and Chemotherapy

Despite the numerous SCLC patients treated with combined modality therapy, the optimal way of combining the chemo- and radiotherapy and the best dose and schedule of radiotherapy are not yet known. Some trials have given irradiation first.[387] Many of the trials have used split course radiotherapy starting 3–7 weeks after the initiation of the chemotherapy.[219,221,222,228,400,420,422,424,426,427,430] Others have used continuous irradiation but are given between the chemotherapy courses.[223,419,425,432] Still others have given the chemo- and radiotherapy concurrently.[220,428,429,433] In comparing non-randomized trials, there is no difference in complete response rate, median survival, or 2-year disease-free survival in limited stage patients (*i.e.*, those expected to benefit the most from combined modality therapy) receiving combined modality therapy whether they received less than 3200 rad, 3500–3600 rad, or over 4000 rad.[392] For both limited and extensive stage disease, there is no significant difference in response or survival for patients receiving continuous or split course radiotherapy.[392] With four and five drug combinations there are no significant differences when the radiotherapy is given first, between the second and third courses of chemotherapy, or simultaneous with the chemotherapy.[432,449] The NCI Radiation Oncology Branch (NCI-ROB) conducted a sequential, rather than randomized, trial of different methods of combining chemo- and radiotherapy and came up with interesting results.[459] They treated 71 consecutive SCLC patients with six different radiation regimens in combination with the same chemotherapy (CTX + VCR + ADRIA). They found that patients treated with concurrent chemotherapy–irradiation experienced better local tumor control than patients treated with sequential chemotherapy–radiation therapy. Life table analysis of the study reveals more patients treated by concurrent therapy in remission at 30 months (25%) compared to those treated with sequential therapy (8%). The optimal concurrent therapy was more toxic than the sequential therapy but resulted in more local control (70% vs. 40%) and more 2-year survivors (50% vs. 20%). The NCI-ROB group also tested whether 3, 6, or 9 weeks of concurrent therapy were better. They found a slight increase in the local control for 9 weeks but a dramatic increase in treatment-related mortality (over 40%) in patients receiving this long treatment period.[459] Maximal survival with the least toxicity was found in patients given a 3-week concurrent course of chemoradiotherapy. This trial still has the greatest reported fraction of 3-year survivors (25%) in limited stage disease. However, it is striking that no extensive stage patient achieved survival over 3 years in the NCI-ROB study even though they were given the same intense combined therapy.[459]

Controlled clinical trials are needed to determine the optimum way to combine chemo- and radiotherapy. However, at present the non-randomized trials suggest the best results come from concurrent therapy given for the first 3 weeks with a dose of 3000 rads.

ROLE OF MAINTENANCE CHEMOTHERAPY

At present, most groups treating SCLC administer the same combination chemotherapy given initially until signs of disease progression or treatment-related toxicities dictate stopping therapy (usually within 2 years). In patients achieving a complete response, the chemotherapy has been stopped arbitrarily at 12 or 24 months. The value of such maintenance therapy is not yet demonstrated. The Cancer and Leukemia Group B (CALGB) randomized complete responders at 6 months to continue or stop additional chemotherapy.[223] The median and 2-year survival of limited disease patients significantly favored maintenance chemotherapy. However, there was no difference in the duration of the initial remission on or off of maintenance chemotherapy making interpretation of this trial difficult. In contrast, three groups at different institutions gave the combination of VCR + ADRIA + CTX (VAC) + chest radiotherapy to limited stage patients and varied the duration of chemotherapy. The radiotherapy was combined with the chemotherapy in different schedules, but most important the NCI group gave chemotherapy for only 3–4 months, the Vanderbilt group gave chemotherapy for 14 months, and the Indiana group gave chemotherapy for 24 months.[220,222,428] There was no significant difference in median survival (18.5, 14+, 17 months respectively), or fraction of 2+ years for disease-free survivors (28%, >10%, and 26% respectively). Recently, the Memorial Sloan Kettering Cancer Center group has also reported on giving four cycles of combination chemotherapy followed by chest radiotherapy to limited disease patients. A large fraction of patients are in an unmaintained complete remission.[460]

The role of maintenance therapy is still an open question. At present, it would appear prudent to continue chemotherapy in partial responders until the time of objective disease progression, at which time the chemotherapy should be changed. For complete responders, it is reasonable to treat for 6–12 months and then stop the chemotherapy after careful restaging has documented the lack of any clinically detectable tumor.

TABLE 14-50. Role of Prophylactic Cranial Irradiation (PCI) in the Treatment of Small-Cell Lung Cancer[218,223,234,322,400,404,424,429,432,433,462,463]

	CNS RELAPSE RATE	
	PCI Given	*PCI Not Given*
# Patients, randomized trials	172	176
% CNS relapse	7%	18%
# Patients, non-randomized trials	422	956
% CNS relapse	8%	22%

(Bunn PA, Ihde DC: Small cell bronchogenic carcinoma: A review of therapeutic results. In Livingston RB (ed): Lung Cancer, vol 1: Advances in Research and Treatment, pp 169–208. The Hague, Martinus Nijhoff, 1981; Ihde DC, Bunn PA: Chemotherapy of small cell bronchogenic carcinoma. In Whitehouse JMA, Williams CJ (eds): Recent Advances in Clinical Oncology, vol. 1. Edinburgh, Churchill Livingston, 1981)

PROPHYLACTIC CRANIAL IRRADIATION AND MANAGEMENT OF CNS METASTASES

Small cell lung cancer metastasizes to the central nervous system (CNS) more frequently than the other types of lung cancer. The CNS is a frequent site of relapse. [234,461,461a] At presentation, CNS metastases are found in 8–10% of patients and patients who live two or more years have an 80% probability of developing a CNS metastasis if prophylactic CNS therapy is not given.[234,238] The results of using prophylactic cranial irradiation (PCI) are shown in Table 14-50 for both randomized and non-randomized trials. Taken as a whole, the data suggest a benefit from PCI with 7–8% of the patients irradiated suffering a CNS relapse while 18–22% of the unirradiated patients relapse in the CNS. However, none of the studies show a benefit in terms of increase in median survival. This is not unexpected since the majority of patients not are yet entering a complete response or living for greater than two years, the groups that should benefit from such prophylactic therapy.

For prophylactic therapy, 3000 rad in 10–15 fractions of whole brain radiotherapy over 2–3 weeks is generally given.[234] Corticosteroids are usually not administered with the radiotherapy. While not generally reported, PCI may cause some toxicity, particularly if it is given concurrently with chemotherapy.[220,429]The patients will all develop alopecia, and a certain fraction will develop desquamation of portions of the ear and otitis. In addition, a transient "CNS syndrome" consisting of memory loss for recent events, tremor, somnolence, slurred speech, and myoclonus in various combinations has been reported in up to 50% of patients in some series when the PCI was given as part of the initial treatment and with the highest doses of chemotherapy. However, the vast majority of series do not report complications from PCI.

The best time to give PCI is not known.[234] At present, the evidence on CNS relapses favor giving PCI to complete responders and it would appear logical to do this at the time patients entered a complete response (in the first 2–6 months). While not formally studied, to avoid reseeding the brain, it would appear prudent to continue maintenance outpatient chemotherapy during this period.

THERAPEUTIC BRAIN IRRADIATION

Patients with brain metastases documented by scan (radionuclide or CT scan), whether they are symptomatic or not, should receive a course of 4,000–5,000 rad given over 4 weeks.[234] For symptomatic patients, dexamethasone (16–100 mg total/day in four divided doses) is also given with the radiotherapy and then tapered to the lowest dosage to relieve symptoms.[234] SCLC patients presenting with CNS metastases at diagnosis and treated with therapeutic cranial irradiation and systemic combination chemotherapy have survivals ranging from 41.5 months.[217,238,464] Despite these poor figures for median survival, there are a subset of patients with CNS metastases that do very well for over one year. Thus, the authors recommend an aggressive treatment approach to patients with brain metastases, particularly at initial presentation.[238]

LEPTOMENINGEAL AND SPINAL EPIDURAL METASTASES

In addition to brain metastases, patients with SCLC experience metastases throughout the neuraxis including the spinal cord and leptomeninges.[238] PCI does not treat these sites, and in patients with longer survival, up to 10% will experience a leptomeningeal or spinal epidural metastasis.[238,466–468] In fact, the probability of having multiple metastases in the brain, spinal epidural space, and leptomeninges increases when metastasis in any one of the sites is found.[238] In the NCI study, 50% of patients with spinal cord compression had a concurrent intracranial metasasis, and 50% had leptominingeal involvement. Conversely, 25% of patients with intracranial metastases had carcinomatous leptomeningitis, and 20% of patients with leptomeningitis had intracranial metastases.[234,238] Thus, the clinical evaluation of patients exhibiting signs and symptoms of a metastasis in one part of the neuraxis demands examination of the other sites as well. The diagnosis and management of spinal cord compression is discussed in detail in Chapter 42 and in the section on common problems in Chapter 14. Response rates of 80% and median survivals over 4 months have been reported in SCLC.[238]

Treatment of carcinomatous leptomeningitis from SCLC consists of intrathecal methotrexate (12 mg total dose) given twice per week until the CSF clears, then 4 mg once per week, then every other week until disease progression. Cranial radiotherapy of 2000 rad in 2 weeks is given if there are no mass lesions. If mass lesions on scan are present in the brain or spinal cord, 4000 rad in 4 weeks is given to the tumor mass or whole brain. If the patient's life expectancy is 3 months or more, it is the authors' policy to have an Omaya reservoir implanted as this makes drug delivery and monitoring for tumor cells much easier on both patient and physician.[234,238] The objective response rate of clearing of SCLC malignant cells from the CSF and relief of neurologic symptoms ranges from 40–80%.[234,465] The median survival is short at 2 months, but a significant fraction of patients will live from 6–12 months.[234] The authors suggest initial use of intrathecal MTX therapy even if the tumor has been previously treated with systemic combination chemotherapy containing MTX because of the relatively high concentrations of MTX achieved in the CSF for long periods. In addition, dexamethasone may initially be used to relieve symptoms, then rapidly tapered with clearing of the CSF.

SMALL CELL CARCINOMA ARISING IN EXTRAPULMONARY SITES

Approximately 4% of small cell carcinoma patients present with no obvious pulmonary primary lesion by chest film or bronchoscopy.[469,470] These cases fall into two groups—those with a localized extrapulmonary lesion (*e.g.*, chest wall, parotid gland, skin nodule, lymph node, uterine cervix, pancreas, prostate, esophagus, or larynx) and those with widespread metastases. Although numbers of treated patients are small, they appear to respond to combination chemotherapy with or without radiotherapy and have median survivals similar to other extensive stage small cell carcinoma patients (8+ months).[469,470] At present, the authors recommend these patients be staged and treated as other extensive stage small cell lung cancer patients. In those patients with only a localized site of extrapulmonary disease it would be reasonable to add local radiotherapy, although there are no data yet to support this.

TOXICITY OF THERAPY IN SMALL CELL CARCINOMA

With the use of three or more drugs given in combination and in high doses, significant myelosuppression with severe granulocytopenia (polymorphonuclear leukocyte count less than 500/μl) occurs in nearly all patients during the initial 6–8 weeks off therapy. The hematologic toxicities approach those achieved with effective therapy for acute myeloblastic leukemia. Thus, the early diagnosis and treatment of granulocytopenic associated fever and infection is mandatory. Patients are either hospitalized or must be closely followed as outpatients during this initial period. The approach and supportive care should be similar to that given to acute leukemic patients during induction therapy (see Chapter 43). Thrombocytopenia usually occurs, but platelet counts less than 25,000/μl requiring platelet transfusion probably develop only 10–20% of the time with the currently used regimens. The acute nonhematologic toxicities such as nausea, vomiting, mucositis, alopecia, and cystitis are similar to those expected for the individual drugs in the doses given.

Chronic toxicities from combination chemotherapy alone also include ADRIA-related cardiotoxicity; interstitial pulmonary disease from several drugs including CTX, MTX, and the nitrosoureas; and chronic marrow suppression from destruction of stem cells.[471–474] Overall, deaths related to therapy toxicity range from 0–10% in currently used, relatively intense, combination chemotherapy programs.[224,229,410,411,454,456] This is the same range as operative mortality for pulmonary resection and re-emphasizes the need for pretherapy evaluation of patients for performance status and various organ function so particularly high-risk candidates can avoid initial intensive therapy, in addition to supportive care of the patients.

Toxicities on normal tissue are increased when combined modality chemotherapy and radiotherapy are given.[475,476] Dysphagia and esophagitis are transient common features of chest radiotherapy; mild esophagitis occurs in 5–50% of cases given sequential chemoradiotherapy.[221,222,427,477] When concurrent chemoradiotherapy is given, esophagitis has been seen in 65–77% of patients, most of which was moderate to severe. In addition, esophageal strictures have been seen in some patients.[220,428,478] In the current NCI trial of chemotherapy plus and minus concurrent radiotherapy, insertion of a spinal cord block posteriorly after 2600 rad dramatically decreases the incidence of severe esophagitis.[434]

Pulmonary fibrosis, pneumonitis, and interstitial pulmonary disease of "unknown etiology" (but presumably related to therapy) is frequently seen with combined modality therapy and has often been severe. Again, the authors stress that pulmonary interstitial disease can be seen with chemotherapy alone and the relative contribution of each treatment modality remains to be determined. Not surprisingly, the combination of bleomycin + CTX + VCR + ADRIA with chest radiotherapy resulted in pulmonary fibrosis in 38% of patients and was fatal in 23% of those treated.[479] However, CTX + ADRIA

+ VCR with concurrent chest radiotherapy but without bleomycin also resulted in pulmonary fibrosis/pneumonitis (often with infection) in 37% of patients; nearly half of these were fatal (17% of the whole group).[220] Analysis of this latter trial revealed the largest fraction of toxicity was associated with concurrent treatment for 6 or 9 weeks (25–50% treatment-related toxic deaths mostly from pulmonary toxicity). However, toxic deaths dropped to 10% when only 3 weeks of concurrent therapy were used.[459] Others have noted less pulmonary toxicity (occurring in only 3% of cases) when the same drugs are used and either given sequentially with the radiotherapy or for only 10 days concurrently rather than for 3 weeks.[438,477] While bleomycin and ADRIA may be expected to potentiate the action of radiotherapy, pulmonary toxicity was also seen when radiotherapy was given concurrently with the combination of CTX + MTX + CCNU.[434] This toxicity was decreased with multiple reshaping of the fields ("shrinking fields") by cutting new blocks to preserve as much normal pulmonary tissue as possible (see Fig. 14-20).[434] All of these features again stress the need to select patients for combined modality therapy and the need for great attention to therapy as the line between mild and severe toxicity appears narrow.

Hematologic toxicity may also increase when combined modality therapy is given. Irradiation of the chest and brain (in PCI) affects 20–25% of the functioning bone marrow.[437] In patients treated on the NCI randomized trial of chemotherapy ± radiotherapy, the addition of radiotherapy produced significantly more myelosuppression than the same chemotherapy alone. This was correlated with a decrease in the peripheral circulation hematopoietic colony-forming units in the blood of the patients.[480] Also, a case of acute erythroleukemia in a long-term survivor treated with chemoradiotherapy has been seen and several of the long-term survivors treated with either combination chemotherapy alone or with radiotherapy have persistent peripheral blood aneuploidy, which may be preleukemic in nature.[493]

Enhanced radiation skin reaction is not a problem; it occurs in 5% or less of cases.[216,222,428,434,477] Cardiac toxicity from adriamycin radiation interaction has not been a problem (occurring in only 2% of cases and in a large series was fatal in only 0.3% of patients).[477] In addition, the total dose of drug rather than the addition of radiation therapy was the significant risk factor for cardiac toxicity.[471] This lack of cardiac toxicity may be a reflection of the relatively short life span of most patients (less than 2 years) and it will be important to evaluate long-term (*e.g.*, 5-year) survivors for this toxicity.

SUMMARY OF THE PRINCIPLES OF PRIMARY TREATMENT OF SMALL CELL LUNG CANCER

It is now useful to summarize the principles of primary treatment of patients with small cell lung cancer incorporating the information from pathology, staging studies, chemotherapy, and combined modality therapy. The first principle is, of course, a correct histologic diagnosis. This is not always easy and it is important to get an adequate tissue sample, correctly processed, for pathologic interpretation. The pathologist should be given the clinical information and then asked to decide if the case is small cell lung cancer, non-small cell lung cancer, or some mixtures of small cell and non-small cell elements. In the case of "undifferentiated," or "poorly differentiated" tumor other options may be needed, and in the future EM studies, biochemical, or immunologic markers may be of use. However, if an experienced pathologist feels that some elements of small cell carcinoma are present the patient should be treated as if pure small cell cancer were found.

The next principle is appropriate staging to determine initial disease extent. While the value of stage-specific therapy has not yet been demonstrated, the prognostic importance of limited stage disease in achieving a complete response and long-term survival remains. If combined modality therapy is being contemplated the determination of limited vs. extensive disease stage is also important. At present the evidence favors only using chest radiotherapy if limited stage disease is found.

Third, the patient should be assessed not only for prognosis based on stage of disease, but also on the basis of performance status, pulmonary function, other underlying medical problems, and various organ system function (*e.g.*, heart, kidney, liver), and weight loss. As previously stated, patients with impaired performance status (particularly PS 3 and 4), and those with severely impaired pulmonary, cardiac, or renal function will tolerate intense combination chemotherapy poorly and are at high risk for therapy-related morbidity and mortality. In those patients deemed able to tolerate it, high dose combination chemotherapy with or without radiotherapy should be given. This must be coupled with good supportive care for infectious, hemorrhagic, and other medical complications. Meticulous attention to the details of therapy and the day-to-day management of the patient through the initial 6–8 weeks of treatment is essential if therapy-related mortality is to remain low. Following the initial intense (or "induction") therapy, patients should be restaged to determine if they entered a "complete clinical remission" (*i.e.*, complete disappearance of all clinically evident lesions and paraneoplastic syndromes), which is prognostically most favorable; a "partial remission" (*i.e.*, objective tumor regression, but tumor still clinically evident); or the 10% or less of cases with "no response" or tumor progression. Besides the history and physical examination, a repeat fiberoptic bronchoscopy with cytologies and biopsy of suspicious areas is needed. Initially positive bone marrow and liver biopsies, as well as initially positive radionuclide liver, brain, bone, and CT scans should be repeated. Abnormal chemistries consistent with paraneoplastic syndromes (*e.g.*, hyponatremia) should revert to normal and be re-evaluated with appropriate studies. Other accessible lesions should be examined or biopsied if appropriate. Following this, maintenance therapy is usually given to complete responding patients for periods of 6–12 months. Then the patients are restaged and if they are still in a complete response, chemotherapy is stopped. Patients with partial tumor regressions are kept on maintenance chemotherapy until the time of objective tumor progression and then switched to new chemotherapy (either with known activity, or on an experimental protocol). Patients not responding should be switched to new chemotherapy, preferably with a non-cross resistant combination, in an attempt to get an objective tumor response. High dose (4000 rad) brain radio-

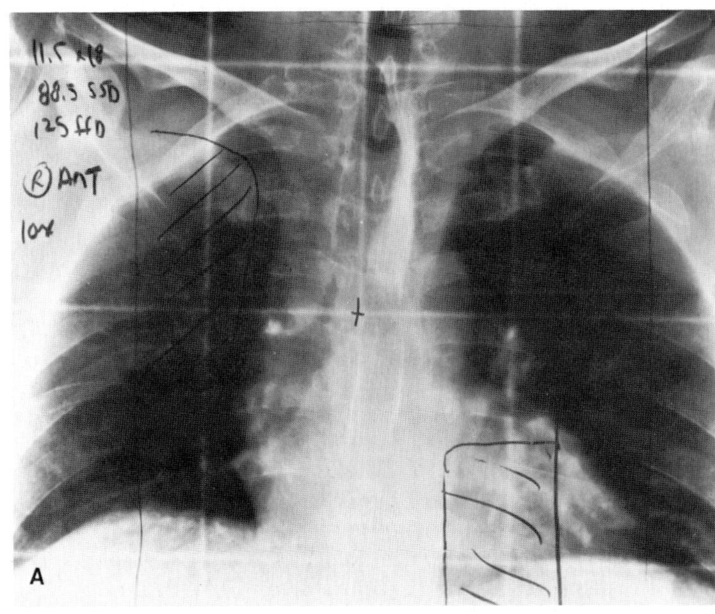

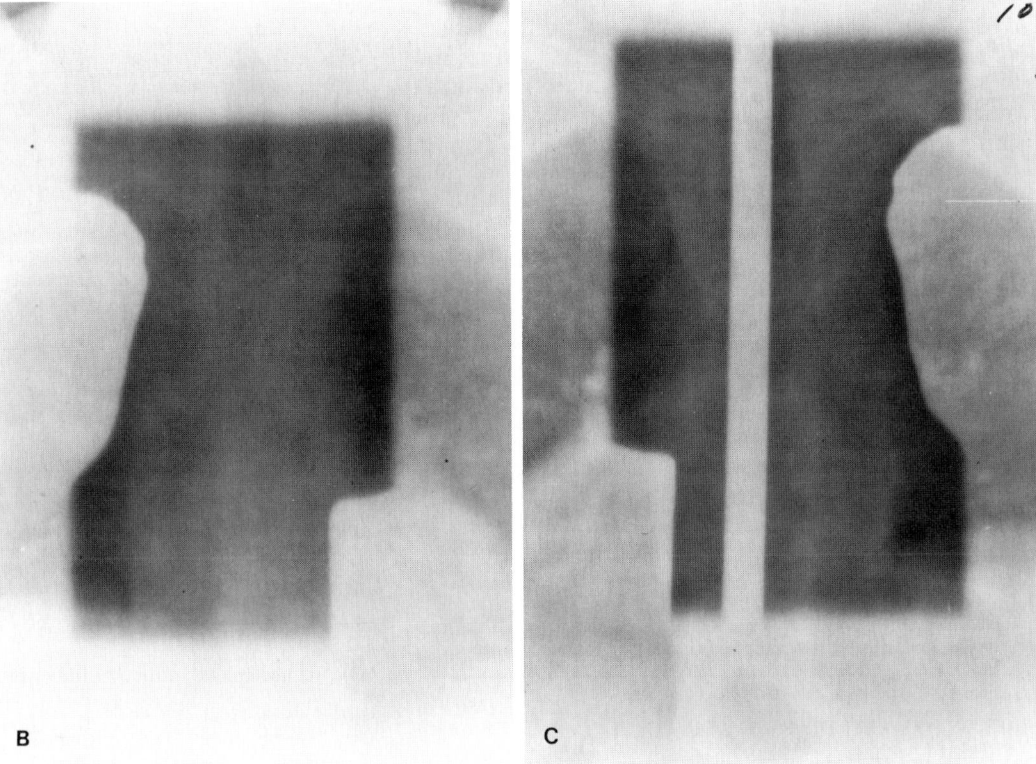

FIG. 14-20. *A*, isocentric simulation of a patient with small cell carcinoma of the lung. Contrast has been placed in the esophagus to identify its location with respect to the central axis of the field (*cross*). This diagnostic quality film has focused blocks outlined in crayon (*cross hatchings*). *B*, anterior port film on the same patient under treatment with a 10 MeV photon beam. Focused blocks reduced the amount of pulmonary parenchyma irradiation as originally drawn. The treatment plan for this patient calls for a midplane tumor dose at the central axis of 4000 rad in 15 fractions over three weeks. A similar field is applied posteriorly. *C*, the posterior field on the same patient, with a spinal cord bar added the last week of treatment on the posterior field only. This bar is added to reduce the overall spinal cord dose to 3000 rad in three weeks, during which time the patient also receives intensive combination chemotherapy. In conjunction with intensive chemotherapy, the bar is felt essential to minimize any risk of radiation injury to the spinal cord. This technique is recommended for high dose irradiation with simultaneous intensive chemotherapy for small cell carcinoma of the lung. For patients with non-oat cell lung cancer, the spinal cord can be protected by shifting to an anterior field plus a posterior oblique field, reducing the volume to minimize the amount of pulmonary parenchyma irradiation, while taking the mediastinal contents to an even higher dose.

therapy should be given to patients with documented brain metastases. Prophylactic cranial radiotherapy may be given to patients with objective tumor responses, particularly those with a complete response. Patients with partial responses may also have PCI although at present it is debatable whether less ambulatory patients should have PCI because of their known short survival and the great possibility for brain reseeding when systemic bulk tumor remains. Finally, at the first unequivocal sign of tumor progression, the current chemotherapy should be stopped and new chemotherapy begun, if this is available, so as to treat the patient at the time of the smallest possible tumor bulk. In the case of progressive lesion on primary therapy in the chest or at other critical sites causing marked symptoms, if radiotherapy has not yet been given, radiotherapy is now appropriate and should be given in full doses (*e.g.*, 4000 rad) to a chest tumor mass.

The current principles of primary chemotherapy may be summarized as follows: first, combination chemotherapy using three or four of the known active agents (*e.g.*, cyclophosphamide, methotrexate, adriamycin, vincristine, VP-16-213, procarbazine, or CCNU) should be used. The agents should be given concurrently in the combination, and probably one of the drugs should be cyclophosphamide. Second, this initial combination chemotherapy should be given in high doses during the first 6–8 weeks of therapy. While this therapy should be intense (such that severe granulocytopenia and moderate to severe thrombocytopenia are to be expected), there is as yet no evidence that very ("super") intense therapy has added benefit. Third, during this induction period, severe leukopenia and thrombocytopenia must be expected, with concomitant risk of infection and bleeding; thus provision of supportive care must be made. Fourth, if a patient goes into a complete remission with the initial combination chemotherapy, the authors would strongly recommend continuing these same drugs. If only a partial response occurs, a second non-cross resistant combination may be tried in an attempt to induce a complete remission. However, it must be recognized that the evidence to date suggests that these later complete responses are not as durable as ones that are achieved early. Next, while randomized trials can justify the use of alternating non-cross resistant combinations, particularly in extensive stage disease, the modest survival and response duration benefits have to be balanced against the potential toxicity from exposing patients to multiple drugs. It is just as reasonable to save one of the non-cross resistant combinations for use at the time of objective tumor progression. Some examples of combination chemotherapy regimens that have been used in the treatment of SCLC at major centers are listed in Table 14-51. An example of the type of dramatic response possible with chemotherapy alone is shown in Fig. 14-19.

In limited stage patients, the benefits of combined modality therapy still need to be proven in prospectively randomized trials from several institutions. However, the retrospective analysis of long-term survivors and an analysis of local failures in the chest following chemotherapy alone are suggestive of

TABLE 14-51. Combination Chemotherapy Regimens Used in the Treatment of Small-Cell Lung Cancer (All doses in mg/m² and given IV unless otherwise stated)

REGIMEN	DOSE	
CMC-VAP REGIMEN (NCI-VA) [229,236]		
INDUCTION OVER 12 WEEKS (NO RADIOTHERAPY GIVEN)		
CMC* (FIRST 6 WEEKS)		
Cyclophosphamide	1,500 mg/m² IV	days 1, 22
Methotrexate	15 mg/m² orally	days 1, 4, 8,11, 22, 25, 29, 32
CCNU	100 mg/m² orally	day 1
VAP SECOND 6 WEEKS		
Vincristine	1.4 mg/m²	days 1, 21 (maximum individual dose not to exceed 2 mg)
Adriamycin	60 mg/m²	days 1, 21
Procarbazine	100 mg/m² orally	days 1 through 10, and 22 through 31 (maximum individual dose = 200 mg)

FOLLOWED BY MAINTENANCE (CMC ALTERNATING WITH VAP)

CMC (one 6-week cycle) doses (all in mg/m²) are CTX 500 IV, MTX 10, CCNU 50 orally with schedule indicated above, alternating with VAP, doses and schedule listed above.

Note: 1) No dose modifications for hematologic toxicity during induction. Platelet and red cell transfusions as needed; appropriate dose reductions for renal and hepatic dysfunction, and omission of methotrexate for severe mucositis. Supportive care given during this period.
2) Total dose of vincristine given at any one time, not to exceed 2 mg.
3) Stop adriamycin at total dose of 450 mg/m².
4) During maintenance therapy, appropriate dose modifications for hematologic toxicity (e.g., 75% dose for white blood counts [WBC] below 4,000/μl, or platelet count less than 100,000/μl, 50% doses for WBC below 3,000 and platelets below 75,000, and 0% dose for WBC below 2,000 and platelets below 50,000 at the time of dose.)
5) Continue for 1 year in complete responders and then stop after appropriate restaging.
6) Continue until time of disease progression or unacceptable toxicity in partial responders.

CAV REGIMEN (VANDERBILT UNIVERSITY)[218,428]		
INDUCTION CAV OVER 18 WEEKS (RADIOTHERAPY ALSO GIVEN)*		
Cyclophosphamide	1000 mg/m² IV	every 21 days for 6 doses
Adriamycin	40 mg/m² IV	every 21 days for 6 doses
Vincristine	1 mg/m² IV	every 21 days for 6 doses
FOLLOWED BY MAINTENANCE #1 GIVEN MONTHLY × 3		
VP-16-213	200 mg/m² IV	days 1, 8
Hexamethylmelamine	8 mg/kg body weight orally	days 1 through 14
FOLLOWED BY MAINTENANCE #2 GIVEN EVERY 3 WEEKS		
Methotrexate	75 mg/m² IM	every 3 weeks for 7 months.

*Radiotherapy to primary tumor of 3000 rad in 300 rad daily fraction was also given starting on day 1. "Doses attenuated" based on WBC and platelet count on day of treatment.

CAVP-16 REGIMEN (BCRC)[413]		
CAVP-16 CYCLE OVER 9 WEEKS (NO RADIOTHERAPY GIVEN)†		
Cyclophosphamide	1,000 mg/m² IV	day 1
Adriamycin	45 mg/m² IV	day 1
VP-16-312	50 mg/m² IV	day 1 through 5

†Repeat CAVP-16 cycle every 3 weeks for 3 doses.

AFTER 3 CYCLES OF CAVP-16 MAY SWITCH TO		
CAVP-16 ALTERNATING WITH ONE 6-WEEK CYCLE OF:		
CCNU	75 mg/m² orally	day 1
Methotrexate	40 mg/m² IV	days 1, 21
Vincristine	1 mg/m² IV	days 1, 21
Procarbazine	75 mg/m² orally	days 1 through 5, 21 through 25

(may be used alone at time of tumor progression)

CCMV 4-WEEK CYCLE (FINSEN INSTITUTE)[414,451,454]		
Cyclophosphamide	1,000 mg/m² IV	day 1
CCNU	70 mg/m² orally	day 1
Methotrexate	20 mg/m² orally	days 18, 21
Vincristine	1.3 mg/m² IV	days 1, 8, 15, 22

SOME PATIENTS ALSO RECEIVED ADRIAMYCIN, VP-16-213 ALTERNATING WITH CCMV OR WERE TREATED AT TIME OF PROGRESSION WITH ADRIAMYCIN, VP-16-213 (4-WEEK CYCLE)

Adriamycin	30 mg/m² IV	day 1
VP-16-213	100 mg/m² IV	days 1 through 4

Appropriate drug dose modifications made for hematologic and other toxicity. Randomized trial ± radiotherapy showed no benefit from adding radiotherapy.

benefit from chest radiotherapy. In contrast to the suggested benefits, there are definite toxicities of both an acute and chronic nature that should be expected with combined modality therapy, particularly if chemotherapy and radiotherapy are given concurrently (the method that appears to produce the best results in combining chemo- and radiotherapy). If radiotherapy is given to the primary lesion, it appears prudent that patients be selected so that the radiotherapy can be given in full doses, by conventional fractionation, and in a manner that will not compromise the needed combination chemotherapy or sacrifice too much lung. This will mean selecting patients of limited stage disease with good initial performance status (PS 0, 1), and good initial pulmonary function. The tumor should be confined to an area that will allow avoiding radiation of the entire heart, entire hemithorax, or contralateral lung. The radiotherapist must have the equipment, staff support, and commitment to deliver tailored radiotherapy with shaping of fields during treatment much the same as that delivered for Hodgkin's disease radiotherapy to the chest. Elderly patients, those with significant heart disease, or those unable to cooperate with the therapy should not be selected. In extensive stage disease, the routine use of chest radiotherapy or radiotherapy to metastatic sites (with the exception of radiation for brain metastases or spinal cord compression) is to be avoided. However, if the chemotherapy is inadequate to relieve local tumor symptoms, a course of radiotherapy can be added. Most of these principles will be incorporated in the planning and execution of clinical trials. However, if new drugs, doses, schedules, drug combinations, or drug-radiotherapy combinations are planned, these should be part of an approved clinical protocol.

LONG-TERM SURVIVORS WITH SMALL CELL LUNG CANCER

Given the intensity and complexity of staging and therapy of SCLC, it is reasonable to ask if any patients can be cured by applying the principles outlined in the previous section. The AJC study revealed less than 1% of all SCLC patients were long-term survivors.[214] The National Cancer Institute established a registry of all potential long-term (30 months plus) survivors to determine whether any patients were actually cured.[482] Slides were reviewed by a central pathology panel; so far, 97 histologically confirmed SCLC cases with long-term survivorship have been accessioned from the U.S., Canada, Japan, and Europe. Of these, 77% had no evidence of recurrent cancer. Over 91% were limited stage disease, but there was no apparent relationship to age, sex, or histologic subtype of small cell cancer (including those with mixture of small cell and large cell tumors). Long-term survivorship was seen with all types of therapy including surgery, radiotherapy, or chemotherapy alone or in combination with one another.

Several institutions have reported long-term survivors in SCLC following treatment with chemotherapy with or without radiotherapy and these series provide estimates of the actual fraction of patients potentially cured (see Table 14-52). All of these trials involved combination chemotherapy, most with early intensive therapy. Overall, 8% of 635 patients were long-term disease-free survivors with a median follow-up to date over 3 years. Significantly, all had entered and remained in an initial complete clinical remission. Some 85% of the long-term survivors had limited stage disease prior to treatment; 15% of all limited stage patients entered this long-term survivor category compared to seven-fold less (2%) of extensive stage patients. Some 79% of these long-term survivors had received combined modality therapy.

These results demonstrate that a significant fraction of all SCLC patients treated can become long-term, potentially cured survivors and indicate an increase in this category of over tenfold compared to prior decades. The data indicate the importance of obtaining an initial complete clinical remisson and the influence of the initial stage of disease on potential cure. However, a small but definite fraction of patients with extrathoracic metastatic disease also enter this category. Because most of the limited stage patients in these initial trials were treated with combined modality therapy and since most of the long-term survivors are limited stage disease, it is not yet possible to ascertain the role of combined chemoradiotherapy in achieving cure. However, the vast majority of long-term survivors now alive were treated with combined modality therapy. The quality of life of survivors has not been discussed. However, in the NCI study, approximately a third of the survivors had signs or symptoms of pulmonary fibrosis related in part to their treatment and in part to chronic underlying cardiopulmonary disease.[484] In addition, 10% of the NCI survivors had died of second (non-lung cancer) malignancies that may have been related to the combined modality therapy. All of these aspects continue to stress the need for controlled trials to test the efficacy of combined modality or other new forms of therapy in SCLC.

TABLE 14-52. Long-Term (30 Month Plus) Disease-Free Survivors with Small-Cell Lung Cancer

INSTITUTION	REFERENCE	# PATIENTS TREATED	% LONG-TERM SURVIVORS*			MEDIAN SURVIVAL MONTHS†
			ALL PATIENTS	LD	ED	
Finsen Institute	(483)	337	6	9	2.3	38+
NCI	(484)	168	11	23	3	46+
SUNY	(426)	72	11	19	2.7	34+
Indiana Univ.	(400)	58	10	32	0	24–38+
Total		635	8	15	2.3	

*LD = limited stage disease; ED = extensive stage disease.
†Median survival reported of long-term disease-free survivors.

EVIDENCE FOR IMMUNE DEFECTS IN LUNG CANCER PATIENTS

Lung cancer patients frequently have severe immunosuppression.[485,486] This is seen in depressed total lymphocyte counts, lowered T-lymphocyte levels, defective ability to respond to DNCB, impaired response to common recall antigens, diminished lymphocyte blastogenesis, impaired macrophage function, and lowered antibody response to bacterial antigens.[487,493] In general, early and regional disease are not associated with the suppression found in more advanced tumors, and reactivity to DNCB is directly related to prognosis, stage of disease, and resectability.[485,486,488,494] Conversion from an anergic to a reactive state can occur and the change in immune status may be associated with improvement in survival.[495,497] Serum-mediated immunosuppression (lymphocyte blastogenesis to PHA and concanavalin A *in vitro*) is seen in lung cancer patients, is correlated with the presence of tumor, and is not present in patients rendered free of clinically evident disease by surgery.[494] This suggests that immunosuppression may be a form of paraneoplastic syndrome associated with lung cancer. In addition, a retrospective review suggested that patients who developed postoperative empyema (and were thus potentially immunostimulated) have better 5-year survival compared to a concurrent historical control who did not get empyema.[498] All of these findings together suggest that one therapeutic strategy would be to reverse the immune suppression in lung cancer patients; this has led into a series of immunotherapy trials.[495,499]

CURRENT RECOMMENDATIONS OF THE USE OF IMMUNOTHERAPY IN NON-SMALL CELL LUNG CANCER

While there is slight suggestive benefit in some trials in terms of increased time to disease recurrence in resected stage I lung cancer patients treated with intrapleural BCG, any difference when all the properly randomized trial data are pooled appears small. There also appears to be significant batch differences in BCG, so even its proponents do not know if a particular batch will work until it has been tested on patients. However, it is possible that with analysis of all the randomized trials, the predictive value of PPD conversion after BCG may prove useful. *C. parvum*, MER-BCG, Freund's adjuvant, and tumor cell vaccines all have no evident benefit while levamisole may actually be detrimental. Because of these results, the authors presently recommend that no patient be given any of these immunotherapies except as part of controlled clinical trials.

IMMUNOTHERAPY OF SMALL CELL LUNG CANCER

Because of the immune suppression that occurs, not only from tumor but also from intensive combination chemotherapy or radiotherapy, it is reasonable to consider immunotherapy in SCLC. A variety of trials have added BCG or *C. parvum* in a nonrandomized fashion to chemotherapy and radiotherapy but the effect of the immunotherapies is, of course, not interpretable. A series of randomized trials has found no survival or response benefit to BCG or MER-BCG added to combination chemotherapy with or without radiotherapy in either limited or extensive stage disease patients. Over 120 patients have been randomized to receive or not receive MER with no effect.[532,533] Some 254 patients were randomized to either receive or not receive BCG by scarification with combined modality therapy. While there was no difference in response rate, response duration, or median survival, there was a significant adverse effect of BCG on long-term survival.[534]

Some 67 SCLC patients were randomized to receive or not to receive calf fraction V thymosin (a modulator of T-cell function capable of correcting T-cell defects in inherited disorders of T cells). Sixty mg/m^2, 20 mg/m^2, or no thymosin therapy was given in 12 doses during the initial 6 weeks of intensive induction combination chemotherapy with or without thoracic radiotherapy.[535] While there was no difference in the complete response rate, patients receiving thymosin 60 mg/m^2 had significantly prolonged survival compared to those receiving thymosin 20 mg/m^2, or no thymosin, even after statistically adjusting for all prognostic imbalances such as performance status. This trial needs to be confirmed by other institutions.

Because of the above results, the current recommendations of the authors are not to use immunotherapy in the treatment of SCLC except as part of approved clinical trials.

REFERENCES

1. Silverberg E: Cancer statistics, 1980. CA 30:2338, 1980
2. Cancer Patient Survival, Report Number 5, DHEW Publ. No. (NIH) 77–992, 1977
3. Rosenow EC III, Carr DT: Bronchogenic carcinoma. CA 29:233–246, 1979
4. Selawry OS, Hansen HH: Lung cancer. In Holland JF and Frei E (eds): Cancer Medicine. Philadelphia, Lea & Febiger, 1974
5. Carbon PP, Frost JK, Feinstein AR et al: Lung cancer: perspectives and prospects. Ann Intern Med 73:1003–1024, 1970
6. Golomb HM, DeMeester TR: Lung cancer: a combined modality approach to staging and therapy. CA 29:258–275, 1979
7. Cohen MH: Diagnosis, Staging, and Therapy. In Harris CC (ed): Pathogenesis and Therapy of Lung Cancer, pp. 653–700. New York, Marcel Dekker, 1978
8. Benfield, JR, Juillar GJF, Pilch YH: Current and future concepts of lung cancer. Ann Intern Med 83:93–106, 1975
9. Israel L, Chaninian AP: Lung Cancer: Natural History, Prognosis, and Therapy. New York, Academic Press, 1976
10. Straus MJ: Lung Cancer: Clinical Diagnosis and Treatment. New York, Grune and Stratton, 1977
11. Harris CC: Pathogenesis and Therapy of Lung Cancer. New York, Marcel Dekker, 1978
12. Muggia FM, Rozencweig M: Progress in Cancer Research and Therapy. Vol. 11: Lung Cancer. New York, Raven Press, 1979
13. Cohen MN: Bronchogenic carcinoma. In Staquet MJ (ed): Randomized Trials in Cancer: A Critical Review by Sites. New York, Raven Press, 1978
14. Zubrod CG, Selawry O: The treatment of lung cancer. Adv Intern Med 23:451–467, 1978
15. Selawry OS, Straus MJ: Lung cancer. Semin Oncol 1:161–287, 1974
16. Cohen MN: Lung cancer: a status report. J Natl Cancer Inst 55:505–511, 1975.
17. Graham EA: A brief account of the development of thoracic surgery and some of its consequences. Surg Gynecol Obstet 36:241–250, 1957

18. Blades B: A case report and miscellaneous comments. J Thorac Surg 36:285–300, 1958
19. Ochsner A: The development of pulmonary surgery, with special emphasis on carcinoma and bronchiectasis. Am J Surg 135:732–746, 1978
20. Ewart W: The bronchi and pulmonary blood vessels. London, Bailliere, Tizdall, and Cox, 1889
21. Jackson CL, Huber JF: Correlated applied anatomy of bronchial tree and lungs with system nomenclature. Dis Chest 9:319–326, 1943
22. Boyden EA: Segmental Anatomy of the Lungs. New York, McGraw-Hill, 1955
23. Martini N: Identification and prognostic implications of mediastinal lymph node metastases in carcinoma of the lung. Prog Cancer Res Ther 11:250–255, 1979
24. Staging of Lung Cancer, 1979. American Joint Committee for Cancer Staging and End-Results Reporting. Task force on lung cancer. (Mountain CF (chairman), DT Carr, N Martini, et al) Chicago, IL. Also: Manual for Staging of Cancer 1978, pp 59–64. Chicago, American Joint Committee for Cancer Staging and End Results Reporting, 1978
25. Kreyberg L: Histologic typing of lung tumors. In Kreyberg L (ed): International Histologic Classification of Tumors, no. 1, pp 19–26. Geneva, World Health Organization, 1967
26. Yesner R, Gerstl B, Auerbach O: Application of the World Health Organization classification of lung carcinoma to biopsy material. Ann Thorac Surg 1:33–49, 1965
27. Matthews MJ: Morphologic classification of bronchogenic carcinoma. Cancer Chemother Rep 3:229–302, 1973
28. Matthews MJ, Gordon PR: Morphology of pulmonary and pleural malignancies. In Straus MJ (ed): Lung Cancer Clinical Diagnosis and Treatment. New York, Grune and Stratton, 1977
29. Mountain CF, Carr DT, Anderson WAD: A system for the clinical staging of lung cancer. Am J Roentgenol Radium Ther Nucl Med 120:130–138, 1974
30. Feinstein AR, Gilfman NA, Yesner R: The diverse effects of histopathology manifestations and outcome of lung cancer. Chest 66:225–229, 1974
31. Hinson KFW, Miller AB, Tall R: An assessment of the World Health Organization classification of the histologic typing of lung tumors applied to biopsy and resected material. Cancer 35:399–405, 1975
32. Auerbach O, Garfinkel L, Parks UR: Histologic type of lung cancer in relation to smoking habits, year of diagnosis and sites of metastases. Chest 67:382–387, 1975
33. Katlic M, Carter D: Prognostic implications of histology, size and location of primary tumors. Prog Cancer Res Ther 11:143–150, 1979
34. Vincent RG, Pickren JW, Lane WW et al: The changing histopathology of lung cancer: a review of 1682 cases. Cancer 39:1647–1655, 1977
35. Soroken SP: The respiratory system. In Greep RO, Weiss L (eds): Histology, 3rd ed, pp 675–712. New York, McGraw-Hill, 1973
36. Tischler AS: Small cell carcinoma of the lung: cellular origin and relationship to other neoplasms. Semin Oncol 5:244–252, 1978
37. Macholda F: Bronchogenic carcinoma: study of growth and evolutionary dynamics of bronchogenic carcinoma its significance for early diagnosis. Acta Univ Carol (Suppl) 41:39–62, 1970
38. Auerbach O, Gere JB, Pawlowski JM: Carcinoma in situ and early invasive occuring in the tracheobronchial tree in cases of bronchial carcinoma. J Thorac Surg 34:298–307, 1957
39. Valaitis JN, McGrew EA, Chomet B: Bronchogenic carcinoma in situ in asymptomatic high risk population of smokers. J Thorac Cardiovasc Surg 57:325–332, 1969
40. Auerbach O, Stout AP, Hammond EG et al: Changes in bronchial epithelium in relation to cigarette smoking and in relation to lung cancer. N Engl J Med 265:253–269, 1961
41. Faumeni JF Jr: Respiratory Carcinogenesis: an epidemiologic appraisal. JNCI 55:1039–1046, 1975
42. Saccomanno G, Archer VE, Auerbach O et al: Histologic types of lung cancer among uranium miners. Cancer 27:515–523, 1971
43. Meyer EC, Liebow AA: Relationship of interstitial pneumonia honeycombing and atypical epithelial proliferation to cancer of the lung. Cancer 18:322–350, 1965
44. Batsakis JG, Johnson HA: Generalized scleroderma involving lungs and liver with pulmonary adenocarcinoma. Arch Pathol 69:633–638, 1960
45. Moolten SE: Scar cancer of lung complicating rheumatoid lung disease. Mt Sinai J Med 40:736–743, 1973
46. Brincker H, Wilbek E: The incidence of malignant tumours in patients with respiratory sarcoidosis. Br J Cancer 29:247–251, 1974
47. Carroll R: The influence of lung scars on primary lung cancer. J Bacteriol 83:293–297, 1962
48. Marq M, Galy P: Bronchoalveolar carcinoma. Clinicopathologic relationships, natural history, and prognosis in 29 cases. Am Rev Respir Dis 107:621–629, 1973
49. Liebow AA: Bronchiolar–alveolar carcinoma. Adv Intern Med 10:329–358, 1960
50. Hewlett TH, Gomez AC, Aronstam EM et al: Bronchiolar carcinoma of lung: review of 39 patients. J Thorac Cardiovasc Surg 48:614–624, 1964
51. Donaldson JC, Kaminsky DB, Elliott RC: Bronchiolar carcinoma. Report of 11 cases and review of the literature. Cancer 41:250–258, 1978
52. Watson WL, Farpour A: Terminal bronchiolar or "alveolar cell" cancer of the lung: Two hundred sixty-five cases. Cancer 19:776–780, 1966.
53. Greenberg SD, Smith MN, Spjut HG: Bronchiolo–alveolar carcinoma, cell of origin. Am J Clin Pathol 63:153–167, 1975
54. Beaver DL, Shapiro JL: A consideration of chronic pulmonary parenchymal inflammation and alveolar cell carcinoma with regard to a possible etiology relationship. Am J Med 21:879–887, 1956
55. Lutwyche VU: Another presentation of fibrosing alveolitis and alveolar cell carcinoma. Chest 70:292–293, 1976
56. Meyer EC, Liebow AA: Relationship of interstitial pneumonia, honeycombing and atypical epithelial preoliferation to cancer of the lung. Cancer 18:322–351, 1965
57. Mulvihill JJ: Host factors in human lung tumors: an example of oncology. J Natl Cancer Inst 57:3–7, 1976
58. Joishy SK, Cooper RA, Rowley PT: Alveolar cell carcinoma in identical twins. Similarity in time of onset, histochemistry, and site of metastasis. Ann Intern Med 87:447–450, 1977
59 Katzenstein AA, Priolequ PG, Askin FG: The histologic spectrum and significance of clear-cell change in lung carcinoma. Cancer 45:943–947, 1980
60. Ihde DC, Cohen MH, Bernath AM et al: Serial fiberoptic bronchoscopy during chemotherapy of small cell carcinoma of the lung. Chest 74:531–536, 1978
61. Gazdar AF, Carney DN, Guccion JE et al: Small cell carcinoma of the lung: cellular origin and relationship to other tumors. In Greco FA, Oldham RK, Bunn PA (eds): Small Cell Lung Cancer. New York, Grune and Stratton (in press, 1981)
62. Ihde DC, Simms EG, Matthews MJ et al: Bone marrow metastases in small cell carcinoma of the lung: frequency, description, and influence on chemotherapy toxicity and prognosis. Blood 53:667–686, 1979
63. Mountain CF, Carr DT, Martini N et al: Staging of lung cancer 1979. American Joint Committee for Cancer Staging and End Results Reporting. Task Force on Lung Cancer, Chicago, Ill, 1980
64. Harley HRS: Cancer of the lung in women. Thorax 31:354–264, 1976
65. Rilke F, Carbone A, Clemente C et al: Surgical pathology of resectable lung cancer. Prog Cancer Ther Res Ther 11:129–142, 1979
66. Tao LC, Delarue NC, Sanders D et al: Bronchiolo-alveolar carcinoma. Cancer 42:2759–2767, 1978
67. Kanhouwa SB, Matthews MJ: Reliability of cytologic typing of lung cancer. Acta Cytol 20:229–232, 1976
68. Cagneten CB, Geller CE, Saenz MDC: Diagnosis of broncho-

genic carcinoma through the cytologic examination of sputum, with special reference to tumor typing. Acta Cytol 20:530–536, 1976
69. Feinstein AR, Gelfman NA, Yesner R: Observer variability in the histopathologic diagnosis of lung cancer. Am Rev Resp Dis 101:671–684, 1970
70. Hirsch FR, Matthews MJ, Yesner R: Problems in the histopathologic classification of small cell carcinoma of the lung. In Hensen HH, Dombernowski P (eds): Abstracts II World Conference on Lung Cancer. An interobservatorial examination, p 177. Amsterdam, Oxford-Princeton, Exerpta Medica, 1980
71. Burdon JGW, Sinclair RA, Henderson MM: Small cell carcinoma of the lung: Prognosis in relation to histologic subtype. Chest 76: 302–304, 1979
72. Hansen HH, Dombernowsky P, Hansen M et al: Chemotherapy of advanced small cell anaplastic carcinoma. Ann Intern Med 89:177–181, 1978
73. Flower CD, Verney GI: Percutaneous needle biopsy of thoracic lesions: an evaluation of 300 biopsies. Clin Radiol 30:215–218, 1979
74. Yesner R: Observer variability and reliability in lung cancer diagnosis. Cancer Chemother Rep 4:55–57, 1973
75. Cuttitta F, Rosen S, Gazdar A et al: Monoclonal antibodies which demonstrate specificity for several types of human lung cancer. Proc Natl Acad Sci USA (in press)
76. Matthews MJ: Personal Communication, 1980.
77. Carney DN, Matthews M, Ihde DC et al: Influence of histologic subtype of small cell carcinoma of the lung on clinical presentation, response to therapy and survival. JNCI 65:1225–1230, 1980
78. Radice PA, Matthews MJ, Ihde DC et al: Characterization of mixed histology large cell/small cell lung cancer and its response to combination chemotherapy. Proc AACR–ASCO 20:409, 1979
79. Matthews MJ: Effects of therapy on the morphology and behavior of small cell carcinoma of the lung—a clinicopathologic study. Prog Cancer Res Ther 11:155–165, 1979
80. Abeloff MD, Eggleston JC, Mendelsohn G et al: Changes in morphologic and biochemical characteristics of small cell carcinoma of the lung. A clinicopathologic study. Am J Med 66:757–764, 1979
81. Gazdar A, Carney D, Baylin S et al: Small cell carcinoma of the lung: altered morphological, biologic and biochemical characteristics in long term cultures and heterotransplanted tumors. Proc AACR–ASCO 21:51, 1980
82. Bell CE, Seetharam S: Expression of endodermally derived and neural crest derived differentiation antigens by human lung and colon tumors. Cancer 44:13–18, 1979
83. Bohm N, Sandritter W: DNA in human tumors: a cytophotometric study. Curr Top Pathol 60:151–219, 1975
84. Nasiell MG, Kato H, Auer G et al: Cytomorphological grading and feulgen DNA-analysis of metaplastic and neoplastic bronchial cells. Cancer 41:1511–1521, 1978
85. Bunn P, Schlam M, Gazdar A: Comparison of cytology and DNA content analysis by flow cytometry in specimens from lung cancer patients. Proc AACR–ASCO 21:40, 1980
86. Cohen MH: Signs and symptoms of bronchogenic carcinoma. In Straus MJ (ed): Lung Cancer Clinical Diagnosis and Treatment, pp 85–94. New York, Grune and Stratton, 1977
87. Byrd RB, Carr DT, Miller WE et al: Radiographic abnormalities in carcinoma of the lung as related to histological cell type. Thorax 24: 573–575, 1969
88. Matthews MJ, Kanhouwa S, Pickner J et al: Frequency of residual and metastatic tumors in patients under going curative surgical resection of lung cancer. Cancer Chemother Rep 3:63–67, 1973
89. Coy P, Kennelly GM: The role of curative radiotherapy in the treatment of lung cancer. Cancer 45:698–702, 1980
90. Pancoast HK: Superior pulmonary sulcus tumor. JAMA 99:1391–1396, 1932
91. Paulson DL: Superior sulcus tumors. Results of combined therapy. NY State J Med 71: 2050–2052, 1971
92. Doehner GA, Marcus SS, Wolff WI: Pancoast's tumor. Five-year survival after combined radiotherapy and surgery. NY State J Med 67:2378–2380, 1967
93. Paulson DL: Carcinomas in the superior pulmonary sulcus. J Thorac Cardiovasc Surg 70:1095–1104, 1975
94. Henderson RD, Boszko A, Van Nostrand AWP: Pharyngoesophageal dysphagia and recurrent laryngeal nerve palsy. J Thorac Cardiovasc Surg 68, 507–512, 1974
95. Salsali M, Cliffton EE: Superior vena cava obstruction with lung cancer. Ann Thorac Surg 6:437–442, 1968
96. Lokich JJ, Goodman R: Superior vena cava syndrome. Clinical management. JAMA 231:58–61, 1975
97. Rubin P, Hicks GL: Biassociation of superior vena cava obstruction and spinal cord compression. NY State J Med 73:2176–2182, 1973
98. Strauss BL, Matthews MJ, Cohen MH et al: Cardiac metastases in lung cancer. Chest 71:607–610, 1977
99. Katz RJ, Simms EB, DiBianco R et al: Pericardial tamponade in lung cancer: Diagnosis, management and response to treatment. Am J Med (in press)
100. Rigler LG: Bronchiolo–alveolar carcinoma of lung with report on new roentgenologic sign. International Congress of Radiology, 1965
101. Homma H, Kira S, Takahasi Y et al: A case of alveolar cell carcinoma accompanied by fluid and electrolyte depletion through production of voluminous amounts of lung liquid. Am Rev Respir Dis 111:857–862, 1975
102. Matthews MJ: Problems in morphology and behavior of bronchopulmonary malignant disease. In Israel L, Chahanian P (eds): Lung Cancer: Natural History, Prognosis, and Therapy, pp 23–62. New York, Academic Press, 1976
103. Odell WD, Wolfsen AR: Humoral syndromes associated with cancer. Ann Rev Med 29:379–406, 1978
104. Blackman MR, Rosen SW, Weintraub BD: Ectopic hormones. Adv Intern Med 85–113, 1978
105. Ayvazian LF: Extrapulmonary manifestations of tumors of the lung. Postgrad Med 63:93–99, 1978
106. Rassam JW, Anderson G: Incidence of paramalignant disorders in bronchogenic carcinoma. Thorax 30:86–90, 1975
107. Goldstraw P, Walbaum PR: Hypertrophic pulmonary osteoarthropathy and its occurrence with pulmonary metastases from renal carcinoma. Thorax 31:205–211, 1976
108. Green N, Kurohara SS, George FW III et al: The biologic behavior of lung cancer according to histologic type. Radiol Clin Biol 41:160–170, 1972
109. Byrd RB, Divertie MB, Spittell JA: Bronchogenic carcinoma and thromboembolic disease. JAMA 202:1019–1022, 1967
110. Sack GH, Levin J, Bell WR: Trousseau's syndrome and other manifestations of chronic disseminated coagulopathy in patients with neoplasms. Medicine 56:1–37, 1977
111. Greenfield GB, Schorsch HA, Shkolnik A: The various roentgen appearance of pulmonary hypertrophic osteoarthropathy. Am J Roentgenol Radium Ther Nucl Med 101:927–931, 1976
112. Croft PB, Wilkinson M: Carcinomatous neuromyopathy: its incidence in patients with carcinoma of the lung and breast. Lancet 1:184–188, 1965
113. Tyler HR: Paraneoplastic syndromes of nerve, muscle and neromuscular junction. Ann NY Acad Sci 230:348–357, 1974
114. Cahan WG, Castro EB, Hajdu SI: The significance of solitary lung shadow in patients with colon carcinoma. Cancer 33:414–426, 1974
115. Berg JW, Schottenfeld D: Multiple primary cancers at Memorial Hospital 1949–1962. Cancer 40:1954–1960, 1977
116. Cahan WG: Multiple primary cancers of the lung, esophagus, and other sites. Cancer 40:1954–1960, 1977
117. Wynder EL, Muskinski MH, Spivak JC: Tobacco and alcohol consumption in relation to the development of multiple primary cancers. Cancer 40:1872–1878, 1977
118. Enstrom JE, Austin DF: Interpreting cancer survival rates. Science 195:847–851, 1977
119. Fontana RS: Early diagnosis of Lung cancer. Am Rev Resp Dis 116: 399–402, 1977. (Also Fontana RS: The usefulness of screening for lung cancer. Personal communication, 1979)

120. Nash FA, Morgan JM, Tomkin JG: South London lung cancer study. Br Med J 2:715–721, 1968
121. Brett GZ: Earlier diagnosis and survival in lung cancer. Br Med J 4:260–262, 1969
122. Weiss W, Boucot KE, Cooper DA: The Philadelphia pulmonary neoplasm research project. Survival factors in bronchogenic carcinoma. JAMA 216:2119–2123, 1973
123. Grzybowski S, Coy P: Early diagnosis of carcinoma of lung: simultaneous screening with chest x-ray and sputum cytology. Cancer 25:113–120, 1970
124. Melamed M, Flehinger B, Miller D et al: Preliminary report of the lung cancer detection program in New York. Cancer 39:369–382, 1977
125. Neel HB III, Woolner LB, Sanderson DR: Sputum cytologic diagnosis of upper respiratory tract cancer. Ann Otol Rhinol Laryngol 87:468–473, 1978
126. Lung cancer mortality appears unaffected by roentgenographic and sputum screening in asymptomatic persons: report from the NIH. JAMA 241:1582, 1979
127. Wolfsen AR, Odell WD: PROACTH: use for early detection of lung cancer. Am J Med 66:765–772, 1979
128. Vincent RG, Chu TM, Lane WW et al: Carcinoembryonic antigen as a monitor of successful surgical resection in 130 patients with carcinoma of the lung. Prog Cancer Res Ther 11:191–198, 1979
129. Baker RR, Ball WC J, Carter D et al: Identification and treatment of clinically occult cancer of the lung. Prog Cancer Res Ther 11:243–249, 1979
130. Sanderson DR, Fontana RS, Woolner LB et al: Bronchoscopic localization of radiographically occult lung cancer. Chest 65:608–612, 1974
131. Martini N, Beattie EJ, Flifften EE et al: Radiologically occult lung cancer. Report of 26 cases. Surg Clin N Am 54:811–823, 1974
132. Fontana RS: Editorial: The needle in the haystack. Mayo Clin Proc 53: 616–617, 1978
133. Kinsey JH, Cortese DA, Sanderson DR: Detection of hematoporphyrin fluorescence during fiberoptic bronchoscopy to localize early bronchogenic carcinoma. Mayo Clin Proc 53:594–600, 1978
134. Cortese DA, Kinsey JH, Woolner LB et al: Clinical application of a new endoscopic technique for detection of in situ broncial carcinoma. Mayo Clin Proc 54:635–642, 1979
135. Bell JW: Positive sputum cytology and negative chest roentgenogram, a surgeon's dilemma. Ann Thorac Surg 9:149–157, 1970
136. Sanderson DR, Fontana RS: Early lung cancer detection and localization. Ann Otol Rhinol Laryngol 84:583–589, 1975
137. Ikeda S, Yanai, Ishikawa S: Flexible bronchofiberscope. Keio J Med 17:1–18, 1968
138. Khan MA, Whitcomb ME, Snider GL: Flexible fiberoptic bronchoscopy. Am J Med 61:151–155, 1976
139. Dvale PA, Bode FR, Kini S: Diagnostic accuracy in lung cancer. Comparison of techniques used in association with flexible fiberoptic bronchoscopy. Chest 69:752–757, 1976
140. Saltzstein SL, Harrell JH II, Cameron T: Brushings, washings or biopsy? Obtaining maximum value from flexible fiberoptic bronchoscopy in the diagnosis of cancer. Chest 71:630–632, 1977
141. Radke JR, Conway WA, Eyler WR et al: Diagnostic accuracy in peripheral lung lesions. Factors predicting success with flexible fiberoptic bronchoscopy. Chest 76:176–179, 1979
142. Mohsenifar Z, Chopra SK, Simmons DH: Diagnostic value of fiberoptic bronchoscopy in lung cancer presenting as mediastinal mass(es). Cancer 44:1894–1896, 1979
143. Richardson RH, Zavala DC, Jukerjee PK et al: The use of fiberoptic bronchoscopy and brush biopsy in the diagnosis of suspected pulmonary malignancy. Am Rev Respir Dis 109:63–66, 1974
144. Solomon DA, Sollida NH, Gracey DR: Cytology in fiberoptic bronchoscopy. Comparison of bronchial brushings, washings and postbronchoscopy sputum. Chest 65: 616–619, 1974
145. Ellis JH: Transbronchial lung biopsy via the fiberoptic bronchoscope. Experience with 107 consecutive cases and comparison with bronchial brushing. Chest 68:534–531, 1975
146. Wallace RJ Jr, Cohen A, Awe RJ et al: Carcinomatous lung abscess. Diagnosis by bronchoscopy and cytopathology. JAMA 242:521–522, 1979
147. Sargent, EN, Turner AF, Gordonson J et al: Percutaneous pulmonary needle biopsy: Report of 350 patients. Am J Roentgenol Radium Ther Nucl Med 122:758–768, 1974
148. Sinner WN: Pulmonary neoplasms diagnosed with transthoracic needle biopsy, Cancer 43:1533–1540, 1979
149. Sinner WN, Sandstedt B: Small-cell carcinoma of the lung. Cytological, roentgenologic, and clinical findings in a consecutive series diagnosed by fine needle aspiration biopsy. Radiology 121:269–274, 1976
150. Sagel SS, Ferguson TB, Forrest JV et al: Percutaneous transthoracic aspiration needle biopsy. Ann Thorac Surg 26:399–405, 1978
151. Trunk G, Gracey DR, Byrd RB: The management and evaluation of the solitary pulmonary nodule. Chest 66:236–239, 1974
152. Steel SJ, Winstanley DP: Trephine biopsy of the lung and pleura. Thorax 24:576–584, 1969
153. Mountain DC, Carr DT, Anderson WA: A system for the clinical staging of lung cancer. Am J Roentgenol Radium Ther Nucl Med 120:130–138, 1974
154. Carr DT, Mountain CF: The staging of lung cancer. Semin Oncol 1:229–234, 1974
155. Mountain CF, Hermes KE: Management implications of surgical staging studies. Prog Cancer Res Ther 11:233–242, 1979
156. Mountain CF: Biologic, physiologic, and technical determinants in surgical therapy for lung cancer. In Straus MJ (ed): Lung Cancer: Clinical Diagnosis and Treatment, pp. 185–198. New York, Grune and Stratton, 1977
157. Study Group. Evaluation of the clinical TNM compared with the TNM in lung cancer. Jpn J Cancer Clin 25:181–189, 1979
158. Henney J, Ishikawa S, Jacobs EM: Surgical aspects: overview. Lung Cancer: Prog Cancer Res Ther 11:231–233, 1979
159. Mountain CF: Surgery of lung cancer including adjunctive therapy. In Hansen HH, Rorth M (eds): Lung Cancer 1980, pp 71–92. Amsterdam-Oxford-Princeton, Excerpta Medica, 1980.
160. Shields TW, Higgins GA, Keehn R: Pathologic stage grouping of the patients with resected carcinoma of the lung. Ann Thorac Surg (in press)
161. Mountain CF: Assessment of the role of surgery for control of lung cancer. Ann Thor Surg 24:365–373, 1977.
162. Higgins GA, Beebe GW: Bronchogenic carcinoma: factors in survival. Arch Surg 94:539–549, 1967.
163. Fennessy JJ: The radiology of lung cancer. Med Clin N Am 59:95–119, 1975.
164. Ikeda S, Tsuuboi E, Ono R et al: Flexible bronchofiberscope. Jap J Clin Oncol 1:55–65, 1971.
165. Robbins HM, Morrison DA, Sweet ME et al: Biopsy of the main carina: staging lung cancer with the fiberoptic bronchoscope. Chest 75:484–486, 1979
166. Conn JH, Fain WR, Chavez CM et al: A critical evaluation of scalene lymphadenectomy in 500 patients. Am Surg 35:125–129, 1969
167. Brantigan JW, Brantigan CO, Brantigan OC: Biopsy of nonpalpable scalene lymph nodes in carcinoma of the lung. Am Rev Respir Dis 107:962–974, 1973
168. Harken DE, Block H, Clauss R et al: A simple cervico-mediastinal exploration for tissue diagnosis of intrathoracic disease. N Engl J Med 251:141–1044, 1954
169. Carlens E: Mediastinoscopy: a method for inspection and tissue biopsy in the superior mediastinum. Dis Chest 36:343–352, 1959
170. Fishman NH, Bronstein MH: Is mediastinoscopy necessary in the evaluation of lung cancer? Ann Thorac Surg 20:578–585, 1975
171. James EC, Ellwood RA: Mediastinoscopy and mediastinal roentgenology: a clinical correlation. Ann Thorac Surg 18:531–538, 1974

172. Jolly PC, Hill LO III, Lawless PA et al: Parasternal mediastinotomy and mediastinoscopy: adjuncts in diagnosis of chest disease. J Thorac Cardiovasc Surg 66:5490556, 1973
173. Ellis JH Jr: Transbronchial lung biopsy via the fiberoptic bronchoscope: experience with 107 consecutive cases and comparison with bronchial brushing. Chest 68:534–532, 1975
174. Goldberg EM: Mediastinoscopy in assessment of lung cancer. In Straus MJ (ed): Lung Cancer: Clinical Diagnosis and Treatment, pp 113–127. New York, Grune & Stratton, 1977
175. Pearson FG, Nelems JM, Henderson RD: The role of mediastinoscopy in the selection of treatment for bronchial carcinoma with involvement of superior mediastinal lymp nodes. J Thoracic Cardiovasc Surg 44:382–390, 1972
176. Goldberg EM, Shapiro CM, Glicksman AS: Mediastinoscopy for assessing mediastinal spread in clinical staging of lung carcinoma. Semin Oncol 1:205–215, 1974
177. Jepson O, Rahbek SH: Mediastinoscopy. Copenhagen, Munksgaard, 1970
178. Fishman NH, Bronstein MH: Is mediastinoscopy necessary in the evaluation of lung cancer? Ann Thorac Surg 20:678–686, 1975
179. Larsson S: Mediastinoscopy in bronchogenic carcinoma. A study of 486 cases with special reference to the indications and limitations of the method. Scand J Thorac Cardivasc Surg (Suppl) 19:1–23, 1976
180. Mintz U, DeMeester TR, Rezai K et al: Sequential staging in primary lung carcinoma: a study of 115 patients. Proc AACR–ASCO 20:9, 1979
181. Baker RR, Lillemoe KD, Tockman MS: The indications for transcervical mediastinoscopy in patients with small peripheral bronchial carcinoma. Surg Gynecol Obstet 148:860–862, 1979
182. DeMeester TR, Bekerman C, Joseph JG et al: Gallium 67 scanning for carcinoma of the lung. J Thorac Cardiovasc Surg 72:699–708, 1976
183. Alazraki NP, Ramsdell JW, Taylor A et al: Reliability of gallium scan and chest radiography compared to mediastinoscopy for evaluating mediastinal spread in lung cancer. Am Rev Respir Dis 1117:415–420, 1978
184. McLoud TC, Wittenberg J, Ferrucci JT: Computed tomography of the thorax and standard radiographic evaluation of the chest: a comparative study. J Comput Assist Tomogr 3:70–180, 1979
185. Mintzer RA, Malave SR, Neiman HL et al: Computed vs convential tomography in evaluation of primary and secondary pulmonary neoplasms. Radiology 132:653–659, 1979
186. Underwood GH Jr, Hooper RG, Axelbaum SP et al: Computed tomographic scanning of the thorax in the staging of bronchogenic carcinoma. N Engl J Med 300:777–778, 1979
187. Benfield JE, Bonney H, Crummy AB et al: Azygograms and pumonary arteriograms in bronchogenic carcinoma. Arch Surg 99:406–409, 1969
188. Mcleod RA, Brown LR, Miller WE et al: Evaluation of the pulmonary hila by tomography. Radiol Clin North Am 14:51–83, 1976
189. Macumber HH, Calvin JW: Perfusion lung scan patterns in 100 patients with bronchogenic carcinoma. J Thorac Crdiovasc Surg 72:299–302, 1976
190. Cunningham JJ: Gray scale echography of the lung and pleural space. Current applications of oncologic interest. Cancer 41:1329–1339, 1978
191. Hansen HH, Muggia FM: Staging of inoperable patients with bronchogenic carcinoma with special reference to bone marrow examination and peritoneoscopy. Cancer 30:1395–1401, 1972
192. Muggia FM, Chervu LR: Lung cancer: diagnosis in metastatic sites. Semin Oncol 1:217–228, 1974
193. O'Mara RE: Skeletal scanning in neoplastic disease. Cancer 37:480–486, 1976
194. Hansen HH, Muggia FM, Selawry OS: Bone marrow examination in 100 consecutive patients with bronchogenic carcinoma. Lancet 2:443–445, 1971
195. Newman SJ, Hansen HH: Frequency, diagnosis and treatment of brain metastases in 247 consecutive patients with bronchogenic carcinoma. Cancer 33:492–496, 1974
196. Ransdell JW, Peters RM, Taylor AT et al: Multiorgan scans for staging lung cancer. Correlation with clinical evaluation. J Thorac Cardiovasc Surg 73:653–659, 1977
197. Bell JW: Abdominal exploration in one-hundred lung carcinoma suspects prior to thoracotomy. Ann Surg 167:199–203, 1969
198. Yashar J: Transdiaphragmatic exploration of the upper abdomen during surgery for bronchogenic carcinoma. J Thorac Cardiovasc Surg 52:599–603, 1966
199. Hansen HH, Muggia FM: Staging of inoperable patients with bronchogenic carcinoma with special references to bone marrow examination and peritoneoscopy. Cancer 30:1395–1401, 1972
200. Mittman C, Bruderman I: Lung cancer: to operator or not? Am Rev Respir Dis 116:477–496, 1977
201. Tarhan S, Moffitt EA: Principles of thoracic anesthesia. Surg Clin North Am 53:813–826, 1973
202. Stanley KE: Prognostic factors for survival in patients with inoperable lung cancer. J Natl Cancer Inst 65:25–32, 1980
202a. Golebiowski A: Pulmonary resection in patients over 70 years of age. J Thorac Cardiovasc Surg 61:265–270, 1971
203. Watson WL, Schottenfeld D: Survival in cancer of the bronchus and lung, 1949–1962; comparison of men and women patients. Dis Chest 53:65–72, 1968
204. Ederer F, Mersheimer WL: Sex differences in the survival of lung cancer patients. Cancer 15:425–432, 1962
205. Connelly RR, Cutler SJ, Baylis P: End results in cancer of the lung: comparison of male and female patients. J Natl Cancer Inst 36:277–287, 1966
206. Harley HRS: Cancer of the lung in women. Thorax 31:254–264, 1976
207. Tarhan S, Moffitt EA, Taylor WF: Myocardial infarction after general anesthesia. JAMA 220:1451–1454, 1972
208. Miller RD: Preoperative pulmonary evaluation of the dyspneic surgical candidate. Surg Clin North Am 53:8050811, 1973
209. Parker FB Jr: Surgery in chronic lung disease. Surg Clin North Am 54:1193–1202, 1974
210. Olsen GN, Block AJ, Swenson EW et al: Pulmonary function evaluation of the lung resection candidate. A prospective study. Am Rev Respir Dis 111:379–387, 1975
211. Legge JS, Palmer KNWV: Effect of lung resection for bronchial carcinoma on pulmonary function in patients with and without chronic obstructive bronchitis. Thorax 30:563–565, 1975
212. Neuhaus H, Cherniack NS: A bronchospirometric method of estimating the effect of pneumonectomy on the maximum breathing capacity. J Thorac Cardiovasc Surg 55:144–148, 1968
213. Lindell SW: ^{133}Xe radiospirometry. Prediction of lung function after pulmonary resection. Scand J Clin Lab Invest 34:289–292, 1974
213a. Page WF, Kuntz AJ: Racial and socioeconomic factors in cancer survival. A comparison of Veteran's Administration results with selected studies. Cancer 45:1029–1040, 1980
213b. Weiss GB, Danils JC: A reevaluation of the association between prolonged survival in lung cancer and HLA antigens AW19 and BS. Clin Res 26:687A, 1978
214. Mountain CF: Clinical biology of small cell carcinoma: relationship to surgical therapy. Semin Oncol 5:272–279, 1978
215. Zelen, M: Keynote address on biostatistics and data retrieval. Cancer Chemother Rep 4(2;):31–42, 1973
216. Bunn PA Jr, Cohen MH, Ihde DC et al: Advances in small cell bronchogenic carcinoma. Cancer Treat Rep 61:333–342, 1977
217. Ihde DC, Makuch RW, Carney DN et al: Prognostic implication of sites of metastases in patients with small cell carcinoma of the lung given intensive combination chemotherapy. Am Rev Respir Dis Chest (in press)
218. Greco FA, Richardson RL, Schulman SF et al: Treatment of oat cell carcinoma of the lung: complete remissions, acceptable complications, and improved survival. Br Med J 2:10–11, 1978
219. Holoye PY, Samuels ML, Lanzotti VJ et al: Combination chemotherapy and radiation therapy for small cell carcinoma. JAMA 237: 1221–1224, 1977
220. Johnson RE, Brerton HD, Kent C: "Total" therapy for small cell carcinoma of the lung. Am Thorac Surg 25:509–515, 1978
221. Livingston BR, Moore TN, Heilbrun L et al: Small cell carcinoma

of the lung: combined chemotherapy and radiation. Ann Intern Med 88:194–199, 1978
222. Einhorn LH, Bond WH, Hornback N et al: Long-term results in combined modality treatment of small cell carcinoma of the lung. Semin Oncol 5:309–313, 1978
223. Maurer LH, Tulloh M, Weiss RB et al: A randomized combined modality trial in small cell carcinoma of the lung: comparison of combination chemotherapy–radiation therapy versus cyclophosphamide radiation therapy, effects of maintenance chemotherapy and prophylactic whole brain irradiation. Cancer 45:30–39, 1980
224. Israel L, Depierre A, Choffel C et al: Immunochemotherapy in 34 cases of oat cell carcinoma of the lung with 19 complete remissions. Cancer Treat Rep 61:343–347, 1977
225. Edmonson JH, Lagako SW, Selawry OS et al: Cyclophosphamide and CCNU in the treatment of inoperable small cell carcinoma and adenocarcinoma of the lung. Cancer Treat Rep 60:925–932, 1976
226. Lowenbraun S, Bartolucci A, Smalley RV et al: The superiority of combination chemotherapy over single agent chemotherapy in small cell lung carcinoma. Cancer 44:406–413, 1979
227. Livingston RB: Treatment of small cell carcinoma: evolution and future directions. Semin Oncol 5:299–308, 1978
228. Eagan RT, Carr DT, Lee RE et al: Phase II studies of polychemotherapy regimens in small cell lung cancer. Cancer Treat Rep 61:93–96, 1977
229. Cohen MH, Ihde DC, Bunn PA et al: Cyclic alternating combination chemotherapy of small cell bronchogenic carcinoma. Cancer Treat Rep 63:163–170, 1979
230. Hansen HH, Dombernowsky P, Hirsch FR: Staging procedures and prognostic features in small cell anaplastic bronchogenic carcinoma. Semin Oncol 5:280–287, 1978
231. Dombernowsky P, Hirsch F, Hansen HH et al: Peritoneoscopy in the staging of 190 patients with small-cell anaplastic carcinoma of the lung with special reference to subtyping. Cancer 41:2008–2012, 1978
232. Hirsch FR, Hansen HH, Hainau B: Bilateral bone-marrow examinations in small-cell anaplastic carcinoma of the lung. Acta Pathol Microbiol Scand 87:59–62, 1979
233. Hirsch F, Hansen HH, Dombernowsky P et al; Bone-marrow examination in the staging of small-cell anaplastic carcinoma of the lung with special reference to subtyping. An evaluation of 203 consecutive patients. Cancer 39:2463–2567, 1977
234. Bunn PA Jr, Nugent JL, Matthews MJ: Central nervous system metastases in small cell bronchogenic carcinoma. Semin oncol 5:314–322, 1978
235. Dunnick NR, Ihde DC, Johnston-Early A: Abdominal CT in the evaluation of small cell carcinoma of the lung. Am J Radiol 133:1085–1088, 1979
236. Cohen MH, Fossieck BE, Ihde DC et al: Chemotherapy of small cell carcinoma of the lung: results and concepts. Prog Cancer Res Ther 11:559–566, 1979
236a. Wittes RE, Yeh SDJ: Indications for liver and brain scans. Screening tests for patients with oat cell carcinoma of the lung. JAMA 238:506–507, 1977
237. Nugent JL, Bunn PA Jr, Matthews MJ et al: CNS metastases in small cell bronchogenic carcinoma. Increasing frequency and changing pattern with lengthening survival. Cancer 44:1885–1893, 1979
238. Paulson DL: Carcinomas in the superior pulmonary sulcus. J Thorac Cardiovasc Surg 70:1095–1104, 1975
239. Matthews MJ, Rozencweig M, Staquet MJ et al: Long-term survivors with small cell carcinoma of the lung. Eur J Cancer 16:527–531, 1980
240. Higgins GA, Shields TW, Keehn RJ: The solitarty pulmonary nodule: Ten-year follow-up of veterans Administration—Armed Forces Cooperative Study. Arch Surg 110:570–575, 1975
241. Churchill ED, Sweet RH, Soutter L et al: The surgical management of carcinoma of the lung. J Thorac Surg 20:349–365, 1956
242. Johnson J, Kirby CK, Blakemore WS: Should we insist on "radical pneumonectomy" as a routine procedure in the treatment of carcinoma of the lung? J Thorac Surg 36:309–315, 1958
243. Shields T, Higgins GA: Minimal pulmonary resection in the treatment of carcinoma of the lung. Arch Surg 108:420–422, 1974
244. Jensik RJ, Faber LP, Milloy FJ et al: Segmental resection for lung cancer: A 15 year experience. J Thorac Cardiovasc Surg 66:563–572, 1973
245. Naef AP: New techniques in the surgical treatment of lung cancer. Prog Cancer Res Ther 11:257–260, 1979
246. Jensik RJ, Faber LP, Brown CM et al: Bronchoplastic and conservative resectional procedures for ronchial adenoma. J Thorac Cardiovasc Surg 68:556–565, 1974
247. Shields TW, Higgins GA, Keehn RJ: Factors influencing survival after resection for bronchial carcinoma. J Thorac Cardiovasc Surg 64:391–399, 1972
248. Higgins GA, Shields TW: Experience of the Veterans Administration Surgical Adjuvant Group. Prog Cancer Res Ther 11:433–442, 1979
249. Paulson DL, Reisch JS: Long-term survival after resection for bronchogenic carcinoma. Ann Surg 184:324–332, 1976
250. Wilkins WE Jr, Scannell JG, Craver JG: Four decades of experience with resection for bronchogenic carcinoma at the Massachusetts General Hospital. J Thorac Cardiovasc Surg 76:364–368, 1978
251. Ashor GL, Kern WH, Meyer BW et al: Long-term survival in bronchogenic carcinoma. J Thorac Cardiovasc Surg 70:581–589, 1975
252. Kirsh MM, Rotman H, Argenta L et al: Carcinoma of the lung: results of treatment over ten years. Ann Thorac Surg 21:371–377, 1976
253. Martini N, Beattie EJ: Results of surgical treatment in Stage I Lung Cancer. J Thorac Cardiovasc Surg 74:499–506, 1977
254. Soorae AS, Stevenson HM: Survival with residual tumor on the bronchial margin after resection for bronchogenic carcinoma. J Thorac Cardiovasc Surg 78:175–180, 1979
255. Shields TW: The fate of patients after incomplete resection of bronchial carcinoma. Surg Gyneocol Obstet 139:569–572, 1974
256. Jeffry RM: Survival in bronchial carcinoma. Tumor remaining in the bronchial stump following resection. Ann R Coll Surg Engl 51:55–59, 1972
257. McNeil BJ, Weichselbaun RR, Parker SG: The fallacy of the five year survival in lung cancer. N Engl J Med 299:1397–1400, 1978
258. Hilton G: Present position relating to cancer of the lung: Results with radiotherapy alone. Thorax 15:17–18, 1960
259. Smart J: Can cancer of the lung be cured by radiation alone? JAMA 195–1034–1035, 1966
260. Caldwell WL, Bagshaw MA: Indications for and results of irradiation of carcinoma of the lung. Cancer 22:999–1004, 1968
261. Guttman RJ: Results of radiation therapy in patients with inoperable carcinoma of the lung whose status was established at exploratory thoractomy. Am J Roentgenol Rad Ther Nucl Med 93:99–103, 1965
262. Guttman RJ: Radical supervoltage therapy in inoperable carcinoma of the lung. In Deeley TJ (ed): Carcinoma of the Bronchus (Modern Radiotherapy), p 193. New York, Appleton-Century-Crofts, 1971
263. Deeley TJ, Singh SP: Treatment of inoperable carcinoma of the bronchus by megavoltage x-rays. Thorax 22:562–566, 1967
264. Abramson N, Cavanaugh PJ: Short course radiation therapy in carcinoma of the lung—a second look. Radiology 108:685–687, 1973
265. Salazar OM, Rubin P, Brown JC, et al: The assessmet of tumor response to irradiation of the lung cancer. Int J Rad Oncol Biol Phys 1:1107–1118, 1976
266. Eisert DR, Cox JD, Komaki R: Irradiation for bronchial carcinoma: Reasons for failure. Analysis of local control as a function of dose, time, and fractionation. Cancer 37:2665–2670, 1976
267. Billingham ME, Bristow MR, Glatstein E et al: Adriamycin cardiotoxicity: endomyocardial biopsy evidence of enhancement by irradiation. Am J Surg Pathol 1:17–23, 1977

268. Sweany SK, Moss WT, Haddy FJ: Effects on chest irradiation on pulmonary function. J Clin Invest 38:587–593, 1959
268a. Moss WT, Haddy FFJ, Sweany SK: Some factors altering the severity of acute radiation pneumonitis: variation with cortisone, heparin, and antibiotics. Radiology 75:50–54, 1960
269. Bloedorn FG, Cowley RA, Cuccia CA et al: Combined therapy: irradiation and surgery in the treatment of bronchogenic carcinoma. Am J Roentgenol Rad Ther Nucl Med 85:175–181, 1961
270. Warren J: Pre-operative irradiation of cancer of the lung; final of a therapeutic trial. Cancer 36:914–925, 1975
271. Shields TW, Higgins GA, Lawton R et al: Pre-operative x-ray therapy as an adjuvant in the treatment of bronchogenic carcinoma. J Thorac Cardiovasc Surg 59:49–56, 1970
272. Sherman DM, Neptune W, Weichselbaum RR et al: An aggressive approach to marginally resectable lung cancer. Cancer 41: 2040–2045, 1978
273. Green N, Kuroharra SS, George FW et al: Post resection irradiation for primary lung cancer. Radiology 116:405–407, 1975
274. Choi NCH, Grillo HC, Gardiello M et al: Basis for new strategies in postoperative radiotherapy of bronchogenic carcinoma. Int J Rad Oncol Biol Phys 6:31–35, 1980
275. Hilaris BS, Martini N, Batata M et al: Interstitial irradiation for unresectable carcinoma of the lung. An Thorac Surg 20:4891–500, 1975
276. Pancost HK: Superior pulmonary sulcus tumor: tumor characterized by pain, Horner's syndrome, destruction of bone and atrophy of hand muscles. JAMA 99:1391–1396 1932
277. Paulson DL , Shaw RR, Kee JL et al: Combined pre-operative irradiation and resection for bronchogenic carcinoma. J Thorac Cardiovasc Surg 44:281–294, 1962.
278. Paulson DL: Carcinomas in the superior pulmonary sulcus. J Thorac Surg 70:1095–1104, 1975
279. Paulson DL: Carcinoma in the superior pulmonary sulcus. Ann Thorac Surg 28:3–4, 1979
280. Miller JI, Mansour KA, Hatcher CR: Carcinoma of the superior pulmonary sulcus Ann Thorac Surg 28:44–47, 1979
281. Higgins GA, Shields TW: Experience of the Veterans Administration Surgical Adjuvant Group Prog Cancer Res Ther 11:433–442, 1979
282. Slack HH: Bronchogenic carcinoma: nitrogen mustard as a surgical adjuvant and factors influencing survival. University Surgical Adjuvant Lung Cancer Project. Cancer 25:987–1002, 1970
283. Brunner KW, Marthaler T, Muller W: Adjuvant chemotherapy with cyclophosphamide (NSC-26271) for radically rsected bronchogenic carcinoma: 9-year follow-up. Prog Cancer Res Ther 11:411–420, 1979.
284. Pirogov AI, Trakhtenberg AK: Results and prospects of combined surgery and antitumor chemotherapy for lung cancer. Cancer Treat Rep 60:1489–1491, 1976
285. Stott H, Stephens WF, Roy DC: 5-year follow-up of cytotoxic chemotherapy as an adjuvant to surgery in carcinomas of the bronchus. Br J Cancer 34:167–173, 1976.
286. Crosbie WA, Kamdar HH, Belcher JR: A controlled trial of vinblastine sulphate in the treatment of cancer of the lung. Br J Dis Chest 60:28–35, 1966
287. Mountain CF, Vincent RG, Sealy R et al: A clinical trial of CCNU as surgical adjuvant treatment for patients with surgical stage I and stage II non-small cell lung cancer: Preliminary findings. Prog Cancer Res Ther 11:421–431, 1979
288. Karrer K, Prindun N, Zwintz E: Chemotherapy studies in bronchogenic carcinoma by the Austrian Study Group. Cancer Chemother Rep 4:207–213, 1973
289. Israel L, Bonadonna G, Sylvester R et al: Controlled study with adjuvant radiotherapy, chemotherapy, immunotherapy, and chemoimmunotherapy in operable squamous carcinoma of the lung. Prog Cancer Res Ther 11:421–431, 1979
290. Higgins GA, Humphrey EW, Hughes FA et al: Cytoxan as an adjuvant to surgery for lung cancer. Surg Oncol 1:211–228, 1969
291. Shields TW, Humphrey EW, Eastridge CE et al: Adjuvant cancer chemotherapy after resection of carcinoma of lung. Cancer 5:2057–2062, 1977
292. Wingfield HV: Combined surgery and chemotherapy for carcinoma of the bronchus. Lancet 1:470–471, 1970
293. Katsuki H, Shimada K, Koyama A et al: Long-term intermittent adjuvant chemotherapy for primary, resected lung cancer. J Thorac Cardiovasc Surg 70:590–599, 1975
294. Dolton EG: Combined surgery and chemotherapy for carcinoma of bronchus Lancet 1:40–41, 1970
295. Buyze EAC, Nelemans FA: A study of postoperative cytostatic medication in patients with operable carcinoma of the lung. Arzneim Forsch 23:860–862, 1973
296. Sealy R: Combined radiotherapy and chemotherapy in non-small cell carcinoma of the lung. Prog Cancer Res Ther 11:315–323, 1979
297. Brouet D: Results of a trial using radiotherapy and chemotherapy in bronchial cancer. Eur J Cancer 4:437–445, 1968
298. Host H: Cyclophosphamide (NSC 26271) as an adjuvant to radiotherapy in the treatment of unresectable bronchogenic carcinoma. Cancer Chemother Rep 4:161–164, 1973
299. Kaung DT, Wolf J, Hyde L et al: Preliminary report on the treatment of nonresectable cancer of the lung. Cancer Chemother Rep 58:359–364, 1974
300. Holsti LR: Alternative approaches to radiotherapy alone and radiotherapy as part of a combined therapeutic approach for lung cancer. Cancer Chemother Rep 4:165–169, 1973
301. Hall TC, Dederick MM, Chalmers TC et al: A clinical pharmacologic study of chemotherapy an X-ray therapy in lung cancer. Am J Med 43:186–193, 1967
302. Benninghoff DL, Alexander LL: Treatment of lung carcinoma: Radiation versus radiation combined with 5-fluorouracil. NY State J of Med (Part 1) 68:532–534, 1967
303. Krant MJ, Chalmers TC, Dederick MM et al: Comparative trial of chemotherapy and radiotherapy in patients with nonresectable cancer of the lung. Am J Med 35:363–373, 1963
304. Durrant KR, Ellis F, Black JM et al: Comparison of treatment policies in inoperable bronchial carcinoma. Lancet 1:715–719, 1971
305. Landgren RC, Hussey DH, Samuels ML et al: A randomized study comparing irradiation alone to irradiation plus procarbazine in inoperable bronchogenic carcinoma. Radiology 108:403–406, 1973
306. Coy P: A randomized study of irradiation and vinblastine in lung cancer. Cancer 26:803–80, 1970
307. Bergsagel DE, Jenkin RDT, Pringle JF et al: Lung cancer: clinical trial of radiotherapy alone vs. radiotherapy plus cyclophosphamide. Cancer 30:621–627, 1972
308. Sandison AG, Falkson G, Fichardt T et al: A statistical evaluation of the treatment of 215 patients with advanced bronchial cancer managed by telecobalt therapy alone and in combination with various cancer chemotherapeutic agents. S Afr J Radiol 5:21–27, 1967
309. Carr DT, Childs DS Jr, Lee RE: Radiotherapy plus 5FU compared to radiotherapy alone for inoperable and unresectable bronchogenic carcinoma. Cancer 29:375–380. 1972
310. Cox JD, Yesner R, Mielowski W et al: Influence of cell type on failure pattern after irradiation for locally advanced carcinoma of the lung. Cancer 44:94–98, 1979
311. Eagan RT, Lee RE, Frytak S et al: Randomized trial of thoracic irradiation plus combination chemotherapy for unresectable adenocarcinoma and large cell carcinoma of the lung. Int J Radiat Oncol Biol Phys 5:1401–1405, 1979
312. Reynols RD, O'Dell S: Combination modality therapy in lung cancer: a survival study showing beneficial results of AMCOF (Adriamycin, Methotrexae, Cyclosposphamide, Oncovin and 5-Fluorouracil). Cancer 42: 385–389, 1978
313. Hansen HH, Muggia FM, Andres R et al: Intensive combined chemotherapy and radiotherapy in patients with non-resectable bronchogenic carcinoma. Cancer 30:315–324, 1972
314. Samuels ML, Barkley HT Jr, Holeoye PY et al: Combination chemotherapy with bleomycin (NSC-125066), vincristine

(NSC-67574), and methotrexate (NSC-740), plus split-course radiotherapy in the treatment of non oat-cell bronchogenic carcinoma. Cancer Chemother Rep 59:377–383, 1975

315. Bitran JD, Desser RK, DeMeester T et al: Combined modality therapy for Stage III MO non-oat cell bronchogenic carcinoma. Cancer Treat Rep 62:327–322, 1978
316. Schultz HP, Overgaard M, Sell A: X-ray therapy and combination chemotherapy in non-small cell carcinoma of the lung—A pilot study. In Hansen HH, Dombernowsky P (eds): Abstracts II World Conference on Lung Cancer, Copenhagen, p 137. Amsterdam-Oxford-Princeton, Excerpta Medica, 1980
317. Bitran J, Golomb H, DeMeester T et al: Combined modality therapy for stage IIIMO non-small cell bronchogenic carcinoma. Proc AACR-ASCO 21:446, 1980
318. Weshler Z, Sulkes A, Fuks Z et al: Combined modality treatment with radiation and chemotherapy in locally advanced bronchogenic carcinoma. In Hansen HH, Dombernowsky P (eds): Abstracts II World conference on Lung Cancer Copenhagen. Amsterdam-Oxford-Princeton, Excerpta Medica, 1980
319. Wils JA: Sequential combination chemotherapy and radiotherapy in metastatic non-small cell lung cancer. In Hansen HH, Dombernowsky P (eds): Abstracts II World conference on Lung Cancer, p 126, Copenhagen. Amsterdam-Oxford-Princeton, Excerpta Medica, 1980
320. Takita H, Hollingshead AC, Rizzo DJ et al: Treatment of inoperable lung carcinoma: a combined modality approach. Ann Thorac Surg 28:363–368, 1979
321. DeMeester T, Golomb H, Griem M et al: Preliminary results of multimodal therapy for Stage III carcinoma of the lung. In Hansen HH, Domerbowsky P (eds): Abstract II World conference on Lung Cancer, p 130, Copenhagen. Amsterdam-Oxford-Princeton, Excerpta Medica, 1980
322. Cox JD, Stanley K, Petrovich Z et al: Cranial irradiation in cancer of the lung of all cell types. In Hansen HH, Dombernowsky P (eds): Abstracts II World conference on Lung Cancer, p 262, Copenhagen. Amsterdam-Oxford-Princeton, Excerpta Medica, 1980
323. Hyde L, Wolf J, McCracken S et al: Natural course of inoperable lung cancer. Chest 64:309–312, 1973
324. Brashea RE: Should asymptomatic patients with inoperable bronchogenic carcinoma receive immediate radiotherapy? North Am Rev Respir Dis 117:411–414, 1978
325. Phillips TL, Miller RJ: Should asymptomatic patients with inoperable bronchogenic carcinoma receive immediate radiotherapy? Yes. Am Rev Respir Dis 117:405–410, 1978
326. Slawson RG, Scott RM: Radiation therapy in bronchogenic carcinoma. Radiology 132:175–176, 1979
327. Line D, Deeley TJ: Palliative therapy. In Deeley TJ (ed): Carcinoma of the Bronchus (Modern Radiotherapy), pp. 298–306. New York, Appleton, Century, Crofts 1972
328. Perez CA, Presant CA, Van Ambury AL: Management of superior cava syndrome. Semin Oncol 5:123–134, 1978
329. Bruckman JE, Bloomer WD: Management of spinal cord compression. Semin Oncol 5:135–140, 1978
330. Raichle ME, Posner JB: The treatment of extradural spinal cord compression. Neurol 20:391–396, 1970
331. Gilbert RW, Kim JH, Posner JB: Epidural Spinal cord compression from metastatic tumor: Diagnosis and treatment. Ann Neurol 3:40–51, 1978
332. Thomas JE, Colby MY Jr: Radiation-induced or metastatic brachial plexopathy? A diagnostic dilemma. JAMA 222:1392–1395, 1972
333. Lagakos SW, Zelen M: Statistical considerations in the planning and analysis of inoperable non-small cell lung studies. Prog Cancer Res Ther 11:393–397, 1979
334. Ruckdeschel J, Metha C, Creech R: Chemotherapy of advanced non-oat cell bronchogenic carcinoma: The Eastern Cooperative Oncology Group Experience. In Hansen HH, Dombernowsky P (eds): Abstracts II World Conference on Lung Cancer, p. 237. Copenhagen, Amsterdam-Oxford-Princeton, Excerpta Medica, 1980
335. Eagan RT, Fleming TR, Schoonover V: Evaluation of response criteria in advanced lung cancer. Cancer 44:1125–1128, 1979
336. Livingston RB: Combination chemotherapy of bronchogenic carcinoma. I. Non-oat cell. Cancer Treat Rev 4:153–1651 1977
337. Wolf J, Jyde L, Philips RW et al: Recent comparative systemic therapy in non-small cell carcinoma of the lung. Prog Cancer Res Ther 11:374–382, 1979
338. Eagan RT, Ingle JN, Frytak S et al: Platinum-based polychemotherapy versus dianhydrogalactitol in advanced non-small cell lung cancer. Cancer Treat Rep 61:1339–1345, 1977
339. Galla RJ, Cvitkovic E, Golby RB: Cis-dichlorodiammine-platinum (II) in non-small cell carcinoma of the lung. Cancer Treat Rep 63:1585–1588, 1979
340. Egan RT, Frytak S, Creagan ET et al: Phase II study of cyclophosphamide, adriamycin and cis-dichlorodiamine platinum (II) by infusion in patients with adenocarcinoma and large cell carcinoma of the lung. Cancer Treat Rep 63:1589–1591, 1979
341. Evans WK, Feld R, Deboer G et al: Cyclophosphamide, adriamycin, and cis-platinum in the treatment of non-small cell lung cancer. Proc AACR-ASCO 21:447, 1980
342. Richards F II, White DR, Muss HB et al: Combination chemotheapy of advanced non-oat cell carcinoma of the lung: Cancer 44:1576–1581, 1979
343. Bitran JD, Desser RK, DeMeester N et al: Metastatic non-oat cell bronchogenic carcinoma: Therapy with cyclophosphamide, doxorubincin, methotrexate and procarbazine (CAMP), JAMA 240:2743–2746, 1978
344. Butler TP, Macdonald JD, Smith FP et al: 5-fluorouracil, adriamycin, and mitomycin-C (FAM) chemotherapy for adenocarcinoma of the lung. Cancer 43:1183–1188, 1979
345. Mason BA, Catalano RB: Mitomycin, vinblastine, and cisplatin combination chemotherapy in non-small cell lung cancer. Proc AACR-ACSO 21:447, 1980
346. Lanzotti VJ, Thomas DR, Boyle LE et al: Survival with inoperable lung cancer. An integration of prognostic variables based on simple clinical criteria. Cancer 39:303–313, 1977
347. Cohen MH, Perevodchikova NI: Single agent chemotherapy of lung cancer. Prog Cancer Res Ther 11:343–374, 1979
348. Faulkner SL Adkins RB Jr, Reynolds VH: Chemotherapy for adenocarcinoma and alveolar cell carcinoma of the lung. Ann Thorac Surg 18:578–583, 1974
349. Brugarolas A, LaCaue AT, Ribas A et al: Vincristine in non-small cell broonchogenic carcinoma. Results of a phase II Clinical Study. Eur J Cancer 14:501–505, 1978
350. Casper ES, Gralla RJ, Kelson DP et al: Phase II studies in non-small cell lung cancer. In Hansen HH, Dombernowski P (eds): Abstracts II World Conference on Lung Cancer, p 225. Copenhagen, Amsterdam-Oxford-Princeton, Excerpta Medica, 1980
351. Furnas B, Einhorn LH, Rohn RJ: A phase II trial of vindesine in non-small cell lung cancer. Proc AACR-ASCO 21:448, 1980
352. Samson MK, Comis RL, Baker LH et al: Mitomycin C in advanced adenocarcinoma and large cell carcinoma of the lung. Cancer Treat Rep 62:163–165, 1978
353. Koons LS, Harris DT, Engstrom PF: Mitomycin C chemotherapy in advanced squamous cell cancer of the lung. Proc AACR-ASCO 19:326, 1978
354. DeJager R, Libert P, Michel J et al: Phase II clinical trials with high dose cisplatin with mannitol induced diuresis in advanced bronchogenic cancer. Proc AACR-ASCO 21:363, 1980
355. Panettiere FJ: Effects of the two dose SWOG cis-platinum program in non-oat cell lung cancer. Proc AACR-ACSO 21:450, 1980
356. Berenzweig M, Vogel SE, Kaplan BH et al: Phase II trial of cis-diamminedichloroplatinum in patients with non-small cell bronchogenic carcinoma not exposed to prior chemotherapy. Proc AACR-ASCO 21:457, 1980
357. Blum RH: An overview of studies with adriamycin in the United States. Cancer Chemother Rep 6:247–251, 1975
358. Rozencweig M, Kenis Y: European studies with adriamycin in lung cancer. Cancer Chemother Rep 6:343–347, 1975
359. Eagan RT, Ingle JN, Creagan ET et al: VP-16-213 chemotherapy

for advanced squamous cell cacinoma and adenocarcinoma of the lung. Cancer Treat Rep 62: 843–844, 1978

360. Costanzi JJ, Gagliano R, Loukas D et al: Ifosfamide in the treatment of recurrent or disseminated lung cancer. A phase II study of two dose schedules. Cancer 41:1715–1719, 1978

361. Eagan RT: Recent Developments in combination chemotherapy of non-small cell lung cancer. Prog Cancer Res Ther 11:383–391, 1979

362. Bodey GP, Lagakos SW, Gutierrez AC et al: Therapy of advanced squamous carcinoma of the lung. Cyclophosphamide versus "COMB". Cancer 39:1026–1031, 1977

363. Bearden JD III, Cotman CA Jr, Moon TE, et al: Combination chemotherapy using cyclophosphamide, vincristine, methotrexate, 5-fluorouracil, and prednisone in solid tumors. Cancer 39:21–26, 1977

364. Livingston RB, Fee WH, Einhorn LH et al: BACON (Bleomycin, adriamcin, CCNU, Oncovin, Nitrogen Mustard) in squamous lung cancer. Cancer 37:1237–1242, 1976

365. Livingston RB, Heilbrun L, Lehane D et al: Comparative trial of combination chemotherapy in extensive squamous carcinoma of the lung: a southwest oncology group study. Cancer Treat Rep 61:1623–1629, 1977

366. Chahinian AP, Mandel EM, Holland JF et al: MACC (Methotrexate, adriamycin, cyclophophamide, and CCNU) in advanced lung cancer. Cancer 43:1590–1597, 1979

367. Vogl SE, Mehta CR, Cohen MH: MACC chemotherapy for adenocarcinoma and epidermoid carcinoma of the lung. Low response rate in a cooperative group study. Cancer 44:864–868, 1979

368. Britell JC, Eagan RT, Ingle IN et al: Cis-dichlorodiammineplatinum (II) alone followed by adriamycin plus cyclophosphamide at progression versus cis-dichlorodiammineplatinum (II), adriamycin and cyclophosphamide in combination for adenocarcinoma of the lung. Cancer Treat Rep 62:1207–1210, 1978

369. Eagan RT, Creagan ET, Ingle JN et al: VP-16, cyclophosphamide, adriamcin and cis-platinum (V:CAP-I) in patients with metastatic adenocarcinoma of the lung. Tumori 65:105–109, 1978

370. Kelsen DP, Gralla RJ, Stoopler MB et al: Combination chemotherapy of non-small cell lung cancer with cisplatin, adriamycin, cyclophosphamide, and vindesine. In Hansen HH, Dombernowsky P (eds): Abstracts II World Conference on Lung Cancer, p 133. Copenhagen, Amsterdam-Oxford-Princeton, Excerpta Medica, 1980, and Proc AACR-ASCO 21:457, 1980

371. Whitehead R, Crowley J, Carbone PP: Cis-dichlorodiammineplatinum, adriamcin, cyclophosphamide, CCNU, and vincristine (PACCO) combination chemotherapy in advanced nonsmall cell bronchogenic carcinoma. Proc AACR-ASCO 21:458, 1980

372. Takita H, Marabella PC, Edgerton F et al: cis-dichlorodiammineplatinum (II), adriamycin, cyclophosphamide, CCNU, and vincristine in non-small cell lung carcinoma: a preliminary report. Cancer Treat Rep 63:29–33, 1979

373. Vogelzang NJ, Bonomi PD, Rossof AH et al: Cyclophosphamide, adriamycin, methotrexate, and procarbazine (CAMP) treatment of non-oat cell bronchogenic carcinoma. Cancer Treat Rep 62:1595–1597, 1978

374. Lad T, Sarma PR, Diekamp V et al: "CAMP" combination chemotherapy unresectable non-oat cell bronchogenic carcinoma. Cancer Clin Trials 2:321, 1979

375. Gralla RJ, Casper ES, Kelsen DP et al: Vindesine and cisplatin combination chemotherapy in non-small cell lung cancer. In Hansen HH, Dombernosky (eds): Abstracts II World Conference on Lung Cancer, p 229. Copenhagen, Amsterdam-Oxford-Princeton, Excerpta Media, 1980

376. Myers JW, Livingston RB, Coltman CA Jr: Combination chemotherapy of advanced adeno and large cell undifferentiated carcinoma of the lung with 5FU, vincristine and mitomycin-C (FOMi). Proc AACR-ASCO 21:453, 1980

377. Miller TP, McMahon LJ, Livingston RB et al: Extensive adenocarcinoma and large cell undifferentiated carcinoma of the lung treated with 5-fluorouracil, vincristine, and mitomycin C (FOMi). Proc AACR-ASCO 21:453, 1980

378. Issel BF, Valdivieso M, Bodey GP: Chemotherapy for adenocarcinoma and large cell anaplastic carcinoma of the lung with Ftorafur, adriamcin, and cis-dichlorodiammineplatinum (II). Cancer Treat Rep 62:1089–1091, 1978

379. Belgian EORTC Lung Cancer Working Party: Combination chemotherapy with cisplatin and VP16 in non-small cell bronchogenic carcinoma. In Hansen HH, Dombernowsky P (eds): Abstract II World Conference on Lung Cancer. Copenhagen, p 116. Amsterdam-Oxford-Princeton, Excerpta Medica, 1980, and Proc AACR-ASCO 21:368, 1980

380. Joss R, Goldhirsch A Cavalli F et al: Cisplatinum and VP 6-213 combination chemotherapy for non-small cell lung cancer, p 233. In Hansen HH, Dobernowsky P (eds): Abstract II World Conference on Lung Cancer. Copenhagen, Amsterdam-Oxford-Princeton, Excerpta Medica, 1980

381. Estape J, Milla, Agusti A et al: VP16-213 (VP–16) and cyclophosphamide in the treatment of primitive lung cancer in phase M 1. Cancer 43:72–77, 1979

382. Weissman CH, Ruckdeschel JC, Reilly C et al: Cyclophosphamide, adriamycin and VP16-213 chemotherapy in the management of advanced non-oat cell bronchogenic carcinoma. Proc AACR-ASCO 21:459, 1980

383. Krauss S, Tornyos K, DeSimone P et al: Cis-dichlorodiammineplatinum (II) and hexamthlemelamine in the treatment of non-oat cell lung cancer: Pilot study of the southeastern cancer study group. Cancer Treat Rep 63:391–393, 1979

384. Fraile RJ, Samson MK, Baker LH et al: Combination chemotherapy with mitomycin C, adriamycin, and cyclophosphamide in advanced adenocarcinoma and large cell carcinoma of the lung. Cancer Treat Rep 63:1983–1987, 1979

385. Dedikian AY, Staab R, Livingston R et al: Chemotherapy for adenocarcinoma of the lung with 5-fluorouracil, cyclophosphamide, and CCNU (FCC). Cancer 44:959–863, 1979

386. Robert F, Omura G, Bartolucci AA: Combination chemotherapy with cyclophosphamide, adriamycin, intermediate dose methotrexate, and folinic acid rescue (CAMF) in advanced lung cancer. Cancer 45:1–5, 1980

387. Trowbridge RC, Kennedy BJ, Vosika GJ: CCNU-adriamycin therapy in bronchogenic carcinoma. Cancer 41:1704–1709, 1978

388. Richards F II, Cooper MR, White DR et al: Advanced epidermoid lung cancer. Prolonged survival after chemotherapy. Cancer 46:34–37, 1980

389. Livingston RB, Heilbrun LH: Patterns of response and relapse in chemotherapy of extensive squamous carcinoma of lung. Cancer Chemother Pharmacol 1:225–227, 1978

390. Vosika GJ: Large cell bronchogenic carcinoma-prolonged disease-free survival following chemotherapy. JAMA 241:594–595, 1979

391. Greco FA, and Einhorn LH: Small Cell Lung Cancer. Semin Oncol 5:233–335, 1978

392. Bunn PA Jr, Ihde DC: Small cell bronchogenic carcinoma: A review of therapeutic results. In Livingston RB (ed): Lung Cancer: Advances in Research and Treatment, vol 1, pp 169–208. The Hague, Martinus Nijhoff, 1981

393. Ihde DC, Bunn PA Jr: Chemotherapy of small cell bronchogenic carcinoma. In Whitehouse JMA, Williams CJ (eds): Recent Advances in Clinical Oncology, vol 1. Edinburgh, Churchill Livingston (in press, 1981)

394. Fox W, Scadding JG: Medical Research Council comparative trial of surgery and radiotherapy for primary treatment of small-celled or oat-celled carcinoma of bronchus. Ten year follow-up. Lancet 2:63–65, 1973

395. Broder LE, Cohen MH, Selawry OS: Treatment of bronchogenic carcinoma. II. Small cell cancer. Cancer Treat Rev 4:219–260, 1977

396. Weiss RB: Small-cell carcinoma of the lung: Therapeutic management. Ann Intern Med 88:5322–531, 1978

397. Medical Research Council Working Party: Study of cytotoxic chemotherapy as an adjuvant to surgery in carcinoma of the bronchus. Br Med J 2:421–428, 1971

398. Karrer K, Pridun N, Denck H: Chemotherapy as an adjuvant to surgery in lung cancer. Cancer Chemother Pharmocol 1:145–159, 1978

399. Meyer JA, Comis RL, Ginsberg SJ et al: Selective surgical resection in small cell carcinoma of the lung. J Thorac Cardiovasc Surg 77:243–248, 1979
400. Mandelbaum I, Williams SD, Hornback NB et al: Combined therapy for small cell undifferentiated carcinoma of the lung. J Thorac Cardiovasc Surg 76:292–296, 1978
401. Tucker RD, Sealy R, van Wyk C et al: A clinical trial of cyclophosphamide (NSC-26271) and radiation therapy for oat cell carcinoma of the lung. Cancer Chemother Rep 4(2):159–160, 1973
402. Ling A, Berry R: Treatment of small cell carcinoma of bronchus. Lancet 1:129–132, 1975
403. Petrovich Z, Mietlowski W, Ohanian M et al: Clinical report on the treatment of locally advanced lung cancer. Cancer 40:72–77, 1977
404. Medical Research Council Lung Cancer Working Party: Radiotherapy alone or with chemotherapy in the treatment of small-cell carcinoma of the lung. Br J Cancer 40:1–10, 1979
405. Matthiessen W: Controlled clinical trial of radiotherapy alone, against radiotherapy plus chemotherapy in small cell carcinoma of the lung: comparison of radiation damage. Scand J Respir Dis (Suppl) 192:209–211, 1978
405a. Green RA, Humphrey E, Close H et al: Alkylating agents in bronchogenic carcinoma. Am J Med 46:516–525, 1969
406. Eagan RT, Carr DT, Frytak S et al: VP-16-213 versus polychemotherapy in patients with advanced small cell lung cancer. Cancer Treat Rep 60:949–951, 1976
407. Alberto P, Brunner KW, Martz G et al: Treatment of bronchogenic carcinoma with simultaneous or sequential combination chemotherapy, including methotrexate, cyclophosphamide, procarbazine, and vincristine. Cancer 38:2208–2216, 1976
408. Cohen MH, Creaven PJ, Fossieck BE et al: Intensive chemotherapy of small cell bronchogenic carcinoma. Cancer Treat Rep 61:349–354, 1977
409. Hansen HH, Selawry OS, Simon R et al: Combination chemotherapy of advanced lung cancer: A randomized trail. Cancer 38:2201–2207, 1976
410. Abeloff MD, Ettinger DS, Khouri NF et al: Intensive induction therapy for small cell carcinoma of the lung. Cancer Treat Rep 63:519–524, 1979
411. Ettinger DS, Karp JE, Abeloff MD et al: Intermittent high-dose cyclophosphamide chemotherapy for small cell carcinoma of the lung. Cancer Treat Rep 62:413–242, 1978
412. Minna JD, Ihde D, Bunn P et al: Extensive stage small cell carcinoma of the lung: Effect of increasing intensity of induction chemotherapy. Proc AACR-ASCO 21:448, 1980
413. Aisner J, Whitacre M, Van Echo DA et al: Alternating non-cross resistant combination chemotherapy for small cell carcinoma of the lung. Proc. AACR-ASCO 21:453, 1980
414. Dombernowsky P, Hansen HH, Soren S et al: Sequential versus nonsequential combination chemotherapy using 6 drugs in advanced small cell carcinoma: A comparative trial including 146 patients. Proc AACR-ASCO 29:277, 1979
415. Livingston R, Mira J: Non-cross resistant combinations in patients with extensive small-cell lung cancer. Proc AACR-ASCO 21:449, 1980
416. Daniels JR, Chak L, Alexander M et al: Oat-cell carcinoma. Alternating compared with sequential combination chemotherapy. Proc AACR-ASCO 21:346, 1980
417. Cavalli F, Jungi WF, Sonntag RW et al: Phase II trial of cisdichlorodiammineplatinum (II) in advance malignant lymphoma and small cell lung cancer: preliminary results. Cancer Treat Rep 63:1599–1603, 1979
418. Natal RB, Gralla RJ, Wittes RE: Phase II trials of vindesine, AMSA and PCNU in patients with small cell lung cancer. In Hansen HH, Dombernowsky P (eds): Abstract II World Conference on Lung Cancer, p 235. Copenhagen, Amsterdam-Oxford-Princeton, Exerpta Medica, 1980
419. Hattori S, Matsudu M, Ikegami H et al: Small cell carcinoma of the lung: Clinical and cytomorphologic studies in relation to its response to chemotherapy. Gann 68:321–331, 1977
420. Holoye PY, Samuels ML: Cyclophosphamide, vincristine and sequential split-course radiotherapy in the treatment of small cell lung cancer. Chest 67:675–679, 1975
421. Eagan RT, Carr DT, Lee RE et al: Phase II studies of polychemotherapy regimens in small cell lung cancer. Cancer Treat Rep 61:93–95, 1977
422. Greco FA, Einhorn LH, Richardson RL et al: Small cell lung cancer: Progress and perspectives. Semin Oncol 5:323–335, 1978
423. Herman TS, Jones SE, McMahon LG et al: Combination chemotherapy with adriamycin and cyclophosphamide (with or without radiation therapy) for carcinoma of the lung. Cancer Treat Rep 61:875–879, 1977
424. McMahon LJ, Herman TS, Manning MR et al: Patterns of relapse in patients with small cell carcinoma of the lung treated with adriamycin cyclophosphamide chemotherapy and radiation therapy. Cancer Treat Rep 63:359–362, 1979
425. King GA, Comis R, Ginsberg S et al: Combination chemotherapy and radiotherapy in small cell carcinoma of the lung. Radiology 125:529–530, 1977
426. Ginsberg SJ, Comis RL, Gottlieb AJ et al: Long-term survivorship in small-cell anaplastic lung carcinoma. Cancer Treat Rep 63:1347–1349, 1979
427. Hornback NB, Einhorn L, Shidnia H et al: Oat cell carcinoma of the lung. Early treatment results of combination radiation therapy and chemotherapy. Cancer 37: 2658–2664, 1976
428. Greco FA, Richardson RL, Snell JD et al: Small cell lung Cancer: complete remission and improved survival. Am J Med 66:625–630, 1979
429. Johnson RE, Brereton HD, Kent CH: Small-cell carcinoma of the lung: Attempt to remedy causes of past therapeutic failure. Lancet 2:289–291, 1976
430. Holoye PY, Samuels ML, Smith T et al: Chemoimmunotherapy of small cell bronchogenic carcinoma. Cancer 42:34–40, 1978
431. Nixon DW, Crey RW, Suit HD et al: Combination chemotherapy in oat cell carcinoma on the lung. Cancer 36:867–872, 1975
432. Wittes RE, Hopfan S, Hilaris B et al: Oat cell carcinoma of the lung: Combination treatment with radiotherapy and cyclophosphamide, adriamycin, vincristine, and methotrexate. Cancer 40:654–659, 1977
433. Jackson DV, Richards F, Cooper MR et al: Prophylactic cranial irradiation in small cell carcinoma of the lung. A randomized study. JAMA 237:2730–2733, 1977
434. Cohen MH, Lichter AS, Bunn PA Jr, et al: Chemotherapy-radiation therapy versus chemotherapy in limited small cell lung cancer. Proc AACR-ASCO 21:448, 1980
435. Wittes RE: Cis-dichlorodiammine-platinum (II) and VP-16-213: an active induction regimen of small cell carcinoma of the lung. Cancer Treat Rep 63:1593–1597, 1979
436. Israel L, Depierre A, Choffel C et al: Immunochemotherapy in 34 cases of oat cell carcinoma of the lung with 19 complete remissions. Cancer Treat Rep 61:343–347, 1977
437. Seydel HG, Creech RH, Mietiowski W et al: Radiation therpay in small cell lung cancer. Semin Oncol 5:288–298, 1978
438. Choi CH, Carey RW: Small cell anaplastic carcinoma of the lung. Reappraisal of current management. Cancer 37:2651–2657, 1976
439. Salazar OM, Rubin P, Brown JC et al: Predictors of radiation response in lung cancer. A clinico-pathobiologic analysis. Cancer 37:2636–2650, 1976
440. Alexander M, Glatstein EJ, Gordon DS et al: Combined modality treatment for oat cell carcinoma of the lung. A randomized trial. Cancer Treat Rep 61:1–6, 1977
441. Eagan RT, Maurer H, Forcier RJ et al: Combination chemotherapy and radiation therapy in small cell carcinoma of the lung. Cancer 32:371–379, 1973
442. Bitran J, Golomb HM, Desser RK et al: Prolonged survival of patients with extensive oat cell carcinoma treated with radiotherapy and cyclophosphamide (NSC-27271), vincristine (NSC-67574), and methotrexate (NSC-740). Cancer Treat Rep 60:221–223, 1976
443. Cox JD, Byhardt RW, Wilson JF et al: Dose-time relationships and control of small cell carcinoma of the lung. Radiology 128:205–207, 1978
444. Cox JD, Byhardt R, Komaki R et al: Interaction of thoracic irradiation and chemotherapy on local control and survival in

small cell carcinoma of the lung. Cancer Treat Rep 63:1251–1255, 1979
445. Abeloff MD, Ettinger DS, Baylin SB et al: Management of small cell carcinoma of the lung. Therapy, staging and biochemical markers. Cancer 38:1394–1401, 1976
446. Osieka R, Schmidt CG, Makoski HB et al: The combined modality approach in the treatment of inoperable small-cell anaplastic carcinoma of the lung. Z Krebsforsch 89:9–18, 1977
447. Burdon JGW, Henderson MM, Moan WJ et al: Combined chemotherapy and radiotherapy for the treatment of small cell carcinoma of the lung. Med J Aust 1:353–355, 1978
448. Burdon JGW, Sinclair RA, Henderson MM: Small cell carcinoma of the lung. Chest 76:302–304, 1979
449. Gilby ED, Bondy RK, Morgan RL et al: Combination chemotherapy for small cell carcinoma of the lung. Cancer 39:1959–1966, 1977
450. Stevens E, Einhorn L, Rohn R: Treatment of limited small cell lung cancer. Proc AACR-ASCO 20:435, 1979
451. Hansen HH, Dombernowsky P, Hansen HS et al: Chemotherapy versus chemotherapy plus radiotherapy in regional small cell carcinoma of the lung. A randomized trial. Proc AACR-ASCO 20:277, 1979
452. Straus MJ: Cytokinetic chemotherapy design for the treatment of advanced lung cancer. Cancer Treat Rep 63: 767–773, 1979
453. Trowbridge RC, Kennedy BJ, Vosika GJ: CCNU-adriamycin therapy in bronchogenic carcinoma. Cancer 41:1704–1709, 1978
454. Hansen HH, Dombernowsky P, Hansen M et al: Chemotherapy of advanced small cell anaplastic carcinoma: Superiority of a four-drug combination to a three-drug combination. Ann Intern Med 89:177–181, 1978
455. Saiontz HI, Dalton RJ, Eagan RT: Cyclophosphamide, adriamcin, and DTIC polychemotherapy in advanced small cell lung cancer. Cancer Treat Rep 61:481–483, 1977
456. Einhorn LH, Fee WH, Farber MO et al: Improved chemotherapy for small cell undifferentiated lung cancer. JAMA 235:1225–1229, 1976
457. Alberto PL: Remission rates, survival, and prognostic factors in combination chemotherapy for bronchogenic carcinoma. Cancer Chemother Rep 4(2):199–206, 1973
457a. Williams C, Alexander M, Glatstein EJ et al: The role of radiation therapy in combination with chemotherapy in extensive oat cell cancer of the lung. A randomized study. Cancer Treat Rep 61:142–143, 1977
458. Sarna GP, Lowitz BB, Haskell CM: Chemo-immunotherapy for unresectable bronchogenic carcinoma. Cancer Treat Rep 62:681–687, 1978
459. Catane R, Lichter A, Lee YJ et al: Cell lung cancer: analysis of treatment factors contributing to prolonged survival cancer. (in press)
460. Natale R, Hilaris B, Wittes R: Prolonged remission of small cell lung carcinoma with intensive chemotherapy induction and high dose radiation therapy without maintenance. Proc AACR ASCO 21:;452, 1980
461. Newman SJ, Hansen HH: Frequency, diagnosis and treatment of brain metastases in 247 consecutive patients with bronchogenic carcinoma. Cancer 33:492–496, 1974
461a. Hansen HH: Should initial treatment of small cell carcinoma include systemic chemotherapy and brain irradiation? Cancer Chemother Rep 4(2):239–241, 1973
462. Hirsch FR, Hansen HH, Paulson OB et al: Development of brain metastases in small cell anaplastic carcinoma of the lung. In Kay J, Whitehouse J (eds): CNS complications of Malignant Disease, p 175–184. London, MacMillan Press, 1979
463. Cox JD, Petrovich Z, Paig C et al: Prophylactic crainial irradiation in patients with inoperable carcinoma of the lung. Cancer 42:1135–1140, 1978
464. Van Hazel G, Scott M: The effects of CNS metastases on survival of patients with small cell lung cancer. Proc AACR-ASCO 21:446, 1980
465. Posner JB: Management of central nervous system metastases. Semin Oncol 4:81–91, 1977
466. Brereton HD, O'Donnell JF, Kent CH et al: Spinal meningeal in small-cell carcinoma of the lung. Ann Intern Med 88:517–519, 1978
467. Greco FA, Fer MF: Oat-cell carcinoma of the lung with carcinomatous meningitis. N Engl J Med 298:1146, 1978
468. Fox RM: Spinal cord metastasis after combination chemotherapy and prophylactic whole-brain irradiation in small cell carcinoma of the lung. Lancet 2:136, 1977
469. Levenson RM, Ihde DC, Matthews MJ et al: Small Cell carcinoma arising in extrapulmonary sites: response to chemotherapy. Proc AACR-ASCO 2:143, 1980
470. Fer MR, Oldham RK, Richardson RL et al: Extrapulmonary small cell carcinoma. Proc AACR-ASCO 21:475, 1980
471. Von Hoff DD, Tayard MV, Basa P et al: Risk factors for doxorubicin induces congestive heart failure. Ann Intern Med 91:710 –717, 1979
472. Glode LM, Hartmann D, Robinson WA: The acute and cumulative marrow toxicity of chemotherapy in small cell carcinoma of the lung with and without bone marrow support. Proc AACR-ASCO 21:448, 1980
473. Costman HD, Matthay RA, Putman CE: Cytotoxic drug-induced lung disease. Am J Med 62:608–615, 1977
474. Brandman J, Ruckdeschel JC, O'Donnell M et al: Unexpected pulmonary complications of intensive therapy for small cell cancer of the lung. Proc AACR-ASCO 21:459, 1980
475. Phillips TL, Fu KK: Quantification of combined radiation therapy chemotherapy effects on critical normal tissues. Cancer 37: 1186–1200, 1976
476. Phillips TL, Fu KK: Acute and late effects of multimodal therapy on normal tissues. Cancer 40:489–494, 1977
477. Moore TN, Livingston R, Heilbrun L et al: An acceptable rate of complications in combined doxorubicin-irradiation for small cell carcinoma of the lung: A Southwest Oncology Group Study. Int J Radiat Oncol Biol Phys 4:675–680, 1978
478. Chabora BM, Hopfan S, Wittes R: Esophageal complications in the treatment of oat cell carcinoma with combined irradiation and chemotherapy. Radiology 123:185–187, 1977
479. Einhorn L, Krause M, Hornback N et al: Enhanced pulmonary toxicity with bleomycin and radiotherapy in oat cell lung cancer. Cancer 37:2414–2416, 1976
480. Abrams RA, Lichter A, Johnston-Early A et al: Enhanced suppression of peripheral blood CFU, white blood cell and platelet counts by regional radiotherapy in adult patients with nonhematologic malignancy. Proc AACR-ASCO 20:114, 1979
481. Bradley EC, Schechter GP, Matthews MJ et al: Erythroleukemia, pancytopenia, and peripheral blood anenploidy as complications of therapy in long term survivors of small cell carcinoma of the lung. Cancer (in press)
482. Matthews MJ, Rozencweig M, Staquet MJ et al: Long-term survivors with small cell carcinoma of the lung. Eur J Cancer 16:527–531, 1980
483. Hansen M, Hansen HH, Dombernowsky PL: Long-term survival in small cell carcinoma of the lung. JAMA 244:247–250, 1980
484. Minna J, Lichter A, Brereton H et al: Small cell lung cancer: Long-term, potentially cured survivors in National Cancer Institute Trials. Clin Res 28:419A, 1980
485. Holmes EC: Immunology and lung cancer. Ann Thorac Surg 21:250–258, 1976, and Chest 71:643–644, 1977
486. Price Evans DA: Immunology of bronchial carcinoma. Thorax 31:493–506, 1976
487. Krant MJ, Manskopf G, Brandrup CS et al: Immunologic alterations in bronchogenic cancer. Cancer 21:623–631, 1968
488. Wanebo HJ, Rao B, Mizaqawa N et al: Immune reactivity in primary carcinoma of the lung and its relation to prognosis. J Thorac Cardiovasc Surg 72:340–350, 1976
489. Brugarolas AN, Takita H: Immunologic status in lung cancer. Chest 64:427–430, 1973
490. Han T, Takita H: Immunologic impairment in bronchogenic carcinoma: A study of lymphocyte response to phytohemagglutinin. Cancer 30:616–620, 1972
491. Goldsmith HS, Levin AG, Southam CM: A study of cellular responses in cancer patients by qualitative and quantitative rebuck tests. Surg Forum 16:102–04, 1965

492. Lee AK, Rowley M, Mackay IR: Antibody capacity in human cancer. Br J Cancer 4:454–463, 1970
493. Wagner V, Janku O, Wagnerova M et al: The production of complete and incomplete antibodies in patients with neoplastic disease. Neoplasma 19:75–87, 1972
494. Giuliano AE, Rangel D, Golub SH et al: Serum-mediated immunosuppression in lung cancer. Cancer 43:917–924, 1979
495. Mikulski SM, McGuire WP, Louis AC et al: Immunotherapy of lung cancer. I. Review of clinical trials in non-small cell histologic types. Cancer Treat Rev 6:177–190, 1979
496. McKneally MF, Maver CM, Kausel HW: Regional immunotherapy of lung cancer using postoperative intrapleural BCG. Prog Cancer Res Ther 6:161–171, 1978, and McKneally M, Maver C, Bennett J et al: Evaluation of regional bacillus-Calmette Guerin (BCG) in lung cancer. In Terry WD, Windhorst D (eds): Immunotherapy of Cancer: Present Status of Trials in Man. New York, Raven Press, 1980
497. Wright PW, Hill LD, Perterson AV et al: Preliminary results of combined surgery and adjuvant bacillus Calmette-Guerin plus levamisole treatment of resectable lung cancer. Cancer Treat Rep 62:1671–1675, 1978, and Wright PW, Hill LD, Perterson AV et al: Adjuvant immunotherapy in with intrapleural BCG and levamisole in patients with resected, non-small cell lung cancer. In Terry WD, Windhorst D (eds): Immunotherapy of Cancer; Present Status of Trials in Man. New York, Raven Press, 1980
498. Ruckdeschel JC, Codish SD, Stranahan A et al: Postoperative empyema improves survival in lung cancer. Documentation and analysis of a natural experiment. N Engl J Med 287:1013–1017, 1972
499. Mikulski SM, McGuire WP, Louie AC et al: Immunotherapy of lung cancer. II Review of clinical trials in small cell carcinoma. Cancer Treat Rev 6:125–130, 1979
500. Terry WD, Windhorst D: Immunotherapy of Cancer: Present Status of Trials in Man. Second International Conference. New York, Raven Press, 1980
501. Holmes EC (for The National Lung Cancer Study Group): Surgical Adjuvant studies in resectable non-oat cell lung cancer. In Terry WD, Windhorst D (eds): Immunotherapy of Cancer: Present Status of Trials in Man. New York, Raven Press, 1980
502. Iles PB, Shore DF, Langman MJ et al: Second interim report on the intrapleural BCG study in the treatment of operable lung cancer. Rec Res Cancer Res 68:292–296, 1978, and Lowe J, Iles PB, Shore DR et al: Intrapleural BCG in operable lung Cancer. In Terry WD, Windhorst D (eds): Immunotherapy of Cancer: Present Status of Trials in Man. New York, Raven Press, 1980
503. Miller AB, Taylor HE, Baker MA et al: Oral administration of BCG as an adjuvant to surgical treatment of carcinoma of the bronchus. Can Med Assoc J 121:45–54, 1979
504. Edwards FR, Whitwell F: Use of BCG as an immunostimulant in the surgical treatment of carcinoma of lung: a five-year follow-up report. Thorax 33:250–252, 1978
505. Herberman RB, Weese JL, Oldham RK et al: Prospect for immunotherapy of lung cancer with specific immunoadjuvants. Prog Cancer Res Ther 11:521–529, 1979 and Perlin E, Weese JL, Heim W et al: Immunotherapy of lung cancer. In Terry WD, Windhorst D (eds): Prolonged disease free interval with systemic BCG immunotherapy in resectable carcinoma of the Lung. New York, Raven Press, 1980
506. Pouillart P, Palangie T, Huguenin P et al: Adjuvant nonintrapleural BCG. Prog Cancer Res Ther 11:477–481, 1979
507. Roscoe P, Pearce S, Ludgate S et al: A controlled trial of BCG immunotherapy in bronchogenic carcinoma treated by surgical resection. Cancer Immunol Immunother 3:115–118, 1977
508. Miyazawa N, Suemasu K, Ogata T et al: BCG immunotherapy as an adjuvant to surgery in lung cancer: A randomized prospective clinical trial. Jpn J Clin Oncol 9:19–26, 1979
509. Yamamura Y, Sakatani M, Ogura T et al: Adjuvant immunotherapy of lung cancer with BCG cell wall skeleton (BCG-CWS). Cancer 43:1314–1319, 1979.
510. Yasumoto K, Manabe H, Yanagawa E et al: Nonspecific adjuvant immunotherapy of lung cancer with cell wall skeleton of Mycobacterium bovis Bacillus Calmette-Guerin. Cancer Res 39:3262–3267, 1979
511. Matthay RA, Mahler DA, Mitchell MS et al: Intratumoral BCG immunotherapy prior to surgery for lung cancer. In Terry WD, Windhorst D (eds): Immunotherapy of Cancer: Present Status of Trials in Man. Hew York, Raven Press, 1980
512. Holmes EC, Ramming KP: Immunotherapy of lung cancer using levamisole and intralesional BCG. Prog Cancer Res Ther 11:483–488, 1979
513. Amery WK: Final results of multicenter placebo-controlled levamisole study of resectable lung cancer. Cancer Treat Rep 62:1677–1683, 1978, and Amery WK: Randomized levanisole study in resectable lung cancer: 4 year results. In Terry WD, Windhorst D (eds): Immunotherapy of Cancer: Present Status of Trials in Man. New York, Raven Press, 1980
514. Anthony M: Presentation at II International Conference on Immunotherapy of Cancer. In Terry WD, Windhorst D (eds): Immunotherapy of Cancer: Present Status of Trials in Man. New York, Raven Press, 1980
515. Wright PW, Hill LD, Peterson AV et al: Levamisole results in immunosuppression and lacks anti-tumor activity when combined with intrapleural BCG in patients with resected non-small cell lung cancer. Proc AACR-ASCO 21:452, 1980
516. The Ludwig Lung Cancer Study Group: Adjuvant immunotherapy in operable lung cancer. In Terry WD, Windhorst D (eds): Immunotherapy of Cancer: Present Status of Trials in Man. New York, Raven Press, 1980
517. Fox RM, Woods RL, Tattersall MH et al: A randomized study of adjuvant immunotherapy with levamisole and parvum in operable non-small cell lung cancer. Abstracts of a symposium on progress and perspectives in lung cancer, p 37. Brussels, European Organization for Research on Treatment of Cancer, 1979
518. Takita H, Takada M, Minowada J et al: Adjuvant immunotherapy of Stage III lung carcinoma. In Terry WD, Windhorst D (eds): Immunotherapy of Cancer: Present Status of Trials in Man. New York, Raven Press, 1980
519. Stewart THM, Hollinshead AC, Harris JE et al: Specific active immunochemotherapy in lung cancer: A survival study. Rec Res Cancer Res 68:278–285, 1979, and Stewart THM, Hollinshead AC, Harris JE et al: Specific active immunochemotherapy of Stage I lung cancer patients. In Terry WD, Windhorst D (eds): Immunotherapy of Cancer: Present Status of Trials in Man. Second International Conference. New York, Raven Press, 1980
520. Takita H, Hollinshead AC, Edgerton F et al: Adjuvant Active immunotherapy of squamous cell lung carcinoma. In Terry WD, Windhorst D (eds): Immunotherapy of Cancer: Present Status of Trials in Man. Second International Conference. New York, Raven Press (in press)
521. Kerman R, Stefani S: Radio and immunotherapy of lung cancer: a preliminary report. In Crispen RG (ed): Neoplasm Immunity: Solid Tumor Therapy, pp 29–35. Proceedings of Chicago Symposium, 1977
522. Pines A: A 5-year controlled study of BCG and radiotherapy for inoperable lung cancer. Lancet 1:380–381, 1976
523. Warren S, Crispen R, Nika B: BCG adjuvant immunotherapy of stage II, III and IV bronchogenic carcinoma. In Crispen RG (ed): Neoplasm Immunity: Solid Tumor Therapy, pp 49–53. Proceedings of Chicago Symposium, 1977
524. Robinson E, Bartal A, Cohen Y et al: Treatment of lung cancer by radiotherapy, chemotherapy, and methanol extraction residue of BCG (MER). Clinical and immunological studies. Cancer 40:1052–1059, 1977
525. Bjornsson S, Takita H, Kuberka N et al: Combination chemotherapy plus Methanol extracted residue of bacillus Camette-Guerin or Corynebacterium parvum in stage II lung cancer. Cancer Treat Rep 62:505–510, 1978
526. Sarna GP, Lowitz BB, Haskell C et al: Chemo-immunotherapy for unresectable bronchogenic carcinoma. Cancer Treat Rep 62:681–687, 1978

527. Issell BF, Valdivieso M, Hersh EM et al: Combination chemoimmunotherapy for extensive non-oat cell lung cancer. Cancer Treat Rep 62:1059–1063, 1978
528. Dimitrov NV, Conroy J, Suhrland LG et al: Combination therapy with Corynebaterium parvum and doxorubicin hydrocloride in patients with lung cancer. Proc Cancer Res Ther 6:181–189, 1978
529. Chahinian AP, Mandel EM, Jaffrey IS et al: Chemotherapy with or without immunotherapy in bronchogenic carcinoma. Proc AACR-ASCO 18:333, 1977
530. Richards F, II, Muss H, White D et al: Combination chemotherapy ± methanol-extracted residue of Bacillus Calmette-Guerin in advanced non-small cell lung cancer. Proc ASCR-ASCO 21:454, 1980
531. Livingston RB, Heilbrun LH, Thigpen T et al: Adriamycin and chlorambucil versus adriamycin and thiabendazole in the treatment of extensive, non-small cell carcinoma of the lung: a southwest oncology group pilot study. Cancer Treat Rep 62:1215–1217, 1978
532. Paschal B, Richards F II, Muss HB et al: Immunotherapy of small cell carcinoma of the Lung: a randomized study. Proc AACR-ASCO 21:461, 1980
533. Aisner J, Esterhay RJ Jr, Wiernik PH: Chemotherapy vs. chemoimmunotherapy for small cell carcinoma of the lung. Proc AACR-ASCO: 18:310, 1977
534. McCracken JD, White JE, Samson MK et al: Adverse effect of BCG immunotherapy combined with chemotherapy/radiotherapy in metastatic small cell carcinoma of the lung. Proc ASCR-ASCO 21:446, 1980
535. Cohen MH, Chretien PB, Ihde DC et al: Thymosin fraction V and intensive combination chemotherapy. Prolonging the survival of patients with small cell lung cancer. JAMA 241:1813–1815, 1979, and Cohen MH, Chretien PB, Early AJ et al: Thymosin fraction V prolongs survival of intensively treated small cell lung cancer patients. In Terry W, Windhorst D (eds): Immunotherapy of Cancer: Present Status of Trials in Man. Second International Conference. Raven Press, New York, 1980

CHAPTER 15

Jerry C. Rosenberg

Neoplasms of the Mediastinum

Mediastinal masses are asymptomatic in at least half the patients who are discovered to have them. The range is from 28% to 65% depending upon the patient population studied.[1] Under these circumstances, the mass is usually detected when a chest roentgenogram is obtained for a reason unrelated to the mediastinal tumor. One can expect asymptomatic patients to harbor a benign lesion since 90% of benign lesions occur in asymptomatic patients (Fig. 15-1).[2,3] Symptoms occur in 28% to 41% of patients with malignant lesions. The most common symptoms produced by mediastinal masses are listed in Table 15-1.

Some patients with benign tumors of the mediastinum are at risk of disability or death if the lesion's size or position interferes with cardiopulmonary function. Because of the high incidence of malignant tumors, and the potential hazards of harboring a benign tumor in the mediastinum, a mass lesion in this location cannot be "passively observed or treated by radiation without benefit of a specific diagnosis," as was occasionally the practice.[4] The lesion must be diagnosed with precision and treated appropriately.

ANATOMICAL CONSIDERATIONS

The boundaries of the mediastinum are the diaphragm inferiorly, the parietal pleura laterally, the sternum anteriorly, the vertebral column and adjacent ribs posteriorly, and the thoracic outlet superiorly. The thoracic outlet is the area encompassed by the superior extent of the thoracic cage, i.e., at the level of the first thoracic vertebra and the first ribs. Because of the constancy with which structures are located within specific areas of the mediastinum and the predilection of different lesions to occur within these mediastinal areas, it is practical to divide the mediastinum into compartments (Fig. 15-2).

The superior mediastinum is that area between the thoracic outlet, as defined above, and a line drawn from the sternal angle of Louis (the junction of the manubrium and body of the sternum) to the fourth intervertebral disc. Since the mediastinum is pyramidal in shape, with the top chopped off,

FIG. 15-1. Symptomatic mediastinal masses are often malignant neoplasms. Half of all new growths of the mediastinum are malignant.

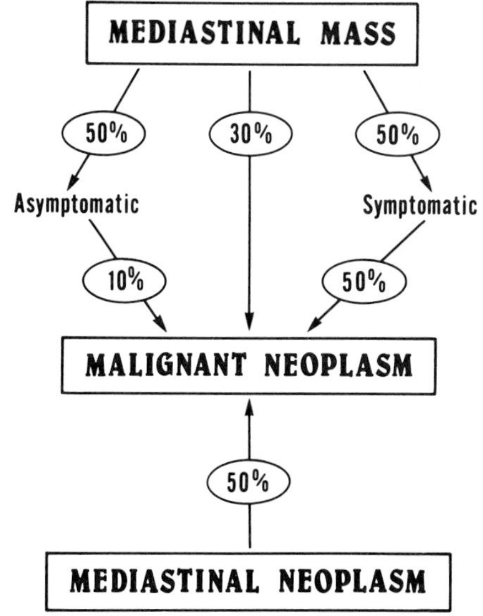

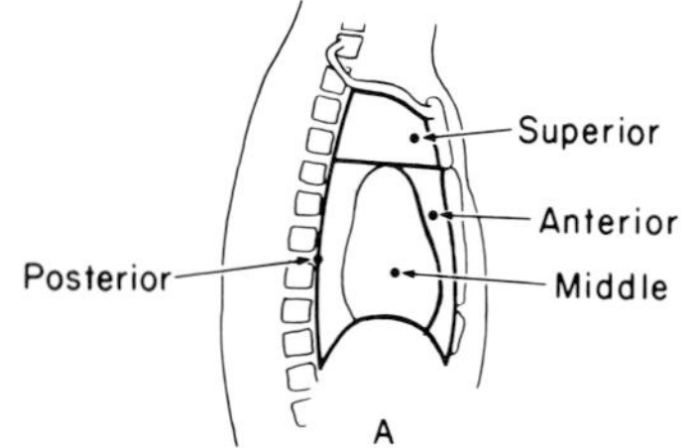

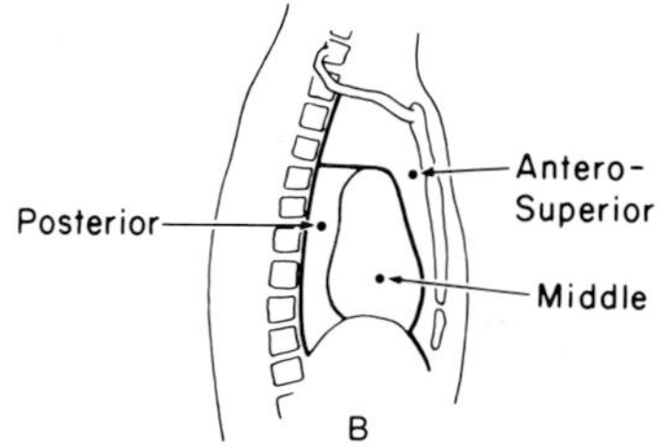

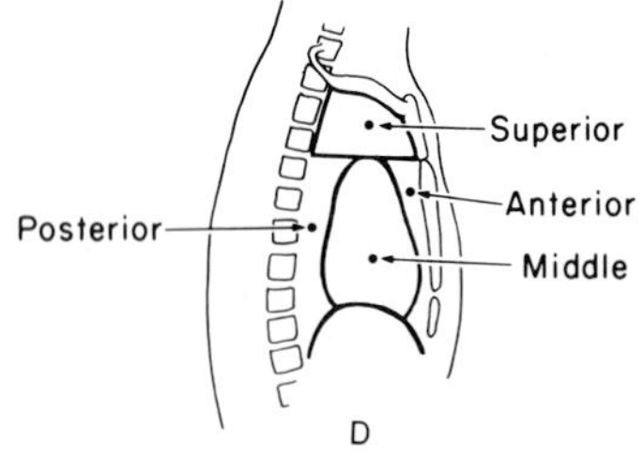

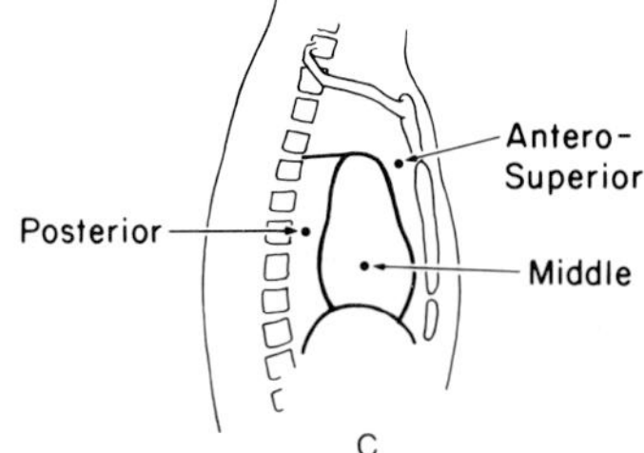

FIG. 15-2. The limits of the mediastinal compartments vary from author to author. The most commonly suggested borders for the divisions are illustrated in this figure. (See the text for details.) (*A*) Division of the mediastinum into four compartments. (*B*) The anterior and superior compartments are combined so that only three divisions of the mediastinum are recognized. (*C, D*) Correspond to *A* and *B*, respectively, with the difference being the posterior extent of the posterior mediastinum.

TABLE 15-1. Mediastinal Masses: Signs and Symptoms

NONSPECIFIC
- Chest discomfort—fullness, tightness, pain
- Anorexia
- Weight loss
- Malaise

SECONDARY TO COMPRESSION OR DISPLACEMENT OF ADJACENT MEDIASTINAL STRUCTURES
- Tracheo-bronchial compression—
  - cough, wheezing, stridor, dyspnea, recurrent respiratory infections
- Esophageal compression—dysphagia
- Superior vena cava syndrome
- Horner's syndrome
- Vocal cord paralysis—dysphonia
- Pulmonic stenosis—murmers
- Cardiac tamponade or arrhythmias

SECONDARY TO ENDOCRINE FUNCTION
- Cushing's disease
- Gynecomastia
- Hypertension
- Hypoglycemia

SYSTEMIC SYNDROMES
- Thymoma*
  - Myasthenia gravis
  - Red cell aplasia
  - Hypogammaglobulinemia
  - Autoimmune diseases
- Carcinoid of thymus
  - Multiple endocrine abnormalities (Type I)
  - Cushing's syndrome
- Neurofibroma
  - Osteoarthritis
- Lymphoma
  - Alcohol-induced pain
  - Fever
- Teratoma
  - Hypoglycemia—insulin producing tumor

* See Table 15-7 for a complete list of systemic syndromes associated with thymomas.

the superior mediastinum is narrowed by the approximation of its lateral boundaries and cannot easily be subdivided further. However, the remainder of the mediastinum can be readily subdivided into anterior, middle, and posterior divisions.

The anterior mediastinum extends from the sternum to the pericardium and great vessels. The posterior mediastinum is bounded by the posterior rib cage and extends anteriorly for a variable distance. Some authors define the posterior mediastinum as extending up to the pericardium (Fig. 15-2C

FIG. 15-3. A cross-section of the thorax demonstrating the limits of the anterior, middle, and posterior compartments of the mediastinum. The posterior mediastinum may be considered to encompass the entire area posterior to the pericardium (see Figs. 15-2*C* and *D*) or only that area posterior to a line drawn anterior to the vertebral body as in Figs. 15-2*A* and *B*).

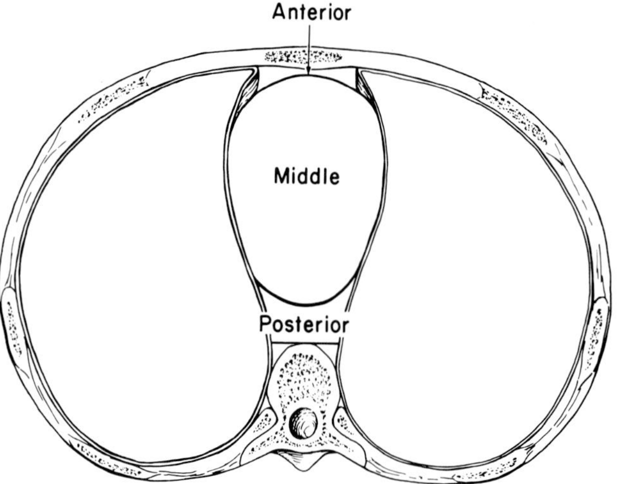

and *D*). Others set it at a line drawn along the anterior borders of the bodies of the vertebrae (Fig. 15-2*A* and *B* and Fig. 15-3). In the latter case the posterior mediastinum would consist of the costovertebral (or paravertebral) areas.

The middle mediastinum includes the section between the anterior and posterior compartments. It is also referred to as the hilar or visceral area since it contains the heart and great vessels.

Burkell and colleagues have suggested a different map of the mediastinum.[5] They speak of only three areas, the anterosuperior, posterior, and middle mediastinal divisions (Fig. 15-2*B*). They consider it impractical to designate the superior mediastinum as a distinct division of the mediastinum since many lesions which are found in the superior mediastinum are also found in the anterior mediastinum, and superior mediastinal masses tend to extend down into the chest and also occupy the anterior mediastinum. Many posterior mediastinal lesions extend upwards, also occupying the superior mediastinum. Thus there is merit to combining the anterior and superior mediastinal compartments into one division as they suggest.

The anatomic structures normally found in the different medisastinal compartments are listed in Table 15-2. Many of the lesions outlined in Table 15-3 can be derived from the list in Table 15-2. In addition to tumors arising from structures normally found in the mediastinum, abnormalities found in the mediastinum may also arise from adjacent anatomical areas such as the abdomen, neck, lungs (e.g., Fig. 15-4), chest wall (Fig. 15-5) and also from tissues not normally located within the mediastinum.

As Table 15-3 indicates, there is an overlap in the distribution of lesions within the mediastinal divisions. Lesions occur predominantly in one or another of the anatomic divisions of the mediastinum, not exclusively in the area under which they are listed. The closest exception to this statement is the very high frequency of teratomas in the anterior mediastinum. Approximately 90% of thyroid masses and thymomas are located anteriorly and superiorly, 80% of neurogenic tumors are located in the posterior mediastinum, and 50% of mediastinal lymphomas occur in the middle mediastinum.[6]

Mediastinal tumors and cysts in the adult are fairly equally distributed throughout the mediastinal compartments. Twenty percent are in the anterior compartment, 20% in the superior division, 20% in the middle mediastinum, and 30% posteriorly. The remaining 10% cannot be localized because

TABLE 15-2. Location of Anatomic Structures within the Mediastinal Compartments

SUPERIOR MEDIASTINUM
- Transverse aorta and great vessels
- Thymus gland

ANTERIOR MEDIASTINUM
- Ascending aorta
- Vena cava and azygos vein
- Thymus gland
- Lymph nodes
- Fat and connective tissue

POSTERIOR MEDIASTINUM
- Sympathetic chain
- Vagus
- Esophagus
- Thoracic duct
- Lymph nodes
- Descending aorta

MIDDLE MEDIASTINUM
- Heart and pericardium
- Trachea and major bronchi
- Pulmonary vessels
- Lymph nodes
- Fat and connective tissue

TABLE 15-3. Mediastinal Masses and their Distribution

SUPERIOR	ANTERIOR	MIDDLE	POSTERIOR
Lymphomas	Lymphomas	Lymphomas	Neurogenic tumors
Thyroid masses	Teratomas	Bronchogenic cysts	Lymphomas
Thymic tumors or cysts	Thymic tumors or cysts	Pericardial cysts	Bronchogenic cysts
Thymoma	Thyroid masses	Sarcoidosis	Enteric cysts
Thymolipoma	Parathyroid tumors	Lipomas	Xanthogranulomas
Carcinoid	Germinal cell neoplasms	Lung cancers	Esophageal masses and diverticula
Lung cancers	Lung tumors	Plasma cell myeloma	Lung cancers
Parathyroid tumors	Lipomas	Vascular tumors	Thyroid masses
Aneurysm or ectasia of innominate or subclavian arteries	Lymphangiomas	Epicardial fat pads	Hiatal hernias
Myxomas	Fibromas	Hiatal hernias	Paravertebral abscesses
Cylindromas of trachea	Hemangiomas		Fibrosarcomas
Bronchogenic cysts	Chondromas		Meningoceles
Tumors arising in posterior mediastinum	Rhabdomyosarcomas		Myxomas
	Morgagni hernias		Chondromas
	Paragangliomas from carotid body		Pheochromocytomas
	Pericardial cysts		Aneurysms of descending aorta
			Enlargement of azygous and hemiazygous veins
			Thoracic duct cysts
			Tumors of spinal column

of their large size or indistinct margins.[6] In children, the posterior mediastinum will contain 63% of the lesions; 26% in the anterior mediastinum, and 11% in the middle compartment.[7]

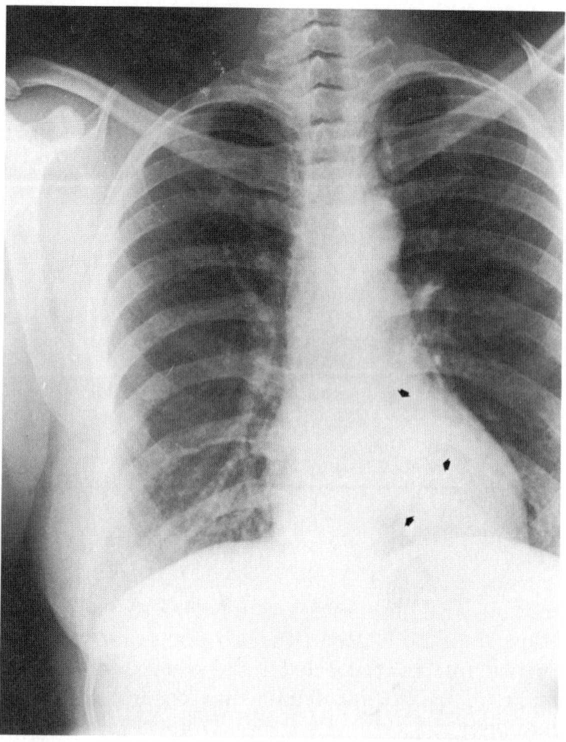

FIG. 15-4. The *arrows* delineate a posterior mediastinal mass which was proven at thoracotomy to be a "benign" metastasizing leiomyoma of the lung which protruded from the surface of the left lower lobe into the posterior mediastinum.

INCIDENCE OF PRIMARY MEDIASTINAL TUMORS

Tables 15-3 and 15-4 are fairly comprehensive lists of the lesions one might encounter in the mediastinum. All of the possibilities are not included in these lists. The odd lesions will inevitably occur when they are least expected (Figs. 15-4 and 15-5).

Since primary tumors of the mediastinum are infrequent and not readily classified in a tabulation of malignancies, the best approximation of their general incidence is to determine how often a major referral center with an interest in mediastinal masses encounters these lesions. Approximately one in every 3400 admissions to Duke University Medical Center was found to have a primary mediastinal tumor or cyst.[1] At the University of Wisconsin, seven to ten patients with all kinds of mediastinal lesions were seen yearly.[5]

Sabiston and his colleagues find that in the adult population, less than one-fourth of mediastinal masses are malignant.[1,3] However, in children they found an incidence of 50%. Overall, the incidence is estimated at 30%.[3] Among mediastinal neoplasms, about half are malignant (Fig. 15-1). The relative incidence of tumors and cysts in a large combined group of 1881 patients is shown in Table 15-5. In a series of 354 children, Hammon and Sabiston found the relative frequency to be somewhat different. No thymomas were encountered, an indication of the rarity of this tumor in patients under the age of 20 years. On the other hand, Hasse, in a collected series of 1189 mediastinal tumors and cysts in children, found that 29% were neurogenic in origin and 12% were thymic.[8]

The Mayo Clinic series (1064 patients from 1929 to 1968) noted that the incidence of malignant tumors in children was approximately the same as that encountered in adults (25%).[9] Most of the cancers in children were of neurogenic, teratomatous or vascular origin. The types of benign lesions found

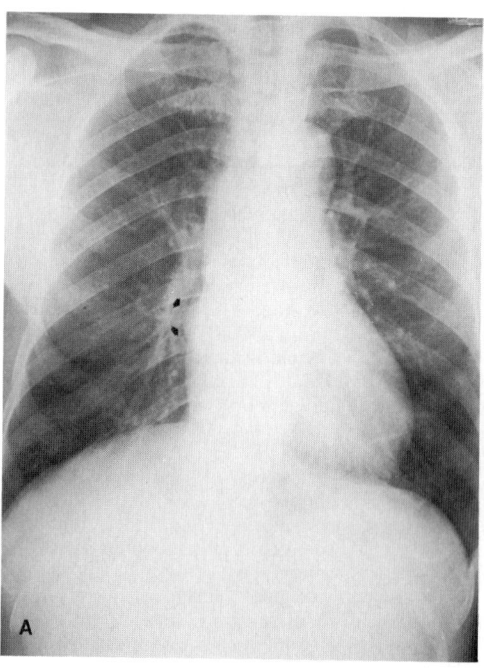

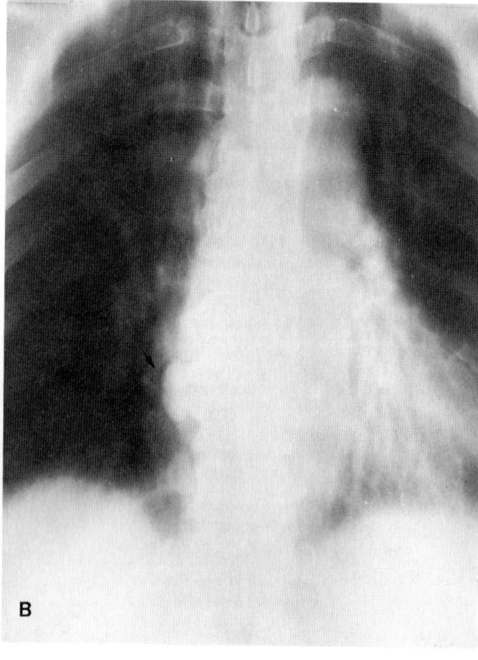

FIG. 15-5. A posterior mediastinal mass seen on a posteroanterior chest roentgenogram (*A*) was found to be an osteophyte when tomograms were obtained (*B*).

TABLE 15-4. Classification of Mediastinal Tumors

NEUROGENIC	MESENCHYMAL TUMORS
Arising from peripheral nerves	Fibroma and fibrosarcoma
Neurofibroma	Lipoma and liposarcoma
Neurilemnoma (Schwannoma)	Mysoma
Neurosarcoma	Mesothelioma
Arising from sympathetic ganglia	Leiomyoma and leiomyosarcoma
Ganglioneuroma	Rhabdomyosarcoma
Ganglioneuroblastoma	Xanthogranuloma
Neuroblastoma	Mesenchymoma
Arising from paraganglionic tissue	Hemangioma
Pheochromocytoma	Hemangioendothelioma
Chemodectoma (paraganglioma)	Hemangiopericytoma
	Lymphangioma
THYMIC	Lymphangiomyoma
Thymoma	Lymphangiopericytoma
Benign	
Malignant	ENDOCRINE TUMORS
Carcinoid	Thyroid
Thymolipoma	Parathyroid
LYMPHOMA	CYSTS
Hodgkin's disease	Pericardial
Histiocytic lymphoma	Bronchogenic
Undifferentiated	Enteric
	Thymic
GERM CELL TUMORS	Thoracic duct
Seminoma	Meningoceles
Nonseminomatous tumors	
Pure embryonal cell	HERNIAS
Mixed embryonal cell	Hiatal
with seminomatous elements	Morgagni
with trophoblastic elements	ANEURYSMS
with teratoid elements	
with entodermal sinus elements (yolk sac tumors)	LYMPHADENOPATHY
	Inflammatory
Teratoma, benign	Granulomatous
	Sarcoid

in children also differed from those seen in adults. Neurogenic and teratomatous tumors and enterogenous cysts made up approximately 78% of the mediastinal masses seen in the pediatric age group. Vascular tumors and cystic hygromas occurred more frequently in infants and children than in adults. Only one of 206 patients with thymoma in the Mayo Clinic series was younger than 20 years of age.[9] Pericardial cysts and intrathoracic goiters were also rare in children.

It should also be noted that the figures presented in Table 15-5 differ significantly from those presented in earlier publications on this subject. In a series of 2251 mediastinal tumors collected from the literature from 1946 to 1971, neurogenic tumors were most frequently found (38%), followed by thymoma and thymic cysts (13.5%). Currently, the incidences of both are about 20%. This change is thought to be the result of the recent, more assiduous search for thymomas in patients with myasthenia gravis and autoimmune disorders.[1] Another factor which may distort these statistics is the criteria used for including lymphomas in tabulations of mediastinal tumors. Lymphomas presenting as a mediastinal mass should be included but not all lymphomas with mediastinal involvement qualify as primary neoplasms.

In this chapter we will discuss tumors of the thymus gland, including germ cell tumors, in some detail. The special characteristics of neurogenic and mesenchymal tumors as they occur in the mediastinum will also be reviewed briefly. They are treated in greater detail in Chapters 29 and 33. Lymphomas have been covered in Chapter 35. Their treatment will not be repeated here.

DIAGNOSTIC APPROACHES TO THE MEDIASTINAL MASS

ROENTGENOGRAMS AND RELATED IMAGING TECHNICS

Roentgenographic examinations constitute the most important diagnostic studies that can be performed to define the location and extent of a mediastinal mass. Chest roentgeno-

TABLE 15-5. Relative Incidence of Mediastinal Tumors and Cysts

	ALL PATIENTS	CHILDREN
Thymomas	21%	–
Neurogenic tumors	20%	38%
Lymphomas	12%	19%
Germs cell neoplasms	11%	12%
Mesenchymal tumors	7%	10%
Endocrine tumors	6%	–
Primary carcinoma	3%	4%
Cysts	19%	17%

(Hammon JW Jr, Sabiston DC Jr: The mediastinum. In Ellis HE, Goldsmith HS (eds): Thoracic Surgery, Hagerstown, Maryland, Harper and Row, 1979)

grams in posteroanterior, lateral, and oblique projections will identify most lesions and localize the bulk of the mass to one of the mediastinal compartments (Fig. 15-6). The shape, size, and density of the mass as it is seen on the chest roentgenogram do not help differentiate whether it is benign or malignant. Most malignant primary lesions are located in the anterior and superior compartments of the mediastinum. The value of comparing current films with previously obtained chest roentgenograms cannot be overemphasized. Growth rates can be estimated and indistinct lesions more clearly defined.

Small lesions located in front of or behind the heart may be missed on a rountine roentgenographic examination of the chest, especially in those patients with a large amount of fat. Penetrated supine views of the chest can be helpful in defining an indistinct mediastinal mass; especially those that deform the so-called para-lines: the paraspinal, paraesophageal, paraaortic, paracardiac, paravenous, and paratracheal lines.

If the lesion is located in the posterior mediastinum, roentgenograms of the spine in various projections should be obtained, looking for erosion of the vertebral bodies, pedicles, and transverse processes and for erosion of the posterior ribs. Coned views of the spine may be of further help. Bony abnormalities can be found with neurogenic tumors as well as with meningoceles and neurenteric cysts. Bone tumors, metastatic lesions, and the lesions of multiple myeloma may also be detected by these technics (Fig. 15-5).

Tomograms are necessary for further delineation and characterization of mediastinal tumors. Middle mediastinal masses can be differentiated more clearly from normal hilar structures by this technic.Frontal and lateral tomograms should be obtained. These films supplement the information obtained by conventional radiographic technics and often reveal changes which would not otherwise be detected, such as the presence of calcifications, cavitations suggesting necrosis, and additional small satellite lesions.

Barium contrast studies may detect intrinsic lesions of the esophagus which present as a mediastinal mass. Esophagograms may also reveal displacement of the esophagus by an extrinsic lesion. The paraesophageal hiatal hernia which presents as a mass in the lower middle mediastinum is also best defined by a barium contrast study. The sliding hiatal hernia, often located in the posterior mediastinum, is also readily diagnosed by a barium study of the upper gastrointestinal tract.

Fluoroscopy may help determine whether a lesion is attached to the diaphragm or the lung if it is seen to move with respiration. If the mass moves with swallowing, it may be a thyroid lesion attached to the larynx. A pulsating mass would suggest an aneurysm and require angiography for further clarification. However, pulsating masses need not be aneurysms. They may represent richly vascularized tumors or transmitted pulsations. Conversely, absence of pulsations does not exclude an aneurysm. Thrombus along the wall of an aneurysm may dampen pulsations.

Aortograms, pulmonary arteriograms, and venograms all have a place in the evaluation of the mediastinal mass (Fig. 15-7). In addition to delineating aneurysms, aortograms may reveal vascular tumors (Fig. 15-8) or displacement of vessels by tumors or cysts. Angiograms are mandatory for lesions in the region of the great vessels prior to attempting a resection or biopsy. Vena cavograms may reveal obstruction or displacement by a mass. Azygography is occasionally helpful if there is involvement or displacement of the posterior chest wall by a tumor which occludes the azygos vein. Selective thymic venography has been recommended to aide in the diagnosis of thymomas.[10]

Angiocardiography was advocated in the 1960s as a valuable diagnostic procedure for the detection of vascular abnormalities which may present as a mediastinal mass, the so-called "pseudo-tumor."[11] Angiocardiography has been replaced by the more sophisticated technics of selective angiography and computerized tomography. However, computerized subtraction technics may result in a revitalization of this technic.[12] Pneumomediastinograms are now also rarely utilized. This procedure is performed by the retrotracheal insufflation of about 400 ml of oxygen or carbon dioxide.[13,14] Pneumomediastinography had its widest application in children in differentiating an enlarged thymus from a tumor. It can also be used to estimate the size and weight of the thymus.[15]

FIG. 15-6. A posteroanterior (*A*), lateral (*B*), and oblique (*C*) view of an anterior mediastinal mass which was found to be an encapsulated thymoma on exploration of the mediastinum (see Figs. 15-10 and 15-15).

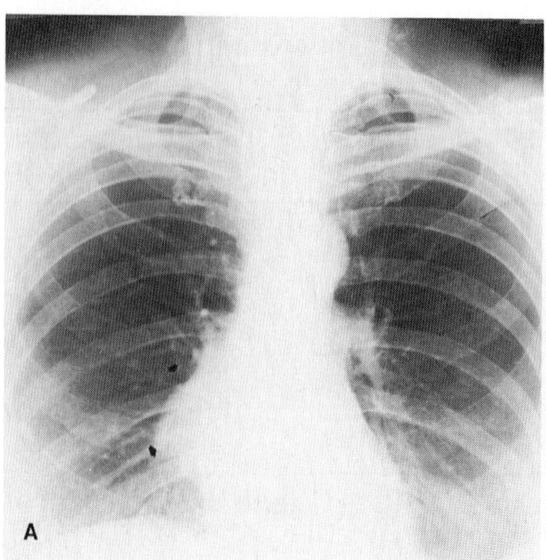

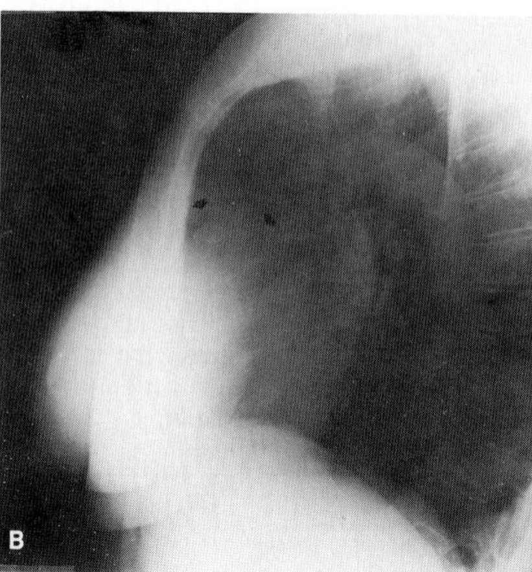

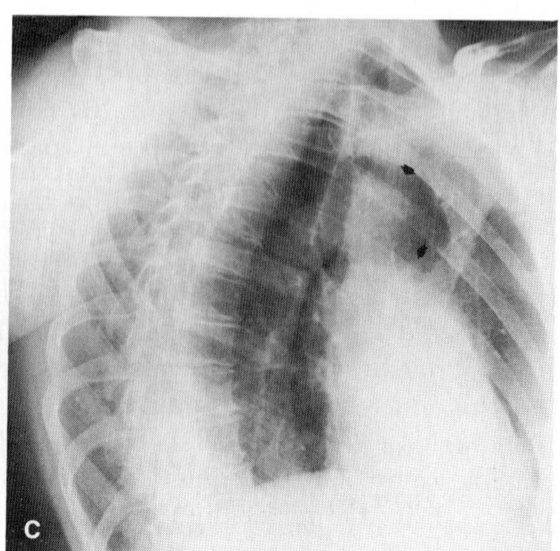

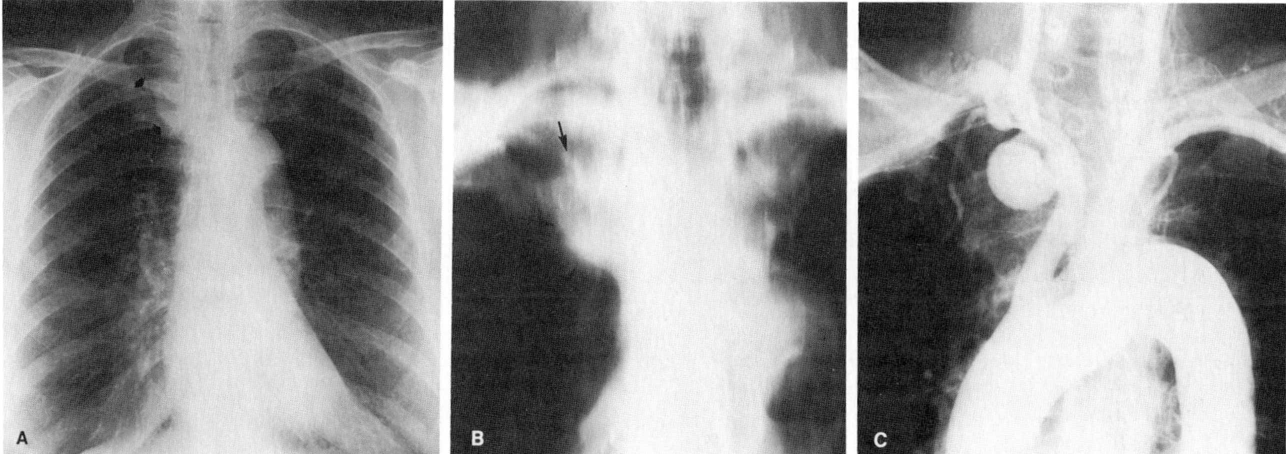

FIG. 15-7. An anterosuperior mediastinal mass seen on a plain film of the chest (*A*) and by tomography (*B*) is revealed to be a saccular aneurysm of the innominate artery when an arteriogram was obtained (*C*).

Myelograms should be performed when a posterior mediastinal mass is accompanied by neurologic abnormalities. Extradural defects or obstruction may be present when a dumbbell-shaped tumor is present, as with a tumor growing into the mediastinum and into the spinal canal. Widening of the intervertebral foramina may be present. These bony abnormalities would require that a myelogram be performed even in the absence of neurologic symptoms.

Nuclide imaging procedures can be helpful. Thyroid scans for superior and anterior masses must be carried out with ^{131}I rather than with technetium pertechnetate.[16] The latter will not identify mediastinal masses because of the high background of this nuclide in the vascular structures of the chest (Fig. 15-9). Iodine ^{131}, on the other hand, will localize in the thyroid in most patients with mediastinal thyroid tissue. Since as many as 10% of mediastinal masses may be goiters, with as many as 25% in the posterior mediastinum, this study should be highly considered in the evaluation of a mediastinal mass. A bone scan may be helpful in determining the nature and extent of posterior mediastinal abnormalities. A gallium scan would be helpful if the lesion is composed of lymphatic tissue, that is, a lymphoma or thymoma. Selenomethionine scans have been recommended for the same purpose.[17]

Ultrasound may occasionally be useful in separating cystic from solid lesions. It should be emphasized that the differentiation of a cystic from a solid mass does not indicate whether it is benign or malignant. Echocardiography may be indicated if the mass is in the vicinity of the heart.

The most recent (1975) innovation in radiographic imaging technics which has been successfully applied to the investigation of mediastinal masses is computerized axial tomography (CT). [18-21] CT of the mediastinum offers two great

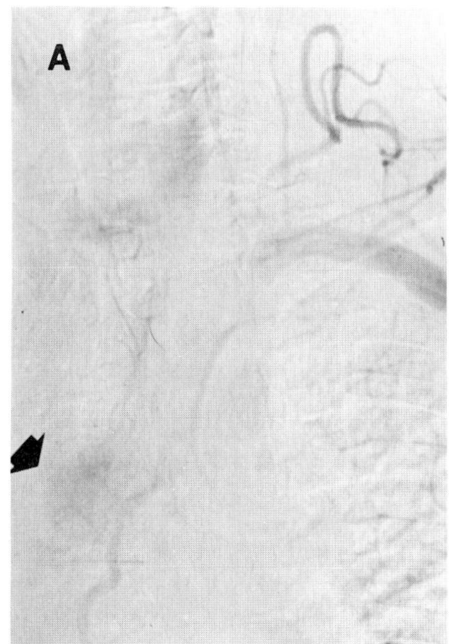

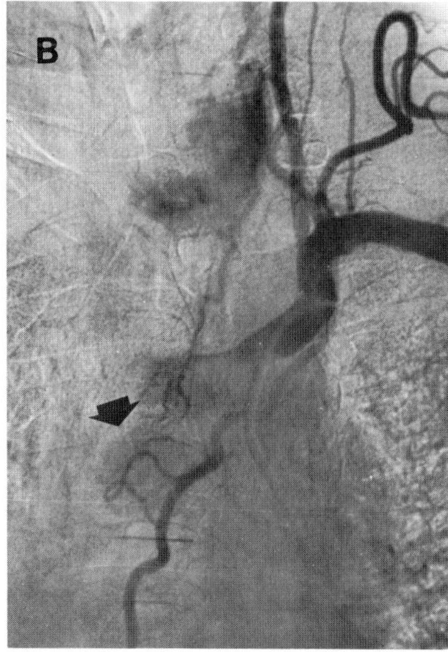

FIG. 15-8. Arteriograms delineate a parathyroid adenoma located within the thymus gland. Using subtraction technics (*A*), the mass seen in *B* can be more easily visualized.

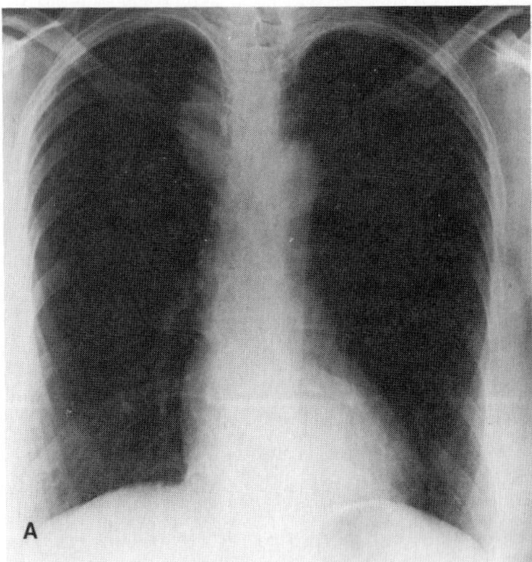

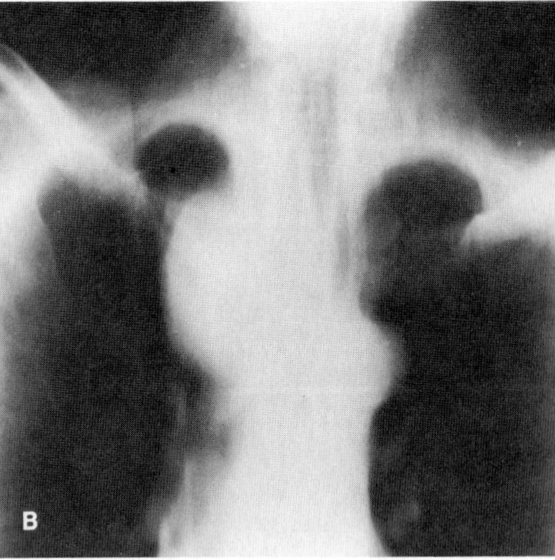

FIG. 15-9. A substernal thyroid goiter presenting as a mediastinal mass in the superior compartment (*A*) with displacement of the trachea on tomography (*B*). The esophagus was also displaced. In this patient, neither the ^{131}I nor the technetium scan identified the lesion as thyroid tissue.

advantages over conventional radiographic procedures. First is the ability to examine the mediastinum's cross sectional anatomy. CT is better than lateral or oblique views to visualize the mediastinum (Fig. 15-10). Some mediastinal tumors may blend in with adjacent mediastinal structures when visualized by chest roentgenograms. CT can more precisely identify the margins between the tumor and adjacent anatomic structures. Based on these features, anatomy heretofore not visible by noninvasive technics can be examined by the clinician.

Widening of the mediastinum because of physiologic fat deposition or by dilation or ectasia of the great vessels can be readily detected by CT. Cystic areas and areas of calcification in the mediastinum can be precisely identified (Fig. 15-11). The extent of involvement by a tumor or structures within the mediastinum can also be assessed by CT.

FIG. 15-10. Computed tomography of patient with the thymoma depicted in Fig. 15-6 (see also Fig. 15-15). The thymoma (*T*) is located immediately anterior to the base of the heart (*H*).

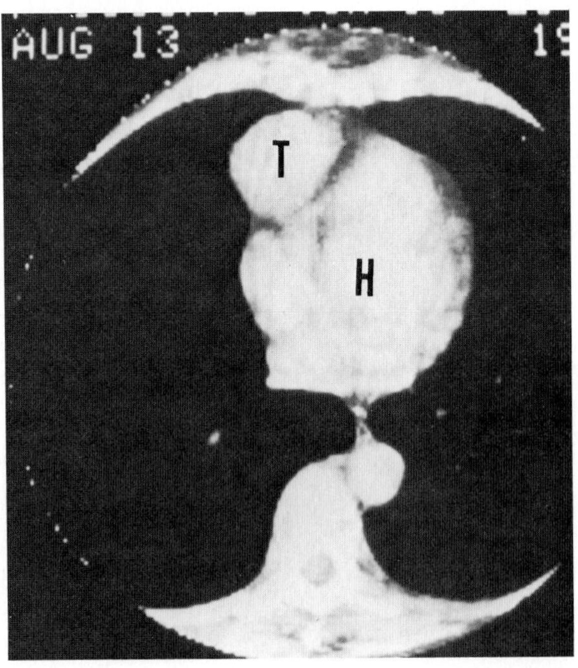

The following indications for obtaining CT of the mediastinum were suggested recently after a study of the efficacy of computed tomography in visualizing anatomic structures in the mediastinum:[18]

1. To evaluate questionable or partially hidden masses within the mediastinum. Conventional radiographic technics will often reveal subtle and ill-defined mediastinal masses. These lesions are seen more clearly by CT.
2. To evaluate tissue density by determining its attenuation coefficient (a measure of the capacity of tissue to transmit roentgen rays). Although this feature of CT has several pitfalls, the following substances can be identified with a fair degree of certainty: iodinated contrast media, blood, fat, air, clear fluids such as cyst contents or cerebrospinal fluid, and calcuim;
3. To determine if a widened mediastinum is caused by fatty infiltration, by widened or tortuous vessels or by lymphadenopathy or a lymphoma;
4. To evaluate the extent and localization of a mediastinal tumor or extension from a lung or esophageal cancer. Pleural or subpleural metastases may be undetected by plain roentgenograms but can be more easily visualized by CT scans.

ENDOSCOPY

Bronchoscopy and esophagoscopy should be performed whenever the radiographic abnormality could, in any way, be caused by a lung or esophageal tumor. The frequency of lung cancer requires that this diagnosis be considered in patients who are 40 years of age and over with a smoking history.

BIOPSY PROCEDURES

Procedures short of thoracotomy are limited in scope and are of little value. If cervical or supraclavicular nodes are palpable, they should be biopsied. Scalene node biopsy in the absence of palpable nodes is rarely rewarding except when one suspects sarcoidosis or lymphoma. Mediastinoscopy and anterior mediastinotomy are worthwhile when the mediastinal mass consists of enlarged lymph nodes secondary to sarcoidosis or a lymphoma. Otherwise, these procedures do not yield a high percentage of positive diagnoses. Whenever lymph node biopsies are obtained, it is important that portions of the node are kept in sterile saline for culture and sensitivity studies, for the determination of T and B cells and for direct imprints.

Bone marrow biopsies should be considered when the mediastinal mass could be a thymoma or lymphoma. Aplastic anemia may be associated with the former and malignant cells may be found in the bone marrow of patients with lymphoma.

Ultimately, many mediastinal masses have to be removed. Thoracotomy will be required using a median sternotomy or posterolateral incision. However, even under these circumstances, biopsy of a mass which cannot be completely removed occasionally leaves the pathologist confused if light microscopy alone is relied upon. Electron microscopy may help differentiate among four kinds of tumors which can be confused with each other: lymphoma, seminoma, thymoma, and mediastinal carcinoid.

If the patient with a mediastinal mass can not tolerate a thoracotomy because of cardiopulmonary insufficiency, one of the aforementioned limited biopsy procedures or a needle biopsy of the mass may be employed. However, before this is done one must be sure the structure being biopsied is not of vascular origin.

HORMONAL ASSAYS AND TUMOR MARKERS

Hormonal assays and the determination of tumor markers such as alphafetoprotein and carcinoembryonic antigen may be of value in selected instances. Pheochromocytomas and some neurogenic tumors will be accompanied by elevated urinary catecholamine, homovanillic acid, and vanillyl mandelic acid levels. Germ cell tumors, teratomas, and some carcinomas will also elaborate glycoproteins (oncofetal antigens) such as carcinoembryonic antigen and alpha-fetoprotein. Chorionic gonadotrophin levels may be elevated in some patients with germ cell tumors. These markers are valuable in the follow-up of patients as well as for diagnosis.

SUMMARY AND CONCLUSIONS

The lists presented in Tables 15-3, 15-4, and 15-6 should be of help in the differential diagnosis of a mediastinal mass.[22] The differential diagnosis will, in turn, indicate which of the aforementioned diagnostic procedures would be most rewarding to perform.

It is currently possible to identify some mediastinal masses without resorting to a major operative procedure such as a thoracotomy. Lesions which do not require exploration are non-neoplastic in nature, such as ectatic vessels, calcified lymph nodes (Fig. 15-11), and fat pads. Those lesions which can be diagnosed by lesser operative procedures such as mediastinoscopy or mediastinotomy are those which usually involve lymph nodes: inflammatory conditions (tuberculosis, histoplasmosis), granulomatous processes (sarcoidosis), or neoplasms (lymphoma or metastatic cancers). The remaining lesions require surgical exploration in order to establish a precise diagnosis. It is to be hoped that definitive therapy can also take place at the operation.

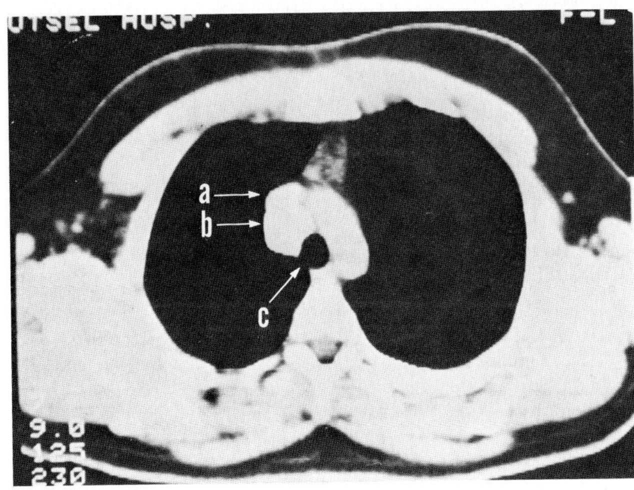

FIG. 15-11. Computed tomography demonstrating a calcified lymph node (*b*) located behind the superior vena cava (*a*) and the right main stem bronchus (*c*).

Patients who undergo thoracotomy require the same detailed diagnostic studies as the patients who do not undergo a major operative procedure. The surgeon should be aware of the exact location and extent of the lesion as well as know whether or not the lesion is vascular in nature and its relationship to the vital structures located in the mediastinum.

THYMIC NEOPLASMS

DEVELOPMENTAL, ANATOMICAL, AND FUNCTIONAL ASPECTS OF THE THYMUS GLAND

Although the fully developed thymus is considered a lymphatic organ, embryologically it originates as epithelial outgrowths of the lower portion of the third pharyngeal pouches on each side. The upper part of the third pharyngeal pouches gives rise to the parathyroid glands. The latter migrate into the neck whereas the right and left thymic anlage descend into the mediastinum to become a bilobed glandular structure which varies greatly in both shape and size.[23–25]

The cords of epithelial cells which initially make up the thymus grow out into the surrounding mesenchyma. These cords subsequently constitute the medullary areas of the future lobules of the thymus (Fig. 15-12).[26] The epithelial cells in the cords eventually spread out to form a reticulum but never lose contact with each other. In some areas the epithelial cells pile up and undergo keratinization and degeneration, forming distinctive structures known as Hassall's corpuscles. These structures are found in the medulla of the lobules.

TABLE 15-6. Differential Diagnostic Features of Mediastinal Masses

LESIONS COMMONLY FOUND INFERIORLY IN THE MEDIASTINUM
- Diaphragmatic hernias
- Pericardial cysts
- Epiphrenic diverticula

LESIONS COMMONLY FOUND IN CARDIOPHRENIC ANGLES ANTERIORLY
- Pericardial cysts (mostly on right)
- Morgagni hernias
- Epicardial fat pad

LESIONS COMMONLY CERVICOMEDIASTINAL IN TYPE
- Thyroid masses
- Lymphatic or vascular tumors
- Innominate artery aneurysms
- Parathyroid lesions

LESIONS CONTAINING FAT
- Lipomas
- Liposarcomas
- Teratomas
- Omental herniations
- Epicardial fat pads

LESIONS CONTAINING CALCIFICATIONS
- Teratomas
- Thymomas
- Thyroid masses
- Mesotheliomas
- Vascular tumors
- Cartilaginous and bone tumors
- Aneurysms of aorta and innominate artery
- Lymph node granulomas

LESIONS COMMONLY FOUND AROUND THE BASE OF THE HEART
- Thymic tumors and cysts
- Teratomas
- Aortic body tumors

LESIONS COMMONLY ASSOCIATED WITH PULMONARY INFILTRATES
- Lymph node enlargement secondary to infection or metastatic disease
- Lymphoma
- Leukemia
- Megaesophagus

LESIONS WHICH MAY CONTAIN AIR OR AIR AND FLUID
- Pharyngeal diverticula
- Epiphrenic diverticula of esophagus
- Megaesophagus
- Hiatal hernias
- Morgagni hernias containing hollow viscera
- Mediastinal abscesses
- Neurenteric cysts
- Bronchogenic cysts
- Enteric cysts

LESIONS WHICH MAY BE ACCOMPANIED BY PLEURAL FLUID
- Mesotheliomas
- Lung cancer
- Lymph node enlargement secondary to primary or metastatic malignancy or inflammation
- Teratomas
- Tumors of nervous tissue, fibrous tissue, fat or muscle

LESIONS WHICH MAY HAVE ASSOCIATED CONGENITAL DEFORMITIES OF THE SPINE OR RIBS
- Neurenteric cysts

LESIONS WHICH ERODE OR DESTROY BONE
- Aneurysms
- Neurogenic tumors
- Meningoceles
- Cartilaginous and bone tumors

LESIONS WHICH MAY BE HUGE WHEN INITIALLY DISCOVERED
- Neurilemmomas
- Neurofibromas
- Ganglioneuromas
- Meningoceles
- Fibromas
- Lipomas
- Mesotheliomas

LESIONS WHICH MAY HAVE ASSOCIATED SPLENOMEGALY
- Lymphomas
- Lymphadenopathy secondary to sarcoidosis or certain inflammatory conditions, e.g., histoplasmosis
- Extramedullary hematoporesis

LESIONS COMMONLY LOCATED AROUND THE TRACHEA
- Tracheal tumors
- Bronchogenic cysts
- Lymphadenopathy of paratrachial nodes secondary to tumor or inflammation

LESIONS WITHIN OR AROUND THE ESOPHAGUS
- Tumors
- Cysts
- Hernias

LESIONS SECONDARY TO TRAUMA
- Aneurysms
- Mediastinitis
- Hematomas
- Pneumomediastinum

LESIONS PROJECTING INTO THE MEDIASTINUM FROM THE ABDOMEN
- Hernias

(Leigh TF: Mass lesions of the mediastinum. Radiologic Clin N Am 1:377, 1963)

As the epithelial cords proliferate and send out side branches into the mesenchyma, lymphocytes appear within the spaces between the epithelial cells of the cortex of the lobules. These lymphocytes are thought to be derived from hematopoietic stem cells which arise in the bone marrow and migrate to the thymus. The stem cells are concentrated in the periphery of the cortex of the thymic lobules. They give rise to the smaller lymphocytes which are located in the deeper cortex of the lobule and fill the spaces between the epithelial cells. Medullary areas of the lobules in the mature thymus contain few lymphocytes and are largely epithelial in character. Germinal centers and lymphoid follicles are normally not found in the thymus.[25]

The process of differentiation into mature thymocytes requires a humoral factor produced by the epithelial cells. One preparation of this hormone, (thymosine) is a polypeptide which can support the development of precursor lymphocytes into thymocytes.[27] This preparation and others, such as the thymic humoral factor of Trainin, are common to all mammals studied thus far.[28]

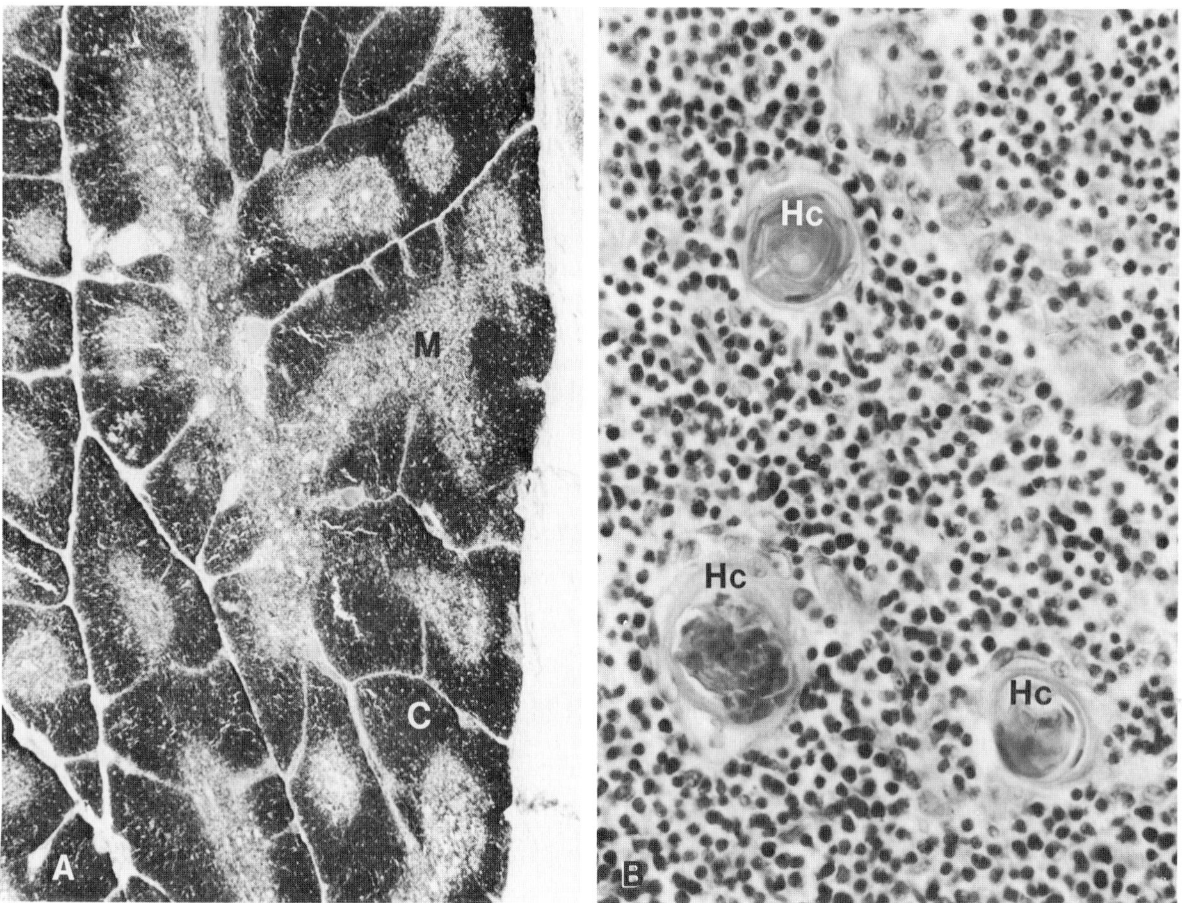

FIG. 15-12. (*A*) Very low-power photomicrograph of the thymus gland. Septa appear as clear lines. The cortex (*S*) of the lobules is dark; the medulla (*M*) is light. (*B*) High-power photomicrograph of an area of the medulla. Three Hassall's corpuscles (*He*) are shown. (Ham AW, Cormack DH: Histology, 8th ed. Philadelphia, JB Lippincott, 1979)

The differentiation of lymphoblasts into thymocytes in humans takes place in fetal and early post-natal life. The thymocytes in the deeper cortex of the thymic lobules then enter the circulation, without passing through the medulla of the lobules, and populate all of the lymphatic tissue. These lymphocytes are referred to as thymus-derived lymphocytes or T-lymphocytes. They have characteristic surface markers and specialized immunological functions, but are morphologically similar to the other major class of lymphocytes, the bone-marrow–derived lymphocytes (B-lymphocytes). A detailed account of the characteristics and functions of these lymphocyte populations relative to the immune response is beyond the scope of this chapter but is discussed in Chapter 48, Section 1. It will suffice here to state that T-lymphocytes are responsible for cellular immunity, such as cell-mediated cytotoxicity, suppressor cell activity, and the interaction with B-lymphocytes to generate humoral immune responses.

T-cells which mature in the thymus are distributed to the T-dependent areas of peripheral lymphoid tissues and to the recirculating pool of lymphocytes. Thus, the main function of the thymus gland is the processing of precursor cells into T-lymphocytes, a function which is completed in humans shortly after birth. Congenital absence of the thymus (Di George syndrome) or its removal early in life, results in a deficiency of cellular immune function. Thymectomy in the adult will also result in a decrease in immunologic competence. However, since the half-life of thymus-derived lymphocytes in man is quite long (several years) the decrease in immunologic function due to the loss of T-lymphocytes is gradual and less evident than when the thymus is removed at birth or shortly thereafter.

Although the mature thymus gland varies greatly from individual to individual with respect to size and shape, it follows a relatively predictable pattern with respect to its size and the age of the patient.

The thymus gland reaches a maximum size of 30 g to 40 g in the adolescent (Fig. 15-13) but its greatest size relative to the rest of the body is attained at about four years of age.[25] Following puberty, the thymis gradually involutes, with the disappearance of its lymphoid component. The parenchyma is largely replaced by fat. Hassell's corpuscles remain to identify the gland. The thymus never completely disappears.

A study of the morphology of the adult thymus by Bell and colleagues quantitated the variation in the dimensions and configuration of the thymus (Fig. 15-14).[23] The gland is generally situated beneath the upper part of the sternum. Its

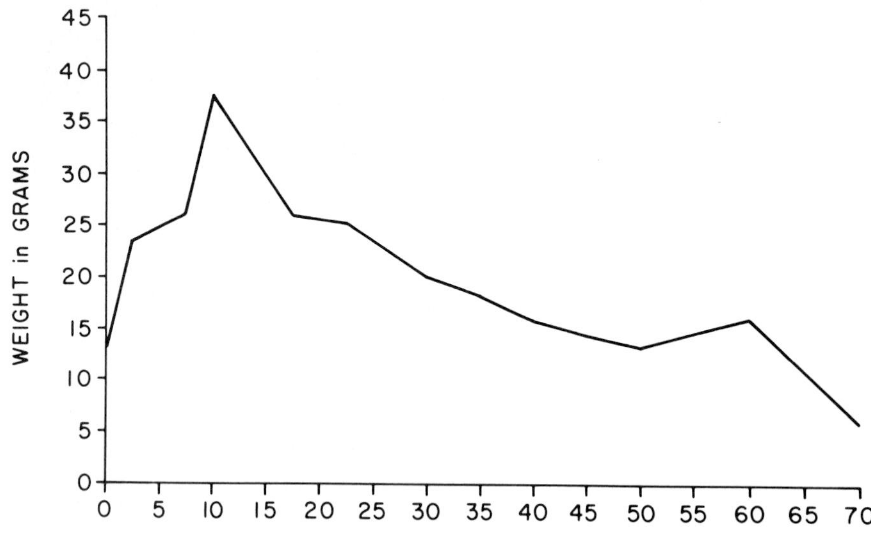

FIG. 15-13. The weight of the thymus gland peaks at about 11 years of age, then begins to decrease in size. (Rosai J, Levine GD: Tumors of the thymus. In Atlas of Tumor Pathology, Second Series, Fascicle 13. Washington, DC, Armed Forces Institute of Pathology, 1976)

lower tip may end at any point between the first intercostal space and the coastal cartilage of the seventh rib. In two-thirds of the cases studied by Bell and colleagues, the caudal extremity of the thymus was between the third and fourth ribs. The thoracic portion of the thymus is usually thickest where it rests on the pericardium. The cervical extent of the thymus is usually the least distinct of the gland's margins. The upper end of the thymus blends imperceptibly into the cervical fat and may extend up to the level of the sixth cervical vertebra.

FIG. 15-14. The caudal tip of thymus gland was found between the third and fourth ribs in 66% of the 125 cadavers studied by Bell and colleagues.[23] Almost all of the glands terminated at some point above the xyphoid.

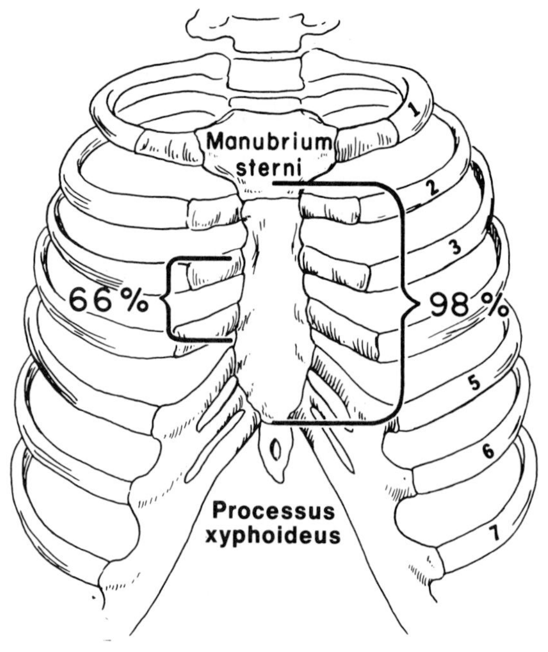

The following neoplasms have been postulated to arise from the thymus gland: thymomas, lymphomas, carcinoid tumors, germ cell tumors, and primary carcinomas. These lesions, other than lymphomas, are discussed below.

THYMOMA

Although the thymus gland is classified as a lymphoid organ, its origin, as we have pointed out, is the epithelium of the third pharyngeal pouches. It is the epithelium of the thymus gland which may undergo neoplastic change to constitute a thymoma. Lymphocytic elements may be present and even dominate the histologic appearance of a thymoma. Nonetheless, a neoplasm of the thymus is not considered to be a thymoma unless the epithelial component is the neoplastic element. Thymomas are strictly tumors of thymic epithelium.

Both Hodgkins and non-Hodgkins lymphomas may involve the thymus gland and must be differentiated from true thymomas. The term "granulomatous thymoma" is a misnomer which has been used to designate Hodgkin's disease of the thymus; it should be discarded. Hodgkin's disease involving the thymus is the same as Hodgkin's disease in any other tissue. It should not be considered a thymoma even though it may occur primarily in the thymus gland.[29–30] Similarly, small cell undifferentiated tumors from the lung, carcinoid tumors, and germ-cell tumors such as seminomas may involve the thymus and may be difficult to differentiate from thymomas.[25]

Pathology

Grossly, thymomas have fibrous septae on cut section. Cystic areas are seen in 40% to 60% of specimens.[25] Several classifications of thymomas have been devised, based on the histopathology of these tumors. Rosai and Levine have reviewed this aspect of thymomas completely in their monograph.[25] The simplest classification designates three types, based on the predominant cell type comprising the tumor:

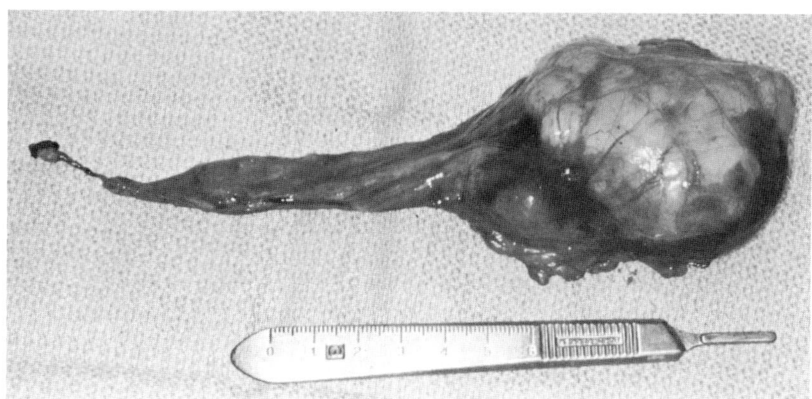

FIG. 15-15. A benign well-encapsulated thymoma removed with the entire thymus gland. This is the lesion seen in Fig. 15-6.

lymphocytic, epithelial, and mixed (lymphoepithelial) A cell type is considered predominant by Bergh and colleagues if more than 80% of the tumor is made up the that cell.[31] By their standards, 23% of 43 thymomas were lymphocytic, 35% were lymphoepithelial, and 42% were epithelial.

The pathologists at the Mayo Clinic reviewed 197 thymomas and classified then into four types: lymphocytic (35% of the tumors), epithelial (18%), mixed (25%), and spindle cell (22%).[32] Spindle cell thymomas are considered variants of epithelial thymomas. Another variant of the epithelial thymoma is the pseudo-rosette type characterized by a predominant pattern of pseudo-rosette formation by the neoplastic epithelial cells.

The Mayo Clinic group found that patients with spindle cell or predominantly lymphocytic cell types had a much higher survival rate than those with mixed or predominantly epithelial cell types.[9] At the University of Michigan, epithelial thymomas also tended to be more extensive and pursue a more aggressive course.[32] Most authors fail to find a correlation between the histopathology of thymomas and their malignant potential.[25] Nor is there a correlation between the histopathology of a thymoma and the coexistence of associated systemic syndromes.[25] The malignant potential of thymomas correlates with their invasive characteristics rather than the microscopic appearance of the tumor. The number of mitotic figures seen is low in all thymomas regardless of the invasiveness of the tumor.[25,31–37]

A benign thymoma is a tumor which is well encapsulated and does not invade adjacent mediastinal structures (Fig. 15-15). Fifty percent to 65% of the thymomas fit this definition (Fig. 15-16). The surgeon is usually in the best position to determine whether a thymoma has infiltrated the surrounding tissue. Frozen section analyses of dense fibrous attachments between the thymoma and surrounding tissue may be necessary to be sure that the tumor is truly confined by its capsule. The capsule should be carefully examined for signs of discontinuity since the latter may represent an area of local invasion. The most common form of metastatic involvement is the occurrence of pleural or pericardial implants. They are thought to result from the shedding of tumor cells from the primary thymoma.

Staging of thymomas as to their extent is therefore based on invasiveness. The following staging system has been suggested by Bergh and colleagues:[31]

Stage I: Intact capsule or growth within the capsule;
Stage II: Pericapsular growth into the mediastinal fat tissue;
Stage III: Invasive growth into the surrounding organs, intrathoracic metastases or both.

In their series, from the University of Goteborg in Sweden, 40% were Stage I, 19% Stage II, and 41% Stage III. The Stage I thymomas ranged in weight from 20 to 440 g; Stage II tumors from 30 g to 375 g; and Stage III from 85 g to 1700 g. Pleural metastases occurred in half of the Stage III patients. Metastases to regional nodes or distant organs are very rare. Malignant thymomas are almost always confined to the thorax. Only 30 instances of blood borne metastases to extrathoracic sites were reported up till 1976.[1] The organs involved have been the liver, bone, colon, kidney, brain, and spleen. Epithelial thymomas gave rise to these metastases more often than other tumors. Thymomas in children appear to run a more malignant course than in adults.[38,39]

FIG. 15-16. Although figures vary from series to series, it is generally found that two-thirds of thymomas are benign. The recurrence rate following removal of these tumors is low, in contrast to the higher recurrence rate following resection of invasive (malignant) thymomas.

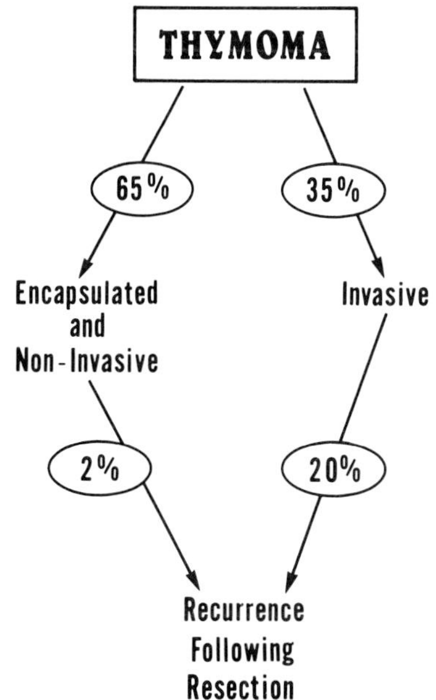

TABLE 15-7. Syndromes and Diseases Associated with Thymomas

AUTOIMMUNE OR IMMUNE PHENOMENA
Myasthenia gravis
Cytopenias
Hypogammaglobulinemia
Polymyositis
Systemic lupus erythematosus
Rheumatoid arthritis
Thyroiditis
Sjogren's syndrome
Chronic ulcerative colitis
Pernicious anemia
Raynaud's disease
Regional enteritis
Rheumatic endocarditis
Sarcoid
Dermatomyositis
Scleroderma
Takayasu syndrome
ENDOCRINE DISORDERS
Hyperthyroidism
Addison's disease
Macrogenitotomica precox
Panhypopituitarism
CANCER (non-thymic)
SEVERE INFECTIONS AND MISCELLANEOUS DISEASES
Myocarditis
Megaesophagus
Other

Clinical Findings

Fortuitous discovery of a thymoma when a chest roentgenogram is obtained for reasons unrelated to the tumor occurs in 30% or 40% of patients with this neoplasm (Fig. 15-17). Patients are usually between 40 years and 60 years of age. No more than 10% of thymomas are found in patients less than 20 years of age.[36] Only 22 malignant thymomas in children were found in the literature by 1979.[38] It is possible that some of these neoplasms were erroneously diagnosed and should be classified as germ cell tumors. Bowie and colleagues could only collect 19 well-documented cases of thymoma from the literature which involved children 18 years of age and under.[39] Men and women are affected equally.

Vague, nonspecific symptoms related to the chest may be present, such as cough, dyspnea, dysphagia, chest tightness, and chest pain. The latter may be a sign of an advanced malignant lesion. Advanced lesions may produce superior vena cava syndrome.

The systemic syndromes which may be associated with a thymoma are listed in Table 15-7. The three most common will be discussed below. The occurrence of these syndromes often leads to the discovery of a thymoma. In reported series of thymomas, 15% to 50% of the tumors are found in patients who present with myasthenia gravis. This wide variation in frequency is a function of the degree to which thymomas are looked for in patients with myasthenia gravis by performing thymectomy or an autopsy. A previously unsuspected gross or microscopic thymoma is found in at least 15% of patients with myasthenia gravis when the thymus is surgically removed.

FIG. 15-17. Symptoms related to a thymoma may be nonspecific or related to one of the many systemic syndromes associated with this tumor. As many as 10% of patients with thymomas will have neoplasms in organs other than the thymus (see Table 15-7).

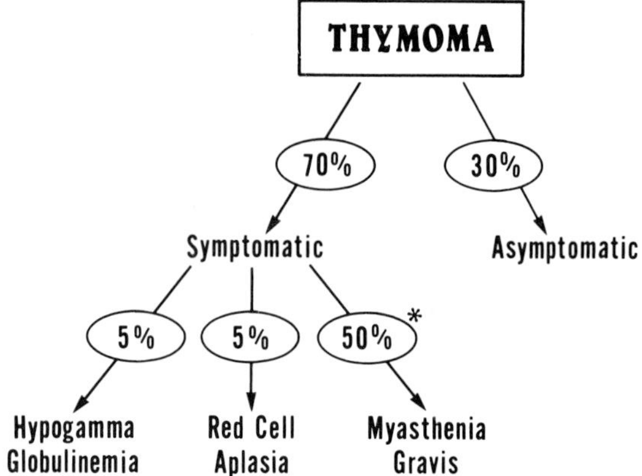

Systemic Syndromes Associated with Thymomas

Since both the parathyroid and thymus glands are derived from the third pharyngeal pouches, the group at the Mayo Clinic thought it would be reasonable to compare the incidence of diseases associated with thymomas and parathyroid adenomas, the latter acting as a control to the former.[40] They reviewed 146 of their own patients with thymoma and 452 found in the literature with sufficient data to evaluate whether or not an associated disease occurred. The incidence of other diseases with thymomas was 71%, compared to a 12% incidence in 177 patients with parathyroid adenomas. The diseases found associated with thymomas could be classified into categories presented in Table 15-7. In some patients more than one disease was associated with the thymoma, such as myasthenia gravis and a cancer or myasthenia gravis and thrombocytopenia. Close to 70% of the patients with thymoma and other diseases will have disorders related to immunologic phenomena. About 10% will have a malignancy and 5% will have an endocrine disorder. The remaining 15% will have a severe infection or another seemingly unrelated condition such as megaesophagus. The most frequent association is between thymoma and myasthenia gravis. Some 40% to 50% of patients with syndromes associated with thymoma have myasthenia gravis (Fig. 15-17). As will be pointed out in greater detail below, some of the endocrine disorders such as Cushing's syndrome are concomitants of carcinoid tumor of the thymus which may be mistakenly diagnosed as as a thymoma.

MYASTHENIA GRAVIS. Pathophysiologically, this disease is characterized by rapid exhaustion of voluntary muscular contractions with a slow return to a normal state. In patients with myasthenia gravis repetitive stimulation of the motor nerve to a muscle results in a progressive decrement of muscle action potentials. Thus, the major symptoms of patients with myasthenia gravis are weakness and fatigability. Another characteristic of myasthenia is that these symptoms are relieved by drugs which inhibit acetylcholinesterese. This enzyme is located within the synaptic junction between the motor neuron and striated muscle. This junction is known as the end plate (Fig. 15-18). Because of these features of myasthenia gravis, the disease is considered an abnormality of neuromuscular transmission.[41]

Prior to 1973, many theories were presented to explain the etiology of this neuromuscular disorder. Since then, it has been widely accepted that myasthenia gravis is an autoimmune disease directed against acetylcholine receptors in voluntary muscle. A myasthenic state can be produced in rabbits by immunizing them with a purified protein having the properties of acetylcholine receptors.[42] The effect of the immune response is to eliminate acetylcholine receptors and impair postsynaptic structure and function. It has been determined that patients with myasthenia gravis have 70% to 90% fewer acetylcholine receptors per neuromuscular junction than do normal people.[41] Since there is a decreased number of acetylcholine receptors present within the end plate of patients with myasthenia gravis, acetylcholine, which is responsible for neuromuscular transmission across the synaptic junction, is less effective in transmitting the signal from nerve to muscle.

Decreased availability of acetylcholine receptors in patients with myasthenia gravis appears to be the result of increased degredation of receptors. This decrease comes about when antibodies of the IgG immunoglobulin class interact with the receptors. Occasionally, skeletal muscle from patients with myasthenia will reveal local collections of lymphocytes. This finding might be taken as an expression of a cellular immune reaction. However, evidence for a humoral autoimmune response is currently stronger than any data which would suggest that myasthenia gravis is caused by cell-mediated effector mechanisms. The known role of T-cells in antibody production, and the salutory response to measures which are known to affect cell-mediated immunity, leave this aspect of the immunopathology of myasthenia gravis somethat unresolved.

An association between the thymus and myasthenia was first suspected when pathologic changes were found in the thymus gland of 75% to 85% of patients with this neuromuscular disease. (Fig. 15-19) Germinal centers are not normally present in the thymus gland; yet 70% of patients with myasthenia gravis and thymic abnormalities demonstrate this form of "thymic lymphoid (follicular) hyperplasia."[43] It is characterized by germinal center proliferation in the medullary areas of the thymus without necessarily increasing the gross appearance or weight of the thymus. Furthermore, 10% to 30% of patients with myasthenia will have gross or microscopic thymomas, depending upon the frequency with which patients with myasthenia gravis have thymectomy or an autopsy to search for this lesion. Follicular hyperplasia of the non-neoplastic thymus may accompany a thymoma.

Thymectomy in patients with myasthenia gravis can be effective in producing a remission of the disease in 20% to 36% of patients. An additional 57% to 86% will be improved (Fig. 15-20).[41] The presence of a thymoma in a patient with myasthenia carries a poorer prognosis than myasthenia patients without thymoma. Improvement in muscle strength following thymectomy can be anticipated in only 25% of patients with myasthenia and a thymoma. A 40% to 60% response rate may result when myasthenic patients have a thymectomy and do not have a thymoma. Female patients under 40 in whom myasthenia gravis is twice as common as older men (70% of patients with myasthenia gravis under age 40 are females) have a 60% response rate to thymectomy in contrast to the 25% therapeutic benefit found for men. The age of patients with myasthenia gravis and thymoma is generally older than myasthenic patients without thymoma (15 to 35 years of age versus 30 years to 60 years of age) (Fig. 15-21). On the other hand, more thymomas accompanied by

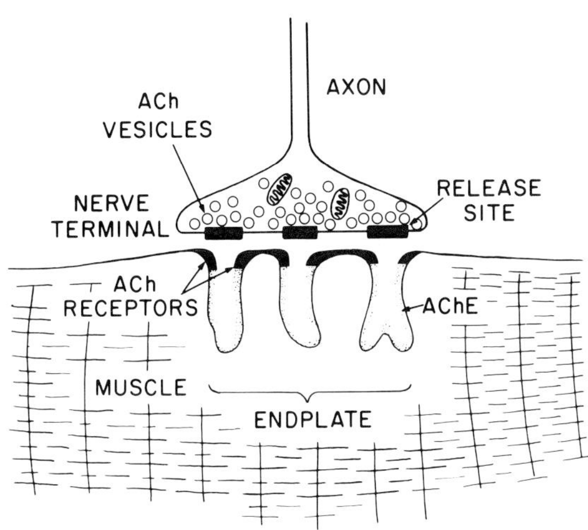

FIG. 15-18. Diagrammatic representation of the neuromuscular junction (endplate) as described by Drachman.[41] Antibody to acetylcholine (A-Ch) receptors eliminate them and impair postsynaptic function in myasthenia gravis. (Drachman DB: Myasthenia gravis. New Engl J Med 298:136 and 186, 1978)

FIG. 15-19. Thymic abnormalities are frequent in patients with myasthenia. Both thymic lymphoid hyperplasia and thymoma may be present in the same patient.

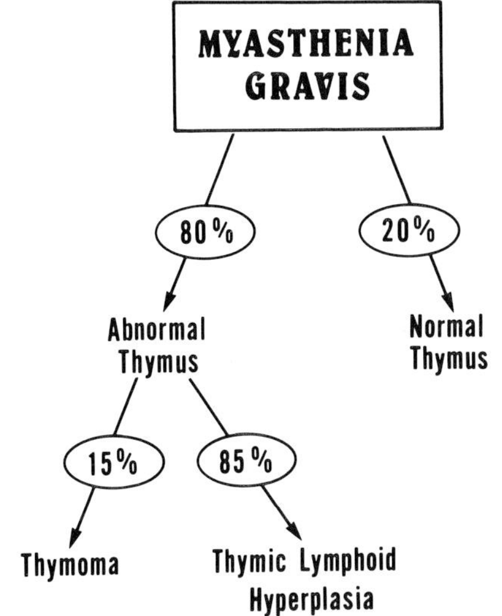

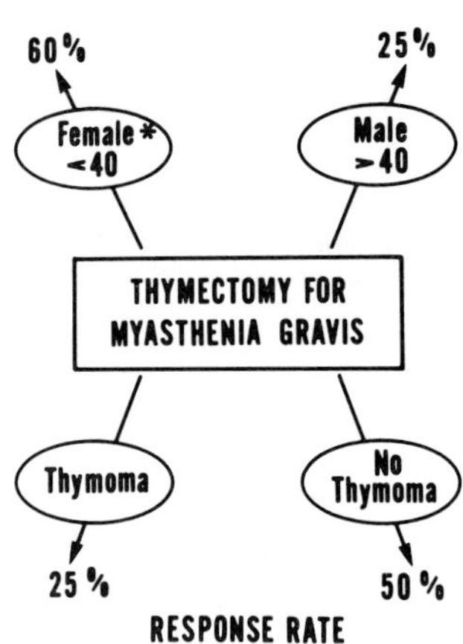

FIG. 15-20. The response to thymacotomy varies depending upon the age and sex of the patient and whether or not a thymoma is present.

myasthenia gravis present in younger individuals than non-myasthenic tumors.

Thymomas in patients with myasthenia gravis are usually smaller than those found in non-myasthenic patients. This finding may be explained by the fact that they are diagnosed earlier. Invasive (malignant) thymomas are found in 35% to 40% of both myasthenic and non-myasthenic patients.

There is no morphologic parameter in a thymoma that is specific for the concomitant or subsequent occurrence of myasthenia gravis but some morphologic features of thymomas are more frequently associated with myasthenia.[43] For example, spindle cell thymomas are rarely associated with myasthenia gravis. Another feature of thymomas and myasthenia gravis is the high frequency of lymphoid follicles with germinal centers in the thymic tissues surrounding the thymoma.[25]

FIG. 15-21. The age incidence of myasthenic patients with and without thymoma are depicted in this graph. Patients with myasthenia gravis and thymoma are generally older than those without this tumor. (Data taken from Castelman as depicted in Rosai J, Levine GD: Tumors of the thymus. Atlas of Tumor Pathology, Second Series, Fascicle 13. Washington, DC, Armed Forces Institute of Pathology, 1976)

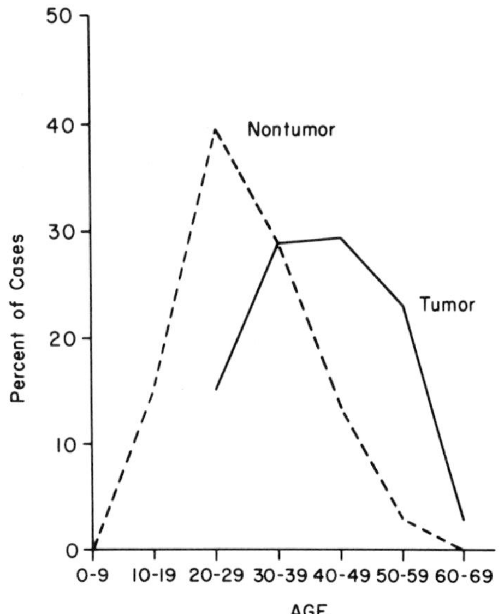

The association of the thymus, thymomas, and myasthenia gravis remains an enigma despite all that has been learned about these structures and the syndrome in the past decade. There are data to suggest that "myoid" or muscle-like cells in the thymus and thymomas which cross-react with anti-muscle antibodies may be responsible for initiating the autoimmune reaction leading to anti-acetylcholinesterase receptor antibodies.[41,44] It has been suggested that a virally-induced "thymitis" could trigger the process whereby antigenic components within the thymus are recognized by the T-lymphocytes and that these antigens cross-react with acetylcholinesterase receptors.[41]

There is evidence that patients with myasthenia have altered immune responsiveness with changes in the relative proportion of B and T lymphocytes in the circulation. Myasthenic patients may also show significant improvement after receiving immunosuppressive drugs such as corticosteroids and azathioprine.[41,45] The salutory effect of thymectomy may also be explained by the immunosuppressive effect of extirpation of this gland.

The complexities of treating patients with myasthenia gravis do not fall within the province of this discussion. Drachman's outline is presented as an indication of how one could proceed (Table 15-8).

Two important aspects with respect to thymectomy for patients with thymomas and myasthenia gravis deserve mention. First, the entire thymus must be removed, along with the thymoma, and an aggressive surgical approach taken to the wide resection of invaded structures whenever possible. The occurrence of myasthenia after thymectomy for thymoma has been shown to be related to recurrent disease or residual thymus tissue. Second, the intricacies of managing the myasthenic patient's respiratory problems following general anesthesia requires an experienced, well-trained team. Improved management of this phase of the procedure is responsible for reducing the mortality from 10% to 27% in the past to 0% to 6% at present.[41]

RED CELL APLASIA. Pure red cell aplasia is also considered an autoimmune disorder and can be found in 5% of patients with thymoma.[1] One-third to half of all patients with red cell aplasia will have a thymoma.[46] An associated decrease in the number of platelets or leukocytes will be found in 30% of patients with red cell aplasia. This syndrome appears after the age of 40 in 96% of the patients who develop it. The diagnosis is made on examination of the bone marrow. Red cell precursors are absent whereas platelet and leukocytic elements are normal. In 66% of the patients with thymoma, a spindle cell tumor will be found.[25] Thymectomy will result in a 25% to 30% remission of the disease.[46] As with the association between thymoma and myasthenia gravis, one can only speculate what the nature of the relationship is.

HYPOGAMMAGLOBULINEMIA. This abnormality is present in 5% to 10% of patients with thymoma.[40] Patients with hypogammaglobulinemia have a 10% incidence of thymoma. More than a third of those patients also have red cell hypoplasia. Combined humoral and cellular immunodeficiencies are present. Practically all patients are over the age of 40 years. Thymectomy has not proven to be beneficial in this condition.

Roentgenographic Features of Thymomas

The tumors are almost always located completely or partially in the anterior mediastinum and are the most frequent neoplasms found in this compartment (Fig. 15-6 and 15-22). Approximately 15% occupy both the anterior and superior mediastinum and 6% are primarily in the superior mediastinum. No more than 5% to 10% of thymomas may occur in other locations, such as the neck and middle and posterior mediastinum. The lesion is characteristically located anterior to the junction of the great vessels. The latter may be displaced posteriorly by the tumor. Thymomas are round or oval with smooth or lobulated margins. The mass may protrude to one or both sides of the mediastinum. Calcifications may be seen in as many as 20% of thymomas, either at the periphery of the tumor or throughout its substance.[25] Califications are best visualized by overpenetrated films, laminograms or by CT (Fig. 15-22). As mentioned previously, the latter studies allow precise definition of the extent of involvement and the nature of the tumor mass, whether solid or cystic. Pleural metastases are also more easily identified by CT than by conventional roentgenograms or laminograms of the chest.

Treatment of Thymoma—Results

Thymomas are slow-growing tumors. Some have been recorded to stay the same size for as long as 15 years.[25] Extrathoracic metastases occur rarely. Thymomas express their malignant potential by invading surrounding tissues and by developing local recurrences and implants in the chest. These features undoubtedly account for the fact that the most effective therapy is complete removal of the tumor. When the thymoma is encapsulated and is removed with the entire thymus, without disturbing the integrity of the capsule, virtually all patients will be cured of the tumor. No more than 2% will develop recurrences.[37] The latter take the form of pleural, pericardial, or diaphragmatic implants or of a localized mediastinal tumor (Fig. 15-23). Another important prognostic determinant, in addition to encapsulation of the tumor versus invasiveness, is the presence or absence of an associated syndrome such as myasthenia gravis.[35,47] The latter is present in half of all patients who develop a recurrence following surgery. Fortunately, 65% of thymomas are well encapsulated and not associated with myasthenia gravis.

TABLE 15-8. Treatment of Myasthenia Gravis

INITIAL THERAPY
Anticholinesterase medication (pyridostigmine bromide, Mesantoin). Adjust dosage for optimal effect.
Corticosteroids, if results with anticholinesterase drugs are unsatisfactory.
THYMECTOMY—INDICATIONS
Thymoma—Postoperative radiation and corticosteroids if thymoma is invasive.
Unsatisfactory response after 6 months to 12 months of drug therapy in patients less than 50 years of age.
IMMUNOSUPPRESSIVE DRUGS
For patients resistant to anticholinesterase medication, thymectomy and corticosteroids.

(Modified from Drachman DB: Myasthenia gravis. New Engl J Med 298:136 and 186, 1978)

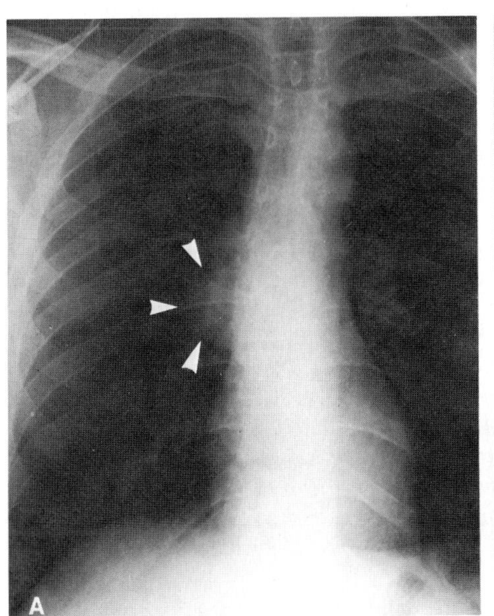

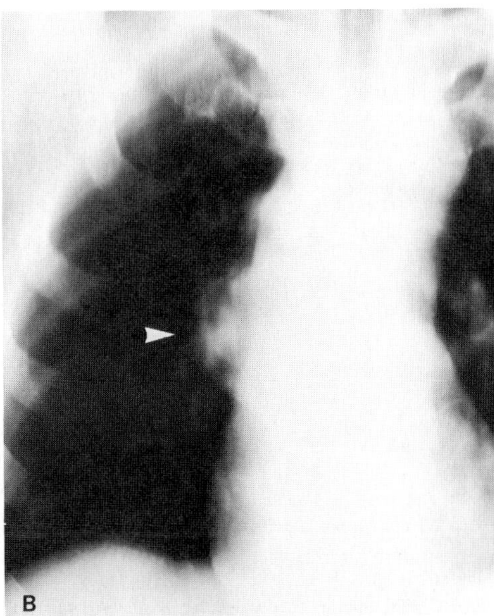

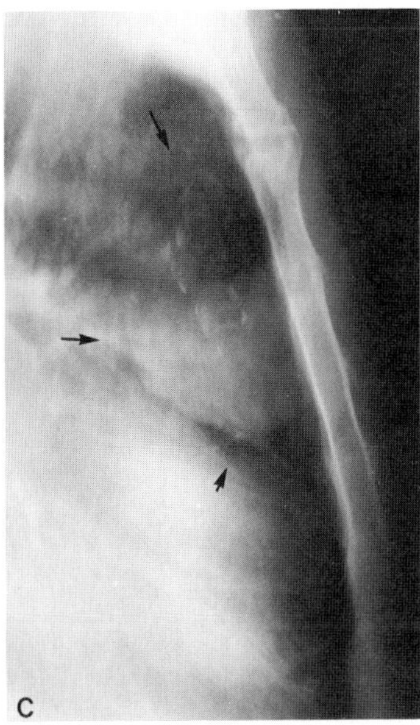

FIG. 15-22. A posteroanterior chest roentgenogram (*A*) of a patient with an invasive thymoma which is best visualized by frontal laminograms (*B*). Calcifications are seen in the lateral laminograms (*C*).

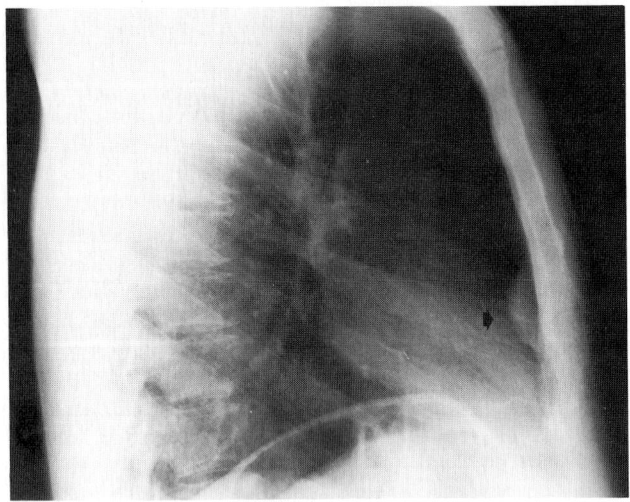

FIG. 15-23. Pleural implant found five years after removal of the invasive thymoma shown in Figure 15-22. Resection was carried out followed by radiation therapy.

As one would expect of patients with a neuromuscular disorder, survival following resection of encapsulated thymomas is also poorer when myasthenia gravis is present (Fig. 15-24). However, recent experiences have noted that patients with thymoma and myasthenia gravis do as well as those without myasthenia.[48]

The operation is best carried out using a midline sternal splitting incision. A bilateral submammary incision transecting the sternum may provide a more cosmetic result. However, the exposure this incision provides is not optimal and it may be more difficult to deal with invasive lesions should they be encountered. The poor exposure provided by a cervical incision renders this approach unsatisfactory. Standard right or left thoracotomies have been performed where the tumor appears to be present largely on one side or another.

Resection of encapsulated non-invasive thymomas presents few problems to the surgeon, since they are easily removed.[34] Invasive tumors, on the other hand, can be difficult and challenging. An aggressive surgical approach should be adopted since these tumors are slow-growing and remain localized in the chest for long periods of time. In order to obtain sufficient exposure to resect all of the tumor, the median sternotomy may have to be combined with a thoracotomy. Pericardium, phrenic nerve, pleura, diaphragm, and lung should be resected if these structures are involved. Lobectomy and even pneumonectomy may be required, depending upon the specific circumstances and extent of involvement. Resection of the innominate vein and portions of all or part of the superior vena cava has been performed when these vessels are invaded.[49] A patch graft of autogenous vein or prosthetic material or a vascular graft of Teflon or Dacron can be used to bridge the resulting venous defect with expectation of a good functional result. When extensive involvement precludes complete resection, such as with invasion of the heart, great vessels, or trachea, as much tumor as can be safely resected should be removed to prevent cardiac tamponade or tracheal occlusion and asphyxiation.

FIG. 15-24. Bernatz found that patients with thymoma with accompanying myasthenia gravis had a poorer prognosis than those without myasthenia gravis (MG). (Bernatz PE, Khonsari S, Harrison EG et al: Thymoma: Factors influencing prognosis. Surg Clin N Am 53:885, 1973)

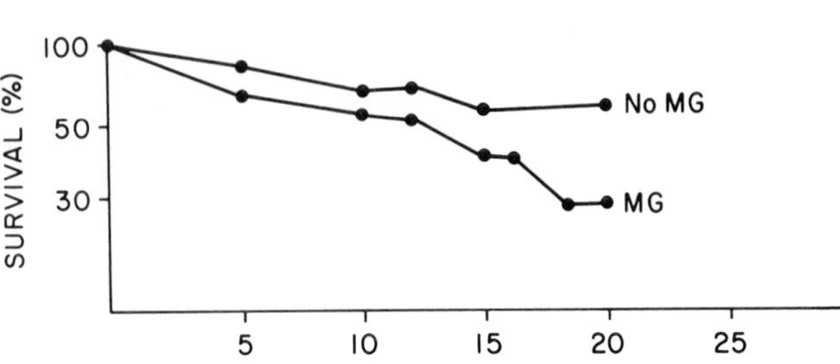

In addition to being tumors that lend themselves to aggressive surgical therapy, thymomas are relatively radiosensitive. Radiation therapy constitutes excellent adjuvent therapy and is considered mandatory for all patients with invasive thymomas, whether or not a complete resection is performed.[50,51] The surgeon should therefore mark off the extent of the resected tumor and thymus with metallic radio-opaque clips in order to facilitate treatment planning by the radiotherapist. Preoperative radiation therapy has been utilized by several groups and has not been found helpful.[52]

There is some disagreement concerning the role of adjuvant radiotherapy for patients with encapsulated non-invasive thymomas. Since the recurrence rate is only 2% and radiotherapy carries some morbidity, Rosai and Levine oppose the use of postoperative radiotherapy when these tumors are removed in toto.[25] At the other extreme is the view that no patient with thymoma can be considered to have been adequately treated unless they receive radiotherapy. It is reasonable to adopt either course depending upon the circumstances. Where long-term follow-up may not be possible or likely, and experienced radiotherapists are able to treat the area with minimal side effects, patients with non-invasive thymomas may be advised to undergo postoperative radiotherapy. On the other hand, patients with small, encapsulated tumors, which were removed with the entire thymus, can be followed closely and receive radiation if recurrences appear. Re-resection should also be considered. In the absence of a prospective controlled randomized study, no definitive statement can be made concerning the role of adjuvant radiotherapy for Stage I thymomas.

Patients with invasive thymomas that can be completely removed have a poorer prognosis than patients with encapsulated non-invasive tumors. At the Mayo Clinic, the ten year survival rate for non-invasive tumors was 65% compared to 30% for invasive tumors.[47] The five-year survival at the Memorial Hospital for encapsulated and invasive tumors was 83% and 54% respectively.[36] Less than half of the patients with invasive thymomas who survived for five years were free of disease. These data are the bases for recommending that patients with invasive thymomas receive post-operative radiotherapy.

Among the options available for the treatment of recurrences are surgical excision, radiotherapy, and chemotherapy. Reresection can often successfully remove local recurrences and pleural and pericardial implants.

Radiotherapy as adjuvant therapy for the treatment of recurrences or to treat unresectable primary thymomas usually consists of 3500 to 4500 rads given over 3 weeks to 6 weeks. Dosages over this range do not significantly increase response rates and increase the risk of post-radiation complications when large fields are used. If the tumor is small, Penn and Hope-Stone recommend using two large anterior oblique wedge fields.[51] Field size in their experience was about 15 cm by 8 cm. More extensive lesions are treated with large parallel opposed fields which might be supplemented with a wedge pair or an additional direct anterior field. Field sizes up to 20 cm by 15 cm are used. These technics minimize exposure to the spinal cord. In addition to irradiating the tumor, it is also often important to treat the entire thymus gland which extends from the sixth cervical vertebra to the level of the fourth to seventh costal cartilage. Skeggs recommends a single anterior and two postero-oblique fields to provide satisfactory dose distribution.[53]

Pneumonitis is a frequent (40%) side effect of radiotherapy when large fields are used.[51] In order to minimize radiation damage to the lungs in patients with pleural implants, Ariaratnam and colleagues utilize a moving strip technique.[50] Mediastinitis, pericarditis, and myocarditis are additional infrequent complications of thymic radiation when unresectable or residual thymomas require large fields and high doses. However, if unresectable or residual tumor is carefully marked out at operation by the surgeon, it should be possible to treat a small tumor volume to a high dose without undue complications.

Corticosteroids have been reported to cause regression of some thymomas and should be utilized in patients with unresectable thymomas that do not respond to radiotherapy.[45] Chemotherapy for thymomas should be reserved for those patients with advanced disease who do not respond to radiation or steroids. Effective single drugs are cis-diamminedichloroplatinum and adriamycin.[54] Responses have also been reported with the use of alkylating agents.[45]

THYMOLIPOMA

This tumor is a curious mixture of fat and hyperplastic thymic tissue. Both components are present in increased amounts, resulting in an enlargement of the thymus gland so that its weight usually exceeds 500 g (normal is one-tenth that).[25] A quarter of these tumors weigh over 2000 g. This lesion is not merely a lipoma involving the thymus gland, since the normal thymic tissue is also hyperplastic and is interspersed within the fat. However, the thymic component has none of the characteristics of a thymoma. Myasthenia gravis has not been reported to occur in association with this tumor. Nor have there been reports of invasion of adjacent structures, metastases, or recurrence following its removal.

CARCINOID OF THE THYMUS

Until 1972, many carcinoid tumors of the thymus were not recognized as distinct lesions and were mistakenly labeled as variants of thymomas.[25,55–57] The fact that they have a similar morphology and similar biologic characteristics with respect to their malignant potential and respond to the same therapy (resection and radiation) might also account for the confusion between carcinoids and thymomas. Significant morphological and biochemical differences exist between these two tumors so that they should be readily differentiated.

Thymic carcinoids develop from cells of neural crest origin which differentiate into Kultschitzky cells. They can undergo malignant change to become carcinoid tumors. No more than 100 thymic carcinoids have been reported in the literature as of 1980.[57] Their gross appearance is similar to that of thymomas. The tumors may be encapsulated or invade adjacent structures. Invasiveness is seen in 50% of thymic carcinoids, compared to 35% of thymomas. Furthermore, thymomas rarely have extrathoracic metastases whereas thymic carcinoids metastasize to bone and other sites in 20% to 30% of patients with this tumor. Fibrous compartmentalization and cystic changes as seen in thymomas do not occur with thymic carcinoids. The two tumors may have similar appearances by light microscopy but electron microscopy can accurately differentiate carcinoid tumors from thymomas. Carcinoids are characterized by numerous cytoplasmic neurosecretory granules, as are other foregut carcinoids. Thymomas will have desmosones, tonofilaments, and elongated cytoplasmic processes not seen in carcinoids. The latter will also contain argyrophil cells when appropriate staining technics are used.

Thymic carcinoids have been classified among the "amine precursor uptake and decarboxylation" tumors (APUD-omas) which are known to have the potential of elaborating peptides, amines, kinins, and prostaglandins. The only endocrine syndrome which has been reported to be directly caused by thymic carcinoids is Cushing's syndrome. In these instances, the carcinoid elaborates ACTH. Patients with carcinoid syndrome secondary to thymic carcinoids have not been reported. However, other endocrine tumors have been reported to occur with thymic carcinoids. Approximately one-third of thymic carcinoids have been associated with paraneoplastic syndromes. Although most of these have been Cushing's syndrome, patients with thymic carcinoids have been described with Type I multiple endocrine neoplasias (pituitary, parathyroid, and pancreatic islet cell tumors). In two-thirds of these patients, the carcinoids have been malignant. Carcinoid tumors of the thymus have also been reported to coexist with medullary carcinomas of the thyroid.

Carcinoid tumors of the thymus are treated by wide excision of the thymus containing the tumor. The resection should be carried out along with contiguous invaded structures which can be sacrificed or replaced. Postoperative radiation therapy has been helpful in patients with persistent or recurrent tumor. As with thymomas, carcinoids of the thymus may recur as long as 10 years after their initial resection. The mortality at 10 years is greater in patients with endocrine abnormalities (50–69%) than in those without endocrine problems (30%).

GERM CELL TUMORS

Much of the material covered in Chapter 24 on testicular tumors applies to this section as well. Except for the difference in anatomic location, testicular and mediastinal germ cell tumors share many characteristics. All types of germinal tumors found in the testes have been reported in the mediastinum.[25] Extragonadal germ cell tumors are usually situated along the body midline, from the cranium to the mediastinum, and in the retroperitoneal and presacral areas. The histogenesis of these tumors is not clear. Those arising within the thymus presumably originate from germ cells which may have migrated into this gland during embryogenesis. Since the urogenital ridge extends from C6 to L4, its juxtaposition to the thymic anlage would favor such a possibility. Alternatively, germ cell tumors may arise from a maldevelopment of thymic anlage during embryogenesis; or from potentially biphasic germ cells left within the thymus.

These tumors are considered under the heading of thymic neoplasms since there is little doubt that they arise within this gland. Many studies have been performed demonstrating that they do not represent metastases from a primary gonadal site. Autopsies of patients with these tumors have enabled pathologists to examine multiple sections of the patient's gonads. No evidence of testicular or ovarian involvement with the germinal tumor has been found in the vast majority of patients with mediastinal germ cell tumors.[25] Other autopsy studies of patients with germ cell tumors of the testes have shown that metastases solely to the anterior mediastinum do not occur.[58] If anterior mediastinal metastases are present, middle and posterior mediastinal nodes are also involved.[59]

It is also convenient to consider these tumors under the heading of thymic neoplasms so that they can be clearly differentiated from thymomas, carcinoid tumors of the thymus, lymphomas, and primary carcinomas of the mediastinum. These tumors may have a similar microscopic structure. Because of the morphologic similarities among these four thymic neoplasms, they may be confused with each other. Electron microscopy has been helpful in differentiating them.[25]

Several classifications of germ cell tumors have been devised. Mediastinal germ cell tumors often are difficult to fit into any classification because they contain mixtures of various types. Rosai and Levine divide mediastinal germ cell tumors into germinomas (seminomas), adult teratomas, embryonal carcinoma, teratocarcinomas, choriocarcinomas, and yolk sac tumors (endodermal sinus tumors).[25] A simpler system of classification is one which considers tumors as either pure seminomas or nonseminomatous carcinomas.[59] The latter may be pure embryonal carcinomas or embryonal carcinomas containing seminomatous, teratoid (teratocarcinomas), trophoblastic (choriocarcinoma), entodermal sinus elements. The wide variation in terminology and the mixed composition of these malignant tumors make it reasonable to classify them as seminomatous and nonseminomatous types. This division separates the tumors on the basis of their treatment and also as to their prognosis. Seminomas have a better prognosis and are more responsive to therapy than the other malignant germ cell tumors of the mediastinum.

Benign (Adult) Teratomas

These tumors frequently occur in young adults with equal incidence in both sexes. Approximately 80% of all mediastinal teratomatous tumors are benign.[1] In adults, mediastinum is the second most frequent location of a teratoma, the first being the gonads. In children, the sacrococcygeal area is the most frequent site of teratomas, followed by the mediastinum.

Teratomas are found almost exclusively in the anterosuperior mediastinum, at the junction of the heart and great vessels. Calcifications are present in 75% of the lesions. Occasionally, they may be found in the pericardium or posterior mediastinum. The tumors contain representations of all three germ layers in a rather mature state. When the lesions are cystic and contain hair and teeth, they have been referred to as "dermoid cysts." This term is a misnomer since these tumors, like the ovarian "dermoids," are not of ectodermal origin.

Most patients with teratomas are asymptomatic. Those with symptoms have them due to the size of the tumor. They have been reported to reach 30 cm in diameter. Erosion into a bronchus is an uncommon complication as is rupture into the pericardium. Insulin production by a teratoma may produce hypoglycemia.

Benign teratomas are easily excised after exposing them through a sternal-splitting or standard thoracotomy incision.

Seminoma (Germinoma) of the Mediastinum

This tumor can be confused with thymoma, lymphoma, and carcinoid because of the similarity of their microscopic structure. Seminomas of the mediastinum occur in men 20 years to 40 years of age. Up to 5% of these tumors may occur in women.[60] They usually cause symptoms by virtue of the structures they impinge upon in the anterior mediastinum. In a small percentage of cases, endodermal sinus tumor elements are present in the malignancy, resulting in elevated serum levels of alpha-fetoprotein. Radioimmunoassays may be required to detect this increase. Immunodiffusion technics are usually not sufficiently sensitive.

Gonadal exploration of patients with mediastinal seminoma is only indicated when testicular abnormalities are discovered or when lymphangiography demonstrates involvement of pelvic or retroperitoneal lymph nodes.[61]

Most patients with mediastinal seminoma have extensive involvement of the great vessels when they are first seen. Only 20% could be completely excised in the ten patients reported by Martini and colleagues.[59] However, because this tumor is one of the most radiosensitive tumors one can encounter, local disease can usually be controlled. The response of seminomas to radiation therapy is in marked contrast to the nonseminomatous germ cell tumors which are radioresistant.

Treatment is based on the experience garnered from the treatment of patients with similar tumors of the testes. Surgery plays a vital role in diagnosis and tumor reduction ("debulking"). Radiotherapy should be given to all patients. When tumor is present, regression can be seen after 2000 rads to 3000 rads over 2 weeks to 3 weeks. Since the supraclavicular, infracleavicular and low cervical lymph nodes can be easily included in the field of radiation, it is recommended that these areas be treated as well.[62] Prophylactic irradiation of the abdominal para-aortic lymph nodes is not necessary. The combination of surgery and radiotherapy will result in a 58%

to 81% five-year survival rate.[62,63] Martini and colleages reported that the local component of mediastinal seminomas could be controlled by resection and radiation in all patients with this tumor regardless of the extent of mediastinal involvement.[59] The majority of patients in their series had disseminated disease which caused the patient's demise. For this reason they recommended early systemic chemotherapy even if there is no disease evident outside the mediastinum.

Reynolds and colleagues reviewed the status of chemotherapy for mediastinal seminomas and concluded that the effectiveness of chemotherapy as an adjuvant to surgery and radiation therapy is unknown.[63] However, chemotherapy can be effective in the control of seminomas. Alkylating agents have been recommended. A patient treated exclusively with chlorambucil and actinomycin-D was free of disease 11 years after diagnosis. These observations, and the results obtained in the treatment of testicular seminomas, provide an encouraging outlook for patients with mediastinal seminoma.

Nonseminomatous Pure and Mixed Germ-Cell Carcinomas of the Mediastinum

The following discussion applies to pure nonseminomatous germ cell tumors and mixed germ cell carcinomas with seminomatous, embryonal endodermal sinus, teratomatous, or trophoblastic elements. The latter have the appearance and functional characteristics of a choriocarcinoma. Teratocarcinomas can be cystic or solid. All of these tumors have a definite predilection for men. Of 20 patients with mixed germ-cell carcinomas of the mediastinum of various kinds treated at Memorial Sloan-Kettering Cancer Center from 1949 through 1971, 14 were male and 6 were female.[59] In many smaller series, all of the patients have been males. The majority of patients are 15 to 35 years of age. Pleuritic or substernal pain with dyspnea, cough, and hemoptysis are frequent presenting symptoms. Gynecomastia is present in one-half to one-third of men with choriocarcinoma. Elevated levels of the beta subunit of immunoreactive human chorionic gonadotrophin may also be present in patients with choriocarcinoma and can be used to evaluate the efficacy of therapy and detect early recurrences and metastases. Serum levels of alpha-fetoprotein and carcinoembryonic antigen may also be helpful in identifying some of these tumors preoperatively. These markers can also be used to follow the tumor's response to therapy and to detect recurrences. Patients with Klinefelter's syndrome may be predisposed to the development of extragonadal germ cell tumors and should be followed carefully with this in mind.[64]

Teratocarcinomas usually contain elements of embryonal cell carcinoma, but other malignant components may be present such as adenocarcinoma, squamous cell carcinoma, and sarcoma.[65] Beattie has vividly described the course of one patient with this lesion who gained widespread attention because of his football playing career prior to developing this disease.[66] Brian Piccolo's death within a year of his diagnosis was memorialized as a book and on the screen. The rarity of this kind of tumor can be gauged from the experience at Memorial Hospital where, in 1969, this was the only patient with this tumor that they had ever seen.

It is currently the Memorial Hospital's view that mediastinal germ cell tumors of this type (nonseminomatous mixed germ cell tumors) should be treated as Stage III germ cell tumors of the testes. Treatment consists of resecting as much of the tumor as possible followed by combination chemotherapy consisting of vinblastine, actinomycin-D, bleomycin (VAB) and *cis*-diamminedichloroplatinum (*cis*-DDP). The latter may be combined with cyclophosphamide and adriamycin (CAP). Vinblastine, bleomycin, and *cis*-DDP (VBP) may also be effective. When the diagnosis is made by needle biopsy, chemotherapy may precede resection. The role of radiation therapy for control of local and metastatic disease is questionable. Neither irradiation nor surgery can control the local disease for a significant length of time.

Prior to the advent of aggressive combination chemotherapy protocols in the early 1970s, nonseminomatous germ cell tumors of the mediastinum were lethal within a year. Since the introduction of effective VAB and VBP combinations with *cis*-DDP or cyclophosphamide for testicular nonseminomatous cancer, the outlook for patients with these same tumors of the mediastinum has also improved. An objective response rate of 53% was reported by Reynolds and colleagues (10 of 19 patients with mediastinal germ cell tumors).[63] Two patients had complete remission. Beattie predicts that the 60% five-year survival rate for Stage III germ cell tumors of testes can be duplicated for these same malignancies of the mediastinum by the use of multimodality therapy.[66] The poor prognosis of patients with mediastinal germ cell tumors does not appear to result from a difference in malignant potential of these tumors as compared to their testicular counterparts. The delay in diagnosis and subsequent extensive involvement seems to be the basis of the poor results obtained with mediastinal germ cell tumors.

PRIMARY CARCINOMA OF THE MEDIASTINUM

The origin of these rare tumors is indeterminate.[1] About half are highly undifferentiated. The others may have adenocarcinomatous or squamous cell appearance. Since they are most common in the anterosuperior compartment, they may arise from thymic epithelium or embryonic nests within the thymus.

NEUROGENIC TUMORS

Much of the material on neurogenic tumors is covered in Chapter 33 and is applicable to neurogenic tumors of the mediastinum. Only those aspects of the various neoplasms that are peculiar to their mediastinal location will be discussed here.

Neurogenic tumors vie with thymoma as the most common primary neoplasm of the mediastinum in adults and are the most common neoplasms in children. (Table 15-5). They usually arise from the intercostal nerves or the sympathetic ganglia in the posterior mediastinum (Fig. 15-25).[1-6,9,67,68]

Tumors arising from the vagus and phrenic nerves are rarely seen, as are tumors derived from paraganglion cells. The neoplasms may originate from the sheath cells of the nervous system, the neurones themselves or both. Approximately 10% to 20% of mediastinal neurogenic tumors are malignant.

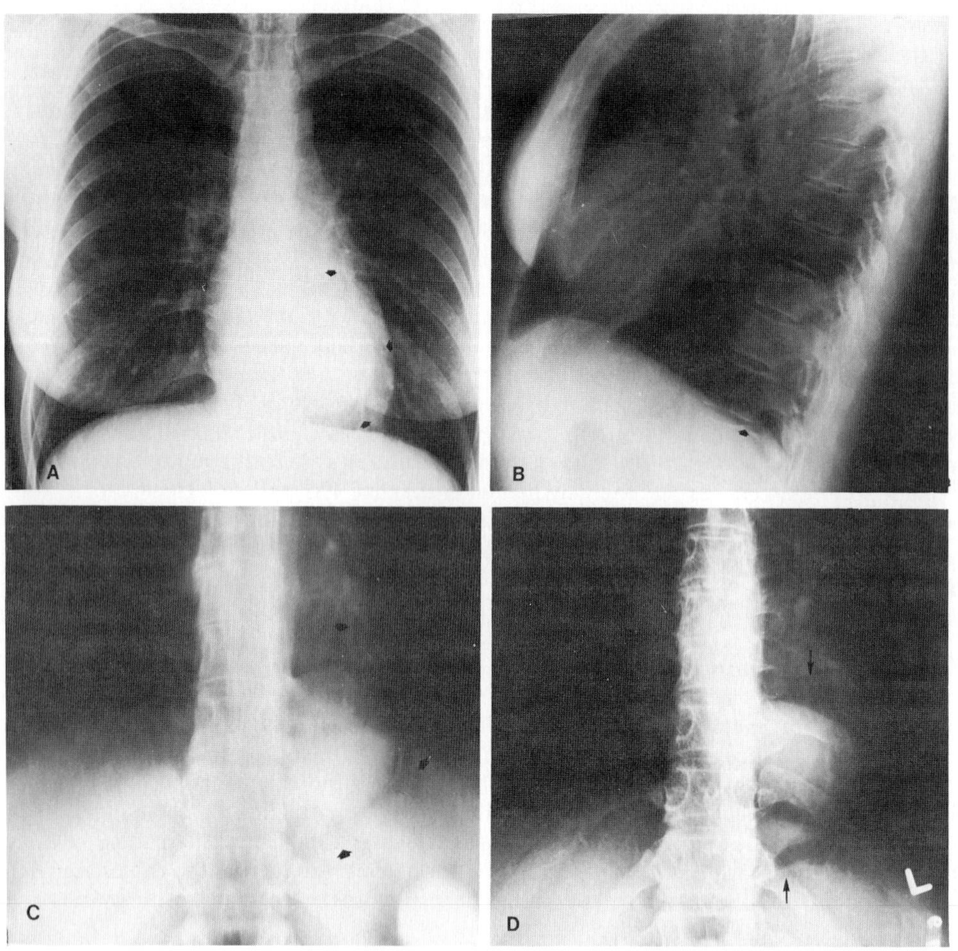

FIG. 15-25. A ganglioneuroma was removed from this 49-year-old woman after a mass lesion was visualized in the posteroanterior (*A*), lateral (*B*), and overpenetrated (*C*) views of the chest and by tomography (*D*).

One unique aspect of neurogenic tumors of the posterior mediastinum is the possibility that they may extend through an intervertebral foramen to assume a dumbbell shape.[67] Among 706 patients with mediastinal neurogenic tumors seen at the Mayo Clinic, 10% presented in this manner. Sixty percent of patients with dumbbell shaped neurogenic tumors have symptoms of spinal cord compression. Roentgenologic studies demonstrating erosion of vertebral pedicles or enlargement of the intervertebral foramina adjacent to a mediastinal mass should suggest the possibility of a dumbbell tumor. A myelogram will establish whether or not there is an intraspinous component of the posterior mediastinal neurogenic tumor. If such is the case, a one-stage combined intra-thoracic and intraspinal approach can be undertaken to completely excise the tumor. The spinal component should be dealt with first to minimize bleeding into the spinal canal. If a dumbbell shaped tumor is inadvertently found during a thoracotomy, a two-stage procedure can be effective. Dumbbell tumors carry the same 10% to 20% malignancy rate that other neurogenic tumors of the posterior mediastinum do.

The most common neurogenic tumors are neurilemomas (Schwannomas), derived from the Schwann cells of the peripheral nerves, and neurofibromas which contain neuronal elements as well as cells derived from the supporting cells. Both tumors can arise from either the intercostal nerves or the sympathetic chain. Patients with neurofibromatosis (von Recklinghausen's disease) more frequently have meningoceles in their posterior mediastinum than neruofibromas when they present with a posterior mediastinal mass. Neurofibrosarcoma (malignant Schwannoma) or neurosarcomas may develop in both types of tumor and carry a poor prognosis.

Ganglioneuromas, and their malignant counterparts, ganglioneuroblastomas and neuroblastomas, arise from the sympathetic ganglia. The benign tumors are easily excised at the time of thoracotomy. The malignant tumors are often unresectable. Their treatment is the same as those encountered elsewhere in the body.

Intrathoracic pheochromocytomas do not differ from those arising in the abdomen. Chemodectomas (paragangliomas) of the thorax may be locally invasive, involving the aorta and its branches and the pulmonary artery.

MESENCHYMAL TUMORS

Most of the connective tissue tumors found in the soft tissues and discussed in Chapter 29 can also be found in the mediastinum. They constitute 6% to 7% of mediastinal neoplasms.[1] About half are malignant. Benign tumors are permanently eradicated by surgical excision. Malignant mesenchymal tumors should be treated as all soft tissue sarcomas with combined modality therapy, that is, resection, radiation, and chemotherapy.

Seventy-five percent of mediastinal lipomas are located anteriorly and may present the same roentgenographic appearance as a pericardial cyst in the right cardiophrenic angle. Large lipomas extend into adjacent mediastinal compartments in an unpredictable manner. Liposarcomas on the other hand tend to occur in the posterior compartment where they may be confused with neurogenic tumors and the rare xanthogranulomas. Lipomatous tumors can be readily recognized by CT.

Mediastinal lymphangiomas can prove to be difficult tumors to completely excise since they grow in a budding fashion and become densely adherent to the great vessels and other mediastinal structures. They are most often found in the anterior mediastinum.

Mesotheliomas may also present as mediastinal masses arising from parietal or pericardium. When they are localized, resection is curative. Diffuse invasive lesions have a poorer prognosis. Histologic criteria cannot differentiate benign from malignant lesions.

REFERENCES

1. Silverman NA, Sabiston DC Jr: Primary tumors and cysts of the mediastinum. In Curr Probl Cancer, Vol. 11, Chicago, Year Book, 1977
2. Oldham HN Jr: Mediastinal Tumors and Cysts. Ann Thorac Surg 11:246, 1971
3. Hammon JW Jr, Sabiston DC Jr: The mediastinum. In Ellis HE, Goldsmith HS (eds): Thoracic Surgery, Hagerstown, Maryland, Harper and Row, 1979
4. Lyons HA, Calvy GL, Sammons BP: The diagnosis and classification of mediastinal masses: 1. A study of 782 cases. Ann Int Med 51:897, 1959
5. Burkell CC, Cross JM, Kent HP et al: Mass lesions of the mediastinum. In Curr Prob Surg Chicago, Year Book, 1969
6. Herlitzka AJ, Gale JW: Tumors and cysts of the mediastinum, Arch Surg 76:697, 1958
7. Grosfeld JL, Weinberger M, Kilman JW et al: Primary mediastinal neoplasms in infants and children. Ann Thorac Surg 12:179, 1971
8. Hasse W: Die Geschwuelste des Mediastinums in Kindesalter. Arch chir 322:1235, 1968
9. Wychulis AR, Payne WS, Clagett OT et al: Surgical treatment of mediastinal tumors. J Thorac Cardiovasc Surg 62:379, 1971
10. Kreel L: Selective thymic venography: New method for visualization of the thymus. Br Med J 1:406, 1967
11. Oldham HN, Sabiston DC Jr: Primary tumors and cysts of the mediastinum. Arch Surg 96:71, 1968
12. Strother CM, Schett JS, Crummy AB et al: Clinical application of computerized fluoroscopy; the extracranial carotid arteries. Radiology 136:781, 1980
13. Sone S, Higashihara T, Morimoto S et al: Normal anatomy of thymus and anterior mediastinum by pneumomediastinography. Am J Roentgenol 134:81, 1980
14. Lissner J: Value of pneumomediastinum in the differential diagnosis of mediastinal lesions. Fortschr Roentgenstrahl 91:445, 1959
15. Hare WSC, Mackay IR: Thymic size in systemic lupus erythematosus. Arch Intern Med 124:60, 1969
16. Irwin RS, Braman SS, Arvanitidis AN et al: Thyroid scanning in preoperative diagnosis of mediastinal goiter. Ann Intern Med 89:73, 1978
17. Masadka A, Kyo S: Selenomethionine scintigraphy in mediastinal diseases. J Thorac Cardiovasc Surg 75:419, 1978
18. Heitzman ER, Goldwin RL, Proto AV: Radiologic analysis of the mediastinum utilizing computed tomography. Radiol Clin N Am 15:309, 1977
19. Livesay JJ, Mink JH, Fee HJ et al: The use of computed tomography to evaluate suspected mediastinal tumors. Ann Thorac Surg 27:305, 1979
20. McLoud TC, Wittenberg J, Ferrucci JT: Computed tomography of the thorax and standard radiographic evaluation of the chest: A comparative study. J Computer (Assit) Tomography 3:170, 1979
21. Goldwin RL, Heitzman ER, Proto AV: Computed tomography of the mediastinum: Normal anatomy and indications for the use of CT. Radiology 124:235, 1977
22. Leigh TF: Mass lesions of the mediastinum. Radiologic Clin N Am 1:377, 1963
23. Bell RH, Knapp BI, Anson BJ et al: Form, size, blood-supply and relations of the adult thymus. Quart Bull Northwest Univ Med Sch 28:156, 1954
24. Sloan HE Jr: The thymus in myasthenia gravis. Surgery 13:154, 1943
25. Rosai J, Levine GD: Tumors of the thymus. Atlas of Tumor Pathology, Second Series, Fascicle 13. Washington DC, Armed Forces Institute of Pathology, 1976
26. Ham AW, Cormack DH: Histology 8th ed. Philadelphia, J.B. Lippincott 1979
27. Schulof RS, Goldstein AL: Thymosin and the endocrine thymus. Adv Int Med 22:121, 1977
28. Trainin N: Thymic hormones and the immune response. Physiol Rev 54:272, 1974
29. Katz A, Lattes R: Granulomatous thymoma or Hodgkin's disease of thymus? Cancer 23:1, 1969
30. Keller AR, Castleman B: Hodgkin's disease of the thymus gland. Cancer 33:1615, 1974
31. Bergh NP, Gatzinsky P, Larsson S et al: Tumors of the thymus and thymic region: I. Clinicopathological studies of thymomas. Ann Thorac Surg 25:91, 1978
32. LeGolvan DP, Abell MR: Thymomas. Cancer 39:2142, 1977
33. Gray GF, Gutowski WT: Thymoma: A clinicopathologic study of 54 cases. Am J Surg Pathol 3:235, 1979
34. Gerein AN, Srivastava SP, Burgess J: Thymoma: A ten year review. Am J Surg 136:49, 1978
35. Salyer WR, Eggleston JC: Thymoma: A clinical and pathological study of 65 cases. Cancer 37:229, 1976
36. Batata MA, Martini N, Huvos AG et al: Thymomas: Clinicopathologic features, therapy, and prognosis. Cancer 34:389, 1974
37. Fechner RE: Recurrence of noninvasive thymomas. Cancer 23:1423, 1969
38. Welch KJ, Tapper D, Vawter GP: Surgical treatment of thymic cysts and neoplasms in children. J Ped Surg 14:691, 1979
39. Bowie PR, Teixeira OHP, Carpenter B: Malignant thymoma in a nine-year-old boy presenting with pleuropericardial effusion. J Thorac Cardiovasc Surg 77:777, 1979
40. Souadjian JV, Enriquez P, Silverstein MN et al: The spectrum of diseases associated with thymoma. Arch Intern Med 134:374, 1974
41. Drachman DB: Myasthenia gravis. New Engl J Med 298:136 and 186, 1978
42. Lindstron J: Autoimmune response to acetylcholine receptors in myasthenia gravis and its animal model. Adv Immunol 27:1, 1979
43. Alpert LI, Papatestas A, Kark A et al: Histologic reappraisal of thymus in myasthenia gravis. Arch Path 91:55, 1971
44. vanderGeld HWR, Strauss ALJ: Myasthenia gravis: Immunological relationship between striated muscle and thymus. Lancet 1:57, 1966
45. Shellito J, Khandekar JD, McKeever WP, et al: Invasive thymoma responsive to oral corticosteroids. Cancer Treat Reports 62:1397, 1978
46. Zeok JV, Todd EP, Dillon M et al: The role of thymectomy in red cell aplasia. Ann Thorac Surg 28:257, 1979

47. Bernatz PE, Khonsari S, Harrison EG, et al: Thymoma: Factors influencing prognosis. Surg Clin N Am 53:885, 1973
48. Wilkins EW, Castleman B: Thymoma: A continuing survey at the Massachusetts General Hospital. Ann Thorac Surg 28:252, 1979
49. Tanabe T, Kubo Y, Hashimoto M, et al: Patch angioplasty of the superior vena caval obstruction (case reports with long fellow-up results). J Cardiovasc Surg 20:519, 1979
50. Ariaratnam LS, Kalnicki S, Mincer F et al: The management of malignant thymoma with radiation therapy. Int J Radiat Oncol Biol Phys 5:77, 1979
51. Penn CRH, Hope-Stone HF: The role of radiotherapy in the management of malignant thymoma Br J Surg 59:533, 1972
52. Sellors, TH, Thackray AC, Thomson AD: Tumors of the thymus. Thorax 22:193, 1967
53. Skeggs DBL: Complications associated with the radiotherapy of thymic tumors. Proc Roy Soc Med 66:155, 1973
54. Boston B: Chemotherapy of invasive thymoma. Cancer 38:49, 1976
55. Levine GD, Rosai J: Thymic hyperplasi and neoplasia: A review of current concepts. Hum Patho 9:495, 1978
56. Salyer WR, Salyer DC, Eggleston JC: Carcinoid tumors of the thymus. Cancer 37:958, 1976
57. Wick MR, Scott RE, Li C-Y et al: Carcinoid tumor of the thymus. Mayo Clin Proc 55:246, 1980
58. Luna MA, Valenzuela-Tamariz J: Germ-cell tumors of the mediastinum, postmortem findings. Am J Clin Pathol 65:450, 1976
59. Martini N, Golbey RB, Hajdu SJ et al: Primary mediastinal germ cell tumors. Cancer 33:763, 1974
60. Polansky, SM, Barwick KW, Ravin CE: Primary mediastinal seminoma. Am J Roentgenol 132:17, 1979
61. Medini E, Levitt SH, Jones TK et al: The management of extratesticular seminoma without gonadal involvement. Cancer 44:2032, 1979
62. Schantz A, Sewall W, Castleman B: Mediastinal germinoma. Cancer 30:1189, 1972
63. Reynolds TF, Yagoda A, Vugrin D et al: Chemotherapy of mediastinal germ cell tumors. Semin Oncology 6:113, 1979
64. Sogge MR, McDonald SD, Cofold PB: The malignant potential of the dysgenetic germ cell in Klinefelter's syndrome. Am J Med 66:515, 1979
65. Fox RM, Woods RL, Tattersall MH, et al: Undifferentiated carcinoma in young men: The atypical teratoma syndrome. Lancet 1:1316, 1979
66. Beattie EJ Jr: Mediastinal germ cell tumors (surgery). Semin Oncology 6:109, 1979
67. Akwari OE, Payne WS, Onofrio BM et al: Dumbbell neurogenic tumors of the mediastinum. Mayo Clin Proc 53:353, 1978
68. Gale AW, Jelihovsky T, Grant AF et al: Neurogenic tumors of the mediastinum. Ann Thorac Surg 17:434, 1974

Jerry C. Rosenberg
James G. Schwade
Vainutis K. Vaitkevicius

CHAPTER 16

Cancer of the Esophagus

Avenzoar (Ibn Zuhr), practicing medicine during the 12th century, described the manifestations of what must have been a cancer of the esophagus. He wrote about a condition, "beginning with mild pain and difficulty in swallowing, and going on gradually to its complete prevention." Avenzoar treated these patients with silver sounds and nutritive enemas, palliative measures which were not improved upon for close to 750 years.[1]

Through the centuries, pathological studies have made reference to cancers of the esophagus. Nicholas Tulp of Amsterdam (the central figure in Rembrandt's *School of Anatomy*) recorded, "a tumor like carcinoma" of the esophagus which narrowed the lumen to such a degree that he could barely pass a probe through it. Descriptions of the clinical manifestations of esophageal cancer have been attributed to two other famous physicians of the Netherlands, Hermann Boerhaave and his student, Gerhard van Swieten.[1]

More aggressive attempts than those of Avenzoar at improving the lot of patients with malignant obstruction of the esophagus were undertaken in the middle of the 19th century. Sèdillot of Strassbourg is credited with performing the first gastrostomy upon a human in 1849.[2] The patient suffered from severe dysphagia. At autopsy, an epithelial tumor of the esophagus was found. Unfortunately, the patient succumbed less than 24 hours after the operation. In 1877 Czerny resected a carcinoma of the cervical esophagus without attempting to restore continuity of the esophagus.[3]

The first successful resection of a thoracic esophageal malignancy was performed in 1913 in New York City by Franz Torek.[4] He did not attempt to reconstruct the gastrointestinal tract, choosing to allow the patient, a 67-year-old woman, to use an external rubber tube to connect a cervical esophagostomy to a gastrostomy tube while eating. The patient survived for 13 years following this procedure. Kirschner proposed an esophagogastrostomy to reconstruct the esophagus after esophagectomy in 1920.[5] The latter form of reconstruction in an intrathoracic position, following esophagectomy, was first reported in Japan by Ohsawa in 1932.[6] It was first performed in the United States by Adams and Phemister in 1938.[7]

Because of the high mortality following resection of the esophagus during the third and fourth decades of the 20th century, radiation therapy was often chosen as a means of controlling the growth and spread of these malignancies. Radiation therapy for esophageal carcinoma was introduced in the 1920s using radium bougies and external radiation. For the latter, equipment in the 250 KeV range was used. Radium bougies were applied intermittently with disappointing results.[8] Deep seated lesions such as carcinomas of the esophagus were poorly handled by external radiation using orthovoltage therapy. Skin reactions and damage to structures close to the esophagus were frequent. In 1945, Nielsen reported on the use of radiation as primary treatment for esophageal cancer and introduced the use of a rotating chair to limit the side effects of the roentgen beam.[9]

Progress in the development of thoracic surgery after World War II stimulated more vigorous operative therapy for esophageal cancer. However, by the 1950s, the poor results obtained by surgical procedures and the development of radiotherapy units in the megavoltage range persuaded many clinicians to resort to radiotherapy rather than surgery for the treatment of this disease. These two forms of therapy have competed for patients with neither of them demonstrating clear-cut superiority over the other.

Despite all that surgeons have accomplished in recent years and the advances that have been made in radiation therapy, the outlook for patients with cancer of the esophagus remains poor. The five year survival for a white population from 1965 to 1969, adjusted for normal life expectancy, was 2% for men and 6% for women.[10]

Lack of progress in curative approaches to cancer of the esophagus has led to a great deal of pessimism when considering the treatment of this disease. Many oncologists, be they surgical, radiation or medical, emphasize palliation rather than cure. Palliation is an important consideration with this malignancy since patients suffer greatly with malignant esophageal obstruction and tracheoesophageal fistulae. However, it is not often necessary to separate objectives of management into palliation and cure; these two objectives can be integrated into a plan of management which will hopefully accomplish both without one compromising the other. A general plan of management which incorporates curative and palliative measures in the treatment of cancer of the esophagus is shown in Fig. 16-1. This type of approach was most succinctly and precisely stated by Burdette who advocated a plan of management for carcinoma of the esophagus, ". . . in which palliative measures were a part of the sequence leading to cure rather than a separate route of management."[11] As Fig. 16-1 indicates, the three major cancer treatment modalities play an important role in the curative and palliative treatment of esophageal cancer.

ETIOLOGIC AND EPIDEMIOLOGIC CONSIDERATIONS

The incidence of cancer of the esophagus in the United States is low (6:100,000 in men and 1.6:100,000 in women).[12]

FIG. 16-1. A flow chart that outlines treatment options for patients with esophageal cancer. Both curative and palliative measures are integrated into this plan of therapy, which utilizes a combined modality approach to the cure and palliation of esophageal cancer.

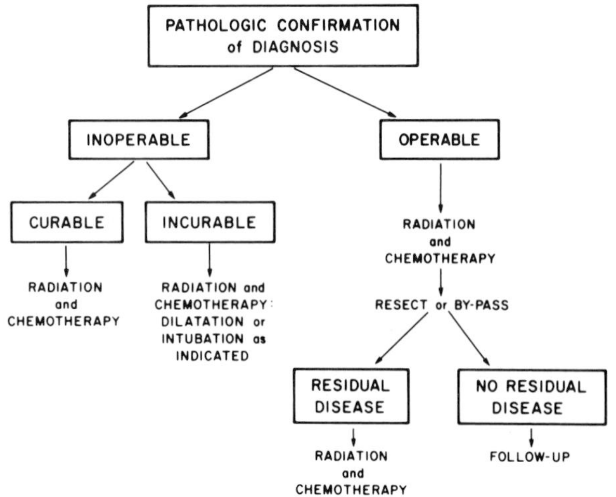

Esophageal cancer is responsible for 7000 to 8000 deaths per year. It constitutes 1.5% of all cancers and 7% of all gastrointestinal carcinomas. These data apply to the United States only and are by no means representative of the incidence of this disease throughout the world or among different groups within a given country. Geographic variations in incidence are greater for squamous cell carcinoma of the esophagus than for any other tumor. Furthermore, many areas of high incidence are located in close proximity to areas of low incidence. In China, the highest rates were found in the mountainous northern provinces where rates, adjusted for age and sex, were 139:100,000. Not far from this area an incidence of 1.4:100,000 was found.[13] In the course of this study, chickens in the county where esophageal cancer was frequent were also found to have this tumor. This observation led to the discovery of nitrosamine compounds in food samples from areas of high incidence.[13]

In Curacao, where esophageal cancer is the most common malignant tumor for both men and women, cocarcinogens have been extracted from the shrub *Croton flaveus*.[14] The leaves and roots of this plant are chewed or used to brew tea.

Examples of variations in the geographic distribution of esophageal cancer can also be found in Africa, where it has been noted that the incidence has changed with time.[15] The incidence of esophageal cancer increased dramatically between 1940 and 1950 in the Transkei region of the Cape Province in South Africa. Prior to 1940, the disease was unknown. The incidence among black males 35 to 64 years of age is now 246:100,000. In Nigeria (West Africa), the comparable incidence is 3:100,000. The sex ratio (males:females) is also much higher among the black population of Cape Province than among the white people (9:1 for blacks versus 4:1 for whites). Environmental factors, rather than genetic, are responsible for these phenomena. Certain alcoholic drinks (home brewed beer) and tobacco or snuff may be responsible for the increased incidence. The etiologic relationships in the Transkei, as well as in China and Curacao are by no means clear.

Perhaps the area of the world with the highest incidence and most obscure etiologic relationships is in Iran and the U.S.S.R. around the Caspian Sea.[16] There is no significant alcohol consumption among the Moslem population in this area; nor is tobacco consumption of great consequence. Dietary factors are most suspect. The Caspian littoral forms part of an "Asian esophageal cancer belt" which extends up through China (Fig. 16-2). However, within this area there are striking variations in the frequency and sex incidence. The age-standardized incidence rates in Gorgan and Gonbad in the northeastern parts of the province of Mazandaran in Iran, is approximately 108:100,000 for males and 174:100,000 for females.[16]

Cancer of the esophagus is common in France, Switzerland, Finland, Iceland, and Puerto Rico (Fig. 16-3). The disease is less frequently seen in Norway, Britain, and Australia, and among the white population of the United States. Alcohol consumption is thought to be related to cancer of the esophagus in the U.S.A., Britain, France (Brittany), Sweden, and Japan. Tobacco consumption may be related to the etiology of this tumor in the U.S.A., France, Britain, Sweden, India, and South Africa.

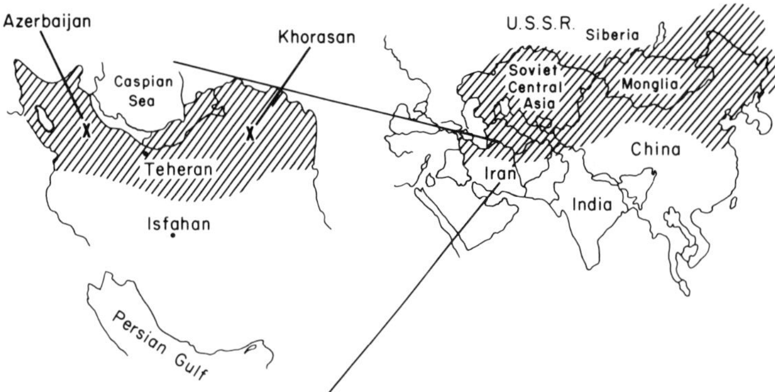

FIG. 16-2. An "esophageal cancer belt" extends across Asia from the southern shore of the Caspian Sea in Iran, through Soviet Central Asia and Mongolia, to Northern China. The incidence of cancer of the esophagus in the area around the Caspian Sea is higher than any other area in the world. (Kmet J, Mahboubi E: Esophageal cancer in the Caspian littoral of Iran: Initial studies. Science 175:846, 1972)

Tobacco and excessive alcoholic intake are widely accepted as two factors which contribute to the development of squamous cell carcinoma of the esophagus in many western countries. Racial and genetic factors have been studied with inconclusive results. Esophageal cancer is more frequent and aggressive in blacks depending upon the geographic area and is independent of whether the disease is common or rare.[17]

The incidence of cancer of the esophagus in blacks in the United States is at least three times greater than in whites (Table 16-1).[17-19] It is also more frequently seen in poorer socioeconomic groups. In the past 25 years the mortality rate for esophageal cancer in blacks has increased 105%.[17] Mortality from cancer of the esophagus in blacks 35 to 54 years of age is second only to lung cancer.[19] It has been postulated that increased tobacco and alcohol consumption among blacks or nutritional factors may account for this increased risk. However, other factors, possibly ethnic, may be involved.[17,20,21]

FIG. 16-3. Age-adjusted mortality rate for esophageal cancer in various countries in the years from 1966 to 1967. (Levin DL, Devesa SS, Goodwin ID et al: Cancer Rates and Risks, 2nd ed. Washington, DC, National Institutes of Health, 1974)

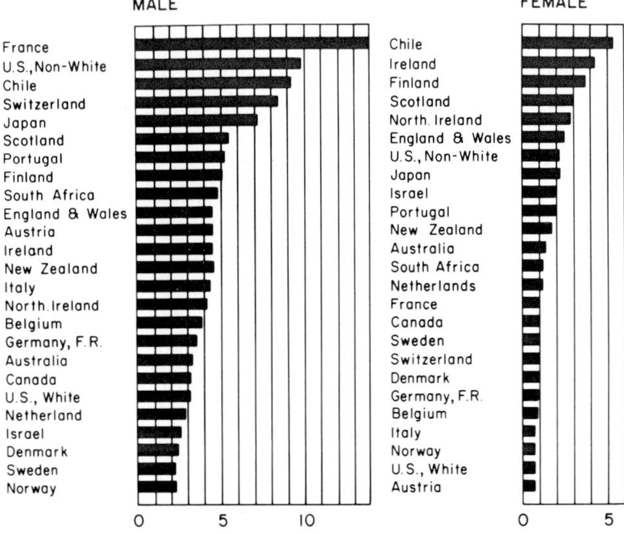

Attempts at correlating genetic factors with an increased incidence of esophageal cancer have failed to reveal a significant relationship. The one exception to this statement pertains to patients with tylosis.[22] Tylosis is a rare syndrome characterized by hyperkeratoses of the palms and soles and papillomata of the esophagus. Its occurrence is determined by an autosomal dominant gene. Seventy percent of patients with tylosis will develop squamous cell carcinoma of the esophagus.

Achalasia of 25 years duration or longer is another disease associated with an increased incidence of squamous cell carcinoma of the esophagus.[23,24] The incidence is about 7% of all patients with this condition. At least half of the cancers are located in the middle third of the esophagus.

Adenocarcinoma of the esophagus is often a direct extension from adenocarcinoma of the stomach. When adenocarcinoma is primary in the esophagus, it usually arises in a columnar epithelium-lined esophagus (Barrett's esophagus). The latter is most often the consequence of prolonged reflux esophagitis. It has been estimated that of the infrequent primary adenocarcinomas of the esophagus, 86% arise from a columnar epithelium-lined mucosa.[25,26]

Nutritional factors have been implicated as etiologic agents. The nitrosamines found in high concentration in the food in North China may be related to the etiology of esophageal cancer in this part of the world, but they have not been found to be significant elsewhere. Further suspicion of nutritional factors involved in this disease are derived from the observation that there is a wide variation in incidence rates for men and women (from 5:1 to 1:1). Since sideropenic anemia, glossitis, and esophagitis (Plummer-Vinson or Patterson-Kelly syndrome) is associated with 10% incidence of esophageal or pharyngeal cancer and is more frequent in women, nutritional

TABLE 16-1. Incidence of Cancer of Esophagus by Race

	WHITE	BLACK
MALE	6.0	19.5
FEMALE	1.6	4.2

1969, Third National Cancer Survey, Incidence per 100,000

deficiencies have been sought as predisposing factors. No clear cut relationships have been found. Heavy seasoning of foods, hot foods, and liquids have been implicated, as have the use of betel nut, tanin-rich foods, contamination of food with silica particles, trace metal deficiencies and excesses, and vitamin deficiences. Consideration has been given to poor oral hygiene, air pollution, radiation, exposure to asbestos, and previous gastric surgery as etiologic factors. These are speculations with little evidence to support them.

The patient with a lye stricture of the esophagus has a 5% chance of developing esophageal cancer.[27] An increased incidence of cancer of the esophagus has also been suspected in patients with epiphrenic diverticula of the esophagus and in patients with esophageal webs.

ANATOMIC CONSIDERATIONS OF CLINICAL SIGNIFICANCE

The esophagus begins at the level of C6, below the cricoid cartilage, where the cricopharyngeus muscle separates it from the pharynx. As it passes through the neck and the superior and posterior mediastinum, the esophagus follows the vertebral column, veering toward the left, passing in front of the aorta, to join the stomach beneath the diaphragm. The length of the esophagus, from pharynx to stomach, ranges from 23 cm to 30 cm.

Endoscopists localize lesions in the esophagus by measuring the lesion's distance from the central incisor teeth. By this method of measurement the esophagus begins 15 cm from the central incisors and terminates 38 cm to 45 cm distally beneath the diaphragm. The thoracic inlet, the dividing line between the cervical and thoracic esophagus, is located 20 cm from the central incisors at the level of T1 (Fig. 16-4).

The cervical esophagus is about 5 cm long. It extends down to the thoracic inlet at the level of T1. The first 3 cm are located behind the larynx. This segment is referred to as the postcricoid portion of the cervical esophagus. Malignancies in this area present a special problem and are fully discussed in Chapter 13 (Cancer in the Head and Neck). The anatomic

FIG. 16-4. Anatomic relationship and major subdivisions of the esophagus.

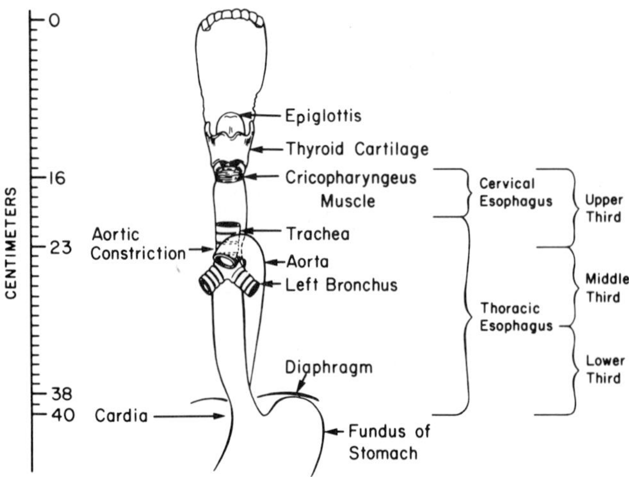

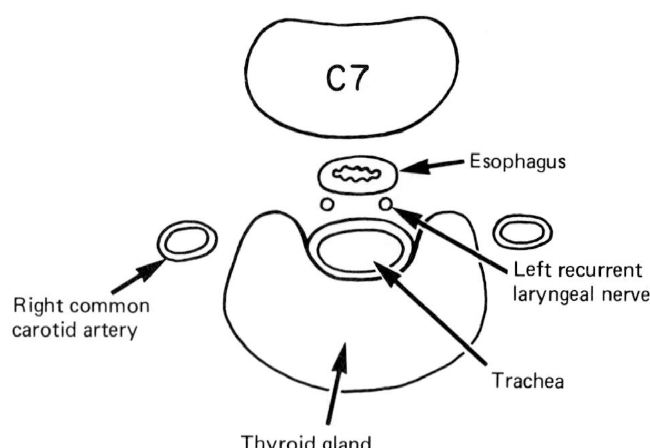

FIG. 16-5. Diagramatic cross-sectional anatomic depiction of the relationship of the distal cervical and proximal thoracic esophagus.

relationships of the distal portion of the cervical esophagus and proximal thoracic esophagus are shown in Fig. 16-5.

The thoracic esophagus begins at the thoracic inlet at the level of the clavicles, and ends at T10. As the esophagus passes down the posterior mediastinum toward the left of the mid-line, it lies close behind the tracheal bifurcation and left main stem bronchus. This occurs at the level of T4 or T5, about 23 cm from the central incisors. The arch of the aorta passes in front of the left side of the esophagus at this level, producing a shallow depression which can be seen to pulsate during endoscopy. These close anatomic relationships are demonstrated in Fig. 16-6. Because of the juxtaposition of these organs, malignant lesions in this area of the esophagus have the potential of involving vital structures early in the course of the disease. Tracheo-esophageal fistulae are the most common problems encountered. These anatomic relationships contribute significantly to the higher operative mortality following resection of lesions at the mid-esophageal level.

The esophagus has been arbitrarily subdivided into more sections than just the cervical and thoracic portions. The American Joint Committee for Cancer Staging and End Results Reporting divides the esophagus into three principal regions: (1) The cervical esophagus, from the pharyngoesophageal junction to the level of the thoracic inlet. They consider the latter to be 18 cm from the upper incisor teeth. (2) The upper and midthoracic esophagus, extending from the thoracic inlet to a point 10 cm above the esophagogastric junction. The latter is usually located at T8, 31 cm from the upper incisor teeth. (3) The lower thoracic esophagus, the distal 10 cm of esophagus.[28] The Japanese Society for Esophageal Diseases has a similar system of dividing the esophagus into regions but further subdivides the upper and midthoracic esophagus and the lower esophagus each into two further subdivisions (Fig. 16-7).[29]

Alternatively, the thoracic esophagus can be divided into upper, middle, and lower portions. The upper thoracic esophagus is about 5 cm long, the middle thoracic esophagus about 10 cm long, and the lower thoracic esophagus comprises the distal portion of this organ. One can also subdivide the esophagus into thirds (Fig. 16-4).[30] The cervical esophagus and upper thoracic esophagus would consist of the upper

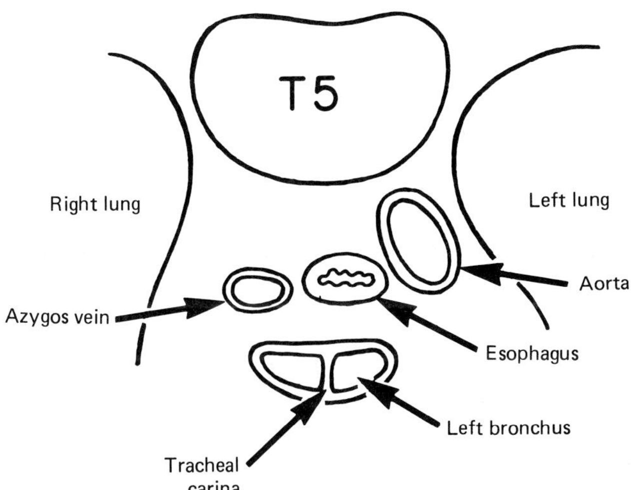

FIG. 16-6. Diagrammatic cross-sectional anatomy depicting the close relationship of the thoracic esophagus to the aorta, trachea, left main stem bronchus, and azygos vein at the mid-thoracic (T4 and T5) level, 23 cm from the central incisors.

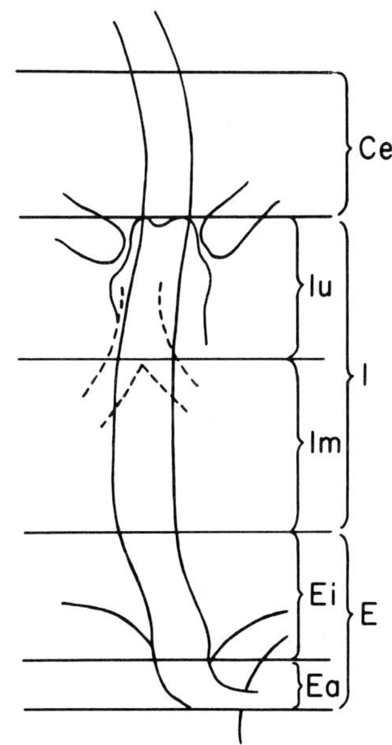

FIG. 16-7. The subdivisions of the esophagus according to the Japanese Society for Esophageal Diseases. *Ce*, cervical esophagus; *I*, thoracic esophagus; *Iu*, upper thoracic esophagus; *Im*, middle thoracic esophagus; *E*, lower esophagus; *Ei*, lower thoracic esophagus; *Ea*, abdominal esophagus. (Japanese Society for Esophageal Diseases: Guidelines for the clinical and pathologic studies on carcinoma of the esophagus. Jap J Surg 6:69, 1976)

third, the middle thoracic esophagus is the middle third, and the lower thoracic esophagus is the lower third. This classification may be most practical since it is the simplest. All subdivisions are arbitrary and malignant lesions often extend beyond the limits of a designated portion of the esophagus. The above discussion is presented to point out the need to define the exact location of an esophageal tumor and its extent, rather than to designate in which portion of the esophagus it is located, since there is wide variation in designating the subdivisions of the esophagus. This recommendation notwithstanding, it has been estimated that 15% of esophageal cancers occur mainly in the upper third of the esophagus (cervical esophagus and upper thoracic esophagus), 50% in the middle third, and 35% in the lower third. These numbers vary from series to series. In some reports, lower third lesions are most common. If operative mortality is excluded, the site of the malignancy in the esophagus does not influence survival.[31]

LYMPHATIC DRAINAGE OF THE ESOPHAGUS

This aspect of esophageal anatomy must be understood in order to explain the pattern of spread of esophageal cancer.[32] Small lymphatic vessels arise within the mucosa and the external muscular coat of the esophagus. These vessels drain into larger lymphatics located in the submucosa and muscular layers of the esophagus respectively (Fig. 16-8). The draining lymphatic channels extend throughout the length of the esophagus and intercommunicate with each other (Fig. 16-9). Thus, lymphatic fluid can follow any one of a great number of pathways before emerging from the esophagus through lymphatic vessels to drain into a lymph node. Tumor cells within the lymphatics have many options with respect to which lymph node system they will drain into. Because of the longitudinal course of the lymphatics and the interconnections between the submucosal and muscular lymphatics draining the esophagus, the pattern of flow to lymph nodes is unpredictable. Flow may be in the direction of adjacent lymph nodes or through the aforementioned network to more distant nodes.

Afferent lymphatics leaving the esophagus to drain into a lymph node tend to follow the arteries which, as a rule, course longitudinally rather than radially. The blood supply to the

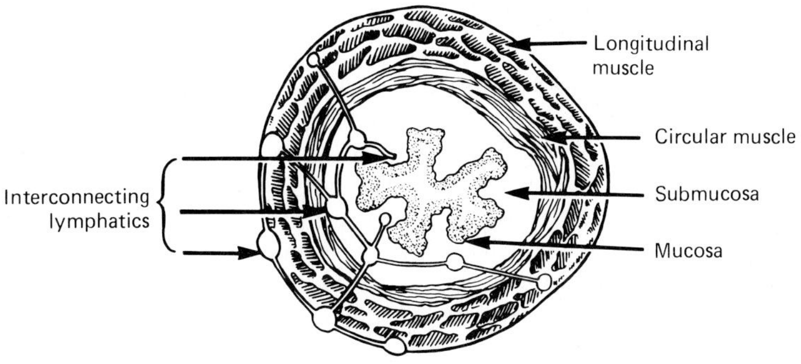

FIG. 16-8. An exaggerated cross-sectional diagrammatic representation of the esophagus, illustrating the disposition of the interconnecting network of submucosal and muscular lymphatics that course the length of the esophagus.

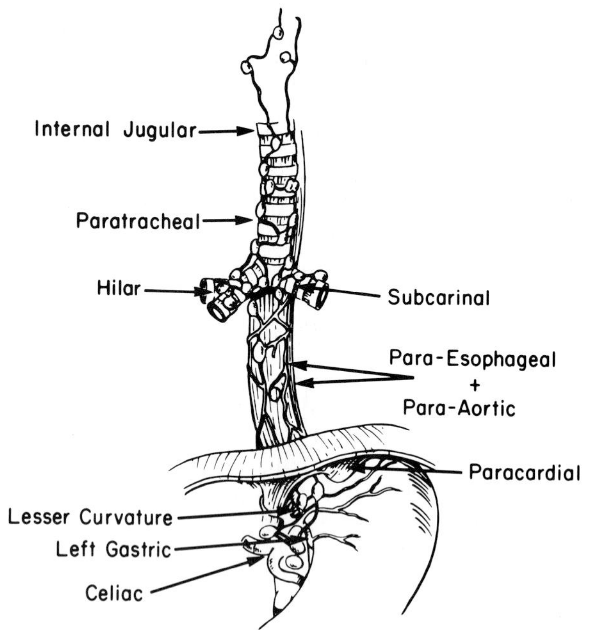

FIG. 16-9. Lymphatics extend throughout the esophagus, draining the esophageal wall (Fig. 16-8) and passing to collections of lymph nodes extending from the neck to the abdomen. Lymph node chains, which may also receive lymphatics from the esophagus, that are not illustrated are the cervical and supraclavicular lymph nodes.

esophagus is not segmental. The primary arteries supplying the esophagus are the inferior thyroid artery, bronchial and esophageal arteries from the aorta, and the left gastric artery.[33] The lymphatics accompanying these arteries drain into the following lymph node chains: internal jugular, cervical, supraclavicular, paratracheal, hilar, subcarinal, paraesophageal, paraaortic, paracardial, lesser curvature, left gastric, and celiac (Fig. 16-9). Involvement of the paratracheal nodes on the right is more common than involvement of those on the left. The lowest right paratracheal lymph node is the azygos node. The posterior hilar lymph nodes are more frequently involved than the other hilar nodes. The paraesophageal and paraaortic group of nodes are part of a chain of lymphatics which extend from the inferior pulmonary vein to the diaphragm. Similarly, the celiac nodes are part of an extensive group of retroperitoneal lymph nodes.

The major lesson to be taken from this brief review of the lymphatic drainage of the esophagus is that there is a longitudinal dual interconnecting system of lymphatics within the esophagus which drain, in a relatively unpredictable manner, into a large number of widely separated collections of lymph nodes. A striking example of this important anatomic feature is the incidence of celiac node involvement with respect to the location of the cancer within the esophagus. An incidence of celiac node involvement of 10% can be found when the esophageal cancer is located in the cervical and upper thoracic esophagus (up to the tracheal bifurcation). The middle third of the esophagus (up to the distal 10 cm of esophagus) may have celiac node involvement in 44% of patients.[34] Another example of the importance of understanding the lymphatic drainage of the esophagus is the phenomena of "skip areas" of involvement.[35] A distance of as much as 8 cm of normal esophagus may be interposed between the site of gross tumor and micrometastases within lymphatic vessels or the esophageal wall.

PATHOLOGY

Non-neoplastic tumors of the esophagus may consist of small islands of gastric heterotopia, cysts of various types (inclusion cysts, retention cysts or duplication cysts) or granulomatous (fibrovascular) polyps.[36]

Benign neoplasms of epithelial origin are rare; the only known one is the squamous cell papilloma. Half the patients with squamous cell papillomas have multiple lesions, as in patients with tylosis. Most patients are asymptomatic. Except for patients with tylosis, it is not clear that these lesions are precursors of squamous cell carcinoma. However, the squamous cell papilloma of the esophagus must be differentiated from the verrucous squamous cell carcinoma (see below). The latter has a similar gross appearance but definite histologic signs of malignancy. Verrucous squamous cell carcinomas have not been shown to arise in benign papillomatous precursor lesions.

The most common benign neoplasm of the esophagus is the leiomyoma, which accounts for 75% of all benign esophageal tumors.[37] Fibromyomas and lipomyomas have also been described. The ratio of leiomyomas to leiomyosarcomas is 100:1. Leiomyomas are found in men two times more often than in women and are most often located in the lower third of the esophagus. In half the patients they are asymptomatic. Treatment of choice is submocosal enucleation. Resection may be required for larger lesions. Under this circumstance, morbidity is increased; however, recurrences are rare. Other benign nonepithelial neoplasms which have been reported to occur in the esophagus are fibromas, lipomas, neurofibromas, giant cell tumors, and osteochondromas.

A list of malignant primary esophageal neoplasms based on the World Health Organization classification is presented in Table 16-2.[36] More than ninety percent of malignant esophageal tumors are squamous cell carcinomas. They arise from the squamous cell epithelium lining the lumen of the esophagus. The well differentiated cancers have the characteristic features of keratin formation (epithelial pearls), intercellular bridges, and minimal pleomorphism. Poorly differentiated tumors do not contain keratin nor demonstrate intercellular bridges and have marked nuclear and cellular pleomorphism. The moderately differentiated tumors are intermediate between these two. The degree of differentiation has not been found to affect the patient's survival, nor does it correlate with lymph node involvement. Thus, the distinction among the different degrees of differentiation does not appear to be of clinical significance.

Spindle-cell carcinoma is a variant of a poorly differentiated squamous cell carcinoma. It is characterized by spindle-shaped cells resembling fibroblasts which may give the tumor the appearance of a sarcoma. When the tumor contains nests of squamous cells with a spindle cell stroma, the term pseudosarcoma has been applied to the cancer. The pseudosarcoma and the carcinosarcoma have been grouped together by recent authors because of their common polypoid

TABLE 16-2. Malignant Esophageal Tumors

EPITHELIAL TUMORS
- Squamous cell carcinoma
  - Well differentiated
  - Moderately differentiated
  - Poorly differentiated
- Variants of squamous cell carcinoma
  - Spindle cell carcinoma
  - Pseudosarcoma and Carcinosarcoma
  - Verrucous carcinoma
  - *In situ* carcinoma
- Adenocarcinoma
  - Adenoacanthoma
- Adenoid cystic carcinoma (cylindroma)
- Mucoepidermoid carcinoma
- Adenosquamous carcinoma
- Carcinoid
- Undifferentiated carcinoma
  - Oat cell carcinoma

NON-EPITHELIAL TUMORS
- Leiomyosarcoma
- Malignant melanoma
- Rhabdomyosarcoma
- Myoblastoma
- Choriocarcinoma

structure on gross examination and the similarity of their histologic appearance.[38]

Verrucous carcinoma is a third variant of squamous cell carcinomas which is well differentiated and is characteristically papillary in appearance.

Areas of dysplasia of the esophageal mucosa, that is, atypical epithelium, should be differentiated from areas *in situ* carcinoma. The former have been found in the esophagus of patients who are predisposed to developing squamous cell carcinoma by way of heavy cigarette smoking.

Primary adenocarcinomas may arise from the sparse submucosal glandular elements within the esophagus or, more frequently, from the columnar epithelium lining of the distal esophagus. It may have a papillary appearance. When small foci of squamous metaplasia are present, the lesion is called an adenoacanthoma.

Cylindromas (adenoid cystic carcinomas) have a characteristic cribriform structure, with glandular and myoepithelial elements, as is seen in the salivary glands and the bronchus. It is rare in the esophagus, as is the mucoepidermoid carcinoma, a tumor comprised of squamous cells and mucus-secreting cells. It is distinguished from the adenosquamous carcinoma which also has adenocarcinomatous and squamous carcinomatous components.

Undifferentiated tumors resembling oat cell carcinomas (APUDomas) have been identified in the esophagus and seem to be increasing in frequency. They arise from argyrophil cells in the esophageal mucosa, predominantly in the lower and middle esophagus of men.[39] This is a highly malignant tumor which occasionally produces paraneoplastic syndromes.

The leiomyosarcoma is the most frequently reported malignant non-epithelial tumor of the esophagus. Metastases occur in 25% of patients with this tumor. Resection is usually effective therapy for the primary lesion. Rhabdomyosarcomas, choriocarcinomas, and myoblastomas of the esophagus have also been reported. Malignant melanoma of the esophagus is more common than these latter lesions, albeit infrequent compared to other malignant tumors of the esophagus. Esophageal melanomas are usually bulky tumors associated with ulceration in most cases.[40,41]

Less than 100 cases of carcinomas metastatic to the esophagus have been reported in the literature. Primary sites have been the breast (most common), pharynx, tonsil, larynx, lung, stomach, liver, kidney, prostate, testicle, bone, and skin.[42]

MALIGNANCIES AT OTHER SITES ASSOCIATED WITH CANCER OF THE ESOPHAGUS

Since cigarette smoking and the excessive consumption of alcoholic beverages are etiologically related to a variety of malignancies, of which cancer of the esophagus is only one, it is understandable that patients with cancer of the esophagus have a higher incidence of other cancers that share the predisposing factors of cigarette smoking and heavy alcoholic consumption. The former increases the risk of developing cancer of the mouth, pharynx, larynx, esophagus, lung, kidney, and bladder. One can expect to see a synchronous or metachronous malignant tumor in 5% to 12% of patients with cancer of the esophagus.[43,44] The oral cavity, pharynx, larynx, and lung are the most frequent sites. About half can be found in the head and neck areas, on the floor of the mouth, the tongue, tonsil, and larynx. Other observers have found that oral and pharyngeal cancers are most often associated with cancer of the esophagus whereas laryngeal cancers are most often associated with cancer of the lung.

At the Memorial Sloan-Kettering Cancer Center 25% of patients with two primary cancers of the oral cavity, pharynx, larynx, and esophagus had the cancers appear synchronously.[43] In 68% they appeared within 2 years of each other. The 60 patients with the multiple primaries came from a pool of 7000 patients seen during the same period of time for one of the aforementioned malignancies.

CLINICAL PRESENTATION AND DIAGNOSIS

The patient with an esophageal cancer is usually between 55 and 65 years of age, with a long-standing history of cigarette smoking and heavy alcohol intake. Dysphagia and weight loss are the initial symptoms of carcinoma of the esophagus in over 90% of patients. It has been observed that difficulty swallowing does not occur until the circumference of the esophagus is narrowed to one-half to one-third of normal. At first the patient has difficulty swallowing coarser foods such as raw vegetables or meat. Finally, liquids are difficult to swallow. Occasionally, the onset is sudden; Most often symptoms have been present for 3 months to 4 months. Pain on swallowing (odynophagia) is seen in about half the patients with cancer of the esophagus. When the pain radiates to the back, spinal column involvement should be suspected. Regurgitation or vomiting and discomfort in the throat, substernal area, or epigastrium may be additional symptoms. Aspiration pneumonia can be another presenting or concomitant feature of the disease. Advanced lesions may present with hematemesis, hemoptysis or melena (10%), persistent cough secondary to an esophagotracheobronchial fistula, dysphonia caused by involvement of the left recurrent laryngeal nerve with laryngeal paralysis, Horner's syndrome, or superior vena caval obstruction. Exsanguinating bleeding may occur when the aorta is involved and a communication is established between the esophagus and the aorta. Other ominous findings are pleural effusion, palpable cervical or supraclavicular lymph nodes, and hepatomegaly. Hematuria can occur with renal involvement. Bone pain is prominent when there are metastases to these structures.

Occasionally a paraneoplastic syndrome is produced by an esophageal tumor. The most common is hypercalcemia unrelated to bone involvement.[45] Gonadotropin and ACTH producing tumors have been described but they are rare.[46]

The gross appearance of an advanced carcinoma of the esophagus is accurately reflected by its radiographic appearance (Fig. 16-10). There are few lesions which can simulate an esophageal carcinoma. Most confusion arises with lesions at the distal end of the esophagus. Adenocarcinomas of the esophagus or stomach, benign tumors, other malignant tumors, peptic strictures, and achalasia may have an appearance similar to squamous cell carcinoma both radiographically and by direct visualization with the esophagoscope.

Obtaining tissue for histopathologic confirmation of the diagnosis may not be easy when visualizing an esophageal tumor through an esophagoscope. Often, the submucosal extension of the tumor will push normal mucosa in front of it and the biopsy forceps will not bite deeply enough to reach the malignant tissue. It is the experience of most endoscopists that brushings of the tumor are more often diagnostic than biopsies (90% versus 70%).[47,48] When both technics are employed and multiple biopsies are obtained, a pathological diagnosis can most often be established. Exfoliative cytology has also been shown to be diagnostically valuable. A careful procedure outlined by the group at the University of Chicago was positive for malignancy in close to 90% of patients with squamous cell carcinoma of the esophagus. In the absence of an esophageal tumor, a negative cytology report was accurate in 98% of the patients.[49]

Small esophageal carcinomas (less than 3.5 cm in length) are not easily identified as malignant lesions by esophagograms. Diagnostic accuracy approaches only 60% under these circumstances. A thickened posterior stripe or band (wider than 4.5 mm) can be identified on the lateral chest x-rays of patients with carcinoma of the esophagus. It has been shown to be caused by peri-esophageal lymphatic involvement and can be seen as early as 6 months prior to the development of symptoms.

FIG. 16-10. An esophagogram. Note the constricting carcinoma of the mid-esophagus.

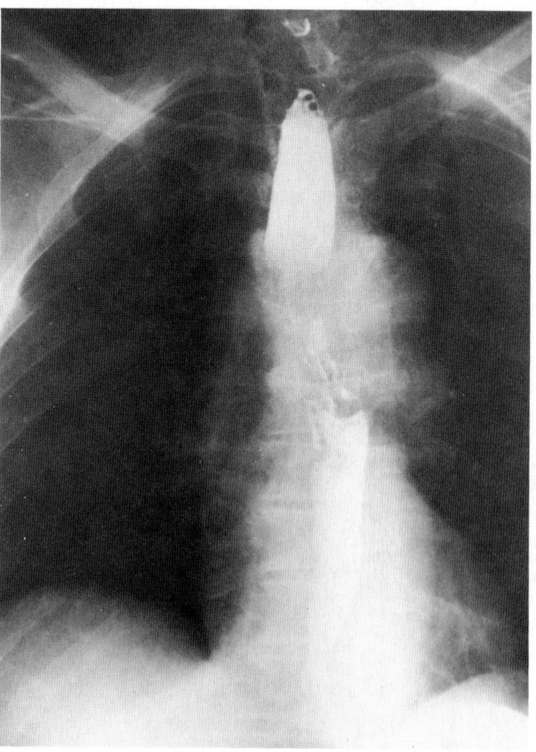

NATURAL HISTORY AND PATTERNS OF SPREAD OF SQUAMOUS CELL CARCINOMA OF THE ESOPHAGUS

Esophageal cancers are characterized by extensive local growth and lymph node involvement before becoming widely disseminated. The unique lymphatic drainage of the esophagus (Figs. 16-8 and 16-9) and the long interval during which the tumor is asymptomatic accounts for the extensive involvement of lymph nodes and structures adjacent to the esophagus at the time of diagnosis. Another anatomic factor responsible for the poor prognosis of patients with esophageal cancer is the close proximity of the aorta and trachea to tumors in this area (Figs. 16-5 and 16-6).

Autopsy studies of the length of esophagus involved by the neoplasm can be correlated directly with the extent of involvement and inversely with curability. The same is true if one examines the resected esophagus. If the tumor is 5 cm long or less, approximately 40% of specimens will demonstrate localized disease, 25% will be locally advanced and 35% will have distant metastases or will be unresectable for cure. If the size of the tumor, that is, its length of involvement, exceeds 5 cm as determined by pathologic examination, only 10% will be localized, 15% will be locally advanced and 75% will have distant metastases or be beyond the limits of a curative resection.[50–52] It is not possible to accurately assess the length of involvement by radiographic means.[31,53,54] Barium contrast and air (double) contrast studies are currently the best clinical methods of determining the size of an esophageal cancer and its extent of involvement. Since it is not possible to accurately assess the size of the tumors by the length of the deformed barium column, the latter does not correlate well with the resectability of the cancer, the degree of lymph node involvement and the pattern of spread.

As expected, lymph node involvement carries a poor prognosis. A five year survival of 10% to 15% is reported following esophagectomy when the lymph nodes are positive. A five year survival two to three times these figures is obtained when the lymph nodes are not involved.[55,56]

Distant metastases rarely dominate the clinical course of esophageal cancer. However, at autopsy, distant metastases are found in up to 90% of patients. Esophageal carcinoma has the ability to spread to virtually any site, including lung, pleura, stomach, peritoneum, kidney, adrenal gland, brain, and bone. The most common visceral metastases are those to the lung and liver.

EVALUATING THE PATIENT WITH SQUAMOUS CELL CARCINOMA OF THE ESOPHAGUS

Prior to treating a patient with squamous cell carcinoma of the esophagus, information should be obtained to answer several questions, viz: Are metastases present? Are other malignancies present? Is the malignancy locally advanced so as to preclude resection? What is the status of the patient's cardiopulmonary function? Can the patient withstand an operation, curative radiotherapy, or chemotherapy?

The history and physical examination can provide important clues with respect to the local extent and metastatic involvement of a cancer of the esophagus. The findings produced by advanced esophageal cancers were described above and are listed in Table 16-3.

Attempts have been made to derive information from the esophagus with respect to resectability. The length of involvement as determined by the esophagogram is not of prognostic significance. Nor is the radiologic type of tumor. However, the degree of deformity of the esophagus produced by the tumor may be predictive of incurability. When the esophageal axis is deformed, mediastinal invasion by the tumor may be present. The deformed axis results from fixation and distortion of the esophagus by the locally invasive cancer. Seventy-five percent to 80% of locally invasive cancers will have a deformed esophageal axis.[57] Since the latter may also result from inflammatory changes, false positives are encountered in 10% and false negatives are seen in 8% of patients with locally invasive tumors (Fig. 16-11).

The high frequency of metastases to the lungs, liver, adrenals, kidney, and bone justifies the use of bilateral whole lung tomograms, liver scan, intravenous pyelography, a bone scan, and a skeletal survey in evaluating patients with esophageal tumor.

Computerized axial tomography (CT) of the mediastinum has proven useful to radiotherapists in planning therapy.[58] CT may also be a more accurate way of assessing length of involvement of the esophagus than the esophagogram. CT

TABLE 16-3. Signs and Symptoms Produced by Advanced Carcinoma of Esophagus

Pain radiating to the back on swallowing
Dysphonia (laryngeal paralysis)
Diaphragmatic paralysis (involvement of phrenic nerve)
Coughing when swallowing (tracheoesophageal fistula)
Superior vena cava syndrome
Palpable superclavicular or cervical nodes
Malignant pleural effusion
Malignant ascites
Bone pain

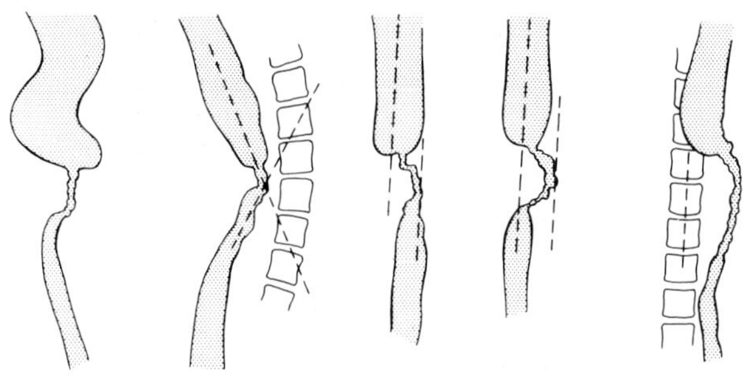

FIG. 16-11. Five types of deformities of the esophageal axis may be produced by an esophageal carcinoma. (Akiyama H: Surgery for carcinoma of the esophagus. Curr Probl Surg, Vol 17. Chicago, Year Book Medical Publishers, 1978)

may be able to detect lymph node enlargement also, both above and below the diaphragm, and involvement of adjacent mediastinal structures.

Gallium scans have been recommended to screen for extramural extension of the tumor and lymph node involvement. With respect to the latter, the sensitivity of this study in the mediastinum and abdomen was reported to be only 27%. The accuracy was 100%.[59]

Azygos venography (azygography) can provide invaluable information with respect to extraesophageal spread and resectability.[54,60] When the azygos vein is obstructed, the lesion is usually unresectable (Fig. 16-12). This study should be considered most highly with lesions of the upper thoracic esophagus. Occasionally, an obstructed azygos vein will respond to radiation and the tumor can be resected with prospects of cure.

Both flexible and rigid esophagoscopy should be used to evaluate esophageal cancers. The rigid esophagoscope can be used to manipulate the tumor and determine its degree of fixation. Because of the high frequency of other malignancies within the upper and lower respiratory passageways, a careful examination of the mouth, pharynx, larynx, and tracheobronchial tree must be performed. Another compelling reason for performing laryngoscopy and bronchoscopy is the frequency of extension into the tracheobronchial tree of mid-esophageal lesions. Special attention should be given to the posterior wall of the left main stem bronchus and trachea where the esophagus crosses these structures. Narrowing in this area or infiltration of tumor, as evidenced by edema, prominent longitudinal folds, and bleeding upon contact, are ominous findings.

Mediastinoscopy has been used to stage esophageal cancers. If the paratracheal or sub-carinal lymph nodes are involved, mediastinoscopy can be revealing.[61,62] Laparoscopy is helpful in identifying patients with malignant ascites, liver metastases and extensive involvement of the stomach. All palpable cervical or supraclavicular lymph nodes deserve biopsy. Bilateral scalene node biopsies will be found positive in some patients with advanced disease even when the nodes are not palpable.[62,63]

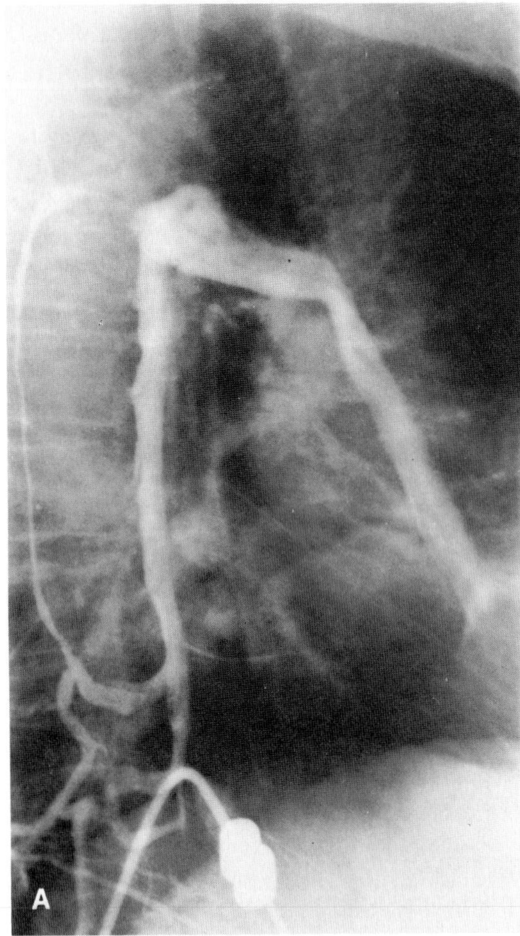

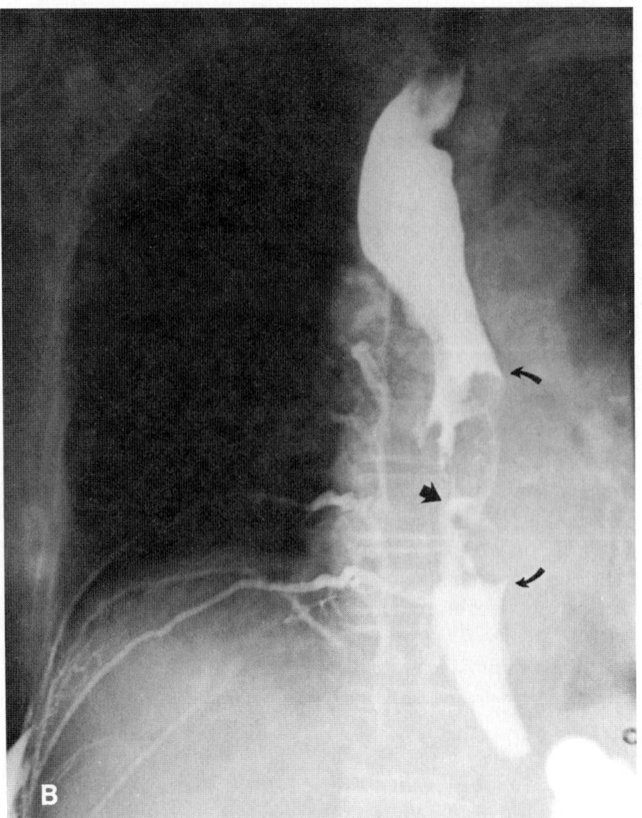

FIG. 16-12. A normal azygogram (*A*) compared to one that was obtained with barium in the esophagus (*B*). The esophagogram delineates a cancer of the esophagus that is obstructing the azygos vein. (Courtesy of Dr. A. Crummy)

Biopsy of the celiac and lesser curvature lymph nodes is of great significance in planning therapy and providing prognostic data. Therefore, biopsy of these lymph nodes at laparotomy should be part of every therapeutic plan. Celiac node involvement can occur in 10% of patients with upper esophageal malignancies. With lower esophageal cancers, the incidence increases at least five-fold.[34]

A summary of the studies which should be performed prior to instituting therapy is presented in Table 16-4.

DETERMINATION OF OPERABILITY

The purpose of obtaining a complete evaluation of patients with carcinoma of the esophagus is to determine what would be the most appropriate and effective therapy for that patient. As was indicated at the outset of this chapter, a plan of therapy should attempt to achieve a cure whenever possible and always try to alleviate the suffering produced by the esophageal cancer (Fig. 16-1). Since operative therapy plays a prominent role in both cure and palliation, it must be established whether or not the patient can withstand a thoracotomy and laparotomy. Several aspects of the patient's general condition must be taken into consideration. Cardiopulmonary function is the most important. It is often impaired by the prolonged alcohol abuse and cigarette smoking that are characteristic of patients with esophageal cancer. A full discussion of this aspect of the patient's evaluation is not within the scope of this chapter. Only the highlights will be mentioned.

Patients with congestive heart failure, significant angina pectoris, and severely impaired respiratory function are not suitable candidates for operative therapy. In order to determine

TABLE 16-4. Evaluation of Patients with Cancer of the Esophagus

STANDARD
History and physical examination
Esophagogram
Chest radiograph and bilateral whole lung tomograms
Electrocardiogram
Pulmonary function studies
Laryngoscopy, bronchoscopy, and esophagoscopy
Computerized tomography of mediastinum and upper abdomen
Bone scan and skeletal survey
Liver function tests and liver scan
Laparotomy and biopsy of celiac lymph nodes
OPTIONAL (for suspected advanced lesions)
Gallium scan
Mediastinoscopy and mediastinotomy
Azygography
Laparoscopy
Scalene node biopsy
Intravenous pyelogram

the presence of cardiac disease that would contraindicate an operation, a history and physical examination, chest roentgenogram, and electrocardiogram should be obtained. Occasionally, non-invasive studies of myocardial function are required, such as post-exercise myocardial scanning or gated cardiac blood pool scanning.

Respiratory function can also be assessed by relatively simple pulmonary function tests. Severe dyspnea, wheezing, and the signs and symptoms of advanced obstructive pulmonary disease are reflected in abnormal pulmonary function tests. Arterial blood gases and exercise tests should also be routinely obtained. Often it is helpful to have diffusion capacity studies. A detailed evaluation of pulmonary function is important not only for the evaluation of operability. Radiation therapy and chemotherapy may also adversely affect pulmonary function. If combined thereapy is utilized, more than one insult may be inflicted upon the already compromised lungs.

STAGING FOR CANCER OF THE ESOPHAGUS

Careful characterization of the extent of involvement of a cancer of the esophagus is necessary in order to plan its treatment. The information gained from this determination can also be used to "stage" the patient, that is, classify the extent of the disease in such a way that patients with similar degrees of involvement can be grouped together. This grouping or staging of patients allows one to compare different therapies on homogeneous populations of patients. It is obviously invalid to compare two forms of therapy on a group with limited disease and another with extensive involvement; the treatment given to the latter group will surely suffer by such a comparison.

The most common method used for staging is the TNM system. Since the esophagus is not an accessible organ, its clinical evaluation leaves a great deal to be desired. The use of invasive technics, including biopsy procedures, is more appropriate. However, they should be carried out before radiotherapy or chemotherapy is used if they are to be reliable, since these therapeutic maneuvers will distort the findings. Since many esophageal cancers are being treated with preoperative radiation or chemotherapy, post-surgical evaluation may also not accurately define the stage of the cancer as it was when it was first diagnosed. The TNM staging system for the cervical and thoracic esophagus is outlined in Table 16-5. Stage grouping is given in Table 16-6.[28,64]

The Japanese Society for Esophageal Diseases has devised a far more detailed staging system, which is too extensive to recount here.[29] Its main advantage is that it provides an excellent means of staging esophageal cancers for clinical investigators and end results reporting. The staging system based on operative findings utilizes extension of the tumor to the adventitia of the esophagus rather than the length of involvement as an index of the primary tumor. Lymph node involvement, distant metastases, and pleural involvement are also used as bases of stage grouping in Japanese centers.

Another means of "staging" or classifying patients is one which is largely clinically oriented. Patients can either be operable or inoperable and either curable or incurable. Patients are operable when they can undergo a combined thoracotomy and laparotomy. The tumor is incurable if there is fixation to neighboring structures, proven growth into the tracheobronchial tree, broadening of the carina with positive bronchial cytology, recurrent laryngeal nerve paralysis, or distant metastases. The Rotterdam Working Group on Esophageal Cancer found 42% of their patients were operable–curable and 35% were inoperable–curable. The remainder were incurable.[65]

TABLE 16-5. TNM Staging for Esophageal Cancer

PRIMARY TUMOR (T)	
T0	No demonstrable tumor
TIS	Carcinoma *in situ*
T1	Tumor involves 5 cm or less of esophageal length with no obstruction nor complete circumferential involvement nor extra esophageal spread.
T2	Tumor involves more than 5 cm of esophagus and produces obstruction with circumferential involvement of the esophagus but no extraesophageal spread.
T3	Tumor with extension outside the esophagus involving mediastinal structures.
REGIONAL LYMPH NODES (N)	
Cervical esophagus (cervical and supraclavicular lymph nodes)	
N0	No nodal involvement
N1	Unilateral involvement (moveable)
N2	Bilateral involvement (moveable)
N3	Fixed nodes
Thoracic esophagus (nodes in the thorax, not those of the cervical, supraclavicular or abdominal areas)	
N0	No nodal involvement
N1	Nodal involvement
DISTANT METASTASES	
M0	No metastases
M1	Distant metastases. Cancer of thoracic esophagus with cervical, supraclavicular, or abdominal lymph node involvement is classified as M1.

SURGICAL THERAPY FOR SQUAMOUS CELL CARCINOMA OF THE THORACIC ESOPHAGUS

PREOPERATIVE PREPARATIONS

In assessing the patient with an esophageal cancer, it must be determined if the patient is a candidate for an operation. Operability is determined by an evaluation of the patient's cardiopulmonary status. Advanced age is not a contraindication to surgical therapy. Debilitation from nutritional deficits must be corrected before considering surgery or any other therapy. The amount of weight loss should be determined. Protein and electrolyte derangements indicate gross nutritional derangement and require immediate attention. Skin testing to determine if the patient is anergic may be worthwhile. However, intense nutritional therapy with restoration of positive nitrogen balance may not suffice to correct anergy.[66] A weighted fine bore feeding tube should be passed through the area of malignant obstruction if possible and positioned in the stomach. If trouble is experienced in passing the tube transnasally, it may be possible to get it through the area of obstruction with the help of an esophagoscope or following dilatation of the tumor. If the alimentary tract cannot be used

TABLE 16-6. Stage Grouping for Esophageal Cancer

STAGE I	
T1N0M0	Tumor that involves less than 5 cm of esophagus without obstruction and no circumferential nor extra esophageal nor nodal involvement and no metastases.
STAGE II	
T1N1M0 T1N2M0 T2N0M0 T2N1M0 T2N2M0	Cervical esophagus: No extraesophageal involvement with moveable regional lymph nodes but no metastases or a tumor more than 5 cm in size without lymph node involvement.
T2N0M0	Thoracic esophagus: Any tumor which is greater than 5 cm in length or produces obstruction or involves the entire circumference of the esophagus without extraesophageal spread.
STAGE III	
Any M1 Any T3	Any esophageal cancer with extraesophageal spread or distant metastases. Cervical esophagus: fixed nodes (Any N3) Thoracic esophagus: regional lymph node involvement (Any N1)

for nutritional support, intravenous hyperalimentation should be employed. Gastrostomy should be avoided since this organ is often used to replace or bypass the esophagus. A striking result has been reported following nutritional replenishment using a feeding jejunostomy: the patient subsequently underwent an operation and survived 31 years after resection of an esophageal cancer.[67]

In addition to nutritional care, other pre-operative measures should be adopted. Pulmonary function can be improved by eliminating cigarette smoking, chest physiotherapy, respiratory therapy (intermittent positive pressure breathing and incentive spirometry), bronchodilators, antibiotics, and eliminating aspiration of oral secretions by placing a nasogastric tube above the malignant obstruction and attaching it to suction. Digitalization may be required, along with diuretics, to correct congestive heart failure.

OPERATIVE CONSIDERATIONS

The above measures, vigorously applied, and equally effective post-operative care, undoubtedly account for the fact that at least 50% of patients with cancer of the esophagus are currently considered operative candidates. Not all of these patients can be resected for cure. However, up to 90% can be found to be resectable for either palliation or cure.

Patients who are operable should all undergo a laparotomy to determine the extent of lymph node involvement and local (extraesophageal) spread. This information is vital in the planning of further therapy. Whenever possible and reasonable, the surgeon should try to remove as much tumor as possible, leaving radiotherapy and chemotherapy the task of eliminating tumor that defies surgical removal. Radiopaque clips should be placed around the site of the tumor. The basis for such an optimistic approach resides in anecdotal data, that is, isolated case reports or the experience of surgeons who have struggled with the problem of esophageal cancer for many years. Wangensteen reports an 11 year cure for a patient with a cancer of the esophagus who had involvement of a lymph node on the greater curvature of the stomach.[3] Sweet described a 16 year survivor of a cancer of the esophagus who had tumor cells present at the margin of the resected specimen.[55] Recent results reported by Ong and colleagues indicate that a 10 year survival is possible even when a bronchoesophageal fistula is present from a lobar bronchus to the esophagus. Ong's patient had an esophagectomy and lobectomy.[68]

Ong cautions that if the main bronchus, trachea, or aorta is infiltrated by the malignancy, resection carries a high mortality and should not be performed. Patching the trachea or bronchus with pericardium is rarely successful. Most often the repair breaks down or infection causes the patched pericardium to slough.

A rationale for leaving tumor behind and reconstructing the gastrointestinal tract by bypassing this area and subsequently irradiating it can also be derived from another single experience provided by Ong and colleagues. They had a patient who survived four years after bypassing a malignant esophagobronchial fistula by esophagogastrostomy and irradiating the tumor.[68] Marcial and coworkers treated a patient with supraclavicular and axillary metastases with radiation and obtained a five year survival, indicating that there is still hope despite widespread disease.[69] It has been emphasized that lymph node involvement following esophagectomy results in half the five-year survival rate of patients with negative regional lymph nodes. Equal emphasis should be given to the fact that even with positive regional lymph nodes, 10% to 15% of patients who have survived esophagectomy can be cured. However, five-year survival rates may not be valid as the basis of deciding whether or not a patient with esophageal cancer is cured. After five years as many as 78% of survivors may succumb to recurrences.[70] Another cogent argument for proceeding with an esophageal resection whenever operable criteria are met is that this operation constitutes excellent palliation. Operative mortality for esophageal resection has been reported to vary from 5% to 30%.[71] More recent reports have indicated that an operative mortality of less than 5% can be attained.[72]

The major components of an operation designed to cure the patient of an esophageal cancer should include a thorough assessment of the abdominal viscera and lymph nodes and the local extension of the tumor, a subtotal or total esophagectomy and reconstruction of the gastrointestinal tract. The reconstructive procedure should allow for normal swallowing and avoid reflux of gastric secretions.

ESOPHAGECTOMY

Because of the many special features of the lymphatic drainage of the esophagus, malignant cells can be found as far as 8 cm from the site of gross tumor with intervening skip areas free of tumor.[35] Lymph node involvement can also occur some distance from the site of the primary. The anatomic bases for these phenomena were described above and deserve re-emphasis here. They are responsible for the generally accepted principle that the only adequate resection for a carcinoma of the thoracic esophagus is its complete removal, that is, a subtotal or total esophagectomy. Esophagectomy should include a cuff of stomach and extend as high up into the chest

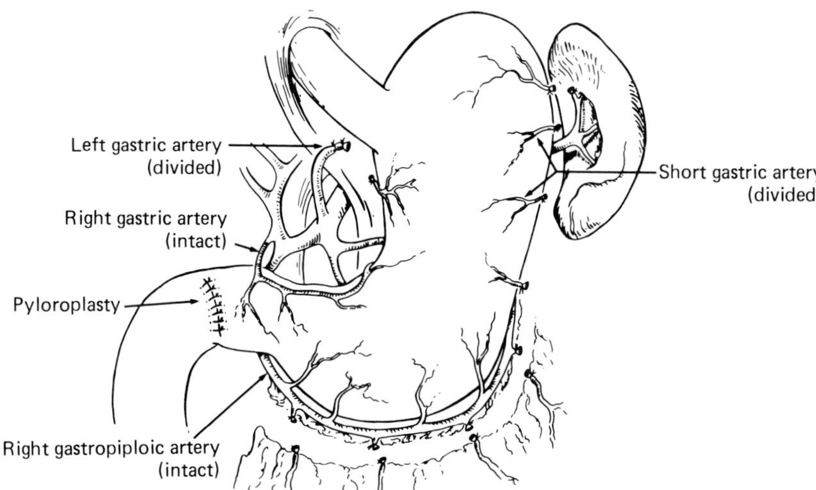

FIG. 16-13. Mobilization of the stomach for reconstruction of the esophagus involves division of the short gastric and left gastric arteries. The right gastric and gastroepiploic artery suffice to adequately vascularize the stomach. Since the vagus nerves are divided when the esophagus is resected, a pyloroplasty is required for adequate gastric drainage.

as is feasible. Higher thoracic esophageal lesions should include a portion of the distal cervical esophagus. If necessary, gastrointestinal continuity should be reconstituted by performing an anastomosis in the neck. Watson's papers in the mid-1950s adequately documented the "case against segmental resection for esophageal carcinoma" and emphasized these principles.[35] Scanlon reported a 45% incidence of recurrence at the anastomotic site when a segmental resection of the esophagus was performed for carcinoma.[73] Thus, a resection which is less than a subtotal esophagectomy is inadequate.

In addition to longitudinal resection of an esophageal cancer, a wide margin of surrounding normal tissues and as many as possible of the regional lymphatic channels including the lymph nodes should be removed. This principle is difficult to adhere to in the upper thoracic esophagus. Because of the proximity of vital structures including the aorta, the heart, the left main bronchus, and the inferior pulmonary veins, it may not be possible to obtain a sufficiently wide excision of the tissues around the esophageal cancer.[55] This deficiency of esophageal resection of the upper esophagus provides a rationale for the use of radiotherapy as an adjunct to local control of the tumor.

There are three approaches to esophageal resection which are practiced currently: (1) through a right thoracotomy, usually combined with a laparotomy; (2) through a left thoracotomy, using a thoracoabdominal incision; and (3) without thoracotomy, using separate abdominal and cervical incisions.

Esophagectomy through the right chest is the most widely accepted approach. It is preceded, during the same anesthetic, by a laparotomy during which the celiac and lesser curvature lymph nodes are biopsied and the stomach mobilized so that it can be used to reconstruct the esophagus (Fig. 16-13).[74] However, when dealing with distal esophageal lesions and those involving the cardio-esophageal junction, a left thoracoabdominal incision may have merit. The aortic arch can be mobilized and the esophagus resected high in the chest if necessary.

The newest and most exciting approach to esophagectomy is the removal of this structure through abdominal and cervical incisions, thus avoiding thoracotomy (Fig. 16-14). This operation was first described in England during the 1930s and was re-introduced by Kirk in 1974.[75] It has also been used in the United States with acceptable results.[76,77] Skepticism exists as to the true place of this form of esophagectomy in the treatment of cancer of the esophagus since it does not allow for a wide resection of adjacent tissues.[78] It may be that esophagectomy without thoracotomy will suffice as a low-risk tumor reductive procedure, allowing radiotherapy and chemotherapy to eliminate the cancer that is left behind.

RECONSTRUCTION FOLLOWING ESOPHAGECTOMY

Table 16-7 outlines the options available for reconstruction of the esophagus following thoracic esophagectomy. Eso-

FIG. 16-14. Esophagus can be bluntly and blindly dissected free of surrounding structure through the esophageal hiatus and a cervical incision, and thus removed.

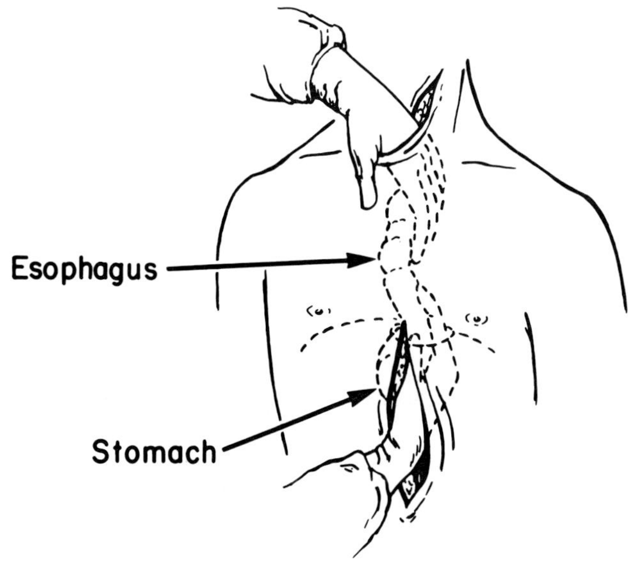

TABLE 16-7. Reconstructive Procedures Following Thoracic Esophagectomy

Esophagogastrostomy
Colon interposition
- left (antiperistaltic)
- right (isoperistaltic)
- transverse

Reverse gastric tube
Jejunal interposition

phagogastrostomy as described by Lewis is the most acceptable, effective and widely practiced form of reconstructive procedure. The operation begins with exploration of the abdomen and assessment of visceral and lymph node involvement. If extensive intra-abdominal metastases are present, precluding a curative resection, a palliative resection should be considered. Similarly, if an unresectable tumor is encountered in the chest, a palliative bypass procedure can be performed. The stomach is mobilized as demonstrated in Fig. 16-13. The right chest is then opened and the tumor removed. (Fig. 16-15 and 16-16). The stomach is then anastomosed to the esophagus.[74,79,80]

Emphasis should be placed on the anastomosis between the esophagus and stomach, since this frequently breaks down and is a major cause of the morbidity and mortality following esophagogastrostomy. In addition to anastomotic disruption, strictures can occur at the anastomotic site. Gastroesophageal regurgitation through the anastomosis can cause a great deal of discomfort and disability due to aspiration. The anastomosis should be performed high in the chest, or in the neck as described by McKeown.[81] The latter procedure is preferred if there is insufficient length of esophagus in the chest; an end-to-end anastomosis stapling device can sometimes be utilized for this anastomosis (Fig. 16-17).[82] Suture technics are standard (Fig. 16-18). After completing the anastomosis, a portion of the stomach should be wrapped around the anastomotic site in the form of a fundoplication whenever possible. This procedure diminishes the possibility of gastroesophageal reflux.[83] Gastroesophageal reflux can be easily controlled after the stomach is brought up into the chest by avoiding recumbency and eating small meals.[84] Thus, a fundoplication may not be always necessary. The anasto-

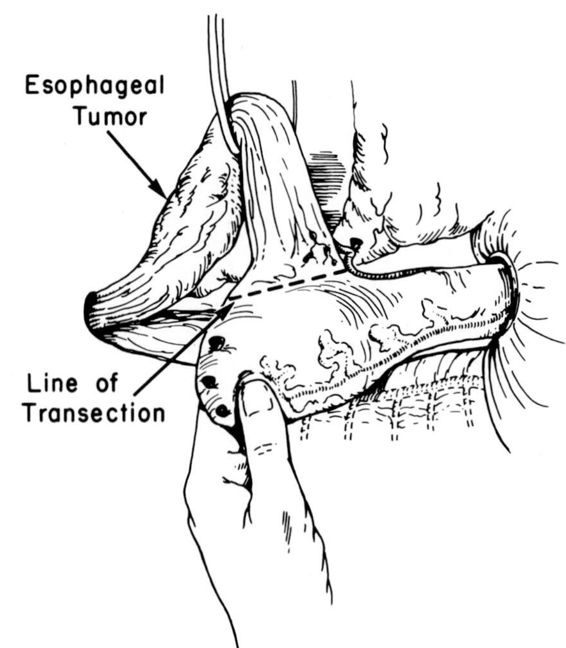

FIG. 16-16. The esophagus is resected along with a cuff of stomach. A stapling device is used to close the stomach.

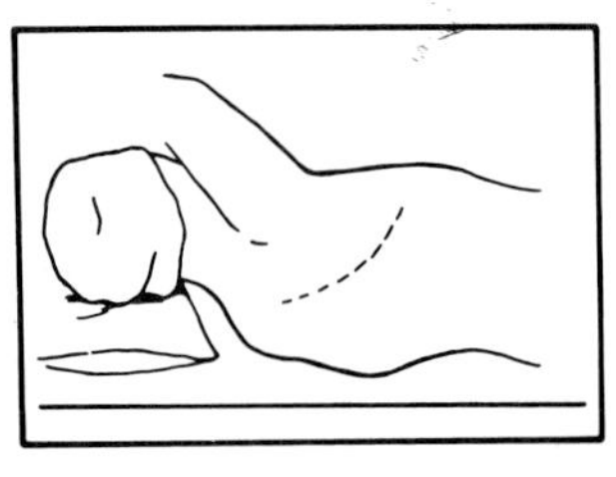

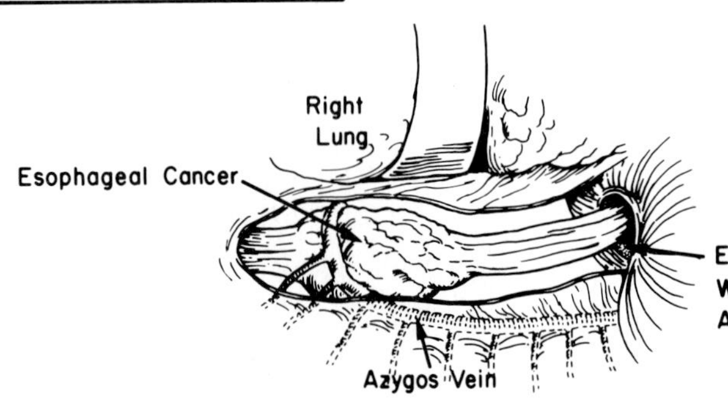

FIG. 16-15. Through a posterolateral incision in the fifth interspace, the esophagus is exposed. The esophagus and tumor are freed from surrounding structures and mobilized. The stomach is brought into the chest through the esophageal hiatus.

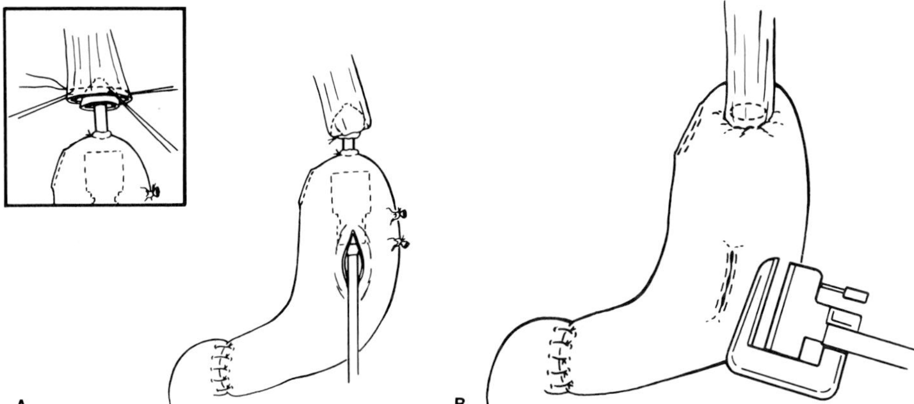

FIG. 16-17. The esophagogastrostomy is performed using an end-to-end anastomosis stapler. The completed anastomosis is shown in *B*. (Steichen FM, Ravitch MM: Mechanical sutures in esophageal surgery. Ann Surg 191: 373, 1980)

mosis should be free of tension. In order to assure this, the stomach should be tacked to the prevertebral fascia. A pyloroplasty should also be performed because a vagectomy is inevitable when removing the esophagus. Not all surgeons believe a pyloroplasty is necessary.[85] The completed procedure constitutes an acceptable functional reconstruction of the esophagus (Fig. 16-19).

If the patient has had a previous gastrectomy, an esophagogastrostomy cannot be performed following esophagectomy. In such instances, a colon interposition will be required to provide a conduit to the stomach (Fig. 16-20).[86] A barium enema pre-operatively is mandatory if a colon interposition is to be employed. Colon carcinoma has been occasionally found in such instances. A mesenteric arteriogram may also be helpful in deciding which portion of the colon will best reach the proximal esophagus. The left colon is best suited for this procedure but the right or transverse colon can also be used. Two surgical teams should be employed to limit operative time, one team working in the abdomen while the other team works in the chest. Because this procedure requires three anastomoses and involves the colon, which has a less adequate blood supply than the stomach, the incidence of anastomotic leaks are higher than after esophagogastrostomy.

Two other options exist for reconstruction of gastrointestinal continuity following subtotal esophagectomy. A gastric tube can be fashioned from the greater curvature of the stomach (Fig. 16-21) [87–88] or a jejunal loop can be used to bridge the esophageal defect (Fig. 16-22).[89] They have no advantages over esophagogastrostomy and carry a higher rate of complications.

POST-OPERATIVE CARE

The following applies to a patient who has had a laparotomy followed by a right thoracotomy and esophagectomy. The patient may have had a cervical incision also with the esophagogastrostomy performed in the neck. Large-bore chest tubes are placed close to the anastomosis if it is in the chest.

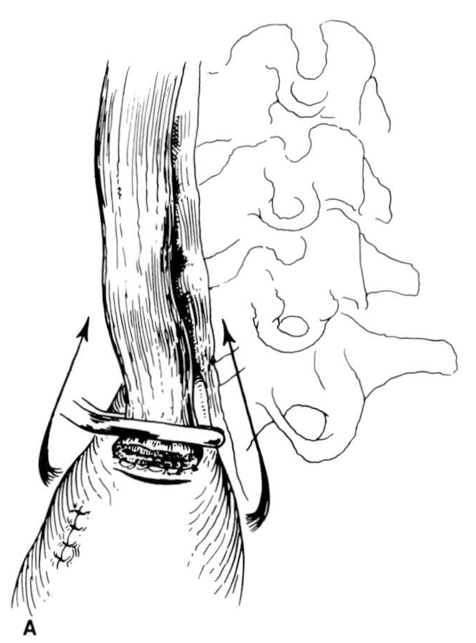

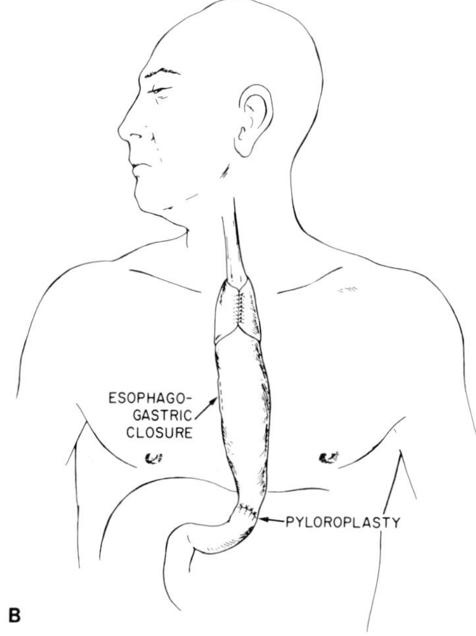

FIG. 16-18. A two-layered end-to-side anastomosis is performed. After completing the anastomosis, the stomach is wrapped around the esophagogastrostomy (arrows). *A*, The stomach is also sutured to the prevertebral fascia to prevent tension on the anastomosis. *B*, The finished operation.

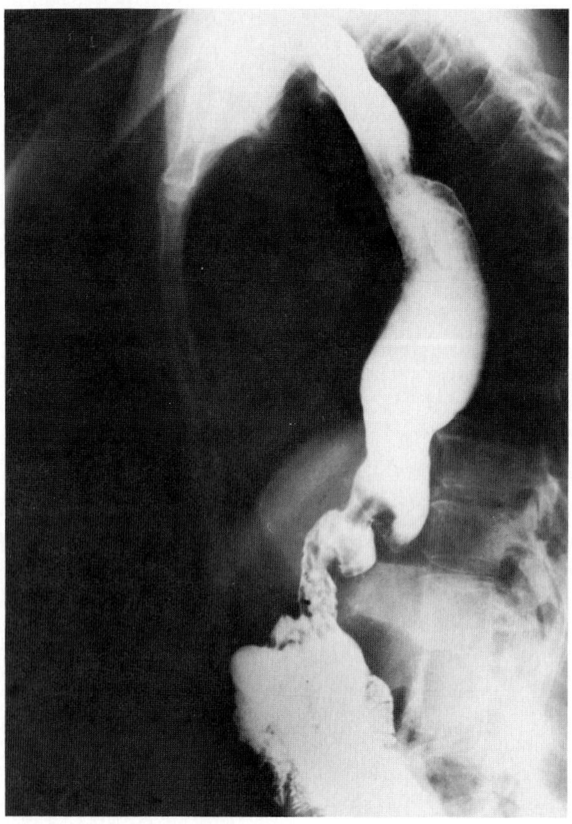

FIG. 16-19. A barium contrast study following esophagogastrostomy.

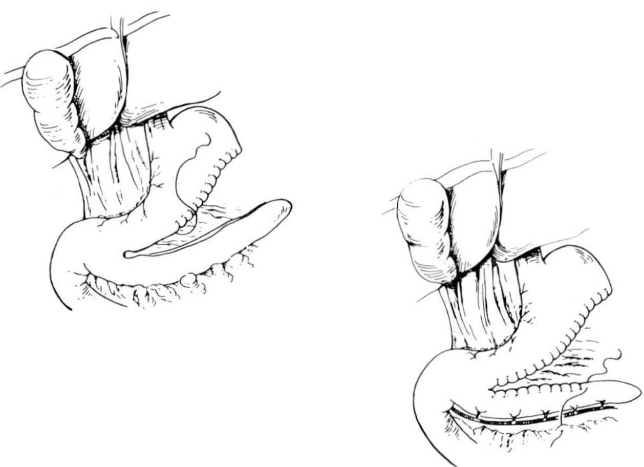

FIG. 16-21. A gastric tube constructed from the greater curvature of the stomach can be used to reconstruct or bypass the esophagus. The gastric tube depicted here is isoperistaltic with the blood supply coming from the right gastroepiploic artery. A reverse gastric tube can be fashioned with the blood supply based at the fundus. (Postlethwait RW: Technique for isoperistaltic gastric tube for esophageal bypass. Ann Surg 189:673, 1979)

An anastomosis in the neck is drained. The patient is kept on a respirator for the first 24 to 48 hours, using an FiO_2 as low as is necessary to maintain an arterial PO_2 of at least 60 mm Hg. Antibiotics, which are started pre-operatively, are continued. Underhydration is far better tolerated than overhydration in these weak and aged patients. Intravenous

FIG. 16-20. Mobilization of the right colon to form an isoperistaltic conduit to the stomach (*A*) or the left colon to form an antiperistaltic esophageal substitute (*B*).

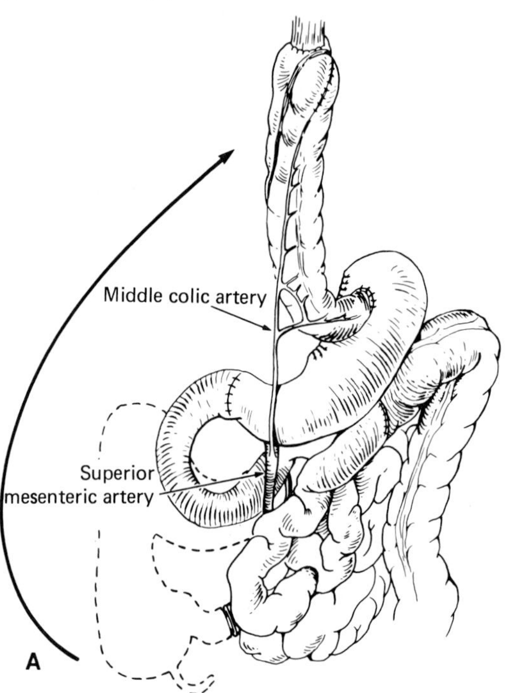

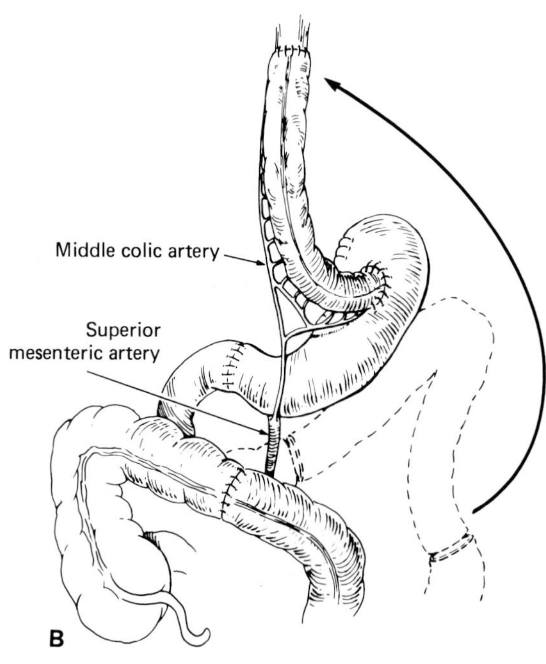

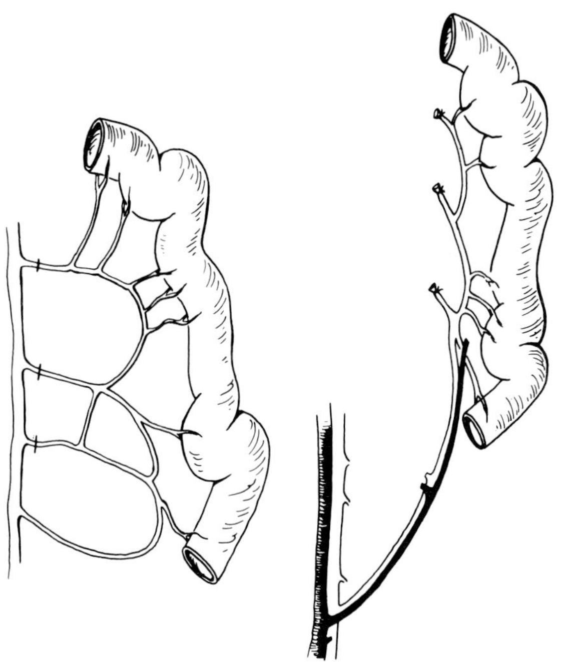

FIG. 16-22. Mobilization of a jejunal loop and its transposition into the chest as an esophageal substitute. The length of jejunum available to reconstruct the esophagus is very limited because of the tenuous blood supply. (*A*) Blood supply of jejunum. (*B*) Blood supply to a jejunal loop to be used as an esophageal replacement.

administration of excessive amounts of sodium containing fluids can be lethal.

Oral feedings are begun as soon as gastrointestinal motility is evident. The chest tubes and drains are left in place in case the anastomosis leaks. If this disastrous complication occurs, intravenous hyperalimentation is begun. After the patient is extubated, chest physiotherapy and incentive spirometry are instituted.

Survival Following Resection

In the absence of prospective randomized trials of therapy comparing like groups of patients, no one can reasonably claim that one form of therapy is better than another. The variation in the results reported for a variety of surgical procedures from different groups is comparable to the variation in results reported for operative and radiation therapy.

Based on a review of several surgical series, 5-year survivors following resection vary from 2% to 21%.[71] Survival after operation ranges from 7 to 28 months. Results are generally better the more distal the site of the cancer.

The operative mortality with esophagogastrostomy ranges from 4% to 30%.[71] Cardiopulmonary complications and anastomotic leaks lead the list of causes of postoperative deaths. Colon interposition procedures have an operative mortality ranging from 10% to 44%. Anastomotic leaks tend to be higher in this group of patients. Other possible complications are listed in Table 16-8.

TABLE 16-8. Causes of Morbidity Following Esophageal Resection

Anastomotic leak
Anastomotic stricture
Respirator insufficiency
Congestive heart failure
Pulmonary embolism
Obstruction at esophageal hiatus
Wound infection or dehiscence
Ruptured spleen
Phlebitis
Subphrenic abscess
Torsion, gangrene or rupture of gastrointestinal replacement
Hemorrhage

RADIATION THERAPY FOR ESOPHAGEAL CANCER

Radiation therapy is used in the curative and palliative treatment of cancer of the esophagus. It is used alone or in combination with surgery or chemotherapy or with both modalities. As a definitive treatment, the rationale for the use of irradiation rests in its ability to treat not only the primary lesion, but also gross or microscopic tumor in para-esophageal tissues. It is frequently not possible to resect these sites completely or they may be resected only with great difficulty or morbidity. The ability of radiation to provide relief of symptoms with relatively low morbidity and the disappointing results obtained with radical therapy of esophageal cancer have influenced many physicians to recommend radiation therapy as the primary treatment.

PATIENT SELECTION AND PROGNOSTIC FACTORS

Nearly all patients with squamous cell or undifferentiated carcinoma of the esophagus are appropriate for radiation therapy. Patients with lesions 5 to 10 cm in length with no evidence of metastatic disease and no evidence of tracheo-esophageal fistula are suitable for treatment with curative intent.[90-93] Patients with lesions greater than 10 cm or with distant metastases are candidates for palliative irradiation. While there is no favorable presentation for patients with carcinoma of the esophagus, upper esophageal lesions have been associated with higher 5-year survivals than distal lesions. Some authors find no difference by site.[56,69,91,92,94-97]

The results obtained by radiation therapy of esophageal cancer in women is better than in men. In one series, the mean survival for women was 12.2 months, whereas it was 8.8 months for men.[97] Another group found that both survival and response rates were higher for females than males.[90] Ninty-one percent of the women responded to radiotherapy, compared to only 53% of the men. On the other hand, a better prognosis for females was not observed in the 1647 cases reported from India.[92] This may represent some biologic difference between European and Asian varieties of the disease, necessitating caution in interpretation of data from different populations.

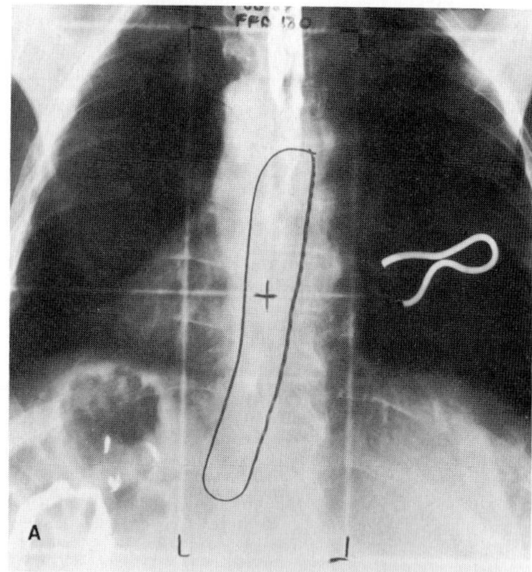

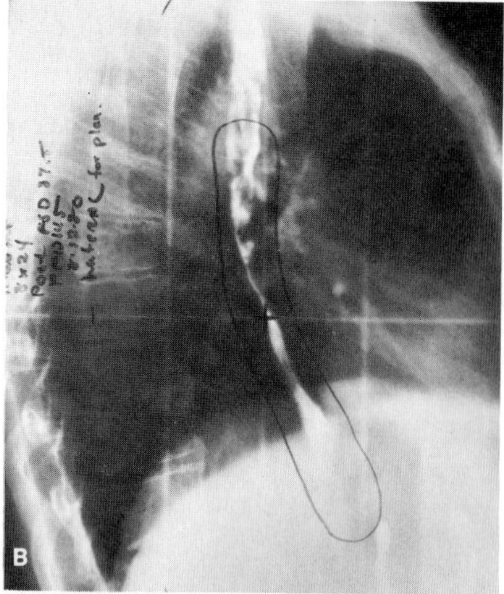

FIG. 16-23. *A*, Posteroanterior and *B*, lateral localization films taken on a treatment simulator. The wire grid outlines the treatment field. The isocenter is indicated by the cross-lines. The tumor volume is outlined with proximal and distal 5 cm margins. The lateral field film is taken to localize the isocenter only, and thus no attempt is made to completely include the tumor volume. *C*, A port film taken on 6 MVX linac for a patient undergoing pre-operative irradiation of a 6 cm lesion. Note the use of shaped blocks to protect the lungs.

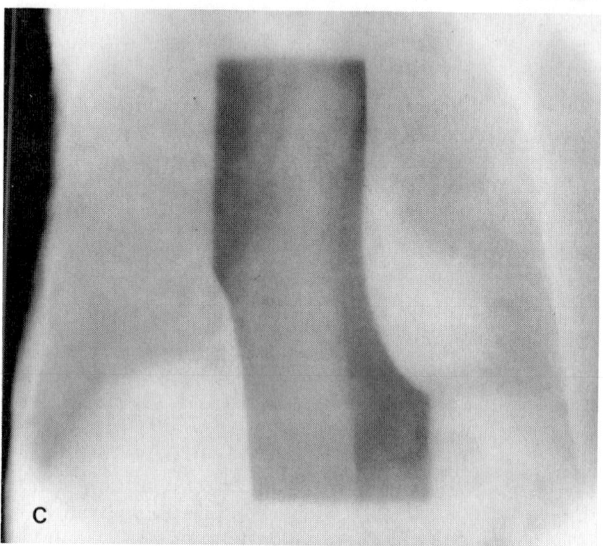

Absence of nodal or distant metastases is also associated with longer survival.[90,91,97] Patients with tracheoesophageal fistulae or endobronchial involvement have a very poor prognosis and generally are not benefited by irradiation. Patients with tracheoesophageal fistulae are palliated best by other modalities. While some radiotherapists believe that endobronchial involvement invariably precedes fistulization, this is not always the case. Marcial and colleagues reported that using lower daily doses (150R) minimized the risk of excessively rapid tumor regression in the wall of the bronchi or aorta. Rapid destruction of tumor in these locations is assumed responsible for fistula formation.[69] Fistulization has been reported to occur in 5% to 18% of irradiated patients, despite exclusion prior to therapy of patients with known tracheoesophageal fistulae.[95,97] Similarly, Pinto and colleagues recommended that patients with fistulae not be irradiated.[92] Fistulization into the aorta may also occur with exsanguinating hemorrhage. The treatment of these patients is extremely discouraging.

TECHNIC

Many technics can be used for treating esophageal carcinoma. Careful treatment planning must take place at the beginning of therapy to avoid excessive dose to the heart, lungs, or spinal cord.

Like the surgeon, the radiation oncologist plans treatment to encompass a specific tumor volume. The treatment should be planned to deliver a tumoricidal dose of radiation to the volume of tumor, while avoiding radiation doses which would exceed normal tissue tolerance. In order to accomplish this goal, the radiation therapist must carefully evaluate pretreatment studies, including esophageal and upper gastrointestinal contrast roentgenograms, mediastinal and lung tomograms, chest roentgenograms, and chest CT scans. Other studies, to determine the absence or presence of metastatic disease, must be viewed in order to decide whether the intent of treatment will be curative or palliative.

Treatment planning begins with fluoroscopy and localization films on the treatment simulator (Fig. 16-23). The patient is placed prone on the treatment simulator to effect maximum separation of the esophagus from the spinal cord.[98] The patients are simulated with a water-soluble contrast material in the esophagus. Some radiotherapists prefer simulation with a nasogastric tube, which either contains a contrast material or is made of a radioopaque substance.[99]

Field length is selected with the aid of the treatment simulator. Cephalad–caudad margins of the volume to be treated are defined. Sometimes treatments start with fields which encompass the entire esophagus, but, as a minimum, fields should be long enough to encompass the known extent of the tumor with at least a 5 cm margin both proximally and distally. It is preferred not to extend pre-operative treatment for a mid or lower esophageal lesion above the aortic arch, thus avoiding the performance of an anastomosis in an irradiated field. Lower lesions will usually necessitate a larger subdiaphragmatic extension to cover celiac nodes adequately. The latter are involved in over half such patients.[100]

A contour or outline of the patient is next obtained with the patient in the treatment position. Contours are obtained at the upper and lower margins of the field as well as through the central plane. These can be obtained with either a solder wire, plaster of Paris strip, or commercially available contouring device. The contour is traced onto a piece of paper, onto which the accurate location of organs of interest, such as lungs, spinal cord, and heart are drawn with the aid of pretreatment studies and postanterior and lateral simulator films. If available, CT is obtained for localization of organs within the treated area ("target volume"). It is an excellent alternative to the technic of mapping the contours and organs (Fig. 16-24). CT obtained for radiotherapy planning must be performed in the precise treatment position. This is essential to keep the relative position of the anatomic structures constant between scanning, planning, and treatment. For this same reason, CT should be performed on a flat surface, similar to the flat surface of a treatment table. Posterior and lateral marks are necessary. This can be accomplished with radio-opaque markers, such as angiograph catheters.

The CT scanner can be interfaced with a treatment planning computer either directly, through the use of magnetic storage devices, or by enlarging the CT scan and tracing the desired outlines using a photographic enlarger. With the latter technique, or when CT is not used for localization, the location of the organs of interest is entered into the computer manually.

Next, utilizing pretreatment studies, as well as simulator films and CT, the tumor volume is outlined on multiple planes, and entered into the computer. Various field arrangements are then used to obtain a desirable dose distribution on the central plane contour. An appropriate plan is selected and the treatment prescription indicated to an isodose curve totally encompassing the tumor volume. Effort is made to maintain no more than 10% difference between the minimum and maximum dose within the tumor volume, and to keep normal tissues to acceptable dose levels. The plan selected for the central plane is then examined in the other planes to insure adequate coverage of tumor and acceptable lung and spinal cord doses at all levels.

After an appropriate treatment plan is selected, it is verified on the simulator. The patient is placed back on the simulator in the treatment position, and the appropriate fields are set. Using a low-melting-temperature alloy, the outline for lung and spinal cord blocks are drawn on simulator films. Appropriate blocks are then cut and their placement verified on the simulator (Fig. 16-25).

Often, because of severe symptoms or rapid progression of disease, it is necessary to begin treatment as soon as possible, before a complete treatment plan is obtained. In most situations it is appropriate to begin treatment using parallel opposed anterior and posterior fields. The patient is simulated as described previously, with anterior and posterior fields of the appropriate width placed at that time. Treatment is started through these fields, but shifted to a complete treatment plan when ready. At the National Cancer Institute, a 3-field plan is preferred, utilizing a direct anterior field and left posterior oblique and right posterior oblique fields with the patient prone (Fig. 16-26).

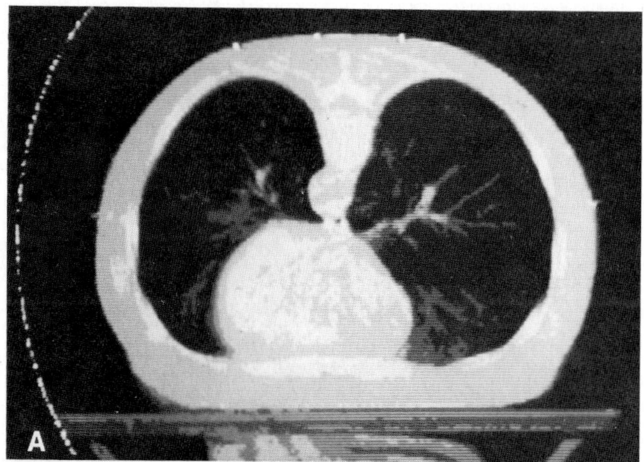

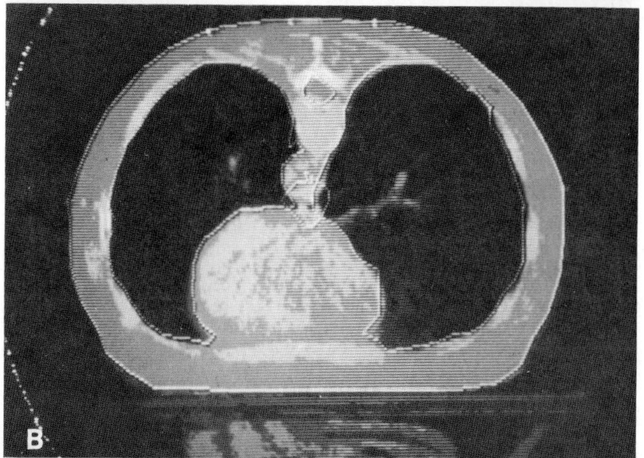

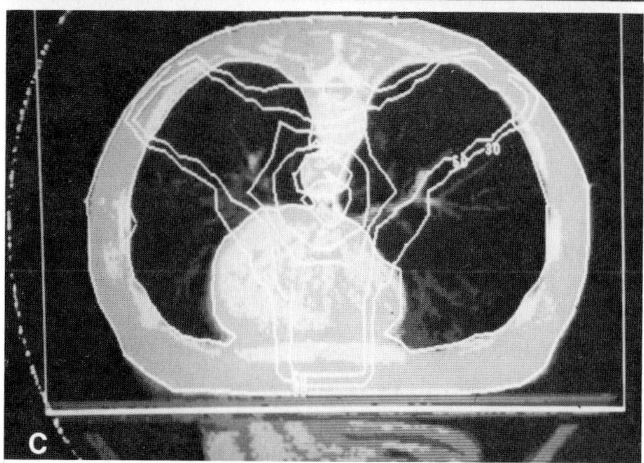

FIG. 16-24. Computerized tomography (CT) is used for localizing tumor volume to develop treatment plans, *A*, CT of a patient in the supine treatment position on flat surface. Lateral and posterior radiopaque markers (angiography tubing) were used to mark the isocenter coordinates, as well as the borders of the parallel opposed anterior and posterior fields through which this patient's treatment was initiated. Markers were placed on the simulator. *B*, Patient contour, tumor volume, and outline of volumes of special interest are indicated. Here, the lungs and spinal cord were localized. Inhomogeneity corrections for transmission through the air-filled lungs can then be utilized, and the treatment plan devised to minimize spinal cord dose. The central plane CT is shown, but the plan should involve scans on multiple planes. *C*, The isodose distribution for the three-field plan (AP, LPO, and RPO) is shown overlying the CT scan.

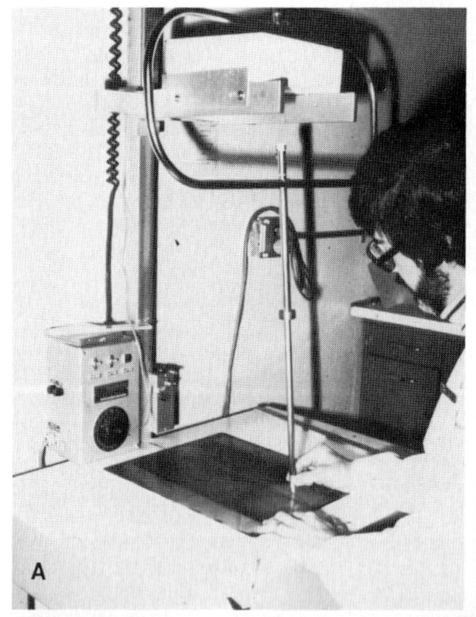

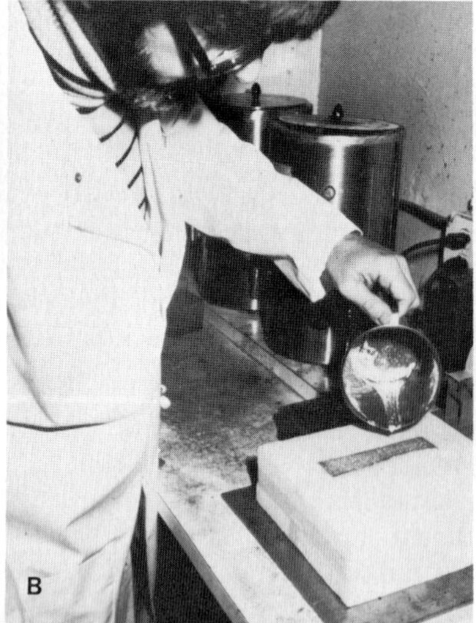

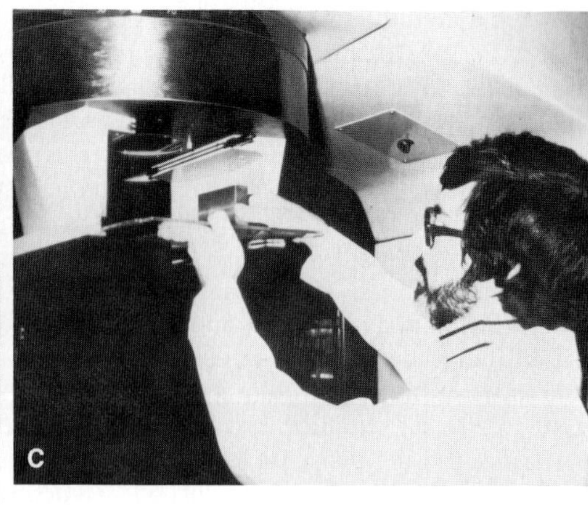

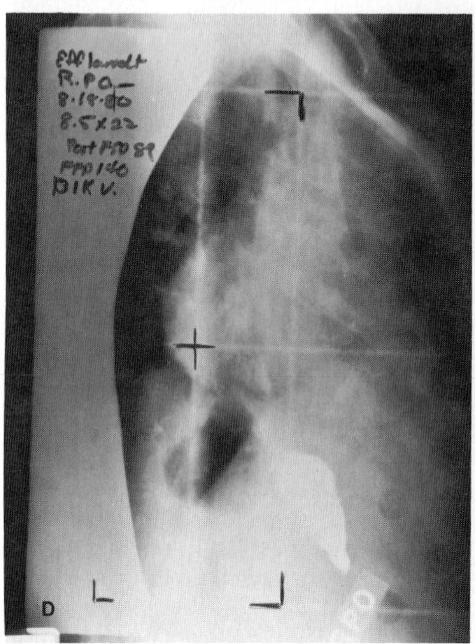

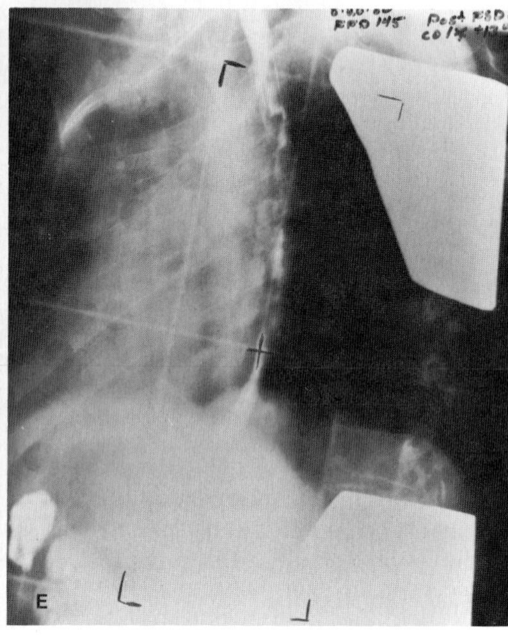

FIG. 16-25. Individually shaped blocks are used to protect normal tissue. Molds for blocks are cut using an apparatus which cuts the styrofoam mold with an electrified wire. *A*, The stylus is traced over the simulator x-ray where blocking is indicated. The electrified wire cuts the styrofoam at an angle matching the beam divergence. *A*, A low melting temperature (158°F) alloy is poured into the styrofoam mold. *C*, Blocks are fastened to lucite trays, and inserted into specially fitted holders on the head of the linear accelerator. *D*, Localization film taken on simulator with spinal cord block in place on right posterior oblique field. The isocenter (+) is localized over the primary lesion. *E*, Another localization film taken on a simulator with spinal cord blocks in place on a left posterior oblique field. In this case, good localization of the esophagus has been confirmed using swallowed contrast material. The collimator has been angled at 13°.

RADIATION DOSES

Experience with other tumors suggests that doses of at least 4500 rads to 5000 rad are necessary to control microscopic squamous cell carcinoma of the esophagus with a high degree of probability. At least 6000 rad to 7000 rad or more with conventional fractionation (180–225 rad per day) is needed to control gross disease.[101,102] A multicenter retrospective review of 2400 patients from 22 European countries concluded that radiation doses less than 3000 rad were ineffective in influencing the course of either pre- or postoperatively irradiated patients.[103] Doses above that level are felt to decrease recurrence from 50% to 36% and metastatic rate from 40% to 30% when applied postoperatively. The lack of detail of radiotherapeutic techniques or number of patients irradiated, however, warrants caution in interpretation of these data. Appelqvist noted an increased survival from 3.7% to 6.4% among 1430 patients treated with 5000 rad or more.[63] Other evidence is scanty that doses beyond 5000 to 6000 rad significantly influence results for this disease. The frequency of significant late esophageal damage in the form of ulceration or stricture is estimated to be 5% of patients treated to a Nominal Standard Dose (NSD) of 1850 ret (6300 rad, 30 fractions, 6 weeks). As many as 50% of patients treated to 2000 ret (6650 rad, 30 fractions, 6 weeks) will have these complications. Thus, a high degree of morbidity will be encountered when treating to very high doses (Table 16-9).[104]

Except for the most extreme cases, there is little difference between a curative or palliative regimen. The evidence from Beatty and colleagues indicated an optimum response at a Nominal Standard Dose (NSD), ranging between 1602 ret to 1714 ret (median 1679 ret).[90] Some physicians prefer to deliver an additional "boost" dose by intracavitary techniques. Inability to achieve significant doses at a useful distance from the source within the paraesophageal tissues limits this technique.[99,105–107]

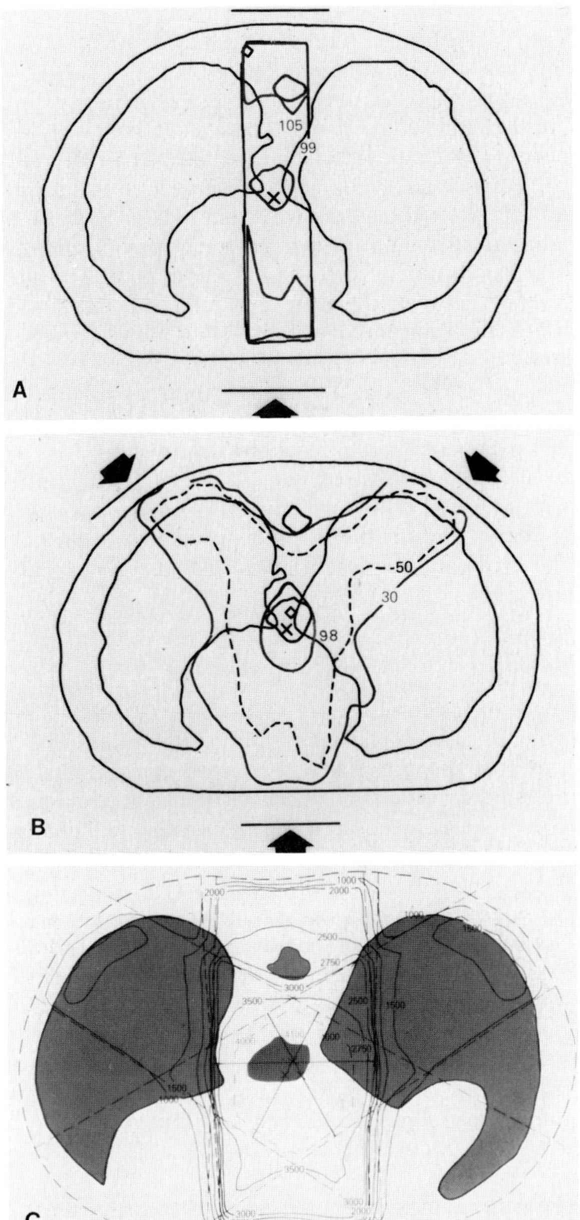

FIG. 16-26. *A,* Isodose curve for a patient with a mid-esophageal lesion treated with parallel opposed anterior and posterior fields (7 × 24 cm, at SAD, 100 cm, 6 MVX). The isodose plot is normalized to the isocenter. Notice that the spinal cord will receive a dose 5% higher than the isocenter, and 6% higher than the volume encompassed by the 99% isodose line. *B,* In contrast, using a 3-field arrangement with a combination of a direct anterior (gantry angle 180°), left posterior oblique (gantry angle 300°), and right posterior oblique (gantry angle 60°) field (7 × 24 cm, at SAD, 100 cm, 6 MVX) a more favorable dose distribution is obtained. The spinal cord receives only 30% of the dose delivered to isocenter. Generally a combination of AP/PA and oblique fields can be used. Rotational fields should be confined to "boost" fields, if used, since the shape of the esophagus does not conform sufficiently to a cylindrical volume. *C,* Using a combination of these two techniques (4 treatments AP/PA, 6 treatments by "3-fields"), at 400 rad minimum tumor dose per fraction, two fractions per week, the central plane dose distribution is as shown. The major portion of the irradiated lung receives only 1000 rad, with maximum spinal cord dose about 2800 rad. The isocenter on this plane is located so that the tumor volume also receives 4000 rad on more cephalad and caudad planes (8 × 21 cm at SAD, 100 cm, 6 MVX).

TABLE 16-9. A. Radiation Tolerance of Normal Esophagus

DOSE (rads)	NORMAL STANDARD DOSE (rets)	INCIDENCE OF COMPLICATIONS*
6300	1850	5%
6650	2000	50%

B. Recommended Maximum Tolerated Dose to the Esophagus

DOSE PER FRACTION (rads)	FRACTIONS PER WEEK	TOTAL (rads)	TIME (weeks)
180–200	5	5000–6800	5–6
400	2	4400–4800	5½–6

* Incidence of clinically significant late esophageal damage (ulceration or stenosis)—30 fractions, 6 weeks (105).

Generally, squamous cell carcinomas of the esophagus are moderately radiosensitive. Local control can be obtained with 20% to 50% of esophageal cancers. Even large lesions can show responses, but the response is poorer for lesions greater than 10 cm in length. Occasional cures occur with 8 cm to 9 cm lesions, justifying aggressive attempts in patients with large localized lesions.[90,91,107]

The importance of tumor grade has been infrequently addressed in the literature. Some authors claim more rapid regression with poorly differentiated tumors.[69] Palliative doses at 4000 rad in ten 400-rad fractions (2 fractions per week over 5 weeks) have also been employed. Curative doses are carried to 4400 rad to 4800 rad, with the last 400 rad to 800 rad being given through a reduced field. The initial treatment is carried out with parallel opposed anterior and posterior portals for 1600 rad, with the remainder given through a 3-field technique (direct anterior, left posterior oblique, and right posterior oblique).

Preoperatively, 4500 rad to 5000 rad are recommended with conventional fractionation (180–200 rad per day). When preoperative radiation is elected, careful coordination and discussion between the radiation oncologist and surgeon are particularly necessary.

Treatment is carried out on megavoltage radiotherapy units. While treatment on a cobalt apparatus or 4 MV linear accelerator is acceptable, higher energy roentgen rays result in more favorable dose distributions.

PALLIATIVE IRRADIATION

Responses to radiation are common, either radiographic or symptomatic. Other than patients with tracheo-esophageal fistulae, most patients are likely to benefit from radiation therapy. Generally, 5000 rads are given by parallel opposed anterior and posterior portals encompassing the entire esophagus for palliation. Resolution of symptoms, particularly dysphagia and pain, can be expected in approximately 80% of patients. Local symptoms and complications of tumor can also be controlled in patients with metastatic disease.

Wara reported that 92 of 103 patients had relief of dysphagia with radiation therapy alone.[97] The average length of palliation was 6 months, with a median of 3 months. Only 11% of these patients were palliated for 6 to 12 months. However, 26% of patients without metastases or with only minor symptoms were palliated for one year as opposed to only one of 35 patients with major symptoms and metastases. While median palliation was almost identical (3.0 versus 2.5 months) in both groups, mean length of palliation was 9.1 as opposed to 3.1 months.

Elkon and colleagues reported partial resolution of dysphagia in 84% and complete resolution in 63% of patients treated by irradiation.[93] Similarly, Marcial reported 77% of patients had relief of dysphagia, but that a significant proportion became reobstructed.[69] In the experience at the National Cancer Institute, symptomatic response was observed in nearly 80% of patients with 400 rad twice weekly to a total of 4000 to 4800 rad.[108] Most patients showed obvious radiographic improvement, and the only patient with total obstruction resumed oral feeding. Other symptoms, such as pain, weight loss, and anorexia are also often relieved with irradiation alone. Even when obstruction results, irradiation may prevent symptoms secondary to nerve or bronchial involvement.[107]

CLINICAL COURSE

During a course of radiation therapy to the esophagus, the patient generally will notice some slight dysphagia or odynophagia in the second and third week of treatment. This esophagitis, characterized by a burning sensation, is the result of epithelial desquamation. Discomfort reaches its peak toward the end of treatment, and usually diminishes within a few weeks after completion.

Some improvements in swallowing may be noticed as early as 1 week to 2 weeks after starting irradiation.[107] This occurs with either conventional doses, or with twice weekly 400 rad doses. At the NCI, the experience with minimum tumor doses of 400 rad twice weekly had yielded very satisfactory results, with frequent improvement in swallowing and only minimal dysphagia from treatment. Acute side effects with this fractionation are usually less severe than conventional fractionated doses (5000–6000 rad in 5–6½ weeks), when doses of 4400 rad are not exceeded. Use of systemic analgesics or local agents, such as 4% viscous lidocaine, are infrequently needed with 400 rad twice weekly to 4400 rad total minimum tumor dose. With any fractionation, nausea, emesis, reflux with burning, and increased mucus formation can occur. When coughing is noticed, particularly after eating or drinking, tracheo-esophageal fistula should be suspected. Persistent fever and chest pain should alert the physician to possible mediastinitis from perforation.

RESULTS OF RADIATION ALONE

As primary treatment, results with radiation therapy have generally been as discouraging as those obtained by surgery. One review of major radiation series between 1964 and 1970 concluded that only 2.7% of 10,024 patients survived five years.[63] A review of 14 series comprising 3637 patients showed a 5-year survival rate ranging from 0 to 20%.[65,69,90–93,97,109–115]

The best results, a nonrandomized series of patients from Edinburgh, have not been duplicated elsewhere.[114] A comparative historical group of 363 patients treated with surgery between 1948 and 1962 achieved only 11% survival at 5 years. Patients receiving radical irradiation in this series had relatively favorable lesions with tumors less than 10 cm in length (mean 6 cm), no evidence of tracheo-esophageal fistula, and no more remote metastases or lymphatic spread. The difference between the results of radiation and surgery is ascribed by Pearson to operative morbidity. Exclusion of patients greater than 75 years old from the surgical series raises the 5-year survival from that group of patients to 23%. A more recent report from the same author stated that 17% of 288 patients radically treated by radiotherapy were alive 5 years after treatment as opposed to 11% of 432 patients treated by surgery.[91] One criticism of these data has been that patients who did not complete the course of radiation were not included in the analysis, thus leading to a bias in favor of radiation therapy.[116]

COMPLICATIONS AND SIDE EFFECTS

The possible side effects of esophageal irradiation include esophagitis, pneumonitis, myelitis, and carditis. The latter two are rarely seen, probably because of short survival. Other rare complications are radionecrosis of the spinal column and pericarditis leading to pericardial constriction. Pneumonitis is also infrequent if attention is paid to keeping the pulmonary dose and volume acceptable. Pulmonary fibrosis may be a long-term sequel of excessive pulmonary radiation.[106]

The low percentage of long-term survivors in this disease does not justify abandonment of careful radiotherapeutic technique. Myelitis in the occasional survivor represents a pathetic and pyrrhic victory. While most quoted doses do not correct for the decreased attentuation of roentgen rays in the air-filled lungs, this factor should be taken into account when planning treatment. Mediastinal and lung doses are often 20% to 30% higher when the fields are directed through lung.[117]

The dangers of precipitating a tracheoesophageal fistula or aortic rupture during radiotherapy of tumors involving these structures has been alluded to. Post-radiation esophageal stricture at the site of an adequately treated tumor may also occur.[30]

FUTURE PROSPECTS FOR RADIATION THERAPY

Local control remains a critical problem with esophageal carcinoma. Since the ultimate development of effective systemic agents will likely emphasize the importance of local control of bulk tumor, improvements in radiation therapy will be necesary. Among the avenues currently under investigation, electron affinic hypoxic cell radiosensitizers, particularly misonidazole (Ro-07-0582) and metronidazole (Flagyl), may increase the effect of irradiation on tumors in preference to normal tissue.[118] Another group of radiosensitizers are the thiaxamethenones, actinomycin-D and lucontone (Nilodin). Since the rate of tumor cell death is 2.5 to 3 times higher in the presence of oxygen than under hypoxic conditions, these agents may render radiotherapy more effective in the treatment of esophageal cancer. Hyperthermia has also been used to potentiate the effects of radiation therapy. Conversely, agents selectively protective of normal tissue but not tumors, such as the phosphorothioate WR 2721, are also under clinical trial.

Charged particles or neutrons hold some theoretical, though yet untested, promise. Meanwhile, conventional photon irradiation remains as the mainstay in the management of this disease.

TREATMENT OF SQUAMOUS CELL CARCINOMA OF THE CERVICAL ESOPHAGUS

Additional material on the treatment of cervical esophageal lesions can be found in Chapter 13.

SURGERY

Resection of a squamous cell carcinoma of the cervical esophagus usually requires removal of portions of the pharynx, the entire larynx and thyroid, and the proximal esophagus.[119] If cervical lymph nodes are involved and the lesion is localized to that, a unilateral radical neck dissection may be included. This is a formidable procedure, leaving a large defect that is difficult to reconstruct. Table 16-10 outlines the technics that can be employed to reconstruct pharyngoesophageal continuity. The operation of choice is currently a pharyngogastrostomy.[120] The stomach is brought up through the posterior mediastinum after it is adequately mobilized as was described for reconstruction of the thoracic esophagus. The entire thoracic esophagus is bluntly dissected free of the surrounding mediastinal structure and resected (Fig. 16-14). Alternatively, a gastric tube may be constructed from the greater curvature of the stomach to re-establish gastrointestinal continuity (Fig. 16-21). These extensive reconstructive procedures further compromise the patient who has already been stressed by the resection of the carcinoma.

The surgical treatment of cervical esophageal malignancies can be summarized by stating that the procedures carry a significant morbidity, leave the patient with a great disability and provide little hope for cure. Most recent reports cite a 20% 2-year survival rate. However, if an esophagogastrostomy is uncomplicated, significant palliation is achieved and the patient may swallow food and saliva without difficulty.

TABLE 16-10. Reconstructive Procedures Following Cervical Esophagectomy

Pharyngogastrostomy
Reverse gastric tube
Skin tubes and skin grafts
Wookey procedure
deltopectoral flap (Bakamjian)
others
Intestinal grafts with vascular anastomoses
jejunum
sigmoid
gastric antrum
Colonic interposition

RADIATION THERAPY

Lesions in the cervical esophagus represent a particularly vexing problem. Generally these lesions are too low to allow good coverage with parallel opposed lateral fields, since irradiation would take place through the patient's shoulders. Conversely, they are often too high to allow treatment with posterior oblique fields. However, it is possible to utilize anterior oblique fields, often with wedges, to obtain satisfactory treatment. It must be stressed again that the proximity of such dose-limiting structures as the spinal cord to the esophagus makes treatment of this disease technically challenging in virtually all patients. Treatment planning technics and radiation dosages are as described in the previous section.

CHEMOTHERAPY OF ESOPHAGEAL CANCER

Because it is difficult to control the primary lesion in patients with esophageal carcinoma, local problems dominate the course of this tumor. Esophageal obstruction causing nutritional deficiency and aspiration pneumonia are the most common problems encountered and must be dealt with before instituting chemotherapy. Invasion of adjacent structures occurs frequently and generally results in fistula formation, connecting the esophagus to the bronchus or trachea. These fistulae usually make any antineoplastic therapy of dubious benefit since successful reduction of the tumor size leads to the enlargement of the fistula and further increases the risk of aspiration pneumonia, mediastinitis, and empyema.

Distant mestatases may present clinical problems in patients whose primary disease has not been controlled, but this happens infrequently. However, in patients whose survival has been prolonged by successful surgery or radiation therapy of the primary tumor, distant metastases acquire increasing clinical significance. In patients with controlled primary disease, distant metastases account for most of the symptoms and present the most common indication for systemic chemotherapy. The paraneoplastic syndromes which are occasionally produced by esophageal cancers may also require systemic chemotherapy.

Since local complications of the uncontrolled esophageal cancer, such as aspiration pneumonia, tracheoesophageal fistulae, and severe cachexia, make the use of cytotoxic therapy in these patients hazardous and, because of the relative infrequency of well-defined measurable metastatic deposits, there is little useful published information on chemotherapy of this disease (Table 16-11). Many of the studies do not provide the precise methods used to determine tumor regression. For this reason, one must evaluate the data with caution. For example, the reported response rates for bleomycin range between 0% and 60%.

At Wayne State University, we developed a set of criteria to determine the degree of tumor response to non-resective therapy. Local disease is particularly difficult to assess, since tumor ulceration and intraluminal necrosis without actual

TABLE 16-11. Single Drugs in the Treatment of Esophageal Cancer

REFERENCE	NUMBER OF PATIENTS EVALUATED	NUMBER OF PATIENTS RESPONDING	RESPONSE RATE	DOSE SCHEDULE
5-FLUOROURACIL				
(121)	26	4	15%	500 mg/m² IV for 5 days every 5 weeks
(122)	14	2	14%	15 mg/kg IV for 4–5 days, then 7.5 mg/kg every 2–3 days to toxicity; repeated monthly
(122)	1	1	100%	1 gm IV for 4 days, then 0.5 gm every 2 days to toxicity
(122)	3	0	0%	15 mg/kg IV weekly for 4 days, then 20 mg/kg weekly for 4 weeks if tolerated
METHOTREXATE				
(121)	27	2	7%	40 mg/m² IV weekly
ADRIAMYCIN				
(121)	18	1	5%	60 mg/m² IV every 3 weeks
(123)	18	6	33%	40 mg/m² for 2 days every 3 weeks
CIS-PLATINUM				
(124)	19	5	26%	50 mg/m² IV days 1 and 8 every 4 weeks
VINDESINE				
(125)	22	3	13%	3 mg/m² IV starting dose, increased by 0.5 mg/m² to maximum dosage of 4.5 mg/m² weekly for 7 weeks, then every 2 weeks thereafter
METHYL GAG				
(126)	2	1	50%	500 mg/m² IV weekly, increased by 100 mg/m² weekly in absence of toxicity
(127)	21	10	47%	5 mg/kg IV daily for 20 days
(128)	3	2	66%	3–4 mg/kg IM twice weekly
CCNU				
(129)	19	3	16%	
HEXAMETHYLMELAMINE				
(130)	3	1	33%	
BLEOMYCIN				
(131)	10	5	50%	15 mg IV daily for 20 days or 30 mg every other day for 10 days
(132)	15	4	26%	15 mg/m² IV twice weekly to total dose of 220–400 mg
(133)	14	0	0%	20 mg/m² IV daily to total dose of 280 mg
(134)	42	7	16%	15 mg/m² IV twice weekly to total dose of 300 mg
(135)	4	0	0%	15 mg IV/IM starting dose followed by 30 mg twice or thrice weekly depending on tolerance, for total dose of 300 mg
(136)	5	1	20%	10–20 mg/m² IV daily for 10–38 days for maximal total dose of 300 mg; in some patients, 20 mg/m² IV was given twice weekly
(137)	3	2	66%	30 mg/m² twice weekly for 4 weeks, repeated after one month
(137)	3	1	33%	15 mg/m² IV for 8 days, repeated after one month
(137)	3	0	0%	15 mg/m² IV for 5 days, repeated two more times at 3 week intervals
(137)	3	0	0%	15 mg/m² IV twice weekly for 4 weeks repeated after one month
(137)	17	1	5%	10 mg/m² IV twice weekly for 4 doses, repeated after one month
(138)	4	4	100%	0.25 mg/kg IV daily to toxicity
(139)	10	6	60%	15 mg/m² IV twice weekly per 4 weeks
(140)	4	0	0%	dose ranging between 1.25 mg/m² to 35 mg/m² IV twice weekly for total of 12 doses

response can mimic tumor response and actually can be followed by transient symptomatic response. Therefore, we classified tumor response as only symptomatic when a patient's swallowing improved and when the esophageal lumen clearly enlarged on barium study. The term "partial tumor response" was confined to patients with unequivocal radiographic improvement when it was accompanied by histological proof of tumor disappearance from a previously histologically documented involved site. In order to classify local response as complete, we demand that the surgically removed primary tumor site contain no histologically recognizable tumor.

The objective evaluation of metastatic tumor represents less difficulty. Liver metastases and retroperitoneal or paraesophageal masses can often be accurately measured by CT, a technic not available to older investigators. Lung metastases are most often discrete and nodular and can be followed by chest roentgenograms.

As in other neoplasms, we generally required that the product of the diameters of such clearly measurable lesions would shrink by at least 50% to qualify a patient for partial tumor response status. Patients classified as having complete tumor response would have to demonstrate complete disappearance of previously documented tumors. To date, in patients treated with systemic therapy alone, we have not seen complete response in this tumor using these criteria.

Agents with some documented activity against carcinoma of the esophagus include 5-fluorouracil (5-FU), mitomycin-C, bleomycin, and *cis*-diamminedichloroplatinum (*cis*-DDP). The effects of methotrexate and of the alkylating agents are not as well documented.[141,142]

Bleomycin is probably the single most effective available drug in the treatment of esophageal cancer. It has been explored in preoperative regimens alone and in combination with radiation.[131,132,143] The tumor responses observed were encouraging. However, the enthusiasm for these combinations must be tempered by the high rate of pulmonary complications observed in these patients. Radiated lung is unusually prone to develop bleomycin-induced pneumonia. Patients with esophageal cancer, with their common episodes of aspiration and frequent history of smoking-related lung disease, do not tolerate this complication well.

Methyl-GAG, a recently rediscovered antineoplastic agent, has produced some encouraging responses in esophageal tumors. However, while the data justify further studies, at the time this is being written, they should be viewed only as representing preliminary observations.[126-128]

COMBINATION CHEMOTHERAPY OF ESOPHAGEAL CARCINOMA

In a large study designed to compare a nitrosourea (methyl CCNU) to mitomycin-C in gastrointestinal malignancies when used in combination with a non-myelosuppressive infusion schedule of 5-FU, the Southwest Oncology Group treated 19 patients with disseminated esophageal cancer.[144] Four out of ten treated patients responded to mitomycin-C and 5-FU, but none of the nine patients so treated responded to the methyl CCNU combination. All of these patients received 5-fluorouracil as a continuous daily infusion of 1000 mg/m^2 for four days repeated every four weeks. In the mitomycin-C containing arm, patients received 20 mg/m^2 mitomycin-C intravenously every eight weeks. In the other arm, 175 mg/m^2 methyl CCNU was administered, also at eight week intervals. Other combination chemotherapy regimens with greater or lesser degrees of success are listed in Table 16-12.

Kelsen and colleagues were encouraged by the results of bleomycin and *cis*-DDP in the treatment of patients with squamous cell carcinoma of the head and neck. Therefore, they utilized this combination for patients with advanced squamous cell carcinoma of the esophagus.[142,145] A 25% response rate (complete and partial remissions) was obtained in 12 patients with measurable metastatic disease. Median

TABLE 16-12. Combination Chemotherapy in the Treatment of Esophageal Cancer

DRUGS	RESPONSE RATE	REFERENCE
5-Fluorouracil and Mitomycin-C	4/10	(144)
Methotrexate, Bleomycin and *cis*-Platinum	5/8	(141)
Bleomycin and *cis*-Platinum	12/65	(142, 145)
Vincristine, Methyl CCNU and 5-Fluorouracil	1/1	(146)

survival was 4 months from onset of chemotherapy. Minor regressions with symptomatic improvements were noted in an additional 50% of patients.

Hentek and colleagues were also encouraged by the results they obtained with a combination of methotrexate, bleomycin and cis-DDP in head and neck cancers.[141] They used this combination in the treatment of advanced esophageal cancer. A response rate of 50% was seen.

The current status of the role of chemotherapy for esophageal carcinoma can be summarized as follows: Only patients with locally controlled disease suffering from distant metastases are good candidates for systemic chemotherapy. Bleomycin, *cis*-DDP (alone or in combination), and 5-FU and mitomycin-C combinations appear to be the best available therapies for these patients. Responses in 20% of patients can be expected with a duration of 2 months to 3 months. The main role of chemotherapy in the management of this tumor will probably be in pre-operative and adjuvant use when combined with radiotherapy. Pulmonary toxicity of otherwise effective drugs like bleomycin and, to a lesser extent, mitomycin-C, makes them difficult to use in this setting. A great deal of work remains to be done in establishing effective protocols using drugs such as *cis*-DDP, 5-FU, and methotrexate in combination with radiation.

COMBINED MODALITY THERAPY OF CARCINOMA OF THE ESOPHAGUS

PREOPERATIVE RADIATION THERAPY

Several groups of radiation therapists and surgeons have recognized that it might be possible to significantly improve the results of therapy of carcinoma of the esophagus by treating patients with radiotherapy prior to resection (Table 16-13). Such efforts arose out of a realization that the advantages of radiation therapy and operative therapy would complement each other. The former carries a low mortality and morbidity and can produce a marked regression in tumor bulk as well as sterilize microscopic disease in areas not resected. It is possible to treat a wider area surrounding the esophageal cancer by radiation therapy than can be reasonably accomplished by surgical means (Fig. 16-27). On the other hand, esophagectomy can treat a greater length of esophagus and contribute to minimizing the possibility of local recurrence. It is hoped that the reduction in tumor bulk resulting from pre-operative radiation therapy would also increase

TABLE 16-13. Preoperative Radiation Therapy

REFERENCE	RADIATION THERAPY	RESECTABILITY	SURGICAL MORBIDITY	SURVIVAL 2 YEAR	SURVIVAL 5 YEAR
(147)	4500 r/4½ wk	47/85 (55%)	15%		2/47 (4%)
(148)	4500 r/½ wk	101/332 (30%)	18%	23/101 (23%)	14/101 (14%)
(149)	2000–2500 r/3–4 day	281/?	4%	41/107 (38%)	3/8 (37.5%)
(150)	5000–6000 r/5–6 wk	76/117 (65%)	21%		(25%)
(151)	5000–6000 r/5–7 wk	22/40 (57%)	33%		2/22 (9%)
(152)	2400 r/3 day	46/70 (66%)	20%	5/46 (10%)	
(153)	5000–6000 r/6–8 wk	12/18 (67%)	6%		4/18 (22%)
(65)	4000 r/4 wk	81/133	21%		18/81 (21%)

resectability rates and decrease operative mortality. Another potential benefit of preoperative radiation is the prevention of metastases and local recurrence of tumor resulting from the operation because of the sterilizing effect of radiation on malignant cells. Finally, it might be possible to use lower radiation doses which would control smaller tumor masses but not the major bulk of tumor.[107] The latter would be reduced in size and, it is to be hoped, resected.

Generally, one-half to three-fourths of the sterilizing dose of radiation is given prior to the operation. The latter should be timed to take place after the early hyperemia secondary to radiation resolves and before fibrosis and scarring occur. The ideal time is between 4 weeks and 6 weeks after completion of radiation therapy.

It is postulated that the difficulties encountered in operating in areas which have received radiation would not increase morbidity and mortality when the aforementioned principles are followed. This has often been true. However, in some instances the morbidity of preoperative radiation has been as high as either operative or radiation therapy alone. Mortality has ranged from 4% to 33%.

One of the earliest groups to institute a treatment protocol of radiation and resection was the one at the Memorial Hospital in New York (Table 16-13). In 15% of cases, there was no evidence of cancer in the resected specimen. Prolongation of the treatment period was considered a disadvantage of preoperative radiation by this group. They concluded that preoperative irradiation would not affect the 5-year survival rate but that it would increase the resectability rate.[147]

FIG. 16-27. Portions of esophagus and adjacent tissues best treated by radiation and resection. (Adapted from Pearson JG: The present status and feature potential of radiotherapy in the management of esophageal cancer. Cancer 39:882, 1977)

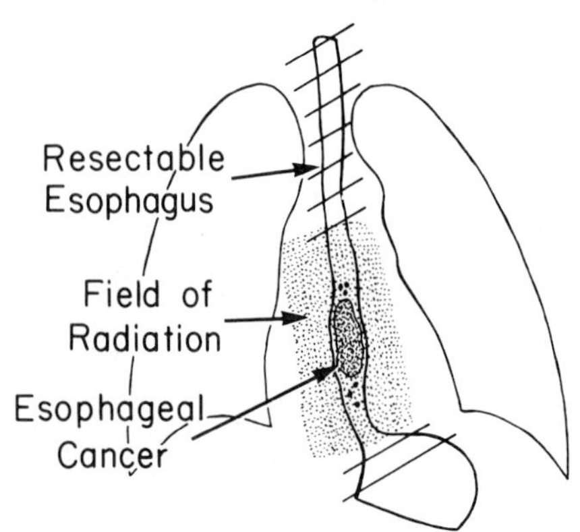

At about the same time the Memorial Hospital group began utilizing preoperative radiotherapy, the group in Charleston, South Carolina adopted a similar approach.[148,154] Fourteen to 30 days after completing the radiotherapy 30% of this group subsequently underwent esophagectomy with either stomach or colon replacement; the former was the procedure of choice. No tumor could be found in 3% of the resected patients. The tumor was reduced to an *in situ* carcinoma in another 10% of 101 resected patients. None of the additional 36 unresectable patients, or the 13 of 101 resected patients who had positive subdiaphragmatic nodes, survived 5 years. The resected patients had tumors which averaged only 4.2 cm in length. This may indicate that pre-operative irradiation should be utilized in a select group of patients when aggressively attempting to cure them of esophageal cancer.[148] When Parker and colleagues compared their initial experiences (1957–1960) to the 1962 to 1967 experience (consisting of 135 and 138 patients respectively) they found that there was an increase in the operability rate from 22% to 34% and an increase in resectability from 70% to 87%.[154] Tumor bulk was reduced by preoperative irradiation. Restoration of the ability to swallow was achieved in most cases, followed by improvement in the patient's nutritional state.

In Japan, where cancer of the esophagus occurs more frequently than in the United States, Nakayama instituted a regimen of preoperative radiation therapy in 1958.[112,149] He and his colleagues adopted a plan of therapy which differed appreciably from other centers utilizing this approach. Nakayama performed a laparotomy and gastrostomy 7 to 10 days prior to irradiation of 2000 rad to 2500 rad in four to five fractions using megavoltage equipment. Three to five days later an esophagectomy and cervical esophagostomy was performed; the latter was connected to the gastrostomy by means of an external rubber tube. Reconstruction consisted of an antethoracic cervical esophagogastrostomy at a third operation. A 37.5% 5-year survival (3 of 8 patients at risk) appears to be an artifact of the exclusion of patients from the analysis who did not complete the planned treatment.[149]

Akakura and his colleagues at the Keio University Hospital instituted a program of preoperative irradiation in 1963.[150] A report of their results in 110 patients with squamous cell carcinoma of the thoracic esophagus revealed that they could resect 82% of the patients. Only 65% could be resected for cure. They found that the resectability rate doubled with preoperative radiation and almost tripled the rate of resection for cure. The resection was found to be easier with less blood loss in the preoperatively irradiated group of patients when compared to patients who had undergone resection without prior radiation. Occasionally, esophagopleural and esophagobronchial fistulas closed during radiation therapy, making resection possible.

At Stanford University a similar approach was instituted in 1962.[151] Only 77% of patients survived esophageal resection and reconstruction. Survival was not improved over the use of either radiation or operation alone. If supraclavicular or epigastric nodes were positive on biopsy, 6100 rad were given to these areas and 4400 rad to the esophagus and uninvolved epigastrium. This intensive pre-operative radiation regimine resulted in aorto-esophageal and tracheo-esophageal fistulae, radiation pneumonitis, and radiation carditis. The high incidence of adverse radiation effects was matched by frequent (7 of 23) elimination of the malignancy in the resected specimen. Only two patients survived 5 years.

In Rotterdam 41% of 328 patients seen completed a course of preoperative radiotherapy for esophageal cancer.[65] Thirty-nine percent of this group could not be resected for cure because of distant metastases or local extention. Only a quarter of all the patients seen completed the combined treatment protocol. Pre-operative radiation was not judged to have contributed to postoperative morbidity and mortality. Postoperatively, patients received an additional 2500 rad to 2600 rad if the surgeon had any doubt about the complete removal of the tumor or if the tumor was present in or close to the resection margins. The 5 year actuarial survival rate of the 81 patients completing this protocol was 21%.

An important conclusion emerges from this review of pre-operative radiation for esophageal cancer. It is not proven that the combination of pre-operative radiation and resection is an improvement over each treatment modality used alone. The higher survival rates reported with combined therapy may represent a process of selection whereby those patients with incurable disease are eliminated as the pre-operative radiation proceeds and the patients are prepared for resection. Only well-controlled prospective clinical trials will be able to determine the true value of pre-operative radiation therapy in the treatment of esophageal carcinoma.

POSTOPERATIVE RADIATION THERAPY

When an exploratory thoracotomy or laparotomy reveals an unresectable advanced carcinoma of the thoracic esophagus, postoperative radiotherapy is often utilized to control the cancer, whether or not a palliative bypass is performed. Radiation therapy under these circumstances should be considered palliative therapy also. An unresectable lesion is unlikely to be cured by radiation therapy, but such a possibility always exists.

The rationale for radiation therapy following curative resections of esophageal cancers resides in the hope that irradiation will eradicate residual disease. The latter could be located within the unresected esophagus, despite the absence of tumor at the margins of resection, or as micrometastases in regional lymphatics and lymph nodes that were not removed. Postoperative radiation may also be effective in controlling implantation or seeding of tumor, which may have occurred at the operation.

More effective radiation might be possible postoperatively. The surgeon can demarcate the extent of the tumor with radiopaque clips at the time of the operation and thus allow the radiotherapist to more accurately direct the treatment to the involved area. However, if the stomach or colon is brought up into the area formerly occupied by the esophagus, radiation therapy must be limited to 4500 rad to 5000 rad because of the greater sensitivity of these viscera to radiation injury.

Postoperative radiation therapy is most often employed when (1) there is tumor found at the margins of the resected esophagus, (2) if tumor was known to be left in the mediastinum, (3) when lymph nodes are involved, or (4) when recurrences become manifest. Of seven patients who underwent esophagectomy and postoperative radiation for the reasons enumerated above, Fraser and colleagues reported two 10-year survivors.[153] Both had tumor present at the resected margins of the esophagus. Goodner reported 25 patients who had esophagectomy and esophagogastrostomy with postoperative irradiation.[147] Two patients survived for 5 years; the average survival was 9.9 months. At the Mayo Clinic, 14 patients with cancer of the upper thoracic esophagus were treated with postoperative radiation. Five of these patients were 3-year survivors.[56]

In summary, there is a paucity of data on the efficacy of postoperative radiation as adjuvant therapy. The advantage to this approach over pre-operative radiation is that an accurate anatomic staging of the disease is possible. On the other hand, if the esophageal reconstruction using stomach or colon is located in the posterior mediastinum, lower doses of radiation are required. This combination of radiation and operation deserves greater consideration as an approach to the curative therapy of cancer of the esophagus.

RESECTION AND CHEMOTHERAPY

There are very few studies recorded in which pre- or post-operative chemotherapy has been combined with resection in order to cure cancer of the esophagus. Fujimaki and colleagues treated 19 patients with pre-operative intramuscular bleomycin (15 mg daily or 30 mg every other day for a planned total dose of 300 mg).[131] Actual dosage ranged from 30 mg to 600 mg. Ten patients underwent resection; one patient did not survive the procedure. Side effects were seen in two of the patients, consisting of fever, skin changes, epilation, and pulmonary changes. In the brief follow-up, 60% of patients had died. Half the patients had histologic changes that were deemed to be effected by the chemotherapy.

Wada and colleagues used a similar regimen in 20 patients with carcinomas of the esophagus.[155] They reported radiographic improvement in 11 of 18 patients and believed that bleomycin had the greatest effect on highly differentiated squamous cell carcinomas.

Kelsen and coworkers employed a combination of preoperative *cis*-DDP and bleomycin for patients with Stage I and Stage II disease.[142] This combination was continued postoperatively. Radiation was used postoperatively if the lesion was Stage III.

Postoperative administration of bleomycin into the paraesophageal posterior mediastinum has been recommended to treat micrometastases in the upper mediastinal and cervical lymph nodes.[156] These nodes tend to be left at surgery, while the lower paraesophageal and paracardial nodes are removed. The efficacy of this form of adjuvant chemotherapy is unproven.

RADIATION AND CHEMOTHERAPY

In addition to their cytotoxic effect on malignant cells, some chemotherapeutic agents can potentiate the cancerocidal action of radiation therapy; *cis*-DDP is one such agent. 5-FU has radiosensitizing properties also. Byfield and colleagues have reported excellent preliminary results with the combination of biweekly infusion of 5-FU (20 μg/kg/24 hours for 5 days) combined with biweekly radiotherapy (250 rad/day for 4 days).[157] Four of six patients with unresectable lesions survived 6 to 21 months.

Roussel and coworkers treated patients with methotrexate before irradiation and found that survival was improved.[158] They gave 10 mg/day intramuscularly for 8 days prior to therapy. One- and three-year survival rates of 35% and 11% have been reported with this combination in inoperable cancer of the esophagus.

Kolaric combined bleomycin with radiation and obtained a response rate of 62%.[132] Kolaric and colleagues also utilized adriamycin alone and in combination with radiotherapy in a randomized study of inoperable esophageal cancer.[123] Eighteen patients were treated with six cycles of adriamycin (40 mg/m^2 for 2 days) with a three week rest period between cycles. Fifteen patients received 4500 to 5200 rad. Response rates increased from 33% to 60% when chemotherapy and radiation therapy were employed in combination. The duration of the response averaged 3.2 months in the adriamycin treated group and 8.6 months in the patients treated with combined therapy. The latter also resulted in more severe side effects (leukopenia, esophagobronchial fistulae, and weight loss). Perhaps because the port utilized for administering the radiation avoided exposing the heart, cardiac toxicity was the same in both groups.

There is a great need to develop adjuvant therapy with curative radiation therapy. To a large extent, radiation failures are due to persistence of malignancy, both locally and at a distance from the primary tumor.

RESECTION, RADIATION, AND CHEMOTHERAPY

If there is validity to the concept of multimodality therapy for esophageal carcinoma, the combination of resection, radiation, and chemotherapy should be most effective. The appeal of this approach, and the enthusiasm with which it is espoused, is not matched by hard data to support it. There are preliminary studies which indicate that a combination of chemotherapy, radiotherapy, and surgical treatment is effective. We must look to the experiences of those who have utilized these combinations in order to determine which treatment protocol would be most worthwhile to test in randomized prospective studies.

At Wayne State University, 54 patients with cancer of the esophagus were treated with 5-FU, mitomycin, and radiotherapy pre-operatively. Radiotherapy and chemotherapy were repeated postoperatively if cancer was found in the resected specimen. Mitomycin was given as a bolus injection on day 1. At the same time, radiation therapy (1000 rad per week for 3 weeks) and a continuous infusion of 5-FU (1000 mg/m^2/day for 4 days) was begun. One week after completing radiation therapy, the 5-FU infusion was repeated. Esophageal resection was undertaken 4 to 6 weeks after completing radiation therapy. Postoperative radiotherapy (2000 rad) and an additional course of chemotherapy were employed if tumor was present in the resected specimen. An esophagectomy using the combined abdominal–thoracic approach with reconstruction by esophagogastrectomy was the procedure of choice.

All patients treated by the above protocol showed significant diminution of tumor size.[159] In 25 patients treated for cure, 23 were successfully resected. Six patients showed no residual tumor in the resected specimens. Sixteen of 26 patients were successfully treated for palliation of their disease. Because pulmonary toxicity induced by mitomycin-C has recently been described and was observed in three patients in the Wayne State University series, an attempt to substitute cis-DDP for mitomycin-C is being attempted with initially encouraging results (Fig. 16-28).[160]

Werner and colleagues combined methotrexate, radiotherapy, and resection in curable patients. A similar approach without surgery was used for palliative care.[161] A relatively low mortality was seen. Kolaric and coworkers have combined adriamycin with radiation and resection.[123]

Fujimaki and colleagues treated 76 patients with a combination of bleomycin and radiation pre-operatively.[131] Their latest protocol called for chemotherapy (intramuscular bleomycin, 7.5 mg/day for 10 days) and radiation (200 rad/day for 15 days) to begin simultaneously. Histologic changes of the primary lesions were used to assess the effectiveness of bleomycin and irradiation. "Favorable changes" were induced in 69% of primary lesions. The authors were enthusiastic about this combination but were concerned about the effect of higher doses of bleomycin (circa 300 mg) on the lungs. Nygaard and coworkers reported a postoperative mortality of 50% among eight patients treated with pre-operative radiation (3000 rad) and bleomycin (120 mg total dose over a prolonged period).[162] They attributed three of the four deaths to respiratory failure. Surviving patients also had varying degrees of pulmonary infiltrates. The authors postulate that bleomycin sensitizes the lungs to radiation damage and the surgical trauma triggers a reaction which leads to respiratory failure. All the patients who died demonstrated interstitial pneumonitis.

Kelsen and coworkers treated 21 patients with pre-operative chemotherapy consisting of *cis*-DDP on day one (3 mg/kg as a rapid intravenous infusion after prehydration, followed by a mannitol-induced diuresis) and bleomycin on day 3 (10 to 15 units/m^2 as a loading dose and 10 to 15 units/m^2 as a 24 hour infusion for 3 days).[142] Two weeks after a single course of chemotherapy, esophagectomy was performed. Postoperatively, a second course of chemotherapy was given as soon as possible and every 6 to 8 weeks thereafter. In Stage III patients, radiation therapy (400 R twice a week for 4 weeks) was given after the second course of chemotherapy. The latter

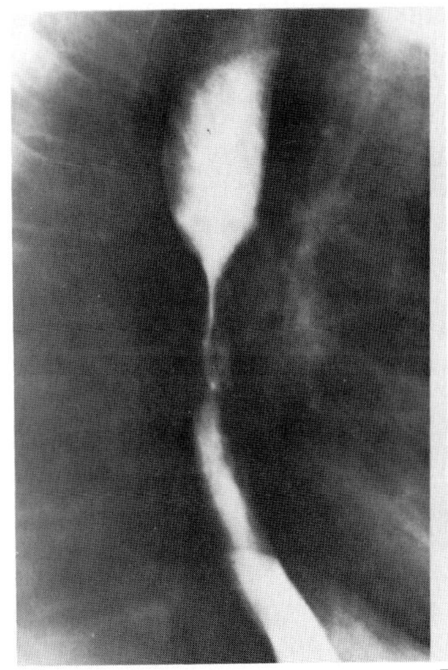
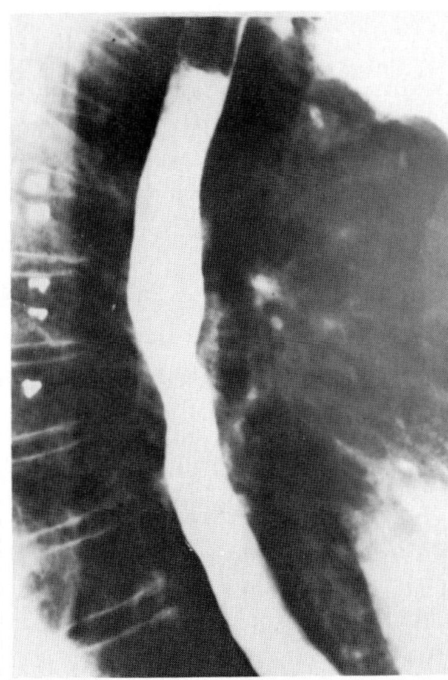

FIG. 16-28. Response of an esophageal cancer to radiation therapy (3000 rad) and 5-FU and *cis*-platinum therapy. (*A*) Preoperative esophagogram. (*B*) Esophagogram after preoperative treatment.

was also continued after radiation for a total of 5 courses to 8 courses in one year. Twelve of the 21 patients had resectable lesions. Eight were alive 4 to 16 months after onset of therapy; 66.6% of these patients had partial responses or minor regressions with the pre-operative chemotherapy. Alopecia, nausea and vomiting, diarrhea, fever, transient tinnitus, chills, ototoxic effects, renal dysfunction, and myelosuppression were among the toxic manifestations of the chemotherapy. The authors conclude that, "Further work is needed before recommending *cis*-DDP and bleomycin as an adjunct to surgery in patients with esophageal carcinoma."

SURGICAL PALLIATION OF SQUAMOUS CELL CARCINOMA OF THE THORACIC ESOPHAGUS

The palliative procedures available for patients with advanced squamous cell carcinoma of the esophagus are outlined in Table 16-14.

RESECTION

The circumstances under which one should perform a palliative esophagectomy are those which have a minimal morbidity and mortality and at least a year of reasonable survival. Patients who are not good candidates for palliative resection are those with the findings outlined in Table 16-15.

The rationale for esophageal resection to palliate esophageal cancer resides in the hope that the procedure can contribute to the patient's cure as well as palliation. If doubt exists as to whether an esophageal lesion can be removed for cure, and the patient is judged to be a good surgical risk, the esophagus should be resected. As pointed out previously, the justification for this philosophy is twofold: occasionally, residual tumor may be successfully eliminated by radiotherapy and chemotherapy, and esophageal resection constitutes satisfactory palliative therapy. As stated by Payne, ". . . most efforts in the management of this condition (esophageal cancer) are palliative for most patients but not prejudicial to cure for the few."[163]

At the Mayo Clinic, more than 90% of patients undergoing resection had unobstructed swallowing throughout their subsequent survival.[163] Hankins and colleagues performed a

TABLE 16-14. Palliative Procedures for Carcinoma of the Esophagus

- Resect and reconstruct
  - Intrathoracic
  - Extrathoracic
    - Presternal
    - Retrosternal
- Bypass
  - Intrathoracic
  - Extrathoracic
    - Presternal
    - Retrosternal
  - Colon
  - Stomach
- Intraluminal intubation
- Gastrostomy and cervical esophagogastrostomy with or without an external tube
- Dilatation

TABLE 16-15. Contraindications to Palliative Esophagectomy for Cancer of Thoracic Esophagus

- Advanced inanition and debilitation
- Inadequate cardio-pulmonary function
- Widespread (visceral) metastases
- Malignant pleural effusion
- Malignant ascites
- Recurrent laryngeal, phrenic or sympathetic nerve involvement.
- Superior vena caval obstruction.
- Tracheoesophageal fistula.
- Extension into the aortic wall or spinal column.

resection for palliation in 11 patients with middle third lesions.[164] All had tumor left behind. There were no operative deaths. At the time of their report five patients had died an average of 7 months postoperatively. Those that were still living had survived an average of 8 months. Similar satisfactory results were obtained following resection of lower third lesions in five patients. Wilson and coworkers performed 20 consecutive esophagogastrectomies with esophagogastrostomy for palliation with a 50% mortality.[165] Mean survival time was 11 months. Piccone and colleagues reported a 93% resectability rate with a 7% mortality. Mean survival time was also 11 months.[166]

At the other end of the spectrum is the series reported by Belsey and Hiebert.[167] The philosophy of these authors was also one which entailed esophagectomy for palliation. An exclusively right-sided thoracotomy approach was used without an abdominal incision. The stomach was mobilized through the esophageal hiatus. During the last 5 years of the study, 97% of all patients with mid-esophageal cancers underwent esophagogastrectomy. Of 119 patients operated upon for palliation, 25% lived one year or more; 8% lived between 2 years and 17 years. However, unlike the aforementioned series, the operative mortality was 28%. At the Duke University Medical Center, palliative resections carried a 20% mortality.[168] Herein lies the major problem with resection of the esophagus for palliation: it can carry a forbidding mortality rate. Morbidity is also high. In 5% to 10% of instances, palliation is not achieved because of anastomotic strictures or fistulae. Variations in the mortality rate are difficult to explain. In a single experience, Ong experienced an increase in the operative mortality rate from 13% to 21.8% in one year.[68]

FIG. 16-29. Mobilization of stomach for esophageal bypass. Note differences here with Fig. 16-13.

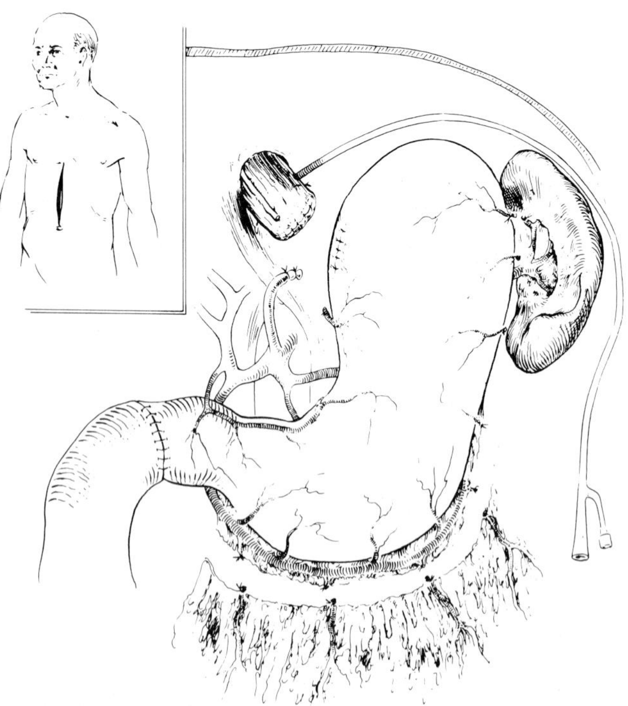

The prognosis of patients with advanced esophageal cancer is so poor that one might validly question whether an undertaking of the magnitude of an esophageal resection is reasonable. A bypass procedure is indicated when the conditions in Table 16-15 exist.

BYPASS

When esophageal resection would carry a prohibitive risk to the patient with concomitant cardiopulmonary disease or when resection cannot be performed because of technical reasons, the better palliative procedure would be one which bypasses the malignant esophageal obstruction. With this philosophy, one would not look upon bypass procedures as competitive to resection. The bypass procedure is reserved for those patients who are not candidates for resection.

Bypass procedures need not be thought of as exclusively palliative procedures. They may be used as the first stage of a curative plan of therapy, recognizing that, like esophageal resection, the bypass is at least palliative if not curative. Burdette employed this strategy, performing a right ileocolonic retrosternal esophagogastric bypass whenever possible.[11] Eight of 25 patients subsequently underwent a second stage procedure which consisted of an esophagectomy.

Currently, the bypass procedure most often recommended is the esophagogastrostomy. It has been well described in great detail by Orringer and Sloan who used it in ten patients with such advanced disease that resection was not possible.[169] The stomach is mobilized and then brought up behind the sternum and anastomosed to the cervical esophagus (Figs. 16-29 and 16-30). Because these patients had advanced malignant disease, postoperative complications were common and the mortality rate high (four deaths).

Steiger and colleagues were able to achieve a 7.4% operative mortality in 54 patients using gastric bypass to exclude the thoracic esophagus.[170] In approximately half of their patients, the stomach was brought up through the hiatus and the anastomosis was performed in the chest. The colon can also be used to bypass the obstructed esophagus (Fig. 16-31).

INTRALUMINAL INTUBATION

Intubation of the esophagus with a prosthetic tube has been used for many years in order to allow patients with malignant esophageal obstruction to swallow. The efficacy of this procedure varies from 40% to 85% and has a duration of approximately 4 months.[71]

Patients who are candidates for this procedure are those who have such advanced cancer of the esophagus that no other therapy is possible. These are patients who are very debilitated and who have tracheo-esophageal fistulae or invasion of the trachea, bronchus, or aorta. Patients who have recurrence after a course of radiotherapy and are not candidates for operative palliation may also benefit from intraluminal esophageal tubes.

There are two types of tubes that can be employed: those that depend entirely upon being pushed blindly through the area of obstruction, and those that are pulled by a guide wire or string through the esophagus into the stomach (Table 16-16). The "push through" tubes are limited to short (10 cm)

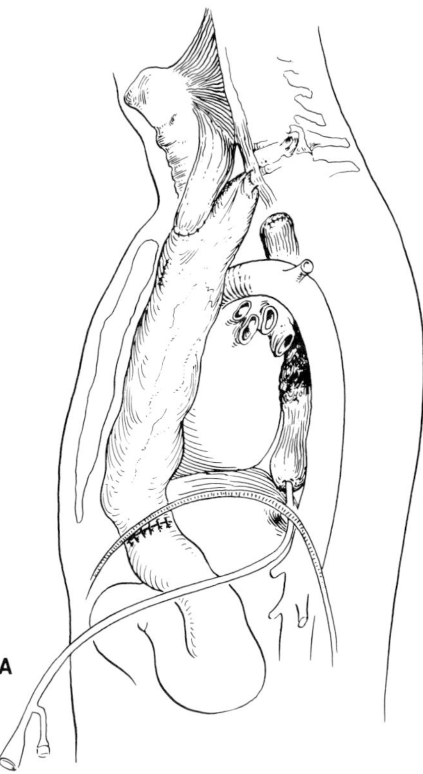

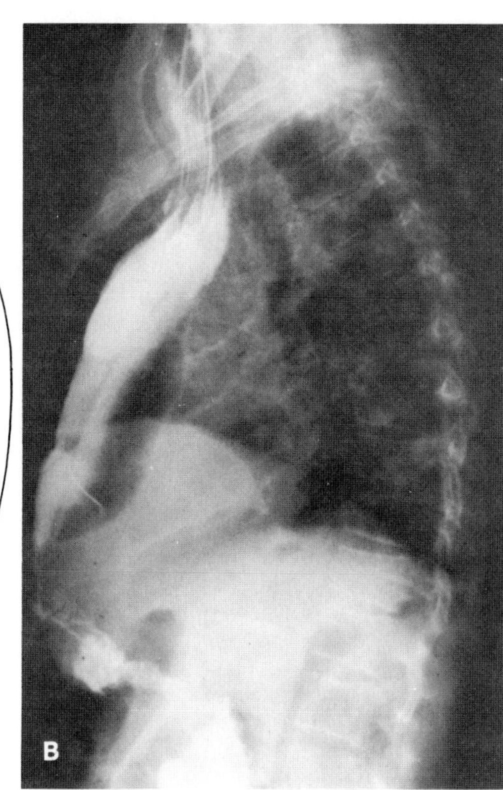

FIG. 16-30. *A*, The stomach is brought up behind the sternum and anastomosed to the esophagus. *B*, Radiographic appearance of a retrosternal gastric bypass.

segments and are best suited for middle and upper third lesions. "Pull through" tubes are most frequently used (Fig. 16-32). This type is best suited for middle or lower third lesions. They are anchored to the stomach by a suture after being placed in proper position.

FIG. 16-31. Colon interposed between cervical esophagus and stomach to bypass an esophagus occluded by a squamous cell carcinoma.

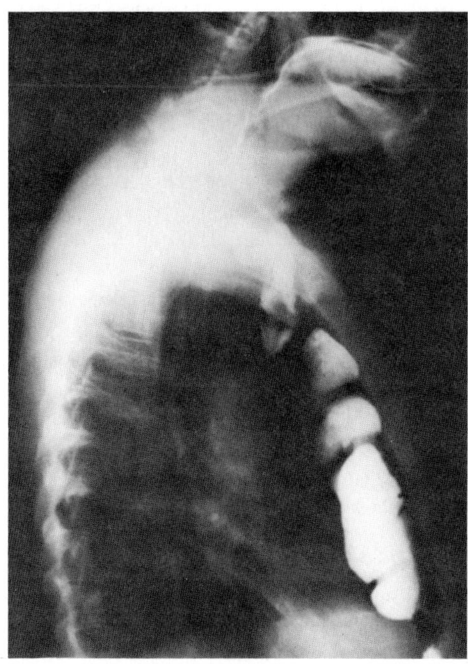

Endo-esophageal tubes have several drawbacks as palliative procedures. A mortality of 10% to 40% accompanies placement of intraluminal tubes.[71] Perforation of the esophagus with mediastinitis may occur. Aspiration of gastric contents is frequent, because the lower esophageal sphincter mechanism is eliminated when the tube passes through the esophagus into the stomach. Patients with this type of tube must be instructed to sleep with the head of the bed elevated. The tubes become dislodged and migrate in about 25% of instances. They also frequently become obstructed and patients must be instructed to chew their food well or confine their diet to semisolid (puréed) foods.

GASTROSTOMY AND CERVICAL ESOPHAGOSTOMY

The least satisfactory of the palliative procedures are those which create a gastrostomy to supply nutrition and a cervical esophagostomy to prevent aspiration of upper airway secretions. The latter procedure is of marginal benefit to the

TABLE 16-16. Intraluminal Intubation for Carcinoma of the Esophagus

PUSH-THROUGH TUBES
Mackler tube
Soutter tube
PULL-THROUGH TUBES
Celestin tube
Mousseau-Barbin tube
Fell tube
Haering tube

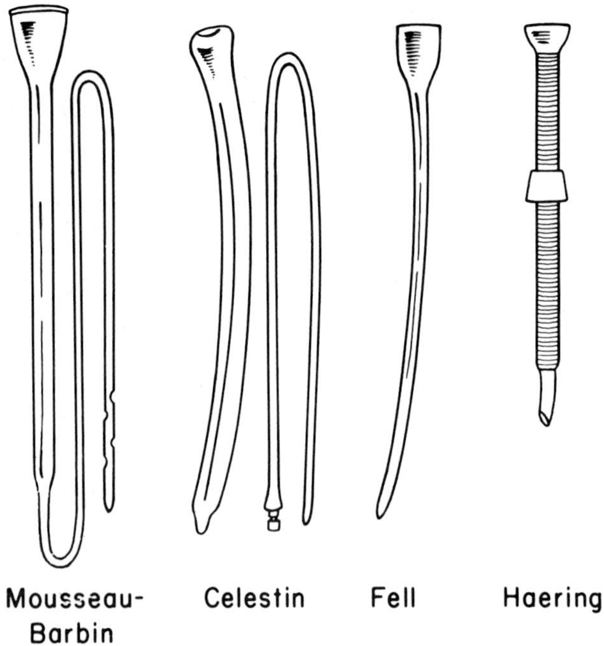

FIG. 16-32. Diagrammatic depiction of four commonly used intraluminal tubes.

patient, in that there is a constant trickle of material through the esophagostomy which is difficult to collect. Personal hygiene and appearance are difficult to maintain. Eating or drinking is not possible with this form of palliation, unless a tube is fashioned to connect the cervical esophagostomy with the gastrostomy; devices to accomplish this are not very effective.

DILATATION

A reasonable alternative to intubation of the esophagus or gastrostomy and cervical esophagostomy is dilatation of the malignant stricture with bougies. Boyce prefers to use the Eder–Preston dilator if the stricture is very tight. When the lumen can take a 15 mm dilator, Maloney bougies (tapered rubber tubes filled with mercury) are employed. When a 15 mm dilator can be passed, the patient will no longer experience dysphagia. Dilatation with the mercury filled bougies are continued daily or on alternate days for from a week to 10 days until the lumen of the esophagus will accept a 17 mm bougie. Radiation can be given in conjunction with this method of palliation. There was no increased incidence of perforation of the esophagus when radiation was combined with esophageal dilatation. During a 3-year period 26 patients were treated by this technic with successful palliation in 24 patients.[171]

Several precautions must be observed if dilatation of a malignant esophageal obstruction is to be used. When using a guide wire, as is required with the Eder–Preston dilator, the guide wire should be passed under fluoroscopic control. Dilatation should not be carried out too rapidly. It is recommended that one should never use more than three different-sized dilators during a single session. Patient discomfort with this procedure is brief. Once the lumen is stretched to 17 mm, redilatation may be required no more than weekly to monthly. Intubation is necesssary when dilatation cannot maintain a patent lumen for more than a day or so.

REFERENCES

1. Long ER: A History of Pathology, Baltimore, Williams and Wilkins, 1928
2. Wangensteen OH, Wangensteen SD: The Rise of Surgery: From Empiric Craft to Scientific Discipline, Minneapolis, University of Minnesota Press, 1978
3. Wangensteen OH: Cancer of the Esophagus and Stomach, 2nd ed. New York, American Cancer Society, 1956
4. Torek F: The first successful case of resection of the thoracic portion of the esophagus for carcinoma. Surg Gynec Obstet 16:614, 1913
5. Kirschner H: Ein neues Verfahren der Oesophagsplastick. Arch Klin Chir 114:606, 1920
6. Ohsawa T: The surgery of the esophagus. Arch Jpn Chir 10:605, 1933
7. Adams WE, Phemister DB: Carcinoma of the lower thoracic esophagus. Report of successful resection and esophagogastrostomy. J Thorac Surg 7:621, 1939
8. del Regato JA, Spjut HF: Cancer: Diagnosis, Treatment and Prognosis 5th ed. St. Louis, Missouri, C.V. Mosby 1977
9. Nielsen J: Clinical results with rotation therapy in cancer of the esophagus. Acta Radiol 26:361, 1945
10. Levin DL, Devesa SS, Goodwin JD et al: Cancer Rates and Risks, 2nd ed. Washington DC, National Institutes of Health, 1974
11. Burdette WJ: Palliative operation for carcinoma of cervical and thoracic esophagus. Ann Surg 173:714, 1971
12. Cutler SJ, Devesa SS: Trends in cancer incidence and mortality in the USA. In Doll R, Vodopija I (eds): Host Environment Interactions in the Etiology of Cancer in Man. Lyon, France, World Health Organization International Agency for Research Cancer, 1973
13. Editorial: Oesophageal cancer in China. Br Med J 3:61, 1975
14. Weber J, Hecker E: Co-carcinogens of the diterpene ester type from *Croton flaveus L.* and esophageal cancer in Curacao. Experientia 34:679, 1978
15. Gilder SSB: Carcinoma of the esophagus. Ann Int Med 87:494, 1977
16. Kmet J, Mahboubi E: Esophageal cancer in the Caspian littoral of Iran: Initial sutdies. Science 175:846, 1972
17. Schoenberg BC, Bailar JC, Fraumeni JF: Certain mortality patterns of esophageal cancer in the United States, 1930–67. J Natl Cancer Inst 46:63, 1971
18. Cutler SJ, Young JL: Third National Cancer Survey: Incidence data. Natl Cancer Inst Monogr 41:1, 1975
19. Garfinkel L, Poindexter CE, Silverberg E: Cancer in black Americans. CA 30:39, 1980
20. Wynder EL, Mabuchi K: Etiological and environmental factors. JAMA 226:1546, 1973
21. Petit HS: Carcinoma of the esophagus: A statistical study. Am J Roentgenol 77:818, 1957
22. Howel-Evans W, McConnell RB, Clarke CA et al: Carcinoma of the oesophagus with keratosis palmaris et plantaris (tylosis): A study of two families Q J Med 27:413 1958
23. Wychulis AR, Woolam GL, Anderson HA et al: Achalasia and carcinoma of the esophagus. JAMA 215:1638, 1971
24. Just-Viera JO, Haight C: Achalasia and carcinoma of the esophagus. Surg Gynec Obstet 128:1081, 1969
25. Poleynard GD, Marty AT, Birnbaum WB et al: Adenocarcinoma in the columnar-lined (Barrett) esophagus. Arch Surg 112:997, 1977
26. Naef AP, Savary M, Ozzello L: Columnar-lined lower esophagus: An acquired lesion with malignant predisposition. J Thorac Cardiovasc Surg 70:826, 1975
27. Gerami S, Booth A, Pate JW: Carcinoma of the esophagus engrafted on lye stricture. Chest 59:226, 1971
28. Manual for Staging of Cancer, Chicago, American Joint Committee for Cancer Staging and End-Results Reporting, 1978

29. Japanese Society for Esophageal Diseases: Guidelines for the clinical and pathologic studies on carcinoma of the esophagus. Jap J Surg 6:69, 1976
30. Rosenberg JC, Franklin R, Steiger Z: Squamous cell carcinoma of the thoracic esophagus: An interdisciplinary approach. Curr Probl Cancer, May 1981
31. Younghusband JD, Aluwihare APR: Carcinoma of the oesophagus: Factors influencing survival. Br J Surg 57:422, 1970
32. McCort JJ: Radiographic identification of lymph node metastases from carcinoma of the esophagus, Radiology 59:694, 1952
33. Shapiro AL, Robillard GL: The esophageal arteries. Ann Surg 131:171, 1950
34. Guernsey JM, Knudsen DF: Abdominal exploration in the evaluation of patients with carcinoma of the thoracic esophagus. J Thor Cardiovasc Surg 59:62, 1970
35. Watson WL, Goodner JT, Miller TP et al: Torek esophagectomy: The case against segmental resection for esophageal cancer, J Thor Surg 32:347, 1956
36. Ota K, Shin LH: Histological Typing of Gastric and Oesophageal Tumors, Geneva, World Health Organization, 1977
37. Seremetis MG, Lyons WS, deGuzman VC et al: Leiomyomata of the esophagus: An analysis of 838 cases. Cancer 38:2166, 1976
38. Matsusaka T, Watanabe H, Enjoji M: Pseudosarcoma and carcinosarcoma of the esophagus. Cancer 37:1546, 1976
39. Imai T, Sannohe Y, Okano H: Oat cell carcinoma (apudoma) of the esophagus: A case report. Cancer 41:358, 1978
40. Kurzban JD, Marshak RH, Maklansky D: Primary malignant melanoma of the esophagus: A case report. Am J Gastroenterol, 65:464, 1976
41. Wood CB, Wood RH: Metastatic melanoma of the esophagus. Am J Diges Dis 20:786, 1975
42. Nussbaum M, Grossman M: Metastases to the esophagus causing gastrointestinal bleeding. Am J Gastroent 66:467, 1976
43. Cahan WG: Multiple primary cancers of the lung esophagus and other sites: Cancer 40:1954, 1977
44. Goldstein HM, Zornoza J: Association of squamous cell carcinoma of the head and neck with cancer of the esophagus. Am J Roentgenol 131:791, 1978
45. Stephens RL, Hansen HH, Muggia FM: Hypercalcemia in epidermoid tumors of the head and neck and esophagus. Cancer 31:1487, 1973
46. Lohrenz FN, Custer GS: ACTH producing metastases from carcinoma of the esophagus. Ann Int Med 62:1017, 1965
47. Kobayashi S, Kasugai T: Brushing cytology for the diagnosis of gastric cancer involving the cardia of the lower esophagus. Acta Cytologica 22:155, 1978
48. Winaiwer SJ, Sherlock P, Belladonna JA et al: Endoscopic brush cytology in esophageal cancer. JAMA 232:1358, 1975
49. Prolla JC, Taebel DW, Kirsner J: Current status of exfoliative cytology in diagnosis of malignant neoplasm of the esophagus. Surg Gynec Obstet 121:743, 1965
50. Fleming JAC: Carcinoma of thoracic esophagus: Some notes on its pathology and spread in relation to treatment. Br J Radiol 16:212, 1943
51. Merendino KA, Merk VJ: An analysis of 100 cases of squamous cell carcinoma. II. With special references to its theoretical curability. Surg Gynec Obstet 94:110, 1952
52. Clayton ES: Carcinoma of the esophagus. Surg Gynec Obstet 46:52, 1928
53. Sefton GK, Cooper DJ, Grech P et al: Assessment and resection of carcinoma at the gastroesophageal junction. Surg Gynec Obstet 144:563, 1977
54. Mori S, Kasai M, Watanabe T et al: Pre-operative assessment of resectability for carcinoma of the thoracic esophagus: Part I. Esophagogram and azygogram. Ann Surg 190:100, 1979
55. Sweet RH: The results of radical extirpation in the treatment of carcinoma of the esophagus and cardia: With five year survival statistics. Surg Gynec Obstet 94:46, 1952
56. Gunnlaugsson GH, Wychulis AR, Roland C et al: Analysis of the records of 1657 patients with carcinoma of the esophagus and cardia of the stomach. Surg Gynec Obstet 130:997, 1970
57. Akiyama H: Surgery for Carcinoma of the Esophagus. Curr Probl in Surg, Vol 17, Chicago, Year Book Medical Publishers, 1978
58. Lane FW: Cancer of the esophagus: The case for irradiation, Hospital Practice 11:68, 1976
59. Kondo M, Hashimoto S, Kubo A et al: Ga scanning in the evaluation of esophageal carcinoma. Radiology 131:723, 1979
60. Crummy AB, Wegner GP, Flaherty TT et al: Azygos venography: An aid in the evaluation of esophageal carcinoma. Ann Thor Surg 6:522, 1968
61. Murray GF, Wilcox BR, Starek JK: The assessment of operability of esophageal carcinoma. Ann Thor Surg 23:393, 1977
62. Just-Viera JO, Silva JE: Esophageal carcinoma. Ann Thor Surg. 19:688, 1975
63. Appelqvist P: Carcinoma of the oesophagus and gastric cardia. Acta Chir Scand Suppl 430, 1972
64. Clinical staging system for carcinoma of the esophagus. CA 25:50, 1975
65. vanAndel JG, Dees J, Dijkhuis CM et al: Carcinoma of the esophagus: Results of treatment. Ann Surg 190:684, 1979
66. Haffejee AA, Angorn IB: Nutritional status and the nonspecific cellular and humoral immune response in esophageal carcinoma. Ann Surg 189:475, 1979
67. Franklin RH: Long term survival after resection of carcinoma of the esophagus. Br Med J 2:1268, 1978
68. Ong, GB, Lam KH, Wong J et al: Factors influencing morbidity and mortality in esophageal carcinoma. J Thor and Cardiovasc Surg 76:745, 1978
69. Marical, VA, Tome JM, Ubinas J et al: The role of radiation therapy in esophageal cancer. Radiology 87:231, 1966
70. Cedarqvist C, Nielsen J, Berthelsen A et al: Cancer of the esophagus. II. Therapy and outcome. Acta Chir Scand 144:233, 1978
71. Cukingnam, RA, Carey JS: Carcinoma of the esophagus. Ann Thor Surg 26:274, 1978
72. Ellis FH, Gibb SP: Esophagectomy for carcinoma: Current hospital mortality and morbidity rates. Ann Surg 190:699, 1979
73. Scanlon EF, Morton DR, Walker JM et al: The case against segmental resection for esophageal carcinoma. Surg Gynec Obstet 101:290, 1955
74. Lewis I: The surgical treatment of carcinoma of the esophagus: With special reference to a new operation for growths of the middle thrid. Br J Surg 34:18, 1946
75. Kirk RM: Palliative resection of esophageal carcinoma without formal thoracotomy. Br J Surg 61:689, 1974
76. Orringer MB, Sloan H: Esophagectomy without thoracotomy. J Thor Cardiovasc Surg 76:643, 1978
77. Szentpetery S, Wolfgang T, Lower R: Pull-through esophagectomy without thoracotomy for esophageal carcinoma. Ann Thor Surg 27:399, 1978
78. Postlethwait RW: Esophagectomy without thoracotomy. Ann Thor Surg 27:395, 1979
79. Akiyama H, Miyazono H, Tsurumaru M et al: Use of the stomach as an esophageal substitute. Ann Surg 188:606, 1978
80. Carey JS, Pleste WG, Hughes RK: Esophagogastrectomy: Superiority of the combined abdominal–right-thoracic approach (Lewis operation). Ann Thor Surg 14:59, 1972
81. McKeown KC: Total three-stage oesophagectomy for cancer of the oesophagus. Br J Surg 63:259, 1976
82. Steichen FM, Ravitch MM: Mechanical sutures in esophageal surgery. Ann Surg 191:373, 1980
83. Pearson FG, Henderson RD, Parrish RM: An operative technique for the control of reflux following esophagogastrostomy. J Thor Cardiovasc Surg 58:668, 1969
84. Ward AS, Collis JL: Late results of oesophageal and oesophagogastric resection in the treatment of oesophageal cancer. Thorax 26:1, 1971
85. Angorn IB: Oesophagogastrostomy without a drainage procedure in oesophageal carcinoma. Br J Surg 62(8):601, 1975
86. Wilkins EW, Burke JF: Colon esophageal bypass. Am J Surg 129:394, 1975
87. Gavriliu D: Aspects of esophageal surgery. In Curr Probl Surg, Vol 12, Chicago, Year Book Medical Publishers, 1975
88. Postlethwait RW: Technique for isoperistaltic gastric tube for esophageal bypass. Ann Surg 189:673, 1979
89. Nicks R, Green D, McClatchie G: A clinico-pathological study of some factors influencing survival in cancer of the oesophagus: A survey of ten years' experience. Aust NZ J Surg, 43:1, 1973

90. Beatty JD, DeBoer G, Rider WD: Carcinoma of the esophagus. Cancer 43:2254, 1979
91. Pearson JG: The present status and feature potential of radiotherapy in the management of esophageal cancer. Cancer 39:882, 1977
92. Pinto JM, Bhalavat RL, Nagaraj Rao D et al: Radiotherapy in carcinoma of the oesophagus. Ind J Cancer 12:380, 1975
93. Elkon D, Lee MS, Hendrickson FR: Carcinoma of the esophagus' sites of recurrence and palliative benefits after definitive radiotherapy. Int J Rad Onc Biol Phys 4:615, 1978
94. Jacobson F: Carcinoma of hypopharynx: a clinical study of 332 cases treated at Radiumhemmet from 1939 to 1947. Acta Radiol 35:1, 1951
95. Schuchmann GF, Heydron WH, Hall RV et al: Treatment of esophageal carcinoma: A retrospective review. J Thorac Cardiovasc Surg 79:67, 1980
96. Earle J, Gelber R, Moertel C et al: A controlled evaluation of combined radiation and belomycin therapy for squamous cell carcinoma of the esophagus. Int J Rad Onc Biol Phys 6:821, 1980
97. Wara WM, Mauch PM, Thomas AN et al: Palliation for carcinoma of the esophagus. Radiology 121:717, 1976
98. Smoron G, O'Brien C, Sullivan C: Tumor localization and treatment technique for cancer of the esophagus. Radiol 111:735, 1974
99. Bloedorn F: Esophagus. In Feltcher G (ed): Textbook of Radiotherapy, New York, Lea and Febiger, 1973
100. Doggett R, Guernsey J, Bagshaw M: Combined radiation and surgical treatment of carcinoma of the thoracic esophagus. In Vaeth J (ed): Front Radiation Ther Onc, Basal/Munchen/Paris/New York, Karger, 1970
101. Fletcher GH: Basic principals of radiobiology—clinical parameters. In Textbook of Radiotherapy, 2nd ed. Philadelphia, Lea & Febiger, 1973
102. Gilbert EH, Goffinet DR, Bagshaw MA: Carcinoma of the oral tongue and floor of mouth: fifteen years experience with linear accelerator therapy. Caneer 35:1517, 1975
103. Giuli R, Gignoux M: Treatment of carcinoma of the esophagus—retrospective review of 1400 patients. Ann Surg (7):44, 1980
104. Phillips TL, Margolis LM: Radiation pathology and the clinical response of lung and esophagus. In Vaeth JM (ed): Radiation Effects and Tolerance of Normal Tissues, Baltimore, University Park Press, 1972
105. Dickson RJ: Radiation therapy in carcinoma of the esophagus. Am J Med Sci 241:662, 1961
106. Rider WD, Diaz Mendoza R: Some opinions on the treatment of cancer of the esophagus. Am J Roentgenol 105:514, 1969
107. Moss W, Brand W, Gattifora A: The esophagus. In Radiation Oncology-Rationale, Technique, Results, 5th ed. St Louis, C. V. Mosby, 1979
108. Schwade JG, Johnston M, Dunnick R et al: Abstract: Twice weekly radiation therapy in carcinoma of the esophagus. Dallas, Am Society of Therapeutic Radiology, 1980
109. Leborgne R, Leborgne JF, Barlocci L: Cancer of the esophagus, results of radiotherapy. Br J Radiology 36:806, 1963
110. Krishnamurthi S: Cobalt-60 beam treatment in cancer of the thoracic esophagus. Indian J Ca 2:115, 1965
111. Pierquin B, Wambirsie A, Tubiana M: Cancer of the thoracic esophagus: two series of patients treated by 22 MeV betatron. Br J Radiol 39:189, 1966
112. Nakayama K, Orihata H, Yamaguchi K: Surgical treatment combined with preoperative concentrated irradiation for esophageal cancer. Cancer 20:778, 1967
113. Millburn L, Hendrickson FR, Faber P: Curative treatments of epidermoid carcinoma of the esophagus. Am J Roent 103:291, 1968
114. Pearson JG: The value of radiotherapy in the management of esophageal cancer. Am J Roent 105:500, 1969
115. Marks RD, Scruggs HJ, Wallace KM: Preoperative radiation therapy for carcinoma of the esophagus. Cancer 38:84, 1976
116. Ellis FH Jr, Salzman FA: Carcinoma of the esophagus: Surgery versus radiotherapy. Postgrad Med 61:167, 1977
117. Young MEJ, Gaylord JV: Experimental tests of correction in tissue in homogeneities in radiotherapy. Br J Radiol 43:349, 1970
118. Chapman JD: Hypoxic sensitizers—implications for radiation therapy. NE J Med 301:429, 1979
119. Silver CE: Surgical management of neoplasms of the larynx, hypopharynx, and cervical esophagus. Curr Probl Surg 19:1, 1977
120. Stell PM: Esophageal replacement by transposed stomach. Arch Otolaryng 91:166, 1970
121. Desai D et al: Chemotherapy of advanced esophageal carcinoma. Proc Am Soc Cl Onc 20:381, 1979
122. Livingston RB, Carter SK: Single Agents in Cancer Chemotherapy, New York, Plenum, 1970
123. Kolaric K et al: Adriamycin alone and in combination with radiotherapy in the treatment of inoperable esophageal cancer. Tumori 63:485, 1977
124. Panettiere F: Personal communication
125. Kelsen, DP et al: Vindesine in the treatment of esophageal carcinoma. Proc Am Soc Cl Onc 20:338, 1979
126. Knight WA et al: Methyl-glyoxal bis-guanylhydrazone (methyl GAG MGBG) in advanced human malignancy. Proc Am Soc Cl Onc 20:319, 1979
127. Falkson G: Methyl-gag (NSG-32946) in the treatment of esophagus cancer. Cancer Chemother Rep 55:209, 1971
128. Shnider BI et al: Effectiveness of methyl GAG (NSC-32946) administered intramuscularly. Cancer Chemother Rep 58:689, 1974
129. Moertel CG, Schmitt AJ, Reitemeier RJ et al: Therapy of gastrointestinal cancer with the nitrosoureas alone and in drug combination. Cancer Treat Rep 60:729, 1976
130. Wesserman TH, Conis RL, Goldsmith M et al: Tabular analysis of the clinical chemotherapy of solid tumors. Cancer Chemother Rep (part 3) 6:399, 1975
131. Fujimaki M et al: Role of preoperative administration of bleomycin and radiation in the treatment of esophageal cancer. Japanese J Surg 5:48, 1975
132. Kolaric K et al: Therapy of advanced esophageal cancer with bleomycin, irradiation and combination of bleomycin with irradiation. Tumori 62:255, 1976
133. Ravry M et al: Treatment of advanced squamous cell carcinoma of the gastrointestinal tract with bleomycin. Cancer Chemother Rep 57:493, 1973
134. Blum RH et al: A clinical overview of bleomycin—a new antineoplastic agent. Cancer 31:903, 1973
135. Shastri S et al: Clinical study with bleomycin. Cancer 28:1142, 1971
136. Clinical Screening Group. Study of the clinical efficiency of bleomycin in human cancer. Br Med J 1:643, 1970
137. Tancini G et al: Terapia con bleomicina da sola o in associazione con methotrexate nel carcinoma epidermoide dell'esofago. Tumori 60:65, 1974
138. Yagoda A et al: Bleomycin, an antitumor antibiotic. Clinical experience in 274 patients. Ann Int Med 77:861, 1972
139. Bonadonna G et al: Clinical trials with bleomycin in lymphomas and in solid tumors. European J Ca 8:205, 1972
140. Ohnuma T et al: Clinical study with bleomycin: tolerance to twice weekly dosage Cancer 30:914, 1972
141. Hentek V et al: Combination chemotherapy of advanced esophageal cancer with methotrexate, bleomycin, and diamminedichloroplatinum. Proc Am Soc Cl Onc 20:400, 1979
142. Kelsen DP et al: *cis*-Dichlorodiammineplatinum (II) and bleomycin in the treatment of esophageal carcinoma. Cancer Treat Rep 62:1041, 1978
143. Kolaric K, Maricic Z, Roth A et al: Combination of bleomycin and Adriamycin (doxorubicin) with and without radiation in the treatment of inoperable esophageal cancer. Cancer 45:2265, 1980
144. Buroker TR: Unpublished data
145. Kelsen DP et al: *cis*-Diamminedichloroplatinum and bleomycin in the treatment of esophageal carcinoma. Proc Am Soc Cl Onc 19:352, 1978

146. Stone LA et al: Combination chemotherapy of disseminated GI adenocarcinoma with vincristine, methyl-CCNU and 5-Fluorouracil. Proc Am Soc Cl Onc 18:326, 1977
147. Goodner JT: Surgical and radiation treatment of cancer of the thoracic esophagus. Am J Roentgenol Rad Therap Nuc Med 105:523, 1969
148. Marks RD, Scruggs HJ, Wallace KM: Pre-operative radiation therapy for carcinoma of the esophagus. Cancer 38:84, 1976
149. Nakayama K, Kinoshita Y: Surgical treatment combined with preoperative concentrated irradiation. JAMA 227:178, 1974
150. Akakura J, Nakamura Y, Kakegawa T et al: Surgery of carcinoma of the esophagus with preoperative radiation, Chest 57:47, 1970
151. Guernsey JM, Doggett RLS, Mason GR et al: Combined treatment of cancer of the esophagus. Am J Surg 117:157, 1969
152. Groves LK, Rodriguez-Antuney A: Treatment of carcinoma of the esophagus and gastric cardia with concentrated preoperative irradiation followed by early operation. A progress report. Ann Thorac Surg 15:333, 1973
153. Fraser RW, Wara WM, Thomas AN et al: Combined treatment methods for carcinoma of esophagus. Radiology 128:461, 1978
154. Parker EF, Gregoire HB: Carcinoma of the esophagus: Long term results. JAMA 235:1018, 1976
155. Wada T, Matoumoto Y, Amano T: Chemotherapy of esophageal cancer with bleomycin. Prog Antimicrob Anticancer Chemother 2:696, 1970
156. Iwamoto M, Yatsuka K, Ozasa T et al: On selective continuous administration of anti-cancer agents into the paraesophageal space—as an adjuvant therapy with operation of esophageal cancer. J Jpn Soc Cancer Ther 12:207, 1975
157. Byfield JE, Barone RM, Mendelsohn J et al: Combined 5-fluorouracil and x-ray therapy in esophageal and other gastrointestinal cancers. Am J Radiat Oncol Biol Phys 4 (Suppl 12): 136, 1978
158. Roussel A: Treatment of nonoperable cancer of the esophagus. Digestion 16:271, 1977
159. Franklin R, Buroker TR, Vaishampayan GV et al: Combined therapies in esophageal squamous cell cancer. Proc Am Assoc Cancer Res 20:223, 1979
160. Martino S et al: Pulmonary toxicity of mitomycin. In Carter SK, Crooke ST (eds): Mitomycin-C: Current Status and New Developments. New York, Academic Press, 1979
161. Werner ID, Silber W, Madden PCU et al: Carcinoma of the thoracoabdominal esophagus. S Afr Med J 49:653, 1975
162. Nygaard K, Smith-Ericksen N, Hatleroll R et al: Pulmonary complications after bleomycin irradiation and surgery for esophageal cancer. Cancer 4:17, 1978
163. Payne WS: Palliation of esophageal carcinoma. Ann Thor Surg 28:208, 1979
164. Hankins JR, Cole FN, Ward A et al: Carcinoma of the esophagus: The philosophy for palliation. Ann Thor Surg 14:159, 1972
165. Wilson SE, Plested WG, Carey JS: Esophagogastrectomy versus radiation therapy for midesophageal carcinoma. Ann Thorac Surg 10:195, 1970
166. Piccone VA, LeVeen HH, Ahmed N et al: Reappraisal of esophagogastrectomy for esophageal malignancy. Am J Surg 137:32, 1979
167. Belsey R, Hiebert CA: An exclusive right thoracic approach for cancer of the middle third of the esophagus. Ann Thor Surg 18:1, 1974
168. Postlethwait RW: Carcinoma of the Esophagus. Current Problems in Cancer, Vol. 11, Chicago, Year Book Publishers, 1978
169. Orringer MB, Sloan H: Substernal gastric bypass of the excluded thoracic esophagus for palliation of esophageal carcinoma. J Thor Cardiovasc Surg 70:836, 1975
170. Steiger Z, Nickel WD, Wilson RF, et al: Improved surgical palliation of advanced carcinoma of the esophagus. Am J Surg 135:782, 1978
171. Heit HA, Johnson LF, Siegel SR et al: Palliative dilatation for dysphagia in esophageal carcinoma. Ann Intern Med 89:629, 1978

John S. Macdonald
Leonard L. Gunderson
Isidore Cohn, Jr.

CHAPTER 17

Cancer of the Stomach

Cancer of the stomach represents an intriguing challenge to the clinical scientist. This tumor is the sixth most common cause of cancer deaths in the United States, with 24,000 new cases occurring in 1980. Although gastric cancer still remains a major health problem in the United States, the death rate from this disease has decreased from 30:100,000 in 1930 to 8:100,000 in 1980.[1] This decline is steepest in older persons and in whites.[2] There has been no adequate explanation for the decreasing death rate from stomach cancer in the United States.

This unexplained decrease in a highly lethal malignancy has intrigued and stimulated epidemiologists. The decline in gastric cancer in the United States is particularly striking when considered in the context of the very high rates of gastric cancer in such countries as Japan (78/10,000) and Chile (70/100,000).[3] The fact that migrant populations from high- to low-incidence countries show a significant decrease in the occurrence of the disease clearly suggests that the cause of this cancer must be related to the environment.[3] The first generation of migrants have higher risk of stomach cancer than do natives of the host country. This finding suggests an etiologic factor that may be persistent in the migrant population for some time.[4,5] This factor may be a learned dietary practice that disappears as migrant groups are assimilated into the host culture.

In the United States and Western Europe, stomach cancer is twice as frequent in the lower as in the highest socioeconomic groups. Increased stomach cancer rates have been associated with a number of occupational groups, including coal miners, farmers (in Japan), and nickel refinery workers (in the U.S.S.R.). Rubber workers and workers who process timber have also been reported to have increased risk of stomach cancer. Whether these occupations are truly associated with increased gastric cancer risk or merely reflect the socioeconomic characteristics of these employees is not clear.[6] Stomach cancer is also more common in asbestos workers, and it is likely that this increase is due to exposure to asbestos fibers.[7]

Familial occurrence of gastric cancer is rare, and associations between gastric cancer and blood group A[8] and intestinal metaplasia[9] will be discussed in subsequent sections of this chapter. There appears to be no increased risk of gastric cancer in persons using alcohol or tobacco.

PATHOLOGY

Of the malignant neoplasms of the stomach, 95% are adenocarcinoma and, generally, when the term gastric cancer is used, it refers to adenocarcinoma of the stomach. Although adeno-acanthoma, squamous cell carcinoma, and carcinoid tumors do occur in the stomach, they each represent less than 1% of gastric malignancies.[10] Leiomyosarcomas of the stomach may account for 1% to 3% of malignant gastric tumors.[11,12]

In evaluating the pathology of gastric cancer, several factors have important clinical significance. The gross appearance, site, and degree of local invasion of the tumor all bear on prognosis, as does the histology of the cancer. The macroscopic appearance of gastric cancer has been described according to several schemes.[10,13] Fifty years ago, the German pathologist Bormann developed a classification scheme that divided the macroscopic appearance of gastric cancer into five types.[13] Type 1 represented polypoid or fungating cancers; type 2 encompassed ulcerating lesions surrounded by elevated borders; type 3 contained ulcerating lesions that were infiltrating the gastric wall; type 4 tumors were diffusely infiltrating carcinomas; and type 5 contained unclassifiable cancers. In the United States, a less formalized descriptive classification of gastric cancers is generally used.[10] This schema divides the gross pathologic features of stomach cancer into four categories. The majority of lesions will be ulcerative. The lesions may have the appearance of a benign gastric ulcer or they may demonstrate the findings classically attributed to malignant ulcers in the stomach. These include lesions of size greater 2 cm in diameter and "heaped up" borders, giving the ulcer the appearance of being raised above the level of the surrounding stomach. Approximately 10% of gastric cancers can grossly be classified as polypoid. These lesions may be quite large without showing evidence of significant invasion or metastases. This may result from the fact that, histologically, these tumors are well differentiated. In the European literature, such well differentiated types of stomach cancers have been classified as being of the intestinal type and have been shown to have a superior prognosis to tumors with diffuse anaplastic histopathology.[14] The third type of gross appearance of gastric cancer is the scirrhous pattern. Approximately 10% of cancers fall into this category. Scirrhous tumors result in thickening and rigidity of the gastric wall owing to diffuse infiltration with anaplastic cancer cells. These malignant cells produce a marked fibrous reaction in the gastric wall leading to stiffened stomach, giving the appearance of linitus plastica. Scirrhous carcinoma has great prognostic significance since this type of tumor is almost uniformly fatal. In a series of 504 patients with resectable gastric cancer reported by the Veteran's Adminstration Surgical Oncology Group, the postgastric resection 5-year survival of patients with scirrhous carcinoma was 2%.[15] The fourth type of gastric cancer is uncommon in this country. This is the superficial variety. This tumor is found in less than 5% of surgical specimens and is characterized by sheet-like collections of cancer cells replacing the normal mucosa.

Gastric cancer does not arise from all sites within the stomach with the same frequency.[10,16] If the stomach is divided into thirds, most tumors develop in the antrum, or lower third. Cancers are less common in the body of the stomach and least common in the cardia. Tumors also are more common in the lesser than in the greater curvature of the stomach. Berkson, in reviewing the site of origin in 587 cases of gastric cancer, noted that the lesser curvature gave rise to the tumor 18% of the time, whereas tumor arose from the greater curvature in only 3% of cases.[17] Multicentric invasion of the stomach has also been reported in patients with stomach cancer. Moertel reported that 2.2% of 1835 patients with gastric cancer showed gross evidence of having more than one primary gastric tumor.[10] If the stomach of a patient with gastric cancer is carefully examined histologically for the presence of multicentric tumor, as many as 22% of cases can be found to have tumors arising from several sites.[18] This phenomenon is more common in patients presenting with gastric cancer after having had pernicious anemia.

Adenocarcinoma occurring in the stomach may be classified according to degree of histologic differentiation. Although not an independent prognostic variable, this is important since the prognosis is worse in the poorly differentiated lesions.[19] If the Broder's classification is used, which grades cells from 1 (well differentiated) to 4 (anaplastic), it is found that patients with unresectable stomach cancer having well differentiated lesions (grades 1 and 2) have a median survival of 7 months. In patients with grades 3 and 4 tumor histology, the survival is only 4 months. It should also be emphasized that histologic grade of tumor and gross pathology are not independent variables. For example, linitus plastica is never seen with well differentiated tumors and only occurs with the more undifferentiated cancer. Conversely, polypoid tumors, as noted previously, are very likely to have well differentiated histology.

ANATOMICAL RELATIONSHIPS OF THE STOMACH

From the standpoint of oncology, the important features of the stomach relate to the other viscera with which it comes in contact, its vascular supply, its lymphatic supply, and what surgical procedures can be performed on the stomach without endangering patient survival (Fig. 17-1).

Since the stomach begins at the gastro–esophageal junction and ends at the pylorus, direct or incontinual spread to the esophagus or the duodenum are each situations which must be taken into account when dealing with lesions in these portions of the stomach. In addition, the stomach is in contact with the diaphragm, the anterior wall, the liver, the transverse colon, the spleen, the left adrenal, the left kidney, the pancreas, the splenic flexure of the colon, the greater omentum, and various loops of small intestine.

The blood supply to the stomach is derived from the celiac axis with the major vessels being the left gastric, the right gastric and the gastro–duodenal, each being a branch of the hepatic; the right and left gastro–epiploic vessels and the short gastric or vasa brevia, which are branches of the splenic artery. Additional arteries of concern in terms of spread of gastric carcinoma or in terms of operative procedures upon the stomach include the splenic, the hepatic, and the middle colic, any one of which might be involved by an extensive tumor arising within the stomach or might be involved in surgical procedures removing these lesions.

In general, the venous drainage of the stomach parallels the arterial supply. The major additional vein is the coronary vein, which runs along the lesser curvature of the stomach and eventually drains into the portal vein.

The lymphatics of the stomach have been described in greater detail by Rouviere, and reference to his work is essential for anyone interested in the routes of potential spread from carcinoma of the stomach (Table 17-1).[16] While there is a rich interconnecting lymphatic network within the stomach, the more important pathways from the standpoint of gastric carcinoma are those that deal with the collecting trunk, and Rouviere has divided these into three major systems: (1) the region of the left gastric chain, (2) the region of the splenic chain, and (3) the region of the hepatic chain. The lymphatic pathways are complex and highly interconnected but, in general, follow the pathways of the major

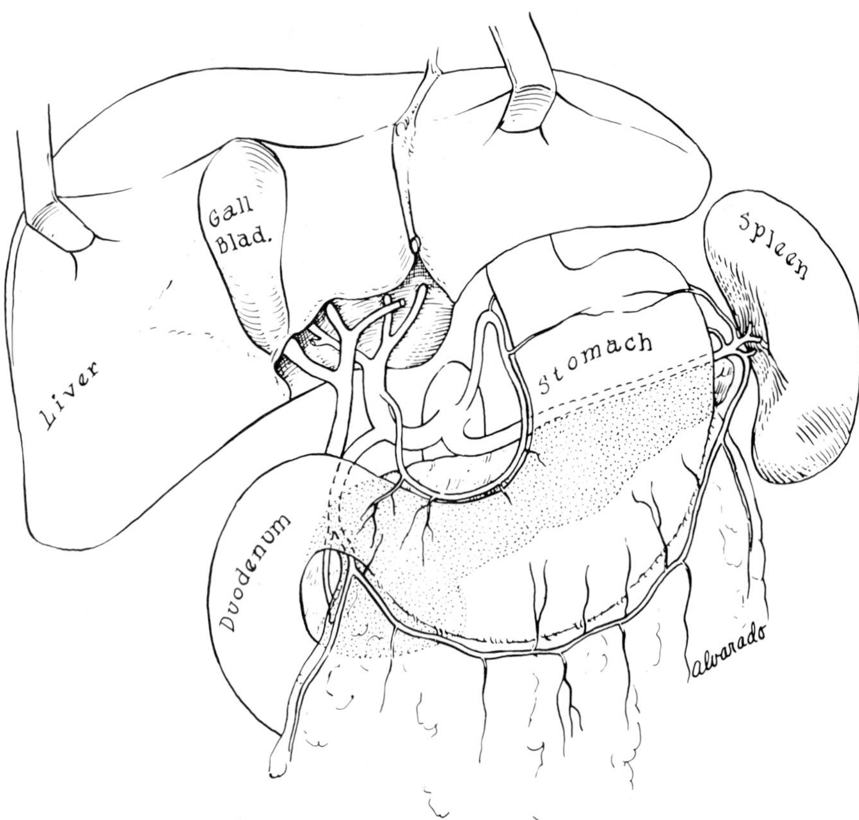

FIG. 17-1. Major anatomical relationships of the stomach, showing its blood supply and the other organs most likely to be involved by primary malignant lesions in the stomach.

vascular supply to the stomach. It is clear from this that lymphatics can be involved along both the lesser and the greater curvature of the stomach, extending to the hilum of the spleen on the left, extending up the portal triad on the right, and across the surface of the pancreas, and down along the course of the duodenum inferiorly. The highly complex nature of the lymphatic pathways explains, to a certain extent, the problems with early and extensive spread of tumors from the stomach to other areas.

TABLE 17-1. Lymphatic Drainage of the Stomach

A. The Lymphatic Networks
   1. The mucous network
   2. The submucous network
   3. The muscular network
   4. The subserous or subperitoneal network
B. The Collecting Trunks
   1. Left gastric chain
      a. Left gastro–pancreatic fold
      b. Lesser curvature nodes
      c. Parietal group
      D. Juxtacardiac nodes
   2. Splenic chain
      a. Suprapancreatic nodes
      b. Infrapancreatic nodes
      c. Afferent and efferent lymph vessels
   3. The hepatic chain
      a. Hepatic group
      b. Gastroduodenal group
      c. Right gastro-epiploic and infrapyloric group
      d. Right gastric group; suprapyloric nodes
      e. Pancreaticoduodenal group
      f. Afferent and efferent vessels

While, in general, the lymphatic pathways have been outlined to show that lesions in particular areas of the stomach generally follow a given direction, it is also clear that this is not an invariable rule, and that if there is early blockage of the normal pathway, that lymphatic drainage can then go in an different direction and, thus, cause even more extensive retrograde lymphatic blockage. It should be emphasized that the relatively rich lymphatic supply of the stomach makes accurate prediction of lymphatic spread of tumor more difficult than in, for example, colon or rectal cancer.

The observation that lesions in the lower portion of the stomach do not usually cause involvement of the lymphatics along the splenic chain or up toward the esophagus has helped to determine that the procedure of choice for low-lying gastric lesions is not a total gastrectomy, and that splenectomy is not routinely indicated for lesions in this area. By the same line of reasoning, the type of resection indicated for lesions in other areas can be plotted from a knowledge of the lymphatics and the natural history of observed cases.

Once a tumor has spread beyond the immediate lymphatics, there can then be lymphatic involvement along the aorta, through the thoracic duct to the cervical nodes, or there can be retrograde spread to other areas within the abdomen and within the peritoneal cavity, including direct implantation in the pelvis.

NATURAL HISTORY

PREMALIGNANT LESIONS

The histology of the normal stomach may have an important influence on the occurrence of gastric cancer. It has been demonstrated that intestinal metaplasia of the stomach is more frequent in countries where the incidence of stomach cancer is high.[20–22] This lesion is defined as the replacement of stomach epithelium by intestinal epithelium containing goblet and paneth cells. In Japan, where gastric cancer causes 40% of all deaths from malignancy, there is intestinal metaplasia in 80% of stomachs resected for gastric cancer.[23] Furthermore, the type of stomach cancer associated with intestinal metaplasia is well differentiated.[24] In cases where metaplasia is not observed, the tumor is poorly differentiated, and frequently presents a scirrhous carcinoma pattern.[23] This last histology is more common in western countries, where intestinal metaplasia is seen less frequently than in Japan.

There is experimental evidence to suggest that the metaplastic change is a carcinogen-induced precursor lesion of gastric cancer.[25,26] In studies done in rats, Japanese workers have shown that nitro-N-nitrosoguanidines, known gastric carcinogens, first induce gastric intestinal metaplasia that is subsequently followed by gastric cancer. Tumors did not occur in rats that did not develop intestinal metaplasia after carcinogen exposure. The relationship between a well-defined premalignant pathologic finding (intestinal metaplasia) induced by a known carcinogen and predisposing the stomach to a specific type of adenocarcinoma (well-differentiated intestinal type) clearly deserves further exploration and implies that intestinal metaplasia is capable of malignant transformation when exposed to a promoting agent.

Although the majority of gastric cancer appears to be carcinogen-induced, there are some conditions predisposing patients to neoplasia of the stomach. The firmest and most convincing evidence relates to the association between pernicious anemia and gastric cancer.[10,27] The incidence of gastric cancer in patients with pernicious anemia had been reported to be between 5% and 10%. It has been estimated that gastric cancer is 20 times more common in patients with pernicious anemia than in an age-matched control population.[28] These results indicate the need to carefully monitor patients with chronic pernicious anemia for the development of gastric malignancy.

The relationship between gastric polyps and gastric ulcers and malignancy has been debated in the literature for many years.[10,29–31] In general, it can be said that polyps are rarely precursor lesions to gastric cancer.[30,32] There are three histologic types of gastric polyps. These are hyperplastic, hemartomatous adenomatous polyps, and villous adenomas. The hyperplastic adenomatous polyps are the most common and it appears that there is no malignant potential associated with these polyps. The hemartomatous adenomatous polyps are composed of normal gastic mucosal cells and are identical to the lesions seen in the Peutz-Jeghers syndrome. These polyps are the rarest form of gastric polyps and do not become malignant. The lesion that does appear to have malignant potential is the villous adenoma.[30,33,34] These polyps are ten times less frequent than hyperplastic polyps, but they are clearly premalignant, since foci of carcinoma are found in approximately 40% of these lesions.

The experience at the Aichi Cancer Center in Japan confirms the importance of histology of polyps in relationship to malignant potential.[34] One-hundred-ninety-eight consecutive cases of gastric polyps were analyzed. Histologic examination revealed that 87.8% of the polyps were hyperplastic and only 2% were villous adenomas. In ten of 198 cases in which cancers of the stomach were present, nine were associated with villous adenoma pathology and only one was associated with hyperplastic polyps. These data indicate that 69% of the villous adenoma and only 0.6% of the hyperplastic polyps were associated with malignancy.

There is controversy between U.S. and Japanese investigators concerning the association between gastric ulcer and malignancy.[10,29–31] The U.S. data can be shown to support the hypothesis that gastric cancer may commonly ulcerate but benign gastric ulcers rarely, if ever, become cancers. In the United States, carcinoma has been found in only 3% of resected gastric ulcers.[35] Conversely, in Japan, the experience at the Yokohama Cancer Hospital initially suggested a very high correlation between chronic gastric ulcer and cancer.[36] In the 1950s, 70% of the early cancers resected showed a deep chronic ulcer surrounded by a narrow cancerous lesion suggesting a preexisting chronic ulcer with malignancy developing at its border. It is of interest that this pathological entity has progressively decreased in Japan coincident with the introduction of fiberoptic gastroscopy. In 1974, only 10% of gastric cancers were associated with chronic gastric ulcers, whereas 75% of resected tumors showed a primary malignant tumor with ulceration. This finding may in part be explained by the fact that the frequency of chronic gastric ulcer also decreased in Japan by 50% during the period 1958 to 1974.[36]

In general, it appears that now even in Japan the risk of gastric cancer occurring in conjunction with gastric ulcer disease is small. This is born out by the experience of Larson and associates in America.[37] These workers followed the course of 664 patients with clinically benign gastric ulcers of less than 4 cm in diameter. All patients were treated with medical management. It is of interest that only 21% of these patients experienced healing and 40% eventually required surgery for persistent symptoms or acute problems such as hemorrhage. The overall incidence of gastric cancer in this group after 5 years to 10 years of follow-up was small. Malignancy was demonstrated in 60 of 664 (9%) cases. It would seem prudent to carefully follow patients with apparently benign gastric ulcer and to consider prompt surgical intervention if healing does not rapidly occur. The clinician should understand, however, that the likelihood of finding malignancy is small.

There are several conditions which were thought to be associated with gastric cancer that now appear to have a tenuous, at best, relationship with stomach cancer. For example, a number of epidemiologic studies have suggested that gastric cancer is more common in persons with blood group A than blood group O.[8,10] Over 55 studies reported from around the world have supported this finding. However, the risk ratio for gastric cancer in persons with blood group A compared to blood group O is only a modest 1/2. Also, several large studies from the Scandinavian countries have found no correlation between gastric cancer and blood group A.

For many years, a relationship between atrophic gastritis and gastric cancer has been postulated.[10,30] It appears that atrophic gastritis is very commonly associated with gastric malignancy. However, it does not follow that atrophic gastritis is a precursor lesion to gastric carcinoma. In the older age group in which gastric cancer occurs, approximately 80% to 95% of individuals exhibit some degree of atrophic gastritis. Thus, a larger percentage of older patients without stomach cancer have atrophic gastritis, making untenable the hypothesis that atrophic gastritis is a precursor of gastric cancer.

PATTERN OF SPREAD

The choice of treatment for any given lesion of the stomach depends upon a knowledge of the natural history of the disease and the more common routes of spread. The TNM staging system which is gaining wider acceptance all the time should be utilized as a baseline to permit appropriate comparisons between series reported from different institutions or at different times. There is, of course, some previously recorded information that continues to be important because of the background it provides for evaluation of the current stage of any disease process.

The routes of spread for gastric carcinoma are similar to those for other gastrointestinal lesions.[38] They include (1) direct spread within the involved stomach and into the adjacent esophagus or pylorus or both, (2) spread to adjacent viscera (3) spread through lymphatic chains, (4) spillage of tumor cells either from the serosal surface of the stomach or from the lumen at the time of an operative procedure, and (5) blood-borne metastases (Table 17-2).

In a study of 423 patients at Charity Hospital at New Orleans, the lesion was grossly limited to the stomach only in 11% of the patients.[39,40] In an additional 11%, the only evidences of disease beyond the stomach were clinically positive nodes. Contiguous extension was documented in 27% and distant metastatic disease was present in 31%. Histologically positive nodes were present in 52% of this entire series. These gross findings at either operation or autopsy can be compared with the final diagnoses based on histological examination to demonstrate that the surgeon's or the pathologist's gross observations do not give sufficient information about the extent of spread (Table 17-3).

TABLE 17-2. Patterns of Spread of Gastric Cancer

A. Direct Extension
   1. Lesser and greater omentum
   2. Liver
   3. Pancreas
   4. Spleen
   5. Biliary tract
   6. Transverse colon
B. Nodal Metastases
   1. Local
   2. Distant
      a. Virchow's node
      b. Left axillary (Irish's) node
      c. Umbilical node
C. Vascular Metastases
   1. Liver
   2. Pulmonary
   3. Bone
   4. Brain
D. Peritoneal Metastases
   1. Disseminated
   2. Pelvic
      a. Krukenburg tumor—ovary
      b. Blumer's rectal shelf

Studies by Arhelger and associates and Coller and associates have demonstrated that neither the size of the lesion nor the location of the primary tumor had a significant bearing on which lymph nodes were involved or how often lymph nodes were involved.[41,42]

The pattern of distant organ involvement was recorded in our own experience with 348 patients subjected to autopsy, and this experience is tabulated along with the reports of Clarke and co-workers, Warren, and Warrick in Table 17-4.[43–45] This study shows that the liver is the most frequently involved organ, being involved almost twice as frequently as the peritoneum or omentum, which are the next two in sequence. The most commonly involved distant organ is the lung, followed by the adrenals. Histologic involvement of the spleen is relatively uncommon, comprising less than 10% of the entire series, which is in contrast to a commonly accepted idea that the spleen is involved in a large proportion of the patients with gastric carcinoma.[10] The infrequent involvement of the spleen indicates that routine splenectomy is not necessary and, as a matter of fact, for lesions originating in the distal stomach without gross involvement of either the spleen or the lymph nodes adjacent to it, suggests that splenectomy is of no real value in this particular circumstance.

The large number of patients with extensive disease as determined by autopsy, and further study of patients with disseminated cancer shortly after an operative procedure, indicate that either the disease is multifocal, that there has been rapid spread induced by the operative procedure, that microscopic spread was present at the time of operation even though it was not detected, or that the operative procedure seeded tumor cells more extensively than has been appreciated. Since it is not possible to document either spillage or microscopic metastatic disease at the time of operation, it is clear that long-term cures will depend upon some type of therapy which attacks a wider base than the primary tumor alone.

Although as documented in Table 17-4, disseminated disease can be documented in 75% of patients at autopsy, the importance of local–regional (LR) failure should not be underestimated. McNeer and associates present complete information on 92 patients autopsied after "curative" subtotal gastrectomies.[46] Some component of local failure was found in 74 (80.4%) as follows: 46 of 92 patients (50%), stomach wall or site of gastroenterostomy; 14 of 92 patients (15.2%), tumor in the duodenum, with five of the 14 associated with recurrence in the gastric remnant; 48 of 92 patients (52.2%), perigastric lymph nodes and stomach bed. Thomson and Robins analyzed 28 cases with previous subtotal resection.[47] Patterns of failure were as follows: gastric stump alone, five of 28 patients (17.8%); duodenal stump, three of 28 patients (10.7%); gastric bed, 13 of 28 patients (46.4%); gastric bed and gastric stump, six of 28 patients (21.4%). Gunderson and Sosin approached the problem of defining sights of recurrence in a different fashion.[48] These workers analyzed the recurrences occurring in a prospective study in which patients undergoing gastric resection were subjected to periodic re-operation at the University of Minnesota. Following their initial operative procedure, 109 patients had single or multiple re-operations. Since two had residual disease after the first procedure, 107 were evaluable for failure purposes. All patients had been treated by operation alone without any pre- and postoperative adjuvants. Extent of the operative procedure was mainly by the era in which the procedure was performed rather than the extent of disease, with a large group of patients having splenectomy, omentectomy, and radical lymph node dissections in addition to some form of gastrectomy.

Of the 107 evaluable patients, 86 (80.4%) had later evidence of cancer. Incidence and patterns of failure were analyzed in detail (Tables 17-5 and 17-6). Distant metastases (DM) alone were uncommon, but occurred as some component of failure in 29.3% of the failure group. Nearly half of the peritoneal failures were localized. Of those that had a diffuse component, nearly all also had a fairly massive local recurrence. Local failure and regional lymph node metastases (LF–RF) occurred as the only failure in 29.3% of the failure group (53.4%, if localized peritoneal seeding was included) and as any component of failure in 87.8%. Extent of operative procedure had little if any effect on either the incidence or type of subsequent failure. The local–regional failures were primarily in lymph nodes and organs and structures of the gastric bed, with a smaller but significant number of failures in the anastomoses, gastric remnant, or duodenal stump. Very few failures occurred in the abdominal incision or stab wounds. Lymph node failures were found in a fairly high percentage of patients who supposedly had radical lymph node dissections. Distant metastases were primarily to the liver.

TABLE 17-3. Histologically determined extent of primary gastric cancer (Hoerr Classification, 462 Patients, Charity Hospital, 1963–1973)

		NO.	(%)
A.	No metastasis	58	(12.7)
B.	Regional metastasis	182	(39.2)
C.	Distant metastasis	164	(35.6)
I.	Inner gastric layer involvement	52	(10.9)
II.	Serosal involvement	75	(16.2)
III.	Contiguous structure involvement	258	(55.8)

(Dupont JB Jr, Cohn I Jr: Gastric adenocarcinoma. Curr Prob Cancer 4:10, 1980).

TABLE 17-4. Metastasis—Autopsy or Operation

NO. PATIENTS	176	348	67	250
	% of patients			
Liver	38	54	34	40
Peritoneum	20	24	28	17
Omentum	13	21	–	–
Lungs	12	22	9	19
Mesentery	9	–	–	–
Pleura	8	–	4	–
Pancreas	7	29	10	–
Adrenals	5	15	3	12
Intestine	4	–	6	–
GU tract	–	3	–	8
Spleen	2	13	1	–
Gallbladder/biliary tract	2	4	6	–
Bone	6	1	6	9
Central nervous system	1	0.2	–	2
No metastasis	23	11	24	22

TABLE 17-5. Patterns of Failure:* University of Minnesota Reoperation Series—86 patients had failure, 82 are evaluable

PATTERN OF FAILURE	ONLY FAILURE	ANY COMPONENT
LOCAL–REGIONAL FAILURE	24%–29.3% (22.4)	72%–87.8% (67.3)
a. + localized PS (20 patients)	44%–53.7% (41.1)	
PERITONEAL SPREAD	3%–3.7% (2.8)	44%–53.7% (41.1)
a. localized		20%–24.4% (18.7)
b. diffuse		†24%–29.3% (22.4)
DISTANT METASTASES	‡5%–6.1% (4.7)	§24%–29.3% (22.4)

* Open figures represent number and percent of the failure group of 82 patients and those in parentheses represent the percent of the total group of 107 patients.

† Additional five patients did not have evidence of PS until third or later look (18/82 = 23.2% diffuse PS if these five are deleted).

‡ One patient had a liver nodule at first operation—liver was involved at reoperation.

§ Total of three patients had DM at first operation—therefore, 21/82 (25.6%) had DM as a new manifestation.

(Gunderson LL, Sosin H: Adenocarcinoma of the stomach—areas of failure in a reoperation series (second or symptomatic looks). Clinicopathologic correlation and implications for adjuvant therapy. Int J Rad Oncol Rad Biol (in press))

TABLE 17-6. Patterns of Local Failure and Regional Failure. Reoperation and Autopsy Series

	INCIDENCE—ANY COMPONENT (%)		
FAILURE AREA	U MINN *(Re-Open)*	McNEER ET AL *(Autopsy)*	THOMPSON AND ROBINS *(Autopsy)*
Gastric bed	54.2% (58/107)	52.2% (48/92)	67.9% (19/28)
Anastomosis or stumps	26.2% (28/107)	59.8% (55/92)	53.6% (15/28)
Abdomen or stab wound	4.7% (5/107)	–	–
Lymph nodes	42% (45/107)	52.2% (48/92)	–

Thus, all these data suggest that although systemic therapy is clearly important, the development of an effective local therapy as an adjuvant to surgery could significantly benefit at least 20% of patients.

CLINICAL PRESENTATION

Almost every article on cancer of the stomach stresses the vague nondiagnostic symptomatology and the fact that patients are likely to be unaware of their disease, as well as presenting a picture that fails to trigger the proper diagnostic impressions in the physician's mind. Article after article stress the "vague," "indefinite," "non-specific" symptoms and then proceed to list such things as epigastric uneasiness, mild anemia, fatigability, ulcer history, weight loss, and so forth. Clearly, none of these symptoms unequivocably indicates gastric cancer, and unless the clinician is alert to that possibility, it is entirely possible that the patient will be treated empirically for ulcer disease, not treated at all, or allowed to think there is no serious problem.[49–53]

Five different reviews covering the span from 1950 to 1970 show essentially no change in the incidence of the key symptoms, and show the vague, nonspecific nature of all of the findings in each individual study (Table 17-7).[43,49–53]

The fact that the major presenting finding in some series could be a palpable mass in one-third of the patients, ascites or the less frequent findings of metastases to superficial nodes or jaundice all suggest the extensive disease that can exist before the patient seeks medical help.

One study compared the incidence of the various symptoms in resectable *versus* nonresectable cases and found very little difference under these circumstances.[54] This same study evaluated the extent of weight loss, duration of symptoms, and location of the tumor in the stomach with regard to the symptoms. There were no differences in any of these parameters except for the relative incidence of dysphagia and regurgitation as related to the location of the lesion within the stomach. Specific symptoms may indicate to the clinician complicating factors in individual cases. For example, a patient with dysphagia may have a cardio–esophageal junction lesion with partial obstruction from involvement of the distal esophagus. Patients with persistent nausea and vomiting, indicating bowel obstruction, may have several syndromes associated with gastric cancer.[10] An antral carcinoma may produce obstruction and gastric dilatation. Occasionally gastric cancer may directly invade the transverse mesocolon and result in transverse colon obstruction. Patients who develop peritoneal dissemination with gastric cancer may manifest distal bowel obstruction. A Blumer's shelf resulting from metastatic gastric carcinoma can result in rectal obstruction.

By the time physical signs of gastric cancer are present, patients are incurable. The commonly found physical findings with stomach cancer are direct manifestations of the pattern of spread of this disease as outlined in Table 17-2. Gastric

TABLE 17-7. Gastric Carcinoma Symptoms

NO. PATIENTS	1112	501	270	250	245
			% of patients		
Weight loss	85	24	58	68	56
Pain	69	38	48	67	56
Vomiting	43	24	21	47	–
Bowel symptoms	41	–	5	–	–
Anorexia	30	4	21	–	–
Dysphagia	20	13	17	–	9
Nausea	20	–	4	65	–
N & V	–	–	–	–	38
Weakness	19	17	–	–	–
Eructation	17	–	–	–	–
Hematemesis	6	16	13	18	–
Regurgitation	6	–	–	–	–
Rapid satiation	5	–	2	–	–
No symptoms	0.4	–	–	5	6

adenocarcinoma disseminates by both lymphatic and hematogenous routes. The earliest sites of lymphatic metastases are to regional nodes and clearly cannot be detected by physical examination. However, three sites of nodal metastases are detectable by examination. Careful evaluation of the supraclavicular fossae is necessary in the patient suspected of gastric cancer. The finding of a firm left supraclavicular (Virchow's) node may allow for tissue diagnosis without abdominal exploration. Two less common sites of nodal metastases are worth noting. Patients with systemic symptoms consistent with stomach cancer should have careful digital examination of the periumbilical area and left axilla. Gastric cancer has been reported to metastasize to nodes in both these areas.[10] The umbilical nodal metastases and left axillary nodes (Irish's node) should be assiduously searched for, since their presence allows for a simple tissue diagnosis in the patient with gastric cancer.

The most common site of hematogenous metastases in stomach cancer is the liver. Firm, smooth or nodular hepatomegaly may be apparent on physical examination as an indication of hepatic metastases. Patients with stomach cancer with locally extensive disease may present to the physician with a palpable epigastric mass that may be mistaken for the left lobe of an enlarged liver when it actually represents the gastric tumor itself.

Rarely does the patient with gastric carcinoma present with significant bleeding. Although mild blood loss that may be detected as occult blood in the stool is common with gastric cancer, massive upper gastrointestinal bleeding is uncommon. In fact, the patient with a gastric mass and upper gastrointestinal hemorrhage is more likely to have gastic leiomyosarcoma than adenocarcinoma of the stomach.[10] Hemorrhage without the presence of mass suggests benign gastric ulcer.

Syndromes of remote effects of carcinoma are rare with stomach cancer. This disease, however, does represent the most common visceral malignancy associated with acanthosis nigricans.[10] In this syndrome, patients exhibit hypertrophic pigmented skin lesions, particularly noted in the axillae. Glucose intolerance may also be present. The syndrome of thrombotic non-bacterial endocarditis has also been associated with gastric cancer, but is not specific and may be seen in any patient with advanced wasting from malignant disease.

STAGING

As more sophisticated combined modality approaches have been utilized in the treatment of gastric cancer, staging has became more important. In the past, an informal staging scheme was used by physicians treating this disease. Thus the surgeon at the time of operation determined the stage of the cancer and this stage determined which treatment option might be useful. Therapy was dictated by stage: (1) completely resectable, (2) locally unresectable indicating the use of radiation therapy and (3) disseminated disease requiring chemotherapy.

Attempts at developing more formal staging plans have been carried out during the last 40 years. In 1941, Coller, Kay, and McInture reviewed 53 cases in detail to attempt to correlate lymphatic metastases and other features of primary lesions in the stomach. They divided the lymphatics into four zones, all four of which they recommended should be removed in all resectable cases. Their lymph node classification has served as the background for much that has been written about the staging of gastric cancer.[42]

A suggestion for gross surgical classification of lesions of the stomach was advocated by Hoerr (Table 17-3).[55,56] His original presentation plus the subsequent reviews based upon that classification have provided an additional means for studying the significance of lesions in the stomach. This classification is based upon the extent of invasion of the wall of the stomach and adjacent viscera, plus the extent of lymph node and distant involvement. Overall classification by this technique assists in determining whether or not a tumor is likely to be resectable and also whether or not there is clear-cut evidence of distant spread.

More recently, the TNM classification (Table 17-8) has been established, and a review by Kennedy (Table 17-9) of 1241 patients demonstrated correlations between lymph node involvement and survival, the depth of penetration of the stomach by the lesion, and the presence of distant metastasis.[57,58] Similar observations have been made by the large Japanese studies, which divide the lymphatics in a much more complex fashion.[59,60] This system serves the Japanese as a basis for their operative and adjuvant treatment of patients with gastric cancer, but the Japanese system has not had wide exposure in the United States.

Desmond reviewed the experience with 1363 cases and divided lymphatic drainage into seven different groups, with recommendations regarding appropriate surgical measures to be employed for lesions which involved any or all of these groups.[61] Although, conceptually, the simple staging of "resectable," "locally advanced," and "disseminated" still has value, it is clear that use of a formalized staging plan such as the TNM approach will allow for much more accurate comparison of different treatment results in the future.

PROGNOSIS

The prognosis of gastric cancer depends both upon extent of disease and treatment. As detailed in the previous section on staging, local and regional extension of disease adversely affects survival. Up until the very recent past, the only patients with any potential for long-term survival were those who underwent complete excision of localized cancer.

Experience with 1497 cases at Charity Hospital provided the background for a number of different evaluations of survival based upon various forms of operative treatment.[39,40] The 5-year survival rate for all patients observed 5 or more years in this study was 7.35%. The best 5-year survival figure of 30.3% obtained in the entire study was for the relatively small group of 149 patients found to have localized disease. Table 17-10 shows the relative 5-year survival rates for a series of different studies and indicates that survival figures are disappointing.

A detailed statistical study of the large experience at the Mayo Clinic by ReMine, Priestly, and Berkson demonstrates relationships between survival, size of lesion, age of patient, operative mortality, age at operation, year of operation, path-

TABLE 17-8. TNM Classification, Definitions

PRIMARY TUMOR (T)

TX	Degree of penetration of stomach wall not determined
T0	No evidence of primary tumor
T1	Tumor limited to mucosa and submucosa, regardless of its extent or location
T2	Tumor involves the mucosa, the submucosa (including the muscularis propria), and extends to or into the serosa, but does not penetrate through the serosa
T3	Tumor penetrates through the serosa without invading contiguous structures
T4	Tumor penetrates through the serosa and invades the contiguous structures

NODAL INVOLVEMENT (N)

NX	Metastases to intra-abdominal lymph nodes not determined (e.g., laparotomy not done)
N0	No metastases to regional lymph nodes
N1	Involvement of perigastric lymph nodes within 3 cm of the primary tumor along the lesser or greater curvature
N2	Involvement of the regional lymph nodes more than 3 cm from the primary tumor, which are removed or removable at operation, including those located along the left gastric, splenic, celiac, and common hepatic arteries
N3	Involvement of other intra-abdominal lymph nodes which are not removable at operation, such as the para-aortic, hepatoduodenal, retropancreatic, and mesenteric nodes

DISTANT METASTASIS (M)

MX	Not assessed
M0	No (known) distant metastasis
M1	Distant metastasis present
	Specify ________
	Specify sites according to the following notations:

Peritoneal (PER)	Bone marrow (MAR)
Pulmonary (PUL)	Pleura (PLE)
Osseous (OSS)	Skin (SKI)
Hepatic (HEP)	Eye (EYE)
Brain (BRA)	Other (OTH)
Lymph nodes (LYM) (above diaphragm or non-abdominal)	

STAGE GROUPING

Stage	Clinical-Diagnostic Staging	Postsurgical Treatment–Pathologic Staging
I	cT1 N0 M0	pT1 N0 M0
II	cT2 N0 M0*	pT2 N0 M0
	cT3 N0 M0	pT3 N0 M0
III	cTX-3 N1-3† M0	pT1-3 N1 M0
		pT1-3 N2 M0
		pT1-3 N3 M0 (resected for cure)
IV	cT4 NX-3† M0 (probably not resectable)	pT1-3 N3 M0
		pT4 N0-3 M0 (not resectable)
	cTX-4 NX-3 M1	pT1-4 or pTX or N0-3 or NX M1

RESIDUAL TUMOR (R)

R0	No residual tumor
R1	Microscopic residual tumor
R2	Macroscopic residual tumor
	Specify ________

*Not applicable—at present there is no reliable clinical method of determining the extent of T2 lesions.

† Established by clinical criteria (e.g., echogram, computerized tomography).

(American Joint Committee for Cancer Staging and End-Results Reporting: Manual for Staging of Cancer 1978, pp 75–76. Chicago, American Joint Committee, 1978)

ologic stage of the disease and other features.[62] Prognosis is also clearly related to resectability rate and hospital mortality. Resectability has been increasing in most hands, but still is not as high as would be desirable. The major key to significant improvements in survival will be reliable diagnostic tests that will allow the diagnosis to be established at a time when the disease is still confined to the stomach and the application of aggressive combined modality therapy. The effects of the various forms of therapy on prognosis in gastric cancer will be dealt with in detail in the treatment section of this chapter.

DIAGNOSIS

Several procedures may be used in making the diagnosis of stomach cancer. These diagnostic steps and a suggested sequence in diagnosis are outlined in Table 17-11. The keystone procedure in the diagnosis of stomach cancer has been the barium upper gastrointestinal series.[10,63,64] Although the majority of patients with gastric cancer present with relatively advanced disease, which should be detected by the conventional upper gastrointestinal series, recently reported studies indicate this not to be the case. A review of contemporary series, comparing the correlation of roentgenographic findings with those of endoscopic biopsy demonstrated that 9% to 40% of endoscopically positive lesions were not detected by previous barium studies.[64] These results suggest that on the average, 10% of symptomatic carcinomas are missed in barium studies. An older study raised the question of faulty interpretation of abnormal findings on upper gastrointestinal roentgenography.[63] This series reported data showing that 15% of malignant abnormalities may be misinterpreted as benign findings.

The diagnostic accuracy of barium roentgenography may be improved by the use of a double contrast technique (Figures 17-2, 17-3).[64,65] This procedure makes use of high density barium combined with an effervescent agent and glucagon administration to induce gastric atony. A double contrast study allows for careful evaluation of the proximal stomach where malignant lesions are most likely to be missed by conventional barium studies.

With the advent of the flexible fiber optic gastroscope, the preferred way to make a tissue diagnosis of gastric cancer has been by endoscopy to obtain either tissue biopsy or exfoliative cytology (see Fig. 17-4). Older studies have reported wide variation in the success rate of endoscopic biopsy and cytology in gastric cancer.[10] In a review of several series, Backus reported positive cytologic examination in 37% to 97% of gastric cancer patients with false positive rates of 0.5% to 13%.[66] With improvement in technique of both endoscopic procedures and pathologic examination, the success rate has improved. Winawer and colleagues have pointed out several factors that bear on the likelihood of making a successful endoscopic tissue diagnosis.[67,68] If the tumor mass is exophytic, endoscopy is usually successful in establishing a tissue diagnosis. In 24 of 26 such patients (92%), the authors obtained positive biopsy or cytologic brush pathology.[68] However, in 24 patients with infiltrative gastric cancer, the diagnoses were made in only 12 (50%). Other factors mitigating against the success of endoscopic biopsy include tumor

TABLE 17-9. 5-Year Survival and Initial Stage of Gastric Cancer

EXTENT OF DISEASE	5-YEAR SURVIVAL (%)
LYMPH NODES (−)	
1. Mucosa only	85
2. Mucosa and gastric wall	52
3. Through gastric wall	47
LYMPH NODES (+)	
Extent of lymph node involvement	
a. Regional only	17
b. Other areas	5

TABLE 17-10. 5-Year Survival

SOURCE	NUMBER OF PATIENTS	5-YEAR SURVIVAL (%)
Cancer Prognosis Manual	10,115	9.0
Keller (1965)	574	4.7
Gilbertsen (1969)	1,983	10.2
Crumb (1970)	123	5.1
Nielson (1974)	385	12.0
Inberg (1975)	2,590	5.8
Kenter (1975)	238	16.9
Cassell (1976)	827	8.8
Svennevig (1976)	209	10.0
Costello (1977)	226	8.5
CHNO	1,497	7.4

(Dupont JB Jr, Lee JR, Burton GR et al: Adenocarcinoma of the stomach: Review of 1497 cases. Cancer 41:941, 1978)

less than 3 cm in diameter, tumor location at the cardia or on the lesser curvature, and recurrent tumors. In such unfavorable situations, lavage cytology may increase the accuracy of brush cytology or biopsy.[67]

The recommended manner (Table 17-11) in which to proceed to establish a tissue diagnosis in the patient suspected of having gastric cancer is the following: (a) careful physical examination for pathologic findings amenable to biopsy (nodes, liver) (b) UGI with double contrast to establish site of abnormality in the stomach (c) endoscopy with biopsy and cytology (d) diagnostic/therapeutic laparotomy.

There are other procedures which may be of ancillary use to the physician dealing with patients with suspected gastric cancer. These include CT scanning, ultrasonography, and plasma tumor markers. In contrast to pancreatic cancer, CT scanning and ultrasonography are of little use in the primary

TABLE 17-11. Sequence of Diagnostic Procedures in Suspected Gastric Cancer

I.	Physical examination ? Lymph node metastasis → biopsy ? Hepatomegaly → biopsy ? Abdominal mass
II.	Double contrast barium upper gastrointestinal series
III.	Fiberoptic endoscopy with biopsy and cytology
IV.	Diagnostic/therapeutic laparotomy

FIG. 17-2. *A*, Normal appearance of the gastric antrum and body on double contrast upper gastrointestinal study. *B*, Normal appearance of gastric fundus. (Laufer I: Double contrast radiology in the diagnosis of gastrointestinal cancer. Jerzy Glass GB (ed): Progress in Gastroenterology, p. 649. New York, Grune & Stratton, 1977)

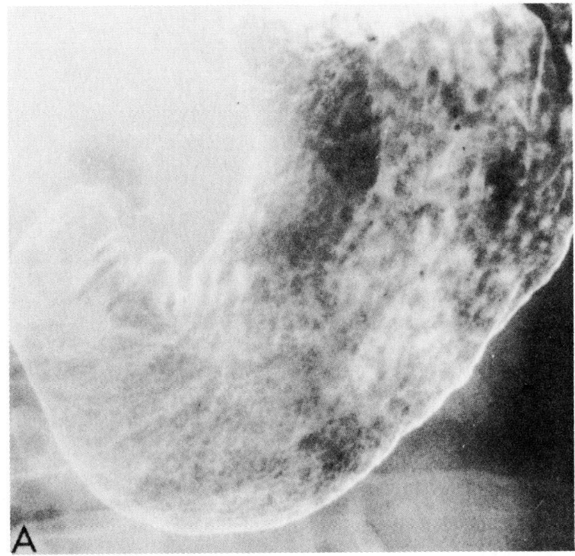

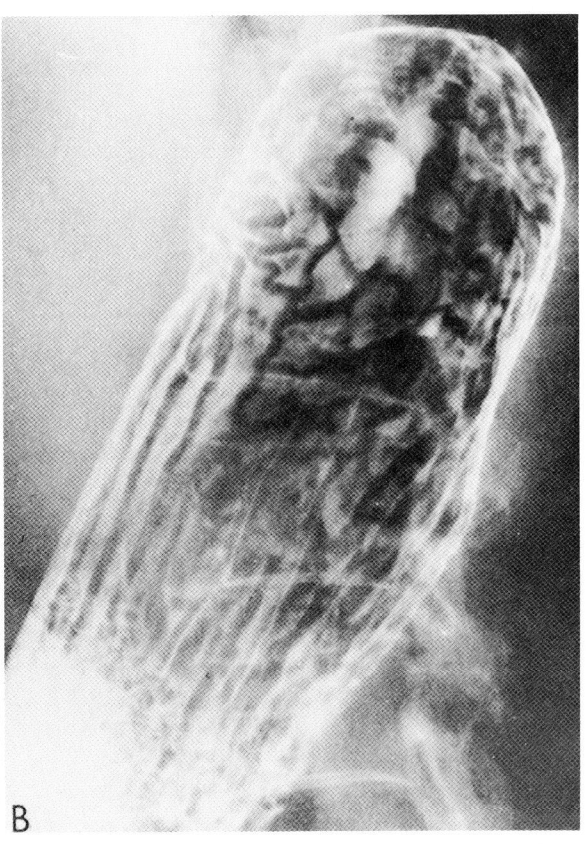

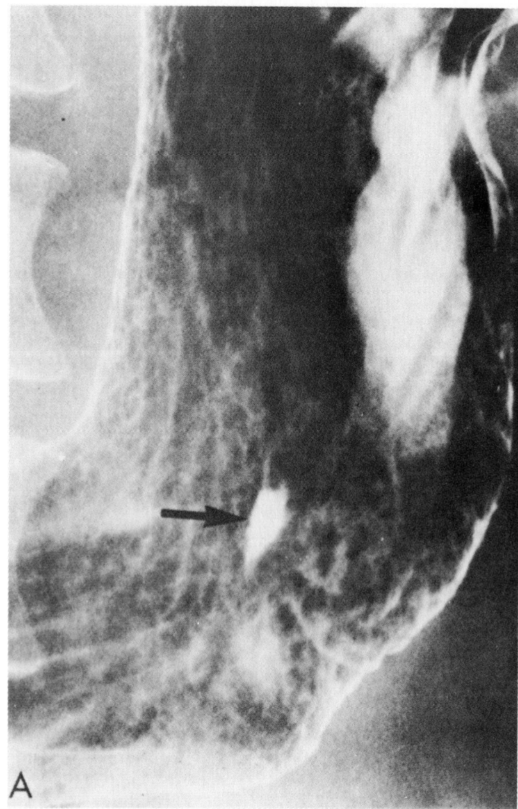

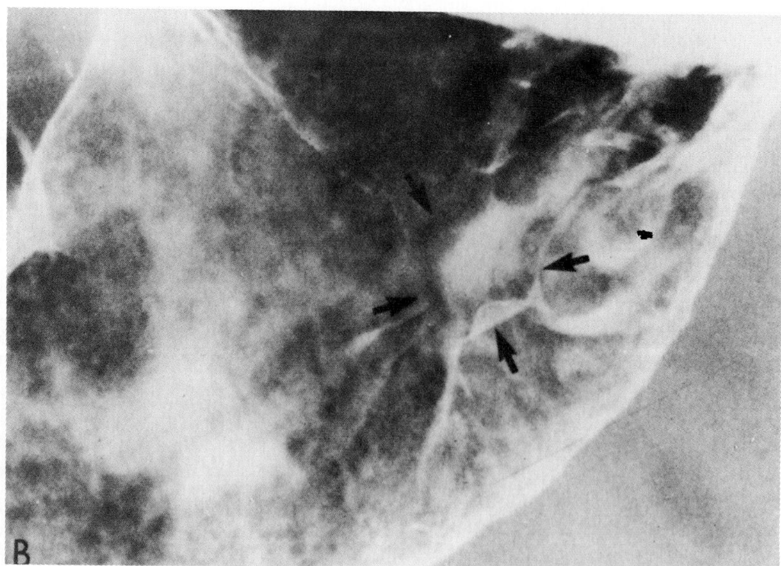

FIG. 17-3. *A*, Benign gastric ulcer on double contrast UGI. The ulcer crater has smooth, sharply defined borders. *B*, Malignant gastric ulcer. Elevated irregular borders are present and the ulcer crater is poorly circumscribed. (Laufer I: Double contrast radiology in the diagnosis of gastrointestinal cancer. In Jerzy Glass GB (ed): Progress in Gastroenterology, p. 652. New York, Grune & Stratton, 1977. By permission)

diagnosis of stomach cancer. This is predominately because the stomach is so accessible to barium roentgenographic studies and to endoscopy. However, both CT and ultrasound scanning may be helpful in defining sites of metastases and extragastric extension. For example, the liver may be evaluated by these techniques, along with radionuclide scanning, to elucidate suspected metastases. Also, peritoneal spread of gastric carcinoma can be demonstrated by CT scanning and ultrasonography. Pelvic masses resulting from either the Krukenberg tumor or pelvic peritoneal dissemination (Blumer's shelf) potentially may be detected by these techniques.

Plasma tumor markers are of limited use in gastric can-

FIG. 17-4. *A*, Endoscopic view of early slightly ulcerated gastric cancer. Lesion shows hemorrhage from two biopsy sites. The gastric antrum is in upper left of photograph. *B*, Nodular gastric cancer with multiple areas of minor hemorrhage.

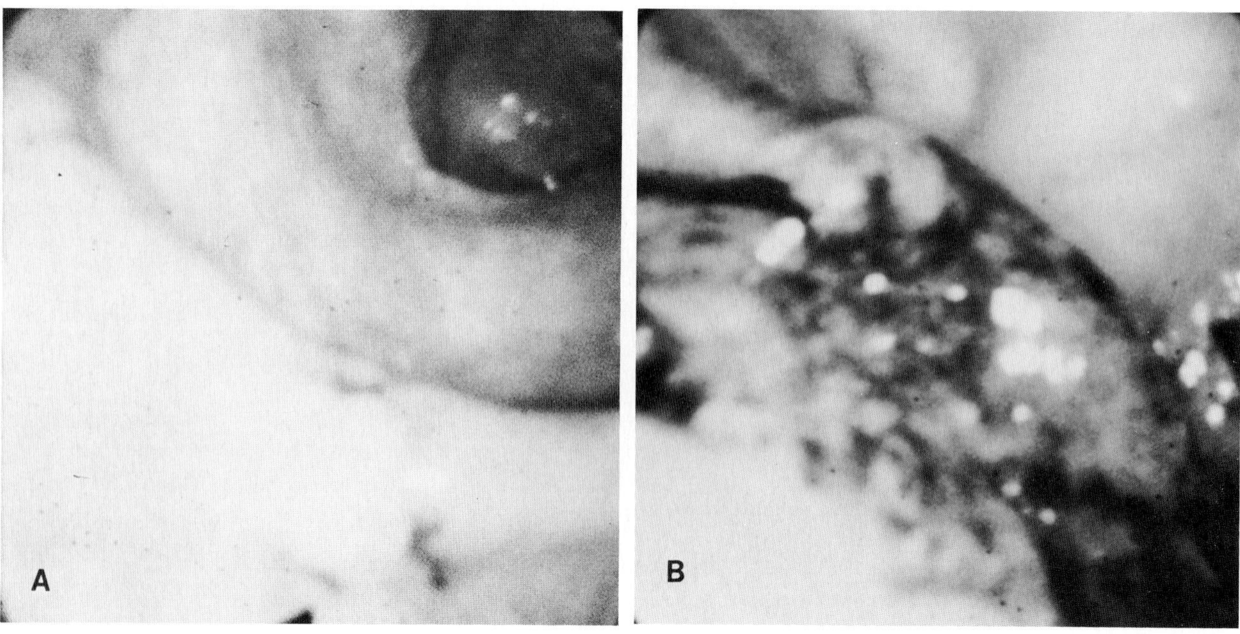

cer.[69,70] Carcinoembryonic antigen (CEA) is frequently elevated in the plasma of patients with gastric cancer and is of no diagnostic value. This marker is increased in 60% of advanced gastric cancer cases but is frequently abnormal in patients who already have other manifestations of tumor. α-Fetoprotein (AFP), another oncofetal protein, also does not assist the clinician in the early diagnosis of stomach cancer. This protein is found elevated in only 15% to 20% of patients with gastric cancer, but is is also elevated in patients with various benign diseases, including cirrhosis and hepatitis, and thus is associated with both false-negative and false-positive errors in regard to gastric cancer.

SCREENING

Because of the extent of the gastric cancer problem in some countries other than the U.S., there has been interest in developing techniques of screening to detect early lesions. This approach has been most highly developed in Japan.

The Japanese have demonstrated the value of mass surveys for gastric carcinoma in their particular population. They have detected cases earlier by the use of mass UGI surveys and the gastro-camera than have been found by the means more commonly used in this country. In order for these techniques to be useful, one needs a cancer-prone population such as exists in Japan, and one needs access to the endoscopic and radiologic techniques that are so widely used there.[71]

The ultimate aim of screening programs would be to decrease the mortality of gastric cancer. The Japanese have succeeded in this endeavor. Operative attempts are highly successful when gastric cancer is limited to the mucosa but the incidence of such early lesions is less than 5% in most U.S. series. In Japan, the incidence of lesions initially confined to the mucosa or submucosa was only 3.8% in the years from 1955 to 1956, but because of screening procedures, this had increased to 34.5% with a corresponding survival rate of 90.9% by 1966.[72]

TREATMENT

SURGERY

The necessary surgical procedures for gastric cancer should be based on anatomical considerations, prior experience, knowledge of the natural history of the disease, and the needs of the particular case. Since the stomach is not vital to a relatively normal life span, the surgical procedure (Fig. 17-5) can involve anything up to and including a total gastrectomy, removal of the omentum, removal of the spleen, removal of the distal portion of the esophagus, removal of the proximal portion of the duodenum, and even simultaneous removal of a portion of the transverse colon. While such an extensive procedure is certainly not recommended as a routine, experience has indicated that any or all of these structures can be removed without jeopardizing the patient's long-term survival. Lesser resections of the stomach are anatomically, surgically, and oncologically possible, and the extent of the resection of the stomach can be determined partly by the extent of the lesion and partly by knowledge of its usual pathways of extension.

For most of the 20th century the preferred treatment for gastric carcinoma has been some form of radical subtotal gastrectomy (Fig. 17-6). There have been significant swings in opinion toward and away from total gastrectomy as the treatment of choice, and this has been coupled with various extensions of total gastrectomy which have been advocated from time to time.[73–78] Some form of subtotal gastrectomy has been returned to after most of the swings of opinions, and our

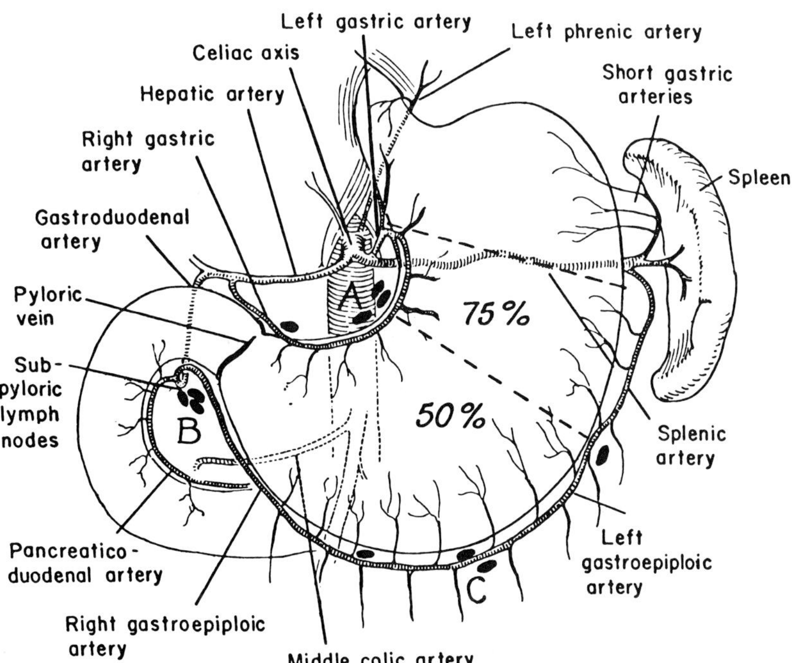

FIG. 17-5. Vascular supply and lymphatic drainage of the stomach in relation to the extent of gastrectomy commonly utilized in gastric cancer. Proximal resection margins for 50% and 75% subtotal gastrectomies are indicated. (Zollinger RM, Zollinger RM Jr: Atlas of Surgical Operations, 4th Ed. Plate XIX No. 1. New York, Macmillan, 1977. Copyright ©, 1975 by Macmillan Publishing Co., Inc.)

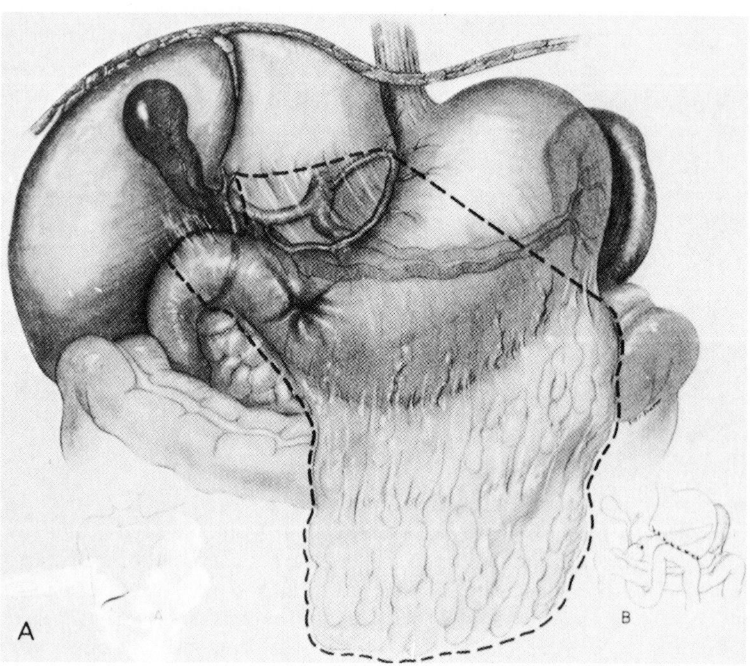

FIG. 17-6. Extent of resection margins of radical subtotal gastrectomy for distal gastric carcinoma. *A*, Surgical incision; *B*, completed resection illustrating gastrojejunostomy. (McNeer G, Pack GT: Neoplasms of the Stomach, p 286. Philadelphia, JB Lippincott, 1967)

own experience with the large Charity Hospital population has convinced us that this is the preferred method of treatment.[39,40,79]

The known propensity of carcinoma of the stomach to cross both the gastroesophageal junction and the pylorus, depending upon the location of the primary tumor within the stomach, has made it essential that any procedure designed to cure should involve resection of enough of the appropriate adjacent end of the stomach to be sure to include whatever segments of the lesion have extended beyond the anatomic boundaries of the stomach. Appreciation of the usual routes of lymphatic spread and of the key adjacent viscera are essential to the proper management of these patients. The frequency with which the transverse colon or its blood supply or both may be involved makes it mandatory that the colon be appropriately prepared prior to any elective procedure on a patient suspected of having carcinoma of the stomach.

Almost every retrospective study of the surgical care of patients with carcinoma of the stomach demonstrates that the morbidity and mortality are higher than expected, and these studies emphasize the importance of careful pre-operative evaluation and preparation of these patients. In addition to all the standard studies that one should do before any major abdominal procedure, there are certain other considerations which are of major importance in the patient with gastric cancer. Appropriate studies, beyond history and physical examination, should be completed to determine if there is any evidence of distant metastases. Chest roentgenograms and physical examination for hepatic and splenic enlargement should be followed by scans of the liver or spleen if there is any suggestion of involvement of either of these organs. Since anemia and weight loss are common accompaniments of gastric cancer, appropriate blood counts, serum protein studies, and evaluations of liver function should be completed. Replacement of blood volume, red cell mass, and protein stores should be accomplished in so far as possible. Depending upon the patient's needs and the time available, hyperalimentation should be considered as part of the pre-operative preparation of the patient. If there is evidence of hepatic dysfunction, attempts should be made to correct this, unless it is believed due to metastatic replacement of normal hepatic tissue or tumor blockage of the biliary tract.

The patient whose stomach is fixed on roentgenographic examination, one with evidence of widespread metastatic involvement, or one with ascites on the basis of peritoneal carcinomatosis should be considered inoperable. The presence of a Virchow node or other evidence of lymphatic permeation does not make the patient inoperable, although we are likely to find the patient incurable with present methods of therapy. The lesion should not be considered unresectable until this can be demonstrated at the time of operation. As long as the stomach is mobile, or the stomach and the organs to which it has become adherent can all be removed without compromising the patient's survival, every attempt should be made to resect the primary lesion regardless of its size and the other organs involved. Leaving behind a mass lesion in the stomach is an open invitation to bleeding, perforation, or further obstruction, as well as significantly diminishing the opportunities for success from adjuvant therapy.[80] Not only can removal of the primary tumor reduce the bulk and thereby improve the chances for chemotherapy, but it also diminishes the likelihood of the other complications just named. Thus, whenever possible, a lesion in the stomach should be removed, even if this is done for purposes of palliation. Both the surgeon and the patient or the patient's family should be aware of the difference between an attempted curative procedure and a palliative one but, nevertheless, a vigorous attempt at palliation is justified.

The large experience at Charity Hospital has documented, once again, the failure of various bypass procedures if the patient's major problem is gastric outlet obstruction and the lesion cannot be resected.[39,40] The urge "to do something" and the performance of some form of gastroenterostomy fail to relieve the obstruction and carry risks that are unwarranted, even though both patient and family—as well as surgeon—are likely to believe the "do nothing" approach is inappropriate. A recent study of the Charity Hospital experience concluded, "Palliative bypass procedures do not increase survival and any hope of improving the quality of life is highly questionable."

The major procedures utilized for curative attempts in gastric cancer are total gastrectomy or some modification of a radical subtotal gastrectomy. A brief outline of the operative and postoperative problems associated with either of these procedures follows.

A total gastrectomy should involve removal of the entire stomach, as much of the adjacent duodenum or esophagus as is indicated by the location of the primary and the obvious evidence of its spread into the appropriate organ, all of the greater omentum, the spleen in the majority of cases and certainly if the lesion is in the proximal half of the stomach, dissection of the celiac axis as completely as possible with ligation of the major vessels at as high a level as possible, and dissection of the hepatic artery as far as possible. Reconstruction of gastrointestinal continuity can be achieved by any one of a variety of techniques, depending upon the way in which the patient is responding to the operative procedure, the time the operative procedure has consumed, and the perceived importance of providing a substitute gastric pouch or reservoir at the time of the initial procedure. If a decision is to not make a pouch, then an end-to-end esophagoduodenostomy can be fashioned in some cases, or if this appears to put too much tension on the anastomosis, then either an end-to-end esophagojejunostomy or an end-to-side esophagojejunostomy with or without a Roux-Y loop. If a decision is made at the outset to fashion a pouch, there are a number of pouches which can be utilized, some of which are illustrated in Figure 17-7. If the patient is tolerating the procedure well, a number of surgeons prefer to fashion the pouch at the time of the primary operation. Others believe that it is better to give the patient some time to recover from the primary procedure and then fashion the pouch at a later date when it is determined that the patient is responding to removal of the primary lesion.

Since all of these procedures involve an anastomosis, one side of which is esophageal, a major problem is a breakdown at this anastomosis. This would be the major postoperative complication that differs in any way from those following a subtotal gastrectomy, and is a problem that needs to be taken into consideration in the decision to do a total gastrectomy.

If the lesion involves a sufficient portion of the stomach to require a total gastrectomy, then this is the procedure of choice. The long-term survival following curative total gastrectomy, however, has not demonstrated superior results.[39]

A total gastrectomy should not be undertaken as a palliative procedure, since the palliation from a total gastrectomy is not good, and the mortality and morbidity of the procedure are too high to justify this as a palliative procedure.

The preferred treatment for gastric carcinoma, particularly for a lesion located in the distal half of the stomach, is a radical subtotal resection of the stomach (Fig. 17-6), which includes removal of 80% to 85% of the stomach, the omentum,

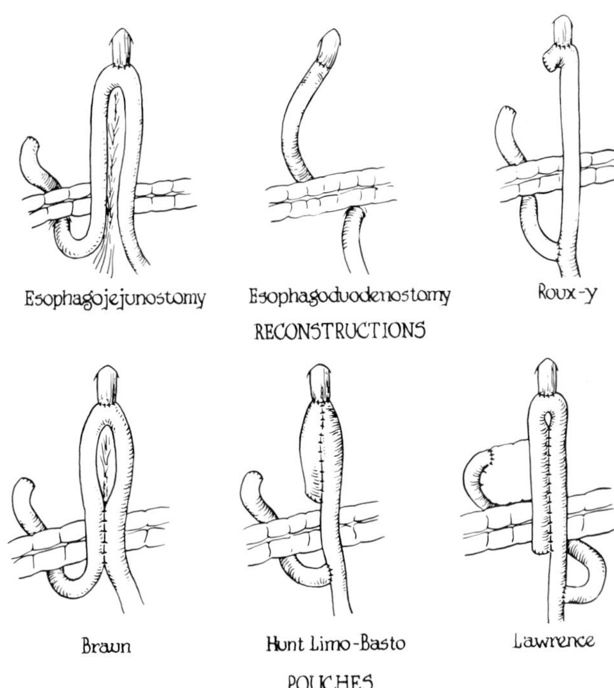

FIG. 17-7. Major variations in types of reconstructions possible after total gastrectomy. Examples of gastric reservoir pouches that can be employed to increase the capacity of the substitute stomach after a total gastrectomy.

first portion of the duodenum, and node-bearing tissue of the hepatico–duodenal pedicle, the gastrohepatic omentum, and the gastrocolic omentum. The spleen should be removed only if there is direct evidence of spread to the spleen or to the splenic nodes, or if the lesion is encroaching upon the proximal half of the stomach.

The experience at Charity Hospital indicates that radical subtotal gastrectomy gave the best survival (Fig. 17-8) and, therefore, this is the procedure which we would recommend.[39] Improved survival in patients undergoing subtotal, as opposed to total, gastrectomy was also noted in a series of 503 patients undergoing "curative" gastric resection.[15] Higgins and associates, in reporting on this group of patients, noted 5-year survival of 15.9% for total gastrectomy, 13.6% for proximal gastrectomy, and 30.1% for subtotal gastrectomy. Although both this experience and the Charity Hospital experience suggest improved results with the subtotal procedure, it is not possible to know with certainty whether the operation results in improved survival or whether the type of patient who is a candidate for a curative subtotal procedure (usually a patient with distal or antral primary) has an intrinsically better prognosis than the patient who requires total gastrectomy (that is, a patient with diffuse involvement of the stomach or a proximal cancer).[39,40] Thus, although radical subtotal gastrectomy remains the procedure of choice *when it can be performed,* and is associated with improved survival, the clinician is cautioned not to assume that survival benefit *results* from the operation. All of the usual complications which accompany any form of gastric resection are potential problems in the patient with carcinoma undergoing either a

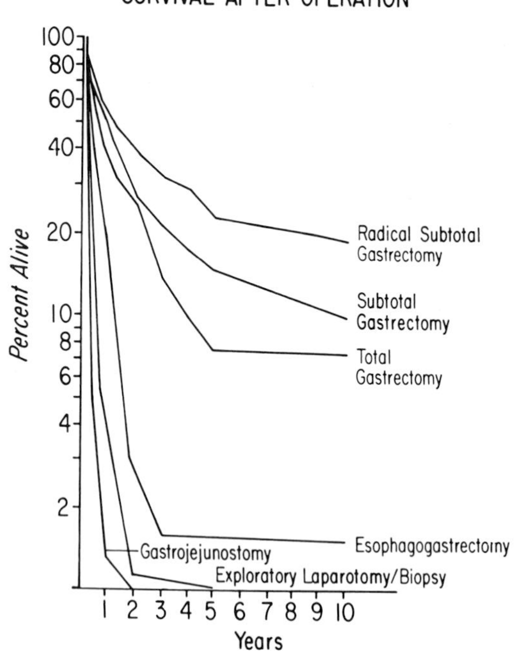

FIG. 17-8. Survival, computed by the life-table method, after various procedures for adenocarcinoma of the stomach. (Dupont JB, Cohn I: Gastric adenocarcinoma. Curr Probl Cancer 4:25, 1980)

total or subtotal gastrectomy. The most common complications are outlined in Table 17-12.

Since there is often involvement of the transverse colon or its blood supply, and since this kind of involvement does not contra-indicate resection, it is essential that every patient being subjected to an elective procedure for cancer of the stomach should have adequate mechanical and antibiotic preparation of the large bowel prior to the operative procedure.

The pancreas is also involved in a fair proportion of patients, and there are those who believe simultaneous resection of the distal pancreas is an appropriate maneuver.

For those patients with actual or impending gastric outlet obstruction, in whom the stomach cannot be removed, our experience and that of others have indicated that a bypass procedure is not of any real value, and we do not recommend this procedure.[39,40,57] All too frequently a gastroenterostomy does not function, the patient does not have restoration of normal gastrointestinal flow, and no real palliation is achieved. This heightens the risk and mortality, lengthens the hospital stay, and does not provide patient or family with any real relief.

If one does not remove all the tumor or if there are known involved lymph nodes left behind, then all of these areas must be carefully marked with radiopaque clips so as to guide the radiotherapist both in treating the patient and in evaluating prognosis.

MEDICAL MANAGEMENT OF PATIENTS WITH GASTRIC RESECTION

Patients with stomach cancer have all had major disruptions of the gastrointestinal tract. Patients with significant gastric resection may have special metabolic problems. The syndromes associated with gastric resection have been reviewed by Lawrence.[83] The most common complication of total gastric resection is the "dumping syndrome." This symptom complex results from lack of antral function and includes epigastric fullness, hyperperistalsis, borborygmi, cramps, and occasional nausea, vomiting, and diarrhea. Other subjective postprandial complaints include diaphoresis, tachycardia, weakness, and dizziness. The mechanisms of the dumping syndrome are due to major fluid shift-out of the intravascular space and into the bowel after the sudden "dumping" of hypertonic foodstuff into the small bowel in gastrectomized patients.

TABLE 17-12. Postoperative Complications after Gastric Resection, 1963–1973 (Charity Hospital Series)

NUMBER COMPLICATION	TOTAL GASTRECTOMY; 18 PATIENTS (%)	SUBTOTAL GASTRECTOMY; 70 PATIENTS (%)	RADICAL SUBTOTAL; 42 PATIENTS (%)
Atelectasis	50	34	43
Pneumonia	33	9	24
Anastomotic leakage	28	3	14
Congestive heart failure	6	9	14
Fistula	11	10	5
Sepsis	22	6	7
Abscess	17	6	7
Wound infection	6	6	7
Hemorrhage	6	4	7
Renal failure	6	4	5
Urinary tract infection	0	3	5
Prolonged ileus	6	1	5
Pulmonary embolus	17	3	0
Gastric outlet obstruction	0	3	0
No complications	11	34	33

High carbohydrate meals, which are most likely to be hyperosmolar, increase symptoms. Many of the symptoms of the dumping syndrome may be produced by the release of seratonin, and antiseratonin agents may occasionally ameliorate the syndrome. Symptomatic therapy for the patient exhibiting the dumping syndrome centers on decreasing the osmotic load presented to the small bowel. Small, frequent feedings of low carbohydrate, high protein meals will usually improve symptoms. A high fat content in the diet is useful because the high caloric value of fat makes it easier to provide the patient with adequate calories.

Patients who have had gastric resection will all eventually become deficient in vitamin B_{12}, since the stomach produces the intrinsic factor necessary for distal ilial absorption of this vitamin. Because of liver storage of vitamin B_{12}, megaloblastic anemia may not occur for up to 4 years after gastric resection. The administration of 100 μg every month of this vitamin will prevent deficiency.

Less commonly, patients with gastrectomy may manifest malabsorption from the afferent or "blind loop" syndrome.[83] A blind loop of bowel is one that allows ingress of bowel contents but not adequate egress. Bacterial overgrowth may occur, with bacterial metabolism of bile acids resulting in malabsorption. Antibiotic therapy may be of help in this situation.

All patients with gastric cancer who are undergoing active treatment either by surgery, radiation therapy, or chemotherapy and are manifesting significant malnutrition (> 10% weight loss, albumin < 2.5 gm/100 ml) should be considered for nutritional support. It should be emphasized that it makes no sense to nutritionally support a patient with advanced gastric cancer who has failed to respond to accepted therapy. However, the patient whose poor nutritional status may prevent the optimal application of a potentially useful treatment should be supported. Either parenteral or enteral hypernutrition may be utilized and are described in detail elsewhere in this book.

It should be emphasized that well-planned, aggressive surgical resection is the only approach that currently results in significant numbers of cures in patients with gastric cancer. Careful patient selection combined with thoughtful pre-operative evaluation and preparation can allow for the safe performance of radical subtotal and total gastrectomy. With this approach, up to 30% of patients with localized disease will be cured. This is hardly an adequate cure rate in resected patients, but may be improved through the careful use of combined treatment with surgery, radiation, and chemotherapy as will be described in subsequent sections.

RADIATION THERAPY

The effective use of radiation in patients with gastric cancer depends on both defining in which clinical situation this modality will be most useful and also developing plans of treatment that are associated with tolerable morbidity. This section will first discuss considerations in planning and executing the radiotherapeutic management of gastric cancer, then will review the results of existing studies.

RADIATION PLANNING

The patterns of the local regional failures in the University of Minnesota re-operative group were in a distribution suitable for inclusion within a shaped radiation portal (Fig. 17-9), which should be modified depending on initial extent of disease.[48] In Fig. 17-10, these portals are superimposed on the limiting organs of tolerance. With accurate field definition, aided by clip placement in the splenic hilum and porta hepatis, one-half to two-thirds of the left kidney could be spared in many patients, and inclusion of the porta hepatis and retroduodenal areas would include only a minor portion of the right kidney.

Dose-limiting organs and structures in the upper abdomen (stomach, small intestine, liver, kidneys, and spinal cord) are numerous. In view of the posterior extent of the gastric fundus, it becomes impractical to use lateral portals to spare spinal cord or kidney as can be done in pancreatic cancer. Since parallel opposed portals are, therefore, the most practical, one must limit either the volume of normal tissue included or the upper dose level.

Exact tolerance of kidneys, when including portions of both, is somewhat uncertain. When including both in entirety, Luxton and Kunkler prefer to limit the dose to the upper one-third of each to 1700 rad but feel their experience suggests that a dose of 2300 rad over 5 weeks to the whole of both kidneys may be acceptable.[84] When including portions of both kidneys, the preference at Stanford and Massachusetts General is to exclude two-thirds to three-fourths of one kidney.[85,86] With this philosophy, problems with radiation nephritis have not been encountered. For proximal gastric lesions, at least one-half of the left kidney is usually within the XRT portal (Fig. 17-11) and the right kidney must be appropriately spared. For distal lesions with narrow or positive duodenal margins, a similar amount of right kidney is often included (Fig. 17-12) and then every effort must be taken to spare enough left kidney.

The most commonly utilized dose schemes of 4000 rad to 5000 rad in 4 weeks to 5 weeks continuous irradiation for various upper abdominal malignancies have been shown to be tolerable by stomach and small intestine with a complication rate ranging from 0% to 8.3% in recent series.[82,87] Roswit and associates summarize the older Walter Reed Hospital testicular data which showed a higher incidence of gastric and intestinal complications, but might have been caused by the following: lower voltage irradiation (maximum 1 MeV), short fractionation schedules (4500 rad to 5400 rad/3 weeks to 4 weeks) and treatment of one field per day.[88]

Daily doses of 170 rad to 180 rad are better tolerated in the upper abdomen than 200 rad or above. Weekly weights should be followed closely. When using daily doses of 170 rad to 180 rad, only about 50% of patients require pretreatment antiemetics. Most patients with intact stomachs, however, have some degree of anorexia and need encouragement to eat adequate amounts. Patients with partial or subtotal gastrectomies seem to tolerate upper abdomen irradiation better than those without resection. Use of oral hyperalimentation should be encouraged, and if weight loss greater than 10% occurs during treatment, admission and intravenous hyperalimentation should be considered.

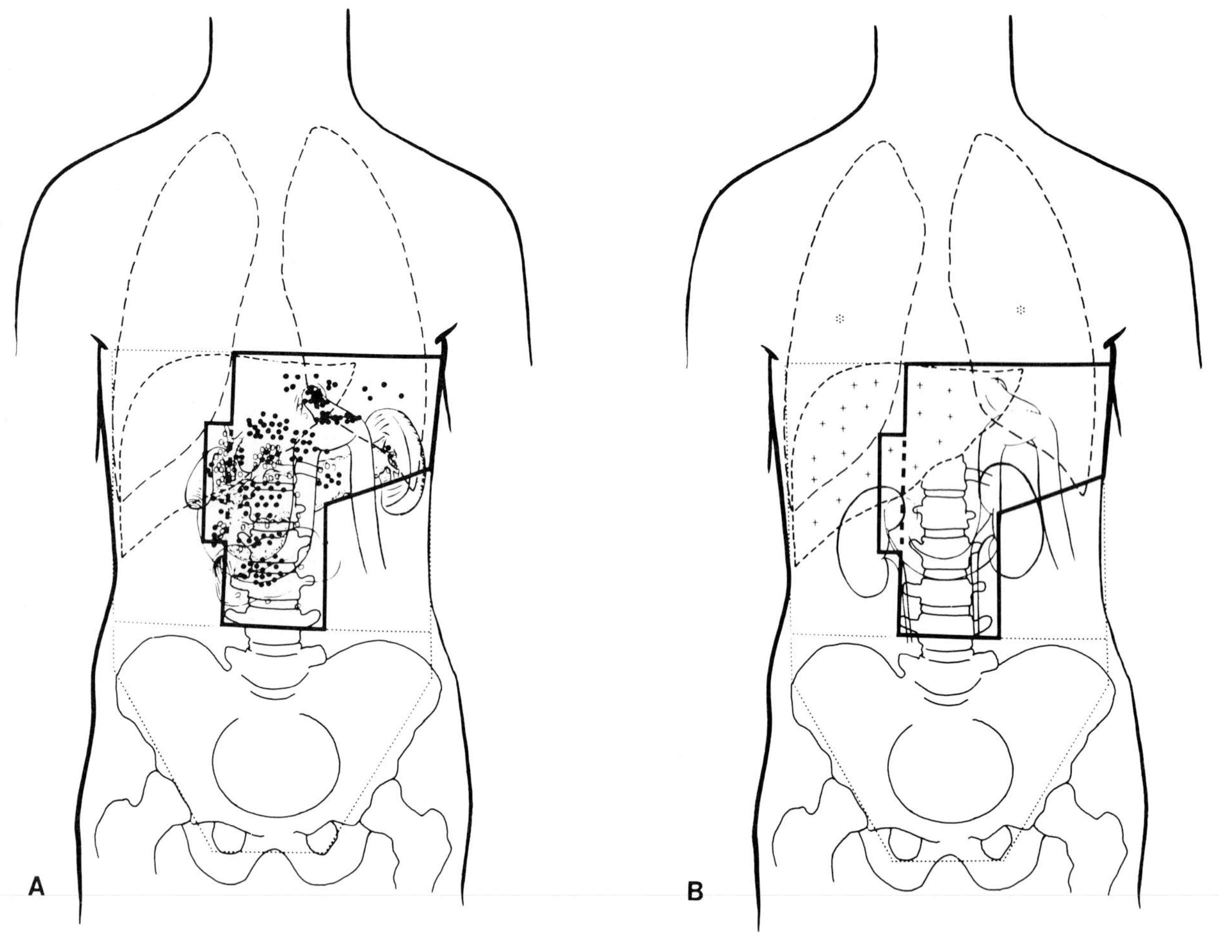

FIG. 17-9. Patterns of failure in the University of Minnesota reoperation series of 82 evaluable patients with evidence of gastric carcinoma after the initial operative procedure. Superimposed radiation portals: postsurgical gastric remnant, anastamoses, duodenal stump, gastric bed structures, and primary and secondary areas of lymph node drainage—*solid lines;* upper or total abdomen fields—*interrupted lines;* A, • = local failures in surrounding organs or tissues; *B*, 0 = lymph node failures; * = lung metastasis; + = liver metastasis. Each marking indicates a single instance of such failure occurring alone or as any component except for lymph node failures where each major area of involvement is indicated.

With proximal gastric lesions or lesions at the esophago–gastric junction, inclusion of a major portion of the left hemidiaphragm is indicated when a lesion extends through the entire alimentary wall. In these circumstances, cerrobend blocking can be useful in decreasing cardiac volume irradiated. This may be of importance since adriamycin is an important chemotherapeutic agent in this malignancy.

METHOD OF IRRADIATION

Differences of opinion might exist regarding the preferred way to combine surgery and irradiation for gastric carcinoma. Pre-operative, intra-operative, and postoperative radiation therapy have been used to some degree in the past, although mainly in Japan.[89–93] The main problem with intra-operative irradiation as the sole method of radiation therapy (XRT) is that the pathologic extent of disease is not known, and irradiation portals cannot be individualized. A possible advantage is that dose-limiting tissues, such as small intestine, colon, and liver, can be retracted outside the radiation field. Such retraction, however, might result in a significant number of marginal failures, since a significant number of local–regional failures involved those organs in the Minnesota re-operative series. A preferred method may be to combine external beam and intra-operative irradiation.

The direct controversy of pre- *versus* postoperative radiation therapy *versus* a combination thereof is probably of greatest interest since intra-operative irradiation is not feasible in most institutions. Theoretical considerations are discussed in the section on colo–rectal cancer. Since 30% to 50% of gastric lesions are technically unresectable, use of some degree of pre-operative radiation to alter implantability or shrink disease or both would be attractive. However, our present diagnostic techniques often reveal only the "tip of the iceberg" regarding extent of disease, and pre-operative fields would, therefore, need to be fairly extensive to ensure inclusion of all disease in most cases. If such fields were used in an attempt to shrink

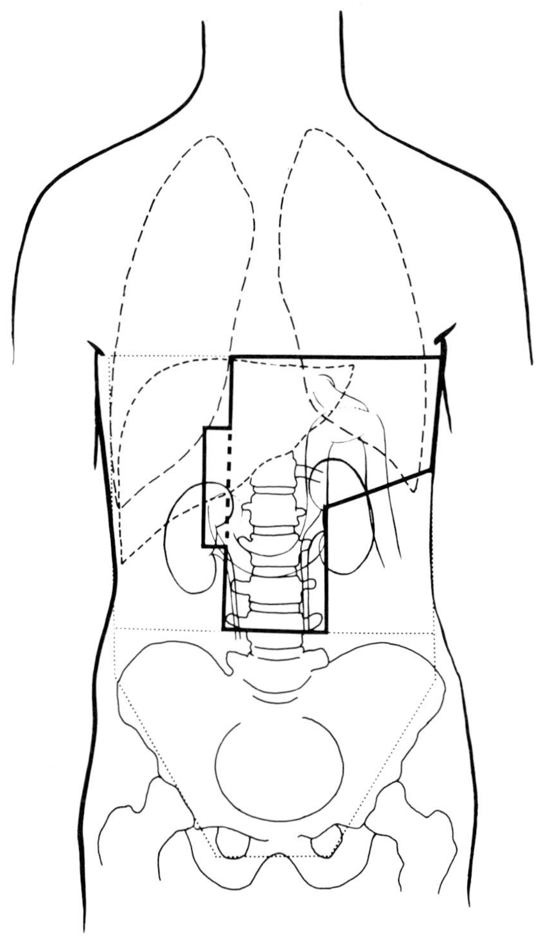

FIG. 17-10. Potential radiation portals are superimposed upon organs and structures of tolerance (gastric remnant, duodenal stump, jejunum, liver, kidneys, spinal cord, and spinal and pelvic marrow).

disease to improve resectability (that is, 4500 rad to 5000 rad), risks of anastomotic leaks would probably increase unless resections were wide, and unless at least one of the limbs of the anastomosis was unirradiated.

With postoperative irradiation, field setup (portals) and dose could be individualized to some degree, with potential portals by extent of disease as follows: (1) LN −, through mucosa but within wall: small field irradiation to the anastomotic area, to include duodenal stump if was a distal lesion. If only a small number of lymph nodes were sectioned, should consider inclusion of primary lymph nodes. (2) LN −, extension through the wall: moderate field radiation to cover the stomach bed structures with or without nodal areas. The entire left hemidiaphragm should be considered for inclusion especially in proximal lesions. (3) LN +, within the wall: cover both the primary and secondary nodal drainage areas—do not need to include the entire left hemidiaphragm and therefore treat less lung and heart. (4) LN +, extension through the wall: cover entire gastric bed plus primary and secondary lymph node drainage areas (major solid line field as shown in Figs. 17-9 and 17-10).

As discussed in patterns of spread, nodal areas considered at risk for primary spread include gastric and gastro–epiploic (usually resected) and the entire celiac axis, including porta hepatis, subpyloric, gastroduodenal, splenic–suprapancreatic, and retropancreatico–duodenal (para-esophageal if with proximal lesions). Secondary nodal chains at risk include superior mesenteric and para-aortic.

The usual dose aim is 4500 rad to 5000 rad in 5 weeks to 6 weeks delivered in 170 rad to 180 rad fractions to the initial field. A boost field is occasionally carried to a maximum of 5000 rad to 5500 rad. Some European and Scandinavian centers utilize upper dose levels of 6000 rad in 6 weeks to 9 weeks, but these centers have provided only minimal information on long-term tolerance. Parallel opposed fields are usually necessary for the initial large field to tumor or tumor bed ± LN areas. Doses greater than 4500 rad to 5000 rad are discouraged with treatment energies 4 MeV or less unless multifield techniques can be utilized for a portion of treatment. If residual or unresected disease is marked with clips, that possibility exists. On rare occasion, residual disease in LN or tumor bed could possibly be boosted to 6000 rad if clips are placed and an upper GI study is done to define residual gastric pouch and small intestine.

Treatment Results

Radiation alone has been shown to have curative potential in a small percentage of patients with resected but residual or unresectable but localized disease.[89,93,94] Its greatest benefit has been when used in combination with chemotherapy, as noted for some time in studies from Mayo and a number of foreign centers.[87,90,95–98]

FIG. 17-11 Portals for radiation showing inclusion of the gastric bed plus 70% of the left kidney but excluding 75% or more of the right kidney.

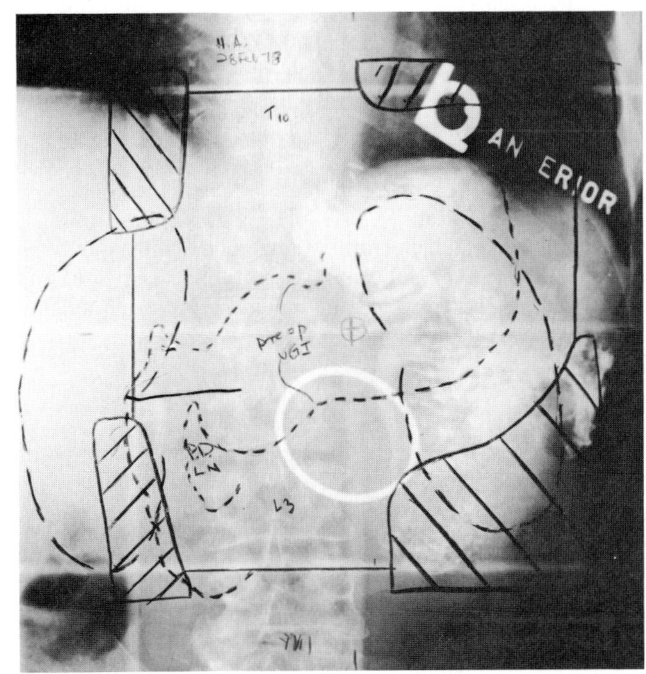

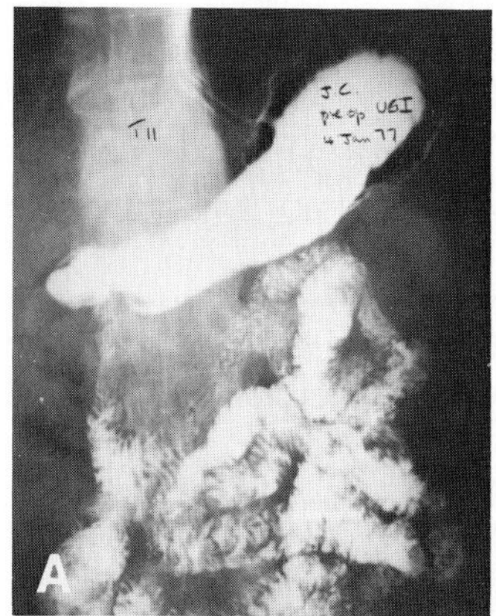

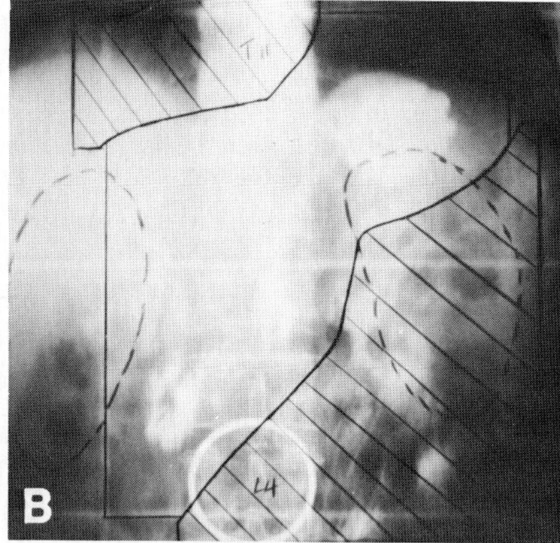

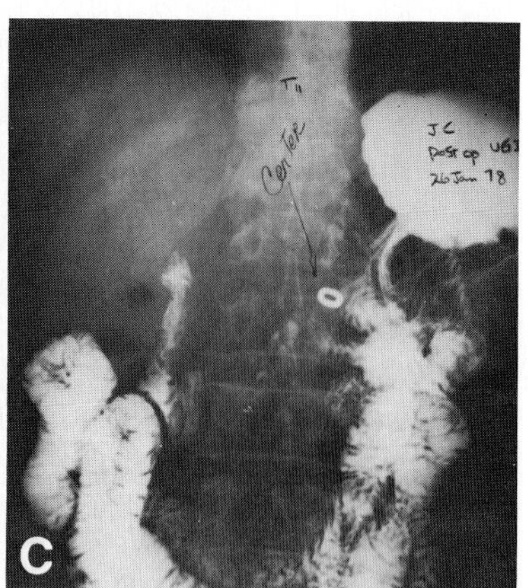

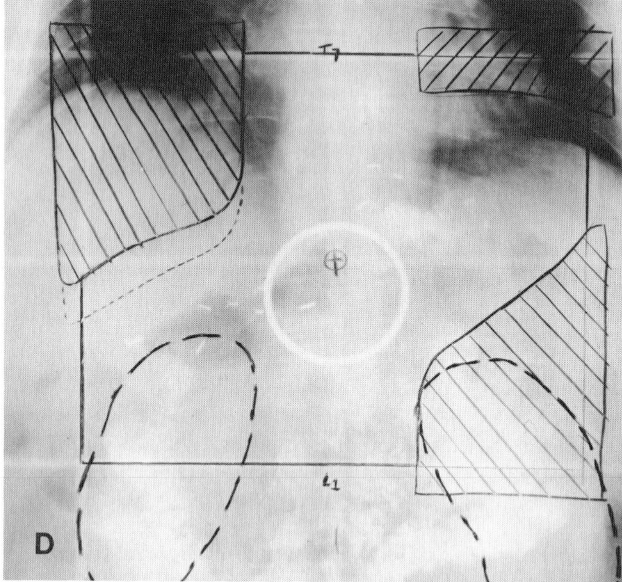

FIG. 17-12. Patient J.C. (*A–C*) had a subtotal gastrectomy with gastro-jejunostomy for adenocarcinoma of the stomach and was referred to MGH for post-op radiation. The initial intent was inclusion of the duodenal stump, a portion of the duodenal loop, the tumor bed and nodal areas, yet sparing 75+% of the left kidney with blocks (*cross-hatched areas*). *A*, Position of the duodenum in the pre-op UGI. *B*, *C*, Good visualization of both the duodenal stump and gastric pouch in both the radiation planning film (*B*) and the post-op diagnostic UGI (*C*).

Patient A.X. had an unresectable carcinoma of the stomach. *D*, The lesion's extent was marked with clips at exploratory laparotomy. Since the radiation therapy portal included nearly 50% of the right kidney, cerrobend blocking was used to exclude the left kidney. Other blocks (*cross-hatched areas*) were used to exclude portions of liver and heart. Additional liver blocking was added after 3500 rad. (Parts *A–C* from Gunderson L: Part IX. In Alimentary Tract Radiology, p 606. St. Louis, CV Mosby, 1979)

Combined therapy would be attractive for the high-risk subgroups with gastric carcinoma. Operative failures have been previously discussed. Although some cures have been obtained with irradiation alone, this is not a viable alternative as the sole treatment method due to the limited tolerance of the stomach and surrounding organs and the initial bulk of disease, which prevent a suitable therapeutic ratio between cure and complications.[93,94] The preferred use of radiation, as an aid to local regional control, would be in combination with operative removal of all gross disease in the primary area and lymph nodes—utilizing radiation for microscopic or subclinical residual disease.

RADIATION AND SURGERY

Available literature supports the concept that adenocarcinoma of the stomach is a radiosensitive lesion. Wieland and Hymen utilized 6000 rad when feasible (150 rad to 200 rad daily) with 11% (nine of 82 patients) 3-year and 7% (five of 72 patients) 5-year survival rates.[94] Takahashi compared historical controls with patients who were inoperable or had palliative procedures and received postoperative radiation (no mention of chemotherapy).[93] The average survival for the irradiated group was longer by 9 months to 10 months with 74.4% (32 of 43 patients) 1-year and 27.9% (12 of 43 patients) 2½-year survival rates. Abe and associates cured three of ten patients with intra-operative radiation in whom operation excision was incomplete.[89] In pre-operative series, Hoshi and co-workers found histologic changes in 28% of patients at doses less than 2000 rad, 74% with 2000 rad, and 88% with higher doses.[92] Asakawa and associates found a greater than 50% decrease in the size of tumor in 60% of patients and total regression in 10% of 40 patients treated with radiation alone or in combination with chemotherapy.[90,91]

RADIATION AND CHEMOTHERAPY

Most reports on combined treatment deal with results in the inoperable patient and show suggestive improvement for radiation plus 5-FU over either radiation alone or 5-FU alone.[87,95–98] In the Mayo series, 5-FU was utilized during the first 3 days of radiation (3500 rad to 4000 rad at 900 rad/wk to 1200 rad/wk).[95,97] For the combined *versus* radiation groups, mean survival was 12 months *versus* 5.9 months and 5-year survival was three of 25 patients (12%) *versus* zero of 23 patients. This was a randomized double-blind study on patients with unresectable disease. Asakawa and co-workers reported a series of 54 patients of whom 42 received some 5-FU.[90,91] At the 2-year interval, three of 33 patients treated without any resection and four of eight with partial resection were alive (6000 rad, 6 week to 9 week was the aim).

In a recent report of the randomized GITSG study 8274, including 90 patients with unresectable or residual disease, the combination of radiation plus 5-FU, followed by maintenance 5-FU-Me CCNU, was statistically superior to 5-FU + Me CCNU alone regarding long-term survival with a plateau of 20% between years 2 and 3 ($p < 0.05$).[99] The short-term advantage to 5-FU ± Me CCNU (median survival 70 weeks *versus* 36 weeks) was felt to be due to early tumor-related and toxicity deaths with the 5-FU + radiation combination during the first 26 weeks of treatment. Irradiated patients received 5000 rad in 8 weeks in split course fashion (2500 rad/3 wk—2-wk rest—2500 rad/3 wk) receiving 5-FU 500 mg/m² days 1 through 3 of each radiation sequence followed by 5-FU + Me CCNU maintenance chemotherapy.

In a series of 46 patients with localized gastric cancer treated with radiation alone (six patients) or in combination with chemotherapy (40 patients) at Massachusetts General Hospital, toxicity-related deaths were not encountered.[86] Categories of patient presentation were as follows: recurrent—4, medically inoperable—4, surgically unresectable—9, resected but residual—15, resected but high risk for local recurrence—14. Patients treated with radiation plus chemotherapy followed two sequences: (1) XRT plus 3 days 5-FU followed by maintenance 5-FU or combined drugs—26 patients; (2) single course of 5-FU + BCNU or FAM + XRT + maintenance combined chemotherapy—14 patients. Irradation with 10 MeV or 25 MeV photons was delivered to tightly contoured portals sparing as much bone marrow and bowel as possible giving 4500 rad to 5200 rad/25–29 fractions/5–6 weeks. Only four patients (8.7%) had poor tolerance with two of those completing XRT. Hematologic parameters delayed the XRT or CT course in 11 patients. The difference in treatment-related toxicity in the GITSG *versus* MGH series may be due in part to the use of tightly contoured portals in the latter series, which is more difficult to coordinate in a multi-institutional study.

The major role for radiation therapy today in gastric cancer is in the management of the patient with locally unresectable, partially resectable, or recurrent disease. The recommended therapy would be the radiation + 5-FU + methyl-CCNU regimen previously outlined in this chapter. With this program, 5-FU + methyl-CCNU are given in the following schedule: 5-FU 325 mg/m² days 1–5, 375 mg/m² days 36–40, Me CCNU 150 mg/m² day 1. The schedule is repeated every 9 weeks to 10 weeks, depending on tolerance, and is not initiated until radiation has been completed and radiation-associated acute toxicities have cleared. It should be emphasized that there is active investigation in the use of combined radiation plus chemotherapy. It is clear that chloroethyl nitrosoureas such as Me CCNU have been associated with long-term toxicities such as nephrotoxicity and second tumors (leukemias). It is possible that more active combinations of drugs such as FAM (to be described in detail) will supplant the less active 5-FU + Me CCNU.

CHEMOTHERAPY OF GASTRIC CANCER

Although surgery remains the only documented curative treatment for gastric cancer, chemotherapy in this disease has aroused considerable interest.[80,100,101] This is because of several studies which have documented response rates of 40% to 50% with combination chemotherapy. Some of these therapies have also been shown to result in improved survival for treated patients.

In evaluating the reported results of chemotherapy in advanced gastric cancer, several prognostic factors are important. There are data available to suggest that patients, who have a good performance status and are only minimally symptomatic and who have followable disease confined to the abdomen, are more likely to respond to chemotherapy than patients with either widely disseminated metastatic disease or poor performance status.[80] Therefore, it becomes very important in evaluating the results of chemotherapy studies that data on performance status and sites of metastatic disease be carefully analyzed. It is clear that any chemotherapy regimen used in totally asymptomatic patients with limited disease would appear to be more effective than a treatment program that was used in heavily symptomatic patients with widely disseminated cancer.

In evaluating the results of chemotherapy trials in gastric cancer, the following criteria for response are used: complete response occurs when all objective evidence of cancer has disappeared. Partial responses (PR) are defined as greater than 50% decrease in the products of the two largest perpendicular diameters of the most clearly measurable metastatic lesion. There can be no increase in size of other metastatic lesions the patient may have. An alternative, "stricter" interpretation of partial response requires a greater than 50% decrease in *all* metastatic lesions. A minimal response is defined as a less than 50% but greater than 25% decrease in measurable metastatic lesions. In general, measurable metastatic disease is either physically measurable or may be measured on a roentgenograph. Liver scans may be used if perfusion defects are greater than 3 cm in diameter.[101] Similarly, large abnormalities on CT or ultrasound scanning are occasionally used as measurable disease, but the use of these techniques for judging the effectiveness of chemotherapy requires more information on clinical correlations. When response to chemotherapy is referred to in this chapter, reference will be made only to partial and complete responses. Minimal responses will not be considered as objective disease regression.

Study design is another factor that must be carefully evaluated when assessing results of chemotherapy trials in patients with stomach cancer. This is particularly important when claims of improved survival are made. The only proper way in which improved survival can be demonstrated for a chemotherapy regimen is to prospectively evaluate that treatment program in a Phase III trial. In advanced gastric carcinoma, a disease in which complete remissions secondary to chemotherapy are exceedingly rare, it is difficlt to sustain the claim that chemotherapy improves survival in partially responding patients. It may be entirely possible that response to a chemotherapy program does not result in prolongation of survival, but rather that the patients who will have the longest survival if untreated are the ones most likely to respond to chemotherapy. Thus, response to chemotherapy may merely be another indication of good prognosis, as other factors such as good performance status, relatively minimal disease, and well-differentiated histology.[80]

One should always also keep in mind that when improved survival is demonstrated for responding patients in a Phase II trial, this result could possibly be from an adverse effect of chemotherapy on non-responding patients, rather than a beneficial effect on responding patients. With the above caveats firmly established, this section will review the results of single agent chemotherapy, combination chemotherapy, and surgical adjuvant chemotherapy of gastric cancer.

SINGLE AGENT CHEMOTHERAPY

The use of systemic chemotherapy for disseminated gastric cancer has depended upon documentation of antitumor activity of a variety of single agents in this disease. Table 17-13 reviews objective response rates reported for single agents in patients with stomach cancer. Many other agents have been reported anecdotally in the literature, but Table 17-13 reports studies in which 14 or greater patients were evaluated.

The fluorinated pyrimidine 5-fluorouracil, which has been tested in close to 400 patients, is the most completely evaluated single agent.[102] The dosage schedule most frequently used is the loading course method in which the drug is administered intravenously for 4 days to 5 days followed by half-doses every other day until toxicity is produced. Various maintenance schedules have been used. The most common are weekly intravenous doses or repeated loading courses at monthly intervals. The objective partial response rate with 5-FU is a disappointing 21%. Complete responses are exceedingly rare and the median durations of 5-FU response can be expected to range from 3 months to 6 months.

The antibiotic mitomycin-C, which was first developed in Japan, has been evaluated in gastric cancer. The original reports of Japanese clinical trials suggested an overall objective response rate of 35%.[103] The initial experience in the United States was considerably less impressive, however. Administration of mitomycin-C on a daily schedule was found to produce significant delayed myelosuppression and a cumulative and persistent bone marrow injury.[104] In addition, inadvertent extravasation during intravenous administration resulted in a severe inflammatory reaction with potential skin slough. Drug-related deaths occurred in 11% of the patients and the objective response rate was only 18%. More recent experience has shown an overall response rate for mitomycin-C in gastric cancer of 15% to 30%[105] There has been renewed interest in the use of this drug with the demonstration that single treatments of 10 mg/m^2 to 20 mg/m^2, at 6 week to 8 week intervals, result in manageable hematological toxicity while retaining therapeutic activity.[106]

The anthracycline antibiotic, adriamycin, is a drug with a wide range of antitumor activity in human solid tumors that has recently been evaluated in gastric cancer. Early trials reported a response rate of 36% for adriamycin.[107] More recently, the Gastrointestinal Tumor Study Group[108] and the Eastern Cooperative Oncology Group have performed Phase II trials testing the efficacy of adriamycin.[109] Both of these studies confirm the activity of this drug. Adriamycin was administered at 60 mg/m^2 every 3 weeks to 4 weeks. Objective responses were demonstrated in four of 17 cases (24%) and eight of 37 cases (22%).[108,109] The median duration of responses to adriamycin was 4 months. These studies have demonstrated that adriamycin is at least as active as the fluorinated pyrimidines and indicate a need to test this drug in combination chemotherapy regimens.

The chlorethylnitrosoureas, BCNU and methyl-CCNU, are representative of another class of single agents evaluated in advanced gastric cancer patients.[80,100] BCNU has been actively tested for efficacy against advanced gastric cancer at the Mayo Clinic. Objective remissions were observed in six of 33 patients treated for a response rate of 18% with a 4-month duration of response.

The methyl-nitrosourea, MeCCNU, has also been tested by ECOG and found to produce responses in 3 of 37 (8%) patients.[80] Median survival of patients receiving this drug was less than 15 weeks. Other single agents which have been reported to have minimal activity (< 20%) in gastric cancer include hydroxyurea, DTIC, and the alkylating agents, meclorethane and chlorambucil.[81,102,119,123]

All the single agents used in gastric cancer have the shared liability of low response rates and short duration of response (3 months to 5 months). Therefore, the single agent chemotherapy of this disease is of minimal practical benefit to the patient. For this reason, the polychemotherapy of stomach cancer is being pursued with increasing intensity.

TABLE 17-13. Single Agent Activity in Gastric Cancer

DRUG	NO. RESPONSES/ NO. PATIENTS	PERCENT RESPONSES	REFERENCE
Adriamycin	5/14	36	107
	4/17	24	108
	8/37	22	109
5-Fluorouracil	84/392	21	102
Mitomycin-C	63/211	30	102
Hydroxyurea	6/31	19	122
BNCU	6/33	18	100
Chlorambucil	3/18	17	123
DTIC	2/15	13	81
Mechlorethane	3/23	13	119
Methyl-CCNU	3/37	8	80

COMBINATION CHEMOTHERAPY

There have been numerous attempts to develop effective combination chemotherapy regimens utilizing both single agents documented to be active and also agents that have not been evaluated for single agent activity. Table 17-14 reviews the published results of combination chemotherapeutic regimens that have been tested in more than ten patients.

Two of the most extensively evaluated regimens in the United States have used 5-FU in combination with either BCNU or methyl-CCNU.[80,100] The combination of 5-FU and BCNU was compared to each drug used as a single agent in a randomized Phase III trial. All drugs were given intravenously in the following doses: 5-FU alone, 13.5 mg/kg/day for 5 days; BCNU alone, 50 mg/m²/day for 5 days; 5-FU plus BCNU, 10 mg/kg/day and 40 mg/m²/day, respectively. The drugs were given for 5 days. Objective responses to therapy were 29% for 5-FU alone, 17% for BCNU alone, and 41% for 5-FU plus BCNU. Median survival for patients treated with the combination was 7 months and was not significantly different from that seen with the single agents alone. However, there was a significant improvement in survival at 18 months for the patients treated with 5-FU plus BCNU. At this point, 25% of the group receiving combination chemotherapy were alive compared to less than 10% of those receiving either single agent.

The Eastern Cooperative Oncology Group has conducted a controlled randomized trial in advanced gastric cancer comparing the combination of 5-FU and methyl-CCNU with methyl-CCNU used alone.[80] The dosages in the combination were the following: 5-FU at 300 mg/m²/day intravenously for 5 days with methyl-CCNU at 175 mg/m² given orally on the first day; this regimen was repeated at 7-week intervals. The dosage of methyl-CCNU alone was 200 mg/m² given in a single oral dose and repeated at 7-week intervals. The combination produced a 40% response rate and was definitely superior to methyl-CCNU alone, which produced an 8% response ($p = 0.05$).[80]

There was significant survival benefit reported for the patients treated with 5-FU plus methyl-CCNU in this trial. The median survival of patients treated with the combination was 20 weeks, whereas the patients treated with methyl-CCNU lived a median of 13 weeks. It is very possible that the differences in survival may reflect the inferior response rate produced by methyl-CCNU (8%). It is of interest in this study that a trial of cyclophosphamide induction followed by the 5-FU plus methyl-CCNU combination not only reduced the response rate of the combination to 20% but also enhanced the toxicity of the subsequently administered 5-FU plus methyl-CCNU.

As illustrated in Table 17-14, other studies have failed to confirm the 40% response rate of 5-FU plus methyl-CCNU. Baker and associates reporting the results of a Southwest Oncology Group Phase III study comparing 5-FU to 5-FU plus methyl-CCNU, noted that the objective response rate in 29 patients with gastric cancer treated with the combination was only 20.7%.[110] This was not different from the response produced by 5-FU alone in this study. However, one must be cautious in interpreting the Southwest Group study since this group used 5-FU in a relatively low dose (400 mg/m²) weekly intravenous schedule rather than an intravenous loading dose schedule.

A recently reported ECOG study also brings into question the high response rate originally reported for 5-FU plus methyl-CCNU.[109] This study compared 5-FU plus methyl-CCNU, 5-FU plus mitomycin-C, and adriamycin used as a single agent. The 5-FU plus methyl-CCNU was used in a dosage schedule identical to that which had earlier produced a 40% response.[80] That response rate was not confirmed in this more recent study. Twelve of 49 (24%) patients receiving methyl-CCNU responded in this study. This compared to 17 of 53 (32%) responses with 5-FU plus mitomycin-C. The patients in all arms of this study were similar regarding sites of disease, extent of disease, and performance status. The survival curves for all arms were identical with median survival of 17 weeks.

The data in Table 17-14 suggest that the most consistently high response rates were seen with the combination of 5-FU plus adriamycin plus mitomycin-C. This is the FAM regimen (Table 17-15) developed at the Vincent T. Lombardi Cancer Center at Georgetown University. A Phase II evaluation of FAM revealed an overall response rate of 42% in 62 patients with advanced measurable gastric cancer.[101] There was significant response in patients with major metastatic liver disease and also large abdominal masses. Responding patients had marked improvement in performance status and in this

TABLE 17-14. Combination Chemotherapy Regimens in Gastric Cancer

DRUG REGIMEN	NO. RESPONSE/ NO. PATIENTS	PERCENT RESPONSE	REFERENCE
5-FU + Adriamycin + Mitomycin-C	6/11	55	111
	26/62	42	101
	8/20	40	112
5-FU + BCNU	14/34	41	100
5-FU + Methyl-CCNU	12/30	40	80
	12/49	24	109
	6/29	21	110
Ftorafur + Adriamycin + Mitomycin-C	3/15	20	124
5-FU + Mitomycin-C	17/53	32	109
5-FU + Adriamycin + Methyl-CCNU	7/15	47	108
5-FU + Cytosine Arabinoside + Mitomycin-C	15/27	55	120
	6/16	38	118
	3/18	17	108

TABLE 17-15. The FAM Regimen

DRUG AND DOSAGE	WEEK 1	2	3	4	5	6	7	8	9
5-Fluorouracil 600 mg/m² IV	X	X			X	X			X
Adriamycin 30 mg/m² IV	X				X				X
Mitomycin-C 10 mg/m² IV	X								X

Phase II trial the survival of responding patients was a median of 13 months compared with 3 months for nonresponding patients. FAM was well tolerated with the only significant toxicity being moderate myelosuppression.

The activity of the FAM regimen has been confirmed in both Phase II and Phase III trials.[111,112] Bitran and co-workers in a small series found that 6 of 11 patients (55%) responded to FAM. In a large Phase III trial, the Southwest Oncology Group compared two dose schedules of FAM. This trial revealed that the drugs given in the simultaneous schedule developed at Georgetown were superior to the same drugs given sequentially.[101] In the simultaneous schedule, eight of 20 patients (40%) responded. When the drugs were given sequentially, the response rate was four of 26 patients (11%). There were not significant differences in survival between these two treatment regimens. It is of interest that the substitution of the furanyl derivative of 5-FU, Ftorafur, which may have less myelosuppressive toxicity than the other fluorinated pyrimidines, decreased the activity of FAM. Woolley and associates[124] reported three of 15 responses (20%) in patients with advanced gastric cancer treated with this regimen. It should also be noted that the toxicity seen with the Ftorafur-substituted FAM was significant and qualitatively different since the Ftorafur caused major transient cerebellar dysfunction.

The most important observation concerning the combination chemotherapy of advanced gastric cancer is the high order of activity evidenced by several regimens in this disease.[80,100,101,109,111,112] Response rates of 40% to 50% are distinctly uncommon in advanced gastrointestinal adenocarcinomas and the apparent responsiveness of gastric cancer has encouraged active investigation of polychemotherapy. Table 17-16 lists some of the trials now ongoing in combination chemotherapy of gastric cancer. It is hoped that relatively active chemotherapy regimens in advanced disease will translate into effective surgical adjuvant chemotherapy.

TABLE 17-16. Ongoing Chemotherapy Trials in Gastric Cancer

REGIMEN	INVESTIGATORS
5-FU + Adriamycin + Mitomycin-C (FAM) *vs.* 5-FU + Adriamycin + Methyl-CCNU (FAMe) *vs.* 5-FU + Methyl-CCNU (FMe)	Gastrointestinal Tumor Study Group (GITSG)
5-FU (F) *vs.* 5-FU + Adriamycin (FA) *vs.* FAM	North Central Cancer Treatment Group (NCCTG)
{ FAM *vs.* FAM + Vincristine *vs.* Chlorozotocin } AMSA	Southwest Oncology Group (SWOG)
FAM *vs.* Adriamycin + Mitomycin-C (AM)	Cancer and Acute Leukemia Group B (CALGB)
FAM *vs.* FAMe *vs.* FMe	Eastern Cooperative Oncology Group (ECOG)
Ftorafur + Adriamycin *vs.* BCNU + Adriamycin	Northern California Oncology Group (NCOG)
Platinum	European Organization for Cancer Treatment Research (EORTC)
FA + Platinum	Georgetown University
FA + Platinum	Mayo Clinic

TABLE 17-17. Surgical Adjuvant Chemotherapy of Gastric Cancer

GROUP	NO. OF PATIENTS	TREATMENT	RANDOMIZED UNTREATED CONTROLS	SURVIVAL BENEFIT FOR TREATED GROUP	REFERENCE
VASOG*	194	1. Thiotepa *vs.* Control	Yes	No 5-year survival Treated 25.5% Control 33.7%	114
	276	2. FudR† *vs.* Control	Yes	No 5-year survival Treated 23.9% Control 21.3%	115
	110	3. 5-FU + Methyl-CCNU *vs.* control	Yes	in progress	–
GITSG*	165	5-FU + Methyl-CCNU *vs.* Control	Yes	chemotherapy improves recurrence-free interval ($p<0.02$)	125
ECOG*	144	5-FU + Methyl-CCNU *vs.* control	Yes	in progress	–
CALGB*	10	FAM *vs.* Control	Yes	in progress	–
SWOG*	24	FAM *vs.* Control	Yes	in progress	–
NCCTG*	6	5-FU + Adriamycin *vs.* control	Yes	in progress	–
Stomach Cancer Study Group (Japan)	209	1. Mitomycin-C *vs.* Thiotepa *vs.* Control	Yes	No	121
	472	2. Mitomycin-C	Yes	No	121
	350	3. Mitomycin-C *vs.* Cyclophosphamide + Chromomycin A_3 *vs.* Control	Yes	No	121
	476	4. 5-FU *vs.* Mitomycin-C + Cyclophosphamide *vs.* Control	Yes	No	121
	460	5. Mitomycin-C + 5-FU *vs.* Mitomycin- (Pre-op) + 5-FU (Post-op) *vs.* Control	Yes	No	121

* Group Abbreviations: VASOG—Veterans' Administration Surgical Oncology Group
GITSG—Gastrointestinal Tumor Study Group
CALGB—Cancer and Acute Leukemia Group B
ECOG—Eastern Cooperative Oncology Group
SWOG—Southwest Oncology Group
NCCTG—North Central Cancer Treatment Group

† FudR—Fluorodeoxyuridine

ADJUVANT CHEMOTHERAPY

The adjuvant chemotherapy of patients undergoing surgical resection is of great interest since a successful chemotherapy treatment has the potential of improving long-term survival. It is important to re-emphasize the clinical and pathologic factors that bear on the probability of recurrence in patients undergoing curative resection for gastric cancer.[15,113] The Veterans' Administration Surgical Oncology Group (VASOG) has examined prognostic factors in 503 patients undergoing gastrectomy for stomach cancer. Performance status before operation is of significant importance, since patients with weight loss, anorexia, and weakness have a higher likelihood of dying of recurrent cancer after operation than patients without these factors. As described previously in this chapter, patients with locally advanced disease, as evidenced by cancer through the gastric serosa, blood vessel, or lymphatic invasion or involvement of perigastric lymph nodes, have a poor prognosis. Patients with any of these evidences of local invasion have less than 20% probability of being cured by gastric resection. Proximal position of the primary tumor in the stomach, necessitating a total gastrectomy, is an adverse prognostic factor. In the Veterans' Administration studies, only 15% of patients requiring proximal or total gastrectomies for resectable gastric cancer survived 5 years, as opposed to 27% survival for those having distal gastrectomies. The pathologic characteristics of the primary tumor constitute very important information in predicting survival. Of patients with linitis plastica, only 2% survived 5 years after resection.

The vast majority of well-designed adjuvant chemotherapy studies that have been reported have failed to show significant benefit for treatment with chemotherapy. Table 17-17 describes a series of studies in which more than 2500 patients were evaluated. It is clear that in an adjuvant therapy study it is exceedingly important that a prospectively randomized design be utilized. Only in this way can one be assured of balancing prognostic factors between treated and control groups. All of the studies detailed in Table 17-17 were prospectively randomized controlled trials of chemotherapy *versus* treatment with surgery alone. In the United States, the Veterans' Administration Surgical Oncology Group was a pioneer in performing these studies. The data derived from this group has shown that single agent chemotherapy with Thiotepa or fluorodeoxyuridine (FUdR) failed to influence disease-free survival at 5 years after resection.[114,115] In the Thiotepa study, it appears that treatment with chemotherapy adversely influenced survival; however, this difference is not significant.[114] Recently the GITSG has reported that 5-FU plus methyl-CCNU as an adjuvant to surgery improves recurrence-free interval ($P < 0.02$) but does not significantly improve overall survival ($P > 0.05$).[125]

Because of the very high incidence of gastric cancer in Japan, there has been great interest in the surgical adjuvant therapy of the disease in that country. Table 17-17 describes a series of five randomized controlled trials in which over 1950 patients have been entered. It can be seen that in no instance was chemotherapeutic treatment superior to surgery alone. The majority of patients in this study were treated with single agent chemotherapy and, as has been previously described, there is now clear evidence that combination chemotherapy is superior to single agent treatment in advanced gastric cancer. It is presumed that the combinations would also be more active in the surgical adjuvant situation.

Adjuvant chemotherapy studies using the moderately active 5-FU plus methyl-CCNU regimen and the highly active FAM regimen are now being pursued in well-designed trials by the VASOG, the GITSG, the SCOG, the CALGB, and the SWOG (Table 17-17). The results of these studies will have major impact on the appropriate postoperative management of patients undergoing gastric resection for cancer.

The studies presented in Table 17-17 should serve as examples of well-planned and conducted studies in this area of investigation. If positive results of similar trials are to be considered valid, it will be increasingly important for clinicians to critically question the design of adjuvant therapy studies in gastric cancer. For example, historically or nonrandomized controlled studies are not acceptable. Also, stratification for significant pathologic and prognostic factors should be an important aspect of a well-designed study.[15,113] For it is only from such well-designed and managed clinical trials that useful information on the appropriate use of surgical adjuvant therapy will emerge.

RECOMMENDATIONS

In the therapy of advanced gastric cancer, it is clear that combination chemotherapy is superior to single agent treatment. Because of the excellent tolerance of patients to the FAM regimen, this program should be the initial treatment for cases not being entered into experimental protocols.

Since there is minimal documentation from well-designed studies that adjuvant chemotherapy is useful in gastric cancer, patients with a high risk of recurrence after complete tumor resection should be entered onto controlled trials. Within the near future, the results of the several studies testing FAM in the adjuvant situation will be available.

FUTURE CONSIDERATIONS

DIAGNOSIS

A major effort towards early diagnosis of gastric cancer is a necessity in countries with a high incidence rate of this disease. This chapter has described the success the Japanese have had with such an approach.[72] However, in the United States, where stomach cancer is not a major public health problem and, if anything, has been decreasing in incidence, massive screening programs for early diagnosis would hardly be cost-effective. Therefore, the future direction in gastric cancer management that the American clinician will deal with will concern attempts to improve therapy of this disease.

TREATMENT

Use of Re-Operations for Carcinoma of the Stomach

The curative benefit of planned re-operations for carcinoma of the stomach was minimal in the University of Minnesota series—four conversions to disease-free status but three operative deaths in the "second look" group.[48] In the "symptomatic look" group, there was one possible conversion to disease-free status but five operative deaths. Griffen and coworkers commented that although the percentage of conversions is small, the use of "second look" procedures with carcinoma of the stomach appears applicable, since even a small increase in cure rate is good in this disease entity.[116] In the future, the use of "second look" procedures might be justifiable for patients who initially have operation without adjuvant therapy but are at high risk for later disease. The reoperation would have a potential of locating such failures early, allowing possible excision of the gross tumor with randomization of the patient to post-excision adjuvants. Use of "symptomatic looks" might be justifiable on the same basis.

Chemotherapy with and without Irradiation

In view of the patterns of failure with this malignancy, it appears that innovative combinations of chemotherapy and irradiation *versus* combined chemotherapy alone may be necessary to alter both short- and long-term survival in resectable as well as unresectable disease. Even after "curative" resections, local regional failures comprise a significant problem, as noted in both the University of Minnesota reoperative series as well as autopsy series.[46–48] This knowledge must be tempered, however, by the fact that distant failures (DM + PS) occur more commonly than with colo–rectal cancer and the natural history is much shorter, perhaps owing to the much higher incidence of poorly differentiated lesions. In view of these combined findings, the time-honored sequence of surgery–XRT–chemotherapy should probably be discarded, as it has been with oat cell cancer of the lung and selected other malignancies. Early tumor-related deaths in the GITSG 8274 study may be related to the fact that combined drug chemotherapy did not begin until at least day 71 from onset of treatment which may have been 4 weeks to 6 weeks after operative resection or exploration (overall interval from diagnosis 13 weeks to 17 weeks or more). If one saves the best chemotherapy for 3 months to 4 months from time of diagnosis in such a disease, the systemic component, if present, may then be beyond control. One approach that will allow earlier chemotherapy is the use of rapid fractionation of irradiation (2 fractions per day, for example). With this technique rapid completion of irradiation will allow the timely initiation of chemotherapy.

A number of institutions are currently involved in pilot studies utilizing drug combinations prior to and after XRT (MGH, with 5-FU–BCNU and FAM; Georgetown University, with FAM) or concomitant with XRT (SWOG, with FAM). In the MGH series, treatment delay due to hematologic problems occurred in nearly one-third of the 5-FU–BCNU group, but were not seen with the FAM combination in preliminary analyses.[86]

Irradiation Techniques with and without Dose Modifiers

The limited tolerance of the stomach and surrounding organs and tissues prevents a major increase in dose levels above 5000 rad to 5500 rad. With residual, unresectable, or recurrent disease, the most likely gains will come from combined XRT–CT (CT–RT–CT), dose modifiers (sensitizers, protectors, hyperthermia, and so on), or the selected cases where dose localization and increased dose with external beam or intra-operative irradiation may be of value.

The Japanese experience of achieving some long-term cures after partial resection by the addition of a single large dose of intra-operative XRT supports continuance of the use of intraoperative irradiation alone or in combination with fractionated external beam irradiation in Japan and other countries. In the latter circumstance, a dose of 1000 rad to 1500 rad could be delivered as a boost field (1) to the area of the primary lesion prior to resection with retraction of appropriate dose-limiting organs with anastamoses done with tissues outside of the irradiation portal, (2) to the tumor bed and primary nodal areas after resection, or (3) to areas of residual disease after resection. Postoperative radiation would then deliver 4500 rad to 5000 rad to the areas at risk, based on both operative findings and pathologic reconstruction.

If the incidence of diffuse peritoneal seeding is not lowered by combined drug chemotherapy alone or in combination with local field irradiation, such failures could possibly be prevented by extending radiation portals to include the entire upper abdomen or total abdomen for a portion of treatment in patients with initial extragastric or extranodal involvement. An upper abdomen portal has an advantage over total abdomen in that it potentially alters both peritoneal and hematogenous failures (liver) but does not increase the amount of bone marrow included. However, since gastric cancer is very similar to ovarian cancer, with the vast majority of cancer failures being abdominal, the encouraging results of total abdominal radiation and pelvic boost for resected Stage II and early Stage III ovarian cancer at Princess Margaret Hospital cannot be overlooked.[117] A similar total abdominal approach with a boost to gastric bed and lymph node areas may have a future role in gastric cancer, realizing that utilization of that technique together with combined drug chemotherapy would be extremely difficult and the risks of radiation hepatitis and nephritis may be increased.

The future directions in chemotherapy depend on two factors. One will be the progressive development of new drugs which may be useful for inclusion in combination treatment, and the second factor will be the innovative use of new and currently available agents.

REFERENCES

1. Silverberg E: Cancer Statistics 1980. CA–A Journal for Clinicians 30:23, 1980
2. Devesa SS, Silverman DT: Cancer incidence and mortality trends in the United States: 1935–74. Journal of the National Cancer Institute 1978; 60:545–571
3. Dunham LJ, Bailar JC III. World maps of cancer mortality rates and frequency ratios. Journal of the National Cancer Institute 1968; 41:155–203
4. Staszewski J. Migrant studies in alimentary tract cancer. Recent Results in Cancer Research 1971; 39:85–97.
5. Haenszel W, Kurihara M, Segi M, Lee RKC. Stomach cancer among Japanese in Hawaii. Journal of the National Cancer Institute 1972; 49:969–988
6. Haas JF, Schottenfeld D. Epidemiology of gastric cancer. In

Lipkin M, Good RA, eds. Gastrointestinal Tract Cancer. Sloan-Kettering Cancer Series. Plenum Medical, New York, 1978
7. Selikoff IJ. Cancer risk of asbestos exposure, pp. 1765–1784. In Hiatt HH, Watson JD, Winsten JA, eds. Origins of Human Cancer, Book C. Cold Spring Harbor Laboratory, 1977
8. Aird I, Benthall HH, Roberts JAF. A relationship between cancer of the stomach and the ABO blood groups. British Medical Journal 1953; 1:799–801
9. Imai T, Kubo T, Watanabe H. Chronic gastritis in Japanese with reference to high incidence of gastric carcinoma. Journal of the National Cancer Institute 1971; 47:179–195
10. Moertel CG: The stomach. In Holland JH, Frei E III (eds): Cancer Medicine, pp 1527–1541. Philadelphia, Lea and Febiger 1973
11. Pack GT: Unusual tumors of the stomach. Ann NY Acad Sci 114:985, 1964
12. Phillips JC, Linsay JW, Kendall JA: Gastric leiomyosarcoma: Roentgenologic and clinical findings. Am J Digest Dis 15:239, 1970
13. Piper DW (ed): Stomach Cancer in UICC Technical Report Series, p 41. Geneva, 1978
14. Morson BC: Carcinoma arising from areas of intestinal metaplasia in the gastric mucosa. Br J Cancer 9:377, 1955
15. Higgins GA, Serlin O, Amadeo JH, McElhinney J, Keehn J: Gastric cancer factors in survival. Surg Gastroentest 10:393, 1976
16. Rouvier H: Anatomy of the Human Lymphatic System, pp 183–187. Ann Arbor, Edwards Bros, 1938
17. Berkson J: Statistical summary In Remine JH, Priestly JT, Berkson J, eds: Cancer of the Stomach. p 207. Philadelphia, WB Saunders Co, 1964
18. Collins WT, Gall EA: Gastric carcinoma, multicentric lesion. Cancer 5:62, 1952
19. Moertel CG, Reitemeier RJ: Advanced gastrointestinal cancer: Clinical management and chemotherapy, pp 3–21. New York, Harper and Row, 1969
20. Correa P: IAP Maude Abbott Lecture. Geographic pathology of cancer in Colombia. Intern Pathol 11:16, 1970
21. Correa P, Cuello C, Duque E: Carcinoma and intestinal metaplasia of the stomach in Colombian migrants. J Natl Cancer Inst 44:297, 1970
22. Piper DW (ed): Stomach Cancer in UICC Technical Report Series, p 16. Geneva, 1978
23. Kawachi T, Sugimura T: Abnormal differentiation of stomach epithelium: Intestinalization as the possible beginning of neoplastic change. In Ebert J, Okada T (eds): Mechanisms of Cell Change. New York, John Wiley, 1979
24. Piper DW (ed): Stomach Cancer in UICC Technical Report Series, p 27. Geneva, 1978
25 Matsukura N, Kawachi T, Sasajima K, Sano T, Sugimura T, Hirota T: Induction of intestinal metaplasia in the stomach of rats by N-methyl-N′-Nitro-N-Nitrosoguanadine. J Natl Cancer Inst 61:141, 1978
26. Sasajima K, Kawachi T, Matsukura N, Sano T, Sugimura T: Intestinal metaplasia and adenocarcinoma induced in the stomach of rats by N-propyl-N′-Nitro-N-Nitrasoguanidine. J Cancer Res Clin Oncol 94:201, 1979
27. Hofman NR: The relationship between pernicious anemia and cancer of the stomach. Geriatrics 25:90, 1970
28. Hitchcock CR, Scheiner SL: Early diagnosis of gastric cancer. Surg Gynecol Obstet 113:665, 1961
29. Kuru M: On cancers developed upon ulcerative lesions of the stomach; a study of the regeneration of the mucous membrane of the stomach with special reference to its malignant transformation. Gann 44:47, 1953
30. Ming SC: Histogenesis and premalignant lesions. JAMA 228:886, 1974
31. Oota K: On the nature of the ulcerative changes in early carcinoma of the stomach. Gann Monogr 3:141, 1968
32. Tomaslo J: Gastric polyps. Histologic types and their relationship to gastric carcinoma. Cancer 27:1346, 1971
33. Ming SC, Goldman H: Gastric polyps: A hystogenetic classification and its relation to carcinoma. Cancer 18:721, 1965
34. Piper DW (ed): Stomach Cancer in UICC Technical Report Series, p 30. Geneva, 1978
35. Thunold S, Wetteland P: Ulcer–carcinoma of the stomach in a 10-year biopsy series: A followup study of 19 patients. Arch Pathol Microbiol Scand 56:155, 1962
36. Piper DW (ed): Stomach Cancer in UICC Technical Report Series, p 31. Geneva, 1978
37. Larson NE, Cain JC, Bartholomew LG: Prognosis of the medically treated small gastric ulcer: Comparison of followup data in two series. N Engl J Med 164:119, 1961
38. Cohn I Jr: The meaning of lymph nodes and their effective treatment as related to stomach, pancreas, and small bowel. In Weiss L, Gilbert H, Ballon S (eds): Metastasis in the Lymphatic System. Boston, GK Hall (in press)
39. Dupont JB Jr, Cohn I Jr: Gastric adenocarcinoma. Curr Probl Cancer 4:25, 1980
40. Dupont JB Jr, Lee JR, Burton, GR et al: Adenocarcinoma of the stomach: Review of 1497 cases. Cancer 41:941, 1978
41. Arhelger SW, Lober PH, Wangensteen OH: Dissection of the hepatic pedicle and retropancreaticoduodenal areas for cancer of the stomach. Surgery 38:675, 1955
42. Coller FA, Kay EB, McIntyre RS: Regional lymphatic metastases of carcinoma of the stomach. Arch Surg 43:748, 1941
43. Clarke JS, Cruze K, El Farra S, Longmire WP Jr: The natural history and results of surgical therapy for carcinoma of the stomach. An analysis of 250 cases. Am J Surg 102:143, 1961
44. Warren S: Studies on tumor metastasis. IV. Metastases of cancer of the stomach. N Engl J Med 209:825, 1933
45. Warwick M: Analysis of one hundred and seventy-six cases of carcinoma of the stomach submitted to autopsy. Ann Surg 88:216, 1928
46. McNeer G, Vandenberg H, Donn FY, Bowden LA: A critical evaluation of subtotal gastrectomy for the cure of cancer of the stomach. Ann Surg 134:2, 1951
47. Thomson FB, Robins RE: Local recurrence following subtotal resection for gastric carcinoma. Surg Gynecol Obstet 95:341, 1952
48. Gunderson LL, Sosin H: Adenocarcinoma of the stomach—areas of failure in a reoperation series (second or symptomatic looks). Clinicopathologic correlation and implications for adjuvant therapy. Int J Rad Oncol Rad Biol (in press)
49. Adashek K, Sanger J, Longmire WP Jr: Cancer of the stomach. Review of consecutive ten-year intervals. Ann Surg 189:6, 1979
50. Goldsmith HS, Ghosh BC: Carcinoma of the stomach. Am J Surg 120:317, 1970
51. Kelsey JR Jr: Cancer of the Stomach. A Clinical Guide for Diagnosis and Treatment. Springfield, Il, Charles C Thomas, 1967
52. LaDue JS, Murison PJ, NcNeer G, Pack GT: Symptomatology and diagnosis of gastric cancer. Arch Surg 60:305, 1950
53. Shahon DB, Horowitz S, Kelly WD: Cancer of the stomach. An Analysis of 1,152 cases. Surgery 39:204, 1956
54. McNeer G, Pack GT: Malignant tumors of the stomach. In Pack GT, Ariel IM (eds): Treatment of Cancer and Allied Diseases, vol 5, pp 111–268. New York, PB Hoeber, 1962
55. Hoerr SO: Prognosis for carcinoma of the stomach. Surg Gynecol Obstet 137:205, 1973
56. Hoerr SO, Hodgman RW: Carcinoma of the stomach. An interpretive review. Am J Surg 107:620, 1964
57. American Joint Committee for Cancer Staging and End-Results Reporting: Manual for Staging of Cancer 1978, pp 75–76. Chicago, American Joint Committee, 1978
58. Kennedy BJ: TNM classification for stomach cancer. Cancer 26:971, 1970
59. Japanese Research Society for Gastric Cancer: The general rules for the gastric cancer study in surgery. Jpn J Surg 3:61, 1973
60. Okajima K: Surgical treatment of gastric cancer with special reference to lymph node removal. Acta Med Okayama 31:369, 1977
61. Desmond AM: Radical surgery in treatment oif carcinoma of the stomach. Proc R Soc Med 69:867, 1976

62. ReMine WH, Priestley JT, Berkson J: Cancer of the Stomach. Philadelphia, WB Saunders, 1964
63. Cooley RN: The diagnostic accuracy of upper gastrointestinal radiologic studies. Am J Med Sci 242:628, 1961
64. Laufer I: Double contrast radiology in the diagnosis of gastrointestinal cancer. In Glass J (ed): Progress in Gastroenterology, pp 643–669. New York, Grune and Stratton, 1977
65. Laufer I: A simple method for routine double contrast study of the upper gastrointestinal tract. Radiology 117:513, 1975
66. Backus HL: Gastroenterology 2nd ed, vol I, pp 743–801. Philadelphia, WB Saunders, 1963
67. Winawer SJ, Melamed M, Sherlock P: Potential of endoscopy, biopsy, and cytology in the diagnosis and management of patients with cancer. Clinics in Gastroenterol 5:575, 1976
68. Winawer SJ, Sherlock P, Hajdu SI: The role of upper gastrointestinal endoscopy in patients with cancer. Cancer 37:440, 1976
69. Nathanson L: Remote effects of cancer in the host. In Horton J, Hill L (eds): Clincial Oncology, pp 49–85. Philadelphia, WB Saunders, 1977
70. Schein PS: Tumor markers. In Beeson P, McDermott W, Wyngaarden J (eds): Textbook of Medicine, pp 1411–1413. Philadelphia, WB Saunders, 1979
71. Kaneko E, Nakamura T, Umeda N, Fujino M, Niwa H: Outcome of gastric carcinoma detected by gastric mass survey in Japan. Gut 18:626, 1977
72. Prolla JC, Kobayashi S, Kirsner JB: Gastric cancer: Some recent improvements in diagnosis based upon the Japanese experience. Arch Intern Med 124:238, 1969
73. Longmire WP Jr: Total gastrectomy for carcinoma of the stomach. Surg Gynecol Obstet 84:21, 1947
74. Miwa K: Advances in treatment of stomach carcinoma in Japan. In Hirayama T (ed): Epidemiology of Stomach Cancer: Key Questions and Answers, pp 105–110. Tokyo, WHO, 1977
75. Pack GT, McNeer G: Total gastrectomy for cancer. A collective review of the literature and an original report of twenty cases. Internatl Abstr Surg 77:265, 1943
76. Paulino F, Roselli A: Carcinoma of the stomach. With special reference to total gastrectomy. Curr Probl Surg pp 1–72, December 1973
77. Ransom HK: Cancer of the stomach. Surg Gynecol Obstet 96:275, 1953
78. Rush BF Jr, Brown MW, Ravitch MM: Total gastrectomy: An evaluation of its use in the treatment of gastric cancer. Cancer 13:643, 1960
79. Lumpkin WM, Crow RL Jr, Hernandez CM, Cohn I Jr: Carcinoma of the stomach: Review of 1,035 cases. Ann Surg 159:919, 1964
80. Moertel CG, Mittelman JA, Bakermeier RF, Engstrom P, Hanely J: Sequential and combination chemotherapy of advanced gastric cancer. Cancer 38:678, 1976
81. Goldsmith MA, Friedman MA, Carter SK: Clinical brochure, 5-(3-3-dimethyl-l-triazeno) imidazole carboxamide (DTIC, DIC). National Cancer Institute, Bethesda, Maryland, 1972
82. Goldstein HM, Rogers LF, Fletcher GH, Dodd GD: Radiological manifestations of radiation-induced injury to the normal upper gastrointestinal tract. Radiology 117:135, 1975
83. Lawrence W: Nutritional consequences of surgical resection of gastrointestinal tract for cancer. Cancer Res 37:2379, 1977
84. Luxton RW, Kunkler PB: Radiation nephritis. Acta Radiol 2:169, 1964
85. Goffinet DR, Glatstein E, Zuks Z, Kaplan HS: Abdominal irradiation in non-Hodgkin's lymphoma. Cancer 37:2797, 1976
86. Gunderson LL, Hoskins B, Cohen A, Kaufman S, Wood W, Carey R: Combined modality treatment of gastric cancer. Proc ASTR Int J Rad Oncol 5:118, 1979
87. Nordman E, Kauppinen C: The value of megavolt therapy in carcinoma of the stomach. Strahlentherapie 144:635, 1972
88. Roswit B, Malsky SJ, Reid CB: Radiation tolerance of the gastrointestinal tract. In J (ed): Vaeth Front. Radiation Ther Onc 6 pp 160–181. Baltimore, Karger, Basel and University Park Press, 1972
89. Abe M, Yabumoto E, Takahashi M, Adachi H, Yoshi M, Mori K: Intra-operative radiotherapy of gastric cancer. Cancer 45:40, 1980
90. Asakawa H, Otawa K, Watarai J: High energy X-ray therapy for the stomach carcinoma, second report: The evaluation of radiotherapy for the early and the inoperable stomach carcinoma. Nippon Acta Radiol 31:505, 1971 (English tables and extended summary)
91. Asakawa H, Takeda T: High energy x-ray therapy of gastric carcinoma. J Jpn Soc Cancer Ther 8:362, 1973
92. Hoshi H: Histologic study on the effect of preoperative irradiation on gastric cancer. Tokohu J Exp Med 96:293, 1968
93. Takahashi T: Studies on preoperative and postoperative telecobalt therapy in gastric cancer. Nippon Acta Radiol 24:129, 1964 (English tables and abstract)
94. Wieland C, Hymmen U: Megavoltage therapy for malignant gastric tumors. Strahlentherapie 140:20, 1970 (abstr)
95. Childs DS, Moertel CG, Holbrook MA, Reitemeier RJ, Colby M: Treatment of unresectable adenocarcinomas of the stomach with a combination of 5-fluorouracil and radiation. Am J Roentgenol 102–541, 1968
96. Falkson G, Falkson HC: Fluorouracil and radiotherapy in gastrointestinal cancer. Lancet 2:1252, 1969
97. Holbrook MA: Radiation therapy in current concepts in cancer. In Rubin P (ed): #44—Gastric Cancer: Treatment Principles JAMA 228:1289, 1974
98. Lagunova IG, Cybulskij BA, Kornev II, Minaeva OD, Sakaja IS: Aufeinander Folgende Strahlentherapie mit einem 25-MeV betatron und chemotherapie mit fluoruraxil zur behandlung von kranken mit Fortgeschrittenem krebs des oberen magenabschnittes (abstr). Radiobiol Radiother (Berlin) 13:307, 1978
99. Schein PS, Novak J, for GITSG: Combined modality therapy (XRT-chemo) vs chemotherapy alone for locally unresectable gastric cancer. Proc Am Soc Clin Oncol 21:419, 1980
100. Kovach JS, Moertel CG, Schutt AJ: A controlled study of combined 1,3-bis(2-chloroethyl)-1-nitrosourea and 5-fluorouracil therapy for advanced gastric and pancreatic cancer. Cancer 33:563, 1974
101. Macdonald JS, Schein PS, Woolley PV et al: 5-Fluorouracil, mitomycin-C, and adriamycin (FAM): A new combination chemotherapy program for advanced gastric carcinoma. Ann Intern Med 93:533, 1980
102. Comis RL, Carter SK: Integration of chemotherapy into combined modality treatment of solid tumors. III. Gastric cancer. Cancer Treat Rev 1:221, 1974
103. Frank W, Osterberg AE: Mitomycin-C (NSC 26989): An evaluation of the Japanese reports. Cancer Chemother Rep 9:114, 1960
104. Jones R: Mitomycin-C–A preliminary report of studies of human pharmacology and initial therapeutic trial. Cancer Chemother Rep 2:3, 1959
105. Moore GF, Bross IDJ, Ausman R: Effects of mitomycin-C (NSC 26980) in 346 patients with advanced cancer. Cancer Chemother Rep 52:675, 1968
106. Baker IH, Caoili EM, Izbick VK: A comparative study of mitomycin-C and profiromycin. Proc Am Soc Clin Oncol 15:182, 1974
107. Moertel CG: Chemotherapy of gastrointestinal cancer. Clin Gastroenterol 5:777, 1976
108. Gastrointestinal Tumor Study Group: Phase II–III chemotherapy studies in advanced gastric cancer. Cancer Treat Rep 63:1871, 1979
109. Moertel CG, Lavin PT: Phase II–III chemotherapy studies in advanced gastric cancer. Cancer Treat Rep 63:1863, 1979
110. Baker LH, Talley RW, Matter, Lehane DG, Ruffner BW, Jones Se, Morrison FS, Stephens RL, Gehan EA, Vaitkevicius VK: Phase III comparison of the treatment of advanced gastrointestinal cancer with bolus weekly 5-FU vs methyl-CCNU plus bolus weekly 5-FU. Cancer 38:1, 1976
111. Bitran JD, Desser RK, Kozloff MF, Billings AA, Shapiro CM: Treatment of metastatic pancreatic and gastric adenocarcinomas with 5-fluorouracil, adriamycin, and mitomycin-C (FAM). Cancer Treat Rep 63:2049, 1979
112. Panettiere FJ, Heilbrun L: Experiences with two treatment

schedules in the combination chemotherapy of advanced gastric carcinoma. In Carter SK (ed): Mitomycin-C, pp 145–157. New York, Academic Press, 1979

113. Serlin O, Keehn RJ, Higgins GA, Harrower HW, Mendeloff GL: Factors related to survival following resection for gastric carcinoma. Cancer 40:1318, 1977
114. Dixon WJ, Longmire WP, Holden WD: Use of triethylenethiophosphoramide as an adjuvant to the surgical treatment of gastric and colorectal carcinoma: Ten year followup. Ann Surg 173:16, 1971
115. Serlin O, Wolkoff JS, Amadeo JM, Keehn RJ: Use of 5-fluorodeoxyuricine (FUDR) as an adjuvant to the surgical management of carcinoma of the stomach. Cancer 24:223, 1969
116. Griffen WO, Humphrey L, Sosin H: The prognosis and management of recurrent abdominal malignancies. Curr Probl Surg April:1, 1969
117. Dembo AJ, Bush RS, Beale FA, Bean HA, Pringle JF, Strageon JFG: The Princess Margaret Hospital study of ovarian cancer: Stages I, II, and asymptomatic III presentations. Cancer Treat Rep 63:249, 1979
118. DeJager GB, Magill GB, Golbey RB, Krakoff IH: Mitomycin-C, 5-fluorouracil, and cytosine arabinoside (MFC) in gastrointestinal cancer. Proc Am Assoc Cancer Res Am Soc Clin Oncol 15:178, 1974
119. Hurley JD, Ellison EH, Carey LL: Treatment of advanced cancer of the gastrointestinal tract with antitumor agents. Gastroenterology 41:557, 1961
120. Kazua O, Junita S, Nishimura M: Combination therapy with mitomycin-C (NSC 26980), 5-fluorouracil (NSC 19893), and cytosine arabinoside (NSC 63878) for advanced cancer in man. Cancer Chemother Rep 56:373, 1972
121. Koyama Y, Kimura T: Controlled clinical trials of chemotherapy as an adjuvant to surgery in gastric carcinoma, pp 1–21. Proc II Int Cancer Congr, Buenos Aires, 1978
122. Livingston RB, Carter SK: Single agents in cancer chemotherapy. New York, IFI/Plenum, 1970
123. Moore G, Bross I, Ausman R, Nadler S, Jones R, Slack N, Rimm AA: Effects of chlorambucil (NSC 3088) in 374 patients with advanced cancer. Cancer Chemother Rep 52:661, 1968
124. Woolley PV, Macdonald JS, Smythe T, Haller DG, Hoth DF, Rosanoff S, Schein P: A phase II trial of Ftorafur, adriamycin, and mitomycin-C (FAM II) in advanced gastric adfenocarcinoma. Cancer 44:1211, 1979
125. Douglass HO, Stablein DM, Bruckner H et al: Randomized controlled trial by the Gastrointestinal Tumor Study Group of adjuvant chemotherapy in gastric cancer. Proc Am Soc Clin Oncol 22:430, 1981

John S. Macdonald
Leonard L. Gunderson
Isidore Cohn, Jr.

CHAPTER 18

Cancer of the Pancreas

Cancer of the exocrine pancreas is a disease that is gaining increasing importance as a cause of cancer-related morbidity and mortality in this country. Over 21,000 patients per year develop this disease and it currently ranks as the fourth most common cause of cancer-related mortality in the U.S.[1,2] The increasing incidence of pancreatic carcinoma takes on even more significance since the disease is highly lethal with less than 2% of patients surviving for 5 years.[1] This chapter deals exclusively with the diagnosis and management of carcinoma of the exocrine pancreas. Other tumors of the pancreas including islet cell carcinomas, carcinoids, and uncommon tumors, such as lymphomas and metastatic malignancies, will be discussed in other chapters in this text.

Carcinoma of the exocrine pancreas has long been recognized as a significant cause of morbidity and death.[3,4] In the past, however, primary emphasis has been placed on the dismal nature of this disease and the difficulties of treating it. It was recognized 45 years ago that operative treatment of pancreatic cancer is exceedingly difficult and that the morbidity and mortality associated with surgical therapy is very high.[3] Although this assessment has been slow to change over the years, oncologists have recently begun to approach this disease in a more hopeful and aggressive manner. This chapter will emphasize these recent developments in the diagnosis and treatment of pancreatic cancer.

PATHOLOGY OF CANCER OF THE PANCREAS

The vast majority of carcinomas of the pancreas are adenocarcinomas.[4,5] The gross morphologic pathology of pancreatic carcinoma has recently been reviewed by Cubilla and Fitzgerald.[5-8] These workers reviewed the pathology of pancreatic cancer in 757 patients treated at Memorial Hospital between 1949 and 1972 and were able to assemble adequate clinical and pathologic data on 508 of these patients.[5] This careful review reveals important information concerning the gross and microscopic pathology of pancreatic cancer.

GROSS PATHOLOGY

Cancer of the pancreas tends to be disseminated at the time of diagnosis. Cubilla and Fitzgerald's review revealed that only 14% of patients had disease confined to the pancreas when initially evaluated.[5] This contrasts with 65% of patients in whom the disease presented with advanced local dissemination or distant metastases. The remaining 21% of the series had localized disease with spread to the regional lymph nodes. The location of the primary tumor within the pancreas obviously is of critical importance to the entire problem since symptoms, diagnosis, and therapy are all significantly affected by whether the primary is in the head or other parts of the pancreas. A review of several large series shows the consistently predominant location of lesions within the head and the relatively similar proportion of tumors located elsewhere in the pancreas (see Table 18-1).[9-14]

The gross size of the lesion in the pancreas varies with location. Carcinoma in the head of the pancreas averages 5 cm in the largest diameter; lesions in the body and tail are 10 cm in diameter.[7] This discrepancy most likely results from the fact that lesions located in the head of the pancreas more frequently presented symptoms (*i.e.*, obstructive jaundice) at an earlier stage than body and tail lesions.

TABLE 18-1. Cancer of the Pancreas Observed in 7145 Patients

HEAD (6223 patients)	BODY (1679 patients)	TAIL (654 patients)
73.2%	19.9%	6.8%

Adapted from Howard JM, Jordan JL Jr: Cancer of the pancreas. Current Probl Cancer 2:25, 1977

MICROSCOPIC PATHOLOGY

It is beyond the scope of this chapter to extensively review detailed information on pancreatic cancer morphology and histology. What will be conveyed, however, is an overview of pancreatic cancer histology with emphasis on the features that may be important to the clinician making decisions on the management of patients with this disease.

Table 18-2, adapted from Cubilla and Fitzgerald, reviews the different cellular histology of pancreatic cancer seen in the Memorial Hospital series.[5] Several general points can be made concerning the microscopic pathology of pancreatic cancer. First, the vast majority of tumors are duct cell adenocarcinomas (see Table 18-2). In the Memorial series, 75% of patients' tumors fall into this category and this correlates well with Moertel's review.[4] Tumors arising in large ducts can be differentiated from those arising in smaller ducts (ductules) by histochemical staining for mucin. Ductular carcinomas do not contain mucin, whereas duct cancers do contain mucin. A second important point is the high incidence of desmoplastic reaction and pancreatitis associated with pancreatic cancer. Virtually all the tumors in the Memorial series were associated with fibrosis.[5] Moertel made the point that frequently less than one-third of the gross pancreatic mass is malignant tissue with the majority of the visible tumor being pancreatitis or fibrosis. The presence of fibrosis and pancreatitis are important considerations for surgeons attempting to make a histologic diagnosis at surgery. It is important for the oncologist managing the patient with primary carcinoma of the pancreas to realize that there is a significant likelihood that occult disease exists in clinically normal areas of the gland. Cubilla and Fitzgerald documented carcinoma *in situ*, remote from the gross malignancy, in ductal epithelium of 24% of patients with pancreatic cancer.[7,8] The data documenting a significant probability of multifocality in apparently localized pancreatic cancer require that the physician treating such patients develop a management plan that will effectively treat the whole pancreas and not just the apparent site of disease.

Specific comments should be made concerning two types of pancreatic cancer histology. Patients with these tumors may exhibit unique clinical courses. Acinar cell carcinomas, which represent less than 5% of pancreatic tumors and do not arise from ducts, are occasionally associated with an unusual systemic syndrome. Patients with this type of cancer and high tumor and serum lipase levels may have a distinct constellation of symptoms.[15] Patients with this carcinoma may demonstrate symptoms similar to a connective tissue disorder with widespread panniculitis associated with eosinophilia, arthralgias, and arthritis.

Cystadenocarcinoma of the pancreas accounts for approximately 1% of pancreatic neoplasms. However, it is of importance because of its unusually good prognosis.[4,5,16,17] This tumor commonly involves the tail of the pancreas and presents as a large mucous-containing mass in the abdomen.[5] Surgical resection may result in long-term survival of 30–60% of these patients.[5,16,17]

TABLE 18-2. Histology of Pancreatic Carcinoma

Type	% of patients
Duct cell adenocarcinoma	75
Giant cell carcinoma	4
Adenosquamous carcinoma	4
Mucinous cystadenocarcinoma	1
Acinar cell adenocarcinoma	1
Others	15

ANATOMICAL RELATIONSHIP OF THE PANCREAS

The deep "silent" location of the pancreas is responsible in large measure for the lack of symptoms, the difficulty in diagnosis, and the technical difficulties related to surgical extirpation of pancreatic lesions. The anatomic consideration in this disease is also critically important in planning radiotherapy. The pancreas is either in contact or in close proximity with stomach, duodenum, colon, liver, gallbladder, common duct, aorta, vena cava, portal vein, superior mesenteric vessels, spleen, kidney, and adrenals (see Figure 18-1). The fact that the common duct traverses the head of the pancreas is responsible for both the few cases with relatively early symptomatology (*e.g.*, the early onset of obstructive jaundice in patients whose primary lesions arise here) and also for the complexity of surgical procedures upon the pancreas. The position of the pancreas directly overlying the portal vein and mesenteric vessels increases the danger of operative procedures on the pancreas and, at the same time, serves as a final determining factor regarding resectability of the pancreas. The tendency of lesions in the head of the pancreas to invade the portal vein has deterred surgeons from attempting resections in most cases.

Knowledge of the normal arterial and venous supply of the pancreas has been extremely helpful to the earlier diagnosis of pancreatic lesions in the hands of expert angiographers. Distortions of vascular supply, encasement of vessels, or abnormalities in distribution of the vascular supply are landmarks that angiographers use to make preoperative determinations of inoperability for lesions in the pancreas.

The close proximity of the duodenum and the pancreas and the interrelationship of the arterial supply to the two viscera determines the operative procedure that must be employed for lesions of the pancreas. It is critical that the pancreas and duodenum be considered together in any discussion of resective procedures.

The recent studies by Cubilla and Fitzgerald have shed new light on the lymphatic spread of tumors from the pancreas, and have focused attention on the regional lymph

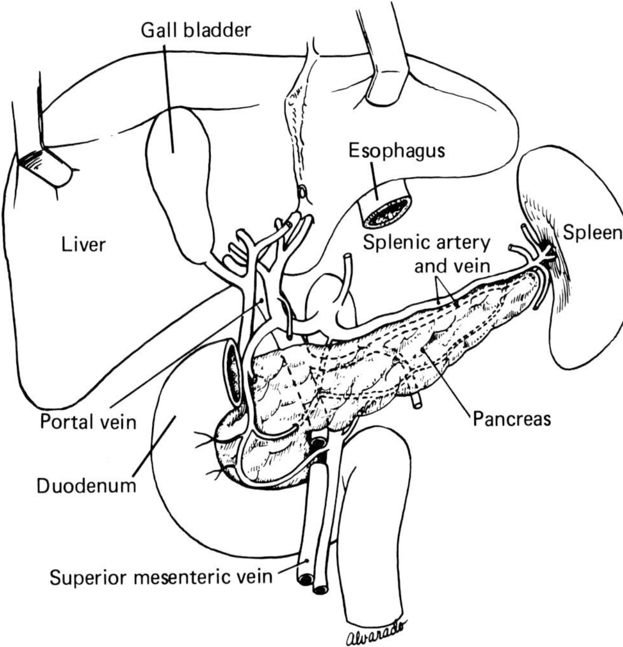

FIG. 18-1. Major anatomic relationships of the pancreas, showing its relationship to other viscera and its blood supply.

node drainage of tumors arising in the pancreas.[5,18,19] Their classification of pancreatic lymph nodes is as follows:

1. Superior
   Superior head
   Superior body
   Gastric
2. Inferior
   Inferior head
   Inferior body
3. Anterior
   Anterior pancreaticoduodenal
   Pyloric
   Mesenteric
4. Posterior
   Posterior pancreaticoduodenal
   Common bile duct
5. Splenic
   Hilum of the spleen
   Tail of the pancreas

In addition to the standard anatomic and surgical texts, there are a number of major articles dealing with the surgical anatomic features of the pancreas, as well as those dealing with the lymphatics.[18,20–24]

NATURAL HISTORY OF PANCREATIC CANCER

PATTERNS OF SPREAD

To understand the varied clinical presentations of pancreatic cancer, one must first be familiar with its patterns of spread. DieGoyanes, Pack, and Bowden emphasized three anatomic characteristics of the pancreas that favor dissemination of cancer:

1. The rich lymphatic drainage and absence of valves in the lymphatic capillaries
2. The rich venous drainage by broad, short vessels that drain into the splenic vein
3. The position of the organ in the abdomen, facilitating intraabdominal spread by peritoneal seeding once the posterior peritoneum is invaded[25]

Their observations were based on a large experience with both clinical cases and detailed autopsy experience.

The direct invasion of other organs from a lesion arising in the pancreas has been documented in Cubilla and Fitzgerald's autopsy studies of 75 patients.[18] The duodenum, the area most commonly involved, was involved in 67% of patients whose lesions arose in the head of the pancreas. The stomach was the next area most commonly involved, being involved in 40% of patients whose lesions arose in the body. However, it is interesting to note that there was direct invasion in at least one patient each of spleen, left adrenal, transverse colon, left kidney, jejunum and right ureter (see Table 18-3).

TABLE 18-3. Organ Directly Invaded (at autopsy) by Pancreas Duct Cancer (in 75 Patients)

ANATOMICAL SITE INVADED	TOTAL NO. PATIENTS	PRIMARY SITE					
		HEAD		BODY		TAIL	
		No.	*(%)*	*No.*	*(%)*	*No.*	*(%)*
Duodenum	30	24	(67)	6	(24)	0	(0)
Stomach	20	9	(25)	10	(40)	1	(7)
Spleen	8	0	(0)	3	(12)	5	(36)
Left adrenal	5	0	(0)	1	(4)	4	(29)
Transverse colon	6	1	(3)	3	(12)	2	(14)
Left kidney	2	0	(0)	1	(4)	1	(7)
Jejunum	3	1	(3)	1	(4)	1	(7)
Ureter (right)	1	1	(3)	0	(0)	0	(0)
Total (%)	75	36	(48)	25	(33)	14	(19)

Cubilla AL, Fitzgerald PJ: Metastasis in pancreatic duct adenocarcinoma. In Day SB, Meyers WPL, Stanley P et al (eds): Cancer Invasion and Metastasis: Biologic Mechanisms and Therapy, pp 81–94. New York, Raven Press, 1977

TABLE 18-4. Sites of Metastases in Carcinoma of the Pancreas

SITE OF METASTASIS	LOCATION OF TUMOR: HEAD (%) (Total patients–5233)	BODY AND TAIL (%) (Total patients–1912)
Regional nodes	75	76
Liver	65	71
Lungs	30	14
Peritoneum	22	38
Duodenum	19	5
Adrenals	13	24
Stomach	11	5
Gallbladder	9	0
Spleen	6	14
Kidney	6	5
Intestines	4	5
Mediastinal nodes	4	5
Other	19	28
No metastasis	13	0

Howard JM, Jordan JL Jr: Cancer of the pancreas. Current Probl Cancer 2:20, 1977

Several different studies (see Table 18-4) have demonstrated the areas that are most likely to be involved by metastatic lesions from pancreatic cancer.[9,11,13,18,26] The liver is the organ most commonly involved, but it is interesting to note the frequent involvement of lungs, adrenals, kidney, spleen and other viscera. The incidence of "other organ" involvement is another explanation for the poor results observed with pancreatic lesions, and again demonstrates the extent to which lesions arising in the pancreas can grow without resulting in local signs or symptoms.

CLINICAL PRESENTATION

The clinical presentation of adenocarcinoma of the pancreas has been extensively reviewed.[4,10,27] The vague nature of the symptoms, except for jaundice, explains, to a degree, the difficulty in making a diagnosis at an appropriate time.[28–31] Collective review of several large series shows that the symptoms related to lesions in the pancreas, regardless of whether the primary is in the head or the body and tail, relate to weight loss, pain, anorexia, nausea, vomiting or weakness, all of which could be symptoms for a variety of other nondescript lesions. Unfortunately, unless jaundice is present or unless the clinician is sufficiently alert, these findings may be missed (see Table 18-5).[9,11,13] Because of the nonspecific nature of many symptoms of pancreatic cancer, an early diagnosis of this tumor requires a high index of suspicion on the part of the physician and a willingness on the part of the patient to undergo extensive diagnostic procedures.

Pain is the single most important symptom in bringing these patients to medical attention. Essentially, all patients have pain at one time or another during their course. Typically, the pain is in the epigastrium, is gnawing and visceral in character, and is worse at night. Patients may report change in pain intensity with change in posture. Although the pain is typically in the epigastrium and hypochondrium, it may radiate to the back in some 25% of patients. However, pain limited to the back is distinctly unusual with less than 5% of patients exhibiting such a clinical presentation.[4] Although pain is associated with lesions of the head, body and tail of the pancreas, it may be more of a severe problem in body and tail lesions (see Table 18-5) since tumors may grow to larger sizes in these areas before diagnosis. This entails a higher likelihood of retroperitoneal invasion and infiltration of splanchnic nerves.

Anorexia and weight loss are also very common nonspecific manifestations of pancreatic cancer (see Table 18-5) and may result in major debilitation. Occasionally, frank malabsorption

TABLE 18-5. Clinical Features of Cancer of the Pancreas

HEAD: SYMPTOMS AND SIGNS	% PATIENTS (Total patients–5223)	BODY AND TAIL: SYMPTOMS AND SIGNS	% PATIENTS (Total patients–1912)
Symptoms		Symptoms	
Weight loss	92	Weight loss	100
Jaundice	82	Pain	87
Pain	72	Weakness	43
Anorexia	64	Nausea	43
Dark urine	63	Vomiting	37
Light stools	62	Anorexia	33
Nausea	45	Constipation	27
Vomiting	37	Food intolerance	7
Weakness	35	Jaundice	7
Pruritus	24	Signs	
Signs		Palpable liver	33
Jaundice	87	Abdominal mass	23
Palpable liver	83	Ascites	20
Palpable gallbladder	29	Jaundice	13
Ascites	14		
Abdominal mass	13		

Adapted from Howard JM, Jordan JL Jr: Cancer of the pancreas. Current Probl Cancer 2:23, 1977

and diarrhea may result from failure of pancreatic exocrine function; however, this is unusual. There are no adequate data to suggest how frequently some degree of subclinical malabsorption occurs with pancreatic cancer and whether such a mechanism could contribute to the wasting syndrome commonly seen with this disease.[27]

Jaundice is a common manifestation of carcinoma of the head of the pancreas. At least 75% of such patients will be icteric during the course of their illness.[27] This results from obstruction of the pancreatic duct and extension of tumor into the common bile duct. Although painless jaundice has been traditionally felt to be an important manifestation of pancreatic cancer, this is, in fact, distinctly unusual. The jaundice of true pancreatic cancer is almost always associated with pain. Painless jaundice is more likely to be a symptom of primary bile duct or ampullary carcinoma.[4] Likewise, Courvoisier's sign (*i.e.*, a palpable gallbladder) is also unusual in pancreatic cancer. Although the gallbladder is frequently seen distended at surgery in patients with pancreatic head neoplasms, less than 30% of patients will have a palpable gallbladder on physical examination.[4]

Patients with carcinoma of the body and tail of the pancreas may present with upper gastrointestinal bleeding due to varices. Esophageal and gastric varices develop in these patients from tumor compression of the portal vein. Likewise, splenomegaly is occasionally seen in such patients secondary to tumor extension and encasement of the splenic vein.

Some 20% of patients with pancreatic cancer have a palpable abdominal mass.[27] In cases presenting with metastatic disease, nodular hepatomegaly and palpable supraclavicular lymph nodes may commonly be present.

Much has been made in the past of psychiatric disturbances being common in patients with pancreatic cancer. Fras and coworkers reported symptoms of depression in 63% of patients with documented pancreatic cancer; this was confirmed by Pietri and coworkers, who noted depressive symptoms in 75% of patients retrospectively interviewed after diagnosis of pancreatic cancer.[32,33] These data were generated by interviewing patients when the diagnosis of pancreatic cancer was either highly suspected or had been established. Patients were evaluated after several months of a clinical course that frequently involved progressive weight loss, anorexia, and pain. Frequently, the patients had seen many physicians and undergone a number of diagnostic tests without an adequate diagnosis being established. Under these circumstances, perhaps the "normal" response is to be depressed. Indeed, as noted by Moertel, it may be more appropriate to question the mental health of the 25% of patients who denied depressive symptoms.[4]

Although venous thrombosis may be increased in patients with pancreatic cancer,[34] particularly if the tumor arises in the body or tail of the pancreas, there is no convincing evidence that the development of superficial or deep venous thrombosis in an otherwise healthy person correlates with the presence of an underlying pancreatic cancer.[4,34]

STAGING

In the past, the staging of pancreative cancer has not received much emphasis for a variety of reasons. This disease was frequently diagnosed only in a relatively advanced stage so that refinement of defining various stages of pancreatic cancer was of little importance. Also, staging of a malignant disease only has importance when relevant treatment decisions depend on a carefully defined stage. Since pancreatic cancer was almost always fatal no matter what therapy was used, staging was of little relevance. However, now with the aggressive use of combined modality approaches in the treatment of pancreatic cancer, accurate staging has gained importance since it can define the patients suitable for surgical resection, radiation therapy, and chemotherapy. Table 18-6 defines two commonly used staging systems.

PROGNOSIS

The prognosis of adenocarcinoma of the pancreas is grave. One major reason for this is the fact that of all the major cancers for which figures are available, cancer of the pancreas has the lowest incidence of diagnosis at the time the lesion is confined to the primary organ.[2] This statement is true regardless of whether patients are divided by age, sex, race, or in almost any other fashion. If the lesion has already spread

TABLE 18-6. Definitions of TNM Categories for Cancer of the Pancreas, Surgical–Evaluative Assessment

T: PRIMARY TUMOR		
	T1:	No direct extension of the primary tumor beyond the pancreas.
	T2:	Limited direct extension (to duodenum, bile ducts, or stomach), still possibly permitting tumor resection.
	T3:	Further direct extension, incompatible with surgical resection.
	Tx:	Direct extension not assessed or not recorded.
N: REGIONAL LYMPH NODE INVOLVEMENT		
	N0:	Regional nodes not involved.
	N1:	Regional nodes involved.
	Nx:	Regional node involvement not assessed or not recorded.
M: DISTANT METASTASIS		
	M0:	No distant metastasis.
	M1:	Distant metastatic involvement.
	Mx:	Distant metastatic involvement not assessed or not recorded.

STAGE	TNM CATEGORY
I	T1 N0 M0 T1 Nx M0 T2 N0 M0 T2 Nx M0 Tx N0 M0 Tx Nx M0 T1,2, x N0, x M0
II	T3 N0 M0 T3 Nx M0 T3 N0, x M0
III	T1 N1 M0 T2 N1 M0 T3 N1 M0 Tx N1 M0 T- N1 M0
IV	T- N- M1
Stage Unknown	T- N- Mx

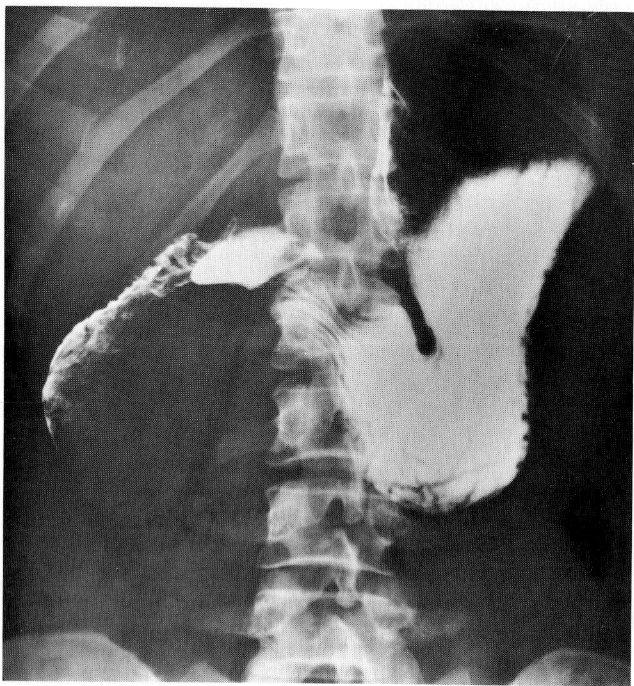

FIG. 18-2. A large carcinoma in the head of the pancreas has expanded the duodenal loop and is invading and effacing duodenal mucosa.

beyond the confines of the primary organ at the time of diagnosis, then it is clear that the likelihood of cure is extremely rare and, for all practical purposes, every patient with unresectable pancreatic cancer dies of the disease. In Moertel's series, the median survival varied from 3–6 months after diagnosis of unresectability; less than 2% of patients were alive at two years.[4] In the 20% of resectable patients, 85% will be dead within 3 years of operation.[4,27] The studies by Cubilla and Fitzgerald demonstrated correlations between the stage of disease and the median survival, with stage 1 lesions having a median survival of 11 months, stage 2, 5 months, and stage 3, 3 months.[18]

DIAGNOSIS

The diagnosis of pancreatic cancer has traditionally centered around the use of radiographic techniques; the conventional upper gastrointestinal series (UGI) has low diagnostic accuracy.[35] Most often it only detects a large carcinoma that is displacing or invading the duodenum (see Fig. 18-2). Patients with such lesions are beyond hope of surgical cure. The common abnormalities that may be seen in the UGI include displacement of the posterior gastric wall, antrum, and duodenal loop. It was hoped that hypotonic duodenography, a modification of the UGI, would increase the sensitivity of this procedure in detecting pancreatic cancer.[35-37] Hypotonic duodenography does have a sensitivity of 90% in detecting ampullary carcinoma and up to 75% in demonstrating carcinoma of the head of the pancreas. However, most patients evaluated with this procedure are already symptomatic and surgically incurable. Hypotonic duodenography is only useful when evaluating lesions of the head of the pancreas; it is not sensitive enough to be used to detect body and tail lesions.

Ultrasonography has undergone recent development as a useful technique in the diagnosis and follow-up of patients with pancreatic cancer (see Fig. 18-3).[38] Ultrasonography can detect the difference between solid and cystic masses in the abdomen and can readily distinguish between pancreatic tumors and pseudocysts.[38-41] Typical echo patterns have been defined for acute pancreatitis, fibrosis, and tumors of the head, body, and tail of the pancreas.[42,43,43a] Ultrasonography may be most useful if used in combination with roentgenography and computerized tomography (CT) when evaluating the patient with suspected pancreatic cancer. The procedure should not be relied upon as a single diagnostic technique since false negative examinations can result from either air, bone, or barium overlying the pancreas.[44]

CT, in combination with ultrasonography, may be a useful technique in diagnosing, following, and planning radiotherapy treatment for patients with pancreatic cancer. Several findings on CT may indicate the presence of pancreatic cancer (see Fig. 18-4). For example, it may be possible to define obliteration of the peripancreatic fat line.[45] This indicates extension of a pancreatic mass into the peripancreatic fat and is helpful in suggesting unresectability of a pancreatic neoplasm. The pancreas distal to the neoplasm may show evidence of atrophy, edema, or pseudocyst formation.[46] There may also be dilatation of the pancreatic duct.[46] CT may also be helpful in delineating other secondary signs of pancreatic cancer, such as enlarged peripancreatic lymph nodes, dilatation of the biliary tree, liver metastases, and ascites.[45,47]

The combination of ultrasonography and CT may be useful in making a preoperative tissue diagnosis of pancreatic cancer.[48-52] Fine needle aspiration of pancreatic masses for cytology can be achieved under CT and ultrasonic monitoring.[53,54] The depth of the lesion to be aspirated may be precisely defined by CT; a 23-gauge needle may then be passed into the lesion under ultrasonography control.[48-54] As many as 4–5

FIG. 18-3. Longitudonal abdominal ultrasound study demonstrating mass in the head of the pancreas. The echo dense area in the head of the pancreas is enlarged and represents a carcinoma of the head of the pancreas.

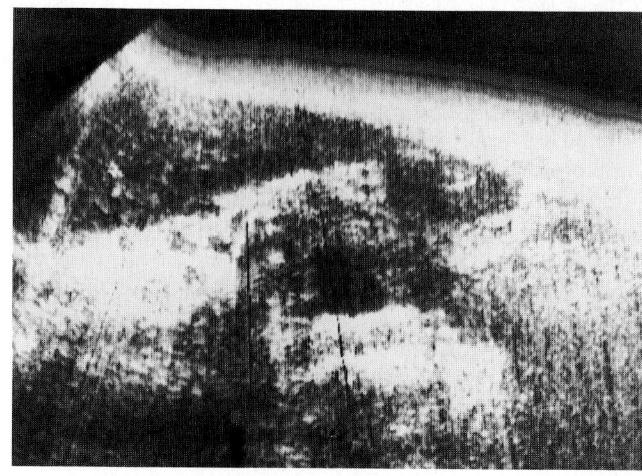

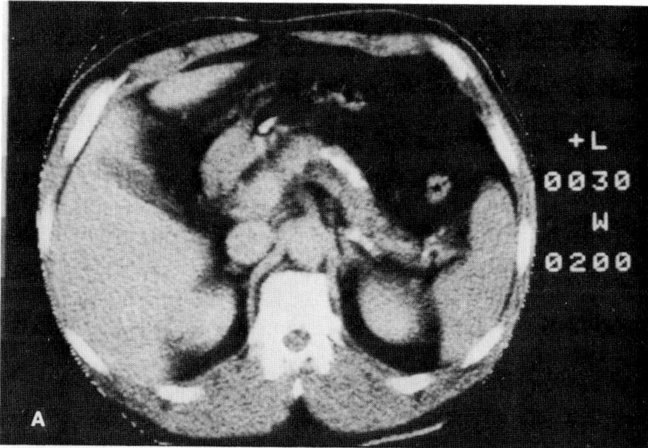

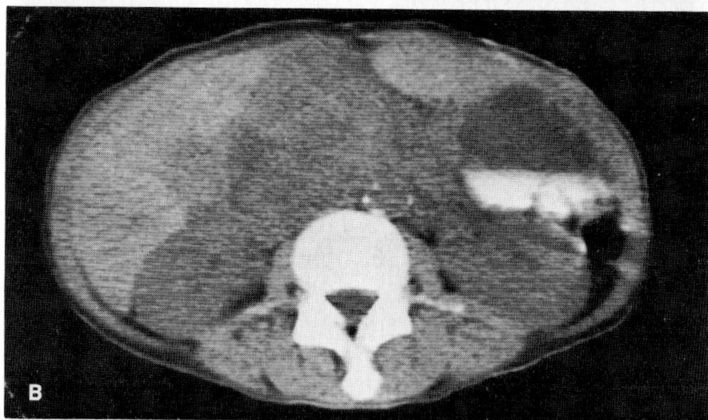

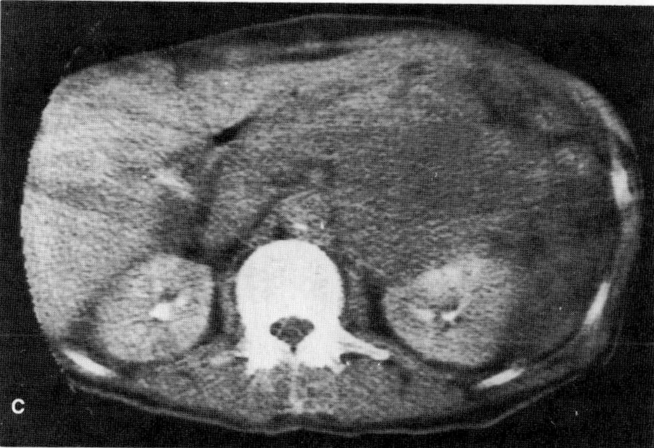

FIG. 18-4. *A*, Normal abdominal computed tomography of the pancreas. The head, body, and tail of the organ are well defined. The calcification in the pancreas represents a calcified splenic artery. *B*, Large carcinoma of the head of the pancreas extending to the anterior abdominal wall. Note the calcification in the abdominal aorta. *C*, Carcinoma in the tail of the pancreas directly compressing the left kidney.

needle passes may be made.[44] Then, cytologic specimens may be prepared and examined within 30–60 minutes. This procedure is very safe and with no significant complications reported in a recent series of patients undergoing aspiration biopsy for suspected abdominal neoplasms.[48] All patients in this series whose tumors were eventually documented pathologically had positive needle aspirations.

Properly performed arteriography may be very effective in detecting pancreatic neoplasm (see Fig. 18-5).[55,56] When the only techniques used are selective celiac and superior mesenteric angiograms, the accuracy of diagnosis of pancreatic cancer is approximately 60%.[57] Large carcinomas are easily detected, but small tumors will frequently be missed. The incidence of detecting small carcinomas of less than 2 cm in diameter when superselective angiographic techniques are used is over 90%.[57] With injection into secondary and tertiary aortic branches and directly into pancreatic arteries including the gastroduodenal, superior and inferior pancreaticoduodenal, and dorsal pancreatic arteries, good visualization of the intrapancreatic arteries may be obtained.[57] Modern radiographic techniques including magnification and photographic substraction help define areas of minimal abnormality.[58–60] The major contraindication to attempting superselective angiography is severe abdominal atherosclerosis.[57]

Pharmaco-angiography with vasoconstrictors and vasodilators may also increase the diagnostic accuracy of the angiogram.[61–63] Vasoconstrictors cause constriction of normal abdominal vascular beds and thus result in preferential shunting of contrast material to the intrapancreatic vessels. Vasodilators, such as tolazoline and papaverine, will enhance visualization of the portal circulation. Secretin has also been used as an agent for pharmacoangiography since it enhances the capillary phase of the pancreatic angiogram.[57]

Many angiographic features of carcinoma have been described.[35,55,64] These include arterial narrowing and encasement, which suggests compression or invasion of the vessels by the neoplasm; neovascularity, an uncommon finding consisting of small, tortuous vessels in fine network; and arterial obstructions of the celiac, superior mesenteric, hepatic, splenic, gastroduodenal, or small intrapancreatic branches.[65,66] Tumor opacification (*i.e.*, tumor blush) is rare. The splenic, portal, and superior mesenteric veins are often involved, especially in tumors of the body and tail of the pancreas, which may grow to large sizes before diagnosis because of a paucity of early symptoms. Vascular displacement does not commonly occur since the carcinoma infiltrates rather than displaces surrounding tissue.[64] Hepatic metastases and gallbladder enlargement can be evaluated by configuration of the hepatic and cystic arteries. In addition to its diagnostic value, pancreatic angiography is useful for predicting tumor resectability.[55,67,68] Patients with encasement limited to intrapancreatic arteries and tumor vessels, in addition to involvement of the gastroduodenal artery but not the extrahepatic arteries, are amenable to surgical exploration and possible resection.

Since pancreatic cancer so commonly results in obstructive jaundice, it is frequently mandatory to rapidly evaluate the biliary tract. Two techniques that have gained wide acceptance for biliary tract evaluation are transhepatic thin-needle cholangiography and endoscopic retrograde choledochopancreatography (ERCP).

Transhepatic cholangiography is performed by the introduction of a fine (23-gauge) needle into distended intrahepatic bile ducts after lateral transcutaneous puncture of the liver (see Fig. 18-6).[69,70] When a bile duct has been identified by aspiration of bile, contrast is injected to evaluate the site of

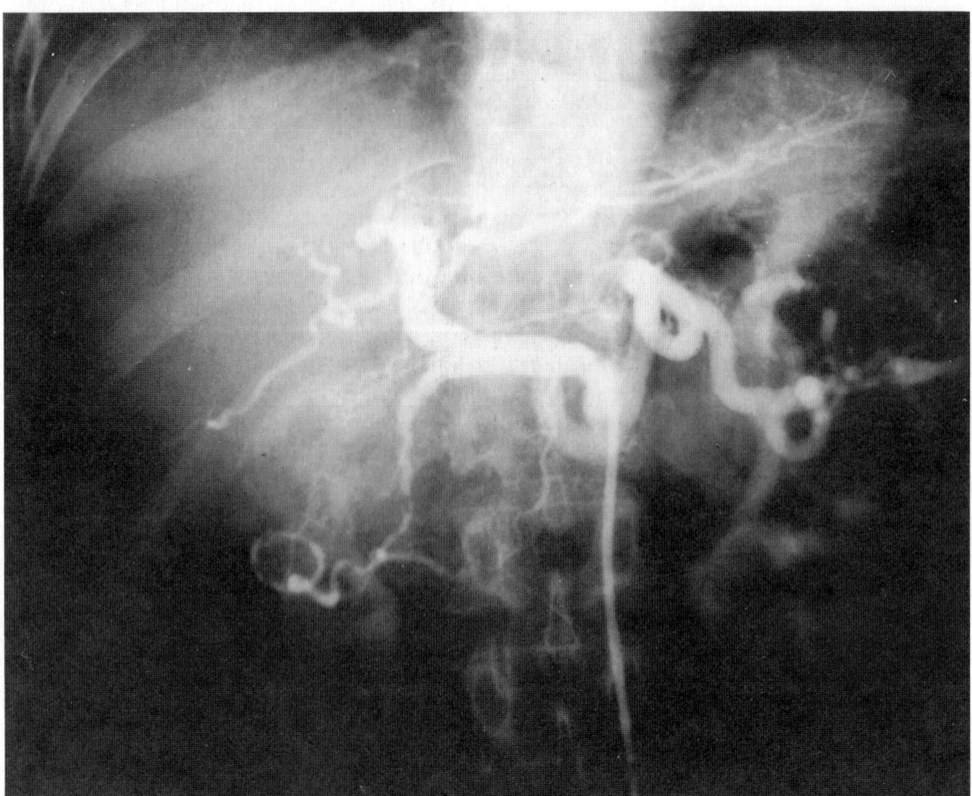

FIG. 18-5. Celiac axis injection in a patient with carcinoma of the head of the pancreas. A normal and typically convoluted splenic artery is seen. An abnormality typical of pancreatic cancer is apparent in the pancreaticoduodenal artery. This vessel (center left of figure) rapidly tapers as it proceeds inferiorly and is indented and encased by a poorly vascularized carcinoma of the pancreatic head.

obstruction. In carcinoma of the pancreatic head, complete or partial obstruction will be noted in the distal common bile duct.[57] A more proximal obstruction would suggest metastases to the hepatic hilum or primary cholangiocarcinoma or choledocholithiasis.

ERCP (see Fig. 18-7), performed with a fiberoptic duodenoscope with cannulation of the ampulla of Vater and retrograde injection of contrast material into the pancreatic ducts, may be a highly accurate technique in diagnosing pancreatic cancer.[71] The major findings of pancreatic cancer by ERCP include pancreatic duct stenosis (solitary or multiple), delayed contrast outflow, ductal occlusion or displacement, necrotic cavity formation, and deformity of the common bile duct by a tumor in the pancreatic head.[72–75] Combined with ERCP, investigators have added carcinoembryonic antigen (CEA) determinations on pancreatic juice; cytology of duodenal juice, pancreatic juice, and bile; secretin testing with collection of ductule fluids; and analysis of bicarbonate levels.[76–78]

ERCP may fail to accurately differentiate chronic pancreatitis from pancreatic cancer in approximately 20% of cases.[29] This reflects the similarity in alteration of pancreatic duct anatomy that may be present in both diseases. Partial or complete intrapancreatic duct obstruction may be secondary to tumor or pancreatitis.

ERCP may be used to obtain tissue to diagnose pancreatic cancer. Cytology brushes can be endoscopically directed into the pancreatic duct and malignant cells can be obtained from lesions of the pancreatic head by this technique.[79] It is also possible to perform direct punch biopsies for diagnosis if the neoplasm involves the distal portion of the main duct.[79]

The accuracy of ERCP in the diagnosis of pancreatic cancer has been reported to be very high. Kawanishi and Pollard reported a series of 28 patients with 89% accuracy in diagnosing pancreatic cancer using ERCP.[29] When this procedure was combined with secretin-stimulated pancreatic juice cytology, the accuracy was 93%. This high level of accuracy will assure continued development and refinement of the well-tolerated ERCP technique.

Circulating tumor markers have been examined in patients with pancreatic cancer. Ona and colleagues demonstrated that CEA levels were elevated (>2.5 ng/ml) in the majority of patients with adenocarcinoma of the pancreas.[80] This correlated with extent of disease, since 70% of patients with metastatic disease had CEA levels greater than 10 ng/ml. All patients with localized cancer had CEA levels less than 9 ng/ml. It should be noted that although CEA is elevated in many patients with pancreatic cancer, it is not a sufficiently specific marker for pancreatic carcinoma since this marker is also elevated in greater than 40% of patients with pancreatitis.[81]

Other tumor markers have been associated with pancreatic cancer. For example, McIntire demonstrated that α-fetoglobulin was elevated (>40 ng/ml) in 25% of patients with pancreatic malignancy.[82] However, this oncofetal antigen is not a specific tumor marker and has been reported to be elevated in several other tumors, most notably embryonal cell carcinoma and primary hepatoma.

Both CEA and α-fetoglobulin are nonspecific markers; the ideal tumor marker would be a specific tumor antigen circulating in patients with pancreatic malignant disease. In 1974, Banwo and coworkers demonstrated evidence for an

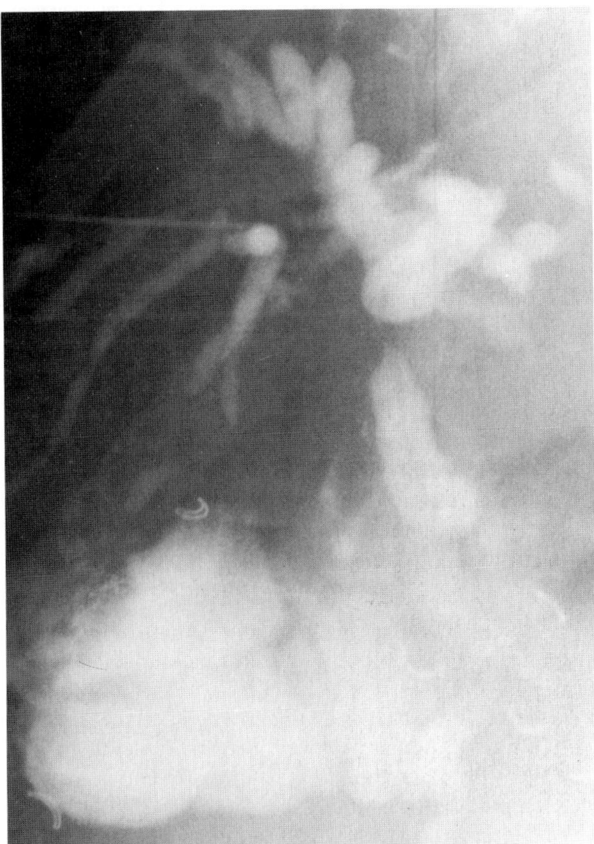

FIG. 18-6. Trans-hepatic cholangiogram illustrating skinny needle in dilated hepatic ducts in a patient with partial obstruction of the common bile duct. Carcinoma in the head of the pancreas caused this obstruction.

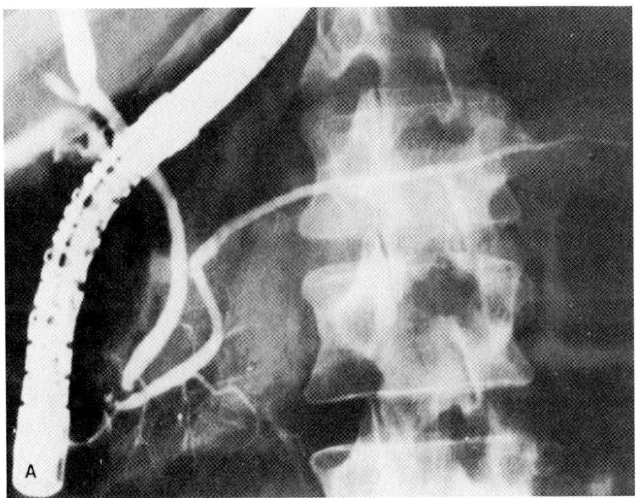

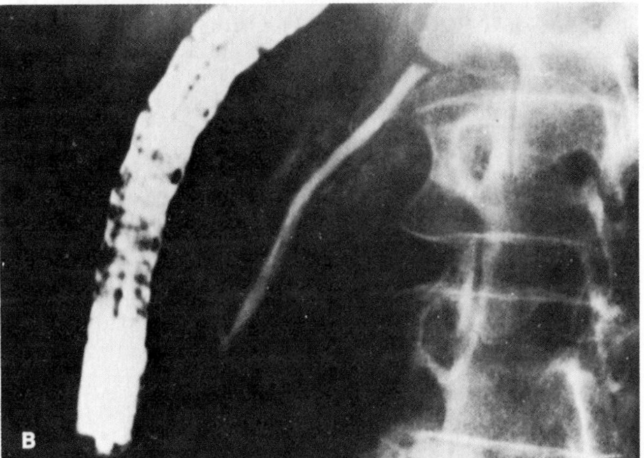

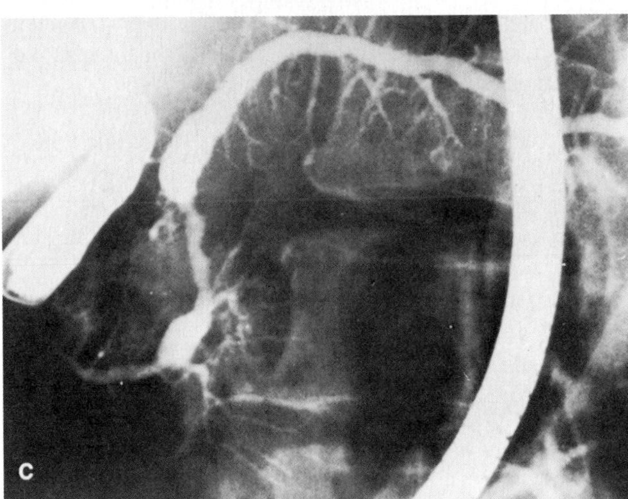

FIG. 18-7. *A*, Normal endoscopic cholangiopancreatography study demonstrating full extent of the pancreatic duct and the common bile duct. *B*, Complete obstruction of the pancreatic duct due to carcinoma. *C*, Narrowing of the pancreatic duct from primary pancreatic carcinoma. Note lack of branching from the stenotic area and distal dilatation of pancreatic duct. (Jerzy Glass GM (ed): Progress in Gastroenterology, pp 634, 969, 975. New York, Grune & Stratton, 1968. By permission)

oncofetal antigen circulating in the sera of patients with pancreatic cancer.[83] Homogenates of fetal pancreas were used to immunize rabbits; the resultant antisera were absorbed with human albumin and adult pancreas. With Ouchterlony gel diffusion techniques, the absorbed antisera formed precipitin lines with the sera of 36 of 37 patients with pancreatic carcinoma. No precipitin lines were seen in 38 controls, including patients with pancreatitis, obstructive jaundice, cirrhosis, carcinoma of the colon, gastric carcinoma, and hepatoma.

The material described by Banwo has now been designated *pancreatic oncofetal antigen* (POA), and has been further characterized by Gelder and co-corkers.[83,84] POA is a glycoprotein with a molecular weight between 800,000 and 900,000 daltons. Gelder and his associates confirmed that POA is found in the fetal pancreas and in pancreatic cancer tissue, but not in the normal adult pancreas. However, POA is not specific for pancreatic adenocarcinoma. Although Gelder and coworkers demonstrated POA in the sera of 20 out of 26 patients (77%) with pancreatic carcinoma, they also detected the antigen in 2 of 11 patients (18%) with carcinoma of the colon, 3 of 4 patients (75%) with carcinoma of the biliary tract, and 2 of 12 patients (17%) with pancreatitis.[84] POA is a tumor-associated rather than a tumor-specific antigen, thus is similar to CEA. Therefore, it is likely that POA will not prove helpful in early diagnosis of pancreatic carcinoma. Following the levels of POA in monitoring the treatment of patients with pancreatic carcinoma must be proved useful in clinical trials.

Although CEA, α-fetoglobulin, and POA have received the majority of clinical interest as markers in pancreatic cancer, there are several other substances that have undergone initial evaluation but require examination to define clinical value. These include RNAase, galactosyltransferase II, polyamines, serum fucose, and a tissue peptide antigen.[85–87]

There are many relevant diagnostic procedures in the patient with suspected adenocarcinoma of the pancreas. Almost all of the various techniques described suffer from lack of sensitivity, or specificity, or both. The most sensitive and specific techniques, such as angiography and ERCP, are invasive procedures with risks of morbidity. The clinician may well ask: Are there combinations of diagnostic tests that significantly increase the probability of accurately diagnosing pancreatic cancer? Several groups of investigators have examined this problem.

DiMagno and associates attempted to prospectively define the efficacy of combinations of diagnostic tests to detect pancreatic cancer.[88] These workers tested 70 patients with suspected pancreatic cancer by using ultrasonography, pancreatic function tests (cholescystokinin-stimulated enzyme outputs), [^{75}Se]methionine scanning, thermography, endoscopic retrograde pancreatography (ERCP), and selective arteriography. Thermography lacked sensitivity and was abnormal in only 15% of patients with pancreatic disease. Pancreatic scanning had an unacceptably high degree of false positives (30%). The combination of ultrasonography, pancreatic function testing, and ERCP was the most sensitive and specific combination for detecting or excluding pancreatic disease. These three tests correctly identified 90% of all patients with pancreatic disease and 80% of the patients with pancreatic cancer.

Another study aimed at evaluating diagnostic techniques for pancreatic cancer has been reported by Moosa and Levin.[31] These workers at the University of Chicago evaluated 186 patients clinically suspected of having carcinoma of the pancreas. All patients underwent the following testing procedures:

1. Secretin-stimulated duodenal drainage studies. Duodenal juice collected was examined for bicarbonate concentration, pancreatic enzymes, and CEA levels; cytologic preparations were also analyzed.
2. Gray scale ultrasonography.
3. Pancreatic scanning; initially [^{75}Se]methionine scans were used. During the latter two years of this 4-year study, longitudinal multiplane emission tomography (LMET) was also used.[52]
4. CT scanning.
5. Selective and superselective arteriography.
6. ERCP with pancreatic duct irrigation for cytology.
7. Sera assayed for gastrin, calcitonin, parathormone, human chorionic gonadotropin, insulin, C-peptide, glucagon, ribonuclease, CEA, α-fetoprotein, and POA.

Moosa and Levin analyzed their results according to specificity, sensitivity, and prediction values of a positive or negative test.[31] The findings from this study are outlined in Table 18-7. The specificity addresses the ability of a given test to exclude pancreatic cancer when patients investigated do not have pancreatic cancer. Sensitivity defines the ability of the test to detect pancreatic cancer in patients eventually documented to have the disease. The predictive value of a positive test is the proportion of patients with disease compared to all patients with a positive test. The converse is true for negative predictive tests. It is useful to analyze these results according to whether the tests are invasive or not. Of the non-invasive tests, ultrasonography is clearly superior. This procedure has high specificity and sensitivity along with high prediction values for both positive and negative tests. CT was useful in this study. However, as demonstrated by a positive test predictability of 73%, CT has a 27% false positive rate. Pancreatic scanning was found unacceptable with a false positive rate of 46%, although the recently developed tech-

TABLE 18-7. Relative Value of Diagnostic Testing in Pancreatic Cancer

TEST	TECHNICAL FAILURE RATE	SPECIFICITY	SENSITIVITY	PREDICTIVE VALUE	
				POSITIVE TEST	NEGATIVE TEST
Ultrasonography	11%	84%	82%	77%	88%
CT	11%	82%	77%	73%	85%
Pancreatic scan	0%	64%	65%	54%	74%
LMET	0%	80%	78%	71%	85%
Duodenal juice analysis for					
a) Low bicarbonate + low volume	9%	99%	10%	94%	63%
b) Cytology	9%	99%	68%	99%	83%
ERCP with Pancreatography Cholangiography Cytology	21%	90%	86%	85%	91%
Angiography	0%	72%	73%	63%	81%

nique of LMET increases sensitivity and specificity to close to 80% and decreases false positives to 29%.[89]

Of the invasive tests, duodenal juice analysis and cytology are very specific since positive tests have an essentially 100% probability of excluding patients without pancreatic cancer. However, the sensitivity of these tests is inadequate.

In this series, ERCP with performance of pancreatography, cholangiography, and cytology is the most valuable invasive test. This procedure has high sensitivity and specificity and a false negative rate of 15%. It should be noted, however, that even highly experienced and skilled endoscopists will fail in 20% of these procedures. Angiography was disappointing in this study. The procedure overpredicted pancreatic cancer in 37% of patients evaluated. This may be because the decision to attempt supraselective arteriography was left to the individual angiographer; thus, patients may not have been as aggressively studied as patients in other series.[66] Also, there are no data presented addressing whether or not pharmacoangiographic techniques were attempted.

Moosa and Levin note that their study may have resulted in an increased percentage of surgically resectable pancreatic cancer patients detected at the University of Chicago.[31] During the period, diagnostic techniques studied were being carried out and the resection rate of patients diagnosed using the techniques studied was 38%. This compared to a historic control resection rate of 12%.

Is there enough information available to define a rational, safe, and cost-effective approach to evaluation of the patient suspected of having pancreatic cancer? The answer is a qualified yes. It would appear that ultrasonography is the best initial test. This may be supplemented by LMET when available. CT may be particularly helpful if ultrasonography is inconclusive. When an abnormality is noted by the noninvasive tests, the first invasive procedure should be ERCP with cytology, pancreatography, and cholangiography. Abnormal ERCP should be followed by angiography in preparation for laparotomy. If ERCP fails and obstructive jaundice is present, transhepatic cholangiography with a Chiba needle may be used to define biliary tract obstruction. Angiography and assessment for laparotomy may follow the transhepatic cholangiogram.

TREATMENT OF PANCREATIC CANCER

SURGICAL THERAPY

One of the first problems that may face the surgeon dealing with a patient with suspected carcinoma of the pancreas is obtaining a tissue diagnosis of malignancy. Although several diagnostic procedures were presented previously, few of them actually aim at obtaining cytology or tissue for a histologic diagnosis. Thus, the surgeon may be left with responsibility of operating on a patient with symptoms and findings consistent with pancreatic cancer without tissue diagnosis of the disease. There are those surgeons who would proceed with a radical resection on the basis of their clinical evaluation. Even the surgeon with sufficiently broad experience with pancreatic lesions, with pancreatic resections, and with a thoroughly acceptable morbidity and mortality rate for pancreatic resection is rarely justified in following this approach. Since the vast majority of surgeons who operate on pancreatic lesions do not fulfill all the criteria just described and since the risk of the operative procedure rises in the hands of surgeons who do only an occasional radical procedure on the pancreas, it is important for the majority of surgeons to do everything possible to obtain a histologic diagnosis prior to proceeding with a major resection.

Needle biopsy can be obtained through the duodenum so that if a fistula does result, it drains into the simultaneously-created opening into the bowel. Skinny (Chiba) needle aspiration biopsy requires the assistance of a pathologist who is interested in and willing to read this different kind of a slide, and also requires a surgeon who is knowledgeable about the difference in technique required to obtain a specimen under these circumstances.

Wedge biopsies are recommended by some when none of the preceding measures are successful in obtaining histologic diagnosis.[90] Recent literature suggests that under some circumstances, wedge biopsies may have a margin of safety. However, the authors' own experience at Louisiana State University has not been good with this form of biopsy; the likelihood of bleeding, abscess, and fistula formation if the pancreas is not resected is so high that the authors prefer not to do a wedge biopsy. Also, if the lesion is positive, the possibility exists that the wedge biopsy may spill tumor cells through the operative field and lead to potential complications.

Additional problems with the wedge biopsy are related to the difficulty in establishing a diagnosis even after the pathologist has the specimen under the microscope. The histologic similarities between some forms of chronic pancreatitis and pancreatic cancer are such that even with the biopsy—and sometimes even with the entire pancreas available—the pathologist may have significant difficulties in arriving at a diagnosis. Thus, if the pathologist cannot provide

FIG. 18-8. Anatomic location of resection required by the Whipple procedure for carcinoma of the head of the pancreas. (Warren KW, Braasch JW, Thum CW: Carcinoma of the Pancreas. Surg Clin North Am 48:601, 1968)

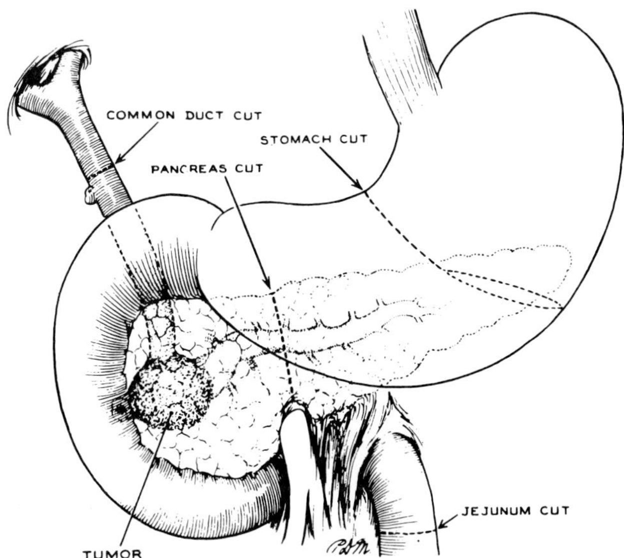

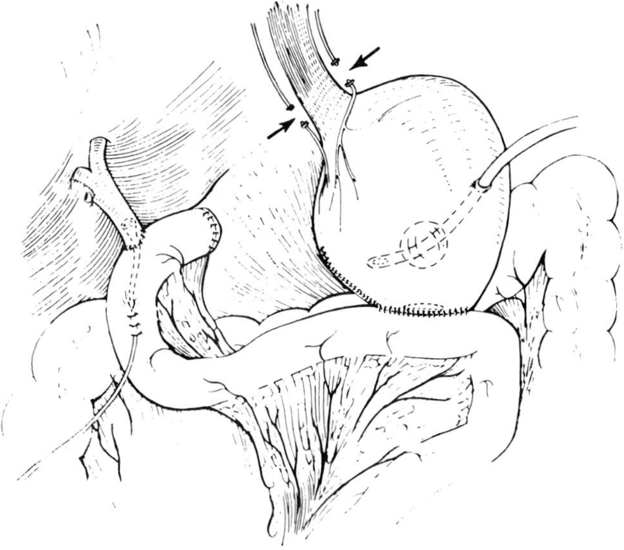

FIG. 18-9. Surgical anatomy after total pancreatectomy for pancreatic cancer. Note choledochojejunostomy, gastrojejunostomy, and vagotomy (*arrows*). (Hicks RE, Brooks JR: Total pancreatectomy for ductal carcinoma. Surg Gynecol Obstet 133:16, 1971. By permission)

a diagnosis or if the surgeon is going to have some hesitancy in accepting the pathologist's opinion, the procedure loses some of its value. It should, however, be emphasized that every effort consistent with patient safety should be made to establish a tissue diagnosis before pancreatic resection since, as noted earlier, most pancreatic cancers are surrounded by areas of chronic pancreatitis and it is impossible by gross inspection to be sure a malignancy coexists with the inflammatory reaction.[4] Thus, there is risk of performing a cancer operation for benign disease if a histologic diagnosis is not obtained.

RADICAL RESECTION

The two surgical approaches most commonly employed today are the Whipple (pancreaticoduodenectomy) (see Fig. 18-8) and total pancreatectomy (see Fig. 18-9).

The 1935 article by Whipple, Parsons, and Mullins described the procedure which, with its modifications, has been the one most widely used in this country.[91] Since its presentation, the major variations have been related to converting this to a one stage procedure and altering the types and sequence of anastomoses.[92-97] From a physiologic standpoint, the anastomoses of common duct and pancreatic duct to small bowel proximal to the gastrojejunostomy has been the most satisfactory solution. As experience has enlarged, a more extensive gastrectomy and vagotomy have been advocated so as to minimize the incidence of marginal ulcer. There have also been suggestions that the pancreatic remnant should be closed without anastomosis to the small bowel, since the major and most devastating complication following a pancreaticoduodenectomy has been related to fistula formation from the pancreatic duct. In 1946, Whipple provided an excellent historic review of the development of pancreatic surgery.[98]

Total pancreatectomy was advocated as early as 1943 by Rockey and then in 1948 by both Waugh and Gaston.[99-101] It is only recently, however, that there has been a swing toward total pancreatectomy to obviate some of the problems that developed with the Whipple procedure, and also to take advantage of the current knowledge about the spread of the disease.[102-109] The advocates of total pancreatectomy give four major reasons for employing this procedure rather than a Whipple resection:

1. The multicentric nature of the tumors and the need to do a total pancreatectomy to remove all of them
2. The presence of tumor in the pancreatic duct at the line of resection
3. The danger of a new tumor arising in the pancreatic tissue left *in situ*
4. The dangers of a pancreatic fistula from any anastomosis

Even though sufficient time has not elapsed to permit evaluation of total pancreatectomy, more and more surgeons are using this approach.

The major deterrent to total pancreatectomy is the management of both the endocrine and exocrine problems that follow total removal of the pancreas. As more experience is gained, the significance of these problems seems to be diminishing, but there is still a very real problem with regard to digestion as well as with control of blood sugar and the other effects of total pancreatectomy.

Even more recently, a further radical approach has been proposed. Fortner and colleagues have employed a "regional pancreatectomy," which is not only a total pancreatectomy and extensive lymph node dissection, but also includes removal of the portal vein, transverse mesocolon, and the adjacent soft tissue.[22,110,111] The total experience with this procedure is not very large and has not been employed in many places. Further information is needed before this procedure can be widely recommended.

Since it is clear that any one of these procedures is a major operation, particularly for a patient who has been subjected to any significant preoperative debilitation, it is imperative that the patient be in optimum condition. Also, there must be clear criteria for what is and what is not a resectable lesion. Resection is contraindicated in the presence of overt metastasis; this is fairly easy to determine. Obvious gross spread of the tumor into any of the adjacent viscera, transverse mesocolon, stomach, duodenum, etc., are all contraindications to attempts at resection.

The difficult determining factors are whether or not there is infiltration posteriorly into the inferior vena cava, portal vein, or superior mesenteric vessels. These determinations will sometimes not be made until relatively late in the operative procedure and at a time when steps have been taken to make continuation of the operation necessary. If there were some way to make these determinations early, much time, effort, and potential blood loss would be saved. Although some preoperative diagnostic studies may provide some of this information, they all are fraught with false positive and false negative results. Currently, the only 100% reliable approach is the operative exploration of these areas to determine resectability. The internist, referring physician, or members of the family, any one or combination of whom have not been properly prepared, may not understand the length of time necessary in the OR to determine resectability and also may not be aware that a final determination of resectability may not be made until very late in the operative procedure. This is likely to give rise to considerable concern on the part of both lay and medical personnel not familiar with the complexities of operative therapy for pancreatic cancer.

Up to this point, little has been said about the diagnostic confusion that may arise in relation to lesions in the ampulla, duodenum, or common duct. While all of these lesions have a distinctly different prognosis from that of a lesion arising in the head of the pancreas, this differential may not be possible preoperatively, and, for that matter, may not even be possible at the time of operation. Since these other diagnostic possibilities do exist and since resection of ampullary lesions leads to relatively good results, one should persevere in attempts to determine resectability even though the precise origin of the tumor is not identified.

It is important that a patient about to undergo pancreatic resection be appropriately prepared medically to decrease the likelihood of complications.

If the patient is jaundiced, which raises the operative morbidity and mortality and decreases the probability of resectability, then efforts should be made to decompress the biliary tree preoperatively. A catheter passed percutaneously into a dilated intrahepatic duct will permit internal or external biliary drainage if no other means of decompression is available.[112] In some instances, it is possible to place a catheter into the common duct endoscopically, and thus decompress the biliary tree. The original description of a two-stage procedure, the first stage of which was designed to provide biliary decompression, is not an ideal procedure.[91] It complicates the second procedure in which pancreatic resection is to be attempted and, for reasons which are not explained, seems to enhance the spread of the tumor between the first and second stages of the operation.

Restoration of normal hemoglobin, hematocrit, blood volume, and electrolytes are all essential. If there is evidence of liver dysfunction, with or without jaundice, efforts should be made to determine the etiology of this insofar as possible.

Reconstruction of gastrointestinal continuity following resection of the pancreas and duodenum has been accomplished in almost as many as there are possible combinations of the various anastomoses (see Fig. 18-10). Agreement is almost universal that the anastomosis of the stomach to the small bowel should be distal to the anastomosis of bile duct and pancreatic duct to provide some alkaline neutralization of gastric acid and to minimize the potential for marginal ulcer. If a pancreatic anastomosis of some kind is made, it should be proximal to the gastroenterostomy, but if a pancreatic anastomosis is not made either because the duct is ligated or because a total pancreatectomy is performed, then the biliary–enteric anastomosis should be proximal to the gastroenterostomy. The anastomoses of common duct and pancreas have been done by such a variety of techniques that it would be difficult, if not impossible, to list them all. There does not seem to be any particular reason for favoring one sequence over another or one specific type of anastomosis over another. The anastomoses that can be accomplished most easily and with which the surgeon is most familiar should be the ones utilized.

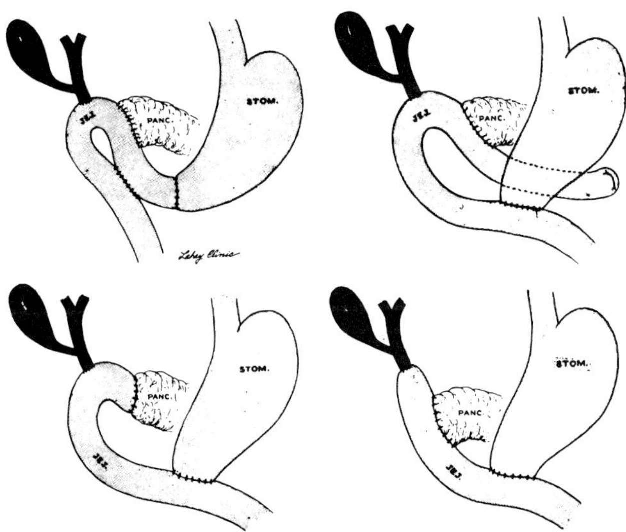

FIG. 18-10. Various methods to establish biliary drainage and gastrointestinal tract continuity after resection of the duodenum and pancreatic head for carcinoma. (Cattell RB, Warren KW: Surgery of the Pancreas, p. 316. Philadelphia, WB Saunders, 1953)

A recent report by Traverso and Longmire suggests that it might be desirable to preserve the pylorus and, thereby, minimize the gastrointestinal difficulties that follow its removal.[113] A small series of 15 patients have been subjected to this procedure for pancreatic carcinoma, and the authors appear to be satisfied with the results. Longer observation and repetition of these results in other hands will give more information about the value of this approach to pancreatic cancer.

Radical pancreatic resection, whether it be the Whipple procedure or the total pancreatic resection, is high-risk surgery. Review of surgical series shows that the operation mortality varies between 5% and 30%.[103,114] This mortality reflects the extent of surgery, the age of the patients operated on, and the potential for preoperative debilitation in patients with pancreatic cancer. It is probable, however, that with a highly skilled and experienced surgeon, careful patient selection, and the most modern and obsessive postoperative care, pancreatic resection can be performed with relative safety.

Postoperative complications associated with the Whipple procedure (see Table 18-8) have been principally related to the pancreatic anastomosis or stump, as has been indicated earlier. Regardless of the way the pancreatic duct is handled, a high incidence of fistula has been noted in the hands of almost everyone who has had any extensive experience with this procedure. The tremendously deleterious effects of pancreatic juice have complicated the problem over and above that which might be associated with fistulae from other parts of the GI tract. The fistula itself may be the only complication—and this can be lethal in itself—or the fistula may lead to breakdown of other anastomoses, massive hemorrhage, or the ultimate cause of wound infection, evisceration, intraabdominal abscesses, and other intestinal fistulas, all major problems following a Whipple procedure. Some of these complications may be related to the debilitated condition of the patient, long-

TABLE 18-8. Postoperative Complications after Pancreaticoduodenectomy 1964–1977: 1,365 Pancreaticoduodenectomies (Collected)

COMPLICATIONS	% OF 1,365 CASES
Pancreatic leak	14.9
Hemorrhage	14.2
Biliary leak	9.6
Cardiopulmonary system	7.4
Intra-abdominal infection	6.9
Pneumonia	4.5
Renal failure	3.5
Wound infection	3.5
Sepsis	1.7
Gastric leak	1.5
Other	3.0

TABLE 18-10. Postoperative Complications after Total Pancreatectomy 1970–1977: 133 Total Pancreatectomies (Collected)

COMPLICATION	% OF 133 CASES
Hemorrhage	11.5
Anastomotic problems	10
Hypoglycemia	5
Cardiopulmonary system	4.5
Bile duct-jejunal leak	3
Hepatic failure	2.2
Renal failure	1.5
Intestinal gangrene	1.5
Wound rupture	1.5
Intra-abdominal abscess	1.5
Septicemia	1.5
Other	5.3

standing biliary obstruction, length of operative procedure, multiple openings in the gastrointestinal tract, or any combination of these factors.

Hemorrhage has been a major problem in the postoperative period. This may be related to the biliary obstruction, but it is also related to the highly vascular bed of the pancreas and to leakage from a pancreatic anastomosis. Marginal ulcer is a long-term complication; modern techniques for handling the stomach tend to eliminate this major complication. The causes of operative and perioperative deaths after the Whipple procedure are detailed in Table 18-9.

The major complications following total pancreatectomy (see Table 18-10) are usually those related to pancreatic endocrine or exocrine deficiency. These patients will all be insulin-dependent diabetics and the management of blood sugar must be handled with some care. Initially, it is best to loosely control a blood sugar to avoid swings in insulin dose and blood sugar levels in the postoperative period. Subsequently, patients may be managed as insulin-dependent diabetics with fractional urines and periodic blood sugars. Replacement of pancreatic exocrine exzymes will be a necessity; all commercially available enzyme preparations, such as pancrelipase (Viokase), should be given with each meal. It will be necessary to increase the dose from two tablets, three times a day, to an appropriate dose for each patient that controls signs of malabsorption. There will still be the possibility of complications related to the various GI anastomoses and to hemorrhage. However, the significant complication of pancreaticojejunostomy leak that can occur in patients subjected to a Whipple procedure is avoided in total pancreatectomy.

TABLE 18-9. Cause of Death after Pancreaticoduodenectomy 1964–1977: 605 Pancreaticoduodenectomies (Collected)

CAUSE OF DEATH	% OF 94 DEATHS
Cardiopulmonary complications	18
Hemorrhage	17
Sepsis	12.7
Hepatorenal failure	12.6
Hemorrhage and fistula	10.6
Sepsis and fistula	9.6
Pancreatic fistula	5.3
Mesenteric thrombosis	4.2
Mesenteric thrombosis and hemorrhage	3
Fluid and electrolyte imbalance	3
Hemorrhage, myocardial insufficiency	1
Pancreatitis	1
Thrombophlebitis, pneumonia	1
Pneumonia, septicemia	1

PALLIATIVE SURGERY

If the tumor is not resectable or if tumor is left behind during a resection, then it is incumbent on the surgeon to place radio-opaque metal clips to outline the tumor in all three dimensions. This gives the radiotherapist clear delineation of the exact area to be treated, which is of increasing importance as the various new radiotherapeutic techniques come into use. It also provides an easily accessible, objective measurement of changes in tumor size, which can be used to follow therapy or determine when experimental adjuvant therapy may be indicated.

A single or double bypass procedure has been recommended by some surgeons as an appropriate palliative measure when resection of the primary tumor is not possible. The major purposes of the bypass procedures are to decompress the biliary tree and eliminate some of the severe pruritis that accompanies the jaundice. Secondly, it is to relieve the duodenal obstruction that either exists or is anticipated. With the advent of endoscopic placement of catheters into the common duct—which may be very difficult in the presence of a malignant lesion—and with the advent of percutaneous decompression of the biliary tree, the need for this type of procedure to relieve jaundice is less apparent.[114] Bypass of the duodenum is often not successful; this is another procedure that cannot be recommended. Unfortunately, the intact obstructed duodenum often serves to complicate the functioning of the gastroenterostomy and even though no actual block can be found on endoscopic or radiologic examination, the bypass frequently fails to work. In addition to this, the added risk of the single or double bypass in a patient who is jaundiced and malnourished creates operative complications that the patient may not tolerate well. Therefore, these procedures usually are not recommended.

The need for, or the desirability of, doing the various bypass procedures may be altered in the patient who is being treated by one of the newer means of radiotherapy, which appear to be providing prolonged survival without extirpation of the tumor.[115–119] If the early promise of these various forms of either intraoperative radiotherapy, intra-tumor implantation of radioactive sources, or postoperative high-energy forms of therapy all continue to show promise, then the need for either GI or biliary bypass may be greater than it has been in the past. Thus, a new justification may be provided for re-evaluating these procedures. If, indeed, a prolonged survival can be obtained without resection of the lesion but with adjunctive high-energy therapy, then it would be important to bypass potential duodenal obstruction and allow the patient to eat, both during and after the course of radiotherapy.

Effect of Surgery on Survival

Although the survival of patients with pancreatic cancer remains poor, survival has been altered more by surgical procedures than by any other approach to therapy.[96,97,102,114] Specific survival curves show a distinct difference between survival of patients with resections compared to those treated by any other method operative or not (see Fig. 18-11). Those subjected to nonoperative treatment had a poorer outlook, which may be a reflection of far advanced disease that did not permit operation. Those who oppose any operative procedure argue from a shaky foundation, even though the overall survival of patients with or without surgical procedures is admittedly not good. No other method of therapy has provided better survival to date or as good a survival. The outcome of the patient with a known pancreatic cancer for whom no therapeutic attempts are made is certain death.[4] Accepting this outcome as the best one can hope for does not follow the best concepts of medicine. At the present state of ability to treat pancreatic cancer, it is clear all patients must be carefully evaluated as candidates for surgical resection. Although many of these patients will not be candidates for resection, those who are are the only ones with potential for long-term survival.

FIG. 18-11. Survival rates according to management. (Gray LW, Crook LN, Cohn Jr. I: Carcinoma of the pancreas. In: Seventh National Cancer Conference Proceedings, pp 503–510. New York, American Cancer Society, 1973)

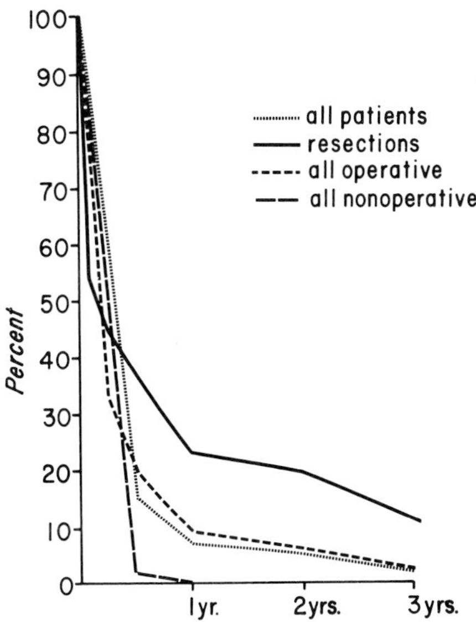

RADIOTHERAPY

Conceptually, carcinoma of the pancreas would represent an ideal tumor to apply radiation therapy for two reasons. First, as already described, many patients present with unresectable but localized cancer. This disease could easily be included in a radiation field. The second clinical problem that radiation therapy has potential to solve is the adjuvant therapy of pancreatic cancer. It is now clear that local failure is a significant problem after radical pancreatic resection. Failures after radical "curative" operations have been analyzed in detail in a series of 31 patients from Massachusetts General Hospital (MGH), in which survival was equivalent to other surgical series. The incidence of local-regional failure (LR-RF) was 50%, which is a minimum figure as local status was unknown in five.[119A] Thus, an effective local modality of therapy applied after radical surgery has the potential to prevent tumor recurrence in 50% of patients.

Radiation Therapy in Unresectable Pancreatic Cancer: Philosophy and Results

EXTERNAL BEAM XRT. Most previously reported series indicate there is at least a palliative role to be gained by radiation therapy. This is of importance since a significant number of patients have exploration only without even an attempt at a palliative bypass. The achievement of palliation, though, appears to depend to some degree on the level of dose delivered. In 1958, Billingsly, Bartholomew, and Childs reported that there was no appreciable palliative benefit in their small series of 13 cases treated with an average dose of 3000 rad (700–4000) at Mayo Clinic.[120] Moertel and coworkers updated the Mayo experience with unresectable pancreatic cancer and concluded that survival of matched untreated patients did not differ from patients treated with XRT alone (see Table 18-11).[4,121] Miller and Fuller, in addition to Green and coworkers, reported good palliation, however, using higher doses and variable technique (doses up to 5000–6000 rad).[122,123] When the Medical College of Wisconsin data were analyzed based on delivering less than vs. greater than 4500 rad (± chemotherapy), the difference in median survival was 7 vs. 13 months; 3/13 patients (21.4%) were alive at 2 years in the high-dose group (see Table 18-11).[124] Similar early differences were seen by dose level in the randomized Gastrointestinal Tumor Study Group (GITSG) study evaluating 4000 rad/6 weeks and 5-FU vs. 6000 rad/10 weeks and 5-FU (6.9 vs. 8.7 month median survival).[125]

The first data to suggest potential radiocurability with external beam technique were reported from Duke University by Haslam, Cavenaugh, and Stroup in 1973 and are summarized in Table 18-11.[126] Some 29 patients presenting with unresectable carcinoma, six of whom had widespread disease, were evaluated. Of the 23 with locally advanced cancer, 20 received their planned course of radiation, which varied from 5040–6680 rad in 6–14 weeks. The average dose was 6000–6100 rad given over a 10-week period in three series of 2000 rad, each delivered in ten fractions and spaced by intervals of 2 weeks. Two-year survival rates for the entire series and median survivals for the 20 patients with curative radiation (11 also had chemotherapy) were equal to the radical resection group reported by MGH.

Dobelbower and coworkers from Thomas Jefferson University postulated that even higher doses of external beam irradiation were necessary to control pancreatic cancer.[127] They described a variety of techniques employing combinations of high energy electron and photon beams and multiple field techniques with beam shaping to deliver high doses to biopsy-proven unresectable pancreatic tumors while sparing normal tissues as much as possible (6000–7000 rad 7–9 weeks with 180 rad fractions). In a recent review that summarizes the entire history of XRT for pancreatic cancer, Dobelbower updated results on their initial 40 patients.[117] Some 90% completed treatment as planned. Only two patients developed delayed tissue reactions (gastritis, bleeding) felt to be due to irradiation. Objective and symptomatic palliation was achieved. Overall survival was superior to that reported from any previous radiation series; after 36 months of follow-up survival was comparable to a group of patients treated with radical operation for cure at MGH. One patient survived 69 months but died of liver metastases. In spite of the high doses used, Dobelbower estimates local control to be less than 50%.

COMBINED RADIATION AND CHEMOTHERAPY

Data from both retrospective and prospective nonrandomized as well as prospective randomized series support the hypothesis that the combination of radiation and chemotherapy produced survival superior to radiation alone (see Table 18-11). In the Duke series, 11 of 20 patients treated with curative intent received chemotherapy with an advantage in median survival of 10 vs. 8 months.[126] In an earlier analysis of the initial 18 patients in the Philadelphia series, 7 of 18 patients received chemotherapy; again, median survival was better than for the group receiving radiation alone (13 vs. 7.5 months).[118] Of the group treated with radiation therapy alone, 7 of 11 survived less than 12 months and 6 of 7 died of disease. In the radiation therapy and chemotherapy group, only 1 of 7 died before one year. Falkson, Falkson, and Fichardt, in addition to Lemon and coworkers, also reported improved palliation with combined radiation and chemotherapy and indicated that the radiation dose also greatly influenced the duration of palliation.[126,129]

The results of the Duke high dose XRT ± chemotherapy series were somewhat paralleled in the lower dose Mayo Clinic randomized study of 64 patients having locally unresectable pancreatic carcinoma reported in 1969 by Moertel and coworkers.[121] An increased median survival (10.4 months vs. 6.3 months; $P < 0.05$) was found when a brief course of 5-FU (15 mg/kg) given during days 1–3 of XRT was added to supervoltage radiation therapy of 3500 rad for 4 weeks (see Table 18-11).

Based on the earlier Mayo and Duke studies, the gastrointestinal tumor study group (GITSG) instituted a randomized prospective trial to study both dose levels of XRT as well as the presence or absence of chemotherapy for patients with unresectable but localized pancreatic cancer. The three treatment arms were as follows: 6000 rad for 10 weeks as per the Duke regimen with and without 5-FU (500 mg/M^2 on days 1–3 of each 2-week cycle of XRT) or 4000 rad plus 5-FU. After irradiation, 5-FU was given weekly on an indefinite basis. Based on an early analysis, short-term survival in the

TABLE 18-11. Comparison of Results: Cancer of the Pancreas—Varied Series and Techniques

SERIES	*No. of Patients*	MEDIAN SURVIVAL (MONTHS) *Total Group*	*Radiotherapy*	*Radiotherapy and Chemotherapy*
Radical operation—MGH	31	10.5	–	–
LOCALLY, UNRESECTABLE				
1. Mayo				
Untreated	67	6.0	–	–
3500 rads for 4 weeks ± 5-FU	64	–	6.3	10.4
2. Medical College of Wisconsin				
< 4500 rads ± chemotherapy	6	7	–	–
> 4500 rads ± chemotherapy	14	13	–	–
3. GITSG				
4000 rads for 6 weeks + 5-FU	79	–	–	6.9
6000 rads for 10 weeks ± 5-FU (XRT: 25 patients; XRT + chemotherapy: 75)	100	–	5.1	8.7
4. Duke (curative group)				
6000 rads for 10 weeks + chemotherapy (Radiation therapy: 9 patients; radiation + chemotherapy: 11 patients)	20	–	8	10
5. Thomas Jefferson				
6300–6700 rads 7–9 weeks ± chemotherapy (Radiation therapy: 11 patients; radiation + chemotherapy: 7 patients)	18	11.8	7.5	13

arm without 5-FU was statistically inferior.[130] That arm was discontinued with a total of 25 evaluable patients. At the latest published analysis, both arms with chemotherapy were statistically superior to the radiation alone arm according to median survival (35 weeks vs. 17.8 weeks; P <0.001); 6000 rad + 5-FU was superior to 4000 + 5-FU (median survival rate 39 vs. 31 weeks and time to progression 31 vs. 22 weeks; P <0.09).[125] By week 60, however, the two survival curves intercepted, implying that the higher XRT dose had a therapeutic benefit in median survival but was not sustained much beyond one year (40% vs. 33% one-year survival for 6000 + 5-FU vs. 4000 + 5-FU). At two years, the survival rates approached 0% in all arms. Toxicity was reasonably comparable in the three treatment groups with the exception that patients receiving 6000 rad + 5-FU required twice as many (24%) radiotherapy modifications than the group receiving 4000 rad + 5-FU (10%).

Recommendations for Radiation Therapy

There are many studies of various types of irradiation being carried out in patients with panceatic cancer. It is clear that this modality of therapy may be useful in the management of patients with locally advanced disease. The most appropriate treatment program in these patients is the well-tolerated 4000–6000 rad of split course radiation plus 5-FU. This regimen had been used in the previously described GITSG study and is capable of producing improved survival along with palliation of symptoms. It should be stressed, however, that almost all patients being treated with this regimen die within 2 years so that it is of great importance to continue to enter patients into clinical studies aimed at improving survival.

Radiation as an Adjuvant to Surgery

While justification for adjuvant treatment is seen in the MGH analysis of patterns of failure after radical operation, published data on results of adjuvant therapy are non-existent.[119A] The GITSG has an ongoing randomized controlled study comparing operation alone to operation plus 4000 rad for 6 weeks plus 5-FU (given as in the unresectable group). Case accession thus far is extremely low since resected pancreatic cancer patients appropriate for this study are uncommon.

Pilepich and coworkers reported the Tuft's series using preoperative radiation in 17 patients with unresectable or borderline resectable lesions (16 of 17 were explored and the main cause of unresectability was vascular adherence or invasion).[131] Lesion size was less than 5 cm in 4 patients and ≥5 cm in 13. Radiation was delivered in 200 rad fractions to a total of 4000–5000 for 4–6 weeks with re-exploration usually in 6 weeks. Of the 17 patients, 11 were re-explored. Radical surgery was done in six, all with lesions in the head. Three of six (50%) are alive; two patients are NED at 5 years and two have known recurrence.

Specialized Methods of Radiation

A number of institutions are using specialized techniques or beams in an attempt to optimize dose distribution even more precisely than done by Dobelbower and coworkers, to minimize effects of hypoxia by using high LET beams or both. These methods include intraoperative irradiation with implantation or external beam techniques (usually electrons but occasionally Co^{60} or orthovoltage), or the use of specialized beams (helium, pi-mesons, neutrons, protons, etc.).

The largest reported *interstitial* series was that of Hilaris and Rousis from Memorial Hospital.[132] Twenty-nine patients were declared unsuitable for resection at laparotomy based on direct tumor spread or nodal metastases (14 patients) and were implanted with encapsulated radionuclides. Twelve with advanced disease received supplementary external radiation with an average dose of 3000–4000 rad in 3–4 weeks. Nine patients presented with liver metastases (31%) and five patients had omental and peritoneal involvement (17%). The five survivors for one or more years had the common feature of absence of liver or nodal metastases. Seven of the 29 had autopsies; three had severe fibrosis but no evidence of residual cancer in the implanted pancreas. Operative mortality was much less than most reported operative series—1/29 (3%) due to a cardiovascular accident. Immediate postoperative complications that might have been related to the implant were found in two patients—peritonitis in one and subdiaphragmatic abscess in the other. Late complications and GI bleeding occurred in four patients; this was associated with a gastric fistula in two out of four patients, leading to death at 15 and 31 months, respectively.

Shipley and coworkers reported the MGH experience in 12 patients judged unsuitable for resection using an I^{125} implant to the tumor, followed by 4000–5000 rad to the tumor and nodal areas with a 4-field technique (see Fig. 18-12).[133] Results were compared with a concurrent group of patients with resectable lesions treated with radical operation. Two patients in each group developed pancreatic fistulae postop-

FIG. 18-12. Operative exposure and needle placement for interstitial treatment of a carcinoma in the head of the pancreas. (Shipley W, Nardi GL, Cohen AM et al: Iodine-125 implant and external beam irradiation in patients with localized pancreatic cancer. (Cancer 45:709,1980)

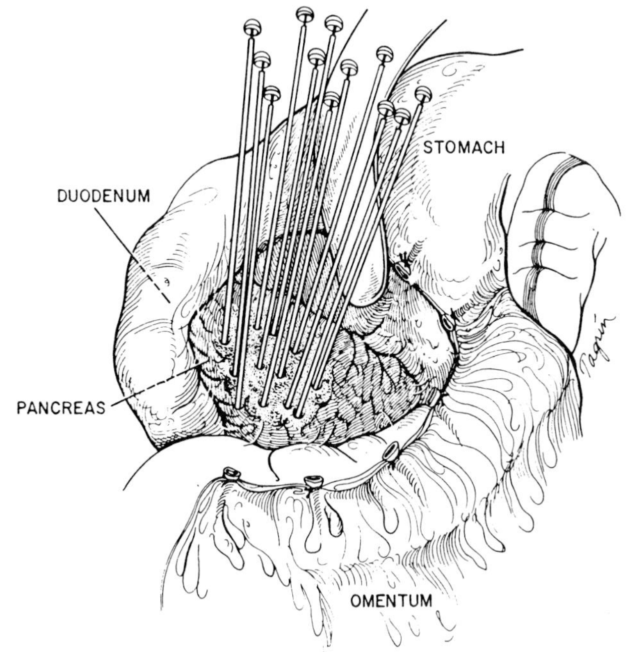

eratively that healed with conservative treatment. Three additional patients in the implant group developed problems that were also resolved with conservative management. Only three implant patients were alive and NED at the report interval. One patient (8.3%) developed recurrence within the implant volume and two additional within the nodal portion of the external beam field (total LF-RF 3 out of 12 or 25%). Of the nine patients with failure, seven (77.7%) had a component of distant failure; 6 of 7 with distant metastases alone (4 liver; 1 lung and pleura; 1 diffuse peritoneal spread). At publication, results in the unresectable XRT group were better than results in the concurrent group with radical resection (median survival 11 vs. 6 months with no survivors in the operative group) and equal to the previously reported MGH group with radical resection (median survival: 10.5 months). With further follow-up all of the implant group have died of disease. (Shipley W: Personal communication.) The longest survivor lived 30 months, but local recurrence was diagnosed at 22 months.

Two Japanese centers report the use of *single dose intraoperative electrons or Co^{60}*. Abe and coworkers treated six patients with unresectable or residual disease, five with 2000–3000 rad with Co^{60}, and the sixth with 2000 rad and 12 MeV electrons.[115] All were dead within 8 months. Lesion size varied from 5–7 cm. Abe commented that "while palliation was obtained, such large tumors can hardly be eradicated by a single dose of radiation, and the potential for combining external beam and intraoperative electron beam therapy will be examined."[115] Hiraoka and coworkers treated 21 patients with unresectable lesions giving 3000–4000 rad with 10–12 MeV electron beams.[135] They found little improvement in survival although definite palliation was achieved.

Three U.S. centers have reported preliminary results with intraoperative irradiation alone, in combination with external beam XRT, or radical resection.[119,136,137] Goldson reported 15 patients treated with 9–15 MeV electrons with a single dose of 1500–3000 rad. Since this was considered a Phase I tolerance study, patients with liver metastases were not excluded (10 of 15 patients or 67%). Median survival was 5.5 months (ranging from 1½–15 months). Serious complications occurred in three patients. MGH has treated 10 patients with unresectable but localized disease with a combination of external beam photons and intraoperative electrons. Patients received 1000–2000 rad in 1–2 weeks preoperatively to the tumor and nodal areas with re-exploration in 1–10 days for an intra-operative electron boost of 1500–1750 rad with 15–29 MeV electrons. Patients received an additional 3000–4000 rad with 4-field photon techniques. One patient developed a postoperative gastric stump leak that prevented delivery of the postoperative segment of radiation. She died of disease at 6 months. The remaining 9 completed the entire radiation sequence. Only one of 9 has died (at 10 months). Here, persistent pancreatic tumor was found at autopsy (she received a 1500 rad intraoperative boost plus external beam). An additional patient is alive with disease at 20 months. Neither patient accepted the recommendation of post-XRT chemotherapy. The remaining eight patients are alive and without evidence of disease progression—the three longest at 30, 20, and 12 months, the rest with shorter follow-up. The two long-term survivors both had portions of stomach within the intraoperative field. One developed distal gastric obstruction requiring gastroenterostomy and the second developed a benign gastric ulcer requiring vasopressin (Pitressin) infusion, cimetidine, and antacids. Subsequent patients have had elective gastroenterostomy and mobilization of the stomach out of intraoperative field. MGH plans to randomize to treatment with external beam plus intraoperative electron boost and chemotherapy vs. high-dose external beam with chemotherapy. (Further consideration is given to intraoperative radiation therapy in the section concerned with newer methods of treatment.) Tepper and coworkers reported preliminary results on five patients combining 1200–2000 rad with radical resection and IV Misonidazole, a radiation sensitizing drug.[137] Two of the five had pancreatic lesions; one has recurred at the common bile duct resection margin. None of the three U.S. series report any problems with postoperative infection in the pancreas group, except for the one MGH patient with leakage of a transected distal gastric stump.

The preliminary Middle Atlantic Neutron Therapy Association (MANTA) experience with fast neutrons for locally advanced adenocarcinoma (19 patients) or islet cell carcinoma (1 patient) was recently reported.[138] Patients received 1716 neutron rad alone or in combination with 5-FU. Median survival was 6 months with five of 20 alive at 1 year and two at 2 years. Late toxicity included hemorrhagic gastritis in five of 20 (one required hemigastrectomy); hepatopathy in ten, but severe in only one; and myelopathy and esophagitis in one patient at 2 years. It was concluded that fast neutrons used in this manner did not produce survival advantages over fractionated photon beam XRT + 5-FU and toxicity was greater.

The TAMVEC experience combined fast neutrons and 25–32 MeV photons aiming at a tumor dose of 6000 rad equivalent (range 5800–6200 rad).[139] Fifteen patients with unresectable lesions were treated, 12 in split course fashion and three with a continuous regimen. Two patients treated with neutrons only survived 7 and 5 months. The mean survival of the entire group was 14.5 months (range 5–42 months with the longest survivor NED at laparotomy). Survival was compared with 31 locally advanced cases treated with photon beams (mean 10.4 months with range 2–79 months) and 25 cases treated with Au^{198} implant (mean 14.7 months with range 1 day to 56 months). One patient in the mixed beam group died of a perforated duodenum 6 months after treatment (involved by tumor). Six patients treated with Au^{198} seeds died with postoperative peritonitis and septicemia. These investigators concluded that a mixed beam of fast neutrons and photons gave good palliation and local control with a minimum of complications and morbidity.

The experience with helium ions was reported by Quivey and coworkers from the University of California, Berkeley Lab.[140] A total of 49 patients were treated; 30 had biopsy proven, locally-advanced disease without evidence of metastases. At latest report, five of 30 were alive 6–51 months after treatment (five of 16 lesions confined to the head of the pancreas; 0 of 14 with extension elsewhere in the pancreas). Chronic toxicity was observed in nine of 49 patients including GI bleeding, diabetes mellitus, pancreatic insufficiency, and gastric outlet obstruction secondary to radiation fibrosis. This study provided the data base for a Phase III randomized

RTOG/NCOG study comparing helium ions with conventional external beam therapy for treatment of unresectable, localized pancreatic carcinoma (6000 rad/10 wk + 5-FU as used in the GITSG study versus Helium + 5-FU). Both the use of hypoxic sensitizers and high LET radiation are discussed in Chapter 48.

TREATMENT PLANNING

DOSE-LIMITING TISSUES

For upper abdominal lesions, including the pancreas, significant short- and long-term palliation and rare cures have been obtained. The dose-limiting organs (*i.e.*, small intestine, stomach, liver, kidneys, and spinal cord), however, are numerous. The use of split-course regimes or precision multi-field standard fraction techniques have allowed delivery of higher external beam radiation doses than were previously accepted as tolerable (Duke split-course regime of 6000 rad for 10 weeks and Thomas Jefferson University precision radiation techniques using 6000–7000 rad for 7–9 weeks). While the precision techniques can allow appropriate sparing of the liver, kidney, and spinal cord, portions of the stomach and small bowel remain within the field. Since the percentage of patients with long-term survival is small, the actual number of patients at long-term risk for small bowel or gastric complications is also small. It is probably inappropriate at present to assume that these dose levels are well-tolerated chronically as well as acutely, although that possibility exists due to inclusion of a much smaller volume of small bowel and stomach within the high dose field.

TREATMENT VOLUMES AND DOSES

Before delivering 6000–7000 rad in 7–9 weeks to the upper abdomen, Dobelbower and coworkers preferred to define tumor volumes by judicious clip placement and requested reoperations, if necessary, to allow them to use precision radiation techniques with multiple field radiation portals (see Fig. 18-13).[117,127] They are currently evaluating the value of ultrasound and especially CT in treatment planning. The conflicts between clip placement and CT studies are distortion and can be overcome for initial treatment planning by doing the CT prior to explanation; however, interference would still exist for the follow-up studies. The University of Wisconsin group achieved tumor localization for radiotherapy planning with an arteriogram at the time of CT. With this combination, they feel they get the best definition of the primary lesion and, in addition, can rule out the possibility of liver metastases. While the University of Wisconsin group has a functioning ultrasound unit in the radiotherapy department and strive to use it for treatment planning, they have not felt it was that useful in pancreatic tumors.

Areas at risk include tumor bed or unresected tumor as well as areas of potential microscopic lymph node involvement. The pancreaticoduodenal lymph nodes are easily included with the primary lesion; the authors extend the fields to

FIG. 18-13. Contour and isodose distribution of a patient with carcinoma of the pancreas using a three-field mixed electron and photon beam technique. (Dobelbower RR Jr, Borgelt BB, Suntharalingam N et al: Pancreatic carcinoma treated with high-dose, small-volume irradiation. Cancer 41:1088, 1978)

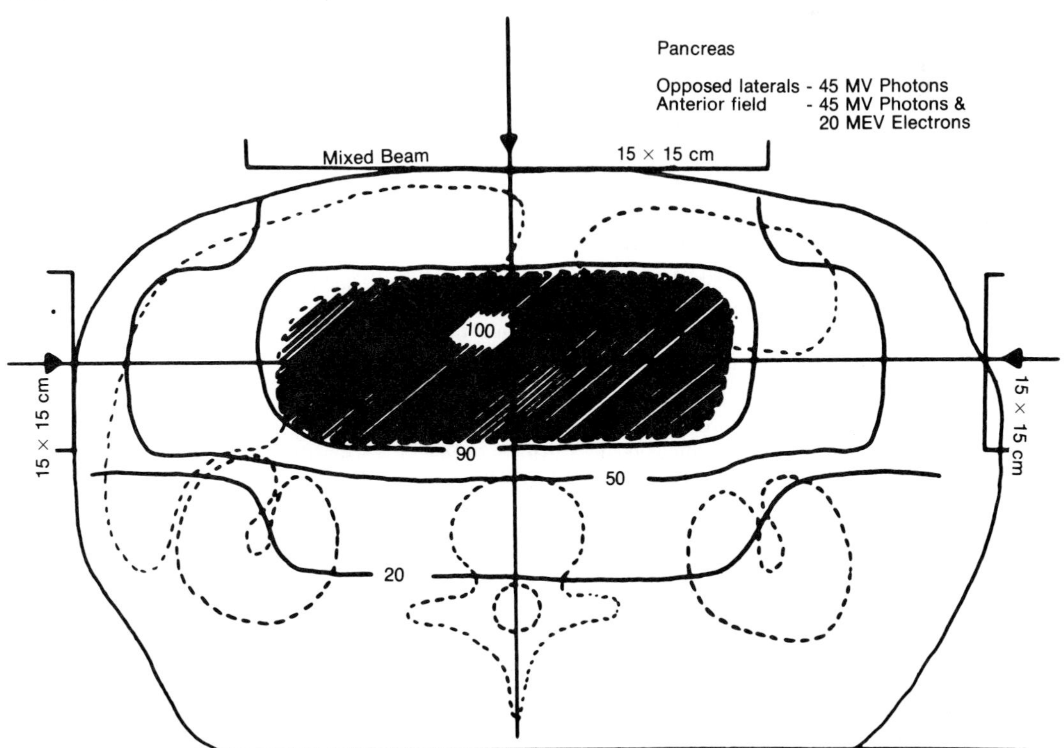

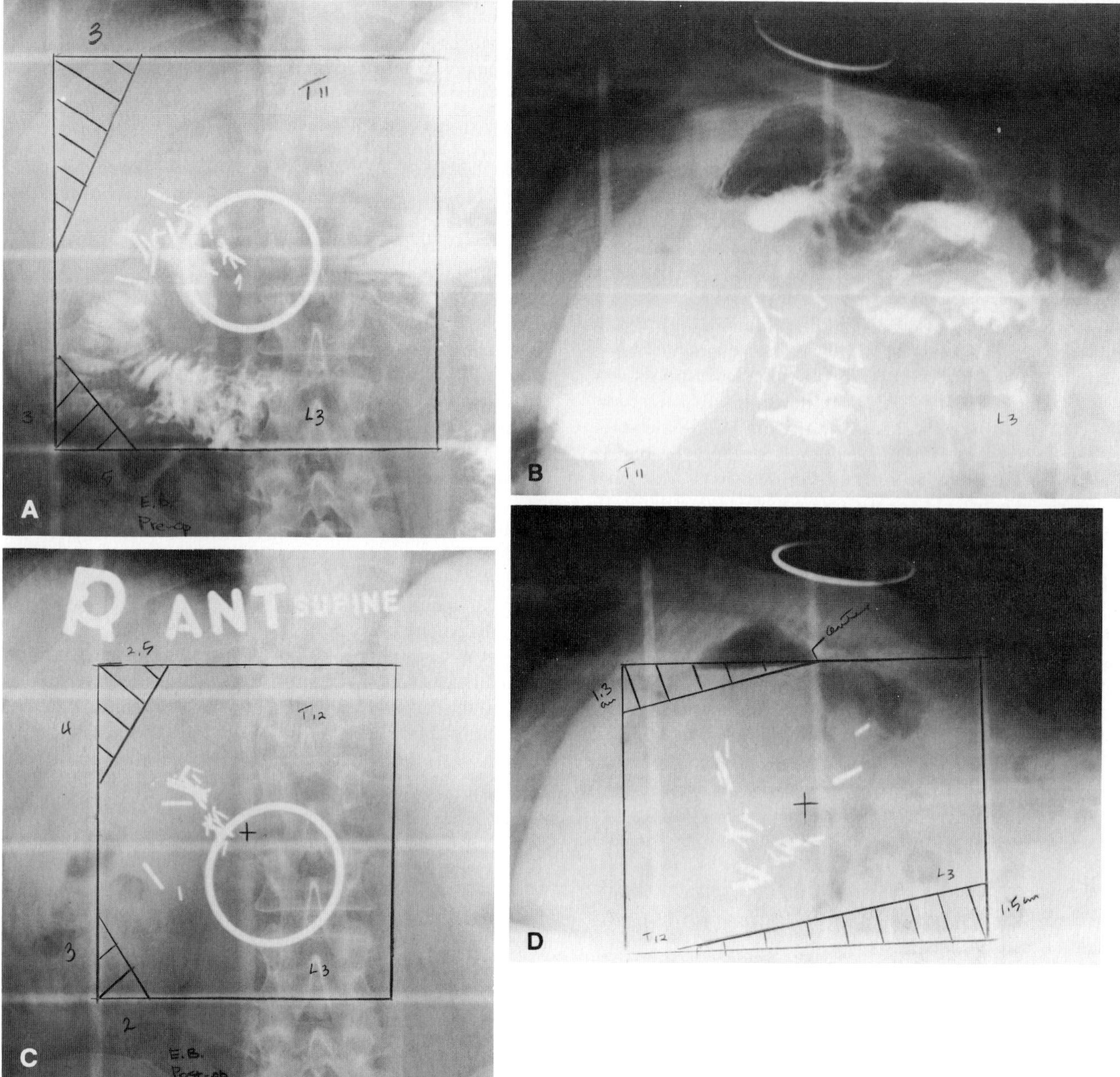

FIG. 18-14. Patient E.B. had an exploratory and was found to have an unresectable carcinoma of the head of the pancreas. The patient received 2000 rad/10 fractions via AP-PA portals. (*A*) Contrast shows the position of the stomach and duodenum on AP and lateral films. (*B*) The patient was re-explored one week later and received 1500 rad to the 90% isodose with 29 MeV electrons with a 7-cm cone (500 of the 1500 rad was delivered with lead blocking behind the pancreas to protect the spinal cord). Starting 5 weeks postoperatively, the patient received an additional 2700 rad/15 × 180 rad via a four-field isocentric technique. The AP-PA (*C*) superior and lateral borders were reduced to exclude more liver and the medial border to exclude more stomach. On the lateral field (*D*) the spinal cord and portions of stomach and liver were excluded. The patient is alive and NED 25 months after the initial exploration.

include the porta hepatis and celiac axis. Suprapancreatic lymph nodes are included to some degree, but in view of the need to spare approximately two-thirds of the left kidney, that coverage is compromised. An intravenous pyelogram (IVP) should be done at the start of treatment to define left renal function, as $\frac{1}{2}$ of the right kidney is usually included. After initial simulation, films are done to outline any surgical clips; contrast in the duodenum helps to define nodal volumes.

The initial large field volume is included to 4500–5000 rad in 170–180 rad fractions five days per week by way of a three or four field plan (AP and laterals or AP:PA and laterals) with high energy photons or mixed photon electron beams (see

Figs. 18-13 and 18-14). Blocking should be used to exclude unnecessary stomach, small intestine, liver and kidney. Use of lateral field for part of the treatment allows decreased dose to the spinal cord, right kidney, and portions of the liver. Our upper dose level within the boost field to gross tumor (primary ± LN, preferably outlined with clips) is 5500–6000+ rad for 6½–7 weeks, using the latter dose only if the boost volume is carefully defined.

If high energy linear accelerators are available (≥8 MeV), parallel opposed AP:PA techniques can be decently well-tolerated to 4500–5000 rad both on an acute and chronic basis. Beyond that level, the risk of symptomatic fibrosis and spinal cord damage increase progressively. The authors prefer multi-field techniques for the purpose of long-term normal tissue tolerance and realize the inherent danger of marginal recurrence if wisdom is not used in field design. Multi-field or rotation techniques are necessary with supervoltage energy 4 MeV or lower if one is planning to go above 4000–4500 rad.

CHEMOTHERAPY

The development of chemotherapy in the management of pancreatic cancer has proceeded slowly due to several factors. First, there has been a general consensus among oncologists that pancreatic cancer is resistant to nonsurgical modes of management, such as radiation therapy and chemotherapy.[141,142] Secondly, there have been relatively few single chemotherapeutic agents evaluated in this disease.[27,30,143,144] Thirdly, the active chemotherapeutic agents may be difficult to evaluate in pancreatic cancer since it may be quite difficult to identify objective parameters of followable disease in patients with this tumor.[88,145] The definition of response to chemotherapy may be particularly difficult with pancreatic cancer as followable lesions may be defined only by techniques such as CT, ultrasonography, and radionuclide liver scanning. A complete response is defined as normalization of all abnormalities related to tumor with no clinical or laboratory evidence of residual tumor. In general, a partial response occurs when there is a greater than 50% decrease in the diameter of a clearly measurable lesion. Liver scans may be used if there are measurable lesions on the scan greater than 3 cm in diameter. The same criterion applies to CT and ultrasound examinations, although clinical correlation must still be interpreted carefully with these techniques.

There is another characteristic of the patient with advanced pancreatic cancer that makes treatment evaluation with chemotherapy difficult. Patients in the advanced stages of pancreatic cancer are frequently debilitated, having poor performance status.[4] These patients have anorexia, severe pain, and weight loss. Obstructive jaundice and hepatic dysfunction from metastatic disease may also be present and alter the pharmacokinetics of drugs that are primarily removed by biliary excretion.[146] In general, in patients with solid tumors, those with a poor performance status have poorer survival and response rates to chemotherapy than patients with a good performance status.[147,148] It is important to keep in mind the difficulties just described when reviewing the results of single agent and combination chemotherapy studies in pancreatic cancer.

SINGLE ANTINEOPLASTIC AGENTS

Table 18-12 lists the single agents that have been evaluated in pancreatic cancer. Several comments can be made concerning this table. First, no column is present describing the effect of single agent treatment on patient survival. This is because many of the studies cited did not include these data. It is clear, however, that none of these drugs could be expected to affect median survival since response rates in excess of 50% are not achieved. Any favorable effect on patient survival could only be expected in the small number of patients achieving partial response. The second factor readily apparent in this table is the small number of patients reported in several of the series. It is clear, for example, that the alkylating agents chlorambucil, mechlorethamine, and cyclophosphamide can hardly be considered to have been adequately evaluated in pancreatic cancer when a total of nine patients have been treated with these drugs.

The most completely evaluated drug in adenocarcinoma of the pancreas has been 5-fluorouracil. The review of Macdonald and coworkers emphasized wide variation in response rates reported in the literature for this drug.[27] Responses have been reported ranging from 0–67%. This wide variation almost certainly reflects differences in patient selection, response criteria, and 5-fluorouracil dosage and schedule between series. Carter and coworkers, in reviewing collected series, reported a response rate of 28%, which may be slightly high since the most recent and carefully done studies have reported approximately 20% partial responses.[143,146]

The two agents that have been adequately evaluated and appear to have activity comparable to 5-fluorouracil are the antibiotic mitomycin-C and the naturally-occurring nitrosourea, streptozotocin.[143,144] Mitomycin-C produced objective regression in 12 of 44 patients (27%) in a collected series. This is analogous to the response rates seen with 5-fluorouracil, but mitomycin-C has the potential for more severe bone marrow toxicity than the fluorinated pyrimidines. When initially used in this country in a loading dose schedule, severe cumulative myelosuppression was common.[149] However, if the drug is given in an intermittent schedule analogous to

TABLE 18-12. Activity of Single Agents in Pancreatic Cancer

DRUG	NUMBER OF RESPONSES	RESPONSE RATE	REFERENCE
5-Fluorouracil	60/212	28%	143
Mitomycin-C	12/44	27%	143
Streptozotocin	8/22	36%	143
Doxorubicin (Adriamycin)	2/15	13%	157
MeCCNU	3/34	9%	155
BCNU	0/20		154
CCNU	2/4		146
Actinomycin-D	1/28		157
Methotrexate	1/25		157
ICRF-159	1/18		156
Galactitol	1/20		156
β-2TGdR	1/26		156
Chlorambucil	4/6		27
Mechlorethamine	1/1		27
Cyclophosphamide	1/2		27

that used with chloroethyl nitrosoureas, many of these problems are obviated and the drug combines well with other myelosuppression agents in combination chemotherapy programs.[150]

Streptozotocin has been reported to result in partial remission in eight of 22 patients (30%).[143] This response rate is a compilation of results from three small series in which response rates ranging from 31% to 50% were reported.[151–153] Although these response rates may be unrealistically high, streptozotocin demands continued careful evaluation in pancreatic cancer since it possesses the property of having minimal myelosuppressive toxicity in the doses used.

The myelosuppressive chlorethyl nitrosoureas BCNU, methyl CCNU, and to a lesser extent, CCNU, have all been evaluated as single agents in pancreatic cancer; when adequate numbers of patients have been studied, response rates have ranged between 0 and 9%.[154,155]

Recently GITSG has developed a randomized Phase II trial to evaluate chemotherapeutic agents in pancreatic cancer.[156,157] This group has done an excellent job of carefully studying the response to chemotherapy in well-characterized patients with advanced pancreatic malignancy. Some 126 patients have been evaluated by the GITSG. These patients have been randomly allocated to therapy with six drugs: doxorubicin (adriamycin), actinomycin-D, methotrexate, ICRF-159, galactitol, and β-2TGdR).[156,157] The only drug of this group demonstrating significant response was doxorubicin. Two of 15 patients (13%) responded to therapy with this drug.[157] All of the other drugs under evaluation by the GITSG were inactive.

Further evaluation of classic alkylating agents needs to be performed in pancreatic cancer. There is one current study being carried out by the Eastern Cooperative Oncology Group which compares L-phenylalanine mustard to combination chemotherapy regimens. The results of this well-controlled study will be of interest in defining the role L-phenylalanine mustard in this disease.

It should be clear that there are relative paucities of single agent chemotherapy data in patients with pancreatic adenocarcinoma. There are only three drugs reported in the literature in which response rates greater than 20% were seen when greater than 20 patients were evaluated.[143] It is, therefore, incumbent on oncologists to continue well-designed Phase II single agent trials in this disease, such as those being carried out by the GITSG.

COMBINATION CHEMOTHERAPY STUDIES

Even with the small numbers of active single agents available, there has been continued interest in combination chemotherapy trials in pancreatic adenocarcinoma. This subject has been well reviewed recently.[27,146] Table 18-13 gives an overview of the more recently reported results of combinations of antineoplastic agents in pancreatic cancer.

Two Phase II trials are of considerable interest. Wiggans and coworkers combined the three most active single agents, 5-FU, mitomycin-C, and streptozotocin (SMF) into a well-tolerated combination regimen.[158] The mitomycin-C was used as a single dose every 8 weeks; the regimen was generally well tolerated (*i.e.,* response rate of 43% was obtained in 23 patients on this regimen). It should be noted that the patients in this series had good performance status with 20 of 33 (87%) being ambulatory. Of significance was the finding of complete regression of biopsy proven liver metastases in one of Wiggans' patients. This patient was reported to be alive, free of disease, and off therapy $3\frac{1}{2}$ years after diagnosis.[158] The major toxicities associated with the regimen were nausea, vomiting, and nephropathy from the streptozotocin.

Partially in response to the nephrotoxicity induced by streptozotocin, a regimen substituting doxorubicin for streptozotocin was developed. This program of 5-FU, doxorubicin, and mitomycin-C (FAM) produced objective responses in ten of 25 patients (40%).[159] One-quarter of these patients had poor performance status and were bed-ridden greater than 50% of the time, a category of patients that normally does very poorly with chemotherapy. The FAM and SMF regimens are currently being evaluated in Phase III trials by the GITSG.

There are several other moderately active combination regimens in pancreatic cancer. 5-FU and BCNU have been evaluated in Phase II and Phase III trials.[154,160] In a Phase III trial, Kovach and coworkers found the combination of 5-FU + BCNU produced responses in ten of 30 patients (33%).[154] This was superior to 5-FU or BCNU used alone. However, there was no improvement in survival of patients treated with combination compared to the survival of those treated with the single agents. Lokich confirmed the activity of 5-FU + BCNU in a Phase II trial.[160] Four of 15 patients (27%) in this series had evidence of partial response to the combination.

Combinations of 5-FU and methyl-CCNU or mitomycin-C have been evaluated by Buroker and coworkers.[161] These workers administered 5-FU by continuous IV infusion. Bu-

TABLE 18-13. Combination Chemotherapy in Pancreatic Cancer

COMBINATION	NUMBER OF RESPONSES	RESPONSE RATE	REFERENCE
Streptozotocin + Mitomycin-C + 5-FU	10/23	43	158
5-FU + Doxorubicin + Mitomycin-C	10/25	40	159
5-FU + BCNU	10/30	33	154
5-FU + BCNU	4/15	27	160
5-FU + Streptozotocin + Mitomycin-C	5/16	31	162
5-FU + MeCCNU	–	17	161
5-FU + Mitomycin-C	–	30	161
5-FU + Spironolactone	80	–	165
5-FU + Testolactone	10/13	77	163

roker and coworkers did not report the number of patients evaluable for response and only reported response rates with the two regimens being treated. The combination of 5-FU + mitomycin-C induced objective regression in 30% of patients whereas the 5-FU + methyl-CCNU regimen caused objective regression in 17% ($p = 0.03$) of patients. These data, obtained in a randomized trial of 143 patients, confirm the relatively high order of activity of 5-FU + mitomycin-C containing regimens.

Another study suggesting a high order of activity of a 5-FU + mitomycin-C containing regimen has been published by Aberhalden and coworkers.[162] In this study, a 5-FU, streptozotocin, and mitomycin-C regimen was evaluated in 16 patients with advanced pancreatic cancer. The scheduling of this SMF regimen was different from that reported by Wiggans and coworkers and five of 16 patients (31%) responded.[162]

In 1973, Waddell reported a ten of 13 (77%) response rate in patients treated with a combination of 5-FU + testolactone or testolactone and spironolactone.[163] There was preclinical evidence suggesting that testolactone had the potential to synergize with 5-FU.[164] The lactones can inhibit the enzyme aspartate transcarbamylase, an enzyme catalysing an early step in pyrimidine biosynthesis. Waddell's study was a Phase II study in a small number of patients and compared survival to a historic control group treated with 5-FU + warfarin (Coumadin). However, the median survival of patients treated with 5-FU + lactone was reported in excess of 31 months; for this reason, a Phase III trial was mounted by the Eastern Cooperative Oncology Group. The results of this trial, published in 1978 by Moertel and colleagues, showed that lactones add nothing to the efficacy of combination chemotherapy in pancreatic cancer.[165] The median survival of treatment groups, whether or not they received lactone, was only 15 weeks.

It is now clear that useful data are to be obtained from carefully performed combination chemotherapy studies in patients with advanced pancreatic cancer. It is obvious that the state of the art of chemotherapy, either by single agent or combination of agents, will not make dramatic advances until more active drugs are developed. However, it is also evident that adequate data are available to suggest that combinations of 5-FU + mitomycin-C have a relatively high order of activity in this disease and variation on this theme should be pursued.

RECOMMENDED THERAPY

Since it is likely that combination chemotherapy is superior to single agent treatment in response rate in advanced pancreatic cancer, patients should be treated with combinations of known activity when not entered into clinical trials. The combination of 5-FU, doxorubicin, and mitomycin-C (FAM) represents a well-tolerated combination chemotherapy program that produces objective remission in 40% of patients.[159] The dose and schedule of this regimen are outlined elsewhere (see Chapter 17). Since many patients with pancreatic cancer will have had previous abdominal radiation therapy, it is important to be aware that prior irradiation decreases the hematologic tolerance to FAM. Irradiated patients should be started at a 25% decreased FAM dosage.

FUTURE DIRECTIONS

DIAGNOSIS

It must clearly be understood that although advances have been made in the therapy of pancreatic cancer, the disease is still poorly treatable. In a malignancy such as carcinoma of the pancreas that is difficult to treat at time of diagnosis, it is obviously critical to attempt to develop methods of diagnosis that will allow the clinician to discover disease at an earlier and hopefully more curable stage. Since all the imaging techniques discussed in this chapter depend on alteration of the pancreatic contour or disturbances in pancreatic vascular physiology and anatomy, it is apparent that such techniques depend on the tumor being grossly apparent before it will be detected. True early detection will depend on work aimed at detecting marker substances produced by early-stage pancreatic cancer. The work of POA is an initial step in this direction.[84]

TREATMENT

Resectable Lesions

For lesions that are theoretically resectable, data from MGH and other surgical series indicate that operation alone is inadequate treatment in a majority of patients. The protocols under study by the GITSG and other study groups may determine whether adjuvant radiation or chemotherapy can alter failure patterns and improve survival rates in this group, provided an adequate number of cases can be accrued. If the use of specialized beams (helium, mixed neutron and photon, pi-meson, proton) or techniques (intra-operative implant or electrons alone or in combination with external beam irradiation) yield superb results in the unresectable group, there is a definite possibility that some of these methods should be randomized against radical operation ± adjuvant radiochemotherapy for even potentially resectable lesions.

Unresectable Localized Lesions

Both chemotherapy and radiotherapy options are improving. Two three-drug regimens now exist that produce promising response rates in advanced disease. Radiation for localized but unresectable disease has resulted in excellent palliation and some long-term cures in a variety of series, as previously described. Survival in most randomized and nonrandomized series is best in patients treated with a combination of XRT + 5-FU.

Analysis of patterns of failure and complications after treatment may give direction to future treatment options regarding disease control and improved therapeutic ratios of disease control vs. complications. Local regional control was only approximately 50% even in the 6000–7000 rad in 7–9 week group reported by Dobelbower and coworkers (distant metastases ≃ 25%).[127] This was increased to 75% in the MGH series, combining I^{125} implant followed by external beam; however, seven patients had already developed distant metastases at the time of the report (58.3% of the entire group of 12; 77.7% of the nine with failure).[133] Shipley felt the I^{125}

implant may be increasing the incidence of distant metastases by tumor manipulation and recommends some degree of preoperative XRT to decrease implantability as well as the use of systemic chemotherapy to those groups who would pursue this technique. Dobelbower has an ongoing pilot study combining an I^{125} implant with his previous 6000–7000 rad external beam dose in an attempt to improve local control. Since his previous external beam dose may border on or exceed long-term tolerance (were a larger percentage of patients to survive 18 to 36 months), this pilot study must be watched very carefully. Future studies will undoubtedly attempt to fine tune local control with the various techniques including implants, high LET radiation, radiation + sensitizing drugs, and intra-operative radiation.

However, with the best local control, unacceptable percentages of distant failure (25–50%) exist. While some of these may result from persistent local disease, a large percentage undoubtedly exist as undiagnosed micrometastases in the liver or peritoneal cavity at initial operation. If combined drug chemotherapy alone, or preferably in combination with aggressive local-regional radiation, does not alter the systemic course of the disease, the option of using upper abdominal or even total abdominal irradiation for a portion of treatment may be evaluated, since pancreas failures are primarily abdominal, and, more specifically, upper abdominal if the initial lesion is in the head. In an attempt to decrease distant metastases and improve patient survival, studies evaluating the sequencing of combination chemotherapy and radiation should be pursued.

Newer approaches to radiation treatment may decrease therapy-associated complications. Gastric and some duodenal complications were seen in most series that reported some long-term survivors. While external beam techniques can minimize the amount of stomach within the field, total exclusion is impossible since the risk of marginal recurrence would increase. With the combined external beam-intraoperative techniques, the dose-limiting structures can be included within a tumor-nodal volume to 4500–5000 rad for 5–6 weeks. One can then exclude stomach from the final boost with intraoperative electrons and can minimize the dose with I^{125} by developing an omental flap between the posterior gastric wall and the pancreatic implant to increase distance and decrease dose. Gastroenterostomies are usually done electively to reduce the risk of symptomatic long-term duodenal problems.

Many treatment options exist that were not available 5–10 years ago. The bulk of disease that exists with the unresectable lesions may still limit the amount of gain, but it appears that discernable gains should be attainable with an acceptable risk of morbidity. If these same tools could be applied to earlier disease, the amount of therapeutic gain should be even more striking.

REFERENCES

1. Silverberg E: Cancer statistics. CA 30:23, 1980.
2. Young JL Jr, Asire AJ, Pollack ES: SEER Program: Cancer Incidence and Mortality in the United States 1973–1976. Bethesda, United States Department of Health, Education, and Welfare, 1978
3. Handley WS: Pancreatic cancer and its treatment by implanted radium. Ann Surg 100:215, 1934
4. Moertel CG: Exocrine pancreas. In Holland JF, Frei E III (eds): Cancer Medicine, p 1559. Lea & Febiger, Philadelphia, 1973
5. Cubilla AL, Fitzgerald PJ: Cancer of the pancreas (non-endocrine): a suggested morphologic clarification. Semin Oncol 6:285, 1979
6. Cubilla AL, Fitzgerald PJ: Morphological patterns of non-endocrine human carcinoma. Cancer Res 35:2246, 1975
7. Cubilla AL, Fitzgerald PJ: Duct cell adenocarcinoma. In Sommers SC, Rosen PP (eds): Pancreas Cancer: Pathology Annual, Part I, p 241. New York, Appelton-Century-Crofts, 1978
8. Cubilla AL, Fitzgerald PJ: Morphologic lesions associated with human primary invasive non-endocrine pancreas cancer. Cancer Res 36:2690, 1976
9. Bell ET: Carcinoma of the pancreas; I. A clinical and pathologic study of 609 necropsied cases, II. The relation of carcinoma of the pancreas to diabetes mellitus. Am J Pathol 33:499, 1957
10. Coutsofitides T, Macdonald J, Shibata HR: Carcinoma of the pancreas and periampullary region: a 41-year experience. Ann Surg 196:730, 1977
11. Gray LW Jr, Crook JN, Cohn I Jr: Carcinoma of the pancreas. In Seventh National Cancer Conference Proceedings, pp 503–510. New York, American Cancer Society, 1973
12. Gudjonsson B, Livstone EM, Spiro HM: Cancer of the pancreas: diagnostic accuracy and survival statistics. Cancer 42:2494, 1978
13. Howard JM, Jordan GL Jr: Cancer of the pancreas. Current Probl Cancer 2:1, 1977
14. Nakase A, Matsumoto Y, Uchida K et al: Surgical treatment of cancer of the pancreas and the periampullary region: cumulative results in 57 institutions in Japan. Ann Surg 185:52, 1977
15. Robertston JC, Eeles GH: Syndrome associated with pancreatic acinar cell carcinoma. Br J Med 2:709, 1970
16. Campagno J, Oertel J: Mucinous cystic neoplasms of the pancreas with overt and latent malignancy (cystadenocarcinoma and cystademona). Am J Clin Pathol 69:573, 1978
17. Cullen PK Jr, Remine WH, Dahlin DC: A clinical pathologic study of cystadenocarcinoma of the pancreas. Surg Gynecol Obstet 117:189, 1963
18. Cubilla AL, Fitzgerald PJ: Metastasis in pancreatic duct adenocarcinoma. In Day SB, Myers WPL, Stansly P et al (eds): Cancer Invasion and Metastasis: Biologic Mechanisms and Therapy, pp 81–94. New York, Raven Press, 1977
19. Cubilla AL, Fortner J, Fitzgerald PJ: Lymph node involvement in carcinoma of the head of the pancreas area. Cancer 41:880, 1978
20. Evans BP, Ochsner A: The gross anatomy of the lymphatics of the human pancreas. Surgery 36:177, 1954
21. Falconer CWA, Griffiths E: The anatomy of the blood vessels in the region of the pancreas. Br J Surg 37:334, 1950
22. Fortner JG: Regional resection of cancer of the pancreas: a new surgical approach. Surgery 73:307, 1973
23. Pierson JM: The arterial blood supply of the pancreas. Surg Gynecol Obstet 77:426, 1943
24. Rouviere H: Anatomy of the Human Lymphatic System, pp 197–205. Ann Arbor, Edwards Brothers, 1938
25. DieGoyanes A, Pack GT, Bowden L: Cancer of the body and tail of the pancreas. Rev Surg 28:153, 1971
26. Cohn I Jr: The meaning of lymph nodes and their effective treatment as related to stomach, pancreas, and small bowel. In Metastasis in the Lymphatic System. Boston, GK Hall, (in press)
27. Macdonald JS, Widerlite L, Schein PS: Biopsy, diagnosis, and chemotherapeutic managemen of pancreatic malignancy. Adv Pharmacol Chemother 14:107, 1977
28. Go VL, DiMagno E: Efforts at early diagnosis of pancreatic cancer: the Mayo Clinic experience. International Meeting on Pancreatic Cancer, New Orleans, LA, March 10–11, 1980
29. Kawanishi H, Pollard HM: Endoscopic evaluation of cancer of the pancreas. Semin Oncol 6:309, 1979
30. Levin B, ReMine WH, Herman RE et al: Cancer of the pancreas. Am J Surg 135:185, 1978

31. Moossa AR, Levin B: Collaborative studies in the diagnosis of pancreatic cancer. Semin Oncol 6:298, 1979
32. Fras I, Litin EM, Bartholomew LG: Mental symptoms as an aid in the early diagnosis of carcinoma of the pancreas. Gastroenterology 55:191, 1968
33. Pietri H, Sahel J, Scules H: Diagnosis of cancer of the pancreas by echotomography, endoscopic pancreatography, arteriography and other means. In Jerzy Glass GB (ed): Progress in Gastroenterology, Vol III, p 617. New York, Grune & Stratton, 1977
34. Sack GH, Levin J, Bell WR: Trousseau's syndrome and other manifestations of chronic disseminated coagulopathy in patients with neoplasms: clinical pathophysiologic and therapeutic features. Medicine 56:1, 1977
35. Rosch J: Radiological diagnosis of pancreatic cancer. J Surg Oncol 7:121, 1975
36. Rennell CL: Diagnostic value of hypotonic duodenography. Am J Roentgenol Radium Ther Nucl Med 121:256, 1974
37. Shirley DV: Hypotonic duodenography in suspected pancreatic disease. Br J Radiol 47:437, 1974
38. King DL: Diagnostic Ultrasound, pp. 31–35. St Louis, C.V. Mosby, 1974
39. Birnholz JC: Sonic differentiation of cysts and homogeneous solid masses. Radiology 108:699, 1978
40. Carlsen EN: Ultrasound physics for the physician: a brief review. J Clin Ultrasound 3:69, 1975
41. Johnson ML, Mack LA: Ultrasonic evaluation of the pancreas. Gastrointest Radiol 3:257, 1978
42. Burger J, Blauenstein UW: Current aspects of ultransonic scanning of the pancreas. Am J Roentgenol 122:406, 1974
43. Filly RA, Freimanis AR: Echographic diagnosis of pancreatic lesions. Radiology 96:575, 1970
43a. Ostrum BJ, Goldberg BB, Isard HJ: A-mode ultrasound differentiation of soft-tissue masses. Radiology 88:745, 1967
44. Robbins AH, Gerlof SG, Pugatch RD: Newer imaging techniques for the diagnosis of pancreatic cancer. Semin Oncol 6:332, 1979
45. Sheedy PF II, Stephens DH, Hattery RR: Computed tomography in the evaluation of patients with suspected carcinoma of the pancreas. Radiology 124:731, 1977
46. Stanley RJ, Sagel SS, Levitt RG: Computed tomographic evaluation of the pancreas. Radiology 124:715, 1977
47. Marshall WH, Brieman RS, Harell GS: Computed tomography of abdominal paraaortic lymph node disease: preliminary observations with a 6 second scanner. Am J Roentgenol 128:759, 1977
48. Ferrucci JT Jr, Wittenberg J: CT biopsy of abdominal tumors: aids for lesion localization. Radiology 129:739, 1978
49. Haaga JR, Alfidi RJ: Precise biopsy localization by computed tomography. Radiology 118:603, 1976
50. Haaga JR, Reich NE, Havrilla TR et al: CT guided biopsy. Cleve Clin Q 44:27, 1977
51. Hancke S, Holm HH, Kock F: Ultrasonically guided percutaneous fine needle biopsy of pancreas. Surg Gynecol Obstet 140:361, 1975
52. Smith EH, Bartrum RJ, Chang YC et al: Percutaneous aspiration biopsy of the pancreas under ultrasonic guidance. N Engl J Med 292:825, 1975
53. Goldstein HM, Zornoza J, Wallace S et al: Percutaneous fine needle aspiration biopsy of pancreatic and other abdominal masses. Radiology 123:319, 1977
54. Kline T, Neal HS: Needle aspiration biopsy: a critical appraisal. JAMA 239:36, 1978
55. Goldstein HM, Neiman HL, Bookstein JJ: Angiographic evaluation of pancreatic disease. Radiology 112:275, 1974
56. Paul RE, Miller HH, Kahn PG et al: Pancreatic angiography, with application of subselective angiography of the celiac or superior mesenteric artery to the diagnosis of carcinoma of the pancreas. N Engl J Med 272:283, 1965
57. Rosch J, Keller FS, Bilbao MK: Radiologic diagnosis of pancreatic cancer. Semin Oncol 6:318, 1979
58. Eisenberg H: Angiography of the pancreas. In Hilal SK (ed): Small Vessel Angiography, pp 405–433. St Louis, C.V. Mosby, 1973
59. Herlinger H, Finlay DBL: Evaluation and follow-up of pancreatic arteriograms: a new role for angiography in the diagnosis of carcinoma of the pancrease. Clin Radiol 29:277, 1978
60. Reuter SR: Superselective pancreatic angiography. In Anacker H (ed): Efficiency and Limits of Radiologic Examination of the Pancreas, pp 149–158. Stuttgart, G. Thieme, 1975
61. Kaplan JH Bookstein JJ: Abdominal visceral pharmacoangiography with angiotensin. Radiology 103:79, 1972
62. Kaude JW, Wirtanen GW: Celiac epinephrine enhanced angiography. Am J Roentgenol 110:818, 1970
63. Uden R: Secretin and epinephrine combined in celiac angiography. Acta Radiol [Diagn] (Stockh) 17:17, 1976
64. Tylen U: Accuracy of angiography in the diagnosis of carcinoma of the pancreas. Acta Radiol [Diagn] (Stockh) 14:449, 1973
65. Bookstein JH, Reuter SB, Martel W: Angiographic evaluation of pancreatic carcinoma. Radiology 93:757, 1969
66. MacGregor AM, Hawkins IF: Selective pharmacodynamic angiography in the diagnosis of carcinoma of the pancreas. Surg Gynecol Obstet 137:917, 1973
67. Suzuki T, Kawabe K, Imamura M et al: Survival of patients with cancer of the pancreas in relation to findings on arteriography. Ann Surg 176:37, 1972
68. Tylen U, Arnesjo B: Resectability and prognosis of carcinoma of the pancreas evaluated by angiography. Scand J Gastroenterol 8:691, 1973
69. Ferrucci JT, Wittenberg J, Sarno RA: Fine needle transhepatic cholangiograph: a new approach to obstructive jaundice. Am J Roentgenol 127:403, 1976
70. Pereiras R Jr, Chiprut RO, Greenwald RA: Percutaneous transhepatic cholangiography with the "skinny" needle. Ann Intern Med 86:562, 1977
71. Zimmon DS, Breslaw J, Kessler RE: Endoscopy with endoscopic cholangiopancreatography. JAMA 233:447, 1975
72. Anacker H, Weiss HD, Kramann B et al: Experience with endoscopic retrograde pancreatography. Am J Roentgenol Radium Ther Nucl Med 122:375, 1974
73. Belsito AA, Cramer GG, Dickinson PB: Delayed ductal drainage: an endoscopic pancreatographic sign of carcinoma of the head of the pancreas. Am J Roentgenol Radium Ther Nucl Med 119:109, 1973
74. Ogoshi K, Masajuki N, Hara Y et al: Endoscopic pancreatocholangiography in the evaluation of pancreatic and biliary disease. Gastroenterology 64:210, 1973
75. Stadelmann P, Safrany A, Loffler A et al: Endoscopic retrograde cholangiopancreatography in the diagnosis of pancreatic cancer: experience with 54 cases. Endoscopy 6:84, 1974
76. Kawanishi H, Sell JE, Pollard HM: Carcinoembryonic antigen and cytology of pancreatic fluid. Gastroenterology 68:923, 1975
77. Endo Y, Moril T, Tamura H et al: Cytodiagnosis of pancreatic malignant tumors by aspiration, under direct vision, using a duodenal fiberscope. Gastroenterology 67:944, 1974
78. Nakano S, Horiguchi Y, Takeda T et al: Comparative diagnostic value of endoscopic pancreatography and pancreatic function tests. Scand J Gastroenterol 9:383, 1974
79. Osnes M, Serck-Hanssen A, Myren J: Endoscopic retrograde brush cytology (ERBC) of the biliary and pancreatic ducts. Scand J Gastroenterol 73:1381, 1976
80. Ona F, Dhar P, Moore TL: Carcinoembryonic antigen (CEA) in the diagnosis of pancreatic cancer. Cancer 31:324, 1973
81. Delwiche R, Zamcheck N, Marcon N: Carcinoembryonic antigen in pancreatitis. Cancer 31:328, 1973
82. McIntire KR, Waldmann TA, Moertel CG et al: Serum α-fetoprotein in patients with neoplasms of the gastrointestinal tract. Cancer Res 35:991, 1975
83. Banwo O, Versey J, Hobbs JR: New oncofetal antigen for human pancreas. Lancet 1:643, 1974
84. Gelder FB, Reese CJ, Moosa AR et al: Purification, partial characterization, and clinical evaluation of a pancreatic oncofetal antigen. Cancer Res 38:313, 1978
85. Reddi KK, Holland JF: Elevated serum ribonuclease in patients with pancreatic cancer. Proc Natl Acad Sci USA 73:2308, 1976
86. Podolsky DK, Weiser MM: Galactosyltransferase isoenzyme II:

correlation with extent of gastrointestinal malignancy and prediction of recurrence. Gastroenterology 74:1140, 1978
87. Holyoke ED, Douglass HO, Goldrosen MH et al: Tumor markers in pancreatic cancer. Semin Oncol 6:347, 1979
88. DiMagno EP, Malagelada JR, Taylor WF et al: A prospective comparison of current diagnostic tests for pancreatic cancer. N Engl J Med 297:737, 1977
89. Hall TJ, Cooper M, Hughes RG: Pancreatic cancer screening-analysis of the problem and the role of radionuclide imaging. Am J Surg 134:544, 1977
90. Isaacson R, Weiland LH, McIlrath DC: Biopsy of the pancreas. Arch Surg 109:227, 1974
91. Whipple AO, Parsons WB, Mullins CR: Treatment of carcinoma of the ampulla of Vater. Ann Surg 102:763, 1935
92. Cattell RB, Warren KW: Surgery of the Pancreas. Philadelphia, WB Saunders, 1953
93. Forrest JR, Longmire WP Jr: Carcinoma of the pancreas and periampullary region: a study of 279 patients. Ann Surg 189:129, 1979
94. Jordan GL Jr: Benign and malignant tumors of the pancreas and the periampullary region, II. Malignancies of the pancreas. In Howard JM, Jordan GL (eds): Surgical Diseases of the Pancreas, pp 451–498. Philadelphia, JB Lippincott, 1960
95. Longmire WP Jr: The technique of pancreaticoduodenal resection. Surgery 59:344, 1966
96. Longmire WP Jr: The Whipple procedure and/or other standard operative approaches to pancreatic cancer. International Meeting on Pancreatic Cancer, New Orleans, March 10–11, 1980
97. Monge JJ, Judd ES, Gage RP: Radical pancreatoduodenectomy: a 22-year experience with the complications, mortality rate, and survival rate. Ann Surg 160:711, 1964
98. Whipple AO: Observations on radical surgery for lesions of the pancreas. Surg Gynecol Obstet 82:623, 1946
99. Rockey WE: Total pancreatectomy for carcinoma: case report. Ann Surg 118:603, 1943
100. Waugh JM: Radical resection of head of pancreas and total pancreatectomy. JAMA 137:141, 1948
101. Gaston EA: Total pancreatectomy. N Engl J Med 238:345, 1948
102. Brooks JR, Culebras JM: Cancer of the pancreas: palliative operation, Whipple procedure, or total pancreatectomy? Am J Surg 131:516, 1976
103. Hicks RE, Brooks JR: Total pancreatectomy for ductal carcinoma. Surg Gynecol Obstet 133:16, 1971
104. Holyoke ED: New surgical approaches to pancreatic cancer. International Meeting on Pancreatic Cancer, New Orleans, March 10–11, 1980
105. Ihse I, Lilja P, Arnesjo B et al: Total pancreatectomy for cancer: An appraisal of 65 cases. Ann Surg 186:675, 1977
106. Matsui Y, Aoki Y, Ishikawa O et al: Ductal carcinoma of the pancrease: rationales for total pancreatectomy. Arch Surg 114:722, 1979
107. ReMine WH: Total pancreatectomy for pancreatic cancer. International Meeting on Pancreatic Cancer, New Orleans, March 10–11, 1980
108. ReMine WH, Priestley JT, Judd ES et al: Total pancreatectomy. Ann Surg 172:595, 1970
109. Tryka AF, Brooks JR: Histopathology in the evaluation of total pancreatectomy for ductal carcinoma. Ann Surg 190:373, 1979
110. Fortner J: Regional pancreatectomy and other radical surgical approaches to pancreatic cancer. International Meeting on Pancreatic Cancer, New Orleans, March 10–11, 1980
111. Fortner JG, Kim DK, Cubilla A et al: Regional pancreatectomy: en block pancreatic, portal vein, and lymph node resection. Ann Surg 186:42, 1977
112. Hansson JA, Hoevels J, Simert G et al: Clinical aspects of nonsurgical percutaneous transhepatic bile drainage in obstructive lesions of the extrahepatic bile ducts. Ann Surg 189:58, 1979
113. Traverso LW, Longmire WP Jr: Preservation of the pylorus in pancreaticoduodenectomy: a followup evaluation. American Surgical Association Annual Meeting, Atlanta, April 23–25, 1980
114. Brooks JR: Operative approach to pancreatic carcinoma. Semin Oncol 6:357, 1979
115. Abe M, Takahashi M, Yabumoto E et al: Clinical experiences with intraoperative radiotherapy of locally advanced cancers. Cancer 45:40, 1980
116. Dobelbower RR Jr: Current radiotherapeutic approaches to pancreatic cancer. International Meeting on Pancreatic Cancer, New Orleans, March 10–11, 1980
117. Dobelbower RR Jr: The radiotherapy of pancreatic cancer. Semin Oncol 6:378, 1979
118. Dobelbower RR Jr, Borgelt BB, Suntharalingam N et al: Pancreatic carcinoma treated with high-dose, small-volume irradiation. Cancer 41:1087, 1978
119. Goldson A: The role of operative radiotherapy for pancreatic cancer. International Meeting on Pancreatic Cancer, New Orleans, March 10–11, 1980
119a. Tepper J, Nardi G, Suit H: Carcinoma of the pancreas. Review of MGH experience: Indications for radiation therapy. Cancer 37:1519, 1976
120. Billingsley JS, Bartholomew LG, Childs DS Jr: A study of radiation therapy in carcinoma of the pancreas. Staff Meetings of the Mayo Clinic 33:426, 1958
121. Moertel CG: Childs DS, Reitemeier RJ et al: Combined 5-fluorouracil and supervoltage radiation therapy of locally unresectable gastrointestinal cancer. Lancet 2:865, 1969
122. Miller TR, Fuller LM: Radiation therapy of carcinoma of the pancreas: report on 91 cases. Am J Roentgenol Rad Ther Nucl Med 80:787, 1958
123. Green N, Beron E, Melbye RW et al: Carcinoma of the pancreas: palliative radiotherapy. Am J Roentgenol Rad Ther Nucl Med 117:620, 1973
124. Komaki R, Wilson JF, Cox JD: Carcinoma of the pancreas: results of conventional irradiation for unresectable lesions (abstr). Int J Radiat Oncol Biol Phys 4:138, 1978
125. Gastrointestinal Tumor Study Group: Comparative therapeutic trial of radiation with or without chemotherapy in pancreatic carcinoma. Int J Radiat Oncol Biol Phys 5:1643, 1979
126. Haslam JB, Cavanaugh PJ, Stroup SL: Radiation therapy in the treatment of irresectable adenocarcinoma of the pancreas. Cancer 32:1341, 1973
127. Dobelbower RR Jr, Strubler KA Suntharalingam N: Treatment of cancer of the pancreas with high-energy photons and electrons. Int J Radiat Oncol Biol Phys 1:141, 1977
128. Falkson G, Falkson HC, Fichardt T: Combined telecobalt and 5-fluorouracil therapy in carcinoma of the pancreas: a report of 97 cases. S Afr Med J 44:444, 1970
129. Lemon HM, Foley JF, Paustian FF et al: Improved palliation of pancreatic carcinoma. Cancer 31:17, 1973
130. Moertel CG, Lokich JJ, Childs DS et al: An evaluation of high dose radiation and combined radiation and 5-flourouracil (5-FU) therapy for locally unresectable pancreatic carcinoma (abstr). Proc Am Soc Clin Oncol 17:244, 1976
131. Pilepich MV, Miller HH, McCauley SE: Preoperative radiotherapy in carcinoma of the pancreas (abstr). Int J Radiat Oncol Biol Phys 4:116, 1978
132. Hilaris BS, Roussis K: Cancer of the pancreas. In Hilaris B (ed): Handbook of Interstitial Brachytherapy, pp 251–262. Acton, Publishing Sciences Group, 1975
133. Shipley WU, Nardi GL, Cohen AM et al: Iodine-125 implant and external beam irradiation in patients with localized pancreatic carcinoma: a comparative study to surgical resection. Cancer 45:709, 1980
134. Abe M, Takahashi M, Yabumoto E et al: Techniques, indications and results of intraoperative radiotherapy of advanced cancers. Radiology 116:693, 1975
135. Hiraoka T, Nakagawa I, Tashiro S et al: Intraoperative irradiation therapy for unresectable pancreatic cancer. J Jpn Soc Cancer Ther 13:146, 1975
136. Gunderson LL, Shipley WU, Suit HD et al: Intraoperative irradiation: a pilot study combining external beam photons with "boost" dose intraoperative electrons: 1979 ASTR Proceedings. Int J Radiat Oncol Biol Phys 5:95, 1979
137. Tepper J, Sindelm W, Glatstein E: Phase I study of intraoperative radiation therapy combined with radical surgery for intra-abdominal malignancies. Proc Am Soc Clin Oncol 21:395, 1980
138. Smith F, Woolley P, Rogers C et al: Fast neutron therapy (FN)

for locally advanced pancreatic carcinoma (LAP). Proc Am Soc Clin Oncol 21:367, 1980

139. Al-Abdulla ASM, Hussey DH, Olson MH et al: Preliminary results of pancreatic carcinoma treated with combined x-ray and fast neutrons: 1979 ASTR Proceedings. Int J Radiat Oncol Biol Phys 5:163, 1979
140. Quivey JM, Castro JR, Chen GTY et al: Helium ion radiotherapy in the treatment of pancreatic carcinoma. Proc Am Soc Clin Oncol 12:416, 1980
141. Childs DS: Role of radiation therapist in palliative management. In Moertel CG, Reitermeier RJ (eds): Advanced Gastrointestinal Cancer: Clinical Management and Chemotherapy, p 58. New York, Harper & Row, 1979
142. Moertel CG: Chemotherapy of gastrointestinal cancer. N Engl J Med 299:1049, 1978
143. Carter SK, Comis RL: Adenocarcinoma of the pancreas, prognostic variables, and criteria of response. In Staquet MJ (ed): Cancer Therapy: Prognostic Factors and Criteria of Response, p 237. New York, Raven Press, 1975
144. Macdonald JS, Widerlite L, Schein PS: Current diagnosis and management of pancreatic carcinoma. JNCI 56:1093, 1976
145. Fitzgerald PJ: The value of diagnostic aids in detecting pancreas cancer. Cancer 41:868, 1978
146. Smith FP, Schein PS: Chemotherapy of pancreatic cancer. Semin Oncol 6:368, 1979
147. Zelen M: Keynote address of biostatistics and data retrieval. Cancer Chemother Rep 4 (part 3):31, 1973
148. Moertel CG, Mittelman JA, Bakemeir RF et al: Sequential and combination chemotherapy of advanced gastric cancer. Cancer 38:678, 1976
149. Moertel CG, Reitemeier RJ, Hahn RG: Therapy with mitomycin-C. In Moertel CG, Reitemeier RJ (eds): Advanced Gastrointestinal Cancer: Clinical Management and Chemotherapy, p 168. New York, Harper & Row, 1969
150. Macdonald JS, Woolley PV, Smythe T et al: 5-fluorouracil, adriamycin and mitomycin-C (FAM) combination chemotherapy in the treatment of advanced gastric cancer. Cancer 44:42, 1979
151. Broder LE, Carter SK: Streptozotocin: Clinical Brochure. Bethesda, Therapy Evaluation Program, National Cancer Institute, 1971
152. Dupriest RW, Hintington M, Massey WH et al: Streptozotocin therapy in 22 cancer patients. Cancer 35:358, 1974
153. Stolkinoky DC, Sadoff L, Braunwald J et al: Streptozotocin in the treatment of cancer. Cancer 30:61, 1972
154. Kovach JS, Moertel CG, Schutt AJ et al: A controlled study of combined 1,3-Bis (2-chloroethyl)-1-nitrosourea and 5-fluorouracil therapy for advanced gastric and pancreatic cancer. Cancer 33:563, 1974
155. Douglass HO Jr, Lavin PT, Moertel CG: Nitrosoureas: useful agents for treatment of advanced gastrointestinal cancer. Cancer Treat Rep 60:769, 1976
156. Kaplan RS: Phase II trial of ICRF-159, β-deoxythioguanosine, β-2TGdR and galactitol in advanced measurable pancreatic carcinoma: A study of the GITSG. Proc Am Soc Clin Oncol 19:335, 1978
157. Schein PS, Lavin PT, Moertel CG: Randomized phase II clinical trial of adriamycin in advanced measurable pancreatic carcinoma: a Gastrointestinal Tumor Study Group report. Cancer 42:19, 1978
158. Wiggans G, Woolley PV, Macdonald JS et al: Phase II trial of streptozotocin, mitomycin-C and 5-fluorouracil (SMF) in the treatment of advanced pancreatic cancer. Cancer 41:387, 1978
159. Smith FP, Macdonald JS, Woolley PV et al: Phase II evaluation of FAM, 5-fluorouracil (F), adriamycin (A) and mitomycin-C (M) in advanced pancreatic cancer. Proc Am Soc Clin Oncol 20:415, 1979
160. Lokich JJ, Skarin AT: Combination therapy with 5-fluorouracil (5-FU) and 1,3-Bis(2-chlorethyl)-1-nitrosourea (BCNU) for disseminated gastrointestinal carcinoma. Cancer Chemother Rep 56:653, 1973
161. Buroker T, Kim PN, Heilbrun L et al: 5-FU infusion with mitomycin-C (MMC) vs 5-FU infusion with methyl CCNU (Me) in the treatment of advanced upper gastrointestinal cancer. Proc Am Soc Clin Oncol 19:310, 1978
162. Aberhalden RT, Bukowski RM, Groppe CW et al: Streptozotocin (STZ) and 5-fluorouracil (5-FU) with and without mitomycin-C (Mito) in the treatment of pancreatic adenocarcinoma. Proc Am Soc Clin Oncol 18:301, 1977
163. Waddell WR: Chemotherapy for carcinoma of the pancreas. Surgery 74:420, 1973
164. Van Rymenant M, Keymolen P, Procheret J et al: Action of testosterone and testolactone on isocitric dehydrogenase, aspartate transcarbamylase and gluconate. Acta Endocrinol (Copenh) 66:498, 1971
165. Moertel CG, Lavin PT: An evaluation of 5-FU, nitrosourea and lactone combinations in the therapy of upper gastrointestinal cancer. Proc Am Soc Clin Oncol 18:344, 1977

John S. Macdonald
Leonard L. Gunderson
Martin A. Adson

CHAPTER 19

Cancer of the Hepatobiliary System

Primary cancers of the liver and biliary passages are relatively uncommon tumors in the United States. It was estimated that these diseases would account for 11,600 new cases in 1980.[1] Although this number is less than 10% of the patients seen each year with new cases of either breast or lung cancer, tumors of the liver and biliary tract are significant because they are highly lethal. The fatality/case ratio with this group of diseases is 0.9.[1] Because primary liver cancers and tumors of the gallbladder and bile ducts are frequently considered collectively for incidence, it is difficult to present totally accurate figures on the occurrence of these tumors. It appears, however, that gallbladder cancer is the most common of these tumors and causes 4000 to 6000 deaths per year.[2,3] The next most common disease is hepatocellular cancer, causing 3000 to 4000 deaths per year; the least common hepatobiliary cancer is cholangiocarcinoma.[4]

We discuss here three clinical tumor sites within the hepatobiliary system: hepatocellular carcinoma, biliary duct carcinoma, and primary carcinoma of the gallbladder. Recent advances have occurred in the management of these neoplasms. There is increased understanding about the etiology and epidemiology of these tumors. Newer diagnostic techniques have allowed a more precise diagnosis. These tumors, which are staged by surgical exploration, have lent themselves to experimental combined modality approaches in which surgeons, radiation oncologists, and medical oncologists have collaborated in therapeutic efforts.

PATHOLOGY

HEPATOCELLULAR CARCINOMA

Gross abnormalities of hepatocellular carcinoma can be classified into three major categories.[4] Two thirds of cases are of the nodular form in which the liver appears to be studded with multiple nodules of hepatocellular carcinoma. The massive form of hepatoma is defined by a large dominant cancer mass that may be associated with multiple satellite lesions; this form accounts for 30% of hepatomas. Five percent of hepatocellular carcinomas are of the diffuse form and always occur in association with cirrhosis. Grossly, very small tumors are scattered diffusely across the surface of the liver.

There is another gross pathologic variation of hepatocellular carcinoma that appears to have significant prognostic value: the encapsulated form, seen in 10% of cases in Japan and 4% of cases in the United States.[5,6] A capsule surrounds the hepatocellular carcinoma and may be grossly visible. This variety of primary hepatic tumor has a less aggressive course than do most hepatocellular cancers. The median survival of patients with encapsulated hepatomas was 17.3 months in a series of 25 patients, and two patients in this series survived for more than 5 years.[6]

Microscopic abnormalities of hepatocellular cancer can vary widely.[4] Well-differentiated tumors may be difficult to distinguish from regenerative nodules. There may be only slight cellular atypia, and diagnosis of well-differentiated hepatoma may depend on these changes and other subtle histologic characteristics, including nuclear abnormalities, absence of bile ductules, and absence of Kupffer cells. More anaplastic hepatocellular cancers may be so undifferentiated that the distinction between an epithelial malignancy and a mesenchymal tumor is difficult.

Two benign tumors of the liver—hepatocellular adenomas and focal nodular hyperplasia—are imporant because they may produce critical illness in young people and are induced by drugs that may induce hepatocellular cancer.[7] The principal difference between these lesions is that focal nodular hyperplasia is a benign proliferation of hepatic parenchymal cells and bile ductules, whereas hepatocellular adenoma consists of hepatic parenchymal cells only.[7] The details of pathology of the benign hepatic neoplasm are not of importance since there is debate about the exact interrelationships between these histopathologic pictures. The important fact to keep in mind is that these tumors have been associated with exogenous hormone administration. Benign hepatic tumors may present as masses within the liver and have been associated with oral contraceptive uses.[8] They have also been the cause of acute surgical emergencies because of rupture and intraperitoneal hemorrhage.[8]

GALLBLADDER CARCINOMA

Primary carcinoma of the gallbladder arises most commonly in the body of the organ. It rarely develops in the cystic duct, and in the series of Arnaud and colleagues occurred there in only 4% of patients.[2] Tumor may infiltrate the gallbladder locally or diffusely and cause thickening and rigidity of the wall.

Microscopic abnormalities of the gallbladder are most commonly adenocarcinomas. In the series of Arnaud and associates, 88% of patients had adenocarcinomas; in the collected series of Strauch, 85% of patients had adenocarcinomas.[2,9] The less common forms of gallbladder carcinoma include anaplastic carcinoma (6%), squamous cell carcinoma (3%), and adenoacanthoma (3%).[2,9]

BILE DUCT CANCER

The most important aspect, grossly, of bile duct carcinoma is the location of the tumor. Location bears directly on presentation and therapy. For example, tumors of the common bile duct may present as obstructive jaundice and occasionally gallbladder distention. Common hepatic duct cancers are proximal to the gallbladder but may infiltrate the right or left hepatic ducts and require partial hepatic resection if curative surgery is to be attempted. Of all bile duct neoplasms, 15% to 20% occur proximally in the area of the porta hepatis, and 50% develop in the distal common bile duct. About 30% of lesions are found in the proximal common bile duct and in the common hepatic duct.[10]

Microscopically, these tumors are almost always adenocarcinomas.[11] Squamous cell cancer and mesenchymal tumors are highly unusual. Bile duct cancers are usually well differentiated, with mucus production being common; about one third are associated with fibrosis and are termed scirrhous carcinomas. As with gallbladder cancer, local extension is common to regional lymph nodes, and the lesion may extend proximally along the bile ducts.[11] Experience with choledochoscopy has suggested that some bile duct cancers may be multicentric in origin.[12] With this new technique, however, it is difficult to know whether multiple lesions within the bile ducts represent multiple primary tumors or intraluminal spread of tumor from a single primary.

ANATOMICAL RELATIONS

PRIMARY HEPATOCELLULAR CANCER

The anatomical associations of hepatocellular carcinoma are important because they bear on surgical resectability. The liver has two lobes of nearly equal size, a division based on primary branchings of the hepatic afferent circulation (hepatic artery and portal vein) and the right and left hepatic biliary ducts (Figs. 19-1 and 19-2).[13] Each lobe has two segments served by secondary arborizations of the afferent vessels and the paralleling ducts. The four segments (anterior and posterior on the right and left medial and lateral divisions) are anatomically separate. Even though the planes of separation are vascular, thick, and not clearly evident (and thus not surgically convenient), segmental, lobar, or trisegmental resections are possible by this arrangement.

Hepatic efferent vessels (the hepatic veins) that run intersegmentally may complicate resection technically but do not preclude it. Thus, three of the four segments of the liver can be removed if the tumor spares blood vessels that supply or biliary ducts that drain the segment to be saved (Figs. 19-1 and 19-2).

The relation of the inferior vena cava and the liver is also anatomically relevant, for the liver rests as a saddle upon the cava. Three major veins and many minor veins drain directly into this large vessel. Tumors that encroach on or invade these veins usually can be removed, but such resections do entail significant technical problems with hemostasis.

GALLBLADDER CARCINOMA

In view of the gallbladder's normal position on the inferior surface of the right lobe of the liver, direct extension is a common mode of spread. Direct invasion may also involve the cystic and common ducts, with resultant obstruction, or may spread to stomach, omentum, colon, pancreas, duodenum, and the anterior abdominal wall.

Initially lymph drainage is into cystic and common bile duct nodes, then into the pancreaticoduodenal system, with later potential spread into the rest of the celiac axis or the superior mesenteric or aortic nodes. Vaittinen[14] reported combined data from a number of series that showed regional nodal involvement in 42% of 1611 patients at exploration and 52% of 400 patients at autopsy.[14] Retroperitoneal nodal involvement was found in 23% and 26% of patients respectively.

Veins within the gallbladder drain into the hepatic division of the portal vein. Hepatic metastases are common, but separating hematogenous metastases from direct extension of tumor to the liver is difficult. The next most frequent area of metastatic involvement is peritoneal, occurring in 19% to

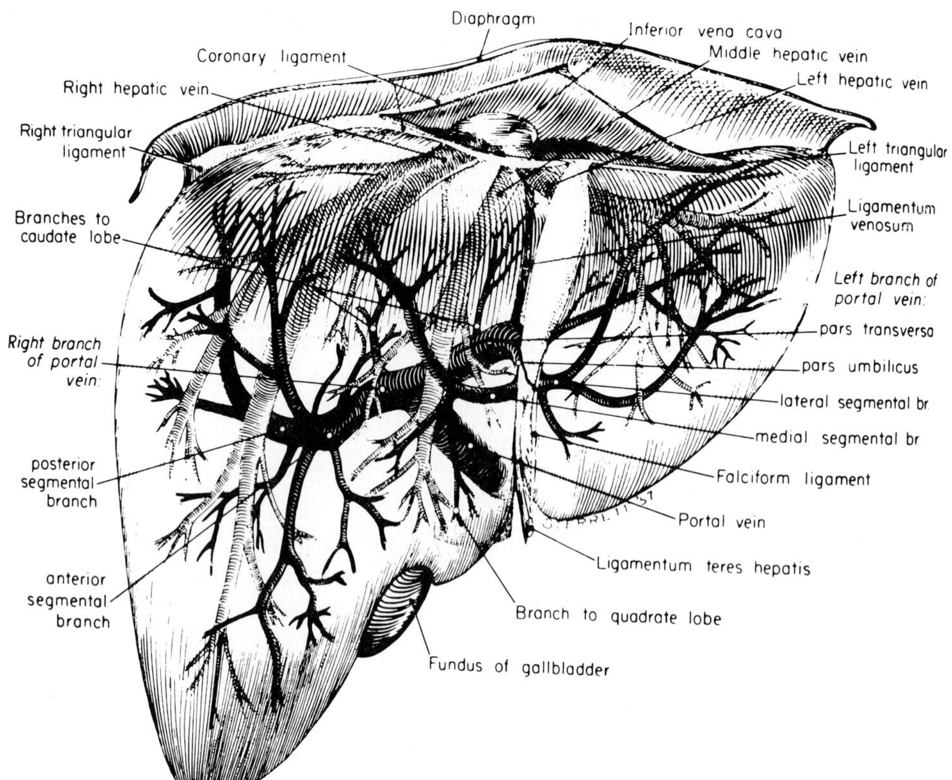

FIG. 19-1. The liver in transparency showing branching and relative position of the parts of the portal and hepatic veins. (Goldsmith NA, Woodburne RT: The surgical anatomy pertaining to liver resection. Surg Gynecol Obstet 105:310, 1957)

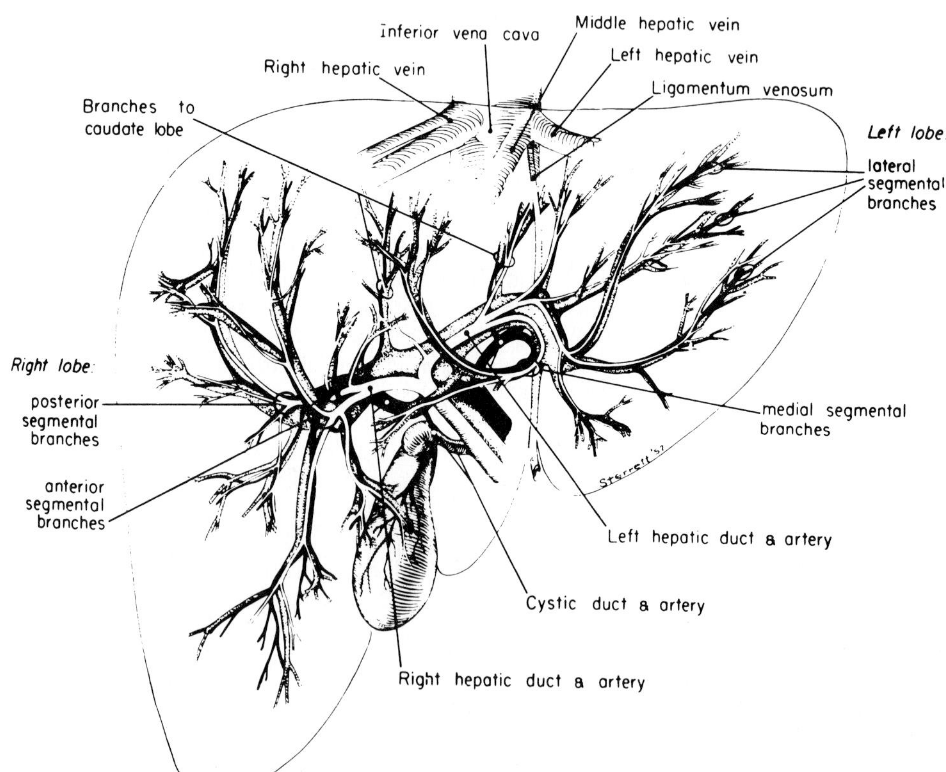

FIG. 19-2. Common branching pattern of the portal vein, hepatic artery, and bile duct radicles in the liver. Portal vein, *stippled;* hepatic artery, *black;* bile duct, *white.* (Goldsmith NA, Woodburne RT: The surgical anatomy pertaining to liver resection. Surg Gynecol Obstet 105:310, 1957)

20% of the 1611 cases at exploration and 400 cases at autopsy reviewed by Vaittinen.[14] Pulmonary metastases were reported by Vaittinen in 8% of the patients at exploration and 17% of the patients at autopsy. Occasionally, spread of tumor will involve the ovaries, spleen, bones, and other distant organs.

EXTRAHEPATIC BILIARY SYSTEM

The extrahepatic bile ducts vary considerably in length, structure, course, and relation to one another, making it difficult grossly at surgery to distinguish normal from abnormal. Lesions commonly spread by direct extension either within the duct structure or with extraductal involvement of surrounding organs, which include liver, portal vein, hepatic artery, duodenum, and head of the pancreas.

The extrahepatic bile ducts have a rich lymphatic network in their thin outer walls. Extension through the duct wall, submucosally, and to lymph nodes in the porta hepatis and celiac axis occurs early. The pancreaticoduodenal nodes are involved more frequently than with primary gallbladder cancers. A review of 11 surgical and autopsy series found that 41% of 376 patients had positive lymph nodes.[15] Of 77 cases studied at Lahey Clinic in Boston (in which primary tumors in the ampulla or diffuse biliary tumors were excluded), 35 patients had spread beyond the ducts (45%). Of these 35 patients, periductal nodes were positive in 25 (71%), and celiac axis nodes were positive in 12 (34%).[16]

Intra-abdominal spread involving peritoneal surfaces or ovaries is uncommon, with death usually occurring from the local obstructive phenomenon. Of the cases studied at Lahey Clinic, only 7 of 77 (9%) patients had a component of peritoneal spread. The combined incidence of distant extra-abdominal spread at either presentation or exploration was only 6% in two series.[15,16] Diffuse involvement of the bile duct with carcinoma has been reported in 40 of 250 (16%) patients in two consecutive series from Lahey Clinic.[16,17]

NATURAL HISTORY

PREMALIGNANT CONDITIONS

Clinicians must be aware of special conditions that predispose patients to hepatobiliary cancer, since this knowledge may result in special observation of individual patients and potentially earlier diagnosis of malignancy. Hepatocellular carcinoma is frequently associated with pre-existing liver disease.[4] In the United States, 50% of patients with hepatocellular cancer have cirrhosis. A minimum of 5% of patients with cirrhosis may eventually develop hepatocellular cancer.[4] Although hepatoma has a higher frequency of association with postnecrotic than with nutritional cirrhosis, higher absolute numbers of patients are seen in the United States with hepatoma and Laennec's cirrhosis because of the high frequency of Laennec's cirrhosis secondary to alcohol abuse. Hepatitis B antigen positivity has been associated with primary hepatocellular cancer.[18] In some countries, there has been a particular correlation between hepatitis B antigen positivity and the presence of liver cell cancer. However, this has generally occurred in areas where the presence of hepatitis B infection is high and a causal relation between hepatitis B infection and hepatoma has not been firmly documented, although probable.[4,18] The major etiologic role that hepatitis infection has in hepatocellular cancer may be through causation of liver injury and cirrhosis, with these two conditions predisposing patients to malignancy.

Evidence suggests that in cirrhosis associated with hepatic cell dysplasia, the risk of eventual development of hepatocellular carcinoma is higher. Anthony and colleagues described cases of cirrhosis and dysplasia in patients with a higher incidence of hepatoma than in those with cirrhosis and no cellular atypia.[19] This work needs confirmation by increasing the length of follow-up, but from a practical viewpoint clinicians caring for cirrhotic paients with dysplasia should be aware of possible malignant transformation.

Recently, steroids have been implicated as possible causes of hepatocellular carcinoma. Mays and associates reported 13 cases of hepatic neoplasms in young women taking oral contraceptives.[8] Although nine of these tumors were benign, four were malignant hepatocellular carcinomas. Androgens have also been associated with hepatic cancer, and Farrell and coworkers reported three cases of hepatocellular carinoma that developed in men taking androgenic steroids.[20] Although the numbers of hepatic tumors associated with steroid ingestion are small, clinicians should be aware of possible neoplasms in patients receiving sex steroids who have right upper quadrant pain or other symptoms referrable to the liver.

Cholelithiasis is a well-defined, pre-existing pathologic condition that predisposes patients to gallbladder carcinoma. Factors that promote this condition are also associated with gallbladder cancer, including the female sex, age greater than 55 years, obesity, abnormalities in lipid metabolism, and ileal disease.[3] In collected series of cases of gallbladder carcinoma, the incidence of cholelithiasis varies between 70% and 90%.[2] To clinicians, the implication of a well-defined premalignant condition in gallbladder carcinoma should be clear. It is reasonable to perform elective cholecystectomy in patients with symptomatic cholelithiasis whose general medical condition allows. This approach is to be particularly stressed in patients with a calcified or porcelain gallbladder secondary to chronic cholelithiasis. In this group of patients, the incidence of gallbladder carcinoma has been estimated to be as high as 60%.[21]

Throughout the world, the largest number of bile duct carcinomas results from liver fluke infestation.[3] A number of different parasites, including *Clonorchis sinensis, Opisthorchis felineus*, and *Opisthorchis viverrini*, have been associated with bile duct cancer in Asian countries.[3] The mechanism by which liver fluke infestation results in bile duct carcinoma is unclear. One hypothesis is that the inflammatory reaction in the bile duct from the parasitic infection serves as a promoting condition for carcinogens secreted in the bile.[3]

Bile duct cancer has been associated with ulcerative colitis.[22] The incidence of biliary tract cancer in patients with ulcerative colitis is estimated to be 0.4%.[22] This tumor is more common in patients with ulcerative colitis than in persons of similar age without ulcerative colitis.[3] Of 103 cases of proximal biliary tract cancer, 8% of patients had coexisting ulcerative colitis, strongly suggesting an association between ulcerative colitis and bile duct carcinoma.[23] The mechanism responsible for this association is unknown, although clinicians caring for patients with ulcerative colitis must be aware that biliary tract disease, either sclerosing cholangitis or bile duct carcinoma, is a possible complication.

CLINICAL PRESENTATION

HEPATOCELLULAR CARCINOMA

Symptoms and findings in patients with hepatocellular cancer depend largely on whether cirrhosis is present. In cirrhotic patients, the presence of hepatoma may be manifested only by a rapid deterioration of hepatic function, leading to liver failure and death.[4] Deterioration of the condition of cirrhotic patients with hepatocellular cancer is highlighted by the fact that these patients have a median survival from diagnosis to death of only 2 months.[24] Symptoms and findings that may be associated with this illness include rapid development of cachexia and wasting, occurrence of right upper quadrant pain, development of jaundice or worsening of pre-existing jaundice, and sudden development of ascites. The last manifestation may be particularly dramatic when it results from involvement of the hepatic vein with tumor. Hepatic vein thrombosis can occur, with resultant Budd-Chiari syndrome producing rapid developing ascites. Hemorrhagic phenomena may be prominent in patients with hepatoma, including gastrointestinal bleeding from varices and the development of hemorrhagic ascites from rupture of a hepatocellular carcinoma into the peritoneal space. Hemorrhage of one sort or another has been implicated in the cause of death of 50% of patients with hepatocellular cancer.[5]

In patients developing hepatoma without pre-existing cirrhosis, all of the above described symptoms and findings may occur. Presentation, however, will frequently be more subtle because these patients have normal livers, and thus small amounts of tumor encroachment will not result in significant impairment of hepatic function. Pain in the right upper quadrant that is frequently of a dull, aching quality is usually the first symptom.[4] There may be a pleuritic quality to the pain, with radiation to the right scapula probably representing tumor approximating or involving the diaphragm. Patients without cirrhosis may also develop a Budd-Chiari syndrome if tumor causes hepatic vein obstruction or thrombosis. With these patients the syndrome may be full-blown, with rapid development of tender hepatomegaly, jaundice, and intractable ascites. Jaundice may develop if both major intrahepatic bile ducts are obstructed with tumors. Although most patients with hepatocellular carcinoma will have initial symptoms referrable to the liver, occasionally distant metastatic disease will be the first indication of tumor.[4] In this event, patients may present with pulmonary metastases or symptomatic bone metastases.

The remote effects of cancer are discussed in detail elsewhere in this book; however, readers should be aware that hepatoma has been one of the tumors most commonly associated with remote neuroendocrine and hematologic syndromes, including polycythemia, thrombocytosis, dysfibrinogenemia, hypercalcemia, hypoglycemia, hypercalcitonemia, ectopic adrenocorticotropic hormone production, and ectopic gonadotrophin production.[4]

GALLBLADDER CANCER

Symptoms and findings in primary gallbladder cancer are the same as those associated with benign disease of the gallbladder.[2,3] The most common symptom is pain in the right upper quadrant or epigastrium, occurring in 80% of patients.[2] Nausea and vomiting and weight loss are the next most common symptoms, found in about 60% of patients. One half of patients will manifest jaundice owing to direct invasion of the liver and biliary ducts. Jaundice is a particularly ominous sign because it correlates with more advanced disease not surgically resectable. Because of the high correlation between gallbladder carcinoma and cholelithiasis, one would assume that some of the jaundice in these cases would be due to choledocolithiasis, not cancer. In the study by Arnaud and colleagues, only 25% of jaundiced patients had biliary tract stones as a cause of icterus, whereas 75% of patients were jaundiced because of direct tumor involvement.[2]

The duration of symptoms in gallbladder cancer presents an interesting clinical problem. In various series, duration of symptoms has varied between periods of only a few weeks to more than 5 years.[2,25] This disparity is likely due to the fact that symptoms of the malignant disease of the gallbladder are very similar to those of the pre-existing benign disease. Thus, clinicians managing patients with gallbladder disease must be alert to the nuances of symptoms and be willing to investigate what might appear to be slight changes in symptoms in an attempt to detect carcinoma.

BILE DUCT CANCER

The clinical presentation of bile duct cancer is analogous to that of gallbladder carcinoma in the sense that symptoms of malignant disease are the same as those of benign disease.[3,26] Cancer of the bile duct can present in only three ways: by obstruction of a major duct, leading to jaundice; by local invasion of the liver, causing symptoms; and, rarely, by metastases. All of these mechanisms of presentation make early detection difficult. Because of its detergent properties, bile will flow very well through partially obstructed ducts, and symptoms of obstruction will occur only when the process is nearly complete and the tumor relatively advanced.[26] The most common symptoms of bile duct cancer are those related to jaundice. The first symptom may be pruritis, preceding clinical jaundice.[3] Tender hepatomegaly may also be present as bile duct obstruction proceeds. The gallbladder may be distended and palpable (Courvoisier's sign) if the carcinoma is in the common bile duct. This, however, is an unusual clinical finding.[3] Fever and pain with jaundice are unusual unless the bile duct cancer is associated with sclerosing cholangitis, as is seen with ulcerative colitis.

PROGNOSIS

HEPATOCELLULAR CARCINOMA

The overall prognosis for patients with hepatocellular carcinoma is poor.[27] In patients with cirrhosis and diffuse hepatoma, the 5-year survival rate is zero.[4] In patients with resectable hepatoma, the prognosis is somewhat better, with occasional 5-year survival times being reported.[4,28] In a series of 137 patients with primary hepatocellular cancer, 32 (27%) were resected with curative intent.[28] In this group of resected patients, the operative mortality was 13%, and five patients (16%) of those resected survived 5 years. There are no data to suggest that unresected patients have the potential of surviving 5 years. The only exception to this is the rare patient with encapsulated hepatoma.[6] (This pathologic variation is described earlier in this chapter.)

GALLBLADDER CANCER

Patients with gallbladder cancer whose tumors are an incidental finding at cholecystectomy done for cholelithiasis are more fortunate.[2,3] Such cases have an excellent prognosis with simple cholecystectomy. In the 70% to 90% of cases coming to surgery with invasive cancer, the prognosis is very poor. In a collected series of more than 1700 patients, the 5-year survival rate after surgical exploration or resection was 2.6%.[29] Even in patients selected for radical surgical procedures frequently including hepatic lobectomy, the 5-year survival rate was only 6%.[29] Chemotherapy and radiation therapy may palliate the symptoms of patients with unresectable gallbladder cancer, but there is no evidence that these procedures produce long-term survival.

BILIARY DUCT CANCER

The prognosis of bile duct cancer, like that of hepatocellular and gallbladder carcinoma, is also poor. This relates to some already described aspects of the natural history of bile duct carcinoma. First, symptoms of the disease only present after almost complete occlusion of the bile duct. Second, this tumor has a propensity for early local invasion, making surgical curative resection difficult or impossible. These unfortunate characteristics of bile duct cancer are reflected in the poor survival rates reported by various authors.[11,16] Warren and colleagues reported that 1 of 7 patients survived more than 3 years, and Longmire, in a large series of 63 patients with carcinoma of the bile ducts, reported that 4 (6%) patients survived more than 4 years.[16,30] The median survival of patients with surgically unresectable disease is 5 months, although some patients with surgically unresectable disease may have a relatively indolent disease and survive more than 3 years.[11] It remains to be ascertained whether new surgical treatments will produce long-term survival in patients with bile duct cancer.

DIAGNOSIS

HEPATOCELLULAR CARCINOMA

Clinical presentation and some aspects of physical signs that may be present in patients with hepatocellular carcinoma have already been reviewed. In patients with moderately advanced hepatoma, physical examination findings may suggest the correct diagnosis. A clearly palpable abdominal mass arising from the liver may be detected in some patients with hepatoma.[4] In patients thought to have this disease and complaining of right upper quadrant pain, careful examination of the right upper quadrant for an audible or palpable friction rub should be done. The presence of a friction rub in connection with a hepatic mass lesion is more common with primary hepatocellular cancer than with metastatic tumor.[4]

Laboratory tests may be helpful in diagnosis but are frequently nonspecific. The most common abnormal laboratory finding is an elevated serum alkaline phosphatase level.[4] This is common in all infiltrative processes in the liver and certainly does not help in differentiating primary from metastatic tumors of the liver, since it is elevated in 70% to 80% of patients with hepatic metastases.[31] The most useful aspect of an elevated alkaline phosphatase finding may be that in asymptomatic patients it may direct physicians to investigate further the possibility of liver disease and thus diagnose a hepatocellular cancer at an early stage.

The alpha-fetoprotein (AFP) assay is one serum test that may be useful in the diagnosis and following-up of cases of hepatocellular carcinoma. Alpha-fetoprotein is strongly associated with hepatocellular carcinoma. When a radioimmunoassay technique is used to measure AFP, 75% to 90% of patients with primary hepatic cancer have levels above the normal value of 20 to 40 ng/ml.[32] Although increased AFP levels are associated with malignancies other than primary hepatocellular cancer, including embryonal cell carcinomas, pancreatic carcinomas, and gastric cancers, the very common elevation of AFP in patients with primary hepatic cancer makes the AFP assay an appropriate test in patients thought to have this disease.[32] The data from Chen and Jung on AFP levels in patients with hepatocellular cancer and other benign and malignant liver diseases showed that serum AFP was greater than 400 ng/ml in 69% of patients with hepatoma.[33] In none of 66 patients with cancer other than hepatocellular carcinoma was the AFP level greater than 400 ng/ml. In 211 patients with nonmalignant liver disease, an AFP level greater than 400 ng/ml was seen in only 1 patient, a person with chronic aggressive hepatitis. These data suggest that in patients thought to have hepatocellular cancer on clinical grounds, AFP levels greater than 400 ng/ml should strongly influence clinicians to confirm the presence of hepatocellular cancer by a tissue diagnosis. Clinicians should remember, however, that some patients with primary hepatic cancer will have normal AFP levels, and normal or moderately elevated levels should not be used to exclude the diagnosis of hepatocellular cancer. Although the usefulness of AFP levels in the follow-up of patients under treatment for hepatoma has not been systematically examined, McIntire and associates did show that elevated AFP levels promptly fell in patients who had undergone hepatic resections. In all patients who had recurrences of disease after surgery, this event was preceded by a rise in serum AFP.[34] Thus, this marker may be useful in following the clinical course of patients with hepatocellular cancer.

Several radiologic and nuclear medicine techniques are useful in the diagnosis of primary hepatocellular cancer. Posteroanterior and lateral chest films may be useful in patients thought to have hepatic neoplasm. Elevation or an uneven appearance of the right diaphragm on x-ray film has been associated with hepatoma, resulting from direct tumor invasion of the diaphragm by tumor.[4] The chest film may also reveal multiple pulmonary metastases. Radionuclide liver scanning is a logical early step in the diagnosis of patients thought to have hepatic neoplasms. This procedure is simple and relatively inexpensive, causes no major morbidity, and can indicate whether the liver has an abnormality consistent with hepatoma.[4,35] The finding on liver scan in patients with hepatoma varies according to whether cirrhosis is present. In patients without cirrhosis, liver scans will frequently reveal single or multiple filling defects (Fig. 19-3).[4] This finding is similar to that found in metastatic disease in the liver and results from the absence of Kupffer cells in primary hepatocellular carcinoma. Kupffer cells of the reticuloendothelial system normally accumulate the technetium sulfur colloid commonly used in liver scanning.[36] In patients with cirrhosis, the interpretation of the liver scan is more difficult because of patchy isotope uptake throughout the liver that may obscure an abnormality due to tumor.

In patients who have clinical and laboratory profiles consistent with hepatoma and who have positive liver scans, a biopsy may be considered to establish a tissue diagnosis. If preoperative evaluation has clearly indicated that the patient is a candidate for potential surgical exploration with resection of a hepatic tumor, a tissue diagnosis may be obtained at the time of exploration. In potentially resectable lesions it is wise to avoid percutaneous liver biopsy since this procedure may potentially seed and spread tumor. If percutaneous liver biopsy is to be performed it should be directed at areas of the liver known to be abnormal on hepatic scan. This biopsy, however, may fail to yield abnormal tissue, and further diagnostic efforts may be needed.[4] Peritoneoscopy with directed needle biopsy of the liver can be a useful procedure, although there is little published experience on its use in primary hepatocellular cancer.[37] This procedure is well tolerated, allows inspection of the liver and other abdominal organs, and allows multiple visually directed biopsies of hepatic abnormalities. In patients in whom percutaneous biopsy has failed, it is reasonable to attempt peritoneoscopy-directed biopsy to obtain a tissue diagnosis of a hepatic mass.

FIG. 19-3. Radionuclide liver scan showing large filling defect in the inferior aspect of the right lobe caused by a hepatocellular carcinoma.

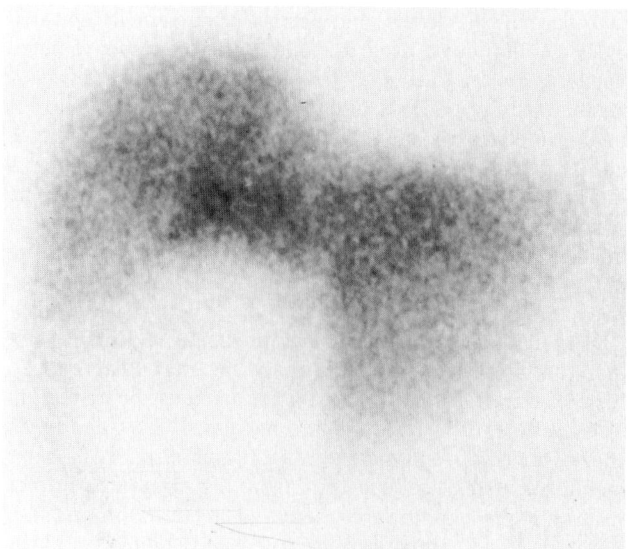

Angiography may be a useful adjunct in the diagnosis and management of patients with hepatocellular cancer.[4,38,39] In unusual cases in which hepatocellular cancer or hepatic metastases are suspected and patients have equivocal or normal liver scans, hepatic angiography can be a useful diagnostic test.[39] In general, however, angiography is most useful in the preoperative assessment of patients scheduled for potential hepatic resection.[4] Hepatocellular carcinoma has a characteristic angiographic appearance. Frequently the arteries feeding the tumor are dilated, with multiple tumor vessels throughout the lesion. Abnormal arteriovenous anastomoses lead to an abnormally early venous phase of the angiogram (Fig. 19-4).[39] This increased vascularity and the presence of tumor vessels represent differences from the angiographic appearance usually seen with metastatic disease to the liver, where markedly increased vascularity is unusual. Angiography may also be useful in suggesting that a hepatic mass is a benign tumor[7,8] and not a malignant hepatocellular neoplasm. When hepatic angiograms are used preoperatively, surgeons are given valuable information. They can define the vessels feeding the tumor, assess multiplicity of tumors or spread throughout the liver, and define any venous invasion by tumor. Such information may be critical in planning hepatic resection or in defining unresectability. Diagnostic tests, including computed tomography scanning and ultrasonography, have little specific value in diagnosis of hepatoma, although they may be useful in defining equivocal results from liver scanning. CT scanning may also allow differentiation of cavernous hemangioma from other hepatic tumors.

The recommended approach for the diagnosis of hepatocellular cancer is as follows: history and physical examination, with emphasis on factors discussed earlier; liver function tests; alpha-fetoprotein assay; liver scan; and surgical exploration or biopsy, either percutaneous or peritoneoscopy–

FIG. 19-4. Arterial phase of hepatic angiogram in patient with hepatocellular carcinoma. Note large tumor blush caused by increased vascularity in the hepatic neoplasm.

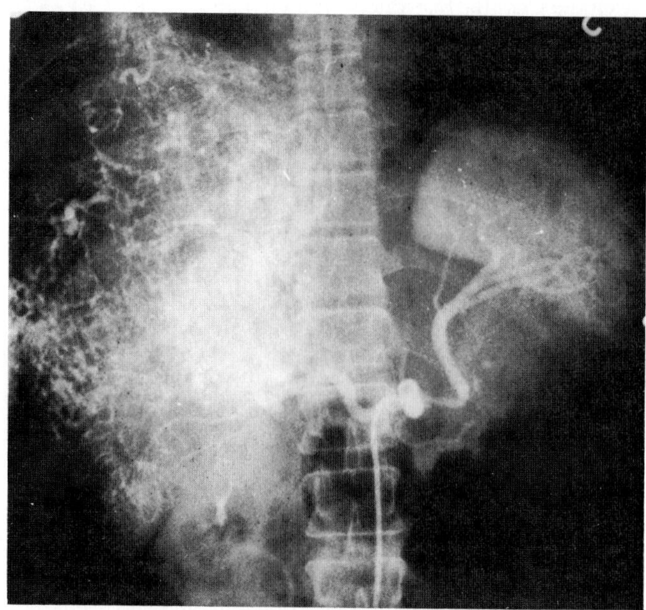

directed. If liver scan is not consistent with hepatic neoplasm, ultrasonography or computed tomography scanning may further define hepatic abnormalities. Angiography should be done for patients scheduled for open biopsy or resection.

GALLBLADDER CARCINOMA

The diagnosis, particularly the early diagnosis of gallbladder cancer as distinct from benign gallbladder disease, is difficult, because symptoms, signs, and laboratory abnormalities are similar in both diseases.[2,40] Although hepatomegaly and jaundice with palpable right upper quadrant mass have been reported in as many as 80% of cases in older series, these findings are clearly associated with advanced disease.[40] Also, with locally advanced gallbladder cancer, a palpable or audible right upper quadrant friction rub may be present.

Liver function test findings are abnormal in from 20% to 75% of patients at presentation.[2,40] The most common abnormality is an elevated alkaline phosphatase level. A nonspecific finding of anemia has been reported in 30% of patients.[2]

Radiographic studies are of little use in differentiating benign from malignant gallbladder disease. Cholecystography revealed a nonfunctioning gallbladder in 75% of patients in the series of Arnaud and coworkers, and in a series of 43 patients Tanga and Ewing found the gallbladder nonfunctioning in 66% of patients.[2,41] In this latter series, only 12% of patients had abnormalities of the duodenum (extrinsic pressure defects) on upper gastrointestinal study, and 4.5% had abnormal liver scans. Angiography is not commonly used in assisting with a primary diagnosis of gallbladder cancer but occasionally will indicate tumor vascularity in the area of the gallbladder.[2]

Although both ultrasonography and computed tomography scanning can define the presence of the gallbladder and the pathologic changes of cholelithiasis, their use in the diagnosis of gallbladder carcinoma is undefined.

In most cases, the diagnosis of gallbladder cancer is not made clinically.[2,42] In Litwin's review of 76 cases of this tumor, the most common preoperative diagnosis was benign biliary tract disease (76%).[42] In 24% of patients in Litwin's series believed preoperatively to have malignant disease, the tumor was assumed to be in the bile ducts or pancreas.

The appropriate diagnostic approach for gallbladder cancer depends not on laboratory or roentgenographic investigation but on the individual physician's clinical judgment, experience, and a high index of suspicion. As indicated earlier in this chapter, the best way to treat gallbladder cancer is to prevent it. Certainly, a physician treating a known benign biliary tract condition should be alert to any change in symptoms in the patient, including increased pain, increased frequency of attacks of cholecystitis, and abnormal liver function test findings. The physician must be willing to consider early operative intervention. Only in this way may symptoms be palliated and the presence of gallbladder cancer be ruled out.

BILE DUCT CANCER

In carcinoma of the extrahepatic bile ducts, jaundice is the symptom that brings the patient to the physician's attention most commonly. Jaundice may be preceded by pruritis, although other symptoms, including weight loss and anorexia, may be present.[3,43] The evaluation of cases of bile duct cancer is essentially the same as that of other cases of obstructive jaundice.

Tender hepatomegaly is frequently present, along with increased bilirubin levels.[3] Alkaline phosphatase level is almost always elevated. Anemia, leukocytosis, and fever may be present. These last two findings suggest mild cholangitis with obstructive jaundice.

Ultrasonography of the liver is a sensitive method of differentiating between obstructive and nonobstructive jaundice and has no morbidity.[3] In patients with obstructive jaundice, ultrasonography will reveal dilated hepatic bile ducts (Fig. 19-5). The next task is to define the anatomical site and nature of the obstruction. Thin-needle (Chiba) transhepatic cholangiography is the simplest and safest way to do this. This procedure is associated with morbidity in only 2% of cases and will nearly always define the area of obstruction (Fig. 19-6).[3] If a skilled endoscopist is available and transhepatic cholangiography has not given adequate

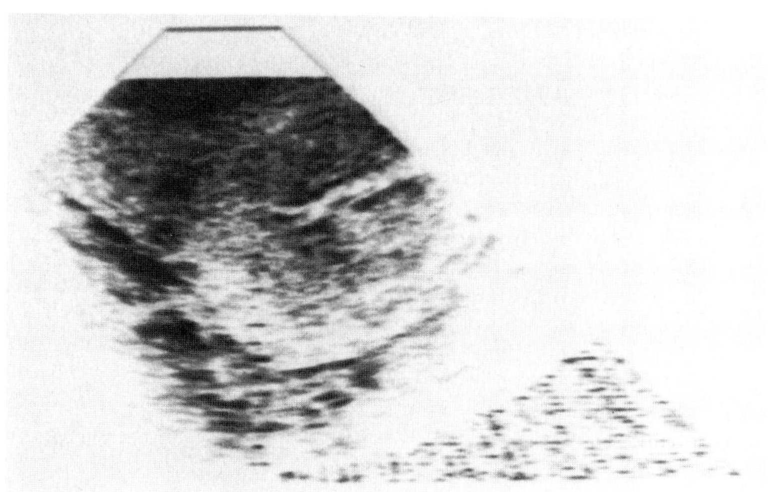

FIG. 19-5. Ultrasonography of the liver in patient with obstructive jaundice caused by bile duct cancer. Note clearly defined dilated intrahepatic duct in the upper right-hand corner.

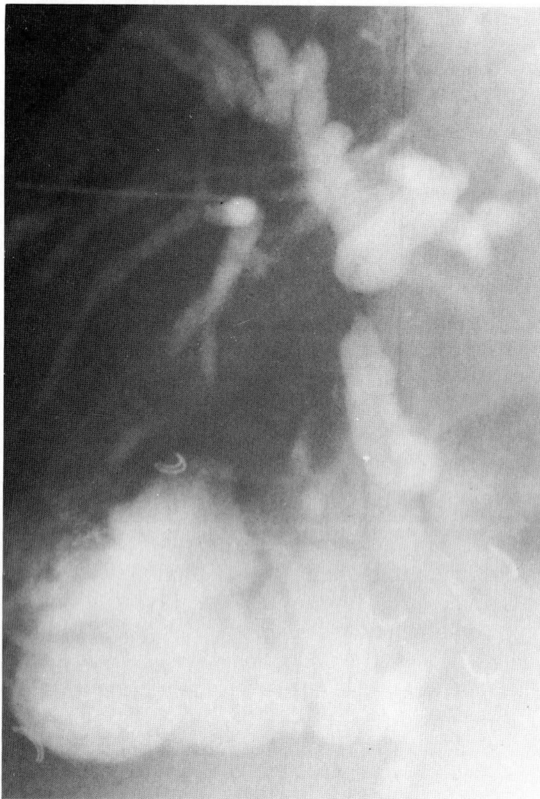

FIG. 19-6. Transhepatic cholangiogram in patient with partially obstructing biliary tract cancer. Note Chiba needle in dilated intrahepatic duct. The common bile duct has an area of construction, and dye has also entered the small bowel.

information, endoscopic retrograde choledocopancreatography (ERCP) may be performed. This procedure may define the lower extent of a completely obstructing lesion, and occasionally brushing of the lesion for cytologic study may provide a pathologic diagnosis.[37] The success of ERCP depends on the skill and experience of the endoscopist. This procedure has been reported to successfully visualize the bile ducts radiographically in 75% to 95% of patients with obstructive jaundice.

In most patients with a complete or high-grade partial obstruction of the bile ducts, operation is the next step and is required for diagnosis, palliation, or cure. With the advent of transhepatic cholangiography, however, another option is open to physicans who have reason to believe that surgical exploration is a high-risk procedure for individual patients. New, safe methods of transhepatic biliary drainage exist in which a drainage tube can be passed through a tract defined by a Chiba needle into a dilated bile duct and subsequently through an obstructing lesion.[44] Safe internal drainage of the obstructed biliary tract into the duodenum is possible (Fig. 19-7). This approach may allow time for patients to be carefully prepared for definitive surgery or may serve as the only palliative treatment necessary for patients who are not surgical candidates.[3]

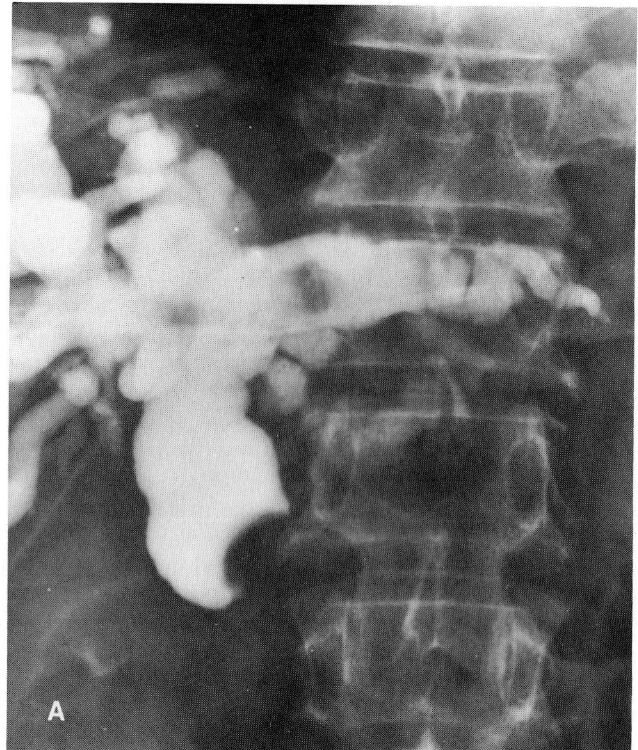

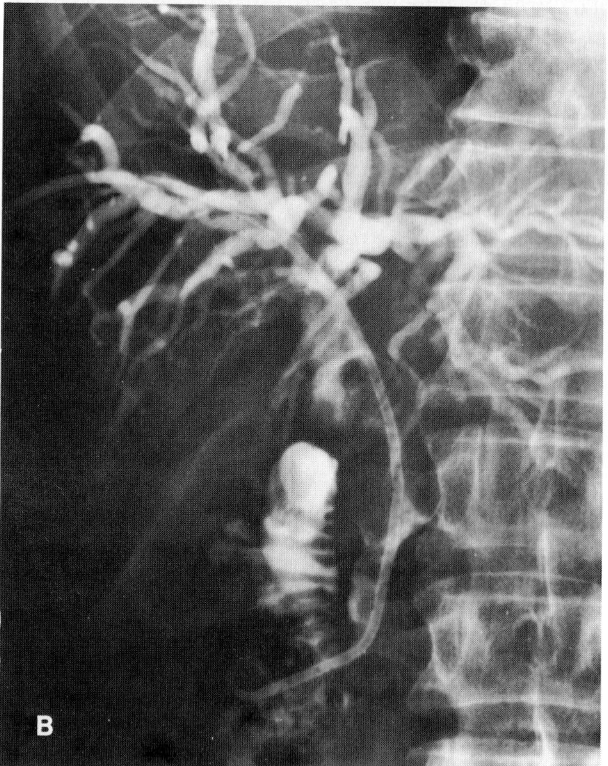

FIG. 19-7. *A*, Transhepatically passed catheter in dilated hepatic duct. Note tumor filling defect completely obstructing the bile duct. *B*, Transhepatic catheter has now been moved past obstructing tumor, and internal biliary drainage has been provided. Note contrast material in small bowel and decompression of the biliary system.

In managing patients with obstructive jaundice, possibly secondary to bile duct cancer, diagnostic procedures should follow a pattern as outlined above: liver function tests; sonogram to establish biliary tract obstruction; transhepatic cholangiography (preferred). If a skilled and experienced endoscopist familiar with ERCP is available, then this procedure may be done as an adjunct to transhepatic cholangiography if the latter procedure has not adequately defined the site of bile duct obstruction. The final procedures include diagnostic/therapeutic laparotomy or transhepatic internal biliary drainage.

SURGICAL TREATMENT

HEPATOCELLULAR CARCINOMAS

The preoperative assessment of patients with hepatocellular carcinoma has been described in the section on diagnosis and may lead to the ascertainment of unresectability. Evaluation of unresectability at the time of exploratory surgery may disclose small bilateral multicentric tumors, unsuspected involvement of regional lymphatics, or direct extension of tumors undetected during preoperative evaluation. Rarely, however, will involvement of hilar structures, the vena cava, or hepatic veins that might preclude resection be found at operation that has not already been revealed by preoperative angiographic evaluation done by an experienced radiologist. Only rarely, also, will unresectable extensions of tumor to contralateral biliary ducts be found in this group of patients, for almost all who have "passed" preoperative evaluation will have no jaundice. Jaundiced patients should have been evaluated before operation by percutaneous transhepatic cholangiographic study, which would have revealed bile duct extension.

The operative assessment of resectability, in summary, entails appreciation of extension across interlobar or intersegmental planes, involvement of the hepatic hilus, and growth encroaching on the vena cava.

SURGICAL TECHNIQUES

The specifics of surgical technique essential to safe resective surgery are relevant here because they give physicians some concept of what can or cannot be done by surgeons.

Because most liver cancers are relatively differentiated and thus are "pushers" that increase in size by expanding, not invading, encroachment on the hepatic hilus, vena cava, or hepatic veins can usually be managed safely if proper exposure is obtained and care is used when dissecting near these vital structures. Thus, patterns of growth and modes of spread of most primary hepatic malignancies do facilitate resective surgery. Although invasion of the diaphragm is common and minimal invasion of adjacent organs is seen at times, usually both can be managed by *en bloc* extensions of the liver resection.

Personal preferences for some techniques relate to operative risk.[45] Because most of these tumors are large and many do encroach on or displace the vena cava or hilar structures, comfort and safety exist in wide operative exposure, best afforded for the management of right-sided tumors by the use of a thoracoabdominal incision. The thoracic extension of an upper abdominal oblique incision is made only after resectability has been confirmed through a limited abdominal incision.

Although resection of some lesions that lie away from the hepatic hilus can be accomplished by large segmental or wedge resections, three fourths of the 60 primary solid tumors that have been resected by one of us (M.A.) required either formal lobectomy or trisegmental resection, since most tumors were large, varying in size from 6 cm to 19 cm (average, 13 cm).

The safety of such resections is increased by preidentification, predivision, and ligation of hepatic veins and branched structures at the hilus (Fig. 19-8) before transection of hepatic parenchyma. The preference for incision with thoracoabdominal extension on the right relates to the need to provide adequate exposure of the vena cava, thus allowing preligation

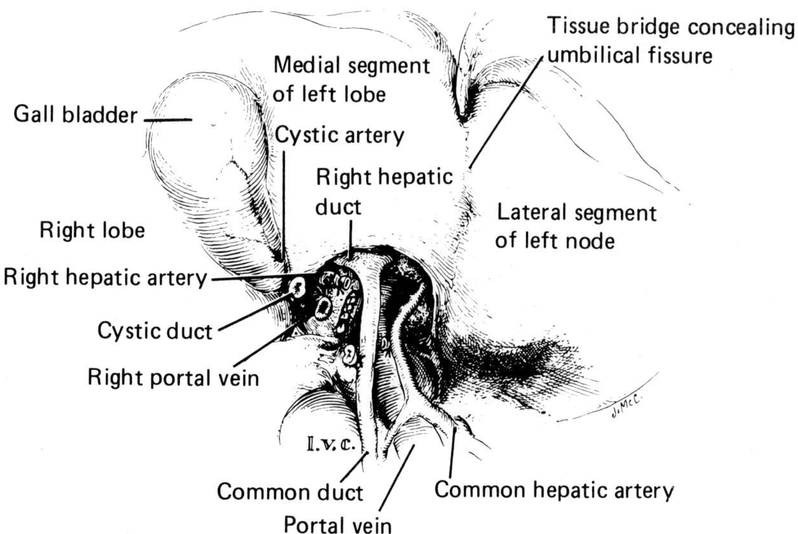

FIG. 19-8. Devascularization of the true right lobe. The cystic artery and cystic duct are ligated and divided to aid in the dissection. Of the structures of the portal triad, the bifurcation of the duct is almost always the most superior, that of the portal vein intermediate, and that of the hepatic artery most inferior. (Starzl TE, Bell RH, Beart RW et al: Hepatic trisegmentectomy and other liver resections. Surg Gynecol Obstet 141:429, 1975)

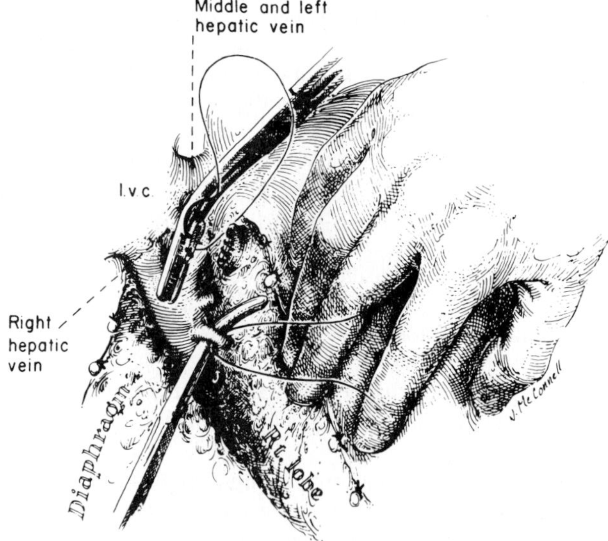

FIG. 19-9. Division of the right hepatic vein. With the right lobe of the liver retracted anteriorly and to the left, the vein is divided between Pott's clamps and oversewn with vascular sutures. Several smaller hepatic veins must be ligated because they enter the retrohepatic vena cava more inferiorly. (Starzl TE, Bell RH, Beart RW et al: Hepatic trisegmentectomy and other liver resections. Surg Gynecol Obstet 141:429, 1975)

of the right hepatic vein (Fig. 19-9) as well as the smaller hepatic veins that drain directly into the cava. On the left, thoracic extension offers no advantage, and surgeons must contend uncomfortably with limited exposure only when tumors are found to involve the caudate lobe. Parenchymal transection, most safely done after preligation of vessels serving the lobe to be resected, is greatly facilitated by use of hemostatic clips (Fig. 19-10).

Cirrhosis associated with cancer of the liver does increase operative risk and postoperative morbidity and mortality. Hemostasis during transection of the firm cirrhotic parenchyma may be a major problem, and limited hepatic reserve may compromise the patient's convalescence.[46]

RESULTS

After resection of 46 primary hepatic malignancies in the personal series of one of us (M.A.), two patients died postoperatively during hospital convalescence. No deaths occurred after standardized "routine" resections, despite their magnitude, and the two deaths relate to special circumstances. One occurred after attempted completion of trisegmentectomy, which followed previous right lobectomy (the left hepatic vein was compromised); and another operative death related to caval invasion by a large tumor thrombus that escaped before it could be removed. The 10-, 5-, and 3-year survival rates of patients who survived resection of malignant lesions were 33%, 36%, and 65%, respectively.

Aggressive surgical management of hepatic malignancies appears to be justified by acceptable operative risk and extended survival of patients found to have clearly resectable lesions. The resection of 14 large benign tumors resulted in one operative death from a caval tear that occurred during removal of a large tumor of the caudate lobe. The remaining 13 patients (8 of whom have been followed-up for more than 5 years) have been living from 1 to 18 years without evidence of new or recurrent tumors. Experience with these benign tumors is included here because aspects of surgical technique and potential complications in surgical treatment of benign hepatic tumor are relevant to the management of primary malignant tumors of the liver.

Results of hepatic resection in the author's (M.A.) Mayo Clinic series of benign and malignant liver tumors are similar to those reported in other surgical series.[46–48]

GALLBLADDER CARCINOMA

SURGICAL EVALUATION

Most often the surgical evaluation of suspected cases of gallbladder carcinoma is simple. Direct extensions of tumor beyond the limits of resection generally are obvious, and lymph nodes beyond the limits of practical lymphadenectomy

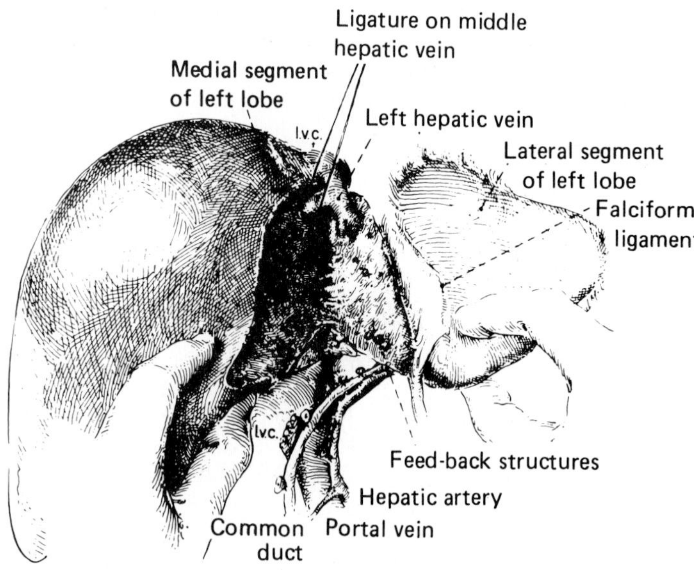

FIG. 19-10. Liver transection nearly completed along exact line of color change demarcated by viable and cyanotic liver tissue. Intersegmental veins are left attached to the lateral segment if possible. The last major structure to be encountered is the middle hepatic vein. (Starzl TE, Bell RH, Beart RW et al: Hepatic trisegmentectomy and other liver resections. Surg Gynecol Obstet 141:429, 1975)

may easily be excised. Such selective biopsies taken from a site most relevant to a tumor's stage will make the patient's needs more objective. At times, the use of silver clips to mark the peripheral extensions of the lesion may help therapeutic radiologists in their efforts whenever unresectable extensions are found.

When unresectable tumor is found in jaundiced patients, the practicalities of biliary decompression must be considered. Decisions on palliation of jaundice (discussed above) will be simplified if the need for percutaneous transhepatic cholangiography has been foreseen preoperatively.

Surgeons and surgical pathologists have special responsibilities whenever a cholecystic cancer of limited extent is found at operation. The surgeon's appreciation of gross pathologic change in the gallbladder should lead to selective biopsy, and suspicious lymph nodes are best excised for study by frozen section, since the detection of lymphatic involvement of limited extent will lead one to perform the proper initial extended operative procedure. Problems do arise when today's pathologist does his work tomorrow. However, when a surgical pathologist able to interpret frozen sections is at hand, removal of additional lymph nodes in the hepatoduodenal ligament, along the hepatic artery, and behind the duodenum is indicated. The lack of such involvement is indicative of a more favorable prognosis, and removal of nodes involved by tumor may offer chance of cure.

Pathologists must determine whether cancer has spread through the wall of the gallbladder to invade its fossa. Such invasion calls for resection of about 2.5 cm of normal liver tissue beyond gross extensions of tumor.

Operative assessment of tumors that involve the hepatic hilus or hepatoduodenal ligament is more complex. The risks and limitations of resection to be considered are greater, and experience and exact knowledge of anatomy may play a special role. Surgeons unfamiliar with such things cannot be criticized so much for inaction in this circumstance as for lack of common sense and clinical wariness that might have led to proper preoperative referral. The chance to help such patients in the course of a second surgical procedure, after tumor has been seeded by misdirected efforts, is greatly reduced.

SURGICAL TECHNIQUE

Operative techniques essential to *what* surgeons should do to assess resectability have been discussed above. *How* surgeons may remove tumors of limited extent can be considered now.

Wedge resection of the gallbladder bed disregards segmental planes and anatomically is not attractive to the surgeon. Efforts to remove invaded liver substance with a margin of unaffected tissue may be limited by hepatic hilar structures vulnerable to damage during blind *en bloc* dissection. Therefore, wedge resection properly is started medial to the fossa only after identification of the right hepatic artery, the right branch of the portal vein, and the right hepatic duct (which may be cannulated temporarily from below to protect it during this dissection). After this is done, blunt dissection of the liver substance will expose vascular and biliary tributaries for their division between hemostatic clips. Major vessels or ducts will not be encountered in developing the wedge laterally beyond the fundus of the gallbladder, unless the tumor is so large that this dissection must be extended to the interlobar plane where the peripheral portion of the right hepatic vein may need to be transected.

Occasionally, when direct invasion from the fundus or body of the gallbladder dominates, more extensive removal of the liver substance may be required, and so-called "middle lobectomy" (a useful misnomer) can be justified. This involves extended resection of hepatic parenchyma with preservation of vessels and ducts that serve both the right lobe and the lateral segment of the left hepatic lobe.

Seldom is right hepatic lobectomy indicated for treatment of a cancer of the gallbladder, for rarely will such cancers involve structures essential to the function of the right hepatic lobe without involving either major vessels in the hepatoduodenal ligament, the left hepatic duct, or unresectable distant lymph nodes.

Regional lymphadenectomy that should be done with any curative extended cholecystectomy entails stepwise dissection to skeletonize the hepatoduodenal ligament, with extension of this dissection along the hepatic artery to include nodes adjacent to the celiac axis and the aorta. Lymph nodes and intervening lymphatic vessels are removed in continuity to the extent possible. Posteriorly, the dissection is carried down along the portal vein and common bile duct well behind the duodenum and pancreas. From this point onward, lymphatic drainage relates so intimately to the superior mesenteric vessels and inaccessible retroperitoneal structures that the addition of pancreatoduodenectomy involves risks not justified by diminishing returns.

RESULTS OF TREATMENT

The results of surgical treatment of cancers of the gallbladder relate mostly to a tumor's stage; at times, however, they may depend on the surgeon's choice of operation.

Surgical results must be considered in relation to three stages of tumor. At one extreme are advanced tumors for which curative operations cannot be done. Although palliation is difficult to assess, patients who suffer most from obstructive jaundice, rather than from systemic effects of disseminated cancer, may be helped by biliary decompression for many months.[49] At the other extreme are the early cancers of the gallbladder removed fortuitously in the management of calculous disease. These cancers, confined to the gallbladder wall, may be cured inadvertently by the surgeon. The gross and microscopic pathologic characteristics of such tumors, which account for about 10% of cholecystic cancers seen at the Mayo Clinic, were reported in 1963.[50,51] Of 21 patients who survived from 5 to 35 years after cholecystectomy alone, about half had papillary, polypoid, or multicentric cancers, and half had cancers that invaded completely through the wall of the gallbladder but did not invade the liver substance. That study showed that some cancers of the gallbladder may be removed completely at an early stage of growth but gave no indication of whether prognosis could be improved by more radical surgical excision in those instances in which adjacent structures are involved.

In 1962, Fahim and colleagues studied the modes of spread

of gallbladder cancer and concluded that "the poor prognosis which attends cancer of the gallbladder is not necessarily due to the biologic nature of the tumor, but rather may well be due to inadequate surgical therapy."[52] Ten years later a review of subsequent experience at the Mayo Clinic was undertaken.[53] Clearly the contentions of Fahim and coworkers had not been properly tested because results in a series of 112 patients[53] showed that despite Fahim's rational analysis, more patients were managed using rationalization than reason.

In this study, 12 of 112 patients who had cancer of the gallbladder evaluated surgically were found to have lesions that extended outside the gallbladder but apparently not beyond resectable structures.[53] Unfortunately, 8 of these 12 patients were managed only by simple cholecystectomy. The rationale for compromise was not always clearly stated, but limited operations were justified by age, obesity, concomitant disease, or regional infection. Importantly, all but one of these 8 patients died within 15 months, not from age, obesity, coexistent disease, or infection, but from cancer. This showed only that tumor residua left behind will grow and kill.

Of the 12 patients, only 4 were treated by wedge resection of the gallbladder fossa and regional lymphadenectomy. Two died 3½ and 6 years after operation. Of the other two, one died (at age 86) 14 years after operation without evidence of recurrent cancer, and the other is living and well without evident recurrence of disease 8 years after operation.

The enhanced survival of this small sample of patients may be attributable to the more radical operation. Thus, this safe and simple extension of cholecystectomy is recommended for the management of that small proportion (15%) of cholecystic cancers theoretically resectable.

Unfortunately, the opportunity for proper surgical treatment often is missed when the surgeon is insensitive to gross evidence of cancer, or when a pathologist skilled in interpretation of frozen section is not at hand. Then, the presence of cancer is recognized a day or a week after simple cholecystectomy. In most of these instances, surgical re-evaluation reveals either extension of tumor unappreciated by the primary surgeon or seeding and implantation of cancer related to the initial operative procedure.

For simplicity, our consideration of cancer of the gallbladder has been based primarily on personal review by one of us (M.A.) of institutional experience. Piehler and Crichlow's collective review provides an in-depth review of the biologic aspects and management of this disease.[50]

BILE DUCT CARCINOMA

OPERATIVE EVALUATION

Gross pathologic changes of ductal tumors may be subtle, and histopathologic features are difficult to interpret by even the most experienced surgical pathologist. These factors and the relative infrequency of such tumors may lead inexperienced surgeons to misadventure. In some reported series, one third of such tumors have been overlooked during initial operation before proper referral.[3,54] Experienced surgeons will know that in patients who did not have previous operations, which might have caused a benign ductal stricture, they must hope to differentiate only between ductal cancer and benign sclerosing cholangitis.

Operative evaluation is simplified when a dilated duct proximal to a mid-duct or distal duct tumor can be exposed for cholangiographic study, but easy access to dilated ducts at or above the ductal bifurcation may be precluded by an infiltrating hilar mass. The unwary surgeon will then appreciate the value of preoperative transhepatic cholangiography. At such times, if the stricture cannot be breached with a Ferris filiform catheter, with a Bakes dilator, or by needle aspiration, transhepatic aspiration and injection may be tried, or the left hepatic duct may be exposed in the left intersegmental plane (umbilical fissure) by way of the so-called round ligament approach.[55]

Further operative evaluation involves differentiation of benign from malignant lesions. Focal benign lesions are truly rare without a patient's having a history of operative trauma. The differentiation between diffuse, benign, and malignant sclerosing changes may be difficult or impossible because of the risk of obtaining large samples from small ducts and of problems with histopathologic study. Surgical therapeutic options and limitations are such, however, as to minimize the importance of certain diagnosis, for the management of benign and malignant lesions differs little surgically when mural involvement is extensive. Therefore, diffuse ductal abnormalities clearly unresectable must be biopsied cautiously to avoid subsequent biliary fistulization.

The assessment of resectability of more focal lesions involves their dissection from identifiable adjacent structures, hoping to isolate the tumor and expose uninvolved ducts above and below the tumor. Biopsy becomes particularly important (to aid the medical oncologist and therapeutic radiologist) when unresectability is confirmed. Still, tissue should be sought and taken cautiously, mindful of postoperative biliary fistulae.

Before resorting to palliative procedures, seek objective evidence of unresectability. Generally, this relates to intrahepatic ductal involvement beyond secondary bifurcations; to invasion of blood vessels essential to hepatic function; to peritoneal seeding; to spread to distant lymphatic nodes; or, in the case of distal ductal tumors, to involvement of the superior mesenteric artery or vein. Unfortunately, microscopic mural invasion beyond gross limits of tumor is common.[56] This accounts for the fact that about one half of ductal tumors resected with hope of cure prove to be only palliative after review of permanent microscopic slides.[54,56,57]

SURGICAL TECHNIQUE

The specifics of surgical technique vary with the site of ductal involvement. Tumors upstream of the primary ductal bifurcation are anatomically and surgically hepatic tumors, the management of which already has been discussed. Three sites of involvement remain to be considered.

Bifurcation tumors

The management of tumors that arise at or near the confluence of the right and left hepatic ducts requires special knowledge of anatomic relations of the hepatic trinity (hepatic artery, portal vein, bile duct) at the hilus. Because the hepatic ducts usually bifurcate outside the liver, the need for resection of hepatic substance along with involved ductal tissue varies with the site and extent of invasion of cancers sited there.[30,58–60] Often, only portions of the adjacent liver substance need to be removed with little regard for knowledge of segmental anatomy. When more extensive parenchymal involvement is found, however, the surgeon must resort to formal lobectomy and also contend with the need to save the blood vessels that serve the hepatic substance. Seldom is formal lobectomy needed to get clear of tumor laterally, but removal of a lobe may be unavoidable when perihilar extensions of tumor encase vessels or ducts that serve an hepatic lobe minimally involved by tumor. Thus, usually it is the proximity of the hepatic ducts and hepatic afferent blood vessels that determines the extent of resection needed for the management of periductal extensions of tumor. This is a key to surgical evaluation and to techniques for removal of such tumors. If the tumor is not clearly (obviously) unresectable, begin dissection by isolating the portal vein within the hepatoduodenal ligament well below the tumor, gaining access through the thin, avascular visceral peritoneum that forms the anterior border of the foramen of Winslow. If the portal venous bifurcation can be freed from tumor, then the uninvolved common hepatic artery is freed and followed up to the tumor, where the extent of arterial involvement can be ascertained. In these close quarters, ascertain whether the arterial supply of one or both hepatic lobes may be spared, a surgical exercise greatly facilitated by preoperative angiographic study. The resection of lesions that do not involve both hepatic arteries may be done by transecting parenchyma using blunt dissection to identify small vessels and ducts that may be occluded and divided between hemostatic clips. When a right or left hepatic artery must be sacrificed, the corresponding lobe should be removed. Ductal drainage is best established by suture anastomosis to a defunctionalized Roux limb.

Mid-Ductal Tumors

Although some authors in their study of ductal tumors have divided the extrahepatic duct into two parts in relation to the point of entry of the cystic duct, this arbitrary separation has no practical anatomical or surgical significance.[36] The cystic duct may enter high or low, and the relation of vessels and ducts between the superior border of the pancreatic head and the primary ductal bifurcation does not differ with respect to surgical techniques involved in resective surgery. Resection of ductal tumors in the hepatoduodenal ligament involves isolation of the hepatic arteries (or sacrifice of one), similar management of the portal vein, regional lymphadenectomy, *en bloc* cholecystectomy, and dissection of tumor that involves hepatic substance or major biliary ducts so that margins grossly uninvolved with tumor are obtained. A competent surgical pathologist who can confirm tumor-free margins by study of frozen sections is essential.

Distal Duct Tumors

The technique of radical pancreatoduodenectomy has been discussed in Chapter 18. It may be modified at times when dealing with well-differentiated distal bile duct tumors by preservation of the stomach, pylorus, and a cuff of duodenum. Such conservatism may minimize postoperative bowel, pancreatic, and biliary tract dysfunction.[59]

Biliary-intestinal continuity must be restored after resection of any ductal tumor. Duct-to-duct anastomosis seldom is feasible, and biliary-intestinal anastomosis generally is needed to re-establish continuity. Techniques for such anastomoses are numerous and varied, but basic surgical principles are few. When possible, duct-to-mucosal anastomoses are favored because they are less disposed to stricture, and the use of defunctionalized Roux limbs will minimize the consequence of any anastomotic leakage. Stents may have value in conjunction with the "mucosal graft" technique, and transhepatic tubular stents placed at operation may have value later for management of recurrent malignant anastomotic stricturing or may find value as routes for administration of interstitial postoperative radiation therapy.[61,62]

RESULTS OF SURGICAL TREATMENT

Judgments about the efficacy of various modes of surgical treatment of biliary cancer are precluded by the paucity of studies involving long-term survivorship. Moreover, analysis of therapeutic results is hampered by the failure of most authors to define carefully the various pathologic types of tumors treated, which is important because of the variation of natural history among these tumors. Thus, one cannot easily learn whether aggressive efforts to resect biliary ductal cancers (with the attendant increased operative risk) can be justified by increased survival of treated patients. Nor can one learn whether reported long-term survivals relate to the choice of operative procedure or to the natural history of disease.

To better assess the natural history and results of surgical therapy in biliary tract cancer, the Mayo Clinic staff has reviewed the results of 1060 surgically evaluated patients treated at the Mayo Clinic and other institutions. Only 26 (less than 3%) lived for 5 years or more after their operations. This small number cannot be viewed as 5-year survivorship of patients managed surgically, for only a small proportion of patients treated had been observed for more than 1 year after "surgical" treatment.

Also of the 1060 patients managed by surgeons, only 10% to 15% had tumors resected with hope of cure. This figure too must be viewed in perspective, for reported rates of resectability likely were ascertained solely by the willingness of an individual surgeon to perform aggressive surgery. Operative mortality (11% to 28% for so-called curative resections) and survival after such treatment (mean survival, 10 to 24 months) must be considered more seriously, even though reported survival rates cannot be analyzed critically for lack of long-term observation of treated patients.

Separate review of the Mayo Clinic institutional experience differed from experiences reported in the general surgical literature only with respect to significant periods of postoperative observation. The study of Farnell and Adson involved 221 patients who had tumors of the hilar (50%), middle (30%), or lower ducts (15%) at the Mayo Clinic between 1950 and 1976.[63] Five percent of tumors were multicentric or diffuse. Only 15% of tumors were resected with hope of cure, with a 15% operative mortality; mean survival after "curative" resection was 30 months.

Only 8 of the 221 patients survived for 5 years or more after surgical management. Significantly, half of the patients had only palliative, nonresective procedures, evidence for the influence of the natural history of their disease rather than the effect of aggressive, resective treatment on their survival.

Thus, from review of the surgical literature and from study of the Mayo Clinic institutional experience, evidence suggests that anatomical and pathologic factors severely limit the resective treatment of biliary-ductal tumors.[64] Nevertheless, more may be accomplished by aggressive surgical management, an approach that has not been used effectively in the past.

This hope can be justified by two observations: Farnell and Adson found, in addition to the 15% of cases of ductal cancers resected with hope of cure, another 10% of the 221 patients who had lesions that, from the surgeon's description, might well have been resected—a finding that correlates well with an earlier institutional analysis.[63,65] This small but significant proportion of patients was denied what might have been optimal treatment by surgical reluctance, borne either of philosophic attitudes (which may well be justfied) or by lack of experience in hepatic surgery.

Hope for some reward from aggressive resective surgery also is found in more recent surgical literature. Now, surgeons more familar with hepatobiliary anatomy are able to resect a greater proportion of cancers that arise in or near the confluence of the hilar ducts.[54,56–58] Whether palliative resections done for 60% or more of patients, and "curative" resections done for 30% or more of patients, can be justified will be known only after longer observation of treated patients.

In competition with surgical extirpation are the palliative measures introduced by Goetze and Schwabe and properly tested by Terblanche.[36,66] Although the success of this method combined with the use of radiation therapy may in part be attributable to the natural history of some biliary ductal cancers, the lesser risk of such treatment must be viewed fairly since it eliminates the greater operative risk involved in resective surgery.

Cancers of the biliary duct may differ in kind. Papillary, protuberant, nodular, or rounded lesions by whatever name are assessable preoperatively by cholangiographic study. Proper referral to surgeons who more frequently deal with complex hepatobiliary problems therefore seems appropriate. They too will find decisions difficult, but there is still a greater chance that initial surgical evaluation (really the patient's only chance) will be appropriate. Certainly this will be true for the management of distal ductal tumors. Survival rates after resection of these tumors by radical pancreatoduodenectomy are similar to the more favorable prognoses associated with such management of ampullary tumors.[65,67] It does seem likely that the greater proportion of ductal cancers are resectable with hope of cure than has been reported in all but the most recent surgical literature.[54,57,58]

Because technologic advances make earlier, more specific diagnosis possible, the risks, limitations, and possible benefits of resective surgery done by experienced surgeons may be properly evaluated in the next decade. In this regard, Todoroki's report of very high resectability rates of less invasive tumors and improved survival after such resections must be viewed as a valuable contribution.[57] There is also evidence that radiation therapy applied externally or locally through transhepatic tubes in conjunction either with resective or palliative surgery may have value.[62]

As with other cancers of the hepatobiliary system, the major determinant of prognosis is, at present, the natural history of the disease. Nevertheless, for patients who have localized or regional disease, proper treatment will involve proper surgical perspective and judgment and detailed knowledge of anatomy and technical complications.

SURGERY FOR PALLIATION

Patients who suffer from incurable cancer may still, at times, be helped by surgery. Although decisions about surgical palliation can be based, in part, on today's technology, more often proper judgments depend on the surgeon's wisdom and perspective, humanity and reason. It is also apparent that anatomical considerations, surgical techniques, and principles of management for palliation are much the same whether patients have hepatoma, gallbladder carcinoma, or bile duct cancer. Surgeons must distinguish sensibly between systemic deterioration caused by disseminated cancer and a tumor's localized effects, and thus distinguish between operations that may prolong the act of dying and those that may extend a tolerable but limited span of life. Moreover, surgeons must take into account the expense, discomfort, time, and convalescence involved in their effort, and then subtract those things from what they hope to do. At times, they should ". . . have the grace to let the sick man die in peace."[68]

Seldom can the systemic effects of disseminated cancer (malaise, anorexia, nausea, or loss of hope) be relieved by surgery. However, surgeons may still help some patients with extensive cancer by relieving pain or jaundice.

Unfortunately, their role in relieving pain caused by hepatobiliary tumors is limited because, most often, pain is caused by unresectable extensions of malignancy to retroperitoneal nerves. Resection then is irrelevant and ineffective. The liberal use of narcotics or splanchnic blocks with alcohol is better.

Only when pain is caused specifically by a lesion's mass may "debulking" have palliative value. Seldom are such heroic efforts justified in dealing with cancers of the gallbladder or biliary ducts. However, palliative extirpation of some very large, incurable, slow-growing, hepatic malignancies may benefit the patient.

The surgeon's role in relieving jaundice must also be considered in perspective. First, the contribution of jaundice to the patient's total disability must be assessed. If the effects of biliary obstruction are overshadowed by other ravages of disease, biliary decompression may be irrelevant or meddlesome. At other times, however, the patient who is systematically well may be offered respite from pruritis or progressive hepatic dysfunction by biliary decompression of a focal but unresectable obstructing lesion.

Not long ago, only surgeons could decompress the obstructed biliary tract. But, in recent years, radiologists have had more to offer. For patients known to have an unresectable malignancy, percutaneous transhepatic decompression may relieve obstructive jaundice as safely and effectively as can surgeons.[49] This procedure has been described in this chapter under diagnosis.

Surgical and radiologic techniques may appear to be competitive, but they are not (even though some surgeons and some radiologists may wish to make them so). When malignancy is known to be incurable, radiologists should prevail in their efforts to decompress the biliary tract. When there is uncertainty, however, about the nature or extent of an obstructing lesion, surgeons in their retreat from an unresectable lesion must look for ways to decompress the obstructed biliary tract.

Biliary decompression may be simple when ductal obstruction is found distal to the ductal bifurcation. In this circumstance, biliary-intestinal anastomoses or stenting of malignant strictures with transhepatic tubes is feasible.[36] Also, more proximal obstructions may be stented, or, at times, decompression of hilar obstruction may be effected best by intrahepatic access to the left hepatic duct.[55] Some authors claim that palliative resection of hilar tumors offers better palliation than stenting or bypassing procedures, but that contention is debatable.[54,58,60] Obstructions above this level, however, most often can be relieved better by radiologists than by surgeons.

RADIATION THERAPY

PHILOSOPHY AND TOLERANCE

Radiation has a significant role in symptomatic hemangiomas, a definite palliative role with metastatic disease, and a possible palliative role in primary unresectable liver tumors. Most questions on liver irradiation center around how high a dose the liver can tolerate. For many years, portions of the liver have been included in the treatment of esophageal cancer or of nodal chains in other malignancies. The major limiting factor seems to be the amount of total organ radiation.

The factors involved in hepatic tolerance to radiation have been discussed in some detail by Ingold and associates and Phillips and colleagues (Table 19-1).[69,70] Metastatic carcinoma was present in the 36 patients from the Memorial series, whereas in the Stanford series, patients with ovarian carcinoma or lymphoma were treated prophylactically.[69,70] Both institutions treated at a dose rate of 1000 rad per week or greater, usually treating one field a day. In the combined series, only four cases of radiation hepatitis occurred at or below 3500 rad: three were at the 3500-rad level and one at 3000 rad. Kaplan and Bagshaw subsequently reported two cases of radiation hepatitis at doses between 2500 to 3000 rad.[71] None of the cases of either fatal or persistent radiation hepatitis have occurred at a dose less than 3850 rad, delivered at the rate of 1000 rad per week.

Suggested dose for whole-organ radiation varies by institution and whether the organ is being treated prophylactically or for involvement (Table 19-2).[69–75] Whole-organ radiation tolerance concomitant with or preceded by chemotherapy is also gaining better definition (Table 19-2).[76–79] Because of the low doses tolerated by the entire liver, use of any supervoltage machine is probably acceptable.

PRIMARY LIVER TUMORS

Little information exists on the value of radiation for primary malignant tumors of the liver. In 1971, El-Domeiri and coworkers discussed a series of 137 patients treated over a 20-year interval at Memorial Hospital in New York.[28] Advanced disease precluded resection in 105 patients, with the following results: 44 patients—no treatment, all dead within 6 months; 31 patients—radiation doses of 1000 to 3600 rad, 70% dead within 6 months, 1 patient survived more than 1 year; 11 patients—radiation and chemotherapy, all dead in less than 1 year; 19 patients—treated with chemotherapy, 13 treated with systemic agents died within 1 year, but 2 of 6 with infusion lived 2 and 3 years. Phillips and Murikami had analyzed in detail 26 cases treated with irradiation at Memorial.[80] In four cases the dose was less than 2000 rad and was ineffective. In 22 cases the average dose was 2956 rad/23 days with the following results: marked regression, 9 cases; measurable regression, additional 5; excellent symptomatic relief, 11; some relief, 5. Average duration of life after radiation therapy was 12 months (range, 1 to 45 months).

Radiation combined with chemotherapy has received dif-

TABLE 19-1. Radiation Hepatitis: Incidence Versus Dose

RADIATION DOSE	PATIENTS WITH RADIATION HEPATITIS		PERSISTENT DAMAGE	TOTAL RECOVERY	INADEQUATE FOLLOW-UP
	Number	*Deaths*			
3000 *rad* or less	1/9 (0/19)	0	0	0	1
>3000–3500	2/9 (1/11)	0	0	1	1
>3500–4000	7/18 (0/6)	1 (3850)*	2 (3900, 3975)*	3	1
4000+	3/4	2 (4000, 5100)*	0	1	0
TOTALS	13/40 (1/36)	3	2	5	3

(Modified from Ingold JA, Reed GB, Kaplan HS et al: Radiation hepatitis. Am J Roentgenol Radium Ther Nucl Med 93:200, 1965 (open numbers) and Phillips R, Karnofsky DA, Hamilton LD et al: Roentgen therapy of hepatic metastases. Am J Roentgenol Radium Ther Nucl Med 71:826, 1954 (numbers in parentheses))

* Dosage in rads at which problems occurred in Stanford series.

TABLE 19-2. Liver Radiation Tolerance: Total Organ

AUTHOR	MAXIMUM SUGGESTED DOSE	REFERENCE	YEAR
Prophylactic or uninvolved			
Fuller	3000 rad/4 wk	72	1975
Ingold et al	3000–3500/3½ wk	69	1965
Kaplan and Bagshaw	2500 rad/2½ wk	71	1968
Organ involved			
Radiation therapy alone			
Henschke	3000 rad/4 wk	74	1975
Whitely et al	3500 rad/3½–4 wk	75	1969
Radiation therapy with or without chemotherapy			
Sherman et al (31/50 had concomitant systemic chemotherapy)	1800–3000 rad/6–10 treatments	76	1978
Webber et al (infusion 5-FUDR,* 25 patients)	2500 rad/10 × 250/2 wk	77	1978
Friedman et al (infusion 5 FU‡ + adriamycin, 35 patients)	1500–2400 rad/5–8 fractions	78	1979

* FU = 5-Fluorouracil
‡ FUDR = Fluorodeoxyuridine

fering reviews by series. Cochrane and colleagues compared results in 10 patients treated with quadruple chemotherapy of 5-fluorouracil, (5-FU), cyclophosphamide, methotrexate, and vincristine versus radiation therapy (3000 rad/15 × 200/3 weeks) followed in 2 months by the same chemotherapy.[81] At 28 weeks, 4 of 10 of the chemotherapy group were still alive versus none of the radiation and chemotherapy group (chemotherapy: median survival 21 weeks, range 4 to 72 weeks; radiation therapy chemotherapy: median survival 12 weeks, range 2 to 28 weeks). Friedman and associates reported results of a Northern California Oncology Group (NCOG) Phase I and II trial combining intrahepatic arterial adriamycin and 5-FU with whole liver radiation therapy (1500 to 2400 rad/5 to 8 fractions) in 13 patients.[78] Objective regression occurred in 6 for 4 to more than 15 months, and an additional 5 had stable disease for more than 1 to 7 months. Symptomatic improvement was noted in 11 patients.

Order and coworkers (at Johns Hopkins) presented Phase I and II data on eight patients using external beam radiation therapy in combination with alternating doses of adriamycin and a radiation sensitizer, metronidazole.[82] Patients with a Karnofsky performance status score of 60% or greater were then prepared for ^{131}I-labeled anticarcinoembryonic antigen (CEA) or antiferritin antibody for hepatoma and anti-CEA for intrahepatic biliary carcinoma. Two patients given the immunoglobulin had tumor targeting with significant remission at 1 year and 5 months, respectively.

HEMANGIOMAS

Radiation can play a significant role in the therapy of symptomatic hemangiomas of the liver. Park and Phillips irradiated five patients who had unresectable lesions with doses varying from 1300 rad in 15 days to 1900 rad in 27 days.[83] Four had excellent results, with preservation of normal function, and were disease-free at intervals varying from 8 to 14 years. Issa presented two cases and reviewed the literature.[84] He advocated radiotherapy as the treatment of choice in massive sessile hemangiomas, with a dose of 2000 to 3000 rad in 3 to 4 weeks.

RADIOTHERAPY: GALLBLADDER PLUS EXTRAHEPATIC BILE DUCT CARCINOMA

PHILOSOPHY AND RESULTS

An increasing number of authors document a significant palliative role for radiation with both primary tumors and metastases to the portahepatitis.[73,85–94] Radiotherapy plays an occasional curative role even when primary lesions recur or cannot be resected. Data on patterns of failure after "curative" operative procedures underscore the potential value of adjuvant irradiation.[94]

Before the last decade, most sources commented that these lesions were radioresistant without reporting experience to support this pessimism. Undoubtedly, because of these comments, the number of patients even referred for consideration of palliation was extremely small. Ackerman and del Regato presented a single case, with invasion through and beyond the gallbladder wall and blood vessels, of a patient given intensive postoperative radiation who remained well at 5 years.[95]

Green and associates reported one of the earliest series of external beam radiation for biliary duct cancers.[88,89] They produced significant palliation in 6 of 8 patients using low-dose schemes, with regression of jaundice and corresponding laboratory values and improvement in quality of life. One of the nonresponders was moribund and really not a candidate; the other had a 13-cm diameter lesion. Of the four cases discussed in detail in the literature, total bilirubin concentration before treatment varied from 15 to 30 mg/dl, and after treatment from 1.0 to 2.9 mg/dl. Duration of jaundice remission was from 4 to 9 months and duration of survival after surgery from 7 to 17 months. Smoran reported similar results in 13 patients treated with 1500 to 6000 rad (usually 4500 rad/25 × 180/5 weeks) for unresectable adenocarcinoma of the gallbladder and biliary tract.[93] Symptomatic relief was achieved in 1 of 5 gallbladder and 4 of 8 biliary duct lesions.

RADICAL PRIMARY RADIATION

Some reports now document the potential value of radical irradiation. Pilepich and Lambert described 11 cases from Tufts, including those of two patients given 6000 rads alone for common bile duct lesions.[92] Both had no evidence of disease 6 and 26 months later. Thirteen patients with biliary tree carcinomas were treated with "curative" intent at Harvard Joint Center (4000 to 5840 rad). Short-term local control was achieved in 5 of 13; 4 cases were controlled for 12 or more months.[87] Hanna and Rider presented results of "radical" radiation therapy at Princess Margaret Hospital (average dose 4000 rad/4 weeks; range 3488 to 6000 rad) on 18 patients with gallbladder or extrahepatic bile duct lesions.[90] Median survival was about 11 months, as opposed to 5 months in patients without radiation therapy (nonrandomized). Seven of the 18 cases reported by Hanna and Rider had initial whole abdominal radiation (2000 rad) before a right upper quadrant boost, but patterns of failure after irradiation were not discussed to document whether the whole abdominal irradiation was of value in preventing peritoneal seeding.[90] None of the preceding series stated whether chemotherapy was used in any patients.

RADIATION AND CHEMOTHERAPY

Although the combination of radiation and chemotherapy appears better than either alone for most unresectable lesions of the gastrointestinal tract, little information exists in the literature on their role for this location. Kopelson and associates presented the results of 13 cases treated at Columbia–Presbyterian Hospital.[15] Twelve of 13 had unresectable or recurrent lesions of the gallbladder or extrahepatic bile duct carcinoma. Adjuvant 5-FU chemotherapy was used in 6 (12.5 to 15 mg/kg): before radiation therapy in 1, concomitant with the first 3 days of radiation therapy in 3, and after radiation therapy in 2. All received 5-FU therapy monthly thereafter, and one also received streptozotocin therapy. Survival from initiation of radiation therapy in the unresectable or recurrent group was as follows: radiation therapy alone, 2 of 7 patients for more than 7 months but none of 7 at 12 months; radiation therapy and chemotherapy, 4 of 5 patients for more than 7 months and 2 of 5 for more than 12 months. Both had no evidence of disease at 12 and 16 months.

ADJUVANT PREOPERATIVE OR POSTOPERATIVE RADIATION THERAPY

Vaittinen reported 31 cases of curative surgery for localized gallbladder cancer (most with simple cholecystectomy).[14] Median survival in the 24 patients treated with operation alone was 29 months, in contrast to 63 months in the 7 who received postoperative radiation therapy. In the Tufts series, 3 patients received postoperative radiation therapy (4400 to 5000 rad/5 to 7 weeks), and 1 received preoperative radiation therapy (4100 rad/21 fractions).[92] Of the postoperative group, 1 of 3 was free of disease 17 months later, and the remaining 2 died of disseminated disease. The preoperative patient had a lesion of the ampulla of Vater, had a Whipple procedure 6 weeks after completion, and was NED at 4.5 years.

RADIATION: SPECIALIZED METHODS

Use of intraoperative electrons, 2500 to 4000 rad in a single fraction, has been reported for unresectable gallbladder and biliary duct lesions by two Japanese centers. Iwasaki and associates treated 8 patients with 11 to 18 MeV electrons (2 of 8 died of liver metastases, and the remaining 6 were alive NED 1 to 11 months after radiation therapy (at the time of the report).[91] Abe and colleagues treated 3 patients who died 2, 6, and 10 months after treatment without assessment of local disease status.[85]

Interstitial techniques have been described in a small number of series. Ariel and Pack reported on the treatment of 14 cases of inoperable cancer of the biliary system with radioactive rose bengal.[86] Some degree of palliation was experienced by 9 patients, and life span was believed to be prolonged in at least 3 instances. In the report by Goebel and colleagues, 2 of 13 patients received some degree of treatment with interstitial techniques with unknown results.[87] Ikeda and coworkers described the insertion of an ^{192}Ir wire through a percutaneous transhepatic catheter, but this technique would be applicable only for lesions of extremely small diameter.[73]

RADIATION THERAPY METHODS: DOSE LEVELS

DOSE-LIMITING STRUCTURES

A major deterrent to improved results is the limited tolerance of the liver, duodenum, stomach (Fig. 19-11A), and spinal cord and lack of clear definition of the lesion's location relative to these dose-limiting structures. Whereas superior and inferior extent of disease can often be outlined by a percutaneous cholangiogram or endoscopic retrograde cholangiopancreatography (ERCP) (Fig. 19-11B), the amount of extraductual disease will have to be defined by other modalities, such as ultrasound and computed tomography. Clip placement may have a potentially significant role in distant ductual lesions (Fig. 19-11C) and the bed of the gallbladder. The potential of long-term palliation and cure should increase if shrinking field techniques can be used to spare as much normal tissue as possible.

TUMOR VOLUME AND DOSE

Definite areas at risk (Fig. 19-11C, 19-11D) include the tumor bed or unresected tumor and areas of potential microscopic lymph node involvement along the porta hepatis, pancreaticoduodenal system, and celiac axis. An intravenous pyelogram should be done at the start of treatment to be certain of left renal function. This is important as one half to two thirds of

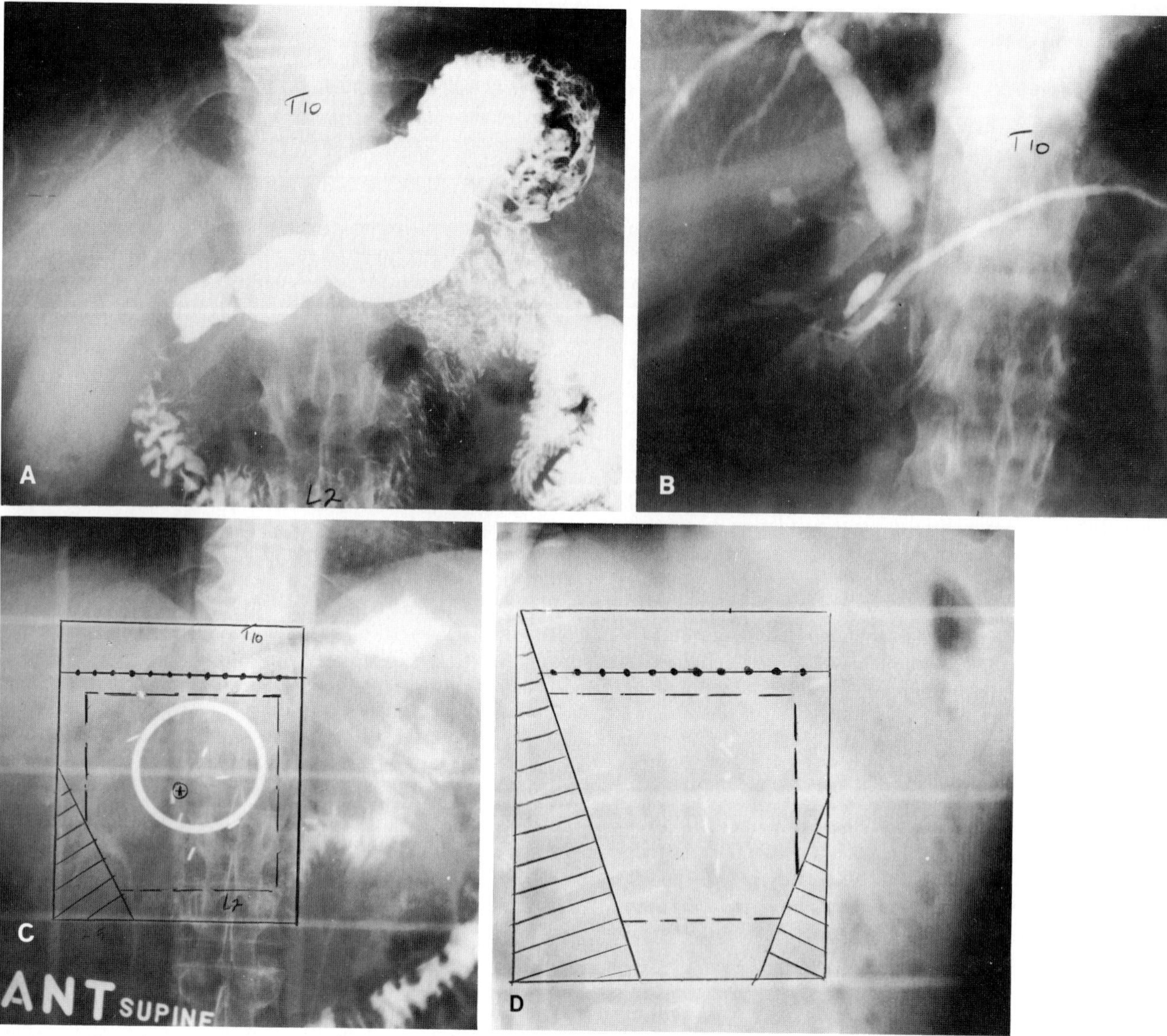

FIG. 19-11. Patient with distal biliary duct lesion unresectable based on adherence to the portal vein. A decompressing bypass procedure was done. Tumor margins were somewhat indistinct. The maximum tumor extent was marked with clips for postoperative radiation. *A*, Preoperative normal upper gastrointestinal series. *B*, Preoperative endoscopic retrograde cholangiopancreatography revealed a normal pancreatic duct. The distal common bile duct is normal for about 3 cm, but just proximal to that is a smooth, tapered narrowing about 1½ cm long. *C*, Anterior and *D*, lateral planning films were done with contrast material in the stomach and kidneys; 30% to 40% of the right kidney was within the initial radiation AP-PA portal, but the left kidney was totally excluded. The most anterior–superior clip does not represent tumor. The patient was treated with a fourfield technique (AP:PA:laterals) at 180 rad/fraction 5 days a week. Large fields (*solid lines with blocks in cross-hatched area*) received 3600 rads, after which the superior field extent was reduced (•—•—•) and the dose increased to 4500 rads. A total dose of 6200 rads was received in the final boost field (---). (Modified from Gunderson L: Hepatic tumors. In Margulis A (ed): Alimentary Tract Radiology, p. 604. St. Louis, CV Mosby, 1979)

the right kidney is usually included in the radiation field, and normal renal function may therefore depend upon a functioning left kidney. After initial simulation films are done to outline surgical clips, contrast in the duodenum helps to define nodal volumes.

The initial large field volume can be included to 4000 to 4500 rad in 170- to 200-rad fractions 5 days/week through a three- or four-field plan (anteroposterior and laterals or anteroposterior:posteroanterior (AP:PA) and laterals) using blocks when possible to exclude unnecessary bowel, kidney, and liver. Use of lateral fields (Fig. 19-11D) for part of the treatment allows decreased dosage to the spinal cord, right kidney, and portions of the liver. Wedge pair or arc techniques can be used during large or boost fields to alter dose distribution. Because of liver tolerance, we usually do our first field reduction after 3500 to 4000 rad and a second reduction after

4500 to 5000 rad if gross disease exists. Our upper dose level within the second boost field (preferably as small as 7 × 7 or 8 × 8) is 5500 to more than 6000 rad/6½ to 7 weeks, using the latter dose only if the boost volume is carefully defined.

If high-energy linear accelerators are available (≥ 8 MeV), parallel-opposed AP:PA techniques can be well tolerated to 4500 to 5000 rad on a short-and long-term basis. Although the Tufts study went to 6000 rads AP:PA by shrinking the medial margin off the spinal cord, the risk of symptomatic fibrosis increases. We prefer multifield techniques for long-term normal tissue tolerance and realize the inherent danger of marginal recurrence if wisdom is not used in field design (computed tomography and ultrasound studies, lateral films done with transhepatic cholangiogram or ERCP studies, and clip placement can help minimize this risk). Multifield or rotation techniques are needed with supervoltage energy 4 MeV or lower if going above 4000 to 4500 rad.

CHEMOTHERAPY

Chemotherapeutic management of gallbladder and biliary tract cancer has rarely been studied systematically because of inadequate numbers of patients at individual institutions.[37, 97–99] Therefore, in reviewing the chemotherapy for these diseases, rely on case reports and small series for evidence of appropriate therapy.

Table 19-3 gives an indication of the small numbers of patients with primary biliary tract cancer that have reportedly undergone therapy with various single agents and combinations of drugs. As can be seen, there is little information available that would allow the clinician to choose a clearly appropriate drug treatment regimen. It appears that mitomycin C is the most active single agent (Table 19-3), although only 15 cases are reported.[37] Only in rare series has combination chemotherapy been used in these diseases (Table 19-3), and fewer still report more than 10 cases.[37] The Southeastern Cancer Study Group has reported a clinical trial in which adriamycin and bleomycin were used in the therapy of patients with hepatocellular and biliary tract cancer.[99] Only 3 patients with biliary tract tumor were entered into the study, and 1 responded. A larger study has been reported by the group at Georgetown with the use of FAM (5-fluorouracil, adriamycin, mitomycin-C) in hepatobiliary tract cancer.[97] Of 13 evaluable cases of cholangiocarcinoma, 4 patients responded to chemotherapy, with partial regression of tumor. The median duration of response was 8.5 months, with a range of 5 to 16 months. Additionally, 6 of 13 patients with previously progressive disease stabilized on FAM therapy without achieving objective response.

Oncologists managing patients with advanced biliary tract cancer should be aware that there are no firmly documented "standard" chemotherapeutic regimens for gallbladder and cholangiocarcinoma; thus patients with these diseases should be entered into clinical trials whenever possible. If patients are to be treated off protocol, the FAM regimen is a reasonable choice. (This program is decribed in detail in the chapter Cancer of the Stomach.) In patients with biliary tract cancer, clinicians should very carefully monitor hepatic function tests when administering FAM chemotherapy. Patients with elevated bilirubin or alkaline phosphatase levels should have the adriamycin doses decreased or eliminated, because this drug depends on biliary excretion for clearance.

HEPATOCELLULAR CARCINOMA

More information is available on the chemotherapy of hepatocellular cancer than on the chemotherapy of gallbladder and bile duct cancers. Two general approaches to chemotherapy have been explored in patients with hepatoma: One is the systemic administration of single and multiple chemotherapeutic drugs, and the other approach is hepatic artery infusion of cytotoxic drugs. The latter strategy has appeal because of the relative ease of placing hepatic artery catheters either at operation or percutaneously.[31] Recently, as reviewed in the radiotherapy section of this chapter, there has been interest in combining hepatic artery infusional chemotherapy with whole liver irradiation.

The systemic chemotherapy of hepatocellular cancer has been extensively reviewed.[37,100] In general, many of the studies cited in these reviews suffer from several defects in protocol design and execution. Many have small numbers of patients (frequently fewer than 10). Patient selection may be an important factor because most studies are not randomized, and it is not clear what criteria may have been used to select patients for inclusion. Moreover, there are differences in criteria used to ascertain objective responses among the various studies.Table 19-4 lists clinical studies on more than 10 patients using various single drugs and combinations of agents and lists ongoing chemotherapeutic studies of hepatocellular cancer. As can be ascertained from Table 19-4, few

TABLE 19-3. Chemotherapy for Primary Biliary Tract Cancer

DRUG	PATIENTS	PARTIAL RESPONSE		REFERENCE
	No.	*No.*	%	
Mitomycin	15	7	(42)	Haskell (37)
5-FU*	17	4	(23)	Haskell (37)
BCNU†	4	2		Haskell (37)
Adriamycin + bleomycin	3	1		Ravry and Hester (99)
5-FU + adriamycin + mitomycin-C (FAM)	13	4	(31)	Cambareri et al (97)

* 5-FU = 5-Fluorouracil
† BCNU = 1,3-Bis(2-Chlorethyl)-1-Nitrosourea

TABLE 19-4. Systemic Chemotherapy of Hepatocellular Carcinoma

DRUG*	EVALUABLE CASES	RESPONSE		AUTHOR OR GROUP†	REFERENCE
Single agent	*No.*	*No.*	*%*		
Adriamycin	13	2	(15)	Idhe et al	101
Adriamycin	11	11	(100)	Olweny et al	102
Adriamycin	41	7	(17)	Vogel et al	103
Adriamycin	14	2	(14)	Falkson et al	104
5-FU (p.o. + i.v.)	21	0	(0)	Link et al	105
5-FU (p.o.)	12	6	(50)	Kennedy et al	106
5-FU (p.o.)	30	7	(23)	Falkson et al (ECOG)	104
Neocarzinostatin	30	7	(23)	Falkson et al (ECOG)	107
Combination chemotherapy					
5-FU + BCNU	19	7	(37)	Moertel	24
5-FU + BCNU	14	1	(7)	McIntire et al	34
5-FU + adriamycin	38	5	(13)	Baker et al (SWOG)	108
5-FU + mitomycin-C	13	5	(38)	Umsawasdi et al	96
5-FU + streptozotocin	13	3	(2)	Falkson et al (ECOG)	104
5-FU + methyl CCNU	26	2	(8)	Ravry and Hester (SEG)	99
Adriamycin + bleomycin	26	5	(19)	Ravry and Hester (SEG)	99
Ongoing studies					
AMSA versus adriamycin versus neocarzinostatin	. . .	. . .		ECOG	. . .
AMSA	. . .	. . .		SWOG	. . .
VP-16	. . .	. . .		EORTC	. . .

* p.o. = orally; i.v. = intravenously; BCNU = 1,3 Bis (2-Chloroethyl)-1-Nitrosourea; CCNU = 1-(2-Chloroethyl)-3-Cyclohexyl-1-Nitrosourea; 5-FU = 5-Fluorouracil; AMSA = 4′-9(Acridinylamino)-Methan-Sulfan-M-Anisidide; VP-16 = Epipodophyllotoxin.

† ECOG = Eastern Cooperative Oncology Group; SWOG = Southwest Oncology Group; SEG = Southeastern Cancer Study Group; EORTC = European Organization for Research on Cancer Treatment.

drugs or combination of drugs have been evaluated in adequate numbers of patients with hepatocellular cancer. Adriamycin, 5-FU, and neocarzinostatin are the only single agents studied in sufficiently large series. The response rates for these agents vary widely between individual series. With adriamycin, for example, reported responses have ranged between 13% and 100%. The study in which 100% response was reported was from Africa, whereas studies on adriamycin's effectiveness in American patients have shown less than a 20% response rate.[101–103] At least in American patients, it appears that good performance status is an important factor favoring response to chemotherapy. In the study by Ihde and colleagues, only 2 of 13 patients responded.[101] Of the 4 fully ambulatory patients, however, 2 responded. In the study by Vogel and associates in which both African and American patients were treated, 7 of 41 patients responded; however, the response rate both in African and American patients with good performance status was 25%.[103]

5-Fluorouracil as a single agent has minimal activity (Table 19-4). This drug has been given intravenously and orally; the largest series found no patient response to this drug.[105] In a small group of 12 patients, Kennedy and coworkers did report a 50% response rate, but these results need to be confirmed by other studies.[106] There were no obvious anomalies in patient performance status, bulk of disease, or criteria of response that would favor high response rates in the Kennedy series.

Results with combination chemotherapy in hepatocellular cancer have also been variable (Table 19-4); 5-FU and BCNU combinations have produced variable response rates. Although a Mayo Clinic study[24] reported a 37% response rate in 19 patients, the Southwest Oncology Group reported that only 5 of 38 (13%) patients responded with this combination.[34] A small study from Thailand by Umsawasdi and coworkers indicated that 5-FU plus mitomycin-C produced a response in 5 of 13 patients (38%).[96] This study needs confirmation. In conclusion, there is no single agent or combination drug program of systemic chemotherapy for hepatocellular cancer that can be considered to be "standard." Certainly, all patients with hepatocellular cancer should be potential candidates for experimental chemotherapy protocols.

Although data on combination chemotherapy in hepatocellular cancer are limited, the quality of responses attained by individual patients may be excellent. Figure 19-12 shows the sequence of liver scan and AFP improvement in a 58-year-old woman with hepatoma treated at the Vincent T. Lombardi Cancer Center at Georgetown University. This woman presented with extensive hepatic tumor involvement and an AFP level of 16,500 ng/ml (normal < 40 ng/ml). She was treated with a combination of 5-FU, mitomycin-C, and streptozotocin (FMS), with progressive improvement in liver scan findings and AFP level over an 18-month period. Figure 19-12 shows the marked resolution of abnormalities on liver scan until, after 1 year of therapy, the scan was normal. The patient was asymptomatic and clinically was a complete responder, although the AFP level never decreased below 500 ng/ml, indicating persistent disease. After 18 months of FMS therapy, the patient's tumor progressed rapidly, leading to death from hepatic failure within 4 months. This case shows the excellent quality of response in patients with hepatocellular cancer and also indicates the usefulness of AFP as a marker of disease progression and regression.

Hepatic artery perfusion with chemotherapeutic agents has

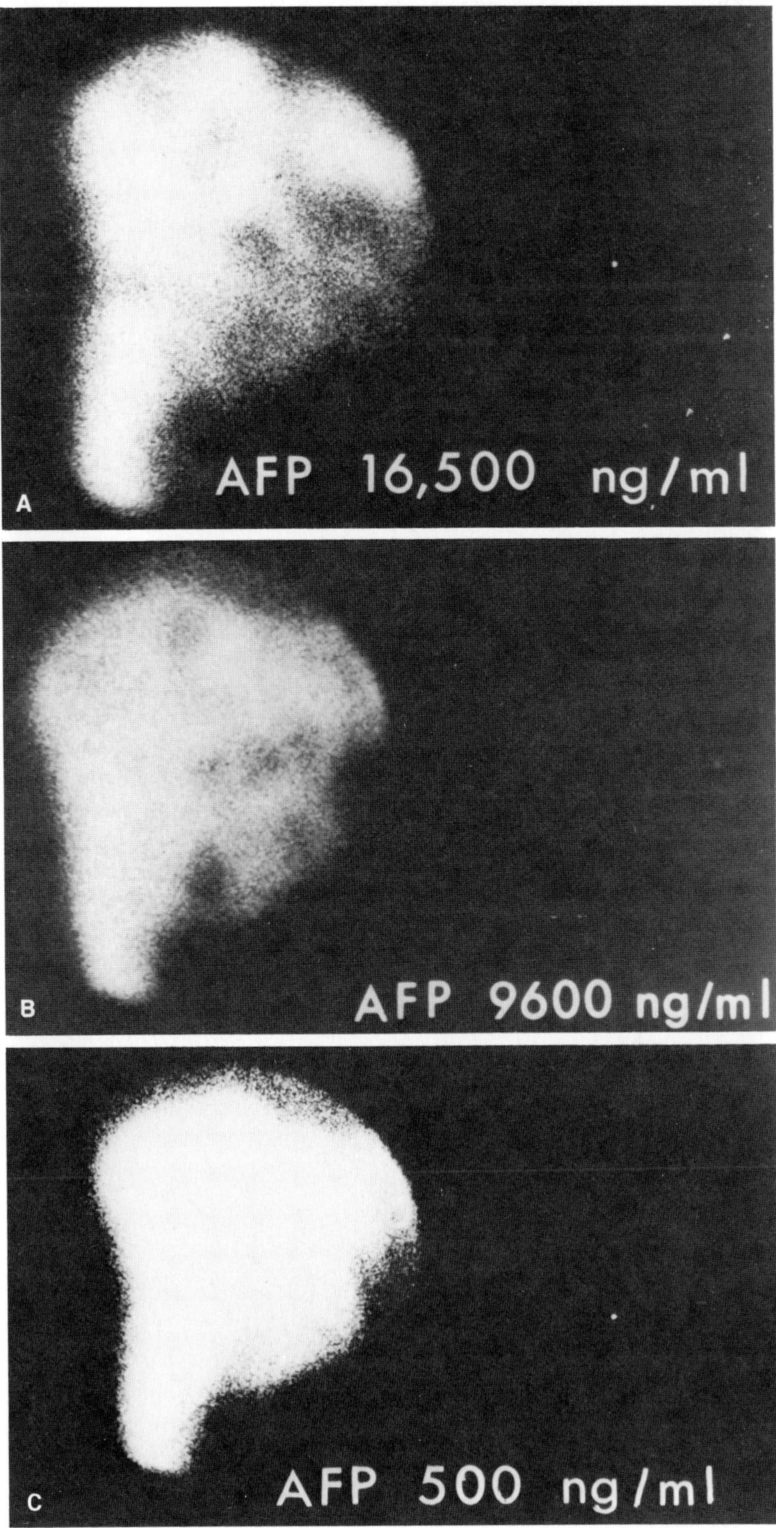

FIG. 19-12. *A*, Liver scan at presentation shows multiple deposits of hepatocellular carcinoma. *B*, After 4 months of chemotherapy, the patient shows improvement on liver scan and decreased alpha fetoprotein (*AFP*). *C*, After one year of therapy, the patient has a normal liver scan, although AFP levels remain elevated, indicating persistent hepatocellular cancer.

also been used in the therapy of patients with hepatocellular carcinoma. This treatment approach has much theoretical attractiveness because hepatocellular carcinoma frequently remains localized to the liver, and hepatic artery perfusion should markedly increase the drug concentration deliverable to the hepatic tumor. However, no controlled trial comparing hepatic artery perfusion with systemic administration of the same chemotherapy has been completed in hepatocellular cancer. Thus, all reports of hepatic artery perfusion chemotherapy are phase II studies and cannot be considered to have proved efficacy superior to that of intravenous treatment.

The number of patients in whom hepatic artery perfusion

has been used is small. In the extensive review of this subject by Haskell, 18 references to clinical experience with hepatic artery perfusion in hepatocellular carcinoma were cited.[37] Of these, only 4 studies included more than 10 patients, and the maximum number of patients included in any one series was 19. This paucity of cases results from the fact that hepatocellular cancer is rare, and also because catheter perfusion of hepatic tumors through the hepatic artery is logistically complicated, since it requires skilled catheter placement, treatment periods lasting from several days to several months, and careful catheter maintenance.[31]

Current data on intra-arterial chemotherapy of hepatocellular carcinoma are reviewed in Table 19-5. The fluorinated pyrimidines 5-FU and FUDR (fluorodeoxyuridine) have been used in the treatment of more than 100 patients. In collected series (in most instances, individual reports contained less than 10 patients), 5-FU produced partial response in 18% of patients, whereas FUDR was effective in 50% of patients. Median survival of all patients treated with fluorinated pyrimidines by the intra-arterial route is about 8.5 months; occasionally such patients experience prolonged survival.[37] Whether FUDR is indeed superior to 5-FU is debatable. No randomized trials between the two drugs given by arterial perfusion have been done, and the FUDR results come from studies performed 5 to 15 years ago when criteria for objective response may not have been as rigorous as at present.

In general, hepatic artery catheterization is well tolerated, with minimal toxicity even after long periods of catheter perfusion.[31] Occasionally, hepatic artery thrombosis will occur as a result of hepatic artery catheterization, and rarely catheter-associated sepsis can occur, although it is usually well managed by systemic antibiotics and catheter removal.

Ongoing studies using hepatic artery perfusion are also described in Table 19-5. The Southwest Oncology Group is doing a phase II study of FUDR plus adriamycin plus streptozotocin. The Sidney Farber Cancer Center is pursuing a phase II and III study comparing various single agents to the combination of methotrexate and thymidine. An interesting phase III multimodality study by the Northern California Oncology Group is being done that compares hepatic radiation alone with hepatic radiation with intra-arterial or intravenous 5-FU, adriamycin, and mitomycin-C. These studies should all be useful in pointing towards the future direction of hepatocellular cancer therapy.

Although all patients with primary liver cancer should be considered candidates for investigative protocols, treatment programs can be recommended for patients who, for whatever reason, are not to be treated in clinical trials. The combination of low-dose hepatic radiation (2100 rad at 300 rad/day;), 5-FU (10 mg/kg/day by constant intra-arterial infusion throughout radiation therapy), and adriamycin (5 mg/m^2 1 hour to 2 hours before each radiation treatment) is well tolerated and produces objective response in up to 40% of patients.[78] If hepatic irradiation and intra-arterial chemotherapy cannot be used, treatment with the FAM regimen (described in detail in the chapter Cancer of the Stomach) may be used. In patients who have had hepatic irradiation plus intra-arterial chemotherapy, FAM may be used as maintenance chemotherapy. The FAM regimen should be started at a maximum of 50% of projected doses to ascertain each individual patient's

TABLE 19-5. Chemotherapy by Hepatic Artery Perfusion in Patients with Hepatocellular Cancer

TREATMENT*	PATIENTS	RESPONSE		AUTHOR OR GROUP†	REFERENCE
	No.	*No.*	*%*		
5-FU	56	10	(18)	Collected series	Haskell (37)
FuDR	48	27	(56)	Collected series	Haskell (37)
Ongoing studies					
FuDR + adriamycin + streptozotocin	...	...		SWOG	...
FuDR versus methotrexate + thymidine versus neocarzinostatin versus BCNU versus dichloro-methotrexate with radiation therapy	...	...		SFCC	...
Whole liver irradiation + 5-FU, adriamycin + mitomycin-C (FAM) i.v. versus whole liver irradiation + FAM by hepatic artery infusion	45	...		NCOG	...

* i.v. = intravenously; FU = 5-Fluorouracil; FuDr = Fluorodeoxyuridine; BCNU = 1,3-bis (2-Chloroethyl)-1-Nitrosourea

† SWOG = Southwest Oncology Group.
NCOG = Northern California Oncology Group.
SFCC = Sidney Farber Cancer Center.

hematologic tolerance to systemic chemotherapy after hepatic irradiation.

FUTURE CONSIDERATIONS

HEPATOCELLULAR CANCER

With the advent of more sophisticated diagnostic techniques, a role may exist for more aggressive liver radiation when isolated single metastases or primary liver tumors are documented in patients in whom operative removal is not appropriate because of the lesion's location or the patient's medical condition. In such instances, whole-organ radiotherapy could be complemented by a boost to the defined gross tumor volumes with shrinking field techniques. In a Radiotherapy Oncology Group (RTOG) pilot study for metastatic disease, about 3000 rads is given to the total liver in 160- to 200-rad fractions, with a 2000-rad boost to the solitary lesion with conventional beams. With specialized beams, such as pi mesons and protons, the boost volume could be localized precisely and even higher boost doses considered.

Another newer modality of therapy that must be evaluated is regional hyperthermia. With the localized nature of many hepatocellular cancers, hyperthermia could be effectively applied and may be appropriate to combine with chemotherapy or radiation therapy.

GALLBLADDER AND EXTRAHEPATIC BILE DUCT CARCINOMA

In view of the large number of patients who are not candidates for radical resection, the combination of radiation and chemotherapy, as used in other nonresectable gastrointestinal carcinomas, should be evaluated more extensively. An aggressive approach is warranted because a large percentage of patients with biliary duct carcinoma die with localized disease. Although occasional local control will be achieved with high-dose precision irradiation to 5500 to more than 6000 rad, most lesions are too large for permanent control at that dose level. Radiation dose modifiers may ultimately play some role. The intraoperative electron beam method used by the Japanese appears likely to result in fibrosis and obstruction even if the lesion is controlled. A preferable approach would be to give an intraoperative boost (about 1500 rad) to the gross lesion at exploration, do a left intrahepatic bypass to the jejunum, or leave in a permanent indwelling tube to prevent later obstruction owing to fibrosis. One could deliver an additional 4500 to 5000 rad/5 to 6 weeks postoperatively with or without chemotherapy. An alternative approach would be to combine external irradiation with a boost dose of interstitial irradiation via an indwelling catheter (2000–3000 rad with iridium or microcesium sources).

Even in patients with resected lesions, the resultant survival rate is significantly less than 50%. Because most failures are in the surrounding organs, tissues, or lymph nodes, preoperative, postoperative, or preoperative plus postoperative adjuvant radiation with or without chemotherapy should strongly be considered in controlled studies rather than just extending the operative procedure, as suggested by Gradisar and Kelly.[109] For gallbladder lesions, because abdominal components of failure are more common, a portion of the radiation treatment may have to be by a total abdominal approach, as for ovarian cancer, if the lesion extends to the serosal surface.[110] However, it should be emphasized that total abdominal irradiation will severely limit the ability to subsequently administer aggressive combination chemotherapy.

REFERENCES

1. Silverberg E: Cancer statistics 1980. Cancer 30:39, 1980
2. Arnaud JP, Graf P, Gramfort JL, et al: Primary carcinoma of the gallbladder: review of 25 cases. Am J Surg 138:403, 1979
3. Bismuth H, Malt RA: Carcinoma of the biliary tract. N Engl J Med 301:704, 1979
4. Moertel CG: The liver. In Holland JF, Frei E III (eds): Cancer Medicine, pp 1541–1547. Philadelphia, Lea & Febiger, 1973
5. Case Records of the Massachusetts General Hospital. N Engl J Med 302:1132, 1980
6. Okuda K, Musha H, Nakajima Y, et al: Clinicopathologic features of encapsulated hepatocellular carcinoma. Cancer 40: 1240, 1977
7. Sorensen TIA, Baden H: Benign hepatocellular tumors. Scand J Gastroenterol 10:113, 1975
8. Mays ET, Christopherson WM, Mahr MM, et al: Hepatic changes in young women ingesting contraceptive steroids. JAMA 235:730, 1976
9. Strauch GO: Primary carcinoma of the gallbladder. Surgery 47:368, 1960
10. Orloff MJ, Charters AC: Tumors of the gallbladder and bile duct. In Bockus HL, Berk JE, and Haubrich WS (eds): Gastroenterology, Vol 3, 3rd ed, pp 831–842. Philadelphia, WB Saunders, 1976
11. Moertel CG: The extrahepatic bile ducts. See Reference 4, pp 1551–1556
12. Tompkins RK, Johnson J, Storm FK: Operative endoscopy in the management of biliary neoplasms. Am J Surg 132:174, 1976
13. Goldsmith NA, Woodburne RT: The surgical anatomy pertaining to liver resection. Surg Gynecol Obstet 105:310, 1957
14. Vaittinen E: Carcinoma of the gallbladder: a study of 390 cases diagnosed in Finland 1953–1967. Ann Chir Gynaecol Fenn 29, Suppl 168:7, 1970
15. Kopelson G, Harisiadis L, Tretter P: The role of radiation therapy in cancer of the extra-hepatic biliary system: an analysis of thirteen patients and a review of the literature of the effectiveness of surgery, chemotherapy, and radiotherapy. Int J Radiat Oncol Biol Phys 2:883, 1977
16. Warren KW, Mountain JD, Lloyd-Jones W: Malignant tumors of the bile ducts. Br J Surg 59:501, 1972
17. Braasch JW, Warren KW, Kune GA: Malignant neoplasms of the bile ducts. Surg Clin North Am 47:627, 1967
18. Fisher RL, Schever PJ, Sherlock S: Primary liver cell carcinoma in the presence or absence of hepatitis B antigen. Cancer 38:901, 1976
19. Anthony PP, Vogel CL, Barker LF: Liver cell dysplasia: a premalignant condition. J Clin Pathol 26:217, 1973
20. Farrell GC, Uren RF, Perkins RW, et al: Androgen induced hepatoma. Lancet 1:540, 1975
21. Polk HC: Carcinoma of the calcified gallbladder. Gastroenterology 50:582, 1966
22. Levin B, Riddell RH, Kirsner JB: Management of precancerous lesions of the gastrointestinal tract. Clin Gastroenterol 5:827, 1976
23. Ross AP, Braasch JW: Ulcerative colitis and carcinoma of the proximal bile duct. Gut 14:94, 1973
24. Moertel CG: Clinical management of advanced gastrointestinal cancer. Cancer 36:675, 1975
25. Keill RH, DeWeese MS: Primary carcinoma of the gallbladder. Am J Surg 119:726, 1973
26. Okuda K, Kubo Y, Okazaki N: Clinical aspects of intrahepatic

bile duct carcinoma including hilar carcinoma: a study of 57 autopsy proven cases. Cancer 39:323, 1977
27. Moertel CG, Reitemeier RJ: Advanced Gastrointestinal Cancer: Clinical Management and Chemotherapy. New York, Harper, 1969
28. El-Domeiri AA, Huvos AG, Goldsmith HS, et al: Primary malignant tumors of the liver. Cancer 27:7, 1971
29. Dowdy GS Jr: The Biliary Tract. Philadelphia, Lea & Febiger, 1969
30. Longmire WP: Tumors of the extrahepatic biliary radicals. Curr Probl Surg 1, No. 2:1, 1976
31. Ramming KP, Sparks FC, Eilber FR, et al: Management of hepatic metastases. Semin Oncol 4:71, 1977
32. Waldmann TA, McIntire KR: The use of a radioimmunoassay for alpha-beta-protein in the diagnosis of malignancy. Cancer 34:1510, 1974
33. Chen DS, Jung JL: Serum alpha-beta-protein in hepatocellular carcinoma. Cancer 40:779, 1977
34. McIntire KR, Vogel CL, Primack A, et al: Effect of surgical and chemotherapeutic treatment on alpha-beta-protein levels in patients with hepatocellular carcinoma. Cancer 34:677, 1976
35. Spencer RF: Radionuclide liver scans in tumor detection. Cancer 37:475, 1976
36. Terblanche J: Carcinoma of the proximal extrahepatic biliary tree: definitive and palliative treatment. Surg Annu 11:249, 1979
37. Haskell CM: Cancer of the liver. In Haskell CM (ed): Cancer Treatment, pp 319–357. Philadelphia, WB Saunders, 1980
38. Ramming KP, Haskell CM, Tesler AS: Gastrointestinal tract neoplasms. See Reference 37, 327
39. Reuter SR: The current status of angiography in the evaluation of cancer patients. Cancer 37:532, 1976
40. Moertel CG: The gallbladder. See Reference 4, pp 1547–1551
41. Tanga MR, Ewing JB: Primary malignant tumors of the gallbladder: review of 52 cases. Am J Surg 113:738, 1967
42. Litwin MS: Primary carcinoma of the gallbladder: a review of 78 patients. Arch Surg 95:236, 1967
43. McDermott WV, Peinert RA: Carcinoma in the superampillary portion of the bile ducts. Surg Gynec Obstet 149:681, 1979
44. Ozaki H, Hojo K, Miwa K: A safe method of intrahepatic biliary drainage in obstructive jaundice. Am J Surg 133:379, 1977
45. Adson MA, Beart RW: Elective hepatic resections. Surg Clin North Am 57:339, 1977
46. Lin TY: Results of 107 hepatic lobectomies with a preliminary report on the use of a clamp to reduce blood loss. Ann Surg 177:413, 1973
47. Fortner JG, Kim D, MacLean BJ: Major hepatic resection for neoplasia: personal experience in 108 patients. Ann Surg 188:363, 1978
48. Starzl T, Koep LJ, Weil R, et al: Right trisegmentectomy for hepatic neoplasms. Surg Gynecol Obstet 150:208, 1980
49. Berquist TH, May GR, Johnson CM, et al: Percutaneous biliary decompression. Am J Roentgenol (in press)
50. Piehler JM, Crichlow RW: Primary carcinoma of the gallbladder (collective reviews). 147, Surg Gynecol Obstet 6:929, 1978
51. Appleman RM, Morlock CG, Dahlin DC: Longterm survival in carcinoma of the gallbladder. Surg Gynecol Obstet 117:459, 1963
52. Fahim RB, McDonald JR, Richard JC, et al: Carcinoma of the gallbladder: a study of its modes of spread. Ann Surg 156:114, 1962
53. Adson MA: Carcinoma of the gallbladder. Surg Clin North Am 53:1203, 1973
54. Iwasaki Y, Ohto M, Todoroki T, et al: Treatment of carcinoma of the biliary system. Surg Gynecol Obstet 144:219, 1977
55. Dudley SE, Adson, MA: Biliary decompression in hilar obstruction. Arch Surg 114:519, 1979
56. Koep LJ: Personal communication
57. Todoroki T, Okamura T, Fukao K: Gross appearance of carcinoma of the main hepatic duct and its prognosis. Surg Gynecol Obstet 150:33, 1980
58. Evander A, Fredlund P, Hoevels J, et al: Evaluation of aggressive surgery for carcinoma of the extrahepatic bile ducts. Ann Surg 191:23, 1980
59. Traverso LW, Longmire WP: Preservation of the pylorus in pancreaticoduodenectomy: a followup evaluation. Ann Surg 192:306, 1980
60. White TT, Hart MJ: Central hepatic resection and anastomosis for strictures or carcinoma. Presented at the American Surgical Association Meeting, Atlanta, April 1980
61. Smith R: Hepaticojejunostomy with transhepatic intubation: a technique for very high strictures of the hepatic ducts. Br J Surg 51:186, 1964
62. Cameron JL, Gayler BW, Zuidema GD: The use of silastic transhepatic stents in benign and malignant biliary strictures. Ann Surg 188:552, 1978
63. Farnell MB, Adson, MA: Unpublished data
64. Akwari OE, Kelly KA: Surgical treatment of adenocarcinoma. Arch Surg 114:22, 1979
65. van Heerden JA, Judd ES, Dockerty MB: Carcinoma of the extrahepatic bile ducts. Am J Surg 113:49, 1967
66. Goetze O, Schwabe H: Alte und neve Operationen der hohen Gallengangsstenose. Langenbecks Arch Klin Chir 270:97, 1951
67. Akwari OE, van Heerden J, Adson MA, et al: Radical pancreatoduodenectomy for cancer of the papilla of Vater. Arch Surg 112:451, 1977
68. Buchan J: Witch Wood, p 195. London, Hodder & Stoughton, 1927
69. Ingold JA, Reed GB, Kaplan HS, et al: Radiation hepatitis. Am J Roentgenol Radium Ther Nucl Med 93:200, 1965
70. Phillips R, Karnofsky DA, Hamilton LD, et al: Roentgen therapy of hepatic metastases. Am J Roentgenol Radium Ther Nucl Med 71:826, 1954
71. Kaplan HS, Bagshaw MA: Radiation hepatitis: possible prevention by combined isotopic and external radiation therapy. Radiology 91:1214, 1968
72. Fuller L: Personal communication, 1975
73. Ikeda H, Kuroda C, Uchida H, et al: Intraluminal irradiation with Iridium-192 wires for extrahepatic bile duct carcinomas. Nippon Igaku Hoshasen Gakkai Zasshi 39:1356, 1979
74. Henschke U: Personal communication, 1975
75. Whiteley HW, Stearns MW Jr, Leaming RH, et al: Radiation therapy in the palliative management of patients with recurrent cancer of the rectum and colon. Surg Clin North Am 49:381, 1969
76. Sherman DM, Weichselbaum R, Order SE, et al: Palliation of hepatic metastases. Cancer 41:2013, 1978
77. Webber BM, Soderberg CH, Leave LA, et al: A combined treatment approach to management of hepatic metastases. Cancer 42:1087, 1978
78. Friedman MA, Volberding PA, Cassidy MJ, et al: Therapy for hepatocellular cancer with intrahepatic arterial adriamycin and 5-fluorouracil combined with whole liver radiation: an NCOG Study. Cancer Treat Rep 63:1885, 1979
79. Volberding PA, Friedman MA, Phillips TL: Hepatoma treated with intraarterial (IA) polychemotherapy plus whole liver radiation (abstr). Proc Am Soc Clin Oncol Am Assoc Cancer Res 21:481, 1980
80. Phillips R, Murikami K: Primary neoplasms of the liver: results of radiation therapy. Cancer 13:714, 1960
81. Cochrane AMG, Murray-Lyon IM, Brinkley DM, et al: Quadruple chemotherapy versus radiotherapy in treatment of primary hepatocellular carcinoma. Cancer 40:609, 1977
82. Order SE, Leibel S, Klein JL, et al: A phase I–II study of radiolabeled antibody integrated in multimodal treatment of primary hepatic malignancies: Proceedings of the American Society of Therapeutic Radiology, 1979. Int J Radium Oncol Biol Phys 5:120, 1979
83. Park WC, Phillips R: The role of radiation therapy in the management of hemangiomas of the liver. JAMA 212:1496, 1970
84. Issa P: Cavernous haemangioma of the liver: the role of radiotherapy. Br J Radiol 41:26, 1968
85. Abe M, Takahashi M, Yabumoto E: Clinical experiences with intraoperative radiotherapy of locally advanced cancer. Cancer 45:40, 1980
86. Ariel IM, Pack GT: The treatment of inoperable cancer of the

biliary system with radioactive I[131] rose bengal. Am J Roentgenol Radium Ther Nucl Med 83:474, 1980
87. Goebel RH, Levene MB, Weischselbaum RR, et al: Techniques for localized radiation of carcinoma of the biliary tree (abstr). Int J Radiat Oncol Biol Phys 5:80, 1979
88. Green N: Personal communication, 1975
89. Green N, Mikkelsen WP, Kernen JA: Cancer of the common hepatic bile ducts—palliative radiotherapy. Radiology 109:687, 1973
90. Hanna SS, Rider WD: Carcinoma of the gallbladder or extrahepatic bile ducts: the role of the radiotherapy. Can Med Assoc J 118:59, 1978
91. Iwasaki Y, Ohto M, Todoroki T, et al: Treatment of carcinoma of the biliary system. Surg Gynecol Obstet 144:219, 1977
92. Pilepich MV, Lambert PM: Radiotherapy of carcinomas of the extrahepatic biliary system. Radiology 127:767, 1978
93. Smoron GL: Radiation therapy of carcinoma of gallbladder and biliary tract. Cancer 40:1422, 1977
94. Kopelson G, Galdabini J, Warshaw AL et al: Patterns of failure after curative surgery for extrahepatic biliary tract carcinoma: Implications for adjuvant therapy. Int J Rad Oncol Biol Phys 7:413, 1980
95. Ackerman LV, del Regato JA: Cancer of the digestive tract. In Cancer: Diagnosis, Treatment and Prognosis, 4th ed, pp 408–605. St Louis, CV Mosby, 1970
96. Umsawasdi T, Chainuvati T, Viranuvatti V: Combination chemotherapy of hepatocellular carcinoma with fluorouracil and mitomycin-C (abstr). Proc Am Soc Clin Oncol Am Assoc Cancer Res 19:193, 1978
97. Cambareri RJ, Smith FP, Kales A, et al: 5-fluorouracil, adriamycin and mitomycin-C in cholangiocarcinoma (abstr). Proc Am Soc Clin Oncol Am Assoc Cancer Res 21:418, 1980
98. Moertel CG: Chemotherapy of gastrointestinal cancer. Clin Gastroenterol 5:777, 1976
99. Ravry MJR, Hester M: Combination chemotherapy of hepatocellular and biliary tract cancer with adriamycin plus bleomycin (abstr). Proc Am Soc Clin Oncol Am Assoc Cancer Res 21:366, 1980
100. Lee YTN: Systemic and regional treatment of primary carcinoma of the liver. Cancer Treat Rev 4:195, 1977
101. Ihde DC, Kane RH, Cohen MH, et al: Adriamycin therapy in American patients with hepatocellular carcinoma. Cancer Treat Rep 61:1385, 1977
102. Olweny CLM, Toya T, Katongole-Mbidde E, et al: Preliminary communication: treatment of hepatocellular carcinoma with adriamycin. Cancer 36:1250, 1975
103. Vogel CL, Bayley AC, Brocker RJ, et al: A Phase II study of adriamycin in patients with hepatocellular carcinoma from Zambia and the United States. Cancer 39:1923, 1977
104. Falkson G, Moertel CG, Lavin PT: Chemotherapy of primary liver carcinoma: A parallel study in American and African Bantu patients (abstr). Proc Am Soc Clin Oncol Am Assoc Cancer Res 17:21, 1976
105. Link JS, Bateman JR, Paroly WS, et al: 5-fluorouracil in hepatocellular carcinoma. Cancer 39:1936, 1977
106. Kennedy PS, Lehane DE, Smith FE, et al: Oral fluorouracil therapy of hepatoma. Cancer 39:1930, 1977
107. Falkson G, Von Hoff D, Klassen D, et al: A Phase II study of neocarzinostatin in malignant hepatoma. Cancer Chemother Pharm 4:33, 1980
108. Baker LH, Saiki JA, Jones SE, et al: Adriamycin and 5-fluorouracil in the treatment of advanced hepatoma: a Southwest Oncology Group Study. Cancer Treat Rep 61:1595, 1977
109. Gradisar IA, Kelly TR: Primary carcinoma of the gallbladder. Arch Surg 100:232, 1970
110. Dembo AJ, Bush RS, Beale FA, et al: The Princess Margaret study of ovarian cancer stages I, II, and asymptomatic III presentations. Cancer Treat Rep 63:249, 1979

CHAPTER 20

William F. Sindelar

Cancer of the Small Intestine

Neoplasms of the small intestine are uncommonly encountered. Although the small bowel accounts for over 75% of the length and over 90% of the mucosal absorptive surface area of the entire GI tract, only approximately 5% of all GI neoplasms arise in the small intestine.[1-2] Small intestinal cancers average about 1% of all GI tract malignancies.[3-5]

The diagnosis of small intestinal neoplasm is often difficult to establish because symptoms may be vague and nonspecific.[6-7] In malignant small bowel tumors, metastatic disease is often present at the time of diagnosis, and overall prognosis is not favorable.[7-8] Surgical resection has salvaged some patients with small bowel cancers.[7-10] However, radiotherapy and chemotherapy have proved to be of little benefit in the treatment of small intestinal malignancies.[7-8,11-15]

HISTORICAL CONSIDERATIONS

The first mention of small intestinal tumor dates back to 1655.[16] The first clinically reported small bowel neoplasm was a duodenal carcinoma described in 1746.[17] Wesner reported the first small intestinal leiomyosarcoma in 1883.[18] The first successful resection of a small intestinal tumor was reported by Fleiner in 1885.[19]

An early review of small intestinal neoplasms was performed in 1899 by Heurtaux.[20] The entire early literature of small bowel neoplasms was reviewed by King in 1917; his work provides a convenient reference for the review of early cases.[21] Several modern major reviews have been published on the subject of small intestinal tumors as well.[1,3-4,6-10,14-16,22-29]

EPIDEMIOLOGY

The age range for reported small intestinal tumors is from 1 to 84 years, with a mean age of 59 years.[1,7,8,23] The average age of presentation of benign tumors is 62 years, while malignant tumors present at a mean age of 57 years.[30]

There appears to be a slight predominance of small intestinal neoplasms in males and among blacks. The age-adjusted incidence for clinically diagnosed small bowel tumors in the U.S. per 100,000 in the white population is 1.2 for males and 0.8 for females.[31] The incidence per 100,000 blacks in the U.S. is 1.6 for males and 0.7 for females.[31] The incidence rates translate into approximately 700 cases in males and 500 cases in females of clinically diagnosed small intestinal neoplasms.[5,31] There appears to be a uniform worldwide incidence of small intestinal neoplasms.[5,8]

The autopsy incidence of small intestinal tumors is 0.2%, with many being benign.[32] The operative incidence of neoplasms of the small bowel is under 0.01%, with an approximately equal distribution of benign and malignant lesions, suggesting that most benign tmors are clinically innocent and asymptomatic while malignant tumors progress to symptomatology requiring surgical intervention.[8,33-36] Most clinical series report an approximately equivalent distribution between

TABLE 20-1. Benign and Malignant Small Bowel Neoplasms in Clinical Series

AUTHOR	REFERENCE	YEAR	NUMBER OF NEOPLASMS		
			Benign	*Malignant*	*Total*
Darling et al	24	1959	46	86	132
Krouse et al	33	1961	24	12	36
Skandalakis et al	9	1962	340	257	597
Botsford et al	30	1962	71	44	115
Sawyer et al	34	1963	23	27	50
Schmutzer et al	35	1964	59	41	100
Ebert et al	10	1965	48	29	77
Ostermiller et al	36	1966	77	122	199
Spratt	37	1966	11	19	30
Freund et al	38	1978	37	79	116
Miles et al	39	1979	11	31	42
Mittal et al	7	1980	15	39	54
Herbsman et al	8	1980	20	54	74
Totals			782 48%	840 52%	1622

benign and malignant small bowel tumors.[7-10,30,33-39] See Table 20-1 for summary of distribution of benign and malignant small bowel neoplasms.

Small intestinal neoplasms are associated in increased frequency with certain inherited disorders of the gastrointestinal tract including familial polyposis, Gardner's syndrome, Peutz-Jeghers syndrome, Crohn's disease, celiac disease, and neurofibromatosis.

ETIOLOGIC CONSIDERATIONS

No factors have been definitely implicated in the etiology of small intestinal neoplasms. However, because of the rarity of small bowel tumors compared to neoplasms in the remainder of the GI tract, there have been frequent speculations that local factors in the small intestine may function in the prevention of neoplasia or in the clearance or deactivation of potential GI tract carcinogens (see Table 20-2).

The alkalinity of the small bowel content has been suggested to be protective against neoplasia.[8-9] Higher tumor incidences are found throughout the GI tract where the content is generally acid. It is known in small bowel regions where the content is frequently acid, such as the duodenum, there is a higher incidence of malignancy.[9,14,23] It is known that nitrosamines, which have been shown to be potent experimental GI carcinogens, are formed within the GI tract only in acid environments.[40]

TABLE 20-2. Possible Protective Factors Resulting in Low Incidence of Small Intestinal Neoplasia

Alkalinity of small bowel content may prevent formation of potential carcinogens.
Rapid transit of small bowel content may minimize exposure to potential carcinogens.
Liquid content of small intestine may be less irritating to mucosal surfaces than content with particulate material.
Small intestinal hydroxylases may inactivate potential carcinogens.
High concentration of immunoglobulin (IgA) may be protective.
Absence of bacteria in small intestine may be protective by minimizing exposure to bacterial-produced potential carcinogens.

The relatively rapid movement of the small bowel content, compared to the remainder of the GI tract, has been thought to be protective, perhaps by minimizing the time of mucosal exposure to potential carcinogenic agents.[41] Also, it has been proposed that the liquid small bowel content may be less abrasive or irritating to the mucosa than food particles in the esophagus, chyme in the stomach, or fecal material in the colon.[42]

A high level of benzopyrene hydroxylase has been found in small bowel mucosa that has been postulated to be a mechanism of detoxification of potential carcinogens.[8,43] The high concentration of immunoglobulin (IgA) in the small intestine has been considered to be protective against neoplasia, perhaps by neutralizing possible oncogenic viruses.[28] Evidence for a protective effect of intestinal immunoglobulin includes observations of increased incidence of small intestinal neoplasia in immunoglobulin deficiencies and in immunosuppressed patients.[28]

The relative absence of bacteria in the small intestine as compared to other portions of the intestinal tract has been considered to be a protective factor against neoplastic transformation resulting from bacterial-produced carcinogens from substances in the intestinal content.[28]

ANATOMIC CONSIDERATIONS

EMBRYOLOGY

The small intestine develops from the embryonic endodermal primitive gut tube. Yolk sac elements differentiate into GI elements beginning at about 14 days of gestation. The yolk sac then resorbs by 5 weeks, leaving a primitive intestinal cylinder suspended to the dorsal portion of the coelomic cavity by a mesentery that carries the developing blood supply to the gut. A rapid elongation of the gut then takes place to form an intestinal loop, which rotates in a counterclockwise direction as the intestinal tract increases in length. Intestinal rotation takes place at about 10 weeks of embryonic life, leaving the developing small intestine surrounded by the embryonic colon. The intestinal mesentery attaches to the dorsal abdominal wall by 20 weeks, forming the mesenteric root obliquely across the dorsal wall of the abdominal cavity and providing the vascular and lymphatic supply to the small bowel. The yolk sac remnant, or vitelline duct, communicates with the developing small bowel in the region, which ultimately gives rise to the ileum. More proximal intestine forms jejunum. Persistence of the vitelline duct gives rise to Meckel's diverticulum.

The stomach and duodenum develop from the proximal gut tube, which is supported by dorsal and ventral mesenteries. During development, a counter-clockwise 90 degree rotation takes place, drawing the dorsal mesentery anteriorly to form the greater omentum and moving the ventral mesentery posteriorly to produce the omental bursa and the lesser omentum. The duodenum develops caudal to the stomach, and the duodenal endoderm gives rise to dorsal and ventral diverticula, which form primordia of the pancreatic ducts. Rotation of the duodenum by 8 weeks of gestation moves dorsal and ventral pancreatic primordia together where fusion takes place to form a single developing pancreas. The bile duct arises from a duodenal diverticulum, which enters the developing liver and is moved, by duodenal rotation, into proximity with the pancreatic duct. The developing duodenum comes to lie in the dorsal portion of the coelomic cavity by 12 weeks of gestation and assumes a largely retroperitoneal position.

ANATOMIC RELATIONS

The small intestine measures more than 6 m in length and extends from the gastric pyloric ring to the colonic ileocecal

FIG. 20-1. Anatomy of the small intestine. *A*, Mesentery of the small intestine; *B*, vascular supply of the small intestine; *C*, relationships of the duodenum. (Healey JE: A Synopsis of Clinical Anatomy, p. 179. Philadelphia, WB Saunders, 1969)

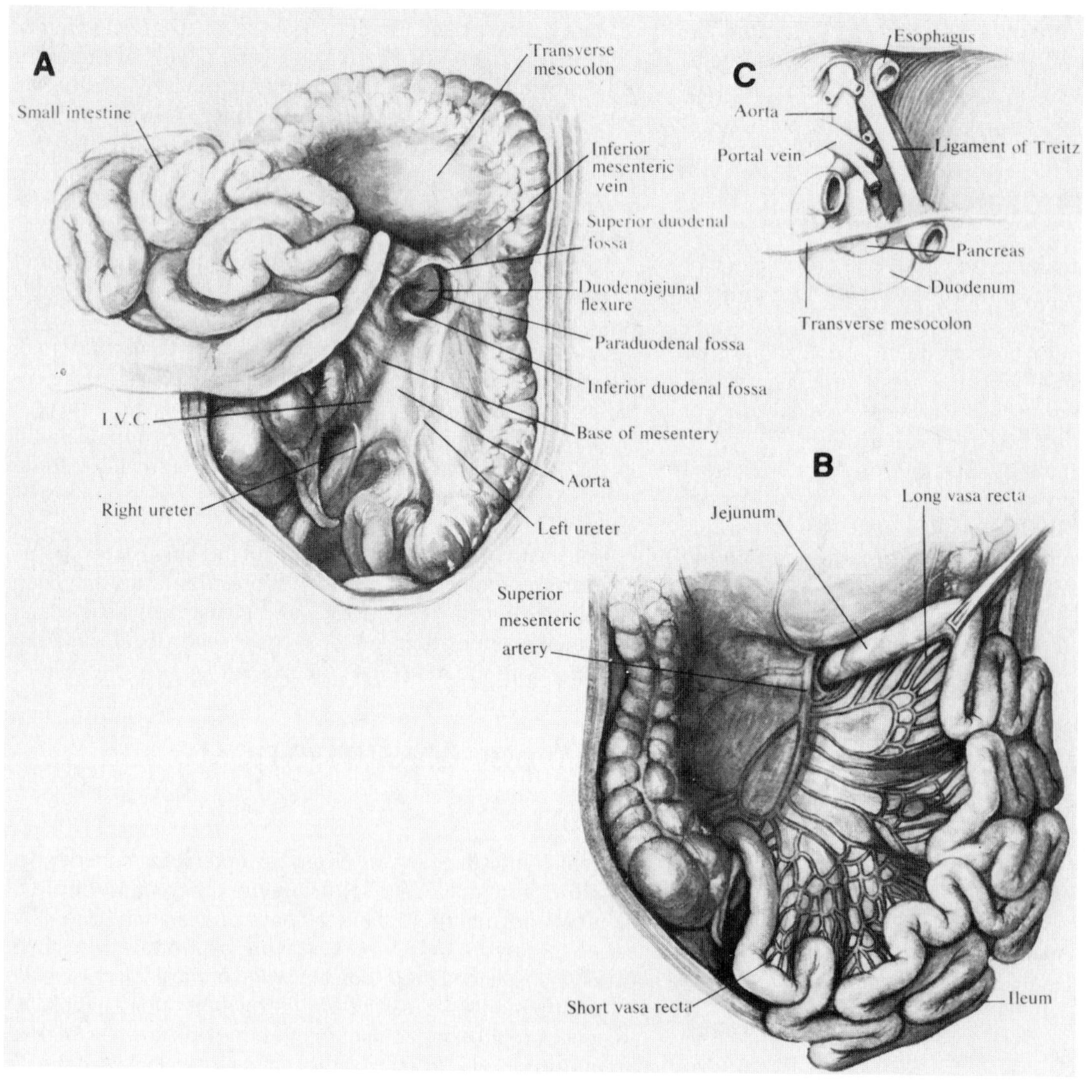

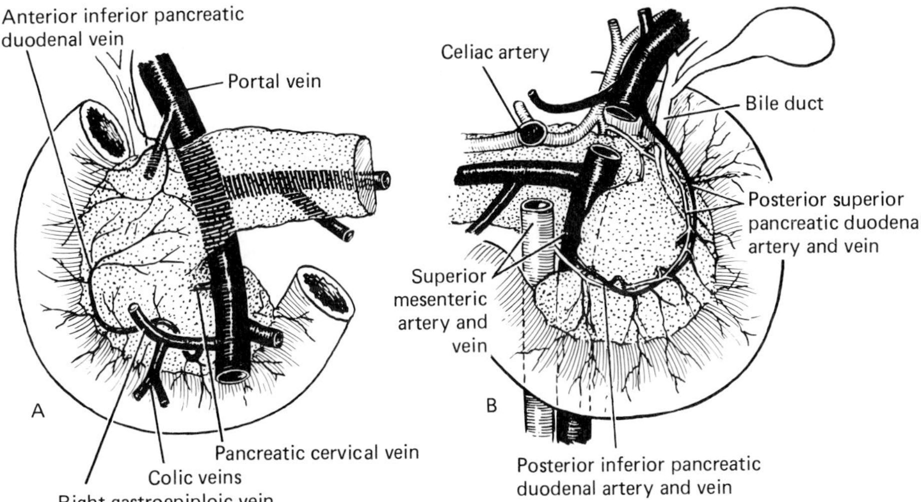

FIG. 20-2. Anatomy of the duodenum. *A*, Anterior view with pancreaticoduodenal vessels; *B*, posterior view with posterior vascular arcades. (Edwards EA, Malone PD, MacArthur JD: Operative Anatomy of Abdomen and Pelvis, p. 127. Philadelphia, Lea & Febiger, 1975)

valve. It consists of duodenum, jejunum, and ileum. (See Fig. 20-1 for the anatomy of the small intestine.)

The duodenum extends to the right from the pyloric ring as an intraperitoneal structure and then turns caudally to become retroperitoneal, surrounding the head of the pancreas. Here it receives the openings of the biliary and pancreatic ducts at the papilla of Vater on its medial portion. The duodenum then extends horizontally to the left, passing beneath the superior mesenteric vessels before turning superiorly and emerging as an intraperitoneal structure at the ligament of Treitz. The duodenum derives its arterial supply from both the celiac axis and superior mesenteric artery through the anterior and posterior pancreaticoduodenal arteries. Venous drainage is into the portal system through pancreaticoduodenal veins. (See Fig. 20-2 for vascular anatomy in the region of the duodenum.) Duodenal lymphatics drain behind the head of the pancreas into the pancreaticoduodenal lymph nodes and to the celiac nodes.

The jejunum begins at the ligament of Treitz, situated to the left of the second lumbar vertebra, and extends caudally from the free border of the mesentery. Arterial supply is through branches of the superior mesenteric artery that pass through the mesenteric border and anastomose freely. Venous drainage is through mesenteric tributaries that terminate in the portal system through the superior mesenteric vein. Lymphatic drainage follows mesenteric vessels, with numerous nodes found in the mesentery.

The ileum is continuous with the jejunum, and the division is indistinct between the distal jejunum and proximal ileum. Arterial branches supply the ileum from the ileocolic artery, arising as an extension of the superior mesenteric artery. Venous drainage into the portal system is through the superior mesenteric vein. Lymphatic drainage is through the mesentery, with lymph nodes located along the vascular channels.

The mesentery inserts onto the dorsal abdominal wall in an oblique line measuring approximately 20 cm and extending from the left side of the second lumbar vertebra to the right iliac fossa (see Fig. 20-1). The free mesenteric border spreads like a fan measuring over 6 m and allowing convolutions of the small intestine within the abdominal cavity. The mesentery supports the arterial supply, venous drainage, and lymphatic drainage of the small intestine. Blood vessels anastomose freely in the mesentery in broad arcades and supply the intestine segmentally.

MICROSCOPIC ANATOMY

The small intestine is an elongated cylinder containing an innermost mucosal layer supported by a submucosa of connective tissue, a middle smooth layer consisting of an inner circular and outer longitudinal layer of muscle fiber arrangement, and an outer serosal layer of peritoneum and connective tissue (see Fig. 20-3). The mesentery supports the intestine to supply mechanical attachment to the dorsal abdominal wall as well as to carry blood vessels and lymphatics.

The mucosal surface of the small intestine is increased in area by circular folds, the valvulae conniventes, which are prominent in the duodenum and jejunum, and become less developed distally in the ileum. The valvulae consist of all mucosal layers. Villi are formed by foldings of the epithelium. The lining epithelium is made up of the columnar epithelial cells, goblet cells, and enterochromaffin cells.

The submucosa contains connective tissue and lymphatics, and carries the intestinal blood supply in both longitudinal and circular directions in a submucosal plexus. The submucosa contains considerable amounts of lymphatic tissue throughout the small intestine, with increasing concentrations distally. In the ileum, lymphatic tissue aggregates into large follicles designated as Peyer's patches.

The muscular portion of the small intestine is formed of smooth muscle with small amounts of connective tissue, blood vessels, and lymphatics. The thick, inner, circularly-oriented layer is opposed to the thin, outer, longitudinal layer by an attenuated layer of connective tissue. Contained in this layer is the myenteric nerve plexus.

The serosa is composed of a layer of peritoneal epithelium overlying a subserosa of loose connective tissue. The serosal coat covers the circumference of the intestine, except at the point of mesenteric attachment where the intestinal serosa is continuous with the peritoneal epithelium of the mesentery.

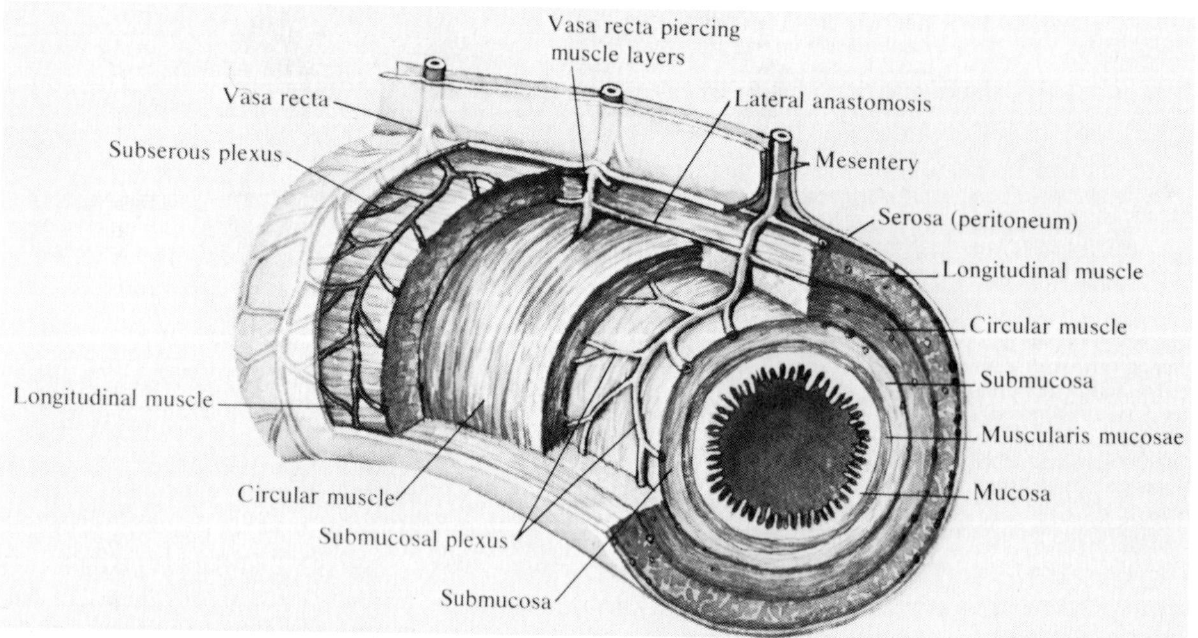

FIG. 20-3. Structural arrangement of the small intestine. (Healey JE: A Synopsis of Clinical Anatomy, p. 179. Philadelphia, WB Saunders, 1969)

PATHOLOGIC CONSIDERATIONS

Neoplasms can arise from any of the tissues comprising the small intestine, with both benign and malignant tumors seen. A classification of benign and malignant small intestinal tumors is given in Table 20-3.

Among benign tumors of the small intestine, the most frequently encountered are adenomas, leiomyomas, and lipomas.[44-45] Fibromas and neurofibromas are uncommon small bowel tumors. Intestinal neurofibromas can sometimes be seen in clinical neurofibromatosis. Vascular tumors, such as hemangiomas and lymphangiomas, are rare. Hamartomas of the small intestine are associated with the Peutz-Jeghers syndrome. Lymphoid hyperplasia in the small intestine can lead to polypoid masses; small intestinal pseudolymphoma has been described.[5] Distribution of benign neoplasms in the duodenum, jejunum, and ileum is given in Table 20-4.

Malignant small bowel neoplasms are chiefly adenocarcinomas, comprising approximately half of small bowel cancers.[3] Carcinoid tumors account for about 20% of malignant small intestinal lesions while leiomyosarcomas are the most common among the small intestinal sarcomas, with angiosarcoma and liposarcoma only rarely seen.[46] Neurofibrosarcomas occur and are occasionally associated with neurofibromatosis. Malignant lymphomas are rare as primary lesions in the small intestine. Lymphoma may involve the small bowel in association with systemic lymphomatous involvement. The distribution of malignant neoplasms in the duodenum, jejunum, and ileum is given in Table 20-5.

TABLE 20-3. Classification of Small Intestinal Neoplasms

TISSUE OF ORIGIN	BENIGN	MALIGNANT
Epithelium	Adenoma	Adenocarcinoma
Enterochromaffin cells		Carcinoid
Connective tissue	Fibroma	Fibrosarcoma
Vascular tissue	Hemangioma Lymphangioma	Angiosarcoma
Lymphoid tissue	Pseudolymphoma	Lymphoma
Smooth muscle	Leiomyoma	Leiomyosarcoma
Nerve and nerve sheath	Neurofibroma Neurilemoma	Neurofibrosarcoma Malignant schwannoma
Fat	Lipoma	Liposarcoma

del Regato JA, Spjut HJ: Ackerman and del Regato's Cancer. Diagnosis, Treatment, and Prognosis, 5th ed, pp 493–506. St Louis, CV Mosby, 1977

TABLE 20-4. Distribution of Benign Neoplasms in the Small Intestine

TYPE OF NEOPLASM	NUMBER AND PERCENTAGE BY REGION Duodenum	Jejunum	Ileum	TOTAL
Adenoma	167 33%	127 25%	211 42%	505
Fibroma	12 7%	28 17%	125 76%	165
Hemangioma, lymphangioma	18 8%	99 47%	95 45%	212
Pseudolymphoma	0 0%	1 17%	5 83%	6
Leiomyoma	86 19%	188 41%	180 40%	454
Neurofibroma, neurilemoma	12 15%	25 32%	41 53%	78
Lipoma	72 24%	54 18%	175 58%	301
Totals	367 21%	522 30%	832 49%	1721

Wilson JM, Melvin DB, Gray GF et al: Benign small bowel tumor. Ann Surg 181:247–250, 1975

TABLE 20-5. Distribution of Malignant Neoplasms in the Small Intestine

TYPE OF NEOPLASM	NUMBER AND PERCENTAGE BY REGION Duodenum	Jejunum	Ileum	TOTAL
Adenocarcinoma	399 40%	381 38%	222 22%	1002
Carcinoid	42 6%	73 10%	599 84%	714
Lymphoma	4 16%	12 48%	9 36%	25
Leiomyosarcoma	41 10%	156 37%	224 53%	421
Fibrosarcoma, angiosarcoma, neurofibrosarcoma, malignant schwannoma, liposarcoma	2 29%	0 0%	5 71%	7
Totals	488 22%	622 29%	1059 49%	2169

Wilson JM, Melvin DB, Gray GF et al: Primary malignancies of the small bowel: A report of 96 cases and review of the literature. Ann Surg 180:175–179, 1974; Loehr WJ, Mujahed Z, Zahn FD et al: Primary lymphoma of the gastrointestinal tract: A review of 100 cases. Ann Surg. 170:232–238, 1969

CLINICAL FEATURES

SYMPTOMS

Benign small bowel tumors may cause no symptoms, incidentally being found at autopsy.[24,30] Lack of symptomatology may be due to the easy distensibility of the small intestine and the low viscosity of the fluid content that require substantial occlusion of the intestinal lumen before any obstruction is produced.[8] It is estimated that approximately half of all benign small bowel tumors eventually become symptomatic.[24] Pain is the usual presenting complaint in benign tumors of the small intestine producing clinical symptoms.[2] This pain may be related to partial or complete intestinal obstruction, which is present in more than 50% of symptomatic cases.[29] Intussusception is frequently the cause of intestinal obstruction, with the tumor acting as the lead point. The most frequent cause of adult intussusception is a benign small bowel neoplasm.[24] Intestinal obstruction often is chronic and intermittent, probably due to the distensibility of the small bowel in allowing passage of fluid content around an obstructing lesion of substantial size.[1-2,8,13-15] Symptoms produced by proximal obstruction, including duodenum and proximal jejunum, are usually unrelenting nausea and vomiting with epigastric crampy pain. Distal obstruction, in the distal jejunum and ileum, typically results in intermittent vomiting, abdominal distension, and periumbilical crampy pain. Hemorrhage may occur from benign small intestinal tumors and results from mucosal involvement of the neoplastic process, being present in approximately 25% of symptomatic patients.[9-10,35] Hemorrhage is usually slow and chronic resulting in anemia, weakness, and debilitation.[36] Severe bleeding sufficient to warrant surgical intervention is unusual in benign small bowel tumors.[24] Symptoms of benign small intestinal neoplasms are summarized in Table 20-6.

Malignant tumors of the small intestine produce symptoms in over 75% of patients.[7-9,14-15,21,24-28,46-47] Pain is the most common presenting symptom, occurring in over 65% of cases of malignant small bowel tumors.[8,14,24-25,34,47] The pain is usually variable in character, occurring as cramps or as diffuse dull aches that may radiate through the abdomen or to the back. Weight loss is quite common in malignant small intestinal neoplasms, being present in over 50% of patients.[28,34,47] The most profound weight loss typically occurs in the lymphomas. Symptoms of intestinal obstruction develop in approximately 35% of the patients with malignant lesions.[8] Obstruction is generally incomplete, owing to the distensibility of the small intestine and its ability to pass its liquid content around large obstructive lesions.[15] Obstruction is often due to actual tumor invasion of the bowel wall and only rarely to intussusception, unlike benign small intestinal tumors that rarely infiltrate and frequently result in intussusception. Hemorrhage may occur with small bowel malignancies.[10,36] Bleeding is often chronic and occult, leading to anemia. Rarely, massive hemorrhage may be the presenting complaint and is usually associated with intestinal sarcomas. Malignant small bowel tumors may present as an acute abdomen, with bowel perforation and peritonitis. Approximately 10% of small bowel malignancies perforate, usually lymphomas or sarcomas.[24] Frequently, symptoms may be vague and nonspecific, often leading to difficulties in diagnosis and not suggesting a neoplastic process.[48-49] Diarrhea or steatorrhea may occur, particularly with lymphomas involving the duodenum or jejunum.[50] Carcinoids can produce the symptom complex termed the carcinoid syndrome and characterized by cutaneous flushing, cyanosis, chronic diarrhea, and intermittent respiratory distress.[51-52] The carcinoid syndrome is manifest only in the presence of metastatic disease. A summary of clinical symptoms occurring with small intestinal malignancies is given in Table 20-6.

SIGNS

Clinical examination in patients with benign small intestinal tumors is often unrewarding, with many patients presenting with no abnormal findings. Benign tumors are not papable unless they are very large. If palpable, benign tumors are typically freely movable.[5,10] Distension and visible peristaltic waves may be present in the case of clinical intestinal obstruction. Intussusception may cause the formation of a palpable tender mass; grossly bloody stool may be present. Benign tumors may cause intestinal bleeding, which produces anemia and stools positive for gross or occult blood. See Table 20-7 for outline of signs in benign small intestinal neoplasms.

Small intestinal malignancies may present with no obvious clinical findings. Signs of weight loss are common as presenting findings; cachexia may be present if the disease is advanced.[30] An abdominal mass may be palpable, occurring in approximately 25% of cases; distension can be present with intestinal obstruction; and clinical obstruction develops in about 25% of patients.[4,8,30,53] Gross or occult blood may be present in the stool if there has been hemorrhage from the tumor; signs of anemia are frequently present. Clinical jaundice is routinely seen with duodenal and periampullar malig-

TABLE 20-6. Clinical Symptoms of Small Intestinal Neoplasms

SYMPTOM	BENIGN	MALIGNANT
Asymptomatic	Frequent	Unusual
Pain	Common, often vague	Usual
Weight loss	Unusual	Frequent
Intestinal obstruction	Frequent, often intermittent, often due to intussusception	Frequent, often intermittent, intussusception rare
Intestinal hemorrhage	Frequent, usually mild and chronic	Frequent, usually chronic, sarcomas may produce massive hemorrhage
Acute abdomen	Rare	Unusual, can occur in sarcomas and lymphomas
Diarrhea	Unusual	Common in lymphomas
Malabsorption	Rare	Common in lymphomas
Jaundice	Rare	Common in duodenal and periampullary lesions
Flushing	Rare	Seen in carcinoid syndrome

TABLE 20-7. Physical Findings in Small Intestinal Neoplasms

FINDING	BENIGN	MALIGNANT
No abnormal findings	Common	Frequent
Palpable mass	Rare	Infrequent, common in sarcomas
Distension	Frequent, if intestinal obstruction	Frequent, if intestinal obstruction
Signs of weight loss	Unusual	Frequent
Icterus	Rare	Common in duodenal and periampullary lesions
Lymphadenopathy	Rare	Common in lymphomas
Hypertension and flushing	Rare	Seen in carcinoid syndrome

nancies. Signs of peritonitis can also occur with tumors that have perforated the intestinal wall. Steatorrhea and malabsorption can be present with small intestinal malignancies, especially the lymphomas, where there can be villous atrophy of the intestinal mucosa.[49,54–57] Peripheral lymphadenopathy may be present in disseminated lymphomas. Hypertension and cutaneous hyperemia may be present as a consequence of advanced carcinoid. A summary of the physical findings and signs in malignant small bowel tumors is given in Table 20-7.

DIAGNOSTIC EVALUATION

General Considerations

The diagnosis of benign or malignant small intestinal tumors prior to surgical exploration is difficult because of lack of specificity of symptoms and signs. A correct preoperative diagnosis can be expected in less than half of the symptomatic patients.[36,46]

Laboratory Studies

Routine laboratory studies rarely show specific abnormalities in the presence of small intestinal neoplasms. A hypochromic, microcytic anemia is often present, resulting from chronic blood loss due to hemorrhage from tumor ulceration of the intestinal mucosa. Elevations of bilirubin and hepatic enzymes routinely result from duodenal neoplasms that obstruct the ampulla of Vater. Serum tumor markers (*i.e.*, carcinoembryonic antigen or alpha-fetoprotein) are rarely elevated in small bowel tumors unless metastatic disease is present in the liver. Carcinoid tumors commonly result in elevated urinary levels of 5-hydroxyindoleacetic acid.

Radiologic Studies

Roentgenographic examinations are the diagnostic tests of greatest utility in the diagnosis of small intestinal neoplasms (abdominal films are generally nonspecific). If intestinal obstruction is present, air-fluid levels and intestinal dilatation are observed. In the case of bulky intestinal tumors, such as sarcomas, a mass may be visible on roentgenograph.

Contrast radiography is the most valuable roentgenographic modality for diagnosing small intestinal tumors. Upper GI series with small bowel follow-through have been successful in demonstrating small intestinal tumors, particularly in obstructing malignant lesions where diagnostic accuracy as high as 50% has been reported.[27] The GI series can, at times, distinguish various types of small bowel lesions.[8] Intraluminal masses typically represent benign lesions such as polyps or leiomyomas; intramural masses that thicken the intestinal wall but cause little or no mucosal change are consistent with mural sarcomas or malignant lymphoma; and ulcerative mucosal lesions generally result from carcinomas. When interpreting GI roentgenograms particular attention should be paid to bowel caliber, mucosal pattern, ulcerations, filling defects, and bowel loop displacements, which can all suggest the presence of a neoplasm. GI series may demonstrate intussusception. Hypotonic duodenography may improve visualization of the duodenum and small intestine by arresting intestinal motility at the time of contrast radiography through the administration of glucagon or anticholinergics.[58] Selective intubation of the small intestine may be possible, allowing detailed study of particular intestinal segments through the instillation of contrast material and air directly into the intestinal segment. The distal ileum is frequently poorly visualized through upper GI contrast studies. However, the ileum can frequently be demonstrated through barium enema where the contrast material is refluxed through the ileocecal valve from the colon into the distal small intestine.

Angiography may be of benefit in the diagnosis and localization of small intestinal tumors. Tumor blush may be noted on angiogram in vascular neoplasms such as hemangiomas or carcinoids, and displacement of normal bowel vascular architecture can occur with hypovascular tumors such as carcinomas. Vascular malformations of the small intestine may be demonstrated angiographically. Bleeding intestinal neoplasms may be localized by angiographic examination if the rate of bleeding from the lesion is greater than 1 ml/min.

Chest roentgenography should always be performed in the evaluation of small intestinal tumors to examine for possible metastatic tumor deposits and to look for possible pulmonary pathology that might influence the decision as to whether a patient should undergo operation. Lung tomography may be performed to evaluate any questionable pulmonary metastatic lesions.[59]

The development of CT body scans has considerably improved roentgenographic accuracy and sensitivity in diagnosing intra-abdominal neoplasms. However, body scans are not frequently helpful in the diagnosis of small intestinal neoplasms. The presence of fluid and gas in the small intestine can obscure mass effects in the bowel wall. Small intestinal tumors are seldom sufficiently large to be distinctly resolved on body scan. In the obstructed small intestine, artifacts produced by large volumes of intraluminal air and fluid are likely to obscure any intestinal mass lesions that could be resolved on CT. Body scans may, however, be of benefit in the definition of large tumors extending beyond the bowel wall. CT may aid in the demonstration of advanced metastatic malignant disease of the small intestine by resolving liver metastases as hepatic filling defects or by demonstrating mesenteric or retroperitoneal masses representing metastatic lymphadenopathy or peritoneal implantation.

Diagnostic ultrasound is useful in the evaluation of certain intra-abdominal masses, particularly in distinguishing solid from cystic lesions. Ultrasound has little role, however, in the diagnosis of small intestinal neoplasms since the fluid content of the small bowel assumes the same sonic density as intestinal wall or intramural lesions. The fluid content of the small bowel, therefore, obscures the ultrasonic detection of small intestinal lesions. Also, the presence of small bowel gas blocks the transmission of sound waves and thereby eliminates the possibility of ultrasonic detection of small intestinal masses in regions of gaseous bowel distension. Large tumors extending outside of the intestine may be detected on ultrasonographic examination. Ultrasound may detect the presence of disseminated malignant disease, particularly hepatic metastases.

Radioisotopic Scans

Radionuclide scans have little role in the diagnosis of small bowel neoplasms. Tumors rarely take up imaging agents selectively. For example, nonspecific intestinal incorporation of imaging material may obscure visualization of neoplasms in gallium scans. Radioisotopic scans may be of benefit, however, in the detection of metastatic malignancies of the small bowel. Liver scan may show metastatic foci as hepatic filling defects and bone scan may demonstrate uptake of osseous metastases.

Endoscopy

Endoscopy can be used to examine the duodenum. Using flexible fiberscopes, the entire duodenum and the proximal jejunum at the ligament of Treitz can be visualized. Direct biopsies and cytologic samples can be obtained endoscopically as well. Ampullary lesions can be evaluated directly by endoscopic cannulation of the biliary and pancreatic ducts through the papilla of Vater and by injecting contrast material to obtain roentgenographic visualization of the biliary and pancreatic drainage. The distal ileum can sometimes be endoscopically examined with the colonoscope by passing the fiberoptic colonoscope through the ileocecal valve and viewing the ileum retrograde. Although experimental fiberscopes capable of being passed through the entire small intestine exist, currently no endoscopic instruments or techniques are available for the routine examination of the entire jejunum and ileum.

TREATMENT CONSIDERATIONS

Therapy for small bowel neoplasms is dependent on the type of tumor. Specific therapies are discussed with each particular tumor classification. However, certain general comments can be made concerning the treatment of tumors of the small intestine.

Surgery is the indicated treatment for virtually all symptomatic primary tumors of the small intestine. Benign tumors can be removed by local excisions. Small tumors, particularly pedunculated neoplasms, may be adequately removed by enterotomy and simple excision. Large sessile tumors may require segmental resection of the involved portion of intestine, with re-establishment of bowel continuity by end-to-end

FIG. 20-4. Segmental resection of small intestine. *A*, Isolation of loop of intestine containing lesion and determining margins of resection; *B*, isolation of mesenteric vessels; *C*, division of mesentery; *D*, division of bowel. (Halverson JD, Harper FB, Ballinger WF: Small intestine. In Nora PF (ed): Operative Surgery. Principles and Techniques, 2 ed, p 447. Philadelphia, Lea & Febiger, 1980)

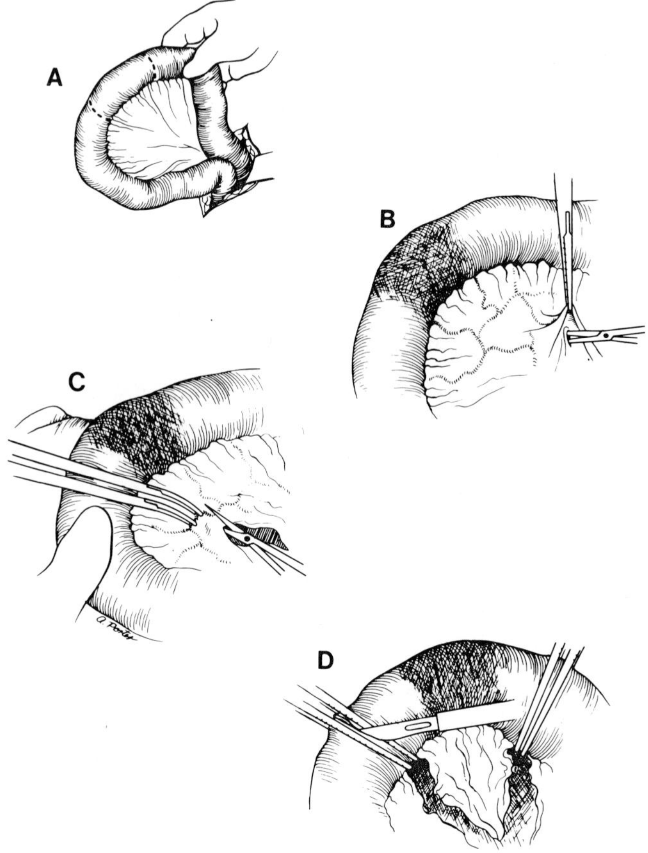

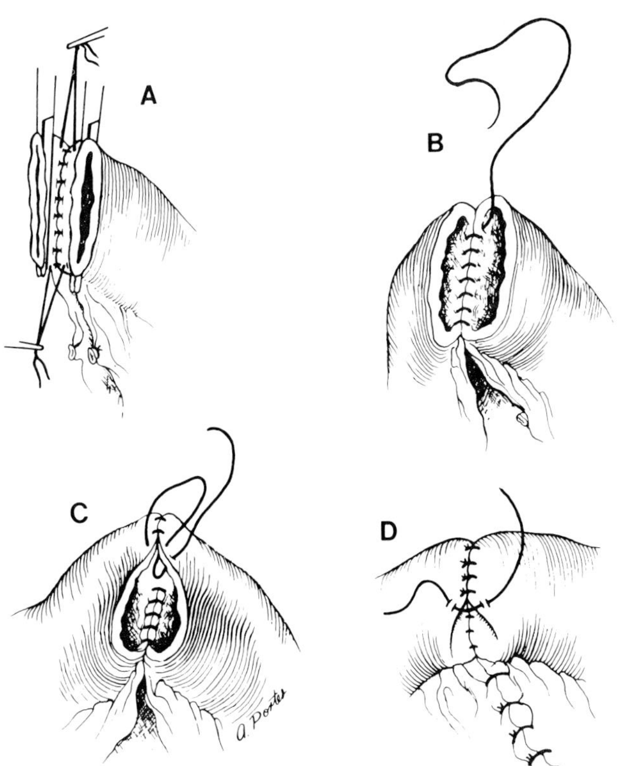

FIG. 20-5. End-to-end anastomosis of small intestine. *A*, Posterior row of outer interrupted seromuscular sutures; *B*, posterior row of inner continuous through-and-through sutures; *C*, anterior row of inner continuous Connell sutures; *D*, anterior row of outer interrupted seromuscular sutures. (Halverson JD, Harper FB, Ballinger WF: Small intestine. In Nora PF (ed): Operative Surgery. Principles and Techniques, 2 ed, p 448. Philadelphia, Lea & Febiger, 1980)

FIG. 20-6. Extent of pancreaticoduodenal resection. Shaded areas are resected. (Howard JM, Jordan GL: Cancer of the pancreas. Curr Probl Cancer 2:1–52, 1977)

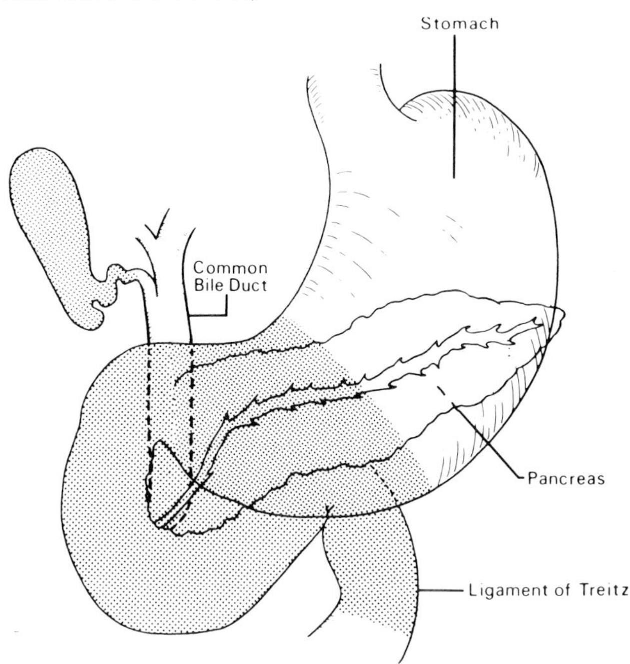

anastomosis (see Figs. 20-4 and 20-5). Malignant tumors require wide surgical excision involving segmental resection of the involved bowel with wide margins around the neoplasm, including the vascular and lymphatic pedicle. The portion of mesentery supplying the involved intestinal segment is thereby removed. Lesions in the jejunum and ileum are also amenable to wide segmental resection. However, difficulties in wide resection of neoplasms are posed in the duodenum because of the retroperitoneal location and the proximity to pancreas, biliary system, portal venous system, and stomach. Segmental resection of the duodenum is possible only in the distal portion; adequate resection of lesions in the proximal portion and C-loop require pancreaticoduodenectomy or Whipple operation (see Figs. 20-6 and 20-7, in addition to Chapter 18). For nonresectable tumors, surgical palliation is indicated if intestinal obstruction is present. Usually, obstruction is palliated through bypass, anastomosing the intestine proximal to the lesion to the bowel located distal to the obstruction.

Radiation therapy has little role in the treatment of primary small bowel tumors except in the palliation of advanced disease. Chemotherapy is generally used only in the treatment of metastatic small intestinal malignancies. Adjuvant radiotherapy and chemotherapy are controversial in small bowel tumors and are hence the subject of current investigation.

FIG. 20-7. Reconstruction after pancreaticoduodenal resection. (Nardi GL: The pancreas. Neoplastic diseases. In Nora PF (ed): Operative Surgery. Principles and Techniques, 2 ed, p 618. Philadelphia, Lea & Febiger, 1980)

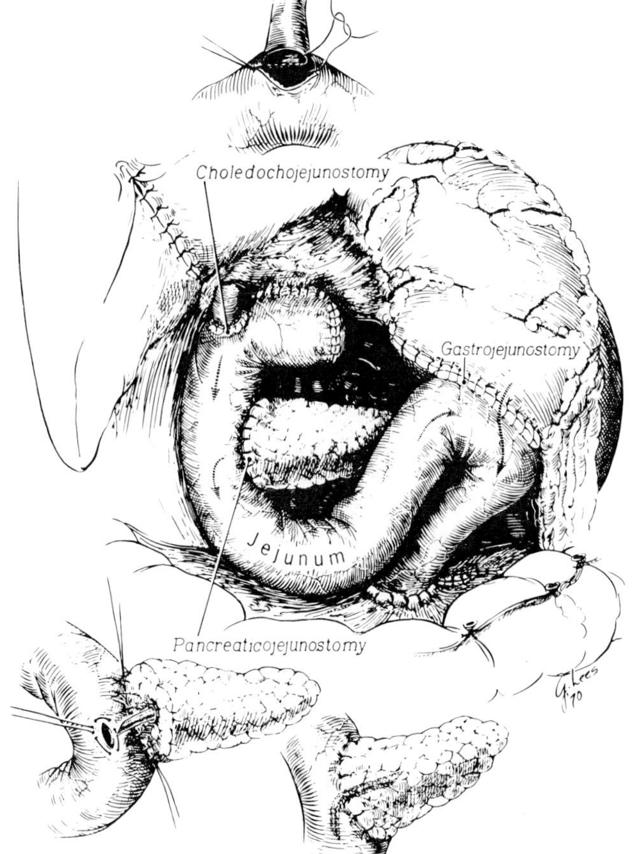

BENIGN TUMORS

ADENOMAS

Adenomas represent benign proliferations of epithelium arising from the mucosa or the mucosal glands. Adenomas comprise approximately 35% of all benign small intestinal neoplasms.[8,27,34] Most lesions are polypoid, although sessile adenomas are occasionally found.[60-61] Adenomas can occur as adenomatous polyps, villous adenomas, and Brunner's gland adenomas.

Adenomatous Polyps

Adenomatous polyps can be found throughout the small intestine. They are generally most commonly located in the duodenum, but are also found with regular frequency in the jejunum and ileum.[8,23-24,27,47] They are usually solitary, but multiple polyps through the small bowel are occasionally present.[23,34] Rarely, the entire GI tract may contain adenomatous polyps in a polyposis syndrome.[62] Familial colonic polyposis does not typically involve the small intestine. Adenomatous polyps are typically pedunculated with the adenoma attached to the surrounding normal intestinal mucous membrane by a pedicle. Sessile, non-stalked adenomatous polyps are also found.

Adenomatous polyps are often asymptomatic and can be found incidentally at autopsy or at laparotomy performed for causes other than small intestinal neoplasms.[24,30] Symptomatic polyps most frequently present with intestinal obstruction, commonly due to intussusception. The obstructive symptoms often are intermittent, with repetitive bouts of intestinal obstruction.[2,13-15] Polyps may result in intestinal bleeding, which is usually chronic, leading to anemia and occult blood in the stool.[10] Rarely will small intestinal adenomatous polyps cause profuse hemorrhage.[36]

Indications for the treatment of small intestinal adenomatous polyps are obstruction or hemorrhage. (It is not known whether small intestinal adenomatous polyps are premalignant.) If found incidentally, the potential complications of bleeding, obstruction, and intussusception require immediate treatment, that is, surgical removal. Pedunculated polyps may be simply excised at the base of the stalk by enterotomy. Some duodenal polyps can be endoscopically removed. For sessile polyps, excision around the base is required for removal, and segmental intestinal resection may be necessary to prevent narrowing of the bowel lumen by mucosal closure after removal of a sessile lesion. For cases of intussusception, the intussuscepted bowel segment must be reduced and segmental resection performed on any portion of the intestine suspected to have sustained vascular compromise. If no compromised bowel is present after intussusception reduction, simple enterotomy and polyp excision is sufficient for treatment.

Villous Adenoma

Villous adenomas of the small intestine have been recognized since 1893 and have been described as benign neoplasms in early clinical reports.[63-65] Villous adenomas are rare in the small bowel, occasionally occurring in the jejunum and ileum, but most frequently in the duodenum.[66] The duodenum has been reported as the site of more than half of all small bowel villous adenomas.[66] Of all small intestinal neoplasms, villous adenomas comprise less than 1%.[67] The lesions are sessile polyps with exhuberant villous fronds; they may attain large size before becoming symptomatic, but most lesions are under 5 cm.[68-70] Malignant degeneration has been reported in up to half of these lesions.[70-71]

Symptoms produced by villous adenomas are typically pain (usually of intermittent, crampy, epigastric character) and intestinal bleeding.[8,72] Bouts of partial intestinal obstruction can be seen in approximately 35% of patients.[70] When present, intestinal obstruction is usually intermittent. Intestinal hemorrhage is relatively common with villous adenomas, being present in about half of symptomatic patients.[70] Bleeding is usually mild or occult; however, massive bleeding has been reported.[62] Hemorrhage is almost always present with malignant degeneration. Small intestinal villous adenomas are not heavily secretory and do not produce electrolyte loss or diarrhea.[8]

Diagnosis of villous adenomas can be established by contrast radiography in as many as 75% of cases.[67,73-74] Villous adenomas characteristically produce filling defects with striated patterns, where contrast material infiltrates between the villous fronds. For duodenal lesions, endoscopic examination and biopsy can confirm a diagnosis.

Treatment of small intestinal villous adenomas is surgical. Lesions should be removed because of their high tendency toward malignant transformation. Although some small duodenal lesions may be amenable to endoscopic resection, the vast majority of lesions require laparotomy for removal. Small lesions can be simply excised locally through an enterotomy incision. Large lesions may require segmental bowel resection. For villous adenomas with evidence of malignant transformation, bowel resection with wide margins should be performed. In the jejunum and ileum, resection for malignant villous adenoma should include the intestinal segment containing the lesion with at least 10 cm margins proximally and distally, as well as the portion of intestinal mesentery containing the lymph nodes draining the lesion. For duodenal malignant lesions, a segmental resection may be possible for small tumors, but large neoplasms may require pancreaticoduodenal resection.

Adenoma of Brunner's Glands

Brunner's glands are exocrine glands located in the submucosa of the duodenum that produce an alkaline mucous. Adenomas of Brunner's glands are rare lesions.[27,75] They are typically pedunculated, solitary, and found only in the duodenum. Usually the adenomas are less than 1 cm in diameter, although large tumors have been reported.[75-77] Malignant transformation has not been recognized.

Adenomas of Brunner's glands can cause duodenal obstructive symptoms, including upper abdominal distension, nausea, and vomiting.[75] The tumors may cause hemorrhage.[75] Clinically, Brunner's gland adenomas may mimic peptic ulcer disease, with epigastric pain, vomiting, and upper GI hemorrhage.[8] Diagnosis of Brunner's gland adenoma may be made by contrast roentgenography, showing a characteristic duodenal polypoid lesion. Endoscopy and biopsy may establish the diagnosis.

Symptomatic Brunner's gland adenomas should be treated surgically by simple excision. However, large tumors that are not amenable to local excision should be bypassed by gastroenterostomy rather than performing an extensive resection for a benign neoplasm with no known potential for malignant degeneration.

FIBROMA

Fibromas are benign neoplasms of connective tissue. They can arise in the subserosa of the GI tract. Small intestinal fibromas are rare, constituting less than 8% of all benign neoplasms of the small bowel.[78] They are typically located within the bowel wall, with intraluminal extension. Rarely, the tumor may extend extraluminally into the mesentery. Tumors are usually small, under 2 cm in diameter.[79] They can be pedunculated lesions, but most are sessile.[78–79]

Most fibromas are asymptomatic and discovered incidentally at autopsy or laparotomy for causes other than small bowel tumor. Occasionally, fibromas can cause symptoms of hemorrhage from ulceration of the mucosa overlying the lesion or from intestinal obstruction, chiefly intussusception. Symptomatic fibromas should be treated by surgical excision. Simple local excision can suffice for small tumors; large lesions may require segmental bowel resection.

BENIGN TUMORS OF VASCULAR TISSUES

Hemangioma

Hemangiomas represent tumors arising from a proliferation of blood vessels. They are thought to represent developmental malformations but are usually classified as neoplasms.[78] Hemangiomas are rare in the small intestine, accounting for approximately 5% of all benign tumors in the small bowel.[23,80] These tumors typically arise from the submucosal vascular plexus, although hemangiomas of the subserosa have been reported.[78] The lesions are polypoid and usually have intraluminal extension. Large tumors may be annular, causing bowel constriction.[81] Ulceration may develop in mucosa overlying hemangiomas. Approximately 40% of small intestinal hemangiomas are solitary; these solitary lesions can be small (under 1 cm) or can involve major segments of the bowel as long as 30 cm or more.[78,82] Multiple lesions can occur, accounting for about 60% of small intestinal hemangiomas.[78,82–84] The hemangiomas are commonly found throughout the entire GI tract, with some instances of involvement only in the small intestine. The jejunum is most extensively affected, with fewer lesions in the ileum and least in the duodenum.[78,85]

Multiple hemangiomas in the GI tract are commonly designated as multiple phlebectasia. The tumors grossly appear as congested small submucosal nodules ranging up to 5 mm in diameter. Often, hemangiomas are found in the skin when intestinal hemangiomas are present. Although most cases of multiple GI phlebectasia are sporadic, a hereditary form exists and is known as the Olser-Weber-Rendu syndrome, where long segments of the small intestine can be involved with telangiectatic lesions.[80]

Most patients with intestinal hemangiomas develop clinical manifestations. Symptoms are present in approximately 70% of patients, and the chief clinical presentation is diffuse intestinal bleeding.[8,78,82–85] Rarely, vague abdominal pain, intestinal obstructive symptoms, or intussusception may characterize the clinical presentation.

Diagnosis of intestinal hemangioma may be difficult. The diagnosis may be suspected if hemangiomatous lesions are detected in the skin or by an examination of the esophagus, stomach, or rectum on endoscopy. Contrast roentgenographic studies may reveal large hemangiomas of the small intestine, but small lesions are usually not visible on roentgen ray studies. Occasionally, hemangiomas may be thrombosed and calcified, which may be apparent on abdominal films.[86] Visceral angiography is the most successful diagnostic modality for confirming and locating intestinal hemangiomas when active bleeding is present.[87] Occasionally, angiography may detect arteriovenous malformations in hemangiomas in the absence of hemorrhage.[87]

The treatment of symptomatic hemangiomas of the small intestine is surgical excision. Generally, the involved segment of bowel must be removed to ensure complete extirpation of the abnormal vessels giving rise to the tumor; obstructing lesions should be segmentally resected. Most instances of surgical intervention are for intestinal hemorrhage. Unless preoperative angiography can localize the point of hemorrhage, operative identification of the site of bleeding can be difficult. If a single lesion is present in the intestine, it may be identified by palpation of the intestine or by inspection for fullness in the bowel wall. However, when multiple hemangiomas are present, localization of the bleeding lesion may be difficult. Transillumination of the bowel wall for hemorrhagic lesions, engorgement of mesenteric vessels in the region of bleeding, division of the intestine and examination of the direction of bleeding in the lumen to determine whether hemorrhage is proximal or distal to the point of division, and multiple enterotomies to directly examine possible bleeding sources have been used in surgery for bleeding hemangiomas of the small intestine.[8,82–85,88] Even if the bleeding site can be identified and resected, the patient has the potential for subsequent hemorrhage at a later time if multiple phlebectasia is present.

Lymphangioma

Lymphangiomas of the small intestine are rare tumors, accounting for under 2% of benign small bowel lesions.[78] They arise from masses of dilated lymphatic vessels in the submucosa. It is believed that lymphangiomas represent developmental lymphatic malformations. The lesions are usually small (diameters under 1 cm), but large lesions have been reported.[78,89] Lymphangiomas may occur throughout the intestinal tract. They are usually solitary intramural lesions, with occasional multiple lymphangiomas reported.[90]

Most intestinal lymphangiomas are asymptomatic and discovered incidentally at autopsy or surgery for problems unrelated to intestinal tumor. Rarely, lymphangiomas produce intussusception and intestinal obstruction. Symptomatic lymphangiomas should be treated by surgical segmental excision of the involved bowel segment.

OTHER BENIGN TUMORS OF THE INTESTINE

Pseudolymphoma

Pseudolymphoma of the small intestine refers to hyperplasia of lymphoid tissue in the small bowel wall that can occur with infectious stimuli such as systemic viral illnesses or bacterial enteritis. Hyperplasia has also been reported with hypoglobulinemia.[91] In addition, lymphoid polyposis has been reported to precede the development of leukemia or lymphoma.[92] Occasionally, intestinal lymphatic hyperplasia can progress sufficiently so that the enlarged lymphoid aggregates can cause abdominal pain or symptoms of intestinal obstruction. Usually, the enlarged lymphoid tissue collections are located in the ileum but significant hypertrophy of lymphoid patches can also rarely occur in the jejunum and duodenum. Contrast radiologic studies may demonstrate the enlarged lymphoid aggregates, giving the impression of intestinal tumor. The aggregates are formed of normal lymphoid elements, in distinction to the atypical lymphoid elements present in malignant lymphoma of the small intestine. Pseudolymphoma is a benign condition which resolves after removal or treatment of the infectious stimulus.

Leiomyoma

Leiomyomas of the small intestine are benign neoplasms of smooth muscle, arising from the muscularis. They are relatively common, comprising approximately 20% of all benign small bowel neoplasms.[9,29,93] They are found throughout the small intestine with approximately equal frequency in the jejunum and ileum and a slightly diminished incidence in the duodenum.[8,29,78] The tumors can occur at any age, but frequency increases with advancing age.[23,78,94] Leiomyomas occur with equal frequency in males and females.[9,23,93–94]

Leiomyomas grow as intramural masses that expand the intestinal wall. Tumor growth usually causes compression of the lumen and subserosal bulging.[29] The tumors may vary in size (1 cm–10 cm), with the usual lesion averaging approximately 2 cm diameter.[9,78] A characteristic growth feature of leiomyomas involves central ulceration, probably from compression of feeding blood vessels and resultant necrosis. The tumors frequently erode the small blood mucosa. They are typically well-circumscribed but lack a true capsule.

Most leiomyomas produce clinical symptoms.[9,23,29] More than 70% of patients present with clinical signs and symptoms, which can be prominent.[78] Patients usually suffer from fatigue and weakness; weight loss may be present. Abdominal pain is a presenting complaint in at least 65% of patients, with the character of the pain being crampy and intermittent. Intestinal obstructive symptoms are present in about 30% of cases, with the obstruction being chronic.[29] Intussusception develops in approximately 15% of patients.[9,29] A palpable abdominal mass is present in up to 25% of patients with symptomatic leiomyomas.[9] Intestinal bleeding is a common clinical feature; intermittent episodes of bleeding typically occur and are manifested as melena in tumors located throughout the small intestine.[94] Hematemesis can occur with lesions in the duodenum. However, massive intestinal hemorrhage from leiomyoma is rare.[78] Intestinal bleeding frequently results from the tendency of leiomyomas to develop necrotic centers and to ulcerate intestinal mucosa, thus producing bleeding into the gut lumen.

Diagnosis of small intestinal leiomyoma can sometimes be clinically established. Detection of occult blood in the stool is possible in more than 50% of symptomatic patients.[8,23] Anemia is frequently present.[16] Contrast radiography may identify an intestinal neoplasm, and ulcerations in the intestinal mucosa can sometimes be seen at the site of the neoplasm. For leiomyomas in a subserosal location, contrast roentgenography may show no abnormalities. Plain abdominal films show dilated bowel loops; air-fluid levels of obstruction are present. Occasionally, leiomyomas contain calcifications visible on an abdominal film, but the findings are not specific. Angiography can be helpful in localizing lesions in the unusual case of massive intestinal hemorrhage.

Small intestinal leiomyomas should be treated surgically. Lesions should be removed by segmental bowel resection with margins of surrounding normal tissue, since at the time of surgery it may not be possible to pathologically distinguish the tumor as benign.

Neurogenic Tumors

NEUROFIBROMA. Benign tumors of neuroectodermal origin occur with low frequency in the small intestine. Neurofibromas are composed of nerve elements and appear in the small intestine as nonencapsulated intramural tumors. Neurofibromas account for less than 10% of all benign small bowel neoplasms.[23,29] They can occur at any age and be single isolated lesions or multiple neoplasms. Multiple small intestinal neurofibromas are associated with clinical neurofibromatosis; among patients with multiple intestinal neurofibromas, clinically apparent von Recklinghausen's disease is present in 15%.[23,95–97] The entire small intestine can be involved with multiple neurofibromas. When neurofibromas are solitary, they usually occur in the ileum but have been reported in the jejunum and duodenum as well.[8] Neurofibromas are usually under 1 cm in diameter.

Neurofibromas can be asymptomatic, but an estimated 70% of patients develop symptoms.[97] Pain occurs as the presenting symptom in about 40% of patients; intestinal bleeding in 35%.[29] Intermittent intestinal obstruction can occur, often with intussusception.[78]

Diagnosis of neurofibromas of the small intestine can be suspected in a patient with clinical manifestations of von Recklinghausen's disease including cutaneous neurofibromas, axillary freckling, and cafe-au-lait spots. Stool is usually positive for occult blood. Abdominal films can show signs of intestinal obstruction, and contrast roentgenography may demonstrate small bowel filling defects.

Symptomatic intestinal neurofibromas can be treated by surgical excision. Segmental intestinal resections are usually necessary in bleeding lesions or when obstruction has taken place. Small pedunculated tumors can be removed by local excision.

NEURILEMOMA. Neurilemomas are benign tumors of nerve sheath. They are quite rare in the small intestine, accounting for considerably less than 1% of all benign small bowel tumors in clinical series.[78] In autopsy studies, intestinal neurilemomas are found in less than 0.01% of cases.[78,98] The tumors are small, encapsulated, and reported in all areas of the small intestine. Neurilemomas of the small bowel can cause pain, hemorrhage, and intestinal obstruction. Symptomatic tumors should be surgically excised.

Lipoma

Lipomas are neoplasms of mature adipose tissue found throughout the GI tract, occurring as well-circumscribed tumors in the submucosa. Fifty percent of all GI lipomas are found in the small intestine where they account for approximately 20% of all benign neoplasms of the small bowel.[29,78] They occur chiefly in the distal small intestine, with 60% of lesions in the ileum.[24,29,99] Lipomas can develop in the jejunum (20%) and duodenum (20%) in approximately equal frequency; they increase in frequency in advancing age and are slightly more frequent in men than in women.[8] They are usually single, but may occur as multiple lesions. Lipomas of the small bowel are asymptomatic in at least 35% of cases, being discovered at autopsy or surgery performed for indications other than intestinal tumors.[94] In about 60% of symptomatic cases lipomas that cause clinical symptoms usually produce intestinal obstruction.[29] Intussusception is frequent. Bleeding from intestinal lipomas is uncommon and pain is usually crampy and associated with intermittent intestinal obstruction.

Diagnosis of intestinal lipoma can occasionally be made on a GI series where a small bowel filling defect is produced. Lipomas frequently occur at the ileocecal valve, where a filling defect can often be demonstrated on barium enema.

Treatment for symptomatic intestinal lipomas is excision. Local surgical excision is sufficient for small lesions. For large or obstructing tumors, segmental intestinal resection is recommended to avoid bowel vascular compromise or stricture of lumen following removal of a large segment of bowel wall with the neoplasm.

Hamartoma

Small intestinal polyps may be formed from developmental overgrowths of portions of the bowel wall, resulting in lesions containing myoepithelial elements.[5,8,47] These are known as polypoid hamartomas and can occur singly or in multiple polyposis patterns. The polyps can result in pain, intestinal obstruction, or bleeding and may also remain asymptomatic.

Small intestinal hamartomatous polyps can occur as a manifestation of clinical syndromes. Multiple hamartomas have been identified with adenomatosis of the entire GI tract.[62] A well-recognized clinical entity associated with multiple small intestinal hamartomas is the Peutz-Jeghers syndrome.[100-102] The disease is a hereditary condition carried as a simple mendelian dominant trait characterized by multiple small intestinal polyps, circumoral pigmentation, and perianal mucosal melanosis. GI polyps in the Peutz-Jeghers syndrome are concentrated in the jejunum but also occur in the ileum, duodenum, stomach, and occasionally the colon. Polyps can produce pain, intestinal obstruction, intussusception, and bleeding. Most cases of Peutz-Jeghers syndrome can be managed conservatively; however, symptomatic polyps may require surgical exploration and excision. Since polyps are multiple, it can be a difficult clinical problem to distinguish the area of the small intestine producing symptoms of pain, intermittent obstruction, or bleeding. Preoperative localization of obstructed points or hemorrhage by roentgenographic studies may be helpful. Frequently, patients with symptomatic Peutz-Jeghers intestinal polyps require multiple operations for recurrent clinical difficulties. Surgically, simple excision of symptomatic polyps is sufficient, unless compromise of the bowel wall or vasculature occurs and requires segmental resection. Although reports exist of malignancy in the Peutz-Jeghers syndrome, malignant transformation of the polyps is quite unlikely.[2,102-105]

MALIGNANT TUMORS

ADENOCARCINOMA

General Considerations

Adenocarcinomas are the most common of malignant small intestinal tumors, accounting for more than 50% of all malignancies of the small intestine in most series.[3,24,27-28,38-39,106-110] Adenocarcinomas increase in frequency with advancing age, with peak incidence in the 70's.[29] Incidence of adenocarcinomas is slightly higher in males than in females.

The distribution of adenocarcinomas in the small intestine tends to be greatest proximally in the duodenum, with lessening frequency more distal in the jejunum, and lowest incidence in the ileum and distal small intestine.[8,15,24,28,32,34-35,107-110] The duodenum is the site of approximately 40% of small bowel carcinomas, the jejunum 35%, and the ileum 25%. Considering the average length of the duodenum as 50 cm, the jejunum as 300 cm, and the ileum as 300 cm, the frequency of occurrence of small bowel carcinomas in relation to intestinal length is highest in the duodenum, less in the jejunum by a factor of approximately 7-fold, and least in the ileum by a factor of 10-fold. In the duodenum, approximately 65% of carcinomas occur in the region of the ampulla of Vater (periampullary), 20% proximal to the ampulla (supra-ampullary), and 15% distal to the ampulla (infra-ampullary).[78] Carcinomas of the jejunum tend to occur proximally, with 70% being present within 100 cm of the ligament of Treitz.[78] Ileal carcinomas are chiefly distal, 70% being found within 100 cm of the ileocecal valve.[78]

Small intestinal carcinomas are adenocarcinomas, derived from the glandular epithelium. They tend to grow through the intestinal mucosa to form ulcerative lesions as well as infiltrate the bowel wall to penetrate through surrounding serosa. Adenocarcinomas tend to metastasize routinely to regional lymph nodes as well as hematogenously to liver, lungs, peritoneum, bone, and other sites.

Clinical Features

The clinical manifestations of small intestinal carcinoma depend upon the location of the tumor.[5,8,32,94] Clinical presentations may include abdominal pain, weakness, weight loss, nausea and vomiting, bowel obstruction, GI hemorrhage, anemia, or intestinal perforation.

Duodenal carcinomas produce jaundice in over half of patients.[78] Periampullary lesions result in a presenting complaint of jaundice in more than 75% of cases.[8,111] The jaundice results from obstruction of the ampulla of Vater. Jaundice is usually intermittent and fluctuating but sometimes may reflect complete biliary tract obstruction and be unremitting. Hemorrhage is common with duodenal carcinomas, resulting in anemia and the presence of occult blood in the stool in over 75% of cases.[32,94] Pain is often present, usually epigastric in location, with a burning character that may mimic an ulcer diathesis.[8] Intestinal obstruction is unusual in duodenal carcinomas. A palpable mass is present in only 25% of cases.[8]

Carcinomas of the jejunum produce complaints of vague, cramping abdominal pain, weight loss, and weakness. Hemorrhage is common, resulting in anemia and stools positive for occult blood. Intestinal obstruction occurs in approximately 25% of patients.[28] A mass is palpable in about 30% of cases, and is frequently mobile.[8,78]

Ileal carcinomas present clinically as cramping pain, chiefly in the lower abdomen. Weakness and weight loss are common and hemorrhage from the tumor frequently occurs, producing anemia and stools positive for occult blood. Obstructive symptoms develop in 35% of patients. Tumors usually occur distally in the ileum and frequently grow circumferentially around the bowel. Approximately 35% of patients present with a palpable abdominal mass that is often mobile.[8,78] In addition, some association has been reported between Crohn's disease and the development of adenocarcinomas of the ileum.[112-114]

Diagnosis

Duodenal carcinomas may be diagnosed by upper GI series, which may demonstrate filling defects, mucosal ulceration, or displacement suggestive of neoplasm (see Fig. 20-8). In cases of jaundice, transhepatic cholangiography may reveal malignant obstruction in the ampullary area. CT of the abdomen may reveal a duodenal mass, particularly when

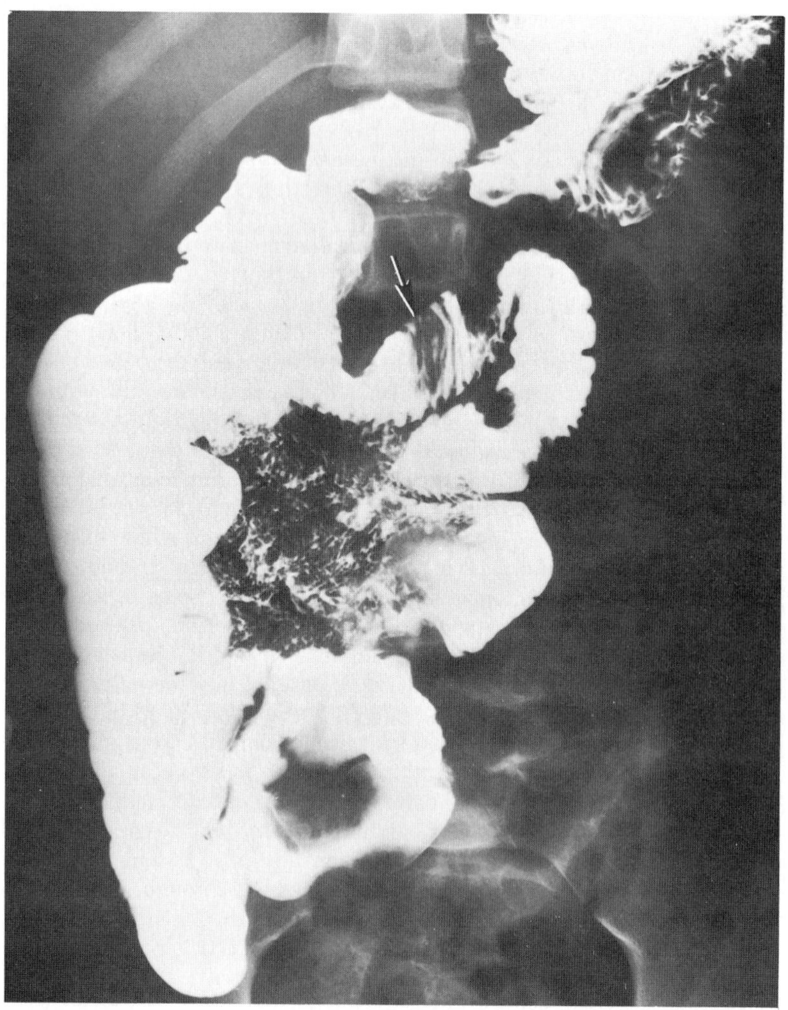

FIG. 20-8. Adenocarcinoma of duodenum. Note filling defect in duodenum proximal to ligament of Treitz.

associated with the pancreas, and can show the site of biliary obstruction when jaundice is present. Diagnostic ultrasound can be helpful in demonstrating a duodenal mass or in confirming biliary obstruction if jaundice is indeed present. Endoscopy enables duodenal carcinomas to be directly visualized and biopsied. Endoscopic retrograde cholangiopancreatography (ERCP), with endoscopic cannulation of pancreatic and biliary ducts through the ampulla of Vater for the injection of radiographic contrast material, can be helpful in differentiating neoplasms causing obstructive jaundice from biliary lithiasis or inflammatory pancreatic masses. Occasionally, duodenal carcinomas can be diagnosed from cytologic specimens obtained from the duodenum by intubation and aspiration or by endoscopic brushings.[8] Percutaneous needle aspiration of material for cytologic examination has also proved valuable in diagnosing malignancies in the region of the duodenum and head of pancreas.[115–116]

Jejunal carcinomas may be diagnosed by barium contrast radiography. Upper GI series with small bowel follow-through may demonstrate filling defects, intramural lesions, mucosal abnormalities, or bowel displacement suggestive of neoplasm. Arteriography may be helpful in delineating jejunal neoplasms suspected of hemorrhage. CT body scan is not generally helpful since resolution of the small bowel is poor because of shadow artifacts caused by intraluminal air and fluid. However, large tumors may be visible on body scan, as may enlarged regional metastatic lymph nodes or metastatic disease in the liver. Ultrasound is not helpful since resolution is limited by the inability of sound waves to pass through intestinal air or gas. Large tumors or metastatic deposits may occasionally be detected by ultrasonic examination. Endoscopy is not routinely possible beyond the ligament of Treitz and is not helpful in the diagnosis of carcinoma of the jejunum.

Carcinomas of the ileum are best demonstrated roentgenographically. GI series may show filling defects, ulcerations, or bowel loop displacement, and barium enema with reflux of contrast material through the ileocecal valve may identify ileal lesions; arteriography may detect carcinomas of the ileum presenting with intestinal bleeding. Carcinomas occurring in the distal ileum and ileocecal valve may occasionally be directly visualized endoscopically through colonoscopy and retrograde examination through the ileocecal valve. Usually, CT body scans and diagnostic ultrasound are not helpful in the diagnosis of tumors of the ileum, except for possibly detecting metastatic deposits in the liver.

Treatment and Prognosis

SURGERY. The treatment of choice for carcinomas of the small intestine is surgical resection. The resection should be radical to ensure complete tumor removal and removal of surrounding tissue at risk for tumor invasion or involvement. Surgical resection of small intestinal carcinomas should include the segment of bowel containing the tumor, giving wide margins of surrounding normal tissue, including the regional draining lymph nodes. In advanced nonresectable or metastatic disease, local resection or tumor bypass may be necessary for the palliation of obstructive symptoms.

Duodenal carcinomas found to be localized should be treated by radical resection. Although wide segmental resections may occasionally be possible for tumors occurring proximally or distally in the duodenum away from the pancreas, most duodenal tumors require wide resection of duodenum and head of pancreas to remove tissue at risk for tumor involvement. Duodenal carcinomas are best treated by pancreaticoduodenal resection (Whipple operation) comprising duodenectomy, antrectomy, resection of head of pancreas, and resection of distal common bile duct, with reconstruction of the GI tract after resection by pancreaticojejunostomy, choledochojejunostomy, and gastrojejunostomy. Although the surgical procedure is quite major in scope, the operative mortality in experienced hands is under 10%.[117–119] Radical resection for duodenal carcinoma has resulted in 5-year survivals as high as 50% in patients with lesions favorable for resection, although the overall survival experience in most series averages about 20%.[111,119–126] See Table 20-8 for a summary of collected series of survival rates following resection of duodenal carcinomas.

Localized resections for duodenal carcinomas have led to prompt tumor recurrences and no significant patient survivals.[8] Patients with metastatic disease or with lesions not amenable to radical surgical resection should receive palliative bypass to correct or prevent biliary or gastric obstruction if they are operative candidates. Survival following palliative surgery is short, averaging 4 months.[125] Survival in untreated duodenal carcinoma is typically less than 3 months from diagnosis.[78]

TABLE 20-8. Survival in Carcinoma of the Duodenum

AUTHOR	YEAR	NUMBER PATIENTS	RESECTABILITY RATE	OPERATIVE MORTALITY	MEAN SURVIVAL (MONTHS)	5-YEAR SURVIVAL
Spinazzola et al[121]	1963	12	50%	0%	16.3	0%
Mongé et al[122]	1964	25	100%	24%	10.0	39%
Cortese et al[123]	1972	32	44%	29%	45.9	28%
Warren et al[124]	1975	39	100%	21%	31.4	22%
Shulka et al[111]	1976	8	50%	25%	9.0	0%
Nakase et al[125]	1977	50	62%	16%	19.0	7%
Coutsoftides et al[126]	1977	14	79%	0%	78.0	36%

Carcinoma occurring in the jejunum should be treated by radical surgical resection that includes the segment of intestine containing the primary tumor, wide margins of normal bowel around the tumor, and segmental resection of the mesentery supporting the involved intestine to include all draining lymph nodes down to the mesenteric root. Tumor extension into the mesentery may involve mesenteric blood vessels that could require excision and consequent removal of bowel supplied by the excised vessels but not directly involved by the neoplasm. Tumor involvement of mesenteric vessels at the root of the mesentery, where vascular branches to all portions of the small bowel take origin, may prohibit radical resection of all potentially tumor-contaminated tissues since total sacrifice of the small intestine or its blood supply is not feasible. Prognosis for resected jejunal tumors is not particularly favorable, with tumor recurrence likely following treatment. The 5-year survival rates of most series average approximately 20%.[8,14,25,28,47,78,106–110,127–128] See Table 20-9 for summary of survivals of collected series following resection of jejunal adenocarcinomas.

For metastatic carcinomas or lesions that are unable to be resected for cure, palliative segmental bowel resection or bypass may be necessary to relieve or prevent obstruction. Survival following palliation is usually under 6 months; survival of untreated cases is under 4 months.[8,78]

Adenocarcinomas in the ileum are best treated by radical resection of the involved bowel segment, wide margins of normal tissue, and mesentery containing draining lymph nodes. Frequently, radical resection for ileal lesions may require right colectomy, since resection of the mesentery containing the lymph nodes draining the ileum may require sacrifice of the blood supply to the right colon. Tumor extension in the mesentery may require wide excision of vasculature requiring sacrifice of normal intestine. Extensive tumor at the root of mesentery may prevent radical extirpation by involving the entire small bowel blood supply that cannot be sacrificed. For patients with carcinomas of the ileum who have had successful radical resection, 5-year survivals average approximately 20%.[8,14,28,106–110] Table 20-10 summarizes survival following resection of carcinomas of the ileum.

Palliative segmental intestinal resection or bypass may be required to relieve or prevent obstruction in patients with metastatic carcinoma or in patients with lesions too extensive for curative resections. Survival following palliation is usually under 6 months; survival in untreated cases is usually less than 4 months.[8,78]

RADIATION THERAPY. Carcinomas of the small intestine may be treated with radiation therapy if curative surgical resection is not possible. Radiotherapy has been reported to occasionally produce remissions and to prolong survival in patients with advanced disease; palliative radiotherapy may cause partial relief of pain or obstructive symptoms.[5,8,129] However, many GI carcinomas are radioresistant, and the overall results of the role of radiation therapy in the treatment of small intestinal cancer is discouraging.[8] Radiotherapy to the intestinal tract is poorly tolerated, resulting in malaise, nausea, vomiting, and enteritis. Radiation toxicity may often prevent delivery of sufficient dosage to control tumor growth. A combination of radiation therapy and surgery may be of benefit in situations where surgical resection is likely to leave behind microscopic residual tumor that can be subsequently sterilized by radiation therapy. The use of intraoperative radiation may ultimately prove useful, where, at the time of surgical resection, a single large dose of radiation is given to the tumor bed and areas at risk for tumor contamination and recurrence.[130–131] Normal tissues not at risk for tumor contamination may be operatively removed from the radiation beam path or shielded to minimize radiation exposure to normal tissues and to reduce toxicity. The exact role of radiation therapy as an adjunct to surgical resection in GI carcinomas is uncertain and is presently undergoing evolution and evaluation.

CHEMOTHERAPY. Chemotherapy may be used in the treatment of small intestinal carcinomas where curative surgical resection is not possible. It occasionally has been useful in advanced intestinal cancers, resulting in some objective tumor regressions and perhaps improving survival.[13–15,26,28,128] The principal chemotherapeutic agents used in small intestinal carcinomas have been 5-fluorouracil and the nitrosoureas. Combination chemotherapy regimens have been shown in various GI cancers to have improved response rates when compared to single agents.[132–133] Combination chemotherapy is likely to evolve to be of therapeutic benefit in the treatment of intestinal carcinomas. The role of chemotherapy following surgical resection or in combination with radiotherapy is unknown but is presently under investigative evaluation and ultimately may prove to be a useful treatment adjunct.

CARCINOID

Carcinoids represent malignant neoplasms arising from argentaffin cells.[134] These are rare tumors located throughout

TABLE 20-9. Survival in Carcinoma of the Jejunum

AUTHOR	YEAR	NUMBER PATIENTS	RESECTABILITY RATE	5-YEAR SURVIVAL
Darling et al[24]	1959	16	44%	14%
Rochlin et al[3]	1961	9	67%	17%
McPeak[15]	1967	17	100%	6%
Silberman et al[27]	1974	5	80%	50%
Wilson et al[28]	1974	16	88%	21%

TABLE 20-10. Survival in Carcinoma of the Ileum

AUTHOR	YEAR	NUMBER PATIENTS	RESECTABILITY RATE	5-YEAR SURVIVAL
Darling et al[24]	1959	4	75%	0%
Rochlin et al[3]	1961	4	75%	33%
McPeak[15]	1967	3	100%	0%
Silberman et al[27]	1974	4	75%	33%
Wilson et al[28]	1974	13	85%	0%

the GI tract and occasionally in the respiratory tract or gonads.[135-136] The appendix and small intestine are the sites most frequently affected. Carcinoids account for over 25% of all small intestinal malignancies.[137] The clinical features and treatment of carcinoid tumors in general are discussed in detail in Chapter 28. The present section outlines the features of carcinoids of the small intestine.

Carcinoids of the small intestine typically occur as small submucosal nodules under 1 cm in diameter.[137-138] They are usually solitary, although multiple small intestinal carcinoids are seen in approximately 30% of cases.[139] They are infrequent in the duodenum, occur more commonly in the jejunum, and are most frequent in the ileum.[136-141] Often, the tumors produce a marked desmoplastic reaction in the intestinal wall that can lead to intestinal obstruction from formation of adhesions or a sclerotic mass.[138] Small bowel carcinoids usually have a slow rate of growth and as many as 70% remain asymptomatic, being discovered at autopsy or at operation performed for problems unrelated to carcinoid.[36,136-137] When carcinoids of the small intestine produce symptoms, the clinical features can be vague and nonspecific. Abdominal pain is the chief symptom; nausea and vomiting may also be features.[140-141] Intestinal obstruction may occur from fibrosis around the tumor or from intussusception. Occasionally, an abdominal mass is palpable. By the time patients present with symptoms, metastatic disease has developed in as many as 90%.[137,142] Despite the high incidence of metastatic disease, the overall 5-year survival rate of intestinal carcinoid is reasonable, averaging 20%.[136]

The carcinoid syndrome is an infrequent but well-recognized clinical entity occuring in under 10% of patients with carcinoids of the small bowel.[140,143] Because of their derivation from argentaffin cells, carcinoids produce serotonin, 5-hydroxytryptamine (in large amounts), along with histamine, kinins, and catecholamines which are released into the circulation and produce vasoactive manifestations.[136,144-145] Clinical features of the carcinoid syndrome include cutaneous flushing, episodic watery diarrhea, and paroxysmal dyspnea or asthma (see Chapter 28). The syndrome is manifest only in advanced disease when hepatic metastases are present. Circulating serotonin is metabolized and excreted in the urine as 5-hydroxyindoleacetic acid, which can serve as a chemical diagnostic marker for the carcinoid syndrome.

Diagnosis of carcinoid of the small bowel may be difficult to establish prior to surgical exploration. Contrast roentgenography may reveal small bowel filling defects, obstructing lesions, mural thickening, or kinking of the bowel. Lesions in the ileum can sometimes be demonstrated retrograde by barium enema. Angiography may reveal a tumor blush, as carcinoids can be highly vascular. Urinary excretion of 5-hydroxyindoleacetic acid can be elevated, particularly in advanced disease.

Treatment of carcinoids of the small intestine is dependent on the extent of disease. Curative surgical removal is possible for localized disease. Tumors of the jejunum should be treated by wide segmental bowel resection. Lesions in the ileum may require right hemicolectomy in addition to resection of the involved small bowel segment. Duodenal carcinoids often require pancreaticoduodenal resection. Surgical treatment of advanced cases of intestinal carcinoid is indicated if the patient can clinically tolerate surgery, since resection of bulk disease, including intra-abdominal metastases, can result in prolonged survival.[25,136,146] Treatment of advanced cases with carcinoid syndrome may consist of the pharmacological management of such symptoms as flushing, diarrhea, and dyspnea with antiserotonin and antibradykinin agents.[147-148] Although radiation therapy is of little benefit in carcinoids of the small intestine, palliative liver radiation has benefited some patients with extensive hepatic metastatic carcinoid.[136,149] Chemotherapy of intestinal carcinoid has had limited success. Streptozotocin has shown some efficacy against carcinoids, in addition, intra-arterial chemotherapy for hepatic metastatic disease has been of palliative benefit for some patients.[150-151]

SARCOMAS

General Considerations

Sarcomas are malignant tumors arising in tissues of mesodermal origin. They are found in all body regions and can occur as primary tumors of the small intestine. There are numerous histologic types of sarcomas, deriving from connective tissue, muscle, vascular tissue, neural elements, fat, and other tissues. However, in spite of a broad spectrum of histogenesis, sarcomas generally have similar clinical behavior and can be considered as a single class of malignant neoplasms for purposes of diagnosis and management.

Sarcomas account for approximately 25% of all malignant primary small bowel tumors.[9,16,24,28,35-36,106] Small intestinal sarcomas have been reported at all ages, with a general increase in frequency with advancing age. Most tumors present after age 50.[8] Small bowel sarcomas tend to occur in approximately equal frequency in males and females. They may develop in all regions of the small intestine. Sarcomas are least common in the duodenum, with collected series averaging 10% duodenal lesions.[9,24,28,35] The jejunum accounts for approximately 40% of intestinal sarcomas, with the ileum being the most frequent site of sarcomas of the small intestine, collected series averaging approximately 50%.[9,24,28,35]

Small intestinal sarcomas typically develop intramurally and grow predominantly toward the serosal surface, so that the tumor often extends outside the bowel wall where it can invade surrounding structures. Growth of tumor toward intestinal mucosa can take place, producing ulceration. Intestinal sarcomas frequently develop into tumors of large size, with more than 75% being in excess of 5 cm in diameter.[106] Because of their relatively large size, sarcomas often outgrow their vascular supply and develop ischemic central necrosis.

Sarcomas of the small intestine typically spread by direct extension into surrounding tissues such as mesentery, abdominal wall, retroperitoneum, and adjacent intestine or other viscera. Intestinal sarcomas disseminate chiefly by the hematogenous route, with the most frequent sites of metastasis being the lungs and liver.[9,24,28,35–36] Lymphatic metastases of intestinal sarcomas have been reported, but are unusual.[8,78]

Histologic Types and Characteristics

FIBROSARCOMA. Fibrosarcomas are derived from malignant change in connective tissue elements. Fibrosarcomas occurring in the small intestine are rare, accounting for less than 10% of small intestinal sarcomas.[24] Fibrosarcomas have been reported in both males and females and typically occur in persons beyond age 50. They are most frequently reported in the ileum, with moderate distribution in the jejunum, and rare in the duodenum. Fibrosarcomas often develop and grow slowly. Average 5-year survival is 35%.[78]

ANGIOSARCOMA. Angiosarcomas develop from vascular elements and are extremely rare in the small intestine.[78] They are typically aggressive, rapidly-growing lesions with a poor prognosis. Angiosarcomas have occurred in all areas of the small intestine in both males and females. The lesions are typically intramural with mucosal extension and extensive ulceration. They are highly vascular and often clinically present with GI hemorrhage.

LEIOMYOSARCOMA. Leiomyosarcomas are considered to arise from malignant degeneration of smooth muscle elements. In the small intestine, leiomyosarcomas are the most common malignant neoplasm derived from connective tissue, comprising approximately 20% of all malignant small bowel tumors.[8–9,16,35–36] They have been reported at all ages, but with a general increase in frequency with advancing age and a peak incidence in the 60-year age group.[8] There is a slight male predominance, with most series reporting an approximately 1.2:1 ratio of males:females.[9] Intestinal leiomyosarcomas occur predominantly in the ileum, with a moderate incidence in the jejunum, and a low frequency of occurrence in the duodenum. Leiomyosarcomas usually grow intramurally in the small bowel with serosal extension, and the tumors often develop into large masses that invade outside of the intestine. The tumors often develop ischemic necrotic centers, which can lead to abscess or fistula formation. Leiomyosarcomas often exhibit slow growth over a protracted course, with approximately 50% of patients surviving 5 years after diagnosis.[8,106]

LIPOSARCOMA. Liposarcoma is a malignant neoplasm derived from lipoblasts. Liposarcomas are commonly found in the abdomen and retroperitoneum, but primary liposarcoma of the small intestine is quite rare.[78] Intestinal liposarcomas typically arise in the bowel serosa and develop into masses that cause extrinsic bowel compression leading to symptoms of intestinal obstruction. They usually grow slowly and can achieve large size.[8] Intestinal liposarcomas are found chiefly in the ileum but can less commonly occur in the jejunum. They are extremely rare in the duodenum.

NEURAL SARCOMAS. Neurofibrosarcomas are malignant derivatives of neural elements. In the small intestine, neurofibrosarcomas are rare, accounting for less than 1% of malignant small bowel neoplasms. Intestinal neurofibrosarcoma tends to be an aggressive neoplasm exhibiting rapid growth and early dissemination. The tumor develops intramurally with both serosal and mucosal extension. It occurs in all regions of the small bowel with approximately equal frequency in the duodenum, jejunum, and ileum. Intestinal neurofibrosarcoma occurs in equal frequency in males and females with an increased incidence in patients with von Recklinghausen's disease.[78] Malignant schwannomas are derived from cells of the nerve sheaths. Schwannomas of the intestinal tract are rare, comprising under 1% of small bowel malignancies.[78] The tumor generally develops in the intestinal wall and extends subserosally, although mucosal invasion and ulceration may occur. They occur chiefly in the ileum, with lesser frequency in the jejunum, and rarely in the duodenum. Most grow reasonably slowly; patient survival of more than 2 years following diagnosis is frequent, even in the presence of metastatic disease.

Clinical Features

Most patients with small intestinal sarcoma complain of abdominal pain that is usually intermittent and crampy. Less commonly, the pain may be steady discomfort or feeling of fullness. Pain is a feature at clinical presentation in more than 65% of most clinical series.[4,16,24,28,106] Weight loss is reasonably common, seen in at least 30% of patients, and nausea and vomiting, although often intermittent, are common and are part of the clinical presentation of approximately 40% of cases.[24,28] GI hemorrhage is present in about 50% of patients presenting with leiomyosarcoma of the small bowel.[8–9,24,28] Bleeding is usually chronic, resulting in melena and anemia; hematemesis is occasionally present in tumors of the proximal intestine, and profuse GI hemorrhage can occur in some cases.[8] Intestinal obstruction can occur from direct tumor occlusion of the bowel, of bowel kinking around tumor, or from intussusception. Clinically significant intestinal obstruction, however, is relatively uncommon, developing in less than 20% of patients.[9,28,36] Intestinal perforation can occur as a result of tumor necrosis, resulting in clinical presentation as an intra-abdominal catastrophe. An abdominal mass is palpable in more than half of patients at the time of clinical presentation.[8–9,28]

Diagnosis

Diagnosis of small intestinal sarcoma made prior to treatment is an infrequent occurrence. However, the diagnosis may be suggested by the presence of an abdominal mass on radiograph. If extensive necrosis is present within the tumor, air-fluid levels may be visible within the area of the mass. Radiographic contrast studies may show intestinal filling defects, ulcerative lesions, or displacement of bowel loops. Barium enema may show colon displacement by a large abdominal mass, and reflux of contrast through the ileocecal valve may demonstrate neoplasms in the distal small bowel in a retrograde manner. Arteriography may show a tumor mass or blush and may reveal areas of necrosis within the mass.

CT may delineate the extent of an abdominal mass and identify areas where the tumor may have invaded surrounding structures. Diagnostic ultrasound may show cystic necrotic areas within a mass. Metastatic disease in the liver, peritoneum, or retroperitoneum may be revealed by body scan or ultrasound. In addition, liver scan may show hepatic metastatic disease, and gallium scintigraphy may occasionally reveal the extent of the primary intestinal tumor, particularly if areas of necrosis are present within the neoplasm.

Endoscopy may provide a diagnosis of sarcoma located proximally in the intestine within reach of the fiberoptic gastroscope or distally within viewing distance of the colonoscope passed retrograde through the ileocecal valve. Since many sarcomas grow in subserosal directions and spare the mucosa, even if the intramural mass is endoscopically visible, biopsies may be negative for neoplasm unless the tumor has invaded into the mucosa.

Treatment and Prognosis

SURGERY. Surgical excision should be attempted in primary sarcomas of the small intestine. Resection should include the intestinal segment giving rise to the tumor along with wide areas of surrounding tissue in areas of potential contiguous spread. Wide resection may require sacrifice of, besides the involved intestine, portions of adjacent viscera such as liver, retroperitoneum and retroperitoneal viscera, or portions of the abdominal wall. Because lymphatic metastases are unusual in sarcomas, extensive dissections of the nodal drainage beds are not typically performed. Five-year survivals as high as 50% are reported following curative resections.[8,106]

In the case of nonresectable tumor, palliative segmental bowel excision or bypass of the tumor should be performed to relieve or prevent obstruction. Nearly all unresectable patients are dead of their disease within 1 year.[106]

Pulmonary metastases, in the absence of disseminated metastatic sarcoma, are best treated by thoracotomy and wedge excision if all metastatic disease is removable from the lung. In many sarcomas, salvage rates as high as 20% are seen following aggressive surgical excision of pulmonary metastatic disease.[152–154] If hepatic metastases are present, they should be considered for excision. Accessible hepatic metastases should be removed by wedge excision if the metastatic deposits can be extirpated with reasonable morbidity. Particularly if solitary hepatic metastases are present, serious contemplation should be given for operative removal if there are no other sites of metastatic disease. Although overall survival in the case of metastatic hepatic disease is poor, occasional patients may derive long-term benefit from the removal of liver metastases.[155]

RADIATION THERAPY. Although many sarcomas have been considered to be radioresistant, nonresectable intestinal sarcomas may benefit from radiotherapy for palliation.[8,24,156] Various histologic types of sarcomas occasionally respond well to radiation therapy in high dose, with long-term cures resulting even in the presence of gross tumor.[157]

Radiation therapy should seriously be considered as an adjunct following surgical resection of intestinal sarcoma, particularly if extra-intestinal tissue invasion was present with the possibility of microscopic residual tumor remaining at surgical margins following resection. Surgical resection combined with radiation therapy has achieved good disease control in various intra-abdominal sarcomas, even when resected with positive surgical margins.[158–159]

CHEMOTHERAPY. Chemotherapy can be of benefit in the palliation of advanced sarcomas.[160–161] Doxorubicin is the current agent with the greatest activity against sarcomas. In metastatic sarcoma, objective response rates in excess of 65% have been reported using combination chemotherapy including doxorubicin, cyclophosphamide, vincristine, and imidazole carboxamide.

Adjuvant chemotherapy following surgical resection of sarcomas has been suggested to be of benefit in decreasing the chance of disease recurrence.[158–159] Adjuvant chemotherapy following surgery and sometimes given in combination with radiation therapy is presently being evaluated for a possible role in improving treatment results with various sarcomas.

SMALL BOWEL LYMPHOMA

Lymphoid cells are found throughout the small intestine, and the small bowel can become involved in malignant disease of the lymphoid system.[162] Malignant lymphoma may originate in the small bowel as a primary neoplasm. The small intestine may also become secondarily involved with lymphoma as a manifestation of systemic lymphoid malignancy. The clinical features and treatment of lymphoma are discussed in detail in Chapter 25. The present section reviews the manifestations and management of malignant lymphoma confined to the small intestine.

Primary lymphoma of the small intestine is typically localized to a single segment of bowel, although multiple separate lesions are present in approximately 20% of cases.[162–163] All areas of the small intestine may develop lymphoma; however, the frequency is lowest in the duodenum, moderately frequent in the jejunum, and most frequent in the ileum, consistent with the relative increase in the concentration of lymphatic tissue progressing from the duodenum through the jejunum into the ileum.[163-164] Intestinal lymphoma comprises approximately 5% of all lymphoid malignancies and accounts for about 1% of small bowel neoplasms.[8,50,163] There appears to be an association between chronic celiac disease with malabsorption and an increased frequency of intestinal lymphoma.[165-166] In addition, a high incidence of intestinal lymphoma occurs in natives of the Middle East.[167] Patients with immune deficiency disease may have an increased frequency of intestinal lymphoma.[8,168]

Intestinal lymphoma represents the most common GI tumor in children below the age of 10 years.[169] GI lymphoma is, however, more common in the adult. There appears to be an increased incidence below the age of 10, a low incidence to approximately age 50, then a dramatically increased incidence of intestinal lymphoma above 50.[8,162] There is a slight male predominance, with the male:female ratio being approximately 1.5:1. In areas of the Middle East where the incidence of intestinal lymphoma is high, males and females are equally affected, and the disease tends to become manifest in the 30-year age group.[167]

In intestinal lymphoma, the neoplasm arises in the lymphoid tissue of the submucosa. The tumor expands the bowel wall, invades and ulcerates the mucosa to produce ulceration, and may penetrate through the bowel wall into the serosa. Histologic architecture of the neoplasm may be nodular with aggregations of lymphoid cells or diffuse with a uniform infiltration of malignant lymphoma. Involvement of mesentery and regional lymph nodes in the area of small bowel lymphoma is common. The area of bowel involvement may be localized or extend for considerable distances along the intestine. Most intestinal lymphomas are large, with 70% of the lesions exceeding 5 cm in diameter.[106]

Clinically, intestinal lymphoma manifests signs and symptoms attributable to the presence of a small intestinal mass that may be ulcerated or obstructing.[162] Abdominal pain is common, usually crampy in character, and may be associated with nausea and vomiting. Frequently, the lymphoma causes intestinal obstruction that is typically partial and intermittent. Complete obstruction can occur, but is unusual. GI hemorrhage is frequent and usually chronic, leading to anemia and the presence of occult blood in the stool. Massive intestinal bleeding can occur with acute ulceration of the tumor, but is rare. Fever may be present, usually indicating extensive lymphoma. Occasionally, GI lymphomas cause perforation with the clinical presentation of an acute abdomen. A palpable abdominal mass is frequently present. Diffuse lymphadenopathy or abdominal organomegaly suggests advanced disseminated disease. Ascites can be present when there is extensive intra-abdominal or retroperitoneal tumor spread.

In many instances, the diagnosis of intestinal lymphoma may be made roentgenographically. GI contrast studies may show infiltration of the bowel wall with ulceration or alteration of the mucosa (see Fig. 20-9). Segmental intestinal constriction may be present. If large necrotic masses are present that slough into the GI tract lumen, areas of bowel dilatation may appear. Displacement of bowel loops may be present with extensive bulky disease. Barium enema may show colonic displacement with large tumors, or may reveal abnormalities of the distal ileum by retrograde filling of the small intestine. Lymphangiography may be useful in determining lymphomatous involvement of intra-abdominal and retroperitoneal nodes. CT body scans can be helpful in delineating the extent of large intra-abdominal masses.

Treatment of primary lymphoma of the small intestine is surgical and should involve wide resection of the involved bowel segment and surrounding tissues as well as draining regional lymph nodes. Disease too extensive for complete resection may require palliative tumor resection or bypass to relieve or prevent intestinal obstruction. Prognosis for resected cases of intestinal lymphoma is reasonably favorable, with most series reporting 5-year survival rates of approximately 40%.[106,162,164] Patients with nonresectable disease have an overall 5-year survival rate of 25%.[8] Radiotherapy is of benefit in the palliation of extensive nonresectable intestinal lymphoma, and chemotherapy is indicated for the treatment of intestinal lymphoma patients who are not able to have curative resections.[8,162,170] Chemotherapeutic agents with activity against malignant lymphomas include methotrexate, vincristine, cyclophosphamide, and 6-mercaptopurine.[171]

There is considerable debate over the possible roles of adjuvant radiation therapy and adjuvant chemotherapy following complete surgical excision.[12] Although resection of isolated primary lymphoma of the small bowel can be curative in almost half of patients, studies are currently underway to evaluate whether adjuvant radiation therapy and chemotherapy after operation may result in improved patient salvage.[171]

Prognosis of nodular histologic patterns of lymphoma is generally better than that of diffuse lymphoma. Overall 5-year survival of patients with nodular lymphoma is approximately 50%, while survival in the diffuse lymphomas is in the range of 25%.

METASTATIC TUMORS

INVOLVEMENT OF SMALL INTESTINE BY DIRECT INVASION

The small intestine may be involved by malignant tumors that originate outside of the bowel and secondarily invade the intestine. The duodenum may be involved by tumor extension from cancers of the colon, stomach, pancreas, or kidney.[172-175] Metastatic tumor involving retroperitoneal lymph nodes, such as tumors of the ovary or testis, may enlarge and directly invade the bowel.[176] The jejunum may be directly invaded by malignancies of the colon, stomach, pancreas, kidney, or retroperitoneum.[8,177] The ileum may be involved by cancers arising in the colon, pelvis, or retroperitoneum.[8,177]

Direct tumor extension into the small intestine can produce clinical symptoms of intestinal obstruction or intestinal hemorrhage if tumor invasion causes mucosal ulceration.

Diagnosis of small bowel involvement by direct tumor extension may be made by radiologic contrast studies that may illustrate compression, displacement, or ulceration of the small intestine. However, diagnosis of the primary tumor first must be established. A GI series may demonstrate gastric or pancreatic malignancies, barium enema may reveal colonic neoplasms, IV pyelography may reveal renal carcinomas, or lymphangiography may localize retroperitoneal malignant

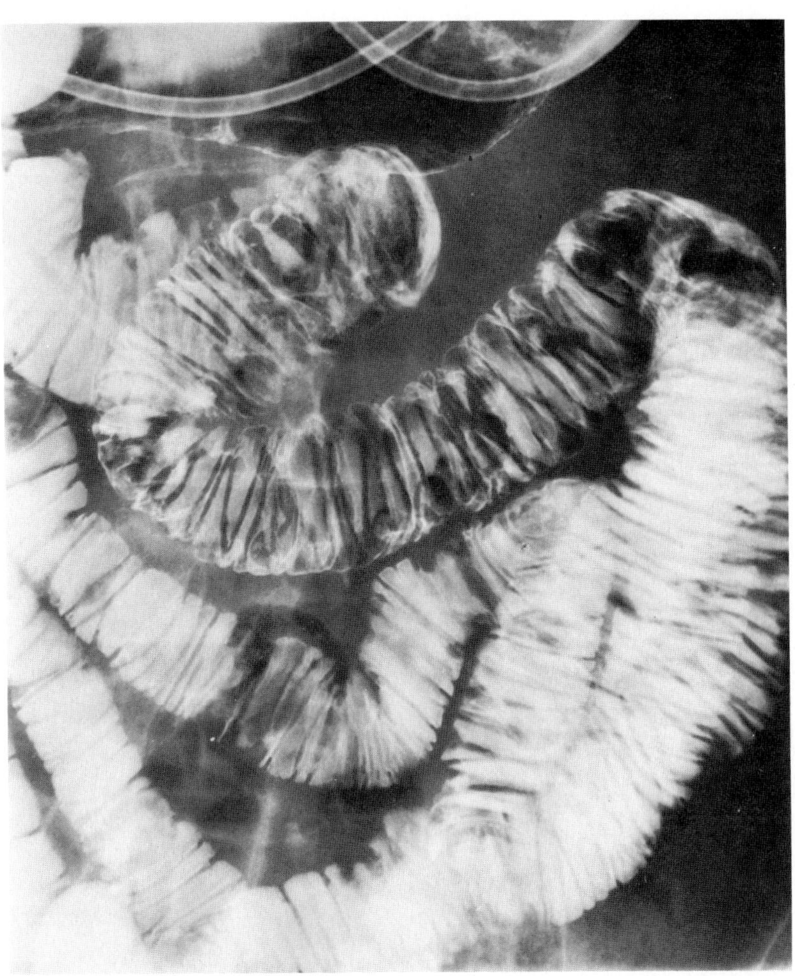

FIG. 20-9. Primary lymphoma of jejunum. Note extensive involvement of proximal jejunum by multiple filling defects.

adenopathy. CT body scans may be helpful in demonstrating intra-abdominal tumor masses and may indicate areas of bowel invasion.

Treatment of tumors invading the small bowel should be by wide surgical resection of the primary tumor including the bowel segment invaded. Resection may need to be quite extensive to include all areas at risk for tumor extension.[175,177–178]

METASTASES TO SMALL INTESTINE

The small intestine may be the site of metastatic deposits from tumors arising outside of the small bowel.[179–180] Although the incidence of metastatic involvement of the small bowel is low, tumors reported to give rise to small intestinal metastases include carcinoma of the cervix, malignant melanoma, carcinoma of the lung, esophageal carcinoma, and malignancies of the ovary.[8,175–176,179–182] In a review of tumors metastatic to the small intestine, carcinoma of the cervix was found to be the most frequent in producing bowel metastases, followed in frequency by melanoma, and then colonic neoplasms.[179] Metastases may be manifested late, wtih the time of diagnosis of melanoma metastatic to the intestine sometimes being more than 8 years following treatment of the primary tumor.[179]

Metastatic deposits in the small bowel typically develop in the submucosa to produce intramural lesions. The metastases may form masses in the intestinal wall leading to obstruction, ulcerated lesions penetrating mucosa to give intestinal hemorrhage, or polypoid masses producing the possibility of intussusception. The most common presenting clinical complaint of patients with metastatic lesions to the small bowel is partial intestinal obstruction.[179] Chronic intestinal bleeding may be present, with resultant anemia and stools positive for occult blood.[179–180]

The diagnosis of metastatic involvement of the small intestine may be difficult. Roentgenographic contrast studies may reveal masses or filling defects in the small intestine (see Fig. 20-10). However, in approximately 50% of cases of small bowel metastases, no roentgen ray abnormalities can be demonstrated.[8]

Treatment of metastases to the small intestine that produce symptoms of obstruction or hemorrhage should be surgical resection. The involved portion of intestine is best treated by segmental resection, with intestinal continuity established by end-to-end anastomosis. Frequently, multiple bowel metastases are present and the operative procedure is consequently palliative to relieve obstruction or hemorrhage. If multiple metastases are present, care must be taken to adequately identify and treat the lesions causing the obstruction or hemorrhage for which the surgery was undertaken. Large lesions are best excised by segmental bowel resection, but local excision may be possible if the tumors are small or

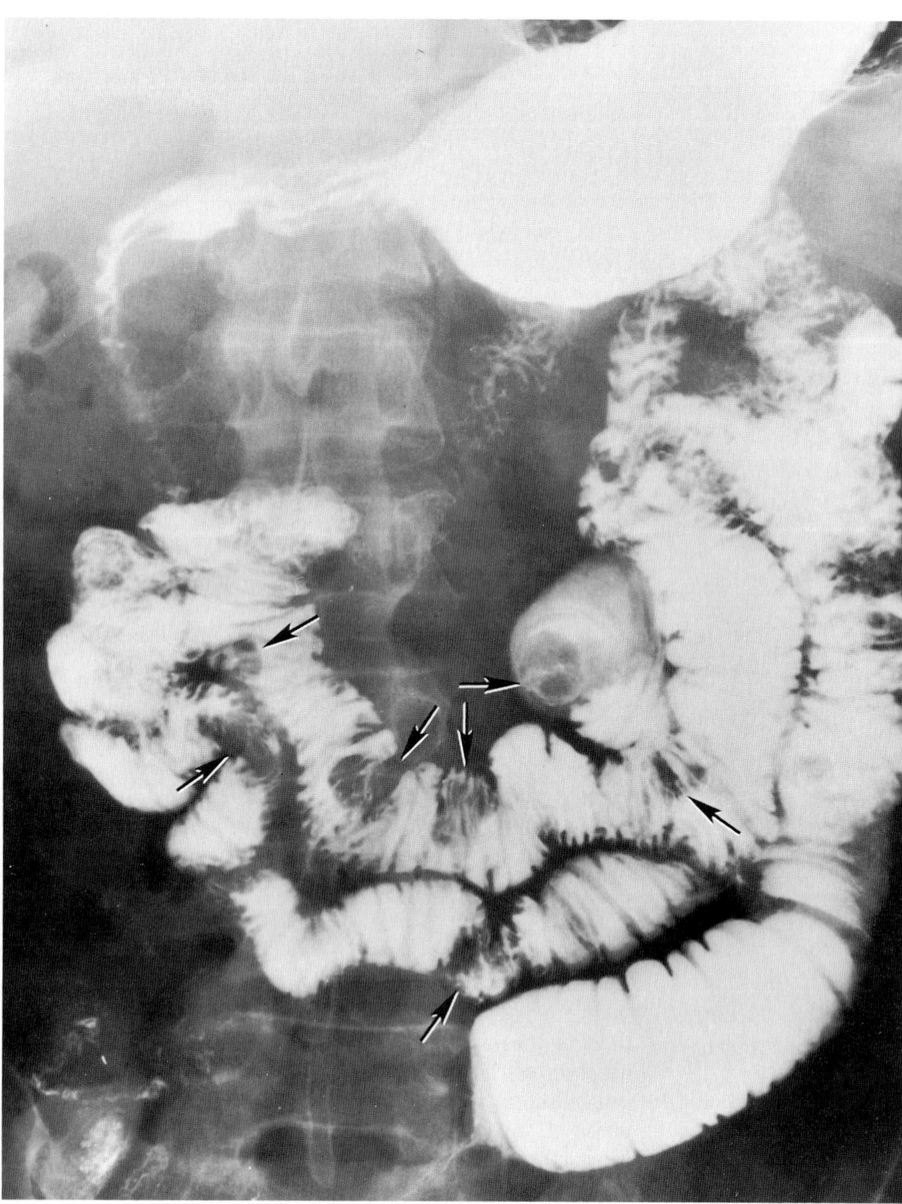

FIG. 20-10. Metastatic melanoma in small intestine. Note multiple small bowel filling defects.

pedunculated. If the lesions are not resectable, intestinal bypass for palliation is usually indicated. If a solitary metastasis is present, it should be segmentally resected. If the small bowel solitary metastasis is the only demonstrable site of disseminated tumor, there is a small chance that adequate resection of the metastatic deposit will be curative with no further disease developing.[180] Serious consideration should be given to a complete curative resection of the metastatic focus, including removal of the involved intestinal segment with the wide tissue margins, along with the surrounding normal tissues. In resections for cure of metastatic melanoma to the small intestine, it may be important to resect the nodal drainage basin supplying the involved bowel segment since the draining nodes from metastatic melanoma frequently contain tumor.[180]

REFERENCES

1. Braasch JW, Denbo HE: Tumors of the small intestine. Surg Clin North Am 44:791–809, 1964
2. Schier J: Diagnostic and therapeutic aspects of tumors of the small bowel. Int Surg 57:789–792, 1972
3. Rochlin DB, Longmire WP: Primary tumors of the small intestine. Surgery 50:586–592, 1961
4. Good CA: Tumors of the small intestine. Am J Roentgenol 89:685–705, 1963
5. del Regato JA, Spjut HJ: Ackerman and del Regato's Cancer. Diagnosis, Treatment, and Prognosis, 5 ed, pp 493–506. St Louis, CV Mosby, 1977
6. Croom RD, Newsome JF: Tumors of the small intestine. Am Surg 41:160–167, 1975
7. Mittal VK, Bodzin JH: Primary malignant tumors of the small bowel. Am J Surg 140:396–399, 1980

8. Herbsman H, Wetstein L, Rosen Y et al: Tumors of the small intestine. Curr Probl Surg 17:121–184, 1980
9. Skandalakis JE, Gray SW, Shepard D et al: Smooth Muscle Tumors of the Alimentary Tract. Leiomyomas and Leiomyosarcomas—A Review of 2525 Cases, pp 1–468. Springfield, IL, Charles C Thomas, 1962
10. Ebert PA, Zuidema GD: Primary tumors of the small intestine. Arch Surg 91:452–455, 1965
11. Sternlieb P, Mills M, Bellamy J: Hodgkin's disease of the small bowel. Am J Med 31:304–309, 1961
12. Weaver DK, Batsakis JG: Primary lymphomas of the small intestine. Am J Gastroenterol 42:620–625, 1964
13. Rochlin DB, Smart CR, Silva A: Chemotherapy of malignancies of the gastrointestinal tract. Am J Surg 109:43–46, 1965
14. Dorman JE, Floyd CE, Cohn I: Malignant neoplasms of the small bowel. Am J Surg 113:131–136, 1967
15. McPeak CJ: Malignant tumors of the small intestine. Am J Surg 114:402–411, 1967
16. Starr GF, Dockerty MB: Leiomyomas and leiomyosarcomas of the small intestine. Cancer 8:101–111, 1955
17. Hamberger GE: Propempticum Auspicale quo Dissertationem Solennem. Indicit et de Ruptura Intestini Duodeni Disserit, pp 1–8. Jena, Litteris Ritterianis, 1746
18. Wesner F: Beiträge zur casuistik der geschwülste. I. Ueber ein telangiectatisches myom des duodenum von ungewöhnlicher grösse. Virchows Arch [Pathol Anat] 93:377–386, 1883
19. Fleiner W: Zwei fälle von darmgeschwülsten mit invagination. Virchows Arch [Pathol Anat] 101:484–523, 1885
20. Heurtaux A: Note sur les tumeurs benignes de l'intestin. Arch Prov Chir 8:701–712, 1899
21. King EL: Benign tumors of the intestines with special reference to fibroma. Surg Gynecol Obstet 25:54–71, 1917
22. Shallow TA, Eger SA, Carty JB: Primary malignant disease of the small intestine. Am J Surg 69:372–383, 1945
23. River L, Silverstein J, Tope JW: Benign neoplasms of the small intestine. A critical comprehensive review with reports of 20 new cases. Int Abstr Surg 102:1–38, 1956
24. Darling RC, Welch CE: Tumors of the small intestine. N Engl J Med 260:397–408, 1959
25. Brookes VS, Waterhouse JAH, Powell DJ: Malignant lesions of the small intestine. A ten-year survey. Br J Surg 55:405–410, 1968
26. Reyes L, Talley RW: Primary malignant tumors of the small intestine. Am J Gastroenterol 54:30–43, 1970
27. Silberman H, Crichlow RW, Caplan HS: Neoplasms of the small bowel. Ann Surg 180:157–161, 1974
28. Wilson JM, Melvin DB, Gray GF et al: Primary malignancies of the small bowel: A report of 96 cases and review of the literature. Ann Surg 180:175–179, 1974
29. Wilson JM, Melvin DB, Gray GF et al: Benign small bowel tumor. Ann Surg 181:247–250, 1975
30. Botsford TW, Crowe P, Crocker DW: Tumors of the small intestine. A review of experience with 115 cases including a report of a rare case of malignant hemangio-endothelioma. Am J Surg 103:358–365, 1962
31. Cutler SJ, Young JL: Third National Cancer Survey: Incidence data. Natl Cancer Inst Monogr 41:1–454, 1975
32. Spiro HM: Clinical Gastroenterology, 2 ed, pp 571–590. New York, Macmillan, 1977
33. Krouse JM, Eyerly RC, Babcock JR: Tumors of the small bowel. Am J Surg 101:121–127, 1961
34. Sawyer RB, Sawyer KC, Sawyer KC et al: Benign and malignant tumors of the small intestine. Am Surg 29:268–272, 1963
35. Schmutzer KJ, Holleran WM, Regan JF: Tumors of the small bowel. Am J Surg 108:270–276, 1964
36. Ostermiller W, Joergenson EJ, Weibel L: A clinical review of tumors of the small bowel. Am J Surg 111:403–409, 1966
37. Spratt JS: Prevalence of neoplastic and pseudoneoplastic lesions of the small intestine. Geriatrics 21:231–238, 1966
38. Freund H, Lavi A, Pfeffermann R et al: Primary neoplasms of the small bowel. Am J Surg 135:757–759, 1978
39. Miles RM, Crawford D, Duras S: The small bowel tumor problem. An assessment based on a 20 year experience with 116 cases. Ann Surg 189:732–740, 1979
40. Schmahl D: Carcinogenic substances and carcinogens—Their clinical significance. In Herfarth C, Schlag P (eds): Gastric Cancer, pp 15–18. New York, Springer-Verlag, 1979
41. Wattenberg LW: Carcinogen-detoxifying mechanisms in the gastrointestinal tract. Gastroenterology 51:932–935, 1966
42. Lowenfels AB: Why are small-bowel tumours so rare? Lancet 1:24–25, 1973
43. Wattenberg LW: Studies of polycyclic hydrocarbon hydroxylases of the intestine possibly related to cancer. Effect of diet on benzpyrene hydroxylase activity. Cancer 28:99–102, 1971
44. Barnett WO: Benign tumors of the duodenum. Am Practit 13:625–632, 1962
45. Stassa G, Klingensmith WC: Primary tumors of the duodenal bulb. Am J Roentgenol 107:105–110, 1969
46. Everson TC: Carcinoma of the small intestine. In Everson TC, Cole WH (eds): Cancer of the Digestive Tract. Clinical Management, pp 75–85. New York, Appleton-Century-Crofts, 1969
47. Lowe WC: Neoplasms of the Gastrointestinal Tract, pp 125–144. Flushing, NY, Medical Examination Publishing, 1972
48. Hancock RJ: An 11-year review of primary tumours of the small bowel including the duodenum. Can Med Assoc J 103:1177–1179, 1970
49. Haghighi P, Nasr K: Primary upper small intestine lymphoma (so-called Mediterranean lymphoma). Pathol Annu 8:231–255, 1973
50. Loehr WJ, Mujahed Z, Zahn FD et al: Primary lymphoma of the gastrointestinal tract: A review of 100 cases. Ann Surg 170:232–238, 1969
51. Cassidy M: Abdominal carcinomatosis associated with vasomotor disturbances. Proc R Soc Med 27:220–221, 1934
52. Thorson A, Biörck G, Björkman G et al: Malignant carcinoid of the small intestine with metastases to the liver, valvular disease of the right side of the heart (pulmonary stenosis and tricuspid regurgitation without septal defects), peripheral vasomotor symptoms, bronchoconstriction, and an unusual type of cyanosis. A clinical and pathologic syndrome. Am Heart J 47:795–817, 1954
53. Montgomery GE, Liechty RD: Malignant small-bowel tumors. J Iowa Med Soc 56:249–251, 1966
54. Lee FD: Nature of the mucosal changes associated with malignant neoplasms in the small intestine. Gut 7:361–367, 1966
55. Brzechwa-Ajdukiewicz A, McCarthy CF, Austad W et al: Carcinoma, villous atrophy, and steatorrhoea. Gut 7:572–577, 1966
56. Jinich H, Rojas E, Webb JA et al: Lymphoma presenting as malabsorption. Gastroenterology 54:421–425, 1968
57. Brunt PW, Sircus W, Maclean N: Neoplasia and the coeliac syndrome in adults. Lancet 1:180–184, 1969
58. Chernish SM, Miller RE, Rosenak BD et al: Hypotonic duodenography with the use of glucagon. Gastroenterology 63:392–398, 1972
59. Sindelar WF, Bagley DH, Felix EL et al: Lung tomography in cancer patients. Full-lung tomography in screening for pulmonary metastases. JAMA 240:2060–2063, 1978
60. Morson BC, Dawson IMP: Gastrointestinal Pathology, pp 352–377. London, Blackwell Scientific Publications, 1972
61. Muto T, Bussey HJR, Morson BC: The evolution of cancer of the colon and rectum. Cancer 36:2251–2270, 1975
62. Ravitch MM: Polypoid adenomatosis of the entire gastro-intestinal tract. Ann Surg 128:283–298, 1948
63. Perry EC: Papilloma of the duodenum. Trans Pathol Soc London 44:84–85, 1893
64. Wechselmann L: Polyp und carcinom im magen-darmkanal. Beitr Klin Chir 70:855–904, 1910
65. Joyeux R: Tumeur adenomato-villeuse du duodenum. J Chir (Paris) 66:437–448, 1950
66. Steinberg LS, Shieber W: Villous adenomas of the small intestine. Surgery 71:423–428, 1972
67. Kutin ND, Ransom JHC, Gouge TH et al: Villous tumors of the duodenum. Ann Surg 181:164–168, 1975

68. Golden R: Non-malignant tumors of the duodenum. Report of two cases. Am J Roentgenol 20:405–413, 1928
69. Hoffman BP, Grayzel DM: Benign tumors of the duodenum. Am J Surg 70:394–400, 1945
70. Shulten MF, Dyasu R, Beal JM: Villous adenoma of the duodenum. A case report and review of the literature. Am J Surg 132:90–96, 1976
71. Bremer EH, Battaile WG, Bulle PH: Villous tumors of the upper gastrointestinal tract. Clinical review and report of a case. Am J Gastroenterol 50:135–143, 1968
72. Meltzer AD, Ostrum BJ, Isard HJ: Villous tumors of the stomach and duodenum. Radiology 87:511–513, 1966
73. Waters CA: The roentgenologic diagnosis of papilloma of the duodenum. Am J Roentgenol 24:544–557, 1930
74. Ring EJ, Ferrucci JT, Eaton SB et al: Villous adenomas of the duodenum. Radiology 104:45–48, 1972
75. Silverman L, Waugh JM, Hiuzenge KA et al: Large adenomatous polyp of Brunner's glands. Am J Clin Pathol 36:438–443, 1961
76. Deutschberger O, Tchertkoff V, Daino J et al: Benign duodenal polyp: Review of the literature and report of a giant adenomatous polyp of the duodenal bulb. Am J Gastroenterol 38:75–84, 1962
77. de Silva S, Chandrasoma P: Giant duodenal hamartoma consisting mainly of Brunner's glands. Am J Surg 133:240–243, 1977
78. Wood DA: Atlas of Tumor Pathology. Tumors of the Intestines, section VI, fascicle 22, pp 19–120. Washington, DC, Armed Forces Institute of Pathology, 1967
79. Rankin FW, Newell CE: Benign tumors of the small intestine. Report of twenty-four cases. Surg Gynecol Obstet 57:501–507, 1933
80. Gentry RW, Dockerty MB, Clagett OT: Vascular malformations and vascular tumors of the gastrointestinal tract. Int Abstr Surg 88:281–323, 1949
81. Moore RM, Schmeisser HC: Benign tumors of the small intestine. South Med J 27:386–393, 1934
82. Sivula A: Intestinal haemangioma. Observation on two cases treated surgically. Acta Chir Scand 131:485–491, 1966
83. Bilton JL, Riahi M: Hemangioma of the small intestine. Am J Gastroenterol 48:120–124, 1967
84. Hyun BH, Palumbo VN, Null RH: Hemangioma of the small intestine with gastrointestinal bleeding. JAMA 208:1903–1905, 1969
85. Brown AJ: Vascular tumors of the intestine. Surg Gynecol Obstet 39:191–199, 1924
86. Nys A, Buyssens N: Diffuse cavernous hemangiomatosis of the small intestine. Gastroenterology 45:663–666, 1963
87. Alfidi RJ, Esselstyn CD, Tarar R et al: Recognition and angiosurgical detection of arteriovenous malformations of the bowel. Ann Surg 174:573–582, 1971
88. Calem WS, Jimenez FA: Vascular malformations of the intestine. Their role as a source of hemorrhage. Arch Surg 86:571–579, 1963
89. Arnett NL, Friedman PS: Lymphangioma of the colon: Roentgen aspects. A case report. Radiology 67:882–885, 1956
90. Puppel ID, Morris LE: Lymphangioma of the jejunum. Arch Pathol 38:410–412, 1944
91. Hermans PE: Nodular lymphoid hyperplasia of the small intestine and hypogammaglobulinemia: Theoretical and practical considerations. Fed Proc 26:1066–1611, 1967
92. Shaw EB, Hennigar GR: Intestinal lymphoid polyposis. Am J Clin Pathol 61:417–422, 1974
93. Golden T, Stout AP: Smooth muscle tumors of the gastrointestinal tract and retroperitoneal tissues. Surg Gynecol Obstet 73:784–810, 1941
94. O'Brien TF: Primary tumors and vascular malformations. In Sleisenger MH, Fordtran JS (eds): Gastrointestinal Disease. Pathophysiology—Diagnosis—Management, 2 ed, pp 1124–1137. Philadelphia, WB Saunders, 1978
95. Shaw RC: Von Recklinghausen's disease of the small intestine associated with skin lesions. Am J Surg 80:360–363, 1950
96. Brasfield RD, Das Gupta TK: Von Recklinghausen's disease: A clinicopathological study. Ann Surg 175:86–104, 1972
97. Hochberg FH, Dasilva AB, Galdabini J et al: Gastrointestinal involvement in von Recklinghausen's neurofibromatosis. Neurology (Minneap) 24:1144–1151, 1974
98. Cedermark J: Neurinomas of the gastrointestinal tract. J Int Coll Surg 12:5–11, 1949
99. Smith FR, Mayo CW: Submucous lipomas of the small intestine. Am J Surg 80:922–928, 1950
100. Jeghers H, McKusick VA, Katz KH: Generalized intestinal polyposis and melanin spots of the oral mucosa, lips and digits. A syndrome of diagnostic significance. N Engl J Med 241:993–1005, 1949
101. Dormandy TL: Gastrointestinal polyposis with mucocutaneous pigmentation (Peutz-Jeghers syndrome). N Engl J Med 256:1093–1102, 1141–1146, 1186–1190, 1957
102. Reid JD: Duodenal carcinoma in the Peutz-Jeghers syndrome. Report of a case. Cancer 18:970–977, 1965
103. Williams JP, Knudsen A: Peutz-Jeghers syndrome with metastasizing duodenal carcinoma. Gut 6:179–184, 1965
104. Humphries AL, Shepherd MH, Peters HJ: Peutz-Jeghers syndrome with colonic adenocarcinoma and ovarian tumor. JAMA 197:296–298, 1966
105. Payson BA, Moumgis B: Metastasizing carcinoma of the stomach in Peutz-Jeghers syndrome. Ann Surg 165:145–151, 1967
106. Pagtalunan RJG, Mayo CW, Dockerty MB: Primary malignant tumors of the small intestine. Am J Surg 108:13–18, 1964
107. Goel IP, Didolkar MS, Elias EG: Primary malignant tumors of the small intestine. Surg Gynecol Obstet 143:717–719, 1976
108. Rich JD: Malignant tumors of the intestine: A review of 37 cases. Am Surg 43:445–454, 1977
109. Sager, GF: Primary malignant tumors of the small intestine. A twenty-two year experience with thirty patients. Am J Surg 135: 601–603, 1978
110. Coutsoftides T, Shibata HR: Primary malignant tumors of the small intestine. Dis Colon Rectum 22:24–26, 1979
111. Shukla SK, Elias EG: Primary neoplasms of the duodenum. Surg Gynecol Obstet 142:858–860, 1976
112. Morowitz DA, Block GE, Kirsner JB: Adenocarcinoma of the ileum complicating chronic regional enteritis. Gastroenterology 55:397–402, 1968
113. Tyers GFO, Steiger E, Dudrick SJ: Adenocarcinoma of the small intestine and other malignant tumors complicating regional enteritis: Case report and review of the literature. Ann Surg 169:510–518, 1969
114. Frank JD, Shorey BA: Adenocarcinoma of the small bowel as a complication of Crohn's disease. Gut 14:120–124, 1973
115. Smith EH, Bartrum RJ, Chang YC et al: Percutaneous aspiration biopsy of the pancreas under ultrasonic guidance. N Engl J Med 292:825–828, 1975
116. Goldman ML, Naib ZM, Galambos JT et al: Preoperative diagnosis of pancreatic carcinoma by percutaneous aspiration biopsy. Am J Dig Dis 22:1076–1082, 1977
117. Howard JM: Pancreatico-duodenectomy: Forty-one consecutive Whipple resections without an operative mortality. Ann Surg 168: 692–640, 1968
118. Gilsdorf RB, Spanos P: Factors influencing morbidity and mortality in pancreaticoduodenectomy. Ann Surg 177:332–337, 1973
119. Howard JM, Jordan GL: Cancer of the pancreas. Curr Probl Cancer 2:1–52, 1977
120. Brunschwig A, Tiholiz IC: Surgical treatment of malignant tumors of the duodenum exclusive of those arising from the papilla of Vater. Surg Clin North Am 26:163–175, 1946
121. Spinazzola AJ, Gillesby WJ: Primary malignant neoplasms of the duodenum: Report of twelve cases. Am Surg 29:405–412, 1963
122. Mongé JJ, Judd ES, Gage RP: Radical pancreatoduodenectomy: A 22-year experience with the complications, mortality rate, and survival rate. Ann Surg 160:711–722, 1964
123. Cortese AF, Cornell GN: Carcinoma of the duodenum. Cancer 29:1010–1015, 1972
124. Warren KW, Choe DS, Plaza J et al: Results of radical resection for periampullary cancer. Ann Surg 181:534–540, 1975

125. Nakase A, Matsumoto Y, Uchida K et al: Surgical treatment of cancer of the pancreas and the periampullary region: Cumulative results in 57 institutions in Japan. Ann Surg 185:52–57, 1977
126. Coutsoftides T, MacDonald J, Shibata HR: Carcinoma of the pancreas and periampullary region: A 41 year experience. Ann Surg 186:730–733, 1977
127. Vuori JVA: Primary malignant tumors of the small intestine. Analysis of cases diagnosed in Finland, 1953–1962. Acta Chir Scand 137:555–561, 1971
128. Morgan DF, Busuttil RW: Primary adenocarcinoma of the small intestine. Am J Surg 134:331–333, 1977
129. Cavanaugh PJ: Considerations appropriate to a clinical trial of definitive radiation therapy in adenocarcinoma of the pancreas. J Surg Oncol 7:135–137, 1975
130. Abe M, Takahashi M, Yabumoto E et al: Techniques, indications and results of intraoperative radiotherapy of advanced cancers. Radiology 116:693–702, 1975
131. Abe M, Takahashi M, Yabumoto E et al: Clinical experiences with intraoperative radiotherapy of locally advanced cancers. Cancer 45:40–48, 1980
132. Bunn PA, Nugent JL, Ihde DC et al: 5-Fluorouracil, methyl-CCNU, adriamycin, and mitomycin-C in the treatment of advanced gastric cancer. Cancer Treat Rep 62:1287–1293, 1978
133. Higgins GA: Chemotherapy in advanced gastric cancer. In Herfarth C, Schlag P (eds): Gastric Cancer, pp 361–366. New York, Springer-Verlag, 1979
134. Pearse AGE: The APUD cell concept and its implications in pathology. Pathol Annu 9:27–41, 1974
135. Ritchie AC: Carcinoid tumors. Am J Med Sci 232:311–328, 1956
136. Marks C: Carcinoid Tumors. A Clinicopathologic Study, pp 1–154. Boston, GK Hall, 1979
137. Moertel CG, Sauer WG, Dockerty MB et al: Life history of the carcinoid tumor of the small intestine. Cancer 14:901–912, 1961
138. Horsley BL, Baker RR: Fibroplastic response to intestinal carcinoid. Am Surg 36:676–680, 1970
139. Cunningham PJ, Norman J, Cleveland BR: Malignant carcinoid associated with thoraco-abdominal aneurysm and analysis of thirty-one cases of gastrointestinal carcinoid tumors. Ann Surg 176:613–619, 1972
140. Ostermiller WE, Joergenson EJ: Carcinoid tumors of the small bowel. Arch Surg 93:616–619, 1966
141. Sterling JA, Jayasanker MR, Galvez M: Carcinoids of the gastrointestinal tract. Am J Gastroenterol 47:373–378, 1967
142. Dockerty MB: Carcinoids of the gastrointestinal tract. Am J Clin Pathol 25:794–796, 1955
143. Diffenbaugh WG, Anderson RE: Carcinoid (argentaffin) tumors of the gastrointestinal tract. Arch Surg 73:21–37, 1956
144. Sjoerdsma A, Weissbach H, Udenfriend S: A clinical, physiologic and biochemical study of patients with malignant carcinoid (argentaffinoma). Am J Med 20:520–532, 1956
145. Kowlessar OD: The carcinoid syndrome. In Sleisenger MH, Fordtran JS (eds): Gastrointestinal Disease. Pathophysiology—Diagnosis—Management, 2 ed, pp 1190–1201. Philadelphia, WB Saunders, 1978
146. Chandler JJ, Foster JH: Malignant carcinoid syndrome treated by resection of hepatic metastases. Am J Surg 109:221–222, 1965
147. Melmon KL, Sjoerdsma A, Oates JA et al: Treatment of malabsorption and diarrhea of the carcinoid syndrome with methysergide. Gastroenterology 48:18–24, 1965
148. Tilson MD: Carcinoid syndrome. Surg Clin North Am 54:409–423, 1974
149. Herbsman H, Hassan A, Gardner B et al: Treatment of hepatic metastases with a combination of hepatic artery infusion chemotherapy and external radiotherapy. Surg Gynecol Obstet 147:13–17, 1978
150. Schein P, Kahn R, Gorden P et al: Streptozotocin for malignant insulinomas and carcinoid tumor. Report of eight cases and review of the literature. Arch Intern Med 132:555–561, 1973
151. Sparks FC, Mosher MB, Hallauer WC et al: Hepatic artery ligation and postoperative chemotherapy for hepatic metastases: Clinical and pathological results. Cancer 35:1074–1082, 1975
152. Thomford NR, Woolner LB, Clagett OT: The surgical treatment of metastatic tumors in the lungs. J Thorac Cardiovasc Surg 49:357–363, 1965
153. Ochsner A, Rush V: Treatment of pulmonary metastatic disease. Surg Clin North Am 46:1469–1473, 1966
154. Fallon RH, Roper CL: Operative treatment of metastatic pulmonary cancer. Ann Surg 166:263–265, 1967
155. Foster JH, Berman MH: Solid Liver Tumors, pp 209–234. Philadelphia, WB Saunders, 1977
156. McNeer GP, Cantin J, Chu F et al: Effectiveness of radiation therapy in the management of sarcoma of the soft somatic tissues. Cancer 22:391–397, 1968
157. Suit HD, Russell WO, Martin RG: Management of patients with sarcoma of soft tissue in an extremity. Cancer 31:1247–1255, 1973
158. Rosenberg SA, Kent H, Costa J et al: Prospective randomized evaluation of the role of limb-sparing surgery, radiation therapy, and adjuvant chemoimmunotherapy in the treatment of soft-tissue sarcomas. Surgery 84:62–69, 1978
159. Rosenberg SA, Sindelar WF: Surgery and adjuvant radiation-chemo-immunotherapy in soft tissue sarcomas: Result of treatment at the National Cancer Institute. In van Oosterom AT, Muggia FM, Cleton FJ (eds): Therapeutic Progress in Ovarian Cancer, Testicular Cancer and the Sarcomas, pp 397–412. Boston, Martinus Nijhoff, 1980
160. Jacobs EM: Combination chemotherapy of metastatic testicular germinal cell tumors and soft part sarcomas. Cancer 25:324–332, 1970
161. Gottlieb JA: Combination chemotherapy for metastatic sarcoma. Cancer Chemother Rep 58:265–270, 1974
162. Trier JS: Lymphoma. In Sleisenger MH, Fordtran JS (eds): Gastrointestinal Disease. Pathophysiology—Diagnosis—Management, 2 ed, pp 1115–1124. Philadelphia, WB Saunders, 1978
163. Rosenberg SA, Diamond HD, Jaslowitz B et al: Lymphosarcoma: A review of 1269 cases. Medicine (Baltimore) 40:31–84, 1961
164. Naqvi MS, Burrows L, Kark AE: Lymphoma of the gastrointestinal tract: Prognostic guides based on 162 cases. Ann Surg 170:221–231, 1969
165. Harris OD, Cooke WT, Thompson H et al: Malignancy in adult coeliac disease and idiopathic steatorrhoea. Am J Med 42:899–912, 1967
166. Dutz W, Asvadi S, Sadri S et al: Intestinal lymphoma and sprue: A systematic approach. Gut 12:804–810, 1971
167. Eidelman S, Parkins RA, Rubin CE: Abdominal lymphoma presenting as malabsorption: A clinico-pathologic study of nine cases in Israel and a review of the literature. Medicine (Baltimore) 45:111–137, 1966
168. Whitehead R: Primary lymphadenopathy complicating idiopathic steatorrhoea. Gut 9:569–575, 1968
169. Mestel AL: Lymphosarcoma of the small intestine in infancy and childhood. Ann Surg 149:87–94, 1959
170. Treadwell TA, White RR: Primary tumors of the small bowel. Am J Surg 130:749–755, 1975
171. McGovern VT: Lymphomas of the gastrointestinal tract. In Yardley, JH, Morson BC, Abell MR (eds): The Gastrointestinal Tract, pp 184–205. Baltimore, Williams & Wilkins, 1977
172. Grinnell RS: Lymphatic metastases of carcinoma of the colon and rectum. Ann Surg 131:494–506, 1950
173. Lawson LJ, Holt LP, Rooke HWP: Recurrent duodenal haemorrhage from renal carcinoma. Br J Urol 38:133–137, 1966
174. Treitel H, Meyers MA, Maza V: Changes in the duodenal loop secondary to carcinoma of the hepatic flexure of the colon. Br J Radiol 43:209–213, 1970
175. Veen HF, Oscarson JEA, Malt RA: Alien cancers of the duodenum. Surg Gynecol Obstet 143:39–42, 1976
176. Ngan H: Involvement of the duodenum by metastases from tumours of the genital tract. Br J Radiol 43:701–705, 1970
177. Van Prohaska J, Govostis MC, Wasick M: Multiple organ

resection for advanced carcinoma of the colon and rectum. Surg Gynecol Obstet 97:177–182, 1953

178. Ellis H, Morgan MN, Wastell C: "Curative" surgery in carcinoma of the colon involving duodenum. A report of 6 cases. Br J Surg 59:932–935, 1972
179. de Castro CA, Dockerty MB, Mays CW: Metastatic tumors of the small intestines. Surg Gynecol Obstet 105:159–165, 1957
180. Das Gupta TK, Brasfield RD: Metastatic melanoma of the gastrointestinal tract. Arch Surg 88:969–973, 1964
181. Farmer RG, Hawk WA: Metastatic tumors of the small bowel. Gastroenterology 47:496–504, 1964
182. Beckly DE: Alimentary tract metastases from malignant melanoma. Clin Radiol 25:385–389, 1974

Paul H. Sugarbaker
John S. Macdonald
Leonard L. Gunderson

CHAPTER 21

Colorectal Cancer

Cancer of the colon and rectum is one of the commonest internal malignancies in the United States for males and females combined. It will occur in approximately 5% of U.S. born males and 6% of females. The incidence rates of this tumor and survival following surgical resection have not improved in the last 40 years except that mortality following surgery has decreased with improvements in anesthetic techniques, blood transfusion, and antibiotics in the management of septic complications. However, knowledge of the natural history of colorectal cancer has increased markedly during this time. With this new knowledge a strategy for the control of large bowel cancer in the 1980s may be formulated as: (1) identification of large bowel carcinogens and their elimination from the environment, (2) screening the general population over the age of 50 years, (3) identification of high risk groups for careful followup, (4) adequate primary surgical treatments coupled with controlled clinical trials to test new adjuvants, and (5) careful follow-up after surgical resection with aggressive therapy for localized recurrence.

ANATOMY

GROSS ANATOMY OF THE LARGE BOWEL

The anatomic segments of the large bowel are shown in Fig. 21-1. It begins at the ileo–cecal valve and ends at the anal canal. The most distinguishing feature of the peritoneal surface of the colon is its taenia; these are three concentrations of longitudinal musculature that form narrow bands puckering the colon surface into haustrations. The taenia come together at the base of the cecum as if pointing to the appendix. In the rectosigmoid area the taenia coalesce to provide a thick longitudinal muscular coat for the rectum. In the anal area this circular muscle coat becomes the internal anal sphincter. Between taenia the longitudinal muscular coat is thinned, but not absent. Other distinguishing features of the peritoneal surface of the colon are the epiploic appendages and the greater omentum which arises off the transverse colon.

The ascending and descending colon, as well as splenic and hepatic flexures, are similar to the rectum in that they are relatively immobile structures which lack a mesentery and usually lack a peritoneal covering (serosa) on the posterior and lateral surfaces. A lesion that extends through the entire bowel wall in these areas has the potential, as does rectal carcinoma, of compromised operative margins—especially with posterior or lateral extension. In contrast, the transverse and sigmoid colon are freely suspended on a mesentery and consequently are freely mobile except for their proximal and distal segments. For carcinomas that involve a mobile portion of the colon, the risk of peritoneal seeding of malignant cells may be as great or greater than the risk of local recurrence. In these bowel locations, the risk of inadequate operative removal is probably greatest when there is tumor adherence to or invasion of surrounding organs or tissues. Patients with cecal cancer may be at risk for retention of malignant cells within the retroperitoneum or for seeding into the free peritoneal cavity and adjacent structures, for the cecal mesentery is variable.

The rectum can be conveniently divided into three sections and treatment of carcinoma located in different sections varies greatly. Fig. 21-2 shows the division of the rectum by the upper, lower, and middle valves of Houston. It should be noted that two valves are located on the left and one on the right. The right middle valve is generally the most prominent and is situated at the same level as the peritoneal reflection. Below the middle valve of Houston the rectum expands as the rectal ampulla. In the adult the middle valve of Houston is 10 cm to 12 cm from the anal verge; this distance to the peritoneal reflection is important to remember, for cancer or

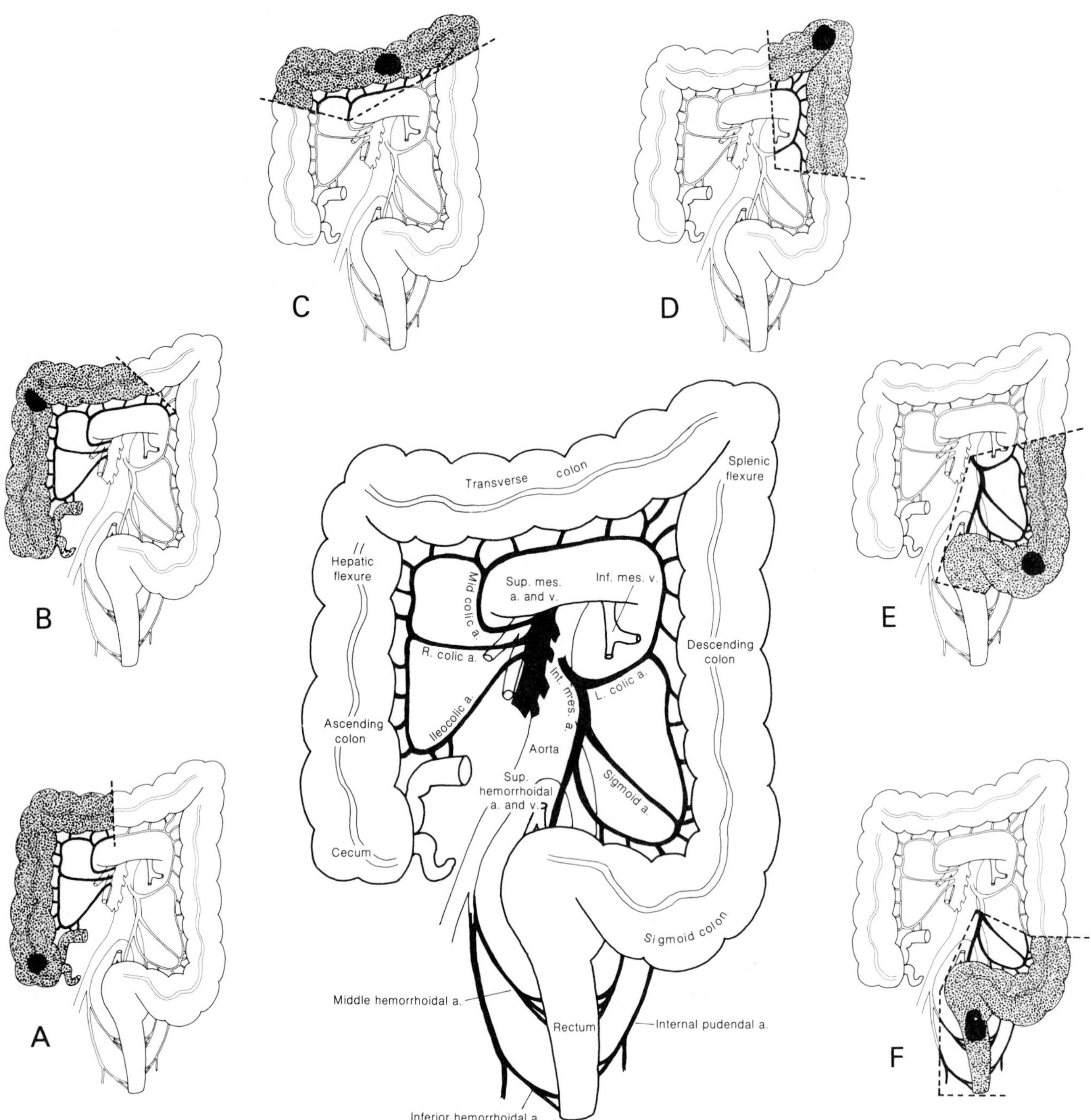

FIG. 21-1. Anatomic segments, arterial and venous blood supply, and surgical resections of the colon and rectum. (Modified from Jones T, Shepard WC: A Manual of Surgical Anatomy. Philadelphia, WB Saunders, 1945; and Coller JA: Cancer of the Colon and Rectum. New York, Am Cancer Soc Inc, 1956)

other rectal diseases tend to obscure definite location of Houston's valves. Fulguration of invasive tumors cannot be safely performed above this point, for the upper third of the rectum is within the free peritoneal cavity. Once beneath the pelvic peritoneum the rectum is bounded by the sacrum posteriorly and fits closely to the curve of the sacrum. The contour between rectum and sacrum seen on lateral roentgenogram with a barium-filled bowel is important in assessing possible recurrent cancer following anterior resection. A thickening or irregularity seen here can occasionally indicate recurrent disease when palpation and inspection of this segment of bowel seems completely normal. Anterior to the rectum in the female is the vagina; in the male, the trigone of the bladder, seminal vesicles, prostate gland, and urethra are anterior.

The rectum ends at the pectinate line which is 1 cm to 2 cm below the muscular anorectal ring. Between the anorectal ring and the pectinate line are the rectal columns of Morgagni.

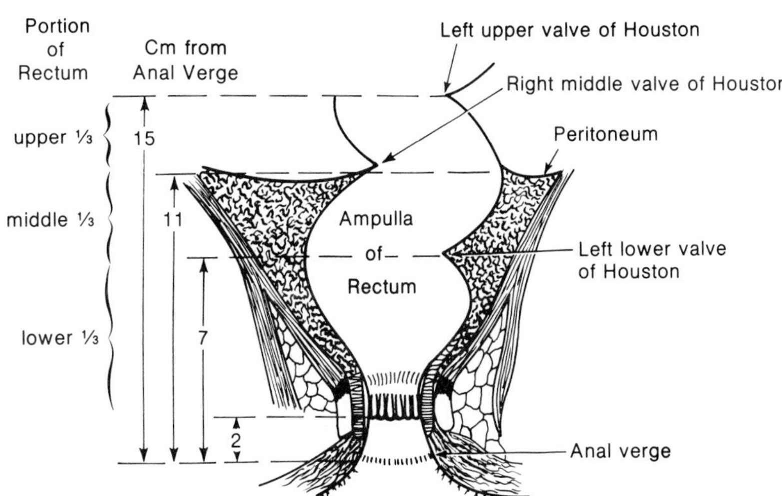

FIG. 21-2. Division of the rectum into upper, middle and lower thirds. (Modified from Goligher JC: In Turrell R (ed): Diseases of the Colon and Ano-rectum. Philadelphia, WB Saunders, 1959)

The major anatomic landmark of this area is the pectinate line, where large bowel mucosa and squamous epithelium meet. Some anatomists refer to this transition zone as the dentate line. The anal canal lies between the pectinate line and the anal verge. The anal verge marks another transition zone between nonkeratinized and keratinized stratified squamous epithelium. Below the anal verge is perianal skin (see Chap. 22, Cancer of the Anal Region).

Bacon has emphasized that although lymphatic and arterial supply is well divided by the pectinate line, the venous system is rich in collateral channels between superior, middle and inferior hemorrhoidal veins.[4] This pelvic venous plexus is one of the major pathways for collateral portal venous flow and unpredictable spread of hematogenous metastases.

ARTERIAL BLOOD SUPPLY TO THE LARGE BOWEL

The dual blood supply to the colon through the superior and inferior mesenteric arteries is shown in Fig. 21-1. Also shown are the anatomic resections of large bowel that can be performed based primarily on this arterial network.

A question is sometimes raised as to the adequacy of the marginal artery of Drummond to supply a portion of the left colon if the inferior mesenteric artery is taken at its origin. Goligher presents evidence to suggest that the marginal artery is adequate to supply the descending colon in a majority of patients; however, exceptions are seen.[5] From a practical standpoint it is usually best in performing a sigmoid colectomy to divide the descending colon in its upper portion or mid-portion; prior to performing the anastomosis one should check to see that the color of the bowel is good and that a pulse in the marginal artery is palpable.

The rectum is supplied by three hemorrhoidal arteries. The superior hemorrhoidal artery is the lowest branch off the inferior mesenteric artery. The middle and inferior hemorrhoidal arteries come off the internal iliac artery. The middle hemorrhoidal arteries are well developed in only 25% of persons and this undoubtedly is why they are not always located while performing a low anterior or abdomino–perineal resection. Because the arterial blood supply to the lower one-third of the rectum and anal canal is from the internal iliac, some surgeons have used ligation of this artery as a first step in performing the pelvic portion of an abdominoperineal resection.[6]

VENOUS DRAINAGE OF THE LARGE BOWEL

The venous drainage of the colon differs markedly from the arterial supply. The superior mesenteric vein drains directly into the portal system. The inferior mesenteric vein enters into the splenic vein just beneath the ligament of Treitz and from there empties into the portal system. The upper and middle thirds of the rectum also drain to the portal system. However, the lower third of the rectum has a dual venous drainage to portal system by way of the superior hemorrhoidal vein and to the inferior vena cava by way of the middle hemorrhoidal veins. Therefore, primary metastases filtered out in the first capillary bed occur in the liver for cancers in the colon and upper two-thirds of the rectum. Carcinomas in the lower third of the rectum may metastasize to either liver or lung. As we shall see in the section on treatment of metastases these anatomical facts may help determine if a hepatic or pulmonary lesion should be resected.

LYMPHATIC DRAINAGE OF THE LARGE BOWEL

The lymphatics of the colon have been classified as epicolic (on the wall of the colon), paracolic (along the marginal artery and between it and the bowel), intermediate (along the colic and sigmoid arteries), and principal (at the origins of the superior and inferior mesenteric vessels and their middle and left colic branches). The lymphatics tend to follow the arterial supply much closer than veins and the intermediate nodes are named for the artery they accompany (Fig. 21-3).

The lymphatic drainage of the colon is nearly always convergent toward major arterial trunks; an exception to this occurs when nodes become blocked by tumor and an unpredictable retrograde lymphatic drainage occurs.[9] Retrograde lymphatic flow, even with extensive lymph node metastases, is rare and occurs in only about 1% of cases (see section on lymphatic spread). This is an important factor which makes

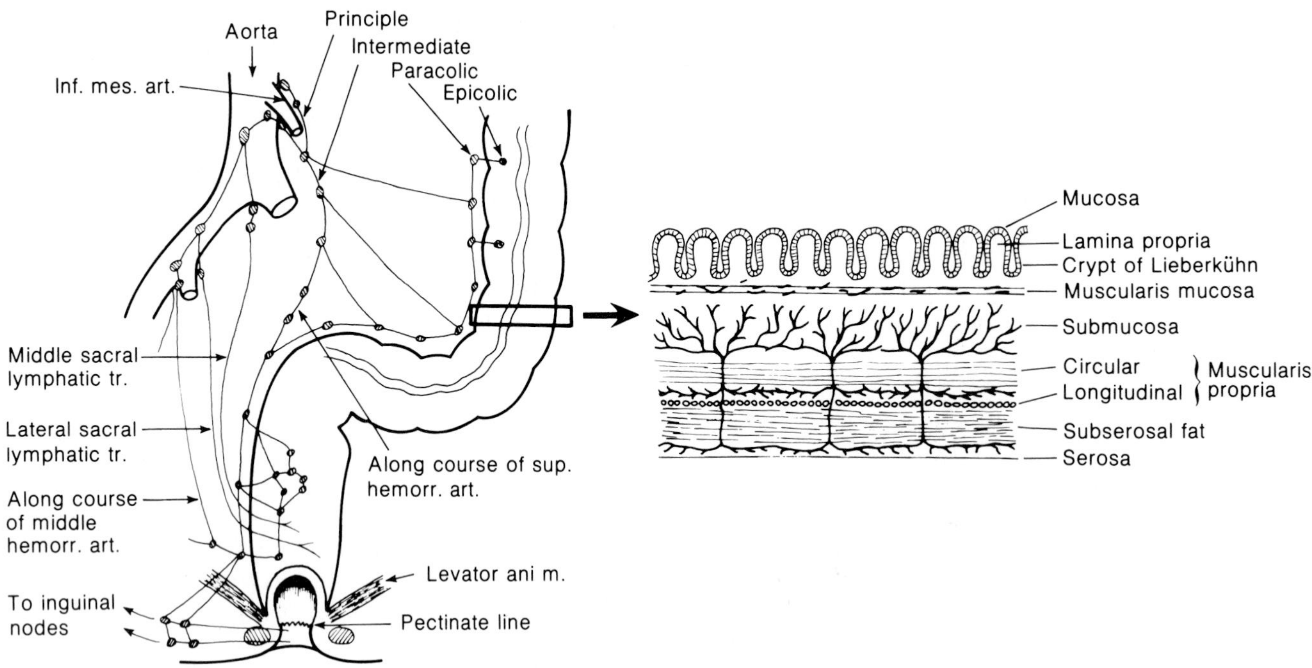

FIG. 21-3. Lymphatic drainage of the large bowel, including the colon wall. (Modified from Villemin F, Huard P, Montague M: Rechetches anatomiques surles lymphatics du rectum, et de l'anus. Rev Chir 63:39–80, 1925; and Cole PP: The intramural spread of rectal carcinoma. Br Med J 1:431–433, 1913)

anterior resection a reasonable operation for most cancers of the rectosigmoid and upper two-thirds of the rectum.

The lymphatic drainage of the right colon joins that from the small bowel and pancreas to drain into superior mesenteric nodes. From here lymph follows along into the celiac nodes and then into a major lymphatic trunk, usually the left lumbar lymphatic trunk or directly into the cisterna chyli. The relative proportion of lymph passing upward along the superior mesenteric artery as compared to that along the portal vein is unknown. The major flow apparently accompanies the arterial system. However, metastatic colon cancer within lymph nodes at the porta hepatis is not uncommon and is evidence of portal lymphatic drainage of the colon.

Lymphatic drainage of the left colon, sigmoid colon, and upper two-thirds of the rectum is primarily along branches of the inferior mesenteric artery; again a lesser flow is along the inferior mesenteric vein to nodes in the porta hepatis.

The pectinate line serves as an anatomic division for lymphatic flow in the anorectal area; the flow of lymph, and therefore the migration of tumor cells, is upwards into the superior hemorrhoidal system from rectal wall above the pectinate line. Lymphatic flow from the area immediately adjacent to the pectinate line is in three directions: upwards into the superior hemorrhoidal system, lateral along the middle hemorrhoidal vessels, and downward into the inferior hemorrhoidal system. Migration of tumor cells along the middle hemorrhoidal system may result in metastases in obturator, internal iliac, and common iliac lymph nodes. Tumor cells going along the inferior hemorrhoidal system result in metastases in the superficial and occasionally deep inguinal lymph nodes. Lymphatic flow from below the pectinate line is primarily to inferior hemorrhoidal lymphatics and then inguinal lymph nodes.

The studies of Inquist and Block suggested that lymphatic drainage of the rectum courses anteriorly and posteriorly much more extensively than has been previously recognized.[10] They injected dye (direct sky-blue) into the anus or lower, middle, and upper third of the rectum. If injections were in the lower two-thirds of the rectum, dye in females went up along the rectovaginal septum and was seen within vaginal lymphatics. Only with dye injection into the upper rectum did lymphatics go only to the superior hemorrhoidal vessels. They suggested that in carcinoma of the middle and lower thirds of the rectum the lower half of the posterior vaginal wall should be included in the operative specimen.

PHYSIOLOGY OF THE LARGE BOWEL

The function of the larger bowel is to receive 800 ml to 1000 ml of ileal contents per day, absorb water and electrolytes, and act as a reservoir to fecal matter until it is discharged. Mucus must be secreted in large amounts to lubricate the mucosal surface and allow the dehydrated feces to move along. The major function of the right colon is reabsorption of water and that of the left colon storage of feces.

HISTOLOGY OF THE LARGE BOWEL

The histology of the large bowel directly reflects its principal function of elimination of wastes. The colon wall consists of mucosa, submucosa, muscularis, and serosa; in the rectum no serosa is present but a generous layer of fat is adherent to the muscular coat. The inside surface of the colon is smooth, for there are no plicae or villi as in the small bowel. Long, straight, tubular glands extend down from the surface through the entire thickness of the mucosa. These glands are the crypts of Lieberkuhn. The surface epithelium is composed primarily of tall columnar absorbing cells that have a striated border. Goblet cells are interspersed among the columnar absorbing cells at the surface, but are far more numerous within the walls of the glands. Cells at the base of the crypts appear more undifferentiated with multiple mitoses. They are rapidly dividing to push new cells to the surface to replace those which are constantly being exfoliated at the surface. Rarely, enterochromaffin cells are seen at the base of a crypt.

The lamina propria extends up between the glands; it is delicate because tubules are packed close together. The muscularis mucosa consists of an inner circular and outer longitudinal layer of smooth muscle and the base of the crypts of Lieberkuhn almost rest on the muscularis mucosa. The lymphatics that accompany the muscularis mucosa do not extend up into the lamina propria or epithelium of the mucosa.[11] This fact is of great importance in deciding the surgical management of polyps that contain foci of malignancy (see section on treatment of polyps).

The submucosa is composed of loosely arranged connective tissue. It is the strongest layer of the bowel wall and, if transected, colonic perforation is much more likely with much less internal pressure. Solitary lymph follicles from the lamina propria project into the submucosa. The muscularis propria is arranged into two layers, an inner circular layer and an outer longitudinal layer.

The vascular anatomy of the colon wall is circular in its arrangement. From the marginal artery, short and long branches of the vasa recti course around the colon. Goligher has shown that vasa recti may be occluded if an epiploic appendage is picked up using traction and then tied off.[5] Cole described the lymphatic anatomy of the colon wall by following microscopic extensions of tumor in lymphatic channels around the colon wall.[8] Lymphatics were found to course circularly in the submucosa, then radially penetrate the inner circular muscle. Between the two muscle layers further circular lymphatic channels were identified. These drained through the longitudinal muscle to epi- and paracolic lymph nodes (Fig. 21-3). The fact that lymphatic drainage of the colon is of circular arrangement accounts for the annular growth of a majority of tumors. Almost invariably the transverse diameter of tumors exceeds their longitudinal measurement, showing the circular spread within the colon wall.

EPIDEMIOLOGY

Within the past decade it has become clear that the incidence of colonic and rectal cancers is shifting from a predominance in the rectum to a predominance in the colon.[12-14] The cause for this change in incidence is not known. About 70% of the incident cases and 80% of the deaths from large bowel cancer are due to tumors in the colon; the remainder are in the rectum. There is some reason to think that tumors of the rectum and colon are etiologically different in some respects. Thus, tumors of the colon are slightly more frequent in females than in males, whereas the reverse is true of rectal tumors. On the other hand, many of the epidemiologic features of the two cancers are similar and some differences may be attributed to differences in classification of tumors at the colorectal junction. At the present time the epidemiologic patterns are not yet distinct enought to warrant describing the two conditions separately.

There have been no remarkable changes in incidence or mortality from colon and rectum cancer in the last 50 years.[15] Up until about 1950, rates for blacks were substantially lower than those for whites, but subsequently, the former have risen and the latter remained constant, so that rates are now approximately the same in the two races.

There are very substantial international variations in rates, the most notable being the low rates seen in Japan and in the black populations of sub-Saharan Africa. Japanese migrants to the United States acquire, within the same generation, rates that are very much higher than those in Japan.[16] Further, the children of emigrants from low-risk countries of Europe have rates just as high as other U.S. whites.[17] It is clear, therefore, that the causes of the international differences in rates are environmental, not genetic. There has been considerable speculation that the responsible factors are dietary in origin and a great deal of work has been undertaken to evaluate the various hypotheses that have been proposed. These include the following:

1. Diets that are low in "fiber" (a loose term used to cover a variety of indigestible carbohydrate dietary components) lead to low-bulk stools and slow transmission of dietary components through the gut. The slow transit time may permit a longer time for the formation of carcinogens in the gut and a longer period during which carcinogens are in contact with the gut wall. The low-bulk stool may lead to carcinogens being present in higher concentrations than in a high fiber stool.[18] There may, in addition, be binding of carcinogens to pectins and other specific components.
2. Diets high in fat, particularly unsaturated fat, appear to be associated with high colon cancer rates.[19] Metabolism of fat in the lumen of the gut is associated with the production of acid and neutral steroids and their metabolites, some of which have a structural similarity to known carcinogens. Bile acids may also play a role. It is known that the fecal concentration of bile acids and neutral steroids is influenced by the intake of fat and, in one case-control study, high fecal bile-acid concentrations were found in 82% of the cancer patients but only 17% of the controls.[20,21] The possibility that the tumor itself changes the metabolism of the gut contents complicates studies of the latter type.
3. Bacterial fauna of the gut, and particularly the anaerobes capable of deconjugation of bile salts, varies with diet and will be an important determinant of the chemical composition of gut content. It is likely that some microorganisms can metabolize fat or bile acids to carcinogens.[22]

A great deal of work is now in progress to evaluate the several components of these hypotheses. It has been fully reviewed recently by Rowland.[23] No body of research better illustrates the importance of integration of epidemiologic and laboratory work in endeavoring to unravel the etiology of a disease.

Recent geographic correlations have suggested the possibility of a link between beer consumption and cancer of the large bowel.[24] These are almost certainly spurious, since association with beer or other alcoholic beverage has not been found in case-control studies or in follow-up studies of heavy beer drinkers.[25]

NATURAL HISTORY OF SURGICALLY TREATED COLORECTAL CANCER

Colorectal cancer presents as a wide variety of lesions, from large, fungating tumors to small, malignant foci in the head of a pedunculated polyp.[26] Throughout this discussion of the natural history of colon and rectal cancer we assume that rectal and colonic adenocarcinoma are really the same malignancy in two different anatomic parts of the large bowel. Grinnell and more recently, Wood, compared growth patterns and prognostic variables of colon and rectal disease; their studies suggested marked similarities, although there are differences.[27,28]

ORIGIN OF LARGE BOWEL CANCER—*DE NOVO* CARCINOMA OR AN ADENOMATOUS POLYP TO CANCER TRANSITION

An important question for those interested in screening for large bowel malignancy concerns the origin of the primary tumor. Do a majority of malignancies arise in benign polyps or do cancers come *de novo* from formerly normal colonic epithelium? Perhaps both processes occur? If all cancers arise slowly over the course of years in an identifiable benign lesion (polyp), then it is possible that a screening test for this lesion may virtually eliminate the disease. Polyps can be expeditiously removed by way of a colonoscope and the carcinogen–polyp–cancer sequence can be interrupted.

Historically, many clinicians and pathologists have assumed that large bowel cancers arose from benign polyps. Indeed, there is much circumstantial evidence to suggest that adenomatous polyps are a precursor of colorectal cancer. One might expect that a direct answer to this question should be available by careful follow-up of unresected polypoid lesions. However, one cannot exclude the presence of malignancy in a polyp by simple biopsy. Because of sampling error, cancerous change cannot be excluded from a particular polyp without a complete histologic examination of the entire specimen. Such examinations would require excision of the polyp itself and, therefore, excision for exact diagnosis would destroy the clinical experiment. Furthermore, some evidence suggests that an adenoma to cancer transition exists at least in some individuals, so that failure to completely excise a lesion may subject the patient to an undue risk.

Arguments in support of an adenoma to colorectal cancer transition are listed in Table 21-1. It seems likely that remnants of adenomatous tissue within cancers should be evident if polyps degenerate into malignancy. Dukes stated that this transition was seen, but he did not determine the frequency of this observation.[29] Indeed, contrary to what might be expected, remnants of adenomatous tissue at the site of a large bowel cancer is not a routine finding. Spratt, Ackerman, and Moyer could find no tissue resembling adenomatous polyp in a study of 323 carcinomas of the colon.[30] Similarly, Castleman and Krickstein state that "in the hundreds of frank cancers of the colon, either polypoid or ulcerating, seen at the Massachusetts General Hospital, we have not found a single one with a remnant of adenomatous polyp."[31] Spratt and Ackerman studied 20 colon and rectal cancers 2 cm or less in diameter by serial sectioning, thinking that in these small lesions one would be most likely to see residual adenomatous tissue.[32] No remnant of adenomatous polyp was found. Kjeldsberg and Altschuler report a patient with three small foci of *in situ* adenocarcinoma of the transverse colon without associated adenomatous remnants.[33]

Quite different observations have been reported by Morson in a study of 76 patients selected out of a total of 2305 who had "early cancer."[34] In 56.6% of this early group, Morson found evidence within the specimen of tissue thought to be left from a pre-invasive process. The frequency with which benign tissue could be detected histologically varied with the extent of spread. Morson thought that this was to be expected, for cancerous tissue would outgrow and then overgrow the benign tissue from which it arose. When a large number of cancers was examined, if the primary tumor was limited to the bowel wall, persistence of benign tumor was found in 18.3% of specimens; if spread in continuity involved extramural tissues, the incidence dropped to 7.6%.

Several other investigators have sought to check Spratt, Ackerman, and Moyer's findings by searching thoroughly within primary adenocarcinomas for areas of adenoma. Enterline and co-workers studied 666 colorectal cancers; areas of adenomatous polyp were found in six.[35] Enterline and co-workers were working retrospectively from scattered random

TABLE 21-1. Arguments for an Adenomatous Polyp to Cancer Transition (with reference numbers)

1. Residual adenomatous tissue is observed quite commonly in small cancers (34).
2. Patients kept polyp free also remain cancer free (40, 41).
3. Small foci of intramucosal cancer are commonly seen in polyps but extremely rare in normal mucosa (43).
4. Some apparently benign adenomatous polyps have developed into cancer (44–48).
5. There is an increasing incidence of cancer in polyps of increasing size (42, 48).
6. There is an increasing incidence of cancer as the number of polyps increases (48).
7. There are no good criteria by which adenomatous polyps can be classified as a different biologic entity from villous adenomas, a lesion with definite malignant potential (49).
8. The adenomatous-polyp to cancer transition has been seen in familial polyposis (50).
9. The adenomatous-polyp to cancer transition has been seen in experimental animals (51).
10. A presumed transition from a precancerous state to invasive malignancy is seen in several other epithelial tissues.
11. The peak age at which polyps are diagnosed precedes that for cancer by about 5 years (48).
12. There is a similar distribution of polyps and cancer within the large bowel (54–56).

sections, although all cases studied included sections showing the junction of carcinoma with normal mucosa. Lesions that showed remnants of villous adenoma were not included. Therefore, the incidence of 1% must be considered a minimal one. Turell and Broadman found adenomatous tissue within adenocarcinomas in 16 of 150 consecutive colorectal cancer specimens.[36] Also, Blatt found that four of 465 colon and rectal polyps contained both areas of benign adenomatous tissue and cancer.[37]

Lane and co-workers attempt to resolve the discrepant observations of Spratt and Ackerman and Morson.[38] They point out that only two of the 20 carcinomas Spratt and Ackerman studied were 5 mm or less in diameter, while the majority of them were between 1 cm and 2 cm. All the lesions had already become invasive. They suggest that a 1 cm to 2 cm cancer is a large lesion and that a more accurate study would need to include lesions of 5 mm in size. Lane and co-workers suggest that colon and rectal cancers do arise in adenomas, but that these adenomas may be extremely small.

Lipkin, Sherlock, and Bell point out that cell division and therefore turnover of colonic epithelium is extremely rapid; complete regeneration of the entire intestinal mucosa occurs every 48 hours.[39] Therefore, it is possible that cancer can overgrow adenomatous tissue quite rapidly.

Perhaps the most significant clinical experiment testing the polyp-to-cancer transition hypothesis was reported by Gilbertsen and co-workers.[40,41] In Gilbertsen's study, 21,150 individuals underwent proctosigmoidoscopic examinations on an annual basis. Polyps found were removed. Twenty-five adenocarcinomas were detected on the initial examination. However, over the subsequent 92,650 patient-years of followup, only 13 additional cancers were detected by sigmoidoscopy. Epidemiologic data predicted one cancer per thousand patient-years, or about 90 cancers. Only 13 of 90 (15%) of the expected cancers appeared. Also, the cancers were at an early stage of development and all had an excellent chance for cure.

Up to 30% of large bowel adenomas contain areas of *in situ* or invasive malignancy; also, the incidence of malignant change increases as the size of the polyp increases.[42] However, as Fenoglio and Lane point out, early carcinoma does not seem to occur unassociated with adenoma.[43] They reason that since colorectal cancer is so common, one should often find small malignant foci of carcinoma that arose from areas of normal-appearing epithelium. Fenoglio and Lane state that the "apparent nonexistence of small intramucosal carcinoma in normal mucosa, and its common occurrence in adenomas are two fundamental pathologic facts. They would seem to disprove the proposition that cancer cells arise *de novo* from the normal cells of the crypt of Lieberkuhn without the interposition of a stage in the neoplastic process that we recognize as adenoma."

Colorectal cancer has been found to arise at the site where a presumably benign adenoma was located. Buie and Brust report four patients in whom carcinoma was superimposed on the site of a previously noted adenoma.[44] Jackman and Mayo related the course of two patients with benign adenoma by biopsy.[45] These lesions were not removed and 16 years and 19 years later, carcinomas were present at the site of the previous polyp. Scarborough reviewed a personal experience with 1088 cases to find ten in which presumptively benign polyps when not removed, progressed to become cancer.[46] Knoernschild reviewed the growth of 213 asymptomatic presumably benign polyps for a 3-year to 5-year period.[47] Most lesions stayed the same size, but two polyps changed in appearance and were proven by biopsy to have developed into cancer. Finally, Muto, Bussey, and Morson reported three adenomatous polyps of the rectum that did not receive any surgical treatment for 5 years, 6 years, and 13 years after their discovery; at the previous polyp site adenocarcinoma was detected. In a fourth patient, an adenomatous polyp remained benign over an 11-year time period.[48] Of course, as mentioned above, these reports cannot be used as definite evidence of a polyp-to-cancer transition, for the presence of cancer in the original lesion cannot be ruled out.

Muto, Bussey, and Morson in a review of an 11-year experience with polypoid lesions at St. Mark's Hospital, show that there is an increasing incidence of cancer in polyps of increasing size.[48] Adenomatous polyps under 1 cm had a 1.0% incidence of invasive malignancy, 1 cm to 2 cm had a 10.2% incidence; and over 2 cm, 34.7%.

Muto, Bussey, and Morson also showed that the risk of cancer, either synchronous or metachronous in patients who have adenomatous or villous polyps, increased as the number of polyps in the large bowel increased.[48] Presumably, the greater the number of polyps present, the more likely malignant transformation of adenomatous tissue becomes.

Even the most outspoken critics of the adenomatous polyp-to-cancer transition will agree that villous polyps do often undergo malignant transformation. Neither Spratt, Ackerman, and Moyer nor Castleman and Krickstein argue against villous polyps as frequent origin of carcinoma.[30,31] However, there are no good criteria by which one can separate the two morphologic entities. Rather, adenomatous and villous polyps seem to include a spectrum of lesser and greater potential for malignant change. Indeed, Fung and Goldman found, using a dissecting microscope and multiple sections, focal villous change in 35% of solitary adenomatous polyps and 75% of lesions larger than 1 cm in diameter.[49] Most likely, adenomatous and villous polyps are histologic variants of the same neoplastic process.

Bussey reviewed the St. Mark's experience with 199 cancers in patients with familial polyposis.[50] Histological examination showed adenomatous tissue in continuity with the invasive cancer in 72 (36%) of cancers. Apparently, in this clinical situation where a large number of polyps will, if not removed, result in cancer in 100% of the patients, a transition from polyp to cancer is also seen. The polyps seen with familial polyposis are almost exclusively adenomatous.

Lipkin and his associates have shown in the colon of experimental animals treated with colonic carcinogens a spectrum of histologic changes which can be compared to changes seen in humans.[51] Mucosal lesions form by a confluence of hyperplastic crypts; with time, adenomas and adenocarcinomas were observed.

Several other arguments have been offered to support an adenomatous polyp to cancer transition: colonic epithelium would be expected to undergo change from a precancerous to cancerous state similar to that seen with other tissues. Esophagus, stomach, bladder, cervix, oral cavity, and skin cancers are reported to be associated with premalignant processes. Muto, Bussey, and Morson report the peak age at which polyps are found precedes the peak age for colorectal cancer by about 5 years.[48] This suggests a polyp-to-cancer transition which takes 5 years.

Finally, some arguments suggest an association of adenomatous polyps and cancer and therefore hint at a polyp-to-cancer transition. There is a tendency for polyps and cancer to occur together in an individual's colon. Prager and co-workers from the Lahey Clinic followed up patients known to have had adenomatous polyps removed; the number of cancers that developed in these patients was twice that expected in an unaffected population.[52] Rider and co-workers have tabulated the numerous reports which show the frequent association of carcinoma with polyps.[53] Also, some authors have been impressed with the similar anatomic distribution of polyps and carcinoma.[54–56]

In summary, there is good evidence for a transition of adenomatous polyps to carcinoma. Certainly, not all polyps undergo malignant change but it seems that the more polyps allowed to grow for a longer time to larger size, the greater the likelihood of cancer developing from them. The big question that does remain is, *how often* does colorectal cancer arise in a previously benign polyp?

VILLOUS POLYP-TO-CANCER TRANSITION

The relative number of cancers preceded by villous polyps in relation to adenomatous polyps, or those with an intermediate histology is not definitely known. However, Muto, Bussey, and Morson found remnants of polypoid tissue in 278 of 1961 colorectal carcinoma specimens (14.2%); of these tissue remnants 32.7% were adenomatous, 31.3% were intermediate type, and 36% were villous type.[48] However, only 10% of polypoid lesions are of villous histology and 15% of intermediate type. If the number of cancers arising in each is about equal, villous polyps have 10 times the malignant potential and intermediate type 6.7 times the malignant potential that adenomatous polyps possess.

RATE OF GROWTH

The first quantitation of the rate of growth of a primary cancer of the large bowel was recorded by Spratt and Ackerman.[57] They reported the slowly progressive growth of a transverse colon cancer that was studied nine times by double contrast barium enema over a period of seven-and-one-half years. The cancer was finally removed from the patient and was shown to be a not unusual constricting adenocarcinoma of the transverse colon. Spratt and Ackerman calculated that the cancer grew with a doubling time of 636 days. It was first thought that this particular tumor was exhibiting abnormally slow growth. However, Welin, Youker, and Spratt reported the doubling time for 20 additional carcinomas serially studied in Mahmo, Sweden, to be 620 days.[58] These authors conclude that large bowel tumors must have very long periods of silent growth before they become large enough to produce symptoms. Even the fastest-growing cancer they observed would have required 6 years to 8 years to grow from glandular size to a diameter of 60 mm.

However, the growth rate of pulmonary metastasis (and presumably hepatic metastasis, although the studies have not been done) is much more rapid than the growth of the primary tumor within the bowel wall. Collins reported that the average doubling time for 25 separate patients with pulmonary metastasis was 116 days.[59] Confirming this, Welin, Youker and Spratt reported the median doubling time of 43 pulmonary metastases in 36 patients to be 109 days.[58] Apparently, the mean growth rates of metastases in lung from colonic and rectal cancers are five-fold to six-fold faster than the mean rates of growth of the primary cancers growing in the colon or rectum. It may be that ulceration of tumor and exfoliation of tumor cells into the colonic lumen accounts for the slower growth of the primary.

DUKES' HYPOTHESES CONCERNING THE SPREAD OF COLORECTAL CANCER

Concepts related to the growth and spread of colorectal cancer were largely formulated by Cuthbert Dukes, pathologist at St. Marks' Hospital, London, England through a meticulous gross and microscopic study of thousands of rectal cancer specimens. They can be summaried by three basic hypotheses: First, concerning local progression, Dukes found that cancer of the rectum advanced locally by progressively increasing the depth of penetration of the bowel wall. Lymphatic metastases were rarely found before the carcinoma had spread by direct continuity through the muscularis propria into the extra-rectal tissues.[29] Second, concerning progression of lymphatic metastases, he was impressed by the orderly and predictable course of lymphatic spread. The first glands to receive metastases are those situated in the perirectal tissues on the same level or immediately above the primary growth. The next to be affected are the chain of glands accompanying the superior hemorrhoidal vessels.[60] Third, concerning the rate of progression of disease, histologic grading was regarded as an approximate method of measuring the pace of growth of a tumor and the A, B, and C classification (see section on staging) was regarded as a measurement of the distance reached.[29]

Although Dukes' hypotheses go far to explain the natural history of large bowel adenocarcinoma they fail to explain why approximately 50% of patients with recurrence succumb to persistent local disease with tumors that are by all criteria completely removed surgically. We would add a fourth hypothesis to Dukes' three hypotheses. In some patients, tumor cells penetrating through interstitial tissue or leaking from lymphatic channels at the time of surgical extirpation implant within the abdominal cavity, usually in the raw surface left at the resection site. Eventually, these implants result in locally recurrent tumor and treatment failure. In our further discussion of the natural history of colorectal cancer we will present data to support these four hypotheses. Also, notable exceptions to these generalizations will be pointed out.

ROUTES OF SPREAD

The routes of spread of colorectal cancer are shown in Table 21-2.

Local Spread

Percival Cole, in 1913, reported his studies of the gross and microscopic features of 20 rectal cancer specimens.[8] He traced microscopically the course of carcinomatous deposits extending from the primary tumor within the bowel wall to determine whether spread was parallel or perpendicular to the course of the bowel. He made the important gross observation that the long axis of the ulcerating tumor was, in every specimen, transverse; that is, the lesions showed a tendency to involve the bowel circularly rather than longitudinally. Consequently, the tumors tended to narrow and constrict the bowel lumen. Cole suggested that the circular distribution of lymphatics (see section of anatomy) was largely responsible for the circular distribution of carcinomatous growth. Cole concluded that recurrence from rectal cancer could not be explained by persistence of tumor that had grown along the bowel wall as Miles had suggested, but thought that recurrence was due to extramural deposits of tumor cells that were not removed by local excision.

The findings of Cole were in direct contradiction to those of Miles who observed longitudinal spread along the rectal wall in a majority of specimens he resected.[61] However, review of Miles' data suggests that his patients had far-advanced disease with retrograde spread of tumor along paracolic lymphatics. The type of tumor spread he described and which comprised Miles' major rationale for abdomino–perineal resection only occurs with far-advanced tumors which are nearly always uncurable (see below).

Black and Waugh sought to determine by pathologic studies the extension of colon carcinoma in the long axis of the bowel.[62] By microscopic examination of 103 specimens of left colon cancer, they showed that spread along the long axis of the bowel was very limited. Confirming the observations of Cole, spread through the muscular layer was characterized by columns of carcinoma cells radiating out through the muscle bundles. Spread was greatest in the submucosa, but even in this layer it was very limited in a longitudinal dimension. The greatest extension along the course of the bowel in any specimen was 12 mm and in only four of the total number of specimens was the spread 5 mm or more. No appreciable differences were noted in the extension above or below the lesion.

Numerous studies performed on rectal cancer specimens to establish the rationale for low anterior resection also have shown limited spread of cancer along the long axis of the bowel. Grinnell reported the distal intramural spread of carcinoma of the rectum and rectosigmoid seen in 126 specimens.[63] In 67 of 76 curative resections there was no retrograde spread and a margin of 5 cm would have been adequate in all. When retrograde spread did occur, tumors were nearly always advanced invasive lesions of high grade malignancy. Retrograde spread occurred by way of lymphatics in the subserosa and perirectal fat. No intramural lymphatic spread of any significance was seen.

Studies cited to this point would indicate that extension of the primary tumor parallel to the long axis of the bowel rarely occurs; however, spread circularly around the course of the bowel occurs within the bowel wall. Extension of colorectal cancer perpendicular to the long axis of the bowel was recognized by Dukes and associates as the route for further local, lymphatic, or hematogenous dissemination. By Dukes first hypothesis, only after extension through the bowel wall did tumor spread to involve local lymph nodes or metastasize hematogenously. Cases where metastases had been found at an earlier stage were recorded by Miles but were thought by Dukes to be exceedingly rare.[61] No metastases in tumors that did not penetrate the muscular coats of the bowel were found in 38 cases reported in 1932.[64] In lesions where lymph nodes were involved, as a rule, the tumor had extended through the bowel wall. Grinnell found only two of 69 tumors with lymph node involvement before complete penetration of the bowel wall had occurred.[27]

Dukes himself recognized an exception to his first hypothesis. Poorly differentiated tumors may metastasize hematogenously or lymphatically much earlier than expected. In 14 of 400 (3.5%) of specimens reported by Dukes in 1940 this occurred.[29] Morson substantiated this finding; he identified 46 of 2084 tumors in which growth was limited to the mucosa and submucosa.[34,65] Five instances of lymphatic spread were seen; three of the five were of Broders grade IV and two were of grade III. That lymphatic or hematogenous metastases can occur from poorly differentiated carcinoma in the head of a pedunculated polyp is further evidence of metastases occurring earlier than predicted by Dukes' first hypothesis.[26,66,67]

If lymphatic metastases are related to tumor penetration of the bowel wall, then one might expect the incidence of metastases to increase as local extension of tumor increased. As seen in Table 21-3, Dukes and Bussey showed a direct

TABLE 21-2. Spread of Colorectal Cancer

Local routes
- Circularly within bowel wall
- Parallel to bowel wall
- Perpendicular to bowel wall
- Perineural
- Adjacent organs or structures

Lymphatic routes

Hematogenous routes
- Colon to liver
- Rectal to liver and lung
- Batson's plexus to spine

Implantation
- Wound
- Anastomotic
- Intraperitoneal

TABLE 21-3. Relation of Extent of Local Spread to Lymphatic Metastases

EXTENT OF LOCAL SPREAD	NUMBER OF PATIENTS	NUMBER WITH METASTASES	PERCENT
none	302	43	14.2
slight	516	223	43.2
moderate	273	155	56.8
extensive	641	478	74.6
TOTAL	1732	899	51.9

(Dukes CE, Bussey HJR: The spread of rectal cancer and its effect on prognosis. Br J Cancer 12:309–320, 1958)

relationship of the extent of local spread to the incidence of lymphatic metastases.[68] Also, Grinnell found that tumor limited to the submucosa and muscularis propria, metastasized to nodes in 13% of cases (23 of 183 cleared specimens), whereas tumors which had penetrated beyond the muscularis propria had node metastases in 50%.[69] The more extensive lymphatic network beyond the muscularis propria afforded the cancer greater opportunities for metastases from its enlarged periphery. The fact that stage C1 tumors by the Astler and Coller classification are unusual (see section on staging) would also support progression of disease as suggested by Dukes.[70]

Dionne showed that the extent of penetration of the bowel wall was found to control the incidence of hematogenous metastases, as well as lymph node metastases.[71] However, because hematogenous spread is only rarely seen in the absence of lymphatic spread, there must be a tendency for metastasis to occur by the lymphatic route slightly earlier.[72]

Another pathway for local extension of tumor was studied by Seefeld and Bargen and concerns the spread of tumor along perineural spaces.[73] In a pathologic study of 100 resected rectal cancer specimens, they found perineural involvement in 30. Pain reported to be "aching," "boring," "gnawing," "constant" was recorded in the history of 80% of patients with perineural involvement and 34% of the time in patients without perineural involvement. The incidence of perineural involvement increased, as might be expected, in groups with lymphatic involvement, with higher degrees of malignancy by Broder's grading and with venous invasion. Of clinical importance was the local recurrence rate which was two-and-one-half times more frequent in cases with nerve invasion than in cases in which it was not observed.

Finally, colorectal cancer may extend to and invade adjacent organs. The effect this growth may have on prognosis and surgical approach is discussed below.

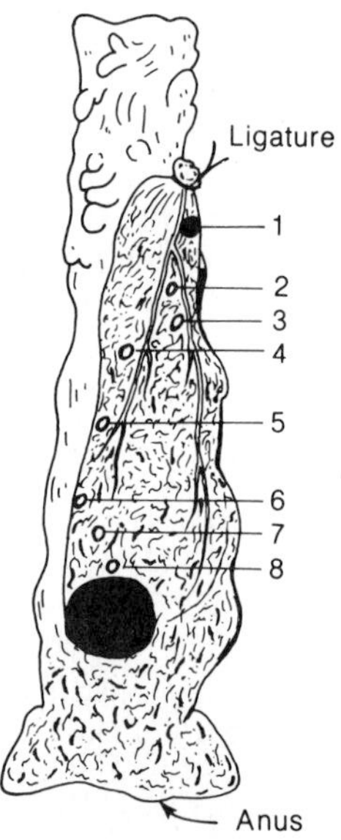

FIG. 21-4. Aberrant lymphatic metastases. Metastases from this primary rectal cancer skipped over seven nodes and implanted in one just below the highest ligature. (From Gabriel WB, Dukes C, Bussey HJR: Lymphatic spread in cancer of the rectum. Br J Surg 23:409, 1935)

Lymphatic Extension

It is important to determine the pathways of spread of lymphatic metastases, for this will influence the surgeon's plan in removal of the primary tumors and potentially involved lymphatics. Gabriel, Dukes, and Bussey reported findings in 62 specimens in which lymphatic metastases were found.[60] One-half of these patients had three or less glands affected and one-half had four or more glands affected. Dukes reasoned that glandular dissemination must proceed slowly from gland to gland. If lymphatic spread had been rapid, one should find cases falling mostly into groups with no glands or with several glands involved. As mentioned earlier (Dukes' second hypothesis) the course of lymphatic dissemination was thought to be a stepwise process along the lymphatic arcade draining the primary tumor. The first glands to receive metastases were those situated in the perirectal tissues on the same level or immediately above the primary growth. The next to be affected were the chain of glands accompanying the superior hemorrhoidal vessels. As a rule, these were invaded in sequence from below upwards. In an advanced case, the metastases formed an unbroken chain from the regional lymph nodes to the glands situated at the point of ligature of the inferior mesenteric vessels. Gilchrist and David also found through their careful study of 200 specimens evidence for an orderly progression of tumor through the lymphatic network.[74]

However, exceptions to this orderly progression of lymphatic metastases do occur. An exception to Dukes second hypothesis is illustrated in Fig. 21-4. This occurs with aberrent lymphatic channels which may be traced from the rectum directly to the inferior mesenteric artery. These direct lymphatic routes were described in 1925 by Villemin, Huard and Montague.[7] Skip metastases occurred in six of 51 specimens with lymph node metastases studied by Wood and Wilkey, one of 62 specimens reported by Gabriel, Dukes, and Bussey and four of 118 specimens reported by Grinnell.[27,60,75] Stearns and Deddish found evidence for skip metastases in three of 122 patients undergoing abdomino–pelvic lymph node dissection plus left colectomy for rectal cancer.[76]

A second exception to Dukes' second hypothesis is seen with atypical retrograde lymphatic metastases that occur when there is blockage of lymphatics by tumor (Fig. 21-5). When this occurs, the inter-connection of lymphatic channels allows lymph nodes at a considerable distance from the relevant arcade to become involved by tumor. In a review of clinical data of 913 cleared specimens, 34 patients (3.7%) were shown by Grinnell to have this type of atypical spread.[9] This lymphatic obstruction accounts for the retrograde extension of tumor below the primary lesion in carcinoma of the rectum.

It is important to remember that there is a dual lymphatic drainage to the lower rectum. The major drainage system is up along the superior hemorrhoidal vessels, but drainage laterally along the middle hemorrhoidal vessels may occur. The problem of lateral lymphatic spread is discussesd in the section on principles of surgery.

Duke's third hypothesis concerning the spread of rectal cancer concerns the relationship of histologic grade of tumor to the pace of tumor growth. Dukes suggested that the

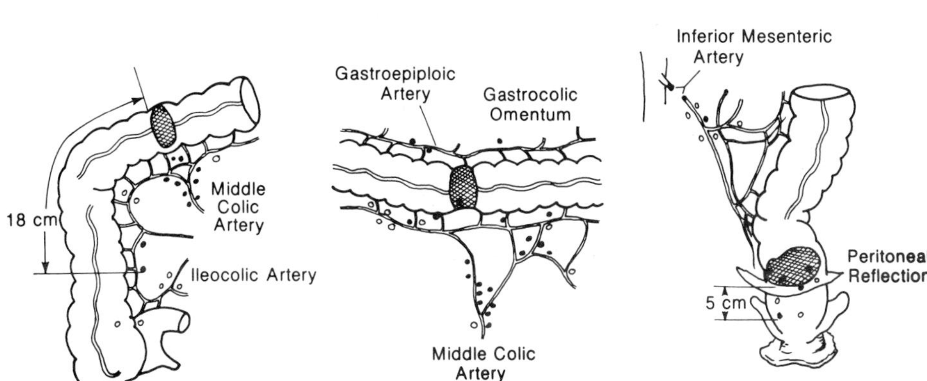

FIG. 21-5. Retrograde lymphatic metastases. Lymph nodes other than in the relevant lymphatic area may become involved with metastatic cancer if proximal lymph flow is blocked by tumor (From Grinnell RS: Lymphatic block with atypical and retrograde lymphatic metastasis and spread in carcinoma of the colon and rectum. Ann Surg 163:274, 276, 1966)

histologic grade could be used to estimate the rate of growth the tumor had undergone to reach a particular size.[29] Dukes divided 985 rectal cancers into four grades of tumor depending on their degree of atypia. Grade I tumors were extremely well differentiated while Grade IV tumors were anaplastic (see section on prognosis). Dukes found a close connection between the histologic grade and the extent of local spread, the incidence of lymphatic metastases, and the incidence of venous spread. This correlation of higher grade of malignancy with an increased incidence of lymphatic and hematogenous metastases has been reported by several other workers.[72,77–79]

Hematogenous Metastases

Approximately one-third of patients at the time of initial presentation of a large bowel cancer have clinical evidence of hematogenous metastases. The most common site of visceral disease is the liver, but lung metastases are also seen prior to or at the time of diagnosis of the primary tumor. Brown and Warren carefully tabulated the sites of visceral metastases from rectal cancer in a retrospective study of 70 autopsies.[78] They found metastasis to the liver alone 23 times and to the lung alone 6 times. In all patients with lung metastases alone, the local lesion was in the *lower* 9 cm of the rectum.

Tumor deposits in other locations in the absence of liver or lung metastasis were extremely rare. Apparently, the progression of visceral metastases is in an orderly fashion with this tumor—similar to the orderly progression of lymphatic metastases along lymph node networks. Distant metastases in the absence of tumor deposits in the liver or lung occurred in only three of 70 patients with hematogenous metastases. One of these patients had a cerebral lesion and the other two patients had nodules in the lumbar and thoracic vertebrae. The origin of vertebral metastasis will be discussed further below.

These important observations document the dual pathways of hematogenous spread for rectal cancer; upwards along the superior hemorrhoidal veins to the liver or laterally along the middle hemorrhoidal system to the lungs. This has clinical significance in patients who develop pulmonary metastases following resection of rectal carcinoma. There may be a chance for cure by resection of pulmonary metastasis from *rectal* cancer if the liver is clinically free of disease. However, pulmonary metastases from a colon primary, with few exceptions, originate from liver metastases. The liver seems to be an effective filter for most tumor emboli; 73% of Dionne's 506 patients with hematogenous spread had metastases to the liver only.[71]

Dionne in a study of 506 patients with "blood-borne" metastases could not substantiate Brown and Warren's finding that pulmonary metastases with upper rectal or colon cancer indicated the presence of hepatic metastases.[71] Dionne claimed that of 44 patients with only lung metastases, the primary lesion had its origin in the *upper* rectum in 13 instances. However, the presence of metastases in Dionne's study was determined by "routine clinical examination during follow-up" in 246 of the 506 patients studied. Many instances of subclinical hepatic metastases may have gone undetected. The data of Brown and Warren from autopsied cases must be considered more accurate.

Both Brown and Warren and Dionne found that the further advanced the primary tumor, the greater the incidence of hematogenous metastases.[71,78] Brown and Warren separated all their cases into three groups; those with primary tumors limited by the muscularis propria, those penetrating through the muscularis propria and those penetrating into adjacent organs. Incidence of visceral metastasis in each group was 24%, 46%, and 48%, respectively. Dionne's observations were similar, with 12% hematogenous metastases found with tumors showing "no local spread," 27% found with tumors of "moderate extension," and 43% with tumors of "extensive local spread." Dionne also found that the incidence of blood-borne metastases increased concomitantly with lymphatic metastases. In patients with lymph node positive primary tumors, the incidence of vascular metastases was three times higher than in the group of cases without lymphatic spread. As noted by Gordon-Watson the high survival rate of patients without lymphatic spread is strong evidence that venous metastases do not often precede lymphatic invasion.[80] A correlation of high grade of tumor with an increased incidence of vascular spread was reported. Brown and Warren report that Grade I tumors were associated with hematogenous spread in 23% of patients, Grade II in 49%, and Grades III and IV in 56%. Dionne similarly found that tumors the histopathology of which was designated as low grade had a 22% incidence of metastasis, as compared to 29% with average grade tumors, and 40% with high grade tumors. Dionne observed a relationship between gross pathology of the primary tumor and the incidence of hematogenous metastases. In fungating tumors, the incidence of hematogenous spread was 23%. Ulcerating tumors had a 31% incidence while stenosing lesions resulted in hematogenous spread in 45% of patients. This correlation likely reflects the same relationship of depth of penetration of the bowel wall by tumor and incidence of either lymphatic or hematogenous metastases. Fungating tumors often do not penetrate the bowel wall but grow almost entirely into the lumen. Ulcerating tumors extend into the bowel wall and, with progressive growth, constrict the lumen and cause a stenosing lesion.

Careful histopathologic study of the primary tumor almost invariably shows evidence of invasion of capillaries or veins by tumor if visceral metastases occur. Brown and Warren found that the absence of intravascular tumor invasion "nearly always rules out visceral metastases." Dionne found a 47% incidence of hematogenous metastases when the pathologist found evidence of venous invasion and 27% when veins were free. Grinnell reports that 27 of 30 patients with visceral metastases showed venous invasion; only three patients (10%) failed to show it.[81]

The pathways of hematogenous spread to the spine and pelvis deserves special comment. Dionne found 6% of patients with spread to pelvis and lumbosacral spine while Brown and Warren report 14% with vertebral involvement.[71,78] Of course, in some of these patients, spread from rectal cancer may be by direct extension to the pelvis or spine along nerve roots as described by Seefeld and Bargen or as tumor emboli from established deposits of tumor in the liver or lung (metastases from metastases).[73] Interestingly, Brown and Warren describe isolated metastases in lumbar and thoracic vertebrae in one patient and lumbar vertebrae in another. These metastases almost undoubtedly result from tumor embolization from the portal venous system to paravertebral veins. These portal–vertebral communications described by Batson likely result in the early spinal metastasis occasionally seen with colon or rectal cancer.[82]

Implantation

There seems to be little doubt that cancer can be spread from the primary site to distant tissues through exfoliation of tumor (either single tumor cells or clumps of tumor cells) and subsequent implantation and growth of these tumor cells. Ackerman and Wheat discussed this phenomenon and pointed out the numerous ways that surgical manipulations could be responsible for the phenomen.[83] Implants may grow from tumor cells that are within the bowel lumen, from tumor cells within lymphatic channels, or from the serosal surface if a tumor has penetrated the bowel wall.[84] Reports of spread of tumor cells by implantation of malignant cells from within the bowel lumen are listed in Table 21-4.[85-94] Hemorrhoidectomy performed with an unrecognized tumor above accounts for numerous instances of intraluminal spread.

An important example of tumor cell implantation is that which may occur at an anastomotic site following colon or rectal resection for cancer. Gordon-Watson was aware of the danger of suture line recurrence and reported a case.[80] He cautions that "handling and pressure on the growth from without, before division of the bowel, may explain early recurrence at the anastomotic line." Borema showed that free carcinoma cells do persist in the lumen of the large bowel.[95] He washed out the specimen lumen and distal loop of large bowel in patients undergoing resection and demonstrated tumor cells in the mucous and bowel contents in most cases of ulcerative carcinoma. McGrew and co-workers searched

TABLE 21-4. Spread of Colorectal Cancer by Implantation of Cells from Within the Bowel Lumen

AUTHOR (Reference Number)	DATE	IMPLANTATION SITE	PRIMARY TUMOR SITE	NUMBER OF PATIENTS
Laurie (85)	1906	Abdominal incision	Sigmoid	1
Rial (86)	1907	Abdominal incision	–	1
Mayo (87)	1913	Colostomy site	Rectum	1
Goligher, Dukes, and Bussey (88)	1951	Abdominal incision	Rectum	1
Cole (89)	1952	Perineal incision	Rectum	1
		Colostomy site	Rectum	3
Quer, Dahlen, and Mayo (90)	1953	Hemorrhoidectomy scar	Sigmoid	1
Guiss (91)	1954	Fistula in ano	Sigmoid	1
Beahrs, Phillips, and Dockerty (92)	1955	Hemorrhoidectomy scar	Rectum & Sigmoid	4
LeQuesne and Thompson (93)	1958	Hemorrhoidectomy scar	–	1
		Perineal incision	–	1
Boreham (94)	1958	Abdominal incision	–	6
		Colostomy site	–	2

for free malignant cells in the lumen of 50 specimens of carcinoma of the colon at varying distances from the tumor.[96] They found that the percentage of positive smears for tumor cells varied inversely with the distance from the tumor. Positive smears were found in 42% of proximal ends and 65% of distal ends of resected large intestines; this was at an average distance of 21 cm and 10 cm respectively from the primary tumor. The unavoidable conclusion is that viable tumor cells do exist within the lumen of the colon and their implantation must be surgically avoided. The reported incidence of suture line recurrence before and after the institution of precautionary techniques to rid the bowel lumen of viable cells is shown in Table 21-5.[88,97–109]

Beal and Cornell make the interesting point that anastomotic recurrence is much more common in left colon cancer than in right colon cancer.[101] They found 19 of 91 patients (21%) having anastomotic recurrences with left colon cancer where only two of 49 (4%) had an anastomotic recurrence with right colon cancer. Factors operating to produce this discrepancy may include more operative manipulation of left-sided tumors, a closer proximity of the suture line to the carcinoma in rectosigmoid tumors and better bowel preparation and reduction of colon flora with left-sided lesions than with right-sided lesions. Wright, Thomas, and Cleveland similarly noted two of 272 (0.7%) patients with ileocolic suture line recurrences as opposed to 69 of 566 (12%) with colocolic suture lines.[105]

The data shown in the lower portion of Table 21-5 suggests that precautionary techniques may reduce suture line recurrences. Keynes looked at the incidence of local recurrence after anterior resection following the institution of mercury bichloride 1:500 treatment.[103] In the 12 years following the institution of this therapy, the suture line recurrence rate fell from 13% to 2.6%; 229 patients were followed for more than two years. Southwick, Harridge, and Cole used buffered sodium hypochlorite (Dakin's solution, 0.25%) to irrigate the proximal and distal bowel lumen.[109] They followed 101 patients operated on between 1954 and 1960 with all patients undergoing at least 1 year of follow-up after surgery. In the entire group in which recurrent disease had developed (26 patients with recurrent disease) they were unable to find a single instance of recurrence at the suture line.

It is not likely that tumor implantation only occurs within the bowel lumen on abraided mucosal surfaces and within abdominal or perineal incisions. Implantation within the abdominal cavity also occurs. Cole, in 1959, reported a patient with intraperitoneal seeding of tumor in the suture line of the floor of the pelvis; in almost every point where the suture penetrated the peritoneum an implant of tumor was present.[110] Other evidence for the intraperitoneal implantation of colorectal cancer tumor cells comes from the study of ovarian metastases found at the time of colon or rectal resection. Burt calls attention to the fact that 30% of ovarian tumors are actually metastatic.[111] In 493 cancers of the colon and rectum in women, 17 cancers of the ovaries secondary to colorectal cancer were observed (incidence 3.4%). Nine of these 17 cancers were in the sigmoid colon, but others were at a considerable distance from the ovary in the hepatic flexure, ascending colon, and descending colon. In 13 instances the tumor in the ovary was completely separate from the primary bowel cancer. Twelve patients had Dukes' C tumors. Stearns and Deddish report six patients with ovarian or fallopian tube metastases in a series of 122 (incidence 5%) patients undergoing abdomino–perineal resection.[76] All but one of these patients with ovarian metastases had extensive lymph node metastases. It seems impossible to incriminate a lymphatic route of metastases in all cases. Direct implantation within the peritoneal cavity seems to be the most reasonable explanation. Knoepp, Ray, and Overly report ten ovarian metastases from colorectal primary tumors; they emphasize that ovarian metastases may be considerably larger than the primary tumor and that they indicate a poor prognosis.[112]

TABLE 21-5. Anastomotic Recurrences Prior to and After the Institution of Precautionary Techniques

AUTHOR (Reference Number)	DATE	INCIDENCE	PERCENT
RECURRENCES PRIOR TO PRECAUTIONARY TECHNIQUES			
Lloyd-Davis (97)	1948	16/65	25
Wagensteen and Toon (98)	1948	7/63	14
Garlock and Ginsberg (99)	1950	18/151	12
Golligher, Dukes, and Bussey (88)	1951	15/162	9
Cole (89)	1952	9/55	16
Southwick and Cole (100)	1955	11/114	10
Beal and Cornell (101)	1956	21/140	15
Wheelock et al (102)	1959	10/90	11
Keynes (103)	1961	3/23	13
Floyd et al (104)	1965	18/50	36
Wright et al (105)	1969	71/838	8
Slanetz et al (106)	1972	22/234	9
Mason et al (107)	1976	16/152	11
RECURRENCES AFTER PRECAUTIONARY TECHNIQUES			
Morgan (108)	1959	2/148	1
Keynes (103)	1961	6/229	3
Southwick et al (109)	1962	0/101	0

PATTERNS OF RECURRENCE

Evidence for Implantation or Persistence of Tumor Cells at the Resection Site as a Cause of Treatment Failure

This section is an attempt to generate data supporting a hypothesis concerning the spread of colorectal cancer following surgical resection. The hypothesis is as follows: at the time of colorectal cancer resection, tumor cells are present on the serosal surface, in the interstitial spaces, or lymphatic channels immediately adjacent to the tumor. Prior to or at the time of surgical resection, these tumor cells can be dislodged by trauma; the more advanced the primary tumor, the more likely is this local dissemination to occur. When a large raw surface is created by surgical resection, free tumor cells may implant and, over the course of months and years, produce local recurrence.

Presumptive evidence to support this mechanism of spread comes from the study of recurrence patterns for carcinoma of the rectum and colon. Several authors have shown that for both rectal and colon cancer, the most common site for recurrence is at the resection site. The most direct evidence for this comes from the experience with "second-look surgery" performed by Wangensteen and co-workers in Minneapolis.[113] Six months to 12 months after the initial curative surgery, the first reoperation or second look was performed; the operation consisted of a careful search of the abdomen and pelvis with systematic examination of both the previous operative area and likely sites of spread. Tumor, when localized, was excised if at all possible and biopsies were taken from any suspicious areas. When tumor was not found, repeat explorations were performed at 6 month to 12 month intervals (third and fourth look, and so forth) until no disease was found or the tumor has obviously spread beyond surgical control. Other patients underwent "symptomatic second look;" this group was reoperated when symptoms suggested locally recurrent cancer. Gunderson and Sosin analyzed the data from the University of Minnesota reoperative series.[114] Seventy-four patients with complete bowel wall penetration, with or without involved lymph nodes at the time of initial curative surgery, had single or multiple reoperations. Tumor due to recurrent or metastatic carcinoma was found in 52 of 74.

TABLE 21-6. Summary of Sites of Recurrence Found at Second Look Surgery for Rectal Cancer in 52 Patients with Recurrent Disease*

PATTERN OF RECURRENCE	ONLY RECURRENCE	COMBINED RECURRENCE
Local–Regional†	25/52 (48%)	48/52 (92%)
Disseminated (hematogenous)	4/52 (8%)	26/52 (50%)
Peritoneal seeding	0 –	3/52 (6%)

* Fifty-two of 74 patients after initial curative operation had evidence of recurrent disease at second-look surgery.

† Included as local–regional recurrences were patients with para-aortic lymph node metastases.

(Modified from Gunderson LL, Sosin H: Areas of failure found at reoperation (second or symptomatic look) following "curative surgery" for adenocarcinoma of the rectum. Cancer 34:1278–1292, 1974)

Distant metastasis alone was uncommon (8%), but occurred as some component of failure in 50% of the group with failure. Peritoneal seeding was rare. Local failure and regional lymph node metastases including aortic nodes occurred in 48% of patients as the only failure or in combination with distant metastases in 92% (see Table 21-6).

Lofgren, Waugh, and Dockerty itemized their experience with local recurrence of rectal and rectosigmoid cancer after anterior resection.[115] They divided their patients, all of whom had locally recurrent disease, into two groups. One group of 47 patients had no lymph nodes positive for tumor and the other group of 51 patients had tumor in lymph nodes at the time of pathological examination of the resected specimen. In their group with no lymph node involvement, 41 of 47 recurrences were within the operative field and adjacent or involved with the suture line. In the 51 patients who had positive lymph nodes and locally recurrent disease, 45 patients had recurrent disease confined to the resection site. This seemed remarkable to Lofgren and co-workers. They reasoned that if residual tumor left in lymph nodes were growing out and causing local recurrence after anterior resection, the incidence of recurrence at the site of anastomosis should be less in the group with lymphatic metastases than the group without. The lymphatic drainage and nodes at risk extend over a considerably wider area than that around the suture line; therefore, lesions caused by metastases to lymph nodes would be situated at a distance from the suture line. Lofgren and co-workers suggest that malignant tissue broken into, left behind, and disseminated at the time of the removal of the primary lesion was the cause of a majority of the local recurrences that they studied.

Gilbertsen studied the incidence and locations of recurrent tumor following curative operations for adenocarcinoma of the rectum.[116] Eighty-nine of these patients had abdomino–perineal resection, and 36 patients had other types of excisions, including low anterior resection, posterior excision, or pull-through procedure. Ninety-three patient had recurrences and 47 (51%) were identified as having local recurrence. Gilbertsen makes several pertinent observations: In women the area of local recurrence was most often in the vagina and cul-de-sac area. This was, he thought, related to the continuity of the lymphatics of these organs with the lymphatics of the rectum. In men, the prostate gland, base of the bladder and distal ureter area was the site for recurrence. It was the anterior/posterior dimension of the surgical resection which seemed to be at greatest risk for local recurrence.

In 1959, Stearns and Deddish reported on the results of abdomino–pelvic lymph node dissection plus left colectomy for rectal cancer.[76] Of the patients who died of residual or metastatic carcinoma, the charts of 37 contained sufficient data for a reasonably accurate appraisal of the condition within the pelvis. Twenty-three of these 37 (60%) had residual carcinoma in the pelvis.

Taylor did an autopsy study on 125 patients who died of cancer of the colon and rectum to determine what the lesion was that actually killed the patient.[117] Seventy-two percent died of intra-abdominal causes of death, either intestinal obstruction, or intercurrent infection. Only 3% of patients died of lung metastases and 25% of liver metastases. It should be noted that autopsies reveal only the end patterns of failure and the site of earliest recurrence may be missed. However, if tumor is at the site of cancer resection, it most likely has been there since the time of operation for it would be unusual for the tumor to metastasize hematogenously back to, or, by local extension, regrow at the resection site. Floyd, Corley, and Cohn did a study of 50 patients that were either reexplored or underwent autopsy examination for recurrence of carcinoma of the colon or rectum.[118] They found local recurrence of carcinoma in 18 of the 50 patients (36%). Thirty-three of the 50 patients had lesions which were classified as Dukes A or B with no lymph node spread. When they sought to determine cause of death, in 24 of the 41 patients who underwent autopsy examination, local recurrence was either the primary cause of death or a highly contributory factor to the patient's death. Distant metastases were responsible for only nine of 41 deaths. Salanetz, Herter and Grinnell in reviewing 524 patients with cancer of the rectum and rectosigmoid reported that two of every three patients dying of cancer had persistent tumor in the pelvis.[106] They comment that it must be assumed that in those patients with local recurrence occult cancer present in the perirectal fat or lymphatics at the time of initial resection failed to be included in the operative specimen. Ree and co-workers studied 72 patients who underwent abdomino–perineal resection.[119] They found 19 local recurrences: 5 were in the vagina, 3 in the pelvis, 2 were perineal, and 2 were in the abdominal wall. These authors suggest that if local control could be improved, even if overall survival could not be prolonged, this would markedly improve care. Prevention of local recurrence would improve the quality if not the length of life.

Cass, Million, and Pfaff retrospectively evaluated 165 patients who developed recurrent cancer.[120] Sixty-three of the 105 (60%) had local recurrence alone, 15 of 105 (14%) had distant metastases alone. Ninety-two percent of the local recurrences developed in structures contiguous with the operative site. Through 5 years, local recurrence without clinical evidence of distant metastases was the most common cause of death. They found that the cecum and rectosigmoid had higher local recurrence rates than did the transverse or descending sigmoid colon, perhaps owing to the greater number of contiguous structures and lesser length of mesentery in the areas of colon fixed to the retroperitoneum. Ten of 11 cecal recurrences were local only, and 42 of 45 rectal and rectosigmoid recurrences were local only. The transverse colon which has a long mesentery associated with it had only 26% local recurrence rate.

Increased Local Recurrence with Increased Penetration of Primary Tumor Through the Bowel Wall

Cass, Million, and Pfaff also found that the degree of tumor anaplasia and depth of penetration through the bowel wall influenced the rate of local recurrence.[120] Other groups have reported that the incidence of local recurrence increases as the depth of penetration of the bowel wall by primary tumor increases. The University of Chicago rectal cancer series noted subsequent evidence of pelvic recurrence in 56.7% of patients with the operative finding of extension through the entire rectal wall *versus* 11.4% if bowel wall penetration were not present.[121]

Rich and co-workers correlated the rate of pelvic recurrence and survival in 130 rectal and rectosigmoid cancer patients with depth of penetration of the bowel wall.[122] These data reflect minimum 5-year followup. Although the number of patients in some subcategories is small, the data support the concept that with each degree of extension through the entire wall, operative margins are increasingly compromised and the incidence of pelvic recurrence rises accordingly (Table 21-7). In the subgroups with nodes negative, the incidence of local treatment failures nearly doubled with each degree of extra rectal involvement.

At this closing point in our discussion of the natural history of surgically treated colorectal cancer, we again ask; why do so many of these patients whose tumors seem completely and adequately excised eventually develop recurrence? Several possibilities may be advanced: first, distant metastases in the lymphatic system may result in unrecognized residual tumor left after surgery. This is not likely to often be the case, for lymphatic metastases almost invariably follow a gradual pro-

TABLE 21-7. Tumor Extension Through Bowel Wall Correlated with Pelvic Recurrence and Survival of 130 Rectal and Rectosigmoid Patients After Curative Resection

INITIAL EXTENSION	TOTAL FAILURE	PELVIC RECURRENCE	ABSOLUTE SURVIVAL*	DETERMINANT SURVIVAL*
LYMPH NODE NEGATIVE				
A Mucosa only	0/3	0/3	2/3	2/2
B1 Within wall	7/33 (21%)	3/33 (9%)	29/33 (88%)	29/32 (91%)
B2 (m) microscopically through wall	3/13 (23%)	2/13 (15%)	9/13 (69%)	9/12 (75%)
B2 (m+g) grossly through wall	15/31 (48%)	9/31 (29%)	11/31 (36%)	11/26 (42%)
B3 involves adjacent structure(s)	6/10 (60%)	5/10 (50%)	4/10 (40%)	4/10 (40%)
LYMPH NODE POSITIVE				
C1 Within wall	1/4	1/4	2/4	2/3
C2 (m) microscopically through wall	2/5	1/5	3/5	3/5
C2 (m+g) grossly through wall	18/27 (67%)	12/27 (44%)	6/27 (22%)	6/25 (24%)
C3 involves adjacent structure(s)	4/4	4/4	0/4	0/4

* Minimal 5 year follow up

(Rich T, Gunderson LL, Goldabin J et al: Clinical and pathologic factors influencing local failure after curative resection of carcinoma of the rectum and rectosigmoid. Int J Radiat Oncol Biol Phys 4(2):135, 1978)

gression. If lymph nodes at the margin of resection are negative, skip metastases would be expected in only a few percent of patients. The studies of Lofgren, Waugh, and Dockerty also argue against this suggestion (see above).

A second possibility may be that patients are dying of hematogenously disseminated tumor cells exfoliated from the primary tumor into veins prior to or at the time of surgical resection. One would expect the site of first recurrence, then, to be at sites distant from the primary tumor in liver, lung and bone. This explanation is not likely, for studies innumerated here strongly suggest that distant disease alone is an uncommon recurrence pattern.

A third possibility is that tumor cells persisting at the resection site may be the major source of first recurrence for colorectal cancer. The local resection site may, therefore, be a major focus for adjuvant therapies in an attempt to improve survival in patients undergoing potentially curable surgery.

PATHOLOGY

In the section on the natural history of colorectal cancer, data were presented which related the focus for malignant change within the colorectum to adenomatous and villous polyps. It was suggested that cancers may arise within a polyp, gradually destroy the polyp by invasive growth, and then proceed to penetrate into, around, and then through the bowel wall. The greater the depth of penetration, the more likely were lymphatic and hematogenous spread to occur. Our task now is to describe the gross and histologic appearance of these events. We start with studies that trace the development of polyps from an irregular growth pattern within the colonic mucosa. Then, a description of the various types of polypoid lesions and their malignant potential is presented. The muscularis mucosa is identified as an important morphologic structure that can be used to separate *in situ* malignancy from invasive malignancy. Finally, the various gross and histologic types of colorectal malignancy are presented and discussed.

POLYPS AND THEIR MALIGNANT POTENTIAL

Four different types of polyps constitute the majority of polypoid lesions seen within the colorectum. They have a widely varied spectrum for malignant change. The hyperplastic polyp probably never undergoes malignant degeneration, while adenomas not infrequently do. By histologic study, adenomas may be classified as of adenomatous, villous or intermediate type (Table 21-8).

Hyperplastic Polyps

The hyperplastic polyp or areas of mucosal hyperplasia often originate in mucosa that is exposed to chronic irritation; the stoma of a colostomy is a common site. Occasionally, areas of hyperplasia may take on an adenomatous histologic appearance and are then referred to as areas of adenomatous hyperplasia. However, Lane, Kaplan, and Pascal in studying 2136 hyperplastic and adenomatous polyps found no transition from hyperplastic to adenomatous mucosa.[123] Their conclusion was that only adenomatous polyps are of significance in colon carcinogenesis and that there exists a fundamental biologic difference between adenomatous and hyperplastic polyps.

By gross appearance, areas of mucosal hyperplasia are slightly raised up from surrounding mucosa or are obviously polypoid. The lesions are very similar in color and surface texture to normal mucosa, so that their detection by gross inspection may be difficult. Microscopically, it appears that there are excessive numbers of cells in the crypts resulting in papillary infoldings of the epithelium. This gives a typical serrated or corkscrew appearance of the glands. Both at the epithelial surface and within the glands the cells appear enlarged, increased in numbers, and more closely packed than usual. Cells lining hyperplastic glands usually show no multilayering and very often cells appear overstuffed with mucus. The basement membrane upon which the epithelial cells rest is often more prominent. Hyperchromatic cells or cells undergoing mitosis are seen only at the base of the crypts of Lieberkuhn.

Adenomas

As adenomatous polyps grow they may remain sessile, usually become pedunculated or present intermediate variations. Often a polyp that appears sessile will upon closer inspection be pedunculated. A midsagittal section of a supposed sessile lesion often reveals a short central stalk with tumor overhanging the margins. The color of an adenomatous polyp is much redder (raspberry-like) than the surrounding normal mucosa. Its texture is more velvety or granular; occasionally, shaggy gray areas that may spontaneously bleed represent areas of ulceration or early carcinoma.

TABLE 21-8. Adenomas—Colorectal Polyps with Malignant Potential

TYPE (alternate names)	HISTOLOGY	INCIDENCE	INVASIVE MALIGNANCY	PEAK AGE INCIDENCE
Adenomatous polyp (tubular adenoma, adenoma)	Branching tubules embedded in lamina propria	75%	5%	58 ± 1.6 years
Villous polyp (villous adenoma, villous papilloma)	Finger-like projections of epithelium over delicate lamina propria	10%	40%	65.2 ± 3.3 years
Intermediate type polyp (tubulo–villous adenoma, villo–glandular adenoma, papillary adenoma)	Mixture of adenomatous and villous patterns	15%	22%	58 ± 1.6 years

By light microscopic examination, adenomatous polyps markedly resemble the rapidly proliferating tissue in the lower one-third of a crypt of Lieberkuhn. Glandular spaces are lined by columnar epithelial cells. Neither mucus distention nor appreciable multilayering of the cells is present. Nuclei are basally situated; some may be hyperchromatic. Numerous mitotic figures may be noted especially if multilayering of glandular lining is prominent.

The stalk of a pedunculated adenomatous polyp is made up of a central fibrous stalk which radiates out to support the glandular tissue in the head of the polyp. Blood vessels often of respectable caliber, along with strands of smooth muscle from the muscularis mucosa, are within the stalk. The stalk itself is covered by normal-appearing mucosa. Adenomatous polyps (often from older patients or large lesions) frequently contain a papillary (villous) component and are then classified as intermediate type polyps. This is especially true if multiple sections are taken throughout the lesion.[49]

Villous polyps may become pedunculated but more often remain sessile. Their color is purplish compared to surrounding mucosa and their texture is extremely soft. Their papillary stalk usually lacks the fibromuscular stroma that adenomatous polyps possess. Foci of atypia are frequent; such foci or areas of carcinoma-*in-situ* are frequently present in polyps where invasive carcinoma has also developed and signal the need for a careful histologic search for invasive disease.[48] Welin and co-workers showed that the rate of growth of villous polyps is usually many times that of adenomatous polyps and is essentially the same as for adenocarcinoma.[58]

Morphologically, villous polyps usually have multiple finger-like projections of lamina propria that may arise from an extensive surface area of mucosa. Each stalk is likely to support a papillary arborization. The epithelial covered papillary projections may reach down to abut the muscularis mucosa. This penetration of the mucosal layer of the bowel may account for the frequent recurrence of villous polyps following fulguration for removal. Eosinophils, plasma cells, and mononuclear cells usually infiltrate the center of papillary projections, but a rich vascular stroma as in the stalk of an adenomatous polyp is not present. Mitoses are frequent but are not significant in the absence of signs of atypia or malignant change.

GROWTH PATTERNS OF NORMAL AND ABNORMAL COLONIC MUCOSA

Studies on the replication and migration of colonic epithelial and mesenchymal tissues have shown fundamental differences between benign epithelium and the adenoma. By electron microscopic and autoradiographic studies, Kay, Pascal, and Lane established that in normal colonic mucosa cell division is very active, but is restricted to the deep one-half or one-third of the crypts of Lieberkuhn.[124] Cells produced by replication within the crypts migrate toward the colonic lumen and differentiate into two principal cell types—the goblet cells and the absorptive cells. Mitotic figures are present in the lower one-third of the crypts as is the uptake of tritiated thymidine; also, in normal mucosa the mitotic activity ceases as cells move from within the crypts to surface mucosa (Figure 21-6). Fibroblasts which make up the pericryptal fibroblast sheath also migrate from within the crypts towards the colonic lumen and in so doing undergo maturation and differentiation.[125] In an area of normal colonic mucosa this dynamic process of cell division within the crypts of Lieberkuhn and migration to the mucosal surface is perfectly balanced. Cells regularly exfoliate from the free surface into the lumen as fast as they are produced.

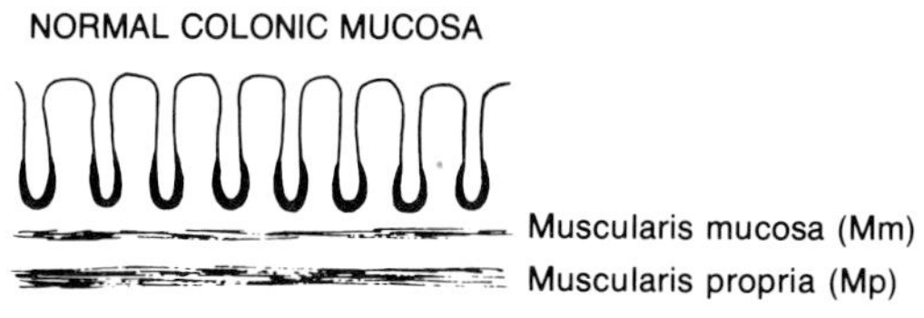

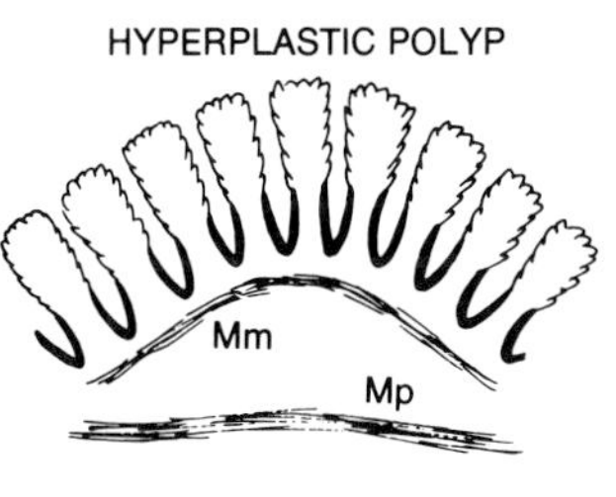

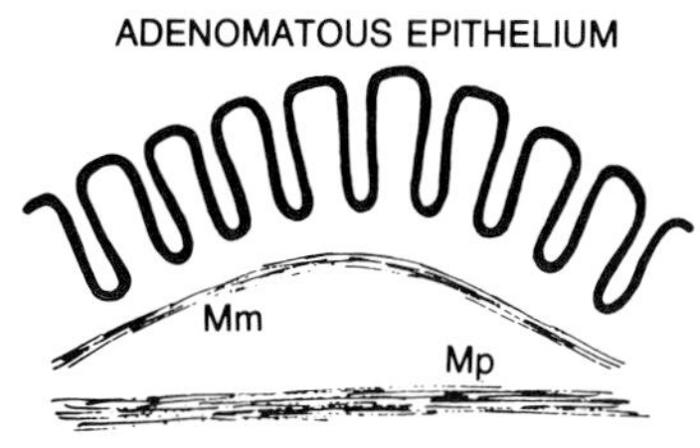

FIG. 21-6. Epithelial replication in *normal, hyperplastic,* and *adenomatous* epithelium. The area of cell replication is indicated by *heavy shading*. In contrast to normal mucosa and hyperplastic polyps, cell replication occurs in all regions of adenomatous epithelium. The loss of control of replication demonstrates the neoplastic nature of adenomas. (Modified from Lane N. Fenoglio CM, Kaye GI: et al: Defining the precursor tissue of ordinary large bowel cancer: Implications for cancer prevention. In Lipkin M, Good R (eds): Gastrointestinal Tract Cancer, pp. 298, 300, 304. New York, Plenum Press, 1978)

In a hyperplastic polyp there is an excessive proliferation of epithelial cells within the crypts of Lieberkuhn. However, as cells migrate out the neck of the crypt toward the mucosal surface, differentiation into goblet and absorptive cells is completed as normal. Mitotic activity at the mucosal surface is not present. Because cell differentiation is complete and restriction of cell division is similar to normal, hyperplastic polyps are considered non-neoplastic tissue.

In either adenomatous, villous, or intermediate polyps, the dynamic process of production and exfoliation of cells is not maintained. Cell division takes place at all levels within the tissue. Also, cells which at the lumenal surface appear as goblet cells or absorptive cells in normal tissue do not appear to be differentiating. Both morphologically and dynamically, cells at the surface of an adenomatous polyp look just like the partially differentiated cells which normally constitute the lower one-third of a crypt of Lieberkuhn.

Abnormalities in fibroblast replication and differentiation similar to that seen in the epithelium have also been described.[125] Normally, the epithelial cells within a crypt are tightly invested by a sheath of fibroblasts: this is referred to as the pericryptal fibroblast sheath. Deep in the crypt there is minimal collagen between the fibroblasts and epithelial cells. However, at the lumenal surface under the free surface of epithelium a prominent and uniform band of collagen is observed. This appears to be supporting the epithelium and is referred to as the collagen table. Fibroblasts at the base of the crypts are actively proliferating in normal mucosa; also, similar to epithelial cell replication patterns, as fibroblasts migrate toward the lumenal surface, replication ceases. In adenomas the fibroblasts beneath surface epithelium remain immature in appearance and continue to show thymidine incorporation. Also, the fibroblasts apparently do not function as differentiated cells by producing collagen, for the collagen table is thinner than normally present. In contrast, the collagen table in hyperplastic polyps is characteristically thicker than in normal epithelium.

In summary, adenomatous tissue is thought to result from a continuation of cell proliferation from within the crypt of Lieberkuhn onto the epithelial surface. Exfolation of tissue cannot keep up with tissue replication so that an accumulation of tissue that protrudes into the bowel lumen results. This failure of tissue to show site specific restriction of replication may be responsible for neoplastic growth.

FREQUENCY OF VARIOUS TYPES OF POLYPS

Hyperplastic polyps occur at least ten times as frequently as do all adenomas combined.[126] Also, small adenomas less than 1.5 cm in diameter and with a low incidence of invasive malignancy are about ten times as common as large adenomas.[34] Thus, the clinically significant lesion represents only about 1% of all large bowel polyps.

According to Muto, Bussey, and Morsen, adenomatous polyps represent about 75% of all adenomas.[48] Intermediate type polyps represent approximately 15%, and pure villous lesions 10% of the total number of adenomas (Table 21-8). As polyps increase in size and as the patient's age increases, so does the incidence of intermediate and villous polyps. The malignancy rate differs markedly for the three types of adenomas. Muto, Bussey, and Morsen found "unequivocal evidence of invasion" by 5% of adenomatous polyps, 22% of intermediate type polyps, and 40% of villous polyps. Therefore, although villous lesions are much less common, they are much more likely to contain invasive malignancy. The peak age incidence for hyperplastic polyps is 8 years before adenomatous polyps. Adenomatous polyps occur on the average 5 years before carcinoma and has led some to suggest that several years are required for an adenomatous polyp to become a symptomatic malignancy. The peak age incidence for villous adenomas is 65.2 years; suprisingly older than the peak incidence for cancer. The distribution of all types of adenoma within the colorectum is quite similar to that for adenocarcinoma.[54-56] About half the lesions are in the sigmoid and rectum and half in the remainder of the colon.

MUSCULARIS MUCOSA AS A HISTOLOGIC ENTITY TO SEPARATE *IN SITU* FROM INVASIVE MALIGNANCY

Lane and Kay established the muscularis mucosa as a discrete morphologic structure by which invasive and *in situ* malignancy can be distinguished.[13] Adenocarcinomatous glands which invade, but do not pass across the muscularis mucosa, can be classified as *in situ* malignancy and present no danger for the development of metastases. From the clinician's point of view, these are malignant-appearing lesions with totally benign behavior (see section on treatment of polyps).

GROSS TYPES OF ADENOCARCINOMA

Dionne reviewed 1592 patients treated at St. Mark's for carcinoma of the rectum; 1376 of these patients had the gross pathology of their primary tumor described.[71] Twenty-five percent were fungating, 61% were ulcerating, 7% were stenosing, and 7% had some other gross configuration. Jackman and Beahrs found 25% of adenocarcinomas a fungating type and 65% "crateriform".[127] In the right colon, polypoid lesions are more common; stenosing lesions are more common within the left colon.

HISTOLOGIC TYPES OF COLORECTAL MALIGNANCY

Malignant epithelial tumors of the large intestine may be divided into five major morphologic types: the adenocarcinomas, mucinous or colloid adenocarcinomas, signet ring adenocarcinoma, scirrhous tumors and carcinoma simplex. The prognosis that accompanies each of these histologic types is discussed in the section on prognosis. Also, adenocarcinomas are identified and classified histologically as to their grade of malignant appearance. As discussed later, this also has prognostic significance.

In many ways, adenocarcinoma of the large bowel resembles colonic epithelium, cut in cross section. Cells are columnar to cuboidal with irregular attempts at multilayering and glandular differentiation. The stroma varies from scant in polypoid lesions to abundant in stenosing lesions. Most tumors have a imperfect acinar architecture.

Mucinous adenocarcinomas possess the same basic structure as adenocarcinoma, but differ in that there is abundant extracellular mucus. Most all adenocarcinomas produce some mucin, so mucinous tumors are those with a great amount of mucin production. Symmonds and Vickery classified tumors as mucinous if over 60% of the surface area of microscopic sections was occupied by mucus.[128]

Signet ring adenocarcinoma is a mucin-producing tumor in which the majority of mucin remains intracellular. This results in the nucleus being pushed to the side of the cell and a signet ring appearance. As documented in the section on prognosis and staging, survival with this tumor is extremely poor.

In 1965, Woolam and associates at the Mayo Clinic studied clinical and pathologic features of scirrhous carcinoma.[129] Morphologically the tumor shows very little glandular formation; there is, however, a marked desmoplasia which surrounds the glandular structures. Grossly, there is a firm, rubbery stricture rather than a prominent ulcer crater or polypoid lesion. The abrupt change from normal mucosa to a malignant process is not obvious. By proctoscopy the lesion often appears as an inflammatory stricture. Woolam and associates claim that most scirrhous tumors are in the rectum and rectosigmoid.

Carcinoma simplex includes tumors with the least amount of differentiation. Aggregates of pleomorphic epithelial cells differ markedly in size and form solid cords and masses. The tumor may be so anaplastic that it is difficult to distinguish from sarcoma. Submucosal lymphatics are freely permeated by tumor and metastases to regional nodes occur early.

STAGING

Perhaps the most confusing aspect of large bowel cancer to both clinician and student alike is the staging of this disease. Historically, numerous classification systems have arisen (Fig. 21-7). The Dukes' system, now often employed, is simple and easy to use, yet may fail to separate patients into prognostic groups accurately enough. In some newer systems, complex classification of a patient becomes laborious and may be confusing. In our discussion of staging, let us first historically review the systems of classification to discover what aspect of the natural history of this disease a particular system emphasizes.

SURGICAL CLASSIFICATION AS CURATIVE OR PALLIATIVE

Perhaps the oldest staging system employed is that which a surgeon offers at the time of resection, based on experience with the disease. Indeed, every cancer surgeon in the formal operative note gives an opinion regarding the likelihood for cure from the procedure performed. Later, in reviewing the pathologic findings with the pathologist, a more accurate statement regarding the likelihood for cure in this individual patient can be made. Surgical experience has shown that if the primary tumor cannot be removed *en bloc,* or if tumor cells are spilled into the peritoneal cavity, a curative resection is unlikely. Such palliative efforts are, however, necessary and often offer excellent short term benefits to the patient.

A precautionary note should be given concerning assessment of a procedure as palliative because of enlarged lymph nodes at the margin of lymphatic resection. Gabriel, Dukes, and Bussey compared the gross characteristics of lymph glands (what the surgeon sees) with subsequent microscopic examination. Of 1242 glands, 905 were considered from gross examination to be negative; later microscopic examination showed 18 to contain metastases—an error of only 2%.[60] However, in 337 glands which were judged positive from their gross examination, metastases were present in only 132, a mistake being made in 205 nodes or 61% of the total. Therefore, a surgeon's conjecture with respect to metastases within enlarged nodes may be more often wrong than right. The local sepsis produced by a tumor that erodes the mucosal surface in the midst of a fecal stream accounts for the enlarged

FIG. 21-7. Staging systems for colorectal cancer.

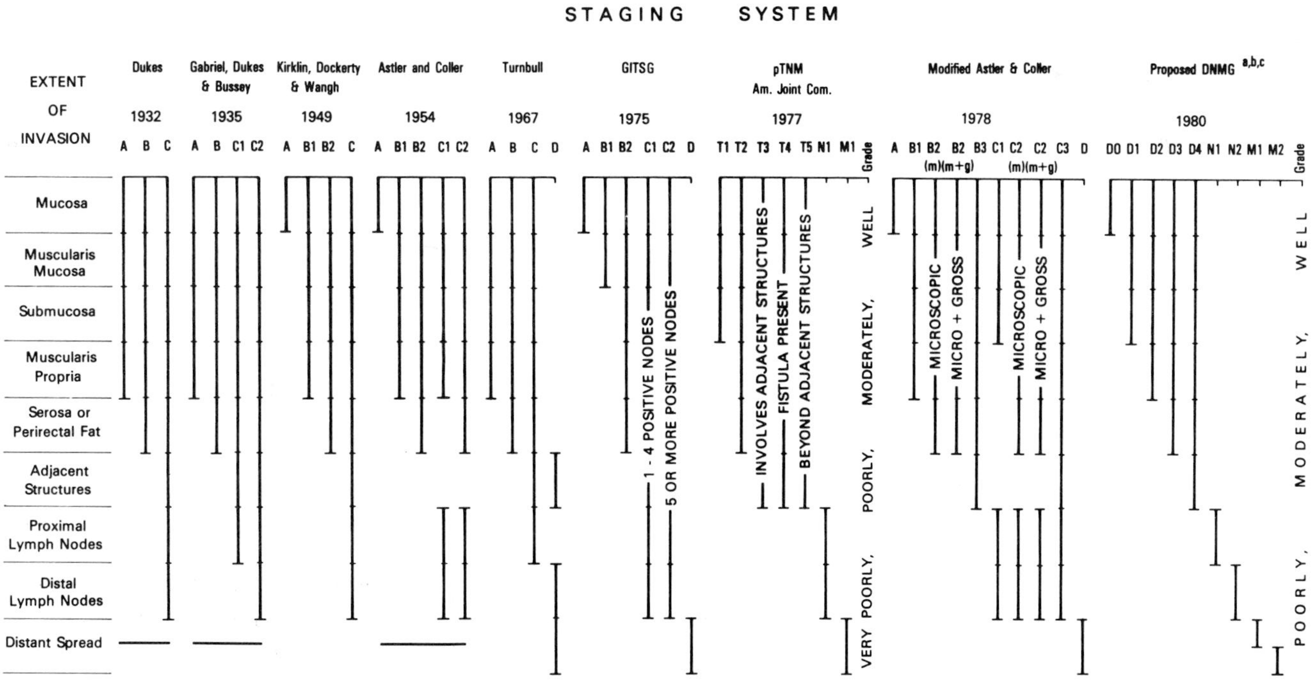
STAGING SYSTEM
EXTENT OF INVASION
Dukes 1932 A B C
Gabriel, Dukes & Bussey 1935 A B C1 C2
Kirklin, Dockerty & Wangh 1949 A B1 B2 C
Astler and Coller 1954 A B1 B2 C1 C2
Turnbull 1967 A B C D
GITSG 1975 A B1 B2 C1 C2 D
pTNM Am. Joint Com. 1977 T1 T2 T3 T4 T5 N1 M1 Grade
Modified Astler & Coller 1978 A B1 B2 B2 B3 C1 C2 C2 C3 D (m)(m+g) (m)(m+g)
Proposed DNMG a,b,c 1980 D0 D1 D2 D3 D4 N1 N2 M1 M2 Grade
Mucosa
Muscularis Mucosa
Submucosa
Muscularis Propria
Serosa or Perirectal Fat
Adjacent Structures
Proximal Lymph Nodes
Distal Lymph Nodes
Distant Spread
1 - 4 POSITIVE NODES
5 OR MORE POSITIVE NODES
INVOLVES ADJACENT STRUCTURES
FISTULA PRESENT
BEYOND ADJACENT STRUCTURES
WELL
MODERATELY,
POORLY,
VERY POORLY
MICROSCOPIC
MICRO + GROSS
WELL
MODERATELY,
POORLY,

a - D for DEPTH of penetration
b - M1 metastases are resectable; M2 are not resectable
c - Proximal nodes - epi and parocolic; Distal nodes - intermediate and principal

lymph nodes. The amount of lymphoid hypertrophy does correlate with the size of the primary tumor, but not with the extent of spread (or lack of spread) either within the bowel wall or in lymphatics.[130] Therefore, there is no suggestion that the lymphoid hypertrophy is in response to tumor, but more likely a response to local sepsis associated with tumor growth. McVay and Coller, Kay and MacIntyre, and Grinnell likewise found that size of lymph nodes did not correlate with their involvement with tumor.[81,131,132]

CLASSIFICATION BY DEPTH OF INVASION OF BOWEL WALL AND PRESENCE OR ABSENCE OF LYMPHATIC METASTASES—THE A, B, C SYSTEM OF LOCKHART-MUMMERY

On the basis of clinical observations, Lockhart-Mummery at Saint Mark's Hospital in London divided rectal cancers into three "classes."[133] Class A included cases where the growth was small and had not apparently invaded the muscular coat, and no glands were involved. Class B cases involved the muscular coat, but where the growth was not unduly fixed and there was no extensive involvement of glands. In class C cases, the growth was large and fixed, or there was evidence of extensive involvement of glands. Eighty-two patients so classified and observed 5 years survived 74%, 44%, and 44% of the time in Class A, B, and C, respectively.

DUKES' CLASSIFICATION OF RECTAL CARCINOMA

The meticulous gross and microscopic studies of over 2000 rectal cancer specimens confirmed beyond doubt that the prognosis of patients with rectal cancer is significantly correlated with the depth of invasion of the primary tumor into the bowel wall and with the presence or absence of lymph node spread.[68,134] In the original classification system proposed by Gordon-Watson and Dukes, the depth of penetration of the bowel wall was assessed by noting the degree of involvement of the normal layers of the bowel wall.[135] In A cases, tumor extended into the submucosa, but not into the muscularis propria. In B cases, tumor spread into the muscularis propria, but not by direct continuity into the perirectal tissue. B cases were further subdivided as B1 or B2 depending on whether or not the outer longitudinal muscle of the rectal wall had been reached. In C cases the tumor had spread by direct continuity into the perirectal tissues. C cases were also subdivided into C1 or C2 to indicate the absence or presence of nodal metastases. Simpson and Mayo used a modification of Dukes' 1929–1930 classification system to help analyze factors that affect survival in carcinoma of the colon above the rectosigmoid.[136]

However, it soon became clear to Dukes that the 1929–1930 classification system was unnecessarily complex for the advanced rectal cancers usually seen at St. Mark's Hospital. In 1932 he proposed the classification system that is currently in use.[64] A cases lumped together A, B1, and B2 cases from the previous classification: "A cases are those in which the carcinoma is limited to the wall of the rectum, there being no extension into the extrarectal tissue and no metastases in lymph nodes." B cases included the previous C1 class: "B cases are those in which the carcinoma has spread by direct continuity to the extra-rectal tissues but has not yet invaded the regional nodes." C cases included the previous C2 class: "C cases are those in which metastases are present in the regional lymph nodes." Dukes thought that the A, B, C classification system reflected the natural evolution of cancer of the rectum, in that spread through the rectal wall was itself an important feature of disease progression and led to lymphatic and hematogenous dissemination of disease (see section on natural history). The system also divided patients into groups of more nearly equal size. Of 215 rectal cancers, 18% were A cases, 35% were B cases, and 47% were C cases. In the previous classification system only one of 100 patients was classified as an A case. Dukes also saw a "striking difference in the probability of survival of A, B, and C patients after excision of the rectum."

In 1935, Gabriel, Dukes, and Bussey proposed their only modification to the A, B, C classification system.[60] Those cases in which the regional lymph glands only were involved, or at least spread had not reached glands at the point of ligature of the blood vessels were classified as C1. Those cases in which the glandular spread had reached up to the point of ligature of the blood vessels were classified as C2. The value of the C1 and C2 subdivision was shown in 1958 by a comparison of survival rates in over 1000 patients; 5-year survival for C1 cases was 40.9% and for C2 cases was 13.6%.[68]

MODIFIED DUKES' CLASSIFICATION OF KIRKLIN, DOCKERTY, AND WAUGH

In 1949, Kirklin, Dockerty, and Waugh introduced a modification of the Dukes' classification; A lesions were limited to the mucosa; B1 lesions extended into the muscularis propria but did not penetrate it; B2 lesions penetrated through the muscularis propria; and C lesions were those of either types B1 or B2 with lymph node involvement.[137] This classification system did two important things. First, it excluded patients from classification unless a "curative" operation had been performed. Dukes had made "no distinction between those cases in which the growth was incompletely removed (palliative operations) and those where a cure could be hoped for (radical operations)."[68] Second, this classification identified the non-invasive cancers as a separate group with little or no chance for lymph node involvement and an excellent prognosis.

ASTLER–COLLER MODIFICATION OF THE DUKES' CLASSIFICATION

In 1954, Astler and Coller proposed a modification of the Kirklin, Dockerty, and Waugh classification system; C lesions were those that contained lymph node metastases but they were subdivided into C1 and C2 categories.[70] C1 lesions were limited to the bowel wall with positive nodes and C2 lesions penetrated all layers with positive nodes. Several important features of this classification system should be noted. First, Astler–Coller's C1 and C2 tumors were completely different from C1 and C2 tumors of Dukes. The Astler–Coller C1 and C2 subdivision was made to separate tumors with lesser or greater penetration of the bowel wall; Dukes' C1 and C2 subdivision was made to separate tumors with lesser or greater lymphatic involvement. Second, the extremely small proportion of C1 cases (14 of 351, 3.98%) substantiated Dukes' first hypothesis that lymph node metastases are unlikely unless penetration of the bowel wall has first taken place. Third, Astler and Coller did re-emphasize in their classification system an important point: the survival of patients with colon or rectal cancer progressively declines in proportion to the depth of penetration of the tumor through the bowel wall, and this is an independent variable to be used in assessing prognosis in addition to lymph node involvement. The difference in survival in Astler and Coller's study for B1 *versus* B2 lesions was 11% and for C1 *versus* C2 lesions was 22%. Because of small numbers, there was no statistically significant survival between groups with similar node status, but different degrees of bowel wall invasion. Subsequent studies of Dukes and Bussey and Copeland, Miller, and Jones convincingly showed that depth of invasion of bowel wall was a prognostic variable independent of node status.[68,138]

STAGING ACCORDING TO TURNBULL AND ASSOCIATES

In 1967, Turnbull and co-workers divided patients into four clinico–pathologic stages: Stage A, tumor confined to the colon and its coats; Stage B, tumor extension into pericolic fat; Stage C, tumor metastases to regional mesenteric lymph nodes, but no evidence of distant spread; Stage D, tumor metastases to liver, lung, bone, seeding of tumor, tumor irremovable because of parietal invasion, or adjacent organ invasion.[139] This clinico–pathologic staging system was useful in that it separtated (as had Kirklin, Dockerty, and Waugh) A, B, and C lesions from those having a variety of other more extensive and probably incurable tumors. However, it was confusing in that the clinical features that led to a D stage were left incompletely undefined. Did distant spread to lymph nodes mean para-aortic node involvement? Would lesions thought irremovable because of adjacent organ involvement by one surgeon be considered curable by *en bloc* dissections by other surgeons? Clearly, if a Stage D category is to be added, criteria for D classification must be clearly defined and rigidly adhered to.

Gilbertsen noted that the effect of adding the D category does markedly improve the survival statistics expected in the A, B, and C categories by eliminating on clinical grounds poor prognosis patients.[140] Finally, in discussing a D category that indicates far advanced disease, both a D1 and D2 class might be suggested. D1 would include tumors that are possibly surgically curable (adjacent organ involvement, solitary hepatic or pulmonary metastases) and D2 would include unresectable disease (multiple hepatic or hepatic plus pulmonary metastases, bone marrow metastases, and so forth).

TNM CLASSIFICATION

In an attempt to bring together a greater number of variables that may impact on survival, the International Union Against Cancer and the American Joint Committee for Cancer Staging and End Result Reporting have each proposed a TNM classification for colon and rectal cancer.[141,142] In the TNM staging system important prognostic variables are collected concerning the size of the primary tumor (T), the lymph nodes (N), and the presence or absence and location of metastatic deposits (M). This is to be done before surgery is performed as a combined *clinical surgical* evaluation (csTNM) and then as a *postsurgical* treatment (pTNM) evaluation. Several points should be made regarding the clinical surgical evaluation. First, the size of a primary colon or rectal malignancy has no correlation with prognosis (see section on prognosis).[130,131,132,143] Certainly an attempt to predict survival on the basis of primary tumor size is unwarranted; however, the depth (D) of penetration of the bowel wall is an important prognostic factor (see Figure 21-7).

Second, enlarged lymph nodes do not indicate glandular involvement.[60,130,131] Attempts by finger palpation to detect pararectal lymphadenopathy or lymphangiography to see para-aortic lymphatic disease is unwarranted.

Finally, the most common site for metastatic disease is the liver, but detection of subclinical metastasis with liver function tests or liver imaging studies is far from accurate (see section on diagnosis of metastases). In summary, a clinical surgical TNM classification is probably not worthwhile; a possible exception to this rule is some rectal tumors, where an estimate of prognosis through careful physical examination of the primary tumor may be possible (see section on diagnosis of rectal cancer).

Figure 21-7 shows the pTNM staging system as proposed by the American Joint Committee in 1977. There may be some good reasons for adoption of a TNM type system, especially in a research setting. However, the general acceptance of the Dukes' A, B, C system is so widespread and its use so simple that strong arguments for a new system must be offered before the Dukes' system is abandoned.[144] Some reasons for adoption of a TNM type system may be listed as follows. (1) The Dukes' systems have been so changed and modified and consequently confused that it is difficult or impossible to know exactly to which A, B, or C one refers. Adoption of a TNM system would result in a fresh start and avoid further confusion. (2) More accurate staging of the primary tumor is required. Early lesions seen much more frequently than in earlier years require that more staging categories be available. The Dukes' ABC system puts all lesions from mucosa to muscularis propria into a single category. (3) Histopathologic grading should be worked into the system. (4) Clinical data regarding involvement of adjacent structures (including peritoneal implants, perforation, and fistula formation), location of involved lymph nodes (proximal as epicolic and paracolic nodes and distal as intermediate and principal nodes), and the presence or absence and type (resectable or nonresectable) of metastasis are required. A proposed DNMG (depth, nodes, metastases, grade) system is shown in Figure 21-7.

PROGNOSIS

In discussing the prognostic variables that may affect survival with large bowel cancer, clinical and anatomic features that can be determined from history, physical examination, radiologic examination, or endoscopic examination are considered first (Table 21-9). Pathologic variables determined from a

TABLE 21-9. Clinical Features of Primary Large Bowel Cancer and Their Effect on Prognosis

CLINICAL FEATURE	EFFECT ON PROGNOSIS
Diagnosis in asymptomatic patients	Improved
Long duration of symptoms	No effect, possibly improved
Age less than 30 years	Diminished
Age greater than 70 years	Improved
Pre-operative CEA	
Greater than 5 ng/ml	Diminished
Less than 5 ng/ml	Improved
Less than 5 ng/ml (poorly differentiated tumor)	Not evaluable
Obstruction	Diminished
Free perforation	Markedly diminished
Localized perforation with abscess formation	Diminished
Hemorrhage as a presenting symptom	Improved
Adjacent organ involvement	Diminished
Fistula formation	Diminished
Size of the primary tumor	No effect
Configuration of the primary tumor	
Ulcerated	Diminished
Polypoid	Improved
Location of the primary tumor	
Rectum	Diminished
Rectum below peritoneal reflection	Diminished
Circumferential bowel lumen involvement	Diminished

study of the resected specimen are then examined (Table 21-14).

CLINICAL FEATURES AND THEIR EFFECT ON PROGNOSIS

Diagnosis in Asymptomatic Patients

Diagnosis of large bowel cancer before symptoms have developed improves survival consistently. Hertz, Deddish, and Day followed 58 patients in whom sigmoidoscopic examination in the asymptomatic state detected invasive adenocarcinoma.[145] Only 15% of these patients had positive lymph nodes and the five-year survival rate was 88%. Gilbertsen and Nelms report 25 adenocarcinomas detected in asymptomatic patients by an initial sigmoidoscopic examination.[41] Sixteen of these 25 patients (64%) were five-year survivors. The authors believe that this is at least twice the absolute survival rate for rectal cancer patients. Thirteen tumors were detected by the Minnesota Detection Clinic on annual recheck sigmoidoscopic examination, resulting in a 92% absolute five-year survival rate.

Sanfelippo and Beahrs studied 391 patients treated in 1964 for colorectal cancer at the Mayo Clinic.[146] The most important factor in assessing prognosis with operable cancers was the status of the lymph nodes; however, the next most important prognostic factor was the patients' symptoms. When the patient was asymptomatic the 5-year survival rate was 71% compared to 49% when symptoms were present. Corman, Coller, and Veidenheimer and Dabs and colleagues also report improved survival when cancer was detected by sigmoidoscopic examination.[147,148]

Recently, screening with the hemoccult test has resulted in detection of colon and rectal adenocarcinomas in "asymptomatic individuals."[149] The 5-year survival rates of these patients are not yet available. However, the incidence of lymph node positivity was reduced when tumors were found using hemoccult screening in asymptomatic individuals. Of 23,500 participants returning hemoccult slides, 525 had one or more positive tests. Evaluation of 415 participants was completed at the University of Minnesota Hospital and 42 primary cancers of the colorectum were detected. Seventy-three percent were Dukes A, 11% were Dukes B, 9% were Dukes C and 7% were Dukes D. Generally, near 50% of patients are Dukes C, so that a marked increase in survival is expected for this group of patients.

Long Duration of Symptoms

One would expect that the longer a patient with symptoms delayed in seeking medical help, the more advanced a tumor would become, and hence a poorer prognosis. However, for colorectal cancer patients numerous studies have shown no correlation of a short duration of symptoms and improved survival or long duration of symptoms and poorer prognosis.[138,150–160] Indeed, those patients whose acute onset of symptoms brings them to the hospital on an emergency basis have a poorer prognosis.[151,155,156] An important relationship between duration of symptoms and prognosis was presented by Devlin, Plant, and Morris.[158] These authors showed that individuals presenting with early symptoms are a subset of poor prognosis patients. First, in 61 patients with colicky abdominal pain, 36 presented early with acute obstruction and poor prognosis that accompanies nearly circumferential involvement of the bowel lumen by tumor (see below). Second, there was an association between short duration of symptoms and high histologic grade of the tumor. Only one of 26 undifferentiated tumors went longer than 1 year with undiagnosed symptoms while 32 of 108 and 25 of 95 moderately differentiated and well differentiated tumors did so. These were statistically significant differences.

Rowe-Jones and Aylett, in a study of 100 colon and 100 rectal cancer patients, contrary to the reports cited above, did find a statistically significant increased proportion of Dukes stage C patients in a group of patients in whom diagnosis was delayed.[161] This important study's results differ from those cited above for the following reasons: first, only two of 200 patients presented with intestinal obstruction; and second, this is the only paper in which the important distinction is made between patient-induced delay and medically-induced delay. Delay in diagnosis resulting from external factors other than the patient's symptoms was important in diminishing prognosis.

One may summarize the available data on delay in diagnosis and treatment of large bowel cancer and its effect on prognosis as follows: for a population of individuals, patient-delay in seeking medical advice is not associated with an unfavorable prognosis. This is because patients who seek help early often have aggressive tumors; they are a subset of patients with annular constricting lesions and poorly differentiated tumors who are compelled to seek medical help without delay. Any improvement in treatment results this group may enjoy by electing to seek medical attention early is more than offset by the aggressive biologic nature of their tumor. Patients with less acute symptoms as a whole have less virulent tumors. However, for the individual patient with an average grade tumor, early diagnosis and treatment may significantly improve survival. One final point; delay in diagnosis cannot be considered unimportant medically, because with delay more patients fail to benefit the short-term effects of non-curative resection and more patients must undergo emergency surgical procedures with much higher morbidity and mortality rates.[159]

Age Less than 30 Years

Recio and Bussey, from St. Mark's Hospital, reported that approximately 1% of 4430 colon and rectal cancers occurred before the age of 30 years.[162] The 5-year survival in this group of patients was markedly reduced, with 19.5% patients surviving 5 years. Survival rate at St. Mark's in an unselected rectal cancer population was 34.7%. It should be pointed out that these tumors did not occur in patients with ulcerative colitis or with familial polyposis. Fifty-three percent of the young patients had tumor histology showing high grade malignancy; only 20.2% had such tumors in the general series. Also, Recio and Bussey note that there were an increased number of mucoid tumors in this young group of patients. Table 21-10 shows that a larger proportion of poorly differentiated tumors, more mucinous tumors, and a lesser number of potentially curative resections combine to make the prognosis with colorectal cancer in young patients very poor.[162–170]

Age 70 Years or Greater

Block and Enker studied 111 patients 70 years of age and older in the Chicago area who had a diagnosis of rectal cancer.[171] Sixty-four patients underwent abdomino–perineal or anterior resection. The postoperative mortality was 15%. When operative deaths were excluded, survival was 67.2%; survival for rectal cancer patients 69 and under receiving definitive treatment was 60.9%. Block and Enker conclude that "for elderly patients surviving orthodox operation, the relative 5-year survival exceeds that of the general population." Jensen, Nielsen, and Balslev report similar findings for colon cancer.[172]

Calabrese, Adam, and Volk studied 226 patients 80 years of age or older with colorectal cancer.[173] Of these, 156 underwent surgery; operative mortality was 32.6% and 5-year survival rate for those 156 patients was 22.4%. Age-corrected survival was 53.3%. Calabrese and co-workers conclude that prognosis from cancer following successful surgery was "more favorable" in the aged than unselected patients. The operative mortality was, of course, extremely high.

Finally, it should be mentioned that in a larger number of patients there is a trend for a lower grade of tumor to occur at an older age. Dukes and Bussey report low, average, and high grade malignancy to occur at an average age of 61.9 ± 0.6 years, 60.5 ± 0.3 years, and 57.0 ± 0.7 years, respectively, in males and 61.3 ± 0.9 years, 58.3 ± 0.5 years, and 53.8 ± 1.1 years in females.[68]

Preoperative Carcinoembryonic Antigen (CEA) Determination

CEA is a circulating glycoprotein molecule produced in variable amounts by most colorectal cancers (see section on tumor markers). Wanebo and co-workers showed a correlation of pre-operative CEA levels with subsequent recurrence for Dukes B and C cancer as shown in Figure 21-8.[174] Also, a correlation between mean pre-operative level and estimated time to recurrence was found. Band and associates, with 2 years follow-up of 36 patients with colorectal cancer, report four of 14 patients with recurrence who had pre-operative CEA of less than 2.5 ng/ml (normal range is 0 to 2.5 ng/ml). However, 17 of 22 patients with elevated pre-operative CEA levels had recurrence.[175] Goslin and co-workers also found a relationship between pre-operative CEA and disease recur-

TABLE 21-10. Colorectal Cancer (Exclusive of Ulcerative Colitis and Familial Polyposis)

AUTHOR (Reference Number)*	YEAR	TOTAL NUMBER OF PATIENTS	NUMBER OF YOUNG PATIENTS	AGE	POORLY DIFFEREN-TIATED (%)	MUCIN-OUS (%)	5-YEAR NED (%)	CURATIVE RESEC-TIONS
YOUNG ADULT PATIENTS								
Hall and Coffey (163)	1961	718	50	16–40	35	20	18	66
Johnson et al (164)	1962	–	169	16–29	47	–	21	86
Mayo and Pagtalunan (165)	1963	–	67	<30	36	–	35	75
Recio and Bussey (162)	1965	4435	52	<30	53	increased	19.5	50
Rosato et al (166)	1969	1084	35	≤35	27	–	40	94
Lagenberg and Ong (167)	1972	582	21	13–25	43	–	0	67
Recalde et al (168)	1974	2156	38	≤35	13	32	13	87
Sanfelippo and Beahrs (169)	1978	4% of all colorectal cancer patients	118	<40	–	–	39	–
PEDIATRIC PATIENTS								
Cain and Longino† (170)	1970	–	97	<18	–	51	<10	–

*Exclusive of ulcerative colitis and familial polyposis patients.
†Literature review of all reported patients with colorectal cancer under age 18 years.

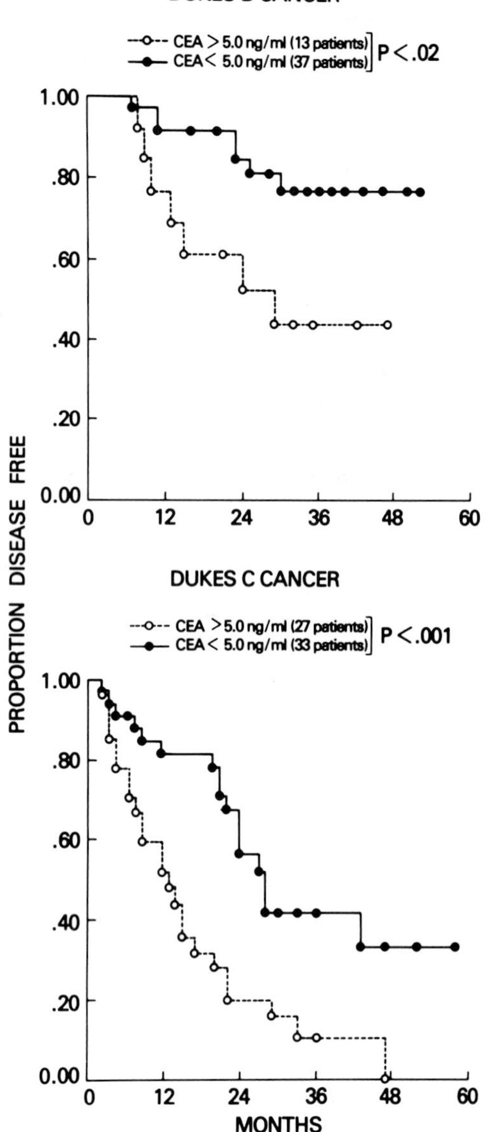

FIG. 21-8. Preoperative CEA levels and post-resection recurrence of Dukes' B and C cancer (Wanebo HJ, Rao B, Pinsky C et al: Preoperative carcinoembryonic antigen (CEA) level as a prognostic indicator in colorectal cancer. N Engl J Med 299:449, 450, 1978)

rence in Dukes' C patients.[176] An important caveat noted from their study concerns tumors with poorly differentiated histology. These tumors produce relatively little CEA as compared to more well-differentiated tumors and therefore a normal pre-operative CEA with poorly differentiated tumor histology does not suggest a more favorable prognosis.

Obstruction

Colorectal cancer with intestinal obstruction is associated with a poorer prognosis than are non-obstructing lesions.[177–188] Table 21-11 shows the results of treatment for obstructing cancer and establishes the dismal prognosis expected in association with this clinical entity. Several factors combine to produce the very limited 5-year survival. First, only about 50% of patients are candidates for potentially curative surgery at the time of exploratory laparotomy. Second, the surgery is accompanied by a high morbidity and mortality rate. Surgical complication rates occur in one-third to one-half of patients. Operative mortality ranges from 5% to 20%. Unfortunately, even if a patient can be resected for cure and has no complications resulting from surgery, the 5-year survival is still markedly reduced. Five-year survival following curative surgery is rarely greater than 30%. Ragland, Londe, and Spratt make the interesting observation that survival with even one positive lymph node is extremely poor.[185] When all lymph nodes were negative, the 5-year survival rate was 58.8% in resected cases. With one to five positive nodes the 5-year survival rate dropped to 16.7%. There were no survivors in the Ellis Fischel series with six or more lymph node metastases.

Ackerman studied the effects of increased intraluminal pressure in dogs on lymph flow.[189] Both an increase in intraluminal pressure induced by an insufflation or hyperperistalsis stimulated by electrical current increased intestinal lymph flow four to six times normal. Ackerman suggests that decreased survival rate in patients with obstructing cancers, may at least in part be related to higher flow of lymph from the area of the carcinoma causing an increased dissemination of cancer cells.

Perforation

Perforative carcinoma of the colorectum for this discussion is defined as either free perforation into the abdominal cavity or localized perforation with abscess formation; the results of treatment are summarized in Table 21-12.[177,182,186–188,190–192] The problem of fistula formation and adjacent organ involvement will be discussed later in this section. Glenn and McSherry reported 99 of 1815 patients (5.5%) with colorectal cancer who had perforations of the colon due to carcinoma.[186] In 58 patients the perforation was localized and in 41 the perforation was free into the peritoneal cavity. Sixty-five of 99 patients had curative operations with a mortality rate of 19.2%; 33% had palliative procedures with a mortality rate of 27.3%. The 5-year survival rate for 41 patients with free perforation of the carcinoma into the peritoneal cavity was 7.3%. In contrast, the 5-year survival rate for 58 patients with localized perforations was 41.4%. It is clear that perforative carcinoma of the colorectum carries with it a dismal prognosis. The almost negligible survival rate after free perforation is likely due to implantation of tumor cells within the abdominal cavity.

Obstruction and Perforation

Glenn and McSherry report 30 patients with obstruction and perforation.[186] In 29, both obstruction and perforation occurred at the location of the cancer. One patient with an obstructing tumor of the transverse colon had a perforation of the cecum, presumably as a result of pressure necrosis from overdistention.[193,194] Operative mortality rate was 31% and only two patients (6.7%) survived 5 years.

TABLE 21-11. Obstructive Colorectal Cancer

AUTHOR (Reference Number)	YEAR	TOTAL PATIENTS	PATIENTS OBSTRUCTED	CURATIVE SURGERY (%)	HOSPITAL MORTALITY (%)	OVERALL 5 YEAR SURVIVAL (%)	5-YEAR SURVIVAL CURATIVE SURGERY (%)
Goligher and Smiddy (177)	1957	1664	290	44.1	34.1	–	–
Ulin and Ehrlich (178)	1962	1005	227	–	17	33	–
Chang and Burnett (179)	1962	465	106	–	22.6	18.9	–
Minster (180)	1964	145	26	–	11.0	27	–
Loefler and Hofner (181)	1964	573	87	–	39.0	10.3	–
Hickey and Hyde (182)	1965	444	43	41.9	27.9	11.5	27.8
Floyd and Cohn (183)	1967	1741	512*	–	24.0	17.0	–
Watters (184)	1969	343	84	69.0	13	30.9	44.8
Ragland et al (185)	1971	1137	73†	47.8	18.0	15.1	34.4
Glenn and McSherry (186)	1971	1815	210	46.6	15.2	19.5	41.8
Welch and Donaldson (187)	1974	1566	124	71.7	15.0	28.0	40.0
Clark et al (188)	1975	–	136	62.5	31.0	–	–

*Includes patients with partial and complete obstruction, survival in both groups similar.
†Complete intestinal obstruction in 73 patients studied, total number with obstruction 227.

TABLE 21-12. Perforative Colon Cancer

AUTHOR (Reference Number)	YEAR	TOTAL NUMBER OF PATIENTS	NUMBER OF FREE AND LOCALIZED PERFORATIONS	CURATIVE SURGERY (%)	HOSPITAL MORTALITY (%)	OVERALL 5-YEAR SURVIVAL (%)	5-YEAR SURVIVAL CURATIVE SURGERY (%)
Goligher and Smiddy (177)	1957	1644	free 57*	19.0	73.9	–	–
			localized 38				
Miller et al (190)	1966	1102	free 7	71.4	42.9	14.3	20.0
			localized 64†	87.5	20.3	26.6	30.3
Crowder and Cohn (191)	1967	1687	free 24‡	42.2	53.3	2.2	5.0
			localized 21§				
Glenn and McSherry (186)	1971	1815	free 71	64.3	20.1	7.0	34.9
			localized 58†			41.4	
Welch and Donaldson (192)	1974	2004	free 51‖	55.3	29.7	9.8	33
			localized 51†			19.6	35

*Twenty of 57 perforations above an obstructing colon or rectal cancer.
†Localized perforation with abscess or fistula formation.
‡Twelve of 24 perforations above an obstructing colon or rectal cancer.
§Excludes patients with fistulas.
‖Seventeen of 51 perforations above an obstructing colon or rectal cancer.

Hemorrhage as a Presenting Symptom

As might be expected from the discussions on delay in diagnosis, obstruction, and perforation, the symptoms which force patients to seek medical attention suggest a diminished prognosis. Hemorrhage is a symptom that carries an improved prognosis. For example, Thomas reporting on 267 patients with cancer of the right colon found a 54% 5-year survival rate for patients presenting with hemorrhage, 28% for patients presenting with obstruction, and 11% for patients with perforation.[195]

Involvement of Adjacent Organs or Structures

Involvement of adjacent organs or structures by the primary tumor is not a rare occurrence and occurs in 10% to 20% of patients. The survival statistics that accompany tumors that involve adjacent organs or structures are shown in Table 21-13.[196–208] The patients presented were selected because some other structure besides colon or rectum required removal for an *en bloc* resection of the primary colon or rectal cancer. In each series, extended resections done for palliation were not included; therefore, this is a rather select group of patients. Yet, accepting that these are retrospective studies, that there has been considerable patient selection, and that there is incomplete 5-year follow-up in some groups of patients, there is an appreciable 20% to 50% patient salvage.

From studying these reports it is not possible to determine the sites of treatment failure. The incidence of lymph node metastasis was not usually included in the reports. El Domeri and Whiteley do mention that five of ten patients with involvement of the anterior abdominal wall had lymphatic metastases.[205] Many of these patients are undoubtedly examples of a type of colorectal tumor described by Spratt, "The

TABLE 21-13. Involvement of Adjacent Organs and Structures Treated by *en bloc* Resection

AUTHOR (Reference Number)	YEAR	TOTAL PATIENTS	OPERATIONS ADJACENT ORGANS INVOLVED	PROLONGED SURVIVAL	OPERATIVE MORTALITY
Grey and Turner (196)	1929	241	22 (9%)	*8 (36%)	18%
Sugarbaker (197)	1946	220	42 (19%)	*19 (44%)	19%
Gilchrist and David (198)	1947	200	35 (18%)	14 (40%)	20%
Van Prohska et al (199)	1953	225	21 (9%)	*10 (48%)	5%
Cooke (200)	1955	–	12	*7 (58%)	8%
Taylor et al (201)	1955	–	18	6 (33%)	10%
Rosi (202)	1962	–	24	14 (64%)	8%
Aldrete and Remine† (203)	1966	–	42	11 (24%)	12%
Jensen and Nielsen (204)	1970	–	60	28 (47%)	22%
El-Domeri and Whiteley‡ (205)	1970	–	10	6 (60%)	10%
Polk§ (206)	1972	437	24 (5%)	*10 (42%)	4%
Ellis et al‖ (207)	1975	–	6	3 (50%)	0%
Davis and Ellis¶ (208)	1975	198	24 (12%)	*13 (54%)	0%
Welch and Donaldson (192)	1974	2004	164 (8%)	56 (34%)	6%
Rich et al (122)	1978	130	**10 (8%)	4 (40%)	0%
			††4 (3%)	0 (0%)	0%

*Complete 5-year survival statistics unavailable.
†All patients with vesicocolic fistulas, one patient had a colonic leiomyosarcoma.
‡All patients with anterior abdominal wall involvement.
§Five patients with recurrent colorectal malignancy included.
‖All patients with duodenal involvement.
¶Nineteen patients with palliative resections involving adjacent organs or structures not included.
**Patients without lymph node involvement.
††Patients with lymph node involvement.

non-metastasizing variant."[143] Spratt believes these tumors may grow very large, invade locally, but only rarely result in hematogenous or lymphatic metastases.

Size of the Primary Tumor

For nearly every human cancer the size of the primary tumor is related to that tumor's tendency to spread by lymphatic or hematogenous pathways (see chapter on diagnosis and staging). Colorectal cancer is an exception to this rule; for this tumor the size of the malignancy that the clinician sees has little or no relationship to prognosis.[28,131,132,143,156,208,210] Rather, as Dukes has established, it is the depth of penetration of the bowel wall that is related to that tumor's tendency to metastasize (Fig. 21-9). McSherry and co-workers reviewed 908 large bowel cancers; diameter of tumors in patients surviving 5 years was 4.9 cm and in those patients who died of disease it was 5.1 cm.[210] Spratt and Spjut found no relationship of the greatest longitudinal dimension of the primary tumor and 5-year or 10-year survival. There was a slight tendency of very large tumors to have an improved prognosis.[143]

One study by Grinnell of a large number (941) of specimens did show a statistically significant correlation of tumor size as measured by the greatest linear diameter of the tumor and the incidence of lymph node metastases.[69] However, this relationship was observed only in tumors 1.5 cm to 6.9 cm in diameter; in larger tumors (7.0 cm to 15.9 cm) the prognosis improved as size increased. It is not clear why the carefully prepared data of Grinnell differs from the other reports. Grinnell's specimens were subjected to the clearing technique, so more minute foci of glandular cancer may have been found. Possibly, Grinnell's measurements were taken from within the bowel lumen or from a cut section of the tumor; if taken from a cut section of the bowel, size measurements could reflect depth of invasion. Also, it is possible that there were fewer polypoid tumors.

Configuration of the Primary Tumor

Numerous authors have commented that tumor configuration seems to reflect the biologic nature of the primary tumor. Polypoid tumors project into the bowel lumen and tend not to invade deeply into the bowel wall. Ulcerating tumors are usually found to penetrate the bowel wall and therefore are associated with a poorer prognosis. Grinnell classified the primary tumors as projecting, intermediate, and infiltrating; 83% (19 of 23) of patients with projecting tumors survived 5 years; 45% (19 of 42) of patients with intermediate tumors survived 5 years; and 38% (six of 16) with infiltrating tumors survived.[27] Coller, Kay, and MacIntyre found that in both rectal and colon tumors, projecting lesions which appeared to be growing into the lumen metastasized to lymph nodes less frequently than sessile tumors.[131] For rectal cancer specimens, 54% (15 of 28) of polypoid tumors had glandular spread, whereas 81% (17 of 21) of sessile lesions had lymphatic metastasis.[79] Also, Dionne observed that the gross configuration of the primary tumor influenced the venous spread of disease.[71] Fungating, ulcerating, and stenosing tumors resulted in hematogenous metastases 23% (80 of 342), 31% (265 of 844) and 45% (44 of 98) of the time. Clearly, the gross anatomical configuration of the primary tumor is of value in assessing prognosis.

Location of the Primary Tumor

Most, but not all, reports suggest that survival with rectal cancer is poorer than with colon cancer; furthermore, survival diminishes as rectal tumors are located more distally in the bowel. Dwight, Higgins, and Keehn found the 5-year survival of 633 colon cancer patients to be 60.9% while with 430 rectal cancer patients survival was 42.8%.[211] The differences between survival of colon and rectal cancer patients in other series, although present, was less marked.[143,146]

The position of the primary rectal tumor in relation to the peritoneal reflection has been the subject of several investigations. If local recurrence is an important cause of treatment failure as postulated in the section on natural history, then tumors below the peritoneal reflection with one less covering layer (serosa) and more difficult surgical removal should recur more frequently. The lower the tumor in the rectum, the closer to bony pelvis laterally and posteriorly and to vagina or prostate anteriorly. An alternative explanation for the poorer prognosis with low lying lesions is the differing lymphatic drainage. Upper lesions would be expected to metastasize only by a superior hemorrhoidal lymphatic channel. Lower lesions could metastasize not only by way of this route but also by way of the middle and inferior hemorrhoidal lymphatics. Gilchrist and David reviewed the 5-year survival of rectal cancer patients with negative and positive nodes.[198] Survival with tumor below the peritoneal reflection without involved nodes was 89% (32 of 36 patients) while above the reflection without nodes was 100% (18 of 18 patients); also, survival with tumor below the peritoneal reflection with involved nodes was 49% (26 of 53 patients) while above the reflection with nodes was 60% (18 of 30 patients). Survival was about 10% poorer with tumors below the peritoneal reflection than above, independent of lymph node status. Likewise, others have reported a greater proportion of patients free of disease at 5 years with lesions at greater distances from the dentate line.[99,208,212–214]

An interesting relationship between the level of the rectal lesion and the incidence of local recurrence was noted by Wangensteen and Toon, Von Oppolzer and Nietsehe, and Morrison, Vaughn, and Bussey.[98,211,212,215,216] One study by Kirklin, Dockerty, and Waugh failed to find a relationship of the tumor's location above or below the peritoneal reflection and survival.[137]

Proportion of Circumference of Bowel Lumen Involved

As documented above, obstructing tumors carry a poorer prognosis; therefore, one might expect that the greater the proportion of the bowel lumen involved by tumor, the worse the prognosis. Grinnell showed higher frequencies of metastasis to lymph nodes and venous invasion and lower survival rates when tumors were completely annular as compared to those that were not completely annular.[27,72,81] Also, Dunning, Jones, and Hazard found a definite decrease in survival rates with increasing circumferential involvement.[217] Coller, Kay, and MacIntyre found an increase in the likelihood of lymph node metastasis as more of the bowel circumference is involved by primary tumor.[79] Percival Cole was apparently correct in postulating a circumferential route of spread of tumor within the bowel wall along circular lymphatic channels.[8] A single paper by Gilchrist and David did not find a correlation of lymph node involvement and proportion of circumference of bowel wall involved by tumor.[74]

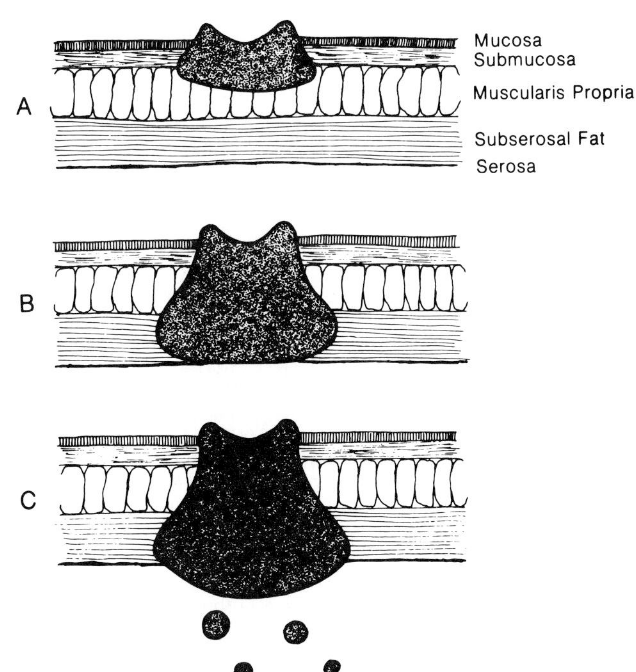

FIG. 21-9. Lack of correlation between intraluminal tumor size and depth of bowel wall penetration.

Paracolic Lymphadenopathy by Rectal Examination

McVay; Gabriel, Dukes, and Bussey; Grinnell; and Coller, Kay and MacIntyre all report their inability to determine the presence or absence of metastases from the size of lymph nodes. This, along with the difficulty of appreciating lymphadenopathy through the rectal wall, makes this an unreliable means by which to assess prognosis.[26,60,131,132]

PATHOLOGIC FEATURES AND THEIR EFFECT ON PROGNOSIS (Table 21-14)

Assessment of Prognosis by Histologic Grading

The earliest efforts of pathologists to predict from examination of a specimen the likelihood for cure involved studies of tumor histopathology. Broders, in 1915, began his well-known system of grading tumors according to the degree of differentiation.[218] Rankin and Broders were able to find a direct correlation between tumor grade, lymph node metastases, and survival in 589 patients with rectal carcinoma.[219] The variable morphologic criteria used in different grading systems is shown in Table 21-15.[27,29,68,219,220,221]

TABLE 21-14. Pathologic Features of Primary Large Bowel Cancer and Their Effect on Prognosis

PATHOLOGIC FEATURE	EFFECT ON PROGNOSIS
Histologic grade	
Well differentiated	Improved
Moderately well differentiated	No effect
Poorly differentiated	Diminished
Infiltrating deep margin of tumor	Diminished
Mucoid adenocarcinoma	Diminished
Signet ring adenocarcinoma	Diminished
Scirrhous carcinoma	Diminished
Penetration of bowel wall	Diminished
Lymph node involvement	Diminished
Lymphatic invasion	Diminished
Venous invasion	Uncertain effect; increased hematogenous spread
Perineural invasion	Increased local recurrence rate
Distal margin less than 5 cm	Diminished
Inflammatory response surrounding primary tumor	
None	Diminished
Intense	Improved
Lymph node histology	
Paracortical immunoblasts	Improved
Sinus histiocytosis	Improved
Germinal center activity	No effect

Undoubtedly, the most disciplined study of histologic grading was reported by Grinnell.[27] He correlated survival of colon and rectal cancer patients with eight different histologic grading criteria. Gradations of glandular arrangement, invasiveness, loss of nuclear polarity, and number of mitosis correlated with survival, while papillary character, mucin secretion, size of nucleus, and variation in size of nuclei could not be correlated with survival.

There seems little doubt that histologic grading does have value in assessing prognosis. However, the grading of colorectal cancer is severely handicapped for several reasons. First, there is no uniform system of grading. With the exception of Grinnell, the roles that differentiation, mitotic figures, nuclear polarity, glandular architecture, and thickness of glandular walls should play in estimating prognosis has never been determined. Indeed, the advantages of more complex grading schema over the Broders' system of determining the proportion of differentiated cells have never been established. Perhaps as suggested by Spratt and Spjut the only important criteria is invasiveness seen at the deep margins of the tumors.[143]

A second major limitation of grading is its lack of discriminatory power except at the extremes of grades. Treatment of Grade I tumors is likely to result in cure, whereas treatment of Grades III and IV is likely to result in failure. Unfortunately, only about 40% of tumors are graded at those extremes. Grade II tumors account for at least 60% of the total and no predictability is found within this large group.

Third, no means of integrating grading with other important

TABLE 21-15. Histologic Grading of Colorectal Cancer

SYSTEM (Reference Number)	DATE	CRITERIA FOR GRADING	GRADES	PERCENT PATIENTS PER GROUP	SURVIVAL
Rankin and Broders (219)	1928	"Cellular differentiation and mitoses"	I	18	56
			II	50	38
			III	23	25
			IV	9	15 (n = 598)
Stewart and Spies (220)	1929	"Glandular structure, nuclear polarity, mitotic activity"	I	11	–
			II	56	–
			III	24	–
			IV	9	–
Grinnell (27)	1939	"Glandular arrangement, invasiveness, nuclear polarity, number of mitoses"	I	39	66
			II	37	48
			III	24	25 (n= 204)
Dukes (29)	1940	"Arrangement of glandular tissue"	I	7	–
			II	57	–
			III	23	–
			IV	1	–
			Mucoid	12	– (n= 985)
Dukes and Bussey (68)	1958	"Cellular arrangement and differentiation"	Low grade adenoca	16	77
			Average grade adenoca	52	60
			High grade adenoca	17	28
			Carcinoma simplex	2	–
			Colloid	13	–
Wood (221)	1967	"Organoid appearance"	Well differentiated		
			Moderately differentiated		
			Poorly differentiated		
			Mucoid		
			Scirrhous		

pathologic variables such as depth of invasion and lymph node involvement has been achieved.

Finally, as studied by Qualheim and Gall, the cytologic and structural variation of the tumor from one portion to another is marked.[222] Since such variation was exhibited, they questioned if the utilization of microscopic grading as a means of determining prognosis was profitable. However, Grinnell makes two important points: (1) the area of most poorly differentiated tumor within the specimen must be used for grading, and (2) the deep margins of the tumor mass are likely to be the areas of highest grade and must be studied.[27]

Many studies would suggest that histologic grading does give an estimate of the degree of malignancy and is a useful indication of prognosis. Colorectal cancers of a higher grade have: (1) less chance for cure than those of lower grades[27,64,68,156,209,217,223] (2) is associated with greater local extent.[27,68] (3) increased frequency of venous invasion.[29,73,81,223,224] (4) distant metastases.[71,78] (5) perineural invasion.[73] and (6) metastases to lymph nodes.[27,29,68,73,78,79,131,219,225]

Histologic Grading of Biopsy Specimens of Primary Tumor

With the development of fiberoptic colonoscopy and sigmoidoscopy it is now possible to biopsy nearly every colon and rectal cancer prior to surgical resection. If certain precautions are regarded, histologic grading may in some patients help determine prognosis. Grinnell performed a study comparing the grading of biopsy specimens to grading of the complete specimen.[27] In 58 of 74 cases (78%) the biopsy was given the same grade as the tumor on later examination. In all 16 discrepant cases, the biopsy was rated less malignant than was the tumor. In 1958, Dukes and Bussey softened their prior harsh criticism of the use of biopsy specimens to assess prognosis.[64,68] They reviewed their experience with 2447 operative specimens of rectal cancer: "Microscopic examination of a biopsy fragment and grading the tumor if it proved to be malignant was not much help if the tumor was reported as being of an average grade of malignancy; but it had a definite value in the other two grades because if the tumor is well differentiated it is probably slow growing, whereas if it is undifferentiated it is more likely to have given rise to lymphatic metastases." It seems that reliable information from a biopsy specimen can be obtained from those specimens which are at the extremes of the grading system.

Pushing or Infiltrating Tumor Borders

Grinnell in a search for histologic criteria by which to grade colorectal carcinoma found invasiveness to be of the greatest prognostic value.[27] In correlating survival in 126 patients with slight, moderate, or marked invasiveness, 71%, 55% and 23% of patients were alive, free of disease, at 5 years. Invasiveness was a "term used to describe the tendency of tumor cells to appear to stream out singly or in small groups into surrounding tissues." Grinnell repeatedly emphasized that invasiveness was best assessed at the deep advancing edge of the tumor.

Spratt and Spjut likewise studied histologically the deep margins of the primary tumor.[143] The margin was characterized as pushing, infiltrating, or mixed. Five-year survival in operable patients with pushing margins was 46%, with infiltrating margins, 28%, and with mixed margins, 54%. From these studies it seems clear that an invasive character of the deep margin of the primary tumor carries with it a poorer prognosis.

Mucoid Adenocarcinoma

Parham, Trimpi and Bacon, and Symonds and Vickery made a special study of colon and rectal carcinomas that secreted large amounts of mucus.[128,222,223,226,227] In all studies, survival was reduced when compared to tumors producing an average amount of mucoid material. Symonds and Vickery report a 34% 5-year survival in patients with mucoid adenocarcinoma compared to 53% in controls.[128] These tumors had a particularly bad prognosis in the rectum with an 18% 5-year survival; control non-mucus producing tumors had a 49% survival. Grinnell noted that this poor prognosis occurs even if the tumor is well differentiated and nodes uninvolved; with lymph node positivity, few patients have prolonged survival.[27] Wood, in an AFIP monograph, suggests that the overall prognosis for patients with mucoid adenocarcinoma is poor even though the disease-free interval from initial resection until diagnosis of recurrent disease may be great; these tumors often seem to be slow, but relentless in their recurrence pattern.[221]

Signet Ring Adenocarcinoma

When the accumulation of large amounts of mucoid material is intracellular, individual cells have a signet ring appearance. Survival with this tumor is unusual and its biologic character seems akin to poorly differentiated tumors. Mucoid and signet ring adenocarcinoma occurs in a higher proportion of young colorectal cancer patients and is largely responsible for their poor prognosis.

Scirrhous Carcinoma

Woolam and associates at the Mayo Clinic reviewed their experience with 93 patients with scirrhous carcinoma of the terminal 25 cm of the large bowel.[129] Only 18% of this group survived 5 years. Symptoms seemed to occur late in the course of the disease from stenosis or obstruction of the bowel lumen; bleeding was an unusual symptom, occurring in only three patients. Diagnosis was occasionally difficult to establish; an ulcerating tumor was seen in only 16% as compared to 50% of non-scirrhous controls. Often, repeat biopsy was necessary to obtain a positive biopsy from "leathery" tumor. The histologic grade of the tumors was more poorly differentiated than usual. Forty percent of scirrhous tumors were Grades III or IV by Broders' grading; only 27% are usually Grades III or IV.[228] Also, 75% of tumors were Dukes C classification; usually, less than 50% of cases are Dukes C. Finally, at exploratory laparotomy, 47% of patients, because of extensive local disease, received only palliative surgical procedures. Usually, palliative surgery must be performed in less than half this percentage of patients. In summary, the clinical and pathologic diagnosis of scirrhous carcinoma of the large bowel carries with it a very poor prognosis.

Penetration of Bowel Wall

As noted in the section on natural history, the depth of penetration of the bowel wall is important prognostically for two reasons. First, lymphatic metastases only rarely occur before the primary tumor has grown through the bowel wall. Secondly, as shown in Table 21-16, penetration and the extent of penetration of the bowel wall is associated with a reduced prognosis independent of lymph node status.[68,70,138]

Lymph Node Involvement

Undoubtedly, the most important prognostic variable for colorectal cancer is the presence or absence of lymph node involvement. Also, as shown in Table 21-17, as the number of involved nodes increases, survival diminishes.[138] Dukes and Bussey found a corrected 5-year survival of 83.7% in patients without lymph node involvement and a survival of 32.0% with lymph nodes involved.[68] They point out that "if lymphatic spread is still at an early stage the prognosis may still be relatively good." If only regional lymph nodes contained metastases (C1 cases) corrected survival was 40.9%. If there was more extensive lymphatic spread, involving the nodes at the point of ligature of the blood vessels (C2 cases), survival was 13.6%.

Lymphatic Invasion

Spratt and Spjut reported a 5-year survival of 20% with lymphatic invasion and 47% in its absence.[143] Of course, many of the patients with lymphatic invasion may also have lymph node invasion. Data to show that lymphatic invasion is an independent prognostic variable is not available.

TABLE 21-16. Relationship Between Local Spread and 5-year Survival Rates After Surgical Treatment, Cases without Lymphatic Metastases

	NUMBER OF CASES	CORRECTED 5-YEAR SURVIVAL RATE (%)
Slight extra-rectal spread	266	89.7
Moderate extra-rectal spread	109	80.0
Extensive extra-rectal spread	148	57.0

(Dukes CE, Bussey HJR: The spread of rectal cancer and its effect on prognosis. Br J Cancer 12:309–320, 1958)

Distal Margin of Resection Less than 5 cm

Lofgren, Waugh, and Dockerty studied 108 patients who, after undergoing anterior resection for cancer of the rectum and sigmoid, developed recurrent disease.[115] These patients with a control group for comparison were studied in an attempt to determine factors which result in subsequent recurrent disease. Fixed specimens from the recurrent group had a lesser length of normal mucosa distal to the base of the primary tumor; 45% of specimens from the recurrent group had a distal margin of 1.5 cm or less whereas 23% of specimens from the survivors had this distal margin. In a similar group of patients, Copeland, Miller, and Jones found a poorer prognosis with a margin of resection less than 5 cm.[138] If the local resection margin was less than 5 cm, only 38.4% of patients were alive without disease at 5 years; if the margin was greater than 5 cm, 51.1% were alive without carcinoma.

The cause for a reduced prognosis when there is a lesser margin of resection is unclear. Goligher, Dukes, and Bussey reported that downward spread three-fourths of an inch or more was noted in only 2% of 1500 rectal cancer specimens studied at St. Mark's.[88] Lofgren, Waugh, and Dockerty suggested that the closer the lesion is to the distal resection margin and the lower the lesion is within the pelvis "the more difficult it is to remove it, and hence the greater the likelihood of traumatic dispersal of viable malignant cells along the raw surfaces of the operative site." Apparently an adequate margin of resection as seen by pathologic study of the resected specimen may not be an adequate margin of resection for optimal 5-year survival.

A report by Wilson and Beahrs failed to find a relationship between a narrow margin of resection and diminished prognosis.[227]

Venous Invasion

There is no question that the presence of venous invasion within a colorectal cancer specimen correlates with an increased incidence of hematogenous metastases and reduced survival. Brown and Warren, in their autopsy study of 170 cases of rectal cancer, make the following pertinent obser-

TABLE 21-17. Correlation of Nodal Involvement and 5-Year Survival of Patients with Carcinoma of the Colon

STATUS	NO NODES INVOLVED (584 patients)	ONE NODE INVOLVED (112 patients)	TWO NODES INVOLVED (68 patients)	THREE NODES INVOLVED (40 patients)	FOUR NODES INVOLVED (24 patients)	FIVE OR MORE NODES INVOLVED (110 patients)
Alive with no carcinoma	48.5%	26.8%	25.0%	15.0%	29.1%	9.1%
Alive with carcinoma	3.0%	3.5%	2.9%	2.5%	4.2%	0.9%
Dead with no carcinoma	17.6%	6.2%	5.9%	2.5%	4.2%	4.5%
Dead with carcinoma	31.9%	63.5%	66.2%	80.0%	62.5%	85.5%

(Copeland EM, Miller LD, Jones RS: Prognostic factors in carcinoma of the colon and rectum. Am J Surg 116:875–880, 1968)

vations: (1) The incidence of venous invasion and visceral metastasis increases as the histologic grade becomes more undifferentiated; (2) Mucinous carcinomas rarely metastasize by way of the bloodstream; (3) The more the primary tumor penetrates the bowel wall, the greater are the chances of blood-borne metastases; (4) Visceral metastases are extremely unusual if a careful study of the resected specimen does not show local intravascular invasion. Only one patient in 70 had visceral metastases and no demonstrable vascular invasion.[78] Grinnell pointed out that visceral metastases usually occurred in patients with nodal spread. Only 25% (8 of 32 patients) with visceral metastases failed to also have nodal metastases.[27,68,71,73,78,81,138,143,223,224]

Recently, Khankhanian and co-workers have suggested that venous invasion is not in itself an independent pathologic variable.[230] They correlated vascular invasion "within the bowel wall" in the surgical specimen with postoperative tumor-free interval and survival. Dukes' B colorectal cancer patients with vascular invasion had nearly identical free interval and survival to patients without vascular invasion. The discrepancy of Khankhanian and co-workers with other investigators undoubtedly is due to the type of examination. Other investigators have looked for venous invasion into the superior or middle hemorrhoidal venous systems, not within the bowel wall. Vascular invasion of mural vessels is apparently not of prognostic significance, while invasion of extravascular veins is.

The data of Grinnell suggest that venous invasion does operate independently of lymph node involvement as a prognostic variable.[72] As Table 21-18 shows, Dukes' B patients with vein invasion have approximately the same chance of cure as cases that have node metastases (Dukes C) but no vein involvement. Also, C cases with vein invasion have a significantly poorer prognosis than those without vein invasion.

Perineural Invasion

Seefeld and Bargen studied the clinical and prognostic effects associated with perineural invasion seen on histopathologic study.[73] Definite local recurrences were found in 81.2% of patients in whom perineural invasion was seen, whereas in those without perineural invasion local recurrence was seen in 30.4%. Only two of 29 (6.9%) traceable patients survived 5 years with perineural invasion; 18 of 51 (35.3%) patients without perineural invasion survived.

Inflammatory Response Surrounding the Primary Tumor

Spratt and Spjut assayed microscopically the inflammatory reaction surrounding 802 colorectal cancers.[143] A complete absence of inflammation at the tumor margin was associated with a poor prognosis with only 20% of 127 patients surviving 5 years. A moderate inflammatory response was associated with a 36% survival (439 patients) and an intense response with abscess formation with a 41% (223 patients) survival. Thirteen patients were not classifiable.

Lymph Node Histology

Patt and co-workers studied histologic parameters within lymph nodes thought to reflect immunologic responses and correlated these with survival of 36 patients with sigmoid colon adenocarcinoma.[231] They examined nodes for sinus histiocytosis, paracortical activity, and germinal center activity. Both sinus histiocytosis and paracortical immunoblastic activity correlated with a significantly improved ($p < 0.05$) survival. If both sinus histiocytosis and abundant paracortical immunoblasts were present, survival was improved further. The presence or absence of germinal center activity was not associated with a significantly different survival. Pihl and co-workers and Tsakraklides have also correlated improved survival with immunoreactivity of regional lymph nodes in colorectal cancer patients.[232-234]

SCREENING FOR CANCER IN ASYMPTOMATIC PATIENT POPULATIONS

Several facts suggest that survival from colorectal cancer would be significantly improved if adequate screening tests were to be generally employed. First, this is an extremely common malignancy, with approximately 100,000 new cases in the United States each year. Every man and woman in the United States has approximately one chance in 25 of developing colorectal cancer in his or her lifetime. Second, there is ample time for detection; colorectal cancer is slow to grow from a small focus of malignancy to an incurable process. The doubling time is approximately two years (see section on natural history). Perhaps as many as 5 years pass between the occurrence of a detectable mass lesion and the presence of symptoms. Third, the presence of a tumor may be preceeded

TABLE 21-18. Five-Year Survival Results: Vein Invasion and Mural Penetration: Colon and Rectum

	NO VEIN INVASION			VEIN INVASION		
TOTAL CASES	*Total*	*5-Year Survival*	*Percent Survival*	*Total*	*5-Year Survival*	*Percent Survival*
A: 17	17	16	94	–	–	–
B: 47	32	28	88	15	9	60
C: 69	33	18	55	36	10	28
133	82	62		51	19	

(Grinnell RS: Lymphatic metastases of carcinoma of the colon and rectum. Ann Surg 131:494–506, 1950)

by many years by a malignant precursor—the adenoma. If adenomas are removed, the polyp-to-cancer sequence may be interrupted, full function preserved, and the disease completely prevented. Finally, as discussed in the section on prognosis, when tumors are detected early in an asymptomatic state, the cure rate is greatly improved. Survival is between 80% and 100% in patients in whom a diagnosis was made in the asymptomatic state.

At the present time the most efficient approach to colorectal cancer screening seems to be (1) the identification of high risk groups, (2) the employment of currently available screening tests in these groups, and (3) a thorough workup of patients with positive screening tests to find or exclude colorectal pathology.

HIGH RISK GROUPS FOR COLORECTAL CANCER

The high risk groups for colorectal malignancy are listed in Table 21-19.

Age Greater than 40 Years

The risk for men and women is approximately the same and begins to rise significantly between age 40 and 45. There is approximately a two-fold increase in each decade reaching a peak at age 75.[235] It is important to remember that cancer of the colon does occur below the age of 40 years, and when it does, the survival is much reduced (see section on prognosis).

Ulcerative Colitis as an Associated Disease

In patients with ulcerative colitis the risk of malignant change is greater when ulcerative colitis begins in childhood, has been present more than 10 years, involves the entire colon, has continuous rather than intermittent symptoms, and was of severe onset. The incidence of cancer is twice as high if colitis began before the age 25.[236] In all patients with ulcerative colitis compared to a normal population, the colorectal cancer risk is 5 to 11 times higher.[237–240]

TABLE 21-19. High Risk Groups for Colorectal Cancer

Age
Over 40 years in asymptomatic men and women
Associated disease
Ulcerative colitis
Granulomatous colitis
Past History
Colorectal adenomas
Colorectal cancer
Female genital cancer
Female breast cancer
Family history
Familial polyposis
Gardner's syndrome
Turcot's syndrome (CNS tumors)
Oldfield's syndrome (extensive sebaceous cysts)
Colorectal cancer
Colorectal polyps
Cancer family syndrome
Generalized gastrointestinal juvenile polyposis

Granulomatous Colitis as an Associated Disease

Weedon and co-workers showed that patients with granulomatous bowel disease (Crohn's disease) with onset of disease before age 21 had a 20 times greater risk of developing colorectal cancer.[241] Involved areas of both the small and large bowel are at increased risk. Cancer occurs at an earlier age than in a normal population and was frequently found in bypassed segments of intestine as well as in fistulous tracts.

History of Colorectal Adenomas

Prager and co-workers at the Lahey Clinic followed 305 patients who by proctosigmoidoscopy were shown to have adenomas. After a followup period of 15 years the incidence of cancer in this population was twice that expected in a normal population; this was a statistically significant ($p < 0.05$) increased incidence.[52] Rider and co-workers reviewed their experience with carcinoma of the colorectum in patients with and without polyps.[53] In 7086 patients without polyps, the incidence of carcinoma was 2.1%. The incidence of invasive malignancy in 401 polyp patients was 10.7%. In 14 of the 43 polyp patients (33%) the polyp itself was the site of invasive malignancy. In the other 29 patients the carcinoma developed before (nine patients) at the same time, (13 patients) or after, (7 patients) the polyp and in a different area of the large bowel. Rider and associates also showed that patients with multiple polyps are twice as likely to develop carcinoma as individuals with a single polyp. They found 33 carcinomas in 352 patients with a single polyp (9.4%) and 10 carcinomas in 49 patients with multiple polyps (20.4%).

Copeland, Miller, and Jones presented additional data to support the concept that a colon that develops an adenoma is also prone to undergo malignant degeneration at some time; 23% of patients with a single colon cancer had associated polyps.[138] The incidence of polyps in the general population is only 5.4%.[53] In patients who had second primary large bowel cancer, 50% of synchronous lesions and 60% of metachronous lesions had associated polyps. Also, in patients with multiple polyps in the primary cancer specimen the incidence of second primary large bowel cancer was 2.5 times greater than in patients with single polyps.

History of Colorectal Cancer

There can be no doubt that patients with previous colorectal cancer must be considered at increased risk for subsequent large bowel cancer even though a substantial part of this organ is resected with the first cancer. Schottenfeld, Berg, and Vitsky reported the annual incidence of subsequent primary cancer of the large bowel to be 3.5 per 1000 patients at risk, which represents a threefold excess over that expected in the general population.[242] Similar increased risk for a second primary large bowel cancer has been reported.[243]

History of Female Genital or Breast Cancer

Women with female genital tract or breast cancer have an increased large bowel cancer risk.[244] It is not clear whether this association exists only within the "cancer family syndrome" or whether these combinations of multiple primary cancer can occur as isolated cases.

History of Radiation Therapy for Cervical Cancer

MacMahon and Rowe and Castro, Rosen, and Quan have suggested that prior radiation therapy for cervical or uterine cancer was etiologically related to the development of sigmoid colon cancer.[245,246] No data regarding the overall incidence of rectosigmoid cancer in patients receiving pelvic radiation was available in these studies and more study of this problem needs to be done before a definite correlation of rectosigmoid cancer and prior pelvic irradiation can be made.

Familial Polyposis Syndromes

Familial polyposis is a disease in which the colon of affected individuals becomes by age 15 to 25 covered by innumerable adenomatous polyps. The disease is inherited as an autosomal dominant trait with 90% penetrance. Unless colectomy is performed in early adulthood, death from colon cancer approaches 100% by age 55. By age 37, over 50% of patients will develop adenocarcinoma; patients often manifest multiple cancers.[50] After age 50, individuals in a polyposis family who have not yet developed polyps are unlikely to ever manifest the disease.[247]

Familial polyposis may arise *de novo* in a population as a genetic mutation. More commonly, a family history with autosomal dominant inheritance is discovered. It becomes extremely important to identify these families so that family members can be examined frequently to determine whether they are in the unlucky 50% to develop polyposis. In the past, two-thirds of patients when first seen with polyposis also had evidence of cancer. In carefully followed family groups this has been reduced to 9%.[248] Only a very small number of all patients with colorectal cancer occur in polyposis families. In Michigan, Reed and Neel found the incidence to be 1 in 8300; in Kentucky, Pierce found it to be 1 in 6850.[249,250] However, in this clinical situation early diagnosis and treatment can eliminate the risk of cancer.

Gardner's syndrome is a second polyposis syndrome.[251] About one in seven families with a polyposis syndrome has one or several of the associated features of Gardner's syndrome. These are sebaceous cysts, desmoid tumors, fibromas, facial bone osteomas, and abnormal dentition. Turcot described a variant polyposis syndrome in which malignant tumors of the central nervous system were associated with familial polyposis.[252] Also, Oldfield described a syndrome in which multiple sebaceous cysts were found in patients with polyposis coli and colorectal adenocarcinoma.[253] In the Peutz–Jeghers syndrome multiple polyps throughout the gastrointestinal tract are associated with melanin pigmentation of the buccal mucosa, lips, face, fingers, toes, vagina, and anus.[254] However, in this syndrome the intestinal polyps are not adenomas, but hamartomas and there is no good evidence for an increased risk of intestinal cancer.

There is increasing evidence that the genetic defect in the polyposis syndromes is not limited to the adenomas that develop.[255] The colonic epithelial cells throughout the colon lose their ability to repress DNA synthesis. Cutaneous epidermal cells are also apparently abnormal. When grown in culture, cutaneous fibroblasts grow with criss-cross orientation and in multilayers rather than the usual growth pattern of monolayers. Also, fibroblasts in culture from patients with polyposis coli are comparatively more susceptable to viral transformation by murine sarcoma virus.[256] Also, metabolic abnormalities are suggested by higher amounts of undergraded cholesterol in the stool of familial polyposis patients.[257] These systemic variations seen in association with familial polyposis syndromes offer great promise in screening families and perhaps even the fetus for disease.

Family History of Colorectal Cancer

Independent of polyposis syndromes and cancer families, colon cancer shows a "modest familial aggregation."[258] This familial susceptibility is not synonymous with genetic causation but may be due to environmental factors. Whatever the causation, family members who have a relative with large bowel cancer have three to four times the risk of this disease. Lovette obtained detailed family histories on 209 patients treated at St. Mark's in London for cancer of the large bowel.[248] Forty-two cancers of the large bowel were found in mothers, fathers, brothers, or sisters of colorectal cancer patients. Only 11.65 such cancers would be expected in a general population. This was not just an increase in all cancers for those families, but seemed to be largely specific for colon and rectum. In male relatives, carcinoma of the large bowel was recorded more than twice as frequently as cancer of the bronchus. Among females, colorectal cancer was recorded more than twice as frequently as breast cancer. Also, large bowel malignancy occurs at an earlier age in relatives of patients with large bowel cancer.[259]

Hereditary Colorectal Cancer

Lynch and Lynch have reviewed the multiple reports of hereditary colon cancer occurring without a polyposis syndrome.[260] The syndrome is characterized by autosomal dominant inheritance, a low mean age (41 years) for the occurrence of colon cancer, and a marked increase proportion of tumors in the proximal colon. Sixty-five percent of large bowel cancers in this syndrome occur in the proximal colon (above the sigmoid) whereas only 35% occur in this portion of the colon in a general population.[261] Finally, in this syndrome solitary adenomatous polyps may occur in a large proportion of family members in either the presence or absence of colorectal cancer.[262]

Cancer Family Syndrome

In these families there is an increased risk of adenocarcinomas of all varieties with a particular predominance of carcinoma of the colon and endometrium.[263,264] Cancers occur at an early mean age and multiple primary malignant neoplasms in one individual frequently occurs. The inheritance is autosomal dominant. Williams has emphasized the need for serial diagnostic tests and education in cancer families.[265]

Familial Juvenile Polyposis

Haggitt and Pitcock described two patients with juvenile polyposis of the colon accompanied by a family history of colonic cancer at a young age.[266] The patients did not have a typical familial polyposis syndrome for the polyps were not numerous enough (30 in one patient and 80 in the other) and were typical juvenile polyps rather than adenomas. Stemper, Kent, and Summers emphasized that the juvenile polyps could occur throughout the gastrointestinal tract and that malignancy in the family occurred unusually frequently in the stomach and right colon.[267] No cases of primary rectal or sigmoid cancer were seen. These authors suggest that persons with a gene for juvenile polyps may express this gene in more than a single fashion; malignant foci within the gastrointestinal tract would be an alternate mode of gene expression.

SCREENING TECHNIQUES FOR COLORECTAL CANCER

After one identifies the groups at high risk for colorectal cancer, the appropriate screening test to employ needs to be identified.

Stool Test for Blood, Hemoccult

Success with the hemoccult test to screen a general population for cancer must be attributed in large part to the persistent efforts of Greegor.[268,269] He developed a test that utilized guaiac-impregnated paper on which a small quantity of stool could be smeared. This slide of paper was contained in a cardboard envelope; by this method the testing of stool for occult blood is esthetically tolerable for most individuals. By adjusting the sensitivity of the test, the number of false-positive and false-negative tests has been minimized. Christensen, Anker, and Mondrup compared the sensitivity and reproducibility of five different methods of testing the stool for occult blood and concluded that the hemoccult method was the best available.[270]

To further help eliminate false-positive tests, patients are asked to refrain from eating meat, fish, and chicken for at least 24 hours before stool specimens are collected. Also, large quantities of vegetables, fruit and cereal are to be consumed for a high residue diet. This roughage in the diet is designed to cause an ulcerated or necrotic area of tumor to bleed slightly and, in so doing, help eliminate false negative examinations. Deyhle and co-workers presented data suggesting that a high roughage diet did decrease false-negative tests.[271] Also, to help eliminate false-negative examinations, two samples of stool from different areas of a fecal mass are to be collected on three consecutive days (total of 6 specimens). Winawer and co-workers call attention to the fact that a single positive slide is as likely to reveal neoplasia as multiple positive slides.[272] Therefore, careful follow-up studies are required if only one slide is positive, the same as if all slides are positive.

With experience in using the hemoccult test to date, several problems have been identified. Miller pointed out that responses to mass screening were from "cancer oriented" populations.[273] In five different mass screening projects just under 10,000 individuals returned slides. Twenty-two cancers were found; however, only three to five would be expected in a general population. It seems likely that not all patients participating were actually asymptomatic. It is not surprising therefore that the stage of disease in the early hemoccult studies was not much different than would be found in a group of symptomatic patients. A second consistent finding is the low proportion of a population participating in a mass screening project. Only 1% to 3% of individuals in a study population participate.[274,277] In contrast to the low proportion of participants, the compliance of individuals who do enroll is 85%.

Undoubtedly, the greatest problem with the hemoccult method as used today is false-negative results. Even with the most cautious interpretation of the results, a negative test for cancer implies that malignancy has been ruled out—especially to the patient. Unfortunately, nearly as many adenomas are missed as are found and some cancers (about 20%) are not detected when individuals completing the hemoccult test undergo sigmoidoscopy or fiberoptic sigmoidoscopy.[277-279] The various causes of false-positive and false-negative hemoccult tests are shown in Table 21-20. Many of these undesirable results can be avoided by careful patient instruction.

In an ongoing study at the Strang Clinic in New York City, data on the utility of the hemoccult method in large number of truly asymptomatic persons is being accumulated.[279] In 9709 hemoccult tests in men and women, aged 40 years and over, 1% of patients had at least one positive slide. Half of the hemoccult positive patients had, upon workup, neoplastic lesions. Neoplastic lesions were defined as polyps greater than 5 mm in diameter (38%) and cancers (12%). The other 50% of hemoccult-positive patients had diverticulosis only, polyps less than 5 mm, or no pathology was found. This meant that the hemoccult method had a very respectable predictive value of 50%. Also, the false-positive ratio was 0.5%; this is probably a tolerable number of negative follow-up studies that must be completed.

Gilbertsen and co-workers have emphasized that proper follow-up examination of hemoccult-positive patient populations is required if early potentially curable carcinomas are to be detected.[280] At the time of Gilbertsen's report, 72 primary carcinomas had been detected through hemoccult screening.

TABLE 21-20. Causes of False-Positive and False-Negative Tests Using the Hemoccult Method

FALSE-POSITIVE TESTS	FALSE-NEGATIVE TESTS
Meat in diet	Failure to employ high residue diet
Diverticulosis	Vitamin C in diet
Minor anorectal problems hemorrhoids fissures proctitis	Time lag between specimen collection and specimen examination Failure to properly prepare slides or complete all six slides
Peroxidases in skins of vegetables and fruits (tomatoes and cherries)	Followup examinations which failed to detect lesion
Upper gastrointestinal pathology gastritis from ASA ingestion ulcer disease hiatus hernia gastric malignancy	Lesion not bleeding at the time of stool collection Outdated Hemoccult slides or reagent

Sixteen were in the rectum and found by endoscopy. Fifty-six of the carcinomas were in the colon, 33 were suspected by barium enema. No evidence for the presence of cancer in the remaining 19 was found by careful roentgenographic examinations. These cancers were detected by subsequent colonoscopic examination. Roentgenographic examination missed only one of 11 Dukes C and D carcinomas, but missed 19 of 45 more likely curable Dukes A and B carcinomas. Gilbertsen and colleagues conclude that colonoscopy was superior to barium enema in the diagnostic evaluation of hemoccult-positive patients. Their present routine is to recommend barium enema only if colonoscopy is not complete.

The most encouraging results from studies utilizing the hemoccult method are those showing patients with an early stage of disease when cancer is detected by hemoccult screening.[149] Seventy-seven percent were Dukes A or B lesions, 16% were Dukes C, and only 7% Dukes D. The improved prognosis one expects from cancer diagnosis in the asymptomatic state is apparently true for the hemoccult method of testing.

Winawer and co-workers have itemized the "debits and credits" of the hemoccult method of testing for fecal occult blood to detect colorectal cancer.[276] A revised list is given in Table 21-21.

Digital Rectal Examination

Although digital rectal examination is a standard part of every physical examination and proctosigmoidoscopic examination, few studies have singled out the utility of rectal examination for screening. Miller and Knight provided rectal examination as an optional part of their hemoccult screening project.[276] Patients with a "rectal mass" were subsequently studied by sigmoidoscopy and barium enema. Of 2332 patients, 28 rectal masses were noted; two carcinomas and four adenomatous polyps were among these 28. False-positive examinations included hemorrhoids, hypertrophic papillae, postoperative tear, fissure, and normal examination. Digital rectal examination does detect significant numbers of neoplasms and should be a part of a screening program if logistically possible.

Sigmoidoscopy

There seems little doubt that sigmoidoscopy used as a screening test can detect reasonable numbers of rectal and rectosigmoid cancers. The real question is whether the expenditures of time and money are best spent on sigmoidoscopy or on other health care programs. Between two and five cancers will be found by sigmoidoscopy in each 1000 asymptomatic men and women over the age of 40.[41,145] The tumors identified in asymptomatic patients will also result in a markedly improved prognosis (see section on prognosis).

There is a second benefit to the patients from sigmoidoscopic examination. Adenomas are seen and removed and this apparently interrupts the polyp to cancer sequence. This led Gilbertsen to postulate that large bowel cancer was a "preventable disease."[40]

Bolt questioned if "routine sigmoidoscopy was the final answer to cancer of the rectosigmoid."[281] His reasoning was as follows: for each 10,000 examinations about 20 cancers would be detected in an asymptomatic state. From the data of Hertz, Deddish, and Day, 88% 5-year survival would be expected in these patients; with symptoms 50% survival would be expected.[145] Therefore, 17 of 20 rather than ten of 20 of these patients would survive their malignancy. If the cost of each sigmoidoscopy examination is 50 dollars, the screening program for the 10,000 patients would cost 500,000 dollars. Each life spared a cancer death would cost about 70,000 dollars.

Because of the expense of routine sigmoidoscopic examination, Corman, Coller, and Veidenheimer suggested that screening should not begin until age 50.[147] Also, because of the growth rate of adenomas and carcinomas, repeat examinations could be done every 2 years rather than annually. In 2500 sigmoidoscopic examinations at the Lahey Clinic in asymptomatic patients 50 years of age or under, no cancers were found.

Flexible Fiberoptic Sigmoidoscopy

Recently, interest in a flexible fiberoptic instrument to examine the entire rectum and sigmoid colon has been renewed. This instrument, about 60 cm in length, can be navigated from anus to junction of sigmoid and descending colon; biopsy channels allow biopsy and polyp removal on an outpatient basis.

Several groups have shown, as would be expected, that with visualization of about three times the length of bowel, about three times the number of adenomas and carcinomas are detected.[277,278,282,283]

Credits as a screening device for flexible sigmoidoscopy include the following points. First, a greater number of lesions are detected as compared to rigid sigmoidoscopy. Recent epidemiologic data suggest that there has been a proximal migration of carcinoma of the colon.[12–14] Second, patient tolerance of the examination with the flexible instrument is the same or better than with the rigid instrument.[278,282] Finally, photographic recording of lesions is possible, and biopsy and polypectomy are safer and speedier with the fiberoptic instrument than with the rigid sigmoidoscope; this is especially true if polyps are above the peritoneal reflection.

TABLE 21-21. Credits and Debits of Fecal Occult Blood Testing

CREDITS
1. Good patient compliance (85%)
2. Manageable percentage of positive slides (approximately 1%)
3. High percentage of neoplastic lesions in patients with positive slides (approximately 50%).
4. Favorable pathological staging of detected cancers in asymptomatic screened patients (86% localized)

DEBITS
1. Low participation by general population
2. False-positive rate for both colorectal cancers and adenomas (approximately 0.5%).
3. Demonstrated false negativity for neoplastic lesions in rectosigmoid area, especially with adenomas.
4. Conversion of positive slides to negative.

(Modified from Winauer SJ, Andrews M, Flehinger B: Progress report on controlled trial of fecal occult blood testing for the detection of colorectal neoplasia. Cancer 45:2959–2964, 1980)

Debits of the flexible fiberoptic instrument include: (1) greater time requirement for the procedure; (2) more involved patient preparation; (3) a requirement for more highly trained personnel; (4) greater cost for the instrumentation; and (5) still about one-third of colonic lesions (those above junction of sigmoid and descending colon) not detected.

Further trials with the flexible fiberoptic sigmoidoscope are needed to fully assess its utility.

DIAGNOSIS OF COLORECTAL CANCER IN THE SYMPTOMATIC PATIENT

Early carcinoma of the colorectum is an asymptomatic process. The common symptoms are relatively late manifestations of the disease. Also, unfortunately, the colon has a minimal number of ways that it can respond to a great variety of neoplastic infectious, vascular or traumatic processes. Symptoms which usually accompany a harmless process may mask similar symptoms produced by a malignant tumor.

Jones studied the "normal bowel habit" of 112 New Zealand men and women over age 40 and randomly selected from the population.[284] Six percent of persons reported continuous trouble with constipation. Over half of them reported blood *per* rectum, 24% on the feces and 32% on the toilet paper. Twenty-two percent had noted weight loss. Jones concludes that "one factor which greatly impairs the diagnostic process is the familiarity of the symptomatology when it occurs." Blood *per* rectum, for example, was found so common as to be considered normal. He questioned the value of educational programs which remind the public of symptoms they have repeatedly experienced.

The five most common symptoms of colorectal cancer are shown in Table 21-22.[285] It should be emphasized that nearly any symptom can occur from a cancer in any region of the colorectum. Abdominal pain is the most common symptom of colon cancer. In right colon cancer, pain is ill-defined; it may be confused with gallbladder or peptic ulcer disease. The characteristic feature of this pain is that it has no distinguishing features. In left colon cancer, pain is usually of an intermittent nature and secondary to constriction of the bowel lumen. The patient will often complain of gas cramps. In patients with rectal cancer, local pain and a sense of incomplete evacuation is common; pain in the low back or radiating down the legs is a sign of locally advanced disease.

Rectal bleeding from a right colon cancer is usually brick red with blood and stool mixed. With tumors in the left colon, blood coats the stool and is brighter red. Anemia may result from chronic blood loss more commonly with right colon cancer. A change in bowel habit is seen with cancer at any site but a change in the caliber of the stool is characteristic of left colon cancer.

In a patient that complains of symptoms possibly related to colon or rectal cançer, a careful history is very important. In the review of symptoms direct questioning about other symptoms of possible colorectal pathology should be done: general complaints (fatigue, weight loss) or site-specific complaints (pneumaturia from sigmoidovesical fistula) can be valuable clues suggesting the need for definitive workup. Personal history of other malignancy (especially breast or endometrial) or previous adenoma or large bowel cancer should greatly increase one's index of suspicion. A positive family history will also place the patient in a higher risk category.

In performing the physical examination one should train himself or herself to look for and recognize any external signs of colorectal malignancy. External inspection of the eyes and skin should be thorough. Is there pallor caused by anemia, is the skin thin? Does the patient appear fatigued, tired, depressed, suggesting nutritional deprivation from an internal malignancy? What about the skin color; are there areas of brown discoloration, especially at flexures, which may be acanthosis nigricians? Dermatomyositis and pruritus have been associated with large bowel cancer.[286,287]

In the remainder of the physical exam, suspicious findings must be recognized and noted. The lymph nodes especially the left supraclavicular (Virchow's nodes) and inguinal areas are at risk for metastatic disease. The liver size should be carefully determined. Abdominal masses may be felt, especially with right colon cancer. Abdominal distention and hyperactive bowel sounds may suggest partial obstruction from a constricting lesion. On rectal examination the presence or absence of a mass must be determined; also, a rectal shelf or nodularity along the pelvic sidewall can occasionally be felt. Although a random stool sample should not be used to rule out large bowel cancer, the presence or absence of blood in the stool should be determined.[288] If the gloved finger returns containing flecks of blood and pieces of necrotic debris, carcinoma or villous adenoma of the rectum is likely present. Upon performing the rectal examination, one must not suspect all tumors to be hard and either polypoid or ulcerated. Villous adenomas, because they lack a well-developed stroma, can be extremely soft to the touch. Also, some tumors arise as plaque-like growths; if one is feeling for a polypoid or ulcerated tumor, such plaque-like tumors may be missed. In females, pelvic examination is important; if pos-

TABLE 21-22. A Comparison of the Five Most Frequent Symptoms in Rectal, Left Colon and Right Colon Cancer

RECTUM AND RECTOSIGMOID (258 Patients)	LEFT COLON (99 Patients)	RIGHT COLON (984 Patients)
Melena (85%)	Abdominal pain (72%)	Ablominal pain (74%)
Constipation (46%)	Melena (53%)	Weakness (29%)
Tenesmus (30%)	Constipation (42%)	Melena (27%)
Diarrhea (30%)	Nausea (25%)	Nausea (24%)
Abdominal pain (26%)	Vomiting (23%)	Abdominal mass (23%)

(Postlethwait RW: Malignant tumors of the colon and rectum. Ann Surg 129:34–46, 1949)

sible, the size of each ovary should be determined to rule out ovarian metastases.

If any of the major symptoms or signs of large bowel malignancy are present, sigmoidoscopy and barium enema are definitely indicated; even though rectal bleeding is accompanied by hemorrhoids, or anemia accompanied by a poor dietary history, further workup is indicated. Major symptoms cannot be attributed to a benign process until malignancy is ruled out.

The sigmoidoscopic examination should be the first special test performed. About one-third of colorectal neoplasia can be seen with this instrument. If a flexible fiberoptic instrument is available, even better, for nearly two-thirds of problems can be diagnosed with it. A digital rectal examination precedes introduction of the well-lubricated sigmoidoscope. The sigmoidoscope should be advanced as far as possible without severe discomfort. The initial 10 cm are straight along the anterior surface of the sacrum. When the rectosigmoid junction is reached, advancement under direct vision is required. Jackman has emphasized that withdrawal of the sigmoidoscope and redirection using the anus as a fulcrum, allows passage around the rectosigmoid.[127] Once around the impasse, complete examination to 25 cm is customary, but this part of the examination is usually somewhat painful and should be completed as quickly as possible. Careful observation is done as the sigmoidoscope is withdrawn.

If a polyp is visualized, it is biopsied; removal usually is best performed at a second examination when the possible hazards of electrosurgery have been explained to the patient and the bowel is more thoroughly prepared to prevent possible explosion. If a carcinoma is detected, important information to characterize the lesion should be recorded. The following should be noted in the patient's permanent record: [1] An anatomic description of the tumor as ulcerated (crateriform) polypoid or plaque-like; [2] degree of fixation to the bowel wall and to surrounding structures (Figure 21-10). When the lesion is palpated or nudged by the sigmoidoscope tip, does it move freely without moving the surrounding mucosa? If it does, the lesion is not invasive and may even possess a short stalk. When the lesion is nudged, does the surrounding bowel move with the cancer? If it does, the lesion has invaded bowel wall but is not fixed to other pelvic structures.[289] What about transmission of motion to the uterus and vagina when the cancer is manipulated? If, in attempting to move the mass, it seems adherent to pelvic side wall, sacrum, or abdominal contents, advanced adjacent organ involvement must be suspected; [3] the location of the tumor within the circumference of the bowel lumen and the percent of the circumference involved should be noted carefully. This is best done generally by describing the tumor as extending from one number to another as on a clock face (*i.e.*, 12 to 3:00 o'clock); and [4] the distance of the upper and lower edge of the tumor from the anal verge should be noted. A biopsy should be taken for tissue confirmation of malignancy and to histopathologically grade the tumor.

Barium enema is needed to rule out a large bowel neoplasm if suggested by the patient's history. If the sigmoidoscopy has been positive, the barium enema is needed to help further characterize the lesion and to rule out other colorectal pathology. If a biopsy was performed in doing the sigmoidoscopy,

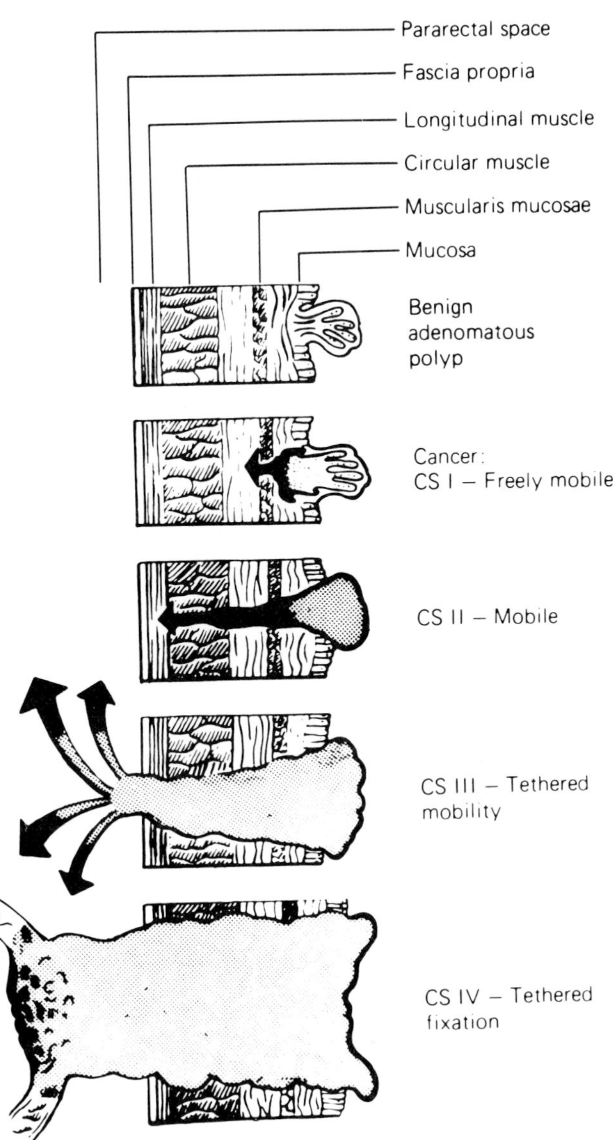

FIG. 21-10. Determination of the depth of penetration of rectal cancer by tumor mass mobility. (Mason AY: Transsphincteric surgery for lower rectum cancer. Surg Tech Illust. 2:73, 1977

the barium enema should be delayed 10 days to allow healing of the mucosa and submucosa. This will help prevent inadvertent submucosal dissection of barium or bowel perforation during the barium enema examination.

A great improvement in the diagnostic accuracy of the barium enema examination is the double contrast enema. In this examination, barium coats the large bowel lumen that is insufflated with air. Therefore, not only large filling defects within a column of barium are detected, but also small lesions coated by barium in an air-filled bowel are seen directly. Colonoscopy is an important tool that needs to be used in the preoperative work-up of all large bowel cancer patients. The high incidences of two synchronous primary large bowel cancers and of concomitant polyps (*see* section on screening) require that preoperative colonoscopy be done. Careful examination of the entire large bowel before surgery is needed if all malignant and precancerous lesions are to be consistently removed; this probably can be done most accurately with colonoscopy.[290-296]

CONSTRICTING LESIONS FROM LARGE BOWEL CANCER

By barium enema, colorectal cancer is seen as either a filling defect within the bowel lumen or as a constricting lesion. The filling defects may be flat or polypoid; these lesions may progress to become constricting.[297] Filling defects, especially the flat type, may be difficult to detect radiologically. Constricting cancer produces a segmental narrowing of the bowel lumen. Two important radiologic features of the colorectal malignancy may help in differentiating it from other constricting processes. First, there is usually an *abrupt* change from normal caliber to narrowed bowel lumen. This occurs because the tumor usually grows vertically from the epithelial (inside) surface into the bowel lumen, giving the proximal and distal edge of the lesion the appearance of a "shoulder." Other processes that tend to constrict do so from outside the bowel lumen and cause a tapering effect. Second, in lesions caused by colorectal cancer, the mucosa within the constricting lesion is almost invariably ulcerated. In most other causes of constriction the mucosa is intact.

Table 21-23 lists the processes other than colorectal cancer that may cause colonic constriction.[298-322] Some of these are easily differentiated from large bowel cancer by history and physical examination, for the constricting lesion is accompanied by other manifestations of the disease process. Other conditions may be differentiated from colorectal cancer only when a high index of suspicion prompts one to search for other causes of bowel constrictions.

TABLE 21-23. Differentiation of Colorectal Cancer from other Constricting Lesions*

PROCESSES INTRINSIC TO THE LARGE BOWEL
Inflammatory
Diverticulitis (298,299)
Diverticulosis (300)
Chronic ulcerative colitis (301)
Acute ulcerative colitis (302)
Granulomatous colitis
Infarction of appendices epiploical (303)
Foreign body (304)
Abcess from perforated walled off appendicitis (305)
Actinomycosis (306)
Tuberculosis (307)
Ameboma (308)
Vascular
Acute ischemis (309–311)
Chronic ischemia (310,311)
Other
Colitis cystica profunda (312)
Physiologic sphincters (313)
Idiopathic muscular stricture (314)
Mucocele of the appendix (305)
PROCESSES EXTRINSIC TO THE LARGE BOWEL
Inflammatory
Pancreatitis (315)
Gastrojejunostomy site (316)
Neoplastic
Renal cell carcinoma (317,318)
Lymphoma (318)
Ovarian carcinoma (318)
Other
Endometriosis (319–322)

* Reference numbers in parentheses

DIAGNOSIS OF RECURRENT COLORECTAL CANCER

Polk and Spratt studied the symptoms and physical signs of recurrent colorectal cancer.[323] The symptoms of recurrent colon cancer were nonspecific and contributed little to diagnosis. Crampy abdominal pain and constipation were complaints as frequently in those who remained tumor free as in those who recurred. One symptom, weight loss, was seen in 23 of 121 patients with recurrence. For rectal cancer, symptoms of dull aching perineal discomfort aggravated by sitting preceded detection by 1 month to 9 months in 16 of 20 patients developing recurrent cancer in the perineal scar. Sugarbaker, Zamcheck, and Moore performed a prospective study attempting to determine the most sensitive objective test by which to detect recurrent disease.[324] Monthly serial CEA assays, 3 monthly physical examinations, and a battery of laboratory and radiologic tests were employed on a monthly basis on 34 patients. Serial CEA assay was the earliest indication of recurrence in 58% of patients, physical examination in 25%, and CEA assay simultaneous with physical exam in 8%. The laboratory and radiologic tests did not detect recurrence in any patients, but barium enema did detect new polyps in two.

TREATMENT OF COLORECTAL POLYPS

Before the development of colonoscopy and snare polypectomy by Wolff and Shinya, each patient with a polypoid lesion above the reach of the sigmoidoscope was an individual problem in management.[325] An important surgical equation had to be constructed in which the surgical risk of colotomy had to be weighed against the risk of invasive malignancy. Polyps 1 cm or greater in size were estimated to have a 3% incidence of invasive malignancy; this was thought to match the risk of surgical removal.[69,326] Therefore, in patients who were reasonable candidates for surgery, polyp resection was recommended for lesions 1 cm or greater in size. Patients who might tolerate surgery less well were followed by serial (initially six-monthly and then yearly) barium enema examinations.[327] The rate of growth of the lesion was assumed to indicate the risk of nonoperative management; indeed many lesions were watched for many years with little or no growth of the lesion and no harmful sequelae.

The colonoscope and the techniques developed by Shinya for colonoscopic polypectomy have revolutionized the treatment of colonic polyps.[325] At the present time even the smallest of polyps (1 mm-5 mm) in diameter can be visualized and biopsied. Destruction of these minute lesions using the hot biopsy technique can be safely accomplished in experienced hands.[328] Larger polyps (5 mm and greater) can be removed *in toto* for complete histopathological examination using the snare technique. The risk of this procedure is extremely low. Complications occur with diagnostic examination in about 0.1% of procedures and, if electrosurgery is used, 1.0% or less. Death from complications of the procedure is exceptionally rare, with only a few cases reported to date. The surgical equation is now markedly in favor of polyp resection unless the patient has a limited life expectancy.

The difficult decision in treating colonic polyps now occurs when a resected lesion contains a malignant foci. When should colectomy be recommended? The work of Lane and Kaye is of great help in determining the best answer in this clinical situation.[26] Their studies have shown that the muscularis mucosa is of great importance in determining the potential for spread a polyp may possess. If the carcinomatous tissue is restricted to the zone superficial to the boundary indicated by bundles of the muscularis mucosa, it is an *in situ* malignancy (Fig. 21-11). If the malignant foci have penetrated into the muscularis mucosa, it must be considered invasive. Fenoglio and co-workers showed by light and electron microscopic studies, that there is a lymphatic plexus associated with the muscularis mucosae, but there are no lymphatics above this level.[11] They suggest that this explains why lymphatic metastases from superficial intramucosal foci of carcinoma in adenomas do not occur.

In constructing a surgical equation to decide if further treatment is indicated following colonoscopic polypectomy, the six questions presented in Table 21-24 must be considered. It is important to determine at the time of colonoscopic polypectomy if a lesion is sessile or pedunculated, for the management plan is quite different for the two lesions. Often a polyp that initially appears sessile is really pedunculated on a short stalk with an overgrowth of adenomatous tissue that rests on normal mucosa. However, often both adenomatous and villous polyps may be sessile; colonoscopic removal is reasonable and may require resection by a piecemeal technique. After resection of a sessile polyp the endoscopist should attempt to reconstruct the lesion and orient the pathologist so that vertical histopathologic sections can be taken. A special burden is put on the pathologist if *in situ* malignancy is seen in a sessile lesion. Does the foci of malignancy cross the muscularis mucosa (Fig. 21-11*B*)? This may be very difficult or impossible to determine, especially if the lesion is friable or has been traumatized in resection. If the lesion can confidently be categorized as *in situ* no further therapy is indicated. A check colonoscopy in 6 months to observe the resection site would be all that is indicated. If the lesion shows invasive malignancy in a sessile polyp, colonic resection of the tumor and its relevant lymphatic arcade should be performed.

FIG. 21-11. Determination of *in situ* or invasive malignancy in polyps using the muscularis mucosa. (*A*) Pedunculated polyp. (*B*) Sessile polyp. (Modified from Lane N, Kaye GI: Pendunculated adenomatous polyp of the colon with carcinoma, lymph node metastasis, and suture-line recurrence: Report of a case and discussion of terminology problems. Am J Clin Pathol 48:172, 1967)

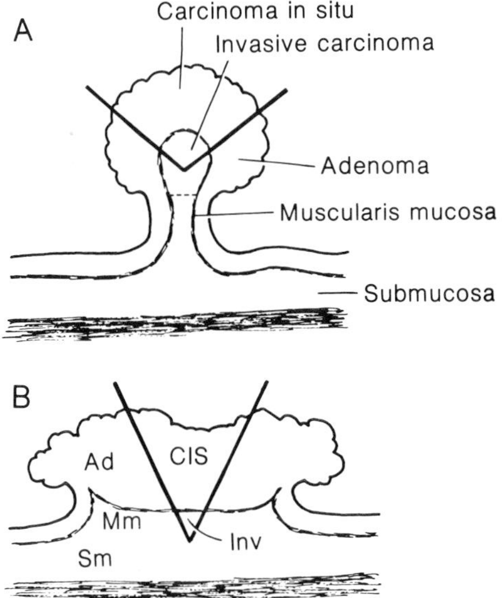

TABLE 21-24. Construction of a "Surgical Equation" for Treatment of Colonic Polyps Removed by Colonoscopic Polypectomy

1. Is the excised polyp sessile or pedunculated?
2. Is the focus of carcinoma *in situ* or invasive?
3. Was the margin of resection clear?
4. Is the focus of carcinoma poorly differentiated?
5. What is the patient's operative risk?
6. Will close endoscopic follow-up be possible?

If the resected polyp is pedunculated, the surgical approach can be somewhat less aggressive. Of course, as with sessile lesions, if the foci of malignancy are *in situ*, no further treatment but only followup is indicated. If the foci of malignancy are invasive, an assessment of the adequacy of the margin of resection must be made. If there is danger of malignant tissue being left behind, resection of that portion of bowel is indicated. Also, if the foci of invasive malignancy are poorly differentiated, spread to lymphatics is possible. At present, the incidence of lymphatic or hematogenous metastases from poorly differentiated cancer confined to the head or stalk of a pedunculated polyp is not known. That it does occur has been definitely established and must usually weigh the surgical equation in favor of colectomy.

In this approach to colonic polyp management, bowel resection is not recommended in malignant pedunculated polyps that have a generous margin of resection and that contain no poorly differentiated cancer. This approach has been adopted by Knutson and Max, Wolff and Shinya, Shatney and co-workers and Sugarbaker and co-workers.[325,329–331] Recently, Hedberg has questioned the wisdom in this approach to invasive malignancy. He found five of nine colonoscopically resected pedunculated polyps with foci of invasive malignancy to have lymph node metastases at the time of colonic resection (personal communication 1979). Perhaps other relative criteria for colectomy should be included until further follow-up of the conservative approach is available. If the patient is young and an excellent operative risk, resection may be recommended. If the foci of invasion are not limited, involve part or all of the head of the polyp or even extend into the stalk, resection should be further considered. Lymphatic invasion within the head of a pedunculated polyp has been associated with lymp node metastases and local intramural recurrence and may also suggest the need for surgical resection.[330,332]

Not infrequently, broad-based or extremely large polyps within the colon that cannot be safely resected by colonoscopic surgery are encountered. These lesions should be removed by colectomy plus a limited resection of the lymphatic arcade. The rate of invasive malignancy in these large polyps approaches 50%; colonoscopy with biopsy and brush cytology may help determine the malignant character of these lesions prior to their surgical removal.[333] Colotomy, polypectomy, and histopathological determination of malignancy or benignancy by cryostat sectioning does not carry a lesser morbidity and mortality than does simple segmental resection of the colon.

In the rectum the treatment of large broad-based lesions is more of a problem, for adequate resection of a segment of bowel may require a permanent colostomy. Lockhart-Mummery and Dukes reviewed the pathology and results of treatment of malignant rectal polyps and concluded that the important factors in deciding about further radical surgery after local removal were histological grade of malignancy in the polyp and the presence of absence of a free margin of excision.[334] Carden and Morson followed up on patients treated at St. Mark's Hospital and were guided by these principles.[332] Forty patients received local excision alone and seven of these (17.5%) developed a recurrence. In five of these seven cases, review of the pathology suggested that a more aggressive surgical approach should have been taken. One patient had high-grade malignancy and four others had deeply invasive malignancy (of average grade) to the limits of resection. In the other two cases, anterior resection for local recurrence resulted in a 7-year survival free of disease in one patient and in another, rectal resection of a Dukes C tumor resulted in postoperative death. Carden and Morson conclude that local removal can be justified if: (1) the tumor is not poorly differentiated; (2) multiple histological sections of the whole tumor confirmed that local excision is complete; and (3) regular followup is employed.

Large villous tumors of the rectum present several special problems. First, because of sampling error, it may be difficult or impossible to determine if a lesion is benign or malignant. If initial biopsies show only villous polyp but the lesion is clinically suspicious for malignancy, repeat deeper biopsies obtained with the patient under general anesthesia are indicated. Otani has suggested that foci of malignant transformation are usually central in location.[335] Of course, if malignancy is found, a low anterior resection, abdomino–perineal resection, or other alternative operation for rectal cancer should be recommended (see section on treatment of rectal cancer). However, if on repeat biopsy, no invasive malignancy can be found, wide local excision, if possible, should be recommended. There may be large lesions that, even though benign, cannot be safely removed short of abdomino–perineal resection. Several approaches to local excision have been advocated; however the use of fulguration in this clinical setting should not be used for two reasons. First, this frequently results in local recurrence and, second, it causes the specimen to be destroyed so that a complete histopathologic search for invasive malignancy is impossible.[336]

Several approaches to surgical excision of benign villous adenomas of the rectum have been advocated. Undoubtedly if the tumor is in the upper or middle thirds of the rectum, low anterior resection of the segment and relevant lymphatic arcade is the treatment of choice. In the lower third of the rectum a transanal approach may allow an adequate margin.[337] For larger lesions a trans-sphincteric approach or trans-sacral approach may be used.[338-340] A transsacral approach has been used with good results.[241,242]

Careful followup is mandatory in the treatment of all villous tumors. Recurrence may appear to be a more aggressive lesion than initially suspect.[336] Raymond and co-workers from Lyon advocate surgical excision as initial treatment, but have found contact radiation therapy of use for recurrence or if the excised lesion is found upon histopathological study to contain invasive malignancy.[343]

PRINCIPLES OF SURGICAL TREATMENT OF COLORECTAL CANCER

It cannot be emphasized too strongly that nearly all patients with colorectal cancer will have particular problems in diagnosis or management that need careful individual attention. However, there are features common to every patient's workup, preoperative care, operation, postoperative care, and followup that can be identified. This next section is to discuss principles of surgical management in patients in whom a colon or rectal cancer has been identified and for whom resection is contemplated.

PREOPERATIVE WORKUP

Prior to scheduling the patient for colon or rectal resection several diagnostic tests are useful. A full set of laboratory data including liver function tests and a CEA assay is in order. A liver scan may alert the physician to the presence of hepatic metastases; if the metastases appear limited, this may warn the surgeon and patient of the possible need for hepatic resection. With colon tumors multiple metastases seen on liver scan usually do not change the need for resection of the primary tumor. However, with rectal cancer, in the presence of multiple hepatic matastases it may save the patient an operation and preserve function if radiation therapy and fulguration are used to control the primary tumor. A liver scan done pre-operatively can be used as a baseline study by which to compare studies postoperatively.

A final test useful in the pre-operative workup is the intravenous pyelogram. It tells the surgeon the number of ureters present on the right and left and serves as a baseline examination should urologic complications arise intra-operatively or in followup. Cystoscopy and a cystogram are indicated if the patient has a recent history of urinary infection, pneumaturia or pyuria by urinalysis.

PREOPERATIVE CARE

Preparation of patients for colon and rectal surgery may be as important in terms of prevention of complication as are the techniques employed intra-operatively. The psychological preparation of the patient should not be neglected, especially if a temporary or permanent colostomy is contemplated. In preparing the large bowel, thorough mechanical cleansing is the most essential part of pre-operative care. This should be done through a diet of clear fluids, purgatives such as magnesium citrate, and, occasionally, high colonic enemas. An alternative lavage method has been described which works well, but should only be used in younger patients with no compromise of cardiac or renal function.[344,345] By this routine, 8 liters to 10 liters of Ringer's lactate solution administered by NG tube produces an intestinal lavage, which is continued until the effluent *per* rectum is clear.

The use of oral antibiotics to reduce septic complications of colorectal surgery has for many years been a controversy. Studies using sulfathalidine alone, neomycin alone, or kanamycin alone have not consistently shown better results for antibiotic treated groups. However, Condon, in a review, points out that single agents are likely to fail.[346] Human colonic flora is composed of two broad classes of organisms; aerobes and anaerobes. *Escherichia coli* is the most common aerobic organism and *Bacteroides fragilis* is the most common anaerobic organism. Therefore, an effective regimen should include antibiotics effective for both groups of organisms. Clark and co-workers reported the results of a Veterans' Administration cooperative study of 106 patients undergoing elective colon or rectal surgery.[347] Neomycin was given orally to control aerobic bacteria and erythromycin base was given orally to control the growth of anaerobic organisms. All patients in this study had thorough mechanical bowel preparation, but half were randomly allocated to receive oral antibiotics. The overall rate of septic complications was 43% in the placebo group and 9% in the group receiving oral neomycin and erythromycin base. Wound infection rates were 35% and 9% in the two groups. Workers in this cooperative study concluded that oral administration of neomycin and erythromycin base together with vigorous mechanical cleansing reduces the risk of septic complications after elective colorectal operations. Table 21-25 outlines the bowel preparation recommended by Condon and co-workers.[348]

If preoperative use of oral antibiotics to combat aerobic and anaerobic colonic organisms is effective, does the additional use of systemically administered antibiotics bring about a further reduction in the incidence of wound infection and other septic complications? Most probably systemic antibiotics used for a short time pre-operatively and postoperatively are effective in reducing infectious complications.[349]

Some problems may result from bowel preparation. If, for diagnostic tests and preparation for surgery, a long period of clear fluid diet is needed, the patient may become weak from nutritional depletion. A "space food" diet plus generous vitamin supplementation will help keep the patient's mental and physical strength up. The administration of vitamin K is wise to avert bleeding from hypoprothrombinemia, and supplemental oral or intravenous potassium may be needed. The mechanical bowel preparation may cause dehydration. So that hypotension does not occur on induction of anesthesia, intravenous hydration the evening before surgery is recommended.

Another possible hazard of antibiotic bowel preparation is increased suture line implantation of tumor as studied by Vink.[350] He innoculated Brown and Pearce tumor into the colon of rabbits in whom a colonic anastomosis had been recently prepared. In animals whose bowels had been prepared using sulphasuxidine and streptomycin, suture line recurrence was three times more common. Cohn and Atrik, using a similar model, found an increase in tumor implantation at the anastomosis in rabbits in whom there was a reduction in gastrointestinal flora by either antibiotics or lavage.[351] They also observed that tumor cells spilled into the peritoneal cavity while a colonic anastomosis was being done would grow in various areas within the abdominal cavity. Also, trauma to the colon was thought to increase the incidence of tumor growth in an anastomosis.

TABLE 21-25. Bowel Preparation Recommended by Condon and Coworkers

Day 1	Low-residue diet. Bisacodyl, 1 capsule at 6 P.M.
Day 2	Continue low-residue diet Magnesium sulfate, 30 ml of 50% solution (15 gm) at 10 A.M., 2 P.M. and 6 P.M.
Day 3	Neomycin, 1 gm, and erythromycin base, 1 gm. orally at 1 P.M., 2 P.M. and 11 P.M. Clear liquid diet Magnesium sulfate, 30 ml of 50% solution at 10 A.M. and 2 P.M. No enemas IV maintenance fluids started if clinically indicated
Day 4	Operation at 8 A.M.

(Condor RE, Nyhus LM: Manual of Surgical Therapeutics, 3rd ed. Boston, Little, Brown and Co, 1975)

POSTOPERATIVE CARE

Postoperatively, after colon or rectal resection, the course is usually uncomplicated. Problems that do arise most often occur as a result of compromised cardiac, respiratory, or renal function known to be present pre-operatively. Nasogastric suction should be used until the patient passes flatus showing that ileus has passed and the anastomosis is open. After a colon resection, when the patient is fully ambulatory, Foley catheter drainage can be discontinued. After rectal resection, even a week of catheter drainage may still not be enough time for recovery of sufficient bladder tone for complete emptying of the bladder. Early ambulation and leg exercises in bed should be used to diminish thromboembolic complications.

LYMPH NODE RESECTION

Surgical resection of a primary colon or rectal cancer must be considered standard treatment; the objective of an operation is removal of the primary tumor and any regional spread that may have occurred without allowing any further dissemination of tumor. Through the operative procedure the surgeon maps out, dissects up and carefully preserves a specimen of tumor and surrounding tissues.

Since approximately half the patients presenting with colon or rectal adenocarcinoma have involved lymph nodes, only a few surgeons do not always insist on removal of lymph nodes draining the primary tumor. A few advocates of local removal of primary rectal cancer argue that the cost to patients of abdomino–perineal resection does not equal the improvements in survival that operation affords those with positive nodes (for a more complete discussion see the section on fulguration of rectal cancer). However, with this single exception, all agree that a lymph node dissection around the primary tumor is indicated; the controversy focuses on the extent of this lymphatic dissection. As an example of this controversy, consider the operation indicated for cancer of the sigmoid colon. Should the resection include a segment of colon 10 cm to 15 cm on either side of the tumor, plus a wedge of mesentery that would include relevant paracolic and intermediate lymph nodes surrounding sigmoidal arteries and veins? Or, should the surgeon set out to resect the entire left hemicolon and its mesentery, including lymphatics, arteries, and veins back to their origin on the aorta and splenic branch of the portal vein? In addition, some would include in this dissection the left retroperitoneal lymph nodes.

The rationale for this radical approach came from the meticulous studies of lymphatic metastases observed in resected specimens. It was found that regional spread to lymphatics proceeds from paracolic to intermediate to primary lymph nodes, usually in an orderly fashion, and before any systemic dissemination of disease is evident. In an occasional patient, skip metastasis from the primary tumor directly to primary lymph nodes was seen. An unpredictable retrograde lymphatic spread that occurred when the main routes of lymphatic flow were blocked was reported in a few patients. Also, in 1938, Gilchrist and David examined on autopsy eight patients who died in the postoperative period following a resection of a large bowel cancer.[198] In four of these eight patients residual cancer in lymph nodes was present. In all four patients, an additional 2 cm to 3 cm of dissection would have rendered these patients disease-free.

However, after examining the series of patients shown in Table 21-26, one must conclude that no data currently available would strongly suggest improved survival with radical or supraradical resections of colon or rectal cancer as compared to segmental resection.[6,76,202,211,352,353] However, as suggested by Morgan, if by radical lymphatic resection one can convert some C2 lesions to the C1 category, a few patients may benefit.[108] Certainly, a great many patients need to receive the radical operation and not benefit at all for a very few patients to be salvaged. With this limited improvement of survival, any possible increase in morbidity and mortality would weigh one's surgical equation in favor of segmental resection. If the patient's age or physical condition are at all compromised making them a less than good operative risk, a limited segmental resection of the colon and relevant lymphatic arcade should be recommended.

Harvey and Auchincloss collected important data from the Presbyterian Hospital, New York, that showed the infrequent success of surgical therapy when large bowel carcinoma is not confined to a few lymph nodes that would be removed by segmental resection.[354] In 442 survivors of colon cancers, only 3.2% had more than five lymph nodes involved, and for 183 rectal cancer survivors only 2.8% had greater than five nodes involved. In the few instances in which multiple (more than five) nodes were found in a survivor, nodes were clustered close to the tumor. Also, when metastases were found in fewer than five nodes, the nodes seldom lay far from the tumor. Harvey and Auchincloss suggest that extensive resections may be indicated for large bowel cancer only if minimal added risk or disability results from the radical procedure. A minimal added risk could be considered commensurate with the limited additional survival radical procedures offer.

LATERAL LYMPHATIC SPREAD WITH RECTAL CANCER

Enker and co-workers have suggested that *en bloc* dissection of all lymphatic tissue accompanying the internal iliac artery and vein should be a routine addition to the specimen preserved in an abdomino–perineal resection.[353] The lateral lymphatic spread along middle hemorrhoidal vessels is to lymph nodes close to tumor; also this dissection gives a better soft tissue margin for the specimen. Enker and co-workers found local recurrence in two of 11 (18.2%) C2 rectal cancers resected with an internal iliac lymph node dissection as part of an abdomino–perineal resection and three of three patients who had a conventional abdomino–perineal resection. Waugh and Kirklin, and Guernsey, Waugh, and Dockerty suggested that the poorer survival seen with low rectal cancer was due

TABLE 21-26. Results of Extended Lymph Node Dissections for Left Colon and Rectal Cancer

AUTHOR	DATE	NUMBER PATIENTS	SURVIVAL ADVANTAGE	MORTALITY	STATISTICAL SIGNIFICANCE
Bacon et al (6)	1958	80	5%	0	N.S.
*Stearns and Deddish (76)	1959	122	8%	3%	N.S.
Rosi et al (202)	1962	137	6.8%	2.2%	N.S.
Grinnell (352)	1965	179	5.7%	6.2%	N.S.
Dwight et al (311)	1969	345	None	–	–
Enker et al (353)	1979	216	Not evaluable	6.4%	–

* Noted increased morbidity especially urinary tract complications.

to lateral lymphatic spread from tumors near the level of the levator ani muscle.[213,214] The actual incidence of lymph node metastases along the middle hemorrhoidal vessels is somewhat controversial. Gabriel, Dukes, and Bussey found no lateral lymphatic spread in 62 specimens of rectal cancer.[60] They suggested that it may occur only if there was lymphatic blockage by extensive metastases within superior hemorrhoidal lymphatics. Grinnell agreed with this, finding only one example of lateral spread in 118 rectal cancer specimens.[72] Gilchrist and David saw lateral spread in four of 27 rectal cancers.[74] Coller, Kaye, and MacIntyre found six of 53 rectal cancer specimens to have lateral spread.[79] All six occurred in rectal cancers within the anal canal and low rectum (six of 18 cases). Sauer and Bacon performed internal iliac node dissections in 17 patients and found two with positive pelvic nodes.[355] Stearns and Deddish found lymph node involvement in and around the pelvis in 11 of 122 patients who underwent abdominopelvic lymph node dissection for rectal cancer.[76] In eight of these patients, widespread metastases to mesenteric nodes were also found, suggesting a retrograde mechanism of lateral spread to pelvic nodes. All in all, the incidence of spread laterally along the middle hemorrhoidal vessels to internal iliac nodes does not seem great; but it does occur in low rectal cancers and the incidence increases if retrograde lymphatic spread from lymphatic blockage has occurred.

It must be remembered that the margin a histopathological examination of the specimen reveals as adequate may not be adequate for cure. As was seen in the section on prognosis, downward spread from rectal cancer is almost never seen more than 2 cm from the lower edge of the tumor; yet a distal margin less than 5 cm in length adversely affects long-term survival. The same type of situation may exist for lateral lymphatic spread. Even though lymph nodes along the middle hemorrhoidal vessels are seldom found to be positive histopathologically, nevertheless their removal may impact favorably upon 5-year survival. It is difficult to see how questions such as, "Should *en bloc* removal of internal iliac lymph nodes be a routine part of the abdominoperineal resection?" can be answered short of a controlled and randomized clinical trial.

TECHNICAL DETAILS OF LARGE BOWEL RESECTIONS

Several surgical groups have emphasized technical details to be followed in the course of a large bowel resection which they suggest improve survival. None of these techniques have been shown in a clinical trial to improve survival; however, for purely theoretical reasons, most should be practiced. If adherence to one or several of these techniques presents an added risk to the patient, one should avoid that particular step of the procedure.

In 1966, Cole, Roberts, and Strehl summarized the precautionary measures they thought essential for large bowel resection for cancer.[356] These techniques were designed to prevent dissemination of tumor cells within the peritoneal cavity, within the bowel lumen, and into the lymphatic and venous system. To prevent intra-peritoneal dissemination of tumor, Cole and associates advocated minimal manipulation of the tumor mass at the time of surgical exploration of the abdomen. To prevent tumor cell dissemination within lymphatics and veins, ligation of vascular trunks prior to dissection around the tumor was advocated. Wound edges were to be kept covered to prevent implantation in the incision. If dissection around a tumor was required, it was to be kept covered by gauze packs and instruments and gloves discarded from the operative field following any dissection close to the tumor. To prevent dissemination of tumor cells throughout the bowel lumen, ligatures above and below the tumor were advocated. Therefore, as malignant cells were dislodged from the tumor surface during the course of the operation, they would be contained. To eliminate intraluminal malignant cells at the site of the anastomosis, proximal and distal ends of the bowel were to be irrigated with distilled water, Dakins solution, or bichloride of mercury. Following irrigation before performing the anastomosis, re-excision of the proximal and distal ends of the bowel was advocated to remove any tumor cells deeply implanted within the colon wall by a crushing clamp.

Turnbull's philosophy of large bowel resection was similar to that of Cole's group. He advocated that a "non-manipulative" method of resection replace the "manipulative" conventional technique.[139] The essential feature of Turnbull's technique was ligation of the vascular channel as the first step in the resection of the tumor and was to occur before the tumor bearing segment was manipulated or handled in any way. This "no-touch isolation technique" was suggested by Turnbull as the reason for greatly improved survival in a group of personally operated patients.

Stearns and Schottenfield suggested that there are multiple differences between the no-touch technique and conventional colon resection; not just early ligation of vascular channels.[357] Stearns suggested that the essential feature of optimal colorectal cancer surgical technique was "wide removal of the cancer-bearing segment of bowel and its mesentery." Steps to minimize cancer emboli through vascular channels by early ligation or minimal manipulation of the tumor were to be followed so far as feasible, but should not interfere with wide resection.

Cohn thought that an essential technical detail in colon cancer surgery was the elimination of tumor implantation from the bowel lumen to suture line or peritoneal cavity.[358] In a review of published series, Cohn showed that recurrence at the suture line occurred in 3% to 50% of patients. His experimental studies showed that anastomotic recurrence did not occur from implantation on the mucosal surface; rather, implantation is onto the serosal surface at the anastomotic site. Alternatively, malignant cells can be innoculated into the bowel wall by suture during the anastomosis. To prevent anastomotic implantation, Cohn advocated the use of iodized suture or a closed anastomosis. To prevent peritoneal implants Cohn suggested immediate postoperative radiation therapy, irrigation with low molecular weight dextran or injection of 90Yt-tagged ceramic microspheres into the abdominal cavity.

Another approach to the problem of suture line recurrence is intra-operative colonic lavage. In this technique a large volume of fluid (usually water) is flushed into the large bowel through the rectum after the patient is anesthetized. Then while the abdomen is being opened, this lavage is emptied by sump suction. As soon as resection is begun and before tumor cells can repopulate the colon and rectum clamps are placed across the upper and lower margins of resection. This technique may be less apt to result in tumor or bacterial contamination that may occur if open ends of bowel are to be swabbed or irrigated.

Recently, Gunderson and Cohn have suggested that careful attention should be directed to the surgical specimen.[359] Cooperative efforts of the surgeon, pathologist, and radiation therapist were advocated to focus further therapy on areas likely to fail surgical treatments alone. During the course of resection the surgical specimen is to be carefully preserved and marked. Also, within the patient, margins of resection are to be marked with metallic clips so they can be accurately localized radiologically in the postoperative period. If the pathologist, in his examination of the specimen, finds a minimal or inadequate margin of resection, this area should receive supplemental treatment with radiation therapy in the postoperative period. In this approach, the removal of lymph nodes is seen as the surgeon's job; control of local extensions of tumor growth is a combined task for surgeon and radiation therapist.

A RATIONAL SURGICAL APPROACH

Resection of a reasonable segment of large bowel and adjacent mesentery, as shown in Fig. 21-1, should be the surgeons goal; more extensive resections of bowel plus retroperitoneal lymph node dissections are not thought to be indicated. Their potential benefits probably do not match the added risks. Emphasis should be on wide local margins around the tumor with adipose and fibroareolar tissues sharply dissected away from the patient and left on the specimen. Tearing of tissues should not occur, so that the integrity of the specimen and its margins is preserved. These authors would de-emphasize the need for extensive lymphatic dissection and emphasize the need for wide local excision around the primary tumor. In patients who are not a good surgical risk, an even more limited resection may be indicated; a minimal operation in a poor risk patient would include 5 cm or more of bowel on either side of the tumor and a wedge of paracolic and intermediate lymph nodes in the vascular arcade draining the tumor.

If a left colon or rectal tumor is being removed, the large bowel is lavaged with water. After an adequate incision, the abdomen is thoroughly explored and adhesions lysed; it may be necessary to occlusively cover the tumor intermittently, but a gauze or rubber wrapping secured to the tumor is discouraged, for this tends to make the tumor a convenient handle by which to manipulate the bowel. Identification of the extent of colonic resection plus clamping, dividing, and occlusively covering the cut ends of the bowel is the next step. If the cut ends of the bowel are not covered at this time, it may be incovenient to stop the dissection later on to do so.

Next, isolation of the arterial, lymphatic, and venous blood supply should be accomplished. Ligatures within the mesentery, but not at the highest point of vascular transection as advocated by Cole, should not be used.[356] This may be associated with bleeding or a cancerous node may be traumatized. If accurate ligation of vascular structures at the limits of the dissection cannot be identified, mesenteric attachments should be divided until the vascular anatomy is clear, and then vessels ligated. On the specimen side, large ligatures that incorporate a vessel and all the surrounding lymphatics are recommended. This helps prevent leakage of tumor cells from lymphatics of the specimen into the operative field. To prevent slippage of ligatures, on the patient side, large vessels should be isolated, tied, and then suture ligated. If adjacent structures are adhesed to the specimen, they should be resected *en bloc* with the tumor.

Reanastomosis should be accomplished without tension or a colostomy constructed. Extensive saline irrigation of the operative site and then entire abdomen should be performed. Before closure of the abdomen, the margins of resection and major anatomic structures are marked with metal clips. Also, the surgeon is responsible to mark and orient the specimen for the pathologist so that margins of resection and level of positive lymph nodes can be determined. The peritoneum and fascia are reapproximated with the skin and subcutaneous tissue left open for a delayed primary closure.

COMPLICATIONS OF COLORECTAL SURGERY

Dwight, Higgins, and Keehn examined characteristics of 1171 patients and their postoperative course following resections for colorectal cancer.[211] The early postoperative (30 day) mortality was 9.6%. In this group of patients pulmonary complications were associated with 44 postoperative deaths, cardiovascular complications (excluding pulmonary embolism) with 40 deaths, and pulmonary embolism with 10 deaths. Technical complications of wound dehiscence occurred in 14 patients who died, peritonitis in 12, and intestinal obstruction in 8.

Hughes and co-workers from Australia reported 94 (6.7%) postoperative deaths in 1395 rectal resections.[360] Mortality following abdomino—perineal resection, pull-through procedure, or anterior anastomosis was very similar. This report points out the rapid increase in operative mortality as the patient's age increases (Table 21-27). Calabrese, Adam, and Volk found the operative mortality in 156 patients 80 years of age or older was 32.6%.[173] These high operative mortality rates for aged colon and rectal cancer patients must be considered when formulating a management plan. For colon cancers in patients over 70 years of age, a conservative resection rather than a hemicolectomy is almost always

TABLE 21-27. Operative Mortality and Age of Patient

AGE (years)	NUMBER	NUMBER OF DEATHS	PERCENT
0–9	0	0	0.0
10–19	1	0	0.0
20–29	18	2	11.1
30–39	62	1	1.6
40–49	182	6	3.3
50–59	350	9	2.6
60–69	450	26	5.8
70–79	276	41	14.9
80–81	56	9	16.0
TOTAL	1395	94	6.7

(Hughes ES, McDermott FT, Masterton JP et al: Operative mortality following excision of the rectum. Br. J Surg 1:49–51, 1980)

TABLE 21-28. Complications Following Abdominoperineal Resection in 300 Patients

COMPLICATION	NUMBER OF PATIENTS	PERCENT OF PATIENTS
Urinary tract problems	81	27
Cardiovascular	26	9
Pulmonary	3	1
Sepsis	28	9
Small bowel obstruction	17	6
Colostomy problems	62	20

(Colcock BP, Jarpa S: Complications of abdominoperineal resection. Dis Colon Rectum 1:90–96, 1958)

indicated. For rectal cancers in aged patients, if a local excision that has adequate margins can be performed it should be strongly considered.

In a study of 300 patients undergoing abdomino–perineal resection, Colcock reported that 58% of patients had at least one complication and 21% had multiple complications.[361] The problems Colcock encountered are itemized in Table 21-28. Urinary tract problems were the most common complication, occurring in 27% of patients. Lapides and Tank made a special study of urinary complications following abdomino-perineal resection.[362] They attributed the majority of problems to loss of good detrusor contraction. The trauma to bladder, urethra, and associated nerve and blood supply resulted in temporary decompensation of the bladder muscle. Persistent problems continuing three weeks postoperatively were found associated with previously existing prostatism in the male and atonic, large bladder in the infrequent voiding female.

In the studies of Dwight, Higgins, and Keehn, Ginzberg and associates, and Hughes and associates, sepsis followed cardiopulmonary complications as a cause of postoperative mortality.[211,360,363] Septic complications were noted to be especially common in the group of patients undergoing low anterior resection. Manson and co-workers at the Lahey Clinic studied factors that were related to anastomotic complications.[364] These investigators determined that atherosclerotic disease, anemia, obstruction and perforation, an anastomosis below the peritoneal reflection, diabetes, and the use of drains were associated in a statistically significant way with obstruction, sepsis, or fistula from a low anterior anastomosis. Interestingly, in patients in whom the anastomosis was below the peritoneal reflection, an open peritoneum seemed to protect the patient against the development of anastomotic complications ($p = 0.005$). Also, the use of drains placed near the anastomosis increased the complication rate ($p < 0.05$). Berliner, Burson, and Lear and Akwari and Kelly also reported a higher incidence of anastomotic leakage with a pelvic drain in place.[365,366] Berliner and co-workers concluded that an intraperitoneal drain will not protect a suture line from leakage, does not prevent a diffuse peritonitis, and may, by interposition between omentum and anastomotic site, prevent the omentum from sealing a leak.

Sexual dysfunction, a major problem in males undergoing abdominoperineal resection, is discussed in Chapter 45 (Gonadal Dysfunction).

PRINCIPLES OF RADIATION THERAPY OF COLORECTAL CANCER

Radiation therapy has been employed for primary colorectal cancer as the initial treatment, as an adjuvant for those at high risk for recurrence following surgery or those known to have residual disease left after resection. It has also been used in patients with rectal cancer thought to be locally inoperable because of tumor fixation to the pelvis. In addition, it has been shown to be of marked palliative benefit to patients with local problems caused by recurrent disease.

COMBINED APPROACH OF SURGERY PLUS RADIATION THERAPY

Several recent developments have led to marked interest in a combined approach, utilizing radiation therapy plus surgery for treatment of rectal and selected colonic carcinomas. Proponents of this approach emphasize the need for prevention of local recurrence within the operative field. This has been identified as a significant problem in spite of potentially curative surgery[367] (see section on natural history). Although palliation of such recurrences can sometimes be obtained with radiation alone or in combination with chemotherapy, the duration of palliation is often limited and the curative potential is 5% or less. Therefore, prevention of local recurrence is a necessity.

Possible radiation therapy/surgery sequences are pre-operative irradiation, postoperative irradiation or combined pre- and postoperative (sandwich technique) irradiation.

Pre-operative irradiation may be given for two important reasons. Perhaps the major advantage of preoperative irradiation is the potential damaging effect on tumor cells that may otherwise disseminate locally or distantly at the time of operation. Both human and animal data suggest this may be as low as 500 rad in a single fraction or doses of 1000 rad or less in 3 to 5 fractions.[368,369] The favorable effects of this low dose pre-operative irradiation are thought to be very short-lived and resection should follow it within a few hours.[370] The usual pre-operative dose should be small enough to allow immediate operative intervention and permit bowel anastomoses to be done safely.

A second objective of pre-operative irradiation may be to bring about tumor regression and thus convert questionable margins of resection to adequate margins.[371,372]

The major advantage of postoperative irradiation is the ability to select groups of patients at high risk for local recurrence on the basis of operative and pathologic findings but to delete patients with a low risk for local recurrence or with operative finding of previously undiagnosed metastatic disease.

Well-designed combinations of pre- and postoperative irradiation (sandwich technique) could in fact combine the theoretical advantage of both other techniques. In the sandwich technique the pre-operative dose and field size should be of a magnitude suitable for theoretically preventing the implantation and growth of cells that might be disseminated at the time of operation. Regression of tumor and altered tumor extent should not be required for adequate margins of resection. Then, following surgery, based on surgical findings and the pathologist's reports, patients at high risk for local recurrence would receive additional radiation to individualized portals postoperatively.[373]

Results From Studies Using Pre-operative Irradiation

A number of groups have utilized pre-operative irradiation for resectable rectal or rectosigmoid lesions with a variety of dose levels and portal arrangements. Some have demonstrated proof of tumoricidal responsiveness in the resected specimen by partial or total regression of the primary tumor or by finding of a lower incidence of lymph node involvement than would have ordinarily been anticipated; others, using low dose irradiation pre-operatively, evaluate survival statistics only. Data available to date are summarized in Table 21-29 and allow some tentative conclusions.[371,372,374-378] First, local recurrence rates are reduced appreciably when pre-operative radiation therapy was used. This was true in all studies except that of Rider and colleagues; in this study patterns of failure relative to local recurrence or distant metastases have not yet been published. Second, some tumors disappear completely by histopathologic examination with adequate doses of irradiation. Third, some inoperable lesions may be converted to operable ones with adequate dose. Finally, two studies suggest improved survival when low dose pre-operative irradiation is combined with curative resection. This effect may be more pronounced with low rectal cancers requiring abdominoperineal resection.

Results from Studies Using Postoperative Irradiation

Gunderson and Romsdahl and Withers in two major prospective, but nonrandomized, postoperative radiation therapy trials have subdivided their patients into those with curative resections and those with noncurative resections in whom there was evidence after surgery of residual disease.[379,380] Both series utilized similar fields and dose levels (4500 rad to 5500 rad over 5 weeks to 6.6 weeks). Since only those patients at high risk for local recurrence were treated, end results cannot be compared directly to pre-operative irradiation series. For all groups of patients, local recurrence decreased from 37% to 48% with operation alone down to 6% to 8% in patients receiving surgery followed by postoperative radiation therapy; similar decreases were seen for each respective stage of disease. Distant metastases in both series continue to be a problem in 20% to 30% of patients.

Selection of Pre-operative, Postoperative, or Sandwich Techniques

The radiation therapy/surgery sequencing options and radiation dosages perferred are outlined in Table 21-30. Patients who receive either low dose or moderate dose preoperative radiation are usually those with rectal or rectosigmoid lesions. For patients who receive moderate dose pre-operative radiation therapy (4500 rad to 5000 rad) the operation which follows usually has been limited to abdomino–perineal resection. If low anterior resections are performed after the higher doses of irradiation, one should follow the recommendations of Stevens and co-workers and utilize both an unirradiated segment of colon for the proximal portion of the anastomosis and a temporary diverting colostomy.[381] Usually, patients undergoing a sphincter saving operation receive low dose pre-operative irradiation. Doses used are 500 rad in a single fraction with the operation the same or following day or 1000 rad in four to five fractions with operation in 1 day to 3 days.

TABLE 21-29. Results of Pre-Operative Radiation Therapy

AUTHOR (Reference Number)	DATE	RAD	TECHNIQUES	NUMBER OF PATIENTS IRRADIATED	RESULTS
Quan, Deddish, and Stearns (374)	1960	not stated (variable)	not stated (variable)	447	Retrospective study showed statistically significant 5 and 10 year improved survival in treated Dukes C rectal cancer patients.
Stearns, Deddish, and Quan (375)	1968	not stated	not stated	194	Patients randomized by birthdate, no differences in survival in any groups. Decreased local recurrence rate.
Ruff et al (371)	1961	not stated	implant 2/3 patients, others implant plus external beam	99	Ten patients no residual cancer in operative specimen. Ten lesions converted from operable to inoperable.
Kligerman et al (376)	1972	4400–4600	External beam	15	Half the expected number of Dukes C specimens with irradiation
Stevens, Allen and Fletcher (372)	1976	5000–6000 in 5½-8 weeks	External beam	97	Ten percent complete disappearance of tumor, ten percent inoperable lesion converted to operable. Negligible local recurrent rate.
Roswit, Higgins, and Keehn (377)	1975	2000–2500 in 12 days	External beam	350	Randomized controlled trial suggested improved 5 year survival and lower incidence of local recurrence in treated patients undergoing abdominoperineal resection (results not statistically significant).
Rider et al (378)	1977	500	Single dose of cobalt irradiation four hours before surgery	60	Randomized controlled trial showed significant differences in survival, 40 vs 20 percent.

TABLE 21-30. Radiation Therapy/Surgery Sequencing Options

SEQUENCE	LESIONS TREATED	RAD	TIMING OF RADIATION THERAPY WITH RESPECT TO SURGERY
Pre-operative low dose	rectum and rectosigmoid	500 × 1 or 200 × 5 fractions	Irradiation same day or 1–3 days pre-operatively
Pre-operative moderate dose	rectum and rectosigmoid	4500 to 5000	Irradiation complete 4–6 weeks before surgery
Postoperative	extrapelvic colon, rectum and rectosigmoid	4500–5500	Irradiation starts 2–4 weeks postoperatively
Sandwich technique	rectum and rectosigmoid	500 × 1 or 200 × 5 fractions	Irradiation same day or 1–3 days pre-operatively
		4000–4500	Irradiation starts 2–4 weeks postoperatively

For lesions that are clinically resectable (as opposed to borderline resectable), there may be a definite advantage of low dose over moderate dose pre-operative irradiation. In the Massachusetts General Hospital series, only 42% of patients (16 of 38) ultimately required a full course of irradiation on the basis of operative and pathologic findings. With moderate dose pre-operative irradiation, almost 50% of patients who are irradiated may not require it.[373,382]

Indications for Postoperative Radiation Therapy

Selection of patients for postoperative irradiation depends on the position of the tumor and its depth of penetration through the bowel wall. Tumors within portions of the bowel which contain a mesentery are not usually considered for irradiation treatment unless they are adhesed to unresectable structures (retroperitoneum, duodenum, anterior abdominal wall). However, portions of the colorectum fixed to the retroperitoneum (cecum and descending colon) or pelvis (rectosigmoid and rectum) have definite pathologic criteria for postoperative irradiation. These include: (1) known inadequate margins of resection; (2) adherence to retroperitoneum, sacrum, or pelvic sidewalls; (3) transmural tumor penetration of a macroscopic degree; and (4) extensive microscopic tumor penetration with the presence of positive lymph nodes.

Occasionally patients with lymph node metastasis near the highest surgical ligature may be candidates for radiation therapy to the remaining intermediate, principal, or para-aortic lymph nodes. In general, however, elimination of lymph node spread is a surgical responsibility. Irradiation of lymphatic areas includes treatment to a large volume of small bowel.

There may be clinical indications for abdominal irradiation if the danger of intraperitoneal tumor seeding is great. Moving-strip total abdomen techniques have been utilized in some institutions.[383] Such fields are probably warranted on a theoretical basis, but even then, the therapeutic gain is uncertain owing to the treatment volumes.

CONSTRUCTION OF A THERAPEUTIC RATIO

For radiation therapy to be successfully employed the beneficial effects of treatment must outweigh the harmful effects. A number of techniques exist to help achieve both acceptable local control rates and minimize small bowel complications. They are (1) improved tumor and normal tissue localization; (2) operative attempts to decrease adhesions and displace all or part of dose limiting organs out of a potential irradiation field; and (3) optimal radiation equipment, techniques, and dosage schedules (Table 21-31).

Improved tumor and normal tissue localization can be accomplished with precise descriptions of operative findings, accurate clip placement, judicious use of non-operative diagnostic techniques such as CT, ultrasound, and barium studies, including special small bowel films to determine position and degree of mobility.[359]

Precise description of the operation, careful labeling of the operative specimen, and accurate clip placement around residual or inoperable tumor or areas of adherence are vital exercises at the time of the initial exploration. The physical presence of the responsible radiation therapist in the operating room may be indispensable for optimal radiation treatment planning. Although metal clips may interfere with subsequent computerized body tomography, this practice is essential in patients who are explored and found to have residual or inoperable tumor. It is advantageous to obtain PA and lateral films in the early postoperative period that are centered over the location of the clips so that the surgeon and radiotherapist can reconstruct the position of the tumor. Increasingly so-

TABLE 21-31. Minimizing Small Bowel Radiation Injury

A. Careful case selection by interaction of surgeon, pathologist, and radiation therapist
B. Surgical considerations
   1. "Clipping" of highest risk areas
   2. Pelvic reconstruction
      a. Reperitonealize pelvic floor
      b. Omental sling or pedicle flap
      c. Retrovert uterus into pelvis
      d. Other pelvic organ reconstruction or temporary devices
C. Diagnostic considerations
   1. Define location and mobility of small bowel with postoperative small bowel series
   2. Computerized tomography
   3. Ultrasound
D. Radiation considerations
   1. Use of lateral fields (large and boost)
   2. Shrinking or boost field techniques
   3. Treat prone with bladder distended (rectum), or on side (extra + peritoneal colon)

phisticated ultrasound and computerized tomography techniques should be complementary to the use of metal clips.

Small bowel films should be obtained to help define dose limits. Doses greater than 5000 rad in 180 rad fractions, 5 days per week, are rarely utilized unless there is a good small bowel mobility or a minimal amount of small bowel within the field. Doses above 6000 rad, in similar daily fractions, are not allowed unless the small bowel is completely out of the boost field.

The CT scan has proved useful in defining residual, recurrent, or inoperable lesions as well as tumor bed contours in patients who have had a "curative resection," but are at high risk for local recurrence. Sophisticated shaped treatment portals may be used with subsequent inclusion of less normal tissue.

In some patients, surgical techniques can help displace small bowel from within the radiation portals. An omental flap sutured into the pelvis may keep small bowel from entering a pelvic field of irradiation. Sometimes the uterus can be retroverted into the pelvis to prevent small bowel from lodging here. Usually, careful reconstruction of the pelvic floor after abdomino–perineal resection is the most appropriate surgical maneuver. Further research attempts to decrease postoperative adhesions and displace normal tissue out of the operative field are indicated. While operative displacement of normal tissues is of interest in an adjuvant setting, it is even more important with residual, inoperable, or recurrent lesions where higher irradiation doses are needed.

After a dose has been delivered which is adequate for control of subclinical or microscopic foci of disease (4500 rad to 5000 rad over five to six weeks) fields are reduced to include known gross or microscopic tumor as defined by the metal clips and diagnostic radiography. These boost fields are usually treated with 3-field (PA and lateral) or 4-field techniques (lateral and paired posterior obliques). Field shaping of the lateral boosts portals is often helpful in deleting additional irradiation to the small intestine anteriorly and superiorly. The concept of utilizing shrinking field techniques to a maximum dose of 6000 rad to 7000 rad has been utilized for pelvic lesions, but can also be used within the abdominal cavity for colonic cancer. In some patients, the use of lateral portals is a major factor in avoiding the more anterior loops of small intestine, especially when high risk tumor beds are marked with clips. Patients may have their bladders distended during radiation therapy treatments, since this maneuver may be extremely useful in displacing small bowel superiorly and anteriorly out of both large and boost fields. In some elderly patients, bladder catheterization and distention is occasionally necessary. In some instances, the radiotherapist must limit his dose to conform to small bowel tolerance. Alternatively, more surgery to displace the small bowel must be performed or the delivery of intra-operative radiation therapy while the small bowel is displaced may be required.

The increasing availability of high energy supervoltage equipment results in improved dose distribution and delivery. Specialized beams (modulated protons, pi-mesons, intra-operative electrons) may allow even more precise distribution of radiation dose and effectiveness. Such sophistication is of value only if the means to define the tumor and normal tissue volumes are as precise as the methods of dose delivery. Failure to define tumor volume and extent could lead to marginal recurrence.

COMPLICATIONS OF RADIATION THERAPY

Both moderate and high dose pre- and postoperative radiation might increase the rate of complications, but this possibility must be considered in perspective by weighing potential benefits against risk. At present, 50% to 70% of patients with tumor extension through the bowel wall with or without lymph node involvement suffer from recurrence, metastases, and death if treated by operation alone.

In the reports from University of Oregon, M.D. Anderson Hospital, and Latter Day Saints Hospital, with doses in the range of 4500 rad to 5000 rad in 5 weeks to 6.5 weeks, small bowel adhesions requiring operative intervention occurred in approximately 10% of patients.[372,379,380] However, 2% to 15% of patients having operation alone may develop similar complications.[381] At such dose levels, the incidence of radiation specific small bowel damage with small bowel obstruction, perforation, or fistulization is approximately 5%. Such doses, however, can increase bowel friability. Therefore, even if adhesions which cause an obstruction are not due to irradiation therapy, surgical options may be limited, or operative complications increased, if large volumes of small bowel are included in the field of irradiation. If the surgeon attempts to dissect out adhesions in irradiated loops of small bowel the incidence of fistulization increases; if a bypass procedure is performed excluding large amounts of small bowel, malabsorption syndromes may result. In the Veterans Administration Hospital, low dose pre-operative series radiation-related complication rates are reported to be minimal, but that series reports a local recurrence rate of 29% in an autopsy subgroup. This recurrence rate is, in itself, a major complication.[384,385]

PRINCIPLES OF CHEMOTHERAPY FOR COLORECTAL CANCER

The chemotherapeutic management of advanced colorectal cancer has been disappointing up to the present time. Oncologists interested in this field have written numerous reviews of this subject over the last 15 years.[386–396] All the information generated by chemotherapy of advanced colorectal cancer can be succinctly summarized as follows. First, of the over 40 single chemotherapy drugs tested in this disease, only three classes of agents have been documented to have consistent activity.[393] These are represented by the fluorinated pyrimidines, the nitrosoureas, and mitomycin-C. Second, there is no evidence that single agent chemotherapy significantly improves the survival of treated patients.[386–396] Third, although there have been some promising results in combination chemotherapy of this disease, recent reviews fail to confirm these effects.[391–397] Currently, there is little evidence that aggressive combination chemotherapy is superior in response rate or improved survival compared to single agent chemotherapy.

SINGLE AGENT CHEMOTHERAPY IN ADVANCED DISEASE

The most commonly used chemotherapy agent in colorectal cancer is 5-fluorouracil (5-FU). Large numbers of patients have been treated with this drug and Carter reported in a compilation of series containing over 2000 patients that the response rate for 5-FU was 21%.[391] Although the 20% figure is generally accepted as valid, a wide variation in response rates to 5-FU has been reported. Objective regression rates varying between 8% and 85% have been published owing to differences in patient selection and in criteria for assessment of response.[387]

There has been much interest in various dose routes and schedules for administration of 5-FU. The originally reported method of 5-FU administration involved intravenous injection of 15 mg/kg body weight per day for 5 days.[387] This was followed by half doses on alternate days for four more doses. This schedule produced significant toxicity with gastrointestinal symptoms in the form of nausea, vomiting, and stomatitis being present in 50% to 90% of patients.[388,398] Bone marrow suppression was present in at least 70% of patients.

Other approaches to 5-FU administration have been examined. These have included lower doses of 5-FU given in a loading course schedule, weekly intravenous injection, and continuous intravenous administration. [391,398–400] The use of continuous infusion 5-FU was of interest because there was less myelosuppression when the drug was given in this manner.[401] In the comparative study of Seifert and associates, the response rate was 44% with infusion and 19% with the loading dose schedule, but the duration of response was not different between the two groups.[401] Other studies have confirmed the decreased myelosuppression associated with prolonged infusion but have failed to demonstrate a therapeutic advantage over loading-dose therapy.[398,399]

Oral usage of 5-FU has been evaluated in colorectal cancer because of ease in administration and on the assumption that oral drugs will enter the portal circulation and be delivered to the liver in high concentration. Theoretically, this would represent a therapeutic advantage in treating hepatic metastases. This premise is flawed, however, in that hepatic metastases usually draw their blood supply from the hepatic artery and not the portal vein.[402,403] Three controlled trials have been performed comparing oral to intravenous 5-FU.[404–406] All have shown superiority for intravenous drug in response rate and duration of response. Also, no benefit in treating liver metastases was seen with oral 5-FU. The inferiority of the oral route of administration is due to inconstant absorption from the gastrointestinal tract.[405]

A prospective study comparing all the commonly used 5-FU schedules has been performed by the Central Oncology Group. This group examined the influence of schedule and route of administration of 5-FU in 462 patients with breast and colorectal cancer.[406] Four regimens were evaluated: (1) a daily loading schedule of 12 mg/kg/day for 5 days, (2) weekly intravenous therapy at 15 mg/kg, (3) a low-dose intravenous loading regimen of 500 mg/day for 4 days, and (4) oral 5-FU 15 mg//kg for 6 days followed by 15 mg/kg orally once weekly. The loading regimen had the greatest response rate (33%), while the others had 12% to 18% response rates. However, the loading-dose regimen was significantly more toxic with 18% of patients experiencing severe or life-threatening toxicity. It was projected that the loading-dose schedule would result in 4 months to 6 months greater survival than the other regimens. This difference is not statistically significant ($p = .09$). Although the loading dose schedule appears to be marginally superior, the price for that minimal superiority is significantly increased toxicity.

Many single agents other than fluorinated pyrimidines have been evaluated in colorectal cancer.[388–394] Most attention has been received by the chloroethyl nitrosoureas, BCNU, CCNU, and methyl-CCNU. These drugs have demonstrated response rates of 10% to 15% in patients with advanced colon cancer.[388,394,407] In a controlled trial, Moertel demonstrated that methyl-CCNU had activity equivalent to 5-FU.[408] As a result of this activity, methyl-CCNU has come to be the most commonly used nitrosourea in colorectal cancer.

Several studies have shown that mitomycin-C has reproducible activity in this disease.[388,394,407] Objective regression of tumor in 12% to 16% of patients has been documented with this drug. However, as with all single agents, the response duration was short (less than three months). Chronic myelosuppression and severe local tissue reactions after extravasation limited the usefulness of mitomycin-C.

COMBINATION CHEMOTHERAPY IN ADVANCED DISEASE

Even with the modest efficacy of single agents in colorectal cancer, there has been active investigation of combination therapy.[408–420] Clinical studies carried out at Mayo Clinic evaluating various combinations of 5-FU, BCNU, mitomycin-C, CCNU, actinomycin-D, and cyclophosphamide showed no superiority in response to 5-FU alone.[415] The first combination of drugs that appeared to be more active than 5-FU was reported by Falkson and co-workers in 1974.[409] These workers compared 5-FU to the combination of 5-FU, BCNU, vincristine, and the imidazole carboxamide derivative, DTIC. The combination resulted in a 43% response rate compared to a 25% response in patients receiving 5-FU alone; however, this was not a significant difference in response. Subsequently, Moertel and colleagues reported a similarly high response rate for the combination 5-FU plus methyl-CCNU plus vincristine.[410] In a Phase III trial, 43% of patients treated with the combination responded compared to 19% treated with 5-FU alone. These results were statistically significant ($p < .05$). There was, however, no benefit in survival for patients treated with the combination.

5-FU plus methyl-CCNU has been combined with drugs other than vincristine. Table 21-32 illustrates the number of regimens that have been evaluated. As can be seen, the addition of DTIC does not improve response rates. However, it should be noted that the series of Kemeny and co-workers suggests some benefit for the addition of streptozotocin to 5-FU, methyl-CCNU, and vincristine.[420] This four-drug regimen is currently being evaluated in a prospectively randomized trial compared with 5-FU, methyl-CCNU, and viscristine.

The response rates of 5-FU compared to 5-FU plus methyl-

TABLE 21-32. 5-FU Plus Methyl-CCNU Combination Regimen in Advanced Colon Cancer

TREATMENT	NUMBER OF PATIENTS	NUMBER OF PARTIAL RESPONSES (%)	SURVIVAL SUPERIOR TO 5-FU ALONE	REFERENCE NUMBERS
5-FU + Methyl-CCNU	489	98 (20)	no	394 415–418
5-FU: + Methyl-CCNU + Vincristine	358	82 (23)	no	394, 408, 413–414
5-FU + Methyl-CCNU + DTIC	83	14 (14)	no	414
5-FU + Methyl-CCNU + Vincristine	71	11 (15)	no	414
5-FU + Methyl-CCNU + vincristine + streptozotocin	54	15 (27)	not done	420

CCNU regimens have been investigated as outlined in Table 21-32. One should remember when examining this table that the generally accepted response rate for 5-FU alone in colorectal cancer is 20%. Although initial studies with 5-FU plus methyl-CCNU and 5-FU plus methyl-CCNU plus vincristine reported response rates of 30% to 43%, further evaluation has failed to confirm this. In a randomized Phase II study performed by the ECOG, no 5-FU plus methyl-CCNU containing regimen had a response rate greater than 15%.[412] Also, a randomized study of 5-FU, methyl-CCNU, and vincristine performed at Memorial New York showed this program to produce objective responses in only 11% of patients.[413] Finally, a large Phase II study of 5-FU plus methyl-CCNU reported by Lokich and co-workers[419] demonstrated a 4% response rate.[422] All these data clearly indicated that combination chemotherapy with 5-FU plus methyl-CCNU regimens cannot be considered superior to 5-FU in either response rate or improvement in patient survival. It should be apparent that the 5-FU plus nitrosourea combination must be considered suboptimal and certainly is not a standard approach to the therapy of advanced colorectal cancer.

Progress in the chemotherapy of advanced colorectal cancer depends on several factors. It is apparent that the array of drugs available at present do not possess adequate activity in adenocarcinoma of the colon. It is unlikely that major benefits will be obtained by continued attempts to produce new combinations of these drugs. There must, therefore, be a major emphasis placed in new drug development in the hopes of being able to produce single agents with improved activity in metastatic colon cancer. One possible way in which the currently available drugs may be used to advantage is to capitalize on the possibility of producing drug interactions based on the principles of biochemical and pharmacologic modulation of drug action. For example, studies are currently being performed utilizing combinations of 5-FU plus methotrexate, 5-FU plus thymidine and 5-FU plus N-(phosphonacetyl-L-aspartate) (PALA) in the chemotherapy of colorectal cancer.[421–424] All of these combinations are based on preclinical evidence documenting biochemical mechanism of synergistic antitumor activity. Although it is too early to draw any conclusions concerning human efficacy of these combinations, it is clear that the principle of maximizing the potential for effective chemotherapy by basing treatment on documented preclinical findings of drug interactions is a rational approach to the problem.

TREATMENT OF PRIMARY COLORECTAL CANCER

TREATMENT OF CANCER OF THE RIGHT COLON

A one-stage right hemicolectomy must be considered the standard treatment for right colon cancer. The abdomen may be opened through a generous right subcostal or midline incision (Fig. 21-12*A*). After a gentle but thorough exploration of the abdomen, lysis of any adhesions should be performed. If peritoneal implants are seen, attempts are made to incorporate these within the specimen. If adjacent organs or structures are adhesed to the tumor or if liver metastases are seen, steps outlined in the section on special problems should be taken.

The first step in resection is to remove all large and small bowel from within the abdominal cavity; the small bowel should be placed on gentle traction to the patient's left and the transverse colon and greater omentum pulled superiorly and the ascending colon moved to the patient's right (Fig. 21-12*B*). Very often the tumor will be immobile; if so, the tumor and adjacent colon should not be dissected up at this time. With the bowel displayed on the anterior abdomen, the branches of the superior mesenteric artery are identified. The terminal ilium is divided between crushing clamps 3 inches to 4 inches from the ileocecal valve and the transverse colon is divided just proximal to the mid-colic artery. Gauze sponges are secured to the transected ends of bowel to prevent bacterial or tumor contamination. Throughout these steps the tumor is kept covered with a moist gauze.

In some asthenic individuals it may be possible at this point in the procedure to localize the right colic and ileocolic

RIGHT HEMICOLECTOMY

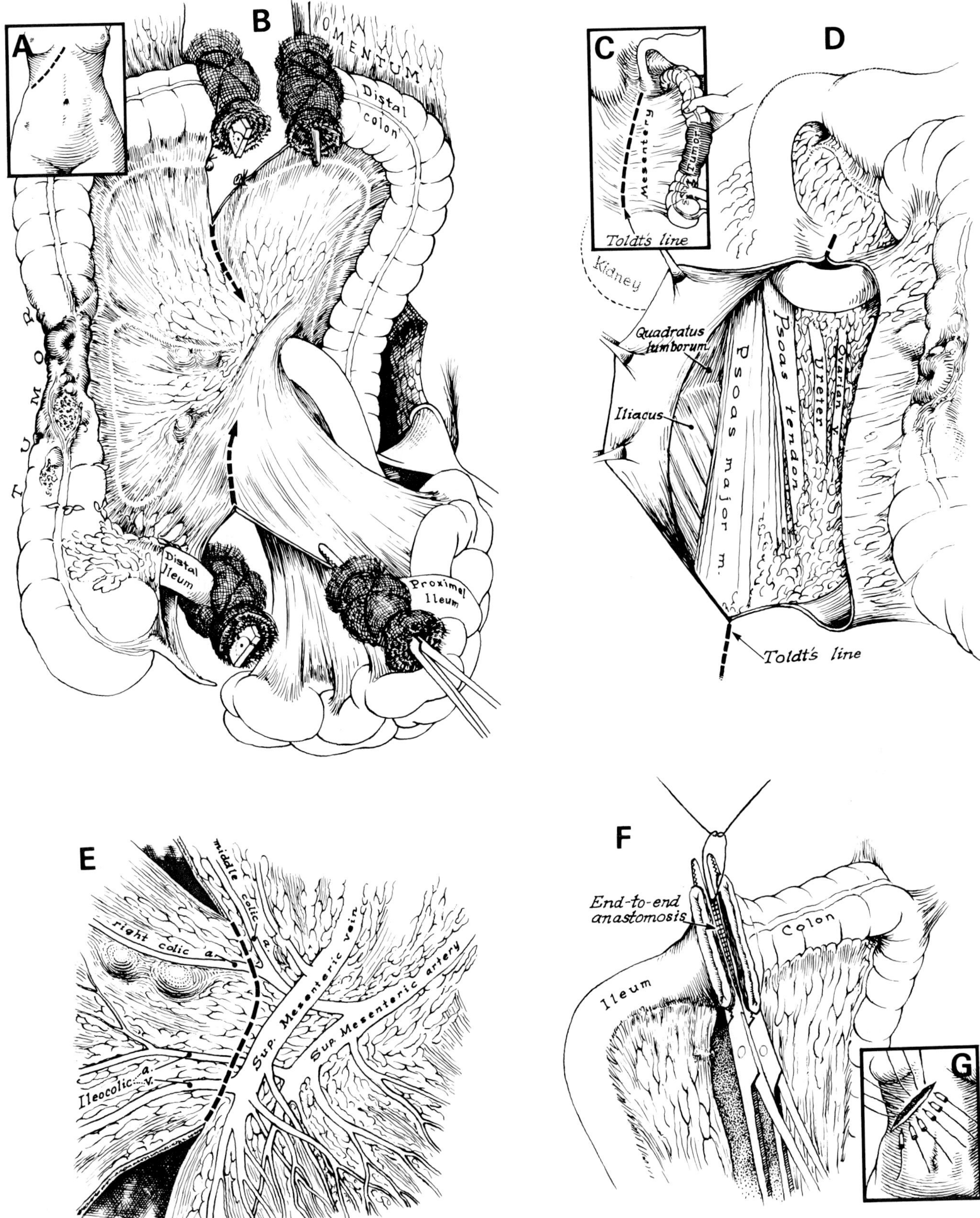

FIG. 21-12. Right hemicolectomy.

branches of the superior mesenteric artery and vein and ligate and divide them. However, this step is best delayed until the right mesocolon has been dissected up. To do this and not traumatize the tumor or open tissue planes adjacent to the tumor may be the most important technical feature of the resection. To dissect up the right mesocolon, the ascending colon is placed on gentle traction to the patient's left (Fig. 21-12*C*).

Toldt's white line is incised opening up the right retroperitoneum. The normal tissue planes are not used; rather a plane that skeletonizes psoas and iliacus muscle plus right ureter and testicular or ovarian vein is created using sharp dissection. All fibroareolar tissue over the right kidney (including Gerota' fascia over the lower pole of the right kidney), and duodenum stay with the tumor specimen (Fig. 21-12*D*). After dissecting up the right mesocolon the surgeon can palpate arterial structures between fingers above and below the specimen. Right colic and ileocolic artery and vein can be ligated at their highest point without danger of trauma to the superior mesenteric vein. As mentioned earlier, large ligatures around major vessel and all the surrounding soft tissue should be used on the specimen side to prevent leakage of malignant cells out of lymphatics. On the patient's side, individual vessels should be tied and suture ligated (Fig. 21-12*E*).

After excising the tiny segment of bowel that was within the crushing clamps an end-to-end anastomosis is performed and mesentery closed (Fig. 21-12*F*). The operative site is copiously irrigated with saline and then the entire abdomen with an antibiotic solution. The abdomen is closed in layers with the skin and subcutaneous tissue loosely packed with gauze to be closed in a delayed primary fashion on the fifth to seventh postoperative day (Fig. 21-12*G*).

Therapy for Right Colon Cancer

Postoperative radiation therapy may often be indicated in patients with right colon cancer in an attempt to decrease local recurrence rates. As emphasized in the section on anatomy, the cecum and ascending colon lack a mesentery; therefore, tumors on the lateral or posterior wall of the bowel which penetrate through the colon wall are likely to result in residual tumor cells at the resection site. Adequate doses (4000–4500 rad) of postoperative radiation therapy should minimize the problem of local recurrence.

TREATMENT OF CANCER OF THE TRANSVERSE COLON AND SPLENIC FLEXURE

As shown in Fig. 21-1, cancer of the transverse colon is resected with the entire transverse colon and middle colic artery in the specimen. Cancer of the splenic flexure is resected as a left hemicolectomy in a good risk patient. In a less than good risk patient, segmental resection of the splenic flexure with the left colic artery and lymphatic arcade is recommended. Super-radical excisions (in the absence of tumor adhesions) of the splenic flexure including spleen and tail of pancreas have no rationale. If an adjacent organ or structure is adhesed to the tumor (such as left lobe of liver) it should be removed with a generous margin *en bloc* with the specimen.

TREATMENT OF CANCER OF THE LEFT AND SIGMOID COLON

Standard treatment for carcinoma of the descending, sigmoid, and rectosigmoid colon including the upper one-third of the rectum is left hemicolectomy. As soon as the patient is anesthesized, a large volume of distilled water is run into the colon through the rectum; and, while the abdominal incision is being made, the water is removed by sump suction. This sump suction should remain on throughout the procedure to remove any intracolic debris or gas that may accumulate. A generous midline abdominal incision is followed by a thorough exploration of the peritoneal cavity (Fig. 21-13*A*). To expose the major vascular structures and to select the areas of colon to transect, the small and large bowel are removed from the peritoneal cavity. The small bowel is pulled to the patient's right, the transverse colon and greater omentum superiorly and the left colon to the patient's left (Fig. 21-13*B*). The ligament of Treitz is located and the peritoneum opened; the left ovarian or testicular vein coming off the left renal vein, the inferior mesenteric vein coming off the splenic vein, and the inferior mesenteric artery coming off the aorta are ligated and divided. All soft tissue surrounding the superior mesenteric artery and vein in the specimen are ligated with heavy ties to prevent a possible lymphatic leak of malignant cells into the operative field. The colon is transected between crushing clamps proximally and distally and the cut ends of bowel covered by gauze sponges. If the cancer is located within the pelvis, an adequate distal margin cannot be obtained until Toldt's line is incised and the peritoneum opened down into the pelvis (Fig. 21-13*C*). Care should be taken to avoid the left ureter and left common iliac vein.

If dissection to this point has been time consuming and repositioning of the tumor mass repeatedly required to maintain exposure in the pelvis, a second irrigation of the distal bowel with water is indicated. Transection of the bowel distally frees the specimen of all major attachments (Fig. 21-13*D*).

At this point the splenocolic ligament is divided so that the splenic flexure and left portion of the transverse colon are released (Fig. 21-13*E*). If the inferior mesenteric artery and vein have been transected, the colon has excellent mobility and even transverse colon can be anastomosed deep within the pelvis without tension. If the inferior mesenteric artery was left intact, the left colic branch may tether the proximal colon so that the anastomosis is made under tension. To avoid this danger it is usually wisest to ligate the inferior mesenteric artery at the aorta and rely on the middle colic artery through the marginal artery to nourish the bowel proximal to the anastomosis.

When the inferior mesenteric artery is ligated, the blood supply to the rectosigmoid and sigmoid colon is retrograde through the middle and inferior hemorrhoidal vessels. If a low rectal resection is performed the bowel distal to the anastomosis is nourished by inferior hemorrhoidal or inferior plus middle hemorrhoidal vessels. However, if the tumor is higher up in the sigmoid colon, the bowel is transected through an area normally supplied by the superior hemorrhoidal or lowest sigmoid artery. This may result in devascularization of a segment of sigmoid colon below the anastomosis, for a marginal artery closely opposed to the colon

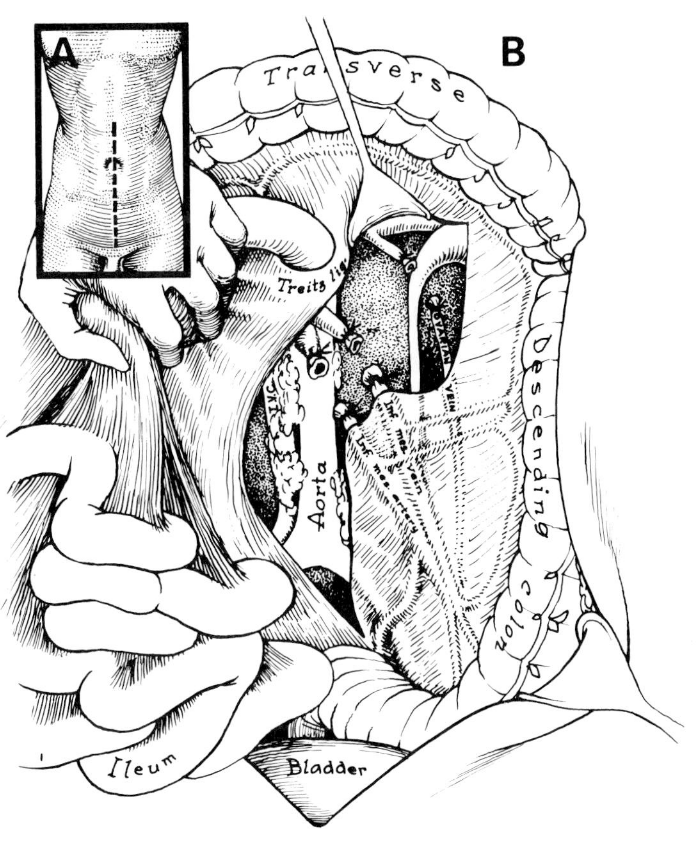

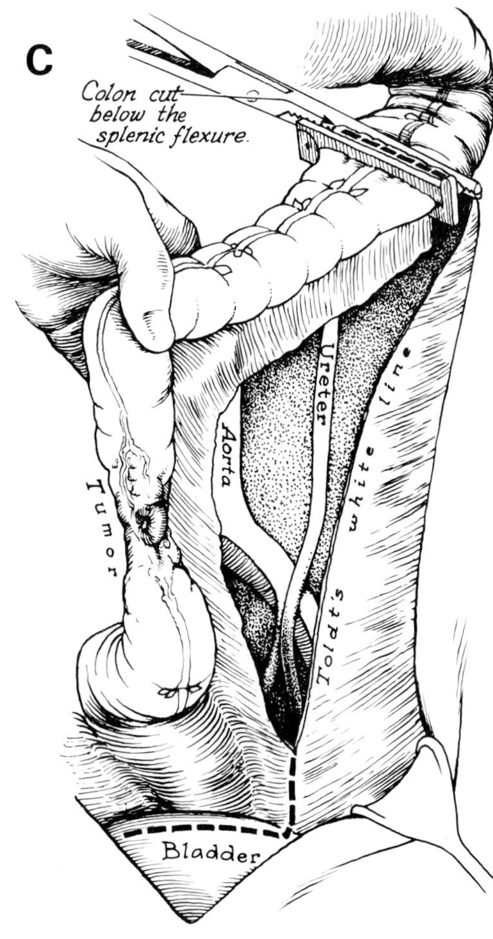

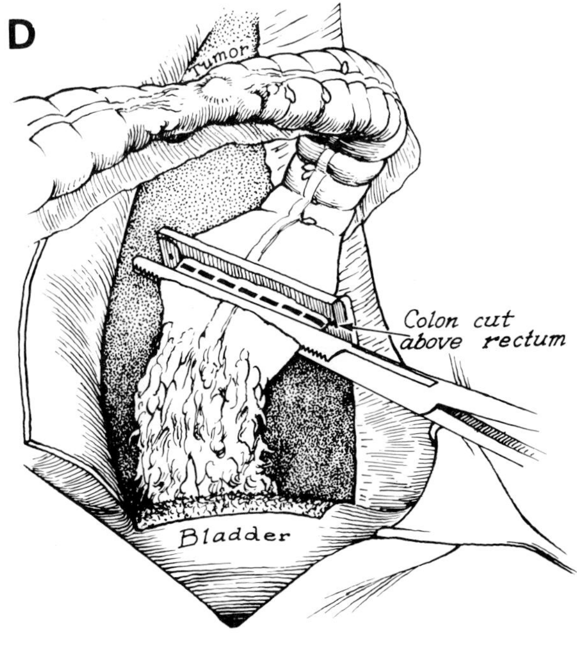

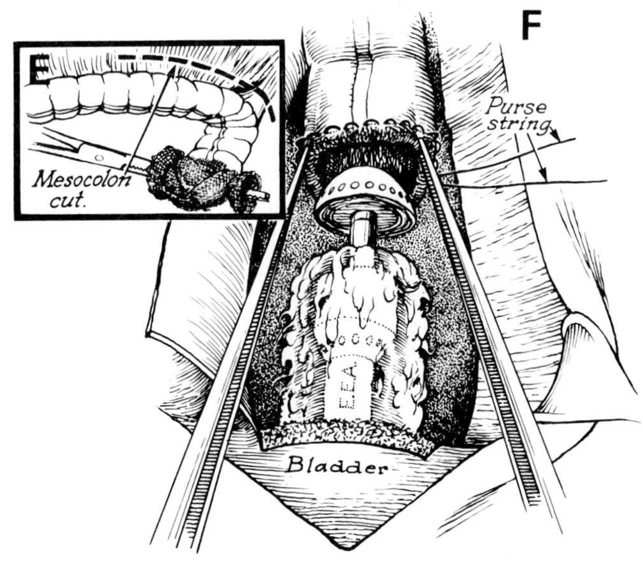

FIG. 21-13. Left hemicolectomy.

wall is not usually present in the rectosigmoid colon (Sudek's critical point). A marginal artery between superior hemorrhoidal and lowest sigmoid artery may be present in less than 50% of patients. Therefore, retrograde vascular supply from middle and inferior hemorrhoidal arteries along the lower sigmoid colon cannot be relied on. If the inferior mesenteric artery is to be ligated, the sigmoid colon must be sacrificed down to the peritoneal reflection and the anastomosis carried out using rectosigmoid distally.

An anastomosis is performed between proximal and distal segments of colon (Fig. 21-13*F*). If the colon was transected through the rectosigmoid a routine end-to-end anastomosis can be carried out. If the distal bowel must be transected below the peritoneal reflection to insure an adequate distal margin of resection, a technique for low anterior anastomosis may be required.

Following completion of the colorectal anastomosis, the operative site is copiously irrigated with saline and then the entire abdominal cavity with an antibiotic solution. The peritoneum should not be closed over the pelvis. The abdominal fascia is closed in layers while the skin and subcutaneous tissue are left open for a delayed primary closure.

RADIATION THERAPY FOR CANCER OF THE LEFT COLON

Seldom does postoperative radiation therapy need to be employed in left colon cancer. Occasionally tumors penetrating through the bowel wall on the posterior or lateral aspect of the descending colon may be selected. Another indication would be tumor adhesions to vital structures severed during the surgical procedure.

TREATMENT OF RECTAL CANCER

Potential treatments for rectal cancer are best discussed by dividing the rectum into upper, middle, and lower thirds. Invasive cancer in the upper third of the rectum is best treated by low anterior resection. The problems in treatment planning come with cancers of the middle and lower third of the rectum. In cancer of the middle one-third, low anterior resection (not possible with all patients or all tumors), abdomino–perineal resection, local excision, or radiation therapy may be selected. In cancer of the lower one-third of the rectum, resection and anastomosis is impossible so the choice is abdomino–perineal resection, a local excision, or radiation therapy. Not only the age and operative risk of the patient, but also the extent of the local tumor should be considered in selecting an appropriate management plan for a particular patient with rectal cancer.

THE CHOICE OF LOW ANTERIOR RESECTION OR ABDOMINO–PERINEAL RESECTION AS A TREATMENT FOR CANCER OF THE MIDDLE THIRD OF THE RECTUM

The selection of low anterior resection or abdomino–perineal resection is based on two factors: (1) adequate exposure within the pelvis and (2) an adequate margin of bowel and soft tissue distal to the primary tumor. Exposure is best in the thin female and most difficult in the mesomorphic male. With an anastomotic clamp or staple gun available, the technical difficulties of performing an anastomosis deep within the pelvis are minimized. To get the longest possible distal margin the dissection may be carried right down to the puborectalis muscle. The rectum may be transected flush with the surrounding levator ani musculature, but in so doing the mucosa below the hemorrhoidal ring should not be pulled up to be included with the specimen. If the mucosa that lies within the anorectal ring is sacrificed, specialized nerve endings are lost that are necessary to preserve perfect continence. With this limitation in mind the surgeon must set out to adequately resect the rectal tumor with safe distal and lateral margins.

Best and Blair collected histological evidence from six reports; retrograde extension in the rectal wall or through lymphatic channels beyond 2 cm from the lower margin of the tumor occurred in less than 1% of over 600 specimens.[425] Goligher, Dukes, and Bussey and Grinnell have observed that retrograde spread of tumor within the wall of the rectum or in lymphatics occurs only in patients whose tumor is "incurable by any operation".[63,88] Grinnell advised that a margin of bowel beyond 5 cm is unprofitable; patients whose tumor is so extensive that they may benefit from a distal margin greater than 5 cm will almost surely succumb to disseminated lymphatic metastases.

Cullen and Mayo suggest that sometimes the surgeon must delay the choice of anterior resection or abdominoperineal resection until the specimen has been dissected free within the pelvis and the length of bowel and surrounding soft tissue below the tumor mass determined.[426] Butcher has proposed a "rule of thumb" which if applied to the usual patients, will result in a good cancer operation, will not sacrifice anal function unnecessarily, and will not be associated with excessive complication rates.[427] Butcher's Rule was stated as follows: If the lesion is easily palpated with the examining finger, abdomino–perineal resection is indicated; however, if at the time of resection the tumor, after mobilization of the rectum to the level of the levator ani muscles, can be brought to the level of the abdominal incision, an adequate anterior resection may be performed.

Certainly, numerous studies that have compared the 5-year survival of anterior resection with that of abdomino–perineal resection show very similar results.[99,102,106,107,229,426,428–442] The studies of Glover and Waugh and Gilbertsen stand alone as reports of a large number of patients showing diminished survival in those receiving anterior resection for carcinoma of the rectum as compared to abdominoperineal excision.[443,444]

Survivals for both operations are very near 50%. The somewhat increased survival rates reported by some for anterior resection over abdomino–perineal excision are likely due to two factors. First, in selecting to use anterior resection the surgeon may instinctively choose anterior resection to treat the favorable lesions while the more advanced cancers are treated by abdomino–perineal resection. Second, in any series of patients with tumors in the mid-third of the rectum, the tumors that are deeper in the pelvis are more likely to be treated by abdomino–perineal excision. As reviewed in the section on prognosis, the deeper a lesion within the pelvis the poorer the prognosis. Therefore, the abdomino–perineal group may contain patients with slightly worse prognosis tumors because they are the patients in the group with slightly lower tumors.

SURGICAL TECHNIQUES FOR LOW RECTAL RESECTION PLUS ANASTOMOSIS

Several different techniques for low rectal resection plus anastomosis have been described and results published. Six different techniques are illustrated in Fig. 21-14. Anterior resection is the least traumatic of the techniques described, for it does not involve a second incision in the anus, as does the pull-through procedure, or a sacral incision, as in the abdomino–transsacral procedure.[439,445,446] Because of an unpredictable sloughing of distal sigmoid and not infrequent fecal incontinence, the pull-through procedure is seldom used nowadays.[447,448] If the rectal wall is too thick for the safe use of a staple gun, an anastomotic instrument or a single layer anastomosis with a diverting right transverse colostomy should be used.[449–451] If a marked size discrepancy between proximal and distal segments of bowel exists, an end-to-side rectosigmoid anastomosis may be ideal.[452]

ABDOMINO–PERINEAL RESECTION FOR CANCER OF THE MIDDLE AND LOWER THIRD OF THE RECTUM

Standard therapy for cancers in the lower one-third of the rectum is abdomino–perineal resection. The technique of this procedure is illustrated in Fig. 21-15. First, double-puncture laparoscopy is performed looking for hepatic metastases or peritoneal carcinomatosis.[453] If multiple hepatic metastases are seen, fulguration plus radiation therapy is usually recommended to control the primary tumor and preserve anal function. If a solitary metastasis is observed and the patient is a good risk, resection of both the liver and rectal lesions may be considered. Prior to making the abdominal incision, the left colon is irrigated with a large volume of distilled water and suctioned dry by sump suction.

The abdomen is opened through a midline incision that extends down to the symphysis pubis (Fig. 21-15*A*). After a thorough exploration of the abdominal cavity with palpation of the liver, the small bowel is removed from the abdominal cavity and pulled to the patient's right. The transverse colon and greater omentum are placed superiorly and the descending colon and sigmoid colon pulled to the patient's left (Fig. 21-15*B*). The peritoneum beneath the ligament of Treitz and

(*Text continues on p. 700.*)

FIG. 21-14. Techniques of low anterior resection. EEA = end-to-end anastomosis.

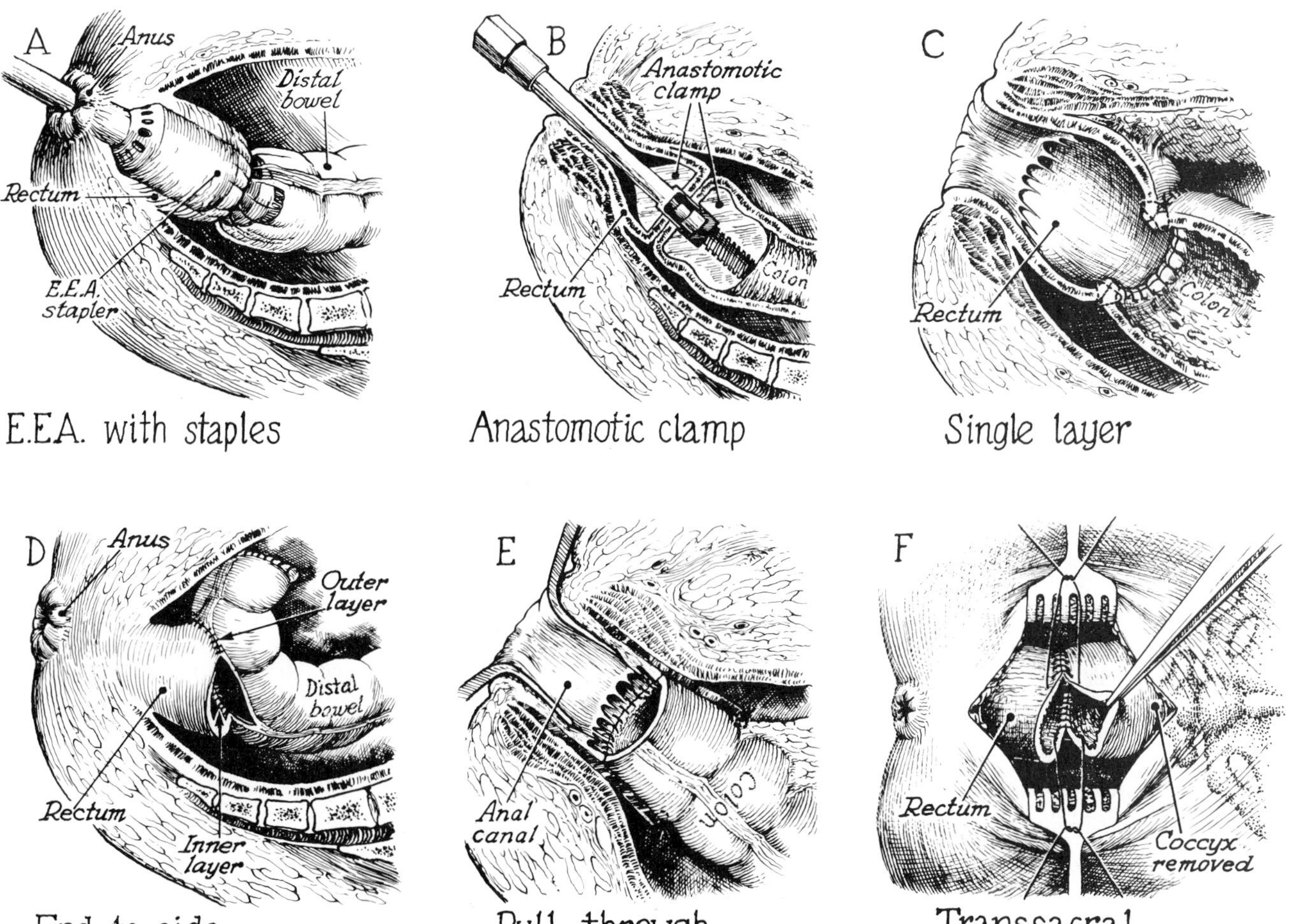

ABDOMINOPERINEAL RESECTION

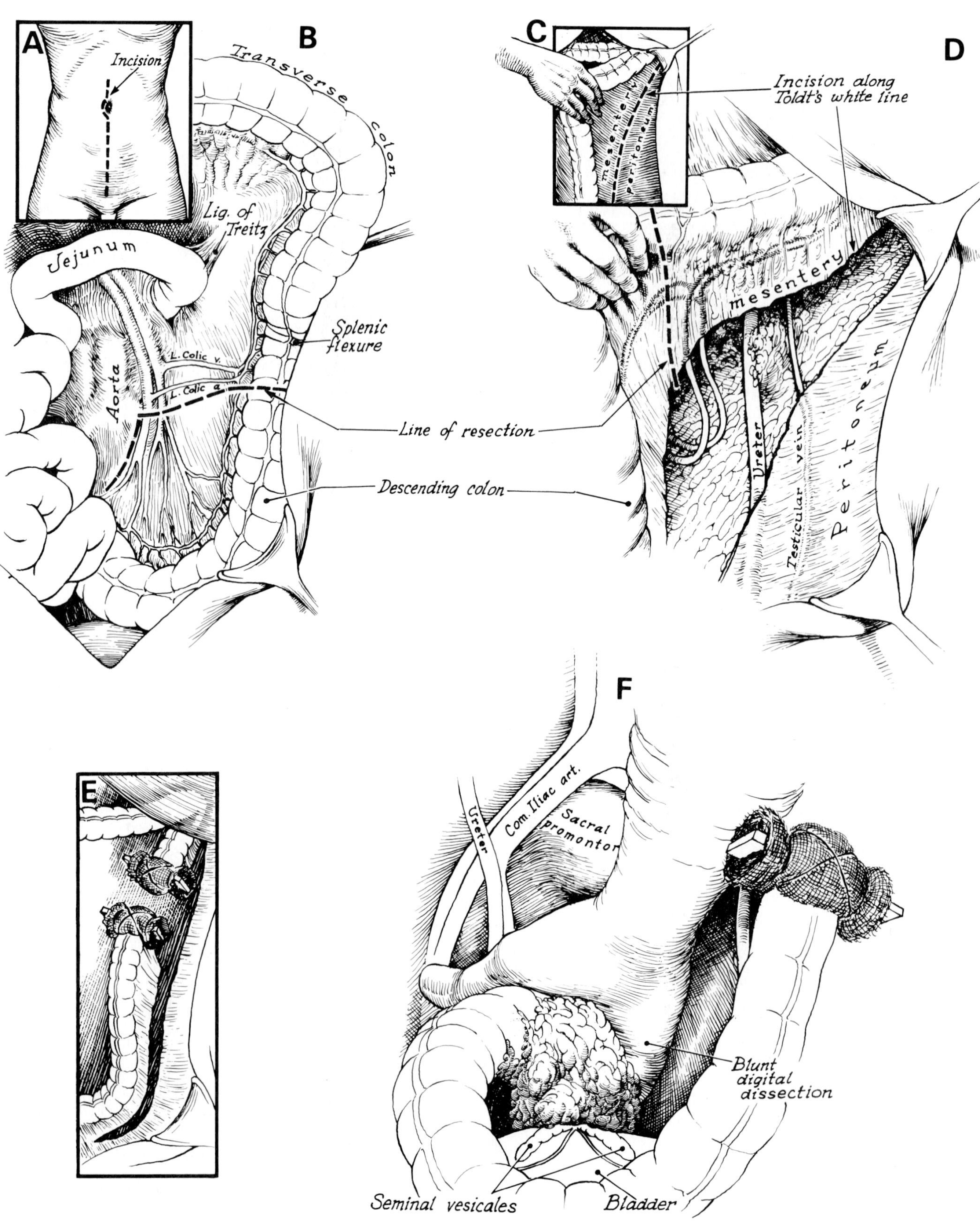

FIG. 21-15. Abdominoperineal resection.

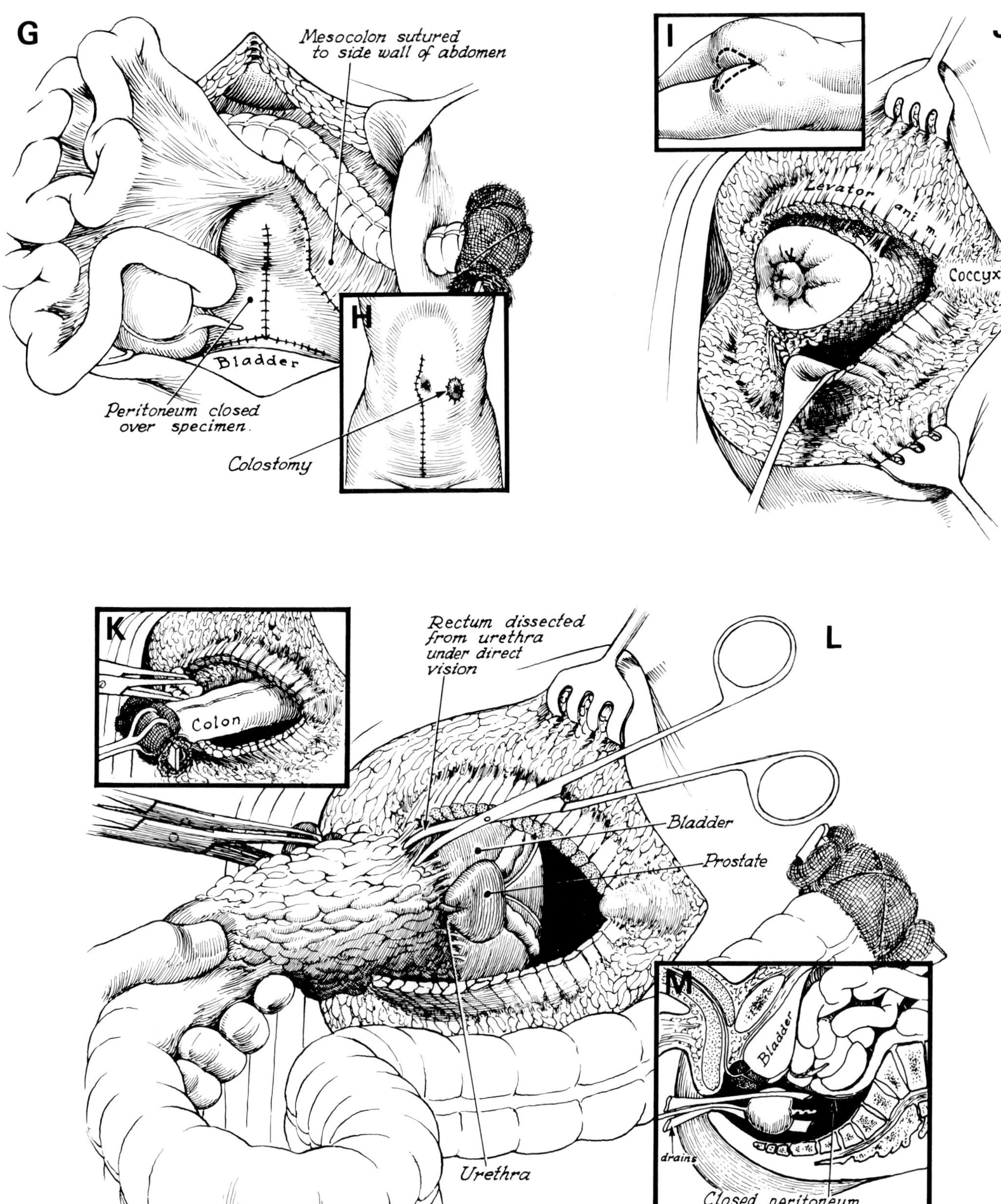
G
Mesocolon sutured to side wall of abdomen
Bladder
Peritoneum closed over specimen.
H
Colostomy
I
J
Levator ani m.
Coccyx
K
Colon
Rectum dissected from urethra under direct vision
L
Bladder
Prostate
Urethra
M
Bladder
drains
Closed peritoneum

over the inferior mesenteric vein and artery is opened and the left colic vein and artery are identified. Just below their left colic branch, the inferior mesenteric vein and artery are ligated in continuity and then divided. All small and large bowel except that which is to be resected is packed into the upper abdomen.

Traction on the descending colon is changed from the patient's left to the right (Fig. 21-15*C*). Toldt's line is opened laterally avoiding the left ureter and the testicular or ovarian vein (Fig. 21-15*D*). These peritoneal incisions are continued along the base of the sigmoid mesocolon to join just beneath the bladder. Leaves of peritoneum should be preserved for later reconstruction of the pelvic floor. The descending colon is divided just below the left colic artery between clamps and the cut ends of the bowel occlusively covered by gauze sponges (Fig. 21-15*E*). Using sharp and some blunt dissection the rectum is freed from the sacrum and pelvic side walls (Fig. 21-15*F*). If the tumor seems close or adherent to either pelvic side wall, the internal iliac artery and vein should be severed at their origin from the common iliac and an internal iliac lymph node dissection performed. When the levator ani muscles have been reached and the middle hemorrhoidal vessels and lateral rectal ligaments severed, the specimen is closed beneath the newly created pelvic peritoneal floor (Fig. 21-15*G*). The descending mesocolon is sutured to the left abdominal side wall to prevent small bowel from herniating down lateral to the colon. The anterior abdominal wall is closed and the colostomy brought out through the abdominal wall and matured primarily (Fig. 21-15*H*).

The patient is now turned on his side, right side down in a modified Sims position (Fig. 21-15*I*). Tape is used to hold the buttocks open and the rectum is stitched shut. An elliptical incision is made around the anus into ischiorectal fat aiming the incision for the medial edges of the ischial tuberosity (Fig. 21-15*J*). By sharply incising just below the coccyx, the pelvis is entered; the levator ani muscles are divided above a finger placed within the pelvis. The specimen is delivered from within the pelvis (Fig. 21-15*K*). Under direct vision the specimen is sharply dissected free of urethra (Fig. 21-15*L*). The fascia overlying levator muscles is reapproximated as much as possible and the skin closed over a soft drain plus a large Foley catheter containing sterile saline to fill the space within the pelvis. The catheter is placed to suction (Fig. 21-15*M*).

Postoperatively, the patient is kept at bedrest and with Foley catheter drainage for 1 week. Leg exercises are performed to help prevent thromboembolism. When the patient is ambulatory, a cystometrogram is obtained and if bladder function has begun to return, the Foley catheter is removed from the bladder. Fluid is removed from the perineal balloon so that the perineal space is obliterated within 10 days to 2 weeks. Irrigation of a perineal sinus tract may be required for several weeks especially if pre-operative radiation therapy was used.

FULGURATION FOR THE TREATMENT OF CANCER OF THE MIDDLE AND LOWER THIRD OF THE RECTUM

Beginning with the works of Strauss, several surgeons have investigated the use of fulguration for the treatment of rectal cancer below the peritoneal reflection.[454–469] Crile and Turnbull treated 62 patients by electrocoagulation and compared the results to those of abdomino–perineal resection; 46% of 226 patients undergoing abdomino–perineal resection survived 5 years while 68% of patients treated by electrocoagulation survived 5 years.[468] As discussed by Baker it is impossible to find a matched group of patients treated by abdomino–perineal resection or electrocoagulation outside of a randomly controlled clinical trial.[470] Nevertheless, the number of 5-year survivors in patients treated by electrocoagulation is impressive. Proponents of this technique argue in the following manner that most cancers in the middle or lower third of the rectum can be electively treated by electrocoagulation. First, local tumor can be controlled by fulguration as well as by abdomino–perineal resection. Second, although regional lymph node metastases are present in at least one-third of patients, those rendered free of disease following abdomino–perineal resection are so few that *cures are offset by the operative mortality*. Abdomino–perineal resection must be performed in all patients to benefit that small group with one to four positive lymph nodes.[471]

Although this simplified approach of electrocoagulation for all patients with carcinoma of the extraperitoneal rectum sounds enticing, in reality, electrocoagulation should be reserved for poor risk patients. Problems with the general use of electrocoagulation are as follows:

1. Local control by fulguration is far from 100%. Stearns and Baker have both reported serious problems with uncontrolled local cancer growth.[439,470] Also, Madden and Kandalaft report repeat fulguration sessions (average 3.5 sessions per patient) needed in 87% of patients.[469] Eleven of 131 (8.4%) of their patients required subsequent abdomino–perineal resection. Crile and Turnbull report 8 of 62 (13%) patients requiring radical resection because of uncontrolled local growth of tumor.[468] In this series seven of eight were 5-year survivors after radical resection for persistent cancer; however, in the Madden and Kandalaft series only one of 11 survived. Wanebo and Quan report that only three of 14 patients needing radical surgery for fulguration failure survived 5 years.[472]
2. More than one-third of patients with rectal cancer have disease in lymph nodes. Using cleaning techniques and multiple sections of lymph nodes, nearly 50% of patients have spread to lymph nodes.[60]
3. An operative mortality for abdomino–perineal resection of 10% is too high. This may be near the proper figure for patients over age 70, but not for younger patients.[360,439] (see section on complications)
4. Approximately half the cancers in the middle third of the rectum that are candidates for fulguration could be treated by low anterior resection with excellent results expected even in some lymph node positive patients.[439] Although fulguration is certainly possible in the middle one-third of the rectum, it may be indicated only in patients who are a poor operative risk.
5. Finally, electrocoagulation of rectal cancer presents a problem because it destroys the specimen as the cancer is removed. No data regarding prognosis and no indication for the need of postoperative radiation therapy can be gained.

In summary, a treatment equation for selection of abdomino–perineal resection or fulguration may be constructed as follows: The further advanced the tumor by digital rectal and sigmoidoscopic examination (Fig. 21-10) and the higher the grade by biopsy, the greater the indication for radical surgery. The older the patient and the greater the operative risk of the patient the stronger the indication for fulguration. Certainly, young patients with far advanced tumors are candidates for radical surgery and old, infirm patients with polypoid cancers are candidates for fulguration.

LOCAL EXCISION OF RECTAL CANCER

An approach to local excision of selected rectal cancer shown to give good results was advocated by Jackman, Morson and colleagues, and Deddish.[473–476] The criteria by which these authors selected patients for local procedures or radical surgery are similar to those shown in Table 21-33. A conservative approach to *selected* cases of rectal cancer is justified.

The techniques for local excision of favorable rectal cancers are numerous.[337–342] Perhaps the most popular is that described by Kraske.[477] Through a longitudinal skin excision the coccyx is removed and the muscle fibers of the levator ani split. If a lesion is on the anterior wall of the rectum, it is approached by an incision through the posterior rectal wall. If the tumor is lateral or posterior, an elliptical incision of the tumor with a margin of rectal wall is made. Mason has described a trans-sphincteric approach for removal of selected rectal cancers and Olsen a trans-anal approach.[337,338]

A comment should be made about the advantages of local excision of selected early cancers as compared to destruction of the lesions by electrocautery or cryosurgery. If a clean excision of the specimen is performed, the margins of resection and the depth of invasion of the lesion can be determined. From this information a rational decision about the possible need for further radical surgery can be made and the need for postoperative radiation therapy determined.

ENDOCAVITARY IRRADIATION (PAPILLON TECHNIQUE)

Treatment of carefully selected patients with low and mid-rectal lesions by a technique of low kilovoltage endocavitary irradiation is one of the acceptable sphincter saving options available. Treatment selection is based on both tumor and equipment factors.[478–481] Tumors with the following features are required for this technique:

1. Perfect accessibility. Tumors should be less than 12 cm above the anal verge.
2. Small or moderate size. The maximum acceptable lesion size is 3 cm × 5 cm which can be covered in overlapping fields with the treatment cone of 3 cm diameter.
3. Negligible infiltration with ulcerative invading lesions; if the lesion is crateriform, endocavitary radiation must be supplemented with an implant.
4. Moderate to well differentiated tumors to decrease the risk for lymph node involvement.

Patients are treated on an outpatient basis using a Phillips 50 KV superficial x-ray unit with rapid output (1000 rad/minute to 2000 rad/minute). The treatment proctoscope is inserted after gradual dilation of the anus (Fig. 21-16).

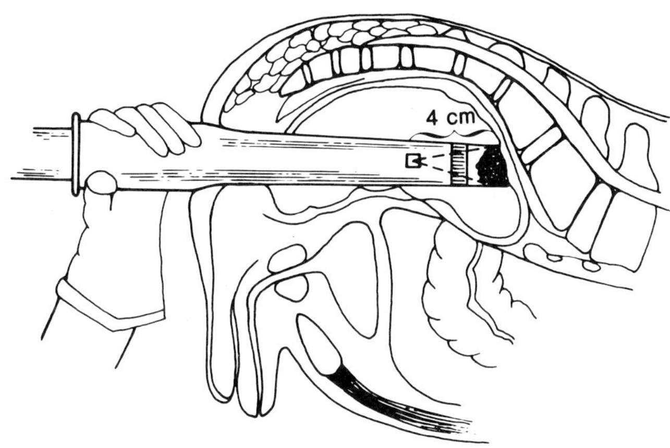

FIG. 21-16. Technique for irradiation of selected rectal cancers. The applicator containing the x-ray tube is inserted with the proctoscope. The 4 cm focal length of the x-ray beam is indicated. (Sischy B, Remington J: Treatment of carcinoma of the rectum by intracavitary radiation. Surg Gynecol Obstet 141:562–564, 1975)

Patients receive 2500 rad to 4000 rad per treatment to a total maximum dose of 8000 rad to 15,000 rad. Treatment fractions are usually separated by 2 weeks to 3 weeks. By the third treatment, visualization of the original lesion is often difficult. While the total dose seems excessive, it should be realized that at a depth of 6.25 mm only 50% of the surface dose is delivered. Therefore, the first and second treatments are essentially absorbed in the exophytic portion of the tumor to cause shrinkage so that the third and fourth treatments can treat the tumor bed and bowel wall.

There are some potential advantages of this technique over treatment of similar select lesions with fulguration:

1. Ambulatory outpatient treatment
2. Colostomy or anesthesia not required
3. No danger of bleeding and negligible risk of perforation
4. Easier to follow clinically in that associated induration is less; therefore local recurrence is easier to diagnose early when surgical salvage with abdominoperineal resection is still feasible

TABLE 21-33. Prognostic Factors Important in the Physical and Sigmoidoscopic Examination of Primary Rectal Tumors of the Mid- and Lower Third of the Rectum

PROBABLY CURABLE BY LOCAL EXCISION (GOOD PROGNOSTIC FEATURES)*	POSSIBLY CURABLE BUT ONLY BY RADICAL RESECTION (POOR PROGNOSTIC FEATURES)†
polypoid	crateriform
mobile	immobile
less than 25% circumference involved	more than 25% circumference involved
tumor grade well differentiated	poorly differentiated
CEA normal	CEA elevated

* Local excision favored in as many patients as possible over the age of 70 years.

† If advanced tumor is suspected in a good-risk patient, hypogastric lymph node dissection may be indicated, otherwise standard abdomino-perineal resection indicated.

Papillon in a personal communication reported 186 cases treated with curative intent with endocavitary irradiation alone or in combination with implant. The overall local failure rate was only 7.5%. Of 133 patients at risk for 5 years, 104 (78%) were alive and free of disease and only 12 (9%) had died from their malignancy. Local recurrence had occurred in 11 (8.3%) and surgical salvage was possible in six. Sischy and Remington report 39 patients treated with curative intent; local recurrence occurred in only two patients (5.1%).[481]

RADIATION THERAPY AND SURGERY AS COMBINED TREATMENT FOR CANCER OF THE RECTUM

Selection of patients for radiation therapy following surgical resection was discussed in the section on principles of radiation therapy. Treatment plans which maximize the therapeutic ratio utilize large fields with moderate doses (4500 rad over 5 to 6 weeks), followed by boost fields (5000 rad to 5500 rad). The large field arrangement depends on the structure of the pelvis, location of the primary tumor, presence or absence of adjacent organ involvement, and the area and number of lymph nodes involved. The width of AP:PA ports should be sufficient to cover the pelvic inlet. Lateral margins extending 1 cm to 2 cm beyond the widest point of the bony pelvis are usually sufficient, depending on treatment energy and penumbrum. The superior margin should be at least 1.5 cm above the level of the sacral promontory. Occasionally mid-L5 to L4 and infrequently, peri-aortic coverage to L1 or T12 may be wise depending on the extent of mesenteric and

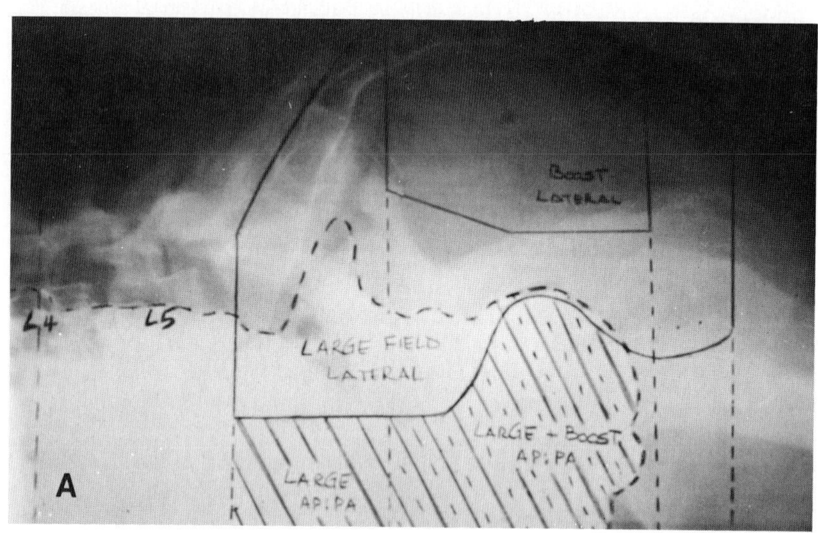

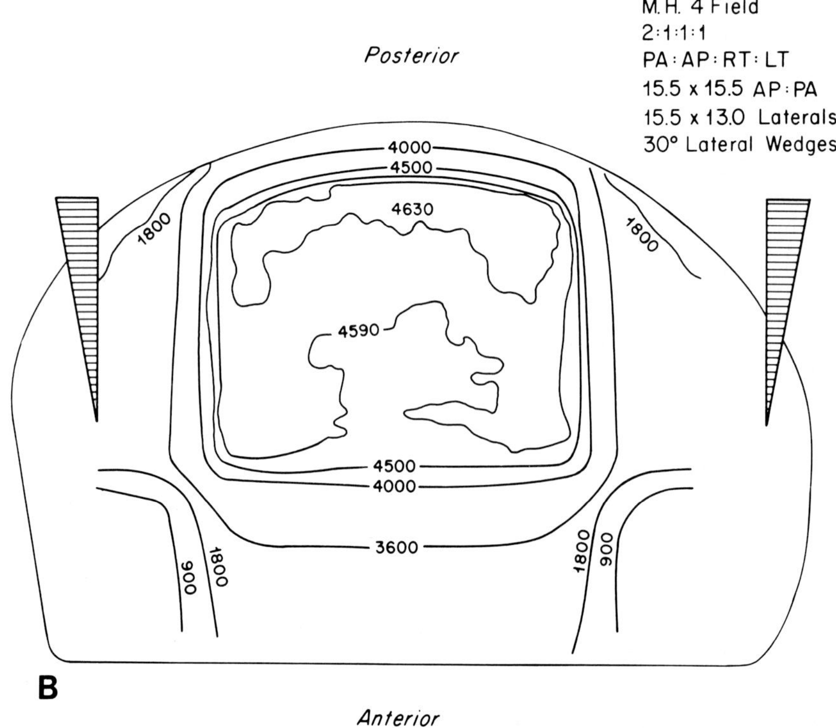

FIG. 21-17. Postoperative pelvic irradiation following a low anterior resection for an adenocarcinoma on the posterior wall of the mid to upper rectum with gross extra-rectal extension and positive lymph nodes. Radiation treatment to cover the tumor bed as well as internal iliac and presacral nodes was accomplished with a 4-field set-up using lateral large field portals in conjunction with PA-AP fields. This was used to deliver a dose of 4500 rads. The tumor bed was then boosted with an additional 500 rads using a 3 field set-up of PA, right lateral, and left lateral portals. *A*, a lateral radiograph of the sacral area with superimposed lateral fields. A small amount of small intestine is present within the antero-superior portion of the large lateral field but is totally out of the boost field portal. (Note that the patient is in a prone treatment position.) The *cross-hatched area* shows the additional amount of small bowel that would receive full radiation dose if only PA-AP portals were used. *B*, the isodose contours through a cross-section of the patient at mid-sacrum. (Modified from Gunderson LL, Cohen AM, Welch CE: Residual, inoperable or recurrent colorectal cancer: Surgical–radiotherapy interaction. Am J. Surg 139:518–525, 1980)

iliac nodal involvement. After anterior resection, the inferior extent may be somewhat variable; the usual intent is coverage of the obturator foramina. The minimal extent should be 2 cm to 5 cm below the gross tumor (pre-operative) or below the most inferior extent of dissection or mobilization of the distal colon (postoperative), which ideally would be marked with surgical clips. The posterior field margin is vital since the rectum and perirectal tissue lie just anterior to the sacrum and coccyx. Accordingly, dependent on treatment energy, the posterior field margin should be a minimum of 1 cm to 1.5 cm behind the anterior bony sacral margin to allow for some daily patient movement and can be shaped with cerrobend or similar blocks to spare posterior muscle and soft tissues.

Following abdomino–perineal resection, the perineum with its anteroposterior and inferolateral limits of operative dissection must be included within the large field. Lead shot or wire should be used to mark the entire extent of the perineal scar when localization films are obtained; field edges should be 1.5 cm to 2 cm beyond the scar as marked. Anteriorly, the lower third of the rectum abuts the posterior vaginal wall and prostate and these structures should be included. In female patients adequate coverage of the posterior vagina is assured if a contrast soaked gauze pad or tampon is placed within the vagina when localization films are taken.

Internal iliac lymph node dissections are not a standard part of rectal cancer surgery and should therefore be included in the initial irradiation field. External iliac nodes are not a primary nodal drainage site and are not included unless pelvic organs with major external iliac drainage (bladder, prostate, cervix, vagina) are involved by direct extension or the pelvic side wall itself is involved.

The perineum is included to a dose level of 4500 rad in 5 weeks in most patients with multiple field techniques including lateral fields. To boost the perineal scar, the buttocks may be taped apart and toward the end of treatment, using controlled thickness and width, a bolus of irradiation used to cover the perineal scar. For male patients the penis and scrotum should be elevated cephalad behind the symphysis during treatment.

Boost fields are occasionally as small as 8 cm by 8 cm in postoperative cases, with targets precisely demarcated by clips, or with good reconstruction from diagnostic barium enema studies. Boost fields more frequently should be 10 cm by 10 cm to 12 cm by 12 cm to insure adequate coverage to at least 5000 rad.

EMPLOYMENT OF SMALL BOWEL ROENTGENOGRAMS

In an effort to minimize both acute toxicity and chronic complications of pelvic and abdominal radiotherapy for colorectal malignancies, small bowel contrast studies should be utilizied to influence both design of portals and radiation doses. Studies are performed preferably after the first week of treatment to allow the study to reflect current anatomy.

These studies demonstrate considerable variability in the localization and mobility of the small intestine following extensive intraabdominal procedures. The advantage of 4-field extended (PA:AP and lateral) or 3-field boost portals (PA and laterals) over AP:PA techniques in sparing the small intestine becomes apparent when radiation portals are superimposed over small bowel films and isodose contours are compared (Figure 21-17A, B).

For pelvic lesions, the value of bladder distention to displace small bowel has been useful. The amount of small bowel that can be displaced by bladder distention is seen in Fig. 21-18. Since the technique is simple and effective, it can be utilized

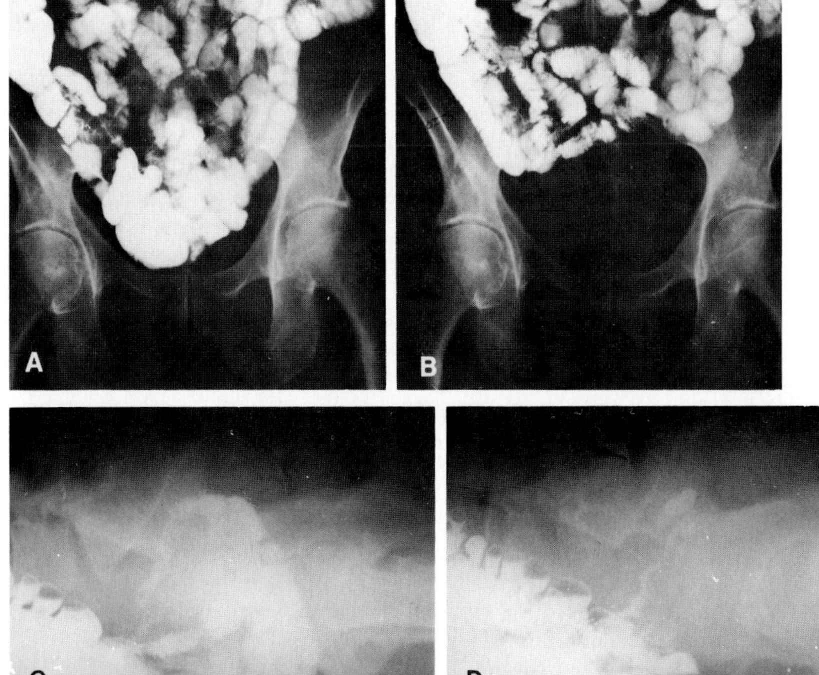

FIG. 21-18. Bladder distention for displacement of the small intestine out of pelvic irradiation portals for postoperative radiation after curative abdominoperineal resection. A marked difference in the inferior extent of the small intestine is seen with the bladder empty (*A, C*) vs. distended (*B, D*) on both AP and prone cross-table lateral views. As seen on lateral radiographs, a single loop of small bowel remains in the presacral space. (From Gunderson LL, Dosorety D, Blitzer DH et al: Low dose preoperative irradiation, surgery and elective postoperative irradiation for resectable rectal and recto sigmoid carcinoma. 1980 Am Rad Soc Proc. Int J Radiat Oncol Biol Phys 6(1):38, 1980)

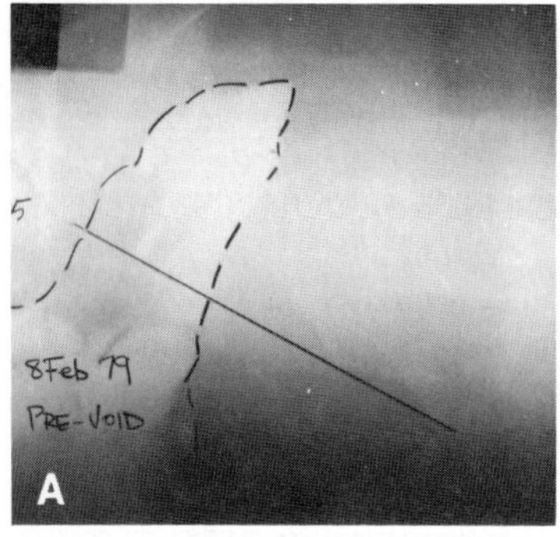

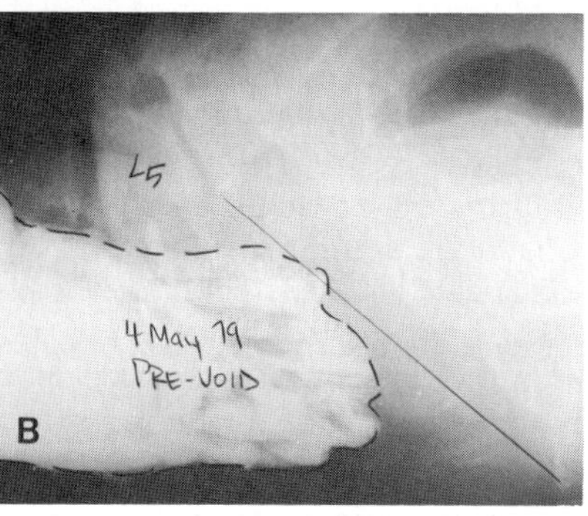

FIG. 21-19. Small bowel displacement with an "omental sling." In this patient, some displacement of the small intestine out of the irradiation field was seen with bladder distention. However, some loops of bowel remained adjacent to tumor (*A*). Displacement of small bowel out of the pelvis was accomplished by laparotomy and construction of the omental sling (*B*).

in virtually all patients with pelvic colon lesions. An exception is the category of patients with tumor adherence to or invasion of the dome of the bladder in whom bladder distention could displace not only small bowel (Fig. 21-19), but also the necessary tumor volume out of the irradiation field.

ADJUVANT CHEMOTHERAPY

Even though chemotherapy appears to be of, at best, limited value in advanced colorectal cancer, there have been many efforts to apply this treatment at earlier stages of the disease as an adjuvant to surgery.[483-488] Selection of cases for adjuvant chemotherapy is based upon the ability to determine the likelihood of relapse in patients who have undergone surgical therapy for primary colon cancer and have a relatively poor survival after resection with curative intent.

The most extensively investigated adjunctive chemotherapies have been single agents. The Veterans Administration Surgical Oncology Group (VASOG) utilized thiotepa and subsequently floxuridine (FUDR) given at the time of operation and in the immediate postoperative period.[483,484] In these prospectively randomized trials, neither drug improved 5-year survival. The next drug the VASOG chose to investigate was 5-FU. Five-year and, in some cases, 7-year survival data are available in these trials.[487]

The results of this trial showed evidence of minimal benefit from 5-FU treatment. Although within the curative resection group, the 5-year survival was 58% among 152 patients receiving 5-FU *versus* 49% for 146 control patients, these differences were not statistically significant. The trend toward better survival with 5-FU therapy was seen in the clinically and histologically proven palliative resection groups, although again statistical significance was not attained.

TABLE 21-34. Controlled Trials of Fluorinated Pyrimidines in Colorectal Cancer by the Veterans Administration Surgical Oncology Group

DRUG	NUMBER OF PATIENTS	STATISTICAL SURVIVAL BENEFIT WITH TREATMENT	REFERENCE NUMBER
FUDR	548	None	(484)
5-FU	308	None	(483)
5-FU	522	None	(487)
5-FU	156	None	(485)
5-FU	210	None	(489)

The next study by VASOG evaluated prolonged intermittent 5-FU therapy in poor prognosis patients with colorectal cancer.[487] Randomization was between 5-FU treatment after surgery and surgery alone. A drug course consisted of 5-FU 12 mg/kg body weight intravenously daily for 5 days and courses were repeated at 6 week to 8 week intervals. Follow-up is now complete in excess of 4 years. Actuarial survival at 7 years shows some benefit for the treated group. Thirty-three percent of patients receiving 5-FU and 26% of control patients are alive at 7 years. These differences are not statistically significant. For those patients undergoing palliative resection, the 18-month survival is 38% for 5-FU treated cases *versus* 26% for controls. These results are not significantly different.

The Central Oncology Group has examined the effect of 5-FU on disease-free interval and survival in 210 patients who had curative resections for colorectal cancer.[488] Fifty-seven of 113 controls (50%) and 54 of 97 treated patients (56%) are surviving free of disease. These results are not significantly different. However, in the patients with Dukes C lesions, there was statistically significant ($p = .04$) prolongation of disease-free interval in the patients receiving 5-FU therapy. In a small group of 29 patients with rectal cancer on this study, 5-FU therapy was associated with significant prolongation in survival ($p = .011$).

Table 21-34 summarizes the results obtained with controlled trials of adjuvant therapy with fluorinated pyrimidines. As can be seen when overall survival of all patients in any one trial is examined there is no evidence of statistical benefit in survival from fluorinated pyrimidine therapy. It should, however, be noted that these trials all show some small benefit for 5-FU therapy and when subgroups are examined or when the results of patients undergoing palliative and curative resections are analyzed together statistical significance has been claimed.[487] In any event, the maximum 5-year survival benefit that has been demonstrated in controlled trials is only 5% to 10% greater than controls. These results have to be considered of marginal biologic and clinical significance and clearly continued clinical trials with new approaches to surgical adjuvant therapy must proceed.

There are a number of uncontrolled studies of adjuvant therapy originally reported to show significant benefit over historical controls.[486,488,490] These trials illustrate the risks of using historical controls since they have not been confirmed in prospectively randomized trials. The Li and Ross study utilized the 5-FU regimen used in the first VASOG study and as noted previously, that study demonstrated no significant benefit from this treatment. The novel approach of using intraluminal 5-FU at the time of surgery reported by Rousselot and co-workers has been tested in a randomized control trial by Lawrence and colleagues and found to represent no improvement on surgery alone.[485]

The study of Mavligit et al deserves special mention because it is a widely reported study using immunotherapy with BCG.[488] In this two-armed study, patients with Dukes C disease were either treated with BCG (52 patients) or BCG + 5-FU (69 patients). The disease free interval and survival of these patients were compared to these parameters in a historical control group of patients treated with surgery only. With a minimum follow-up of 30 months, the treated patients had benefit in survival compared to the controls. The 75% survival time of adjuvant therapy patients was 34 months *versus* 20 months for controls (p = .01). This study will require confirmation in controlled trials and currently is being evaluated by the SWOG and the NSABP. At the present time in situations where the expected differences between treatments are small, as is the case in the adjuvant therapy of colorectal cancer, the controlled clinical trial appears to be the only appropriate mechanism for study.[491]

With the advent of significant interest in combination chemotherapy of colorectal cancer in the last several years, trials of combination regimens have been tested in the adjuvant situation. These studies have all been recent in origin and analysis is not complete. The results have yet to be published in these studies, their design is illustrated in Table 21-35. The total number of patients to be evaluated in all the studies listed in Table 21-35 will be in excess of 2500 and the majority have a prospectively randomized surgery-only arm. This study design should allow for clear definition of the role of 5-FU plus methyl-CCNU and nonspecific immunostimulants in the surgical adjuvant therapy of colorectal cancer.

The Gastrointestinal Tumor Study Group (GITSG) is in the process of analyzing a Phase III trial testing combined modality therapy in resected rectal cancer. In this protocol patients with Dukes B2, C1 and C2 rectal cancer are randomly allocated after surgery to: (1) no further therapy, (2) treatment with postoperative radiation therapy (4000 rad–4800 rad), (3) postoperative chemotherapy with 5-FU plus methyl-CCNU, or (4) combined modality therapy with radiation therapy plus 5-FU and methyl-CCNU. One hundred and eighty-seven patients are evaluable in this protocol and the results of treatment are demonstrated in Table 21-36. A personal communication of results from the GITSG shows the inferiority

TABLE 21-35. Chemoimmunotherapy Trials Now in Progress in an Adjuvant Setting

REGIMEN	NUMBER OF PATIENTS (years studied)	DURATION OF THERAPY (Months)	CONCURRENT UNTREATED CONTROL	PATIENTS ELIGIBLE	GROUP
A. 5-FU B. 5-FU + Methyl CCNU	866 (3/76–9/78)	18 18	No	Dukes' B + C	ECOG
A. 5-FU + methyl CCNU B. Surgery only control	588 (8/73–79)	12	Yes	Dukes' B + C	VASOG
A. 5-FU + methyl CCNU B. MER C. 5-FU + methyl CCNU + MER D. Surgery only control	550 (7/75–8/79)	12	Yes	Dukes' B + C	GITSG
A. 5-FU + methyl CCNU B. 5-FU + methyl CCNU + oral BCG	573 (8/75–79)	12	No*	Dukes' B + C	SWOG
A. 5-FU + methyl CCNU B. BCG C. Surgery only control	292 (11/77)	12	Yes	Dukes' B + C	NSABP
A. Levamisole B. Levamisole + 5-FU C. Surgery only control	87 (5/78)	12	Yes	Dukes' B + C	NCCTG

* Untreated control arm begun after initiation of study

TABLE 21-36. Relapse Rates in Rectal Cancer

	TREATMENT			
	Control	*Chemotherapy + Radiation*	*Chemotherapy*	*Radiation*
FRACTION RECURRED	28/54 (52%)*	8/39 (21%)	19/47 (39%)	15/47 (36%)
MEDIAN TIME TO RECURRENCE (WEEKS)	52	92	72	40
LOCAL RECURRENCE	10/54 (19%)	1/39 (3%)	11/47 (23%)	7/47 (15%)

* $p < .05$

of the surgery only treatment arm compared to the other treatments. Twenty-eight of the 54 patients receiving no postoperative treatment relapsed in a median time of 52 weeks. This was statistically inferior ($p. < .05$) to the 21% relapse rate observed in patients treated with combined chemotherapy and irradiation. This treatment approach was also very effective in preventing local recurrences since only 1 of 39 patients (3%) developed local relapse after combined modality therapy.

These results demonstrate that postoperative treatment is superior to no treatment. It is not yet clear which treatment arm is superior and accrual is continuing to determine the most appropriate treatment program. It should be emphasized that although no survival differences are now apparent among the various treatment arms of this protocol, survival benefits will eventually be seen in patients in which postoperative treatment has prevented relapse.

A problem with the GITSG study at present is that the true relapse patterns are impossible to discern, since only first patterns of failure have been tabulated. If asymptomatic liver metastases are suspected on the basis of frequent screening with liver chemistries and CEA and confirmed with liver scan, that patient is coded as distant metastasis only—even if a symptomatic or asymptomatic pelvic recurrence is found at a later interval. Only if the distant metastases and local recurrence occurred simultaneously, would both be coded. The same is true in reverse if a pelvic recurrence is diagnosed prior to a failure in the liver. Therefore, until further data is generated, it is difficult to accurately compare the relative incidence of local recurrence or distant metastasis by treatment arm.

Because 30 to 50% of patients eventually have the liver as a site of metastases in colon cancer it would seem reasonable to develop therapies aimed at specifically prophylactically treating the liver as an adjuvant therapy in colon cancer (see section on hematogenous spread). The efficacy of 5-FU administered via portal vein infusion after colectomy requires confirmation. Taylor and co-workers reported a randomized trial in which 154 patients were randomized to either receive 5-FU by portal vein infusion (66 patients) or be treated with surgery alone (73 patients).[492] At latest analysis, 20 of the 73 patients in the surgery-only group had died of metastases compared to five of the 66 patients in the 5-FU group. With follow-up now in excess of one year, only two of the treated group developed liver metastases. Attempts to confirm this exciting early result are in order.

The GITSG is now examining the value of prophylactic therapy to the liver. Patients will be randomized between surgery only and surgery plus 2100 rad of hepatic radiation followed by 5-FU. The results of this study will be awaited with interest. The only way progress will be made in the treatment of this disease is if all patients are considered candidates for well-designed and controlled clinical trials.

SPECIAL PROBLEMS IN MANAGEMENT

A standard approach to diagnosis and treatment does not apply in a variety of special problems discussed in this section. The entities to be discussed include ulcerative colitis, familial polyposis syndromes, multiple adenomas, obstructing carcinoma, perforating carcinoma, and involvement by tumor of adjacent organs or structures within both the abdomen or pelvis.

SURGICAL MANAGEMENT OF ULCERATIVE COLITIS

Because of the increased risk of cancer in patients with ulcerative colitis some groups have recommended prophylactic total colectomy after the tenth anniversary of the onset of disease. Dennis and Karlson found four cancers per 100 patient-years occurring after 10 years of colitis.[492] They suggested that this figure (4% per year) is higher than the risk of proctocolectomy (under 2%) so that after 10 years, surgical removal of the colon and rectum was indicated. Other investigators agree that one criteria for prophylactic colectomy is 10 years of disease, but emphasize that total involvement of the colon is a second criteria.[236,237,233,234,236,239]

However, in the past few years two developments have occurred that impact greatly on the selection of ulcerative colitis patients for colectomy. First, flexible fiberoptic colonoscopy has been developed (see section on endoscopy). Second, the association of epithelial dysplasia and carcinoma in colitis has been established. Clinical studies have shown that the presence of dysplasia identifies a subgroup of colitis patients at ultra-high risk for developing or having carcinoma. Riddell presented a concept of dysplasia in which the polyp–cancer sequence in the noncolitic large bowel was compared to the dysplasia–cancer sequence in ulcerative colitis.[494] Riddell suggested that in neither the noncolitic nor ulcerative colitis colorectum does invasive carcinoma arise from morphologically normal mucosa. Rather, cancer arises from a morphologically identifiable precursor; in the noncolitic large bowel, this is the adenoma and in the ulcerative colitis bowel, areas of mucosal dysplasia.

It should be noted that the histopathological entity called "precancer" had long been recognized as a frequent accompaniment of cancer in ulcerative colitis.[495-497] The conceptual breakthrough that Morson and Pang put forward in 1967 involved the predictive value that the changes of precancer had for the stimultaneous presence of invasive cancer in a colitic colon.[498] A goodly number of retrospective studies of colectomy specimens confirmed the frequent association of the epithelial changes of precancer in the rectum and colon with invasive cancer.[499-509]

Dobbins, Stock, and Ginsberg collected data from all reports on this subject prior to their report.[510] They summarize the incidence of cancer and precancer in colectomies of 453 patients with ulcerative colitis. In 66% of specimens containing invasive carcinoma, precancer was identified; precancer was not identified in 12% of specimens in which an invasive carcinoma was identified. Clinical trials will be necessary to determine how accurate the presence or absence of precancer is in predicting the presence of invasive malignancy.

Riddell and Morson have called attention to an important clinical feature of precancerous changes in the rectum.[509] There is a marked variability in the proportion of rectal mucosa involved by dysplastic changes even in those patients with carcinoma. They caution that because of the possibility of false-negative biopsies due to sampling error, multiple biopsies from different areas of the rectum should be taken to detect dysplasia.

Yardley and Keren have pointed up an additional caveat.[502] Active colitis (acute inflammation) artificially increased the number of biopsies showing changes suspicious of precancer. Chronic inflammation usually caused no difficulty even if marked. However, in colons that showed significant acute inflammation of the lamina propria, they found areas with a striking viliform pattern associated with atypia. Such areas, thought to be areas of "atypical reactive hyperplasia" were especially common in markedly inflamed and ulcerated specimens removed for toxic megacolon.

Riddell makes the following suggestions for followup of patients with ulcerative colitis:

1. Because of the focal nature of dysplastic change, multiple carefully anatomically identified biopsies from throughout the colon should be obtained.
2. Endoscopic and radiologic (double contrast barium enema) identification of suspicious areas should be attempted and these areas biopsied. This is, in reality, any area raised slightly (plaque-like) or markedly (polypoid lesion) above the surrounding mucosa.
3. If suspicious areas are not present, and even if they are, random biopsies every 10 cm along the colon should be taken.
4. With the exception of adenomas, lesions that by endoscopic biopsy yield dysplasia are best treated as carcinoma.[494]

If on the basis of clinical history and precancerous changes, colectomy is to be recommended, what procedure should be advised? Should total proctocolectomy with ileostomy be selected as the operation of choice or is sphincter preservation with colectomy plus ileoproctostomy sufficient? The study of Baker and coworkers would seem to confirm the necessity for proctocolectomy and ileostomy as the only reasonable treatment if resection is required.[511] They found 22 cancers occurring in the rectum of 374 patients with ileorectal anastomosis. Surprising, comparison of the incidence of cancer in the group of patients with ileorectal anastomosis to that of colitis patients with intact bowel, showed the risk of cancer to be of the same order. Since only the rectum remained in these patients, the risk per unit area of bowel must have been great. Also, the results of surgical treatment of carcinoma in the retained rectal segment was extremely poor. Four patients were inoperable, nine had died and nine were alive 2 months to 10 years after rectal excision. In five patients yet living, prognosis was guarded for Dukes C poorly differentiated cancer was resected. Several other authors have agreed that proctocolectomy with ileostomy is a proper surgical treatment should resection be required.[239,240,512] Others continue to advocate ileorectal anastomosis[513–517]

SURGICAL MANAGEMENT OF FAMILIAL POLYPOSIS SYNDROMES

In patients with a familial polyposis syndrome, unlike with ulcerative colitis, the physician does not need to worry if colectomy is indicated. However, a relevant clinical question is *when* should colectomy be performed. In families known to carry the polyposis gene the offspring should be studied by proctosigmoidoscopic examination every 6 months. Colonoscopy is usually unnecessary. Of 170 patients with active polyposis seen at St. Mark's Hospital, London, none had the rectum completely free of polyps.[247] This screening should start in early adolescence, for eleven instances of carcinoma have been reported complicating familial polyposis in children 16 years of age or younger.[518] When over 100 polyps are apparent by sigmoidoscopy and barium enema, the diagnosis is definitely established and surgery should not be unduly delayed.

Some controversy exists regarding the proper choice of surgical procedures. Moertel, Hill, and Adson strongly recommend proctocolectomy with ileostomy in nearly all patients.[519] Their experience at the Mayo Clinic with ileorectosigmoidostomy showed a high incidence of cancer in the retained segment of large bowel. Cancer occurred in 5% of patients by 5 years and in 59% of patients followed 23 years. They concluded that ileorectosigmoidostomy was inadequate treatment for familial polyposis; only in patients who did not have rectal polyps initially should this sphincter-saving procedure be considered.

Bussey reporting the experience from St. Mark's Hospital in London had much different data.[247] At 5 years cancer occurred in 1.5% of patients and remained at 3.6% up to more than 20 years follow-up. Schaupp and Volpe and De Cosse and colleagues report favorable results with the ileorectosigmoid anastomosis.[520,521]

Ravitch and Sabiston reported the construction of an anal ileostomy with preservation of the sphincter mechanism.[522] Ferrari and Fonkalsrud revised the technique by adding an ileal reservoir proximal to the ileal segment that is pulled through the rectal segment from which mucosa was stripped.[523] No long-term results with this procedure in adults have been reported.

Perhaps, at this point in time the safest operation for familial polyposis is proctocolectomy with ileostomy. However, most young patients will not accept this alernative; colectomy with ileorectosigmoid anastomosis is the usual procedure. Sixmonthly follow-up with excision of polyps as they occur must be continued for the remainder of the patient's lifetime. If malignant degeneration of polyps occurs or if polyps become confluent, rectal excision is required.

MULTIPLE COLORECTAL NEOPLASMS

Lillehei and Wangensteen suggested that subtotal colectomy with cecorectal anastomosis or total colectomy with ileoproctostomy was indicated in patients with multiple polyps in several different segments of the colon and in patients with cancer and polyps.[524] Teicher and Abrahams advocated subtotal colectomy for multiple polyps of the colon and Peabody and Smithwick advocated an extensive three-quarter colectomy if one or more polyps were identified in addition to cancer.[525,526]

The assumed advantages of this radical approach were:

1. Unsuspected adenomas and carcinomas in other segments of the large bowel would not be missed. Several studies have shown that more polyps or cancers are

present in the colon than are identified by barium enema.[290–295]

2. Subtotal colectomy was recommended as a means of cancer prophylaxis.
3. Subtotal colectomy was not found to be associated with a high mortality or morbidity; and hospital mortality rate of 5.5% was reported by Lillehei and Wangensteen. Also, bowel function with subtotal colectomy was normal unless more than 30 cm of terminal ileum were resected along with the colon.

Grinnell reported that 21 patients having one large bowel cancer had a subsequent second colon primary, and eight of these patients died as a result of their second cancer (see also section on high risk groups). However, 1083 subtotal colectomies would have had to be performed to salvage these eight patients (0.73%). Certainly, performing subtotal colectomies on all colorectal cancer patients would increase operative mortality more than 0.73% so that routine subtotal colectomy is not indicated.[527] However, Grinnell also identified 67 patients with multiple polyps or one or more polyps plus a cancer; seven patients (10%) had a second cancer develop which would have been avoided if subtotal colectomy had been done initially.

Peabody and Smithwick suggest that if cancer of the large bowel is associated with one or more adenomas in distant segments of the colon, a strong potential for malignant change within the entire colorectum has been demonstrated.[526] In these patients, if they present favorable operative risks, an extensive colon resection should be performed. If terminal ileum and large bowel below rectosigmoid are preserved, function should be normal and the only contraindication to such a procedure is the slightly higher operative mortality an extensive colectomy carries.

Today, pre-operative colonoscopy can help solve some clinical problems in management. In a patient with multiple adenomas, if all polyps can be adequately resected, careful surveillance with repeat colonoscopy may be all that is required. If polyps plus cancer are present or if two cancers are diagnosed colonoscopically in different areas of the large bowel, subtotal colectomy is indicated.

OBSTRUCTIVE OR PERFORATIVE COLORECTAL CANCER

The operative approach to obstructive cancer in each individual case must vary with (1) the site of obstruction, (2) the presence or absence of strangulation, (3) the presence or absence of acute cecal dilatation, (4) the general condition of the patient, and (5) the patient response to decompressive procedures.

In obstructive carcinoma of the right colon, emergency treatment with intravenous fluid and electrolytes plus adequate bowel decompression should be instituted. In a majority of patients this will alleviate acute obstruction and allow complete decompression plus adequate bowel preparation. Then on an elective basis, right colectomy and primary ileotransverse colostomy should be performed. If, at the time of surgery, the bowel wall is edematous or the distal colon poorly prepared, resection plus exteriorization of terminal ileum and midtransverse colon should be performed. Even with right colon cancer, extremely high complication rates may be expected unless the conditions under which an anastomosis is performed are optimal.[188]

In obstructive carcinoma of the transverse, descending, or sigmoid colon the urgency of surgical intervention depends on the presence or absence of accompanying problems. If strangulation from volvulus or acute dilatation of the cecum is present, then rapid surgical decompression by colostomy construction above the cancer must be accomplished. However, if the patient can be stabilized and bowel dilatation reduced by nasogastric or long tube suctioning, it is possible that resection plus exteriorization of bowel can be safely accomplished. Resection and anastomosis of dilated colon should never be attempted because of the prohibitively high rate of suture line dehiscence.[187] Several weeks after the resection exteriorization procedure, bowel continuity can be reestablished with low risk.[528]

If obstruction occurs low in the sigmoid or in the rectum an end-sigmoid colostomy should be performed. Then after decompression and bowel preparation, an anterior resection or abdomino–perineal resection performed.

With free perforations through cancer, the segment of bowel leaking stool and tumor cells must be excised or there is almost no chance for survival.[177] The proximal and distal segments of colon are exteriorized without anastomosis. At the time of exteriorization the abdominal cavity should be copiously irrigated. The fascia of the abdominal wall should be closed with a monofilament nonresorbable suture and the skin and subcutaneous tissue should be left open for a delayed primary closure. If the perforation is walled off those structures adherent to tumor should be resected *en bloc* if at all possible with the tumor.

An especially lethal combination of an obstructing cancer with proximal perforation (usually of the cecum) has been described by several authors.[177,182,186,187,191] Aggressive management with exteriorization of the perforated segment must be performed. Later resection of the primary tumor plus anastomosis can be completed. In hospital mortality in this group of patients has consistently been reported as over 50%. It cannot be emphasized too strongly that an expectant (nonoperative) approach or diverting transverse colostomy above a perforation only is associated with nearly a 100% mortality in all reported series of perforative colorectal cancer.

INVOLVEMENT OF ADJACENT ORGANS OR STRUCTURES

What is the approach to treatment of locally advanced colorectal cancer that will provide the greatest incidence of survival at a reasonable cost in morbidity and mortality? The data presented in Table 21-37 show that lysis of the adhesions between a cancer and adhesed structures will result in dissemination of tumor cells and residual malignancy left behind on the adjacent tissues. The principle of management is *en bloc* resection of tumor and adjacent adhesed structures.

This generalization may be tempered in some instances by surgical judgement. One exception noted by Sugarbaker and Wiley are lesions lightly fixed to the bladder base.[197] In this situation the chance for spread probably does not equal the morbidity and mortality involved in an anterior exenteration.

TABLE 21-37. Nature of Adhesions at Interface of Primary Tumor and Adjacent Organ or Structure

AUTHOR (Reference Number)	YEAR	NUMBER OF PATIENTS	CARCINOMATOUS ADHESIONS	INFLAMMATORY ADHESIONS
Sugarbaker and Wiley (529)	1950	*100	57 (57%)	43
Merrill, Dockerty and Waugh (530)	1950	30	†12 (40%)	12
Van Prohaska et al (199)	1953	21	21 (100%)	0
Taylor, Dockerty and Dixon (201)	1955	54	20 (38%)	34
Phillips, Dockerty and Waugh (531)	1955	‡47	36 (51.4%)	34
Jensen, Bolslev and Nielsen (204)	1970	60	42 (70%)	18
El Domeri and Whitley (205)	1970	10	8 (80%)	2
Davies and Ellis (208)	1975	43	30 (74%)	26

* Includes 52 patients in whom primary tumor was freely movable and 48 patients with fixed tumor
† Nature of adhesions not stated for six patients
‡ Forty-seven patients had 70 sites of organ fixation to a cancer at the hepatic flexure

One should in this situation clearly mark with metal clips the structures at risk for local recurrence intra-operatively (Figure 21-20). Then in the postoperative period, radiation therapy can be accurately delivered. A second clear indication for postoperative radiation therapy is duodenal involvement from right colon or hepatic flexure cancer.

It should be emphasized at this point that fixed adhesions to the base of the bladder or trigone do not make a patient surgically incurable. If the patient is a suitable operative risk, primary carcinoma of the rectum involving the base of the bladder may be an indication for total pelvic exenteration; if the primary tumor is in the sigmoid or rectosigmoid area an anterior exenteration may be performed. With this approach Kiselow, Butcher, and Bricker reported a 30% 5-year survival rate in 43 patients.[532] However, they found exenteration an "unsuitable operation" for locally recurrent disease following abdomino–perineal resection.

A technical point should be made for dealing with adhesions between sigmoid colon and the dome of the bladder. A decision concerning the amount of bladder to be resected may be difficult. With bladder and colon and often other involved structures stuck together down in the pelvis, resection without spillage of tumor cells from disruption of tissue planes may be difficult. If a three-way Foley catheter is inserted into the bladder prior to operation, at the proper time in the procedure the bladder can be distended with fluid. At this time an adequate cuff of bladder to be excised *en bloc* with the colon or rectal tumor can be determined. If the detrusor muscle is not expanded, an unnecessarily large portion of bladder may be sacrificed with the *en bloc* resection.

Jensen, Balslev, and Neilsen make the important point that in a palliative resection, *en bloc* resections are usually not indicated.[204] If distant metastases are identified, adhesions should be lysed and the smallest possible resection undertaken for speedy postoperative recovery.

Rectal Cancer Fixed Within the Pelvis

Not infrequently, rectal cancers are fixed within the pelvis upon initial presentation. These tumors cannot be resected

FIG. 21-20. Use of metalic clips in postoperative radiation therapy following abdominoperineal resection for adenocarcinoma of the rectum. Gross residual disease in the posterior aspect of the pelvis was marked with metalic clips. *A*, The uterus was sutured into the presacral space in an attempt to displace the small intestine out of the irradiation field during postoperative irradiation. *B*, the radiation fields used. The field shown (*solid lines*) received a dose of 5040 rads. The boost field (*dotted lines*) received a total dose of 7040 rads. (Modified from Gunderson LL. Cohen Am, Welch CE: Residual, inoperable or recurrent colorectal cancer: Surgical–radiotherapy interaction. Am J Surg 139:518–525, 1980)

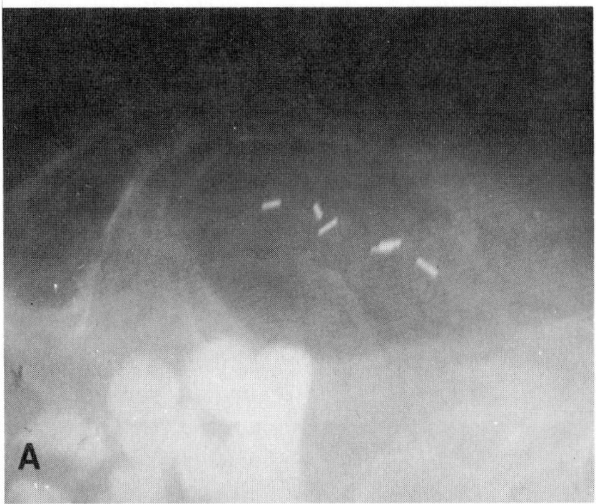

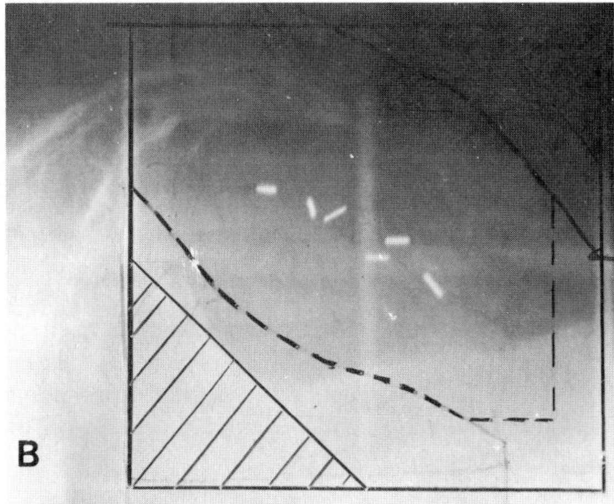

for cure using surgery alone; positive margins of resection and traumatic dissemination of tumor cells at the time of operation will almost invariably result in early and widespread recurrence. To minimize these problems radiation therapy has been used.

Preoperative Irradiation Designed to Make Fixed Rectal Lesions Resectable

Although some cures have been obtained in initially unresectable lesions by combining moderate dose preoperative radiation (4500 rad to 5000 rad over 4 weeks to 5 weeks) with later resection, results vary little from those attained with radiation alone.[371,372,533–538] An exception may be the recent report by Pilepich and colleagues in which 22 of 44 patients (50%) were disease free with median followup of 27 months.[540] Of the 27 patients with curative resection after preoperative radiation therapy, one died postoperatively and three have thus far developed pelvic recurrences. Fourteen of 43 patients (32.6%) had local tumor persistence or developed recurrence with short term followup. An analysis from the Princess Margaret Hospital was made of 34 patients followed approximately 2 years.[535] Of 21 patients who had presented with tumor fixation, two were alive free of disease, five had persistent local tumor, and two had distant metastases. Of 13 patients who presented with mobile lesions, local control was achieved in 11 of 13 (85%); eight of the 11 with local control were clinically free of disease.

Combination Radiation and Chemotherapy for Locally Inoperable Rectal Cancer

Moertel reported a randomized series of 65 patients with locally unresectable or recurrent colorectal carcinoma treated with 4000 rad for 4 weeks plus placebo *versus* 4000 rad plus 15 mg/kg of 5-FU on the first 3 days of treatment.[387] Average survival time was 16.8 months in the placebo group compared to 23 months in the 5-FU group ($p < .05$). Since radiation doses in this study were fairly low, it is possible that an increase in radiation may have achieved the same results.

Postoperative Irradiation of Known Residual Colon or Rectal Cancer After Resection

Temporary palliation can be achieved with radiation dose levels as low as 2000 rad but prolonged tumor control requires dose levels of 4000 rad to 5000 rad or higher.[553] At or above the 5000 rad level, the potential of permanent small bowel injury alters the ability to achieve a suitable therapeutic ratio for prolonged palliation. However, with careful treatment planning long term control with acceptable morbidity has been reported.[379,540,541] Satisfactory results have not been achieved if prolonged local control of tumor is followed by one to three years of radiation induced small bowel damage with perforation and fistulization terminating in death from nonmalignant causes.

TREATMENT OF RECURRENT AND DISSEMINATED DISEASE

DURATION OF SURVIVAL FOLLOWING DIAGNOSIS OF DISSEMINATED DISEASE

Pestana and co-workers at the Mayo Clinic found average survival after diagnosis of inoperable carcinoma in 583 patients to be 9.8 months.[542] In patients initially presenting with a primary tumor plus incurable spread, survival was nine months. Longer survival was seen in females, in patients with tumors of low Broder's grade, and in patients with only local spread. In Pestana and coworkers' study, 353 patients with liver metastases had an average survival of 9.0 months; the studies of Bengmark and Hafstrom revealed a mean survival of 7.8 months, and the studies of Morris and co-workers, a median survival of 11.4 months.[542,543,544]

RECURRENT DISEASE

Careful followup of colorectal cancer patients after resection is important for several reasons: a second primary large bowel cancer will occur in 3–15% of patients. Also, patients who have had colorectal cancer are at high risk for another primary cancer in other organs (see section of high risk groups). Finally, follow-up may in some instances diagnose recurrent disease when it is localized, and amenable to further curative therapy. Griffen, Humphrey, and Sosin report eight of 83 (10%) patients with recurrent colon cancer were converted to a cancer-free status by second look surgery and two of 44 (5%) rectal cancer patients were likewise converted.[545] Ellis reported 12 good results in 42 patients with colorectal cancer re-explored suspecting recurrent cancer. Four of the 12 had recurrent disease resected and five of the 12 had a metachronous cancer removed.[546] Polk and Spratt selected 12 of 62 patients for reoperation; they thought on clinical grounds that recurrent disease was limited.[323] Indeed in six of these 12, all colorectal cancer was eliminated by reoperation and patients died four years to ten years later free of large bowel carcinoma.

The major problem with the second look approach as originally described by Wangensteen was the operative morbidity and mortality (about 10%) that accompanied the difficult and repetitive procedures.[113] A great number of patients had to endure the risks of repeat exploratory laparotomy for a few patients to benefit. To overcome this problem some groups have used serial postoperative carcino-embryonic antigen assays to select patients for second-look surgical procedures. It has been established that CEA can detect recurrent disease at a time when surgical resection is possible. However, what the long term salvage of patients will be had not been determined (see section on tumor markers).

RADIATION THERAPY FOR RECURRENT CANCER

An expanding volume of literature reveals the marked palliative and occasional curative value of radiation for residual, inoperable and recurrent colorectal lesions.[379,531,533,536,537,546,547] The overall response except in a report by Rao and co-workers of the recurrent group is least favorable, which is not surprising, since the tumor has often regrown in poorly vascularized scar tissue.[536]

Results with recurrent disease have been fairly similar from series to series, that is, good palliation but infrequent cure. The Memorial Hospital group reported 80% good or excellent palliation in 102 patients with local disease treated with low radiation doses; 200 rad to 2500 rad were used in eight to twelve fractions.[547] Williams treated 155 patients, utilizing doses of 6000 rad over six weeks when possible with 5.8% 5-year survival.[537] Significant pain relief was achieved in 85% and complete in 57%. Wang and Schulz achieved palliation in 84% of 111 patients; 25 of the 111 had inoperable or residual disease and the remainder recurrent cancer.[533]

Radiation Dose Levels for Treatment of Inoperable Rectal Cancer

Clinical data from Wang and Schulz for residual, inoperable, or recurrent lesions suggest that the percentage of patients who received palliation for 6 months or more increased as radiation dose increased (2100 rad to 3000 rad: three of 24 or 12%; 3100 to 4000 rad: five of 28 or 31%; 4100 to 5000 rad: seven of 12 or 58%).[533] Correlation of response and dose level was also seen in the series reported by Rao and co-workers and Hindo and co-workers on groups of patients treated for palliation.[536,548]

Data from other tumor systems would indicate that the incidence of permanent local control and possible cure might improve if doses of 6000 rad to 7000 rad could be safely delivered in 7 weeks to 8 weeks.[549] At such levels, the incidence of specific radiation therapy-induced small bowel damage will be prohibitive unless information is available regarding the relative position of tumor and small bowel and is used to modify irradiation doses and portals.[550]

CHEMOTHERAPY FOR DISSEMINATED CANCER

From the practical point of view, there are two important questions in the management of patients with advanced colorectal cancer: (1) When should chemotherapy be initiated? and (2) Which treatment regimen should be used? In dealing with the first question, it must be understood that chemotherapy is not curative in this disease. Therefore, it is most appropriate that when a patient is discovered with asymptomatic metastatic disease, treatment be withheld and this patient be carefully followed to obtain an assessment of the pace of the individual's metastatic disease. If it becomes clear that metastases are steadily increasing in size or are threatening important structures then treatment should be initiated. However, if an individual has relatively stable metastatic disease and good performance status, it is reasonable to withhold therapy until clear disease progression occurs.

In regard to choice of treatment, there are two options. As noted previously, there is no standard combination chemotherapy regimen for this disease. Thus, patients with advanced colorectal cancer should be encouraged to enter well-designed experimental treatment protocols. If this is not appropriate, 5-FU as a single agent may be administered. The drug should be started at 500 mg/m^2 intravenously for 4 consecutive days. White blood count and platelet count should be monitored weekly. One should strive to produce white blood cell counts of 2000/mm^3 to 3000/mm^3 with this regimen and doses should be escalated to obtain this degree of leukopenia. The treatment may be repeated every 3 weeks to 4 weeks depending on tolerance. Patients having received previous radiation therapy should receive 5-FU 400 mg/m^2 as initial dosage.

PALLIATIVE SURGERY FOR INCURABLE CANCER

If unresectable liver metastases are encountered at the time of primary resection of colon cancer, intestinal obstruction from the primary tumor must be averted by resection and anastomosis, bypass or colostomy construction. Bacon and Martin and Stearns and Binkley found palliative resection associated with improved survival and therefore recommend resection rather than bypass in this group of patients.[551,552] Modlin and Walker, and Bengmark and Hafstrom found survival rates not influenced by the type of palliative large bowel procedure performed.[553,543] Jaffe and co-workers correlated the extent of hepatic metastases with the operation performed.[554] They found that the extent of hepatic metastases influenced the decision of the surgeon. When groups were controlled for the amount of hepatic involvement, a palliative resection or merely a colostomy yielded comparable survival rates.

For rectal cancer present along with hepatic metastases, several treatment alternatives also exist. Abdomino–perineal resection is an effective means by which to control local tumor.[553,555–557] Madden and Kandalaft and Ramsey had good results with simple fulguration.[469,558] Ramsey's technique seemed especially appropriate in this situation. As an outpatient procedure the rectal cancer's intraluminal growth was kept in check using fulguration. Complications were few and obstructions did not occur. If the primary lesion is not circumferential and less than 10 cm from the anal verge, control by electrocoagulation should be attempted. If resection is thought to be required, an anterior resection with low anastomosis should be performed; if at all possible an abdomino–perineal resection should be avoided.

LIVER METASTASES

Quite often liver metastases occur early in the course of this disease; at the time of initial exploration, Bengmark and Hafstrom reported 24% of patients with liver metastases, Oxley and Ellis reported 18%, and Morris and colleagues 14.5%.[543,544,559]

Surgical Treatment of Liver Metastases

Metastases that arise in the first capillary network proximal to a tumor mass may be resectable for cure. Several reports have indicated that limited hepatic metastases from colorectal cancer can be resected with a reasonable (20% to 30%) chance for cure.[560–566] Also a prolongation of survival in patients not cured has been suggested.[566] The results of surgical resection of liver metastases are more completely discussed in Chapter 41.

Ackerman and colleagues showed that the blood supply to small hepatic metastases in experimental animals was from both hepatic artery and portal vein.[402,403,567] However, large metastases were nourished mainly by the hepatic artery. This led some groups to attempt to treat symptomatic hepatic metastases by hepatic artery ligation.[568] However, the promptness of revascularization by collateral arterial flow suggests that any effects must be temporary.

Chemotherapeutic Treatment of Liver Metastases by Way of the Hepatic Artery

Because of the frequency of liver metastases in colorectal cancer, fluorinated pyrimidines have been administered via hepatic artery catheter in patients with metastatic colon cancer.[569-572] The delivery of high concentration of drug by way of the hepatic artery was thought to potentially give a therapeutic advantage in treating liver metastases. Ansfield and co-workers reported 50% to 60% response rates with this approach.[569,570] However, the percutaneous or surgical placement of a hepatic artery catheter may be difficult and many patients require hospitalization for 15 days to 30 days while the infusion is in progress. Also, significant complications, including hepatic artery thrombosis, hemorrhage, and infection, have been reported with this technique.[570]

A controlled randomized trial of intravenous *versus* hepatic artery perfusion was carried out by the Central Oncology Group. This study showed no differences in response rate and survival between the two treatment arms. The intraarterial route was associated with significantly more morbidity than intravenous therapy. This study indicates that intra-arterial therapy with 5-FU is unlikely to result in significant benefit.[573]

PULMONARY METASTASES

Pulmonary metastases occur in approximately 15% of patients with colorectal metastases and in two percent these metastases are solitary.[574] A surprisingly good survival has been reported following resection. Mountain and co-workers at the M. D. Anderson Hospital found a 28% 5-year survival rate in 28 patients who had pulmonary resections for metastatic colon or rectal cancer.[575] Cahan, Castro and Hajdu reported a 35% 5-year survival in 25 patients with metastatic colon carcinoma.[576] McCormick and co-workers found a 13% survival of 40 patients undergoing pulmonary resection at Memorial Hospital, New York.[577] Half of these patients had multiple metastases.

Cahan and co-workers established an important principle in the clinical management of patients with a solitary lung shadow.[576] In 54 colon cancer patients with a synchronous or metachronous solitary lung shadow, 25 had colon carcinoma metastases, and 29 had separate primary lung cancers. The malignancy prone nature of the colorectal cancer patient is evident from Cahan and co-workers' study.

Collins performed clinically relevant calculations regarding the time of occurrence of pulmonary metastases from carcinoma of the colon and rectum.[578] His objective was to estimate the duration of silent growth of pulmonary metastases. Collins assumed that the growth rate of the pulmonary metastases was exponential and at a constant rate. He estimated that distant metastases occurred, on the average, about 10 years before the diagnosis of primary carcinoma is made. Whether those calculations and their assumptions are correct or not remains to be corroborated. Certainly efforts to improve survival by early diagnosis of malignancy may be less successful if metastatic spread can occur at such an early time.

REFERENCES

1. Jones T, Shepard WC: A Manual of Surgical Anatomy. Philadelphia, WB Saunders, 1945
2. Coller JA: Cancer of the Colon and Rectum. New York, Am Cancer Soc Inc, 1956
3. Goligher JC: In Turrell R (ed): Diseases of the Colon and Anorectum. Philadelphia, WB Saunders, 1959
4. Bacon HE: Anus, Rectum, Sigmoid Colon, 3rd ed. Philadelphia, JB Lippincott, 1949
5. Goligher JC: Surgery of the Anus, Rectum and Colon, p 27. London, Bailliere Tindall, 1975
6. Bacon HE, Dirbas F, Myers TB et al: Extensive lymphadectomy and high ligation of the inferior mesenteric artery for carcinoma of the left colon and rectum. Dis Colon Rectum 1:457–465, 1958
7. Villemin F Huard P, Montague M: Recherches anatomiques sur les lymphatiques du rectum et de l'anus. Rev Chir 63:39–80, 1925
8. Cole PP: The intramural spread of rectal carcinoma. Br Med J 1:431–433, 1913
9. Grinnell RS: Lymphatic block with atypical and retrograde lymphatic metastasis and spread in carcinoma of the colon and rectum. Ann Surg 163:272–280, 1966
10. Enquist IF, Block IR: Rectal cancer in the female: Selection of proper operation based upon anatomic studies of rectal lymphatics. Prog Clin Cancer 2:73–85, 1966
11. Fenoglio CM, Kaye GI, Lane N: Distribution of human colonic lymphatics in normal, hyperplastic, and adenomatous tissue: Relationship to metastasis from small carcinoma in pedunculated adenomas, with two case reports. Gastroenterology 64:51–66, 1973
12. Cady B. Persson AV, Monson DO et al: Changing patterns of colorectal carcinoma. Cancer 33:433-426, 1974
13. Axtell LM, Chiazze L: Changing relative frequency of cancers of the colon and rectum in the United States. Cancer 19:750–754, 1966
14. Rhodes JB, Holmes FF, Clark GM: Changing distribution of primary cancers in the large bowel. JAMA 235:1641–1643, 1977
15. Devesa SS, Silverman DT: Cancer incidence and mortality trends in the United States: 1935–74. JNCI 60:545–571, 1978
16. Haenszel W, Kurihara M: Studies of Japanese migrants: 1. Mortality from cancer and other diseases among Japanese in the United States. JNCI 40:43–68, 1968
17. Haenszel W, Correa P: Cancer of the colon and rectum and adenomatous polyps: A review of epidemiologic findings. Cancer 28:14–24, 1971
18. Burkitt DP: Some neglected leads to cancer causation. JNCI 47:913–919, 1971
19. Wynder EL, Shigematsu T: Environmental factors of cancer of the colon and rectum. Cancer 20:1520–1561, 1967
20. Hill MJ: The effect of some factors on the faecal concentration of acid steroids, neutral steroids and urobilins. J Pathol 104:239–245, 1971
21. Hill MJ, Draser BS, Williams REO et al: Faecal bile-acids and clostridia in patients with cancer of the large bowel. Lancet 1:535–539, 1975
22. Hill MJ: Bacterial metabolism and colon cancer. Nutrition and Cancer 1:46–50, 1979
23. Rowland IR: Diet and cancer of the colon. Food Cosmet Toxicol 14:209–212, 1976

24. Breslow NE, Enstrom JE: Geographic correlations between cancer mortality rates and alcohol-tobacco consumption in the United States. JNCI 53:631–639, 1974
25. Jensen OM: Cancer morbidity and causes of death among Danish brewery workers. Int J Cancer 23:454–463, 1979
26. Lane N, Kaye GI: Pedunculated adenomatous polyp of the colon with carcinoma, lymph node metastasis, and suture-line recurrence: Report of a case and discussion of terminology problems. Am J Clin Pathol 48:170–182, 1967
27. Grinnell RS: The grading and prognosis of carcinoma of the colon and rectum. Ann Surg 109:500–533, 1939
28. Wood DA, Robbins GF, Zippin C et al: Staging of cancer of the colon and cancer of the rectum. Cancer 43:961–968, 1979
29. Dukes CE: Cancer of the rectum: An analysis of 1000 cases. J Path and Bact 50:527-539, 1940
30. Spratt JS, Ackerman LV, Moyer CA: Relationship of polyps of the colon to colonic cancer. Ann Surg 148:682–698, 1958
31. Castleman B, Krickstein HI: Do adenomatous polyps of the colon become malignant? N Engl J Med 267:469–475, 1962
32. Spratt JS, Ackerman LV: Small primary adenocarcinomas of the colon and rectum. JAMA 179:337–346, 1962
33. Kjeldsberg CR, Altshuler JH: Carcinoma *in situ* of the colon. Dis Colon Rectum 13:376–381, 1970
34. Morson BC: Factors influencing the prognosis of early cancer of the rectum. Proc Roy Soc Med 59:607–608, 1966
35. Enterline HT, Evans GW, Mercado-Lugo R et al: Malignant potential of adenomas of colon and rectum. JAMA 179:322–339, 1962
36. Turell R: Diseases of the Colon and Anorectum. Philadelphia, WB Saunders, 1959
37. Blatt LJ: Polyps of the colon and rectum: Incidence and distribution. Dis Colon Rectum 4:277–282, 1961
38. Lane N, Fenoglio CM, Kaye GI et al: Defining the precursor tissue of ordinary large bowel cancer: Implications for cancer prevention. In Lipkin M, Good R (eds): Gastrointestinal Tract Cancer. New York, Plenum, 1978
39. Lipkin M, Sherlock P, Bell B: Cell proliferation kinetics in the gastrointestinal tract of man. Gastroenterology 45:721–729, 1963
40. Gilberstein VA, Knatterud GL, Lober PH et al: Invasive carcinoma of the large intestine: A preventable disease? Surgery 57:363–365, 1965
41. Gilbertsen VA, Nelms JM: The prevention of invasive cancer of the rectum. Cancer 41:1137–1139, 1978
42. Grinnell RS, Lane N: Benign and malignant adenomatous polyps and papillary adenomas of the colon and rectum: An analysis of 1,856 tumors in 1,335 patients. Internat Abstr Surg 106:519–538, 1958
43. Fenoglio CM, Lane N: The anatomical precursor of colorectal carcinoma. Cancer 34:819–823, 1974
44. Buie LA, Brust JCM: Solitary adenomata of the rectum and lower sigmoid. Tr Am Proct Soc 36:57–67, 1935
45. Jackman RJ, Mayo CW: The adenoma-carcinoma sequence in cancer of the colon. Surg Gynecol Obstet 93:327–330, 1951
46. Scarborough RA: The relationship between polyps and carcinoma of the colon and rectum. Dis Colon Rectum 3:336–342, 1960
47. Knoernschild HE: Growth rate and malignant potential of colonic polyps: Early results. Surg Forum 14:137–138, 1963.
48. Muto T, Bussey HJR, Morson BC: The evolution of cancer of the colon and rectum. Cancer 36:2251–2270, 1975
49. Fung CH, Goldman H: The incidence and significance of villous change in adenomatous polyps. Am J Clin Pathol 53:21–25, 1970
50. Bussey HJR: Familial Polyposis Coli. Baltimore, Johns Hopkins University Press, 1975
51. Lipkin M: Biology of large bowel cancer: Present status and research frontiers. Cancer 36:2319–2324; 1975
52. Prager ED, Swinton NW, Young JL et al: Follow-up study of patients with benign mucosal polyps discovered by proctosigmoidoscopy. Dis Colon Rectum 17:322–324, 1974
53. Rider JA, Kusner JB, Moeller HC: Polyps of colon and rectum. JAMA 170:633–638, 1959
54. Jackman RJ, Mayo CW: The adenoma-carcinoma sequence in cancer of the colon. Surg Gynecol Obstet 93:327–342, 1951
55. Welch CE, Hedberg SE: Polypoid lesions of the gastrointestinal tract, p 9–10. Philadelphia, WB Saunders, 1975
56. Berge T, Ekelund TBG, Mellner C et al: Carcinoma of the colon and rectum in a defined population. Acta Chir Scand 438:11–86, 1973
57. Spratt JS, Ackerman LV: The growth of colonic adenocarcinoma. Am Surg 27:23–28, 1961
58. Welin S, Youker J, Spratt JS et al: The rates and patterns of growth of 375 tumors of the large intestine and rectum observed serially by double contrast enema study (Malbo technique). Am J Roentgenol, Rad Therapy & Nuclear Med 90:673–687, 1963
59. Collins VP, Loeffler RK, Tivey H: Observations on growth rates of human tumors. Am J Roentgenol 76:988–1000, 1956
60. Gabriel WB, Dukes C, Bussey HJR: Lymphatic spread in cancer of the rectum. Br J Surg 23:395–413, 1935
61. Miles WE: The spread of cancer of the rectum. Lancet 1:1218–1219, 1925
62. Black WA, Waugh JM: The intramural extension of carcinoma of the descending colon, sigmoid, and rectosigmoid: A pathologic study. Surg Gynecol Obstet 87:457–464, 1948
63. Grinnell RS: Distal intramural spread of carcinoma of the rectum and rectosigmoid. Surg Gynecol Obstet 99:421–430, 1954
64. Dukes CE: The classification of cancer of the rectum. J Path and Bact 35:323–332, 1932
65. Morson BC: Precancerous lesions of the colon and rectum. JAMA 179:316–331, 1962
66. Krause FT: Pedunculated adenomatous polyp with carcinoma in the tip and metastasis to lymph nodes. Dis Colon Rectum 8:283–286, 1965
67. Manheimer LH: Metastasis to the liver from a colonic polyp: Report of a case. N Engl J Med 272:144–145, 1965
68. Dukes CE, Bussey HJR: The spread of rectal cancer and its effect on prognosis. Br J Cancer 12:309–320, 1958
69. Grinnell RS: The chance of cancer and lymphatic metastasis in small colon tumors discovered on x-ray examination. Ann Surg 159:132–138, 1964
70. Astler VB, Coller FA: The prognostic significance of direct extension of carcinoma of the colon and rectum. Ann Surg 139:846–852, 1954
71. Dionne L: The pattern of blood-borne metastasis from carcinoma of rectum. Cancer 18:775–781, 1965
72. Grinnell RS: Lymphatic metastases of carcinoma of the colon and rectum. Ann Surg 131:494–506, 1950
73. Seefeld PH, Bargen JA: The spread of carcinoma of the rectum: Invasion of lymphatics, veins and nerves. Ann Surg 118:76–90, 1943
74. Gilchrist RK, David VC: Lymphatic spread of carcinoma of the rectum. Ann Surg 108:621–642, 1938
75. Wood WQ, Wilkie DPD: Carcinoma of the rectum: An anatomico-pathologic study. Edinberg Med J 40:321–331, 1933
76. Stearns MW, Deddish MR: Five-year results of abdominopelvic lymph node dissection for carcinoma of the rectum. Dis Colon Rectum 2:169–172, 1959
77. Buckwalter JA, Kent TH: Prognosis and surgical pathology of carcinoma of the colon, Surg Gynecol Obstet 136:465–472, 1973
78. Brown CE, Warren S: Visceral metastasis from rectal carcinoma. Surg Gynecol Obstet 66:611–621, 1938
79. Coller FA, Kay EB, MacIntyre RS: Regional lymphatic metastasis of carcinoma of the rectum. Surgery 8:294–311, 1940
80. Gordon-Watson C: Origin and spread of cancer of the rectum. Lancet 1:239–345, 1938
81. Grinnel RS: The lymphatic and venous spread of carcinoma of the rectum. Ann Surg 116:200–215, 1942
82. Batson OV: The function of the vertebral veins and their role in the spread of metastases. Ann Surg 112:138–149, 1940
83. Ackerman LV, Wheat MW: The implantation of cancer: An avoidable surgical risk? Surgery 37:341–355, 1955
84. Pomeranz AA, Garlock JH: Postoperative recurrence of cancer of colon due to desquamated malignant cells. JAMA 158:1434–1436, 1955

85. Lawrie H: Cancer contagion and inoculation. Br Med J 1:198–199, 1906
86. Ryall C: Cancer infection and cancer recurrence: A danger to avoid in cancer operations. Lancet 1:1311–1312, 1907
87. Mayo WJ: Grafting and traumatic dissemination of carcinoma in the course of operations for malignant disease. JAMA 60:512–513, 1913
88. Goligher JC, Dukes CE, Bussey HJR: Local recurrences after sphincter-saving excisions for carcinoma of the rectum and rectosigmoid. Br. J surg 39:119–211, 1951
89. Cole WH: Recurrence in carcinoma of the colon and proximal rectum following resection for carcinoma. Arch Surg 65:264–270, 1952
90. Quer EA, Dahlin DC, Mayo CW: Retrograde intramural spread of carcinoma of the rectum and rectosigmoid: Microscopic study. Srug Gynecol Obstet 96:24–30, 1953
91. Guiss RL: The implantation of cancer cells with a fistula in ano: Case report. Surgery 36:136–139, 1954
92. Beahrs OH, Phillips JW, Dockerty MB: Implantation of tumor cells as a factor in recurrence of carcinoma of the rectosigmoid: Report of four cases with implantation at dentate line. Cancer 8:831–838, 1955
93. LeQuesne LP, Thomson AD: Implantation recurrence of carcinoma of rectum and colon. N Engl J Med 258:578–582, 1958
94. Boreham P: Implantation metastases from cancer of the large bowel. Br J Surg 46:103–108, 1958
95. Boerema I: (Quoted by Vink) Arch Chir Neth 2:129, 1950
96. McGrew EA, Laws JF, Cole WH: Free malignant cells in relation to recurrence of carcinoma of the colon. JAMA 154:1251–1254, 1954
97. Lloyd-Davies OV: Restorative resections performed for rectal cancer. Proc Soc Lond 43: 706–719, 1950.
98. Wagensteen OH, Toon TW: Primary resection of the colon and rectum with particular reference to cancer and ulcerative colitis. Surgery 75:384–404, 1948
99. Garlock JH, Ginzburg L: An appraisal of the operation of anterior resection for carcinoma of rectum and rectosigmoid. Surg Gynecol Obstet 90:525–534, 1950
100. Southwick HW, Harridge WH, Cole WH: Recurrence at the suture line following resection for carcinoma of the colon. Am J Surg 103:86–89, 1962.
101. Beal JM, Cornell GN: A study of the problem of recurrence of carcinoma at the anastomotic site following resection of the colon for carcinoma. Ann Surg 143: 1–7, 1956
102. Wheelock FC, Toll G, McKittrick LS: An evaluation of the anterior resection of the rectum and low sigmoid. N Engl J Med 260:526–530, 1959
103. Keynes WM: Implantation from the bowel lumen in cancer of the large intestine. Ann Surg 153:357–364, 1961
104. Floyd CE, Corley RG, Cohn I: Local recurrence of carcinoma of the colon and rectum. Am J Surg 109:153–159, 1965
105 Wright HK, Thomas WH, Cleveland JC: The low recurrence rate of colonic carcinoma in ileocolic anastomoses. Surg Gynecol Obstet 129:960–962, 1969
106. Slanetz CA, Herter FP, Grinnell RS: Anterior resection versus abdomino–perineal resection for cancer of the rectum and rectosigmoid. Am J Surg 123:110–117, 1972
107. Mason AY: Cancer of the colon and rectum: Carcinoma of the lower two thirds of the rectum. Dis Colon Rectum 19:11–14, 1976
108 Morgan CN: The comparative results and treatment for cancer of the rectum. Postgrad Med 26:135–141, 1959
109. Southwick HW, Harridge WH, Cole WH: Recurrence at the suture line following resection for carcinoma of the colon. Am J Surg 103:86–89, 1962
110. Cole WH: Recurrence in carcinoma of the colon and prexımal rectum following resection for carcinoma. Arch Surg 65:264–268, 1952
111. Burt CAV: Carcinoma of the ovaries secondary to cancer of the colon and rectum. Dis Colon Rectum 3:352–357, 1960
112. Knoepp LF, Ray JE, Overby I: Ovarian metastases from colorectal carcinoma. Dis Colon Rectum 16:305–311, 1973
113. Gilbertsen VA, Wangensteen OH: A summary of thirteen years' experience with the second look program. Surg Gynecol Obstet 114:438–442, 1962
114. Gunderson LL, Sosin H: Areas of failure found at reoperation (second or symptomatic look) following "curative surgery" for adenocarcinoma of the rectum. Cancer 34:1278–1292, 1974
115. Lofgren EP, Waugh JM, Dockerty MB: Local recurrence of carcinoma after anterior resection of the rectum and the sigmoid. Arch Surg 74:825–838, 1957
116. Gilbertsen VA: Adenocarcinoma of the rectum: Incidence and locations of recurrent tumor following present-day operations performed for cure. Ann Surg 151:340–348, 1960
117. Taylor FW: Cancer of the colon and rectum: A study of routes of metastases and death. Surgery 52:305–308, 1962
118. Floyd CE, Corley RG, Cohn I: Local recurrence of carcinoma of the colon and rectum. Am J Surg 109:153–159, 1965
119. Ree PC, Marks JE, Moosa AR et al: Rectal and Rectosigmoid Carcinoma: Physician's prediction of local recurrence. J Surg Res 18:1–7, 1975
120. Cass AW, Million RR, Pfaff WW: Patterns of recurrence following surgery alone for adenocarcinoma of the colon and rectum. Cancer 37:2861–2865, 1976
121. Moosa AR, Ree PC, Marks JE et al: Factors influencing local recurrence often abdominoperineal resection for cancer of the rectum and rectosigmoid. Br J Surg 62:727–730, 1975
122. Rich T, Gunderson LL, Goldabini J et al: Clinical and pathologic factors influencing local failure after curative resection of carcinoma of the rectum and rectosigmoid. Int J Radiat Oncol Biol Phys 4(2):135, 1978
123. Lane N, Kaplan H, Pascal RR: Minute adenomatous and hyperplastic polyps of the colon: Divergent patterns of epithelial growth with specific associated mesenchymal changes. Gastroenterology 60:537–551, 1971
124. Kaye GI, Pascal RR, Lane N: The colonic pericryptal fibroblast sheath: Replication, migration, and cytodifferentiation of a mesenchymal cell system in adult tissue: III Replication and differentiation in human hyperplastic and adenomatous polyps. Gastroenterology 60:515–536, 1971
125. Pascal RR, Kaye GI, Lane N: The colonic pericryptal fibroblast sheath: Replication, migration, and cytodifferentiation of a mesenchymal cell system in adult tissue: 1. Autoradiographic studies of normal rabbit colon. Gastroenterology 54:835–851, 1968
126. Arthur JF: Structure and significance of metaplastic nodules in the rectal mucosa. J Clin Pathol 21:735–743, 1968
127. Jackman RJ, Beahrs OH: Tumors of the Large Bowel. Philadelphia, WB Saunders Co, 1969
128. Symonds DA, Vickery AL: Mucinous carcinoma of the colon and rectum. Cancer 37:1891–1900, 1976
129. Woolam GL, Jackman RJ, Ramirez RJ et al: Scirrhous carcinoma of the lower intestine. Surg Gynecol Obstet 121:753–755, 1965
130. Dukes CE: The surgical pathology of rectal cancer Proc R Soc Lond 37:131–144, 1944
131. Coller FA, Kay EB, MacIntyre RS: Regional lymphatic metastasis in carcinoma of the colon. Ann Surg 114:56–63, 1941
132. McVay JR: Involvement of the lymph-nodes in carcinoma of the rectum. Ann Surg 76:755–767, 1922
133. Lockhart-Mummery JP: Two hundred cases of cancer of the rectum treated by perineal excision. Br J Surg 14:110–124, 1926–1927
134. Dukes CE, Bussey HRJ, Lamb GW: The examination and classification of operation specimens of intestinal cancer. Bul Int Assoc Med Museums 28:55–65, 1948
135. Gordon-Watson C, Dukes C: The treatment of carcinoma of the rectum with an introduction on the spread of cancer of the rectum. Br J Surg 17:643–669, 1930
136. Simpson WC, Mayo CW: The mural penetration of the carcinoma cell in the colon: An anatomic and clinical study. Surg Gynecol Obstet 68:872–877, 1939
137. Kirklin JW, Dockerty MB, Waugh JM: The role of the peritoneal reflection in the prognosis of carcinoma of the rectum and sigmoid colon. Surg Gynecol Obstet 88:326–331, 1949
138. Copeland EM, Miller LD, Jones RS: Prognostic factors in carcinoma of the colon and rectum. Am J Surg 116:875–880, 1968

139. Turnbull RB, Kyle K, Watson FR et al: Cancer of the colon: The influence of the no-touch isolation technic on survival rates. Ann Surg 166:420–427, 1967
140. Gilbertsen VA: Adenocarcinoma of the large bowel. Factors seemingly responsible for unrealistically optimistic appraisals of current curative achievements and a suggestion for improvement of therapeutic results. JAMA 174:1789–1793, 1960
141. Donegan WL, DeCosse JJ: Pitfalls and controversies in the staging of colorectal cancer. In Enker WE: Carcinoma of the colon and rectum, p 60. Chicago: Year Book Medical Publishers, 1978
142. American Joint Committee for Cancer Staging and End Results Reporting: Manual for Staging of Cancer 1978. Chicago, National Cancer Institute, 1978
143. Spratt JS, Spjut HJ: Prevalence and prognosis of individual clinical and pathologic variables associated with colorectal carcinoma. Cancer 20:1976–1985, 1967
144. Goligher JC: The Dukes' A, B and C categorization of the extent of spread of carcinomas of the rectum. Surg Gynecol Obstet 146:793–794, 1976
145. Hertz REL, Deddish MR, Day E: Value of periodic examination in detecting cancer of the rectum and colon. Postgrad Med 27:290–294, 1960
146. Sanfelippo PM, Beahrs OH: Factors in the prognosis of adenocarcinoma of the colon and rectum. Arch Surg 104:401–406, 1972
147. Corman ML, Coller JA, Veidenheimer MC: Proctosigmoidoscopy—age criteria for examination in the asymptomatic patient. Cancer 25:286–290, 1975
148. Schottenfeld D: Patient risk factors and the detection of early cancer. Prev Med 1:335–351, 1972
149. Gilbertsen V: Colon cancer screening: The Minnesota experience. Gastrointest Endosc 26:315–325, 1980
150. Welch CE, Burke JF: Carcinoma of the colon and rectum. N Engl J Med 266:211–216, 1962
151. Irvin TT: Delay in diagnosis of symptomatic colorectal cancer. Lancet 1:489, 1979
152. Keddie N, Hargreaves A: Symptoms of carcinoma of the colon and rectum. Lancet 2:749–750, 1968
153. Clarke AM, Jones IS: Diagnostic accuracy and diagnostic delay in carcinoma of the large bowel. Aust NZ J Med 71:341–347, 1970
154. MacAdam DB: Delay in diagnosis of symptomatic colorectal cancer. Lancet 1:489–490, 1979
155. Speck RL, Thomas WH, Larson RA: Analysis of 860 patients with carcinoma of the transverse and descending colon. Surg Gynecol Obstet 130:259–262, 1970
156 Osnes S: Carcinoma of the colon and rectum: A study of 353 cases with special reference to prognosis. Acta Chir Scand 110:378–388, 1955
157. Irvin TT, Greaney MG: Duration of symptoms and prognosis of carcinoma of the colon and rectum. Surg Gynecol Obstet 144:883–886, 1977
158. Devlin HB, Plant JA, Morris D: The significance of the symptoms of carcinoma of the rectum. Surg Gynecol Obstet 137:399–402, 1973
159. Holliday HW, Hardcastle JD: Delay in diagnosis and treatment of symptomatic colorectal cancer. Lancet 1:309–311, 1979
160. MacLeod JH, Chipman ML, Gordon PC et al: Survivorship following treatment for cancer of the colon and rectum. Cancer 26:1225–1231, 1970
161. Rowe-Jones DC, Aylett SO: Delay in treatment in carcinoma of colon and rectum. Lancet 2:973–976, 1965
162. Recio P, Bussey HJR: The pathology and prognosis of carcinoma of the rectum in the young. Proc R Soc Lond 58:789–790, 1965
163. Hall A, Coffey RJ: Cancer of the large bowel in the young adult. Am J Surg 102:66–72, 1961
164. Johnson JW, Judd ES, Dahlin DC: Malignant neoplasms of the colon and rectum in young persons. Arch Surg 79:365–372, 1962
165. Mayo CW, Pagtalunan JG: Malignancy of colon and rectum in patients under 30 years of age. Surgery 53:711–718, 1963
166. Rosato FE, Frazier TG, Copeland EM et al: Carcinoma of the colon in young people. Surg Gynecol Obstet 129:29–32, 1969
167. Langenberg AV: Carcinoma of large bowel in the young. Br Med J 3:374–376, 1972
168. Recalde M, Holyoke ED, Elias EG: Carcinoma of the colon, rectum and anal canal in young patients. Surg Gynecol Obstet 139:909–913, 1974
169. Sanfelippo PM, Beahrs OH: Carcinoma of the colon in patients under forty years of age. Surg Gynecol Obstet 148:169–170, 1978
170. Cain AS, Longino LA: Carcinoma of the colon in children. J Pediatr Surg 5:527–532, 1970
171. Block GE, Enker WE: Survival after operations for rectal carcinoma in patients over 70 years of age. Ann Surg 174:521–527, 1971
172. Jensen HE, Nielsen J, Balslev I: Carcinoma of the colon in old age. Ann Surg 171:107–115, 1970
173. Calabrese CT, Adam YG, Volk H: Geriatric colon cancer. Am J Surg 125:181–184, 1973
174. Wanebo HJ, Rao B, Pinsky C et al: Preoperative carcinoembryonic antigen level as a prognostic indicator in colorectal cancer. N Engl J Med 299:446–451, 1978
175. Band PR, Beck IT, Dinner PJ et al: Two year follow-up study of patients with known serum concentrations of carcinoembryonic antigen. Can Med Assoc J 117:657–659, 1977
176. Goslin R, Steele G, MacIntyre J et al: The use of preoperative plasma CEA levels for the stratification of patients after curative resection of colorectal cancer. Am Surg 192:747–751, 1980
177. Goligher JC, Smiddy FG: The treatment of acute obstruction or perforation with carcinoma of the colon and rectum. Br J Surg 450:270–274, 1957
178. Ulin AW, Ehrlich EW: Current views related to management of large bowel obstruction caused by carcinoma of the colon. Am J Surg 104:463–467, 1962
179. Chang WYM, Burnett WE: Complete colonic obstruction due to adenocarcinoma. Surg Gynecol Obstet 114:353–356, 1962
180. Minster JJ: Comparison of obstructing and nonobstructing carcinoma of the colon. Cancer 17:242–247, 1964
181. Loefler I, Hafner CD: Survival rate in obstructing carcinoma of colon. Arch Surg 89:716–718, 1964
182. Hickey RC, Hyde HP: Neoplastic obstruction of the large bowel. Surg Clin North Am 45: 1157–1163, 1965
183. Floyd CE, Cohn I: Obstruction in cancer of the colon. Ann Surg 165:721–731, 1967
184. Watters NA: Survival after obstruction of the colon by carcinoma. Can J Surg 12:124–128, 1969
185. Ragland JJ, Londe AM, Spratt JS: Correlation of the prognosis of obstructing colorectal carcinoma with clinical and pathologic variables. Am J Surg 121:552–556, 1971
186. Glenn F, McSherry CK: Obstruction and performation in colorectal cancer. Ann Surg 173:983–992; 1971
187. Welch JP, Donaldson GA: Management of severe obstruction of the large bowel due to malignant disease. Am J Surg 127:492–499, 1974
188. Clark J, Hall AW, Moossa AR: Treatment of obstructing cancer of the colon and rectum. Surg Gynecol Obstet 141:541–544, 1975
189. Ackerman NB: The influences of mechanical factors on intestinal lymph flow and their relationship to operations for carcinoma of the intestine. Surg Gynecol Obstet 138:677–682, 1974
190. Miller LD, Boruchow IB, Fitts WT: An analysis of 284 patients with perforative carcinoma of the colon. Surg Gynecol Obstet 123:1212–1218, 1966
191. Crowder VH, Cohn I: Performation in cancer of the colon and rectum. Dis Colon Rectum 10:415–420, 1967
192. Welch JP, Donaldson GA: Perforative carcinoma of colon and rectum. Ann Surg 180:734–740, 1974
193. Rack FJ: Obstructive perforation of the cecum: Report of eight cases. Am J Surg 84:527–533, 1952
194. Albers JH, Smith LL, Carter R: Perforation of the cecum. Ann Surg 143:251–255, 1956
195. Thomas WH, Larson RA, Wright HK et al: An analysis of patients with carcinoma of the right colon. Surg Gynecol Obstet 127:313–318, 1968
196. Turner GG: Cancer of the colon. Lancet 1017–1023, 1929
197. Sugarbaker ED: Coincident removal of additional structures in

resections of carcinoma of the colon and rectum. Ann Surg 123:1036–1046, 1946
198. Gilchrist RK, David VC: A consideration of pathological factors influencing five-year survival in radical resection of the large bowel and rectum for carcinoma. Ann Surg 126:421–438, 1947
199. VonProhaska J, Govostis MC, Wasick M: Multiple organ resection for advanced carcinoma of the colon and rectum. Surg Gynecol Obstet 97:177–182, 1953
200. Cooke RV: Advanced carcinoma of the colon with emphasis on the inflammatory factor. Ann R Coll Surg Engl 18:46–61, 1955
201. Taylor EF, Dockerty MB, Dixon CF: The prognosis in carcinoma of the colon perforating into the urinary bladder. Surg Gynecol Obstet 96:193–199, 1955
202. Rosi PA, Cahill WJ, Carey J: A ten-year study of hemiocolectomy in the treatment of carcinoma of the left half of the colon. Surg Gynecol Obstet 114:15–24, 1962
203. Aldrete JS, ReMine WH: Vesicocolic fistula—a complication of colonic cancer: Long-term results of its surgical treatment. Arch Surg 94:627–637, 1966
204. Jensen HE, Bolslev I, Nielsen J: Extensive surgery in treatment of carcinoma of the colon. Acta Chir Scand 136:431–434, 1970
205. El-Domeiri A, Whiteley HW: Prognostic significance of abdominal wall involvement in carcinoma of cecum. Cancer 26:552–556, 1970
206. Polk HC: Extended resection for selected adenocarcinomas of the large bowel. Ann Surg 175:892–899, 1972
207. Ellis H, Morgan MN, Wastell C: "Curative" surgery in carcinoma of the colon involving duodenum: A report of 6 cases. Br J Surg 59:932–935, 1972
208. Davies GC, Ellis H: Radical surgery in locally advanced cancer of the large bowel. Clin Oncol 1:21–26, 1975
209. Rankin FW, Olson PF: The hopeful prognosis in cases of carcinoma of the colon. Surg Gynecol Obstet 56:366–374, 1933
210. McSherry CK, Cornell GN, Glen F: Carcinoma of the colon and rectum. Ann Surg 169:502–512, 1969
211. Dwight RW, Higgins GA, Keehn RJ: Factors influencing survival after resection in cancer of the colon and rectum. Am J Surg 117:512–522, 1969
212. Judd ES, Bellegie NJ: Carcinoma of rectosigmoid and upper part of rectum. Arch Surg 64:697–706, 1952
213. Waugh JM, Kirklin JW: The importance of the level of the lesion in the prognosis and treatment of carcinoma of the rectum and low sigmoid colon. Ann Surg 129:22–33, 1949
214. Guernsey DE, Waugh JM, Dockerty MB: Carcinoma of the rectum: Prognosis based on the distance of lesion from, or involvment of, the levator ani muscle, and involvement of the anal sphincters. Surg Gynecol Obstet 92:529–538, 1951
215. Oppolzer R, Nitsche L: Ergebnisse und erfahrungen mit der chirurgischen therapie des mestdarmkrebses. Arch Klin Chir 203:159–2–5, 1942
216. Morson BC, Vaughn EG, Bussey HJR: Pelvic recurrence after excision of rectum for carcinoma. Br Med J 2:13–18, 1963
217. Dunning EJ, Jones TE, Hazard JB: Carcinoma of the rectum: A study of factors influencing survival following combined abdominoperineal resection of the rectum. Ann Surg 133:166–173, 1951
218. Broders AC: Carcinoma: Grading and practical application. Arch Pathol 2:376–381, 1926
219. Rankin FW, Broders AC: Factors influencing prognosis in carcinoma of the rectum. Surg Gynecol Obstet 46:660–667, 1928
220. Stewart FW, Spies JW: Biopsy histology in the grading of rectal carcinoma. Am J Pathol 5:109–115, 1929
221. Wood DA: Tumors of the intestines. In Armed Forces Institute of Pathology: Atlas of Tumor Pathology, Sec 4, pp 161–168, Fasicle 22. Washington, 1967
222. Qualheim RE, Gall EA: Is histologic grading of colon carcinoma a valid procedure? Arch Pathol 56:466–472, 1953
223. Sunderland DA: The significance of vein invasion by cancer of the rectum and sigmoid. Cancer 2:429–437, 1949
224. Carroll SE: The prognostic significance of gross venous invasion in carcinoma of the rectum. Can J Surg 6:281–288, 1963
225. Kay EB: Regional lymphatic metastases of carcinoma of the gastrointestinal tract. Surgery 12:553–562, 1942
226. Parham D: Colloid carcinoma. Ann Surg 77:90–105, 1923
227. Trimpi HD, Bacon HE: Mucoid carcinoma of the rectum. Cancer 4:597–609, 1951
228. Broders AC, Buie LA, Laird DR: Prognosis in carcinoma of the rectum: A comparison of the Broders and Dukes methods of classification. JAMA 115:1066–1971, 1940
229. Wilson SM, Beahrs OH: The curative treatment of carcinoma of the sigmoid, rectosigmoid, and rectum. Ann Surg 183: 556–565, 1976
230. Khankhanian N, Mavligit GM, Russell WO et al: Prognostic significance of vascular invasion in colorectal cancer of Dukes' B class. Cancer 39:1195–1200, 1977
231. Patt DJ, Brynes RK, Vardiman JW et al: Mesocolic lymph node histology is an important prognostic indicator for patients with carcinoma of the sigmoid colon: An immunomorphologic study. Cancer 35:1388–1397, 1975
232. Pihl E, Nairn RC, Nind AP et al: Correlation of regional lymph node *in vitro* antitumor immunoreactivity histology with colorectal carcinoma. Cancer Res 36:3665–3670, 1976
233. Phil E, Malahy MA, Khankhanian N et al: Immunomorphological features of prognostic significance in Dukes' Class B colorectal carcinoma. Cancer Res 37:4145, 1977
234. Tsakraklides V, Wanebo HJ, Sternberg SS et al: Prognostic evaluation of regional lymph node morphology in colorectal cancer. Am J Surg 129:174–180, 1975
235. Burdette WJ (ed): Carcinoma of the colon and anticident epithelium. Springfield, Charles C Thomas, 1970
236. Hinton JM: Risk of malignant change in ulcerative colitis. Gut 7:427–432, 1966
237. Edwards FC, Truelove SC: The course and prognosis of ulcerative colitis. Gut 5:1–22, 1964
238. Morson BC: Cancer in ulcerative colitis. Gut 7:425–426, 1966
239. MacDougall IPM: The cancer risk in ulcerative colitis. Lancet 2:655–658, 1964
240. De Dombal FT, Watts J McK, Watkinson G et al: Local complications of ulcerative colitis: Stricture, pseudopolyposis, and carcinoma of colon and rectum. Br Med J 1:1442–1447, 1966
241. Weedon DD, Shorter RG, Ilstrup DM et al: Crohn's disease and cancer. N Engl J Med 289:1099–1104, 1973
242. Schottenfeld D, Berg JW, Vitsky B: Incidence of multiple primary cancers: 11. Index cancers arising in the stomach and lower digestive system. JNCI 43:77–86, 1969
243. Warren S, Gates O: Multiple primary malignant tumors: A survey of the literature and a statistical study. Am J Surg 16:1358–1414, 1932
244. McGregor RA, Bacon HE: Multiple cancers in colon surgery: Report of 162 cases. Surgery 44:828–833, 1958
245. MacMahon CE, Rowe JW: Rectal reaction following radiation therapy of cervical carcinoma: Particular reference to subsequent occurrence of rectal carcinoma. Ann Surg 173:264–269, 1971
246. Castro EB, Rosen PP, Quan SH: Carcinoma of large intestine in patients irradiated for carcinoma of cervix and uterus. Cancer 31:45–52, 1973
247. Bussey HJR: Gastrointestinal polyposis. Gut 11:970–978, 1970
248. Lovett E: Familial factors in the etiology of carcinoma of the large bowel. Proc R Soc Lond 67:751–752, 1974
249. Reed TE, Neel JV: A genetic study of multiple polyposis of the colon (with an appendix deriving a method of estimating relative fitness). Am J Hum Genet 7:236–259, 1955
250. Pierce ER: Some genetic aspects of familial multiple polyposis of the colon in a kindred of 1,422 members. Dis Colon Rectum 11:321–329, 1968
251. Gardner EJ: Follow-up study of a family group exhibiting dominant inheritance for a syndrome including intestinal polyps, osteomas, fibromas and epidermal cysts. Am J Hum Genet 14:376–390, 1962
252. Turcot J, Despres JP, St. Pierre F: Malignant tumors of the central nervous system associated with familial polyposis of the colon: Report on two cases. Dis Colon Rectum 2:465–468, 1959
253. Oldfield MC: The association of familial polyposis of the colon with multiple sebaceous cysts. Br J Surg 41:534–541, 1954

254. Jeghers H, McKusick VA, Katz KH: Generalized intestinal polyposis and melanin spots of the oral mucosa, lips and digits. New Engl J Med 241:993–1005, 1949
255. Lipkin M: The identification of individuals at high risk for large bowel cancer. Cancer 40:2523–2530, 1977
256. Kopelovich L, Pfeffer LM, Bias N: Growth Characteristics of human skin fibroblasts in vitro. Cancer 43:218–223, 1979
257. Reddy BS, Mastromarino A, Gustafson C et al: Fecal bile acids and neutral sterols in patients with familial polyposis. Cancer 38:1694–1698, 1976
258. McKusick VA: Genetics and large-bowel cancer. Am J Dig Dis 19: 954, 1964.
259. Moertel CG, Bargen JA, Dockerty MB: Multiple carcinomas of the large intestine: A review of the literature and a study of 261 cases. Gastroenterology 34:85–98, 1958
260. Lynch HT, Lynch PM: Heredity and gastrointestinal tract cancer. In Lipkin M, Good RA (eds): Gastrointestinal Tract Cancer. New York, Plenum, 1978
261. Lynch PM, Lynch HT, Harris RE: Hereditary proximal colonic cancer. Dis Colon Rectum 20:661–668, 1977
262. Richards RC, Woolf C: Solitary polyps of the colon and rectum: A study of inherited tendency. Am Surg 22:287–294, 1956
263. Lynch HT, Swartz M, Lynch J et al: A family study of adenocarcinoma of the colon and multiple primary cancer. Surg Gynecol Obstet 134:781–786, 1972
264. Dubosson JD, Klein D, Pettavel J et al: Syndrome du cancer familial avers 4 generations. Schweiz Med Wochenschr 107:875–881, 1977
265. Williams C: Management of malignancy in "cancer families." Lancet 1:198–199, 1978
266. Haggitt RC, Pitcock JA: Familial juvenile polyposis of the colon. Cancer 26:1232–1238, 1970
267. Stemper TJ, Kent TH, Summers RW: Juvenile polyposis and gastrointestinal carcinoma: A study of kindred. Ann Intern Med 83:639–646, 1975
268. Greegor DH: Diagnosis of large-bowel cancer in the asymptomatic patient. JAMA 201:943–945, 1967
269. Greegor DH: Occult blood testing for detection of asymptomatic colon cancer. Cancer 28:131–134, 1971
270. Christensen F, Ankerk N, Mondrup M: Blood in faeces: A comparison of the sensitivity and reproducibility of five chemical methods. Clin Chim Acta 57:23–27, 1974
271. Deyhle P, Nuesch HJ, Kobler E et al: Der Haemoccultest in der vorsorge des dickdarmkarzinoms. Schweiz Med Wochenschr 106:297, 1976
272. Winawer SJ, Miller DH, Schottenfeld D et al: Screening for colorectal cancer with fecal occult blood testing. Front Gastrointest Res 5:28–34, 1979
273. Miller SF: Colorectal cancer: Are the goals of early detection achieved? Cancer 27:338–343, 1977
274. Hastings JB: Mass screening for colorectal cancer. Am J Surg 127:228–233, 1974
275. Sterchi JM: Screening for colorectal cancer. South Med J 72:1144–1146, 1979
276. Miller SF, Knight AR: The early detection of colorectal cancer. Cancer 40:945–949, 1977
277. Lipshutz GR, Katon RM, McCool MF et al: Flexible sigmoidoscopy as a screening procedure for neoplasia of the colon. Surg Gynecol Obstet 148:19–22, 1979
278. Winawer SJ, Leidner SD, Boyle C et al: Comparison of flexible sigmoidoscopy with other diagnostic techniques in the diagnosis of rectocolon neoplasia. Dig Diseases and Sciences 24:277–281, 1979
279. Winawer SJ, Andrews M, Flehinger B et al: Progress report on controlled trial of fecal occult blood testing for the detection of colorectal neoplasia. Cancer 45:2959–2964, 1980
280. Gilbertsen VA, Williams SE, Schuman L: Colonoscopy in the detection of carcinoma of the intestine. Surg Gynecol Obstet 149:877–878, 1979
281. Bolt RJ: Sigmoidoscopy in detection and diagnosis in the asymptomatic individual. Cancer 28:121–122, 1971
282. Crespi M, Casale V, Grassi A: Flexible sigmoidoscopy: a potential advance in cancer control. Gastrointest Endosc 24:291–292, 1978
283. Winnan G, Berci G, Panish J et al: Superiority of the flexible to the rigid sigmoidoscopy. N Engl J Med 302:1011–1012, 1980
284. Jones ISC: An analysis of bowel habit and its significance in the diagnosis of carcinoma of the colon. Am J Protol 27:45–56, 1976
285. Postlelhwait RW: Malignant tumors of the colon and rectum. Ann Surg 129:34–46, 1949
286. Bartholomew LG, Schutt AJ: Systemic syndromes associated with neoplastic disease including cancer of the colon. Cancer 28:170–174, 1971
287. Rosato FE, Shelley WB, Fitts WT et al: Nonmetastatic cutaneous manifestations of cancer of the colon. Am J Surg 117:277–281, 1969
288. Ostrow JD, Mulvaney CA, Hansell JR et al: Sensitivity and reproducibility of chemical tests for fecal occult blood with an emphasis on false-positive reactions. Am J Dig Dis 18:930–940, 1973
289. Mason AY: Transsphincteric surgery for lower rectal cancer. Surg Tech Illust 2:71–90, 1977
290. Coller JA, Corman ML, Veidenheimer MC: Colonic polypoid disease: Need for total colonoscopy. Am J Surg 131:490–494, 1976
291. Watanabe H, Numazawa M, Shoji K et al: Diagnosis of early cancer of the colon and rectum. Tohoku J Exp Med 129:183–195, 1979
292. Marks G: Guidelines for use of flexible fibroptic colonoscopy in management of patients with colorectal neoplasia. Dis Colon Rectum 22:302–305, 1979
293. Appel MF: Preoperative and postoperative colonoscopy for colorectal carcinoma. Dis Colon Rectum 19:664–666, 1976
294. Wolff WI, Shinya H: Earlier diagnosis of cancer of the colon through colonic endoscopy (Colonoscopy). Cancer 34:912–931, 1974
295. Knutson CO, Max MH: Value of colonoscopy in patients with rectal blood loss unexplained by rigid protosigmoidoscopy and barium contrast enema examinations. Am J Surg 139:84–87, 1980
296. Laufer I, Smith NCW, Mullens JE: The radiological demonstration of colorectal polpys undetected by endoscopy. Gastroenterology 70:167–170, 1976
297. Kriss N: Analysis of morphological and projection factors in nodular lesions of the colon. Radiol Clin Biol 34:221–235, 1965
298. Dean ACB, Newell JP: Colonsocopy in the differential diagnosis of carcinoma from diverticulitis of the sigmoid colon. Br J Surg 60:633–635, 1973
299. Sugarbaker PH, Vineyard GC, Lewicki AM et al: Colonoscopy in the management of diseases of the colon and rectum. Surg Gynecol Obstet 139:341–349, 1974
300. Morson BC: The muscle abnormality in diverticular disease of the sigmoid colon. Br J Radiol 36:385–392, 1963
301. Goulston SJM, McGovern VJ: The nature of benign structures in ulcerative colitis. N Engl J Med 281:290–295, 1969
302. Morris SJ, Greenwald RA, Tedesco FJ: Acute ulcerative colitis mimicking an obstructive carcinoma of the colon. Am J Gastroenterol 70:194–196, 1978
303. Shehan JJ, Organ C, Sullivan JF: Infarction of the appendices epiploicae. Am J Gastroenterol 46:469–476, 1966
304. Mapelli P, Sead LH, Conner WE et al: Perforation of colon by ingested chicken bone diagnosed by colonscope. Gastrointest Endosc 26:20–21, 1980
305. Phillips WM, ReMine WH, Beahrs OH et al: Benign lesions of the cecum simulating carcinoma. JAMA 172:1465–1468, 1960
306. Cowgill R, Quan SHQ: Colonic actinomycosis mimicking carcinoma. Dis Colon Rectum 22:45:46, 1979
307. Couropmitree C, Rhatigan RM, Walklett WR: Intestinal tuberculosis mimicking carcinoma of the colon. J Fla Med Assoc 57:18–20, 1970
308. Balikian JP, Garabedian MM: Ameboma of the transverse colon simulating carcinoma. Lebanese Med J 18:259–263, 1965
309. Hagihara PF, Ernst CB, Griffen WO: Incidence of ischemic colitis following abdominal aortic reconstruction. Surg Gynecol Obstet 149:571–573, 1979
310. Schwartz S, Boley SJ, Robinson K et al: Roentgenologic features

of vascular disorders of the intestines. Radiol Clin North Am 2:71–87, 1964
311. Farman J: Vascular lesions of the colon. Br J Radiol 39:575–582, 1966
312. Stolar J, Silver H: Differentiation of Pseudoinflammatory colloid carcinoma from colitis cystica profunda. Dis Colon Rectum 12:63–69, 1969
313. Templeton AW: Colon sphincters simulating organic disease. Radiology 75:237–241, 1960
314. Roesch W: Idiopathic muscular structure of the sigmoid colon simulating carcinoma. Acta Hepatogastroenterol 19:210–211, 1972
315. Abcarian H, Eftaiha M, Kraft AR et al: Colonic complications of acute pancreatitis. Arch Surg 114:995–1001, 1979
316. Lefrak EA, Roehm JOF, Henly WS: Pseudotumor of the transverse colon. Postgrad Med 49:55–57, 1971
317. Morin ME, Marsan RE, Baker DA: Renal carcinoma simulating colon carcinoma. JAMA 239:2476, 1978
318. Khilnani MT, Marshak RH, Eliasoph J et al: Roentgen features of metastases to the colon. Am J Roentgenol Rad Ther Nuc Med 96:302–310, 1966
319. Jenkinson EL, Brown WH: Endometriosis: A study of one hundred and seventeen cases with special reference to constricting lesions of the rectum and sigmoid colon. JAMA 122:349–354, 1943
320. Siegal HA: Endometriosis simulating carcinoma of the colon. Am J Proct 20:192–201, 1969
321. Elhence IP, Goldberg HM: Endometriosis of the pelvic colon presenting as intestinal obstruction. Int J Surg 54:132–134, 1970
322. Meyers WC, Kelvin FM, Jones RS: Diagnosis and surgical treatment of colonic endometriosis. Arch Surg 114:169–175, 1979
323. Polk HC, Spratt JS: Recurrent colorectal carcinoma: Detection, treatment and other considerations. Surgery 69:9–23, 1971
324. Sugarbaker PH, Zamcheck N, Moore FD: Assessment of serial carcinoembryonic antigen (CEA) assays in postoperative detection of recurrent colorectal cancer. Cancer 38:2310–2315, 1976
325. Wolff WI, Shinya H: A new approach to colonic polyps. Ann Surg 178:367–378, 1973
326. Spratt JS, Ackerman LV: Pathologic significance of polyps of the rectum and colon. Dis Colon Rectum 3:330–335, 1960
327. Figiel LS, Figiel SJ, Wietersen FK: Is surgical removal of every colonic polyp necessary? Am J Roentgenol 88:721–732, 1962
328. Williams CB: Diathermy biopsy: A technique for the endoscopic management of small polyps. Endoscopy 5:215–218, 1973
329. Knutson CA, Max MH: Diagnostic and therapeutic colonoscopy. Arch Surg 114:430–435, 1979
330. Shatney CH, Lober PH, Gilbertsen VA et al: The treatment of pedunculated adenomatous colorectal polpys with focal cancer. Surg Gynecol Obstet 139:845–850, 1974
331. Sugarbaker PH, Vineyard GC, Lewicki AM et al: Colonoscopy in the management of diseases of the colon and rectum. Surg Gynecol Obstet 139:341–349, 1974
332. Carden ABG, Morson BC: Recurrence after local excision of malignant polyps of the rectum. Proc R Soc Med 57:559–561, 1964
333. Winawer SJ, Leidner SD, Hajdu SI et al: Colonoscopic biopsy and cytology in the diagnosis of colon cancer. Cancer 42:2849–2853, 1978
334. Lockhart-Mummery HE, Dukes CE: The surgical treatment of malignant rectal polpys. Lancet 2:751–755, 1952
335. Otani S: Large sessile mucosal polyps of the colon: The problem of repeatedly negative biopsies. Mt Sinai J Med (NY) 39:39–47, 1972
336. Wheat MW, Ackerman LV: Villous adenomas of the large intestine. Clinicopathologic evaluation of 50 cases of villous adenomas with emphasis on treatment. Ann Surg 147:476–487, 1958
337. Olsen WR: Transanal excision of sessile rectal polyps. Surg Gynecol Obstet 140:766–768, 1975
338. Mason AY: The place of local resection in the treatment of rectal carcinoma. Proc R Soc Lond 63:1259–1262, 1970
339. Oh C, Kark AE: The transsphincteric approach to mid and low rectal villous adenoma. Ann Surg 176:605–612, 1972
340. Crowley RT, Davis DA: A procedure for total biopsy of doubtful polypoid growths of the lowest large bowel segment. Surg Gynecol Obstet 93:23–26, 1951
341. Wilson SE, Gordon HE: Excision of rectal lesions by the Kraske approach. Am J Surg 118:213–217, 1969
342. O'Brien PH: Kraske's posterior approach to the rectum. Surg Gynecol Obstet 142:412–414, 1976
343. Raymond A, Horiot JC, Guillaud M et al: Les tumeurs villeuses coliques et rectales: Analyse comparative du traitement chirurigical et du traitement radiotherapique: A propos de 104 observations. J Chir (Paris) 114:153–186, 1977
344. Crapp AR, Pouis SJA, Tillotson P et al: Preparation of the bowel by whole gut irrigation. Lancet 2:1233, 1975
345. Chung RS, Gurll NJ, Berglund EM: A controlled clinical trial of whole gut lavage as a method of bowel preparation for colonic operations. Am J Surg 137:75–81, 1979
346. Condon RE: Preparation of the bowel for colon and rectal operations. J Surg Practice 8:10–28, 1979
347. Clarke JS, Condon RE, Bartlett JG et al: Preoperative oral antibiotics reduce septic complications of colon operations: Results of prospective, randomized, double-blind clinical study. Ann Surg 186:251–259, 1977
348. Condon RE, Nyhus LM: Manual of Surgical Therapeutics, 3rd ed. Boston, Little, Brown and Co, 1975
349. Barber MS, Herschberg BC, Rice CL et al: Parenteral antibiotics in elective colon surgery: A prospective controlled clinical trial. Surgery 86:23–32, 1979
350. Vink M: Local recurrence of cancer in the large bowel: The role of implantation metastases and bowel disinfection. Br J Surg 41:431–435, 1954
351. Cohn I, Atik M: The influence of antibiotics on the spread of tumors of the colon: An experimental study. Ann Surg 151:917–929, 1960
352. Grinnel RS: Results of ligation of inferior mesenteric artery at the aorta in resections of carcinoma of the descending and sigmoid colon and rectum. Surg Gynecol Obstet 120:1031–1036, 1965
353. Enker WE, Laffer UT, Block GE: Enhanced survival of patients with colon and rectal cancer is based upon wide anatomic resection. Ann Surg 190:350–260, 1979
354. Harvey HD, Auchincloss H: Metastases to lymph nodes from carcinomas that were arrested. Cancer 21:684–691, 1968
355. Sauer I, Bacon HE: Influence of lateral spread of cancer of the rectum on radicability of operation and prognosis. Am J Surg 81:111–120, 1951
356. Cole WH, Roberts SS, Strehl FW: Modern concepts in cancer of the colon and rectum. Cancer 19:1347–1358, 1966
357. Stearns MW, Schottenfeld D: Techniques for the surgical management of colon cancer. Cancer 28:165–169, 1971
358. Cohn I, Gonzales EA, Floyd CE et al: Influence of nitrogen mustard on tumor implantation. JAMA 185:575–577
359. Gunderson LL, Cohen AM, Welch CE: Residual, inoperable or recurrent colorectal cancer: Surgical–radiotherapy interaction. Am J Surg 139:518–525, 1980
360. Hughes ES, McDeremott FT, Masterton JP et al: Operative mortality following excision of the rectum. Br J Surg 1:49–51, 1980
361. Colcock BP, Jarpa S: Complications of abdominoperineal resection. Dis Colon Rectum 1:90–96, 1958
362. Lapides J, Tank ES: Urinary complications following abdominal perineal resection. Cancer 28:230–235, 1971
363. Ginzburg L, Freund S, Dreiling DA: Mortality and major complications following resection for carcinoma of the large bowel. Ann Surg 150:913–927, 1959
364. Manson PN, Corman ML, Coller JA et al: Anterior resection for adenocarcinoma: Lahey clinic experience from 1963 through 1969. Am J Surg 131:434–441, 1976
365. Berliner SD, Burson LC, Lear PE: Intraperitoneal drains in surgery of the colon: Clinical evaluation of 454 cases. Am J Surg 113:646–647, 1967
366. Akwari OE, Kelly KA: Anterior resection for adenocarcinoma of the distal large bowel. Am J Surg 139:88–94, 1980
367. Morson BC, Bussey HJR: Surgical pathology of rectal cancer in relation to adjuvant radiotherapy. Br J Radiol 40:161–169, 1967

368. Houge RC, Smith RR: The effectiveness of small amounts of preoperative irradiation in preventing the growth of tumor cells disseminated at surgery: An Experimental study. Cancer 14:284–295, 1961
369. Inch WR, McCredie JA: Effect of small dose of X-radiation on local recurrence of tumors in rats and mice. Cancer 16:595–598, 1963
370. Powers WE, Tohmach LJ: Preoperative radiation therapy: Biological basis and experimental investigation. Nature 201: 172–204, 1964
371. Ruff CC, Dockerty MB, Frickle RE: Preoperative radiation therapy for adenocarcinoma of the rectum and rectosigmoid. Surg Gynecol Obstet 112:715–723, 1961
372. Stevens KR, Allen CV, Fletcher WS: Preoperative radiotherapy for adenocarcinoma of the rectosigmoid. Cancer 37:2866–2874, 1976
373. Gunderson LL, Dosorety D, Blitzer DH et al: Low dose preoperative irradiation, surgery and elective postoperative irradiation for resectable rectal and rectosigmoid carcinoma. Am Rad Soc Proc. Int J Radiat Oncol Biol Phys 6(1):38, 1980
374. Quan SHQ, Deddish MR, Stearns MW: The effect of preoperative roentgen therapy upon the 10 and 5 year results of the surgical treatment of cancer of the rectum. Surg Gynecol Obstet 111:507–508, 1960
375. Stearns MW, Deddish MR, Quan SHQ: Preoperative irradiation for cancer of the rectum and rectosigmoid: Preliminary review of recent experience (1957–1962). Dis Colon Rectum 11:281–284, 1968
376. Klingerman MM, Urdaneta N, Knowlton A et al: Preoperative irradiation of rectosigmoid carcinoma including its regional lymph nodes. Am J Roentgenol Rad Ther Nucl Med 114:498–503, 1972
377. Roswit B, Higgins GA, Keehn RJ: Preoperative irradiation for carcinoma of the rectum and rectosigmoid colon: Report of a National Veterans Administration randomized study. Cancer 35:1597–1602, 1975
378. Rider WD, Palmer JA, Mahoney LJ et al: Preoperative irradiation in operable cancer of the rectum: Report of the Toronto trial. Can J Surg 20:335–338, 1977
379. Gunderson LL: Combined irradiation and surgery for rectal and sigmoid cancer. In Hickey R (ed): Emerging roles of radiotherapy in four selected areas. Curr Probl Cancer 1:40–53, 1976
380. Romsdahl M, Withers HR: Radiotherapy combined with curative surgery. Arch Surg 113:446–453, 1978
381. Stevens KR, Fletcher WS, Allen CV: Anterior resection and primary anastomosis following high dose preoperative irradiation for adenocarcinoma of the recto-sigmoid. Cancer 41:2065–2071, 1978
382. Gunderson LL: Radiation Therapy of colorectal carcinoma. In Thatcher N (ed): Digestive Cancer: XII International Cancer Congress Proceedings. New York, Pergamon Press. 9:29–38, 1979
383. Turner SS, Vieira EF, Ager PJ et al: Elective postoperative radiotherapy for locally advanced colorectal cancer. Cancer 40:105–108, 1977
384. Higgins GA, Conn JH, Jordan PH et al: Preoperative radiotherapy for colorectal cancer. Ann Surg 181:624–631, 1975
385. Gilbert SB: The significance of symptomatic local tumor failure following abdomino-perineal resection. Int J Radiat Oncol Biol Phys 4:801–807, 1978
386. Moertel CG: Natural history of gastrointestinal cancer. In Moertel CG, Reitemeier RJ (eds): Advanced Gastroinestinal Cancer/Clinic Management and Chemotherapy, p 3414. New York, Harper and Row, 1969
387. Moertel CG: Large bowel. In Holland JF, Frie E III (eds): Cancer Medicine, p 1597–1626. Philadelphia, Lea & Febiger, 1973
388. Moertel CG: Clinical management of advanced gastrointestinal cancer. Cancer 36:675, 1975
389. Schein PS, Kisner D, Macdonald JS: Chemotherapy of large intestinal carcinoma. Cancer 36:2418–2420, 1975
390. Moertel CG: Chemotherapy of gastrointestinal cancer. Clin Gastroenterol 5:777–793, 1976
391. Carter SK: Large bowel cancer: The current status of treatment. JNCI 56:3–10, 1976
392. Woolley PV, Macdonald JS, Schein PS: Chemotherapy of malignancies of the gastrointestinal tract. Prog Gastroenterol 3:671–700, 1977
393. Heal JM, Schein PS: Management of gastrointestinal cancer. Med Clin North Am 61:991–999, 1977
394. Moertel CG: Chemotherapy of gastrointestinal cancer. N Engl J Med 299:1049–1052, 1978
395. Schutt AJ: Chemotherapy of gastrointestinal neoplasms. In: Brodsky J, Kahn SB, Conroy JE (eds): Cancer Chemotherapy, p 135. New York, Grune & Stratton, 1978
396. Bergevin PR: Gastrointestinal tract. In Bergevin PR, Blom J, Tormey DC (eds): Guide to Therapeutic Oncology, p 315. Baltimore, Williams & Wilkins, 1979
397. Macdonald JS, Neefe J: Chemotherapy in the management of gastrointestinal cancer. Abdom Surg 21:126–131, 1979
398. Moertel CG, Reitemeier RJ, Hahn RG: Therapy with the fluorinated pyrimidines. In Moertel CG, Reitemeier RJ (eds): Advanced Gastrointestinal Cancer, p 86. New York, Koeber, 1969
399. Jacobs EM, Reeves WJ, Wood DA et al: Treatment of cancer with weekly intravenous 5-fluorouracil. Cancer 27:1302–1305, 1971
400. Leone LA: The chemotherapy of colorectal cancer. Cancer 34:972, 1974
401. Seifert P, Baker LH, Reed ML: Comparison of continuously infused 5-fluorouracil with bolus injection in treatment of patients with colorectal adenocarcinoma. Cancer 36:123–128, 1975
402. Ackerman NB, Lein WM, Kondi ES et al: The blood supply of experimental liver metastases: 1. The distribution of hepatic artery and portal vein blood to "small" and "large" tumors. Surgery 66:1067–1072, 1969
403. Mann JD, Wakim KG, Baggenstoss AH: The vasculature of the human liver: a study by injection-cast method. Mayo Clin Proc 28:227–231, 1953
404. Bateman J, Irwin L, Pugh R et al: Comparison of intravenous and oral administration of 5-fluorouracil for colorectal carcinoma. Proc Am Assoc Cancer Res 16:242, 1975
405. Hahn RG, Moertel CG, Schutt AJ et al: A double-blind comparison of intensive course 5-FU by oral vs intravenous route in the treatment of colorectal carcinoma. Cancer 35:1031, 1975
406. Ansfield R, Klotz J, Nealon T et al: A Phase III study comparing the clinical utility of four regimens of 5-fluorouracil. Cancer 39:34–40, 1977
407. Wasserman TH, Comis RL, Goldsmith M et al: Tabular analysis of clinical chemotherapy of solid tumors. Cancer Chemother Rep 6:399, 1975
408. Moertel CG: Therapy of advanced gastrointestinal cancer with the nitrosoureas. Cancer Chemother Rep (Pt 3) 3, 4:27, 1973
409. Falkson G, Van Eden EG, Falkson HC: Fluorouracil, imidazole carboximide dimethyltriazeno, vincristine and bis-chloroethyl-nitrosourea in colon cancer. Cancer 33:1207–1208, 1974
410. Moertel CG, Schutt AJ, Hahn RG et al: Therapy of advanced colorectal cancer with a combination of 5-fluorouracil, methyl-1,3-cis(2-chloroethyl)-1-nitrosourea and vincristine. JNCI 54:69–71, 1975
411. Falkson G, Falkson HC: Fluorouracil, methyl-CCNU, and vincristine in cancer of the colon. Cancer 38:1468–1470, 1976
412. Macdonald JS, Kisner DF,Smythe T et al: 5-Fluorouracil (5-FU), methyl-CCNU and vincristine in the treatment of advanced colorectal cancer: Phase II study utilizing weekly 5-FU. Cancer Treat Rep 60:1597–1600, 1976
413. Kemeny N, Yagoda A, Golbey R: Randomized study of 2 different schedules of methyl CCNU (MeCCNU), 5-flururacil (5-FU), and vincristine (VCR) for metastatic colorectal carcinoma. Proc Am Assoc Cancer Res and Am Soc Clin Oncol 18:336, 1977
414. Engstrom P, MacIntyre J, Douglass H Jr et al: Combination chemotherapy of advanced bowel cancer. Proc Am Assoc Cancer Res and Am Soc Clin Oncol 19:384, 1978
415. Moertel CG, Reitemier RJ, Hahn RG: Combination chemotherapy in advanced gastrointestinal cancer. Cancer Res 30:1425–1428, 1970
416. Baker LH, Talley RW, Matter R et al: Phase III comparison of the treatment of advanced gastrointestinal cancer with bolus

weekly 5-FU vs. methyl-CCNU plus bolus weekly 5-FU: A Southwest Oncology study. Cancer 38:1–7, 1976
417. Posey LE, Morgan LR: Methyl-CCNU versus methyl-CCNU and 5-fluorouracil in carcinoma of the large bowel. Cancer Treat Rep 61:1453–1458, 1977
418. Buroker T, Kim PN, Heilbrun L et al: 5-FU infusion with mitomycin C vs. 5-FU infusion with methyl CCNU in the treatment of advanced colon cancer: A Phase III Study. Proc Am Assoc Cancer Res and Am Soc Clin Oncol 18:271, 1977
419. Lokich JJ, Skarin AT, Mayer RJ et al: Lack of effectiveness of combined 5-fluorouracil and methyl-CCNU therapy in advanced colorectal cancer. Cancer 49:2792–2796, 1977
420. Kemeny N, Yagoda A, Golbey R: Methyl-CCNU, 5-fluorouracil, vincristine and streptozotocin for metastatic colorectal cancer. Proc Am Assoc Cancer Res and Am Soc Clin Oncol 19:354, 1978
421. Friedman MA, Ignoffo RJ, Resser KJ: Combination 5-FU + moderate dose methotrexate + leukovorin: A Phase I-II study of patients with disseminated colorectal cancer. Proc Am Assoc Cancer Res and Am Soc Clin Oncol 20:24, 1979
422. Kirkwood JM, Frei E III: 5-Fluorouracil with thymidine: A Phase I trial. Proc Am Assoc Cancer Res and Am Soc Clin Oncol 19:159, 1978
423. Nayak R, Martin D, Stolfi R et al: Pyrimidine nucleosides enhance the anticancer activity of FU and augment its incorporation into nuclear RNA. Proc Am Assoc Cancer Res and Am Soc Clin Oncol 19:63, 1978
424. Dixon WJ, Longmire WP, Holden WD: Use of triethylenethiophosphoramide as an adjuvant to the surgical treatment of gastric and colorectal cancer: Ten-year follow-up. Ann Surg 173:26–39, 1971
425. Best RR, Blair JB: Sphincter preserving operations for rectal carcinoma as related to the anatomy of the lymphatics. Ann Surg 130:538–556, 1949
426. Mayo CW, Cullen PK: An evaluation of the one-stage, low anterior resection. Surg Gynecol Obstet 111:82–86, 1960
427. Butcher HR: Carcinoma of the rectum: Choice between anterior resection and abdominoperineal resection of the rectum. Cancer 28:204–207, 1971
428. Dixon CF: Anterior resection for malignant lesions of the upper part of the rectum and lower part of the sigmoid. Ann Surg 128:425–442, 1948
429. Judd ES, Bellegie NJ: Carcinoma of rectosigmoid and upper part of rectum: Recurrence following low anterior resection. Arch Surg 64:697–706, 1952
430. Morgan CN: Trends in the treatment of tumors of the rectum, rectosigmoid and left colon. J R Coll Surg Edinb 1:112–125, 1955
431. Deddish MR, Stearns MW: Anterior resection for carcinoma of the rectum and rectosigmoid area. Ann Surg 154:961–966, 1961
432. Beahrs OH: Low anterior resection for rectal carcinoma. Surg Gynecol Obstet 23:593–594, 1966
433. Vandertoll DJ, Beahrs OH: Carcinoma of the rectum and low sigmoid: Evaluation of anterior resection of 1,766 favorable lesions. Arch Surg 90:793–798, 1965
434. Waugh JM, Block MA, Gage RP: Three- and five-year survivals following combined abdominoperineal resection with sphincter preservation, and anterior resection for carcinoma of the rectum and lower part of the sigmoid colon. Ann Surg 142:752–757, 1955
435. Williams RD, Yurko AA, Kerr G et al Comparison of anterior and abdominoperineal resections for low pelvic colon and rectal carcinoma. Am J Surg 111:114–119, 1966
436. Best RR, Rusmussen JA: Sphincter-preserving operations for cancer of the rectum. Arch Surg 72:948–956, 1956
437. Doci R, Bozzetti F, Gennari L: Anterior vs. abdominoperineal resection for cancer of the rectum and rectosigmoid. Front Gastrointest Res 5:182–187, 1979
438. Palumbo LT, Sharpe WS: Anterior versus abdominoperineal resection: Resection for rectal and rectosigmoid carcinoma. Am J Surg 115:657–660, 1968
439. Stearns MW: The choice among anterior resection, the pull-through, and abdominoperineal resection of the rectum. Cancer 34:969–971, 1974
440. Glenn F, McSherry CK: Carcinoma of the distal large bowel: 32-year review of 1,026 cases. Ann Surg 163:838–849, 1966
441. Bacon HE, Gutierrez RR: Cancer of the rectum and colon: Review of 2,402 personal cases. Dis Colon Rectum 10:61–64, 1967
442. Floyd CE, Stirling CT, Cohn I: Cancer of the colon, rectum and anus: Review of 1,687 cases. Ann Surg 163:829–837, 1966
443. Glover RP, Waugh JM: The retrograde lymphatic spread of carcinoma of the "rectosigmoid region." Its influence on surgical procedures. Surg Gynecol Obstet 82:434–448, 1946
444. Gilbertsen VA: Adenocarcinoma of the rectum: A fifteen-year study with evaluation of the results of curative therapy. Arch Surg 80:135–143, 1960
445. Localio SA, Eng K: Sphincter-saving operations for cancer of the rectum. N Engl J Med 300:1028–1030, 1979
446. Donaldson GA, Rodkey GV, Behringer GE: Resection of the rectum with anal preservation. Surg Gynecol Obstet 123:571–580, 1966
447. Black BM, Walls JT: Combined abdominoendorectal resection: Reappraisal of a pull-through procedure. Surg Clin North Am 47:977–982, 1967
448. Attiyeh FF: Proctosigmoidectomy with pull-through for adenocarcinoma of the rectum. Clin Bull 6:147–150, 1976
449. Goligher JC, Lee PWR, Macfie L et al: Experience with the Russian model 249 suture gun for anastomosis of the rectum. Surg Gynecol Obstet 148:517–524, 1979
450 Nance FC: New techniques of gastrointestinal anastomoses with the EEA stapler. Ann Surg 189:587–600, 1979
451. Sugarbaker ED: Low anterior proctosigmoidectomy using an anastomotic instrument. Am J Surg 108:64–68, 1964
452. Baker JW: Low end to side rectosigmoidal anastomosis: Description of technique. Arch Surg 61–143–156, 1950
453. Sugarbaker PH: Double puncture laparoscopy. Surg Gynecol Obstet 152:
454. Kiger WH: The Percy method of treating cancer of the uterus applied in the treatment of cancer of the rectum. Tr Am Proc Soc 23:102–109, 1923
455. Henschen C: Regeln und instrumentarium zur peranalen elektrokoagulation des rectumcarcinoms. Archiv Klin Chir 180:264–270, 1934
456. Strauss AA, Strauss SF, Crawford RA et al: Surgical diathermy of carcinoma of the rectum JAMA 104:1480–1484, 1935
457. Santos RP: Electrocoagulation of rectal cancer. Am J Dig Dis Nutrition 4:390–392, 1937–1938
458. Pruitt MC: Electrocoagulation of cancer of the rectum. J Med Assoc Ga 27:229–230, 1938
459. Hayes HT, Burr HB: The use of electrocoagulation in the treatment of tumors of the rectum. Texas State Med J 35:292–295, 1939
460. Kergin FG: Diathermy fulgurization in the treatment of certain cases of rectal cancer. Can Med Assoc J 69:14–17, 1953
461. Wassink WF: The curative treatment of carcinoma recti by means of electro-coagulation and radium. Arch Chir Neerl 8:813–829, 1956
462. Rosenthal II, Turrell R: Surgical diathermy (electrothermia) of cancer of the rectum. JAMA 167:1602–1605, 1958
463. Klok PAA: The treatment of some forms of rectal cancer by electrocoagulation. Arch Chir Neerl 16:173–183, 1964
464. Poirier A, Poirier JP: Electro-destruction dans les cancers du rectum. Archives Francaises des Maladies de l'Appareil Digestif 58:37–48, 1969
465. Madden JL, Kandalaft S: Electrocoagulation in the treatment of cancer of the rectum: A continuing study. Ann Surg 174:530–540, 1971
466. Swerdlow DB, Salvati EP: Electrocoagulation of cancer of the rectum. Dis Colon Rectum 15:228–232, 1972
467. Kratzer GL, Ohsanit T: Fulguration of selected cancers of the rectum: Report of 27 cases. Dis Colon Rectum 15:431–435, 1972
468. Crile G, Turnbull RB: The role of electrocoagulation in the treatment of carcinoma of the rectum. Surg Gynecol Obstet 135:391–396, 1972

469. Madden JL, Kandalaft S: Electrocoagulation in the treatment of cancer of the rectum. In Nylrus L (ed): Surgery Annual. New York, Appleton-Century Crofts, 1974.
470. Baker AR: Local procedures in the management of rectal cancer. Semin Oncol 7:385–391, 1980
471. Viedenheimer MC: Alternatives to surgery in treatment of carcinoma of the rectum. Surg Clin North Am 3:815–824, 1971
472. Wanebo HJ, Quan SHQ: Failures of electrocoagulation of primary carcinoma of the rectum. Surg Gynecol Obstet 138:174–176, 1974
473. Wittoesch JH, Jackman RJ: Results of conservative managment of cancer of the rectum in poor risk patients. Surg Gynecol Obstet 107:648–650, 1958
474. Jackman RJ: Conservative management of selected patients with carcinoma of the rectum. Dis Colon Rectum 4:429–434, 1961
475. Morson BC, Bussey HJR, Samoorian S: Policy of local excision for early cancer of the colorectum. Gut 18:1045–1050, 1977
476. Deddish MR: Local excision. Surg Clin North Am 54:877–880, 1974
477. Kraske P: Zur exstirpation hochsitzender mast darm krebse. Verh Dtsch Ges Chir 14:464–474, 1885
478. Papillon J: Endocavitary irradiation in the curative treatment of early rectal cancers. Dis Colon Rectum 17:172–180, 1974
479. Papillon J: Intracavitary irradiation of early rectal cancer for cure: A series of 186 cases. Cancer 36:696–701, 1975
480. Sischy B, Remington J: Treatment of carcinoma of the rectum by intracavitary radiation. Surg Gynecol Obstet 141:562–564, 1975
481. Sischy B, Remington JH, Sokel SH: Treatment of rectal carcinomas by means of endocavitary irradiation: A progress report. Cancer 46:1957–1961, 1980
482. Sischy B, Remington JH, Sobel SH, et al: Treatment of carcinoma of the rectum and squamous carcinoma of the anus by combination chemotherapy, radiotherapy and operation. Surg Gynecol Obstet 151:369–371, 1980
483. Dwight RW, Higgins GA, Keehn RJ: Factors influencing survival after resection in cancer of the colon and rectum. J Surg Oncol 5:243, 1973
484. Dwight RW, Humphrey EW, Higgins GA et al: FUDR as an adjuvant to surgery in cancer of the large bowel. J Surg Oncol 5:243, 1973
485. Lawrence W Jr, Terz JJ, Horsley S: Chemotherapy as an adjuvant to surgery for colorectal cancer. Ann Surg 181:616, 1975
486. Li MC, Ross ST: Chemoprophylaxis for patients with colorectal cancer: Prospective study with five-year follow-up. JAMA 235:2825–2828, 1976
487. Higgins GA, Lee LE, Dwight RW et al: The case for adjuvant 5-fluorouracil in colorectal cancer. Cancer Clin Trials 1:35–41, 1978
488. Mavligit GM, Burgess MA, Seibert GB et al: Prolongation of postoperative disease free interval and survival in human colorectal cancer by BCG or BCG plus 5-fluorouracil. Lancet 1:871–875, 1976
489. Grage TB, Hill GJ, Cornell GN et al: Adjuvant chemotherapy in large bowel cancer: An updated analysis of single agent chemotherapy. In Jones SE, Salmon SE (eds): Adjuvant Chemotherapy of Cancer, 2nd ed, pp 587–594. New York Grune & Stratton, 1979
490. Rousselot LM, Cole DR, Grossi CE: Adjuvant chemotherapy with 5-fluorouracil in surgery for colorectal cancer: Eight year progress report. Dis Colon Rectum 15:169, 1972
491. Moertel CG, Freireich EJ: Final Overview. In Jones SE, Salmon SE (eds): Adjuvant Chemotherapy of Cancer, 2nd ed, pp 631–636. New York, Grune & Stratton, 1979
492. Taylor I, Brooman P, Rowling JT: Adjuvant liver perfusion in colorectal cancer: Initial results of a clinical trial. Br Med J 2:1320–1322, 1977
493. Dennis C, Karlson KE: Cancer risk in ulcerative colitis: Formidability per patient-year of late disease. Surgery 50:568–571, 1961
494. Riddell RH: Dysplasia in inflammatory bowel disease. Clin Gastroenterol 9:439–458, 1980
495. Dawson IMP, Pryse-Davies: The development of carcinoma of the large intestine in ulcerative colitis. Br J Surg 47:113–128, 1959
496. Goldgraber MB, Kirsner JB: Carcinoma of the colon in ulcerative colitis. Cancer 17:657–665, 1964
497. Bargen JA: Chronic ulcerative colitis associated with malignant disease. Arch Surg 17:561–576, 1928
498. Morson BC, Pang LSC: Rectal biopsy as an aid to cancer control in ulcerative colitis. Gut 8:423–434, 1967
499. Evans DJ, Pollock DJ: In-situ and invasive carcinoma of the colon in patients with ulcerative colitis. Gut 13:566–570, 1972
500. Fenoglio CM, Pascal RR: Adenomatous epithelium, intraepithelial anaplasia, and invasive carcinoma in ulcerative colitis. Am J Dig Dis 18:556–562, 1973
501. Myrvold HE, Knock NG, Ahren C: Rectal biopsy and precancer in ulcerative colitis. Gut 15:301–304, 1974
502. Yardley JH, Keren DF: "Precancer" lesions in ulcerative colitis. A retrospective study of rectal biopsy and colectomy specimens. Cancer 34:835–844, 1974
503. Hulten L, Kewenter J, Ahren C: Precancer and carcinoma in chronic ulcerative colitis: A histopathological and clinical investigation. Scand J Gastroenterol 10:663–669, 1975
504. Cook MG, Goligher JC: Carcinoma and epithelial dysplasia complicating ulcerative colitis. Gastroenterology 68:1127–1136, 1975
505. Gewertz BL, Dent TL, Appleman HD: Implications of precancerous rectal biopsy in patients with inflammatory bowel disease. Arch Surg 111:326–329, 1976
506. Crowson TD, Ferrante WF, Gathright JB: Inefficacy for early carcinoma detection in patients with ulcerative colitis. JAMA 236:2651–2652, 1976
507. Lennard-Jones JE, Morson BC, Ritchie JK et al: Cancer in colitis: Assessment of the individual risk by clinical and histological criteria. Gastroenterology 73:1280–1289, 1977
508. Nugent FW, Haggitt RC, Colcher H et al: Malignant potential of chronic ulcerative colitis: Preliminary report. Gastroenterology 76:1–5, 1978
509. Riddell RH, Morson BC: Value of sigmoidoscopy and biopsy in detection of carcinoma and premalignant change in ulcerative colitis. Gut 20:575–580, 1979
510. Dobbins WO, Stock M, Ginsberg AL: Early detection and prevention of carcinoma of the colon in patients with ulcerative colitis. Cancer 40:2542–2548, 1977
511. Baker WNW, Glass RE, Ritchie JK et al: Cancer of the rectum following colectomy and ileorectal anastomosis for ulcerative colitis. Br J Surg 65:862–868, 1978
512. Daly DW: The outcome of surgery for ulcerative colitis. Ann R Coll Surg Engl 42:38–57, 1968
513. Griffen WO, Lillehei RC, Wangensteen OH: Ileoproctostomy in ulcerative colitis: Long-term follow-up, extending in early cases to more than 20 years. Surgery 53:705–710, 1963
514. Jagelman DG, Lewis CB, Rowe-Jones DC: Ileorectal anastomosis: Appreciation by patients. Br Med J 1:756–767, 1969
515. Sprechler M: Ileorectal anastomosis for ulcerative colitis. Br Med J 1:527, 1971
516. Gruner OPN, Flatmark A, Naas R et al: Ileorectal anastomosis in ulcerative colitis: Results in 57 patients. Scand J Gastroenterol 10:641–646, 1975
517. Jones PF, Munro A, Ewen SWB: Colectomy and ileorectal anastomosis for colitis: Report on a personal series, with a critical review. Br J Surg 64:615–623, 1977.
518. Peck DA, Watanabe KS, Trueblood HW: Familial polyposis in children. Dis Colon Rectum 15:23–29, 1955
519. Moertel CG, Hill JR, Adson MA: Surgical management of multiple polypsis. Arch Surg 100:521–526, 1970
520. Schaupp WC, Volpe PA: Management of diffuse colonic polyposis. Am J Surg 124:218–222, 1972
521. DeCrosse JJ, Condon RE, Adams MB: Surgical and medical measures in prevention of large bowel cancer. Cancer 40:2549–2552, 1977
522. Ravitch MM, Sabiston DC: Anal ileostomy with preservation of the sphincter: A proposed operation in patients requiring total colectomy for benign lesions. Surg Gynecol Obstet 84:1095–1098, 1947

523. Ferrari BT, Fonkalsrud EW: Endorectal ilea: pullthrough operation with ileal reservoir after total colectomy. Am J Surg 136:113–120, 1978
524. Lillehie RC, Wangensteen OH: Bowel function after colectomy for cancer, polyps and diverticulitis. JAMA 159:163–170, 1955
525. Teicher I, Abrahams JI: The treatment of selected cases of multiple polyps, familial polyposis and diverticular disease of the colon by subtotal colectomy and ileoproctostomy. Surg Gynecol Obstet 103:136–146, 1956
526. Peabody CN, Smithwick RH: Practical implications of multiple tumors of the colon and rectum. N Engl J Med 261:853–855, 1961
527. Grinnell RS: The rationale of subtotal and total colectomy in the treatment of cancer and multiple polyps of the colon. Surg Gynecol Obstet 106:288–292, 1958
528. Nayman J: Primary resection without anastomosis for carcinoma of the sigmoid colon with obstruction. Aus NZ J Surg 33:222–226, 1964
529. Sugarbaker ED, Whiley HM: The significance of fixation in operable carcinoma of the large bowel. Surgery 27:343–347, 1950
530. Merril JG, Dockerty MB, Waugh JM: Carcinoma of the colon perforating into the anterior abdominal wall. Surgery 28:662–671, 1950
531. Phillips JW, Dockerty MB, Waugh JM: Carcinoma of the hepatic flexure. Cancer 8:151–157, 1955
532. Kiselow M, Butcher HR, Bricker EM: Results of the radical treatment of advanced pelvic cancer: A fifteen-year study. Ann Surg 166:428–436, 1967
533. Wang CC, Schulz MD: The role of radiation therapy in the management of carcinoma of the sigmoid, rectosigmoid and rectum. Radiology 79:1–5, 1962
534. Rider WD: Is the Miles operation really necessary for the treatment of rectal cancer? J Can Assoc Radiol 26:167–175, 1975
535. Rider WD, Hawkins NV, Cummings BJ et al: Radiation for the cure of rectal cancer (abstr). Int J Radiat Oncol Biol Phys 4(2):114, 1978
536. Rao AR, Kagan AR, Chan PYM et al: Effectiveness of local radiotherapy in colorectal carcinoma. Cancer 42:1082–1086, 1978
537. Williams IG: Radiotherapy of carcinoma of the rectum. In Dukes C (ed): Cancer of the Rectum, pp. 210–219. Edinburgh, Churchill Livingstone
538. Sklaroff D: Radiation as a primary therapy for rectal carcinoma. Am Fam Physician 8:81–85, 1973
539. Urdaneta-Lafre N, Kligerman MM, Knowlton AH: Evaluation of palliative irradiation in rectal carcinoma. Radiology 104:673–677, 1972
540. Pilepich MY, Munzenrider JE, Tak WK et al: Preoperative irradiation of primarily unresectable colorectal carcinoma. Cancer 47:1077–1081, 1978
541. Samala E, Boseworten JL, Gerorsein NA: Results of postoperative radiotherapy in patients who had incomplete resection of a colorectal cancer (abstr). Int J Radiat Oncol Biol Phys 5(2): 121, 1979
542. Pestana C, Reitemeier RJ, Moertel CG et al: The natural history of carcinoma of the colon and rectum. Am J Surg 108:826–829, 1964
543. Bengmark S, Hafstrom L: The natural history of primary and secondary malignant tumors of the liver: 1. The prognosis for patients with hepatic metastases from colonic and rectal carcinoma by laparotomy. Cancer 23:198–202, 1969
544. Morris MJ, Newland RC, Pheils MT et al: Hepatic metastases from colorectal carcinoma: An analysis of survival rates and histopathology. Aust NZ J Surg 47:365–368, 1977
545. Griffen WO, Humphrey L, Sosin H: The prognosis and management of recurrent abdominal malignancies. Current Probl Surg, 1969
546. Ellis H: Is a "second look operation" justified in suspected recurrences after abdominal cancer surgery? Br J Surg 62:830–832, 1975
547. Whiteley AW, Steams MW, Leaming RH et al: Radiation therapy in the palliative management of patients with recurrent cancer of the colon and rectum. Surg Clin North Am 49:381–387, 1969
548. Hindo WA, Soleimani PK, Miller WA et al: Patterns of recurrent and metastatic carcinoma of the colon and rectum treated with radiation. Dis Colon Rectum 15:436–440, 1972
549. Fletcher GH: Clinical dose-response curves of human malignant epithelial tumors. Br J Radiol 46:1–12, 1973
550. Freund H, Gunderson L, Krause R et al: Prevention of radiation enteritis after abdominoperineal resection and radiotherapy. Surg Gynecol Obstet 149:206–208, 1979
551. Bacon HE, Martin PV: The rationale of palliative resection for primary cancer of the colon and rectum complicated by liver and lung metastasis. Dis Colon Rectum 7:211–217, 1964
552. Stearns MW, Binkley GE: Palliative surgery for cancer of the rectum and colon. Cancer 7:1016–1019, 1954
553. Modlin J, Walker HSJ: Palliative resections in cancer of the colon and rectum. Cancer 2:767–776, 1949
554. Jaffe BM, Donegan WL, Watson F et al: Factors influencing survival in patients with untreated hepatic metastases. Surg Gynecol Obstet 127:1–11, 1968
555. Bordos DC, Baker RR, Cameron JL: An evaluation of palliative abdominoperineal resection for carcinoma of the rectum. Surg Gynecol Obstet 139:731–733, 1974
556. Martin RG, Soriano SJ, Clark RL: Abdominoperineal resection as palliation for advanced rectal carcinoma. Cancer Bulletin 2:28–31, 1966
557. Lockhart-Mummery HE: Surgery in patients with advanced carcinoma of the colon and rectum. Dis Colon Rectum 2:36–39, 1959
558. Ramsey WH: Treatment of inoperable cancer of the rectum by fulguration. Dis Colon Rectum 5:114–117, 1962
559. Oxley EM, Ellis H: Prognosis of carcinoma of the large bowel in the presence of liver metastases. Br J Surg 56:149–152, 1969
560. Wilson SM, Adson MA: Surgical treatment of hepatic metastases from colorectal cancers. Arch Surg 111:330–334, 1976
561. Wanebo HJ, Semoglou C, Attiyeh F et al: Surgical management of patients with primary operable colorectal cancer and synchronous liver metastases. Am J Surg 135:81–85, 1978
562. Fortner JG, Kim DK, MacLean BJ et al: Major hepatic resection for neoplasia: Personal experience in 108 Patients. Ann Surg 188:363–371, 1978
563. Attiyeh FF, Wanebo HJ, Stearns MW: Hepatic resection for metastasis from colorectal cancer. Dis Colon Rectum 21:160–162, 1978
564. Foster JH: Survival after liver resection for secondary tumors. Am J Surg 135:389–394, 1978
565. Foster JH, Berman MM: Solid Liver Tumors. Philadelphia, WB Saunders, 1977
566. Adson MA, VanHeerden JA: Major hepatic resections for metastatic colorectal cancer. Ann Surg 191:576–583, 1980
567. Breedis C, Young G: The blood supply of neoplasms in the liver. Am J Pathol 30:969–954, 1954
568. Madding GF, Kennedy PA: Hepatic artery ligation. Surg Clin North Am 52:719–728, 1972
569. Ansfield FJ, Ramirez G, Skibba J et al: Intrahepatic arterial infusion with 5-fluorouracil. Cancer 28:1147, 1971
570. Ansfield FJ, Ramirez G, Davis HL: Further clinical studies with intrahepatic arterial infusion with 5-fluorouracil. Cancer 36:2413, 1976
571. Grage TB, Vassilopoulos P, Schingleton WW et al: Results of a prospective randomized study of hepatic artery infusion with 5-fluorouracil versus intravenous 5-fluorouracil in patients with hepatic metastases from colorectal cancer: A central oncology group study. Surgery 86:550–555, 1979
572. Buroker T, Samson M, Correa J et al: Hepatic artery infusion of 5-FUdR after prior systemic 5-fluorouracil. Cancer Treat Rep 60:1227, 1976
573. Grage TB, Vassilopoulos PP, Shingleton WW et al: Results of a prospective randomized study of hepatic artery infusion with 5-fluorouracil versus intravenous 5-fluorouracil in patients with

hepatic metastases from colorectal cancer: A central oncology group study. Surgery 86:550–555, 1979
574. Schulten MF, Heiskell CA, Shields TW: The incidence of solitary pulmonary metastasis from carcinoma of the large intestine. Surg Gynecol Obstet 146:727–729, 1976
575. Mountain CF, Khalil KG, Hermes KE et al: The contribution of surgery to the management of carcinomatous pulmonary metastases. Cancer 41:833–840, 1978
576. Cahan WG, Castro EB, Hajdu SI: The significance of a solitary lung shadow in patients with colon carcinoma. Cancer 33:414–421, 1974
577. McCormack PM, Bains MS, Beattie EJ et al: Pulmonary resection in metastatic carcinoma. Chest 73:163–166, 1978
578. Collins VP: Time of occurrence of pulmonary metastasis from carcinoma of colon and rectum. Cancer 15:387–395, 1962

Paul H. Sugarbaker
Leonard L. Gunderson
John S. Macdonald

CHAPTER 22

Cancer of the Anal Region

Epidermoid carcinoma of the anal region (also called squamous cell cancer) is a less frequently occurring tumor than adenocarcinoma of the colon and rectum. It accounts for only two to four percent of all tumors of the distal alimentary tract. Also, Stearns and Quan found that one-third of all tumors of the anal and perianal skin are epidermoid cancer.[1] Because of the complexity of the anatomy of this region of the body, the great variations in stage of disease encountered and the relatively few patients encountered by any one physician or group, management decisions are often very difficult.

EPIDEMIOLOGY

As a whole, this disease is equally as common in males as it is in females. However, over this short segment of anatomy referred to as the anal region, there are marked differences in occurrence by sex. Cancers of the anal margin are three times more common in males whereas cancer of the anal canal is slightly more common in females.[2]

The frequent association of epidermoid carcinoma with other conditions of this region deserves mention. Nearly any condition which causes chronic irritation of the anal canal or perianal region has been associated with this disease. Brennan and Stewart, reporting on 39 patients with epidermoid carcinoma, found five (13 percent) with condylomata, four (10 percent) with fistulae, three (8 percent) with fissures, three with abscesses, and three with hemorrhoids.[3] In this series of patients, approximately half had associated anorectal pathology. Bretlan collected some 75 cases of squamous cell carcinoma arising in anal fistulae; a majority of these fistulae were of long standing.[4] McAnally and Dockerty estimated the incidence of carcinoma in anal fistulae at 0.1 percent.[5] Wolfe and Bussey also reported leukoplakia of the anus and prior irradiation as associated conditions.[2]

ANATOMICAL CONSIDERATIONS

Epidermoid cancer of the anal region occurs over a very limited area; the anal canal is only 2.5 to 3 cm in length and the perianal area measures 6 cm from the anal verge. The anatomic landmarks for physical examination of this region are the anorectal ring, the pectinate line, and the anal verge; each marks an area of transition of the epithelium (Figure 22-1).

Above 1.5 cm above the pectinate line in the area of the rectal columns, the columnar mucosa of the rectum changes to a cuboidal pattern. This transitional epithelium closely resembles the lining of the urinary tract and is thought to be a remnant of the cloacal membrane. Cloacogenic carcinoma arises from this epithelium. However, it is not unusual for stratified squamous epithelium to extend upward into the area of anal valves replacing a portion of the transitional epithelium and giving rise to squamous cell carcinoma within the rectum.[6] Also, at the base of the columns of Morgagni (anal crypts) the anal glands arise. These not only give rise to fistula *in ano,* but according to Morson, mucoepidermoid tumors.[7] Below the pectinate line the smooth stratified squamous epithelium of the anal canal is seen. At the anal verge this squamous epithelium becomes pigmented and supports numerous hair follicles. The keratinized stratified squamous epithelium below the anal verge is the perianal area. It constitutes an area about 12 cm in diameter which is char-

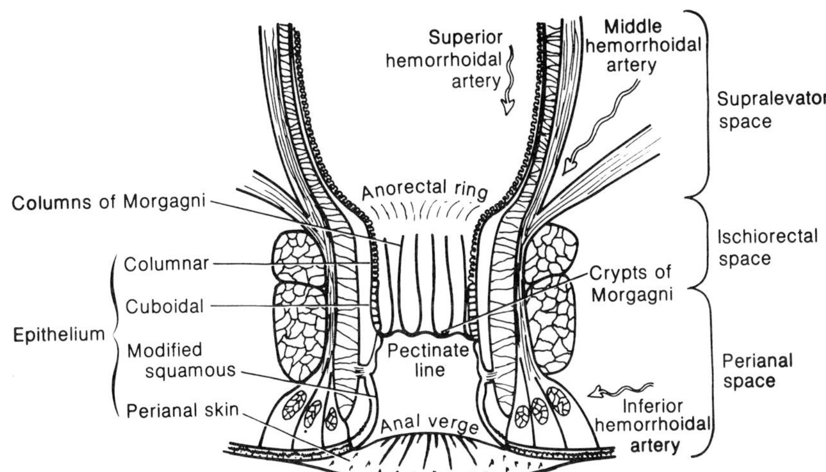

FIG. 22-1. Anatomy of the anal region. (Modified from Harkins HN: Anorectum. In Moyer CA, Rhoads JE, Allen JG, Harkins HN (eds): Surgery, Principles and Practice, 3rd ed, p 1124. Philadelphia, JB Lippincott, 1965)

acterized by hyperpigmentation, large numbers of hair follicles, and skin folds radiating out from the anal verge.

Lymphatic spread with this disease is unfortunately diffuse. From the pectinate line and within the anal canal, spread may go three directions; upward to the superior hemorrhoidal system, lateral along the middle hemorrhoidal system and downward to the inguinal nodes. At the anal verge and perianal area, lymphatic flow is to the inguinal nodes.

PATHOLOGY

Morson lumped all tumors that arise in the anal canal and perianal region into two groups, keratinizing and nonkeratinizing tumors.[7] Tumors derived from the transitional epithelium are usually of the nonkeratinizing variety; they are also called basosquamous, basaloid, and cloacogenic carcinoma. Tumors arising below the anal canal show keratin production 84 percent of the time while those from within the anal canal form keratin in only 45 percent of patients. Morson suggested that keratin production is a rough guide to the grade of malignancy of these tumors. Therefore, the prognosis of anal margin disease after surgical treatment is somewhat better than anal canal carcinoma. Further simplifying the pathology, Stearns and Quan suggested that all the pathological variants of epidermoid carcinoma be considered together in discussions concerning treatment.[1] The cell type has little or nothing to do with treatments while clinical characteristics are extremely important.

One final precautionary note regarding basal cell (basaloid) cancer of the anal canal: These tumors may appear as a low grade malignancy and do carry a better prognosis;[1] however, they are metastasizing tumors and should be treated as such.[7] They do not behave as do the common basal cell cancers of skin.

NATURAL HISTORY

The routes of spread of epidermoid carcinoma of the anal region depend in large part on the location of the tumor in relation to the anatomy of the anorectum. Figure 22-2 shows the location of 189 epidermoid cancers.[8] Two percent were in the rectum and most likely resulted from malignant change in stratified squamous epithelium that may extend up along the columns of Morgagni. The greatest number, 58 percent, were abutting the pectinate line. Fourteen percent were within the anal canal and 11 percent abutted the anal verge. Fifteen percent were totally within perianal skin.

Local spread occurs by invasion of perineal tissues. The sphincter ani muscles are first to be involved. The muscular coat surrounding the anal canal is many times thicker than that of the colon or rectum because of the sphincter muscles. Wolfe and Bussey found spread along the submucosa above the sphincter muscles occurring for a distance of six to seven cm; therefore, longitudinal spread of this tumor along the bowel wall is quite different for squamous cell carcinoma of the anal area than for adenocarcinoma of the colon and rectum.[2] Spread of squamous cell carcinoma of the anus may

FIG. 22-2. Areas and percent of tumor occurrence in the anal region. (Adapted from Kuhn PG, Eisenberg H, Reed JF: Epidermoid carcinoma of the perianal skin and anal canal. Cancer 22:932–938, 1968)

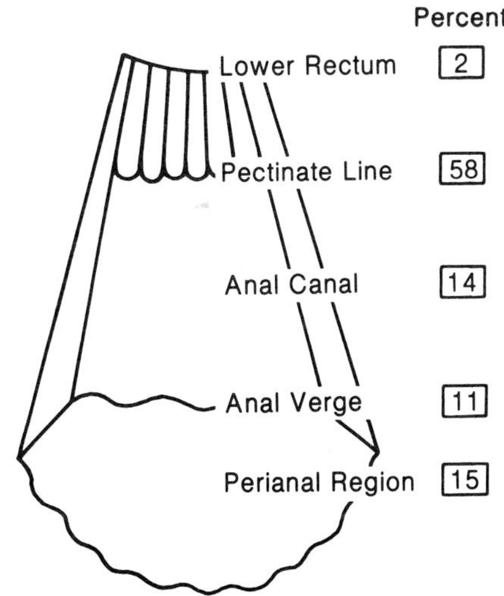

TABLE 22-1. Mesenteric Lymph Node Involvement in Epidermoid Carcinoma of the Anal Margin and Anal Canal

		ANAL MARGIN		ANAL CANAL	
AUTHORS	YEAR	*Number of Patients*	*Mesenteric Nodes*	*Number of Patients*	*Mesenteric Nodes*
Dillard, Spratt, and Ackerman[11]	1963	10	4 (40%))	37	14 (38%)
Sawyers, Herrington, and Main[10]	1963	16	1 (6%)	26	7 (27%)
Wolfe and Bussey[2]	1968	12	0	102	39 (38%)
Hardy, Hughes, and Cuthbertson[12]	1969	18	9 (50%)	23	10 (44%)
Total		53	14 (26%)	200	86 (43%)

be analogous to the longitudinal spread of esophageal carcinoma.

If the sphincter muscles are penetrated, the prostate, urethra, and bladder in the male, the vagina in the female, and the sacrum and ischial tuberosities in both sexes may be involved. Welch and Malt documented vaginal invasion in eight of 34 (24 percent) of the female patients.[9]

Wolfe and Bussey reported that the location of the primary tumor determines in large part the direction of lymphatic metastases.[2] In reviewing major resection specimens, 44 percent of carcinoma of the anal canal had spread to hemorrhoidal glands. In contrast, none of 12 patients with anal margin cancer had upward spread. However, as shown in Table 22-1, Wolfe and Bussey stand alone with these data. Sawyers and coworkers, Dilliard and coworkers, and Hardy and coworkers showed approximately one-third of patients with anal margin cancer had mesenteric nodal involvement.[10,11,12]

Stearns and Quan studied the routes of lymphatic spread documented in their patients with epidermoid carcinoma of the anal canal and perianal skin. Groin metastases (downward spread) developed in 40 percent (44 of 109 patients), mesenteric nodal metastases (upward spread) in 24 percent (16 of 24 patients), and pelvic lymph node metastases (lateral spread) in 33 percent (15 of 45 patients).[1] The incidence of spread was not correlated with the position of the primary tumor within the anorectal area. The large proportion of patients with lateral spread may be of significance in planning treatments.

Hematogenous spread to the liver was reviewed by MacLean, Murray, and Bacon.[13] Metastases to the liver via the portal system occurred in 24 of their collected series of 869 patients or 2.8 percent. Lung metastases occurred in six of 200 (3 percent) patients in Kuehn's 1968 series.[8] Certainly, hematogenous spread is much more unusual in squamous cell carcinoma of the anorectum than in adenocarcinoma of the colorectum.

DIAGNOSIS

Rectal bleeding is by far the most common symptom and was present in 60 percent of the patients reviewed by Richards, Beahrs, and Woolner.[14] The bleeding was in small amounts, rarely resulted in anemia and was often confused with symptoms of benign anorectal conditions. Thirty-nine percent of patients complained of pain or pressure in the perineal region. Seventeen percent noted a mass. Other less common symptoms included change in bowel habits, pruritus, and anal discharge. Six percent of patients had no symptoms at all, the lesion being picked up by biopsy of a lesion seen on a routine physical examination.

Delay in diagnosis is a common feature of many tumors, presumably because the symptoms of this disease are often confused with those of common benign conditions. However, the disease may be obscured by the presence of a fistula or a painful fissure which may make examination difficult. Examination under general anesthesia may frequently be required for accurate diagnosis.

ASSESSMENT OF PROGNOSIS

Clinicopathological features of this disease and their effect on prognosis are shown in Table 22-2. Diagnosis of epidermoid

TABLE 22-2. Clinicopathologic Features and Their Effect on Prognosis of Epidermoid Carcinoma of the Anal Region

Diagnosis in the asymptomatic patient	Improved
Long duration of symptoms	Diminished
Carcinoma in a fistulous tract	Diminished
Large size	Diminished
Location at anal margin	Improved
Able to be locally excised	Improved
Low (versus high) Broder's Grade	Improved
A, B, C classification	
A	Improved
B	Diminished
C	Diminished
Pushing (versus infiltrating) character of margin	Improved
Involvement of sphincter muscle	Diminished
Perirectal node involvement	Further diminished
Inguinal node involvement occurring after treatment of the primary tumor	Further diminished
Inguinal node involvement at the time of diagnosis of the primary tumor	Further diminished

carcinoma of the anal region in the asymptomatic patient carries a favorable prognosis.[15,16] With a wide margin taken at the time of reexcision survival is near 100 percent. A long duration of symptoms and presence of carcinoma in a fistulous tract are poor prognostic variables.[3,8]

Contrary to adenocarcinoma of the colorectum, prognosis with epidermoid carcinoma is directly related to size of the primary lesion. Dillard and coworkers found 75 percent five-year survival in 12 patients with tumor size less than 8 square cm, but only 47 percent survival in 38 patients with tumor size greater than 8 cm.[11] Keuhn, Eisenberg, and Reed reported no survivors with the primary tumor over 6 cm in diameter.[8]

Tumors at the anal margin present a slightly better prognosis than those of the anal canal. These tumors being more external may be diagnosed somewhat more readily. Also, they tend to be more well-differentiated.[2] However, Paradis, Douglass, and Holyoke found no difference in survival rates between tumors arising within the anal canal and in the perianal region.[17]

Morson found the amount of keratin formation could be used to classify tumors as differentiated or undifferentiated, but did not find further histologic grading of value.[7] Anal margin cancer usually shows more keratin production than anal canal cancer. Morson thought this was the main reason that prognosis of anal margin disease after surgical treatment is better than for anal canal carcinoma. In the studies of Paradis, Douglass, and Holyoke, prognosis of perianal and anal canal lesions was the same.[17] Richards, Beahrs, and Woolner found that Broders' Grades were a good prognostic indicator.[14] Dillard and coworkers also found grading of value in assessing prognosis.[11] Unfortunately, breaking the small sample of patients into four subgroups results in unreliable analysis; using Morson's two grades is preferred.

STAGING

Richards, Beahrs, and Woolner classified 41 patients by the A,B,C method: the proportion of patients in each class and the five-year survival are shown in Table 22-3.[14] Unfortunately, the anatomic limits of the various classes were not given. Were Class B tumors those that penetrated through the entire sphincter muscles that are the muscular coat of the anal canal?

Paradis, Douglass, and Holyoke proposed a staging system based primarily on the involvement of the sphincter ani muscles and spread to various regional lymph node groups.[17] Involvement of perirectal nodes was not as ominous a prognostic sign in their series as was inguinal involvement (Table 22-3).

TREATMENT

SURGICAL APPROACH

Until recently, the standard therapy for epidermoid carcinoma of the anus has been surgical. Not only was radiation treatment usually ineffective in eradicating disease, but its long term effects on anal function were undesirable.[18] Damage to the perianal skin and anal sphincter necessitating colostomy was not unusual following curative radiation therapy.

The surgical treatment of this tumor depends in large part on the location plus degree of invasion of the primary tumor and presence or absence of inguinal adenopathy. Tumors of the perianal skin are treated like epidermoid tumors elsewhere.[15] They should be widely excised; if inguinal lymphadenopathy suggestive of metastases is present initially or develops upon followup the involved groin nodes should be excised *en bloc*.

The treatment of epidermoid tumors at the anal verge is not so widely agreed upon. Wolfe and Bussey justify the local excision of anal margin cancer saying that upward metastases are rare; they were found in zero of 12 of their patients undergoing abdominoperineal resection.[2] However, as noted in Table 22-1, other groups have found upward metastases in at least one-third of patients. There may be an explanation to partially explain this discrepancy; patients at different stages of their disease may be being compared.

TABLE 22-3. Staging Systems for Epidermoid Carcinomas of the Anal Region

CLASS		PROPORTION OF PATIENTS (%)	FIVE-YEAR SURVIVAL (%)
	A,B,C Classification (Richards, Beahrs and Woolner, Surg Gynecol Obst, 114:475–482, 1962)		
		n = 60	n = 41
A		27	83.3 (10/12)
B		35	71.4 (10/14)
C		38	40.0 (6/15)
	Roswell Park Classification (Paradis, Douglass and Holyoke, Surg Gynecol Obst, 141:411–416, 1975)		
		n = 47	n = 47
0	Carcinoma *in situ*	4	100 (2/2)
I	Sphincter muscle not involved	26	100 (12/12)
II	Sphincter muscle involved	30	50 (7/14)
III	Regional metastases		
IIIA	Perirectal nodes only	19	56 (5/9)
IIIB	Inguinal nodes	6	0 (0/3)
IV	Distant metastases, para-aortic nodes, sacrum	15	0 (0/7)

Dillard and coworkers at the Ellis Fischel Hospital, based on a study of 79 epidermoid carcinomas of the anal area, suggested treatment by abdominoperineal resection in all but a select few patients with anal margin cancer.[11] Nine of ten of their patients treated by radical resection survived five years, whereas only three of ten treated by local excision survived a similar period. This was in spite of the fact that cancers treated by local excision were better differentiated and were smaller than cancers treated by abdominoperineal resection. These investigators suggested strict criteria by which anal margin cancer could be treated by local excision. The tumor should be 2 by 2 cm or less, of well-differentiated histological grade, and not fixed to deeper tissues. Of course, all *in situ* cancers in the anal region should be treated by local excision.[19]

If there is some difference of opinion about treatment of carcinoma of the anal verge, there is little disagreement about the need for radical treatment of invasive carcinoma of the anal canal. Lymphatic metastases to three lymph node drainage areas are frequent. With approximately one-third of patients having lateral spread, Paradis, Douglass, and Holyoke, and Stearns and Quan have suggested the addition of a pelvic lymph node dissection to abdominoperineal resection in good-risk patients.[1,17] Stearns and Quan had two of seven long-term survivors with metastases to hypogastric or obturator nodes. This additional lymphatic dissection, when confined to the pelvis, adds morbidity to abdominoperineal resection but may improve the operative results.

Kuehn, Eisenberg, and Reed, Welch and Malt, and Sawyers have emphasized the need for wide excision of perineal tissue in performing the abdominoperineal resection.[8,9,15] Lesions on the anterior portion of the anal canal in females should be excised *en bloc* with the posterior portion of the vagina. Kuehn and coworkers had ten of 94 patients, whose initial treatment was abdominoperineal resection, fail locally with inadequate vaginal or bladder resections. Total pelvic exenteration should be performed if lesions involve the bladder or urethra.[20]

Of course, if inguinal nodes are involved, they need to be excised; even though chances for cure are few, radiation therapy infrequently controls gross inguinal disease. For clinically negative inguinal nodes at presentation, most groups justify the watch and wait policy for the following reasons: First, these nodes are readily accessible to physical examination so that metastatic deposits may be detected early by the physician or a carefully instructed patient. Second, if positive at the time of initial presentation, early death from cancer is the rule. A review of data from the major series showed 11 of 67 (16 percent) long term survivors from groin dissection done to eradicate inguinal disease present at the time of presentation (Table 22-4). Spread to inguinal nodes often indicates a tumor of high-grade malignancy and carries a most dismal prognosis. Third, the "morbidity" from the combined procedures is almost prohibitive in itself. Immediate problems with wound healing and long term problems with lymphedema occur in nearly half of the patients. Fourth, only about one-third of patients ever need even unilateral groin dissection. If prophylactic bilateral groin dissections were done, Stearns and Quan estimate that 61 of 96 patients would have had bilateral groin dissection without benefit.[1] Finally, the watch and wait policy seems to give acceptable results. Stearns and Quan report 12 of 20 (60 percent) survivors free of disease if groin dissections were done when inguinal nodes became palpable; Kuehn and coworkers reported seven of 16 (44 percent) survivors. A review of the literature is presented in Table 22-5.

Golden and Horsley and Ely and Sullivan collected survival statistics on locally and radically excised tumors of both anal margin and anal canal.[25,26] In both collections of data, survival after local excision was about 65 percent, whereas survival following abdominoperineal resection was about 50 percent. Of course, the patients treated by local excision were a select group of early, low grade tumors thought suitable by the responsible surgeon for limited surgery. It is, therefore, somewhat disconcerting that results were not better. Only in patients whose prognosis is favorable by the criteria suggested in Table 22-2 should local excision be recommended.

Dillard has suggested that an absolute contraindication to wide local excision is carcinom in a fistula *in ano*.[11] None of eight of their patients with this combination problem survived five years with local excision.

RADIATION THERAPY

Epidermoid anal cancers are generally as radiosensitive as other epidermoid carcinomas. External irradiation is somewhat limited by the problem of perineal reaction and requires

TABLE 22-4. Five-Year Survival of Patients with Epidermoid Carcinoma of the Anal Region with Synchronous Inguinal Metastases

AUTHORS	YEAR	NUMBER OF PATIENTS	NED AT 5 YEARS
Sedgwick and Wainstein[21]	1959	6	2
Wolfe and Bussey[2]	1961	19	5
Richards, Beahrs, and Woolner[14]	1962	1	1
Brown and McKenzie[22]	1963	1	0
Dillard, Spratt, and Ackerman[11]	1963	6	2
Kuehn et al[8]	1968	6	0
Martin, Miller and Thorpe[23]	1967	5	1
Stearns and Quan[1]	1970	15	0
Brennan and Steward[3]	1973	2	0
Paradis, Douglass, and Holyoke[17]	1975	6	0
Total		67	11 (16%)

TABLE 22-5. Five-Year Survival of Patients with Epidermoid Carcinoma of the Anal Region with Metachronous Inguinal Metastases

AUTHORS	YEAR	NUMBER OF PATIENTS	NED AT 5 YEARS
Lone, Berg and Sterns[24]	1960	2	2
Wofe and Bussey[2]	1968	9	5
Dillard, Spratt, and Ackerman[11]	1963	3	3
Kuehn et al[8]	1968	16	8
Martin, Miller, and Thorpe[23]	1967	11	4
Hardy, Hughes, and Cuthbertson[12]	1969	1	1
Stearns and Quan[1]	1970	21	12
Paradis, Douglas, and Holyoke[17]	1975	7	1
Total		70	36 (51%)

protraction of treatment to avoid untoward effects. Indications for combining pre- or postoperative irradiation with surgery are difficult to derive, since surgical series rarely report local recurrence figures. For anal canal lesions, local recurrence risks would theoretically be similar to those after abdominoperineal resection for adenocarcinoma.

Implant and External Beam Using Orthovoltage

In the past, primary radiation therapy (irradiation without operation) was given largely with implantation due to limitations of orthovoltage. Although it achieved cure rates varying from 20 to 53 percent, it has been much maligned as a sole modality due to high complication rates including stricture, infection, necrosis, hemorrhage, and problems of severe post-irradiation pain.[27,28] Papillon reviewed his own series with minimum 5-year followup and states such complications are the result of overdosage or faulty technique.[29] He discussed methods used to combine external and interstitial irradiation as well as the use of interstitial irradiation alone in the treatment of 98 patients with selected anal malignancies. Of 64 patients at risk for five years, 44 (68 percent) were alive and free of disease. If those dying from nonmalignant causes are excluded, the determinant five-year survival rate was 80 percent. Four of the 98 (4.1 percent) had radical operative procedures for severe radionecrosis—all occurred within the first two years of treatment. Milder ulceronecrotic reactions occurred in 20 cases which were treated by antibiotic ointment and steroid therapy. All healed in less than four months without colostomy, sequelae, or discomfort and sphincteric function was preserved.

Papillon attributes his high cure and low necrosis rates to the use of more fractionated schemes. For early lesions which are treated with implant alone, he uses two or three implantations spaced at intervals of about two months. For advanced lesions, a combination of 3000 rad in three-week external irradiation with supervoltage is utilized, followed in five to eight weeks by an interstitial implant.

Papillon's recommendations are as follows: (1) *Tumors of External Margin*. Small tumors can be treated conservatively by local excision, radium implant or external irradition. Large tumors may at times be treated by external irradiation combined with an interstitial implant which is preferable to abdominoperineal resections. (2) *Anal Canal*. Small tumors may be treated by radium implant alone with proper fractionation and resultant preservation of sphincteric function. Advanced tumors, when not too infiltrating, are suitable for either a fractionated radium implant, combination of external and implant, or abdominoperineal resection. If extensive infiltration is present, abdominoperineal resection is recommended. External beam pre- or postoperative irradiation should also be considered in situations dependent on the operative and pathologic extent of disease.

External Beam Using Supervoltage

A number of recent papers report treatment plans utilizing carefully fractionated supervoltage external beam irradiation. Results suggest that such techniques, alone or in combination with operation or implant, can achieve good survival and local control with minimal morbidity.[30-32] Svenson and Montague reported a group of 23 patients with transitional cloacogenic carcinoma treated from 1958 to 1976 with abdominoperineal resection alone (15 patients), irradiation alone (two patients with small lesions) or abdominoperineal resection plus pre- or postoperative irradiation (six patients). Operation alone failed to control perineal and pelvic disease in one of six patients with negative nodes (tumor >2 cm diameter) and six of nine with positive nodes (66.7%). In the six patients with more advanced disease who received pre- or postoperative irradiation, no local failures have occurred and all six are alive and free of disease. Patients in the postoperative radiation therapy group received 5000 rad/5 weeks with 22 to 25 MeV photons to the pelvis and perineum followed by a boost to residual disease (upper dose not given).

Green and coworkers reported a group of 33 patients who received a major component of external beam irradiation for various histology carcinomas of the anus from 1966 to 1979. Surgical therapy was delayed until maximal effects of irradiation were completed. Twenty-one of 33 patients presented with lesions 5 cm or less in diameter; 19 were within the anal canal and two at the anal margin. The latter were treated with localized perineal fields and the rest with both pelvis and perineal fields. Seventeen of 21 were treated definitely with irradiation (4500–9000 rad). No local recurrences have occurred in the entire group of 12. One died free of disease at 4½ years and the remaining 11 are alive and well from 10 months to 9 years. Only one patient had required anal dilation for partial stenosis of the anal canal and no colostomies were required for treatment related causes.

Preoperative Radiation and Chemotherapy

Recently multimodality protocols for the treatment of squamous cell carcinoma in a research setting have been proposed.[33-36] In these studies, radiation therapy to 3000 rad plus 5-FU and mitomycin C chemotherapy are given prior to surgical intervention. Nigro reported experience with 19 patients:[36] twelve of the 19 went on to abdominoperineal resection; in eight no tumor could be found at the primary cancer site. Sischy, Remington and coworkers treated ten patients with anal carcinoma with similar chemotherapy but larger irradiation doses (4000 rad over 5 weeks to pelvis AP:PA plus 1000 rad concomitant perineal boost at 100 rad/day). Of the four undergoing abdominoperineal resection none had residual disease.[35] Six others with biopsy but no resection are also free of disease. Further follow-up and controlled trials of these studies are needed to confirm the seemingly favorable results. Long term undesirable side effects from radiation plus chemotherapy in the anorectal area must be carefully evaluated.

Adjuvant Radiation Therapy

For patients with infiltrative lesions of the anal margin or anal canal who are referred for pre- or postoperation irradiation, dose levels and techniques are essentially the same as for patients with cancer of the rectum referred after abdominoperineal resection utilizing 4500 to 5000 rad in 5 to 6 weeks with multiple field techniques to include the primary as well as internal iliac and pelvic mesenteric nodes. Disagreement exists as to whether clinically uninvolved inguinal nodes should be included within irradiation ports. Papillon and Green suggest that surgical or irradiation salvage of inguinal disease should it occur is so good that prophylactic treatment is not warranted.[29,32]

Primary Irradiation

In this situation irradiation doses are necessarily increased to 6000 to 7000 rad to areas of persistent tumor remaining after the initial pelvic field of 4500 to 5000 rad. It is perhaps unwise to give the lower external beam dose level of 3000 rad/3 weeks used by Papillon, as this would be inadequate in many patients for sterilization of microscopic nodal disease. A treatment break of 2 to 3 weeks will often be required before the boost can be given with implant or further external beam. If the lesion involves less than the full circumference of the anal region, one should attempt to spare a portion of the circumference above the dose level of 6000 rad to lessen the chance of long term stenosis although Green and coworkers saw no problems while including the entire circumference.[32]

For select early lesions that can be treated with implantation alone, (local excision usually an alternative) the techniques of Papillon are recommended.[29] In essence, this means use of fractionated implants instead of a single implant as used by Dalby and Pointon.[28]

REFERENCES

1. Stearns MW, Quan SHQ: Epidermoid carcinoma of the anorectum. Surg Gynecol Obstet 131:953–957, 1970
2. Wolfe HRI, Bussey HJR: Squamous cell carcinoma of the anus. Br J Surg 55:295–301, 1968
3. Brennan JT, Stewart CF: Epidermoid carcinoma of the anus. Ann Surg 176:787–790, 1972
4. Bretlau P: Carcinoma arising in anal fistula. Acta Chir Scand 133:496–500, 1967
5. McAnally AK, Dockerty MB: Carcinoma developing in chronic draining cutaneous sinuses and fistulas. Surg Gynecol Obstet 88:87–96, 1949
6. Comer TP, Beahrs OH, Dockerty MB: Primary squamous cell carcinoma and adenoacanthoma of the colon. Cancer 28:1111–1117, 1971
7. Morson BC: The pathology and results of treatment of squamous cell carcinoma of the anal canal and margin. Proc Roy Soc Med 53:414–420, 1960
8. Kuehn PG, Eisenberg H, Reed JF: Epidermoid carcinoma of the perianal skin and anal canal. Cancer 22:932–938, 1968
9. Welch JP, Malt RA: Appraisal of the treatment of carcinoma of the anus and anal canal. Surg Gynecol Obstet 145:837–841, 1977
10. Sawyers JL, Herrington JL, Beachley F: Surgical considerations in the treatment of epidermoid carcinoma of the anus. Ann Surg 157:817–824, 1963
11. Dillard BM, Spratt JS, Ackerman LV, Butcher HR: Epidermoid cancer of anal margin and canal. Arch Surg 86:100–105, 1963
12. Hardy KJ, Hughes ESR, Cuthbertson AM: Squamous cell carcinoma of the anal canal and anal margin. Aust N Z J Surg 38:301–305, 1969
13. MacLean MD, Murray FH, Bacon HE: Hepatic metastasis of squamous cell carcinoma of the anal canal: review of literature and case report. Dis Colon Rectum 4:51–55, 1961
14. Richards JC, Beahrs OH, Woolner LB: Squamous cell carcinoma of the anus, anal canal and rectum in 109 patients. Surg Gynecol Obstet 114:475–482, 1962
15. Sawyers JL: Squamous cell cancer of the perianus and anus. Surg Cl N Am 52:935–941, 1972
16. Grodsky L: Unsuspected anal cancer discovered after minor anorectal surgery. Dis Colon Rectum 10:471–478, 1967
17. Paradis P, Douglas HO, Holyoke ED: The clinical implications of a staging system for carcinoma of the anus. Surg Gynecol Obstet 141:411–416, 1975
18. Binkley GE: Epidermoid carcinoma of the anus and rectum. Am J Surg 79:90–95, 1950
19. Ruiz-Moreno F: Carcinoma in situ of the anal canal: report of a case. Dis Colon Rectum 6:218–221, 1963
20. Grinnell RS: Squamous cell carcinoma of the anus in Turrell: Diseases of Colon and Norectum, pp. 1019–1028. Philadelphia, Saunders, 1959
21. Sedgwick CE, Wainstein E: Epidermoid carcinoma of the anus and rectum. Surg Cl N Am 39:759–773, 1959
22. Brown DA, McKenzie AD: Squamous cell carcinoma of the anus. Can J Surg 6:45–50, 1963
23. Martin RG, Miller LS, Thorpe RG: Treatment for squamous cell carcinoma of the anus. In Cancer of the Gastrointestinal Tract, Chicago, Year Book Medical Publishers, 1967
24. Lone F, Berg JW, Stearns MW: Basaloid tumors of the anus. Cancer 13:907–911, 1960
25. Golden GT, Horsley JS: Surgical management of epidermoid carcinoma of the anus. Am J Surg 131:275–280, 1976
26. Eby LS, Sullivan ES: Current concepts of local excision of epidermoid carcinoma of the anus. Dis Colon Rectum 12:332–337, 1969
27. Moertel CG: The Anus Chapter XXIV-13 in Alimentary Tract Cancer. In Holland J, Frei E (eds): Cancer Medicine, pp 1627–1631. Philadelphia, Lea & Febiger, 1973
28. Dalby JE, Pointon JS: The treatment of anal carcinoma by interstial irradiation. Am J. Roentgen 85:515–520, 1961

29. Papillon J: Radiation therapy in the management of epidermoid carcinoma of the anal region. Dis Col Rect 17:181–187, 1974
30. Svenson EW, Montague ED: Results of treatment in cloacogenic carcinoma. Cancer 46:826–830, 1980
31. Ager P, Samala E, Bosworth J, Rubin M, Ghossein NA: The conservative management of anorectal cancer by radiotherapy. Am J Surg 137:228–230, 1979
32. Green JP, Schaupy WC, Cantril ST, Scholl G: Anal carcinoma: current therapeutic concepts. Am J Surg 140:151–155, 1980
33. Buroker TR, Nigro N, Bradley G, Pelok L, Chomchai C, Considine B, Vaitkevicius VK: Combined therapy for cancer of the anal canal: a follow-up report. Dis Colon Rectum 20:677–678, 1977
34. Newman HK, Quan SHQ: multi-modality therapy for epidermoid carcinoma of the anus. Cancer 37:12–19, 1976
35. Sischy B, Remington JH, Schel SH, Savlov ED: Treatment of carcinoma of the rectum and squamous carcinoma of the anus by combination chemotherapy, radiotherapy and geration. S G & O 151:369–371, 1980
36. Nigro N: Personal communication

SELECTED READING

1. Stearns MW, Urmacher C, Sternberg SS, Woodruff J, Attiyeh F: Cancer of the anal canal. Curr Probl in Cancer 4:4–44, 1980
2. Grodsky L: Rare nonkeratinizing malignancies of anal region. Arch Surg 90:216–221, 1965

David F. Paulson
Carlos A. Perez
Tom Anderson

CHAPTER 23

Genito-Urinary Malignancies

RENAL ADENOCARCINOMA

Renal cell carcinoma is the most common malignancy involving the kidney. It is most common in the fifth decade of life but can be observed in other age groups. The incidence is three times higher in males than in females.[1-3]

ETIOLOGY

There is considerable evidence that renal adenocarcinoma, both in animal and human systems, follows the principles of carcinogenesis previously discussed. Ionizing radiation can induce renal adenocarcinoma in animals and in humans. An increased incidence of renal neoplasia can be shown in mice treated with 690 rad of external radiation 3 hours after unilateral nephrectomy as compared with mice treated with external radiation alone or with nonirradiated but unilaterally nephrectomized animals.[4] Irradiation alone induces no kidney tumors and uninephrectomy without irradiation provokes no renal neoplasia. The appearance of renal neoplasia in these roentgen-irradiated mice is increased greatly as a consequence of unilateral nephrectomy, which produces a specific stimulus for cellular growth in the remaining kidney. The necessity for active cell metabolism and replication in the residual kidney at the time of the oncogenic stimulus is similar to the induction and promotion phenomenon of chemical carcinogenesis and reflects the sensitivity of the cell to oncogenic stimuli during periods of enhanced DNA synthesis. In humans, an increased incidence of renal adenocarcinoma has been shown in patients exposed to thorotrast, a 2.5% solution of thorium dioxide used in the 1920s as a constant medium for renal and liver visualization.[3,5,6,7,8] Thorium is a radioactive element with the nuclear disintegration manifesting itself in the form of ionizing radiation producing alpha rays, beta rays, and gamma rays; the increased tumor incidence is felt to be due to the chronic exposure to ionizing radiation.

Hormonal manipulation can be shown to produce renal adenocarcinoma in animals.[9] Implantation of pellets of diethylstilbestrol in hamsters will lead to the formation of estrogen-dependent renal adenocarcinomas histologically similar to the human malignancy. These tumors initially were shown to be hormonally dependent with cessation of growth after withdrawal of stilbestrol. They, however, would metastasize if hormonal treatment were continued. These tumors could be transplanted to other animals that were estrogen-treated and would lose their estrogen-dependence after several transplantations, with subsequent ability to grow in nontreated hamsters. The observations show that apparently nonendocrine tissues have latent endocrine properties that can be expressed during carcinogenesis, but these properties may be lost during the progression of the tumor as other control mechanisms are also discarded. These observations of Horning and Clayson are the basis for the treatment of human renal adenocarcinoma by hormonal manipulation.[9,10] Tobacco and tobacco products have been associated statistically with an increased incidence of renal adenocarcinoma. Epidemiologic studies have shown a definite relationship between renal adenocarcinoma and exposure to cigarette, pipe, or cigar smoking, or tobacco chewing.[11]

PATHOLOGY

Grawitz originally postulated that these tumors arose from adrenal rests due to their microscopic resemblance to adrenal tissues. This prompted him to establish the name hypernephroma, a term which has persisted until today.[12] It was later established that the tumors were of renal tubular origin.[12–17] Immunologic data supports this concept as it has been demonstrated that antibodies specific for the microvilli of the convoluted proximal tubular cells will cross-react with cells both of renal adenomas and carcinomas.[18] Renal adenomas are segregated from renal adenocarcinomas on the basis of size, those lesions being less than 2 centimeters being identified as adenomas, those lesions larger than 2 centimeters being termed carcinomas. Whether renal adenomas are small renal carcinomas with the potential for growth and metastasis is a subject of debate. Grossly, the renal cell carcinoma varies from yellow to gray-white on cut sections with multiple cystic and hemorrhagic areas. A false capsule can be identified between the renal parenchyma and tumor, but no true capsule exists. Three cell types can be identified in the malignancies: (a) *clear cell carcinoma*. This tumor is composed of large polyhedral cells with distinct margins and clear to lightly vasculated cytoplasm. The cytoplasm contains large amounts of triglycerides and phospholipids that are removed during histologic processing providing the "empty cell" appearance; (b) *granular cell carcinoma*. Granular cells are smaller in size and are round or cuboidal. With progressive anaplasia, these cells become more irregular in shape. They possess numerous mitochondria with a highly developed Golgi apparatus. (c) *sarcomatoid*. Sarcomatoid cells are spindle-shaped and resemble the fibrosarcoma. These cells often are arranged in papillary or tubular structures. Mitotic figures are rare. The stroma associated with these cellular patterns is richly vascularized and cholesterol deposits and inflammatory cells are seen frequently in areas of necrosis.

Kidney tumors often are given a pathologic grade of I, II, or III, based on the degree of cellular anaplasia with Grade I being least anaplastic and Grade III showing the greatest degree of anaplasia.

Metastatic Sites

Spread occurs both by direct extension and through lymphatic and hematogenous routes. The most common sites of metastases are lungs (55%), lymph nodes (34%), liver (33%), bone (32%), adrenal (19%), contralateral kidney (11%), brain (6%), heart (5%), spleen (5%), bowel (4%), and skin (3%).

SIGNS AND SYMPTOMS

The classic clinical presentation is one of pain, hematuria, and a flank mass. This complex, however, is the expression of advanced disease and usually reflects incurable disease. The disease may remain clinically silent during early stages and, in over 50% of patients, metastatic disease is present at the time of diagnosis.

Renal cell carcinoma may present with a wide variety of symptomatic patterns. (Table 23-1). A review of the survivorship patterns would indicate that only in two instances was either an adverse or a favorable prognosis associated with the clinical presentation. Irrespective of the clinical presentation, only 37% of all patients survived 5 years with the exception of patients who presented with symptoms referrable directly to metastatic disease at the time of diagnosis, in which case, only 3% of the patients survived 5 years. If the cancer was identified incidentally within the kidney at the time of screening for other disease, 65% of the patients survived five years. A symptom complex of reversible hepatosplenomegaly with hepatic dysfunction without evidence of liver metastases has been identified in some 10% of patients with renal cell carcinoma.[19–21]

TABLE 23-1. Presenting Symptoms, Laboratory Abnormality, or Abnormality on Physical Examination and Its Relation to Survival Rate in 309 Consecutive Patients Undergoing Nephrectomy for Renal Cell Carcinoma

PRESENTING SYMPTOM, ABNORMAL LABORATORY FINDING, OR ABNORMALITY ON PHYSICAL EXAM	NUMBER OF PATIENTS; AND PERCENT OF TOTAL (309)	NUMBER OF PATIENTS SURVIVING 5 YEARS
Classic triad (gross hematuria, abnormal mass, pain)	29 (9%)	9 (of 29) 31%
Hematuria	183 (59%)	74 (of 183) 40%
Pain	127 (41%)	56 (of 127) 44%
Abdominal mass	139 (45%)	49 (of 139) 35%
Fever	21 (7%)	8 (of 21) 38%
Weight loss	85 (28%)	29 (of 85) 39%
Anemia	64 (21%)	24 (of 64) 38%
Erythrocytosis	10 (3%)	4 (of 10) 40%
Hypercalcemia	11 (3%)	4 (of 11) 35%
Acute varicocele	7 (2%)	3 (of 7) 43%
Tumor calcification on x-ray film	39 (13%)	18 (of 39) 46%
Symptoms for metastases	31 (10%)	1 (of 31) 3%
Cancer, an incidental finding (silent)	20 (7%)	13 (of 20) 65%

(Modified from Skinner DG, Colvin RB, Vermillion CD et al: Diagnosis and management of renal cell carcinoma: A clinical and pathologic study of 309 cases. Cancer 28:1165–1177, 1971)

Liver functional parameters will improve with disappearance of hepatosplenomegaly following nephrectomy. A humeral factor has been implicated in initiation of this syndrome, although the specific etiology is unknown. Hypertension has been associated with renal cell carcinoma in 14 to 40% of all patients with neoplasm.[22-24] Elevated peripheral renin levels may be identified in these patients and these elevated levels are associated with high grade and high stage lesions.[9] No information exists as to whether the renin is produced by the tumor itself or is secondary to ischemia of adjacent renal parenchyma produced by the expanding renal mass lesion. It has been postulated that these elevated peripheral renin levels may be due to decreased rates of renin degradation peripherally, or to renin production by non-renin sources. Nephrectomy will result in lowering of elevated plasma renal levels.[23]

DIAGNOSIS OF RENAL MASS LESIONS

The evaluation of the asymptomatic or symptomatic mass related lesion of the renal parenchyma identified by intravenous pyelography should be conducted by a series of sequential steps. Sequential, orderly, and thoughtful approach to the diagnosis of the renal mass lesions will prevent superimposition of a large number of unneeded and unnecessary studies. Using a symptomatic approach to identification of renal mass lesions, 85% of renal mass lesions can be identified by combination of only two sequential examinations (Fig. 23-1).

Asymptomatic space-occupying lesions of the kidney often are best evaluated first by nephrotomography. Seventy percent of renal mass lesions identified by nephrotomography in the asymptomatic patient will be benign renal cysts, while only 5.5% will be malignant neoplasms (Table 23-2).[25] The most common asymptomatic renal neoplasm is the metastatic tumor with carcinoma of the breast being the most common.[26,27] Only 2% of asymptomatic space-occupying lesions of the kidney are renal cell carcinomas. Cystic, necrotic, and hypovascular tumors are more common in the asymptomatic patient than hypervascular tumors. Fifty percent to 65% of all renal cell carcinomas presenting as asymptomatic space occupying lesions are hypovascular.

Cysts will demonstrate a sharply defined interface against adjacent defined renal parenchyma. The lesions will be thin-walled in those areas of the mass lesion which project outside of the renal borders and may demonstrate a cortical spur. Ultrasonography will confirm the lesion as being cystic or solid. Cyst puncture and aspiration can establish the accuracy of diagnosis of benign renal cyst with accuracy close to 100%.[28-30]

Benign cysts contain fluid which is clear, lightly straw colored, and low in fat, protein, lactic acid dehydrogenase, and amylase content. In contrast, cystic tumors have a dark or cloudy cystic fluid, high in fat, protein, and lactic acid dehydrogenase.[31,32] If the urea nitrogen content of the cyst fluid is greater than 40 mg/100 ml, the cyst will have a tendency to reform. A cyst fluid pressure of less than 80 mm of water is an indicator that the cyst will probably regress following aspiration. However, if the opening pressure is greater than 160 mm of water, the cyst is likely to reform following aspiration. Inflammatory cysts have either clear or

FIG. 23-1. CPATC (computerized axial tomography). (Modified from Lang EK: Diagnosis of renal and parenchymal tumors. In Skinner DG, deKernion JB (eds): Genitourinary Cancer. Philadelphia, WB Saunders, 1978)

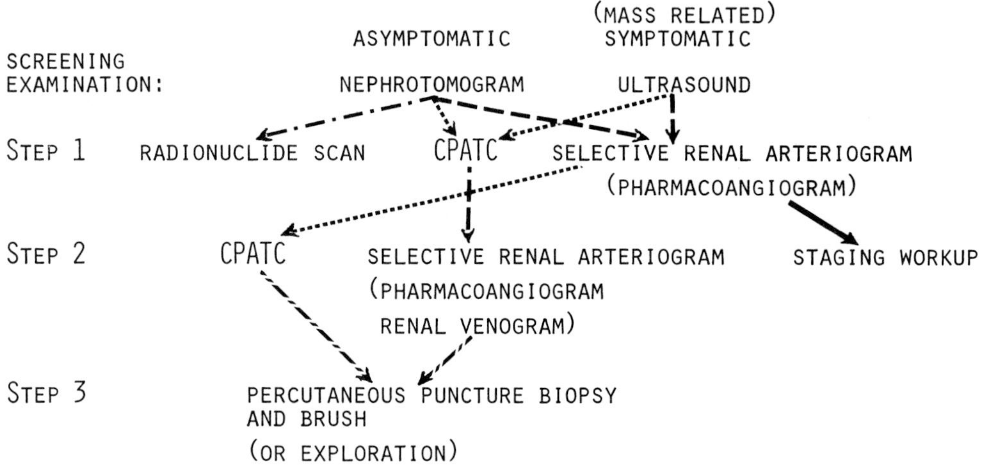

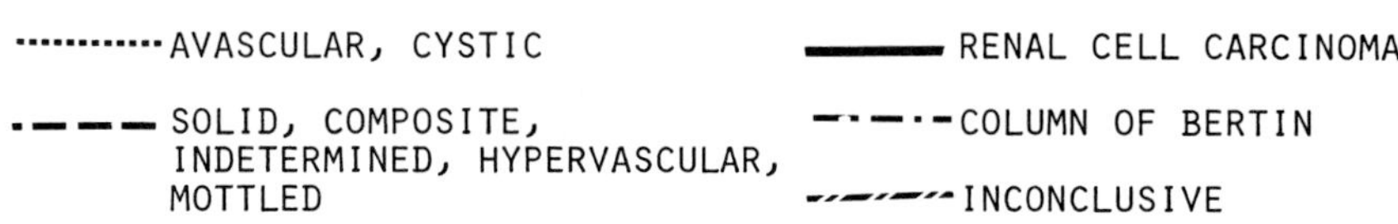

cloudy fluid with mild elevation of lactic acid dehydrogenase and amylase content. Benign hemorrhagic cysts contain a dark aspirate high in fat, protein, and lactic acid dehydrogenase content. Double contrast studies may be misleading, owing to the presence of fibrin or blood clots on the cyst wall.[33]

When the intravenous pyelogram demonstrates a hypervascular or a mottled appearance, or when the ultrasound study is indeterminate or represents a solid lesion, the patient should undergo arteriography. Approximately 85% of renal cell carcinomas are hypervascular by angiography. Hypervascular renal cell carcinomas classically demonstrate tumor neovascularity and arteriovenous shunts. Also, as the tumor vessels consist of a vascular epithelium without accompanying smooth muscle cells or elastic fibers, pseudo-aneurysms with extravasation of contrast material are common. The lack of smooth muscle accounts also for the failure of vasoactive agents to alter flow in the tumor vessels.[34-36]

Renal cell adenocarcinomas can be hypovascular, with the overall incidence of hypovascular tumors ranging from 10% to 26%. The papillary tubular adenocarcinoma comprises about 5% of all renal adenocarcinomas and classically is hypovascular.[37] The remaining hypovascular renal cell carcinomas are clear cell or granular cell adenocarcinomas, usually with extensive areas of necrosis.[38]

The biologic hazard of the avascular papillary tubular adenocarcinoma is less than that of hypervascular renal adenocarcinomas. The less aggressive tendency of this hypovascular tumor is evident in that only 18% of papillary tubular renal cell carcinomas show capsular invasion, in contrast to 50% of the non-papillary tumors.[39]

TABLE 23-2. Underlying Pathologic Conditions in 940 Asymptomatic Space-Occupying Lesions of the Kidney

TYPE OF LESION		PERCENT OF TOTAL NUMBER OF LESIONS
Cystic Lesions		58
Benign cysts	515	
Benign hemorrhagic cysts	4	
Hydronephrosis	8	
Cystic dysplastic kidney	3	
Polycystic kidney	17	
Malignant neoplasms		5.5
Hypernephromas	21	
Other malignant neoplasms	31	
Benign neoplasms	40	4.2
Inflammatory lesions (pyelonephritis, abscess)	213	23
Intrarenal hematoma	7	0.7
Pseudotumors	81	8.6

(Modified from Lang EK: Diagnosis of renal and parenchymal tumors. In Skinner DG, deKernion JB (eds): Genitourinary Cancer, p 42. Philadelphia, WB Saunders, 1978)

FIG. 23-2. Staging system for renal adenocarcinoma. (Modified from Skinner DG, Vermillion CD, Colvin RB: The surgical management of renal cell carcinoma. J Urol 107:705–716, 1972)

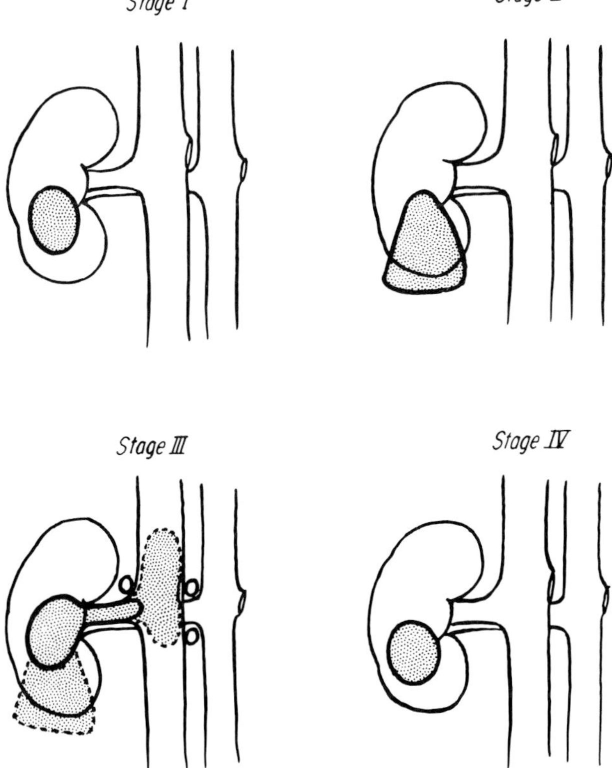

STAGING OF RENAL ADENOCARCINOMA

The accepted clinical staging of renal adenocarcinoma is as given in Fig. 23-2 and Table 23-3. The TMN classification, however, provides an accurate method of disease assessment (Table 23-4). This staging system should be modified by consideration of information identified by Skinner, Osner, and Mittleton.[40-43] Renal vein involvement or vena cava extension when there is no involvement of the perinephric fat or regional lymph nodes does not alter prognosis when compared with tumors confined to the kidney.

SURGICAL TREATMENT

Surgical therapy is directed towards removal of the kidney and the associated tumor, the adrenal gland, the surrounding perinephric fat and Gerota's fascia, along with the regional lymph nodes.

Surgical dissection can be established through one of several incisions: either through transabdominal, modified

TABLE 23-3. Staging System of Renal Adenocarcinoma

- Stage I. Tumor confined to the kidney
- Stage II. Tumor locally invasive but confined to Gerota's fascia.
- Stage III. Regional invasion.
  - A. Invasion of renal vein or vena cava or both
  - B. Metastases to regional lymph nodes.
  - C. Combination of A and B.
- Stage IV.
  - A. Invasion of surrounding organs (other than adrenal glands).
  - B. Distant metastases.

(Robson CJ, Churchill BM, Anderson W: The results of radical nephrectomy for renal cell carcinoma. J Urol 101:297–301, 1969)

TABLE 23-4. TNM Classification—Kidney

Primary Tumor (T)

TX	Minimum requirements cannot be met
T0	No evidence of primary tumor
T1	Small tumor, minimal renal and calyceal distortion or deformity. Circumscribed neovasculature surrounded by normal parenchyma
T2	Large tumor with deformity and/or enlargement of kidney and/or collecting system
T3a	Tumor involving perinephric tissues
T3b	Tumor involving renal vein
T3c	Tumor involving renal vein and infradiaphragmatic vena cava

Note: Under T3, tumor may extend into perinephric tissues, into renal vein, and into vena cava as shown on cavography. In these instances, the T classification may be shown as T3a, b, and c, or some appropriate combination, depending on extension—for example, T3a,b is tumor in perinephric fat and extending into renal vein.

T4a	Tumor invasion of neighboring structures (e.g., muscle, bowel)
T4b	Tumor involving supradiaphragmatic vena cava

Nodal Involvement (N)

The regional lymph nodes are the para-aortic and paracaval nodes. The juxtaregional lymph nodes are the pelvic nodes and the mediastinal nodes.

NX	Minimum requirements cannot be met
N0	No evidence of involvement of regional nodes
N1	Single, homolateral regional nodal involvement
N2	Involvement of multiple regional or contralateral or bilateral nodes
N3	Fixed regional nodes (assessable only at surgical exploration)
N4	Involvement of juxtaregional nodes

Note: If lymphography is source of staging, add "1" between "N" and designator number; if histologic proof is provided "+" if positive, and "−" if negative. Thus, $N1^{+}$ indicates multiple positive nodes seen on lymphography and proved at operation by biopsy.

Distant Metastasis (M)

MX	Not assessed
M0	No (known) distant metastasis
M1	Distant metastasis present Specify Specify sites according to the following notations:

Pulmonary—PUL	Bone Marrow—MAR
Osseous—OSS	Pleura—PLE
Hepatic—HEP	Skin—SKI
Brain—BRA	Eye—EYE
Lymph Nodes—LYM	Other—OTH

Note: Add "+" to the abbreviated notation to indicate that the pathology (p) is proved.

flank, full flank, or thoracoabdominal routes. Irrespective of the incision made to gain access to the tumor, once the incision has been made, immediate access to the vascular supply of the tumor and kidney should be established. This may be achieved either by incising the posterior peritoneum and Gerota's fascia over the vessels at the site of origin of the aorta and vena cava, or by establishing a plane of dissection between the peritoneal envelope anteriorly and Gerota's fascia posteriorly, and continuing this dissection medially until the vessels are identified at their site of origin. Early vascular control should be sought in order to reduce the possibility of tumor dissemination with the dissection, and to permit mobilization of the tumor mass with minimal blood loss. It is not uncommon to encounter large renal tumors with minimal lymphatic involvement around the vasculature, permitting uncomplicated and early vascular control. After the vasculature has been controlled, the renal tumor with its encompassing fat should be removed without transgressing Gerota's fascia. The fascial envelope can be separated both from the posterior body wall with blunt dissection and from the anteriorly placed peritoneal envelope with blunt dissection. The superior aspect of Gerota's fascia will be sharply divided from the inferior aspect of the diaphragm. Once this has been accomplished, the fascial envelope containing the renal tumor can be lifted from the operative bed and dissection proceed distally (Fig. 23-3). The ureter will be encountered distally and should be divided. Right-sided renal tumors may require mobilization of the second portion of the duodenum to expose the vena cava and the origin of the renal vein.

In securing the vascular origins, every effort should be made to interrupt the arterial supply prior to occlusion of the vein. The exact location of the artery or the presence of multiple renal arteries can be established by preoperative angiography. The vasculature should be controlled by suture ligation with nonabsorbable suture where appropriate. Simultaneous mass ligature of the artery and vein within the vascular pedical should be avoided, but may be necessary owing to unavoidable intraoperative conditions.

The incidence of right-sided caval extension is significant. Accordingly, when preoperative studies indicate extension of the tumor thrombus into the renal vein or vena cava, the vena cava should be mobilized above and below the entrance of the renal vein. The cava can be controlled by these tapes and a cavotomy established for adequate tumor removal. Margins of the incision should be monitored by frozen section to insure that infiltration of the vessel wall has not occurred at the level of transection. After the vascular pedicle is controlled, there is usually minimal bleeding from the extensive vascular plexus which converges over the surface of the tumor. The relative benefits of regional lymph node dissection for this tumor have not been established. Nodal spread has been established in approximately 22% of patients.[44,45] It has been recommended that node dissection be conducted from the diaphragm to the bifurcation of the aorta.[45,46] The dissection may be accomplished in continuity with the nephrectomy or established after the nephrectomy has been accomplished. The dissection should include, at a minimum, a distance of 4 cm to 6 cm above and below the renal vessels and should include the nodes behind the vessels and the inter-aortico–caval nodes. Several factors mitigate against a therapeutic value of lymphadenectomy: the profuse lymphatic drainage from renal carcinoma, the difficulty in removing all involved nodes, the frequency with which regional nodes are bypassed with drainage directly to the cisterna chyli, and the frequency with which blood-borne metastases accompany lymphatic metastases. While an occasional patient with a single involved node near the hilum may be cured by lymphadenectomy, the therapeutic value of extensive lymph node dissection is questionable and may increase morbidity.

Radical nephrectomy with or without node dissection provides an enhanced cure over that established by simple nephrectomy (Table 23-5).[40,47] There is no hard data to indicate that lymphadenectomy in the presence of positive lymph nodes provides an enhancement of cure. Patients with only regional lymph node involvement may experience a 33% 5-year survival with only 17% surviving 10 years (Table 23-6).

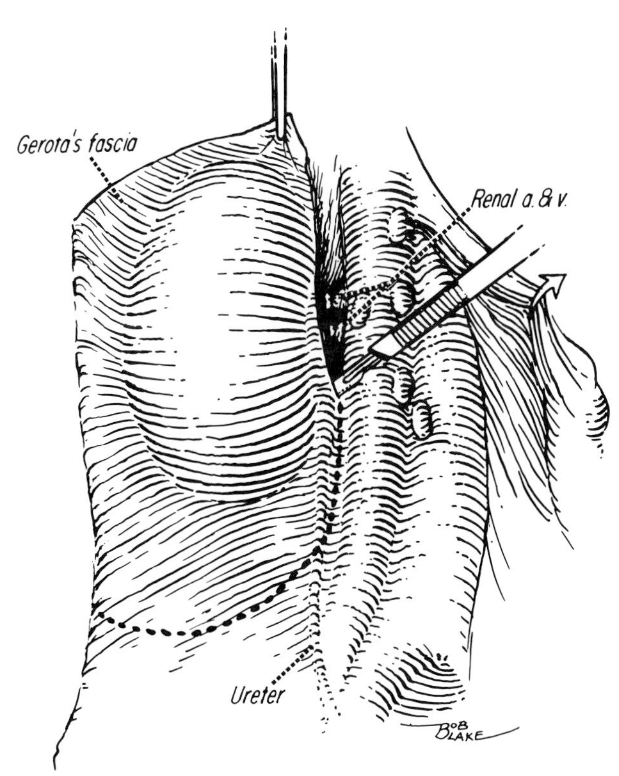

FIG. 23-3. Radical nephrectomy. Kidney is removed within its investing fascia.

TABLE 23-5. Survival Relating to Grade and Therapy

	GRADE I	GRADE II	GRADE III
Incidence of lymph node involvement	12%	28%	34%
5-year survival following simple nephrectomy	77%	31%	8%
5-year survival following radical nephrectomy	87%	64%	40%

(Modified from Robson CJ, Churchill BM, Anderson W: The results of radical nephrectomy for renal cell carcinoma. Trans Am Assoc Genitourin Surg 60:122, 1968 and from Skinner DG, Colvin RB, Vermillion CD et al: Diagnosis and management of renal cell carcinoma: A clinical and pathologic study of 309 cases. Cancer 28:1165–1177, 1971)

TABLE 23-6. Survival Rate According to Specific Extent of Histologic Involvement by Tumor

		SURVIVAL RATE	
PATHOLOGIC INVOLVEMENT	HISTOLOGIC EXTENT	5 YEARS (PERCENT)	10 YEARS (PERCENT)
Stage I—kidney only	Confined	65	56
Renal vein	Alone	66	49
	+ Vena cava	55	43
	+ Perinephric fat	50	33
	+ Regional nodes	0	0
Perinephric fat	Alone	47	20
Regional nodes	Alone	33	17
Direct extension to contiguous visceral structure		0	0

(Modified from Skinner DG, Pfister FG, Colvin R: Extension of renal cell carcinoma into the vena cava: The rationale for aggressive surgical managment. J Urol 107:711, 1972)

Whether these survivorship figures reflect the impact of regional lymphadenectomy or the biology of the tumor alone remains speculative. The decrease in survival rate between 5 and 10 years would indicate that there is lack of tumor control established in at least half of those 5-year survivors by lymphadenectomy and that half of these 5-year survivors survive with tumor. Despite the enhanced operative mortality of radical nephrectomy (3.8%) over that of simple nephrectomy (1.4%) the more extensive procedure obviously provides enhanced survivorship in patients without nodes. This probably reflects the enhanced salvage established in patients who have involvement through the renal capsule or in the pararenal tissues.

NEPHRECTOMY WITH METASTATIC DISEASE

The role of nephrectomy in metastatic renal carcinoma is controversial. It has been argued that nephrectomy in the face of metastatic disease will provide control of symptoms referrable to the local lesion as pain, fever, hematuria, hepatomegaly, anemia, or hypercalcemia, that it will reduce the likelihood of further dissemination of the disease, that it may prolong life without spontaneous progression of metastases, that it will enhance the hormonal or drug response of residual disease, and that that it will reduce the psychological impact of disease on the patient by removal of the primary tumor. No difference in the quality of life has been established between nephrectomy and non-nephrectomy patients with metastatic disease. The systemic symptoms which may accompany renal cell carcinomas may be perpetuated by the metastatic disease and not the renal primary. Much palliation can be established by pharmaceutical means or by less extensive intervention. No data exist to establish that response to hormonal therapy or chemotherapy is enhanced by prior nephrectomy. Similarly, there is no evidence to establish that nephrectomy without therapy enhances survivorship. Middleton, in reporting on 141 patients with multiple metastases had no survivors beyond 2 years despite nephrectomy having been established in 33 patients.[48] Johnson and coworkers reported a survivorship of 11.3 months in 43 patients undergoing nephrectomy prior to initiation of hormonal therapy or chemotherapy with a survivorship of 7.9 months in 50 patients who received similar therapy without nephrectomy.[49]

Survival time is not altered by the site of metastatic disease but it may be influenced by the number of metastatic sites and the time of appearance of the metastatic lesion.[50-52] Conflicting reports have appeared regarding the enhanced survival seen with bony metastases as opposed to parenchymal disease. Initial reporting indicated that approximately 35% of patients with only osseous metastases could be expected to survive longer than 12 months as opposed to only 18% of those with parenchymal disease.[50,51] However, it would appear that patients with osseous metastases do not define a select group who have the potential for prolonged survival owing to slower progression of disease within the bone, as others have reported that the survivorship for patients with parenchymal disease approximates that for patients with only bony disease.[52] The number of metastases and not the site of metastatic disease may impact significantly on survivorship.[53,54]

Pursing radical nephrectomy in hopes of establishing spontaneous regression of metastatic disease seems inappropriate. Fifty-one cases of spontaneous regression have been recorded to occur after nephrectomy for the primary disease. The incidence of spontaneous regression has been established at 0.8%; with the operative mortality after nephrectomy in patients with metastatic disease between 2.3% and 10%.[50,51,53] There therefore seems little justification in conducting nephrectomy in hopes of producing spontaneous regression.

Bilateral Renal Adenocarcinomas or Tumors in Solitary Renal Units

Approximately 100 cases of renal cell cancer have been reported in a solitary kidney.[55-57] Accumulated data would indicate that survivorship is dependent on the condition of the contralateral kidney. If the contralateral kidney had been removed for carcinoma, the appearance of disease in the residual kidney is felt to reflect the appearance of metastatic disease as the 5-year survivorship is 37%, with the mean survival being 26 months. These survival times are similar to those seen in patients with isolated metastatic lesions at other parenchymal sites. The length of survivorship is directly related to the interval between the original nephrectomy for malignant disease and its appearance in the residual kidney. When the opposite kidney was agenetic or removed for other than malignant disease the 5-year survival rate following partial nephrectomy approximates that seen in patients with malignancy in one of two kidneys when compared by staging. Stage I renal cell carcinomas treated by partial nephrectomy in patients having the opposite kidney removed for benign disease will have 65% to 70% five year survival rate.

Twenty-five cases of simultaneously appearing bilateral renal cell carcinoma have been reported, with 72% of the patients dead within 6 months and only five remaining alive for 21 months.[53-57] All of these patients were treated by unilateral nephrectomy, contralateral partial nephrectomy. The survival data are similar to that seen in patients with renal cell carcinoma in a single kidney and who have a simultaneously identified distant metastatic site. It is felt, therefore, that the simultaneously appearing bilateral renal adenocarcinoma represents the appearance of a primary lesion with a metastatic contralateral implant.

Nephrectomy and Resection of Metastasis

Although much enthusiasm exists to support the aggressive management of patients with identified metastatic disease at the time of presentation, no hard data exist to support the pursuit of such an aggressive surgical approach (Table 23-7). It has been argued that patients with an apparent solitary metastasis would benefit from simultaneous removal of the metastatic site at the time of radical nephrectomy. One percent to 39% of patients will present with an isolated metastatic site. Thirty-three percent of the patients who have undergone simultaneous removal of one or two metastatic foci excluding bone at the time of radical nephrectomy can be anticipated to survive 5 years.[53] This 33% 5-year survival rate is similar to that seen in patients who have regional nodal disease only. Until it can be demonstrated that the survivorship

TABLE 23-7. Results of Excision of Metastatic Lesions of Renal Cell Carcinoma According to Location of Metastasis

METASTATIC SITE	NUMBER OF PATIENTS TREATED	NUMBER OF RESECTIONS	DEAD WITHIN 2 YEARS	DEAD WITHIN 2–5 YEARS	NUMBER OF PATIENTS AND PERCENT ALIVE AFTER 5 YEARS	DEAD AFTER 5 YEARS OF METASTATIC RENAL CELL CARCINOMA
Lung	17	19	8	4	5 (29%)	1
Lung plus other site	4	8	1	0	3 (75%)	2
Opposite kidney	6	6	5	1	0 (0%)	0
Brain	1	1	0	0	1 (100%)	0
Retroperitoneum (renal fossa)	6	6	2	1	3 (50%)	0
Bone	6	6	5	0	1 (17%)	1
TOTAL	40	46	21	6	13 (13%)	4

(Modified from Skinner DG: In Brenner BB, Rector F (eds): The Kidney. Philadelphia, WB Saunders, 1976)

represents other than the natural history of the disease it seems unreasonable to proceed with attempted surgical control. Patients who have excision of a solitary metastasis at an interval after nephrectomy survive longer than those who have a metastatic site removed at the time of initial surgery.

Surgery does appear indicated in patients with isolated pulmonary lesions that stabilize or undergo only partial regression with chemotherapy.[58]

Renal Adenocarcinoma and Renal Transplantation

Seventy-three patients have been reported to have undergone renal transplantation after nephrectomy for a primary renal neoplasm. These patients can be divided into three distinct groups. Thirty-four patients (Group One) underwent antineoplastic therapy for one year or less prior to transplantation. Fifty-three percent of these 34 patients developed metastases or local recurrences. Fifteen patients (Group Two) had a waiting period of at least fifteen months between nephrectomy and transplantation. None of these patients developed malignant disease, emphasizing the value of a lengthy waiting period between treatment of the neoplasm and the performance of the transplantation with associated immunosuppressive therapy. Twenty-four patients (Group Three) had incidentally discovered renal malignancies during the workup of chronic renal failure or after bilateral nephrectomy in preparation of renal transplantation. None of these 24 patients developed recurrence or metastases.[59] This data would indicate that nephrectomy and delayed transplantation are reasonable in patients who have a first and primary renal adenocarcinoma in a single kidney.

Transcatheter Arterial Occlusion

Renal artery embolization in patients with renal cell carcinoma may be indicated preoperatively to decrease blood loss in hypervascular lesions with extensive collateral vascularization, to reduce bleeding and control pain in patients with inoperable tumors, and to reduce tumor bulk in patients who are receiving chemotherapy.[60–63]

Many substances have been employed to produce venous occlusion, including autogenous clot and tissue, clot modified with thrombin, Gelfoam, cell, silastic spheres, silicone rubber, cyanoacrylates, balloon catheters, and stainless steel coils. Autogenous clot may produce obstruction for hours to days until the clot is lysed or recannulated. Gelfoam establishes a framework for future thrombus formation with the occlusion lasting for weeks to months. However, autogenous clot or Gelfoam produces only a temporary occlusion and should be used only for short term preoperative management. However, a more permanent solution can be established with the stainless steel coil or the removable balloon. Intra-arterial occlusion is not without complications. Flank pain will occur with occlusion, last 24 hours to 48 hours and may require narcotics for control. Fever of up to 40°C can occur without infection being present. The fever usually appears within 12 hours to 18 hours and may last three to five days. Symptomatic management of anorexia, nausea, and vomiting occurring within 24 hours after occlusion and lasting 3 days to 5 days may be necessary. Paralytic ileus may occur. Hypertension may occur immediately with embolization and last several hours following embolization. Renal abscess is rare, occurring in less than 2% of patients. Gas formation in the infarcted tissues has been observed after renal embolization with no clinical evidence of abscess. The appearance of gas in the infarcted kidney is part of the post-infraction syndrome and is analogous to the appearance of gas in fetal tissues after intra-uterine death.[64,65]

ROLE OF RADIATION THERAPY

As stated previously, the management of renal cell carcinoma is primarily surgical. Radiation therapy has been used pre- or postoperatively in combination with a nephrectomy. A number of reports have been published in the past suggesting that the addition of irradiation to a nephrectomy may improve survival and local tumor control (Table 23-8).[53,66] Radiation therapy alone has been used in unresectable tumors or in patients with widespread metastatic disease for relief of pain, to decrease the size of renal masses or to stop bleeding. In 1935, Walters reported that renal cell carcinoma was responsive to irradiation and that even inoperable lesions could be rendered operable. Doses ranging from 1600 rad to 3500 rad were delivered with 200 KV roentgen rays. Riches advocated preoperative irradiation after demonstrating in a small group of patients that survival was higher and local recurrences

TABLE 23-8. Summary of the Published Results of Treatment of Renal Cell Carcinoma

SERIES	NO. CASES	5-YEAR SURVIVAL						10-YEAR SURVIVAL					
		NEPHRECTOMY ALONE		NEPHRECTOMY PLUS IRRADIATION		OVERALL		NEPHRECTOMY ALONE		NEPHRECTOMY PLUS IRRADIATION		OVERALL	
Flocks and Kadesky 1926–1950	96	27/56	48%	21/40	52%	48/96	50%	9/39	23%	9/27	33%	18/66	27%
Riches et al. 1935–1950	398	105/345	30%	26/53	59%	131/398	33%	30/177	17%	4/15	27%	34/192	17%
Peeling 1940–1965	164	50/96	52%	17/68	25%	67/164	40%						
Hand and Broders 1901–1923	193	44/193		0		44/193	23%						
Foot et al 1926–1949	104	33/81	40%	0		33/81	40%	9/40	22%			9/40	22%
Myers 1940–1955	479	259/479	54%	0		259/479	54%	183/479	38%			183/479	38%
Middleton 1932–1965	334			25% received radiation		112/320	35%			25% received radiation		19/108	18%
Kaufman and Mims 1966	79	37/79	47%	0		37/79	47%	27/79	34%	0		27/79	34%
Robson et al 1949–1964	70	40/70	57%	0		40/70	57%	18/34	53%	0		18/34	53%
Skinner et al 1935–1965	232	109/190	57%	9/18	50%	118/208	57%	61/139	44%	0		61/139	44%

(Modified from Skinner DG, Colvin RB, Vermillion CD et al: Diagnosis and managment of renal cell carcinoma: A clinical and pathologic study of 309 cases. Cancer 28:1165–1177, 1971)

decreased after administration of a dose of 3000 rad followed by a nephrectomy in 3 weeks.[68] However, van der Werf-Messing observed no improvement in 5-year survival with preoperative irradiation, even though this may be of value in reducing the probability of local recurrence.[40] Rost and Brosig advocated preoperative radiation to facilitate and reduce the scope of a radical nephrectomy.[70]

Postoperative irradiation has been used by some, particularly when there is tumor extension into the renal capsule, pelvis, or vein. Rafla, in a nonrandomized study of 244 patients, noted that the administration of 3000 rad to 4000 rad in 3 weeks to 4 weeks after nephrectomy resulted in an overall 5-year survival rate of 56% in 81 patients at risk in comparison to those with surgery alone (37% in 94 patients at risk).[71] The 10-year tumor-free survival was 34% and 19% respectively. In patients with involvement of the renal capsule the 5-year survival rate was 57% in the irradiated group and 28% in those treated with surgery alone. When involvement of the renal pelvis and capsular tissues was present, the tumor-free 5-year survival was 85% in the postoperative radiation group and 33% in the surgery alone group. Patients with renal vein invasion showed less benefit from postoperative radiation, with a 40% 5-year survival rate in comparison to 30% for those treated with surgery alone. In contrast, a randomized clinical trial reported by Finney utilizing postoperative radiation (dose not stated) quoted a 5-year survival rate of 36% in 51 patients receiving postoperative radiotherapy in comparison to 44% in 49 patients treated with nephrectomy alone.[72] The incidence of distant metastasis was the same (approximately 30%) in both groups. In the radiotherapy group there were eight local recurrences with nine local recurrences in the surgical group. No significant improvement was noted in the irradiated group when there was involvement of the renal capsule or renal vein. It is interesting that four of the irradiated patients died within 5 months of completion of therapy, probably because of liver failure, secondary to inclusion of large volumes of the liver in the irradiated portals. In summary, there are conflicting reports on the value of pre- or postoperative radiation in the management of resectable renal cell carcinoma.

Radiation threapy alone has been reported to yield a 6% 5-year survival rate in 83 inoperable patients, in contrast to 9.5% survival rate in 362 inoperable patients who received no treatment.[73] Irradiation can be used for palliation to decrease pain, size of large masses, or hematuria from a renal cell carcinoma. Doses in the range of 4500 rad to 5000 rad delivered in about 5 weeks will yield more satisfactory results, although doses in the range of 3000 rad in 2 weeks for patients in poor general condition may provide short relief of symptoms.

Metastatic tumors from other primary sites, such as lung, breast, stomach, and contralateral kidney may produce renal metastasis. Radiotherapy may relieve significantly the local symptoms in these patients.[74] Doses in the range of 4000 rad to 5000 rad are recommended, depending on the general condition of the patient.

Malignant lymphomas also can be treated with irradiation of the renal bed and the regional lymph nodes. Doses in the range of 4000 rad in 4 weeks to 5 weeks are recommended, although it must be realized that this dose will cause irreversible severe radiation nephritis.

CHEMOTHERAPY OF HYPERNEPHROMA

In contrast to the demonstrable antitumor activity of a variety of agents in Wilms' tumor, no clearly effective chemotherapeutic regimen has yet been demonstrated for hypernephromas. There has been an obvious lack of careful systematic clinical trials in this relatively unusual tumor. Attempts to analyze a particular drug's efficacy require compilation of multiple reports on small series of patients, which tend to have variations in patient selection, drug dose and schedule, definitions of response, and so forth. As recently as 1975, a review of data in the literature, together with information filed with Clinical Trials Evaluation Program at the NCI, stated that only seven chemotherapeutic agents had been felt to have an adequate trial.[75] The classic alkylating agents such as cyclophosphamide, chlorambucil, and phenylalanine mustard all appeared to either lack activity or had not yet been adequately tested in spite of their availability for almost 2 decades. Similarly, antimetabolites such as 5-fluorouracil, the anthracycline cycline derivative adriamycin, antibiotics such as bleomycin, and 5-(3,3-dimethyl-1-triazino)-imidazole-4-carboxamide (DTIC) all lack significant antitumor activity when used as a single agent.[75-80] These include hydroxyurea, vinblastine, and cyclohexylchloroethylnitorourea (CCNU); however, the data demonstrating antitumor efficacy of these compounds are scanty and not convincing. Given the difficulty in objectively verifying tumor response, and the short-lived nature of the responses reported, one must conclude that there is no proven effective single agent chemotherapy for hypernephroma; the only possible exception is the potential efficacy of vinblastine.[79,80]

These observations have prompted a number of investigators to develop combination chemotherapy regimens in an attempt to augment the meager responses noted with single agent therapy. These combinations have included hydroxyurea plus vincristine, CCNU plus bleomycin, and CCNU plus vinblastine.[78,81-83] Not surprisingly, little if any augmented response has been noted. Only in a single small series of patients treated with CCNU plus vinblastine has any meaningful data been produced. While not obtaining a higher response rate (7 of 29 patients = 24%), two patients had a complete response and five patients had partial responses lasting from 2 months to 9 months.[83] This response rate was lower than a preliminary report that four of six patients had responded to this regimen.[82] The toxicity was moderate, using doses of vinblastine 0.1 mg/kg on days one and eight, together with CCNU at a dose of 120 mg/m^2 on day one of each 6 week to 8 week treatment cycle.

Paulson and co-workers, evaluating the impact of the combination adriamycin and cytoxan on metastatic renal adenocarcinoma were able to identify characteristics which predicted for response to therapy.[84] Prognostic factor analysis yielded four characteristics with a significant bearing on survival—sex, initial alkaline phosphatase, initial hematocrit, and site of metastasis. The 20 men in the study had a median survival of 7.1 months compared to that of only 2.5 months for women (Fig. 23-4, p = 0.001). Elevated alkaline phosphatase predicted a poor survival, with a median survival of 2.9 months for those patients with values above 200 I.U. at study entry versus 6.9 months for those with values below 200 I.U. (Fig. 23-5, p = 0.01). Elevation of alkaline phosphatase was not correlated significantly with presence of either liver or bone metastases. Patients who were anemic (hematocrit less than 36) at study entry had a median survival of 2.9 months, whereas that of patients with normal hematocrits was 7.1 months (p = 0.003). The only site of metastasis portending a particularly poor survival was bone. The relationship of bone metastasis to survival was apparent only after adjustment for the other prognostic factors by multivariable analysis.

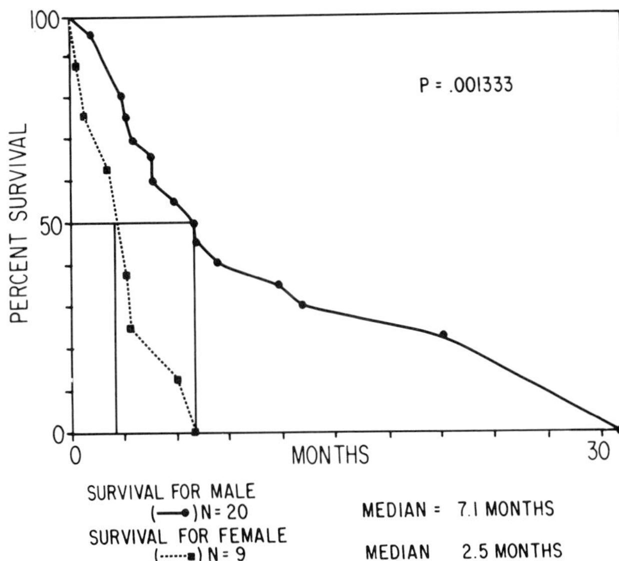

FIG. 23-4. Survival by sex for patients with metastatic renal adenocarcinoma receiving chemotherapy.

HORMONAL MANIPULATION

This tumor has proven to be one of the least responsive tumors to systemic therapy. Hormonal manipulation previously had been one of the main stages in therapy in advanced disease, as these treatments carry little serious toxicity and as reported response rates were inaccurately high. The early

FIG. 23-5. Survival by alkaline phosphatase levels for patients with renal adenocarcinoma receiving chemotherapy.

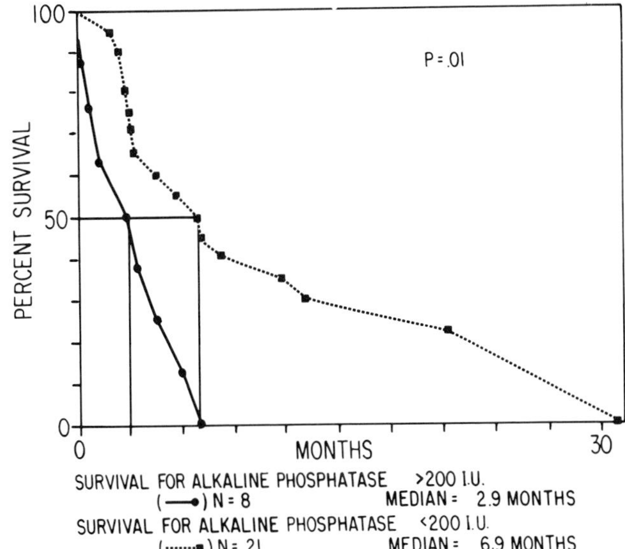

enthusiasm for androgenic and progestational therapy was generated by reports which seldom clearly separated response criteria in subjective categories. In addition, the objective response criteria were poorly defined. Later studies, which have used standardly acceptable response criteria, have identified response rates to hormonal therapy which range from 0.09% to 6.09%. A 1976 study by the Eastern Cooperative Oncology Group treated patients with either chemotherapy or chemotherapy plus Depo-Provera and showed no additional benefit among any of the 166 patients who received hormone.[85,86,87]

CARCINOMA OF THE RENAL PELVIS

Carcinoma of the renal pelvis constitutes 5% of all renal tumors. The peak incidence is in the fifth and sixth decade of life with a progressive increase in incidence with advancing age. Incidence in males predominates two to one.

ETIOLOGY

Transitional epithelium lining the calyceal system and renal pelvis are subject to the potential carcinogenic influences of environmental carcinogens discussed in the section on transitional cell carcinoma of the bladder. There are, however, two specific instances in which chemical carcinogens may play a role in the generation of carcinoma of the renal pelvis above and beyond that of the bladder. The first is an enhanced incidence of renal pelvic malignancy in patients with a longstanding history of phenacetin ingestion, there is an enhanced incidence of papillary necrosis, and transitional cell carcinoma is undetermined. There is a strong relationship between the metabolites of phenacetin and those compounds which produce malignant transitional cell carcinoma of the bladder. N-hydroxylate metabolites are increased in the urine in patients ingesting phenacetin. The primary metabolite is 4-acetoaminophenol, a compound structurally similar to the known urothelial carcinogens.[88]

An association has been established also between carcinoma of the renal pelvis and Danubian endemic familial nephropathy (Balkan nephropathy). The etiology of Balkan nephropathy and the reason for the enhanced incidence of renal pelvic tumor in this patient population is unknown, although exogenous environmental factors are felt to be causative,[89,90] There is no evidence that viruses play a role in the initiation of transitional cell carcinoma of the human renal pelvis.[91]

PATHOLOGY

No specific premalignant lesions have been identified. Transitional cell carcinoma of the renal pelvis may undergo squamous or a glandular metaplasia response to chronic urethelial inflammation. There is no known relationship between the various forms of metaplasia and malignancy, although malignancy is frequently associated with these abnormalities. Squamous metaplasia frequently is associated with calculus disease. It is characterized by large clear polygonal cells with dark pyknotic nuclei. Glandular metaplasia may occur simultaneously with squamous metaplasia or may appear as an isolated phenomenon. The histology will demonstrate hyperplastic islets of cells appearing to invade the lamina propria. Nests of epithelial cells may lose their contact with surface epithelia and, with mucus secretion, form cysts. When this occurs, these types of changes give rise to pyelitis or ureteritis cystica.

Malignant lesions of the renal pelvis can be segregated into transitional cell carcinomas, squamous cell carcinomas, adenocarcinomas, and connective tissue tumors. Approximately 90% of all cancers of the renal pelvis are transitional cell tumors. The distinction between papillary transitional cell carcinomas and transitional cell papillomas is blurred. It is often best to view transitional cell papillomas as one end of the spectrum of malignant transitional cell disease. Papillomas do not show histologic invasion and the epithelial cells cannot be distinguished from those of normal transitional epithelium. They are, however, associated with the appearance of tumors elsewhere in the urinary tract, they may be multiple and they may be associated with the subsequent development of invasive disease. Approximately 25% of patients with solitary renal pelvic papillomas will develop malignancy at some other site in their urinary tract at a future date. Patients with multiple papillomas have a 50% probability of the delayed appearance of invasive carcinoma.[92,93]

The transitional cell carcinomas spread both by direct extension and by blood and lymphatics. Eighty-five percent of the transitional cell carcinomas of the renal pelvis are papillary, with 15% being sessile. Approximately 50% of the papillary tumors demonstrate muscle invasion at the time of resection and approximately 80% sessile tumors show muscle invasion at the time of resection. Approximately 7% of renal pelvic tumors are squamous cell carcinoma. These tumors are sessile and often associated with a great degree of inflammation. As these tumors seldom produce obstruction, they often are identified late in their disease course and the simultaneous appearance of metastatic disease is not uncommon. Squamous cell carcinoma of the renal pelvis, as adenocarcinoma of the renal pelvis, is commonly associated with renal calculi and chronic urinary tract infection.

Much debate exists on the potential of transitional cell carcinomas of the upper tract to seed the lower urinary tract. It is now felt that the appearance of lower tract malignancy occurs due to the exposure of the entire urethelial surface to the promoting carcinogens with the appearance of multifocal areas of disease. Thirty percent to 50% of patients with carcinoma of the renal pelvis will have other urinary tract cancers with 3% to 4% having malignant disease in the contralateral renal pelvis or ureter.

CLINICAL PRESENTATION

Hematuria, either gross or microscopic, appears in 80% to 90% of patients with renal pelvic tumors. The appearance of pain is precipitated by ureteral or uretero-pelvic junction obstruction secondary to a tumor mass. A palpable flank mass in a patient with transitional cell carcinoma classically signifies massive extrarenal extension or hydronephrotic renal destruction secondary to obstruction. The diagnosis is promoted by the appearance of a defect in the collecting system or renal pelvis on excretory pyelography (Table 23-9).

Ureteral pelvic junction obstruction with hydronephrosis may produce some disease in renal function. Nonvisualization is most commonly produced by obstruction rather than by renal parenchymal invasion. Urinary cytologies may be helpful in confirming the diagnosis.[94,95] However, only approximately 60% of patients with carcinoma of the renal pelvis will have malignant cells identified in the urine. The difficulty rests in the well-differentiated nature of many tumors of the upper urinary tract and their resemblance to normal cells using standard cytologic techniques. If tumor fragments can be obtained either by brush biopsy of the lesion or by lavage of the renal pelvis, the diagnosis can be confirmed. Renal arteriography is usually nondiagnostic in establishing the presence or absence of renal pelvic tumors. If, however, there is invasion of the renal parenchyma, there may be encasement or invasion of the arteriolar system rather than hypervascularity. Renal phlebography frequently shows venous encasement.[96,97] Staging is as in Table 23-10.

TREATMENT

The classic management of renal pelvic tumors is nephroureterectomy with excision of a cuff of bladder and bladder mucosa. The removal of the entire ureter is recommended, as approximtely 20% of patients with residual ureteral stumps will develop tumor in these ureteral stumps. Although regional lymph node dissection at the level of the renal hilum has been advocated, there are no data to indicate that this additional dissection provides enhanced cure. Given the theoretical possibility of dislodging cells with manipulation of the tumor and the possibility of bladder seeding, it is recommended that the mucosa around the ureteral orifice be mobilized and the ureter closed by sewing this mucosa over the ureteral orifice. It is advisable to isolate the potential areas of wound seeding by placing the skin margins behind a cytotoxic barrier. Abdominal pads soaked in concentrated nitrofurazone will provide an adequate barrier. As there are no reported benefits to conduct of the operation through either one or two incisions, the surgical approach should be established to encompass both the skills of the surgeon and the body habitus of the patient.

In those instances in which it is desirable to preserve the renal unit and in which a tumor can be identified only as a single calyx, it is possible to do a partial nephrectomy with isolation of the calyx before transection to prevent wound seeding. The potential for cure of interpelvic tumor by electrocoagulation has not been established.

FOLLOW-UP AND SURVIVAL

Due to the high incidence of recurrent transitional cell tumors within the bladder, the patient would be managed with cystoscopy at 2 month to 3 month intervals for the first 2 years. Urinary cytologies will also monitor the appearance of disease within the contralateral kidney and within the bladder. This is important, as about 5% of renal pelvic tumors are bilateral. The survival of patients with renal pelvic carcinoma is poor. Five-year survival rates range between 30% and 40%, regardless of the grade of the disease.[98]

TABLE 23-9. Differential Diagnosis of Cancer of the Renal Pelvis

INTRINSIC LESIONS
Calculus
Blood clot
Cholesteatoma
Malakoplakia
Inflammatory lesions of urothelium (pyelitis cystica, etc.)
Benign ureteropelvic junction obstruction
Benign (connective tissue) tumors of renal pelvis
Renal cell carcinoma
Suburothelial hemorrhage
EXTRINSIC LESIONS
Vascular impressions
Parapelvic cyst

(Modified from Fraly EE: Cancer of the renal pelvis. In Skinner DG, de Kernion JB (eds): Genitourinary Cancer, p 141. Philadelphia, WB Saunders, 1978

TABLE 23-10. Renal Pelvic Cancer

Stage I	Papillary or planar (nonpapillary) carcinoma with no evidence of invasion.
Stage II	Papillary or planar carcinoma. Superficially invasive but with invasion limited to the lamina propria.
Stage III	Papillary or planar carcinoma, extending to the level of the muscularis (may extend beyond the muscularis in intrarenal portions of the renal pelvis if confined to the kidney.)
Stage IV	Papillary or planar carcinoma extending to the adventitial surface and either involving adjuvant structures or metastatic or both.

(Modified from Bennington JL, Beckwith JB: Armed Forces Institute of Pathology, 2nd ed, Fasc 12, 1975)

CARCINOMA OF THE URETER

Carcinoma of the ureter is most common in the older age group, being rare before 30 years of age. Incidence in males predominates at a ratio of 2/1.

HISTOLOGY

Over 70% of transitional cell carcinomas of the ureter are primary transitional cell malignancies with only 8% being pure squamous cell tumors. (Table 23-11).

CLINICAL PRESENTATION AND DIAGNOSIS

Approximately 50% of all patients with ureteral tumors will present with urinary frequency or dysurea as opposed to only 10% of patients with renal pelvic tumors.[99] The characteristic ureteral dilation associated with ureteral tumors was described by Bergman and said to distinguish ureteral papillary tumors from ureteral calculi.[100] (Fig. 23-6). It is felt that the dilation is the response of the ureter to accommodate a slowly expanding tumor mass and reflects the absence of ureteral spasm produced by the presence of irritative calculus.The ureteral malignancy may present as a diffuse, stricture-like

TABLE 23-11. Classification of Tumors of the Ureter

PRIMARY TUMORS
- Epithelial
  - Malignant
    - Transitional cell carcinoma (71%)
    - Transitional cell carcinoma with differentiation (20%)
      - Squamous differentiation
      - Glandular differentiation
      - Mixed
    - Squamous cell carcinoma (pure) (8%)
    - Adenocarcinoma (1%)
    - Undifferentiated carcinoma (1%)
  - Benign
    - Papilloma
- Mesodermal
  - Malignant
    - Leiomyosarcoma
  - Benign
    - Fibroepithelial polyp
    - Leiomyoma
    - Neurilemmoma
    - Angioma

SECONDARY TUMORS (All Malignant)
- Drop metastases
- Metastases via blood or lymph
- Direct extension

(Modified from Bennington JL, Beckwith JB: Armed Forces Institute of Pathology, 2nd ed, Fasc 12, 1975)

obstructive lesion rather than a dilation of the ureter above an intralumenal mass. Differential diagnosis of the radiologic abnormalities include non-opaque calculi, blood clots, ureteritis cystica, ureteral varicosities, non-specific ureteritis, extramarrow malignancy with ureteral depression, preureteral fibrosis, and endometriosis.[101-103]

Antegrade pyelography may delineate the upper tract when ureteral obstruction produces a non-functioning kidney and precludes appropriate renal pelvic definition.[104] During the time of conduct of this maneuver, aspiration may be conducted for cytologic examination. Twenty percent of patients may have false-negative urinary cytologies in the presence of tumors of the renal pelvic and ureter.[105]

FIG. 23-6. Retrograde ureteropyelogram showing ureteral dilation about a filling defect in the lower ureter.

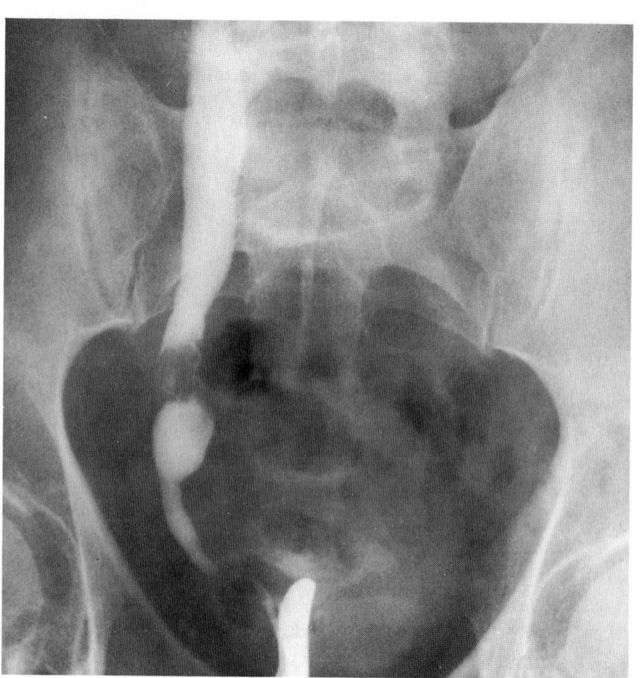

Nuclear cytologic characteristics may indicate the histologic grade of the tumor, but there is no correlation between histologic grade and the presence or absence of invasion.[106,107] In patients with surgically confirmed upper tract urothelial malignancy, positive urinary cytologies will be identified in approximately 30% to 50% of patients with invasive tumors, and in 60% of patients with Grade III or Grade IV invasive tumors. Staging of ureteral tumors is based on the modification of Hewitt's criteria of 1963 Table 23-12).[108] There is an apparent correlation between the degree of cellular anaplasia and staging. One hundred percent of Grade I tumors and 85% of Grade II tumors were non-invasive, with 30% of Grade III and only 8% of Grade IV being non-invasive.[99]

The ultimate clinical course of patients seems based on cell type, tumor grade, and tumor stage. Those patients with squamous cell carcinoma or undifferentiated malignancy have a poor prognosis.[99] Survival can be correlated with grade and stage of the disease with low stage tumors rarely showing invasion (Table 23-13).

TREATMENT

Nephroureterectomy has been traditionally the treatment of choice for ureteral transitional cell carcinomas. This philosophy is based on the likelihood of disease in the segment above the ureteral tumor in up to 30% of patients with an apparent isolated lower ureteral lesion.[109] There is, however, rising sentiment for preservation of the renal unit by local resection of the lesion. The relative advantages and disadvantages to these operative philosophies remain undefined. It is, however, well established that should the renal unit be removed at the time of operation for ureteral cancer, the entire ureter, including a cuff of bladder, should be removed. Recurrence of tumor in the remaining ureteral stump has been reported in more than one-third of patients treated by nephrectomy with partial ureterectomy.[109] The argument for less than nephroureterectomy springs from the interpretation that the salvage rate is dependent upon the biologic aggressiveness of the tumor, rather than the surgical therapy chosen. Patients with a high-grade or advanced lesions have little chance for cure with radical surgery, while patients with low-grade lesions have an excellent chance of cure only with a regional resection.

NEPHROURETERECTOMY

The surgical technique for radical nephroureterectomy includes an en bloc removal of the kidney, ureter with cuff of bladder, and the surrounding lymphatic structures. The addition of lymphadenectomy at the time of surgical resection may not provide any enhanced disease control, but does provide information with regard to the staging of the disease and may select patients for adjunctive chemotherapy at the time that appropriate agents have been identified. Batata and co-workers have reported that 12 of 41 patients had initial or subsequent metastases, with 17 or those 22 involving the regional nodes, and 5 involving distant metastatic site.[110] Ninety percent of the lymphatic metastases were unilateral, involving the adjacent pelvic nodes with the perioaortic nodes involved in 60% of the patients. The high incidence of unilateral regional node involvement makes lymphadenectomy at the time of nephroureterectomy an appropriate surgical addition. It is felt by most surgeons that removal of a cuff of bladder should include opening the bladder with sharp excision of the ureteral orifice. Attempt to remove the distal ureter by the extravesical maneuver often leaves a short stump of extravesical or intramural ureter behind.

Operative procedures to conserve the renal unit by removal of the localized tumor may encompass: (1) excision of the tumor only with an end-to-end ureteroureterostomy; (2) excision of the tumor with a uterercutaneous diversion; (3) excision of the local tumor with ureteral reimplantation; (4) replacement of the ureters with an isolated ileal segment and ureteroileocystostomy; and (5) resection of the involved segment with renal auto-transplantation. Local resection must establish adequate margins on both sides of the tumor with resection until normal ureter is identified. *Carcinoma-in-situ* should not be left at the surgical margins. Lower third ureteral tumors may be removed by distal third ureterectomy with a simultaneous unilateral lymph node dissection. The ureter can be transplanted directly into the bladder by use of a psoas hitch.

TABLE 23-12. Ureteral Staging

Stage 0	Limited to mucosa
Stage A	Lamina propria invasion
Stage B	Confined to the muscularis
Stage C	Invasions through the muscularis with involvement of adjacent structures or metastases.

TABLE 23-13. Correlation of Survival Rate with Pathologic Characteristics of Ureteral Cancer

	5-YEAR SURVIVAL RATE (Percent)	
	Bloom and Associates (1970) (54 Patients)	*Batata and Associates (1975) (41 Patients)*
HISTOLOGIC GRADE		
I	83.0	78.0
II	52.0	50.0
III	18.0	0
IV	12.0	0
PATHOLOGIC STAGE		
0, A	62.0	91.0
B	50.0	43.0
C	33.3	23.0
D	0	0

RESULTS OF TREATMENT

The rate of survival is influenced by the grade and stage of the tumor. The overall survival rate is approximately 40%, with a 5-year survival rate for well-differentiated malignancy (Grade I, Grade II) of 56%, as opposed to 16% for poorly differentiated lesions (Grade III, Grade IV). Sixty percent of patients with non-invasive disease survive 5 years, as compared to 28% of those with invasive tumors.[99]

CHEMOTHERAPY OF TRANSITIONAL CELL CARCINOMA OF THE RENAL PELVIS AND URETER

Little experience has been gathered in either systemic or intralumenal chemotherapy of the renal pelvis and ureter. The accumulative experience would indicate that the systemic agents and intralumenal agents which are most effective in management of transitional cell carcinoma of the bladder are also most effective in the management of transitional cell carcinoma of the renal pelvis and ureter. Refer to the section on Chemotherapy of Transitional Cell Carcinoma of the Bladder.

CARCINOMA OF THE BLADDER

Epidemiologic studies showing a high incidence of bladder transitional cell carcinoma in relationship to certain industrial exposures have led to the identification of many carcinogenic agents previously unsuspected. Whereas a detailed discussion of these is beyond the scope of this presentation, these compounds have provided important leads in defining the mechanisms of chemical carcinogens. In addition, there is some evidence to suggest that a substance or substances present in urine may play a role at least some time during bladder carcinogenesis. Chapman and co-workers created a bladder patch in mice by ligating the midportion of the bladder.[111] Before ligation, a paraffin pellet was inserted into each pouch and the mice were observed for 40 weeks for development of bladder carcinoma. Bladder tumors developed only in the lower pouch, which was always in contact with the urine. No tumors developed in the upper, isolated pouches. When the urine was in contact with the pouch, stone formation was evident in one-half of the pouches, and in those pouches with stone formation, the incidence of tumors approximately doubled. It was concluded that there are at least two factors necessary for the presence of bladder tumors: an unidentified substance or factors related in the urine and the presence of a foreign body. The influence of chronic irritation of the bladder mucosa is seen also in relationship to shistosoma hematobia infection.[112]

There is other evidence to support the contention that urine contains a growth-promoting substance. Hashimoto and Kitagawa successfully induced *in vitro* neoplastic transformation of epithelial cells of rat bladder using nitrosamines.[113] They used butyl-(4-hydroxybutyl)-nitrosamine (BBN) and an active metabolite of dibutyl nitrosamine (DBN) and butyl-(3-carbosypropyl)-nitrosamine (BCPN), which are major urinary metabolites in rats and are carcinogenic exclusively for bladder mucosa.[114–116] Furthermore, BBN can be converted to BCPN upon incubation with bladder mucosa or liver tissue, although the metabolic conversion with bladder mucosa is approximately one-tenth of that observed for liver tissue. These

TABLE 23-14. TNM Classification

Primary Tumor (T)

The suffix "m" should be added to the appropriate T category to indicate multiple lesions. Papilloma is classified as "GO."

TX	Minimum requirements cannot be met
T0	No evidence of primary tumor
TIS	Sessile carcinoma in situ
Ta	Papillary noninvasive carcinoma
T1	On bimanual examination a freely mobile mass may be felt; this should not be felt after complete transurethral resection of the lesion and/or there is papillary carcinoma without microscopic invasion beyond the lamina propria
T2	On bimanual examination there is induration of the bladder wall, which is mobile. There is no residual induration after complete transurethral resection of the lesion and/or there is microscopic invasion of superficial muscle of bladder
T3	On bimanual examination there is induration or a nodular mobile mass is palpable in the bladder wall which persists after transurethral resection
T3a	Microscopic invasion of deep muscle
T3b	Invasion through the full thickness of bladder wall
T4	Tumor fixed or invading neighboring structures and/or there is microscopic evidence of invasion of the prostate and in the other circumstances listed below at least muscle invasion
T4a	Tumor invading substance of prostate uterus, or vagina
T4b	Tumor fixed to the pelvic wall and/or infiltrating the abdominal wall

Nodal Involvement (N)

The regional lymph nodes are the pelvic nodes just below the bifurcation of the common iliac arteries. The juxtaregional lymph nodes are the inguinal nodes, the common iliac, and para-aortic nodes.

NX	Minimum requirements cannot be met
N0	No involvement of regional lymph nodes
N1	Involvement of a single homolateral regional lymph node
N2	Involvement of contralateral bilateral or multiple regional lymph nodes
N3	There is a fixed mass on the pelvic wall with a free space between this and the tumor
N4	Involvement of juxtaregional lymph nodes

Note: Subsequent data regarding the histologic assessment of the regional lymph nodes may be added to the N category thus: "N – " for nodes with no microscopic evidence of metastases, or "N + " for those with microscopic evidence of metastasis, for example, N0 +, etc.

Distant Metastasis (M)

MX	Not assessed
M0	No (known) distant metastasis
M1	Distant metastasis present Specify ___________ Specify sites according to the following notations:

Pulmonary—PUL	Bone Marrow—MAR
Osseous—OSS	Pleura—PLE
Hepatic—HEP	Skin—SKI
Brain—BRA	Eye—EYE
Lymph Nodes—LYM	Other—OTH

Note: Add " + " to the abbreviated notation to indicate that the pathology (p) is provided.

findings suggest that BCPN is responsible for carcinogenesis of the bladder by BBN or that both BCPN and BBN are directly carcinogenic to the bladder epithelium. Hashimoto and Kitagawa showed that when bladder epithelial cells were exposed to plain culture medium, or to plain culture medium containing BCPN, they died after 4 weeks to 5 weeks.[116] However, in tissue culture medium containing 0.05% urea and PCPN, or urea and BBN, some cells survived and after a 4 week to 8 week period, the cells began dividing to form several colonies per flask. After formation of focal monolayers, the cells finally grew without contact inhibition to form a confluent monolayer after 13 weeks to 15 weeks. The cells could be successfully passed *in vitro* in plain culture medium. The cells also formed squamous cell carcinoma when injected intraperitoneally, subcutaneously, or intravesically. These studies would indicate two points: (a) the key to success apparently lay in the addition of a small amount of urea to the culture medium, and (b) culture conditions reflected in the *in vivo* condition for induction of bladder tumor by BBN inasmuch as the concentration with nitrosamine in the medium was compatible to that of BCPN excreted in the urine when a carcinogenic concentration of BBN is administered to the drinking water. The observations suggest that urine contains a growth-promoting factor. One of these may be urea, and the other may be glycoprotein.[117]

Urinary bladder tumors in cattle may be associated with either a filterable agent (a virus), or with chronic ingestion of bracken fern (a carcinogen). Of 16 naturally occurring bovine bladder tumors, six were found to be transmissible as cell-free suspensions.[118] Suspensions of these six tumors produced fibropapillomas of the skin and vagina, as well as polypoid growths with fibroma formation in the urinary bladder of test calves. The inducation period in these studies ranged from 11 days to 25 days. The infective agents subsequently isolated resembled the bovine papilloma virus in behavior in these test calves and the lesions produced with this infective agent were similar to those induced with the bovine cutaneous papilloma suspension.[118,119] There are, however, bladder tumors seen in cattle that do not seem to be associated with viruses. Epidemiologic studies of cattle in Turkey suggest that the chronic ingestion of bracken fern (eteris aquilina) can produce bladder lesions after several months. Furthermore, urinary extracts of cows fed bracken fern from Turkey will produce bladder hemangiomas in the dog and cutaneous papillomas in mice.[119] Topical application of bracken fern extracts to mouse urinary bladder epithelium will also produce a high incidence of bladder carcinoma.[120,121] The nature of the carcinogenic substance or substances of bracken fern has not yet been established.

PATHOLOGY

Ninety percent of urothelial bladder tumors are transitional cell tumors. They are usually papillary and often multicentric, the latter characteristic reflecting the "field change" phenomena so often observed in transitional cell malignancies. Squamous cell carcinoma accounts for 6% to 8% of bladder tumors with 2% being adenocarcinomas, excepting adenocarcinomas of urachal origin, are felt to arise through a process of transitional cell metaplasia and, as do transitional cell tumors, occur most often in the most dependent part of the bladder and in the trigone. Urachal origin adenocarcinoma characteristically arises from the dome of the bladder.

Tumors are graded by the degree of cellular atypia and nuclear abnormalities and the number of mitotic figures. Border's classification segregates tumors on a scale of 1 to 4, based on the degree of anaplasia. Tumor extension and survival of the treatment can be related to increasing tumor grade. Bladder tumors are staged by the depth of invasion (Tables 23-14, 23-15). Survival after treatment decreases with increasing tumor penetration.

Two variants of urothelial neoplasia deserve special comment. Bladder papillomas are felt by some to be Stage I bladder cancers. These benign transitional cell lesions have a recurrence rate of 47% and 10% of patients will progress to invasive bladder cancer. In addition, there is a high incidence of cancer at other sites in these patients, with one-third of men and one-half of women either having had or subsequently developing malignancy at a non-urologic site. Carcinoma-*in-situ* may be found alone or in association with an existing bladder cancer. If carcinoma-*in-situ* is found adjacent to an existing low-grade or low-stage tumor, 80% of these patients will ultimately develop an invasive neoplasm; if found in an individual with a previous history of bladder malignancy, 40% will develop an invasive tumor; if found as an isolated phenomenon, 13% of patients will develop invasion.

CLINICAL PRESENTATION AND DIAGNOSIS

Hematuria, with or without symptoms of detrusor irritability, occurs in 75% of patients. Approximately 30% of patients have an associated urinary tract infection and the presenting symptom complex is dismissed often as "hemorrhagic cystitis." Vesical irritability alone is the persisting symptom in 30% of patients and usually signifies muscle invasion. Advanced cases may present with symptoms of rectal obstruction, pelvic pain from local extension or nerve root involvement, or lower extremity edema secondary to lymphatic or venous occlusion. A presumptive diagnosis may be supported by urinary cytology. As low-grade tumors tend to shed cells which appear little different from normal exfoliated transitional epithelium, approximately 20% of urinary cytologies will be falsely negative. The diagnosis of bladder tumor is confirmed by cytoscopic examination and trans-urethral biopsy of the suspected area. At the time of biopsy, bimanual examination should be

TABLE 23-15. Staging of Bladder Cancer

		JEWETT & STRONG (1946)	JEWETT (1952)	MARSHALL (1952)	TNM (1974)*	
					Clinical (T)	*Pathological (P)*
O.	Confined to mucosa			0	T0NxM0+	P0N0M0
Ps.	Carcinoma-*in-situ*				TIS	PIS
A	Infiltration of submucosa	A	A	0	T1NxM0	P1N0M0
B	Infiltration of:					
	Superficial muscle		B1	B1	T2NxM0	P2N0M0
	+	B				
	Deep muscle		B2	B2	T3aNxM0	P3aN0M0
	Perivesical infiltration	C	C	C	T3bNxM0	P3bN0M0
	Prostate				T4aNxM0	P4aN0M0
	Uterus/vagina				T4bNxM0	P4bN0M0
	Adjacent organ			D1		
					Pelvic abdominal wall	
	Nodes + (pelvic only)			D1	T(any)NxM0	P(any)N1–3M0
	Distant metastases			D2	T(any)NxM1a	T(any)N(4)M1a
	Nodes + (above aortic bifurcation)					
	Pelvic, abdominal wall fixation					

*T—primary tumor; N—nodal involvement; M—distant metastases; x—cannot be assessed.

conducted to assess the extent of the tumor and the presence or absence of fixation to adjacent pelvic structures. Even with the greatest care in staging of the disease, inaccurate staging occurs in 30% to 45% of patients. At the time of evaluation of tumor extent, care should be taken to determine the depth of muscle invasion, the size and extent of the tumor mass, the presence or absence of fixation, the presence or absence of adjacent or distant *carcinoma-in-situ,* and the condition of the mucosa at the bladder neck and the prostatic urethra. The information so acquired is necessary for treatment selection and failure to acquire this information as carefully as possible results in selection of treatment inappropriate for the stage of disease.

TREATMENT

Philosophic Considerations

Treatment of transitional cell carcinoma of the bladder should be selected so as to prevent death from malignancy in the host. Current methods rely heavily on surgical intervention to achieve this goal. Tumors which are confined to a single site within the bladder conceivably can be controlled by either transurethral resection or partial cystectomy. However, the propensity for malignant change not yet manifest as a visible tumor provides hesitancy in relying on these methods for tumor control. An assessment of the changes that have occurred within the bladder provides an indication of the likelihood of success of local control procedures. Tumors less than 1 cm in diameter are associated with a recurrence frequency of 35%, while tumors over 3 cm in diameter are associated with a recurrence frequency of 80%. If a single superficial tumor is present at the time of initial resection, only 4% of patients will develop delayed muscle invasion. If there are multiple initial tumors, the incidence of future invasion rises to 40%. If *carcinoma-in-situ* is present in association with an existing bladder tumor, 80% of the patients will develop a new cancer. If *carcinoma-in-situ* is identified in a patient with a past history of bladder cancer, 40% will develop subsequently invasion disease. Total cystectomy, therefore, is considered when it is doubtful that the tumor can be controlled by local resection alone.

SURGERY OF BLADDER CARCINOMA

Stage 0 (*in situ*) tumors are frequently treated with *transurethral resections* or *fulguration*. Many of these lesions are papillary and can be locally controlled with conservative therapy in over 80% of the cases. However, some lesions are more infiltrating and less differentiated and recurrences in over 50% of the patients have been reported. It is important for the urologist to remove the base of the lesion with an adequate margin and to examine the resected tissues by frozen section to make sure that the margin resections are negative. Wider resections may be necessary if the margins are positive. It is extremely important to place an indwelling bladder catheter and to drain the bladder in the postoperative period to prevent distension, which may lead to extravasation and postoperative complications. Transurethral resection of non-infiltrating bladder carcinoma may in and of itself be an etiologic factor in recurrence rates. Page and co-workers have demonstrated a difference in the distribution within the bladder of primary and recurrent tumors.[122] Whereas three-quarters of the primary tumors were confined to a restricted area and near the ureteric orifices, only one-fifth of recurrent tumors were found in this site. The most common sites for recurrent tumors were the postero–superior wall of the bladder and in the air bubble region, sites in which primary tumor was not found. The posterio–superior wall of the bladder is subject to mild trauma and abrasion by the tip of an endoscope and the air bubble region is traumatized by hot gas produced by the diathermy. This local trauma is felt to encourage tumor formation, either by producing a raw surface which allows implantation of tumor cells or by producing local susceptibility to a primary carcinogenic factor.

Similar observations have prompted the use of post-operative intravesical chemotherapy to reduce the rate. Thiotepa, 60 mg in 60 cc of water retained for 20 minutes daily for 3 days, then weekly for 4 weeks, beginning on the day of surgery has been shown to reduce recurrence rates.

CARCINOMA-*IN-SITU*

Management of carcinoma-*in-situ* may present specific problems in patients with transitional cell carcinoma. Carcinoma-*in-situ* is noninvasive but has a high potential for subsequent invasion. Carcinoma-*in-situ* is multifocal and diffuse and reflects the potential for the entire urethelial surface to undergo exposure to potential carcinogens. Approximately 90% of patients with carcinoma-*in-situ* will present with frequency, dysuria, urgency, and hematuria. The extent of severity of this symptom complex is directly related to the extent of the involvement of bladder mucosa. There is a direct relationship between the intensity of these symptoms and the occurrence of microscopic invasion.[123,124]

If the lesion involves only a small portion of the bladder, less than 5 cm, and is reasonably well delineated, does not involve the prostatic urethra, vesical neck, or either ureteral orifice, and there is no evidence of positive cytologies from the upper urinary tract, thorough electrofulguration of the involved areas followed by a course of intravesical thiotepa for 6 months may be employed. The patient should be followed post treatment with cystoscopy and urinary cytologies at 2-month to 3-month intervals for the first year and at 4-month intervals for the second year, and at 6-month intervals thereafter. If the lesion does not respond, and cytologies do not convert to negative and the irritative bladder symptoms remain after treatment, cystoprostatectomy with urinary diversion is recommended. In patients who have diffuse lesions, involvement of the prostatic urethra, or severe irritative bladder symptomatology, radical cystectomy is warranted. The terminal 6 cm of each ureter should be removed with the proximal cut surface monitored for extension of carcinoma-*in-situ*. It is rare to have involvement of the terminal ureters of a distance more than 5 cm.

Involvement of the prostatic urethra with carcinoma-*in-situ* should prompt incontinuity urethrectomy.

The initiation of aggressive treatment of carcinoma-*in-situ* is prompted by the previous experience of Utz and co-workers.[123,124] In their initial series in which carcinoma-*in-*

situ was treated primarily by transurethral electroresection and fulguration, subsequent invasion developed in 73% of patients, with 57% of these patients dying of their disease in 5 years. The experience following more aggressive approach in the management of this disease in which 15 patients who had cystectomy after diagnosis of carcinoma-*in-situ* demonstrated no deaths. Three of these patients had microinvasion with more than 80% of the bladder replaced by *in-situ* cancer at the time of pathologic examination.[124]

The role of segmental resection in the management of transitional cell carcinoma of the bladder remains controversial.[125-127] However, this operative option presents an attractive alternative for carefully selected patients. Selection of the patients for partial cystectomy is complicated by the tendency of the entire vesicourethelium to be unstable in the presence of an isolated and well defined lesion, and because of the probability of undetected microinvasion and carcinoma-*in-situ* in areas distant to the bladder. The additional problem of wound seeding at the time of partial cystectomy must not be underemphasized.

A series of specific criteria must be established in order to select the appropriate patient for surgery. The grade of the tumor should be II, III, or IV. Grade I cancers are classically papillary and often can be resected trans-urethrally unless they are too great in size. The tumor should be invasive. Transitional cell carcinomas have a better response to partial cystectomy than do squamous cell carcinomas owing to the tendency of squamous cell carcinomas for intramural extension via lymphatics and venous plexus of the bladder wall.[126,127] The tumors should be less than 6 cm to 8 cm in size to permit resection to have sufficient tumor-free margins with a residual acceptable functional bladder capacity.

The lesion should be solitary and primary and is ideally in the upper part of the bladder or on the posterior wall. Invasion of the vesical neck or the prostate is a contradiction.

The appearance of carcinoma-*in-situ* adjacent or distant to the lesion, itself, indicates urethelial instability and is a contraindication to partial cystectomy. Prior to partial cystectomy to devitalize the tumor cells and prevent wound seeding, preoperative radiotherapy in the form of a minimum dose of 1000 rad in three days or 2000 rad in 5 days should be established.[136,138,139] Prior to opening of the bladder, the bladder should be irrigated with sterile water. When laterality of the lesion can be established, a unilateral pelvic node dissection should be established in continuity.

The necessity for rigid patient selection makes segmental resection appropriate for only 5% of patients with bladder cancer.[126,127] Five-year survival rates in patients with Stage 0, A, or B bladder cancer treated by partial cystectomy ranges from 65% to 81% (Table 23-16).[126,127]

Radical cystectomy is advised for most patients whose tumors demonstrate muscle invasion, for patients with recurring Grade II lesions who have failed to respond to more conservative treatment and who return with a higher tumor grade, and for all patients with Grade III and Grade IV tumors irrespective of stage.[128] Radical cystectomy in the male includes the bladder, prostate, seminal vesicles, and and the immediately adjacent perivesical tissue. In women, radical cystectomy includes the bladder, uterus, tubes, ovaries, anterior vagina, and urethra.[129,130] Pelvic lymphadenectomy is advocated by some, however, the poor survival when pelvic nodal metastases exist makes the potential benefit of this additional procedure questionable (Table 23-17).[131,132]

SURGICAL TECHNIQUE

The patient is best approached through an incision slightly to the left of the midline. An inverted V incision is then made into the anterior peritoneum beginning at the umbilicus and continuing bilaterally to the internal rings. The lateral margins of this incision should be the inferior epigastric vasculature. The inferior portion of the peritoneal envelope is incised and the incision is carried cephalad in posterior peritoneum using the testicular vasculature as the lateral margins of dissection. This defines the limits of the dissection and exposes the pelvic vasculature, lymphatics, and ureters. When pelvic lymphadenectomy is to be considered, it should begin at the level of the common iliac bifurcation and include the node-bearing tissue surrounding the external iliac vasculatures, obturator nerves, and hypogastric vasculature.

Radical cystectomy requires institution of an acceptable method of urinary diversion. This can be done either by uretero–enteric conduit, uretero–sigmoidostomy or cutaneous ureterostomy. The enteric conduit is preferred by most as it effectively separates the urinary and fecal streams (Fig. 23-7). The primary consideration in construction of an enteric conduit is that the bowel tube created be sufficiently short to function merely as a conduit and not as a repository for urine. This will keep absorption of excretory products to a minimum and prevent the electolytic disturbances which accompany the absorption of urine.

If a small-bowel conduit is being considered, any segment of small bowel may be used. It is felt that the distal ileum is ideal and there is minimal risk of producing damage to the bowel vasculature during isolation of the intestinal segment. However, pre-operative radiation may produce sufficient dam-

TABLE 23-16. Comparison of Five Year Study in Patients Treated by Radium Implant or Segmental Resection

TREATMENT	STAGE A	STAGE B_1	STAGE B_2C
Radium Implantation (van der Werf-Messing)			
Alone	50%	80%	12.5%
+ Postoperative radiotherapy (1500 Rad)	91%	55%	21%
+ Preoperative radiotherapy (1050 Rad)	80%	67%	47%
Segmental Resection (Utz)	68%	47%	35%
Segmental Resection (Resnick)	71% (O + A)	76.9%	15.6%

TABLE 23-17. Patient Survival Following Cystectomy and Preoperative Radiotherapy

SERIES	B_1	B_2	C	D_1	D_2	NO TUMOR	OPERATIVE MORTALITY	NO. OF RADS
Reid	28/43 (64.1%)	38/92	(34.5%)	5/24 (25.8%)			13% (135)	2000
Whitmore	4/9 (44.4%)	8/18 (45%)	2/8 (25%)	2/9 (22%)	1/16 (6%)	10/19	11% (119)	4000
Whitmore	8/16 (50%)	9/14 (64.4%)	6/12 (50%)	3/12 (21%)	1/16 (6%)	2/4	9% (86)	2000
Van der Werf-Messing	10/21 (48%)	24/54	(44%)	2/7 (29%)				4000
Wallace	– –	34/98	(33%)	–	–		7.8% (77)	4000
Miller	– –	18/35	(51%)	–	–			5000
TOTALS	50/89 (56%)	139/331	(42%)	14/84	(17%)	12/23		
			Patient Survival Following Cystectomy Alone					
Whitmore	18/30 (60%)	8/31 (26%)	2/19 (16%)	2/16	0/18		14%	
Riches	– –	3/33 (9%)	1/28 (4%)	–	–		12.5%	
Jewett	2/4 (50%)	2/12 (16%)	5/45 (12%)	–	–		–	
Bowles & Cordonnier	11/17 (63%)	5/10 (50%)	4/20 (20%)	0/3			5.4%	
Pearse	7/14 (50%)	5/12 (42%)	2/15 (13%)	0/11			19%	
TOTALS	38/65 (58%)	20/65 (30%)	14/125 (11%)					
Subtotal:	B_2C	34/190 (18%)						

age to the intestine to make it necessary to select a segment proximal to the distal ileum, occasionally needing to proceed as high as the jejunum. A segment of distal ileum approximately 15 cm in length should be isolated and the continuity of the bowel reestablished with either a single layer or double layer ileo–ileostomy. The proximal end of the isolated segment is then closed with an inverted running absorption suture. The left ureter is then led through a tunnel beneath the sigmoid mesocolon to lie in the right retroperitoneum along-

FIG. 23-7. Ileal loop urinary diversion.

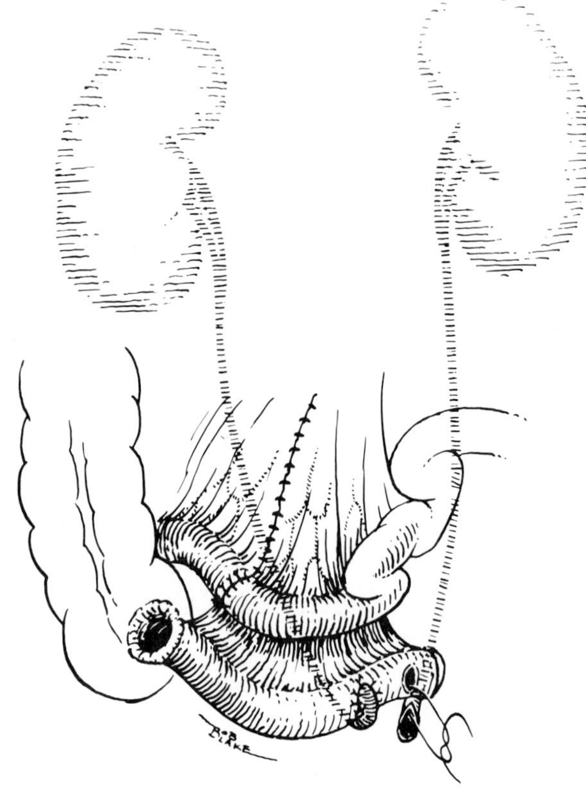

side the right distal ureter. Both ureters are spatulated and are anastomosed to the proximal end of the isolated ileal segment on the antimesenteric border using a mucosal-to-mucosal anastomosis with absorbable suture. Both distal ureters are optimally spatulated to prevent postoperative stricture. In addition, many technicians advise conducting the anastomosis over a stenting catheter to provide drainage for 5 days to 7 days.

After the ileoureteral anastamoses have been completed, the proximal end of the isolated ileal segment is fixed to the retroperitoneum with multiple interrupted sutures of 2-0 chromic catgut. The distal end of the isolated ileal segment is then led out through a defect in the right lower abdominal wall, usually placed one-half of the distance between the anterior superior iliac spine and the umbilicus. An everted mucocutaneous anastomosis is established again with absorbable suture material. The isolated ileal segment ideally will lay beneath the cecum, however, when anatomy does not permit this, it may be lead anteriorly to the cecum.

The necessity for simultaneous urethrectomy in all males undergoing radical cystectomy remains in debate. Only 7% of all patients subjected to radical cystectomy will subsequently develop urethral malignancy. However, this figure will double when diffuse *in situ* changes exist within the bladder or prostatic urethra, or when the primary tumor is at the level of the bladder neck.[133–135] These patients should undergo simultaneous incontinuity urethrectomy with removal also of the fossa navicularis and glandular meatus. Patients whose urethras are not removed should be followed with urethral cytologies obtained by washing or by direct swabbing of the retained urethra.

RADIATION THERAPY

Radiation therapy, alone, has fallen from favor as a single treatment modality for bladder cancer, just as radical surgery, alone, is felt to be less beneficial than the treatments in combination. Radiation therapy, alone, suffers, as not all bladder cancers are radio-sensitive and radiation therapy does not reverse premalignant urethelial changes which may have occurred in the bladder at sites distant from the tumor under treatment.

Radiation therapy is used, therefore, in combination with surgery for the treatment of infiltrating lesions (Stage B and C), and used alone for the management of inoperable patients with the above stages as well as those with more advanced unresectable tumors (Stage D1). The main rationale for pre-operative radiation has been to inactivate tumor cells that may be disseminated at the time of an operation, to eradicate the tumor micro-metastases and, in more extensive lesions, to reduce the size of the mass to improve the opportunity for removal.

TECHNIQUES OF IRRADIATION

The classical method for irradiation of carcinoma of the bladder has been external beam. Some authors have described the use of interstitial radium or tantalum, delivering high doses of irradiation to volume of interest, usually with insertion of the sources through a suprapubic cystostomy.[136,137]

Most authors recommend 15 cm × 15 cm or 18 cm × 15 cm ports to encompass the entire pelvic contents, including the common iliac lymph nodes and the prostatic urethra in men or the entire urethra in women. Smaller portals, 10 cm × 10 cm or 12 cm × 12 cm have been used by some authors, but as pointed out by Whitmore and coworkers, a higher incidence of recurrence has been noted in these patients in comparison with those treated with larger portals.[138] With high energy beams it is possible to deliver high doses of irradiation, pre-operatively or alone through AP and PA portals. However, with ^{60}Co or photons below 8 MV, lateral portals utilizing the box technique of two posterior oblique fields are necessary in order to minimize the dose to the small intestine and rectum.

RESULTS OF TREATMENT

Survival rates appear dependent on the stage, grade, and cell type. Low grade tumors have a better prognosis than high grade tumors. The major prognostic determinant, however, is the stage of the disease at the time of diagnosis. Stages 0 and A can be expected to have a 75% 5-year-survival rate after transurethral resection alone. Stages B1 through stage C patients have an expected 5-year survival rate of 35% to 40% after radical cystoprostatectomy (with radiation therapy pre-operatively). Stage D1 disease can be expected to have a minimal 5-year survival rate (16%–17% if only a few nodes in the pelvis are involved). In Stage D2 disease there are no survivors with any form of treatment. Much confusion occurs when survival rate data is compared between series. Some authors report survival rate as a function of clinical stage, others as a function of pathologic stage. As clinical staging inaccuracy can occur in up to 50% of patients, any attempt to compare survival rates between patients clinically staged and those pathologically staged is hazardous. Furthermore, the reader must be aware that certain forms of therapy, as partial cystectomy, are used only in highly selected patients, making comparisons of results of partial cystectomy and radical cystectomy selectively biased.

Dosages in pre-operative irradiation have ranged from 1000 rad in 2 fractions to 5000 rad in 5 weeks to 6 weeks. The 5-year survival rate in 46 nonrandomized patients with Stages B and C receiving 1000 rad pre-operatively was 50% and 28%, respectively. Miller treated 125 patients with pre-operative radiation (5000 rad in 5 weeks) and a radical cystectomy.[139,140] Twenty of 54 patients available for 10-year observation survived. The local failure rate was 16% with 30% failing with distant metastases.

In contrast, of 348 primary cases of similar stage (280 patients available for ten year survival analysis) treated by irradiation alone, only 8% survived. The incidence of pelvic recurrence was 4%, with 22% failing at distant sites. A decreasing incidence of local recurrence occurs with higher doses of irradiation; however, there is a marked increase in complications with tumor doses over 5000 rad.[141]

Whitmore and co-workers have compared the survival rates in patients treated pre-operatively with either 2000 rad or 4000 rad.[138] A group of 119 patients were treated with 4000 rad from 1959 to 1965, showing a 5-year tumor-free survival in 43% and mortality from recurrence of bladder cancer in 44%. Eighty-six patients were treated from 1966 to 1970 with 2000 rad and demonstrated a 5-year tumor-free survival rate of 42% and a pelvic recurrence rate of 42%. The incidence of pelvic recurrence was 22% (19 of 86 patients) in the 200 rad group and 25% (30 of 119 patients) in the 4000 rad group. It is of interest that in both groups, those patients treated with 15 cm × 15 cm portals had a pelvic recurrence rate of 28% to 29% in contrast with 44% to 50% in patients treated with smaller portals (12 cm × 12 cm). The authors observed decreasing survival with more advanced stages or higher degrees of undifferentiation of the tumor. In deeply invasive tumors in the two irradiated groups, the 5-year survival rate was twice as high as that seen at the same institution for similar tumors (historical controls) treated by radical cystectomy alone.

Van der Werf-Messing treated 89 patients with Stage T3NxM0 carcinoma of the bladder with 4000 rad pre-operatively in 4 weeks followed by a total cystectomy within a week after completion of radiotherapy and documented an uncorrected actuarial 5-year survival rate of 50%.[142,143] Initially, the portals covered the true pelvis, but after 1972, the fields were extended to include the common iliac lymph nodes to the fifth lumbar vertebra. Two-thirds of the patients experienced a reduction in the depth of infiltration of the tumor, with lesser stages being present at the time of the surgery. In patients on whom a T reduction was noted, the 5-year survival rate was 70%.

A trial in which patients with Stage B_2 and C were randomized to either surgery alone, or 4500 rad pre-operatively followed in 4 weeks to 8 weeks by surgery has demonstrated an actuarial five year survival of 40% in 99 irradiated patients as compared to 27% in 129 non-irradiated patients.[144] Furthermore, the survival was 51% in a group of 10 patients who showed no residual tumor.

Ellingwood and co-workers treated a small group of patients with an initial exploratory staging laparotomy and construction of an ileal conduit followed by 5000 rad preoperative radiation delivered in 30 fractions.[145] Four weeks to 6 weeks after completion of radiotherapy a total cystectomy was performed.

Preliminary analysis showed local control in 21 of 22 previously untreated patients and the actuarial 4-year survival rate was 54%. No treatment related deaths have occurred, only 12 of 22 specimens had viable tumor at the time of cystectomy and only two major complications are reported. Barnhouse and Mahoney have reported similar satisfactory results.[145-147] Postoperative radiation for patients whose tumor is found beyond the surgical margins does not seem advised.

COMPLICATIONS

The short course pre-operative irradiation may produce a radiation enteritis requiring aggressive parental support in the postoperative period. Residual bowel and skin damage is similar to that seen after irradiation for prostatic adenocarcinoma and is similarly controlled.

CHEMOTHERAPY OF METASTATIC BLADDER CANCER

Carcinoma of the bladder represents an intriguing and frustrating paradox of advantages and disadvantages in exploring the efficacy of chemotherapy. In the patient who has not had a total cystectomy or urinary diversion, it is a tumor which has the theoretical advantage that relatively high concentrations of select drugs can be presented to the superficial surface of the tumor, which may be relatively avascular, at the same time that drug can be delivered hematogenously as is applicable to other tumor sites. Drugs such as *cis*-dichlorodiammine platinum-II, methotrexate, bleomycin, and, to some extent, the metabolites of 5-fluorouracil and cyclophosphamide are all excreted *via* renal mechanisms. As such, significant amounts of drug can be delivered to the surface of a bladder carcinoma if not previously resected or the urine stream diverted. Such a theoretical advantage is supported by the clinical experience with intravesical chemotherapy using thiotepa, mitomycin-C, and bleomycin for superficial, early stage disease.[148,149] At the same time that one enjoys these theoretical advantages, a number of practical disadvantages exist in treating this patient population. Most patients are over the age of 50 years, indeed many are over the age of 60 years. Many patients with advanced disease have compromised renal function, and many have had a radical cystectomy or urinary diversion or both, which obviates the advantages alluded to above. An ever-increasing proportion of patients have had radiotherapy, thus introducing at least some element of bone marrow compromise. Finally, it has historically been difficult to document objective responses in patients who have recurrent pelvic or abdominal disease because of the difficulties in measuring tumor masses in these sites. The introduction of ultrasonography and computerized axial tomography, however, may well overcome this latter deficiency.

Systemic chemotherapy for bladder carcinoma (as well as transitional cell carcinoma of the renal pelvis or ureter) has not been systematically studied. As pointed out in a review article by Carter and Wasserman, among the 16 most common tumors, the systematic evaluation of chemotherapy for bladder carcinoma ranks at the bottom of the list. This is in spite of the fact that there is at least some demonstrable antitumor activity with a wide variety of chemotherapeutic agents. Although these data tend to be fragmented among many reports with small numbers of patients, they are complicated by the difficulties in evaluability of patient responses and compromised by the overall poor performance status and complicating medical illnesses of the patients entered into such trials.[150-152] In spite of this, there is clearcut antitumor activity demonstrable by a variety of agents. The most effective agent is *cis*-dichlorodiammine platinum-II (DDP) with objective response rates ranging from 33% to 45% of patients, depending upon their overall performance status and whether or not they had received previous chemotherapy.[153,154] A variety of combination therapy regimens have also been tested including DDP plus cyclophosphamide (47% response rate), DDP plus adriamycin (50% response rate), cyclophosphamide plus adriamycin (17–50% response rate), adriamycin plus 5-FU (35% response rate), adriamycin plus VM 25 (19% response rate), DDP plus adriamycin plus 5-FU (46% response rate), DDP plus cyclophosphamide plus adriamycin (33%–90% response rate) Table 23-18).[151,152,155-160]

With such a wide diversity of chemotherapeutic regimens and reported response rates, it is important to place such data in perspective. It is clear that overall performance status and previous therapy (including surgery or radiotherapy or chemotherapy or some combination) have profound effects upon subsequent responses to chemotherapeutic regimens. It is also obvious that response rates vary dependent upon the stage of patients entered into the trial, the site of recurrent disease (lung metastases appear to be the most responsive), and the definitions of an objective response employed by the authors. The data of Sternberg and co-workers are highly encouraging with a 90% response rate.[160] However, it is not clear that this apparently improved response rate is due to this intensive and toxic combination regimen or whether this was a fortuitous observation based on a small number of patients. In a sequence of studies performed by Yagoda and colleagues and in reports by Stoner and Williams and colleagues there is no clearcut evidence that combination chemotherapy is superior to single agent therapy with DDP alone.[152,158,159] It is, however, clear that such regimens are more toxic. Until more definitive studies are performed, the recommended chemotherapeutic regimen for a patient with recurrent or metastatic bladder carcinoma should be intermittent chemotherapy with DDP at a dose of 70 mg/m^2 as a single dose or 20 mg/m^2 per day over 5 days. Both regimens should be administered every 3 weeks to 4 weeks. Utilization of the single dose regimen requires hydration and diuresis with either 12.5 mg to 25 mg of mannitol and/or 20 mg to 40 mg of IV furosemide 1 hour prior to the administration of DDP. The latter regimen can be administered with hydration alone (1000 ml of appropriate intravenous fluid daily with each dose of DDP) but requires 5 days of administration. These hydration and diuretic regimens will minimize renal toxicity and prevent the subsequent development of azotemia in greater than 95% of patients. DDP should be administered with caution to any patient with creatinine clearance of 60 ml/min. Modified doses should be utilized. In all cases, renal function must be reevaluated prior to the next cycle of therapy. Toxicity includes bone marrow suppression, manifested predominantly as a persistent anemia, nausea, and vomiting, which usually becomes the dose limiting toxicity and peripheral neuropathy or ototoxicity or both; the incidence and

TABLE 23-18. Chemotherapy of Bladder Carcinoma

AGENT	RESPONSE	RANGE
Single Agent Therapy		
Cis-dichlorodiammine Platinum (II) (DDP)	11/33 (33%)	33–57%
Methotrexate	22/88 (25%)	17–36%
Adriamycin	54/235 (23%)	0–37%
Cyclophosphamide	17/41 (41%)	0–53%
5-Fluorouracil	24/116 (25%)	0–75%
Mitomycin-C	25/75 (33%)	16–33%
NEWER AGENTS WITH POSSIBLE ACTIVITY		
Hexamethylmelamine	6/16 (38%)	–
Two-Drug Regimens		
DDP + Cyclophosphamide	15/32 (47%)	5 months (median)
DDP + Adriamycin	14/28 (50%)	5 months "
Cyclophosphamide + Adriamycin	13/50 (26%)	4 months "
Adriamycin + 5-FU	7/20 (35%)	7–17 months "
Adriamycin + VM 26	5/27 (19%)	17.8 months (Median)
Three-Drug Regimens		
DDP + Cyclophosphamide + Adriamycin	9/10 (90%)	?
DDP + Cyclophosphamide + Adriamycin	9/16 (57%)	5+ Months
DDP + Cyclophosphamide + Adriamycin	11/33 (33%)	168 days
DDP + 5-Fluorouracil + Adriamycin	18/39 (46%)	6.1 months

severity of the latter toxicity are as yet not clearly defined—subclinical ototoxicity may be frequent but severe debilitating ototoxicity is fortunately relatively rare. Systemic reactions are observed in an occasional patient and are manifested as flushing, pruritus, anxiety, agitation, and occasionally dyspnea. Such systemic reactions usually, but do not always, preclude further administration of DDP. Several recent reports have also indicated unusual toxicity, including hemolytic anemias with hemoglobinuria and selective renal tubular toxicity producing hypomagnesemia and secondary hypocalcemia.[161,162] This latter complication has been most predominantly noted in patients receiving combination chemotherapy containing DDP, but has been observed in patients receiving DDP alone. The incidence of hypomagnesemia may be as high as 50%, but can usually be managed with oral magnesium supplementation.

Responses to DDP therapy have been observed in all metastatic sites except for CNS metastases. Responses are invariably rapid in onset, with most patients having a demonstrable response within 10 days to 14 days. If a patient with measurable disease does not have an objective response with the first two cycles of DDP (probably even with the first) the regimen should be discontinued. The median duration of response is only 4 months to 6 months, but occasional patients have had their disease controlled for 12 months to 18 months.

The role of adjuvant systemic chemotherapy is only currently being explored. The National Bladder Cancer Collaborative Group A is testing the efficacy of adjuvant DDP in patients undergoing preoperative radiotherapy and subsequent radical cystectomy. This randomized trial compares the results of DDP versus observation and therapy at the time of relapse. As yet, no definitive data are available with this trial. High-dose methotrexate at a dose of 1 g to 2 g/m^2 with leucovorin rescue is also undergoing investigation. A preliminary report suggests that this regimen may dramatically increase or decrease relapse rates.[163] However, this is not a prospective randomized trial, and must be confirmed before such a logistically complicated and expensive chemotherapeutic regimen can be administered to patients outside of a therapy trial.

In the patient who has multiple recurrent noninvasive transitional cell carcinoma of the bladder or who has diffuse *carcinoma-in-situ*, it is theoretically advantageous to use intravesical chemotherapeutic agents in order that a relatively high concentration of these drugs can be presented to the superficial surface of the tumor that effects tumor destruction. Multiple agents such as thiotepa, mitomycin, and bleomycin have been used for superficial early stage disease.[148,149] The largest experience has been gathered with thiotepa. Among all patients, it would appear that thiotepa will produce tumor control in approximately one-third of patients, produce a decrease in the rate of recurrence in approximately one-third of patients and produce no treatment and no disease control in the remaining third. There are no predictors for selection. Thiotepa seemingly has little impact in the management of carcinoma-*in-situ*, however, preliminary unpublished results would indicate that mitomycin-C may be effective in the management of carcinoma-*in-situ*. Patients who are to be treated with thiotepa should receive 60 mg of drug and 60 cc of water intravesically, once weekly, for 4 weeks and then once monthly for an additional 4 months. They should be monitored prior to each treatment with a hematologic profile. Tumor response can be monitored cystoscopically. The dose level for mitomycin-C is 40 mg and 40 cc of water intravesically each week for 4 weeks and then each month for 4 months. Treatment response is monitored in the similar manner.

PROSTATE CANCER

EPIDEMIOLOGY

The incidence of prostatic cancer is estimated to be 48 per 100,000 person-years with approximately 47,500 white and 8,500 black new cases recorded each year.[163] The reported incidence of prostate cancer is rising.[164,165] For whites, the incidence rate has risen from 30 per 100,000 person-years in 1937 to 46 in 1971; the corresponding rate for blacks was 31 in 1937 and 78 in 1971. Overall 5-year survival is projected to be 57% in whites and 49% in blacks.

The several studies examining the relationship between socioeconomic status and prostate cancer to determine whether or not black–white socioeconomic differences contribute to the observed racial difference in incidence have yielded inconsistent results.[166–170] Although the relationship between socioeconomic status and prostate cancer is still unclear, it appears unlikely that the black–white difference in prostate cancer incidence is attributable to socioeconomic differences.

International Variation

A 40-fold difference in prostate cancer incidence is observed between U.S. blacks, who have the highest rate in the world, and residents of Japan, one of the low-incidence areas.[171] Interestingly, immigrants from low-risk countries to the U.S. have incidence rates between those of their country of origin and the U.S.[172,173] The considerable variations observed and the change in incidence with migration from low- to high-risk countries suggest an important role for unidentified environmental factors.

The sexual activity of prostate cancer patients was first examined by Steele and co-workers, who identified an increased number of sexual partners and a higher occurrence of venereal diseases in the case group than in the controls, prompting the authors to suggest a viral-venereal relationship with prostatic cancer.[174] Three additional studies confirm a higher frequency of history of venereal disease in the prostate cancer patients.[175–177] There is little agreement as to the possible roles of coital frequency or number of sexual partners. Conflicting reports both confirm and deny an increased incidence of prostatic cancer in males whose sexual partners have cervical cancer.[178] Although epidemiologic support for the viral-venereal hypothesis is meager, urologic and serologic studies appear to support the hypothesis. A strain of cytomegalovirus (CMC-Mj) isolated from human prostate tissue has been reported to transform human prostate cell lines.[179] Moreover, higher antibody titers against herpes virus type 2 and cytomegalovirus have been found in prostatic cancer patients than in controls.[176,179]

No viral etiology for human prostatic carcinoma has been established. Tannenbaum reported the appearance of filamentous ultrastructural features in human prostatic carcinoma that resembled similar features seen in the Lueke virus-induced frog kidney tumor.[179] Although it is now clear that these filamentous structures are not the oncogenic agent in the frog tumor as originally proposed, their significance in both the Leuke tumor and carcinoma of the prostate is undetermined. Further, there has been little effort to isolate viruses from prostatic tissue or from prostatic secretions. The investigations of carcinoma of the cervix would promote herpes genitalis as one of the prime virus suspects. Herpes genitalis has been isolated from the prostatic secretions of men with prostatitis. In addition, antibodies to cytomegalovirus have been shown in high titer in the serum of men with prostatitis. Herpes virus has been isolated from cells of a human prostatic adenocarcinoma. This virus has been shown to be a herpes virus Type II and will cause *in vitro* transformation of hamster cells.[180–182] Rapp has shown a long-term persistence of the cytomegalovirus genome in cultured human cells of prostatic origin.[180]

The second hypothesis, that man's hormonal profile determines his risk of prostate cancer, is based on the following: (1) no prostate cancer has been found in castrated men, and (2) latent prostate cancer is less frequent in cirrhotics who tend to have hyperestrogenism.[183–186] Epidemiologic data suggest that prostate cancer patients have a later onset of development of secondary sex characteristics; however, the differences are not statistically significant.[177] The lack of clearly identifiable landmarks in the male sexual maturation process (as compared to menarche, child-bearing, and menopause in females) makes the investigation of the role of these hormonal factors difficult. Familial aggregation of prostatic adenocarcinoma has been identified, the mortality from prostate cancer being up to three times more frequent in relatives of prostate cancer propositi than in those of controls.[174,176,186]

Since both prostate cancer and BPH are common in older men and often are found concurrently, two epidemiologic studies have examined the relationship between BPH and prostate cancer.[187–189] Greenwald and co-workers followed 838 BPH cases and 802 age-matched controls for an average of 10 years and did not find any difference in the incidence of prostate cancer between the two groups.[187] However, Armenian and co-workers followed 296 BPH cases diagnosed either histologically or clinically and 299 age-matched controls for from 7 years to 27 years and found the incidence of prostate cancer to be 3.7 times higher in the BPH group than in controls.[189]

PATHOLOGY

Adenocarcinoma accounts for over 95% of prostatic cancer. The degree of malignancy is based on the degree of dedifferentiation and can be shown to correlate with both metastatic spread and survival. Although multiple systems for the histologic grading of prostatic cancer have been proposed, the Gleason classifying system is felt by many to be the pathologic reference point for classifying patients. The Gleason system is based upon the degree of glandular differentiation and the growth pattern of the tumor in relation to the prostatic stroma. The pattern may vary from a well-formed and crusty malignant Grade I to an undifferentiated Grade V. The Gleason system assigns a histologic grade both to the predominate primary pattern and to any secondary patterns. In this regard, it differs from all other systems which judge the histologic grade on the basis of the most undifferentiated portion or on the basis of the most representative (majority) portion of the material. The Gleason experience would suggest that the histologic pattern of the tumor remains the same throughout the life of the host and recent published data would indicate that the Gleason system accurately predicts the absence of metastatic nodal disease. Prostatic adenocarcinoma spreads by direct extension to the seminal vesicles, bladder, membraneous urethra, and pelvic sidewalls. The rectum is protected by Denonvilliers' fascia and is invaded rarely by prostatic

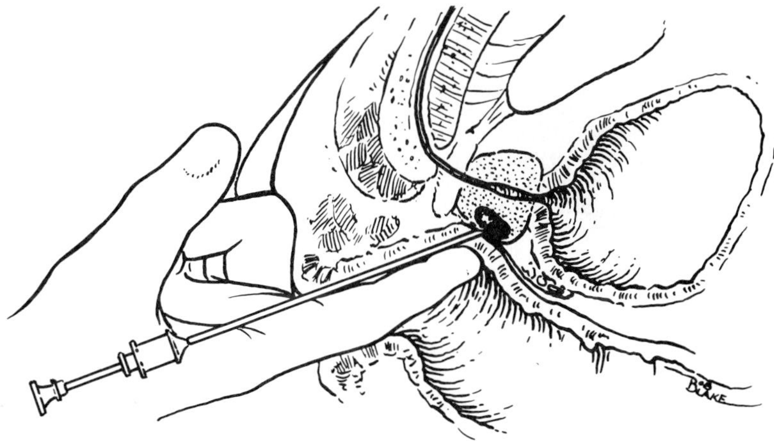

FIG. 23-8. Transrectal needle biopsy of the prostate.

cancer. Prostatic adenocardinoma spreads by lymphatic and hematogenous routes to involve the pelvic lymphatics and adjacent bones. The bone lesion is unique in that it appears radiographically as an osteoblastic, not an osteolytic, lesion. The increased radiographic density is produced not by an increase in calcium deposition, but in noncalcified osteoid which replaces the air spaces within the bone, producing the paradoxical appearance of increased bone density in areas of calcium loss.

CLINICAL PRESENTATION

The majority of patients present with symptoms of bony metastasis, of back pain, stiffness, and occasionally with pathologic fractures. Not infrequently, the disease is erroneously treated as degenerative arthritis. Local prostatic growth produces symptoms of urethral outflow obstruction. Occasional patients may present with severe irritative bladder symptoms in the absence of clinical evidence of infection. Isolated hematuria or hematospermia is rare.

DIAGNOSIS AND STAGING

Rectal examination will frequently provide the diagnosis. Prostatic cancer produces an area of firmness within the prostate which is increased over that of the surrounding tissue. Approximately 10% of patients with prostatic carcinoma will have a normal-feeling prostate by rectal examination with the disease being identified only by pathologic examination of tissue removed for what was felt to be benign prostatic disease. A working diagnosis of prostatic cancer should be confirmed by either transrectal or transperineal needle biopsy (Fig. 23-8).

Confirmation of the clinical diagnosis of prostatic adenocarcinoma must be accomplished by histologic review of tissue from the area under suspicion. Closed needle biopsy of the tumor will provide histologic confirmation of the presence of disease. Closed needle biopsy can be accomplished either *via* the perineal or the transrectal route. The transrectal needle biopsy has the advantage of allowing the surgeon to guide the point of the biopsy needle into the areas suspicious for malignant disease. Prophylactic, pre-biopsy, broad spectrum antibiotic coverage has reduced the hazard of post-biopsy prostatitis to less than 1%.

Treatment selection in prostatic adenocarcinoma is based on the extent of the disease. Multiple staging systems have been proposed. (Fig. 23-9, Table 23-19). These staging systems are similar in that they designate the disease as either being confined to the organ of origin, having local spread involving either regional or distant lymph nodes or involving other bone or parenchymal sites (Table 23-20). The disease extent of prostatic cancer is best assessed by sequential application of routine chest and pelvic roentgenograms, radioisotopic bone scanning, and staging pelvic lymphadenectomy. Bipedal lymphangiography and pathologic grading of the primary prostatic tumor can be predictive of nodal extension in a small population of patients.

The recently reported study by the Uro-oncology Research Group clearly defines the impact of radioisotopic bone scanning, lymphangiography, and staging pelvic lymph node dissection in assessing the disease extent of prostatic adeno-

FIG. 23-9. Staging of prostatic adenocarcinoma.

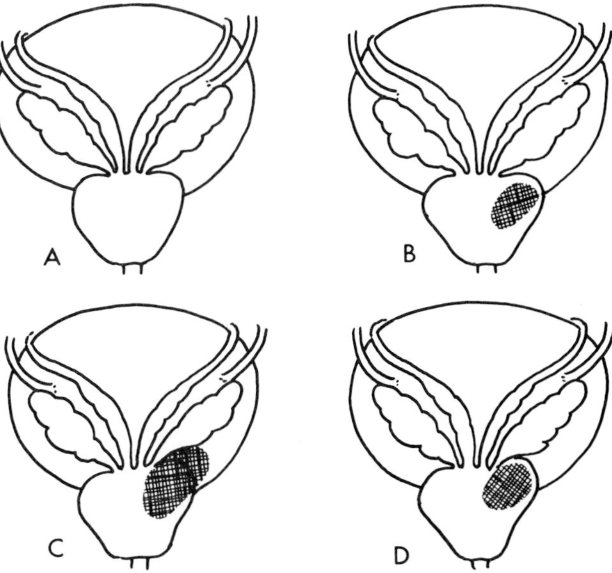

TABLE 23-19. TNM Classification

Primary Tumor (T)
- TX Minimum requirements cannot be met
- T0 No tumor palpable; includes incidental findings of cancer in a biopsy or operative specimen. Assign all such cases a G, N, or M category
- T1 Tumor intracapsular surrounded by normal gland
- T2 Tumor confined to gland, deforming contour, and invading capsule, but lateral sulci and seminal vesicles are not involved
- T3 Tumor extends beyond capsule with or without involvement of lateral sulci and/or seminal vesicles
- T4 Tumor fixed or involving neighboring structures. Add suffix (m) after "T" to indicate multiple tumors (e.g., T2m)

Nodal Involvement (N)
- NX Minimum requirements cannot be met
- N0 No involvement of regional lymph nodes
- N1 Involvement of a single regional lymph node
- N2 Involvement of multiple regional lymph nodes
- N3 Free space between tumor and fixed pelvic wall mass
- N4 Involvement of juxta-regional nodes

Note: If N category is determined by lymphangiography or isotope scans, insert "1" or "i" between "n" and appropriate number (e.g., N12 or Ni2). If nodes are histologically positive after surgery, add "+," if negative, add "−."

Distant Metastasis (M)
- MX Not assessed
- M0 No (known) distant metastasis
- M1 Distant metastasis present
  Specify ____________
  Specify sites according to the following notations:

Pulmonary—PUL	Bone Marrow—MAR
Osseous—OSS	Pleura—PLE
Hepatic—HEP	Skin—SKI
Brain—BRA	Eye—EYE
Lymph Nodes—LYM	Other—OTH

Note: Add "+" to the abbreviated notation to indicate that the pathology (p) is proved.

TABLE 23-20. Preliminary Stage Classification

STAGE	STAGE	AJC CLASSIFICATION	LOCAL LESION	PROSTATIC ACID PHOSPHATASE	BONE METASTASES BY BONE ROENTGENOGRAM
A, Focal	IA	$T_0N_xM_0$	Not palpable, focal	Not elevated	No
A, diffuse	IB	$T_0N_xM_0$	Not palpable, diffuse	Not elevated	No
B	II	$T_1T_2N_xM_0$	Confied to prostate	Not elevated	No
C	III	$T_3N_xM_0$	Local extension	Not elevated	No
D	IVA	$T_{any}N_xM_0$	Any	Elevated	No
D	IVB	*$T_{any}N_{1\text{-}4}M_0$	Any	Any	No
D	IVC	$T_{any}N_{any}M_1$	Any	Any	Yes

* IVB patients can not be assigned a stage classification until after node dissection as this category is reserved for patients with lymph node extension.

carcinoma.[189] In this study, 509 men presenting with newly diagnosed prostatic adenocarcinoma were assigned a preliminary clinical stage based on the results of physical examination, routine bone survey, and serum acid phosphatase. Patients then received in sequence a radioisotopic bone scan, lymphangiogram, and a staging pelvic node dissection, and were assigned a final clinical stage. Technetium-99 medronate bone scanning demonstrated bony metastases in approximately 25% of all patients judged free of disease by a routine bone survey.

Patients believed to be free of bone disease after isotopic scanning were then subjected to pedal lymphangiography and a staging pelvic node dissection. Lymphangiography was accurate in identifying those patients with positive nodal extension. There was only a 12% false-positive rate, but a 22% false-negative rate. The impact of isotopic bone scanning and lymph node biopsy is that over 50% of patients were shifted to a higher disease category following these two staging maneuvers. The impact was greatest in the preliminary clinical stages of I-B, II, and III. Failure to determine the presence of bone or nodal extension by these studies would have resulted in inappropriate treatment selection.

SURGICAL EVALUATION OF DISEASE EXTENT

It is felt necessary to determine whether the malignancy with the prostate is focal or diffuse. Byer and co-workers reported on 148 patients with Stage A focal carcinoma treated conservatively or not at all.[190] Only 6.8% of these patients showed progression of disease. A literature review demonstrated that the death rate from Stage A-1 cancer was only 1.9% in 262 patients. The conclusion is therefore drawn that Stage A-1 carcinoma is best treated by only conservative measures. Stage A-2 or diffuse prostatic adenocarcinoma has a survival rate, however, approaching that of Stage B diffuse carcinoma.

Transurethral resection may be of benefit in differentiating between occult focal and diffuse prostatic adenocarcinoma and may be necessary to establish a national therapy. McMillen and Wettlaufer subjected 27 patients with Stage A adenocarcinoma of the prostate to repeat transurethral resection 3 months after the initial diagnosis.[191] Seven of 27 patients (26%) were found to have significant residual tumor at the time of repeat resection and were reclassified as Stage A-2. Three additional patients had a single focus of adenocarcinoma on a repeat biopsy.

The lymphatic spread of prostatic carcinoma occurs *via* the vasculature which exists from the posterior aspect of the prostate with subsequent extension to the hypogastric (primary), obturator (secondary), external iliac (tertiary), and presacral (quadranary) lymphatics (Fig. 23-10).[192–196] The nodes which are readily opacified by pedal lymphangiography are those nodes of the external iliac, common iliac, and para-aortic lymphatics. This accounts for the relatively low false-positive rates (10%–17%) when the lymphograms are confirmed by node dissection. However, the difficulty in visualizing nodes of the hypogastric and obturator lymphatics, those lymphatics early involved in nodal extension, accounts for the relatively high incidence of false-negative lymphangiography (22%–40%).[189,191,198,199]

The limits of dissection of pelvic lymphadenectomy for staging of prostatic adenocarcinoma vary from author to author. The limits of dissection are variable, some surgeons promoting dissection to the bifurcation of the aorta. The accrued data would indicate that extending the dissection further may increase the amount of nodal material removed, but does not alter significantly the identification of patients with node-positive disease. The preferred method for node dissection is as below.[189,196,200–204]

The pelvis may be entered through the midline or transverse lower abdominal incision. The bladder should be mobilized laterally, and common and external iliac vasculature identified. Dissection may be begun at the bifurcation of the common iliac vessels, carried down the medial inferior margin of the external iliac vasculature to the pelvic floor, medially across the pelvic floor to the inferior border of the prostate, and then superiorly along the hypogastric vessels back to the bifurcation of the common iliac vessels. The tissues surrounding the obturator nerve should be incorporated in the specimen. The obturator artery and vein may be sacrificed. The limitation of node dissection to this area has minimal morbidity without sacrificing accuracy. Comparison of the incidence of identified nodal spread by clinical stage is similar whether the dissection is limited, as described above, or whether it is more extensive. The more extensive dissection which encompasses all the lymphatic vessels around the external iliacs or which goes above the bifurcation of the common iliacs is associated with delayed lower extremity edema and genital edema, particularly in those who subsequently receive full pelvic external beam radiotherapy.[205–209] Pre-sacral and pre-sciatic node dissection adds little to the identification of metastatic disease.[197] Out of 30 patients who were subjected to extensive pelvic node dissection, including the pre-sacral and pre-sciatic areas, only two patients had pre-sacral or pre-sciatic nodal metastasis when there was not also involvement of the external iliac, obturator, or internal nodes.

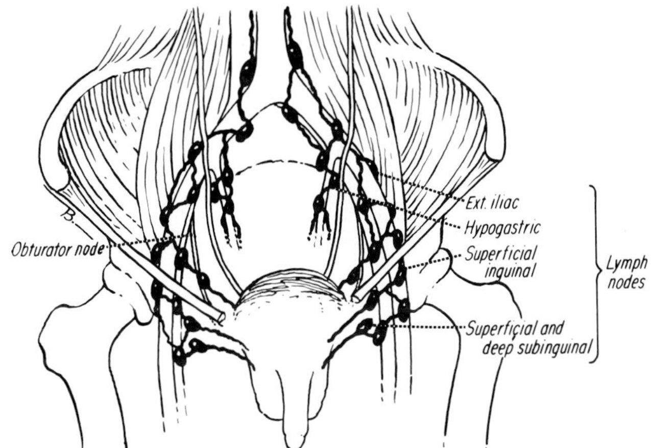

FIG. 23-10. Lymphatic drainage of the prostate.

There is no documented necessity to remove para-aortic lymph nodes to detect nodal spread if the pelvic nodes are negative at the time of dissection. Unpublished data of the UORG have demonstrated that the paralumbar (para-aortic) nodal groups were involved in 12 of 54 (22%) of patients when the external and internal iliac nodes were positive, but in another 54 patients with negative pelvic nodes, all had negative para-aortic nodes. These observations substantiate the earlier studies of Spellman and associates that para-aortic nodal metastases occur only when the pelvic nodes are involved.[210]

Pelvic lymph node dissection is associated with moderate morbidity and occasional mortality. Therefore, it is reasonable to examine methods for identifying nodal disease which avoid node dissection. Pedal lymphangiography has false-positive and false-negative rates which preclude its use as the ultimate predictor. Serum acid phophatase elevation in the presence of a negative isotopic bone scan is associated with an increased incidence of positive pelvic nodes as identified by nodal dissection; however, the accuracy of this predictor is not sufficient to exclude node dissection in this population. The pathologic Gleason sum of the primary prostatic tumor may permit the clinician to predict the presence or absence of positive lymph nodes in a significant portion of the patients.[211] Histopathologic specimens of prostatic biopsies can be classified using the Gleason grading system of tumor differentiation. Primary and secondary patterns of malignant growth may be identified and their numerical sums combined to provide a final overall grade between 2 and 10. Paulson and

TABLE 23-21. Comparison of Gleason Sum with Node Biopsy

GLEASON SUM	NODE BIOPSY *Positive*	*Negative*	*N/Group*	
2–5	13.9%	86.1%	36	
6	32.4%	67.6%	34	
7	49.9%	50.1%	21	$X^2 = 28.2$
8	75.0%	25.0%	12	p .0005
9–10	100.0%	0%	7	
No Diagnosis	33.3%	66.7%	12	

(Modified from Paulson DF, Piserchia PV, Gardner W: Predictions of lymphatic spread in prostatic adenocarcinoma: Uro-oncology Research Group study. J Urol 123:697–699, 1980)

associates demonstrated that patients with low Gleason sums of 2 to 5 had a 14% chance of having positive nodes, while those with a Gleason sum of 9 or 10 had a 100% incidence of positive nodes (Table 23-21). The occurrence of a normal or elevated acid phosphatase level did not enhance discrimination. A corroborating study in another population demonstrated that 93% of patients with a Gleason sum of 8, 9, or 10 had regional nodal metastases regardless of the preliminary clinical stage and that no patient with a Gleason sum of 2, 3, or 4 had nodal disease (Table 23-22). In both series the incidence of positive pelvic nodes in those patients with intermediate sums of 5, 6, or 7 increased progressively as the numbers rose. This data would indicate that histopathologic grading of prostatic adenocarcinoma using the Gleason classification system permits identification of those patients at least or greatest risk for having nodal spread and may provide a methodology for selecting patients in whom staging pelvic lymphadenectomy could be eliminated as a diagnostic maneuver.

The value of serum acid phosphatase elevation to aid in staging prostatic adenocarcinoma has both detractors and supporters.[212–214] It has been proposed that serum acid phosphatase elevation, as determined by the coloremetric assays, occurs only when extension from the primary site has occurred. It is not known whether the radiolabelling technology using either the radioimmunoassay or counter immunoelectrophoresis permits the early detection of metastatic disease or detection of clinically unsuspected local disease. Counter immunoelectrophoresis is reliable and can detect as little as 20 ng/ml to 30 ng/ml of prostatic acid phosphatase. The false-positive rates may be as low as 5%; however, it is felt that this is accomplished at the expense of sensitivity.[213,214] The radioimmunoassay is a more sensitive method, but sensitivity is achieved at the expense of specificity, 10% to 20% false-positive rates being observed.[213,215]

The significance of bone marrow acid phosphatase in patients with prostatic carcinoma is doubtful. The levels of bone marrow acid phosphatase using total and tartrate stable acid phosphatase indicates that the level of bone marrow acid phosphatase gives no supplemental diagnostic information in any patient with prostatic carcinoma. It is doubtful that elevated levels of bone marrow acid phosphatase are diagnostic of early metastases of prostatic carcinoma.[215]

TREATMENT OF PROSTATIC ADENOCARCINOMA

At the present time, multiple modalities are used in the treatment of prostatic adenocarcinoma, with the treatment selection being based on the stage of the disease and the patient and physician bias. The basic therapeutic approaches are (a) radical prostatectomy, (b) interstitial irradiation with ^{125}I combined with pelvic lymphadenectomy, (c) external irradiation to the prostate only, (d) external irradiation to the prostate and pelvic lymph nodes and (e) hormonal manipulation and chemotherapy.

RADICAL PROSTATECTOMY

The philosophy of radical prostatectomy is removal of the primary disease. The anatomic location of the prostate presents technical difficulties in removal of the organ and has led to the development of several approaches for radical prostatovesiculectomy (Fig. 23-11).[216–220] Prostatoseminovesiculectomy consists of radical removal of the prostate and its

TABLE 23-22. Comparison of Gleason Patterns as a Predictor of Nodal Metastatic Disease

PELVIC LYMPHADENECTOMY	NO. PTS.	GLEASON PATTERNS *(2, 3, 4)*	*(5, 6, 7)*	*(8, 9, 10)*
Positive	53	$\frac{0}{31}$ (0%)	$\frac{26}{84}$ (31%)	$\frac{27}{29}$ (93%)
Negative	91	$\frac{31}{31}$ (100%)	$\frac{58}{84}$ (69%)	$\frac{2}{29}$ (7%)

(Modified from Kramer SA, Spahr J, Brendler CB, et al: Experience with Gleason Histopathologic Grading in Prostatic Cancer. J Urol 124:223–225, 1980)

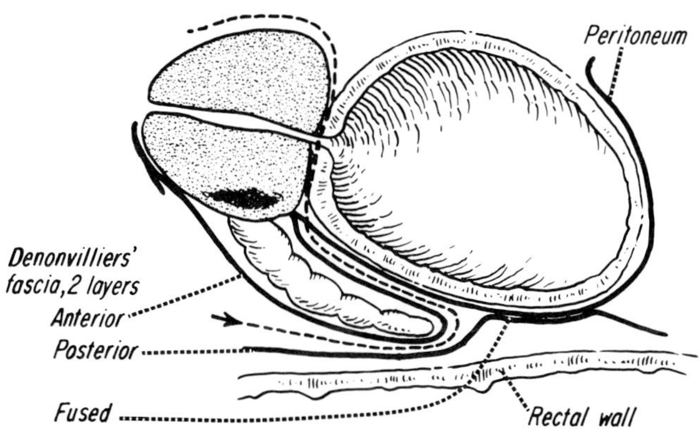

FIG. 23-11. Limits of dissection for radical prostatectomy

investing capsule together with the seminal vesicles, the ampulla, the vas deferens, and the cuff of the bladder in continuity. Carcinoma which is confined to the prostate can be well controlled through this operative procedure. In radical prostatectomy, the prostate should be excised at its junction with the membraneous urethra. No residual of prostatic tissue should be left at the apex. While some authors advocate dissecting the urethra from the distal prostate to decrease the possibility of damage to the membraneous urethrea, no well defined plane exists in this area and a clean line of incision distal to the prostatic apex is more in keeping with the principles of cancer surgery.

The anterior layer of Denonvilliers' fascia, that extension of the obliterated peritoneal layers which separates the rectum from the prostate and provides a posterior barrier to the extension of the prostatic carcinoma, should be removed with the specimen. Although this potential space can be opened to permit development of a hypovascular cleavage plane and diminution of the possibility of rectal injury, it is not necessary, as the posterior layer of Denovilliers' fascia will peel off the rectum without difficulty and provide an additional barrier of fascial investment around the malignancy. The fascia which extends between the bladder and seminal vesicles should be carried with the specimen despite the potential danger of damage to the posterior bladder wall and ureters. These two fascial layers do provide an area for containment of local growth of the tumor.

The vascular supply to the prostate arises from the inferior vesicle artery; both venous and arterial structures course together with their fascia at the vesicoprostatic junction posterior–laterally. The vascular supply of the seminal vesicles also arises from the inferior vesicle plexus and routinely is controlled during the division and ligation of the vascular pedicles of the prostate.

Arterial bleeding often will cease spontaneously, however, branches of the internal pudendal artery adjacent to the prostate may be difficult to control as they retract into the fat surrounding the rectum. In addition, troublesome bleeding may occur if the muscular bulb of the penis is entered or the bladder wall is entered. Venous bleeding usually provides the major blood loss during prostatovesiculectomy. The capsular vein generally drains at the three anterolateral plexus which communicate with veins from the penis. Surgical injury to the rectum or bladder may occur due to the anatomic approximation of these structures to the prostate. If the rectum is entered, the likelihood of fistula formation between the bladder and rectum is enhanced should the operation proceed. The ureters may be damaged if there is dissection within layers of the trigone while attempting to define a cleavage plane between the bladder and seminal vesicles.

Perineal prostatoseminovesiculectomy has the advantage of providing a relatively avascular field for dissection, good exposure for reconstruction of the vesicourethral anastomosis, and postoperative drainage. It has the additional advantage in that it is well tolerated in the elderly patients in whom an intra-abdominal approach may very well compromise pulmonary function. The principal disadvantage is that it does not afford simultaneous exposure of the pelvic lymphatic drainage to the prostate and thus requires a second operative procedure. The primary contraindications to the surgery are ankylosis of the hips and previous prostatic surgery which fixes the prostate and bladder in the pelvis and makes reconstruction of the vesico–urethral junction difficult.

The retropubic route to prostatoseminal vesiculectomy is chosen by many surgeons due to their increased familiarity with the pelvis. The operation has additional appeal in that a simultaneous pelvic lymphadencectomy can be accomplished at the time of surgery, including ureteral reimplantation or cystectomy with urinary diversion, should that operation be necessary during the primary procedure. The disadvantages of the retropubic approach are related to the enhanced vascularity encountered during this route and the difficulty in establishing a direct vesico–urethral anastomosis beneath the pubis. It has been advocated that the symphysis be removed. This does not increase instability of the pelvis post-surgically, but may enhance the degree of post-operative incontinence.

RADIATION THERAPY FOR PRIMARY TREATMENT

At present time, there is no consensus as to the optimal volume to be irradiated in patients with carcinoma of the prostate. In patients with Stage B, intersititial techniques deliver adequate doses of radiation to the prostate only. With interstitial ^{125}I the minimal tumor dose is in the range of 14,000 rad to 15,000 rad. This high dose can be delivered

FIG. 23-12. Isodose curves for interstitial ^{125}I implant. A high dose is delivered to the prostate with rapid fall-off in the adjacent tissues.

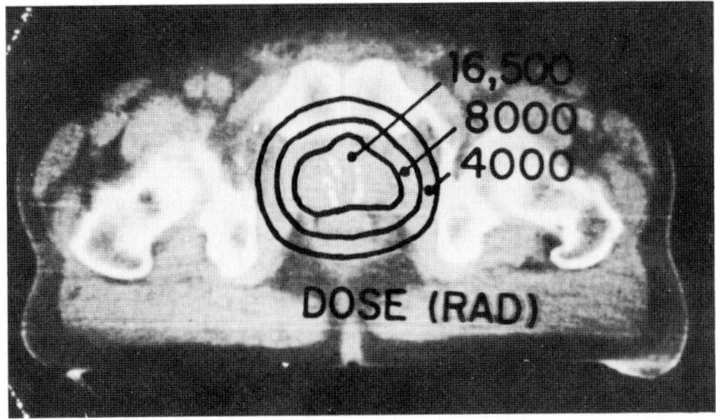

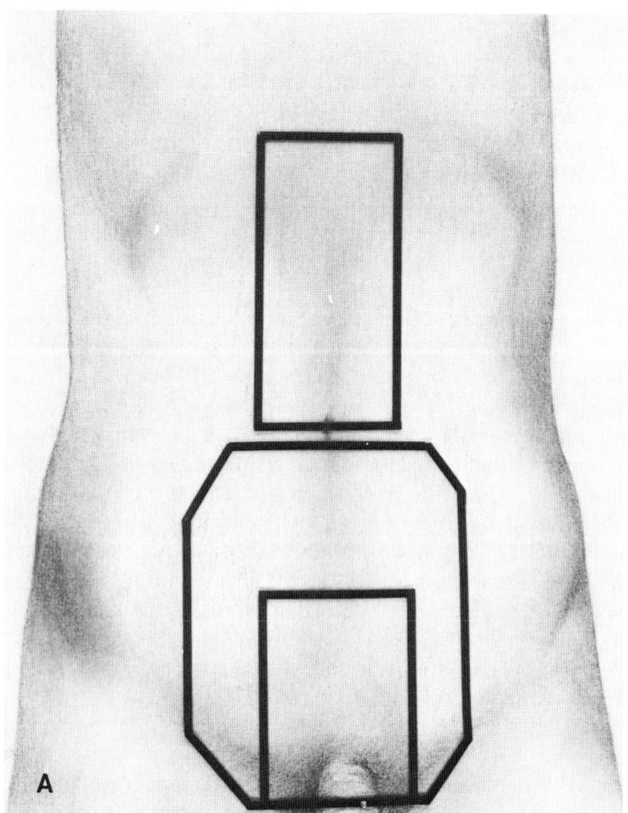

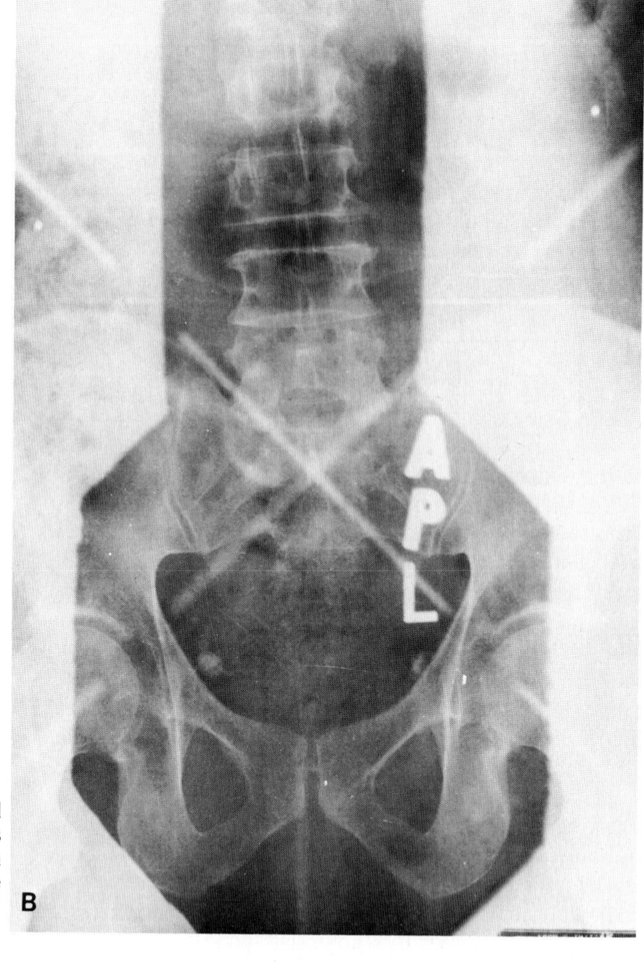

FIG. 23-13. Example of diagram of ports for pelvic lymph nodes and prostate boost. Example of portal for periarotic lymph nodes is illustrated. *B*, Portal for periaortic and lymph node irradiation when a large field is available. This arrangement avoids the juncture of the periarotic nodes and pelvic portals.

because of the rapid fall of brachytherapy and the low energy of the ^{125}I (average 30KV). The bladder and rectum receive doses in the range of 6000 rad with external beam irradiation and 4000 rad to 5000 rad with interstitial therapy (Fig. 23-12). Bagshaw has reported over 80% control of the tumor with relatively localized ports to the prostate and periprostatic tissues, without specific attempts to cover the pelvic lymph nodes.[221] Similar results have been reported by Perez and co-workers in patients receiving at least 5000 rad to the pelvic lymph nodes in addition to a prostatic boost.[222,223] This observation may stem from the fact that patients without lymph node metastases will not benefit from elective irradiation of those lymph nodes and that survival will be the same as in patients treated to the prostate only. In patients with metastatic lymph nodes, as reported by Hilaris and co-workers there is a high incidence of distant metastasis, and irradiation of grossly metastatic lymph nodes may not increase survival either.[224] Thus, we must hypothesize that only a small number of patients with limited metastatic disease in the lymph nodes and without distant micrometastasis will benefit from regional lymph node therapy. Lipsett and co-workers reported similar results in 44 patients with various stages of prostatic carcinoma treated to the periaortic nodes (4500 rad split course) in comparison with 42 similar patients receiving irradiation to the pelvis and prostate only.[225]

The portals for irradiation of the prostate only are usually 8 cm × 10 cm to 10 cm × 12 cm, depending on the size of the gland and periprostatic extensions. At Washington University and other institutions, when the pelvic lymph nodes are irradiated the portals are 15 cm × 15 cm for Stage B and 18 cm × 15 cm for Stages C and D1. The lower margin of the portals should cover the prostatic, membraneous, and bulbous urethra and the upper margin should extend up to the bifurcation of common iliac in Stage B and the proximal iliac lymph nodes in Stage C. The lateral margins are approximately 1 cm lateral to the bony pelvis (Fig. 23-13A). When using small fields localized to the prostate it is important to remember that the seminal vesicles project above the horizontal pubic ramus and the upper margin of the portal should be designed to cover this tissue (Fig. 23-13B).

An example of dose distribution with AP-PA ports including the pelvic lymph nodes and an anterior 270° arc through reduced parts localized to the prostate is shown in Fig 23-14.

In patients with metastatic periaortic lymph nodes, either by lymphangiogram or surgical exploration, it is common practice to irradiate these lymph nodes. The technique may involve a separate peri-aortic port to be placed above the pelvic fields. Calculations for an appropriate gap should be carried out (Fig 23-15A). If the available field size allows it, it is more convenient to use a single field including periaortic and pelvic

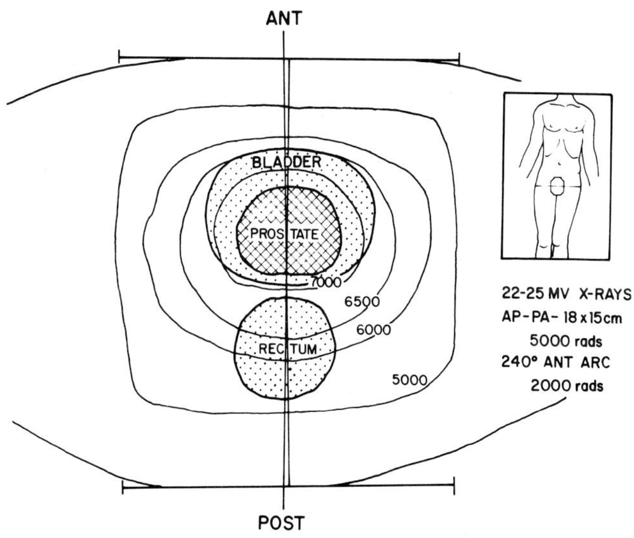

FIG. 23-14. Isodose distribution for external irradiation delivering 500 rad and 2000 rad with 240° anterior arc to the prostate.

volume (Fig. 23-15B). In that case the daily dose should be 160 rad to 170 rad to improve tolerance.

RESULTS OF TREATMENT

A major difficulty in assessing the impact of treatment for cancer localized to the prostate is that many of the studies which have been published did not use the radioisotopic bone scan or pelvic lymphadenectomy to stage the extent of disease. Table 23-23 gives the accumulated survival rate figures at 15 years for patients with localized prostatic carcinoma treated by surgery. The incidence of patient loss at 5 years approximates the incidence of positive pelvic nodes in the patient population for a given clinical stage of disease. All survival figures deteriorate with the increasing pathologic grade. This observation is in keeping with the previous observation that patients with high grade pathologic tumors have a higher incidence of nodal extension, and consequently would seemingly not be controlled by surgical therapy directed at a single anatomic site.

In general, in Stage B, tumor doses of 6500 rad will produce 90% to 100% tumor control in the prostate; in patients with Stage C a tumor dose of 7000 rad has been reported to control the tumor in 80% to 85% of the patients.[205,222,223,226]

At Washington University there were only three local pelvic recurrences in 42 patients with Stage B (7%) and 24 in 141 patients with Stage C (19%). Correlation of the tumor control and dose showed a decreasing number of pelvic recurrences

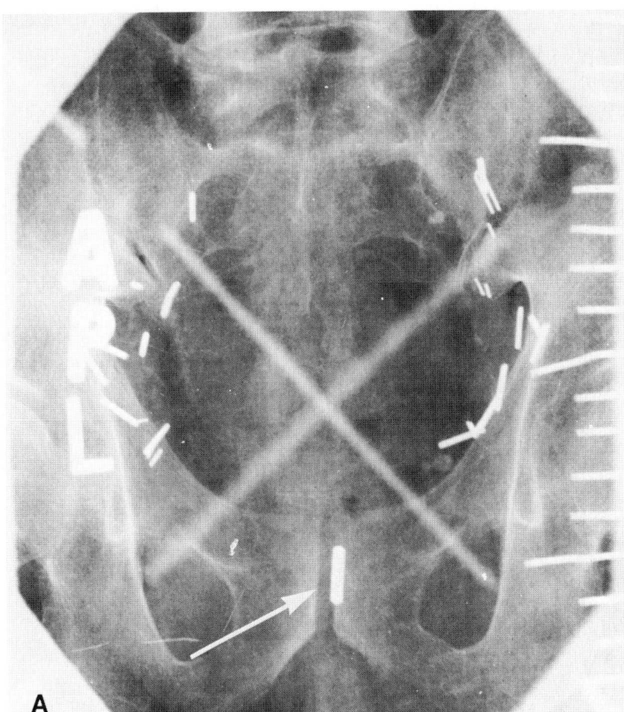

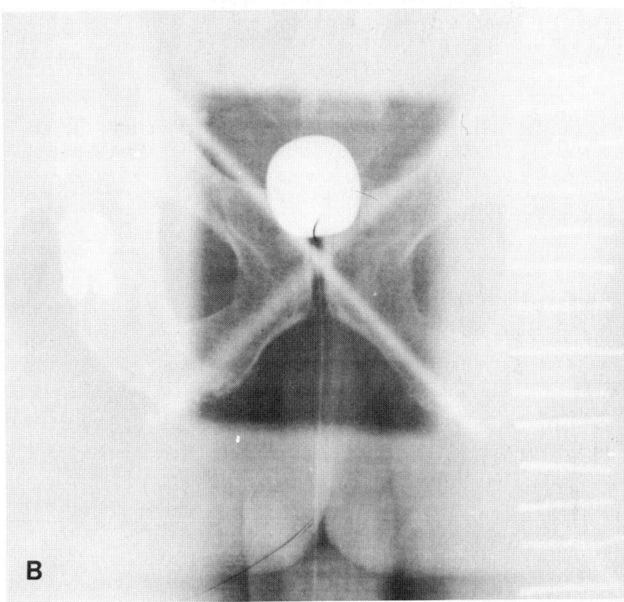

FIG. 23-15. Localization film of the pelvis with eclipse outlining the periaortic nodes and the common iliac lymph nodes and a marker (*arrow*) on the prostate. *B*, Reduced portal for irradiation for prostate and prostatic tissue. Foley balloon with contrast material is outlined in the bladder neck.

TABLE 23-23. Cancer-Free Survivorship 15 Years or Longer After Radical Perineal Prostatectomy

AUTHOR	CLINICAL STAGE	PATHOLOGIC STATE	NUMBER OF PATIENTS	NUMBER SURVIVING	PERCENT SURVIVING
Berlin (1968)		B	116		38.6
Jewett (1968)		B	103	28	27
Culp (1973)	B_1		86	28	33

with higher dose of irradiation (Fig. 23-16). In more extensive lesions, with fixation to the pelvic wall (Stage C), local tumor control was demonstrated in 17 patients treated with 6500 rad and 75% of 36 patients treated with 7000 rad. The tumor-free 5-year survival rate reported after definitive irradiation is about 75% to 80% for Stage B and 55 to 60% for Stage C (Fig. 23-17).

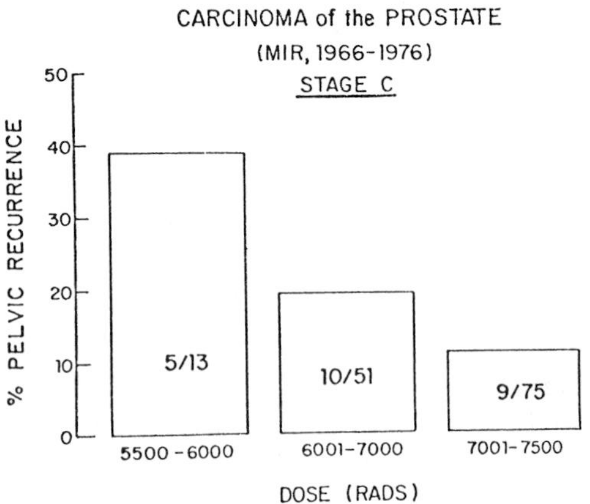

FIG. 23-16. Correlation of pelvic recurrence and doses of irradiation in stage C adenocarcinoma of the prostate. MIR = Mallinckrodt Institute of Radiology.

FIG. 23-17. Tumor-free actuarial survival for patients at the Mallinckrodt Institute of Radiology (MIR) with various stages of disease.

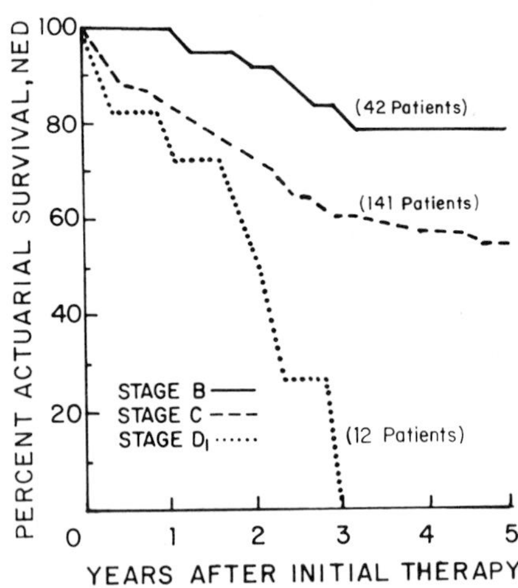

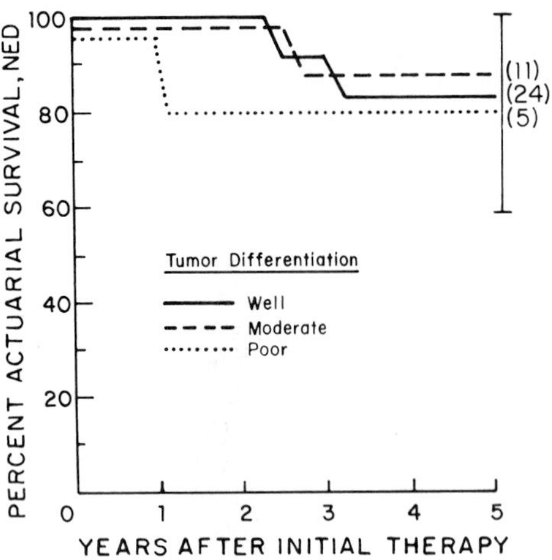

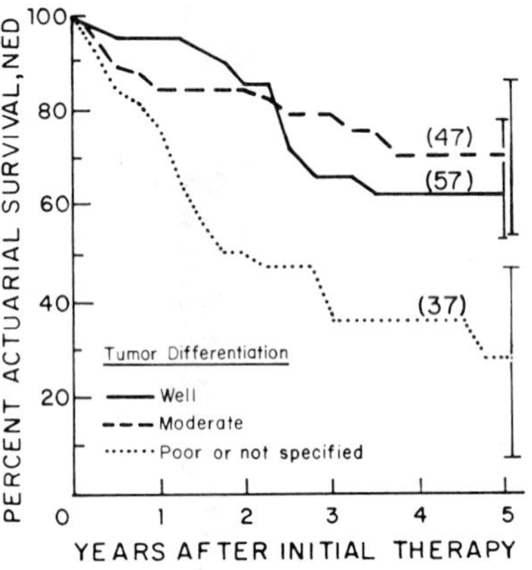

FIG. 23-18. *A* Tumor free actuarial survival in patients with stage B carcinoma of the prostate according to histologic differentiation of the tumor. Two patients on whom slides were not available for review are not included. *B* Tumor-free actuarial survival in patients with stage C carcinoma of the prostate according to histological differentiation of the tumor.

In 40 Stage B patients there was no significant influence of the degree of differentiation of the tumor on survival. However, in 141 patients with Stage C tumors, those with well or moderately differentiated tumors have a 5-year survival rate (Fig. 23-18) of 70% in comparison to only 25% in those with poorly differentiated lesions. Gleason, using a prognostic indicator system which encompasses both the stage and histological differentiation of the tumor, has shown a significantly higher survival rate (over 80%) in patients with small, well differentiated lesions and only about 20% in patients with poor prognostic features.[211]

The time for institution of radiation therapy in relation to the initial diagnosis has been reported by Harisiadis and coworkers and Perez and co-workers to have had some prognostic significance.[222,223] The latter noted that 116 patients with Stage C on whom radiotherapy was instituted immediately after the initial diagnosis had a 5-year survival rate of 65%, as opposed to 45% in 11 patients delayed for from 4 months to 12 months and of 23% in a group of 14 patients with delay greater than 12 months. The majority of the patients on whom irradiation was delayed received hormonal therapy for some months prior to the institution of the irradiation. Several studies comparing the survival after irradiation alone or combined with hormones have shown no significant benefit from this combination. (Fig.23-19)[221,225–227]

When there is severe lower urinary tract obstruction because of prostatic enlargement a trans-urethral resection (TUR) may be necessary prior to irradiation. The incidence of urinary incontinence is high (13%, 8/60) in patients on whom this procedure was performed in comparison with 4.4% (6/135) when the TUR was not necessary. Therefore, it is advisable to wait for from 4 weeks to 6 weeks after the TUR prior to initiation of radiotherapy to allow healing of the tissues.

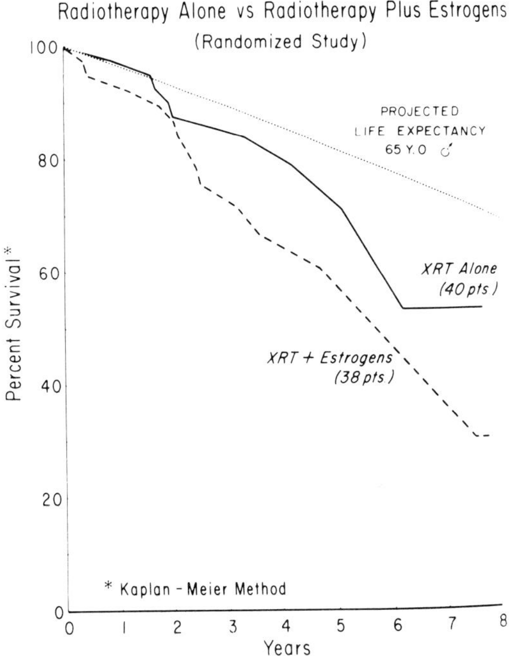

FIG. 23-19. Randomized trial comparing radiation therapy alone or with estrogens. The difference is not statistically significant. (Modified by Neglia WJ, Hussey DH, Johnson DE: Int J Radiat Oncol Biol Phys 2:878, 1977)

COMPLICATIONS OF TREATMENT

Radical surgery will produce erective impotence in virtually 100% of the patients with another 3% to 7% experiencing urinary incontinence of varying degree. All patients treated with irradiation to the pelvis will develop transient symptoms related to the irradiation effects in the small intestine, urinary bladder, and rectosigmoid. Diarrhea, frequency, nocturia, and some bladder spasms, as well as rectal irritation and tenesmus, are common.

These symptoms can be significantly improved with diet, kaolin, pectin compounds, and opiate derivates, and Lomotil and other parasympathiocolytic drugs, to decrease the mobility of the small intestine. Also, we advise the patients to take an abundant amount of fluids (at least 2 quarts daily) to maintain satisfactory bladder capacity. It is important to prevent urinary tract infection. Also, old pyridium, 100 mg to 200 mg three to four times daily, urisep and Mandelamine are useful to decrease bladder irritability. Urispas, 100 mg four to six times daily may be useful to decrease bladder neck spasm. Major complications, which occur in about 3% of the patients, include small bowel obstruction due to fibrosis, severe proctitis with stricture and hemorrhagic cystitis, both of which may require surgical correction (colostomy or urinary diversion). Less severe complications, seen in about 15% of the patients, include chronic cystitis and proctitis (not requiring surgical procedures), persistent diarrhea due to malabsorption syndrome, and edema of the scrotum or the leg. The incidence of leg edema is significantly higher (about 20%) in patients on whom a staging laparotomy is done in comparison to an incidence of less than 2% in those treated with radiation alone. Erectile impotence occurs in about 30% of the patients, the etiology not being definitely established.

Areas of Controversy

Two areas of specific concern are the efficacy of current treatments in managing patients with identified nodal spread and the clinical importance of biopsy-proven disease within the prostate after irradiation.

The practice of obtaining post-irradiation biopsies of the prostate is felt by some to have limited value.[228,229] The probability of observing persistent tumor or microscopic sections seems related to the time after irradiation at which the specimen is obtained. Cox and Kagan noted that in 37 patients on whom serial biopsies were done, it took between 12 months and 18 months to decrease the number of positive biopsies to 20%.[228] Kagan and co-workers reported their experience with biopsy and clinical evaluation in 20 patients with carcinoma of the prostate treated with radiation therapy.[229] Eleven patients had negative biopsies; 17 of the 20 (85%) had a negative clinical examination between 2 years and 7 years after therapy. Three patients had clinical recurrence of tumor and a positive post-irradiation biopsy; however, there were several patients with residual tumor in microscopic sections who never developed pelvic tumor recurrence. Whether persistence of biopsy-proven disease after irradiation represents treatment failure remains speculative. Prostatic adenocarcinoma would be unique among the human tumors if histologic evidence of persistent disease after radiation did not represent treatment failure. The low demonstrated lethality associated with persistent disease may reflect the biology of that disease and not the impact of treatment.

Recent studies have indicated that no treatment may impact significantly in patients with node-positive disease.[230] Forty-four patients with regional node metastasis and negative bone scans after pelvic lymphadenectomy were assigned to treatment with either radical prostatectomy, external beam radiation therapy (5000 rad) to the full pelvic and periaortic nodes

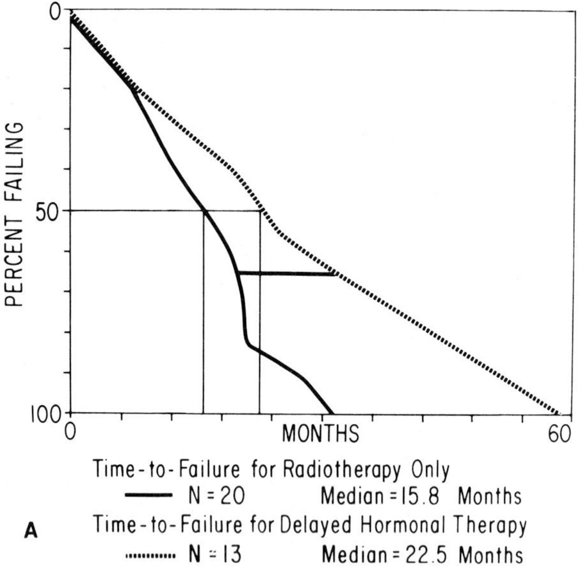

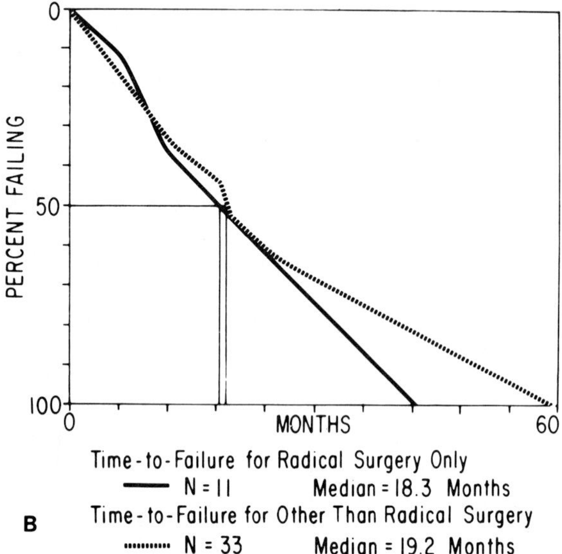

FIG. 23-20. Results of treatment of patients with prostatic carcinoma and regional lymph node metasteses. (Kramer SA, Cline WA Jr, Farnham R et al: Radical prostatectomy in patients with advanced prostatic carcinoma. J Urol (in press))

with a 2000 rad boost to the prostate, or delayed hormonal therapy.

Eleven patients underwent radical perineal prostatectomy, 20 patients received 5000 rad to the full pelvis and peri-aortic nodes to the level of the diaphragm with an additional 2000 rad to the prostate. Thirteen patients were assigned to delayed hormonal therapy with treatment being withheld until progression of the disease was noted. Kaplan-Neier survival curves demonstrated a median survival time of 31.6 months for the entire patient group. Time-to-failure curves were used to permit early identification of treatment effect unencumbered by interposition of a second treatment. Time to first evidence of treatment failure was similar for each of the treatment groups (Fig. 23-20). Comparison of times to treatment failure between the groups showed no disease control benefit of either of the three treatments. The median time of first evidence of failure was just less than 2 years for all treatment groups.

An 8-month difference in time-to-failure (not statistically significant) could be identified in patients having only one positive lymph node compared with those having more than one positive lymph node (Fig. 23-21). Although Barzell and associates reported a better prognosis in patients having only microscopic evidence of lymph node extension, and although the potential for cure in the occasional patient with an isolated nodal metastasis exists, the accumulated data would support the statement that nodal involvement presents a patient at enhanced risk for treatment failure.[231] Therefore, use of local or regional treatments in patients with nodal disease must be tempered by the high failure rate of those treatments. The systematic nature of the disease once nodal spread has occurred should encourage development of treatments which are otherwise directed to systemic control.

MANAGEMENT OF METASTATIC PROSTATIC ADENOCARCINOMA

The observation that adult prostatic epithelium atrophies when the sustaining physiologic effect of androgenic hormones is removed has led to the therapeutic application of androgen ablation or suppression in management of metastatic prostatic adenocarcinoma.[232–235]

Hormonal treatment of prostatic adenocarcinoma is based on the assumption that malignant prostatic epithelium is androgen-dependent as is non-malignant prostatic tissue. Reduction of androgenic support of prostatic epithelia can be accomplished therapeutically by (a) removal of the primary source of circulating androgens, (b) removal or suppression of hypothalamic luteinizing hormone-releasing factor, thereby reducing the release of pituitary leutenizing hormone and reducing testicular testosterone production, (c) direct

FIG. 23-21. Influence of the number of nodal metasteses on time to treatment failure in patients with prostatic carcinoma.

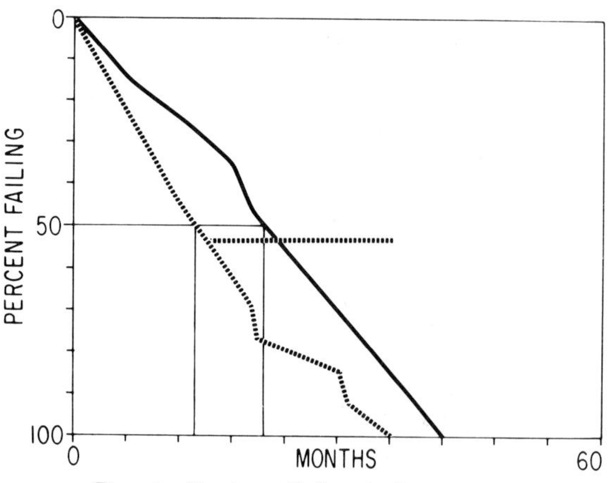

Time-to-Treatment Failure for Patients with One Positive Node
N = 17 Median = 21.5 Months
Time-to-Treatment Failure for Patients with More Than One Positive Node
N = 18 Median = 13.7 Months

inhibition of androgen synthesis at the cellular level, and (d) blocking of androgens or their effect at a cellular level.

Removal of the Primary Androgen Source

Serum testosterone levels in the normal male range between 400 and 1000 ng-percent. Bilateral orchiectomy will reduce plasma testosterone levels by 90%.[236-239] In the adult human male, there is no detectable increase in plasma testosterone levels from activation of secondary androgen sources following orchiectomy. The appearance of endocrine-unresponsive symptomatic disease after bilateral orchiectomy is not associated with demonstrated increases in circulating plasma androstenedione, dehydroepiandosterone or testosterone, indicating that symptomatic recurrence is not associated with an increase in circulating androgens or their metabolic end products.[239]

These studies would indicate that estrogen rescue of patients who progress after orchiectomy on low dose estrogens is unlikely. The published experience of high-dose estrogen-dosage trials supports these observations.

Hypothalamic Suppression

Estrogens establish their major effect at the hypothalamic level by occupying the hypothalamic binding site of testosterone and thus inhibiting the release of luteinizing hormone-releasing factor with subsequent suppression of luteinizing hormone release by the pituitary and reduction in testosterone production by the testes.

Plasma testosterone levels in males treated with 1 mg/day of stilbestrol or its equivalent show variation not only between subjects, but also with respect to serial values obtained during longitudinal observations with a single subject. Serum testosterone levels may not reach anorchid levels. Three milligrams per day of stilbestrol suppresses testosterone levels to the castrate range and doses exceeding 3 mg/day have no additional effect.

Inhibitors of Androgen Synthesis at the Cellular Level

Selective inhibitors of androgen synthesis should produce pharmaceutical orchiectomy, and while certain of these agents are available for clinical trial, none has yet been released with specific indication. Aminoglutethimide will block side-chain cleavage of cholesterol and subsequent hydroxylation, thus inhibiting production of both cortisone and aldosterone.[236] Cyproterone acetate blocks 17, 20-desmolase and thus interferes with androgen synthesis.[240,241] Walsh and Sitteri, using spironolactone, found that plasma testosterone levels were suppressed by 40% to 60%.[240] All three agents have been evaluated in the treatment of endocrine-unresponsive prostatic malignancy, and none has been found effective in reversing the clinical course of this patient population.[236,237]

Antiandrogens

Antiandrogens block the effectiveness of androgens at the target level by interfering with the intracellular events that mediate androgenic action. These agents are capable of inhibiting both endogenously-secreted and exogenously-administered androgens.[244-246] All effective compounds tested to date act through a common mechanism by inhibiting the formation of the receptor-dihydrotestosterone complex, interrupting the binding of a dihydrotestosterone-receptor complex to nuclear chromatin and thereby suppressing RNA formation and protein synthesis. Cyproterone acetate is the most potent of the steroidal antiandrogens. It is well absorbed locally and it not only produces target organ inhibition, but also interferes with gonadotrophin release and inhibits steroidogenesis.

Area of Controversy

The controversy with regard to hormonal treatment of prostatic carcinoma has been engendered by the clinical observation that hormonal manipulation may provide dramatic symptomatic relief and disease regression and the statistical observation that survival of the prostatic cancer patient may not be enhanced by endocrine intervention.[247-251] The resulting uncertainty has focused on the form of endocrine intervention selected, the dose level of exogenous estrogen administered, and the timing of therapeutic intervention in the course of disease. The accepted clinical assumption is that survival must necessarily be prolonged as a consequence of any treatment which appears to effective in reducing the debilitating symptoms of disease progression.

The wide variation in estrogen dosage and in disease staging in the majority of publications to date prevents a rational assessment of the relative benefits and hazards of estrogen control. The randomized study of the Veterans Administration Cooperative Urologic Research Group was established specifically to examine questions raised by the previous publications.[249] Randomized application of four treatments: placebo, placebo plus orchiectomy, diethylstilbestrol 5 mg daily, and orchiectomy plus diethylstilbestrol 5 mg daily was evaluated in 1903 Stage III and IV prostatic cancer patients. In Stage III disease, placebo and orchiectomy plus placebo were significantly better than orchiectomy plus estrogen with respect to overall survival rates. However, less than a 10% difference between the worst and the best treatment groups could be detected 9 years after initiation of treatment. In Stage IV disease, where the competing risk from cancer was significant, no differences in overall survival rates between any of the four treatment groups could be detected at any one time. When Stage III and IV disease were combined and survival curves established, dependent upon death from prostatic cancer alone, diethylstilbestrol, 5 mg daily, and orchiectomy plus estrogen were both more effective than orchiectomy plus placebo or placebo alone.

Subsequent studies by this same group indicated that 1 mg of diethylstilbestrol daily was as effective as 5 mg daily in controlling cancer deaths in either Stage III or Stage IV disease, but that in Stage III disease, where there was less competing risk of death from malignancy, there were fewer cardiovascular deaths on the 1 mg dose than on the 5 mg does. These higher doses were both superior to placebo or 0.2 mg of diethylstilbestrol daily in controlling death from malignant disease. Thus, it would appear that there is a dose-dependent association between the negative effects of diethylstilbestrol on the cardiovascular system and the therapeutic effect in controlling malignancy.

The minimal impact on overall survival rate produced by the various endocrine treatments would indicate that the predictors determining the relative cardiovascular and cancer risks within a specific patient have not yet been established. In recognition of this dilemma of patient selection, it has been recommended that there is little advantage in giving hormonal therapy prior to the onset of symptoms of bone pain or such evidence of active progression as weakness, anemia, progressive outflow, or ureteral obstruction. Considerable controversy exists as to the form that hormonal therapy should take.

It would seem ideal to select a level of hormonal intervention which (a) provides least risk and (b) establishes adequate disease control. Advocates of orchiectomy argue that this maneuver insures removal of the source of continuing testosterone production and negates the necessity for faithful estrogen consumption. Diethylstilbestrol, 1 mg daily, does not produce uniformly anorchid levels of serum testosterone but has less cardiovascular hazard than 5 mg daily. Diethylstilbestrol, 3 mg daily, does produce anorchid levels of serum testosterone; however, the relative cardiovascular hazard of this dose level has not been determined.[236,237] Diethylstilbestrol, 5 mg daily, also produces anorchid levels of serum testosterone but is associated with cardiovascular hazard greater than the 1 mg dose.[237,248,249]

Orchiectomy seems the most sure way of reducing serum testosterone while providing the least cardiovascular hazard. Simultaneous administration of diethylstilbestrol, 1 mg daily, or its equivalent is postulated but unproven to provide additional control at the cellular level. When estrogen therapy with or without orchiectomy is administered, certain biologic effects can be anticipated. Gynecomastia uniformly occurs and may be both physiologically and psychologically painful. Radiation of the breasts (300–400 rad) in a single or divided dose prior to estrogenization will prevent this problem and should be considered in each male before initiation of therapy. Fluid retention and dependent edema usually can be managed with salt restriction and diuretics. Prophylactic anticoagulation with either coumadin or aspirin to reduce the thromboembolic hazards of estrogen control is an attractive treatment adjunct but is unproven.[236–239,249]

CHEMOTHERAPY OF PROSTATIC CARCINOMA

Knowledge regarding the efficacy of chemotherapy in prostatic carcinoma is similar to that noted for urothelial tumors and hypernephroma. In spite of the fact that prostatic carcinoma is a significant contributor to causes of death from cancer, and that more than half the patients have disease extending beyond the prostatic capsule at the time of diagnosis, the knowledge regarding efficacy of chemotherapy for prostatic cancer is quite sparse. Undoubtedly, the advanced age of patients, complicating concurrent medical illnesses, difficulties in monitoring disease responses, and relatively effective (albeit transient) alternative modalities of therapy have contributed to minimizing the experience with chemotherapy for metastatic prostatic carcinoma. The 1970s, however, have seen a change in attitude towards therapy of prostatic carcinoma, and in the 1980s substantial experience in treating this disease will undoubtedly be accrued and will help resolve some of the discrepancies in experience with therapy that have been noted by other authors.

Only approximately 10% of the currently available antitumor drugs have been adequately tested in patients with prostatic carcinoma, as compared to the 34% experience in testicular carcinoma and perhaps as high as 90% or more of currently available drugs having been tested in colon and lung cancer.[252] Evaluation parameters for responses to therapy have been difficult to agree upon, but are now relatively well accepted and include the criteria elaborated by the National Prostatic Cancer Project (Table 23-24). Criteria of an objective response is a 50% reduction in a measurable or palpable soft tissue tumor mass when present, return of a previously elevated acid phosphatase to normal, and the reclassification of some of the osteolytic lesions if present. Criteria of objective progression include significant deterioration in symptoms, weight decrease, or decrease in performance status, appearance of new areas of involvement by malignant disease, and increase in any previously measurable lesion (either soft tissue and lung, but excluding bone) by more than 50% in two perpendicular diameters; however, an increase in acid or alkaline phosphatase alone is not considered a reliable indicator of progression.[252] These criteria have been identified in an attempt to standardize response criteria, since this is a disease which tends to involve predominantly osseous structures and so it has been difficult to clarify responses.

Using the criteria noted above, a number of chemotherapeutic agents have been identified as having demonstrable antitumor activity. In a study of patients with Stage D hormone-resistant prostatic carcinoma, the NPCP prospectively studied the effects of cyclophosphamide or 5-FU compared to a wide variety of conventionally available nonchemotherapeutic agents. Objective responses noted were only in the range of 10% to 15% for both agents; an additional 20% to 30% of patients appeared to have at least stabilization of their disease; if these patients were included in an analysis with the partial responders as having "benefitted," the treatments appeared to be better than the standard secondary or tertiary hormonal management programs.[252] Survival of responders was significantly longer than that of non-responders in these chemotherapy trials; these patients were also noted to live longer than patients treated with further hormonal therapy, but no statistics were reported to verify this statement. Subsequent follow-up protocols from the NPCP included a prospective protocol comparing Estracyt (estramustine phos-

TABLE 23-24. Evaluable Criteria in Prostatic Cancer

A. *Objective Regression*
   1 ⩾50% reduction in two perpendicular diameters in measurable soft tissue tumor mass or masses
   2 Return of an elevated acid phosphatase to normal
   3 Recalcification of osteolytic bone lesions if present

B. *Objective Progression*
   1 Significant deterioration in symptoms, decrease in weight or decrease in performance status
   2 Appearance of new areas of malignant disease
   3 ⩾50% increase in two perpendicular diameters in any measurable lesion (bone excluded)

N.B. An increase in acid or alkaline phosphatase *alone* is not considered an indication of progressive disease

(Bell ET: Renal Diseases, 2nd ed, p 435. Philadelphia, Lea and Febiger, 1950)

TABLE 23-25. Effective Single Agent Chemotherapy for Prostatic Cancer

DRUGS	RESPONSE RATE	EVALUABLE PATIENTS	REFERENCES
5-Fluorouracil	23%	107	329 330
Cyclophosphamide	11%	98	329 330
Nitrosoureas	18%	44	329 260
Adriamycin	29%	42	329 254
Streptozotocin	0%	38	252
Nitrogen mustard	39%	31	329
Vincristine	9%	22	329
Cis-platinum	43%	21	259
Hydroxyurea	46%	13	261

phate) or streptozotocin to standard salvage hormonal management. Response or stabilization rates noted were 19% for standard salvage hormonal therapy, 30% for the estramustine phosphate, and 32% for streptozotocin. However, the only true partial responders noted in the study were in the estramustine phosphate arm.[252] A subsequent follow-up protocol was a prospective study comparing procarbazine, DTIC, and cyclophosphamide. Response rates were 27%, 48%, and 29% respectively, but again included the category of stable patients.[252] Other investigators have reported that adriamycin produces at least a 25% objective response rate.[253,254]

Estramustine phosphate represents a new conceptual approach to prostatic carcinoma, being the nitrogen mustard derivative of estradiol, estradiol-3-N-bis (2-chloroethyl)-carbamate 17-phosphate. This compound is designed to utilize the estrogenic portion of the molecule to promote uptake of the cytotoxic nitrogen mustard moiety. This is based on the assumption that prostatic carcinoma contains an estrogen receptor. Indirect laboratory evidence indicates that estramustine phosphate does indeed compete for estrogen receptors in mammalian tissue.[255] Clinical reports indicate that estramustine phosphate may produce response rates as high as 30% to 55%, but it is not clear whether this would be better than a regimen that included combination therapy with an estrogenic compound and an alkylating agent simultaneously.[256-258] Such a comparative study has not been done. Estracyt is interesting because its dose-limiting toxicity is usually due to the estrogenic effects rather than the alkylating effects of the compound. While now currently available in other countries as an accepted mode of therapy, Estracyt is still under investigation in the United States. An analogous compound, Prednimustine (Sterocyt, LEO 1031) is also undergoing investigation. Using Estracyt as a model, Prednimustine is an ester of prednisone and the alkylating agent chlorambucil. As yet, the data are too preliminary to make any definitive conclusions.[252] Other drugs which have been reported to have effect in prostatic carcinoma include cis-dichlorodiammine platinum II, nitrogen mustard, adriamycin, 5-fluorouracil, and the nitrosureas (Table 23-25).[252,259,260]

The data presented in Table 23-29 represent a collation of a variety of reports which are reasonably convincing in terms of their definition of disease state, treatment regimens, and criteria for response rates.

Several reports now exist regarding the efficacy of combination chemotherapy for prostatic carcinoma. These include the combination of cyclophosphamide and 5-FU (6% objective response rate), Cytoxan and adriamycin (6% response rate), adriamycin and DDP (48% response rate), 5-FU-methotrexate-vincristine-melphalan and prednisone (24% response rate), Cytoxan, 5-FU, and adriamycin (50% stabilization, no objective response data given), and Cytoxan, methotrexate, 5-FU, vincristine and prednisone (37.5% response rate) (Table 23-26).[261-265]

Much of the above noted data has accrued by a collation of a number of series usually containing small numbers of patients with slightly differing criteria of response. As noted, this difficulty relates to the behavior of prostatic carcinoma. The usual criteria for response utilized in chemotherapy trials

TABLE 23-26. Efficacy of Combination Chemotherapy for Prostatic Cancer

DRUGS	RESPONSE RATE	EVALUABLE PATIENTS	REFERENCES
Cytoxan, 5-FU	6%	46	331, 332
Cytoxan, Adriamycin	6%	31	331, 262
Adriamycin, DDP	48%	23	333, 263
5-FU, MTX, Vincristine, Melphalan, Prednisone	24%	25	265
CTX, 5-FU, Adriamycin	50% stabilization	12	334
CTX, MTX, 5-FU, Vincristine, Prednisone	37.5%	16	264

TABLE 23-27. Prognostic Value of Initial Patient Characteristics

VARIABLE	TRAIT A (Number)		MEDIAN SURVIVAL (Weeks)	TRAIT B (Number)		MEDIAN SURVIVAL (Weeks)	p
Race	White	(64)	39.2	Black	(22)	44.2	.789
Age	65	(43)	28.8	65	(45)	57.0	.014
Prior radiation	No	(39)	39.0	Yes	(49)	39.6	.653
Sites of metastases	Bone + other organ	(22)	28.9	Bone only	(63)	45.6	.012
Malignant pleural effusion	Yes	(9)	24.5	No	(79)	41.9	.041
Liver scan	Abnormal	(13)	27.0	Normal	(75)	40.3	.058
LDH	200 U	(63)	29.1	200 U	(35)	62.7	.003
SGOT	50 U	(21)	27.2	50 U	(67)	48.5	.006
Alkaline phosphatase	110 U	(71)	35.4	110 U	(17)	75.9	.013
Acid phosphatase	5 U	(32)	26.5	5 U	(56)	51.7	.010

depends upon patterns of disease which facilitate reproductive measurement of primary or metastatic lesions. Unfortunately, prostatic carcinoma does not readily lend itself to such an analysis. Indeed, in a series of patients reported by Paulson and co-workers, only seven of 85 patients (12%) had either pulmonary nodules or palpable lymph nodes which could be measurable. This group did a multifactorial analysis to determine what other parameters could be reliably utilized in measuring objective responses to prostatic carcinoma.[265–267] Their group approach was to prospectively follow a large number of parameters while treating a group of patients with relatively standard combination chemotherapy. Each parameter was then analyzed statistically to determine whether a change in that parameter, in what would be assumed to be a favorable direction, could in fact ultimately be correlated with any change in the survival of that group of patients.

As had been recognized before by other reports of evaluation of osteoblastic lesions by roentgenogram or scan, intensity of bone pain, or measurements of LDH or SGOT, all fail to have any statistical correlation with subsequent improved survival and can be assumed to be unreliable parameters of response. (Table 23-27).

In contrast, weight gain equal to or greater than 10% original body weight, normalization of previously elevated acid phosphatase, 50% or greater decrease in alkaline phosphatase, and normalization of carcinoembryonic antigen (CEA) levels all had a statistical correlation with improved subsequent survival (Fig. 23-22). Since in virtually all disease, responders to therapy live longer than nonresponders, this prospective analysis to define reliable predictors of survival can be utilized to identify parameters of a biologically important objective response. Note that this important prospective analysis correlates closely with the criteria elucidated by the NPCP noted in Table 23-24; specific comments regarding recalcification of osteolytic lesions were not made in this study because of the limited number of patients presenting with this variant of disease, but extends the concept in terms of utilization of other tumor markers such as acid phosphatase and weight gain. In this study, changes in performance status failed to correlate with subsequent survival. It is hoped that in the future all therapeutic reports will utilize these kinds of criteria, even though to date there is still some controversy as to the reliability of such markers as acid phosphatase.

Recommendations regarding chemotherapy for prostatic carcinoma to date rest upon the data from single agent therapy (Table 23-28). Patients who are candidates for prospective scientific trials should be entered into such trials whenever possible. With the variety of agents that show some degree

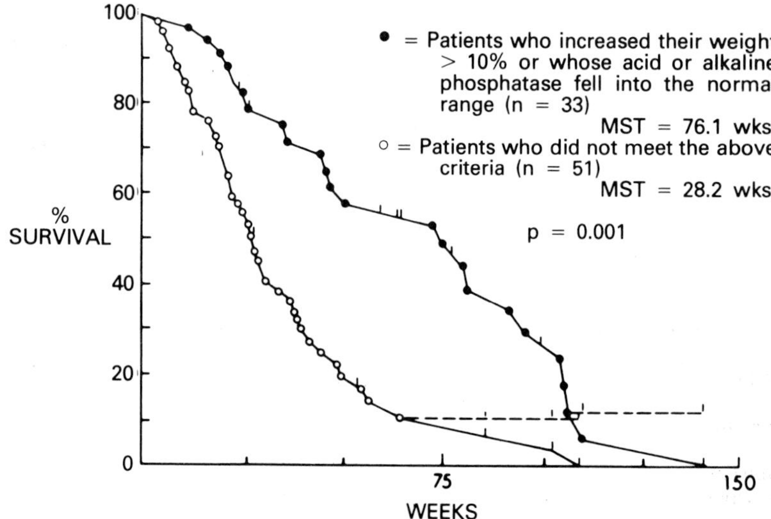

FIG. 23-22. Survival for patients whose acid or alkaline phosphatase values fell to normal or who increased their weight by at least 10% compared to patients who met none of these criteria. MST = median survival time. (Berry W, Laszlo J, Cox E et al: Prognostic factors in metastatic and hormonally unresponsive carcinoma of the prostate. Cancer 44:763–775, 1979)

TABLE 23-28. Recommended Chemotherapy Regimens for Prostatic Cancer

DRUGS	DOSAGE	SCHEDULE	MODIFICATIONS
Cyclophosphamide	1 gm/m^2 IV	q. 3–4 weeks	75% dosage recommended for patients with extensive bony involvement and/or previous radiotherapy
Nitrogen mustard	0.2 mg/kg/day × 1–2 IV	q. 3–4 weeks	Same as above
Cis-platinum	30 mg/m^2/day × 3 or 70 mg/m^2 single dose, IV	q. 3–4 weeks	50% doses recommended for patients with creatinine clearance in range of 50%–60% predicted, should not be utilized except with great caution for patients with creatinine clearance less than 50% of predicted
Hydroxyurea	1–1.5 qm/m^2 per day, p.o. modifications administer daily	Dose schedules to be modified downward based upon CBC results.	
Adriamycin	40–60 mg./m^2 I.V.	q. 3 weeks	Should be used with great caution and/or at reduced doses in people with established active cardiac disease.
5-Fluorouracil	10 mg/k/day × 3 or 15 mg/k	q. 3 weeks q. weekly	Dose modifications *as per* GI tolerance and CBC and bone marrow parameters.
? Drug combinations	?	?	?

of activity, the potential exists for the identification of a combination chemotherapeutic regimen which may have both enhanced efficacy and minimally increased toxicity as compared to standard single agent therapy. To date, however, no such convincing reports exist. Chemotherapy of prostatic carcinoma at this time should consist of a series of sequential single agent treatments, utilizing alkylating agents, *cis*-dichlorodiammine platinum II, hydroxyurea, adriamycin, and 5-FU. Decisions regarding which agents to utilize initially must be made based upon the individual patient. It is highly likely that within the next few years convincing trials will demonstrate the efficacy of combination regimens containing alkylating agents, adriamycin, *cis*-platinum, and antimetabolites such as 5-FU and hydroxyurea. Similar regimens, while toxic, can effectively be given to patients with breast carcinoma, in similar age groups. While such patients usually have less bone marrow involvement than patients with prostatic carcinoma, they often have more pulmonary and hepatic involvement. Thus, carefully designed and administered combination regimens have the potential to improve upon the response rate and survival of patients with prostatic carcinoma.

CARCINOMA OF THE PENIS

Squamous cell carcinoma of the penis accounts for less than 1% of malignancies in men in the United States; however in populations where circumcision is not a common practice and personal hygiene is not well established, squamous cell carcinoma of the penis accounts for 10% to 12% of all malignancies of males.[268,269] Premalignant lesions of the penis have been identified (Table 23-29). Malignant lesions other than squamous cell carcinoma have been identified (Table 23-30). Prognosis correlates well with the stage of disease at the time for initial diagnosis. Unfortunately, although the

TABLE 23-29. Premalignant Lesions of the Penis

	CHARACTERISTICS	TREATMENT
Busche-Lowenstein	Large venacous lesion, histologically benign; may undergo malignant degeneration	Local excision with negative margins. Topical therapy doubtful. Radiotherapy has limited effectiveness, may precipitate malignant degeneration.
Erythroplasia of Querat	Raised, red, velvet lesion; cellular disorientation with multiple mitoses; identical to carcinoma-*in-situ* of skin; 10% to 20% may develop areas of invasive squamous cell carcinoma	Topical 5-fluorouracil twice daily (normal histology, no recurrence up to 70 months); Local excision good, extent of lesion may preclude nonlocal control; radiotherapy is associated with a high recurrence rate.
Paget's disease	Red, locally inflamed area	Local excision
Leukoplakia	White plaque	Local excision

TABLE 23-30. Malignant Lesions of the Penis

	CHARACTERISTICS	TREATMENT
Melanoma	Blue-black or dark brown plaque; neous cells with atypical junctional activity on histologic section	A surgical excision provides good local control, but there remains a high incidence of systemic dissemination—total penectomy with bilateral *en bloc* dissection is advanced but not established as curative.
Sarcoma	Rare: arise from neural or mesenchymal elements; tendency for local growth only.	Wide local excision
Metastatic carcinoma	Usually from bladder, prostate, rectum, or kidney	Local control only: cure usually not obtained, owing to wide metastatic spread of primary.
Leukemic or lymphomatous infiltrate	Rare	Treatment of the systemic disorder.

penis is readily visible, the lesion frequently is ignored when it first appears. This presumably results from patients' reluctance to identify the potential disease in such a psychologically charged organ site. The most common presenting symptoms are phimosis, the presence of a mass, or a nonhealing ulcer.

Many staging systems have been proposed for classification of the disease. The most commonly accepted staging system is that recommended by Jackson: Stage 1: tumors limited to the gland and prepuce; Stage 2: invasion involving the shaft or corpora, but without nodal or distant node metastases; Stage 3: tumor confined to the shaft, but with proven regional node metastases; and Stage 4: tumor invasive from the shaft with inoperable regional node metastases or with distant metastases(Table 23-31).[269] Comparison with the TMN system is recommended (Table 23-32). It is estimated that 50% to 60% of patients are diagnosed as a Clinical Stage 1 at the time of presentation; however, some isolated series report an incidence as low as 30% for Stage 1 disease.[149,269-272]

SURGICAL TREATMENT

Two primary problem areas exist in disease management. The first is the selection of the appropriate treatment for the primary lesion, the second area is evaluation of nodal extension and treatment for patients with identified nodal disease.

Treatment of the Primary Lesion

If cure is to be expected, adequate control of the primary tumor must be accomplished. Surgical therapy involves removal of the lesion with adequate margins to insure failure of local recurrence. Small tumors which are limited to the prepuce are best treated by circumcision alone. Lesions which are felt on physical examination to involve the skin only without involvement of the underlying structures may be controlled by excisional biopsy. Following removal of the primary lesion, margins peripheral to the initial line of incision or deep to the visible tumor must be obtained to exclude invasion beyond the surgical margins. Penectomy, either partial or total, is indicated for lesions which, by the nature of their size, invasiveness, or location on the shaft, are not amenable for more conservative treatment. Partial penectomy requires that a 2 cm margin of grossly normal shaft be available proximal to the primary lesion. For lesions which approach the base of the shaft or for extensive lesions, total penectomy should be accomplished with excision both of the corpora and creation of a perineal urethrostomy.

TABLE 23-31. Carcinoma of the Penis

JACKSON	TMN
I	$T_1,T_2N_0M_0$
II	T_1,T_2,N_0,M_0
III	T_1,T_2,T_3N_1,N_2,M_0
IV	$T_1,T_2,T_3,T_4,N_0,N_3,N_4,M_0,M_1$

(Modified from Jackson SM: The treatment of carcinoma at the penis. Br J Surg 53:33, 1966)

Partial Penectomy

Following prepartion of the patient for surgery, the lesion should be excluded from the operative field by placement of a thick gauze or a condom over the primary site. A bloodless field may be obtained by placement of a tourniquet in the form of a small Penrose drain or a small red rubber catheter around the base of the shaft (Fig. 23-23). The skin should then be incised circumferentially 2 cm proximal to the margin of the tumor. The corpora may then be amputated to the level of the urethra. The dorsal vasculature should be controlled by ligation. The urethra may be dissected distally for a length of .5 cm to 1 cm to provide a margin for reconstruction, care being taken to maintain adequate distance from the primary tumor. The cut margins of the tunica albuginea surrounding the corpora cavernosum should then be approximated using an interrupted mattress suture. Redundant urethra should be spatulated on the dorsal surface and a mucocutaneous closure established with interrupted 4-0 chromic suture. The skin of the shaft is then brought over the repaired ends of the corpora cavernosum to complete the repair. An indwelling Foley catheter should be left for 5 days to 7 days to permit initial healing.

Total Penectomy

After surgical preparation of the patient and isolation of the primary lesion, an eliptical incision is made around the base

TABLE 23-32. Squamous Carcinoma of the Penis TNM Classification*

T		N		M	
TX	Minimum requirements cannot be met	NX	Minimum requirements cannot be met	MX	Minimum requirements cannot be met
TO	No evidence of primary tumor	NO	No evidence of involvement of regional lymph nodes	MO	No evidence of distant metastases
TIS	Carcinoma *in situ* (Bowen's disease, erythroplasia of Queyrat)	N1	Involvement of a single regional node	M1	Distant metastases present
T1	Tumor not more than 1 cm in largest dimension and clearly superficial	N2	Involvement of single bilateral inguinal nodes or multiple unilateral nodes	M1a	Evidence of occult metastases based on biochemical and/or other tests
T2	Tumor 1 cm in any dimension and clearly superficial	N3	Fixation of regional nodes or ulceration of skin over involved regional nodes	M1b	Single metastasis in a single organ site
T3	Tumor of any size invading underlying tissues	N4	Involvement of juxtaregional lymph nodes	M1c	Multiple metastases in a single site
T4	Tumor invading adjacent structures, that is, corpus, urethra, symphysis, perineum			M1d	Metastases in multiple organ sites

* Minimal requirements for tumor (T) include clinical examination with biopsy; for nodes (N) clinical examination, lymphography, and/or urography; for distant metastasis (M) clinical examination, chest x-ray film, lymphography and/or metastatic bone studies. The regional nodes are those of the superficial inguinal region. Juxtaregional nodes are those of the external iliac chain below the bifurcation of the common iliac artery and those of the hypogastric region.

of the penis. Suspensory ligament should be identified and divided and the vasculature controlled at the level of egress from the perineal diaphragm. The corpora should then be dissected sharply from the ischium until a minimum of a 3 cm gross tumor margin is established. The urethra may be divided 2 cm proximal to the tumor margin itself. The urethral stump then is mobilized for creation of perineal urethrostomy. An Allis clamp may then be placed on the perineal body and a 1 cm eliptical bud of skin removed. With alternating sharp and blunt dissection, a direct tunnel may be established to permit placement of the urethra without angulation. The urethra should be spatulated on either the dorsal or ventral surface to prevent meatal contracture with healing. Local recurrence is rare in patients treated in this manner. Tumors of the glans penis itself should not be locally excised as malignancies in this area have a tendency for broad local spread due to early involvement of the vascular plexus of the glans. Forty percent of locally excised lesions of the glans will recur and either partial penectomy or radiation must be considered for lesions in this area.

MANAGEMENT OF REGIONAL LYMPH NODE EXTENSION

A primary problem in management of carcinoma of the penis is the treatment of the regional lymphatics. The freely anastomosing lymphatics of the prepucial skin and the skin of the shaft converge at the base of the shaft itself. The lymphatics thereafter drain bilaterally to the superio–medial group of superficial inguinal nodes. Superficial inguinal nodes are located within the deep membraneous portion of Camper's fascia superficial to the deep fascia of the thigh, the fascia lata (Fig. 23-24)[273–276] Lymphatics thereafter drain into the deep inguinal lymphatics which accompany the femoral

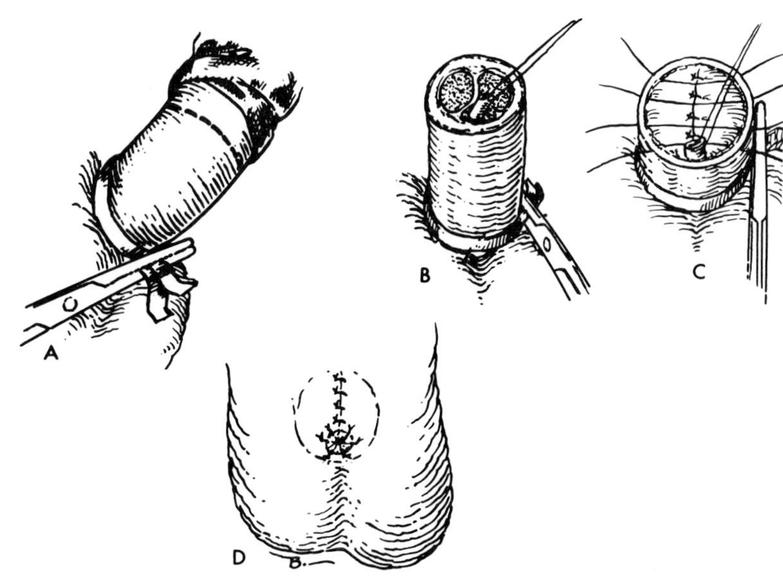

FIG. 23-23. *A*, Base controlled by tourniquet; *B*, guillotine amputation of shaft with preservation of urethral segment; *C*, closure of fascia of corpora cavernosa; *D*, final skin closure.

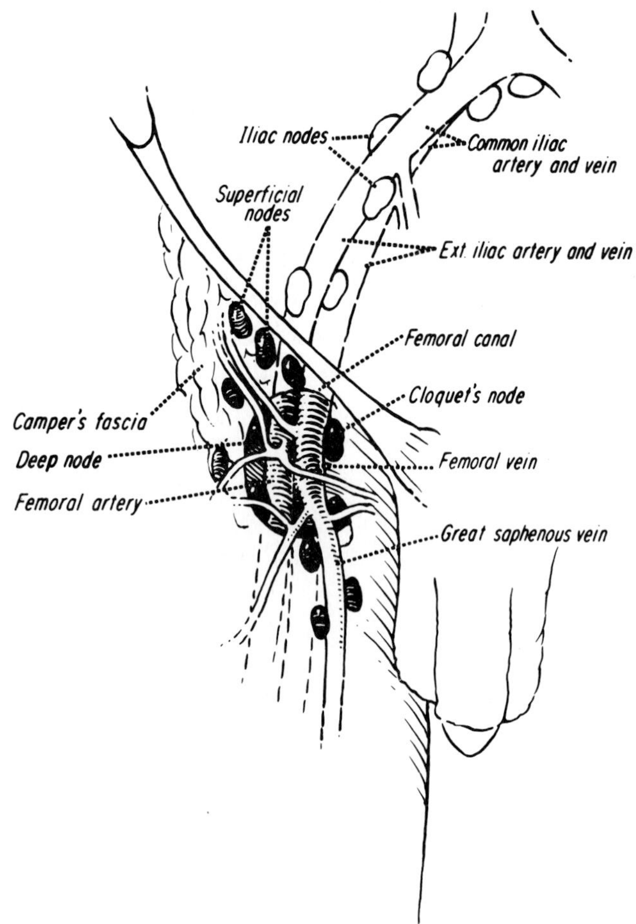

FIG. 23-24. Lymphatic drainage of penis.

vessels and extend to the external iliac, common iliac, and peri-aortic lymphatic channels. Invasion of the corpora convernosum or the posterior portion of the urethra also implies early involvement of the deep pelvic lymphatic structures of the hypogastric and obturator node chain.

Controversy surrounding management of lymphatics concerns the philosophy of treatment intervention in the face of clinically positive nodes *versus* treatment intervention in the face of no identifiable nodal disease. Much of the controversy revolves around clinical assessment of regional nodes. Clinical evaluative assessment of regional nodes is particularly perplexing in penile carcinoma. The incidence of palpable nodes in patients presenting with carcinoma ranges between 35% and 60%.[270,277] Approximately 35% of these patients will fail to demonstrate positive nodes if node dissection is undertaken.[270,278] The staging error is also compounded when one examines a population of patients with clinically positive nodes, who, after a negative node biopsy, subsequently develop regional nodal disease. Approxmiately 10% of patients with clinically positive nodes that are negative on node biopsy subsequently will demonstrate regional disease.[270,279,280,281]

This data would argue that biopsy, alone, of a clinically positive node is not sufficient, but that a patient should have, as a minimum, a superficial inguinal node dissection. When the nodes are clinically positive, node dissection is subsequently advised. Approximately 40% to 55% of patients with positive nodes have disease control after node dissection, whereas progressive disease with death occurs in approximately 2 years to three years in those patients who fail to undergo treatment.[278,282–285] The present controversy concerns the issue of early node dissection for patients with clinically negative nodes *versus* operation only after identification of clinically positive nodes. Regional metastaic disease is seldom seen in lesions which fail to invade the corpora.[270,278] However, the presence of inguinal adenopathy is common, and usually reflects inflammation at the site of the primary tumor. Only nodes which are enlarged at 3 weeks to 5 weeks following adequate local excision should be considered clinically positive.[270,283,284]

Only 25% to 35% of those patients with pathologic Stage I primary lesions will have persistent adenopathy 3 weeks following surgical excision of their primary lesions.[270,279] The late development of nodal extension to the groin after adequate excision of non-invasive primaries occurs only in 5% to 11% of patients. The low incidence of metastatic nodal disease therefore, makes routine ileoinguinal node dissection difficult to justify for Stage 1 tumors.[270] However, pathologic invasion of the corpora cavernosum is associated with a higher possibility of nodal extension. Two-thirds of those patients with invasive primary disease will have proven nodal extension at some time during their follow-up period.[270,279,283] When the primary lesion invades the corpora, 70% to 75% of clinically positive nodes persisting 3 weeks to 5 weeks after removal of the primary will be pathologically positive. However, there is no evidence that "prophylactic" node dissection in the presence of clinically negative disease produces enhanced survival. Although some reports indicate that with invasive disease, 16% to 20% of patients with surgically negative nodes will develop positive nodes, other reports give incidence figures as low as 2%.[274,277,279,280]

There also is evidence to indicate that delaying surgery until regional metastases clinically are palpable does not decrease the chance for surgical control.[285,286] Extrum and Elsmyr identified a 50% disease control rate in patients who had node dissection delayed until adenopathy was evident on followup.[285] Few and co-workers identified no cancer deaths in patients in whom lymph node extension was deferred until the presence of clinical node disease was evident.[286] The controversial report of Breggs and Spratt indicated that the mortality of lymphadenectomy of 1% was approximately equal to that of patients who died of cancer due to delayed nodal excision.[277] Given this background, it seems appropriate to establish a policy for the management of penile carcinoma. Patients with pathologic Stage I disease, those who do not show evidence of invasion, and who have no clinically palpable disease 3 to 5 weeks after primary section, can be safely monitored with careful clinical evaluation of nodal extension with the intention of delayed resection should such extension be evident. Patients who demonstrate invasion of the corpora at the presentation are at a greater risk for developing nodal extension. However, it seems reasonable to delay dissection 3 to 5 weeks to permit inflammatory changes to resolve and permit a more accurate assessment of nodal disease. The clinically positive nodes should be biopsied to determine the presence of nodal disease. The incision should be chosen so as not to compromise a formal node dissection. In the presence of nodal disease, attention should then be turned immediately to the external iliac and internal iliac node-bearing chains. If no deep gross pelvic adenopathy is present, following completion of a bilateral deep pelvic node dissection, a superficial and deep unilateral dissection on the side of the positive biopsy should be conducted.

Initial bilateral dissection should be established if metastatic disease can be documented in either regional node group at the time of initial evaluation, as bilateral positive adenopathy can be demonstrated in up to 60% of patients who so present.[285] However, unilateral node dissection in the patient who is managed by delayed or interval lymphadenectomy is reasonable, as the contralateral spread in these patients is less than 10%.

TECHNICAL ASPECTS OF LYMPHADENECTOMY

Three weeks to 5 weeks after resection of the primary tumor or in the patient who subsequently develops clinically positive disease, the side in question should be biopsied. As mentioned previously, the primary area of drainage is to the superiomedial nodes of the superficial inguinal lymphatic chain. The skin incision should be chosen in such a way so as not to compromise subsequent superficial inguinal node dissection. The preferred incision is a single oblique incision inferior to the inguinal ligament. The vasculature of the inguinal region is such that the vessels that supply the inferior and superior skin flaps are parallel to the inguinal ligament. The oblique incision reduces the possibility of transection of these vessels, which are necessary for adequate vascularization during healing. The incidence of skin sloughs and wound disruption is lower in patients who are treated with oblique incisions rather than with vertical or S-shaped incisions.[286,287] Following skin incision, the node in question and any surrounding nodes should be removed in an excisional biopsy. In the face of negative nodes, a superficial inguinal node dissection should be accomplished.

The patient should be placed supine with the leg on the operative slightly abducted and externally rotated. A small sandbag may be placed beneath the knee. The scrotum may be sutured to the contralateral thigh to facilitate exposure. The major anatomic landmarks of the umbilicus, pubic tubercle, and anterio-superior iliac spine must be within the surgically prepared operative field. The skin flaps should be 2 mm to 4 mm in thickness, carried to the inguinal ligament superiorly with the distal margin being approximately 8 cm to 10 cm from the inguinal ligament. The prepubic node should be considered in this area of dissection. The skin margins should be manipulated with either traction suture or skin rakes to minimize devascularization. At the limits of the dissection, the subcutaneous tissue is sharply incised down to the fascia lata. The saphenous vein is ligated at the distal margin of the dissection and at the site of its entrance into the femoral vein. It is reasonable to place interlocking mattress sutures at the borders of the dissection to control lymphatic drainage. When a superficial and deep inguinal node dissection is being considered, the subcutaneous tissue is incised through the fascia lata down to the muscle using the margins

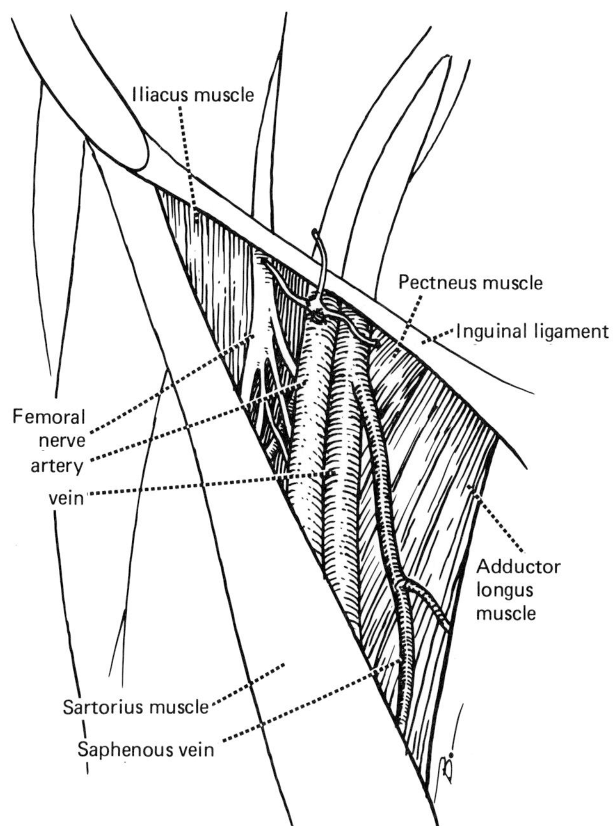

FIG. 23-25. Anatomic limits of deep groin dissection.

of the femoral triangle indicated in Fig. 23-25 as the limits for the deep dissection. The floor of the femoral triangle is formed by the iliopsoas and pectineus muscles and its roof by the fascia lata. The femoral triangle contains the nodes of the deep inguinal lymphatics and these nodes must be removed completely to satisfy the demands of a radical ileoinguinal lymphadenectomy. After completion of mobilization of the superficial lymphatic package, the lymphatics within the femoral triangle are kept in continuity with superficial specimen and the femoral vessels are stripped of all surrounding tissues, including the vascular adventitial tissues. The lymphatic bearing tissues are dissected off the pectineas and a specimen is dissected free to the level of the femoral canal. At this point, the specimen can be transected and the deep and superficial dissections delivered separately or the deep pelvic and superficial inguinal dissections can be done in continuity. At the completion of the dissection, Poupart's ligament should be sutured to the transversalis fascia to prevent femoral herniation in the postoperative period.

The femoral vessels should be protected postoperatively. The sartorious may be sectioned at its origin near the anterior superior iliac spine and transposed to cover the femoral vessels. The transected end of the muscle may then be sutured to the medial aspect of the inguinal ligament with the borders of the muscle sutured to the adjacent musculature. An alternative method is to approximate the pectorius and abductor longus over the femoral vessels.

TABLE 23-33. Ilioinguinal Node Dissection

COMPLICATIONS	INCIDENCE	PERIOPERATIVE COUNTERMEASURES
Skin flap necrosis	14–65%	Oblique inguinal incision Skin flap thickness Care in tissue handling Transposition of sartorius muscle Excision of ischemic flap margins
Wound infection	10%	Interval resolution of region inflammation Mechanical bowel preparation Prophylactic antibiotics
Sarcoma/lymphedema	19–45%	Ligation of transected lymphatics Transposition of sartorius muscle Closed catheter suction drainage Immobilization of dissected extremity Elastic support stockings

The skin margins should be closed without tension over large suction catheters to prevent lymphatic accumulation. The patient should be kept at bedrest during the postoperative period for a minimum period of 7 days to 10 days with the thigh slightly flexed to reduce tension on the suture line. Compression dressing should be maintained on the lower extremity for at least 7 days following surgery. Mobilization should be deferred until the wound suction has been withdrawn.

Pelvic Lymphadenectomy

The pelvic lymphadenectomy should be accomplished through a midline incision with the superior margin of the dissection being bifurcation of the common iliac bilaterally.

The technique of dissection is similar to those described elsewhere and the reader is referred to that section.

Complications

A recent complication of inguinal lymphadenectomy is necrosis of the skin flap, reported as high as 60% (Table 23-33). Necrosis usually is first noted in the midportion of the wound and occurs between the fourth and twelfth postoperative days. This should be managed by careful debridement of the involved area, and skin grafting as appropriate. Lymphedema is the most common delayed complication. Lymphedema rarely occurs following superficial inguinal dissection alone; however, after radical ileal-inguinal lymphadenectomy, it is seen in up to 40% of patients. During the early postoperative period, lymphedema can be reduced with compression stockings. In anticipation of this complication, patients pre-operatively should be fitted for elastic stockings. Continued lymphatic drainage may result if the transected lymphatics are not ligated. Small collections of lymphatic fluid beneath the flaps should be managed by aspiration and pressure dressings and by continued elevation and immobilization of the involved extremities.

IRRADIATION OF PENILE CARCINOMA

Radiation therapy can be used for the treatment of small primary squamous cell carcinoma of the penis or for palliation in advanced non-resectable tumors or lymph node metastasis.[289,290] Irradiation alone will control the tumor in a significant number of patients, thus avoiding anatomical and functional deficits that may produce devastating psychological effects on the patients.[291-300] In addition, if radiation therapy fails, a surgical procedure may control the recurrence if it is not too extensive and metastases are not present. In general, because of poor tolerance, irradiation is not frequently used for the elective treatment of inguinal lymph nodes. However, in patients with recurrent or inoperable metastatic lymph nodes, effective palliation can be achieved with relatively high doses of irradiation (5500–6000 rad in 5–6 weeks).

The techniques of irradiation can be divided into three groups.[2]

1. *Low energy orthovoltage* (60–150 KVp) has been used for the treatment of relatively superficial invasive carcinoma or for carcinoma-*in-situ* (including the erythoplasia of Queiralt). The lesion is treated with a margin of 1 cm to 2 cm beyond visible or palpable tumor. Higher energy beams with filtration, 4 mm to 8 mm (aluminum or .25 mm copper) can be used, depending on the thickness of the lesion. Doses in the range of 6000 rad in 5 weeks to 6 weeks will produce local control in most instances.
2. *Megavoltage irradiation* is necessary for infiltrating tumors with thickness greater than .5 cm. It is also required for the irradiation of inguinal lymph nodes. When the tumor in the lymph nodes is infiltrating the skin, bolus should be used to avoid skin-sparing effect.

   For the treatment of the primary lesion, the entire penis should be included in the irradiated volume. This can be done with appositional portals using special positioning devices. The doses of irradiation should be 6500 rad to 7000 rad, five weekly fractions, in 5 weeks to 7 weeks depending on the volume treated.

3. *Interstitial implants* with ^{226}Ra, ^{137}Ce, ^{192}Ir, or other radioactive materials has been used for superficial tumors or for those with limited infiltration (less than .5 cm). With larger lesions a combination of megavoltage, external irradiation, and interstitial implants to increase the dose to residual tumor should be used. Doses in the range of 6000 rad in 6 days are usually delivered with interstitial therapy.

Another method for treating primary tumors of the penis is surface molds containing radioactive sources.[299] This modality should be limited to superficial tumors in the distal portion of the organ. The doses of irradiation are similar to those given with interstitial therapy (6000 rad in 6 days, dividing several fractions during the week).

Haile and Delclos reported on 20 patients with carcinoma of the penis primarily treated by radiotherapy and 16 by preoperative irradiation and partial or total penectomy.[293] In the 20 patients treated by radiation alone, there were two failures requiring partial amputation. In addition, two radiation complications required partial amputation. Thus, 80% of the patients had conservation of this organ. In the 16 patients treated with pre-operative radiation and surgery, there was tumor control in all patients, but with loss of penis.

The authors advocated elective irradiation of the inguinal pelvic lymph nodes for patients in high-risk groups (large lesions or undifferentiated tumors) when no clinically palpable nodes were present. A dose of 4500 rad to 5000 rad in 4.5 weeks to 5 weeks was delivered. This procedure controlled the tumor in a few patients treated. Irradiation of clinically positive nodes was not as effective even when combined with a node dissection. Patients without clinically palpable nodes, in general, were not treated, since prophylactic groin dissection has no value in these cases because of the relatively low incidence of subsequent metastatic lymph node development. Only one of 16 patients without treatment had an inguinal lymph node failure.

In cases in which irradiation is used to treat the lymph nodes, both inguinal and pelvic nodes to the common iliac bifurcation should be irradiated with paralleled AP and PA portals. Because of the anterior position of the lymph nodes, an unequal loading favoring the anterior portals can be used. For elective treatment, without clinical evidence of metastatic tumor doses in the range of 5000 rad in 5 weeks are adequate. In patients with metastatic unresectable or recurrent lymph node the same portals can be used to deliver doses in the range of 6500 rad in 6 weeks. As was indicated previously, bolus should be used if there is infiltration of the skin or the superficial subcutaneous tissues by the tumor. Special skin care must be instituted in order to prevent moist epidermitis and serious discomfort to the patient. The prevention of infection is critical in the satisfactory completion of the radiation therapy.

Jackson reported on 79 patients treated by radiation therapy and 51 treated by surgery.[294] The 5-year survival rate following irradiation was 61% in comparison to 53% for those treated with surgery. However, the patients treated in the surgical groups had more advanced lesions in a larger proportion. Also, irradiation controlled the primary tumor in 40 of the patients and amputation was necessary for the irradiation failures. Jackson reported inguinal lymph nodes developing in 20% of the patients initially treated with radiotherapy to the penis and that 10% of the patients died because of the inguinal lymph node metastasis.[294] Almgard and Edsmyr described the results in 16 patients treated with irradiation alone, usually orthovoltage (140–150 Kv, the total dose not stated in their publication).[289] There were four local recurrences which were treated with a local radical excision and all survived after salvage therapy. Of the 16 patients, two developed small necrosis of the glans and one, a urethral stricture. In 17 patients local radiotherapy was followed by amputation of the penis, four of them for suspected recurrence. Sixteen of the 17 patients were reported tumor-free from 5 years to 32 years after therapy.

Palliation

Palliation can be achieved in patients with advanced ulcerated or infiltrating tumors, which sometimes may involve the entire penis, adjacent scrotum, and abdominal wall. A direct appositional port may be adequate and doses in the range of 4000–6000 rad may provide temporary tumor regression with decreased pain, bleeding and healing of neoplastic ulceration.

Postoperative Irradiation

In patients on whom complete resection of the gross tumor is carried out, but there is question or evidence of inadequate margins at the primary tumor or the lymph nodes, postoperative radiation may be utilized. Doses in the range of 5000–6000 rad in 6 weeks should be delivered using the portal and beam arrangements described previously.

CARCINOMA OF THE MALE URETHRA

Carcinoma of the urethra in men is extremely rare, with only approximately 450 cases being recorded in the world's literature. The majority of patients are over 50 years of age with a peak instance at 58 years.[301] Etiologic factors have not been identified. Chronic inflammation is felt to play a role in initiation of this disease, based on the observation that the majority of these patients have an antecedent history of venereal disease with urethritis, urethral stricture, or repeated urethral dilations for stricture. The incidence of urethral stricture ranges from 24% to 76% with the most frequent site of urethral stricture being also the most frequent site of malignancy.[301–305]

However, the relationship between inflammation and carcinoma is tenuous at best. The lesion is usually insidious in onset with the symptom complex being contributed primarily to benign stricture rather than to malignant disease. The interval between symptom initiation and diagnosis ranges up to 15 years, with an average of 5 months.[306]

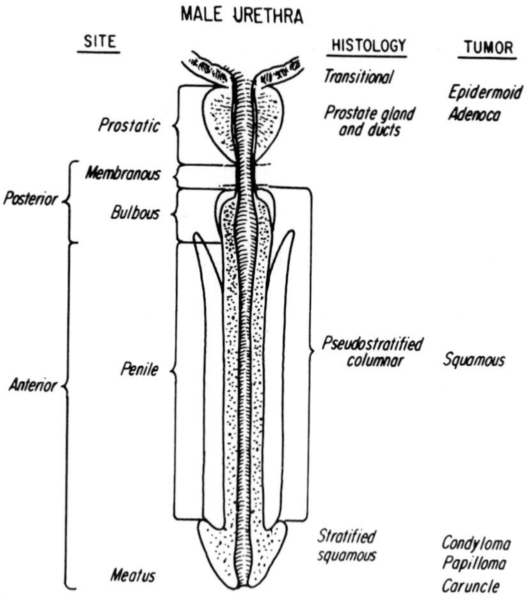

FIG. 23-26. Anatomy and pathology of urethral carcinoma.

TABLE 23-35. Presenting Symptoms of Carcinoma of the Male Urethra

SYMPTOM	TOTALS (23 Cases)
Urethral mass	15/23 (65%)
Obstructive symptoms (with or without retention)	13/23 (57%)
Urethral fistula or periurethral abscess	5/23 (22%)
Pain	6/23 (26%)
Hematuria	5/23 (22%)
Hemospermia	1/23 (4%)

(Modified from Ray B, Canto AR, Whitmore W. Experience with Primary Carcinoma of the Male Urethra. J Urol 117:591–594, 1977)

PATHOLOGY

Tumors of the male urethra may be categorized according to histology of the cells lining the various anatomic regions (Fig. 23-26). The transitional epithelium of the prostatic urethra produces transitional cell malignancies that are histologically and clinically distinct from the adenocarcinoma commonly associated with prostatic malignancy (Table 23-34). Squamous cell carcinomas arise from the bulbous and membraneous urethra, with the distal penile urethra, meatus, and perimeatal regions harboring condyloma accumanata and benign papilloma.

The early lesions tend to spread by direct invasion of adjacent structures with involvement of the vascular structures of the corpora cavernosum and periurethral tissues being common. Symptoms reflect local involvement (Table 23-35). Tumors of the bulbomembraneous urethra often invade the deep structures of the perineum, including the penile and scrotal skin, urogenital diaphragm, and prostate. As will be described, treatment must therefore be directed to the lymphatics which drain these specific areas. Lymphatic drainage of the anterior urethra is to the superficial and deep inguinal lymphatics with occasional extension to the external iliac lymphatic chains where the lymphatic drainage from the posterior is to the external iliac, obturator, and hypogastric lymphatic node chains.[307,308] In general, tumors of the anterior urethra tend to metastasize to the inguinal nodes while tumors of the posterior urethra metastasize to pelvic nodes. Staging is as in Table 23-36.

TUMORS OF THE PROSTATIC URETHRA

Primary transitional cell carcinomas of the prostatic urethra do occur; however, when transitional cell tumors of the prostatic urethra are seen in association with histologically similar bladder carcinomas, they are felt to result from implantation following transurethral resection of the primary vesical malignancy and reflect direct extension of the primary tumor.[309] Transitional lesions of the prostatic urethra are felt to begin as carcinoma-*in-situ* of the ductal epithelium with subsequent invasion of the substance of the prostate itself. No characteristic symptomatology heralds this lesion at a clinical level. In patients with infiltrating transitional cell carcinoma, the prostate frequently has palpably hard areas. The age range of these affected patients is between 60 years and 78 years. The serum acid phosphatase is normal. The tumors feature complete resistance to endocrine therapy with a poor response to radiation therapy and a poor response to surgery once the disease has infiltrated the prostatic stroma. If the tumors are superficially infiltrating, they may be tumors of the urethra and can be controlled in over 50% of the patients by transurethral resection alone.[310] However, in most instances, the primary prostatic transitional tumors involve

TABLE 23-34. Carcinoma of the Male Urethra: Type *versus* Sites

TYPE	LOCATION			
	Penile	*Bulbo–Membranous*	*Prostatic*	*Total*
Squamous	27 (29%)	40 (43%)	2 (2%)	69
Transitional	3 (3%)	4 (4.5%)	12 (13%)	19
Adenocarcinoma		4 (4.5%)		4
Undifferentiated		1 (1%)		1
TOTAL	30 (32%)	49 (53%)	14 (15%)	93

(Modified from Ray B, Guinan PD: Primary carcinoma of the urethra. In Javadpour N (ed): Principles and Management of Urologic Cancer, p 448. Baltimore, Williams & Wilkins, 1979)

TABLE 23-36. Staging System for Carcinoma of the Male Urethra

O	Confined to mucosa only (*in situ*)
A	Into but not beyond lamina propria
B	Into but not beyond substance of corpus spongiosum or into but not beyond prostate
C	Direct extension into tissues beyond corpus spongiosum (corpora cavernosa, muscle, fat, fascia, skin, direct skeletal involvement), or beyond prostatic capsule
D_1	Regional metastasis including inguinal and/or pelvic lymph nodes (with any primary tumor)
D_2	Distant metastasis (with any primary tumor)

(Modified from Ray B, Canto AR, Whitmore W: Experience with primary carcinoma of the male urethra. J Urol 117:591–594, 1977)

the bulk of the prostate so that one must consider radical prostatectomy or radical cystoprostatectomy with simultaneous pelvic lymph node dissection, as an appropriate form of aggressive therapy. The frequency of lymph node involvement is not known. It is unlikely that if the deep pelvic lymph nodes are involved, the patient may be salvaged. Aggressive radiation therapy to the prostate at dose levels of 6000 rad to 7000 rad has produced an occasional long-term survivor. It is, therefore appropriate to consider aggressive external beam radiation therapy as an initial form of treatment with biopsy monitoring up to 6 months following completion of radiation therapy. Patients failing to have tumor-free biopsies at this time should be considered for radical cystoprostatectomy. Absolute recommendations regarding therapy are not possible due to the small series which are available on the multiple treatments which have been applied to various tumor experiences. However, the experiences with transitional cell tumors of the bladder would indicate that a course of radiotherapy may very well produce the modification of the tumor biology and therefore either immediate or delayed radical surgery in conjunction with pelvic lymph node dissection should be deemed appropriate.

CARCINOMA OF THE DISTAL URETHRA

Epidermoid carcinoma of the bulbo-membraneous urethra is the most common urethral malignancy encompassing approximately 75% of carcinomas of the male urethra. In a large series by Kaplan, 30% of the patients had antecedent venereal disease, 35% had strictures, 60% had urethral trauma. The most frequently presenting symptom complex is obstruction, seen in up to 47% of the patients, with 30% of patients presenting with a palpable mass, 31% with a periurethral abscess, 20% with a fistula, and 22% with urethral discharge.[311] It is not uncommon to have a suspicion of malignancy without confirmation of a diagnosis, as biopsy of the involved area usually reveals only chronic inflammatory disease until deep tissue bites can be secured.[312] Differentiation between malignancy and periurethral abscess is difficult and the physician is aided most by a high index of suspicion. Retrograde urethrography may define the extent of disease and indicate spread to the surrounding tissue. Survival rates are poor (Table 23-37).

TREATMENT

Untreated patients can anticipate a median survival of 3 months with a range of from 1 week to 15 months. Only 16% of these patients will survive more than 5 years.

Treatment Group 1

For lesions localized on the distal half of the urethra, partial amputation of the urethra with pathologically controlled margins 2 cm proximal to the lesion is a recognized and established form of treatment. Radical amputation of the penis with perineal urethrostomy as described previously may be performed for more extensive lesions which preclude salvage of sufficient penile length to effect voiding in the erect position.[313]

Radical penectomy gives no increased survival rate over that afforded by partial penectomy. Emasculation with total penectomy-scrotectomy and orchiectomy is indicated only when there is extensive local scrotal involvement and an attempt is made to minimize local recurrence.

Group II Lesions

Early lesions of the bulbomembraneous urethra have been treated successfully by transurethral resection or by resection of the involved segment of the urethra with end-to-end anastomosis, but these cures are rare.[314,315] Poor survival figures have been recorded with any form of treatment. However, the recorded series would indicate that radical excision offers the best opportunity for long-term disease control with the lowest incidence of local recurrence. The reported benefits of incontinuity resection of the pubic ramus is not substantiated. Management of regional lymphatics for distal urethral lesions implies the same guidelines as those

TABLE 23-37. Carcinoma of the Male Urethra: Type and Site vs Survival

	LOCATION			
TYPE	*Penile*	*Bulbo–Membranous*	*Prostatic*	TOTAL
Squamous	12/27 (44%)	4/40 (10%)	0/1 (0%)	16/68 (24%)
Transitional	1/3 (33%)	0/4 (0%)	4/13 (31%)	5/20 (25%)
Adenocarcinoma	–	1/4 (25%)	–	1/4 (25%)
Undifferentiated	–	0/1 (0%)	–	0/1 (0%)
TOTAL	13/30 (43%)	5/49 (10%)	4/14 (29%)	22/93 (24%)

(Modified from Ray B, Canto AR, Whitmore W: Experience with primary carcinoma of the male urethra. J Urol 117:591–594, 1977)

established for carcinoma of the penis. Lesions of the posterior urethra, as treatment will most commonly involve radical cystoprostatectomy or radical prostatectomy, should have simultaneous deep pelvic node dissection and should determine the presence of gross nodal extension. There is no evidence that cure can be established in the patients with gross pelvic disease.

CARCINOMA OF THE FEMALE URETHRA

Malignant carcinoma of the urethra is twice as common in the female urethra as in the male.[316] Tumors most commonly occur in older menopausal women, with 75% of the women being over 50 years of age. The racial distribution is such that the disease is more prevalent in Caucasians.

HISTOLOGY AND PATHOLOGY

Stratified squamous epithelium lines the distal two-thirds of the female urethra with the proximal one-third being lined with transitional epithelium (Fig. 23-27).[301] Classification of the malignant disease in the female urethra reflects the histology. The predominant type of tumor is the squamous cell carcinoma; adenocarcinoma ranks second, with scattered patients having myeloma, sarcoma, and other miscellaneous types. The female urethra should be considered pathologically as being separated into segments, the distal third and the proximal two-thirds.[301] Tumors are classically classified as anterior when they are limited to the distal one-third of the urethra and entire when more than the anterior one-third is involved. Of the reported tumors of the female urethra, 46% are situated in the anterior urethra and 54% in the entire urethra.

The presence of the three types of epithelium within the urethra explains the main histologic types of carcinoma of the female urethra: epidermoid or squamous, transitional cell, and adenocarcinoma. It is felt that the adenocarcinoma arises from periurethral glands which are found near the external orifice, sometimes within the mid portion of the urethra, and occasionally near the internal orifice. Rarely, mucoid adenocarcinomas have been reported. Distribution of the histologic type of tumor according to age and site are given in Table 23-38. Carcinomas of the anterior urethra are usually low-grade, whereas carcinomas of the entire urethar are of higher grade.

FIG. 23-27. Anatomy and pathology of the female urethra.

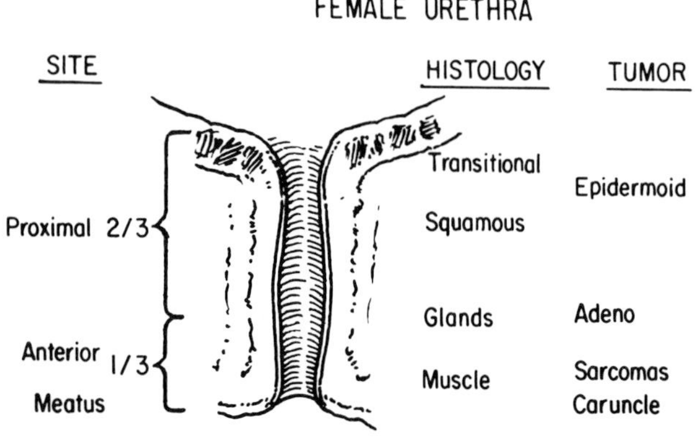

ETIOLOGIC RELATIONSHIPS

The etiology of urethral carcinoma in the female has not been established although a causal relationship is reported between chronic irritation and malignancy, as proliferative lesions, caruncles, papillomas, adenomas, and polyps are reported in high incidence in association with malignancy.[316,317] Marshall and co-workers identified carcinoma in nine of 376 patients with clinically diagnosed urethral caruncles, an incidence rate of 2.4%. The association of malignancy and caruncles has been as high as five of 47 and 13 of 29.[317,318] The high incidence of urethral caruncle and malignancy may be erroneous, as caruncles are common and malignancy is rare. No identified relationship exists between urethral stricture and malignancy; however, the reported occurrence of urethral malignancy in patients with persistent and resistant strictures indicates that the index of suspicion should be high in patients with a history of resistant urethral strictures. Leukoplakia of the urethra should be considered a premalignant change and treated accordingly.

The tumor usually appears as a small papillary growth and usually progresses to become a soft fungating mass that bleeds easily. Ulcerative lesions may produce a diffuse serosanguineous which becomes foul-smelling after bacterial involvement. Spread from the primary lesion is by local extension and infiltration with subsequent involvement to the bladder neck and vulva with ultimate urethrovaginal fistulation. It may be difficult on initial physical examination to differentiate malignant tumors of the urethra from those of malignant vulvar tumors. Late regional node extension in large tumors is common. Lymphatic drainage of the various segments of the urethra is poorly defined, however, it is generally accepted that lymphatics of the distal urethra usually drain into the inguinal lymphatics with only minor distribution. The lymphatic drainage from the proximal urethra is to the obturator and external and internal iliac nodes with late involvement of the common iliac nodes. Between 25% and 50% of cases will have inguinal node involvement at the time of initial diagnosis.[301,319–322] An additional 15% of patients will develop nodes during the time of follow-up. In contradistinction to carcinoma of the penis, clinically positive nodes are considered positive in women with urethral carcinoma.

TREATMENT OF CANCER OF THE FEMALE URETHRA

Treatment of tumors of the female urethra should be based primarily on the tumor stage and to a lesser extent on pathology. Squamous cell carcinoma of the anterior urethra is treated preferably by partial urethrectomy. The incidence of lymph node metastases with distal urethral tumors is low and partial urethrectomy alone is often sufficient for cure. Squamous cell carcinoma of the entire urethra has a poor prognosis irrespective of the form of treatment whether surgery, radiotherapy, or a combination. Treatment of patients with adenocarcinoma involving the entire urethra is similarly dismal. In a large series reported by Zeigerman, 27 patients

TABLE 23-38. Carcinoma of the Female Urethra: Pathologic Type *versus* Age

TYPE	AGE (Years) 20–39	40–49	50–59	60–69	70–79	80+	TOTAL
Squamous	6	17	29	28	13	1	94
Transitional		2		4	2	3	11
Adenocarcinoma	1	4	7	6	2		20
TOTAL	7	23	36	38	17	4	125

(Modified from Ray B, Guinan PD: Primary carcinoma of the urethra. In Javadpour N (ed): Principles and Management of Urologic Cancer, p 461. Baltimore, Williams & Wilkins, 1979)

with carcinoma of the entire urethra received various forms of treatment.[323] The average survival was 8 years in patients receiving radiation therapy, 11.6 years in those receiving surgical therapy. Bracken and co-workers reported 81 cases of carcinoma of the female urethra with the overall 5- and 10-year survival rates of the entire group being 32%.[324] The survival expectations for patients with squamous carcinoma, transitional cell carcinoma, and adenocarcinoma are similar when analyzed according to stage, and all cell types appear to respond equally well with radiotherapy. There is a high incidence of local recurrence for all forms of single modality therapy, which ranges between 46% and 64%. This suggests the need for exploring combination forms of therapy.

No correlation can be identified between the size of the primary lesion and the incidence of nodal extension. However, there is a correlation between location of the primary and the incidence of nodal disease. Thirteen percent of patients with tumors of the anterior urethra can be expected to evidence nodal extension, as compared to 30% of patients with carcinoma of the entire urethra.[325] Distant metastatic disease is rare, occurring in less than 5% of all patients at the time of presentation. The common sites of distant nodal disease are lung, liver, bone, and brain, with distant metastases being diagnosed clinically in only approximately 14% of patients at any time during the course of their disease. Death can usually be expected to occur in 12 months to 18 months in nontreated patients and approximately 75% of unsuccessfully treated patients die within 12 months and 94% within 2 years.[326,327] Death usually is secondary to regional spread with subsequent sepsis and urinary obstruction (note staging diagram).

RADIATION THERAPY

In small tumors, less than 2 cm in diameter, interstitial implantation alone may be adequate. However, the majority of the patients are treated with a combination of interstitial and external beam irradiation, which results in improved survival. The tumor doses for the primary tumor should range from 6000 rad to 8000 rad depending on the extent of the lesion. Uninvolved lymph nodes can be adequately treated with doses of 5000 rad, whereas gross metastatic nodes will require 6500 rad to 7000 rad.[328] The interstitial implant is done with needles (^{226}Ra, ^{137}Ce, ^{192}Ir) to deliver a specified dose at least 0.5 cm from the gross margin of the tumor. Whether a single or double plane or volume implant is used will depend on the extent of the lesion and dose of irradiation to be delivered. Computer calculations should always be performed to determine the dose distribution. External beam irradiation should preferably be delivered with high energy photons, although 4 Mv to 8 Mv photons or even ^{60}Co may be used. In the latter situation, in addition to anterior and posterior parallel portals, lateral fields may be necessary to deliver the desired dose. With the small lesions the local control is good and the 5-year disease-free survival rates are approximately 75% to 80%. Better results are obtained with lesions in the anterior urethra in women. Patients with involvement of the bladder neck or, in women, with tumor extension to the vulva, have poor prognoses, with less than 10% surviving 5 years. All patients with bladder neck or periurethral tissue involvement should receive external irradiation to a dose of 4000 rad in 4 weeks to 5 weeks, combined with an interstitial implant to deliver additional 3000 rad to 4000 rad in 3 days to 4 days. In these patients a suprapubic cystostomy may be required at the time of the radium implant to properly insert the needles.

Patients with more extensive lesions or gross evidence of metastatic lymph nodes should receive at least 5000 rad external irradiation with parallel opposing AP PA or lateral fields or both and additional dose to be delivered with reduced ports or interstitial therapy. Electron beams can be extremely useful in boosting the local dose to a relatively superficial urethral primary or for inguinal lymph node metastasis.

The most common complication of this therapy is soft tissue necrosis, which may take place at the site of the primary tumor or where higher doses of irradiation are delivered. Urethral strictures also may appear after irradiation. Pelvic abscess or fistula is uncommon.

REFERENCES

1. Bell ET: Renal Diseases, 2nd ed, p 435. Philadelphia, Lea & Febiger, 1950
2. Nause MH, Yurdin DH: Renal cell carcinoma in children. J Urol 82:21, 1959
3. Bennington JL, Kradjiann RM: Renal Carcinoma, pp 38–42, 180–196. Philadelphia, WB Saunders, 1967
4. Rosen VJ, Cole LJ: Accelerated induction of kidney neoplasms in mice after X-radiation (690 rads) and unilateral nephrectomy. J Natl Cancer Inst 28:1031, 1962
5. Rijnders WP, Donker PJ, Ybema HJ et al: Renal changes following retrograde pyelography using thorotrast. Arch Chir Neerl 15:157, 1963
6. Laetsch F, Klug W: Strahlenschaden and tumorentwicklung nach thorotrastpyelographie. Z Urol 57:505, 1964
7. Swarm RL: Introduction. Experience with colloidal thorium dioxide. Ann NY Acad Sci 145–525, 1967

8. Wenz, W: Tumors of the kidney following retrograde pyelography with colloidal thorium dioxide. Ann NY Acad Sci 145:806, 1967
9. Horning ES: Observations on hormone-dependent renal tumors in the golden hamster. Br J Cancer 10:678, 1956
10. Clayson DB (ed): Chemical Carcinogenesis. London, Churchill, 1962
11. Bennington JL, Laubsche FA: Epidemiologic studies on carcinoma of the kidney: Association of renal adenocarcinoma with smoking. Cancer 21:1069, 1968
12. Grawitz PA: Die sogenannten Lipome der Niere. Virchows Arch Pathol Anat 93:39–63, 1883
13. Stoerk O: Zur Histogenese der Grawitzschen Nierengeschwulste. Beitr Pathol Anat 43:393–437, 1908
14. Sudek P: Zwei Falle Bon Adenosarcom der Niere. Virchows Arch Pathol Anat 133:558–562, 1893
15. Trinkle AJ: The origin and development of renal adenomas and their relation to carcinoma of the renal cortex. Am J Cancer 27:676, 1936
16. Pearse R: Malignant adenomas of the kidney. J Urol 59:553, 1948
17. Leary T: Crystalline ester cholesterol and adult cortical renal tumors. Arch Pathol 50:151, 1950
18. Wallace AC, Nairn RC: Renal tubular antigens in kidney tumors. Cancer 29:977–981, 1972
19. Creevy CD: Confusing Clinical manifestations of malignant renal neoplasms. Arch Intern Med 55:895, 1935
20. Hanash KA, Uts DC, Ludwig J et al: Syndrome of reversible hepatic dysfunction associated with hypernephroma: an experimental study. Invest Urol 8:399, 1971
21. Ramon CU, Taylor HB: Hepatic dysfunction associated with renal carcinoma. Cancer 20:1287, 1972
22. Sufrin G, Mirand EA, Moore RH et al: Hormones in renal cancer. J Urol 117:443, 1977
23. Hollifield JW, Page DI, Smith C et al: Renin-secreting clear cell carcinoma of the kidney, Arch Intern Med 135:859, 1975
24. Chisholm GD: Nephrogenic ridge tumors and their syndromes. Ann NY Acad Sci 230:403, 1974
25. Lang FK: Roentgenographic assessment of asymptomatic renal lesions. Radiology 109:257–269, 1973
26. Butnick, B: Carcinoma simulated by xanthogranulomatous pyelonephritis. J Urol 106:815–817, 1971
27. Bennington JL, Beckwith JB: Tumors of the Kidney, Renal Pelvis and Ureter. Bethesda, Air Force Institute of Pathology, 1975
28. Lang ED, Johnston B, Chance HL et al: Avascular renal mass lesions; the use of nephrotomography, arteriography, cyst puncture double contrast study and histochemical and histopathologic examination of the aspirate. South Med J 65:1–10, 1972
29. Pedersen JS, Haneke S, Christensen AK: Renal carbuncle antibiotic therapy governed by ultrasonically guided aspiration. J Urol 109:777–778, 1973
30. Pfister RC, Shae TE: Nephrotomography; performance and interpretation. Radiol Clin North Am 9:41–62, 1971
31. Pollack HM, Goldberg BB, Morales JO et al: Systematized approach to differential diagnosis of renal masses. Radiology 113:653–659, 1974b
32. Raskin MM, Boens S, Scrafini AN: Renal cyst puncture combined flouroscopic and ultrasonic technique. Radiology 113:425–427, 1974
33. Lang ED: Asymptomatic space occupying lesions of the kidney; a programmed sequential approach and its impact on quality and cost of health care. South Med J 70:277–285, 1977
34. Ekelund L, Lunderquist A: Pharmacoangiography with angiotensin. Radiology 110:553, 1974
35. Ekelund L, Johnsson N, Lunderquist A: Tumor vessels, angiographic histopathologic correlation. Radiologe 17:3:95–102, 1977
36. Kauffman G, Meyer P, Bammert J: Morphometrisehe Differenzierung von Tumor and Entzundung im Angiogram. Radiology 17:3103–11, 1977
37. Becker JA, Kinkhabwala M, Pollack H et al: Augiomyolipoma (hamartoma) of the kidney. Acta Radiol 14:561–568, 1973
38. McLaughlin AP, Talner LB, Leopold GR et al: Avascular primary renal cell carcinoma; varied pathologic and angiographic features. J Urol 111:587–593, 1974
39. Blath RA, Manci-la-Jimenez R, Stanley RJ: Clinical comparison between vascular and avascular renal carcinoma. J Urol 115: 514–519, 1976
40. Middleton RG, Presto AJ III: Radical thoracoabdominal nephrectomy for renal cell carcinoma. J Urol 110:36, 1973
41. Ochsner MG, Brannan W, Pond HS III et al: Renal cell carcinoma: Review of 26 years experience at the Ochsner Clinic. J Urol 110–643, 1973
42. Robson CJ: Radical nephrectomy for renal cell carcinoma. J Urol 89:37, 1963
43. Skinner DG, Pfister FG, Colvin R: Extension of renal cell carcinoma into the vena cava: The rationale for aggressive surgical management. J Urol 107:711, 1972a
44. Angervall L, Carlstrom E, Wahlquist L et al: Effects of clinical and morphological variables on spread of renal carcinoma in an operative series. Scand J Urol Nephrol 3:134–140, 1969
45. Robson CJ, Churchill BM, Anderson W: The results of radical nephrectomy for renal cell carcinoma. J Urol 101:297–301, 1969
46. Hulten L, Rosencrantz M, Seeman T et al: Occurrence and localization of lymph node metastases in renal carcinoma: Lymphographic and histopathologic investigation in connection with nephrectomy. Scand J Urol Nephrol 3:129–133, 1966
47. Robson CJ, Churchill BM, Anderson W: The results of radical nephrectomy for renal cell carcinoma. Trans Am Assoc Genitourin Surg 60:122, 1968
48. Middleton RG: Surgery for metastatic renal cell carcinoma. J Urol 97:973–977, 1967
49. Johnson DE, Swanson DA: The role of nephrectomy in metastatic renal carcinoma. In Johnson CE, Samuels ML (eds): Cancer of the Genitourinary Tract, pp 27–32. New York, Raven Press, 1979
50. Montie JE, Stewart BH, Stratton RA et al: The role of adjunctive nephrectomy in patients with metastatic renal cell carcinoma. J Urol 117:272–275, 1977
51. Johnson DE, Kaesler KE, Samuels ML: Is nephrectomy justified in patients with metastatic renal carcinoma? J Urol 114:27–29, 1975
52. Klugo RCM, Detmers RE, Stiles RW et al: Aggressive versus conservative management of stabe IV renal cell carcinoma. J Urol 118:244–246, 1977
53. Skinner DG, Colvin RB, Vermillion CD et al: Diagnosis and management of renal cell carcinoma: A clinical and pathologic study of 309 cases. Cancer 28:1165–1177, 1971
54. Tolia BM, Whitmore WF Jr: Solitary metastasis from renal cell carcinoma. J Urol 114:836–838, 1975
55. Wickham JEA: Conservative renal surgery for adenocarcinoma. The place of bench surgery. Br J Urol 47–25, 1975
56. Kaufman JJ, Skinner DG: The treatment of renal cell carcinoma in the solitary kidney. J Int Soc Urol 2:160–175, 1976
57. Palmer JM, Swanson DA: Conservative surgery in solitary and bilateral renal carcinoma: Indication and technical considerations. J Urol 120:113–117, 1978
58. McCormack PM, Martini N: The changing role of surgery for pulmonary metastases. Ann Thorac Surg 28(2):139–45, 1979
59. Penn I: Transplantation in patients with primary renal malignancies. Transplantation 24(6):424–34, 1977
60. Rosch JCT, Dotter CT, Brown MJ: Selective arterial embolization. Radiology 102:303–306, 1972
61. Almgard LE, Fernstrom I, Haverling M: Treatment of renal adenocarcinoma; embolic occlusion of the renal circulation. Br J Urol 45:474–479, 1973
62. Anderson JH, Wallace S, Gianturco C: Transcatheter intravascular coil occlusion of experimental arteriovenous fistulas. Am J Roentgenol 129:795–798, 1977
63. Goldstein HM, Medellin H, Beydoun MT et al: Transcatheter embolization of renal cell carcinoma. Am J Roentgenol 1237:557–562, 1975
64. Bergreen PW, Woodside J, Paster SB: Therapeutic renal infraction. J Urol 118(3):372–4, 1977

65. Rankin RN: Gas formation after renal tumor embolization without abscess: A benign occurrence. Radiology 130(2):317–20, 1979
66 Rubin P: Comment: National Cooperative Studies, Adjuvant Radiotherapy, Current Concepts in Cancer, pt. IX, pp 128–129. *In* Rubin P (ed): Urogenital Tract: Kidney. Chicago, AMA Publisher, 1974
67. Walters CA: Preoperative irradiation of cortical renal tumors. AM J Roentgenol Rad Ther 33:149–164, 1935
68. Riches E: The place of irradiation. JAMA 204(3):138–140, 1968
69. van der Werf-Messing B: Carcinoma of the kidney. Cancer 32:1056–1061, 1973
70. Rost A, Brosig W: Preoperative irradiation of renal cell carcinoma Urology 10:414–417, 1977
71. Rafla S: Renal cell carcinoma. Natural history and results of treatment Cancer 24:26–60, 1970
72. Finney R: The value of radiotherapy in the treatment of hypernephroma: A clinical trial. Br J Urol 45:258–269, 1973
73. Riches EW, Griffiths IH, Thackray AC: New growths of kidney and ureter. Br J Urol 23:138–140, 1951
74. Wagle DG, Moore RH, Murphy GP: Secondary carcinomas of the kidney. J Urol 114:30–32, 1975
75. Carter SK, Wasserman TH: The chemotherapy of urologic cancer. Cancer 36:729–747, 1975
76. Johnson DE, Chalband RA, Holoye PY et al: Clinical trial of bleomycin (NSC 125066) in the treatment of metastatic renal carcinoma. Cancer Chemotherapy Rep 59:433–435, 1975
77. Lokich JJ, Harrison JH: Renal cell carcinoma: Natural history and chemotherapeutic experience. J Urol 114:371–374, 1975
78. Merrin CC, Murphy GP: Chemotherapy of urogenital cancer. Surg Annu 8:391–412, 1976
79. Hrushesky WJ, Murphy GP: Current status of the therapy of advanced renal carcinoma. J Surg Oncol 9:277–288, 1977
80. Hahn DM, Schimpff SC, Ruckdeschel JC et al: Single agent chemotherapy for renal cell carcinoma: CCNU, Vinblastine, thioTEPA or bleomycin. Cancer Treat Rep 61:1585–1587, 1977
81. Johnson DE, Rodriguez L, Holoye PY: et al: Combination vincristine (NSC 67574) and hydroxyurea (NSC 32065) for metastatic renal carcinoma. Cancer Chemotherapy Rep 59:1159–1160, 1975
82. Merrin C, Mittleman A, Fanour N et al: Chemotherapy of advanced renal cell carcinoma with vinblastine and CCNU J Urol 113:21–23, 1975
83. Davis TE, Manalo FB: Combination chemotherapy of advanced renal cell cancer with CCNU and vinblastine. Proc Am Soc Clin Oncol 19:316, 1978
84. Paulson F, Lastinger B, Cox EB: Metastatic renal adenocarcinoma: Predictors of treatment response. J Urol (in press)
85. Talley RW: Chemotherapy of adenocarcinoma of the kidney. Cancer 32:1062–1065, 1973
86. Alberto P, Senn HJ: Hormonal therapy of renal carcinoma alone and in association with cytostatic drugs. Cancer 33:1226–1229, 1974
87. Hahn RG, Brodovsky H: Methyl CCNU, Velban and Depo-Provera treatment trials in advanced renal cancer (abstr) Proc Am Assoc Cancer Res Am Soc Clin Oncol 17:246, 1976
88. Johansson S, Angervall L, Bengtsson U: Uroepithelial tumors of the renal pelvis associated with abuse of phenacetin-containing analgesics. Cancer 33:743–753, 1974
89. Apostolov K, Spasic P, Bojanic N: Evidence of a viral actionology in endemic (BALKAN) nephropathy. Lancet 2:1271–1273, 1975
90. Craciun EC, Rosculescu I: On Danubian endemic familial nephropathy (Balkan nephropathy). Some problems. Am J Med 49:774–779, 1970
91. Elliott AY, Fraley EE, Cleveland P et al: Isolation of an RNA virus from papillary tumors of the human renal pelvis. Science 179:393–395, 1973
92. Bennington JL, Beckwith JB: Tumors of the kidney, renal pelvis, and ureter. In Atlas of Tumor Pathology, 2nd Series, Fasc 12. Washington, DC Armed Forces Institute of Pathology, 1975
93. Grabstald H, Whitmore WF, Melamed MR: Renal pelvic tumors. JAMA 218:845–854, 1971
94. Cullen TH, Popham RR, Voss HJ: Urine cytology and primary carcinoma of the renal pelvis and ureter. Aust N Z J Surg 41:230–236, 1972
95. Sarnacki CT, McCormack LJ, Kiser WS et al: Urinary cytology and the clinical diagnosis of urinary tract malignancy. A clinicopathologic study of 1400 patients. J Urol 106:751–764, 1971
96. Lang EK: The arteriographic diagnosis of primary and secondary tumors of the ureter or ureter and renal pelvis. Radiology 93:799–805, 1969
97. Pontes JD, Christensen LC, Pierce JM Jr: Angiographic aspects of tumors of renal pelvis and ureter. Urology 7:334–336, 1976
98. Riches EW, Griffiths IH, Thackery A: New growths of kidney and ureter. Br J Urol 23:297, 1951
99. Bloom NA, Vidone RA, Lytton B: Primary carcinoma of the ureter: A report of 102 new cases. J Urol 103:590, 1970
100. Bergman H, Friedenerg RM, Sayegh V: New roentgenologic signs of carcinoma of the ureter. Am J Roetgenol 86:707, 1961
101. Finby N, Begg CF: Carcinoma of the ureter. Coiled catheter sign. NY J Med 63:2397, 1963
102. McIntyre D, Pyrah LN, Raper FP: Primary ureteric neoplasms, with a report of forty cases. Br J Urol 37:160, 1965
103. Samellas W: Varices of the ureter: A rare cause of hematuria. J Urol 94:55, 1965
104. Casey WC, Goodwin WE: Percutaneous antegrade pyelography and hydronephrosis. J Urol 74:164, 1955
105. Cullen TLHL, Popham RR, Voss HJ: Urine cytology and primary carcinoma of the renal pelvis and ureter. Aust N Z J Surg 41:230, 1972
106. Eriksson O, Johansson S: Urothelial neoplasms of the upper urinary tract. A correlation between cytologic and histologic findings in 43 patients with urothelial neoplasms of the renal pelvis or ureter. Acta Cytol 20:20, 1976
107. Batata MA, Grabstald H: Upper urinary tract urothelial tumors. Urol Clin North Am 3:79, 1976
108. Hewitt CB: Nephrourecterectomy with bladder cuff in the treatment of transitional cell carcinoma of the upper urinary tract. In Scott R (ed): Current Controversies in Urologic Management. Philadelphia, WB Saudners, 1972
109. Strong DW, Pearse HD: Recurrent urothelial tumors following surgery for transitional cell carcinoma of the upper urinary tract. Cancer 38:2178, 1976
110. Batata MA, Whitmore WF Jr, Hilaris BS et al: Primary carcinoma of the ureter. A prognostic study. Cancer 35:1626, 1975
111. Chapman WH, Kircheim D, McRoberts JW: Effect of the urine and calculus formation on the incidence of bladder tumors in rats implanted with paraffin wax pellets. Cancer Res 33:1225, 1973
112. Ferguson AR: Associated Bilharziosis and primary malignant disease of the urinary bladder, with observations on a series of 40 cases. J Pathol Bacteriol 16:76, 1911
113. Hashimoto Y, Kitagawa HS: In vitro neoplastic transformation of epithelial cells of rat urinary bladder by nitrosoamines. Nature 252:497, 1974
114. Bertram JS, Craig AW: Specific induction of bladder cancer in mice by Butyl-(4 hydroxybutyl)-nitrosoamine and effects of hormonal modifications on the sex difference in response. Eur J Cancer 8:487, 1972
115. Okada M, Suzuki E: Metabolism of butyl-(4-hydroxybutyl)-nitrosoamine in rats. Gann 53:391, 1972
116. Hashimoto Y, Suzuki E, Okada M: Induction of urinary bladder tumors in ACI/N rats by butyl-(e-carboxyprophyl) nitrosoamine, a major urinary metabolite of butyl-(4-hydroxybutyl) nitrosoamine. Gann 63:637, 1972
117. Metcalf D, Stanley ER: Quantitative studies on the stimulation of mouse bone marrow colony growth in vitro by normal human urine. Aust J Exp Biol Med Sci 47:453, 1969
118. Olson C, Pamukcu AM, Brobst DF: Papilloma-like virus from bovine bladder tumors. Cancer Res 25:840, 1965
119. Olson C, Pamukcu AM, Brobst DF et al: A urinary bladder tumor induced by a cutaneous papilloma agent. Cancer Res 19:779, 1959
120. Georgiev R, Vrigasov A, Antonov WS et al: Determination of the presence of carcinogenic substances in urine of cows fed

hay from hematuria regions. Wien Tierarztl Monatsschr 58:589, 1963
121. Pamukcu AM, Price JM, Bryan GT: Assay of fractions of bracken fern (Pteris aquilina) for carcinogenic activity. Cancer Res 30:902, 1970
122. Page BH, Levison VB, Curwen MP: The site of recurrence cf noninfiltrating bladder tumors. Br J Urol 50(4):237–42, 1978
123. Farrow GM, Utz DC, Rife CC et al: Clinical observations on 69 cases of in situ carcinoma of the urinary bladder. Cancer Res 37:2794–2798, 1977
124. Utz DC, Hanash KA, Farrow GM: The plight of the patient with carcinoma in situ of the bladder. J Urol 103:160–164, 1970
125. Johnson DE, Schoenwald MB, Ayala AG et al: Squamous cell carcinoma of the bladder. J Urol 115:542–544, 1975
126. Marshall VF, Holden J, Ma, KT et al: Survival of patients with bladder carcinoma treated by simple segmental resection. Cancer 9:568–571, 1956
127. Masina F: Segmental resection for tumors of the urinary bladder: Ten-year follow-up. Br J Surg 52:279–283, 1965
128. Cordonnier JJ: Cystectomy for carcinoma of the bladder. J Urol 99:172–173, 1968
129. Kaufman JJ: The management of tumours of the bladder. Practitioner 197:611–619, 1966
130. Whitmore WF Jr: Bladder cancer: Combined radiotherapy and surgical treatment. JAMA 207:349–350, 1969
131. Bowles WT, Cordonnier JJ: Total cystectomy for carcinoma of the bladder. J Urol 90:731–735, 1963
132. Whitmore WF Jr, Marshall VF: Radical total cystectomy for cancer of the bladder: 230 consecutive cases in 5 years later. J Urol 87:853–868, 1962
133. Wolinska WH, Melamed MR, Schellhammer PF et al: Urethral ctyology following cystectomy for bladder carcinoma. Am J Surg Pathol 1(3):225–34, 1977
134. Schellhammer PF, Whitmore WF Jr: Urethral meatal carcinoma following cystourethrectomy for bladder carcinoma. J Urol 115(1):61–4, 1976
135. Schellhammer PF, Whitmore WF Jr: Transitional cell carcinoma of the urethra in men having cystectomy for bladder cancer. J Urol 115(1):56–60, 1976
136. van der Werf-Messing B: Cancer of the urinary bladder treated by interstitial radium implant. Int J Radiat Oncol Biol Phys 4:373–378, 1978
137. Bloom HJG: Treatment of carcinoma of the bladder; a symposium—I Treatment by interstitial irradiation using tantalum 182 wire. Br J Radiol 33:471–479, 1960
138. Whitmore WF Jr, Batata MA, Hilaris BS et al: A comparative study of two preoperative radiation regimens with cystectomy for bladder cancer. Cancer 40:1077–1086, 1977
139. Miller LS: Bladder cancer: superiority of preoperative irradiation and cystectomy in clinical stages B2 and C. Cancer 30:973–980, 1977
140. Walz BJ, Perez CA, Risch J et al: Small dose preoperative irradiation in carcinoma of the bladder. Presented at meeting of the American Society of Therapeutic Radiology, 1975
141. Morrison R: The results of treatment of cancer of the bladder—A clinical contribution to radiobiology. Clin Radiol 26:67–75, 1980
142. van der Werf-Messing B: Carcinoma of the bladder T3NxMo treated by preoperative irradiation followed by cystectomy. Cancer 36:178–722, 1975
143. van der Werf-Messing B: Preoperative irradiation followed by cystectomy to treat carcinoma of the urinary bladder category T3Nx, 0-4MO. Int J Radiat Oncol Biol Phys 5:394–401, 1979
144. Prout GR Jr, Slack NH, Broxx IDJ: Preoperative irradiation and cystectomy for bladder carcinoma, IV: Results in a selected population, pp 783–791. In Seventh National Cancer Conference Proceedings, Biltmore Hotel, Los Angeles, CA, September 26–29. Philadelphia, JB Lippincott, 1972
145. Ellingwood KE, Drylie DM, DeTure FA et al: Post diversion precystectomy irradiation for cancer of the bladder. Cancer 43:1032–1036, 1979
146. Barnhouse DH, Reed WG, Johnson SH III et al: Staged treatment of invasive bladder cancer. Urology 5:606–609, 1975
147. Mahoney EM, Weber ET, Harrison JH: Post-diversion precystectomy irradiation for carcinoma of the bladder. J Urol 114:46–69, 1975
148. Anderson T: Chemotherapy of urologic cancer. In Javadpour N (ed): Principles and Management of Urologic Cancer. Baltimore, Williams & Wilkins, 1979
149. Anderson T: Developmental concepts: Effective chemotherapy for bladder cancer. Semin Oncol 6:240–248, 1979
150. Carter SK, Wasserman TH: The chemotherapy of urologic cancer. Cancer 35:729–747, 1975
151. Yagoda A: Future implications of phase II chemotherapy trials in 95 patients with measurable advanced bladder cancer. Cancer Res 37:2775–2780, 1977
152. Yagoda A, Watson RC, Whitmore W: Cis-platinum (DDP) regimens in bladder cancer. Proc Am Soc Clin Oncol 20:237, 1979
153. Hahn RG: Bladder cancer treatment considerations for metastatic disease. Semin Oncol 6:236–239, 1979
154. DeKernion JB: Chemotherapy of advanced bladder carcinoma. Cancer Res 37:2771–2774, 1977
155. Merrin C, Cartagena R, Wajsman Z et al: Chemotherapy of bladder carcinoma with cyclophosphamide and adriamycin. J Urol 114:884–887, 1975
156. Cross RJ, Glashan RW, Humphrey CS et al: Treatment of advanced bladder cancer with adriamycin and 5-fluorouracil. Br J Urol 48:609–615, 1976
157. Rodriguez LH, Johnson DE, Holoye PY et al: Combination VM-26 and adriamycin for metastatic transitional cell carcinoma. Cancer Treat Rep 61:87–88, 1977
158. Williams SD, Einhorn LH, Donohue JP: Cis-platinum combination chemotherapy for bladder cancer: an update. Cancer Clin Trials 2:335–338, 1979
159. Troner MB: Cyclophosphamide, adriamycin and platinum CAP in the treatment of urothelial malignancy. Proc Assoc Cancer Res 20:117, 1979
160. Sternberg JJ, Bracken RB, Handel PB et al: Combination chemotherapy (CISCA) for advanced urinary tract carcinoma; a preliminary report. JAMA 238:2282–2287, 1977
161. Getaz EP, Beckley S, Fitzpatrick J et al: Cis-platinum induced hemolysis. N Engl J Med 302:334–335, 1980
162. Schilsky RL, Anderson T: Hypomagnesemia and renal magnesium wasting in patients receiving Cisplatin. Ann Intern Med 90:929–931, 1979
163. Third National Cancer Survey: Incidence Data: NCI mongraph 41. Bethesda, DHEW Publication (NIH) pp 75–787, 1975
164. Hutchison GB: Epidemiology of prostatic cancer. Semin Oncol 3(2):151–159, 1976
165. Axtell LM, Ardyce JA, Myers MH (eds.): Cancer Patient Survival Report No. 5 Bethesda, U.S. Department of Health, Education and Welfare, 1976
166. Graham S, Levin M, Lilienfeld AM: The socioeconomic distribution of cancer of various sites in Buffalo, NY, 1948–1952. Cancer 13:180–191, 1960
167. Seidman H: Cancer death rates by site and sex for religious and socioeconomic groups in New York City. Environ Res 3:234–250, 1970
168. Enster VL, Selvin S, Sacks ST et al: Prostatic cancer: Mortality and incidence rates by race and social class. Am J Epidemiol 107:311–320, 1978
169. Ross RK, McCurtis JW, Henderson BE et al: Descriptive epidemiology of testicular and prostatic cancer in Los Angles. Br J Cancer 39:284–292, 1979
170. Wynder EL, Mabuchi K, Whitemore WF: Epidemiology of cancer of the prostate. Cancer 28:344–360, 1971
171. Doll R: Geographic variation in cancer incidence: A clue to causation. World J Surg 2:595–602, 1978
172. Staszewshi J, Haenszel W: Cancer mortality among the Polish-born in the U.S. J Nat Cancer Inst 35:291–297, 1965
173. Haenszel W, Kurihara M: Studies of Japanese migrants. I.

Mortality from cancer and other disease among Japanese in the United States. J Natl Cancer Inst 40:43–68, 1968
174. Steel R, Lees REM, Kraus AS et al: Sexual factors in the epidemiology of cancer of the prostate. J Chron Dis 24:29–37, 1971
175. Krain LS: Some epidemiologic variables in prostatic carcinoma in California. Prev Med 3:154–159, 1974
176. Schuman LM, Mandel J, Blackard C et al: Epidemiologic study of prostatic cancer: Preliminary report. Cancer Treat Rep 61(2):181–186, 1977
177. Rotkin ID: Studies in the epidemiology of prostatic cancer; expanding sampling. Cancer Treat Rep 61(2):173–180, 1977
178. Feminella JG, Lattimer JK: An apparent increase in genital carcinomas among wives of men prostatic carcinomas: An epidemilogic survey. Pirq Bull Clin Med 20(6):3–10, 1973
179. Sanford EJ, Geder L, Laycock A et al: Evidence for the association of cytomegalovirus with carcinoma of the prostate. J Urol 118:789–792, 1977
180. Sanford EJ, Geder L, Laychock A et al: Evidence for the association of cytemogalovirus with carinoma of prostate. J Urol 118:789, 1977
181. Sanford EJ, Dagen JE, Gedar L et al: Lymphocyte reactivity against virally-transformed cells in patients with prostatic carcinoma. J Urol 118:809, 1977
182. Geder L, Sanford EJ, Rohner TJ Jr et al: Cytomegalovirus in carcinoma of the prostate: In vitro transformation of human cells. Cancer Treat Rep 61(20):139, 1977
183. Moore RA: Benign hypertrophy and carcinoma of the prostate. Surgery 16:152–167, 1944
184. Glantz GM: Cirrhosis and carcinoma of the prostate gland. J Urol 91 (3):291–293, 1964
185. Robson MC: Cirrhosis and prostatic neoplasms. Geriatrics 21(12):150–154, 1966
186. Woolf CM: An investigation of the familial aspect of carcinoma of the prostate. Cancer 13:739–744, 1960
187. Greenwald P, Kirmas V, Polan AK et al: Cancer of the prostate among men with benign prostatic hyperplasia. J Natl Cancer Inst 53:335–340, 1974
188. Sommers SC: Endocrine changes with prostatic carcinoma. Cancer 10:345–358, 1957
189. Paulson DF, Uro-Oncology Research Group. The impact of current staging procedure in assessing disease extent of prostatic adenocarcinoma. J Urol 121:300–302, 1979
190. Byar DP, Veterans Administration Cooperative Urological Research Group: Survival of patients with incidentally found microscopic cancer of the prostate: Results of a clinical trial of conservative treatment. J Urol 108:908, 1972
191. McMillen SM, Wettlaufer JN: The role of repeat transurethral biospy in Stage A carcinoma of the prostate. J Urol 116(6):759–60. 1976
192. Gray H: Anatomy of the Human Body, 27th ed. Philadelphia, Lea & Febiger, 1959
193. Rouviere H: Anatomy of the Human Lymphatic System. Translated by MJ Tobias. Ann Arbor, Edwards Brothers, 1938
194. Flocks RH, Culp D, Porto R: Lymphatic spread from prostatic cancer. J Urol 81:194, 1975
195. Smith MJV: The lymphatics of the prostate. Invest Urol 3:439, 1966
196. Golimbu M, Morales P, Al-Askari S et al: Extended pelvic lymphadenectomy for prostatic cancer, J Urol 121:617, 1979
197. Cern JC, Farah R, Rian R et al: An evaluation of lymphangiography in staging carcinoma of prostate. J Urol 113:367, 1975
198. Ray GR, Pistenma DA, Castellino RA et al: Operative staging of apparently localized adenocarcinoma of the prostate: Results in fifth unselected patients. I. Experimental design and preliminary results. Cancer 38:73, 1976
199. Freiha FS, Pistenma DA, Bagshaw MA: Pelvic lymphadenectomy for staging prostatic carcinoma: Is it always necessary? J Urol 122:176, 1979
200. Ardinno LJ, Glucksman MA: Lymph node metastases in early carcinoma of the prostate. J Urol 88:91, 1962
201. Whitmore WF Jr, Hilaris B, Grabstald H et al: Implantation of I^{125} in prostatic cancer. Surg Clin North Am 54:887, 1974
202. McLaughlin AP, Saltzstein SL, McCullough DL et al: Prostatic carcinoma: Incidence and location of unsuspected lymphatic metastases. J Urol 115:89, 1976
203. McCullough DL, Prout GR Jr, Daly JJ: Carcinoma of the prostate and lymphatic metastases. J Urol 111:65, 1974
204. Wilson CS, Dahl DS, Middleton RG: Pelvic lymphadenectomy for the staging of apparently localized postatic cancer. J Urol 117:197, 1977
205. Bagshaw MA: Radiation therapy for cancer of the prostate. In Skinner, DG, deKernion JB: Genitouriuary Cancer p 360. Philadelphia, WB Saunders, 1978
206. Carlton CE, Jr: Radioactive isotope implantation for cancer of the prostate. In Skinner, DG, deKernion JB (eds.): Genitourinary Cancer Philadelphia, WB Saunders, 1978
207. Barzell W, Bean MA, Hilaris BS et al: Prostatic adrenocarcinoma: Relationship of grade and local extent to the pattern of metastases. J Urol 118:278, 1977
208. Pistenma DA, Bagshaw MA, Freitha FS: Extended-field radiation therapy for prostatic adenocarcinoma: Status report of a limited prospective Trial. In Johnson, Samuels (eds): Cancer of the Genitourinary Tract 229. New York, Raven Press, 1979
209. Whitemore WF, Batata M, Hilaris B: Prostatic irradiation: Iodine-125 implantation. In Johnson DE, Samuels ML (eds): Cancer of the Genitourinary Tract, p 195. New York, Raven Press, 1979
210. Spellman ML, Costellino RA, Ray GR et al: An evaluation of lymphangiography in localized carcinoma of the prostate. Radiology 125:737, 1977
211. Gleason DF, Mellinger FT, Veterams Administration Cooperative Urological Research Group: Prediction of prognosis for prostatic adenocarcinoma by combined histological grading and clinical staging. J Urol 111:58–64, 1974
212. Pontes JE, Chose B, Rose N et al: Reliability of bone marrow acid phosphates a parameter of metastalic prostatic cancer. J Urol 122:178, 1979
213. Chu TM, Wang MC, Scott WW et al: Immunochemical detection of serum prostatic acid phosphatase methodology and clinical evaluation. Invest Urol 15:319, 1978
214. Foti AG, Cooper JF, Herschman H, Malvaez RR: Detection of prostatic cancer by solid-phase radioimmunoassay of serum prostatic acid phosphates. N Engl J Med 297:1357, 1977
215. Fossa SD, Sokolowski J, Theodorsen L: The significance of bone marrow acid phosphatase in patients with prostatic carcinoma. Br J Urol 50(3) 185–9, 1978
216. Hutch JA: A new theory of the anatomy of the internal urinary sphincter and the physiology of micturition. IV. The urinary sphincteric mechanism, J Urol 97:705–712, 1967
217. Vickery AL Jr, Kerr WS Jr: Carcinoma of the prostate treated by radical prostatectomy. A clinicopathological survey of 187 cases followed for 5 years and 148 cases followed for 10 years. Cancer 16:1598–1608, 1963
218. Weyrauch HM: Surgery of the Prostate. Philadelphia, Saunders, 1959
219. Hanash KA, Utz DC, Cook EN et al: Carcinoma of the prostate: A 15-year followup. J Urol 107:450, 1972
220. Whitmore WF Jr: The rationale and results of ablative surgery for prostatic cancer. Cancer 16:1119—1132, 1963
221. Bagshaw MA, Ray GR, Pistenma DA et al: External beam radiation therapy of primary carcinoma of the prostate. Cancer 36:723–728, 1975
222. Perez CA, Bauer W, Garza R et al: Radiation therapy in the definitive treatment of localized carcinoma of the prostate. Cancer 40:1425–1433, 1977
223. Perez CA, Walz BJ, Zivnuska FR et al: Irradiation of carcinoma of the prostate localized to the pelvis: Analysis of tumor response and prognosis. Int J Radiat Oncol Biol Phys 6:555–563, 1980
224. Hilaris BS, Whitmore WF, Batata MA et al: ^{125}I implantation of the prostate: Dose-response considerations. Front Radiat Ther Oncol 12:82–90, 1978

225. Lipsett JA, Cosgrove MD, Green N et al: Factors influencing prognosis in the radiotherapeutic management of carcinoma of the prostate. Int J Radiat Oncol Biol Phys 1:1049–1058, 1976
226. Neglia WJ, Hussey DH, Johnson DE: Megavoltage radiation therapy for carcinoma of the prostate. Int J Radiat Oncol Biol 2:773–783, 1976
227. Harisiadis L, Veenema FJ, Senyszyn JJ et al: Carcinoma of the prostate. Treatment with external radiotherapy. Cancer 41:2131–2142, 1978
228. Cox JD, Stoffel TJ: The significance of needle biopsy after irradiation for stage C adenocarcinoma of the prostate. Cancer 40:156–160, 1977
229. Kagan AR, Gordon J, Cooper JR et al: A clinical appraisal of postirradiation biopsy in prostatic cancer. Cancer 39:637–641, 1977
230. Kramer SA, Cline WA Jr, Farnham R: Radical prostatectomy in patients with advanced prostatic carcinoma. J Urol (in Press)
231. Barzell WE, Bean MA, Hilaris BS et al: Prostatic adenocarcinoma: Relationship of grade and local extent to the pattern of metastases. J Urol 118:278–282, 1977
232. Huggins C, Stevens RE, Hodges CV: Studies on prostatic cancer II. The effects of castration on advanced carcinoma of the prostate gland. Arch Surg 43:209, 1941
233. Huggins, C: Anti-androgenic treatment of prostatic carcinoma in man, Approaches to tumor chemotherapy, pp 379–383. Washington, DC, Am Assoc Adv Sci 1947,
234. Birk C, Franksson D, Planton LD: Estrogen therapy in carcinoma of prostate. Acta Chir Scand 109:1, 1955
235. Blackard CE, Byar DP, Jordan WP: Orchiectomy for advanced prostatic carcinoma. Urology 1:553, 1973
236. Robinson MRG, Thomas BS: Effect of hormonal therapy on plasma testosterone levels in prostatic carcinoma. Br Med J 4:391, 1971
237. Shearer RJ, Hendry WF, Sommerville IF et al: Plasma testosterone: An accurate monitor of hormone treatment in prostatic cancer. Br J Urol 45:668, 1973
238. Young HH II, Kent JR: Plasma testosterone levels in patients with prostatic carcinoma before and after treatment. J Urol 99:788, 1968
239. Mackler MA, Liberti JP, Smith MJV et al: The effect of orchiectomy and various doses of stilbestrol on plasma testosterone levels in patients with carcinoma of the prostate. Invest Urol 9:423, 1972
240. Walsh PC, Siteri PK: Suppression of plasma androgens by spironolactone in castrated men with carcinoma of the prostate. J Urol 114:254, 1975
241. Goldman AS: Further studies of steroidal inhibitors of ^{5}-3-hydroxysteroid dehydrogenase and ^{5}-3-ketosteroid isomerase in pseudomonas testosteroni and in bovine adrenals. J Clin Endocarinol 29:1538, 1968
242. Schoones R, Schalach DS, Murphy GP: The hormonal effects of anti-androgen (SH-714) treatment in man. Invest Urol 4:635, 1971
243. Smith RB, Walsh PC, Goodwin WE: Cyproterone acetate in the treatment of advanced carcinoma in the prostate. J Urol 110:106, 1973
244. Fang S, Liao S: Antagonistic action of anti-androgens on the formation of a specific dihydrostestosterone-receptor protein complex in rat ventral prostate. Mol Pharmacol 5:428, 1969
245. Walsh PC, Korenman SG: Mechanism of androgenic action: Effect of specific intracellular inhibitors. J Urol 105:850, 1971
246. Neri R, Florence K, Koziol P et al: A Biological profile of a nonsteroidal antiandrogen SCH 13521 (4-nitro e′-trifluoromethylisobutyranilide). Endocrinology 93:427, 1972
247. Nesbit RM, Baum WC: Endocrine control of prostatic carcinoma. JAMA 143:1317, 1950
248. Emmett JL, Greene LF, and Papantoniou A: Endocrine therapy in carcinoma of the prostate gland: 10-year survival studies. J Urol 83:471, 1960
249. Koontz WW: Intravesical chemotherapy in chemoprevention of superficial, low grade, low stage bladder carcinoma. Semin Oncol 6:217–219, 1979
250. Birke G, Granksson C, Plantin L-O: Estrogen therapy in carcinoma of the prostate. ACTA Chir Scand 109:1, 1955
251. Brendler H: Therapy with orchiectomy or estrogens or both. JAMA 210:1074, 1969
252. Murphy GP (ed) Prostatic Cancer. Littleton, Ma, PSG Publishing Co., Inc. 1979
253. Eagan RT, Hahn RG, Myers RP: Adriamycin (NSC-123127) versus 5-flourouracil (NSC-19893) and cyclophosphamide (NSC-226271) in the treatment of metastatic prostatic cancer. Cancer Treat Rep 60:115–117, 1976
254. O'Bryan RM, Baker LH, Gottlieb, JE et al: Dose response evaluation of adriamycin in human neoplasia. Cancer 39:1940–1948, 1977
255. Kadohama N, Kirdani RY, Murphy GP et al: Estramustine phosphate: Metabolic aspects related to its action in prostatic cancer. J Urol 119:235–239, 1977
256. Nilssen T, Jonssan G: Primary treatment of prostatic carcinoma with estramustine phosphate: Preliminary report. J Urol 114:168, 1976
257. Andersson L., Edsmyr F, Jonssan G et al: Estramustine phosphate therapy in carcinoma of the prostate. Recent Results Cancer Res 60:73–77, 1977
258. VonHoff DD, Rozencweig M, Slavik M et al: Estramustine phosphate: A specific chemotherapeutic agent? J Urol 117:464–466, 1977
259. Merrin C: Treatment of advanced carcinoma of the prostate (Stage D) with infusion of cis-diammine-dichloroplatinum (II NCS 119875): A pilot study. J Urol 119:522–524, 1978
260. Tejada F, Eisenberg MA, Broder LA et al: 5-Fluorouracil versus CCNU in the treatment of metastatic prostatic cancer. Cancer Treat Rep 61:1589–1590, 1977
261. Lerner H, Malloy T, Cromie W et al: Hydroxyurea in Stage D carcinoma of the prostate: A pilot study. J Urol 114:425–429, 1975
262. Lloyd RE, Jones SE, Salmon SE et al: Combination chemotherapy with adriamycin (NSC 123127) and cyclophosphamide (NSC 25271) for solid tumors: A phase II trial. Cancer Treat Rep 60:77–83, 1976
263. Perloff M, Ohnuma T, Holland JF et al: Adriamycin (ADM) and diamminedichloroplatinum (DDP) in advanced prostatic carcinoma (PC). Proc. Am Soc Clin Oncol 18:333, 1977
264. Buell GV, Saiers JH, Saiki JH et al: Chemotherapy trial with COMP-F regimen in advanced adenocarcinoma of prostate. Urology XI:247, 1978
265. Kane RD, Stocks LH, Paulson DF: Multiple drug chemotherapy regimen for patients with hormonally-unresponsive carcinoma of the prostate: A preliminary report. J Urol 117:467–471, 1977
266. Berry W, Laszlo J, Cox E et al: Prognostic factors in metastatic and hormonally-unresponsive carconoma of the prostate. Cancer 44:763–775, 1979
267. Paulson DF, Berry WR, Cox EB et al: Treatment of metastatic endocrine-unresponsive carcinoma of the prostate with multi-agent chemotherapy; Indicators of response to therapy. MNCI 63:615–622, 1979
268. Kyolwazi SK: Carcinoma of the penis. A review of 153 patients admitted to Mulago Hospital, Kaysala, Uganda. East Afr Med J 43:415–421, 1966
269. Jackson SM. The treatment of carcinoma of the penis. Br J Surg 53:33–35, 1966
270. deKernion JB, Tyneberg P, Persky L et al: Carcinoma of the penis. Cancer 32:1256–1262, 1973
271. Dean AL Jr: Epithelioma of the penis. J Urol 33:252–283, 1935
272. Furlong JH, Uhle RA: Cancer of the penis—A report of eighty-eight cases. J Urol 69:550–555, 1953
273. Cabanas RM: An approach for the treatment of penile carcinoma. Cancer 39:456, 1977
274. Colon JE: Carcinoma of the penis. J Urol 67:702, 1952
275. Rouviere H: Anatomy of the Human Lymphatic System. MJ Tobias (trans): Ann Arbor, Michigan, Edwards Brothers, 1938
276. Sen AK, Tagore JK, Sen D et al: Study of the lymphatic drainage from the growth in the penis by radioactive colloidal gold. Indian J Cancer 4:295, 1967
277. Beggs JH, Spratt JS: Epidermoid carcinoma of the penis. J Urol 91:166–172, 1964
278. Gregl A, Heitmann D, Truss F: Life expectancy in penile

carcinoma (statistical evaluation of 150 penile carcinomas in the period 1912–1979). Urology 15:107–109, 1977
279. Hardner GJ, Bhanalaph T, Murphy GP et al: Carcinoma of the penis—Analysis of therapy in 100 consectuive cases. J Urol 428–430, 1972
280. Hanash K, Furlow W, Usz D et al: Carcinoma of the penis—A clinicopathologic study. J Urol 104:291–297, 1970
281. Whitmore WF Jr: Tumors of the penis, urethra, scrotum and testis. In Campbell MF, Harrision JH, (eds): Urology, pp 1190–1229. Philadelphia, WB Saunders, 1970
282. Da'nczak-Ginalska Z: Treatment of penis carcinoma with interstitially administered iridium; comparison with radium therapy. Recent Results Cancer Res 60:127–134, 1977
283. Skinner DG, Leadbetter WF: The surgical management of squamous cell carcinoma of the penis. J Urol 107:273–277, 1972
284. Doeven JJ, Oldhoff J, Boer PW et al: Penile cancer. Arch Chir Neeri 27:41–52, 1975
285. Ekstrom T, Elsmyr F: Cancer of the penis. Acta Chir Scand 115:25, 1958
286. Frew JD, Jeffries JD, Swinney J: Carcinoma of the penis. Br J Urol 39:398–404, 1967
287. Fraley EE, Hutchens HC: Radical ileo-ingunal node dissection: The skin bridge technique. J Urol 108:279–282, 1972
288. Uehling, DT: Staging laparotomy for carcinoma of the penis. J Urol 110:213–215, 1973
289. Almgard LE, Edsmyr F: Radiotherapy in treatment of patients with carcinoma of the penis. Scand J Urol Nephrol 7:1–5, 1973
290. Bloedorn FA: Penis and male urethra. In Fletcher GH (ed): Textbook of Radiotherapy, 2nd ed., pp 772–779. Philadelphia, Lea & Febiger, 1973
291. Combes PF, Daly N, Regis H: Fifty cases of penile tumors treated at the Claudius Regaud Center from 1958 to 1973. J Radiol Electrol Med Nucl 56:773–778, 1975
292. Duncan W, Jackson S: The treatment of early cancer of the penis with megavoltage X-rays. Clin Radiol 23:246–248, 1972
293. Haile K, Delclos L: The place of radiation therapy in the treatment of carcinoma of the distal end of the penis. Cancer 46:1980–1984, 1980
294. Jackson SM: The treatment of carcinoma of the penis, Br J Surg 53:33–35, 1944
295. Knudsen O, Brennhovd I: Radiotherapy in the treatment of the primary tumor in penile cancer. Acta Chir Scand 133:69–71, 1967
296. Lutolf VM, Glanzmann C, Harst W: Radiation therapy of carcinoma of the penis: Indications and results. Stralhentherapie 152:333–337, 1976
297. Marcial VA, Figueroa-Coln J, Marcial-Rojas RA et al: Carcinoma of the penis. Radiology 79:209–220, 1962
298. Newaishy G, Deeley T: Radiotherapy in the treatment of carcinoma of the penis. Radiology 41:519–522, 1968
299. Paterson R: Treatment of Malignant Disease by Radiotherapy, pp 390. Baltimore, Williams & Wilkins, 1963
300. Prasasvinichai S, Schneider H, Brady LW: Carcinoma of the penis. Int J Radiat Oncol Biol Phys 1:1069–1073, 1976
301. Grabstald H: Tumors of the urethra in men and women. Cancer 32:1236–1255, 1973
302. Kaplan GW, Bulkey GJ, Grayhack JT: Carcinoma of the male urethra. J Urol 98:365–371, 1967
303. King LR: Carcinoma of the urethra in male patients J Urol 92:555–559, 1964
304. Ray B, Canto AK, Whitmore WF Jr: Experience with primary carcinoma of the male urethra. J Urol 117:591–594, 1977
305. Zaslow J, Priestley JT: Primary carcinoma of the male urethra. J Urol 58:207–211, 1947
306. Mandler JT, Pool TL: Primary carcinoma of the male urethra. J Urol 96:67–72, 1966
307. Flocks RH: The treatment of urethral tumors. J Urol 75: 514–526, 1956
308. Hotchkiss RS, Amelar RD: Primary carcinoma of the male urethra. J Urol 72:1181–1191, 1954
309. Johnson DE, Hogan JM, Ayala AC: Transitional cell carcinoma of the prostate—A clinical morphological study. Cancer 29:287–293, 1972
310. Shenasky JH, Gillenwater JY: Management of transitional cell carcinoma of the prostate. J Urol 108:462–465, 1972
311. Kaplan GW, Buckley GI, Grayhack JT: Carcinoma of the male urethra. J Urol 98:354–371, 1957
312. Mandler JI, Pool TL: Primary carcinoma of the male urethra. J Urol 96:67–72, 1966
313. Pointon RCS, Pool-Wilson DS: Primary carcinoma of the urethra. Br J Urol 40:682–693, 1968
314. Lower WE, Hausfeld KF: Primary carcinoma of the male urethra: Report of ten cases. J Urol 58;192—206, 1947
315. McCrea LE, Furlong JH Jr: Primary carcinoma of the male urethra. Urol Surv 1:1–30, 1951
316. Marshall FC, Uson AC, Melicow MM: Neoplasms and caruncles of the female urethra. Surg Gynecol Obstet 110:723–733, 1960
317. Hess E: Primary carcinoma of the female urethra with special reference to the lesion known as urethral caruncle. Penn Med J 48:1150–1155, 1945
318. Walther HWE: Caruncle of the urethra in the female with special reference to the importance of histological examination in the differential diagnosis J Urol 50:380–388, 1943
319. Desai S, Libertino JA, Zinman L: Primary carcinoma of the female urethra. J Urol 110:693–695, 1973
320. Monaco AP, Murphy GB, Dowling W: Primary cancer of the female urethra. Cancer 11:1215, 1221, 1958
321. Ritter DW: Primary malignancy of the female urethra. West J Surg Obstet Gynecol 51:420–429, 1953
322. Staubitz WJ, Carden LM, Oberkircher OJ et al: Management of uretheral carcinoma in the female. J Urol 73:1045–1053, 1955
323. Zeigerman JH, Gordon SF: Cancer of the female urethra—A curable disease. Obstet Gynecol 35:785–789, 1970
324. Bracken RB, Johnson DE, Miller LS et al: Primary carcinoma of the female urethra. J Urol 116:188–192, 1976
325. Grabstald H, Hilaris B, Henschke U et al: Cancer of the female urethra. JAMA 197:835–842, 1966
326. Ruch, RM, Frerichs JB, Arneson AN: Cancer of the female urethra. Cancer 5:749–753, 1952
327. Seng M, Siminovitch M: Carcinoma of the urethra in the female. Can Med Assoc J 58:29–33, 1948
328. Chu AM: Female urethral carcinoma. Radiology 107:627–630, 1973
329. Carter SK, Wasserman TH: The chemotherapy of urologic cancer. Cancer 36:729, 1975
330. Scott WW, Gibbons RP, Johnson DE et al: The continued evaluation of the effects of chemotherapy in patients with advanced carcinoma of the prostate. J Urol 116:211, 1976
331. Merrin C, Etra W, Wajsman Z et al: Chemotherapy of advanced carcinoma of the prostate with 5-fluorouracil, cyclophosphamide and adrimycin. J Urol 115;86, 1976
332. Kuss R, Khoury S, Richard F et al: Cancer de la prostate resistant aux estrogenes avec metastases osseuses: Chimiotherapie palliative par le 5-fluouracil et la cyclophosphamide. Nouv Press Med 7:2478, 1978
333. Mills RC, Maurer LH, Forcier RJ et al: Clinical trial of combined therapy with adrimycin and cis-dischlorodiammine-platinum (II). Cancer Treat Rep 61:477, 1977
334. Chlebowski RT, Hertorff R, Sadoff L et al: Cyclophosphamide (CTX) versus 5-fluorouracil (5-FU), adriamycin (ADR), and CTX in the treatment of metastatic prostatic carcinoma. Proc Am Soc Clin Oncol 19:68, 1978

CHAPTER 24

David F. Paulson
Laurence Einhorn
Michael Peckham
Stephen D. Williams

Cancer of the Testis

Testicular tumors are rare, comprising approximately 1% of all cancers occurring in men, with an annual incidence of 2.3/100,000 and an annual death rate of 0.64% in the adult male population.[1-4] These tumors are of major clinical importance since they occur in young men, and are a leading cause of cancer deaths (11%–13%) in men in the second and third decades of life. Classification and staging of testicular malignancy is important, as treatment selection should be based on the pathologic classification, on the presence or absence of residual disease following surgical intervention, and on the presence of extended disease beyond the area of local control. Accurate clinical and surgical–pathologic staging is therefore critical in diagnosis, prognosis, and selection of treatment modalities. Tumors of germinal cell origin comprise approximately 90% of all neoplasms of the testes.[5] They occur slightly more frequently on the right than on the left and are bilateral in only 2% of patients.[6] Four classic histologic types of testicular malignancy exist: seminoma, embryonal carcinom, teratoma, and choriocarcinoma.[1,2,7,8] Each cell type can occur in pure form or two or more cell types can be coexistent (Table 24-1). Each basic pattern has multiple variations and it is convenient to describe the various histologic patterns individually. For the purposes of treatment selection, it is valuable to select the histologic pattern which carries the most ominous prognosis.

HISTOLOGIC PATTERNS

SEMINOMA

The cells are polyhedral with fine, definite cytoplasmic membranes, finely granular or clear cytoplasm, and centrally placed nuclei with well-dispersed chromatin and one-to-two-nuclei (Fig. 24-1).[7,8] Two variations of seminoma exist. The anaplastic seminoma is characterized by nuclei with irregularly clumped chromatin and prominent nucleoli.[7,8] Mitotic figures are frequent and giant tumor cells, which resemble trophoblastic giant cells, are frequent. The anaplastic seminoma represents one end of the histologic spectrum of seminoma and has no prognostic significance. The anaplastic pattern may comprise all or any part of the histologic sections. The spermatocytic seminoma is rare, comprising between 4% and 7% of all seminomas.[9-11] It is so named because the cells of the spermatocytic seminoma have round nuclei with coarsely granular and dense chromatin and resemble the nuclei of spermatozoa and spermatocytes. This pattern has not been reported associated with either other seminoma cell types nor with other forms of germinal neoplasia. No specific prognostic significance can be given to the appearance of this pattern.

TABLE 24-1. Cell Types

Tumors showing a single cell type
1. Seminoma
2. Embryonal carcinoma
3. Teratoma
4. Choriocarcinoma

Tumors showing more than one histologic pattern
1. Embryonal plus teratoma without seminoma
2. Embryonal plus teratoma with seminoma
3. Embryonal carcinoma plus seminoma
4. Teratoma plus seminoma
5. Any combination with choricarcinoma

EMBRYONAL CARCINOMA

The embryonal carcinoma has both epithelial and stromal elements with mitoses frequent in both elements (Fig. 24-2).[8,12] Although well-differentiated areas of epithelium exist, necrosis and hemorrhage are common in the least differentiated areas. Glands of varying shape may be present and are lined by cuboidal or columnar epithelium.

TERATOMA

The teratoma is characterized by the presence of differentiated or partially differentiated somatic tissues.[5,8,13] The most common elements are glial tissue, gastrointestinal or respiratory epithelium, cartilage, bone, and smooth muscle. Teratomas containing only fully-differentiated tissues occur rarely in the testes of adults, but with increased frequency in the testes of infants and young children. Occasionally, even when extensive sampling of the original mass fails to reveal undifferentiated foci, subsequent metastases may demonstrate that fully malignant components were present but undetected in the primary tumor (Fig. 24-3).

CHORIOCARCINOMA

Choriocarcinoma in the testis resembles choriocarcinoma of uterine origin. Two cell types are present, the cytotrophoblast and the syncytiotrophoblast (Fig. 24-4).[8,14] The cytotrophoblast is small and polyhedral with a distinct cell membrane and clear cytoplasm. The nuclei are small and central and have small nucleoli. The syncytiotrophoblast is a giant cell with eosinophilic cytoplasm. Nuclei number three or more and are variable in size, shape, and appearance.

The proposed World Health Organization classification of these tumors and their multiple components provides guidelines for pathologic segregation (Table 24-1).[14]

ETIOLOGY AND EPIDEMIOLOGY

Testicular tumors may be segregated into germinal and non-germinal tumors. The germinal tumors are thought to arise from cells of the germinal series while the non-germinal tumors (interstitial-cell tumors, sarcomas) arise from non-germinal epithelium (Fig. 24-5). The germinal cell tumors

FIG. 24-1. Seminoma. Note the characteristic large cells with clear cytoplasm, well-defined nucleus, and prominent nucleolus.

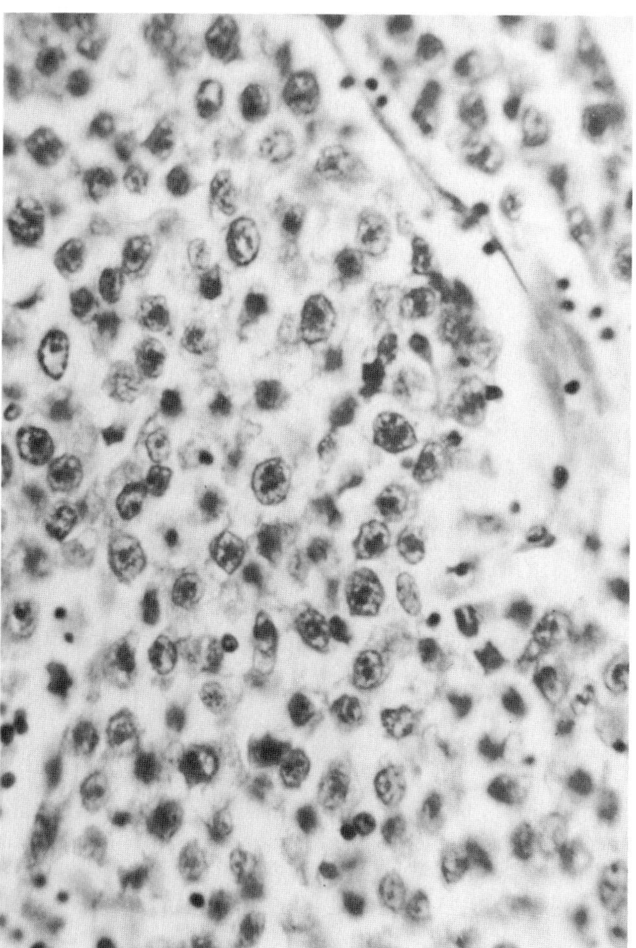

FIG. 24-2. Embryonal cell carcinoma. Note the considerable cellular and architectural variation. There are areas of closely packed, large, highly anaplastic cells without definite cell borders. The nucleoli are prominent and the differentiated areas are glandular.

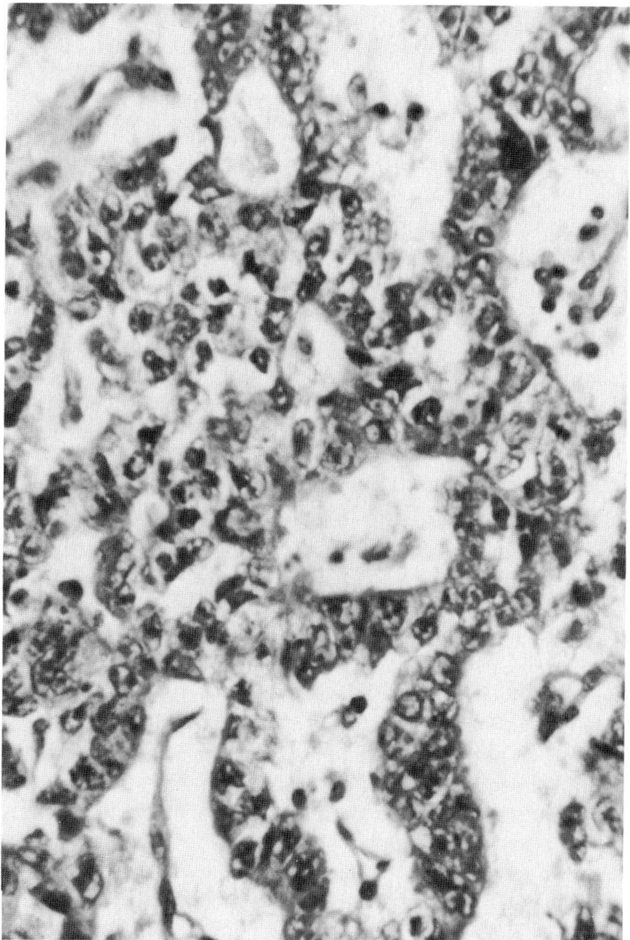

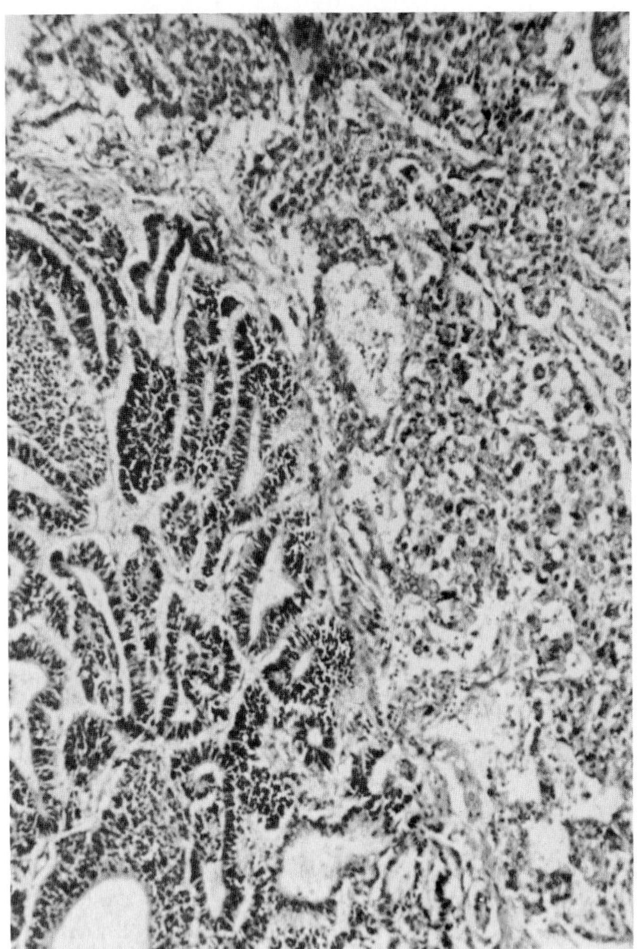

FIG. 24-3. Teratoma. These tumors reveal a disorderly arrangement of fetal and adult structures originating from ectoderm, endoderm, and mesoderm mingled with malignant cells recognized as seminoma, embryonal carcinoma, and, occasionally, sarcomatous elements.

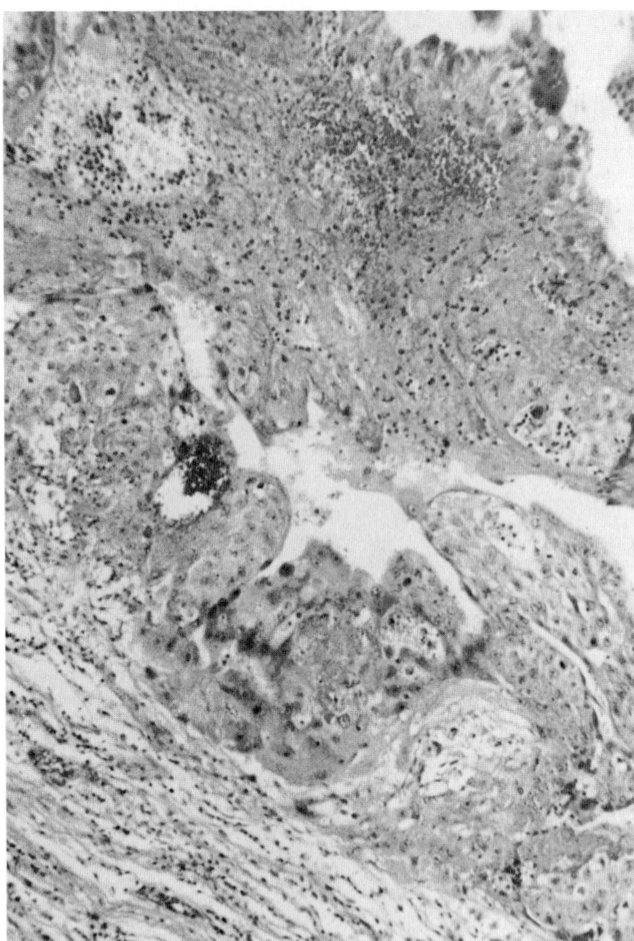

FIG. 24-4. Choriocarcinoma. Microscopically, this carcinoma contains two types of cells: cytotrophoblasts and syncytiotrophoblasts. These cells, in addition to the villus-like structures, are characteristic of the tumor.

are believed to be derived from totipotential primordial germ cells.[15,16] Under oncogenic stimulus, development of the primordial germ cell proceeds in either somatic, trophoblastic, or combined directions. An embryonal carcinoma is believed to arise when differentiation occurs before teratoid or choriocarcinomatous structures have formed. Further trophoblastic differentiation results in choriocarcinoma whereas somatic differentiation produces teratomatous elements. The stimulus which produces these changes is unknown. However, there are certain pathologic conditions which are associated with an increased appearance of testicular tumor. There seems to be an increased incidence of testicular tumors in the atrophic testicle. Gilbert, in reviewing 5500 cases of testicular malignancy identified 80 tumors (1.5%) which had arisen in an atrophic testis and an additional 24 which occurred in testes atrophied secondary to mumps orchitis.[17] The association is sufficiently strong to prompt recommendation of close follow-up upon identification of an asymptomatic atrophic testis in the young male.[18,19] Testicular tumors also are found in higher incidence in patients with a cryptorchid testis, between 3.6% and 11.6% of these tumors arising in the cryptorchid testis.[15,20,21] Orchidopexy may not prevent subsequent development of malignancy, particularly if surgery is performed after puberty.[21,22] Testicular tumors are rarely reported in patients who undergo orchidopexy prior to 10 years of age, indicating that orchidopexy may have a protective effect if accomplished prior to the pubescent hormonal surge. There is evidence to suggest that an inherent germinal defect within the germinal epithelium may be responsible for both maldescent and tumor formation. An increased incidence of dysgenetic tissue has been identified in the cryptorchid testes and this may account for the susceptability to subsequent malignant degeneration.[23,24]

Should dysgenesis be a factor in tumor formation, the contralateral testis would contain dysgenetic tissue in a significant number of patients with unilateral cryptorchidism and would be at increased risk for tumor formation. About one of every five tumors developing in a patient with an antecedent history of maldescent arise in the contralateral normal scrotid testis.[21]

It now is recommended that if testicular function is to be preserved and the risk of malignant degeneration reduced, then orchidopexy should be performed prior to the pubescent hormonal surge and preferably prior to 6 years of age.[25–27] The undescended testis, under the influence of the hormonal surge of follicle-stimulating hormone and luteinizing hormone, undergoes progressive involution and degeneration. The increased risk of tumor formation after puberty has prompted many to advocate orchiectomy rather than orchidopexy. However, the rarity of testicular malignancy even in the testis brought down after puberty prompts recommendation of orchidopexy with careful follow-up of both scrotal compartments.

CLINICAL PRESENTATION

The common clinical presentation is that of the young male with a painless scrotal mass.[28,29] The mass may, however, have become acutely tender or be recognized only after scrotal trauma (Table 24-2). The differentiation from varicocele, hydrocele, spermatocele, torsion, or epididymitis may be difficult and doubt should prompt early biopsy confirmation of the working diagnosis.[30] A history of trauma can be elicited in 6% to 21% of patients presenting with testicular tumors. However trauma has no documented role in the generation of these tumors. A history of mild testicular pain is given by 30% to 50% of patients but acute pain is uncommon. Acute pain with or without the sudden appearance of a scrotal mass prompts suspicion that hemorrhage, necrosis, or infection has occurred within the tumor. Acute onset of abdominal pain in a patient with a cryptorchid testis may indicate torsion of or hemorrhage within an intra-abdominal testicular tumor. Although between 14% and 34% of patients may have metastatic disease at the time of presentation, only 5% to 10% of these patients present with symptoms due only to metastatic disease.[31–35] Back pain, usually lumbar in location, is noted in 7% to 10% of patients and usually is due to retroperitoneal node metastases. The remaining symptoms of nausea, abdominal pain and distension, anorexia, weight loss, or skeletal pain are sufficiently infrequent so as to deserve mention in passing only.

PHYSICAL EXAMINATION

The patient should be examined in both the erect and supine positions with attention directed to the intrascrotal contents. If the mass can be separated from the body of the testicle,

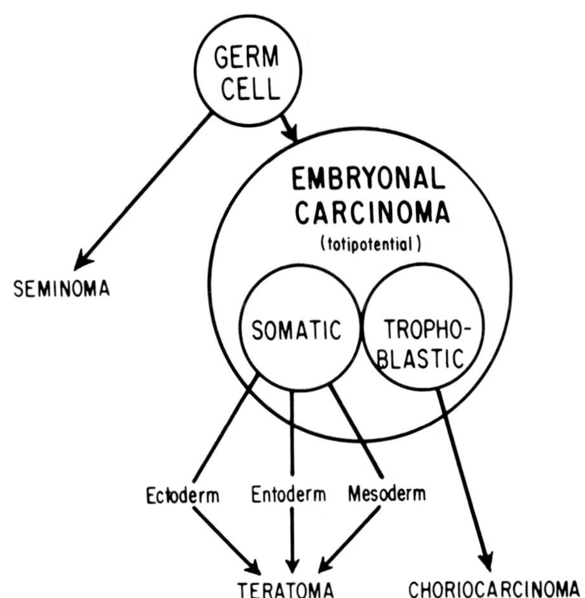

FIG. 24-5. Proposed scheme for the development of germinal tumors.

then the diagnosis of a germinal cell tumor can be discarded. The intrascrotal contents should be examined in an orderly fashion, beginning with the normal testicle to provide a point of reference for abnormality. Attention should be directed to the body of the testis, noting its relationship to the tunica vaginalis, the head, body and tail of the epididymis, and the cord structures to the external ring. The normal testicle is uniform in consistency and any area of induration, nodularity, or irregularity should be considered a tumor. The mature testis may be replaced by tumor producing uniform firmness throughout the testis. Hydroceles occur in 5% to 10% of patients with testicular tumors and the presence of a hydrocele in the young male should prompt suspicion of malignancy. If the tumor cannot be defined by palpation or transillumination, inguinal exploration with ablation of the hydrocele is warranted. Should the hydrocele fluid be bloody and not clear, either invasion of the tunica albuginea or infiltration of the epididymis has occurred. The epididymis can usually be separated from the body of the testicle. Inflammatory lesions of the epididymis usually produce an associated thickening of the vas deferens; in testicular lesions, the vas remains unchanged.

TABLE 24-2. Presenting Symptoms (2926 Patients)

STUDY	NO. OF CASES	TESTICULAR MASS/SWELLING	TESTICULAR PAIN	SYMPTOMS OF METASTATIC DISEASE	NO SYMPTOMS	HISTORY OF TRAUMA
Patton et al (1960)	491	74%	23%	10%	5%	7%
Thompson et al (1961)	178	76%	33%	–	–	21%
Collins & Pugh (1964)	858	91%	32%	14%	2%	10%
Robson et al (1965)	360	80%	26%	5%	4%	19%
Vechinski et al (1965)	112	88%	13%	11%	4%	–
MacKay & Sellers (1966)	731	78%	15%	4%	1%	6%
Kurohara et al (1967)	196	85%	49%	10%	8%	7%

TABLE 24-3. Errors In Diagnosis

Epididymitis	Hematoma
Epididymo-orchitis	Torsion
Hydrocele	Spermatocele
Inguinal hernia	Varicocele
Hematocele	Gumma

Initial physical examination should seek evidence of local extension, clinically positive adenopathy, or residue of previous surgery in the groin or scrotum.[30,36,37] Initial physical examination should assess the possibility of distant spread. Careful attention should be given to determining the presence or absence of enlarged lymph nodes, particularly in the supraclavicular, cervical, and inguinal areas. While it is more common for the subdiaphragmatic lymphatics to drain to the left supraclavicular lymph nodes, anomalous lymphatic drainage into the right or into both supraclavicular regions can occur. The abdomen should be examined for the presence of intra-abdominal or large retroperitoneal masses. The scrotum should be carefully examined for evidence of direct extension to the scrotal tunics or skin, as such involvement carries an adverse prognosis.

CONFIRMATION OF A WORKING DIAGNOSIS OF TESTICULAR MALIGNANCY

The differential diagnosis of testicular malignancy is as presented in Table 24-3. If error is to be made, it should be to incorrectly diagnosis a lesion as malignant and to push for surgical confirmation. The working diagnosis is confirmed by open surgical biopsy. The testicular lymphatics receive no branches from the surrounding scrotal tissues. The surgical approach advocated for biopsy and excision of the primary tumor has been designed to prevent disruption of the lymphatic drainage. The high inguinal approach allows delivery of the testicle and its tunics without contamination of adjacent scrotal tissue.[29,38,39] The incision for radical inguinal orchiectomy is that employed for hernia repair and lies in a line from the anterior–superior iliac spine to the pubic tubercle (Fig. 24-6). The cord should be isolated and controlled with a non-crushing clamp during manipulation of the testicle. The mass then can be delivered into the operative field for inspection. If the mass is identified as malignant, the cord then should be transected and doubly ligated at the level of the external ring. Identification and ligation of the separate arteries, veins, and the ductus deferens will insure that all vascular structures released in the retroperitoneal space are controlled adequately. The residual portion of the proximal stump of the spermatic cord should be cauterized. It is of benefit to tie and transfix the stump with a non-absorbable suture some 2 cm to 3 cm in length to enhance subsequent identification at the time of retroperitoneal lymph node dissection.

FIG. 24-6. Surgical approach for inguinal orchiectomy. The cord structures are exposed after incision of the external oblique fascia.

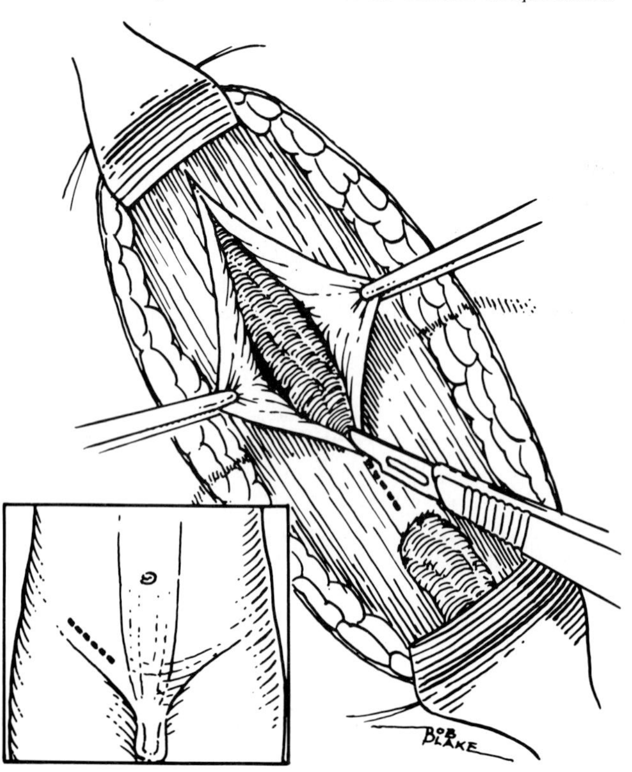

Inadequate, improper initial management at the time of diagnosis is not uncommon. Diagnosis often is established incorrectly by needle biopsy or transcrotal wedge biopsy, with local treatment then being either a scrotal orchiectomy or a low inguinal orchiectomy.[40]

When the testicular malignancy has been managed initially by other than inguinal orchiectomy, immediate and aggressive steps should be taken to remove the contaminated field.[40] Subsequent operation for inappropriate, initial diagnostic biopsy or orchiectomy should include wide local incision of the scrotal incision with excision of the ipsilated intrascrotal contents and removal of the cord structures to the level of the internal ring. Inguinal node dissection should be delayed until adenopathy is evident clinically.

STAGING OF TESTICULAR MALIGNANCY

Following identification of the malignancy, accurate definition of the extent of the disease in the individual patient is necessary for appropriate selection of treatment. While metastases from testicular malignancy may occur by direct extension or by hematogenous routes, the majority of the germinal cell tumors metastasize by way of the lymphatic system with the exception of choriocarcinoma, which extends primarily by way of hematogenous routes. The identification of extended disease and the frequency with which it occurs is dependent upon the morphology of the tumor and the completeness of the staging procedures. The documented incidence of metastatic disease at presentation increases from seminoma-to-embryonal cell carcinoma to teratoma-to-choriocarcinoma.[36]

Clinical staging of the disease is accomplished by (a) PA and lateral chest roentgenograms, (b) intravenous pyelography, (c) pedal lymphangiography, abdominal ultrasound or computerized axial tomography and (d) post-orchiectomy levels of serum α-fetoprotein and B-subunit HGG. These studies are chosen in order to detect spread of disease beyond the testicle. The chest roentgenogram screens for metastatic pulmonary spread. The metastatic pulmonary deposit is round, dense, and well demarcated (Fig. 24-7). Chest tomography is indicated rarely. Woodhead and co-workers subjected 76 patients with testicular malignancy to chest tomography.[41] The laminograms failed to detect a single lesion not evident on routine chest roentgenogram. Tomography may aid in the definition of lesions poorly defined on routine chest films. Chest tomography should be done in all patients in whom biologic marker elevation indicates extension of disease not identified by non-invasive retroperitoneal imaging. The urogram will provide a simple assessment of the retroperitoneal area and may identify, when displacement or obstruction of the kidneys or ureters is present, the presence of peri-aortic or hilar lymph node involvement (Fig. 24-8).

EVALUATION OF THE RETROPERITONEAL LYMPHATICS

The testicular lymphatics are relatively "pure" and there is no communication with the surrounding scrotal tissue.[42] Surgical procedures in the groin (herniorrhaphy or orchidopexy) will interrupt the original lymphatic distribution and redirect some drainage to the groin lymphatics with important consequence to the planned surgical management.[43–46]

The embryologic origin of the testis from the urogenital ridge, with subsequent migration through the retroperitoneum into the scrotum, accounts for the primary area of nodal extension. The testicular lymphatics accompany the internal spermatic artery and vein and drain into the lumbar nodes which lie between the level of the aortic bifurcation and the renal vasculature (Fig. 24-9).[47–49] The left testicular lymphatics drain into the peri-aortic nodes near the left renal vein in approximately two-thirds of all patients. The lymphatics draining into the left testicle tend less frequently to cross to the right testicle. The propensity of testicular tumors to metastasize by way of the lymphatic system requires evaluation of the retroperitoneal nodes. The initial metastases will occur in the retroperitoneal nodes 85% of the time. In only 15% of patients will there be metastases which have bypassed the retroperitoneal nodes. Unilateral or bilateral pedal lymphangiography will identify the character of the retroperitoneal nodes with confidence limits ranging from 15% to 35%, depending on the experience of the local lymphangiographer (Fig. 24-10).[50–53] Testicular lymphangiography, while it will more accurately identify the drainage of the involved testis, routinely does not provide sufficient extra information to rationalize the additional expenditure of effort. There is lymphatic drainage from the epididymis, tunica vaginalis, and ductus deferens to the lymphatic system inferior to the bifurcation of the common iliac. Identification of such extension in the radical orchiectomy specimen warrants both staging and treatment efforts at that level.

The relative advantages or disadvantages of computerized axial tomography over lymphangiography in detection of retroperitoneal disease remains in debate. Computerized axial

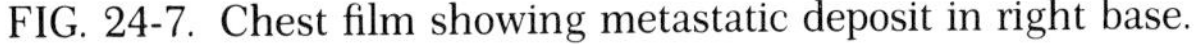
FIG. 24-7. Chest film showing metastatic deposit in right base.

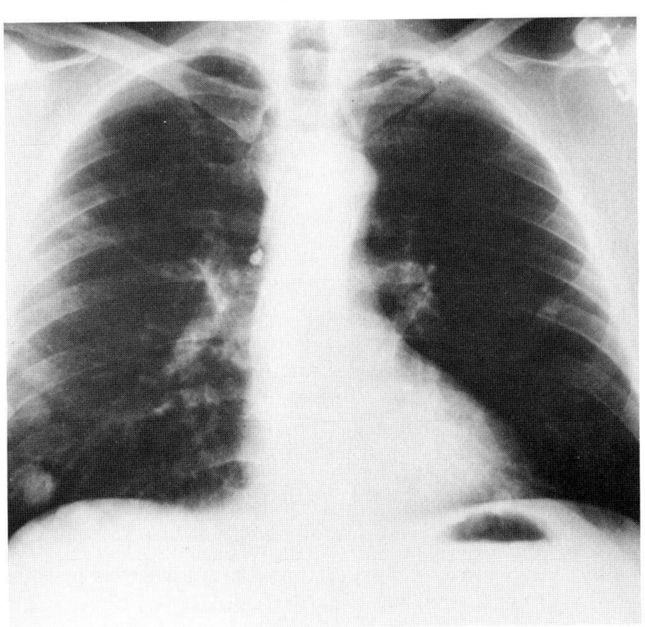

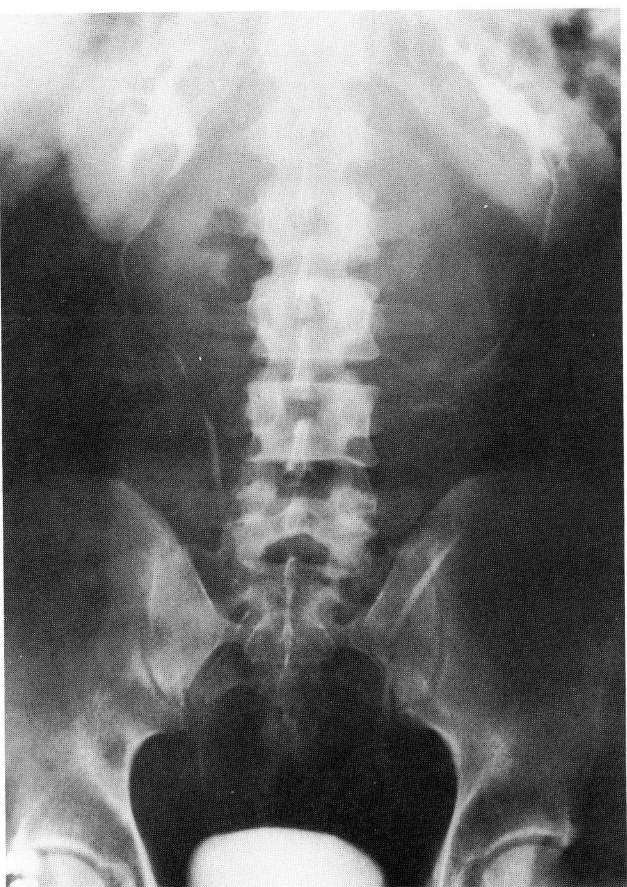

FIG. 24-8. Excretory urogram showing displacement of left lower pole and both ureters because of the retroperitoneal extension of the tumor.

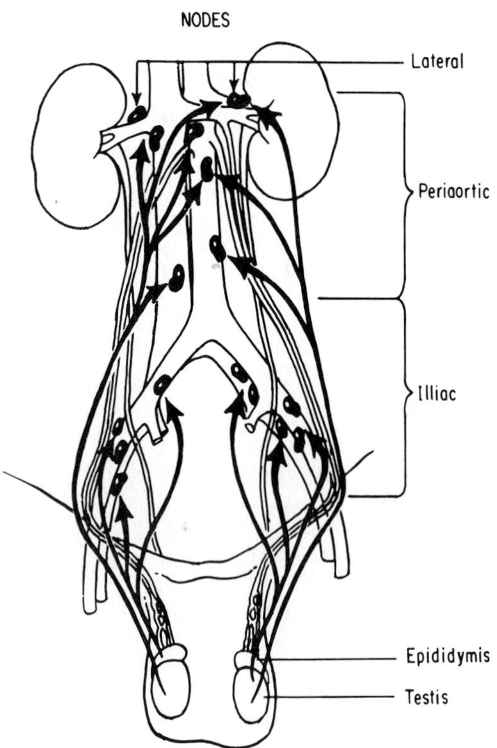

FIG. 24-9. Lymphatic drainage of the testicles.

tomography (CT) does have the benefit of providing an assessment of the relationship of possible metastatic sites to the retroperitoneal structures. However in the thin patient with little retroperitoneal fat, detection of metastatic nodes can be difficult (Fig. 24-11). As will become evident in the discussion to follow, it seems reasonable to use lymphangiography for the staging of seminomatous disease as smaller nodal deposits, which will prompt alteration in radiation treatment fields, can be detected than can be identified by CT scanning. CT scanning in non-seminomatous disease will give evidence as to whether the retroperitoneal disease is treated initially by surgery or chemotherapy as CT scanning can assess with moderate accuracy whether the disease is resectable or not resectable. Disease which is not resectable should be converted to resectable by preoperative chemotherapy.

SERUM MARKER PROTEINS

The recent identification of α-fetoprotein and B-subunit HCG production, either one or both, by the majority of non-seminomatous germinal cell tumors has provided a serum marker by which the presence of testicular malignancy can be determined.[54-59]

Urinary gonadotropin as an indicator of disease activity now has been replaced by the more sensitive radio-immunoassays of serum α-fetoprotein and β-subunit human chorionic gonadotropin.[37-42] Two polypeptide chains, α and β, constitute the gonadotropin molecule. The β chain is responsible for the biologic activity of the hormone and is not present in normal

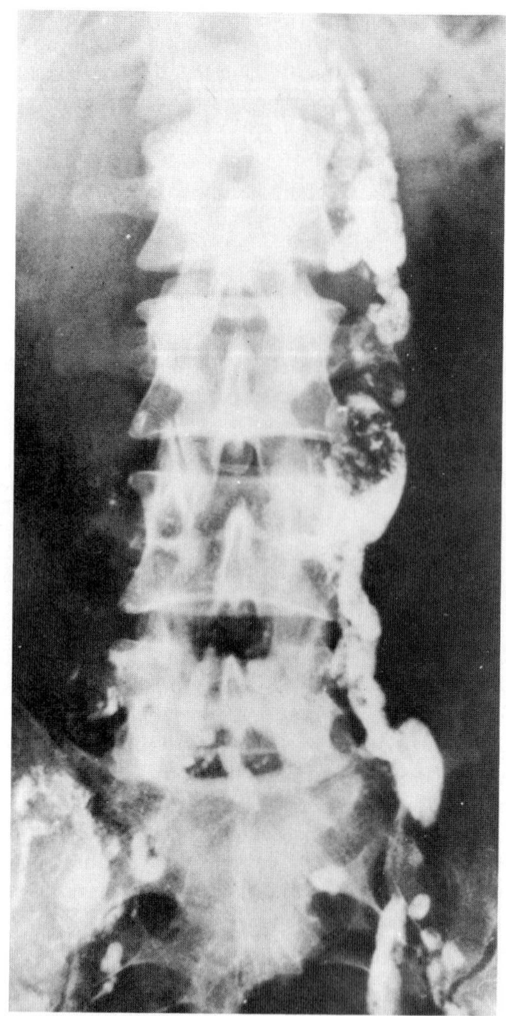

FIG. 24-10. Pedal lymphangiogram showing the moth-eaten appearance of the lymph nodes, indicating tumor extension.

FIG. 24-11. Computed tomography scan showing massive retroperitoneal tumor anterior to the psoas musculature.

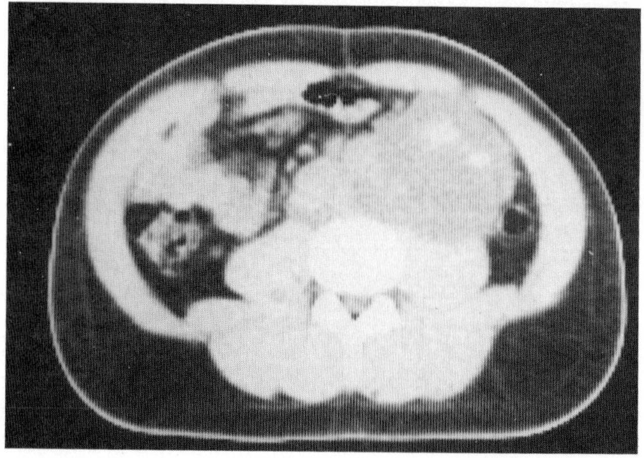

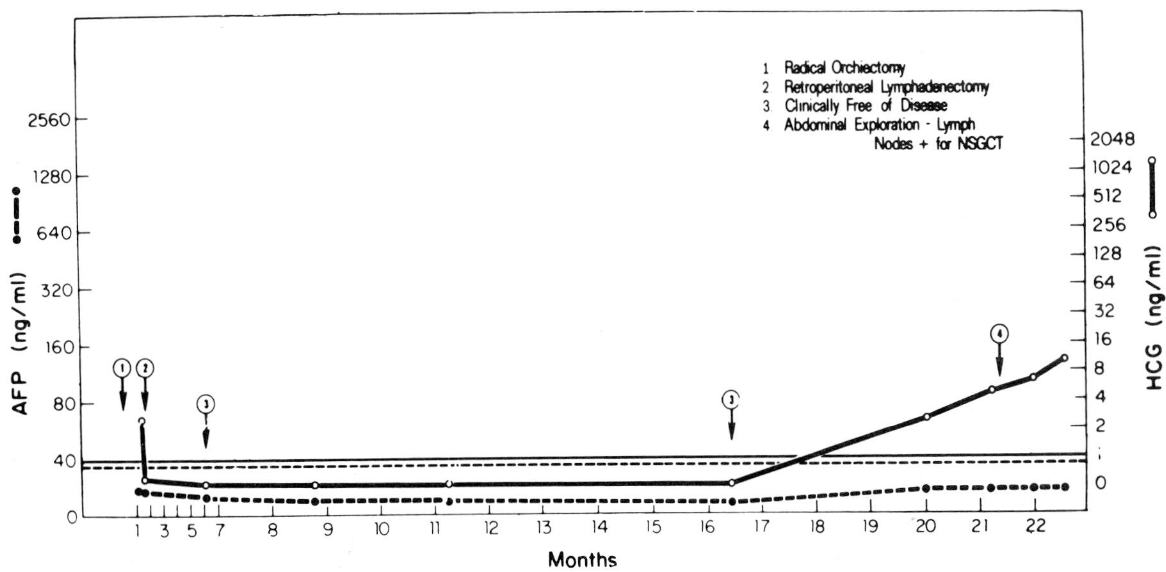

FIG. 24-12. Clinical progression of marker proteins after surgery and with disease progression.

adult males.[60-62] The production of β-HGG by trophoblastic elements within testicular tumors provides the potential for identification of small tumor volumes not recognized by routine screening methods. Radioimmunoassay techniques have been developed which permit detection of serum β-HGG in the presence of high levels of luteinizing hormone. Alpha-fetoprotein, an α-1-globulin occurs in adults only in disease states.[63,64] It is found in patients both with hepatocellular and testicular malignancies. When found in patients with testicular tumors, embryonal elements have uniformly been identified with the tumor. Radioimmunoassay techniques permit detection of serum α-fetoprotein as low as 4 ng/ml. Serum for assay of these marker proteins should be obtained prior to orchiectomy. Considering the persistence of disease, it is important to have knowledge of the half-life of those markers in order to correctly interpret the meaning of elevated levels. The half-life of α-fetoprotein is 5 days and that of human chorionic gonadotropin is about 16 hours. Therefore, half-life curves may need to be drawn to insure that marker substance measured is not from tumor previously removed. Elevated marker proteins after orchiectomy and prior to lymphadenectomy indicate persistent disease. Elevated marker proteins after lymphadenectomy indicate residual postoperative disease. The delayed appearance of markers indicates disease (Fig. 24-12). It should be recognized that not all testicular tumors release marker proteins and that tumors may lose their ability to produce marker proteins with time.

STAGING OF TESTICULAR TUMORS

The staging of testicular malignancy, as based on the principles defined above, can be segregated into clinical and surgico–pathological divisions (Table 24-4). Treatment selection should be based on the information accessed by the second, third, and fourth columns, which permits patients to be placed in a preoperative clinical stage. Present treatment philosophy tends to emphasize that treatment option which establishes effective local control and permits accurate surgico–pathologic staging. Patients whose clinical staging

TABLE 24-4. Clinical and Surgico-Pathological Divisions

CLINICAL STAGE	HISTORY, PHYSICAL CHEST X-RAY FILM	LYMPHANGIOGRAM IVP	SERUM MARKERS	LAPAROTOMY	SURG. PATH. STAGE
I	Negative	Negative	Negative	Negative	I negative nodes
	Negative	Negative	Negative	Microscopic nodes positive	IIa microscopic nodes positive
II	Negative	Negative	Elevated	Microscopic nodes positive	IIb macroscopic nodes clearly resected IIc macroscopic nodes not clearly resected IId macroscopic nodes not resected
IIIa IIIb	Positive	Positive/ Negative	Positive/ Negative	Positive/ Negative	Any of the above possibilities

clearly indicates that surgical resection will not establish effective local control should have pre-operative cytoreductive therapy to downstage the tumor mass and permit subsequent total excision. Patients with surgico–pathologic Stage II disease are at greater disease risk than patients with Stage I disease, with the risk increasing with increasing tumor load. The TNM classification system (Table 24-5) accurately describes the anatomic distribution of the tumor and attempts to establish prognostic categories based on local and retroperitoneal disease extension. The two staging systems are not totally compatible. The TNM staging system does not use the newly acquired biologic marker information but does weigh the adverse prognostic importance of extended local disease (T_2, T_3) and the volume and number of retroperitoneal nodes, those patients with more than five positive nodes or a single node greater than 2 cm in volume having been demonstrated to be in a high risk category.

A comparison of the two staging systems can be made and the relative benefits of each becomes readily apparent (Table 24-6). Either staging system can be utilized for patient stratification as long as internal consistency is maintained. The TNM staging system is emphasized by the U.I.C.C. and the modification of their TNM system as seen in Table 24-5 is supported by the American Joint Committee for Cancer Staging and End Results Reporting. (Staging forms using their classification system are available from American Joint Committee, 55 East Erie Street, Chicago, Illinois 60611.)

TABLE 24-5. Staging Definitions

T_1—Tumor limited to testis and testicular end of spermatic cord.
T_2—Spermatic cord histologically positive at inguinal ring.
T_3—Normal tissue barriers broken as by scrotal orchiectomy or invasion through testicular capsule by tumor.
N_1—Lymph nodes not visibly enlarged at surgery but microscopic disease found on pathologic exam.
- N_{1A}— Five or fewer nodes are positive
- N_{1B}— More than five nodes positive.

N_2—Lymph nodes enlarged and microscopically contain tumor but no extension beyond the lymph nodes into the areolar tissue.
- N_{2A}— Largest node is 2 cm and five or fewer nodes are involved (both criteria).
- N_{2B}— Largest nodes are 2 cm or more than five nodes are involved (either criterion).

N_3—Extension from lymph nodes into adjacent areolar tissue (microscopic as well as gross). No gross residual tumor remaining after surgery.
N_4—Tumor present in retroperitoneal lymph nodes, retroperitoneal areolar tissue with gross residual tumor remaining after surgery.

TABLE 24-6. Comparison of Staging Systems

I	T_1	N_0	M_0
II			
IIa	T_1	N_{1a},N_{1b}	M_0
IIb	T_1	N_{2a}, N_{2b}, N_3	M_0
IIc	T_1 (T_2, T_3)	N_4	M_0
IId	T_1 (T_2, T_3)	N_4	M_0
IIIa	Any T	Any N	M_+
IIIb			

CLINICAL MANAGEMENT OF TESTICULAR MALIGNANCY

The clinical management of testicular malignancy is based on the cell type and the extent of disease. As will become evident in the discussion to follow, surgery, radiotherapy, and chemotherapy each, singly and in combination, contribute to control of the disease. The discussion will focus first on the treatment of seminoma by clinical stage and then on the relative benefits of surgery, radiotherapy, and chemotherapy in the management of non-seminomatous germinal cell tumors.

SEMINOMA

Seminoma is a highly radiosensitive tumor which tends to present at an early stage. High cure rates are achieved with orchiectomy and radiotherapy to the regional lymphatics.

STAGE I

The incidence of occult retroperitoneal node metastases in Stage I seminoma is unknown as, for the last 25 years to 30 years, patients have been treated by regional radiation after non-invasive staging. The accepted incidence of occult metastases is 10% to 15%.[65,66] Following orchidectomy, routine radiotherapy is delivered to the para-aortic and ipsilateral pelvic lymph nodes. A midplane dose of 2500 rad to 3000 rad is given in 3 weeks using daily fractionation and opposed anterior and posterior fields. The techniques of radiation therapy are presented in the section in non-seminomatous disease. If there is no history of orchidopexy, scrotal involvement, or inappropriate surgery, the lower border of the treatment volume is placed at the mid-obturator foramen, the contralateral testis being shielded.

If there is a scrotal incision, it is included in the treatment field together with the inguinal lymphatics. Prophylactic irradiation of the mediastinum and supraclavicular areas is not indicated in Stage I disease. Only one of 62 Stage I patients electively treated only to the iliac and peri-aortic areas subsequently developed disease in the mediastinal or supraclavicular areas. The 3-year NED rates achieved with irradiation to the iliac and periaortic lymphatics (95.2%) equals that achieved when additional treatment to the mediastinum and supraclavicular areas is delivered (90.9%).[36]

Table 24-7 summarizes the results of treatment of 190 previously untreated patients with seminoma seen at the Royal Marsden Hospital between 1963 and 1975.[66a]

Of 121 Stage I patients only one had died of seminoma and this was due to metastases arising from a second testicular tumor. Four of 21 patients (3.3%) relapsed but three were satisfactorily controlled with further radiation therapy. It is of interest that 7/121 (5.8%) of Stage I seminoma patients developed contralateral testicular tumors and six of these remain disease-free after additional treatment. Thirteen patients were lost to follow-up, all beyond the 2 year follow-up period. All 13 were in complete remission at their last follow-up examination.

TABLE 24-7. The Results of Treatment by Stage of 190 Previously Untreated Patients with Seminoma Testis (Royal Marsden Hospital 1963–1975)

STAGE	TOTAL PATIENTS	LOST TO FOLLOW-UP	RELAPSED	DIED OF INTERCURRENT DISEASE	DIED SEMINOMA	DIED TERATOMA	DEVELOPED SECOND TUMOR
I	121	13	4	4	1 (second tumor)	0	7
IIA	38	1 (42 months)	6	4	6	0	0
IIB	16	0	4	1	3	–	0
III	8	1 (67 months)	1/1 NC*	0	2	2	2 (both died teratoma)
IV	7	1 (9 months)	0/4 NC	0	1	1	1 (died teratoma)

* NC—Never controlled by therapy.

STAGE II

In patients with small or moderate volume Stage II disease (IIA, IIB) radiotherapy is given as for Stage I (Table 24-7). If involvement extends to the lower para-aortic chain and there is a risk of retrograde spread, the contralateral pelvic nodes are included. A midplane dose of 2500 rad to 3500 rad is delivered in 3.5 weeks. Elective irradiation of the mediastinum and left supraclavicular areas is advocated by many (2500 rad to 3500 rad in 3 weeks); however, the demonstrated effectiveness of chemotherapy in controlling disease which recurs above the diaphragm has prompted many to limit radiotherapy to the subdiaphragmatic lymphatics, with chemotherapy being reserved for the 20% to 25% with Stage II disease that recurs above the diaphragm. Large volume (Stage IIB) retroperitoneal disease can be managed by a dose boost to 4000 rad total to the area of the mass, taking care to limit the renal dose to 1500 rad, or to use pre-radiation chemotherapy to secure volume reduction prior to radiation.

As summarized in Table 24-7, Stage II was subdivided into two subgroups, IIA (metastases < 5 cm maximum diameter) and IIB (metastases > 5 cm). A more recent analysis described below uses the staging subclassification described for non-seminoma tumors (IIA, B, and C).

Stage IIA (Corresponds to Non-seminoma Categories IIA and IIB)

Between 1962 and 1975, 38 patients in this category were treated by irradiation, including treatment to the mediastinal and supraclavicular lymph nodes. Thirty-two patients (82%) showed no evidence of relapse but six died of disseminated seminoma. Two patients developed recurrent disease, initially in the scrotal sac and inguinal nodes. Neither had received local irradiation as part of initial management despite the presence of locally advanced primary tumors.

Stage IIB (Corresponds to Non-seminoma Category IIC)

Between 1962 and 1975, 16 Stage IIB patients were treated with radiotherapy (Table 24-7). One patient developed a second primary tumor (malignant teratoma) and died of disseminated disease. Three relapsed with seminoma and have died. Thirteen (81.%) patients showed no evidence of seminoma relapse although one has subsequently died of intercurrent disease. The relapse rate of 15.8% and 25% for the Royal Marsden Hospital series of small- and large-volume Stage II patients, respectively, indicates that the patient with bulky intra-abdominal disease is at a higher risk from developing recurrent tumor. The causes of treatment failure seem two-fold: (a) failure to include all tumor within the irradiated volume so that marginal recurrence occurs, and (b) the subsequent appearance of extralymphatic metastases. Two measures can be taken to correct this deficiency: more precise delineation of the tumor and the use of chemotherapy before irradiation to achieve tumor volume reduction and to eliminate sub-clinical metastases outside the treatment volume.

Influence of Tumor Volume in Stage II Seminoma

A more detailed analysis of patients with Stage II disease seen at the Royal Marsden Hospital between 1962 and April 1979 demonstrates the impact of tumor volume on survival.[66b] In this study the results of radiotherapy were considered in relation to the size of the retroperitoneal lymph node metastases (Table 24-8). There is a striking relationship between tumor volume and probability of relapse following irradiation (Fig. 24-13). The sites of initial relapse in this group of patients are summarized in Table 24-9. All first relapses were outside the abdominal lymph node chain. One patient developed mediastinal adenopathy in conjunction with pulmonary

TABLE 24-8. Results of Treatment in Stage II Seminoma Testis (Royal Marsden Hospital, 1962–1979)

STAGE	SIZE OF RETROPERITONEAL NODE METASTASES (cm)	TOTAL PATIENTS	TOTAL RELAPSING	DEAD OF SEMINOMA	DEAD OF INTERCURRENT DISEASE
IIA	2 cm	31	3 (9.7%)	2	5
IIB	<5 cm	11	2 (18%)	1	0
IIC	>5 cm	21	8 (38%)	6	3
TOTAL		63	13 (21%)	9 (14.3%)	8 (12.7%)

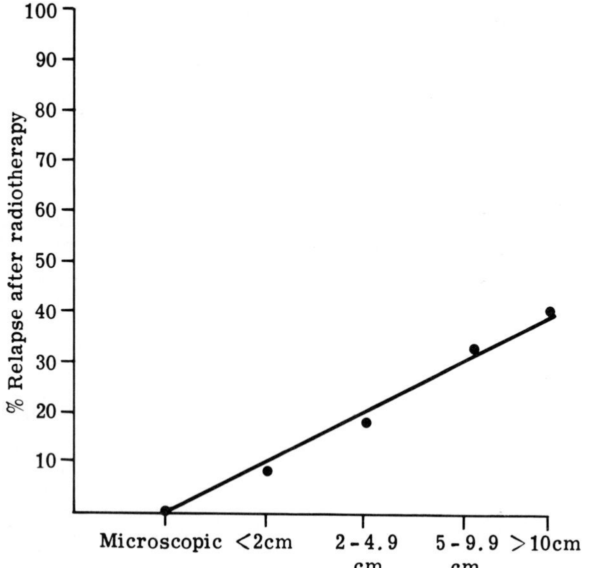

FIG. 24-13. Relationship of size and response to radiation.

spread and two developed cervical nodes. The remainder relapsed outside the lymphatic system. If the sites of second or subsequent relapses are examined, then intra-abdominal disease in association with treatment failure becomes apparent in 6 patients (Table 24-10). Since the retrospective analysis extends back to 1962, it is likely that the proportion of treatment failures in the retroperitoneum may have been minimized. This also is suggested by the documentation of intra-abdominal tumor later in the course of the disease when it became more clinically obvious.

A major factor predisposing to treatment failure in seminoma is the volume of metastatic tumor, with 8/21 (38%) of patients with retroperitoneal metastases of >5 cm in diameter relapsing after radiotherapy. Clearly, in the period during which patients included in the above analysis were treated, clinical staging procedures improved markedly and the extent to which these improvements might contribute to improved local control within the irradiated volume is unknown. Prior to the introduction of CT scanning, staging laparotomies were carried out in a limited number of patients to determine the extent of nodal involvement accurately and to exclude extra-lymphatic dissemination. Six of 7 Stage IIC patients (85%) undergoing laparotomy prior to irradiation are alive and disease-free (Table 24-11). This procedure now has been abandoned in favor of routine CT scanning in seminoma patients with lymphographic evidence of metastases.

Eighty percent of relapses occur within the first 2 years after treatment, although late relapse is a well-recognized occurrence in the occasional patients (Fig. 24-14).

STAGE III

Aggressive treatment may salvage many Stage III patients. Radiotherapy as outlined above to the subdiaphragmatic and supradiaphragmatic lymphatics fails to control disease outside the designated treatment areas. Consequently, a program of combined multi-agent chemotherapy and radiation now is advocated for these patients. Of eight patients with Stage III disease, two died of seminoma and two of malignant teratoma metastasizing from second primary tumors.

STAGE IV

Chemotherapy is the treatment of choice although radiotherapy is employed to treat sites of initial bulky disease. Only one of seven patients with Royal Marsden series remains alive three years after initial therapy (Table 24-7).

Nine deaths from intercurrent disease occurred in 183 patients with Stage I–III seminoma (Table 24-7). Of 54 Stage II patients where the mediastinum was electively irradiated there have been five deaths from intercurrent disease; two of these (3.7%) were due to cardiovascular disease. As seminoma tends to be quite radiosensitive these figures suggest that the treatment is associated with no significant long-term morbidity.

CHEMOTHERAPY OF SEMINOMA

A discussion on the chemotherapy of metastatic seminoma must begin with the realization that what appears to be

TABLE 24-9. Stage II Seminoma Testis: Sites of Initial Relapse after Radiotherapy (Royal Marsden Hospital, 1962–1979)

			SITES OF FIRST RELAPSE					
STAGE	SIZE OF RETROPERITONEAL NODE METASTASES (cm)	TOTAL PATIENTS	*Lung ±Mediastinum*	*Cervical*	*Scrotum or groin nodes**	*Liver*	*Extradural*	*Multiple sites*
IIA	2	31	1	0	2	0	0	0
IIB	2–4.9	11	0	0	1	0	1	0
IIC	5–9.9	9	2	0	0	1	0	0
IID	>10	12	1	2	0	0	0	2
TOTAL		63	4	2	3	1	1	2

* Two of three patients who had scrotal interference prior to orchidectomy and who did not receive scrotal and groin node irradiation suffered local relapses.

TABLE 24-10. Stage II Seminoma Testis: Sites of Second or Subsequent Relapse Following Irradiation (Royal Marsden Hospital, 1962–1979)

			ABDOMEN*				
MEDIASTINUM	LUNG	CERVICAL	*ITV*	*OTV*	LIVER	BONE	MARROW
4	6	3	2	4	4	1	2

* ITV—inside irradiated volume; OTV—outside irradiated volume.

TABLE 24-11. Staging Laparotomy Prior to Radiotherapy for Bulky State II/III Seminoma Testis (Royal Marsden Hospital, 1972–1977)

PATIENT	STAGE	ELECTIVE OTHER TREATMENT PRIOR TO IRRADIATION*	OUTCOME† (Months)
1	II		NED 91
2	II		NED 74
3	II		NED 37
4	II		DOD 20
5	II	CY, VAM	NED 56
6	II		NED 40
7	II	Melphalan	NED 25
8	II	PVB	NED 20

*CY—cyclophosphamide; VAM—vinblastine, actinomycin-D, and methotrexate; PVB—cis-platinum, vinblastine, and bleomycin.
†NED—No evidence of disease; DOD—Died of disease.

metastatic seminoma may in reality be nonseminomatous disease. Patients who were initially treated with orchiectomy and irradiation for pure seminoma and later develop metastases may possibly have a different cell type than their original presentation, as most metastases are not rebiopsied, especially osseous or pulmonary metastases.

Nineteen patients with disseminated seminoma were treated at Indiana Unviersity with the VPB regimen to be described. The median age of these 19 patients was 38 years (range 16–63), and only three were under 30 years. This is 10 years older than the median age of patients treated during the same time period with disseminated nonseminomatous germ cell tumors. The median follow-up was 19 months (range 12–37 months). Seven patients (37%) had anaplastic seminoma and the other 12 had "typical" seminoma. Three patients had primary mediastinal seminoma and one had primary retroperitoneal seminoma. Three of these four extragonadal seminomas had been previously treated with extensive prior irradiation. Nine patients (47%) had elevated serum HCG levels, and two of these patients also had elevated α-fetoprotein at the initiation of platinum combination chemotherapy. As will be demonstrated, marker protein elevation in patients with "pure" seminoma may well document nonseminomatous metastatic disease. Fourteen patients with disseminated seminoma were treated with platinum + vinblastine + bleomycin, and adriamycin. The patient population is described in Table 24-12. The therapeutic results are depicted in Table 24-13. Twelve of 19 patients (63%) achieved complete remission (C.R.), and the other seven patients had partial remission (P.R.) with a greater than 50% reduction. All patients have been followed for at least 1 year. There were no relapses, but one patient died of Klebsiella pneumonia while still in complete remission. This patient was a chronic alcoholic and had been off all chemotherapy for 4 months at the time he developed Klebsiella pneumonia. He had no gross or microscopic evidence of tumor at autopsy. Thus, 11 patients of 19 (58%) remain alive and disease free from over 12 months to 36 months. These results in metastatic seminoma are quite comparable to the results in disseminated nonseminomatous tumors with the same chemotherapy.

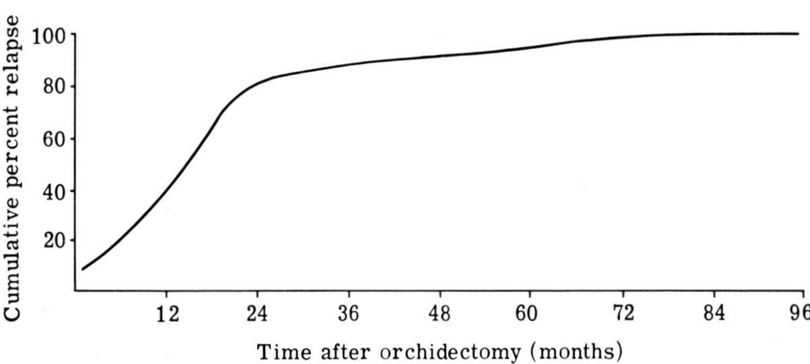

FIG. 24-14. Cumulative percent relapse in seminoma.

Five of six patients with no prior radiotherapy achieved complete remission. The only failure in this group was a patient with massive hepatic metastases. The toxicity in the six patients without prior irradiation was considerably less than that seen in the 13 patients with prior radiotherapy. Ten patients had negative HCG and α-fetoprotein levels at the initiation of platinum combination chemotherapy. Six of these ten patients (60%) achieved complete remission and all six remain continuously disease free.

These results in metastatic seminoma are quite comparable to the results with the same chemotherapy in nonseminomatous tumors. There are no present data to indicate a difference in response rate or potential curability of metastatic seminoma compared to nonseminomatous tumors. The chemotherapeutic strategy for disseminated seminoma should parallel that employed for nonseminomatous germ cell tumors.

TUMOR MARKERS AND SEMINOMA

The occasional elevation of chorionic gonadotrophin in histologically pure seminoma is of interest. Recent studies using an immunocytochemical approach have demonstrated HCG-containing syncytial cells in some patients with testicular seminoma.[67] The relationship of these cells to subsequent outcome is unclear at the present time, although there are no data to suggest that they are an adverse prognostic indicator.

Friedman and Pearlman, in 1970, described a variant of seminoma called "seminoma with trophocarcinoma" which is associated with elevated HCG levels, which is more aggressive and more radioresistant than classical seminoma, and which these authors considered to be distinct from combined tumors of the testis.[68] In the earlier series of Royal Marsden patients with pure seminoma primary tumors (Table 24-7), two patients (9%) showed histological evidence of nonseminomatous components at autopsy. It is probable that metastasis occurred from a small undetected focus of teratoma present in the original tumor. When found in combination with nonseminomatous tumors, the seminomatous component frequently forms discrete nodules of tumor, suggesting separate development. While it has been postulated that seminoma could evolve into nonseminomatous disease and that this might explain the presence of histologically confirmed nonseminomatous disease identified in relapse in some patients with an apparently pure primary seminoma, it is likely that the metastatic deposit arose from nonsemitomatous elements not detected in the "pure" primary. No patient in the Royal Marsden seminoma series had an elevated serum α-fetoprotein level. In those cases where there was an elevated α-fetoprotein level, a nonseminomatous component invariably has been demonstrated at autopsy or by biopsy (Fig. 24-15). Gynecomastia in nonseminomatous disease tends to be associated with an elevated HCG level, but in the Royal Marsden

TABLE 24-12. Patient Population

PATIENT	AGE (Years)	HISTOLOGY	PRIOR THERAPY*	TREATMENT†	METASTATIC SITES
1	33	Anaplastic	RND	PVB	Retroperitoneal nodes
2	30	Seminoma	XRT; chlorambucil + methotrexate + actinomycin-D + vincristine	PVB	Liver, lungs, abdominal nodes, ascites
3	45	Retroperitoneal Seminoma	XRT; chlorambicil	PVB	Liver, abdominal mass, lungs
4	45	Seminoma	RND + XRT	PVB	Lungs
5	41	Seminoma	XRT	PVB	Abdominal nodes, bone
6	23	Anaplastic	None	PVB	Lungs, abdominal mass, bone
7	34	Seminoma	XRT	PVBA	Elevated HCG + α-fetoprotein
8	43	Seminoma	XRT	PVB	Lungs, brain
9	33	Anaplastic	RND	PVB	Supraclavicular nodes
10	38	Seminoma	XRT	PVB	Adbominal nodes
11	16	Anaplastic	None	PVB	Liver, lungs, abdominal mass
12	45	Anaplastic	RND	PVBA	Abdominal nodes
13	40	Anaplastic Mediastinal Seminoma	XRT	PVB	Liver
14	44	Anaplastic	XRT	PVBA	Suprasternal mass
15	63	Seminoma	XRT	PVB	Lungs
16	43	Mediastinal Seminoma	XRT	PVB	Abdominal mass
17	37	Seminoma	XRT; cyclophosphamide + vincristine + prednisone	PVB	Liver, abdominal mass
18	29	Seminoma	XRT; RND	PVBA	Lungs, abdominal mass
19	32	Mediastinal Seminoma	None	PVBA	Mediastinal mass

* RND = retroperitoneal node dissection; XRT = radiotherapy.
† PVB = platinum, vinblastine and bleomycin; PVBA = platinum, vinblastine, bleomycin, and adriamycin.

TABLE 24-13. Treatment Results

PATIENT	HCG*	AFP†	RESPONSE	DURATION (Months)	SURVIVAL (Months)
1	N	N	C.R.	36+	37+
2	53	N	P.R.	4	5
3	86	N	P.R.	7	8
4	153	N	C.R.	9‡	10
5	N	N	C.R.	32+	34+
6	N	N	C.R.	30+	32+
7	73	86	C.R.	28+	29+
8	1320	N	P.R.	6	22+
9	N	N	C.R.	19+	20+
10	20	N	C.R.	18+	19+
11	N	N	P.R.	3	6
12	870	675	C.R.	16+	17+
13	N	N	C.R.	14+	15+
14	N	N	C.R.	14+	15+
15	N	N	P.R.	3	4
16	N	N	P.R.	3	4
17	N	N	P.R.	4	5
18	360	N	C.R.	11+	12+
19	64	N	C.R.	11+	12+

* Human chorionic gonadotropin: N—normal (less than 1.5 mIU/ml)
† α-fetoprotein: N—normal (less than 20 ng/ml)
‡ Died of Klebsiella pneumonia; no tumor at autopsy

Hospital series gynecomastia was detected in five seminoma patients in the absence of an elevated HCG level and was of no prognostic significance in four.

Javadpour and colleagues, in 1978, reported elevation of serum HCG in ten of 130 seminoma patients (7.6%) but no patient had an elevated AFP level.[69] In the latter series, stage of disease correlated with the probability of HCG elevation (Table 24-14). Survival following radiotherapy of seminoma patients with elevated HCG levels is summarized in Table 24-15. The excellent survival in patients with elevated B-HCG levels suggests that this finding is not associated with an adverse prognosis. However, many observers feel that marker protein elevation indicates nonseminomatous elements.

In summary, seminoma patients generally present with Stage I disease. The prognosis with radiotherapy after orchidectomy is excellent. Abdominal node metastases require careful attention regarding tumor localization and treatment planning. Abdominal node irradiation in patients with Stage IIA and IIB disease controls almost 80% of patients. Chemotherapy is not indicated in this group. Patients with more bulky Stage II disease (>5 cm) experience a relapse rate significantly higher owing to the increased probability of

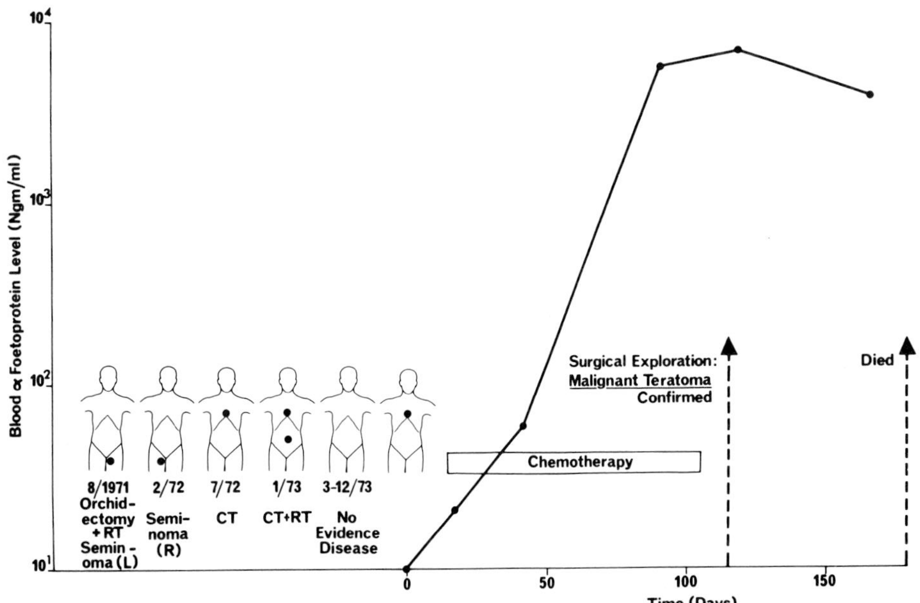

FIG. 24-15. α-Fetoprotein level and the appearance of malignant teratoma metastases in a patient with apparently pure bilateral testicular seminomas. RT = radiation therapy; CT = chemotherapy.

TABLE 24-14. Elevated HCG Serum Levels in Seminoma Testis

STAGE	TOTAL PATIENTS	NUMBER WITH RAISED HCG LEVELS	PERCENT
I	109	4	3.6
II	18	7	39
III	3	0	
TOTAL	130	11	8.4

(Javadpour N, McIntire KR, Waldman TA: Human chorionic gonadotropin (HCG) and alpha-fetoprotein (AFP) in sera and tumor cells of patients with testicular seminoma: A prospective study. Cancer 42:2768–2772, 1978)

TABLE 24-15. Survival after Radiotherapy of Patients with Histologically Pure Seminoma Testis and Elevated Serum–HCG Levels

SERIES	TOTAL PATIENTS	DISEASE FREE
Javadpour et al, 1978	11*	11
Mauch et al, 1979	6	6
Royal Marsden Hospital	9	9†

* One patient treated by surgery alone

† One patient had cyclophosphamide and one patient Melphalan prior to irradiation

extranodal metastases. Chemotherapy is advocated in bulky Stage II and in Stage III disease, followed by irradiation to sites of initial disease. The combination of *cis*-platinum, vinblastine, and bleomycin (PVB) seems appropriate. There is no rationale for single agent chemotherapy. A similar chemotherapeutic approach is advocated in Stage IV patients with subsequent irradiation of bulky, unresponsive disease sites. There is moderate controversy regarding a routine policy of supradiaphragmatic irradiation in Stage II patients and it is advised that this may compromise subsequent chemotherapy because of the extensive bone marrow irradiation. Elevated serum α-fetoprotein levels probably indicate nonseminomatous disease and these patients should be managed as if they had nonseminomatous elements only. The concept of anaplastic seminoma does not contribute to clinical management and stage-by-stage analysis does not indicate that the histological criteria proposed for the diagnosis of anaplastic seminoma confers an adverse prognosis.

CLINICAL MANAGEMENT OF NON-SEMINOMATOUS TUMORS

The goal of treatment programs designed for control of nonseminomatous testicular tumors is eradication of all disease. The programs presently designed employ surgery, radiotherapy and chemotherapy in various combinations. While proponents of radiotherapy state that radiotherapy is as effective as surgery in controlling retroperitoneal disease, the current trend in the United States is to use surgery as the primary form of tumor control for disease that is confined to a single anatomic region, reserving chemotherapy for patients with microscopic residual or delayed distant disease. Disease felt not resectable by initial surgical intervention is presently treated by cytoreduction chemotherapy followed by surgical excision of residual disease. Currently, radiotherapy is not used as a first line of control of retroperitioneal disease owing to concern regarding potential compromise of chemotherapy secondary to radiation-induced marrow damage. The discussion to follow will present the case for surgical and radiotherapeutic management of retroperitoneal disease, followed by a discussion of chemotherapy and the impact of current programs in control of residual or disseminated disease.

SURGICAL MANAGEMENT OF TESTICULAR CANCER—STAGE I AND STAGE II

Surgical management of testicular malignancy should be directed toward local control. Appropriately selected, surgery can effectively control testicular cancer both at the primary site and at metastatic retroperitoneal sites. However, surgery should be considered only a local control modality. While there is considerable opinion that cytoreductive surgery may contribute to subsequent chemotherapeutic or radiotherapeutic control, there is a large body of evidence demonstrating that pre-operative cytoreductive radiotherapy or chemotherapy may transform unresectable lesions into resectable lesions and that this should be the initial step in management of bulky lesions to preserve tissue planes and prevent surgical dissemination of malignancy. The controversy surrounding retroperitoneal lymphadenectomy focuses on the relative benefits of bilateral *versus* ipsilateral retroperitoneal node dissection and of infrarenal *versus* suprarenal node dissection.[70–72] The rationale for ipsilateral node dissection is based on the observation that rarely do contralateral metastatic nodes appear when the ipsilateral nodes are negative. A secondary purpose for limiting the dissection to the unilaterally affected side is to preserve ejaculatory function.[73] Nonetheless, the majority of patients who undergo unilateral dissection continue to have difficulty in ejaculation.[74] Similarly, the extreme rarity of suprahilar nodal disease in the face of negative infrahilar nodes supports the merits of an infrahilar dissection in the presence of negative nodes.[75–77] An unpublished report by Donohue indicates that suprahilar nodes were present in only two of 60 patients with negative infrahilar nodes. However, if the rationale for surgical retroperitoneal node dissection is to totally remove the nodal drainage pathways of the testicle within an area that is surgically approachable and comparable to that area encompassed by external beam therapy, and thus to establish total retroperitoneal lymphatic control, one can readily argue both for bilateral and suprahilar dissection. Suprahilar or infrahilar, ipsilateral or bilateral node dissection can be accomplished either by way of the thoracoabdominal or transperitoneal approach.[78,79] The transabdominal retroperitoneal lymphadenectomy can be accomplished through a midline vertical incision from the xiphoid to below the umbilicus (Fig. 24-16). The root of the small bowel is incised running from the right lower quadrant to the ligament of Treitz. Exposure can be increased by dividing the inferior mesenteric vein and artery. Dissection should be carried from the level of the renal vessels. A useful guide for determining the lateral boundary of the dissection is the angle formed by the joining of the spermatic and left renal vein. As the left posterior aspect of the aorta is exposed, the posterior layer of Gerota's fascia must be incised in order to expose the retroaortic lymph nodes.

Should it be necessary, additional exposure can be obtained by further mobilization of the bowel. The large bowel should be mobilized with the meso-colon incised from the foramen of Winslow to the cecum. The posterior peritoneal incision must be extended through the base of the foramen of Winslow, which covers the anterior surface of the vena cava, as later dissection must extend above this area. As the incision is carried across the root of the small bowel mesentery, the inferior mesenteric vein will be encountered and can be divided in order to carry the incision in an oblique manner further cephalad into the left upper quadrant paralleling the inferior border of the pancreas. Failure to divide the inferior mesentric vein may restrict exposure in this area. After division of the inferior mesenteric vein, the pancreas can be fully mobilized and retracted off the anterior surface of Gerota's fascia. The anterior surface of Gerota's fascia can be separated bluntly and sharply from the under surface of the bowel, the pancreatic head and body, as well as the duodenum and cecum. The abdominal contents then can be reflected out of the wound and placed on the chest.

Routinely the dissection is started at the superior mesenteric artery and proceeds distally. Dissection of the right renal hilum is carried to the bifurcation of the renal vessels. Left hilar dissection is carried laterally several centimeters past the entrance of the left spermatic vein. For bilateral dissection, the lateral borders of the dissection are the ureters. The gonadal vessels on the involved side should be taken at their origin and carried with the specimen. They should be followed distally to their termination at the internal ring. The vas, when encountered, is clipped and divided so that the distal vas can be submitted with the spermatic vessels and stump of the residual cord. On the left side, tunnelling under the left colon mesentery will be necessary. The iliac dissection should extend several centimeters beyond the takeoff of hypogastric artery on either side. At this level, it may be necessary to mobilize the psoas, as the nodes may not be visible without mobilization of the psoas from the paravertebral musculature.

The anatomy of the testicular lymphatic drainage dictates the area of surgical dissection. The lymphatic drainage of the right testicle is predominantly to the interaorticocavel nodes at the level of insertion of the right spermatic vein into the vena cava.[50] Ray and associates identified contralateral left-sided nodal involvement in 15 of 61 Stage II right testicular tumors with the primary ipsilateral nodes involved in all but one patient.[47] The primary area for drainage of left testicular tumors is to the pre-aortic and para-aortic nodes just below the renal pedicle. Twenty percent of patients with Stage II tumor had contralateral nodes, and having also ipsilateral primary nodal disease. Contralateral metastases from left-sided tumors usually are found just lateral to the vena cava in an area extending from the renal pedicle to the insertion of the right spermatic vein, with contralateral metastases from right-sided tumors occurring predominately in an area between the renal pedicle and the inferior mesentery artery. This area of lymphatic drainage identifies the anatomic boundaries of dissection advocated for control of disease. It is not necessary to conduct the dissection as an *en bloc* dissection; it often is possible to remove nodal blocs by anatomic region and so designate them for review by the pathologist. Complete removal of nodal material between and around both great vessels is necessary and it may be necessary to divide the lumbars to achieve total mobilization of the vasculature and access to the nodes (Fig. 24-17). Although no spinal cord complications have been recorded using this maneuver, careful dissection often can accomplish nodal control without resorting to division of the lumbars.

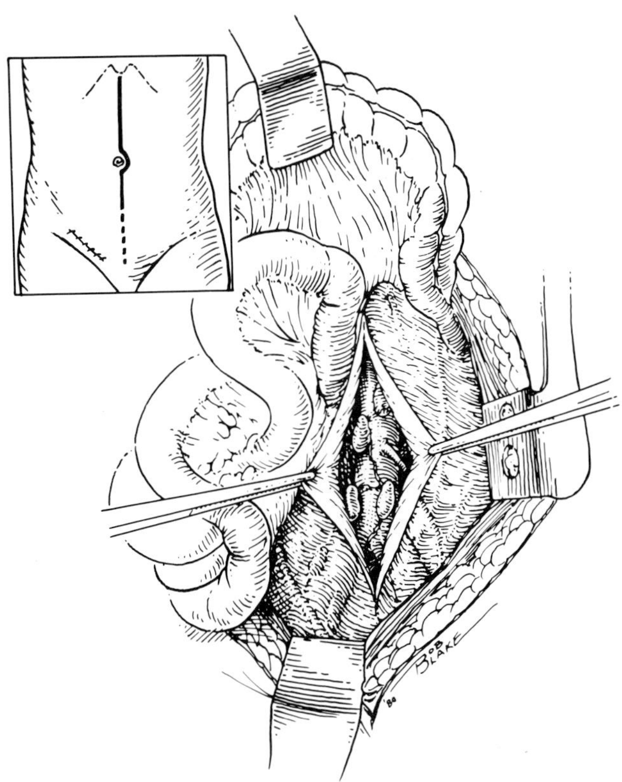

FIG. 24-16. Transperitoneal approach to the retroperitoneum.

Transthoracic retroperitoneal lymphadenectomy probably provides optimum exposure of the ipsilateral suprahilar region.[80,81] Modification of the standard transthoracic lymphadenectomy will provide access also to the contralateral nodes. The modified transthoracic procedure, as described by Fraley, originates with the patient in the flank position and hyperextended.[71] The incision should begin between the eighth and ninth rib and be carried medially across the ipsilateral rectus if necessary. A separate vertical incision can be made from the midpoint of the upper incision just lateral to the rectus muscle to a point close to the inguinal orchiectomy incision in the lower quadrant. Using this incision, the lymphatics and peri-adventital connective tissue can be removed over the entire length of the great vessels from the point where the vessels pass through the crus of the diaphragm to the level of the inferior mesenteric artery. The tissues may be dissected free from the underside of the great vessels after

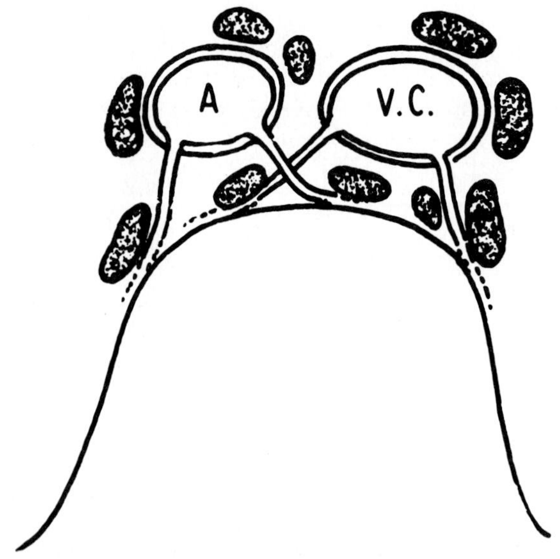

FIG. 24-17. Development of nodes around the great vessels necessitates dissection beneath the vessels for complete tumor removal. A = aorta; VC = vena cava.

retraction tapes have passed beneath them so that the vessels can be held upward to facilitate dissection. Once the ipsilateral renal hilum has been dissected, the contralateral suprahilar tissues can be exposed to remove nodal tissue. Dissection is carried unilaterally from the inferior mesenteric artery to the bifurcation of the common iliac vessels unless gross nodal disease is present. In the presence of extensive nodal metastases, bilateral dissection below the inferior mesenteric artery down to the bifurcation of the common iliacs should be conducted.

Prior to retroperitoneal node dissection, irrespective of the technical approach chosen, attention should be directed to preparation of the patient. Mechanical bowel preparation should be established several days prior to the scheduled surgery. Vigorous intravenous hydration should be begun the night before surgery. Intra-operative diuresis with mannitol is recommended to prevent or reduce the oliguria often seen with extensive bilateral renovascular dissection and vascular spasm. Intra-operative colloid will be needed to replace the large third space losses which occur during and after dissection. If these third space losses are not replaced, falsely high misleading hematocrits will occur during the postoperative period.

Careful conduct of surgery will provide local disease control in a high number of patients. Stage I, node-negative patients have an 85% 5-year survival rate following lymph node dissection alone (Table 24-16). Stage II patients treated by surgery alone have a 48% 5-year survival rate. Control of retroperitoneal disease can be accomplished by surgical lymphadenectomy. The relative survival benefits of suprahilar *versus* infrahilar, unilateral *versus* bilateral dissection on survival rates has yet to be established; however, the accumulated experience would indicate that those centers which advocate the more aggressive approach experience the best survival rates.

THE ROLE OF ADJUNCTIVE POSTOPERATIVE CHEMOTHERAPY IN STAGE I AND STAGE II DISEASE TREATED INITIALLY BY SURGERY

The criteria for successful application of adjuvant therapy are (1) poor prognosis for cure with primary therapy alone and (2) evidence that the proposed adjuvant therapy is effective in metastatic disease. Stage I nonseminomatous testicular cancer has an 80% to 100% cure rate with surgery alone, and very few institutions recommend any form of adjuvant therapy. Although such patients are treated and "surgically staged" with a retroperitoneal node dissection, in reality, the only therapy that was necessary was an orchiectomy. Clearly, survival is not enhanced by removal of multiple histologically normal abdominal nodes. Approximately one-half of patients undergoing a retroperitoneal node dissection will be found at surgery to have negative nodes (Stage I). It may be appropriate to examine abandonment of node dissection with its attendant morbidity, including sterility, in patients with Stage I disease. One should be concerned that patients with clinical Stage I disease (normal lymphangiography) might in reality still harbor positive abdominal nodes, and that failure to remove such carcinomatous deposits might ultimately cause the demise of the patient. However, the current staging methodology permits progressively accurate definition of the patient population with no nodal extension. The availability of radioimmunoassay α-fetoprotein and beta-subunit human chorionic gonadotropin, abdominal CT scanning, and ultrasound permit assay of disease extension. Patients who have normal HCG, AFP, abdominal ultrasound, and abdominal CT scan are unlikely to have a positive node dissection; however, hard figures are not available. It is probable that about 85% of retroperitoneal node dissections on such patients would find only histologically benign nodes. It has been suggested that the patient population with clinical Stage I disease (normal HCG, AFP, abdominal ultrasound, and computed tomography of abdomen) should not receive a radical bilateral retroperitoneal node dissection, but instead should be treated with orchiectomy alone. Close follow-up with monthly HCG, AFP, and chest roentgenograms once a month for 1 year and every

TABLE 24-16. Disease-Free Survival at 3 Years

	HISTOLOGIC STAGE I		HISTOLOGIC STAGE II	
SERIES	*Number of Patients*	*% Disease free (3 years)*	*Number of Patients*	*% Disease free (3 Years)*
Staubitz et al	17	88	8	87
Skinner	40	92	16	81

other month the second year of observation would detect the majority of those patients who were not pathologic Stage IV. Should recurrent disease become manifest, the probability of cure with effective chemotherapy could be exceedingly high. The European Organization for the Research and Treatment of Cancer (EORTC) is currently embarked upon a study for clinical Stage I disease in which half of such patients will be randomized to receive no further therapy after orchiectomy. This is a very important study, and the results will be eagerly anticipated. However, until the accuracy of the non-invasive staging maneuvers described above is documented, the current standard of care should prompt retroperitoneal lymphadenectomy from identification of nodal extension.

Patients with Stage II disease have a considerably more ominous prognosis for surgical cure. Generally speaking, patients with microscopically positive nodes, with nodes fewer than five in number, will have a 60% to 80% cure rate with surgery alone. Patients with grossly positive nodes surgically resected have only a 20% or 60% cure rate with surgery alone. The bulkier the retroperitoneal involvement, and the more positive nodes found pathologically, the worse the prognosis.

Although adjuvant chemotherapy for patients with Stage II disease appears attractive, and clearly would reduce the surgical relapse rate, it may not be capable of improving survival. Although a high percentage of State II patients will ultimately relapse, such patients are eminently curable with present-day chemotherapy administered at the time of relapse.

Following a retroperitoneal lymphadenectomy, whether the nodes were positive or negative, there is a definable probability for relapse. Postoperative patients with testicular cancer should be followed monthly the first year and every other month the second year with physical examination, HCG, AFP, and chest roentgens. The majority of Stage I or II patients who relapse will do so within 1 year of lymphadenectomy and a smaller number will relapse the second year. Relapses beyond 2 years are distinctly unusual. Postoperative radiotherapy for such patients probably does not decrease the relapse rate, and may be deleterious because of inability to give full dose chemotherapy at the time of relapse. Radiotherapy instead of retroperitoneal lymphadenectomy may be capable of producing equivalent results in selected patients with Stage I or Stage II disease. Sandwich radiotherapy (preoperative irradiation, retroperitoneal lymphadenectomy, and postoperative irradiation) may be capable of minimally improving the results obtained with surgery alone, although this is highly questionable. However, 10% to 20% of Stage I and 20% to 60% of Stage II patients will ultimately relapse after initial therapy, and those patients that received prior radiotherapy may be in a distinct disadvantage because of the difficulty in administering subsequent curative chemotherapy.

One-hundred-twelve patients with Stage I or II nonseminomatous testicular cancer treated with orchiectomy followed by a bilateral retroperitoneal lymphadenectomy have been treated at Indiana University. None of these patients received pre- or postoperative irradiation. These patients have been followed from 16 months to 76 months, with a median of 40 months. There were 57 surgical Stage I patients in this series and none of these patients received postoperative therapy. Four (7%) have relapsed; however, they all went into complete remission with platinum plus vinblastine plus bleomycin and all 57 Stage I patients are presently alive and disease free. There were 55 Stage II patients, and 26 of those patients had grossly positive nodes. Eighteen patients (33%) have relapsed. Initially, it was treatment policy to treat surgical Stage II patients with monthly courses of actinomycin-D for one year following lymphadenectomy. Thirty-one patients were given adjuvant actinomycin-D, and 14 relapsed (45%). However, these 14 patients then received platinum plus vinblastine plus bleomycin for recurrent Stage III disease, and all achieved complete remission. One of these Stage III patients later relapsed and subsequently succumbed to metastatic testicular cancer. As experience with platinum plus vinblastine plus bleomycin for Stage III disease increased, and the therapeutic results became apparent, adjuvant actinomycin-D was discontinued. The primary treatment philosophy in the past several years for Stage II disease has been to administer no adjuvant chemotherapy, but instead follow such patients at monthly intervals for the first postoperative year with HCG, AFP, and chest roentgenogram rays and obtain the same studies every 2 months the second year of observation. Twenty-four patients with Stage II, completely resected disease were thus followed and 4 have relapsed. However, all of these patients again achieved complete remission with platinum plus vinblastine plus bleomycin.

Clearly, the only way to determine the value of adjuvant platinum combination chemotherapy would be with a carefully designed random prospective clinical trial. As mentioned above, the experience at Indiana primarily has been without aggressive adjuvant chemotherapy, and 111 of 112 patients are presently alive and disease free. The adjuvant actinomycin-D did not have any apparent effect on lowering the relapse rate, so essentially those are all patients who received no effective adjuvant therapy. These data re-emphasize the belief that the cure rate for properly managed Stage I and Stage II, completely resected disease should approach 100%. The treatment program is as below:

1. Monthly follow-up for 1 year after retroperitoneal lymphadenectomy (whether Stage I or II) with HCG, AFP, and chest roentgenogram rays and the same studies every 2 months during the second year of observation. Surgical relapses beyond this point are uncommon, and the same studies should be done only every 4 months to 6 months thereafter;
2. Avoid pre-operative and postoperative radiotherapy in nonseminomatous testicular cancer, as this may compromise chemotherapy and increase drug morbidity and mortality in those patients who relapse and subsequently require chemotherapy;
3. Use effective chemotherapy if and when recurrent disease becomes manifest.

RADIOTHERAPY FOR TREATMENT OF NONSEMINOMATOUS TUMORS

Metastases from nonseminomatous germinal cell tumors (NSGCT) of the testis are moderately radiosensitive and may be eradicated when the tumor volume is small. In this section

TABLE 24-17. Histologically Proven Metastases from Testicular Teratoma in Negative Lymphogram Patients

SERIES	NUMBER PATIENTS WITH NEGATIVE LYMPHOGRAMS	POSITIVE HISTOLOGY
Fein & Taber (1969)	30	10
Wallace & Jing (1970)	49	8
Hussey (1977)	73	13
Maier & Schamber (1972)	24	6
Hulten et al (1973)	16	4
Jonsson et al (1973)	10	2
Safer et al (1975)	21	3
Durant & Barrat (1977)	14	6
Kademian & Wirtanen (1977)	16	4
Lasser et al (1965)	11	4
Cook et al (1965)	12	4
Seitzman & Halaby (1964)	12	6
Storm et al (1977)	28	10
TOTAL	316	80 (24.7%)

it is proposed to review the results of radiotherapy in relation to clinical stage and to consider the potential future role of radiotherapy in combination with chemotherapy and surgery.

RESPONSE OF SUBCLINICAL METASTASES TO RADIATION

Clinical Stage I patients routinely have been treated by irradiation of the ipsilateral pelvic nodes and the para-aortic lymph node area. Three-hundred-sixteen patients with negative lymphograms subsequently had histological examination of the nodes to assess the accuracy of lymphography (Table 24-17). Approximately 25% of patients had pathologic evidence of tumor despite the negative lymphogram. Analysis of the sites of relapse following irradiation for clinical Stage I disease shows that relapse in the irradiated abdominal nodes is a rare event (Fig. 24-18). It therefore has been concluded that subclinical deposits of tumor are eradicated by nodal irradiation.

RESPONSE OF CLINICALLY DETECTABLE LYMPH NODE METASTASES

The incidence of histologically negative nodes in lymphogram-positive patients undergoing surgery is low. Even allowing for the variability in criteria for lymphographic interpretation, it is clear that the large majority of patients with clinical Stage II disease may be assumed to have nodal metastases. Approximately 50% of patients in Stage II are cured by orchidectomy and radiation therapy with therapeutic response seemingly dependent on metastatic volume (Fig. 24-19, 24-20). Patients with abdominal node metastases less than 2 cm in maximum diameter demonstrated a low local recurrence rate and an overall cure rate of 80% whereas patients with more bulky tumor deposits demonstrate only a 35% survival with local recurrence invariably associated with treatment failure.[82a] These observations, made on a small number of patients, indicate that the small-volume clinically apparent tumor deposit can be eradicated but that radiation therapy alone is inadequate treatment for bulkier disease. Maier and Mittemeyer, in 1977, reported a 3-year disease-free survival in nine of 11 Stage II patients following radiation therapy and noted that the smaller volume metastases tended to fall into this group.[83] Further indirect evidence of the response of nodal deposits to radiation may be deduced from the results of those centers employing pre-operative irradiation before node dissection. Thus, Klein and Maier, in 1977, comparing experience at the Walter Reed and M. D. Anderson Hospitals, reported that the incidence of positive nodes was reduced in patients receiving 2500 rad to 3000 rad before surgery (Table 24-18).[83a]

No firm dose–response data are available for NSGCT. No obvious relationship between nominal standard dose (NSD) and local control can be identified (Fig. 24-21). The observations cited above from Klein and Maier suggest that small aggregates of tumor may be eradicated by moderately low radiation doses.[83a]

THE ROYAL MARSDEN EXPERIENCE

The clinical staging outlined in Table 24-19 describes the extent of tumor, the site(s) of involvement and tumor volume. It is convenient to consider the results of radiotherapy before and since the introduction of effective megavoltage therapy (Table 24-20).

Between 1962 and 1976 radiotherapeutic management was as follows:

FIG. 24-18. Sites of relapse in stage 1 and IIA testicular teratoma patients treated by orchidectomy and nodal irradiation.

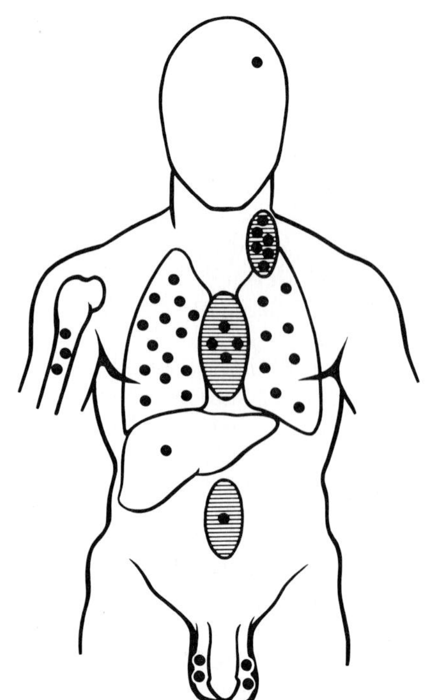

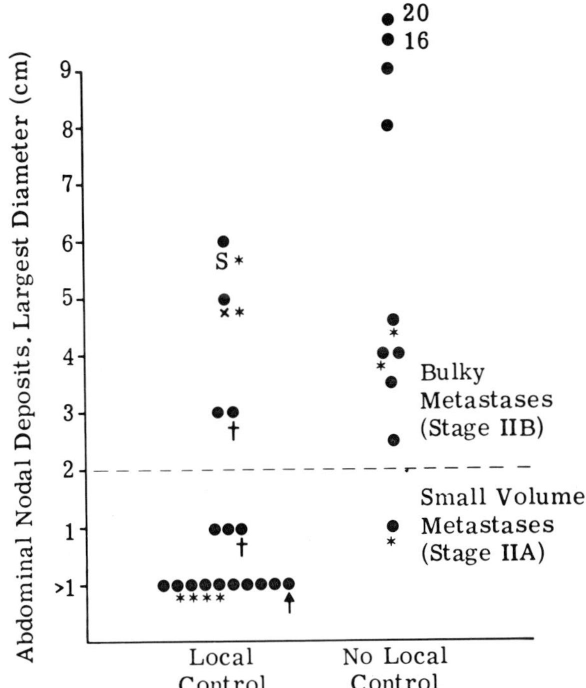

FIG. 24-19. The response to irradiation of retroperitoneal nodal metastases from testicular teratoma according to size of metastasis. †: Subsequent dissection (fully diff. teratoma) not considered as relapses. ↑: Also had and responsed to actinomycin D. ×: Very high dose (5600 rads in split course). S: Deposits thought to be seminomatous. ∅: Combined tumors. Two cases were excluded because of inadequate follow-up of abdominal nodes.

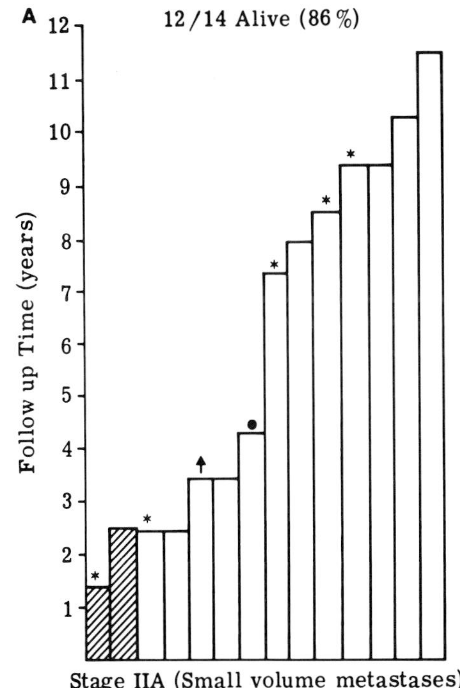

STAGE I	Irradiation of the para-aortic and ipsilateral pelvic lymph node chain.
STAGE II	In addition to infradiaphragmatic lymph node irradiation, supradiaphragmatic irradiation was employed treating the mediastinum and both supraclavicular areas.
STAGE III	Infra- and supradiaphragmatic irradiation.
STAGE IV	In selected patients whole lung irradiation was considered, particularly when disease control at other sites had apparently been achieved and lung disease was minimal.

TREATMENT TECHNIQUE

Mevavoltage radiation has enabled adequate doses to be delivered to the para-aortic and pelvic nodes and, because of the small focal spot, provide a well-defined beam with sharp cut-off at the edges of the field. The latter factor was important since it minimized unnecessary renal irradiation, while allowing adequate coverage of lymph nodes at the renal hilum.

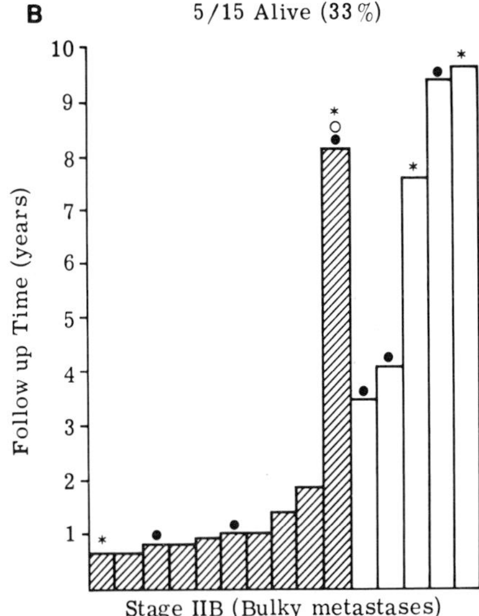

FIG. 24-20. *A*, survival of patients with small volume (2 cm or less in diameter) retroperitoneal node metastases from testicular teratoma treated with postorchidectomy irradiation. *B*, Survival of patients with bulky (> 2 cm in diameter) retroperitoneal node metastases from testicular teratoma treated with postorchidectomy irradiation.

TABLE 24-18. Results of Node Dissection With and Without Pre-operative Irradiation

CLINICAL STAGE	PRE-OPERATIVE RADIATION THERAPY	INCIDENCE OF HISTOLOGICALLY POSITIVE NODES AT DISSECTION			
		M. D. Anderson		*Walter Reed*	
I	–	18/106	(17%)	6/24	(25%)
	+	0/5	(0%)	1/30	(3%)
II	–	20/22	(91%)	32/35	(91%)
	+	15/28	54%)	11/21	(52%)

(Klein, KA, Maier JG: Positive nodes and treatment failures in testicular carcinomas. Int J Radiat Oncol Biol Phys 2: 1229–1231, 1977)

TABLE 24-19. Clinical Staging System

I Lymphogram negative, no evidence of metastases
II Lymphogram positive, metastases confined to abdominal nodes, three sub-groups are recognized:
A. Maximum diameter of metastases—2 cm
B. Maximum diameter of metastases—2–5 cm
C. Maximum diameter of metastases—5 cm
III Involvement of supra and infradiaphragmatic lymph nodes. No extralymphatic metastases.
Abdominal status:
A, B, C as for Stage II
IV Extralymphatic metastases
Suffixes as follows:
0 lymphogram negative
A, B, C as for Stage II
Lung status:
L_1 ≤ 3 metastases
L_2 multiple, none greater than 2 cm diameter
L_3 multiple, one or more greater than 2 cm diameter
Liver status:
H+ liver involvement
Criteria for liver involvement:
Of the four following parameters, three should be positive before liver involvement is diagnosed:
1. Abnormal liver function tests
2. Positive CT scan
3. Positive ultrasonic or isotopic scan
4. Clinical enlargement

An increase in the focal skin distance (F.S.D.) is necessary because of the large field sizes needed. Using an F.S.D. of 142 cm, a maximum field length of 42 cm is achieved. The patient is treated in the prone and supine positions. Anterior and posterior planning films are taken on a simulator with the arms at the side, toes together and heels apart. Two tattoo marks are made on the skin for each field in order that the perspex template can be correctly aligned. A ring of wire is placed over each tattoo and ruler, with 1 cm radiopaque marks placed on the skin. From this the dimensions of the field can be calculated. The lymphogram and intravenous urogram which are routinely carried out as part of the staging procedure provide information about the position of nodes and kidneys for localization on the planning films. In some cases it is preferable to perform a pyelogram by injecting contrast at the time of treatment planning. This ensures that the position of the nodes at the renal hilum can be localized accurately, since the renal pelvis can be visualized. Using the planning films, a template of perspex is made in the mold-room. This is interposed between the treatment head and the patient. The treatment field is outlined on the template in wire and when the skin tattoos are accurately aligned with the corresponding markers on the template, the shadow cast by the template wire defines the field on the skin surface and avoids the use of skin marks. Once the template has been made, a check radiograph is taken on the simulator to check its accuracy. As a final check a film is taken on the accelerator at the time of the first prone and first supine treatment (Fig. 24-22). Parallel opposed, anterior, and posterior fields are employed. The upper border of the field is the lower border of T10 and the lower border, the mid-obturator foramen. In the para-aortic area the field extends laterally to cover nodes at the renal hila, usually between 8 cm and 9.5 cm wide at the skin depending on position of the kidneys and the size of the patient. The pelvic field extends from the medial border of the obturator foramen to 2 cm beyond the pelvic brim. The point of inflexion between the para-aortic and pelvic area is at the lower border of L5 on the medial side and approximately at the transverse process of L4 on the lateral side. This ensures adequate inclusion of the common iliac nodes in the angle between L5 and the sacrum. The remaining testis is protected from scattered radiation by the placement of radiation shields.

If there was prior scrotal interference surgically, such as

TABLE 24-20. Results of Radiotherapy for Testicular Teratoma (Royal Marsden Hospital, 1931–1966)

YEARS	RADIATION FACILITY	TOTAL PATIENTS TREATED	% SURVIVAL	
			3 years	*5 years*
1931–1949	200–400 KV x-rays	32	47%	47%
1950–1961	2 MeV x-rays	52	59%	59%
1961–1966	6 MeV x-rays	16	75%	–

(Smithers DW, Wallace ENK, Wallace DM: Radiotherapy for patients with tumours of the testicle. Br J Urol 43:83–91, 1971)

transscrotal needle biopsy or scrotal orchidectomy, or in those patients where there was tumor invasion of the scrotum or possible altered lymphatic drainage following surgery for testicular maldescent or herniorrhapy, it has been the Royal Marsden policy to irradiate the ipsilateral scrotal sac and to extend the pelvic field to include the inguinal lymph nodes. Orthovoltage roentgen rays (250 KV) have been employed to treat the scrotal sac using a direct field and preparing a lead cut-out to shield the penis and contralateral testis. The position of the shield is maintained by means of a flexible plastic support fitted in the mold-room at the time the lead cut-out is prepared.

In most patients, the ipsilateral pelvic nodes only are irradiated; however, in those rare instances where the patient presents with synchronous bilateral testicular tumors or in those patients where the lower para-aortic nodes are involved with consequent risk of retrograde lymphatic extension, the contralateral pelvic lymph node chain has been irradiated using an "inverted Y" technique. In patients with involved para-aortic nodes a boost dose may be delivered using smaller fields. In some patients the reduced field irradiation has been given through anterior and posterior fields but in others a three-field technique employing lateral wedged fields and an anterior field can be used satisfactorily.

In patients with Stage II and III disease who proceeded to supradiaphragmatic irradiation, a 4-week interval was allowed to elapse after abdominal radiation. It is essential to calculate

FIG. 24-21. Response to irradiation of retroperitoneal node metastases from testicular teratoma according to nominal standard dose (*NSD*).

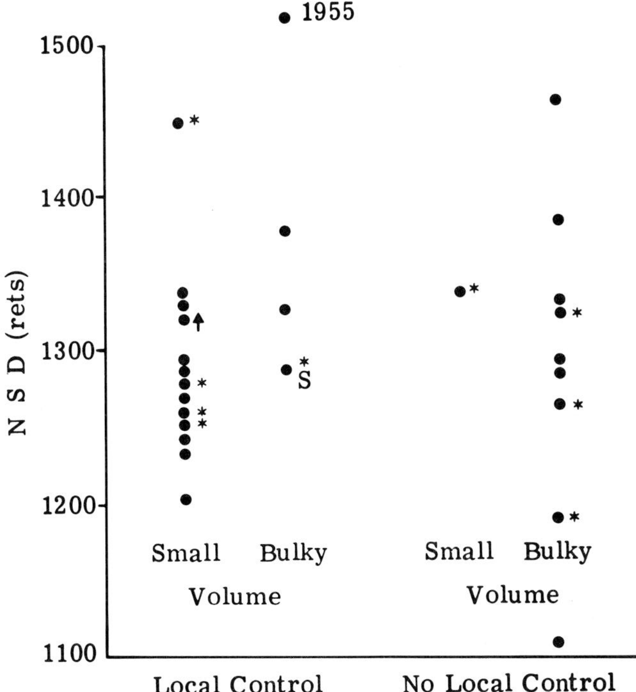

* Combined tumors
↑ Also had and responded to actinomycin D
S Deposits probably seminoma

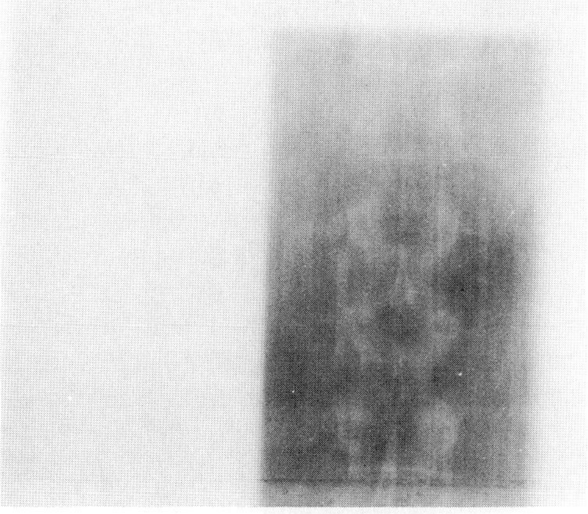

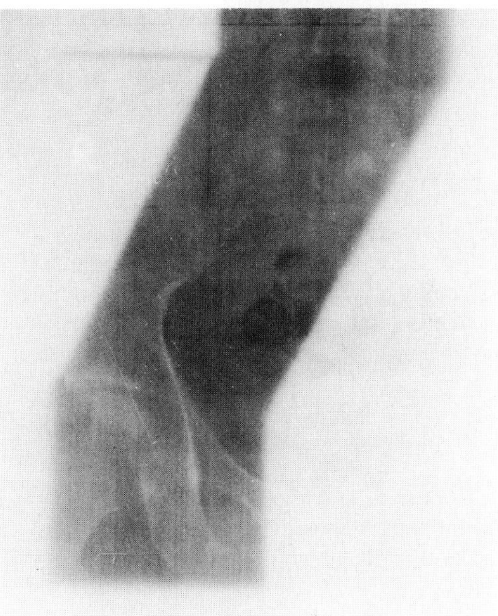

FIG. 24-22. Check film taken with the patient in the treatment position on a 6 MeV linear accelerator.

the gap to be left at the skin surface between the upper border of the abdominal field and the lower border of the supradiaphragmatic field individually for each patient. The upper border of the supradiaphragmatic field is high enough to include adequately both supraclavicular fossae. The upper border of the abdominal field is tattooed at the end of treatment to indure correct placement of the calculated gaps. The gap is calculated from the isodose curves at the field size employed, from anatomical data derived from lateral simulator films. The posterior fields are approximated with a gap calculated to avoid spinal cord overlap so that the fields abut at the level of the lymph node chain. The anterior gap is calculated so that the fields abut at the level of the nodes. The lateral borders of the field are placed so that the supraclavicular fossae are covered adequately. The mediastinal field extends at least 1 cm beyond recognized mediastinal lymph nodes and the inferior border of the supraclavicular component of the field extends along the lower border of the clavicles with the larynx protected throughout treatment. The spinal cord is shielded posteriorly at 1500 rad (mid-plane dose) in seminoma and at 2000 rad in NSGCTs.

Stage I disease is treated with a mid-plane dose of 4000 rad in 20 fractions over 4 weeks. A similar dose is given to the supradiaphragmatic node areas. In patients with positive abdominal nodes (Stages II and III), boost doses of 500 rad to 1000 rad are given, depending upon the volume of tissue irradiated. The toxicity of well-planned abdominal node irradiation is low compared with the reported side-effects and small mortality of radical node dissection. Acute morbidity varies from patient to patient, but is rarely severe enough to interrupt therapy. A degree of anorexia and nausea is common, but vomiting should rarely pose a problem with adequate symptomatic treatment. Diarrhea may occur and require treatment. These symptoms subside promptly following cessation of therapy.

The long-term morbidity has been minimal in the Royal Marsden series. In the few cases of peptic ulcer the tumor dose employed has generally exceeded 4000 rads in 4 weeks and often there has been a history of prior dyspepsia.

RESULTS OF TREATMENT OF NSGCTs AT THE ROYAL MARSDEN HOSPITAL PRIOR TO 1976

The survival results obtained in patients receiving radiotherapy between 1931 and 1966 are summarized in Table 24-20. In 1962, lymphography was introduced as a routine procedure and a linear accelerator became available. The results obtained up to December, 1975, are summarized below (Table 24-21).

Response in The Absence of Documented Metastatic Disease (Stage I)

Between 1962 and the end of 1975, 108 Stage I patients were treated by orchidectomy and radiotherapy as described above. Of this group 89 (82.4%) remain alive and disease free. The survival rate was significantly worse for MTU patients than MTI (Fig. 24-23, Table 24-21). There were only 3 MTT patients and these have all survived. Only one example of retroperitoneal relapse was encountered with the predominant sites of initial relapse in the lungs and supradiaphragmatic nodes (Fig. 24-18). The majority of relapses occurred within the first year after treatment (Fig. 24-24).

TABLE 24-21. Survival of Stage I Testicular Teratoma Patients Treated by Orchidectomy and Radiotherapy Prior to the Introduction of Effective Chemotherapy (Royal Marsden Hospital, 1962–1975)

HISTOLOGY	NUMBER PATIENTS	NUMBER DISEASE FREE	PERCENT DISEASE FREE
MTI	57	52	91
MTU	48	34	70
MTT	3	3	(100)
TOTAL	108	89	82.4

TABLE 24-22. Results of Treatment of Patients with Metastatic Testicular Teratoma Prior to the Use of Effective Chemotherapy (Royal Marsden Hospital, 1962–1975)

STAGE	TOTAL PATIENTS	NUMBER DISEASE FREE	PERCENT DISEASE FREE
IIA	21	17	80.9
IIB, C	24	6	25.1
III	16	5	31.2
IV	112	11	9.8

Response in Documented Metastatic Disease (Stage II)

A retrospective analysis of the Royal Marsden Hospital series demonstrated that abdominal node metastases <2 cm in maximum diameter could be satisfactorily controlled with radiation therapy (Fig. 24-25, Table 24-22). The policy has been to treat as for Stage I, adding a supplementary dose of 500 rad to 1000 rad using small fields to treat the involved nodes. Previously it was policy to treat the mediastinum and neck, but this has been abandoned since the probability of supradiaphragmatic node involvement is low (Table 24-23). Furthermore, when supradiaphragmatic node involvement is present, the probability of extranodal extension is high rendering localized therapy inappropriate. In addition, irradiation of a large volume of bone marrow compromises subsequent chemotherapy should this become necessary. In practice, the Stage IIA category is extremely uncommon.

In patients of Stages IIB, IIC and III, results with radiotherapy alone are poor (*vide infra*) and treatment should be initiated with chemotherapy.

Van der Werf Messing, in 1976, has reported treatment results obtained in 203 patients with nonseminomatous tumors managed between 1950 and 1974.[84] A cure rate of 90% was reported for Stage I patients and 45% for patients with clinical node involvement. Similar results were reported by Hussey and colleagues in 1977, with 3-year disease-free survival rates of 78.2% for Stage I, 46.7% for Stage IIA, and 17.6% for Stage IIB.[85] Maier and colleagues, in 1977, reported the results of a randomized prospective study carried out between 1968 and 1973 comparing radiotherapy with pre- and post-operative irradiation and radical node dissection.[83] These results are summarized in Table 24-24 and show radiotherapy to be as effective as the combined approach.

TREATMENT RESULTS SINCE THE INTRODUCTION OF EFFECTIVE CHEMOTHERAPY

After January, 1976, chemotherapy was the initial treatment for all patients except those in Stages I and IIA who were

TABLE 24-23. Occult Supraclavicular Node Metastases in Teratoma Patients with Abdominal Node Metastases (Stage II)

SERIES	NUMBER PATIENTS SAMPLED	HISTOLOGY POSITIVE
Buck et al (1972)	23	3
Donohue et al (1977)	14	3
TOTAL	37	6 (16.2%)

TABLE 24-24. Teratoma Testis: 3-Year Disease-Free Survival Rates in the Walter Reed Trial

	STAGE I		STAGE II	
	Total Patients	*Percent*	*Total Patients*	*Percent*
Radiotherapy	29	85	11	82
Node dissection plus pre- and postoperative radiotherapy	30	97	21	81

(Maier JG, Mittemeyer B: Carcinoma of the testis. Cancer 39:981–986, 1977)

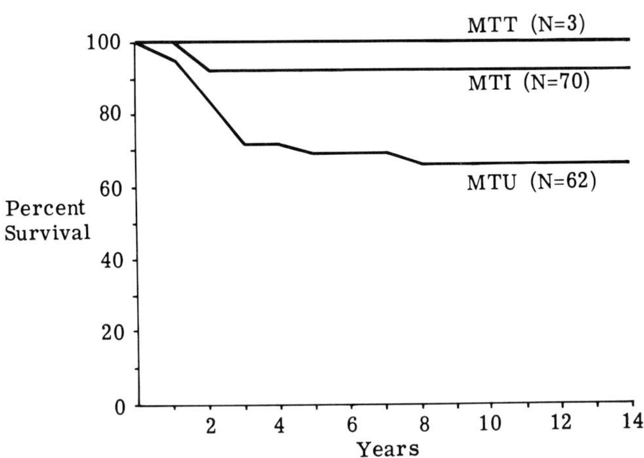

FIG. 24-23. Survival of state I and HA testicular teratoma according to histology. (The Royal Marsden Hospital 1962–1975). MTT = malignant teratoma trophoblastic (British); MTU = malignant teratoma undifferentiated (British); MTI = malignant teratoma intermediate (British).

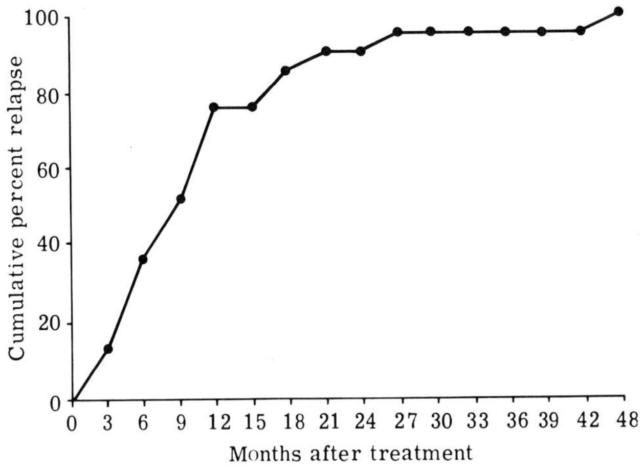

FIG. 24-24. Time to relapse in 32 patients treated for stage I and HA testicular teratoma (Royal Marsden Hospital 1962–1975)

managed as indicated above. Patients relapsing after lymph node irradiation for early stage disease received prompt chemotherapy (Table 24-25). Patients with advanced disease either unassociated with detectable extralymphatic metastases (Stages IIB, IIC, and III) or with small-volume lung disease (Stage IVL_1L_2) received radiotherapy to initial sites of disease after chemotherapy. Selected patients completing chemotherapy and radiotherapy proceeded to node resection if there was evidence of a residual mass. Patients with bulky extralymphatic metastases received only chemotherapy. The rationale of the combined approach is based on the volume dependency of both drug and radiation response in NSGCTs.[85a]

The relationship between tumor volume and drug response seems evident. With these observations in mind it was postulated that chemotherapy would effectively control presumed subclinical extralymphatic metastases (Stages IIB, IIC, III) or demonstrable small-volume lung metastases (Stage

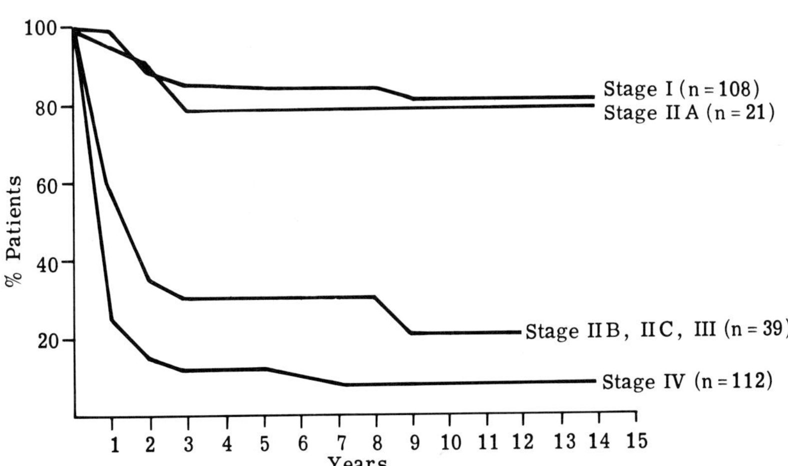

FIG. 24-25. Results of treatment of testicular teratoma by stage. (The Royal Marsden Hospital 1962–1975)

IVL_1L_2), whereas it was more likely to fail in bulky lymph node masses, or when there was advanced extralymphatic disease (IVL_3,IVH+). Furthermore, the influence of tumor volume on radiation response described above indicated that radiotherapy as prior or sole treatment for Stages IIB, IIC, or III would be ineffective but that cytoreduction by prior drug therapy might enable residual tumor foci to be eliminated by irradiation (Fig. 24-26). The approach to management during this period can be summarized as follows:[85b]

Category	*Stage*	*Treatment*	
Early stage disease	I, IIA	Lymph node irradiation	Chemotherapy for relapse
Advanced stage	IIB, IIC III, IVL_1L_2	Chemotherapy, (1) to eliminate small extralymphatic metastasis, (2) to reduce the volume of lymph node masses followed by radiotherapy to eliminate residual tumor in lymph nodes	Surgery for residual masses
Advanced stage Group II	IVL_3 IVH+	Chemotherapy alone	

Patients proceeding through the combined management protocol are assessed after four cycles of chemotherapy and prior to surgery.

Patients were staged as follows: lymphograpy, chest radiography and whole lung tomography, intravenous urography, renal and hepatic function tests, and full blood count. Ultrasonic scanning of the liver and retroperitoneum was employed routinely prior to the availability of CT scanning facilities in mid-1977. Since that time all patients have had

FIG. 24-26. *A*, Royal Marsden Hospital protocols for combined management of selected patients with advanced teratoma testis. *B*, Protocol for patient assessment during combined therapy of advanced testicular teratoma.

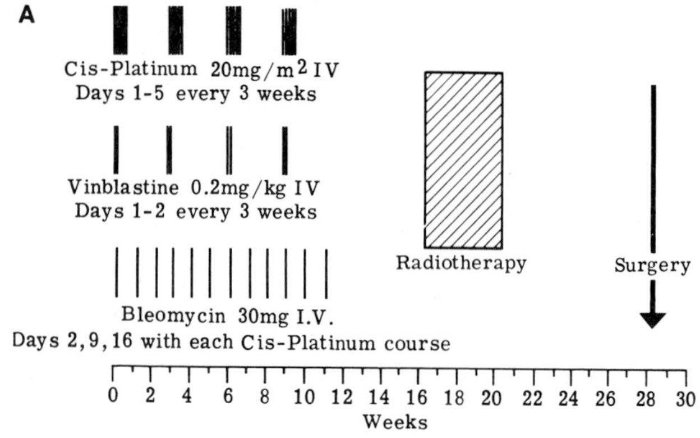

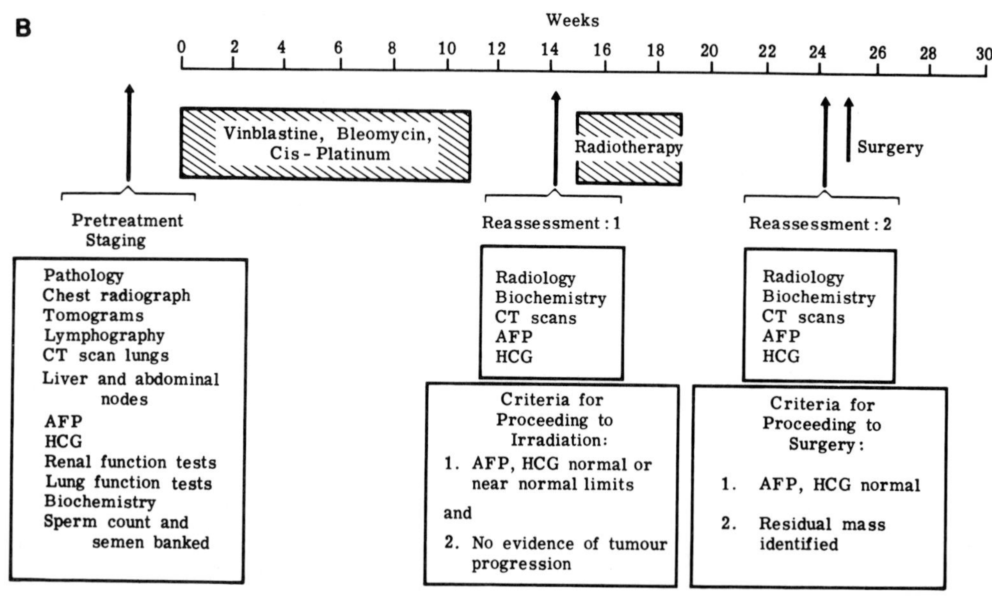

TABLE, 24-25. Outcome of Treatment in 98 Patients with Previously Untreated Teratoma Testis (Royal Marsden Hospital, 1976–1979)

STAGE	TOTAL PATIENTS	DISEASE FREE	ALIVE WITH DISEASE	DEAD OF DISEASE	DEAD OF INTERCURRENT DISEASE OR TREATMENT
I	39	8	37 (95%)	–	2
IIA	4	1	4 (100%)	–	–
IIB–III	17	1	13 (76.5%)	1	1
IVO A L_1 L_2	9	–	9 (11%)	–	–
IVB C L_1 L_2	10	–	6 (60%)	1	1
IVO A L_3	8	–	5 (62.5%)	3	–
IVB C L_3	5	–	1 } (9%)	2	–
IV H^+	6	–		6	–
TOTAL	98	10	75 (76.5%)	13	4

CT scans of the liver, retroperitoneum, and lungs unless the presence of obvious metastatic disease rendered this inessential. All patients have sequential serum sampling for α-fetoprotein (AFP) and β-human chorionic gonadotrophin (B-HCG) levels from the time of presentation.

Patients in the present series were classified according to the criteria of the British Testicular Tumor Panel into malignant teratoma intermediate (MTI), malignant teratoma undifferentiated (MTU) or malignant teratoma trophoblastic (MTT). The presence of associated seminoma or yolk sac components was noted but did not modify the classification.

Between January, 1976, and April, 1979, 98 men with previously untreated nonseminomatous tumors were treated as described above (Table 24-25). A further group was referred with disease relapsing after radiation therapy and will be discussed separately.

TREATMENT RESPONSE OF STAGE I AND IIA

There were 39 patients with clinical Stage I disease, all of whom received abdominal node irradiation after orchidectomy (Table 24-25). Of these, eight (20.5%) relapsed and received chemotherapy. Six are alive and disease free, one man died of uncontrolled gastrointestinal hemorrhage and a second death occurred in a man of 67 years from a cerebrovascular accident 15 months after therapy. Thus 37 patients (95%) are alive and disease free (Fig. 24-27). Seventy-four percent (29/39) of Stage I patients had an MTI primary tumor (Table 24-26). The relapse rates for MTI and MTU were comparable (20.6% and 22.2% respectively).

Stage IIA is an uncommon stage presentation and during the 3-year period under consideration only four patients were treated with both infra- and supradiaphragmatic irradiation. All four are alive and disease free (Table 24-25). One patient who relapsed had been successfully treated with chemotherapy. Forty-one of 43 (95.3%) of the Stage I and IIA men are alive and disease free.

Treatment of early stage patients by orchidectomy and lymph node irradiation, deferring chemotherapy until early relapse is documented, has proved successful with 41 of 43 (95%) patients managed between December, 1976, and April, 1979, alive and free from disease. The increasing precision of clinical staging maneuvers, including the judicious use of serum markers and CT scanning, allows more detailed patient evaluation. Furthermore, since chemotherapy is effective for small-volume disease, deferral of any form of therapy in selected patients undergoing orchidectomy only is rendered a practicable possibility. The objective of such a study would be to define prognostic factors as accurately as possible so that a rational approach to future management could be established. The following sections discuss the evidence bearing upon the constitution of the clinical Stage I group.

False Negative Lymphography

Table 24-17 represents a collected series from the literature in which lymphographic interpretation has been compared with the histology of resected lymph nodes. Approximately 25% of lymphogram-negative patients have occult retroperitoneal lymph node metastases, and since retroperitoneal relapse following radiotherapy has been uncommon in our experience there is a high probability that small-volume metastases are eradicated with radiotherapy.

CT Scanning

Following orchidectomy and prior to radiotherapy, 5 of 21 (19%) clinical "Stage I" patients have been shown to have

FIG. 24-27. State I and IIA non-seminomatous germ cell tumors of the testis. Disease-free survival. (Royal Marsden Hospital 1976–1979)

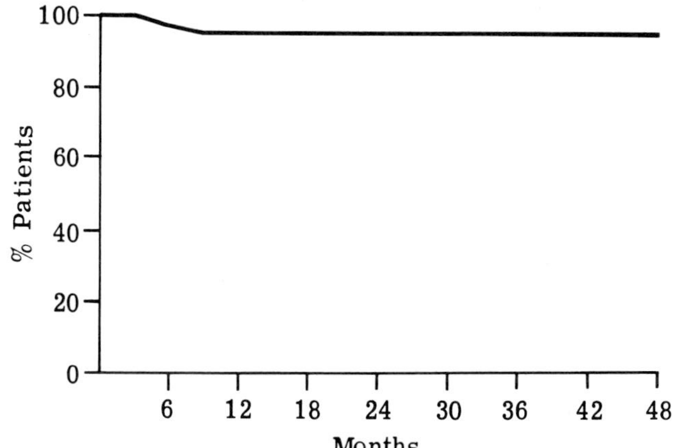

TABLE, 24-26. Early Stage Malignant Teratoma Testis Receiving Orchidectomy, Lymph Node Irradiation, and Chemotherapy for Relapse: Outcome by Histology. (Royal Marsden Hospital, 1976–1979)

STAGE	HISTOLOGY	TOTAL PATIENTS	RELAPSES	CURRENTLY DISEASE FREE	DEATH OF TUMOUR	DEATH OF INTERCURRENT DISEASE
I	MTD	1	–	1	–	–
I	MTI	29	6	28	–	1
I	MTU	9	2	8	–	1
IIA	MTI	2	1	2	–	–
IIA	MTU	2	–	2	–	–
TOTAL		43	9	41 (95.3%)	–	2

TABLE 24-27. Relapse Rate According to Serum Marker Status Following Radiotherapy for Clinical Stage I Teratoma Testis (Royal Marsden Hospital, 1973–1978)

GROUP	TOTAL PATIENTS	NUMBER OF RELAPSES	PERCENT RELAPSES
A	11	7	63.6
B	48 ($p < 0.01$)	7	14.6

TABLE 24-28. Relapse Rate, in Relation to Invasion by Tumor, or the Spermatic Cord in Clinical Stage I Teratoma Testis Treated by Irradiation After Orchidectomy (Royal Marsden Hospital, 1973–1978)

CORD HISTOLOGY	TOTAL PATIENTS	NUMBER OF RELAPSES	PERCENT RELAPSES
Negative	41	9	21.9
Positive	6	3	(50)

Difference not statistically significant

small pulmonary metastases which were not detected by conventional pulmonary radiography.

Tumor Markers in Stage I

Fifty-nine patients treated between 1973 and 1978 were studied in order to better understand the role of serum markers as prognostic indicators in patients treated by elective lymph node irradiation.[85c] The patients were divided into two groups.

Group A patients had elevated serum markers (AFP and/or HCG), which following orchidectomy either remained elevated or fell slower than was compatible with rapid plasma clearance due to production by the primary tumor alone.

Group B patients either had persistently negative markers or marker elevation prior to orchidectomy which cleared rapidly following removal of the primary tumor and before institution of radiation therapy. More than half of Group A patients relapsed with extralymphatic metastases (Table 24-27).

Involvement of the Spermatic Cord

The spermatic cord was examined in 47 patients (Table 24-28). The numbers are too small to permit a satisfactory analysis but suggest that a larger experience would confirm the adverse prognostic significance of cord invasion.

Tissue Markers

Histological sections from the primary tumor were stained by the immunoperoxidase technique for the presence of HCG. HCG-positive cells were identified in 27 tumors but not in 21. There was no difference in relapse rate between these two groups.

The experience quoted above and the observation that between 10% and 20% of patients who have histologically negative nodes at radical node dissection subsequently relapse, usually with pulmonary metastases, prompts a tentative analysis of the constitution of clinical Stage I disease (Fig. 24-28).

ADVANCED STAGE PATIENTS

Thirteen of 17 (76.5%) patients with Stage IIB, IIC, and III disease remain alive and disease free despite initially bulky lymph node disease, hitherto carrying a poor prognosis (Table 24-25). Stage IV results are also summarized in Table 24-25. Patients with bulky abdominal and pulmonary disease and those with liver involvement are designated as Advanced Stage Group II (ASG II). Stages IIB, IIC, III, and Stage IV0–CL_1L_2, are designated as Advanced Stage Group I (ASG I). Patients in the ASG I category are eligible for the sequential chemotherapy–radiotherapy–surgery protocol as described above, whereas patients in the ASG II group are managed with chemotherapy alone. Within the advanced stage categories the importance of substage based on tumor volume needs to be emphasized. The disease-free survival curves for the subgroups described above are shown in Fig. 24-29 and demonstrate that disease-free rates ranging from 100% to <10% can be obtained within the Stage IV category. The implications for the comparison of results from different centers are obvious and unless there is a clear statement of the extent and size of metastatic disease, direct comparisons are impossible to interpret in a meaningful way.

In addition to the 98 previously untreated patients, 33 men were treated with chemotherapy for disease relapsing after prior irradiation (Table 24-29). Twenty-three are alive (69.7%) and 15 (45.5%) are disease free. The disease-free survival curve for the whole series of advanced-stage patients and previously irradiated and unirradiated groups is not signifi-

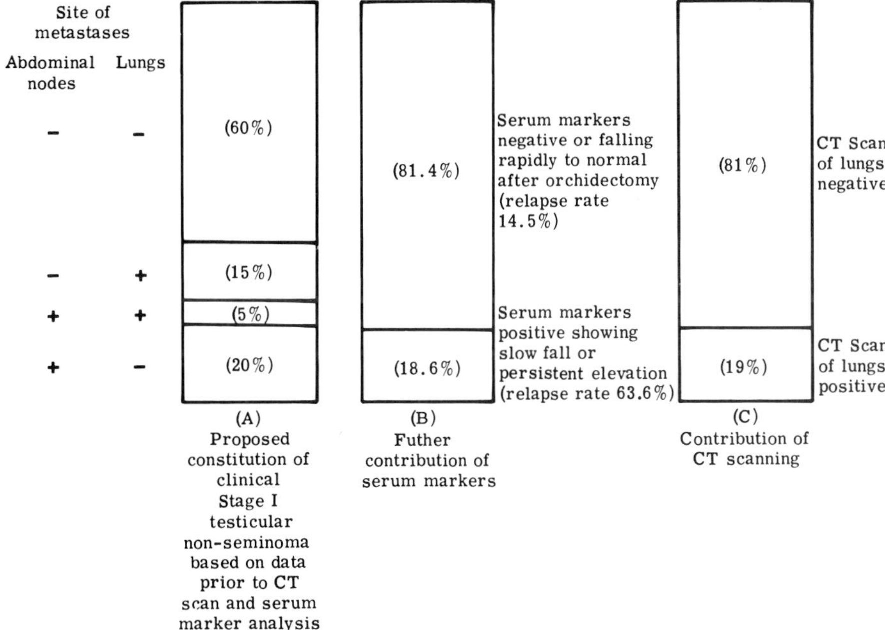

FIG. 24-28. Analysis of clinical stage I testicular non-seminoma.

TABLE 24-29. Chemotherapy for Patients with Testicular Non-Seminoma Relapsing After Radiation Therapy: Outcome of Treatment by Stage (Royal Marsden Hospital, 1976–1979)

STAGE*	TOTAL PATIENTS	DISEASE FREE	ALIVE WITH DISEASE	DEAD OF TUMOUR	DEAD OF INTERCURRENT DISEASE
IIB	9	4 (44%)	2	2	1
IVO A L_1L_2	11	7 (64%)	3	–	1
IV B C L_1L_2	5	2 (40%)	1	1	–
IV B C L_3 H^+	3	0 (0)	–	2	1
TOTAL	33	15 (45.5%)	8 24	6 (18.2%)	4 (12.1%)

* Represents stage at time of initiation of chemotherapy

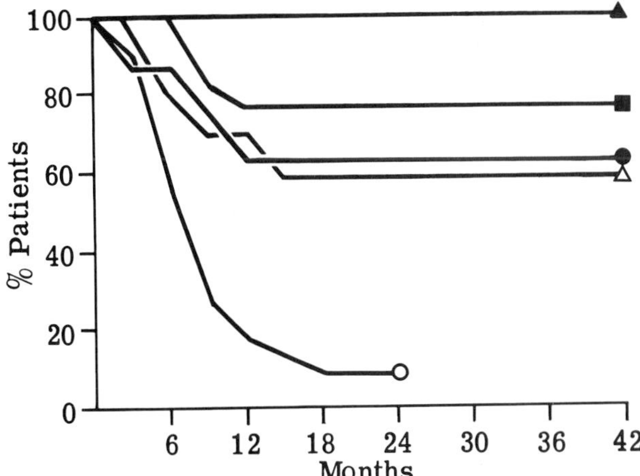

FIG. 24-29. Previously untreated advanced non-seminomatous germ cell tumors of the testis. Disease-free survival by stage. (Royal Marsden Hospital 1976–1979)
The following differences in the chart are significant:

IV O A L_1 L_2	IV B C L_1 L_2	(P = 0.05)
IV O A L_1 L_2	IV B C L_3 H^+	(P = 0.05)
II, III	IV B C L_3 H^+	(P = 0.001)
IV B C L_1 L_2	IV B C L_3 H^+	(P = 0.05)
IV O A L_3	IV B C L_3 H^+	(P = 0.005)

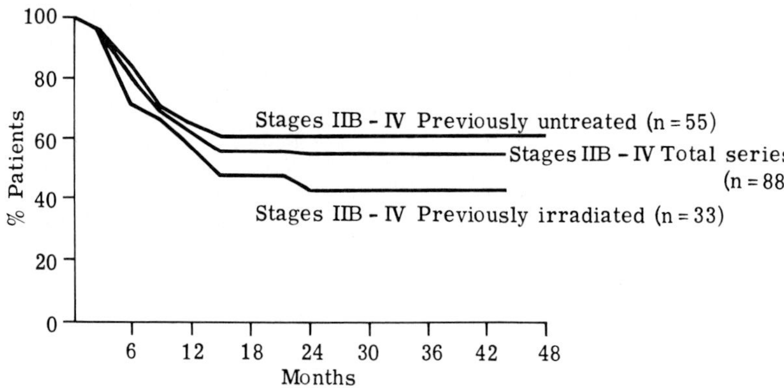

FIG. 24-30. Advanced non-seminomatous germ cell tumors of the testis. Disease-free survival. (Royal Marsden Hospital 1976–1979)

cant. The influence of prior irradiation has been examined in relation to advanced stage grouping (Fig. 24-30). ASG I patients not previously irradiated did considerably better than those relapsing after radiotherapy (Table 24-30, Fig. 24-31). The difference was not significant (P—0.07). One possible explanation for this difference could relate to the difficulty of delivering adequate chemotherapy. No differences were observed in the ASG II patients in relation to prior treatment status.

In the ASG I, previously untreated patients, 26 men after chemotherapy received elective irradiation to sites of initial disease (Table 24-30). Twenty-three of 26 patients (88.4%) are alive, 21 (80.8%) without evidence of tumor. Patients who are alive have been followed from 12 months to 45 months (median 26 months). Of those patients who did not receive irradiation after chemotherapy either because they were referred after prior radiotherapy or because they were treated with chemotherapy ± surgery only, 19 of 35 (54.3%) are currently free from evidence of disease. The tolerance to radiotherapy after chemotherapy has been satisfactory and the two late complications encountered relate to the use in the early phase of the study of high doses of radiation given in an attempt to control residual bulky tumor. One patient is disease free at 40 months, having had surgery for an infarcted segment of bowel at 32 months and a second patient has developed partial cord damage but is stable and disease free at 47 months.

PURPORTED ADVANTAGES OF RADIOTHERAPY

An important advantage of radiotherapy over radical node dissection is the preservation of normal sexual function. Fertility is preserved in a proportion of patients, provided efforts are made to avoid irradiating the remaining testis. The human testis is extremely sensitive to radiation. The effect of single doses of between 8 rad and 600 rad were studied in detail by Rowley and co-workers in 1974.[86] The prompt reduction in sperm count following irradiation is accompanied by a sharp rise in urinary gonadotrophin levels. This coincided with denuding of the germinal epithelium and persisted until histologic recovery occurred. With repopulation of the germinal epithelium the total gonadotrophin levels returned to normal. Urinary LH levels did not change but FSH levels paralleled total gonadotrophins. Rises in plasma FSH levels were dose related and significant increases occurred between 75 rad and 600 rad; plasma LH behaves similarly. Plasma testosterone levels were unchanged. Spermatogonia showed morphological and quantitative changes at all dose levels (except 8 rad, where no samples were taken). Approximately 70 days were necessary for the expression of azoospermia at all dose levels above 80 rad. Moderate oligospermia was observed with 20 rad. Histological recovery was seen at about 6 months to 8 months and the first sperm or sperm number increase in seminal fluid occurred at 6 months following 20 rad and 24 months after 600 rad.

It is well documented clinically that following orchidectomy and abdominal node irradiation, fertility may be preserved, although temporary oligospermia is generally observed. Sandeman, in 1966, reported a total of 18 testicular tumor patients fathering children following radiotherapy.[87] In this study sequential sperm counts were carried out and showed in most men oligospermia, with recovery between 1 year and 2 years.

Amelar and colleagues, in 1971, reported recovery of sperm

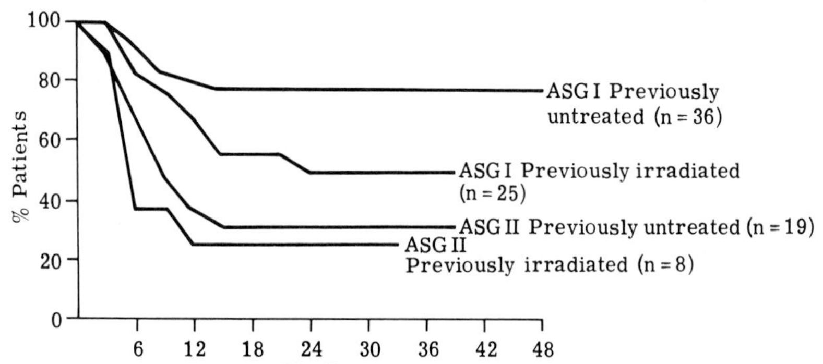

FIG. 24-31. Advanced non-seminomatous germ (*ASG*) cell tumors of the testis. Disease-free survival by prior treatment status. (Royal Marsden Hospital 1976–1979)

TABLE 24-30. Radiotherapy to Sites of Initial Disease After Intensive Chemotherapy for Advanced Testicular Teratoma (Royal Marsden Hospital, 1976–1979)

		NO RADIOTHERAPY AFTER CHEMOTHERAPY	
	ELECTIVE RADIOTHERAPY AFTER CHEMOTHERAPY	*Previously Untreated Patients*	*Previously Irradiated Patients*
TOTAL PATIENTS	26	10	25
NED	21	6	13
PERCENT	80.8	60	52
TOTAL	21/26 (80.8%)	19/35 (54.3%)	

Range 12–45 months (median 32 months)

count in four men with fathering of children subsequently by three.[88] Van de Werf Messing, in 1976, reported that 31 men in her series of patients fathered children after successful radiation therapy.[84] Orecklin and co-workers, in 1973, described 28 patients who attempted to father children following treatment of a testicular tumor.[89] Of these 18 (65%) were successful, 16 of whom had received prior irradiation. In 1971, Smithers and co-workers, reporting on the Royal Marsden Hospital series, described 34 irradiated patients who fathered 52 children.[90] Thermoluminescent dosimetry has shown that employing testicular shielding, and with the sharply defined beam of the linear accelerator, the testicular radiation dose is of the order of 50 rad to 70 rad. If inappropriate surgery, past history, or tumor extent demand scrotal and inguinal node irradiation, a higher testicular dose is inevitable and the chances of preserving fertility correspondingly reduced. The proportion of men with pretreatment sperm counts within the normal range who preserve fertility is unknown.

SURGERY AFTER CHEMOTHERAPY WITH OR WITHOUT RADIOTHERAPY

Retroperitoneal node resection has been carried out in selected patients who have evidence of residual masses after chemotherapy and radiotherapy or who have persistent large-volume abdominal disease after chemotherapy. The value of surgery is clear. Resection of residual viable tumor contributes to patient cure directly or may provide valuable information regarding tumor persistence, indicating the necessity for further chemotherapy. Present evidence indicates that surgery only, carried out in patients with elevated serum markers or who have evidence of residual malignancy fares poorly unless they receive further chemotherapy. Furthermore, apparently completely differentiated structures in the resected specimen do not preclude disease reactivation. Indeed, prompt and rapid tumor growth both locally and in the lungs may occur after the resection of well-differentiated teratoma. In the present series a total of 15 patients underwent surgical resection of residual masses in the retroperitoneum (14) or thorax (1). Eleven patients had had prior irradiation and nine showed no evidence of residual malignancy. Of the 15 men who came to surgery, 12 (80%) are disease free compared with 16 of 21 (76.2%) ASG I patients who did not. More recent data are summarized in Table 24-31. The proportion of patients who had residual malignancy in excised masses is lower in those receiving radiotherapy after chemotherapy than in those patients proceeding directly to surgery after chemotherapy.

Re-exploration seems justified in those patients with persistence of a retroperitoneal mass despite shrinkage after chemotherapy or radiotherapy. The role of re-exploration in clinically negative patients remains to be defined. Re-exploration usually is difficult owing to scarring from the initial surgery. While few keys exist to assist in re-exploration, dissection can be facilitated by selecting a surgical approach that avoids the initial line of incision. If the initial approach was transabdominal, re-exploration should be thoraco–abdominal; if the initial approach was thoraco–abdominal, re-exploration should be extended transabdominal.

Table 24-31. Advanced Testicular Teratoma: Histology of Resected Tissue After Prior Chemotherapy with and without Radiotherapy

	TOTAL PATIENTS	FIBROSIS	MATURE TERATOMA	CARCINOMA
(A) Chemotherapy followed by surgery			12	
Einhorn et al (1980)	40	15	8	13
Garnick et al (1980)	15	2	7	5
Royal Marsden Hospital	14	2		5
TOTAL	69	19 (27.5%)	27 (39%)	23 (33.3%)
(B) Chemotherapy followed by radiotherapy and surgery				
Royal Marsden Hospital	13	9 (69.2%)	2 (15.4%)	2 (15.4%)

CHEMOTHERAPY OF TESTICULAR TUMORS

HISTORICAL PERSPECTIVE

Testicular cancer was a chemosensitive tumor even in the earlier era of single-agent chemotherapy in the 1950s. In 1960, Li and associates introduced the first major thrust of chemotherapy in advanced testicular cancer with the combination of actinomycin-D, chlorambucil, and methotrexate.[91] Subsequent studies confirmed a 50% to 70% response rate.[92,93] During the 1960s, several single agents such as vinblastine, mithramycin, and bleomycin demonstrated similar activity.[93-95] The results of these and other early clinical trials are depicted in Table 24-32. The major significance of these early studies of chemotherapy in testicular cancer was the demonstration that 10% to 20% of these patients achieved a complete remission (C.R.) and that approximately half of the patients achieving C.R. were ultimately proven to be cured of their neoplasm.[92-94,96] Furthermore, most of those patients who relapsed after a chemotherapy-induced complete remission did so within one year of achieving C.R., with a smaller percentage of relapses occurring during the second year. Late relapses (beyond 2 years) have been exceedingly rare.

Although it is encouraging that approximately 50% of these complete remissions were apparent cures, it is expected that modern combination chemotherapy today will have a considerably lower relapse rate for those patients achieving complete remission because of more effective remission induction therapy with platinum combination chemotherapy (*vide infra*) and because of the increased accuracy in defining complete remission today (radioimmunoassay β-HCG, AFP, whole lung tomograms, abdominal CT scan, abdominal ultrasound). Another point of particular interest in these earlier studies was the durability of complete remission with mithramycin despite the absence of maintenance therapy.[94] While the role of mithramycin is not so important as it once was, the drug may be of importance. The details of its use are found in the pharmacology chapter. Kennedy utilized mithramycin for 6 months, and then stopped all therapy. It is quite possible that maintenance therapy is apparently unnecessary.[97]

VINBLASTINE PLUS BLEOMYCIN

Combination chemotherapy with vinblastine plus bleomycin in disseminated testicular cancer was pioneered by Samuels, and represented a major advance in this disease.[98,99] This two-drug regimen is an apparently synergistic regimen, producing higher complete remission rates than would be predicted by the single agent data. A possible explanation for this synergism is that bleomycin, *in vitro*, is most effective in killing Chinese hamster ovary cells in mitosis and vinblastine produces an arrest in the mitotic phase of the cell cycle.[100]

Initial studies with vinblastine plus bleomycin (VB-I) were started by Samuels in 1970, using dosages of 0.6 mg/kg of vinblastine plus bleomycin 15 mg/M^2 twice weekly.[101] There were 17 of 51 (33%) complete remissions with VB-I in disseminated nonseminomatous testicular cancer with a relapse rate of 23%. In 1973, bleomycin therapy was switched from intermittent therapy to continuous infusion (VB-III) (30 units in 1000 cc of 5% glucose and water over a 24-hour period for 5 consecutive days starting on day 2).[101] Therapy was repeated every 28 days to 35 days, as toxicity permitted.

The rationale for continuous infusion bleomycin was based upon the data that the half-life is short (less than 2 hours) and tissue inactivation is rapid, and the drug is a cell-cycle specific drug acting at the G_2-M interphase.[98] Recently updated data for VB-III indicated a 53% complete remission rate (47/89 patients); relapse data were not available.[99] The toxicity of these vinblastine plus bleomycin programs has been well-described in previous publications.[98,101] Bacteriologically proven sepsis was seen in 13% of these patients and was responsible for 4 drug-related deaths. Bleomycin pulmonary fibrosis was seen in 7% of these patients, and half of the patients developing this complication died from pulmonary fibrosis. However, there was no drug-induced mortality in any patient in complete remission.[101]

Although many groups continue to utilize continuous infusion bleomycin in testicular cancer and other malignancies, there is no firm data demonstrating its superiority over the more easily administered intermittent bleomycin. Table 24-33 compares VB-I, which was employed from 1970 to 1973, to VB-III, which has been used since 1973. Although the complete remission rate appears higher for VB-III compared

TABLE 24-32. Results with Early Chemotherapy Trials in Disseminated Testicular Cancer

AUTHOR/ REFERENCE NUMBER	TREATMENT	TOTAL NUMBER OF PATIENTS	COMPLETE REMISSIONS	PROLONGED SURVIVORS*
Wyatt (111)	Methotrexate	10	4 (40%)	4
MacKenzie (93)	Actinomycin-D (alone or with chlorambucil ± methotrexate)	154	24 (16%)	13
Samuels (96)	Vinblastine	21	4 (19%)	2
Kennedy (94)	Mithramycin	23	5 (22%)	5
Mendelson (112)	Cyclophosphamide + vincristine + methotrexate + fluorouracil (COMF)	17	5 (29%)	1

* Refers to those patients remaining alive and disease free at the time of publication.

TABLE 24-33. Continuous *Versus* Intermittent Bleomycin

	VB-I			VB-III		
	Total	*C.R. (%)*	*P.R. (%)*	*Total*	*C.R. (%)*	*P.R. (%)*
Embryonal	26	7 (26%)	13 (50%)	36	21 (58%)	13 (36%)
Teratocarcinoma	24	10 (44%)	5 (21%)	24	7 (33%)	5 (24%)
Choriocarcinoma	1	0	1	4	1 (25%)	0
TOTAL	51	17 (33%)	19 (37%)	61	29 (48%)	21 (34%)

to the historical control VB-I, this possible superiority was only applicable for embryonal carcinoma.[101] It is thus unlikely that there would be a therapeutic advantage to using continuous infusion bleomycin in platinum plus vinblastine plus bleomycin combination chemotherapy because 90% of patients with embryonal cell carcinoma achieve a disease-free status with platinum plus vinblastine plus bleomycin.

Vinblastine plus bleomycin represented a major advance in the early 1970s in the treatment of disseminated testicular cancer. Another major advance was the discovery of the activity of *cis*-diamminedichloroplatinum in germinal neoplasms. *Cis*-diamminedichloroplatinum is one of a group of coordination compounds of platinum identified by Rosenberg, Van Camp, and Krigas that strongly inhibits bacterial replication.[102] This agent has significant activity in refractory advanced testicular cancer and is ideal for combination chemotherapy because of its relative lack of myelosuppression.[103] It is our feeling that platinum is the single most active agent in testicular cancer, and should be an integral part of any combination chemotherapy program for disseminated testicular cancer.

VAB PROGRAMS—MEMORIAL

The Memorial group evaluated combination chemotherapy with vinblastine plus actinomycin-D plus bleomycin (VAB-I) from June, 1972, to April, 1974.[104] This treatment regimen produced only 14% complete and 22% partial remissions in 71 evaluable patients.[105] Although the dosages and method of administration were markedly different from Samuels' vinblastine–bleomycin program, the rather low complete remission rate with VAB-I raises serious questions as to the role (if any) of actinomycin-D in modern-day remission induction chemotherapy in testicular cancer. VAB-II incorporated *cis*-diamminedichloroplatinum and continuous infusion bleomycin into the VAB protocol.[106,107] This protocol was utilized from June, 1974, to January, 1976, and produced a 50% complete and a 34% partial remission rate in 50 evaluable patients.[106] An additional two patients were rendered disease-free by surgical resection of residual disease after a chemotherapy-induced partial remission. There was a 60% complete and a 36% partial response rate in previously untreated patients. The induction phase consisted of vinblastine 0.06 mg/kg and actinomycin-D 0.02 mg/kg on day 1. Bleomycin 0.5 mg/kg was given by continuous infusion for 7 days, and platinum was given in a dosage of 1 mg/kg on day 8. A weekly maintenance of vinblastine and bleomycin with actinomycin-D and platinum on a rotating schedule was given followed by vinblastine, actinomycin-D, and chlorambucil every 3 weeks to 4 weeks. The induction course (vinblastine plus actinomycin-D plus bleomycin plus platinum) was repeated 4 months after the start of therapy. Following this reinduction, maintenance was changed to vinblastine 0.1 mg/kg and actinomycin-D 0.025 mg/kg every 3 weeks and chlorambucil 0.1 mg/kg p.o. daily for a total of 2 years to 3 years in the absence of relapse. There was one drug-related death in this series, and seven instances of allergic reactions to platinum. At the time of publication only 15 of 50 patients remain alive (30%) and only 12 (24%) are presently disease-free from 19 to 35 months following start of therapy.[106] These results are markedly inferior to those achieved at Indiana University with platinum plus vinblastine plus bleomycin during a similar time period (*vide infra*).

The Memorial group next evaluated a rather complicated regimen (VAB-III). Eighty patients were treated from July, 1975, through September, 1976, with a 63% complete and a 35% partial remission rate.[105] With follow-up of 17 months to 31 months, 44% of the VAB-III patients remain free of disease.[108]

Since September, 1976, the Memorial group has been using VAB-IV, using the same drugs and doses of VAB-III but with slight scheduling modifications and with similar therapeutic results to VAB-III.[105] The preliminary analysis of VAB-IV reveals 24 to 28 patients (50%) to be free of disease with a follow-up shorter than for VAB-III.[108]

PLATINUM PLUS VINBLASTINE PLUS BLEOMYCIN

In August, 1974, the Indiana group began studies utilizing platinum plus vinblastine plus bleomycin (PVB) in disseminated testicular cancer. In these initial studies, 50 patients with disseminated germ-cell tumors of the testis were treated with PVB.[109] Three patients died within 2 weeks of initiation of chemotherapy and were considered inevaluable. The term "inevaluable" is no longer used and all subsequent studies included all patients entered on chemotherapy trials. The therapy regimen for this initial PVB study is depicted in Table 24-34. Platimum was dissolved in 50 cc sterile water and given as a 15-minute infusion. Most patients received three courses of platinum; however, if a complete remission was not achieved after three courses, a fourth course was administered. Vinblastine was given 6 hours prior to bleomycin. However, this kinetic scheduling is no longer felt to be necessary, and we now give vinblastine and bleomycin simultaneously. After completion of the 12 weeks of remission induction, maintenance therapy was given with vinblastine

TABLE 24-34. Platinum + Vinblastine + Bleomycin

Platinum 20 mg/M² IV × 5 days every 3 weeks (3–4 courses) Vinblastine 0.2 mg/kg IV × 2 every 3 weeks (4 courses) Bleomycin 30 units IV push weekly × 12 weeks	(REMISSION INDUCTION THERAPY)
Vinblastine 0.3 mg/kg monthly × 21 weeks	(MAINTENANCE THERAPY)

0.3 mg/kg every 4 weeks for a total of 2 years of chemotherapy. Initially, bacillus Calmette–Guerin (BCG) immunotherapy was given if complete remission was achieved in an attempt to augment host cell mediated immunity and prolong the duration of complete remission. However, the value of adding BCG is doubtful and in the past 4 years no form of immunotherapy has been used. Since the relapse rate remains at a very low level despite cessation of BCG, it appears unlikely BCG contributed any therapeutic advantage.

The primary goal was to increase the complete remission rate and potential cure rate. Partial remission was not considered a worthwhile goal unless the patient was left with localized disease that could be surgically removed. Thirty-three of 47 evaluable patients (70%) achieved complete remission (defined as a complete disappearance of all clinical, radiographic, and biochemical evidence of disease, including normal whole lung tomograms, serum β-HCG, and α-fetoprotein). The remaining 14 patients achieved partial remission (greater than 50% decrease of measurable disease). Furthermore, five of these 14 patients were rendered disease-free following surgical removal of residual localized disease after significant reduction of tumor volume with chemotherapy. The therapeutic results are outlined in Table 24-35. These patients now have all been followed for more than 4 years and they are all off chemotherapy. Four patients died in complete remission in the early part of this study. Two of these deaths were due to gram-negative sepsis, one from bleomycin-induced pulmonary fibrosis, and one from multiple small-bowel fistulae and obstruction secondary to previous surgery. One of the septicemia deaths was from Klebsiella pneumonia in a chronic alcoholic who had no evidence of granulocytopenia during this fatal pneumonia. Thus, this regimen was directly responsible for two drug-related fatalities.

Only six of these 33 complete remissions have relapsed. Five of these relapses occurred within 9 months of initiation of complete remissions and the sixth relapse occurred at 17 months.

TABLE 24-35. Results with Platinum + Vinblastine + Bleomycin

Evaluable patients:	47
Complete remission:	33 (70%)
Partial remission:	14 (30%)
Disease free after surgery:	5 (11%)
Number alive:	31 (66%)
Number continuously NED:	26 (55%)
Number presently NED:	28 (60%)

As previously mentioned, five of the 14 partial remissions were rendered free of disease by surgical removal of residual localized disease. It has been treatment policy to do surgery on these patients only if they have persistent localized disease following four courses of platinum + vinblastine + bleomycin. Usually, this clinical situation occurs in patients with Stage III disease who exhibit complete disappearance of pulmonary metastases (confirmed by whole lung tomograms) but still have persistnt abdominal disease (as *per* physical examination, abdominal ultrasound, or CT). It should be noted that those patients who present *de novo* with Stage III disease and achieve complete remission are *not* subjected to a laparotomy (*i.e.*, only those patients with clinical or radiographic evidence of residual abdominal disease receive the operation). We do not feel that patients need a laparotomy and retroperitoneal node dissection merely because they had never had a node dissection originally; rather, we employ laparotomy only if there is evidence of persistent abdominal disease. Furthermore, we do not perform laparotomies on patients achieving chemotherapeutic partial remissions if they have evidence of remaining pulmonary metastases. Using this criteria for laparotomy, about one-third will have transformed to benign mature teratoma, and one-third will have fibrous tissue only.

The toxicity and prognostic variables have been described in detail in a previous publication.[109] With long-term followup of all patients, it is gratifying to note that there have been no second malignancies, progressive azotemia, or pulmonary fibrosis. Late relapses have not been seen. Twenty-eight of 47 patients (60%) were cured of disseminated testicular cancer with this initial PVB regimen.

PLATINUM PLUS VINBLASTINE PLUS BLEOMYCIN PLUS ADRIAMYCIN

Although our original PVB regimen produced very respectable therapeutic results, we have been concerned with the toxicity. Although platinum is potentially nephrotoxic, this nephrotoxicity has not been a clinical problem since the routine utilization of saline hydration. The most important factors are prehydration and the ensuring of adequate urinary excretion of platinum. These goals are usually accomplished by continuous intravenous hydration with normal saline beginning the night before the first day of platinum chemotherapy and continuing at a rate of 100 ml/hour during the 5-day course. Outpatient platinum can be given by prehydrating the patient with 1000 ml of normal saline over 2 hours before and after each dosage of platinum. Mannitol diuresis or furosemide is felt to be unnecessary.

Likewise, clinically significant bleomycin pulmonary fibrosis has been an uncommon complication, although in patients with prior mediastinal irradiation or those above age 50, more caution is necessary. Diffusion capacity (correcting for anemia) is the most valuable pulmonary function test, but basically, the bleomycin is usually continued unless there are inspiratory rales or a respiratory lag on physical examination or roentgenological evidence for pulmonary fibrosis.

The major serious toxicity has been secondary to high dose (0.4 mg/kg) vinblastine. Myalgias, constipation, and paralytic ileus were all troublesome side-effects, but severe granulocytopenia and potential sepsis were the most worrisome toxicity. Thirty-eight percent of the patients on our original PVB required hospitalization for granulocytopenia and fever above 101° F between platinum courses, and 15% had documented sepsis. This toxicity was seen only during the 12-week remission induction therapy with PVB; there were no hospitalizations for toxicity during maintenance therapy with vinblastine (0.3 mg/kg once a month for 21 months).

Therefore, in 1976, we started a random prospective trial comparing our standard PVB with the same regimen using a 25% dosage reduction (0.3 mg/kg) for vinblastine during remission induction. We felt that the reduced vinblastine dosage would reduce the hematological toxicity, but the critical question was whether it would maintain the same excellent therapeutic results. A third arm, adding adriamycin to PVB, was tried in order to see whether the use of adriamycin in combination with PVB (0.2 mg/kg vinblastine) would further improve the C.R. rate. We had previously had encouraging results with platinum plus adriamycin in patients who had developed progressive disease on chemotherapy with vinblastine + bleomycin (Table 24-36).

Seventy-eight patients were entered on this study, and all patients have been followed for over 2 years. The median follow-up is 34 months. The degree of myelosuppression for high-dose vinblastine (0.4 mg/kg) was similar to our original PVB study. The 25% reduction in the vinblastine dosage resulted in the expected decrease in hematological toxicity (Table 24-37). The results of therapy are illustrated in Table 24-38. The overall C.R. rate (68%) and surgical resection rate for localized residual disease (14%) were remarkably similar to our original PVB study. The therapeutic results are almost identical on the 3 separate induction regimens. The relapse rate remains low, with all relapses occurring within 1 year of initiation of platinum combination chemotherapy.

The most important determinant to achieving complete remission was extent of disease (Table 24-39). Advanced pulmonary metastases were defined as pulmonary metastases greater than 2 cm in diameter, and advanced abdominal disease referred to hepatic metastases or a palpable abdominal mass. Four patients had elevated human chorionic gonadotropin (HCG) levels (57 mIU/mL to 4810 mIU/mL) and elevated α-fetroprotein (AFP) (35 ng/mL to 559 ng/mL) as their only manifestation of disease. All four patients had both markers elevated. Thirty of 31 patients with minimal metastatic disease have achieved complete remission; the only patient not achieving a C.R. had a median sternotomy with removal of small residual bilateral pulmonary nodes that were mature teratoma histopathologically. Fifty-three of 78 patients (68%) in this three-armed random prospective study remain continuously free of disease. In addition, five other patients are currently disease free, either with subsequent surgery

TABLE 24-36. PVB Regimens

R A N D O M I Z E	Platinum 20 mg/M² × 5 days q 3 weeks (3–4 courses) Bleomycin 30 units IV weekly × 12 Vinblastine *0.4 mg/kg* q 3 weeks
	Platinum 20 mg/M² × 5 days q 3 weeks (3–4 courses) Bleomycin 30 units IV weekly × 12 Vinblastine 0.3 mg/kg q 3 weeks
	Platinum 20 mg/M² × 5 q 3 weeks (3–4 courses) Bleomycin 30 units IV weekly × 12 Vinblastine *0.2 mg/kg* q 3 weeks Adriamycin *50 mg/M²* q 3 weeks

After completion of 12 weeks of bleomycin, maintenance therapy on all three arms to be vinblastine 0.3 mg/kg monthly for 2 years.

TABLE 24-37. PVB with and without Adriamycin and Sepsis

	GRANULOCYTOPENIC FEVERS	DOCUMENTED SEPSIS
PVB (0.3 mg/kg vinblastine)	4 (15%)	0
PVB (0.4 mg/kg vinblastine)	9 (35%)	3 (12%)
PVB ± adriamycin	6 (24%)	1 (4%)

TABLE 24-38. Therapeutic Results

	PVB (0.4)*	PVB (0.3)†	PVB + ADRIAMYCIN	TOTAL
No. Patients:	26	27	25	78
Complete Remissions:	18 (69%)	17 (63%)	18 (72%)	53 (68%)
Partial Remission:	8 (31%)	10 (37%)	5 (20%)	23 (30%)
NED with Surgery:	5 (19%)	4 (15%)	2 (8%)	11 (14%)
Relapses:	5 (19%)	2 (10%)	3 (15%)	10 (13%)
No. Continuously NED:	18 (69%)	18 (67%)	17 (68%)	53 (68%)

* 0.4 mg/kg vinblastine
† 0.3 mg/kg vinblastine

TABLE 24-39 Extent of Disease and PVB with and without Adriamycin

	NUMBER	C.R.	NED + SURG.
A. Minimal Pulm.:	14	13 (93%)	0
B. Advanced Pulm.:	20	10 (50%)	3 (15%)
C. Minimal Abd. and Pulm.:	13	13 (100%)	0
D. Advanced Abd.:	23	10 (43%)	8 (35%)
E. Elevated Markers only:	4	4 (100%)	0
F. Miscellaneous:*	4	3 (75%)	0

* 2 patients with cervical nodes only, 1 with spinal cord compression and 1 with bone metastases.

after relapse, or with salvage chemotherapy with platinum + VP-16 combination chemotherapy.[110] Fifty-eight patients (74%) are currently alive and disease free.

The role of maintenance therapy in disseminated testicular cancer has never been clearly established. It is quite possible that in a disease where remission induction therapy is so effective and C.R. can be defined so accurately (radioimmunoassay HCG, AFP, lung tomograms, and computed abdominal tomography), maintenance therapy may be unnecessary. To test this hypothesis, patients achieving C.R. are currently randomized to standard maintenance vinblastine (0.3 mg/kg monthly for 21 months) as opposed to no maintenance therapy after the 12 weeks of remission induction therapy. This study is being done as part of a Southeastern Cancer Study Group project. All patients receive four courses of platinum combination chemotherapy to insure uniformity in the remission induction. Fifty patients have been entered on this study at Indiana University and have been followed for a minimum of 1 year, and 40 (80%) are currently disease free. The relapse rate has been only 4%, with or without maintenance vinblastine. Although the results are preliminary, with a small number of patients and inadequate duration of follow-up, this study is already suggesting that maintenance therapy may be unnecessary, and that a routine fourth course of platinum combination chemotherapy may lower the relapse rate of patients achieving a complete remission.

In summary, there is no longer any justification for pessimism in the management of patients with disseminated testicular cancer, and such patients *must* be treated with curative intent. Platinum + vinblastine + bleomycin consistently produces 70% complete remissions and a further 10% of patients will be rendered disease free following surgical excision of residual disease. The relapse rate in such patients remains low (10%–20%), and all relapses have occurred within 9 months of initiation of complete remission, except for one late relapse. The rate may drop below 5% when four courses of platinum combination chemotherapy are employed during remission induction. Toxicity with the lower dosage (0.3 mg/kg) of vinblastine is considerably less than with the higher dosage (0.4 mg/kg), with an equivalent therapeutic response. High dose vinblastine is no longer recommended as part of the platinum + vinblastine + bleomycin regimen. The projected cure rate for patients today with Stage III nonseminomatous testicular cancer is 70%–80%. It is interesting to note that this is higher than the surgical cure rate for Stage II disease. Major progress has clearly been made in the past decade in disseminated testicular cancer, as the projected cure rate in the 1960s was less than 10%. Platinum combination chemotherapy represents a major advance in the treatment of testicular cancer.

Current treatment program for control of testicular tumors should be directed to eradication of all detectable disease at least patient risk. Disease confined to the scrotum is well controlled by orchiectomy alone. The present difficulty arises in detecting disease beyond the scrotum. While studies underway presently are being evaluated to determine their ability to predict disease extent, their accuracy remains undetermined. Until it can be demonstrated that the hazard of failing to detect disseminated disease is less than the hazard of retroperitoneal node dissection with its proven diagnostic and therapeutic benefit, it must remain prominent in the treatment plan. While radiotherapy may be as effective as surgery in controlling retroperitoneal disease, the Royal Marsden data would indicate that this radiotherapy may impair future chemotherapeutic salvage. Volume of disease adversely affects treatment response irrespective of the treatment selected. Treatment of bulky disease should therefore be chosen such that subsequent therapy is not compromised. Bulky retroperitoneal disease seems preferentially treated by chemotherapy followed by surgery of residual disease with radiotherapy reserved for margin positive resection. Initial surgical debulking destroys tissue planes which could be valuable at a second attempt at resection after chemotherapy. Attention to these principles in light of the data presented above will assist in proper selection of a management program for both seminomatous and nonseminomatous germinal cell tumors and permit an understanding of studies presently underway to further improve disease control.

REFERENCES

1. Dixon FJ, Moore RA: Tumors of the male sex organs. Armed Forces Inst Path FASC 32:48–103, Washington, DC 1952
2. Collins DH, Pugh RCB: Classification and frequency of testicular tumours. Brit J Urol 36:1–11 (suppl), 1964
3. Clemmesen J: A doubling in mortality from testis carcinoma in Copenhagen 1943–1962. Acta Path Microbiol Scand 72:348–349, 1968
4. Drain LS: Testicular cancer in California from 1942 to 1969: the California tumor registry experience. Oncology 27:45–51 1973
5. Dixon FJ, Moore RA: Clinicopathologic study. Cancer 6:427–454, 1953
6. Johnson DE, Morneau J: Bilateral sequential germ cell tumors of the testis. Urology 4:567–570, 1974
7. Mostofi FK: Testicular tumors. Epidemiologic, etiologic, and pathologic features. Cancer 32:1186, 1973
8. Mostofi FK, Price EB Jr: Tumors of the male genital system.

Atlas of Tumor Pathology, 2nd series, Fasc 8. Armed Forces Institute, Washington, DC, 1973
9. Pugh RCB (ed): Pathology of the Testis. Oxford, Blackwell Scientific Publications, 1976
10. Rosai J, Khodadoust K, Silber I: Spermatocytic seminoma. II. Ultrastructural study. Cancer, 24:103, 1969
11. Rosai J, Silver I, Khodadoust K: Spermatocytic seminoma. I. Clinicopathologic study of six cases and review of the literature. Cancer, 24:92, 1969
12. Kleinsmith LJ, Pierce GB Jr: Multipotentiality of single embryonal carcinoma cells. Cancer Res, 24:1544, 1964
13. Pugh RCB, Smith JP: Teratoma. In Collins DH, Pugh RCB (eds): The Pathology of Testicular Tumours. Edinburgh and London, E & S Livingstone Ltd, 1964, p 28
14. Bat W, Hedinger C: Comparison of histologic types of primary testicular germ cell tumor—consequences for the WHO and the British nomenclatures? Virchows Arch Pathol Anat 370:41, 1976
15. Collins DH, Pugh RCB: Classification and frequency of testicular tumours. Br J Urol 36:1–11 (suppl), 1964
16. Melicow MM: Classification of tumors of testis. J Int Coll Surg 25:187–201, 1956
17. Melicow MM: New British classification of testicular tumors: a correlation, analysis and critique. J Urol 94:64–68, 1965
18. Hausfeld KF, Schrandt D: Malignancy of testis following atrophy: report of three cases. J Urol 94:69–72, 1965
19. Haines JS, Grabstald H: Tumor formation in atrophic testes. Arch Surg 60:857–860, 1950
20. Campbell HE: The incidence of malignant growth of the undescended testicle: a reply and re-evaluation. J Urol 81:663–668, 1959
21. Johnson DE, Woodhead DM, Pohl DR et al: Cryptorchism and testicular tumorigenesis. Surgery 63:919–922, 1968
22. Dow JA, Mostofi KF: Testicular tumours following orchiopexy. Southern Med J 60:193–195, 1967
23. Sohval AR: Testicular dysgenesis in relation to neoplasm of the testicle. J Urol 75:285–291, 1956
24. Sohval AR: Testicular dysgenesis as an etiologic factor in cryptorchidism. M Urol 72:693–702, 1954
25. Hinman F Jr: The implications of testicular cytology in the treatment of cryptorchidism. Am J Surg 90:381–386, 1955
26. Giarola A: Protection of reproductive capacity as a factor in therapy for undescended testicle. Fertil Steril 18:375–380, 1967
27. Lesson CR: An electron miscroscope study of cryptorchid and scrotal human testes, with special reference to pubertal maturation. Invest Urol 3:498–511, 1966
28. Gordon-Taylor G, Wyndham NR: On malignant tumours of the testicle. Br J Surg 35:6, 1947
29. Markland C: Testicular tumors. Curr Probl Surg, September, 1968
30. Patton JF, Hewitt CB, Mallis N: Diagnosis and treatment of tumors of the testis. JAMA 117:2194, 1959
31. Patton JF, Sietzman DN, Zone RA: Diagnosis and treatment of testicular tumors. A J Surg 99:525–532, 1960
32. Thompson IM: Lymphadenectomy for testicular tumor. Arch Surg 83:746–748, 1961
33. Robson CJ, Bruce AW, Charbonneau J: Testicular tumors: a collective review from the Canadian Academy of Urological Surgeons. J Urol 94:440–444, 1965
34. Vechinski TO, Jaeschke WH, Vermund H: Testicular tumors. An analysis of 112 consecutive cases. Am J Roentgen 95:494–514, 1965
35. MacKay EN, Sellers AH: A statistical review of malignant testicular tumours based on the experience of the Ontario Cancer Foundation Clinics 1938–1961. Can Med Assoc J 94:889–899, 1966
36. Johnson DE: Testicular tumors. 2nd Ed. Flushing, NY, Medical Examination Publishing Co, 1976
37. Markland C: Special Problems in Managing Patients with Testicular Cancer. In Fraley EE (ed): The Urologic Clinics of North America, Vol 4, no 3, Oct 1977. Symposium on testicular tumors. Philadelphia, WB Saunders, pp 427–451
38. Scardino PT, Cos HD, Waldman NT et al: The value of serum tumor markers in the staging and prognosis of germ cell tumors of the testis. J Urol, 118:994, 1977
39. Leadbetter WF: Treatment of testis tumors based on their pathological behavior. JAMA 151:275, 1953
40. Markland C, Kedia K, Fraley EE: Inadequate orchiectomy for patients with testicular tumors. JAMA, 224:1025, 1973
41. Woodhead DM, Johnson DE, Pohl DR, Robison JR: Aggressive management of advanced testicular malignancy: experience with 147 patients. Milt Med 136:634–638, 1971
42. Fraley EE, Clouse M, Litwin SB: The uses of lymphography, lymphadenography and color lymphadenography in urology. J Urol 93:319, 1965
43. Bowles WT: Inguinal node metastases from testicular tumor developing after varicocelectomy. J Urol 88:266, 1962
44. Altman BL, Malament M: Carcinoma of the testis following orchiopexy. J Urol 97:498, 1967
45. Anson BJ, McVay CB: Surgical Anatomy, 5th Ed. Philadlphia, WB Saunders, 1971, p 869
46. Dow JA, Mostofi FK: Testicular tumors following orchiopexy. So Med J 60:193, 1967
47. Ray B, Hajdu SI, Whitmore WF Jr: Distribution of retroperitoneal lymph node metastases in the testicular germinal tumors. Cancer 33:340, 1974
48. Chevassu M: Tumeurs du testicle. Bull Mem Soc Chir 36, 236, Paris, 1910
49. Jamieson JD, Dobson JF: The lymphatics of the testicle. Lancet 1:493, 1910
50. Borski AA: Diagnosis, staging and natural history of testis tumors. Cancer 32:1202, 1973
51. Wallace S, Jing B: Lymphangiography: diagnosis of nodal metastases from testicular malignancies. JAMA 213:94, 1970
52. Safer ML, Green JP, Crews QE, Hill, DR: Lymphangiographic accuracy in the staging of testicular tumors. Cancer 35:1603, 1975
53. Maier J, Schamber O: The role of lymphangiography in the diagnosis and treatment of malignant testis tumors. Am J Roent 114:482, 1972
54. Lange PH, McIntire DR, Qaldmann IA et al: Serum alpha-fetoprotein and human chorionic gonadotropin in the diagnosis and management of non-seminomatous germ-cell testicular cancer. New Engl J Med 295:1237, 1976
55. Lange PH, McIntire KR, Waldmann TA et al: Alpha-fetoprotein and human chorionic gonadotropin in the management of testicular tumors. J Urol 118:593–596, 1977
56. Maier JG, Sulak MH: Radiation therapy in malignant testis tumors. Part 1: Seminoma; Part II: Carcinoma. Cancer 32:1212, 1974
57. McIntire KR, Waldmann TA, Moertel CG et al: Serum alpha-fetoprotein in patients with neoplasms of the gastrointestinal tract. Cancer Res 35:991, 1975
58. Mizejewski GJ, Young SR, Allen RP: Alpha-fetoprotein: Effect of heterologous antiserum on hepatoma cells in vitro. J Natl Cancer Inst 54:1361, 1975
59. Moore MR, Vogel CL, Walton KN et al: The use of human chorionic gonadotropin and alpha-fetoprotein in evaluation of testicular tumors. Am Soc Clin Oncologists (Abstracts No. C-12), 1976
60. Vaitukaitis JL, Ross GT: Recent advances in the evaluation of gonadotropic hormones. In Cruger WP, Coggin CH, Hancock EW (eds): Annual Review of Medicine Palo Alto, Annual Reviews, 1973, Vol 24, pp 295–302
61. Vaitukaitis JL, Braunstein GD, Ross GT: A radioimmunoassay which specifically measures human chorionic gonadotropin in the presence of human leuteinizing hormone. Am J Obstet Gynecol 113:751, 1972
62. Braunstein GD, Vaitukaitis JL, Carbone PP et al: Ectopic production of human chorionic gonadotropin by neoplasms. Ann Internal Med 78:39, 1973
63. Bracken RB, Johnson DE, and Samuels ML: Alpha-fetoprotein determinations in germ cell tumors of the testis. Urology 6:382, 1975
64. Shepheard BGF: Alpha-fetoprotein and teratomas of the testis. Proc Royal Soc Med 67:307, 1974

65. Maier JG, Sulak MH, Mittemeyer BT: Seminoma of the testis: analysis of treatment success and failure. Am J Roentgen 102:596–602, 1968
66. Notter G, Ranudd NE: Treatment of malignant testicular tumours—a report of 355 patients. Acta Radiol NS 2:273–301, 1964
66a. Calman FMB, Peckham MJ, Hendry WF: The pattern of spread and treatment of metastases in testicular seminoma. Br J Urol 51:154–160, 1979
66b. Ball D, Barrett A, Peckham MJ: The management of metastatic seminoma testis. Unpublished data
67. Heyderman E, Neville AM: Syncytiotrophoblasts in malignant testicular tumours. Lancet II: 103, 1976
68. Friedman M, Pearlman AW: Seminoma with trophocarcinoma: A clinical variant of seminoma. Cancer 26: 46–64, 1970
69. Javadpour N, McIntire KR, Waldmann TA: Human chorionic gonadotropin (HCG) and alpha-fetoprotein (AFP) in sera and tumor cells of patients with testicular seminoma: A prospective study. Cancer 42:2768–2772, 1978
70. Cooper JF, Leadbetter WF, Chute R: The thoracoabdominal approach for retroperitoneal gland dissection: its application to testis tumors. Surg Gynecol Obstet 90:486, 1950
71. Fraley EE, Kedia K, Marklan C: The role of radical operation in the management of nonseminomatous germinal tumors of the testicle in the adult. In Varco RL, Delaney JP (eds): Controversy in Surgery, Philadelphia, WB Saunders, 1976, p 479
72. Merrill DC: Modified thoracoabdominal approach to the kidney and retroperitoneal tissue. J Urol 117:15, 1977
73. Blandy J, Chapman R, Pollack D et al: The management of tumors of the testis. In Varco RL, Delaney JP (eds): Controversy in Surgery, Philadelphia, WB Saunders, 1976, p 489
74. Kedia KR, Markland C, Fraley EE: Sexual function following high retroperitoneal lymphadenectomy. J Urol 114:237, 1975
75. Stuabitz WJ, Early KS, Magoss IV et al: Surgival treatment of non-seminomatous germinal testis tumors. Cancer 32:1207, 1973
76. Van Buskirk KE, Young JG: The evolution of the bilateral ategrade retroperitoneal lymph node dissection in the treatment of testicular tumors. Milit Med 133:575, 1968
77. Whitmore WF Jr: Treating germinal tumors of the adult testes. Cont Surg 6:17, 1975
78. Young JD Jr: Retroperitoneal surgery, In Glenn JF, Boyce H (eds): Urologic Surgery, 2nd Ed, New York, Harper & Row, 1975, p 848
79. Skinner DG: Non-seminomatous testis tumors: a plan of management based on 96 patients to improve survival in all stages by combined therapeutic modalities. J Urol 115:65, 1976
80. Skinner DG, Leadbetter WF: The surgical management of testis tumors. J Urol 106:84, 1971
81. Skinner DG: Considerations for management of large retroperitoneal tumors; use of the modified thorabdominal approach. J Urol 117:605, 1977
82. Skinner DG: Management of non-seminomatous tumors of the testis. In Skinner DG, deKernion JB (eds): Genitourinary Cancer. Philadelphia, WB Saunders, 1978
82a. Tyrell CJ, Peckham MJ: The response of lymph node metastases of testicular teratoma to radiation therapy. Br J Urol 48:363–370, 1976
83. Maier JG, Mittemeyer B: Carcinoma of the testis. Cancer 39:981–986, 1977
83a. Klein KA, Maier JG: Positive nodes and treatment failures in testicular carcinomas. Int J Radiat Oncol Biol Phys 2:1229–1231, 1977
84. van der Werf Messing B: Radiotherapeutic treatment of testicular tumors. Int J Rad Oncol Biol Phys 1, 235–248, 1976
85. Hussey DH, Luk KH, Johnson DE: The role of radiation therapy in the treatment of germinal cell tumors of the testis other than pure seminoma. Radiology 123:175–180, 1977
85a. Peckham MJ, Barrett A, McElwain TJ: Combined management of malignant teratoma of the testis. Lancet II: 261–270, 1979
85b. Peckham MJ, Barrett A, McElwain TJ et al: Non-seminoma germ cell tumors (malignant teratoma) of the testis: Results of treatment and an analysis of prognostic factors. Br J Urol 53:162–172, 1981
85c. Raghawan D, Peckham MJ, Heyderman E et al: Prognostic factors in clinical stage I non-seminomatous germ cell tumors of the testis managed by orchiectomy and lymph node irradiation. Unpublished data.
86. Rowley MJ, Leach DR, Warner GA et al: Effect of graded dosesof ionizing radiation on the human testis. Rad Res 59:665–678, 1974
87. Sandeman TE: The effects of x-irradiation on male human fertility. Br J Rad 39:901–907, 1966
88. Amelar RD, Dublin L, Hotchkiss RS: Restoration of fertility following unilateral orchidectomy and radiation therapy for testicular tumors. J Urol 106:714–718, 1971
89. Orecklin JR, Kaufman JJ, Thompson RW: Fertility in patients treated for malignant testicular tumors. J Urol 109:293–395, 1973
90. Smithers DW, Wallace ENK, Wallace DM: Radiotherapy for patients with tumours of the testicle. Br J Urol 43:83–91, 1971
91. Li MC, Whitmore WF, Golbey R, et al: Effects of combined drug therapy on metastatic cancer of the testis. JAMA 174:145–153, 1960
92. Ansfield FJ, Korbitz BD, Davis HL Jr et al: Triple therapy in testicular tumors. Cancer 24:442–446, 1969
93. MacKenzie AR: Chemotherapy of metastatic testis cancer—results in 154 patients. Cancer 19:1369–1376, 1966
94. Kennedy BJ: Mithramycin therapy in advanced testicular neoplasms, Cancer 26:755–766, 1970
95. Blum RH, Carter S, Agre K: A clinical review of bleomycin—a new anti-neoplastic agent. Cancer 31:903–914, 1973
96. Samuels ML, Howe CD: Vinblastine in the management of testicular cancer. Cancer 25:1009–1017, 1970
97. DeVita VT, Canellos G, Hubbard S et al: Chemotherapy of Hodgkin's disease with MOPP: A 10-year progress report (abstr). Proc Am Soc Clin Oncol 17:269, 1976
98. Samuels ML, Johnson DE, Holoye PY: Continuous intravenous bleomycin (NSC-125066) therapy with vinblastine (NSC-49842) in stage III testicular neoplasia. Cancer Chemother Rep 59:563–570, 1975
99. Samuels ML, Lanzotti VJ, Holoye PY et al: Stage III testicular cancer: complete response by substage to velban plus continuous bleomycin infusion (VB-3). Proc Am Assoc Cancer Res 18:146, 1977
100. Barranco C, Humphrey RM: The effects of bleomycin on survival and cell progression in Chinese hamster cells *in vitro*. Cancer Res 31:1218–1223, 1971
101. Samuels ML, Lazotti VJ, Holoye PY et al: Combination chemotherapy in germinal cell tumors. Cancer Treat Rev 3:185–204, 1976
102. Einhorn LH, Donohue JP: *Cis*-diamminedichloroplatinum, vinblastine and bleomycin combination chemotherapy in disseminated testicular cancer. Ann Int Med 87:293–298, 1977
103. Higby DJ, Wallace HJ, Albert DJ et al: Diamminodichloroplatinum: A phase I study showing responses in testicular and other tumors. Cancer 33:1219–1225, 1974
104. Wittes RE, Yagoda A, Silvay O et al: Chemotherapy of germ cell tumors of the testis. Cancer 37:637–645, 1976
105. Cvitkovic E, Cheng E, Whitmore WF et al: Germ cell tumor chemotherapy update. Proc Am Soc Clin Oncol 18:234, 1977
106. Cheng E, Cvitkovic E, Wittes RE et al: Germ cell tumor VAB II in metastatic testicular cancer. Cancer 42:2162–2168, 1978
107. Cvitkovic E, Wittes R, Golbey R et al: Primary combination chemotherapy (VAB II) for metastatic or unresectable germ cell tumors. Proc Am Assoc Cancer Res 19:174, 1978
108. Intergroup Cooperative Study of Testicular Cancer. Chicago, May, 1978
109. Einhorn L, Donohue JP: *Cis*-diamminedichloroplastinum, vinblastine, and bleomycin combination chemotherapy in disseminated testicular cancer. Ann Int Med 87:293–298, 1977
110. Williams SD, Einhorn LH: VP-16-213 salvage therapy for refractory germinal neoplasms. Cancer 44:1514–1516, 1979
111. Wyatt JK, McAninch LH: A chemotherapeutic approach to advanced testicular carcinoma. Can J Surg 10:421–426, 1967
112. Mendelson D, Serpic AA: Combination chemotherapy of testicular tumors. J Urol 103:619–623, 1970

Carlos A. Perez
Robert C. Knapp
Robert C. Young

CHAPTER 25

Gynecologic Tumors

Gynecologic malignant tumors are common, endometrial carcinomas representing 13% of all malignancies in women, ovarian tumors 6%, uterine cervix tumors 6%, and other malignancies 2% to 3%.

Table 25-1 summarizes the estimated number of new cases and deaths for different gynecologic malignancies in 1980 published by the American Cancer Society.[1] The anatomy of the female pelvis is illustrated in Fig. 25-1.

CARCINOMA OF THE UTERINE CERVIX

EPIDEMIOLOGY

Carcinoma of the uterine cervix is one of the most common malignant neoplasias in women, after breast, colo-rectum, and endometrium. It is more common on continents such as Latin America and Africa and less frequent in Jewish European women and Fiji Islanders.[2] Some have attributed the low frequency of cervical carcinoma in Jewish women to the circumcision of Jewish men but this low incidence has not been demonstrated in sexual partners of non-Jewish circumcised men.[3,4] Ackerman and del Regato postulate that perhaps Jewish women have a genetic resistance to this particular tumor.[5]

The incidence of cervical carcinoma is appreciably higher in low socio-economic classes, and perhaps, this factor may explain some of its worldwide distribution. Carcinoma of the uterine cervix is more frequent in women who had first intercourse at an early age, have a history of sexual promiscuity, or a large number of pregnancies.[6–8] In contrast, carcinoma of the cervix is infrequent in nulliparous women, those with inactive sexual lives such as nuns, and in married women without children.[9,10]

Experimentally, carcinoma of the uterine cervix can be induced in animals by application of hormonal or other chemical carcinogens.[11]

A history of diethylstilbestrol (DES) administration to women during pregnancy has resulted in a significant incidence of clear cell adenocarcinoma of the cervix and vagina in their offsprings.[12] In contrast, no definite evidence exists to link the use of oral contraceptives with carcinoma of the uterine cervix.[13–15] Despite many theories, at the present time the causative agents of cervical carcinoma are not known, although predisposing and associated factors have been reported.[16]

The identification of herpes virus type-2 (HVS-2) and high antibody titers against this virus have been reported more often to be elevated in patients with cervical carcinoma than in controls.[17–22] However, a direct etiologic role has not been established.

TABLE 25-1. Gynecologic Cancer: New Cases and Deaths Per Year in the U.S.

	ESTIMATED NEW CASES	ESTIMATED DEATHS
Carcinoma of the endometrium	38,000	3,200
Carcinoma of the ovary	17,000	11,200
Carcinoma of the cervix, invasive	16,000	7,400
Other and unspecified gynecological tumors	4,500	1,000

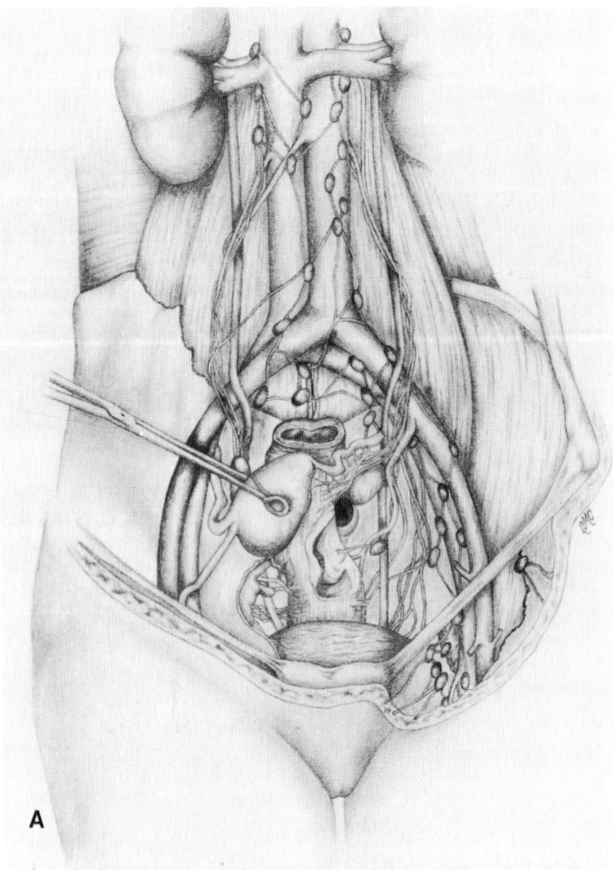

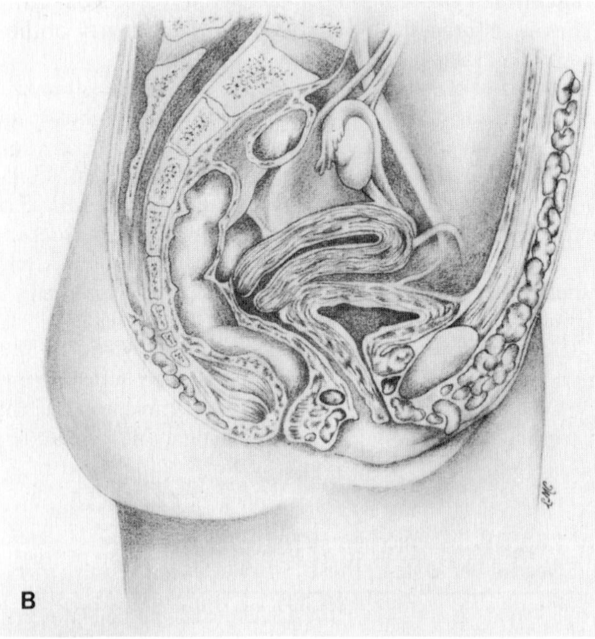

FIG. 25-1. Coronal (*A*) and sagittal (*B*) representation of pelvic anatomy showing spacial relationship of various organs.

NATURAL HISTORY

In most instances, squamous cell carcinoma of the uterine cervix has its origin at the squamous-columnar junction of the endocervical canal and the portio of the cervix. The lesion is frequently associated with a long history of chronic cervicitis, severe dysplasia and carcinoma *in situ*.[23,24] This progression may take from 10 to 20 years.[25-26]

It is generally accepted that invasive carcinoma of the cervix is preceded in the majority of cases by carcinoma *in situ*[27] Petersen reported on 127 patients with untreated carcinoma *in situ* followed for at least three years.[28] By the 10th year of followup, about 30% of the patients had developed invasive carcinoma. After one year of observation only half of the original patients still had carcinoma *in situ;* Koss and coworkers noted that in 67 cases of carcinoma *in situ* followed for a minimum of three years, 17 (25%) regressed after the initial diagnosis, which is an indication that either the original diagnosis was incorrect or that some of the lesions regress spontaneously.[29] Clemmesen and Poulsen later revised this series and concluded that at least 40% of the patients with carcinoma *in situ* subsequently developed invasive lesions.[30] However, in a series of 31 cases of carcinoma *in situ* followed for over 12 years by Kottmeier, 71% developed invasive carcinoma and at 30 years followup, 80% of the cases had become invasive.[31]

The malignant process breaks through the basement membrane of the epithelium and invades the cervical stroma.[32] If the invasion is less than 3 mm, the lesion is classified as microinvasive or superficially invasive and the probability of lymph node metastases is about 1%.[33-35] Invasion may progress, but if the tumor is not grossly visible and the depth of penetration is less than 5 mm, the tumor is classified as occult invasive carcinoma. The incidence of metastatic pelvic lymph nodes is related to the depth of invasion with an overall incidence of 5–8%.[36]

Extension of the lesion in the cervix may eventually be manifested by superficial ulceration, exophytic tumor, or extensive infiltration of the endocervix. The lesion may spread to the adjacent vaginal fornices or to the paracervical and parametrial tissues, with eventual direct invasion of the bladder or the rectum or both.

Carcinoma of the uterine cervix has been found to extend into the lower uterine segment and the endometrial cavity in 10% to 30% of cases.[37,38] In an analysis of 439 patients, Perez and coworkers observed decreased survival and greater incidence of distant metastases in patients with stromal endometrial invasion or replacement of normal endometrium by cervical carcinoma confirming observations previously reported by Mitani and coworkers (see Fig. 25-2).[37,38]

Regional lymphatic or hematogenous spread occurs depending on the stage of the tumor, but dissemination does not always follow an orderly sequence and occasionally a small carcinoma may be seen infiltrating the pelvic lymph nodes, invading the bladder, rectum, or producing distant metastasis.

In addition to stage and volume of tumor, and in some instances the histologic type of the lesion and vascular invasion, there are other factors that affect the prognosis of patients with cervical carcinoma.[39,40] Evans, Bush and coworkers, and Vigario and coworkers have reported a greater incidence of pelvic recurrences and lower survival in patients with anemia (hemoglobin below 10–11 gm%).[41–43] The use of blood transfusions improves the response of the tumor to radiation therapy, decreasing the occurrence of pelvic failures and enhancing the prognosis.

Jenkin and coworkers observed a higher incidence of pelvic recurrences and complications in patients with arterial hypertension (diastolic pressure above 110 mm Hg).[44]

Decreased survival of a group of 260 patients with oral temperature higher than 100°F was reported by Van Herik in a study of 666 patients.[45] In 21.2% of the patients, pelvic inflammatory disease was noted and in 6.9% local infection. However, in 57.3% of the patients no specific etiologic factor could be determined. The prognosis was worse with a longer duration of the fever (more than 7 days).

FIG. 25-2. Percent survival in 439 patients with stage IB, II, and III carcinoma of the cervix with stromal endometrial invasion or tumor only (positive curettings) in endometrium.

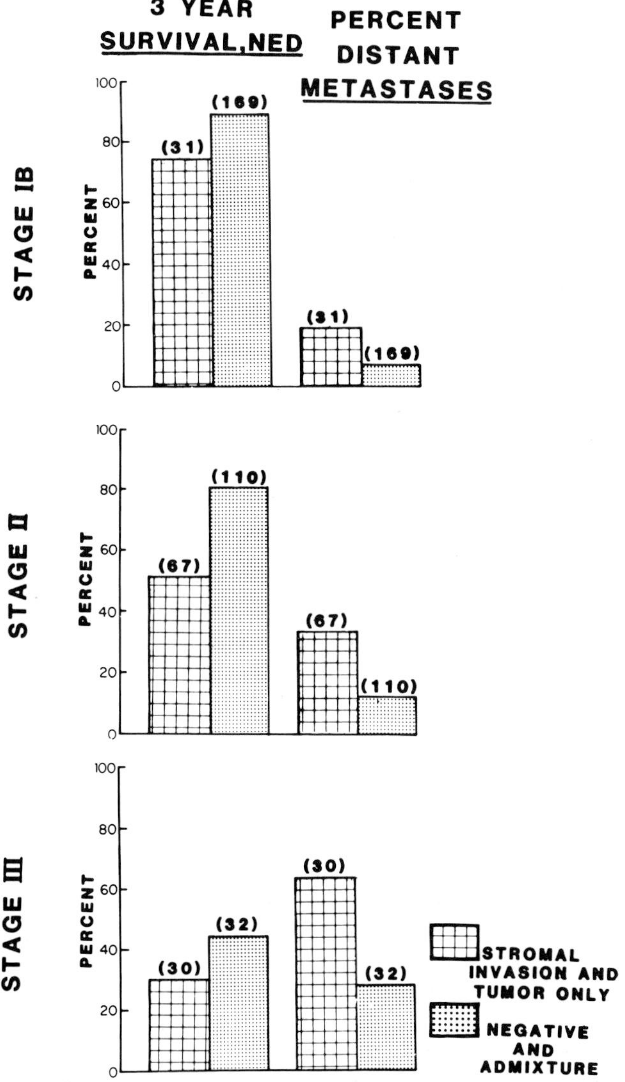

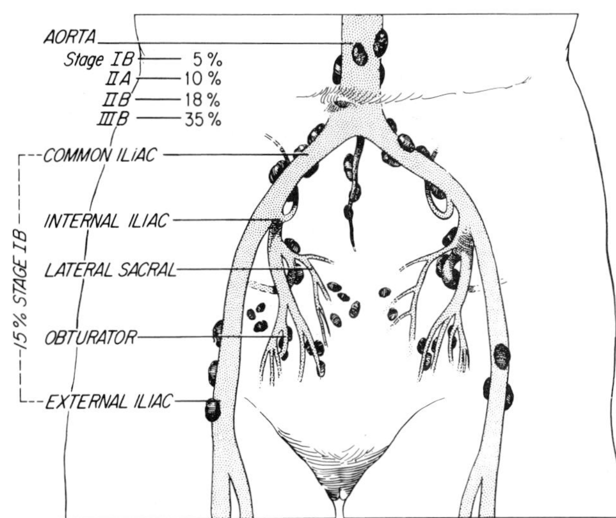

FIG. 25-3. Location and occurrence of metastatic lymph nodes in carcinoma of the cervix. The pelvic nodes most commonly involved are the obturator, often considered a medial group of the external iliac. In order of descending frequency, metastases occur to the internal iliac, external iliac, common iliac, and lateral sacral.

According to some authors, carcinoma of the cervix has the same prognosis in younger and older patients.[46,47]

TUMOR DISSEMINATION

The cervix has a rich lymphatic network that is more abundant in the muscular layers. Once the tumor has invaded these structures there will be a higher probability of dissemination to the regional lymphatics. Carcinoma of the cervix may spread to the paracervical and parametrial lymphatics, metastasizing to the obturator lymph nodes (considered a medial group of the external iliac), to other external iliac and to the hypogastric lymph nodes. From these, there may be tumor metastases to the common iliac or to the para-aortic lymph nodes (see Fig. 25-3).[48,49]

TABLE 25-2. Incidence of Metastatic Pelvic Nodes in Carcinoma of the Uterine Cervix

AUTHOR	STAGE I	STAGE II	STAGE III
NO IRRADIATION			
Morton	16%	32%	47%
Guttman	11%	35%	
Meigs	18%	45%	
Brunschwig	13%	30%	
Christensen	16%	44%	
Graham (collected series)	15%	27%	66%
POST-IRRADIATION LYMPHADENECTOMY			
Morton	9%	21%	17%
Guttman	0%	4%	
Rutledge	3%	14%	13%
Perez	7%	0%	

TABLE 25-3. Metastases to Paraaortic Node in Carcinoma of Uterine Cervix

	STAGE											
	IB		IIA		IIB		IIIA		IIIB		IV	
Sudarsanam	11/153	(7%)	3/21	(14%)	4/22	(18%)	2/3	(66%)	3/16	(19%)	0/3	(0%)
Nelson					5/31	(16%)			13/28	(46%)		
Piver					6/46	(13%)			18/49	(36%)	4/7	(57%)
Wharton	0/21	(0%)	0/10	(0%)	10/47	(21%)			14/42	(33%)		
Lagasse	8/143	(5%)	4/22	(18%)	19/58	(33%)	0/3	(0%)	19/61	(31%)	1/4	(25%)
Buchsbaum	0/23	(0%)	1/12	(7%)					7/20	(35%)	1/2	(50%)
Averette	3/40	(8%)	2/9	(22%)	2/9	(22%)			2/20	(10%)	1/2	(50%)
TOTAL	22/380	(6%)	10/74	(14%)	46/213	(22%)			85/260	(33%)		

Modified from Lagasse LD, Creasman WT, Shingleton HM et al: Gynecol Oncol 9:90, 1980

TABLE 25-4. Distribution by Stages of Distant Metastases in 2,220 Patients with Squamous-Cell Carcinoma of the Cervix Treated Between September 1948 and December 1963

STAGE	NO. OF PATIENTS		PATIENTS IN WHOM DISTANT METASTASES DEVELOPED	
IA	134		1	(0.74%)
IB	337		16	(4.74%)
IIA	456		42	(9.21%)
IIB	414		67	(16.18%)
IIIA	417		85	(20.38%)
IIIB	362		75	(20.71%)
		59*	14	(24.13%)
IV	100			
		41†	41	(100.00%)
TOTAL	2,220		341	(15.37%)

* Classified as stage IV because of local extension to bladder and/or rectum.

† Classified as stage IV because metastasis was present at initial examination.

Carlson V, Delclos L, Fletcher GH: Radiology 88:961, 1967

TABLE 25-5. Sites of Distant Metastases in 2,220 Patients with Squamous-Cell Carcinoma of the Cervix Treated Between September 1948 and December 1963

SITE	SINGLE ORGAN METASTASES (No. of Patients)	MULTIPLE ORGAN METASTASES (No. of Patients)
Nodes	33 (30.0%)	157 (67.9%)
Supraclavicular	9	57
Para-aortic	12	54
Inguinal	8	43
Mediastinal	1	37
Iliac	1	28
Cervical	1	16
Axillary	0	12
Other	1	38
Lung	40 (36.3%)	86 (37.2%)
Bone	18 (16.3%)	67 (29.0%)
Abdomen	8 (7.2%)	97 (41.9%)
Generalized	0	37
Peritoneum	2	11
Liver	6	42
Gastrointestinal Tract	0	24
Other	0	54
Miscellaneous	11	101

Carlson V, Delclos L, Fletcher GH: Radiology 88:961, 1967

The incidence of pelvic or para-aortic lymph nodes according to various stages of the disease are listed in Tables 25-2 and 25-3.

Hematogenous dissemination through the venous plexus and the paracervical veins occurs less frequently, but is relatively high with more advanced stages (see Table 25-4). The most common metastatic sites are the lungs, mediastinal and supraclavicular lymph nodes, bones and liver (see Table 25-5).[50,51]

CLINICAL MANIFESTATIONS

Intraepithelial or early invasive carcinoma of the cervix can be detected before it becomes symptomatic by periodic cytological smears.

In patients with intraepithelial carcinoma *in situ,* no gross abnormality of the cervix may be noted; a small cental superficial ulceration may be the only finding.

Frequently the first manifestation of abnormality in cervical carcinoma is postcoital spotting, which later may increase to limited metrorrhagia (intermenstrual bleeding) that may be observed after exertion. Later, more prominent menstrual bleeding may appear (menorrhagia).

In patients with invasive carcinoma, sero-sanguinous or yellowish vaginal discharge may be noted, particularly with more advanced necrotic lesions. This discharge may be foul smelling and may be intermixed with profuse bleeding. If chronic bleeding occurs, the patients may complain of fatigue or other symptoms related to anemia.

Pain, usually in the pelvis or the hypogastrium, may be noted. This could be due to tumor necrosis or associated pelvic inflammatory disease. Some patients may complain of pain in the lumbosacral area and, in these cases, the possibility of para-aortic lymph node involvement with extension into the lumbosacral roots or hydronephrosis should be considered. Occasionally, epigastric pain may be due to high para-aortic metastatic lymph nodes.

Urinary and rectal symptoms may appear in advanced stages as a consequence of invasion of the bladder or the rectum by the neoplasia. In this situation, hematuria or rectal bleeding may occur.

PATHOLOGIC CHARACTERISTICS

Gross Appearance

On clinical or pathologic examination, invasive lesions of the cervix may appear as small superficial or more extensive ulceration involving one or several quadrants of the portio. Larger lesions have an exophytic appearance or extensive necrotic ulceration. They may take an infiltrating, endophytic appearance extending into the stroma of the cervix and endocervical canal. These lesions may extend upward and concentrically expand the lower uterine segment, constituting the so-called barrel shaped cervix. Perez and coworkers have described extension of carcinoma of the cervix into the endometrial cavity with infiltration of the myometrium.[38]

The tumor may protrude toward the vagina acquiring an exophytic or necrotic appearance.

Infiltration of the adjacent soft tissues in the vagina, parametria, rectum, or bladder can be demonstrated by clinical evaluation and in surgical specimens.

Microscopic Appearance

Figure 25-4 shows the histogenesis of carcinoma of the cervix.

Over 90% of the tumors are of the squamous cell type. Approximately 5% are classified as adenocarcinoma, 1% to 2% are clear cell, mesonephric type.

Wentz and Ragan have divided the squamous cell carcinoma into three types:[52]

1. Keratinizing
2. Non-keratinizing
3. Small cell type

The epidermoid carcinoma is composed of cores and nests of epithelial cells, arranged in random fashion and forming multiple arborescences of different size configurations. The keratinizing cells show foci of keratinization with cornified pearls. The non-keratinizing cells have well-demarcated tumor-stromal borders but no evidence of keratinization or cornified pearls. The small cells have a spindle or small, round appearance and poorly defined tumor-stromal borders.

The connective tissue stroma may be infiltrated by tumor and shows edema of the collagen fibers, infiltration by leukocytes and neovessel formation. The tumor may destroy the basement membrane and grow in large cores throughout the stroma. Electron microscopy may show desmosomes and tonofilaments.

Adenocarcinoma arises from the cylindrical mucosa of the endocervix or the mucus-secreting endocervical glands.[53] Sometimes it is difficult to differentiate a primary endocervical and adenocarcinoma from an endometrial tumor. The endocervical adenocarcinoma may form mucosal glands lined by high columnar cells and producing tubular folds oriented in many directions. The stroma surrounds the epithelial formations. A well-differentiated cervical adenocarcinoma has been improperly designated as "adenoma malignum," when this is truly a malignant tumor that invades adjacent tissues and may produce distant metastasis.[54]

As the tumor becomes less differentiated, the cells are more bizarre, contain more mitoses, and do not have a glandular appearance.

Adenosquamous carcinoma is relatively rare (2–5% of all cervical carcinomas) and consists of intermingled epithelial cell cores and glandular structures. If the squamous component is benign metaplasia, the tumor is called adenoacanthoma.

The glassy cell carcinoma is considered a poorly differentiated adenosquamous tumor, with a distinctive histological appearance. Survival is poor after surgery or irradiation; Littman and coworkers reported only four of 13 patients, the majority with stage II surviving 5 years (six had extrapelvic failures).[55]

Several authors have not found a meaningful correlation between the histopathologic characteristics of the tumor and response to irradiation for comparable stage and volume of tumor.[56,57] In contrast, Wentz and Reagan and Swan and Roddick reported a correlation between histologic grade and survival, particularly after radiation therapy.[52,58] However, other factors that may affect patterns of failure were not analyzed, such as techniques of irradiation, geometric and anatomic placement of intracavitary sources, volume of tumor within a given stage, and so forth.

A small group of adenocarcinomas are of clear type (mesonephric) and may grow in a tubular, glandular, papillary, or solid pattern. It is composed of clear and "hobnail" cells. The clear cell is characterized by a voluminous cytoplasm filled with glycogen and a "hobnail" by single cell apical projections into the neoplastic lumina.[59,60,61]

FIG. 25-4. Histogenesis of carcinoma of the uterine cervix.

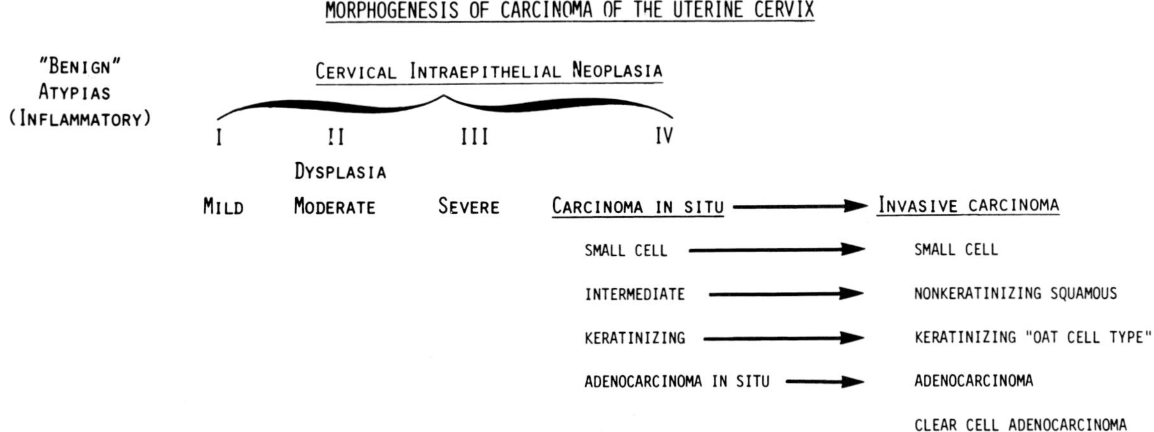

Another uncommon type of adenocarcinoma is the adenocystic carcinoma or cylindroma (less than 1%), which has an appearance similar to that of the counterparts in the salivary gland or the bronchial tree.[62,63]

Small cell carcinoma constituted 14.3% of 1035 cases of grade III–IV cervical carcinoma seen at Mayo Clinic. The 5-year survival was 66%, which was comparable to other subtypes.[64] In contrast, Wentz and Reagan reported only 17% survival 5 years after therapy.[52]

Primary sarcomas of the cervix have been occasionally described (leiomyosaroma, rhabdomyosarcoma, stromal sarcomas, carcinosarcomas).[65,66]

Malignant lymphomas, primary or secondary, in the cervix have been sporadically reported. They should be treated as other lymphomas.[67,68]

DIAGNOSIS AND WORK-UP

Every patient with carcinoma of the cervix should be jointly evaluated and staged by the radiation oncologist and gynecologist. All patients should have a complete physical and detailed pelvic and rectal examination. The techniques have been described in standard textbooks.[69]

Cytology

The ideal is to detect carcinoma of the cervix when it is still a severe dysplasia or carcinoma *in situ*. The detection and proper treatment of carcinoma *in situ* by screening cytology have resulted in a decreased prevalence of invasive carcinoma, lowering the mortality from these tumors.[70,71]

Screening for carcinoma of the cervix represents a significant financial outlay. It has been estimated that 2.5 cases of carcinoma of the cervix may be found for every 10,000 vaginal smears examined. After the first negative examination, many thousands of patients need to be screened to find a single case of invasive carcinoma of the cervix. Fidler and coworkers reported 17 new cases of invasive carcinoma in 357,000 women who had been previously screened. The average time since the last screening was 3.5 years, implying that 75,000 women would have to be screened annually to detect a single case of carcinoma *in situ*.[72] Therefore, it is important to consider optimal screening schedules. The American Cancer Society has recommended that asymptomatic women 20 years of age and older and those under 20 who are sexually active have a Pap smear annually for two consecutive years and at least one every three years until the age of 65. Women who are at high risk of developing cervical carcinoma because of early age at first intercourse, multiple sexual partners, and multiparity should have a yearly Pap smear. A complete gynecologic examination should be performed when the vaginal smears are obtained.[73]

The correlation between the cytologic diagnosis and subsequent histologic examination is over 90%.[74] Vaginal smears have been classified as: I (normal), II (atypical), III (dysplasia), IV (carcinoma *in situ*), or V (invasive carcinoma). However, some pathologists prefer to avoid the "class" system and describe the morphologic diagnosis on the cytologic exam.

The technique for obtaining Pap smears has been described in standard textbooks.[69] If the cytologic smears show atypia or mild dysplasia (class II), the Pap smear should be repeated no sooner than 2 weeks to allow representative cellular exfoliation. Also, the patient should be instructed not to take douches before the examination and specimens should be obtained for studies of trichomonas. If the findings persist, the patient should be followed closely and Pap smears repeated every 6 months.

If the cytologic smear shows dysplasia or malignant cells, directed biopsies using Schiller tests or colposcopy should be carried out immediately. Endocervical curettage must always be obtained. If the biopsies are negative they should be repeated under direct colposcopic observation and, if necessary, a conization should be performed.

Pap smears can be useful in evaluating patients after therapy. However, it must be remembered that there may be dysplasia and bizarre epithelial changes following radiation therapy, which make the interpretation of cytological smears difficult.[75] Marcial and coworkers reported on 342 patients with cervical carcinoma treated with irradiation within 4 months after therapy; approximately 90% had negative cytologic smears.[76] A negative cytologic smear 4–12 months post-irradiation is associated with a good prognosis with stages I and II, but this is not true in stages III and IV. The presence of tumor cells in the smear in the first 4 months after completion of irradiation is of no prognostic significance. However, Koss had previously reported that the presence of tumor cells 4 weeks or more following the completion of irradiation carried an ominous prognosis.[77] The authors believe that the presence of tumor cells in cytologic smears should be of concern 3–4 months after irradiation; in that case, a cervical biopsy and D & C (dilatation and curettage) should be performed.

Colposcopy

Colposcopy may adequately evaluate the exocervix and a portion of the endocervix adjacent to the transition of the squamous and columnar epithelium (T zone). This examination, performed with a colposcope, provides a 10- to 15-fold magnification view of the cervix. A colposcope is essentially an instrument with a light source and a magnifying optical system; an axial or parallax illumination system can be brightened or dimmed at will and a mounting device permits movement of the apparatus so that the cervix may be examined clearly. The focal length is 20–25 cm with visual field of not less than 25 mm. To visualize the vascular system, a green filter is attached. Color photographs or television views can be obtained. Combined with cytologic examination and biopsy of grossly abnormal size, colposcopy may be extremely useful in detecting the majority of early cervical lesions[78,79]

Conization

Conization must be performed in specific situations such as when no gross lesion of the cervix is noted and an endocervical tumor is suspected; the entire lesion cannot be seen with the colposcope; diagnosis of microinvasive carcinoma is made on biopsy; discrepancies are found between the cytologic and the histologic appearances of the lesion; or the patient is not reliable for continuous followup.[80]

Conization involves a conical removal of a large portion of the exocervix and endocervix. Cold biopsies with a scalpel or other appropriate instrument should always be obtained. At least 50% of the endocervical canal should be removed without compromising the internal sphincter. A curettage of the remaining endocervial canal should be carried out.

Hot cones (fulguration) should never be performed since they will distort the tissues and prevent pathologic examination.

Many gynecologists still utilize the application of Lugol's iodine solution (Schiller's test) to delineate abnormal mucosa in the cervix or vagina. Squamous cell epithelium produces glycogen that will result in a dark staining of the normal mucosa. In contrast, the non-glycogen producing malignant cells will not stain.

Biopsy

When a gross lesion of the cervix is present, multiple punch biopsies should be adequate to confirm the diagnosis of invasive carcinoma. The biopsies should be obtained of any suspicious area as well as in all four quadrants of the cervix.

It is important to obtain samples from the periphery of the lesion with some adjoining normal tissue. Biopsies from central ulcerated or necrotic areas may not be adequate for diagnosis.

Areas with abnormal staining on the Schiller test should always be biopsied.

Dilatation and Curettage (D & C)

Because of the possibility of upper extension of the tumor, which may modify the plan of therapy, fractional curettage of the endocervical canal and the endometrium is recommended at the time of initial evaluation or during the first intracavitary insertion if the patients are treated with radiation therapy.

Other Work-up

For invasive carcinoma the patients should have the following workup:

- Laboratory
  - Complete peripheral blood evaluation, including hemogram, white blood count, differential and platelet count
  - SMA-12, with particular attention to BUN, creatinine, uric acid, and liver function parameters
- Radiographic Studies
  - Chest films and IV pyelogram should be obtained on all patients
  - Barium enema should be obtained on patients with stage III and IVA as well as on patients with earlier stages who have symptoms referable to the colon and rectum
  - Lymphangiogram may provide useful information concerning lymph node involvement in the pelvis or periaortic nodes. Unfortunately, not all the lymph nodes where carcinoma of the cervix may metastasize are opacified by pedal lymphangiogram (*i.e.*, obturator, hypogastric). Small metastatic lesions do not produce enough modification of the architecture of the lymph node to be apparent in the lymphangiogram, at times the metastatic tumor completely obliterates the lymph node or obstructs lymphatics preventing visualization of the involved lymph nodes.

    Piver and coworkers reported on 102 patients on whom lymphangiograms were correlated with operative findings.[81] Of 41 positive lymphangiograms, 40 were subsequently confirmed (98% accuracy) by biopsy and laparotomy. In contrast, 12 of 61 lymphangiograms interpreted as negative showed metastases in the lymph nodes at laparotomy (about 20% false negative).

    The initial enthusiasm on the use of the lymphangiogram has been replaced with a more realistic expectation. The lymphangiogram definitely is of value in outlining abnormal lymph nodes that can be included in the irradiated fields or in the case of surgical management that should be removed by the surgeon for pathologic examination.
  - Computed tomography is beginning to be used more frequently and at some institutions attempts are made to replace the lymphangiogram with this procedure.[82] However, at the present time there is no reliable evaluation of the accuracy of this procedure or the contributions that it can make to the staging or to therapeutic decisions.

Other Staging Procedures

Cystoscopy or rectosigmoidoscopy should be performed on all patients with stage IIB, III, and IVA or on patients with earlier stages who have a history of urinary or lower GI disturbances.

It has been emphasized by Griffin and coworkers that these staging procedures may have a low yield of positive findings (see Table 25-6).[83] However, these procedures must be selectively carried out, depending on the stage of the tumor. Even if negative, they have value as a baseline point of reference for evaluation of the patient following therapy.[84,85]

Surgical Staging Procedures

Some gynecologists have advocated the use of pretherapy laparotomy, particularly to evaluate the presence of periaortic lymph nodes.[86] However, it has not been demonstrated that this procedure increases the probability of survival of these patients.[87,88] In addition, a high incidence of complications has been reported when laparotomy and extensive periaortic lymph node dissections are carried out on patients that are subsequently treated with definitive radiation therapy.[89]

Wharton and coworkers reported on 120 patients with squamous carcinoma of the uterine cervix who had a preirradiation celiotomy.[90] Sixty-four patients had metastatic carcinoma in lymph nodes, 33% of them in the pelvis and 20% in the common iliac or periaortic lymph nodes. (There were 16 fatal complications and 32 major intestinal complications, particularly small bowel obstruction and perforation. The

TABLE 25-6. Tumor-related Abnormalities Found

		POSITIVE FINDINGS BY				
CLINICAL STAGE	NO. PATIENTS	CYTOSCOPY	PROCTOSCOPY	BARIUM ENEMA	INTRAVENOUS PYELOGRAM	CHEST X-RAY
I	111	0	0	0	0	0
IIA	123	0	0	0	0	0
IIB	44	0	0	0	2	1
IIIA	8	0	0	0	2	0
IIIB	37	2	5	3	24	1
IV	4	2	4	4	3	0
TOTAL	227	4	9	7	31	2

Griffin RW, Parker RG, Taylor WS: Am J Roentgenol 127:826, 1976

majority of the patients with positive lymph nodes failed because of distant metastasis). Because of this negative experience, pre-irradiation laparotomy has been discontinued at M. D. Anderson Hospital and the status of the lymph nodes is investigated with lymphangiography and verified when possible with percutaneous transabdominal needle biopsy.[91]

Averette and coworkers have reported a disturbingly high lack of correlation between the clinical stage of patients with carcinoma of the cervix and the surgical findings (26% in stage 1B, 45% in stage IIA, 60% in stage IIB, 66% in stage IIIA and 95% in stage IIIB).[92] However, in other series, these differences are considerably lower and the discrepancy may reflect the dexterity of the persons staging the patients and the thoroughness of the presurgical evaluation. In a group of 45 patients with stage IB and 11 patients with IIA treated with low dose preoperative irradiation and radical hysterectomy at Washington University, only three were found to have a more advanced stage of the disease at the time of the operation.[93]

Ketcham and coworkers reported positive scalene fat pad biopsies in seven of 36 patients with stage II, III and IV carcinoma of the cervix and in four of 22 patients with postirradiation recurrences. Twenty-three patients reported by Buchsbaum with positive aortic nodes had left scalene node biopsy and eight (34.8%) had positive nodes.[95] He recommends a scalene node excision prior to any treatment plan when the aortic lymph nodes are found positive.[95] However, this procedure is not routinely carried out at most institutions because of the lower yield of positive specimens. For instance, Perez-Mesa and Spratt reported that in 73 consecutive patients with various stages of cervical carcinoma, the scaling lymph node biopsy failed to demonstrate metastatic tumor in a single instance.[96]

CLINICAL STAGING

It is extremely critical that the gynecologist and radiation oncologist jointly evaluate and stage the tumor in every patient. This should be done after bimanual pelvic and rectal examination under general anesthesia. Ideally, this should be done prior to institution of therapy; however, on occasion, after an initial evaluation the final staging is postponed because of logistic and economic reasons until the first intracavitary radioisotope insertion (which should be done within one week from initiation of the external radiotherapy if the patients are treated with this modality). In surgically treated patients, the clinical staging can be done immediately before the radical hysterectomy is performed.

The initial staging was proposed in 1929 by a subcommittee of the League of Nations, which was subsequently revised in 1937 and 1950. These functions were taken over by the International Federation of Gynecology and Obstetrics (FIGO) in collaboration with the World Health Organization and the International Union Against Cancer. The staging recommendations by this committee were last revised in 1971. Table 25-7 defines the current criteria for the various stages.[97] The FIGO classification should be based on clinical evaluation (inspection, palpation, colposcopy), roentgenographic examination of the chest, kidneys, skeleton, and endocervical curettage and biopsies. Lymphangiogram, arteriograms, CT findings, laparoscopy, or laparotomy findings should not be used for clinical staging.

When there is a disagreement regarding the staging, the earlier stage should be selected for statistical purposes. All histologic types should be included.

When there is invasion of the bladder or the rectum, this should be confirmed by biopsy. Bullous edema of the bladder or swelling of the mucosa of the rectum is not accepted as a definitive criterion for staging.

The tumor should definitely extend to the lateral pelvic wall, although fixation is not required to classify the lesion as stage III.

Patients with hydronephrosis or non-function of the kidney ascribed to parametrial extension of the tumor should be classified as a stage III, regardless of the pelvic findings.

A similar TNM staging system has also been proposed.[98]

GENERAL PRINCIPLES OF MANAGEMENT

Controversy has existed between those who advocate radical surgery and those who support radiotherapy for the treatment of carcinoma of the uterine cervix. Patients should be treated with close communication between the gynecologist and radiation oncologist and an integrated team approach should be vigorously pursued.

A direct comparison of the results obtained with these

modalities is extremely difficult because there is a definite selection of patients, those younger, with better general condition and smaller tumors being treated surgically and the less favorable group with radiation therapy. In addition, surgical exploration eliminates from this group those patients with more advanced disease.[99] It is critical that the results of surgical series be reported based on the initial clinical staging.

TREATMENT OF CARCINOMA *IN SITU*

Patients with carcinoma *in situ,* which may include those with severe dysplasia, are best treated with a total abdominal hysterectomy without or with a small vaginal cuff.[100] The decision to remove the ovaries will depend on the age of the patient and status of the ovaries.

Occasionally, when the patient wishes to have more children, carcinoma *in situ* may be treated conservatively with a therapeutic conization.[101] This procedure should be judiciously selected when the extent of tumor allows it and the patient is reliable for continued follow-up.

Christopherson and coworkers described 124 cases of carcinoma *in situ* diagnosed by biopsy.[102] Of those, 117 showed the same lesion on conization but 14 also had microinvasive carcinoma; three were negative and four showed residual dysplasia.

Kolstad and Klem reported that in 795 patients with carcinoma *in situ* treated with therapeutic conization, 19 (2.3%) developed recurrent carcinoma *in situ* and seven (.9%) invasive carcinoma.[103] A nonrandomized comparable group of 238 patients were treated with a hysterectomy. Three patients (1.2%) developed recurrent carcinoma *in situ* and five (2.1%) invasive carcinoma.

Colposcopy for periodic evaluation plays a major role in the conservation management of patients with carcinoma *in situ* of the cervix.[104]

Irradiation may be useful for the treatment of *in situ* carcinoma, particularly in postmenopausal patients with strong medical contraindications for surgery or when there is extension of the lesion to the vaginal wall or multifocal carcinoma *in situ* both in the cervix and the vagina.[100,103,105]

In a group of 30 patients with carcinoma *in situ* treated at Washington University with intracavitary radium alone [approximately 5000 milligram hours (mgh)], no recurrences were recorded.[106]

Even though some surgeons use frozen sections of the conization to decide whether hysterectomy should be carried out or not, pathologists prefer permanent sections since a more thorough examination of the specimen can be followed through.[107] The therapeutic hysterectomy can be performed 6 weeks after the conization.

Stage IA

The definition of microinvasive (stage IA) carcinoma of the cervix lacks uniformity of diagnostic criteria; depth of invasion and tumor confluence have been identified as prognostic factors that should be taken into consideration when planning therapy.[108,109] Early carcinoma of the cervix (stage IA) can be treated with intracavitary radioactive sources alone (7000–9000 mgh in one or two insertions) or with a radical

TABLE 25-7. Definitions of the Different Clinical Stages in Carcinoma of the Cervix Uteri*

PRE-INVASIVE CARCINOMA	
Stage 0	Carcinoma in situ, intra-epithelial carcinoma. Cases of Stage 0 should not be included in any therapeutic statistics for invasive carcinoma.
INVASIVE CARCINOMA	
Stage I	Carcinoma strictly confined to the cervix (extension to the corpus should be disregarded).
Stage Ia	Microinvasive carcinoma (early stromal invasion).
Stage Ib	All other cases of Stage I. Occult cancer should be marked "occ."
Stage II	The carcinoma extends beyond the cervix, but has not extended on to the pelvic wall. The carcinoma involves the vagina, but not the lower third.
Stage IIa	No obvious parametrial involvement.
Stage IIb	Obvious parametrial involvement.
Stage III	The carcinoma has extended on to the pelvic wall. On rectal examination there is no cancer-free space between the tumor and the pelvic wall. The tumor involves the lower third of the vagina. All cases with a hydro-nephrosis or non-functioning kidney should be included, unless they are known to be due to other cause.
Stage IIIa	No extension on to the pelvic wall.
Stage IIIb	Extension on to the pelvic wall and/or hydro-nephrosis or non-functioning kidney.
Stage IV	The carcinoma has extended beyond the true pelvis or has clinically involved the mucosa of the bladder or rectum. A bullous edema as such does not permit a case to be allotted to Stage IV.
Stage IVa	Spread of the growth to adjacent organs.
Stage IVb	Spread to distant organs.

* Adopted in 1976 by the International Federation of Gynecology and Obstretics (FIGO)

hysterectomy. When the depth of penetration of the stroma by tumor is less than 3 mm, the incidence of lymph node metastasis is 1% or less and a lymph node dissection or pelvic external irradiation is not required. With more extensive lesions, a Wertheim radical hysterectomy with pelvic lymphadenectomy is the preferred treatment. In either case, the tumor control is close to 100%, patients eventually dying of intercurrent disease or other causes.[36,110]

Stages IB and IIA

The choice of definitive irradiation or radical surgery for stage IB and IIA carcinoma of the cervix remains controversial and the preference of one procedure over the other depends on the institution, the gynecologist, or radiation oncologist involved, in addition to general condition of the patient and characteristics of the lesion. An operation has been preferred by some in young women because of the desire to preserve the ovaries and the possibility of more pliable vagina following surgery.[111]

It is generally agreed that surgery and irradiation are equally effective in the treatment of stage I and IIA carcinoma of the cervix. Numerous noncontrolled studies support the merits of either modality.[112-117] Newton and Roddick and Greenlaw reported in prospectively randomized studies comparable survival and pelvic recurrences in patients with stage IB and IIA carcinoma of the uterine cervix treated with a radical hysterectomy or irradiation alone.[118,119]

Kielbinska and coworkers, in a long-term follow-up of 792 women treated by irradiation and 789 women treated with hysterectomy and irradiation for stage I cervical carcinoma, found no difference in survival, general health, incidence of recurrent carcinoma, or appearances of second primary malignancies.[120]

Other reports show no significant difference in survival or pelvic tumor control with either modality (see Tables 25-8 and 25-9).

Bulky endocervical carcinoma (so-called barrel-shaped cervix) has a higher incidence of central recurrence, pelvic and periaortic lymph node metastasis, and distant dissemination.[121,122] Because of the inability of the intracavitary sources to encompass all of the tumor in a high-dose volume, larger doses of external irradiation to the whole pelvis or a surgical procedure to remove the uterus or both are necessary to improve therapeutic results.[123,124]

There are no controlled studies showing improved survival with pelvic radiation following radical surgery in the presence of positive nodes. Postoperative radiation therapy has been recommended in the presence of pelvic node metastasis.[125] However, a recent panel report summarizing the anecdotal experience at several institutions in the U.S. and a review of available literature showed:

1. The lack of controlled studies to evaluate postradical hysterectomy irradiation in patients with early carcinoma of the cervix having metastatic pelvic lymph nodes
2. No difference in survival in irradiated vs. nonirradiated patients (50 to 83% five-year survival)
3. Higher incidence of pelvic failures in the nonirradiated patients (84% in 57 recurrent cases) compared with those irradiated (50% in 18 recurrent patients).[126]

Stages IIB, III, and IVA

Patients with stages IIB and III are treated with irradiation alone. Patients with stage IVA (bladder or rectal invasion) can be treated with either high doses of whole pelvis external irradiation, intracavitary sources, and additional parametrial irradiation or with pelvic exenteration.[127]

At the present time, there are no known chemotherapeutic agents that have proven effectiveness in the adjuvant treatment of patients with advanced disease, which has a higher incidence of distant metastasis.

SURGICAL TECHNIQUES

In 1881, W. A. Freund performed a total abdominal hysterectomy with removal of lymph node metastasis.[128] A similar operation was done by Ries in Chicago and by Clark in Baltimore. Wertheim perfected the operation and developed the technique of removing the parametrium, paravaginal tissue, and pelvic lymph nodes. At the time Wertheim was performing the abdominal radical procedure, Schauta developed the vaginal radical hysterectomy. His operative mortality was only 2.3%, as compared to the operative mortality of Wertheim of 18.6%.[129] The 5-year cure rate for each approach was approximately 40%. In the early 1940's Meigs revitalized

TABLE 25-8. Survival Rates for Stage I and II Carcinoma of the Cervix Treated by Radical Hysterectomy and Pelvic Lymphadenectomy

AUTHOR	STAGE	NUMBER OF PATIENTS	SURVIVORS[a]	PERCENTAGE SURVIVAL
Blaikley *et al.* (1969)	IB	98	64	65.5
	IB & IIA	161	96	50.8
Brunschwig and Barber	IB (A)[b]	173	141	81.5
	IB & IIA(B)[b]	308	231	76.0
Christensen *et al.*	IB	168	137	82.7
	IB & IIA	219	168	77.0
Ketcham *et al.*	IB	28	Actuarial	86.0
	IB & IIA	42		87.0
Litt and Meigs	IB	116	91	78.4
	IB & IIA	165	119	72.1
Masterson	IB	120	105	87.5
	IB & IIA	150	124	82.5
Park *et al.*	IB	126	Actuarial	91.0
AVERAGE	IB			81.9
	IB & IIA			74.2

[a] Patients dead of intercurrent disease were included with survivors when data were available.
[b] Surgical and pathological classification.
Modified from Hoskins WJ, Ford Jr. JH, Lutz MH et al: Gynecol Oncol 4:287, 1976

TABLE 25-9. Survival of Patients with Stage I and II Carcinoma of the Cervix Treated by Radiotherapy

AUTHOR	STAGE	NUMBER OF PATIENTS	SURVIVORS*	PERCENTAGE SURVIVAL
Blaikley *et al.*	I	183	123	67.2
	I & II	551	296	53.7
Dickson	IB	348	249	71.6
	IB & IIA	983	589	60.0
Fletcher	IB	549	Actuarial	91.5
	IB & IIA	973		83.5
Kline *et al.*	IB	45	37	81.4
	IB & IIA	64	47	70.5
Kottmeier	IB	611	547	89.5
	IB & IIA	1576	1244	78.9
Muirhead and Green	I	194	152	78.0
	I & II	208	306	68.0
Wall *et al.*	I	101	87	86.4
	I & II	208	153	73.5
AVERAGE	I			83.5
	I & II			75.6

Hoskins WJ, Ford Jr. JH, Lutz MH et al: Gynecol Oncol 4:285, 1976
* Patients dead of intercurrent disease included with survivors when data available.

the abdominal radical hysterectomy, using modern surgical techniques with a low complication rate as well as significant cure.[130] Brunschwig performed the pelvic exenteration on patients with persistent or recurrent cervical cancer.[131]

The operations that are performed for carcinoma of the cervix consist of:

1. Cervical conization
2. Total abdominal extrafascial hysterectomy
3. Modified radical hysterectomy
4. Radical hysterectomy with bilateral pelvic lymphadenectomy
5. Radical vaginal hysterectomy
6. Pelvic exenteration
7. Pretreatment laparotomy prior to radiation therapy

Cervical Conization

Cervical conization may be diagnostic or therapeutic. A diagnostic cone is necessary if the directed biopsies do not correlate with the cytology, microinvasive carcinoma is found on biopsies, or the entire transformation zone extending into the endocervical canal cannot be visualized. The diagnostic cone is performed with a cold knife rather than electrocautery or laser so as not to destroy cells at the tissue edges.

The therapeutic cone is used in the treatment of carcinoma *in situ* of the cervix. Its use is controversial due to reports of persistent or recurrent carcinoma *in situ*.[132,133]

Total Extrafascial Abdominal Hysterectomy

The type I extrafascial hysterectomy consists of a removal of the cervix and adjacent tissues as well as the upper vagina in a plane outside the pubocervical fascia. There is minimal disturbance of the ureters and the trigone of the bladder, which decreases the risk of urinary complications. When desired, a small vaginal cuff can be removed (1–2 cm) (see Fig. 25-5).

Total abdominal extrafascial hysterectomy has been advocated for treatment of carcinoma *in situ* and stage IA (microinvasive carcinoma),[108,134,135] A total abdominal hysterectomy alone is recommended in the treatment of microinvasive carcinoma when the stroma is invaded to less than a depth of 3 mm, providing there is no lymphatic or blood vascular involvement, and that the tumor volume beneath the basement membrane is minimal. Nelson and co-workers considered microinvasion up to 1 mm of stromal invasion with no demonstrable vascular penetration by malignant cells; Seski, Abell, and Morley defined microinvasion as stromal penetration to a depth of 3 mm, excluding lymphatic and vascular involvement.[80,135] Using this definition, pelvic lymph nodes were negative for tumor metastasis in 37 patients evaluated. Stromal invasion beyond 5 mm is associated with a higher incidence of pelvic lymph node metastases (5–10%).[36,109] The volume of tumor in the stroma may be a more reliable criterion than depth of penetration to arrive at a definition of stage IA.[136]

The use of an extrafacial total abdominal hysterectomy in combination with radiation therapy has been advocated in barrel-shaped endocervical carcinoma of the cervix.[124] In 1976, Rutledge and coworkers reported an increase in the 5-year survival from 59% to 89% in patients with barrel-shaped stage IA and IIB cervical cancers when hysterectomy was added to radiation therapy.[137] In a small series, Van Nagell and coworkers showed the advantage of using radiation followed by simple hysterectomy for bulky cervical cancers more than 5 cm in diameter.[138] Six of seven patients receiving

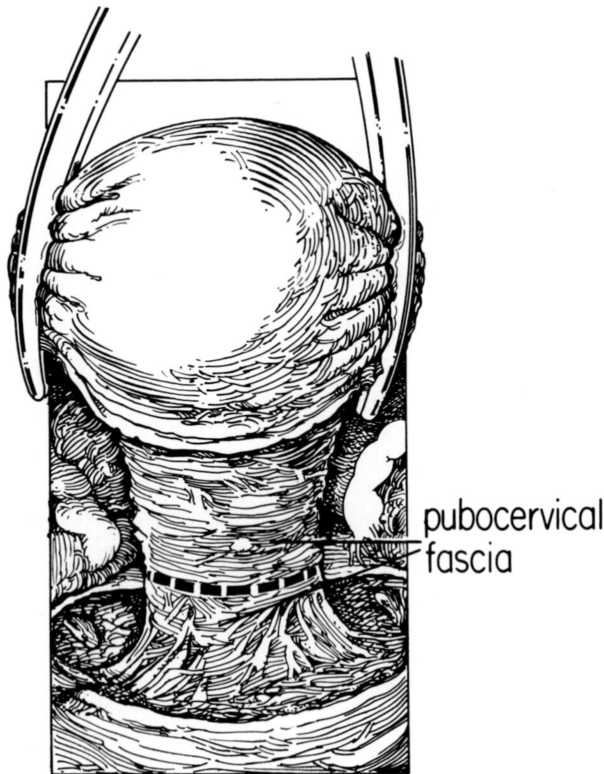

FIG. 25-5. Total extrafascial hysterectomy used for carcinoma *in situ,* stage IA (micro-invasive carcinoma), and in combination with radiation therapy. The *pubocervical fascia* invests the cervix and is not incised with the extrafascial hysterectomy. The fascia is removed in continuity with the cervix.

radiation therapy alone recurred, while with radiation followed by hysterectomy, there were no recurrences among the five patients so treated. The extrafascial total hysterectomy has been used in carcinoma of the cervix with endometrial extension. Pelvic and distant recurrences were approximately the same whether radiation therapy was used alone or in combination with surgery.[38]

Modified Radical Hysterectomy

In this operation, the cervix and upper vagina are removed, including paracervical tissues, and ureters are dissected in the paracervical tunnel to their point of entry into the bladder. Since the ureters are unsheathed, parametrium and paracervical tissue can be safely removed medial to the ureter (see Fig. 25-6).

The modified radical hysterectomy has been used in patients with microinvasive carcinoma. This operation has also advocated by Way for treatment of carcinoma *in situ,* because of a 21% incidence of carcinoma *in situ* in the vaginal cuff.[139] However, the finding is higher than generally reported and with careful followup by cytology and colposcopy, the removal of large vaginal cuff in carcinoma *in situ* is rarely necessary.

Radical Abdominal Hysterectomy with Bilateral Pelvic Lymphadenectomy

In the radical hysterectomy, a wider resection of the paracervical tissues is carried out, with dissection of the ureters and mobilization of the bladder neck as well as the rectum to allow for the more extensive removal of tissues and the bilateral pelvic lymphadenectomy. Also, a vaginal cuff of at least 2–3 cm is always included in the procedure (see Fig. 25-7).

The indications for radical hysterectomy are limited to selected patients with stage IB and IIA carcinomas of the cervix. In young women, it is possible to conserve ovarian function as cervical carcinoma rarely metastasizes to the ovary. According to some gynecologists, treatment with radical pelvic surgery may alter sexual function to a lesser degree than radiation therapy.[140] Another important advantage of surgery is the opportunity to do a thorough pelvic and upper abdominal evaluation since there is a disparity between the clinical and surgical-pathologic stage. However, surgical staging had not been shown to improve overall patient survival.[90,141]

The uretero-vaginal fistula is one of the most significant hazards of the radical hysterectomy and pelvic node dissection. Meticulous surgical technique and the use of drainage reduces the risk of uretero-vaginal fistula to less than 1%. Fifty percent of these fistulae spontaneously heal with a normal urinary tract function. Those fistulae that fail to heal spontaneously can be operated on at 6 months following the original surgery and the ureter reimplanted into the bladder with ease.

Other complications of radical surgery include hemorrhage, infection, bowel obstruction, bladder, and recto-vaginal fistulae. Post-surgical complications are generally more amenable to correction than late complications following radiation.[142]

Pelvic Exenteration

In 1948, Brunschwig introduced this procedure for the en masse excision of all pelvic viscera for presenting stage IVA and recurrent carcinoma of the cervix.[143] In former years, it was used in stage IVA carcinoma of the cervix with extension to the bladder. Modern radiation therapy makes this rarely necessary, since Million and Fletcher reported 18 of 53 patients with bladder involvement surviving NED after definitive irradiation.[144] The operation, which is not done as a palliative procedure, consists of a radical hysterectomy, pelvic lymph node dissection, removal of bladder (anterior exenteration), removal of rectosigmoid (posterior exenteration), or both (total exenteration). The ileum or sigmoid have been the usual means of urinary diversion. Since some of the patients have a pelvic recurrence following radiation therapy, the transverse colon is used for the urinary conduit. Proof that there is no extension of disease beyond the pelvis is mandatory. Metastasis outside the pelvis, including para-aortic lymph nodes, or any viscera are absolute contraindications to the procedure. Bilateral ureteral obstruction secondary to tumor is also a relative contraindication.[145,146]

At laparotomy, if tumor is found in the periaortic nodes or abdominal viscera, the operation is discontinued. The paravesical and pararectal space is also entered to identify tumor fixation to the lateral pelvic walls since this also is a contraindication for an exenteration. The question of operability in the presence of positive pelvic lymph nodes is still not completely answered. One approach is to continue the operation if only a few of the parametrial nodes are positive. Barber, in evaluating 148 patients who had positive pelvic nodes at the time of the exenteration, reported a 5-year survival of only 4.7%.[147]

In 1960, Brunschwig and Daniel reported on 592 exenterations with a 5-year survival of 17% and an operation mortality of 23%.[145] The 5-year survival rate reported in patients on whom exenteration is completed is about 30%.[148-153]

Preoperative Laparotomy

Investigators have performed pretreatment laparotomies to evaluate the presence of metastases to the pelvic or peri-aortic nodes. If periaortic node metastases are present, patients are treated with 5500–6000 rad to the para-aortic area, which unfortunately may result in a high complication rate. Four years following therapy, 50% of the patients reported by Nelson and coworkers with positive para-aortic nodes had distant metastasis; only one of 13 patients was alive.[154] Other investigators throughout the country have confirmed the low survival with the majority of these patients, secondary to distant metastasis and high incidence of complications after extended field irradiation. Chism and Keys concluded that because of the morbidity of the operation, the incidence of pelvic recurrences after initial therapy, and the probability of developing distant metastasis, less than 3% of the patients subjected to staging laparotomy would benefit from the procedure. Nelson and coworkers reported no improvement in survival in a group of patients with stage IIB and stage III who had staging laporatomy in comparison with a similar group treated without exploration (see Table 25-10).[154]

To avoid complications that may result from the laparotomy and radiation therapy, Berman and coworkers performed an extraperitoneal bilateral pelvic and aortic lymphadenectomy.[156] Buchsbaum performed a pretreatment laparotomy with biopsy of the para-aortic nodes in patients with stage IIB invasive carcinoma of the cervix.[157] He documented metastasis in 33% of cases.

RADIATION THERAPY TECHNIQUES

The use of radium therapy was first presented in the treatment of carcinoma of the cervix in 1913 at the Congress at Halle. The techniques described apply, with some individualization, to most patients with cervical carcinoma. Despite a slower regression after irradiation, reflecting the cellular kinetics and a slow growth, no difference in tumor control or survival has been observed in adenocarcinomas when compared with epidermoid carcinoma.[158-162] Because of the predilection for endocervical involvement in adenocarcinoma, a combination of irradiation and conservative hysterectomy has been advocated.[163,164]

At the present time, the two main modalities of irradiation are either external photon beam or brachytherapy.

External irradiation is used to treat the whole pelvis and the parametria including the common iliac lymph nodes, while the central disease (cervix, vagina, and medial parametria) are primarily irradiated with intracavitary sources. External pelvic irradiation is delivered prior to intracavitary insertions in patients with:

1. Bulky cervical lesions to improve the geometry of the intracavitary application
2. Exophytic easily-bleeding tumors
3. Tumors with necrosis or infection

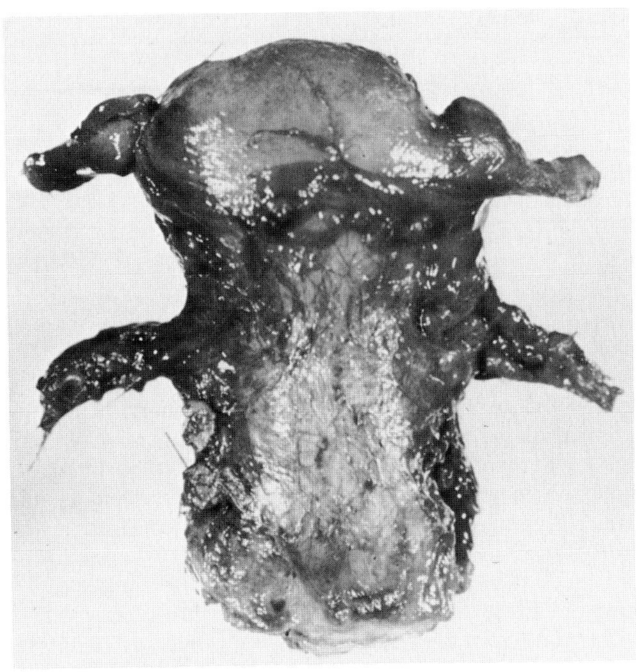

FIG. 25-6. Modified radical hysterectomy advocated for stage IA (microinvasive carcinoma) when an extrafascial hysterectomy is not considered adequate. The ureter is visualized, but not dissected free of the peritoneum except in the paracervical area. Parametrium medial to the ureter, in addition to the upper-third of the vagina, can be removed without injury to the ureter by this technique.

Portals

In the treatment of invasive carcinoma of the uterine cervix, it is important to deliver adequate doses of irradiation to the pelvic lymph nodes. For stages IB and IIA, 15 × 15 cm

FIG. 25-7. Radical abdominal hysterectomy indicated for selected patients with stage IB and IIA carcinoma of the cervix. This figure reveals the removal of parametrium surrounding the uterus and upper-third of the vagina. Parametrial lymph nodes are removed enbloc in the dissection. The remaining pelvic lymph nodes are dissected after the specimen has been removed.

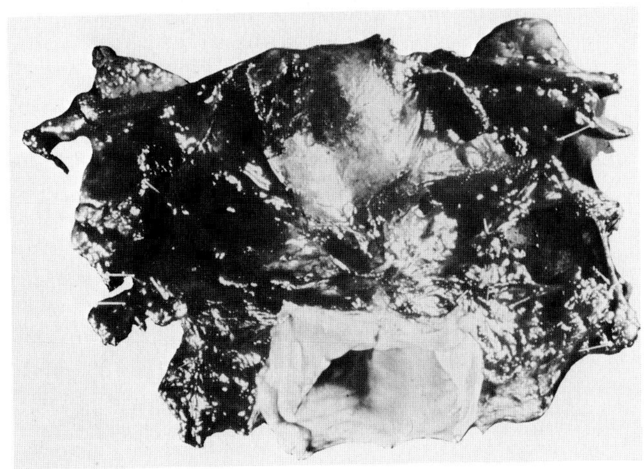

TABLE 25-10. Carcinoma of the Uterine Cervix: Survival after Staging Laparotomy

	EXPLORED		NOT EXPLORED	
STAGE	NO. PATIENTS	PERCENT SURVIVING	NO. PATIENTS	PERCENT SURVIVING
IIB	31	64.5	14	92.8
IIIA–IIIB	28	57.1	10	60

Nelson JH, Macasaet MA, Lu T et al: Am J Obstet Gynecol 118:753, 1974

portals are sufficient. For patients with stages IIB, III, and IVA, somewhat larger portals, 18 × 15 cm, are required to cover all of the common iliac nodes in addition to the cephalad half of the vagina (see Fig. 25-8). A 2 cm margin lateral to the bony pelvis is adequate. If there is no vaginal extension, the lower margin of the port is at the inferior border of the obturator foramen. When there is vaginal involvement, the entire length of this organ should be treated down to the introitus.

If metastatic periaortic lymph nodes are suspected or confirmed, the retroperitoneal tissues need to be irradiated either through a separate portal or with a field that includes both the periaortic nodes and the pelvic tissues (see Fig. 25-9).

Beam Energies

Because of the thickness of the pelvis, high-energy beams are specially suited for this treatment. They decrease the dose of radiation delivered to the peripheral normal tissues and provide a more homogeneous dose distribution in the central pelvis. Figure 25-10 shows the dose profile for anterior/posterior and posterior/anterior parallel ports using different x-ray beam energies. It is evident that with lower-energy beams, higher maximum doses must be given, and more complicated field arrangements used for achievement of the same midplane tumor dose. This, by necessity, delivers more irradiation to the bladder and the rectum, which may result in higher complication rate.

When Cobalt-60, 4 or 6 MV photons are employed, there is a need to use more complex portal arrangements (three fields or pelvic box technique) to minimize the dose to the bladder and the rectum while delivering an adequate dose to the cervix and the parametria (see Fig. 25-11).

FIG. 25-8. Simulation AP film of pelvis showing volume treated with external irradiation, which includes the uterus, upper vagina, parametria, and pelvic lymph nodes.

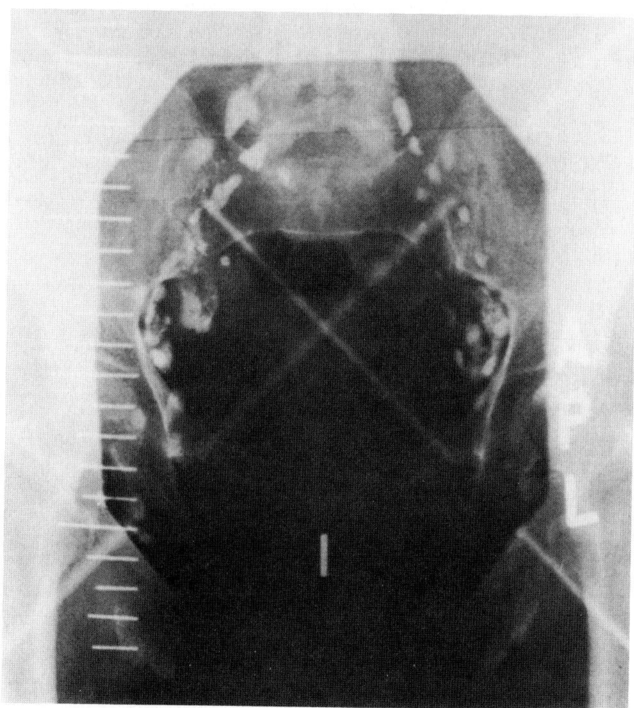

Doses of Irradiation

Optimal dose for invasive carcinoma of the cervix is delivered with a combination of whole pelvis, intracavitary, and, at times, interstitial therapy. Some institutions use lower doses of whole pelvis, external irradiation (1000 rad for stage IB and IIA, and 2000 rad for stage IIB, III, and IVA) in addition to parametrial doses to complete rad in stage IB and IIA and 6000 rad for more advanced stages. An assortment of step wedges designed in accordance with the isodose curves of the intracavitary applications are used to block the midline (see Fig. 25-12). This technique affords a high central dose to the cervix, paracervical tissues, and parametria as well as a moderate homogeneous dose to the external iliac lymph nodes without exceeding the bladder and rectal tolerance doses (see Fig. 25-13).

Other institutions prefer higher doses of whole pelvic external irradiation (usually 4000 rad) with additional parametrial dose to complete 5000 rad in patients with stages IB and IIA and 6000 rad for patients with IIB, III, or IVA tumors. This is usually combined with one or two intracavitary insertions for approximately 5000 to 6000 mgh.

When residual tumor is palpated at the completion of the prescribed course of therapy, an additional 1000 rad through a small 10 × 12 cm field to one parametrium or 12 × 12 cm to both parametria are used to deliver an additional 1000 rad. The midline block is left in place.

Brachytherapy can be delivered with intracavitary techniques using applicators consisting of an intrauterine tandem and vaginal colpostats or, when necessary, with vaginal cylinders. Also, interstitital implants with needles in limited tumor volumes are helpful in specific clinical situations (*i.e.*, localized residual tumor).

The intracavitary therapy, with its rapid dose fall-off as a function of distance, yields a high dose to the uterus and

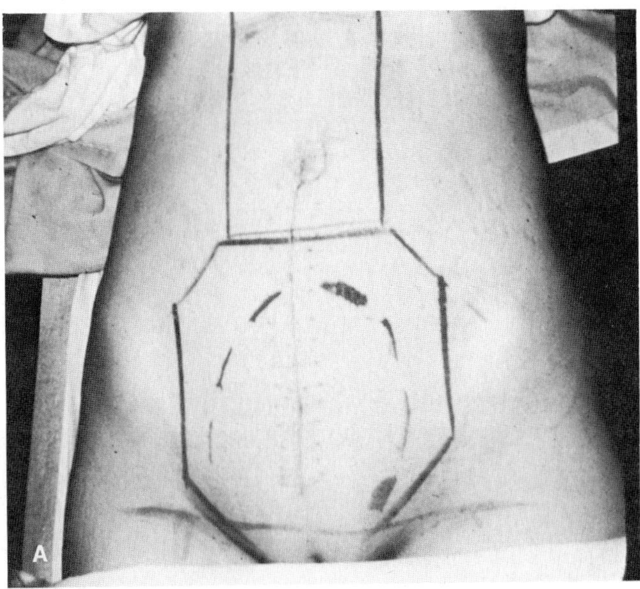

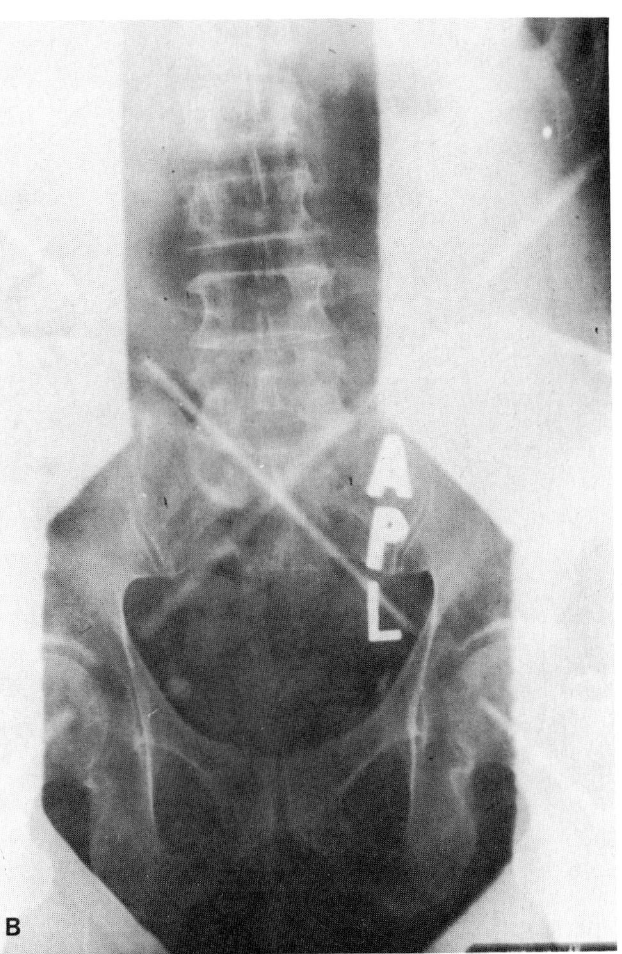

FIG. 25-9. *A*, Example of separate portals for external irradiation of pelvic and periaortic nodes. *B*, "Banjo" or extended fields used for pelvic and periaortic nodes for external irradiation.

paracervical tissues but it is inadequate to treat the pelvic lymph nodes (see Fig. 25-14).

There are several isotopes available, although at the present time ^{137}Cesium and ^{226}Radium are the most popular (see Table 25-11). There are a variety of applicators used for intracavitary therapy, the majority at the present time being after loading (see Fig. 25-15). This allows a better application since the operators are not concerned with radiation exposure; also, the technique can be exploited to achieve more optimal dose distribution with replacement or removal of sources in the tandem or the vaginal ovoids at different times. Radiographs of the application can be obtained using dummy sources, the active sources will only be inserted after the films have been reviewed and the position of the applicators is felt to be satisfactory.

In general, the first intracavitary insertion is scheduled after 1000–2000 rad of external irradiation if an adequate geometry exists in the pelvis. Otherwise, 2000–4000 rad are delivered prior to the first application to decrease the size of the lesion and improve the relationship of the applicators to the cervix and vagina. The second application is performed one or two weeks later after therapy.

Results of Treatment

Using these techniques, the results of therapy in stage IB and IIA are comparable with irradiation alone or combined

FIG. 25-10. Dose profile for parallel, opposing pelvic ports with different energies. Note that significantly greater maximum doses must be delivered with cobalt-60 and 4 MV roentgen rays as compared to higher energy roentgen ray beams to achieve similar midpelvis dose. (Perez CA, Purdy JA, Korba A et al: High-energy x-ray beams in the management of head and neck and pelvic cancers. In Kramer S, Suntharalingam N, Zinninger GF (eds): High-Energy Photons and Electrons p. 230. New York, John Wiley & Sons, 1976)

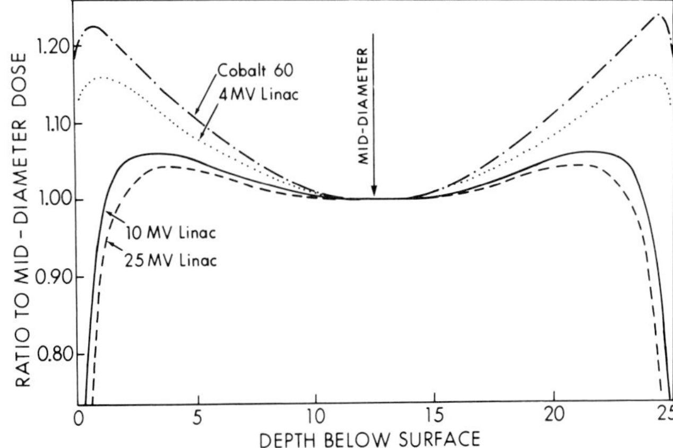

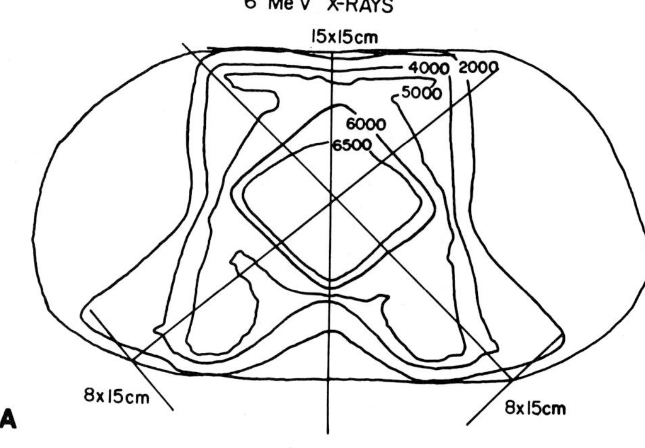

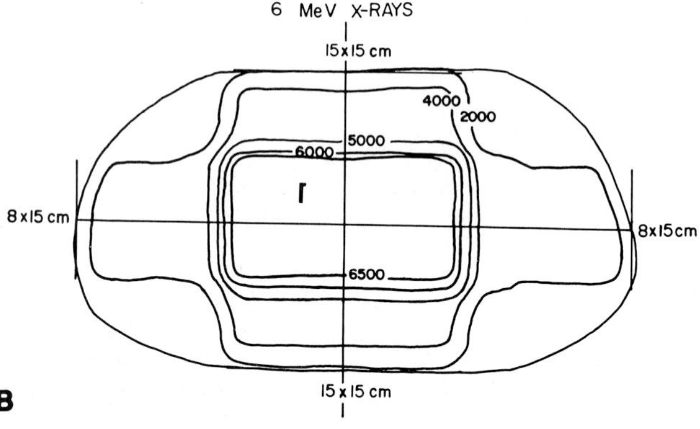

FIG. 25-11. *A*, Example of three-field arrangement (one anterior and two posterior oblique) for treatment of pelvic tumors with low energy photons. *B*, Example of "box technique" with anterior-posterior and lateral portals used for the treatment of pelvic tumors.

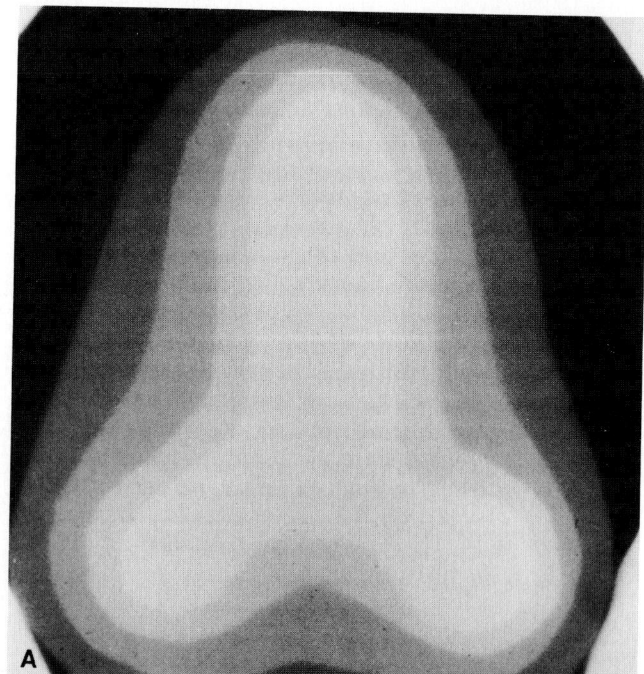

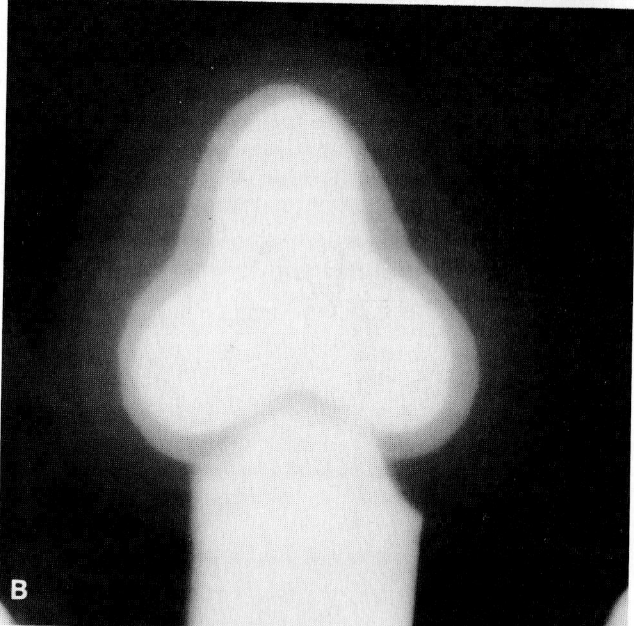

FIG. 25-12. Examples of step wedges used to shield midline structures during external beam irradiation of the pelvis. Wedges are designed according to dose distribution of intracavitary insertion (*A*). In *B*, a block has been added below the wedge to protect the distal rectum.

with a radical hysterectomy (see Fig. 25-16). The usual 5-year survival rate for stage IB is 85–92% and for stage IIA about 75%. In stage 11B, the 5-year survival is 60–65%, and practically all patients are treated with irradiation alone. Occasionally, a hysterectomy is performed. Prior to 1965, a pelvic lymphadenectomy was carried out in some patients but this procedure did not improve the survival over irradiation alone. In stage IIIB, the 5-year survival rates range from 25–40%. This may be related to the socio-economic status of the patients, extent of the disease, techniques of irradiation, and dose delivered to the parametrium (see Fig. 25-17).

Allt and coworkers, and in an update of the same randomized study, Johns reported better pelvic tumor control and survival and less complications in a group of 65 patients with stage IIB and III cervical carcinoma treated with 23 MV photons

TABLE 25-11. Isotopes Used in Intracavitary Therapy of Carcinoma of Cervix

ISOTOPE	HALF-LIFE (Yrs)	E (MeV)	HVL (mm Pb)	K FACTOR (R/hr. at 1 cm)
Radium	1620	.8	8	8.25
Co^{60}	5.27	1.2	12	13.4
Cs^{137}	30	.66	6	3.3
Ir^{192}	.20	.400	2.6	5.5

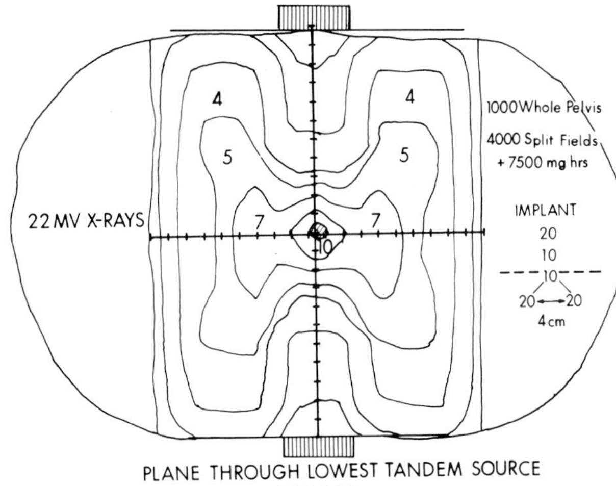

FIG. 25-13. Isodose distribution in the pelvis with combined external and intracavitary irradiation showing doses to be delivered to the cervix and parametria without exceeding irradiation of bladder and rectum.

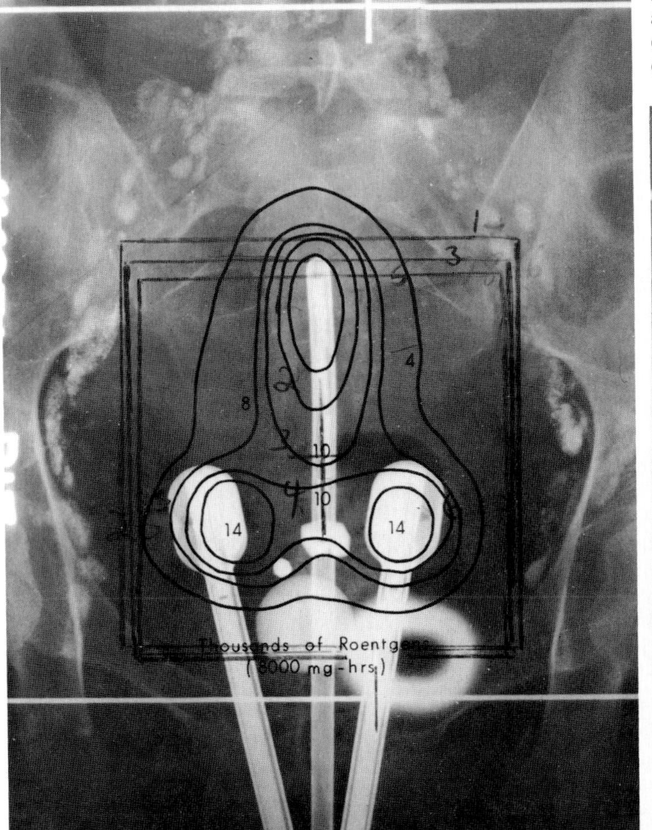

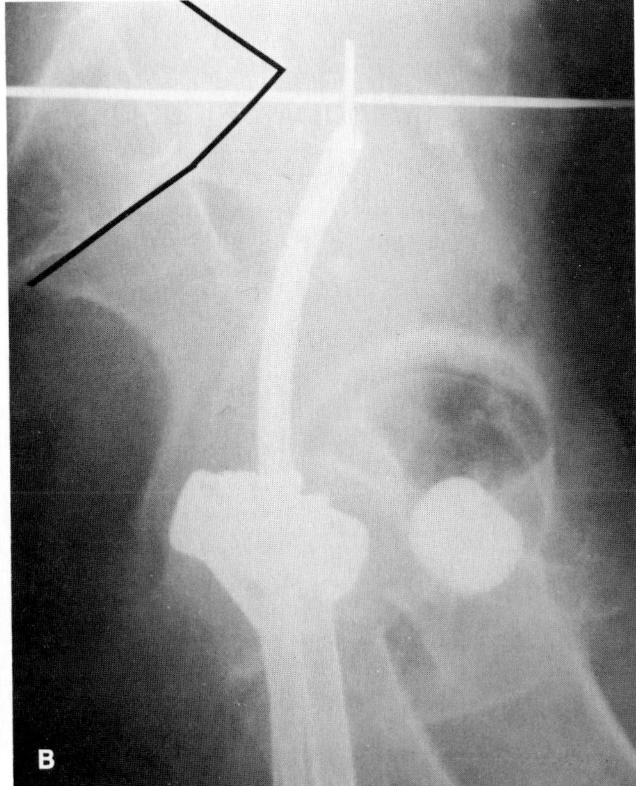

FIG. 25-14. AP (*A*) and lateral (*B*) radiographs of the pelvis showing an intracavitary application with intrauterine tandem and vaginal colpostats. Isodose dose curves on a coronal plane are superimposed on AP port.

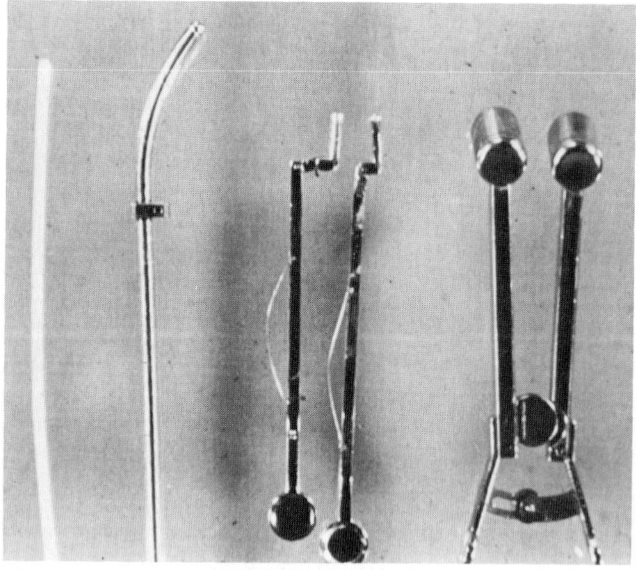

FIG. 25-15. Example of after-loading applicators used for intracavitary therapy (tandem and colpostats) with afterloading inserts.

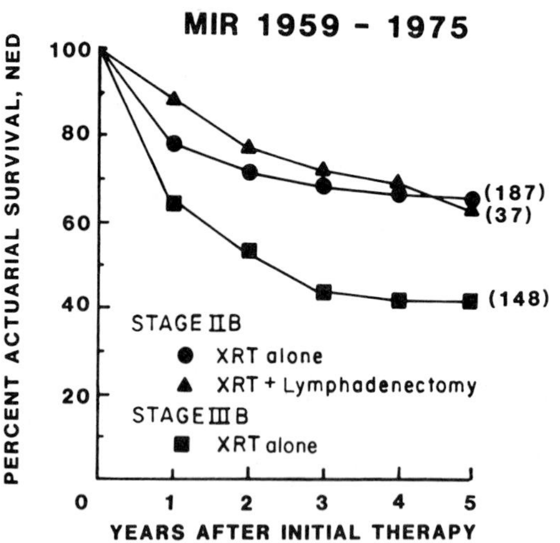

FIG. 25-17. Five-year survival rates for stage IIB and IIIB cancer of cervix patients treated with irradiation alone or a combination of irradiation and surgery.

FIG. 25-16. Comparison of 5-year survival rates for patients with stage IA, IB, and IIA cancer of cervix treated with irradiation alone or irradiation combined with a radical hysterectomy.

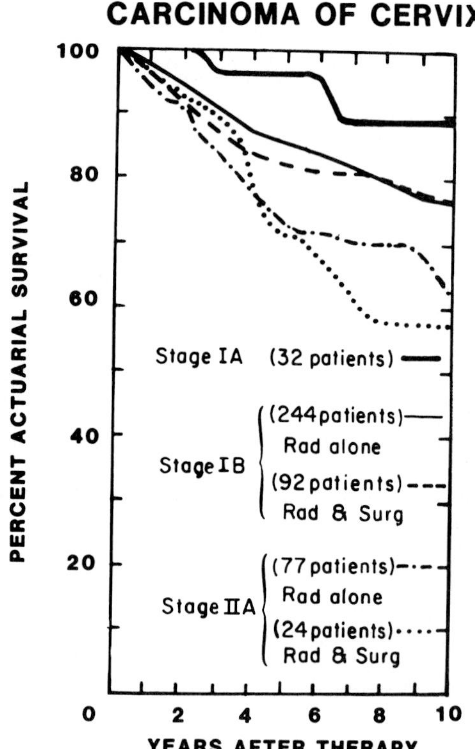

in comparison with 61 patients treated with Cobalt-60 external irradiation and intracavitary insertions (see Fig. 25-18).[165,166]

Patterns of Failure

The anatomic sites of failure in carcinoma of the uterine cervix after irradiation are closely correlated with tumor stage. Cervical or vaginal vault (central) recurrences should always be confirmed by biopsy. When possible, parametrial recurrences should be documented by needle biopsy. However, a clinical diagnosis can be made in the presence of a "triad"

FIG. 25-18. Survival curves for patients with stage III carcinoma of the uterine cervix on a randomized treatment study with either betatron or cobalt-60 external beams in addition to intracavitary insertions.* (Johns HE: Optimization of energy and equipment. In Kramer S, Suntharalingam N, Zinninger GF (eds): High-Energy Photons and Electrons p. 336. New York, John Wiley & Sons, 1976)

* Unpublished data.

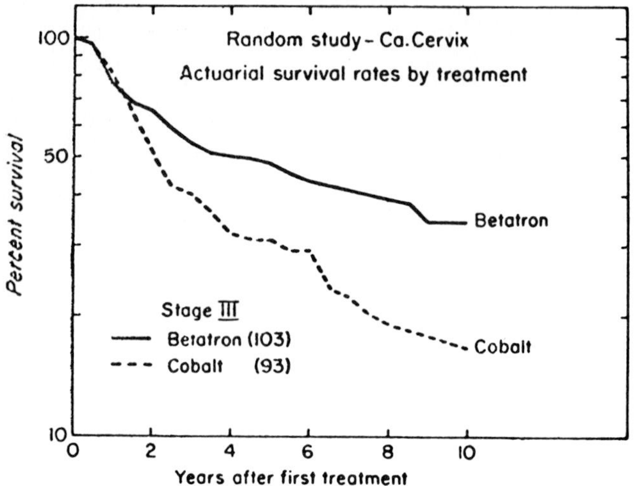

consisting of sciatic pain, leg edema, and hydronephosis. CT or lymphangiography is useful in outlining the tumor in the regional lymph nodes. Extrapelvic metastasis are documented by clinical examination, radiographic, or radionuclide studies and biopsy when indicated. Table 25-12 shows the incidence of pelvic recurrence or distant metastasis in 841 patients treated with definitive radiotherapy at Washington University. Jampolis and coworkers, analyzing the postirradiation recurrences in 916 patients with squamous cell carcinoma of the intact uterus treated at M.D. Anderson, reported similar figures.[167] These authors pointed out that central recurrences were extremely rare in stage IB and IIA (2%) and that in most instances they could be attributed to improper placement of the vaginal colpostats, which could produce low doses of irradiation in the cervix. Parametrial recurrences in stage I, IIA, and IIB were correlated with lateral deviation of the radium system without compensation from the external irradiation in about 75% of the patients. The overwhelming cause of failure in patients with stage IIIB was massive parametrial infiltration that could not be controlled with doses of 7000 rad.

Periaortic lymph node metastases are frequently combined with distant dissemination, but are clinically apparent only in 10–20% of the patients that recur.

It is important to stress the high incidence of distant metastasis in patients with stage III and IV carcinoma of the cervix, which makes imperative the development of adequate adjuvant therapy to improve the prognosis of these patients in the near future. The most common metastatic sites are the lungs, mediastinal lymph nodes, liver, and bones.

Radiation therapy can salvage about 50% of the patients with localized pelvic recurrences after surgery alone.[168,169]

COMBINATION OF IRRADIATION AND SURGERY

At some institutions, preoperative irradiation combined with a radical hysterectomy has been used in the treatment of patients with stages IB and IIA.[128,170–172] Sometimes an intracavitary insertion alone is used (5000–6000 mgh). When metastatic pelvic lymph nodes are found, postoperative irradiation is delivered. If only intracavitary therapy is given preoperatively, 2000 rad to the whole pelvis and 3000 rad to the parametria are administered shielding the midline. If some external therapy is delivered preoperatively, an additional parametrial dose to complete 5500–6000 rad should be given. Others have used a combination of external irradiation (2000–4000 rad to the pelvis) with an intracavitary insertion for 5000 mgh.

The results of several series are comparable to those obtained with irradiation alone. Einhorn and coworkers, in a non-randomized study, reported better survival in 49 patients with stage IB (100% at 5 years) in comparison with 64 patients treated with irradiation alone (81% at 5 years).[173] No difference was observed in 25 patients with stage IIA treated with combined therapy and 40 treated with irradiation alone (about 75% 5-year survival). Patients with metastatic lymph nodes have survival rates that are approximately 50% of those with negative nodes.[174,175]

The rationale for the use of an operation has been the alleged inability of irradiation to completely eradicate the metastatic tumor in the pelvic lymph nodes and the belief of some gynecologists that a more functional vagina in sexually active patients will be left after the surgical procedure.[170,176,177,178]

The dose of irradiation delivered to the lymph nodes, the time of the operation, and the pathologic examination of the specimens are critical in determining the presence of postirradiation residual tumor (see Table 25-13).

Rampone and coworkers reported a 15% incidence of metastatic lymph nodes in a group of 537 patients with stage IB treated with two preoperative intracavitary insertions (total of 6000 mgh), which delivered 1500 rad to the pelvic lymph nodes.[172] All patients with positive nodes in the operative specimen were given postoperative external radiation to the pelvis. The 5-year survival was 92.9% for 456 patients with negative nodes in contrast to 52% in 81 patients with positive nodes.

Rutledge reported only 3.3% metastatic lymph nodes in 30

TABLE 25-12. Carcinoma of Uterine Cervix (MIR: 1959–1975) Treatment with Irradiation Alone

			RECURRENT TUMOR			
STAGE	NUMBER OF CASES	5 YEAR ACTUARIAL SURVIVAL NED*	*Pelvic*	*Pelvic + DM*†	*Total Pelvic Failures*	*DM Only*
IB	281	88%	6 (2.5%)	14 (5.7%)	20 (8.2%)	17 (7%)
IIA	88	74%	1 (1.3%)	6 (7.8%)	7 (9.1%)	10 (13%)
IIB	256	64.8%	16 (10%)	13 (8.1%)	29 (18.1%)	14 (8.7%)
IIIB	201	42%	23 (16.8%)	41 (30%)	64 (46.7%)	25 (18.2%)
IVA	15	7%	—	6 (54.5%)	6 (54.5%)	—

* NED = no clinical evidence of disease.
† DM = distant metastases.

TABLE 25-13. Carcinoma of the Uterine Cervix—Stage IB and IIA: Percent Metastatic Pelvic Lymph Nodes and Dose of Irradiation Delivered to Lymph Nodes

AUTHOR	STAGE IB		STAGE IIA		ESTIMATED DOSE (rads) TO NODES
	Surgery alone	*Preop XRT*	*Surgery alone*	*Preop XRT*	
Christensen *et al*	29/167 (17.4%)	—	27/104 (26%)	—	0
Morley *et al*	18/143 (12.6%)	—	—	—	0
Morton *et al*	9/38 (23.7%)	4/32 (12.5%)	—	—	1800
Sweeney and Douglas	—	5/39 (13%)	—	9/54 (17%)	3500
Rampone *et al*	—	81/537 (15%)	—	—	2000
Decker *et al*	—	5/38 (13.2%)	—	11/45 (24.4%)	4000
Quigley *et al*	—	13/136 (9.6%)	—	—	1800
Parker *et al*	15/95 (16%)	6/73 (8%)	7/16 (44%)	20/71 (28%)	Not stated
Gray *et al*	5/44 (11.4%)	3/58 (5.2%)	6/17 (35.3%)	Incl. with I	4500
Perez *et al*	—	2/43 (4.6%)	—	2/24 (8.3%)	3000–4000
Perez *et al*	—	0/32 (0%)	—	—	4001–5000
Rutledge *et al*	—	1/30 (3.3%)	—	4/39 (10.3%)	5000

Perez CA, Breaux S, Askin F et al: Cancer 43:1062, 1979

patients with stage I and 10.3% in 39 patients with stage IIA carcinoma of the uterine cervix who underwent a bilateral pelvic lymphadenectomy six weeks after completion of definitive radiation therapy.[179] The dose of irradiation to the lymph nodes was in the range of 5000 rad delivered with megavoltage external photon beam and two intracavitary radium insertions. The survival rate in the patients that were treated with irradiation alone or combined with lymphadenectomy was the same (see Fig. 25-19). Complications were somewhat higher in the patients treated with the combination of the two modalities.

In patients with large endocervical lesions (barrel-shaped) or with endometrial extension of cervical carcinoma, Durrance and coworkers and Nelson and coworkers recommended an extrafascial conservative hysterectomy 6 weeks following completion of high dose preoperative radiation (2000 rad to the whole pelvis, 3000 rad split fields and one intracavity insertion of 6000 mgh).[123,180]

Perez and coworkers reported that in patients with primary carcinoma of the uterine cervix who have endometrial stromal invasion or tumor only in the curettings, the addition of a hysterectomy did not improve the survival since most of the patients failed because of distant dissemination.[38]

Van Nagell and coworkers evaluated the recurrence in carcinoma of the cervix after radical hysterectomy or irradiation.[138] They found that the recurrence rate was 5% for tumors less than 2 cm in diameter. It was essentially the same for patients treated with radiation. In lesions 2–5 cm in diameter, the failure rate was 24% for surgery, but only 11% for radiation. The authors recommend radical surgery for patients with tumors of 2 cm or less. Piver and Chung reported an 89% five-year survival rate for Stage IB lesions up to 3 cm in diameter, and only a 66% survival for tumors 4 to 5 cm in diameter in a large series of women treated by radical hysterectomy.[181] They also correlated the incidence of pelvic nodes with the size of the tumor and found in 18% incidence of pelvic nodes in tumors up to 1 cm; 22% with 2–3 cm lesions; and 35% with tumors of 4–5 cm.

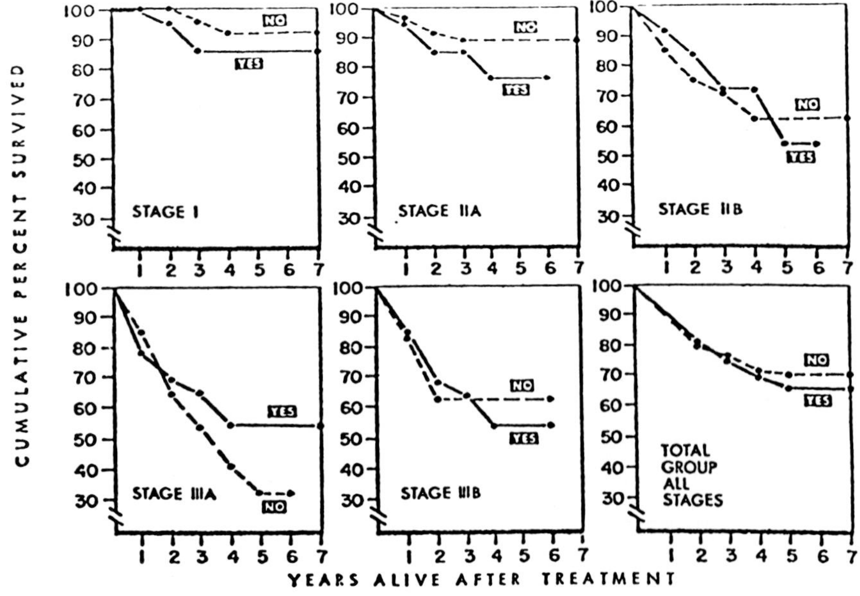

FIG. 25-19. Survival curves of patients treated for squamous cell carcinoma of the cervix, stage I, IIA, IIB, IIIA, and IIIB and all stages combined. Patients who had lymphadenectomy after definitive irradiation to their treatment are represented by *solid line curves*. The *broken line curves* are for patients who had radiation treatment only. Rutledge FN, et al: Am J Roentgenol Radium Ther Nucl Med 93:607, 1965)

Complications

Major complications of radiation therapy for stages I and IIA carcinoma of the cervix range from 3–5% and for stage IIB and III, between 10 and 15%. The most frequent major complications for the various stages are listed in Tables 25-14 and 25-15. Madoc-Jones and coworkers and Kottmeier and others have demonstrated a greater incidence of complications with higher doses of irradiation (see Fig. 25-20).[182,183] Higher doses of external irradiation to the whole pelvis have also been associated with greater number of complications.[184] Injury to the gastrointestinal tract usually appears within the first 2 years after radiotherapy, whereas complications of the urinary tract are seen more frequently 3–4 years after treatment. When preoperative radiation is combined with surgery, the complication rate tends to be somewhat higher (5–10%), particularly because of injury to the ureter or the bladder (ureteral stricture of uretero- or vesico-vaginal fistula).

The dose and techniques of irradiation and the type of surgical procedures performed are important in determining the morbidity of combined therapy. Nelson and coworkers reported an incidence of severe complications of 17.5% in a group of 80 patients treated with radiation and radical hysterectomy in contrast to 7.4% major complications in a group of 95 patients treated with high-dose preoperative radiation and a conservative extrafascial hysterectomy.

The pre-therapy staging laparotomy is frought with a significant number of complications, particularly if irradiation is given (over 5000–5500 rad) when metastatic periaortic lymph nodes are found. The usual operative complications may be noted, such as pneumonia, thrombophlebitis, cardiovascular accident, hepatitis, or evisceration. Late complications include those of combined surgery and irradiation in the abdomen and pelvis, such as small bowel obstruction, stricture and fibrosis of the intestine or rectosigmoid, recto- or vesico-vaginal fistula, and so forth. The incidence of complications has been listed between 5% and 20%, depending on the extent of the periaortic lymph node dissection, the transperitoneal or retroperitoneal approach for the operation, and the dose of irradiation given.[89,90,185]

With improving anesthesia, surgical techniques, and antibiotic therapy the mortality for radical hysterectomy with pelvic lymphadenectomy has decreased to 1% or less.[99] Other complications include ureterovaginal fistula, the incidence of which has decreased to less than 3%.

CHEMOTHERAPY

Chemotherapy has not been extensively evaluated in cervical cancer, primarily because of effective initial therapy with other modalities and because cytotoxic agents used in patients with recurrent cervical carcinoma have shown less than optimal efficacy.[186] Other factors that complicate the effective use of chemotherapy in cervical carcinoma include decreased pelvic vascular perfusion, limited bone marrow reserve, and, at times, poor renal function related to ureteral obstruction from tumor or fibrosis.

TABLE 25-14. Carcinoma of the Cervix Major Complications

			IIB		III	
	I	IIA	*Before 1963*	*After 1964*	*Before 1963*	*After 1964*
No. of cases	86	28	36	37	37	27
No. of complications	5	2	10	4	11	3
Percent	5.8%	7%	27%	11%	29%	11%
Type:						
GI						
Rectovaginal fistula	1*	—	2	1	4	1
Rectouterine fistula	—	—	1	—	—	—
Sigmoid perforation/ stricture	—	1	—	1†	—	—
Rectal ulcer/proctitis	1	1	3	1	3	1
Intestinal obstruction or perforation	2	—	—	—	3	1
G.U.						
Vesico-vaginal fistula	—	—	1‡	—	—	—
Ureteral obstruction	1	—	1	—	—	—
Severe cystitis	—	—	2	—	1	—
Other (not directly related to irradiation)						
Hepatic necrosis	—	—	—	1	—	—
Pulmonary embolism	—	—	1	—	—	—
Thrombophlebitis	1 (non-fatal)	—	—	—	—	—

* Also ureteral stricture (following post-irradiation hysterectomy for pelvic abscess).
† Also ureteral stricture and small bowel obstruction 2 mos. later.
‡ Concomitant rectovaginal fistula.
Madoc-Jones H, unpublished data, 1980

TABLE 25-15. Carcinoma of Uterine Cervix—Stage IB and IIA (MIR—1958–1974): Major Complications of Treatment

	RADIATION ALONE (321 PATIENTS)		RADIATION AND SURGERY (116 PATIENTS)	
Gastrointestinal				
Rectovaginal fistula	2	(1.9%)	3	(5.2%)
Sigmoid perforation	1		—	
Small bowel obstruction	2*		3	
Small bowel perforation	1		—	
Proctitis or sigmoiditis	5 [2*]		1	
Rectal or sigmoid stricture	4		1	
Diverticulitis	1		—	
TOTAL	16 (5%)		8 (6.9%)	
Genitourinary				
Vesico-vaginal fistula	2		2	
Hemorrhagic cystitis*	1		1	
Bladder ulcer*	2		1	
Ureteral stricture	7†		3	
Uretero-vaginal fistula	—		1	
TOTAL	12 (3.7%)		8 (6.9%)	
Other				
Postop shock (tubular necrosis)			1 (.9%)	

* Patients treated with parametrial colloidal gold.

† Five of these patients received single intracavitary insertion for 5400, 5600, 6590, 6600, and 7265 mg/hour, in addition to 2000 rads whole pelvis + 2000 rads to parametria.

Perez CA, Breaux S, Askin F et al: Cancer 43:1062, 1979

Nevertheless, chemotherapy may eventually play an important role in the management of several groups of patients including those with advanced (stage III and IV) disease, disease recurrent after surgery and radiation therapy, and pelvic or para-aortic nodal metastasis with a low potential for cure with current local treatment modalities. In addition, chemotherapy may play a role as a radiosensitizer enhancing conventional irradiation. Finally, the location of cervical carcinoma and regional extension in the pelvis makes the use of chemotherapy by intra-arterial infusion conceptually attractive.

TABLE 25-16. Single Agent Chemotherapy in Cervical Carcinoma

DRUGS	RESPONDING/ TOTAL PATIENTS/ STUDIED	% OVERALL RESPONSE
Alkylating Agents		
Cyclophosphamide	31/228	14
Chlorambucil	11/44	25
Antimetabolites		
5-Fluorouracil	68/348	20
Methotrexate	12/77	16
Mitotic Inhibitors		
Vincristine	10/44	23
Antitumor Antibiotics		
Doxorubicin (Adriamycin)	8/78	10
Bleomycin	17/172	10
Other Agents		
Cis-Platinum	21/52	40
Hexamethylmelamine	11/49	22
CCNU or Methyl CCNU	5/120	4

American Cancer Society: 1980 Facts and Figures. New York, American Cancer Society, 1979

Single Agent Chemotherapy

Table 25-16 lists the single agents that appear to have some activity in cervical carcinoma.[187] These data can only be used to suggest activity because, for the most part, they represent collected information from the literature in which variable criteria for response were used. Significant activity in well-designed studies with adequate patient numbers has been documented only for 5-fluorouracil and cis-platinum.[188,189]

Combination Chemotherapy in Cervical Carcinoma

Since there are several classes of cytotoxic agents with different mechanisms of action that have activity in carcinoma of the cervix, a number of combinations have been used. None of the earlier combinations were more effective than single agents. Recently, several studies show 10–29% objective complete remission rates, suggesting some enhancement of effect. Table 25-17 lists those combination chemotherapy studies in which reasonable numbers of evaluable patients have been studied and the response rates appear to exceed those of single agents. However, the majority of the studies have not compared combination chemotherapy regimens to standard single agents and the toxicity of these combinations is substantial.

TABLE 25-17. Combination Chemotherapy in Cervical Carcinoma

REGIMEN	EVALUABLE PATIENTS	NUMBER OF RESPONSES (%)	COMPLETE RESPONSES (%)
Bleomycin and Methotrexate	20	12 (60%)	0 (0%)
Bleomycin, methotrexate, and phosphamide	70	22 (31%)	4 (6%)
Doxorubicin (Adriamycin) and Methotrexate	59	39 (66%)	13 (22%)
	24	7 (29%)	0 (0%)
Doxorubicin and Methyl CCNU	31	14 (45%)	9 (29%)
Doxorubicin and Cis-Platinum	19	6 (31%)	2 (10%)
Bleomycin and Mitomycin-C	15	14 (93%)	12 (80%)
Mitomycin-C, Vincristine, and Bleomycin	91	46 (51%)	14 (15%)

Intra-Arterial Chemotherapy

Intra-arterial infusions of chemotherapeutic agents in cervical carcinoma have been of considerable theoretical interest for some years based upon the distinct arterial supply to the tumor-bearing area. Unfortunately, the responses have been uncommon and of short duration. The toxicity and complication rates have also been significant. Morrow and coworkers and Swenerton and coworkers each studied 20 patients treated with this technique using bleomycin or a combination of bleomycin, mitomycin C-vincristine respectively.[190,191] Morrow and coworkers observed only two of 16 objective regressions; Swenerton and coworkers reported three of 20.[190,191] Toxicity in both studies was significant, including pulmonary fibrosis from bleomycin and infectious or embolic complications of arterial catheterization. Both investigators concluded that there is little benefit from continuous arterial infusions of chemotherapy in recurrent cervical carcinoma. Slightly more optimistic reports have been published by Japanese investigators when the arterial infusions precede initial radiation management.[192-194] However, randomized comparisons will be required to establish the benefits, if any, of intra-arterial chemotherapy infusions.

Chemotherapy as a Radiosensitizer

Several studies have been published that attempt to enhance the effect of radiation therapy using chemotherapy as a radiosensitizer. The two most provocative studies have used hydroxyurea, a drug with limited single agent activity on its own. Piver studied 130 patients with stages IIB–IIIB cervical carcinoma in a prospective double-blind randomized study in which patients received split-course radiation therapy with or without hydroxyurea.[195] In clinical stage IIB patients, a significant improvement in 2-year survival was achieved for the group receiving hydroxyurea (74%) in comparison with the control group treated with radiotherapy and a placebo (43.5%). In clinically staged IIIB patients, 52.1% of these receiving hydroxyurea were alive at two years compared to 33.3% of those receiving a placebo with radiation ($p = 0.22$).

Hreshchyshyn and coworkers reported a study of the Gynecologic Oncology Group comparing hydroxyurea or placebo combined with irradiation in stages IIIB and IV cervical cancer in 104 evaluable patients randomized to two treatment regimens.[196] The complete response rate was 68.1% for the hydroxyurea treated group and 48.8% for the placebo group ($p < 0.05$). Duration of progression-free intervals and survival were also significantly better in the patients receiving hydroxyurea. However, hematologic toxicity was more common and more severe in those patients receiving hydroxyurea. Results from both of these studies must be qualified because the patients were not all surgically staged and substantial numbers of randomized patients were inevaluable. Also, with more effective radiotherapy alone, Fletcher and coworkers and our own results (see table 25-12) demonstrate survival and tumor control similar to those observed with the addition of hydroxyurea in the two series described.[127] Nevertheless, the two studies do suggest a potential role for radiation sensitizers in cervical carcinoma. Other agents might be more effective. Benjamin and coworkers reported the effects of doxorubicin (adriamycin) and hydroxyurea on human squamous cell carcinoma of the cervix transplanted into nude mice.[197] Comparing the radiosensitizing effects of the two agents, they found doxorubicin superior to hydroxyurea.

HYPERBARIC OXYGEN, HYPOXIC SENSITIZER, AND HYPERTHERMIA COMBINED WITH IRRADIATION

Several reports have been published on clinical trials evaluating the efficacy of hyperbaric oxygen (HPO) combined with irradiation in the treatment of a variety of human tumors, one of them carcinoma of the uterine cervix.[198] Watson and coworkers, in a randomized clinical trial involving 320 patients (stages III and IVA) treated at four institutions, reported a 5-year survival of 33% in the oxygen-treated group in contrast to 27% in the control patient group treated in air ($P = .08$).[199] The greatest improvement in survival was observed in women below the age of 55, in which the 5-year survival for those treated with oxygen was 50% in contrast to 30% for the control group treated in air. The local recurrence rate was 33% in the 161 patients treated with oxygen and 53% in 159 patients treated in air. The difference is statistically significant ($P < 0.001$). The morbidity in the patients treated with oxygen was greater (20 severe and 13 moderate) than in those treated

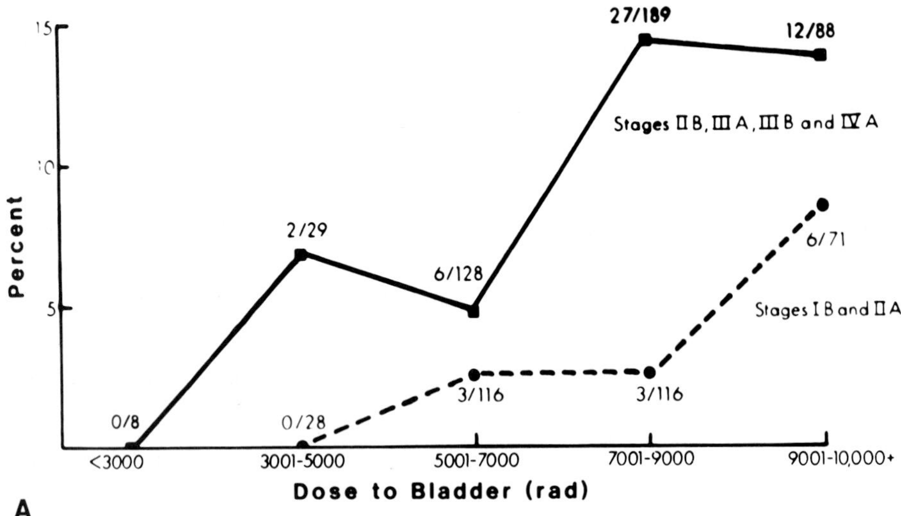

FIG. 25-20. *A*, Incidence of grade II and III genitourinary complications in 850 patients treated with irradiation alone for various stages of carcinoma of the uterine cervix.* *B*, Incidence of grade II and III intestinal complications in 850 patients with various stages of carcinoma of the uterine cervix treated with irradiation alone.

* (Madoc-Jones H: Unpublished data)

in air (six severe and eight moderate). The difference was particularly striking in the bowel (13 vs. two severe complications respectively).

On the other hand, an extensive trial of carcinoma of the cervix reported by Fletcher and coworkers in 233 patients with stage IIB, III, and IV randomized to be treated with conventional irradiation in air or with hyperbaric oxygen demonstrated no significant benefit in survival or tumor control (20 of 109 patients treated with oxygen failing in the pelvis in contrast to 29 of 124 treated in air).[200] Further, the morbidity was greater (26 complications) in patients treated with hyperbaric oxygen compared with the control group (15 complications). A smaller series reported by Glassburn and coworkers showed no benefit in survival but increased morbidity with hyperbaric oxygen.[201] It is evident that no definite conclusions can be drawn concerning the use of hyperbaric oxygen in carcinoma of the cervix but it seems to increase the effect of irradiation both in tumor and normal tissues. It is possible that hyperbaric oxygen administered with fewer high dose fractions may be more efficacious than when combined with conventional dose and fractionation schemes.[202] An important point to be explored is whether higher doses of irradiation may be as effective as HPO in achieving local tumor control without increasing the incidence of major complications.

The trials reported have not shown an increased incidence of distant metastasis, which has been reported in a clinical study and in some animal experiments.[203]

Thomas and coworkers described a Phase I study of metronidazole carried out on 80 patients with various stages of carcinoma of the uterine cervix.[204] The authors suggested that a daily dose of 1.3 gm/m^2 was well tolerated but no tumor response data were reported; Phase III clinical trials were recommended.

Dische reported preliminary observations on the use of misonidazole in the treatment of advanced carcinoma of the cervix in ten patients.[205] The morbidity of this therapy is comparable to that observed with irradiation alone, except for some misonidazole neurotoxicity. All ten patients had over 50% tumor regression, results felt to be very promising. At the present time, randomized studies by the Radiation Therapy Oncology Group are in progress to evaluate the sensitizing effects of misonidazole in stage III and IVA carcinoma of the cervix (daily dose of 400 mg/m^2 for a total of 12 gm/m^2) treated with conventional fractionation.

Because of technological limitations to deliver adequate heat to large parts of the body such as the pelvis, the evaluation of hyperthermia in the treatment of carcinoma of the uterine cervix has been sparse. Hornback and coworkers recently reported on a non-randomized study stating that the combination of microwave hyperthermia and irradiation (433 MHz) resulted in improved pelvic tumor control and survival in a group of 79 patients in comparison with previously irradiated controls.[206]

CARCINOMA OF THE CERVIX AND PREGNANCY

The concurrent presence of carcinoma *in situ* or invasive carcinoma of the uterine cervix and pregnancy poses a therapeutic dilemma to the gynecologist and radiation oncologist. Because of the epithelial changes associated with pregnancy sometimes the diagnosis of intraepithelial carcinomas may be difficult. However, Green and Peckham stressed the validity of the diagnosis of preinvasive carcinoma and the need to treat these patients adequately.[207]

Boutselis reported 134 intraepithelial tumors (.14%) and 71 invasive carcinoma of the cervix (.07%) in 95,000 deliveries.[208] If the pregnancy is to be allowed to full-term, confirmation of the diagnosis by colposcopy and conservative management of carcinoma *in situ* with monthly Pap smears constitutes the best management.[209] Conization has frequently been performed; however, Boutselis reported a 20% incidence of complications, the most frequent being abnormal bleeding.[208,210] Mikuta and coworkers reported four abortions in 20 patients on whom conization was performed and in four others premature deliveries were induced.[211]

Punch biopsies can also be obtained, but the diagnostic accuracy is less reliable. As many as 50% of the patients have residual carcinoma *in situ* after delivery.

Most authors recommend vaginal delivery of a full-term pregnancy and definitive therapy, usually consisting of an abdominal hysterectomy performed after the immediate postpartum period.[207,208,211]

In patients with invasive carcinoma, the lesion is usually clinically apparent. Multiple punch biopsies are adequate to confirm the diagnosis.

Since there is a greater need to institute therapy as soon as possible, the accepted method of treatment in patients in the first 6 months of pregnancy is to carry out definitive surgery or radiotherapy as indicated by the stage of the disease.[212,213] In the third trimester of pregnancy when the fetus may be salvaged, a C-section is preferred followed by definitive treatment. However, several authors report that vaginal delivery does not affect the prognosis deleteriously. Creasman reported on 113 patients, 48 treated by irradiation, 45 by irradiation followed by surgery, and five with a radical hysterectomy alone.[214] The survival was comparable to the non-pregnant patients for similar stages. The survival for patients with stage I was comparable whether the patients were allowed to deliver vaginally or a C-section was performed (about 85% in stage I and 50–64% in stage II). Also, the percentage of infants surviving (over 80%) was the same in both groups.

If it is decided to terminate the pregnancy, the patient is initially treated with external irradiation to the whole pelvis (4000 rad in 4 weeks). Usually an abortion will occur and there will be some involution of the uterus. After this dose of irradiation, an evacuation of the uterus and an intracavitary insertion can be performed under general anesthesia.

If surgery is to be performed, approximately 5000 mgh are given. If not, two intracavitary insertions for a total of 8000 mgh and an additional 1000 or 2000 rad to the parametria with a midline block are delivered.

The usual surgical procedure is a radical hysterectomy with lymphadenectomy except for microinvasive carcinoma in which the lymphadenectomy is not performed.

Kinch, Symmonds, Creasman, and others have reported similar 5-year survival in the pregnant and non-pregnant patients, the stage of the disease at the time of diagnosis being the only determining prognostic factor (see Fig. 25-21).[214–216]

If a radical hysterectomy is performed and positive pelvic lymph nodes are found, the usual postoperative radiation including external beam and intracavitary insertion should be carried out.

The survival is the same regardless of the trimester of the pregnancy in which definitive treatment is instituted.[214,216]

The practice popularized 30 years ago of administering "restraining dose of radium" and deferring definitive radiotherapy until delivery is carried out should be strongly discouraged. Strauss reported two of 11 babies being born with microcephalia in addition to other complications such as alopecia, facial deformity, eye damage, and chromosomal abnormalities.[217]

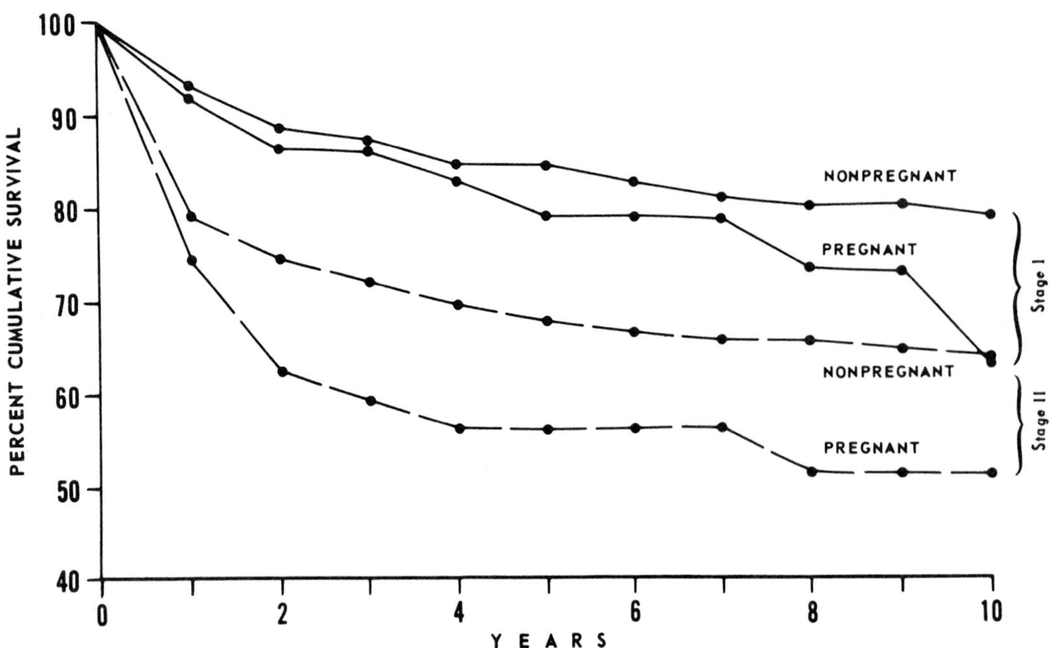

FIG. 25-21. Actuarial survival rates for pregnant and nonpregnant women with carcinoma of the cervix. (Creasman WT, Rutledge FN, Fletcher GH et al: Obstet Gynecol 36:495, 501, 1970)

CARCINOMA OF THE CERVICAL STUMP

Subtotal hysterectomy, a relatively popular procedure for benign conditions of the uterus in past years, is performed rarely today. These patients are, of course, at risk to develop carcinoma of the uterine cervix.

It is important to divide patients with carcinoma of the cervical stump into *true,* when the first symptom occurs three or more years after subtotal hysterectomy, or *coincidental,* when the symptoms are noticed before the third postoperative year.[218] Moss and coworkers recommend two elapsed years after hysterectomy as the time for the classification of these lesions. This distribution is important because the prognosis for carcinoma of the true stump is significantly better than for coincidental lesions, which probably means that carcinoma was present at the time the hysterectomy was performed.

The natural history and patterns of spread of carcinoma of the cervical stump are similar to those of the cervix in the intact uterus. The diagnostic work-up, clinical staging, and basic principles of therapy are the same.

When surgery is performed for stage I tumors, it is somewhat more difficult because of the previous surgical procedures and the presence of adhesions in the pelvis.

When irradiation is administered, the lack of a uterine cavity to insert a tandem containing three or more sources makes intracavitary therapy more difficult. Whenever possible, sources should be inserted in the remaining cervical canal. Occasionally, transvaginal irradiation may be used to boost the dose delivered to central disease in the stump. It is important to deliver more whole pelvis irradiation.

In general, patients with stage I are treated with a combination of 2000 rads to the whole pelvis and 3000 rads to the parametria with midline shielding combined with two intracavitary insertions. The dose of intracavitary therapy depends on the number of sources that can be placed in the cervical canal (1000–3000 mgh for one to three sources). The vaginal vault should receive about a 7000 rad mucosal dose (approximately 2500 mgh).

More advanced stages should be treated with 4000 rad whole pelvis and 2000 rad to the parametria with midline shielding, combined with the same intracavitary inserting doses.

If there is bulky disease present in the cervix, parametrium or vagina interstitial therapy with needles is advisable.

When there is no opportunity to insert any sources in the cervical canal, the whole pelvis dose must be increased to 6000 rad.

When intravaginal cones are used, a 3000–5000 rad air dose is delivered in 2–4 weeks, in 3–5 weekly fractions. Moss limits the dose to the vaginal vault for transvaginal irradiation to 3000 rad in 10 days.[219]

The 5-year survival for carcinoma of the cervical stump is similar to that reported for patients with carcinoma of the intact uterus.[218,220,221]

Creadick and coworkers reported their results on 83 patients, 25 of whom were treated with radical trachaelectomy and pelvic lymphadenectomy.[222] They report a salvage rate of 85.7% in squamous cell carcinoma and 50% in adenocarcinoma (patients with stage I and II disease).

The anatomic site of failure and the incidence of recurrences are similar to those seen in the intact uterus. Distant metastasis follow the same distribution as those in the intact uterus.

Because of the close proximity of the bladder, rectum, and small intestine to the intracavitary sources and due to the often higher doses of whole pelvic external beam irradiation given, complications are somewhat more frequent than in the carcinoma of the intact uterus. Wimbush and coworkers reported five fistula, six severe proctosidmoiditis, and 12 vault necrosis in 238 patients treated with definitive radiotherapy.

CARCINOMA OF THE CERVIX INADVERTENTLY TREATED WITH A SIMPLE HYSTERECTOMY

Occasionally, because of inadequate preoperative work-up, a simple or total abdominal hysterectomy is performed and invasive carcinoma of the cervix is incidentally found in the surgical specimen. It is critical that these patients receive radiation therapy immediately when their postoperative status allows it.

When carcinoma is detected following an abdominal or vaginal hysterectomy, the prognosis is worse if postoperative irradiation is not administered.

However, Durrance and coworkers and Andras and coworkers have reported survival rates similar to those of the intact uterus when these patients are treated appropriately.[223,224] If only microinvasive carcinoma is found and an extrafascial hysterectomy with wide cuff is performed, no additional therapy is necessary. If a less comprehensive dissection was carried out, an intracavitary insertion with vaginal colpostats should be performed to deliver a 6000 rad mucosal dose to the vault. The usual therapy in patients with microscopic residual disease or gross tumor that is incompletely removed consists of 2000 rad to the whole pelvis and 3000 rad to the parametria, combined with an intracavitary insertion to the vaginal vault for a 6000 rad mucosal dose. If there is residual tumor present in the vaginal vault, the whole pelvis dose should be increased to 4000 rad and the parametrial dose to an additional 2000 rad. An intracavitary insertion (as outlined above) should be carried out. If there is residual tumor, interstitial implants with needles should be carried out to increase the dose to this volume. Durrance and coworkers pointed out that patients with tumor at the margin of resection or gross residual tumor have a less favorable prognosis than those without residual tumor.

Green and Morris reported nine of 30 patients (30%) who survived five years after definitive radiotherapy for the treatment of invasive cervical carcinoma after inadvertent simple hysterectomy.[225] The same authors noted that 14 of 32 patients treated with resurgical procedure, usually a Wertheim hysterectomy, died within five years. Eight of nine patients with negative nodes survived and one died of postoperative complications. The same authors pointed out that the five year cure rate was 30% in the patients treated within one year after the hysterectomy, in contrast to 16% for those treated after one year. Thus, the time at which the patients are treated, in addition to the bulk of tumor, is an important prognostic factor.

CARCINOMA OF THE ENDOMETRIUM

This is the most common malignant tumor in the female genital tract, comprising about 13% of all malignant tumors in women.

EPIDEMIOLOGY

The prevalence of carcinoma of the endometrium has increased over the past 20 years, perhaps related to the fact that the life-span of women in the U.S. has increased and less carcinoma of the uterine cervix is diagnosed.[5]

Carcinoma of the endometrium has been observed more frequently in Jewish women than in other nationalities; it also may be associated with obesity, hypertension, and diabetes.[226]

Smith and coworkers have related the development of carcinoma of the endometrium to an abnormal estrogen balance such as is observed in patients with feminizing ovarian tumors, or with cortical stromal hyperplasia or in women that have received estrogen therapy for prolonged periods of time. Some recent reports strongly suggest that the prolonged administration of exogenous hormones may be correlated with a greater risk of developing carcinoma of the endometrium, although controversy still surrounds this subject.[227–229]

Most cases are diagnosed in the 60- and 70-year age group.[230]

CLINICAL MANIFESTATIONS

The most frequent complaint is unexpected postmenopausal vaginal bleeding or abnormal menometrorrhagia in premenopausal age. The patients may also complain of yellowish or serosanguineous vaginal discharge. Hypogastric or pelvic pain is occasionally reported, which could be due to the concomitant presence of myomata in the uterus.

Pyometria and hematometria may be present in patients with an enlarged uterus with blockage of the cervical canal.

Occasionally, lumbosacral pain may be noted in the presence of periaortic lymph node metastasis.

NATURAL HISTORY

The appearance of endometrial carcinoma may be preceded by adenomatous hyperplasia in some patients.[231] It is not exactly known what etiological factors induce the malignant changes. However, the tumor may start in one of several locations in the endometrial cavity, usually in the fundus, and may spread to involve the endometrium extensively. Depending on the degree of differentiation of the tumor, there is a greater propensity of the carcinoma to infiltrate the myometrium, starting at the surface and extending all the way through the serosa. Whereas, myometrial extension is rare in well-differentiated tumors (less than 5%), it is seen in approximately one-third of the patients with poorly differentiated lesions (see Table 25-18). The presence of myometrial invasion has a direct effect on the frequency of pelvic lymph node metastasis and has a negative impact on survival.[233]

The tumor may involve the lower uterine segment and extend into the endocervical canal (5–10% of patients). The involvement of the cervix may be microscopic or there may be gross infiltration and ulceration of the exocervix.[234,235]

Particularly in patients with myometrial infiltration the carcinoma may extend into the broad ligament and invade the parametrium.[236] Also, metastasis or extension to the tubes

TABLE 25-18. Relationship of Pelvic Node Metastasis to Myometrial Penetration and Histologic Grade

DEPTH OF INVASION	HISTOLOGIC GRADE 1 No.	(%)	2 No.	(%)	3 No.	(%)	TOTAL No.	(%)
≤ 1/3	1/60	(1.6)	4/42	(9)	4/14	(28)	9/116	(7.8)
≥ 1/3	1/5	(20.0)	2/8	(25)	4/11	(36)	7/24	(29.0)
TOTAL	2/65	(3.0)	6/50	(12)	8/25	(32)	16/140	(11.4)

Morrow CP: Int J Radiat Oncol Biol Phys 6:365, 1980

or ovaries has been reported in 5–10% of patients, correlated with the grade of tumor differentiation.[237]

Metastatic dissemination to the pelvic and periaortic nodes has been correlated with the stage of the disease, the degree of differentiation of the tumor, and myometrial invasion. Fig. 25-22 illustrates the percentage of positive nodes reported in a group of patients treated with definitive surgery.

Extension to the vagina is rare (seen in less than 5% of the patients) but when it occurs, it is more frequently noted in the suburethral region. The incidence of vaginal cuff recurrence has been reported to be 5–10% without preoperative radiation, but can be reduced to 1–3% with adjuvant radiotherapy. The incidence of vaginal metastasis is dependent on the stage and degree of tumor differentiation.[238–240]

Metastases in the peritoneal cavity and omentum are occasionally seen; spread through the fallopian tube has been postulated.[241,242] Inguinal lymph node metastases are rarely seen in patients that have extensive parametrial involvement or distal vaginal involvement.

Malignant tumors of the uterus, particularly of mesenchymal origin, have a tendency to spread through the bloodstream, causing metastases to the lungs, liver, bones, brain, and so forth.

Hormonal receptors to progesterone and estrogens have been identified in the endometrium and about 40% of the tumors are hormone responsive.[243–247]

FIG. 25-22. Reported incidence of pelvic node metastasis and intermediate and deep myometrial invasion by histologic grade in endometrial cancer. (Boronow RC: Obstet Gynecol 47:630, 1976)

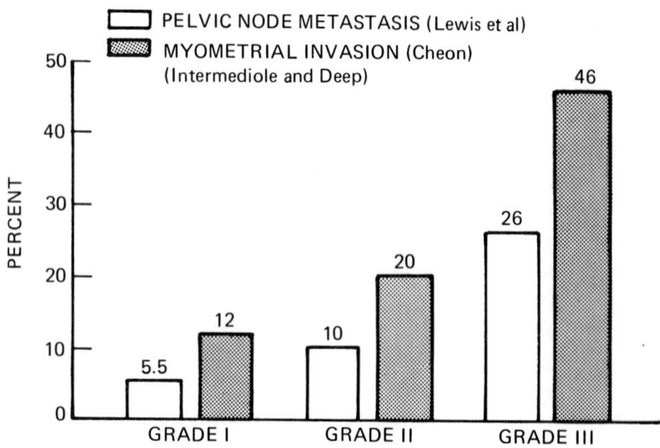

PATHOLOGY

Over 90% of the malignant tumors of the uterine corpus are adenocarcinomas. Grossly these lesions may have a polypoid or exophytic appearance or may infiltrate the endometrial mucosa, which appears thick and indurated. The tumor may infiltrate the myometrium, with resulting increased thickness of the wall and uterine enlargement.[230]

The microscopic appearance is that of numerous glands lined by cylindrical epithelium, the cells of which disclose nuclear atypia and mitosis that will vary according to the degree of tumor differentiation. In general, the tumor is well vascularized and may contain abundant connective tissue stroma. Infiltration with leukocytes, histiocytes, and microphages may be present. Foci of benign cartilaginous or osseous metaplasia may rarely be noted. Occasionally the diagnosis of hyperplasia of the endometrium, carcinoma *in situ,* or early well-differentiated carcinoma may be difficult.

Well-differentiated carcinoma has numerous glands, similar to those of the normal endometrium, separated by thin bands of stroma. As the tumor becomes more undifferentiated, the glands show an irregular pattern, atypia, and eventually the endometrium is replaced with cells disposed in nests or large sheets with bizarre forms, irregular nuclei, and abundant mitosis.

Endometrial carcinoma is classified as grade I, II, or III, depending on the degree of tumor differentiation. Approximately 60% of the patients have grade I, 20% grade II, and 20% grade III lesions.[230]

Sometimes the adenocarcinoma has squamous elements that can either be benign (in which case the tumor is called adenocanthoma) or malignant (in which case it is called adenosquamous carcinoma). Ng and Silverberg and coworkers described these lesions in detail that comprised 6.9–17.6% of the adenocarcinomas.[248,249] They reported a more aggressive behavior with increasing myometrial infiltration, higher incidence of lymph node and distant metastases and lower survival in comparison with adenocarcinoma. Silverberg and coworkers and Salazar and coworkers showed that adenosquamous carcinoma has a prognosis related to the degree of differentiation of the adenocarcinoma (see Fig. 25-23).[249,250]

A second group of tumors found in the endometrial cavity, of mesenchymal origin, are the mixed mullerian tumors. Fig. 25-24 shows the various types of lesions.

The mixed mullerian tumors may have a polypoid appearance with a yellow-tan necrotic mass projecting through the cervix into the vagina. These lesions have closely packed

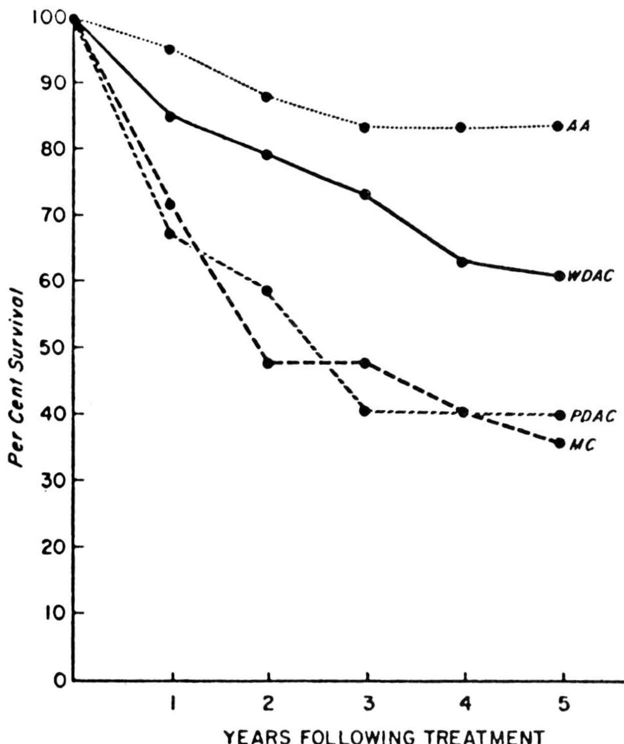

FIG. 25-23. Actuarial survival data for adenocanthoma (*AA*), mixed adenosquamous carcinoma (*MC*), and well-differentiated and poorly differentiated adenocarcinoma (*WDAC* and *PDAC*). (Silverberg SG, Bolin NG, DeGiorgi LS et al: Cancer 30:1307, 1972)

spindle-shaped stromal cells with prominent vesicular nuclei and scant cytoplasm. The reticular network of the endometrial stromal may be noted. In the endometrial stromal sarcoma, the cells are less differentiated, the nuclei larger and hyperchromatic, and mitoses more frequent. Occasionally, benign glandular inclusions are noted, resembling undifferentiated carcinomas that may acquire sarcomatoid appearance.[230,251–254]

The carcinosarcoma has a more pleomorphic appearance and is composed of a mixture of spindle cell, stromal, sarcoma cells and adenocarcinoma. If only tissues normally present in the endometrium are found, the carcinosarcoma is classified as homologous; if other mesenchymal tissues, such as bone, cartilage or striated muscle are identified, the tumor is classified as heterologous. The prognosis in carcinosarcoma is poor—only patients with stage I exhibiting 5-year survival of 60–70% and stage II about 50%. The prognosis is the same for homologous and heterologous groups.[235–255]

These lesions have a great propensity to metastasize to the abdominal cavity and to develop hematogenous metastasis to the liver and lungs.

The endolymphatic stromal myosis has a good to intermediate prognosis. Although histologically it has a well-differentiated pattern, this tumor invades lymphatic spaces and may develop distant metastases. The endometrial stromal sarcoma is associated with poor prognosis; commonly the patients show hematogenous tumor dissemination.[256]

Leiomyosarcomas derived from the uterine smooth muscle represent less than 1% of the malignant tumors of the body of the uterus. This tumor may originate in a leiomyoma or, less frequently, *de novo*. The prognosis depends on the degree of tumor differentiation. The number of mitosis per 10 high-power fields have been used to separate benign from malignant smooth muscle tumors (5 mitosis per [10]HPF being the dividing line). Also, the atypia of the cells, presence of bizarre nuclei, necrosis, and invasiveness of the tumor are important criteria.[230,257–260]

Other unusual primary tumors of the body of the uterus may derive from the vascular tissue (hemangioendothelioma, hemangiopericytoma, liposarcoma, rhabdomyosarcoma, or osteogenic sarcoma).[230] Occasionally, malignant lymphoma may be observed.[261]

Primary clear cell carcinoma of the endometrium is rare and characterized, as in the cervix, by the presence of large cells with abundant clear cytoplasm that contain glygocen and alternate with "hobnail" cells projecting into the lumina of the gland.[262]

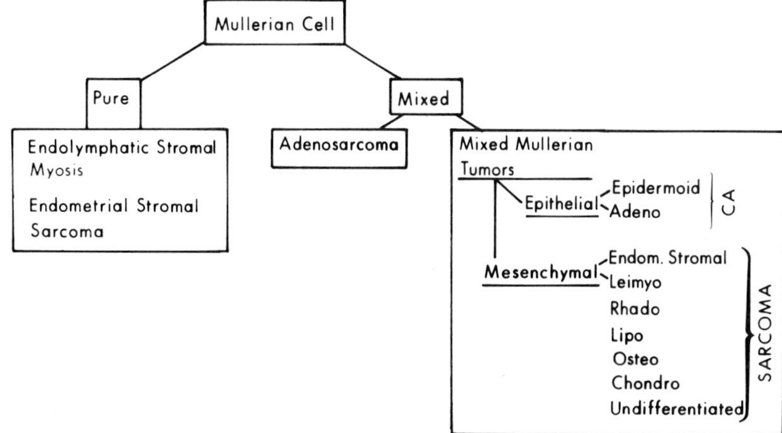

FIG. 25-24. Pathologic classification of mesenchymal tumors of the uterus. (Perez CA, Askin F, Baglan RS et al: Cancer 43:1274, 1979)

Occasionally, uterine polyps may be associated with adenocarcinoma.

Epidermoid carcinoma of the endometrium is extremely rare and probably originates from benign squamous metaplasia. The coexistence of invasive epidermoid carcinoma of the cervix must carefully be ruled out.[263]

DIAGNOSTIC WORK-UP

As in patients with carcinoma of the uterine cervix, a complete history and physical examination should be performed. In addition, a detailed bimanual pelvic and rectal examination should be carried out, preferably under general anesthesia. On the pelvic examination, it is extremely important to examine the entire vagina, particularly the suburethral meatus and introitus since this is a frequent area for metastasis.

Routine laboratory work-up should include hemogram, blood chemistry profile (SMA-12), and urinalysis.

A Pap smear is inadequate to screen for endometrial carcinoma; less than 50% of the patients have abnormalities on smears obtained from the cervix and vagina.[264] More reliable, however, is the use of endometrial biopsy either with a Novack curette or a biopsy clamp[265,266]

The Gravlee's jet washer was popularized about 10 years ago.[267] However, it has not gained the acceptance that was initially reported by some gynecologists and has largely been replaced by endometrial biopsies.[268]

Fractional dilatation and curettage (D & C) should always be performed if endometrial pathology is suspected. In addition to sounding and curetting of the uterine cavity including the lower segment of the uterus, it is imperative to obtain a separate endocervical curetting. Preferably the endocervical sample should be obtained before the internal os is dilated to prevent contamination with endometrial material. Punch biopsies of the cervix should be obtained. Pathologists discourage frozen sections because of the difficulty in making the diagnosis with the small amount of material many times available.

Other diagnostic work-up procedures include chest film and IV pyelogram, which should be performed routinely. Barium enema is indicated if there is suspected large bowel pathology or tumor extension.

Lymphangiogram is useful only to detect periaortic lymph nodes in high risk patients (undifferentiated tumors or lesions beyond stage II).[269]

Hysterography has been used at some institutions to detect the extent and location of the lesion in the uterine body.[270]

Cystoscopy or sigmoidoscopy is recommended only when there is suspicion of bladder or rectal involvement by the tumor

CLINICAL STAGING

As in the other gynecologic tumors, staging should be done jointly by the gynecologist and radiation oncologist; bi-manual pelvic examination under general anesthesia should be an integral part of the examination.

The two classifications most commonly used are the one proposed by the International Federation of Gynecology and Obstetrics (FIGO) or the International Union Against Cancer (UICC). Both are shown in Table 25-19.

TABLE 25-19. Staging Criteria for Carcinoma of the Endometrium

Stage		
Stage O	(TIS)	Carcinoma in situ
Stage I	(T1)	Carcinoma confined to the corpus
IA	(T1a)	Uterine cavity 8 cm or less in length
IB	(T1b)	Uterine cavity greater than 8 cm in length Stage 1 should be subgrouped by histology as follows: G1-highly differentiated, G-2 moderately differentiated, G3-undifferentiated
Stage II	(T2)	Extension to cervix only
Stage III	(T3)	Extension outside the uterus but confined to true pelvis
Stage IV	(T4)	Extension beyond true pelvis or invading bladder or rectum

Rubin P (ed): Clinical Oncology for Medical Students, 5th ed, p 109. American Cancer Society, 1978

It is important to subclassify the stage I lesions according to the degree of tumor differentiation. The authors recommend that this practice be applied to stage II tumors as well. The stage II lesions (corpus et colum), as reported by Madoc-Jones and coworkers, have a better prognosis when there is only microscopic involvement of the cervix (80% five-year survival in contrast to only 50% with gross tumor extension).[235]

GENERAL PRINCIPLES OF MANAGEMENT

As in other gynecologic tumors, integrated management with close consultation between the radiotherapist and the gynecologist is mandatory. The therapeutic approach will be determined by the stage of the tumor, size of the uterus, histologic type and degree of differentiation, and the medical condition and potential operability of the patient.[236,271–273] Kempson and Pokorny reported that younger women with endometrial carcinoma have a better prognosis than older patients.[274] Most of the tumors in 22 young patients were well-differentiated carcinoma. In seven cases, the diagnosis was revised to endometrial hyperplasia. These authors recommended that if the diagnosis is unclear, the lesion is well-differentiated, and childbearing is an issue, the patient be treated with progestational agents and repeated curettages (every 2 months initially until a negative specimen is obtained). Hysterectomy would be reserved for persistent tumor.

Even though the survival for stage I carcinoma of the endometrium is 85–95% after adequate therapy, it is important to realize that this disease may be serious and that efforts should be made to treat these patients optimally.[275] Boronow illustrated in a collected series that the survival of patients with endometrial carcinoma is similar to that of carcinoma of the uterine cervix (see Fig. 25-25).[275]

The indications for surgery, irradiation, or a combination of both have not been clearly established and vary with the prognostic characteristics of the tumor, medical condition of the patient, and institutional treatment policies.[236,271,276,277]

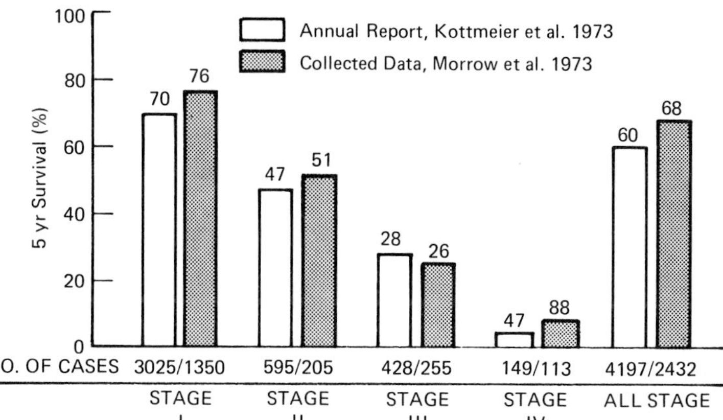

FIG. 25-25. Endometrial cancer 5-year salvage rate by clinical stage. (Boronow RC: Endometrial cancer: Not a benign disease. Obstet Gynecol 47:630–634, 1976)

Stage IA

From the management viewpoint, patients with stage IA carcinoma can be subdivided into two groups:

1. Those with well and moderately differentiated adenocarcinoma who may be treated with a wide cuff hysterectomy. Pelvic lymph node dissections are not indicated. If the tumor invades the myometrium only superficially, postoperative irradiation is not necessary because of the low incidence of vaginal recurrences after hysterectomy (less than 5%).[278] With involvement of the middle third of the myometrium, irradiation of the vaginal cuff with intracavitary ovoid insertions should be given (8000 rad mucosal dose). With extensive myometrial invasion, in addition to the vaginal cuff irradiation, it is necessary to treat the remaining pelvic tissues and lymph nodes with external irradiation. Usually a dose of 2000–3000 rad whole pelvis and additional parametrial irradiation with midline block to deliver about 5000 rad to the pelvic lymph nodes is used.
2. Patients with poorly differentiated tumors are infrequent in the stage IA group and should be treated with pre- or postoperative irradiation as described for stage IB.[278,279]

Stage IB

All patients with stage IB adenocarcinoma of the endometrium should receive preoperative radiation therapy, although with well-differentiated tumors the indication for preoperative irradiation is controversial.[236,278,280]

There is general agreement that with moderately differentiated lesions at least one intracavitary insertion for 5000–6000 mgh should be delivered. In general, about 3000–3500 mgh is delivered to the body of the uterus and 7000 rad to the vaginal mucosa.

Patients with poorly differentiated tumors, because of the high incidence of pelvic lymph node metastases and increasing parametrial failures, are treated with a combination of external irradiation (2000 rad whole pelvis and 3000 rad split field) combined with a intracavitary insertion for about 6000 mgh.

Elective irradiation of the periaortic lymph nodes is not justified in endometrial carcinoma. Patients with known periaortic nodes in addition to the pelvic therapy described above receive periaortic lymph node irradiation (a total dose of 5000 rad in 5–6 weeks) and hormonal therapy. An occasional long-term survival is reported.

Stage II

Patients with stage II endometrial carcinoma can be divided into those with microscopic or gross involvement of the cervix. Several reports strongly suggest that when there is microscopic involvement of the cervix with tumor being detected only in the curettings, reoperative intracavitary therapy (5000–6000 mgh) and a wide cuff hysterectomy will yield satisfactory results in over 85% of the patients.[235,281] However, in the presence of gross cervical involvement, a more aggressive management is necessary. High-dose preoperative irradiation (2000 rad whole pelvis and 3000 rad split field combined with an intracavitary insertion for 6000 mgh) should precede the hysterectomy. Some authors advocate postoperative irradiation and report similar results.[282]

Stages III and IVA

These patients with more extensive tumors are considered technically inoperable and should be treated by radiotherapy alone.[277,283] The usual treatment consists of a combination of whole pelvis external irradiation (2000–4000 rad) with additional irradiation delivered to the parametria with a midline block to complete 5000–6000 rad. This is combined with two or more intracavitary insertions for a total of approximately 8000 mgh. If there is persistent parametrial induration or if vaginal lesions are present, interstitial implantation with needles should be considered for a dose supplement.

In the treatment of patients with stage IVA (bladder or rectal involvement), the techniques of irradiation are similar, but special care must be directed to avoid major injury to the bladder or rectum that may result in a vesico- or recto-vaginal fistula.

SURGERY

In 1900, Cullen described the treatment of endometrial cancer by abdominal hysterectomy and bilateral salpingo-oophorectomy and recommended the vaginal hysterectomy only in the very obese or medically indigent patient.[284] Healy was one of the first to describe the combination of radiation therapy with surgery for the treatment of endometrial carcinoma.[285] Arneson compared radiation plus surgery, surgery alone, and radiation alone and found that the combination therapy did yield improved 5-year survival as compared to the other groups. However, the differences in results were not statistically significant.

Total Abdominal Hysterectomy and Bilateral Salpingo-Oophorectomy

Prior to performing the hysterectomy, peritoneal cell washings of the pelvis and abdomen should be obtained for cytologic studies, as the peritoneum is the most frequent site of distant metastasis in adenocarcinoma of the endometrium.[287] The liver and bowel should be carefully examined and with a grade 3 lesion; pelvic and aortic nodes must be sampled.

The hysterectomy should always be extrafascial and the adnexa removed because of the risk of ovarian metastasis. In an effort to prevent vaginal vault recurrences, gynecologists have used a variety of techniques to close the cervical os prior to the hysterectomy.[288] However, it has not been demonstrated that these techniques prevent vaginal recurrences or improve survival.[236] Similarly, to prevent vaginal vault recurrences, the upper third of the vagina has often been excised with the hysterectomy specimen. To remove the upper third of the vagina while avoiding ureteral injury, a modified radical hysterectomy is performed. This operation requires the unsheathing of the ureters from the bladder. With the ureters under direct visualization, the upper third of the vagina can safely be removed. However, the use of pre- or postoperative radium or external radiation precludes the necessity for removal of the upper third of the vagina.

The vaginal hysterectomy for endometrial cancer has generally been selected for those patients who are obese or poor medical risks. This procedure increases operability over the abdominal procedure. However, due to the inability to explore the abdomen and the difficulty of removing the adnexae, the vaginal hysterectomy for endometrial cancer is not generally recommended.

In the late 1940's, Brunschwig popularized the use of radical hysterectomy for endometrial cancer. His rationale was to remove possible lymph node metastasis, paravaginal tissue, and the upper portion of the vagina. Although the results were good, the morbidity was high. The radical hysterectomy is still being used in some institutions for stage II endometrial cancer, although Kottmeier believes it is not indicated.[276]

In the collected series of Jones, the overall 5-year survival rate for patients treated with radical hysterectomy for all stages was 76.7%.[236] However, the 5-year survival rate fell to 24.3% with positive pelvic nodes. Many of the patients with positive nodes developed extrapelvic recurrence, suggesting that distant metastases were present at the time of the original surgery.

The radical hysterectomy and pelvic lymphadenectomy have been used as treatment for stage II endometrial cancer.[290] In the multiple series reporting the use of radical hysterectomy and bilateral pelvic lymphadenectomy for stage II disease, the 5-year survival rates varied from 9–70%.[291] Kinsella and coworkers evaluated combination radiation and total abdominal hysterectomy for stage II endometrial cancer and found a disease-free survival of 83% at 10 years.[292] Therefore, better survival statistics with much less morbidity can be obtained with the use of combination radiation and total abdominal hysterectomy than with the use of radical hysterectomy and pelvic lymphadenectomy for stage II endometrial cancer.

There is no difference in the survival, whether pre- or postoperative external radiation is used. The advantage of surgery prior to radiation therapy is that the upper abdominal exploration can identify metastasis and therapy can be altered, if necessary; myometrial penetration of tumor can be best determined in the non-radiated uterus.

EXENTERATION

Pelvic exenteration has rarely been performed in patients with recurrent endometrial cancer.[293,294] However, this ultraradical approach has not been as satisfactory as it has for carcinoma of the cervix. Brunschwig reported only a 14.5% five-year survival.[294] Recurrences must be central and limited to the pelvis if the exenteration is to be successful. The manner of spread of endometrial cancer to peritoneum and upper abdomen limits this possibility to only a few selected cases.

Techniques of Irradiation

As in the cervix, external beam or brachytherapy irradiation, or combinations of both, are used in the treatment of these patients.

The techniques of external beam irradiation, volume to be treated, and portals used are similar to those used in the treatment of carcinoma of the uterine cervix.

For the intracavitary insertions, in addition to afterloading tandem and vaginal ovoids, it is common practice to pack the uterine cavity with Heyman or afterloading Heyman-Simon capsules (see Fig. 25-26). This technique allows the placement of sources in the body of the uterus around the tumor and, at the same time, some pressure can be exerted on the uterine wall, hopefully with some reduction in its thickness. These two effects may result in higher doses of irradiation delivered to the serosa of the uterus and immediately adjacent paracervical tissues.

The lower segment of the uterus and the endocervical canal can be treated with capsules or with a tandem. The vaginal vault is always irradiated with vaginal colpostats. If there is tumor extension into the vagina, the entire length of this organ should be treated with a cylinder or special applicator (*i.e.*, Burnett, Bloedorn, Delclos) to include the suburethral regions and introitus because of the propensity of advanced endometrial adenocarcinoma to metastasize to this site through submucosal venous and lymphatic plexuses.

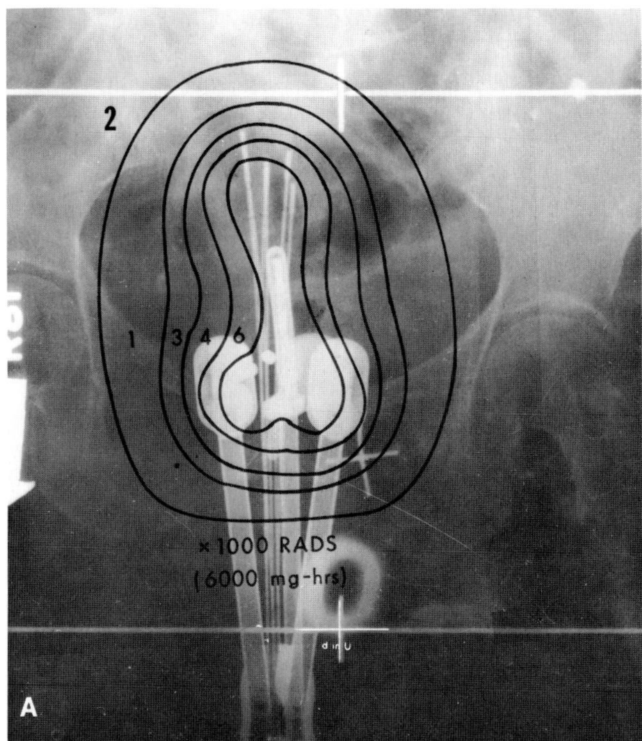

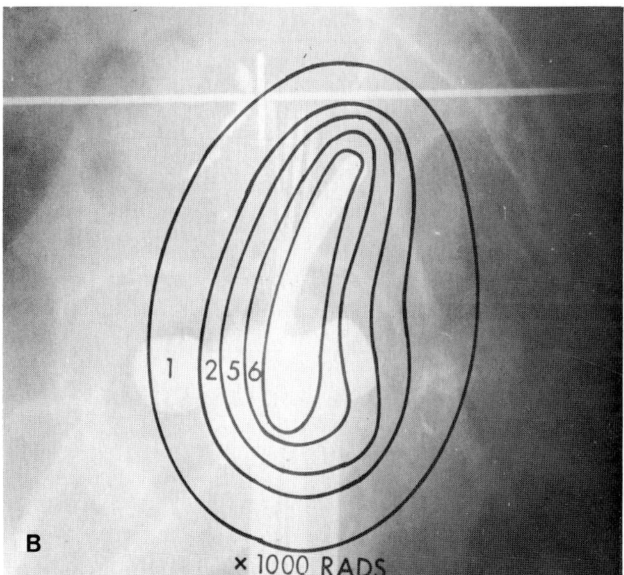

FIG. 25-26. Frontal (*A*) and lateral (*B*) radiographs of intracavitary insertion in patient with carcinoma of the endometrium showing Heyman-Simon after loading capsule in the uterine fundus, tandem in the lower segment, and ovoids in the vaginal vault.

PATTERNS OF FAILURE

Approximately 20% of the patients with endometrial carcinoma eventually die of the disease. High-risk groups include patients with stage III and IV disease; recurrent disease including those with isolated vaginal recurrences; clinical stages I and II disease when positive para-aortic nodes are found, who might benefit from postoperative adjuvant therapy; and positive pelvic nodes, deep myometrial invasion, or poorly differentiated (high grade) tumors.

The incidence of tumor recurrence or distant metastasis in endometrial carcinoma is correlated with the stage of the disease with surgery alone. In stage I, approximately 10–15% of the patients fail, in stage II, 25%, and in stage III, 75%. Of the recurrences, about 50% occur in the pelvis, half of them in the vaginal vault or distal vagina.[295]

Table 25-20 summarizes the anatomic site of failure in 364 patients, according to clinical stage and method of treatment. Those treated with surgery alone had 18% vaginal and pelvic failure, but this was reduced to 4% with preoperative irradia-

TABLE 25-20. Endometrial Carcinoma Analysis of Failures by Stage

TREATMENT	CLINICAL STAGE	ORIGINAL NO. PTS	NO. OF FAILURES (%) VAGINA	PELVIS INCL. VAGINA	DISTANT MET.	TOTAL OVERALL	AVERAGE TIME FOR FAILURE (Months)
Initial Surgery	I	106	10 (9)	16 (15)	10(9)	23 (22)	26.3
	II	12	3 (25)	1 (8)	2 (17)	4 (33)	10.3
	III–IV	8	5 (63)	6 (75)	5 (63)	8 (100)	16.1
	All	126	18 (14)	23 (18)	17 (14)	35 (28)	22.1
Preoperative radiation	I	176	0 (0)	6 (3)	12 (7)	15 (9)	23.2
	II	20	0 (0)	1 (5)	3 (15)	4 (20)	38.3
	III–IV	5	2 (40)	2 (40)	2 (40)	2 (40)	22.0
	All	201	2 (1)	9 (4)	17 (8)	21 (10)	26.0
Radiation alone	I	25	2 (8)	4 (16)	8 (32)	12 (48)	19.0
	II	8	1 (13)	2 (25)	2 (25)	4 (50)	10.0
	III–IV	4	1 (25)	2 (50)	1 (25)	3 (75)	3.7
	All	37	4 (11)	8 (22)	11 (30)	19 (51)	14.7

Salazar OM, Feldstein ML, DePapp EW et al: Int J Radiat Oncol Biol Phys 2:1101, 1977

TABLE 25-21. Distant metastases and nodal failure in endometrial carcinoma*

DISTANT METASTASES (48 patients) METASTATIC SITE	NO.	%	NODAL METASTASES (48 patients) METASTATIC SITE	NO.	%
Lung	17	35	Pelvic	15	38†
Liver	14	29	Paraaortic	9	19
Omentum and peritoneum	12	25	Common iliac	6	13
GI Tract	10	21	Cervical and supraclavical	5	10
Bone	7	15			
Kidney and adrenal	5	10	Inguinal	2	4
Brain	3	6			
Breast	2	4			

* All Stages, all treatments.
† Calculated on the basis of 40 pelvic failures. This value may be higher since nodal status was not documented in every failure.
Salazar OM, Feldstein ML, DePapp EW et al: Int J Radiat Oncol Biol Phys 2:1101, 1977

tion. Patients treated with radiotherapy alone had the highest pelvic failure rate (22%), probably reflecting more advanced stage of the disease. No difference in failure rates was noted in stage I, grade 1 or 2 lesions; however, patients with grade 3 tumors had significantly more pelvic failures and distant metastasis. In patients without myometrial invasion, the failure rate was 10–12%, whereas with myometrial involvement 40–50% failed.

Periaortic lymph node metastases account for clinical manifestation of distant dissemination in 25% of the patients that fail after treatment. Distant metastases occur mostly in the lungs, liver, peritoneal cavity, and bone (see Table 25-21).

Approximately 90% of all recurrences take place within three years from initial therapy.

Rubin and colleagues and Salazar and coworkers have reported that 35% of the patients with isolated pelvic or vaginal recurrences can be salvaged by appropriate irradiation (external beam to the pelvis and intracavitary insertion).[240,295]

RESULTS

In stage I, the 5-year survival rate of surgery alone or combined with pre- or postoperative radiation therapy has varied from 80–95%.[278,280,286,296] Statistically valid data is not available to support the impact of adjuvant radiotherapy in survival. However, in a randomized study, Graham reported better 5-year survival with the combination therapy as opposed to hysterectomy alone, although the difference between the pre- and postoperation irradiation group was not statistically significant (see Table 25-22).[297] Nolan, in a nonrandomized study, also demonstrated improved survival with combined therapy in patients with stage I in high risk groups (large uterus or less differentiated lesions).[280]

TABLE 25-22. Adenocarcinoma of Endometrium Stage I, Group I Randomly Assigned Treatment

	5 YEAR SURV., NED	VAGINAL RECURRENCE
Hysterectomy alone	21/33 (64%)	6/49 (12%)
Pre-op Radiation and Hysterectomy	45/59 (76%)	2/82 (3%)
Hysterectomy and Post-op Radiation	25/31 (81%)	0/51 –

Graham J: Surg Gyn Obst, 32:855, 1971

Nevertheless, there has been a significantly decreased incidence of vaginal recurrences in patients treated with irradiation (1–3%), in contrast to those treated with hysterectomy alone (15%). Several authors have reported a greater incidence of vaginal pelvic recurrences and distant metastases in patients with poorly differentiated (grade III tumors) or in those with advanced stage.[297] However, radiation therapy has been shown to decrease the incidence of pelvic recurrences.

Uterine size in stage I correlates with prognosis only if the enlargement is related to tumor infiltration in the myometrium (see Table 25-23). Wade and Javert noted that often benign conditions such as myomata and adenomyosis may contribute to uterine enlargement and have no significant impact on prognosis.[298,299] Myometrial invasion decreases the 5-year survival from 80% to 85% when it is absent to 60% or less when involvement is more than half-way through the myometrium.[236] Similar findings are reported according to the degree of tumor differentiation (Table 25-24).

A few reports have compared the effectiveness of external irradiation or intracavitary radium without conclusive results. Sala and del Regato compared the survival after 4000 rad external irradiation to the pelvis on two patients or a radium implant for 6000 mgh (48 patients).[300] The 3-year survival rate was 87% and 77% respectively. No vaginal recurrences were noted in either group. The survival was comparable whether residual tumor was present in the surgical specimen or not. Similar findings were reported by Silberberg and Degiorgi in 76 patients treated with preoperative irradiation and hysterectomy.[301] Weigensberg observed a 75% five-year actuarial disease-free survival in 53 patients treated with intracavitary irradiation and hysterectomy and 48% in 38 patients treated with external beam irradiation in a randomized study.[302] Patients treated with intracavitary radium received 5400 mgh and with external beam irradiation, 4000 rad. Only two of the intracavitary therapy patients had pelvic recurrences in contrast to nine in the external beam group.

TABLE 25-23. Five Year Survival Rates Correlated with Depth of Myometrial Invasion

	NO INVASION		SUPERFICIAL INVASION		DEEP INVASION	
AUTHOR	*No. pts.*	*5-year survival*	*No. pts.*	*5-year survival*	*No. pts.*	*5-year survival*
Anderson (1965)	12	100%	22	86%	7	43%
Gusberg (1964)	245	67%	96	70%	94	34%
Climie (1965)	56	87%	20	80%	23	56%
Austin (1969)	133	91%	239	95%	163	81%
Cheon (1969)	181	81%	91	77%	73	42%
Nilsen (1969)			205	89%	131	76%
Lewis (1970)	16	93%	41	88%	22	54%
Ng (1970)	129	88%	48	72%	22	27%
Sall (1970)			75	92%	16	75%
Nahhas (1971)	75	85%	33	82%	28	56%
Frick (1973)	63	79%	101	77%	42	45%
TOTAL PATIENTS	910		971		621	
TOTAL SURVIVORS	736		827		376	
AVERAGE 5-YEAR SURVIVAL		80%		85%		50%

Jones HW III: Obstet Gynecol Survey 30:149, 1975

Uterine size and degree of tumor differentiation were similar in both groups.

The patients treated with irradiation alone, in earlier stages because of medical reasons or in stage III and IV because surgery has no place in the treatment of these lesions, have survival rates lower than the surgical patients. However, Landgren and coworkers reported on 124 medically inoperable patients treated with irradiation alone, with a 5-year survival of 75–80% in patients with stage I and 60% in stage II.[277]

The patients who are technically inoperable and treated with irradiation alone have extensive pelvic disease and a high incidence of metastatic lymph nodes. The survival rate ranges from 24–27%.[276,277,303]

Landgren and coworkers observed 89% pelvic tumor control in stage IA, 78% in stage IB, 82% in stage IIA, and 62% in stage III tumors treated with irradiation alone.[304]

HORMONAL THERAPY

The most commonly used systemic treatment in recurrent endometrial carcinoma has been synthetic progestational agents with response rates ranging from 30–37%.[305–307] Responses are associated with prolonged survival; mean survivals for patients responding to progesterone therapy have been 23–29 months compared to 6 months for patients without an objective response.[227,308] Response to hormonal therapy seems

TABLE 25-24. Relationship Between Tumor Differentiation and 5-year Survival

	GRADE I		GRADE II		GRADE III	
AUTHOR	*No. pts.*	*5-year survival*	*No. pts.*	*5-year survival*	*No. pts.*	*5-year survival*
Webb (1955)	32	84%	155	52%	37	30%
Lindgren (1957)	120	88%	153	82%	56	80%
Gusberg (1960)	204	62%	85	53%	65	32%
Boutselis (1963)	81	75%	42	64%	49	14%
Anderson (1965)	14	100%	51	82%	26	65%
Climie (1965)	56	93%	24	75%	18	44%
Dobbie (1965)	147	81%	74	78%	45	73%
Roman (1967)	47	87%	105	78%	113	51%
Wade (1967)	65	84%	150	78%	50	42%
Austin (1969)	126	96%	239	96%	163	75%
Cheon (1969)	196	81%	72	78%	77	44%
Ng (1970)	91	86%	101	75%	62	37%
Nahhas (1971)	106	84%	57	75%	35	48%
Beiler (1972)	54	83%	130	65%	67	40%
Frick (1973)	218	79%	76	54%	54	30%
TOTAL PATIENTS	1558		1515		917	
TOTAL SURVIVORS	1267		1124		462	
AVERAGE 5-YEAR SURVIVAL		81%		74%		50%

Jones HW III: Obstet Gynecol Survey 30:150, 1975

to be related to the histologic grade of the tumor; well-differentiated tumors respond more frequently than those with poorly differentiated histologies. Other factors that influence hormonal therapy response include disease-free interval, age, and presence of areas of squamous metaplasia within the tumor. Recent studies of the progesterone receptor content of endometrial cancers suggest a more effective means of predicting response.[244] Although the number of patients studied thus far is small, endometrial cancers with high progesterone affinity responded, while only 13% of those with low affinity had objective tumor regression.[309] The study also found the progesterone binding affinity to correlate with histologic grade; 85% of grade 1 tumors had high affinity while only 50% of grade 3 tumors were positive. These receptor studies may allow more rational selection of hormonal management in a manner analogous to that of the estrogen receptor assay in breast cancer.

Systemic hormonal therapy with progestogens has been well-established as first line systemic therapy for patients with recurrent or disseminated disease. The most commonly used progestogens have been hydroxyprogesterone (Delalutin) and medroxyprogesterone (Provera). Recent reports indicate that the oral agent megestrol (Megase) produces similar results. The usual dose is 1–3 gm/week IM for the initial dose, followed by maintenance doses of 400–800 mg weekly for indefinite time, until recurrence or distant metastasis develop.

More controversial is its use as a prophylactic therapy in earlier stages. In one large adjuvant trial, stage I patients received either adjuvant Depo-Provera or a placebo.[310] In spite of unbalanced stratification with regard to prognostic factors and frequent unevaluability, there was no difference in 5-year survivals. Similar experience was recently reported from the Mayo Clinic in a study of 35 stage IA and IB patients treated with surgery with or without subsequent treatment with 6-methyl-17α-hyroxy-progesterone. In spite of this, several investigators have advocated the use of prophylactic progestational agents in high-risk patients.[312–314] However, the worth, if any, of adjuvant progesterone therapy in any stage of endometrial carcinoma at present must be considered unproven.

TABLE 25-25. Single Agent Chemotherapy in Endometrial Carcinoma

DRUGS	PATIENTS RESPONDING/ TOTAL TREATED	RESPONSE RATE (%)
Alkylating Agents		
Cyclophosphamide	7/33	21%
Nitrogen Mustard	3/11	27%
Antimetabolites		
5-Fluorouracil	10/43	23%
Antitumor Antibiotics		
Doxorubicin (Adriamycin)	33/92	36%
Bleomycin	3/8	37%
Miscellaneous Agents		
Hexamethylmelamine	2/8	25%
Piperazinedione	1/20	5%

American Cancer Society: 1980 Facts and Figures. New York, American Cancer Society, 1979

CHEMOTHERAPY

Single Agent Chemotherapy

Non-hormonal chemotherapy has not been systematically studied in any detail. Table 25-25 lists the apparently active single agents reported in a few studies that have included relatively small numbers of patients.[308,315] This information can only be taken to suggest activity of the listed agents. Of these, only doxorubicin has been well evaluated in adequate numbers of patients and has shown established activity in advanced endometrial cancer. Thigpen and coworkers recently reported the experience of the Gynecology Oncology Group, which treated 43 patients with advanced or recurrent disease.[316] Using 60 mg/m^2 IV doxorubicin every 3 weeks, they reported a 37% response rate (16/43) and 26% (11/43) had clinical complete regressions of disease. Median survival was 14 months for patients achieving a complete response, 6.8 months for those with a partial regression, and 3.5 months for patients with progressive disease. Of interest is the fact that age, time to first recurrence, histologic grade of primary, site of metastasis, and previous therapy had no effect on probability of response. Toxicity was similar to that in other studies in which doxorubicin was used as a single agent.

Combination Therapy

Combination chemotherapy for advanced endometrial carcinoma has been studied to a very limited degree. Available information is fragmentary. Unfortunately, few studies have been completed and these generally have evaluated small numbers of patients.[317,318] Other studies have added combination chemotherapy and progestogens, but the independent contribution of the drugs and the hormone cannot be assessed in these single arm studies.[319,320]

Whether combination approaches will be more effective than single agents is not yet known and should be the subject of well-controlled clinical trials.

TREATMENT OF MIXED MESODERMAL TUMORS

The primary treatment of this lesion, as in the adenocarcinoma, is a wide cuff hysterectomy. Lymphadenectomy is not indicated since these patients fail mostly because of hematogenous tumor dissemination.

The role of radiation therapy in the management of these patients has been highly controversial. Perez and coworkers reported on 54 patients and suggested that the use of adjuvant radiotherapy decreases the incidence of pelvic and vaginal recurrences.[254] However, whether this improves the survival has not been demonstrated.

In stage I, preoperative irradiation consisting of an intracavitary insertion with packing of the endometrial cavity, tandem, and colpostats to deliver approximately 6000 mgh has been used. For stage II, a combination of external irradiation (2000 rad to the whole pelvis and 3000 rad to the parametria with a midline shield) and an intracavitary insertion for 5000–6000 mgh have been employed. Patients with stage III tumors are treated with irradiation alone in a manner similar to endometrial carcinoma. Table 25-26 shows the 3-year survival in 54 patients. Approximately 60% of the patients with stage I and 30% with stage II survived. All patients with stage III and IV died with persistent or metastatic tumor.

Perez and coworkers demonstrated that a lower number of specimens contained tumor as higher doses of irradiation were delivered.

With adequate irradiation and surgery, the sites of failure in these patients are less often the pelvis (20–30%) than in the abdomen or at distant sites (over 50% of the patients). In contrast, Edwards and coworkers reported eight recurrences in 10 patients treated with surgery alone; Norris and Taylor described pelvic extension in 16 of 25 patients dying of tumor in a group of 31 initially treated by hysterectomy.[321,322] Vaginal metastases were noted in about 20% of patients.

DiSaia and coworkers in 75 patients usually treated with a combination of irradiation and surgery reported local control in 14 of 17 patients with stage I, 10 of the patients surviving over 2 years (treated with preoperative irradiation and hysterectomy).[323] Of seven patients treated with hysterectomy and postoperative irradiation, four survived 2 years and five had local tumor. Vongtama and coworkers reported eight of 29 patients (27.6%) treated with surgery alone surviving 5 years in contrast to 10 of 19 patients (52%) treated with surgery and irradiation.[324]

TREATMENT OF UTERINE SARCOMAS

As in adenocarcinoma, the primary treatment is a total abdominal hysterectomy, usually with salpingo-oophorectomy. Irradiation may have some value in reducing pelvic failures, but no definite increase in survival rates has been reported.[325]

Salazar and coworkers reviewed 81 patients collected from several institutions who failed after treatment of uterine leiomyosarcoma: only eleven had a pelvic recurrence alone, 49 pelvic failure combined with distant metastases, and 21 distant metastases only.[326] Thus, both pelvic recurrence and distant dissemination are almost as frequent after surgical therapy. The overall incidence of failure was not stated, but seven of 20 patients treated at the author's institution recurred after treatment (35%).

Belgrad and coworkers reported on 12 patients with leiomyosarcoma.[327] No significant correlation was noted in prognosis with the mitotic rate, increased pleomorphism, invasiveness, or presence of giant cells. Four of the patients received postoperative radiotherapy, but unfortunately the patients are intermixed with other stromal sarcomas, so that the effects of irradiation in leiomyosarcoma cannot be determined. Gilbert and coworkers reported on 40 patients with stage I leiomyosarcoma treated with total abdominal hysterectomy and bilateral salpingo-oophorectomy.[328] Radiation therapy (5000 rad to the pelvis) was given pre- or postoperatively. Seventeen of the patients recurred (six in the pelvis, four in the abdomen, and 13 with distant metastasis). Because of the high incidence of distant metastases, no significant effect on survival was observed. However, in 12 patients with stage III leiomyosarcoma, radiation therapy provided palliative benefit. In an analysis of 22 patients with stage I and II leiomyosarcomas, Vongtama and coworkers concluded that adjunctive radiotherapy was of no therapeutic value.[324] Eight of 18 patients (46%) treated with hysterectomy alone survived 5 years without tumor.

Some uncontrolled clinical trials are in progress to evaluate the potential application of pelvic irradiation and multiagent chemotherapy in the treatment of these patients.[329] At Washington University a combination of 5000 rad to the pelvis and 8–10 cycles of cyclophosphamide (Cytoxan) and doxorubicin administered every 4 weeks is under investigation. In operable patients, two cycles are administered prior to the surgery.

TABLE 25-26. Mixed Mullerian Tumors of the Uterus: 3-Year Survival (NED) According to Clinical Stage

	STAGE					
	I		II		III	IV
Surgery alone	3/6	(50%)	0/3		0/3†	0/2
Pre-operative intracavitary insertions (Co^{60})	6/10	(60%)	2/3	(66%)	—	0/1
Pre-operative intracavitary and external XRT	5/7	(71%)	1/5	(20%)	0/1	0/1
Irradiation alone (external and intracavitary)	—		0/1*		0/8	0/2
No radiation	1/0		—		0/1	0/1
TOTAL	14/24	(58%)	3/10	(30%)	0/13	0/7

* Inoperable, metastatic peri-aortic nodes at exploration
† Two postoperative deaths
Perez CA, et al: Cancer 43:1274, 1979

POSTIRRADIATION GYNECOLOGICAL MALIGNANCIES

Several reports have been published on the incidence of malignant tumors of the endometrium or other pelvic organs in patients treated with irradiation for benign or malignant pelvic conditions.

Smith and Doll reported an increased incidence of leukemia (seven deaths observed against 2.3 expected) and cancers of the heavily irradiated sites (59 observed vs. 40.1 expected) 5 or more years after irradiation to the pelvis for benign metrapathia haemorrhagica.[330] The mean dose of radiation to the bone marrow was estimated to correlate with the projected excess rate of leukemia, which is about 1.1 case/woman/rad/year. However, other authors such as Hutchinson have not observed this increased incidence (three cases observed vs. 16 expected).[331]

Dickson reported two deaths from leukemia whereas only 1.1 were expected.[332] Wagoner observed no excess of leukemia among 7,835 women treated with radium and roentgen rays for primary uterine cancer.[333] Arneson and Schellhas and Spratt and Hoag observed no significant increase of malignancy in patients treated with irradiation for carcinoma of the uterine cervix.[334,335]

Lee and coworkers reviewed 1150 patients treated with irradiation for carcinoma of the uterine cervix at Washington University.[336] Table 25-27 shows the observed and expected incidence of malignancy in several series. Thus, the current data fail to support the suggestion that irradiation may increase the incidence of malignancy in patients irradiated for gynecologic cancer.

Wagoner also studied 1803 patients treated for benign gynecologic disorders with radium and observed 10 deaths from leukemia against 3.6 expected; in a similar series in Connecticut, nine cases of leukemia were seen against 2.8 expected.[337] A decreased death rate from carcinoma of the breast has been observed by Smith and Doll and others with an artificial inducement of menopause.[330,338,339] In the patients treated for carcinoma of the cervix at Washington University, a similar lower mortality from breast cancer was noted. It is possible that the castration induced by irradiation in younger women may influence the subsequent development of carcinoma of the breast. Villasanta and Rubel reported 15 cases of pelvic malignancy in 174 patients irradiated for benign uterine bleeding in contrast to only three malignant tumors in 147 non-randomized control patients that were not irradiated.[340] The majority of the tumors developed in the endometrium or the ovary. The dose of irradiation was relatively small (2000–2400 mgh). In contradistinction, the same authors observed only 19 patients developing a second pelvic malignancy in 569 with malignant tumors of the gynecological tract treated with doses of irradiation above 5000 rad and followed for 4 years or longer. Dickson pointed out that the incidence of malignancy after irradiation for benign uterine bleeding was significantly less in patients treated with external irradiation than those treated with intracavitary radium.[332] As reported by Thomas and coworkers, the majority of the postirradiation malignancies of the uterus are adenocarcinomas of the endometrium, followed by mixed Müllerian tumors and sarcomas of the uterine cervix.[341] The prognosis of these patients after treatment was similar to those of patients without history of previous irradiation.[341]

The principles of management for these patients are similar to those who receive no previous irradiation.

Most authors agree that the primary treatment of these patients is surgical. There is some controversy as to whether preoperative or postoperative irradiation should be delivered. However, the number of patients is small and no definite conclusions can be drawn.

TABLE 25-27. Incidence of Post-Irradiation Gynecological Malignancy

	AVG. AGE	NO. OF PATIENTS	No. 2 NDI°	MAN YRS. OBSERV.	CA PER MAN YR.	RATE PER 100,000
Perez	52	1053	49	6244	.00785	785
Arneson	49	874	36	6142	.00586	586
Spratt	54	1853	36	6264	.00574	574

Lee J, Perez CA, Tarlow D: Unpublished data, 1980

CARCINOMA OF THE FALLOPIAN TUBE

Primary carcinoma of the fallopian tube is the least frequent of all malignant tumors of the female genital tract, comprising between .5–1.1% of all gynecologic malignancies.[342] Hu and coworkers reviewed 466 cases in 1950 and Sedlis reported on an additional 230 cases collected over the next 10 years[342,343] An additional 200 cases have subsequently been described.[344–348] The most recent review was reported by Henderson and coworkers in 1977.[349]

Sometimes it is difficult to differentiate a primary tubal carcinoma from metastatic disease of adjacent organs. Finn and Javert and Hu and coworkers established rigid criteria for the diagnosis of primary tubal carcinoma which require that the tumor be grossly located within the tube and that the ovaries and uterus have either no malignancy present or malignancy that is different from that found within the tube. The tubal malignancy must also involve the mucosa with transition from benign to malignant epithelium clearly demonstrated.

EPIDEMIOLOGY

Tubal carcinoma occurs most frequently in the 50- and 60-year age group, with the median age in the late 50's. Family history, exposures to carcinogens, or hormones do not appear to be significant etiologic factors in primary tubal cancer. Between 25% and 50% of the patients are nulliparous. Infertility is associated with many of the reported cases. These observations suggest a possible association of chronic salpingitis with tubal carcinoma. Lofgren and Dockerty noted chronic salpingitis in almost every patient that they evaluated with tubal carcinoma.[351] However, the high frequency of tubal salpingitis as contrasted to the rarity of tubal carcinoma makes the possibility of an inflammatory process as an etiologic factor highly questionable.

PATHOLOGY

Gross Characteristics

The usual appearance of the tumor is associated with fusiform swelling that may involve primarily the distal portion or the entire length of the tube; often, this cannot be distinguished from other benign lesions of the tube or even hydrosalpinx. The consistency of the tumor may be soft initially, although later when infiltration takes place the mass will feel firm and nodular. Eventually there is infiltration of the serosa of the tube and there may be extension to adjacent pelvic structures. Occasionally, instead of diffuse swelling, the tumor is visualized as a well-circumscribed solid or partially cystic nodular mass. In gross sections, the tumor shows a soft grey to pink color. Areas of degeneration with hemorrhage and necrosis are frequently observed.[344]

In a few patients with extensive disease, a tumor may involve both the tube and the adjacent ovary, in which case it is impossible to determine the exact primary site of the tumor, thus they are classified as tubo-ovarian carcinoma.

It is unclear whether bilateral tubal involvement is of multicentric or metastatic origin. Novak and Woodruff found bilateral involvement in one half of the primary cancers of the tube, and noted that this represents tumor arising in "paired organs" and not an example of lymphatic or direct extension.[352] Sedlis, in his review of 176 cases, reported bilateral involvement in 26 cases (15%).[342] Green and Scully noted that all of their cases were unilateral, except in one of six patients with tubo-ovarian carcinoma.[344] Henderson and coworkers, in their recent review of 12 cases of primary carcinoma of the tube, reported bilateral involvement in one.[349] The absence of extratubal metastasis in the presence of bilateral tubal carcinoma lends evidence to the concept of independent development of these cancers.[353]

Adenocarcinoma is the most common histologic type of primary carcinoma of the tube. Rare tumors, such as sarcoma, mixed mesodermal tumors, lymphomas, and carcinosarcomas have been reported. Choriocarcinoma of the tube usually follows an ectopic pregnancy. Recently, Weiss and coworkers described a case of intraepithelial epidermoid carcinoma of cervix, endometrium, and fallopian tube.[354]

Hu, Taymor, and Hertig have related histologic grade of tumor differentiation to prognosis.[343] Hu and coworkers classified their tumors into grade 1, papillary; grade 2, papillary-alveolar; grade 3, alveolar-medullary.[343] The more anaplastic the cancer, the greater the propensity for invasion and dissemination. However, once the tubal serosa had been involved, metastasis develops irrespective of the histologic grade. Hu and Momtazee and Kempson have reported 50–60% five-year survival with grade 1, 40% with grade 2, and 16.7% with grade 3 tumors.[343,345]

TUMOR DISSEMINATION

Tubal carcinoma may disseminate by transluminal migration of tumor cells, direct implantation or contiguous invasion, and lymphatic and hematogeneous dissemination. The most frequent site of dissemination is the pelvic peritoneum including the broad ligament and omentum.[342,349,352,355]

Many of the patients have relatively early lesions at the time of diagnosis; widespread peritoneal dissemination at this time is uncommon, being reported in approximately 15% of the patients.

Next in order of frequency is ovary, followed by uterus. Other distant sites of metastases are intestine, lung, and liver. Since the pattern of intraperitoneal spread of tubal cancer is similar to that of ovary, the diaphragm should also be evaluated for metastasis.[356] The peritoneal dissemination may occur through direct invasion through the thin tubal walls or through the ostium of the tubes. Plentl and Friedman described in detail the lymphatics of the fallopian tube, which leave the tubal wall within the mesosalpinx where they join efferent lymphatics from the ovary and uterus, and follow the ovarian vessels to terminate in the aortic lymph nodes.[355] Other lymphatics course within the broad ligament and terminate in the interiliac nodes, and a separate lymphatic channel from the ampulla of the tube travels within the broad ligament to terminate in the superior gluteal lymph nodes. Henderson and coworkers report four of their patients with primary tubal cancer having para-aortic or mesenteric lymph node metastasis. Plentl and Friedman noted metastasis to regional lymph nodes, especially in iliac and aortic, and occasionally to inguinal nodes.[355]

CLINICAL MANIFESTATIONS

The diagnosis of tubal carcinoma is made prior to surgery in only 5% of the reported cases.[357] Preoperative diagnosis and clinical staging are extremely difficult to accomplish and a surgical exploration is required for accurate determination of the extent and pathologic characterization of the tumor.

Abnormal vaginal bleeding is the most common symptom, along with pelvic and abdominal pain. Henderson and coworkers noted lower abdominal pain in eight of 12 cases, and intermenstrual or postmenopausal bleeding in six.[349] A serosaguineous discharge is frequently associated with tubal carcinoma. Hydrops tubae profluens is a rare symptom in which the patient describes lower pelvic pain, which is relieved by a sudden release of vaginal discharge. In advanced tubal cacinoma, there may be enlargement of the abdomen, evidence of intestinal obstruction, or weight loss.

In all these situations it is extremely important to rule out the more common gynecologic neoplasias, such as cervix, endometrium, and ovary. However, with a patient experiencing intermittent vaginal bleeding or discharge, abdominal pain with an adnexal mass, or localized tenderness in the pelvis and negative endometrial curettage, the possibility of ovarian or tubal neoplasia must be strongly considered.

Infrequently, cervical cytology is positive, particularly if there is spread to uterus and cervix. Cytologic smears from the cervix and vagina and dilatation and curettage performed on six patients showed no histological evidence of malignancy.[344] Green and Scully reported adenocarcinoma cells detected in vaginal smears in one of five patients evaluated by this method.[344]

All patients with suspected tubal carcinoma should undergo a complete physical and pelvic examination, including rectal exam.

When an adnexal mass is palpated, it may be difficult to distinguish tubal from ovarian carcinoma or a subserous myoma. Laparoscopy may be helpful, but unless there is perforation of the serosa, the laparoscope may reveal only tubal enlargement, which may be confused with salpingitis.

Radiographic studies should include chest roentgenogram, IV pyelogram, ultrasound studies, or CT of the abdomen and pelvis (with special attention to the retroperitoneal lymph nodes). If a large mass is palpated in the pelvis, a barium enema should be carried out to rule out colorectal pathology or involvement by the tumor.

STAGING

Staging of carcinoma of the fallopian tube is determined at laparotomy, where the presence or absence of ascites must be noted. If there is no ascites, 500 ml of saline is added to the peritoneal cavity for 5 minutes, then withdrawn from both right and left gutters and cul-de-sac and sent for pathologic diagnosis. The diaphragm should be carefully assessed for the presence of tumor.[356] The omental apron should be removed, even if there is no gross evidence of metastasis. If no upper abdominal disease is demonstrated, the periaortic nodes should be sampled. Dodson and coworkers and Erez modified the staging for ovarian tumors for tubal cancer as illustrated in Table 25-28.[348,358]

TABLE 25-28. Criteria for Staging Carcinoma of the Fallopian Tube*

Stage O	Carcinoma is confined to the epithelium on the fallopian tube.
Stage I	Carcinoma is confined to the fallopian tube.
Stage IA	Disease is confined to one fallopian tube with no ascites.
Stage IB	Disease is confined to both fallopian tubes with no ascites.
Stage IC	Disease is confined to one or both fallopian tubes; ascites are present with malignant cells in the fluid.
Stage II	The carcinoma extends to other intraperitoneal organs or tissue within the true pelvis.
Stage IIA	Disease extends only to the uterus or ovaries or both.
Stage IIB	Disease extends to the uterus or ovaries and to other intraperitoneal organs or tissues within the true pelvis.
Stage III	The carcinoma extends to the uterus or ovaries and to other intraperitoneal organs and tissues beyond the true pelvis (*e.g.*, the omentum, the small intestine, or mesentery).
Stage IV	The carcinoma metastasizes to organs or tissues outside the peritoneal cavity.

* Criteria for staging carcinoma of the ovary Dodson MG, Ford JH Jr, Averette HE: Clinical aspects of the fallopian tube carcinoma. Obstet Gynecol 36:935–939, 1970; Erez S, Kaplan AL, Wall JA: Clinical staging of carcinoma of the uterine tube. Obstet Gynecol 30:547–550, 1967.

The authors agree with Plentl and Friedman's criticism of this staging in that the number of cases available in any single series is small.[355] The limited number of cases makes evaluation of results in any series statistically invalid. Accuracy of staging information often times is further complicated by the lack of clear data to substantiate surgical assessment (*i.e.*, biopsies of the diaphragms, periaortic nodes, and omentum).

However, stage is an important prognostic indicator.[342,344,349,353,359] The 5-year survival according to stage for combined series is approximately 70% for stage I, 45% in stage II, 15% in stage III, and 0 in stage IV.

GENERAL PRINCIPLES OF MANAGEMENT

Surgery

The primary treatment of carcinoma of the fallopian tube is surgical, consisting of a total abdominal hysterectomy (TAH) with bilateral salpingo-oophorectomy (BSO). If the tumor invades adjacent pelvic organs or is extending directly into the lower abdomen with separate metastases, an en bloc excision of all tumor in addition to the TAH and BSO is indicated.

A unilateral salpingo-oophorectomy may be adequate surgical treatment for a small, well-differentiated tubal carcinoma. Cytoreductive surgery, leaving tumor deposits no greater than 2 cm in any location, may be of value when followed by multiple agent chemotherapy or pelvic-abdominal radiation. Although there are isolated instances in which radical surgery is reported to have increased survival, in view of the manner of spread of tubal carcinoma, there appears to be little justification for radical hysterectomy or pelvic exenteration. Based on limited experience, a total abdominal hysterectomy and bilateral salpingo-oophorectomy combined with pelvic irradiation have been the accepted treatment in stage II disease.

Radiation Therapy

The role of radiation therapy in the treatment of these patients has not been documented.

Based on results reported by Erez and co-workers, Kneale and Atwood, Sedlis, and Green and Scully, postoperative irradiation probably offers some benefit to patients with stage I tumors with evidence of wall infiltration or serosal excrescences.[342,344,348,360] Further, Phelps and Chapman reported on 15 patients, nine of them with stage I and II and six with stage III lesions.[361] Fourteen of the patients received postoperative pelvic irradiation (between 3000 and 5000 rad). In addition, six were treated with upper abdominal irradiation and six with IP installation of radioactive colloidal Au^{198} or P^{32}. Eight of the nine patients with stage I and II survived, six of the eight having been followed for at least five years. None of the patients with stage III tumors survived. These authors felt that tumor spillage at the time of surgery, regardless of the stage of the tumor, may be associated with poor prognosis.

Therefore, postoperative pelvic irradiation (5000 rad tumor

dose in 5–6 weeks) is recommended for patients with more aggressive stage I and all stage II tumors. In patients with stage III disease, it is necessary to treat the entire abdomen in addition to the pelvis. The techniques are similar to those described for ovarian tumors. In Henderson's series, postoperative pelvic radiation combined with total hysterectomy and bilateral salpingo-oophorectomy resulted in a 50% survival as compared to a 25% five-year survival with surgery alone.[349]

In the series of 18 patients reported by Green and Scully, of eight who received postoperative radiation, survival ranged from nine months to 4½ years.[344] In contrast, of eight patients who received no irradiation, none survived for more than one year after exploration. Cohn, Rossano, and Fenton reported an overall survival rate of 40% with a combination of surgery and radiation.[346]

Chemotherapy

It is possible that chemotherapeutic agents may have a role in the management of these patients. Griffiths used chlorambucil as an adjuvant to pelvic irradiation following total abdominal hysterectomy and bilateral salpingo-oophorectomy and reported some long-term survivors.[362] Henderson and coworkers employed triple drug therapy, consisting of cyclophosphamide, actinomycin-D, and 5-fluorouracil in one patient with stage IIB and another with stage III.[249] One patient survived 6 months and the other 13.5 months without evidence of disease.

CARCINOMA OF THE VAGINA

Carcinoma of the vagina accounts for less than 2% of all gynecologic malignancies.[363–365] Plentl and Friedman reported 1,777 cases of vaginal cancer in 85,461 genital malignancies (2.08%).[366] Carcinoma of the vagina is defined as a malignant lesion, primarily arising in the vagina that does not involve the cervix nor the vulva. Negative biopsies of the cervix are mandatory.

In recent years, most series report a downward trend in this tumor which may be due, in part, to early detection with cervical cytology; or, more rigid diagnostic criteria, eliminating cancer arising from adjacent organs as cervix or vulva or metastases from endometrial cancer. Although primary vaginal cancers are historically squamous in origin, recent interest has focused on adenocarcinoma of the vagina, which has been encountered in young women who were exposed to diethylstibestrol (DES) in utero.

EPIDEMIOLOGY

There are no clear epidemiological predisposing factors to invasive squamous cell carcinoma of the vagina. Pride and co-workers noted that nine of 43 patients (20.9%) with invasive squamous cell carcinoma of the vagina had a prior history of radiation therapy to the pelvis (seven to 20 years previously).[367]

Local irradiation has been suggested as a possible causative factor for primary squamous cell carcinoma of the vagina.[368] Herbst and co-workers, reviewing the literature for possible etiological factors of primary squamous cell carcinoma, noted that the disease occurred primarily in the elderly population, but that no apparent etiology or associated factors were uncovered that predisposed a patient to this malignancy.[365] Herbst and co-workers noted that in their series, one-half of the patients (47.1%) were 60 years of age or older, with a peak incidence occurring in the 50–70-year age group. Pride and co-workers, in their review reported that the mean age for invasive squamous cell cancer was 62 years.[367] The medium age of the DES-exposed with clear cell adenocarcinoma of the vagina was 19 years.

In 1971, the sudden increase in the occurrence of clear cell adenocarcinoma of the vagina in women in their late teens and early twenties was found to be related to the use of DES by their mothers during pregnancy. Herbst and coworkers showed that the annual incidence of clear cell adenocarcinoma of the vagina and cervix had been found to correspond closely to the estimated usage of DES for pregnancy support in the U.S.[369] The annual incidence of the DES-associated cases appears to have decreased in 1978 and 1979, in comparison to 1973–1975. There is an association between the risk of developing cancer and the time of first exposure; the greatest risk was for females exposed early in pregnancy and declined for those whose exposure began in the 17th week or later. Although total dosage of DES ranged from 131 to 21,400 mg during pregnancy, precise information on dosage and duration of treatment was not available to evaluate the relation of these factors to the occurrence and location of the clear cell adenocarcinoma.

NATURAL HISTORY AND ANATOMIC CONSIDERATIONS

Vaginal cancers occur most commonly on the posterior wall of the upper third of the vagina. Plentl and Friedman, in an extensive review of the literature, noted that 51.7% of primary vaginal cancers occurred in the upper third of the vagina and 57.6% on the posterior wall.[366]

TUMOR DISSEMINATION

Vaginal cancer may spread along the vaginal wall to involve the cervix or vulva. However, if the cervix is involved the tumor must be considered a primary cervical lesion. The anterior vaginal cancers penetrate into the vesicovaginal septum early, giving the characteristic bullous edema of the bladder mucosa. The posterior lesions tend to distend and displace the vaginal mucosa and only after a considerable growth of tumor are the deep recto-vaginal layers invaded. The tumor spreads by continuity, invading the paracolpal and parametrial tissues with extension into the obturator fossa, cardinal ligaments, lateral pelvic walls, and uterosacral ligaments.

The lymphatic drainage of the vagina consists of an extensive intercommunicating network. The lymphatics in the upper portion of the vagina primarily drain by way of the lymphatics of the cervix, while the lowest portion of the vagina drains either cephalad to cervical lymphatics or following drainage patterns of the vulva into femoral and inguinal nodes. The anterior vaginal wall cancers drain most commonly into the deep pelvic nodes, with the interiliac and parametrial nodes being the first involved. However, due to the complex lymphatic system of the vagina, drainage may occur to any of the many nodal groups regardless of the location of the lesion.[366] The incidence of lymph node metastasis is directly proportional to the stage of the vaginal cancer. Plentl and Friedman, in their review of the literature, reported 141 of 679 patients with positive nodes (20.8%).[366] Metastases to the lungs or supraclavicular nodes in squamous cell carcinoma of the vagina tend to occur in the more advanced stages. However, Robboy and coworkers noted that in clear cell carcinoma in young women metastases to the lungs or supraclavicular lymph nodes accounted for a third of the recurrences, a proportion much greater than for squamous cell carcinoma of the cervix or vagina.[370]

PATHOLOGY

Over 90% of all vaginal tumors are epidermoid carcinoma. Primary carcinoma *in situ* or invasion of the vagina following treatment for carcinoma of the uterine cervix has been diagnosed in a small number of patients.[371,372] The possibility of a marginal recurrence of the cervical lesion cannot be excluded. However Perez and coworkers reported that when the vaginal tumor was detected more than 5 years after treatment of the cervical carcinoma, without evidence of local recurrence in the cervix, the results after therapy were comparable to those of *de novo* primary vaginal carcinoma.[373] Adenocarcinoma of the vagina accounts for approximately 5%. However, during the past eight years, there has been a marked increase in the number of patients with vaginal adenocarcinoma (almost all of the clear cell type) reported in young women with a history of intrauterine exposure to DES.

Clear cell adenocarcinoma of the vagina in the young female may affect any region of the vagina. Robboy and coworkers reported that 75% of tumors have a surface area of less than 12 cm^2, and of these, the majority are located in the anterior wall, usually in the upper third.[374] Most of the tumors are polypoid or nodular and the majority tend to penetrate less than 3 mm into the vaginal stroma. The most common microscopic features are cells with abundant cytoplasm, filled with glycogen and "hobnail" cells, which are characterized by bulbous nuclei that protrude into the lumen of tubules and cysts. Robboy notes that no squamous differentiation has been observed in these tumors.

Tavassoli and Norris reviewed the clinical and pathologic features of 60 smooth muscle tumors of the vagina, the most common mesenchymal tumor of the vagina in the adult woman.[375] They state that a neoplasm with moderate to marked atypia and greater than five mitotic figures per ten high power fields (HPF) merits the designation of leiomyosarcoma. Five neoplasms recurred in the 60 patients, and these were all larger than 3 cm in diameter, with greater than 5 mitosis per ten HPF and various degrees of atypia.

Rare cases of malignant melanoma have occasionally been reported in the literature. This cancer may arise from remnants of the urogenital sinus-containing pigment that may undergo malignant change. The tumors have the characteristic deep pigmentation of melanoma, forming an ulcerative lesion which bleeds easily. The tumor readily invades adjacent organs, involving bladder, rectum, and spreads to vulva and cervix with infiltration into the parametrium. Both hematogenous and lymphatic dissemination frequently occur.[376-378]

Sarcoma botryoides is generally found as a cancer of the vagina in childhood. It is a lesion of mesodermal origin with rhabdomyoblast elements present but rarely, if ever, cartilage and bone. The tumor rapidly fills the vagina and can be noted protruding from the introitus with the characteristic grape-like appearance externally. The tumor is locally invasive and may involve femoral, parametrial, and periaortic lymph nodes. Hematogenous metastases are common predominantly to the lung, liver, and bones. Primary leiomyosarcoma of the vagina has been occasionally reported.[379]

CLINICAL MANIFESTATIONS

Most invasive squamous cell carcinomas of the vagina present with vaginal bleeding. This may be in the form of dysfunctional bleeding or postcoital spotting. Vaginal discharge is common. Only in more advanced stages, with tumor spread to adjacent organs, are these symptoms associated with dysuria and pelvic pain.[380]

DIAGNOSIS AND STAGING

The clinical diagnosis of carcinoma of the vagina is best made by a careful speculum examination and palpation of the vagina. Since many of the cancers originate from the posterior wall of the vagina, speculum must be carefully rotated in all positions and levels during the exam so not to obscure the lesion by the blades of the speculum. Cytology is most helpful in detecting early squamous cell carcinoma of the vagina, but is not as useful in the clear cell adenocarcinomas, which often grow in a subepithelial location. Colposcopy is particularly suited for directed biopsies in abnormal sites in the vagina. Once the diagnosis of invasive carcinoma has been confirmed pathologically the patient should undergo a metastatic evaluation, including cystoscopy and proctosigmoidoscopy. The patient is best staged under anesthesia by the gynecologist and radiation therapist. Further biopsies of the vagina are taken at various sites to delineate the limits of abnormal vaginal mucosa. Multiple biopsies of the cervix are mandatory. The patients are staged using the FIGO staging system (see Table 25-29).

TABLE 25-29. Carcinoma of the Vagina Staging Classification FIGO Nomenclature

Stage O	Carcinoma *in situ;* intraepithelial carcinoma
Stage I	Carcinoma is limited to the vaginal wall
Stage II	Carcinoma has involved the subvaginal tissue but has not extended to the pelvic wall
Stage III	Carcinoma has extended to the pelvic wall
Stage IV	Carcinoma has extended beyond the true pelvis or has involved the mucosa of the bladder or rectum. Bullous edema as such does not permit a case to be allotted to stage IV
Stage IVA	Spread of the growth to adjacent organs
Stage IVB	Spread to distant organs

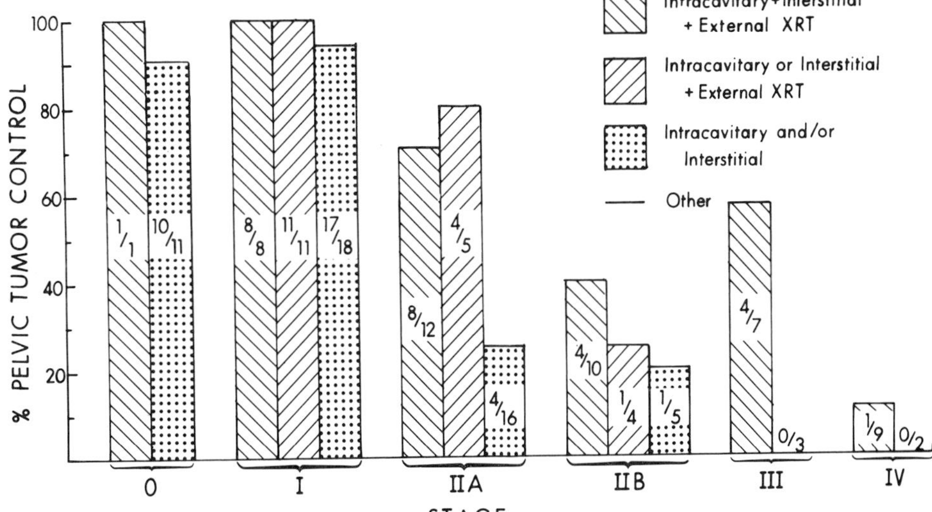

FIG. 25-27. Tumor control in the vagina and pelvis as a function of type of treatment used and anatomic stage of disease. There is a critical need for the addition of external beam irradiation in patients with tumor beyond stage I to improve tumor control. (Perez CA, Korba A, Sharma S et al: Int J Radiat Oncol Biol Phys 2:639–649, 1977)

GENERAL PRINCIPLES OF MANAGEMENT

Early reports suggested that tumors of the vagina had a poorer prognosis than those in the uterine cervix, the cure rates for the former ranging from 20% to 50%. However, several authors in recent publications have pointed out the complexity of management of these patients and the need for careful radiotherapeutic techniques, which has resulted in survival similar to that for carcinoma of the uterine cervix.[381] Perez and coworkers have suggested that a correlation can be drawn between the doses of irradiation given to various stages of carcinomas and probability of local tumor control.[382]

Radiation therapy is the treatment of choice for most carcinomas of the vagina even though some authors advocate a surgical approach.[383] However, operations should be discouraged because of the excellent tumor control and good functional results obtained with adequate radiation therapy. Surgical procedures may be reserved for the treatment of irradiation failures.

Brown and coworkers, Rutledge, and Perez and coworkers have reported excellent tumor control and survival in patients with carcinoma *in situ* and stage I invasive carcinoma.[363,373,385] These authors have cautioned against an overly aggressive therapy in these early lesions because of the possibility of producing mucosal injury and interference with sexual function. Carcinoma *in situ* and the majority of patients with stage I superficial tumors can be treated adequately with intracavitary and interstitial sources alone. If the carcinoma is less than .5 cm thick, intracavitary irradiation with a vaginal cylinder to deliver 8000 rad to the mucosa will yield excellent results (over 90% tumor control). If the lesion is thicker or localized to one of the walls of the vagina, the addition of an interstitial single plane implant will deliver an adequate dose of irradiation to the tumor limiting the exposure to the uninvolved normal tissues.

In the patients with more extensive stage I lesions, external irradiation should be administered to treat the paravaginal tissues as well as the regional lymph nodes, in addition to intracavitary and interstitial therapy.

Perez and coworkers described approximately the same tumor control in the pelvis of carcinoma *in situ* and stage I with or without the addition of external beam irradiation.[383] However, better tumor control (75–80%) was observed in stage IIA with the addition of external irradiation in comparison with 25% with brachytherapy only (see Fig. 25-27).

Patients with stage II require a more comprehensive approach which should include external beam irradiation and brachytherapy. In general, doses of 2000 rad to the whole pelvis are delivered followed by a supplemental dose to the parametria with a midline shielding block (3000 rads). This is combined with interstitial and intracavitary therapy to deliver a minimum of 5500–7000 rad to the base of the tumor and 5000 rad to the pelvic lymph nodes.

In the more advanced lesions (stages III and IVA) the results with irradiation have been less than satisfactory, with only 25–30% pelvic tumor control and survival. Therefore, higher doses with a greater contribution from the external irradiation are used. Several authors have suggested a combination of irradiation and surgery in an effort to improve therapeutic results. Rhabdomyosarcoma of the vagina is generally treated with a combination of surgical resection, irradiation and systemic chemotherapy.[385] Melanoma and leiomyosarcoma are treated primarily with radical surgical resection.

Techniques of Irradiation

The pelvic portals should encompass the entire vagina down to the introitus and the pelvic lymph nodes to the upper

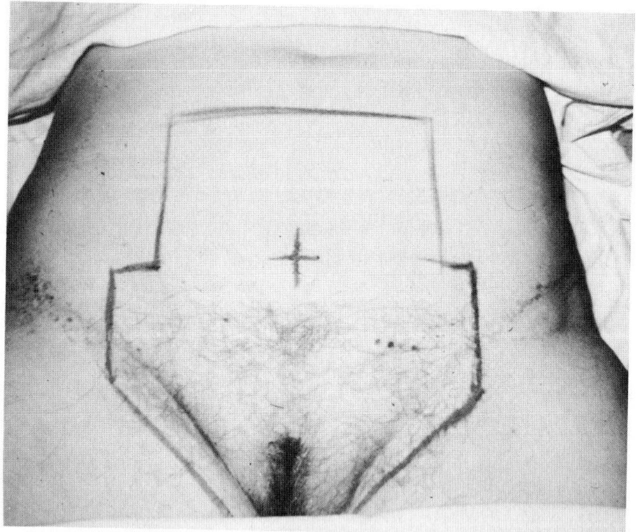

FIG. 25-28. Portal for external beam irradiation of the pelvis, including inguinal lymph nodes.

portion of the common iliac chain. Portals of 15 × 15 cm or 15 × 18 cm are usually adequate.

In lesions of the lower two-thirds of the vagina, it is necessary to electively include the inguinal lymph nodes in the irradiated field even when no palpable lymph nodes are present (see Fig. 25-28).

Intracavitary therapy is carried out with varying diameter vaginal cylinders, such as the Burnett or the Bloedorn or Delclos applicators. The largest possible diameter should be used to improve the ratio of mucosa/tumor dose (see Fig. 25-29).

Interstitial therapy with ^{137}Cesium, ^{226}Radium needles or after loading ^{192}Iridium needles have been employed. Single plane, double plane, or volume implants should be planned depending on the extent and thickness of the tumor.

When the lesion is in the upper third, it is the authors practice to treat the upper vagina with the same intracavitary arrangement as in carcinoma of the uterine cervix, including an intrauterine tandem and vaginal colpostats. The middle and distal vagina are treated in a subsequent insertion with

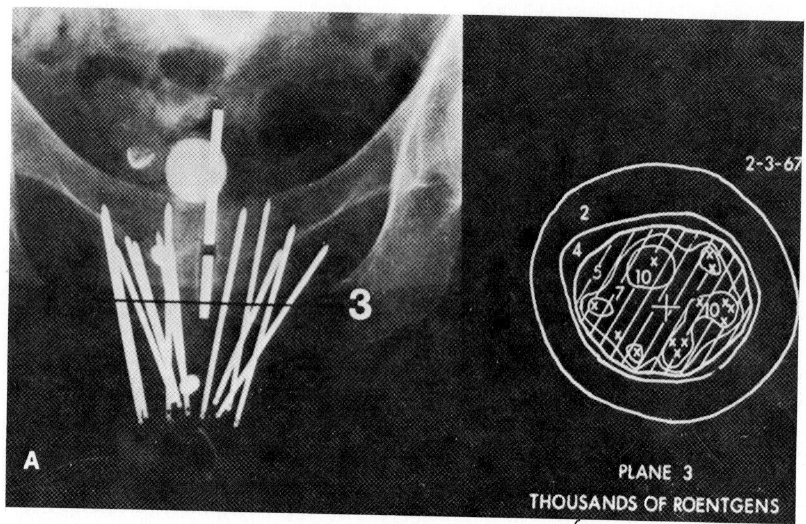

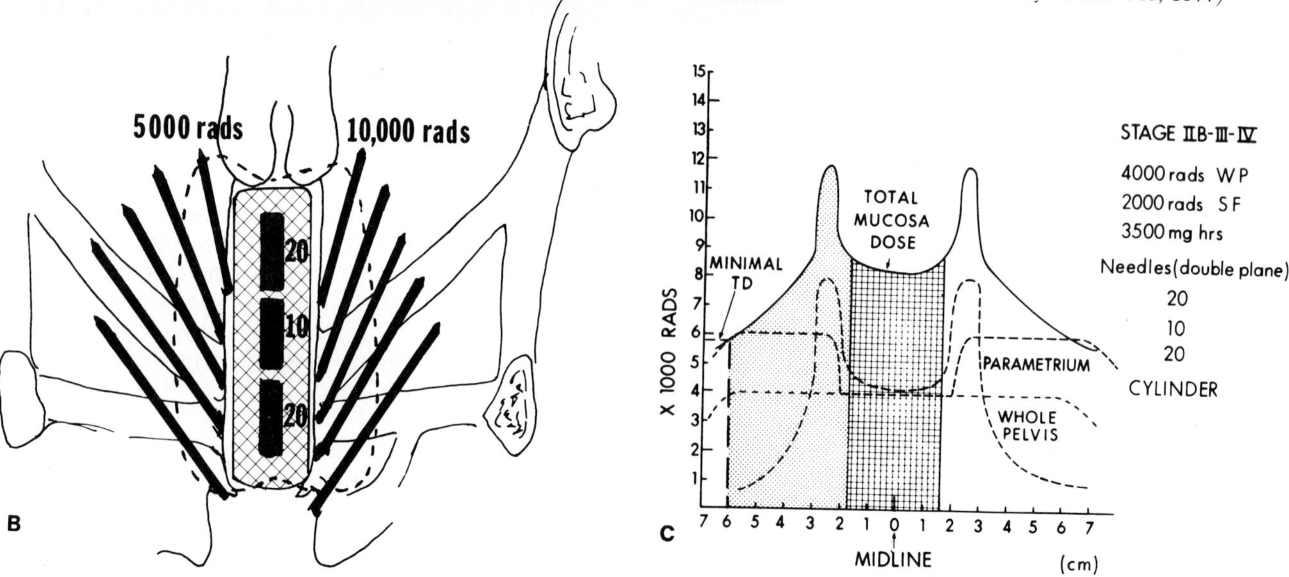

FIG. 25-29. *A*, Example of an intracavitary and double plane interstitial implant used to treat an extensive carcinoma of the vagina. This was combined with external beam 22 MV photon irradiation (4000 rad whole pelvis and additional 2000 rad parametrial dose). *B*, Distribution of radioactive sources and minimal tumor doses around primary tumor. *C*, Dose profile for patients with advanced vaginal carcinoma, using a combination of whole pelvic (*WP*) and parametrial external irradiation (*SF*), and intracavitary and double plane interstitial implant. (Perez CA, Korba AA, Sharma S et al: Int J Radiat Oncol Biol Phys 2:639–649, 1977)

TABLE 25-30. Carcinoma of the Vagina: Absolute 5-year Survival, NED* Patients Treated by Irradiation

	ALIVE AT 5 YEARS, NED		DEAD WITH TUMOR, ANY SITE		DISTANT METASTASIS	
STAGE	# PATIENT	%	# PATIENTS	%	# PATIENTS	%
O	10/12	83	0	0	0	0
I	26/32	81	4	10	2	5.4
IIA	17/33	57	15	45	6	18
IIB	5/19	26	14	73	5	26
III	3/10	30	7	70	4	40
IV	1/11	9	10	90	6	54

* NED: No evidence of disease.
Perez CA, Korba A, Sharma S et al: Int J Radiat Oncol Biol Phys 2:639, 1977

a vaginal cylinder. If the entire dose has been delivered to the upper vagina, a blank source can be used in the cylinder. Other wise, a lower intensity source can be inserted to deliver the desired dose.

For small lesions (carcinoma *in situ* and stage I), a dose of 6000 rad .5 cm under the mucosa is adequate. For larger lesions, doses in the range of 7000–8000 rad are necessary. In general, the vaginal mucosa receives an estimated 8000–10,000 rad, which usually is well-tolerated. The pelvic lymph nodes usually receive 5000–6000 rad with whole pelvis and split fields.

Results of Treatment

Welton and Kottmeier reported an overall 5-year survival of 26.5% in 117 patients treated primarily by radiation therapy.[286] Fifty-seven patients (48.8%) had persistent or recurrent primary tumor.

Rutledge reported a 35% five-year survival in patients with stage I or II carcinoma with some patients dying of intercurrent disease.[363] At Washington University, 11 of 12 patients with stage 0 carcinoma of the vagina treated by various techniques had control of the tumor at least 3 years after initial irradiation. In stage I, the tumor control was over 95% (38 of 39 patients treated). In more advanced patients the pelvic control decreased significantly (about 40–50% depending on tumor extent and techniques used). Table 25-30 shows the 5-year tumor-free survival in the group of patients treated at Washington University with radiation therapy alone.

The incidence of pelvic lymph nodes varies with the stage and location of the primary tumor. Welton and Kottmeier reported eight of 117 with clinically palpable inguinal nodes, four of them having metastatic tumor confirmed by biopsy.[386] Brown and coworkers observed five of 76 patients with metastatic inguinal nodes on admission and six additional patients who developed metastases in the lymph nodes sometime after the initial treatment.[384] Perez and coworkers reported six of 113 patients (5.1%) with invasive carcinoma who had clinical evidence of metastatic inguinal lymph nodes at the time of diagnosis.[382] In all but one the tumor was located near the introitus or at the fourcette.

Since vaginal carcinoma can be effectively treated with surgery after postirradiation local failure, meticulous and regular follow-up examinations are important to detect the recurrence early. The surgical procedure may range from a wide local excision or partial vaginectomy to a posterior or total pelvic exenteration.

Complications of Therapy

Major complications are noted in less than 5% of the patients treated for stages I and II and in about 6–10% of the patients with more advanced lesions. At Washington University there were three rectal strictures and two rectovaginal fistulae noted in 113 patients treated. Hemorrhagic cystitis occasionally develops (3–5%).

The most frequent minor complications are fibrosis of the vagina and small areas of mucosal necrosis that are noted in about 10% of the patients.

Treatment of Clear Cell Carcinoma

Stage I lesions of the cervix or vagina can be treated either with surgery or radiation therapy.[369,387] All other stages should be treated with radiation therapy.

Surgery for stage I clear cell carcinoma may have the advantage of ovarian preservation and better vaginal function following skin graft. Yet, Wharton and coworkers advocate intracavitary or transvaginal irradiation for the treatment of small tumors, since this may yield excellent tumor control with a functional vagina and preservation of ovarian function.[387]

Vaginal clear cell carcinoma would require removal of most of the vagina. Since the tumor often spreads subepithelially, it is important that the surgeon obtain frozen section biopsies of the distal margins of resection to determine the lower limits of the surgery. The vagina is dissected first before the abdominal procedure. A radical hysterectomy and lymph node dissection is necessary both for vaginal or cervical clear cell carcinoma. This procedure is necessary to encompass the parametria and paracopus to the side walls of the pelvis. Para-aortic node should be sampled prior to the procedure to determine whether there is lymphatic disease beyond the pelvis. Fletcher and coworkers reported the results in 24 young women treated with irradiation alone (two combined with surgery), 15 of them followed for over 2 years.[388] Eighteen of the patients are surviving, 17 of them tumor free. One patient with an extension lesion has a vaginal recurrence and one patient died of a pulmonary embolus after removal of radium needles.

CARCINOMA OF THE VULVA

The skin and mucosa of the vulva are prone to a variety of malignancies, which due to the extensive lymphatics, can result in an early node metastases.[389,390] The modern concept of their pathogenesis, dissemination, and therapy was defined by Taussig in the classic text *Diseases of the Vulva* in 1923.[391] The frankly malignant carcinoma of the vulva comprises about 3–4% of all female primary genital malignancies. Ninety percent of vulvar cancers are of the squamous type. Basal cell cancer, although the most common malignancy of the skin, accounts for only 3% of vulvar cancer. Other malignancies encountered on the vulva are adenocarcinoma of the Bartholin duct and gland, Paget's disease, which may be associated with adenocarcinoma of the sweat glands, melanoma, sarcoma, and verrucous carcinoma (see Fig. 25-30).

Stanley Way described the surgical management of carcinoma of the vulva and defined the lymphatic drainage pathways.[392] Collins, McKelvey, and Green increased knowledge of carcinoma of the vulva by their clinical investigations.[393–394]

EPIDEMIOLOGY

The median age for carcinoma *in situ* and early invasive squamous cell carcinoma of the vulva is 48 years.[396,397] Invasive carcinoma of the vulva is a disease of the elderly, rarely occuring below the age of 40 (the median age is 60). Other vulvar lesions are frequently present in patients with invasive carcinoma of the cervix. Associated medical illnesses include hypertension, cardiovascular disease, obesity, and venereal diseases.[395,398–400] Diabetes is the single most important medical condition associated with vulvar carcinoma although it does not appear to be solely related to advanced age; in Green's series, only 18% of the younger age group were reported to have diabetes along with their vulvar malignancy.[395] Associated malignancies reported are breast, endometrial, and cervical carcinoma.

FIG. 25-30. Lymphatic drainage of the vulva by major channels. The lymphatics form an extensive network that is divided into the superficial and deep inguinal and femoral nodal groups. Efferents drain primarily to the deep femoral nodes along the femoral artery and to Cloquet's node at the upper end of the femoral canal. The insert shows the lines of surgical incision.

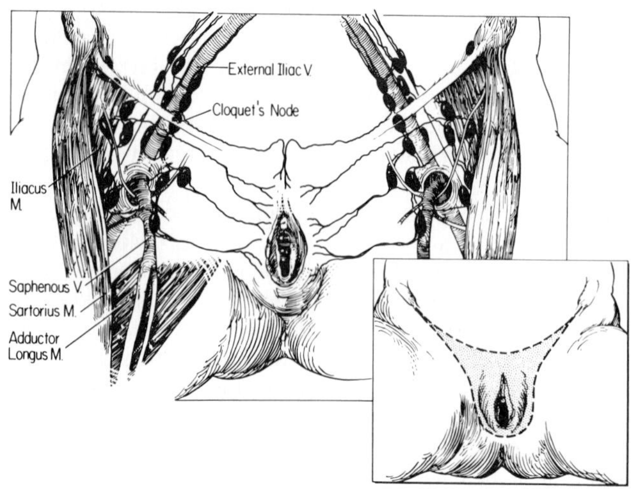

PATHOLOGY

No discussion of carcinoma of the vulva is complete without proper reference to the premalignant lesions of the vulva. Leukoplakia (white lesion) has been considered a pre-cancerous lesion and Taussig reported finding leukoplakia vulvitis in about one-half of his patients with carcinoma.[401] The white epithelium may result from a thick layer of keratin, while the epithelium underneath is atrophic and inactive. It is the underlying epithelial cells that are significant in the development of neoplasia. Magrina and coworkers noted 70% of their patients with vulvar dystrophy (atrophic in 9, hypertrophic in 41, and unspecified when no previous biopsies were available in 24).[398]

In an effort to better define the various skin lesions seen on the vulva, a classification of vulva dystrophies was adopted in 1976 by the International Society for the Study of Vulvar Disease.[402] The gross changes seen on the vulva may be diffused or localized, may be thick or thin, white or red. The classification as noted below is based on histopathologic features according to the microscopic changes:

1. Hyperplastic dystrophy
   Without atypia:
   Epithelial hyperplasia is present; varying degree of hyperkeratosis; chronic inflammation may be present; no atypia is noted.
   With atypia:
   Mild, moderate, or severe.
2. Lichen sclerosis
   Variable degree of hyperkeratosis and thinning of the squamous epithelium; the dermis may be infiltrated with lymphocytes and plasma cells.
3. Mixed dystrophy (lichen sclerosis with foci of epithelial hyperplasia)
   Without atypia
   With atypia
4. Paget's disease of the vulva
   A distinct clinicopathologic entity with characteristic large pale cells present in the epithelium and skin adnexal; adenocarcinoma of the underlying sweat glands may be associated with Paget's disease in about 20% of cases.
5. Carcinoma *in situ*
   May present clinically as papules or macules coalescent or discrete, single or multiple. The histologic appearance is characterized by loss of epithelial architecture, which extends through the full thickness of the epithelium. Mytotic figures, giant cells and multinucleated cells are present throughout the epithelium.

Basal cell carcinoma constitutes about 3% of all vulvar malignancies.[403] Metastases do not occur in the pure form of the tumor and the lesion can be cured by wide local excision.

Verrucous carcinoma of that vulva is a rare lesion that presents as a cauliflower-like growth that is locally destructive and often difficult to differentiate microscopically from benign epithelial proliferating lesions. Lucas and coworkers described these lesions as soft, warty, with branching papillary stalks causing local destruction.[404] Lymph nodes, although enlarged from inflammation, are free of metastasis and vascular invasion is not demonstrated.

Tavassoli and Norris reviewed cases of smooth muscle tumors of the vulva and noted that the sarcomas were leiomyosarcomas.[405] They state that neoplasms should be regarded as sarcomas if they are greater than 5 cm, have infiltrating margins, and 5 or more mytotic figures per 10 HPF.

Malignant melanoma is a particularly aggressive tumor of the vulva. In two reported studies, the primary site of occurrence involved mucosal sites, particularly the labia minora and clitoris.[406,407] Chung and coworkers noted that no patient with either level I or II depth of penetration had lymph node metastasis.[406]

NATURAL HISTORY

About 7% of the 128 patients with vulvar dystrophy reported by Kaufman and coworkers had a histologic diagnosis of squamous dysplasia. It appears that 20% of vulva dysplasias will result in invasive epidermoid carcinoma if left untreated.[408] These lesions may coexist either as invasive cancer, carcinoma *in situ*, or vulva dystrophy.

Plentl and Friedman, in their review of the literature, noted that the labia is the usual site of carcinoma in 70% of cases, with the labia majora three times more frequently involved than the labia minora.[409] The clitoris is involved in 13% of cases and Bartholin's gland in 1%.

Seeding by contact has been considered as a means of the development of contiguous foci. The extensive and free anastomosis of lymphatics of the vulva is probably a more plausable explanation for the often multicentric origin of these tumors.[392] The well-differentiated lesions tend to spread slowly on the surface and invade the underlying stroma less readily than the more anaplastic lesions. Increase in size of the lesion, invasion below the basement membrane, and the degree of anaplasia of tumor are related to lymph node metastasis.[410] Squamous carcinoma may also spread by continuity and involve adjacent organs such as vagina, urethra, and anus. The squamous carcinoma spreads rapidly in the lymphatic system and involves the inquinal lymph nodes with subsequent involvement of femoral and deep inguinal nodes. Rarely are tumor emboli found in the lymphatic channels.[410] It is rare for vulvar cancer to spread hematogenously except for melanoma. Only in advanced disease are blood vessels invaded, and usually the large veins are involved.

PATTERNS OF SPREAD

The lymphatics of the vulva form an extensive and diffuse network which Way described as a superficial inguinal nodal group along the inguinal ligament.[392] He also noted superficial femoral nodes in the femoral triangle around the saphenous vein and deep femoral nodes along the femoral vessels terminating in lymph nodes under the inguinal ligament, at the upper end of the femoral canal. The latter is referred to as the node of Cloquet or Rosenmuller. Subsequent drainage occurs into the deep pelvic nodes, mainly along the external iliac, obturator, and hypogastric chain and along the course of the round ligament. A group of nodes are located in the lower portion of the mons veneris and around the root of the clitoris. Drainage from this area is to Cloquet's node, around the bladder neck or the lymphatic channels on the inner aspect of the pubic symphysis, which communicates directly with the deep pelvic nodes. Plentl and Friedmann noted that the collecting trunks from the prepuce and the anterior portion of the labia drain into the superficial inguinal and femoral nodes and then into deep inguinal and femoral nodes.[409] The lymphatics of the clitoris may bypass the femoral nodes and enter directly into the pelvis accompanying the dorsal vein of the clitoris. The lymphatics of the vulva may also enter the pelvis directly between the insertion of the rectus muscle at the superior aspect of the symphysis and drain into the deep pelvic nodes. The drainage from the lower portion of the labia and fourchette drains directly into the superficial femoral nodes, and superficial inguinal nodes, particularly those lying below the inguinal ligament. The lymphatics from the posterior portion of the vulva are medial to the crural fold.

The overall incidence of positive lymph nodes in vulvar malignancy is about 40%. Clinically, it is difficult to assess the presence of tumor in inguinal and femoral nodes. The nodes may be enlarged by inflammation while nonpalpable nodes may actually contain cancer. Way has emphasized the fact that if Cloquet's node contains no tumor, the chance of deep pelvic nodal involvement is slight.[392] Most series report that less than 2% of all women, regardless of the stage and location of the tumor, will have pelvic node metastasis in the absence of positive inguinal or femoral nodes. The overall incidence of positive pelvic nodes is about 10%.

CLINICAL PRESENTATION

The symptoms of carcinoma of the vulva are variable and insidious. Buscema and coworkers found that 20% of their patients were asymptomatic and the lesion was found only on pelvic examination. Carcinoma of the vulva is one condition in which both patient and physician delay often occur. However, Green noted earlier diagnoses of vulvar cancer in recent years, probably due to educational efforts both on the part of the patient and the physician.[395] The most common complaint is the presence of a mass or growth in the vulvar area.[400] Pruritus vulvae, bleeding, and pain are often noted as presenting symptoms.

The diagnosis of vulvar neoplasia is made only biopsy. An initial sample of tissue can be obtained by a rotating punch biopsy as an out-patient procedure. Colposcopy has not been found to be particularly helpful in identifying areas to biopsy. The use of toluidine blue has been advocated to help localize areas to biopsy; the stain may reveal areas of increased nuclear activity thus defining a lesion at risk for biopsy. The use of topical 5-FU is also of help in delineating areas to biopsy. In approximately one week after the use of topical 5-FU, the lesions at risk are red and clearly defined.

TABLE 25-31. Staging of Carcinoma of the Vulva*

Stage O	Carcinoma *in situ*
Stage I	Tumor confined to vulva, 2 cm or less in diameter. Nodes are not palpable or are palpable in either groin, not enlarged, mobile (not clinically suspicious of neoplasm).
Stage II	Tumor confined to the vulva, more than 2 cm in diameter. Nodes are not palpable or are palpable in either groin, not enlarged, mobile (not clinically suspicious of neoplasm).
Stage III	Tumor of any size with adjacent spread to the urethra and any or all of the vagina, the perineum, and the anus; or, the nodes are palpable in either or both groins (enlarged, firm, and mobile, not fixed but clinically suspicious of neoplasm).
Stage IV	Tumor of any size infiltrating the bladder mucosa or the rectal mucosa or both, including the upper part of the urethral mucosa; or, fixed or ulcerated nodes in either or both groins.

* FIGO nomenclature

If invasive carcinoma is not found on the directed biopsy, the suspected lesion should be biopsied under general anesthesia. A large biopsy should be obtained so that normal surrounding tissue is included in the biopsy. Multiple sites should also be biopsied as indicated due to the multicentric origin of these lesions. The vagina, cervix, and pelvis should be carefully examined, including bimanual palpation and D & C. Metastatic evaluation includes chest film, proctosigmoidoscopy, and cystoscopy.

STAGING

The FIGO nomenclature has been adopted (see Table 25-31). The rules for classification are similar to those at the other gynecologic sites. Tumors present in the vulva as secondary growths from either a genital or extragenital site should be excluded. Malignant melanoma should be separately reported.

The accuracy of clinical staging is limited as in other malignancies. Plentl and Freidman, reviewing the data on 605 patients, noted that 38% of patients with clinically palpable nodes were free of tumor.[409] Among patients with clinically normal nodes, 35% showed microscopic invasion. This staging system makes no reference to the histology nor to the depth of invasion below the basement membrane of the epithelium. Wharton and coworkers reviewed 45 patients with invasive squamous cell carcinoma of the vulva, 2 cm or less in diameter.[411] Twenty-five of the 45 patients had carcinomas that invaded the stroma to a depth of 5 mm or less. None of these patients had positive lymph nodes. Therefore, it is essential to include the degree of anaplasia and depth of stromal penetration in any therapeutic decision. Furthermore, the size of the lesion does not necessarily correlate with nodal involvement. Collins and coworkers found positive nodes in 20% of small vulvar lesions.[343] An analysis of any series of vulvar cancer must include, in addition to the clinical staging, the surgical and pathologic stagings.

PRINCIPLES OF TREATMENT

Historically, the treatment of carcinoma of the vulva has been surgical. Radiation therapy has not been found effective in its management. The results of treatment with this modality have shown poorer survival when compared to the results of surgical treatment. However, this may not be entirely due to its effectiveness, but to biased case selection (*i.e.*, patients who are not medically able to tolerate surgery or have extensive inoperable lesions).

Stage O (Carcinoma in situ *of the Vulva)*

The diagnosis of carcinoma *in situ* (CIS) must be confirmed before treatment. Although the histopathology of CIS of the vulva varies greatly, it does not influence the treatment modality. The time-honored treatment for CIS is a simple vulvectomy. This operative procedure has been predicated because of the multicentric location of these tumors. The survival rate with simple vulvectomy approaches 100%.[412]

Collins and coworkers have advocated radical vulvectomy for CIS.[413] In 4 of their 41 patients, an unsuspected invasive lesion was found to co-exist with the CIS in the final vulvectomy specimen. Therefore, if invasion is found in the final specimen, proper initial therapy would have been administered prior to nodal dissection.

Some investigators have recently evaluated the use of less radical surgical procedures for CIS of the vulva since even the simple vulvectomy causes disfigurement that can be detrimental to normal sexual activity. If the CIS is discrete and localized and the rest of the vulva appears normal, wide local excision may be performed. Buscema and coworkers evaluated 106 patients with carcinoma *in situ* of the vulva, treated by simple vulvectomy or wide local excision.[396] The incidence of recurrence was essentially the same in both groups. Inasmuch as CIS involves only the skin and not the stroma, Rutledge has devised a technique that excises the vulvar skin, conserving the fat, muscle, and glandular structures below the skin. A split thickness graft from the inner thigh is then applied to cover the denuded area. This technique has been shown to yield better cosmetic results than vulvectomy.[414]

Treatment of stage 0 cancer of the vulva with topical 5% 5-FU over a 2–3 month period has been advocated by some investigators as effective treatment of CIS. However, some find this inadequate. Dinitrochlorobenzene (DCNB) has also been used experimentally with some success.

Paget's disease of the vulva, although considered a carcinoma *in situ*, is often difficult to irradicate. The tumor extends subepithelially and requires a wide excision around the entire vulva. It is often necessary to take frozen sections in the remaining skin tissue to make sure that the tumor has not extended to these sites. The lesion may extend into the anal canal requiring dissection in this area. If Paget's disease is associated with an adenocarcinoma of the sweat glands, the treatment should be radical vulvectomy and bilateral groin dissection. Recurrent or persistent Paget's disease may respond topically to bleomycin.[415]

Stage I

Treatment of stage I squamous cell cancer of the vulva has recently been the subject of re-evaluation in an effort to minimize the extent of surgery. Wharton and coworkers, evaluating 25 patients with invasive squamous cell cancer 2 cm or less in diameter (and less than 5 mm of stromal invasion) found no patient with positive lymph nodes, no recurrences, and no deaths as a result of vulvar cancer.[411] They felt that the term microinvasive carcinoma of the vulva is justified and that patients with lesions of this type may be treated by vulvectomy without lymph node dissection. Parker and coworkers recommended radical vulvectomy without lymphadenectomy if the lesion is less than 2 cm, stromal invasion is 5 mm or less in depth, if there is no vascular channel invasion, and the tumor is well-differentiated.[416] However, there are series that report lymph node metastasis in which the tumor depth of invasion was no greater than 5 mm.[417] In an effort to determine the presence of lymph node involvement in early cancer of the vulva, Di Saia and coworkers developed an operative procedure that removes the superficial inguinal lymph nodes bilaterally for frozen section.[397] If the nodes are negative, no further groin dissection is done and a radical vulvectomy is performed.

The definition of microinvasive carcinoma of the vulva remains controversial. Until it is clear that microinvasive carcinoma of the vulva is a separate entity, radical vulvectomy and lymph node dissection must be advocated as the treatment of choice as with other patients with stage I carcinoma of the vulva. The radical vulvectomy and lymph node dissection need not be as extensive in stage I as in the more advanced stages.

The operation for squamous cell carcinoma of the vulva is a radical vulvectomy with dissection of the groin nodes as outlined by Rutledge, Smith, and Franklin.[418]

Stages II and III

In these stages, the operation must be more extensive than that for stage I. If the distal urethra is involved, it may be necessary to excise as much as 2 cm of the urethra. The urethra is plicated to prevent urinary incontinence. Extension into the vagina may require vaginal resection to allow for clear margins. Rarely does anal extension require a posterior exenteration. It may be necessary to section the anal sphincter to remove adequate tissue. In order to prevent wound breakdown, suction drainage is used and pressure on the skin flaps is avoided. The patient should remain in bed approximately 5 days postoperatively. Wound breakdown may occur with the extensive resection required in the stage II and III lesions. Usually this is allowed to granulate but at times it is necessary to resort to a gracilis muscle graft. The results of the muscle graft are particularly gratifying as a split thickness graft from a donor's site is not used.

The inclusion of an extraperitoneal node dissection is controversial. Way has recommended evaluating Cloquet's node as the indicator of pelvic node involvement.[392] Green showed no instance of deep pelvic node metastasis in the absence of superficial inguinal-femoral node involvement.[395] Piver and Xynos reviewed 33 patients with carcinoma of the clitoris and found no patients with positive pelvic node metastasis without inguinal node involvement.[419] Even with the addition of a pelvic node dissection, the survival rate for patients with pelvic lymph node metastasis is only 20%.[409] Therefore, the pelvic node dissection should be limited to those patients who demonstrate inguinal or femoral node involvement and should not be performed as a routine procedure. An anterior lesion may be at greater risk for deep pelvic node involvement than a posterior vulvar lesion.

Plentl and Friedman, in their extensive review, showed an overall survival of 75% in patients with negative nodes and a 41.5% survival in patients with positive nodes.[409] Green, in his series, showed an 87% five-year survival in patients with negative nodes and a 33% in patients with positive nodes.[395] He defined his results by clinical stage and found an 87% five-year survival for stages I and II, a 56% for stage III, and 8% for stage IV. Morley reported a corrected 5-year survival rate of approximately 80% for patients treated with radical vulvectomy and groin lymphadenectomy.[400] If the regional lymph nodes were negative, it was approximately 93%.

Stage IV

Tumors that infiltrate the bladder or rectal mucosa are best treated with radical vulvectomy and the addition of an exenteration. Those patients with stage IV who have fixation to the bone or distant metastasis must be treated palliatively for control of symptoms.

MALIGNANT MELANOMA OF THE VULVA

Malignant melanoma of the vulva is generally treated by radical vulvectomy, bilateral groin node dissection, and often the addition of pelvic lymphadenectomy. Morrow and Rutledge reported a 5-year survival of 50% in patients treated in this manner.[407] In their series, the vagino-urethral margin of resection is the most frequent site of recurrence. They further state that prognosis is related to the stage of the vulvar cancer. Chung and others, in their series, also recommend a similar operation with the use of pelvic node dissection if the inguinal nodes are positive.[406] They further evaluated their cases as to the level of invasion and noted that in level I and II no patient has lymph node involvement. Positive lymph nodes were found only with levels III, IV, and V. Despite radical surgery, the mortality was 60% at level III and IV and 80% at level V. It would appear that a wide local excision may be adequate for lesions up to level II and the radical procedure should be reserved for levels III through V.

SITES OF FAILURE

The most frequent failure is local persistence or recurrence.[393,420] This may indicate inadequate operative resection.

Early recurrences tend to involve the pelvis or distant organs, usually concomitantly.[409] These recurrences relate to the presence of nodal involvement and correlate with the size of the lesion and degree of anaplasia. Local recurrences following radical vulvectomy tend to be late, often after 3 or more years. These may be new primaries developing in the field of the previous vulvectomy.[418] The size of the initial malignancy correlates with both persistence and recurrent disease. Collins and others noted a 76.5% survival with initial lesions of less than 3 cm and 38.2% with larger tumors.[393]

COMPLICATIONS OF TREATMENT

Wound breakdown is the most frequent complication and skin grafting may be necessary in such cases. About one-third of the patients complain of leg edema, which may be transient or chronic. The use of elastic stockings is recommended for 6 months postoperatively. Rupture of the femor artery has occasionally been reported. The occasional use of the sartorius muscle graft over the femoral vessel has decreased this complication. The use of pressure dressings is not recommended as this creates necrosis at the edges of the skin flap.

FUTURE CONSIDERATIONS

There are certain specific areas that require a reassessment in vulvar cancer as to future consideration for management and treatment. The first is an emphasis on early diagnosis. This requires education on the part of both patient and physician. Green, in comparing his two 25-year series, has shown a dramatic decrease in patients in which only palliation could be given from 27% in 1927 through 1950, to only 5% in 1951 through 1976.[395] The definition of microinvasive carcinoma needs further clarification and study. Since the groin dissection is the most morbid portion of the surgical treatment, radiation therapy could be considered in lieu of the groin dissection. Elective radiation therapy to the groin (4500–5000 rad in 5 weeks) may be adequate to treat nodes that are not palpable and contain only microscopic tumor. If there are palpable nodes, a radical groin dissection would be necessary rather than radiation therapy. Postoperative irradiation has been advocated by some to decrease the probability of local recurrence. Because of the sensitive skin, perspiration, friction of clothes, and bacterial contamination, irradiation of the vulvar and perineal area should carefully be done, emphasizing hygiene and skin care.

TROPHOBLASTIC TUMORS

Choriocarcinoma is characterized by anaplastic trophoblastic tissue composed of cyto- and syncytio-trophoblast that has lost its capacity to form a normal villous structure.

Trophoblastic tumors most commonly develop following a molar pregnancy, (50% of cases) but may be seen after an antecedent term pregnancy, abortion, or ectopic gestation. After a molar pregnancy, the tumor may consist either of a hydatidiform mole or choriocarcinoma. However, after a nonmolar antecedent pregnancy, all trophoblastic tumors show the histologic pattern of choriocarcinoma. The natural history of persistent trophoblastic tumor can follow three paths: spontaneous regression, local invasion, and distant dissemination.

The trophoblastic tumor may remain locally invasive in 15% of patients following evacuation of molar pregnancy, and less commonly following termination of a term pregnancy or abortion. The trophoblastic tumor is often an invasive mole (chorioadenoma destruens) when it follows a molar gestation and a locally invasive choriocarcinoma following a term pregnancy or abortion.

Prior to the use of chemotherapy, the only effective treatment for gestational trophoblastic neoplasms was surgery and occasionally for palliation, radiation therapy. Even when the tumor was apparently confined to the uterus, only a 40% cure rate could be achieved by hysterectomy.[421] If metastasis occurred in patients with gestational trophoblastic neoplasms (GTN), survival was less than 10% in one year in the prechemotherapeutic era. In 1956, Li, Hertz, and Spence reported complete regression of metastatic choriocarcinoma in three women treated with methotrexate.[422] Five years later, Hertz and coworkers showed a 47% complete remission rate in 63 patients with metastatic GTN treated with chemotherapy.[423]

EPIDEMIOLOGY

The incidence of hydatidiform mole and gestational trophoblastic neoplasms varies significantly throughout the world; it is 7–10 times more frequent in Asia than the reported incidence in Europe and North America. Nutritional and socioeconomic factors have been cited as possible etiological factors in the high incidence of GTN in the Orient. Acosta-Sison assessed the dietary history of patients with molar pregnancies.[424] She noted that the wealthy Philippinos had a greater quantity of meat protein in their diet. The poorer Philippinos, whose diet consisted mostly of rice with fish, had an incidence of hydatidiform mole of one per 200 pregnancies.

Trophoblastic tumors also appear to be increased in women over 40; Teoh and coworkers noted that in Singapore the frequency of trophoblastic tumors in women over 45 was 12 times greater than among younger women.[425]

PATHOLOGY

Hertig and Sheldon divided hydatidiform mole into six pathologic groups based on cellular differentiation, mitotic activity, quantity of trophoblast, pattern of growth, and stromal and vascular invasion.[426] While they were able to correlate histologic appearance with clinical outcome, this was neither absolute nor constant. Some anaplastic tumors had an indolent course, while some well-differentiated tumors behaved aggressively. Recently, Deligdisch and coworkers correlated the pathology of GTN with therapeutic response and showed that trophoblastic tumors with increased mitotic activity, nuclear atypia, and compact cytotrophoblastic growth required more intensive chemotherapy to obtain complete sustained remission.[427] Absence of a fibrinoid layer and lymphocytic infiltration correlated well with resistance to chemotherapy.

Originally, trophoblastic tumors were categorized on the basis of morphology, such as hydatidiform mole, invasive mole (chorioadenoma destruens), and choriocarcinoma.

All trophoblastic tumors produce human chorionic gonadotropin (hCG), which is roughly proportional to the number of viable tumor cells.[428] Therefore, hCG titers can be used as a sensitive indicator of therapeutic response and the presence or absence of viable tumor cells. Initially, a radioimmune assay for LH was developed, which was used for diagnosis and monitoring patients with trophoblast tumors.[429] However, the crossreaction between LH and hCG posed difficulty in monitoring patients with minimal disease. Vaitukaitas and others described a radioimmunoassay method presently employed in most centers that was specific for the beta subunit of hCG and could therefore selectively measure hCG in the presence of LH.[430]

The hCG titers usually regress in 8–10 weeks following

evacuation of a benign trophoblast tumor.[431] However, in approximately 25% of patients with molar pregnancy, the hCG titer will regress over a longer period of time in a step-by-step manner with frequent plateaus. In these patients, a decrease of the hCG to normal levels may take 14–16 weeks. During that time, the remaining trophoblastic tissue may undergo slow regression due to immunologic mechanisms that destroy the residual tissue.

Tumor Dissemination

The tumor remains localized within the uterus, but viable trophoblastic cells may invade into the myometrium and perforate through the serosa of the uterus. The uterus subinvolutes and vaginal bleeding persists with elevated hCG titers. Complications of intraperitoneal hemorrhage or erosion through uterine vessels may occur with the local invasive trophoblastic tumors.

Distant dissemination may occur in 5% of patients following evacuation of a molar pregnancy, and in about 1:40,000 abortions, term, or ectopic pregnancies. The presence of metastatic disease is generally associated with choriocarcinoma. Choriocarcinoma disseminates by the hematogenous route. At the New England Trophoblast Disease Center, the common metastatic sites are as follows: lungs 80%, vagina 30%, pelvis 20%, brain 10%, liver 10%, bowel, kidney and spleen less than 5%, other less than 5%, undetermined with persistent hCG titer following hysterectomy less than 5%.[432]

Clinical Manifestation

The most common symptom of trophoblastic tumor is abnormal vaginal bleeding. One should be alerted to the possibility of trophoblastic tumor in a patient with a suspected threatened abortion with evidence of early toxemia or a uterus whose size is out of proportion to gestation. Occasionally, patients may present with evidence of systemic metastasis. The diagnosis is based on pathology of the obtained tissue; radiologic diagnosis including ultrasound isotope scan; and hCG determinations.

STAGING

Since it was difficult to correlate pathology with prognosis, the International Union Against Cancer recommended that patients be classified as to whether there was evidence of nonmetastatic or metastatic involvement. Investigators in the field further classified patients into low-risk and high-risk based on the extent and duration of disease and recommended therapy according to these risk factors.[433]

Recently, the New England Trophoblast Disease Center, adopted a new staging system outlined in Table 25-32.[432] Stage 0 refers to molar pregnancy and is divided into low-risk and high-risk groups. The low-risk molar pregnancies are characterized by serum hCG levels less than 100,000 IU/ml, uterine size equal to or smaller than dates, ovarian cyst smaller than 6 cm, and absence of other associated metabolic or epidemiologic factors.[434] Patients with high-risk molar pregnancies are characterized by a serum hCG over 100,000 IU/ml, uterine size larger than dates, ovarian size larger than 6 cm, and associated metabolic and epidemiologic factors (*e.g.*, molar pregnancy or trophoblastic tumor, maternal age over 40, toxemia, coagulopathy, trophoblastic embolization, and hyperthyroidism). Stage I defines patients with persistently elevated hCG titers in whom the trophoblast tumor is localized to the uterine corpus. In the New England Trophoblast Disease Center, approximately 75% of patients with stage I have invasive mole (chorioadenoma destruens) and 25% have locally invasive choriocarcinoma. Stage II includes patients with evidence of disease outside the uterus localized to the vagina or pelvic structures including adnexa and pelvic peritoneum. At the New England Trophoblast Disease Center, 60% of these patients have metastatic choriocarcinoma and 40% have metastatic mole. Stage III includes patients with radiographic evidence of pulmonary metastasis with or without uterine, pelvic, or vaginal lesions. Stage IV patients have involvement of the brain, liver, kidney, spleen, or GI tract. All of these patients have choriocarcinoma. All patients with stage IV disease are considered to be at high risk because of their relative resistance to chemotherapy.

TABLE 25-32. Staging of Gestational Trophoblastic Neoplasms

Stage O	Molar pregnancy A low risk B high risk
Stage I	Confined to uterine corpus
Stage II	Metastases to pelvis and vagina
Stage III	Metastasis to lung
Stage IV	Distant metastases

Goldstein DP, Berkowitz RS: The management of gestational trophoblastic neoplasms. In Current Problems in Obstetrics and Gynecology, p 20. Chicago, Year Book Medical Publisher, 1980

TREATMENT

The following treatment policies for each of the stages are used at the New England Trophoblast Disease Center of the Department of Obstetrics and Gynecology, Boston Hospital for Women, Harvard Medical School.

Treatment for Stage I

All patients, regardless of risk factors, are treated initially with single agent chemotherapy or hysterectomy, depending on their fertility desires. Methotrexate with leucovorin (Citrovorum) rescue is the chemotherapeutic agent of choice, unless the liver function tests are abnormal, in which case actinomycin-D is used instead of methotrexate.[435] Four doses of methotrexate are given over an 8 day period, 1 mg/kg IM followed on alternate days by leucovorin 0.1 mg/kg IM. If hysterectomy is selected as the primary treatment, one course of either methotrexate with leukovorin rescue or actinomycin-D is used to decrease the chance of dissemination of viable tumor cells at surgery. Actinomycin-D is given over a 5-day period, at a dose of 12 mcg/kg/day. After the initial course of chemotherapy, the hCG level is monitored three times per week. With an hCG level fall of 1 log within 18 days after the initial treatment, additional chemotherapy is withheld and the hCG titer is followed.[435] If the hCG titer does not fall by 1 log or reaches a plateau for three consecutive weeks or if it rises after the initial fall, a second course of chemotherapy is administered. Therapy is continued until the hCG titer becomes undetectable (less than 10 mU/ml) for three consecutive weeks. The patient is followed for 12 consecutive months and contraception is maintained. With normal hCG titers after 12 months, pregnancy is permitted. The majority of patients with stage I respond to sequential single agent chemotherapy or hysterectomy. Resistance developed in 0.5% of patients at the New England Trophoblast Disease Center and multiple agent therapy or hysterectomy was used successfully.

Stage II Disease

Patients with low-risk factors are treated in an identical manner as outlined for patients with stage I. If the patient does not respond to single agent therapy, combination chemotherapy should be instituted immediately.[432] Cases with high-risk factors are treated initially with combination chemotherapy. Treatment with each protocol is continued until the patient has three consecutive weeks of normal hCG titers. Hysterectomy or local resection of tumor masses is advisable in the presence of serious bleeding or infection.

High-risk patients are managed initially with a combination regimen including methotrexate, actinomycin-D, and either cholorambucil or cyclophosphamide. Response is achieved in approximately 80% of patients but only 40%–50% of those with hepatic or cerebral metastasis.[436] Moderate dose methotrexate (16 hour infusions of 1 gm) followed by leukovorin rescue has been studied in patients with metastasis in sites other than lung. A 70% complete response rate was reported and the toxicity was less severe than with the conventional methotrexate regimen.[437] Several reports of the successful use of aggressive six to seven drug combinations in patients who have been refractory to triple drug chemotherapy have been published; however, the number of patients treated is small.[438,439] Newlands and Bagshawe have recently published their experience with high dose (120 mg/M^2) cis-platinum, vincristine, and methotrexate with leukovorin rescue in 17 patients refractory to extensive previous therapy.[440] Of the 17, 6 (35%) achieved a complete remission and were off therapy 10–25 months. The toxicity was tolerable and only one patient experienced significant but reversible renal toxicity. Two new agents, cis-platinum and VP-16, have recently been reported to produce regressions in some patients resistant to conventional therapy.[441,442] The role of these new agents and combinations as first line approach to bad prognosis patients or in refractory disease remains to be fully elucidated.

Stage III Disease

The preferred treatment for patients with pulmonary metastasis and low-risk factors is methotrexate and leucovorin factor.[443] The high-risk patients are treated with combination methotrexate-CF, actinomycin-D, and cyclophosphamide as outlined for stage I. Rarely, local resection of an unresponsive lung lesion may be necessary if the hCG titer is persistently elevated with no other apparent metastatic sites or the patient has developed resistance or excessive toxicity to available chemotherapeutic agents.

Stage IV Disease

Patients with distant organ involvement by choriocarcinoma are at the highest risk. Patients with proven brain lesions or elevated cerebrospinal fluid hCG should receive whole head irradiation at a dose of 3000 rad. At times, surgery is indicated for acute intracranial bleeding. Chemotherapy at the New England Trophoblast Disease Center for stage IV disease consists of the CHAMOCA (Bagshawe) regimen. This protocol includes hydroxyurea, actinomycin-D, vincristine, methotrexate, and Cytoxan. Table 25-33 outlines the drug regimen.

Bagshawe has treated brain lesions with intrathecal administration of MTX.[433] Liver lesions are best diagnosed with hepatic arteriography. At times, actinomycin-D may be infused into the liver by way of a hepatic artery catheter. With initial multiple agent chemotherapy and selective radiation therapy and surgery, two-thirds of the stage IV patients are now surviving.

Because trophoblastic tumors are rare and life-threatening, it is essential that these patients be treated by persons with experience in this disease process. Patients with trophoblastic tumors deserve full benefit of modern chemotherapy and advanced technology.

LATE CONSEQUENCES OF CHEMOTHERAPY

At present, there is no evidence of increased maternal complications or fetal abnormalities during pregnancy and delivery of women who have been treated and cured of choriocarcinoma.[444] Two recent publications also support this conclusion.[445,446]

TABLE 25-33. Chamoca (Bagshawe)

DAY	TIME	THERAPY
1	0700 hours	Hydroxyurea 500 mg PO
	1300 hours	Hydroxurea 500 mg PO
	1900 hours	Actinomycin-D 0.5 mg IV
2	0100 hours	Hydroxyurea 500 mg PO
	0700 hours	Vincristine 1 mg/M^2 IV
		Hydroxyurea 500 mg PO
	1900 hours	Methotrexate 100 mg/M^2 IV push
		Methotrexate 200 mg/M^2 IV over 12 hours
		Actinomycin-D 0.5 mg IV
3	1900 hours	Actinomycin-D 0.5 mg IV
		Cytoxan 500 mg/M^2 IV
		Folinic Acid 14 mg IM*
4	0100 hours	Folinic Acid 14 mg IM
	0700 hours	Folinic Acid 14 mg IM
	1300 hours	Folinic Acid 14 mg IM
	1900 hours	Folinic Acid 14 mg IM
		Actinomycin-D 0.5 mg IV
5	0100 hours	Folinic Acid 14 mg IM
	1900 hours	Actinomycin-D 0.5 mg IV
6	No treatment	
7	No treatment	
8		Cytoxan 500 mg/M^2 IV
		Doxorubicin (Adriamycin) 30 mg/M^2

* Folinic acid = citrovorum factor

Goldstein DP, Berkowitz RS: The management of gestational trophoblastic neoplasms. In Current Problems in Obstetrics and Gynecology, pp 25–26. Chicago, Year Book Medical Publishers, 1980

REFERENCES

1. American Cancer Society: 1980 Facts & Figures. New York, American Cancer Society, 1979
2. Hochman A, Ratzkowski E, Schrieber H: Incidence of carcinoma of cervix in Jewish women in Israel. Br J Cancer 9:358–364, 1955
3. Terris M, Wilson F, Nelson JH Jr: Relation of circumcision to cancer of the cervix. Am J Obstet Gynecol 117:1056–1066, 1973
4. Stern E, Dixon WJ: Cancer of the cervix—a biometric approach to etiology. Cancer 14:153–160, 1961
5. Ackerman LV, delRegato JA (eds): *Cancer: Diagnosis, Treatment, and Prognosis*, pp 717–819. St. Louis, C.V. Mosby, 1977
6. Christopherson WM, Parker JE: Relation of cervical cancer to early marriage and childbearing. N Engl J Med 273:235–239, 1965
7. Keighley E: Carcinoma of the cervix among prostitutes in a women's prison. Br J Vener Dis 44:254–255, 1968
8. Rotkin ID: Adolescent coitus and cervical cancer associations of related events with increased risk. Cancer Res 27:603–617, 1967
9. Rotkin ID: Sexual characteristics of a cervical cancer population. Am J Publ Health 57:815–829, 1967
10. Taylor RS, Carroll BE, Lloyd JW: Mortality among women in 3 Catholic religious orders with special references to cancer. Cancer 12:1207–1223, 1959
11. Joneja MG, Coulson DB: Histopathology and cytogenetics of tumors induced by application of 7,12-dimethybenz (a)anthracene (DMBA) in mouse cervix. Eur J Cancer 9:367–374, 1973
12. Herbst AL, Cole P, Norusis MJ et al: Epidemiologic aspects and factors related to survival in 384 registry cases of clear cell adenocarcinoma of the vagina and cervix. Am J Obstet Gynecol 135:876–886, 1979
13. Boyce JG, Lu T, Nelson JH Jr et al: Cervical carcinoma and oral contraception. Gynecol Invest 40:139–146, 1972
14. Drill VA: Oral contraceptives: Relation to mammary cancer, benign breast lesions and cervical cancer. Am Rev Pharmacol 15:367–385, 1975
15. Melamed MR, Flehinger BJ: Early incidence rates of precancerous cervical lesions in women using contraceptives. Gynecol Oncol 1:290–298, 1973
16. Nahmias AJ, Naib ZM, Josey WE: Epidemiological studies relating genital herpetic infection to cervical carcinoma. Cancer Res 34:1111–1117, 1974
17. Adam E, Rawls WE, Melnick JL: The association of herpes virus type-2 infection and cervical cancer. Prev Med 3:122–141, 1974
18. Fridell GH, Hertig AT, Younge PA: Carcinoma *in situ* of the uterine cervix. Springfield, IL, Charles C Thomas, 1960
19. Kessler II: Perspectives on the epidemiology of cervical cancer with special reference to the herpes virus hypothesis. Cancer Res 34:1091–1109, 1974
20. Melnick JL, Adams E, Rawls WE: The causative role of herpesvirus type 2 in cervical cancer. Cancer 34:1375–1385, 1974
21. Nahmias AJ, Naib ZM, Josey WE et al: Prospective studies of the association of genital herpes simplex infection and cervical anaplasis. Cancer Res 33:1491–1497, 1973
22. Rawls WE, Gardner HL, Kaufman RL: Antibodies to genital herpes virus in patients with carcinoma of the cervix. Am J Obstet Gynecol 107:710–716, 1970
23. Reagan JW, Wentz WB: Genesis of carcinoma of the uterine cervix. Clin Obstet Gynecol 10:883–921, 1967
24. Richart RM: Natural history of cervical intraepithelial neoplasia. Clin Obstet Gynecol 10:748–784, 1967
25. Barron BA, Richart RM: Statistical model of the natural history of cervical carcinoma. II. Estimates of the transition time from dysplasia to carcinoma *in situ*. J Natl Cancer Inst 45:1025–1030, 1970
26. Kashigarian M, Dunn JE: The duration of intraepithelial and preclinical squamous cell carcinoma of the uterine cervix. Am J Epidemiol 92:221–222, 1970
27. Kolstad P: Carcinoma of the cervix, stage 0; diagnosis and treatment. Am J Obstet Gynecol 96:1098–1111, 1966
28. Petersen O: Spontaneous course of cervical pre-cancerous conditions. Am J Obstet Gynecol 72:1063–1071, 1956
29. Koss LG, Stewart FW, Foote FW et al: Some histological aspects of behavior of epidermois carcinoma in situ and related lesions of the uterine cervix. Cancer 16:1160–1211, 1963
30. Clemmesen J, Poulsen H: Report of the Ministry of the Interior, Document 3, Copenhagen, 1971
31. Kottmeier HL: Evolution et traitment des epitheliomas. Rev Fr Gynec Obstet 56:821–826, 1961
32. Christopherson WM, Parker JE: Microinvasive carcinoma of the uterine cervix. A clinical-oathological study. Cancer 17:1123–1131, 1964
33. Way S: Microinvasive carcinoma of the cervix. Acta Cytol (Baltimore) 8:14–15, 1964
34. Bohm JW, Krupp PJ, Lee FYL et al: Lymph node metastases in microinvasive epidermoid cancer of the cervix. Obstet Gynecol 48:65–67, 1976
35. Kolstad P: Carcinoma of the cervix stage IA. Am J Obstet Gynecol 104:1015–1022, 1969
36. Ruch RM, Pitcock JA, Ruch WA Jr.: Microinvasive carcinoma of the cervix. Am J Obstet Gynecol 125:87–92, 1976
37. Mitani Y, Yukinari S, Jimi S et al: Carcinomatous infiltration into the uterine body in carcinoma of the uterine cervix. Am J Obstet Gynecol 89:984–989, 1964
38. Perez CA, Zivnuska F, Askin F et al: Prognostic significance of endometrial extension from primary carcinoma of the uterine cervix. Cancer 35:1493–1504, 1975
39. Piver MS, Chung WS: Prognostic significance of cervical lesion size and pelvic node metastases in cervical carcinoma. Obstet Gynecol 46:507–510, 1975
40. van Nagell JR Jr, Donaldson ES, Wood EG et al: The significance of vascular invasion and lymphocytic infiltration in invasive cervical cancer. Cancer 41:228–234, 1978
41. Evans JC, Bergsjo P: The influence of anemia on the results of radiotherapy in carcinoma of the cervix. Radiology 81:709–716, 1965
42. Bush RS, Jenkin RDT, Allt WEC et al: Definitive evidence for hypoxic cells influencing cure in cancer therapy. Br J Cancer 37:302–306, 1978
43. Vigario G, Kurohara SS, George FW III: Association of hemoglobin levels before and during radiotherapy with prognosis in uterine cervix cancer. Radiology 106:649–652, 1973
44. Jenkin RDT, Stryker JA: The influence of the blood pressure on survival in cancer of the cervix. Br J Radiol 41:913–920, 1968
45. Van Herik M: Fever as a complication of radiation therapy for carcinoma of the cervix. Am J Roentgenol Radium Ther Nucl Med 43:104–109, 1965
46. Berkowitz RS, Ehrmann RL, Lavizzo-Mourey R et al: Invasive cervical carcinoma in young women. Gynecol Oncol 8:311–316, 1979
47. Kyriakos M, Kempson RL, Perez CA: Carcinoma of the cervix in young women. Obstet Gynecol 39:930–944, 1971
48. Henricksen E: The lymphatic spread of carcinoma of the cervix and of the body of the uterus. A study of 420 necropsies. Am J Obstet Gynecol 58:924–942, 1949
49. Beyer FD Jr, Murphy A: Patterns of spread of invasive cancer of the human cervix. Cancer 18:34–40, 1965
50. Badib AO, Kurohara SS, Webster JH et al: Metastasis to organs in carcinoma of the uterine cervix; influence of treatment on incidence and distribution. Cancer 21:434–439, 1968
51. Carlson V, Delclos L, Fletcher GH: Distant metastases in squamous-cell carcinoma of the uterine cervix. Radiology 88:961–966, 1967
52. Wentz WB, Reagan JW: Survival in cervical cancer with respect to cell type. Cancer 12:384–388, 1959
53. Abell MR, Gosling JRG: Gland cell carcinoma (adenocarcinoma) of the uterine cervix. Am J Obstet Gynecol 83:729–755, 1962
54. Silverberg SG, Hurt WB: Minimal deviation adenocarcinoma ("adenoma malignum") of the cervix: A reappraisal. Am J Obstet Gynecol 121:971–975, 1975
55. Littman P, Clement PB, Henriksen B et al: Glassy cell carcinoma of the cervix. Cancer 37:2238–2246, 1976
56. Gunderson LL, Weems WS, Hervertson RM et al: Correlation of histopathology with clinical results following radiation therapy

for carcinoma of the cervix. Am J Roentgenol Radium Ther Nucl Med 120:74–87, 1974
57. Finck FM, Denk M: Cervical carcinoma: Relationship between histology and survival following radiation therapy. Obstet Gynecol 35:339–343, 1970
58. Swan DS, Roddick JW: A clinical-pathological correlation of cell type classification for cervical cancer. Am J Obstet Gynecol 116:666–670, 1973
59. Hameed K: Clear cell carcinoma of the uterine cervix. Am J Obstet Gynecol 101:954–958, 1968
60. Hart WR, Norris HJ: Mesonephric adenocarcinomas of the cervix. Cancer 29:106–113, 1972
61. Noller KL, Decker DG, Dockerty MB et al: Mesonephric (clear cell) carcinoma of the vagina and cervix. Obstet Gynecol 43:640–644, 1974
62. Gordon HW: Adenoid cystic (cylindromatous) carcinoma of the uterine cervix: Report of two cases. Am J Clin Path ,58:51–57, 1972
63. Ramzy I, Yuzpe AA, Hendelman J: Adenoid cystic carcinoma of uterine cervix. Obstet Gynecol 45:679–683, 1975
64. Field CA, Dockerty M, Symmonds RE: Small cell cancer of the cervix. Am J Obstet Gynecol 88:447–451, 1964
65. Blaustein A, Immerman B: Leiomyosarcoma of the cervix. Obstet Gynecol 22:224–227, 1963
66. Schade FF: Sarcoma botryodes of the cervix uteri. Report of a case in an adult with survival. Obstet Gynecol 26:731–733, 1965
67. Retikas DG: Hodgkin's sarcoma of the cervix. Report of a case. Am J Obstet Gynecol 80:1104–1107, 1960
68. Stransky GC, Acosta AA, Kaplan AL et al: Reticulum cell sarcoma of the cervix. Obstet Gynecol 41:183–187, 1973
69. Novak ER, Jones GS, Jones HW (eds): Novak's Textbook of Gynecology. Philadelphia, Williams & Wilkins, 1970
70. Breslow L: Cytology and the decline in uterine cervix mortality in California. In Clark RL, Cumley RW, McCay JE et al (eds): Oncology 1970 (Proceedings of the Tenth International Cancer Congress), vol IV. Diagnosis and Management of Cancer: Specific Sites, Chicago, Year Book, 1971
71. Guznick DS: Efficacy of screening for cervical cancer: A review. Am J Public Health 68:125–134, 1978
72. Fidler HK, Boyes DA, Worth AJ: Cervical cancer detection in British Columbia. J Obstet Gynaecol Br Comm 75:392–404, 1968
73. American Cancer Society: ACS Report on the Cancer-Related Health Checkup CA 30:194–240, 1980
74. Kern WH, Zivolich MR: The accuracy and consistency of the cytologic classification of squamous lesions of the uterine cervix. Acta Cytol 21:519–523, 1977
75. Wentz WB, Reagan JW: Clinical significance of post-irradiation dysplasia of the human cervix. Am J Obstet Gynecol 106:812–817, 1970
76. Marcial VA, Blanco MS, DeLeon E: Persistent tumor cells in the vaginal smear during the first year after radiation therapy of carcinoma of the uterine cervix: Prognostic significance. Am J Roentgenol Radium Ther Nucl Med 102:170–175, 1968
77. Koss LG: Recurrent carcinoma and presence of radiation cell changes. Acta Cytologica 3:418, 1959
78. Dolan TE, Boyce J, Rosen Y et al: Cytology, colposcopy, and directed biopsy: What are the limitations? Gynecol Oncol 3:314–324, 1975
79. Nyberg R, Tornberg B, Westin B: Colposcopy and Schiller's iodine test as an aid in the diagnosis of malignant and premalignant lesions of the cervix uteri. Acta Obstet Gynecol Scand 39:540–556, 1960
80. Nelson JH, Averette HE, Richart RM: Detection, diagnostic evaluation and treatment of dysplasia and early carcinoma of the cervix. Cancer 25:134–151, 1975
81. Piver MS, Wallace S, Castro JR: The accuracy of lymphangiography in carcinoma of the uterine cervix. Am J Roentgenol Radium Ther Nucl Med 111:278–283, 1971
82. Walsh JW, Amendola MA, Konerding KF et al: Computed tomographic detection of pelvic and inguinal lymph-node metastases from primary and recurrent pelvic malignant disease. Radiology 137:157–8166, 1980
83. Griffin TW, Parker RG, Taylor WJ: An evaluation of procedures used in staging carcinoma of the cervix. Am J Roentgenol Radium Ther Nucl Med 127:825–827, 1976
84. Cunningham JJ, Fuks ZY, Castellino RA: Radiographic manifestations of carcinoma of the cervix and complications of its treatment. Radiol Clin North Am 12:93–108, 1974
85. Parker RG, Friedman RF: A critical evaluation of the roentgenologic examination of patients with carcinoma of the cervix. Am J Roentgenol Radium Ther Nucl Med 96:100–107, 1966
86. Lagasse LD, Creasman WT, Shingleton HM et al: Results and complications of operative staging in cervical cancer: Experience of the Gynecologic Oncology Group. Gynecol Oncol 9:90–98, 1980
87. Kademian MT, Bosch A: Is staging laparotomy in cervical cancer justified? Int J Radiat Oncol Biol Phys 2:1235–1238, 1977
88. Piver MS, Barlow JJ: Para-aortic lymphadenectomy in staging patients with advanced local cervical cancer. Obstet Gynecol 43:544–548, 1974
89. Lepanto P, Littman P, Mikuta et al: Treatment of para-aortic nodes in carcinoma of the cervix. Cancer 35:1510–1513, 1975
90. Wharton JT, Jones HW III, Day TG Jr et al: Preirradiation celiotomy and extended field irradiation for invasive carcinoma of the cervix. Obstet Gynecol 49:333–338, 1977
91. Zornoza J, Lukeman JM, Jing BS et al: Percutaneous retroperitoneal lymph node biopsy in carcinoma of the cervix. Gynecol Oncol 5:43–51, 1977
92. Averette HE, Ford JH Jr, Dudan RC et al: Staging of cervical cancer. Clin Obstet Gynecol 18:215–232, 1975
93. Perez CA, Camel HM, Kao MS et al: Randomized study of preoperative radiation and surgery or irradiation alone in the treatment of stage IB and IIA carcinoma of the uterine cervix: Preliminary analysis of failures and complications. Cancer 45:2759–2768, 1980
94. Ketcham AS, Sindelar WF, Felix EL et al: Diagnostic scalene node biopsy in the preoperative evaluation of the surgical cancer patient. Cancer 38:948–952, 1976
95. Buchsbaum HJ: Extrapelvic lymph node metastases in cervical carcinoma. Am J Obstet Gynecol 133:814–824, 1979
96. Perez-Mesa C, Spratt JS: Scalene node biopsy in the pretreatment staging of carcinoma of the cervix uteri. Am J Obstet Gynecol 125:93–95, 1976
97. Kottmeier HL (ed): Annual Report on the Results of Treatment in Carcinoma of the Uterus, Vagina and Ovary, Vol 15. Stockholm, Internation Federation of Gynecology and Obstetrics, 1973
98. Tarlowski L, Lukawaska K, Mielcarzewicz A et al: Comparison of the FIGO and TNM staging systems for uterine cervix cancer based on classification of 6,193 cases. Gynecol Oncol 4:270–277, 1976
99. Hoskins WJ, Ford JH Jr, Lutz MH et al: Radical hysterectomy and pelvic lymphadenectomy for the management of early invasive cancer of the cervix. Gynecol Oncol 4:278–290, 1976
100. Creasman WT, Rutledge FN: Carcinoma *in situ* of the cervix. Obstet Gynecol 3:373–380, 1972
101. Bjerre B, Eliasson G, Linell F et al: Conization as only treatment of carcinoma *in situ* of the uterine cervix. Am J Obstet Gynecol 125:143–152, 1976
102. Christopherson WM, Gray LA, Parker JE: Microinvasive carcinoma of the uterine cervix. Cancer 38:629–632, 1976
103. Kolstad P, Klem V: Long-term follow-up of 1,121 cases of carcinoma *in situ*. Obstet Gynecol 48:125–129, 1976
104. Channen W, Hollyock VE: Colposcopy and the conservative management of cervical dysplasia and carcinoma *in situ*. Obstet Gynecol 43:527–534, 1974
105. DelRegato JA, Cox JD: Transvaginal roentgentherapy in the conservative management of carcinoma *in situ* of the uterine cervix. Radiology 84:1090–1095, 1965
106. Perez CA, Tarlow D: Unpublished data, 1980
107. Kaufman RH: Frozen section evaluation of cervical conization specimen. Clin Obstet Gynecol 10:838–852, 1967

108. Benson, WL, Norris HJ: A clinical review of the frequency of lymph node metastasis and death from microinvasive carcinoma of the cervix. Obstet Gynecol 49:632–638, 1977
109. Hasumi K, Sakmoto A, Sugano H: Microinvasive carcinoma of the uterine cervix. Cancer 45:928–921, 1980
110. Creasman WT, Parker RT: Microinvasive carcinoma of the cervix. Clin Obstet Gynecol 16:261–275, 1973
111. Webb GA: The role of ovarian conservation in the treatment of carcinoma of the cervix with radical surgery. Am J Obstet Gynecol 122:476–484, 1975
112. Brunschwig A: The surgical treatment of cancer of the cervix stage I and II. Am J Roentgenol 102:147–151, 1968
113. Park RC, Patow WE, Rogers RR et al: Treatment for stage I carcinoma of the cervix. Obstet Gynecol 41:117–122, 1973
114. Parker RT, Wilbanks GD, Yowell RK et all: Radical hysterectomy with and without preoperative radiotherapy for cervical cancer. Am J Obstet Gynecol 99:933–943, 1967
115. Pilleron JP, Durand JC, Lenoble JC: Carcinoma of the uterine cervix, stages I and II, treated by radiation therapy and extensive surgery (1000 cases). Cancer 29:593–596, 1972
116. Sall S, Pineda AA, Calanog A et al: Surgery treatment of stages IB and IIA invasive carcinoma of the cervix by radical abdominal hysterectomy. Am J Obstet Gynecol 135:422–446, 1979
117. Surwit E, Fowler WC Jr, Palumbo L et al: Radical hysterectomy with or without preoperative radium for stage IB squamous cell carcinoma of the cervix. Obstet Gynecol 48:130–133, 1976
118. Newton M: Radical hysterectomy of radiotherapy for stage I cervical cancer. Am J Obstet Gynecol 123:535–542, 1975
119. Roddick JW Jr, Greenlaw RH: Treatment of cervical cancer. Am J Obstet Gynecol 19:754–764, 1971
120. Kielbinska S, Ludwika T, Fraczek O: Studies of mortality and health status in women cured of cancer of the cervix uteri; comparison of long-term results of radiotherapy and combined surgery and ratiotherapy. Cancer 32:245–252, 1973
121. Lu T, Macasaet M, Nelson JH Jr: The barrel shaped cervix. Am J Obstet Gynecol 124:596–600, 1976
122. Fletcher GH (ed): *Textbook of Radiotherapy*, 2 ed, pp 620–665. Philadelphia, Lea & Febiger, 1973
123. Durrance FY, Flecher GH, Rutledge FN: Analysis of central recurrent disease in stages I and II squamous cell carcinomas of the cervix on intact uterus. Am J Roentgenol Radium Ther Nucl Med 106:831–838, 1969
124. O'Quinn AG, Fletcher GH, Wharton JT: Guidelines for conservative hysterectomy after irradiation. Gynecol Oncol 9:68–79, 1980
125. Guttman R: Significance of postoperative irradiation in carcinoma of the cervix; a ten-year study. Am J Roentgenol Radium Ther Nucl Med 108:102–108, 1970
126. Morrow CP: Panel Report: Is pelvic radiation beneficial in the postoperative managment of stage IB squamous cell carcinoma of the cervix with pelvic node metastasis treated by radical hysterectomy and pelvic lymphadenectomy? Gynecol Oncol 10:105–110, 1980
127. Fletcher GH: Cancer of the uterine cervix. Janeway Lecture. Am J Roentgenol Radium Ther Nucl Med 111:225–242, 1971
128. Christensen A, Lange P, Neilsen E: Surgery and radiotherapy for invasive cancer of the cervix: Surgical treatment. Acta Obstet Gynecol 43:59–87, 1964
129. Plentl AA, Friedman EA: Lymphatic System of the Female Genitalia: The Morphologic Basis of Oncologic Diagnosis and Therapy, pp 85–115. Phliladelphia, WB Saunders, 1971.
130. Liu W, Meigs JV: Radical hysterectomy and pelvic lymphadenectomy: A review of 473 cases including 244 for primary invasive carcinoma of the cervix. Am J Obstet Gynecol 69:1–32, 1955
131. Brunschwig A, Barber HRK: Surgical treatment of carcinoma of the cervix. Obstet Gynecol 27:21–29, 1966
132. Schulman H, Cavanagh D: Intraepithelial carcinoma of the cervix. The predicatability of residual carcinoma in the uterus from the microscopic study of the margins of the cone biopsy specimen. Cancer 14:795–800, 1961
133. Silbar EL, Woodruff JD: Evaluation of biopsy, cone and hysterectomy sequence in intraepithelial carcinoma of the cervix. Obstet Gynecol 27:89–97, 1966
134. Fennell RH: Microinvasive carcinoma of the uterine cervix. Obstet Gynecol Survey 33:406–411, 1978
135. Seski JC, Abell MR, Morley GW: Microinvasive squamous carcinoma of the cervix. Definition, histologic analysis, late results of treatment. Obstet Gynecol 50:410–414, 1977
136. Burghardt E, Holzer E: Diagnosis and treatment of microinvasive carcinoma of the cervix uteri. Obstet Gynecol 49:641–653, 1977
137. Rutledge FN, Wharton JT, Fletcher GH: Clinical studies with adjunctive surgery and irradiation therapy in the treatment of carcinoma of the cervix. Cancer 38:596–602, 1976
138. Van Nagell JR, Rayburn W, Donaldson ES et al: Therapeutic implications of patterns of recurrence in cancer of uterine cervix. Cancer 44:2354–2361, 1979
139. Way S, Henninger M, Wright VC: Some experiences with preinvasive and microinvasive carcinoma of the cervix. J Obstet Gynaec Br Comm 75:593–602, 1968
140. Siebel M, Freeman MG, Graves WL: Carcinoma of the cervix and sexual function. Obstet Gynecol 55:484–487, 1979
141. Nelson JH, Macasaet MA, Lu T et al: The incidence and significance of para-aortic lymph nodes metastases in late invasive carcinoma of the cervix. Am J Obstet Gynecol 118:749–756, 1974
142. Symmonds RD: Morbidity and complications of radical hysterectomy with pelvic lymph node dissection. Am J Obstet Gynecol 94:663–668, 1966
143. Brunschwig A: Complete excision of the pelvic viscera for advanced carcinoma. Cancer 1:177–183, 1948
144. Million RR, Fletcher GH, Rutledge F: Stage IV carcinoma of the cervis with bladder invasion. Am J Obstet Gynecol 113:239–246, 1972
145. Brunschwig A, Daniel WW: Pelvic exenteration operations. Ann Surg 151:571–576, 1960
146. VanDyke AH, Van Nagell JR Jr: The prognostic significance of ureteral obstruction in patients with recurrent carcinoma of the cervix uteri. Surg Gynecol Obstet 141:371–373, 1975
147. Barber HRK: Relative prognostic significance of preoperative and operative findings in pelvic exenteration. Surg Clin North Amer 49:431–447, 1969
148. Barber HRK, Graber EA: Treatment of advanced cancer of the cervix by pelvic exenteration. Bull NY Acad Med 49:870–886, 1973
149. Bricker EM, Modlin J: The role of pelvic evisceration in surgery. Surgery 30:76–94, 1951
150. Deckers PJ, Ketcham AS, Sugarbaker EV et al: Pelvic exeneration for primary carcinoma of the uterine cervix. Obstet Gynecol 37:647–659, 1971
151. Ingersoll FM, Ulfelder H: Pelvic exenteration for carcinoma of the cervix. N Eng J Med 274:648–651, 1966
152. Kiselow M, Butcher HR Jr, Bricker EM:: Results of the radical surgical treatment of advanced pelvic cancer: A fifteen year study. Ann Surg 166:428–436, 1967
153. Ulfelder H: Extended radical surgery for recurrent and advanced cervical cancer. Clin Obstet Gynecol 10:940–957, 1967
154. Nelson JH, Boyce J, Macasaet M et al: Incidence, significance and followup of para-aortic lymph node metastases in late invasive carcinoma of the cervix. Am J Obstet Gynecol 128:336–340, 1977
155. Chism SE, Park RC, Keys HM: Prospects for para-aortic irradiation in treatment of cancer of the cervix. Cancer 35:1505–1509, 1975
156. Berman ML, Lagasse LD, Ballon SC et al: Modification of radiation therapy following operative evaluation of patients with cervical carcinoma. Gynecol Oncol 6:328–332, 1978
157. Buchsbaum H: Para-aortic lymph node involvement in cervical carcinoma. Am J Obstet Gynecol 113:942–947, 1972
158. Cuccia CA, Bloedorn FG: Treatment of primary adenocarcinoma of the cervix. Am J Roentgenol Radium Ther Nucl Med 99:371–375, 1967
159. Rutledge FN, Gutierrez AG, Fletcher GH: Management of stage

I and II adenocarcinomas of the uterine cervix on the intact uterus. Am J Roentgenol Radium Ther Nucl Med 102:161–164, 1968

160. Sala JM Gleason JA, Spratt JS: Adenocarcinoma of the cervix uteri: Report of 104 cases. Mo Med 59:1168–1173, 1962
161. Ubinas J, Marcial V: Adenocarcinoma of the cervix: A review of cases; Dr. I. Gonzalez-Martinez Oncologic Hospital, J Am Med Women Assoc 21:571–574, 1966
162. Weiner S, Wizenberg MJ: Treatment of primary adenocarcinoma of the cervix. Cancer 35:1514–1516, 1975
163. Rutledge FN, Gutierrez AG, Fletcher GH: Management of stage I and II adenocarcinomas of the uterine cervix on intact uterus. Am J Roentgenol Radium Ther Nucl Med 102:161–164, 1968
164. Rutledge FN, Galakatos AE, Wharton JT et al: Adenocarcinoma of the uterine cervix. Am J Obstet Gynecol 122:236–245, 1975
165. Allt WEC: Supervoltage radiation treatment in advanced cancer of the uterine cervix. Can Med Ass J 100:792–797, 1969
166. Johns HE: Optimazation of energy and equipment. In Kramer S, Suntharalingam N, Zinninger GF (eds): High-Energy Photons and Electrons: Clinical Applications in Cancer Management, pp 333–345. New York, John Wiley & Sons, 1976
167. Jampolis S, Andras J, Fletcher GH: Analysis of sites and causes of failure of irradiation in invasive squamous cell carcinoma of the intact uterine cervix. Radiology 115:681–685, 1975
168. Deutsch M, Parsons JA: Radiotherapy for carcinoma of the cervix recurrent after surgery. Cancer 34:2051–2055, 1974
169. Friedman M, Pearlman AW: Carcinoma of the cervix; radiation salvage of surgical failures. Radiology 84:801–811, 1965
170. Morton DG, Lagasse LD, Moore JG et al: Pelvic lymphadenectomy following radiation in cervical carcinoma. Am J Obstet Gynecol 88:932–938, 1964
171. Quigley MM, Knab DR, McMahan ER: Carcinoma of the cervix. A third treatment. Obstet Gynecol 45:650–655, 1975
172. Rampone JF, Klem V, Kolstad P: Combined treatment of stage IB carcinoma of the cervix. Obstet Gynecol 41:163–167, 1973
173. Einhorn N, Bygdeman M, Sjoberg B: Combined radiation and surgical treatment for carcinoma of the uterine cervix. Cancer 45(4):720–723, 1980
174. Pilleron JP, Durand JC, Hamelin JP: Prognostic value of node metastasis in cancer of the uterine cervix. Am J Obstet Gynecol 119:458–462, 1974
175. Morley, GW, Seski JC: Radical pelvic surgery versus radiation therapy for stage I carcinoma of the cervix (exclusive of microinvasion). Am J Obstet Gynecol 126:785–798, 1976
176. Leveuf J, Godord H: L'exerese chirugicales des ganglions pelviens complement de la curtherapie des cancers du col de 'uterus, J Chir 43:177–187, 1934
177. Taussig FJ: Iliac lymphadenectomy with irradiation in the treatment of cancer of the cervix. Am J Obstet Gynecol 28:650–667, 1934
178. Abitbol NM, Davenport JH: Sexual dysfunction after therapy for cervical carcinoma. Am J Obstet Gynecol 119:181–189, 1974
179. Rutledge FN, Fletcher GH, MacDonald EJ: Pelvic lymphadenectomy as an adjunct to radiation therapy in treatment for cancer of the cervix. Am J Roentgenol Radium Ther Nucl Med 93:607–614, 1965
180. Nelson AJ, Fletcher GH, Wharton T: Indications for adjunctive conservative extrafascial hysterectomy in selected cases of carcinoma of the uterine cervix. Am J Roentgenol Radium Ther Nucl Med 123:91–99, 1975
181. Piver MS, Chung WS: Prognostic significance of cervical lesion size and pelvic node metastases in cervical carcinoma. Obstet Gynecol 46;507–510, 1975
182. Madoc-Jones: Unpublished data, 1979
183. Kottmeier HL: Complications following radiation therapy in carcinoma of the cervix and their treatment. Am J Obstet Gynecol 88:854–866, 1964
184. Strockbine MF, Hancock JE, Fletcher GH: Complications in 831 patients with squamous cell carcinoma of the intact uterine cervix treated with 3000 rads or more whole pelvis irradiation. Am J Roentgenol Radium Ther Nucl Med 108:293–304, 1970
185. Piver MS, Vongtama V, Barlow JJ: Para-aortic lymph node irradiation for carcinoma of the uterine cervix using split-course technique. Gynecol Oncol 3:168–175, 1975
186. Smith JP, Rutledge F, Burns BC Jr et al: Systemic chemotherapy for carcinoma of the cervix. Am J Obstet Gynecol 97:800–807, 1967
187. Young RC: Gynecologic malignancies. In Pinedo HM (ed): Cancer Chemotherapy, pp 340–375. Oxford, Excerpta Medica, 1979
188. Malkasian GD, Decker DG, Jorgensen EP: Chemotherapy of carcinoma of the cervix. Gynecol Oncol 5:109–120, 1976
189. Thigpen T, Shingleton H, Homesley H: Phase II trial of cispaltinum as first or second line treatment for advanced squamous cell carcinoma of the cervix. Proc Am Assoc Cancer Res 20:388, 1979
190. Morrow CP, DiSaia PJ, Mangan CF et al: Continuous pelvic arterial infusion with bleomycin for squamous carcinoma of the cervix recurrent after irradiation therapy. Cancer Treat Rep 61:1403–1405, 1977
191. Swenerton KD, Evers JA, White GW et al: Intermittent pelvic infusion with vincristine, bleomycin and mytomycin-C for advanced recurrent carcinoma of the cervix. Cancer Treat Rep 63:1379–1381, 1979
192. Miura T, Oku T, Iwasaki M et al: Surgical chemotherapy for advanced carcinoma of the cervix uteri. J Jpn Soc Cancer Ther 254, 1977
193. Ohta A: Basic and clinical studies on the simultaneous combination treatment of cervical cancer (especially advanced cases) with a carcinostatic agent and radiation. J Tokyo Med Coll 36:529, 1978
194. Oku T, Iwaskaki M, Tojo S: Study on surgical chemotherapy for advanced cancer of the uterine cervix—particularly on the problem of clinical effect and drug concentration. Acta Obstet Gynaec Jpn 31:1833, 1979
195. Piver MS, Varlow JJ, Vongtama V et al: Hydroxyurea and radiation therapy in advanced cervical cancer. Am J Obstet Gynecol 120:969–972, 1974
196. Hreshchyshyn MM, Aron BS, Boronow RC et al: Hydroxyurea or placebo combined with radiation to treat stages IIIB and IV cervical cancer confined to the pelvis. Int J Radiat Oncol Biol Phys 5:317–322, 1979
197. Banjamin I, Xynos FP, Rana MW: Effects of adriamycin and hydroxyurea on human squamous cell carcinoma of cervix transplanted into nude mice. Fed Proc 28:1319, 1979
198. Fowler JF: Radiobiological considerations from the hyperbaric oxygen trials. A personal view. Br J Radiol 51:68–69, 1978
199. Watson ER, Halnan KE, Dische S et al: Hyperbaric oxygen and radiotherapy: A Medical Research Council trial in carcinoma of the cervix. Br J Radiol 51:879–887, 1978
200. Fletcher GH, Lindberg RD, Caderao JB et al: Hyperbaric oxygen as a radiotherapeutic adjuvant in advanced carcinoma of the uterine cervix. Preliminary results of a randomized trial. Cancer 39:617–623, 1977
201. Glassburn JR, Damsker JI, Brady LW et al: Hyperbarix oxygen and radiation in the treatment of advanced cervical carcinoma. In *Fifth International Hyperbaric Congress Proceedings, II*, pp 813–819. Simon Fraser University, 1974
202. Dische S: Hyperbaric oxygen: The Medical Research Council Trials and their clinical significance. Br J Radiol 51:888–894, 1979
203. Johnson RJR, Walton RJ: Sequential study on the effect of the addition of hyperbaric oxygen on the 5 year survival rates of carcinoma of the cervix treated with conventional fractional irradiations. Am J Roentgenol Radium Ther Nucl Med 120:111–117, 1974
204. Thomas GM, Rauth AM, Bush RS et al: A toxicity study of daily dose metronidazole with pelvic irradiation. Cancer Clin Trials 3:223–230, 1980
205. Dische S: Misonidazole in the clinic at Mount Vernon. Cancer Clin Trials 3:175–178, 1980
206. Hornback NB, Shidnia H, Shupe RE et al: Results comparing hyperthermia and radiation versus radiation alone in treatment of 79 patients with stage IIIB carcinoma of the uterine cervix. Int J Radiat Oncol Biol Phys 6:1384, 1980

207. Greene RR, Peckham BM: Preinvasive cancer of the cervix and pregnancy. Am J Obstet Gynecol 75:551–564, 1958
208. Boutselis JG: Intraepithelial carcinoma of the cervix associated with pregnancy. Obstet Gynecol 40:657–666, 1972
209. DePetrillo AD, Townsend DE, Morrow CP et al: Colposcopic evaluation of the abnormal Papanicolau test in pregnancy. Am J Obstet Gynecol 121:441–445, 1975
210. Averette HE, Nasser N, Yankow SL et al: Cervical conization in pregnancy. Analysis of 180 operations. Am J Obstet Gynecol 106:543–549, 1970
211. Mikuta JH, Enterline HT, Braun TE Jr: Carcinoma *in situ* of the cervix associated with pregnancy. JAMA 204:763–766, 1968
212. Dudan RC, Yon JL Jr, Ford JH Jr et al: Carcinoma of the cervix and pregnancy. Gynecol Oncol 1:283–289, 1973
213. Thompson JD, Caputo TA, Franklin EW et al: The surgical management of invasive cancer of the cervix in pregnancy. Am J Obstet Gynecol 121:853–863, 1975
214. Creasman WT, Rutledge FN, Fletcher GH: Carcinoma of the cervix associated with pregnancy. Obstet Gynecol 36:495–501, 1970
215. Kinch RAH: Factors affecting the prognosis of the cervix in pregnancy. Am J Obstet Gynecol 82:45–51, 1961
216. Symmonds RE: Carcinoma of the cervix associated with pregnancy. Clin Obstet Gynecol 6:964–974, 1963
217. Strauss A: Irradiation of carcinoma of the cervix uteri in pregnancy. Am J Roentgenol Radium Ther Nucl Med 43:552–566, 1940
218. Sala JM, deLeon AD: Treatment of carcinoma of the cervical stump. Radiology 81:300–306, 1963
219. Moss WT, Brand WN, Battifora H (eds): Radiation Oncology. Rationale, Technique, Results, pp 408–453. St. Louis, CV Mosby, 1973
220. Wimbush PR, Fletcher GH: Radiation therapy of carcinoma of the cervical stump. Radiology 93:655–658, 1969
221. Wolff JP, Lacour J, Chassagne D et al: Cancer of the cervical stump. A study of 173 patients. Obstet Gynecol 39:10–16, 1972
222. Creadick RN: Carcinoma of the cervical stump. Am J Obstet Gynecol 75:564–574, 1958
223. Durrance FY: Radiotherapy following simple hysterectomy in patients with stage I and II carcinoma of the cervix. Am J Roentgenol Radium Ther Nucl Med 102:165–169, 1968
224. Andras EJ, Fletcher GH, Rutledge F: Radiotherapy of carcinoma of the cervix following simple hysterectomy. Am J Obstet Gynecol 115:647–655, 1973
225. Green TH, Morse WJ: Management of invasive cervical cancer following inadvertent simple hysterectomy. Obstet Gynecol 33:763–769, 1969
226. Moss WT: Common peculiarities of patients with adenocarcinoma of the endometrium; with special reference to obesity, body build, diabetes and hypertension. Am J Roentgenol Radium Ther Nucl Med 58:203–210, 1947
227. Smith JP: Hormone therapy for adenocarcinoma of the endometrium. In: Cancer of the Uterus and Ovary, p 73. Chicago, Year Book 1969
228. Ziel HK, Finkle WD: Increased risk of endometrial carcinoma among users of conjugated estrogen. N Engl J Med 293:1167–1170, 1975
229. Shapiro S, Kaufman DW, Slone D et al: Recent and past use of conjugated estrogens in relation to adenocarcinoma of the endometrium. N Eng J Med 303:485–489, 1980
230. Gumpel C, Silverberg SG (eds): Pathology in Gynecology and Obstetrics, 2 ed. Philadelphia, JB Lippincott, 1977
231. Gusberg SG, Kaplan AL: Precursors of corpus cancer. IV. Adenomatous hyperplasia as stage 0 carcinoma of the endometrium. Am J Obstet Gynecol 87:662–678, 1963
232. Morrow CP: Endometrial carcinoma stages I and II: Is surgery adequate? Int J Radiat Oncol Biol Phys 6:365–366, 1980
233. Creasman WT, Boronow RC, Morrow CP et al: Adenocarcinoma of the endometrium: Its metastatic lymph node potential. Gynecol Oncol 4:239–243, 1976
234. Tak WK: Carcinoma of the endometrium with cervical involvement (stage II). Cancer 43:2504–2509, 1979
235. Madoc-Jones, H: Adenocarcinoma of the endometrium, stage II: Problems in definition and management. Int J Radiat Oncol Biol Phys 6:887–890, 1980
236. Jones HW III: Treatment of endometrial carcinoma. Obstet Gynecol Survey 30:147–169, 1975
237. Berman ML, Ballon SC, Lagasse LD et al: Prognosis and treatment of endometrial cancer. Am J Obstet Gynecol 136:679–688, 1980
238. Brown JM, Dockerty MB, Symmonds RE et al: Vaginal recurrence of endometrial carcinoma. Am J Obstet Gynecol 100:544–549, 1968
239. Ingersoll FM: Vaginal recurrences of carcinoma of the corpus. Management and prevention. Am J Surg 121:473–477, 1971
240. Rubin P, Gerle RD, Quick RS et al: Significance of vaginal recurrence in endometrial carcinoma. Am J Roentgenol Radium Ther Nucl Med 89:91–100, 1963
241. Creasman WT, Lukeman J: Role of the fallopian tube in dissemination of malignant cells in corpus cancer. Cancer 29:456–457, 1972
242. Lynch RC, Dockerty MB: The spread of uterine and ovarian carcinoma with special reference to the role of the fallopian tube. Surg Gynecol Obstet 80:60–65, 1945
243. Rao BR, Weist WG, Allen WM: Progesterone "receptor" in human endometrium. Endocrinology 95:1275–1281, 1975
244. Rao BR, Wiest WG: Receptors for progesterone. Gynecol Oncol 2:239–248, 1974
245. Anderson DG: The possible mechanisms of action of progestins on endometrial adenocarcinoma. Am J Obstet Gynecol 113:195–211, 1972
246. Reifenstein EC: The treatment of advanced endometrial cancer with hydroxyprogesterone caproate. Gynecol Oncol 2:377–414, 1974
247. Rozier JC, Underwood PB: Use of progestational agents in endometrial adenocarcinoma. Obstet Gynecol 44:60–64, 1974
248. Ng AB, Reagan JW, Storaasli JP et al: Mixed adenosquamous carcinoma of the endometrium. Am J Clin Pathol 59:765–781, 1973
249. Silverberg SG, Bolin MG, DeGiorgi LS: Adenoacanthoma and mixed adenosquamous carcinoma of the endometrium. A clinicopathologic study. Cancer 30:1307–1314, 1972
250. Salazar OM, DePapp EW, Bonfiglio TA et al: Adenosquamous carcinoma of the endometrium: An entity with an inherent poor prognosis? Cancer 40:119–130, 1977
251. Williamson EO, Christopherson WM: Malignant mixed mullerian tumors of the uterus. Cancer 29:585–592, 1972
252. Mortel R, Koss LG, Lewis JL et al: Mixed mesodermal tumors of the uterine corpus. Obstet Gynecol 43:246–252, 1974
253. Norris HJ, Roth E, Taylor HB: Mesenchymal tumors of the uterus—II. A clinical and pathological study of 31 mixed mesodermal tumors. Obstet Gynecol 28:57–63, 1966
254. Perez CA, Askin F, Baglan RJ et al: Effect of irradiation on mixed mullerian tumors of the uterus. Cancer 43:1274–1284, 1979
255. Chuang JT, Van Velden DJJ, Graham JB: Carcinosarcoma and mixed mesodermal tumors of the uterine corpus: Review of 49 cases. Obstet Gynecol 35:769–780, 1970
256. Norris HJ, Taylor HB: Mesenchymal tumors of the uterus. I. A clinical and pathological study of 53 endometrial stromal tumors. Cancer 19:755–766, 1966
257. Abell MR, Ramirez JA: Sarcomas and carcinosarcomas of the uterine cervix. Cancer 31:1176–1192, 1973
258. Christopherson WM, Williamson EO, Gray LA: Leiomyosarcoma of the uterus. Cancer 29:1512–1517, 1972
259. Kempson RL, Bari W: Uterine sarcomas. Hum Pathol 1:331–348, 1970
260. Silverberg SG: Leiomyosarcoma of the uterus; a clinicopathologic study (views and reviews). Obstet Gynecol 38:613–628, 1971
261. Wright CJE: Solitary malignant lymphomas of the uterus. Am J Obstet Gynecol 117:114–120, 1973
262. Silverberg, SG, DeGiorgi LS: Clear cell carcinoma of the endometrium. Clinical, pathologic, and ultrastructural findings. Cancer 31:1127–1140, 1973

263. Kay S: Squamous-cell carcinoma of the endometrium. Am J Clin Pathol 61:264–269, 1974
264. Hecht EL, Oppenheim A: The cytology of endometrial cancer. Surg Gynecol Obstet 122:1025–1029, 1966
265. Baitlon D, Hadley JO: Endometrial biopsy; pathologic findings in 3,600 biopsies from selected patients. Am J Clin Pathol 63:9–15, 1975
266. Hofmeister FJ: Endometrial biopsy: Another look. Am J Obstet Gynecol 118:773–777, 1974
267. Lukeman JM: An evaluation of the negative pressure "jet washing" of the endometrium in menopausal and postmenopausal patients. Acta Cytol (Baltimore) 18:462–471, 1974
268. Vassilakos R, Wyss R, Wenger D et al: Endometrial cytohistology by aspiration technic and by Gravlee jet washer. Obstet Gynecol 45:320–324, 1975
269. Wallace S, Jing B-S, Medellin H: Endometrial carcinoma: Radiologic assistance in diagnosis, staging, and management. Gynecol Oncol 2:287–299, 1974
270. Zsolnai B, Hyiro L: Hysterography in corpus carcinoma. Zentralbl Gynaekol 90:273–279, 1968
271. Gusberg SB, Chen SY, Cohen CJ: Endometrial cancer: Factors influencing the choice of treatment. Gynecol Oncol 2:308–313, 1974
272. Malkasian GD Jr: Carcinoma of the endometrium: Effect of stage and grade on survival. Cancer 41:996–1001, 1978
273. Keller D, Kempson RL, Levine G et al: Management of the patient with early endometrial carcinoma. Cancer 33:1108–1116, 1974
274. Kempson RL, Pokorny GE: Adenocarcinoma of the endometrium in women 40 years of age and younger. Cancer 21:650–662, 1968
275. Boronow RC: Endometrial cancer: Not a benign disease. Obstet Gynecol 47:630–634, 1976
276. Kottmeier HL: Individualization of therapy in carcinoma of the corpus. In Cancer of the Uterus and Ovary, M.D. Anderson Hospital, pp 102–108. Chicago, Yearbook Medical Publication, 1969
277. Landgren RD, Fletcher GH, Delclos L et al: Irradiation of endometrial cancer in patients with medical contraindication to surgery or with unresectable lesions. Am J Roentgenol Radium Ther Nucl Med 126:148–154, 1976
278. Wharam MO, Phillips TL, Bagshaw MA: The role of radiation therapy in clinical stage I carcinoma of the endometrium. Int J Radiat Oncol Biol Phys 1:1081–1089, 1976
279. Monson RR, MacMahon B, Austin JH: Postoperative irradiation in carcinoma of the endometrium. Cancer 31:630–632, 1973
280. Nolan JF, Dorough ME, Anson JH: The value of preoperative radiation therapy in stage I carcinoma of the uterine corpus. Am J Obstet Gynecol 98:663–674, 1967
281. Surwit EA, Fowler WC, Rogoff EE et al: Stage II carcinoma of the endometrium. Int J Radiat Oncol Biol Phys 5:323–326, 1979
282. Kottmeier HL: Corpus et colli. What is the disease? What is the treatment? Clin Obstet Gynecol 16:276–285, 1973
283. Antoniades J, Brady LW, Lewis GC: The management of stage III carcinoma of the endometrium. Cancer 38:1838–1842, 1976
284. Cullen TH: Cancer of the Uterus. Philadelphia, WB Saunders, 1900
285. Healy W, Brown R: Experience with surgical and radiation therapy in carcinoma of the corpus uteri. Am J Obstet Gynecol 38:1–13, 1939
286. Arneson A: Clinical results and histologic changes following the radiation treatment of cancer of the corpus uteri. Am J Roentgenol Radium Ther Nucl Med 36:461–476, 1936
287. Plentl AA, Friedman EA: Lymphatic System of the Female Genitalia: The Morphologic Basis of Oncologic Diagnosis and Therapy, pp 123–152. Philadelphia, WB Saunders, 1971
288. Copenhaver EH, Barsamian M: Management of adenocarcinoma of the endometrium. Surg Clin North Am 47:723–735, 1967
289. Brunschwig A, Murphy A: The rationale for radical panhysterectomy and pelvic node excision in carcinoma of the corpus uteri. Clinical and pathological data on the mode of spread of endometrial carcinoma Am J Obstet Gynecol 68:1482–1488, 1954.
290. Homesley HD, Boronow RC, Lewis JL Jr: Stage II endometrial carcinoma. Memorial Hospital for Cancer, 1949–1965. Obstet Gynecol 49:604–608, 1977
291. Rutledge F: The role of radical hysterectomy in adenocarcinoma of the endometrium. Gynecol Oncol 2:331–347, 1974
292. Kinsella TJ, Bloomer WD, Lavin PT et al: Stage II endometrial carcinoma: Ten year followup of combined radiation and surgical treatment. Gynecol Oncol 10:290–297, 1980
293. Barber HRK, Brunschwig A: Treatment and results of recurrent cancer of the corpus uteri in patients receiving anterior and posterior pelvic exenteration (1947–1963). Cancer 22:949–955, 1968
294. Brunschwig A: Some reflections on pelvic exenterations after twenty years' experience. In Sturgis SH, Taymor ML (eds): Progress in Gynecology, vol 5, pp 290–297. New York, Grune & Stratton, 1970
295. Salazar OM, Feldstein ML, DePapp EW et al: Endometrial carcinoma: Analysis of failures with special emphasis on the use of initial preoperative external pelvic radiation. Int J Radiat Oncol Biol Phys 2:1101–1107, 1977
296. Underwood PB, Lutz MH, Kreutner A et al: Carcinoma of the endometrium: Radiation followed immediately by operation. Am J Obstet Gynecol 128:86–98, 1977
297. Graham J: The value of preoperative or postoperative treatment by radium for carcinoma of the uterine body. Surg Gynecol Obstet 132:855–860, 1971
298. Wade ME, Kohorn EI, Chir M et al: Adenocarcinoma of the endometrium. Evaluation of preoperative irradiation and factors influencing prognosis. Am J Obstet Gynecol 99:869–876, 1967
299. Javert CT: The spread of benign and malignant endometrium in the lymphatic system with a note on coexisting vascular involvement. Am J Obstet Gynecol 64:780–806, 1952
300. Sala JM, DelRegato JA: The treatment of carcinoma of the endometrium. Radiology 79:12–17, 1962
301. Silverberg SG, DeGiorgi LS: Histopathologic analysis of preoperative radiation therapy in endometrial carcinoma. Am J Obstet Gynecol 119:698–704, 1974
302. Weigensberg IJ: Preoperative radiation therapy in endometrial carcinoma: Preliminary report of a clinical trial. Am J Roentgenol Radium Ther Nucl Med 127:391–323, 1976
303. Lampe I: Endometrial carcinoma. Am J Roentgenol Radium Ther Nucl Med 90:1011–1015, 1963
304. Landgren RD, Fletcher GH, Gallager S: Treatment failure sites according to irradiation technique and histology in patients with endometrial cancer. Cancer 40:131–135, 1977
305. Donovan JF: Nonhormonal chemotherapy of endometrial adenocarcinoma: A review. Cancer 34:1587–1592, 1974
306. Karlstedt K: Progesterone treatment for local recurrence and metastases in carcinoma corporis uteri. Acta Radiol (Ther) Stockh) 10:187–192, 1971
307. Malkasian GD Jr, Decker DG, Mussey E et al: Progestogen treatment of recurrent endometrial carcinoma. Am J Obstet Gynecol 110:15–21, 1971
308. Reifenstein EC: Hydroxprogesterone caproate therapy in advanced endometrial cancer. Cancer 27:485–502, 1971
309. Ehrlich EC, Cleary RE, Young ELM: The use of progesterone receptors in the management of recurrent endometrial cancer. In Brush MG, King RLB, Taylor RW (eds): Endometrial Cancer, pp 258–264. London, Bailliere Tindall, 1978
310. Lewis GC Jr, Slack NH, Mortel R et al: Adjuvant progestogen therapy in the primary definitive treatment of endometrial cancer. Gynecol Oncol 2:368–376, 1974
311. Malkasian GD Jr, Decker DG: Adjuvant progesterone therapy for stage I endometrial carcinoma. Int J Gynaecol Obstet 16:48–49, 1978
312. Beck RP: Experience in treating two hundred and eighty-eight patients with endometrial carcinoma from 1968 to 1972. Am J Obstet Gynecol 133:260–267, 1979
313. Gusberg SB: Current concepts in cancer: The changing nature of endometrial cancer. New Engl J Med 302:729–731, 1980
314. Kucera VH, Gerstner G, Michalica W, Weghaupt K: Hormon-

prophylaxe bel der strahlenbehandlung des korpuskarzinomas mit hochdosierten gestagenen. Weiner Medizinsche Wochenschrift 129:395–399, 1979

315. LaGasse L, Thigpen T, Morrison F: Phase II trial of piperazinedione in treatment of advanced endometrial carcinoma, uterine sarcoma, and vulvar carcinoma. Proc Am Assoc Cancer Res 20:388, 1979
316. Thigpen JT, Buchsbaum HJ, Mangan C et al: Phase II trial of Adriamycin in the treatment of advanced or recurrent endometrial carcinoma: A Gynecologic Oncology Group Study. Cancer Treat Rep 63:21–27, 1979
317. Muggia FM, Chia G, Reed LJ et al: Doxorubicin cyclophosphamide: Effective chemotherapy for advanced endometrial adenocarcinoma. Am J Obstet Gynecol 128:314–319, 1977
318. Ramirez G, Weiss A, and the Central Oncology Group: A phase II study of Adriamycin-5-fluorouracil given weekly in the treatment of solid tumors. Proc Am Soc Clin Oncol 17:248, 1976
319. Bruckner HW, Deppe G: Combination chemotherapy of advanced endometrial adenocarcinoma with Adriamycin, clyclophosphamide, 5-fluorouracil and medroxyprogesterone acetate. Obstet Gynecol 50:10S–12S, 1977
320. Cohen CJ, Deppe G, Bruckner HW: Treatment of advanced adenocarcinoma of the endometrium with melphalan, 5-fluorouracil and medroxyprogesterone acetate. A preliminary study. Obstet Gynecol 50:415–417, 1977
321. Edwards DL, Sterling LN, Keller RH et al: Mixed heterologous mesenchymal sarcomas (mixed mesodermal sarcomas) of the uterus. Addition of 7 cases. Am J Obstet Gynecol 85:1002–1011, 1963
322. Norris HJ, Taylor HB: Mesenchymal tumors of the uterus. III. A clinical and pathologic study of 31 carcinosarcomas. Cancer 19:1459–1465, 1966
323. DiSaia PJ, Castro JR, Rutledge FN: Mixed mesodermal sarcoma of the uterus. Am J Roentgenol Radium Ther Nucl Med 117:632–636, 1973
324. Vongtama V, Karlen JR, Piver SM et al: Treatment, results and prognostic factors in stage I and II sarcomas of the corpus uteri. Am J Roentgenol Radium Ther Nucl Med 126:139–147, 1976
325. Badib AO, Vongtama V, Kurohara SS et al: Radiotherapy in the treatment of sarcomas of the corpus uteri. Cancer 24:724–729, 1969
326. Salazar OM, Feldstein ML, DePapp EW et al: The proper management of endometrial carcinoma. Cancer 41:230–240, 1978
327. Belgrad R, Elbadawi N, Rubin P: Uterine sarcoma. Radiology 114:181–188, 1975
328. Gilbert HA, Kagan AR, Lagasse L et al: The value of radiation therapy in uterine sarcoma. Obstet Gynecol 45:84–88, 1975
329. Buchsbaum HJ, Lifshitz S, Blythe JG: Prophylactic chemotherapy in stages I and II uterine sarcoma. Gynecol Oncol 8:346–348, 1979
330. Smith PG, Dool R: Late effects of X irradiation in patients treated for metropathia haemorrhagica. Br J Radiol 49:224–232, 1976
331. Hutchinson GB: Leukaemia in patients with cancer of the cervix uteri treated with radiation. A report covering the first five years of an international study. J Natl Cancer Inst 40:951–982, 1968
332. Dickson RJ: The late results of radium treatment for benign uterine haemorrhage. Br J Radiol 42:582–594, 1969
333. Wagoner JK: Radiation Therapy for Gynecological Disorders and Subsequent Leukaemia, Uterine Sarcoma, and Other Malignancies. Thesis submitted to Faculty, Harvard School of Public Health, 1970
334. Arneson AN, Schellhas HF: Multiple primary cancers in patients treated for carcinoma of the cervix. Am J Obstet Gynecol 106:1155, 1970
335. Spratt JS, Hoag MG: Incidence of multiple primary cancers per man year of follow-up: 20 year review from Ellis Fischel State Cancer Hospital. Ann Surg 164:775–784, 1966
336. Lee JY: Unpublished data, 1980
337. Wagoner JK: Leukaemia and other Malignancies Following Radiation Therapy for Benign Gynecological Disorders. Presented before the Radiological Health and Epidemiology Section, American Public Health Association, 1969
338. Feinleib M: Breast cancer and artificial menopause: A cohort study. J Natl Cancer Inst 41:315–339, 1968
339. Trichopoulos D, Macmahon B, Cole P: Menopause and breast cancer risk. J Natl Cancer Inst 48:605–613, 1972
340. Villasanta U, Rubel H: Radium treatment of benign uterine bleeding. Long-term follow-up. Obstet Gynecol 33:813–817, 1969
341. Thomas WO Jr, Harris HH, Enden JA: Postirradiation malignant neoplasms of the uterine fundus. Am J Obstet Gynecol 104:209–219, 1969
342. Sedlis A: Primary carcinoma of the fallopian tube. Obstet Gynecol 16:209–226, 1961
343. Hu CY, Taymor ML, Hertig AT: Primary carcinoma of the fallopian tube. Am J Obstet Gynecol 59:58–67, 1950
344. Green TH, Scully RE: Tumors of the fallopian tube. Clin Obstet Gynecol 5:886–906, 1962
345. Momtazee S, Kempson RL: Primary adenocarcinoma of the fallopian tube. Obstet Gynecol 32:649–656, 1968
346. Cohn S, Rossano RW, Fenton AN: Primary carcinoma of the fallopian tube. NY State J Med 69:1321–1328, 1969
347. Jones OV: Primary carcinoma of the uterine tube. Obstet Gynecol 26:122–129, 1965
348. Erez S, Kaplan AL, Wall JA: Clinical staging of carcinoma of the uterine tube. Obstet Gynecol 30:547–550, 1967
349. Henderson SR, Harper RC, Salazar OM et al: Primary carcinoma of the fallopian tube. Difficulties of diagnosis and treatment. Gynecol Oncol 5:168–179, 1977
350. Finn WF, Javert CT: Primary and metastatic cancer of the fallopian tube. Cancer 2:803–814, 1949
351. Lofgren KA, Dockerty MB: Primary carcinoma of the fallopian tubes. Surg Gynecol Obstet 82:199–206, 1946
352. Novak ER, Woodruff JD: In Novak's Gynecologic and Obstetric Pathology, pp 314–318. Philadelphia, WB Saunders, 1974
353. Woodruff JD, Pauerstein CJ (eds): Malignant Tumors of the Fallopian Tube, pp 66–306. Baltimore, Williams & Wilkins, 1969
354. Weiss PD, MacDougall MK, Reagan JW et al: Primary adenosquamous carcinoma of the fallopian tube. Obstet Gynecol 55:88S–89S, 1980
355. Plentl AA, Friedman EA: Lymphatic System of the Female Genitalia: The Morphologic Basis of Oncologic Diagnosis and Therapy, pp 153–167. Philadelphia, WB Saudners, 1971
356. Feldman GB, Knapp RC: Lymphatic drainage of the peritoneal cavity and its significance in ovarian cancer. Am J Obstet Gynecol 119:991–994, 1974
357. Frick MC: Cancer of the fallopian tube. In Gusberg SG, Frick MD (eds): Corscaden's Gynecologic Cancer, pp 368–374. Baltimore, Williams & Wilkins, 1978
358. Dodson MG, Ford JH Jr, Averette HE: Clinical aspects of the fallopian tube carcinoma. Obstet Gynecol 36:935–939, 1970
359. Hayden GE, Potter EL: Primary carcinoma of the fallopian tube. Am J Obstet Gynecol 79:24–31, 1960
360. Kneale BLG, Atwood HD: Primary carcinoma of the fallopian tube. Am J Obstet Gynecol 94:840–848, 1966
361. Phelps HM, Chapman KE: Role of radiation therapy in treatment of primary carcinoma of the uterine tube. Obstet Gynecol 43:669–673, 1974
362. Griffiths CT: Ovary and the fallopian tube. In Holland JF, Frei E III (eds): Cancer Medicine, pp 1718–1720. Philadelphia, Lea Febiger, 1972
363. Rutledge F: Cancer of the vagina. Am J Obstet Gynecol 97:635–655, 1967
364. Daw E: Primary carcinoma of the vagina. J Obstet Gynecol Br Commonwealth 78:853–856, 1971
365. Herbst AL, Green TH Jr, Ulfedler H: Primary carcinoma of the vagina. Am J Obstet Gynecol 106:210–218, 1970
366. Plentl AA, Friedman EA: Lymphatic System of the Female Genitalia: The Morphologic Basis of Oncologic Diagnosis and Therapy, pp 51–74. Philadelphia, WB Saunders, 1971
367. Pride GL, Schultz AE, Chuprevich TW et al: Primary invasive squamous carcinoma of the vagina. Obstet Gynecol 53:218–225, 1979

368. Way S: Primary carcinoma of the vagina. J Obstet Gynecol Br Emp 55:739–755, 1948
369. Herbst AL, Robboy SJ, Scully RE et al: Clear-cell adenocarcinoma of the vagina in girls: Analysis of 170 registry cases. Am J Obstet Gynecol 119:713–724, 1974
370. Robboy SJ, Herbst AL, Scully RE: Clear cell adenocarcinoma of the vagina and cervix in young females: Analysis of 37 tumors that persisted or recurred after primary therapy. Cancer 34:606–614, 1974
371. Kanbour AI, Klionsky B, Murphy AI: Carcinoma of the vagina following cervical cancer. Cancer 34:1838–1841, 1974
372. Schiffer MA, Markles AM, Greene HJ: Carcinoma *in situ* of the vagina after hysterectomy. Surg Gynecol Obstet 134:652–654, 1972
373. Perez CA, Arneson AN, Dehner LP et al: Radiation therapy in carcinoma of the vagina. Obstet Gynecol 44:862–872, 1974
374. Robboy SJ, Scully RE, Herbst AL: Pathology of vaginal and cervical abnormalities associated with prenatal exposure to diethylstilbesterol. J Reprod Med 15:13–18, 1975
375. Tavassoli FA, Norris HJ: Smooth muscle tumors of the vagina. Obstet Gynecol 53:689–693, 1979
376. Desai S, Cavanagh D: Malignant melanoma of the vagina. Cancer 19:632–636, 1966
377. Norris HJ, Taylor HB: Melanomas of the vagina. Am J Clin Pathol 46:420–426, 1966
378. Ragni MV, Tobon H: Primary malignant melanoma of the vagina and vulva. Obstet Gynecol 43:658–664, 1974
379. Malkasian GD Jr, Welch JS, Soule EH: Primary leiomyosarcoma of the vagina. Am J Obstet Gynecol 86:730–736, 1963
380. Livingstone RC: Primary Carcinoma of the Vagina. Springfield, IL, Charles C Thomas, 1950
381. Chau PM: Radiotherapeutic management of malignant tumors of the vagina. Am J Roentgenol Radium Ther Nucl Med 89:502–523, 1963
382. Perez CA, Korba A, Sharma S: Dosimetric considerations in irradiation of carcinoma of the vagina. Int J Radiat Oncol Biol Phys 2:639–649, 1977
383. Underwood RB, Smith RT: Carcinoma of the vagina. JAMA 217:46–52, 1971
384. Brown GR, Fletcher GH, Rutledge FN: Irradiation of '*in situ*' and invasive squamous cell carcinomas of the vagina. Cancer 28:1278–1283, 1971
385. Piver MS, Barlow JJ, Wang JJ et al: Combined radical surgery, radiation therapy, and chemotherapy in infants with vulvovaginal embryonal rhabdomyosarcoma. Obstet Gynecol 42:522–526, 1973
386. Welton J, Kottmeier HL: Primary carcinoma of the vagina. Acta Obstet Gynecol Scand 41:22–40, 1962
387. Wharton JT, Rutledge FN, Gallager HS et al: Treatment of clear cell adenocarcinoma in young females. Obstet Gynecol 45:365–368, 1975
388. Fletcher GH (ed): Textbook of Radiotherapy, 3 ed, pp 821–824. Philadelphia, Lea & Febiger, 1980
389. Gussenbauer C: Uber die entwicklung der secundaren lymphdrusengeschwulste. Z Heilk 2:17–19, 1881
390. Kustner O: Zur pathologie und therapie des vulva carcinoma. Z Geburtsk Gynak 7:70–76, 1882
391. Taussig FJ: Diseases of the Vulva. New York, Appleton, 1923
392. Way S: The anatomy of the lymphatic drainage of the vulva and its influence on the radical operation for carcinoma. Ann Roy Coll Surgeons of England 3:187–209, 1948
393. Collins CG, Collins JH, Barclay DL et al: Cancer involving the vulva: A report on 109 consecutive cases. Am J Obstet Gynecol 87:762–772, 1963
394. McKelvey JL: Carcinoma of the vulva: Treatment and prognosis. Obstet Gynecol 5:452–455, 1955
395. Green TH: Carcinoma of the vulva: A reassessment. Obstet Gynecol 52:462–468, 1978
396. Buscema J, Woodruff JD, Parmley TH et al: Carcinoma *in situ* of the vulva. Obstet Gynecol 55:255–230, 1980
397. DiSaia PJ, Creasman WT, Rich WM: An alternate approach to early cancer of the vulva. Am J Obstet Gynecol 133:825–832, 1979
398. Magrina JF, Webb MJ, Gaffey TA et al: Stage I squamous cell cancer of the vulva. Am J Obstet Gynecol 134:453–459, 1979
399. Collins CG, Lee FYL, Ramon-Lopez JJ: Invasive carcinoma of the vulva with lymph node metastasis. Am J Obstet Gynecol 109:446–451, 1971
400. Morley GW: Infiltrative carcinoma of the vulva: Results of surgical treatment. Am J Obstet Gynecol 124:874–888, 1976
401. Taussig FJ: Late results in the treatment of leucoplakic vulvitis and cancer of the vulva. Am J Obstet Gynecol 31:746–754, 1936
402. International Society for the Study of Vulvar Disease: New nomenclature for vulvar disease. Report of the Committee on Terminology. Obstet Gynecol 47:122–124, 1976
403. Schueller EF: Basal cell cancer of the vulva. Am J Obstet Gynecol 91:199–208, 1965
404. Lucas WE, Benirschke K, Lebherz TB: Verrucous carcinoma of the female genital tract. Am J Obstet Gynecol 119:435–440, 1974
405. Tavassoli FA, Norris HJ: Smooth muscle tumors of the vulva. Obstet Gynecol 53:213–217, 1979
406. Chung AF, Woodruff JM, Lewis JL: Malignant melanoma of the vulva. Obstet Gynecol 45:638–646, 1975
407. Morrow CP, Rutledge FN: Melanoma of the vulva. Obstet Gynecol 3:745–752, 1972
408. Kaufman RH, Gardner HL, Brown D Jr et al: Vulvar dystrophies: An evaluation. Am J Obstet Gynecol 120:363–367, 1974
409. Plentl AA, Friedman EA: Lymphatic System of the Female Genitalia: The Morphologic Basis of Oncologic Diagnosis and Therapy, pp 15–50. Philadelphia, WB Saunders, 1971
410. Cherry CP, Glucksmann A: Lymphatic embolism and lymph node metastasis in cancer of the vulva and the uterine cervix. Cancer 8:564–575, 1955
411. Wharton JT, Gallagher S, Rutledge FN: Microinvasive carcinoma of the vulva. Am J Obstet Gynecol 118:159–162, 1974
412. Boutselis JG: Intraepithelial carcinoma of the vulva. Am J Obstet Gynecol 113:733–737, 1972
413. Collins CG, Ramon-Lopez JJ, Lee FYL: Intraepithelial carcinoma of the vulva. Am J Obstet Gynecol 18:1187–1191, 1970
414. Rutledge FN: Premalignant and malignant disease of the vulva. Contemp Obstet Gynecol 7:73–79, 1976
415. Watring WG, Roberts JA, Lagasse LD et al: Treatment of recurrent Paget's disease of the vulva with topical bleomycin. Cancer 41:10–11, 1978
416. Parker RT, Duncan I, Rampone J et al: Operative management of early invasive epidermoid carcinoma of the vulva. Am J Obstet Gynecol 123:349–355, 1975
417. Yazigi R, Piver MS, Tsukada Y: Microinvasive carcinoma of the vulva. Obstet Gynecol 51:368–370, 1978
418. Rutledge F, Smith JP, Franklin E: Carcinoma of the vulva. Am J Obstet Gynecol 106:1117–1129, 1970
419. Piver MS, Xynos FP: Pelvic lymphadenectomy in women with carcinoma of the clitoris. Obstet Gynecol 49:592–594, 1977
420. Franklin EW III, Rutledge FD: Prognostic factors in epidermoid carcinoma of the vulva. Obstet Gynecol 37:892–901, 1971
421. Brewer JI, Rinehart JJ, Dunbar R: Choriocarcinoma. Am J Obstet Gynecol 81:574–583, 1961
422. Li MC, Herz R, Spence DB: Effect of methotrexate therapy upon choriocarcinoma and choirioadenoma. Proc Soc Exp Biol Med 93:361–366, 1956
423. Hertz R, Lewis J Jr, Lipsett MB: Five years' experience with the chemotherapy of metastatic choriocarcinoma and related trophoblastic tumors in women. Am J Obstet Gynecol 82:631–645, 1961
424. Acosta-Sison, H: Statistical study of chorionepithelioma in the Philippine General Hospital. Am J Obstet Gynecol 58:125–132, 1949
425. Teoh ES, Dawood MY, Ratnam SS: Epidemiology of hydatidiform mole in Singapore. Am J Obstet Gynecol 110:415–420, 1971
426. Hertig AT, Sheldon WH: Hydatidiform mole—a pathologico-clinical correlation of 200 cases. Am J Obstet Gynecol 53:1–36, 1947
427. Deligdisch L, Driscoll SG, Goldstein DP: Gestational tropho-

blastic neoplasms: Morphologic correlates of therapeutic response. Am J Obstet Gynecol 130:801–806, 1978
428. Goldstein DP: Endocrine assay in chorionic tumors. Clin Obstet Gynecol 18:41–60, 1975
429. Aona T, Goldstein DP, Taymor ML: A radioimmunoassay method for human pituitary leuteinizing hormone (LH) and human chorionic gonadotropin (hCG) using 125-I-labelled LM. Am J Obstet Gynecol 98:996–1001, 1967
430. Vaitukaitis JL, Bruanstein GD, Ross GT: A radioimmunoassay which specifically measures human chorionic gonadotropin in the presence of human luteinizing hormone. Am J Obstet Gynecol 113:751–758, 1972
431. Goldstein DP: Chorionic gonadotropin. Cancer 38:453–457, 1976
432. Goldstein DP, Berkowitz RS: The management of gestational trophoblastic neoplasms. Cur Prob Obstet Gynecol 4:1–42, 1980
433. Bagshawe KD: Risk and prognostic factors in trophoblastic neoplasia. Cancer 38:1373–1385, 1976
434. Goldstein DP, Berkowitz RS, Cohen SM: The current management of molar pregnancy. Cur Prob Obstet Gynecol 3:1–39, 1979
435. Berkowitz RS, Goldstein DP: Methotrexate with citrovorum factor rescue for nonmetastatic gestational neoplasms. Obstet Gynecol 54:725–728, 1979
436. Ballon SC, Berman ML, Lagasse LD et al: The unique aspects of gestational trophoblastic disease. Obstet Gynecol Survey 32:405–415, 1977
437. Aitken S, Dembo A, Quirt I et al: Moderate dose methotrexate with folinic acid rescue (MX-MTX-FAR) in gestational trophoblastic disease (GID). Ann R Coll Physicians Surg Can 12:61, 1979
438. Bagshawe KD: Treatment of trophoblastic tumours. Ann Acad Med 5:273–279, 1976
439. Surwit EA, Suciu TN, Schmidt HJ et al: A new combination chemotherapy for resistant trophoblastic disease. Gynecol Oncol 8:110–118, 1979
440. Newlands ES, Bagshawe KD: Activity of high dose cis-platinum (NCI 119875) in combination with vincristine and methotrexate in drug resistant gestational choriocarcinoma. A report of 17 cases. Br J Cancer 40:943–945, 1979
441. Amiel JL, Droz JP, Tursz T: Placental tumors resistant to usual chemotherapy: Treatment using cis-diaminedichloroplatinum. Two cases. Nouv Presse Med 7:1933–1935, 1978
442. Newlands ES, Bagshawe KD: Epipodophyllin derivative (VP-16-213) in malignant teratomas and choriocarcinomas. Lancet 2:87, 1976
443. Berkowtiz RS, Goldstein DP, Jones MA et al: Methotrexate with citrovorum factor rescue: Reduced chemotherapy toxicity in the management of gestational trophoblastic neoplasms. Cancer 45:423–426, 1980
444. Ross GT: Congenital anomalies among children born to mothers receiving chemotherapy for gestational trophoblastic neoplasms. Cancer 37:1043–1047, 1976
445. Kuten A, Cohen Y, Tatcher M et al: Pregnancy and delivery after successful treatment of epidural metastatic choriocarcinoma. Gynecol Oncol 6:464–466, 1978
446. Theobald P, Pfau P: Three cases of choriocarcinoma. Geburtsh u Frauenheilk 38:212, 1978

Robert C. Young
Robert C. Knapp
Carlos A. Perez

CHAPTER 26

Cancer of the Ovary

Ovarian cancer is the fourth most frequent cause of cancer death in women and is the leading cause of gynecologic cancer death in the United States. Incidence and mortality estimates for 1980 indicate that 17,000 new patients will be diagnosed and 11,200 women will die from ovarian cancer.[1] A steady increase in the age-adjusted cancer death rates has been observed over the past 25 years and similar increases in other industrialized nations as well.[2]

EPIDEMIOLOGY AND STATISTICS

The highest ovarian cancer rates are reported from the highly industrialized countries with age-adjusted mortality rates that range from 3.02/100,000 in Italy, to 7.04/100,000 in the U.S., and 11.02/100,000 in Denmark. A notable exception to this association is Japan where rates of death from ovarian cancer are 1.69/100,000—among the lowest in the world. Studies of migrant populations also suggest significant environmental influences. Japanese migrants to Hawaii and their first generation offspring in the U.S. have an incidence that is significantly higher than those in Japan, but lower than in the indigenous Caucasian population of the U.S.[3],[4] Ovarian cancer is uncommon in developing nations perhaps, in part, because the disease is not always diagnosed.

In the U.S., the common epithelial neoplasms are most frequent in adult Caucasian populations and are rarely seen before menarche. However, they tend to increase significantly thereafter, with peak incidence in the 40–70 year-old age group. In contrast, germ cell ovarian tumors are primarily seen in children and young women, and are more frequent in nonwhite populations.

Several epidemiologic studies suggest that disordered endocrine function may contribute to the development of ovarian cancer. Higher incidences of epithelial tumors are seen in women with lower mean number of pregnancies, in those never pregnant, and those with a history of difficulties in conception.[5,6,7] Although a clear-cut association between ovarian cancer and administration of synthetic estrogens has not been established, it has been suggested that there may be an increased risk in patients receiving stilbestrol for menopausal symptoms.[8] Epidemiologic studies also suggest that cancer of the breast and ovary share some common etiologic factors. For example, women with breast cancer have twice the expected risk of developing subsequent ovarian carcinoma. Women with ovarian cancer have a three- to fourfold increase in the frequency of subsequent breast cancer.

Retrospective studies searching for some kind of viral association have generally been negative. Paradoxically, a lower than expected frequency of mumps and other viral exanthems is reported for women with ovarian cancer.[9]

Familial and genetic associations have been reported as well but are rare. Ovarian cancer has been reported in multiple members of the same or succeeding generations.[10] In addition, several unusual genetic disorders seem to predispose to ovarian neoplasms although the tumors are usually benign and stromal in origin. Females with Peutz–Jeghers syndrome (mucocutaneous pigmentation and intestinal polyps) have a 5–14% chance of developing ovarian tumors. Women with the inherited basal cell nevus syndrome develop benign fibromas or, rarely, other tumors. Patients with gonadal dysgenesis (46 XY genotype or mosaic) are prone to develop gonadoblastomas. Interestingly, patients with Turner's syndrome (45 XO) and undeveloped gonads have no such tendency. An increased frequency of ovarian thecomas has been described in patients on long-term anticonvulsant therapy. It is believed to be related to variations in the ability to metabolize anticonvulsant drugs.[11]

Although epidemiologic evidence strongly suggests that environmental factors are important, few, if any, associations have firmly been established. There is no good evidence to prove that either diagnostic or therapeutic irradiation increases the frequency of this malignancy. Likewise, there is no established association with known chemical carcinogens. However, there is still some concern about the association of asbestos and talc exposure with ovarian carcinoma in humans since talc and asbestos-like birefringent bodies have been identified in ovarian cancer tissue.[12] Studies indicate a higher-than-expected frequency of ovarian and peritoneal neoplasms in asbestos workers. Passage of such materials through the bowel wall or, in retrograde fashion, through the female reproductive tract has been described and could explain the access of such agents to the ovarian epithelium. Therefore, due to the above and other evidence further investigation of these two potential co-carcinogens should be undertaken.

PATHOGENESIS

The epithelial carcinomas of the ovary account for 80–90% of ovarian malignancies. They appear to have a common origin arising from the serosal mesothelial layer of the gonads. In the embryo, the coelomic epithelium overlies the mesoderm of the urogenital ridge and becomes the serosal mesothelial layer of the gonads or the paramesonephric coelomic epithelium. It is this epithelium that also develops into the müllerian duct, differentiating into the epithelium of the fallopian tube, endometrium, endocervix, and the squamous epithelium of the vagina. Since the paramesonephric coelomic epithelium has a multipotential capability of differentiating into endometrioid, mucinous, or serous epithelium, the common epithelial tumors in the ovary may give rise to malignancies having these characteristics.[13] These tumors disseminate primarily by surface implantation or lymphatic spread and rarely metastasize hematogenously.

The most common mechanism of spread is by continuity and intraperitoneal dissemination.[14] To clearly understand this mechanism, the spread of material introduced into the peritoneal cavity and its dissemination must be described. When a suspension of red blood cells, india ink, colloidal silver, or radiographic contrast media is injected into the peritoneal cavity of humans or experimental animals, it is removed almost exclusively by lymphatic capillaries lining the diaphragmatic peritoneum.[15] These capillaries form a diffuse plexus on the diaphragm's pleural surface. They are concentrated in the muscular portion of the right diaphragm. The rolling motion of the intestines and the fluctuating intra-abdominal pressure associated with respiration appear to be responsible for the cephalad movement of material toward the undersurface of the diaphragm, especially in the area over the liver. In turn, the lymphatic capillaries of the diaphragm that arise in the submesothelial plexus intercommunicate with a comparable plexus arising on the pleural surface. From the diaphragm, lymphatic drainage primarily occurs to the anterior mediastinal lymph nodes that also communicate with the supraclavicular nodes on the left side. Efferent lymphatics of the anterior mediastinal nodes enter into the right subclavian vein. This pathway is quantitively the most significant, accounting for 80% of the clearance from the peritoneal cavity. Based on the physiology of particulate matter removal from the peritoneal cavity by the diaphragmatic lymphatics, diaphragmatic metastasis may occur in patients with ovarian carcinoma without gross intra-abdominal disease.[16]

Studies using an ovarian carcinoma mouse model have revealed ovarian tumor cells filling diaphragmatic lymphatics well in advance of clinical ascites.[17] Studies from the National Cancer Institute (NCI) have evaluated the presence of diaphragmatic metastasis in patients with presumptive Stage I and II ovarian cancer and reported an incidence of 44%.[18,19] Piver and associates reviewed the overall incidence of diaphragmatic metastasis and noted an 11.3% incidence for Stage I and a 23.0% for Stage II.[20] Based upon current information, the spread of ovarian carcinoma and its major pathways are presented in Figure 26-1.

Ascites formation in ovarian cancer appears to be related to impaired diaphragmatic drainage. This correlates histologically with the presence of tumor cells obstructing the diaphragmatic lymphatics. Studies with mediastinal lymphoscintigraphy suggest that blockage of the normal lymphatic pathways draining the peritoneal cavity may be one of the mechanisms involved in the ascites accumulation of malignant disease.[21]

Although intraperitoneal dissemination is the most commonly observed modality of spread, the ovarian lymphatics are also an important pathway of dissemination. The ovary contains an extensive lymphatic network in the theca externa and corpus luteum. The ovarian efferents from the subovarian

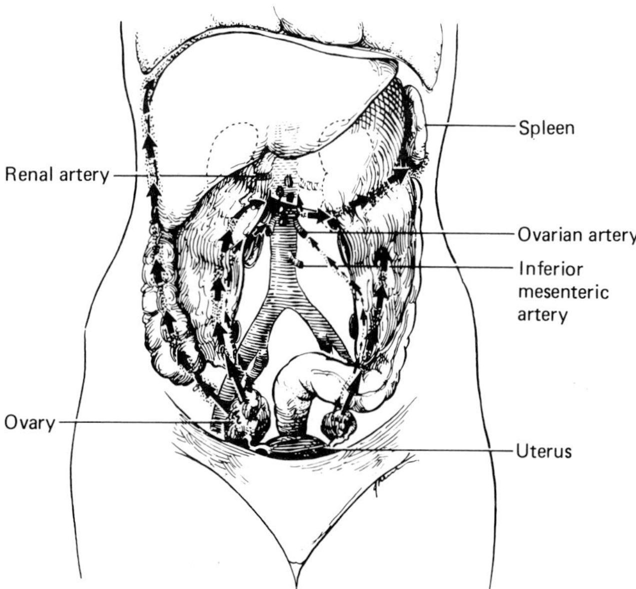

FIG. 26-1. Schematic drawing representing the patterns of dissemination of ovarian carcinoma. (Courtesy of Knapp RC, Berkowitz RS, Leavitt Jr. T: Natural history and detection of ovarian cancer. In Bushsbaum HJ (ed): Gynecology and Obstetrics, vol IV—Oncology, pp 1–14. Hagerstown, Harper and Row, 1980)

TABLE 26-1. World Health Organization Classification of Malignant Ovarian Tumors

COMMON EPITHELIAL TUMORS

- Malignant Serous Tumors
  - Adenocarcinoma, papillary adenocarcinoma, papillary cystadenocarcinoma
  - Surface papillary carcinoma
  - Malignant adenofibroma, cystadenofibroma
- Malignant Mucinous Tumors
  - Adenocarcinoma, cystadenocarcinoma
  - Malignant adenofibroma, cystadenofibroma
- Malignant Endometrioid Tumors
  - Carcinoma
    - Adenocarcinoma
    - Adenoacanthoma
    - Malignant adenofibroma, cystadenofibroma
  - Endometrioid stromal sarcomas
  - Mesodermal (Mullerian) mixed tumors: homologous and heterologous
- Clear Cell (mesonephroid) Tumors
  - Malignant
  - Malignant: carcinoma and adenocarcinoma
- Brenner Tumors
  - Malignant
- Mixed Epithelial Tumors
  - Malignant
- Undifferentiated Carcinoma
- Unclassified Epithelial Tumors

SEX CORD—STROMAL TUMORS

- Granulosa–Stromal Cell Tumors
  - Granulosa cell tumor
  - Tumors in the thecoma–fibroma group
  - Fibroma
  - Unclassified
- Androblastomas: Sertoli–Leydig Cell Tumors
  - Well differentiated
    - Tubular androblastoma, Sertoli cell tumor (tubular adenoma of Pick)
    - Tubular androblastoma with lipid storage, Sertoli cell tumor with lipid storage (folliculome lipidique of Lecene)
    - Sertoli–Leydig cell tumor (tubular adenoma with Leydig cells)
    - Leydig cell tumor, hilus cell tumor
  - Of intermediate differentiation
  - Poorly differentiated (sarcomatoid)
  - With heterologous elements
- Gynandroblastoma
- Unclassified

LIPID (LIPOID) CELL TUMORS

GERM CELL TUMORS

- Dysgerminoma
- Endodermal Sinus Tumor
- Embryonal Carcinoma
- Polyembryoma
- Choriocarcinoma
- Teratomas
  - Immature
  - Mature dermoid cyst with malignant transformation
  - Monodermal and highly specialized
    - Struma ovarii
    - Carcinoid
    - Struma ovarii and carcinoid
    - Others
- Mixed forms

GONADOBLASTOMA

- Pure
- Mixed with dysgerminoma or other form of germ cell tumor

(Modified from Serov SF, Scully RE, Solvin LH: International histological classification of tumors, No. 9. Histological Typing of Ovarian Tumors. Geneva, World Health Organization, 1973)

plexus follow the ovarian blood vessels in the infundibulopelvic ligament. They cross the ureter and external iliac artery and travel cephalad with the ovarian vessels, close to the psoas muscle along the lateral aspect of the ureter. At the lower pole of the kidney, the lymphatics turn medially, cross the ureter a second time, and terminate in the para-aortic nodes.

A recent review of the incidence of aortic and pelvic lymph node metastasis in Stage I and II ovarian cancer reported an incidence of approximately 10%.[20] At surgery, it is often difficult to distinguish aortic lymph node metastases from benign glandular inclusions.[22] Biopsy of these nodes must be performed to establish the accurate stage. Bergman reviewed the autopsies of patients who died from ovarian cancer and showed an incidence of aortic nodal involvement of 78%.[23] He noted that ovarian carcinoma in this autopsied group spread primarily and predominantly by direct peritoneal involvement and lymphatic dissemination irrespective of the histologic type and grade of carcinoma.

Although peritoneum, omentum, and bowel surfaces are the most frequent sites of spread of metastatic ovarian cancer, other organs are at risk for metastasis. Of the genital organs, the uterus is the most frequent site of involvement, particularly the posterior serosal surface of the uterus and the cul-de-sac. The coexistence of ovarian and uterine adenocarcinoma is not infrequent. The primary site of origin is difficult to ascertain, particularly in endometrioid ovarian carcinoma where one-third are associated with endometrium carcinoma.[24]

The fallopian tube is not infrequently involved in ovarian cancer. It appears that involvement is a direct extension rather than lymphatic permeation. The involvement of the opposite ovary has been reported by Woodruff to occur in more than 50% of all cases of epithelial ovarian cancer and this involvement is often related to the grade and histologic tumor type.[25] Serous carcinomas of the ovary are generally reported to be bilateral in almost two-thirds of all cases.[24] About 25% of the mucinous adenocarcinomas are bilateral. The spread from one ovary to the other is often by way of retrograde lymphatic extension caused by tumor blockage in the efferent lymphatics. Among the distant organs that may be involved with ovarian carcinoma (in order of decreasing frequency) are: liver, lung, pleura, kidney, bone, adrenal, bladder, and spleen.[14]

PATHOLOGY

HISTOLOGIC TYPES

Several comprehensive reviews of the pathology of ovarian cancer have been published recently. These provide detailed pathologic descriptions for each of the individual tumor types.[26–28] The World Health Organization (WHO) and the International Federation of Gynecology and Obstetrics (FIGO) have adopted a unified classification of the common epithelial tumors, the sex cord–stromal tumors, and the germ cell tumors (see Table 26-1). The vast majority (85–90%) of malignant ovarian tumors seen in the U.S. are of the epithelial type and their approximate overall frequency is as follows: serous cystadenocarcinoma, 42%; mucinous cystadenocarcinoma, 12%; endometrial carcinoma, 15%; undifferentiated carcinoma, 17%; and clear cell carcinoma, 6%. The remaining 8% of primary tumors are the sex cord–stromal and germ cell tumors.

TUMORS OF BORDERLINE MALIGNANCY

Epithelial tumors are generally classified according to whether they are benign, malignant (invasive), or "carcinomas of low malignant potential" (tumors of borderline malignancy). The latter group is characterized pathologically like tumors that have neoplastic epithelial cells, detached cellular clusters from sites of origin, increased mitotic activity, and nuclear abnormalities. However, they *lack* obvious invasion of the supporting stroma. These tumors clearly possess a different natural history; they progress and metastasize slowly. Nevertheless, patients do die from these tumors of low malignant potential and the issue of what constitutes optimal therapy is controversial and unresolved. It is, however, important to recognize their different natural history. This group is to be considered an important stratification factor when analyzing survival data from clinical trials. Many investigators advocate therapeutic approaches similar to those used for more invasive tumors, for in spite of the fact that these tumors grow more slowly, approximately 15% of these patients will die of disease within the first five years.

In invasive epithelial carcinomas, significant independent correlation of survival with histologic type has been difficult to establish since some investigators have reported such a correlation while others have not.[29,30,31] The current consensus is that there is limited prognostic significance to the histologic type of malignant epithelial ovarian cancer independent of clinical stage, extent of residual disease, and histologic grade. Published response rates for the three major epithelial tumors (serous, mucinous, and undifferentiated) treated with single alkylating agents are similar to the complete remission rates.[32,33] Median durations of complete remission are longer for mucinous (46.5 months) than for serous (20 months) or undifferentiated (16.5 months), but these differences may relate to histologic grade or extent of residual disease more than to histologic type.[33]

HISTOLOGIC GRADING

In contrast to histologic type, the degree of cellular differentiation of epithelial cancers (histologic grade) appears to be an important independent prognostic factor. It helps to determine response to treatment and survival.[34–37] The influence of grading has been more prognostically significant for patients with Stage I and II disease. For example, studies from the Mayo Clinic using the Broder's classification in Stage II, serous cystadenocarcinoma demonstrate an 80% survival for patients with grade 1 tumors, 47% for grade 2, and 10% for grade 3 and 4 tumors.[38] Anderson has made similar observations using the pattern system of grading.[39] In Stage I and II serous carcinoma of the ovary, patients with grade 1 tumors had a 78% seven year survival, compared to 35% for grade 2, and 0% for grade 3. Although early studies demonstrated this prognostic impact more dramatically for patients with early stage disease, more recent studies suggest it is an important factor even in more advanced disease. Using grading systems based upon cytologic detail (Broder's) or the pattern-grading classification based upon the degree to which the tumor forms papillary structures or glands versus solid tumor, NCI investigators were able to show survival significance to grading systems for patients with advanced disease treated with chemotherapy.[40] Similar conclusions using another grading scheme from patients treated with radiation therapy in recent studies from the Princess Margaret Hospital have also been shown.[41] Furthermore, recent information suggests that grading systems may even predict for responses to different chemotherapy approaches. Analysis of NCI chemotherapy studies in advanced disease indicates that combination chemotherapy produces a more impressive survival effect in patients with modified Broder's grade 2 and 3 tumors compared to single alkylating agent treatment.[42]

Histologic grading of ovarian tumors has not been accepted enthusiastically by pathologists, primarily because no standardized and easily reproducible objective classification exists. In spite of the different classifications used, virtually every published study thus far indicates an important survival impact of grading these tumors. Grading of epithelial ovarian tumors is now a necessary requirement in every carefully designed clinical study. Therefore, an easily reproducible, uniformly accepted classification should be established.

STROMAL AND GERM CELL TUMORS

Stromal Tumors

Less than 10% of all ovarian tumors fall into this category. These include tumors containing granulosa, theca, Sertoli, Leydig, and collagen-producing stromal cells or their embryonic precursors.[28,43] Only one of the many stromal tumors listed in Table 26-1 is seen with significant frequency—the granulosa cell tumor. This tumor is composed of granulosa cells, with or without an admixture of theca cells, and may contain folliculoid structures known as Call–Exner bodies. These tumors can be associated with feminizing effects and precocious puberty due to tumor-related estrogen secretion. Presenting signs and symptoms are similar to epithelial ovarian tumors with the exception of those related to hyperestrogenism. These tumors tend to be discovered at earlier stages and have a more indolent course than the epithelial tumors. Late recurrences can sometimes be effectively treated with repeated cytoreductive surgery. There is no convincing evidence that the tumor is particularly responsive to radiation therapy. In addition, chemotherapy has been limited but responses to alkylating agents and adriamycin have been published.

Sertoli–Leydig cell tumors are characterized by differentiation toward testicular structures. These contain various mixtures of Sertoli and Leydig cells and tissues similar to the fetal testis.

Gonadal stromal tumors occasionally contain granulosa cell elements combined with tubules and Leydig cells characteristic of the arrhenoblastoma. Thus, they are then termed gynandroblastomas.

Germ Cell Tumors

Although germ cell tumors comprise less than 5% of all ovarian malignancies they form an important group. They are more apt to occur in young women, display vastly different natural histories, and often require different therapeutic approaches. Of these tumors, dysgerminoma, endodermal sinus tumor, and embryonal carcinoma are most often encountered. The dysgerminomas comprise less than 2% of all ovarian malignancies, are cytologically similar to seminoma of the testis, and display a very similar natural history. These tumors are frequently unilateral, tend to be localized with secondary spread by way of the lymphatics to the para-aortic nodes. The tumor is highly radiosensitive. Primary management is surgery and radiation. Five year survival rates with effective conventional therapy approach 80–90%.

The terms *endodermal sinus tumor* and *embryonal carcinoma* have, in the past, often been used interchangeably to describe highly malignant germ cell tumors of the ovary. However, there is now evidence to prove that the two disorders are different.[43] Embryonal carcinoma, with the different patterns typical of embryonal carcinoma of the testis and associated with elevations of hCG or alpha fetoprotein, is rarely seen in the ovary. Endodermal sinus tumors are more commonly seen and are similar morphologically to the infantile orchioblastoma of the testis. The endodermal sinus tumor, also called yolk sac tumor, is characterized by reticular patterns, papillary formations known as Schiller–Duval bodies, and both intracellular and extracellular hyaline droplets. This tumor is derived from extra-embryonic rather than embryonic tissues. Both tumors are highly aggressive, metastasize hematogenously, and are poorly controlled even with radical surgery and irradiation. Chemotherapy is highly effective and will be discussed in a later section.

Lipid Cell Tumors

Lipid, or lipoid, cell tumors are a heterogenous group composed of polygonal cells containing lipid. They are the rarest of the functioning ovarian tumors and are usually virilizing, although 25% have been associated with estrogen secretion. They are usually unilateral and benign.

Teratomas

These tumors are comprised of elements from all three germ cell layers—ectoderm, mesoderm, and endoderm. They are cystic or solid, and composed of admixtures of immature and adult tissues. The malignant potential of these tumors is related to the presence of immature embryonal tissues rather than their gross appearance.

Gonadoblastomas

Gonadoblastomas are rare tumors characterized by germ cells admixed with sex cord elements resembling immature granulosa and Sertoli cells. Bilateral involvement occurs in about one-third of all cases. These tumors occur almost exclusively in genetically abnormal persons with the majority of cases being sex chromatin negative. In addition, approximately one-half of all reported cases have been associated with dysgerminomas.

DIAGNOSIS AND STAGING

PRESURGICAL STAGING

Symptoms related to ovarian malignancy are usually manifestations of advanced disease. Kent and McKay reviewed 349 patients and reported that the initial presenting symptom in patients with ovarian cancer was pain in 57% and abdominal distention in 51%.[36] Pearse and Behrman reported that 25% of patients with ovarian cancer had dysfunctional or postmenopausal bleeding as their presenting symptom.[44] This bleeding may be due to metastatic involvement of the endometrium, a concurrent primary endometrial malignancy, or a sex cord mesenchymal tumor with a functionally active stroma.

During the early course of its natural history, ovarian cancer tends to remain asymptomatic and silent. Since no peritoneal covering on the ovary exists, pain is elicited by stretching of the ovarian ligaments. Pain may also be caused by torsion of the ovary. Rupture of an ovarian malignancy can cause pain, eliciting the signs of generalized peritoneal irritation. As the ovarian cancer grows, it may invade or compress adjacent pelvic organs causing abdominal distress and bladder and bowel irritability. Since the growth and involvement of adjacent structures is often insidious, symptoms of nausea, dyspepsia, and vague lower abdominal discomfort are frequently ignored by the patient or the doctor. It is essential that perimenopausal or postmenopausal women with gastrointestinal or pelvic complaints have a thorough physical and pelvic examination with particular attention to the adnexal area. The physical examination must be guided by the knowledge of patterns of spread of ovarian cancer. For example, examination for the presence of lymphadenopathy should be part of the initial physical examination, as an enlarged left supraclavicular lymph node may be the first clinical sign of ovarian malignancy.

Since the clinical assessment of ascites is often difficult, a needle paracentesis is often helpful in obtaining a definitive diagnosis of malignant ascites.

Still the best method of evaluating possible ovarian cancer is the pelvic examination. This bimanual examination should evaluate uterine position, size, and the presence of any adnexal masses. The recto–vaginal examination is the best method of determining the presence of adnexal pathology and, at the same time, assessing nodularity in the cul-de-sac and obtaining stool for occult blood. Often, fecal material, particularly in a redundant sigmoid, can be confused with adnexal nodular masses. If occult blood is noted in the stool of older patients, a diagnosed adnexal mass may be due to a colonic malignancy or diverticulitis. For the preoperative evaluation of a patient with a suspected ovarian malignancy, both sigmoidoscopy and barium enema are necessary.

When an adnexal mass is palpated, associated physical

findings that suggest a malignant process may exist. When the adnexal mass is fixed to adjacent structures ovarian cancer should be suspected. (Ovarian malignancy frequently involves both ovaries.) Painless nodules in the cul-de-sac or along the uterosacral ligaments may also be linked to cancer. At initial presentation, physical examination will reveal pelvic nodularity or a frozen pelvis in one-third of all patients with ovarian cancer.[44]

If an ovarian enlargement is noted during the reproductive years, the most likely diagnosis is a functional ovarian cyst. Under the age of 30, 90% of ovarian neoplasms are benign. When a follicular or luteal cyst is suspected based on physical findings, a re-examination in six to eight weeks is indicated. Most functional cysts will undergo spontaneous regression in one or two menstrual cycles. The patients may also be placed on oral contraceptives for ovarian suppression to facilitate resolution of the functional cyst. Concern for ovarian cancer is heightened when an adnexal mass is detected in a perimenopausal female or when the ovary is greater than 5 cm in diameter. Approximately one-third of perimenopausal neoplasms are malignant. The differential diagnosis from the subserosal myoma is often difficult. After cessation of the menstrual cycles, the ovary atrophies from 3½ × 2 × 1½ cm to a size of approximately 2 × 1 × ½ cm. Therefore, it should not be palpable on pelvic examination. The presence of a palpable postmenopausal ovary must alert the physician to possible underlying malignancy.[45]

Cervical and vaginal pool cytology is rarely positive for the detection of ovarian cancer. Needle culdocentesis is used as a possible aid in detecting early ovarian cancer. Cell samples can be obtained readily by culdocentesis and malignant cells in peritoneal fluid from early ovarian cancer can be identified.[46] However, it is not likely that the widespread use of peritoneal fluid sampling for the early detection of ovarian cancer is clinically applicable. Further, 1,123 asymptomatic women were evaluated by this method and no ovarian cancers were detected.

Laparoscopy may be of value in ovarian cancer diagnosis when used to differentiate uterine leiomyoma from a solid ovarian neoplasm or endometriosis.

Ultrasound

Refinements in technology and increased sophistication in interpretation have made ultrasonic evaluation of pelvic masses helpful in the pre-staging evaluation of suspected ovarian cancer. The use of gray scale and B-scanning along with dynamic scanning permits greater discrimination and more precise evaluation of adnexal pathology than older, more conventional equipment. The presence of solid elements and prominent papillary projections and the involvement of adjacent viscera may suggest a malignant neoplasm. Ultrasound may be used to distinguish ascites from a large ovarian cyst. A mass separate from the uterus associated with internal echoes of normal sensitivity may indicate ovarian cancer. Ultrasound has also been used as a diagnostic tool.[47,48] Ultrasound may also be used to direct percutaneous aspiration of suspected metastasis or aspiration biopsies of aortic nodes in ovarian cancer.[49]

Lymphangiography

Lymphangiography has been reported to be useful in the prestaging evaluation of patients with known or suspected ovarian cancer.[50,51] In a series from Stanford University, 21% of patients classified as Stage I or Stage II at laparotomy had positive lymphangiograms.[52] Musumeci and coworkers reported on the use of the lymphangiogram in 289 patients with epithelial ovarian cancer.[53] Aortic node dissection was performed in 68 patients to assess the validity of lymphangiographic interpretation. In 20 patients with positive preoperative lymphangiograms, aortic node dissection confirmed the presence of nodal involvement in all 20 patients. In 48 patients with negative preoperative lymphangiograms, microscopic nodal involvement was demonstrated in eight patients for a false negative rate of 19% The overall accuracy of lymphangiographic diagnosis in their study, compared to aortic node dissection, was 87%. Athey and associates reported a 90% incidence of metastasis to aortic nodes in patients with germ cell tumors and 30% incidence to iliac nodes.[51] They noted that ovarian cancers of epithelial cell origin metastasized to iliac lymph nodes in 73%, to aortic lymph nodes in 60%, and to the inguinal lymph nodes in 41%.

Computerized Tomography

The diagnostic accuracy of computerized tomography (CT) is currently being compared with ultrasound, lymphangiography, and surgery in several prospective studies. CT may clearly delineate liver and pulmonary nodules, abdominal and pelvic masses, and retroperitoneal nodal involvement. CT has been particularly useful in ovarian carcinoma when therapeutically produced bowel ileus due to pelvic and abdominal masses makes ultrasound impossible to interpret.[54] Recently, CT has been used to detect subcutaneous metastasis in patients with ovarian cancer.[55]

SURGICAL STAGING

The initial operation for ovarian cancer determines the stage of the disease and the future management of the patient. Surgical treatment is the keystone for all subsequent therapy. The surgeon must carefully record the location of tumor spread, note whether the residual tumor is greater than 2 cm in any single location, and approximate the remaining tumor volume. In 1976, revisions of early staging classifications brought the TMN and the classification of the International Federations of Gynecology and Obstetrics (FIGO) into complete conformity. The Manual for Staging of Cancer states, "Staging is based on the findings of clinical examination and surgical exploration. The final histologic findings (and cytologic when available) after surgery are to be considered in the staging."[56] Stages based on the FIGO nomenclature are listed in Table 26-2.

The abdominal incision for surgical staging should be vertical and of adequate length to insure proper exploration of the abdominal contents. A horizontal low abdominal incision below the pubic hair line (Pfannenstiehl) is not adequate for proper exploration in the staging of ovarian cancer. If a

TABLE 26-2. FIGO Stage Grouping for Primary Carcinoma of the Ovary (1976)

STAGE I	Growth limited to the ovaries
STAGE IA	Growth limited to one ovary; no ascites
STAGE IAi	No tumor on the external surface; capsule intact
STAGE IAii	Tumor present on the external surface, or capsule(s) ruptured, or both
STAGE IB	Growth limited to both ovaries; no ascites
STAGE IBi	No tumor on the external surface; capsule intact
STAGE IBii	Tumor present on the external surface, or capsule(s) ruptured, or both
STAGE IC	Tumor either stage IA or IB, but with ascites present or with positive peritoneal washings
STAGE II	Growth involving one or both ovaries with pelvic extension
STAGE IIA	Extension and/or metastases to the uterus and/or tubes
STAGE IIB	Extension to other pelvic tissues
STAGE IIC	Tumor either Stage IIA or IIB, but with ascites present or with positive peritoneal washings

(Uldfelder H (Chairman): Staging system for cancer at gynecologic sites. Manual for staging of cancer, pp. 94–97, 1978)

TABLE 26-3. Staging Laparotomy in Ovarian Cancer

EVALUATION
Unilateral or bilateral disease
Tumor on external surface of ovary
Capsule intact
Spill

BIOPSIES
Any suspicious lesions
Pelvic peritoneum (three biopsies)
Cul-de-sac peritoneum
Right and left abdominal gutter
Under surface of right diaphragm
Partial omentectomy
Para-aortic nodes
Peritoneal washings

transverse incision has been performed and ovarian cancer has been discovered, the incision should be extended and the rectus muscles divided. Even then, upper abdominal exploration is more difficult than if the vertical incision was made. The presence, amount, and character (*i.e.*, bloody) of ascites should be noted and samples of the ascitic fluid sent for cytologic evaluation of malignant cells. The status of the tumor capsule should also be determined for the presence of rupture or excrescence on the external surface of the tumor. Webb and coworkers reported that the five-year survival of 111 patients with Stage I ovarian carcinoma in whom the tumor capsules were intact was 90%; in 108 patients with capsular penetration or rupture, the five-year survival was 57%.[57] If no ascites is present, approximately 200 ml of saline should be instilled in the abdomen and allowed to circulate for approximately 3–5 minutes prior to aspiration for cytologic examination. The washings should be placed in separate containers so that sites of positive tumor cells can be identified relative to particular locations for further therapy.

Prior to any dissection of the pelvic organs, the upper abdomen must be carefully explored. Particular attention should be paid to both the manual and visual examination of the diaphragm to detect the presence of tumor nodules, particularly on the right leaf of the diaphragm. Tumor seedings on the diaphragm can usually be felt. These seedings should be biopsied for accurate staging using a flexible pinch forceps. All liver nodules should be biopsied for histologic confirmation. The omentum should be inspected starting at its attachment of the lower border of the stomach and a partial omentectomy performed to detect the presence of nonpalpable metastatic omental involvement. Parker has suggested removal of the omental apron from the transverse colon to improve survival in patients with Stage I ovarian cancer.[58] However, it is difficult to determine if omentectomy contributes to increased survival or merely eliminates patients with micrometastasis from Stage I.

Both paracolic gutters must be inspected, particularly on the right side. The entire small and large bowel must be examined for metastatic spread. Suspected cancer on both bowel and mesentery surfaces should be biopsied. Since the root of the small bowel mesentery, the rectosigmoid, and cul-de-sac are often early sites of metastatic spread, it is important that careful attention be directed to these areas. Finally, evaluation is made of the pelvic peritoneum, including the peritoneum over the bladder, serosa of the uterus, and fallopian tubes.

Even if no tumor is detected outside the pelvis, the aortic nodes should be sampled to prove the presence or absence of cancer in the upper abdomen. Aortic nodes should be biopsied on the same level as the insertion of the ovarian arteries, whether or not they are clinically suspicious. Metastatic deposits are often present in clinically nonsuspicious aortic lymph nodes. Aortic node sampling is essential in patients with Stages I and II disease during the operative procedure, particularly if frozen section has shown the tumor to be poorly differentiated. The 60–65%, five-year survival reported for Stage I disease may be due in part to failure in detecting unsuspected aortic lymph node involvement. One would assume that if all tumor had, in fact been confined to one or both ovaries, survival would be considerably higher. In obvious Stage III disease sampling of aortic nodes is not always necessary.

The surgical exploration for staging must be thorough. Areas as remote as the splenic pedicle must be checked for any evidence of metastasis. Thorough exploration yields proper staging. Thus, the treatment can be planned accordingly. Routine evaluation of all intra-abdominal areas at high risk should be undertaken along with biopsies of appropriate sites as outlined in Table 26-3.

Staging is incomplete without emphasizing the prognostic importance of the size of residual tumor remaining after the surgical procedure. Surgical staging should note the size and exact sites of residual tumor, as this information is crucial to planning of the therapeutic regimen and prognosis of the patient. Accurate staging has important prognostic implications. Tobias and Griffiths showed the correlation between stage and five-year survival in a collected series shown in Table 26-4.[59]

The operative procedure for Stage I ovarian carcinoma in the perimenopausal or menopausal woman is a total abdominal hysterectomy and bilateral salpingo–oophorectomy.

Since 10% of malignant epithelial cancers occur in patients below the age of 35, the surgeon must make a judgment decision at the initial operation to perform either a unilateral salpingo–oophorectomy or to take the more radical approach of removing both ovaries and the uterus. Unless there is unequivocal evidence on frozen section of poorly differentiated cancer, the initial operation should be as conservative as possible. Cell washings are obtained, the abdomen carefully surveyed for metastatic disease, and omentectomy performed for diagnostic evaluation of metastasis. Since the common epithelial cancers may be bilateral, adequate wedge biopsy of the opposite ovary should be obtained. Scully reviewed the results of three major series in which the cancer was limited to a single ovary.[24,28] He noted a 78% survival among 72 patients treated conservatively and a 79% survival among 67 treated more radically. He analyzed Munnell's data in which 28 patients were treated conservatively and 105 treated radically and the survival was 75% in each instance. Kottmeier recommends conservative treatment of the unilateral mucinous and endometrioid tumors, whether borderline or invasive. The serious and undifferentiated tumors, which have a greater propensity for bilaterality, are to be treated by removal of both adnexae. Young women with poorly differentiated cancer proven on permanent section require reoperation if the conservative approach has been used at the initial operation. At the time of the second operation, a total abdominal hysterectomy and bilateral salpingo–oophorectomy should be performed as well as sampling of the aortic lymph nodes.

Surgical therapy of malignant germ cell tumors requires special consideration. In the patient with dysgerminoma and a unilateral encapsulated tumor, it is essential to evaluate pelvic and aortic lymph nodes, as these tumors have a propensity to spread by way of the lymphatics. The opposite ovary should be adequately biopsied at the initial operation. Several experts recommend conservative therapy if the opposite ovary is found to be negative, the lymph nodes reveal no metastasis, and there is no demonstrable intraperitoneal spread. Nevertheless, these patients should be followed closely during the first two postoperative years when the majority of recurrences take place.

The endodermal sinus tumor limited to one ovary is well-treated with an oophorectomy, biopsy of the opposite ovary, aortic node sampling, and omentectomy. There appears to be no advantage to radical surgery in Stage I endodermal sinus tumors since chemotherapy has been responsible for effective disease control after more conservative surgery.

Stage II ovarian cancer is treated by total abdominal hysterectomy, bilateral salpingo–oophorectomy, and removal of all pelvic tumor, so that no tumor greater than 2 cm remains in any single location. Meticulous care must be taken to be sure that the cancer is limited to the pelvis.

CYTOREDUCTIVE SURGERY

Recently, cytoreductive surgery for ovarian cancer has gained popularity. The purpose of cytoreductive surgery in ovarian cancer is to decrease the total body burden of tumor cells. Theoretically, it would appear essential for the surgeon to remove as much tumor as possible to reduce the total number of malignant cells. However, studies have indicated that simply reducing the tumor mass and leaving bulk tumor does not seem to be sufficient.

TABLE 26-4. Relation of Stage to Prognosis*

STAGE	NUMBER OF PATIENTS	% FIVE YEAR SURVIVAL
I	751	61
Ia	528	65
Ib	130	52
Ic	80	52
II	401	40
IIa	40	60
IIb	205	38
III	539	5
IV	101	3

*collected series
(Tobias JS, Griffiths CT: N Engl J Med 294:818–823, 1976)

For several decades, surgeons have made an effort to remove bulk disease in ovarian cancer. It has been apparent that patients without palpable or gross residual cancer survive appreciably longer in comparison to patients with more extensive disease. Delclos and Quinlan first reported improvement in four-year survival when patients are categorized by the amount of disease remaining after surgery.[60] When surgery was followed by radiation therapy, survival was better when small tumor nodules, less than 2 cm in diameter, remained than when larger tumor masses remained after surgery. Griffiths and Fuller have estimated that in Stage III ovarian carcinoma, the volume of solid tumor usually exceeds 1 kilogram in weight, which is in excess of 10^{12} cells, and represents 40 tumor doublings from the initial single neoplastic cell.[61] The removal of 50% of the tumor bulk only reduces tumor growth by one doubling or 2.5%. Thus, reducing the tumor bulk by 50% is of little value.

Griffiths did a retrospective evaluation to determine the significance of cytoreductive surgery in ovarian cancer using a multilinear regression equation with survival as the dependent variable.[62] The diameter of the largest residual tumor below 1.5 cm was highly significant as an independent determinant of survival. Survival time was decreased if the diameter of the largest residual tumor exceeded 1.0 ± 0.5 cm regardless of other prognostic factors. He further evaluated a group of patients with Stage III ovarian carcinoma in whom tumor size was surgically reduced to less than 1.5 cm. The survival of these patients was similar to those patients whose largest metastases were below 1.5 cm prior to surgery. Survival in both groups was 20% at 80 months, as compared to a 0% survival at 38 months in patients whose residual tumor exceeded 1.5 cm. Smith and Day reviewed the records of 2,115 patients with ovarian cancer and noted that the single most important prognostic factor was a residual tumor nodule of less than or equal to 1 cm.[63] Patients with tumor masses of greater than 1 cm remaining after surgery had a poor five-year survival. From their analysis, it appears that stage or amount of abdominal spread is less important than the size of the largest residual nodule after surgery, particularly if the nodule is 2 cm or larger.

The maximal effectiveness of cytoreductive surgery, in which the largest residual tumor nodule is less than 2 cm, can only be achieved by further therapy with effective chemotherapy or radiation. The induction of a complete response from chemotherapy is more likely in patients who have residual tumor of no greater than 2 cm in any single location. The necessity to follow cytoreductive surgery with the most effective chemotherapy is emphasized in a study by Young and coworkers.[64] They prospectively evaluated melphalan versus hexamethylmelamine, cyclophosphamide, methotrexate, and 5-fluorouracil (HexaCAF). In the melphalan arm there was a greater proportion of responses in patients with masses under 2 cm than in those with larger masses. In the HexaCAF arm there were complete responses in all eight patients with masses under 2 cm. However, only five of 32 patients with larger masses had complete responses. Parker and coworkers reviewed 60 patients with Stage III–IV ovarian adenocarcinoma in which adriamycin and cyclophosphamide were employed after surgical treatment.[65] In 11 of 12 patients in whom the lesions were less than 2 cm in size, a complete response was noted as opposed to one of 24 patients with tumors greater than 2 cm. Griffiths and associates evaluated 28 patients treated with adriamycin–cyclophosphamide.[66] When cytoreductive surgery was followed with postoperative combination chemotherapy, the median survival was 18+ months; in those patients in whom chemotherapy was followed by surgery, the median survival was only 6+ months; in those with operations for recurrence, the median survival was 12 months.

The improved survival following cytoreductive surgery is not solely limited to chemotherapy. Dembo and coworkers showed that the survival of patients receiving whole abdominal radiation was significantly better than that of patients receiving pelvic irradiation plus chemotherapy, but only when the comparison was among patients who had minimal residual disease, following bilateral salpingo–oophorectomy and hysterectomy.[67]

It is apparent that initial cytoreductive surgery, which will reduce the tumor burden to less than 2 cm in diameter in any single location, followed by effective combination chemotherapy or abdominal radiation, can increase survival of patients with advanced ovarian cancer. To remove part of the tumor, leaving more than 2 cm residual masses, is of little value. Reducing the tumor burden to less than 2 cm appears to be more significant than stage of the disease.

Evidence now indicates that the extent of residual disease at initial surgery directly correlates with the incidence of negative second-look operations. In a followup of patients from M. D. Anderson, Smith and Schwartz found negative "second-looks" in approximately 30% of those with minimal residual disease compared to 16.7% for patients who started with residual disease greater than 2 cm.[68] Residual tumor resection at second-look surgery also improves survival. Two and five year survivals for patients who had the complete tumor resected at second-look were 47.5 and 27% respectively. In their study, patients treated with chemotherapy (in most instances, single agent melphalan) had better survival than those subsequently treated with radiation.

It is obvious that cytoreductive surgery is not feasible in all situations. A short course of combination chemotherapy, followed by cytoreductive surgery, and then continuing chemotherapy may be of value in those cases where optimal primary surgery is not possible. However, it is important to reserve as much of the chemotherapy to the postoperative period as possible. It is still not clear why patients with similar grade and stage are operable and others are not. It appears to be primarily related to the method of the tumor spread. If the tumor extends into the lesser sac around the pancreas, or the splenic pedicle, cytoreductive surgery may not be possible.

The operative technique and the need for nutritional support have been well described.[61] Knapp and coworkers have described a method of dissecting parauterine tissue planes and lateral pelvic wall structures to effect a rapid, simple, and relatively bloodless exposure in situations where the ovarian cancer has completely obliterated all tissue planes in the pelvis.[69] The paravesical space is entered by incising the round ligament some distance from the uterine incision (dissection must be done on the lateral side of the hypogastric artery). The space is entered with a finger or blunt instrument; the peritoneum over the psoas muscle is extended cephalad to the pelvic brim; the ureter is identified by displacing tissue bluntly in a medial direction; and the ovarian vessels in the infundibulopelvic ligament are divided. Using this technique, the operation can then proceed from a lateral to medial direction, with the ureter now clearly visualized and all pelvic peritoneum freely and simply removed.

POSTSURGICAL STAGING

If the upper abdomen was not correctly evaluated at the initial operation, postoperative re-evaluation by either laparotomy or laparoscopy may be necessary even before initial treatment is begun. Understaging as a result of inadequate initial surgery is unfortunately common. Of 16 patients with clinical Stage I and II ovarian carcinoma sent to the National Cancer Institute (NCI) for treatment and evaluation by laparoscopy, seven (44%) were found to have more advanced disease than originally reported.[18,19] Piver and coworkers, in reviewing the literature, found one of 27 patients to have omental metastases in suspected Stage I disease.[20]

The use of laparoscopy in patients with ovarian carcinoma has been shown to be of value both for initial staging and as a means of surveillance for therapeutic response.[18,19] The NCI experience in the routine use of peritoneoscopy in staging and restaging of 99 patients with ovarian cancer has recently been summarized.[70] In 42 patients, peritoneoscopy documented new involved sites undetected by conventional radiologic and isotopic procedures. In addition, it provided the only evidence for followable disease in 25 patients (38%). Some 21% of patients referred with Stage I–II disease were upstaged to Stage III based on diaphragmatic disease detected at peritoneoscopy. In the 66 restaging peritoneoscopies, residual disease was found in 33 (50%); peritoneoscopic findings were the only evidence for disease in 24 patients (36%). These patients were spared an unnecessary second look laparotomy. Those patients (33) with negative peritoneoscopies went on to laparotomy. Residual ovarian cancer was found in 12 (55%), mainly in the pelvis and mesentery. Therefore, a negative peritoneoscopy must be followed by a laparotomy before a patient with ovarian cancer can be considered disease-free.

Peritoneoscopy was found a safe and feasible procedure even in patients who had prior laparotomies. Only 6% of patients had technical problems that precluded complete evaluation. There were few serious complications in the 159 procedures; only 2.5% of the cases required medical therapy to deal with a complication. Complications included pneumothorax (1 case), bleeding requiring transfusion (1 case), wound infection (1 case), and hypotension (2 cases). Other complications (not requiring therapy) were pneumomediastinum and subcutaneous, or mesenteric, emphysema. There were no deaths or viscus perforations; no patient required surgical exploration because of a peritoneoscopy complication.

Other institutions have had similar experiences. Berek, Griffiths, and Leventhal, in an unpublished series, reviewed 112 laparoscopies on 57 patients with all stages of ovarian carcinoma and none had clinical evidence of disease. In 80 (71%) of the procedures, the entire peritoneal cavity was visualized; visualization was totally inadequate in only 16. Similar complications occurred in this series, but none were serious. For patients under therapy laparoscopy proved a useful tool in monitoring subclinical disease.

Second Look Operation

The "second look operation" describes a variety of procedures performed under several different circumstances. This confusion in terminology has resulted in difficulty when evaluating efficacy.[71] The procedures often called "second look operations" in ovarian surgery have been performed for the following indications:

1. Accuracy in staging when the initial operation has not clearly defined spread of disease
2. Cytoreductive surgery after a course of radiation therapy or chemotherapy
3. Excision of recurrent disease
4. Removal of retained ovaries after complete tumor disappearance by clinical evaluations
5. Removal of residual tumor following reduction of tumor mass by chemotherapy or radiation therapy
6. Assessment of tumor status in patients who have completed an initial course of treatment and demonstrate no clinical evidence of tumor by non-operative means (It is the latter situation to which the term "second-look operation" should be applied.)

The second look procedure is usually performed immediately after completion of chemotherapy or radiation therapy. The same abdominal exploration outlined for staging should be performed for second look procedure. This includes washings, close inspection, and biopsy of suspicious areas of the pelvis, bowel, mesentery, diaphragm, and retroperitoneal lymph nodes. Only by this careful second-look evaluation can a second line treatment be instituted and the patient given a chance for cure.

Smith and Rutledge evaluated second-look operations in patients with epithelial cancers of the ovary treated with chemotherapy at the M.D. Anderson Hospital and Tumor Institute.[72] In those patients who demonstrated a complete or near complete response to chemotherapy, the second-look operation was performed to remove all residual tumor, determine the status of the residual tumor, and modify subsequent treatment according to surgical findings. Among 103 patients who had the second-look surgery, 65 survived an additional two years and 34 survived five years. Chemotherapy was discontinued in 23 patients without evidence of cancer; 17 survived 5 years. Tepper reported a series of 17 patients with advanced ovarian carcinoma receiving radiation therapy and thio-*TEPA* who subsequently underwent a second-look procedure. Four patients survived three years.

Berek, Griffiths, and Leventhal used laparoscopy for surveillance during treatment and also as a second-look procedure following intensive chemotherapy. This helped to determine early recurrence and provided an opportunity to reinstate new therapy. Laparoscopy with negative biopsies and washings at six months were highly predictive of survival. Predictability increased with each subsequent laparoscopy.

If the laparoscopy has been used for surveillance during treatment, it can be employed as a second-look procedure; laparotomy would not be necessary if positive tumor is found. However, if a complete evaluation is not possible, laparotomy should be performed. In addition, it should be considered if the laparoscopy demonstrates no tumor, or if the laparoscopy has not been used for surveillance during treatment.

TUMOR MARKERS IN OVARIAN CANCER

A rigorous effort has been undertaken to identify tumor markers capable of detecting early ovarian cancer. This has been done because the majority of patients are diagnosed when they already have advanced disease. These markers have often been helpful in monitoring the more rare germ cell malignancies; however, they have not been very helpful thus far in detecting early epithelial ovarian malignancies.

The serial measurement of alpha fetoprotein has facilitated the post-surgical evaluation of therapy for patients with endodermal sinus tumors. Kurman and Norris reported on the clinicopathologic characteristics of this tumor in 71 patients.[74] After surgical resection of endodermal sinus tumors, serum alpha fetoprotein levels progressively declined. With tumor recurrence, the alpha fetoprotein became elevated prior to clinically palpable disease. The use of alpha fetoprotein as a tumor marker is also helpful in the diagnosis of an endodermal sinus tumor in a young female with a rapidly enlarging, solid ovarian mass.

Human chorionic gonadotropin (hCG) or its beta subunit has been a valuable tumor marker in the postsurgical evaluation of patients with ovarian choriocarcinoma. Human chorionic gonadotropin and its beta subunit are also sensitive tumor markers for germ cell tumors with choriocarcinoma elements.[75] Serial determination of hCG and its beta subunit may aid in the diagnosis and management of these ovarian malignancies. These determinations may act as a sensitive monitor of the effectiveness of anticancer therapy.

Measurable levels of carcinoembryonic antigen (CEA) have been reported in 58% of patients with Stage III epithelial ovarian cancer.[76] The frequency of elevated CEA levels in ovarian cancer progressively increases with advancing stage and bulk of tumor. CEA appears to be particularly elevated in the serum and cyst fluid of patients with mucinous cystadenocarcinoma. Electron microscopy studies of mucinous cystadenocarcinoma cells have demonstrated ultrastructural similarities to malignant colonic epithelium. However, since serum levels of CEA have also been elevated in patients with cirrhosis, chronic pulmonary disease, inflammatory bowel disease, and a history of heavy cigarette smoking, it is a limited diagnostic tool in the detection of ovarian cancer. Nevertheless, in patients with elevated CEA levels prior to therapy, serial CEA measurements may be valuable in monitoring patients with subclinical ovarian cancer.

Following the original work of Levi and coworkers several investigators have attempted to isolate tumor specific antigens that could be used for both serologic diagnosis and monitoring of patients under therapy.[77] Work from several laboratories suggests that ovarian carcinoma cells possess a distinct surface membrane antigen that is not shared by normal tissue.[78–81] Bhattacharya and Barlow isolated and purified an ovarian cystadenocarcinoma-associated antigen and developed a radioimmunoassay test using the Farr technique.[82] About 70% of ovarian carcinoma patients with advanced disease have ovarian cystadenocarcinoma-associated antigen levels above 10 ng/ml serum. Knauf and Urbach reported the development of a double antibody radioimmunoassay using Iodine–125 labeled ovarian cancer antigen, isolated and purified from human ovarian serous and mucinous cystadenocarcinomas.[83] Using the test for serial monitoring, a positive level of ovarian cancer antigen occurred in patients with progressive disease.

To improve specificity and to obtain an adequate quantity of antibody to be used for a radioimmunoassay test, monoclonal antibodies against human ovarian carcinoma have been prepared by Kohler and Milstein's in the laboratory of Knapp and Bast.[84]

MANAGEMENT OF MINIMAL RESIDUAL DISEASE

Historically, the treatment of ovarian cancer has been discussed in the context of FIGO staging, that is, separating early disease (FIGO Stage I and II) from advanced disease (FIGO Stage III and IV). However, recent analysis of long-term survival results from several major institutions indicates that the natural history and the selection of appropriate therapy is dependent upon the extent of residual disease as well as the stage. Because the therapeutic options are similar for all patients with minimal residual disease, these patients will be discussed as a group. Patients in this category include those with Stage IA, IB, IC, as well as Stage II and III with minimal or no residual disease after initial surgery. The rationale for this approach is based upon the following data. As previously noted, the extent of residual disease remaining after initial surgery is an important prognostic factor in the outcome of subsequent treatment and eventual survival. After initial surgery, an improved survival for patients with less than 2 cm diameter of the largest residual tumor nodule has been documented, based on the analysis of over 2000 patients from the M.D. Anderson Hospital. So important is this factor that patients left after surgery with either no residual disease or less than 1 cm have essentially the same prognosis regardless of the initial tumor stage.[85] In the M.D. Anderson Hospital study, patients with limited or no residual disease had a five year survival of approximately 40% when all subsequent treatment methods were combined. Recently, this group has submitted prognostic factors in 278 patients with Stage III and IV epithelial ovarian cancer to logistic regression analysis.[86] Survival at 24 months was 52.7% for those patients with less than or equal to 2 cm residual compared to 29.2% for those with greater than 2 cm; at 48 months, the survival figures were 25% and 13.2% respectively.

Similar observations have been made where radiation therapy has been the primary modality of therapy. Studies from the Princess Margaret Hospital indicate the principal prognostic factors were the ability to complete bilateral salpingo-oophorectomy and hysterectomy (BSOH), the histologic grade of the tumor, and the amount of residual tumor following surgery.[41] Actuarial five year survival for 190 patients with Stages IB, II, and asymptomatic III when BSOH could be completed was 65.7% compared with 23.7% when BSOH was incomplete.

These and other studies must take into consideration this important prognostic factor when analyzing therapeutic results and comparing different modalities and studies.

Since tumor volume is a particularly important question in treatment, it is important to discuss stages I, II, and III with minimal residual disease separately from the more frequent patients with bulky residual tumor and advanced Stage III and IV disease. Management of ovarian cancer patients with minimal or no residual disease can include either radiation therapy, radioisotopes, or chemotherapy.

RADIATION THERAPY

Traditionally, radiation therapy has been used to treat resectable ovarian carcinoma beyond Stage IA in combination with a surgical resection. In most instances, radiation therapy has been administered postoperatively. Initially, external orthovoltage irradiation or intraperitoneal installation of radioactive colloidal gold (^{198}Au) or phosphorus (^{32}P) were employed. This was later replaced by megavoltage irradiation.[37,87–91]

There is no evidence that the various histologic types of epithelial ovarian carcinoma have different responses to irradiation. However, the histologic tumor grade is critical in determining the prognosis since well-differentiated tumors have a five year survival of approximately 75% in contrast to 20% or less in patients with poorly differentiated tumors.[31]

Irradiation Techniques

Several irradiation techniques have been used in patients with ovarian carcinoma. Currently, megavoltage irradiation is the preferred method because of the better depth dose delivered and the sparing of skin and superficial normal tissues (see Fig. 26-2).

With external irradiation, the whole abdomen is treated with anterior and posterior portals, using either open fields

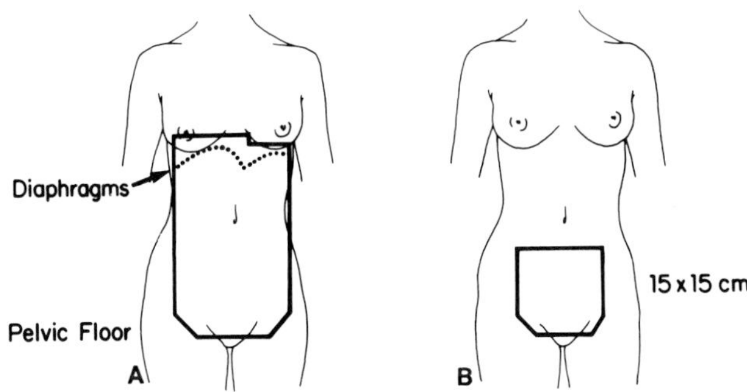

FIG. 26-2. Volume covered with megavoltage irradiation. *A*, Parallel opposing fields to the whole abdomen with open fields including both diaphragms. A dose of 3000 rads in 5–6 weeks can be given with proper shielding of the kidneys and liver. *B*, Pelvic irradiation (15 × 15 cm fields). Lower border at midpubis for adequate coverage of pelvic floor. (Delcos L: Tumors of the evary. In Fletcher GH (ed): Textbook of Radiotherapy, pp 690–702. Philadelphia, Lea and Febiger, 1973)

or the strip technique. Open fields are technically easier; however, the strip technique presumably allows the delivery of higher, biologically equivalent doses. This technique, designed in Manchester and adapted to cobalt 60 by Delclos, divides the abdomen in strips 2.5 cm wide (see Fig. 26-3).[92,93] As indicated by Bush, and Glatstein and coworkers, it is extremely important that the entire pelvis, and both domes of the diaphragm, and the lateral peritoneal gutters be included in the irradiated volume because of the pathways of dissemination in ovarian carcinoma (see Fig. 26-2).[94,95] Initially, two, three, and four strips are treated daily as therapy progresses. When the number of strips treated daily reaches four, a new strip is added to the volume treated every day. A strip that has completed four treatments on the frontal and four treatments on the posterior portals is excluded from the irradiated field. Thus, at any time, only four anterior posterior (AP) or posterior anterior (PA) strips are irradiated. This sequence progresses until the entire abdomen has been treated, at which time the number of strips is decreased to 3,2,1. At the end of therapy every 10 cm segment of abdomen should have received a total of eight treatments (4AP and 4PA). The details of the technique and the isodose curves are illustrated in Fig. 26-4A and B.

Khan and coworkers described the more complicated physics of this technique with linear accelerators since the scattered dose is not as high as with cobalt 60.[96] These authors reported that with 10 MeV roentgen rays, the variation in depth dose across the strips in the sagittal plane was about 10% at the strip junctions but only 3% in the middle of the strips. Other factors that may influence dose distribution are the collimator design, flattening filter, or beam compensator of the accelerator and the thickness of the patient. The unavoidable variations when repositioning the patient from day to day, the natural intra-abdominal movement of both tumor and normal tissues, and the fact that not all volume of the abdomen is being irradiated at any given time are criticisms leveled against the moving strip technique. Also, Smoron, with the use of 4 MeV linear accelerators and to a lesser extent with cobalt 60, pointed out a decrease in dose along the transverse centers of the strips at the midplane of the abdomen. This was due to the divergence of the beam and lack of contiguity at the surface. He suggested that the strip lines be staggered so that the posterior surface lines fall in the center of the anterior strip projections to reduce the area underdosed to a clinically insignificant width.

In a recent publication Bush presents a critical review of results reported with the moving strip technique at a number of institutions.[94] He points out the need to adequately treat the entire peritoneal cavity and pelvis to improve present therapeutic results.

The dose of irradiation selected varies with the institution. The abdomen is usually treated with 2250 to 3000 rad in 3–4 weeks. An additional 2250 to 3000 rad are delivered to the pelvis through smaller ports.

It should be stressed that the tolerance dose of irradiation for the kidneys is about 1800 rad. For the liver, 3500 rad with conventional fractionation (200 rad per day) is tolerable. However, the maximum is probably 2500 rad when large daily fractions are delivered with strip technique.

Whether the older approach, such as pelvic irradiation (see Fig. 26-2), or total abdominal irradiation is given by the moving strip technique or with open fields, each has advantages and disadvantages. For example, external beam irradiation to the pelvis is inadequate to encompass areas of potential tumor spread, such as the omentum, the retroperitoneal lymph nodes, the diaphragmatic lymphatics or the peritoneum. Also, whole abdomen irradiation cannot be given in doses above 3500 rad; the kidneys and liver must be blocked at lower doses to avoid irreparable damage. Hanks and Bagshaw observed poor tolerance with doses of 4000 rad to the upper abdomen.[98] Wharton and coworkers reported 14 of 65 patients with ovarian cancer treated with strip technique who developed radiation hepatitis after receiving doses ranging from 2450 to 2920 rad in eight fractions over 12 elapsed days. In addition, there is a possibility of small bowel injury; practically all patients have a moderate to severe bone marrow depression requiring four to six months for recovery.[100] Dif-

FIG. 26-3. The total abdominal irradiation approach using the moving strip technique. Volume covered with the megavoltage moving strip technique. Kidneys are shielded from the posterior beam by two half-value layer(s) of lead. The liver is shielded from the anterior beam by two half-value layer(s) of lead. To compensate for the lower dose at both ends of the irradiated volume, treatment is started one strip below the lower margin of the pelvic field and completed one strip above the diaphragm.

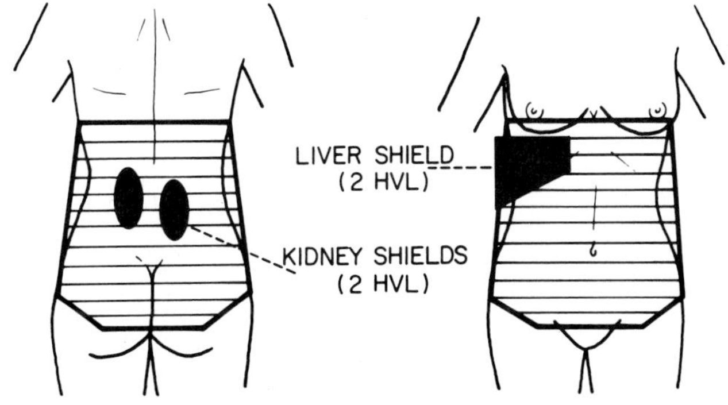

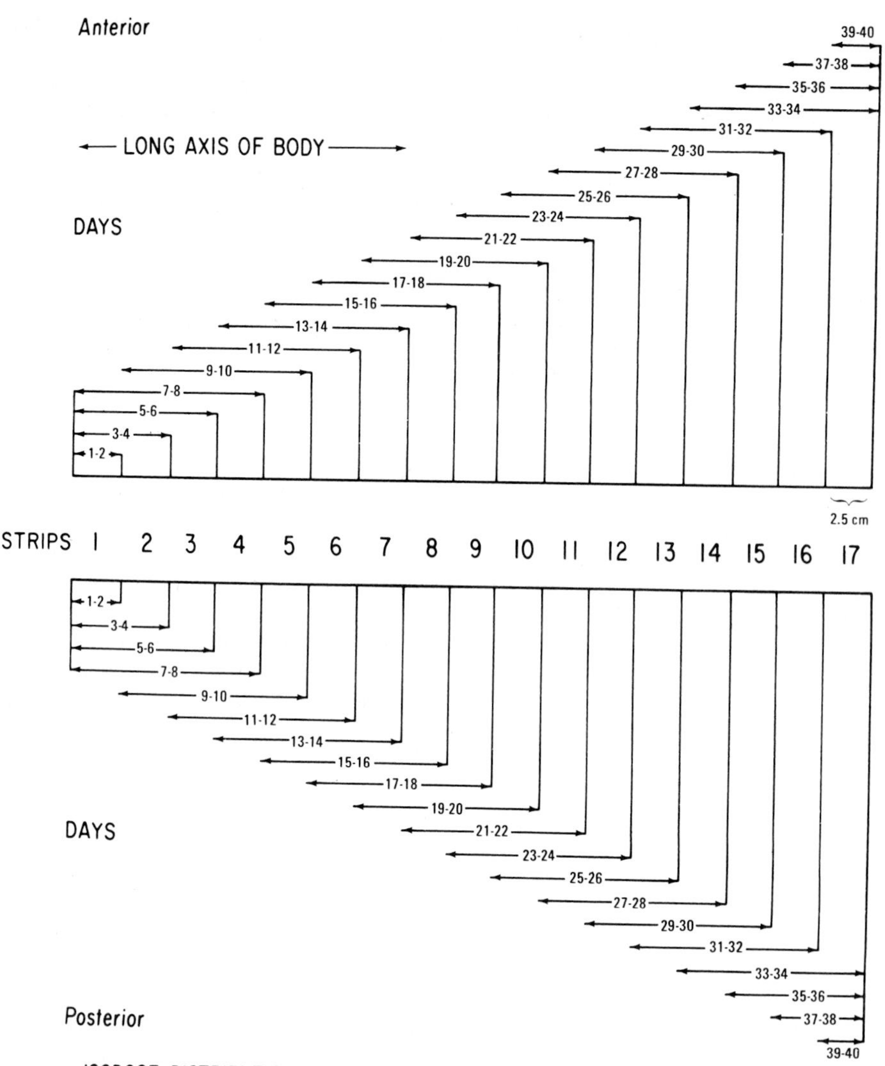

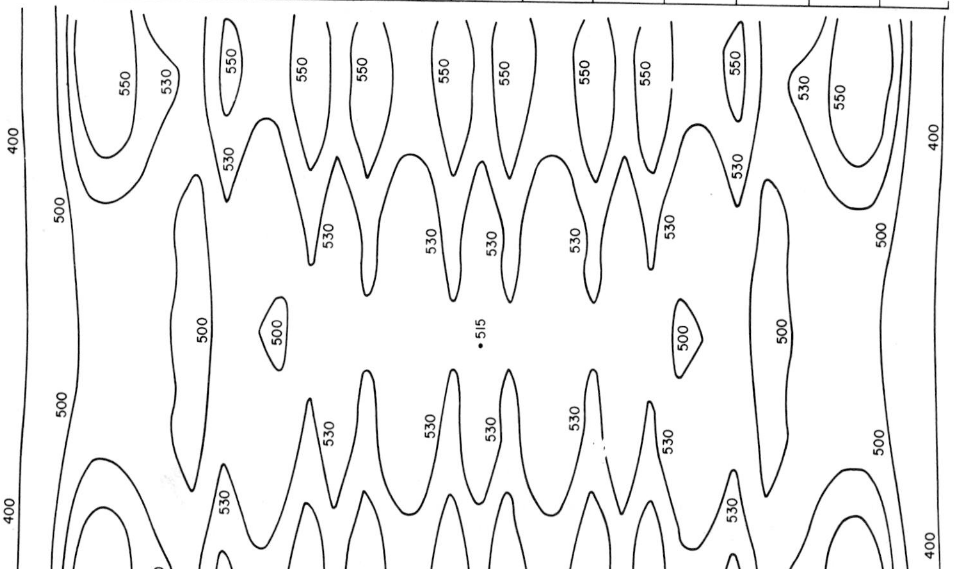

FIG. 26-4. *A*, Strip technique. The treatment sequence to the anterior and posterior surfaces is shown. Half the prescribed given dose is delivered each day to the anterior and posterior strips. *B*, Strip technique. An example of the combined isodose distribution when treatment is completed in the sagittal plane. This includes the longitudinal axis as well. The total dose given to each strip is 100%. This distribution is computer generated for an Eldorado 8 Cobalt Unit, source-skin distance 80 cm, trimmers at 65 cm from the source (except for a 2.5 cm field). (Sampier VA: Radiation measurements and dosimetric practices. In Fletcher GH (ed): Textbook of Radiation, pp 1–30. Philadelphia, Lea and Febiger, 1973)

ferences in effectiveness and tolerance between open fields and the cobalt 60 strip technique for abdominal irradiation have not been established. Fazekas and Maier published a randomized study comparing these two modalities in two similar groups of 25 patients, each with tumors ranging from Stage I to IV.[101] The survival rates were comparable in both groups. The patients treated with the cobalt 60 strip technique tolerated the therapy better; termination of therapy was necessary in only 4000 patients, in contrast to six in the open field group. However, the strip technique patients had slightly more severe gastrointestinal reactions. In addition, poor tolerance to chemotherapy has been reported after radiation therapy to the whole abdomen.[102]

With minimal residual disease patients, irradiation is employed as an adjuvant after complete or nearly complete resection of all gross disease, regardless of the stage of the tumor (except in Stage IA well-differentiated tumors where there is yet no convincing proof of the value of adjuvant radiotherapy). In Stage IA, irradiation is used when there are serosal excrescences of the tumor, spillage of cystic tumor contents in the peritoneal cavity, or in cases where the tumor is poorly differentiated.[103]

In patients with Stage I or II disease, irradiation may be beneficial, although this has not definitely been proven.[31,104] The recent practice at most institutions has been to treat the pelvis *and* abdomen, since about 20–30% of the patients may have clinical recurrence in the retroperitoneal lymph nodes or the upper abdomen.[105,106] Delclos and Quinlan reported no significant difference in survival in patients with Stage I serous adenocarcinoma when the pelvis or abdomen or both were irradiated.[60] However, in patients with Stage II disease, only five out of 12 survived with either the pelvis or the whole abdomen treated. In contrast, nine of 11 patients survived when both volumes were treated with the moving strip technique and a pelvic boost. In Stage III there were no survivors out of 25 patients irradiated to either the pelvis or the abdomen. In contrast, seven of 9 patients survived when both the whole abdomen and pelvis were irradiated.

A randomized study was carried out by the Gynecology Oncology Group on Stage I patients; they were treated with surgery alone, irradiation to the pelvis, or melphalan.[107] With about 35 patients per treatment arm, the study has shown no significant difference in survival. However, in patients treated with surgery alone, there were five pelvic failures combined with abdominal recurrences; in the patients treated with pelvic irradiation, no failures in the pelvis but the same number of recurrences in the abdomen. The lowest relapse frequency thus far is seen in patients treated with chemotherapy. Therefore, it appears that the irradiation of the entire abdomen or systemic chemotherapy may ultimately prove most useful. Both Bush and coworkers, Dembo and coworkers, have reported on a randomized study at the Princess Margaret in which patients with Stage I, II, and completely resected III lesions were treated with either pelvic irradiation alone or pelvic irradiation and chlorambucil* (6 mg/day orally for two years or until relapse), or, a combination of pelvic irradiation and abdominal strip technique.[108,109] Patients with Stage III were not randomized to pelvic irradiation alone. The dose of irradiation was 4500 rad to the pelvis in 20 fractions through 15 x 15 cm AP–PA ports or an abdominal pelvic irradiation of 2250 rad to the midplane in 10 fractions immediately followed by a 2250 tumor dose (TD) to the midplane in 10 fractions to the whole abdomen and pelvis using cobalt 60 strip technique. The kidneys were shielded posteriorly throughout the treatment but no shielding was used for the liver. All patients were treated in the prone position. The results for Stage IB and II (147 patients) clearly indicate better results with the abdomino–pelvic irradiation compared to other techniques.

* A potential criticism of this otherwise excellent clinical trial is that the selection of chlorambucil and the dose given may not be optimal compared with other chemotherapeutic agents used at the present time.

Smith and coworkers from the M.D. Anderson reported the preliminary results of a randomized study comparing pelvic and abdominal cobalt 60 strip technique irradiation with a one year administration of melphalan in 156 patients with Stage I, II, and III disease. None of the patients had residual tumor larger than 2 cm after surgical resection or tumors located in areas in which the radiation dose had to be limited (*i.e.,* the peritoneum in front or behind the kidneys or the inferior surfaces of the diaphragm).

Patients were treated with either abdominal cobalt 60 moving strip technique (2600 to 2800 rad in 2½ weeks) followed by additional 2000 rad to the pelvis in two weeks delivered with 22 MeV photons (15 × 15 cm AP–PA ports). The liver was shielded both front and back with one half value layer of lead; the kidneys were shielded posteriorly with two half value layers of lead. Chemotherapy consisted of melphalan (.2 mg/kg/day in divided doses for five days for a total of 1 mg/kg/five day cycle) every four weeks for a total of 12 cycles. Preliminary analysis of the study showed no significant difference between the two groups in survival or patterns of failure. The actuarial five year survival rate for Stage I is approximately 90%, for Stage II, 60%, and for Stage III, 35% (see Fig. 26-5). The specific sites of recurrences were not specified in this publication.)

However, the pelvis has been the site of recurrence in approximately 10–20% of patients with Stage I and II disease, and about 50% of those with Stage III. The abdomen is the site of recurrence in approximately 20–30% of the patients with Stage I and II respectively, and 75% of those with Stage III. In about 50% of the patients with recurrent tumor, pelvic and abdominal failures are concomitant; the other 50% occur at either site alone.

Preoperative Radiation

Preoperative radiation has been used occasionally in the treatment of ovarian carcinoma. Long and Sala reported eight patients surviving eight years after 4000 rad preoperative radiation and radical surgery for extensive pelvic ovarian carcinoma.[111] Kottmeier reported 34 of 86 patients surviving after three years following preoperative radiation and total hysterectomy with bilateral salpingo-oophorectomy (BSO) in most instances.[112] However, further information on these patients is not available. This approach has not been popular because of several reasons. One is the lack of histologic confirmation of malignancy without a laparotomy. However,

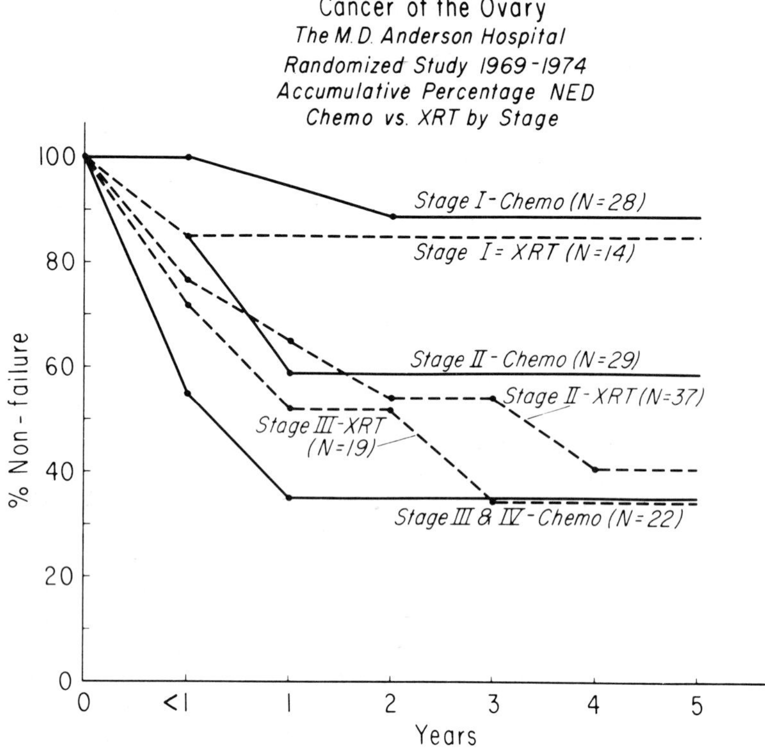

FIG. 26-5. The M. D. Anderson Hospital randomized 1969–1974 study of accumulative percentage NED chemo vs. XRT by stage; percentage of patients without evidence of cancer by treatment plan; stages of cancer divided. *NED* = no evidence of disease. *Chemo* = chemotherapy. *XRT* = irradiation therapy. (Smith JP, Young RC: Natl Cancer Inst Monogr 42:149–153, 1975)

this may be circumvented with needle aspiration biopsies as reported by Kjellgren and coworkers who, in 80 patients with palpable ovarian tumors (52 of them carcinomas), found a 93–95% diagnostic accuracy with fine needle biopsy in comparison with histological sections obtained at subsequent operations. Another reason is that after irradiation, the full extent of the disease is not known. Finally, there may be technical difficulties in carrying out the surgery following these high doses of preoperative irradiation.

RADIOISOTOPES

The intraperitoneal instillation of radioactive colloidal ^{198}Au or ^{32}P to irradiate the peritoneal cavity was employed widely until 1965.[114,115] The colloidal particles increase isotope uptake by the mesothelial peritoneal cells and lymph nodes, and decrease systemic radioisotope elution. Radioactive gold has a half-life of 2.7 days; 90% of its radiation is delivered by beta-rays (.96 MeV) and 10% by roentgen rays (.41 MeV). Radioactive phosphorous (chromic phosphate) has a half-life of 14.2 days and emits only beta particles (1.7 MeV maximum energy). The range of beta particles in tissues is only 3–5 mm; thus, radioisotopes ^{198}Au or ^{32}P may sterilize microscopic peritoneal implants but they are inadequate to treat large masses because of the limited range of the beta particle. Because of adhesions or loculation, poor distribution in the peritoneal cavity may occur. This can be avoided by careful assessment of the distribution, injecting a radiopaque material and taking radiographs, or installing a small amount of radioactive material in the peritoneal cavity, then scanning the patient before the therapeutic dose is administered. The subsequent surgical treatment of these patients may be more difficult because of reactive fibrosis in the peritoneal cavity and serosal surface of the intestine. Also, there are always possible radiation safety hazards. The usual doses delivered to the abdomen were 150 mc of radiogold or 20–25 mc of radiophosphorus. Both were diluted with sterile saline (1000 ml) and properly distributed throughout the entire peritoneal cavity. If the average peritoneal surface is estimated at 30,000^2 cm, the dose of irradiation delivered to the peritoneum is 6000 rad and 7000 rad to the omentum.[115]

Various methods for the administration of the isotopes and verification of adequate distribution in the peritoneal cavity have been published.

Because of safety considerations and the relatively frequent complications (particularly small bowel obstruction), these isotopes have been used less of late. However, some institutions have maintained an interest in the application of this therapeutic method. Bushbaum and coworkers, and Decker have reported on a significant number of patients treated with this modality.[103,116] In addition, Order and coworkers have recently described an innovative technique consisting of irradiation of the abdomen with external beam, intraperitoneal administration of radioactive phosphorus, and systemic administration of I^{125}-labeled specific antitumor immunoglobulins.

The most common complication with the use of intraperitoneal colloidal radioisotopes is small bowel obstruction and stenosis. Pezner and coworkers reported on a group of 104 patients treated in this fashion.[118] Eleven of these patients required surgery for adhesions or fibrosis of the small intestine with severe chronic diarrhea; one with partial small bowel obstruction was treated conservatively. In the patients with radioactive colloidal gold, only one of 45 (2.2%) developed small bowel complications in contrast to 12 of 50 (24%) treated with this technique in addition to pelvic external radiotherapy (about 4000 rad in four weeks with cobalt 60 or 2 MeV photons). Complications tend to be slightly higher in patients who have uneven distribution of the radio-active material in the peritoneal cavity.

CHEMOTHERAPY

Three studies have looked at alternative therapies for patients with "early" ovarian cancer and minimal residual disease. The Gynecologic Oncology Group, in a study mentioned earlier, has presented updated data on patients with Stage IA and IB epithelial ovarian cancer, randomized after surgery to receive either no additional therapy, pelvic irradiation, or intermittent oral melphalan.[120] Although there is no difference yet in survival, the frequency of relapse is highest for pelvic irradiation alone (36.4%) and lowest (6.7%) for melphalan.

The updated results of the Princess Margaret Hospital study mentioned earlier randomized 190 patients with Stage IB, II, and asymptomatic III disease to receive either pelvic irradiation alone (PEL), pelvic irradiation plus chlorambucil (P + Ch), or total abdominal irradiation (P + AB).[41] Only the patients who had a BSOH complete showed any survival differences according to therapy. In BSOH completed patients, P + AB was significantly better than either PEL or P + Ch at five year followup. The improved survival is apparently related to a reduction in relapses occurring in the upper abdomen.

Both this study and that from the Gynecologic Oncology Group suggest little benefit from pelvic irradiation alone in "early" ovarian cancer. The recognized high frequency of intra-abdominal metastasis provides little rationale for localized irradiation volume in "early" disease.

The M.D. Anderson group has published a prospective randomized trial of patients with minimal residual disease. This study compares single agent melphalan with total abdominal irradiation by moving strip in a slightly different dose and schedule.[85,121] The two and five year survivals for the groups are 86.5% and 71.5% respectively for radiation and 90% and 78% for melphalan. They conclude that chemotherapy is as effective as irradiation, has fewer serious side effects, and is less expensive.

Combination chemotherapy has also been used for patients with minimal residual disease. There is evidence that such patients respond more completely and experience improved survival. In a prospective trial comparing L–PAM with the four drug combination HexaCAF (hexamethylmelamine, cyclophosphamide, methotrexate, and 5–fluorouracil), the overall response rate was better for those patients with minimal residual disease; the frequency of complete remission was also higher (see Table 26-5).[64] Of the eight patients with minimal residual disease treated with HexaCAF, six are alive at 5-year followup. Single arm studies with both hexamethylmelamine alone and in combination with adriamycin-Cytoxan also demonstrate a higher overall response and complete remission rate in patients with minimal residual disease.

The Mayo Clinic group compared cyclophosphamide alone with cyclophosphamide-adriamycin in 111 patients with advanced disease. While there was no difference between the two regimens in patients with bulky disease, there was a significant increase in response rate and improved survival in those patients with minimal residual disease treated with the combination.

TABLE 26-5. Response to Chemotherapy by Extent of Residual Disease

REGIMEN	NO. PATIENTS	OBJECTIVE RESPONSE %	COMPLETE RESPONSE %
Hexa-CAF			
<2 cm	8	100	100
>2 cm	32	69	16
L-PAM			
<2 cm	11	73	18
>2 cm	26	46	15

These studies provide convincing evidence that patients with minimal residual disease are responsive to a variety of therapies, including chemotherapy. Prospective comparisons between combinations and single agents provide strong evidence for the increased effectiveness of combination chemotherapy in this group of patients. Prospective comparisons are clearly needed of appropriate total abdominal irradiation and combination chemotherapy in patients with minimal residual disease.

Unique techniques for delivering chemotherapy to the patient with peritoneally-dispersed minimal residual disease are now being investigated. The pharmacologic basis for high volume intraperitoneal chemotherapy ("belly bath") in ovarian cancer has recently been published describing initial results with methotrexate.[124] Demonstration of the clinical effectiveness of intraperitoneal adriamycin in a murine ovarian cancer model has established a rationale for intraperitoneal chemotherapy with that drug in ovarian cancer patients.[125] Initial clinical trials have been performed with the attainable concentration of adriamycin in the ascites being assayed against human ovarian carcinoma cells in the human tumor stem cell assay.[126,127] Further studies will be necessary before this technique can be proposed for widespread clinical use.

SUMMARY OF THERAPEUTIC OPTIONS FOR PATIENTS WITH MINIMAL RESIDUAL DISEASE

For patients with Stage IA and IB disease where the tumor is well-differentiated and a complete staging procedure has been performed, no additional therapy may be needed. For those patients with Stage I disease, but poorly differentiated histology and for those with Stage IC, II, and III disease with minimal or no residual disease, it is impossible to conclude that one specific approach. However, acceptable approaches include single agent melphalan, total abdominal and pelvic irradiation as outlined by the Princess Margaret Group, or combination chemotherapy. Intraperitoneal radioisotopes (^{32}P in the form of chromic phosphate) have been used in such patients, but no randomized comparison of alternative treatments has been performed.

At present, three commonly used approaches to such patients are clearly inadequate:

1. No therapy (in light of the high frequency of unappreciated intra-abdominal metastasis in inadequately staged patients)
2. Pelvic irradiation alone (for the same reason and based upon the results of the two studies mentioned previously)
3. Total abdominal irradiation (this shields the liver and does not include the domes of the diaphragm)

MANAGEMENT OF MACROSCOPIC RESIDUAL DISEASE

As emphasized in the previous section, therapy has traditionally been selected based upon FIGO staging alone. It is now clear that other factors contribute to proper selection of therapy and therefore must be considered. There are several options available for patients with "advanced" (FIGO Stage III and IV) disease who have minimal or no residual disease after initial surgery. These have been discussed in the previous section.

At present, the unfortunate reality is that out of approximately two-thirds of women with advanced ovarian cancer at the time of diagnosis, approximately 75% have such extensive disease that cytoreductive surgery cannot be performed. The patient is left with advanced disease with extensive residua. These patients have responded poorly to conventional therapies of all types. The major challenge for the future lies in the development of successful management approaches for this large group of women. In recent years the mainstay of therapy for this group has been systemic chemotherapy; however, there are several groups of patients with unique presentations for whom radiation therapy may be appropriate.

RADIATION THERAPY

It is worthwhile to separate patients with gross abdominal tumor from those with only retroperitoneal lymph node metastasis since they may have a different prognosis due to the varying cell burden. Hintz and coworkers, reporting on testing at Stanford University, noted that patients that have retroperitoneal lymph nodes as the only site of extra pelvic disease have a survival rate of about 55% at five years in contrast to 10% in patients with peritoneal spread.[119]

Radiation therapy has been utilized less successfully in the treatment of patients with unresectable or partially resected tumors with bulky residual disease.[102,110] Techniques have varied from extended pelvic ports in combination with chemotherapy to encompass gross disease to abdomino–pelvic irradiation using the moving strip technique.[60,90,100]

Doses in the range of 5000–6000 rad are delivered in six to seven weeks to those areas of gross disease through large local ports. Occasionally, 2500–3000 rad are administered to the entire abdominal cavity, as described previously, with a boost to the bulky tumor (2500 rad).

Unfortunately, survival is very poor in those patients who have large lesions remaining after surgery. In a 20-year experience using a variety of radio-therapeutic approaches, Delclos reported that 17.2% of patients with 4–6cm residual disease were free of disease at five years and no patients with 6–10cm residual were alive at five years.[89]

In the randomized study from Princess Margaret Hospital, the patients who had completed bilateral salpingo–oophorectomy and hysterectomy in Stage IB, II, and symptomatic III had a five year survival of approximately 65% in contrast to 25% who had an incomplete surgical procedure. In the same series, in patients who had a complete BSO and abdominal hysterectomy, the incidence of recurrences after treatment was significantly greater than in the patients known to have residual tumor (8/18 vs. 3/32).

Griffiths and coworkers described a median survival of 26 months in 19 patients with Stage III disease who had complete resection of the tumor and received postoperative irradiation and chemotherapy; in comparison, a median survival of 9.5 months occurred in 26 patients with Stage III having residual masses after surgical resection.

Complications of Radiation Therapy

Five to ten percent of these patients have major complications depending on the technique, doses, or irradiation and volume treated. With megavoltage irradiation, small bowel perforation or fibrosis with obstruction have been described in 2–4% of the patients. Smith and coworkers reported that seven patients in a group of 70 treated with the moving strip technique required surgery because of a small bowel injury; in some of these patients, a bypass of a long segment of small intestine was required resulting in malabsorption and chronic weight loss.[110] Six of the seven patients with small bowel injury were irradiated to the pelvis immediately followed by abdominal irradiation. In contrast, only one of 17 patients treated with the strip technique to the abdomen first starting at the pelvis followed by the pelvic irradiation developed this complication. In a previous report from the M.D. Anderson Hospital, seven of 166 patients treated with the strip technique followed by pelvic boost developed a small bowel injury requiring surgery. Perez and coworkers also reported on one case each of necrotizing colitis, rectal ulcer, ureteral stricture, chronic severe cystitis, and pubic bone necrosis in 52 patients treated with pelvic irradiation followed by abdominal strip technique (3000 rad to the pelvis and 3000 rad to the abdominal strips).[100]

Wharton and coworkers reported severe or fatal radiation hepatitis in 14 of 65 patients who received doses between 2450 and 2950 rad to the entire liver with the moving strip technique.[99] Because of this, the technique has been modified at that institution to shield the liver with one-half value layer (HVL) both in the frontal and posterior portals.

Occasionally, symptoms of intermittent partial small bowel obstruction, hemorrhagic cystitis, proctitis, or sigmoiditis may appear, but they do not often require a surgical procedure and usually improve with prolonged conservative management.

Other complications of less severity include bone marrow depression, particularly with lymphopenia and some thrombocytopenia. In the M.D. Anderson series, three of 70 patients required that their radiation therapy be interrupted for one week or more due to myelosuppression.

Dembo and coworkers, in contrast, have reported myelosuppression in about 8–20% of patients.[41] About 20% required some interruption of therapy because of low peripheral blood counts. Only one out of 76 required a surgical procedure for repair of a small bowel injury. These researchers feel that with the modification of the technique used at the Princess Margaret Hospital (treating the pelvis first to 2250 rad, followed by the abdominal pelvic strip irradiation of 2250 rad starting at the diaphragm) there is no need to shield the liver or the kidneys, a practice that may result in underdosage to areas containing tumor, such as the diaphragm or the peritoneum in front of the kidneys.

CHEMOTHERAPY

Chemotherapy has ordinarily been employed as initial treatment in those patients with advanced disease (FIGO Stages III and IV) and, in the past, for patients who were not considered to be appropriate candidates for radiation therapy.[88] Recently, with the discovery of more active chemotherapeutic agents, combination drug treatment is often used as initial therapy in advanced disease.

Alkylating agents have been used more extensively in patients with advanced ovarian cancer than any other class of chemotherapeutic agents. Published reports of more than 1000 patients treated with melphalan, chlorambucil, cyclophosphamide, and thiotepa have produced similar objective response rates (35–65%).[32] The median survival of patients in these trials is approximately 10–14 months; the median survival of those responding to chemotherapy is 17–20 months; and for those not responding, 6–13 months. The five-year survival of patients treated with chemotherapy alone is reported to be 0–9% (mean 7%). The five-year survival of the largest single series of patients treated with melphalan was 9%; approximately 20% of the responders in that series were alive at five years with some patients alive and free of disease for periods in excess of 7.5 years. Second-look studies indicate that patients with no residual tumor at second look laparotomy have a five-year survival in excess of 80% without further therapy.[68] Consequently, it is clear that some women with advanced ovarian cancer have been cured of their disease with single alkylating agent therapy alone. Other classes of antitumor agents have been less thoroughly tested, primarily in small numbers of patients who have initially failed with alkylating agents or radiotherapy (*i.e.*, settings in which the responses are known to be diminished). A summary of the activity of some of the single agents in advanced ovarian cancer is listed in Table 26-6. In many instances, alternative

TABLE 26-6. Single Agents Active in Advanced Ovarian Adenocarcinoma

DRUG	SCHEDULE	NO. OF PATIENTS	RESPONSE RATE (%)
Alkylating Agents			
Melphalan	0.2 mg/kg/day × 5 PO or IV q3–5 wk	494	47 (20 complete)
Chlorambucil	0.2 mg/kg/day PO	280	50
Thiotepa	10 mg/day × 15 courses IV	144	65
Cyclophosphamide	50–150 mg/day PO	126	49
	400 mg/day × 4 days IV Then, 50–150 mg/day PO	104	37
Mechlorethamine	0.2 mg/kg/day × 2 IV Then, chlorambucil 8–14 mg/day PO	81	35
Antimetabolites			
5–Fluorouracil	15 mg/kg/day × Then, 7.5 mg/kg q.o.d./ 34 wk	81	32 (18–20)
	15 mg/kg IV/wk	21	33
Methotrexate	5 mg/day × 5–10 PO or IV 3–4 wk	16	25
	1–7.5 gm/m² IV wk with leukovorin rescue	23	13
Vinca Alkaloids			
Vinblastine	0.1–0.15 mg/kg/day × 1–3 IV	16	13
Miscellaneous			
Hexamethylmelamine	8 mg/kg/day PO or 6 mg/kg/day PO × 14 days q 4 wk	53	41
Doxorubicin (Adriamycin)	30 mg/m²/day × 3 IV	18	28
	50 mg/m² IV q 3 wk	33	36
Progestogens	200–600 mg/wk IM	50	10
Cisplatin	30 mg/m² daily IV × 3 q 28 days	34	27

schedules have been used with equivalent response rates and altered toxicity. Since the schedules listed were those initially reported and may not be optimal, the reader is advised to carefully review alternative schedules available for the particular drug in question before using any of the listed drugs.

In addition to the alkylating agents, recently three of the drugs (hexamethylmelamine, doxorubicin (Adriamycin), and cis–platinum) have been fairly extensively studied and their potential roles more carefully defined. A prospective randomized trial comparing melphalan, doxorubian, hexamethylmelamine, and 5–fluorouracil has been performed in previously untreated patients with Stage III or IV disease. Objective response was strictly defined and had to persist for three months or longer. The response rates achieved were 30% for melphalan, 17% for 5–fluorouracil, 33% for hexamethylmelamine, and 29% for adriamycin. Two studies on the use of hexamethylmelamine in patients resistant to alkylating agents have demonstrated an objective response rate of approximately 28%.[128,129] Although few of these responses were complete and the durations were short (approximately five months), these studies suggest that hexamethylmelamine is not invariably cross-resistant to alkylating agents and has some utility as a second-line agent after initial therapy failure. A comprehensive study of hexamethylmelamine used in 54 previously untreated patients has been completed.[122] The overall response rate was 31.8%. The drug was given orally continuously in this study and there was significant gastrointestinal, hematologic, and neurologic toxicity. Recent studies suggest reduced toxicity with intermittent 14 day per month schedules. The pharmacokinetic distribution of hexamethylmelamine indicates that peak plasma levels are reached in one-half to four hours but that the drug, when orally administered, is erratically absorbed. A search is underway for the other active drugs in the melamine family that can be administered parenterally (e.g., pentamethylmelamine).

Doxorubicin is an active first-line agent in advanced ovarian cancer. Collected experience indicates a response rate of approximately 30%. Unfortunately, several studies indicate that the drug has very little activity when used as a second or third-line agent with only three of 56 patients (5%) responding to the drug after failing initial chemotherapy.[130,131]

Cis–diaminedichloroplatinum (DDP) is one of the more active agents in ovarian cancer. Information on the single agent activity of the drug indicates an overall response rate of 25% (40 of 161 patients).[132] Patients responding to treatment survive longer than those who fail to respond (9 months versus 3.2 months); ($p = 0.014$). Toxicities are significant and include nausea and vomiting, nephrotoxicity, and bone marrow suppression. The latter two toxicities are seen more frequently in those patients who were previously treated extensively. Forced diuresis with or without mannitol is necessary to minimize the renal toxicity of the drug.

Unique techniques for delivering chemotherapeutic agents to patients with ovarian cancer are now under study. Because the disease usually remains confined to the intra–abdominal space, the use of large-volume continuous exchange intraperitoneal administration is being tested. The pharmacologic basis for this "belly bath" therapy in ovarian cancer is based on the observation that peritoneal permeability of many anticancer drugs is less than plasma clearance. In addition, when administered in large volumes to insure adequate distribution, significantly greater concentrations of the drug may be maintained in the peritoneal space than in the plasma.[133] Studies using methotrexate, 5–fluorouracil, and doxorubicin are underway and initial trials with methotrexate have been reported.[124] Initial clinical trials with doxorubicin have also been performed with the attainable concentration of the drug in the ascites being assayed against the clonogenicity of human ovarian cancer cells.[126]

Approaches like this may result in greater local antitumor effect and reduced systemic toxicity. However, further studies will be necessary before this technique can be proposed for widespread clinical use.

For many years, attempts have been made to define the activity of potentially useful chemotherapeutic agents using a variety of *in vitro* screening techniques. Although these have not been particularly useful in the past, recent studies show more promise. An *in vitro* tumor colony assay that evaluates clonogenic potential after exposure to chemotherapy has been used in a variety of tumors and has received considerable study in ovarian carcinoma.[127] The possible uses of an assay such as this include the selection of second-line agents active against a patient's particular tumor; the screening and identification of new drugs appropriate for Phase II trials in ovarian carcinoma; and the study of biochemical and pharmacologic mechanisms of drug resistance in human ovarian cancer cells.

An updated summary of the human tumor stem cell assay in ovarian cancer has recently been published that presents data on 80 patients.[134] Some 75% of specimens provided sufficient colony growth to permit drug activity assessment. Forty-four patients have now been studied *in vitro* and *in vivo* and the assay predicted *in vivo* sensitivity with 64% accuracy, and *in vivo* resistance with 97% accuracy. Screening newer drugs in the assay produced evidence for activity of vinblastine, pentamethylmelamine, and AMSA.

Combination Chemotherapy

In the past, relatively few combination chemotherapy studies were published involving only a few patients with ovarian cancer. For example, early studies with a combination known as *ActFuCy* (actinomycin D, 5–fluorouracil, and cyclophosphamide) in patients refractory to melphalan were encouraging. However, when prospective trials were performed at the same institution the overall response rate was similar to melphalan (45% versus 42%) and the toxicity of the combination was greater.[33] Even in nonrandomized trials of combinations where higher initial response rates were seen, significantly longer remission durations or survivals than those achieved with alkylating agents alone could not be demonstrated. The worth of any particular combination will only be established when directly compared with alkylating agents alone in a comparable group of patients. Then, important prognostic factors of stage must be considered, along with the histologic grade and extent of residual disease in the randomization and data analysis.

Unfortunately, the majority of available combination chemotherapy studies on advanced ovarian cancer do not include these vital considerations. Consequently, a wide variety of combination chemotherapy studies are now being reported in which responses vary from 22–85% and complete remission rates vary from 10–65%, depending on the type of patients included and the criteria used for assessing response. Only a very few of the studies are randomized comparisons where adequate analysis of prognostic factors are available. The great variation in patient selection, prognostic factors, and response criteria make it difficult, if not impossible, to compare most of these studies. Furthermore, the differences in patient characteristics may, in many of the studies, have a more important influence on survival than the therapies being reported. In general, the recently published studies can be divided into three major groups: 1) studies comparing single agents with combinations; 2) studies on patients who have failed previous alkylating agent and/or radiation therapy; and 3) studies done on previously untreated patients.

Single Agents Versus Combination Chemotherapy

The first study that demonstrated significantly improved survival with any combination in a prospective comparison with a standard alkylating agent was published in 1978.[64] Eighty previously untreated patients were randomized to receive either melphalan in conventional doses, or Hexa–CAF (hexamethylmelamine, cyclophosphamide, methotrexate, and 5-fluorouracil). Treatment with the four-drug combination achieved a significantly increased overall response rate (75% versus 54%, p less than 0.05), more complete remissions (33% versus 16%, p = 0.06), and significantly longer median survival (29 versus 17 months, p less than 0.02). However, Hexa–CAF was most effective in patients with minimal residual disease where a higher overall response was achieved than in patients with extensive residual disease (84% versus 53%, p less than 0.05). Emphasis was placed on important stratification factors such as extent of residual disease and histologic grade, as well as age, stage, and histologic type. Careful reassessment of complete remission using peritoneoscopy or "second-look" laparotomy was crucial to proper management. Patients achieving complete remission, which was documented by restaging, had a long survival and 60% of these women continued to survive in excess of four years. The toxicity of the combination was greater than that of the single agent with hematologic toxicity primarily included along with nausea, vomiting, and alopecia. A dose modification scheme is necessary to tailor the regimen to individual patient tolerance.

Dutch investigators have confirmed the activity of the Hexa–CAF combination in previously untreated patients (overall response rate 57% with 30% complete remission).[135] They have also demonstrated that in previously treated patients, Hexa–CAF has a much lower overall response rate, 3/13 (25%), no complete remissions, and increased toxicity. Their study emphasizes the marked reduction of activity of any regimen used as second-line therapy in advanced ovarian cancer and, in addition, the lack of success of initiating therapy with an alkylating agent, then later attempting to salvage relapsing patients with a more aggressive combination chemotherapy approach.

Several other prospective comparisons in previously untreated patients between combinations and single alkylating agents suggest enhanced activity of the combinations. A recent trial of 24 previously untreated patients compared single agent L–PAM with CHF (cyclophosphamide, hexamethylmelamine, and 5-fluorouracil).[136] The overall response rate was 83% for the combination and 58% for L–PAM. Median duration of remission was 14 months for CHF and 9 months for L–PAM. Median survival for L–PAM was 11 months compared to 14 months for patients treated with CHF. In a Mayo Clinic study mentioned earlier, 111 patients were randomized to receive either cyclophosphamide alone or cyclophosphamide and doxorubicin. While there was no difference between the two regimens in patients with bulky disease, there was a significant increase in response rate and survival in those patients with minimal residual disease treated with the doxorubicin-cyclophosphamide combination.[123] A list of the combination chemotherapy regimens with improved results when prospectively compared to single alkylating agents in previously untreated patients is shown in Table 26-7.

TABLE 26-7. Combination Chemotherapy Regimens When Compared to an Alkylating Agent in Advanced Previously Untreated Ovarian Carcinoma

REGIMEN	DOSES	SCHEDULE	RESPONSE RATE: RESPONDERS/ TOTAL PATIENTS	REFERENCE
Hexa–CAF				
Hexamethylmelamine	150 mg/m² PO qd × 14	Every 4 wk	30/40 (75%)	64
Cyclophosphamide	150 mg/m² PO qd × 14			
Methotrexate	40 mg/m² IV, days 1,8			
5–Fluorouracil	600 mg/m² IV days 1,8			
A–C				
Cyclophosphamide	500 mg/m² IV	Every 4 wk	45/99 (45%)	123
(Adriamycin)	40 mg/m			
Doxorubicin				
CHF				
Cyclophosphamide	100 mg/m² PO qd × 14	Every 4 wk	10/12 (83%)	136
Hexamethylmelamine	150 mg/m² PO qd × 14			
5–Fluorouracil	600 mg/m² IV days 1,8			

Combination Chemotherapy After Alkylating Agent Failure

The use of combinations after alkylating agent failure has been reported. Details on these regimens are presented in Table 26-8. Unfortunately, none of these trials really established any regimen as particularly successful in managing radiation or chemotherapy failures. In spite of the high overall response reported for many of these combinations, the number of patients included in each is small with the majority of the responses partial and of very short duration (4–6 months). The toxicity, when reported, appears to be substantial. Very few of these patients, regardless of the regimen, are alive at one year. With the currently available drugs and regimens, the use of combination chemotherapy fails after initial treatment. The cure rate in this disease is not likely to improve

TABLE 26-8. Combination Chemotherapy After Alkylating Agent Failure

REGIMEN	REFERENCE	SCHEDULE	NO. OF PATIENTS STUDIED	RESPIRATORY RATE %	(CLIN. CR%)	DURATION OF REMISSION	SURVIVAL	TOXICITY
Hexamethlymelamine + 5–Fluorouracil	137	8 mg/kg PO qd × 21 12 mg/kg IV days 1,8,15–22	9	33	22	N.S.*	9 months	Excessive—GI, neurologic, and hematopoietic
Doxorubicin (Adriamycin) + Cis–platinum	138	60 mg/m² IV q 3–4 wk 60 mg/m² IV q 3–4 wk	20	42	0	3–14 months	N.S.	Severe GI toxicity, alopecia, hematopoietic
	129	50 mg/m² IV q 3–4 wk 50 mg/m² IV q 3–4 wk	11	54	0	6 months	N.S.	Severe nausea and vomiting and anemia, mild nephrotoxicity and leukopenia
Doxorubicin (Adriamycin)– Cis-platinum 5–Fluorouracil Hexamethylmelamine	140	25 mg/m² IV day 1 50 mg/m² IV day 1 300 mg/m³ IV days 1,8 150 mg/m² PO days 1–14	103	48	(N.S.)	5.8 months	12 months	Severe hematopoietic
CHAP Cyclophosphamide Hexamethlymelamine Doxorubicin (Adriamycin) Cis–platinum	141	300 mg/m² IV day 1 150 mg/m² PO days 1–14 40 mg/m² IV day 1 50 mg/m² day 1	35	49	20	6 months	N.S.	Severe-profound leukopenia, thrombocytopenia, and GI intolerance.
HAD Hexamethylmelamine Doxorubicin (Adriamycin) Cis–platinum	142	200 mg/m² PO days 8–22 30 mg/m² IV day 1 50 mg/m² IV day 1	27	67	27	6 months	10 months	Severe hematologic toxicity, anemia
CAP Cyclophosphamide Doxorubicin (Adriamycin) Cis–platinum	143	300 mg/m² IV day 1 q 3 wk 30 mg/m² IV day 1 q 3 wk 50 mg/m² IV day 1 q 3 wk	24	50	8	N.S.	7 months	Severe anemia, hematopoietic toxicity, nausea, and vomiting
Cyclophosphamide + High Dose Methotrexate + CF ± Vincristine	144	250 mg/m² IV days 1–5 750 mg/m² IV as 4–hr infusion with CF 10 mg/m² q 6 hr × 12 doses 1.5 mg/m²+ IV (max 2 mg) 6 hrs before MTX	55	29.8	4	3–9 months	7.5 months	Severe myelosuppression in 24%

*N.S. = Not Stated

and can, at present, be thought of as a way to identify interesting regimens for primary therapy of the untreated patient.

Combination Chemotherapy as Initial Treatment

Several studies report results of combination chemotherapy used as initial treatment in advanced disease. These studies have either been single arm studies or randomized trials in which two or more combinations have been compared. A summary of a representative group of these trials is shown in Table 26-9. Most of these studies contain relatively small numbers of patients and are reported in a preliminary fashion. A few studies contain sufficient information about prognostic factors, response duration, and survival to allow any realistic comparison with currently established combination chemotherapy regimens or single agents. Until a sufficient amount of patients have been studied and follow-up has been at least two and one-half years, these regimens must be considered to be of an experimental nature.

Immunotherapy

Immunotherapy has been investigated in a limited number of studies. However, a good theoretical basis for immunotherapy exists and is based upon: 1) the existence of tumor-associated antigens demonstrated in ovarian cancer; 2) circulating lymphocytes that are reactive to the patient's tumor cells; 3) defects in B-cell function demonstrated in patients with advanced ovarian cancer, although T-cell function appears intact; 4) animal models of ovarian cancer that demonstrate enhanced tumor killing with chemotherapy and either non-specific immunotherapy or specific antibody generated against ovarian tumor cells.

Recently, several studies have been published using immunotherapy in conjunction with chemotherapy in ovarian cancer. In general, most suffer from being single arm studies containing heterogenous populations of patients where data on histologic grade or extent of residual disease are not available. The most provocative study suggesting a role for immunotherapy in advanced disease comes from a Southwest Oncology Group study.[147] Patients were randomized to receive either adriamycin plus cyclophosphamide (AC) or adriamycin plus cyclophosphamide plus BCG given by scarification (AC + BCG). Some 118 evaluable patients have now been randomized. The overall response rate is 36% for the combination chemotherapy alone and 53% for the chemo-immunotherapy arm. There are very few true complete remissions in either arm of the study but there are more (12%) for the AC + BCG group than for the AC group (2%). Survival is also better for the chemo-immunotherapy group (23.5 months versus 13.1 months). Further information from this trial is needed as histologic grading of included patients has not been completed and the extent of residual disease after surgery is not stated.

None of the completed immunotherapy studies has sufficient patient numbers, duration of follow-up, and analysis of known important prognostic factors to allow a definite conclusion as to the independent contribution of immunotherapy in the treatment of ovarian carcinoma. More properly-structured, prospective studies will be required to resolve this matter.

Finally, as therapy for advanced ovarian cancer improves, a variety of late complications are being observed that are related to either the treatment or the altered natural history of the disease. Late occurrence of unusual lesions such as bone metastases or CNS involvement have now been reported.[148] Acute leukemia as a late complication of therapy in ovarian cancer has been reported in several studies. A published survey of 70 institutions with a population of 5455 patients revealed 13 patients who developed leukemia representing a 21-fold increase in risk.[149] Risks were highest in patients who had chemotherapy in excess of two years and approximately two-thirds of the patients had received irradiation as well. Often a prolonged period of pancytopenia antedated frank leukemic transformation. Two-thirds of the leukemic patients who died showed no evidence of ovarian cancer at autopsy. The overall risk of acute leukemia in ovarian cancer is quite small (0.3%).[149] However, techniques for minimizing the risk such as cyclic intermittent chemotherapy rather than continuous daily treatment; avoidance of combined radiation-chemotherapy treatments where possible; and better techniques for defining the complete remissions so that therapy can be discontinued will undoubtedly serve to minimize this risk.

Summary of the Therapeutic Options for Patients with Macroscopic Residual Disease

Patients left with bulky residual disease after initial surgery have a poor prognosis whether they are FIGO Stage II, III, or IV. The currently accepted approach to such patients has been to use systemic chemotherapy either with single alkylating agents or, more recently, with combination chemotherapy. Concomitant or sequential use of local irradiation to sites of bulky residual disease is sometimes possible if the port size is not too extensive.

Those patients with retroperitoneal lymph node metastasis as their only site of spread outside the pelvis are appropriately managed with pelvic irradiation and an inverted Y-port to encompass known sites of disease.

MANAGEMENT OF STROMAL AND GERMINAL OVARIAN TUMORS

Although germ cell and stromal tumors of the ovary only make up about 10% of all ovarian tumors, they are important because of their unusual natural history and clinical manifestations. In addition, it is necessary to utilize different therapies for the various tumor types.[102] These tumors are particularly important because some of the most aggressive of these tumors are now curable with combination chemotherapy and less aggressive surgery and can be separated into three groups:

1. Those with ovarian stromal components, such as the granulosa cell and Sertoli–Leydig cell tumors
2. Tumors derived from germ-cell elements such as malignant teratoma, embryonal carcinoma, and dysgerminoma
3. Choriocarcinoma

TABLE 26-9. Combination Chemotherapy as Initial Treatment

REGIMEN	REFERENCE	SCHEDULE	NO. OF PATIENTS	RESPONSE RATE %	(CLIN. CR %)	DURATION OF REMISSION	SURVIVAL	TOXICITY
CHAD Cyclophosphamide Hexamethylmelamine (Adriamycin) Doxorubicin Cis–platinum	142	600 mg/m² IV day 1 200 mg/m² PO days 8–22 25 mg/m² IV day 1 50 mg/m² IV day 1	26	90	(38)	N.S.*	N.S.	Median followup 6 mos from start of therapy, severe nausea and vomiting, 23%; peripheral neuropathy—4%; azotemia and deafness—significant hematopoietic toxicity
MECY Cyclophosphamide Methotrexate + CF	144	250 mg/m² IV × 5 days 750 mg/m² IV over 4 hrs followed by CF 10 mg/m² q 6 hrs × 12 doses	23	67	(48)	Greater than 15 months	N.S.	10% severe bone marrow suppression
FUCY Cyclophosphamide 5–Fluorouracil	144	250 mg/m² IV × 5 days 280 mg/m² IV × 5 days	23	32	(14)	Greater than 15 months	N.S.	10% severe bone marrow suppression
AP Doxorubicin (Adriamycin) Cis–platinum	145	50 mg/m² IV q 3 wks 50 mg/m² IV q 3 wks	36	70	(40)	N.S.	19+	N.S.
CHAD Cyclophosphamide Hexamethylmelamine (Adriamycin) Doxorubicin Cis–platinum	145	150 mg/m² PO days 2–8 150 mg/m² PO days 2–8 30 mg/m² IV day 1 50 mg/m² IV day 1	N.S.	80	(30)	N.S.	N.S.	N.S.
PAC–1 Cis–platinum Doxorubicin (Adriamycin) Cyclophosphamide	146	20 mg/m² IV d × 5 q 4 wks 50 mg/m² IV day 1 q 4 wks 750 mg/m² IV day 1 q 4 wks	19	58	(39)	N.S.	N.S.	Severe nausea, vomiting, and hematopoietic toxicity—mild nephrotoxicity 46%—severe thrombocytopenia 28%
PAC–5 Cis–platinum Doxorubicin (Ariamycin) Cyclophosphamide	146	20 mg/m² IV d × 5 q 4 wks 50 mg/m² IV day 1 q 4 wks 750 mg/m² IV day 1 q 4 wks	17	65	(35)	N.S.	N.S.	Hematopoietic toxicity more severe than with PAC–1
CHex-UP Cyclophosphamide Hexamethylmelamine 5–Fluorouracil Cis–platinum	132	150 mg/m² PO days 2–8 and 9–16 150 mg/m² PO days 2–8 and 9–16 600 mg/m² IV days 1 and 8 30 mg/m² IV days 1 and 8	29	72	(52)	N.S.	17+	Significant hematopoietic toxicity—severe in 30%; 100% nausea and vomiting—mild nephrotoxicity in 30%

*N.S. = Not Stated

OVARIAN STROMAL TUMORS

Ovarian stromal tumors comprise approximately 1–3% of all ovarian tumors, have a long natural history, and sometimes recur many years after initial therapy. They occur bilaterally in less than 5% of patients. They are sometimes associated with precocious feminization; their association with unopposed estrogen secretion and an increased incidence of concomitant endometrial carcinoma has been emphasized. Stage and Grafton report an incidence of 7.8% in 51 patients with granulosa–theca cell tumors.[150] In their review, 43% of these tumors were theca, 23.5% pure granulosa cell tumors, and 33% mixed granulosa–theca cell tumors. None of the patients with thecomas died as a result of their disease; deaths occurred only in the granulosa cell-containing tumors with metastases.

Stromal tumors are treated with a total hysterectomy and bilateral salpingo–oophorectomy whenever possible. Factors, such as tumor size, degree of differentiation or histologic patterns of the tumor, and tumor spillage are of prognostic importance. Because of their protracted natural history, it is difficult to document the value of postoperative radiation. However, in tumors that are not completely resected, a dose of 5000 to 6000 rad to the pelvis has been advocated.[151] Rutledge reported on 37 patients referred to the M. D. Anderson Hospital for initial therapy.[102] The five year survival rate was about 75% for Stage I and 50%–60% for Stage II and III.

The role of chemotherapy in the granulosa–theca cell tumors has been poorly defined because so few patients have been studied. Alkylating agents have not been particularly noteworthy, although objective tumor regressions and even complete remissions have been documented.[102,152] Disaia and coworkers have reported a complete remission induced with doxorubicin after the patient had failed abdominal irradiation and combination therapy with melphalan and 5-fluorouracil. Adriamycin at 70 mg IV every 3 weeks sustained the remission for one year. In light of this report and an earlier one documenting another complete response, doxorubicin should be considered for further study in patients with recurrent granulosa cell tumor.

Prior to 1968, single agent chemotherapy was used at the M. D. Anderson Hospital to treat recurrent granulosa cell tumors when tolerance doses of irradiation had been administered. No complete responses were observed, although three patients had a partial response. Since 1968, a combination of actinomycin-D, 5-fluorouracil, and cyclophosphamide has been used.

Only nine patients with Sertoli–Leydig cell tumors have been seen at M. D. Anderson Hospital, five at the time of initial therapy and four for recurrent tumor. Two patients with recurrent lesions had a complete response after administration of a combination of vincristine, actinomycin-D, and cyclophosphamide.

The following philosophy of management of ovarian stromal tumors was outlined by Rutledge:[102]

> Patients with Stage IA, under 40 years of age are treated with unilateral oophorectomy if preservation of ovarian function or childbearing is important. Otherwise, patients with early lesions are treated with bilateral salpingo-oophorectomy and a total abdominal hysterectomy.
>
> Patients with more advanced lesions (Stage IB through III) are treated with total abdominal hysterectomy and bilateral salpingo-oophorectomy. In the more advanced patients, as much metastatic tumor as possible is excised.
>
> Patients with residual tumor less than 2 cm in diameter or with complete resection receive abdomino–pelvic irradiation with strip technique and pelvic boost. Patients with residual tumor greater than 2 cm or metastasis beyond the abdominal cavity are treated with combination chemotherapy. Following 12 courses of chemotherapy, and exploratory laparotomy (second-look operation) is carried out and additional resection of tumor is attempted. If there is no residual tumor, chemotherapy is discontinued.
>
> Recurrent stromal tumors are treated with surgical resection and postoperative irradiation or chemotherapy as outlined above. If the residual tumor can be encompassed by external irradiation, this method is preferred to chemotherapy. Otherwise a combination of cytotoxic agents is given; DAC/5-FU/Cy (actinomycin-D, 5-fluorouracil, and cyclophosphamide) for granulosa cell and VAC (vincristine, actinomycin-D, cyclophosphamide) for Sertoli–Leydig tumors.

OVARIAN GERM CELL TUMORS

These tumors may have a mixed histologic pattern within a given lesion. Treatment should be designed to deal with the most malignant component of the tumor. Malignant embryonal carcinoma, endodermal sinus tumors, and malignant teratomas have an extremely poor prognosis and surgery alone offers long term survival in only a small percentage of patients.[154] Jimerson and Woodruff reported on a group of patients submitted to the Ovarian Tumor Registry of the American Gynecological Society with endodermal sinus tumor. Of 34 patients on whom follow-up was available for longer than two years, 31 were dead of disease. Three patients with Stage IA were surviving 2½, 9, and 12 years after treatment.

Major advances in the treatment of these tumors have been made since physicians realized that patients are rarely cured by aggressive surgery and radiation therapy and are highly responsive to combination chemotherapy.

Endodermal Sinus Tumors

Endodermal sinus tumors are unusual and aggressive tumors of germ cell origin and reproduce the extraembryonic structures of the early embryo. The tumor is rarely bilateral. Prior to the use of combination chemotherapy, the tumor was almost invariably fatal.

The general consensus at present is that all patients, regardless of stage, should receive chemotherapy. One of the more effective regimens is the VAC (vincristine, actinomycin-D, cytoxan) program developed by the group at the M. D. Anderson Hospital.

Two recent studies summarize the results of the VAC regimen in a variety of more aggressive germ cell tumors. Cangir and coworkers from the M. D. Anderson Hospital reported on 21 patients treated (eight malignant teratomas, six endodermal sinus tumors, six mixed germ cell tumors, and one Sertoli–Leydig tumor).[156] Fourteen of these 21 patients who had a second-look operation after chemotherapy showed no evidence of malignancy. Therefore, the authors conclude that maximal surgical removal followed by adjuvant VAC is the treatment of choice and that irradiation has no role in initial management of such patients unless radiosensitive elements are histologically present in the tumors. Slayton and coworkers report the experience of the Gynecologic Oncology Group with VAC, as well as other regimens, in aggressive germ cell tumors.[157] Thirty-nine patients were treated (14 endodermal sinus tumors, two embryonal carcinoma, 13 mixed cell tumors, five immature teratomas, and five others). Of the 23 patients with surgically resectable disease, only seven have failed. Of the 16 patients who presented with advanced disease (Stage IIB and III recurrent), eight have responded to chemotherapy. The median follow-up for those remaining free of disease is 26.5 months. In their series, 16 of 27 (58%) patients who received the VAC regimen postoperatively are alive and well, including 69% of those with complete tumor resection before chemotherapy. Eight of 12 (66%) of those who received other combinations also remain alive and well. Gallion and coworkers have reviewed the published literature on 150 cases of pure endodermal sinus tumors.[158] Prior to the use of chemotherapy, the overall 2-year survival of patients with Stage I disease was 27% and did not differ from patients presenting with more advanced disease. Surgery alone was ineffective, producing only a 16% two-year survival. Even total abdominal hysterectomy and bilateral salpingo-oophorectomy for Stage IA disease in one study produced a 13% two-year survival. Pelvic or total abdominal radiation added little to these two-year survival figures.

Combination chemotherapy has dramatically altered survival in this disease. Over 65% of patients are now alive after treatment with one of several combination regimens. The largest experience has been with the VAC combination; however, actinomycin D, 5-fluorouracil, cyclophosphamide seem to produce similar results.

Malignant Teratoma

Malignant teratoma of the ovary is a rare but lethal germ cell tumor. Over half of the patients present under the age of 20. The tumor is rarely bilateral. Prognosis seems to be related to the histologic grade of the tumor. The M. D. Anderson group has recently published their experience with 25 patients.[159] Prior to the use of combination chemotherapy, patients were managed with aggressive surgery followed by irradiation or single-agent chemotherapy. Of the eight patients managed in this manner, none survived although all different grades were represented. In contrast, using the combination chemotherapy regimen VAC without irradiation, ten of 12 patients are surviving with a median of 43 months. This would seem to be the approach of choice at the present time based upon these good results.

Dysgerminoma

Dysgerminoma comprises only about 2% of all ovarian malignancies and is unique among the germ cell tumors because of its high cure rate and sensitivity to radiation therapy. It is also the only ovarian malignancy that occurs bilaterally with significant frequency. While it is the counterpart of testicular seminoma in males, this tumor is more frequent in young girls, and is bilateral in 10% to 15% of the patients. It metastasizes to the regional lymph nodes in about 20% of the patients and can be cured with limited surgical procedures and low doses of radiation therapy.

Other malignant germ cell tumor components should be identified since this influences the prognosis. Asadourian and Taylor reported an admixture of germinal elements in 12 of 117 patients with dysgerminoma reviewed at the Armed Forces Institute of Pathology.[160] However, several studies indicate that extension through the capsule of the tumor, extra ovarian spread, large tumor size, or the presence of bilateral lesions is a poor prognostic sign.[161,162]

At surgery, the contralateral ovary should be carefully examined. If there is any question of involvement, it should be bivalved and wedge frozen biopsies should be obtained. If the tumor is localized to one ovary, a unilateral salpingo-oophorectomy should be performed. Also, the pelvic and periaortic nodes should be evaluated carefully by palpation; biopsies should be taken of any suspicious areas. If the tumor is localized inside the capsule of the ovary, no postoperative irradiation is indicated. Otherwise, a dose of 2000 to 2500 rad should be delivered to the midplane of the hemipelvis on the side of the lesion in addition to the pelvic and periaortic nodes.[162,163] If there is bilateral extension, bilateral salpingo-oophorectomy should be carried out and irradiation to the pelvis, iliac, and periaortic nodes given. If gross metastatic nodes are present, a boost of 500 to 1000 rad should be delivered with reduced fields. High energy linear accelerator beams should be used to decrease the scatter dose to the contralateral ovary.

In five patients with Stage IA disease treated with unilateral salpingo-oophorectomy only at M. D. Anderson Hospital, no recurrences were noted. All patients are alive three to 20 years after initial treatment and three of these patients have had children. The group from the M. D. Anderson Hospital have reported results on 36 patients with pure dysgerminoma.[163] They emphasize the importance of carefully searching for any mixed tumor elements in the tumors which, if found, require different and more aggressive management. Of their patients, 61% were Stage I and 34% had advanced disease (FIGO Stages III and IV). Management was generally with aggressive debulking surgery followed by total abdominal irradiation. Lymphangiography should be used to assess disease in the para-aortic nodes. The overall survival for their group of patients was 86%. This is perhaps the only germ cell tumor which is so radiation-sensitive. Brody reported the results in 56 patients who received radiation therapy at the Radiumhemmet Institute.[162] The overall five-year survival was 75% with 36% of the patients developing a recurrence. As indicated in Table 26-10, the extent of the tumor was a critical factor in determining survival and recurrences. In 40 patients treated initially at the institution, 13 recurrences were noted and of these, eight survived for five years or more after the beginning of therapy. Asadourian and Taylor reported recurrences or metastasis in 23 of 105 patients (24%); additional therapy resulted in the cure of 10 of these patients.[160] They also observed a 96% five year actuarial survival in 78 patients with tumor localized to one or both ovaries in contrast to 63% in 17 patients with extra ovarian extension.

Brody pointed out that low doses of radiation (probably below 1000 rad tumor dose) were not as effective as somewhat

TABLE 26-10. Relation Between Extension of the Disease at the Time of Operation and Prognosis in Dysgerminoma of the Ovary*

Correlation Between Extent of Disease at Operation and Prognosis

EXTENSION OF DISEASE AT OPERATION	NUMBER OF PATIENTS	FIVE-YEAR SURVIVAL RATE (%)	RECURRENCE RATE (% of Living)
Tumor encapsulated and movable	22	95	14
Ascites	5	100	40
Tumor adhesions	8	75	50
Rupture of tumor before or at operation	5	60	0
Metastasis (including bilateral ovarian involvement)	12	33	25

*Only cases treated with combined surgery and radiotherapy five or more years ago have been included in this table.
(Brody S: Acta Radiologica (Ther) 56:217, 1961)

higher doses. There were 18 pregnancies after treatment in ten patients. Fifteen of the babies were normal and one malformed. There were two abortions—one therapeutic and one spontaneous.

Recurrent tumors when more extensive or with distant metastasis have been treated with combination chemotherapy. For example, Cohen and Goldsmith reported the successful treatment of a radiation-resistant patient with vincristine and bleomycin followed by vincristine and methotrexate maintenance for three years. This patient continues to be free of disease two years after therapy was discontinued.

Ovarian Choriocarcinoma

This tumor is extremely rare (less than 1% of ovarian tumors). Chemotherapy, as in trophoblastic lesions, has been the treatment of choice.[165] The prognosis, however, is extremely poor. Rutledge reported a few patients responding to a combination of methotrexate, actinomycin-D, and cyclophosphamide (MAC).[102]

TREATMENT OF OVARIAN CARCINOMA ASSOCIATED WITH PREGNANCY

The association of ovarian carcinoma with pregnancy is unusual.[166] In 1963, Jubb found only 34 reports of primary epithelial carcinoma in pregnancy in the literature. Creasman reported 17 patients treated at M. D. Anderson who were either pregnant or had been pregnant within six months of the diagnosis of ovarian carcinoma. The majority of these patients were asymptomatic and the ovarian mass was found during a routine prenatal examination. In one of the patients, the diagnosis of ovarian pathology was made during the third trimester and in six at the time of delivery. Three of the patients had obstetric complications.

Ten of the 17 patients had Stage IA tumors, five of them being dysgerminoma and two granulosa cell tumor. One patient with granulosa cell tumor was treated with a unilateral salpingo-oophorectomy and the other with total abdominal hysterectomy and bilateral salpingo-oophorectomy with no recurrence five years and 16 years after treatment.

Of the five patients with dysgerminoma, three had recurrent disease when first seen. The majority were treated with a total abdominal hysterectomy, salpingo-oophorectomy, and postoperative irradiation. Four patients with serous adenocarcinoma were treated in the same fashion; two survived. Of 11 patients diagnosed antepartum as having ovarian carcinoma, eight delivered normal infants, seven of which survived the neonatal period.

This study emphasizes the importance of prenatal examination in detecting these lesions and the need for appropriate treatment since many of the tumors are in early stages and histology. Patients with dysgerminoma and granulosa cell tumors can be treated conservatively (salpingo-oophorectomy) and even those with recurrent disease have a 50% probability of survival. Patients with other germ cell tumors have a poor prognosis and require aggressive combination chemotherapy.

Creasman and coworkers advocate an exploratory operation for patients who have an ovarian mass antepartum.[168] If the exploratory laparotomy shows Stage IA dysgerminoma or granulosa cell tumor and there are no lymph nodes or malignant cells in peritoneal washings, a salpingo-oophorectomy is performed and the pregnancy may be allowed to be completed with a vaginal delivery. Following delivery, additional therapy should be administered.

In patients with low grade Stage IA mucinous or serous cystadenocarcinoma in the second or third trimester, the usual management could be instituted after delivery. However, in patients with more malignant tumors, definitive therapy should be carried out at the time of diagnosis and the pregnancy sacrificed.

REFERENCES

1. Cancer Facts and Figures 1980. American Cancer Society Publication, New York, 1980
2. Doll R, Muir C, Waterhouse J (eds): International Union Against Cancer: Cancer incidence in five continents, vol. 2, Berlin, Springer-Verlag, 1970
3. Buell P, Dunn JE: Cancer mortality among Japanese Issei and Nisei of California. Cancer 18:656–664, 1965
4. Haenszel W, Kurihara M: Studies of Japanese migrants I. Mortality from cancer and other disease among Japanese in the United States. J Natl Cancer Inst 40:43–68, 1968

5. Joly DJ, Lilienfeld AM, Diamond EL et al: An epidemiologic study of the relationship of reproductive experience to cancer of the ovary. Am J Epidemiol 99:190–209, 1974
6. Beral V, Fraser P, Chilvers C: Does pregnancy protect against ovarian cancer? Lancet 1083–1086, 1978
7. Lingeman CH: Etiology of cancer of the human ovary: A review. J Natl Cancer Inst 53:1603–1618, 1974
8. Hoover R, Gray LA, Fraumeni JF: Stilbesterol and the risk of ovarian cancer. Lancet ii:533–534, 1977
9. West BO: Epidemiologic study of malignancies of the ovaries. Cancer 19:1001–1007, 1966
10. Fraumeni JF, Grundy GW, Creagan ET: Six families prone to ovarian cancer. Cancer 36:364–369, 1975
11. Schweisguth O, Gerard-Marchant R, Plainfosse B, et al: Bilateral nonfunctioning thecoma of the ovary in epileptic children under anticonvulsant therapy. Acta Paediatr Scand 60:6–10, 1971
12. Longo DL, Young RC: Cosmetic talc and ovarian carcinoma. Lancet ii:349–351, 1979
13. Janovski NA, Paramanandhan TL: Tumors and tumor-like conditions of the ovaries, fallopian tubes and ligaments of the uterus. In Friedman EA (ed): Major Problems in Obstetrics and Gynecology, Vol 4, p 12. Philadelphia, WB Saunders, 1973
14. Plentl AA, Friedman EA: Lymphatic system of the female genitalia: The morphologic basis of oncologic diagnosis and therapy, pp 168–180. Philadelphia, WB Saunders, 1973
15. Feldman GB, Knapp RC: Lymphatic drainage of the peritoneal cavity and its significance in ovarian cancer. Am J Obstet Gynecol 119:991–994, 1974
16. Holm-Hielsen P: Pathogenesis of ascites in peritoneal carcinomatosis. Acta Pathol Microbiol Scand 33:10–21, 1953
17. Feldman GB, Knapp RC, Order SE, Hellman S: The role of lymphatic obstruction in the formation of ascites in a murine ovarian carcinoma. Cancer Res 32:1663–1666, 1972
18. Bagley CM, Young RC, Schein PS, Chabner BA, DeVita VT: Ovarian carcinoma metastatic to the diaphragm: Frequently undiagnosed at laparotomy. J Obstet Gynecol 116:397–400, 1973
19. Rosenoff SH, DeVita VT, Hubbard S, Young RC: Peritoneoscopy in the staging and follow-up of ovarian cancer. Semin Oncol 2:223–228, 1975
20. Piver MS, Barlow JJ, Lele SB: Incidence of sub-clinical metastasis in stage I and II ovarian carcinoma. Obstet Gynecol 52:100–104, 1978
21. Coates G, Bush RS, Aspin N: A study of ascites using lymphoscintigraphy with 99m Tx-sulfur colloid. Radiology 107:577–583, 1973
22. Ehrmann RL, Federschneider JM, Knapp RC: Distinguishing lymph node metastases from benign glandular inclusions in low grade ovarian carcinoma. Am J Obstet Gynecol 136:737–746, 1980
23. Bergman F: Carcinoma of the ovary, a clinicopathological study of 86 autopsied cases with special reference to mode of spread. Acta Obstet Gynecol Scand 45:211–231, 1966
24. Scully RE: Recent progress in ovarian cancer. Human Pathol 1:73–98, 1970
25. Novak ER, Woodruff JD: Novak's Gynecologic and Obstetric Pathology, p 389. Philadelphia, WB Saunders, 1974
26. Serov SF, Scully RE, Solvin LH: International histological classification of tumors, No. 9. Histological Typing of Ovarian Tumors. Geneva, World Health Organization, 1973
27. International Federation of Gynaecology and Obstetrics: Classification and staging of malignant tumors in the female pelvis. Acta Obstet Gynaecol Scand 50:1–7, 1971
28. Scully RE: Ovarian tumors. Am J Pathol 87:686–720, 1977
29. Kottmeier HL: Ovarian cancer with special regard to radiotherapy. J Roentgenol Radium Ther Nucl Med 111:417–421, 1971
30. Aure JC, Høeg K, Kolstad P: Clinical and histologic studies of ovarian carcinoma: long-term followup of 900 cases. Obstet Gynecol 37:1–9, 1971
31. Perez CA, Walz BJ, Jacobson PL: Radiation therapy in the management of carcinoma of the ovary. Natl Cancer Inst Monogr 42:119–125, 1975
32. Young RC, Hubbard SP, DeVita VT: The chemotherapy of ovarian carcinoma. Cancer Treat Rev 1:99–110, 1974
33. Smith JP, Rutledge F, Wharton JT: Chemotherapy of ovarian cancer: new approaches to treatment. Cancer 30:1565–1571, 1972
34. Julian CG, Woodruff JD: The role of chemotherapy in the treatment of primary ovarian malignancy. Obstet Gynecol Surv 24:1307, 1969
35. Munnell EW, Taylor HC: Ovarian carcinoma: a review of 200 primary and 51 secondary cases. Am J Obstet 58:943, 1949
36. Kent SW, McKay DG: Primary cancer of the ovary. Am J Obstet Gynecol 80:430–438, 1960
37. Perez CA, Bradfield JS: Radiation therapy in the treatment of carcinoma of the ovary. Cancer 29:1027–1037, 1972
38. Decker DG, Mussey E, Williams TJ: Grading of gynecologic malignancy: epithelial ovarian cancer. Proc 7th Natl Cancer Congr, p 233–231. Philadelphia, JB Lippincott, 1972
39. Day TG, Gallager HS, Rutledge RN: Epithelial carcinoma of the ovary: prognostic importance of histologic grade. Natl Cancer Inst Monogr 42:15–18, 1975
40. Ozols RF, Garvin AJ, Cost J et al: Histologic grade in advanced ovarian cancer. Cancer Treat Rep 63:255–263, 1979
41. Dembo AJ, Bush RS, Beale FA: Ovarian carcinoma: improved survival following abdominopelvic irradiation in patients with a completed pelvic operation. Am J Obstet Gynecol 134:793–800, 1979
42. Ozols RF, Garvin AJ, Costa J: Advanced ovarian cancer: correlation of histologic grade with response to therapy and survival. Cancer 45:572–581, 1980
43. Scully RE: World Health Organization Classification and Nomenclature of ovarian cancer. Natl Cancer Inst Monogr 42:5–7, 1975
44. Pearse WH, Behrman SJ: Carcinoma of the ovary. Obstet Gynecol 3:32–45, 1954
45. Barber HRK, Graber EA: The PMPO (postmenopausal ovary syndrome). Obstet Gynecol 38:921–923, 1971
46. McGowan L: Peritoneal fluid profiles. Natl Cancer Inst Monogr 42:76–79, 1975
47. Cochrane WJ, Thomas MA: Ultrasound diagnosis of gynecologic pelvic masses. Radiology 110:649–654, 1974
48. Samuels BI: Usefulness of ultrasound in patients with ovarian cancer. Semin Oncol 2:229–233, 1975
49. Berkowitz RS, Leavitt T Jr, Knapp RC: Ultrasound directed percutaneous aspiration biopsy of periaortic lymph nodes in cervical carcinoma recurrence. Am J Obstet Gynecol 131:906–908, 1978
50. Parker BR, Castellino RA, Fuks, ZY, Bagshaw MA: The role of lymphography in patients with ovarian cancer. Cancer 34:100–105, 1974
51. Athey PA, Wallace S, Jing B, Gallagher HS, Smith JP: Lymphangiography in avarian cancer. Am J Roetgenol 123:106–113, 1975
52. Fuks Z: External radiotherapy of ovarian cancer: Standard approaches and new frontiers. Semin Oncol 2:253–266. 1975
53. Musumeci F, Banfi A, Bolis G: Lymphangiography in patients with ovarian epithelial cancer: An evaluation of 289 consecutive cases. Cancer 40:1444–1449, 1977
54. Schaner EG, Head GL, Kalman MA, Dunnick NR, Doppman JL: Whole body computed tomography in the diagnosis of abdominal and thoracic malignancy: Review of 600 cases. Cancer Treat Rep 61:1537–1560, 1977
55. Dunnick NR, Schaner EG, Doppman JL: Detection of subcutaneous metastasis by compute tomography. J Comp Assist Tomogr 2:275–279, 1978
56. Ulfelder H. (Chairman): Staging system for cancer at gynecologic sites. Manual for staging of cancer, pp 94–97, 1978
57. Webb MJ, Decker DG, Mussey E, Williams TJ: Factors influencing survival in stage I ovarian cancer. Am J Obstet Gynecol 166:222–228, 1973
58. Parker RT, Parker CH, Wilbanks GD: Cancer of the ovary. Am J Obstet Gynecol 108:878–888, 1970
59. Tobias JS, Griffiths CT: Management of ovarian carcinoma:

Current concepts and future prospects. N Engl J Med 294:818–823, 887–882, 1976
60. Delclos L, Quinlan EJ: Malignant tumor of the ovary managed with postoperative megavoltage irradiation. Radiology 93: 659–663, 1969
61. Griffiths CT, Fuller AF: Intensive surgical and chemotherapeutic management of advanced ovarian cancer. Surg Clin North Am 58:131–142, 1978
62. Griffiths CT: Surgical resection of bulk tumor in the primary treatment of ovarian carcinoma. Symposium on Ovarian Cancer. Natl Cancer Inst Mongr 42:101–104, 1975
63. Smith, JP, Day TG: Review of ovarian cancer at the University of Texas Center, M. D. Anderson Hospital and Tumor Institute. Am J Obstet Gynecol 135:984–993, 1079
64. Young RC, Chabner BA, Hubbard SP: Prospective trial of melphalan (L-PAM) versus combination chemotherapy (Hexa-CAF) in ovarian adenocarcinoma. N Engl J Med 299: 1261–1266, 1978
65. Parker LM, Griffiths CT, Yankee RA: Combination chemotherapy with adriamycin-cyclophosphamide for advanced ovarian carcinoma. Cancer in press
66. Griffiths CT, Parker LM, Fuller AF: Role of cytoreductive surgical treatment in the management of advanced ovarian cancer. Cancer Treat Rep 63:235–240, 1979
67. Dembo AJ, Bush RA, Beale FA: Ovarian carcinoma: Improved survival following abdominopelvic irradiation in patients with a completed pelvic operation. Am J Obstet Gynecol 134:793–800, 1978
68. Smith JP, Schwartz PE: Second-look laparotomy and prognosis related to extent of residual disease. In Van Oosterom, Muggia (eds): Therapeutic Progress in Ovarian Cancer, Testicular Cancer, and the Sarcomas. The Hague, Martinus Nyhoff Publishers, 1980
69. Knapp RC, Donahue VC, Friedman EA: Dissection of paravesical and pararectal spaces in pelvic operations. Surg Gynecol Obstet 137:758–762, 1973
70. Ozols RG, Fisher RI, Anderson T, Makuch R, Young RC: Peritoneoscopy in the management of ovarian cancer. Am J Obstet Gynecol (in press)
71. Wallach RC, Kabakow B, Blinick G: Current status of the second-look operation in ovarian carcinoma. Natl Cancer Inst Monogr 42:105–107, 1975
72. Smith JP, Rutledge FN: Chemotherapy in advanced ovarian cancer. Natl Cancer Inst Monograph 42:141–143, 1975
73. Tepper E, Sanfilippo LJ, Grey J, Romney SL: Second look surgery after radiation therapy for advanced statges of cancer of the ovary. Am J Roentgenol Radium Ther Nucl Med 112:755–759, 1971
74. Kurman RJ, Norris HJ: Endodermal sinus tumor of the ovary—a clinical and pathologic analysis of 71 cases. Cancer 38:2404–2419, 1976
75. Goldstein DP, Piro AJ: Combination chemotherapy in the treatment of germ cell tumors containing choriocarcinoma in males and females. Surg Gynecol Obstet 134:61–66, 1972
76. DiSaia PJ, Morrow CP, Haverback BJ, Dyce BJ: Carcinoembryonic antigen in cancer of the female reproductive system—serial plasma values correlated with disease state. Cancer 39:2365–2370, 1977
77. Levi MM, Keller S, Mandl I: Antigenicity of papillary serous cystadenocarcinoma tissue homogenate and its fractions. Am J Obstet Gynecol 105:856–861, 1969
78. Bhattacharya M, Barlow JJ: Immunologic studies of human serous cystadenocarcinoma of the ovary. Demonstration of tumor-associated antigens. Cancer 31:588–595, 1973
79. Gall SA, Walling J, Pearl J: Demonstration of tumor associated antigens in human gynecologic malignancies. Am J Obstet Gynecol 115:387–393, 1973
80. Imamura N, Takahasi T, Lloyd KO, Lewis JL, Old, LJ: Analysis of human ovarian tumor antigens using heterologous antisera: Detection of new antigenic system. Int J Cancer 21:570–577, 1978
81. Dorsett BH, Ioachim HL, Stolbach L, Walker J, Barber HRK: Isolation of tumor-specific antibodies from effusions of ovarian carcinoma. Int J Cancer 16:779–786, 1975
82. Bhattachary M, Barlow JJ: Immunodiagnosis of cancer. In Herberman RB, McIntyre KR (eds): pp 632–643. New York, Marcel Dekker, 1978
83. Knauf S, Urbach GI: The development of a double-antibody radioimmunoassay for detecting ovarian tumor-associated antigen fraction OCA in plasma. Am J Obstet Gynecol 131:780–787, 1978
84. Bast RC Jr, Lazarus H, Feeney M, Knapp RC: Reactivity of a monoclonal antibody with human ovarian carcinoma. AACR Abstrat (in press)
85. Smith JP: Treatment of ovarian cancer. In Carter, SK, Goldin A, Kuretroi K et al: (eds): Advances in Cancer Chemotherapy, pp 493–503, Jpn Sci Soc Press Tokyo/Univ Park Press, Baltimore, 1978
86. Wharton JT, Herson J, Edwards CL, Seski J, Hodge MP: Long-term survival following chemotherapy for advanced epithelial ovarian carcinoma. In Van Oosterom AJ, Muggia FM (eds): Therapeutic progress in Ovarian Cancer, Testicular Cancer and the Sarcomas, pp. 95–112. The Hague, Martinus Nijhoff Publishers, 1980
87. Kotstad P. Davy M. Høeg K: Individualized treatment of ovarian cancer. Am J Obstet Gynecol 128:617, 1977
88. Bagley CM Jr, Young RC, Canellos GP, DeVita VT: Treatment of ovarian carcinoma: Possibilities for progress. N Engl J Med 287:856–862, 1972
89. Delclos L, Smith JP: Ovarian cancer, with special regard to types of radiotherapy. Natl Cancer Inst Monogr 43:129–138, 1975
90. Griffiths CT, Grogan RH, Hall TC: Advanced ovarian cancer: Primary treatment with surgery, radiotherapy, and chemotherapy. Cancer 29:1–7, 1972
91. Rubin P, Grise JW, Terry R: Has postoperative irradiation proved itself? Am J Roentgenol Radium Ther Nucl Med 88:849–886, 1962
92. Paterson R: The treatment of malignant disease by radium and x-rays: being a practice of radiotherapy, pp 425–432. Baltimore, Williams & Wilkins, 1948
93. Delclos L, Braun EJ, Herrera JR, Sampiere VA, Van Rossenbeek E: Whole abdominal irradiation by cobalt-60 moving strip technique. Radiology 81:632–641, 1963
94. Bush RS: Problems related to the evaluation of reported results in cancer of the ovary. Int J Radiat Oncol Biol Phys 5:2157–2160, 1979
95. Glatstein E, Fuks Z, Bagshaw MA: Diaphragmatic treatment in ovarian carcinoma: A new radiotherapeutic technique. Int J Radiat Oncol Biol Phys 2:357–362, 1977
96. Khan FM, Moore VC, Johnes TK, Stryker JA, Levitt SH: Dose distribution analysis of moving-strip technique for abdominal irradiation using 10 MV X-rays. Radiology 112:421–424. 1974
97. Smoron GL: Strip-staggering. Elimination of inhomogeneity in the moving-strip technique of whole abdominal irradiation. Radiology 104:675–660, 1972
98. Hanks G, Bagshaw MA: Megavoltage radiation therapy and lymphangiography in ovarian cancer. Radiology 93:649–654, 1969
99. Wharton JT, Delclos L, Gallager S, Smith JP: Radiation hepatitis induced by abdominal irradiation with the cobalt 60 moving strip technique. Am J Roentgenol Radium Ther Nucl Med 117:73–80, 1973
100. Perez CA, Korba A, Zivnuska F, Prasad S, Katzenstein A-K: ^{60}Co moving strip technique in the management of carcinoma of the ovary: Analysis of tumor control and morbidity. Int J Radiat Oncol Biol Phys 4:379–388, 1978
101. Fazekas JT, Maier JF: Irradiation of ovarian carcinomas. A prospective comparison of the open-field and moving-strip techniques. Am J Roentgenol Radium Ther Nucl Med 120:118–123, 1974
102. Rutledge FN, Fletcher GH, Smith JP, Wharton JT, Delclos L, Day T, Gallager HS: Gynecologic cancer. In Clark RL, Howe CD (eds): Cancer Patient Care at M.D. Anderson Hospital and

Tumor Institute, pp 263–308. Chicago, Year Book Medical Publishers, 1976
103. Decker DB, Webb MJ, Holbrook MA: Radiocolloid treatment of epithelial cancer of the ovary. Late results. Am J Obstet Gynecol 115:751–758, 1973
104. Davis BA, Latour JPA, Philpott NW: Primary carcinoma of the ovary, Surg Gynecol Obstet 102:565–573, 1956
105. Fuks Z, Bagshaw MA: The rationale for curative radiotherapy for ovarian carcinoma. Int J Radiat Oncol Biol Phys 1:21–32, 1975
106. Parker BR, Castellino RA, Fuks ZY, Bagshaw MA: The role of lymphography in patients with ovarian cancer. Cancer 34:100–105, 1974
107. Hreshchyshyn MM: Results of the gynecologic oncology group trials on ovarian cancer: Preliminary report. Natl Cancer Inst Monogr 42:155–165, 1975
108. Bush RS, Allt WEC, Beale FA, Bean H, Pringle JF, Sturgeon J: Treatment of epithelial carcinoma of the ovary: Operation, irradiation, and chemotherapy. Am J Obstet Gynecol 127:692–704, 1977
109. Dembo AJ, Van Dyke J, Japp, B et al: Whole abdominal irradiation by a moving-strip technique for patients with ovarian cancer. Int J Radiat Oncol Biol Phys 5:1933–1942, 1979
110. Smith JP, Rutledge FN, Delclos L: Postoperative treatment of early cancer of the ovary: A random trial between postoperative irradiation and chemotherapy. Natl Cancer Inst Monogr 42:149–153, 1975
111. Long RT, Sala JM: Radical surgery combined with radiotherapy in the treatment of advanced ovarian carcinoma. Surg Gynecol Obstet 117:201–204, 1963
112. Kottmeier HL: Carcinoma of the uterine cervix, endometrium and ovary, p 293. Chicago, Year Book, 1962
113. Kjellgren O, Angstrom T, Bergman F, Wiklund D-E: Fine-needle aspiration biopsy in diagnosis and classification of ovarian carcinoma. Cancer 28:967–976, 1971
114. Aure JC, Hoeg K, Kolstad P: Radioactive colloidal gold in the treatment of ovarian carcinoma. Acta Radiol Ther (Stockh) 10:399–407, 1971
115. Moore DW, Langley II: Routine use of radiogold following operation for ovarian cancer. Am J Obstet Gynecol 98:624–630, 1967
116. Bushbaum HJ, Keettel WC: Radioisotopes in treatment of stage IA ovarian cancer. Natl Cancer Inst Monogr 42:123–127, 1975
117. Order SE, Rosenshein NB, Klein JL, Lichter AS, Ettinger DS, Dillon MB, Leibel SA: New methods applied to the analysis and treatment of ovarian cancer. Int J Radiat Oncol Biol Phys 5:861–873, 1979
118. Pezner RD, Stevens KR Jr, Tong D, Allen CV: Limited epithelial carcinoma of the ovary treated with curative intent by intraperitoneal installation of radiocolloids. Cancer 42:2563–2671, 1978
119. Hintz BL, Fuks Z, Kempson RL, et al: Results of postoperative megavoltage radiotherapy of malignant surface epithelial tumors of the ovary. Radiology 114:695–700, 1975
120. Hreshchyshyn MH, Norris GH, Park R et al: Postoperative treatment of resectable malignant and possibly malignant epithelial ovarian tumors with radiotherapy, melphalan or no further treatment (Abstr, 9W57). Proc XII Int Cancer Congress 157, 1978
121. Drouin P, Rutledge FN, Delclos L et al: Comparison of external radiotherapy and chemotherapy in ovarian cancer. Ann R Coll Phys Surg Can 12:61, 1979
122. Wharton JT, Rutledge F, Smith JP et al: Hexamethylmelamine: An evaluation of its role in the treatment of ovarian cancer. Am J Obstet Gynecol 133:833, 1979
123. Edmonson HJ, Fleming TR, Decker DG et al: Different chemotherapeutic sensitivities and host factors affecting prognosis in advanced ovarian carcinoma versus minimal residual disease. Cancer Treat Rep 63:241–247, 1979
124. Jones RB, Myers CE, Guarino AM et al: High volume intraperitoneal chemotherapy ("Belly Bath") for ovarian cancer. Cancer Chemother Pharmacol 1:161–166, 1978
125. Ozols RF, Locker GY, Doroshow HJ et al: Adriamycin treatment of ovarian cancer: pharmacokinetics, tissue penetration and rationale for intraperitoneal administration. Cancer Res 39:3209–3214, 1979
126. Ozols RF, Young RC, Speyer JL: Intraperitoneal adriamycin in ovarian carcinoma, p 425. Proc Am Soc Clin Oncol 21:C-423, 1980
127. Hamburger AW, Salmon SE, Kim MB et al: Direct cloning of human ovarian carcinoma cells in agar. Cancer Res 38:3438–3444, 1978
128. Johnson BL, Fisher RI, Bender RA et al: Hexamethylmelamine in alkylating agent resistant ovarian carcinoma. Cancer 42:2157, 1978
129. Bolis G, D'Incalci M, Belloni C et al: Hexamethylmelamine in ovarian cancer resistant to cyclophosphamide and adriamycin. Cancer Treat Rep 63:1375, 1979.
130. Bolis G, D'Incalci M, Gramellini F et al: Adriamycin in ovarian cancer patients resistant to cyclophosphamide. Europ J Cancer 14:1401, 1978
131. Hubbard SM, Barkes P, Young RC: Adriamycin therapy for advanced ovarian carcinoma after chemotherapy. Cancer Treat Rep 62:1375, 1978
132. Young RC, Von Hoff DD, Gormley P et al: Cis-dichlorodiammineplatinum (II) for the treatment of advanced ovarian cancer. Cancer Treat Rep 63:1539–1544, 1979
133. Dedrick RL, Myers CE, Bungay PM et al: Pharmacokinetic rationale for peritoneal drug administration in the treatment of ovarian cancer. Cancer Treat Rep 62:1, 1978
134. Salmon SE, Soehnlen B, Alberts DS: New drugs in ovarian cancer: In vitro Phase II screening with the human tumor stem cell assay. In van Oosterom A, Muggia FM (eds): Therapeutic Progress in Ovarian Cancer, Testicular Cancer and the Sarcomas. The Hague, Martinus Nyhoff Publishers, 1980
135. Neijt JP, Vanlindert ACM, Vendrijk CPJ et al: Hexa-CAF combination chemotherapy and other multiple drug regimens in advanced ovarian carcinoma: Present and future. Neth J Med 22:28, 1979
136. Delgado G, Schein P, MacDonald J et al: L-PAM vs cyclophosphamide, hexamethylmelamine, and 5-fluorouracil (CHF) for advanced ovarian cancer. Proc Am Assoc Cancer Res 20:434, 1979
137. Kardinal CG, Luce JK: Evaluation of a hexamethylmelamine and 5-fluorouracil combination in the treatment of advanced ovarian carcinoma. Cancer Treat Rep 61:1691, 1977
138. Briscoe KE, Pasmantier MW, Ohnuma T et al: Cis-dichlorodiammineplatinum (II) and adriamycin treatment of advanced ovarian cancer. Cancer Treat Rep 62:2027, 1978
139. Bonomi PD, Slayton RE, Wolter J: Phase II trial of adriamycin and cis-dichlorodiammineplatinum (II) in squamous cell, ovarian, and testicular carcinomas. Cancer Treat Rep 62:1211, 1978
140. Alberts DS, Hilgers RD, Moon TE et al: Combination chemotherapy for alkylator-resistant ovarian carcinoma: A preliminary report of a Southwest Oncology Group trial. Cancer Treat Rep 63:301, 1979
141. Kane R, Harvey H, Andrews T et al: Phase II trial of cyclophosphamide hexamethylmelamine, adriamycin, and cis-dichlorodiammineplatinum (II) combination chemotherapy in advanced ovarian carcinoma. Cancer Treat Rep 63:307, 1979
142. Vogl SE, Berenzweig M, Kaplan BH et al: The CHAD and HAD regimens in advanced ovarian cancer: Combination chemotherapy including hexamethylmelamine, adriamycin and cis-dichlorodiammineplatinum (II). Cancer Treat Rep 63:311, 1979
143. Bruckner HW, Ratner LH, Cohen CJ et al: Combination chemotherapy for ovarian carcinoma with cyclophosphamide, adriamycin, and cis-dichlorodiammineplatinum (II) after failure of initial chemotherapy. Cancer Treat Rep 62:1021, 1978
144. Barlow JJ, Piver MS: High-dose methotrexate plus cytoxan in ovarian cancer. Proc Am Assoc Cancer Res 20:361, 1979
145. Bruckner HW, Cohen CJ, Wallach RC et al: Prospective controlled randomized trial comparing combination chemotherapy of advanced ovarian carcinoma with adriamycin and cis-platinum + or − cyclophosphamide and hexamethylmelamine. Proc Am Assoc Cancer Res 20:414, 1979
146. Ehrlich CE, Einhorn L, Williams SD et al: Chemotherapy for

Stage III–IV epithelial ovarian cancer with cis-dichlorodiammineplatinum (II), adriamycin, and cyclophosphamide: A preliminary report. Cancer Treat Rep 63:281–288, 1979
147. Alberts DS, Moon TE, Stephens RA et al: Randomized study of chemotherapy for advanced ovarian carcinoma: A preliminary report of a Southwest Oncology Group study. Cancer Treat Rep 63:325, 1979
148. Mayer RJ, Berkowitz RS, Griffiths CT: Central nervous system involvement by ovarian carcinoma: A complication of prolonged survival with metastatic disease. Cancer 41:776, 1978
149. Reimer RR, Hoover R, Fraumeni JF: Acute leukemia after alkylating agent therapy in ovarian cancer. N Engl J Med 297:117, 1977
150. Stage AH, Grafton WD: Thecomas and granulosa-theca cell tumors of the ovary: An analysis of 51 tumors. Obstet Gynecol 50:21, 1977
151. Diddle AW: Granulosa and thecal-cell ovarian tumors: Prognosis. Cancer 5:215–228, 1952
152. Lusch CJ, Mercurio TM, Runyeon WK: Delayed recurrence and chemotherapy of a granulosa cell tumor. Obstet Gynecol 51:505, 1978
153. DiSaia PJ, Saltz A, Kagan AR et al: A temporary response of recurrent granulosa cell tumors to adriamycin. Obstet Gynecol 52:355, 1978
154. Woodruff JD, Protos P, Peterson WF: Ovarian teratomas. Am J Obstet Gynecol 102:702–715, 1968
155. Jimerson GK, Woodruff JD: Ovarian extraembryoneal teratoma. I. Endodermal sinus tumor. Am J Obstet Gynecol 127:73–79, 1977
156. Cangir A, Smith J, VanEys J: Improved prognosis in children with ovarian cancers following modified FAC (Vincristine sulfate, dactinomycin, and cyclophosphamide) chemotherapy. Cancer 42:1234, 1978
157. Slayton RE, Hreshchyshyn MM, Silverberg SG et al: Treatment of malignant ovarian germ cell tumors: Response to vincristine, dactinomycin, and cyclophosphamide (preliminary report). Cancer 42:390, 1978
158. Gallion H, VanNagell JR, Powell DR et al: Therapy of endodermal sinus tumor of the ovary. Am J Obstet Gynecol 135:447, 1979
159. Curry SL, Smith JP, Gallagher HS: Malignant teratoma of the ovary: prognostic factors and treatment. Am J Obstet Gynecol 131:845, 1978
160. Asadourian LA, Taylor HB: Dysgerminoma. An analysis of 105 cases. Obstet Gynecol 33:370–379, 1969
161. Pedowitz P, Felmus LB, Grayzel PM: Dysgerminoma of the ovary. Am J Obstet Gynecol 70:1284–1297, 1955
162. Brody S: Clinical aspects of dysgerminoma of the ovary. Acta Radiol (Ther) (Stockh) 56:209–230, 1961
163. Krepart G, Smith JP, Rutledge F, Delclos L: The treatment for dysgerminoma of the ovary. Cancer 41:986–990, 1978
164. Cohen SM, Goldsmith MA: Prolonged chemotherapeutic remission of metastatic ovarian dysgerminoma. Report of a case. Gynecol Oncol 5:299, 1977
165. Goldstein DP, Piro AJ: Combination chemotherapy in the treatment of germ cell tumors containing choriocarcinoma in males and females. Surg Gynecol Obstet 134:61–66, 1972
166. Munnel EW: Primary ovarian cancer associated with pregnancy. Clin Obstet Gynecol 6:983–993, 1963
167. Jubb ED: Primary ovarian carcinoma in pregnancy. Am J Obstet Gynecol 85:345–354, 1963
168. Creasman WT, Rutledge F, Smith JP: Carcinoma of the ovary associated with pregnancy. Obstet Gynecol 38:111–116, 1971

Samuel Hellman
Jay R. Harris
George P. Canellos
Bernard Fisher

CHAPTER 27

Cancer of the Breast

EPIDEMIOLOGY

Cancer of the breast accounts for more deaths of American women than any other malignancy. Each year, in the United States, about 100,000 cases are diagnosed and 30,000 deaths are attributed to the disease. About one American woman in 14 will develop breast cancer during her life and this attack rate may be expected to increase.[1]

Rates of incidence of and mortality from breast cancer are approximately five times as high in North America and Northern Europe as they are in many Asian and African countries. Southern European and South American countries have rates intermediate between these extremes. Migrants from Asia (principally Chinese and Japanese) to the United States do not themselves experience much, if any, change in breast cancer risk, but their first and second generation descendants have rates substantially higher than their ancestors that approach those of the U.S. Caucasian population.[2] Rates in U.S. blacks are little different from those of whites.

The principal risk factors for breast cancer include menstrual and reproductive history, family history, and history of benign breast disease. The menstrual factors comprise a cluster of associations which point to an important role for a functioning ovary in the genesis of ovarian cancer. Most clear is the fact that castration, either by surgery or by radiotherapy, reduces substantially a woman's breast cancer risk.[3,4] The reduction is larger the earlier the castration, and oophorectomy prior to 35 years of age is associated with a reduction of risk to one-third of that experienced by women undergoing a natural menopause. In addition, women with early menarche and those with late natural menopause appear to be at increased risk.

The reproductive characteristic most strongly associated with breast cancer risk is the age at which a woman bears her first child. Women who have a first full-term pregnancy under the age of 18 years have only one-third the breast cancer risk of those whose first child is delayed until age 30 years. Women who bear their first child after age 30 years actually have slightly higher risk than do those who remain nulliparous.[5] In most studies no additional protective effect is seen associated with pregnancies after the first, but, since the earlier a woman has her first child, the higher her total parity is likely to be, there is an overall inverse association between risk and total parity. However, in a few studies, there does appear to be a protective effect of total parity additional to that associated with early first birth.[6]

Women who have a first-degree relative with breast cancer have a risk two or three times that of the general population. There are occasional families in which the risk appears to be substantially higher than this, and in such families the disease is often bilateral and premenopausal in onset.[7]

A history of benign breast disease is associated with a risk of breast cancer approximately four times that of women without such a history and this increase in risk appears to last at least 30 years after the diagnosis of benign disease.[8]

To date, no hypothesis has yet been established as a likely explanation of these associations. It seems likely that some as yet unidentified endocrine profile is associated with increased risk and it may well be that dietary fat plays a role, possibly by altering hormonal profiles. In particular it seems most likely that strong or prolonged estrogen stimulus is associated with increased risk, but the determinants and mechanism of action of such stimulus are poorly understood.[1,2]

There are two known exogenous causes of breast cancer—ionizing radiation and exogenous estrogens used for the relief of menopausal symptoms. Increased risk associated with exposure to relatively large (100 rad and greater) doses of ionizing radiation has been demonstrated in survivors of the atomic bombings of Hiroshima and Nagasaki, women having multiple fluoroscopies in the course of pneumothorax treatment of tuberculosis and women treated with radiotherapy for mastitis.[9–11] The effect of the much smaller, fragmented doses used in diagnostic radiology, particularly mammography, is controversial and will be discussed in the section on screening as related to the risk of mammography.

Data are accumulating to the effect that long-term treatment with estrogens for symptoms of the menopause increases the risk of breast cancer. Among women with intact ovaries, treated with a total estrogen accumulation in excess of 1500 mg, the risk is 2.5 times the risk of women not treated.[12] It is of considerable theoretical, as well as practical, importance that no increase in breast cancer risk has yet been observed in women taking the estrogen–progesterone combinations commonly prescribed for contraception.[13]

A considerable controversy surrounds the question of whether the use of reserpine for control of hypertension increases breast cancer risk. Reviewing the evidence in 1979, Kelsey concluded that the evidence for such an association was not strong.[1] However, there has been a subsequent report showing a positive association with long-term usage of reserpine and a negative association with short-term use.[14] The matter should probably be considered still open.

Association of use of hair dyes with breast cancer risk has been investigated since the demonstration of many ingredients that are mutagenic. Little support for the presence of an association has been found.[15,16]

The relationship of diet to tumor incidence has been suggested by increasing tumor incidence in countries with dietary patterns becoming more westernized and from incidence rates correlated with dietary factors in a number of countries. Although the total dietary fat has been most often suggested as the relative importance of etiological significances of other factors and some inconsistent studies make the importance of diet uncertain at this time.[17]

Histopathologic examination of breast cancer makes available information which (a) establishes the diagnosis of the lesion, (b) aids in determining patient prognosis and (c) leads to a better understanding of the biology of the disease. This section presents a general overview of the subject with emphasis on recent contributions which have enhanced our understanding of the nature of this tumor or which have raised important questions which require resolution. For a more in-depth analysis of the subject the reader is referred to a syllabus and other publications regarding breast cancer pathology obtained from findings of the National Surgical Adjuvant Breast Project (NSABP).[18]

CLASSIFICATION OF TUMOR TYPES

A number of pathologic classifications of mammary carcinomas are in current use. They are frequently confusing. If it is appreciated that morphologic studies are based upon anatomic or structural units present in an organ, and that in the female breast those units consist of large-, medium-, and small-sized ducts from which arise a variety of tumor types, a better understanding of breast tumor pathology may result. Only during pregnancy are acinar units present.

Tumors arising from duct epithelium may be found only within the lumen of the ducts of origin—that is, the carcinomas are intraductal and do not invade surrounding stroma. Most frequently, such tumors arise from large ducts, and they may present as several types. If they grow into the ducts with a papillary configuration, they are recognized as *papillary carcinomas*. Such lesions are rare, comprising about 1% of breast cancers. Pleomorphic duct epithelial cells with disturbed polarity can be demonstrated histologically, as can be their heaping up into papillae. The basement membrane is intact. Considerable difficulty may be encountered in differentiating a papillary carcinoma from benign atypical papillomatosis.

Papillary carcinomas rarely become infiltrating—that is, rarely do they invade the surrounding stroma. A survival rate approaching 100% may be anticipated with complete excision. When such tumors do invade surrounding tissue, they grow rather slowly and attain considerable bulk. Skin and fascial attachments are unusual, and axillary node involvement is a late feature. Clinically non-invasive tumors are found to be movable, circumscribed lesions that have a soft consistency not unlike that of fibroadenomas. The 5-year survival rate of patients with such tumors is better than average.

Infiltrating duct carcinomas, in which no special type of histologic structure is recognized are designated NOS (not otherwise specified) and are by far the most common duct tumors, accounting for almost 70% of breast cancers. They are clinically characterized by their stony hardness to palpation. When transected, a gritty resistance is encountered and the tumor retracts below the cut surface. Yellowish, chalky streaks that represent necrotic foci are observed. Histologically, varying degrees of fibrotic response are present. As a rule they do not reach large size. They frequently metastasize to axillary lymph nodes, and their prognosis is the poorest of the various tumor types.

There are several other types of invasive carcinomas that arise from large ducts, each having its own distinct histopathologic picture. The *medullary carcinoma,* comprising 5% to 7% of all mammary carcinomas, is a circumscribed lesion that attains large dimensions and demonstrates low-grade, infiltrative properties. This tumor is characterized by an extensive infiltration of the tumor by small lymphocytes. The 5-year survival rate following removal of such a tumor is better than average. A tumor in which tubule formation is evident is known as *tubular carcinoma*. This tumor has a high nuclear grade with some polarity of its cells. Its prognosis, while regarded as better than infiltrating duct cancers is less favorable than that of medullary carcinoma, despite the fact that the cells of the latter tumor are more poorly differentiated than are those of tubular carcinoma. Another tumor type, the *mucinous,* or *colloid carcinoma,* comprises about 3% of all mammary carcinomas. This ductal carcinoma is characterized on microscopy by its nests and strands of epithelial cells floating in a mucinous matrix. It is usually slow-growing and can reach bulky proportions. When the tumor is predominantly mucinous, the prognosis tends to be good.

One type of tumor that has been attracting considerable attention in recent years is the *lobular carcinoma,* which arises from the small end-ducts of the breast. The non-invasive variety, the so-called lobular carcinoma-*in-situ,* is characterized by clusters of anaplastic small cells of high nuclear grade that lie within lobules. When this lesion extends beyond the boundary of the lobule or terminal duct from which it arises, it is known as *invasive lobular carcinoma* and may be indistinguishable from the conventional infiltrating duct carcinoma. The true incidence of lobular carcinomas is uncertain. It has been emphasized that *all* non-invasive mammary carcinomas comprise almost 5% of all neoplastic lesions of the female breast, and that lobular carcinoma-*in-situ* accounts for about 50% of these, or 2.5% to 2.8% of all tumors. Lobular carcinoma-*in-situ* will be discussed separately later in this chapter.

TABLE 27-1. Incidence of Histologic Types of Breast Cancer

	PERCENT
Pure tumor groups	
Infiltrating duct NOS (not otherwise specified)	52.6
Medullary	6.2
Lobular invasive	4.9
Mucinous	2.4
Tubular	1.2
Adenocystic	0.4
Papillary	0.3
Carcinosarcoma	0.1
Paget's disease	2.3
With intraductal carcinoma	0.2
Infiltrating duct NOS	1.6
Infiltrating duct NOS + tubular	0.4
Infiltrating duct NOS + mucinous	0.1
Combinations with infiltrating duct NOS	28.0
Infiltrating duct NOS:	
+ Tubular	16.5
+ Lobular invasive	3.3
+ Mucinous	1.6
+ Lobular invasive + tubular	1.6
+ Papillary	1.2
+ Adenocystic	1.0
+ Tubular + adenocystic	0.8
+ Tubular + papillary	0.8
+ Mucinous + papillary	0.4
+ Adenocystic + mucinous	0.2
+ Lobular invasive + adenocystic	0.1
+ Lobular invasive + mucinous	0.1
+ Lobular invasive + papillary	0.1
+ Tubular + mucinous	0.1
+ Adenocystic + papillary	0.1
+ Lobular invasive + tubular + adenocystic + mucinous	0.1
Other combinations of tumor types exclusive of NOS	1.6
Tubular + papillary	0.5
Lobular invasive + tubular	0.4
Tubular + mucinous	0.2
Lobular invasive + mucinous	0.1
Tubular + adenocystic	0.1
Adenocystic + mucinous	0.1
Mucinous + papillary	0.1
Lobular invasive + tubular + adenocystic + papillary	0.1
TOTAL	100.0

Two entities represent special manifestations of mammary carcinomas. *Paget's disease* of the breast occurs in 1% to 4% of all patients with breast cancer. Clinically, the patient presents with a relatively long history of eczematoid changes in the nipple with itching, burning, oozing, or bleeding or some combination of these. The nipple changes are associated with an underlying carcinoma in the breast that can be palpated in about two-thirds of the patients. The subadjacent tumor may be either intraductal or of the invasive duct type. Prognosis is related to the histologic type of the associated tumor. Histologically, the nipple epithelium contains nests of tumor cells. *Inflammatory breast cancer* is characterized clinically by skin redness and warmth, a visible erysipeloid margin and induration of the underlying breast. These criteria in the past were sufficient for the diagnosis. Currently, this must include pathologic corroboration. Biopsies of the erythematous areas, as well as adjacent normal-appearing skin, reveal undifferentiated cancer cells in the subdermal lymphatics causing an obstructive lymphangitis. Inflammatory cells are rarely present. Most patients have signs of advanced cancer, including palpable axillary nodes, supraclavicular nodes, and distant metastases.

There are several other histologic types of mammary carcinoma which have been described but are rarely encountered. Fewer than 100 cases of adenocystic carcinoma have been reported. Because of the small number of cases, no meaningful association with prognosis is available. Carcinosarcomas, pure squamous cell carcinomas, metaplastic carcinomas (carcinoma with osseous or cartilaginous stroma), basal cell carcinomas, and so-called lipid-rich carcinomas have been observed. Again, because of their rarity, clinical correlates are practically non-existent.

The incidence of histologic types of breast cancer in 1000 cases entered into NSABP Protocol B-04 is presented in Table 27-1. More than half (52.6%) are pure infiltrating duct lesions (NOS).

TUMOR CHARACTERISTICS

Attention has been directed to the possible relationship between the behavior of malignant neoplasms and their degree of "anaplasia." Mammary carcinomas have been graded into three *histologic grades* of malignancy, depending upon the degree of tubular formation, size of cells, size of nuclei, and degree of hyperchromatism and number of mitoses. Tumors of low-grade malignancy have been designated as Grade 1 and a high degree of malignancy Grade 3. In the NSABP analysis, 69.6% of tumors were designated as histologic Grade 3; only 2.3% were well-differentiated enough to be classified Grade 1.

Nuclei of tumor cells have been characterized according to their differentiation into three *nuclear grades.* Contrary to conventional methods of grading, Grade 1 represents the most anaplastic nuclear appearance, and Grade 3 the most well differentiated. Black and associates have reported that there exists a relationship between nuclear grade of tumor, sinus histiocytosis of axillary lymph nodes and patient survival.[19-22] In the 1000 NSABP cases only 8.5% exhibited well-differentiated nuclei (Grade 3) and about one-third were considered to be poorly differentiated.

Tumor necrosis of varying degrees was encountered in 60% of 1539 patients with invasive breast cancer in NSABP Protocol B-04. Necrosis, particularly when observed to be of marked degree and of the noncomedo type or a combination of the latter with the comedo form, was positively correlated with increased rates of treatment failure, which were confirmed by life table analyses. Although necrosis was observed to be significantly associated with a number of clinical and histopathologic features purportedly related to an ominous prognosis in this disease, it was not correlated with pathologic nodal status, and multivariate analysis revealed it to influence treatment failure independently of tumor size in those lesions measuring less than 5 cm in greatest diameter. Extrapolation of the data fails to reveal any consistent information that might relate tumor necrosis to tumor growth *per se* in accounting for such a role. Although considerations suggest that this alteration might be a reflection of "dedifferentiation," it appears also to exert its effect independently of the latter, at least in tumors of the highest or most malignant grade.

Mammary carcinomas may be described relative to their *circumscription*. They generally assume either a circumscribed or more infiltrative irregular or stellate configuration. A better prognosis has been ascribed to the former tumor type.

Much significance has been attached to *cell reaction* occurring within a tumor. Such a finding has been ascribed to a host response to the tumor and has been considered to be a favorable prognostic sign. Twenty-four percent of the 1000 NSABP patients had an absence of cell reaction to their tumor, 59% had slight or moderate infiltration, and 17% an intensive reaction. No association with sinus histiocytosis of lymph nodes was observed, as has been suggested.[19-22] The reaction seems to be more closely related to those features indicating the degree of malignancy of the cancer than to a host response, that is, large tumors, blood vessel invasion, and high histologic grade (Grade III).

One-third of the tumors from NSABP patients exhibited *lymphatic* invasion and another 23% were considered questionable. Such a finding was associated with other unfavorable characteristics and was associated with short-term treatment failures. Blood vessel invasion was observed in only 5% of patients and was associated with the finding of four or more positive axillary nodes, lymphatic invasion, and certain other undesirable findings.

Of 36 pathologic and six clinical features evaluated for patients according to their nodal status, only a few were found to relate to treatment failure at 5 years (Table 27-2).[23] Prognosis was worse in individuals whose tumors exhibited all of the undesirable characteristics than in those in whom one or two could be detected. Histologic grade represents a more refined factor of discrimination than nuclear grade alone.[24]

Many, if not all, breast cancers may display *multicentricity*. While several investigators have addressed themselves to this,

TABLE 27-2. Characteristics Related to 5 Year Treatment Failure (from Life Tables)

Absent Nodal Metastases	
Nodal germinal center predominance	($p = .005$)
Tumor necrosis	($p = .03$)
Histologic grade	($p = .05$)
Tumor size (> 4 cm *vs.* ≤ 2 cm)	($p = .04$)
1–3 Positive Nodes	
None with significance	
4 + Positive Nodes	
Tumor necrosis	($p = .002$)
Tumor size (> 4 cm *vs.* ≤ 2 cm)	($p = .005$)
NOS pure type	($p = .04$)
Histologic grade	*

*Trend with multivariate significance

it is difficult to be certain how many multicentric, independent cancers might have been present, since no clear distinction as to actual site or pathologic type of lesion encountered was provided. In examination of 904 NSABP cases, except in those instances in which it was beneath the nipple or in the tail of the breast, data were collected only from quadrants in which the primary was not encountered. This avoided the difficulty in distinguishing a new focus of carcinoma in the quadrant of the primary from an integral part of the primary lesion. Either invasive or non-invasive cancers regarded as independent cancers were found in 13.4% of the 904 patients. The probability of detecting such lesions increased with the number of quadrants available for examination rather than with the study of any particular quadrant. The incidence of invasive and non-invasive cancers encountered were the intraductal (66.7%), lobular carcinoma-*in-situ* (22.6%), and a combination of both (10.7%). All of the invasive forms were of the infiltrating duct NOS type. While the multicentricity of breast cancer is a reality, the clinical significance of such an observation remains enigmatic. The impetus for resolving this enigma comes from the consideration that segmental resections of the breast with or without radiation might be equally as effective in terms of curability, and cosmetically more acceptable than a more radical procedure. One of the major deterrents to accepting such a limited resection is the realization that such an excision may ignore clinically and pathologically undetected *de novo* cancers at sites within the breast remote from the dominant mass.

Similarly, there has appeared evidence to indicate that the incidence of cancer in the contralateral breast may be *much* greater than previously supposed.[25,26] An overall detection rate of 15% in contralateral breasts biopsied has been reported. Despite the significant incidence of multifocal lesions in both breasts of a woman with a primary breast cancer, however, two or more clinically overt primary cancers in the primary breast are extremely rare. Similarly, synchronous bilateral tumors are uncommon and the incidence of a second asynchronous primary tumor in the uninvolved or opposite breast fails to approach the incidence of occult lesions detected by random biopsy or autopsy.[27] It has been noted, for example, that the incidence of clinically latent intraductal carcinomas in breasts of women over the age of 70 years who died from causes other than mammary carcinoma is 19 times greater than the reported incidence of clinical breast cancer.[28] Such findings strongly suggest that all cancers do not progress to overt lesions or may even undergo regression. These conclusions are similar to and gain support from neuroblastomas of the adrenal in children, thyroid carcinomas, and carcinomas of the prostate which are found pathologically more frequently in randomly examined material than clinically in comparable populations.

Lymph Nodes

Attention has been directed to the occurrence and significance of sinus histiocytosis in axillary nodes draining mammary cancers. There has been observed a more or less direct relationship between the intensity of the nodal response and survival.[19-22,29] The reaction has been considered by some to represent a manifestation of the host response to tumor growth. Others have failed to find any correlation between sinus histiocytosis and survival in breast cancer.[30,31] Reported NSABP data have indicated that sinus histiocytosis was consistently found in nodes that were clinically positive but found not to contain tumor pathologically. When sinus histiocytosis was absent there was a greater likelihood that four or more nodes contained metastases. A relationship between the absence of sinus histiocytosis and short-term treatment failure was also noted at the 12-month interval of follow-up observation.

Nonepithelial Neoplasms of the Breast

A variety of nonepithelial neoplasms of the breast have been described. Various types of sarcomas predominate. Fibrosarcomas, leiomyosarcomas, rhabdomyosarcomas, and angiosarcomas are extremely infrequent. They are ominous and usually result in rapid death as a result of widespread dissemination. Liposarcomas originating in the breast also occur rarely. Their prognosis is perhaps more favorable, although the number of cases is too few to be certain. Lymphomas have had their initial onset in breast as well as occurring as a focus of generalized disease. Hodgkin's disease and leukemia have occurred with initial manifestation in the breast. Some have been mistaken for inflammatory carcinoma.

Cystosarcoma phylloides is partially an epithelial and partially a non-epithelial tumor. As Haagensen has pointed out cystosarcoma phylloides "is a tumor of the breast with frightening clinical and microscopic characteristics which have given it prominence beyond its due. For it is in fact not only common but usually benign."[32] Such tumors are fibro-epithelial in character and are often derived from fibro-adenomas. They may achieve a great size and not infrequently demonstrate some invasion of adjacent breast tissue. They are best handled by local excision with a rim of breast tissue. Cystosarcoma phylliodes has been known to metastasize and to kill. Unfortunately, it is difficult to determine from clinical or histologic appearance which tumors will metastasize and behave in malignant fashion.

TABLE 27-3. 5-Year Relapse Rate According to the Location of the Primary and Nodal Status (NSABP)

LOCATION	NEGATIVE NODES	POSITIVE NODES
UOQ	17% (208)	63% (239)
UIQ	25% (75)	59% (37)
LIQ	22% (23)	55% (22)
LOQ	26% (46)	70% (44)

Numbers in parenthesis indicate the number of patients in each subgroup.

Pathologic Characteristics and Estrogen Receptor

Estrogen receptor (ER) status was correlated with a large number of pathological and clinical characteristics of invasive breast cancers in patients in NSABP Protocol B-04. Positive ER was found to be significantly associated with high nuclear and low histologic grades, absence of tumor necrosis, presence of marked tumor elastosis, and older patients. These pathologic parameters enumerated are either directly or indirectly related to tumor differentiation suggesting that ER represents another index of this characteristic. Multivariate analyses disclosed that both age and tumor differentiation are associated with the ER status. Well-differentiated tumors were more frequently ER+ in older women. Inclusion of an estimate of tumor necrosis, as well as patient age, appears to allow for further discrimination of ER status in poorly differentiated lesions.

LOCAL SPREAD OF BREAST CANCER

The primary site of breast cancer is commonly described by its location by quadrant in the breast. In one series of 696 cases 48% were located in the upper outer quadrant, 15% in the upper inner quadrant, 11% in the lower outer quadrant, 6% in the lower inner quadrant, and 17% in the central region (designated as within 1 cm of the areola).[33] An additional 3% were termed diffuse because of multifocal origin or massive involvement of the entire breast. The reason for the increased frequency of breast cancer in the upper outer quadrant is felt to be simply related to the greater amount of breast tissue in that quadrant. In this series of patients, no differences in survival based on quadrant location were noted. The relationship between the location of the breast primary and prognosis was also examined in another large series from the National Surgical Adjuvant Breast Project (NSABP). Even when the location of breast primary was considered relapse and ultimate survival was decided by the pathological status of axillary nodes, no significant differences in prognosis due to primary location were noted (Table 27-3).[34]

The size of the breast mass is an important prognostic factor. This will be discussed below in an attempt to separate its influence from that of lymph node involvement.

The spread of cancer through the breast has been summarized by Haagensen.[35] This spread occurs by:

1. direct infiltration into the breast parenchyma;
2. along mammary ducts;
3. by breast lymphatics.

Direct infiltration of the cancer tends to occur by ramifying projections which give a characteristic stellate appearance on gross examination. If untreated, direct involvement of overlying skin or deep pectoral fascia is commonly seen. Involvement along ducts is frequently observed and may include wide segments of the breast. It is unclear, however, whether this intraductal involvement represents true spread of a primary cancer along previously uninvolved ducts or a field cancerization which results in simultaneous transformation along entire lengths of ducts. It is likely that both processes may occur. Spread can also occur by the extensive network of breast lymphatics. Investigators have emphasized lymphatic spread vertically down to the lymphatic plexus in the deep pectoral fascia underlying the breast. In addition, spread to the central subareolar region has been described. These multiple mechanisms of spread through the breast stress the likelihood for cancer to be present in the breast, well beyond the palpable primary mass.

REGIONAL SPREAD

The most commonly involved routes of spread of breast cancer to regional lymph nodes are to the axillary, internal mammary, and supraclavicular lymph node regions. A knowledge of the likelihood of spread to these areas and their significance is critical to planning treatment for patients with breast cancer.

Axillary Node Involvement

The axillary lymph node region is the major regional drainage for carcinoma of the breast. Approximately 40% to 50% of patients with breast cancer have the cancer spread to axillary nodes. The likelihood of axillary nodal involvement is directly related to the size of the primary as shown in Fig. 27-1. The evidence that the location of the primary in the breast influences the likelihood of axillary lymph node involvement is not clear-cut. Most data, however, tend to support the observation that axillary node positivity is not significantly related to the location of the primary in the breast.

To some extent, the incidence of histological involvement of axillary nodes is dependent on the type of surgery performed and the extent of the pathological analysis of the axillary specimen.

Radical mastectomy allows for the most complete dissection of the axillary contents and yields the greatest number of axillary nodes. Lesser surgical procedures, such as the modified radical mastectomy, give a less complete axillary dissection and fewer axillary nodes. As a result of this variable extent of axillary dissection, the likelihood of histologic involvement must be viewed in terms of the surgical procedure performed. In one pathological study of axillary specimens, it was noted that axillary node involvement would have been reduced by 29% if the axillary dissection was extended only to the lower border of the pectoralis minor muscle.[36] The incidence of histologic involvement is also related to the degree of pathological analysis. Pickren was the first to show that a more thorough clearing and sectioning of the axillary specimen resulted in a greater yield of histologic involvement.[37] Of 51 specimens routinely analyzed and found to be negative 11 (22%) showed evidence of involvement on more careful analysis.

Another NSABP report was directed toward determining whether discovery and examination of more nodes in a resected specimen are more meaningful in terms of prognosis than if only a few are recovered.[38] The recurrence and survival rates of more than 2000 patients with breast carcinoma from 46 institutions have been correlated with the number of lymph nodes obtained and examined in surgical specimens. In all institutions, the range of the number of nodes examined per specimen was remarkably great, the median number varying from a low of seven at one to a high of 28 at another. It was suggested that the great range in the number of nodes per specimen is related to a combination of anatomic differences, errors in identification of all nodes by the pathologist, and possible variation in the extent of surgical dissection. A comparison of methods used for identification of nodes in resected specimens failed to reveal a correlation between the number of nodes found and the technique employed to find them.

The results obtained failed to demonstrate that the discovery and examination of a greater number of nodes in a specimen were more meaningful in determining prognosis than if only a few recovered. It was observed that patients having five or ten nodes reported as negative had essentially the same

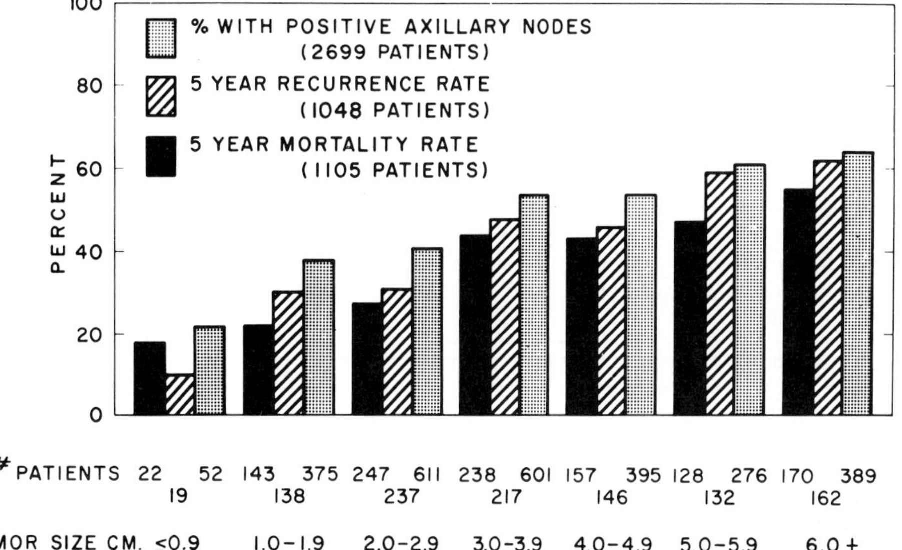

FIG. 27-1. The relationship of tumor size to axillary node involvement, recurrence, and mortality rates. (Fisher B, Slack NH, Borss ID, et al: Cancer of the breast: size of neoplasm and prognosis. Cancer 24:1071–1080, 1969)

TABLE 27-4. Accuracy of Physical Examination in Predicting Histological Involvement of Axillary Nodes

	BUTCHER	HAAGENSON	SCHOOTENFELD	BUCALOSSI
FALSE POSITIVE	25%	24%	26%	29%
FALSE NEGATIVE	32%	32%	27%	29%

recurrence and survival rates as did those with 25 to 30 nodes free of tumor. Likewise, whether specimens from patients with positive nodes contained from one to five, or more than 30, nodes, recurrence and survival rates were similar. The patient with two positive nodes out of five examined was not found to be at greater risk than another having two with tumor out of 30 recovered. In both studies, no association was found between the presence of this occult axillary involvement and a worse prognosis; patients with occult involvement had the same survival as patients without involvement.

Detection of axillary involvement by physical examination has both a high false positive and false negative rate (Table 27-4). When axillary lymph nodes are palpable, histologic evidence of metastatic disease is not found in approximately 25% of cases. One recent series, however, has a 92% correlation of pathological findings and clinical evaluation when the nodes are thought to contain tumor.[39] Conversely, when axillary nodes are not palpable, histological involvement is detected in approximately 30% of cases. These figures indicate the shortcomings of clinical evaluation in predicting histological involvement. These results are of particular importance, since histological involvement of axillary nodes has a high correlation with prognosis. Table 27-5 shows 10-year survival figures related to axillary involvement from six separate series of patients treated by radical mastectomy. Patients with histologically negative axillary nodes have markedly improved survival compared to patients with histological involvement. Furthermore, patients with from one to three positive nodes do better than patients with four or more positive nodes. At the current level of understanding, the presence of spread to the axilla represents the single most important prognostic factor for patients with breast cancer.

For purposes of analysis, the axilla is commonly divided into three levels: (1) proximal—tissue inferior to the lower border of the pectoralis minor muscle; (2) middle—tissue directly beneath the pectoralis minor; and (3) distal—tissue superior to the pectoralis minor. Prognosis has been shown to be related to the level of axillary involvement (Table 27-6). Involvement of upper level nodes carries a worse prognosis than involvement of proximal level nodes alone. In a study of 182 mastectomy specimens examined by clearing, involvement of nodes at the apex of the axilla was found in 15.[49] All 15 patients suffered relapse, indicating the grave prognosis associated with involvement high in the axilla. In this group of 15 patients, the mean number of involved nodes was 16.2 (range, 4–37). In general, involvement of upper level nodes is commonly associated with high total numbers of lymph nodes involved. In another study, axillary node involvement and survival were examined in 385 patients to determine whether the total number of involved nodes or the level of axillary node involvement was a better indicator of prognosis.[36] They found that for any given number of involved nodes, survival was independent of the level of involvement and concluded that prognosis was more directly related to the total number of nodes involved and not the level of involvement.

Prognosis has been shown to be related to both the size of the primary and to axillary node involvement. The question whether or not these two factors independently predict for prognosis is addressed in Table 27-7. When axillary nodes are involved, the size of the primary is still of prognostic value. For example, in the data from Valagussa and colleagues the 5-year relapse rate was 37% for patients with positive nodes and small (0 cm–2 cm) primaries, and 79% for patients with positive nodes and large (greater than 5 cm) primaries.[44] In the data by Fisher and co-workers this relationship was further analyzed by the number of positive axillary nodes (1–3 or 4 more).[50] Within each subgroup of axillary nodes positive the size of the primary was still an independent prognostic factor. When axillary nodes are negative, the relationship is less clear-cut. The prognosis for patients with small (0 cm–2 cm) primaries and negative nodes is exceptionally good, with a 5-year relapse rate of approximately 10%. For primaries larger than 2 cm, the prognosis is not as good as for these

TABLE 27-5. Prognosis Related to Histologic Involvement of Axillary Lymph Nodes for Patients Treated by Radical Mastectomy

	VALAGUSSA (10-YEAR DISEASE-FREE SURVIVAL)	HAAGENSEN (10-YEAR SURVIVAL)	SCHOTTENFELD* (10-YEAR SURVIVAL)	FISHER (10-YEAR DISEASE-FREE SURVIVAL)	SPRATT AND DONEGAN (10-YEAR SURVIVAL)	PAYNE* (10-YEAR ACTUAL SURVIVAL)
HISTOLOGICALLY NEGATIVE	72%	76%	72%	76%	68%	76%
HISTOLOGICALLY POSITIVE	25%	48%	43%	24%	27%	35%
1–3 NODES POSITIVE	34%	63%	–	36%	–	–
≥ 4 NODES POSITIVE	16%	27%	–	14%	–	–

*Significant number of patients received post operative irradiation.

TABLE 27-6. 10 Year Survival (%) Related to Primary Size and Level of Axillary Involvement

AXILLARY STATUS	<2 cm	2–5 cm	>5 cm	TOTAL
Negative	82%	65%	44%	72%
Positive, Proximal Only	73%	74%	39%	65%
Positive, Middle or Distal	*	28%	37%	31%
Positive, All	68%	51%	37%	

*Insufficient data
(Schottenfeld D, Nash AG, Robbins GF et al: Ten-year results of the treatment of primary operable breast carcinoma. Cancer 38:1001–1007, 1976)

smaller primaries. Of note, however, is that the prognosis for patients with large (greater than 5 cm) primaries and negative nodes is not significantly worse than patients with 2 cm to 5 cm primaries and negative nodes. These data imply that axillary sampling is of value for prognostic purposes in patients with large primaries, since those patients with histologically negative axillary nodes do relatively well without further therapy. The 30 year results from Adair support these observations: for negative node patients the 30-year survival rate was 61% when the primary was 0 cm to 2 cm, 46% for 2 cm to 5 cm primaries, and 50% for primaries greater than 5 cm.[52] For patients with involvement of level I axillary nodes, the 30-year survival rate was 40% when the primary was 0 cm to 2 cm, 31% for 2 cm to 5 cm primaries, and 14% for primaries greater than 5 cm.

In summary, the axillary nodal region is the major drainage site for carcinoma of the breast, and a histological analysis of the axilla provides a useful guide for prognosis. The more practical issue of what, if any, treatment is required to the axillary region will be addressed in later sections.

Internal Mammary Node Involvement

The second major drainage area for carcinoma of the breast is to the internal mammary lymph node (IMN) chain. This chain lies at the anterior ends of the intercostal spaces by the side of the internal thoracic artery. Because of their intrathoracic location and their uncommon clinical presentation, the frequency of internal mammary node involvement was not appreciated as early as axillary node involvement. One of the first to document this second route of spread was Sampson Handley, who reported his results of internal mammary node biopsy in 1000 patients in 1975 (Table 27-8).[53] These results illustrate the following two points.

TABLE 27-7. 5-Year Relapse Rate According to the Size of Primary and Axillary Node Involvement

	SIZE OF PRIMARY		
	<2 cm	*2–5 cm*	*5 cm*
AXILLARY NODES NEGATIVE			
Fisher et al	12%	24%	27%
Nemoto et al	13%	19%	25%
Valgussa et al	8%	24%	19%
AXILLARY NODES POSITIVE			
Fisher et al	50%	60%	79%
Nemoto et al	39%	50%	65%
Valagussa et al	37%	64%	74%

TABLE 27-8. Internal Mammary Node Involvement Related to Location of Primary and Axillary Node Involvement

% IM INVOLVEMENT	UIQ	LIQ	CENTRAL	UOQ	LOQ
Total	27% 67/248	33% 20/61	32% 70/216	14% 54/382	13% 12/93
Axilla Not Involved	14% 20/143	6% 2/36	7% 5/76	4% 7/170	5% 2/40
Axilla Involved	45% 47/105	72% 18/25	46% 65/140	22% 47/212	19% 10/53

(Handley RS: Carcinoma of the breast. Ann Roy Coll Surg 57:59–66, 1975)

1. internal mammary node involvement is more common for inner quadrant of central primaries than for outer quadrant primaries, and
2. axillary lymph node involvement is more likely than IMN involvement.

Even in patients with inner or central primaries, axillary involvement was more common than IMN involvement (42% *versus* 28%). Furthermore, if axillary nodes are uninvolved, IMN involvement is uncommon (8%). Another large series of patients reported from Italy has confirmed the Handley results.[54] In addition, the authors stressed the importance of primary size in relation to IMN involvement. Of primaries measuring less than 5 cm, IMN involvement was seen in 19%, compared to 37% for primaries greater than 5 cm.

Supraclavicular Lymph Node Involvement

The major route of spread to the supraclavicular lymph node areas is through the axillary lymph node chain. In one series of patients undergoing routine supraclavicular dissection, involvement of the supraclavicular region was found in 23 of 125 patients (18%) who had involvement of axillary nodes, and in 0 of 149 patients (0%) who did not have involvement of axillary nodes.[55] The significance of supraclavicular node involvement was first shown by Halsted, who performed a supraclavicular dissection in 119 patients. Forty-four of these were found to have involvement of these nodes and only two were free of cancer at 5 years.[56] Supraclavicular node involvement represents a late stage of axillary nodal involvement and carries a grave prognosis.

Intercostal Lymph Involvement

Another area of potential lymph node involvement from carcinoma of the breast is the regional intercostal lymph nodes. The likelihood of involvement of these nodes has not been established in patients with operable breast cancer. It is generally assumed, however, that this involvement is uncommon except in advanced or recurrent cases.

TABLE 27-9. Sites of Metastases From Breast Cancer in Three Collected Series

	160 CASES	43 CASES	100 CASES
Organ	59%	65%	69%
Liver	58%	56%	65%
Bone	44%	–	71%
Pleura	37%	23%	51%
Adrenals	31%	41%	49%
Kidneys	not recorded	14%	17%
Spleen	14%	23%	17%
Pancreases	–	11%	17%
Ovaries	9%	16%	20%
Brain	–	9%	22%
Thyroid	–	–	24%
Heart	–	–	11%
Diaphragm	–	–	11%
Pericardium	5%	21%	19%
Intestine	–	–	18%
Peritoneum	12%	9%	13%
Uterus	–	–	15%
Lymph Nodes	72%	–	76%
Skin	34%	7%	30%
REFERENCE NUMBER	(57)	(58)	(59)

Distant Metastases

Metastatic spread from carcinoma of the breast can be present in a variety of organs. The likelihood of organ involvement has been studied in a number of autopsy series (Table 27-9).

STAGING

Staging refers to the grouping of patients by the extent of their disease. It is useful in determining the choice of treatment for individual patients, estimating their prognosis and comparing the results of different treatment programs. Staging of breast cancer is initially performed on a clinical basis; that is, based on the physical examination as well as laboratory and radiologic evaluation.

The most widely used clinical staging system is the one adopted by both the UICC (International Union against Cancer) and the AJC (American Joint Commission in Cancer Staging and End Results Reporting). It is based on the TNM system (T, tumor; N, nodes; M, metastases) and is given below:

T Primary tumors
T1 Tumor 2 cm or less in its greatest dimension
- a. No fixation to underlying pectoral fascia or muscle
- b. Fixation to underlying pectoral fascia or muscle

T2 Tumor more than 2 cm but not more than 5 cm in its greatest dimension
T3 Tumor more than 5 cm in its greatest dimension
- a. No fixation to underlying pectoral fascia or muscle
- b. Fixation to underlying pectoral fascia or muscle

T4 Tumor of any size with direct extension to chest wall or skin
Note: Chest wall includes ribs, intercostal muscles, and serratus anterior muscle, but not pectoral muscle
- a. Fixation to chest wall
- b. Edema (including peau d'orange) ulceration of the skin of the breast, or satellite skin nodules confined to the same breast
- c. Both of above
- d. Inflammatory carcinoma

Dimpling of the skin, nipple retraction, or any other skin changes except those in T4b may occur in T1, T2, or T3 without affecting the classification.

N Regional lymph nodes
N0 No palpable homolateral axillary nodes
N1 Movable homolateral axillary nodes
- a. Nodes not considered to contain growth
- b. Nodes considered to contain growth

N2 Homolateral axillary nodes containing growth and fixed to one another or to other structures

N3 Homolateral supraclavicular or infraclavicular nodes containing growth or edema of the arm
M Distant metastasis
M0 No evidence of distant metastasis
M1 Distant metastasis present, including skin involvement beyond the breast area

Clinical Stage-Grouping

Stage I	T1a	N0 or N1a	
	T1b	N0 or N1a	M0
Stage II	T0	N1b	
	T1a	N1b	
	T1b	N1b	M0
	T2a or T2b	N0, N1a, or N1b	
Stage III	T1a or T1b	N2	M0
	T2a or T2b	N2	M0
	T3a or T3b	N0, N1 or N2	M0
Stage IV	T4	any N	any M
	any T	N3	any M
	any T	any N	M1

Another clinical staging system, the Columbia Clinical Classification, is at present less widely used, but is of historical importance. Like the UICC–AJC system, patients are grouped by the extent of disease in the primary tumor site, nodal areas, and distant metastases. The Columbia Clinical Classification (CCC) is given below:

Stage A: No skin edema, ulceration, or solid fixation of the tumor to the chest wall. Axillary nodes not clinically involved

Stage B: No skin edema, ulceration, or solid fixation of the tumor to the chest wall. Clinically involved nodes, but less than 2.5 cm in transverse diameter and not fixed to overlying skin or deeper structures of the axilla

Stage C: Any one of the five grave signs of advanced breast carcinoma:

1. edema of the skin of limited extent (involving less than one-third of the skin over the breast)
2. skin ulceration
3. solid fixation of the tumor to the chest wall
4. massive involvement of axillary lymph nodes (measuring 2.5 cm or more in transverse diameter)
5. fixation of the axillary nodes to overlying skin or deeper structures of the axilla

Stage D: All other patients with more advanced breast carinoma, including:

1. a combination of any two or more of the five grave signs listed under stage C
2. extensive edema of the skin (involving more than one-third of the skin over the breast)
3. satellite skin nodules
4. The inflammatory type of carcinoma
5. clinically involved supraclavicular lymph nodes
6. internal mammary metastases as evidenced by a parasternal tumor
7. edema of the arm
8. distant metastases

Both clinical systems are based upon the results of surgery in treating breast cancer. The major points of discrepancy between the UICC–AJC system and the CCC system are: (1) the recognition by the UICC–AJC that primary size by itself is of prognostic importance and (2) the recognition by the CCC that axillary nodes measuring greater than 2½ cm usually indicate extension beyond the lymph node capsule and, therefore, a high risk of local recurrence.

As noted before, clinical evaluation of spread to the axilla has a high false positive and false negative rate. For this reason pathological staging based on the histologic evaluation of the axillary specimen is sometimes preferable. For the individual patient, prognosis is better determined by pathological staging than by clinical staging. This is illustrated in Table 27-10. For patients felt by clinical means to have spread of tumor, but in whom the histologic evaluation is negative, survival (72%) is comparable to the group of patients with the histologically negative nodes (76%) and not to patients with positive nodes (48%). Similarly, if a patient does not have clinical evidence of axillary involvement, but microscopic involvement is detected pathologically, survival (57%) is comparable to the group of patients with microscopic involvement.

Pathologic stage is commonly given as Stage I (axillary nodes not involved) or Stage II (axillary nodes involved). Refinements of this simple staging format have been made. One refinement has been made to subdivide the staging scheme by the number of positive axillary nodes. Since prognosis has been clearly related to the extent of axillary involvement (Table 27-5), it has become convention to subdivide axillary involvement into one to three nodes positive or more than four nodes positive. Another refinement is based on the recognition that micrometastatic involvement of axillary lymph nodes is not associated with the poor prognosis seen with macrometastatic involvement.

A comparison of the significance of axillary nodal micro- and macrometastases has been the object of recent pathologic study. Occult metastases were demonstrated in regional lymph nodes by an extended histopathologic technique in 24% of 78 cases of invasive breast cancer which would have been regarded as pathologic Stage I (absent nodal metastases) after "routine" pathologic examination.[60] Interestingly, no relationship was found between the presence of these occult

TABLE 27-10. 10-Year Survival According to Clinical and Pathologic Assessment of Axillary Nodes

	PATHOLOGICAL ASSESSMENT OF AXILLARY NODES		
CLINICAL ASSESSMENT OF AXILLARY NODES	*N-*	*N+*	*All*
N0	77%	57%	71%
N1	72%	34%	44%
All	76%	48%	

(Haagensen CD: Treatment of curable carcinoma of the breast. Int J Rad Oncol Biol Phys 2:975–980, 1977)

lesions and an average survival of 5 years. Patients in whom the largest nodal metastases measured ≤2 mm in its greatest diameter, regarded as micrometastases, were compared with those in whom the lesions were ≥2 mm, macrometastases (NSABP B-04). Life-table analyses failed to reveal any significant difference in survival between patients with micrometastases and those without nodal metastases. Both of these groups exhibited significantly greater survival than patients with macrometastases. A subset of patients with micrometastases in whom the metastases measured ≤1.3 mm was identified. These patients exhibited survival and treatment failure rates similar to those of the negative-node patients.

In the study by Huvos and co-workers from Memorial Hospital in New York City, prognosis was related to the pathological extent of axillary nodal involvement.[61] For the 62 patients with no involvement of axillary nodes, the 8-year survival rate was 82% (51/62). When micrometastatic involvement (defined as less than 2 mm) of level I axillary nodes was found, the 8-year survival rate was 94% (17/18). In comparison, the survival was 62% (28/45) for patients with macrometastatic involvement of level I axillary nodes. Other refinements are based on the recognition that extension of metastatic involvement beyond the lymph node capsule, or involvement of an axillary node greater than 2 cm have been associated with a worse prognosis, independent of the number of nodes involved.

These refinements have been included in the Post Surgical Treatment Pathological classification given by the UICC–AJC in 1977:

Primary Tumor (T)	
T0	No evidence of primary tumor
T1–T4	Same as UICC–AJC classification except for sub-division of T1 into: i: Tumor less than 0.5 cm ii: Tumor 0.5 cm–0.9 cm iii: Tumor 1.0 cm–1.9 cm
Nodal Involvement (N)	
N0	No metastatic homolateral axillary node
N1	Movable homolateral axillary metastatic nodes not fixed to one another or to other structures
N1a	Lymph nodes with only histologic metastatic growth
N1b	Gross metastatic carcinoma in lymph nodes
i	Micrometastatic smaller than 0.2 cm
ii	Metastasis (larger than 0.2 cm) in one to three lymph nodes
iii	Metastasis to four or more lymph nodes
iv	Extension of metastasis beyond the lymph node capsule
v	Any positive node greater than 2 cm in diameter
N2–N3	Same as clinical UICC–AJC classification

THEORIES ON THE SPREAD OF BREAST CANCER

The relationship between the primary cancer in the breast, its spread to draining lymph nodes and its spread to distant sites has been a matter of practical importance and controversy. It is of interest to review Halsted's concept of the spread of breast cancer. In common with other surgeons at the turn of the century, he believed that all extension of the cancer from the primary was by direct spread (called permeation). At the time, it was believed that cancer did not spread by embolization from the primary, but solely by direct extension. This concept of the spread of the disease was the basis for performing an *en bloc* radical resection of the affected region. In fact, Halsted in his 1907 review, conjectured that even more radical surgery might be indicated.

> Though the area of disease extended from cranium to knee, breast cancer in the broad sense is a local affliction, and there comes to the surgeon an encouragement to greater endeavor with the cognition that the metastases to bone, to pleura, to liver, are probably part of the whole, and that the involvements are almost invariably by process of lymphatic permeation and not embolic by way of the blood. Extension, the most rapid, taking place beneath the skin along the fascial planes . . . it must be our endeavor to trace more definitely the routes traveled in the metastases to bone, particularly to the humerus, for it is even possible in case of involvement of this bone that computation of the shoulder joint plus a proper removal of the soft parts might eradicate the disease. So, too, it is conceivable that ultimately when our knowledge of the lymphatics traversed in cases of former involvement becomes sufficiently exact, amputation at the hip joint may seem indicated.[56]

Beginning with work performed in the 1930s, it has become clear that embolization is the predominant node of spread to draining lymph nodes and to distant sites.[62,63] More recently, debate has centered on the relation of draining lymph node spread to the appearance of distant metastasis. It was originally felt that the spread of breast cancer was sequential: arising in the breast, spreading first to regional lymph nodes, and finally to distant sites. According to this review, the regional lymph nodes act as a filter or barrier to the further spread of the cancer. More recently, it has been suggested that the spread to lymph nodes, and to distant sites represents two independent (but correlated) processes. This latter review has been summarized in the quotation by DeWitt: "Axillary lymph node metastases are an expression of a bad prognosis, not the determinant."[64] Support for the original view has been provided by the observation that a significant proportion of patients with involvement of axillary nodes have apparent cures following radical surgery. It was thereby assumed that in these patients untreated axillary metastasis would have provided a source for the further development of the cancer and the ultimate death of the patient. Some recent clinical observations, however, have cast some doubt on this assumption. As noted before, in patients without axillary lymphadenopathy, 30% to 40% will demonstrate spread pathologically. Nevertheless if an axillary dissection is not performed in this group of patients, only 10% to 15% will ever clinically manifest cancer in their axilla. In addition, Baum and Coyle have recently reported on a series of 25 patients with clinically positive axillary lymph nodes treated by simple mastectomy alone.[65] While it would have been expected that 25% of this group did not have pathological involvement, 13 patients (52%) of the group underwent spontaneous regression of their axillary lymphadenopathy within 3 months of mastectomy. These observations suggest that there may be important (but undefined) host defense mechanisms that are capable of containing or eradicating untreated axillary metastases, and that untreated axillary metastases do not necessarily serve as a focus for the further spread of cancer.

Some investigations have gone further to suggest that treatment of draining lymph nodes may, in fact, be harmful.[66] It has been theorized that immune defenses play a critical role in determining survival in breast cancer and that either surgical or radiotherapeutic treatment of regional lymph nodes may depress these immune defenses and thereby lessen survival. This controversy regarding the spread of breast cancer and the node treatment has recently been addressed in a number of prospective clinical trials.

One such trial, sponsored by the Cancer Research Campaign (CRC) in the United Kingdom, was begun in 1970. Patients with T1 or T2, N0 or N1, M0 carcinoma of the breast were randomized to either simple mastectomy followed by radiotherapy (which is the most common form of "radical" treatment practiced in the United Kingdom) or simple mastectomy alone. Two-thousand-two hundred forty-three evaluable persons entered the study between May, 1970, and April, 1975, and preliminary 8-year results were published in July, 1980.[68] Local–regional recurrence was significantly reduced for irradiated patients. Of the 140 patients treated by simple mastectomy, 30% developed local or regional recurrences compared to 11% for 1103 patients treated by simple mastectomy and radiation therapy ($P \leq 0.001$). Despite this clear-cut improvement in local–regional control, there was not a significant difference in either distant recurrence or survival between the two treatment arms. The rate of distant relapse was 35% for patients treated with simple mastectomy and 33% for patients treated with simple mastectomy and radiation. The 5-year survival rates were 70% and 73%, respectively. Similar results have been obtained in two other trials from Britain in which these same two treatment arms were tested.[69,70]

In 1971, a trial was begun in this country by the National Surgical Adjuvant Breast Project (NSABP) comparing simple mastectomy, radical mastectomy, and simple mastectomy and radiation therapy for patients with clinically negative axillary lymph nodes. One-thousand-six-hundred-sixty-five evaluable patients were randomized by 1974, and 3-year results were reported in 1980.[71] Here again, local and regional control was improved by regional treatment, but no statistically significant differences in survival among these three treatment arms were noted. The 5-year relapse-free survival was 68% for radical mastectomy, 71% for simple mastectomy and radiation, and 63% for simple mastectomy alone. Of interest in this trial is that, while not statistically significant, the survival rate for patients receiving regional treatment was better than for patients not receiving regional treatment. These results are still preliminary and further follow-up may provide a more definite answer.

These studies suggest that treatment of axillary lymph nodes is neither harmful nor beneficial with regard to survival. In this sense, these studies did not confirm the theory that regional treatment depressed immune defenses important to survival in breast cancer. They also failed to confirm the view that regional treatment was a critical part of the initial management of breast cancer.

If these preliminary results are confirmed by longer follow-up, the whole conceptual approach to breast cancer will require revision. The original concept that the cancer begins in the breast, secondarily spreads to axillary (and perhaps internal mammary) lymph nodes, and finally spreads to distant sites will have to be replaced by the concept that breast cancer, for the most part, spreads to the draining lymph nodes and distant sites at approximately the same time. According to this newer concept, treatment of draining lymph nodes will decrease local–regional recurrence but will not improve survival, since the vast majority of patients with lymph node metastases already have distant spread which cannot be affected by regional treatment.

Another interpretation of these studies is possible. Instead of assuming that the entire patient population was identical in terms of their host defenses and tumor biology, one could speculate that there were significant differences between patients. In some patients, treatment of the axillary lymph nodes by either surgery or radiation did improve survival by eradicating the only site of metastatic spread, while in other patients, this treatment did depress host defenses which otherwise, would have been able to suppress metastatic spread. If these two subgroups of patients were approximately the same proportion, it might be possible to improve survival by identifying these separate subgroups and using regional lymph node treatment only in the appropriate subgroups.

Even if these clinical trials confirm that lymph node treatment is not useful in improving survival, axillary dissection may remain an important element in the primary local–regional treatment. For one reason, it can be argued that axillary dissection is a relatively nonmorbid procedure, which is easily performed and is useful in preventing axillary recurrence in about 15% of patients with clinically negative nodes. Of greater importance, perhaps, is that at the current time, axillary node histology is the most important means to identify patients at great risk of having occult distant spread and therefore suitable for adjuvant chemotherapy, to be discussed below. At this writing, the long-term effects of adjuvant chemotherapy have not been determined and, for the most part, the use of this therapy is restricted to patients with histologically proven axillary metastasis. In the future, however, the need for axillary dissection may be obviated. If adjuvant chemotherapy proves to be both efficacious and relatively nontoxic in patients with positive nodes, its use could very well be extended to patients with negative axillary nodes. In this case, axillary dissection would not be required. In addition, if newer means of prognostication became available, which were equally accurate in determining the likelihood of treatment failure, axillary dissection may also be avoided. Recent evidence suggests that the use of estrogen receptor protein studies, perhaps coupled for primary tumor size, might provide such a means of prognostication. Nevertheless, at the present time, axillary dissection provides the most commonly accepted criterion for the use of adjuvant therapy, and for this reason, will likely remain a part of local–regional treatment.

SCREENING FOR BREAST CANCER

There has been much interest in recent years in the early detection of breast cancer by screening asymptomatic women. No controlled trials of screening programs on any malignancy were done until the HIP study done for the detection of breast cancer.[72,73] This study reviewed 31,000 women and compared those offered screening with a control group. The screening included both physical examination and mammography. The results so far in this program indicate a reduced breast cancer mortality in the screening population. It was this study which has stimulated much of the use of screening and formed the frame of reference for considerations of mammography. It is useful to consider the important factors in evaluating any screening program.

In order for such a program to be of value, the possible benefits must include either a decrease in mortality or a decrease in morbidity or both. In the HIP study there was a definite decrease in mortality in those women over the age of 50 years, although no clear benefit was shown in those women between 40 years and 49 years. The morbidity question is not resolved, since it depends on whether women with early breast cancer can be treated with more conservative procedures than those used for more advanced tumors. There is some evidence for such a conservative approach as discussed in the treatment sections of this chapter. There are, of course, risks involved in a screening program.[74] If the procedure has a low sensitivity, and therefore picks up only a small proportion of the asymptomatic patients with the disease, then those other patients may be given false reassurance, perhaps causing them to delay seeking medical advice when the disease becomes symptomatic to later than they would had they not been screened. Second, there may be far too many biopsies if the procedure has a low specificity; that is, if it picks up abnormalities, many of which may turn out not to be cancer. Many women would be exposed to biopsy for inconsequential reasons which never would have been found without the screening procedure. Finally, and perhaps most discussed, is the risk of mammography resulting in the possible induction of secondary breast cancers.[75] There have been a number of studies indicating that radiation can induce breast cancer. These studies have come from a variety of sources, including survivors of the atomic bomb, patients irradiated due to frequent fluoroscopy for tuberculosis, and breast irradiation for benign disease.[8,11,76,77] All of these appear to indicate an increasing risk with increasing dose, although the dose administered in all these reports is far greater than that from a single mammographic examination. This has led to extensive discussion as to whether the risks are linear with dose, so that the findings at higher doses can be extrapolated down to lower doses. This has been excellently reviewed by Boice, Land and their colleagues who suggest that the most reasonable expectation is a linear dose response curve and that a large deviation from this is not consistent with the data.[78-80] Their review also indicates that in all the studies there clearly appears to be a greater risk in irradiation of women under the age of 30 years than in older women. There have been two major governmental reviews of this issue, the BEIR report and a more recent NIH consensus development.[81,82] From all of these studies it seems reasonable to assume that women irradiated in the second decade of life have a higher incidence of breast cancer, but when women are irradiated after the age of 35 or 40 years the risk appears to be about an excess of six cases per million patients per year per rad following a 10-year latency period. With this information, plus a continued reduction in mammographic exposure, there appears to be general agreement that mammography as a screening procedure appears clearly to be of value over the age of 50 years and probably should not be used in the general population under the age of 35 years. The correct approach to the women between 35 years and 50 years is still under discussion and depends on many of the assumptions used. For example, there seems to be as yet no clear evidence that mortality is reduced by screening patients in this age group—thus, whatever your estimation of risk, if there is no clear gain mammography should not be employed. The dose received during mammography has been reduced due to the appreciation of this potential hazard. High-quality mammograms can be made with less than 1 rad administered to the breast and substantially lower doses may be achieved. All these considerations are for women in the general population; special exceptions should be made for patients identified in high-risk groups. These high-risk groups include at the minimum those patients with a very strong family history, especially those whose mother and sister have had the disease. Their likelihood of having the disease under the age of 40 years and bilaterally is extremely high. It should also include those patients who will have already had a breast cancer on the other side, as the incidence of second tumors appears to be approximately 1% per year of risk after the diagnosis of the initial breast cancer. Finally there are women who have had a suspicious biopsy of breast lesions who need careful follow up.

The debate on breast cancer screening has resulted in effective reduction in the mammographic exposure without significant loss in the sensitivity or specificity of the procedure. This appears to be a valuable contribution. Mammography is an important addition, too, but cannot substitute for physical examination in the screening of asymptomatic women for breast cancer. Both procedures may find tumors undetected by other means. In the HIP study, approximately one-third of the tumors were found by mammogram alone, while 40% of the tumors detected were not seen on the mammograms. A screening program including both of these techniques is clearly of value in women over the age of 50 years, although its optimal frequencies is yet not determined. In the HIP study there were four annual screening examinations resulting in an approximately one-third reduction of breast cancer mortality. Another procedure that has been studied is the use of thermography. It appears as though this technique has too low a sensitivity and specificity to be at present of general use in breast cancer screening.

PRE-TREATMENT EVALUATION

There is general agreement that the pre-treatment evaluation of a patient with breast cancer should include a complete medical history and physical examination (Table 27-11), chest roentgenogram (posterior–anterior and lateral views), CBC, and liver chemistries. The utility of other tests (bone scan, liver scan, and mammogram) has been a matter of controversy.

Radionuclide scans are acknowledged as a sensitive test for early bone metastases. The yield of bone scanning, however, in asymptomatic patients with early breast cancer is small. In one study from John Hopkins, only one of 64 patients with Stage I or II breast cancer had a positive pre-operative bone scan. In contrast, 25% of patients with Stage III disease had positive scans preoperatively.[83] In another study from the Peter Bent Brigham Hospital, the yield of bone scanning was 0/37 in Stage I, 4% in Stage II, and 16% in Stage III.[84] In addition, bone scans can also be positive in a number of benign bone conditions and this can result in treatment delay and increased patient anxiety. These data suggest that a scan is warranted in Stage III breast cancer, but its usefulness in early stage disease is less certain. Some clinicians claim that a bone scan should be obtained in all patients as a baseline for future comparison, but this justification has not been established.

The yield of positive pre-treatment liver scans is even smaller than that of bone scans. In a series of 234 patients studied with routine preoperative liver scans at the Mt. Sinai Hospital of Cleveland only 11 (5%) abnormals were obtained.[85] Of further interest, eight of these abnormals were later established as false-positive by further evaluation, so that the ultimate result of the test was only 1%. These findings are not surprising when one considers the observation that metastases greater than 2 cm are required for visualization on liver scans.[86] It is generally recommended that liver scans should be reserved only for those patients with abnormal liver chemistries or hepatomegaly.

It is worth emphasizing that a positive bone or liver scan does not necessarily establish metastatic disease. These tests both commonly have significant false-positives, and the results of a positive scan need to be viewed within the context of the total evaluation of the patient. In many cases, histologic confirmation should be obtained before definitive primary therapy is abandoned.

Bilateral mammograms are frequently recommended prior to a biopsy of a suspicious breast mass. The purpose of the mammogram is to detect any occult lesion that should also be biopsied. The use of mammograms in this setting clearly improves the pre-operative diagnostic accuracy, but a negative mammogram in the presence of a suspicious breast mass is not a justification to avoid biopsy. In some institutions, however, mammograms are not routinely obtained pre-operatively, since the yield is felt to be small in detecting additional lesions. The use of mammography in patients with a positive biopsy is even less clear. Mammography of the opposite breast is commonly recommended to rule out occult contralateral disease.

For patients to be treated by mastectomy, the detection of additional lesions in the involved breast is of limited value. If a patient is to be treated by primary radiation therapy, however, the detection of additional lesions is important. The presence of multicentric gross lesions would influence a decision for additional surgery, an altered radiotherapeutic program, or possibly mastectomy.

Brain scans and CT scans of the head are both sensitive tests to detect early metastatic involvement. The yield of these studies in a pre-treatment setting is very small and is not recommended in the absence of suspicious signs or symptoms.

TABLE 27-11. Pertinent Medical History and Physical Examination For the Patient with Breast Cancer

1. Breast and Axillary Symptoms—first noted and evolution
   Breast mass
   Breast pain
   Nipple discharge
   Nipple or skin retraction
   Axillary mass or pain
   Arm swelling
2. Past Medical History of Breast Disease Including Prior Biopsies
3. Reproductive History
   Age of onset of menses
   Frequency, duration and regularity of menstrual periods
   Number of pregnancies, children, abortions
   Age at first pregnancy
   Age of onset of menopause
   History of hormone use—including birth control pills
   Breast feeding
4. Family History—age of diagnosis and death of family members with breast cancer
5. Review of Symptoms—with particular reference to possible metastatic spread.
6. Physical Examination (a diagnosis is recommended)
   Breast Mass—size
      location (specified by clock position and the distance from edge of the areola)
      shape
      consistency
      fixation to skin, pectoral muscle, or chest wall

   Skin Changes—erythema
      edema (note location and extent)
      dimpling
      satellite nodules

   Nipple changes—retraction
      discoloration
      thickening
      reddening
      erosion

   Nodal Status—axillary nodes–number
      location
      size
      fixation to other nodes or underlying structures
      clinically suspicious or benign
   infraclavicular fullness
   supraclavicular nodes or area swelling

An area of growing interest has been the use of biological markers. A number of substances including CEA, ferritin, and HCG have been suggested as possible markers. In patients with metastatic breast cancer, 70% have been shown to have elevated CEA levels, 50% have elevated HCG levels, and 67% have elevated ferritin levels.[87–91] There is preliminary evidence to suggest that pre-treatment markers can be used as a prognostic indicator. In one study, patients with postoperative CEA levels greater than 2.5 ng/ml had a 2-year recurrence rate of 65% compared to 20% for those with normal CEA levels ($P < 0.001$). The use of serial marker determination in the follow-up period has also been suggested as a means for the early detection of recurrence. This field is undergoing rapid evolution and firm recommendations are not available at this time. Pre-treatment levels, particularly of CEA, are easily obtained and relatively inexpensive.

TREATMENT OF LOCAL AND REGIONAL DISEASE

ENDPOINTS AND DEFINITION OF TERMS

The two most commonly used endpoints to judge the effectiveness of local and regional treatment are: (1) local and regional tumor control and (2) survival. Despite the general acceptance of these two endpoints, each presents difficulties in analyzing the results of treatment. While it is clear that the object of treatment is to eradicate all cancer in the breast, chest wall, and draining lymph node areas, it is not now possible to determine at the end of the treatment if this has been accomplished. As a result, follow-up information on patients is required to detect any reappearance of cancer in these areas. Such a reappearance is termed local or regional recurrence, and is taken as an indication of the failure of the treatment to achieve eradication of the cancer. In contrast, the absence of local or regional recurrence is termed local–regional tumor control and is taken as evidence for the eradication of cancer.

Unfortunately, the assumptions are not always valid. Persistent tumor may not always result in a clinically detectable recurrence during the patient's life; and conversely, reseeding from metastatic tumor deposits elsewhere may result in an apparent local–regional recurrence. There are three lines of evidence for the first objection. First, it is known that while approximately 40% of patients without palpable axillary nodes who undergo axillary dissections have histologically positive axillary nodes, only 15% of those who do not undergo axillary dissection develop recurrence in the axilla.[92] Thus, it may be assumed that two-thirds of patients in whom tumor has spread to axillary nodes fail to develop clinically apparent disease in the axilla. Second, multifocal disease within the breast is found in at least 15% of total mastectomies, but only 5% of patients who undergo partial mastectomy for carcinoma develop recurrent disease in the residual ipsilateral breast tissue.[93] Here, too, at least two-thirds of patients who presumably have residual tumor fail to develop clinical evidence of recurrence. Third, an autopsy study on nonselected patients with breast cancer demonstrated the high frequency with which microscopic deposits of breast cancer are found in the chest wall of patients felt on clinical grounds to be free of local recurrence.[94]

The second possibility, namely reseeding of the chest wall and axilla from distant metastases, is more difficult to document. Many investigators, however, now record only the *first* site of failure to minimize this problem of possible reseeding. In this way, a local and regional failure is scored only if it occurs as the first site of relapse; local and regional failures that occur after the appearance of distant metastases are not scored. Even by this form of analysis, however, it is still possible that some apparent local and regional recurrences may represent reseeding from distant sites of disease. Given these reservations, local and regional recurrence rates still remain the most important endpoint in judging the effectiveness of local and regional treatment, and are used in many of the studies to be quoted later.

In addition to the use of local–regional recurrences as an endpoint, the survival rates of treated patients are commonly given. As will be discussed later, many patients with breast cancer die of their disease at long intervals after primary treatment. For this reason, it is commonly acknowledged that 10-year survival rates are required to assess fully the results of treatment. This requirement of 10 years of follow-up has the disadvantage of considerably slowing the pace of clinical research. Since the great majority of relapses of breast cancer occur within the first 5 years after treatment, some investigators have used the 5-year relapse-free survival rate as a substitute for the 10-year survival rate. The major objection to the use of survival as an endpoint for local–regional treatment is that survival is not primarily determined by this treatment. Survival is more directly related to the presence or absence of subclinical distant metastases at the time of initial treatment. Such metastases cannot be affected by local–regional treatment. In this way, survival is more a reflection of case selection, whereby patients with earlier disease have less likelihood of distant spread and, hence, have better survival. The main advantage to the use of survival is to detect any adverse effects of treatment which may not be immediately obvious.

Taken together, these two endpoints (local–regional tumor control and survival) are the major means of judging the effectiveness of local–regional treatment.

SURGICAL MANAGEMENT OF PRIMARY BREAST CANCER

A few years ago any textbook discussion regarding the surgical management of breast cancer was direct and uncomplicated. It encompassed a description of the technique of performing a radical mastectomy or, in some instances, an extended radical mastectomy. Lesser procedures were either ignored or condemned. The accepted operations were predicated upon "Halstedian" principles described previously based on concepts of the biology of the disease when the "modern" era of breast cancer surgery was formulated around 1890.

As a consequence of these considerations, and in keeping with the understanding of the disease at the time, there arose an anatomical basis for breast cancer surgery. The "proper" cancer operation consisted of removal of the primary tumor together with regional lymphatics and lymph nodes by *en bloc* dissection. Since it was deemed that there was an "orderliness" about tumor spread and that clinical recognizable cancer was in many instances a local–regional disease, it was considered to be more curable if the surgeon would be more expansive in his interpretation of what constituted the "region" and if, above all, he utilized better technique so that he could eradicate the last cancer cell. Local–regional recurrences were considered to be the result of inadequate application of surgical skill rather than a manifestation of systemic disease. The hope was that "one more lymph node dissection would cure more cancers." With the advent of better supportive measures to improve patient survival, such as blood transfusions, anesthesia, correction of physiologic defects resulting from operation, and development of technical skills, super-radical cancer surgery came into being and such procedures as extended radical mastectomy were developed.

The past decade has seen the beginning decline of cancer surgery based on anatomical principles. As a consequence of conceptual changes that have resulted from new information concerning tumor biology, a new basis for cancer surgery is arising. Those factors which have prompted a redefinition of the rationale for breast cancer surgery have been repeatedly reviewed.[71,95] They provide a scientific, rather than an emotional basis for the present controversy concerning the surgical management of breast cancer.

The primary goal of an operation is to effect local–regional disease control. The following provides an overview of those operations that have been employed to achieve that aim.

Radical Mastectomy

Radical mastectomy as described in 1894 by William Halsted and Willy Meyer became the standard operation in the United States for operable breast cancer. A recent survey conducted by the American College of Surgeons has indicated that whereas in 1972, 45% of patients had a radical mastectomy, in 1977, 22% of patients were still treated by that operation. The procedure consists of an *en bloc* dissection of the entire breast and skin overlying the tumor, together with the pectoralis major and minor muscles and the contents of the axilla (Figs. 27-2, 27-3). Not too long ago, discussion concerning this operation centered around the proper incision to employ, the amount of skin to be removed, how thin or thick skin flaps should be, whether skin grafts to the chest wall should be used, what the best approach for removal of the highest axillary node is, and even the importance of the length of the operative time. It becomes obvious from recurrence and survival rates obtained from patients studied by the NSABP 5 years and 10 years after operation that conventional radical operation for the treatment of so-called curable breast cancer is a less than satisfactory form of therapy.[96,97] The finding that 65% of patients having any number of positive axillary lymph nodes at operation, and 79% of those with four or more nodes involved, demonstrated tumor recurrence within 5 years of operation attests to the inadequacy of therapy

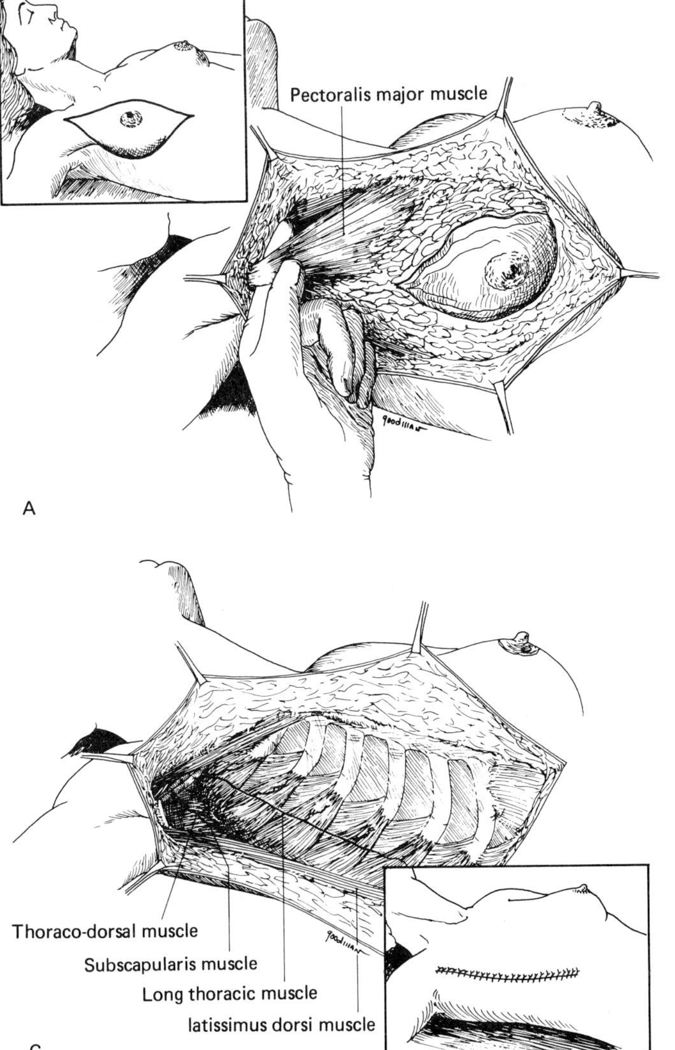

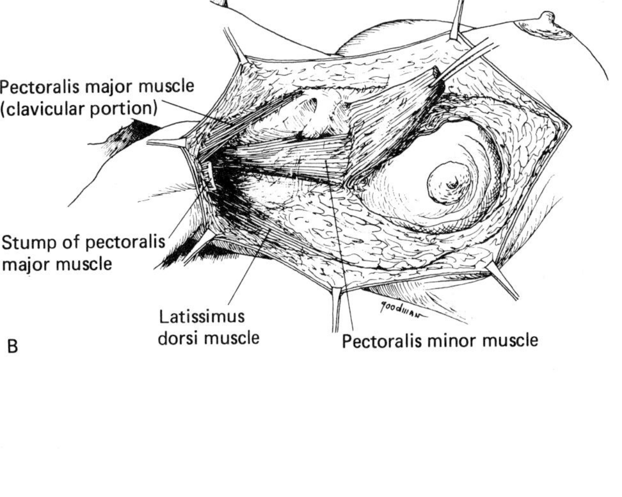

FIG. 27-2. Technique of radical mastectomy. *A*, An eliptical incision is made around the breast mass including overlying skin. The skin flaps are raised medially to the midline, posteriorly to the latissimus dorsi muscle, superiorly to the axillary vein, and inferiorly to a level below the breast. The breast is dissected off the skin flaps and the chest wall. *B*, If the pectoralis major muscle is to be sacrificed, it is to be divided at its insertion. In a modified radical mastectomy, the pectoralis major muscle is not divided, but reflected superiorly to allow access to the axillary contents. The pectoralis minor muscle, which underlies the pectoralis major muscle, can be either excised or left intact in a modified radical mastectomy. The axillary contents are then dissected to the apex of the axilla along the axillary vein. *C*, the appearance of the operative field following a radical mastectomy. All of the breast and the fibroareolar tissue containing lymph nodes in the axilla have been removed. (From Hardy, JD: Surgery. Philadelphia, JB Lippincott, 1977)

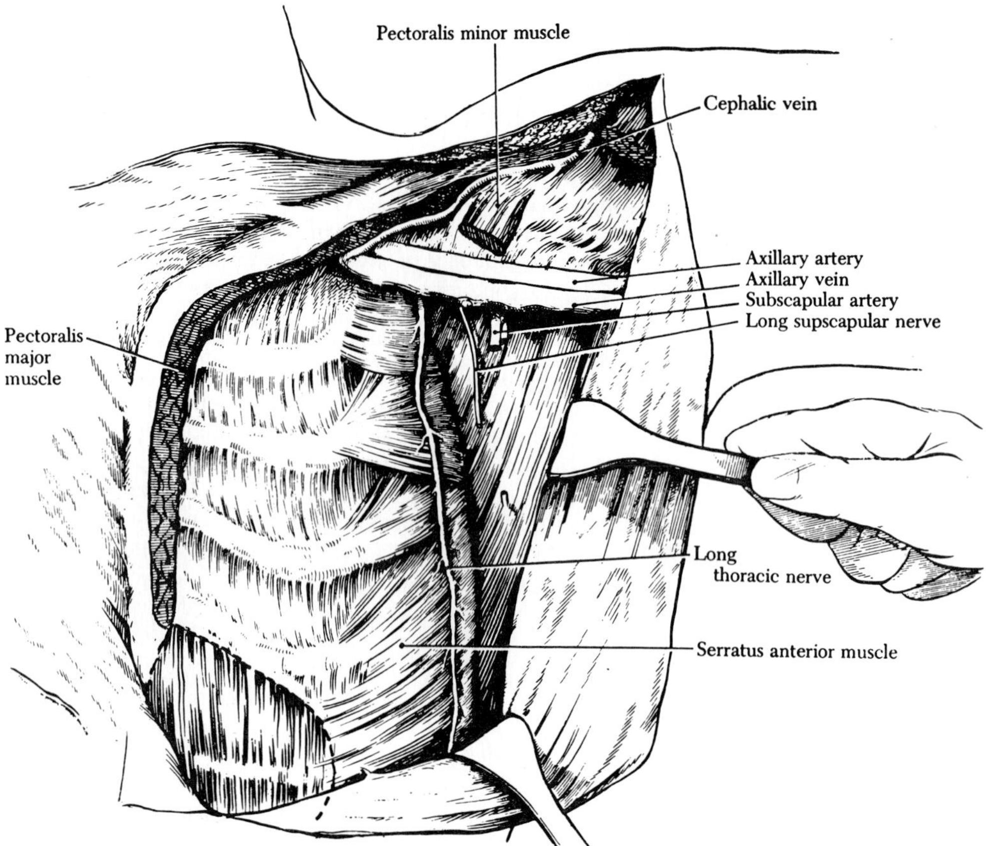

FIG. 27-3. Detailed appearance of the anatomy of the axilla following a radical mastectomy. The outlines of the pectoralis major muscle are shown. It is left intact in a modified radical mastectomy and can be reflected superiorly to reveal the contents of the axilla. Note the long thoracic nerve and the thoraco-dorsal (long subscapular nerve), which should be preserved during this dissection if not involved with tumor. Note the complete dissection of tissue medially from the midline, laterally to the latissimus dorsi muscle, superiorly and the axillary vein (From Warren R (ed): Surgery, Fig. 284. Philadelphia, WB Saunders, 1963)

in such patients. Even women having the smallest sized tumors removed (1.0 cm–1.9 cm), but with four or more positive axillary nodes, had a 65% 5-year tumor recurrence rate.[50] When tumors removed were 3.0 cm or greater in this four-plus positive-node group, the recurrence rate was between 81% and 94%, despite the fact that such patients met generally recognized criteria of operability. That nearly one of every four patients having negative axillary nodes at the time of her operation developed tumor recurrences within 10 years led to dissatisfaction with the operation. Information from a more recent NSABP study indicates from life-table analyses that 7 years after radical mastectomy 17% of axillary node negative patients and 57% of those with any number of positive nodes (44% with 1–3 positive nodes and 70% with ≥4 positive nodes) had a tumor recurrence.

The morbidity associated with radical mastectomy in terms of arm swelling, deformity, and problems with wound healing is not insignificant. Those problems are all the more unacceptable when they occur in women who have failed to be cured of their disease by the procedure.

Extended Radical Mastectomy

If the removal of the entire lymphatic drainage area in every cancer operation is of paramount importance, then the so-called radical operation for cancer of the breast may be considered inadequate, for the evidence is substantial that lymph nodes other than those in the axilla frequently are involved with tumor.

Turner-Warwick, using dye and colloidal gold injection, demonstrated that about 75% of the lymph leaving the breast goes to the ipsilateral axillary nodes and the remainder drains mostly into the ipsilateral internal mammary chain, with a small amount going to the posterior intercostal lymph nodes.[98] Of more importance were his findings that both the axilla and the internal mammary chain receive lymph from all quadrants of the breast and that there is no striking tendency for any particular quadrant to drain in one direction. While such a finding may have validity in so far as lymph is concerned, it is hazardous to conclude from such information that tumor cells behave similarly in their peregrinations. That they probably do so, however, is suggested by numerous observations. In 1946, Handley and Thackray began to do biopsies on internal mammary lymph nodes of consecutive cases undergoing radical mastectomy. Involvement of internal mammary nodes was observed in 31% of patients having inner-quadrant tumors.[99] When tumors were outer-quadrant or central, such nodes were involved in 19% and 47% of patients, respectively. Of women having axillary node involvement, those with inner-quadrant, outer-quadrant, or central lesions had internal mammary node involvement in 51%, 28%, and 59% of cases, respectively. Such findings forced Handley to conclude that the classic radical operation is "not radical at all and will fail in its object in at least 25% of operable cases."

Others have also observed frequent involvement of the internal mammary chain. Dahl-Iversen noted involvement of the parasternal lymph nodes in 30% of medial-half lesions and in only 12% of lateral breast cancers.[55] Of cases in which he performed the conventional radical operation accompanied by extirpation of the parasternal nodes in the upper three intercostal spaces, positive lymph nodes were found in 24%. In an earlier report, Andreassen and Dahl-Iversen reported that in a series of patients with positive axillary nodes, a supraclavicular dissection revealed microscopic evidence of tumor in 33% of instances.[100] Later, Andreassen and associates reported that in 100 patients, 41% had axillary node metastases, 17% internal mammary node involvement, and 3% supraclavicular involvement.[101] More recently, Caceres demonstrated the incidence of metastases in the internal mammary chain, as determined by its removal along with the breast and contents of the axilla, in 600 consecutive cases.[102] In his series, inner-half lesions of the breast resulted in internal mammary node involvement in 28%; tumors centrally located, 21%; and outer-half lesions, 13%. When there was no axillary involvement, the possibility of internal mammary chain involvement was 7%, and when axillary nodes contained tumor, 29% of the internal mammary chain did likewise. Analyzing the latter finding (positive axillary node) according to the location of the tumor, he found that when the tumor was located in the inner half, the incidence of metastases was 44%, and when located in the central portion, 33%. The incidence dropped to 19% when tumors were in the outer half of the breast.

With the accumulation of such evidence, surgeons extended their operative dissections. The extended radical operation has been employed, utilizing a variety of techniques. Margottini was the first to resect the internal mammary nodes as a routine therapeutic attack on breast cancer, beginning in 1948.[103] In 1963, he and his associates reported 5-year and 10-year findings with 900 patients treated, and compared them with those obtained from patients undergoing radical mastectomies.[104] Results were distinctly better for patients treated by extended radical mastectomy. His data, however, give no assurance that case material compared was equivalent. In 1976, Lacour and associates reported results obtained from an international cooperative study carried out to compare standard radical mastectomy with radical mastectomy and internal mammary node dissection in patients with breast cancers classified as T1, T2, or T3 (diameter <7 cm without complete pectoral muscle fixation, without skin involvement, and without inflammatory signs), N0, N1 and M0.[105] While no significant difference was observed in the overall 5-year survival rate between the two groups, when subgroups were evaluated it was reported that those with T1 and T2 tumors occurring in the medial quadrants, and who had positive axillary nodes, benefited from extended radical mastectomy. On the other hand, patients with inner or medial quadrant T3 lesions which had a greater IM node involvement than T1 and T2 lesions failed to benefit from the mammary node dissection. In the United States, only a few surgeons such as Urban and Sugarbaker have advocated the extended mastectomy. That the operation has never been accepted is indicated by the findings in a recent American College of Surgeons Survey indicating that of 15,114 patients treated for primary breast cancer in 1972 only 42 patients (0.3%) had a superradical mastectomy. In 1977 only 5 of 14,554 patients (0.03%) were so treated.[106]

Modified Radical Mastectomy

An operation for breast cancer ignored in the United States for almost 25 years after its description, the modified radical mastectomy, has supplanted radical mastectomy as the "standard" operative procedure for the treatment of primary breast cancer. Whereas in 1972 only 26% of primary breast operations were modified radical mastectomies, in 1977, that operation comprised 58% of all procedures (according to the American College of Surgeons Survey).

Patey and Dyson, influenced by anatomic studies which demonstrated that "the deep fascia is a plane devoid of or very poor in lymphatics and hence not an important potential plane of spread," began to perform an operation that left the pectoralis major intact but removed the breast, pectoralis minor, and the axillary contents.[63] In 1948, they reported their early experiences with this technique and concluded that this modified radical operation, with preservation of the pectoralis major, showed results as good as those of the standard radical operation.[107] Consequently, removal of this muscle was deemed not to add to the value of surgical treatment. Perhaps the most outstanding advocate of the Patey operation has been Handley, of the Middlesex Hospital in London. In 1965, he reported his observations with 200 such procedures.[108] He noted that 76% of 117 Stage A patients were alive at 5 years, although six had recurrent disease. Fifty-seven percent of 75 Stage B patients were alive at that time, but 11 had recurrent disease. From his findings, he concluded that "at this time of doubt and confusion, it appears that conservative radical mastectomy is a very reasonable compromise. It secures the advantages which Halsted first pointed out, without the deformity which sacrifice of the pectoralis major entails."

Increasing numbers of surgeons are now leaving both pectoral muscles intact when performing that operation. While the operation provides superior functional and cosmetic results to those obtained with radical mastectomy, it is of interest to point out that no properly conducted comparison of the two has ever been undertaken to determine their equivalence insofar as disease control is concerned.

Total (Simple) Mastectomy

The term "simple" mastectomy is not advisable since its precise meaning is ambiguous. Many of the operations described as simple mastectomies are indeed no more than partial mastectomies. To carry out a total mastectomy, the resection must extend from the clavicle to the costal margin and from the midline to the latissimus dorsi. The entire axillary tail and the pectoral fascia should be completely removed. Moreover, skin should be excised and skin flaps should be similar to thickness to those in a radical mastectomy. The axilla is not invaded and axillary nodes are not removed. Such an operation should be referred to as a "total" mastectomy.

In 1948, McWhirter, of the Royal Infirmary of Edinburgh, suggested that total mastectomy combined with postoperative radiotherapy might be a better modality to employ in the treatment of breast cancer.[109–114] He reached this conclusion following analysis of results obtained from patients at the Royal Infirmary between 1941 and 1945, whose main method of treatment was total mastectomy followed by roentgen ray therapy. These findings were compared with those in women who were treated at the same institution between 1930 and 1934 with radical mastectomy alone and with those treated between 1935 and 1940 when radical operation followed by postoperative irradiation was the therapy of choice.

McWhirter's rationale for the adoption of this therapeutic regimen was related to his concern that radical operations failed to get rid of all tumor tissue in the operative area and that "at the time of operation tissues actually invaded by tumor must be divided." It was his opinion that, as a result of this trauma, malignant cells would have an increased tendency to disseminate to other sites and, should this occur before the application of radiotherapy, its later use would be ineffective in saving the life of the patient. Although he appreciated the possibility that such cells could still be liberated from the area of operation when a total mastectomy was performed, he was of the opinion that, in contrast to the situation following radical mastectomy, they would be trapped by the intact barrier of the axilla. Moreover, he believed that since healing was likely to take place more rapidly after total mastectomy than after radical mastectomy, during which cells could be disseminated to distant sites. Such views possessed rationality in that they were in keeping with usual simplistic, mechanistic approach toward both tumor dissemination and eradication popular at the time. The demonstration that regional lymph nodes are not barriers to tumor cell dissemination has obtunded the worth of McWhirter's primary rationale for the procedure.[115] Other considerations further led him to support total mastectomy and irradiation. He held that: (a) when the disease is confined to the breast, dissection of the axilla is unnecessary; (b) when the tumor has spread to the axillary nodes, radical mastectomy must frequently fail because occult metastases may be present in the supraclavicular nodes that are beyond the surgical dissection but which can be eradicated by radiation therapy; (c) radical mastectomy alone cannot influence the course of the disease in patients in whom metastases to the internal mammary nodes might disseminate the disease; and (e) edema of the arm would not be as frequent following the less radical procedure.

In the United States, Crile has been a prime champion of total mastectomy. He has upheld the merits of this treatment for breast cancer. His first report in 1961 concluded that: (a) in clinical Stage I cancer of the breast, total mastectomy without prophylactic irradiation appeared to be at least as effective as radical mastectomy with or without irradiation; (b) in those patients with clinical Stage I cancer who were treated by total mastectomy without irradiation and whose disease later reappeared in the axillary nodes and then was removed by axillary dissection, the chances of survival did not seem to be any less than if the axilla had been treated prophylactically by radical mastectomy; and (c) in favorable clinical Stage II cancers, modified radical mastectomy without irradiation was as effective as any other treatment or combination of treatment. The greatest contribution of this study was, as Crile says, "that as a result of it and others, the success of simple treatments is well enough established so that controlled clinical studies can now be done without fear of doing an injustice to the patients receiving the simpler treatments."

In 1968, he reported that the 5-year survival rate of patients whose axillae contained no palpably involved nodes at the time of operation was 13% higher when the nodes were left in place and not irradiated than when they were removed with the breast.[116] He advised that "although both clinical and laboratory evidence indicates that uninvolved regional nodes contribute to the host's immunological resistance to systemic metastases, a large randomized study of patients with operative Stage I breast cancers will have to be done before it can be stated with certainty that removal of uninvolved nodes promotes metastases."

The Results of an NSABP Trial Comparing Alternative Procedures to Radical Mastectomy

By 1970 it was apparent that there was urgent need to implement a prospective randomized clinical trial the findings of which would provide data that would aid in resolving the clinical dilemma concerning the operative management of primary breast cancer. Between August, 1971, and August, 1974, members of 34 institutions in the United States and Canada entered 1765 patients into such a study. Women meeting rigid protocol requirements, who were clinically axillary node-negative, were randomized so that they received one of three distinctly different local–regional treatment regimens. They either had a conventional radical mastectomy (RM), a total (simple) mastectomy followed by local–regional radiation (TM + R), or a total mastectomy alone (TM) with subsequent removal of axillary nodes only if and when they subsequently became positive. Similarly, clinically positive node patients were treated by RM or TM + R. All patients entered the trial between 5 years and 8 years ago and the average time on study at this writing is 76 months.

In clinically negative-node patients there is no significant difference in total treatment failure (TF) between the TM + R and the RM groups, or between the TM and RM groups, as determined by life-table analyses.[71,117] At 5 years the incidence of distant disease in the three groups, that is, those who had nodes removed, radiated, or unremoved, is similar. Such is the case when distant disease occurring as the first site of treatment failure is used in the comparison or when distant disease regardless of the first site, that is, following local recurrences as well as a first site, is employed. Moreover, the time from operation to the detection of distant disease in either circumstance is not appreciably different between RM and TM + R groups. In fact, that time interval is longer for the TM than for the RM patients. The overall survival of the three clinically negative-node groups does not differ significantly in frequency or in time from operation to death.

In the clinically positive-node patients there is no significant difference between the RM and TM + R groups when they are compared relative to total TF or distant TF. There is no significant difference in survival between the groups. In summary, the findings to date from this NSABP study indicate that variation in local–regional treatment, even leaving positive lymph nodes unremoved, failed to influence the incidence of distant disease or survival.

Complications of importance following primary surgery for breast cancer are infrequent. The severe arm edema and restricted shoulder mobility noted with frequency following radical mastectomy, particularly when accompanied by postoperative radiation, is becoming rare, since that form of treatment is less often employed. Its occurrence following total or segmental mastectomy and axillary dissection is almost never observed. When encountered, it is a minor problem requiring no special consideration. The necrosis of skin edges and the accumulation of fluid in the axilla or under the skin flaps are annoying but not serious. The proper use of postoperative suction technique with elimination of "paper-thin" skin flaps has all but abolished skin necrosis as a major problem. Primary wound healing should occur in almost all cases. The infrequent incidence of surgical complications which has accompanied the abandoment of Halstedian principles of radical mastectomy eliminates that consideration as a factor when deciding upon the operation to be employed.

Segmental Mastectomy

The spectrum of surgical modalities to be considered is completed by local excision, which is aimed at preserving the breast and which has been interchangeably referred to as segmental mastectomy, partial mastectomy, lumpectomy, or tylectomy. There are numerous reports that offer suggestive evidence that partial mastectomy with and without irradiation can be an effective procedure under certain circumstances.

In 1954, Mustakallio of Finland first reported that merely removing the tumor, sparing the breast, and roentgen therapy is a satisfactory method of treatment when lymph nodes cannot be palpated in the axilla or the supraclavicular fossa and the primary tumor is no large than a "hen's egg."[118]

Over the ensuing years, reports by Porritt, Peters and Crile have provided retrospective information regarding the worth of the use of this surgical procedure.[119–123] A prospectively randomized clinical trial of segmental mastectomy has been carried out by Atkins and associates at Guy's Hospital, London, and the results have been reported and will be discussed in the section on Primary Radiation Therapy.

When all of the reports are considered *in toto,* there seems to be evidence to suggest that segmental mastectomy might have a place in the management of a certain group of patients having primary breast cancer and a clinical trial to confirm or repudiate that contention is mandatory.

As a consequence, the NSABP implemented a clinical trial in which patients who have potentially curable breast cancers amenable to segmental mastectomy are randomized and they receive one of three treatments. All patients, whether treated by segmental mastectomy with or without radiation of the breast or by total mastectomy, have an axillary dissection. Patients in all groups with positive axillary nodes receive systemic chemotherapy. Such a trial, in addition to determining whether better cosmesis results, will also provide information regarding the clinical significance of the multicentricity of breast cancers—a theoretical objection to this procedure.

In the NSABP protocol (B-06) patients are eligible if (a) the tumor is confined to the breast and axilla, (b) the tumor size is ≤4 cm, (c) the tumor is movable with no skin involvement, (d) the breast is of sufficient size to allow for acceptable cosmesis, and (e) tumors are in a location favorable for cosmesis, that is, *not* subareolar. At present, over 600 patients have been entered into the trial and certain points regarding the operative management have evolved. The procedure does not require an *en bloc* dissection of the primary tumor and the axillary contents. The tumor is removed with only that amount of normal breast tissue encompassing it to permit the pathologist to determine that the margins of resection are free of tumor. A minimal (~ 1 cm in width) ellipse of skin is removed to provide orientation of the specimen for the pathologist and to encompass the biopsy tract. It is not required that the pectoral fascia be removed with the specimen if the lines of reaction are otherwise free of tumor. The most satisfactory management of the breast following tumor removal is to (a) make no attempt to approximate any tissues in order to completely or partially obliterate the cavity in the breast, (b) insert no drains in the cavity, and (c) close the skin with a continuous subcuticular suture. Pressure dressings are not employed. The axillary dissection is almost always carried out through a separate transverse curvilinear incision following skin creases. Even when tumors are in the upper outer quadrant a separate incision is preferable. The axillary dissection performed is as complete as that which the operator carries out when doing a modified radical mastectomy. Such a dissection removes all of the nodes in at least the two levels of the axilla. The axilla following dissection is drained just as when dissection is carried out with breast operations.

A trial of segmental mastectomy was begun at the National Cancer Institute of Milan, Italy, by Veronesi in 1973.[124] Patients in that study are randomized so they receive either a radical mastectomy or a breast resection (quadrantectomy) with an axillary dissection and radiotherapy of the residual breast. The trial applies to patients classified as T1N0M0, with tumors of less than 2 cm in diameter. The resection of the mammary tissue comprises an entire quadrant of the breast together with the overlying skin and the corresponding portion of the fascial sheet of the pectoralis major muscle. Whenever possible, the axillary dissection is performed *en bloc* and in continuity with the breast quadrantectomy, a procedure that is feasible when the tumor is located in the upper or outer quadrants of the breast or both. For tumors of the lower inner quadrants, the axillary dissection is performed with a separate incision. After surgery the patients receive 6000 rad of radiation to the residual breast tissue over 5 weeks to 6 weeks, starting 15 days after operation. From 1973 to the end of 1975 patients with positive lymph nodes were further randomized, 50% receiving radiotherapy to supraclavicular and internal mammary nodes and 50% having no further treatment. At the beginning of 1976 the program was changed and all N+ cases are now submitted to adjuvant chemotherapy.

Special Surgical Problems

A number of special problems require separate comment. Just as with infiltrating duct carcinoma equal or more confusion exists concerning the management of most of them.

PAGET'S DISEASE OF THE NIPPLE. It has been suggested that treatment of this condition is related to whether or not a mass is palpable in the breast. Nance and associates observed that none of 16 patients without a mass had axillary metastases, whereas axillary metastases were present in 50% when a mass was present.[125] Moreover, none of 21 patients without a mass died of cancer, whereas 18 of 32 with a mass died of cancer within 5 years. While a tumor was difficult to find when no mass was present, it was identified in 20 of 21 patients. In 17, the lesion was noninvasive intraductal carcinoma. Consequently, radical mastectomy was recommended for patients with masses and total mastectomy for those without. On the other hand, Maier and co-workers reported that eight of 56 patients without a mass had positive axillary nodes.[126] Consequently, he advocated radical mastectomy in all patients. Total mastectomy and axillary dissection is the present surgical treatment of Paget's disease—particularly if a mass is present.

INFLAMMATORY CARCINOMA. There is no role for operation in the management of this condition other than to obtain a biopsy so as to establish the diagnosis. The use of radiotherapy in combination with chemotherapy is the treatment of choice. Despite the use of local and systemic treatment the prognosis is poor.

MANAGEMENT OF THE UNINVOLVED BREAST. Another facet of the uncertainty that exists today relative to the proper treatment of clinically curable female breast cancer is that concerned with the management of the contralateral breast that does not simultaneously contain clinically recognizable neoplasm. As far back as 1921, Kilgore estimated that 7% to 10% of women who survive the removal of a first cancer will develop another in their other breast.[127] Over the years, numerous investigators have reported their experiences in that regard. The incidence of asynchronous contralateral breast cancers was found by many to be similar to Kilgore's estimation.[128–132] The risk of developing a cancer in the second breast has been reported as being between four and seven times greater than would be the risk of an initial cancer by an equivalent segment of the general population.[132–135] In a prospective study of primary cancer in the opposite breast, Robbins and Berg showed that following mastectomy there was almost a 1% chance per year that a woman would develop a new cancer in the remaining breast.[132] Results from other sources, however, indicate a lower incidence. Lewison found that only 1.5% of his own private patients developed a second nonsimultaneous primary breast cancer during their lifetime.[130] He refers to a similar experience (1.5%) at the Leningrad Postgraduate Institute (2027 patients). Observations of NSABP patients demonstrated the incidence of such tumors to be only 1.9% in 6 years following mastectomy.

Evidence has been presented to indicate that the incidence of cancer in the contralateral breast may be much greater than previously supposed. A review of available data in that regard relative to lobular carcinoma-*in-situ* will be presented separately. Several of Urban's publications have aroused interest concerning this problem.[25,26] He noted that of 337 women who had undergone biopsy of both breasts (either at time of first or during treatment of a second lesion), 20% of those with all types of infiltrating carcinoma as well as noninfiltrating introductal carcinoma had bilateral tumors. If there exists such a high-risk breast cancer in the opposite breast, it is difficult not to advocate that a prophylactic total mastectomy be carried out simultaneously or shortly after mastectomy on the involved side. At least there would seem to be ample reason for generous random biopsy of the unsuspicious contralateral breast, with treatment then determined after noting the microscopic findings. Although such a procedure seems appealing, a more conservative attitude toward management of the opposite breast seems appropriate. It is difficult to explain the dichotomy between the high incidence of tumors found by random biopsy and the number of patients who develop overt cancers in their contralateral breast. If Urban's findings can be confirmed by others then the findings may be highly suggestive that all cancers do not progress to overt lesions—they may undergo regression. Just as was mentioned elsewhere regarding the multicentricity of breast cancer, other cancers are found much more frequently in pathologic examination than ever become clinically significant.

Conservatism is also recommended for the management of other categories of high-risk patients, that is, those with a family history of breast cancer, those exhibiting certain patterns of mammary dysplasia, and those with hyperplasia and atypia. Only rarely should subcutaneous mastectomy be contemplated in such women.

BREAST BIOPSY AND TWO-STAGE PROCEDURES. The days of taking a patient with an unproven diagnosis of her breast lesion to the operating room, carrying out a biopsy, frozen section, and definitive operative procedure, all at one time, are coming to an end. Such a routine is more related to logistics than to sound medical practice. When a palpable mass is present the diagnosis may be established in most instances by one of the following three procedures carried out on an out-patient basis under local anesthesia. Either cytologic examinations of material removed by thin needle aspiration may be employed, or pathologic examination of fixed tissue removed as a core by a biopsy needle or by excisional biopsy can be done. When the latter is employed, it is mandatory that it be carried out in a facility (preferably hospital) where the removed specimen can be immediately examined and if it is tumor, a portion subjected to proper cryo-preservation for subsequent estrogen receptor determination. Estrogen receptor determination must be carried out on all breast cancers removed. Even when the diagnosis has been established by needle biopsy, it is essential that the tumor be removed for such an analysis prior to proceeding with breast removal and axillary dissection. It has been established that during the course of the operation, as a result of the compromise of the blood supply to the breast (and tumor), a tumor initially positive for estrogen receptor may be converted to negative. Negative needle biopsies may not be accepted as final. In such circumstance, excisional biospy should be carried out.

Only upon having established that the diagnosis is positive is it possible to rationally present to the patient her options for management and to intelligently engage in the dialogue with her which has now become an accepted "way of life." Moreover, such a method of diagnosis provides all who might be concerned with her management time for rational decision making.

BREAST RECONSTRUCTION AFTER MASTECTOMY FOR CANCER

All women undergoing mastectomy for cancer should be made aware of the possibilities for breast reconstruction.[136-142] Though attitudes of individual patients towards the psychologic and cosmetic effects of loss of the breast vary greatly, there are patients who find significant comfort in the possibility of future breast reconstruction.

Prior to undertaking surgery for breast reconstruction, careful discussion of the expectations and motivating factors of the patient should be conducted. It is essential that the patient have realistic expectations of the cosmetic and sensory differences that will exist in the reconstructed breast compared to the original breast. It is often helpful to show the prospective patient photographs of typical as well as good and poor results following breast reconstruction. The possibilities of breast reconstruction should be discussed with the patient prior to undertaking the mastectomy. Horizontal mastectomy incisions tend to be most satisfactory for subsequent reconstruction. Another factor to be considered at the time of mastectomy is whether or not the nipple–areolar complex should be restored.

Considerable flexibility exists as to the timing of breast reconstruction. The breast can be reconstructed at the time of mastectomy for cancer although there is considerably less experience with this technique and the complication rates are higher.[137,139,143] Most plastic surgeons advocate a delay of from 4 months to 6 months from the mastectomy to the reconstruction procedure. This provides adequate time for resolution of skin changes and contractures and is thought to lead to a more secure blood supply to the skin and soft tissue around any subsequent implants. The likelihood of locally recurrent disease has also been a factor in timing the reconstructive procedure because of the increased difficulty in detecting subsequent local chest wall recurrences. The rarity of chest wall recurrences in the absence of nodal disease have led most surgeons to abandon this factor as an important one in selecting patients for breast reconstruction who have no evidence of nodal involvement. While the 4 month to 6 month delay after mastectomy is often considered a minimum, breast reconstruction can be performed at any time thereafter and many patients have had reconstruction as late as 10 years or more after a primary mastectomy.

TYPES OF BREAST RECONSTRUCTION

Many different techniques have been developed for reconstruction of the breast following mastectomy and decisions in any individual patient must be individualized, based on the presence of adequate skin coverage, laxity of skin on the anterior chest wall, the presence of the pectoralis major muscle, the thickness of the skin flaps, and the contour of the opposite breast.

When even small amounts of laxity in the skin over the anterior chest exists, direct implants of inorganic material are the treatment of choice for replacing the breast contour.[136,144-147] Silastic gel implants are the most commonly used and in a recent survey by Cocke, 310 of 419 patients had this type of prosthesis placed.[138] Also available are inflatable prostheses and polyurethane-coated prostheses with Dacron patches, although these latter are infrequently used.[136] Although contour–form types of prostheses are available, these tend not to be as satisfactory as round prostheses in the majority of patients. Prostheses come in a variety of sizes that can be individualized to the patient.

If the anterior chest wall is very tight or if skin changes exist because of radiation, then it is necessary to advance both skin and subcutaneous tissue to the area of the breast using one of a variety of flaps.[136-142] Medially based transverse abdominal flaps can be used to replace or add skin to the central or lower portion of the mastectomy defect. Perforating branches of the deep epigastric artery enter this flap near the medial aspect of the rectus abdominus sheath.

The latissimus dorsi myocutaneous island flap is an effective flap for replacing the bulk lost by removal of the pectoralis major muscle and brings a generous amount of skin to the reconstruction site. Skin in this flap is supplied by muscular perforating vessels from the latissimus dorsi muscle originating from the thoraco–dorsal artery. When adequate skin coverage exists and bulk tissue is required to fill the pectoralis major muscle defect, then latissimus dorsi muscle flaps supplied by the thoraco–dorsal branch of the subscapular artery are useful.

A variety of other types of flaps exist, including local skin transfer from surrounding tissue, reconstructions based on taking part of the opposite breast, and the use of distant skin flaps such as elevation of abdominal tube flaps.[136-138] It is also possible to utilize a flap of greater omentum pedicled on a single gastroepiploic artery and vein covered with a skin graft.[149,150] The exact choice of type of reconstruction to be used requires judgement based on experience and must be individualized for each patient.

It is also sometimes necessary to perform plastic reconstructive procedures on the remaining breast, such as reduction or augmentation mammoplasty, because of significant asymmetry that may exist following reconstruction.

NIPPLE–AREOLAR RECONSTRUCTION

Though the procedures mentioned above can reconstruct the breast mound, reconstruction of the areolar–nipple complex is desired by many women for cosmetic reasons. Preservation of the patient's own areolar–nipple conflex is cosmetically superior to other methods for substituting or reconstructing the areola.[136–138,151] It is possible to transplant the areola at the time of the mastectomy to an area on the lower abdomen where the areola is "banked" for the months between the primary operation and the reconstructive procedure. If this procedure is to be undertaken then it is essential that all possible precautions be taken to ensure that the nipple to be saved is not involved with tumor. If the areolar is to be "banked" then careful frozen section examination of the base of the nipple should be performed prior to transplantation of the nipple to an alternate location. There have been cases reported of cancer in transplated areolae and this procedure does involve some risk.[151–153]

Other procedures for reconstructing the nipple–areolar complex involve the use of labia minora grafts.[154] A semicircle of labia minora can be excised and transferred as full thickness grafts to the de-epithelialized site on the breast eminence. Nipple prominence can be created by using purse string sutures at the desired site of the nipple. Techniques have been devised for partitioning the nipple on the remaining breast and transplanting it to the breast eminence on the opposite side.[136–138,155] This results in little cosmetic defect in the remaining breast. It is also possible to simulate the presence of an areola by tattooing the surface of the breast mound and this method is often satisfactory in recreating the appearance of a nipple.

COMPLICATIONS OF RECONSTRUCTIVE PROCEDURES

A variety of complications accompany attempts at breast reconstruction.[136–142] The presence of skin changes due to previous radiation therapy can substantially increase complication rates and some doctors do not accept patients for reconstruction who have had radiation therapy to the chest wall with any clinical stigmata of radiation injury. Complications of breast reconstruction include hematoma, infections, soft tissue ischemia, skin loss, and prostheses extrusion. Tight or heavy capsules sometimes form around breast implants and secondary procedures may be required to release this capsule.

RADIATION THERAPY OF EARLY BREAST CANCER

In 1895, Roentgen, using a primitive cathode ray tube, discovered a new form of radiation that was able to penetrate various materials and darken photographic plates. Within weeks of Roentgen's discovery, Henri Becquerel demonstrated that some naturally occurring materials, such as uranium compounds, emitted a form of radiation similar to these "x-rays." Three years later, in 1898, Marie and Pierre Curie discovered radium and described its strong radioactive properties. These physicists provided the tools to be used in the radiation therapy of cancer: x-rays created by cathode ray tubes; and gamma rays emitted by radium and other radioactive materials. With surprising speed, these tools were used in the treatment of cancer. Within 1 year after Roentgen reported his discovery, patients with cancer were being treated by x-rays.[156–158] These early workers were limited by the rudimentary roentgen-ray machines available prior to 1920 that were in the range of 120–135 kV compared to greater than 4000 kV used today. Roentgen-rays from these older types of machines have their maximal dose at the skin surface with a rapid fall off into deeper tissues. Typically, these older machines delivered 16% of maximal dose at a depth of 5 cm, in contrast to 81% seen with modern equipment. With the poor penetration of those low-energy roentgen rays, radiation therapy was limited by the dose delivered to the skin, with relative sparing of tumor situated at deeper levels. In addition to the poor penetration seen with older equipment, the doses delivered were poorly measured. As a result, physicians using these treatments had to rely on clinical reactions, particularly skin effects, to judge proper dosage. Despite these severe handicaps, the ability to shrink and, occasionally, locally eradicate breast tumors was demonstrated.

POSTOPERATIVE RADIATION

One of the first major uses of radiation therapy in breast cancer treatment was an ancillary therapy following mastectomy. This use of postoperative radiation was based on two considerations. As previously noted, there is a significant incidence of local–regional relapse following mastectomy, especially if axillary nodes are involved (Table 27-12). A second consideration was that radical mastectomy failed to remove internal mammary nodes, one of the major lymph node drainage areas from the breast. Of 1000 patients with operable breast cancer undergoing internal mammary node biopsy by Handley, 223 showed metastatic spread.[53] Taken together, these results indicate that occult residual cancer frequently remains in the local–regional area following radical mastectomy. It was hoped that postoperative radiation could eliminate this occult residual cancer, and, thereby, improve the survival in those patients without disease spread.

There is now an extensive experience with postoperative radiation, and it has clearly demonstrated that moderate dose radiation can eliminate occult residual deposits of breast cancer. If postoperative radiation is not given, 20% to 25% of patients with positive axillary nodes will relapse in the supraclavicular area. Fletcher, at the M. D. Anderson Hospital, demonstrated that low dose radiation (3000 rad–3500 rad in 4 weeks) reduced supraclavicular relapse in axillary node-positive patients to 7%, while moderate dose radiation (4500 rad–5000 rad in 4 weeks) reduced the relapse rate to 1%.[159] These data stress the importance of adequate dose (4500 rad–5000 rad 5 weeks) in eradicating subclinical disease. The results from the Joint Center for Radiation Therapy also demonstrate the effectiveness of postoperative radiation.[160] During the period July, 1968, through December 1972, 354 patients were referred for postoperative radiation. These patients were referred for a variety of reasons, including spread to axillary lymph nodes, inner or central primary cancers, or because the surgeon was concerned about margins of resection. The overall axillary, supraclavicular, or internal mammary node recurrence rate was 1%, and the chest wall recurrence rate was 5%. These results are significantly less than would be expected in the absence of radiation. Results from a variety of other institutions have also demonstrated that moderate dose radiation significantly reduces the likelihood of local–regional relapse.[161-163]

While postoperative radiation has clearly reduced local–regional relapse, its effect on survival remains controversial. In an attempt to address this question, the NSABP conducted a prospective randomized trial in which patients with early breast cancer were treated by radical mastectomy and were then randomly assigned to postoperative radiation to regional lymph node areas, or to a control group.[164] The results of this study are shown in Table 27-13. Postoperative radiation clearly reduced regional relapse, but there was not a statistically significant improvement in survival. More recently, two additional clinical trials testing the value of postoperative radiation have shown similar results.[161,162] The weight of current evidence supports the conclusion that postoperative radiation, in general, does not significantly improve survival. The current understanding is that the large majority of patients with occult residual local–regional cancer following mastectomy, already have occult distant spread. As a result, while postoperative radiation can eliminate the residual local–regional cancer, it does not prevent the appearance of distant metastases or improve survival.

While postoperative radiation is not of value in unselected patients, further study will be required to determine whether or not there are subsets of patients for whom postoperative therapy is of value. There is preliminary evidence that patients with inner or central primaries, and positive axillary nodes may be such a subset.[105,161] In addition, many physicians feel that for high-risk patients, the prevention of local–regional recurrence is sufficient reason to recommend this treatment. Local–regional recurrence can be a highly distressing occurrence to a patient and, once manifest, is only controlled in 50% to 67% of cases.[165,166]

With the demonstration, however, that moderate-dose radiation could eradicate subclinical disease in the supraclavicular and internal mammary node regions, it was logical to ask whether or not radiation could eradicate disease in the axilla. MacWhirter, from Scotland, was one of the first to combine total mastectomy with radiation to the axillary, internal mammary, and supraclavicular lymph node areas as a substitute for radical mastectomy.[110] That retrospective study and the prospective NSABP study discussed indicate that this combination is a satisfactory alternative to radical mastectomy.

TABLE 27-12. Local Regional Relapse Following Radical Mastectomy

STUDY	PATHOLOGIC STATUS	
	Positive Axillary Nodes	*Negative Axillary Nodes*
Valagussa*	27%	8%
Haagenson⁺	19%	3%
Fisher*	25%	4%
Spratt and Donnegan⁺	26%	6.5%

*Only includes first site of relapse
⁺Does not include supraclavicular relapse

The next logical question to ask is whether or not radiation can be combined with even more conservative surgery (namely, a resection of only the primary tumor in the breast) and still achieve adequate local–regional tumor control. If moderate doses of radiation can eradicate subclinical disease in the supraclavicular, internal mammary, and axillary lymph node areas, it is reasonable to assume it can eradicate subclinical cancer in the breast. This approach of conservative surgery for resection of gross cancer, combined with moderate dose radiation to the breast and draining lymph node regions is what is meant by primary radiation therapy for carcinoma of the breast.

PRIMARY RADIATION THERAPY

The concept of combining conservative surgery with radiation as a substitute for more radical surgery is not new. Geoffrey Keynes, a surgeon at St. Bartholomew's Hospital in London, began to treat patients with operable carcinoma of the breast in this fashion as early as 1924.[167,168] Because of the rudimentary external beam radiation equipment available at that time, Keynes treated patients by radium needle implantation of the breast and draining lymph node areas. A 10-year retrospective review from St. Bartholomew's Hospital was published in 1953.[169] For patients with disease clinically confined to the breast, the 10-year survival rate following simple surgery and radium treatment was 49%, compared to 52% for radical surgery. For patients with clinical spread to axillary nodes, the 10-year survival rate following simple surgery and radium

TABLE 27-13. 5-Year Results from the NSABP Trial Testing the Value of Post Operative Radiation Therapy

HISTOLOGIC AXILLARY NODAL STATUS	RELAPSE-FREE SURVIVAL		REGIONAL RECURRENCES	
	Irradiated Patients	*Controls*	*Irradiated Patients*	*Controls*
Negative	78.6%	76.0%	0%	2.1%
1–3 Positive	49.1%	47.8%	0%	4.5%
4 or More Positive	28.4%	18.0%	1.5%	12.5%

treatment was 27%, compared to 26% for radical surgery. Local–regional control following the more conservative treatment, however, was not as good as following radical surgery. The local–regional recurrence index was 13% with conservative treatment and 6% with radical surgery. Subsequent experience has shown that implantation of large and complex volumes, such as the breast and draining lymph node areas, cannot provide the radiation dose homogeneity required for optimal local–regional control. Implantation is now reserved for boosts to localized areas, following more homogeneous radiation to those larger volumes using high energy external beam radiation.

Two early advocates of conservative surgery combined with radiation were Vera Peters and Sakari Mustakallio. Beginning in 1939, Peters at the Princess Margaret Hospital in Toronto, treated patients with T1 or T2, NO breast cancers with excision and radiation.[120,170] In order to compare her results to those achieved by radical surgery, she performed a matched pair analysis in which each of 184 patients treated by excision and radiation were matched by age, size of primary, and year of treatment to three patients treated by radical mastectomy and radiation. These results carried out to 30 years do not show any significant differences in survival.

Mustakallio, in Helsinki, beginning around 1940, similarly employed simple excision with radiation in patients with clinically negative axillary nodes.[171] The radiation therapy given by Mustakallio is considered inadequate by current standards. Using 180 KV–250 KV equipment, he delivered 2100 rad surface dose in six fractions to the breast and lymph node areas. As a result of this technique, 25% of his patients developed local–regional recurrence by 10 years. Despite this high local recurrence rate, he observed a 5-year survival rate of 79% and a 10-year rate of 61%. In a more recent review of Mustakallio's experience, Rissanen and Holsti retrospectively compared the results of local excision and radiation to radical mastectomy and radiation.[172] They found that the 10-year survival rates were similar for the two treatments in patients with T1 primary tumors, but noted an advantage for the more radical surgery in patients with T2 primary tumors. This advantage is, in part, due to the selection of older patients for the conservative surgery. When the results are analyzed by patient age, as well as T stage (Table 27-14) the only subgroup in which the more radical surgery appears to be of benefit is in patients aged 65 years or greater with T2 primaries.

Based on the findings obtained in retrospective studies such as these, a prospective randomized trial was begun in 1961 at the Guy's Hospital in London by Hedley-Atkins and Hayward. In this trial, patients aged 50 years or greater with T1 or T2, NO or N1 carcinoma of the breast were randomized to either radical mastectomy and postoperative radiation, or wide local resection and post-operative radiation. Between 1961 and 1971, 310 patients entered the trial with 188 undergoing radical mastectomy and 182 undergoing wide local resection. This study has been criticized because of the low doses of radiation delivered. Patients undergoing the conservative operation were treated on a 300 KV machine to the axillary and supraclavicular lymph node areas, and received 2500 rad to 2700 rad in 12 days. The breast, including the internal mammary chain, was treated on a 6 MeV linear accelerator and received 3500 rad to 3800 rad in 3 weeks. While the dose delivered to the breast was close to what is required for control of subclinical disease, the dose to the axilla was extremely low. This is especially true for N1 patients (axillary nodes clinically suspicious), many of whom had gross axillary disease. As a result of these low radiation doses, 22% of patients in the conservatively treated group developed axillary recurrences. In comparison, only 1% of patients treated by radical mastectomy developed axillary recurrences. As noted before, with adequate doses to the axilla, recurrences in that area are uncommon. Of interest is that with the higher dose used to treat the breast, only 5% of patients treated by wide excision and radiation developed recurrence in the residual breast tissue.

The 5-year results from the Guy's Hospital trial were published in 1972, and the updated 10 year results in 1977 (Table 27-15).[173,174] The results are subdivided by whether or not axillary nodes were clinically negative (NO) or positive (N1). For NO patients, there was no significant difference in the incidence of distant metastases or in survival confirming the results seen at 5 years. For N1 patients, there was a slight increase in the incidence of distant metastases in the conservatively treated group, and a decrease in survival. While the previously published 5-year results were statistically significant, the updated 10-year results failed to reach statistical significance.

The results of the Guy's Hospital trial clearly indicate that wide local excision and low dose radiation is not an effective means of obtaining local–regional tumor control. As will be indicated, the results with more modern radiotherapeutic

TABLE 27-14. 10-Year Absolute Survival After Local Excision and Radiation and After Radical Mastectomy and Radiation, by Stage and Patient Age

	$T_1N_0M_0$			$T_2N_0M_0$		
	<50	50–64	≥65	<50	50–64	≥65
RADICAL MASTECTOMY AND RADIATION	92%	69%	29%	76%	59%	43%
LOCAL EXCISION AND RADIATION	89%	73%	35%	67%	57%	20%

(Rissanen PM, Holsti P: A comparison between conservative and radical surgery combined with radiotherapy in the treatment of breast cancer stage I: A 10-year follow-up study on 866 patients. Strahlentherapie 147:370–374, 1974)

TABLE 27-15. 10-Year Results from the Guy's Hospital Trial Comparing Wide Excision and Radiation with Radical Mastectomy and Radiation

	(NO) AXILLARY NODES CLINICALLY NEGATIVE		(N1) AXILLARY NODES CLINICALLY POSITIVE	
	Percent Distant Metastases	*Percent Survival*	*Percent Distant Metastases*	*Percent Survival*
WIDE EXCISION AND RADIATION	44%	52%	65%	30%
RADICAL MASTECTOMY AND RADIATION	46%	58%	60%	43%

(Atkins H, Hayward JL, Kligman DJ: Treatment of early breast cancer: A report after 10 years of a clinical trial. Br Med J 2:427–429, 1972)

techniques and adequate radiation dose provide vastly improved local–regional tumor control. Despite the inadequacies in the radiation treatment, the Guy's Hospital 10-year results actually provide support for the use of conservative treatment, especially in patients with clinically negative axilla, by demonstrating no differences in survival or distant metastases.

Beginning in the early 1960s, a number of institutions in France began treating patients with early breast cancer primarily with radiation. This treatment approach was based on the earlier work of Baclesse, who in the 1930s provided histological evidence of breast cancer eradication following adequate doses of radiation using orthovoltage equipment.[175] With the widespread introduction of megavoltage ^{60}Co and ^{137}Ce units in France in the late 1950s, it became possible to treat patients with improved dose homogeneity and with sparing of the uppermost levels of the skin. The experience from these institutions not only provides long-term results following primary radiation, but also illustrates the importance of certain technical factors involved in this treatment. In 1978, Calle and his associates at the Curie Foundation in Paris published their results on 154 patients with operable breast cancer.[176] The treatment protocol at the Curie Foundation depended on the clinical stage of the cancer. If the primary tumor was 3 cm or less, and no suspicious axillary nodes were present, patients were treated by lumpectomy followed by radiation. If the primary tumor was greater than 3 cm, or if suspicious axillary nodes were present, the diagnosis was confirmed by needle biopsy and treatment was given exclusively with external beam radiation. For patients treated by lumpectomy and radiation, the absolute survival, without evidence of disease, was 85% at 5 years and 75% at 10 years. The local–regional recurrence rate in this group was 13% at 5 years, and only 2% of patients had poor cosmetic results. In contrast, the results achieved by exclusive radiation were less satisfactory. 234 of 394 patients (59%) required secondary surgery either for persistent or recurrent disease. In addition, with the higher doses of radiation required to treat gross disease, the cosmetic result was not as good. Only 38% of patients had good to excellent cosmetic results, and 17% had poor results. Salvage of radiation failures by mastectomy was good, so that survival in this group did not appear to be compromised. The experience from the Curie Foundation provides long-term support for the efficacy of conservative surgery combined with radiation, but indicates that lumpectomy is important for maximizing initial local tumor control. Similar 10-year results have also been reported by Amalric and associates at the Marseilles Cancer Institute, France.[177]

Pierquin and co-workers at the Henri Mondor Hospital in France recently published their experience with primary radiation therapy in 177 patients with operable breast cancer.[178] The policy in this series of patients regarding the extent of surgery was similar to that at the Curie Foundation. Only those patients with primary tumors less than 3 cm underwent lumpectomy. Of note in this series, however, was the routine use of interstitial implantation. Treatment was begun in all patients using megavoltage ^{60}Co; 4500 rad in 5 weeks was delivered to the entire breast and draining lymph node areas, and booster doses were delivered to the axillary and internal mammary lymph node areas. An additional 2500 rad to 3700 rad was then delivered to the primary tumor site by interstitial implantation. Fig. 27-4 is a schematic illustration of the radiation doses obtained with interstitial implantation, and demonstrates the high dose of radiation that can be localized to a tumor-bearing volume in the breast, with relative sparing of nearby normal tissues, such as lung and skin. In addition to this advantage in dose distribution, it has also been hypothesized that the constant, low dose-rate radiation delivered with interstitial implantation may have a greater antitumor effect than the intermittent, high dose-rate radiation given with external beam treatment. Pierquin and colleagues chose to use ^{192}Ir as the source for interstitial radiation because of its effective energy (340 keV), half life (74.5 days), and convenience of administration. Using this technique, they observed a 5% 5-year local–regional recurrence rate in T1 tumors, and an 8% rate in T2 tumors. In addition, overall survival and relapse-free survival at 5 years was comparable to that for similarly staged patients treated by radical surgery at that institution. These results suggest that the use of interstitial implantation is an important technique for optimizing local tumor control.

Beginning in 1973, a prospective randomized clinical trial testing the value of primary radiation therapy-segmented mastectomy was begun at the National Cancer Institute of Italy at Milan. In this trial, women with primary tumors less than 3 cm and clinically negative axillary nodes were randomized to either radical mastectomy or to conservative treatment consisting of a wide local resection and full axillary

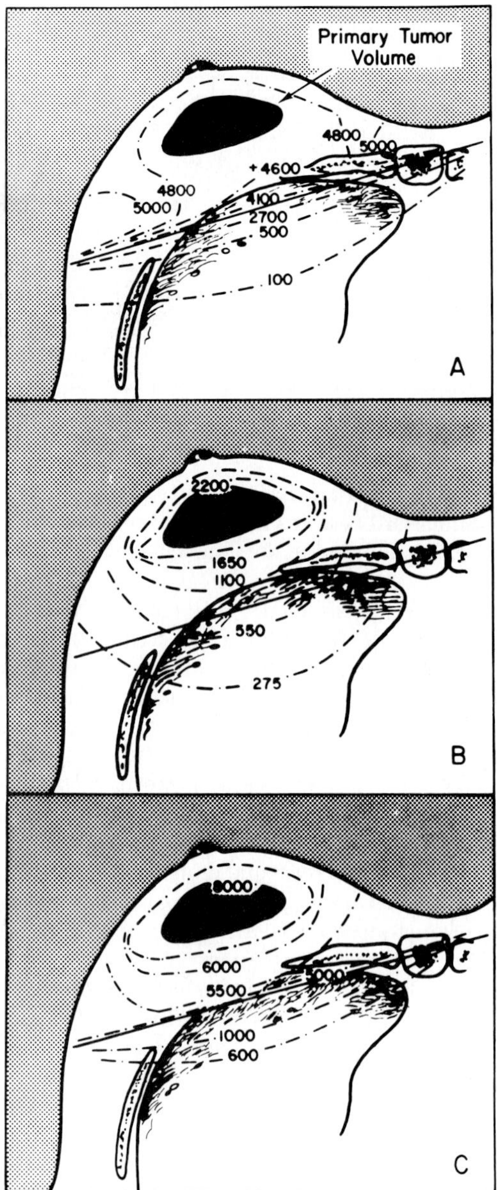

FIG. 27-4. Dose distribution for Joint Center for Radiation Therapy technique for *A*, external beam radiation; *B*, interstitial implantation; *C*, composite both techniques.

dissection, followed by radiation. The radiation consisted of 5000 rad to the residual breast tissue and a 1000 rad boost using orthovoltage to the region of the primary. As of November, 1979, 330 patients were randomized to the conservative treatment and 328 to radical mastectomy. Four patients treated conservatively had developed local–regional recurrence, compared to seven patients treated by radical mastectomy. In this preliminary report, the actuarial probability of survival and relapse-free survival (Fig. 27-5) were comparable for the two treatments.[179]

More recently, a large number of institutions in this country have begun to treat women with early breast cancer with primary radiation therapy.[180–183] The experience at The Joint Center for Radiation Therapy is representative of these recent studies, and illustrates the results that can be obtained.[184] This experience includes 176 consecutive patients with UICC Stage I and II carcinoma of the breast treated between July, 1968 and December, 1977. Eight of these patients had a contralateral breast cancer treated for a total of 184 breasts treated by primary radiation therapy. In all cases, microscopic examination revealed invasive carcinoma. Patients were initially referred for treatment if they refused mastectomy or were considered medically unfit for surgery. Later in the series, patients were referred because of physican or patient preference. Follow-up ranged from 12 months to 117 months with a median of 33 months. The details of the therapy have been described previously.[185]

In presenting these results, we have principally directed our attention to local–regional control rates, because this is the primary objective of local–regional treatment. Since the majority of local–regional failures occur in the first 2 years to 3 years following treatment, these results are considered a good indication of the eventual control rates to be obtained. Of the 184 breast cancers treated, 11 (6%) have had local–regional recurrence. Three of 62 (5%) Stage I cancers recurred locally, while eight of 122 (7%) Stage II recurred locally. Ten of the failures occurred in the breast alone and one occurred in the breast and axilla.

The role of attempted excisional biopsy and interstitial implantation on local–regional recurrence control is considered in Table 27-16. The use of interstitial implantation was associated with a statistically significant improvement in local–regional control ($p < 0.05$, by the 2-tail Fisher Exact test). One of 73 patients (1%) treated by interstitial implantation developed a local recurrence, compared to ten of 111 patients (9%) in whom implantation was not performed. Local–regional control was better in patients having an excisional biopsy compared to patients having less than an excisional biopsy, but the number of patients failing to have

FIG. 27-5. Prospective randomized trial comparing radical mastectomy with conservative surgery and radiation from the National Cancer Institute in Milan. (Veronesi U: The value of limited surgery for breast cancer (in press))

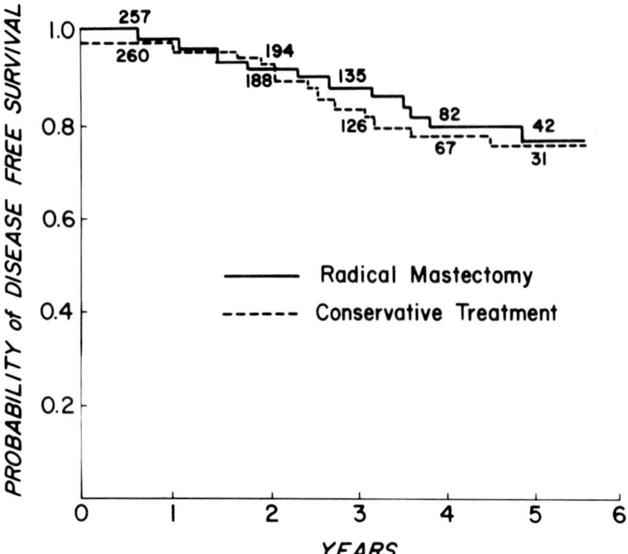

excisional biopsy was small, and the difference in control did not reach statistical significance ($p = .08$). These results corroborate the findings from both Paris groups by demonstrating the importance of both excisional biopsy and interstitial implantation in maximizing local tumor control.

The actuarial 5-year survival rate in this group of patients was 94% for Stage I and 73% for Stage II. While 10 year to 15 year survival rates are required in carcinoma of the breast, these preliminary results are comparable to those seen following mastectomy in similarly staged patients.

While the local control rates in this series are encouraging, local control is not the sole criterion for judging the success of primary radiation therapy. If primary therapy is to be a useful alternative to surgery for early carcinoma of the breast, radiation therapy must not only provide local control rates comparable to surgery, but must also achieve good cosmetic results. Cosmetic evaluation revealed that 66% of treated breasts were judged good or excellent by physician evaluation, and 88% were judged good or excellent by the patients themselves.[186] Three principal treatment factors were identified that influenced the cosmetic outcome: (1) the extent and location of the biopsy procedure; (2) the time–dose factors of the radiation therapy, and (3) the technique of the radiation therapy. Cosmetic results were adversely affected when the biopsy procedure included a wide resection of breast tissue, or when the biopsy scar was obvious. Increasing doses of external beam radiation above 4500 rad to 5000 rad in 5 weeks were associated with greater degrees of retraction and fibrosis of the treated breast. All patients in this series were treated using megavoltage equipment and permanent skin changes secondary to treatment were infrequent. The use of interstitial implantation was not found to diminish the cosmetic outcome. Figure 27-6 shows cosmetic results that are typical of those seen following primary radiation therapy.

In our experience, external beam radiation for breast cancer is well tolerated, with mild fatigue being the most common side-effect. These treatments are given 5 days a week for approximately 5 weeks. Each treatment takes 15 minutes to 20 minutes, with the majority of that time spent on patient set-up. Patients rarely complain of nausea, and cranial hair loss is not seen. At the end of 5 weeks, patients may develop local skin changes varying from dry desquamation and erythema, to areas of moist desquamation. These changes are transient, and they clear within 1 week to 3 weeks. Interstitial implantation is usually performed under general anesthesia, and remains in place for approximately 2 days to 3 days. Following recuperation from the anesthesia, patients are up and about their room and, typically, do not require analgesics. Late reactions in the irradiated volume can occur in the months following treatment. The most common reaction was rib fractures, which occurred in ten of the 184 cases (5%). Five patients (3%) developed a non-productive cough and mild shortness of breath, and chest x-ray films showed evidence of radiation pneumonitis. In all cases, these symptoms were self-limited and did not require hospitalization. Other transient reactions include one patient who developed a pleural effusion following treatment and another patient with paresthesias in her ipsilateral arm. In three patients, more significant side effects occurred. One patient developed

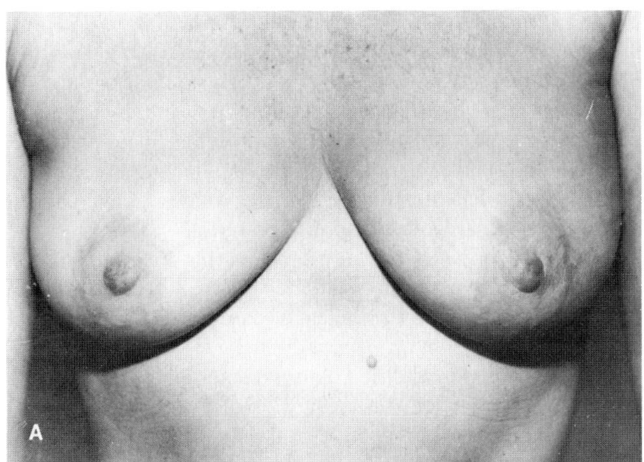

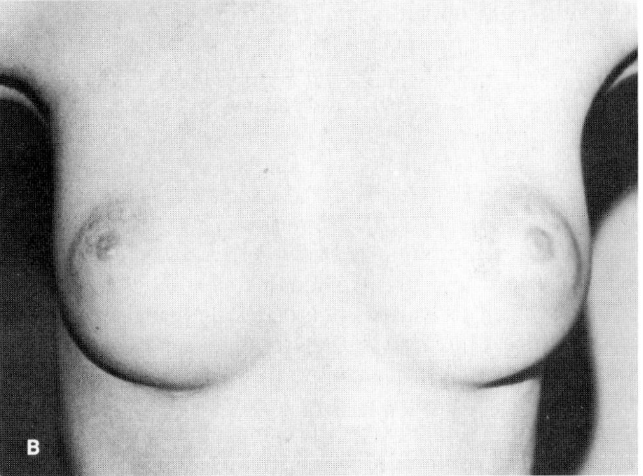

FIG. 27-6. Cosmetic results following primary radiation therapy. *A*, This patient had a tumor of the left breast four years before the photograph. *B*, This patient had a tumor of the right breast four years before the photograph.

TABLE 27-16. Local–Regional Recurrence Related to Biopsy Procedures and Interstitial Implantation (JCRT series)

	IMPLANTATION	NO IMPLANTATION	TOTAL
EXCISIONAL BIOPSY	1/63	7/103	8/166 (5%)
LESS THAN EXCISIONAL BIOPSY	0/10	3/8	3/18 (17%)
TOTAL	1/73 (1%)	10/111 (9%)	11/184 (6%)

marked fibrosis in her treated supraclavicular region and persistent motor weakness in her ipsilateral arm. Another patient developed significant arm edema and a venogram revealed partial obstruction of her innominate vein. The third patient who presented with a synchronous bilateral breast cancer, developed radiation pericarditis following mediastinal irradiation of her internal mammary nodes. This patient required a pericardiectomy, but is now well.

One of the possible complications of this treatment is the induction of tumors in the irradiated volume. While radiation has been clearly identified as a carcinogen, the risk of carcinogenesis following therapeutic levels of radiation has not been adequately defined. A full discussion of this topic is beyond the scope of this review, except to mention two considerations: (1) the dose of radiation, and (2) the age at the time of exposure. The likelihood of tumor induction following therapeutic doses of radiation can *not* be extrapolated from estimates following lower doses of radiation. This is discussed in the chapter on principles of radiation therapy.

In a large Massachusetts study examining the risk of breast cancer in women following repeated fluoroscopic examinations of the chest, there was no increased risk seen for women 30 years of age or older, while a 3.8-fold increased risk was observed for women aged 15 years to 19 years.[87] Similar findings were noted in another fluoroscopic study from Nova Scotia.[188] In a follow-up of women treated at the Radiumhemmet in Sweden for various non-neoplastic conditions of the breast, a 4-fold increase in the breast cancer risk was seen. For women aged 34 or less, the risk was 7.1-times greater than expected, while for women aged 35 or greater, the risk was 2.2-fold.[77] Similarly, the data from the atom bomb experience in Japan indicated an increase in breast cancer in exposed women, but that this risk was significantly greater for younger women.[76]

The available data regarding the risk of tumor induction following radiation for carcinoma of the breast suggests that this risk is small. As noted before, primary radiation therapy for breast cancer was first begun as early as the 1930s, and there have not been any reported second malignancies following this treatment. The experience with postoperative radiation is even more extensive, and with greater follow-up. In a study from Ontario, Canada, the risk of developing a contralateral breast cancer was not increased in patients who received postoperative radiation as compared to unirradiated patients.[189] Soft tissue and bone sarcomas have been seen following postoperative radiation. In a 50-year review of records from the Memorial Hospital in New York City, there were nine cases of sarcomas following radiation for breast cancer.[190] The total number of irradiated patients is not given, although it was common practice for many years at that institution to deliver postoperative radiation in all patients with positive nodes. For comparison, over a similar time span at the Columbia–Presbyterian Hospital, a total of 18 cases of lymphangiosarcoma of the ipsilateral arm were seen as a consequence of radical mastectomy.[191] Here too, the total number of patients at risk is not available, so that the likelihood of developing this complication cannot be calculated. For the most part, however, lymphangiosarcoma has been considered a rare complication, and was not felt to be a contraindication to radical mastectomy.

At the present time, the risk of carcinogenesis following therapeutic doses of radiation for carcinoma of the breast has not been fully clarified, although present evidence suggests this risk is small.

The use of adjuvant chemotherapy following radiation therapy can follow the same guidelines used for patients undergoing mastectomy. These will be discussed below. Patients considered for adjuvant chemotherapy now undergo an axillary sampling prior to treatment. This sampling provides histologic confirmation of axillary node involvement currently required for the use of adjuvant chemotherapy. Review of experience with 177 patients undergoing this procedure has been recently reported.[192] In most cases, a separate incision in the axilla is preferred. Lymph nodes from level one, and sometimes level two, are removed, and typically about ten nodes are recovered. This type of axillary sampling is a useful procedure with minimal morbidity in those patients for whom adjuvant chemotherapy is contemplated. The timing of chemotherapy and radiation is currently under review.

In most patients with early breast cancer, an excisional biopsy is performed for pathologic confirmation of the diagnosis, and for determination of hormone receptor status. At this point, the various options regarding local treatment are discussed with the patient. If a patient decides on a course of primary radiation therapy, and an axillary sampling is indicated, it is convenient and feasible to perform axillary sampling and interstitial implantation of the breast under the same anesthesia. In these patients, the external beam portion of the treatment follows the interstitial implant. Chemotherapy, for the most part, has been used following completion of the radiation. More recently, in some cases, chemotherapy has been started prior to institution of radiation. Further study will be required to determine the optimal sequencing of the radiation and chemotherapy.

The last two decades have seen considerable evolution in breast cancer treatment and, at present, there is uncertainty and controversy regarding the optimal treatment of this disease. Both from a conceptual and practical point of view, breast cancer treatment can be divided into (1) local–regional treatment to the breast and draining lymph node areas, and (2) systemic treatment for metastatic spread. Mastectomy has been the traditional form of local–regional treatment and has provided local–regional tumor control in 85% to 90% of cases. Initially, radiation was used following mastectomy. While this experience with postoperative radiation has not been shown to be of survival value in unselected patients, it has clearly demonstrated that moderate doses of radiation can eradicate subclinical deposits of breast cancer. Further study is required to identify whether or not there are subsets of patients in whom postoperative radiation is of value. Primary radiation therapy is an alternative to mastectomy that combines conservative surgery for removal of gross disease with moderate doses of radiation for control of subclinical disease. Recent results with this treatment have shown local–regional tumor control that is comparable to that achieved by mastectomy. Effective tumor control with radiation depends on the removal of gross disease by surgery and the use of adequate doses and technique of radiation. A booster dose to the involved quadrant of the breast is required for optimal results, and this can be satisfactorily delivered by an interstitial implant. Cosmetic results following primary radiation are typically good to excellent but, here again, the technique of the surgery and radiation are crucial. Survival results at 5 years and 10 years from a number of retrospective studies are also comparable to surgical results. Side-effects from treatment are minimal when good technique is employed, but longer experience will be required to judge more fully any late effects of this treatment. The use of adjuvant chemotherapy, for control of metastatic disease, can be combined with primary radiation therapy. Patients considered for adjuvant chemotherapy currently undergo an axillary sampling prior to radiation in order to judge the need for adjuvant chemotherapy. The sequencing of these various modalities of treatment is currently under review.

TREATMENT OF LOCALLY ADVANCED BREAST CANCER (STAGE III)

Locally advanced carcinoma of the breast refers to those breast carcinomas with significant primary of nodal disease, but where distant metastases cannot be documented. This group of breast cancers has been shown to be poorly managed by radical surgery alone and to have a poor prognosis. Any T3b–T4, N2 or N3–M0 lesion is now regarded as locally advanced inoperable breast cancer. T3a, N0 or N1, M0 cancers are included in the UICC Stage III, because of their poor prognosis, but are generally considered operable.

Following Halsted's popularization of the radical mastectomy at the turn of the century, the operation was performed without an understanding as to which patients were being benefited by its use. Haagensen and Stout reviewed the records of patients undergoing radical mastectomy at the Presbyterian Hospital between 1915 and 1942, and identified various clinical features that were associated with high local recurrence rates and poor survival.[193] Table 27-17 lists those clinical features that they considered categorically inoperative by virtue of local recurrence rates greater than 50% and no 5-year clinical cures. Those features form the basis for classifying patients as Columbia Clinical Class D, or inoperable. In addition, they identified five grave signs that were associated with a somewhat increased likelihood of local recurrence and poor survival (Table 27-18). While a single grave sign was not necessarily felt to indicate inoperability, in the presence of any two grave signs, 42% developed local recurrence and only 1 (2%) was free of disease at 5 years. The presence of a single grave sign forms the basis of Columbia Clinical Class C, while patients with two or more grave signs are included in class D.

Because of this high incidence of local–regional recurrence with surgical treatment, radiation therapy, either alone or in conjunction with surgery, has come to play a major role in this stage of the disease. For radiation therapy to be effective in controlling these locally advanced cancers, however, doses greater than those used in early stage tumors are required. While 5000 rad has been shown to be effective in eradicating microscopic amounts of tumor, doses in excess of 6000 rad are required for gross tumor. Francois Baclesse was one of the first to show that tumor control was achievable using sufficiently high radiation doses.[175] In a more recent study,

TABLE 27-17. Clinical Features of Breast Cancer Associated with Poor Results Following Radical Mastectomy

CLINICAL FEATURE	NUMBER OF PATIENTS	PERCENT LOCAL RECURRENCE	5-YEAR PERCENT CLINICAL CURE
Extensive Edema of Skin Over Breast	51	61%	0
Satellite Nodules	7	57%	0
"Inflammatory" Carcinoma of the Breast	25	60%	0
Distant Metastases	10	20%	0
Parasternal or Supraclavicular Node Mets	16	56%	0
Edema of the Arm	4	50%	0

(Haagensen CD: Diseases of the Breast, rev 2nd ed. Philadelphia, WB Saunders, 1971, p 623)

TABLE 27-18. Grave Signs of Breast Cancer

CLINICAL FEATURE	NUMBER OF PATIENTS	PERCENT LOCAL RECURRENCE	5-YEAR PERCENT CLINICAL CURE
Edema of the skin of the breast (less than one-third)	75	32%	23%
Skin ulceration	14	14%	36%
Solid fixation of the tumor to the chest wall	20	40%	5%
Axillary lymph node greater than 2.5 cm	24	13%	38%
Fixed axillary nodes	8	13%	13%

(Haagensen CD: Diseases of the Breast, rev 2nd ed. Philadelphia, WB Saunders, 1971, pp 625–628)

Fletcher and Montague administered 6000 rad in 8 weeks and obtained local control in 72% of patients with inoperable breast cancers.[196]

In a recent review at the Joint Center for Radiation Therapy the results of primary radiation therapy in 116 patients with locally advanced cancers were analyzed.[197] The 5-year actuarial probability of local tumor control for all 116 patients was 64%. In patients who had either an excisional biopsy or an interstitial implant, local control was 77% and 76% respectively. For the seven patients who had both excisional biopsy and implantation, no local failures were seen. In contrast, patients having neither an excisional biopsy nor an implant had local control in only 41%. When local control was examined according to total dose delivered, patients receiving more than 6000 rad had a local control rate of 78% compared to 39% for patients receiving less than 6000 rad. These results stress the importance of adequate doses of radiation in controlling locally advanced cancer, and indicate that excisional biopsy and interstitial implantation, when feasible, facilitate local control in these patients. In addition, the local control results obtained in patients receiving 6000 rad or greater are comparable to those for patients treated by combined mastectomy and irradiation, suggesting that mastectomy may not be required for optimal treatment. Table 27-19 outlines a local treatment program for Stage III carcinoma of the breast.

Despite this reasonable level of local control, achieved by high dose radiation therapy, the prognosis for these patients is not good. Of the 118 patients treated at the JCRT, the 5-year actuarial relapse-free survival was only 22%, stressing the high likelihood of occult distant metastases and the need for effective systemic therapy in order to improve survival. Of note in the JCRT scores was that 26 patients received adjuvant combination chemotherapy and their 5-year relapse-free survival was 51%. This was compared to a 5-year relapse-free survival of 29% for a group of patients who did not receive chemotherapy and were matched by stage, age, and year of treatment.

The first major study to test the value of adjuvant chemotherapy in locally advanced breast cancers was from the National Cancer Institute, Milan, Italy, and failed to show a significant benefit.[198] In this prospective randomized clinical trial, patients with T3b or T4 breast cancer were treated with four cycles of adriamycin and vincristine (AV) followed by supervoltage radiation therapy (RT); 6000 rad in 6 weeks was delivered to the breast with an additional 1000 rad to the area of residual tumor. Patients achieving a complete response (CR) following this combined treatment were then randomized to no further therapy or six more cycles of chemotherapy.

AV produced objective responses in 89% of patients (complete in 16%, partial in 55% and improvement in 19%). At the end of RT, 81 of 98 patients (83%) responding to AV were classified as having achieved CR. Despite this substantial improvement in CR rate, the 3-year survival rate was only 53%, not substantially different than the survival rate seen in a previous study of patients treated at that institution by RT alone. In addition, they found that a substantial percentage of patients had either recurrence or persistent disease in the breast.

In a subsequent trial from Milan, patients with locally advanced breast cancer were treated with three cycles of AV, then randomized to either RT or radical mastectomy (RM) and followed by additional AV. The results at 3 years failed to show a difference between the two treatment arms, although patients treated by RM had a somewhat better local control rate than those treated by RT. The local control rate was 73% for RM and 59% for RT ($p = 0.36$), the relapse-free survival rate was 39% for RM and 27% for RT ($p = 0.42$), and the overall survival rate was 61% for RT and 59% for RM ($p = 0.66$). Once again these results were not appreciably better than those achieved by RT alone, and indicated the failure of this drug program to prevent relapse in this group of patients.

Despite the failure of this specific drug program to improve survival, it is clear that some form of effective systemic therapy is required for improved results in this group of patients. At this time significant questions remain to be answered. Should treatment be started with systemic therapy, local therapy, or both, simultaneously. Should local therapy be RT, surgery, or a combination of the two? Further studies

TABLE 27-19. Guidelines for the Local and Regional Management of Advanced Carcinoma of the Breast (JCRT)

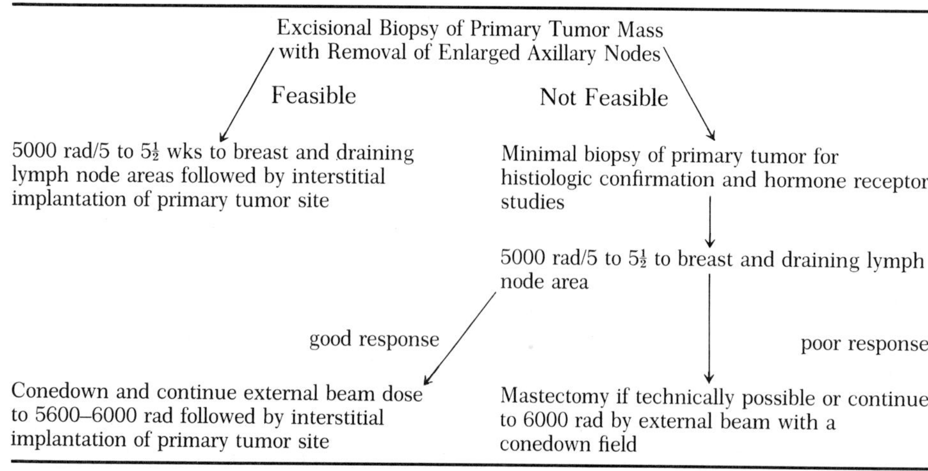

using more effective forms of systemic therapy will be required to provide answers to these questions.

SYSTEMIC THERAPY OF BREAST CANCER

Systemic therapy of breast cancer has evolved to an increasing state of complexity and, in some instances, controversy. Because of the advances in cytotoxic and hormonal therapy over the past 10 years, the clinician is confronted with expanding lists of available treatments including newer antihormonal agents and combination chemotherapy regimens.

Human breast cancer is a heterogenous tumor with widely disparate patterns of growth and metastatic spread. As such, the impact of the therapy on survival is difficult to assess. Lacking an ideal therapy for all patients, the timing, selection, and intensity of hormonal cytotoxic therapy is gauged according to the clinical stage, extent of disease, and biochemical information as to hormonal dependency. However, substantive therapeutic advances have achieved broad acceptance only in the setting of a controlled clinical trial.

HORMONE RECEPTORS

Cytoplasmic proteins act as receptors which bind and transfer the appropriate steroid molecule into nuclei to exert specific hormonal function. The clinically most important and most widely measured is the estrogen receptor protein (ERP). The binding capacity is expressed as femtomoles of ^{3}H-estradiol bound per mg of cytosol protein.[200,201] Values above 10 femtomoles/mg are considered positive while <3 femtomoles/mg is receptor negative.[202] Values in between are borderline. About 50% of all primary tumors are ERP-positive, with a slightly lower percent positivity in metastatic lesions.[203] The extent of positivity is proportional to the degrees of differentiation and the histologic subtype. Approximately 90% or more of well-differentiated ductal tumors and lobular carcinomas are ERP positive. Infiltrating ductal carcinoma is the most common type of breast tumor and is ERP positive in 60% to 70% of cases. Tumors with extensive lymphocytic infiltration tend to have a lower incidence of ERP (30%–50%).[204]

Premenopausal patients have a lower incidence of ERP-positive tumors (30%) compared to 60% in the postmenopausal period. The perimenopausal tumors have the lowest rate (<20%).[205] Sequential studies of ERP in the same patients will usually reveal no significant change in the absence of hormonal therapy, but biopsies of multiple metastatic sites will have a concordance of about 85%. Visceral lesions, especially hepatic metastases, tend to have the lowest ERP values.[206] ERP-negative tumors tend to have higher proliferative activity with a higher tritiated thymidine incorporation index than ERP-positive tumors.[207] This higher mitotic activity associated with ERP-negative tumors is reflected in the fact that ERP-negative cancers tend to relapse sooner than the ERP-positive.[202] Stage I ERP-negative tumors have a prognosis equivalent to or worse than ERP-positive Stage II tumors.[208,209]

Response to hormonal therapy of any type is correlated with the incidence and quantity of ERP. The prior administration of cytotoxic chemotherapy does not influence the ERP content.[205] The rate of response to hormonal treatment in ERP-positive tumors is 50% to 60% and less than 10% in ERP-negative tumors. Refractoriness to prior hormonal therapy can be correlated with a decrease in the ERP, suggesting the emergence of hormonally independent cell lines.[203] The accuracy of ERP as a predictor of subsequent chemotherapy response has been debated. Conflicting reports had the response to chemotherapy correlating with ERP-positive or negative status of the primary tumor.[210,211] At the present time the available information suggests that the ERP does not predict subsequent response to drug therapy.[212] Progesterone receptors (PRP) have been found in about 40% of ERP-positive tumors. Both receptors are found in 46% of cases, with a response rate to hormonal therapy of 77% when both receptors are present. About 20% to 50% are ERP-positive, PRP-negative, and this group has a poorer response to hormonal therapy (20%–30%).[213] Despite the presence of the cytosol receptor for estrogen, at least 40% of patients fail to respond to hormonal treatment. Defects in translocation of cytosol-receptor–estradiol-complex to the nucleus might explain the failure. Nuclei isolated from ERP-positive tumors failed to take up estrogen from the complex in 20% of tumors. In borderline ERP tumors the incidence is 34% and in ERP-negative tumors it reaches 87%.[214] The standard assay for estrogen receptor is the dextran-coated charcoal method. It compares favorably with sucrose gradient centrifugation assay. The latter demonstrates the 8S molecular type of ER which is a characteristic feature of the receptor. The charcoal method permits assay of more specimens, since the sucrose density method is limited because of the centrifugation time.[215]

HORMONAL THERAPY

Castration

Bilateral oophorectomy in premenopausal women was one of the earliest forms of systemic therapy for advanced breast cancer. In patients whose tumors are estrogen-dependent the procedure can be expected to induce a regression lasting 9 months to 12 months. In unselected series almost 30% to 40% of patients will respond. However, the results are considerably better in those with ERP-positive tumors (50% to 60%). Radiation (2000 rad) castration gives comparable results but can take up to 2 months for an effect. Prophylactic castration following mastectomy does not decrease the potential relapse rate or prolong the survival of those who relapse. When performed as an adjuvant, it deprives the assessment of endocrine responsiveness which, in the absence of ERP data, is the only criterion to determine subsequent endocrine treatment. There are a number of clinical criteria which correlate with response to oophorectomy and, by inference, with hormonal dependency. A prolonged disease-free interval, in excess of 2 years, has been thought to predict for response to hormonal treatment, although one large series showed no difference in disease-free interval between responders and non-responders.[216] The metastatic sites likely to respond to oophorectomy and parenthetically to all other hormonal treatments include bone, soft tissue, lymph nodes, and lung. Metastases in liver and brain rarely respond.[217]

Of those who show a response to oophorectomy, the likelihood of subsequent response to another hormonal modality, either ablative surgery or hormonal agents, is in the range of 40% to 50%.[218] Patients responding to a succession of hormonal treatment have historically survived longer than non-responders by 20 months to 24 months.

Hypophysectomy–Adrenalectomy

In 1952 Huggins demonstrated that adrenalectomy could induce regression of metastatic breast cancer.[219] At about the same time, Luft and co-workers introduced surgical hypophysectomy.[220] Both procedures further reduced estrogen production in the castrated or postmenopausal women.

Adrenalectomy has a general response rate of 30% to 40% in most series.[221] The response in previous oophorectomy responders or those with ERP-positive tumors is closer to 50%. As with oophorectomy, responses are seen primarily in those with osseous and soft tissue metastases, although a single visceral site such as lung or pleura is also likely to respond with equal frequency (30% to 40%).[222] Multiple visceral metastases or a single visceral site with bone and soft tissue involvement have a response rate between 20% and 30%. The disease-free interval >2.5 years is generally associated with a higher response rate (50%) as opposed to 30% for those <2.5 years. There is no advantage to premenopausal women in performing adrenalectomy–oophorectomy as a single combined procedure over the sequence of oophorectomy followed by adrenalectomy, even though the response rate to the combined operation is superior to oophorectomy alone.[223] The same authors compared adrenalectomy to primary additive hormone therapy in postmenopausal women. Although the response rate was significantly better with the former (38.6% >20%), the median survival of the groups was similar. This and other comparative studies of hormonal therapy should ideally be stratified according to prognostic criteria for hormonal response or ERP if available. Contraindications to adrenalectomy include metastatic disease to the CNS or liver, advanced lymphangitic pulmonary metastases and a disease-free interval of less than 18 months.[224,225] Replacement therapy for adrenalectomized patients is 50 mg to 70 mg cortisone per day by mouth with 0.1 mg of fluorohydrocortisone. Some patients may malabsorb prednisone and thus cortisone may be necessary.

Hypophysectomy is the ablative procedure alternative to adrenalectomy. The response by way of the transphenoidal approach is about 40%, rising to 65% in patients with ERP-positive tumors. In the postmenopausal state, the response is higher in those who are 10 years or longer from menopause.[226] Replacement therapy, consisting of cortisone 25 mg twice a day and 120 mg of thyroid, is required. Diabetes insipidus, which usually will develop, requires replacement therapy with posterior pituitary hormone.[227]

The completeness of pituitary ablation can be assessed by measurement of basal or stimulated blood levels of pituitary derived polypeptide hormones.[228,229] Levels of follicle stimulating luteinizing hormones and thyrotropin releasing factor–stimulated thyrotropin and prolactin were measured prior to, and following, hypophysectomy. Prolactin levels remained normal following surgery but were stimulated to high levels by thyroid releasing factor in transphenoidal patients. Incomplete ablation of pituitary function as measured by residual circulating polypeptides does not preclude an antitumor response. Transfrontal hypophysectomy appears to offer a more complete hormonal ablation, but not greater antitumor effect than the transphenoidal approach. Hypophysectomy proved to be effective in 40% of patients who had become refractory to previous anti-estrogen therapy. The converse situation also applies; that is, response to antiestrogens by previous responders to hypophysectomy who have measurable levels of serum estrogens. At the present time, the response to hypophysectomy and adrenalectomy are equivalent in postmenopausal women. Prospective comparisons have been rare and have not been performed according to ERP status. A comparison of transphenoidal hypophysectomy with medical adrenalectomy with aminoglutethimide demonstrated a superiority for the latter.[230] The further reduction of plasma estrogens by adding aminoglutethimide to previously hypophysectomized patients underlies the problem of incomplete ablation.

Hormone Profile as a Discriminant Function

Prior to the availability of the estrogen receptor assay, the only biochemical estimate available to predict response to adrenal or pituitary ablation was measurement of urinary steroids. The results of those investigations postulated a higher response rate in those who excrete more urinary androgen metabolites.

The Bulbrook discriminant was based on a calculation in turn based on urinary 17-hydroxycorticoids and etiocholanolone (80–80 [17-hydroxycorticoids mg/24 hrs.] + etiocholanolone μgm/24 hrs.). Patients who excrete large amounts of etiocholanolone relative to 17-hydroxycorticoids have a positive discriminant.[231] A prospective analysis revealed that the discriminant did not reproducibly predict for response to adrenalectomy and was clearly inferior to the ERP assay.[232]

Medical Adrenalectomy

Although 30% to 40% of previously castrated women respond to surgical adrenalectomy, it is not without associated morbidity and mortality and permanent dependence on hormone replacement.

Aminoglutethimide, first developed as an anticonvulsant, is a compound capable of inhibiting adrenal steroid production. It suppresses *de novo* adrenal steroid synthesis by inhibiting the first step in the metabolic pathway, the conversion of cholesterol to pregnenolone (Table 27-20). The inhibition is less than complete, however, for Δ4 type of steroids such as testosterone, progesterone, 17 α-hydroxyprogesterone, dihydrotestosterone, and androstenedione.[233] The last is especially important since the adrenal gland secretes no estrogens *per se* but rather secretes androstenedione, which is converted in extra-adrenal tissues to estrone and estradiol (aromatization reaction). The latter mechanism, which is the principal source of estrogens in postmenopausal or castrated women, is almost completely inhibited by aminoglutethimide.[234] Thus, this drug exerts a dual inhibitory effect.

In addition to the above, it is known to accelerate the metabolism of synthetic glucocorticoids such as dexamethasone.[233] The adrenal suppression with its associated fall in cortisol secretion leads to reflex rise in ACTH, which can

TABLE 27-20. Medical Adrenalectomy with Aminoglutethimide

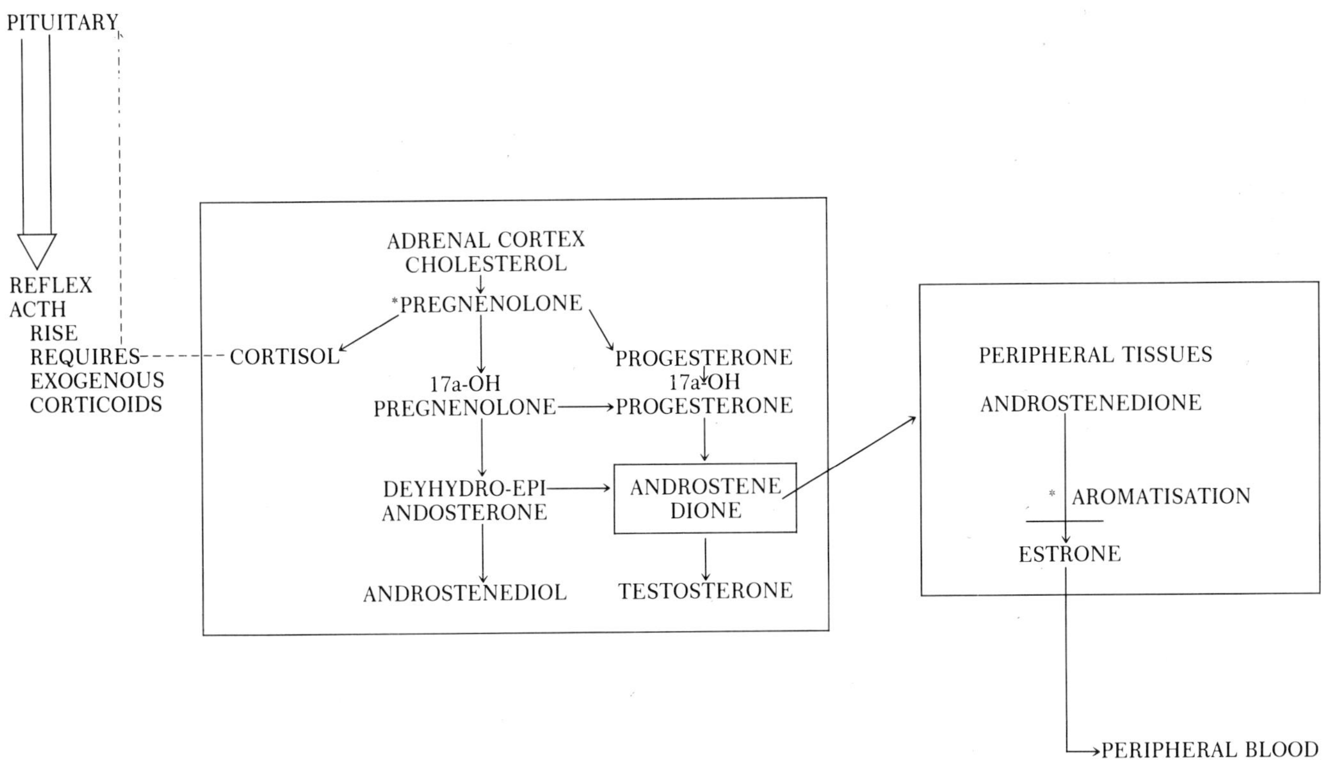

*Sites of inhibition
(Santen RJ, Samojlik E, Lipton A et al: Kinetic, hormonal, and clinical studies with aminoglutethimide in breast cancer. Cancer 39:2948–2958, 1977)

overcome the aminoglutethimide blockade. Added glucocorticoid therapy is required. Maximal estrogen suppression requires that aminoglutethimide be given at 250 mg by mouth four times a day together with 40 mg of hydrocortisone in divided dose (10 mg in A.M., 10 mg at 5:00 P.M., and 20 mg at bedtime). The side-effects are seen at the onset of therapy and include lethargy, dizziness, and visual blurring, which disappear over the succeeding days of treatment. A pruritic maculo-papular rash has also been noted within 10 days of treatment. The predictive factors for and sites of response are similar to those for endocrine ablative surgery. The unselected response rate is about 35%, rising to 50% in ER-positive patients.[235,236] In patients treated with aminoglutethimide–hydrocortisone, the urinary cortisol and plasma estrone, estradiol, fall significantly while on continuous therapy with a median duration of response in the 11 month to 17 month range. Medical adrenalectomy has been prospectively compared to hypophysectomy and surgical adrenalectomy.[230,237] In both instances medical therapy was equal or superior. No permanent adrenal insufficiency or acute crisis was noted. An interesting observation is the fact that two of the four responders to surgical adrenalectomy sustained further antitumor responses with aminoglutethimide.[238] Medical adrenalectomy appears to be an acceptable alternative to surgical ablation.

Additive Hormone Therapy

Estrogens, androgens, and progestational agents have been used to treat advanced breast cancer in postmenopausal women since 1950. The most commonly used hormonal agents are the estrogens. About 30% of unselected postmenopausal patients may show objective response lasting 12 months to 14 months.[238] The presence of the ERP predicts for a response in up to 50% of cases.[239] The antitumor response to estrogens is usually quite slow, requiring several weeks, and is primarily confined to metastatic disease in the skin, lymph nodes, breast, and osseous lesions. The most commonly used preparation is diethylstilbestrol. Anorexia, nausea, and vomiting are the most common problems with this preparation when used in the usual dose of 5 mg t.i.d. The problem can be relieved by changing to other estrogenic preparations such as Premarin 10 mg, 3 times a day, or Estinyl, 3 mg/day.[240] The undesirable side-effects of chronic estrogen administration include stress incontinence (especially in elderly patients), which can be severe enough to require discontinuation of the agent. Pigmentation of the nipples is almost universal. Sodium and fluid retention, increased libido, and withdrawal bleeding can be troublesome complications. Rarely, in patients with extensive metastatic bone disease, a flare of the disease, characterized by increased bone pain or hypercalcemia or both, can occur. This can be treated with hydration, diuresis, or intravenous mithramycin. If possible, the hormone should be continued, since this flare reaction may actually signal a subsequent antitumor response.[240] The mechanism of this flare reaction, which is subsequently beneficial, is unknown. Those patients who respond to estrogen therapy and subsequently become resistant may attain a further regression of the disease upon abrupt cessation of the hormone. This rebound regression can result in responses of up to 30% of treated cases and can predict for subsequent response to other hormonal therapy.[241]

The mechanism of action of high-dose estrogens is unknown. Although some have postulated a direct inhibitory effect on prolactin secretion by the pituitary, there is a body of evidence which would suggest a direct effect of the high-dose estrogens on the malignant cell.[242] Human breast cancer lines (MCF-7) stimulated by low doses of estrogen are inhibited by concentrations of 17 β-estradiol or diethylstilbestrol in excess of 10^{-7}m.[242] It is likely that this inhibition is nonspecific, as it is not mediated through an estrogen receptor. In the clinical situation, however, estrogen responses are confined to ERP-positive patients. The antitumor mechanism of high-dose estrogen remains an unexplained paradox.

Androgens have been commonly used and are considered less effective than estrogens in postmenopausal women with soft tissue metastases. However, they have enjoyed a reputation of being equal or superior to estrogens in the treatment of osseous metastases.[227] The preparations used include testosterone proprionate 100 mg i.m. three times a week or fluoxymesterone 10 mg by mouth twice a day. The side effects are mainly virilization, increased libido in some women, and erythrocytosis. As with the estrogens, the mechanism of action is unknown. Up to 20% of unselected patients in the postmenopausal period respond to androgen therapy. The responses are generally confined to bone and soft tissue metastases and last 12 months to 14 months as with estrogens. The response to both estrogens and androgens increases with years postmenopause up to the eighth year, although premenopausal women who have relapsed after castration may respond briefly to a course of androgens.[227,238,240] Most comparative trials reveal a superiority of estrogens in postmenopausal women (29% > 10%), especially for soft tissue metastases. The sequential use of these agents has shown that failure to respond to androgens does not preclude a response to estrogens. The converse does not apply.[243]

Progestational agents in high dosage have also been used in patients who have previously responded to other additive hormones. The usual preparation is medroxyprogesterone acetate, usually given 100 mg, three times weekly intramuscularly or, as a high dose regimen, 1000 to 1500 mg i.m. per day, which may be associated with a higher response rate.[244–246] Megesterol acetate up to 80 mg per day can produce an equivalent response varying from 10% to 30%.[247] The mechanism of action is unknown; however, it has been shown that progestational agents will compete for androgen and progestational receptor sites on cell membranes. Regressions are noted more frequently in tumor containing large amounts of androgen receptors.[248] Progestational agents do not compete with estradiol for estrogen receptor binding. Responses, when they occur, can last for about 12 months to 14 months, as with other hormones. The combination of estrogens and androgens or progestational agents does not increase the response rate over estrogens alone.[243] It is unlikely that corticosteroids can offer but a transient antitumor effect by virtue of their ability to suppress pituitary ACTH production. Large doses of corticoids should not be used in the routine treatment of metastatic breast cancer because of the toxicity. They are indicated in the supportive treatment of acute hypercalcemia, intracranial metastases, jaundice due to hepatic metastases, and dyspnea due to extensive pulmonary involvement. The use of sex steroid hormones as first line treatment has gradually been replaced by safe and effective antiestrogen therapy with tamoxifen, since the responses achieved are of comparable rate and duration.

Antiestrogens

Antiestrogens are compounds which have been demonstrated to block the uptake of estrogen by target tissues by binding to the estrogen receptor. As a group, antiestrogens are nonsteroid amino–ether derivatives of polycyclic phenols. The structural resemblance to synthetic estrogen-like stilbestrol and chlorotrianisene explains the mild estrogenic effects of high doses of antiestrogens in experimental animals.[249] The three antiestrogens that have had clinical evaluations are clomiphene citrate, nafoxidine, and tamoxifen.[250] All three have been shown to result in antitumor responses in postmenopausal women. Because of toxicity, the first two have essentially been removed from general use. Tamoxifen has had extensive trial and was found to be safe and effective.[251] The drug is given daily by mouth with antitumor responses seen at a daily dose of 20 mg to 80 mg per day. Most trials employ 20 mg p.o. b.i.d. Lack of responses at one dose level rarely can be improved by increasing the dose.[251] Side-effects are rare and withdrawal of the therapy is unusual. As with estrogens, a "flare" of bone pain and hypercalcemia has been noted which is short-lived and usually results in an antitumor response if drug is continued.[252]

The antitumor effect is seen primarily in a setting of a hormonal response; that is, in older age patients, patients with ERP-positive tumors, or patients with a prior response to endocrine therapy. The unselected overall response rate is 40% (Table 27-21).[253] The response rate is higher in the older, postmenopausal patients. Relatively few pre-menopausal patients have been treated and responses have been seen, but it does not appear as yet to be a subsitute for oophorectomy. ERP-positive patients have up to a 75% response rate.[254] Soft tissue and osseous metastases are more likely to respond, sometimes requiring several weeks before becoming apparent. Complete responses are less likely but in most instances a partial antitumor response lasts for a median of 8 months with a range of 4 months to more than 40 months.[251,253,254] Tamoxifen has been compared prospectively with the androgen, fluoxymesterone, in a series of postmenopausal women. Responses occurred more often with tamoxifen (30% / 19%).[255]

TABLE 27-21. Antiestrogen Therapy

	RESPONSE ACCORDING TO ESTROGEN RECEPTOR STATUS			
	Patients	*Response*	*ERP+*	*ERP−*
Manni	113	50 (50%)	31/49	0/6
Morgan	72	28 (38%)	19/36	0/10
Kiang	59	19 (32%)	6/10	0/10
Bloom	25	11 (44%)	11/20	0/5
Others	296	84 (29%)	21/43	3/20
TOTAL	565	198 (35%)	98/158 (62%)	3/51 (6%)

	RESPONSE TO SUBSEQUENT HORMONAL THERAPY ACCORDING TO TAMOXIFEN RESPONSE	
	Responder	*Non-Responder*
Additive hormones	13/23	6/33
Hypophysectomy	8/20	2/24
TOTAL	21/43 (49%)	8/57 (14%)

The responses of bone metastases were equivalent, although the duration of tamoxifen response was superior. Of particular interest is the comparison with hypophysectomy. Remissions were seen with tamoxifen in six of 26 (23%) previously hypophysectomized patients. Similarly, this operation resulted in responses in eight of 20 patients, all of whom had previously responded to tamoxifen.[256] A prospective comparison with a cross-over plan in the trial showed four of seven hypophysectomized patients responding to tamoxifen and two of nine tamoxifen responders responding to hypophysectomy.[257] The mechanism of resistance to antiestrogen therapy is unknown, although a selection of ERP-negative cell lines has been suggested.[203] The mechanism of hypophysectomy response in tamoxifen failures is also unexplained. Whether surgical adrenalectomy or aminoglutethimide can achieve further remission in the same setting is unknown. Tamoxifen has clearly replaced other additive hormones as the primary hormonal treatment of postmenopausal women with ERP-positive tumors or clinical features predictive of a hormonal response. It remains to determine whether medical adrenalectomy combined with tamoxifen will enhance the response rate and duration of response.

Options for Systemic Hormonal Therapy

The clinical features of metastatic breast cancer that predict for response to hormonal therapy have been well defined and consist of long disease-free interval (from mastectomy to metastases) and predominantly osseous and soft tissue disease. In addition, postmenopausal women are more likely to respond than pre-menopausal women. The presence of the estrogen receptor correlates with these clinical features. Since receptor "positivity" represents a wide range of amounts of receptor, likelihood of response tends to parallel the quantity of cytosol receptor. Determination of progesterone receptor will increase the predictability of response, but it is also more frequent in tumors with high estrogen receptor. Thus, the value of measuring the more complicated progesterone receptor has not been established.

Surgical ablation has become a less frequent mode of hormonal ablation. Antiestrogen therapy with tamoxifen has replaced additive hormones as well as adrenalectomy and hypophysectomy as the first-line hormonal treatment by postmenopausal women. Although there is less data available at present, it may replace oophorectomy in pre-menopausal women. At the same time, improved techniques of medical adrenalectomy have permitted its wider application and favorable comparison with surgical ablation of the adrenal and pituitary.

The mechanism of resistance to tamoxifen is not completely understood but could entail selection of estrogen receptor–negative cell lines. However, this may not be the only explanation, for previous tamoxifen responders are known to respond to other subsequent hormonal manipulation, such as hypophysectomy and additive hormones (Table 27-21). It has been established that response to prior hormonal therapy or ERP status does not influence the response to cytotoxic therapy. In fact with the possible exception of rapidly progressive disease, the sequence in which the two forms of treatment are given does not influence survival.

This trial comparing hormonal therapy and chemotherapy had shown that patients with extensive and rapidly evolving metastatic disease rarely respond to endocrine treatment and should be treated with cytotoxic chemotherapy.[258] The vast majority of patients with metastatic breast cancer eventually become candidates for chemotherapy. In addition, a progressively increasing number of women with Stage II disease are receiving chemotherapy as an adjunct to surgery.

CHEMOTHERAPY OF BREAST CANCER

INTRODUCTION

The introduction of cancer chemotherapeutic agents has made a major impact on the survival of patients with leukemia, lymphoma, and testicular cancer. Among the more common malignancies of adults, carcinoma of the breast has been the most responsive to a wide variety of single agents and combination programs.

PROGNOSTIC FACTORS FOR RESPONSE TO CHEMOTHERAPY

Although a single biochemical test is not available to predict for the response to cytotoxic chemotherapy, a variety of clinical factors have been identified which significantly influence the response to chemotherapy. Two series have analyzed over 889 patients and identified important prognostic factors which will predict for initial response to chemotherapy and in most instances, survival. Those factors which predict for a poor response to chemotherapy and consequently survival are: poor performance status, anemia, thrombocytopenia, abnormal liver function studies, decreased serum albumin, prior treatment with cytotoxic chemotherapy or radiation therapy, and extent of disease rather than a dominant site.[259–261]

A number of factors were found to have no influence on response to chemotherapy and they include age, menstrual status, family history of breast cancer, type of surgery, extent of axillary node involvement, and size of primary. There seems to be general agreement on these factors. One study showed that the disease-free interval predicted for a lower response rate and concluded that ambulatory patients with a long disease-free interval and no liver involvement had the best prognosis.[259] If adjustment is made for performance status and liver involvement, then other covariants such as menopausal status, bone involvement, and the number of metastatic sites, duration of metastatic disease was not significantly related to response. In addition, the type of chemotherapy, the frequency of administration and the dose are all factors which will be discussed below.

The combination chemotherapy has a superior response rate to single drugs and the frequency of adminstration of cycles of chemotherapy given every 3 weeks is superior to cycles which are in excess of 4 weeks.[260] The value of estrogen receptor analysis as a predictive for response to chemotherapy has been controversial. In one retrospective analysis of estrogen receptor with response to a variety of chemotherapeutic regimens, there appears to be a significant correlation between response and absence of the receptor.[211] Other workers found exactly opposite relationships.[210] The issue appears to have been clarified in subsequent studies, where the estrogen receptor content of a primary breast cancer sample was found to have no prognostic utility for response to cytotoxic chemotherapy.[212] A series of 136 patients with metastatic carcinoma of the breast who received prior adequate trials of hormonal therapy showed an equivalent complete and partial response rate in hormone responders and non-responders. There was, however, a significantly longer chemotherapy-induced response in those patients who were previously hormonal responsive.[262]

SINGLE AGENTS IN THE TREATMENT OF BREAST CANCER

A wide variety of antineoplastic agents of differing biochemical mechanisms of action are effective in metastatic breast cancer. They include the alkylating agents, cyclophosphamide, phenylalanine mustard (L-PAM), thiotepa, and chlorambucil.[263,264] The most commonly used is cyclophosphamide.

The response to cyclophosphamide appears to be equivalent, regardless of the schedule, used either as a daily oral medication or intermittent, intravenous doses. Other alkylating agents evaluated in the past include isophosphamide, which appears to have no advantage. The nitrosoureas have had some evaluation and are associated with a relatively low response rate of approximately 15%.[264] The two most commonly used antimetabolites are 5-fluorouracil and methotrexate, for with a wide variety of dosage schedules, these agents have been associated with a 25% to 35% response rate.[265,266] Other antimetabolites such as cytosine arabinoside, 6-mercaptopurine, and 6-thioguanine are without effect. The vinca alkaloids have been enigmatic, since objective regression of disease usually requires weekly doses that inevitably result in serious neurotoxicity (Table 27-22). Other vinca alkaloids such as vinblastine and vindesine have recently been evaluated as second-line drugs and have been reported to show responses in 18 out of a total of 51 patients.[267,268] A prospective randomized trial of combination chemotherapy, with or without vincristine, failed to show an advantage to the use of this agent in combination chemotherapy.[269] Thus, there has been

TABLE 27-22. Effect of Single Agents in Metastatic Breast Cancer

AGENT	NUMBER OF PATIENTS	PERCENT ANTITUMOR RESPONSE	MEDIAN DURATION (Months)	REFERENCE NUMBER
Melphalan	131	23%	–	(264)
Cyclophosphamide	529	34%	–	(264)
5-Fluorouracil	1263	26%	–	(264)
Methotrexate	356	34%	–	(264)
Vincristine	226	21%	–	(264)
Adriamycin				
Prior Therapy				
1. 20 mg/M² d. 1, 8 q. 28 d	60	27%	7	(270)
2. 60–75 mg/M² q. 3 wks	40	38%	7	(271)
No Prior Therapy				
1. 75 mg/M² q. 3 wks	32	38%	7.5	(272)
2. 60 mg/M² q. 3 wks	20	50%	8.0	(273)
3. 60 mg/M² q. 3 wks	79	39%	5.0	(274)

a tendency to omit the vinca alkaloids from recently developed combination chemotherapy programs.

The anthracycline antibiotic, adriamycin, is probably the most active single agent available for the treatment of breast cancer. The usual dose of 60 mg/m² to 75 mg/m² given intravenously every three weeks is associated with a response rate varying from 38% to 50% in previously untreated patients with a median duration of response of approximately 5 months to 8 months.[270–274] Prior chemotherapy often reduces the response rate to single agents, but even in that setting 30% of patients would be expected to respond. There have been few studies of dose–response in breast cancer chemotherapy. However, one trial comparing 70 mg every 3 weeks to an every-5-week schedule showed no difference in response.[275] "Low-dose" adriamycin (20 mg/m² i.v. days 1, 8 q. 28 days) resulted in a 27% response rate in patients who progressed on CMF. A trial exploring high-dose methotrexate showed a 29% response rate in previously treated patients.[276] This result is not dissimilar to those with lower doses of methotrexate. Most new agents are investigated as second-line chemotherapy, and on Table 27-23, a listing of newer agents used in that setting is shown. It is clear that with few exceptions, very few patients respond. Single agent chemotherapy is rarely associated with complete response, with a duration of response that is relatively short. For each agent there is a progressive shortening of the period of disease control with the use of succeeding single agents.

The advent of combination chemotherapy in advanced breast cancer was heralded by two early reports in the 1960s. The first was a report on the effect of the combination of thiotepa, methotrexate, and 5-fluorouracil in addition to prednisone and testosterone.[277] The 60% response rate was impressive and went relatively unnoticed until 1969, when Cooper reported a previously unheard of response rate of 90% in 60 hormone-resistant patients.[278] Cooper's regimen is shown on Table 27-24 and is henceforth referred to as CMFVP. These five drugs can be combined in a variety of schedules and doses and have thus been considered in the literature as a "Cooper-type" regimen. Early evaluations of this regimen confirmed the efficacy, but a more realistic response rate in the range of 50% was observed. The CMFVP regimen was modified in dose, composition, and schedule. Most trials using the original Cooper regimen had a consistent 50% response rate with the duration usually less than 8 months.[279–285] Some modifications included deletion of vincristine or prednisone or both, sparing the toxicity without significantly affecting overall response.[286,287] This was confirmed in randomized trials comparing CFP or CMF to CMFVP.[288,289] The continuous weekly schedule of the original regimen proved superior to an intermittent (q 28 days) regimen in a comparative trial.[283] However, for the first time, complete remissions were noted as compared to the previous experience of single agents.

Since the reason for combination chemotherapy is to impart a greater antitumor effect with tolerable toxicity, it was important to compare the results of combination chemotherapy to single agent treatment. These trials are outlined on Table 27-6.[25] The initial trials compared either the three-drug combination to L-PAM or cyclophosphamide compared to the

TABLE 27-23. Breast Cancer Second Line Chemotherapy Patients Refractory to Conventional Agents

DRUG	RESPONSE	REFERENCE NUMBER
Platinum	0/26	(312)
Cyclocytidine	1/36	(313)
Hexamethylmelamine	2/95	(314–316)
Asparaginase Methotrexate	10/33	(317)
Mitomycin-C	12/57	(318)
Rubidozone	0/19	(319)
Maytansine	1/21	(320)
Thioguanine	1/23	(321)
High-dose 6MP	2/17	(322)
ICRF-159	2/40	(323)
Vindesine	6/21	(268)
Anguidine	1/30	(324)
Pyrazofurin	0/17	(325)
Vinblastine (5-day continuous infusion)	12/30	(267)
Vinblastine–Mitomycin	10/22	(237)

TABLE 27-24. Carcinoma of the Breast: Commonly Used Combination Chemotherapy Regimens

1. "Cooper"	
Cyclophosphamide	2 mg/kg/day p.o.
Methotrexate	0.7 mg/kg/wk IV × 8 wks.
5-FU	12 mg/kg/wk IV then q.o.w.
Vincristine	35 μg/kg/wk. × 4–5 wks.
Prednisone	0.75/kg/day. Reduced 1/2 q. 10 days to 5 mg/day for 3 wks.
2. CMF (ECOG), Milan	
Cyclophosphamide	100 mg/M²/day p.o. day 1–14
Methotrexate	30–40 mg/M² IV day 1, 8 q. 28 days
5-FU	400–600 mg/M² IV day 1, 8
3. CFP, Mayo	
Cyclophosphamide	150 mg/M²/day p.o. × 5
5-FU	300 mg/M²/day I.V. × 5 q. 6 wks.
Prednisone	30 mg/day × 7
4. FAC, MDA	
5-FU	400 mg/M² I.V. days 1, 8
Adriamycin	40 mg/M² I.V. day 1 q. 28 days
Cyclophosphamide	400 mg/M² I.V. day 1

CMFVP regimen.[287,290] The results of both trials clearly suggested that the alkylating agents were associated with a 21% to 25% response rate as opposed to a 53% to 63% response rate for the combination program. The L-PAM *versus* CMF trial, however, documented a survival advantage only in those patients with liver involvement or who were non-ambulatory.[287] The obvious criticism of single agent *versus* combination trials is the lack of definition of second-line chemotherapy for those who fail the initial alkylating agents. Three trials, however, were designed to compare combination chemotherapy with the components of the combination used in sequence (Table 27-25). The use of combination chemotherapy not only was associated with a higher response rate in most trials, but median survival for the combination group in one trial was double that of patients treated on sequential chemotherapy.[283] A Western group trial found it extremely difficult to show a survival advantage comparing CMFVP to sequential single agent CMFVP chemotherapy.[284] In that trial, separate analysis of those patients without liver metastases showed no advantage of combination chemotherapy, suggesting that there are a large number of patients who may benefit from less aggressive chemotherapy. There remains a question whether all patients with hormone-resistant, disseminated breast cancer benefit from intensive chemotherapy. It is clear, however, that patients with extensive and rapidly progressive disease with weight loss, poor performance status, and liver and bone marrow functional impairment constitute a high-risk group, requiring rapid and effective reversal of their course. However, liver involvement or extensive metastatic disease contribute to a poor performance status of patients and these require combination chemotherapy to reverse the downhill course.

The introduction of adriamycin was widely greeted as a new and active agent for breast cancer. Its high single drug activity had the promise of even more significant effects when combined with other agents. Table 27-26 indicated, however, that it is difficult to appreciate the significant improvement in the overall response rate between adriamycin combined with another agent and three and four drug adriamycin-containing regimens.[293-297] In one trial, the addition of cyclophosphamide, an active single agent, did not appreciably add to the result of 5-FU and adriamycin alone.[294] These data suggest that tolerable doses of two or three active agents would appear to be optimal therapy for advanced breast cancer. However, the addition of other myelotoxic agents usually compromised the dose of the other drugs. When cytoxan, adriamycin, and fluorouracil (CAF) was compared to CMF or to CMFVP, there appeared to be no gross difference between the two regimens, although the objective response rates to CAF were 82% and 64% compared to 62% and 32% respectively.[285,293] Only the CAF versus CMFVP trial showed a corresponding superiority in duration of response.[285] This same pattern was noted in a trial comparing CAF(VP) with CMF(VP) although the overall response rates were similar.[298] Clear-cut statistical significance, however, was never achieved. The complete response rate in all of these programs varies from 12% to 20%. At the present time, the most effective regimens available for general use are the CMF or

TABLE 27-25. Metastatic Breast Cancer—Single Agents Alone or in Sequence—Compared to Combination Chemotherapy

SINGLE AGENTS	NUMBER OF PATIENTS	PERCENT RESPONSE	REFERENCE NUMBER
1. L-Pam 6 mg/M²/d × 5	91	21%	(287)
CMF	93	53%	
2. Cyclophosphamide 3 mg/kg/day p.o.	27	25%	(290)
CMFVP ("Cooper")	28	63%	
SEQUENTIAL SINGLE AGENTS			
1. 5-FU → Cyxlo → VCR (full dose)	30	53.3%	(291)
C 4 mg/kg IV × 5 F 7.5 mg/kg IV × 5 V .015 mg/kg 1, 8	46	43.5%	
2. 5-FU → Cyclo → Pred → MTX	60	32%	(284)
C 2 mg/kg/d. p.o. F 15 mg/kg q. 2 wks. IV M 30 mg/M²/q. 2 wks. IV P 0.5 mg/M²/kg/day p.o.	61	56%	
3. 5-FU 600 mg/M²/wk → MTX 20/M² b.i.w. Cyclo 100 mg/M² p.o./d → VCR 1.0 mg/M² wk.	34	18%	(283)
CMFVP ("Cooper")	35	46%	

TABLE 27-26. Addition of Adriamycin to Other Agents

	NUMBER OF PATIENTS	PERCENT RESPONSE	PERCENT CR	RESPONSE MEDIAN (Months)	REFERENCE NUMBER
TWO DRUGS (NO PRIOR THERAPY)					
1. Cyclo 1.0 gm/M² q. ADR 40 mg/M²	26	50%	12%	10	(295)
2. Cyclo 200 mg/M²/d. × 4d ADR 40 mg/M² q. 21–28 d.	55	80%	12%	10	(296)
*3. 5-Fluorouracil 500 mg/M² d. 1, 8 ADR 40 mg/M² q. 21 days	105	42%	11%	15	(294)
THREE DRUGS (NO PRIOR THERAPY)					
*4. Cyclo 400 mg/M² q. 21 d. ADR 40 mg/M² 5-FU 400 mg/M² 1, 8	103	43%	14%	15	(294)
5. Cyclo 100 mg/M²/d 1–14 ADR 30 mg/M²/d 1, 8 q. 28 d. 5-FU 500 mg/M² d. 1, 8	38	82%	18%	10	(293)
6. Cyclo 500 mg/M² ADR 50 mg/M² q. 21 d. 5-FU 500 mg/M²	59	64%	20%	8	(285)
FOUR DRUGS (NO PRIOR THERAPY)					
7. ADR 40 mg/M² day 1; Cycl 1.0 gm/M² day 1; MTX 30 mg/M² d. 21, 28, 35; 5-FU 400–600 mg/M² d. 21 28, 35 } q. 6 wks.	22	55%	32%	10	(295)
8. Cycl 50 mg/M² d. 1–14; ADR 20 mg/M² d. 1, 8; MTX 20 mg/M² d. 1, 8; 5-FU 300 mg/M² d. 1, 8 } q. 28 days	39	62%	—	12	(297)

*Randomized trial.

CAF programs (Table 27-24). In the absence of an investigative protocol, either of these programs will offer the patient at least a 50% chance of response.

Responses to combination chemotherapy have been seen in all sites, including bone, liver, soft tissue, and viscera. Likewise, in all these sites, a complete disappearance of all evidence of disease might be seen. The response of bone lesions represents a major impact of combination chemotherapy, since bone metastases rarely responded to single agents. The median duration of response in most trials of combination chemotherapy varies from 12 months to 18 months. At that point, further antitumor effect may be derived from one of the more commonly used agents. However, as mentioned above, second-line chemotherapy has been disappointing. In patients who achieve a complete remission, the median duration of response is 16 months to 18 months, with the median survival approaching 32 months when compared to the 24 months for the partial responders and 17 months for stable disease.[299,300] The goal of achieving a complete remission would appear justified, as it certainly is in lymphoma therapy. However, analysis of most series does not offer a breakdown according to prognostic factors. Therefore, it is possible that patients with relatively early metastatic disease can be treated to complete remission, and these remissions last for a period of time which appears to be superior or in excess of the partial or stable disease status achieved with chemotherapy in patients with far more advanced disease. Thus, the comparison should probably be from the time of initial metastases with stratification according to prognostic factors. In an analysis of patients in complete remission, 79% of the patients had one or two metastatic sites involved.[300] Thus at the present time, it is not clear whether patients who achieve a complete remission are, indeed, achieving a superior survival. Patients who relapse from combination chemotherapy may still be eligible for hormonal treatment if they are estrogen-receptor positive and have not demonstrated previous refractoriness to endocrine therapy, since prior cytotoxic chemotherapy does not compromise the response to subsequent endocrine treatment. The sequence of administration of cytotoxic or endocrine therapy does not influence survival, except in patients with rapidly progressive disease where cytotoxic chemotherapy is the preferred approach.[259]

Sequential administration of non-cross-resistant combination chemotherapy with a fixed crossover to an alternate regimen was investigated in the hope that a more prolonged control of disease could be achieved. Two of the four trials shown on Table 27-27 involve prospective comparison of the sequential administration of two non-cross-resistant regimens.[301,304] The Milan trial compared CMF with adriamycin and vincristine, given in alterating courses of two cycles each.[301] There was no advantage to either arm and the data would appear to be comparable to that previously seen with CMF alone. The duration of disease control barely exceeded 12 months. In all of the trials shown in the table, there was no increase in the complete response rate. There is no advantage to the sequential administration of alternating non-cross-resistant regimens as opposed to using a given regimen until evidence of disease resistance. These observations and those previously outlined which fail to show an advantage to

TABLE 27-27. Sequential Combination Chemotherapy (Fixed Crossover)

	NUMBER OF PATIENTS	PERCENT RESPONSE	PERCENT CR	REFERENCE NUMBER
1. CMF (2 cycles) Alt. with ADR–VCR (2 cycles)	55	60%	18%	(301)
ADR–VCR (2 cycles) Alt. with CMF (2 cycles)	55	53%	20%	
2. Cyclo (700 mg/M²)-ADR (50 mg/M²) q. 3 wks × 4 MTX (25 mg/M² 600 mg/M² q. 2 wks. × 3	34	56%	9%	(302)
3. { Cyclo 100 mg/M² p.o. 1–14 Adriamycin 30 mg/M² 1, 8 5-FU 500 mg//M² 1, 8 q. 28 days	21	63%	13%	(303)
Dibromodulcitol 135 mg/M² 1–10 Adriamycin 45 mg day 1 VCR 1.2 mg/m² 1, 8 Alt. with CMF	25	70.8%	10%	
4. Cyclo 750 mg/M², ADR 50 mg/M² } q. 21 days × 1–3 courses 7–9 VCR 1.5 mg/m² q. wk. followed by 5-FU 500 mg/M² × 5 days q. 28 day × 4–6 courses MTX 30 mg/M² day 1, 8, 15 plus BCG	156	67%	20%	(304)

adding drugs to adriamycin plus another agent suggests an early emergence of cross-resistant cell lines which constitute the clinical relapse. This may explain the limited effectiveness of second-line chemotherapy by agents of widely differing biochemical action.

COMBINED CHEMOTHERAPY AND HORMONAL TREATMENT

The rationale for using combination chemotherapy in sequence with hormonal treatment is that each modality might act through an entirely different mechanism, thus achieving a greater effect (Table 27-28). The Mayo Clinic randomized 75 premenopausal patients to oophorectomy alone or oophorectomy followed by CFP.[305] The same regimen would be used in the oophorectomy-only arm as treatment after progression of metastatic disease. Those patients who received early chemotherapy had an improved response and survival rate. The median duration of disease control was 53 weeks compared to 17 weeks for oophorectomy alone. The median survival of the combined group was 131 weeks compared to 88 weeks in the oophorectomy control group. However, both lines came together at about 150 weeks postoophorectomy. The same improvement in disease-free survival is noted with the use of cyclophosphamide plus oophorectomy compared to oophorectomy alone.[306] All of these trials were performed without the benefit of estrogen receptor analysis.

The Swiss Cooperative Group compared oophorectomy plus the CMFVP chemotherapy *versus* CMFVP alone.[307] In premenopausal patients the advantage to the combined approach was minimal. Although the response rate was higher, the median duration of response did not significantly differ between the two groups. In postmenopausal patients, where estrogen plus CMFVP was compared to chemotherapy alone, the duration of disease-free survival was superior in the chemotherapy group to the combined group.[307] These data show that the response rate to the combination of oophorectomy plus chemotherapy does not appear to be significantly higher than for chemotherapy alone. The advantage, if any, is not translated into an improved response duration. The addition of low-dose CMF to ERP-positive postmenopausal patients responding to tamoxifen demonstrated no additional benefit. The doses of CMF were quite low in this series and might not be expected to impart a major antitumor effect.[308] Chemotherapy contributes a prolongation of the antitumor response of oophorectomy probably as an additive effect and this response is not greater than what might be achieved by chemotherapy alone in a population unselected for estrogen receptor status.

IMMUNOTHERAPY

Immunotherapy has not been well studied in breast cancer. Treatment has been confined to the use of non-specific immunostimulants, usually with chemotherapy. Using historical controls, the FAC combination (Table 27-5) was combined with BCG scarification or levamisole and found to be superior in terms of prolonged remission duration.[309] However, the Mayo Clinic tested the value of MER (methanol-extracted residue of BCG) plus CFP *versus* CFP alone in a randomized trial of 71 patients. The response rate and median survival were not augmented by MER.[310] BCG plus systemic therapy compared to systemic therapy alone as adjuvant in Stage II breast cancer showed no difference in the relapse rate.[311]

ADJUVANT THERAPY

In the last 10 years, one of the most exciting and controversial areas in the management of human breast cancer is the role

TABLE 27-28. Combined Chemotherapy and Hormonal Treatment or Endocrine Ablation

	NUMBER OF PATIENTS	PERCENT RESPONSE	RESPONSE MEDIAN DURATION	MEDIAN SURVIVAL (Months)	REFERENCE NUMBER
1. Mayo Clinic					
↗Oophorectomy + Cyclo 150 mg/M² × 5, 5-FU 300 mg/M² × q. 6 wks., Prednisone 50 mg/d × 7	36	39%	53 weeks	42	(305)
↘Oophorectomy Progression → CFP	37	26%	17 weeks	22	
2. CALGB					
↗Oophorectomy + Cyclo 300 mg/M²/day × 5 day daily oral 2 mg/kgm	56	65%	16 months	23	(306)
↘Oophorectomy	38	18%	5 months	30	
3. Swiss Group (SAKK) Pre-menopausal					
↗Oophorectomy + CMFVP ("Cooper")	19	74%	9.5 months	19.9	(307)
↘CMFVP	23	43%	7.8 months	13.2	
Postmenopausal					
↗Diethylstilbestrol + CMFVP	48	63%	8.4 months	26.7	
↘CMFVP	48	54%	10.6 months	19.2	
4. Univ. of Pennsylvania Postmenopausal (ERP + or unknown)					
TAM × wks (63) ↗continue TAM	34	18%	12.5	N.A.	(308)
TAM × wks (63) ↘low dose CMF +TAM	29	28%	17.0	N.A.	

of adjuvant therapy following optimal local treatment with curative intent. The excitement for this approach was based on the early results of controlled clinical trials which demonstrated an advantage for the early administration of systemic chemotherapy compared to an untreated control group randomized to no therapy. With the passage of time, the differences between the treated and untreated groups became less significant in postmenopausal patients. This observation has raised the issue of a potentially antihormonal effect due to the effect of chemotherapy on ovarian function. The optimal duration and intensity of chemotherapy as well as the impact on long-term overall survival beyond 10 years has yet to be appreciated.

PROGNOSTIC FACTOR FOR RELAPSE

Although a variety of histopathologic characteristics have been defined as possibly correlating with unfavorable prognosis, the most useful prognostic factor in women with operable cancer is the histologic status of the axillary nodes at the time of the initial diagnosis as discussed previously. The likelihood of relapse can be correlated with the number of involved nodes such that the 5-year relapse rate of patients with one to three positive nodes is approximately 50%, but in patients with four or more positive nodes is almost 80%. By 10 years, the relapse rate will be increased by another 10% to 15%, respectively, in both groups.[46] The relapse-free and, furthermore, overall survival are not effected by menopausal status at the time of diagnosis of breast cancer. The pattern of recurrence is such that in node-positive patients, local–regional recurrence is usually seen within the first 3 years following mastectomy.[44] The initial site of recurrence will be the chest wall or local regional area with or without distant metastasis in about 40% of patients. The remainder will show dissemination in distant sites. At least 60% of these patients will have a distant metastasis within 2 years following local regional recurrence. The remainder will have dissemination in the subsequent years.

A biochemical characteristic of the tumor which may predict for early relapse is the absence of the estrogen receptor protein. When estrogen receptor content of tumor cytosol is compared to the frequency of thymidine labeling, there is an inverse correlation between the quantity of estrogen receptor protein and the proliferative activity of the tumor.[207,327] When corrected for tumor size, primary therapy, and axillary node status, most studies show a decreased relapse rate for patients with estrogen-receptor positive tumors.[208,209,328] The data show an early prognostic advantage for estrogen-receptor positive tumors, since most were followed for only 2 years to 3 years. Receptor positive, node positive patients will have a slower rate of relapse compared to ER-negative patients, but this advantage gradually disappears with the increasing interval following mastectomy. In one study, estrogen-receptor negative patients without evidence of axillary lymph node metastases had a prognosis for recurrence within the first 3 years similar to that of all patients with positive axillary nodes.[209] An early relapse pattern reflects the increased proliferative potential of estrogen-receptor negative tumors.

PROPHYLACTIC CASTRATION

The well-established benefit of bilateral oophorectomy in the management of some patients with advanced metastatic breast cancer prompted a number of studies exploring the worth of oophorectomy as an adjunct to radical surgery in pre-menopausal women (Table 27-29). In 1961, the NSABP (National Surgical Adjuvant Breast Project) conducted a randomized prospective clinical trial (Study #3) to address this point. A total of 154 patients were oophorectomized and 203 control patients had no adjuvant therapy of the drug thiotepa. A detailed analysis of the data revealed no difference between the two groups in terms of recurrence rate and survival up to 5 years of follow-up.[329] In patients with four or more positive nodes, the disease-free survival rate between the control and treated groups was 33% and 23% respectively.

Between 1948 and 1955, the Christie Hospital, Manchester, performed a randomized trial incorporating irradiation castration as a form of endocrine ablation. The doses were generally in the range of 450 rad, which is less than the present-day dosage of 1000 rad to 2000 rad.[330] This trial in particular raised the question of adequacy of ablation, since the recurrence of menstrual bleeding occurred in 32% of patients under 40 years of age. A more recent trial (Toronto–London Trial), begun in 1965, offered higher doses of radiation (2000 rad in 5 days) for ovarian ablation following optimal local therapy. This was to be compared to no further therapy in patients aged 35 years to 44 years. Older pre-menopausal patients (>45 years) were randomized to receive no further therapy, ovarian irradiation, or ovarian irradiation and prednisone 7.5 mg/day. There was no stratification according to axillary node status. In addition, patients received postoperative radiation therapy to the regional nodes and chest wall prior to randomization. A total of 705 (Table 27-10) were randomized and followed up to 10 years. In pre-menopausal women age 45 years or more, ovarian irradiation plus prednisone caused a significant delay in recurrence and prolongation of survival at 10 years.[331] This advantage was not seen for those patients treated with ovarian irradiation alone in this age group or in those under 45 years of age.

Interpretation of such data without the benefit of estrogen receptor analyses is difficult since an imbalance in the randomization could produce an advantage for hormonal management in the treated group. However, the fact that advantage persisted for 10 years is of interest. There are no prospective trials of adjuvant bilateral adrenalectomy, but one uncontrolled series of postmenopausal patients with four or more positive axillary nodes were subjected to adjuvant adrenalectomy. Six out of 17 patients are surviving without recurrence 5 years or more since their primary treatment.[332] Adjuvant trials of additive hormone therapy or antiestrogens in postmenopausal women are currently underway, but the impact of antiestrogen therapy on adjuvant chemotherapy has been studied.[311] The addition of the antiestrogen, tamoxifen, demonstrated a clear-cut early advantage in estrogen receptor positive patients over chemotherapy (CMF) alone. The recurrence rate within the first 2 years was decreased by 20% in the CMF plus tamoxifen arm compared to CMF alone. No such differences were noted in estrogen-receptor negative patients. Although the estrogen receptor does not predict for responses to chemotherapy, this trial demonstrated earlier recurrences in estrogen-negative patients treated with adjuvant CMF compared to the estrogen-receptor positive patients.

TABLE 27-29. Adjuvant Treatment Castration Compared to Combination Chemotherapy—Premenopausal (Stage II)

TRIAL		TREATMENT	NUMBER OF PATIENTS	SURVIVAL DISEASE-FREE	OVERALL SURVIVAL	REFERENCE NUMBER
1. NSABP B-03		Surgery	43	227% (5 yrs.)*	40%	(329)
1961		Surgery + Oophorectomy	78	24%	39%	
2. Manchester		Surgery	200	38% (10 yrs.)	47.5%	(330)
1948–55		Surgery + Ovarian Radiation (450r)	203	49.3	55.5%	
3. Toronto		Surgery + RT	58	40% (10 yrs.)	46%	(331)
1965	<45 yrs.	Surgery + RT + Ovarian Radiation (2000r)	61	51%	61%	
	≥45 yrs	Surgery + RT	44	48%	59%	
		Surgery + RT + Ovarian RAD	47	60%	64%	
		Surgery + RT + Ovarian RAD + Prednisone	52	69%	77%	
4. NCI (Milan)		Radical Mastectomy	47	40% (5 yrs.)	61%	(338)
1973–75	<45 yrs.	Radical Mastectomy + CMF × 12 mos.	61	62%	82%	
	≥45 yrs	Radical Mastectomy	39	50%	65%	
		Radical Mastectomyy + CMF × 12 mos.	42	76%	92%	

*( )—time of evaluation in years.

Hormonal ablation has not demonstrated an improvement in the overall survival rate in all trials, except for one subgroup in the Toronto ovarian irradiation trial. Hormonal treatment combined with chemotherapy as an adjuvant continues to be investigated, but even in this circumstance, the advantage would be expected only in those patients who are estrogen-receptor positive.

ADJUVANT CYTOTOXIC CHEMOTHERAPY

The use of cytotoxic antitumor drugs as an adjuvant to radical surgery was initiated in 1957 when the NSABP randomly allocated patients to receive thiotepa in a dose of 0.4 mg/kg at the time of the operation followed by 0.2 mg/kg on each of the first two postoperative days or a placebo.[46] The basis for this was the observation of tumor cells in the circulating blood of patients undergoing surgical operation. A 10-year follow-up of this study employing 826 patients demonstrated that a small amount of systemic chemotherapy can enhance the early disease-free survival rate, but beyond 5 years there was no difference between the treated group and control. There appeared to be an advantage to a subgroup of premenopausal women with four or more positive nodes. This advantage persisted from 18 months to 10 years. It indicated approximately a 20% advantage in disease-free survival and overall survival. The trial confirmed the fact that 80% of treatment failures occurred within the first 5 years of observation. The node-positive patients in particular had an 86% chance of failure by 5 years.

Two major controlled trials exploring single-agent adjuvant treatment employed an alkylating agent because of the early demonstration of antitumor activity and ease of administration (Table 27-30). The succeeding NSABP trial (B-05) employing L-phenylalanine mustard (L-PAM) at a dose of 6 mg/m²/day for 5 days given every 6 weeks for 2 years was compared to a placebo-treated group.[71] L-PAM was initially attractive as an adjuvant chemotherapeutic agent since it was associated with minimal constitutional toxicity except for bone marrow suppression. The trial began in September, 1972, and terminated in February, 1975. With 370 patients admitted, 5-year follow-up indicates a significant disease-free survival difference between the treated and the control group for those patients who are pre-menopausal, that is, less than 49 years of age, with one to three positive nodes. Postmenopausal patients appear to have derived no benefit when compared to the palcebo-treated group. In the second generation trial (protocol B-7) 5-fluorouracil 300 mg/m²/day i.v. for 5 consecutive days was given simultaneously with L-PAM at 4 mg/m²/day p.o. for 5 days. The treatment was repeated every 6 weeks.[145] The patients were randomly assigned to this combination program (PF) or L-PAM 6 mg/m²/day for 5 days every 6 weeks. This trial randomized 741 patients between 1975 and 1976. It showed an overall advantage to adding the fluorouracil to L-PAM. A significant difference in disease-free survival was surprisingly confined to women over the age of 50 years who had four or more positive nodes. Since the follow-up is only four years, these results should be considered preliminary, but the suggestion is that the more intensive regimen was associated with better early disease-free survival advantage. These results were also obtained in the Mayo Clinic study which compared L-PAM with their CFP regimen which employs cyclophosphamide 150 mg/m²/day p.o. for 5 days, fluorouracil 300 mg/m²/day for 5 days, and prednisone 30 mg/day for 7 days given every 6 weeks for ten cycles.[146] This was very similar to the PF regimen in protocol B-7 of the NSABP. Tumor recurred more frequently with a higher mortality in the L-PAM-treated patients than in those on combination chemotherapy (Table 27-30).

A Scandinavian multi-institute trial which did not stratify according to node status compared a short course of cyclophosphamide given immediately postoperatively with a dosage of 30 mg/kg given over 6 days to no further therapy. A total of 507 patients were treated, compared to 519 randomized to no further therapy. The differences in the recurrence rate and death rate are significant and in favor of the treated group at 10 years in follow-up. The differences in recurrence are approximately 10% and have remained steady from 4 years after mastectomy to 10 years.[334] The authors contend that the

TABLE 27-30. Adjuvant Chemotherapy: Breast Cancer—Percent Disease-Free

CONTROLLED TRIALS	NUMBER OF PATIENTS	TIME OF EVALUATION	PREMENOPAUSAL			POSTMENOPAUSAL			REFERENCE NUMBER
			Total	1–3	4 Nodes	Total	1–3	4 Nodes	
1. NSABP (1958)	414	10 yrs.	55%	40%	32%	48%	43%	11%	(46)
→Thiotepa 0.4 mg/kgm post 0.2 mg/kgm × 2d									
→Placebo	406		46%	44%	11%	53%	32%	16%	
2. NSABP (1972–76)	346	5 yrs	60%	75%	40%	48%	60%	35%	(71)
→L-PAM (B-05-07)	505		40%	52%	30%	52%	68%	35%	
→Placebo (B-05-04)									
3. Milan (NCI) (1973–75)	207	4 yrs.	69%	85%	51%	56%		45%	(337)
→CMF × 12 mos.									
→No Treatment	179		41%	50%	23%	53%		43%	
4. Milan (NCI) (1975–78)	160	3 yrs	85%	90%	70%				(341)
→CMF × 12 mos.									
→CMF × 6 mos.	165		82%	89%	71%				
5. →Mayo	51	2 yrs.	58%			75%			(333)
L-PAM									
→CFP	58		85%			76%			

mechanism is probably not only a delay in the onset of clinical recurrence, but an actual reduction in the recurrence rate. Statistical analysis of the data demonstrated that the menstrual state did not influence the effect of chemotherapy in this trial such that the 10% difference occurred in the pre- as well as the postmenopausal patients. In those institutions where chemotherapy was delayed by at least 3 weeks rather than given according to protocol, the disease-free and survival advantage did not occur. The reason for this interesting difference has not been explained. The more dramatic results of adjuvant chemotherapy were seen in controlled trials using combination chemotherapy administered as has been previously shown on Table 27-24. The previously demonstrated superiority of combined drug therapy over single agents in advanced disease predicted for a greater early benefit when compared to no therapy. Cyclophosphamide, methotrexate, and fluorouracil (CMF) had a superior response rate to L-PAM (53% / 22%).[287] Thus, in 1973, NCI (Milan) initiated a trial utilizing CMF in a dosage of cyclophosphamide 100 mg/m²/day for 14 days, methotrexate 30 mg/m² and fluorouracil 400 mg/m² given on days 1 and 8 in each 28-day cycle for 12 cycles.[148–150] This was compared to no treatment in a prospective randomized trial with patients stratified according to menopausal status. This trial ended in 1975 after 386 patients were randomized. The data have been analyzed annually, and at 5 years of follow-up have demonstrated disease-free survival of 48% in the controls to 64% in the CMF-treated group.[338] The differences are most marked in pre-menopausal patients with one to three positive nodes (Table 27-30).

There appears to be no statistical advantage at the present time for disease-free survival for postmenopausal women. The observation that postmenopausal patients did not appear to benefit from adjuvant chemotherapy in the NSABP and Milan trials has been prematurely interpreted as a totally negative observation. However, it is clear that the doses of CMF used in the Milan trial were less than those previously employed in the trial, showing it to be superior to L-PAM, and in fact both series employed lower doses of CMF than in the original NCI (Bethesda) pilot trial in advanced disease.[286] A retrospective analysis of the Milan data with relatively small numbers at risk for 5 years indicates a statistical advantage compared to controls for those patients who received 85% or more of their prescribed dose of CMF.[346] The issue of dosage is important, since it has previously been shown by the same group that maximal doses of CMF were required to show an antitumor response in the setting of advanced disease. Essentially little antitumor effect occurred when less than 65% of the CMF dose was given that would imply an average dose of methotrexate of about 15 mg/m² and 200 mg/m² and 5-FU on days 1 and 8. The assessment of dose-response is retrospective in the Milan data. At least one group has demonstrated a 46% response rate on a "low dose" CMF schedule.[340] Postmenopausal patients who received more than 85% of the dose also demonstrated an advantage over the lower dose levels and controls. The numbers upon which the statistical information was based are quite small, with only nine patients at risk for 5 years who received 85% or more of the dose. These were compared to 38 control patients with the p value of 0.03.[339] It is clear that retrospective analysis of dose is probably not adequate to explain the differences. There, indeed, could be other factors which contribute to the difference. The case for the adjuvant therapy of postmenopausal women has been defended by the fact that uncontrolled trials employing combination chemotherapy showed a superior disease-free survival in postmenopausal women compared to historical controls. These include the two trials as shown in Table 27-31. In addition, the preliminary analysis of the NSABP Protocol 7 which compares L-PAM plus 5-FU shows a disease-free survival advantage at 5 years in postmenopausal women with four or more positive nodes. Postmenopausal women would be expected to benefit from adjuvant chemotherapy, since there does not seem to be a difference in response to cytotoxic drugs according to menstrual status.[260] Clearly, age, prior medical history, and other degenerative illnesses of old age could limit the dose of chemotherapy. A retrospective analysis of the Milan data showed only a total of 20 out of 87 postmenopausal women received 85% or greater of the dose. Despite the uncertain benefit of adjuvant therapy in the postmenopausal period, the Milan data are now showing an overall survival advantage in the pre-menopausal patients. The optimal duration and intensity of chemotherapy has not been established. Based on the early success of adjuvant chemotherapy in pre-menopausal women, the Milan group studied the issue of duration of adjuvant therapy in a prospective randomized trial in pre-menopausal women with positive axillary nodes comparing 6 months *versus* 12 months of CMF as an adjuvant to radical mastectomy.[341] Evaluation at 3 years shows no differences between the two groups. The issue of the intensity of adjuvant chemotherapy is being addressed in several comparative trials. These entail prospective comparisons of L-PAM with combination programs that have been shown to be effective in advanced diseases. These

TABLE 27-31. Adjuvant Chemotherapy: Breast Cancer—Uncontrolled Trials, Percent Disease-Free

	NUMBER OF PATIENTS	TIME OF EVALUATION	PREMENOPAUSAL			POSTMENOPAUSAL			REFERENCE NUMBER
			Total	1–3	4 Nodes	Total	1–3	4 Nodes	
1. Cooper CMFVP ± RT	100	8 yrs.	68%	–	68%	68%	–	68%	(342)
2. MDA FAC ± BCG	222	3 yrs.	70%	80%	65%	83%	91%	78%	(343)
3. UCLA CMF ± BCG	57 (35–50 yrs) patients	2 yrs.	75%	Disease at 2 yrs.					(344)

*See Table 27-5 for details of chemotherapy regimen.

include CMF (Manchester), CFP (Mayo) and CMFVP (SEOG). Preliminary analyses of these trials all show an advantage over L-PAM. Clinical trials without simultaneous controls which employed intensive combination chemotherapy either of the CMFVP type or the combination of fluorouracil, adriamycin, and cytoxan plus BCG have shown an impressive disease-free survivorship at 3 years and 8 years; 65% and 85%, respectively, in patients with four or more positive nodes.[342–344] Further, a retrospective analysis of the Milan data shows a clear-cut relationship between the response and amount of CMF administered. This is also seen in the NSABP trial B-7 where L-PAM plus fluorouracil appears to be superior to L-PAM alone in the postmenopausal patients with over four positive nodes. It is possible to speculate that shorter courses of high dose chemotherapy might be equivalent to the longer, more protracted schedules that have been used in the past. A definitive answer can only come from a carefully designed, prospective randomized trial. The observation that the benefits of the chemotherapy seem to be confined primarily to pre-menopausal women has raised the issue that these are mediated through the effects of these agents on ovarian function. Studies of follicle-stimulating hormone (FSH), luteinizing hormone (LH), and plasma estradiol levels in patients who become amenorrheic on adjuvant chemotherapy support the concept of ovarian failure.[345] However, the analysis of the NSABP and Milan trials would indicate that those patients who benefitted most from adjuvant chemotherapy, that is, younger pre-menopausal women, have the lowest incidence of amenorrhea. Seventy-three percent of the women aged 40 years to 49 years became amenorrheic, as opposed to only 22% of those less than 39 years of age.[346] Although one can conclude that suppression of ovarian function may account for some of the benefit of adjuvant chemotherapy in pre-menopausal women, the major impact comes from a direct cytotoxic effect over and above the induction of ovarian failure. Comparison of the treatment failure rate in adjuvant ovarian ablation trials with the results of adjuvant CMF indicates a clear-cut early superiority of chemotherapy.[347]

The role of immunotherapy in the adjuvant treatment of breast cancer has been poorly evaluated, with a heavy reliance on historical controls.[343,344] In the early evaluation of a prospective trial where BCG plus chemotherapy was compared to chemotherapy alone or chemotherapy plus tamoxifen, no added benefit of BCG scarification could be demonstrated.[311]

The follow-up of patients receiving adjuvant chemotherapy entails periodic evaluation including a physical examination every 4 weeks to 6 weeks during treatment and approximately every 4 months to 6 months after cessation of chemotherapy. The chest roentgenogram and bone scans are repeated on an every 6 month to 8 month basis. A routine liver scan is generally unnecessary unless there are clinical or biochemical findings that justify investigation. The pattern of first relapse does not appear to be substantially changed by adjuvant combination chemotherapy.[348] Bone and lung comprise the major metastatic sites both in the control and treated groups of patients accounting for 50% to 60% of relapsed patients. The relapse following cessation of adjuvant chemotherapy can be retreated with the original regimen.[349] The response rate to regimens such as CMF or FAC in this setting is approximately 40% to 60%—almost the same response rate as noted in those untreated control patients who subsequently relapsed. As has been mentioned previously, cytotoxic chemotherapy does not effect the estrogen receptor status of the recurrent tumor, thus does not compromise the opportunity of a subsequent response to endocrine therapy.

At this point in time, adjuvant chemotherapy appears to have exerted a major effect within the first 5 years on the disease-free survival of patients with Stage II breast carcinoma. In addition, several major randomized controlled trials are demonstrating a survival advantage for pre-menopausal patients treated with adjuvant chemotherapy. The optimal dose and schedule of adjuvant treatment are unknown and are currently under investigation.

GUIDELINES FOR SYSTEMIC THERAPY

General recommendations for the treatment of the various stages of breast cancer are made according to the menstrual state, ERP content, and extent of disease (Table 27-32). There are likely to be many exceptional circumstances; however, these are offered as general guidelines. They include some options which in the future may become the more conventional approach. Antiestrogens may soon be used as the primary treatment of ERP-positive premenopausal women. Stage III pre-menopausal women should be offered the benefits of "adjuvant" chemotherapy after maximal local treatment with surgery and radiation as described earlier. Adjuvant chemotherapy or hormonal therapy can be considered for selected postmenopausal women, despite the absence of sound data to support its use. Ideally, adjuvant therapy of postmenopausal women should be undertaken in the context of a clinical trial. Advanced (Stage IV) disease can be treated with hormonal therapy in ERP-positive patients but pattern of metastatic disease and rate of progression may dictate cytotoxic drugs regardless of ERP status.

Anti-estrogen therapy has replaced additive hormone or endocrine ablation as the first-line hormonal treatment of postmenopausal ERP-positive women. Responders who subsequently relapse might still be responsive to subsequent ablation or other hormones.

Pharmacologic techniques which interfere with adrenal and pituitary secretion have already been introduced, but only medical adrenalectomy with aminoglutethimide and corticoid has shown clinical promise. Patients with advanced disease refractory to endocrine treatment and chemotherapy with "conventional" agents at the present time have few therapeutic options as most of the newer agents have been shown to be ineffective (Table 27-23). Many of the recent regimens do not include vinca alkaloids and some responses to vinblastine have been noted. More recently the combination of vinblastine and mitomycin-C has been used for refractory patients with responses seen in 44% patients.[237]

Further progress in therapeutic research will require the continuing accession of patients to clinical trials. Since systemic therapy in advanced disease is palliative in almost all instances, new and promising agents can be employed early upon symptomatic relapse from the best first-line chemotherapy. It has become increasingly difficult to evaluate new agents in breast cancer because of the extensive prior treat-

TABLE 27-32. Options for Systemic Therapy

PREMENOPAUSAL	
Stage I	
ERP+	No further therapy
ERP−	Adjuvant chemotherapy (optional)
Stage II	
ERP+	Adjuvant chemotherapy +/− antihormone
ERP−	Adjuvant chemotherapy
Stage III	
ERP+ } ERP− }	Maximal local treatment plus combination chemotherapy*
Stage IV	
ERP−	Combination chemotherapy
ERP+	Oophorectomy or antiestrogen therapy
POSTMENOPAUSAL	
Stage I	
ERP+	No further therapy
ERP−	No further therapy
STAGE II	
ERP+	Chemotherapy } Investigational; Antiestrogen } Investigational
ERP−	Chemotherapy Optional
Stage III	
ERP+ } ERP− }	Maximal local control plus antiestrogen or chemotherapy (combination chemotherapy)
Stage IV	
ERP+	Antiestrogen → Ablation → Chemotherapy
ERP−	Combination chemotherapy

*Except where combination chemotherapy–investigational protocols in use. CMF, CMFP or FAC have the most extensive evaluation and are equivalent in effectiveness.

ment most refractory patients will have previously received, including radiation therapy.

SPECIAL CONSIDERATIONS CONCERNING LOBULAR CARCINOMA-*IN-SITU*

In 1941 Foote and Stewart as well as Muir called attention to an *in situ* form of carcinoma of the female breast apparently arising within the end parts of the lobule which they designated as lobular carcinoma-*in situ*.[350,351] Subsequent to their reports, as well as those of others, it becomes recognized that *in situ* carcinoma may develop into, or at least be associated with, a relatively distinct histologic type of invasive carcinoma designated as lobular infiltrating or lobular invasive carcinoma. The frequency or absolute certainty of such a progression is not known, but judgments have been made attesting to its rarity as well as to its prevalence.[352–356] It should be recognized that a substantial number of patients who have received no other treatment than local excision of lobular carcinoma-*in-situ* have failed to develop invasive breast cancer, even after prolonged follow-up.[357,358] Further, it is generally accepted that the presence of *in situ* lobular carcinoma is not essential for the diagnosis of the invasive type although in the study of 1000 cases of invasive breast cancer of all types, *in situ* lobular carcinoma was significantly more frequent in association with the lobular invasive form than other histologic types, although not exclusively limited to it.[18,359]

Of particular interest, both biologically as well as clinically, is the extensive information which indicates that such tumors are multicentric and have a tendency to involve both breasts, either synchronous or asynchronous. The frequency of bilateral involvement is less than certain.[25,129,350,352,354,356,358,360–364]

Early studies suggested an incidence of about 20%.[352,356] More recent reports indicate a greater occurrence. Urban reported that 35% of biopsies of opposite breasts of patients with *in situ* lobular carcinoma demonstrated such lesions and Snyder observed that 33% of his patients had bilateral circinomas-*in-situ*.[25,363] Lewison and Finney obtained similar findings in 47% of their patients subjected to bilateral breast biopsies.[365] Benfield acknowledged a "35% to 59% incidence of bilaterality of lobular carcinoma" and Warner, in summarizing data in that regard, concluded that "combining all results, the overall occurrence of bilaterality in lobular carcinoma appears to be no less than 15%. However, among patients investigated by bilateral biopsy and mammography, the incidence is considerably higher."[361,366] Not all investigators have recorded bilateral tumors so frequently. Hutter and Foote found bilaterality in only 13% of 46 patients followed from 4 to 27 years, and Farrow observed a 10% incidence.[360,367] In a subsequent report he noted that 12.3% of his cases had simultaneous and 6% had non-simultaneous bilateral lobular carcinomas-*in-situ*.[362]

PRE-OPERATIVE DIAGNOSIS

It is virtually impossible to make a diagnosis of lobular carcinoma-*in-situ* by clinical examination. Symptoms are variable and, even if present, are of little value in diagnosis.[362] In most instances the signs and symptoms which lead to clinical examination and biopsy are related to benign lesions, such as fibrocystic mastopathy, which have no relationship to the lobular carcinoma-*in-situ*. Roentgenologic methods (conventional mammography or xeroradiography) are likewise not very helpful. While stippled or linear flecks of calcium may draw attention to the possibility of the presence of a lesion, such findings have been noted in less than 50% of breasts containing these tumors.[363,368,369] The calcifications, when present, are most frequently found in lobules surrounding the *in situ* carcinoma rather than in the tumor itself. Since similar micro-calcifications occur in a variety of benign breast diseases as well, they fail to provide sufficient specificity for making a diagnosis.

PATHOLOGIC FEATURES

Lobular carcinoma-*in-situ* cannot be diagnosed by gross pathologic examination. Occasionally, and retrospectively, one may gain the impression of an ill-defined area of induration within the breast substance. The lesion has most frequently been encountered as an incidental finding in specimens removed for benign disease. They have been identified in specimens of breasts containing calcified fat necrosis, fibroadenomas, abscesses, fibrosis, duct papillomas and papillomatosis, cysts, and sclerosing adenosis—all of which are in no way causally treated.

The microscopic diagnosis of lobular carcinoma-*in-situ* is sometimes difficult because of the mimicry afforded by lobular hyperplasias.[370] This dilemma is analogous to that encountered in the differential diagnosis of proliferative or hyperplastic lesions and intraductal carcinomas of the larger or extralobular ductal system. Such difficulty and uncertainty are frequently reflected by the designation "atypical" lobular hyperplasia. A detailed description of the pathologic features of this *in situ* tumor is available for reference.[371]

SURGICAL MANAGEMENT

The diagnosis of this lesion by frozen section is undesirable and the implementation of schemata of treatment based upon such a procedure may be subject to criticism for several reasons. First, the distinction between *in situ* lobular carcinoma and some instances of lobular hyperplasia, even by those with expertise, often may be extremely difficult. Second, multiple well-prepared sections must be available for examination to exclude the presence of invasive lobular carcinoma even if the *in situ* diagnosis is entertained by the rapid method.

Treatment strategies for the management of a lobular carcinoma-*in-situ* have evolved from considerations relative to (a) its multicentricity, (b) its tendency to occur either synchronously or asynchronously in the other breast, and (c) the popularly held conviction that it represents a stage in the development of lobular invasive cancer. Consequently, surgical management has been related to two basic questions. What procedure should be employed in the treatment of the involved breast? What, if anything, should be done with the contralateral breast? Benfield and associates have suggested that after the diagnosis of *in situ* lobular carcinoma is established, total mastectomy should be performed and the upper outer quadrant of the contralateral breast be biopsied.[352] If the mastectomy specimen reveals invasive carcinoma, a radical mastectomy should be performed. When the biopsy of the contralateral breast reveals *in situ* lobular carcinoma, total mastectomy is advised. Although the authors did not elaborate it might be presumed that should the second breast be found after total mastectomy to have an invasive tumor, a radical mastectomy would also be performed. Benfield and associates subsequently modified their views suggesting that total mastectomy should be performed on the contralateral breast without biopsy.[361] Such a mastectomy would be considered "prophylactic" if it contained no tumor. If the patient refused contralateral mastectomy and mammography demonstrated no abnormality, they recommended biopsy of the upper outer quadrant of that breast. They urged that such patients be examined and have mammograms at periodic intervals for the rest of their lives. A repeat biopsy or total mastectomy is to be carried out if mammograms or physical examination becomes "suspicious." In 1972, they reiterated their position by stating that "contralateral total mastectomy is advised for both *in situ* and for invasive lobular carcinoma because the high incidence of bilaterality warrants this recommendation."[372]

Lewison and Finney have recommended that total mastectomy be the procedure of choice for management of the involved breast.[365] They are more conservative in regard to the contralateral breast and state that "mammography and biopsy of the opposite breast if indicated, as well as careful follow-up examination is absolutely mandatory."

Newman and Farrow have both suggested the use of total mastectomy and axillary dissection for the management of the involved breast.[356,360] The former has advocated a biopsy of the upper outer quadrant of the opposite breast at the time of mastectomy and the latter made no specific recommendation relative to the other breast. Donegan and Perez-Mesa, as well as Dall'Olmo and associates have advocated total mastectomy with elective biopsy of the opposite breast as the preferred method of management.[373,374]

In 1971, Fisher expressed concern about the need for total mastectomy in the management of such non-invasive cancers.[375] Subsequently, others have cautiously indicated a similar reservation.[353,374] For several important reasons, a total or a modified radical mastectomy would seem to be an overly extended operation. Similarly, a segmental mastectomy without recovery of axillary nodes may be less than adequate. A singular lack of information attesting to the significance of multicentric carcinoma suggests that total removal of the breast for the purpose of eliminating multicentric foci of lobular carcinoma-*in-situ* is inappropriate. Evidence suggests that such lesions despite their presence, may be of dubious clinical significance. Local breast recurrence following a relatively large number of segmental mastectomies occurs only rarely and it is not clear whether they are persistencies of the original tumor or the result of multicentric foci.[173] The few recurrences have been satisfactorily treated by mastectomy and such unorthodoxy failed to influence survival.

If lobular carcinoma-*in-situ* is a stage in the development of lobular invasive carcinoma, as has been suggested, then the oversight of remaining undetected foci of *in situ* carcinomas following a segmental mastectomy could be difficult to justify.[354] While apparent progression from the *in situ* to the infiltrating form has been noted, proof of such an occurrence remains inconclusive and has been questioned.[356,376] Moreover, a substantial number of cases subjected to biopsy only have failed to demonstrate invasive tumors after extensive follow-up.[357,358] Recently Dall'Olmo and co-workers reviewed from published papers the fate of patients with lobular carcinoma-*in situ* treated by excisional biopsy alone.[374] From that compilation it is evident there is substantially less risk of progression from the *in situ* to the invasive form than noted by McDivitt and associates.[354] A study by Wheeler and others exemplifies that finding.[377] They noted that of 25 patients treated by excisional biopsy alone and having an average follow-up of 17.5 years, only one patient (4%) developed infiltrating carcinoma. Of particular interest is the fact that of the ten patients in the series of McDivitt and associates who had unilateral lobular carcinoma *in situ* treated by excisional biopsy, and who subsequently developed infiltrating carcinoma, eight of the latter were infiltrating duct and two were infiltrating lobular types.[354,378] Moreover, six of those with infiltrating carcinoma had on previous biopsy been diagnosed as having benign disease. Those diagnoses were changed retrospectively after the invasive cancers were found. The frequent association of invasive tumors of other histologic types with *in situ* carcinomas must result in the conjecture that factors resulting in the development of the latter may also effect the development of the former and that there is not necessarily a causal relationship between the two.

Thus, because of the uncertain significance of multicentricity and because of the questionable relationship of the *in situ* to the invasive form, we fail to be impressed with those circumstances as sufficient justification for the performance of total mastectomy for *in situ* lobular carcinoma. Moreover increasing proficiency with mammographic techniques provides a technical backup to such conservative considerations. In that regard it is of interest that investigators who recommend management of the contralateral breast by biopsy only "in those instances when clinical or roentgenologic evidence suggests a pathologic process" are unwilling to utilize the same procedure following segmental resection of a breast for lobular *in situ* tumors, but proceed at once to total breast removal.[374]

Should the surgical management of lobular carcinoma-*in-situ* include an axillary dissection? Recently Dall'Olmo and associates reported finding no instance of nodal involvement in 24 cases of lobular carcinoma-*in-situ* treated by radical mastectomy.[374] Because of this they recommended total mastectomy without axillary intervention as the proper therapy for this lesion. While theoretically it might be anticipated that the axillary contents would be devoid of tumor in the presence of *in situ* lesions, we have observed positive axillary nodes in a few instances in which the primary tumor was, by conventional light microscopic techniques, of the non-invasive intraductal type.[362,379] The sampling error inherent in the diagnosis of *in situ* or non-invasive carcinomas is likely to result in the occasional case in which invasion is overlooked. Consequently, a low axillary dissection (axillary "sampling") should accompany segmental mastectomy. Certainly such a procedure is cosmetically more desirable than is total mastectomy without axillary dissection. In the rare instance when lymph nodes are found to be tumor-positive, other therapeutic approaches such as total mastectomy, breast radiation, or systemic adjuvant therapy will require consideration.

Insofar as treatment of the contralateral breast is concerned, biopsy should be performed only for those lesions which are suspicious by mammography or clinical examination.[375] Prophylactic mastectomy has no place in the therapeutic approach to this cancer. Interval mammographic examination of both the contralateral and ipsilateral breasts is mandatory.

A recent report by Rosen and associates of findings from 99 patients with *in situ* lobular carcinoma, identified by breast biopsies performed at Memorial Hospital between 1940 and 1950 and not treated by mastectomy, has attracted considerable attention.[380] Those authors have concluded from that retrospective review that low axillary dissection and concurrent biopsy of the opposite breast is the procedure of choice. Their decision is based upon the observation that in that group of patients "when compared with general population data, the frequency of subsequent breast carcinoma was nine times greater than expected and deaths due to breast cancer were 11 times more frequent than expected." Examination of the actual data leads to conclusions not as absolute as that statement would imply. Twelve of 99 patients developed ipsilateral cancers over a 24-year period. Surprisingly, many of the cancers were of the non-lobular type, either completely or partially, and six subsequently died of breast cancer. Despite their conclusions relative to management, those authors acknowledged that "the more we learn about this disease, the less certain it appears at present that any single recommendation for therapy is appropriate for all patients."

CARCINOMA OF THE BREAST IN MALES

Carcinoma of the breast occurs quite infrequently in males. It is estimated to have an incidence of about 1% of the disease in females.[381,382] The average age appears to be about 10 years older than for that of the female breast cancer.[382–385] There have been few epidemiologic studies. There does appear to be some familial distribution with very rare families of multiple males with breast cancer.[386,387] Some families with high likelihood for breast cancer in the females have an occasional associated male with breast cancer. It appears to be associated with disease that causes hyperestrogenism. Bilharziasis appears to be associated with the disease.[388] This damages the liver and causes hyperestrogenism. In Egypt, where this is a common disease, male breast cancer constitutes about 6% of all breast cancer as opposed to the 1% usually described. There is some evidence that gynecomastia also predisposes to the disease. There is a significant elevation of the incidence in patients with Klinefelter's syndrome.[389] The tumor, on pathologic examination, resembles carcinoma of the breast in females with the exception that the lobular carcinoma-*in situ* is not seen in the male. Estrogen receptors have been found on male breast cancer in as many as 84% of the specimens.[340] Clinically, the disease usually presents abnormality of the nipple, including retractive nipple, crusting or discharge from the nipple, and ulceration. The tumor is frequently less well defined than in the female breast cancer and because of the limited breast tissue in males without evidence of lobules the tumor is frequently closely applied to the pectoral fascia and early on can involve the muscle itself.

Distribution of patients by stage of disease indicates that male breast cancer usually presents in a more advanced state.[383,384] Review of breast cancer at the Ellis Fischel State Cancer Hospital revealed a statistical significant difference in the clinical factors shown in Table 27-33. The reported experience has been to use mastectomy, usually a radical mastectomy because of the involvement of the muscle. Occasionally, if the muscle is not involved extensively, then the pectoral muscle can be spared. Use of radiation therapy alone for early carcinoma of the male breast has not been reported in significant numbers. It has been used both as an adjuvant, both postoperatively following mastectomy, and in advanced male breast cancer.[385] Lymph node involvement has the same prognostic significance in males as it does in females.

There is some difference in the literature as to prognosis. Most authors feel that, while male breast cancer presents in a more advanced stage, within each stage prognosis is similar to that in females.[383,384,391] There are some authors who feel that the chance of survival is worse than in female breast cancer even when stage is considered.[392]

The pattern of metastasis is similar to the female with bone (48%), soft tissue (60%), and various visceral sites.[391] The standard therapy for metastatic disease is orchidectomy. The objective remission rate is higher than for female castration (50%–60%).[393,394] The high response rate most likely reflects the high incidence of ERP. The responses last 3 months to 40 months with a median duration of 12 months. Further palliation may be obtained by adrenalectomy. A review of the literature by one author identified 17 cases, of which 12 were evaluable.[395] Nine patients objectively responded for from 5 months to 5 years. Hypophysectomy may also palliate advanced disease. A review of the experience with that operation confirmed objective remissions including complete responses in five of eight patients.[396]

Although there is no experience with antiestrogen, a few responses have been noted with additive hormones.[396] Refractoriness to hormonal management would require chemotherapy of the type used in advanced female breast cancer. Similarly, although no data exists to support it, adjuvant chemotherapy could be offered to those patients with positive axillary nodes.

TABLE 27-33. Clinical Features Found Different in 27 Patients with Male Breast Cancer as Compared to 2370 Patients

CLINICAL FACTOR	FEMALE	MALE
Mean age	60.6 years	71.2 years
History of trauma	11.1%	29.6%
Central lesion	17.8%	85.7%
Ulceration of breast	11.1%	31.6%
Satellite nodules present	7.6%	20.0%
Stage D (Columbia Class)	30.0%	52.4%

(Donegan WL, Perez–Mesa C: Carcinoma of the male breast. Arch Surg 106:273–279, 1973)

REFERENCES

1. Kelsey JL: A review of the epidemiology of human breast cancer. Epidem Rev 1:74–109, 1979
2. MacMahon B, Cole P, Brown J: Etiology of human breast cancer: a review. J Natl Cancer Inst 50:21–42, 1973
3. Trichopoulos D, MacMahon B, Cole P: Menopause and breast cancer risk. J Natl Cancer Inst 41:315–329, 1968
4. Smith PG, Doll R: Late effects of x-irradiation in patients treated for metropathia haemorrhagica. Br J Radiol 49:224–232, 1976
5. MacMahon B, Cole P, Lin TM et al: Age at first birth and breast cancer risk. Bull WHO 43:209–221, 1970
6. Tulinius H, Day NE, Johannesson G et al: Reproductive factors and risk for breast cancer in Iceland. Int J Cancer 21:724–730, 1978
7. Petrakis NL: Genetic factors in the etiology of breast cancer. Cancer 39:2709–2715, 1977
8. Monson RR, Yen S, MacMahon B et al: Chronic mastitis and carcinoma of the breast. Lancet 2:224–226, 1976
9. McGregor DH, Land CE, Choi K et al: Breast cancer incidence among atomic bomb survivors, Hiroshima and Nagasaki, 1950–1969. J Natl Cancer Inst 59:799–811, 1977
10. Boice JD Jr, Monson RR: Breast cancer in women after repeated fluoroscopic examinations of the chest. J Natl Cancer Inst 59:823–832, 1977
11. Shore RE, Hempelmann LH, Kowaluk E et al: Breast neoplasms in women treated with x-rays for acute postpartum mastitis. J Natl Cancer Inst 59:813–822, 1977
12. Ross RK, Paganini-Hill A, Gerkins VR et al: A case-control study of menopausal estrogen therapy and breast cancer. JAMA 243:1635–1639, 1980
13. Brinton LA, Williams RR, Hoover RN, et al: Breast cancer risk factors among screening program participants. J Natl Cancer Inst 62:37–43, 1979
14. Williams RR, Feinleib M, Connor RJ et al: Case-control study of antihypertensive and diuretic use by women with malignant and benign breast lesions detected in a mammography screening program. J Natl Cancer Inst 61:327–335, 1978
15. Hennekens CH, Speizer FE, Rosner B et al: Use of permanent hair dyes and cancer among registered nurses. Lancet 1:1390–1393, 1979
16. Nasca PC, Lawrence CE, Greenwald P et al: Relationship of hair dye use, benign breast disease, and breast cancer. J Natl Cancer Inst 64:23–28, 1980
17. Miller AB, Bullbrook RD: The epidemiology and etiology of breast cancer. New Engl J Med (in press)
18. Fisher ER, Gregorio RM, Fisher B et al: The pathology of invasive breast cancer: A syllabus derived from findings of the National Surgical Adjuvant Breast Project (Protocol 4). Cancer 36:1–85, 1975
19. Black MM, Opler SR, Speer FD: Survival in breast cancer cases in relation to the structure of the primary tumor and regional lymph nodes. Surg Gynecol Obstet 100:543–551, 1955
20. Black MM, Speer FD: Immunology of cancer. Int Abstr Surg 109:105–116, 1959
21. Black MM, Speer FD: Nuclear structure in cancer tissues. Surg Gynecol Obstet 105:97–102, 1957
22. Black MM, Speer FD, Opler SR: Structural representations of tumor–host relationship in mammary carcinoma—biologic and prognostic significance. Am J Clin Pathol 26:250–265, 1956
23. Fisher E, Redmond C, Fisher B et al: Pathologic Findings from the National Surgical Adjuvant Breast Project (Protocol 4) VI. Discriminants for 5-year treatment failure. Cancer 46: 908–918, 1980
24. Fisher ER, Redmond C, Fisher B: Histologic Grading of Breast Cancer. Pathology Annual 15: 234–251, 1980
25. Urban JA: Bilaterality of cancer of the breast. Biopsy of the opposite breast. Cancer 20: 1867–1870, 1967
26. Urban JA: Biopsy of the "normal" breast in treating breast cancer. Surg Clin N Am 49:291–301, 1969

27. Slack NH, Bross IDJ, Nemoto T et al: Experiences with bilateral primary carcinoma of the breast. Surg Gynecol Obstet 136:433–440, 1973
28. Kramer WM, Rush BF: Mammary duct proliferation in the elderly: A histopathologic study. Cancer 31:130–137, 1973
29. Black MM, Speer FD: Sinus histiocytosis of lymph nodes in cancer. Surg Gynecol Obstet 106:163–175, 1958
30. Berg JW: Sinus histiocytosis—A fallacious measure of host resistance to cancer. Cancer 9:935–939, 1956
31. Kister SJ, Sommers SC, Haagensen CD et al: Nuclear grade and sinus histiocytosis in cancer of the breast. Cancer 23:570–575, 1969
32. Haagensen CD: Diseases of the Breast, 2nd ed. Philadelphia, WB Saunders, 1971, p 829
33. Spratt JS, Donegan WL: Cancer of the Breast. Philadelphia, WB Saunders, 1967, pp 133–134
34. Fisher B, Slack NH, Ausman RK, et al: Location of breast carcinoma and prognosis. Surg Gynecol Obstet 129: 705–716, 1969
35. Haagensen CD: Diseases of the Breast, rev 2nd ed. Philadelphia, WB Saunders, 1971, pp 384–390
36. Smith JA, Gamez-Araujo JJ, Gallagher HS et al: Carcinoma of the breast: Analysis of total lymph node involvement *versus* level of metastasis. Cancer 39:527, 1977
37. Pickren JW: Significance of occult metastases. Cancer 14:1266–1271, 1961
38. Fisher B, Slack NH, et al: Number of lymph nodes examined and the prognosis of breast cancer. Surg Gynecol Obstet 131:79–88, 1970
39. Rose CM, Botnick LE, Harris JR et al: The use of axillary sampling to determine nodal status in patients undergoing definitive breast irradiation (abstract). Int J Rad Oncol Biol Phys 4:174, 1978
40. Bretcher H: Radical mastectomy for mammary carcinoma. Ann Surg 170:883–884, 1969
41. Haagensen CD, Cooley E: Radical mastectomy for mammary carcinoma. Ann Surg 170:884–888, 1969
42. Schottenfeld D, Nash AG, Robbins GF et al: Ten-year results of the treatment of primary operable breast carcinoma. Cancer 38:1001–1007, 1976
43. Bucalossi P, Veronesi V, Zingo L et al: Enlarged mastectomy for breast cancer: Review of 1213 cases. Am J Roentgen Rad Ther Nucl Med 111:119–122, 1971
44. Valagussa P, Bonadonna G, Veronesi V: Patterns of relapse and survival following radical mastectomy. Cancer 41:1170–1178, 1978
45. Haagensen CD: Treatment of curable carcinoma of the breast. Int J Rad Oncol Biol Phys 2:975–980, 1977
46. Fisher B, Slack N, Katrych D et al: Ten-year followup results of patients with carcinoma of the breast in a cooperative clinical trial evaluating surgical adjuvant chemotherapy. Surg Gyn Obstet 140:528–534, 1975
47. Spratt JS, Donegan WL: Carcinoma of the Breast. Philadelphia, WB Saunders, 1967, p. 136
48. Payne WS, Taylor WF, Khonsari S, et al: Surgical treatment of breast cancer: Trends and factors affecting survival. Arch Surg 101:105, 1970
49. Haagensen CD: Diseases of the Breast, Rev 2nd ed, Philadelphia, WB Saunders, 1971, p. 405
50. Fisher B, Slack NH, Borss IDJ et al: Cancer and the breast: Size of neoplasm and prognosis. Cancer 24:1071–1080, 1969
51. Nemoto T, Vana J, Bedwani RN et al: Management and survival of female breast cancer: Results of a national survey by the American College of Surgeons. Cancer 45:2917–2924, 1980
52. Adair F, Berg J, Joubert L et al: Long term follow-up of breast cancer patients: The 30-year report. Cancer 33:1145, 1974
53. Handley RS: Carcinoma of the breast. Ann Roy Coll Surg 57:59–66, 1975
54. Bucalossi P, Veronesi D, Zingo L et al: Enlarged mastectomy for breast cancer: Review of 1213 cases. Am J Roent Rad Ther Nucl Med 111:119, 1971
55. Dahl-Iversen E: Recherches sur les metastases microscopiques des cancers du sein dans les ganglions lymphatiques parasternaux et susclavicularies. Mem Acad de Chin 78:651, 1952
56. Halsted WS: The results of radical operations for the cure of cancer of the breast. Ann Surg 46:1–19, 1907
57. Warren S, Witman EM: Studies on tumor metastases: The distribution of metastases in cancer of the breast. Surg Gyn Obstet 57, 81, 1937
58. Saphillo O, Parker ML: Metastases of primary carcinoma of the breast with special reference to spleen, adrenal glands and ovaries. Arch Surg 42:1003, 1941
59. Haagensen CD: Diseases of the Breast, 2nd ed. Philadelphia, WB Saunders, 1971, p 426
60. Fisher ER, Swamidoss S, Lee CH et al: Detection and significance of occult axillary lymph node metastases in patients with invasive breast cancer. Cancer 42:2025–2031, 1978
61. Huvos AG, Hutter RVP, Berg JW: Significance of axillary macrometastases and micrometastasis in mammary cancer. Ann Surg 173:44–46, 1971
63. Gray HJ: Relation of the lymphatic vessels to the spread of cancer. Br J Surg 26:462–495, 1939
64. Dewitt JE: The significance of regional node metastasis in breast cancer. Can Med Assoc J 93:289–293, 1965
65. Baum M, Coyle PJ: Simple Mastectomy for early breast cancer and the behavior of the untreated axillary nodes. Bull Cancer 64:603–610, 1977
66. Crile G Jr: A Biological Consideration of the Treatment of Breast Cancer. Ft. Lauderdale, Charles A. Thomas, 1967
67. Stjernsward J: Decreased survival related to irradiation postoperatively in early operable breast cancer. Lancet II: 1285–1286, 1974
68. Cancer Research Campaign Working Party: Cancer research campaign trial for early breast cancer. Lancet II:55–60, 1980
69. Lythgoe JP, Leck I, Swindell R: Manchester regional breast study: Preliminary results. Lancet 1:744–747, 1978
70. Turnbull AR, Turner DTL, Chant ADB et al: Treatment of early breast cancer. Lancet 2:7–9, 1978
71. Fisher B, Redmond C, Fisher ER et al: The contribution of recent NSABP clinical trials of primary breast cancer therapy to an understanding of tumor biology. Cancer (in press)
72. Shapiro S, Strax P, Venet L et al: Changes in 5-year breast cancer screening program. In Proceedings of Seventh National Cancer Conference, Philadelphia, JB Lippincott, 1973
73. Shapiro S: Evidence on screening for breast cancer from a randomized trial. Cancer 39:2772–2782, 1977
74. Miller AB: Risk–benefit in mass screening programs for breast cancer. Sem Oncol 5:351–359, 1978
75. Bailar JC: Mammography, a contrary view. Ann Intern Med 85:77–84, 1976
76. Tokunaga M, Norman JE, Asano M et al: Malignant breast tumors among atomic bomb survivors, Hiroshima and Nagasaki, 1950–1974. J Natl Cancer Inst 62:1347–1359, 1979
77. Baral E, Larsson LE, Mattson B: Breast cancer following irradiation of the breast. Cancer 40:2905–2910, 1977
78. Boice JD Jr, Land CE, Shore RE et al: Risk of breast cancer following low-dose radiation exposure. Radiology 131:589–597, 1979
79. Land CE, Boice JD Jr, Shore RE, et al: Breast cancer risk from low-dose exposures to ionizing radiation. J Natl Cancer Inst (in press)
80. Land CE: Low dose radiation—a cause of breast cancer? Cancer 46:868–873, 1980
81. Advisory Committee on the Biological Effects of Ionizing Radiations, National Academy of Sciences—National Research Council: The effects of populations of exposure to low levels of ionizing radiation. Washington DC, US Govt Print Off, 1972
82. Thier S: NIH/NCI Consensus Development Meeting on Breast Cancer Screening. Bethesda, Maryland, Sept 14–16, 1977 (submitted to the National Institutes of Health, Oct 18, 1977)
83. Baker ER: The indications for bone scan in the pre-operative assessment of patients with operable breast cancer. Breast Dis 3:43–45, 1977
84. McNeil B, Pace PD, Gray E et al: Pre-operative and follow-up bone scans in patients with primary carcinoma of the breast. Surg Gyn Obstet 147:745–748, 1978
85. Wiener SN, Sachs SH: An Assessment of positive liver scanning in patients with breast cancer. Arch Surg 113:126–127, 1970

86. Casta GNA, Benfield J Jr, Yamama H et al: The reliability of liver scans and function tests in detecting metastases. Surg Gyn Obstet 134:463–469, 1972
87. Steward AM, Nixon D, Zamcheck N et al: Carcinoembryonic antigen in breast cancer patients. Cancer 33:1246–1252, 1979
88. Tormey DC, Wastros TT, Ahmann D et al: Biological markers in breast cancer I. Incidence of abnormalities of CEA, HCG, polyamines and three minor nucleosides. Cancer 35:1095–1100, 1975
89. Tormey DC, Waalkes TP, Semon RM: Biological markers in breast cancer II. Clinical correlation with chorionic gonadotrophin. Cancer 39:2391–2396, 1976
90. Marcus DM, Zinberg N: Measurement of serum ferritin by radioimmunoassay: Results in normal individuals and patients with breast cancer. J Natl Cancer Inst 55:791–845, 1975
91. Waalkes TP, Tormey DC: Biological markers and breast cancer. Sem Oncol 5:434–444, 1978
92. Fisher B: The operative management of primary breast cancer. Int J Rad Oncol Biol Phys 2:989–992, 1977
93. Cooperman AM, Blanchard JM, Esselstyn C Jr: Partial mastectomy. Surg Clin N Am 58:737–741, 1978
94. Roth D, Bayat H: The role of residual tumor in the chest wall in the late dissemination of mammary cancer. Ann Surg 168:887–890, 1968
95. Fisher B: Breast cancer management: Alternatives to radical mastectomy (editorial). N Eng J Med 301:326–328, 1979
96. Fisher B, Moore GE, Ravdin RG et al: Breast Cancer: Early and Late (Thirteenth Annual Clinical Conference on Cancer, 1968, at The University of Texas, MD Anderson Hospital and Tumor Institute), pp 135–153. Chicago, Year Book, 1970
97. Fisher B, Ravdin RG, Ausman RK et al: Surgical adjuvant chemotherapy in cancer of the breast: Results of a decade of cooperative investigation. Ann Surg 168:337–356, 1968
98. Turner-Warwick RT: The lymphatics of the breast. Br J Surg 46:574–582, 1959
99. Handley RS: The early spread of breast carcinoma and its bearing on operative treatment. Br J Surg 51:206–208, 1964
100. Andreassen M, Dahl-Iversen E: Recherches sur le metastases microscopiques des ganglions lymphatiques sus-clavicularis dous de cancer du sein. J Int Chir 9:27, 1949
101. Andreassen M, Dahl-Iversen E, Sorensen B: Glandular metastases in carcinoma of the breast: Results of a more radical operation. Lancet I:176–182, 1954
102. Caceres E: An evaluation of radical mastectomy and extended radical mastectomy for cancer of the breast. Surg Gyn Obstet 125:337–341, 1967
103. Margottini M, Bucalossi P: El metastasi lymphoghiandolari mammario interne nel cancro della mammell. Boll Oncol 23:79, 1949
104. Margottini M, Jacobelli G, Cau M: The end results of enlarged radical mastectomy. Acta Unio Int Contra Cancrum 19: 1555–1559, 1963
105. Lacour J, Bucalossi P, Cacers E et al: Radical mastectomy *versus* radical mastectomy plus internal node dissection. Cancer 37:206–214, 1976
106. Vana J, Bedwani R, Mettlin C, et al: Trends in diagnosis and management of breast cancer in the US. Surveys of the American College of Surgeons (in press)
107. Patey DH, Dryson WH: The prognosis of carcinoma of the breast in relation to the type of operation performed. Br J Cancer 2: 7–13, 1948
108. Handley RS: The technique and results of conservative radical mastectomy (Patey's operation). Prog Clin Cancer 1:462–470, 1965
109. McWhirter, R: Discussion: The treatment of cancer of the breast (abridged). Proc R Soc Med 41:122–129, 1948
110. McWhirter R: Simple mastectomy and radiotherapy in the treatment of breast cancer. Br J Radiol 28:128–139, 1955
111. McWhirter R: Should more radical treatment be attempted in breast cancer? Caldwell lecture, 1963. Am J Roentgenol 92:3–13, 1964
112. McWhirter R: The principles of treatment by radiotherapy in breast cancer. Br J Cancer 4:368–371, 1950
113. McWhirter R: The value of simple mastectomy and radiotherapy in the treatment of cancer of the breast. Br J Radiol 21:599–610, 1948
114. McWhirter R: Treatment of cancer of the breast by simple mastectomy and roentgenotherapy. Arch Surg 59:830–842, 1949
115. Fisher B, Fisher ER: Transmigration of lymph nodes by tumor cells. Science 152:1397–1398, 1966
116. Crile G Jr:Results of simple mastectomy without irradiation in the treatment of operative stage I cancer of the breast. Ann Surg 168:330–336, 1968
117. Fisher B, Montague E, Redmond C, et al: Comparison of radical mastectomy with alternative treatments for primary breast cancer: A first report of results from a prospective randomized clinical trial. Cancer 39:2827–2839, 1977
118. Mustakallio S: Treatment of breast cancer by tumor extirpation and roentgen therapy instead of radical operation. J Fac Radiol 6:23–26, 1954
119. Porritt A: Early carcinoma of the breast. Br J Surg 51:214–216, 1964
120. Peters VM: Wedge resection and irradiation, an effective treatment in early breast cancer. JAMA 200:134–135, 1967
121. Crile G Jr: Treatment of breast cancer by local excision. Am J Surg 109:400–403, 1965
122. Crile G Jr, Hoerr SO: Results of treatment of carcinoma of the breast by local excision. Surg Gynecol Obstet 132:780–782, 1971
123. Crile G Jr: The case for local excision of breast cancer in selected cases. Lancet I: 549–554, 1972
124. Veronesi U: Conservative treatment of breast cancer: A trial at the Cancer Institute of Milan. World J Surg 1:324–326, 1977
125. Nance FC, DeLoach DH, Welsh RA et al: Paget's disease of the breast. Ann Surg 171:864–874, 1970
126. Maier WP, Rosemond GP, Harasym EL et al: Paget's disease in the female breast. Surg Gynecol Obstet 128:1253–1263, 1969
127. Kilgore AR: The incidence of cancer in the second breast. JAMA 77:454–457, 1921
128. Fitts WT Jr, Patterson LT: The spread of mammary cancer. Surg Clin N Am 35:1539–1551, 1955
129. Leis HP Jr, Mersheimer WL, Black MM, et al: The second breast. NY State J Med 65:2460–2468, 1965
130. Lewison EF: The management of the contralateral breast. Hosp Pract 5:101–106, 1970
131. Pack GT: Bilateral mastectomy. Surgery 29:929–931, 1951
132. Robbins GF, Berg JW: Bilateral primary breast cancers: A prospective clinicopathological study. Cancer 17:1501–1527, 1964
133. Hubbard TB Jr: Nonsimultaneous bilateral carcinoma of the breast. Surgery 34:706–723, 1953
134. Kilgore AR, Bell HG, Ahlquist RE Jr: Cancer in the second breast. Am J Surg 92:155–161, 1956
135. Mustacchi P, Pandolfi A, Bucalossi P: Bilateral mammary cancer in Italian women. J Natl Cancer Inst 19:1035–1042, 1957
136. Hohler H: Reconstruction of the female breast after radical mastectomy. In Converse JM (ed): Reconstructive Plastic Surgery. Philadelphia, WB Saunders, 1977, pp 3710–3726
137. Georgiade NG (ed): Reconstructive Breast Surgery. CV Mosby, St. Louis, 1976
138. Cocke WM Jr: Breast Reconstruction Following Mastectomy for Carcinoma. Boston, Little Brown, 1977
139. Hartwell SW Jr, Anderson R, Hall MD et al: Reconstruction of the breast after mastectomy for cancer. Plast Reconstr Surg 57:152–157, 1976
140. Bostwick J III, Vasconez LO, Jurkiewicz MJ: Breast reconstruction after a radical mastectomy. Plast Reconstr Surg 61:682–693, 1978
141. Lewis JR Jr: Reconstruction of the breasts. Surg Clin NA 51:429–440, 1971
142. Edgerton MT: Breast reconstruction after radical mastectomy for cancer. South Med J 60:719–723, 1967
143. Watts GT: Restorative prosthetic mammaplasty in mastectomy for carcinoma and benign lesions. Clin Plastic Surg 3:177–191, 1976
144. Williams JE: Experience with a late series of silastic breast implants. Plast Reconstr Surg 49:253–258, 1972

145. Synderman RK, Guthrie RH: Reconstruction of the female breast following radical mastectomy. Plast Reconstr Surg 47:565–567, 1971
146. Bradley SA: Acceptable Plastic Implants. In Simpson DC (ed): Modern Trends in Biomechanics, Chapter 2.11. London, Butterworths, 1970, pp 25–51
147. Rees TD, Guy CL, Coburn RJ: The use of inflatable breast implants. Plast Reconstr Surg 52:609–615, 1973
148. Birnbaum L, Olsen JA: Breast reconstruction following radical mastectomy, using custom designed implants. Plast Reconstr Surg 61:355–363, 1978
149. Phillips CM: Reconstructive surgery after classical radical mastectomies using omental pedicled grafts and fascia lata. Breast 4:10–18, 1978
150. Arnold PG, Hartrampf CR, Jurkiewicz MJ: One-stage reconstruction of the breast, using the transposed greater omentum (Case report). Plast Reconstr Surg 57:520–522, 1976
151. Hohler H: Reconstruction after mastectomy. In Symposium on Neoplastic and Reconstructive Problems of the Female Breast. St. Louis, CV Mosby, 1973
152. Allison AB, Howorth MB Jr: Carcinoma in a nipple preserved by heterotopic auto-implantation. New Engl J Med 298:1130, 1978
153. Parry RG, Cochran TC Jr, Wolfort FG: When is there nipple involvement in carcinoma of the breast? Plast Reconstr Surg 59:535–537, 1977
154. Smith J, Payne WS, Carney JA: Involvement of the nipple and areola in carcinoma of the breast. Surg Gynecol Obstet 143:546–548, 1976
155. Adams WM: Labial transplant for correction of less of the nipple. Plast Reconstr Surg 4:295–299, 1949
156. Gocht: Therapetusche verwendig der Rontgenstrahlen. Fortschritte auf Gebrete der Rontgenstrahlen. 1:14–22, 1897
157. Johnson W, Merril W: X-rays in the treatment of carcinoma. Phil Med J 234:1138–1140, 1900
158. Grubbe E: Priority in the therapeutic use of X-rays. Radiology 21:156–162, 1933
159. Fletcher GH: Local results of irradiation in the primary management of localized breast cancer. Cancer 29:545–552, 1972
160. Weichselbaum RR, Marck A, Hellman S: The role of postoperative irradiation in carcinoma of the breast. Cancer 37:2682–2690, 1976
161. Høst H, Brennhovd IO: Does postoperative radiation live any place following radical mastectomy? Cancer (in press)
162. Wallgren A: A controlled study: Pre-operative versus postoperative irradiation. Int J Radiat Oncol Biol Phys 2:1167–1169, 1977
163. Bonadonna G, Valagussa P, Rossi A et al: Are surgical adjuvant trials altering the course of breast cancer? Semin Oncol 5:450–464, 1978
164. Fisher B, Slack NH, Cavanaugh PJ et al: Postoperative radiotherapy in the treatment of breast cancer: Results of the NSABP clinical trial. Ann Surg 172:711–730, 1970
165. Chu FCH, Lin FJ, Kim JH et al: Locally recurrent carcinoma of the breast. Results of radiation therapy. Cancer 37:2677–2681, 1976
166. Zimmerman KW, Montague ED, Fletcher GH: Frequency, anatomic distribution, and management of local recurrences after definite therapy for breast cancer. Cancer 19:67–74, 1966
167. Keynes G: The treatment of primary carcinoma of the breast with radium. Acta Radiologica 10:393–402, 1929
168. Keynes G: Conservative treatment of cancer of the breast. Br Med J 2:643–647, 1937
169. Wiliams IG, Murley RS, Curwen MP: Carcinoma of the female breast: conservative and radical surgery. Br Med J 2:787–796, 1953
170. Peters MV: Wedge resection with or without radiation in early breast cancer. Int J Radiat Oncol Biol Phys 2:1151–1156, 1977
171. Mustakalio S: Conservative Treatment of Breast Carcinoma—Review of 25 years follow-up. Clin Radiol 23:110–116, 1972
172. Rissanen PM, Holsti P: A comparison between conservative and radical surgery combined with radiotherapy in the treatment of breast cancer stage I: A 10-year follow-up study on 866 patients. Strahlentherapie 147:370–374, 1974
173. Atkins H, Hayward JL, Klugman DJ: Treatment of early breast cancer: A report after 10 years of a clinical trial. Br Med J 2:423–429, 1972
174. Hayward JL: The Guy's trial of treatments of "early" breast cancer. World J Surg 1:314–316, 1977
175. Baclesse F: Roentgen therapy as the sole method of treatment for cancer of the breast. Am J Roentgenol Radium Ther Nucl Med 62:311–319, 1949
176. Calle R, Pilleron JP, Schlienger P et al: Conservative management of operable breast cancer. Cancer 42:2045–2053, 1978
177. Amalric R, Santamaria F, Robert F et al: Radiation Therapy With and Without Primary Limited Surgery for Operable Breast Cancer: A 20-Year Experience at the Marseilles Cancer Institute (in press)
178. Pierquin B, Owen R, Maylin C et al: Radical radiation therapy of breast cancer. Int J Radiat Biol Phys 6:17–24, 1980
179. Veronesi U: The value of limited surgery for breast cancer (in press)
180. Chu AM, Cope O, Russo R et al: Treatment of early stage breast cancer by limited surgery and radical irradiation. Int J Radiat Oncol Biol Phys 6:25–30, 1980
181. Prosnitz L, Goldenberg IS: Radiation therapy as primary treatment for early stage carcinoma of the breast. Cancer 35:1587–1596, 1975
182. Alpert S, Ghossein NA, Stacy P et al: Primary management of operable breast cancer by minimal surgery and radiotherapy. Cancer 42:2054–2058, 1978
183. Montague ED, Gutierrez AE, Barker J et al: Conservative surgery and irradiation for the treatment of favorable breast cancer. Cancer 43:1058–1061, 1979
184. Hellman S, Harris JR, Levene MB: Radiation therapy of early carcinoma of the breast without mastectomy. Cancer 46:988–994, 1980
185. Harris JR, Levene MB, Hellman S: Role of radiation therapy in the primary treatment of carcinoma of the breast. Semin Oncol 5:403–416, 1978
186. Harris JR, Levene MB, Svensson G et al: Analysis of cosmetic results following primary radiation therapy for stages I and II carcinoma of the breast. Int J Radiat Oncol Biol Phys 5:257–261, 1979
187. Boice JD Jr, Monson RR: Breast cancer in women after repeated fluoroscopic examinations of the chest. JNCI 59:823–832, 1977
188. Myrden JA, Hiltz JE: Breast cancer following multiple fluoroscopies during artificial pneumothorax treatment of pulmonary tuberculosis. Can Med Assoc J 100:1032–1034, 1969
189. McCredie JA, Inch WR, Alderson M: Consecutive primary carcinoma of the breast. Cancer 35:1472–1477, 1975
190. Kim JM, Chu FC, Woodward HQ et al: Radiation-induced soft tissue and bone sarcomas. Radiology 129:501–508, 1978
191. Stout AP, Lattes R: Tumors of the Soft Tissue. Arms Forces Institute of Pathology, Washington DC, 1967
192. Botnick LE, Rose CM, Harris JR et al: Technique and results of axillary sampling in patients undergoing definitive breast irradiation (abstract). Proceedings ASTR, 1980
193. Haagenson CD, Stout AP: Carcinoma of the breast; criteria of operability. Ann Surg 118:859–870, 1032–1051, 1932
194. Haagensen CD: Diseases of the Breast, rev 2nd ed. Philadelphia, WB Saunders, 1971, p 623
195. Ibid, p 625–628
196. Fletcher GH, Montague ED: Radical irradiation of advanced breast cancer. Am J Roentgenol Radium Ther Nucl Med 93:573, 1965
197. Bruckman JE, Harris JR, Levene MB et al: Results of treating stage III carcinoma of the breast by primary radiation therapy. Cancer 43:985–993, 1979
198. DeLena M, Zucali R, Viganotti G et al: Combined chemotherapy–radiotherapy approach in locally advanced (T3b–T4) breast cancer. Cancer Chemother Pharmacol 1:53–62, 1978
199. DeLena M, Zucali R, Varini M et al: Combined modality approach in locally advanced breast cancer (T3b–T4). Proc Am Soc Clin Oncol, 1979
200. Jensen EV, Jacobson HI: Basic guides to the mechanism of estrogen action. Recent Progress Hormone Res 18:387–414, 1962

201. Jensen EV, Suzuki T, Kawashima T et al: A two step mechanism for the interaction of estradiol with rat uterus. Proc Natl Acad Sci 59:632–638, 1968
202. McQuire WL, Horwitz KB, Zava DT et al: Progress Endocrinology and metabolism—hormones in breast cancer: Update, 1978. Metabolism 27:487–501, 1978
203. Allegra JC, Barlock A, Huff KK et al: Changes in multiple or sequential estrogen receptor determinations in breast cancer. Cancer 45:792–794, 1980
204. Parl FF, Wagner RK: The histopathological evaluation of human breast cancers in correlation with estrogen receptor values. Cancer 46:362–367, 1980
205. Kiang DT, Kennedy BJ: Factors affecting estrogen receptors in breast cancer. Cancer 40:1571–1576, 1977
206. Rosen PP, Menendez-Botet CJ, Urban JA et al: Estrogen receptor protein (ERP) in multiple tumor specimens from individual patients with breast cancer. Cancer 39:2194–2200, 1977
207. Silvestrini R, Daidone MG, DiFronzo G: Relationship between proliferative activity and estrogen receptors in breast cancer. Cancer 44:665–670, 1979
208. Hahnel R, Woodings T, Vivian AB: Prognostic value of estrogen receptors in primary breast cancer. Cancer 44:671–675, 1979
209. Cooke T, George D, Shields R: Estrogen receptors and prognosis in early breast cancer. Lancet I:995–997, 1979
210. Kiang DT, Frenning DH, Goldman AI et al: Estrogen receptors and responses to chemotherapy and hormonal therapy in advanced breast cancer. New Engl J Med 299:1330–1334, 1978
211. Lippman ME, Allegra JC, Thompson EB et al: The relation between estrogen receptors and response rate to cytotoxic chemotherapy in metastatic breast cancer. New Engl J Med 298:1223–1228, 1978
212. Hilf R, Feldstein ML, Gibson SL et al: The relative importance of estrogen receptor analysis as a prognostic factor for recurrence or response to chemotherapy in women with breast cancer. Cancer 45:1993–2000, 1980
213. Bloom ND, Tobin EH, Schreibman B et al: The role of progesterone receptors in the management of advanced breast cancer. Cancer 45:2992–2997, 1980
214. MacFarlane JK Fleiszer D, Fazekas AG: Studies on estrogen receptors and regression in human breast cancer. Cancer 45:2998–3003, 1980
215. McGuire WL, De La Garza M, Chamness GC: Evaluation of estrogen receptor assays in human breast cancer tissue. Cancer Res 37:637–639, 1977
216. Puga FJ, Welch JS, Bisel HF: Therapeutic cophorectomy in disseminated carcinoma of the breast. Arch Sur 111:877–880, 1976
217. Schweitzer RJ: Oophorectomy/adrenalectomy. Cancer 46:1061–1065, 1980
218. Kennedy BJ, Fortuny IE: Therapeutic castration in the treatment of advanced breast cancer. Cancer 17:1197–1202, 1964
219. Huggins C, Bergenstal DM: Inhibition of human mammary and prostatic cancer by adrenalectomy. Cancer Res 12:134–141, 1952
220. Luft R, Olivecrona H, Ikkos D, et al: Hypophysectomy in the management of metastatic cancer of the breast. In Currie A (ed): Endocrine aspects of breast cancer. Edinburgh, Livingstone pp 27–35, 1958
221. Moore FD, VanDevanter SB, Boyden CM et al: Adrenalectomy with chemotherapy in the treatment of advanced breast cancer: Objective and subjective response rates: Duration and quality of life. Surgery 76:376–390, 1974
222. Silverstein MJ, Byron RL, Yonemoto RH et al: Bilateral adrenalectomy for advanced breast cancer: A 21-year experience. Surgery 77:825–831, 1975
223. Yonemoto RH, Tan MSC, Byron RL et al: Randomized sequential hormonal therapy vs. adrenalectomy for metastatic breast carcinoma. Cancer 39:547–555, 1977
224. Schmidt M, Nemoto T, Dao T et al: Prognostic factors affecting adrenalectomy in patients with metastatic cancer of the breast. Cancer 27:1106–1111, 1971
225. Harris HS Jr., Spratt JS: Bilateral adrenalectomy in metastatic mammary cancer. An analysis of sixty-four cases. Cancer 23:145–151, 1969
226. Manni A, Pearson OH, Brodkey J et al: Transsphenoidal hypophysectomy in breast cancer. Evidence for an individual role of pituitary and gonadal hormones in supporting tumor growth. Cancer 44:2330–2337, 1979
227. Kennedy BJ: Hormonal therapies in Breast Cancer. Sem Oncol I:119–130, 1974
228. Bates T, Rubens RD, Bulbrook RD et al: Comparison of pituitary function and clinical response after transphenoidal and transfrontal hypophysectomy for advanced breast cancer. Eur J Cancer 12:775–782, 1976
229. LaRossa JT, Strong MS, Melby JC: Endocrinologically incomplete transethmoidal trans-sphenoidal hypophysectomy with relief of bone pain in breast cancer. New Engl J Med I:1332–1335, 1978
230. Harvey HA, Santen RJ, Osterman J et al: A comparative trial of transsphenoidal hypophysectomy and estrogen suppression with aminoglutethimide in advanced breast cancer. Cancer 43:2207–2214, 1979
231. Atkins H et al: Ten years' experience of steroid assays in the management of breast cancer. The Lancet I:7581–1264, 1968
232. Masnyk IJ, Silverman DT, Hankey BF: Prediction of response to adrenalectomy in the treatment of advanced breast cancer. J Natl Cancer Inst 60:271–278, 1978
233. Santen RJ, Samojlik E, Lipton A et al: Kinetic, hormonal, and clinical studies with aminoglutethimide in breast cancer. Cancer 39:2948–2958, 1977
234. Santen RJ, Santner S, Davis B et al: Aminoglutethimide inhibits extraglandular estrogen production in postmenopausal women with breast carcinoma. J Clin Endrocr Metab 47:1257–1265, 1978
235. Smith I.E. et al: Aminoglutethimide in treatment of metastatic breast carcinoma. Lancet I: 646–649, 1978
236. Lawrence BV, Lipton A, Harvey HA, et al: Influence of estrogen receptor status on response of metastatic breast cancer to aminoglutethimide therapy. Cancer 45:786–791, 1980
237. Knoits PH, Aisner J, Van Echo DA et al: Mitomycin-C and vinblastine chemotherapy for advanced breast cancer. Proc AACR and ASCO 21:410, 1980
238. Kennedy BJ: Hormone therapy for advanced breast cancer. Cancer 18:1551–1557, 1965
239. Legha SS, Davis HL, Muggia FM: Hormonal therapy of breast cancer: New approaches and concepts. Ann Int Med 88:69–77, 1978
240. Baker WH, Kelly RM, Sohier WD: Hormonal treatment of metastatic carcinoma of the breast. Am J Surg 99:538–543, 1960
241. Baker LH, Vaitkevicius VK: Reevaluation of rebound regression in disseminated carcinoma of the breast. Cancer 29:1268–1271, 1972
242. Lippman M, Bolan G, Huff K: The effects of estrogens and antiestrogens on hormone-responsive human breast cancer in long-term tissue culture. Cancer Res 36:4595–4601, 1976
243. Kennedy BJ, Brown JH: Combined estrogenic and androgenic hormone therapy in advanced breast cancer. Cancer 18:431–435, 1965
244. Muggia FM et al: Treatment of breast cancer with medroxyprogesterone acetate. Ann Int Med 68:328–337, 1968
245. Klaassen DJ, Rapp EF, Hirte WE: Response to medroxyprogesterone acetate (NSC-26386) as secondary hormone therapy for metastatic breast cancer in postmenopausal women. Cancer Treat Rep 60:251–253, 1976
246. De Lena M, Brambilla C, Valagussa P et al: High-dose medroxyprogesterone acetate in breast cancer resistant to endocrine and cytotoxic therapy. Cancer Chemother Pharmacol 2:175–180, 1979
247. Ansfield FJ, Davis HL, Kamirez G et al:Further clinical studies with megesterol acetate in advanced breast cancer. Cancer 38:53–55, 1976
248. Teulings FAG, van Glise HA, Henkelman MS et al: Estrogen, androgen, glucocorticoid, and progesterone receptors in progestin-induced regression of human breast cancer. Cancer Res 40:2557–2561, 1980

249. Heel RC, Brogden RN, Speight TM et al: Tamoxifen: A review of its pharmacological properties and therapeutic use in the treatment of breast cancer. In: Evaluations on New Drugs 16:1–24, 1978
250. Tagnon HJ: Antiestrogens in treatment of breast cancer. Cancer 39:259–2964, 1977
251. Mouridsen H, Palshof T, Patterson J et al: Tamoxifen in advanced breast cancer. Cancer Treat Rev 5:131–141, 1978
252. Plotkin D, Lechner JJ, Jung WE et al: Tamoxifen flare in advanced breast cancer. JAMA 240:2644–2646, 1978
253. Kiang DT, Kennedy BJ: Tamoxifen (Antiestrogen) therapy in advanced breast cancer. Ann Int Med 87:687–690, 1977
254. Morgan LR Jr, Schein PS, Woolley PV et al: Therapeutic use of tamoxifen in advanced breast cancer: Correlation with biochemical parameters. Cancer Treat Rep 60:1437–1443, 1976
255. Westerberg H: Tamoxifen and fluoxymesterone in advanced breast cancer: A controlled clinical trial. Cancer Treat Rep 64:117–121, 1980
256. Manni A, Trujillo JE, Marshall JS et al: Antihormone treatment of stage IV breast cancer. Cancer 43:444–450, 1979
257. Kiang DT, Frenning DH, Vosika GJ et al: Comparison of tamoxifen and hypophysectomy in breast cancer treatment. Cancer 45:1322–1325, 1980
258. Preistman T, Baum A, Jones V et al: Treatment and survival in advanced breast cancer. Br Med J 2:1673–1674, 1978
259. George SL, Hoogstraten B: Prognostic factors in the initial response to therapy by patients with advanced breast cancer. J Natl Cancer Inst. 60:731–736, 1978
260. Swenerton KD, Legha SS, Smith T et al: Prognostic factors in metastatic breast cancer treated with combination chemotherapy. Cancer Res 29:1552–1562, 1979
261. Rozencweig M, Staquet MJ, Von Hoff DD et al: Prognostic factors for the response to chemotherapy in advanced breast cancer. Cancer Clin Trials 2:165–170, 1979
262. Legha SS, Buzdar AV, Smith TL et al: Response to hormonal therapy as a prognostic factor for metastatic breast cancer treated with combination chemotherapy. Cancer 46:438–445, 1980
263. Hoogstraten B, Fabian C: A reappraisal of single drugs in advanced breast cancer. Cancer Clin Trials 2:101–109, 1979
264. Carter SK: Integration of chemotherapy into combined modality treatment of solid tumors. Cancer Treat Rev 3:141–174, 1976
265. Ansfield FJ, Ramirez G, Mackman S et al: A ten-year study of 5-Fluorouracil in disseminated breast cancer with clinical results and survival times. Cancer Res 29:1062–1066, 1969
266. Vogler WR, Furtado VP, Huguley CM Jr: Methotrexate for advanced cancer of the breast. Cancer 21:26–30, 1968
267. Yap HY Blumenschein GR, Keating MJ et al: Vinblastine given as continuous 5-day infusion in the treatment of refractory advanced breast cancer. Cancer Treat Rep 64:279–283, 1980
268. Smith IE, Hedley DW, Powles TJ et al: Vindesine: A phase II study in the treatment of breast carcinoma, malignant melanoma, and other tumors. Cancer Treat Rep 62:1427–1433, 1978
269. Ahmann DL et al: An analysis of a multiple-drug program in the treatment of patients with advanced breast cancer utilizing 5-fluorouracil, cyclophosphamide, and prednisone with or without vincristine. Cancer 36:1925–1935, 1975
270. Creech RH, Catalano RB, Shah MK: An effective low-dose adriamycin regimen as secondary chemotherapy for metastatic breast cancer patients. Cancer 46:433–437, 1980
271. Nemoto T, Rosner D, Díaz R et al: Combination chemotherapy for metastatic breast cancer. Cancer 41:2073–2077, 1978
272. Ahmann DL, Bisel HF, Eagan RT et al: Controlled evaluation of adriamycin (NSC-123127) in patients with disseminated breast cancer. Cancer Chemo Rep 58:877–882, 1974
273. Hoogstraten B, George SL, Samal B et al: Combination chemotherapy and adriamycin in patients with advanced breast cancer. Cancer 38:13–20, 1976
274. Gottlieb JA, Rivkin SE, Spigel SC et al: Superiority of adriamycin over oral nitrosoureas in patients with advanced breast carcinoma. Cancer 33:519–526, 1974
275. Knight EW, Horton J, Cunningham T et al: Adriamycin: Comparison of a 5-week schedule with a 3-week schedule in the treatment of breast cancer. Cancer Treat Rep 63:121–122, 1979
276. Yap HY, Blumenschein, GR, Yap BS et al: High-dose methotrexate for advanced breast cancer. Cancer Treat Rep 63:757–761, 1979
277. Greenspan, EM: Combination cytotoxic chemotherapy in advanced disseminated breast carcinoma. J Mt Sinai Hosp 33:1–27, 1966
279. Spigel SC, Coltman CA Jr, Costanzi JJ: Disseminated breast carcinoma. Arch Intern Med 132:575–577, 1973
280. Davis HL Jr, Ramirez G, Ellerby RA et al: Five-drug therapy in advanced breast cancer. Factors influencing toxicity and response. Cancer 34:239–245, 1974
281. Lee JM, Abeloff MD, Lenhard RE Jr et al: An evaluation of five drug combination chemotherapy in the management of recurrent carcinoma of the breast. Surg Gyn Obstet 138:77–80, 1974
282. Kaufman S, Goldstein M: Combination chemotherapy in disseminated carcinoma of the breast. Surg Gyn Obstet 137:83–86, 1973
283. Smalley RV, Murphy S, Huguley CM Jr et al: Combination *versus* sequential five-drug chemotherapy in metastatic carcinoma of the breast. Cancer Res 36:3911–3916, 1976
284. Chlebowski RT, Irwin LE, Pugh RP et al: Survival of patients with metastatic breast cancer treated with either combination or sequential chemotherapy. Cancer Res 39:4503–4506, 1979
285. Smalley RV, Carpenter J, Bartolucci A et al: A comparison of cyclophosphamide, adriamycin, 5-fluorouracil (CAF) and cyclophosphamide, methotrexate, 5-fluorouracil, vincristine, prednisone (CMFVP) in patients with metastatic breast cancer. Cancer 40:625–632, 1977
286. Canellos GP, DeVita VT, Gold GL et al: Combination chemotherapy for advanced breast cancer: Response and effect on survival. Ann Int Med 84:389–392, 1976
287. Canellos GP, Pocock SJ, Taylor III SG et al: Combination chemotherapy for metastatic breast carcinoma. Prospective comparison of multiple drug therapy with L-phenylalanine mustard. Cancer 38:1882–1886, 1976
288. Rosner D, Nemoto T: Sequence for developing optimal combination chemotherapy of metastatic breast cancer. Eur J Cancer 15:1197–1201, 1979
289. Muss HB, White DR, Cooper MR et al: Combination chemotherapy in advanced breast cancer. A randomized trial comparing a three- *vs.* a five-drug program. Arch Intern Med 137:1711–1714, 1977
290. Mouridsen HT, Brahm TPM, Rahbek I: Evaluation of single-drug *versus* multiple-drug chemotherapy in the treatment of advanced breast cancer. Cancer Treat Rep 61:47–50, 1977
291. Baker LH, Vaughn CB, Al-Sarraf et al: Evaluation of combination *vs.* sequential cytotoxic chemotherapy in the treatment of advanced breast cancer. Cancer 33:513–518, 1974
292. Hortobagyi GN, Gutterman JD, Blumenschein GR et al: Combination chemoimmunotherapy of metastatic breast cancer with 5-fluorouracinal, adriamycin, cyclophosphamide, and BCG. Cancer 44:1955–1962, 1979
293. Bull JM, Tormey DC, Li SH et al: A randomized comparative trial of adriamycin *versus* methotrexate in combination drug therapy. Cancer 41:1649–1657, 1978
294. Tranum B, Hoogstraten B, Kennedy A et al: Adriamycin in combination for the treatment of breast cancer. Cancer 41:2078–2083, 1978
295. Kennealey GT, Boston B, Mitchell MS et al: Combination chemotherapy for advanced breast cancer. Two regimens containing adriamycin. Cancer 42:27–33, 1978
296. Jones SE, Durie BG, Salmon SE: Combination chemotherapy with adriamycin and cyclophosphamide for advanced breast cancer. Cancer 36:90–97, 1975
297. Creech RH, Catalano RB, Harris DT et al: Low dose chemotherapy of metastatic breast cancer with cyclophosphamide, adriamycin, methotrexate, 5-fluorouracil (CAMF) versus sequential cyclophosphamide, methotrexate, 5-fluorouracil (CMF) and adriamycin. Cancer 43:51–59, 1979
298. Muss HB, White DP, Richards F et al: Adriamycin *versus* methotrexate in five-drug combination chemotherapy for advanced breast cancer. Cancer 42:2141–2148, 1978

299. Decker DA, Ahmann DL, Bisel HF et al: Complete responders to chemotherapy in metastatic breast cancer. Characterization and analysis. JAMA 242:2075–2079, 1979
300. Legha SS, Buzda AV, Smith TL et al: Complete remissions in metastatic breast cancer treated with combination drug therapy. Ann Int Med 91:847–852, 1979
301. Brambilla C, Valagussa P, Bonadonna G: Sequential combination chemotherapy in advanced breast cancer. Cancer Chemother Pharmacol 1:35–39, 1978
302. Abeloff MD, Ettinger DS: Treatment of metastatic breast cancer with adriamycin–cyclophosphamide induction followed by alternating combination therapy. Cancer Treat Rep 61: 1685–1689, 1977
303. Tormey DC, Falkson G, Simon RM et al: A randomized comparison of two sequentially administered combination regimens to a single regimen in metastatic breast cancer. Cancer Clin Trials 2:247–256, 1979
304. Blumenschein GR, Hortobagy GN, Richman SP et al: Alternating noncross-resistant combination chemotherapy and active nonspecific immunotherapy with BCG or MER–BCG for advanced breast carcinoma. Cancer 45:742–749, 1980
305. Ahmann DL, O'Connell MJ, Hahn RG et al: An evaluation of early or delayed adjuvant chemotherapy in premenopausal patients with advanced breast cancer undergoing oophorectomy. New Engl J Med 297:356–360, 1977
306. Falkson G, Falkson HC, Glidewell O et al: Improved remission rates and remission duration in young men with metastatic breast cancer following combined oophorectomy and chemotherapy. A study by cancer and leukemia Group B. Cancer 43:2215–2222, 1979
307. Brunner KW, Sonntag RW, Alberto P et al: Combined chemo- and hormonal therapy in advanced breast cancer. Cancer 39:2923–2933, 1977
308. Glick JH, Creech RH, Torr S et al: Tamoxifen plus sequential CMF chemotherapy *versus* Tamoxifen alone in postmenopausal patients with advanced breast cancer: A randomized trial. Cancer 45:735–741, 1980
309. Hortobagyi GN, Gutterman JV, Blumenschein GR et al: Combined chemoimmunotherapy for advanced breast cancer. A comparison of BCG and levamisole. Cancer 43:1112–1122, 1979
310. Britell JC, Ahmann DL, Bisel HF et al: Treatment of advanced breast cancer with cyclophosphamide, 5-fluorouracil, and prednisone with and without methanol-extracted residue of BCG. Cancer Clin Trials 2:345–350, 1979
311. Hubay CA, Pearson OH, Marshall JS et al: Antiestrogen, cytotoxic chemotherapy, and bacillus Calmette-Guerin vaccination in stage II breast cancer: A preliminary report. Surgery 87:494–501, 1980
312. Yap HY, Salem P, Hortobagyi GN et al: Phase II study of *cis*dichlordiammineplatinum (II) in advanced breast cancer. Cancer Treat Rep 62:405–408, 1978
313. O'Bryan RM, Baker L, Whitecar J et al: Cyclocytidine in breast cancer. Cancer Treat Rep 62:455–456, 1978
314. Legha SS, Buzdar AU, Hortobagyi GN et al: Phase II study of hexamethylmelamine alone and in combination with mitomycin-C and vincristine in advanced breast carcinoma. Cancer Treat Rep 63:2053–2056, 1979
315. Fabian CJ, Rasmussen S, Stephens R et al: Phase II evaluation of hexamethylmelamine in advanced breast cancer: A southwest oncology group study. Cancer Treat Rep 63:1359–1361, 1979
316. Denefrio JM, Vogel CL: Phase II study of hexamethylmelamine in women with advanced breast cancer refractory to standard cytotoxic therapy. Cancer Treat Rep 62:173–175, 1978
317. Yap HY, Benjamin RS, Blumenschein GR et al: Phase II study with sequential L-asparaginase and methotrexate in advanced refractory breast cancer. Cancer Treat Rep 63:77–83, 1979
318. Godfrey TE: Mitomycin-C breast cancer. In Mitomycin-C: Current Status and New Developments. New York, Academic Press, 1979, pp 91–99
319. Ingle JN, Ahmann DL, O'Fallon JR et al: Randomized phase II trial of rubidazone and adriamycin in women with advanced breast cancer. Cancer Treat Rep 63:1701–1705, 1979
320. Cabanillas F, Bodey GP, Burgess MA et al: Results of a Phase II study of maytansine in patients with breast carcinoma and melanoma. Cancer Treat Rep 63:507–509, 1979
321. Pandya KJ, Tormey DC, Davis TE et al: Phase II trial of 6-thioguanine in metastatic breast cancer. Cancer Treat Rep 64:191–192, 1980
322. Esterhay RJ Jr, Aisner J, Levi JA et al: High-dose 6-mercaptopurine in advanced refractory cancer. Cancer Treat Rep 62:1229–1231, 1978
323. Creech RH, Engstrom PF, Harris DT et al: Phase II study of ICRF-159 in refractory metastatic breast cancer. Cancer Treat Rep 63:111–114, 1979
324. Yap HY, Murphy WK, DiStefano A et al: Phase II study of anguidine in advanced breast cancer. Cancer Treat Rep 63:789–791, 1979
325. Nichols WC, Kvols LK, Ingle JN et al: Phase II study of triazinate and pyrazofurin in patients with advanced breast cancer previously exposed to cytotoxic chemotherapy. Cancer Treat Rep 62:837–838, 1978
326. Rossi A, Bonadonna G, Valagussa P et al: CMF adjuvant program for breast cancer: Five-year results. Proc AACR and ASCO 21:404, 1980
327. Meyer JS, Rao BR, Stevens SC et al: Low incidence of estrogen receptor in breast carcinomas with rapid rates of cellular replication. Cancer 40:2290–2298, 1977
328. Bishop HM, Elston CW, Blamey RW et al: Relationship of estrogen-receptor status to survival in breast cancer. Lancet I: 283–284, 1979
329. Ravdin RG, Lewison EF, Slack NH et al: Results of a clinical trial concerning the worth of prophylactic cophorectomy for breast cancer. Surg Gyn Obstet 131:1055–1064, 1970
330. Cole MP: Suppression of ovarian function in primary breast cancer. In Forrest APM, Kunkler PB (eds): Prognostic Factors in Breast Cancer. Edinburgh, E&S Livingstone, 1968, pp 146–156 (Proceedings of First Tenovus Symposium, Cardiff, 1967)
331. Meakin JW, Allt WEC, Beale FA et al: Ovarian irradiation and prednisone following surgery for carcinoma of the breast. In: Salmon SE, Jones SE (eds): Adjuvant Therapy of Cancer. Amsterdam, North-Holland 1977, pp 9–95
332. Dao TL, Nemoto T, Chamberlain A et al: Adrenalectomy with radical mastectomy in the treatment of high-risk breast cancer. Cancer 35:478–482, 1975
333. Ahmann DL, Scanlon PW, Bisel HF et al: Repeated adjuvant chemotherapy with phenylalanine mustard or 5-fluorouracil, cyclophosphamide, and prednisone with or without radiation, after mastectomy for breast cancer. Lancet I:893–896, 1978
334. Meyer RN, Kjellgren K, Malmio K et al: Surgical adjuvant chemotherapy. Results with one short course with cyclophosphamide after mastectomy for breast cancer. Cancer 41:2088–2098, 1978
335. Bonadonna G, Brussamolina M, Vallagussa P et al: Combination chemotherapy as an adjuvant treatment in operable breast cancer. N Engl J Med 294:405–410, 1976
336. Bonadonna G, Rossi A, Valagussa P et al: The CMF program for operable breast cancer with positive axillary nodes. Cancer 39:2904–2915, 1977
337. Bonadonna G, Valagusso P, Rossi A et al: Are surgical adjuvant trials altering the course of breast cancer? Sem Oncol 5:450–464, 1978
338. Rossi A, Bonadonna G, Valagussa P et al: CMF adjuvant program for breast cancer: Five-year results. Proc AACR and ASCO 21:404, 1980
339. Bonadonna G, Valagussa P: Dose–response effect of CMF in breast cancer. Proc AACR and ASCO 21:413, 1980
340. Creech RH, Catalano RB, Mastrangelo MJ et al: An effective low-dose intermittent cyclophosphamide, methotrexate, and 5-fluorouracil treatment regimen for metastatic breast cancer. Cancer 35:1101–1107, 1975
341. Tancini G, Bajetta E, Marchini S et al: Preliminary 3-year results of 12 *versus* 6 cycles of surgical adjuvant CMF in premenopausal breast cancer. Cancer Clin Trials 2:285–292, 1979
342. Cooper RG, Holland JF, Glidewell O: Adjuvant chemotherapy of breast cancer. Cancer 44:793–798, 1979

343. Buzdar AU, Blumenschein GR, Gutterman JU et al: Postoperative adjuvant chemotherapy with fluorouracil, doxorubicin, cyclophosphamide, and BCG vaccine. JAMA 242:1509–1513, 1979
344. Sparks FC, Wile A, Ramming KP et al: Immunology and adjuvant chemoimmunotherapy of breast cancer. Arch Surg 111:1057–1062, 1976
345. Samaan NA, DeAsis DN Jr, Buzdar AU et al: Pituitary–ovarian function in breast cancer patients on adjuvant chemoimmunotherapy. Cancer 41:2084–2087, 1978
346. Fisher B, Sherman B, Rockette H et al: L-Phenylalanine mustard (L-PAM) in the management of pre-menopausal patients with primary breast cancer: Lack of association of disease-free survival with depression of ovarian function. Cancer 44:847–857, 1979
347. Henderson IC, Canellos GP: Medical progress, cancer of the breast: The past decade. New Engl J Med 302:17–30, 78–90, 1980
348. Valagussa P, Tess JDT, Rossi A et al: Has adjuvant CMF altered the patterns of first recurrence in operable breast cancer with N+? Proc AACR and ASCO 21:413, 1980
349. Rossi A, Tancini G, Marchini S et al: Response to secondary treatment after surgical adjuvant CMF for breast cancer. Proc AACR and ASCO 21:190, 1980
350. Foote FW Jr, Stewart FW: Lobular carcinoma-*in-situ*—A rare form of mammary cancer. Am J Pathol 17:491, 1941
351. Muir R: The evolution of carcinoma of the mamma. J Pathol Bacteriol 52:155, 1941
352. Benfield JR, Jacobson M, Warner NE: *In situ* lobular carcinoma of the breast. Arch Surg 91:130, 1965
353. Giordano JM, Klopp CT: Lobular carcinoma-*in-situ*: Incidence and treatment. Cancer 31:105, 1973
354. McDivitt RW, Hutter RVP, Foote FW Jr et al: *In situ* lobular carcinoma. A prospective follow-up study indicating cumulative patient risks. JAMA 201:82, 1967
355. Miller HW Jr, Kay S: Infiltrating lobular carcinoma of the female mammary gland. Surg Gynecol Obstet 102:661, 1956
356. Newman W: Lobular carcinoma of the female breast: Report of 73 cases. Ann Surg 164:305, 1966
357. Berg JW, Robbins GF: 20-year follow-ups of breast cancer. Acta Un Int Cancer 19:1575, 1963
358. Newman W: *In situ* lobular carcinoma of the breast: Report of 26 women with 32 cancers. Ann Surg 157:591, 1963
359. Fechner RE: Infiltrating lobular carcinoma without lobular carcinoma *in situ*. Cancer 29:1539, 1972
360. Farrow JH: Clinical considerations and treatment of *in situ* lobular breast cancer. Am J Roentgen 102:652, 1968
361. Benfield JR, Fingerhut AG, Warner NE: Lobular carcinoma of the breast—1969: A therapeutic proposal. Arch Surg 99:129, 1969
362. Farrow JH: Current concepts in the detection and treatment of the earliest of the early breast cancers. Cancer 25:468, 1970
363. Snyder RE: Mammography and lobular carcinoma-*in-situ*. Surg Gynecol Obstet 122:255, 1966
364. Toker C: Small cell dysplasia and *in situ* carcinoma of the mammary ducts and lobules. J Path 114:47, 1974
365. Lewison EF, Finney GG Jr: Lobular carcinoma-*in-situ* of the breast. Surg Gynecol Obstet 126:1280, 1968
366. Warner NE: Lobular carcinoma of the breast. Cancer 23:840, 1969
367. Hutter RVP, Foote FW Jr: Lobular carcinoma-*in-situ*: Long term follow-up. Cancer 24:1081, 1969
368. Gershon-Cohen J, Berger SM, Curcio BM: Breast cancer with microcalcifications: Diagnostic difficulties. Radiology 87:613, 1966
369. Hutter RVP, Snyder RE, Lucas JC et al: Clinical and pathologic correlation with mammographic findings in lobular carcinoma-*in-situ*. Cancer 21:826, 1969
370. Stewart FW: Tumors of the Breast: Atlas of Tumor Pathology. Washington DC, Armed Forces Institute of Pathology, 1950
371. Fisher ER, Fisher B: Lobular carcinoma of the breast: An overview. Ann Surg 185:377, 1977
372. Benfield JR, Fingerhut AG, Warner NE: A multidiscipline view of lobular breast carcinoma. Ann Surg 176:115, 1972
373. Donegan WL, Perez-Mesa CM: Lobular carcinoma—An indication for elective biopsy of the second breast. Am Surg 176:178, 1972
374. Dall'Olmo CA, Ponka JL, Horn RC et al: Lobular carcinoma of the breast *in situ*: Are we too radical in its treatment? Arch Surg 110:537, 1975
375. Fisher B: Primary breast cancer: Some considerations concerning its management. In Cooper P, Nyhus LM (eds): Surgery Annual. New York, Appleton-Century Crofts, 1971, pp 227–248
376. Kaufmann C, Hamperl H, Baldus F et al: Lobular carcinoma-*in-situ* of the breast-diagnosis, clinical features, and treatment. Germ Med 2:39, 1972
377. Wheeler JE, Enterline HT, Roseman JM et al: Lobular carcinoma-*in-situ* of the breast: Long-term follow-up. Cancer 34:554, 1974
378. Hutter RVP, Foote FW Jr: *In-situ*-lobular carcinoma of the female breast: 1939–1968. In Breast Cancer Early and Late. Chicago, Year Book, 1970
379. Ozello L, Sanpitak P: Epithelial—stromal junction of intraductal carcinoma of the breast. Cancer 26:1186, 1970
380. Rosen PP, Lieberman PH, Braun DW Jr et al: Lobular carcinoma-*in-situ* of the breast. Am J Surg Pathol 2:225, 1978
381. Treves N, Holleb AI: Cancer of the male breast: A report of 146 cases. Cancer 8:1239–1250, 1955
382. Haagenson CD: Diseases of the Breast 2nd ed, pp 779–792. Philadelphia, WB Saunders, 1971
383. Langlands AO, Maclean N, Ken GR: Carcinoma of the male breast: Report of a series of 88 cases. Clin Radiol 27:21–25, 1976
384. Donegan WL, Perez-Mesa C: Carcinoma of the male breast. Arch Surg 106:273–279, 1973
385. Roswit B, Edlis H: Carcinoma of the male breast: A thirty-year experience and literature review. Int J Radiat Oncol Biol Phys 4:711–715, 1978
386. Anderson DE: Genetic considerations in breast cancer. In: Breast Cancer: Early and Late, pp 27–36. Chicago, Year Book Medical Publishers, 1970
387. Everson RB, Li FP, Fraumeni JF et al: Familial male breast cancer. Lancet 1:9–12, 1976
388. El-Gazayerli MM, Abdel-Aziz AS: On bilharziasis and male breast cancer in Egypt. Br J Cancer 17:566–571, 1963
389. Harnden DG, Maclean N, Langlands AO: Carcinoma of the male breast and Klinefelter's syndrome. J Med Genet 8:460–461, 1971
390. Gupta N, Cohen JL, Rosenbaum C et al: Estrogen receptors in male breast cancer. Cancer 46:1781–1784, 1980
391. Yap HY, Tashima CK, Blumenschein GR et al: Male breast cancer: A natural history study. Cancer 44:748–754, 1979
392. Heller KS, Rosen PP, Schottenfeld D et al: Male Breast Cancer: A Clinicopathologic Study of 97 Cases. Ann Surg 188:60–65, 1978
393. Treves N: Treatment of Cancer of the Male Breast by Ablative Surgery and Hormonal Therapy: An analysis of 42 patients. Cancer 12:820–832, 1959
394. Holleb A, Freeman HP, Farrow JH: Cancer of the male breast. NY State J Med 68:544–553; 656–663, 1968
395. Li MC, Janelli DE, Kelly EJ et al: Metastatic carcinoma of the male breast treated with bilateral adrenalectomy and chemotherapy. Cancer 25:678–681, 1970
396. Kennedy BJ, Kiang DT: Hypophysectomy in the treatment of advanced cancer of the male breast. Cancer 29:1606–1612, 1972

CHAPTER 28

Murray F. Brennan

Cancer of the Endocrine System

The Thyroid Gland

with William D. Bloomer

Malignant disease of the thyroid gland arouses great emotion between proponents of aggressive and conservative treatment. This debate arises because of the high probability of long-term survival in patients with small or occult cancers discovered by routine screening. This chapter provides an approach to thyroid cancer that will make decisions involving the extent of investigation and treatment easier. As all thyroid cancers are potentially lethal, the authors believe that a thorough attempt to provide definitive diagnosis of a lesion in the thyroid gland is justified.

HISTORY

The thyroid gland was given its name because of its shape (from the Greek *thyreos*—a shield), as it was thought to shield the larynx, much as the thyroid cartilage did. Hyperthyroidism was described by Parry in 1786, by Graves in 1835, and Von Basedow in 1840. Myxedema was described by Curling in 1850 and Gull in 1875. Thyroidectomy by Reverdin in 1882 produced myxedema which was successfully treated with thyroid extract by Murray and Howitz in 1890.[1,2] Isolation of the hormone thyroxine (T4) was performed by Kendall in 1914.[3]

The first successful thyroidectomy appears to be that performed by the Moor Albucasis about 950 A.D. in Zahra, an Arab city of Spain.[2]

However, the pioneer of thyroid surgery was Theodore Kocher, professor of surgery in Berne. Kocher is thought to have performed approximately 4,000 thyroid operations in his clinic, being well aware of the necessity to spare the parathyroid glands and the recurrent laryngeal nerves. Dr. Kocher was said to have had a 4.5% mortality in 2,000 cases. Kocher confirmed that total thyroidectomy in man resulted in myxedema and that this complication could be prevented by subtotal thyroidectomy. For these, and many other contributions to understanding of diseases and therapy of the thyroid gland, Kocher received the Nobel Prize in 1909. In the U.S. it was Dr. Halsted who, after visiting Kocher on many occasions, evolved his own method of thyroidectomy.[2]

Thyroxin was first synthesized by Harringtron and Barger in 1927 and [3-5-3]tri-iodothyronine was identified by Gross, Pitt-Rivers, and Roche, and Lissitsky and Mitchel almost simultaneously. Thiouracil, the first anti-thyroid drug, was introduced in 1943 by McKenzie and Astwood.

EPIDEMIOLOGY

The incidence of thyroid cancer in women (5.5/100,000) is more than double that of men (2.4/100,000 for 1970), with the majority of cases occurring between 25 and 65 years of age (see Figs. 28-1 and 28-2 and also Table 28-1).

There appears to have been a definite increase in the incidence of thyroid cancer between the Second National Cancer Survey in 1947 and the Third National Cancer Survey in 1969–1971, and again between 1973 and 1977 (see Fig. 28-3).[4] The overall age-adjusted incidence for both sexes, all ages and races combined, increased from 2.4 to 3.9 per

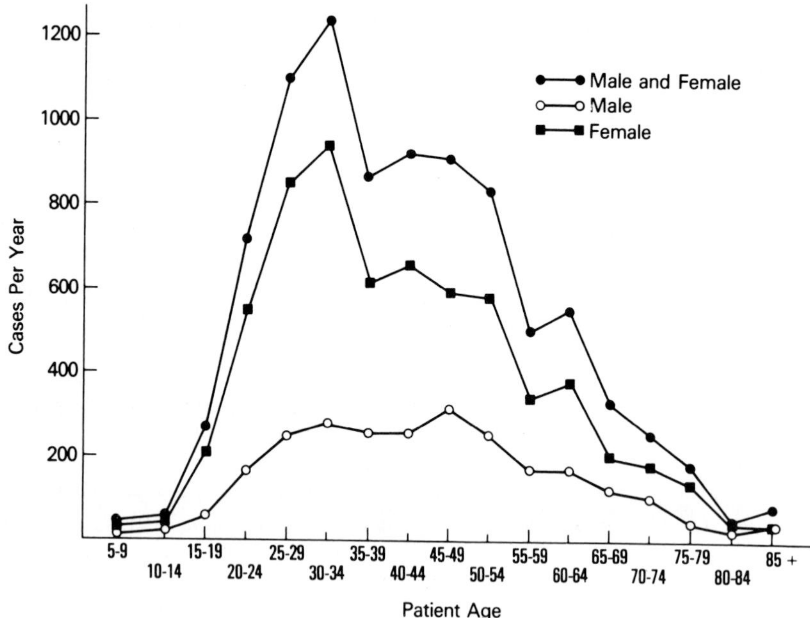

FIG. 28-1. The age distribution of papillary follicular cancer from 1973–1977 for males and females. The figure is drawn from data provided by the SEER program, NCI (see text).

TABLE 28-1. Thyroid Cancer; Age-Adjusted Incidence Rates (1973–1977) per 100,000 Population

All Races	Total	4.0	(5.9)
Male		2.4	(6.2)
Female		5.5	(5.6)
White	Total	3.8	(6.2)
Male		2.3	(6.6)
Female		5.2	(5.9)
Black	Total	2.8*	(0.6)*
Male		1.4*	(0.7)*
Female		4.0*	(0.8)*

( ) = Comparative rates for melanoma from Seer program, NCI.
* Standard error > 5%

TABLE 28-2. Incidence of Thyroid Cancer (per 100,000 Population)

	MALE	FEMALE
Black (San Francisco)	1.4	2.7
(Los Angeles)	0.9	3.7
White		
Australia (New South Wales)	0.7	2.1
New Zealand	1.0	2.0
Hawaii	3.1	9.2
Seattle	1.9	4.0
San Francisco	2.8	6.2
Los Angeles	2.4	6.1

Menck HR, Henderson BE: Cancer incidence rates in the Pacific Basin: Second symposium on epidemiology and cancer registries in the Pacific Basin. NCI Monograph 53: NIH Publication 79-1864, 1979

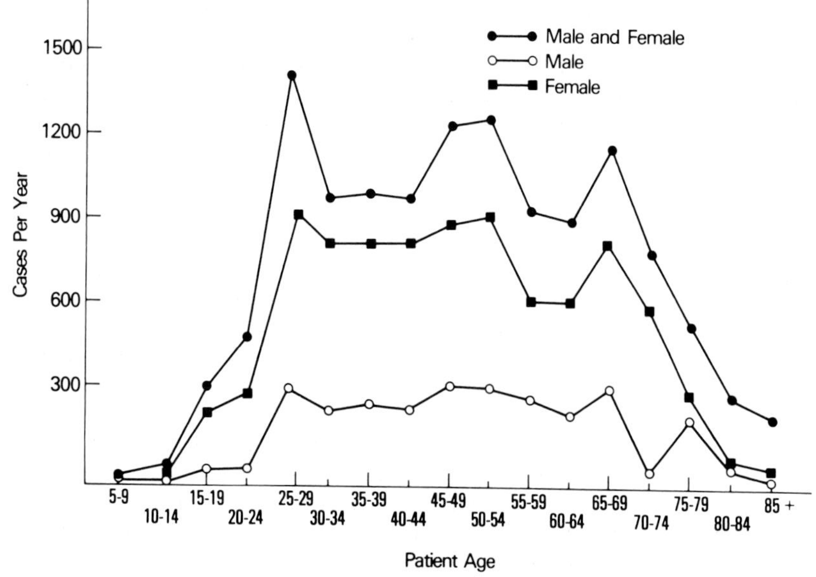

FIG. 28-2. The age distribution of follicular cancer from 1973–1977 for males and females. The figure is drawn from data supplied by the SEER program, NCI (see text).

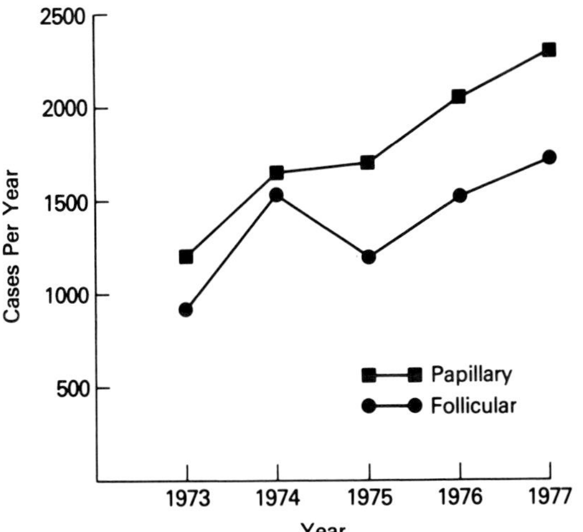

FIG. 28-3. The rising incidence of carcinoma of the thyroid from 1973–1977. The figure is drawn from data supplied by the SEER program, NCI (see text.).

100,000 population between 1947 and 1971. The age-adjusted incidence rate for 1970 is approximately 4/100,000. This data is based on the Surveillance Epidemiology and End Results (SEER) Program of the National Cancer Institute, from 11 population-based registries including five states and six metropolitan areas that make up approximately 10% of the U.S. population.

The prevalence of thyroid cancer at autopsy in patients dying of other diseases has been as high as 5.7%.[5] The incidence in Pacific Basin countries has recently been reviewed (see Table 28-2).[6]

The absolute prevalence of cancer in solitary and multinodular glands is approximately 10–15%.[7–10]

ANATOMIC CONSIDERATIONS

The thyroid gland sits in the midline of the neck, draped on either side of the lower aspect of the thyroid cartilage. It is covered anteriorly by the thyrohyoid and more superficially by the sternohyoid muscles. The nerve supply enters these muscles at varying levels; the nerves to the sternothyroid and the sternohyoid muscles are derived from the superior root of the ansa cervicalis (descendens hypoglossi of the ansa hypoglossi) or the ansa itself. Most commonly, a branch directly from the superior root supplies the upper half of the sternohyoid and sternothyroid, while a branch from the ansa supplies the lower portions of the two muscles. Various claims have been made that by dividing these muscles during thyroidectomy at levels approximately midway between the thyroid cartilage and the suprasternal notch allows for both the superior and inferior branches to enter the muscle and not be damaged by such division. The inconsistency of this point of entrance, however, makes it difficult to guarantee success by this maneuver.

The thyroid gland consists of right and left lobes, lateral to the larynx and trachea and united across the front, usually just below the cricoid cartilage, by an isthmus. From the isthmus, a process of thyroid tissue projects upward as a pyramidal lobe, which may be developed to a varying degree. On rare occasions, it may extend to the hyoid bone. The thyroid gland is surrounded by a thin layer of connective tissue which, between the posterior surface of the anterior "strap" muscles and the thyroid gland itself, is usually referred to as the pretracheal fascia. The connective tissue, which is more densely adherent to the thyroid, is known as the thyroid fascia or false thyroid capsule. There is usually a layer of this fascia that extends posteriorly to embrace the recurrent laryngeal nerve and to extend back behind the esophagus. In this area, however, the tissue is thin and easily distorted. This accounts for the confusion as to whether the parathyroid glands, which are usually thought of as lying between this thyroid fascia and thyroid gland itself, sometimes appear to lie within the false capsule of the thyroid. The true capsule of the thyroid is quite firm, adherent, and sends septa between the lobules of the thyroid gland as an integral part of the gland. Technically, the two fascias, the thyroid capsule, and the thyroid fascia can be distinguished by the ability to readily and bluntly dissect the external fascia, whereas the thyroid capsule requires sharp dissection for its interruption.

The blood supply to the thyroid gland is extensive, with two main arteries on either side (see Fig. 28-4). The superior thyroid artery usually arises as the first or second branch in close approximation, but usually slightly superficial to the external branch of the superior laryngeal nerve. This nerve is, therefore, liable to damage in blindly placing a clamp on the arterial pedicle.

The superior laryngeal nerve, a branch of the vagus at the lower end of the inferior ganglion, divides into a small external and a large internal branch. The external branch runs downward on the lateral surface of the inferior constrictor to which it may give a branch to end in the cricothyroid muscle. The internal branch curves forward, high on the thyrohyoid membrane, and penetrates this membrane to break up into branches distributed within the pharynx and larynx.

As the superior thyroid artery nears the gland, it divides into anterior and posterior branches that distribute numerous branches to the superior aspect of the gland. A common large branch runs across the superior medial aspect of the thyroid lobe to anastomose with the branch on the contralateral side.

The inferior thyroid artery most commonly arises from the thyrocervical trunk. This artery usually runs up in front of the vertebral artery, continuing in the direction of the thyrocervical trunk. At the level of the sixth cervical vertebra, the inferior thyroid artery gives off the ascending cervical branch and then crosses medially and somewhat downward to arch behind the carotid sheath, penetrating the prevertebral fascia to reach the posterior aspect of the thyroid gland. As the artery curves medially, it crosses the cervical sympathetic trunk that may be in front of the artery. As the inferior thyroid artery divides in the posterior lateral aspect of the inferior pole of the thyroid gland it is in close relationship to the recurrent laryngeal nerve.

The thyroid ima artery is occasionally present as an accessory to (or rarely as replacement of) the inferior thyroid artery. This artery is usually a branch from the innominate artery, and ascends in front of the trachea to be at risk during tracheostomy.

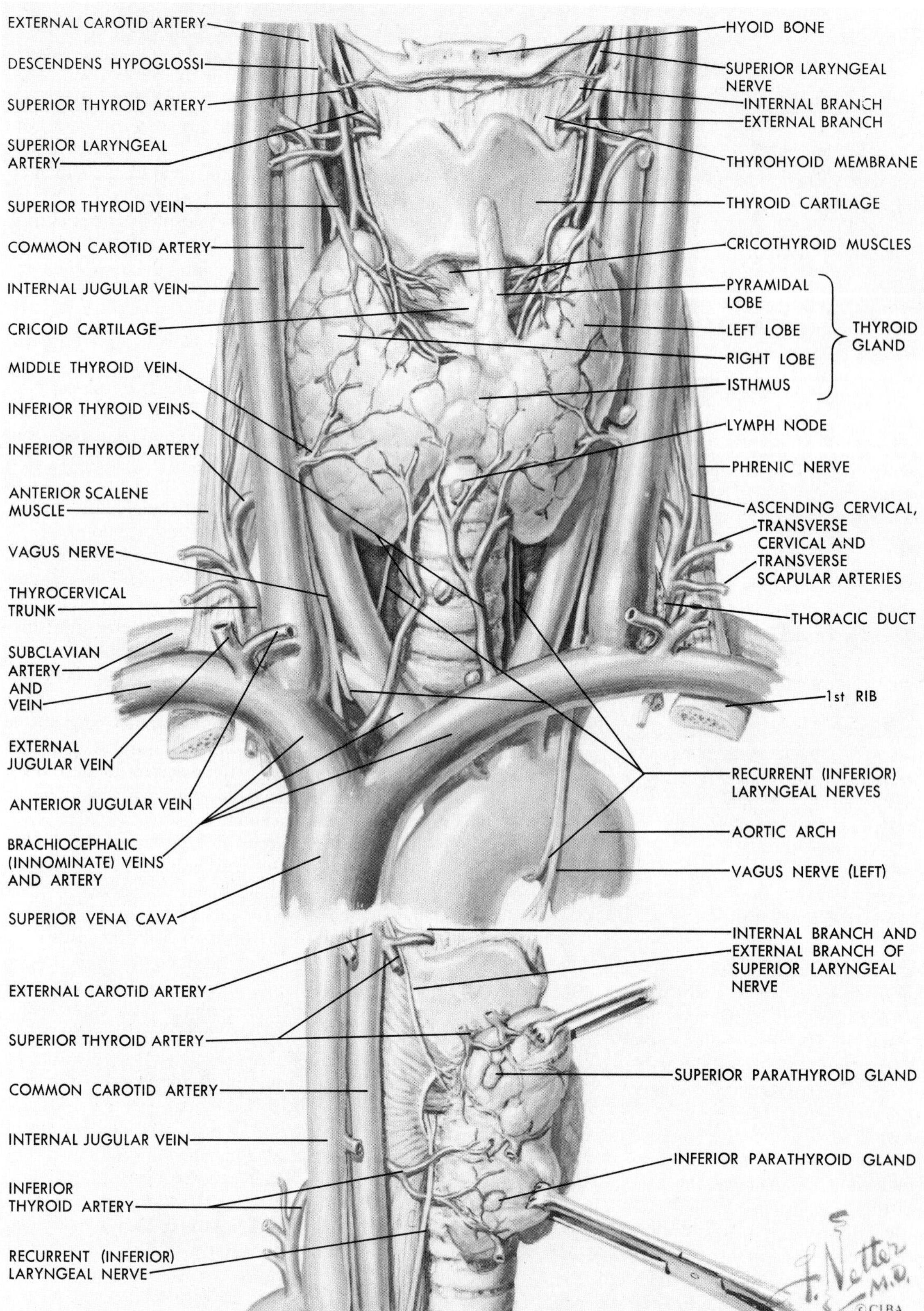

FIG. 28-4. The thyroid gland. (Netter FH (ed): Anatomy of the Thyroid and Parathyroid Glands, Section II, Plate 2. The Ciba Collection of Medical Illustrations, Volume 4: The Endocrine System and Selected Metabolic Diseases. New York, Ciba, 1965)

The recurrent laryngeal nerve arises on the right side from the vagus as it passes in front of the subclavian artery. It then curves below and behind the subclavian and passes upward and medially into the central visceral compartment of the neck. The left recurrent laryngeal nerve rises from the left vagus as this vagus passes in front of the arch of the aorta. The nerve then passes below and upward behind the aorta at the level of the ligamentum arteriosum to pass medially, closely between the trachea and esophagus. Rarely, an anomalous right "recurrent" nerve may pass medially from the vagus at the level of the cricoid. Both recurrent laryngeal nerves cross the inferior thyroid arteries and both are in close relationship to the posterior aspect of the thyroid gland. Unfortunately, the recurrent nerves are not in fixed positions and are, therefore, at increased risk during thyroidectomy. The right recurrent nerve may be quite lateral to the trachea and usually passes between branches of the terminal divisions of the inferior thyroid arteries. However, the nerve can pass in front of or completely behind the inferior thyroid artery. Of particular importance is that at the site where the recurrent nerve is most attached to the thyroid gland, the thyroid gland is itself most densely attached to the larynx by a dense area of connective tissue, the lateral suspensory ligament. On occasion (up to 10% of the time), the nerve may actually penetrate the thyroid gland for a very short distance, putting it at increased risk of injury (see Fig. 28-5). The recurrent laryngeal nerve may penetrate the larynx before or after it has divided. Most often the nerve divides after entrance into the larynx. The nerve enters the larynx just behind the cricothyroid articulation.[11]

INJURY TO THE SUPERIOR AND RECURRENT LARYNGEAL NERVES

Paralysis of the superior laryngeal nerve causes paralysis of the cricothyroid muscle. Since this muscle is responsible for changes in the length of the vocal cords, bilateral damage to these nerves can make it difficult to sing high notes. The patient notices the voice to be somewhat easily tired, with hoarseness and weakness after prolonged talking.

Injury to the recurrent nerve produces a much more disabling injury. Injuries to these nerves, however, are often confusing as interpretation of damage is judged by assessing movements of the vocal cords. Following injury, the cords may appear to be in abduction, adduction, or anywhere in between. The midposition (cadaveric) implies that no muscles are acting on the cord and would be expected only if superior and inferior laryngeal nerves were damaged on that side. The division of one recurrent nerve will usually cause some dyspnea upon exertion, with the cord fixed in the adducted position, but the voice will be good because the contralateral cord can meet in the midline. If the cord is fixed in the abducted position, there will be hoarseness but no dyspnea.

If the voice is hoarse following the operation, improvement in hoarseness may result in increasing dyspnea as gradual adduction takes place. The delayed paralysis, which occasionally occurs a week or two following thyroidectomy, is thought to be due to edema and will rarely be permanent.

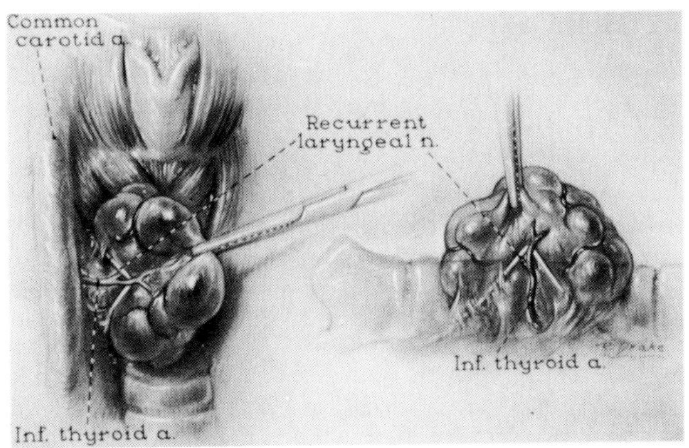

FIG. 28-5. The close association of recurrent nerve, inferior thyroid artery, and thyroid gland increases the risk of nerve damage when the thyroid lobe is pulled forward. (Black, BM: The Cyclopedia of Medicine, Surgery, Specialties, 3rd ed, vol 14, p 173. Philadelphia, FA Davis, 1962)

LYMPHATIC DRAINAGE

The lymph nodes of the neck are intimately contiguous, although for convenience are divided into several groups (see Fig. 28-6).[12]

The lymphatic drainage of the thyroid gland usually accompanies the arterial blood supply. Lymphatic channels on the superior aspect of the thyroid gland and the superior border of the isthmus drain into the upper deep cervical nodes. The inferior aspects of both lobes and the isthmus drain by channels into the lower deep cervical nodes, including supraclavicular nodes and especially the pretracheal and prelaryngeal nodes.

FIG. 28-6. The normal lymphatic drainage of the thyroid gland to the deep cervical and paratracheal nodes. (Mahorner, HR, Caylor, HD, Schlotthauer, CF, Pemberton, J de J: Anat Rec, 36:341, 1927)

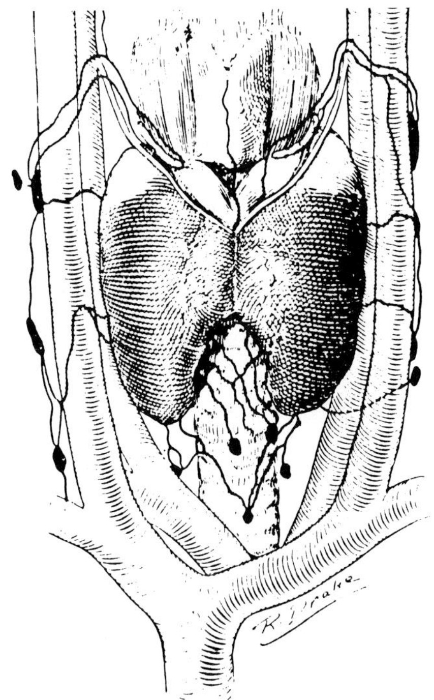

PATHOLOGY

The majority of malignant tumors of the thyroid gland are of glandular–epithelial origin (see Table 28-3). Because of the clinical appreciation that some thyroid cancers grow very slowly and have a rather benign cause, classification is often dependent on the demonstration of invasion rather than on pure cellular morphology.[13]

The problem has been complicated because some lesions that are microscopically identical to benign adenomas (except for the single feature of microscopic blood vessel invasion), have a relatively benign course so aggressive therapy may not be required. These tumors can, however, metastasize; a suitable term is lacking, varying from adenoma with invasion, occult cancer, potentially malignant thyroid tumor, to adenoma with angio-invasive potential.

Multifocality of cancer within the thyroid gland is common with malignant tumors of the thyroid gland: up to 80% multifocality documented when multiple sections are taken from patients with papillary cancer.[14] An important clinicopathologic observation is the presence of direct extension into the adjacent tissues of the neck, which is of more ominous prognostic value than isolated lymph node metastases.

Because of the problem alluded to above, staging of thyroid carcinoma has not been uniformly applied; an acceptable staging classification based on combined surgical and histopathologic interpretation is given in Table 28-4.

TABLE 28-3. Classification of Malignant Tumors of the Thyroid Gland

Well-Differentiated Carcinoma
Papillary or Papillary-Follicular Adenocarcinoma
Follicular Carcinoma
Hurthle Cell Carcinoma
Undifferentiated (Anaplastic) Carcinoma
Small Cell Carcinoma
Giant Cell Carcinoma
Medullary Carcinoma
Other Malignant Tumors
Sarcoma
Lymphoma
Epidermoid Carcinoma
Metastatic Tumor
Malignant Teratoma

TABLE 28-4. Clinicopathologic Staging of Malignant Tumors of the Thyroid Gland

STAGE I	
A	Unilateral
B	Multifocal or Bilateral
STAGE II	
A	Unilateral Lymph Nodes
B	Bilateral or Mediastinal Lymph Nodes
STAGE III	
	Local Cervical Invasion With or Without Positive Lymph Nodes
STAGE IV	
	Distant Metastases

PAPILLARY ADENOCARCINOMA

Papillary carcinoma varies in necrosis and gross appearance, dependent on size. Small lesions (often called occult, sclerosing carcinomas) may be recognizable only by careful, multiple section, histopathologic examination. The larger tumors are usually poorly defined, although some may show attempts at encapsulation. With very large tumors, cystic degeneration is not uncommon and these cysts can contain hemorrhage; associated fibrosis is common and calcium may be deposited in the fibrotic areas.

The classic appearance is of papillary projections formed by the fibrovascular pedicle with its superimposed tumor epithelium. The epithelium is commonly of one layer but can be heaped up, containing homogeneous, cuboidal, amphophilic cells; mitoses are uncommon, squamous metaplasia common, and psammoma bodies of calcific laminations are common. Lymphatic invasion is very common and often occurs throughout the tumor. Venous invasion, however, is quite uncommon. Whether the multiple foci are multiple metastatic foci by lymphatic spread or multicentric has never been proven.

Many of these well-differentiated carcinomas are neither purely papillary nor purely follicular, but admixtures of both in varying proportions. As a consequence, the term mixed papillary and follicular carcinoma has been used; unfortunately, there is no firm agreement about which terms should be included in these mixed categories. Many prefer to consider any tumor containing papillary components to be classified under the papillary neoplasms. A reasonable alternative is to classify the tumor with its dominant pattern including, where appropriate, mention of the less dominant feature.

FOLLICULAR CARCINOMA

Some follicular carcinomas cannot be distinguished from follicular adenomas, a common cause for excision of a thyroid nodule. However, some follicular carcinomas show gross evidence of invasion. The tumors are firm with a fibrous, sometimes calcified, fibrotic center. There may be wide range of hemorrhage and infarction in larger tumors. Occasionally, the blood vessel invasion can be appreciated grossly.

The microscopic pattern is again variable, with tumors being nearly totally solid, without any follicles to being well-differentiated follicles containing colloid. Commonly, there are components of papillary cancer found if a consistent search is made. Pure follicular carcinomas are thought to be relatively uncommon. Again, mitoses are relatively infrequent and pleomorphism minimal; psammoma bodies can occur.

To be defined as a follicular carcinoma, some degree of invasiveness must be recognized; this can vary from minimal to extensive. Blood vessel invasion is more common in follicular than papillary carcinoma and is usually associated with capsule invasion.

MEDULLARY CARCINOMA

This tumor usually presents as a solid, hard, grayish white mass, often with apparent encapsulation; obvious blood vessel invasion is frequent. The tumor is thought to arise from "C" cell. The predominant area of "C" cell aggregation is at the junction of the superior and middle third of the gland and accounts for the preponderance of this site as the site of neoplasia. In sporadic forms of the disease, it is usually unilateral; whereas, in association with a familial, multiple, endocrine neoplasia syndrome, the tumors are uniformly bilateral. Microscopically, the tumor cells are in solid irregular groups, often separated by an amyloid-containing stroma. The tumor cells are variable in size as are the clusters of cells. The actual cells are round and have an eosinophilic granular cytoplasm with the nuclei somewhat hyperchromatic with binuclear cells frequent. Wide variation in cellular type and cellular arrangement occurs. The amyloid may occasionally be seen within the tumor cell and is thought to be formed by the epithelial cells of the tumor. Deposition of calcium within the stroma is frequent and accounts for the calcification identifiable on x-ray. Microscopic vascular invasion is very common.

UNDIFFERENTIATED (ANAPLASTIC) CARCINOMA

These carcinomas form neither papillary nor follicular elements and do not contain amyloid. They are usually highly malignant and can contain several subgroups; most common subclassifications are small-cell and large-cell carcinomas.

The small-cell carcinoma is a highly malignant tumor which, in gross appearance, is extremely suspicious, being poorly defined with extension into adjacent thyroid and often into structures surrounding the thyroid gland. Microscopically, the cells are usually variations between two types: compact, uniform-appearing, small cells or closely packed tumor cells growing in strands or clusters. Mitoses are frequent and the stromas often fibrous and hyaline, not too different from that of medullary carcinoma without the amyloid. The diffuse type of small cell carcinoma can occasionally be mistaken for a lymphoma as the cells grow in a diffuse lymphoma-like pattern.

The giant-cell carcinoma is a highly malignant form of the anaplastic undifferentiated type with large cells and dissociated giant and spindle cells. The tumor cell is again hard, ill-defined, and extensive at the time of presentation, often showing extraglandular invasion. Microscopically, the tumor cells are large, pleomorphism is common, and some cells may resemble those of a fibrosarcoma. The frequent mitoses are often atypical with multinuclear cells.

NATURAL HISTORY OF THYROID CARCINOMAS

PAPILLARY ADENOCARCINOMA

This is the commonest type of thyroid cancer, often presenting with cervical lymph node metastases. Most series report 50–75% of lymph node involvement at presentation. In the cervical lymph node, metastasis can be the presenting complaint with a tumor in the thyroid gland so small that it can only be identified by multiple sectioning. The majority do not metastasize by the bloodstream; however, distant metastases have been reported in as high as 10% of cases at presentation.

FOLLICULAR CARCINOMA

The feature that distinguishes these tumors is the propensity for blood vessel invasion. Like papillary cancer, the metastases may be slow and dormant for some years before progressing. The majority metastasize to the lung and bone.

MEDULLARY CARCINOMA

Medullary carcinoma makes up 5–10% of all thyroid carcinomas, with the majority of the sporadic type occurring in patients over 40 years of age. A progressively younger age group is being diagnosed in those with familial disease as a result of screening for thyrocalcitonin.

UNDIFFERENTIATED CARCINOMA

These tumors are characterized by rapid growth, extensive invasion, and rapid metastases. The prognosis is poor with 5-year survivals, of 20–25%, regardless of type. The tumor usually occurs in the older age group, with rapid progression, metastases, local invasion, and early death. It is common that in these cases, time from diagnosis to death is less than 6 months (see Table 28-5).[15-20]

PATHOGENESIS

RADIATION-INDUCED THYROID CANCER

That radiation given in childhood and infancy for benign conditions of the head and neck can produce thyroid cancer was suggested in 1950 and confirmed later by others.[21-25] In one series, the interval between irradiation and surgery was 27 years, comparable to other radiation-induced tumors.[25] Most commonly, patients have undergone irradiation for acne, thymic abnormalities, or suspected or proven hypertrophy of the tonsils or adenoids[26-28] and have received between 200 and 1,000 rad, although doses as little as 6 rad given for tinea capitis have been incriminated.[26-28] At higher doses (greater than 2,000 rad) the thyroid gland tends to be sterilized with very few cells present to undergo malignant degeneration. Various computations have suggested the incidence of thyroid neoplasia is a function of radiation dose with the dose-response being linear, initially at three per 100 person years at risk per 1,000 rad. Currently, the risk is nine cases of

TABLE 28-5. Five-Year Mortality from Thyroid Cancer

CLINICALLY APPARENT	REF. 15	REF. 16	REF. 17	REF. 18	REF. 19	REF. 20
Papillary cancer	6%	11%	10%	20%	—	—
Follicular cancer	—	33%	41%	40%	—	—
Anaplastic cancer	—	76%	100%	—	81%	99%

cancer per year, per 18,000 people, each with a thyroid dose of 300 rad.[26,29] Risk factors include the following.

Sex–females have increased risk
Age–the younger at irradiation, the higher the risk
Interval after irradiation–increasing risk with increasing interval
Thyroid dose–the risk is linear *i.e.*, 3–3.7 cases/year/rad/million persons exposed up to 1270 REM, after which there is diminishing risk
Patients given irradiation for thymic, tonsillar or adenoidal enlargement have a higher risk than those given x-ray therapy for acne[26]

One study of 100 asymptomatic patients with a history of radiation to head or neck revealed palpable abnormalities of the thyroid in 26%; malignant tumors were confirmed in seven of 15 who had surgery.[30] In larger series, abnormalities of thyroid by palpation and scan were found in 27% of 1,056 irradiated patients; carcinomas were found in 33% of 60 patients who underwent operation.[23,31]

OTHER RISK FACTORS

Some studies have suggested an association of follicular and anaplastic cancer with endemic goiter.[34]

Papillary cancer has increased in the U.S. and Switzerland since iodized salt was introduced and is higher in high iodine than low iodine areas.[32]

The increased incidence of Hashimoto's disease in the U.S. and the alleged increased incidence of cancer in Hashimoto's disease has raised concern that an increase in thyroid cancer would be detected.[33] However this has not been proven on subsequent review.[34]

PATTERNS OF SPREAD

The spread of thyroid neoplasms is dependent upon pathology. The low grade, well-differentiated papillary or papillary-follicular neoplasms tend to spread to regional lymph nodes frequently, but only rarely have disseminated distant metastases, (see Fig. 28-6).

In those papillary-follicular lesions in which vascular invasion can be demonstrated, especially in pure follicular lesions, disseminated metastases are common.

CLINICAL PRESENTATION

The manner in which an incidental thyroid nodule, found by the patient or at examination because of a history of prior radiation, should be evaluated and treated is undergoing active change. Because of the high incidence of thyroid nodules and the relatively infrequent occurrence of cancer, it becomes imperative that accurate diagnosis and staging be made so as to avoid unnecessary surgery, but without missing significant thyroid cancer.

The factors in the history and physical examination that make cancer a high suspicion include a history of previous external radiation therapy; the relatively recent onset of a firm, hard, single nodule in the thyroid; and the obvious presence of cervical lymphadenopathy. Although females are more commonly affected than males, nodules are uncommon in men and are more likely to be cancer. A family history of thyroid cancer should raise the suspicion of a multiple endocrine neoplasia syndrome.

On physical examination, the defined presence of a single, firm, enlarging nodule or cervical lymphadenopathy in an apparently euthyroid state heightens suspicion.

DIAGNOSTIC METHODS

Except for the determination of thyrocalcitonin in medullary carcinoma of the thyroid, the only unequivocal diagnostic tool in thyroid cancer is biopsy. The accuracy of clinical diagnosis of a thyroid nodule varies with the experience of the observer; however, without supportive suspicion it is generally unreliable. The common, clinically accepted aphorism that a single nodule is more worrisome than a multinodular gland must be interpreted in the light of the fact that of those patients coming to surgery for a uninodular lesion some 30–75% will have multinodular change. The prevalence of cancer (10%) reported in both multinodular and uninodular glands, a figure higher than in some series of uninodular glands, makes this distinction further suspect.[8–10]

Many attempts have been made to differentiate between the benign and the malignant nodule preoperatively. These include the following:

THYROID GLAND SUPPRESSION

The use of exogenous thyroid hormone in an effort to suppress thyroid nodules and make them disappear is claimed to be effective. However, firm numbers on this factor are not commonly available and at best, one might expect 20% to disappear. In one study of 230 patients, 30% of goiters completely regressed and 30% decreased in size.[35] Unfortunately, the majority of the "good" results were in diffuse goiters; 40% of solitary nodules failed to respond. In other reports, 2% of all nodules responded and 3.6% of 111 nontoxic nodular goiters regressed.[34,36] In a double-blind study using tri-iodothyronine for 6 weeks, only one of 16 patients with uninodular goiter had 50% regression. In 16 patients who had surgery two had cancer—one had increased and one had decreased in size on thyroxine suppression. This failure to suppress was presumptively due to the independence of most nodules, both benign and malignant, of TSH.[15] If benign and not malignant nodules regressed, then thyroid hormone would not be expected to be of value in suppression of post-thyroidectomy cancer recurrence. However, the authors do employ this test, requiring approximately 6 months to determine whether or not the nodule has decreased or resolved. The authors justify their use of thyroid suppression on the basis that many nodules will be due to a diffuse process involving all the thyroid gland. With careful follow-up, any delay in definitive treatment will not translate into long-term morbidity or mortality.

ULTRASONOGRAPHY

The fact that some benign nodules are cystic, a rare occurrence in the malignant nodule, has led to the use of ultrasonography in an effort to distinguish benignity from malignancy. The presence of a cyst must be confirmed by aspiration; if cystic, a cytologic examination of the aspirated fluid can provide a diagnosis. The prevalance of cancer in cysts has been given as 0.6% and 2%.[37,38] Unfortunately, cysts represent only 10–25% of nodules.[39,40]

FINE NEEDLE ASPIRATION

Fine needle aspiration is a simple and safe technique. A#22 gauge needle is introduced into the lesion and tissue aspirated for cytologic examination. If the lesion is cystic, then the fluid can be spun down and the cells examined. If only a few cells or minimal aspirate is obtained, then they can be expressed onto a glass slide, smeared, and placed in fixative. A recent study found adequate cellular material in 93% of aspirates with an overall incidence of malignant cells in 37%.[41] A high degree of specificity was obtained. In series with subsequent surgical excision, false positives are extremely rare and false negatives occur in 5–10% of cases.[42,43]

PERCUTANEOUS NEEDLE BIOPSY

Percutaneous needle biopsy of the thyroid can provide tissue for histologic analysis.[44] This needle biopsy, however, is not a simple procedure, requiring some expertise to obtain adequate tissue. The concern that tumor can be disseminated along the tract is real and has been reported, although it must be exceedingly rare.[45]

One reason for persisting with the aggressive efforts at preoperative diagnosis is the help that the patient and surgeon receive with a preoperative diagnosis of carcinoma. Explanation as to the type of definitive operation without the need for diagnosis from frozen section can help a great deal.

Fortunately, delay in diagnosis is of less importance in the patient with a papillary or papillary-follicular tumor because of its slow growth rate, low incidence of aggressive malignancy, and efficacy of surgery even at a later stage.

OTHER DIAGNOSTIC MODALITIES

Other diagnostic modalities, such as thermography and lymphography, have been employed but are much less specific.[46,47] They should be reserved for institutions where prospective evaluation of the techniques is being employed.

THYROID SCANNING

Thyroid scanning is performed with 99^{m}Tc-pertechnetate, I^{131}, I^{123}, or 75-Se-selenomethiomine. The preferred agent is 99^{m}TC because it delivers less than one rad to the thyroid and has a short half-life of 6 hours.[48] I^{131} delivers 75 rads to the thyroid and has a half-life of 8.1 days. I^{123} has a half-life of 13 hours and delivers only three rads to the thyroid; although it is the agent of choice when iodination is required, it is not readily available (see Table 28-6). A case report has implicated diagnostic I^{131} as an etiologic factor in the development of carcinoma of the thyroid.[49] The usual dose of I^{131} administered for I^{131} uptake is five microcuries, which results in an irradiation dose to the thyroid of 6.5–9 rads. When an I^{131} scan is to be performed, the common dose is 50 microcuries, which results in an irradiation dose of about 100 rads.

TABLE 28-6. Dosage from Radioisotopes Used in Thyroid Scanning

ISOTOPE	DOSE TO THYROID (rads)
^{131}I Thyroid Scan	10
^{131}I Thyroid Uptake*	75–200
^{99m}Tc Thyroid Scan	<1.0
^{123}I Thyroid Scan	2–3
^{123}I Thyroid Uptake	6–8

(*Assume a 15 gm normal thyroid with 30% uptake and 100 mC dose.)

Weber PM, Jasko IA; Dos Remedios L.V. Thyroid scintophotography in 1000 patients: Rational use of ^{99m}Tc and ^{131}I compounds. J. Nucl Med 12:673–677, 1971

In an analysis of 125 patients with irradiated thyroid glands correlated with pathologic findings, preoperative physical examination, and scans, 88% of the lobes containing carcinoma were abnormal to palpation, whereas only 50% of the same lobes were abnormal on the scan.[25] In large studies of papillary thyroid carcinoma, doubt has been raised concerning the discriminatory value of such scans in the identification of cancer.[50] Most of these suggest that the incidence of hypofunction in cases of benign thyroid modules is similar. It seems reasonable at this point to encourage physical examination of the thyroid rather than repetitive thyroid scanning. The thyroglobulins have been employed to differentiate patients with thyroid carcinoma from patients with benign diseases. Thyroglobulin levels tend to be elevated in the thyroid carcinoma patients. Unfortunately, the overlap between normal subjects and patients with thyrotoxicosis and other head and neck malignancies render this test rather useless for the individual patient. It remains possible that the test may be valuable in long-term follow-up studies of patients with thyroid cancer that have undergone therapy.[51]

STANDARD WORK-UP

A careful history of radiation dose and the reason for it is followed by meticulous physical examination of the thyroid gland to determine the presence or absence of nodules, hoarseness, difficulty in swallowing, cervical lymphadenopathy and indirect laryngoscopy, if indicated.

A radioisotope scan is reasonable, although many would suggest that discrete nodules should be biopsied or removed, regardless of the results.

The authors liberally employ needle aspiration biopsy for cytology in most patients with a single palpable nodule or if thyroiditis is suspected. The objections to needle aspiration can be dismissed if the responsible physician does not allow a negative aspiration to falsely reassure physician and patient.

The next step is thyroid suppression for 3–6 months ensuring that adequate suppression is maintained. When a discrete nodule is revealed that does not suppress on thyroid hormone, surgery is then indicated.

The authors' approach is outlined in Fig. 28-7.

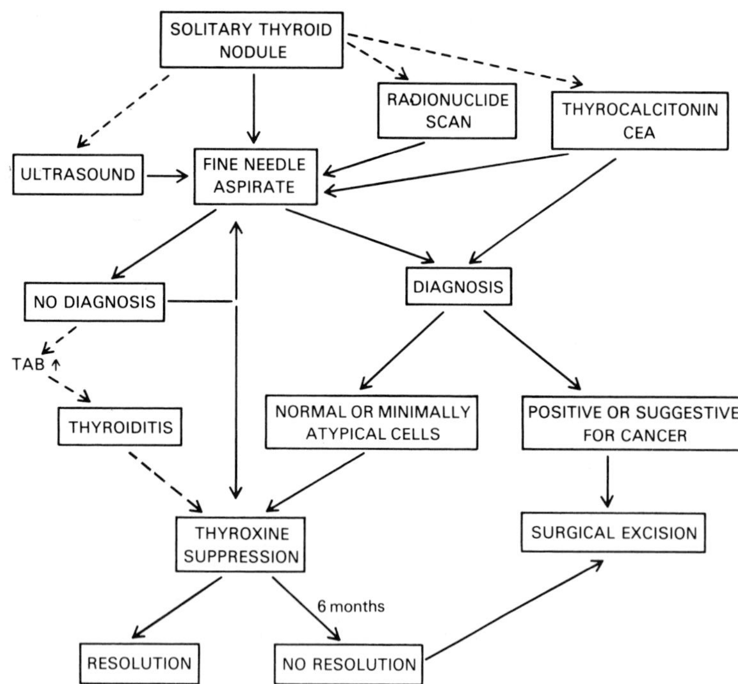

FIG. 28-7. Diagnostic approach to the patient with a thyroid lump.

TREATMENT

SURGICAL APPROACH TO A THYROID NODULE

Once the decision to operate has been made, surgical treatment of the thyroid nodule is performed on the assumption that is represents a potential carcinoma.

In the vast majority of cases, a lobectomy for a nodule confined to one lobe is performed rather than simple nodule excision. This can be modified, on occasion, to nodular excision either for a prominent nodule involving the isthmus or when undue risk to the recurrent nerve exists.

The reason for performing a lobectomy as the first-order preferred procedure is that any reoperation is technically difficult and the recurrence rate will be high because of the multifocality of any carcinoma.

The patient is positioned such that the neck is extended by using a malleable, vacuum pack that provides good head stabilization and firmly arches the neck forward. The table should be flexed so that the patient is in a semi-sitting position, which prevents venous engorgement in the neck and provides a more comfortable dissection position for the surgeon.[52] A horizontal skin crease incision is then made, developing flaps that include skin, subcutaneous tissue, and platysma muscle with the cautery. The flaps are raised to the superior level of the thyroid notch and to the superior aspect of the manubrium and clavicle.

The fascia is divided in the midline with retraction of the strap muscles. This is done in any patient undergoing a primary operation. It is not the routine to divide the strap muscles. This is rather an uncommonly needed procedure. The division of the strap muscles makes it more difficult at any subsequent reoperation. In patients undergoing reoperation it is occasionally efficacious to approach lateral to the strap muscles.

The extent of the operation can be usually appreciated once the strap muscles are mobilized laterally. If the strap muscles are densely adherent to the thyroid gland (a situation that does not normally occur), then part of the strap muscle is taken with the thyroid lobe.

Particular attention must be paid to the recurrent laryngeal nerve and the parathyroid glands. Any lymph nodes in the central cervical neck area that are in any way suspicious are excisionally biopsied. If the nodes are unquestionably involved, a block dissection is preferred, taking the lymphatic tissue along with the thyroid lobe.

Once the lobe is removed and the nodule is confirmed as being carcinoma, a near total thyroidectomy is completed, leaving only that portion of the thyroid gland on the contralateral side that allows preservation of the recurrent laryngeal nerve and the parathyroid glands. A "total" thyroidectomy (*i.e.*, removal of all gross thyroid) is frequently possible. If the parathyroid gland is inadvertently devascularized, then that parathyroid tissue can be autografted.[53,54]

If the nodule is benign on frozen section, the operation is terminated with the one lobe removed. It should be emphasized that the contralateral lobe should be palpated with the finger for any suspicious nodules not seen or appreciated preoperatively.

If permanent histology reveals a carcinoma not appreciated at the time of frozen section, two courses are possible. The preference is to treat the patient with thyroid suppression unless an obvious carcinoma not appreciated at frozen section is identified. In that situation, we would reoperate and remove the majority of the contralateral lobe. Reoperation would not be necessary for an occult carcinoma found incidentally on subsequent permanent histology. Such a patient requires careful follow-up.

SURGERY FOR PROVEN THYROID CANCER

Surgery is the therapy of choice for all primary lesions; recommendations are summarized in Table 28-7.

There is no general agreement concerning the preferred operation. In the hands of a skilled and experienced surgeon, total thyroidectomy or near-total thyroidectomy would be the procedure of choice given the multicentricity of most of these lesions. The prevalance of microscopic foci in the contralateral lobe of patients undergoing total thyroidectomy for a lesion apparently confined to one lobe varies from 38–87%.[14,55] The incidence of recurrence following lobectomy alone varies from 2–40%, with most series reporting 5–10%.[16,55–58] The minimally acceptable procedure is total lobectomy on the side of the lesion. Recurrence occurs more than twice as often in those who had had subtotal thyroidectomy compared to patients who had total thyroidectomy.[50]

A second argument for total or near-total thyroidectomy, which is applicable to follicular cancer as well as to the more commonly multicentric papillary form, is the ease of subsequent diagnosis and treatment of metastatic disease.[31,59–62] Finally, the progression of apparently well-differentiated carcinoma to highly aggressive anaplastic carcinoma at the time of recurrence is well-documented.[15,20,63,64] It should be emphasized that a total thyroidectomy is rarely a 100% thyroidectomy. In most patients, a 2–5% uptake of radioiodine can subsequently be demonstrated after the operation. The relative merits of destroying the residual amount of thyroid tissue by radioactive iodine remains unclear in terms of recurrent thyroid cancer. In a group of patients undergoing postoperative I^{131} and thyroid medication, recurrence occurred in three of 116 patients.[50] Of 413 patients treated with thyroid medication alone, 11% developed recurrent cancer. In neither group were there any deaths. In 32 patients given no postoperative therapy, 37.5% developed recurrence and 12.5% died.[50] As only those who received total thyroidectomy would have required thyroid medication, those given no postoperative therapy must have had at least residual thyroid left behind.

The use of suppressive therapy in the management of thyroid cancer is based on the observation that prolonged stimulation of TSH plays a permissive role in the development of radiation-induced benign and malignant tumors.[65]

MANAGEMENT OF MEDULLARY CARCINOMA OF THE THYROID

The diagnosis of, and screening for, medullary carcinoma is discussed in the section under Multiple Endocrine Neoplasia Type II.

Surgery remains the only effective therapy. The operation of choice is total thyroidectomy, as in the familial cases, the disease is bilateral in 100% of cases. Occasionally, in the sporadic form of the disease, unilateral lesions exist.[45] Unfortunately, about 40–50% of all patients present with nodal metastases.[67–70] This number can be expected to decrease in familial cases with screening, which can be expected to make diagnoses of C cell hyperplasia early in the disease.

TABLE 28-7. Recommended Surgical Approach to Papillary and Follicular Thyroid Cancer

AGE	SIZE	RECOMMENDED SURGERY	
<45	<1 cm	Lobectomy	TT/NTT if nodules in contralateral lobe
<45	1–4 cm	Lobectomy*	TT/NTT
<45	>4 cm	NTT/TT†	I^{131} ablation
>45	1–4 cm	NTT/TT†	I^{131} ablation
<45	+nodes	NTT/TT+MND	I^{131} ablation
>45	>4 cm	NTT/TT	I^{131} ablation
>45	+nodes	NTT/TT+MND	I^{131} ablation

All go on thyroid hormone postoperatively
MND = Modified neck dissection
TT = Total thyroidectomy
NTT = Near total thyroidectomy
* If frozen section confirms cancer
† If uptake >0.5% at scan 3 months postoperatively

The value of nodal dissection is unproven. Without positive nodes, it is unnecessary as all patients with disease confined to the thyroid will be cured.[66,71–74]

In an effort to determine clinically inapparent disease in patients following thyroidectomy with elevated basal or stimulated thyrocalcitonin levels, one group has selectively catheterized the neck and sampled for thyrocalcitonin under pentagastrin stimulation.[75] All patients were confirmed biochemically and, at subsequent modified radical neck dissection, to have nodal metastases. No patient was biochemically "cured" by this procedure. Although some patients had their peripheral basal and stimulated thyrocalcitonin (TCT) levels fall to less than detectable ranges, repeat central vein catheterization with stimulation showed persistent biochemical disease in the neck or mediastinum. The value of such aggressive localization attempts may now be questioned. Without proof of impact on long-term survival, and the ability to predict that, the patient with positive lymph nodes adjacent to the thyroid gland at thyroidectomy and elevated TCT following operation will have residual positive nodes on the same side of the neck; this makes localization unwarranted.[75,76]

MANAGEMENT OF METASTATIC DISEASE

Local Nodal Metastases in Papillary and Follicular Carcinoma

Local nodal metastases are more common in papillary than follicular neoplasms, although nodal metastases have been reported in as many as 25% of the later.[63] The subject is confused by the varying reports that show a worse outcome with nodal metastases or no influence on survival.[18,50,77,78]

Recognized nodal involvement should be removed at initial surgery, but without aggressive morbid radical neck dissections.[79,80] Therapeutic radical neck dissection in the presence of involved nodes may or may not diminish recurrence rate, but has not been shown to improve survival.[50,81] Even in locally extensive disease, the recurrent laryngeal nerve should not be sacrificed deliberately.

Locally Advanced or Recurrent Disease

Locally advanced or recurrent disease presents a difficult problem. Where possible, surgical ablation is the treatment of choice, even including radical extirpation of the underlying larynx.[64] Where the tumor is still able to take up I^{131}, further iodine ablation is indicated. In some situations, external irradiation has been employed in conjunction with doxorubicin (adriamycin).[82]

Metastatic Disease

Cytotoxic chemotherapy has not been widely employed in thyroid cancer (see Table 28-8). Gottlieb and Hill have reported response rates of 50% or greater in 11 of 30 patients treated with doxorubicin.[82] The overall response rate in this series was 11/30 (37%) with median survival of responding patients being 11+ months (range 5+–40+), compared to a 4-month median survival in non-responding patients. Also, three of five patients with medullary carcinoma and 4/14 patients with spindle cell and Hurthle cell carcinoma responded. This degree of responsiveness to doxorubicin was not confirmed in a smaller study in which only one of six patients with medullary carcinoma responded.[83] It should be noted that doxorubicin was given in a different schedule in this study (22.5 mg/m^2 every week until toxicity).

The activity of 4'-epiadriamycin, Vindesine, and *cis*-platinum as single agents is not clearly defined since so few patients have been treated. Bleomycin given at 45–90 mg each week has been used by Japanese workers in a series of 21 patients.[84] In 11 evaluable patients "some improvement" was seen. However, it is not clear how this finding translates into objective criteria for response.

A combination chemotherapy study in patients with anaplastic carcinoma was reported by the EORTC Thyroid Cancer Cooperative Group in 1978.[85] These workers used doxorubicin, vincristine, and bleomycin in a schedule designed to synchronize the cell cycle in hopes of increasing bleomycin activity. Nine of the 14 (64%) patients in this study evidenced partial response to chemotherapy. Toxicity was mild with significant leukopenia seen in 5/14 (36%) and mild bleomycin skin toxicity in four patients. This study clearly requires confirmation.

Two ongoing studies of doxorubicin + *cis*-platinum have not been completed and will require further patient accrual before meaningful results may be obtained. The fact that one study mounted by the Southeastern Cancer Study Group, a large multi-institutional group accrued only 11 patients in 2 years, shows the difficulty in recruiting adequate numbers of patients to thyroid cancer chemotherapy studies.

Doxorubicin (60–75 mg/m^2 q 3 wks) would seem the drug of choice, even though a more recent study has not confirmed the high activity that Gottlieb reported for this agent in medullary carcinoma.[88] Other experience is minimal, although actinomycin D, methotrexate, and bleomycin have been employed.[90–92] More recently, Burgess has shown statistical improvement in survival when partial response was compared to progressive disease.[93]

EXTERNAL BEAM IRRADIATION

Most regimens employ anterior fields using 15–20 MV electrons up to a total dose of 4,000 rads to the residual thyroid bed.

In patients with medullary cancer or large residual thyroid masses, anterior and posterior fields covering the neck and mediastinum with high energy photons (20–25 MV), CO-60, or 4–8 MV x-rays have all been suggested. In most of these regimens spinal cord shielding is required. Doses of 3,600–5,000 rads can be employed; meaningful evaluation of

TABLE 28-8. Chemotherapy of Thyroid Carcinoma

DRUGS	SCHEDULE	NO. EVALUABLE PATIENTS	NO. PARTIAL RESPONSES	INSTITUTION	REFERENCE
Doxorubicin (Adriamycin)	45–75 mg/m^2 q 3 wks	30	11	M.D. Anderson	82
Bleomycin	40–90 mg q wk	11	9*	Japan	84
Doxorubicin (Adriamycin)	22.5 mg/m^2 q wk until toxicity	6†	1	Duke	83
Cis-Platinum	15 mg/m^2 q d × 5	3†	0	Duke	83
4'-Epiadriamycin	60–90 mg/m^2 q 3 wks	2	1	NCI (Milano)	86
Vindesine	3 mg/m^2 q wk	1	0	Rush, Chicago	87
Doxorubicin (Adriamycin) + *Cis*-Platinum	60 mg/m^2 q 4 wks 60 mg/m^2	11	—	Southeastern Cancer Study Group (SEG)	—
Doxorubicin (Adriamycin) + *Cis*-Platinum	75 mg/m^2 q 4 wks 75 mg/m^2	—	—	M.D. Anderson	—
Doxorubicin (Adriamycin) + Vincristine + Bleomycin	60 mg/m^2 2 mg q 3 wks 30 mg (Given 4–6 hrs after adriamycin + vincristine)	14 (Anaplastic cancer only)	9	Royal Marsden	85

* Improvement; not necessarily partial response
† Medullary carcinoma

the results of such therapy is not available. In 1975, the combination of XRT and methotrexate was reported to give six partial and two complete responses in eight patients treated.[91]

In contrast to papillary and follicular carcinoma, medullary carcinoma does not concentrate iodine, and thus cannot be treated with radioactive iodine. On rare occasions where residual tumor lies locally in the thyroid bed, I^{131} therapy can be given with some expectation of effect.[94] Once the tumor is outside the local confines of the thyroid bed, however, this approach is ineffective.

RADIOACTIVE IODINE

Technical Considerations of I^{131} Therapy

Several questions remain to be answered concerning the use of I^{131} ablation of residual normal or neoplastic thyroid. Does ablation of normal tissue prevent recurrence? Does I^{131} therapy for persistent disease prolong life or decrease recurrence? How often will residual disease respond to I^{131} therapy? Is this response reflected in prolonged survival? What is the morbidity of such therapy?

Ablation of disease is usually done 6 weeks after surgery, with the patient off T4 for a minimum of 4 weeks and off T3 for a minimum of 2 weeks.

In patients with residual uptake in the neck, presumably due to incomplete thyroidectomy but not due to residual disease, doses from 75–100 mCi are usually employed.

In patients receiving therapeutic dosage for residual disease in the neck, either moderate (up to 200mCi) or rarely high dose therapy (up to 500 mCi) have been employed.[95] The relative efficacy of these two regimens has yet to be delineated. The aim in the latter high-dose treatment protocol is to limit dosage such that the bone marrow receives less than 200 rads. The amount retained is less than 120 mCi at 48 hours (less than 80 mCi, if lung metastases).

RADIATION-INDUCED THYROID CANCER

The subject of thyroid irradiation and carcinogenesis has recently been reviewed.[96] The use of radioactive iodine to treat goiter has made some worry that this would increase the incidence of thyroid carcinoma. In fact, this has been an extremely rare finding, presumably because in therapeutic doses of I^{131} the cells of the thyroid gland receive a mean dose of 5,000–10,000 rads and the incidence of thyroid cancer is low once 2,000 rads have been exceeded.[99] In children, the risk for the development of thyroid adenomas may be greater when the I^{131} dose is insufficient to ablate the thyroid.[100,101]

RESULTS

In 1979, about 9,000 cases of thyroid cancer and 1,000 deaths from thyroid cancer occurred in the U.S. The survival statistics of 1955–1964 are outlined in Table 28-9. The risk factors that influence such survival are outlined in Table 28-10. For individual patients, sex (male worse than female) can be added, as it is thought to be a major prognostic indicator.[102] Recently, the European Cooperative Group have established a prognostic index that correlates with survival (see Table 28-11).[103]

TABLE 28-9. Survival of Patients with Thyroid Cancer (1955–1964)

	5-YEAR	10-YEAR
Overall survival	76% (82%)	70% (83%)
Localized disease	89% (95%)	83% (95%)
Regional disease	77% (83%)	70% (80%)

( ) = Relative rate
(From Cutler SJ [ed]: Cancer Report #4. Washington, U.S. Government Printing Office, 1972)

TABLE 28-10. Thyroid Cancer Risk Factors for Survival

I Minimal Risk <5% excess 10-year mortality
<45, Papillary-Follicular, up to 4 cm single nodule, or microscopic multifocal only, or microscopic nodal positivity
II Low Risk—5–20% excess 10-year mortality
<45, Papillar-Follicular, >4 cm or gross multifocal, or capsule invasion or macroscopic positive nodes
<45, Papillary-Follicular, <4 cm or multifocal or capsule invasion (micro).
III Moderate Risk—20–60% excess 10-year mortality
>45, Papillary, >4 cm single nodule or extraglandular gross invasion
>45, Follicular single nodule or multifocal, or capsule invasion, or extraglandular
IV High Risk—60–100% excess 10-year mortality
Papillary-Follicular metastases outside the neck

(From National Thyroid Cancer Treatment Cooperative Group)

TABLE 28-11. Survival According to EORTC Prognostic Index

SCORE*	OBSERVED 5-YEAR SURVIVAL (%)
<50	95
50–65	80
66–83	51
84–108	33
>109	5

Prognostic index score obtained by:
Age at diagnosis + 12 for male
+ 10 for medullary, follicular undifferentiated
+ 45 for anaplastic
+ 10 for extrathyroid extension
+ 15 for one distant metastasis
+ 15 for multiple distant metastasis
____ = Total Score

Byar DP, Green SB, Dor P et al: A prognostic index for thyroid carcinoma. A study of the EORTC thyroid cancer cooperative group. Eur J Cancer 15:1033–1041, 1979

INFLUENCE OF THERAPY ON RESULTS

The influence of therapy on outcome is difficult to demonstrate, as rarely are the same stages disease treated by two different methods. Because of the necessity for 10- and 15-year follow-up, randomized series are virtually nonexistent.

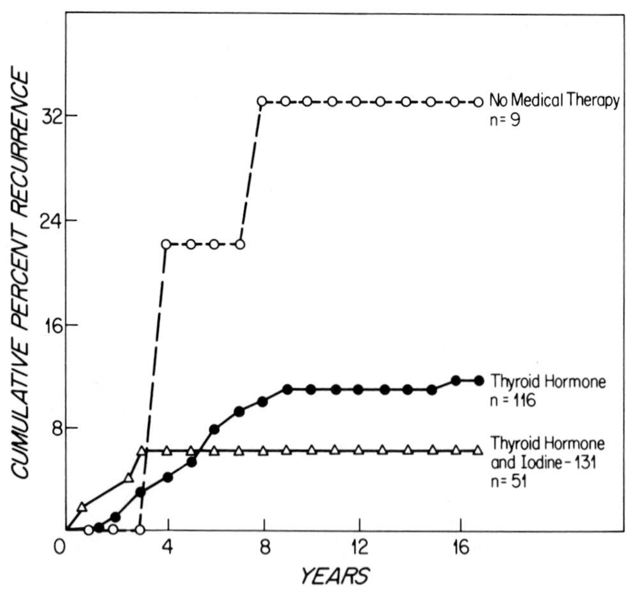

FIG. 28-8. Papillary carcinoma. Cumulative recurrence rate according to type of postoperative therapy. (Mazzaferri EL, Young RL, Oertel JE et al: Medicine 56:183, 1977)

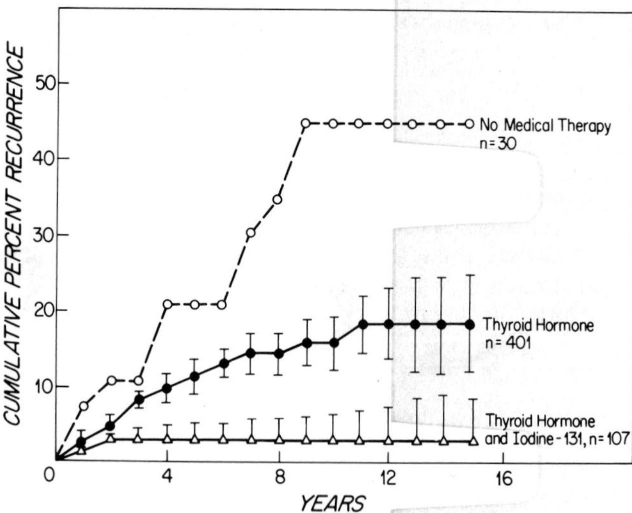

FIG. 28-9. Follicular carcinoma. Cumulative recurrence rate according to type of postoperative therapy. (Young RL, Mazzaferri EL, Rahe AJ et al: J Nucl Med 21:735, 1980)

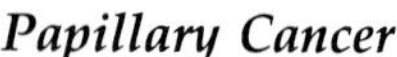

Papillary Cancer

In 106 cases reviewed by Staunton, only one of nine survived 5 years when treated with radiotherapy only.[104] As 83% of these patients had extrathyroidal spread and were an average age of 60 years, this was not surprising.[104]

In patients treated with surgery alone, lobectomy alone fared worst (18%, or 2/11, alive at 20 years). In comparison, subtotal thyroidectomy had a 60% (9/15) 20-year survival; total thyroidectomy had only 67% (8/12) alive at 5 years. Operative deaths were high in total thyroidectomy, and extra-thyroidal spread was highest (40%) in the total thyroidectomy, compared to 28% of the subtotal thyroidectomy group.[104]

Recurrence rates for both papillary and follicular carcinoma are lowest when patients are given both radioactive iodine and thyroid hormone (see Figs. 28-8 and 28-9).

COMPLICATIONS OF TREATMENT

Morbidity and mortality after thyroidectomy have recently been reviewed.[50,105] A retrospective review of 24,108 thyroid operations performed in 1970 (from the records of the Commission on Professional and Hospital Activities) was thought to have included about one-third of the thyroid operations performed in the U.S. Of these patients 89% had partial or subtotal thyroidectomy, 10% had total thyroidectomy, and

TABLE 28-12. Follow-Up of Patients after Thyroidectomy

STAGE I	Every 3 months for 1 year Every 6 months for 2 years Then yearly
STAGE II	No known residual disease: same as stage I Residual disease being ablated by I^{131} every 3 months until ablation completed, then as for stage I
STAGE III	If undergoing external beam irradiation: weekly during therapy, then every 3 months for 2 years, then as for stage I
STAGE IV	Monthly for 1 year, if no progression, then every 3 months

TABLE 28-13. Follow-Up for Patients Following Thyroidectomy for Thyroid Cancer

EACH VISIT
CBC
T4, T3, rT3, TSH
Chest film
Thyroglobulin, CEA, thyrocalcitonin where appropriate
YEARLY FOR 5 YEARS, EVERY 2 YEARS THEREAFTER
DIAGNOSTIC
Discontinue T4 for 4 weeks T3 for 2 weeks
Day 1–3: 10 U TSH q.d.
Day 4: 5 mCi I^{131} orally
Day 6: Whole body scan
THERAPEUTIC
As above, if functioning metastases detected
Day 4: 100–200 mCi I^{131} orally
Day 7–9: Whole body scan
Repeat 6 months until no function
Maintain on thyroid replacement

0.6% had less substantial thyroid operations. Operative mortality was highest in operations for malignancy in patients over 50 years of age (2.8%), and lowest for patients under 50 having an operation for nonmalignant nontoxic lesions (0.02%).

In patients having total (637 patients) or subtotal (7126 patients) thyroidectomy for cancer, the incidence of hypoparathyroidism was 8% and 1.5%, respectively. Vocal cord paralysis occurred in 1% of total thyroidectomies and 0.5% of subtotal procedures for cancer.[105]

In a group of 571 patients undergoing surgery for papillary carcinoma, there were no operative deaths, permanent hypoparathyroidism occurred in 7.8%, and vocal cord paralysis in 1.2%. Hypoparathyroidism was greatest in the 21 patients who had total thyroidectomy and radical neck dissection (20%). Temporary cord damage and transient hypoparathyroidism occurred in 0.8% and 1.9% of all patients.[50]

COMPLICATIONS OF ABLATIVE I^{131} THERAPY

The temporary effects are nausea, vomiting, occasional parotitis, and diminished white blood cell and platelet counts (nadir is at 3–6 weeks).

Permanent side effects (which are rare) include aplastic anemia, pulmonary fibrosis, amenorrhea, leukemia, and prolonged white blood cell and platelet suppression.

FOLLOW-UP

For follow-up, see Table 28-12, based on the staging of Table 28-4. The actual tests to be performed are outlined in Table 28-13. In patients with known residual disease, tests will be dependent on disease progression and site (see section on I^{131} therapy).

The Adrenal Gland

The adrenal glands consists of the adrenal cortex and medulla, and were probably first described by Bartolomeu Eustacchio in 1563. He termed them the "glandulae Renibus Incumbentes." Eustacchio's "Tabulae Anatomicae" was not published until many years after his death, but was finally published in 1714 by the Italian Lancisi.[106] In 1716, the Science Academy of Bordeaux offered a prize for an answer to the question concerning the function and meaning of the suprarenal glands. The judge was unable to award the prize to any of the conflicting and confusing suggestions!

In 1855, Thomas Addison described 11 fatal cases that he and his colleagues at Guy's Hospital had examined.[107] Addison directed the comments to the generalized debility, anemia, and "peculiar change of color in the skin occurring in connection with a disease condition of the suprarenal capsules." Early attempts to link the quite considerable blood supply of the adrenal with some function in detoxification, the ability to respond to some external stimuli, and the rapid death from adrenalectomy in animals led to the adrenals being considered a detoxicating organ. Perhaps the first to support Addison was Wilks in 1862.[108] Confusion was added by the choice of experimental animals, with the rat surviving adrenalectomy whereas other animal species did not. The failure of the rat to invariably die after adrenalectomy has been interpreted as evidence for the presence of accessory adrenal tissue, some of which can be demonstrated.

Early attempts to decide whether the adrenal cortex or medulla was the essential component to life led to confusing results. The destruction of inter-renal "cortical tissue" in fish suggested that the inter-renal organs were responsible for preventing adrenal insufficiency. A unilateral adrenalectomy, followed by destruction of the contralateral medullary tissue, suggested similar results. Finally, in the late 1920's, it was concluded that the adrenal cortex or its resultant function was essential for life, whereas the adrenal medulla was not.

ANATOMIC CONSIDERATIONS OF THE ADRENAL GLANDS

The adrenal glands are well-hidden posteriorly in the retroperitoneum, associated with the upper and anteromedial surface of the corresponding kidney (see Fig. 28-10). Each adrenal has an individual distinct compartment of the renal fascia. The right gland is more pyramidal with a concave base overlying the kidney surface. The left gland is more flattened and intimately related to the left kidney. These special relationships are relatively irrelevant in the presence of a tumor, which will clearly distort the gland. Both the adrenal glands are attached to their own compartment of the renal fascia. Any ptosis of the kidney is not accompanied by adrenal gland migration, and congenital malposition of the kidney is not associated with corresponding malposition of the adrenal gland. The right gland rests against the diaphragm on the anteromedial aspect of the upper end of the right kidney. The right side is crossed by the reflection of the posterior layer of the coronary ligament from the liver to the diaphragm. Because of this, the upper part of the gland will have no peritoneum covering the surface. The medial portion of the lower half of this gland is usually covered or overlapped by the duodenum. On the left side, the gland is only partially covered by peritoneum, the remainder being overlapped by the pancreas and the splenic vessels. On the left, the gland rests medially on the left crus of the diaphragm.

Typically, the adrenal gland has arterial supply from at least three sources. The usual predominant blood supply is derived from multiple branches of the inferior phrenic artery. Like other adrenal arterial vessels, these vessels divide before entering the adrenal, such that the actual number of arterial vessels entering the adrenal gland may be large. They do not enter the hilum where the single adrenal vein exists, and multiple small branches from the aorta and the renal arteries enter throughout the middle and lower portions of the gland. On rare occasions, the adrenal may receive blood supply from other than the three main sources, (*e.g.*, the ureteric artery).

Venous drainage is handled mainly by way of a large central vein that leaves the anterior surface of the gland at the hilum.

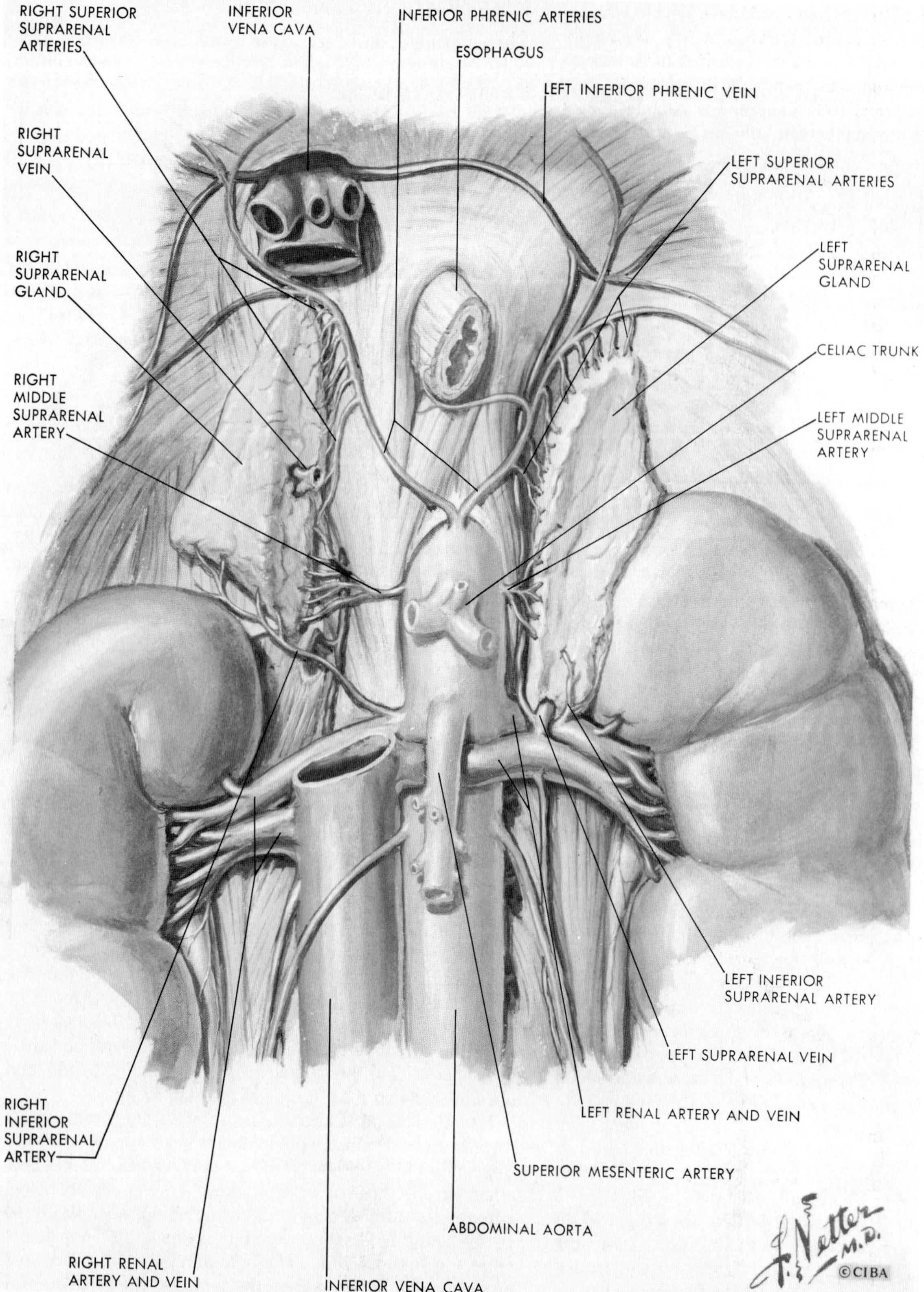

FIG. 28-10. Anatomy of the adrenal glands. Netter FH: The Endocrine System, Section III, Plate 3, p 79 of the Ciba Collection of Medical Illustrations, vol 4.

The tiny capsular veins that accompany arteries are inconsequential as a source of venous drainage. The left adrenal vein passes downward, over the lower part of the anterior surface of the gland to enter the left renal vein. It is often joined before entering the renal vein by the left inferior phrenic vein. On the right side, the adrenal vein drains directly into the inferior cava, almost always separate from the right inferior phrenic vein.

Inclusion of the adrenal gland beneath the capsule of the kidney had been reported, but is extremely rare. Ectopic medullary tissue is difficult to define as it is extremely common, developing in association with the chromaffin cells of the sympathetic nervous system. The largest extra-adrenal mass of chromaffin tissue is characteristically seen in the fetus and the newborn infant; this disappears by adult life. This, the organ of Zuckerkandl, is usually in front of the aorta at the level of the origin of the inferior mesenteric artery. It is in organs such as this and other accessory chromaffin tissue that ectopic pheochromocytoma can occur.

The adrenal cortex and medulla, although in intimate contact, are essentially different organs and will be described as such.

THE ADRENAL CORTEX

HISTORY

Hartman was probably the first to suggest that the function of the adrenal was to produce a general tissue hormone, rather than perform a detoxifying function.[108] In 1927, he was able to demonstrate that extracts from the adrenal extended life in adrenalectomized animals.[109] By 1930, it was demonstrated that lipid extracted adrenal preparations could maintain adrenalectomized cats indefinitely.[110,111] The first clinical trial of the Swingle–Pfiffner extracts was made by Drs. Rountree and Greene at the Mayo Clinic in 1930.[112–114] Earlier experiments at producing syndromes due to excess of adrenal cortical extract had failed. Such attempts were classical examples of the ability of exogenous adrenal cortical extract to inhibit endogenous production. Gradually, it was realized that numerous steroids could be crystallized from extracts of the adrenal. Finally, cortisone and aldosterone were synthesized as a consequence of much work by many people.[115,116]

In 1946, Selye summarized much of the work involving syndromes of response to nonspecific stress.[117] The early attempts, by Hench at the Mayo Clinic, to find the reason for improvement of rheumatoid arthritis during pregnancy led to the thought that it might indeed be due to some anti-rheumatic "substance X" that could be an adrenal hormone. Accordingly, this was first tried with dramatic results using either 17-hydroxy-11-dehydroxycorticosterone (compound E) or ACTH.[116] This discovery led to Nobel Prize Awards for Drs. Kendall, Hench, and Reichstein.

CUSHING'S DISEASE AND SYNDROME

Osler was probably the first (in 1899) to describe a patient with Cushing's syndrome, but the diagnosis or etiology was not determined.[118] Cushing, in describing what became known as Cushing's disease, almost certainly included patients with adrenocortical tumors.[119]

Others had preceded him in the description of pituitary causes of the syndrome (notably Raab in 1924 and Teel in 1931).[120,121] Cushing's syndrome, caused by a confirmed adrenal tumor, was described in 1913 by Turney and in 1926 by Parkes-Weber.[122,123]

EPIDEMIOLOGY AND GENETICS OF ADRENOCORTICAL CARCINOMA

The true incidence and prevalence of adrenocortical carcinoma is difficult to determine. In the Seer 10-state survey, 66 patients with adrenocortical carcinoma were seen in the 5-year period from 1973–1977. This survey, which covers approximately 10% of the U.S. population, would mean that approximately 132 new cases of adrenocortical carcinoma occur in the U.S. each year. The means of confirming malignancy in this group was by histology alone in 20/66 (30%), and by proven invasion or metastases in 39/66 (59%). Seven out of 66 (11%) were unstaged. Given that by histologic examination alone the primary tumor may be incorrectly called malignant (and excluding the unstaged cases) this prevalence may fall to 78 new cases per year.

No data exist for the prevalence of benign tumors of the adrenal cortex. It is commonly accepted that approximately 20–25% of patients with Cushing's syndrome have adrenal tumors, with benign adenomas being slightly more common than carcinomas in the adult. Therefore, the prevalence of adrenal tumors, benign and malignant, as a cause of adrenocortical excess must be 150–300 per year.

Adrenal adenomas are found in 2% of all adult autopsies, in up to 30% of elderly obese diabetics, and in up to 20% of hypertensives.[124] The incidence in patients with known familial multiple endocrine syndromes is at least 33% at autopsy.[124] These latter figures exclude the aldosterone-producing adrenal cortical neoplasms. Malignant aldosterone-producing tumors are exceedingly rare, with only questionable case reports in the world literature.

PATHOLOGY OF THE ADRENAL CORTEX

Adrenocortical hyperplasia can be diffuse or nodular, and is usually bilateral. The hyperplasia usually involves the zona fasciculata and reticularis when adrenal virilism exists. Pure zona reticularis hyperplasia is very unusual. Zona glomerulosa hyperplasia is seen in secondary aldosteronism, but is only rarely a cause of primary aldosteronism. Unilateral nodular hyperplasia can occur as a cause of primary aldosteronism.

Adrenocortical tumors are usually large, single, rounded masses of yellow-orange adrenocortical tissue that may show hemorrhage, cystic degeneration, and calcification. Histologically, the adenomas are composed of relatively regular large cells with uniformly abundant lipid, arranged in nodules and cords with a fasciculate pattern. Giant cells do occur in benign adenomas with prominent nuclei and polymorphism but are not of themselves primary indications of carcinomatous change.[124]

Adrenocortical carcinomas are predominantly functional. Carcinomas are usually large when diagnosed and have considerable hemorrhage, necrosis, and calcification. The atypia, large nucleoli, multinucleated cells, mitosis, and compact cytophilic cells are typical. Malignancy is usually diagnosed on the basis of vascular invasion; however, without metastases the diagnosis is always in doubt. About 50% of adrenal carcinomas are associated with Cushing's syndrome, 20% with virilization, 4% with both, 12% with feminization, and 4% with aldosteronism and other conditions.[124]

NATURAL HISTORY OF ADRENAL CORTICAL TUMORS

Tumors of the adrenal cortex may be functional or non-functional. Non-functional tumors tend to present late by pure mass effect.

The functional tumors present depending on the predominant hormone produced by the tumor. The main hormones synthesized by the adrenal cortex are cortisone, corticosterone, aldosterone, and 11-hydroxyandrostenedione. All of these hormones are derivatives of cholesterol and their physiologic features are well-known. In functional tumors, usually either the glucocorticoid, mineralocorticoid, or sex steroids predominate. These result in the classic syndromes of hyperaldosteronism (Conn's syndrome), adrenocortical excess (Cushing's syndrome), or various forms of precocious puberty or virilization.

PATHOGENESIS

Pathogenesis of the clinical syndrome is highly dependent on the hormone or hormones elaborated. Approximately 10% of adrenal carcinomas are nonfunctional and will be suspected from the effects of local growth and invasion, or unexplained fever. Glucocorticoid excess is the most common presentation and will result in the features of Cushing's syndrome. These signs and symptoms are due to increased gluconeogenesis and glucose intolerance. Amino acid uptake and protein synthesis are both inhibited and protein breakdown is accelerated. This results in the clinical picture of bruising, impaired wound healing, osteoporosis, muscle wasting, and striae. In addition, the immunologic response to an immunologic challenge is altered and a decrease in the inflammatory response occurs. The characteristic redistribution of adipose tissue results from the glucocorticoid excess.

Where only mild virilization and feminization signs are evident, these may be due solely to the corticosteroids that do have some androgenic and estrogenic properties.

CLINICAL PRESENTATION

EXCESS CORTICOSTEROIDS

The characteristic appearance of truncal obesity, redistribution of truncal fat with buffalo hump, rounded facies, striae, and mild hypertension are well-known. In addition, mild glucose intolerance can be demonstrated with alterations in immune function, plethora, thinning of the skin, and osteoporosis. About 10% of patients with adrenal cortical excess develop renal calculi. Not uncommonly, depression and psychotic behavior occur.

TABLE 28-14. Clinical Manifestations of Androgen-Estrogen Excess

VIRILIZATION
- In women:
  - Male pattern baldness
  - Hirsutism
  - Deepening voice
  - Breast atrophy
  - Clitoral hypertrophy
  - Decreased libido
  - Oligomenorrhea
- In prepubertal boys:
  - Precocious puberty

FEMINIZATION
- In men:
  - Gynecomastia
  - Breast tenderness
  - Testicular atrophy
  - Decreased libido
- In prepubertal girls:
  - Precocious puberty

ALDOSTERONE EXCESS

This syndrome, first described by Conn, is manifested by sodium retention, increased total plasma volume, increased renal artery pressure and inhibition of renin secretion.[125–127] Primary and secondary forms occur, and both forms need to be excluded when investigating patients with essential hypertension (Fig. 28-20).[128,129]

EXCESS SEX HORMONES

Normal male and female maturation is under the control of the gonads. When inappropriate or excessive masculinization (virilization) or feminization occurs, an adrenal neoplasm must be suspected. Even though virilization dominates, the possibility of underlying Cushing's syndrome (due to adren-

TABLE 28-15. Tests Employed to Confirm Adrenocortical Functional Excess

TEST	DETERMINATION	ADRENOCORTICAL EXCESS EXPECTED
PM cortisol	Serum cortisol	>15 μg/dl
1 mg dexamethasone at 11 PM	AM serum cortisol	>10 mg/dl
Low dose dexamethasone (0.5 mg q6 for 48 hrs)	Urine 17-OHCS	Failure to suppress to <3 μg/24 hours
	Urine cortisol	Failure to suppress to <25 μg/24 hours
Urine-free cortisol	Urine cortisol	>100 μg/24 hours

TABLE 28-16. Tests to Determine the Etiology of Cushing's Syndrome

TEST	DETERMINATION	NORMAL	PROBABLE SOURCE OF GLUCOCORTICOID EXCESS: PITUITARY	ECTOPIC	ADRENAL
ACTH	Plasma ACTH	Normal	↑	↑ ↑	↓
High-dose Dexamethasone (2 mg q6 for 48 hrs)	Urine cortisol	↓ ↓	↓	↑ ↓	↑ ↓
	Urine 17-OHCS	↓ ↓	↓	↑ ↓	↑ ↓
Metyrapone (750 mg q4 for 48 hrs)	Urine 17-OHCS	↑ ↑	↑	↑ ↓	↑ ↓
Peptide by-products	Plasma $\frac{\text{LPH}}{\text{ACTH}}$	—	↓	↑	—

ACTH = Adrenocorticotropin
LPH = Lipotropin

ocortical excess) should be considered, as therapy will differ.[130] Adrenal hyperplasia may best be treated by cortisol, and pituitary dependent hyperplasia approached directly (see Table 28-14).

METHODS OF DIAGNOSIS AND STAGING OF FUNCTIONAL TUMORS

INVESTIGATION OF THE PATIENT WITH CORTICOSTEROID EXCESS

Adrenocortical excess is readily confirmed using the simple outline in Fig. 28-11 (also see Table 28-15). More elaborate tests are not required unless the present tests are equivocal and suspicion remains high.[131] The value of tests used in screening of patients for Cushing's syndrome has recently been reviewed.[132] Once the diagnosis of Cushing's syndrome has been made, then a clear attempt at elucidation of the etiology must be determined before any meaningful therapeutic approach can begin (see Table 28-16).

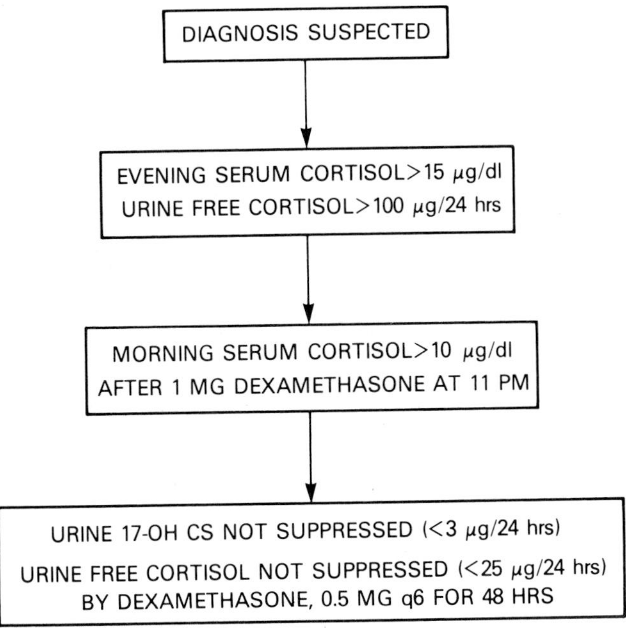

FIG. 28-11. Flow sheet for confirmation of a suspected diagnosis of Cushing's syndrome.

TABLE 28-17. Available Tests for Preoperative Localization of Adrenal Tumors

Dependent on hormone production:	Selective venous sampling
	Radionuclide scanning
Independent of hormone production:	Computed tomography
	Ultrasound
	Selective arteriography
	Retrograde venography

Once the origin of the corticosteroid excess can be confirmed to be arising *de novo* from the adrenal, then attempts to localize the site of excess production can be made (see Table 28-17 and Fig. 28-12).[133]

Computed Tomography (CT)

Rapid advances are being made in the development of CT scanners. The examination of the retroperitoneal adrenal glands has been particularly rewarding. In the use of this noninvasive study, normal adrenal glands can be expected to be identified in virtually all patients.[134] The left adrenal gland is identified as an inverted "V," lying anterior and medial to the upper aspect of the left kidney and lateral to the aorta (see Fig. 28-13). The right adrenal gland is behind the vena cava and medial to the liver. The inverted "V" shape is altered such that one arm is foreshortened to give an appearance similar to the number seven (see Fig. 28-14). Hyperplasia can readily be recognized as bilateral enlargement, which is symmetrical but maintains approximately normal configuration (see Fig. 28-15).[135,136] Tumors are recognized as localized masses in the region of the adrenal gland; malignancy is suspected on the CT scan by either an enlarged tumor or demonstrable venous invasion (see Figs. 28-15 and 28-16).[133,137]

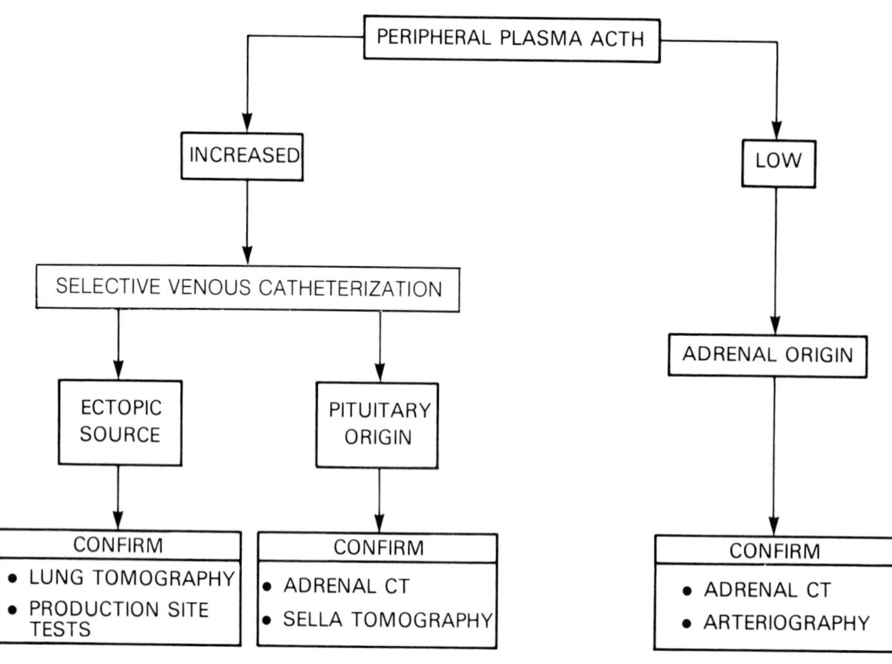

FIG. 28-12. Flow sheet to elucidate the etiology of confirmed Cushing's disease. Confirmatory tests needed for localization.

Ultrasonography

The adrenal gland is envisioned using a gray scale ultrasound unit with digital scan conversion and an internally focused 2.25 or 3.5 mhz transducer. A normal adrenal gland has been identified with ultrasound, but this is much better seen by CT.[138] Reliable identification of adrenal tumors with ultrasound has been limited to lesions 3 cm in diameter or larger.[139,140]

FIG. 28-13. CT of normal left adrenal gland. (Brennan MF, Dunnick NR: Localization of functional adrenal tumors. In Najarian JS, Delaney JP (eds): Breast and Endocrine Surgery. Chicago, Year Book Medical Publishers, 1981)

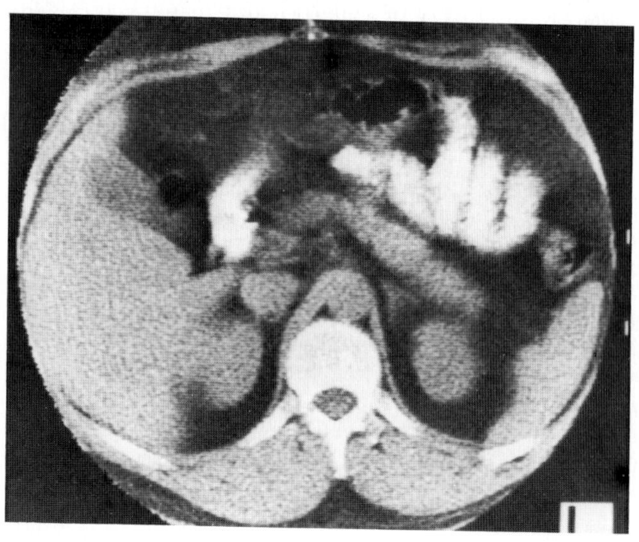

Arteriography

It is important to emphasize that selective injections of at least a renal and an inferor phrenic artery are necessary to accurately identify an adrenal tumor. The normal arterial supply from the aorta by way of the middle adrenal artery should also be looked for. When carcinoma is even suspected, more extensive arteriographic examination is warranted to identify additional abnormal arterial supply, the presence of

FIG. 28-14. CT of normal right adrenal gland. (Brennan MF, Dunnick NR: Localization of functional adrenal tumors. In Najarian JS, Delaney JP (eds): Breast and Endocrine Surgery Chicago, Year Book Medical Publishers, 1981)

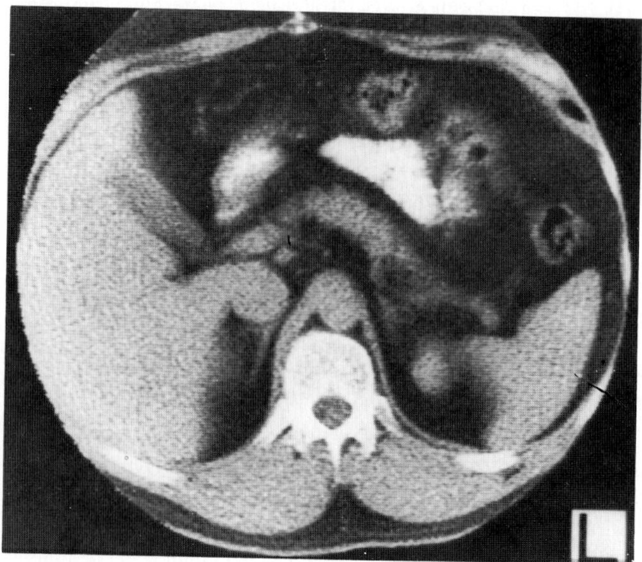

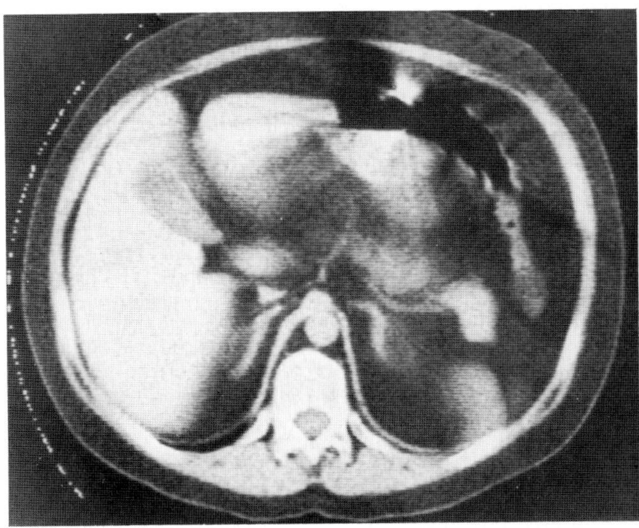

FIG. 28-15. CT of bilateral adrenal hyperplasia. (Brennan MF, Dunnick NR: Localization of functional adrenal tumors. In Najarian JS, Delaney JP (eds): Breast and Endocrine Surgery. 1980. Reprinted from Breast and Endocrine Surgery, Symposia Specialists, Inc., Box 610397, Miami, Florida 33162)

vascular invasion, and the identification of hepatic metastases.[141]

Adrenal Venography

Adrenal venography is less commonly used and is usually only employed at selective venous sampling to insure appropriate positioning of the sampling catheter.

Adrenal Venous Sampling

Adrenal venous sampling requires two catheters, one through each femoral vein to allow bilateral simultaneous sampling. Peripheral samples are obtained from either the arm or the inferior vena cava below the level of the renal veins. After the initial samples are collected, IV infusion of 25 units of ACTH is given; the sampling is repeated 15 minutes later. An example of a selective venous sampling in a patient with a pituitary source of excess ACTH is shown before and after ACTH in Fig. 28-17. When patients with primary aldosteronisms are being studied, simultaneous cortisol concentrations are measured to determine the degree of dilution of the adrenal venous input, thereby correcting for malposition of the catheter.[133,142]

FIG. 28-16. Suspected left adrenal carcinoma. Note enormous size. (Brennan MF, Dunnick NR: Localization of functional adrenal tumors. In Najarian JS, Delaney JP (eds): Breast and Endocrine Surgery. 1980. Reprinted from Breast and Endocrine Surgery, Symposia Specialists, Inc., Box 610397, Miami, Florida 33162)

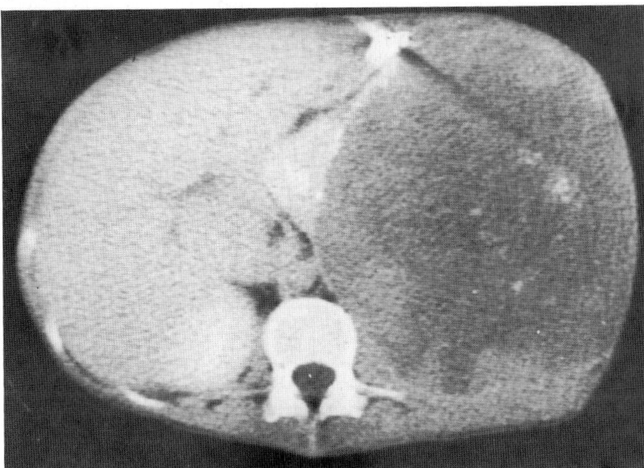

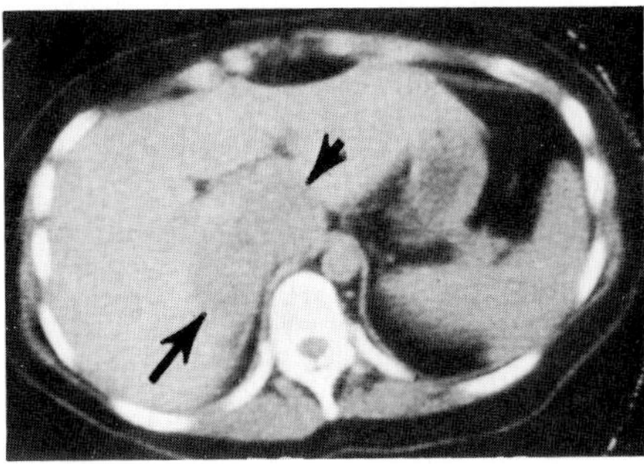

FIG. 28-17. Right adrenal carcinoma (*large arrow*) showing inferior vena cava invasion (*small arrow*). (Javadpoor N, Woltering E, Brennan MF: Adrenal neoplasm. Curr Probl Surg 17:1, 1–52, 1980. Copyright © 1980 by Year Book Medical Publishers, Inc., Chicago)

Radionuclide Scanning

Functional adrenal tumors can be identified by using radionuclide scans.[143] The most commonly employed agent was I^{131}-19-iodocholesterol; 2 μCi in 1.5 cc of volume containing approximately 1 mg of cholesterol are injected IV. To decrease thyroid accumulation of the I^{131}, Lugol's solution is given prior to the injection and continued (three drops twice a day) for 2 weeks. Two or three scans are obtained using a photogamma camera between 4 and 14 days following injection. The percentage uptake of the I^{131}-iodocholesterol in each gland is determined using a minicomputer interfaced with a gamma camera. On occasions, suppression scintograms are obtained while the patient is taking either 0.5 or 1 mg dexamathasone orally every six hours beginning at least 24 hours prior to the radionuclide injection. The radiation dose to the adrenals and the gonads is equivalent to that received during a conventional IVP.[144] Recently, I^{131}-iodocholesterol has been replaced by 6-Iodomethyl-19-Norcholesterol (NP–59).[145,146] The agent is used following one or two days of Lugol's iodine with a 1–2 μCi dose injected. The patients are imaged for 20 minutes (or 50,000 counts). Suppression scans are used as before, but usually while taking a 2 mg q 6 dose of dexamethasone beginning 2 days pre-injection and continuing until imaging is complete. To enhance interpretation, the kidneys can be imaged by a small dose of Technetium Tc 99 m.

RESULTS OF LOCALIZATION STUDIES

The most accurate test for functional tumors is selective venous sampling for hormone production. This can be expected to provide accurate identification in nearly 100% of

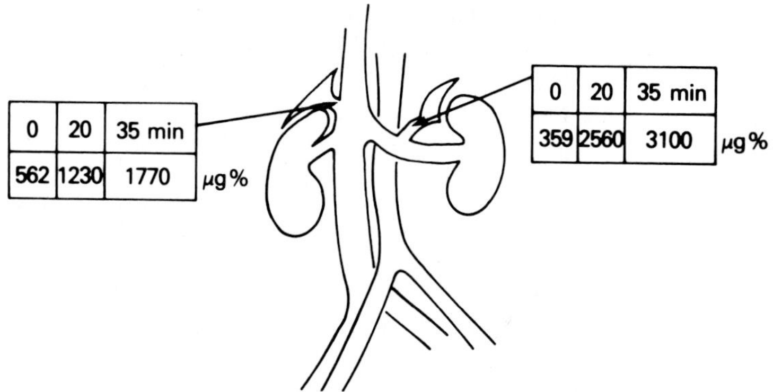

FIG. 28-18. Results of selective venous sampling for cortisol concentration in a female patient with a pituitary adenoma. Note the equivalent bilateral elevated cortisols before and after stimulation with 25 units IV of ACTH.

patients subsequently confirmed as having aldosteronomas.[133,142] In patients randomly selected, localization of even small lesions will be provided in 75% of cases.[143] The rapid development of the CT scanner and the accuracy of identification and of the adrenals make this the non-invasive study of choice.[133,135] Given these results, a CT scan is the initial localization study in suspected adrenal tumors (see Figs. 28-18 and 28-19).

ADRENOCORTICAL CARCINOMA

When an adrenal mass is identified, the factors that raise the suspicion that the lesion is a carcinoma and not an adenoma, are outlined (see Table 28-18). Because benign functional tumors commonly present early because of the associated endocrinopathy, the presence of an adrenal abdominal mass is highly suspicious for adrenocortical carcinoma.

The conventional adrenocortical carcinoma staging system is presented in Table 28-19.

ADRENAL MEDULLA

The adrenal medulla, although in intimate association with the adrenal cortex, has a markedly different embryology and physiology. The adrenal medullary cells arise from the neuroectoderm and fulfill the criteria for an amine presursor uptake and decarboxylation (APUD) cell.

Tumors arising in the adrenal medulla may be either pheochromocytoma (Greek phaios = dusky, chroma = color, the functionally active tumors or neuroblastoma), or ganglioneuroma or sympathogonoma, the functionally inactive tumors. Neuroblastoma is the commonest extracranial solid neoplasm in children and is discussed in Chapter 34. Pheochromocytoma can occur sporadically or as part of a multiple endocrine neoplasia syndrome.

EPIDEMIOLOGY AND GENETICS

The prevalence of tumors in the adrenal medulla are not known. The Seer program has data on the prevalence of

FIG. 28-19. Flow sheet for localization of functional adrenal tumors.

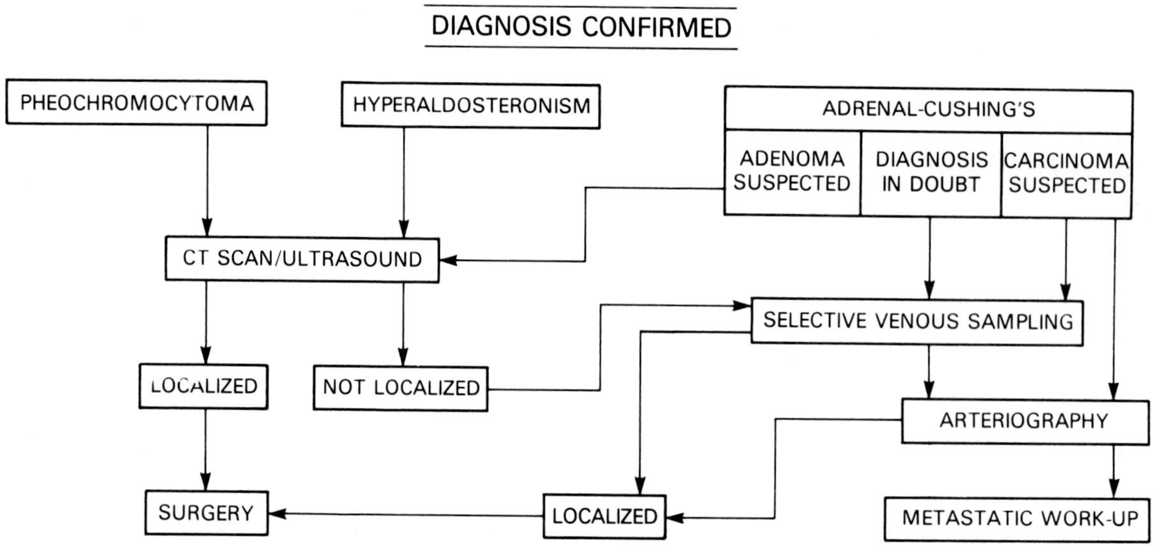

DIAGNOSIS CONFIRMED

PHEOCHROMOCYTOMA

HYPERALDOSTERONISM

ADRENAL-CUSHING'S

ADENOMA SUSPECTED

DIAGNOSIS IN DOUBT

CARCINOMA SUSPECTED

CT SCAN/ULTRASOUND

SELECTIVE VENOUS SAMPLING

LOCALIZED

NOT LOCALIZED

ARTERIOGRAPHY

SURGERY

LOCALIZED

METASTATIC WORK-UP

TABLE 28-18. Factors Raising the Suspicion that an Adrenal Tumor is an Adrenocortical Carcinoma

A. ADRENAL CUSHING'S SYNDROME
1. Palpable mass
2. No suppression with high-dose dexamethasone
3. Patient under 20-years-old
4. Increased urinary 17-ketosteroids

B. VIRILIZATION OR FEMINIZATION SYNDROMES

C. ADULT WITH PALPABLE ABDOMINAL MASS AND
1. CT positive for adrenal tumor
2. Increased urinary 17-keto or 17-OH-corticosteroids
3. Weight loss or fever

TABLE 28-19. Adrenocortical Carcinoma—Staging

Stage 1:	Tumor <5 cm, negative nodes, no local invasion, no metastases
Stage 2:	Tumor >5 cm, negative nodes no local invasion, no metastases
Stage 3:	Positive nodes or local invasion
Stage 4:	Positive nodes and local invasion or distant metastases

malignant pheochromocytoma from their 10-state survey. This suggests that approximately 40 new malignant pheochromocytomas would occur in the U.S. each year. Since a malignant diagnosis was made based on positive histology from a metastasis in 88% of the cases surveyed, this is probably a realistic figure. As in most series the incidence of malignancy is about 10%; 400 new cases of pheochromocytoma probably occur each year in the U.S. (see Table 28-20).[137,147-149]

The adrenal medullary cells have both APUD characteristics and good evidence that they are of neural crest origin.

As best as can be determined, about 1% of severe hypertension can be attributed to pheochromocytoma.[147-153]

PATHOLOGY OF ADRENAL MEDULLARY TUMORS

Histologically, pheochromocytomas show notable variability of cell size, nuclear size, and arrangement. A twisted cell cord pattern, basophilic or cytophilic staining with fine intracytoplasmic pigment granules, and PAS-stained secretory droplets aid in the diagnosis.

By ultrastructure, epinephrine-containing cytoplasmic granules are larger than those seen in the normal medulla. The catecholamines are stored and secreted from osmiophilic cytoplasmic granules. The development of large metastases from a tumor that appeared benign histologically is not infrequent.

Associated syndromes with pheochromocytoma include Von Rechlinghausen's neurofibromatosis, Lindau–von Hippel disease, cerebellar hemangioblastoma, Albright's syndrome, multiple mucocutaneous neuromas, and familiar multiple endocrine neoplasia (MEN) syndromes. In familiar syndromes, the bilateriality of the pheochromocytoma should be assumed until proven otherwise.

NATURAL HISTORY OF PHEOCHROMOCYTOMA

PATHOGENESIS

The adrenal medulla excretes both norepinephrine and epinephrine. Approximately 80% of adrenal vein catecholamine output is epinephrine. Enzymes responsible for formation of epinephrine from norepinephrine are present in the adrenal medulla. Secretion of catecholamines is initiated by the acetylcholine released from the neurons that embrace the secretory cell. This mechanism, probably mediated by increased permeability of the secretory cell to calcium, results in secretion induction. Most catecholamines act for a very short time within the circulation and reduce after oxidation to 3-methoxy-4-hydroxymandelic acid (VMA).

CLINICAL PRESENTATION

Pheochromocytomas present with sporadic hypertension. The patient usually presents with severe headache, paroxysmal or sustained hypertension, excess perspiration, angina, and cardiac arrhythmias related to the output of catecholamine. Symptoms vary little, whether the disease is benign or malignant. Table 28-21 illustrates the dominant symptoms of 22 patients with malignant pheochromocytomas (16 adrenal and six extra-adrenal) seen at the National Institute of Health. The "classical" presentation of episodic hypertension occurring with an attack but showing natural blood pressure at other times probably occurs in no more than 50% of cases.[147,148,154]

Besides having elevated blood pressure, patients with pheo-

TABLE 28-20. Pheochromocytoma, Incidence of Malignancy and Extra Adrenal Tumors

REFERENCE	147	148	149	137	183
YEARS	1950–1975	1926–1970	1950–1975	1953–1977	1957–1977
NUMBER OF PATIENTS	44	138	26	68	58 (72)*
BILATERAL TUMORS	7%	4%	4%	—	10% (8%)
EXTRA ADRENAL	16%	10%	4%	13%	10% (18%)
MALIGNANT	11%	13%	12%	32%	9% (7%)

*( ) = Includes autopsy cases

TABLE 28-21. Presenting Symptoms in Malignant Pheochromocytoma

Sweating	72%
Episodic attacks	63%
Palpitations	59%
Anxiety	50%
Headache	45%

22 patients

TABLE 28-23. Normal Values of Diagnostic Tests for Pheochromocytoma

Test	Normal value
Urine catecholamines	10–100 μgm/24 hours
Norepinephrine	10–70 μgm/24 hours
Epinephrine	0–20 μgm/24 hours
Urine VMA	1.8–7.0 mg/24 hours
Urine normetanephrine and metanephrine	<1.3 mg/24 hours

chromocytomas often have associated nervousness, perspiration, tachycardia, palpitations, and often severe anxiety. Pain in the abdomen and chest, associated with nausea and vomiting are also reported.[155] The presence of postural hypotension with hypertension should increase the suspicion of a pheochromocytoma. The presumptive mechanism is that related to hypovolemia following chronic catecholamine excess.

DIAGNOSIS

Careful attention to details of history suggesting other familial syndromes or stigmata of other neuroectodermal disease such as neurofibromatosis, cafe-au-lait spots, port-wine hemangiomas, or a thyroid mass should be pursued. An abdominal mass, which will occur in about 15% of patients, should carefully be sought.

Definitive diagnosis depends on documentation of excess levels of plasma or uninary catecholamine or their metabolites (see Table 28-22). Currently, there is debate concerning the value of plasma catecholamine assays. One group suggests that plasma epinephrine and metanephrine levels are more accurate than 24-hour urine collections for VMA or metanephrines.[156] Others have been much more adamant about the determination of metanephrines as the most rewarding urinary collection.[152] Still others have suggested that free urinary catecholamine is the best test (see Table 28-23).[153,157]

TABLE 28-22. Evaluation of Patients with Suspected Phaeochromocytoma

I. History
  - Family history of phaeochromocytoma, MEN IIa, IIb
  - Other neuro-ectodermal disease

II. Physical exam
  - Stigmata of neuro-ectodermal disease
    - Neurofibromatosis, port wine hemangioma
    - Oral ganglioneuromatosis

III. Biochemical Determinations
  - Plasma—Catecholamines
  - Urine—Catecholamines
    - Metanephrine, normetanephrine
    - VMA

IV. Blockade
  - α—All patients
  - α—methylparatyrosine (synthesis blocker)—selected patients
  - β—Persistent hypertension, tachycardia

V. Localization
  - CXR
  - CT
  - Ultrasound
  - Arteriography
  - Vena caval catheterization

It is rare to require provocative tests. In the rare occasion where suspicion is high and diagnosis cannot be made, the provocative use of glucagon is preferred under extremely carefully-controlled conditions.

Once the diagnosis has been made, then alpha-adrenergic receptor blockade should be initiated prior to further staging and localization. Phenoxybenzamine is administered orally, 10–40 mg four times a day (1–3 mg/kg/24 hours).[153] This needs to be titrated to reduce the blood pressure and minimize associated symptoms.

This drug has a relatively long half-life, approximately 8–12 hours and is successful in most cases. Should the patient also have considerable beta-adrenergic effects, such as persistent tachycardia or ventricular arrhythmias, then a beta-blocker, such as small doses of propranolol (20 mg three times a day) should be instituted. It is rather uncommon to need to use both alpha- and beta-blockade during a preoperative evaluation.

The authors have had some experience with alpha-methyl paratyrosine, which inhibits tyrosine hydroxylase and the subsequent production of catecholamines. Used in doses of 250–500 mg four times a day, the drug can be remarkably effective in maintaining a symptom-free patient. Naturally, because of its action in blocking catecholamine synthesis, it is important that the diagnosis be confirmed with urine and blood samples prior to drug initiation.[158]

LOCALIZATION AND STAGING

Once the diagnosis is made, consideration as to localization and staging should be determined. Five to 10% of all pheochromocytoma will be bilateral and 10% will be extra-adrenal. In a patient with a familial endocrine neoplasia syndrome, the assumption should initially be made that the tumors are bilateral.

As with most endocrine tumors, the diagnosis of malignancy may be difficult but can be helped by various localization procedures. The incidence of malignancy varies from 11–32%, with the lower number being more likely, as the latter refers to a rather unique referral pattern (see Table 28-20).

Localization and staging begin with chest films for thoracic paravertebral masses, which represent ectopic or metastatic disease. Abdominal CT is the next localization procedure because it is non-invasive, and as most pheochromocytomas are large, this is usually remarkably accurate.[159] If localization with CT is unsuccessful, arteriography is used in the well-

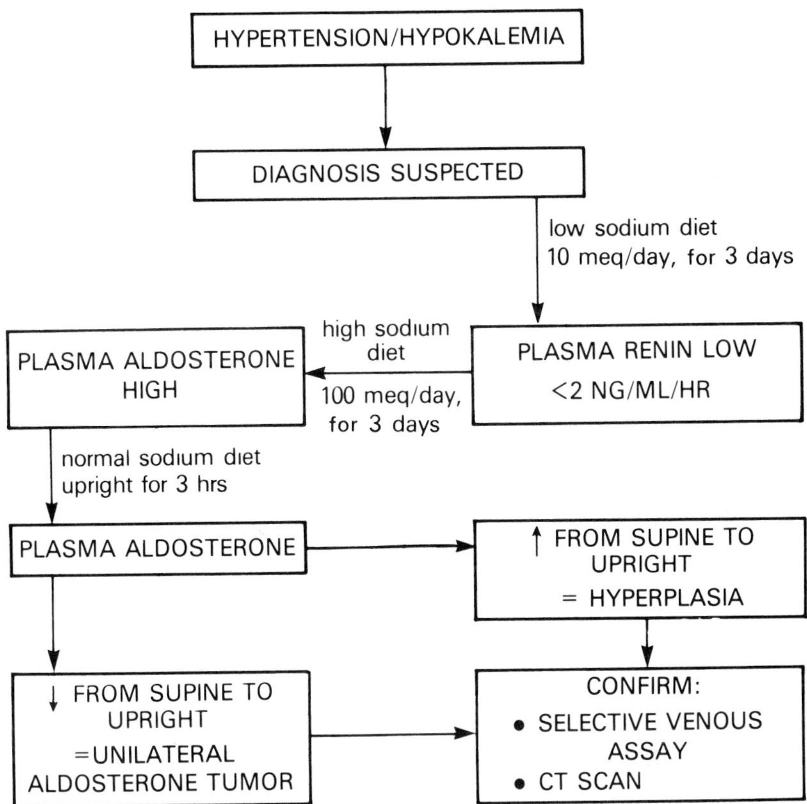

FIG. 28-20. Flow sheet for diagnosis and localization of primary aldosterone excess site.

prepared patient already receiving adrenergic blockade (see Fig. 28-21).

Vena cava catheterization with determination of plasma catecholamine levels at various locations is one of the oldest recorded tests.[159] However, it is only indicated in order to localize a tumor not found by other methods, to evaluate recurrent symptoms following resection, or to evaluate possible metastatic disease (see Fig. 28-22).

TREATMENT OF ADRENAL TUMORS

Surgery is the primary form of treatment of all adrenal tumors.

Benign Localized Lesions

For the small (<10 cm), well-localized benign adenoma producing excess aldosterone or corticosteroid a unilateral posterior surgical approach is preferred (see Fig. 28-23). If the lesion is a little larger, this can be converted to the oblique or posterolateral position, which allows extension if warranted (see Fig. 28-24). For large tumors, the anterior approach becomes necessary and can on occasion be converted to a thoraco-abdominal incision (see Fig. 28-25).

Adrenocortical Carcinoma

A lesion suspected of being an adrenocortical carcinoma should be approached in such a manner that wide local, en

FIG. 28-21. Arteriographic localization of a local recurrence of malignant pheochromocytoma following prior left adrenalectomy for pheochromocytoma in a 44 year-old female patient.

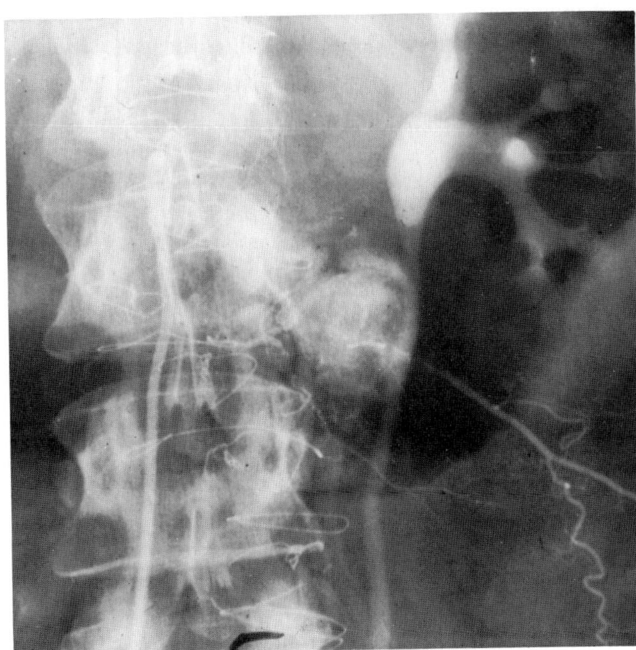

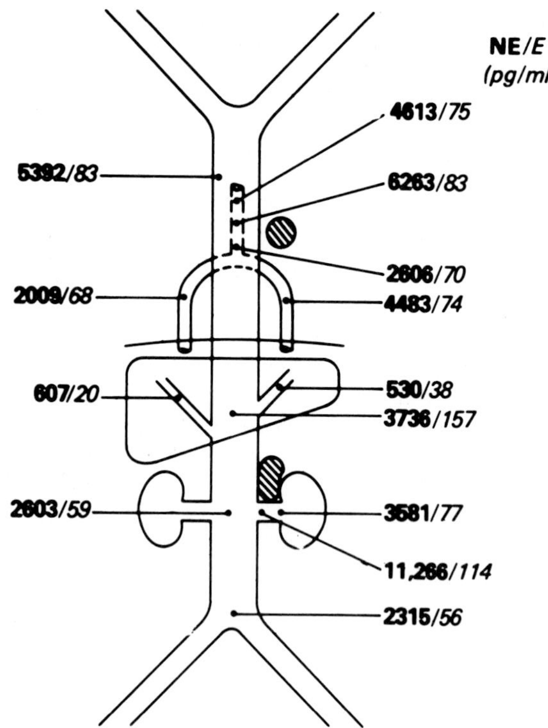

FIG. 28-22. Selective venous sampling for catecholamine in a patient with a local recurrence of a malignant pheochromocytoma (see Fig. 28-21). Note the elevation in the venous azygos system, suggesting a second metastatic lesion in the thoracic paravertebral area. Both lesions were subsequently confirmed and resected at a single operation. The patient is alive and well 3 years later. *NE* = Norepinephrine; *E* = Epinephrine. (Javadpour N, Wollering E, Brennan MF: Adrenal neoplasm. Curr Probl Surg 17:1, 1–52, 1980. Copyright © 1980 by Year Book Medical Publishers, Inc., Chicago)

bloc resection can be performed. This usually means a deliberately planned thoraco-abdominal incision, or an incision that can be extended into either thoracic cavity.

Pheochromocytoma

Surgery is definitive therapy for pheochromocytoma and can be performed safely if considerable preoperative and intraoperative precautions are taken. Patients should come to OR with a well-positioned and functioning central venous line, monitored electrocardiographically throughout the procedure and have an arterial line for blood pressure monitoring. Choice of anesthesia is not restricted, although halothane or a balanced anesthetic with a muscle relaxant are the most

FIG. 28-23. Position for posterior adrenalectomy.

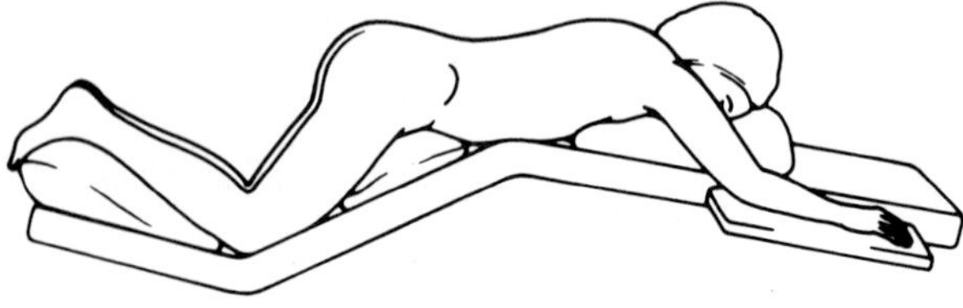

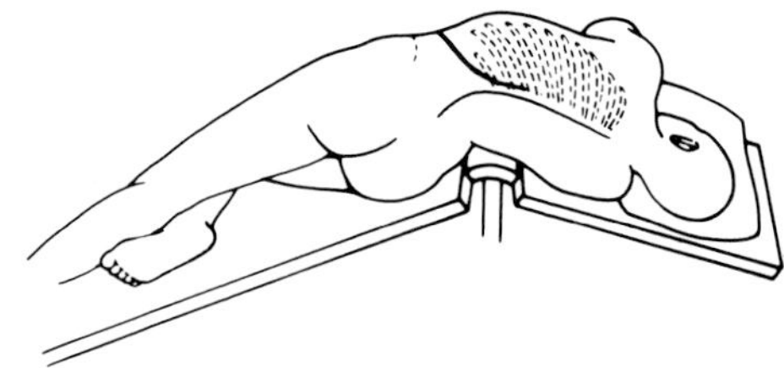

FIG. 28-24. Position and incision for extended posterolateral approach.

frequent choices. In an effort to avoid tachycardias, atropine is not used.

For a long time, blood volume was measured preoperatively; the value of this has been placed in doubt.[150,151] It is felt by Sjoerdsma that the majority of patients with retracted vascular spaces have metastatic disease, but this has not been confirmed. Using preoperative alpha-blockade, the intravascular volume can be expanded to normal prior to surgery.

Small doses of phentolamine intraoperatively or nitroprusside to control wide fluctuations in blood pressure are preferred.[162] Certainly, others have documented the effectiveness of nitroprusside; arrhythmias can be readily treated with blood pressure control or, if needed, small doses of IV propranolol.[163] Immediately following a successful operation, the withdrawal of catecholamine with resultant loss of vascular tone can be associated with the risk of hypotension. This can be prevented by preoperative restoration of blood volume and a sensitivity to the increased intraoperative and postoperative needs for fluid.

Preoperative Steroid Coverage

Corticosteroids are not required unless bilateral adrenalectomy is performed (see Table 28-24). The patients who will require corticosteroids are indicated in Table 28-25. For long-term management, a multitude of preparations are available; the comparative glucocorticoid and mineralocorticoid activity is indicated in Table 28-26. For long-term corticosteroid man-

TABLE 28-24. Perioperative Corticosteroid Coverage

PREOPERATIVE
100 mg hydrocortisome IM or IV with premedication
INTRAOPERATIVE AND DAY OF OPERATION
100 mg hydrocortisone every 8 hours IV as continuous infusion
POSTOPERATIVE
Day 1
75 mg hydrocortisone IV(IM) every 8 hours
Day 2
50 mg hydrocortisone IV (IM) every 8 hours
Day 3
40 mg hydrocortisone IV (IM) or PO every 8 hours
Day 4
20 mg hydrocortisone IV (IM) or PO every 8 hours
Thereafter:
Cortisone acetate 25 mg PO in AM, 12.5 mg PO in PM, or equivalent preparation

TABLE 28-25. Patients Requiring Perioperative Corticosteroid Administration

NONE REQUIRED	PERIOPERATIVE	LONG-TERM
Unilateral aldosteronoma	—	—
Unilateral pheochromocytoma	—	—
	Bilateral adrenalectomy	Bilateral adrenalectomy
	Unilateral adrenalectomy for cortical adenoma or carcinoma	—
		Unilateral adrenalectomy for carcinoma on o,p'DDD

TABLE 28-26. Comparison of Steroid Preparation Potencies

STEROID	DOSE IN MG	RELATIVE GLUCOCORTICOID ACTIVITY	RELATIVE MINERALOCORTICOID ACTIVITY
Cortisol	20	1	1
Cortisone	25	0.75	0.7
Prednisone	5	4	0.7
Prednisolone	5	4	0.7
Dexamethasone	0.75	30	2
Methylprednisolone	4	5	0.5
Aldosterone		—	400
Fludrocortisone	0.1	—	400

agement, cortisone acetate (25 mg AM and 12.5 mg PM), with appropriate adjustment as required is adequate. Mineralocorticoid requirements are variable, depending on the amount and type of corticosteroid preparation employed. With the use of cortisone acetate, fludro-cortisone acetate (0.1 mg) only once daily may be needed. However, many patients on adequate electrolyte and water replacement will require no mineralocorticoid supplementation (see Table 28-26).

Technical Aspects of Surgery—Posterior Approach to the Adrenal

The patient is positioned as shown in Fig. 28-23. An incision paralleling the paraspinous muscles and following the course of the 12th rib is made (see Fig. 28-25). The latissimus dorsi muscle and the lumbodorsal fascia are then divided with the cautery. Laterally, the external and internal oblique muscles

FIG. 28-25. Incision and position for lateral and thoraco-abdominal approach to the adrenal. (Javadpour N, Wollering E, Brennan MF: Adrenal neoplasms. Curr Probl Surg 17:1, 1–52, 1980)

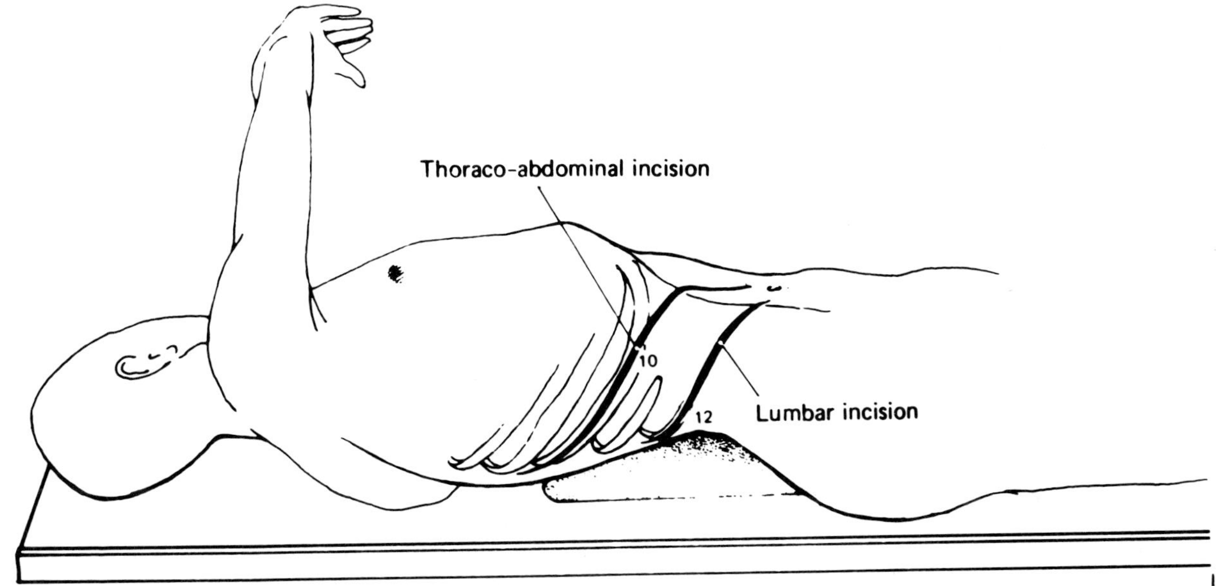

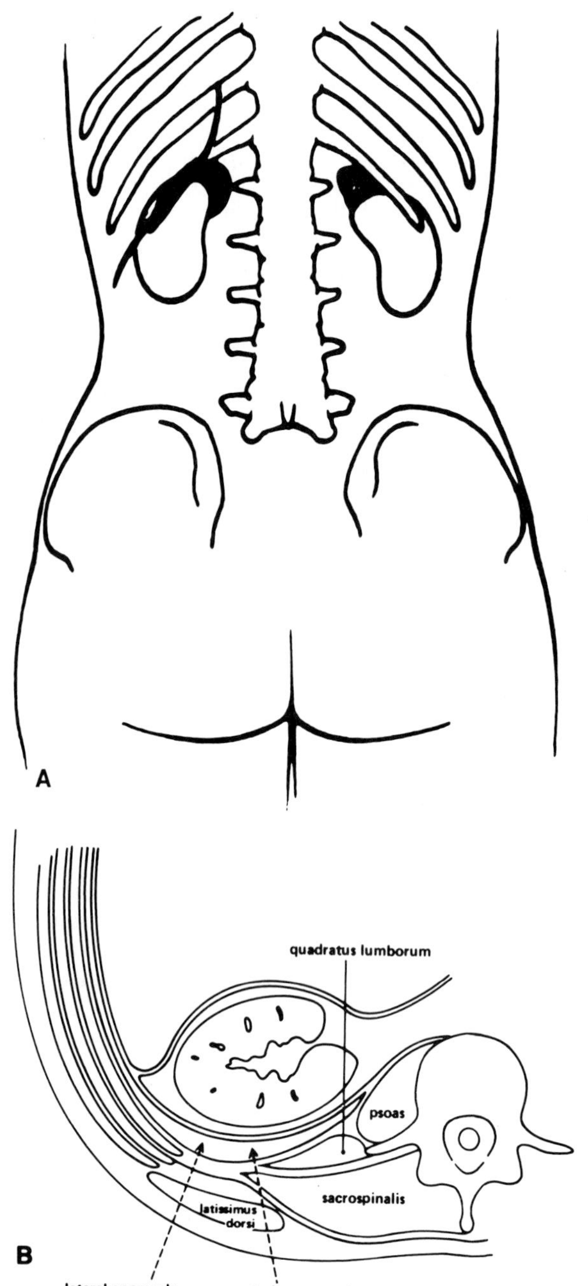

FIG. 28-26. *A*, Incision for posterior approach to the adrenal. *B*, Posterior and lateral approaches to the adrenal. (Saxe A, Brennan MF, Javadpour N: Diagnosis and surgical management of adrenal tumors. Contemp Surg 18:31–40, 1981)

are divided or split. The posterior lumbar fascia is divided and the thoracospinal muscles retracted medially. The 12th rib is removed and the intercostal bundle is swept aside or ligated (see Fig. 28-26). The pleura can then be reflected superiorly and the perirenal fascia delivered into the wound. The fascia can then be opened, a hand placed above the adrenal gland, and the adrenal and kidney drawn toward the wound. The plane between the kidney and adrenal should not be developed initially, since the attachment aids in delivery of the adrenal. With the adrenal and the superior renal pole controlled between the index and second fingers, the periadrenal tissue can be gently swept aside with scissors, ligating the small adrenal arteries. This should be done with clips, paying attention to clearly identifying the main adrenal vein, which is doubly clipped and divided. The adrenal can then be separated from the kidney, again sweeping periadrenal fat toward the gland. Then the adrenal gland with the contained tumor can be removed.

Complications of posterior surgery can involve injury of the inferior vena cava, the renal vein, the pleura, and on the left side the pancreatic tail. Only rarely is the spleen at risk. The wound should not be drained. The incision is closed with absorbable sutures, reconstituting the carefully divided anatomic muscular planes.

Anterior Approach to the Adrenal Glands

An oblique or transverse incision is preferred except for the poorly localized or known pelvic pheochromocytoma; in this instance, a midline incision is employed (see Fig. 28-27A).

The right adrenal is then exposed by mobilization of the hepatic flexure and duodenum (see Fig. 28-27B). The left gland may be approached through the gastric-colic ligament and by incising the inferior border of the pancreatic tail and swept up (see Fig. 28-27C). On occasion, by mobilizing the lateral attachments of the spleen, the spleen can be displaced downward with the pancreas so that a ready approach above the superior border of the pancreas can be made, preserving the spleen and with excellent access to the left adrenal. The spleen and pancreatic tail can be reflected to the right to give additional exposure.

TREATMENT OF METASTATIC DISEASE

METASTATIC ADRENOCORTICAL CARCINOMA

When surgery is no longer feasible, the use of vascular embolization should always be considered. Considerable functional ablation can often be achieved.

As previously noted, most adrenal cortex cancers are functional and produce excess steroids. The antihormonal agents used in the treatment of this disease decrease the production of adrenal steroids. The first drug to be used in patients with this disease was metapyrone (metyrapone), an inhibitor of the 11, β-hydroxylation step in cortical biosynthesis.[164] This drug had been reported to effectively ameliorate symptoms of hypercortisolism in a few anecdotal cases, but was generally found to be ineffective in patients with bulky metastatic disease.[164] Also, since metapyrone inhibits 11, β-hydroxylation, it leads to the production of mineralocorticoids and may precipitate hypertension and hypokalemia.

A commonly used antihormonal medication in functioning adrenal cortex cancer is aminoglutethimide. This drug was initially used as an anticonvulsant; however, it was noted that with continued use, adrenal insufficiency and goitrous hypothyroidism occurred. Further studies demonstrated that the drug produces distinct histologic changes in the adrenal gland

and inhibits the enzymatic conversion of cholesterol to 5-pregnenolone.[165] Aminoglutethimide is an effective, palliative treatment in Cushing's syndrome, secondary to adrenocortical carcinoma, adenoma, and ectopic ACTH production by extra-adrenal carcinomas, and may produce a rapid and sustained suppression of corticosteroid synthesis.[166,167] Because the drug may alter the extra-adrenal metabolism of cortisol, and thus measurement of urinary 17-OH-corticosteroid excretion may overestimate the effectiveness of therapy, assessment of plasma cortisol concentration is the most reliable means of measuring drug effect.[168] The toxicities associated with aminoglutethimide include anorexia, dermatitis, somnolence, ataxia, and decreased thyroid function. Dosage is escalated until a satisfactory fall in plasma cortisol associated with symptomatic improvement is seen or until toxicities are intolerable. The usual dose is 1–2 g/day, although higher doses may be needed in individual cases.

Antitumor Therapy

It is not unexpected that in a disease that occurs in less than 150 patients throughout the U.S. each year chemotherapy data would be sparse. The effects of cytotoxic agents in adrenocortical cancer are basically unknown. The one agent that has been used in this disease is o,p'-DDD (mitotane), a derivative of the insecticide DDT. The use of o,p'-DDD in the treatment of adrenocortical carcinoma originated from the empirical observations of Nelson and Woodward in 1948, that the commercial insecticide DDT produced selective atrophy of the zona fasciculata and zona reticularis of the adrenal cortex of the dog.[169] Biochemically, o,p'-DDD has inhibited dog adrenal glucose-6-phosphate dehydrogenase; this enzyme of the pentose pathway is responsible for the generation of NADPH, an essential cofactor in hydroxylation reactions for steroid synthesis, such as the conversion of cholesterol to 5-pregnenolone.[170] In addition to its direct effects on cortisol synthesis, o,p'-DDD significantly alters the extra-adrenal metabolism of cortisol, making its indirect measurement by 17-hydroxy-corticosteroid excretion invalid. As is the case with aminoglutethimide, direct measurement of plasma cortisol is required for an accurate estimate of the effect of o,p'-DDD on the secretion of this hormone.[171] In 1960, Bergenstal reported that the drug could both inhibit steroid secretion and produce objective tumor regression in metastatic adrenocortical carcinoma.[172]

As a result of this initial experience, two series with more than 100 adrenocortical cancer patients have been treated with o,p'-DDD. In 1966, Hutter and Kayhoe reported results in 138 patients.[173] A 50% decrease in abnormal steroid production was obtained in 79/113 (70%) of patients who initially had elevated steroid levels. A minimum of 4 weeks was required for an adequate test of therapy since, of those patients who ultimately responded, only 37% had responded by 21 days, whereas by 30 days of treatment, 87% of eventual responders had evidence of tumor regression. The average dose required for response was 8.5 gm/day. Biochemical response, as measured by decreased steroid levels, was attained more easily than objective antitumor response. Of 59 patients with measurable disease, objective tumor regression was seen in 20 (34%). The median time on therapy until antitumor response was 6 weeks and the mean duration of response was 10.2 months.

An additional 115 patients with adrenal carcinoma treated with o,p'-DDD between 1965 and 1969 were reported by Lubitz and coworkers in 1973.[174] The measurable disease response in this series was 61%, compared to the previously reported figure of 34%, and the steroid excretion response of 89% demonstrated an improvement over the 72% noted by Hutter and Kayhoe.[173]

The majority of patients treated with o,p'-DDD sustain some form of toxicity when dosage is brought to the therapeutic range of 8–10 g/day. This is usually mild, commonly consisting of GI symptoms including anorexia, nausea, vomiting, or diarrhea. Neuromuscular toxicity has been recorded in 40–60% of cases. This is usually lethargy and somnolence. Dizziness or vertigo and dermatologic toxicity are observed in 15% of cases, while leukopenia and liver function abnormalities rarely occur.[173,174]

Successful treatment of a functioning tumor with o,p'-DDD will result in signs of adrenal insufficiency. This probably is mainly related to the suppressed pituitary adrenal axis secondary to the longstanding massive steroid secretion by the tumor, and to adrenal damage by o,p'-DDD. In patients demonstrating a hormonal response, the need for replacement glucocorticoid therapy should be anticipated.

The clinical options available to the physician dealing with a patient with functioning unresectable adrenal cortical carcinoma are few. Therapy with o,p'-DDD escalating to a daily dose of 8–10 grams is the one approach that may produce both antitumor effect and palliation of symptoms of hypercorticism. Aminoglutethimide may be used to decrease symptoms from hormonal excess and is purely a symptomatic measure. Cytotoxic chemotherapy may be used, but the choice of drug or drugs, doses, and schedules in this disease is empirical at this point. Radiation therapy has shown little benefit other than for occasional palliation of bone pain.[173,175]

MALIGNANT PHEOCHROMOCYTOMA

Surgery

Aggressive surgical resection of single accessible metastases should always be considered.

Cytotoxic Chemotherapy

The majority of reports are single cases or minute "series." A comprehensive overview of the agents used and their "effectiveness" is given in Table 28-27.[176–182]

The definition of "effectiveness" is sufficiently variable as to make any meaningful comments difficult.[182] Virtually no regimen can be suggested with any certainty.

Antihormonal Therapy

The use of catecholamine blocking agents remains the mainstay of therapy, and varies widely from patient to patient (see Table 28-28). The long-term use of the synthesis blocker α-methyl paratyrosine can give significant palliation from the functional effects of the tumor.

TABLE 28-27. Cytotoxic Treatment of Malignant Pheochromocytoma

DRUG	EFFECTIVE		NOT EFFECTIVE	
	Reference	*Year*	*Reference*	*Year*
Cyclophosphamide	176	1967	177	1966
			178	1976
			179	1973
Nitrogen mustard	177	1966		
Thiotepa	177	1966		
Vincristine			178	1976
Doxorubicin (adriamycin)			178	1976
Doxorubicin (adriamycin) and cyclophosphamide	182	1976		
Methotrexate			179	1973
Streptozotocin			181	1977

TABLE 28-28. Therapy for Malignant Pheochromocytoma

OPERATION ALONE	6
α-Methyl-para-tyrosine (AMPT) alone	2
Surgery plus AMPT	5
Surgery plus propranalol (P)	1
Surgery plus dibenzamine (DBZ)	2
Surgery plus AMPT + P	1
Surgery plus AMPT + DBZ	2
Surgery plus AMPT + P + DBZ	1
Surgery plus AMPT + DBZ	1
Surgery plus chemotherapy + AMPT + DBZ	1

RESULTS OF TREATMENT

SURGICAL RESECTION OF BENIGN LESIONS

The surgical resection of benign pheochromocytoma results in a normal life expectancy.[148] The cure of hypertension, however, is not always obtained. The persistence or recurrence of hypertension can occur in as high as 25% of patients thought to be related either to residual, benign pheochromocytoma tissue, unsuspected metastatic malignancy, or pre-existing underlying irreversible renal vascular disease. A 10-year survival rate of 64% has been reported.[183] Increased morbidity and mortality in operation for recurrence of pheochromocytoma has been documented, and increasingly aggressive surgical efforts at resection appear warranted.[137,184–186] The results of surgery for primary aldosterone-producing tumors is dependent on underlying pathology.[187–191] Primary aldosteronism, produced by bilateral adrenal disease, responds poorly to adrenalectomy, complete response rates of 14% and 18% having been reported (see Table 28-29).[192] Fortunately, this distinction can now be made with some accuracy preoperatively with the advent of precise localization techniques.[133,135,142] The complete response rates for adenomas have been 60%, 68%, and 74% respectively.[192–194] Operative response can be predicted by prior treatment with spironolactone, allowing time for preoperative correction of hypokalemia.[193,195] With selection of patients, operative morbidity should be low, mortality zero, and complete response to adrenalectomy present in greater than 90% of cases.

TABLE 28-29. Response to Surgical Treatment of Primary Aldosteronism

	CR	PR	NR
Single adenoma (n=27)	66%	33%	—
Multiple adenomata (n=5)	60%	—	40%
Adenomatous hyperplasia (n=4)	75%	—	25%
Bilateral hyperplasia (n=9)	22%	33%	44%

CR = Complete response
PR = Partial response
NR = No response
Auda SP, Brennan MF, Gill JR: Evolution of the Surgical Management of primary aldosteronism. Ann Surg 191:1–7, 1980

Surgical resection of benign corticosteroid-producing tumors of the cortex should be 100% curative. With the advent of accurate diagnosis and localization, mortality should approach 0% and morbidity should be correspondingly low.

MALIGNANT TUMORS

Malignant tumors producing primary aldosteronism are inordinately rare.

ADRENOCORTICAL CARCINOMA

When surgery alone is employed for adrenocortical carcinoma, 43% of those with a completely resected tumor were alive at an average of 7.2 years postoperatively.[196]

Regardless of whether or not function is present, survival results are similar (see Table 28-30).[137] It should be emphasized, however, that prolonged survival can occur in patients with metastatic disease, although recent reports suggested an average survival of 8 and 10 months.[196,197]

MALIGNANT PHEOCHROMOCYTOMA

Aggressive surgical ablation has been the preferred treatment whenever possible. Unfortunately, as previously mentioned, the diagnosis of malignancy in these tumors is difficult, and four of the 22 had the diagnosis of malignancy made based on histology alone.

With the accepted difficulties of re-establishing an accurate incidence of malignancy without metastasis, the survival in a group of cases treated at the National Institutes of Health

TABLE 28-30. Adrenocortical Carcinoma Survival

	N	MEAN SURVIVAL (Years)	RANGE	5-YEAR SURVIVORS
Functional	49	2.7	1 mo–17 yr	18%
Nonfunctional	9	2.6	2 mo–5 yr	11%

Javadpour N, Woltering E, Brennan MF: Adrenal Neoplasms. Curr Probl Surg XVII (1): 1–52, 1980

TABLE 28-31. Malignant Pheochromocytoma Survival

	N	MEAN SURVIVAL (Years)	RANGE	5-YEAR SURVIVORS
Adrenal	16	6.6	2 mo–16 yr	43%
Extra-adrenal	6	1.2	2 mo–3 yr	0%

is illustrated in Table 28-31. As in adrenocortical carcinoma, prolonged survival can occur, although those patients with extra-adrenal malignancy appear to have a poor prognosis, no patient having survived 5 years. Of the 22 patients, six were treated with surgery alone, 13 with surgery and a blocking agent, two with α-methyl paratyrosine alone, and one with surgery, blockers, and cytotoxic chemotherapy (see Table 28-26). It should again be emphasized that individual patients can achieve long-term significant palliation.[182,185]

FUTURE CONSIDERATIONS

The early diagnosis of small lesions of the adrenal medulla is receiving increasing emphasis.[198] Most of these depend on sensitive plasma nonepinephrine and epinephrine determination applied to familial or MEN Type II kindreds, or hypertensives with borderline increases of urinary Vanillylmandelic Acid (VMA). In these patients, stimulatory tests may be more applicable.[199,200]

The Endocrine Pancreas

with John S. Macdonald

As there are at least five known different endocrine cell types in the pancreas, endocrine syndromes associated with tumors of each individual cell type are increasingly being reported. These include the gastrinoma, the insulin-producing tumors, tumors producing pancreatic polypeptide, vasoactive intestinal peptide, glucagon, and somatostatin, in addition to a syndrome characterized by watery diarrhea of uncertain etiology.[202–214]

Since the islet cells of the pancreas have multiple potential, examples of endocrine pancreas tumors producing other hormones are becoming more frequent. These include ACTH, ADH, parathyroid hormone, 5-OH tryptophan or 5-OH tryptamine, and thyrocalcitonin.[215–217]

An attempt has been made to integrate these cell types with a unifying concept, the "apud" cell system.[218–219] The collective term "apudoma" was initially applied to a medullary carcinoma of the thyroid secreting ACTH; subsequently, it has been widely described.[220–222]

EPIDEMIOLOGY

There is a paucity of information on prevalence and incidence of islet cell tumors. The Seer Program, in their survey of approximately 10% of the U.S. population, documented 127 islet cell carcinomas diagnosed between 1973 and 1977. This would mean approximately 250 new islet cell carcinomas in the U.S. each year. Malignancy in islet cell carcinomas is often difficult to prove, unless unequivocal metastases are present. The manner in which the diagnosis was made in the Seer Survey for 1973–1977 is illustrated in Table 28-32. Because histology alone is unreliable in determining malignancy in endocrine tumors, it is possible that the true incidence is less, but at least 190 new cases per year of islet cell carcinoma do occur in the U.S. This agrees with the 1 in 100,000 of the population reported previously.[223] These tumors are equally distributed between male and female and appear in both black and Caucasian populations.

The true prevalence of benign and malignant islet cell tumors is unknown, but islet cell adenomas may be found in as many as 1.5% of carefully performed autopsies, the great majority of which are not diagnosed antemortem.[224] The finding of an islet cell tumor at autopsy does not equate with the function. Of 44 islet cell tumors found during 10,314 autopsies; eight were associated with hypoglycemia. Somewhere between 200 and 1,000 new endocrine pancreatic tumors are clinically diagnosed each year.

NATURAL HISTORY, CLINICAL PRESENTATION, AND DIAGNOSIS

The presentation, diagnosis, and outcome of patients with pancreatic endocrine tumors are highly dependent on the hormone produced by the predominant cell contained in the tumor. The syndrome produced can be due to a benign

TABLE 28-32. Islet Cell Carcinoma of the Pancreas: Confirmation of Malignancy*

Distant metastases confirmed by histology	68
Distant metastases by radiograph	1
Regional nodes involved by histology	8
Regional extension	19
Localized, but metastatic by histology	18
Unknown or unstaged	12
	127

*1973–77

TABLE 28-33. Endocrine Tumors of the Pancreas

ISLET CELLS	SECRETED ACTIVE AGENT	SNYDROME
Alpha (α)	Glucagon	Glucagonoma
Beta (β)	Insulin	Insulinoma
Delta (Δ)	Somatostatin	Somatostatinoma
D	Gastrin	Gastrinoma
A → D	Vasoactive Intestinal Peptide (VIP)	WHDA
	5HT	Carcinoid
	ACTH	Cushings
	MSH	Hyperpigmentation
	Secretin, VIP	Verner Morrison
INTERACINAR CELLS		
D_1	Pancreatic polypeptide	Multiple
EC	5-HT	Carcinoid

adenoma, a malignant carcinoma, or adenomatous hyperplasia.

As each syndrome varies widely, diagnosis and presentation will be given for each known pancreatic endocrine tumor in sequence, followed by a general comment on management. (This is with the exception of gastrin-producing tumors which, because of their different management, are dealt with separately.) The list of tumors arising from the pancreatic islet cells is inevitably incomplete, and does not reflect the fact that many of these tumors can arise from cells located in the duodenum or other parts of the alimentary tract; in addition, many patients may have multiple tumors and combination syndromes (see Table 28-33). This particular area is developing rapidly with advances in many areas so as to make reviews out-of-date by the time of publication.

THE ANATOMY OF THE PANCREAS

The pancreas lies tranverse across the posterior wall of the abdomen, extending from the epigastrium to the left hypochondrium. The pancreas weighs approximately 80-90 grams and is 12-15 cm long.[226] The right extremity is termed the head and is connected to the main portion of body by a slight constriction, the neck, while the left extremity tapers to form the tail. The head lies in the curve formed by the first, second, and third parts of the duodenum. The angle at the inferior and left lateral aspect of the head forms a prolongation termed the uncinate process. In the grooves between the duodenum and the right lateral border of the head are the superior and inferior pancreaticoduodenal arteries. The anterior surface of the body is covered by the dorsal surface of the stomach, being separated by the omental bursa. The posterior surface lies in direct contact with the left renal vein, left kidney, left adrenal, and the origin of the superior mesenteric artery. The pancreatic duct (duct of Wirsung) runs transversely from left to right through the substance of the pancreas. It terminates by coming into contact with the common bile duct within the head, then passes through the muscular amd mucosal coats of the duodenum to end in an orifice common to it and the common bile duct at the duodenal papilla, approximately 7-10 cm distal to the pylorus. In about 40% of patients, the pancreatic duct and the common bile duct open separately into the duodenum. An accessory duct opens approximately 2.5 cm proximal to the papilla. The arterial supply is mainly from branches of the splenic artery, which form several arcades within the pancreas, the gastroduodenal, and direct branches from the superior mesenteric artery. The veins form tributaries of the splenic and superior mesenteric portions of the portal vein and are important in the elucidation of selective venous sampling to localize hormonal production. The superior mesenteric artery and vein lie posterior to the neck of the pancreas, partially embraced from behind by the uncinate process. The union of splenic vein and superior mesenteric vein to form the portal vein takes place behind the neck of the pancreas.

PATHOPHYSIOLOGY

The cell system termed the 'APUD' system was postulated by Pearse to include cells with common cytochemical attributes of amine precursor uptake and decarboxylation.[218] These cells are neuroectodermal in origin and will secrete either normal or abnormal peptide hormones. Considerable debate exists concerning the exact origin of the apud cells and whether the pancreatic endocrine cells are derived directly from the neural crest. The apud cells of the carotid body, thyroid, adrenal medulla, sympathetic nervous system, and melanocytes are neuroectodermal in origin. Some evidence exists that other cells, including those apud cells of the alimentary tract and endocrine pancreas, are also derived from a neuroectodermal site. However, the removal of the neural fold of 9 day-old rat embryos did not prevent typical islet cells containing secretory granules from appearing in subsequent development.[222]

PATHOLOGY

The pancreatic apudomas may be studied and identified in various ways. The concentrations of polypeptides may be measured in the peripheral blood or in the venous blood draining a tumor. The majority of these methods employ radioimmunoassay. The tumors can be examined by light microscopy, cytochemical methods, electron microscopy, and immunocytochemistry. It is becoming increasingly difficult to attribute these tumors (and their associated syndromes) to a single hormone. When tumors and the adjacent islets are examined by immunofluorescent techniques, several hormones are commonly identified. The clinical syndrome associated with such a tumor or tumors will depend on the quantity and biologic activity of the dominant hormone.

In recent report, five patients with tumors and an associated glucagonoma syndrome were compared to three patients with multiple tumors of the endocrine pancreas.[227] In the five patients with the glucagonoma syndrome, no common diagnostic features were present by electron microscopy, whereas the majority of tumors both with and without the glucagonoma syndrome contained cells intensely positive for glucagon. In a series of 94 pancreatic endocrine tumors studied by immunocytochemistry, 73 (78%) were multicellular.[228] Extracts of the tumors revealed significant amounts of somatostatin in 19 of 94 (20%) and pancreatic polypeptide in 17 of 94 (18%).

THE ZOLLINGER–ELLISON SYNDROME

The Zollinger–Ellison syndrome (ZES) is a syndrome of fulminant ulcer disease, gastric hyperacidity, and a gastrin-producing islet cell tumor.

HISTORY

The description of two patients with fulminant peptic ulcer disease and non-beta islet cell tumors of the pancreas by Drs. Robert Zollinger and Edwin Ellison on April 29, 1955 at the American Surgical Association has been followed by a great number of similar cases.[202,229–233] Drs. Zollinger and Ellison were careful to point out a previous report and the personal communications about four other cases from Drs. Jenkins, Moyer, and Bernard.[202,234] They were able to document three other cases for a total of nine cases and suggested that glucagon might be responsible for the observed syndrome. Gastrin was not implicated until the isolation of a gastrin-like substance in 1960.[235]

EPIDEMIOLOGY

Prior to 1970, diagnosis of the ZES was made by radiography, gastric analysis, and gastrin bioassay. The development of radioimmunoassay and provocative testing has changed this approach to one of more certainty.[236] It is thought that this syndrome accounts for less than 1% of peptic ulcer disease. It is very likely that the occurrence of gastrin-producing tumors is far more common than clinically suspected. Gastrinomas have been reported in childhood and old age, but the majority occur between the third and fifth decade.

ANATOMIC CONSIDERATIONS

It is thought that the gastrin in these pancreatic tumors arises from the pancreatic D cell, although many different types of apudoma can produce excess gastrin and cause variations of the Zollinger–Ellison syndrome. These include the G cell of the stomach and antrum. Most of the tumors are multifocal-within the pancreas and about 60–75% are malignant with metastases at the time of presentation.[237–239] The incidence of malignancy will probably fall as earlier diagnoses are made by using gastrin radioimmunoassay. Approximately 35% are benign adenomas, and 5% present as islet cell hyperplasia. Multiplicity is common (20–40%) and 30–50% will belong to MEN kindreds; as many as 10% may arise in the duodenal wall.[239–241]

PATHOGENESIS

Gastrin is normally stored in the endocrine G cells of the antral gastric mucosa, although smaller quantities have been reported in the duodenum and intestine.[242,243]

Without a tumor, gastrin is not present in the adult pancreas but can be found in the fetal pancreas.[244] Under normal circumstances, antral gastrin is released in response to a protein meal. This release is inhibited by elevated gastric acid and is not controlled by vagotomy or atropine. The primary role of gastrin appears to be the stimulation of acid secretion by the stomach, although some debate exists as to the trophic effect of gastrin on the stomach, small intestine, and pancreas; this seems fairly certain under experimental conditions. This suggested factor has been used to explain the increase in the gastric rugal folds seen in patients with gastrinoma and occasionally permits diagnosis by barium swallow.

Various biologically active forms of gastrin have now been identified. They range from big (G-34), little (G-17), and mini (G-14) gastrins. The biologic half-lives of these G-34 = 40 minutes, G-17 = 6 minutes, respectively. Recently, a larger gastrin called big-big gastrin has been reported.[245,246] The majority of patients with gastrin-producing tumors have a greater quantity of G-34 than G17 in their plasma. The different molecular forms are measured at similar levels by most gastrin antibodies and the detection of an elevated gastrin level is the prime consideration in the diagnosis.

PATTERNS OF SPREAD

Definitive statistics on the localization of metastatic disease are unknown. The liver is the pre-eminent site, while lymph nodes and lung are common sites.

CLINICAL PRESENTATION

The most common presenting feature is severe peptic ulcer disease, manifested by pain in 70–95% of patients. The ulcers are commonly multiple, often with atypical sites and with multiple recurrences.[230,242] The syndromes are commonly associated with diarrhea, which may precede the ulcer or be the dominant feature of presentation in 15–20% of cases. In the presence of diarrhea, concern must be raised as to whether other peptide-producing tumors or multiple hormones from the same tumor may be the cause of the diarrhea.[241] Without diarrhogenic hormone secretion, diarrhea is dependent on the increased gastric acid secretion and can be improved by gastric acid aspiration.[240]

During the interval between onset of symptoms and surgical therapy, there is a high incidence of peptic ulcer disease complications. Hemorrhage occurs in about 30%; perforation in 15%.

The predominant feature is the recurrent nature of the episodic attacks, especially pain. The recurrence is often rapid after conventional medical or surgical therapy for peptic ulcer disease, unless cimetidine is employed.

In 30–50% of patients, associated multiple endocrine syndromes coexist. This number can be expected to increase as screening for multiple hormones becomes more widespread.

With earlier diagnosis, the severity of the disease is less; the incidence of malignancy (before 1970, 44%) is apparently falling (now, 25%).[247]

A recent report of 40 patients has emphasized the changing pattern of presentation.[247] Mean duration of symptoms in unoperated patients was 32 months (2 months–9 years). Approximately 50% of this group had had symptoms for less than 3 months. The predominant symptom was pain, consistent with peptic ulcer disease, with 22 of 40 having had one or more episodes of upper GI bleeding. Acute perforated peptic ulcer had occurred in four patients, two of whom had had prior surgery. Diarrhea was a common symptom in this group (30%). Nine of the 40 patients had features of a MEN syndrome (eight with parathyroid and three with pituitary pathology).[247] The authors of this report emphasize the increased frequency of diagnosis (more than double from 1970–77 compared to 1955–70). The presenting features have changed with more patients having the diagnosis made prior to surgery; other symptoms of bleeding, pain, steatorrhea, and the incidence of associated endocrine abnormalities were all being remarkably similar to the earlier series.[240] The typical sites of peptic ulceration seen in earlier series are less common, with one-third of patients having a single duodenal ulcer, although ulcers were present in 91% of this group of 34 patients. Marked acid hypersecretion was still a feature.[248] In addition, characteristic ulcer craters of the earlier series were replaced by a more superficial mucosal erosive duodenitis.

DIAGNOSIS

Availability of radioimmunoassay has made the diagnosis possible often before symptoms are severe.[247,248] There are, however, multiple forms of gastrin with variations in biologic activity. They are named "big gastrin," "big-big gastrin," "little gastrin," "mini-gastrin," and by specific names for specific immunoassays (see section on Pathogenesis in this chapter). Fortunately, the different molecular forms of gastrin are measured at similar levels by most gastrin antibodies in most screening laboratories. Consequently, regardless of the assay, the detection of a markedly elevated level of gastrin is presumptive evidence for the diagnosis of gastrinoma. Such elevation does not comment on site of origin of the gastrin; in interpreting elevated concentrations of hormone, suspicions of other syndromes that can cause false elevations must be made. In the case of gastrin, renal failure, gastric outlet obstruction, and pernicious anemia may all raise the circulating level. The majority of these syndromes are, however, usually associated with low acid secretion and the absence of severe peptic ulcer disease.

Without radioimmunoassay for gastrin, suspicion can be increased by an unusually sited ulcer or by the rapid return of ulceration following ulcer surgery. The abnormal radiologic changes in the upper small bowel include huge rugal folds in the stomach with an ulcer in the duodenum or post-bulbar area.[249] The abnormally located ulcer, while a classic sign, is present in only a small fraction of ZES patients.

Acid secretory studies have been extensively used in the past with suggestive features being a basal acid output (BAO) of greater than 10 mEq per hour, a basal acid output to maximal acid output (MAO) ratio greater than 0.6, or an overnight 12-hour acid secretion of more than 100 mEq (see Table 28-34).

The combination of elevated BAO and elevated gastrin is almost certainly due to a gastrinoma. However, acid secretory studies may be within the normal range; in up to 50% of patients, the BAO/MAO ratio may be less than 0.6. Some 5% of duodenal ulcer patients and 7% of controls will have values greater than 0.4. The diagnosis rests on a gastrin level that is ten times greater than normal (see Fig. 28-28).[246] Provocative testing with calcium and glucagon shows a considerable overlap and cannot be considered of great value.[248]

The association of elevated levels of other hormones has frequently been reported. In an early observation, the increased levels of thyrocalcitonin in patients with ZES were noted.[250] It was suggested that gastrin may be able to directly stimulate thyrocalcitonin production without an associated medullary carcinoma of the thyroid. In 24 patients with ZES who had pancreatic polypeptide (PP) measured, levels were significantly higher than 72 normal controls. The overlap, however, was large. No correlation between levels of gastrin and PP was identified and the increased PP levels were not related to the presence of an MEN syndrome or metastases.[251] The elevated levels of PP in patients with insulinoma may be due to hypoglycemia, making alternative explanations for the rise seen in ZES possible.[252] In another study, while mean serum PP levels in patients with gastrinoma were significantly greater than in normals, only five of 18 patients with gastrinomas had PP levels above the upper limit of normal.[253] Malignant disease may be suspected preoperatively if levels of alpha or beta hCG are elevated.[254,255] A recent report examining 40 patients prior to gastrectomy suggested that metastatic disease was seen in all patients with serum gastrin greater than 1,500 pg/ml, while levels greater than 8,000 pg/

TABLE 28-34. Gastrinoma—Diagnostic Tests

1. BAO:MAO ≥ 0.6
2. Overnight AO ≥ 100 mmols mEq
3. BAO ≥ 10 mmols/hr mEq
4. Serum gastrin 10× nl, or 500 pg/ml
5. Secretin test: 1 unit/kg IV rapid injection: Positive = 100% increase in gastrin within 10 minutes; 2 units/kg: Positive = 100 pg/ml increase over baseline
6. Calcium infusion: 4 mg/kg/hr for 3 hours: Positive = increase of 400 pg/ml over baseline

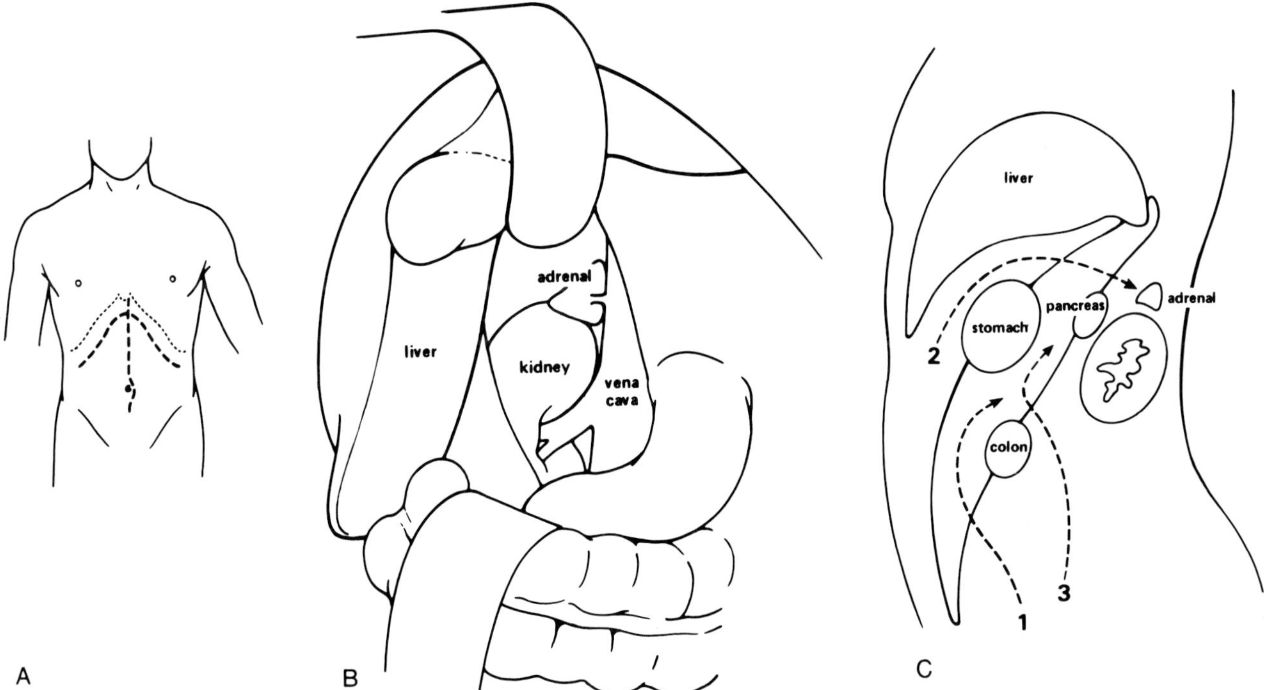

FIG. 28-27. *A*, Anterior incisions to approach the adrenal. *B*, Reflection of colon and duodenum to reveal the right adrenal. *C*, Approaches to the retroperitoneally placed adrenal gland. (Saxe A, Brennan MF, Javadpour N: Diagnosis and surgical management of adrenal tumors. Contemp Surg (18:31–40, 1981) used with permission of Bobit Publishing)

ml were due to massive liver replacement by tumor.[256] In this study, provocative tests with calcium and secretion were of no value in determining malignancy. Alpha hCG was normal in all patients with benign disease and elevated in four of 20 with malignant disease. In another experience, however, six patients thought to have benign disease did have elevated levels, although benignity was not confirmed by surgery in all. Of the seven with malignant disease, six had elevated beta hCG.[255]

LOCALIZATION

In 60–70% of patients, the tumors cannot be localized by radiography.[249] The evaluation of angiography in ZES has recently been reported.[257] Only three of 20 patients with ZES had unequivocally positive angiographic studies for a primary pancreatic tumor, while five others had equivocal findings based on adequate studies. Five patients had clearly identifiable hypervascular liver metastases. These findings are in contrast to many smaller series and case reports that imply ready diagnosis by angiography.[258–261] It should be emphasized that in 25% of these cases hepatic metastases were unequivocally identified; the authors' experience with CT is similar.[262] In 18 cases with ZES examined, four patients had the primary lesion identified and four patients had their hepatic metastases identified. Unfortunately, the smallest primary tumor was 5 cm in diameter; it is expected that other smaller tumors were missed. The referral nature of our institution makes it likely, however, that many of these patients were representative not of early, but of late and extensive disease. Consequently, other radiologic tests, including selective pancreatic venous catheterization through the liver, have been employed. The use of selective venous catheterization in association with a provocative stimulus, such as secretin, may provide much more accurate localization as this method has done for medullary carcinoma of the thyroid gland.[263,264] Clinicopathologic localization of the tumors has previously been reported (see Table 28-35).[240]

MANAGEMENT OF GASTRINOMA

Recent reviews have addressed the problem of management.[265–268] Resection of the tumor or pancreatectomy is not

TABLE 28-35. Location of Gastrin-Producing Tumor in 624 Patients With Zollinger–Ellison Syndrome

Pancreas (n = 426)		
Multiple or metastatic	296/624	(47%)
Coexisting islet cell hyperplasia	21/624	(3%)
Single localized tumor	109/426	(26%)
Duodenal wall (n = 103)		
With metastases	50/103	(49%)
Coexisting islet cell hyperplasia	5/103	(5%)
Localized duodenal wall tumor	45/103	(44%)
Islet cell hyperplasia alone	40/624	(6%)
Metastatic tumor only	55/624	(9%)

(Fox PS, Hoffman JW, Wilson SD et al: Surgical management of the Zollinger–Ellison syndrome. Surg Clin North Am 54:395–407, 1974)

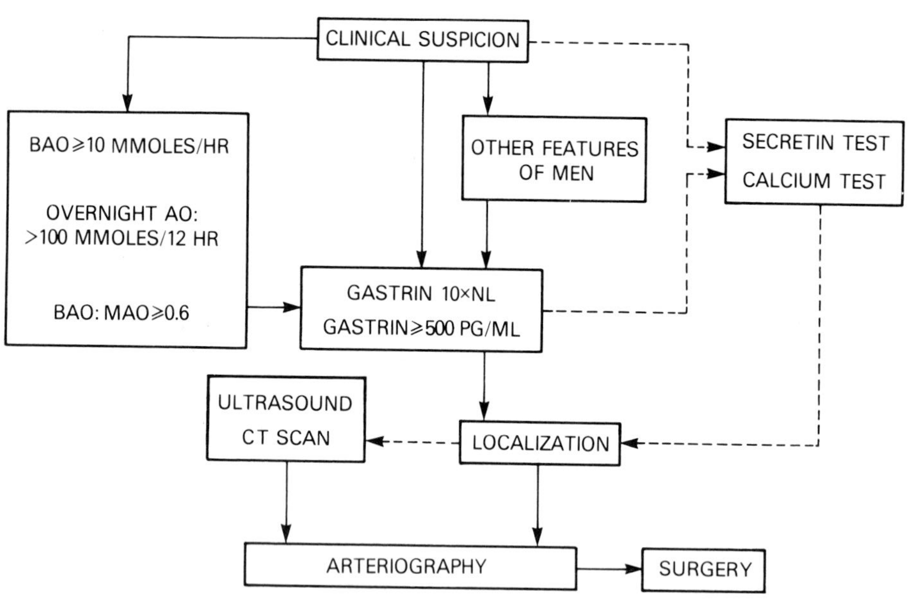

FIG. 28-28. A diagnostic flow chart for suspected Zollinger-Ellison syndrome patients.

a practical issue on most occasions, mainly because of the multifocality and high incidence of malignancy at presentation. Total gastrectomy is believed to be the initial operation of choice.[269]

The use of cimetidine (Tagamet), however, has markedly improved outcome. Now other possibilities should be explored.[270,271]

Once the diagnosis has been made, the concept of a "staging laparotomy" is advocated. The intent in this situation is to briefly control acid output with cimetidine, then at a time when the patient is in excellent condition, an elective exploratory laparotomy should be performed. If a benign or solitary gastrinoma is found, it may be resected. If no solitary tumor is found, or metastases are present, accurate histopathological staging can be performed.

Whether a total gastrectomy should be performed is a matter of considerable debate. Total gastrectomy is not always necessary. However, failure to proceed may mean that at some subsequent time, when and if the patient becomes resistant to cimetidine, total gastrectomy may not be technically possible.[272] The possibility that a lesser operation, such as a highly selective vagotomy, may allow more prolonged and easy management with cimetidine has been suggested. Gastric acid secretion can be reduced by truncal or selective vagotomy such that the ability of cimetidine to reduce basal acid secretions can be improved.[273] The suggested approach is seen in Fig. 28-29.

TABLE 28-36. Survival Results According to Tumor Resection

	N	MEAN SURVIVAL (Years)*	5-YEAR SURVIVAL
Tumor completely resected	22	9	76%
Tumor incompletely or not resected	14	3	21%
No tumor found	6	–	100%

*p=less than 0.01

Zollinger RM, Ellison EC, Fabri PJ et al: Primary peptic ulcerations of the jejunum associated with islet all tumors. Ann Surg 192:422–430, 1980.

SURGICAL MANAGEMENT OF ZES

When complete extirpation of the tumor is possible, a cure can be expected. Dr. Zollinger's recent review emphasizes the improved outcome when surgical extirpation of the tumor can be obtained (see Table 28-36).[266] When cimetidine is not available or not able to be used, total gastrectomy should be performed for unresectable tumors. Because of tumor multicentricity, malignancy, or occult primary, primary tumor ablation is often difficult and unrewarding. The ZES Tumor Registry reports a total of 70% of 268 patients undergoing total gastrectomy survived, compared with 43% of those undergoing lesser procedures.[240] Of the 30% who did not survive total gastrectomy, one-half died of postoperative complications. Interestingly, only 16 patients are reported as dying of progressive disease. In patients with associated hyperparathyroidism, the cervical exploration should be performed first to detect the effect of lowering serum calcium on gastric hypersecretion. This is particularly important as gastrin levels are usually mildly elevated in primary hyperparathyroidism and gastric acid secretory studies may be equivocal in making a ZES diagnosis.[274–276]

SURGICAL TREATMENT

TECHNICAL CONSIDERATIONS

A long midline or an extended right subcostal is the preferred incision. If a known lesion is present in the pancreas that is potentially resectable, the extended subcostal can be employed, rarely with a cephalic extension being required.

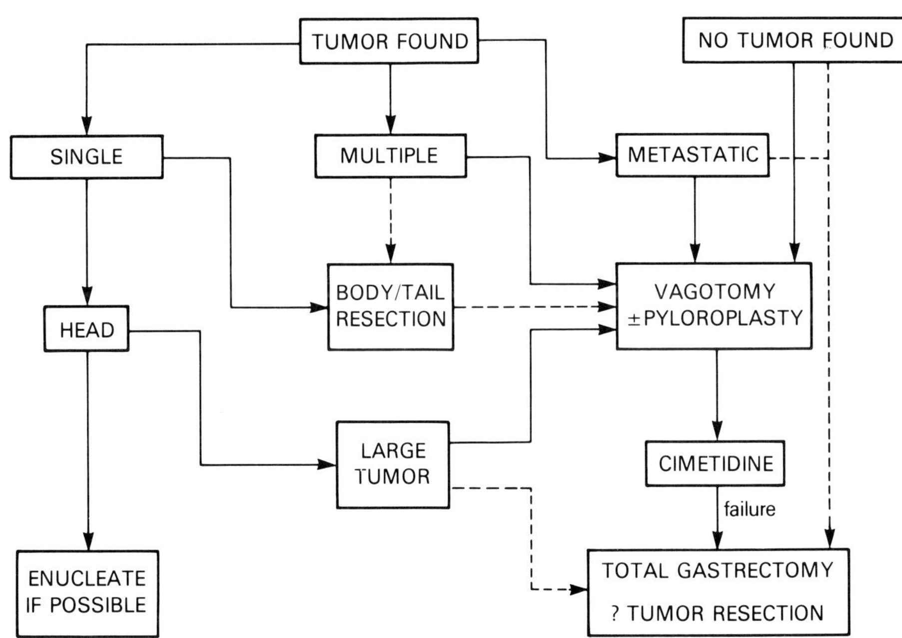

FIG. 28-29. Suggested approach to the intra-operative management of Zollinger-Ellison syndrome.

The exploration then follows as for other endocrine tumors of the pancreas. When total gastrectomy is required, the following approach is taken: Following entry into the abdominal cavity, the careful search of the pancreas having failed to reveal a tumor and any suspicious lymph nodes having been biopsied, gastrectomy can begin with mobilization of the stomach. The gastrocolic and gastrosplenic ligaments should be divided to identify the left and right gastric arteries. The left and right gastric arteries are divided, the duodenum transected and closed. Complete mobilization of the stomach can then be completed and the stomach rolled back to identify the posterior aspect of the esophagus. The esophagus is anastomosed to a loop of jejunum, either in Roux-en-Y fashion, or a double loop is brought up and an entero-enterostomy fashioned or a complete accessory stomach formed by making a Hunt–Lawrence pouch. The Roux-en-Y is preferred, performed by transecting the jejunum distal to the ligament of Trietz bringing the loop up behind the colon, the proximal end closed, and an end-to-side anastomosis made to the esophagus. The proximal jejunum is then anastomosed in an end-to-side fashion to the Roux-en-Y limb about 40–45 cm below the esophageal-jejunal anastomosis (see Figs. 28-30 and 28-31).[277]

FIG. 28-30. Esophageal-jejunal anastomosis following total gastrectomy. *A–C,* With the stomach serving as a retractor, the esophagus is now anastomosed end to side in two layers to a loop of jejunum brought up either by the antecolic or retrocolic route. The stomach is removed. *D,* The completed anastomosis. *E,* The jejunum is sutured to the diaphragm by a third row of interrupted stitches, which provide support for the anastomosis and relieve any tension of the suture line. (Edis AJ, Ayala LA, Egdahl RH: Manual of Endocrine Surgery, p 89. New York, Springer-Verlag, 1975)

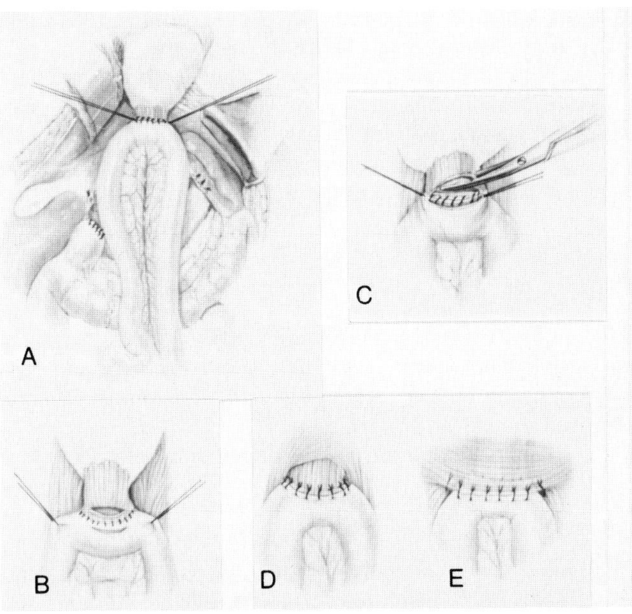

RESULTS

Of 187 survivors of total gastrectomy, 112 are alive up to 5 years, 50 are alive 5–10 years, and 16 are alive greater than 10 years after surgery.[240] Pancreaticoduodenectomy was successful in only 23 of 73 patients, mortality was 30%, and 30% required subsequent total gastrectomy.

Death was due to ulcer diathesis (37%), postoperative complications (26%), and tumor progression (19%). There was little tumor effect of benignity (50% alive) or malignancy (44% alive), the outcome being more dependent on control of acid secretion (see Table 28-37).

TABLE 28-37. Results of Surgical Treatment of Zollinger–Ellison Syndrome

	N	OPERATIVE DEATH	5-YEAR SURVIVAL
Total gastrectomy	268	81	112/268 (42%)
Pancreaticoduodenectomy	73*	26	23/73 (31%)
Tumor excision			
—without gastrectomy	35	—	21/35 (60%)
—with gastrectomy	37	—	31/37 (84%)

* 24 patients needed subsequent total gastrectomy
(Fox PS, Hoffman JW, Wilson SD et al: Surgical management of the Zollinger–Ellison Syndrome. Surg Clin North Am 54:395–407, 1974)

INSULINOMA

HISTORIC ASPECTS

The internal secretion of the pancreas was described by Drs. Banting and Best in 1922 while working in the Department of Physiology at the University of Toronto. Dr. Best was an Assistant in Physiology at Western University, London, Ontario, and based his idea on a resume published by Baron in 1920.[278]

Dr. Banting, who subsequently became an orthopedic surgeon, hypothesized that if, following pancreatic duct ligation, degenerative changes take place in the acini of the pancreas but not the islet tissue, advantage might be taken of this fact to prepare an active extract of islet tissue. The work performed by Dr. Banting was begun under the direction of Prof. J. J. R. Macleod in May, 1921. In their first article, they give due credit to Mering and Minkowski for reporting in 1889 that total pancreatectomy in dogs resulted in severe and fatal diabetes.[279]

They also give credit to Laguesse for first suggesting that the islet might be the source of pancreatic internal secretion in 1911.[279] Opie, in 1901, and Sscobolew, in 1902, independently furnished the first clinical foundation for the belief that the islets were involved in pancreatic diabetes.[280,281] Minkowski first used the pancreas in defects of carbohydrate metabolism, trying to feed the pancreatic tissue orally, but without beneficial results.[281]

Dr. Banting was careful to suggest in his original article that "according to Macleod, there are two possible mechanisms by which the islets might accomplish this [blood sugar] control. One, the blood might be modified while passing through the islet tissue, and two, the islets might produce an internal secretion." Dr. Banting and Prof. Best presented information to address this issue. They performed pancreatic duct ligation on a number of dogs; the dogs were then given a lethal dose of chloroform.[279] The degenerated pancreas was removed and sliced into Ringer's solution. The contents were then partially frozen and complete macerated. The solution was then filtered and the filtrate raised to body temperature and injected IV. They then showed that the injection of this extract causes a sudden fall in blood sugar. They concluded that IV injection of extracts from the dog's pancreas, removed 7–10 weeks after ligation of the ducts, invariably resulted in a reduced percentage of sugar in the blood. This was accompanied by a decrease in glycosuria. Rectal injections were not effective and the extent and duration of the reduction of the blood sugar varied directly with the amount of extract injected. The extract was destroyed by pancreatic juice. They were careful to point out that injections of large quantities of saline and extracts of other tissues did not cause a reduction of blood sugar, and that hemoglobin concentration was left unchanged.[279]

By 1924, other abnormalities of the islet cells were beginning to be suspected.[282] Five patients were described with hyperinsulinism and dysinsulinism, the majority attributed to heredity and too much work!

By 1927, the first case of carcinoma of the islets of Langerhans was reported. In this, the first recorded case of a patient with cancer requiring hourly doses of glucose to prevent fainting and hypoglycemia was documented.[283] At autopsy the cells of the metastatic cancer were similar to islet cells and alcoholic extracts made from the cancer acted like insulin on injection into rabbits. This was followed by a report of a patient who had prolonged episodes of hypoglycemia who underwent an operation on March 15, 1929 at which time an encapsulated tumor found in the middle of the pancreas, approximately 2 cm across, was enucleated.[284] An extract from the tumor was tested by Prof. Best for insulin, which was positive in a mouse assay. The patient recovered well with complete amelioration of symptoms. It was fortunate that the tumor was so obvious, as Finney had performed an operation in a similar case the year before but did not find a tumor. It is of interest that at the time, Dr. Finney resected 22.5 g of the pancreas without alleviating the patient's symptoms.[285]

The subject of hyperinsulinism was reviewed by Dr. Whipple in 1935, emphasizing the existence of islet cell adenomas. Dr. Whipple takes great pains to point out that the first procedure reported by Howland was performed by Dr. Roscoe Graham, although his name did not appear on the authorship.[281,284]

EPIDEMIOLOGY AND INCIDENCE

In 1974, Stefanini was able to gather 1,067 patients with beta islet cell tumors. Of these patients, 40% were male and 68% were between 30–60 years of age, with the youngest being four and the oldest 82-years-old.[286]

No figures exist for annual incidence or prevalence.

ANATOMIC CONSIDERATIONS

Insulinomas are evenly distributed throughout the pancreas, usually between 0.5 and 5 cm in size.[287] The ectopic sites that

TABLE 28-38. Insulinomas

All sites	1018
Head	342
Body	324
Tail	332
Ectopic	20
Wall of duodenum	5
Near tail of pancreas	3
Gastrosplenic omentum	2
Posterior to tail	1
Between head and liver	1
Posterior to head	1
Paraduodenal	2
Adherent to stomach	1
Spleen	1
Not specified	3

Filipi CJ, Higgins GA: Diagnosis and management of insulinoma. Am J Surg 125:231–239, 1973

have been described in the English literature up to 1973 have been reviewed by Filipi.[287] It appears that true ectopic insulinomas not arising in pancreatic tissue must be inordinately rare (see Table 28-38).

PATHOLOGY

In the extensive review by Stefanini, 32% were found in the head, 30% in the body, and 34% in the tail. The majority (83%) were single and benign (84%), and 4% were associated with a MEN syndrome.[286]

As it is extremely difficult to confirm malignancy by histopathologic examination of the primary lesion, the reported incidence of metastatic lesions (5%) would suggest that greater than 90% are benign. In a similar manner, present experience suggests that the association of insulinoma with the MEN syndromes is at least four or five times that suggested by Stefanini's retrospective review.[286]

Four morphologic types have been described: Type I with B granules only; Type II with B granules and atypical granules; Type III with atypical only; and Type IV without granules. The content of granules was associated with increased insulin content and decreased proinsulin content.

PATHOGENESIS

The beta cell of the islets produce the insulin precursor, proinsulin. Proteolytic digestion converts proinsulin to insulin and a connecting peptide, C peptide. The C peptide has 31 amino acids and is a major part of the connection between the A and B chains of insulin within the proinsulin molecule. Once divided, both C peptide and insulin are stored within the beta cells, to be released during exocytosis.

The characteristic syndrome is dependent on an inappropriate insulin secretion for the ambient blood sugar. Hyperinsulinemia, with grossly elevated levels, is not always present. The ability of hypoglycemia to arrest insulin release from insulinoma cells is assumed to be absent, although this is far from proven. In addition, there appears to be a defect in the transformation of proinsulin to insulin, as well as impaired cellular retention.[204]

PATTERNS OF SPREAD

Metastasis occurs predominantly to lymph nodes and the liver. The significance of small nodal micrometastases is unknown, as patients following incidental resection of a small micrometastasis may survive for many years without known recurrence.

CLINICAL PRESENTATION

The clinical presentation is dominated by the neuropsychiatric symptoms of hypoglycemia. The combination of loss of consciousness, confusion, dizziness, and weakness were present in 92% of the 1,067 patients reviewed by Stefanini.[286] The multiple causes for such symptoms account for the delay in diagnosis, 20% after 5 years, and only 34% in the first year of symptoms.[286] The average age at presentation is 42, but the wide range from infancy to the ninth decade make this of little value.[288] The rare manifestation of muscular weakness or neuropathy, although occurring independently, should alert clinicians to the possibility of a MEN syndrome, as these patients have the potential to secrete multiple hormones.[289]

FIG. 28-31. Roux-en-Y reconstruction after total gastrectomy. *A, B,* the jejunum is transected a few inches below the ligament of Treitz, and by progressive division of the mesenteric vascular arcades (*broken line*) an elongated limb of intestine is fashioned. *C,* the proximal end of the Roux limb is closed and a careful anastomosis is then made end-to-side with the esophagus. The proximal jejunum just beyond the ligament of Treitz is anastomosed in an end-to-side manner to the Roux limb about 45 cm below the esophagojejunal anastomosis to complete the Y. Roux-en-Y reconstruction after total gastrectomy effectively prevents reflux alkaline esophagitis. (Edis AJ, Ayala LA, Egdahl RH: Manual of Endocrine Surgery, p 91. New York, Springer-Verlag, 1975)

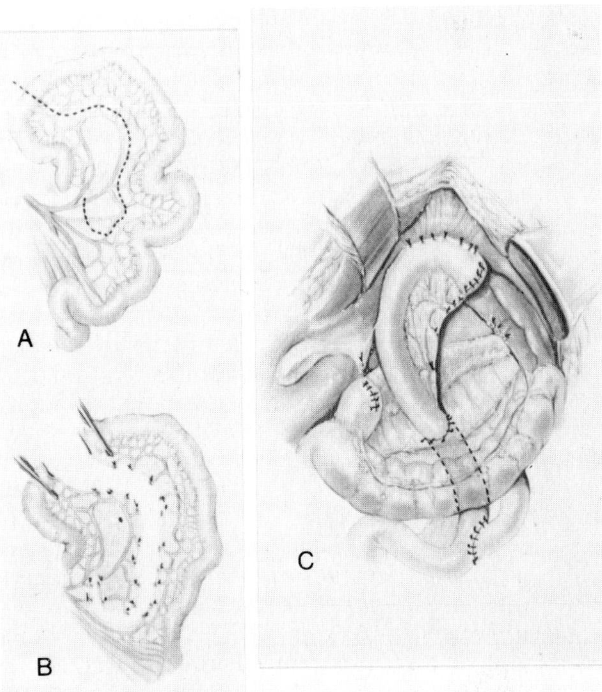

TABLE 28-39. Diagnostic Tests for Insulinoma

TEST	% POSITIVE
Prolonged Fast	95
Tolbutamide Tolerance	80
Glucagon	72
Glucose Tolerance	60
Leucine Tolerance	50

Stefanini P, Carboni M, Patrasi N et al: Beta islet all tumors of the pancreas: Results of a study on 1067 cases. Surgery 75:597–609, 1974

DIAGNOSIS

The presence of fasting hypoglycemia, less than 50 mg%, subsequently confirmed by an associated raised insulin, but relieved by glucose administration is pathognomonic.

Multiple provocative tests are available, including tolbutamide, calcium, alcohol, fish insulin, diazoxide, glucagon, arginine, and leucine, but all need to be reserved for investigative studies of the biology of insulin secretion or for the uncommon situation where a carefully controlled fasting test is equivocal (see Fig. 28-32). The positivity of the tests employed is documented in Table 28-39.[286]

The calcium provocative test has recently been studied in 16 adult patients with hypoglycemia. In nine of 10 patients with proven insulinoma, significant hypoglycemia and hyperinsulinemia occurred 60–90 minutes following the start of a 10 mg/kg calcium infusion over 2 hours. Post-resection testing gave no change in glucose or insulin. Patients with non-insulinoma causes of hypoglycemia were negative by this test.[290]

The measurement of proinsulin has been employed in the diagnosis of insulinoma. Almost all patients with insulinomas have elevated proinsulin and the proinsulin:total insulin ratio is elevated. The highest proinsulin percentages tend to be in patients with carcinoma.[291] The C peptide level can also be measured as a reflector of insulin secretion. The measurement of C peptide is especially valuable in making a diagnosis of insulinoma in the following circumstances:

1. The patient receiving exogenous insulin
2. The detection of the factitious administration of insulin
3. As a suppression test in response to exogenous insulin

Preoperative Localization of Insulinomas

The available studies for preoperative localization of insulin-producing tumors of the pancreas include:

1. Computerized tomography (CT)
2. Ultrasound
3. Selective arteriography
4. Transhepatic selective venous catheterization for insulin concentration
5. Endoscopic retrograde cholangiopancreatography

The most important test is the selective arteriogram. The accuracy of selective arteriography has continuously improved from 66% to 91%.[286,292] The preferred diagnostic approach to localization is illustrated in Fig. 28-33.

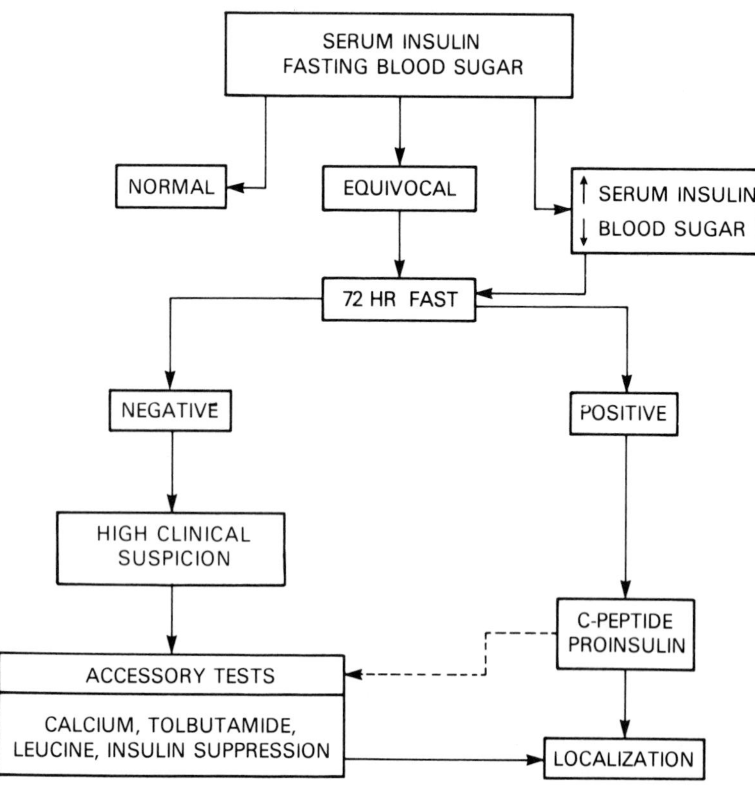

FIG. 28-32. Flow chart for the diagnosis of suspected insulinoma.

GLUCAGONOMA

HISTORY AND EPIDEMIOLOGY

This pancreatic endocrine neoplasm is composed mainly of pancreatic alpha cells, although other cells may be involved, particularly the D cell. The syndrome refers to a characteristic clinical combination of migratory necrolytic erythema in association with weight loss, mild diabetes, anemia, diarrhea, and often stomatitis.[293,294]

The first patient with glucagonoma was described in 1942, but the syndrome was relatively uncommon until more recently.[208,295-297]

A recent report documents 47 reported cases, including some of the authors'.[298] Absolute prevalence is unknown.

ANATOMIC CONSIDERATIONS

Most (90%) of the small numbers of cases in whom information has been documented have had lesions in the body and tail, although most tumors are extensive. Therefore, this information is of questionable value.

PATHOLOGY

The tumor arises in the pancreatic A or alpha cell, although other cell types, especially the D cell, have been incriminated. The majority of tumors are malignant, although the absolute incidence of true malignancy is not clear. It has been suggested to be in the order of 60%.[209]

Hyperplastic lesions can occur, particularly in multiple endocrine neoplasia syndromes, either as a solitary manifestation of the pancreatic endocrine tumor of this disease or in conjunction with other tumors producing other pancreatic endocrine hormones.[289]

NATURAL HISTORY

A majority have metastasized at the time of presentation. Growth, however, is relatively slow, and patients with extensive malignant disease have survived for prolonged periods.

PATHOGENESIS

Glucagon is a single chain polypeptide. In circulating form it can exist in at least four different molecular weight patterns. Symptoms can be explained by the function of glucagon on carbohydrate and protein metabolism.

Glucagon acts to promote glycogenolysis and gluconeogenesis, and acts as a counter-regulatory hormone to insulin. The presence of glucagon prevents hypoglycemia, which would accompany the hyperinsulinemia produced by a large, predominantly protein meal.

PATTERNS OF SPREAD

Spread is predominantly local and to the liver where vascular lesions can be demonstrated.

CLINICAL PRESENTATION

The syndrome of weight loss, glucose intolerance, and the characteristic migratory necrolytic erythemia, when thought of, makes diagnosis obvious. Skin lesions are bullous and edematous, progressing to a characteristic eczema. The skin rash can be intermittent and can move from one area to another. It is associated with low plasma amino acid levels that occur as a consequence of the gluconeogeneic activity of glucagon.[297] This has been reversed by the administration of glucose and amino acids in high doses but not by amino acids given alone.[299]

METHODS OF DIAGNOSIS AND STAGING

The clinical signs and symptoms are sufficiently characteristic so that the primary test (*i.e.* the measurement of plasma glucagon) is indicated. The plasma glucagon levels are often very high so any form of provocative test is rarely required. Numerous functional provocative tests, including IV glucose tolerance tests, arginine infusion, and somatostatin infusion have been employed, but are of minimal value.

Arteriography will confirm the lesion and often demonstrate the presence or absence of vascular lesions in the liver. In rare instances where the tumor is not malignant and is only a small size at diagnosis, then, theoretically at least, pancreatic venous sampling for glucagon levels should be of value.[300]

WDHA SYNDROME

A syndrome of refractory, watery diarrhea and hypokalemia associated with a known insulin-secreting islet cell tumor was described in 1958.[212,213] These tumors have subsequently been called vipomas, although considerable debate exists as to whether or not the VIP (vasoactive intestinal peptide) is the cause of the syndrome.[301,302] More conventionally, it has been referred to as the WDHA syndrome, the watery diarrhea, hypokalemia, and achlorhydria syndrome.[214]

PATHOLOGY

This syndrome, originally thought to be due to pancreatic islet cell tumors or diffuse islet cell hyperplasia, has more recently been associated with tumors of the sympathetic nervous system including the adrenal glands.[303]

PATHOGENESIS

Great debate exists as to whether or not a single cell of origin is the causative agent in these diseases.[302] Multiple hormones, including serotonin, pancreatic polypeptide, secretin, GIP (gastric inhibitory poplypeptide), gastrin, glucagon, and (as with most of these endocrine tumors) prostaglandins have all been suggested as possible causes of the syndrome.[213,304-308] Modlin suggests that VIP is the predominant causative agent.[246,309]

As with glucagonoma, the majority of these tumors are malignant and have metastasized by the time of diagnosis, with spread being predominantly to liver parenchyma.[310]

CLINICAL PRESENTATION

A diagnosis is suspected when a patient has profuse and profound diarrhea to the extent of several liters per day. This diarrhea contains high quantities of potassium and is always of a secretory nature.[311] An important diagnostic feature is that once all intake is removed the diarrhea does not cease. The patients are hypokalemic, presumably due to the loss of potassium in the diarrhea. The secondary effects of low potassium are common with severe weakness and lethargy predominant. As with other pancreatic endocrine tumors, facial flushing can be a prominent feature. As with the glucagonoma syndrome, a mild hyperglycemia and abnormal glucose tolerance can occur, the cause of which is not known. Low gastric acidity is common, extending over a wide range from achlorhydria; hyperchlorhydria has occurred after removal of functional tumors.

SOMATOSTATINOMA

A tentative description of this syndrome makes the association of mild diabetes mellitus, steatorrhea, cholelithiasis, and a pancreatic tumor.[312]

In 1977, three cases of pancreatic somatostatinoma were reported and a projected syndrome defined.[210,211,313] Other reports of patients with malignant islet cell tumors that contain somatostatin have also been described (see Table 28-40).[314–316]

The tumor is extremely uncommon. It will be more readily diagnosed as vigorous attempts to identify somatostatin in islet cell tumors of the pancreas are made.

PATHOLOGY

Of the six reported cases, five have had malignant disease or metastases at diagnosis. Only one patient seems to be cured by resection of the pancreatic tumor with no demonstrated recurrence over four years.[211] The primary tumors tend to consist of solid islet cells and uniformly demonstrate a positive reaction on immunofluorescence with an anti-somatostatin antiserum. Calcitonin has also been identified.

NATURAL HISTORY

Natural history is unknown. Given the high incidence of malignancy, it would be expected that the tumors will be similar to gastrin-producing tumors and present with malignant disease in the liver. Concurrently, three of the six patients died immediately postoperatively.

CLINICAL PRESENTATION

The majority of patients presented with cholelithiasis, with diabetes mellitus being uniform and steatorrhea common. Diarrhea also occurred with invariable weight loss and, on occasion, anemia.

METHODS OF DIAGNOSIS AND STAGING

Clinical suspicion of the associated new onset of mild diabetes with the other clinical symptoms, as mentioned previously, should raise suspicion. Confirmation of a pancreatic islet cell tumor could then be searched for and the plasma somatostatin level measured for confirmation.

PANCREATIC POLYPEPTIDE

Malignant pancreatic islet cell tumors producing only pancreatic polypeptide (PP) have been reported.[317] One was associated with the watery diarrhea syndrome; in another, elevated PP was the only manifestation. Two patients with right upper quadrant pain and hepatomegaly without metabolic or GI abnormalities were studied.[317] Both had vascular pancreatic head tumors and angiographic evidence of hepatic metastases. PP was elevated (6,140 and 2,725 pg/ml; nl less than 512 pg/ml) and hepatic metastases contained PP. All other measured hormones were low (insulin, glucagon, somatostatin, VIP, gastrin). Five-hydroxy-indolacetic acid was normal.

Treatment with streptozotocin resulted in decreased PP and reduction in tumor size associated with patient improvement.

Prospective screening for PP in 12 members of three families with MEN Type I resulted in the detection of three pancreatic tumors in three asymptomatic patients. Two of these patients had the tumors excised, which resulted in normal plasma PP concentrations postoperatively.[318]

TABLE 28-40. Somatostatinoma

FASTING PLASMA GLUCOSE (mg/dl)	FASTING PLASMA INSULIN (IU/ml)	FASTING PLASMA GLUCAGON (pg/ml)	FASTING PLASMA SRIF (pg/ml)	GLUCOSE TOLERANCE TEST	TUMOR SRIF	REF
NR*	NR		2,700	NR	NR	315
NR	NR	NR	8,000	diabetic	+	316
169	5.0	0	NR	diabetic	+	211
NR	NR	NR	NR	NR	+	314
NR	3.0	10	107,000†	diabetic	+	210
163	244.0‡	70	20,000	diabetic	+	312
60–90	4–24	70–200	80	—	—	

* NR = not reported
† Hepatic vein sample
‡ C-peptide insulin was 3.7 ng/ml (nl: 0.9–4.2)
SRIF = Somatostatin

SURGICAL MANAGEMENT OF PANCREATIC ENDOCRINE TUMORS

Once the diagnosis of a hormonally active pancreatic tumor is made, vigorous attempts at localization should be performed and surgery advised (see Fig. 28-34). The approach to tumors producing VIP, glucagon, insulin, ACTH, PTH, somatostatin 5-OH-tryptamine or any other hormone by the pancreatic islets (with the exception of gastrin) should result in a similar surgical approach. The aim is tumor removal with consideration of end-organ ablation reserved for the ZES.

OPERATIVE PHILOSOPHY

When a single tumor is present, the aim is usually to remove this by enucleation (see Fig. 28-35). A frozen section is required under all circumstances to confirm the diagnosis. If the tumor is large, deeply embedded in the pancreas, or associated with local invasion (an uncommon event), then distal pancreatectomy should be performed. Rarely, multiple tumors involving the head of the pancreas will require either a pancreaticoduodenectomy for single tumors or a total pancreatectomy for multiple tumors (see Fig. 28-36). It is the authors' strong belief that the small risk from a pancreatic fistula, when larger tumors are enucleated from the head, is acceptable when the alternative is total pancreatectomy.

With good localization, the risks of being unable to find a tumor have considerably lessened. However, when no tumor can be found and none have been preoperatively localized, then the distal pancreas is resected to the left of the superior mesenteric vessels (see Fig. 28-37). This is then given to the pathologist for multiple sectioning. If still no tumor is present and the diagnosis is unequivocal, then the pancreas is further resected, but not to the extent of a total pancreatectomy. The need for total pancreatectomy should be inordinately rare. If preoperative selective venous catheterization through the liver and the portal vein has been performed, then the expectations of where the tumor might be allows a more definitive operation. Particularly, if venous samples from the head of the pancreas are negative for hormone, while samples from the distal pancreas are positive, then distal pancreatectomy can be performed with a high likelihood of success. Without experienced attempts at preoperative localization, it is better to perform no pancreatic resection if the tumor is not found; refer the patient for more expert localization studies.

FIG. 28-33. Suggested approach to the localization of insulinoma.

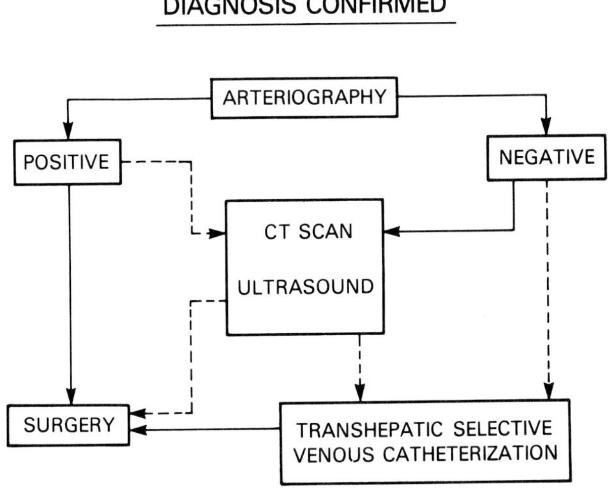

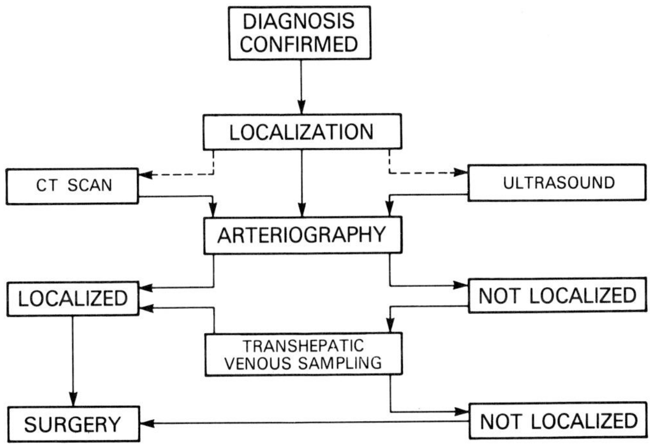

FIG. 28-34. Suggested approach to the localization of functional pancreatic islet cell tumors.

TECHNIQUE AND EXPLORATION FOR PANCREATIC TUMORS

An extended right subcostal incision that extends across to the subcostal margin is the preferred technique. This incision allows division of both recti and ready access to the left chest, if needed. In patients with insulinoma who are also obese, a bilateral subcostal incision can be used (referred to as the subcostal "frown"). Our personal preference is not to employ a midline incision. With the abdomen opened, the pancreas is begun to be exposed. This is done by reflecting the hepatic

FIG. 28-35. Intra-operative approach to single functional pancreatic islet cell tumors.

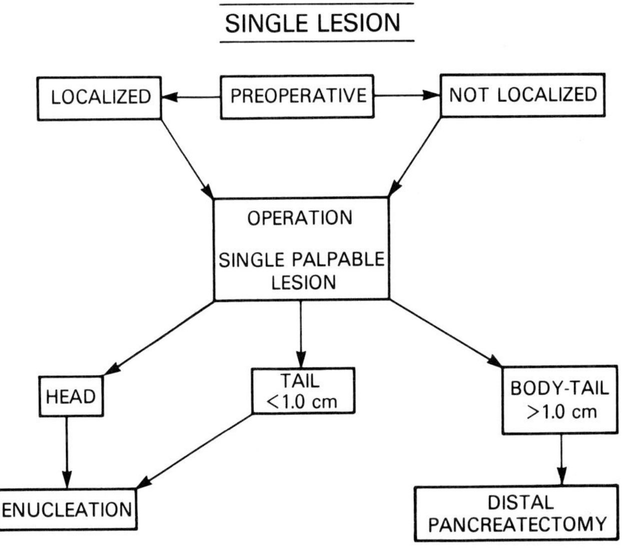

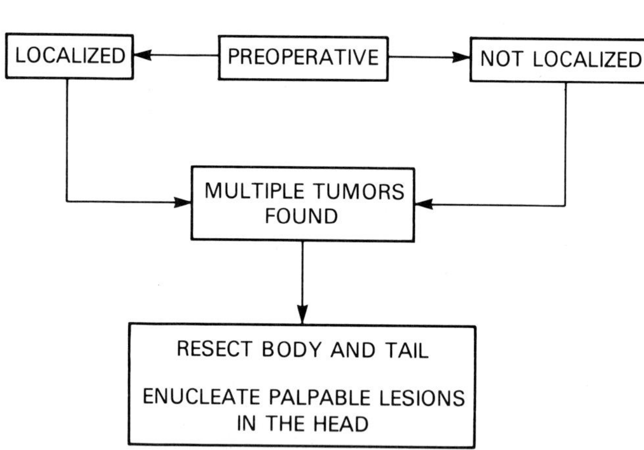

FIG. 28-36. Intra-operative approach to multiple functional islet cell tumors.

flexure of the colon away from the liver with the greater omentum.

If the tumor is localized, then one can proceed directly either to the head or to the body and tail. If the tumor is not localized, the body and the tail of the pancreas should be exposed first. This is done through the lesser sac, with division of the gastrocolic omentum. The splenic flexure of the colon will usually need to be mobilized away from the spleen. With the body and tail of the pancreas now well exposed, any light, filmy adhesions can be dissected free and the stomach reflected superiorly. If the tumor is not visible at this point, then the pancreas can be carefully palpated. This may involve dissecting the inferior and part of the superior border of the pancreas away from the loose retroperitoneal tissue (see Fig. 28-38). The inferior border is much less vascular and should be mobilized first. Careful palpation of both the body and tail of the pancreas can be performed with the hand from below (see Figs. 28-39). Any suspected nodules can then be gently teased free and excised for frozen section. Characteristically, the islet cell adenoma is a little more bluish and dusky in color. The use of methylene blue has not been routinely employed, but it may, on occasion, be helpful.[319]

Mobilization of the head is performed after reflection of the hepatic flexure by the standard Kocher maneuver. This will then allow palpation of the head from the lateral aspect of the duodenum. With the enucleation of a single adenoma, the wound is inspected carefully and the site is marked with one tiny peripheral clip. A soft drain of the Jackson–Pratt type is led down to the body at the site of enucleation.

Distal pancreatectomy can be performed without removal of the spleen; this is preferred in most patients. Removal of the spleen, however, does make the procedure much more simple, as the splenic vein does not need to be so carefully dissected away from the body of the pancreas. If not done meticulously, this dissection will result in brisk bleeding from the splenic vein. The procedure involves further mobilization of the superior and inferior borders of the pancreas to identify the splenic artery and vein superiorly and dissecting the posterior aspect of the pancreas away from them. Once fully mobilized over to the superior mesenteric vessels, the pancreas can be divided. Where possible, the main duct should be identified and individually ligated, but this is not always possible. A fish mouth division of the pancreas should be made such that the anterior and posterior surfaces can be more readily apposed with interrupted, non-absorbable sutures.

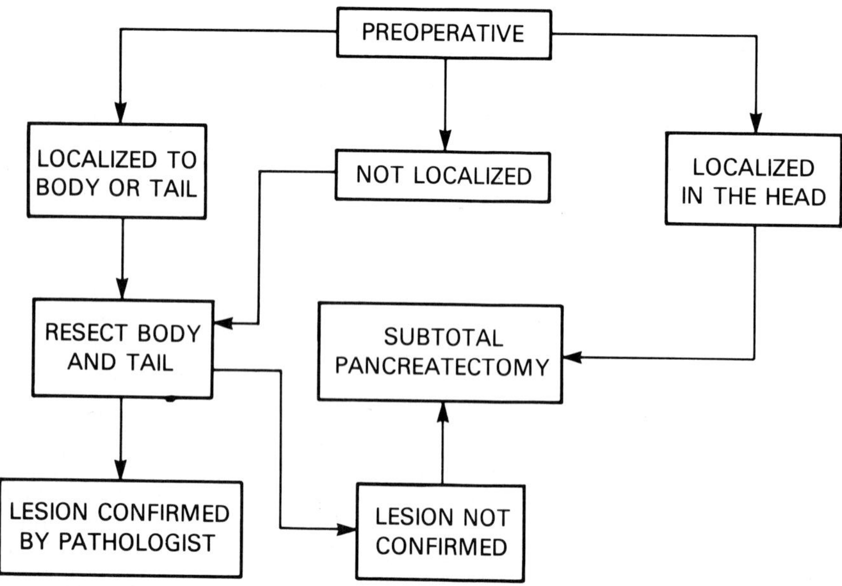

FIG. 28-37. Intra-operative approach to the patient with an unequivocal diagnosis of a functional non-gastrin producing tumor that cannot be found at surgery.

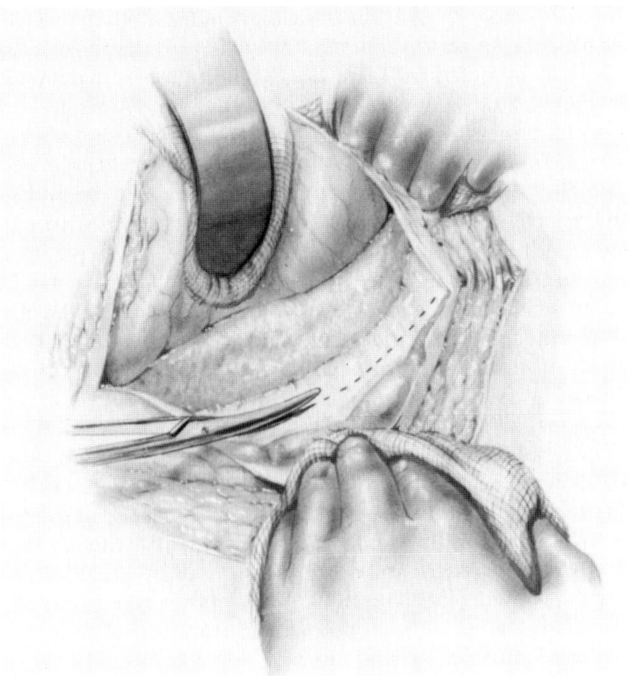

FIG. 28-38. Intra-operative mobilization of the tail of the pancreas, beginning with an exposure through the lesser sac and an incision along the inferior border of the pancreas. (Edis AJ, Ayala LA, Egdahl RH: Manual of Endocrine Surgery, p 87. New York, Springer-Verlag, 1975)

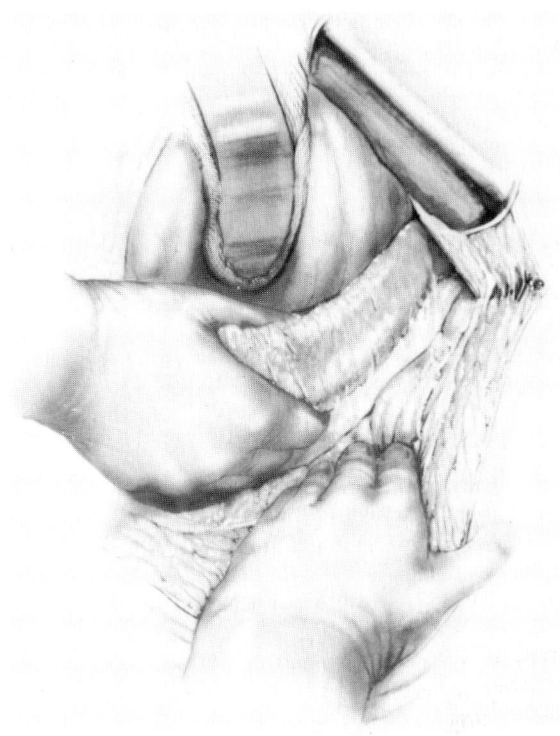

FIG. 28-39. Palpation of the tail of the pancreas to locate a small islet cell tumor. (Edis AJ, Ayala LA, Egdahl RH: Manual of Endocrine Surgery, p 86. New York, Springer-Verlag, 1975)

SUBTOTAL PANCREATECTOMY

The same procedure is performed, only the extension is continued to the right of the mesenteric vessels, with care to preserve the patency of the inferior mesenteric and portal veins.

PANCREATICODUODENECTOMY OR TOTAL PANCREATECTOMY

This should be a rare operation for functional islet cell tumors. It will occasionally be indicated for large benign and malignant non-functional tumors that obstruct duodenum and biliary tree.

TREATMENT OF METASTATIC DISEASE

ABLATION

Surgical resection of functional metastases should be considered. In situations where this is not possible, embolization of functional liver metastases by way of the hepatic artery should certainly be considered.[320]

Chemotherapy can be used with cytotoxic agents or antihormonal agents.

CYTOTOXIC CHEMOTHERAPY

The cytotoxic chemotherapy of islet cell tumors has been a difficult area of clinical oncology to interpret. This has resulted from the rarity of these diseases and the fact that the biological and clinical characteristics of the various islet cell malignant diseases can be quite different. A factor related to islet cell tumors that makes the interpretation of response to chemotherapy difficult is that criteria of response include objective tumor regression, amelioration of hormone-related syndromes, and measurement of decreased circulating hormone levels. Thus, some reported responses may relate to biochemical improvement while others may, in the classic sense, refer to tumor regression.

The chemotherapy of islet cell tumors has centered around the use of one drug—streptozotocin. This drug is an antibiotic isolated from the fermentation cultures of *Streptomyces acromogenes*. Chemically, it is composed of the known anticancer agent, 1-methyl-1-nitrosourea, combined with glucose.[321] The diabetogenic properties of streptozotocin were discovered during its initial preclinical toxicologic evaluation.[322] It was noted that a single IV dose could produce a permanent diabetic state in rodents, dogs, and monkeys by the selective destruction of the pancreatic B cell. Because of its diabetogenic properties, an attempt has been made to use streptozotocin in the treatment of malignant insulinomas.

In a series of 29 cases of insulinoma in which measurable disease was present, 48% of patients had an objective reduction in tumor mass, and 17% were considered to have obtained complete remission status with streptozotocin therapy.[323] Some 60% of patients manifested an objective biochemical response to therapy as measured by decreases in plasma insulin levels. It is clear that treatment with streptozotocin may improve the quality of life in patients with insulinoma.

TABLE 28-41. Chemotherapy for Metastatic Islet Cell Carcinoma—Use of Streptozotocin

Biochemical response	64%
Measurable response	50%
Increased one year survival	
Toxicity—Renal	65%*
Hepatic	67%
Hematologic	20%
Toxicity (nausea and vomiting)	98%
Responders vs non-responders = Doubling in median survival	

*Five deaths from renal failure

(Broder LE, Carter SK: Results of therapy with streptozotocin in 52 patients. Ann Intern Med 79:108–118, 1973)

There is also improvement in survival in responding as opposed to non-responding patients. The survival for responding patients in Broder and Carter's series was a median of 744 days vs a median of 298 for non-responding patients (see Table 28-41).[323] However, clear definition of survival benefits will require Phase III trials.

When streptozotocin is used as a single agent, two schedules are commonly used. The first is 1–2 g/m² IV weekly and the second is 500 mg/m² qd x 5 days repeated every 3–4 weeks. Both schedules must be adjusted if drug toxicity is seen.

The toxicities associated with streptozotocin treatment are well-known. Nausea and vomiting are experienced by almost all patients but with variable severity. These symptoms are partially prevented or controlled by phenothiazine antiemetics, and may diminish if the 5-day schedule is used. Renal tubular damage is the most common serious drug toxicity and its occurrence severely limits the potential for further treatment.[341] The earliest manifestation is the development of proteinuria in the range of 400–1,500 mg/24 hours. With more significant nephrotoxicity, excretion of up to 10 g of protein/24 hours has been documented. If unaccompanied by other renal function abnormalities, proteinuria is usually reversible in 2–4 weeks. Continued treatment may produce pronounced signs of proximal tubular damage, including aminoaciduria, phosphaturia, uricosuria, glycosuria, and renal tubular acidosis, all of which are potentially reversible. Nephrogenic diabetes insipidus, after large doses of the drug, and varying degrees of azotemia have been observed with streptozotocin.[341]

Serious renal toxicity can be avoided by close monitoring of urine for protein excretion and by stopping treatment until full reversal of abnormal renal function has been demonstrated.

Mild abnormalities in liver function may occur after streptozotocin therapy. This is manifested by a transient elevation in serum transaminases observed at the end of each course of treatment in many patients. These biochemical abnormalities have had no apparent clinical significance.[324] Although generally an non-myelosuppressive antitumor agent, streptozotocin has produced mild degrees of leukopenia, which is not dose-limiting. One case of profound bone marrow depression following a dose of 7.5 g/m² in a case of advanced malignant insulinoma previously treated with doses of 2.5 and 3.0 g/m² has been reported.[327,328] The very large dose of streptozotocin (7.5 g/m²) in this case is unique and may have changed the spectrum of qualitative toxicity of streptozotocin.

As can be noted in Table 28-42, the number of patients treated with single agent streptozotocin with non-insulinoma islet cell tumors is exceedingly small. In eight patients with nonfunctioning tumors, Moertel reported five partial responses.[324] In patients with the pancreatic cholera syndrome, two objective antitumor and symptomatic responses in patients with liver metastases were reported.[325] These patients were treated with hepatic artery infusions of streptozotocin; remissions lasted in excess of one year. The experience with streptozotocin in ZES is also anecedotal. However, Stadil and Schein have reported three cases in which objective tumor regression and decreased circulating gastrin levels were documented.[326–328]

The combination chemotherapy of islet cell tumors is now being actively pursued (see Table 28-42).[329,330] In 1973, Moertel reported that six of eight patients responded to the combination of 5-fluorouracil and streptozotocin; that combination was brought into a Phase III trial by the Eastern Cooperative Oncology Group (ECOG).[329,330] In this study, 81 evaluable patients with a variety of metastatic islet cell tumors were randomized between 5-fluorouracil, 400 mg/m² IV every day for five days plus streptozotocin, 500 mg/m² IV every day for five days, and streptozotocin alone, 500 mg/m² IV every day for five days. Both regimens were repeated every 6 weeks. The combination of 5-fluorouracil plus streptozotocin was clearly superior to streptozotocin alone. Twenty-five of 40 patients (63%) receiving the two drugs manifested complete or partial responses. This compared to 14/41 (34%) in the streptozotocin alone arm. This difference was highly significant ($p = 0.01$). Some 33% of patients receiving the combination had a complete response, whereas only 12% of those on streptozotocin showed complete disappearance of disease ($p < .05$). The median survivals were 26 months for the combination and 16 months for the single agent.

A new three-armed study is currently underway in the ECOG (see Table 28-42). The protocol compares the best previous treatment (5-fluorouracil plus streptozotocin) to either streptozotocin plus adriamycin or chlorozotocin as a single agent.

The clinical oncologist managing the patient with unresectable islet tumor has two options in designing a therapeutic program. The currently recommended regimen is 5-fluorouracil, 400 mg/m² IV every day for five days, plus streptozotocin, 500 mg/m² every day for five days. This regimen should be repeated every 6 weeks with appropriate monitoring and dose modification for toxicity. An alternative regimen undergoing evaluation at the National Cancer Institute for non-beta cell tumor is outlined in Table 28-43.

Other agents have been reported as being effective (*e.g.*, DTIC in glucagonoma), but await more extensive evaluation.[342]

ANTIHORMONAL THERAPY

Antihormonal therapy for the hormonal consequences of tumor hormone production has been extensively studied. The

TABLE 28-42. Chemotherapy of Islet Carcinoma

REGIMEN		DISEASE	NO. PATIENTS	NO. RESPONSE (%)	REF
Streptozotocin, 1–2 mg/m² IV q wk or 500 mg/m² IV × 5 days q 4–6 weeks		Insulinoma Nonfunctioning Pancreatic cholera Zollinger–Ellison	29 8 2 3	14 (48) 5 (65) 2 3	323 324 325 326 327
5-fluorouracil (5-FU), various schedules		Insulinoma	12	3 (25)	323
Streptozotocin, 500 mg/m² × 5 + 5-FU 400 mg/m² × 5	q 6 wk	Mixed	8	6 (75)	329
Streptozotocin, 500 mg/m² × 5 + 5-FU 400 mg/m²	q 6 wk	Mixed	40	25 (63)	330
vs Streptozotocin, 500 mg/m² × 5 q 6 wk			41	14 (34)	
Streptozotocin, 500 mg/m² × 5 + 5-FU 400 mg/m² × 5	q 6 wk		31	In progress	(ECOG)
vs (Adriamycin), Doxorubicin 50 mg/m² day 1 and 22 + Streptozotocin, 500 mg/m² × 5	q 6 wk				
vs Chlorozotocin, 150 mg/m²	q 7 wk				

most widely used agents are diazoxide for insulinomas and cimetidine for ZES. However, numerous other hormonal agents have been used (see Table 28-44).

Insulinoma

Diazoxide is a non-diuretic benzothiadiazine with a hypotensive and hyperglycemic action. It was synthesised in 1961 as a hypotensive agent.[331] The recognition of its hyperglycemic effects was made later.[332–334] Diazoxide was probably first used in man as an hyperglycemia agent; it was used for islet cell tumors in 1964.[335,336] In doses of 300–500 mg/day, diazoxide is well tolerated. Side effects such as nausea occur, but are usually tolerable. In children, the dose is 1–5 mg/kg body weight/day.

Diazoxide is thought to act by directly suppressing insulin release, although concomitant increase in plasma catecholamines with consequent insulin suppression and glycogenolysis has also been suggested.[337,338]

Diazoxide, when effective at low dose and without side effects, can be used in the patient suspected of having a benign insulinoma to improve operative risk by weight reduction, pulmonary toilet, and so forth.

TABLE 28-43. Protocol for Chemotherapy in Metastatic Non-Beta Cell Islet Neoplasms

	TREATMENT REGIMEN (Day) 1	8	29	36
5-FU, 600 mg/m²	+	+	+	+
STZ, 1.5 g/m²	+	+	+	+
ADR, 40 mg/m²	+	−	+	−

Repeated until progression, maximal dosage, or toxicity.
5-FU = 5-fluorouracil
STZ = Streptozotocin
ADR = Adriamycin

TABLE 28-44. Antihormonal Therapy for Functional Pancreatic Endocrine Neoplasms

TUMOR HORMONE	ANTI-HORMONAL DRUG	REF	DOSE
Insulin	Diazoxide	288	300–800 mg qd
	Somatostatin	346	—
	Corticosteroids	— 288	100 mg qd of cortisone equivalent
	Glucagon		1 mg
Glucagon	Somatostatin	348	
	Diphenylhydantoin	349	1 gm qd
VIP	Indomethacin	308	—
	Lithium	351	—
	Corticosteroids	350	—
Gastrin	Somatostatin	346,348	—
	Cimetidine	272	2,000–5,000 mg

In patients with metastatic inoperable insulinoma diazoxide can be used in the highest tolerated dose to control symptoms.

Corticosteroids have been widely employed in management and treatment of benign and malignant insulinoma. Their use should be avoided whenever possible. The results are not sustained and the inevitable side effects of hypercorticolism difficult to manage. It is particularly disturbing to see a patient undergo an unsuccessful operation and then be placed on high-dose corticoid therapy, so that by the time of referral for reoperation the patient is another 60 pounds overweight! Dose is variable; when used, it should be the lowest possible dose to prevent symptoms.[339]

Glucagon had been used but has such a short effective life span (less than 8 hr) that it is not of value.[340]

Zollinger–Ellison Syndrome

Cimetidine is the current drug of choice. The initial U.S. experience has been reviewed (see Table 28-45). In other reports, doses of up to 21 gm/day have been employed for as long as 18 months.[345] The optimum dose appears to be between 1.2 and 1.6 g/day.

TABLE 28-45. Use of Cimetidine in Zollinger–Ellison Syndrome

Number of cases treated = 61	
Dosage required	1200 mg qd controls* 66%
	2400 mg controls 25%
	1200 mg and anticholinergic controls 90%
Ulcer healing by endoscopy	22/47 (47%)
Ulcer healing by radiograph	13/45 (29%)
Ulcer healing by both	26/55 (45%)
Pain relief at one month	61/61 (100%)
Side effects	
Gynecomastia	6/61 (10%)
Liver function test abnormal	3/61 (5%)

McCarthy DM: Report on the United States experience with cimetidine in Zollinger–Ellison and other secretory states. Gastroenterology 74:453–458, 1978

*Controls = make normal acid production.

Alternative Hormonal Agonists and Antagonists

The most exciting prospects are the somatostatin analogues.[346,347] Recently, a long-acting analogue of somatostatin has been described. The analogue given subcutaneously suppressed tumor hormonal production in eight patients with insulinomas, glucagonomas, and gastrinomas for up to 8 hours.[348]

In specific cases indomethacin, diphenylhydantoin, and lithium have been claimed to be effective.[349–351]

RESULTS

BENIGN DISEASE

Resection of a benign functional endocrine tumor should result in long-term cure. In a recent review of 72 patients with insulinoma, 63 were biochemically cured, six were malignant. In most cases, enucleation, partial pancreatectomy, or a combination of both were the procedures of choice.[204,223,245,292] Operative mortality is approximately 5% for enucleation or

TABLE 28-46. Insulinoma—Operative Mortality

	NUMBER	% MORTALITY
Extirpation	297	4.7
Distal Pancreatectomy	211	4.7
Whipple	11	9.9
Subtotal Pancreatectomy	13	15.3
Total Pancreatectomy	17	11.7

Filipi CJ, Higgins GA: Diagnosis and Management of insulinoma. Ann J Surg 125:231–239, 1973

TABLE 28-47. Chemotherapeutic Treatment of Functional Islet Cell Carcinoma

29 PATIENTS	
CR	17%
PR > 50%	17%
PR 25–50%	14%

Median duration from start of treatment: 13+ months
CR = Complete response
PR = Partial response
Schein PS: Chemotherapeutic management of hormone secreting endocrine malignancies. Cancer 30:1616–1626, 1972

distal pancreatectomy for insulinomas, but rises to 15% for more extensive resections (see Table 28-46).[286,287]

MALIGNANT DISEASE

The results of varying experiences with chemotherapy for islet cell tumors are outlined in Tables 28-41, 28-42, and 28-47.[343] The most recent report using streptozotocin alone, 0.5–1.5 g/m²/week IV, with an induction dose of 6–8 g followed by a maintenance dose every 4th or 5th week, has emphasized the need for more effective regimens (see Table 28-48).[244]

TABLE 28-48. Use of Streptozotocin in Metastatic Endocrine Pancreatic Tumors

DISEASE	N	TOTAL DOSE STZ–RANGE (g)	PR	CR	FOLLOW-UP RANGE (Monthly)
Insulinoma	6	6–34	5	0	5–64
Gastrinoma	3	6–24	2	0	2–15
Glucagonoma	2	4–8	0	0	2–10
VIP-oma	4	10–17	2	1	12–36
Mixed	6	4–30	2	2	2–30

STZ = streptozotocin
(Oberg K, Lundquist G, Bostrom H: The effects of streptozotocin in the treatment of endocrine pancreatic tumors and carcinoids. In Groesbeck T (ed): Streptozotocin. New York, Elsevier Publishing Co, 1981.)

Carcinoid Tumors

with John S. Macdonald

Carcinoid tumors of the intestinal tract are uncommon neoplasms thought to arise from the basigranular, argentaffin cells in the base of the intestinal crypts.[352] Carcinoid tumors of other sites have since been reported with increasing frequency. They are thought to be neuroectodermal derivations associated with the APUD series.[353]

HISTORIC BACKGROUND OF CARCINOID TUMORS

Langhans is credited with the first description of a carcinoid of the ileum in 1867. Beger was probably the first to describe carcinoma of the appendix, although Lubarsch is classically attributed the first description of the features of the carcinoid tumor, published in 1888.[354] "Karzinoide" was introduced in 1890 by Obendorfer in an effort to stress the benign nature of these tumors. The more malignant nature of the tumors was not emphasized until the late 1940's, although metastases were known in 1890.[355,356]

EPIDEMIOLOGY AND GENETICS

An excess of 4,000 carcinoids in various organs have been described.[357] The incidence in autopsy series of GI carcinoids has been reported from 0.2–1.1%.[354,358–360] The figure is probably much closer to the higher than the lower percentage.

In a compilation of 418,186 surgical cases and 26,401 autopsies from seven hospitals, MacDonald found an incidence of proven carcinoid in 102/418,186 (.02%) surgical cases and 254/26,401 (1.0%) autopsy cases.[360] The disparity in incidence results from the fact that carcinoids are rarely symptomatic, and thus are most commonly discovered incidentally at autopsy rather than as a symptomatic disease in a surgical patient. Moertel noted a similar situation in a study of 209 consecutive cases of carcinoid diagnosed at the Mayo Clinic. In this series, 137 cases of carcinoid were noted at autopsy, 72 were diagnosed at surgery.[301] In the autopsy series, only 4/137 (3.0%) patients had been symptomatic during life whereas 52/72 (72%) of the tumors in the surgical series produced clinically significant symptoms.

Distribution according to site varies widely. It is dependent on whether or not the study is clinical or at autopsy. Clinical carcinoids of the appendix are much more common than their incidence in autopsy series. In the most recent Seer data for 1973–1974 (representing approximately 10% of the U.S. population), the projected new incidence per year of malignant

TABLE 28-49. Organ Distribution of Carcinoid Tumors*

	% OF ALL CARCINOIDS	RANGE
Appendix	41.6%	35 → 45
Small Bowel	26.9%	20 → 33
Rectum and Sigmoid	17.1%	12 → 24
Lung and Bronchi	9.3%	4 → 14
Esophagus and Stomach	2.3%	2 → 3
Ovary	1.5%	0.3 → 0.9
Biliary Tract	0.21%	0.1 → 0.3

* See references 354, 357, 362, and 363

TABLE 28-50. Race, Age, and Sex Distribution of Malignant Carcinoid Tumors

	AGE	% OF TOTAL	% TOTAL, MALE	% TOTAL, FEMALE	% TOTAL, CAUCASIAN	BLACK
	0–4	0	0	0	0	0
	5–9	0	0	0	0	0
	10–14	1.3	1	1.5	1.2	3.9
	15–19	2.6	1	3.6	2.6	2.6
	20–24	4.2	3.9	4.4	3.8	7.8
	25–29	5.1	4.7	5.4	5.2	3.9
	30–34	4.7	3.1	5.8	4.6	5.2
	35–39	4.6	4.9	4.4	4.6	5.2
	40–44	6.4	7.0	5.9	5.9	11.7
	45–49	7.2	7.5	7.0	7.0	6.5
	50–54	7.9	8.0	7.8	7.4	10.4
	55–59	8.7	9.9	8.0	9.9	1.3
	60–64	12.5	11.2	13.4	12.7	11.7
	65–69	11.5	13.2	10.3	11.5	13.0
	70–74	9.4	11.2	8.3	9.8	5.2
	75–79	6.2	6.0	6.3	6.2	6.5
	80–84	4.3	4.4	4.2	4.2	3.9
	85+	3.3	2.8	3.6	3.4	1.3
TOTAL		974 (100%)	385 (100%)	589 (100%)	850 (100%)	77(100%)

From 974 malignant carcinoids documented from 1973–1977 by the SEER program

carcinoids is 2,000 new cases or approximately 1 per 100,000 of populations. The distribution by organ site is similar in collected series and in the end-results section of the Third National Cancer Survey (see Table 28-49).[362]

Carcinoid tumors have been described in the esophagus, stomach, duodenum, jejunum, ileum, bile ducts, pancreas, Meckel's diverticulum, appendix, colon, rectum, ovary, testis, larynx, thymus, and bronchus.[363,364]

The sex distribution of malignant carcinoids in the Seer program was 1.5:1 females:males. The tumors occur in all age groups (see Table 28-50). In terms of absolute incidence of tumors within the organ of origin, carcinoid is by far the most common tumor of the appendix, comprising approximately 77% of all apendiceal tumors, and is the second most frequent tumor of the small bowel, comprising 23% of all small bowel tumors and 47% of all malignant small bowel tumors.[357,361]

PATHOLOGY

Most of the carcinoid tumors are usually small, grayish-white, sometimes yellow nodules often encased by intact mucosa. The appendicular carcinoids are very small, hard, yellow to orange, commonly situated near the tip of the appendix. Carcinoids may ulcerate, particularly in the ileum and colon. Microscopically, the carcinoid tumor exhibits solid nests of malignant epithelial cells separated by a delicate connective tissue stroma. Cells may stain black with silver nitrate.

The distribution and pathologic characteristics of carcinoid tumors bear directly on the clinical manifestations produced. The size of the primary carcinoid correlates with the likelihood of metastases. In one series, only 2% of the tumors less than 1 cm in diameter evidenced metastases.[361] In contrast, 80% of tumors greater than 2 cm in diameter were associated with metastatic disease. The site of origin of carcinoid tumors is an important factor in the likelihood that a given tumor will produce the carcinoid syndrome. Sites of origin of carcinoid tumors are divided according to embryologic development.[365] Foregut carcinoids are in the area from the oral pharynx to mid-duodenum; midgut carcinoids originate in the small bowel and proximal colon; hindgut tumors are seen in the descending colon and rectum. The foregut and midgut carcinoids are commonly associated with the carcinoid syndrome, whereas the hindgut tumors are uncommonly associated with the carcinoid syndrome.

PATHOGENESIS

The most commonly accepted theory explaining the multiple hormonal production and multiple sites of origin of carcinoid tumors is that these tumors belong to the APUD series.[353,366] The hypothesis is that these APUD cells arising from the neural crest travel with the GI entoderm and are incorporated into the primitive gut. This allows for the frequently identified association with other multiple endocrine neoplasia syndromes (MEN).[367]

The carcinoid *syndrome* is infrequent in small intestine carcinoids, occurring in only 10% of all small intestine carcinoids.[368,369] For the syndrome to be manifest metastases must be present.[361] However, in the cases of bronchial carcinoid and carcinoids arising from teratomas of the ovary, the syndrome may be present without evidence of metastatic disease and will be reversed with resection of the localized tumor. This phenomenon is explained by venous drainage of the lung and ovary being systemic and bypassing the liver where the excessive serotonin from GI carcinoids is metabolized by monoamine oxidase.

Carcinoids of the small bowel are usually slow-growing. Because of their small size they may often be asymptomatic and discovered incidentally.[359,363,370]

The symptoms caused by carcinoid may result from three different characteristics of these tumors. First, there may be symptoms relating to the primary tumor. When small bowel lesions present symptoms, they are often nonspecific. Abdominal pain predominates with associated nausea and vomiting.[370] Intermittent obstruction can occur occasionally due to intussusception or to the associated perineoplastic fibrous reaction.[371] Rarely, the extensive desmoplastic reaction results in a palpable mass of obstructed small bowel loops.[372] Gastrointestinal bleeding is unusual.

Diagnostic delay is common, averaging 4 years. By the time of diagnosis, metastatic disease is common (as high as 90% in some series).[359,368,370,372–374] Clinical presentation is then predominantly due to the nature and type of hormone produced by the tumor and its metastases.

Carcinoid tumors most commonly metastasize to the liver, with bone and lung being the next most common sites.[375] Patients with symptomatic metastases may also have symptoms of primary bowel tumor since, as noted previously, metastatic potential correlates with the size of the primary tumor. Large primary lesions are likely to cause bowel symptoms. The symptoms that may be attributable to metastases include tender hepatomegaly, bone pain, and dyspnea.

The carcinoid syndrome is an unusual occurrence even in patients with documented tumors. Of the 209 patients in one series, only 14 (6.7%) manifested carcinoid syndrome.[361] Of all patients with liver metastases, only 45% exhibited symptoms compatible with the carcinoid syndrome. The aggregation of symptoms that may be associated with carcinoid tumor are dependent on the causative hormone or amine produced (see Table 28-51).

Serotonin (5-HT) is derived from the essential amino acid, tryptophan, by hydroxylation to 5-hydroxytryptophan (5-HTP), and then decarboxylation to 5-hydroxytryptamine (5-HT). The breakdown product of 5-HT is 5-hydroxyindole-aceticacid (5-HIAA), which is excreted in the urine as a sulfate and glucuronide conjugate. The rapid acceleration of tryptophan into sertonin synthesis in patients with carcinoid syndromes can lead to protein deprivation. The majority of serotonin produced by carcinoid tumors undergoes rapid catabolism. Less than 2% of systemic venous serotonin is not metabolized with a single passage through the pulmonary circulation.[376] As the half-life of serotonin is extremely short (probably less than one minute) and the hepatic extraction very high, patients need to produce vast quantities of the amine to produce symptoms. Though serotonin is not the solitary agent in many of the manifestations of the carcinoid syndrome, it is thought to be the predominant agent in production of the diarrhea.[377] This observation is supported since the diarrhea can be alleviated by serotonin antagonists such as methysergide, parachlorophenylalanine, and alpha-methyldopa. The breakdown of serotonin can be inhibited by the administration of a monoamine oxidase inhibitor such as iproniazid. The administration of serotonin does not, however, cause the characteristic carcinoid flush, which is thought to be caused predominantly by bradykinins and possibly gastrin.[267,278–281]

Multiple other tumors have been recorded as being produced, including growth hormone, ACTH, calcitonin, and prostaglandins.[382–386] Carcinoids arising from different sites may have different secretion patterns.

TABLE 28-51. Clinical Symptoms of Carcinoid Syndrome and Suspected Etiological Agent

Flushing	Bradykinin Hydroxytryptophan Prostaglandins
Telangiectasia	VIP
Diarrhea	Serotonin Prostaglandins Bradykinin
Bronchospasm	Bradykinin Histamine Prostaglandins
Endocardial fibrosis	Serotonin
Glucose intolerance	Serotonin
Arthropathy	Serotonin
Hypotension	Serotonin

Symptoms seen in the carcinoid syndrome are likely to have multifactorial etiology and there may well be other mediators. For example, although 5-HT is the mediator commonly associated with carcinoid tumors, its precursor compound, 5-hydroxytryptophan, may be produced preferentially by gastric and bronchial carcinoids that lack the enzyme L-amino acid decarboxylase.

Occasionally, significant fibrosing reactions may be seen in patients with carcinoid syndrome. For example, an endocardial fibrosis syndrome may occur.[387] Although the right side of the heart is most commonly involved, the left side is not entirely spared. The most common lesions are tricuspid insufficiency and pulmonary regurgitation. When left-sided cardiac involvement is present, the mitral valve is frequently affected.[387]

The combination of cardiac valvular disease and episodes of hypotension and vascular collapse seen in the carcinoid syndrome can result in high-output cardiac failure. The cause of cardiac valvular fibrosis in the carcinoid syndrome is not clear, although it too has been attributed to serotonin.[388] Fibrosis can also occur in the abdomen with local fibrosis in the bowel and mesentery resulting in intestinal obstruction or infarction.[389]

DIAGNOSIS

A non-functioning carcinoid tumor is diagnosed by biopsy and histologic section.

The diagnosis of the carcinoid syndrome depends on histopathological confirmation of the characteristic histology, associated with the clinical syndrome consistent with excessive hormone production. Intestinal carcinoids are difficult to diagnose prior to onset of symptoms due to metastatic disease. Occasionally, contrast radiography can identify filling defects or angulation due to the fibrous reaction, which may suggest the diagnosis. Obvious or suspected metastatic disease can be identified by liver spleen scan, CT, ultrasound, or by the vascular lesions identified by arteriography.

Patients with functioning carcinoids may have this tumor diagnosed by measuring biologically active products excreted by the tumor. Twenty-four hour urine excretion of 5-hydroxyindoleacetic acid (5-HIAA) is the most useful.[375] If 5-HIAA is greater than 9 mg/24 hours in a patient without malabsorption or greater than 30 mg/24 hours in a patient with malabsorption, the diagnosis is confirmed. False positive tests can be caused by the ingestion of foods such as bananas, pineapples, and some nuts. Therefore, patients should be cautioned to avoid these foods before the test. Medication containing reserpine or glycerol guiacolate should also be avoided. Phenothiazines should not be taken before assaying the urine for 5-HIAA since this class of drug can also produce false negative tests.

In the rare foregut carcinoid tumors that lack L-amino acid decarboxylase, 5-HIAA may not be produced, but instead 5-hydroxytryptophan may be the major product. This may be assayed chromatographically.

TREATMENT

Surgical excision is the treatment of choice. Small tumors confined to the intestinal mucosa and diagnosed incidentally can be effectively treated by local excision.

Because most carcinoids are slow growing, aggressive resection of bulk disease, (as with other hormonally-active tumors) may well improve symptoms and survival. Hepatic resection of accessible lesions should always be considered; palliative procedures to bypass obstructed loops not amenable to resection should be performed.

In patients with unresectable, metastatic, or recurrent carcinoid after resection, two approaches to treatment have been used.[388] These are antihormonal measures to ameliorate symptoms caused by the production of biologically-active mediators by carcinoid tumors and cytotoxic chemotherapy aimed at destroying tumor.

ANTIHORMONAL THERAPY

Anti-endocrine therapies capable of antagonizing the principal pharmacologic mediators of the carcinoid syndrome (serotonin, and bradykinin) have undergone active study.[390] The serotonin-related symptoms of watery diarrhea, abdominal colic, and malabsorption have received the greatest attention and therapeutic investigation by clinical pharmacologists.[391] When of mild or moderate severity, these GI manifestations may successfully be managed with symptomatic treatment, such as opiates and diphenoxylate hydrochloride with atropine (Lomotil). With more severe symptoms, peripheral antagonists of serotonin, such as methysergide and cyproheptadine, have been effective in controlling diarrhea; in some cases they have reversed malabsorption.[392]

In managing patients with carcinoid syndrome, it is important to avoid exacerbating the syndrome by inadvertently placing a patient on drugs that inhibit serotonin degradation. Monoamine oxidase inhibitors, such as iproniazid, which may block the degradation of serotonin to its inactive urinary excretion metabolites should be avoided.

There has been clinical investigation into the use of agents that are known inhibitors of serotonin synthesis. One of the first to undergo clinical trial was alpha-methyldopa. This agent is capable of decreasing serotonin production by inhibiting the decarboxylation of 5-HTP to serotonin. Results with this compound have been disappointing, except for the rarely seen patients with 5-HTP-secreting metastatic carcinoid of foregut origin.

Parachlorophenylalanine (PCAC) inhibits the enzyme tryptophan 5-hydroxylase, which catalizes the conversion of the amino acid to 5-HTP, the immediate precursor of serotonin. PCAC at doses of 2–4 g/24 hours has been demonstrated to reduce the urinary excretion of 5-hydroxyindoleacetic acid (an indirect measurement of 5-hydroxyindole synthesis) by 51–81% in patients with malignant carcinoid tumors.[394,395] This was accompanied by good contol of diarrhea and other GI symptoms. PCAC has several toxicities. In addition to lethargy and headaches, chronic administration may be accompanied by depression, anxiety, and confusional states. An allergic eosinophilia appearing 2–weeks after initiation of treatment with PCAC has been observed in 50% of patients. This abnormality is rapidly reversible with withdrawal of the drug, reappears promptly with rechallenge, and mandates cessation of PCAC therapy. Continued treatment in the face of eosinophilia has lead to the development of urticaria, asthma, and pulmonary infiltrates (Loeffler's syndrome).[379] Carcinoid tumors may synthesize and release the proteolytic enzyme, kallikrein, which acts upon a specific α_2-globulin to generate bradykin in a mediator of the carcinoid flush. Phenothiazines antagonize the peripheral action of kinins and have been marginally effective in controlling flushing in some patients.[396] Corticosteroids have been reported to significantly decrease or prevent the attacks of flushing, particularly in cases of bronchial carcinoid.[397,398] Catecholamines can provoke an attack of flushing, probably based on stimulating the release and activation of bradykinin from carcinoid tumors.[378] Based on this, α-adrenergic blocking agents, such as phentolamine, have been proposed as therapeutic agents for patients with this syndrome.[399]

Although prostaglandins appear to have a role in the pathogenesis of the carcinoid syndrome and may potentiate both diarrhea and flushing, few reports exist evaluating the use of prostaglandin synthetase inhibitors in this disease.[375] It would seem reasonable to study the effect of indomethacin and aspirin or the more recently developed inhibitors of prostaglandin synthetase in patients with carcinoid syndrome and elevated prostaglandin plasma levels. More recently, histamine receptor antagonists such as cimetidine have been used with varying success.[380]

ANTITUMOR THERAPY

Cytotoxic chemotherapy of carcinoid tumors has received little attention. In a significant proportion of patients, the disease may remain indolent and active antitumor management may not necessarily be required.[359,361] However, there are patients with more aggressive tumor growth who will present with progressive liver metastases, signs of partial or impending complete intestinal obstruction, ascites, or severe and uncontrollable symptoms for whom anticancer therapy should be considered. Most chemotherapy data in patients with metastatic carcinoids are isolated case reports. This is related to the relative rarity of this disease in any hospital

TABLE 28-52. Combination Chemotherapy Studies in Carcinoid Tumors

REGIMEN	PATIENTS	RESPONSE (%)	REFERENCE
5-FU plus Streptozotocin vs Cyclophosphamide plus Streptozotocin	42 47	14 (33%) 12 (27%)	408
5-FU plus Streptozotocin	9	6 (66%)	402
5-FU plus Streptozotocin	10	2 (20%)	409
Cyclophosphamide plus Methotrexate	11	6 (55%)	375
5-FU plus Streptozotocin vs Doxorubicin (Adriamycin)	146	in progress	ECOG
5-FU plus Doxorubicin (Adriamycin) plus Cyclophosphamide	—	in progress	M. D. Anderson
5-FU plus Doxorubicin (Adriamycin) plus Streptozotocin plus Cyclophoshamide	—	in progress	SWOG

5-FU = 5-Fluorouracil
ECOG = Eastern Cooperative Oncology Group
SWOG = Southwest Oncology Group

center. Cyclophosphamide, thioTEPA, and nitrogen mustard have all produced objective reductions in tumor mass accompanied by subjective improvement.[393,400] 5-Fluorouracil (5-FU) has produced remissions when administered by either the IV or direct intra-arterial route; Moertel has reported that 6/15 (40%) patients exhibited partial response to 5-FU.[401,402] Streptozotocin has been reported to cause objective tumor regression in 3/6 patients, but these remissions were short-lived.[403] However, no response was documented in eight cases treated at the National Cancer Institute with a comparable streptozotocin schedule.[404,405] Case reports have suggested that doxorubicin (adriamycin) and DTIC (Dacarbazine) may have single agent activity in this disease; both these drugs need further evaluation.[406,407]

The development of combination chemotherapy for malignant carcinoids also has suffered from the relative paucity of cases of this disease (see Table 28-52). Small Phase II studies have reported excellent results with partial responses in 6/11 (55%) patients treated with methotrexate + cyclophosphamide and in 6/9 (66%) patients receiving 5-FU + streptozotocin. However, only one reasonably large cooperative trial has been reported.[408] This Phase III trial was performed by the Eastern Cooperative Oncology Group (ECOG) and compared the combination of 5-FU + streptozotocin with streptozotocin and cyclophosphamide. The 5-FU + streptozotocin regimen was chosen because of promising pilot data reported from the Mayo Clinic in which 6/9 patients with metastatic carcinoid responded to this program.[502] The results of the ECOG study demonstrated that 12/47 (27%) patients responded to cyclophosphamide + streptozotocin and 14/42 (33%) responded to the 5-FU + streptozotocin regimen. These results were not significantly different. In patients with carcinoids primary to the small bowel, the response rates were 45% for 5-FU + streptozotocin compared to 33% for cyclophosphamide + streptozotocin. There were no differences in survival between the two treatment arms. Of note in this study was a marked difference in median survival according to the site of primary tumor. The median survival, according to sites of origin, were as follows: small bowel 29.3 months; pancreas, 21.6 months; lung 14.9 months; colon, 10.1 months; and unknown primary, 8.0 months.

These data emphasize the varied natural history of carcinoid tumors and the necessity of carefully evaluating the need to aggressively manage patients with this disease. The clinician must make important decisions as to whether a given patient should be treated and, if treatment is to be initiated, at what point should it start. The oncologist treating a patient with severe carcinoid syndrome also must be aware that effective chemotherapy could result in a potentially lethal carcinoid crisis secondary to tumor lysis.[402] In general, the patient with clearly progressive metastatic disease with or without symptoms is a candidate for chemotherapy. A patient with the carcinoid syndrome whose symptoms are not controlled by the pharmacologic antagonists previously described should also be considered for chemotherapy. There are a number of combination chemotherapy trials that are in progress that should give valuable information. The currently recommended treatment would be 5-FU + streptozotocin.[408] 5-Fluorouracil (500 mg/m^2) + streptozotocin (500 mg/m^2) are administered daily for 5 consecutive days with cycles repeated every 6 weeks. This regimen is generally well-tolerated, although clinicians must be aware of the potential of streptozotocin to produce nephrotoxicity. If the pre-treatment 24-hour urinary 5-HIAA exceeds 150 mg, or if the symptoms of carcinoid syndrome are profound, a 50% reduced chemotherapy dose should be given during the first cycle. This will lessen the probability of precipitating carcinoid crisis.[409]

RADIATION THERAPY

Radiation therapy is ineffective, although for extensive liver disease some palliation by liver irradiation has been claimed.[410]

RESULTS

In patients with small bowel carcinoid without distant metastases in whom surgical removal of all gross disease is possible, the prognosis is good. In the one series of 72 operated cases, the actuarial 5-year survival in patients undergoing resection of all grossly apparent disease was 90%.[361] Nodal or peritoneal metastases were present in most of these patients. Data developed from this series point out the relatively indolent nature of this disease after surgical resection. In patients recurring after operation, the average time to the development of recurrent tumor was 8 years.

Five-year survivals for stomatch (52%), small intestine (54%), appendix (99–100%), colon (52%), rectum (76–83%), and bronchopulmonary (87%) have been reported.[362,411–413]

SCREENING

Screening should be performed in patients with the characteristic syndrome and in patients with suggestive symptoms within a multiple endocrine neoplasia syndrome.

Multiple Endocrine Neoplasia Syndrome

The multiple endocrine neoplasia (MEN) syndromes are conventionally divided into type I, type II-A, and type II-B. The components of these syndromes are illustrated on Tables 28-53 and 28-54.[414–416]

Type I syndrome mainly involves the parathyroid, pituitary, and pancreatic islet cells. On rare occasions adrenal and thyroid adenomas are also found. Even more uncommonly, the carcinoid syndrome is present.

As efforts are made to identify the islet cell tumors with specific immunohistochemistry, we can expect that other cell types such as somatostatin and glucagon will be more commonly identified. The potential for multiple islet cell tumors of different cell types within the same patient has been clearly identified.

Multiple endocrine neoplasia type II-A involves medullary carcinoma of the thyroid gland. This occurs in 100% of patients, being bilateral in all. Medullary carcinoma of the thyroid can occur in sporadic form, but in the latter situation, it is much less commonly bilateral. The adrenal gland is involved with adrenal medullary pheochromocytoma in about half of the affected kindreds.[417–419] The parathyroid glands are involved, but to a much lesser extent than in the type I syndrome.

Type II-B patients have a characteristic marfanoid habitus, with tumors that involve the thyroid with medullary carcinoma, adrenal pheochromocytoma, and neuronal changes manifested by mucosal neuromas and intestinal ganglioneuromas. All patients in this kindred will have the neuroma manifestations and the majority will have medullary carcinoma. Parathyroid disease, however, is uncommon, occurring in less than 4% of patients.[420–424]

HISTORY

MEN I

The first report of multiple endocrine tumors in an individual patient was recorded in 1903 by Erdheim. This patient had a pituitary tumor with multiple gland parathyroid disease. In

TABLE 28-53. Multiple Endocrine Neoplasia Type I

ORGAN-TISSUE	NEOPLASM	% AFFECTED
Parathyroid	Hyperplasia	90%
Pituitary	Adenoma	65%
Pancreas	Islet cell	75%
	Islet cell (Nonβ)	50%
	Islet cell (β)	25%
Adipocyte	Adenolipomata—	Rare
Adrenal	Cortical adenoma	Rare
Thyroid	Adenoma	Rare
Multiple	Carcinoid	Rare

TABLE 28-54. Multiple Endocrine Neoplasia Type II

ORGAN	NEOPLASM	% AFFECTED
TYPE II A		
Thyroid	Medullary carcinoma (Bilateral in 90–100%)	100%
Adrenal	Pheochromocytoma (30–80% Bilateral)	>50%[417]
Parathyroid	Hyperparathyroidism (Chief cell hyperplasia of four glands)	20%
TYPE II B		
Thyroid	Medullary carcinoma	>76%[418]
Adrenal	Pheochromocytoma	34[2]–56%[419]
Parathyroid	Hyperparathyroidism	<4%
Neuron	Mucosal neuromas, Intestinal ganglioneuromas	100%[420]

1927, Cushing reported a similar patient with an eosinophilic adenoma of the pituitary, two parathyroid "adenomas," and a pancreatic islet cell tumor.[416] In 1953, Underdahl reported eight patients with multiple adenomas involving pituitary islet cells of the pancreas and the parathyroid glands.[425] In 1954, Wermer brought together the familial association of cases involving pituitary, pancreas, and parathyroid.[426] This was the first suggestion that this association was due to some genetic defect. By 1961, Schmid postulated that the Zollinger-Ellison syndrome (ZES) described by Dr. Wermer was probably part of the same genetic defect, but with some degree of differing penetrance.[427] The association of adrenal cortical and thyroid adenomas with the syndrome was suggested by Ballard in 1964.[416]

MEN II

MEN II began with the description by Hazard in 1959 of solid or medullary carcinoma of the thyroid gland.[429] In 1961, Dr. John Sipple from the State University of New York at Syracuse described the association of pheochromocytoma and thyroid cancer, noting that there were six thyroid cancers in 537 patients with pheochromocytoma, 14 times the expected incidence.[430] In 1965, Dr. E. D. Williams of London Hospital associated medullary carcinoma with a family history and bilateral pheochromocytoma.[431] Dr. Williams raised the question of the association of parathyroid disease with this entity and in 1966, he described the parafollicular cell origin of the medullary carcinoma, going on to describe the presence of mucosal neuromas.[431–433] In 1968, Dr. Steiner further divided the MEN II syndromes into a II-B variety, which described the characteristic habitus and neuronal changes that went with Type II.[434] Subsequent reports have expanded knowledge of MEN II.[435–444]

The history of thyrocalcitonin (TCT) is different. In 1962, Dr. Carr postulated the presence of a thyrocalcitonin. In 1964, Ostrow identified the parafollicular cell origin of TCT. In 1966, Anthony Pearse described the C cell.[445] In 1968, Melvin and others made the association of the hypocalcemic effects of TCT.[446] With the development in 1970 by Tashjian of radioimmunoassay for thyrocalcitonin, progress began to move much more rapidly, advanced by increased sophistication of immunocytochemistry.[447–451]

EPIDEMIOLOGY

The true incidence and prevalence of medullary carcinoma of the thyroid are unknown, as it can occur in sporadic or in familial forms. With screening for TCT, the diagnosis can be expected to be more readily made. As best as can be derived from the 10-state survey between 1973 and 1977, we would expect nationwide, approximately 250 new cases of medullary carcinoma, both sporadic and familial, to occur each year. From 1973–1977, there was a 100% increase in the diagnosis of medullary carcinoma. This increase has continued and the true presentation of new lesions, (*i.e.*, new medullary carcinomas of the thyroid) is probably 450–500 cases per year in 1980; the majority of the increase being in familial cases.

NATURAL HISTORY

The natural history of familial medullary thyroid carcinoma has recently been described.[452] This study found that in a kindred numbering 107 patients being screened for TCT, 21 converted from normal to a secretory response during the interval 1970–1977. Initially, the test was a calcium challenge test followed in 1974 by the use of pentagastrin stimulation and, on occasion, both tests combined.[453–456] The combination of pentagastrin and calcium is a better test than either given alone.[454,456–458] In the study by Dr. Graze it was clearly noted that of 21 patients converting to an abnormal response, 20 of 21 showed C cell hyperplasia and 8 of the 20 also showed foci of carcinoma. With progressive earlier diagnosis, the tumors have been smaller and the age of diagnosis has moved from a range of 24 years to 64 years in 1970–71, to age 7–30 in 1971–78. However, the age distribution of the population has not changed. This aspect of the natural history should be emphasized as the results of total thyroidectomy without nodal spread can be translated into long-term normal life expectancy as opposed to 10-year survivals of 60% in those patients who have positive nodes at thyroidectomy.[459]

The occurrence of pheochromocytoma, however, has been identified in only 23% of patients under 20 years of age, but in 90% of those over 20.[420]

CLINICAL PRESENTATION

The clinical presentation of multiple endocrine neoplasia is either as one of the component diseases or as a consequence of a screening program.

SCREENING FOR MEN TYPE I

Once the kindred has been identified, all members should undergo screening for the disease. The initial screening is of serum calcium, parathyroid hormone, and serum phosphorus, in an effort to identify the presence of hyperparathyroidism because nearly all patients in these kindreds will have hyperparathyroidism.[460] Other tests can be performed, searching for pituitary and pancreatic islet cell lesions. The pancreatic islet cell lesions are much more readily diagnosed with the multiple available hormonal markers for insulin, gastrin, glucagon, somatostatin, VIP, and PP.[461]

SCREENING FOR MEN TYPE II

Screening for medullary carcinoma of the thyroid is performed by using a thyrocalcitonin assay, given the high predominance of patients expected to have medullary carcinoma of the thyroid or early C cell hyperplasia, patients who have normal base line levels are given provocative tests. These tests rely mainly on the use of either 15 mg of elemental calcium/kg IV over a 4-hour period or the use of pentagastrin (Peptavlon) in a dosage of 0.5 μg/kg administered as an IV bolus injection over 5 seconds. The combined two tests are apparently more accurate than the single test given alone.[454,457,458,462] The important consideration is to sample shortly after the pentagastrin infusion, as the elevations produced by pentagastrin are rapid and occur within the first few minutes. Using these provocative tests, the diagnosis can be made in young children prior to the development of medullary cancer. In one group of MEN II-B, the mean age at diagnosis of medullary thyroid cancer was 19 years in comparison to the mean age of 53 years for patients with sporadic medullary carcinoma of the thyroid.[420,438] In patients with the MEN II-A syndrome, the mean age for diagnosis in 50 patients with clinically evident medullary carcinoma was 34 years.[457] To improve the sensitivity of the test, some have advocated the use of central venous catheterization and sampling from jugular and innominate vessels during the course of stimulation. This can even further enhance the sensitivity and early diagnosis of patients subsequently shown to have C cell hyperplasia at surgery.[463,464]

TREATMENT

Treatment of each individual component of the MEN syndromes is referred to under the appropriate section of this chapter.

When the diagnosis has been made of more than one component of the syndrome in an individual patient, a decision as to which tumor to treat first will arise. In the MEN II syndrome, the pheochromocytoma should be removed first as it is the most life-threatening. The importance of total thyroidectomy as early as possible following the diagnosis of medullary carcinoma cannot be too highly emphasized, as this will result in long-term cure, provided the tumor is confined to the thyroid, or better still remains C cell hyperplasia.[464,465]

RESULTS

There are very few series of significant size to document the outcome of the MEN syndromes—as distinct from the outcome from each individual component. In one such group of 90 patients with the MEN II-B syndrome, 30% died of pheochromocytoma and 22% died of medullary carcinoma of the thyroid (see Table 28-55).[466]

FUTURE CONSIDERATIONS

With increased sophistication in radioimmunoassay and immunohistochemistry techniques it is likely that many other hormone-producing tumors will be identified within these syndromes. (The pancreatic tumors may be multiple in number and differ in the hormone produced by each, even within the same patient.) Indeed, even the differentiation between sporadic and hereditary forms is being made by immunocytochemical methods.[467,468]

Finally, it should be emphasized that although the MEN I and II syndromes have been presented as distinct entities, overlap can and does occur such that a pure combination may not always occur.[469–472] The elucidation of the genetics and penetrance of such components of each individual syndrome is still being evaluated; the screening for precursor lesions in component organs is also being vigorously pursued.[473] Whether the unifying concept of an APUD precursor cell will remain unscathed is the subject of intense scrutiny.[474]

TABLE 28-55. Multiple Endocrine Neoplasia Type II B

90 reported patients
56 female
28 belong to eight kindreds
Autosomal dominant
76% had MCT or C-cell hyperplasia
22% died of MCT (15/69)
Average age at death: 21 Years
<4% had parathyroid disease
34% had pheochromocytoma
30% (10/31) died of pheochromocytoma

(Carney JA, Sizemore GW, Hayles AB: Multiple endocrine neoplasia type 2B. Pathobiol Annu 8:104–153, 1978)

REFERENCES

1. Halsted WS: The operative story of goiter. Baltimore, Johns-Hopkins Hospital Reports 19:71, 1929
2. Halsted WS: Surgical papers vol II, p 257. Baltimore, The Johns-Hopkins Press, 1924
3. Ingbar SH, Woeber KA: The thyroid gland. In Williams RH (ed): Textbook of Endocrinology, 5th ed. Philadelphia, WB Saunders, 1974
4. Third National Cancer Survey. NCI Monograph 41, 1975
5. Sampson RJ, Woolner LB, Bahn RC et al: Occult thyroid carcinoma in Olmsted County, Minnesota: Prevalence at autopsy compared with that in Hiroshima and Nagaski. Cancer 34:2070–2076, 1974
6. Menck HR, Henderson BE: Cancer incidence rates in the Pacific Basin: Second symposium on epidemiology and cancer registries in the Pacific Basin. NCI Monograph 53:NIH Publication 79–1864, 1979
7. Shimaoka K, Sokal JE: Differentiation of benign and malignant thyroid nodules by scintiscan. Arch Int Med 114:36–39, 1974
8. Groesbeck HP: Evaluation of routine scintiscanning of nontoxic thyroid nodules 1: The preoperative diagnosis of thyroid carcinoma. Cancer 12: 1–5, 1959
9. Cope O, Dobyns BM, Hamlin E: What thyroid nodules are to be feared. J Clin Endocrinol Metal 9:1012–1022, 1949
10. Shimaoka K, Badillo J, Sokal JE et al: Clinical differentiation between thyroid cancer and benign goiter. JAMA 181:179–185, 1962
11. Black BM: The Encyclopedia of Medicine Surgery and Specialties, 3rd ed, vol 14, p 173. Philadelphia, FA Davis, 1962
12. Mahorner HR, Caylor HD, Schotthauer CF et al: Anat Rec 36:341, 1927
13. Meissner WA, Warren S: Tumors of the Thyroid Gland: Atlas of Tumor Pathology. Washington, Armed Forces Institute of Pathology, 1968
14. Clark RL, White EC, Russell WO: Total thyroidectomy for cancer of the thyroid: Significance of intraglandular dissemination. Ann Surg 149:858–866, 1959
15. Frazell EL, Foote FW: Papillary cancer of the thyroid: A review of 25 years of experience. Cancer 11:895–922, 1958
16. Hirabayashi RN, Lindsay S: Carcinoma of the thyroid gland: A statistical study of 390 patients. J Clin Endocrinol Metal 21:1596–1610, 1961
17. Geissinger WT, Horsley JS, Parker FP et al: Carcinoma of the thyroid. Ann Surg 179:734, 1974
18. McKenzie AD: The natural history of thyroid cancer. A report

of 102 cases analyzed 10 to 15 years after diagnosis. Arch Surg 102:274–277, 1971

19. Marchetta FC, Stoll HC, Maxwell WT et al: Carcinoma of the thyroid. Clinical and histologic features which influence the results of therapy. NY State Med J 57:3305–3314, 1957
20. Nishiyama RH, Dunn EL, Thompson NW: Anaplastic spindle cell and giant cell tumors of the thyroid gland. Cancer 30:113–127, 1972
21. Duffy BJ, Fitzgerald PJ: Cancer of the thyroid in children. Cancer 3: 1018–1032, 1950
22. Refetoff S, Harrison J, Karanfilski BT et al: Continuing occurrence of thyroid carcinoma after irradiation to the neck in infancy and childhood. N Engl J Med 292:171–175, 1975
23. Favus MJ, Schneider AB, Stachura ME et al: Thyroid malignancy occurring as a late consequence of head and neck irradiation: Evaluation of 1056 patients. N Engl J Med 294:1019–1025, 1976
24. Southwick HW: Radiation associated head and neck tumors. Am J Surg 134:438, 1977
25. Swelstad JA, Scanlon EF, Murphy ED et al: Thyroid disease following irradiation for benign conditions. Arch Surg 112:380, 1977
26. Scanlon EF, Berk RS, Khandekar JD: Post-irradiation neoplasia. Curr Prob Cancer III 6:1–45, 1978
27. Schneider AB, Favus MJ, Stachura ME et al: Incidence, prevalence and characteristics of radiation induced thyroid tumors. Am J Med 64:243–252, 1978
28. Modan B, Ron E, Werner A: Thyroid cancer following scalp irradiation. Radiology 123:741, 1977
29. Hempelmann LH, Hall WJ, Phillips M et al: Neoplasms in persons treated with x-rays in infancy: Fourth survey in 20 years. JNCI 55:519–520, 1975
30. DeGroot L, Paloyan E: Thyroid carcinoma in radiation JAMA 225:487–491, 1973
31. Arnold J, Pinsky S, Yun Ryo U et al: 99MTc-pertechnetate thyroid scintography in patients predisposed to thyroid neoplasms by prior radiotherapy to the head and neck. Radiology 115:653–657, 1975
32. Williams ED, Doniach MD, Bjornason O et al: Thyroid cancer in an iodine rich area . Cancer 39:215, 1977
33. Hirabayashi RW, Lindsay S: The relationship of thyroid carcinoma and chronic thyroiditis. Surg Gynecol Obstet 121:243, 1965
34. Thompson NW, Nishiyama RH, Harness JK: Thyroid carcinoma: Current controversies. Curr Prob Surg 25:(11), 1–67, 1978
35. Astwood EB, Cassidy CE, Aurbach GD: Treatment of goiter and thyroid nodules with thyroid. JAMA 174:459–464, 1960
36. Glassford GH, Fowler EF, Cole W: The treatment of nontoxic nodular goiter with dessicated thyroid: Results and evaluation. Surgery 58:621, 1965
37. Miller JM, Zafar S, Karo JJ: The cystic thyroid nodule: Recognition and management. Radiology 110:257, 1974
38. Crile G: Treatment of thyroid cysts by aspiration. Surgery 59:210, 1966
39. Blum M, Goldman AB, Herskovic J et al: Clinical applications of thyroid echography. N Engl J Med 287:1164, 1972
40. Walfish PG, Hazani S, Strawbridge HTG et al: Combined ultrasound and needle aspiration cytology in the assessment and management of hypofunctioning thyroid nodule. Ann Int Med 87:270–274, 1977
41. Bodo M, Dobrossy L, Sinkovics I et al: Fine needle biopsy of thyroid gland. J Surg Oncol 12:289–297, 1979
42. Crile G, Esseltyn CB, Hawk W: Needle biopsy in the diagnosis of thyroid nodules appearing after radiation. N Engl J Med 301:997–999, 1979
43. Gershengorn MC, McClung MR, Chu EW et al: Fine needle aspiration cytology in the preoperative diagnosis of thyroid nodules. Ann Int Med 87:205, 1977
44. Wang CA, Vickery AL, Maloof F: Needle biopsy of the thyroid. Surg Gynecol Obstet 143:365, 1976
45. Block MA: Well differentiated carcinomas of the thyroid. Curr Prob Cancer 3:8, 1979
46. Clark OH, Greenspan FS, Coggs GC et al: Evaluation of solitary cold nodules by echography and thermography. Am J Surg 130:206–210, 1975
47. Sachdeva HS, Chowdhary GC, Bose SM et al: Thyroid lymphography. Arch Surg 109:385–387, 1974
48. Weber PM, Jasko IA, Dos Remedios L.V. Thyroid scintophotography in 1000 patients: Rational use of 99MTc and I^{131} compounds J Nucl Med 12:673–677, 1971
49. Pilch BZ, Kahn CR, Ketcham AS et al: Thyroid cancer after radioactive iodine diagnostic procedures in childhood. Pediatrics 51:898, 1973
50. Mazzaferri EL, Young RL, Oertel JE et al: Papillary thyroid carcinoma: The impact of therapy in 576 patients. Medicine (Baltimore) 56:3, 171–196, 1977
51. Logerfo P, Colacchio D, Stillman T et al: Serum thyroglobulin and recurrent thyroid cancer. Cancer 1:881, 1977
52. Saxe AW, Brennan MF: Technique of reoperative parathyroidectomy. Surgery 89:417–423, 1981
53. Brennan MF, Brown EM, Spiegel AM et al: Autotransplantation of cryopreserved parathyroid tissue in man. Ann Surg 189:139–142, 1979
54. Wells SA, Gunnells JC, Leslie JT et al: Transplantation of the parathyroid glands in man. Transplant Proc 9:1, 241, 1977
55. Tollefson HR, DeCosse JJ: Papillary carcinoma of the thyroid. Recurrence in the thyroid gland after initial surgical treatment. Am J Surg 106:728, 1963
56. Crile G: Late results of treatment for papillary cancer of the thyroid. Ann Surg 160:178, 1964
57. Black BM, Kirk TA, Woolner LB: Multicentricity of papillary adenocarcinoma of the thyroid: Influence of treatment. J Clin Endocrinol Metab 20:130–135, 1960
58. Marchetta FC, Sako K: Modified neck dissection for carcinoma of the thyroid gland. Surg Gynecol Obstet 119:557, 1974
59. Banez ML, Russell WO, Albores-Saaredro J et al: Thyroid carcinoma—Biologic behavior and mortality. Cancer 19:1039, 1966
60. Harness JK, Thompson NW, Sisson JC et al: Differentiated thyroid carcinomas. Treatment of distant metastases. Arch Surg 108:410, 1974
61. Woolner LB, Lemmon ML, Beahrs OH et al: Occult papillary carcinoma of the thyroid gland. A study of 140 cases observed in a 30 year period. J Clin Endocrinol Metab 20:89, 1960
62. Block MA, Horn RC, Brush BE: The place of total thyroidectomy in surgery for thyroid carcinoma. Arch Surg 81:236, 1960
63. Tollefsen HR, DeCosse JJ, Hutter RVP: Papillary carcinoma of the thyroid. A clinical and pathological study of 70 fatal cases. Cancer 17:1035, 1964
64. Goldman JM, Goren EN, Cohen MH et al: Anaplastic thyroid carcinoma. Long-term survival after radical surgery. J Surg Oncol 14:389–394, 1980
65. Doniach I: Experimental evidence of etiology of thyroid cancer. Proc Roy Soc Med 67:1103, 1974
66. Chong GC, Beahrs OH, Sizemore GW et al: Medullary carcinoma of the thyroid gland. Cancer 35:695, 1975
67. Corwin TR: Medullary carcinoma of the thyroid. Surg Gynecol Obstet 138:453, 1974
68. Dunn EL, Nishiyama RH, Thompson NW: Medullary carcinoma of the thyroid gland. Surgery 73:848, 1973
69. Hill CS Jr, Ibanez ML, Nagiub A et al: Medullary (solid) carcinoma of the thyroid gland. Medicine 52:141, 1973
70. Ljungberg O: On medullary carcinoma of the thyroid. Acta Pathol Microbiol Scand 231:1, 1972
71. Wells SA Jr, Norton JA: Medullary carcinoma of the thyroid and multiple endocrine neoplasia-II syndromes. In Surgical Endocrinology: Clinical Syndromes, p. 287. Philadelphia, J.B. Lippincott 1978
72. Wells SA Jr, Ontjes DA, Cooper CW et al: The early diagnosis of medullary carcinoma of the thyroid gland in patient with multiple endocrine neoplasia type II. Ann Surg 182:362, 1975
73. Wells SA Jr, Baylin SB, Linehan WM et al: Provocative agents and the diagnosis of medullary carcinoma of the thyroid gland. Ann Surg 188:139, 1978
74. Wells SA Jr, Baylin SB, Gann DS et al: Medullary thyroid

carcinoma: relationship of method of diagnosis to pathological staging. Ann Surg 188:377, 1978
75. Norton JA, Doppman JL, Brennan MF: Localization and resection of clinically inapparent medullary carcinoma of the thyroid. Surgery 87:616–622, 1980
76. Block MA, Jackson EC, Tashijan AH Jr: Management of occult medullary thyroid carcinoma. Arch Surg 113–368, 1978
77. Harwood J, Clark OH, Dunphy JE: Significance of lymph node metastases in differentiated thyroid cancer. Am J Surg 136:107, 1978
78. Woolner LB: Classification and prognosis—thyroid carcinoma. Am J Surg 102:354–387, 1961
79. Buckwalter JA, Thomas CE: Selection of surgical treatment for well differentiated thyroid carcinoma. Ann Surg 176:565, 1972
80. Hutter RVP, Frazell EL, Foote FW: Elective radical neck dissection: an assessment of 1 Fc use in the management of papillary thyroid cancer. Cancer 20:87, 1970
81. Marchetta FC, Sako K, Matsuura H: Modified neck dissection for carcinoma of the thyroid gland. Am J Surg 120:452–455, 1970
82. Gottlieb JA, Hill CS Jr, Ibanez ML et al: Chemotherapy of thyroid cancer. An evaluation of experience with 37 patients. Cancer 30:848, 1972
83. Leight GS, Farrell RE, Wells SA et al: Effect of chemotherapy on calcitonin levels in patients with metastatic medullary thyroid carcinoma. Proceedings American Association for Cancer Research 21:155, 1980
84. Harada T, Nishikawa Y, Suzuki T et al: Bleomycin treatment for cancer of the thyroid. Am J Surg 122:53–57, 1971
85. Sokal M, Harmar Gl: Chemotherapy for anaplastic carcinoma of the thyroid. Clin Oncol 4:3–10, 1978
86. Bonfante V, Villani F, Bonadonna G et al: Phase I study of 4′-epiadriamycin. Proceedings of the American Association for Cancer Research 21:172, 1979
87. Rossof AH, Chandra G, Walter J et al: Phase II trial of vindesine in advanced metastatic cancer. Proceedings of the American Society for Cancer Research 20:146, 1979
88. Husain M, Alsever RN, Lock JP et al: Failure of medullary carcinoma of the thyroid to respond to doxorubicin therapy. Horm Res 9:22–25, 1978
89. Hill CS Jr, Ibanez ML, Samaan NA et al: Medullary (solid) carcinoma of the thyroid gland: an analysis of the M.D. Anderson experience with the tumor, its special features, and its histogenesis. Medicine (Baltimore) 52:141–174, 1973
90. Rogers JD, Lindberg RD, Hill CS et al: Spindle and giant cell carcinoma of the thyroid: A different approach. Cancer 34:1328–1332, 1974
91. Jereb B, Stjernsward J, Lowhagen T: Anaplastic giant cell carcinoma of the thyroid. Cancer 35:1293–1295, 1975
92. Shimaoka K, Reyes J: Chemotherapy of thyroid carcinoma. In Robbins J, Braverman LE (eds) Thyroid Research, pp 586–589. Amsterdam, Excerpta Medica, 1976
93. Burgess MA, Hill CS Jr: Chemotherapy in the management of thyroid cancer. In Greenfield LD (ed): Thyroid Cancer, pp. 233–246. West Palm Beach, C.R.C. Press, 1978.
94. Hellman DC, Kartchner M, van Antwerp JD et al: Radioiodine in the treatment of medullary carcinoma of the thyroid. J Clin Endocrinol Metab 48:451–455, 1979
95. Blahd WH: Treatment of malignant thyroid disease. Sem Nucl Med 9:95–99, 1979
96. Foster RS: Thyroid irradiation and carcinogenesis. Review with assessment of clinical implications. Am J Surg 130:608–611, 1975
97. McDougall IR, Kennedy JS, Thompson JA: Thyroid carcinoma following iodine-131 therapy: Report of a case and review of the literature. J Clin Endocrinol Metab 33:287, 1971
98. McDougall IR: Thyroid cancer after iodine-131 therapy. JAMA 227:438, 1974
99. Dolphin GW: The risk of thyroid cancers following irradiation. Health Phys 15:219, 1968
100. Dobbyns BM, Sheline GE, Workman JB et al: Malignant and benign neoplasms of the thyroid in patients treated for hyperthyroidism. J Clin Endocrinol Metab 38:976, 1974
101. Sheline GE, Lindsay S, McCormack KR et al: Thyroid nodules occurring late after treatment of thyrotoxicosis with radioiodine. J Clin Endocrinol Metab 22:9, 1962
102. Cady B, Sedgwick CE, Meissner WA et al: Changing clinical, pathologic, therapeutic, and survival patterns in differentiated thyroid cancer. Ann Surg 184:541–553, 1976
103. Byar DP, Green SB, Dor P et al: A prognostic index for thyroid carcinoma. A study of the EORTC thyroid cancer cooperative group. Eur J Cancer 15:1033–1041, 1979
104. Staunton MD, Greening WP: Treatment of thyroid cancer in 293 patients. Br J Surg 63:253–258, 1976
105. Foster RS: Morbidity and mortality after thyroidectomy. Surg Gynecol Obstet 146:423–429, 1978
106. Thorn GW: The adrenal cortex. I. Historical aspects. Johns-Hopkins Med J 123:49–77, 1968
107. Addison T: On the constitutional and local effects of disease of the suprarenal capsules. London, S. Highley, 1855
108. Hartman FA: The general physiology and experimental pathology of the suprarenal glands. In Barker LF: Endocrinology and Metabolism, vol 2, p 119. New York, Appleton, 1922
109. Hartman FA, MacArthur CG, Hartman WE: A substance which prolongs the life of adrenalectomized cats. Proc Soc Exp Biol Med 25:69–70, 1927
110. Hartman FA, Brownell KA, Hartman WE: A further study of the hormone of the adrenal cortex. Am J Physiol 95:670–680, 1930
111. Hartman FA, Brownell KA: The hormone of the adrenal cortex. Science 72:76, 1930
112. Swingle WW, Pfiffner JJ: An aqueous extract of the suprarenal cortex which maintains the life of bilaterlly adrenalectomized cats. Science 71:321–322, 1930
113. Swingle WW, Pfiffner JJ: Studies on the adrenal cortex. I. The effect of a lipid fraction upon the life span of adrenalectomized cats. Am J Physiol 96:153–163, 1931
114. Rowntree LG, Greene CH, Swingle WW, et al: The treatment of patients with Addison's disease with the "cortical hormone" of Swingle and Pfiffner. Science 72:482–483, 1930
115. Pfiffner JJ: The adrenal cortical hormones. Adv Enzymol 2:325–356, 1942
116. Gaunt R: History of the adrenal cortex. In Greep RO, Astwood EB (eds): Handbook of Physiology Section 7-Endocrinology, Chapter 1, p 1–12. Am Physiol Soc, vol 6, 1975
117. Selye EH: The general adaptation syndrome and diseases of adaptation. J Clin Endocrinol Metal 6:117–230, 1946
118. Osler W: An acute myxoedematous condition with tachycardia, glycosuria, melaena, mania, and death. J Nerv Ment Dis 26:65–71, 1899
119. Cushing HW: The basophil adenomas of the pituitary body and their clinical manifestations (pituitary basophilism). Bull Johns-Hopkins Hosp 15:137–195, 1932
120. Altschule MD: Occasional notes. N Engl Med J 302:1153–1155, 1980
121. Teel HM: Basophilic adenoma of the hypothysis with associated pleury blandular syndrome: Report of a case. Arch Neurol 26:593–599, 1931
122. Turney HG: Discussion of disease of the pituitary body. Proc R Soc Med 6:119–127, 1913
123. Parkes-Weber F: Cutaneous striae, purpura, high blood pressure, amenorrhea and obesity of the type sometimes connected with cortical tumors of the adrenal glands, occurring in the absence of any such tumor—with some remarks on the morphogenetic and hormonic effects of true hypernephromata of the adrenal cortex. Br J Dermatol Physiol 38:1–19, 1926
124. Sommers SC: Adrenal glands. In Anderson WAD (ed): Pathology, vol 2, 6th ed, 1464–1487. St. Louis, C.V. Mosby, 1970
125. Conn JW: Potassium losing nephritis. Br Med J 2:1414, 1954
126. Conn JW: Primary aldosteronism: a new clinical syndrome, J Lab clin Med 45:6, 1955
127. Conn JW, Louis LH: Primary aldosteronism: a new clinical entity. Trans Assoc Am Physicians 68:215, 1955
128. Conn JW: Aldosteronism and hypertension: primary aldosteronism versus hypertensive disease with secondary aldosteronism. Arch Intern Med 107:813, 1961

129. Conn JW: Aldosteronism in hypertensive disease. Med Times 98:116, 1970
130. Liddle GW In Williams RH (ed): Textbook of Endocrinology, 5th ed p 263. Philadelphia, WB Saunders. 1974
131. Crapo L: Cushing's syndrome: A review of diagnostic tests. Metabolism 28:955–977, 1979
132. Gold EM: The Cushing syndromes: Changing views of diagnosis and treatment. Ann Int Med 90:829–844, 1979
133. Brennan MF, Dunnick NR: Localization of functional adrenal tumors In Nayarian JS, Delaney P (eds): Breast and Endocrine Surgery. Chicago, Year Book Medical Publishers, 1981.
134. Wilms G, Baert A, Machal G et al: Computed tomography of the normal adrenal glands: correlative study with autopsy specimens. J Comput Asst Tomogr 3:467–469, 1979
135. Dunnick NR, Schaner EG, Doppman JL, et al: Computed tomography in adrenal tumors. Am J Radiol 132:43–46, 1979
136. Korobkin M, White A, Kressel HY et al: Computed tomography in the diagnosis of adrenal disease. Am J Roentgenol 132:231–238, 1979
137. Javadpour N, Woltering E, Brennan MF: Adrenal neoplasms. Curr Probl Surg XVII (1):1–52, 1980
138. Sample WF: A new technique for the evaluation of the adrenal gland with gray-scale ultrasonography. Radiology 124:463–469, 1977
139. Bernadino ME, Goldstein HM, Green G: Gray-scale ultrasonography of adrenal neoplasms. Am J Roentgenol 130:741–744, 1978
140. Davidson JK, Morley P, Harley GD, et al: Adrenal venography and ultrasound in the investigation of the adrenal gland: an analysis of 58 cases. Br J Radiol 48:435–450, 1975
141. Hoevels J, Ekelund L: Angiographic findings in adrenal masses. Acta Radiol Diag 20:337–352, 1979
142. Dunnick NR, Doppman JL, Mills SR et al: Preoperative diagnosis and localization of aldosteronoma by measurement of corticosteroids in adrenal venous blood. Radiology 133:331–333, 1979
143. Seabold JE, Cohen EL, Beierwaltes WH, et al: Adrenal imaging with $I^{131}-19-$Iodocholesterol in the diagnostic evaluation of patients with aldosteronism. J Clin Endocrinol Metab 42:41–51, 1976
144. Kirschner AS, Ice RD, Beierwaltes WH: The author's reply. J Nucl Med 16:248, 1975
145. Thrall JM, Freitas JE, Beierwaltes WH: Adrenal scintigraphy. Semin Nucl Med 8:23–41, 1978
146. Miles JM, Wahner HW, Carpenter PC et al: Adrenal scintiscanning with NP 59 a new radio iodonated cholesterol agent. Mayo Clin Proc 54:321–327, 1979
147. Scott HW, Oates JA, Nies AS et al: Pheochromocytoma: Present diagnosis and management. Ann Surg 183:587–593, 1976
148. ReMine WH, Chong GC, Van Heerden JA: Current management of pheochromocytoma. Ann Surg 179:740, 1974
149. Delarue NC, Morrow JD, Kerr JH et al: Pheochromocytoma in the modern context. Canad J Surg 21:387–394, 1978
150. Sjoerdsma A, Engelman K, Waldman TA et al: Pheochromocytoma: Current concepts of diagnosis and treatment. Ann Intern Med 65: 1302–1326, 1966
151. Stackpole RH, Melicow MM, Uson AC: Pheochromocytoma in children. J Pediatr 63:315–330, 1963
152. Gitlow SE, Mendlowitz M, Bertani LM: The biochemical techniques for detecting and establishing the presence of a pheochromocytoma. Am J Cardiol 26:270–279, 1970
153. Harrison TS, Bartlett JD, Seaton JF: Current evaluation and management of pheochromocytoma. Ann Surg 168:701–713, 1968
154. Hume DM: Pheochromocytoma in the adult and in the child. Am J Surg 99:458–496, 1960
155. Gifford M, Kvale WF, Maher FT et al: Clinical features, diagnosis and treatment of pheochromocytoma. A review of 76 cases. Mayo Clin Proc 39:281–302, 1964
156. Bravo EL, Tarazi RC, Gifford RW et al: Circulating and urinary catecholamines in pheochromocytoma. Diagnostic and pathophysiologic implications. N Engl J Med 301:682–686, 1979
157. Van Way C, Scott HW, Page DL et al: Pheochromocytoma. Curr Probl Surg 6, 1974
158. Hengstmann JH, Gugler R, Dengler HJ: Malignant pheochromocytoma. Effect of oral α -methyl p-tyrosine upon catecholamine metabolism. Klin Wochenschr 58:351–355, 1979
159. Stewart BH, Bravo EL, Haage J et al: Localization of pheochromocytoma by computed tomography. N Engl J Med 299:460–461, 1978
160. Von Euler US, Gemzell C, Strom G et al: Report of a case of pheochromocytoma with special regard to preoperative diagnostic problems. Acta Med Scand 153:127–126, 1955
161. Temple WJ, Voitk AJ, Thompson AE et al: Phenoxybenzamine blockade in surgery of pheochromocytoma. J Surg Res 22:59–64, 1977
162. Feldman JM, Blalock JA, Fagraeus L et al: Alterations in plasma norepinephrine concentration during surgical resection of pheochromocytoma. Ann Surg 188:758–768, 1978
163. Nourok DS, Gwinup G, Hamwi GJ: Phentolamine-resistant pheochromocytoma treated with sodium nitroprusside. JAMA 183:841, 1963
164. Daniels H, Van Amstel WJ, Schopman W, Van Dommelen C: Effect of metapyrone in a patient with adrenocortical carcinoma. Acta Endocrinol 44:346–354, 1963
165. Cash R, Brough AJ, Cohen MNP et al: Aminoglutethimide (Elipten-Ciba) as an inhibitor of adrenal steriodogenesis: mechanism of action and therapeutic trial. J Clin Endocrinol Metab 27:1239–1248, 1967
166. Gorden P, Becker CE, Levey GS et al: Efficacy of aminoglutethimide in the ectopic ACTH syndrome. J Clin Endocrinol Metab 28:921–923, 1968
167. Schteingart DE, Cash R, Coon JW: Amino-glutethimide and metastatic adrenal cancer. JAMA 198:1007–1010, 1966
168. Fishman LM, Liddle GW, Island DP et al: Effects of aminoglutethimide on adrenal function in man. J Clin Endocrinol Metab 27:481–490, 1967
169. Nelson AA, Woodward G: Severe adrenal cortical atrophy (cytotoxic) and hepatic damage produced in dogs by feeding 2,2-bis-(parachlorophenyl)-1,1-dichloroethane (DDD or TDE). Arch Pathol 48:387–394, 1949
170. Cazorla A, Moncloa F: Action of 1,1-dichloro-2-p-chlorophenyl-1-2-0-chlorophenylethane on dog adrenal cortex. Science 136:47, 1962
171. Bledsoe T, Island DP, Ney RL et al: An effect of o,p'-DDD on the extra-adrenal metabolism of cortisol in man. J Clin Endocrinol Metab 24:1301–1311, 1964.
172. Bergenstal DM, Hertz R, Lipsett MB et al: Chemotherapy of adrenocortical cancer with o,p'-DDD. Ann Intern Med 53:672–682, 1960
173. Hutter AM, Kayhoe DE: Adrenal cortical carcinoma, results of treatment with o,p'-DDD in 138 patients. Am J Med 41:581–592, 1966
174. Lubitz JA, Freeman L, Okun R: Mitotane in inoperable adrenal cortical carcinoma. JAMA 223:1109–1111, 1973
175. Hajjar RA, Hickey RC, Samaan NA: Adrenal cortical carcinoma. A study of 32 patients. Cancer 5:544,–559, 1975
176. Joseph L: Malignant phaeochromocytoma of the organ of Zuckerkandl with functioning metastases. Br J Urol 39:221–225, 1967
177. Moloney GE, Lowdell RH, Lewis CL: Malignant phaeochromocytoma of the bladder. Br J Urol 38:461–470, 1966
178. Phillips AF, McMurtry RJ, Taubman J: Malignant pheochromocytoma in childhood. Am J Dis Child 130:1252–1255, 1976
179. Schart Y, Ben Arieh Y, Gellei B: Orbital metastases from extra adrenal pheochromocytoma. Am J Ophthalmol 69:638–640, 1970
180. Bunuan HD: Gel form embolization of functioning phaechromocytoma. Am J Surg 136:395–398, 1978
181. Hamilton BPM, Cheikhl E, Rivera LE: Attempted treatment of inoperable pheochromocytoma with streptozotocin. Arch Int Med 137:762–765, 1977
182. Drasin H: Treatment of malignant pheochromocytoma. West J Med 128:106–111, 1978
183. Modlin IM, Farndon JR, Shephard A et al: Phaeochromocytomas

in 72 patients. Clinical and diagnostic features, treatment and long-term results. Br J Surg 66:456–465, 1979
184. Harrison TS, Frier DT, Cohen EL: Recurrent pheochromocytoma. Arch Surg 108:450–454, 1974
185. Frier DT, Eckhauser FE, Harrison TS: Pheochromocytoma. Arch Surg 115:388–391, 1980
186. Rote AR, Flint LD, Ellis FH: Intracaval recurrence of pheochromocytoma extending into right atrium. N Engl J Med 296:1269–1271, 1977
187. Biglieri EG, Schambelan M, Slaton PE et al: The intercurrent hypertension of primary aldosteronism. Circ Res (suppl 1) 195:26–27, 1970
188. Biglieri EG, Slaton PE Jr, Silen WS et al: Postoperative studies of adrenal function in primary aldosteronism. J Clin Endocrinol Metab 26:553, 1966
189. Davis WW, Newsome HH, Wright LD Jr et al: Bilateral adrenal hyperplasia as a cause of primary aldosteronism with hypertension hypokalemia and suppressed renin activity. Am J Med 42:642, 1967
190. Laragh JH, Ledingham JGG, Sommers SC: Secondary aldosteronism and reduced plasma renin in hypertensive disease. Trans Assoc Am Physicians 80:168, 1967
191. Auda SP, Brennan MF, Gill JR: Evolution of the surgical management of primary aldosteronism. Ann Surg 191:1–7, 1980
192. Weinberger MH, Grimm CE, Hollifield JW et al: Primary aldosteronism: diagnosis, localization, and treatment. Ann Intern Med 90:386, 1979
193. Hunt TK, Schambelan M, Biglieri EG: Selection of patients and operative approach in primary aldosteronism. Ann Surg 182:353, 1975
194. Herwig KR: Primary aldosteronism: Experience with 38 patients. Surgery 86:470–474, 1979
195. Spark RF, Melby JC: Aldosteronism in hypertension: the spironolactone response test. Ann Intern Med 69:685, 1968
196. King DR, Lack EE: Adrenal cortical carcinoma. A clinical and pathological study of 49 cases. Cancer 44:239–244, 1979
197. Kelly WF, Barnes AJ, Cassar J et al: Cushing's syndrome due to adrenocortical carcinoma. Acta Endocrinol (Copenhagen) 91:303–318, 1979
198. Brown MJ, Lewis PJ, Dollery CT: Diagnosis of small pheochromocytomas. Lancet i, 1185–1186, 1980
199. Atuk NO, McDonald T, Wood T et al: Familial pheochromocytoma, hypercalcemia and vonHippel-Lindau Disease. A ten year study of a large family. Medicine (Baltimore) 58:209–218, 1979
200. Paton WDM, Zaimes EJ: Paralysis of autonomic ganglia by methonium salts. Br J Pharmacol Chemother 6:155–168, 1955
201. Saxe A, Brennan MF, Javadpour N: Diagnosis and surgical management of adrenal tumors. Contemp Surg 18:31–40, 1981
202. Zollinger RM, Ellison EH: Primary peptic ulcerations of the jejunum associated with islet cell tumors of the pancreas. Ann Surg 142:709, 1955
203. Zollinger RM, Martin EW, Carey LC et al: Observations on the postoperative tumor growth behavior of certain islet cell tumors. Ann Surg 184:515–530, 1976
204. Marks V, Semol SE: Insulinoma: Natural history and diagnosis. Clin Gastroenterol 3:559, 1974
205. Larsson LI: Human pancreatic polypeptide, vasoactive intestinal polypeptide and watery diarrhea syndrome. Lancet 2:149, 1976
206. Schwartz CJ, Kimberg DV, Sheerin HEV et al: Vasoactive intestinal peptide stimulation of adenylate cyclase and active electrolyte secretion in intestinal mucosa. J Clin Invest 54:536, 1974
207. Said SI, Mutt V: Polypeptide with biological activity isolated from small intestine. Science 169:12–17, 1970
208. Becker WS, Kahn D, Rothman S: Cutaneous manifestations of internal malignant tumors. Arch Derm Syph 45:1069, 1942
209. McGavran MH, Unger RH, Recant L: A glucagon like secreting alpha cell carcinoma of the pancreas. N Engl J Med 274:1408, 1966
210. Larsson LI, Hirsch MA, Holst JJ et al: Pancreatic somatostatinoma: Clinical features and pathological implications. Lancet 1:666–668, 1977
211. Ganda OP, Weir GC, Soeldner JS et al: "Somatostatinoma" a somatostatin containing tumor of the endocrine pancrease. N Engl J Med 296:963–967, 1977
212. Verner JV, Morrison AB: Endocrine pancreatic islet disease with diarrhea: Report of a case due to diffuse hyperplasia of non-beta islet tissue with a review of 54 additional cases. Arch Intern Med 133: 492, 1974
213. Verner JV, Morrison AB: Non-beta islet cell tumors and the syndrome of watery diarrhea hypokalemia and hypochlorhydria. Clin Gastroenterol 3:595, 1976
214. Marks IN, Bank S, Louw JH: Islet cell tumor of the pancreas with reversible watery diarrhea and achlorhydria. Gastroenterol 52:694, 1967
215. Sjoerdsma A, Nelmon KL: The carcinoid spectrum. Gastroenterology 47:104, 1964
216. Larsson LI, Grimelius L, Hakanson R et al: Mixed endocrine pancreatic tumors producing several peptide hormones. Am J Pathol 79:271, 1975
217. Oberg K, Loff L, Bostrom H et al: Hypersecretion of calcitonin in patients with Verner Morrison syndrome. Scand J Gastroenterol (in press)
218. Pearse AGE: Common cytochemical and ultastructural characteristics of cells producing polypeptoid hormones (the apud series) and their relevance to thyroid and ultimo-brachial C cells and calcitonin. Proceedings of the Royal Society of London: Biological Sciences 170:71, 1968
219. Bloom SR, Polak JM, Welbourn RB, et al: Pancreatic apudomas. World J Surg 3:587–595, 1979
220. Szijj T, Csapo Z, Lasslo FA et al: Medulalry carcinoma of the thyroid associated with hypercorticism. Cancer 24:167, 1969
221. Welbourn RB: Current status of apudomas. Ann Surg 185:1–12, 1977
222. Pearse AGE: The apud concept and its implications in pathology. Pathol Annu 9:27–41, 1974
223. Moldow RE, Connelly RR: Epidemiology of pancreatic cancer in Connecticut. Gastroenterol 55:667–686, 1978
224. Schein PS, DeLellis RA, Kahn CR et al: Islet cell tumors. Current concepts and management. Ann Int Med 79:239–257, 1973
225. Lopez–Kruger R, Dockerty MB: Tumors of one islets of Langerhaus. Surg Gynecol Obstet 185:495, 1947
226. Gray H: Anatomy of Human Body , 29th ed 1258–1263. Goss CM (ed): Philadelphia, Lea and Febiger, 1973
227. Bordi C, Ravazzola M, Baetens D, Gorden P, Unger RH et al: A study of Chicagonomas by light and electron microscopy and immunofluorescence. Diabetes 28:925–936, 1979
228. Heitz TU, Kasper M, Polak JM et al: Pathology of the endocrine pancreas. J Histochem Cytochem 27:1401–1402, 1979
229. Thompson JC, Reeder DD, Villar HV et al Natural history and experience with diagnosis and treatment of Zollinger–Ellison syndrome. Surg Gynecol Obstet 140:721, 1975
230. Isenberg JL, Walsh JH, Grossman MI: Zollinger-Ellison syndrome. Gastroenterology 65:140, 1973
231. Friesen SR: The Zollinger–Ellison syndrome. Curr Prob Surg 4:1–52, 1972
232. Deveney CW, Deveney KS, Way L: Zollinger–Ellison syndrome: 23 years later. Ann Surg 18:384, 1978
233. Ellison EH, Wilson D: The Zollinger–Ellison syndrome. Ann Surg 110:512, 1964
234. Cunningham L, Howe P, Evans RW: Islet cell tumor with unusual clinicopathologic features. Br J Surg 39:319, 1952
235. Gregory RA, Tracy HJ, French JN, et al: Extraction of a gastrin-like substance from a pancreatic tumor in a case of Zollinger–Ellison syndrome. Lancet i:1045–1048, 1960
236. Yalow RS, Berson SA: Radioimmunoassay of gastrin. Gastroenterology 58:1–14, 1970
237. Martin ED, Potet F: Pathology of endocrine tumors of the GI tract. Clin Gastroenterol 3:511, 1974
238. Creutzfeldt W, Arnold R, Creutzfeldt C et al: Pathomorphologic biochemical and diagnostic aspects of gastrinomas (Zollinger–Ellison syndrome). Hum Pathol 6:47, 1975
239. Bonfils S, Bernades P: Zollinger–Ellison syndrome: Natural history and diagnosis. Clin Gastroenterol 3:539, 1974
240. Fox PS, Hoffman JW, Wilson SD et al: Surgical management

of the Zollinger–Ellison syndrome. Surg Clin North Am 54:395–407, 1974
241. Lamers CBH, Stadh F, VanTongeren J: Prevalence of endocrine abnormalities in patients with Zollinger–Ellison syndrome and in their families. Am J Med 64:607, 1978
242. Grossman MI: Physiology and pathophysiology of gastrin. Clin Gastroenterol 3:533, 1974
243. Solcia E, Cappella C, Vassale G et al: Endocrine cells of the gastric mucosa. Int Rev Cytol, 223–286, 1974
244. Pearse AGE: Cytochemical and ultrastructure of polypeptide hormone producing cells of the apud series and the embryological physiological and pathological implications of this concept. J Histochem Cytochem 17:303, 1969
245. Yalow RS, Berson SA: Size and charge distinctions between endogenous human plasma gastrin in peripheral blood and hepatadecapeptide gastrins. Gastroenterology, 58:609–615, 1970
246. Modlin IM: Endocrine tumors of the pancreas. Surg Gynecol Obstet 149:751–769, 1979
247. Regan PT, Malagelada JR: A reappraisal of clinical , roentgenographic and endoscopic features of the Zollinger–Ellison syndrome. Mayo Clin Proc 53:19–23, 1978
248. Stage JG, Stadil F: The clinical diagnosis of the Zollinger–Ellison syndrome. Scand J Gastroenterol (suppl) 14 (53):79–91, 1979
249. Cope V, Warwick F: The role of radiology in the detection of endocrine tumors in the GI tract. Clin Gastroenterol 3:621, 1974
250. Sizemore GW, Go VLW, Kaplan EL et al: Relations of calcitonin and gastrin in the Zollinger–Ellison syndrome and medullary carcinoma of the thyroid. N Engl J Med 288:641–644, 1973
251. Lamers CB, Diemel J, Roeffen W: Serum levels of pancreatic polypeptide in Zollinger–Ellison syndrome, and hyperparathyroidism from families with multiple endocrine adenomatosis-Type 1. Digestion 18:297–302, 1978
252. Nelson RL, Service FJ, Ilstrup DM et al: Are elevated pancreatic polypeptide levels in patients with insulinoma secondary to hypoglycemia? Lancet 2:659–661, 1980
253. Byrnes DJ, Marjason J, Henderson L et al: Is pancreatic polypeptide estimation of value in diagnosing gastrinomas (Zollinger–Ellison syndrome)? Aust NZJ Med 9(4): 364–366, 1979
254. Kahn CR, Rosen SW, Weintraub BD et al: Ectopic production of chorionic gonadotrophin and its subunits by islet-cell tumors. N Engl J Med 297:565–569, 1977
255. McCarthy DM, Weintraub BD, Rosen SW: Subunits of human gonadotrophin in malignant gastrinoma. Gastroenterology (Abstr) 76:1198, 1979
256. Stabile BE, Braunstein GD, Passaro E: Serum gastrin and human chorionic gonadotrophin in the Zollinger–Ellison syndrome. Arch Surg 115:1090–1095, 1980
257. Mills SR, Doppman JL, Dunnick NR et al: Evaluation of angiography in Zollinger–Ellison syndrome. Radiology 131:317, 1979
258. Boijsen E, Samuelsson L: Angiographic diagnosis of tumors arising from the pancreatic islets. Acta Radiol (Diagn) 10:161–176, 1970
259. White TT, Kavlie H: Hormone producing pancreatic islet cell tumors and hyperplasia. Acta Chir Scand 138:809–815, 1972
260. Alfidi RJ, Skillern PG, Cril G: Arteriographic manifestations of the Zollinger–Ellison syndrome. Cleveland Clin Quart 36:41–45, 1969
261. McKinnon CM, Brant B, Brosch J: Angiography in the diagnosis and management of extrapancreatic islet cell tumors. Ann Surg 177:381–383, 1973
262. Dunnick NR, Doppman JL, Mills SR et al: Computed tomographic detection of non-beta pancreatic islet cell tumors. Radiology 135:117–120, 1980
263. Wells SA, Ontjes Da, Cooper CW et al: The early diagnosis of medullary carcinoma of the thyroid gland in patients with multiple endocrine neoplasia type II. Ann Surg 182:362, 1975
264. Norton JA, Doppman JL, Brennan MF: Localization and resection of clinically inapparent medullary carcinoma of the thyroid. Surgery 87:616–622, 1980
265. Carey LC, Ellison EC: The Zollinger–Ellison syndrome: Update Surgical Rounds 6:53, 1979
266. Zollinger RM, Ellison EC, Fabri PJ et al: Primary peptic ulcerations of the jejunum associated with islet cell tumors. Ann Surg 192:422–430, 1980
267. Deveney CW, Deveney KS, Way LW: The clinical diagnosis of the Zollinger–Ellison syndrome—23 years later. Ann Surg 188:384–393, 1979
268. McCarthy DM: The place of surgery in the Zollinger–Ellison syndrome. N Engl J Med 302:1344–1346, 1980
269. Fox PS, Hofmann JW, DeCosse JJ et al: The influence of total gastrectomy on survival in malignant Zollinger–Ellison tumors. Ann Surg 18:8558, 1974
270. Richardson CT, Walsh JH: The value of histamine H-2 receptor antagonist in the management of patients with Zollinger–Ellison syndrome. N Engl J Med 294:13–39, 1976
271. McCarthy DM, Olinger EJ, May RJ et al: H_2-histamine receptor blocking agents in the Zollinger–Ellison syndrome: experience in seven cases and implications for long term therapy. Ann Intern Med 87:668–675, 1977
272. McCarthy DM: Report on the United States experience with cimetidine in Zollinger–Ellison and other secretory states. Gastroenterology 74:453–458, 1978
273. Richardson CT, Feldman M, McClelland RN et al: Effect of vagotomy in Zollinger–Ellison syndrome. Gastroenterology 77:682–686, 1979
274. Turbey WJ, Passaro EW: Hyperparathyroidism in the Zollinger–Ellison syndrome. Arch Surg 105:62, 1972
275. Dent RI, James JH, Wang CA et al: Hyperparathyroidism: gastric acid secretion and gastrin. Ann Surg 176:360, 1972
276. Jaffe BM, Peskin GW, Kaplan EL: Serum levels of parathyroid horomone in the Zollinger–Ellison syndrome. Surgery 74:621, 1973
277. Edis AJ, Ayala LA, Egdahl RH: Manual of Endocrine Surgery. New York, Springer-Verlag, 1975
278. Baron M: The relation of the islets of Langerhans to diabetes with special reference to cases of pancreatic lithiasis. Surg Gynec Obstet 31:437–448, 1920
279. Banting FG, Best CH: The internal secretion of the pancrease. J Lab Clin Med 7:251–266, 1922
280. Opie EL: The relation of diabetes mellitus to lesions of the pancreas. J Exper Med 5:527, 1901
281. Whipple AO, Frantz VK: Adenoma of islet cells with hyperinsulinism: A review. Ann Surg 101:1299, 1935
282. Harris S: Hyperinsulinism and Dysinsulinism. JAMA 23:729–733, 1924
283. Wilder RM, Allan FN, Power MH et al: Carcinoma of the islands of the pancreas, hyperinsulinism and hypoglycemia. JAMA 89:348–355, 1927
284. Howland G, Campbell WR, Mattby EJ et al: Dysinsulinism: Convulsions and coma due to an islet cell tumor of the pancreas with operation and cure. JAMA 93:674–679, 1929
285. Finney JMJ, Finney JMJ Jr: Resection of the pancreas. Ann Surg 88:584–592, 1928
286. Stefanini P, Carboni M, Patrasi N et al: Beta islet cell tumors of the pancreas: Results of a study on 1067 cases. Surgery 75:597–609, 1974
287. Filipi CJ Higgins GA: Diagnosis and management of insulinoma. Am J Surg 125:231–239, 1973
288. Laurent J, Debry G, Floquet J: Hypoglycemic tumors. Amsterdam, Excerpta Medica, 1971
289. Vance JE, Kitabchi AE, Buchanan KD et al: Hypersecretion of insulin, glucagon and gastrin in a kindred with multiple adenomatosis. Diabetes 17:299, 1968
290. Kaplan EL, Rubenstein AH, Evans SR et al: Calcium infusion—a new provocative test for insulinoma. Ann Surg 190:501–507, 1979
291. Rubenstein AH, Kuzuya H, Horwitz DL: Clinical significance of circulating C-peptide in diabetes and hypoglycemic disorders Arch Intern Med 137:625, 1977
292. Van Heerden JA, Edis AJ, Service FJ: The surgical aspects of insulinomas. Ann Surg 189:677–682, 1979
293. Sweet RD: A dermatosis specifically associated with tumor of pancreatic alpha cells. Br J Dermatol 90:301, 1974
294. Malinson CN, Bloom SR, Warin AP et al: A glucagonoma syndrome. Lancet 2:1–5, 1974

295. Holst JJ, Helland S, Ingemannson S et al: Functional studies in patients with glucagonoma syndrome. Diabetologia 17:151–156, 1979
296. Danforth DN, Triche T, Doppman JL et al: Elevated plasma proglucagon like component with a glucagon-secreting tumor—effect of streptozotocin. N Engl J Med 295:242–245, 1976
297. Pederson NB, Johnson L, Holst JJ: Necrolitic migratory erythema and glucagon cell tumor of the pancreas: the glucagonoma syndrome. Acta Derm Venerol Stockholm 56:391, 1976
298. Higgins GA, Recant L, Fischman AB: The glucagonoma syndrome: surgically curable diabetes. Am J Surg 137:142–148, 1979
299. Norton JA, Kahn CR, Schiebinger R et al: Amino acid deficiency and the skin rash associated with glucagonoma. Ann Int Med 91:213–215, 1979
300. Ingemansson S, Holst JJ, Larsson LI et al: Localization of glucagonomas by pancreatic vein catheterization in glucagon assay. Surg Gynecol Obstet 145:509, 1977
301. Bloom SR: VIP and watery diarrhea in 'Gut hormones'. In Bloom SR: Proceedings of the International Symposium on Gut Hormones, pp 583–588. New York, Churchill-Livingston, 1978
302. Gardner JD, McCarthy DM: Arguments against vasoactive intestinal peptides being the cause of the watery diarrhea syndrome. In Bloom SR (ed): Proceedings of the International Symposium on Gut Hormones. New York, Churchill-Livingston, 1978
303. Swift PGE, Gloom SR, Harris E: Watery diarrhea and ganglioneuroma with secretion with vasoactive intestinal peptide. Arch Dis Child 50:896, 1975
304. Larsson LI, Schwartz T, Lindquist G et al: Occurence of human pancreatic polypeptide in pancreatic endocrine tumors: Possible implications in a watery diarrhea syndrome. Am J Clin Pathol 85:675, 1976
305. Wormsley KG: Response to secretin in man. Gastroenterology 54:197, 1968
306. Elias E, Bloom SR, Welbourn B et al: Pancreatic cholera due to the production of gastric inhibitory polypeptide. Lancet ii:791, 1972
307. Barbezat GO, Grossman MI: Cholera-like diarrhea induced by glucagon plus gastrin. Lancet i:1025, 1971
308. Jaffe B, Koren D, DeSchryvcheer-Kecksmeti K et al: Indomethacin response of pancreatic cholera. N Engl J Med 297:817, 1977
309. Modlin IM, Bloom SR, Mitchell S: Experimental evidence for vasoactive intestinal peptide as a cause of the watery diarrhea syndrome. Gastroenterology 75:1051, 1978
310. Kraft AR, Tompkins RK, Zollinger RM: Recognition and management of the diarrheal syndrome caused by non-beta islet cell tumors of the pancreas. Am J Surg 119:163, 1970
311. Krejs GV, Walsh JH, Morawski SG et al: Intractable diarrhea, intestinal perfusion studies and plasma VIP concentrations in patients with pancreatic cholera syndrome and surreptitious injection of laxatives and diuretics. Am J Dig Dis 22:280, 1977
312. Krejs GJ, Orei L, Conlon JM et al: Somatostatinoma syndrome: Biochemical, morphologic and clinical features. N Engl J Med 301:285–292, 1979
313. Unger RH: Somatostatinoma. N Engl J Med 296:998–1000, 1977
314. Kovacs K, Horvath E, Ezrin C et al: Immunoreactive somatostatin in pancreatic islet-cell carcinoma accompanied by ectopic ACTH syndrome. Lancet i:1365–1366, 1977
315. DeNutte N, Somers G, Gepts W et al: Pancreatic hormone release in tumor associated hypersomatostatinemia. Diabetologia 15:227, 1978
316. Galmiche JP, Conlon JM, Srikant J et al: Measurements of somatostatin like immunoreactivity in plasma. Clin Chim Acta 87:275–283, 1978
317. Glasser B, Vinik AI: Clinical findings in patients with malignant tumors secreting pancreatic polypeptide (PP). Clin Res 27:627a, 1979
318. Friesen SR, Kimmel JR, Tomita T: Pancreatic polypeptide as screening marker for pancreatic polypeptide apudomas in multiple endocrinopathies. Am J Surg 139:61–72, 1980
319. Keaveny TV, Tawes R, Belzer FO: A new method for intraoperative visualization of insulinomas. Br J Surg 58:233–1971
320. Allison D, Modlin IM, Jenkins W: Management of carcinoid hepatic metastases. Lancet ii:1323, 1977
321. Herr RR, Jahnke HK, Argondelis AS: Structure of streptozotocin. J Am Chem Soc 89:4808–4809, 1967
322. Rakieten N, Rakieten ML, Nadkarni MV: Studies on the diabetogenic action of streptozotocin (NSC-37917). Cancer Chemother Rep 29:91–98, 1969
323. Broder LE, Carter SK: Results of therapy with streptozotocin in 52 patients. Ann Intern Med 79:108–118, 1973
324. Moertel CG, Reitemeier RJ, Schutt AJ et al: Phase II study of streptozotocin (NSC-85998) in the treatment of advanced gastrointestinal cancer. Cancer Chemother Rep 55:303–307, 1971
325. Kahn CR, Levy AG, Gardner JD et al: Pancreatic cholera: Beneficial effects of treatment with streptozotocin. N Engl J Med 292:941–945, 1975
326. Stadil F, Stage G, Rehfeld JF et al: Treatment of Zollinger–Ellison syndrome with streptozotocin. N Engl J Med 294:1440–1442, 1976
327. Schein PS, DeLillis RA, Kahn CR et al: Islet cell tumors: current concepts and management. Ann Intern Med 79:239–257, 1973
328. Schein PS: Chemotherapy of gastrointestinal endocrine tumors. Excerpta Medica International Congress Series, No. 403, Endocrinology. Proceedings of the V International Congress of Endocrinology, Hamburg, July 18–24, 1976, 2:453–457, 1976
329. Moertel, CG: Clinical management of advanced gastrointestinal cancer. Cancer 36:675–682, 1975
330. Moertel CG, Hanley JA, Johnson LA: A randomized comparison of streptozotocin alone vs. streptozotocin plus 5-fluorouracil in the treatment of metastatic islet cell odrunoma. Proc ASCO & ASCR 21:415, 1980
331. Rubin AA, Roth FE, Winbury MM et al: New class of antihypertensive agents. Science 133:2067, 1961
332. Okun R, Russel RP, Wilson WR: Enhancement of the hypotensive and hyperglycemic effect of trichlormethiazide by nondieuretic basothiadiazine, diazoxide. Circulation 2:735, 1962
333. Langdon RG, Wolff FW: Action of diazoxide. Br. Med J 2:296, 1962
334. Dollery CT, Pentecost BL, Samaan NA: Drug induced diabetes. Lancet 2:735, 1962
335. Bleicher JJ, Chowdhury F, Goldner MG: Thiazide therapy in hypoglycemia of metastatic insulinoma. Clin Res 12:456, 1964
336. Ernesti M, Mitchell ML, Raben MS et al: Control of hypoglycemia with diazoxide and human growth hormone. Lancet 1:628, 1965
337. Yabo R, Viktora J, Stagnet M et al: Studies concerning the hypoglycemic effects of diazoxide and its mode of action. Diabetes 14:591, 1965
338. Zarday Z, Viktora J, Wolff F: The effect of diazoxide on catecholamines. Metabolism 15:257, 1966
339. Marks V, Rose FC, Samols E: Hyperinsulinism due to metastasizing insulinoma: treatment with diazoxide. Proc Roy Soc Med 58:577, 1965
340. Roth J, Thiers S, Segal S: Zinc glucagon in the management of refractory hypoglycemia due to insulin producing tumors. N Engl J Med 274:493, 1966
341. Sadoff L: Nephrotoxicity of streptozotocin (NSC-85998). Cancer Chemother Rep 54:459, 1970
342. Strauss GM, Weitzman SA, Aoki, TT: Dimethyltriazenoimidazole carboxamide therapy of malignant glucagonoma. Ann Int Med 90: 57–58, 1979
343. Schein PS: Chemotherapeutic management of hormone secreting endocrine malignancies. Cancer 30:1616–1626, 1972
344. Oberg K, Lundquist G, Bostrom H: The effects of streptozotocin in the treatment of endocrine pancreatic tumors and carcinoids. In Groesbeek T (ed): Streptozotocin. New York, Elsevier Publishing Co, 1981
345. Bonfils S, Mignon M, Rigaud D et al: Prolonged treatment of Zollinger–Ellison syndrome by cimetidine. Nouv Presse Med 8: 1403–1407, 1979
346. Gurnow RT, Carey RM, Taylor A et al: Somatostatin inhibition

of insulin and gastrin hypersecretion in pancreatic islet cell carcinoma. N Engl J Med 292:1385, 1975

347. Long RG, Adrian TE, Barnes AJ et al: Des AA 1,-2,-4,-5,-12,-13, D Try 8 Somatostatin: A long-acting inhibitor of pancreatic endocrine tumor and non-tumor derived hormones. Gut 20 (10) A949, 1979
348. Long RG, Adrian TE, Brown MR et al: Suppression of pancreatic endocrine tumor secretion by long-acting somatostatin analogue. Lancet ii:764–767, 1979
349. Kramer S, Machina T, Marcus J: Metabolic studies in the malignant glucagonoma syndrome. Diabetes 25:370, 1976
350. Jaffe, BM: The diarrhoegenic syndrome: Verner Morrison, WDHA syndrome. In Friesen SR (ed): Surgical Endocrinology p. 227. Philadelphia, JB Lippincott, 1978
351. Pandol SJ, Korman LY, McCarthy DM et al: Beneficial effect of oral lithium carbonate in the treatment of pancreatic cholera syndrome. N Engl J Med 302:1403–1404, 1980
352. Wood DA: Atlas of Tumor Pathology, Section, VI. Washington, D.C., Armed Forces Institutes of Pathology, 1967
353. Pearse AGE. The APUD cell concept and its implications in pathology. Pathol Ann 9:27, 1974
354. Wilson H, Cheek RC, Sherman RT, et al: Carcinoid tumors. Curr Probl Surg, 11: 1970
355. Pearson CM, Fitzgerald PJ: Carcinoid tumors: a re-emphasis of their malignant nature. Review of 140 cases. Cancer 2:1005, 1949
356. Ransom WB: Letter to the Editor. Lancet 2:1020, 1890
357. Jager RM, Polk HC: Carcinoid apudomas. Curr Probl Cancer 1:11, 1977
358. Linnell F, Manssonk K: On the prevalence and incidence of carcinoids in Malmo. Acta Med Scand (suppl) 445:377, 1966
359. Moertel CG, Sauer WG, Dockerty MB et al: Life history of the carcinoid tumors of the small intestine. Cancer 14:901, 1961
360. MacDonald RA: A study of 356 carcinoids of the gastrointestinal tract: report of four new cases of the carcinoid syndrome. Am J Med 21:867, 1956
361. Moertel CG. Small intestine. In Holland JF, Frei E (eds): Cancer Medicine, pp 1574–84, Philadelphia, Lea & Febiger, 1973
362. Godwin JD: Carcinoid tumors: an analysis of 2837 cases. Cancer 36:560, 1975
363. Marks C: Carcinoid tumors: a clinicopathologic study. Boston, G.K. Hall, 1979
364. Wick MR, Scott RE, Li CY et al: Carcinoid tumor of the thymus: a clinicopathologic report of seven cases with a review of the literature. Mayo Clin Proc 55:246 1980
365. Williams ED, Sandler M: The classification of carcinoid tumors. Lancet 1:238, 1963
366. Pearse AGE, Polak JM, Heath CM: Polypeptide hormone production by "carcinoid" apudomas and their relevant cytochemistry. Virchows Arch 16:95, 1974
367. Weichert RF: The neural ectodermal origin of the peptide secreting endocrine glands: a unifying concept for the etiology of multiple endocrine adenomatosis and the inappropriate secretion of peptide hormones by non-endocrine tumors. Am J Med 49:232, 1970
368. Ostermiller WE, Joergenson EJ. Carcinoid tumors of the small bowel. Arch Surg 93:616, 1966
369. Diffenbaugh WG, Anderson RE: Carcinoid (argentaffin) tumors of the gastrointestinal tract. Arch Surg 73:21, 1956
370. Sterling JA, Jayasanker MR, Galvez M. Carcinoids of the gastrointestinal tract. Am J Gastroenterol 47:373, 1967
371. Herbsman H, Wetstein L, Rosen Y et al: Tumors of the small intestine. Curr Probl Surg 17:121, 1980
372. Horsley BL, Baker RR: Fibroblastic response to intestinal carcinoids. Am J Surg 36:676, 1970
373. Cunningham PJ, Norman J, Cleveland BR: Malignant carcinoid associated with thoraco-abdominal aneurysm and analysis of thirty-one cases of gastrointestinal carcinoid tumors. Ann Surg 176:613, 1972
374. Dockerty MB: Carcinoids of the gastrointestinal tract. Am J Clin Pathol 25:794, 1955
375. Mengel CE, Shaffer RD: The carcinoid syndrome. In Holland JF, Frei E (eds): Cancer Medicine, pp 1584–1594 Philadelphia, Lea & Febiger, 1973
376. Vane JR: The release and fate of vasoactive hormones in the circulation. Br J Pharmacol 35:209, 1969
377. Misiewicz JJ, Waller SL, Eisner M: Motor responses of human gastrointestinal tract to 5-hydroxytryptamine *in-vivo* and *in-vitro*. Gut 7:208, 1966
378. Smith AS, Greaves MW: Blood prostaglandin activity associated with noradrenaline-produced flush in the carcinoid syndrome. Br J Dermatol 90:547, 1974
379. Oates JA, Sjoerdsma A: A unique syndrome associated with secretion of 5-hydroxytryptophan by metastatic gastric carcinoids. Am J Med 32:333, 1962
380. Frolich JC, Bloomgarten ZT, Oates JA et al: The carcinoid flush. Provocation by pentagastrin and inhibition by somatostatin. N Engl J Med 299:1055, 1979
381. Oberhelman HA, Nelsen TS, Johnson AN et al: Ulcerogenic tumors of the duodenum. Ann Surg 153:214, 1961
382. Dabek FT: Bronchial carcinoid tumor with acromegaly in two patients J Clin Endocrinol Metab 38:329, 1974
383. Isawa T, Okubo K, Konno K et al: Cushing's syndrome caused by recurrent malignant broncial carcinoid. Case report with 12 years observation. Ann Rev Resp Dis 108:1200, 1973
384. Milhaud G, Calmette C, Taboulet J et al: Hypersecretion of calcitonin in neoplastic conditions. Lancet 1:462, 1974
385. Delmont J, Rampal P: Prostaglandins and carcinoid tumours. Br Med J 4:165, 1975
386. Feldmann JM, Plonk JW, Cornette JC: Serum prostaglandin $F_{2}\alpha$ concentration in the carcinoid syndrome. Prostaglandins 7:501, 1974
387. Mengel CE: Carcinoid and the heart. Mod Concepts Cardiovasc Dis 35:75, 1966
388. MacDonald JS, Schein PS: Endocrine tumors. In Bergevin PR, Blom J, Tormey DC (eds): Guide to Therapeutic Oncology, pp 497–518. Baltimore, Williams & Wilkins, 1979
389. Crosder BL, Judd ES, Dockerty MD: Gastrointestinal carcinoids and the carcinoid syndrome: Clinical characteristics and therapy. CA 18:359, 1968
390. Oates JA, Butler TC: Pharmacologic and endocrine aspects of carcinoid syndrome. Adv Pharmacol 5:109, 1967
391. Hill GJ: Carcinoid tumors: pharmacological therapy. Oncology 25:329, 1971
392. Brown RE, Hill SR Jr, Berry KW et al: Studies on several possible antiserotin compounds in the functioning carcinoid syndrome. Clin Res 8:61, 1960
393. Mengel CE: Therapy of the malignant carcinoid syndrome. Ann Intern Med 62:587, 1965
394. Engleman K, Sjoerdsma A. Inhibition of catecholamine biosynthesis in man. Circ Res Suppl 1:102, 1966
395. Sjoerdsma A, Lovenberg W. Engelman K et al: Serotonin now: clinical implications of inhibiting its synthesis with para-chlorophenylalanine. Ann Intern Med 73:607, 1970
396. Roch E, Silva M, Garcia-Lerne J: Antagonists of bradykinin. Med Exp 8:287, 1963
397. Melmon KL, Sjoerdsma A, Mason DT: Distinctive clinical and therapeutic aspects of the syndrome associated with bronchial carcinoid tumors. Am J Med 39:568, 1965
398. Ureles AL, Murray M, Wolf R: Results of pharmacologic treatment in malignant carcinoid syndrome. N Engl J Med 267:435, 1963
399. Adamson AR, Grahame-Smith DC, Peart WS et al: Pharmacological blockade of carcinoid flushing provoked by catecholamines and alcohol. Lancet 2:293, 1969
400. Vroom FQ, Brown RE, Dempsey J et al: Studies on several possible antiserotonin compounds in a patient with the functioning carcinoid syndrome. Ann Intern Med 56:941, 1962
401. Reed ML, Kuipers FM, Vaitkevicius VK et al: Treatment of disseminated carcinoid tumors including hepatic-artery catheterization. N Engl J Med 269:1006, 1963
402. Moertel CG: Chemotherapy of gastrointestinal cancer. Clin Gastroenterol 5:777, 1976
403. Moertel CG, Reitemeier RJ, Schutt AJ et al: Phase II study of

streptozotocin (NSC-85998) int he treatment of advanced gastrointestinal cancer. Cancer Chemother Rep 55:303, 1971
404. Schein PS, Kahn R, Jordan P et al: Streptozotocin for malignant insulinoma and carcinoid tumor. Arch Intern Med 132:555, 1973
405. Schein PS, O'Connell MJ, Blom J et al: Clinical antitumor activity and toxicity of streptozotocin (NSC-85998). Cancer 34:993, 1974
406. Soloman A, Sonada T, Patterson FK: Response of metastatic malignant carcinoid tumor to Adriamycin Cancer Treat Rep 60:273, 1977
407. Kessinger A, Foley FJ, Lemon HM: Use of DTIC (Dacarbazine) in the malignant carcinoid syndrome. Cancer Treat Rep 61:101, 1977
408. Moertel CG, Hanley JA: Combination chemotherapy trials for metastatic carcinoid tumor and the malignant carcinoid syndrome. Cancer Clin Trials 2:327, 1979
409. Chernicoff D, Bukowski RM, Groppe CW et al: Combination chemotherapy for islet cell carcinoma and metastatic carcinoid tumors with 5-fluorouracil and streptozotocin. Cancer Treat Rep 63:795, 1979
410. Herbsman H, Hassan A, Gardner B et al: Treatment of hepatic metastases with a combination of hepatic artery infusion chemotherapy and external radiotherapy. Surg Gynecol Obstet 147:13, 1978
411. Moertel CG, Dockerty MB: Familial occurrence of metastasizing carcinoid tumors. Ann Intern Med 78:389, 1973
412. Moertel CG, Dockerty MB: Carcinoid tumors of the vermiform appendix. Cancer 21:270, 1975
413. Orloff MJ: Carcinoid tumors of the rectum. Cancer 28:175, 1971
414. Newsome HH: Multiple endocrine adenomatosis. Surg Clin N Amer 54:387–393, 1974
415. Tomlinson S, O'Riordan JLH, Grahame–Jones E: Multiple endocrine adenomatosis and peptic ulcer. Proc Roy Soc Med 60:445–446, 1973
416. Ballard HS, Frame B, Hartsock RJ: Familial multiple endocrine adenomatosis—peptic ulcer complex. Medicine 43:481–516, 1964
417. Melvin KEW, Tashjian AH Jr, Miller HH: Studies in familial (medullary) thyroid carcinoma. Recent Prog Horm Res 28:399–470, 1972
418. Melvin KEW, Miller HH, Tashjian AH Jr: Early diagnosis of medullary carcinoma of the thyroid gland by means of calcitonin assay. N Eng J Med 285: 1115–1120, 1971
419. Carney JA, Hayles AB: Alimentary tract manifestations of multiple endocrine neoplasia type 2b. Mayo Clin Proc 52:543–548, 1977
420. Khairi MR, Dexter RN, Burzyski NJ et al: Mucosal neuroma, pheochromocytoma and medullary thyroid carcinoma: Multiple endocrine neoplasia type 3: Medicine (Balt) 5:89, 1975
421. Carney JA, Sizemore GW, Tyce GM: Bilateral adrenal medullary hyperplasia in multiple endocrine neoplasia, type 2: the precursor of bilateral pheochromocytoma. Mayo Clin Proc 50:3–10, 1975
422. Carney JA, Sizemore GW, Lovestadt SA: Mucosal ganglioneuromatosis, medullary thyroid carcinoma, and pheochromocytoma: multiple endocrine neoplasia, type 2b. Oral Surg 41:379–752, 1976
423. Carney JA, Go VLW, Sizemore GW et al: Alimentary-tract ganglioneuromatosis: A major component of the syndrome of multiple endocrine enoplasia, type 2b. N Eng J Med 295:1287–1291, 1976
424. Carney JA, Sizemore GW, Sheps SG: Adrenal medullary disease in multiple endocrine neoplasia, type 2: pheochromocytoma and its precursors. Am J Clin Pathol 66:279–290, 1976
425. Underdahl, LO, Wooner LB, Black BM: Multiple endocrine adenomas, report of eight cases in which parathyroids, pituitary and pancreatic islets were involved. J Clin Endocrinol Metab 13:20, 1953
426. Werner P: Genetic aspects of adenomatosis of endocrine glands. Am J Med 16:363, 1954
427. Schmid JR, Labhart A, Rossier PH: Relationship of multiple endocrine adenomas to the syndrome of ulcerogenic islet cell adenomas (Zollinger–Ellison). Am J Med 31:343, 1961
428. Zollinger RM, Ellison EH: Primary peptic ulcertaion of the jejunum associated with islet cell tumors of the pancreas. Am J Surg 142:709, 1955
429. Hazard JB, Hawk WA, Crile G: Medullary (solid) carcinoma of the thyroid: a clinicopathologic entity. J Clin Endocrinol Metab 19:152, 1959
430. Sipple JH: The association of pheochromocytoma with carcinoma of the thyroid gland. Am J Med 31:163–6, 1961
431. William ED: A review of 17 cases of carcinoma of the thyroid and pheochromocytoma. J Clin Path 18:288,292, 1965
432. Williams ED: Diarrhea and thyroid carcinoma. Proc Roy Soc Med 59:602–603, 1966
433. Williams ED, Pollock DJ: Multiple mucosal neuromata with endocrine tumours: a syndrome allied to von Recklinghausen's disease. J Pathol Bacteriol 91:71–80, 1966
434. Steiner AL, Goodman AD, Powers SR: Study of a kindred with pheochromocytoma, medullary thyroid carcinoma, hyperparathyroidism and Cushing's disease: multiple endocrine neoplasia type 2. Medicine (Baltimore) 47:371–409, 1968
435. Gagel RF, Melvin KEW, Tashjian AH Jr et al: Natural history of the familial medullary carcinoma-pheochromocytoma syndrome and the identification of pre-neoplastic stages by screening studies: a five-year report. Trans Assoc Am Physicians 88:177–191, 1975
436. Gilstrap LC III, Brekken AL, Harris RE: Sipple syndrome and pregnancy. JAMA 235:1136–1137, 1976
437. Gorhn RJ, Sedano HO, Vickers RA et al: Multiple mucosal neuromas, pheochromocytoma and medullary carcinoma of the thyroid—a syndrome. Cancer 22:293, 1968
438. Ibanez ML, Cole VW, Russell WO et al: Solid carcinoma of the thyroid gland. Cancer 20:706, 1967
439. Keiser HR, Beaven MA, Doppman J et al: Sipple's syndrome: medullary thyroid carcinoma, pheochromocytoma, and parathyroid disease: studies in a large family. Ann Intern Med 78:561–570, 1973
440. Norton JA, Froome LC, Farrell RE et al: Multiple endocrine neoplasia type IIb: The most aggressive form of medullary thyroid carcinoma. Surg Clin N Amer 59:109–118, 1979
441. Robertson DM, Sizemore GW, Gordon H: Thickened corneal nerves as a manifestation of multiple endocrine neoplasia. Trans Am Acad Ophthalmol Otolaryngol 79:722–787, 1975
442. Schimke RN: Phenotype of malignancy: The mucosal neuroma syndrome. Pediatrics 52:283, 1973
443. Schimke RN, Hartmann WH, Prout TE et al: Syndrome of bilateral pheochromocytoma, medullary thyroid carcinoma and multiple neuromas: a possible regulatory defect in the differentiation of chromaffin tissue. N Eng J Med 279:1–7, 1968
444. Melvin KEW, Miller HH, Tashjian AH Jr: Early diagnosis of medullary carcinoma of the thyroid gland by means of calcitonin assay. N Engl J Med 285:1115–1120, 1971
445. Pearse AGE: Cytochemical and ultrastructure of polypeptide hormone producing cells of the APUD series, and the embyologic physiologic and pathologic implication of the concept. J Histochem Cytochem 17:303, 1969
446. Melvin KE, Tashjian AH: The syndrome of excessive thyrocalcitonin produced by medullary carcinoma of the thyroid. Proc Nat Acad Sci 59:1216–1222, 1968
447. Tashjian AH Jr, Howland BG, Melvin KEW et al: Immunoassay of human calcitonin: clinical measurement, relation to serum calcium and studies in patients with medullary carcinoma. N Eng J Med 283:890–895, 1970
448. Tashjian AH Jr, Voelkel EF: Radioimmunoassay of human calcitonin: application of affinity chromatography. In (Jaffe BM, Behrman H (eds): New York, Academic Press, 1974, pp 199–214.
449. Tashjian AH Jr, Wolfe HJ, Voelkel EF: Human calcintonin: immunologic assay, cytologic localization and studies on medullary thyroid carcinoma. Am J Med 56:840–849, 1974
450. Tashjian AH Jr: Calcitonin 1976: a review of some recent advances. In James VHT (ed): Endocrinology, vol 2, pp 256–261. Amsterdam, Excerpta Medica, 1977

451. Pearse AGE, Polak JM: Endocrine tumors of neural crest origin, neurolipomas, apudomas and the APUD concept. Med Biol 52:3, 1974
452. Graze K, Spiler IJ, Tashjian AH et al: Natural history of familial medullary thyroid carcinoma: Effect of a program for early diagnosis. N Eng J Med 299:980–985, 1978
453. Bade RK, Smager FR: Comparison of serum calcitonin levels after a one-minute calcium injection and pentagastrin injection in the diagnosis of medullary thyroid carcinoma. J Clin Endocrinol Metab 4:980, 1977
454. Hennessy JF, Gray TK, Cooper CW et al: Stimulation of thyrocalcitonin secretion by pentagastrin and calcium in two patients with medullary carcinoma of the thyroid. J Clin Endocrinol Metab 36:200–203, 1973
455. Hennessy JF, Wells SA Jr, Ontjes DA et al: A comparison of pentagastrin injection and calcium infusion as provocative agents for the detection of medullary carcinoma of the thyroid. J Clin Endocrinol Metab 39:487–495, 1974
456. Sizemore GW, Go VLW: Stimulation tests for diagnosis of medullary thyroid carcinoma. Mayo Clin Proc 50:53–56, 1975
457. Wells SA, Baylin SB, Gann DS et al: Medullary thyroid carcinoma: Relationship of method of diagnosis to pathological staging. Ann Surg 188:377, 1978
458. Wells SA, Baylin SB, Linehan WM et al: Provocative agents and the diagnosis of medullary carcinoma of the thyroid gland. Ann Surg 188:189, 1978
459. Chong GC, Beahrs OH, Sizemore GW et al: Medullary carcinoma of the thyroid gland. Cancer 35:695–704, 1975
460. Betts B, O'Malley BP, Rosenthal FD: Hyperparathyroidism: A prerequisite for Zollinger-Ellison syndrome in multiple endocrine adenomatosis. Type I. Q J Med 99:69–76, 1980
461. Modlin IM: Endocrine tumors of the pancreas. Surg Gynecol Obstet 149:751, 1979
462. Jackson CE, Tashjian AH Jr, Block MA: Detection of medullary thyroid cancer by calcitonin assay in families. Ann Intern Med 78:845–852, 1973
463. Wells SA Jr, Ontjes DA, Cooper CW et al: The early diagnosis of medullary carcinoma of the thyroid in patients with multiple endocrine neoplasia type II. Ann Surg 182:362–370, 1975
464. Miller HH, Melvin KEW, Gibson JM et al: Surgical approach to early familial medullary carcinoma of the thyroid gland. Am J Surg 123:438–443, 1972
465. Leape LL, Miller HH, Graze K et al: Total thyroidectomy for occult familial medullary carcinoma of the thyroid in children. J Pediatr Surg 11: 831–836, 1976
466. Carney JA, Sizemore GW, Hayles AB: Multiple endocrine neoplasia type 2b. Pathobiol Annu 8:104–153, 1978
467. Wolfe HJ, DeLellis RA, Jackson CE et al: Immunocytochemical distinction of hereditary from sporadic medullary carcinoma. Lab Invest 42:161–162, 1980
468. DeLellis RA, Nunnemacher G, Wolfe HJ: C-cell hyperplasia: an ultrastructural analysis. Lab Invest 36:237–248, 1977
469. Hansen OP, Hansen M, Hansen HH: Multiple endocrine adenomatosis of mixed type: Acta Med Scand 200:327–331, 1976
470. Cameron D, Spiro HM, Landsberg L: Zollinger-Ellison syndrome with multiple endocrine adenomatosis type II. N Eng J Med 299:152–153, 1978
471. Janson KL, Roberts JA, Varela M: Multiple endocrine adenomatosis: In support of the common origin theories. J Urol 119:161–165, 1978
472. Alberta WM, McMeekin JO, George JM: Mixed multiple endocrine neoplasia syndromes. JAMA 244:1236–1237, 1980
473. DeLellis RA, Wolfe HJ, Gagel RF et al: Adrenal medullary hyperplasia: A morphometric analysis in patients with familial medullary thyroid carcinoma. Am J Pathol 83:177–196, 1976
474. Polak JM, Stagg B, Pearse AGE: Two types of Zollinger–Ellison syndrome: Immunofluorescent, cytochemical and ultrastructural studies of the antral and pancreatic gastrin cells in different clinical states. Gut 13:501, 1972

Steven A. Rosenberg
Herman D. Suit
Laurence H. Baker
Gerald Rosen

CHAPTER 29

Sarcomas of the Soft Tissue and Bone

The term 'soft tissue' refers to the extraskeletal connective tissues of the body that connect, support, and surround other discrete anatomic structures. This portion of the body mass lying between the epidermis and parenchymal organs includes the organs of locomotion, such as muscles and tendons, as well as a wide variety of 'supportive' tissue structures, such as fibrous tissue, fat, synovial tissue, and so forth. The soft somatic tissues are ubiquitous and comprise over 50% of the body weight. The over 400 muscles in the human body comprise about 40% of adult body weight.

The term 'soft tissue sarcomas' refers to a large variety of malignant tumors arising in the soft tissues that are grouped together because of similarities in pathologic appearance, clinical presentation, and behavior. Though embryologic, functional, and morphologic bases for characterization of the soft tissue sarcomas exist, none alone are complete in their definition of this tumor group.

Virtually all of the tumors included in the 'soft tissue' sarcomas (from the Greek *sarkoma* meaning fleshy growth) arise from a common embryonic ancestry, the primitive mesoderm (see Table 29-1). By the ninth to thirteenth day after fertilization of the ovum the human embryo undergoes a transition from a phase of increasing cell number to a phase of morphologic organization into the endoderm, ectoderm, and mesoderm, the three primary germ layers of the embryo.[1] Within these layers are established commitments to developmental potentials that far precede morphologic differentiation of the cells. The primitive mesoderm gives rise to a variety of organs, such as the kidney, ureter, oviducts, uterus, gonads, and heart, as well as a wide range of hematopoietic, lymphatic, and reticuloendothelial tissues. The primitive mesenchyme, a loose network of cells and intercellular matrix within the mesoderm, is largely responsible for the development of the common connective tissues of the body listed in Table 29-1. Only these latter tissues (when they undergo malignant transformation) are included in the category of soft tissue sarcomas. Because of similarities in morphology and clinical behavior, tumors arising in Schwann cells, a class of cells surrounding peripheral nerves that arise from the neural tube of the primitive ectoderm, are also included in the category of soft tissue sarcomas.

It has been customary to categorize malignant tumors into sarcomas and carcinomas based on whether they arise in connective tissue (sarcomas) or epithelial tissue (carcinomas). This differentiation is imprecise and many sarcomas arise from tissues that fit the morphologic criteria of epithelium. Epithelium is a morphologic, not an embryologic, term that is used to designate cellular structures that cover or line surfaces on or in the body and may arise from either ectoderm, endoderm, or mesoderm. The endothelium, or lining of the blood-vascular and lymphatic channels, and the mesothelium, or lining of the body cavities and visceral organs, are two types of epithelium that arise from the mesoderm. These epithelial structures give rise to malignant tumors that resemble and behave like tumors that develop from connective tissue cells rather than like tumors developing from epithelial cells. For this reason, tumors arising from the endothelium and the mesothelium are included in the category of sarcomas.

In summary, sarcomas arise largely, though not exclusively, from mesodermal structures and largely, though not exclusively, from connective tissue cells. Some sarcomas arise from ectodermal structures and some from epithelium. Therefore,

TABLE 29-1. Embryonic Derivation of the Soft Tissue and Bony Sarcomas

Fertilized ovum
→ Blastoderm (day 9–13)

- Endoderm
  - GI tract
  - Lungs, etc
- Mesoderm
  - Hematopoietic system
  - Genitourinary system
  - Heart
  - Connective tissue and smooth muscle of viscera → Visceral sarcomas
  - Pleura, Peritoneum, Pericardium, Blood vessels (wall, endothelium), Bone, Cartilage, Muscle, Soft connective tissues (fibrous, synovial, etc) → Soft tissue and boney sarcomas
- Ectoderm
  - Skin
    - Mammary gland, etc.
  - Nervous system
    - Brain
    - Spinal cord
    - Adrenal medula
    - Schwann cells → Soft tissue and boney sarcomas

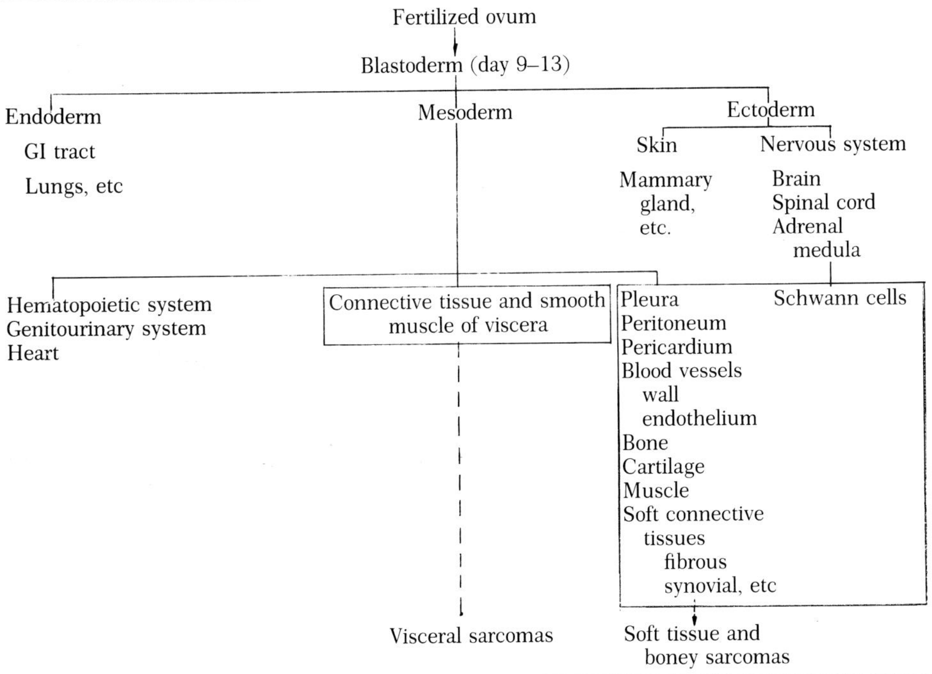

sarcomas are defined as a class of malignant tumors arising largely, though not exclusively, from mesenchymal connective tissues that are characterized by a common morphologic appearance and clinical behavior.

This chapter will deal mainly with the description of the natural history and treatment of the soft tissue and bony sarcomas. All visceral organs contain a connective tissue stroma that can undergo malignant transformation. These 'visceral sarcomas' will be discussed in the chapters dealing with each individual organ system.

INCIDENCE OF SARCOMAS

Approximately 4,500 new cases of soft tissue sarcoma and 1,600 deaths from this disease are reported in the U.S. each year.[2] The annual age-adjusted incidence rate is 2 per 100,000. There is no sex or racial prediliction in the incidence of these cancers.

Soft tissue sarcomas comprise 0.7% of all cancers, though these tumors comprise 6.5% of all cancers in children under the age of 15.[2] Soft tissue sarcomas rank fifth in cancer incidence in children under the age of 15 behind leukemia, central nervous system cancers, lymphomas, and sympathetic nervous system cancers. Soft tissue sarcomas rank fifth as a cause of cancer death in this age group behind leukemia, brain and nervous system cancer, renal cancer, and bone cancer.[2]

EPIDEMIOLOGY

Little is known concerning epidemiologic or etiologic factors of importance in patients with soft tissue sarcomas. There is no proven genetic predisposition to the development of soft tissue sarcomas though Li and Fraumeni have reported four kindreds with pairs of young children (three sets of sibs and one set of cousins) with soft tissue sarcomas.[3] This incidence exceeded that expected on a chance basis ($p = 0.06$). Howard reported two brothers that developed rhabdomyosarcoma of the orbit.[4] Only one in from 100–400 cases of childhood rhabdomyosarcoma are associated with other relatives developing this cancer, however.[3,5]

Several reports have noted an association of childhood sarcomas with a small increased incidence of other familial cancers (most notably, breast cancer) that tended to occur in mothers under 30 years of age.[3,5-11] Other, rather unconvincing evidence for a link between breast cancer and sarcomas was the report of breast cancer as a second primary tumor in 2 of 24 women with liposarcoma.[12] The lymphangiosarcomas of the arm in women following mastectomy and axillary lymph node ablation (Stewart–Treves syndrome) probably does not represent evidence of an etiologic correlation between mammary cancer and sarcoma of soft tissue, but rather development of lymphangiosarcoma in lymphedematous arms.[13]

Though Sloane and Hubbel have reported an increased incidence of congenital defects in children with soft tissue sarcomas, this association was not seen by Li and Fraumeni.[5,14]

Soft tissue sarcomas are thought to occur with slightly increased frequency in patients with a variety of genetically transmitted diseases, such as the basal cell nevus syndrome, multiple neurofibromatosis, tuberous sclerosis, Werner's syndrome, intestinal polyposis, and Gardner's syndrome.[11,15-18]

Though many patients with soft tissue sarcomas present with a recent history of trauma there is no known etiologic relationship and it is likely that minor trauma merely calls a pre-existing lesion to the patients' attention. Chemical carcinogens, such as 3-methylcholanthrene as well as viruses can cause soft tissue sarcomas in experimental animals though there is no convincing link between these factors and sarcomas in humans. Recent reports, however, have linked environmental exposure to phenoxyacetic acids (a class of herbicides) and chlorophenols (wood preservatives) to a six-fold increase in the risk of developing soft tissue sarcoma.[19]

Sarcomas have a higher tendency to occur in areas previously exposed to ionizing irradiation though sarcomas in radiation therapy fields are uncommon.

In 1980, Kim and associates could find only 13 cases in the world literature of fibrosarcoma of the chest wall in women undergoing radiation therapy following mastectomy for breast cancer.[20] The latent period of these lesions ranged from 4–24 years after radiation exposures from 2,000–7,800 rad. Osteosarcomas appear to be the most common sarcomas induced by radiation. Arlen and associates summarized 50 cases of postradiation osteosarcoma and in a long-term follow-up of 455 persons who painted luminous watch dials with radiomesotherium, 26 developed osteosarcoma.[21,22]

Sarcomas are associated with foreign body implantations in rodents. Sporadic reports of this phenomena in humans have also appeared.[23] Ott has tabulated all cases published prior to 1966.[24] In these cases the responsible foreign bodies were mainly metal implants, bullets, shrapnel pieces, bone transplants, and so forth, with latent periods of up to 40 years. The true incidence of foreign body-induced sarcomas is probably minimal since no sarcomas were seen among 11,000 women who underwent augmentation mammoplasty with a variety of materials or in 281 patients who underwent prosthetic replacement for facial defects.[21,26]

SITES OF SOFT TISSUE SARCOMAS

Because of the ubiquitous nature of the connective tissues, soft tissue sarcomas can arise anywhere in the body. Visceral sarcomas can arise from the connective stroma found in all organs; these lesions will not be considered here. The sites of soft tissue sarcomas in four large reported series are presented in Table 29-2.[27-30] About 40% of soft tissue sarcomas occur in the lower extremity, about 75% of these at or above the knee. The upper extremity is the site of about 15% of the soft tissue sarcomas; the trunk accounts for about 30%. Those in the trunk are divided between the retroperitoneum, which accounts for about 10% of these lesions, while most other trunkal sarcomas involve the abdominal or chest wall. The head and neck accounts for about 15% of sarcomas.

PATHOLOGIC CLASSIFICATION

Each of the soft tissues can undergo malignant transformation to a sarcoma. Because of the large number of different soft tissues a variety of distinct but often morphologically similar sarcomas have been identified.[31-35] Each of these tissues can also give rise to benign tumors. While many of these benign growths are easily identifiable, a group of tumors also exist arising from the soft tissues that appear morphologically similar to the sarcomas, but rarely metastasize. Many of these latter tumors (*e.g.* desmoid tumors or aggressive fibromatosis) are capable of aggressively invading local tissues in a fashion characteristic of a true sarcoma. It is important to distinguish these locally aggressive but non-metastasizing lesions from those that are truly 'benign' and those that are 'malignant' because of the obvious differences in therapeutic implications. The response to injury of many of the soft tissues can also give rise to proliferative lesions. These can mimic soft tissue tumors and because of their high mitotic rate can often be difficult to distinguish from malignant lesions; an example of such a benign process is myositis ossificans. The pathologic classification presented in Table 29-3 is based on the putative cell of origin of each tumor. Pathologic classification based on describing the appearance of the predominant cell in the lesion (*i.e.* naming round cell or spindle cell sarcomas) are less useful and should not be employed. In general, each of the sarcomas tends to reflect the morphologic appearance of the cell of origin of most of these tumors and the tendency of these tumors to dedifferentiate results in a variety of overlapping patterns that can make them very difficult to distinguish from one another. Competent pathologists often disagree on the histogenic cell of origin of an individual

TABLE 29-2. Sites of Soft Tissue Sarcomas

	Sheiber et al 1962 (27)*	Russell et al 1977 (28)	Lindberg et al 1977 (29)	Rosenberg et al 1978 (30)	Total
Number of patients	125	1215	166	113	1,619
Site			(% of total cases)		
Head and neck	12.8	15	9.0	4.4	12
Trunk	31.2	32	25.9	34.5	30
(Mediastinum)		(1)		(0.9)	
(Retroperitoneum)		(13)	(9)	(15.0)	
Upper extremity	16.0	13	25.9	10.6	16
Lower extremity	40.0	40	39.2	50.5	42
(At/above knee)		(32)		(38.0)	
(Below knee)		(8)		(12.4)	

*Reference number.

TABLE 29-3. Pathologic Classification of Soft Tissue Tumors

PRESUMED CELL OF ORIGIN	BENIGN TUMORS	BENIGN TUMORS REQUIRING VIGOROUS LOCAL THERAPY	MALIGNANT TUMORS
Fibrous	Fibroma, elastofibroma, palmar and plantar fibromatosis, juvenile aponeurotic fibroma, congenital generalized fibromatosis, fibrous hamartoma of infancy, fibromatosis colli, penile fibromatosis, nodular fasciitis, abdominal desmoid	Extra-abdominal desmoid (aggressive fibromatosis)	Fibrosarcoma
Striated muscle	Rhabdomyoma		Rhabdomyosarcoma
Smooth muscle	Leiomyoma, epithelioid leiomyoma		Leiomyosarcoma
Adipose	Lipoma, atypical lipoma, lipoblastomatosis, hibernoma	Atypical intramuscular lipoma	Liposarcoma
Synovial	Giant cell tumor of tendon sheath, ganglion, villonodular synovitis		Synovial sarcoma
Neural	Neurilemoma, neurofibroma		Neurofibrosarcoma
Vascular and lymphatic	Hemangioma, lymphangioma glomus tumor	Infantile hemangiopericytoma	Angiosarcoma, lymphangiosarcoma, malignant hemangiopericytoma, Kaposi's sarcoma
Histiocytic	Dermatofibroma, fibrous histiocytoma	Atypical fibrous histiocytoma, dermatofibrosarcoma protuberans	Malignant fibrous hystiocytoma, giant cell sarcoma
Mesothelial	Mesothelioma		Malignant mesothelioma
Uncertain	Mesenchymoma, myxoma, granular cell myoblastoma		Alveolar soft part sarcoma, epitheliod sarcoma, malignant mesenchymoma, clear cell sarcoma, malignant granular cell tumor

tumor. The great variation in the reported incidence of various subtypes of soft tissue sarcomas probably reflects differences in pathologic opinion rather than true differences in incidence. Attempts to assign a pathologic grade to an individual tumor in the hope that this might be predictive of clinical behavior is still poorly defined. Although attempts to perform this grading based on mitotic rate, nuclear morphology, and presence of necrosis are predictive of prognosis, no good criteria applicable to all tumors have been described.

In addition to routine light microscopy, histochemistry, electron microscopy, and tissue culture studies can all play a role in distinguishing one tumor subtype from another. In recent years, much progress has been made in the pathologic classification of the soft tissue sarcomas; a variety of new lesions have been identified and characterized.[33] The classification in Table 29-3 distinguishes tumors that are benign, tumors that are benign but with aggressive local growth requiring vigorous local treatment, and malignant tumors. Frequently, it is difficult to assign a definite cell of origin for all benign and malignant tumors. In these instances, the assignment made in the classification in Table 29-3 has been quite arbitrary. Highly undifferentiated tumors may be designated soft tissue sarcoma, type unspecified. For some tumors the cell of origin is unknown even though the tumor is not poorly differentiated, such as epithelioid sarcomas and alveolar soft-part sarcomas. This is indicated in Table 29-3.

MALIGNANT LESIONS

RELATIVE INCIDENCE

In considering the relative incidence of histologic types of soft tissue sarcomas it should be emphasized that competent pathologists will differ significantly in attaching a histogenic label to individual cases. These disagreements also confound attempts to compare series from different institutions with respect to frequency of tumors at different anatomic sites, stage of disease at presentation, frequency of local failure with different treatment modalities, frequency of distant metastasis and other parameters. This is particularly evident in considering Table 29-4, which collates the relative frequency of the various histopathologic types in several series.[27,28,30,36–42] As can be seen, large differences exist in the incidence of the different histopathologic types; these differences almost certainly reflect differences in diagnostic criteria used by the

TABLE 29-4. Relative Incidence of Histologic Types of Soft Tissue Sarcomas

Author	Shieber et al	Hare et al	Pack et al	Martin et al	Ferrell et al	Shiu et al	Simon et al	Russell et al	Lindberg et al	Rosenberg et al	Total
Year	1962	1963	1964	1965	1972	1975	1976	1977	1977	1978	
Reference	(27)	(36)	(37)	(38)	(39)	(40)	(41)	(28)	(42)	(30)	
Sites	All	All	All	All	All	Extremity	Extremity	All	All	All	
Total No. of cases	125	200	717	398	117	297	54	1215	166	113	3,404
Type											
Unclassified	0	28.5	36.4	14.8	0	7.1	5.6	10.0	6.0	17.4	12.5
Liposarcoma	16.0	11.5	14.6	26.9	17.0	27.6	18.5	18.2	12.7	22.6	18.7
Rhabdomyosarcoma	16.0	5.0	13.9	20.6	30.0	17.5	5.6	19.3	9.6	10.4	14.8
Synoviosarcoma	0.8	2.5	8.4	3.0	2.5	14.1	5.6	6.9	10.2	11.3	6.5
Neurofibrosarcoma	3.2	0	6.4	0	0	5.4	0	4.9	19.3	6.1	4.5
Fibrosarcoma	44.0	43.0	5.4	24.1	33.0	20.2	37.0	19.0	13.3	1.7	24.1
Angiosarcoma	4.8	0	2.6	0.3	0	2.0	0	2.7	1.2	1.7	1.5
Leiomyosarcoma	6.4	6.5	0	6.3	4.0	2.4	0	6.5	4.2	11.3	4.8
Mesenchymoma	0	0	0	0	0	0.3	0	0.3	0	0.1	0.1
Malignant fibrous histiocytoma	0	0	0	0	0	1.0	20.4	10.5	17.5	17.4	6.7
Other	8.8	3.0	12.1	4.0	13.5	2.4	7.4	1.7	6.0	0	5.7

involved pathologists. For example, in the series by Sheiber and associates and Ferrell and associates, there are no lesions that are considered as unclassifiable sarcomas.[27,39] In contrast, Hare and coworkers had 28.5% such lesions, Pack and coworkers had 36.4% such lesions and Rosenberg and coworkers 17.4% unclassifiable lesions.[30,36,37] A further example of these disparities is illustrated by the 5.4% incidence of fibrosarcomas in the series by Pack and associates compared to the 37–44% incidence of fibrosarcomas in the series reported by Simon and coworkers, Hare and coworkers, and Sheiber and coworkers.[27,36,37,41] In recent years, changes in histologic classification of these lesions, such as the recognition of a separate category of malignant fibrous histiocytomas, has also lead to wide variations in the reported relative incidence of soft tissue sarcomas. For example, in the five series listed in Table 29-3 published prior to 1972, no cases of malignant fibrous histiocytomas were reported. Since 1972, this lesion has gained increasing recognition and the 20.4% incidence reported in the series by Simon and associates in 1976 is quite comparable to the 18.0% reported by Lindberg and associates and the 17.4% reported by Rosenberg and associates.[30,41,42]

It is clear, therefore, that significant disagreement exists among pathologists concerning the exact diagnosis of individual soft tissue sarcomas. This point should be kept in mind when comparing reported series of individual subtypes of sarcomas. The available evidence indicates that the histopathologic grade is a very powerful indicator of the biologic behavior of soft tissue sarcomas and is of more value to the clinician involved in the management of sarcoma patients than is the knowledge of the exact histopathologic variety of tumor.[28] When histologic grade is accounted for, however, most soft tissue sarcomas have a common biologic behavior. This feature, combined with the difficulties in pathologic classification listed above, make it necessary to consider the treatment of soft tissue sarcomas as a group.

BENIGN TUMORS OF SOFT TISSUE

BENIGN TUMORS OF FIBROUS ORIGIN

There are a large number of variants of fibrous tumors that are non-malignant and do not metastasize. Most are successfully treated by simple excision and do not recur. Some tumors in this categoy, such as nodular fasciitis, can cause difficulty because they can be mistaken for true fibrosarcomas. Others, such as extra-abdominal desmoid tumors, require special attention because aggressive local therapy is necessary to prevent recurrence.

Fibroma

The term *fibroma* has been applied to any benign fibrous growth. Many congenital malformations and reparative tissue growths fall in this category. With an increasing understanding of the variants of fibrous tissue neoplasms, fewer tumors are now referred to as fibromas and the term is now restricted to benign, encapsulated, fibrous nodules that seldom attain size greater than a few centimeters in diameter. Subcutaneous or soft fibroma (fibroma molle) is a pedunculated subcutaneous growth composed of fibrous tissue and fat covered by epidermis. Fibroma durum is a pedunculated lesion often arising in the oral mucosa that may result from malocclusion or malfitting dentures. All of these lesions should be treated by simple excision. They rarely, if ever, recur.

Elastofibroma

This is a rare lesion that usually occurs under the scapular muscles and frequently attaches to the rib cage.[43–46] Many are not appreciated and one series found them present in 10% of 235 autopsy cases.[44] The lesions are totally benign and do not recur after simple enucleation.

Palmar and Plantar Fibromatosis

Tumor-like proliferations of the palmar and plantar aponeuroses can occur and give rise to tumor-like nodules.[47–50] Only the palmar fibromatosis (Dupuytren's contracture) is associated with flexion contractures. Hereditary factors appear to affect incidence, and males predominate over females by 6:1. These lesions grow slowly as localized nodular enlargements that can infiltrate the fascia and involve overlying skin and subcutaneous tissue. The lesions are benign though they have a tendency to recur after simple excision. Consequently, small nodules should be left untouched. When excision is necessary, attempts should be made to widely excise the palmar or plantar fascia.

Juvenile Aponeurotic Fibroma (Keasby Tumor)

This form of fibromatosis effects the palms or soles of children and young adults.[51–53] The lesion can infiltrate and overgrow subcutaneous fat and muscle, though metastases never occur. The lesions invade locally and have a tendency to recur after limited excision. Thus, attempts to acheive negative microscopic margins should be made.

Congenital Generalized Fibromatosis

This generalized condition, generally present at birth, is characterized by multiple, widely scattered nodular and infiltrating fibroblastic lesions, diffusely present in the superficial and deep tissues. viscera, and bone.[54–56] The disease is usually fatal because of vital organ involvement.

Fibrous Hamartoma of Infancy

This lesion occurs predominantly in males and presents in the first year of life with a solitary mass in the axilla, upper extremity, head, or neck.[57] These lesions are situated almost exclusively in the dermis or subcutaneous fat and can acheive large size. Local excision is almost always curative; this lesion does not metastasize.

Fibromatosis Colii

This distinctive form of fibromatosis develops in the sternocleidomastoid muscle of newborn or very young children. In many cases, a small lump in the sternocleidomastoid muscle noticed in the newborn disappears spontaneously.[58,59] If, however, the lesion persists for several months after birth it will increase in size and often lead to the development of neck contractures. Untreated cases can result in very large growths with subsequent spread to the trachea and surrounding organs. These lesions should be excised and often require removal of the entire sternocleidomastoid muscle.

Penile Fibromatosis

This lesion (also called Peyronie's disease) involves a circumscribed fibrous thickening arising in the connective tissue sheath that separates the corpus cavernosum from the tunic albuginea.[60] It causes pain and curvature of the penis on penile erection. Surgical excision of the fibrous tissue is preferred treatment.

Nodular Fasciitis

This is a benign lesion (also termed pseudosarcomatous or proliferative fasciitis) that should be treated by simple excision though its morphologic appearance causes it to be confused with a fibrosarcoma.[61–63] These lesions generally arise in the subcutaneous fascia or the superficial portions of the deep fascia. The growth of these lesions is frequently rapid after they appear. Maximum size is usually achieved within a few weeks and then growth stops. These lesions rarely achieve a size greater than 5 cm and are often asymptomatic. Fewer than 10% recur after simple excision.

Desmoid Tumors

These tumors (also known as aggressive fibromatosis, musculo-aponeurotic fibromatosis) derive primarily from fascial sheaths and musculo-aponeurotic structures throughout the body. They differ from most fibrous growths by their tendency to infiltrate extensively into surrounding structures.[65–67]

The term *abdominal desmoid tumor* refers to lesions found in the muscular aponeurotic structures of the abdominal wall, especially in post-partum women.[68] The lesions are thought to be reparative in nature and to have been initiated by the effects of pregnancy on the abdominal wall musculature. If the lesions are resected with good margin they do not recur. Because of the anatomic location, the lesions are usually seen when they are small. Surgical resection is readily feasible and straightforward. These tumors generally do not recur after simple excision.

Extra-abdominal desmoid tumors may present more difficult problems to the physician because they occur in sites where wide field radical resection is not technically feasible; if attempted, it may be associated with appreciable morbidity. These lesions are not uncommon around the shoulder girdle, inguinal region, and lower extremity; they are also unencapsulated. They infiltrate locally, are destructive, but do not metastasize. Histopathologically, these lesions are primarily fibroblastic with elongated, thin, delicate nuclei, which appear virtually normal. Mitotic figures are most uncommon, usually less than 1 per 50 high power field. The preferred treatment for extra-abdominal desmoid is wide-field resection with care to achieve negative margins in all dimensions. If this is not obtained then efforts should be made to do a wider resection to achieve negative margins. This is true because local recurrence of these lesions where margins are close or margins are positive occurs in the range of 50–75%. In those situations where wide resection is not feasible radiation therapy is an effective treatment modality. James Ewing, in 1928, commented that desmoid tumors did in fact respond to radiation, but slowly, and that this treatment modality could be considered for lesions not amenable to surgical resection.[69] Successful treatment by radiation has been reported in an incidental way in describing results of large surgical series.[70]

More recently, radiation treatment of desmoids has been described.[71] Benninghoff and Robbins described the treatment of four patients with desmoid tumors, three of whom were treated following incomplete surgery and one for frank recurrent tumor. Radiation doses were modest, but good responses were obtained at least in 3 of 4 patients. In 1977, Wara and associates reported on a series of 16 patients with desmoid tumors, 12 of whom were treated for gross tumor (*i.e.* tumor masses greater than 5 cm in dimension). Two of these 12 died of disease but the remaing 10 were alive without tumor 2–6 years post-treatment. Of the four patients treated after incomplete surgical resection (no palpable tumor), there was one local recurrence at 2 years; the other 3 patients were free of evident disease at 2–4 years. Suit and Russell described the results of treatment of four patients with desmoid tumor, two of whom had massive local disease and two of whom were treated post-incomplete surgery.[73] All four have remained disease-free for 5 years. Ten patients have been treated by radiation for desmoid tumors at the Massachusetts General Hospital and followed for more than 18 months (seven had gross palpable tumor and three were post-incomplete surgical resection). For these patients, the radiation dose has been in the range of 5,500–7,000 cGy delivered in 6–8 weeks. Of the seven patients treated with palpable disease, all had complete clearance and six remain free of evident tumor. The one local failure occurred at 1½ years after treatment, involving a 9-year-old boy who presented with disease at multiple sites in the neck (submental region to the superstemal notch) following repeated surgical resections. Because of the age of the patient and extent of involvement, the radiation dose was only 5,500 cGy, the lowest dose employed in this study. However, this is within the range of successfully employed dose levels by Wara and Phillips and higher than that by Benninghoff.

BENIGN TUMORS OF STRIATED MUSCLE

Rhabdomyoma

These are extremely rare benign tumors of skeletal muscle, generally occuring in the tongue, neck muscles, larnyx uvula, nasal cavity, axilla, vulva, and heart.[74,75] These tumors are benign and are treated by simple excision.

BENIGN TUMORS OF SMOOTH MUSCLE

Leiomyoma

Leiomyomas rarely occur outside of the uterus and the GI tract.[76,77] They can occur in the skin and subcutaneous tissues and probably arise from the smooth muscle of small blood vessels in these tissues. These lesions are treated by simple excision.

Epithelioid Leiomyoma

Epithelioid leiomyoma (leiomyoblastoma) are most frequently found in the wall of the GI tract, especially in the stomach. They are similar to other smooth muscle tumors but may become very large in size, hemorrhagic, and exhibit small cystic areas. Simple excision is the treatment of choice and is almost always curative.

BENIGN TUMORS OF ADIPOSE TISSUE

Lipomas

Lipomas are among the most common of all benign neoplasms and arise in any location where fat is normally present. These lesions may occur in deep tissue, although they are usually subcutaneous in origin. They are characteristically multilobulated masses of fatty tissue that may vary in size from small nodules to large masses weighing several kilograms.

There are several variants of the lipomas that deserve mention. Multiple lipomatosis is a conditon of diffuse overgrowths that may occur throughout the body. These are not true tumors and are probably a result of fat metabolism disorders.

Spindle cell lipomas are rare benign tumors that occur almost exclusively in the neck and shoulders of males.[78] The major importance of these tumors is their tendency to be confused with liposarcomas.

Angiolipomas are lipomas that contain a network of many small capillaries that are usually quite painful.[79] Some angiolipomas are of an infiltrating variety and require a wider margin of resection than most normal lipomas.

The treatment for lipomas is simple enucleation. Recurrence is extremely unusual when this limited treatment is used.

Lipoblastomatosis

This rare abnormality (also termed adipose hamartomatosis) is found in infants. It consists of lobular soft tissue growths separated by partitions of loose fibrous tissue.[80,81] About 10% of these lesions recur after simple local excision, but they have no tendency to metastasize.

Atypical Lipoma

Atypical lipomas are a recent designation applied to subcutaneous lipomatous neoplasms that display cytologic atypia of a nature not seen in most lipomas.[82-85] These lesions can occur in either the subcutaneous or deep muscular layers. Simple excision cures virtually all subcutaneous lesions, though simple excision of deep muscular lesions often results in local recurrence that may require re-excision. These lesions have no tendency to metastasize and can most often be controlled by re-excision.

Hibernoma

Hibernomas are an unusual type of lipoma that are thought to arise from vestiges of brown fat similar to the glandular, brown adipose tissue occurring in certain hibernating animal species.[86] These are benign tumors and should be treated by simple excision.

BENIGN TUMORS OF SYNOVIAL TISSUE

Giant Cell Tumor of Tendon Sheath

These benign lesions (also termed localized nodular tenosynovitis) are usually solitary and arise from either the tendon sheath, joints, or bursea of the hand, palm or wrist.[87,88] These soft tissue lesions can produce atrophy of the bony cortex or actual erosion into adjacent bone. Simple excision is the treatment of choice. Villonodular synovitis is probably related to giant cell tumors of tendon sheath but almost always occurs in joints and presents with pain and swelling. This benign tumor-like growth erodes into the bone and appears as a primary bone tumor. The synovium of the effected joint is generally diffusely involved and total synovectomy is the treatment of choice.

Ganglion

Ganglions are multilocular, fibrous, walled cysts usually occurring on the dorsal aspect of the wrist. These lesions appear to form as a result of synovial tissue that has become pinched off and undergoes degeneration. Simple excision is almost always curative.

BENIGN TUMORS OF NEURAL TISSUE

Neurilemoma

These are benign, encapsulated tumors, also called Schwannomas, that almost always occur as solitary lesions.[89,90] The most common site of origin is the eighth cranial nerve (acoustic neurinoma), though cranial peripheral nerves may often be affected. This is also the most common benign neoplasm of the spinal canal. These lesions often grow in continuity with an easily demonstrable flattened nerve seen along its capsule. These lesions rarely recur when resected locally. Every effort should be made to preserve the nerve involved if this nerve is of clinical significance (*e.g.*, the facial nerve). These lesions arise from Schwann cells although they are different from neurofibromas.

Neurofibroma

Neurofibromas are also thought to arise from Schwann cells although they differ from neurilemomas in that they tend not to be encapsulated and have a much softer consistency. [89] They may also occur at multiple different sites. These lesions may be locally infiltrative although simple excision is almost always curative.

Multiple neurofibromas are a feature of Von Recklinghausen's disease.[91-97] In this condition neurofibromas may occur in virtually all sites of the body and be in association with virtually any peripheral nerve as well as intraspinal nerves. Plexiform neurofibromas may result in massive enlargement of an extremity. About 5–10% of patients with Von Recklinghausen's disease develop a malignant schwannoma though these malignant tumors rarely arise in benign, superficial neurofibromas. Neurofibromas in Von Recklinghausen's disease should be removed only for cosmetic reasons and not because of a tendency to degenerate into malignant tumors.

BENIGN TUMORS OF VASCULAR TISSUE

Hemangioma

Hemangiomas are vascular neoplasms that can occur anywhere in the body.[98-100] About 75% are present at birth and about 60% occur in the head and neck area. The majority of hemangiomas of infancy will spontaneously regress. Some lesions grow rapidly during the early months of life and may be a source of some concern though virtually all disappear by about 5 years of age. These lesions may be primarily composed of capillaries or widely dilated veins (cavernous hemangioma). These lesions do not metastasize and simple excision will often be curative, though is not necessary except for cosmetic reasons. In some instances, the angioma may exhibit rapid growth and abut on or compromise vital structures. In these instances, low-dose radiation confined to the hemangioma may be employed. Efforts should be made to use techniques that limit the dose to the vascular process itself. Radiation treatment for these lesions is very rarely indicated and even large centers probably would not see more than three or four cases per decade where radiation treatment would be warranted.

Lymphangioma

These lesions are similar to hemangiomas although the vascular spaces do not contain blood cells. These lesions can occur virtually anywhere in the body. Cystic hygromas are lymphangiomas of the neck.

Glomus Tumors

The normal glomus is a one millimeter end organ arteriovenous anastomosis.[101–104] This organ enlarges into a painful and tender mass. About 15% are present in the subungual regions, though any location in the skin and soft tissue is possible. Local excision is usually curative and metastases do not occur. Glomus tumors may be located along the larger vessels. A common syndrome is that of the glomus tumor near the jugular foramen designated as a glomus jugulari. These lesions are not resectable and are effectively and readily treated by radiation therapy (5,000 cGy delivered over about 5 weeks). Lesions regress slowly but permanent control of the process is regularly achieved.

Infantile Hemangiopericytomas

Although hemangiopericytomas in the adult are more benign in their behavior than most soft tissue sarcomas, these tumors can definitely metastasize and will therefore be considered under the truly malignant lesions.[104,105] However, hemangiopericytomas that occur in infancy appear to be benign lesions without significant metastatic potential. These tumors occur almost exclusively in the skin and may have evidence of infiltrative growth outside the main tumor mass. These lesions generally do not recur after wide local excision.

BENIGN TUMORS OF HISTIOCYTIC TISSUE

In recent years, significant improvement in our understanding and recognition of tumors of presumed histiocytic origin has taken place largely due to the work of Stout and colleagues.[33,34] Variants of these tumors have received over 30 different names in a variety of nomenclature systems. These tumors are composed wholely or in part of cells with the morphologic characteristics of histiocytes but with a varying fibroblastic component as well. It is thought, though evidence is not conclusive, that these tumors are of purely histiocytic origin but that histiocytes in these lesions can differentiate toward fibroplastic morphology.

Dermatofibroma

These are common soft tissue lesions (also called sclerosing hemangioma or fibrous xanthoma of skin) that are generally about 1 cm in diameter and occur in the dermis. Simple excision is always curative.

Fibrous Histiocytoma

Many variants of this lesion (also termed fibrous xanthoma) exist.[34,106] Superficially located histiocytic lesions behave in a very benign manner, though deep benign histiocytomas may invade locally into surrounding tissue. These lesions can occur anywhere in the body. Superficial lesions are always cured by simple excision; a wider margin of normal tissue should be obtained for deep, benign fibrous histiocytomas. Local recurrence is uncommon.

Atypical Fibrous Histiocytomas

Although superficial fibrous histiocytomas are always totally benign and cured by simple excision, deep fibrous histiocytomas may have a more atypical morphologic appearance and are more ominous in their tendency to locally recur.[106-109] Though superficial lesions may occasionally fit the criteria for atypical histiocytoma (three of 18 atypical fibrous histiocytomas reported by Soule and coworkers), almost all are located deep in soft tissue or muscle. Despite the absence of obvious anaplasia a rapidly growing, deeply occurring fibrous histiocytoma may achieve a diameter of 6 cm or greater; over half of these lesions will recur after simple excision. These lesions generally do not metastasize, although very rare reports of metastases following many local recurrences for lesions with this histiology have been reported. Recommended therapy includes wide local excision with an attempt to achieve a negative microscopic margin in all directions. Recurrent local extension of these tumors, especially in the retroperitoneal area, can lead to death, generally as a result of inadequate local treatment at first resection.

Dermatofibrosarcoma Protuberans

These lesions can occur in any part of the body.[110-113] The exact histogenesis is not known, although a histiocytic origin appears likely. These lesions most often begin as indurated nodules in the skin that grow slowly and are therefore often ignored until they achieve a large size. They show an extremely agressive tendency to invade surrounding local tissue; in their local treatment they should be regarded as malignant neoplasms. They do not metastasize, however, even after multiple recurrences. About 50% will recur after simple excision and a wide excision including a wide margin of surrounding tissue should be achieved in therapy. The first resection is of major importance since tumor spread at the inadequate first resection may lead to uncontrollable local growth. These benign lesions may ultimately lead to amputation of extremities or even death because of extensive invasion of vital organs. While surgical excision alone is recommended as initial treatment, surgical treatment of dermatofibrosarcoma protuberans may not be feasible or margins may be inadequate because of anatomic site; in these situations, consideration should be given to combining radiation therapy (high dose) alone or in combination with surgery.

BENIGN TUMORS OF MESOTHELIAL TISSUE

Mesothelioma

The cells lining the pleura, peritoneum, and pericardium are referred to as mesothelial cells. While most tumors of mesothelial tissue are malignant, benign tumors can occur, generally in the pleura. These lesions project outwardly from the viscera or parietal pleura into the adjacent cavity but do not infiltrate aggressively into local tissue. These may grow to quite large size and simple excision is generally curative.

BENIGN TUMORS OF UNCERTAIN TISSUE ORIGIN

Granular Cell Myoblastoma

These small tumors rarely achieve a size greater than 6 cm and can be cured by local excision.[114] When these lesions develop beneath the epidermis or mucus membranes they can lead to squamous tissue proliferation, possibly mimicking a squamous cell carcinoma.

Mesenchymoma

These benign tumors (also referred to as a hamartoma or mixed mesodermal tumor) are composed of at least two different mesenchymal elements.[115] Lesions will often contain smooth muscle, skeletal muscle, fat, angiomatous and osseous tissue in various proportions and combinations. Though most lesions are malignant, rare benign forms have been described. Benign tumors are generally small and none of the individual elements contain cells with atypical or anaplastic appearance.

Myxoma

This tumor is thought to arise from embryonic rests and is composed of spindle cells imbedded in a mucinous intercellular matrix.[116,117] It can occur in any of the soft tissues, bone, or occasionally in the heart and genito-urinary tract. When these lesions develop in the soft tissues, they are generally in close relationship to a large muscle or aponeurosis; they are cured by local excision. Deep tumors can sometimes infiltrate into contiguous structures although even in this situation local resection is almost always curative.

THE DIAGNOSIS OF SOFT TISSUE SARCOMAS

Soft tissue sarcomas most often present as asymptomatic soft tissue masses. Because these lesions arise in compressible soft tissues and are often far from vital organs, symptoms are few until the lesions are quite large in relationship to the anatomic part; for example, 8–15 cm in the thigh or buttock, 3–4 cm in the wrist, but only 0.5–1 cm around the digits. Symptoms generally result from pressure or traction on adjacent nerves or muscles. There are no reliable physical signs to distinguish between benign and malignant soft tissue lesions; consequently, all soft tissue lumps that persist or grow should be biopsied. Even very soft and pliable subcutaneous lumps thought to be lipomas can occasionally prove surprising. Leaving soft tissue lumps in place without biopsy is justified only if they have been present and unchanged for many years prior to being observed by the physician.

The nature of the biopsy of soft tissue sarcomas is an important aspect of the overall management of these patients. Because the biopsy site must be removed in any definitive resection, care should be taken to place the biopsy incision at such a location and orientation so as not to compromise subsequent definitive surgical excision.

Aspiration or needle biopsy should not play a role in the diagnosis of soft tissue sarcoma. Despite careful cytologic delineation of the appearance of sarcomas by Hajdu and Hajdu,[118] the subtle distinctions necessary to distinguish benign from malignant variants of soft tissue sarcomas are often not possible with the small samples obtained by these techniques. Soft tissue sarcomas can be loosely adherent lesions and clean cores of tissues are often not obtained. Needle biopsy artifacts also lead to confusion. A large sample of tissue is often necessary for the accurate diagnosis of soft tissue sarcomas. Special studies (*e.g.* tissue culture and electron microscopy) that may be necessary for accurate diagnosis often cannot be obtained from a core of tissue in a needle biopsy. Because therapy may also be guided by the histologic grade of the lesion, a generous sample of tissue is necessary to enable this distinction as well.

Soft tissue sarcomas grow radially and push surrounding tissue before them. This surrounding tissue forms a pseudocapsule (not a true capsule) and always contains invasive prongs of malignant tissue. For this reason the 'shelling out' of soft tissue sarcomas is never curative. In fact, excision through the pseudocapsule often spreads tumor into surrounding tissue planes and can greatly complicate further surgical treatment. For this reason, excisional biopsy is an inappropriate means of establishing a diagnosis for any but small soft tissue sarcomas less than 3 cm in diameter. The appropriate surgical technique for diagnosing any soft tissue sarcoma greater than 3 cm in diameter is an incisional biopsy. This technique allows for the acquisition of a generous wedge of tissue from the lesion and minimally disrupts the surrounding tissue planes. The incisional biopsy should be performed through a carefully placed incision so as not to compromise subsequent radical excision of the lesion. Care should be taken to obtain excellent hemostasis. Large hematomas resulting from biopsies of soft tissue sarcomas can often lead to spread of tumor far beyond the sites of natural tumor invasion.

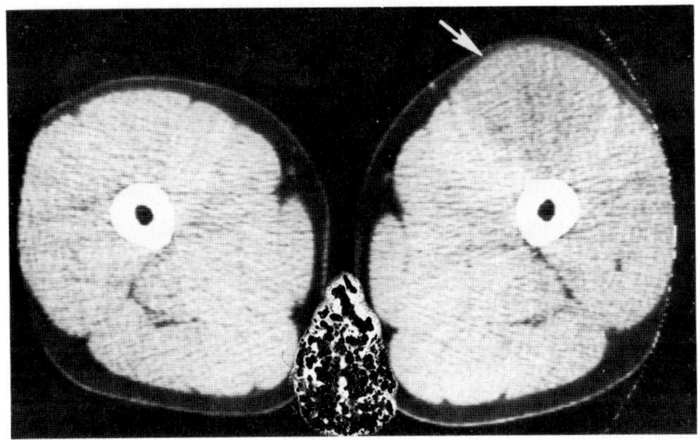

FIG. 29-1. CT of a soft tissue sarcoma of the thigh. (*Arrow* indicates the mass lesion.)

The importance of the adequate placement of the biopsy incision cannot be overemphasized. Improper placement of the biopsy incision may preclude proper radical resection of the lesion and may lead to large increases in the radiation fields necessary to encompass all areas of possible spread. Incisions on the extremities should be placed longitudinally so as not to compromise the muscle group excisions that may subsequently be necessary. Biopsies of lesions in the buttocks should be placed as inferiorly as possible to allow for subsequent development of skin flaps if hemipelvectomy is necessary.

Planning surgical resection or radiation therapy requires a careful and detailed determination of the pattern of local spread and the exact extent of the macroscopic lesion. This must be followed by assessment of the tissues likely to be involved by microscopic disease. The physical examination is of primary importance in determining approximate size of the lesion, attachment to deep or superficial structures, relationship of the tumor to prior biopsy, functional status of the part, and presence of prior injury or concurrent medical disease that would confound the execution of the desired surgery or radiation. The radiographic evaluation of the patient with soft tissue sarcoma should include:

1. Xerogram or soft tissue radiograph of the affected part
2. CT or ultrasound through the affected region
3. Full chest tomogram
4. Arteriogram in certain instances.[119–123]

The most important diagnostic procedure in assessing the pattern of involvement of the primary lesion is computerized axial tomography (see Fig 29-1). It is essential for optimal development of the management strategy that high quality CT scans be obtained and reviewed in detail because this technique permits accurate delineation of the muscle compartment or anatomic structures involved by gross disease.

Arteriography may also be of benefit in delineating the local extent of disease and may be used to supplement the CT scan findings (see Fig. 29-2).[121-123] This is particularly helpful in planning major surgery to estimate the proximity of tumor to major vessels, determine the pattern of displacement or deviation of vessels, and to determine the encasement of a vessel by tumor (resulting in abrupt, irregular change in the caliber of the vessel, which is characteristic of neoplastic involvement). The arteriogram may be of value in demonstrating the relationship of the neoplasm to nearby vascular structures. The late venous phase is of benefit in showing the venous drainage, which should be controlled intra-operatively early in the course of surgery to prevent major embolization of tumor cells. An arteriogram is of minimal benefit in planning the treatment of recurrent tumors or the re-operation of incompletely excised lesions.

Though sarcomas rarely invade bone, assessment of soft tissue "reaction" in the periosteum and at the margin of soft tissues may be estimated by bone scan.[41] A positive scan does not mean that the tumor is directly *adjacent* to bone, but usually that there is a soft tissue "reaction" to tumor *near* the bone. This should serve as a guide to wide resection near the bone or removing a portion of the bone in the area that is positive on scan.

Sarcoma of soft tissue infrequently metastasizes to regional lymph nodes.[124] However, lymphangiogram may be indicated in the evaluation of selected patients, particularly epithelioid sarcomas and synovial sarcoma (the high frequency of metastasis to regional lymph nodes by rhabdomyosarcoma in childhood is well-known but this is covered in Chapter 34).

STAGING OF SOFT TISSUE SARCOMAS

The single most important prognostic factor in patients with soft tissue sarcomas is the histologic grade of the primary lesion. Despite the importance of this factor there is little agreement among pathologists as to objective methods for the grading of these lesions. Grades are assigned from grade I (well-differentiated) to grade III (poorly-differentiated). The histologic grade of an individual soft tissue sarcoma is based on estimates of the number of mitoses present, the presence of necrosis, the degree of cellularity, the nuclear pleomorphism, cell type, capsulation, vascularity, and other ill-defined morphologic qualities. The histogenic cell of origin may also play a role in the grading of soft tissue sarcomas by some pathologists. In the staging system for soft tissue sarcomas proposed by the Task Force on Soft Tissue Sarcoma of the American Joint Committee for Cancer Staging and End Results, the histologic grade is the most important determinant of stage.[28] The system is based on four parameters: G or histopathologic grade, T, N, and M. Details of this staging system are presented in Table 29-5. G1, G2, and G3 lesions

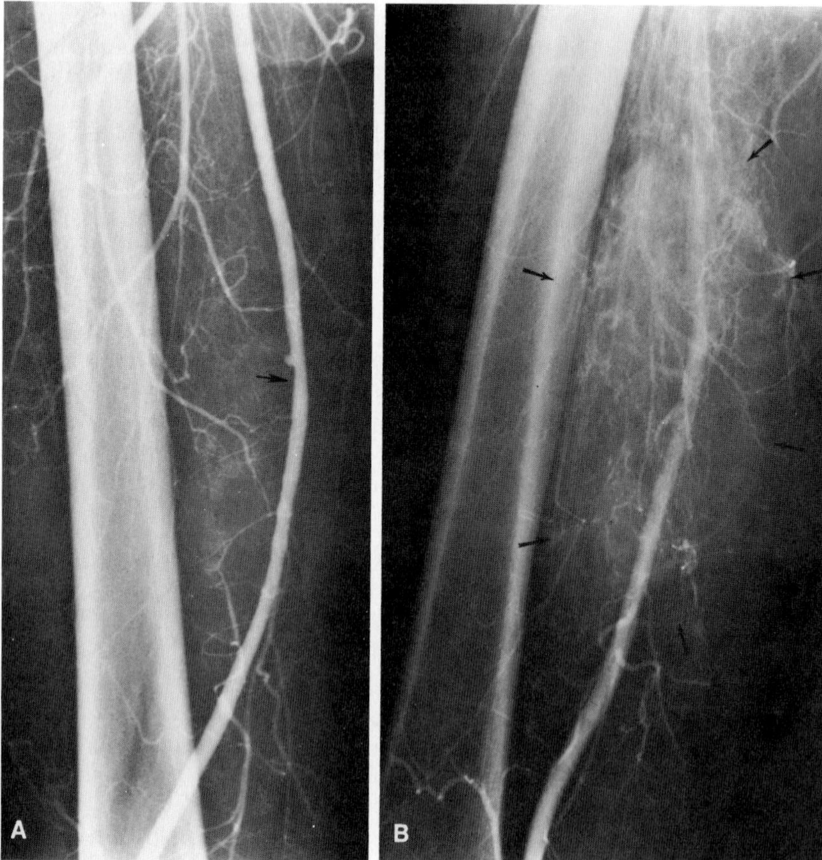

FIG. 29-2. Arteriogram of the proximal thigh in a patient with a large soft tissue sarcoma. Note the displacement of the femoral artery. *A*, arterial phase. *B*, capillary phase.

TABLE 29-5. Schema for Staging Soft Tissue Sarcomas by T N M G

T	Primary tumor T_1=Tumor less than 5 cm T_2=Tumor 5 cm or greater T_3=Tumor that grossly invades bone, major vessel, or major nerve
N	Regional lymph nodes N_0 No histologically verified metastases to regional lymph nodes N_1 Histologically verified regional lymph node metastasis
M	Distant metastasis M_0 No distant metastasis M_1 Distant metastasis
G	Histologic grade of malignancy G_1 Low G_2 Moderate G_3 High
Stage I	
Stage Ia $G_1T_1N_0M_0$	Grade 1 tumor less than 5 cm in diameter with no regional lymph nodes or distant metastases
Stage Ib $G_1T_2N_0M_0$	Grade 1 tumor 5 cm or greater in diameter with no regional lymph nodes or distant metastases
Stage II	
Stage IIa $G_2T_1N_0M_0$	Grade 2 tumor less than 5 cm in diameter with no regional lymph nodes or distant metastases
Stage IIb $G_2T_2N_0M_0$	Grade 2 tumor 5 cm or greater in diameter with no regional lymph nodes or distant metastases
Stage III	
Stage IIIa $G_3T_1N_0M_0$	Grade 3 tumor less than 5 cm in diameter with no regional lymph nodes or distant metastases
Stage IIIb $G_3T_2N_0M_0$	Grade 3 tumor 5 cm or greater in diameter with no regional lymph nodes or distant metastases
Stage IIIc Any $G_{1-3}T_{1-2}N_2M_0$	Tumor of any grade or size (no invasion) with regional lymph nodes, but no distant metastases
Stage IV	
Stage IVa Any $G_{1-3}T_3N_{0-1}M_0$	Tumor of any grade that grossly invades bone, major vessel, or major nerve with or without regional lymph node metastases but without distant metastases
Stage IVb Any $GTNM_1$	Tumor with distant metastases

Russell WO, Cohen J, Enzinger F et al: A clinical and pathological staging system for soft tissue sarcomas. Cancer 40:1562–1570, 1977

are sarcomas which are well-differentiated, moderately differentiated, or poorly differentiated respectively. T1 lesions are less than 5 cm, T2 lesions are greater than or equal to 5 cm, and T3 lesions are of any size that invade bone, major vessles, or nerves. N1 lesions are lesions with metastatic disease in regional lymph nodes; M1 lesions are lesions that have clinical evidence of distant metastasis. In this staging system all patients with soft tissue sarcomas presenting without lymph node involvement or distant metastases with grade I lesions are categorized as stage I, regardless of primary tumor size. Similarly, all grade II lesions without lymph node involvement and distant metastases are categorized as stage II regardless of the size of the primary lesion. Similarly, all grade III lesions are categorized stage III, although patients with nodal involvement are also stage III regardless of grade. The correlation of this staging system with prognosis in over 1,200 patients with soft tissue sarcomas is presented in Figure 29-3.

Factors thought to be of prognostic importance in patients with soft tissue sarcomas are listed in Table 29-6. The site of a soft tissue sarcoma often influences resectability and thus local control. Lesions in the trunk (especially those in the retroperitoneum, mediastinum, and head and neck) often involve vital structures before they become clinically apparent.

In the extremity the exact site of the lesion is also of prognostic importance. Proximal lesions are generally less curable than distal lesions. In the series reported by Simon and coworkers local recurrences in the buttock, groin, thigh and areas below the knee were 38%, 14%, 15% and 0% respectively (see Table 29-7).[41] In the series by Suit and coworkers, seven of 25 (28%) of all thigh lesions recurred locally as did two of five (40%) of upper arm lesions compared to only three of 59 (5%) local failures in patients with lesions in the distal portions in the extremities.[125]

Though size has often been considered a prognostic variable, it is probably not a variable independent of site. Soft tissue sarcomas in the thigh tend to be large before they are diagnosed, though lesions in the distal portion of the extremities are often detected when much smaller. The size of the lesion, however, will often impact significantly on the therapeutic options available for achieving local control.

Soft tissue sarcomas rarely spread to regional lymph nodes. In a review of 374 patients referred to the National Cancer Institute over a 24-year period only three patients (2.6%) had evidence of metastates to draining lymph nodes prior to gross dissemination of disease.[124] In a review of over 2,500 patients in the world literature, Weingrad and Rosenberg analyzed the incidence of lymph node metastases from each of the major histologic types of soft tissue sarcomas (see Table 29-8). In general, only about 5% of patients with soft tissue

TABLE 29-6. Factors of Prognostic Importance in Patients with Primary Soft Tissue Sarcomas

Histologic grade
Site (proximal vs distal)
Size and pattern of local extension
Lymph node involvement

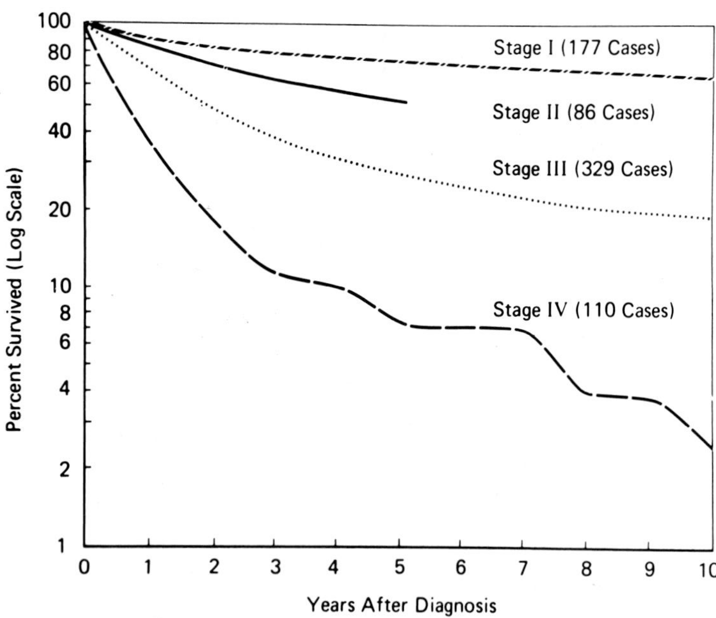

FIG. 29-3. Survival rate of patients with soft tissue sarcomas according to stage of disease. (From Russell WO, Cohen J, Enzinger F et al: A clinical and pathological staging system for soft tissue sarcomas. Cancer 40:1562–1570, 1977)

TABLE 29-7. Anatomic Site Correlated with Local Recurrence Rate in Soft-tissue Sarcomas of the Extremities

	NO. OF PTS.	% TOTAL	NO. WITH RECUR-RENCE	NO. WITHOUT RECUR-RENCE	% RECUR-RENCE
Lower extremity (53)					
Intrapelvic	2	3	2	0	100
Buttock	8	11	3	5	38
Groin	7	10	1	6	14
Thigh	26	37	4	22	15
Knee	3	4	0	3	0
Below knee	7	10	0	7	0
Upper extremity (17)					
Shoulder girdle	4	6	2	2	50
Arm	7	10	0	7	0
Below elbow	6	9	1	5	17

Simon MA, Enneking WF: The Management of Soft-tissue Sarcomas of the extremities. J Bone Joint Surg 58-A:317, 1976

TABLE 29-8. Incidence of Lymph Node Metastases in Patients with Soft Tissue Sarcomas

HISTOLOGY	NO. OF SERIES	NO. OF PATIENTS	INCIDENCE OF LYMPH NODE METASTASES NO.	%
Liposarcoma	7	288	15	5.7
Fibrosarcoma	14	1083	55	5.1
Rhabdomyosarcoma	13	888	108	12.2
Synoviosarcoma	13	535	91	17.0
Unclassifiable	5	125	11	8.8
Neurofibrosarcoma	2	60	0	0

Weingrad DW, Rosenberg SA: Early lymphatic spread of osteogenic and soft-tissue sarcomas. Surgery 84:231–240, 1978

sarcomas developed nodal metastases, although in patients with synovial cell sarcoma and rhabdomyosarcoma the incidence was slightly higher. Patients with involvement of draining lymph nodes had a substantially poorer prognosis than when the lymph nodes were not involved.

The histologic cell or origin of soft tissue sarcomas is not of major prognostic importance if lesions of equivalent grade are compared. Similarly, there appears to be no prognostic importance attached to the age or sex of patients with soft tissue sarcomas.

BRIEF SUMMARY OF THE NATURAL HISTORY OF PATIENTS WITH SOFT TISSUE SARCOMAS

The poor prognosis of most patients with soft tissue sarcomas is due to the tendency of these lesions to invade aggressively into surrounding tissues and to the tendency for early hematogenous dissemination, generally to the lungs. Soft tissue sarcomas have a significant tendency to invade locally along anatomic planes such as nerve fibers, muscle bundles, fascial planes, and blood vessels. It is not unusual for local recurrences to appear up to 12 inches from the margins of obvious gross tumor. Most patients with soft tissue sarcomas present without obvious clinical metastases. In a series from the National Cancer Institute 4% of cases presented with disseminated disease compared to 11% of patients presenting with metastases at Memorial Sloan-Kettering Hospital.[30,126]

Because the appropriate diagnosis is often not appreciated or suspected prior to biopsy, many soft tissue sarcomas are initially treated by 'shelling out' the lesion through the pseudocapsule. Such treatment is inadequate as sole therapy and over 90% of patients so treated will recur locally.

The time of local recurrence is fairly constant in most reported series. Figure 29-4 shows the results of Cantin and coworkers, who demonstrated that approximately 80% of all lesions that will recur will recur by 2 years.[126] In 54 patients treated by Simon and coworkers, all local recurrences that were seen occurred by 30 months following definitive resection.[41] Lindberg and associates also reported that 80% of local recurrences occur in the first 2 years and 100% by 3 years[29] Shiu and associates reported 87% of local recurrences in the first 2 years.[40] Local recurrence following definitive local treatment is a poor prognostic factor and about 1/3 of patients will develop disseminated metastases in close proximity to the local recurrence.[41,126] Wide local excision (*i.e.*, several cm of normal tissue around the pseudocapsule) will result in local recurrence rates of about 50%. Table 29-9 presents local recurrence rates from many reported series for four of the major histologic types of soft tissue sarcomas.[127–145] Patients undergoing amputation or radical local excision (see treatment section for exact definitions) will have local recurrence rates of about 20%.[40,41] In older reported series from Memorial Sloan Kettering Hospital local recurrences of 59% were seen

FIG. 29-4. Time course of local recurrence following definitive treatment for soft tissue sarcomas (data presented as the percentage of local recurrences of those who will ultimately recur) (Cantin J, McNeer GP, Chu FC, et al: Ann Surg 168:47–53, 1947)

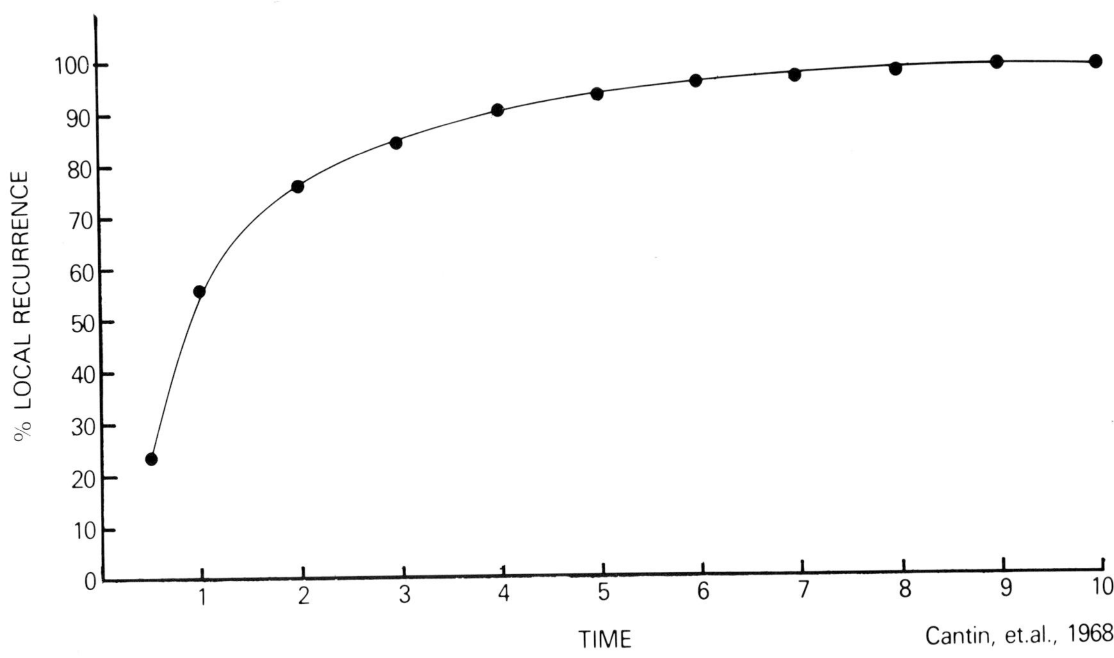

TABLE 29-9. Local Recurrence Rates of Sarcomas*

	%	(Average)
Fibrosarcoma	56.8, 60, 52.5, 56.6, 50.6, 56, 60.4, 55, 29.2, 68	55
Liposarcoma	33.3, 48, 61, 48, 21, 69.6, 63	49
Rhabdomyosarcoma	61, 50, 51, 58	55
Synovial sarcoma	91.5, 28, 46.4, 59	56

*Each number represents a separate reported series.[127–145]

in patients undergoing conservative excision compared to 25% for those undergoing radical excision.[126] At the M. D. Anderson Hospital, patients undergoing conservative excision had a 77% local recurrence rate compared to 28% for those undergoing radical excision.[38] These series were not randomized and these figures are highly influenced by individual patient selection factors. In general, however, the larger the surgical excision in all directions from the tumor the lower the local recurrence rates. The effects on local recurrence of adjuvant radiation therapy and chemotherapy treatments will be presented later.

As previously noted, spread to draining lymph nodes is an uncommon finding in the natural history of patients with soft tissue sarcoma. In a review of over 30 reported series by Weingrad and Rosenberg, 5.8% of almost 3,000 patients reported developed lymph node metastases some time during their course (See Table 29-8)[124] These figures reflect the incidence of lymph node metastases at any time during the course of the disease; spread to lymph nodes in the early stages of the clinical course is less frequent. The incidence of lymph node metastases is somewhat higher in synovial cell sarcoma (17%) and in rhabdomyosarcoma (12%) than for most other histologies.

The lungs are virtually always the first site of dissemination for patients with soft tissue sarcomas of the extremities though patients with retroperitoneal tumors may often spread first to the liver.[146] It is unusual to find evidence of spread to sites other than the lung at the time of first evidence of dissemination. Aggressive pulmonary resection is recommended for the treatment of pulmonary metastases. Approximately 30% of patients with resectable pulmonary metastases can be cured. (see Chapter 41). About 80% of all patients who develop disseminated disease will do so by 5 years following primary tumor resection. Without vigorous resection of pulmonary metastases, the median survival following the onset of pulmonary metastases is about 12 months.[27]

TABLE 29-10. Soft Tissue Sarcomas: 5-Year Survival

GROUP (Ref.)	NUMBER OF PATIENTS	SURVIVAL (%) 5-YEAR	10-YEAR
Task Force, AJC (28)	1,215	41	30
Surgery Branch, NCI (30) (before 1975)	66	48	44
Gerner et al (147)	155	50	26
Shieber et al (27)	125	27	22
Martin et al (38)	183	40	—
Pack et al (37)	717	39	—
Hare et al (36)	200	39	—
Shiu et al (40)	297	55	41

Overall 5-year survival in most reported series of patients with soft tissue sarcoma is about 40% (see Table 29-10 and Fig, 29-5).[27,28,30,36–38,147] At autopsy widespread disease beyond the lungs is often found. Gercouich and coworkers have reported an increase in CNS metastases following chemotherapy in patients with soft tissue sarcomas.[148]

UNIQUE FEATURES OF INDIVIDUAL HISTIOLOGIC TYPES OF SOFT TISSUE SARCOMAS

Despite the common biologic behavior of equivalent grade soft tissue sarcomas, there are some features that are unique to individual histologic types. This section will briefly discuss these unique aspects.

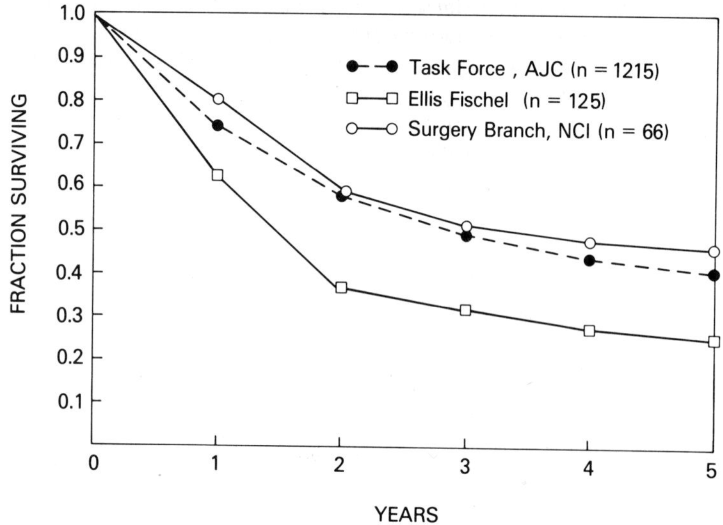

FIG. 29-5. Five-year survival rate of patients with soft tissue sarcomas from three reported series.

FIBROSARCOMA

Prior to about 1965, fibrosarcoma was the most common diagnosis of soft tissue sarcoma.[149,150] Since that time, the recognition of a larger variety of subtypes of soft tissue sarcoma has significantly decreased this diagnosis. As stated by Stout and Lattes, "One should try to restrict the term 'fibrosarcoma' to growths that are composed of cells and fibers derived from fibrocytes and exclude all the fibrous growths derived from other types of cells acting as facultative fibroblasts." Though some pathologists distinguish fibroblastic fibrosarcoma from pleomorphic fibrosarcoma, based largely on the uniformity of the herringbone pattern of the tumor and the number of mitotic figures, this is mainly a reflection of grading.[31] Because of the changing pattern of the term 'fibrosarcoma,' earlier series of fibrosarcomas undoubtedly contain sarcomas that today would be associated with other histologic types.[149–152]

RHABDOMYOSARCOMA

Rhabdomyosarcoma accounts for about 15% of all sarcomas.[153–157] Because the skeletal muscle accounts for approximately 40% of the body weight of most adults, this tumor, on a per weight basis of tissue, is one of the rarest of all tumors. Striated muscle cells are highly differentiated cells that normally do not undergo mitosis in the postnatal period. This probably accounts for the low incidence of malignancies in these tissues.

Three subcategories of rhabdomyosarcoma are generally recognized—pleomorphic, alveolar, and embryonal types. Because the alveolar and embryonal types generally occur in childhood, these are often referred to as juvenile-type rhabdomyosarcomas. The term 'botryoid' indicates the gross appearance of a subset of embryonal rhabdomyosarcomas that have a polypoid or grape-like appearance. Embryonal rhabdomyosarcomas with botryoid features are commonly found in the urogenital tract of infants and children though these tumors have also been noted in the oral and nasal pharynx. Embryonal tumors can be found in the adult and elderly patient; thus, the use of 'juvenile' to refer to these sarcomas is somewhat misleading. Many tumors contain the histologic patterns characteristic of several subtypes of rhabdomyosarcoma. Then the assignment of a specific subtype is often nebulous.

Embryonal rhabdomyosarcomas are the most common soft tissue sarcomas of children. Discussion of these tumors is presented in Chapter 34. Alveolar rhabdomyosarcomas are distinguished from embryonal rhabdomyosarcomas by the presence of slit-like 'alveolar spaces' present in histologic sections of the tumor. Pleomorphic rhabdomyosarcomas generally present in adulthood though they can appear in childhood. The most common site of pleomorphic rhabdomyosarcomas is the extremity. These are often highly anaplastic lesions having both small and large cells with one or many bizzare nuclei. The diagnosis of these tumors has also changed dramatically in recent years and a review by Hajdu of 214 sarcomas originally diagnosed as pleomorphic rhabdomyosarcoma led to a reclassification of 93 of these lesions to other histologic subtypes, mainly malignant fibrous histiocytoma.[31]

LEIOMYOSARCOMA

Leiomyosarcomas are malignant neoplasms that arise from smooth muscle. Since these tumors can arise from the walls of both small and large blood vessels, they can occur anywhere in the body.[158–160] Leiomyosarcomas also occur in the viscera. In these locations they can arise from either smooth muscle in the viscera, (*e.g.*, the uterus), or from vessels in these organs. Leiomyosarcomas commonly arise in the retroperitoneum, where they are highly aggressive neoplasms.

LIPOSARCOMA

Liposarcomas are malignant lesions of adipose tissue.[161–166] The incidence in males exceeds that of females by about 1.5: 1. Multicentric liposarcomas have been described. In a series of 97 patients with liposarcoma reported by Kindbloom and coworkers, 11 patients were found to have a second liposarcoma that developed at a site remote from the first tumor.

Four subtypes of liposarcomas are generally recognized—well-differentiated, myxoid, lipoblastic (or round-cell), and pleomorphic. Some authors also refer to fibroblastic liposarcomas as a fifth subtype. Well-differentiated liposarcomas can exhibit aggressive local invasion, though tend not to metastasize in most cases. Myxoid liposarcomas generally metastasize only later in their course. An 80% 5-year survival can be expected in these lesions. Round-cell (or lipoblastic or epithelioid) sarcomas are comprised of uniform round cells with a highly vascular meshwork of capillaries. These are highly malignant lesions and like the pleomorphic liposarcomas, have only a 20–30% 5-year survival in most reported series.

SYNOVIAL SARCOMA

Synovial sarcomas are malignant neoplasms thought to arise from tendosynovial tissue and occur most commonly in the second through fourth decades.[167–171] The lower extremity is the most common site of synovial sarcoma. It can occur in any muscle, not usually in proximity to joints. Although extremities are the most common site, these can occur in the abdominal wall and in other skeletal muscles of the trunk. Two subtypes of synovial sarcomas are generally recognized; these are the monophasic and biphasic types. Monophasic synovial sarcomas are characterized by sheaths of monotonous spindle cells while the biphasic variety have slit-like spaces or clefts present within the tumor. These clefts are lined by cuboidal or tall columnar epithelial cells and sometimes resemble carcinomas. Calcified areas often appear within the synovial sarcomas and lead to a characteristic x-ray appearance of this type of soft tissue sarcoma. Some authors consider epithelioid and clear-cell sarcomas to be variants of synovial cell sarcoma though these will be considered separately in this chapter.

NEUROFIBROSARCOMAS

Neurofibrosarcomas are malignant tumors of neural sheath origin and have also been referred to as neurogenic sarcomas, malignant schwannomas, and malignant neurilemmomas.[172] These tumors can occur anywhere in the body.

Neurofibrosarcomas are frequently found in association with Von Recklinghausen's disease, a chronic, progressive, hereditary disease inherited as a mendelian dominant trait and associated with multiple neurofibromas and skin pigmentary changes, characterized as cafe-au-lait spots.[91–97] From 15–25% of patients with neurofibromatosis develop sarcomatous changes during their lifetime, often in one of the preexisting, benign masses.

ANGIOSARCOMAS

Hemangiosarcomas and lymphangiosarcomas arise from blood and lymphatic vessels respectively.[173–177] These are almost uniformly high grade lesions. They are uncommon, however, and comprise only approximately 2% of all soft tissue sarcomas. In 1948 Stuart and Treves reported six cases of lymphangiosarcoma in lymphedematous arms following radical mastectomy.[13]

HEMANGIOPERICYTOMA

Malignant hemangiopericytoma is a malignant sarcoma thought to arise from the pericyte cells of smooth muscle origin that lie around small vessels.[105,178–180] Benign and malignant hemangiopericytomas exist and the rarity of these lesions have lead to considerable confusion in distinguishing the benign from malignant variants. Hemangiopericytomas should be treated as other sarcomas. In most series, approximately 50% 5-year survivals are recorded.

KAPOSI'S SARCOMA

In 1872, Kaposi described "multiple idiopathic pigmented sarcoma of the skin" that has since been widely recognized and has a propensity for Jewish and Italian males.[181–182] These tumors are thought to arise from endothelial cells and present as raised, pigmented lesions of the skin. Kaposi's sarcomas tend to evolve slowly although they can metastasize. They are multifocal lesions and can occur anywere in the body. Radiation therapy is the treatment of choice, although remissions with chemotherapeutic agents, including, vinblastine, nitrogen mustard and actinomycin-D, have been reported.

These tumors are over 100 times more frequent in Africa than in North America. Kaposi's sarcomas tend to have a frequent association with malignant lymphoreticular neoplasms, such as Hodgkin's disease, and in patients with Kaposi's sarcoma, death from a second primary is probably as great a threat to life as is mortality from Kaposi's sarcoma itself.[181]

MALIGNANT FIBROUS HISTIOCYTOMA

Malignant fibrous histiocytoma was characterized by O'Brien and Stout as a group of tumors having a common origin from tissue histiocytes.[106,183–187] This diagnosis has achieved great popularity in recent years and many cases previously diagnosed as pleomorphic rhabdomyosarcoma or undifferentiated fibrosarcoma are now categorized as malignant fibrous histiocytoma. A wide spectrum of fibrous histiocytomas exists from those that are benign, to those that are highly atypical, to those that are frankly malignant. In many recent series malignant fibrous histiocytoma is the most common diagnosis attached to soft tissue sarcomas.

ALVEOLAR SOFT-PART SARCOMA

Alveolar soft-part sarcomas were described by Christopherson in 1952.[188–190] These tumors have a unique histiologic appearance but the cell of origin is unknown. These are true malignant sarcomas though they tend to have a more protracted course than most other sarcomas. While most patients will ultimately die of the disease, 5-year survivals of 60% are common. Many patients develop metastatic disease that progresses slowly over the course of 5–15 years before leading to death.

EPITHELIOID SARCOMA

Epithelioid sarcomas are of an unknown cell of origin and occur almost exclusively in the extremities, usually in the hand or foot associated with aponeurotic structures.[191–194] These tumors differ in their natural history from most other sarcomas in that they have a greater propensity to spread to non-contiguous areas of skin, subcutaneous tissue, fat, and bone. In addition, these tumors have a high propensity to spread to draining lymph nodes. In approximately 30% of cases, regional lymph node metastases are found. Long-term survival is similar to or perhaps slightly better than most other soft tissue sarcomas. Recommended therapy for these patients is wide excision often involving amputation of the extremity and regional lymph node dissection.

MESOTHELIOMA

Mesotheliomas are sarcomas arising from the serous lining of the pleural and peritoneal cavities. They spread primarily by local invasion and frequently result in widely diffuse disease with significant effusion. Local control is rarely achieved by surgery or radiation therapy though transient responses to chemotherapy are seen.[303–310]

TREATMENT OF SOFT TISSUE SARCOMAS

The consideration of multimodality approaches to the local treatment of soft tissue sarcomas is an important aspect of the modern management of this disease. A recent emphasis to preserve the limb in patients with soft tissue sarcomas of the extremities has led to a careful exploration of the possible roles of adjuvant radiation therapy and chemotherapy in the treatment of these patients. The role of each individual treatment modality is dependent on the planned use of additional adjuvant treatments. Surgical therapy designed to remove the last cancer cell is different than that treatment approach using surgery to remove gross disease and using concomitant adjuvant radiation therapy designed to eliminate residual microscopic disease. Though the individual treatment modalities will be considered separately, their use in combination is often essential in the successful treatment of these patients.

SURGERY

Because of the tendency of soft tissue sarcomas to invade along anatomic planes, local surgical excision, even with a several centimeter margin of normal tissue surrounding a lesion in all directions, is associated with a local recurrence rate of about 50%.[127–145] The problem of local recurrence following surgical procedures has been well reviewed by Cantin and associates. A summary of numerous individually reported series of local surgical procedures in the treatment of soft tissue sarcomas is presented in Table 29-9. Because the terms 'wide excision' and 'radical excision' have not been precisely used it is difficult to compare the results of surgical treatment of these tumors between treatment centers. A recent categorization of surgical procedures by Enneking and coworkers is useful in carefully defining the nature of the surgical procedure performed.[41] Enneking and associates have divided surgical procedures for soft tissue sarcomas into four types:

1. Incisional biopsy. This surgical procedure involves removal of a small piece of the tumor by directly incising the tumor capsule. Significant tumor remains, thus this procedure is of diagnostic value only.
2. Excisional biopsy. All gross tumor including the pseudocapsule is excised locally. Soft tissue sarcomas tend to grow by radial expansion and compress normal structures around them. This pseudocapsule gives the gross appearance of compartmentalization of the tumor from surrounding structures, but a true capsule does not exist. Invasion of local tissues occurs through the pseudocapsule. Excisional biopsy virtually always leaves residual microscopic tumor.
3. Wide excision. The tumor is removed along with a margin of normal surrounding tissue in continuity with the tumor. This procedure does not, however, imply removal of entire structures within which the tumor may be found.
4. Radical local resection. Tumor is removed along with all tissue in the anatomic compartment occupied by the tumor. The excision takes place by dissecting along planes that are separated from the tumor and its tissues of origin by at least one uninvolved anatomic plane in all directions. The resected specimen includes the origin and insertion of all muscles and any bones or joints that are contained within the anatomic compartment of resection. Such a procedure may involve amputation, though non-ablative procedures can also fulfill the criteria for radical local resection. (See Figs. 29-6, 29-7, 29-8, and 29-9).

Extremity Sarcomas

In the treatment of soft tissue sarcomas of the extremity, a variety of surgical procedures can be employed as detailed below.

1. Amputations of the foot. Though amputations of digits, ray amputations, transmetatarsal amputation, and Syme amputations at the level of the ankle joint are all accepted amputations for ischemic lesions of the foot, they virtually never give an adequate margin for soft tissue sarcomas in the foot and find little use in the treatment of soft tissue sarcomas.
2. Below knee amputation. This amputation is generally performed about ⅓ the distance between the knee and the ankle and involves division of the tibia and fibula. Muscles to the ankle or foot are transected. This amputation is the treatment of choice for any substantive soft tissue sarcoma of the foot. The weight-bearing

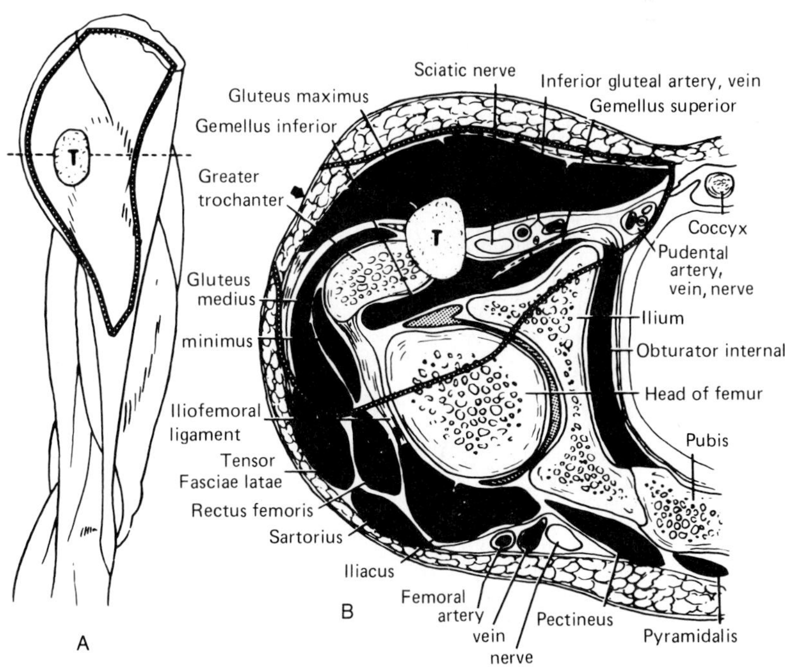

FIG. 29-6. Schematic diagram of the buttock and thigh (*A*) and a transverse section through the hemipelvis (*B*) illustrating the extent (*dotted line*) of a radical resection of a soft tissue sarcoma in the gluteus maximus muscle (*T*). (Simon et al: Surg Annu 11:363–402, 1979)

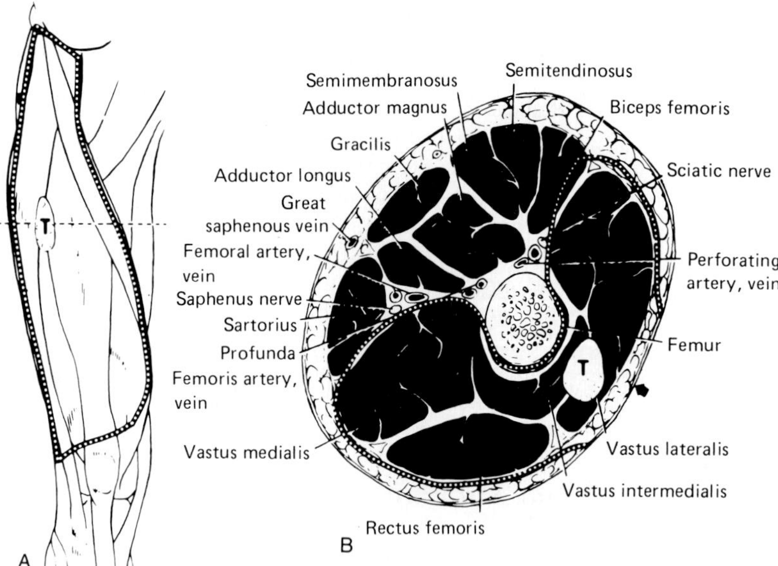

FIG. 29-7. Schematic diagram of the anterior thigh (*A*) and a transverse section through the thigh (*B*) illustrating the anatomic extent (*dotted lines*) of a radical resection, without amputation, of a soft tissue sarcoma in the proximal vastus lateralis muscle (*T*). The origins and insertions of the entire quadriceps muscle and sartorius are resected. (Simon et al: Surg Annu 11:363–402, 1979)

portions of the foot tolerate radiation therapy poorly; therefore, amputation is the treatment of choice for these lesions.

3. Above-knee amputation. Amputation through the thigh can be performed at any level distal to the lesser trocanter. Major muscle groups of the thigh are transected. This amputation is of little value for tumors occurring above the knee and is often indicated for tumors of the leg.
4. Hip disarticulation. This amputation involves disarticulation of the hip joint with complete removal of the femur. Most muscles attaching to the lower extremity are removed in their entirety. It is often suitable for patients with lesions of the middle and distal thigh.
5. Hemipelvectomy. This operation involves removal of the entire lower extremity and hemipelvis with disarticulation of the sacroiliac joint and pubic symphysis.[195-197] All major muscles that attach to the lower extremity with the exception of the iliopsoas are removed. This operation is often applied to the treatment of proximal thigh and buttock lesions. A conventional hemipelvectomy uses a posterior flap of skin and subcutaneous tissue overlying the buttock. For lesions of the buttock, however, it is possible to construct an anterior flap that includes part of the quadriceps muscles as well as the femoral vessels. The use of anterior flap hemipelvectomies has greatly extended the application of this procedure.
6. Modified hemipelvectomy (see Fig, 29-10). Preservation of the iliac wing, when possible, improves patient rehabilitation. This procedure is similar to the standard hemipelvectomy except that the sacroiliac joint is pre-

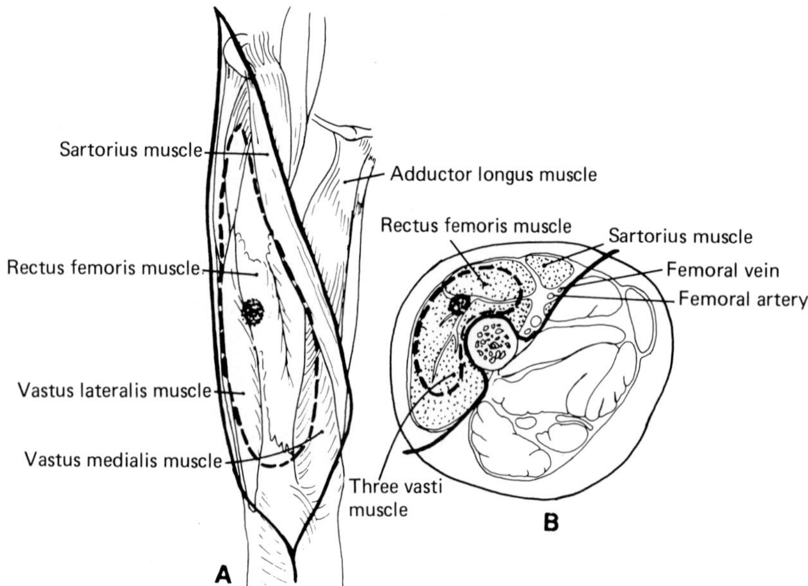

FIG. 29-8. Schematic drawing of the anterior thigh (*A*) and transverse section through the thigh (*B*) illustrating the anatomic extent of a radical resection, without amputation, of a soft tissue sarcoma lying within the rectus femoris muscle. (Courtesy of Dr. Martin Malawer.)

served and the iliac bone is excised from an area below the level of the sciatic notch. This operation does, however, involve transection of muscles in the buttock and is not suitable for lesions in this area.

7. Extended hemipelvectomy. Lesions of the iliac wing may sometimes be situated too close to the sacroiliac joint to permit its disarticulation. Extension of the standard hemipelvectomy to include excision of the sacral ala at the level of the lateral vertebral bodies adds little in morbidity to this procedure and may often provide an added several centimeters of margin from the tumor.
8. Amputations of the upper extremity follow the principles enunciated above for those of the lower extremity. Below elbow amputations are often used for the treatment of tumors of the hand and wrist. Above elbow amputations are used for tumors of the forearm. Disarticulation of the shoulder joint is an operation reserved for distal arm and elbow lesions. Forequater amputation is applied to the treatment of lesions of the shoulder girdle as well as the proximal arm. This operation includes removal of the entire upper extremity including both the scapula and clavicle.

Other non-amputative surgical procedures used in the treatment of patients with soft tissue sarcomas of the extremities should also be known to the oncologist:

1. Muscle group excision. For tumors lying within or invading into muscle, the entire involved muscle or muscle group is excised from its origin to its insertion including overlying soft tissue and any vessels and nerves included in the involved muscle bundles.

FIG. 29-9. Schematic drawing of the posterior leg (*A*) and a transverse section through the leg (*B*) illustrating the anatomic extent (*dotted lines*) of a radical resection, without amputation, of a soft tissue sarcoma (*T*) situated in the soleus muscle. The lateral gastrocnemius muscle, the whole deep posterior compartment with its neurovascular contents, the fibula, and the perineal muscles are resected. (Simon et al: Surg Annu 11:363–402, 1979)

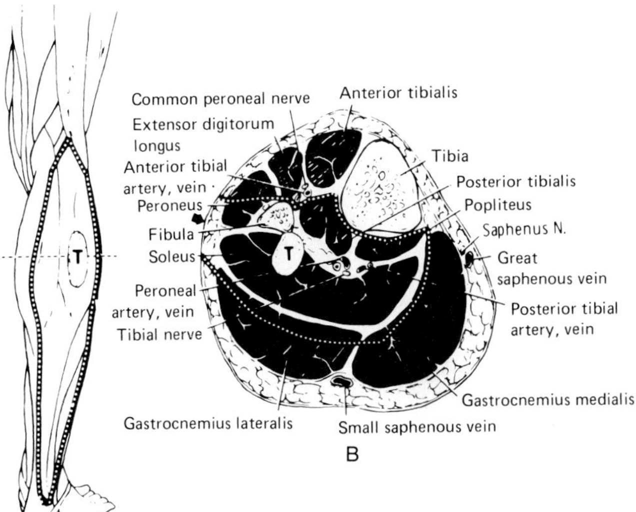

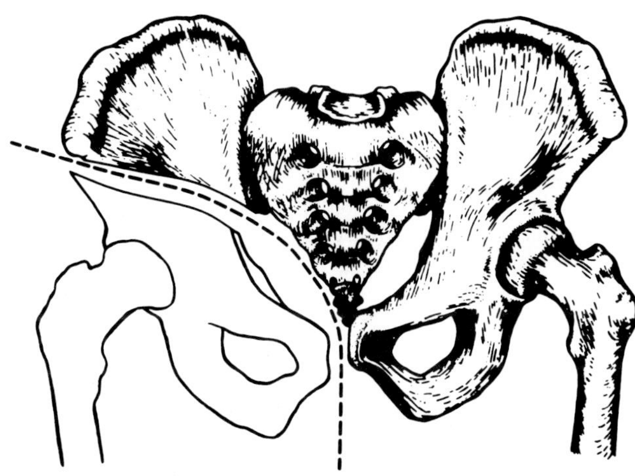

FIG. 29-10. A modified hemipelvectomy with sparing of the wing of the ileum. (Martin RG: In M. D. Anderson Hospital and Tumor Institute (ed): Management of Primary Bone and Soft Tissue Tumors, p 284. Chicago, Year Book Medical Publishers, 1977)

2. Compartmental excision. Some anatomic sites (*i.e.*, the thigh) contain compartments that are bounded by the fascia and its extension. Because it is unusual for sarcomas to transgress these fascial boundaries, excision of the entire anatomic compartment containing the tumor is often successful in irradicating all local tumor. In the thigh there are three major compartments bounded by the fascia lata and its extensions (see Fig. 29-6): the anterior compartment including primarily the quadriceps muscle (see Figs. 29-7 and 29-8); the medial compartment including the adductor muscles; the posterior compartment including the hamstring muscles (see Fig. 29-9).

   The anterior thigh compartment consists of the quadriceps and sartorious muscles and the femoral artery, vein, and nerve. Excision of the anterior compartment leads to significant loss of motion and stability of the knee. In these situations hamstring transfers can be performed to provide needed muscular movement at the knee. The medial thigh compartment consists of the gracilis, adductor brevis, adductor longus, adductor magnus, and the pectineus muscles. The obturator nerve supplies this compartment. In addition, the profunda femorus artery must be sacrificed when this compartment is resected. The posterior compartment consists of the semimembranosus, semitendinosus, and biceps femorus muscles as well as the posterior portion of the adductor magnus muscle and the sciatic nerve.

In performing wide excisions of soft tissue sarcomas sound surgical principles should be adhered to. The more important of these principles are elucidated here:

1. Wide excision of all normal tissue in the tumor area including, if possible, all involved muscle groups
2. Excision of all skin and subcutaneous tissue near the tumor
3. Resection of all previous scars and areas of previous biopsy as well as any areas that may have contained hematoma from previous biopsies

4. Removal of the sarcoma without visualizing the tumor during the surgical excision. Spilling of tumor in a major surgical excision is a serious problem that severely compromises the ability to deliver the local curative radiation therapy.
5. Placement of a tourniquet on the extremity above the lesion. Some workers advocate this modality; it is performed prior to the ligation of the venous outflow as a first part of the surgical procedure. There is no convincing evidence that this maneuver is of any value in reducing the incidence of distant spread from these tumors.
6. Resection of the draining nodes is not recommended for most varieties of soft tissue sarcoma as these tumors rarely metastasize to draining nodes. Lymph node dissection should be confined to those patients with clinically suspicious and biopsy-proven nodal involvement. However, patients with epithelioid sarcoma should have the regional draining lymph nodes resected or treated by appropriate radiation therapy.
7. Placement of metallic clips as a guide to the limits of the surgical dissection. This is essential in all local sarcoma resections for these clips serve as important markers to the radiation therapist, allowing identification of the entire dissected area in the treatment field as the radiation portal is constructed.

From an analysis of published work, the expected incidence of local recurrence following surgery alone for the treatment of soft tissue sarcomas of the extremities, using Enneking's definitions, are 100% following an incisional biopsy, 80–100% using excisional biopsy, about 50% using wide excision, about 10–20% using radical local resection, and about 5% when amputation is performed.

When radical resective surgery is the sole treatment for soft tissue sarcomas of the extremities, local control rates of above 80% can be achieved; however, in the majority of patients amputation will be necessary (Table 29-11).[40,41] In a review of 54 patients by Simon and Enneking, all of whom had resections for extremity lesions, 25 (46%) were capable of having a radical local resection without an amputation and 29 (54%) required an amputation.[41] In this series the local recurrence rate for patients undergoing radical local resection was 12% and 20.7% for patients undergoing amputation. The overall local recurrence rate was 16.7%. Careful pathologic analysis of the resected material revealed that in 46 of the 54 patients a true radical resection as defined above had been performed; in these patients only one recurred. Of the remaining eight patients whose surgical procedures were not adequate to fulfill the requirements of radical resection, all recurred locally. As is clear from the results of Enneking and coworkers, attempts to rely on surgery alone to remove the last tumor cell by removing the complete anatomic compartment containing the tumor will most often require an amputation. When, however, either an amputation or radical local resection is successful in completely removing the involved anatomic compartment, chances of obtaining local control are excellent.

TABLE 29-11. Local Control of Soft Tissue Sarcomas of the Extremities by Radical Surgery

	SIMON ET AL (41)	SHIU ET AL (40)
Total number of patients	54	297
Radical local resection	25 (46%)	158 (53%)
Amputation	29 (54%)	139 (47%)
Local control		
Radical local resection	88%	72%
Amputation	79.3%	93%
Overall	83.3%	82%

Another recent series exemplifying the capabilities of aggressive local surgery alone for the treatment of soft tissue sarcomas of the extremities is that of Shiu and Fortner and their colleagues at Memorial Sloan–Kettering Hospital in New York (see Table 29-11).[40] These workers reported on the results of treatment in 297 patients with soft tissue sarcomas of the lower extremity. With the exception of 18 cases that received radiation therapy, all patients were treated by 'en bloc wide soft part resection.' The surgical management of these patients did not follow defined procedures as closely as that of Enneking and colleagues, but attempts at wide excisions were made. In the report by Shui and coworkers the procedures used are described as follows:

> 'The tumor-bearing structures are removed in monobloc fashion with one tissue plane being beyond the confines of known or suspected tumor. For tumors occurring on or within muscle compartments, whole muscle groups from origin to insertion are resected with their invested fascia. Amputation or major disarticulation has been carried out mostly for bulky lesions involving a major bone, joint, vessel or nerve. The preferred level of exarticulation has been at least one joint above the site of the tumor so as to obviate recurrent disease in tissues contiguous with tumor-bearing area.'

In this series to fulfill the requirements quoted above, 158 (53%) patients underwent soft part resections without amputation and 139 (47%) had major amputations. The local recurrence rate for soft part resections without amputation was 28%, and 7% for patients undergoing amputation. The overall local recurrence rate in this series was 18%.

The low local recurrence rates following amputation for patients with extremity lesions undergoing amputation at or above the joint proximal to the tumor has been demonstrated in the series treated at the National Cancer Institute where no local recurrences have been seen in 31 consecutive patients treated with amputation.

These series are representative of the best attempts to control soft tissue sarcomas of the extremities using surgery alone as therapy (see Table 29-11). When surgery is used alone, amputation will be required in over half of patients if reasonable therapeutic guidelines are followed. When amputations are performed that remove all of the tissue in the anatomic compartments involved, local recurrence rates will probably be as low as 5%.

Attempts to perform less than amputation and still radically excise tumors will be associated with local recurrence rates of about 15–20%. Despite an attempt to apply the careful anatomic principles enunciated by Enneking and his colleagues, misjudgments will be inevitable and local recurrences will be higher than when amputation is performed. To perform less surgery than that described in the two studies considered above would result in local recurrence rates near 50%.

Attempts, therefore, to save the limb and yet achieve suitably low local recurrence rates in a large percentage of patients will thus require the use of adjuvant treatment modalities. The possible effectiveness of adjuvant radiation therapy and chemotherapy are being explored with these goals in mind.

The treatment of locally recurrent sarcomas should follow the same principles as the treatment of the primary tumors though amputation will almost always be necessary if surgery alone is used because of the wide-spread contamination of new tissue planes by the previous surgical procedure.

Truncal Sarcomas

The same general principles guiding the surgical therapy of extremity lesions also apply to truncal sarcomas. There are unique therapeutic features of these lesions, however, that require special consideration. The anatomic location of most truncal sarcomas preclude surgical excision with margins wide enough to ensure local control. This is especially true for sarcomas in the head and neck and for mediastinal and retroperitoneal tumors. For this reason, surgical excision should be aimed at removing all gross tumor with as much marginal tissue in the expected areas of local spread as is compatible with reasonable morbidity. Postoperative radiation therapy should be undertaken in the treatment of virtually all high grade truncal sarcomas. It is especially important that the surgeon outline the margins of resection with metallic clips for all of these lesions.

For tumors of the thoracic or abdominal wall, full thickness excisions except for skin are indicated.[198] Replacement of the abdominal wall with synthetic materials does not preclude the subsequent delivery of radiation therapy.

Sarcomas of the retroperitoneum present a unique surgical challenge.[165,199-201] These tumors tend not to cause symptoms until they are quite large with extensive local invasion. Delamater reported on a patient with an abdominal liposarcoma that reached 275 lb and reports of tumors reaching 60 lb are not rare.[165,202] Most retroperitoneal sarcomas are several pounds when diagnosed and extensively invade local tissues. The most common diagnoses in this location are liposarcoma and leiomyosarcomas.

Evaluation of patients with retroperitoneal sarcomas should include ultrasound studies, computerized axial tomography, IVP, and, when necessary, GI contrast studies. Arteriography is often of use to delineate the extent and blood supply of the tumor. Venacavography should be employed if invasion of the vena cava is suspected.

It is almost always impossible to achieve negative microscopic margins in the excision of these tumors. An attempt should be made to remove all gross tumor even if this involves resection of kidney or other intra-abdominal structures. All patients should be treated by postoperative radiation therapy as will be described in a subsequent section.

Reported 5-year survival following treatment of retroperitoneal sarcomas varies from 0–41% depending on the grade, size, and local extension of the tumor.[165,199-205] A characteristic series of patients has been compiled by Hajdu from the files of Memorial Sloan-Kettering Hospital and is presented in Table 29-12.[31] Some 29% of 86 patients with retroperitoneal sarcomas survived 5 years though many of these ultimately died of their disease. About 60% of patients who died had locally recurrent disease.

RADIATION THERAPY

Radiation therapy is a potent modality in the treatment of soft tissue sarcomas.[29,42,125,126,206-209] Though our strong preference for therapy is the combination of surgery and radiation therapy rather than employing radiation alone, there are occasional patients who are not candidates for surgery because of anatomic location of tumor, medical inoperability, or patient refusal of surgery. For example, of 193 patients at the Massachusetts General Hospital who were accepted for treatment of their soft tissue sarcoma by radiation therapy during 1971–1979, 59 were treated by radiation alone. Fortunately, a worthwhile proportion of these patients may be "cured" and have only minimum to modest degrees of late fibrosis. This may be expected where the lesion is small (<5 cm), sophisticated techniques are employed, radiation doses are high (7,000–8,000 rad in 7–8 weeks), and intensive technical efforts are made. This is to exclude from the treatment volume those tissues not suspected of tumor involvement. Despite the employment of imaginative and high technological treatment methods and radical dose levels, the local failure rate will be higher than after surgical and radiation treatment *vide infra*. A further advantage in the combined treatment is that the radiation dose levels are lower; hence, delayed fibrosis following treatment is diminished.

In 1935, Lecutia reported a patient who was treated by orthovoltage therapy for recurrent fibrosarcoma in the scapula region and survived for more than 10 years without evidence

TABLE 29-12. Retroperitoneal Sarcomas

	NUMBER OF PATIENTS	OPERATIVE MORTALITY (%)	5-YEAR SURVIVAL (%)
Liposarcoma	27	7.4	48.1
Leiomyosarcoma	17	17.6	11.8
Rhabdomyosarcoma	17	5.9	17.6
Fibrosarcoma	15	13.3	20.0
Malignant schwannoma	10	30.0	10.0
TOTAL	86	12.8	29

Hajdu SI: Pathology of Soft Tissue Tumors. Philadelphia, Lea & Febiger, 1979

of tumor.[208] Cade described a series of 22 patients with soft tissue sarcoma who were treated by radiation therapy alone; six survived for 5–26 years with control of primary tumor.[209] McNeer and coworkers reported that of 653 patients treated at Memorial Hospital for soft tissue sarcoma, 25 were treated by radiation alone. Of these, 14 were surviving at 5 or more years without clinical evidence of residual or persistent tumor. At the Massachusetts General Hospital, 26 patients were treated by radiation alone using dose levels of 6500 rad in 6½ weeks (or its equivalent). The actual local control rate at 4 years among these patients is 61%. Five patients are alive with local control at 5–7 years after treatment. Among small and low grade lesions (IB, IIA, IIIA), local failures have been infrequent (2 of 10). Of 28 patients treated at doses less than 6500 rad, only two are alive without tumor at more than 2 years. This demonstrates that prolonged local control after radiation therapy alone requires truly aggressive treatment. When this is done, some fine results may be achieved, particularly for patients with small (<5 cm) lesions.

To achieve these results, the physician should determine the target volume 3-dimensionally; the target volume constitutes the demonstrable tumor mass (by physical examination or by radiographic techniques) and those tissues judged to be involved to a clinically important probability. As defined, this volume constitutes a target for the first component of treatment, namely, a dose of 5,000–6,000 rad. After that dosage level has been achieved the target volume is redefined so as to include only a relatively narrow margin around the demonstrable tumor mass. This second target volume is then treated to a dose of 6,000–7,000 rad. Again, target volume is redefined so as to include only the evident tumor mass. The final or third defined target volume is treated to a total dose of 7,000–8,000 rad. Thus, there is not a single target volume but the target volume is in virtually all instances defined for each of the two to three phases of the treatment. The object here, of course, is to plan a treatment so as to distribute the radiation dose in accordance with the likely number of tumor cells. Probability of tumor eradication increases inversely with tumor volume and tumor cell number; rational planning of radiation therapy takes this fully into account. To achieve the definitions of target volume requires a careful and detailed history and physical examination, review of the histopathology, and exhaustive analysis of various radiographic examinations. Of the latter, the CT scan (employed during actual treatment position) is the most valuable radiographic procedure and should be obtained in all instances. After definition of the position of the diseased tissue and the adjacent normal tissues and organs, the physician and physicist begin treatment planning. The goal is to design a treatment plan that will give a treatment volume or a high-dose volume that closely conforms to each of the 2–3 designated target volumes. To design an optimal treatment plan means that detailed assessment must be made of the several technical approaches feasible for the particular problem. For example, the treatment may use multiple portal roentgen ray beams (using secondary field blocking, shaped fields, wedge filters, compensating filters, stationary or moving gantry or couch, interstitial therapy, electron beam therapy). These modalities may be employed singly or in combination. An essential factor in successful treatment planning is precisely positioning the patient at each treatment so that the treatment volume will be specified with the appropriate allowance for non-reproducibility of set up and patient movement during treatment. At each re-definition of the target volume measurements need to be made of patient contours, in addition to the size and position of tumor. These points are emphasized because it is obviously essential that the entirety of the target volume be included in the treatment volume at each and every session. Further, tissues that are not judged to be involved by tumor should not be irradiated if it is technically feasible to avoid their inclusion in the treatment volume. Hence, the effort at elaborate treatment planning.

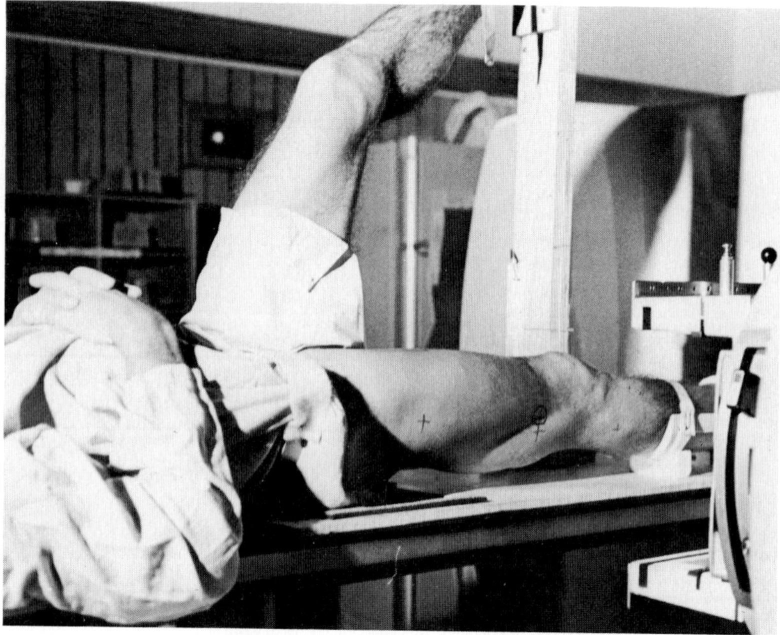

FIG. 29-11. This figure demonstrates an immobilization device employed in the pre-operative radiation therapy of a patient with an extensive liposarcoma of the posterior thigh and popliteal space (Stage IIB, G2T2NOMO). Treatment was given by right and left parallel opposed lateral fields to the posterior compartment of the thigh and a parallel opposed anterior–posterior pair to the upper medial thigh. For the large lateral field approach, the patient's left leg is held out of the beam path as shown. Further, the genitalia are pulled well up out of the field onto the anterior abdominal wall (not shown). The upper field was used only for the first 5000 rad. This particular patient was treated pre-operatively to the obvious tumor mass in the posterior distal thigh to 5600 rad.

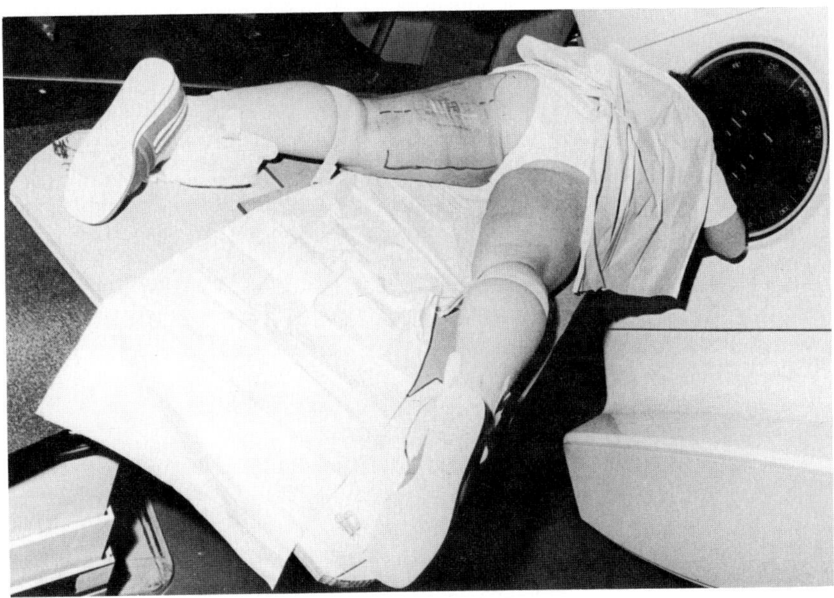

FIG. 29-12. An immobilization device that was used in the post-operative radiation therapy of a patient with a large, (Stage IIIB, G3T2NOMO) malignant fibrous histiocytoma in the posterior mid-portion of the thigh. This lesion was located deeply and was infiltrating muscle; the margins were also positive. The medial and lateral posterior oblique wedge pair were employed so as to encompass the entirety of the posterior compartment of the thigh for the first 5000 rad (because of the length of the field here the dose was 180 rad per fraction). To cover the upper aspect of the posterior compartment and to avoid the problems inherent in using simple front and back fields for such a large volume (irradiation of virtually the entire cross section of the thigh), it is necessary for the thighs to be separated as wide as possible; hence, the employment of the immobilization device to achieve the "spread-eagle" position. By this device, exactly the same separation of the thigh in each and every treatment session is maintained. Of course, after the initial 5000 rad had been given, a much reduced treatment volume was used.

To realize the planned dose distribution in the patient on a day-to-day basis, it is usually essential to prepare a cast or special device for patient immobilization. Figs. 29-11 and 29-12 show patients in such immobilization devices. The patient shown in Fig. 29-11 is being treated for an extensive Grade II liposarcoma in the posterior thigh and popliteal region. Treatment is being given by right and left parallel opposed lateral fields to the posterior compartment of the thigh and a parallel opposed anterior-posterior pair to the upper medial thigh. For the large lateral field approach the patient's left leg is held out of the beam path as is shown. Further, the genitalia are pulled well up out of the field onto the anterior abdominal wall (not shown). The upper field was used only for the first 5000 rad. This particular patient was treated pre-operatively to the obvious tumor mass in the posterior distal thigh to 5600 rad. The patient shown in Fig. 29-12 is in position for treatment of a Stage IIIB malignant fibrous histiocytoma of the mid-portion of the posterior thigh. The treatment plan here is to use an angled wedge pair so as to cover the entirety of the posterior compartment of the thigh. Treatment fields are large because of the fact that this lesion was high grade, arose deep in muscle and was infiltrating muscle tissue. Fig. 29-13 shows the portal film of the right posterior medial oblique field. Dose distribution achieved is shown in Fig. 29-14. For most patients treatments are given at 180–200 rad per day, 900–1,000 rad per week to a total dose of 7,000–8,000 rad. These doses refer to treatment by radiation alone. For radiation combined with surgery, doses are rarely carried to more than 6,600–6,800 rad. These dose levels are large and refer to treatment of lesions of the extremity, torso, and portions of the head and neck region. Clearly, dose aims must be lower for most lesions in the thorax, abdomen, or pelvis. Accordingly, less may be expected in terms of permanent control of those tumors. The general policy for this entire group of tumors where there is a reasonable prospect of cure is to push the dose to the maximum level compatible with a low probability of major complication, say $\leq 3\%$. Planning and execution of these treatments need careful consideration of the patient's general status, pre-existing disease (*e.g.*, diabetes), prior injury, anatomic site, and any other factor that may alter patient tolerance to the intended treatment. Further, the expected compliance by the patient with the recommended post-treatment care is a factor that must be considered. Very heavily irradiated tissue does not heal well following major injury. Thus, treatment will be influenced by patient occupation and life style. To provide these patients

FIG. 29-13. Simulator film of the right medial posterior oblique used in the patient shown in Fig. 29-2.

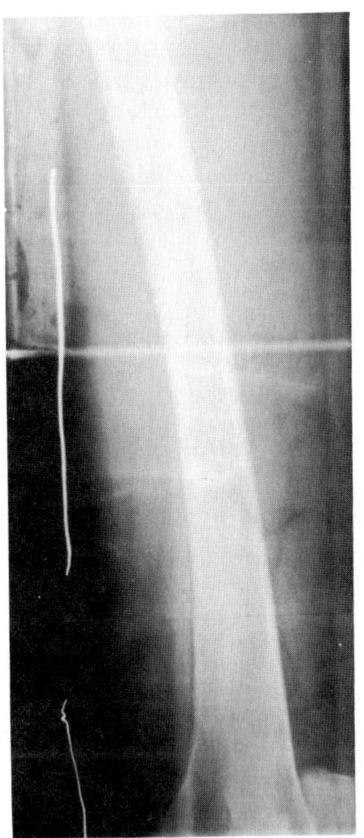

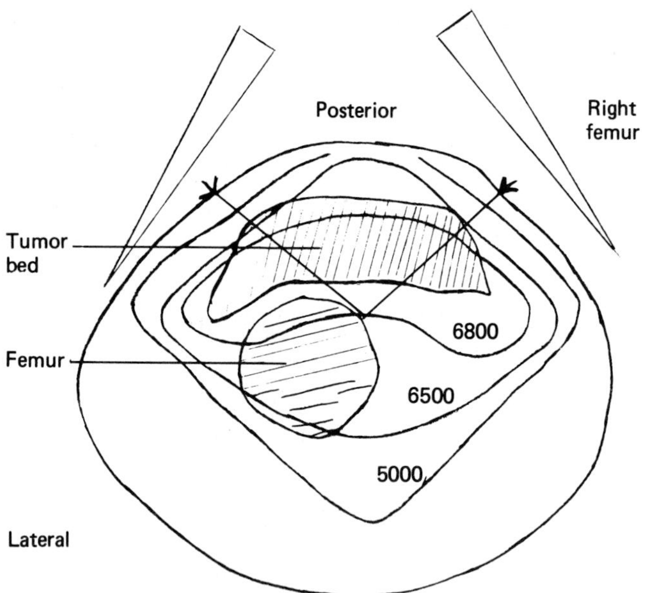

FIG. 29-14. Dose distribution pattern for patient shown in Fig. 29-12.

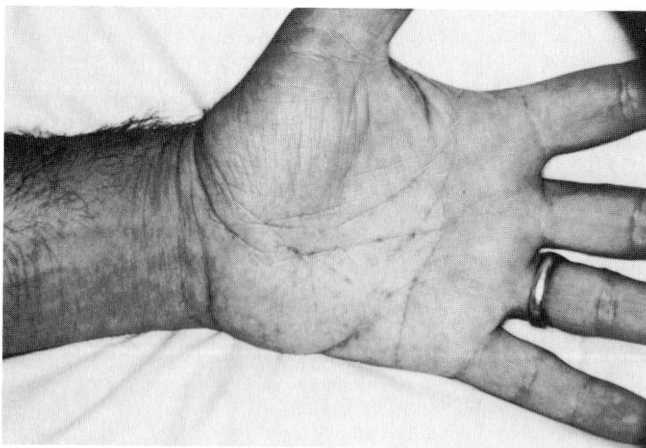

FIG. 29-16. The palmar aspect of the hand 6 years after radiation therapy (6620 rads, 34 fractions, 54 days) given after simple excision of a 3 cm alveolar cell sarcoma of soft parts. Good function is retained and the patient is pain free.

with the best likelihood of a good result, treatment should be undertaken only in large centers with experience in treatment of sarcoma, the full panoply of radiation beam qualities, and a strong active clinical physics group.

SURGERY AND POSTOPERATIVE RADIATION THERAPY

Virtually all patients with soft tissue sarcomas of the extremities that do not receive radical resection (as previously defined) and virtually all patients with truncal sarcomas should receive postoperative radiation therapy. Possible exceptions to this include patients with small, low grade lesions who undergo wide excision.

The amount of surgery to be performed when postoperative radiation therapy is planned is a matter of some controversy. While all gross tumor should be removed some authors advocate minimal excision of surrounding normal tissue while others advocate the maximum wide excision possible compatible with reasonable morbidity and function of the remaining part. Often, larger surgical excisions require the use of wider radiation fields. Recently, several workers have advocated extending local operations to include vascular reconstructive or bone replacement procedures.[210-212]

FIG. 29-15. Portal film of field that covers the medial ⅔ of the palm and the wrist.

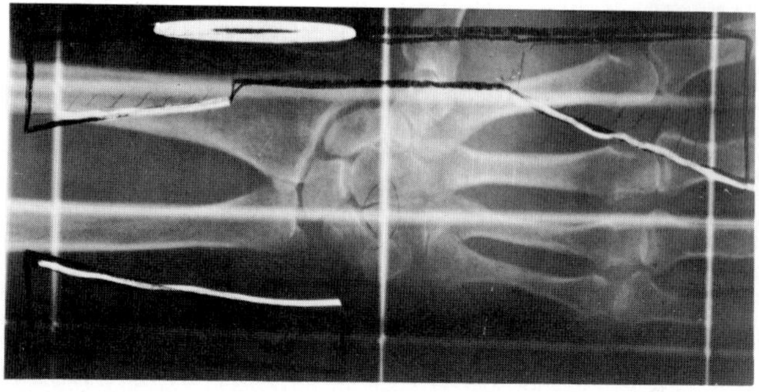

Radiation therapy for these patients is planned during the immediate postoperative period, but is not started until the wound has healed. Planning is significantly aided if the surgeon has carefully placed clips at the outer margins of the surgical field or at the margins of the gross tumor if the procedure was a local excision. Findings of both the gross and microscopic pathologic examination are integrated with the description of the surgical procedure by the physician to aid in design of the optimal treatment plan. The radiation treatment volume encompasses all tissues suspected of involvement by tumor plus those handled in the surgical procedure. Because of the large treatment volumes, complex treatment plans are important in excluding uninvolved tissues to the maximum extent possible. Simple front and back rectangular portals are rarely appropriate. This initial treatment volume should be irradiated to some 5,000 rad in 5–6 weeks; during this component of the treatment, a bolus is placed over the scar. The treatment volume is then reduced to cover only the site of the initial tumor; the dose to this smaller volume is brought to 6,600 rad. Where treatment volumes are unusually large, reduction of daily dose may be required but the final dose is maintained, if feasible. As examples of treatment plans and follow-up results some examples are shown.

Figure 29-15 presents the portal film used for the first component of treatment. This patient is seen post-resection of a 3 cm alveolar cell sarcoma of soft parts of the hypothenar eminence. The plan was to cover the medial two-thirds of the palm and the wrist; the lesion was shown at surgery and histopathologic study to be infiltrating deep structures of the hand. The appearance of the hand at six years after treatment to a dose of 6620 rad in 33 fractions over 54 days medically is an excellent result. He has almost a normal range of function in the hand, only occasional paresthesias in the 4th and 5th finger but this is not a problem (Fig. 29-16). The

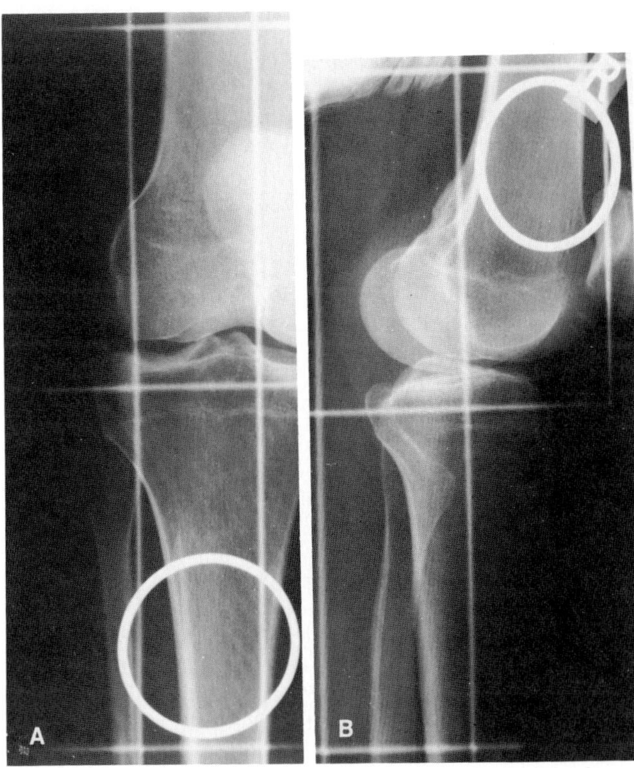

FIG. 29-17. Simulator films showing the anterior (*A*) and right lateral (*B*) coverage of the target area.

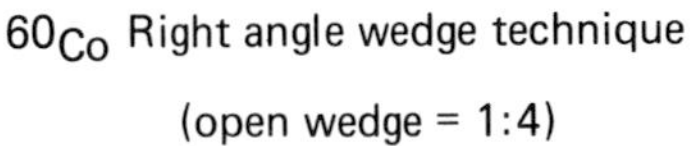

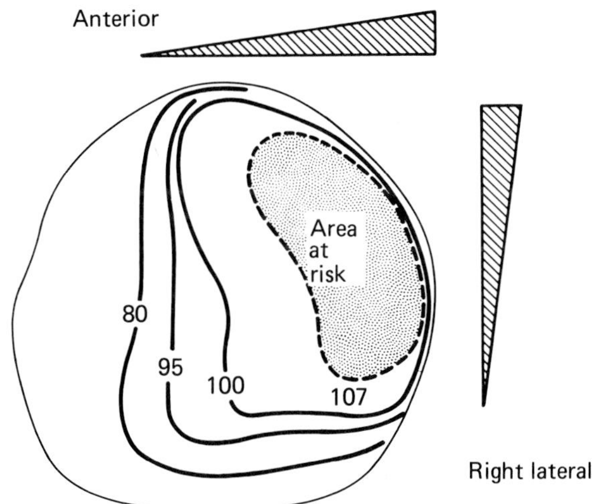

FIG. 29-18. The dose distribution pattern employed for the initial 5800 rads in the post-local excision treatment of a patient with stage IA synovial sarcoma of right lateral knee region.

patient is working regularly as a business executive and is able to use the hand in an almost normal manner. The next case for presentation of a treatment plan is that of a 38 year old woman with a Stage IA synovial sarcoma appearing lateral to the right knee. She was seen status post local excision of a 2 cm. tumor. The treatment plan was to use a right angled wedge pair so as to confine the treatment volume to the lateral aspect of the knee region where the tumor was judged to be. Figures 29-17A and 29-17B show simulation films of the portals employed in this patient. The dose distribution is shown in Fig. 29-18. The treatment volume for the final 1600 rad was smaller than the initial treatment volume. This patient, three years after treatment, with a normal appearing leg, normal range of motion, is free of pain and edema.

There are now data on sufficient numbers of patients from several centers that justify the conclusion that surgery followed by radiation can be an effective treatment strategy for a high proportion of patients with sarcoma of the extremity or trunk. A report from the M. D. Anderson Hospital of 80 patients treated by excision and postoperative radiation gave a local control rate of 80%. Functional results were judged good in 80% of patients. There was no pain, no or minimum edema (if present, it was readily controlled by pressure stocking), a near normal range of motion, and good use of the limb. Results at the Massachusetts General Hospital for local control and disease-free survival at 2 years among 86 patients treated by surgery followed by radiation is presented in Table 29-13. The local control rates at 2 and 5 years for all patients were 92% and 84%, respectively. As noted above in the discussion of results with radiation alone, local failures were more likely in the large and high grade lesions (IIB and IIIB) than in the small or low grade lesions. This accords with the earlier report from the M. D. Anderson Hospital. Disease-free survival rates at 2 years in this group of patients correlated

TABLE 29-13. Two-Year Local Control and Disease-Free Survival Rates (Actuarial) for Patients with Sarcoma of Soft Tissue Treated by Surgery and Post-Operative Radiation According to Histopathologic Type

HISTOPATHOLOGY	NO. PATIENTS	LOCAL CONTROL %	DISEASE-FREE SURVIVAL %
Fibrosarcoma	14	100	90
Spindle cell sarcoma	11	100	78
Synovial sarcoma	10	90	78
Malignant fibrous histiocytoma	11	71	64
Liposarcoma	18	92	85
Rhabdomyosarcoma	6	75	33
Miscellaneous	16	100	85

TABLE 29-14. Results of NCI, Soft Tissue Sarcoma of the Extremity Protocol as of April, 1980

	AMPUTATION	LIMITED SURGERY + RADIATION THERAPY	TOTAL
Number of patients	15	24	39
Local recurrence only*	0	3	3
Local recurrence plus distant metastases	0	1	1
Distant metastases only	2	2	4
Total recurrence	2	6	8
Deaths	0	3	3

* The first site of recurrence is considered

Rosenberg SA, Kent H, Costa J et al: Prospective randomized evaluation of the role of limb-sparing surgery, radiation therapy, and adjuvant chemoimmunotherapy in the treatment of adult soft-tissue sarcomas. Surgery 84:62–69, 1978

well with stage: 100% for stages IA and IB, but 41% for stage IIIB. This same series demonstrates that the histologic type does not exert a major impact on local control or disease-free survival rates. Grade of tumor appears to be an extremely important prognostic guide for both local control and disease-free survival.

It thus appears that the combination of local surgery and radiation therapy can reduce local recurrence rates to about 20% in extremity lesions. This level of local control can be exceeded by radical amputative surgery for extremity lesions. In selecting appropriate treatment the increased risks of local recurrence with local surgery and radiation therapy must be weighed against the evident morbidity of major amputation. Considerations of quality of life play a major role in such decisions.

Rosenberg and coworkers at the National Cancer Institute have conducted a prospective randomized study of patients with soft tissue sarcomas of the extremities in which patients were randomized to receive either amputation at or above the joint proximal to the lesion or wide excision plus radiation therapy.[30] All patients also received adjuvant chemotherapy. Results of therapy as of April, 1980 in this ongoing trial are presented in Table 29-14 with a median follow-up of 41 months. Although these data are preliminary, tentative conclusions can be drawn. Local control is good in both groups; 15 of 15 (100%) for the amputation group and 20 of 24 (83%) for the limited surgery plus radiation therapy group. Of interest is the finding that three of the four local failures in the radiation therapy group occurred in the proximal thigh. Detailed analyses of the quality of life of 24 patients with lower extremity sarcomas have been conducted by Sugarbaker and coworkers in this patient population.* He found little difference between the groups in assessments of economic impact, mobility, pain, 'treatment trauma,' and sexual func-

* Unpublished data

FIG. 29-19. Results of an unpublished study by Sugarbaker and coworkers of the quality of life of patients following either amputation or limb-sparing surgery with irradiation for the treatment of soft tissue sarcomas of the extremities. Patients were assigned randomly to one of the two treatment arms and subsequently assessed for degree of pain, adequacy of sexual relationships, mobility, and psychological treatment trauma. The study detected no significant differences between patients undergoing amputation and those undergoing limb-sparing surgery with radiation therapy.

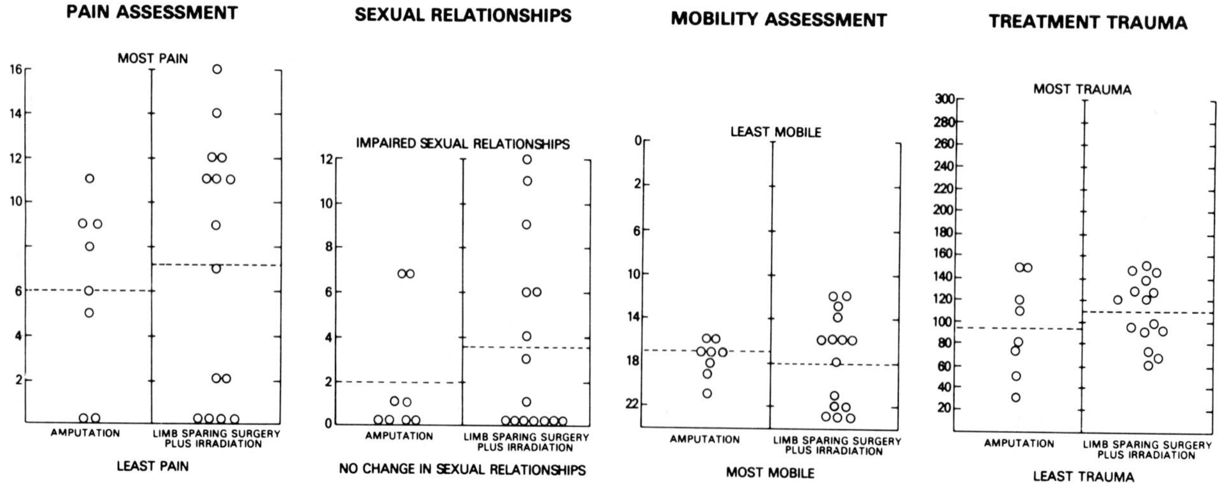

tioning (see Fig. 29-19). Further studies of this kind are necessary to help choose between local treatment alternatives in patients with soft tissue sarcomas.

PREOPERATIVE RADIATION THERAPY

There is now substantial experience with preoperative radiation in the treatment of patients with soft tissue sarcoma. For example, Atkinson reported, in 1963, local control of 14 of 15 patients who were treated by 4,500 rad delivered in 4–5 weeks followed by "block resection."[213] The median follow-up on these patients was almost 3 years. Ten patients with advanced sarcoma of soft tissue were treated by Martin and others and followed for more than one year. No local recurrences were detected among those patients during that follow-up period. Results of this approach for 25 patients treated by radiation followed by resection and followed for 1–8 years at the Massachusetts General Hospital are presented in Table 29-15. There, the radiation therapy was given preoperatively to doses of ≅5600 rad in 5–6 weeks. After a 3-week period a conservative resection was performed and a boost dose of 1,000–1,500 rad administered to the tumor bed intra-operatively. The intra-operative technique was either interstitial therapy or electron beam. The total dose to the tumor bed was usually in the range of 6,600–6,800 rad or its equivalent. For local anatomic reasons where the intra-operative procedure was not readily feasible the boost dose was given post-operatively in a few patients by small field external photon beam technique directed exclusively to the tumor bed as defined by the position of clips placed at the margin of the tumor during surgery. A regular finding at surgery was that the tumor mass was smaller and surrounded by a relatively dense pseudo-capsule. Further, there were usually profound pathologic changes evident. Grossly, the tumor was partially or totally necrotic. Histopathologically, only an occasional area showed residual "intact" tumor cells. In a worthwhile proportion of patients no tumor cells were found. With reference to long-term results in these 25 patients, 24 have local control for the follow-up periods of 1–8 years. The single failure occurred in a patient who was treated for a recurrent tumor in the stump following disarticulation for malignant fibrous histiocytoma. This area had been previously irradiated at the time she was considered for preoperative irradiation and surgery for the recurrence in the disarticulation stump. The treatment of this recurrent tumor was 4,800 rad to the stump region. After a 3-week break there was conservative excision of the residual tumor mass and an ^{192}I implant to the tumor bed. The patient did well for about a year but then local recurrence was detected in the tissue that had received the 4,800 rad but recurrence was not seen in the area that had had the 4,800 rad plus the interstitial implant. As a technical note for implantation, angiocaths or other plastic tubing are inserted into the tumor bed under direct vision. The wound is then closed. Usually, the sources are afterloaded into the angiocaths several days later. These results (*i.e.*, local control rate) of 24 of 25 patients constitute a very satisfactory local success rate. This is especially so considering the fact that nearly all of these lesions were special problems and locally advanced (22 of 25 tumors were >5 cm). Three patients were accepted for this treatment approach but at the time of exploration were found to have a non-resectable lesion because of invasion of major nerves and vessels. Treatment was completed by further radiation. Two of these three have recurred locally. Morton and coworkers employed intra-arterial infusion by doxorubicin (adriamycin) followed by radiation therapy (350 rad × 10 in 2 weeks) followed one week later by en-block resection in the treatment of 17 patients with sarcoma.[212] Recurrences have not been observed with follow-up of 4–34 months.

TABLE 29-15. Local Control and Distant Metastasis in 25 Patients Followed for 1–8 Years

STAGE	PATIENTS TREATED BY RADIATION THERAPY AND RESECTION	
	LOCAL CONTROL	DISTANT METASTASIS
IA	1/1	0/1
IB	4/5*	2/5
IIA	1/1	0/1
IIB	8/8	3/8
IIIA	1/1	0/1
IIIB	9/9	5/9

* Failure in the 4,800 rad-treated volume but not in the operated and boost dose volume

Local control is achieved in an impressively high proportion of patients with locally advanced disease by combination of preoperative radiation (± chemotherapy) followed by resection. The tolerance of patients to this combined approach from these various centers is judged good, with reasonable healing of the wound; three patients have required grafting. These overall satisfactory results with advanced lesions encourage further investigation of this approach and extending it to less advanced lesions. As also shown in Table 29-15, distant failure is predominantly an event in patients with IIB and IIIB lesions, again emphasizing the need for effective adjuvant therapy.

ADJUVANT CHEMOTHERAPY

Despite adequate local surgery with or without radiation therapy, most patients with high-grade soft tissue sarcomas will ultimately recur with distant disease. For this reason, the use of effective systemic adjuvant treatments is desirable. Unfortunately, there are currently no studies that unequivocably demonstrate advantage for the use of adjuvant chemotherapy in the treatment of soft tissue sarcomas. There are, however, a variety of chemotherapeutic agents of proven efficacy in patients with metastatic soft tissue sarcomas. The development of successful adjuvant regimens for the treatment of patients with "local" soft tissue sarcomas is being actively sought.

Between 1973 and 1976, patients with high-grade soft tissue sarcomas at the M.D. Anderson Hospital were randomized to receive either surgery plus postoperative radiation therapy alone or this treatment plus systemic chemotherapy.[214] The chemotherapy (VACAR) consisted of vincristine 1.5 mg/m^2 (maximum 2 mg) IV on day 1 then weekly for nine doses. Doxorubicin (adriamycin) was given at 60 mg/m^2 IV on day 2 and repeated every four weeks for seven doses to a total

TABLE 29-16. Doxorubicin (Adriamycin) in Soft Tissue Sarcomas

SCHEDULE	CR	PR	CASES	%	AUTHOR	REFERENCE
60–75 mg/m² q 3 wk	2	13	49	31	O'Bryan	216
60–90 mg/m² q 3 wk (75 mg/m² infused 72 hrs)	0	44	130	34	Blum	217
20–25 mg/m²/d × 3 q 3 wk	0	2	15	13	Creagan	218
0.4 mg/kg days 1, 2, 3, 8, 9, 10 q 2 wk	1	6	41	15	Cruz	219
70 mg/m² q 3 wk	3	8	39	28	Rosenbaum	220
25 mg/m² vs 50 mg/m² q 3 wk or 45 mg/m² vs 70 mg/m² q 3 wk	1	22	82	28	O'Bryan	221

dose limit of 420 mg/m². Cyclophosphamide was given at a dose of 200 mg/m² orally on days 3, 4, and 5 of each cycle and repeated every 4 weeks with doxorubicin and every 8 weeks while actinomycin-D was being given. Actinomycin-D was substituted for doxorubicin after the dose limitation of this latter drug had been reached and was given at 0.3 mg/m² (dose limit = 0.5 mg/dose) given on days 1–5 of each cycle every 8 weeks. Six courses of actinomycin-D were given over one year. The total time of chemotherapy was 18 months. With follow-up from 9–34 months, there was no statistically significant difference between these two patient groups; 67% of chemotherapy patients were disease-free versus 85% of control patients. While this study demonstrated no efficacy of this adjuvant chemotherapy regimen, follow-up on study was short and only 15 patients had been followed for greater than 24 months.

In 1978, Rosenberg and coworkers reported the results of adjuvant chemotherapy in 49 patients with soft tissue sarcoma treated either by surgery or surgery plus radiation therapy.[30] All patients were treated with a combination of doxorubicin and cyclophosphamide. Adriamycin was given in escalating doses from 50 mg/m²–70 mg/m² on day 1 of a 28-day treatment cycle. Cyclophosphamide was given in escalating doses from 500 mg/m² to 700 mg/m² IV also on day 1 of each 28 day treatment cycle. Patients were treated to a total dose of 530 mg/m² of doxorubicin, at which point they were switched to 6 months of high-dose methotrexate, 250 mg/kg, given once monthly. These patients showed a statistically significant improvement ($p < .001$) in disease-free and overall survival compared to comparable historical control patients treated without chemotherapy. These results have recently been updated. With all patients followed for at least 3 years, the 5-year disease-free survival of patients receiving chemotherapy is 74% compared to 41% in the historical controls. Overall survival in the chemotherapy-treated patients is 84% at 3 years compared to 53% in the historical controls ($p < .001$). While this study did show a statistically significant improvement with the use of adjuvant chemotherapy, these results have been analyzed only with respect to historical controls. A prospective randomized study comparing this adjuvant chemotherapy regimen with no chemotherapy is currently in progress. The severe side effects of doxorubicin-containing regimens (especially cardiomyopathy) in the young patient population that develops soft tissue sarcomas make it essential that prospective randomized studies prove the efficacy of adjuvant chemotherapy before this is widely adopted.

CHEMOTHERAPY OF DISSEMINATED SOFT TISSUE SARCOMA

Until the introduction of doxorubicin into clinical trials, the chemotherapy of soft tissue sarcomas was unrewarding. The standard of practice until 1972 (the introduction of doxorubicin) was either single agents, which had relatively little, if any, activity, or a combination popularized by Jacobs that included vincristine, actinomycin-D, and cyclophosphamide (VAC). In 1970 Jacobs reported eight responses in 17 patients with soft tissue sarcomas.[215] At that time, the VAC regimen began to be appreciated as effective in childhood rhabdomyosarcoma; the assumption was made that it would be effective in adult patients as well. Tables 29-16 through 29-19 demonstrate the single agent activity in patients with soft tissue sarcomas. The data cited in these tables are based on published trials as well as data on file from the cooperative group programs. The data represent a modern interpretation of response in adult patients with disseminated soft tissue sarcomas arising from the soft tissues or internal viscera.

The important role doxorubicin plays in the management of soft tissue sarcomas has been demonstrated predominantly in the cooperative group setting. In 1971, the Southwest Oncology Group performed a phase II trial of doxorubicin in which 49 evaluable patients were treated; complete responses were seen in two and partial responses in 13, for an overall response rate of 31%.[216,283] Two years later, in trying to assess the dose-response relationship of doxorubicin, the Southwest Oncology Group study again confirmed the relatively high response rate with doxorubicin as a single agent. That study of O'Bryan made the initial suggestion that there was a dose relationship in patients with soft tissue sarcomas treated with

TABLE 29-17. DTIC in Sarcomas: Literature Survey

	N	CR	PR	%
Leiomyosarcoma	24	1	5	25
Fibrosarcoma	18	0	1	6
Rhabdomyosarcoma	13	0	2	15
Liposarcoma	7	0	1	14
Synovial cell	1	0	0	0
Angiosarcoma	1	0	0	0
Unspecified	45	0	7	15
TOTAL	109	1	16	16

Dose: 250 mg/m² daily for 5 days every 4 weeks

TABLE 29-18. Other Single Agents: Chemotherapy in Sarcomas

DRUG	EVALUABLE CASES	RESPONSES	AUTHOR (Ref.)
Actinomycin-D	30	5	Golbey (223)
CCNU	19	2	Central Oncology Group (224)
Cyclophosphamide	15	2	Bergsagel (225), Korst (226)
5-Fluorouracil	1	8	Gold (227)
Methotrexate	49	9	Subramanian (228), Andrews (229)
Cis-Platinum	73	6	Karakousis (230), Samson (231), Bramwell (232)
Vincristine	19	1	Selawry (233), Korbitz (234)

adriamycin. This response relationship and survival relationship to dose has been confirmed subsequently in a number of trials.[222,284,285,286] The activity of this drug and its role as the most important drug in the management of disseminated soft tissue is demonstrated in Table 29-16. A phase II trial that actually predated the investigation of the drug was reported by Gottlieb and associates in the study of DTIC (Dimethyl-trianzeno-imidazole-carboxamide), a drug that has been discussed extensively in Chapter 31.[287,288] In this series, a response rate of 17% of 53 patients treated was reported. The response to DTIC was most impressive in Kaposi's sarcoma and leiomyosarcoma. However, since the rate of response to DTIC in the remaining soft tissue sarcomas was at or near 10% and since its use was complicated by severe nausea and vomiting, many investigators did not pursue this lead. Gottlieb, however, then went on to the combination of doxorubicin and DTIC.[289] In this large trial of 218 patients, the response rate to the two drug combination was greater than 30% higher than that seen with doxorubicin alone. The survival for responding patients had doubled compared to the doxorubicin alone-treated patients. However, no randomized prospective trial in disseminated soft tissue sarcomas has been reported to date comparing doxorubicin-DTIC to doxorubicin alone. Currently, Borden and the Eastern Cooperative Group are attempting to answer this question. Following the doxorubicin-DTIC experience, many combinations began to appear. The Southwest group continued to add drugs to their two-drug combinations, including cyclophosphamide, vincristine, and actinomycin-D. The most recent study of Baker and coworkers does not show clear superiority to a three drug combination vs the doxorubicin-DTIC combination. Response rates of doxorubicin-DTIC in this trial were 32% vs 35% with doxorubicin-DTIC and cyclophosphamide vs 24% with doxorubicin-DTIC and actinomycin-D (see Table 29-20). Not only were there no differences in terms of response (complete or partial), but no differences were observed in terms of survival or duration of response.

The most popular and widely studied combination is CY-VADIC (cyclophosphamide, vincristine, doxorubicin and DTIC).[290,291,292] More than 600 patients have been treated with this basic regimen as is reported in the literature. Response rates have varied by author from 30%–57%. Indeed, the necessity of vincristine in this combination may be questioned by careful analysis of the data, which does not seem to reveal any response or survival advantage to the combinations that include or do not include vincristine. Only one doxorubicin-DTIC combination has had a significantly lower response rate than 30% and that was the trial of Creagan and associates in which they reported an 11% response rate of 54 patients treated with vincristine, doxorubicin, and DTIC. However, in this trial patients were re-treated at 5-week intervals; this is almost twice the interval of all other doxorubicin-DTIC schedules.

Another combination therapy approach has been the inclusion of doxorubicin and the nitrosourea, methyl-CCNU. In two trials, the response rate was approximately 50%, although these two trials contain only 63 evaluable patients.[293,294] While the complete response rate from this combination is less than that reported to other combinations, clearly this combination is less toxic than the others as well.

Since there are relatively few randomized prospective trials comparing different therapy regimens in soft tissue sarcomas, it is somewhat difficult and arbitrary to make comparisons among the various combinations and treatment schedules that have been described. Two completed trials, however, do provide useful insight. The trial of Rosenbaum and coworkers compared doxorubicin to the drug combinations vincristine, actinomycin-D, and cytoxan to doxorubicin, cytoxan, and vincristine (VAC) (see Table 29-21). In this trial, the superiority of doxorubicin to the VAC regimen was clearly demonstrated. The recently completed trial of Baker and coworkers comparing doxorubicin and DTIC with or without cyclophosphamide or actinomycin-D does not suggest superiority of the three drug regimen to the two drug regimen (see Table 29-22).[219,223,286,287,290,291,293–300] The third comparative trial of Cruz and coworkers suggests the superiority of doxorubicin alone in comparison to combinations of actinomycin-D and L-Pam; actinomycin-D, L-Pam and vincristine; and actinomycin-D, L-Pam and cycloleucine.[219]

Overall survival from these combination approaches provides a median survival of patients with widely disseminated sarcomas of approximately 11 months. However, duration of remission and survival of responding patients is relatively brief, with median length of remission being approximately 6 months and survival of responding patients approximately 2 years. Nearly 5–10% of all patients entered into these combination therapies will have prolonged and meaningful survival with some patients living disease-free for 5 years.

As mentioned previously, there is a clear dose-response relationship when using doxorubicin. Thus, some of the disparity in the reported trials of doxorubicin combinations may be explained in part by the degree of myelosuppression

TABLE 29-19. Investigational Drugs Studied in Soft Tissue Sarcomas

DRUG	PR	EVALUABLE PATIENTS	AUTHOR (Ref.)
AMSA	2	31	Yap (235) Legha et al (236) Von Hoff et al (237) DeJager et al (238) Schneider et al (239)
Azotomycin	5	25	Chang et al (240) Weiss et al (241) Sooriyaarachchi et al (242)
Baker's Antifol	1	33	Benjamin (243) Rodriguez et al (244) Thigpen et al (245)
Carminomycin	13	48	Perevodchikova et al (246)
Chlorozotocin	3	27	Kovach et al (247) Gralla et al (248) Talley et al (249)
Cycloleucine	22	208	Johnson (250) Aust et al (251) Eastern Cooperative Oncology Group (ECOG) (252) Central Oncology Group (COG) (253)
Cytembena	1	25	Baker et al (254) Matejovsky (255)
Diamino-dichlorophenyl-methylpyrimidine (DDMP)	1	15	Alberto et al (256)
Dibromodulcitol	0	33	ECOG (257)
Dianhydrogalactitol	0	27	Kimball et al (258)
Gallium nitrate	1	22	Samson et al (259) Bedikian et al (260)
Hexamethylmelamine	4	81	Borden et al (261) Blum et al (262)
ICRF 159	1	29	ECOG (263)
Maytansine	0	66	Egan et al (264) Blum et al (265) ECOG (266)
Methotrexate (MTX) (High dose and C.F. rescue)	12	57	Von Hoff et all (267) Isacoff et al (268) Vaughn et al (269) Ambinder et al (270)
Methyl-CCNU	5	85	Creagan et al (271) Tranum et al (272)
Piperazinedione	1	39	Benjamin et al (273) LaGasse et al (274) Southeastern Group (SEG) (275)
Pyrazofurin	0	26	Salem et al (276) Gralla et al (277)
Vindesine	0	11	Currie et al (278) Rossof et al (279) Yap (235)
VM-26	1	33	Radice et al (280) Bleyer et al (281)
VP-16	3	41	Radice et al (280) Bleyer et al (282)

TABLE 29-20. SWOG Study 7613

TREATMENT	COMPLETE RESPONSE	PARTIAL RESPONSE	EVALUABLE PATIENTS	% RESPONSE
Adriamycin + DTIC	11	14	79	32%
Adriamycin + CTX	12	21	95	35%
Adriamycin + ACT-D	9	15	98	24%

acceptable to the treating physician. Patients whose white counts are lowered to 1,000 cells/mm^3 do significantly better than patients who experience little if any myelosuppression. In the most recent SWOG study, response rates in patients who have white count nadirs at or above 3,000 cells/mm^3 have an overall response rate of 18% vs those whose white count nadir is less than 3,000 cells/mm^3 having a response rate of 43%. Another prognostic factor that may be important in these studies is that women tend to survive longer than men. (In the most recent evaluation, median survival of women was 55 weeks vs 36 weeks for men).

Although there is not a definitive answer regarding histologic type of sarcoma and sensitivity to various chemotherapies, a trend begins to emerge. In 46 patients whose pathologic diagnosis was reviewed and suggested leiomyosarcoma, a response rate of 37% is observed vs 32 patients with malignant fibrous histiocytoma having a response rate of 13%. This suggestion is also supported by survival analysis. Therefore, in the leiomyosarcoma group the median survival was 51 weeks vs 25 weeks for the group with malignant fibrous histiocytoma. Thus far in the reported trials, confirmation of the histiologic subtype with all of the difficulties of such a review have not been correlated well with chemotherapy sensitivity. However, many of the currently ongoing trials do consider such pathology subtypes and the relationship to therapy. Thus, definitive statements should be able to be made in the near future regarding this question.

In considering the chemotherapy of soft tissue sarcomas two diseases sometimes included in reviews are Kaposi's sarcoma and mesothelioma. However, Kaposi's sarcoma should not be included since the natural history of this disease is significantly different. Further, the chemotherapy sensitivity of this disease is likewise dissimilar. Vinblastine as a single agent is quite effective in providing long-term control of this disease process.[301,302] Other intensive combination therapies are thus not essential.

Likewise, mesothelioma is often included in reviews but is best separated. Several excellent reviews of chemotherapy sensitivity are available.[303-310] Again, the most important drug is doxorubicin.

BONE TUMORS

The majority of bone manifestations of neoplasia in one large series consisted of patients with multiple myeloma involving bone.[311] However, if this entity were to be excluded from the roster of malignant bone tumors the ratio of malignant to benign bone tumors encountered at a major medical center is approximately 1:7.[311,312]

Of the benign bone tumors encountered, most lesions are of cartilaginous origin. A benign osteochrondroma that usually presents as an osteocartilaginous exostosis is one of the most common benign lesions encountered. Another is the benign chondroma, which is sometimes referred to as a solitary enchondroma or central chondroma. Common benign tumors of osteogenic origin consist of the osteoid osteoma and the benign osteoblastoma. The third most common benign tumor is the benign giant cell tumor.

Of the malignant bone tumors seen at major medical centers, the most common is osteogenic sarcoma. Next in line are chondrosarcoma and Ewing's sarcoma (The usual site of origin of malignant bone tumors is presented in Table 29-23.)

The most common presenting sign of a bone tumor is pain over the lesional area. This may be accompanied by swelling and tenderness. The most helpful diagnostic procedure in a suspected bone tumor patient is the roentgenogram. When examining a film of a bone lesion, the most important consideration is the differential diagnosis between a benign and a malignant bone tumor. In most cases, it will be possible to determine with relative assurance whether or not a lesion is benign or malignant. However, even with the decision that the tumor is benign, surgical intervention is frequently warranted since many benign tumors can go on to give a great deal of local destruction, possibly leading to a pathologic

TABLE 29-21. ECOG Study 2374

TREATMENT	COMPLETE RESPONSE	PARTIAL RESPONSE	EVALUABLE PATIENTS	% RESPONSE
Adriamycin	4	10	50	28%
Adriamycin, vincristine, cyclophosphamide	3	9	56	21%
Actinomycin-D, vincristine, cyclophosphamide (VAC)	2	1	59	5%

TABLE 29-22. Combinations

COMBINATIONS	CR	PR	EVALUABLE	%	AUTHOR	REFERENCES
Actinomycin-D + vincristine + cyclophosphamide q 4 wk	2	1	59	5	Rosenbaum	220
Actinomycin-D + vincristine + cyclophosphamide q 4 wk	1	7	17	47	Jacobs	1
Actinomycin-D + vincristine + cyclophosphamide q 5 wk	1	4	61	8	Creagan	271
Adriamycin + DTIC q 3 wk	25	67	218	42	Gottlieb	289
Adriamycin + DTIC q 3 wk	11	14	79	32	Baker (unpublished data)	295
Adriamycin + DTIC q 3 wk (single dose)	1	5	18	33	Saiki	296
Adriamycin + vincristine + DTIC q 3 wk	10	35	107	42	Gottleib	297
Adriamycin + vincristine + DTIC q 5 wk	1	5	54	11	Creagan	271
Adriamycin + DTIC + vincristine + cyclophosphamide q 3 wk	21	42	125	50	Yap	286
Adriamycin + DTIC + vincristine + cyclophosphamide q 3 wk	8	14	60	37	Pinedo	290
Adriamycin + DTIC + vincristine + cyclophosphamide q 3 wk	27	80	229	45	Benjamin	291
Adriamycin + DTIC + cyclophosphamide q 3 wk	12	21	95	35	Baker	295
Adriamycin + DTIC + cyclophosphamide q 3 wk (continuous infusion)	4	8	21	57	Benjamin	291
Adriamycin + DTIC + cyclophosphamide	4	9	23	45	Blum	285
Adriamycin + vincristine + cyclophosphamide + actinomycin-D q 3 wk	25	55	224	36	Benjamin	291
Adriamycin + DTIC + actinomycin-D q 3 wk	9	15	98	24	Baker	295
Adriamycin + methyl-CCNU	3	17	41	49	Rivkin	293
Adriamycin + methyl-CCNU vincristine	0	10	22	45	Hajdu	294
Adriamycin + streptozotocin	0	2	14	1	Chang	298
Adriamycin + cytoxan + methotrexate	4	38	140	30	Lowenbraun	299
Adriamycin + methotrexate (HD) + vincristine	1	2	14	2	Kaufman	300
Adriamycin + methotrexate (HD) + vincristine + DTIC	0	2	5	4	Kaufman	300
Adriamycin + cytoxan + vincristine	3	9	56	21	Rosenbaum	220
Actinomycin D + L-Pam	0	1	25	4	Cruz	219
Actinomycin D + L-Pam + vincristine	0	0	26	—	Cruz	219
Actinomycin D + L-Pam + cycloleucine	0	0	25	—	Cruz	219
Actinomycin D + chlorambucil	0	5	40	13	Golbey	223
Actinomycin D + chlorambucil + methotrexate	0	8	40	20	Golbey	223

(*Continues on facing page*)

TABLE 29-22. (Continued)

COMBINATIONS	CR	PR	EVALUABLE	%	AUTHOR	REFERENCES
Vincristine + methotrexate + adriamycin + actinomycin D (VMAD)	0	14	32	44	Hajdu	294
Vincristine + methotrexate + adriamycin + actinomycin-D (OMAD) + DTIC + chlorambucil (ALOMAD)	0	13	41	32	Hajdu	294
Vincristine + methotrexate + adriamycin + DTIC + cytoxan (CYVMAD)	0	7	29	24	Hajdu	294

fracture. There are also certain conditions in which the radiologist cannot say with total assurance whether or not the lesion is benign or malignant. In particular, it is sometimes very difficult to tell from the roentgen appearance alone whether or not a diaphyseal tumor in a long bone is osteomyelitis, eosinophilic granuloma, or indeed Ewing's sarcoma.

Most benign bone tumors have a sclerotic rim encompassing the extent of the lesional area in the bone. In addition to this sclerotic rim, it is usually quite evident where the margins of the lesion exist, and the extent of the lesion within the normal bone is usually clearly defined (see Fig. 29-20A). Benign tumors can break through the cortex. Some tumors, such as an aneurysmal bone cyst, can cause considerable thinning and expansion of the cortex; indeed, a pathologic fracture can be a presenting symptom of such a benign bone tumor. However, the roentgen appearance is usually quite characteristic of a long-standing thinning and expansion of the bone cortex. The three major roentgen criteria in determining the diagnosis of a malignant bone tumor are:

1. Diffuse appearance within the bone. This can be either sclerotic or lytic in nature; however, in a malignant bone tumor the margins of the tumor are usually indistinct and difficult to exactly define on the roentgenogram
2. There is usually never a sclerotic rim associated with a malignant bone tumor. However, at times malignant bone tumors that arise in pre-existing benign lesions can give the appearance of having sclerotic proximal or distal borders where the original benign bone cyst or tumor originally existed. However, within the center of the tumor or in one part of it there is usually evidence of more destructive activity, such as breaking through the bony cortex, with the production of a soft tissue mass and subsequent periosteal elevation peripheral to that mass (Codman's triangle).
3. Malignant bone tumors will frequently present with a soft tissue mass. This soft tissue mass is tumor growing through and destroying the cortex. Usually, as the tumor breaks through the cortex it will push out the periosteum causing tenting of the periosteum from the soft tissue growth. This lifted periosteum at its distal and proximal ends away from the tumor is what is sometimes referred to as Codman's triangle. Actually, the angle that the periosteum makes with the cortex of the bone can be distant from the actual tumor tenting the periosteum by its soft tissue growth in the center of the lesion (see Fig. 29-20B).

In general, the sclerosis within a bony cortex can be caused by either neoplastic bone formation or cartilage formation in both benign and malignant tumors, or by intense reactive bone formation to a malignant process or benign process that would otherwise be predominantly a lytic process. The scler-

TABLE 29-23. Usual Site of Origin of Common Malignant Bone Tumors

LONG BONES			FLAT BONES
Epiphyseal	*Metaphyseal*	*Diaphyseal*	
Giant cell Chondrosarcoma	Osteogenic sarcoma Chondrosarcoma	Ewing's sarcoma Hemangioendothelioma	Ewing's sarcoma Osteogenic sarcoma (radiation-induced and in Paget's disease)
	Malignant fibrous histiocytoma	Angiosarcoma	Chondrosarcoma
	Fibrosarcoma Non-Hodgkin's lymphoma	Adamantinoma Hemangiopericytoma	Angiosarcoma Mesenchymal chondrosarcoma Primitive neuroectodermal tumor Non-Hodgkin's lymphoma

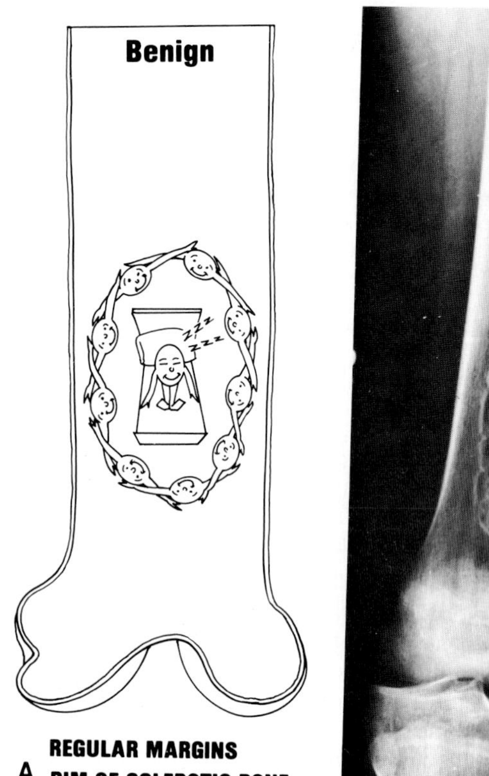

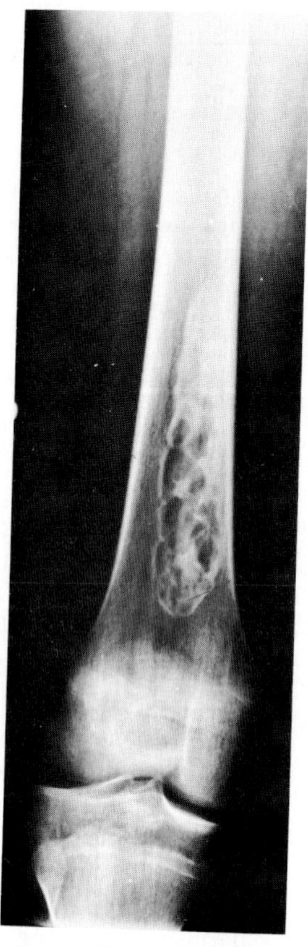

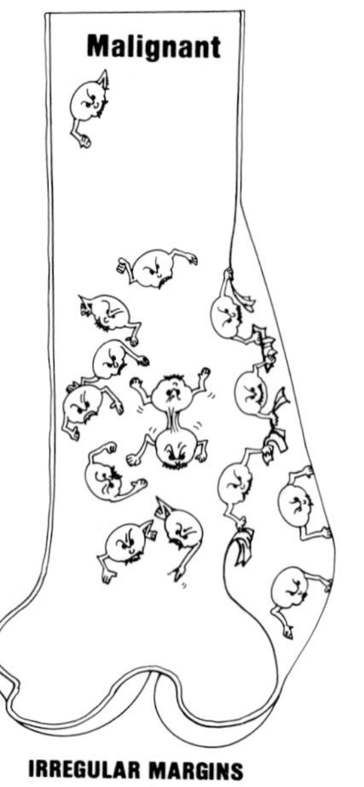

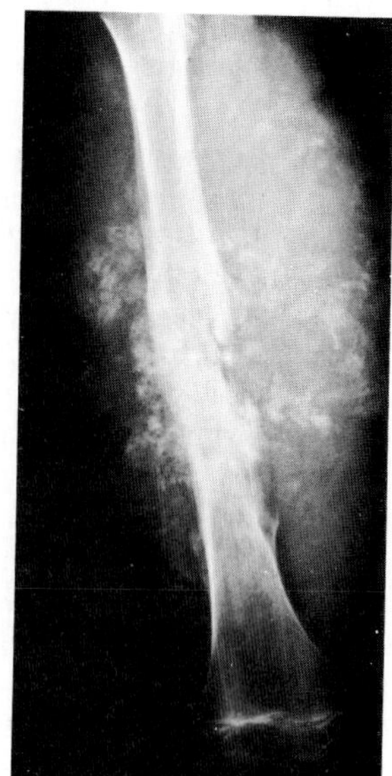

FIG. 29-20. *A*, Benign bone tumors have a characteristic sclerotic rim around the periphery of the lesion. The lesion is usually well defined, and there is no evidence of the erosion of the cortex or soft tissue mass. *B*, Malignant bone tumors can have lytic or sclerotic components. It is frequently difficult to tell the extent of the lesion within the bone, since there is no well-defined sclerotic rim around the tumor. The destructive process is diffuse within the medullary cavity of the bone, and the tumor may break through the cortex of the bone, thus producing a Codman's triangle. Frequently, there is an associated soft tissue mass. Differential diagnosis of this lesion is between an osteogenic sarcoma and chondrosarcoma.

otic rim noted in many benign tumors is reactive bone formation to slow tumor growth. By the same token, one can achieve a sclerotic appearance to a Ewing's sarcoma or a non-Hodgkin's lymphoma of bone, which again is due to reactive bone formation to the tumor. The appearance of calcification in the soft tissue in a patient with a bone lesion is frequently associated with osteoid formation in an osteogenic sarcoma or cartilagenous tissue being laid down by a chondrosarcoma.

BENIGN BONE TUMORS

The majority of benign bone tumors can be treated by biopsy and curettage. In addition to curettage, other orthopedic procedures may be undertaken in an effort to provide stability to the involved bone, particularly if it is one that has to bear weight. Such measures include packing with bone chips, bone grafting, filling the cavity with bone cement, and cryosurgery, as well as postoperative immobilization. The following benign bone tumors can cause potential difficulty. The oncologist may need to respond due to their locally aggressive behavior or their malignant potential, should they recur.

Osteochondromas and Enchondromas

The majority of these lesions are well controlled by simple excision or by curettage and packing with bone chips. However, rarely have they been associated with malignant degeneration into either chondrosarcomas or osteogenic sarcomas. In particular, the hereditary form of multiple exostoses as well as multiple enchondromatosis has been associated with chondrosarcoma and osteogenic sarcoma. In a review of over 500 cases of osteogenic sarcoma at the Memorial Hospital, 11 patients developed osteogenic sarcoma in areas of benign exostoses. All of these patients had hereditary multiple exostoses.[313]

In general, exostoses that are left *in situ* tend to grow particularly at adolescence. Any rapid growth of an exostosis should cause suspicion; what was once an obviously benign lesion should be biopsied if there is sudden onset of pain and growth in the area. In addition, occurrence of pain and sudden onset of swelling in what is thought to be a benign bone cyst or benign enchondroma should also raise suspicion and the lesion should be rebiopsied. Osteogenic sarcoma or chondrosarcoma occuring in these lesions is usually diagnosed rather late; the course of the patient that develops a malignant bone tumor in a pre-existing benign bone cyst is usually rather dismal. In the days prior to effective chemotherapy for the treatment of osteogenic sarcoma, most of the patients developing an osteogenic sarcoma in a pre-existing bone cyst were not curable with radical surgery.[314]

Aneurysmal Bone Cyst

Aneurysmal bone cysts are usually completely benign tumors that can be cured by local surgery consisting of biopsy and curettage. Very rarely has osteogenic sarcoma been noted to occur in an aneurysmal bone cyst. This usually becomes manifest following surgery for what is thought to be a benign aneurysmal bone cyst. The patient may present with swelling in the area, and it may be thought that there is a recurrent aneurysmal bone cyst in the lesional area. However, with further biopsies sometimes osteogenic sarcoma has been diagnosed in the rare patient with aneurysmal bone cyst. Because telangiectatic osteogenic sarcoma can rarely present with roentgenographic appearances of slow growth and expansion of the bone mimicking an aneurysmal bone cyst, it is important to note that extensive biopsy material should be taken from apparently benign aneurysmal bone cyst at surgery. Diagnostic errors can be avoided if the surgeon remembers that the majority of material curetted from the entire cystic cavity should be sent to the pathology laboratory for careful examination.

Eosinophilic Granuloma

Eosinophilic granuloma occurs in two forms—solitary and multiple. The multiple form of eosinophilic granuloma requires systemic chemotherapy. Both require local measures including curettage or low-dose radiation therapy to large lesions in weight-bearing bones that are potential candidates for pathologic fracture. Approximately one-half of patients with eosinophilic granuloma have only solitary disease. It is limited to a primary lesion in one bone and can occur in practically any bone throughout the body. Solitary eosinophilic granuloma usually responds to local therapy only, and seldom gives rise to delayed complications. Local therapy for solitary eosinophilic granuloma consists of biopsy, curettage, and where necessary to prevent impending pathologic fractures in weight-bearing bones, low dose radiation therapy can be given to the lesion to aid in its healing. Multifocal eosinophilic granuloma is usually a progressive disease that can cause considerable morbidity if not treated with systemic chemotherapy.[315]

Eosinophilic granuloma enters into the differential diagnosis of two other important bone lesions; when considering the differential diagnosis of a solitary bone lesion, eosinophilic granuloma must be thought of. It is primarily a disease of childhood and adolescence. However, it can occur in older patients and has been reported in patients as old as 60 to above 65 years of age.[316] It is rare in the older age group, and because of the histologic appearance of eosinophilic granuloma, the physician must always be suspicious of Hodgkin's disease of bone in older patients.

The roentgenographic appearance of eosinophilic granuloma can vary from a cystic-appearing lesion in a bone, to a diffuse lesion with a great deal of destruction, and periosteal new bone formation. Frequently, the differential diagnosis of an eosinophilic granuloma of bone will include osteomyelitis, Ewing's sarcoma, and (in the adolescent and older age group) Hodgkin's disease.

Lesions of eosinophilic granuloma appear to evolve very rapidly. Solitary bone lesions that look like osteomyelitis or Ewing's sarcoma frequently evolve very rapidly producing periosteal new bone formation similar to that which can be seen in Ewing's sarcoma. When such lesions are biopsied, the differential diagnosis between Ewing's sarcoma, osteomyelitis, and eosinophilic granuloma is not distinguished readily on histologic review of the biopsy material. However, in older patients (particularly those in the second decade and above) lesions that appear to be eosinophilic granuloma can actually be metastatic or primary Hodgkin's disease lesions. Hodgkin's disease of bone, a rare primary bone lesion, has previously been reported.[312] Quite frequently when Hodgkin's disease involves bone, typical Reed–Sternberg cells are not found. The presence of solitary or multiple bone lesions that do not have the characteristic "punched-out" look of eosinophilic granuloma, the presence of systemic symptoms such as fever, elevated erythrocyte sedimentation rate, and low serum iron in an older patient should cause suspicion that what is present is Hodgkin's disease manifesting itself in bone. In such situations biopsy of enlarged regional lymph nodes or repeated biopsies of an equivocal lesion may be warranted.

Chondroblastoma

Chondroblastoma is a benign bone lesion that usually arises in the epiphysis. In the Memorial Hospital experience this lesion was most common in the proximal humerus followed by the proximal femur, proximal tibia, and the distal femur, in that order. It is also quite prevalent in and about the ankle and in the pelvis. It is a disease that has its maximum distribution in the second decade of life. Long-standing pain in the lesional area is the usual presenting symptom. All of these symptoms can be present for months before the diagnosis is made.[312]

Roentgenographically, this lesion presents as a lytic round or oval shaped area involving the epiphysis and sometimes extending to the neighboring metaphyseal area. The lesion is usually well-defined by a sclerotic rim giving a clue to its supposed benign nature. On histologic examination, biopsy material shows characteristic polyhedral tumor cells with giant cells present throughout the field. It usually has a scanty matrix and the cellular-appearing polyhedral cells have a worrisome malignant look to them; however, as pointed out by Jaffe these lesions are usually benign.[317]

The local recurrence rate following surgery and curettage alone is somewhere between 20–60% at 5 years. In the Memorial Hospital experience this local recurrence rate following curettage and packing with bone chips was somewhat lower (approximately 20–25%).[318] In addition to the locally aggressive behavior of chondroblastoma, there have been several instances where chondroblastoma has been noted to metastasize.[319–321]

When encountering a benign chondroblastoma it should

be kept in mind that this is a locally aggressive tumor and may have the capacity to metastasize. In those rare patients where metastases have occured some patients have had widespread disease leading to a fatal outcome. Therefore, the local approach to treating chondroblastoma should be with a bit more aggressive treatment than one would normally give to other benign tumors.

MALIGNANT BONE TUMORS

General Considerations

The incidence of primary malignant bone sarcomas is quite rare. With the exception of osteogenic sarcoma, chondrosarcoma, and Ewing's sarcoma, there is little accumulated experience in the successful treatment of rare bone sarcomas with different modalities of treatment. Therefore, by grouping bone sarcomas according to their sensitivity to radiation therapy and chemotherapy it is useful to classify the malignant bone tumors either as spindle cell sarcoma or small-cell sarcoma. Osteogenic sarcoma and chondrosarcoma are examples of the former, and Ewing's sarcoma and reticulum cell sarcoma (non-Hodgkin's lymphoma) being examples of the latter. The reason for this classification is that it is a workable classification for bone sarcomas when considering treatment. In terms of treatment, the spindle cell sarcomas are usually resistant to radiation therapy and relatively resistant to conventional chemotherapeutic agents. On the other hand, the small cell sarcomas are radio-responsive, and usually respond quite well to conventional chemotherapeutic modalities. It is for this reason that the classification considered in Table 29-24 is proposed to the oncologist considering how to treat rare bone sarcoma. In addition, many of the rare bone sarcomas masquerade under different names. Therefore, it is important for the treating oncologist to be aware of the successful treatment modalities for small-cell sarcomas or spindle cell sarcomas. Usually, pathologists can be persuaded to comment whether or not a fully malignant lesion is a spindle cell sarcoma with different degrees of differentiation or an undifferentiated small cell sarcoma.[322–324]

Because of the rarity of some of the bone sarcomas to be considered in this chapter, more time will be spent considering the prototypes in each group. Osteogenic sarcoma will be used as a prototype for spindle cell sarcomas and Ewing's sarcoma, which is extensively discussed in Chapter 34, can be used as a prototype for the treatment of other small-cell sarcomas. Thus, an attempt will be made to describe current thinking on the treatment of the malignant spindle cell sarcomas and on the treatment of the malignant small-cell sarcomas as a group.

Malignant Spindle Cell Sarcomas of Bone

All of the tumors described in this group are relatively radioresistant and require surgery for local control. These tumors all have a high propensity to recur locally if good surgical local control is not achieved at initial surgery. In addition, the local recurrence of a low-grade spindle cell sarcoma can produce recurrent tumors of higher grade histology than those that were originally present at the initial surgical procedure. Spindle cell sarcomas can occur in any grade of malignancy. When dealing with a primary bone tumor the

TABLE 29-24. Classification of Major Malignant Bone Tumors by Treatment Modalities Used

SPINDLE CELL SARCOMAS		SMALL CELL SARCOMAS
Low Grade Histology	*High Grade Histology*	*All High Grade Histology*
Low grade central osteogenic sarcoma	Osteogenic sarcoma	Small cell osteogenic sarcoma
Parosteal osteogenic sarcoma	Parosteal osteogenic sarcoma	
Chondrosarcoma	Chondrosarcoma	Mesenchymal chondrosarcoma
Fibrosarcoma	Fibrosarcoma	
Malignant fibrous histiocytoma	Malignant fibrous histiocytoma	Non-Hodgkin's lymphoma
Giant cell tumor	Giant cell tumor	Ewing's sarcoma
Hemangiopericytoma	Hemangiopericytoma	
Hemangioendothelioma Adamantinoma	Malignant schwannoma	Angiosarcoma Primitive neuroectodermal tumor
Malignant schwannoma (Malignant peripheral nerve tumor)		
Radioresistant-local control by surgery		Radioresponsive-local control by radiation therapy and surgery possible
Rarely metastasize-surgery for solitary metastases	Chemotherapy responsive	Chemotherapy sensitive
	Chemotherapy to prevent metastasis (and shrink primary tumor)	

propensity to metastasize is directly dependent on the histologic grade of malignancy. Low grade tumors need only good local control; high grade tumors need good surgical local control plus systemic chemotherapy since greater than 50% of all high-grade malignant bone tumors have a propensity to metastasize within a few years of surgery for the primary tumor.

Osteogenic Sarcoma

Osteogenic sarcoma is a malignant spindle cell sarcoma usually occurring in bone but can occur as a primary soft tissue tumor. The malignant spindle cell stroma of the tumor forms tumor osteoid. In addition to the formation of tumor osteoid, the tumor can show other forms of differentiation as a predominant feature. However, the presence of osteoid being directly formed by the tumor cells even in tumors that show predominantly fibrous or chondroblastic differentiation as well, still dictates that the tumor be classified as an osteogenic sarcoma. Osteogenic sarcomas whose tumor cells form a great deal of collagen can be classified as fibrosarcomatous types of osteogenic sarcoma or malignant fibrous histiocytomatous osteogenic sarcoma. Large areas of cartilagenous differentiation within an osteogenic sarcoma may cause the tumor to be subclassified as a chondroblastic osteogenic sarcoma. Predominantly lytic tumors that have the histologic appearance of numerous areas of dilated vascular channels are classifed as telangiectatic osteogenic sarcomas.[312]

Approximately 3–4% of all osteogenic sarcomas are what has been called juxtacortical or periosteal osteogenic sarcomas. These tumors originate on the external surface of the bone in close association with the periosteum. Juxtacortical osteogenic sarcomas are thought to be less malignant than the classic osteogenic sarcoma. They typically occur in the posterior aspect of the distal femur (the most common site). Usually the tumor stroma is low grade with few tumor cells and a great deal of collagen matrix, but occasionally a fully malignant tumor with a high-grade stroma is encountered. The prognosis of a periosteal osteogenic sarcoma depends solely on the histologic grade of the malignancy, and not on its location.[325] However, the majority of these lesions do tend to be of low grade.

Approximately 3–4% of children with osteogenic sarcoma present with multiple synchronous primary tumors in the metaphyseal areas of all the long bones and of the pelvis as well.[326] This type of multifocal sclerosing osteogenic sarcoma is quite rare and uniformly fatal even with combination chemotherapy and surgery. It is generally impossible to surgically resect all of the lesions; eventually the patient becomes resistant to therapy and dies of progressive disease.

Osteogenic sarcoma can also arise in Paget's disease. Osteogenic sarcoma arising in Paget's disease is said to be more lethal in its course than classic osteogenic sarcoma. Most patients developing osteogenic sarcoma in Paget's disease develop metastasis within 6 months of diagnosis of the primary lesion.[327]

Osteogenic sarcoma is also a complication of radiation therapy and can occur 10–20 years following radiation therapy for other malignant diseases. Radiation-induced osteogenic sarcomas often occur in the axial skeleton and pelvis, and therefore are usually inoperable at the time the patient presents with a secondary osteogenic sarcoma. Thus, osteogenic sarcoma of the sternum, pelvis, or vertebral body following treatment for Hodgkin's disease usually presents with an inoperable primary that goes on to recur locally after inadequate local therapy, then finally metastasizes.[328] Secondary osteogenic sarcomas arise in the irradiated bones in patients who are apparently cured of retinoblastoma at a much higher frequency than expected in irradiated patients.[329,338]

Classic Osteogenic Sarcoma

Classic osteogenic sarcoma is a malignant tumor of bone composed of proliferating spindle cells that directly form tumor osteoid (see Fig. 29-21). Osteogenic sarcoma (with the exception of multiple myeloma) is the most common primary malignant bone tumor.[312] There are approximately 500 new cases of osteogenic sarcoma diagnosed in the U.S. per year, which makes this tumor approximately twice as prevalent as chondrosarcoma and three times more prevalent than Ewing's sarcoma. Males are affected more frequently than females and in the series at Memorial Hospital the proportion was 1.3:1 (male to female); in the Mayo clinic experience it was reported at 1.6:1.[311,312] Osteogenic sarcoma can occur at any age; however, it is most common in the second decade of life. If one excludes the rare patients in the third, fourth, and fifth decade of life that develop classic osteogenic sarcoma (and the older patients that develop osteogenic sarcoma in irradiated sites or in Paget's disease) the median age for disease development is approximately 14½ years for males and 13½ years for females. Osteogenic sarcoma tends to occur during the adolescent growth spurt. This growth spurt occurs approximately one year earlier in females and may be responsible for the younger median age of the onset of this disease in the female population.

The majority of osteogenic sarcomas occur in and about the knee. The distal femur is the most common site; the proximal tibia, and the proximal humerus are next in frequency.

With the exception of osteogenic sarcoma occurring in familial retinoblastoma patients at a higher incidence, there is no proven familial tendency for this disease to occur within families. However, there are 13 reported cases of osteogenic sarcoma occuring in multiple sibs of a given family.[312] In addition, at Memorial Hospital in the past 5 years, two additional familial cases of primary osteogenic sarcoma without retinoblastoma have been observed in siblings.

PRESENTING SYMPTOMS. Usually, the patient complains of pain in and about the knee or other area involved with osteogenic sarcoma. Pain is the most frequent presenting sign and the tumor may go on to produce rapid soft tissue swelling following the onset of pain. Even if pulmonary metastasis are present at presentation these are usually painless and frequently not suspected until a chest roentgenogram is obtained. Approximately 20% of patients present with evidence of pulmonary metastasis at diagnosis.

Approximately 60% of patients with osteogenic sarcoma (predominantly those with osteoblastic types of osteogenic

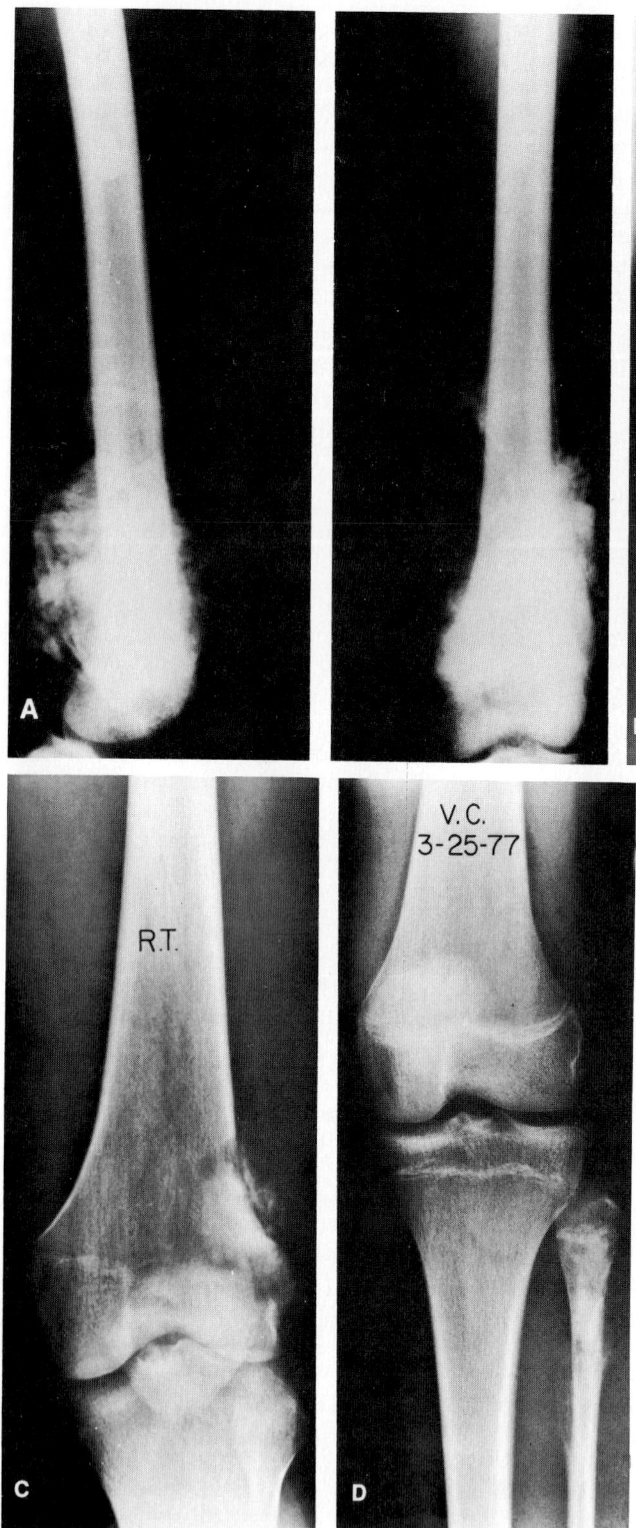

FIG. 29-21. *A*, Osteogenic sarcoma of the distal femur. *B*, Telangectatic osteogenic sarcoma of the proximal humerus. *C*, Osteogenic sarcoma of the distal femur. *D*, Osteogenic sarcoma of the proximal fibula.

sarcoma) present with an elevated serum alkaline phosphatase. The serum alkaline phosphatase can be elevated even in non-osteoblastic lesions. However, when these lesions are examined histologically there is usually evidence of abundant osteoid formation in most tumors. When evaluating an elevated serum alkaline phosphatase it has to be kept in mind that the normal serum alkaline phosphatase for a growing child is somewhere between 2½ and 3 times the upper limit of normal for the adult population.

Rarely, osteogenic sarcoma of the pure lytic or telangiectatic type can present as a pathologic fracture. This type of osteogenic sarcoma grows extremely rapidly at times; however, at presentation with the pathologic fracture there may be no evidence of soft tissue mass. Quite frequently this type of patient has a history of obtaining the fracture after some form of athletic trauma. Although in some instances careful examination of the roentgenogram will yield evidence of abnormal bone erosion around the fracture area, sometimes this finding is missed, and patients are merely treated as if they have a broken bone. The fracture is given a closed reduction and the patient's extremity put in a plaster cast.

DIFFERENTIAL DIAGNOSIS. The classic presentation of a sclerotic lesion with a soft tissue mass in the distal femoral metaphysis usually leaves little doubt as to the diagnosis (see Fig. 29-21). Occasionally, however, fractures occurring in low-grade fibrous benign tumors can cause callous formation. Following biopsy of such a lesion the question of whether or not this is an osteogenic sarcoma can be raised because of reactive bone formation. In this instance, the differential diagnosis between reactive bone formation and neoplastic bone or osteoid production must be accurately made by the pathologist. Failure to make the diagnosis of a lytic or telangiectatic osteogenic sarcoma in a pathologically fractured bone is usually secondary to the fact that a biopsy is not taken.

When a biopsy of an osteogenic sarcoma is performed an attempt should be made to biopsy not only the soft tissue superficially, but to biopsy the bone and medullary contents of the bone as well. Care should also be taken not to make a very large defect in the bone during the biopsy, since fractures at the biopsy site can occur if too large a defect is made at that time. Since pathologic fractures can occur following biopsy, it is imperative that patients be immobilized and made non-weight-bearing on tumors of the lower extremity following biopsy procedures.

Occasionally, when only soft tissue tumor is obtained at biopsy the diagnosis can be obscured. Most osteogenic sarcomas as well as other tumors arising in bone tend to be more differentiated in the tumor center, and the periphery of the soft tissue mass where the tumor is most rapidly growing is sometimes more undifferentiated. Soft tissue specimens obtained from primary bone osteogenic sarcomas may not contain tumor osteoid. At times they may appear to be growing as a malignant fibrous histiocytoma or even as a giant cell tumor. However, on close inspection of the roentgenogram, calcification and sclerosis exist within the tumor center, which most probably represents calcified tumor osteoid. If the serum alkaline phosphatase is elevated this may be a manifestation of osteoblastic activity within the tumor. In such patients the diagnosis of malignant fibrous histiocytoma or even giant cell tumor may be entertained before the fully malignant potential of the osteogenic sarcoma is realized.

Elevation of the serum alkaline phosphatase in a patient who has what appears to be malignant fibrous histiocytoma or fibrosarcoma on biopsy of a soft tissue mass that is coming from a bone should raise suspicion of osteogenic sarcoma. Nevertheless, if a high-grade malignant spindle cell sarcoma is diagnosed, treatment should not differ substantially from treatment of a fully malignant osteogenic sarcoma.

HISTOLOGIC GRADING OF THE TUMOR. Classic osteogenic sarcoma is a fully malignant spindle cell sarcoma. Occasionally, a low-grade lesion will be encountered. It is up to the treating oncologist to decide on whether or not further therapy is indicated. Some low-grade periosteal osteogenic sarcomas carry a prognosis as good as 80–90% disease-free survival following radical surgical resection of the tumor. In other series, the reported 5-year survival of low grade osteogenic sarcomas is only in the vicinity of 50–60%.[325,331] Some tumors can appear low grade in certain areas of the tumor. It is imperative that when dealing with a low grade tumor the pathologist examine multiple sections from all representative tumor areas. If high-grade material is found in any of the sections, this is an indication of a poor prognosis.

CLINICAL PATHOLOGY. There are numerous reports regarding the prognosis in osteogenic sarcoma.[332] Usually, within one to two years 80% of patients will experience pulmonary metastasis. The progression of pulmonary metastasis is the usual cause for death in patients with osteogenic sarcoma. In the majority of series reported, the 5-year disease-free survival for osteogenic sarcoma varies very little from an average of approximately 20%.[333–335] In 210 patients followed at Memorial Hospital with classic osteogenic sarcoma of an extremity only 17% of patients were alive 5 years from diagnosis, the remaining patients succumbing to metastatic disease.[323]

With the ability to keep patients alive longer through the use of thoracic surgery to remove pulmonary metastasis and aggressive chemotherapy to treat metastatic disease, different patterns of metastatic spread have been described.[326] Since the patient is being kept alive longer by treatment of pulmonary metastasis and sometimes aggressive radiation therapy to slow down the growth of life-threatening pulmonary metastasis, patients live long enough to develop manifestations of tumor spreading to different areas. The authors have seen patients develop what seemed to be multiple and more extensive bone metastasis, brain metastasis, extension of pulmonary metastasis down through the diaphragm into the retroperitoneal space, and into the liver and abdominal cavity. In such patients, metastases to adrenal, kidneys, and mesenteric lymph nodes occurred.[337]

Prior to the use of chemotherapy, patients usually died of pulmonary metastases. Metastases to bone occurred in approximately 50% of these patients, in addition to pulmonary metastases. Approximately 50% of patients had subclinical renal metastases, adrenal metastases, and metastases in other visceral organs at autopsy. In addition, at autopsy the frequency of regional nodal involvement in the amputated stump site was 20%, whereas the incidence of regional nodal involvement noted at initial surgery was less than 10%.[313] Local recurrence in an amputated site usually lead to widespread disseminated metastases to lung and other bones.

SURGICAL TREATMENT OF OSTEOGENIC SARCOMA. Local control can be achieved in greater than 90% of patients with osteosarcoma of the extremities if suitable precautions are taken in the selection of the level of amputation.

As in the biopsy of soft tissue sarcomas, it is extremely important to prevent local spread of osteosarcoma in hematomas resulting from the biopsy. Excellent hemostasis must be obtained. Some surgeons prefer to use a tourniquet above the lesion during the biopsy, though most do not, and there is little evidence that the use of a tourniquet is of value.

The level of amputation of extremity sarcomas must be carefully selected after analysis of the standard roentgenogram and the bone scan. The bone scan is of special value in this setting and provides a good approximation of the proximal level of spread as well as the presence of 'skip' metastases in the involved bone. It is often useful to mark the skin with a drop of radionuclide material at the time of bone scan to exactly mark the level of proximal extension of the tumor. Transmedullary amputations should be performed at least 7–10 cm above the proximal extension of tumor.

The possible presence of 'skip' metastases in the involved bone has led some surgeons to advocate removal of the entire involved long bone.[313,338,339] This view has been largely abandoned with careful selection of the level of amputation; cross-bone amputations provide local control in greater than 90% of patients. The bone scan is an effective technique for detecting 'skip' metastases. When these are present, amputation involving the entire length of the long bone is indicated.

Limb sparing surgery for patients with osteogenic sarcoma should be applied with caution only after careful evaluation with bone scans, arteriograms, and computed axial tomography have demonstrated a strong likelihood that the tumor can be resected by such an approach with negative margins in all directions.[340–342] While preoperative chemotherapy may improve the ability to perform local resections of osteogenic sarcoma, experience with use of this approach is limited.[343–346] Local resectional surgery for osteogenic sarcoma can be associated with significant complications and currently should be used only in selected centers experienced with these techniques.

In the Memorial Hospital experience, replacement of a total femur and knee for osteogenic sarcoma of the distal femur was carried out in approximately 30 patients with osteogenic sarcoma. Functional, cosmetic, and psychologic results of treatment were clearly superior to hip disarticulations.[340] However, in the early days of treatment this type of surgery led three of these patients to have a local recurrence of disease, which was ultimately responsible for metastatic disease. In addition, two patients had to undergo amputation due to infection of the endoprosthesis. The majority of the surviving patients that had this type of operation are quite pleased with the end result. However, many of them have arthritis of the hip joint as a result of this early experimental surgery.

The use of a bicentric head on the total femur prosthesis has obviated the occurrence of late arthritis. In recent years the use of an endoprosthesis from the mid-thigh and down including the knee has given even better functional and long-term results. However, the functional results obtained will have to await further evaluation. The cosmetic results are clearly superior, and in recent times there have been no local recurrences and no compromise of survival of patients undergoing such therapy.

Similarly, patients with limited involvement of the proximal femur can undergo *en bloc* resection and replacement of the upper femur with an endoprosthetic device. This can be done where there is minimal soft tissue involvement with tumor.

Resection of the upper humerus and part of the shoulder joint using a modified Tikhoff–Lindberg resection for osteogenic sarcoma can be performed in patients with osteogenic sarcoma of the proximal humerus. These patients have a functioning forearm and hand. The distal humerus is anchored to the chest wall or to the remaining remnants of the shoulder joint with a metallic rod to provide a stable fulcrum at the elbow.[342] These patients have superior functional results since there is no functioning prosthesis for a forequarter amputation. In addition, the use of padding or a plastic device under the shirt produces an almost perfect cosmetic result in such patients.

Finally, in patients with distal femur lesions too young to undergo femur and knee replacement for osteogenic sarcoma of the distal femur because of projected leg length discrepancy a surgical approach called a rotation plasty or turn-up operation is possible. This operation was originally described for displasias of the hip and consists of completely resecting the proximal femur and knee preserving a neurovascular bundle to the remaining lower extremity. The tibia and foot are rotated 180°. The tibia is attached to the femoral stump. This leaves the patient with a long stump with a 180° inversion of the ankle and foot at the end. The patient can be trained to use the ankle as a knee joint when fitted with a proper prosthesis. This type of surgery, done to date on three patients with sarcomas of the distal femur at Memorial Hospital, has resulted in good functional results with the patient ambulating as if he had his amputation at the level below the knee.

CHEMOTHERAPY FOR OSTEOGENIC SARCOMA. Osteogenic sarcoma was classically considered one of the diseases most resistant to chemotherapy. That accounts for the major excitement that took place in the early 1970's when reports of responses of metastatic osteogenic sarcoma to various single agents appeared in the literature. Early single agent chemotherapy in the treatment of evaluable osteogenic sarcoma was excellently reviewed by Friedman and Carter in 1972.[343] The results of single agent chemotherapy in evaluable osteogenic sarcoma is presented in Table 29-25.

Responses in metastatic osteogenic sarcoma to mitomycin-C were initially observed by Evans in the late 1960's.[344] However, a study of mitomycin-C in the treatment of evaluable osteogenic sarcoma that was subsequently undertaken failed to show an appreciable response rate to this agent in a larger group of patients.[345] Indeed, the toxicity encountered with mitomycin-C administration would not seem to justify its use as an adjuvant agent in the treatment of this disease since the response was only approximately 14%.

Other alkylating agents were evaluated in the treatment of osteogenic sarcoma; these included cyclophosphamide, given at various dose schedules, and phenylalanine mustard. Again, the response rates to these various alkylating agents were similar to that seen with mitomycin-C; all were in the vicinity of 15%[346–349]

Doxorubicin (adriamycin), an antitumor antibiotic with apparently more activity in solid tumors than its parent compound daunomycin, was first shown to be effective in the treatment of evaluable osteogenic sarcoma by Cortez and coworkers in the early 1970s. Response rates as high as 50% were reported by Cortez with the use of 90 mg/m^2 per treatment of doxorubicin. However, phase II studies collected in larger groups of patients eventually showed that the response rate to tolerable doses of adriamycin was more in the vicinity of 20% (see Table 29-25).[350–357] Nevertheless, the finding of a significant response rate of osteogenic sarcoma to any chemotherapeutic agent was extremely encouraging. It was at this point that Sutow pioneered the adjuvant treatment of osteogenic sarcoma by combining doxorubicin with (although minimally effective) alkylating agents to treat patients following amputation. Sutow used doxorubicin in combination with cyclophosphamide and phenylalanine mustard in this COMPADRI-I study and very early on was able to demonstrate an increase in the disease-free survival from roughly 15% at the M.D. Anderson Hospital with surgery alone to 55% following COMPADRI-I adjuvant chemotherapy (see Table 29-5).[358]

TABLE 29-25. Single Agent Chemotherapy in Evaluable Osteogenic Sarcoma

AGENT	NO. RESPONSES (COMPLETE + PARTIAL)/ NO. PTS. TREATED	(% RESPONSES)	REFERENCES
Cyclophosphamide	4/28	(14)	346–349
Phenylalanine mustard	5/32	(16)	348
DTIC	1/6	(17)	379
Mitomycin C	11/76	(14)	343–345
Adriamycin	39/183	(21)	350–357
High-dose methotrexate	13/31	(42)	360–364
High-dose methotrexate*	45/66	(68)	365, 366
Cis-platinum	12/48	(25)	367–375

* Previously untreated patients with evaluable primary tumors or pulmonary metastases.

The most excitement and controversy in the field of single agent chemotherapy for osteogenic sarcoma arose in 1972 with the description by Jaffe and Djerassi of objective responses to high-dose methotrexate with citrovorum factor rescue in patients with metastatic osteogenic sarcoma.[359] In over 30 patients treated at various centers with this agent alone the response rate was noted to be 42%.[360–364] Following the use of high-dose methotrexate to treat previously untreated patients with primary tumors prior to *en bloc* resection Rosen and coworkers observed a 68% response rate to high-dose methotrexate with citrovorum factor rescue in 66 patients treated with this modality.[365–366] It should be noted that the doses used in this study were slightly higher than that previously recommended. The initial dosage of high-dose methotrexate recommended by Jaffe was in the vicinity of 200–300 mg/kg. Rosen reported that younger patients treated at this dosage often did not respond to chemotherapy. Indeed, when the dose was escalated in this latter group of patients an increased incidence of responses were observed.[366a] Therefore, the 68% response rate in primary osteogenic sarcoma observed with high-dose methotrexate given as a single agent was achieved with doses of 12 g/m^2 for younger children and 8 g/m^2 for fully grown adolescents and adults. All patients in that study received between 12 and 20 g doses of high dose methotrexate with citrovorum factor rescue.

Toxic episodes following the use of high-dose methotrexate have been reported at doses as little as 5 g or as high as 20 g.[366b] The proper monitoring of blood levels of the drug in patients following massive dose methotrexate made this treatment safe in practically all patients undergoing high-dose methotrexate treatments at centers with experience in its administration and follow-up.[366c,d]

In 1978, Ochs and Friedman reported on the efficacy of *cis*-platinum in the treatment of evaluable osteogenic sarcoma. *Cis*-platinum was given in doses ranging from 90–120 mg/m^2 with mannitol diuresis.[367] In this dose form, the overall response rate of various investigators to *cis*-platinum has been in the range of 20–25%.[368–375] Although this response rate is not as great as that obtained with high-dose methotrexate with citrovorum factor rescue, it was a significant response rate, and indeed the majority of responses observed were clinically significant with almost as many complete responders as partial responders. Thus, by 1978 the armamentarium of single agents capable of causing a regression in evaluable metastatic osteogenic sarcoma was now considerable (see Table 29-3).[376]

COMBINATION CHEMOTHERAPY IN OSTEOGENIC SARCOMA. Combinations of single agents shown to be minimally or moderately effective in the treatment of evaluable osteogenic sarcoma yielded more consistent and higher response rates than single agents alone (see Table 29-25). The combination of mitomycin-C and phenylalanine mustard (two alkylating agents) yielded a response rate of 21% in 28 adequately treated patients; although higher than the response rate compared to single agent alkylating agents, this response rate is probably not significantly different than the response rate to phenylalanine mustard or mitomycin-C alone.[377, 378]

In a study conducted by Gottlieb and coworkers, the combination of doxorubicin and DTIC (± vincristine) showed consistently higher response rates in the majority of the spindle cell sarcomas than had been observed with doxorubicin alone as a single agent.[351] DTIC itself had been studied in only six osteogenic sarcoma patients by Gottlieb; as a single agent DTIC was noted to show a minimal response in one of those six patients.[379] However, in combination with doxorubicin, DTIC appeared to be synergistic, producing a response rate of 35% in 46 adequately treated patients with evaluable osteogenic sarcoma.

Further studies by Gottlieb and the Southwest Oncology Group with the combination CYVADIC (cyclophosphamide, vincristine, adriamycin, and DTIC) showed that the response rate of osteogenic sarcoma to this combination was not significantly different from the response rate of osteogenic sarcoma to the combination of doxorubicin and DTIC.[351] The response rate of metastatic osteogenic sarcoma to CYVADIC was shown to be 24% in 29 adequately treated patients. The most probable reason for no difference or even a slightly lower response rate to this combination was that the dose of doxorubicin used in the CYVADIC regimen had to be lowered to 50 mg/m^2 from 75 mg/m^2, which was used in the prior protocol where doxorubicin and DTIC were the only two drugs employed. Indeed, Cortez and Holland have shown a dose response correlation for the effects of doxorubicin on evaluable osteogenic sarcoma.[40]

In an early study conducted at the Memorial Hospital seven responses were seen in 13 patients with advanced osteogenic

TABLE 29-26. Combination Chemotherapy in Evaluable Osteogenic Sarcoma

AGENTS	NO. RESPONSES (COMPLETE + PARTIAL)/ NO. PTS. TREATED	(% RESPONSES)	REFERENCES
Mitomycin C + phenylalinine mustard + vincristine	6/28	(21)	377, 378
Adriamycin + DTIC + vincristine	16/46	(35)	351
CYVADIC*	7/29	(24)	351
HDMTX† + adriamycin	7/13	(54)	380
HDMTX + vincristine	4/10	(40)	359
HDMTX + vincristine (weekly)	20/27	(74)	360–365
HDMTX + adriamycin + cyclophosphamide	4/16	(25)	363
Bleomycin + cyclophosphamide + dactinomycin (BCD)	8/13	(62)	382
BCD‡	17/21	(77)	343, 383

* CYVADIC = Cyclophosphamide, vincristine, adriamycin, and DTIC
† HDMTX = High dose methotrexate with citrovorum factor rescue
‡ In 21 previously untreated patients with evaluable primary tumors or pulmonary metastases

sarcoma treated with the combination of high-dose methotrexate and citrovorum factor rescue, sequential therapy alternating every 2 weeks with doxorubicin.[380] This 54% response rate obtained was indeed encouraging, however the therapy was given quite frequently. Following 6 months of this sequential chemotherapy most patients received a total cumulative dose of doxorubicin of 540 mg/m^2, which led to the cessation of this combination sequential chemotherapy to prevent cardiomyopathy.

In the initial studies of high-dose methotrexate with citrovorum factor rescue carried out by Jaffe at the Sydney Farber Cancer Center, high-dose methotrexate was given in combination with vincristine. The vincristine was given approximately one hour prior to the 6-hour high-dose methotrexate infusion. The combination of vincristine and high-dose methotrexate with citrovorum factor rescue given every 2–3 weeks produced objective response in four of ten patients treated.[359] This 40% response rate is not significantly different than the response rates obtained with high-dose methotrexate and citrovorum factor rescue without vincristine.

Using vincristine with high-dose methotrexate and citrovorum factor rescue given weekly, Jaffe showed an increased response rate to patients with metastatic osteogenic sarcoma. More importantly, he showed that this modality of chemotherapy could be given safely at weekly intervals. Jaffe used six weekly high-dose methotrexate treatments given with citrovorum factor rescue with vincristine preceding the 6-hour high-dose methotrexate infusion.

Very young patients receiving high doses of methotrexate at weekly intervals may be at a high risk for developing leucoencephalopathy. This entity, a rare form of neurotoxicity, following high-dose methotrexate had been observed at Memorial Hospital in New York in patients receiving this modality of treatment for recurrent brain tumors following radiation therapy. The combined response rate observed by Jaffe and the Memorial Sloan-Kettering group to weekly high-dose methotrexate with or without vincristine was 74% in 27 adequately treated patients.[360–365]

A randomized trial of vincristine, given 24 hours following high-dose methotrexate infusion, was performed based on experimental animal data where Cello and coworkers showed that the effect of conventional and moderate dose methotrexate in solid tumors and leukemia of mice could be greatly enhanced by the administration of a vinca alkaloid 24 hours following the administration of methotrexate.[381] Nevertheless, at this dose schedule high-dose methotrexate proved to be equally effective with and without vincristine in patients with evaluable osteogenic sarcoma.

The sequential combination of high-dose methotrexate with citrovorum factor rescue, doxorubicin, and cyclophosphamide produced objective responses in four of 16 (25%) patients treated by Pratt and associates at the St. Jude's Hospital. The reason for the lower response rate in this small group of patients for this triple combination as compared to high-dose methotrexate and doxorubicin without cyclophosphamide may have been due to the fact that the cyclophosphamide-containing regimen did not use high dose methotrexate at the same high dose as the high-dose methotrexate and doxorubicin schedule previously reported (see Table 29-26).

In 1977, Rosen and coworkers reported on 8 of 13 patients (62%) responding to the combination of bleomycin, cyclophosphamide, and dactinomycin (BCD) in a group of patients resistant to treatment with cyclophosphamide alone given at the dose of 40–60 mg/kg.[382] The dose of cyclophosphamide in the BCD regimen was 600 mg/m^2 day for 2 days.

The BCD combination was subsequently used by Rosen and coworkers as the first drug treatment in a protocol for the treatment of primary osteogenic sarcoma that called for preoperative chemotherapy. Some 21 patients treated on this chemotherapy protocol (T-7) had easily evaluable primary tumors and an elevated serum alkaline phosphatase. Both of these parameters could be rapidly evaluated within 2 weeks of BCD administration prior to the administration of high-dose methotrexate with citrovorum factor rescue. Some 17 of those 21 patients (77%) experienced objective response in their primary tumor as judged by clinical measurement of evaluable soft tissue masses, lowering of the abnormally elevated serum alkaline phosphatase, and, in some patients, reduction in the size of pulmonary metastasis. However, because of the short interval of evaluation, this very encouraging further evaluation of the BCD combination had not been previously reported (see Table 29-26).[343,383]

ADJUVANT CHEMOTHERAPY FOR OSTEOGENIC SARCOMA. The first suggestion of the efficacy of adjuvant chemotherapy in osteogenic sarcoma was reported by Sutow where 10 of 18 patients were long-term disease-free survivors with the regimen of cyclophosphamide, vincristine (Oncovin), phenyalanine mustard, and doxorubicin (adriamycin) (CONPADRI-I) (see Table 29-27).[358] Subsequent use of CONPADRI-I chemotherapy in a larger group of patients yielded the same 2-year disease-free survival.[358] Subsequent COMPADRI protocols that called for the addition of high-dose methotrexate with citrovorum factor rescue failed to increase the disease-free survival over CONPADRI-I.

In 60 patients treated with COMPADRI-II, only 51% were disease-free at 2 years. Sutow has attributed this to the use of less doxorubicin in COMPADRI-II. Similarly, the COMPADRI-III regimen has yielded only a 42% disease-free survival at 2 years.[358] The reason for this lower disease-free survival in the COMPADRI-III regimen may be due to the fact that the effective agents in CONPADRI-I have been diluted by adding high-dose methotrexate with citrovorum factor rescue; indeed, the high-dose methotrexate with citrovorum factor rescue in the COMPADRI-III regimen used rather lower doses of high-dose methotrexate in the beginning of treatment. Thus, patients were started at the dose of 50 mg/kg, which was gradually escalated, although the dose of 250 mg/kg was eventually reached over several months. However, 250 mg/kg may still have been inadequate therapy for very young children receiving this treatment based on the Memorial Hospital experience in treating this patient age population.

Doxorubicin has been the most widely used single agent in the adjuvant chemotherapy of osteogenic sarcoma. In multiple studies using adjuvant doxorubicin alone, the 2-year disease-free survival is approximately 56% in over 130 patients with primary osteogenic sarcoma treated with this single agent chemotherapy.[384–387] The dose of adjuvant doxorubicin used in the treatment for osteogenic sarcoma by Cortez and coworkers was 30 mg/m²/day for 3 consecutive days. This dose is frequently intolerable in many patients and produces severe mucositis. In his study, Cortez eliminated patients who required dose reduction in their doxorubicin dosage if their white count did not go below 1,100 following the prior course of the drug. Many of those patients were considered protocol violators and were eliminated from the overall evaluable results. This may not be a fair evaluation of the drug since the absolute nadir in the total white count alone may not be the only criteria by which subsequent dose reductions should be made.

Nevertheless, the increase in the disease-free survival above 50% with the use of adjuvant doxorubicin alone appeared significant compared to historic controls and is as good as the majority of adjuvant chemotherapy protocols using multiple agents including doxorubicin.[388] This may be due to the

TABLE 29-27. Adjuvant Chemotherapy Regimens for Osteogenic Sarcoma

PROTOCOL	NO. PATIENTS	% DISEASE-FREE AT 2 YEARS	REFERENCES
Adriamycin	132	56	384–387
Vincristine + cyclophosphamide + dactinomycin	11	27	394
Vincristine + cyclophosphamide	14	21	395
Cyclophosphamide	6	50	396
CONPADRI I	44	55	358
COMPADRI II	60	51	358
COMPADRI III	44	42	358
CYVADIC	25	60	388
HDMTX + vincristine	12	42	389
HDMTX + vincristine ± BCG	39	38	390, 391
HDMTX + vincristine + adriamycin	59	62	361, 392
HDMTX + vincristine + adriamycin + cyclophosphamide	83	50	343, 393
HDMTX + adriamycin + bleomycin + cyclophosphamide + dactinomycin ± vincristine (T-7)	61	84	343
Cis-platinum + adriamycin	20	52	397, 398
T-7 ± cis-platinum (T-10)	57	93*	399

* 53/57 patients at 16 months (median)
CONPADRI I = Cyclophosphamide, phenylalinine mustard, adriamycin, and vincristine
COMPADRI II = CONPADRI I + HDMTX
COMPADRI III = CONPADRI I + HDMTX
CYVADIC = Cyclophosphamide, vincristine, adriamycin, and DTIC
HDMTX = High dose methotrexate with citrovorum factor rescue
BCG = Bacillus Calmette Guerin

lowering of the dose when other drugs are given in combination with it, such as in the CYVADIC protocol.[388]

However, the ability to obtain a disease-free survival of 60% in 25 patients treated with the CYVADIC protocol is probably a significant advance over a similar disease-free survival rate for doxorubicin alone, since the lower dose used in the combination chemotherapy protocol (CYVADIC) may lead to a lower incidence of doxorubicin cardiomyopathy in patients so treated.[388] Data confirming this speculation have not yet been published.

In the mid-1970's, there was a proliferation of adjuvant chemotherapy regimens for osteogenic sarcoma. Most of them contained high-dose methotrexate with citrovorum factor rescue and doxorubicin. Some contained cyclophosphamide. Again, the overall disease-free survival rates were approximately 50%. Many of these chemotherapy protocols did not use high-dose methotrexate at what some investigators felt was an effective dose (see Table 29-27).[343,361,389–396]

In 1975 Rosen initiated a protocol using high-dose methotrexate at the dose of 12 g/m^2 for young children and 8 g/m^2 for older (fully grown) adolescents and adults. This dose schedule was derived from observations on previously treated patients who had failed to respond to a lower dose of high-dose methotrexate, and required escalations in the dose of methotrexate to achieve a clinically significant response in evaluable disease. This included both patients undergoing preoperative chemotherapy (whose primary tumor was being evaluated) and patients with evaluable pulmonary and bone metastasis who had failed to respond to lower doses of high-dose methotrexate. The use of high-dose methotrexate and the use of the BCD combination, which was substituted for cyclophosphamide, and the use of doxorubicin at the dose of 75–90 mg/m^2 per course, yielded an 84% disease-free survival in 61 patients treated with the T-7 chemotherapy protocol.[343] All patients had been followed for from 2 years to 56 months (median 36 months). Again, the significantly better results with this chemotherapy protocol have been attributed to the use of 12 g total dose of high-dose methotrexate in the younger patients and the use of the BCD combination in the T-7 protocol.[343]

In 1979, Ettinger reported on the use of adjuvant high-dose *cis*-platinum with mannitol diuresis and doxorubicin sequential chemotherapy in a small group of patients following amputation. His initial results were extremely encouraging, with approximately 90% of 13 patients remaining disease-free.[397] Further follow-up on this group revealed that only 52% of the 20 patients treated with the *cis*-platinum–doxorubicin adjuvant chemotherapy protocol have remained disease-free over 2 years. However, as noted above, *cis*-platinum can produce a clinically significant response in patients with evaluable disease who are resistant to high-dose methotrexate with citrovorum factor rescue, cyclophosphamide, and doxorubicin.

Rosen has reported on a modification of the T-7 chemotherapy protocol in which high-dose methotrexate is given as a single agent prior to primary tumor resection. Patients then receive BCD, high-dose methotrexate, and doxorubicin for 12 weeks postoperatively (see Fig. 29-22). At that time patients are selected to continue to receive the same chemotherapy as maintenance chemotherapy or *cis*-platinum in combination with doxorubicin, alternating with BCD without high-dose methotrexate (T-10 protocol regimen A) (see Fig. 29-22). The selection of maintenance chemotherapy in these patients is based solely on the patient's degree of responsiveness to preoperative chemotherapy with high-dose methotrexate and citrovorum factor rescue as judged from careful histologic examination of the resected primary tumor following preoperative chemotherapy. To date, over 90% of 57 patients are disease-free survivors from 8–26 months (median 16 months) with this individualized approach to maintenance chemotherapy based on the response to preoperative chemotherapy with high-dose methotrexate.[399]

Some disagreement exists concerning the role of adjuvant chemotherapy in osteogenic sarcoma. Rosen, based on his successful experience with the T-7 and T-10 regimen, and many others feel that adjuvant chemotherapy should be an essential part of the management of all patients with osteogenic sarcoma. Others disagree, however, and have embarked on prospective randomized trials to test this question.

Chondrosarcoma

Chondrosarcoma is a malignant tumor containing fully developed cartilage without tumor osteoid being formed by the sarcomatous stroma. Chondrosarcoma is second to osteogenic sarcoma in frequency as a malignant primary tumor of bone. It accounts for approximately 20% of all primary bone tumors.[312] Chondrosarcoma can occur as a malignant tumor of bone, or as a secondary tumor with chondrosarcomatous degeneration of benign bone conditions, such as enchondroma or an osteocartilagenous exostosis. Chondrosarcomas have also been described as occurring more frequently in multiple enchondromatosis (Ollier's disease) and they have also been described in association with Paget's disease.[400,401]

PRESENTING SYMPTOMS. Pain is usually the most common presenting symptom. However, chondrosarcomas of the peripheral skeleton can manifest as relatively painless swellings giving rise to only minor discomfort. Chondrosarcoma is most frequent in the 4th, 5th, and 6th decade; however, it has occurred in younger patients, particularly adolescents and children. When it occurs in this age group it tends to be more malignant.

The most frequent location of chondrosarcoma is the pelvis. In a Memorial Hospital series of 264 cases of chondrosarcoma, 82 (31%) occurred in the pelvis. Some 56 (21%) occurred in the femur with proximal lesions outnumbering those of the distal lesions. The ribs accounted for 9% of the lesions; the cranial facial bones accounted for approximately 9%; the proximal humerus and shoulder girdle accounted for 13%; other skeletal sites were less frequent, but chondrosarcomas have been noted to occur in almost all bones including those of the foot and the hand.[312]

On x-ray examination, the majority of chondrosarcomas show central lucent destructive lesions with blotchy calcifications present throughout the lesion both within the central area of the bone and in the soft tissue. Very frequently calcification in the soft tissue has a flecky appearance to it, and does not have the characteristic sunburst appearance of an osteogenic sarcoma. Flecks of calcification appearing

Induction Chemotherapy for Osteogenic Sarcoma

(T - 10)

HDMTX - 8-12 gm/M² (delete after 12 or 16 doses)

LEUCOVORIN - 10–15 mg po q6h x 10 doses start 20 hours post HDMTX

BCD - Bleomycin 15 mg/M²/day
Cyclophosphamide 600 mg/M²/day
Dactinomycin 600 mcg/M²/day

ADRIAMYCIN (ADR) 30 mg/M²/day

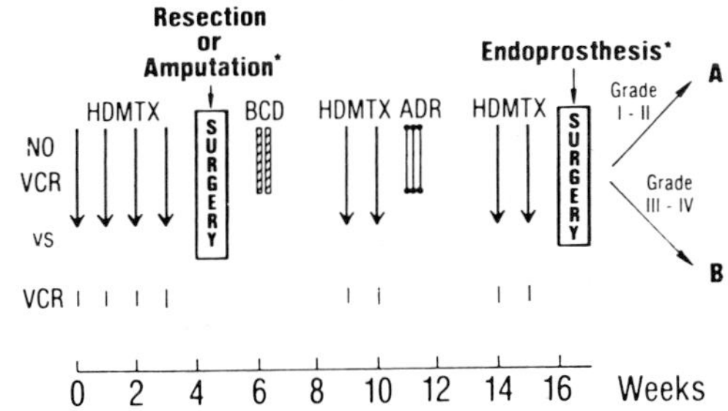

*Patients who are to undergo resection or amputation will have surgery at approximately four weeks; patients who are to undergo endoprosthetic replacement will have surgery at approximately 16 weeks.

A

Maintenance Chemotherapy for Osteogenic Sarcoma

Histologic Response of Primary Tumor

GRADE I - II (T - 10A)

ADR 30 mg/M²/day
CDDP 120 mg/M² or 3 mg/kg

GRADE III - IV (T - 10B)

Bleomycin 15 mg/M²/day
Cyclophosphamide 600 mg/M²/day
Dactinomycin 600 mcg/M²/day

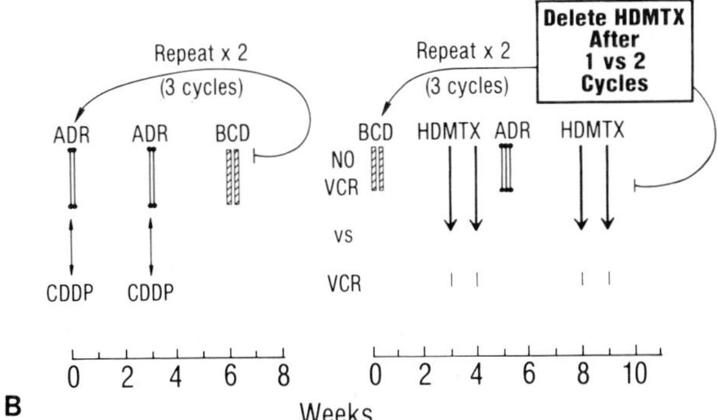

B

FIG. 29-22. *A*, Current chemotherapy protocol used at Memorial Sloan–Kettering Hospital for the treatment of patients with osteogenic sarcoma. All patients received pre-operative high-dose methotrexate with citrovorum factor rescue. Patients undergoing endoprosthetic replacement of the femur at the knee received more pre-operative chemotherapy than did patients with nonfemur lesions. All lesions were evaluated following four high-dose methotrexate treatments given at weekly intervals. The clinical response of femur lesions was evaluated through the use of repeated roentgenograms and bone scans, as well as clinical measurements. Regardless of the amount of pre-operative chemotherapy, all resected lesions were then graded for the histologic effect of pre-operative chemotherapy in the primary tumor. Post-operative chemotherapy depended on the histologic grade of response of the primary tumor to pre-operative chemotherapy. All patients received the 16 weeks of chemotherapy regardless of histologic response. Following the 16 weeks of induction chemotherapy, maintenance chemotherapy was then continued for an additional 30 weeks. *B*, Maintenance chemotherapy. Patients having only a small histologic response to pre-operative induction chemotherapy received a regimen of high-dose *Cis*-platinum combined with adriamycin and BCD. Patients having a better histologic response to pre-operative chemotherapy continued to receive high-dose methotrexate with citrovorum factor rescue, in addition to adriamycin and BCD chemotherapy.

within the soft tissue, particularly in proximal femur lesions, should always make one consider chondrosarcoma.[402]

The prognosis for a patient with a chondrosarcoma is almost directly dependent on two factors. The first is the histologic grade of the chondrosarcoma. Low-grade chondrosarcomas tend to be locally invasive and do not metastasize, however very high-grade chondrosarcomas have a high frequency of metastasizing, particularly to the lungs. In addition, the site of the chondrosarcoma is also of considerable importance since operability may depend on a peripheral location. Many larger pelvic and sacral tumors become inoperable; what may be a low-grade chondrosarcoma in that area can recur or continue to grow with the eventual appearance of metastasis following histologic evolution to a high-grade sarcoma.[403] In a series of a 113 patients with chondrosarcoma, treated by Marcove and coworkers, the average 10-year survival for patients with chondrosarcoma of all types was 40%.[403] There are various histologic subtypes of chondrosarcomas that carry different prognoses.[404]

The mesenchymal chondrosarcoma should not be considered a classic chondrosarcoma since it tends to be a cartilage-producing tumor; however, the stroma of the tumor is usually a small-cell malignant tumor, frequently sensitive to radiation therapy and chemotherapy and behaves in a similar fashion to a Ewing's sarcoma.[405] However, among the true chondrosarcomas there are various subclassifications. Some of the more recently described have been the clear cell type of chondrosarcoma, which is usually of a high grade, tends to recur locally, and metastasizes leading to a poor prognosis.[406]

TREATMENT. Since the majority of chondrosarcomas are of low to medium grade, the primary treatment for chondrosarcoma is that of a low grade spindle cell sarcoma (*i.e.*, radical local therapy is indicated). Usually, systemic chemotherapy is of little value. The recommended treatment for chondrosarcoma is total removal of the entire tumor mass with adequate bone and soft tissue margins.[403,407] This is often quite readily accomplished in peripheral lesions, but becomes more difficult as one approaches the pelvic lesion. An alternative to radical *en bloc* excision of the tumor has been cryosurgery. This has been pioneered by Dr. Ralph Marcove, and the initial results are encouraging in terms of the lack of local recurrence for patients with low-grade chondrosarcomas.[407,408] Other surgical techniques include the Tikhoff–Lindberg resection for chondrosarcomas of the shoulder girdle and *en bloc* excision with bone allografting for distal femur lesions.[409,410]

It is interesting to note that while the 5-year survival for patients above the age of 21 with chondrosarcoma is approximately 50%, this 5-year survival drops to approximately 35% in children below the age of 21. Chondrosarcomas in this age group tend to be of higher grade histology and metastasize

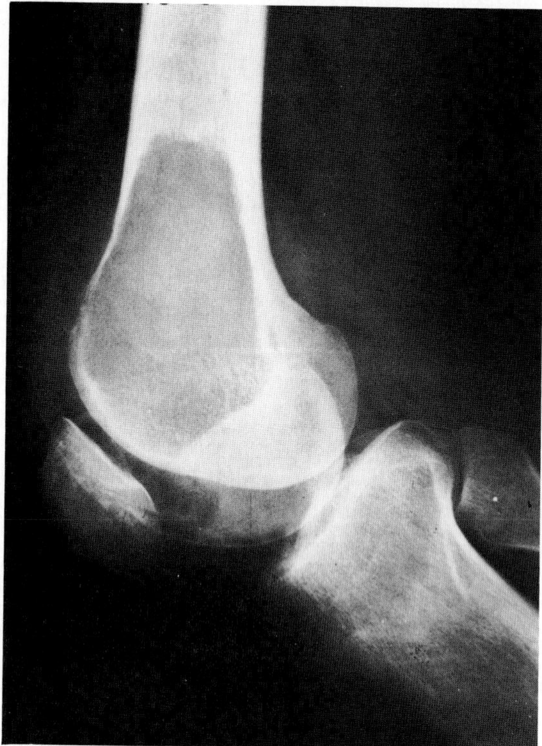

FIG. 29-23. Giant cell tumor arising in the femoral epiphysis.

more frequently. In addition, many lesions classified as chondrosarcomas in the younger age group may indeed be chondroblastic osteogenic sarcomas. The majority of true chondrosarcomas in patients below the age of 21 tend to occur in the ribs and pelvis more frequently then in the long bones.[403]

The role of radiation therapy is quite limited. In mesenchymal chondrosarcoma, radiation therapy and chemotherapy may play a significant role in the treatment of this lesion. However, in the classic chondrosarcoma, which is a spindle cell sarcoma, radiation therapy and chemotherapy are of little proven value. The use of radioactive sulfur (^{35} S) has been tried in the treatment of inoperable malignant chondrosarcomas. Sulfur 35 is incorporated into the chondrocytes and inhibits tumor growth by delivering large doses of radiation over a prolonged period to the tumor cells. This method of treatment has been abandoned, although four patients evidently had meaningful responses to this modality of treatment. Apparently two of the patients developed leukemia that was attributable to the treatment.[411]

Giant Cell Tumor of Bone

Giant cell tumor of bone is a malignant tumor made up of a stroma of plump spindly or ovoid cells, in addition to numerous multinucleated giant cells dispersed throughout the tumor tissue.

This tumor usually presents with pain, swelling, and tenderness at the local site. The most common site of giant cell tumors is in and about the knee with about 50% of all giant cell tumors arising in that area (see Fig. 29-23). Approximately ½ of the lesions occur in the distal femur and ½ of those lesions in the proximal tibia. Other common sites of giant cell tumors include the proximal humerus, the proximal femur, and the sacrum and other pelvic areas.[312]

A giant cell tumor is typically an epiphyseal lesion and presents as a lytic, fairly well-defined lesion arising from the epiphysis. Usually the lesion appears to be well circumscribed and is purely lytic. Sometimes there can be compartmentalization of the lesion by trabeculations that can be noted on the roentgenogram. Metaphyseal giant cell tumors have been reported in the young age group, but when dealing with a metaphyseal lesion, suspicion should arise that a different type of tumor can exist that has a predominant giant cell component to it, such as fibroblastic osteogenic sarcoma or malignant fibrous histiocytoma.[412–414]

Giant cell tumor of bone occurs predominantly in the third and fourth decades of life. It occurs not uncommonly in the second decade of life, but is extremely rare below the age of 10. A great deal of descriptive literature exists about the differential diagnosis of giant cell lesions of bone. Some of the lesions that can mimic a giant cell tumor include non-ossifying fibroma, an aneurysmal bone cyst (which may frequently be accompanied by areas of giant cell tumor), brown tumor of hyperparathyroidism, or a reparative granuloma. (An excellent discussion of the description and differential diagnosis of giant cell tumors can be found in Jaffe's original book on bone tumors.)[317] Giant cell tumors tend to recur locally and metastasize in very rare instances.

The most common form of giant cell tumor is of low-grade histology. Frequently mixed in with this low-grade histology will be areas of what the pathologist may refer to as focally malignant areas. Both of the above lesions, however, should be treated as low-grade tumors with little propensity to metastasize, needing only good local control. Occasionally, however, even low-grade giant cell tumors have been noted to metastasize and the histologic diagnosis of pulmonary nodules that sometimes occur as isolated solitary nodules, is frequently benign giant cell tumor.[415,416] Rarely is a fully malignant giant cell tumor encountered. This lesion, that many pathologists refer to as a grade III malignant giant cell tumor, has a full propensity to metastasize and following surgical local control probably should be treated with chemotherapy. Some of these latter lesions have the appearance of fully malignant spindle cell sarcomas of bone and in many areas the giant cell component is lacking. However, there is also a lack of osteoid formation or other evidence for an osteogenic sarcoma and the tumor may be merely referred to as a fully malignant giant cell tumor. It is estimated that less than 10% of all giant cell tumors are fully malignant at initial diagnosis. However, as many as 20% of giant cell tumors have become malignant after they have recurred locally. In addition, there are many reports of giant cell tumors becoming fully malignant after application of radiation therapy to obtain local control. Whether the giant cell tumor becomes fully malignant when left *in situ* as part of its natural history or whether radiation therapy is truly a oncogenic agent, the occurrence of fully malignant giant cell tumors that metastasize following radiation therapy is an indication that radiation therapy either causes malignant transformation or, in many of these instances, is just not adequate therapy to eradicate a giant cell tumor. The latter would be expected since this is a spindle cell sarcoma that usually does not respond very meaningfully to radiation therapy. Nevertheless, radiation therapy has been used successfully to control inoperable giant cell tumors in patients who might not otherwise have survived long enough to develop "malignant transformation."[417,418]

TREATMENT. The treatment for most giant cell tumors is good surgical control. This usually means *en bloc* excision of the entire tumor. Even with *en bloc* excision there is a considerable local recurrence rate of approximately 30%. With curretage alone the local recurrence rate is in excess of 60%.[413,419,420]

At Memorial Hospital, Marcove and associates have done curettage and cryosurgery through a wide incision in the bone. Marcove's technique includes making a large enough hole in the bone to be able to flush the entire tumor cavity with large amounts of liquid nitrogen. The use of cryosurgery as a supplement to curettage in Marcove's series has reduced the incidence of local recurrence to around 10–15% in approximately 50 consecutive cases of giant cell tumors treated in this way. Follow-up rebiopsy of many of these lesions has failed to reveal any recurrent giant cell tumor. This method of treatment is encouraging and requires continued follow-up to confirm its efficacy.[421]

When encountering the rare fully malignant giant cell tumor of bone, it is recommended that the surgical procedure be more radical and treatment be carried out in a similar way to that of a fully malignant spindle cell sarcoma such as osteogenic sarcoma, including the use of adjuvant chemotherapy. In a limited experience treating giant cell tumor, four patients with inoperable sacral and pelvic giant cell tumors were treated with high-dose methotrexate with citrovorum factor rescue. Although anectodal, two of these four patients had objective evidence of tumor response following treatment.

MALIGNANT FIBROUS TUMORS OF BONE

These spindle cell sarcomas of bone (fibrosarcoma, malignant fibrous histiocytoma, hemangiopericytoma) are more predominant in the 3rd, 4th, and 5th decades of life as opposed to the osteogenic sarcoma, which is more predominant in the younger age group. However, these tumors present in a similar fashion to osteogenic sarcoma with a similar distribution. Most lesions are in the distal femur, followed by the proximal tibia and proximal humerus. The pelvis can be involved more frequently than is seen in osteogenic sarcoma. Tumors of the jaw are not uncommon. These spindle cell sarcomas tend to occur as low-grade fibrosarcomas of bone in a juxtacortical position, such as that of the low-grade juxtacortical osteogenic sarcoma. Very frequently, medullary fibrosarcomas and malignant fibrous histiocytomas of bone, as well as hemangiopericytomas, occur in the mid-shaft and throughout the diaphyseal region and are not as strictly confined to the metaphyseal area as is the classic osteogenic sarcoma.[312,422,423]

In examining a large series of primary fibrosarcoma of bone treated at the Memorial Hospital with surgery alone, Huvos showed that the periosteal variety (which is frequently of a lower histologic grade then the medullary variety of fibrosarcoma) had a better prognosis. Indeed, the 10-year survival of periosteal fibrosarcomas of bone was approximately 50% while it was only about 25% for the medullary lesions.[422]

The treatment of the fibrous tumors of bone is similar to that for other spindle cell sarcomas of bone (*i.e.*, low-grade lesions require adequate local surgical control and high-grade lesions require the latter plus the addition of systemic chemotherapy to prevent distant metastases). These lesions tend to be radio-resistant and if adequate surgical control is not obtained at definitive surgery, local recurrence will almost definitely take place. The management of the malignant fibrous tumors of bone should be similar to that for osteogenic sarcoma.

MALIGNANT SMALL CELL SARCOMAS OF BONE

Malignant small-cell sarcomas of bone make up less than 20% of all malignant bone tumors.[2] The majority of malignant bone tumors are the spindle cell sarcomas.

The characteristics of a malignant small-cell sarcoma of bone are that the stromal component of the tumor is usually made up of undifferentiated small round cells. These tumors differ from the spindle cell sarcomas of bone in that they are usually radio-responsive and more responsive to conventional agent chemotherapy.

Even though they are radio-responsive, some of these small-cell sarcomas (*e.g.*, Ewing's sarcomas) require large doses of radiation therapy for local control. As many as 20% of these tumors will recur following adequate radiation therapy.[424,425] Therefore, whenever feasible, it is desirable to treat these tumors with surgical resection or surgical resection combined with radiation therapy. Many of these tumors can occur in the axial skeleton in which case radiation therapy alone must be relied on for local control.

Most of the small-cell sarcomas are very undifferentiated tumors that have a high propensity to metastasize in the majority of patients even with adequate local control. Therefore, all patients with malignant small-cell sarcomas should be treated with chemotherapy in an effort to prevent distant metastasis to both other bones and lung.[323] The small cell sarcomas make up a heterogenous group of undifferentiated sarcomas occurring in bone that accounts for less than 20% of all primary malignant bone tumors.

Ewing's Sarcoma

Ewing's sarcoma is the most common primary small cell sarcoma of bone accounting for approximately 10% of all primary malignant bone tumors in the population. The treatment of Ewing's sarcoma is fully discussed in Chapter 34.

Non-Hodgkin's Lymphoma of Bone

Non-Hodgkin's lymphoma of bone (or reticulum cell sarcoma of bone) accounts for approximately 5% of primary bone tumors. Although this was once reported as a disease with a favorable prognosis when treated with local therapy alone, reported cases contained patients with "solitary" non-Hodgkin's lymphoma of bone, and the criteria used for a "solitary" non-Hodgkin's of bone was that no evidence of metastatic disease occurred within 6 months of diagnosis and surgical treatment. Thus, patients reported by Shoji and Miller were highly selected; even in that group the cure rate was only about 50% with local treatment.[426,427]

Most non-Hodgkin's lymphomas of bone are not permanently controlled with local therapy since this disease tends to disseminate to other bone and bone marrow.[323,428,429] Primarily in the pediatric population rapid dissemination of disease occurs after local therapy alone. The treatment of non-Hodgkin's lymphoma is discussed extensively in Chapter 35. Primary non-Hodgkin's lymphoma of bone should be treated in the same way as primary non-Hodgkin's of nodal or other extranodal areas.[428-432]

In addition to systemic therapy advocated for non-Hodgkin's lymphoma of bone, the local lesional area is treated with radiation therapy. In the Memorial Hospital experience (of the skeletal distribution of 116 cases on non-Hodgkin's lymphoma of bone), the majority of patients had lesions in the femur that counted for 25% of all lesions and approximately 20% of lesions occurred in the pelvis.[312]

Angiosarcoma

Angiosarcoma of bone is a rare primary bone lesion, accounting for probably less than 0.5% of primary malignant bone tumors.[2] This is not to be confused with the more differentiated hemangioendothelioma, which can be a multi-focal disease in various bones throughout the skeleton or present with multiple lesions within the same bone. This latter tumor has a somewhat more favorable prognosis than angiosarcoma of bone and is frequently cured by surgical resection.[433-435]

However, the angiosarcoma of bone is a rare undifferentiated small-cell sarcoma that tends to metastasize in most patients. Since this is a small-cell undifferentiated tumor, the current treatment approach to the rare patient presenting with this disease is similar to that for patients with Ewing's sarcoma of bone.

Mesenchymal Chondrosarcoma

Mesenchymal chondrosarcoma deserves special consideration, since this lesion is not a typical chondrosarcoma. The mesenchymal chondrosarcoma consists of very undifferentiated cells similar in appearance to those of a Ewing's sarcoma. This entity has been recently described and its exact incidence is not yet known. In addition to areas of malignant small-cell sarcoma, areas of mature cartilage or cartilage that looks like low-grade chondrosarcoma can be seen within the same tumor.

In four patients treated with this entity the tumor has been both radio-responsive and responsive to conventional chemotherapeutic agents used in combination, similar to that used for Ewing's sarcoma. Therefore, in patients presenting with mesenchymal chondrosarcoma, combination chemotherapy and radiation therapy should be used to treat these tumors.

Most mesenchymal chondrosarcomas have occurred in the axial skeleton, such as the pelvis, ribs, or skull (in the periorbital area). However, the occasional mesenchymal chondrosarcoma that occurs in the extremities may be treated surgically or with the combination of surgery and radiation for local control. For some reason there is a propensity for these tumors to occur not only as primary bone tumors, but as primary soft tissue tumors, particularly in and about the meninges. In the latter situation, radiation therapy is the treatment of choice for local therapy.

RADIATION THERAPY FOR SARCOMA OF BONE. The principal indications for definitive radiation therapy in the treatment of patients with bone tumor is limited almost exclusively to the use of radiation therapy in the management of patients with Ewing's sarcoma, primary lymphoma of bone (reticulum cell sarcoma), and solitary myeloma. Management of these tumors is discussed in Chapters 34, 35, and 38. The preferred approach for patients with primary mesenchymal tumors of bone (*e.g.,* osteosarcoma, chondrosarcoma, fibrosarcoma, malignant fibrous histiocytoma, chordoma) should be primary surgery where this is technically and medically feasible. There are, however, patients who present with the mesenchymal tumors at sites where radical surgery is not feasible because of technical or medical reasons. There is one exception to the general rule and this pertains to osteosarcoma of the mandible. There is substantial evidence that warrants recommendation for preoperative radiation therapy prior to radical resection of mandibular or maxillary osteosarcoma. Chambers and coworkers describe results in 33 patients treated by high-dose radiation therapy (either interstitial technique or external beam) followed almost immediately by resection. They obtained 80% survival at 3 years. This is very much higher than has been obtained in other centers by surgery alone. This may be explained by the fact that the surgical margins are very close in dealing with osteosarcoma of the mandible or maxilla. The high-dose levels administered are effective in eradication of the microscopic extension of disease beyond the obvious margin. At other less accessible sites there probably would be similar improvement in local control with radiation therapy and surgery combined.

Sarcomas of the cervical spine and skull are relatively uncommon. They represent about 3–10% of the total incidence of primary sarcoma of bone in humans. The most common varieties of sarcoma of bone in this region are osteosarcoma, chondrosarcoma, or chordoma. Osteosarcomas in the head are limited primarily to the mandible or maxilla and the few osteosarcomas arising in the skull, especially the calverium, are associated with a pre-existing Paget's disease.[437] This means that sarcomas arising in the cervical spine and base of skull are predominantly chordomas and chondrosarcomas. This group of tumors is usually not amenable to surgical resection. In these instances, high-dose ultraprecise radiation therapy may offer the patient a chance for cure. At the Massachusetts General Hospital, 10 patients have been treated for chordomas and chondrosarcomas in this region using complex treatment arrangements combining photons with 160 MV proton beams. The reliance on radiation therapy in these lesions was necessary because sarcomas at these sites are usually non-resectable. Radiation therapy by conventional techniques cannot be administered because high radiation doses are required for permanent control of these tumors and they are in immediate contact or adjacent to sensitive structures of the CNS. Ten patients have been treated with tumor doses in the region of 6300–7800 rad (or its equivalent) with follow-ups from 3 months to 6.5 years. Local control has been achieved to date in all of the 10 patients. Fortunately, no instance of neurologic sequelae from the treatment has been observed. This is a special instance of radiation therapy for bone sarcoma but does emphasize the fact that long-term local control may be achieved in the treatment of these bony tumors where the radiation dose can be quite high. Effective treatments are then almost invariably limited to the treatment of small tumors. In the authors' experience, treatment of chondrosarcoma, fibrosarcoma, malignant fibrous histiocytoma, or osteosarcoma in bone located at usual sites where the tumors are large at presentation is not successful. An occasional patient achieves long-term control, but radiation treatment of large inoperable tumors of the sacrum or sacrum-ilium where hemipelvectomy is not feasible are rarely successful. A reasonable approach to patients with large benign tumors requires a combination of radiation therapy and surgery, if definitive primary surgery cannot be performed.

Radiation therapy may occasionally be required in the treatment of a patient with giant cell tumor because the lesion is located in a site where resection is not feasible or the patient is inoperable for medical reasons. In these instances, doses in the range of 6500–7000 rad should be administered if possible.

REFERENCES

1. Patten BM: Human Embryology. New York, McGraw-Hill, 1968
2. Cancer Patient Survival. Report No. 5, U.S. Department of Health, Education, and Welfare, Publication No. (NIH) 77–992, 1976
3. Li FP, Fraumeni JF Jr: Soft-tissue sarcomas, breast cancer, and other neoplasms. A familial syndrome? Ann Intern Med 71:747–752, 1969
4. Howard GM, Casten VG: Rhabdomyosarcoma of the orbit in brothers. Arch Ophthal 70:319, 1963
5. Li FP, Fraumeni JF Jr: Rhabdomyosarcoma in children: Epidemiologic study and identification of a familial cancer syndrome. J NCI 43:1365–1373, 1969
6. Li FP, Tucker MA, Fraumeni JF Jr: Childhood cancer in sibs. J Pediatr 88:419–423, 1976
7. Miller RW: Deaths from childhood leukemia and solid tumors among twins and other sibs in the United States, 1960–1967. J NCI 46:203, 1971
8. Chabalko JJ, Creagon ET, Fraumeni JF Jr: Epidemiology of selected sarcomas in children. J NCI 53:675, 1974
9. Remzi D, Kendi S: Rhabdomyosarcoma of the prostate in childhood. Turk J Pediatr 8:143–149, 1966
10. Bottomley RH, Condit PT: Cancer families. Cancer Bull 20:22–24, 1968
11. Fraumeni JF Jr, Vogel CL, Easton JM: Sarcomas and multiple polyposis in a kindred. A genetic variety of hereditary polyposis? Arch Intern Med 121:57–61, 1968
12. Enterline HT, Culberson JD, Rochlin DB et al: Liposarcoma. A clinical and pathological study of 53 cases. Cancer 13:932–950, 1960
13. Stewart FW, Treves N: Lymphangiosarcoma in postmastectomy lymphedema: a report of six cases in elephantiasis chirurgica. Cancer 1:64–81, 1948
14. Sloane JA, Hubbell MM: Soft tissue sarcomas in children associated with congenital anomalies. Cancer 23:175–182, 1969
15. Schjweisguth O, Gerard–Marchant R, Lemerle J: Naevomatose baso-cellulaire association a un rhabdomyosarcome congenital. Arch Fr Pediatr 25:1083–1093, 1968
16. Heard G: Malignant disease in von Recklinghausen's neurofibromatosis. Proc Roy Soc Med 56:502–503, 1963
17. Reed WB, Nickel WR, Campion G: Internal manifestations of tuberous sclerosis. Arch Derm 87:715–728, 1963
18. Epstein CJ, Martin GM, Schultz AL et al: Werner's syndrome. A review of its symptomatology, natural history, pathologic features, genetics and relationship to the natural aging process. Medicine (Baltimore) 45:177–221, 1966
19. Hardell L, Sandstrom A: Case-control study: Soft-tissue sarcomas and exposure to phenoxyacetic acids or chlorophenols. Br J Cancer 39:711, 1979
20. Kim K, Tidrick RT, Skeel RT et al: Fibrosarcoma of the chest wall following mastectomy and radiation therapy for mammary carcinoma. Breast, Diseases of the Breast 6:26–30, 1980
21. Arlen M, Higinbotham NL, Huvos AG et al: Radiation induced sarcoma of bone. Cancer 28:1087–1099, 1971
22. Martland HS, Humphries RE: Osteogenic sarcoma in dial painters using luminous paint. Arch Pathol 7:406–417, 1929
23. Brand KG: Foreign body induced sarcomas. In Becker FF (ed): Cancer pp 485–511. New York, Plenum Press, 1975
24. Ott G: Fremd korpersarkome. Exp Med Pathol Klin 32:1, 1970
25. deCholnky T: Augmentation mammaplasty: Survey of complications in 10,941 patients by 265 surgeons. Plast Reconstr Surg 45:573, 1970
26. Rubin LR, Bromberg BE, Walden RH: Long-term human reaction to synthetic plastics. Surg Gynecol Obstet 132:603, 1971
27. Shieber W, Graham P: An experience with sarcomas of the soft tissues in adults. Surgery 52:295, 1962
28. Russell WO, Cohen J, Enzinger FM et al: A clinical and pathological staging system for soft tissue sarcomas. Cancer 40:1562–1570, 1977
29. Lindberg RD, Martin RG, Romsdahl MM: Surgery and postoperative radiotherapy in the treatment of soft tissue sarcomas in adults. Am J Roentgenol Rad Therap Nucl Med 123:123–129, 1975
30. Rosenberg SA, Kent H, Costa J et al: Prospective randomized evaluation of the role of limb-sparing surgery, radiation therapy, and adjuvant chemoimmunotherapy in the treatment of adult soft-tissue sarcomas. Surgery 84:62–69, 1978
31. Hajdu SI: Pathology of Soft Tissue Tumors. Philadelphia, Lea & Febiger, 1979
32. Mirr JM: The Soft Tissues. In Coulson WF (ed): Surgical Pathology. Philadelphia, JB Lippincott, 1978
33. Enzinger FM: Recent developments in the classification of soft tissue sarcomas. In Management of Primary Bone and Soft Tissue Tumors. Chicago, Year Book Medical Publishers, 1977
34. Stout AP, Lattes R: Tumors of the soft tissue. In Atlas of Tumor Pathology, 2nd series. Washington, DC, Armed Forces Institute of Pathology, 1967
35. Enzinger FM: Histological typing of soft tissue tumours. Geneva, World Health Organization, 1969
36. Hare HF, Cerny MF: Soft tissue sarcoma: A review of 200 cases. Cancer 16:1332, 1963
37. Pack GI, Ariel IM: Treatment of Cancer and Allied Diseases. In Tumors of the Soft Somatic Tissues and Bone, vol VIII. New York, Harper and Row, 1964
38. Martin RG, Butler JJ, Albores–Saavedra J: Soft tissue tumors: Surgical treatment and results. In Tumors of Bone and Soft Tissue. Chicago, Year Book Medical Publishers, 1965
39. Ferrell HW, Frable WJ: Soft part sarcomas revisited. Review and comparison of a second series. Cancer 30:475–480, 1972
40. Shiu MH, Castro EB, Hajdu SI et al: Surgical treatment of 297 soft tissue sarcomas of the lower extremity. Ann Surg 182:597, 1975
41. Simon MA, Enneking WF: The management of soft-tissue sarcomas of the extremities. J Bone Joint Surg 58-A:317, 1976
42. Lindberg RD, Martin RG, Romsdahl MM et al: Conservation surgery and radiation therapy for soft tissue sarcomas. In Management of Primary Bone and Soft Tissue Tumors. Chicago, Year Book Medical Publishers, 1977
43. Jarvi OH, Saxen E: Elastofibroma dorsi. Acta Pathol Microbiol Scand (suppl), 144:83–84, 1961

44. Jarvi OH, Lansimies PH: Subclinical elastofibromas in the scapular region in an autopsy series. Acta Pathol Microbiol Scand (A) 83:87–108, 1975
45. Jarvi OH, Saxen AE, Hopsu–Havu VK et al: Elastofibroma; a degenerative pseudotumor. Cancer 23:42–63, 1969
46. Stemmermann GN, Stout AP: Elastofibroma dorsi. Am J Clin Pathol 37:490–506, 1962
47. Conway H: Dupuytren's contracture. Am J Surg 87:10, 1954
48. Luck JV: Dupuytren's contracture. J Bone Joint Surg 41A:635, 1959
49. Skoog T: Dupuytren's contracture: pathogenesis and surgical treatment. Surg Clin North Am 47:433–444, 1967
50. Allen RA, Woolner LB, Ghormley RK: Soft-tissue tumors of the sole: with special reference to plantar fibromatosis. J Bone Joint Surg (Am) 37:14–26, 1955
51. Allen PM, Enzinger FM: Juvenile aponeurotic fibroma. Cancer 26:857–867, 1970
52. Goldman RL: The cartilage analogue of fibromatosis (aponeurotic fibroma): further observations based on 7 new cases. Cancer 26:1325–1331, 1970
53. Keasbey LE: Juvenile aponeurotic fibroma (calcifying fibroma). Cancer 6:338–346, 1953
54. Bartlett RC, Otis RD, Haakso AO: Multiple congenital neoplasms of soft tissues. Report of 4 cases in 1 family. Cancer 14:913–920, 1961
55. Beatty EC: Congenital generalized fibromatosis of infancy. Am J Dis Child 103:620, 1962
56. Teng P, Warden MJ, Cohn WL: Congenital generalized fibromatosis (renal and skeletal) with complete spontaneous regression. J Pediatr 62:748–753, 1963
57. Enzinger FM: Fibrous hamartoma of infancy. Cancer 18:241–251, 1965
58. Chandler A: Muscular torticollis. J Bone Joint Surg 30A:566, 1948
59. Brown JB, McDowell F: Wry-neck facial distortion prevented by resection of fibrosed sternomastoid muscle in infancy and childhood. Ann Surg 131:721–733, 1950
60. Smith BH: Peyronie's disease. Am J Clin Pathol 45:670, 1966
61. Allen PW: Nodular fasciitis. Pathology 4:9–26, 1972
62. MacKenzie DH: The Differential Diagnosis of Fibroblastic Disorders, pp 21, 106. Oxford, Blackwell Scientific Publications, 1970
63. Soule EH: Proliferative (nodular) fasciitis. Arch Pathol 73:437, 1962
64. Hutter RVP, Stewart FW, Foote FW Jr: Fasciitis: a report of 70 cases with follow-up proving the benignity of the lesion. Cancer 15:992–1003, 1962
65. MacKenzie DH: The Differential Diagnosis of Fibroblastic Disorders. Oxford, Blackwell Scientific Publications, 1970
66. Das Gupta TK, Brasfield RD, O'Hara J: Extra-abdominal desmoids. Ann Surg 170:109, 1969
67. Enzinger FM, Shiraki M: Musculoaponeurotic fibromatosis of the shoulder girdle. Cancer 20:113, 1967
68. Brasfield RD, Das Gupta TK: Desmoid tumors of the anterior abdominal wall. Surgery 65:241, 1969
69. Ewing J: Neoplastic Disease. Philadelphia, WB Saunders, 1928
70. Musgrove JE, McDonald JR: Extra-abdominal desmoid tumors: A differential diagnosis and treatment. Arch Pathol 45:513–540, 1948
71. Benninghoff D, Robbins R: The nature and treatment of desmoid tumors. Am J Roentgenol Rad Therap Nucl Med 91:132–137, 1964
72. Wara WM, Phillips TL, Hill DR et al: Desmoid tumors—treatment and prognosis. Radiology 124:225–226, 1977
73. Suit HD, Russell WO: Radiation therapy of soft tissue sarcomas. Cancer 36:759–764, 1975
74. Czernobilsky B, Cornog JL, Enterline HT: Rhabdomyoma: report of case with ultrastructural and histochemical studies. Am J Clin Pathol 49:782–789, 1968
75. Morgan JJ, Enterline HT: Benign rhabdomyoma of the pharynx: a case report, review of the literature, and comparison with cardiac rhabdomyoma. Am J Clin Pathol 42:174–181, 1964
76. Lendrum AC: Painful tumours of the skin. Ann R Coll Surg Engl 1:62–67, 1947
77. Stout AP: Solitary cutaneous and subcutaneous leiomyoma. Am J Cancer 29:435–469, 1937
78. Enzinger FM, Harvey DA: Spindle cell lipoma. Cancer 36:1852–1859, 1975
79. Lin JJ, Lin F: Two entities in angiolipoma. A study of 459 cases of lipoma with review of infiltrating angiolipoma. Cancer 34:720–727, 1974
80. Chung EB, Enzinger FM: Benign lipoblastomatosis. An analysis of 35 cases. Cancer 32:482–491, 1973
81. Chung EB, Enzinger FM: Benign lipoblastomatosis. An analysis of 35 cases. Cancer 32:482–491, 1973
82. Evans HL, Soule EH, Winkelmann RK: Atypical lipoma, atypical intramuscular lipoma, and well differentiated retroperitoneal liposarcoma. A reappraisal of 30 cases formerly classified as well differentiated liposarcoma. Cancer 43:574–584, 1979
83. Dionne GP, Seemayer TA: Infiltrating lipomas and angiolipomas revisited. Cancer 33:732–738, 1974
84. Enzinger FM: Benign lipomatous tumors simulating a sarcoma. In Martin RG, Ayala AG (eds): Management of Primary Bone and Soft Tissue Tumors, pp 11–24. Chicago, Year Book Medical Publishers, 1977
85. Kindblom LG, Angervall L, Stener B et al: Intermuscular and intramuscular lipomas and hibernomas: a clinical, roentgenologic, histologic, and prognostic study of 46 cases. Cancer 33:754–762, 1974
86. Mesara BW, Batsakis JC: Hibernoma of the neck. Arch Otolaryngol 85:95, 1967
87. Jones FE, Soule EH, Coventry MB: Fibrous xanthoma of synovium (giant cell tumor of tender sheath, pigmented nodular synovitis). J Bone Joint Surg 51A:76, 1969
88. Gehwheiler JA, Wilson VW: Diffuse biarticular pigmented villonodular synovitis. Radiology 93:137, 1969
89. Langstadt JR, Javert CT: Sarcoma and myomectomy. Cancer 8:1142, 1955
90. Slooff JL, Kernohan JW, MacCarty CS: Primary intramedullary tumors of the spinal cord and filrim terminale. Philadelphia, WB Sanders, 1964
91. D'Agostino A: Sarcomas of the peripheral nerves and somatic soft tissues associated with multiple neurofibromatosis. Cancer 16:1015, 1963
92. Buck BE: Congenital neurogenous sarcoma with rhabdomyosarcomatous differentiation. J Pediatr Surg 12:581–582, 1977
93. Hammond JA: Detection of malignant change in neurofibromatosis by gallium-67 scanning. Can Med Assoc J 119:352–353, 1978
94. Herman J: Sarcomatous transformation in multiple neurofibromatosis. Ann Surg 131:206, 1950
95. Hunt K: Neurofibrosarcoma complicating Von Recklinghausens disease. J Ky Med Assoc 74:346–349, 1976
96. Lee C: Malignant degeneration of thoracic neurofibromata. NY State J Med 75:347–352, 1972
97. Wander JW, Das Gupta TK: Neurofibromatosis. Curr Probl Surg 14:1–81, 1977
98. Allen PW, Enzinger FM: Hemangioma of skeletal muscle: an analysis of 89 cases. Cancer 29:8–22, 1972
99. Lister WA: The natural history of strawberry nevi. Lancet 1:1429–1434, 1938
100. Modlin JJ: Capillary hemangiomas of the skin. Surgery 38:169–180, 1955
101. Carrol R, Berman A: Glomus tumors of the hand. J Bone Joint Surg 54A:691–703, 1972
102. Carroll RE, Berman AT: Glomus tumors of the hand: review of the literature and report of 28 cases. J Bone Joint Surg 54:691–703, 1972
103. Shugart RR, Soule EH, Johnson EW: Glomus tumor. Surg Gynecol Obstet 117:334–340, 1963
104. Stout AP: Tumors featuring pericytes: glomus tumor and hemangiopericytoma. Lab Invest 5:217–223, 1965
105. Enzinger FM, Smith BH: Hemangiopericytoma. An analysis of 106 cases. Human Path 7:61–82, 1976

106. Soule EH, Enriquez P: Atypical fibrous histiocytoma, malignant fibrous histiocytoma, malignant histiocytoma, and epithelioid sarcoma. A comparative study of 65 tumors. Cancer 30:128, 1972
107. Kempson RL, McGavran MH: Atypical fibroxanthomas of the skin. Cancer 17:1463–1471, 1964
108. Kauffman SL, Stout AP: Histiocytic tumors (fibrous xanthoma and histiocytoma) in children. Cancer 14:469–482, 1961
109. O'Brien JE, Stout AP: Malignant fibrous xanthomas. Cancer 17:1445–1458, 1964
110. Brenner W, Schaefler K, Habrans C et al: Dermatofibrosarcoma protuberans metastatic to a regional lymph node. Report of a case and review. Cancer 36:1897–1902, 1975
111. Burkhardt BR, Soule EH, Winkelman RK et al: Dermatofibrosarcoma protuberans: study of 56 cases. Am J Surg 111:638–644, 1966
112. Taylor HB, Helwig EB: Dermatofibrosarcoma protuberans: a study of 115 cases. Cancer 15:717–725, 1962
113. McPeak CJ, Druz T, Nicastri AD: Dermatofibrosarcoma protuberans; an analysis of 86 cases—five with metastasis. Ann Surg 166:803, 1967
114. Strong EW, McDivitt RW, Brasfield RD: Granular cell myoblastoma. Cancer 25:415–422, 1970
115. Le Ber MS, Stout AP: Benign mesenchymomas in children. Cancer 15:598–605, 1962
116. Stout AP: Myxoma, the tumor of primitive mesenchyme. Ann Surg 127:706–719, 1948
117. Enzinger FM: Intramuscular myxoma. Am J Clin Pathol 43:104, 1965
118. Hajdu SI, Hajdu EO: Cytopathology of sarcomas and other nonepithelial malignant tumors. Philadelphia, WB Saunders, 1976
119. Martel W, Abell MR: Radiologic evaluation of soft tissue tumors. A retrospective study. Cancer 32:352–366, 1973
120. Berger PE, Kuhn JP: Computed tomography of tumors of the musculoskeletal system in children. Clinical applications. Radiology 127:171–175, 1978
121. Levin DC, Watson RC, Baltaxe HA: Arteriography in diagnosis and management of acquired peripheral soft-tissue masses. Radiology 103:53–58, 1972
122. Hudson TM, Haas G, Enneking WF et al: Angiography in the management of musculoskeletal tumors. Surg Gynecol Obstet 141:11–21, 1975.
123. de Santos LA, Wallace S, Finklestein JB: Angiography and lymphangiography in peripheral soft tissue sarcomas. In Management of Primary Bone and Soft Tissue Tumors. Chicago, Year Book Medical Publishers, 1977
124. Weingrad DW, Rosenberg SA: Early lymphatic spread of osteogenic and soft-tissue sarcomas. Surgery 84:231–240, 1978
125. Suit HD, Russell WO, Martin RG: Sarcoma of soft tissue: Clinical and histopathologic parameters and response to treatment. Cancer 35:1478–1483, 1975
126. Cantin J, McNeer GP, Chu FC et al: The problem of local recurrence after treatment of soft tissue sarcoma. Ann Surg 168:47–53, 1968
127. Enzinger FM, Winslow DJ: Liposarcoma—A study of 103 cases. Virchows Arch Path Anat 335:337, 1962
128. Stout AP: Sarcoma of the soft parts. J Missouri State Med Assoc 44:329, 1947
129. Pack GT, Ariel I: End results in the treatment of sarcomas of the soft somatic tissues. In Pack GT, Ariel IM: Tumors of the Soft Somatic Tissues. A Clinical Treatise, pp. 779–796. New York, Paul B Hoeber, 1958
130. Clark RL Jr, Martin RG, White EC et al: Clinical aspects of soft tissue tumors. Arch Surg 74:859, 1957
131. Martin RG, Butler JJ, Albores–Saavedra J: Soft tissue tumors: Surgical Treatment and Results. In Tumors of Bone and Soft Tissue. A Collection of Papers Presented at the Eighth Annual Clinical Conference on Cancer, 1963. Year Book Medical Publishers, 1965
132. Kremitz ET, Shaver JO: Behavior and treatment of soft tissue sarcomas. Ann Surg 157:770, 1963
133. Taylor GW, Nathanson IT: Fibrosarcoma. In Lymph Node Metastases: Incidence and Surgical Treatment in Neoplastic Diseases. New York Oxford University Press, 1942
134. Heller EL, Sieber WK: Fibrosarcoma—A clinical and pathological study of sixty cases. Surgery 27:539, 1950
135. Phelan JT, Nigogosyan G: Fibrosarcoma of superficial soft tissue origin. Arch Surg 86:118, 1963
136. Seel DJ, Booher RJ, Joel RV: Fibrous tumors of musculoaponeurotic origin. Surgery 56:497, 1964
137. Van Der Werf–Messing B, Van Unnik JAM: Fibrosarcoma of the soft tissues. A clinicopathologic study. Cancer 18:1113, 1965
138. Pack GT, Pierson JC: Liposarcoma. Surgery 36:687, 1954
139. Enterline HT, Culbertson JD, Rochlin DB et al: Liposarcoma: A clinical and pathological study of 53 cases. Cancer 13:932, 1960
140. Pack GT, Eberhart WF: Rhabdomyosarcoma of skeletal muscle. Surgery 32:1023, 1952
141. Pack GT, Ariel IM: Tumors of Soft Somatic Tissues. New York, Paul B Hoeber, 1958
142. Cadman NL, Soule EH, Kelley PJ: Synovial sarcoma. An analysis of 134 tumors. Cancer 18:613, 1965
143. Mackenzie DH: Synovial sarcoma. A review of 58 cases. Cancer 19:169, 1966
144. Vieta JO, Pack GT: Malignant neurilemomas of peripheral nerves. Am J Surg 82:416, 1951
145. D'Agostino AN, Soule EH, Miller RH: Primary malignant neoplasms of nerves (malignant neurilemomas) in patients without manifestations of multiple neurofibromatosis (Van Recklinghausen's disease). Cancer 16:1003, 1963
146. Kinne DW, Chu FCH, Huvos AG et al: Treatment of primary and recurrent retroperitoneal liposarcoma. Twenty-five year experience at Memorial Hospital. Cancer 31:53–64, 1973
147. Gerner RE, Moore GE, Pickren JW: Soft tissue sarcomas. Ann Surg 181:803–808, 1975
148. Gercovich FG, Luna MA, Gottlieb JA: Increased incidence of cerebral metastases in sarcoma patients with prolonged survival from chemotherapy. Report of cases of leiomysarcoma and chondrosarcoma. Cancer 36:1843–1851, 1975
149. Pritchard DJ, Soule EH, Taylor WF et al: Fibrosarcoma. A clinicopathologic and statistical study of 199 tumors of the soft tissues of the extremities and trunk. Cancer 33:888–897, 1974
150. Stout AP: Fibrosarcoma: The malignant tumor of fibroblasts. Cancer 1:30–63, 1948
151. Pritchard DJ, Soule EH, Taylor WF et al: Fibrosarcoma: Clinicopathological and statistical study of 199 tumors of soft tissues of extremities and trunk. Cancer 33:880, 1974
152. Castro EB, Hajdu SI, Fortner JG: Surgical therapy of fibrosarcoma of extremities. Arch Surg 107:284, 1973
153. Soule EH, Geitz M, Henderson EH: Embryonal rhabdomyosarcoma of the limbs and limb girdles. A clinico-pathologic study of 61 cases. Cancer 23:1338–1346, 1969
154. Maurer HM, Moon T, Donaldson M et al: The intergroup rhabdomyosarcoma study. Cancer 40:2015, 1977
155. Ariel IM, Briceno M: Rhabdomyosarcoma of the extremities and trunk: Analysis of 150 patients treated by surgical resection. J Surg Oncol 7:269–287, 1975
156. Linscheid RL, Soule EH, Henderson ED: Pleomorphic rhabdomyosarcoma of the extremities and limb girdles: A clinicopathologic study. J Bone Joint Surg 47A:715–725, 1965.
157. Albores–Saavedra J, Martin RG, Smith JL: Rhabdomyosarcoma: A study of 35 cases. Ann Surg 157:186–197, 1963
158. Stout AP, Hill WT: Leiomyosarcoma of the superficial soft tissues. Cancer 11:844–854, 1958
159. Abwasi OE, Dozois RR, Wieland LH et al: Leiomyosarcoma of the small and large bowel. Cancer 42:1375, 1978
160. Kevorkian J, Cento DP: Leiomyosarcoma of large arteries and veins. Surgery 73:390, 1973
161. Enterline HT, Culberson JD, Rochlin DB et al: Liposarcoma. A clinicopathologic study of 53 cases. Cancer 11:932–950, 1960
162. Spittle MF, Newton KA, Mackenzie DH: Liposarcoma. A review of 60 cases. Br. J Cancer 24:696, 1971

163. Kindblom L, Angervall L, Svendsen P: Liposarcoma. A clinicopathologic, radiographic and prognostic study. Acta Pathologica et Microbiologica Scandinavica, 1975
164. Ackerman LV: Multiple primary liposarcomas. Am J Pathol 20:789–793, 1944
165. Enzinger FM, Winslow DJ: Liposarcoma. A study of 30 cases. Virchows Arch Path Anat 335:367–388, 1962
166. Reszel PA, Soule EH, Coventry MB: Liposarcoma of the extremities and limb gridles. A study of 222 cases. J Bone Joint Surg 48A:229, 1966
167. Cadman NL, Soule EH, Kelly PJ: Synovial sarcoma: An analysis of 134 cases. Cancer 18:613–627, 1965
168. Gerner RE, Moore GE: Synovial sarcoma. Ann Surg 181:22–25, 1975
169. Hajdu SI, Shiu MH, Fortner JG: Tendosynovial sarcoma. A clinicopathological study of 136 cases. Cancer 39:1201–1217, 1977
170. Crocker DW, Stout AP: Synovial sarcoma in children. Cancer 12:1123–1133, 1959
171. Mobergen G, Nilsonne U, Friberg S: Synovial sarcoma. Acta Orthop Scand (suppl) 11:3, 1968
172. Storm FK, Eilber FR, Mirra J et al: Neurofibrosarcoma. Cancer 45:126–129, 1980
173. Girard C, Johnson WC, Graham JH: Cutaneous angiosarcoma. Cancer 26:868–883, 1970
174. Gulesserian HP, Lawton RL: Angiosarcoma of the breast. Cancer 24:1021–1026, 1969
175. Dunegan LJ, Tobon H, Watson CG: Angiosarcoma of the breast: A report of two cases and a review of the literature. Surgery 79:57–59, 1976
176. Woodward AH, Ivins JC, Soule EH: Lymphangiosarcoma arising in chronic lymphedematous extremities. Cancer 30:562–572, 1972
177. Rosai J, Sumner HW, Kostianovsky M et al: Angiosarcoma of the skin. A clinicopathologic and fine structural study. Hum Pathol 7:83, 1976
178. Mira JG, Chu FCH, Fortner JG: The role of radiotherapy in the management of malignant hemangiopericytoma. Report of eleven new cases and review of the literature. Cancer 39:1254–1259, 1977
179. Stout AP: Hemangiopericytoma (a study of 25 new cases). Cancer 2:1027–1954, 1949
180. O'Brien PH, Brasfield RD: Hemangiopericytoma. Cancer 14:249–252, 1965
181. O'Brien PH, Brasfield RD: Kaposi's sarcoma. Cancer 19:1497, 1966
182. Taylor JF, Templeton AC, Vogel CL et al: Kaposi's sarcoma in Uganda: a clinicopathological study. Int J Cancer 8:122–135, 1971
183. O'Brien JE, Stout AP: Malignant fibrous xanthomas. Cancer 17:1445–1458, 1964
184. Wasserman TH, Stuart ID: Malignant fibrous histiocytoma with widespread metastases. Autopsy study. Cancer 33:141–146, 1974
185. Kearney MM, Soule EH, Ivins JC: Malignant fibrous histiocytoma. A retrospective study of 167 cases. Cancer 45:167–178, 1980
186. Weiss SW, Enzinger FM: Malignant fibrous histiocytoma. An analysis of 200 cases. Cancer 41:2250–2266, 1978
187. Leite C, Goodwin JW, Sinkovics JG et al: Chemotherapy of malignant fibrous histiocytoma: A Southwest Oncology Group report. Cancer 40:2010–2014, 1977
188. Christopherson WM, Foote FW, Stewart FW: Alevolar soft part sarcomas: structurally characteristic tumors of uncertain histogenesis. Cancer 5:100, 1952
189. Lieberman PH, Foote FW, Stewart FW et al: Aleolvar soft-part sarcoma. JAMA 198:1047–1051, 1966
190. Unni KK, Soule EH: Alveolar soft part sarcoma. An electron microscopic study. Mayo Clin Proc 50:592–598, 1975
191. Bryan RS, Soule EH, Dobyns JH et al: Primary epithelioid sarcoma of the hand and forearm. A review of thirteen cases. J Bone Joint Surg 56A:458–465, 1974
192. Peimer AC, Smith RJ, Sirota RL et al: Epithelioid sarcoma of the hand and wrist: Patterns of extension. J Hand Surg 2:275–282, 1977
193. Prat J, Woodruff JM, Marcove RC: Epithelioid sarcoma. An analysis of 22 cases indicating the prognostic significance of vascular invasion and regional lymph node metastasis. Cancer 41:1472–1487, 1978
194. Enzinger FM: Epithelioid sarcoma. A sarcoma simulating a granuloma or a carcinoma. Cancer 26:1029–1041, 1970
195. Miller TR: 100 cases of hemipelvectomy. A personal experience. Surg Clin North Am. 54:905–913, 1974
196. Douglass HO Jr, Razack M, Holyoke ED: Hemipelvectomy. Arch Surg 110:82–85, 1975
197. Papaioannou AN, Critselis AN, Volk H: Long-term survival after compound hemipelvectomy. Surg Gynecol Obstet 144:175–178, 1977
198. Shiu MH, Flanebaum L, Hajdu SI et al: Malignant soft-tissue tumors of the anterior abdominal wall. Arch Surg 115:152–155, 1980
199. Binder SC, Katz B, Sheridan B: Retroperitoneal liposarcoma. Ann Surg 187:257–261, 1978
200. Kinne DW, Chu FCH, Huvos AG et al: Treatment of primary and recurrent retroperitoneal liposarcoma. Cancer 31:53, 1973
201. Braasch JW, Mon AB: Primary retroperitoneal tumors. Surg Clin North Am 47:663, 1967
202. Delamater J: Mammoth tumor. Cleveland Medical Gazette 1:31, 1859
203. Atkinson L, Garran JM, Newton MC: Behavior and management of soft tissue connective sarcomas. Cancer 16:1552, 1963
204. DeWeerd JH, Dockerty MB: Lipomatous retroperitoneal tumors. Am J Surg 84:397, 1952
205. Enterline HT, Culberson JD, Rochlin DB et al: Liposarcoma. A clinical pathological study of 53 cases. Cancer 13:932, 1960
206. Gilbert HA, Kagan AR, Winkley J: Soft tissue sarcomas of the extremities: Their natural history, treatment, and radiation sensitivity. J Surg Oncol 7:303–317, 1975
207. Hintz BL, Charyulu, KN, Miller WE et al: Adjuvant role of radiation in soft tissue sarcoma in adults. J Surg Oncol 9:329–338, 1977
208. Leucutia T: Radiotherapy of sarcoma of the soft parts. Radiology 25:403–415, 1935
209. Cade S: Soft tissue tumours: Their natural history and treatment. Section of surgery. President's Address. Proc Roy Soc Med 44:19–36, 1951
210. Fortner JG, Kim DK, Shiu MH: Limb-preserving vascular surgery for malignant tumors of the lower extremity. Arch Surg 112:391–394, 1977
211. Imparato AM, Roses DF, Francis KC et al: Major vascular reconstruction for limb salvage in patients with soft tissue and skeletal sarcomas of the extremities. Surg Gynecol Obstet 147:891–896, 1978
212. Morton DL, Eilber FR, Townsend CM Jr et al: Limb salvage from a multidisciplinary treatment approach for skeletal and soft tissue sarcomas of the extremity. Ann Surg 184:268–278, 1976
213. Atkinson L, Garvan JM, Newton NC: Behavior and management of soft connective tissue sarcomas. Cancer 16:1552–1562, 1963
214. Lindberg RD, Murphy WK, Benjamin RS et al: Adjuvant chemotherapy in the treatment of soft tissue sarcomas: A preliminary study. In M. D. Anderson Hospital and Tumor Institute (ed): Management of Primary Bone and Soft Tissue Tumors. Chicago, Year Book Medical Publishers, 1977
215. Jacobs EM: Combination chemotherapy of metastatic testicular germinal cell tumors and soft part sarcomas. Cancer 25:324–332, 1970
216. O'Bryan RM, Luce JK, Talley RW et al: Phase II evaluation of adriamycin in human neoplasia. Cancer 32:1–8, 1973
217. Blum RH: An overview of studies with adriamycin (NSC-123127) in the United States. Cancer Chemother Rep 6:247–251, 1975
218. Creagan ET, Hahn RG, Ahmann DL et al: A clinical trial adriamycin (NSC 123127) in advanced sarcomas. Oncology 34:90–91, 1977
219. Cruz AB Jr, Thames EA Jr, Aust JB et al: Combination

chemotherapy for soft tissue sarcomas: A phase III study. J Surg Oncol 11:313–323, 1979
220. Rosenbaum C, Schoenfeld D: Treatment of advanced soft tissue sarcoma. ASCO Abstr C-81, 1977
221. O'Bryan RM, Baker LH, Gottlieb JE et al: Dose response evaluation of adriamycin in human neoplasia. Cancer 39:1940–1948, 1977
222. Gottlieb JA, Benjamin RS, Baker LH et al: Role of DTIC in the chemotherapy of sarcomas. Cancer Treat Rep 60:199–203, 1976
223. Golbey R, Li MC, Kaufman RF: Actinomycin in the treatment of soft part sarcomas. James Ewing Society Scientific Program (abstr), 1968
224. Central Oncology Group: Unpublished data
225. Bergsagel DE, Levin WC: A prelusive clinical trial of cyclophosphamide. Cancer Chemother Rep 8:120–134, 1960
226. Korst DR, Johnson D, Frenkel EP et al: Preliminary evaluation of the effect of cyclophosphamide on the course of human neoplasms. Cancer Chemother Rep 7:1–12, 1960
227. Gold G, Hall T, Shnider B et al: A clinical study of 5-fluorouracil. Cancer Research 19:935–939, 1959
228. Subramanian S, Wiltshaw E: Chemotherapy of sarcoma—A comparison of three regimens. Lancet 683–686, 1978
229. Andrews N, Wilson W: Phase II study of methotrexate (NSC 740) in solid tumors. Cancer Chemother Rep 51:471–474, 1967
230. Karakousis CP, Holtermann OA, Holyoke ED: *Cis*-dichlorodiammineplatinum (II) in metastatic soft tissue sarcomas. Cancer Treat Rep 63:2071–2075, 1979
231. Samson MK, Baker LH, Benjamin RS et al: *Cis*-dichlorodiammineplatinum (II) in advanced soft tissue and bony sarcomas. A Southwest Oncology Group Study. Cancer Treat Rep 63:2027–2028, 1979
232. Bramwell VHC, Brugarolas A, Mouridsen HT et al: EORTC. Phase II study of cisplatinum in CYVADIC-resistant soft tissue sarcoma. Eur J Cancer 15:1511–1513, 1979
233. Selawry OS, Holland JF, Wolman IJ: Effect of vincristine (NSC-67574) on malignant solid tumors in children. Cancer Chemother Rep 52:497–499, 1968
234. Korbitz BC, Davis HL Jr, Ramirez G et al: Low doses of vincristine (NSC-67574) for malignant disease. Cancer Chemother Rep 53:249–254, 1969
235. Yap BS: Unpublished data
236. Legha SS, Gutterman JU, Hall SW et al: Phase I clinical investigation of 4′-(9-acridinylamino)methanesulfon-m-anisidide (NSC 249992), a new acridine derivative. Cancer Res 38:3712–3716, 1978
237. Von Hoff DD, Howser D, Gormley P et al: Phase I study of methanesulfonamide, N-[4-9-acridinylamino)-3-methoxyphenyl]-(m-AMSA) using a single-dose schedule. Cancer Treat Rep 62:1421–1426, 1978
238. DeJager R, Bodey JJ, Dupont D et al: Phase I study of Oral 4′-(9-acridinylamino)-methanesulfon-m-anisidide (NSC-249992). Proc Am Assoc Cancer Res 20:429, 1979
239. Schneider R, Sklanoff R, Ochoa M: Phase I trial of AMSA (4′-[acrindylamino]-methanesulfon-m-anisidide). Proc Am Assoc Cancer Res 20:114, 1979
240. Chang P, Wiernik PH: Phase II study of azotomycin in sarcomas. Cancer Treat Rep 61:1719, 1977
241. Weiss AJ, Ramirez G, Grage T et al: Phase II study of azotomycin (NSC-56654). Cancer Chemother Rep 52:611–614, 1968
242. Sooriyaarachchi GS, Ramirez G, Roley EL et al: Hemangiopericytoma of the uterus. J Surg Oncol 10:399–406, 1978
243. Benjamin RS: Unpublished data
244. Rodriquez V, Gottlieb J, Burgess MA et al: Phase I studies with Baker's antifol (BAF) (NSC 139105). Cancer 38:690–694, 1976
245. Thigpen JT, O'Bryan RM, Benjamin RS et al: Phase II trial of Baker's antifol in metastatic sarcoma. Cancer Treat Rep 61:1485–1487, 1977
246. Perevodchikova NI, Lichinitser MR, Gorbunova VA: Phase I clinical study of carminomycin: Its activity against soft tissue sarcomas. Cancer Treat Rep 61:1705–1707, 1977
247. Kovach JS, Moertel CG, Schutt AJ: A phase I study of chlorozotocin (NSC 178248). Cancer 43:2189–2196, 1979
248. Gralla RJ, Tan CTC, Young CW: Phase I trial of chlorozotocin. Cancer Treat Rep 63:17–20, 1979
249. Talley RW, Samson MK, Brownlee RW et al: Phase II evaluation of chlorozotocin in advanced human cancers. Eur J Cancer 17:337–343, 1981
250. Johnson R: Preliminary phase II trials with 1-aminocyclopentance carboxylic acid (NSC-1026). Cancer Chemother Rep 32, 1963
251. Aust J, Andrews N, Schroeder J et al: Phase II study of 1-aminocyclopentanecarboxylic acid (NSC 1026) in patients with cancer. Cancer Chemother Rep 54:4, 1970
252. Eastern Cooperative Oncology Group (ECOG): Unpublished data
253. Central Oncology Group (COG): Unpublished data
254. Baker LH, Samson MK, Izbicki RM: Phase I and II evaluation of cytembena in disseminated epithelial ovarian cancer and sarcomas. Cancer Treat Rep 60:1389–1391, 1976
255. Matejovsky Z: Effects of cytembena in the treatment of malignant musculoskeletal tumors. Neoplasma 18:473–480, 1971
256. Alberto P, DeJager RL, Brugarolas A et al: Phase II study of diamino-dichlorophenyl-methylpyrimidine with folinic acid protection and rescue. Proc Am Assoc Cancer Res 20:323, 1979
257. Eastern Cooperative Oncology Group: Unpublished data
258. Kimball JC, Cangir A: Phase II trial of dianhydrogalactitol in advanced soft tissue and bony sarcomas. A Southwest Oncology Group Study. Cancer Treat Rep 63:553–554, 1979
259. Samson MK, Baker L: Personal communication
260. Bedikian AY, Valdivieso M, Bodey GP et al: Phase I clinical studies with gallium nitrate. Cancer Treat Rep 62:1449–1453, 1978
261. Borden EC, Larson P, Ansfield FJ et al: Hexamethylmelamine treatment of sarcomas and lymphomas. Med Pediatr Oncol 3:401–406, 1977
262. Blum RH, Livingston RB, Carter SK: Hexamethylmelamine. A new drug with activity in solid tumors. Eur J Cancer 9:195–202, 1973
263. Eastern Cooperative Oncology Group: Unpublished data
264. Eagan RT, Ingle JN, Rubin J et al: Early clinical study of an intermittent schedule for maytansine (NSC-153858): Brief Communication. NCI 60:93–96, 1978
265. Blum RH, Kahlert T: Maytansine: A Phase I study of an ansa macrolide with antitumor activity. Cancer Treat Rep 62:435–438, 1978
266. Eastern Cooperative Oncology Group: Unpublished data
267. Von Hoff DD, Rozencweig M, Louie AC et al: "Single"-agent activity of high-dose methotrexate with citrovorum factor rescue. Cancer Treat Rep 62:233–235, 1978
268. Isacoff WH, Eilber F, Tabbarah H et al: Phase II clinical trial with high-dose methotrexate therapy and citrovorum factor rescue. Cancer Treat Rep 62:1295–1304, 1978
269. Vaughn C, Baker L: Personal communication
270. Ambinder EP, Perloff M, Ohnuma T et al: High-dose methotrexate followed by citrovorum factor reversal in patients with advanced cancer. Cancer 43:1177–1182, 1979
271. Creagan ET, Hahn RG, Ahmann DL et al: A comparative clinical trial evaluating the combination of adriamycin, DTIC, and vincristine, the combination of actinomycin D, cyclophosphamide, and vincristine, and a single agent, methyl-CCNU, in advanced sarcomas. Cancer Treat Rep 60:1385–1386, 1976
272. Tranum BP, Haut A, Rivkin SE et al: A phase II study of methyl CCNU in the treatment of solid tumors and lymphomas in the Southwest Oncology Group. Cancer 35:1148–1153, 1974
273. Benjamin RS, Keating MJ, Valdivieso M et al: Phase I–II study of piperazinedione in adults with solid tumors and acute leukemia. Cancer Treat Rep 63:939–943, 1979
274. La Gasse L, Thigpen T, Morrison F: Phase II trial of piperazinedione in treatment of advanced endometrial carcinoma, uterine sarcoma and vulvar carcinoma. Proc Am Assoc Cancer Res 20:388, 1979
275. Southeastern Group: Unpublished data
276. Salem PA, Bodey GP, Burgess MA et al: A Phase I study of pyrazofurin. Cancer 40:2806–2809, 1977
277. Gralla RJ, Sordillo PP, Magill GB: Phase II evaluation of

pyrazofurin in patients with metastatic sarcoma. Cancer Treat Rep 62:1573, 1978
278. Currie VE, Wong PP, Krakoff IH et al: Phase I trial of vindesine in patients with advanced cancer. Cancer Treat Rep 62:1333–1336, 1978
279. Rossof AH, Chandra G, Walter J et al: Phase II trial of vindesine (desacetyl vinblastine amide sulfate) in advanced metastatic cancer. Proc Am Assoc Cancer Res 20:146, 1979
280. Radice PA, Bunn PA Jr, Ihde DC: Therapeutic trials with VP-16-213 and VM-26: Active agents in small cell lung cancer, non-Hodgkin's lymphomas, and other malignancies. Cancer Treat Rep 63:1231–1239, 1979
281. Bleyer WA, Krivit W, Chard RL Jr et al: Phase II study of VM-26 in acute leukemia, neuroblastoma, and other refractory childhood malignancies: A report from the Children's Cancer Study Group. Cancer Treat Rep 63:977–981, 1979
282. Bleyer WA, Chard RL, Krivit W et al: Epipodophyllotoxin therapy of childhood neoplasia. A comparative phase II analysis of VM-26 and VP 16-213. Proc Am Assoc Cancer Res 19:373, 1978
283. O'Bryan RM, Baker LH, Gottlieb JE et al: Dose response evaluation of adriamycin in human neoplasia. Cancer 39:1940–1948, 1977
284. Baker LH, Benjamin RS: Histologic frequency of disseminated soft tissue sarcomas in adults. Am Soc Clin Oncol, Washington, DC, 1978
285. Blum RH, Corson JM, Wilson RE et al: Successful treatment of metastatic sarcomas with cyclophosphamide, adriamycin, and DTIC (CAD). Cancer 46:1722–1726, 1980
286. Yap B, Baker LH, Sinkovics JG et al: Cyclophosphamide, vincristine, adriamycin, and DTIC (CYVADIC) combination chemotherapy for the treatment of advanced sarcomas. Cancer Treat Rep 64:93–98, 1980
287. Gottlieb JA, Benjamin RS, Baker LH et al: Role of DTIC (NSC-45388) in the chemotherapy of sarcomas. Cancer Treat Rep 60:199–203, 1976
288. Luce JK, Thurman WG, Isaacs BL et al: Clinical trials with the antitumor agent 5-(3,3-dimethyl-1-triazeno)imidazole-4-carboxamide (NSC-45388). Cancer Chemother Rep 54:119–124, 1970
289. Gottlieb JA, Baker LH, Quagliana JM et al: Chemotherapy of sarcomas with a combination of adriamycin and dimethyl-triazeno-imidazole-carboxamide. Cancer 30:1632–1638, 1972
290. Pinedo HM, Vendrik CPJ, Bramwell VHC et al: Re-evaluation of the CYVADIC regimen for metastatic soft tissue sarcoma. Proc AACR and ASCO (abstr) C-228, 1979
291. Benjamin RS, Gottlieb JA, Baker LH et al: CYVADIC vs CYVADACT-a randomized trial of cyclophosphamide (CY), vincristine (V) and adriamycin (A) plus either dacarbazine (DIC) or actinomycin-D (DACT) in metastatic sarcomas. Proc Am Assoc Cancer Res Am Soc Clin Oncol, 17:256, 1976
292. Baker LH: Unpublished data
293. Rivkin SE, Gottlieb JA, Thigpen T et al: Methyl CCNU and adriamycin for patients with metastatic sarcomas. A Southwest Oncology Group Study. Cancer 46:446–451, 1980
294. Shiv MH, Magill GB, Hopfan S: "Recent trends in treatment of soft tissue sarcomas—Appendix A." In Hajdu SI (ed): Pathology of Soft Tumors, pp 537–542. Philadelphia, Lea & Febiger, 1979
295. Baker LH: Unpublished data
296. Saiki JH: Unpublished data
297. Gottlieb JA, Baker LH, Burgess MA et al: Sarcoma chemotherapy. In Cancer Chemotherapy Fundamental Concepts and Recent Advances, 19th Annual Clinical Conference in Cancer, 1974, M. D. Anderson Hospital, Year Book Medical Publishers, 1975
298. Chang P, Wiernik PH: Combination chemotheapy with adriamycin and streptozotocin. Clin Pharmacol Ther 20:605–610, 1976
299. Lowenbraun S, Moffitt S, Smalley R et al: Combination chemotherapy with adriamycin, cyclophosphamide and methotrexate in metastatic sarcomas. ASCO (abstr) 18:286, 1977
300. Kaufman JH, Catane R, Douglass HO Jr: Combined adriamycin, vincristine, and methotrexate. NY State J Med, 742–743, 1977
301. Scott WP, Voight JA: Kaposi's sarcoma management with vincaleucoblastine. Cancer 19:557–564, 1966
302. Tucker SB, Winkelman RK: Treatment of Kaposi sarcoma with vinblastine. Arch Dermatol 112:958–961, 1976
303. Selikoff IJ: Cancer risk of asbestos exposure. In Hiatt HH, Watson JD, Winsten JA (eds): Origins of Human Cancer, pp 1765–1784. Cold Spring Harbor, NY, Cold Spring Harbor Laboratory, 1977
304. Antman KH, Blum RH, Greenberger JS et al: Multimodality therapy for malignant mesothelioma based on a study of natural history. Am J Med 68:356–362, 1980
305. Oels HC, Harrison EG, Carr DT et al: Diffuse malignant mesothelioma of the pleura: a review of 37 cases. Chest 60:564–570, 1971
306. Elmes PC, Simpson MJC: The clinical aspects of mesothelioma. Q J Med 45:427–449, 1976
307. Antman KH, Blum RH, Greenberger JS et al: Multimodality therapy for malignant mesothelioma based on a study of natural history. Am J Med 68:356–362, 1980
308. Legha SS, Muggia FM: Pleural mesothelioma: clinical features and therapeutic implications. Ann Intern Med 87:613–621, 1977
309. Antman K: Clinical presentation and natural history of benign and malignant mesothelioma. Semin Oncol (in press).
310. Moertel CG: Peritoneal mesothelioma. Gastroenterology 63:346–350, 1972
311. Dahlin DC: Bone Tumors: General Aspects and Data on 3,987 Cases, 2nd ed. Springfield, Ill., Charles C Thomas, 1967
312. Huvos AG: Bone Tumors: Diagnosis, Treatment and Prognosis. Philadelphia, W B Saunders, 1979
313. McKenna RJ, Schwinn CP, Soong KY et al: Sarcomata of the osteogenic series (osteosarcoma, fibrosarcoma, chondrosarcoma, parosteal osteogenic sarcoma, and sarcomata arising in abnormal bone). J Bone Joint Surg (Am), 48:1–26, 1966
314. Rockwell MA, Enneking WF: Osteosarcoma developing in a solitary enchondroma of the tibia. J Bone Joint Surg (Am) 53:341–344, 1971
315. Lieberman PH: Eosinophilic granuloma and relative syndromes. In Beeson PB, McDermott W (eds): Textbook of Medicine, vol 2, 14th ed, pp 1529–1531. Philadelphia, W B Saunders, 1975
316. Lieberman PH, Jones CR, Dargeon HWK et al: A reappraisal of eosinophilic granuloma of bone, Hand-Schuller-Christian syndrome and Letterer-Siwe syndrome. Medicine 48:375–400, 1969
317. Jaffe HL: Tumors and tumorous conditions of bones and joints. Philadelphia, Lea & Febiger, 1958
318. Huvos AG, Marcove RC: Chondroblastoma of bone. A critical review. Clin Orthop 95:300–312, 1973
319. Huvos AG, Higinbotham NL, Marcove RC et al: Aggressive chondroblastoma. Review of the literature on aggressive behavior and metastasis with a report of one new case. Clin Orthop 126:266–272, 1977
320. Green P, Whittaker RP: Benign chondroblastoma. A case report with pulmonary metastasis. J Bone Joint Surg (Am) 57:418–420, 1975
321. Riddell RJ, Lewis CJ, Bromberger NA: Pulmonary metastasis from chondroblastoma of the tibia. Report of a case. J Bone Joint Surg (Br) 55:848–853, 1973
322. Rosen G: Malignant musculoskeletal tumors. The clinical investigative approach to combined therapy. In Care of the Child with Cancer. The American Cancer Society, 73–82, 1979
323. Rosen G: Malignant small-cell sarcomas of bone. Ped. Ann. 7:30–51, 1978
324. Rosen G. Malignant bone tumors: spindle cell sarcomas. Pediatr Ann 7:8–27, 1978
325. Ahuja SC, Villacin AB, Smith J et al: Juxtacortical (parosteal) osteogenic sarcoma. Histological grading and prognosis. J Bone Joint Surg (Am) 59:632–647, 1977
326. Dahlin DC, Coventry MB: Osteogenic sarcoma. A study of 600 cases. J Bone Joint Surg (Am) 49:101–110, 1967
327. McKenna RJ, Schwinn CP, Soong KY et al: Osteogenic sarcoma arising in Paget's disease. Cancer 17:42–66, 1964

328. Kim JH, Chu FC, Woodard HQ et al: Radiation-induced soft-tissue and bone sarcoma. Radiology 129:501–508, 1978
329. Jensen RD, Miller RW: Retinoblastoma—Epidemiologic characteristics. N Engl J Med 285:307–311, 1971
330. Schimke RN, Lowman JT, Kowan GA: Retinoblastoma and osteogenic sarcoma in siblings. Cancer 34:2077–2079, 1974
331. Campanacci M, Giunti A: Periosteal osteosarcoma. Review of 41 cases, 22 with long term follow-up. Ital J Orthop Traumatol 2:23–35, 1976
332. Marcove RC, Mike V, Hajek JV et al: Osteogenic sarcoma under the age of 21. A review of 145 operative cases. J Bone Joint Surg (Am) 52:411–423, 1970
333. Marcove RC, Mike V, Hajek JV et al: Osteogenic sarcoma in childhood. NY State J Med 71:855–859, 1977
334. Sweetnam R, Knowelden J, Seddon H: Bone sarcoma: treatment by irradiation, amputation, or a combination of the two. Br Med J 2:363–367, 1971
335. Weinfeld MS, Dudley HR: Osteogenic sarcoma. A follow-up study of 94 cases observed at the Massachusetts General Hospital from 1920 to 1960. J Bone Joint Surg (Am) 44:269–276, 1962
336. Martini N, Bains MS, Huvos AG et al: Surgical treatment of metastatic sarcoma to the lung. Surg Clin North Am 54:841–848, 1974
337. Nelson JA, Clark R, Palubinskas AJ: Osteogenic sarcoma with calcified renal metastasis. Br J Radiol 44:802–804, 1971
378. Sweetnam R: The surgical management of primary osteosarcoma. Clin Orthop 111:57–64, 1975
339. Enneking WF, Kagan A: "Skip" metastases in osteosarcoma. Cancer 36:2192–2205, 1975
340. Rosen G, Murphy ML, Huvos AG et al: Chemotherapy, en bloc resection and prosthetic bone replacement in the treatment of osteogenic sarcoma. Cancer 37:1–11, 1976
341. Marcove RC: En bloc resection for osteogenic sarcoma. Canad J Surg 20:521–528, 1977
342. Marcove RC, Lewis MM, Huvos AG: En bloc, upper humeral interscapulo-thoracic resection. The Tikhoff-Linberg procedure. Clin Orthop 124:219–228, 1977
343. Friedman MA, Carter SK: The therapy of osteogenic sarcoma. Current status and thoughts for the future. J Surg Oncol 4:482–510, 1972
344. Evans AE: Mitomycin C. Cancer Chemother Rep 14:1–9, 1961
345. Evans AE, Heyn RM, Nesbit ME et al: Evaluation of Mitomycin C (NSC-26980) in the treatment of metastatic osteogenic sarcoma. Cancer Chemother Rep 53:297–298, 1969
346. Pinkel D: Cyclophosphamide in children with cancer. Cancer 15:42–49, 1962
347. Haggard M: Cyclophosphamide in the treatment of children with malignant neoplasms. Cancer Chemother Rep 51:403–405, 1967
348. Sutow WW, Vietti TJ, Fernbach DJ et al: Evaluation of chemotherapy in children with metastatic Ewing's sarcoma and osteogenic sarcoma. Cancer Chemother Rep 55:67–81, 1971
349. Finklestein JZ, Hittle RE, Hammond GD: Evaluation of a high dose cyclophosphamide regimen on childhood tumors. Cancer 23:1239–1242, 1969
350. Cortes EP, Holland JF, Wang JJ et al: Adriamycin (NSC-123127) in 87 patients with osteogenic sarcoma. Cancer Chemother Rep (part 3) 6:305–313, 1975
351. Gottlieb JA, Baker LH, O'Bryan RM et al: Adriamycin (NSC-123127) used alone and in combination for soft tissue and bony sarcomas. Cancer Chemother Rep (part 3) 6:271–282, 1975
352. Wang JJ, Holland JF, Sinks LF: Phase II study of adriamycin (NSC-123127) in childhood solid tumors. Cancer Chemother Rep (part 3) 6:267–270, 1975
353. Bonadonna G, Monfardini S, DeLena M et al: Clinical trials with adriamycin. Results of three years' study. In Carter SK, DiMarco A, Ghione M et al (eds): International Symposium on Adriamycin, pp 139–152. New York, Springer-Verlag, 1972
354. Tan C, Rosen G, Ghavimi F et al: Adriamycin (NSC123127) in pediatric malignancies. Cancer Chemother Rep (part 3) 6:259–266, 1975
355. Pratt CB, Shanks EC: Doxorubicin in treatment of malignant solid tumors in children. Am J Dis Child 127:534–536, 1974
356. Evans AE, Baehner RL, Chard RL et al: Comparison of daunorubicin (NSC-123127) in the treatment of late-stage childhood solid tumors. Cancer Chemother Rep 58:671–676, 1974
357. Ragab AH, Sutow WW, Komp DM et al: Adriamycin in the treatment of childhood solid tumors. A Southwest Oncology Group study. Cancer 36:1567–1576, 1975
358. Sutow WW, Gehan EA, Dyment PA et al: Multi-drug adjuvant chemotherapy for osteosarcoma. Interim report of the Southwest Oncology Group studies. Cancer Treat Rep 62:265–270, 1978
359. Jaffe N: Recent advances in the chemotherapy of metastatic osteogenic sarcoma. Cancer 30:1627–1631, 1972
360. Jaffe N, Frei E, Traggis D et al: Weekly high-dose methotrexate-citrovorum factor in osteogenic sarcoma. Cancer 39:45–50, 1977
361. Jaffe N: High dose methotrexate. A review of adjuvant treatment and limb salvage in osteosarcoma. Cancer Treat Rep (in press)
362. Rosen G, Huvos AG, Mosende C et al: Chemotherapy and thoracotomy for metastatic osteogenic sarcoma. A model for adjuvant chemotherapy and the rationale for the timing of thoracic surgery. Cancer 41:841–849, 1978
363. Pratt CB, Howarth C, Ransom JL et al: High-dose methotrexate alone and in combination therapy for measurable primary or metastatic osteosarcoma. Cancer Treat Rep 64:11–20, 1980
364. Ambinder EP, Perloff M, Ohnuma T et al: High dose methotrexate followed by citrovorum factor reversal in patients with advanced cancer. Cancer 43:1177–1182, 1979
365. Rosen G, Nirenberg A, Caparros B: Evaluation of high dose methotrexate (HDMTX) with citrovorum factor rescue (CFR) single agent chemotherapy in osteogenic sarcoma (OSA). Proc Am Assoc Cancer Res 21:177, 1980
366. Rosen G, Nirenberg A, Juergens H et al: Response of primary osteogenic sarcoma to single-agent therapy with high-dose methotrexate with citrovorum factor rescue. In Nelson JD, Grassi C (eds): Current Chemotherapy and Infectious Disease. Proceedings of the 11th International Congress of Chemotherapy and the 19th Interscience Conference on Antimicrobial Agents and Chemotherapy, vol 2, pp 1633–1635. Washington DC, The American Society for Microbiology, 1980
366a. Rosen G, Marcove RC, Caparros B et al: Primary osteogenic sarcoma. The rationale for preoperative chemotherapy and delayed surgery. Cancer 43:2163–2177, 1979
366b. Catane R, Bono VH, Louie AC et al: High-dose methotrexate, not a conventional treatment. Cancer Treat Rep 62:178–180, 1978
366c. Nirenberg A, Mosende C, Mehta BM et al: High dose methotrexate with citrovorum factor rescue: Predictive value of serum methotrexate concentrations and corrective measures to avert toxicity. Cancer Treat Rep 61:779–783, 1977
366d. Mehta BM, Juergens H, Allen JC et al: Distribution of methotrexate, citrovourm factor, and 5-methyltetrahydrofolate after high-dose methotrexate-leucovorin rescue in osteogenic sarcoma. In Nelson JD, Grassi C (eds): Current Chemotherapy and Infectious Disease. Proceedings of the 11th International Congress of Chemotherapy and the 19th Interscience Conference on Antimicrobial Agents and Chemotherapy, vol 2, pp 1635–1636. Washington DC, The American Society for Microbiology, 1980
367. Ochs JJ, Freeman AI, Douglass HO et al: *Cis*-dichlorodiammine-platinum (II) in advanced osteogenic sarcoma. Cancer Treat Rep 62:239–245, 1978
368. Kamalakar P, Freeman AI, Higby DJ et al: Clinical response and toxicity with *cis*-dichloro-diammineplatinum (II) in children. Cancer Treat Rep 61:835–839, 1977
369. Catane R, Douglass HO, Mittelman A: A phase II study of high-dose *cis*-diammine-dichloroplatinum II (DDP) in non-testicular tumors. Proc Amer Assoc Cancer Res 18:115, 1977
370. Leventhal BG, Freeman A. *Cis*-diamminedichloroplatinum. A phase II study in pediatric malignancies. Proc Am Assoc Cancer Res 20:197, 1979
371. Nitschke R, Starling KA, Vats T et al: *Cis*-diamminedichloroplatinum (NSC-119875) in childhood malignancies. A South-

west Oncology Group study. Med Pediatr Oncol 4:127–132, 1978
372. Rosen G, Nirenberg A, Jeurgens H et al: Phase II trial of *cis*-platinum in osteogenic sarcoma. Proc Am Assoc Cancer Res 20:363, 1979
373. Baum E, Greenberg L, Gaymon P et al: Use of *cis*-diammine-dichloro-platinum in osteogenic sarcoma in children. Proc Am Assoc Cancer Res 19:385, 1978
374. Gaymon P, Baum, E, Greenberg L et al: A phase II trial of *cis*-platinum diammine dichloride (DDP) (NSC-119825) in refractory childhood tumors. A CCSG trial. Proc Am Assoc Cancer Res 20:394, 1979
375. Pratt CB, Hayes FA, Green AA et al: Phase II pharmacokinetic study of *cis*-platinum diamminedichloride (CDDP) in children with solid tumors. Proc Am Assoc Cancer Res 20:361, 1979
376. Pratt CB: Chemotherapy of osteosarcoma. An overview. In Van Oosterom AT, Muggia FM, Cleton FJ (eds): Therapeutic Progress in Ovarian Cancer, Testicular Cancer and the Sarcomas, pp 329–348, The Hague, Martinus Nijhoff Publishers, 1980
377. Jaffe N, Traggis D, Enriquez C: Evaluation of a combination of mitomycin C (NSV 1420) and vincristine (NSC 67574) in the treatment of osteogenic sarcoma. Cancer Chemother Rep 55:189–193, 1971
378. Nathanson L, Hall TC, Dederick MM et al: Initial pharmacologic studies of three types of combination chemotherapy. Cancer Chemother Rep 50: 259–264, 1966
379. Gottlieb JA, Baker LH, Quagliana JM et al: Chemotherapy of sarcomas with a combination of adriamycin and dimethyl triazeno imidazole carboxamide. Cancer 30:1632–1638, 1972
380. Rosen G, Suvanisirikul S, Kwon C et al: High-dose methotrexate with citrovorum factor rescue and adriamycin in childhood osteogenic sarcoma. Cancer 33:1151–1163, 1974
381. Chello PL, Sirotnak DM, Dorick DM et al: Schedule-dependent synergism of methotrexate and vincristine against murine L1210 leukemia. Cancer Treat Rep 63:1889–1894, 1979
382. Mosende C, Guttierez M, Caparros B et al: Combination chemotherapy with bleomycin, cyclophosphamide and dactinomycin for the treatment of osteogenic sarcoma. Cancer 40:2779–2786, 1977
383. Rosen G: Unpublished data
384. Cortes EP, Holland JF, Wang JJ et al: Amputation and adriamycin in primary osteogenic sarcoma. N Engl J Med 291:998–1000, 1974
385. Holland JF, Cortes EP: The role of adriamycin in the treatment of osteogenic sarcoma and future directions for its use. JNCI (in press)
386. Cortes EP, Necheles TF, Holland JF et al: Adriamycin (ADM) alone versus ADM and high dose methotrexate citrovorum factor rescue (HDMTX-CFR) as adjuvant to operable primary osteosarcoma. A randomized study by cancer and leukemic group B (CALGB). Proc Am Assoc Cancer Res 20:412, 1979
387. Fossati–Bellani F, Gasparini M, Gennari L: Adjuvant treatment with adriamycin in primary operable osteosarcoma. Cancer Treat Rep 62:289–294, 1978
388. Murphy WK, Benjamin RS, Eyre HJ et al: Adjuvant chemotherapy in osteosarcoma of adults. In Salmon SE, Jones SE (eds): Adjuvant Chemotherapy of Cancer, p 399. Amsterdam: Elsevier/North Holland Biomedical Press, 1977
389. Jaffe N, Frei E, Watts H et al: High-dose methotrexate in osteogenic sarcoma. A 5-year experience. Cancer Treat Rep 62:259–264, 1978
390. Rosenberg SA, Chabner BA, Young RC et al: Treatment of osteogenic sarcoma. Effect of adjuvant high-dose methotrexate after amputation. Cancer Treat Rep 63:739–751, 1979
391. Rosenberg SA, Flye MW, Conkle D et al: Treatment of osteogenic sarcoma. Aggressive resection of pulmonary metastases. Cancer Treat Rep 63:753–756, 1979
392. Jaffe N: Personal communication
393. Etcubanas E, Wilbur JR: Adjuvant chemotherapy for osteogenic sarcoma. Cancer Treat Rep 62:283–287, 1978
394. Sutow WW, Sullivan MP, Wilbur JR et al: A study of adjuvant chemotherapy in osteogenic sarcoma. J Clin Pharmacol 7:530–533, 1975
395. Pratt CB, Shanks EC, Hustu HO et al: Adjuvant multiple drug chemotherapy for osteogenic sarcoma of the extremity. Cancer 39:51–57, 1977
396. Shepp M, Nechelec TF, Banks HH et al: Adjuvant treatment of osteogenic sarcoma with high-dose cyclophosphamides. Cancer Treat Rep 62:295–296, 1978
397. Ettinger LJ, Douglass HO, Higby DJ et al: Adriamycin (Adr) and cis-diammine-dichloroplatinum (CDDP) as adjuvant therapy in primary osteosarcoma (OS). Proc Am Assoc Cancer Res 20:438, 1979
398. Ettinger LJ: Personal communication
399. Rosen G: Current management of malignant bone sarcomas. In Burchenal JH, Oettgen HF (eds): Cancer. Achievements, Challenges and Prospects for the Future. New York, Grune & Stratton, (in press)
400. Lichtenstein L, Jaffe HL: Chondrosarcoma of bone. Am J Pathol 19:553–573, 1943
401. Grabias S, Mankin HJ: Chondrosarcoma arising in histologically proved unicameral bone cysts. Case report. J Bone Joint Surg (Am) 1501–1509, 1974
402. Pendergrass EP, Lafferty JO, Horn RC: Osteogenic and chondrosarcoma with special reference to the roentgen diagnosis. Am J Roentgenol Rad Ther Nucl Med 54:234–256, 1945
403. Marcove RC, Mike V, Hutter RVP et al: Chondrosarcoma of the pelvis and upper end of the femur—an analysis of factors influencing survival time in 113 cases. J Bone Joint Surg (Am) 54:561–572, 1972
404. Evans HL, Ayala AG, Romsdahl MM: Prognostic factors in chondrosarcoma of bone—a clinical pathologic analysis with emphasis on histologic grading. Cancer 40:818–831, 1977
405. Salvador AH, Beaubout JW, Dahlin DC: Mesenchymal chondrosarcoma—observations on 30 new cases. Cancer 28:606–615, 1971
406. Unni KK, Dahlin DC, Beaubout JW et al: Chondrosarcoma: clear cell variant—a report of 16 cases. J Bone Joint Surg (Am) 58:676–683, 1976
407. Marcove RC. Chondrosarcoma: diagnosis and treatment. Orthop Clin North Am 8:811–820, 1977
408. Marcove RC, Stovell PB, Huvos AG et al: The use of cryosurgery in the treatment of low and medium grade chondrosarcoma—a preliminary report. Clin Orthop 122:147–156, 1977
409. Marcove RC, Lewis MM, Huvos AG: En bloc upper humeral interscapulothoracic resection. Tikhoff–Lindberg procedure. Clin Orthop 124:219–228, 1977
410. Smith WS, Simon MA: Segmental resection for chondrosarcoma. J Bone Joint Surg (Am) 57:1097–1103, 1975
411. Mayer K, Pentlow KS, Marcove RC et al: Sulfur-35 therapy of chondrosarcoma and chordoma. In Spencers RP (ed): Therapy in Nuclear Medicine, pp 185–192. New York, Grune & Stratton, 1978
412. Dahlin DC, Cupps RE, Johnson EW Jr: Giant cell tumor: a study of 195 cases. Cancer 25:1061–1070, 1970
413. Goldenberg RR, Campbell CJ, Bonfiglio M: Giant cell tumor of bone—an analysis of 218 cases. J Bone Joint Surg (Am) 52:619–664, 1970
414. MacIntyre RS, Latourette HB, Hodges FJ: Radiologic aspects of giant cell tumor of bone. Clin Orthop 7:82–92, 1956
415. Jewell JH, Bush LF: "Benign" giant cell tumor of bone with a solitary pulmonary metastases—a case report. J Bone Joint Surg (Am) 46:848–852, 1964
416. Kutchemeshgi AD, Wright JR, Humphrey RL: Pulmonary metastases from a well-differentiated giant cell tumor of bone—report of a patient with apparent response to cyclophosphamide therapy. Johns Hopkins Med J 134:237–245, 1974
417. Laddaga M, Calderazzi A, Ducci F et al: Radiotherapy of giant cell tumor of the vertebral column. Radiol Med (Torino) 62:609–622, 1976
418. Eilers H, Habighorst LV, Alpers P et al: Radiation therapy of an inoperable giant cell tumor. Strahlentherapie 153:103–105, 1977
419. Johnson EW Jr, Dahlin DC: Treatment of giant cell tumor of bone. J Bone Joint Surg (Am) 41:895–904, 1959
420. Hutter RVP, Worcester JN Jr, Francis KC et al: Benign and

malignant giant cell tumors of bone—a clinical pathological analysis of the natural history of the disease. Cancer 15:653–690, 1962

421. Marcove RC, Weis LD, Vaghaiwalla MR et al: Cryosurgery in the treatment of giant cell tumors of bone—a report of 52 consecutive cases. Cancer 41:957–969, 1978
422. Huvos AG, Higginbotham NL: Primary fibrosarcoma of bone—a clinical pathologic study of 130 patients. Cancer 35:837–847, 1975
423. Huvos AG: Primary malignant fibrous histiocytoma of bone—clinico-pathologic study of 18 patients. NY State J Med 76:552–559, 1976
424. Rosen G, Caparros B, Nirenberg A et al: Ewings sarcoma: 10 year experience with adjuvant chemotherapy. Cancer (in press).
425. Perez CA, Razek A, Tefft M et al: Analysis of local tumor control in Ewing's sarcoma. Cancer 40:2864–2873, 1977
426. Shoji H, Miller TR: Primary reticulum cell sarcoma of bone—significance of clinical features upon the prognosis. Cancer 28:1234–1244, 1971
427. Coley BL, Higinbotham NL, Groesbeck HP: Primary reticulum cell sarcoma of bone—summary of 37 cases. Radiology 55:641–658, 1950
428. Reimer RR, Chabner BA, Young RC et al: Lymphoma presenting in bone—results of histopathology, staging and therapy. Ann Int Med 87:50–55, 1977
429. Wollner N, Burchenal JH, Lieberman PH et al: Non-Hodgkins lymphoma in children. Med Pediatr Oncol 1:235–263, 1975
430. Canellos GP, Lister TA, Skarin AT: Chemotherapy of non-Hodgkins lymphomas. Cancer 42:932–940, 1978
431. Harrison DT, Neiman PE, Sullivan K et al: Combined modality therapy for advanced diffuse lymphocytic and histiocytic lymphomas. Cancer 42:1697–1704, 1978
432. Elias L, Portlock CS, Rosenberg SA: Combination chemotherapy of diffuse histiocytic lymphoma with cyclophosphamide, adriamycin, vincristine and prednisone (CHOP) Cancer 42: 1705–1710, 1978
433. Hartman WH, Stewart FW: Hemangioendothelioma of bone—unusual tumor characterized by indolent course. Cancer 15:846–854, 1962
434. Unni KK, Ivins JC, Beabout JW et al: Hemangioma, hemangiopericytoma and hemangioendothelioma (angiosarcoma) of bone. Cancer 27:1403–1414, 1971
435. Otis J, Hutter RVP, Foote FW Jr et al: Hemangioendothelioma of bone. Surg Gynecol Obstet 127:295–305, 1968
436. Chambers RG, Mahoney WD: Osteogenic sarcoma of the mandible. Current management. Am Surg 36:463, 1970
437. Caron AS, Hajdu SI, Strong EW: Osteogenic sarcoma of the facial and cranial bones. Am J Surg 122:719–725, 1971

Martin B. Levene
Harley A. Haynes
Robert M. Goldwyn

CHAPTER 30

Cancers of the Skin

HISTORICAL BACKGROUND OF SKIN CANCER

Basal and squamous cell carcinoma are commonly grouped together and referred to as non-melanoma skin cancer. They share both an origin from the epidermal cell and many common features of epidemiology and carcinogenesis, albeit with significant differences. Many features of therapy are similar, and the prognoses in both are excellent in most cases. Although basal cell carcinoma almost never metastasizes, squamous cell carcinoma has a low incidence of metastatic disease.

There are several proven causes of non-melonoma skin cancer. These include:

1. Chemical carcinogenesis
2. Ultraviolet light
3. Ionizing radiation
4. Immunologic deficiency, or suppression.

A fifth category, genetic defects, can be considered separately, although it probably operates through enhancement of one of the four factors listed above. Viral carcinogenesis is known only in the genetic immunodeficiency disease, epidermodysplasia verruciformis. Scars, including burn scars, and chronic inflammation are also carcinogenic, although the operant stimuli are unknown. The most important carcinogenic stimulus for skin is clearly ultraviolet (UV) light. The cutaneous phenotype of a person determines the extent of deliterious effects from exposure to UV light; that is, ease of sunburning, poor tanning ability, and freckling are correlated with increased risk of skin cancer.

CHEMICAL CARCINOGENESIS

While chemical carcinogenesis of skin does not seem to be nearly as frequent a cause of cancer of the skin as UV light, it was described over a century earlier. The early history of chemical carcinogenesis has been summarized elsewhere.[1] Sir Percivall Pott was the first to describe an occupational chemical carcinogenesis when he noted the high incidence of carcinoma of the scrotal and penile skin in chimney sweeps. He attributed this to soot and chronic irritation. Approximately 100 years later the observation was made of the increased frequency of skin cancer in workers exposed to paraffin, pitch, and shale oil tar. In 1915, Yamagiwa and Ichikawa first produced skin cancer experimentally by the prolonged and repeated application of tar to the skin of the ears of rabbits.

That chemical carcinogenesis may have more than one stage was first suggested by Rous and associates in 1941.[2] Papillomas produced by the repeated application of pitch would regress if the exposure to pitch was discontinued soon enough; subsequent application of a non-specific irritant such as turpentine would cause the papillomas to reappear. Thus, it appeared that the production of the tumor was initiated by the carcinogen, but its subsequent development could be promoted non-specifically. Berenblum further elucidated the two-stage process of carcinogenesis in 1964 using croton oil as the promoting agent.[3] A single application of a potent carcinogen such as benzopyrene or dimethylbenzanthrene applied in quantity unable to produce tumors, did allow tumor development after subsequent repeated applications of croton oil, which by itself produced no tumors at all. Initiation seems to be more or less permanent and irreversible, whereas promotion, up to a point, is reversible.[4,5] To relate this concept of chemical carcinogenesis to UV light carcinogenesis it appears that UV light is both an initiator and a promotor for carcinoma of skin.[6]

ULTRAVIOLET LIGHT

Despite the ubiquitous nature of UV light, it was not until the 1890's that much interest was displayed in sun exposure as a cause of carcinoma of the skin. In 1894, Unna (and Shield in 1899) both mentioned a relationship of skin cancer and UV light.[7-9] Hyde published an article in 1906 entitled "On the Influence of Light in the Production of Cancer of the Skin".[10] In this publication he noted that certain persons were hypersensitive to the action of sunlight, the accelerated appearance of this hypersensitivity in patients with xeroderma pigmentosum, and the protection afforded by the physiologic pigmentation of skin in colored races. In 1928, Finlay produced skin cancer experimentally in mice by exposure to UV light from a mercury vapor lamp. In addition, Finlay also made the important observation that skin cancers appeared more quickly when tar was applied to the skin followed by exposure to UV light.[11] In the 1930s, Roffo expanded these observations by producing skin cancer in rats by exposure to natural sunlight, and demonstrated that clear window glass was able to prevent skin cancer from both mercury arc lamps and natural sunlight, placing the upper limit of UV photocarcinogenesis at 320 nanometers.[14] These observations were further refined by Blum in the 1940's and 1950's.[12,13] The experiment of nature in which different intensities of UV radiation occur at different global latitudes has provided the opportunity for epidemiologic studies to show an increased incidence of nonmelanoma skin cancer in the white population at latitudes closer to the equator as compared to latitudes farther from the equator. The work of Macdonald and Scotto shows an unequivocal inverse relationship between latitude and non-melanoma skin cancer.[15,16] For example, the incidence of non-melanoma skin cancer is 379/100,000 in the Dallas/Fort Worth, Texas area (latitude 32.8n), but only 124/100,000 in Iowa (latitude 42 n). On this geographic relationship to skin cancer, individual phenotypes are noted to be more susceptible to skin cancer within any given geographic area. The susceptible persons tend to have poor tanning ability with easy sunburning and, in addition, often have fair skin, light hair, and blue eyes.[17] In addition to this general phenotype susceptibility, it has been observed that Celtic ancestry tends to predispose to the development of non-melanoma skin cancer.

That man could perturb the stratospheric ozone that filters out much of the carcinogenic wavelengths was first emphasized by McDonald in 1971 in relation to emissions from high-flying airplanes.[18] Subsequently, other man made pollutants, such as chlorofluoromethanes and certain nitrogen fertilizers, are of even greater danger to the ozone filter.[19,20]

The two major effects of UV radiation on the skin which seem likely to be responsible for the carcinogenic effects are: photochemical alteration of DNA and alterations in immunity. In the 1940s and 1950s, Blum worked on the wavelengths and dose-response characteristics of UV carcinogenesis.[12,13] A remarkable degree of conformity was observed in the wavelengths affecting and causing erythema (sunburn), absorption by DNA, and carcinoma of skin. In 1968, Cleever reported the defective repair replication of DNA in xeroderma pigmentosum fibroblasts.[21] In 1969, Setlow showed that xeroderma pigmentosum cells failed to repair UV damage to DNA by failing to excise the thymine dimers.[22] This defect in DNA repair was observed *in vivo* in the skin of patients with xeroderma pigmentosum by Epstein in 1970.[23] Since most persons with skin cancer do not have xeroderma pigmentosum and do have normal (or nearly normal) ability to repair UV light-damaged DNA, other factors may be involved as well. It is now clear that certain immunologic defects, both in skin and in lymphocytes, can be induced by UV radiation. UV-induced fibrosarcomas in mice are more antigenic than tumors induced by other agents. In 1974, Kripke found that these tumors were so highly antigenic that they were immunologically rejected when transplanted into normal non-UV irradiated syngeneic animals.[24] This lead to the discovery that UV radiation causes three immunologic alterations in mice:

1. It destroys the lymphocyte-activating structures (1a) antigens on the surface of lymphoid cells following *in vitro* UV irradiation
2. It temporarily impairs the processing of certain antigens
3. It induces suppressor cells that prevent the rejection of UV-induced tumors[25-26]

Recent attention has been focused on the Langerhans cell. The Langerhans cells appear to be of bone marrow origin and of macrophage-like parentage. They migrate to the epidermis and assume a dendritic shape, coming in contact with a large number of epidermal cells. In that location they appear to act as the sentinel cells for contact dermatitis and other types of delayed hypersensitivity. Exposure to UV light temporarily depletes the epidermis of Langerhans cells and renders it unable to be sensitized to potent allergens.[27] Skin showing signs of chronic UV light radiation damage is less easily sensitized to potent allergens (DNCB) than adjacent non-exposed skin in the same person, but the immunopathology of this defect has not yet been elucidated.[28] Some of these immunologic events related to UV exposure may be important in permitting UV carcinogenesis in humans.

IONIZING RADIATION

Ionizing radiation is carcinogenic for skin as it is for many other tissues. Upton has described the early history of ionizing radiation carcinogenesis.[29] Roentgen radiation-induced squamous cell carcinoma of skin was first reported by Frieben in 1902, soon after the discovery of x-rays. This report involved those who worked with the machines. Shortly, however, cutaneous carcinoma appeared in patients who had been exposed to roentgen radiation. Before the development of modern dosimetry, radiation therapy of lymph nodes and such resulted in a significant skin dose; thus, complications of ulceration and carcinoma occurred. With modern techniques, the skin dose is significantly lower and complications seem very infrequent. As the use of ionizing radiation of benign skin disease has recently been significantly curtailed and industrial and occupational exposure very well controlled, it would appear that ionizing radiation at present is not responsible for much cutaneous carcinogenesis.

MAGNITUDE OF THE PROBLEM

It is estimated that the present annual incidence of non-melanoma skin cancer in Caucasians in the U.S. is 165/100,000 population. This translates into about 300,000 cases of skin cancer in Caucasians in the U.S. each year. The direct

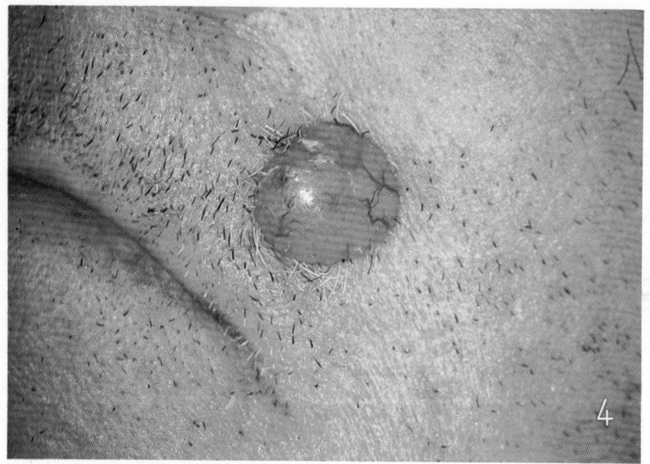

COL. FIG. 30-1. Nodular basal cell carcinoma.

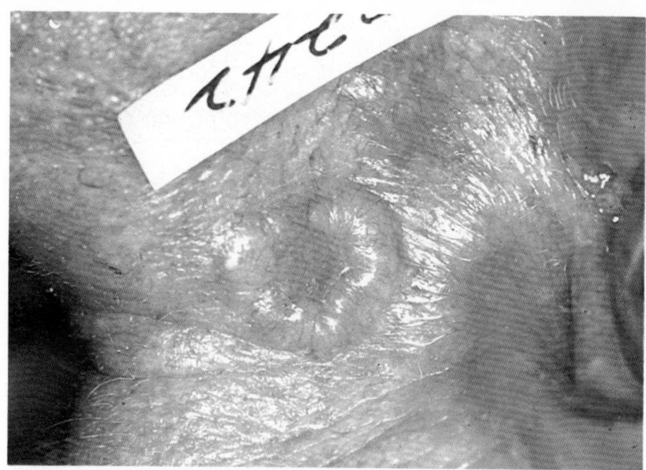

COL. FIG. 30-2. Nodulo-ulcerative basal cell carcinoma.

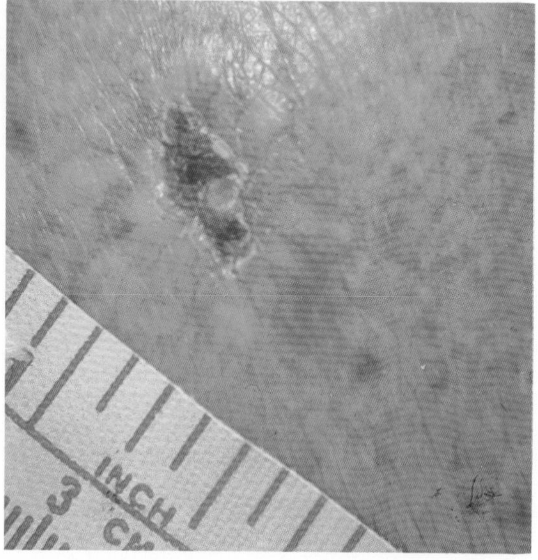

COL. FIG. 30-3. Ulceration with crusting in nodulo-ulcerative basal cell carcinoma.

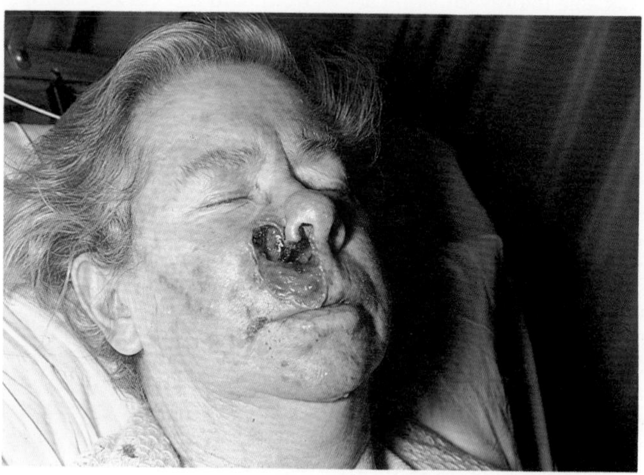

COL. FIG. 30-4. Ulcerating and deeply invasive basal cell carcinoma. The patient has had this carcinoma for many years.

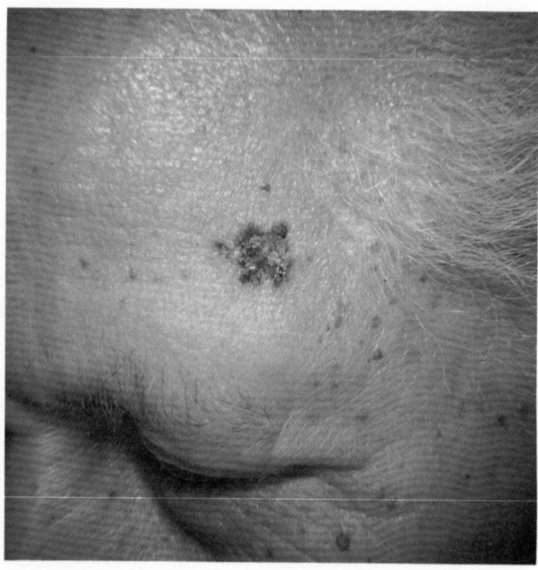

COL. FIG. 30-5. Pigmented basal cell carcinoma.

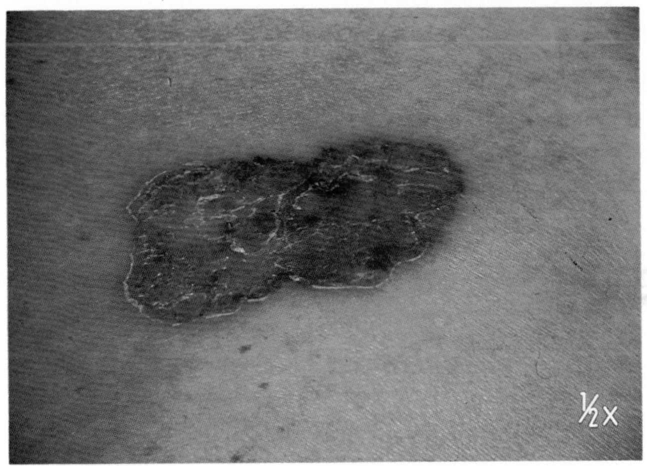

COL. FIG. 30-6. Pigmented basal cell carcinoma.

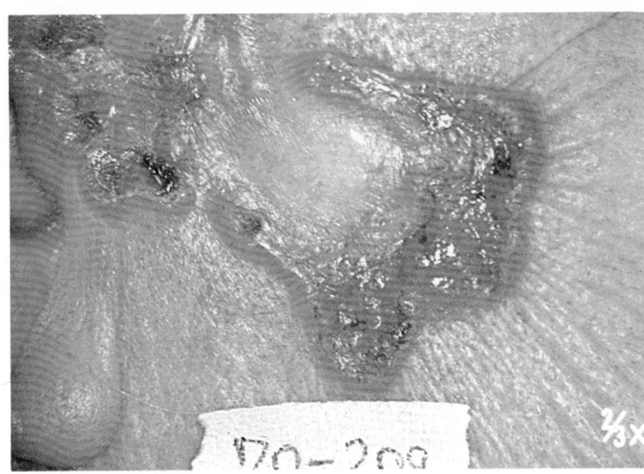

COL. FIG. 30-7. Sclerosing basal cell carcinoma that damaged the facial nerve.

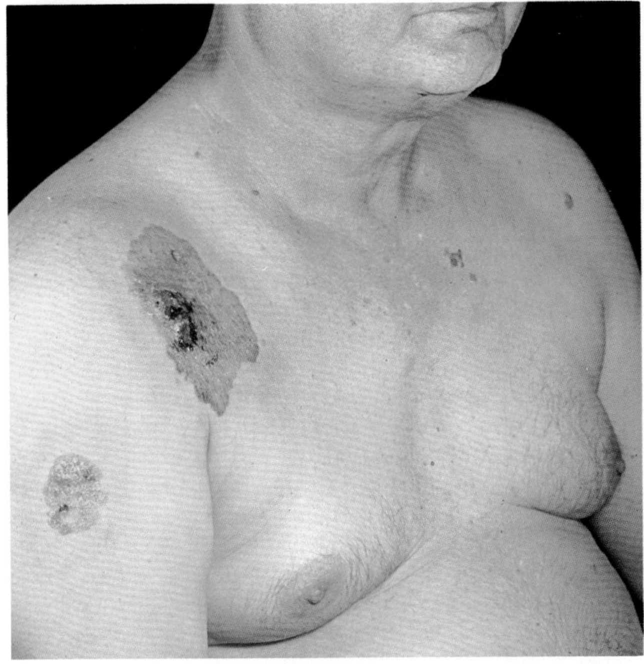

COL. FIG. 30-8. Superficial "multicentric" basal cell carcinomas.

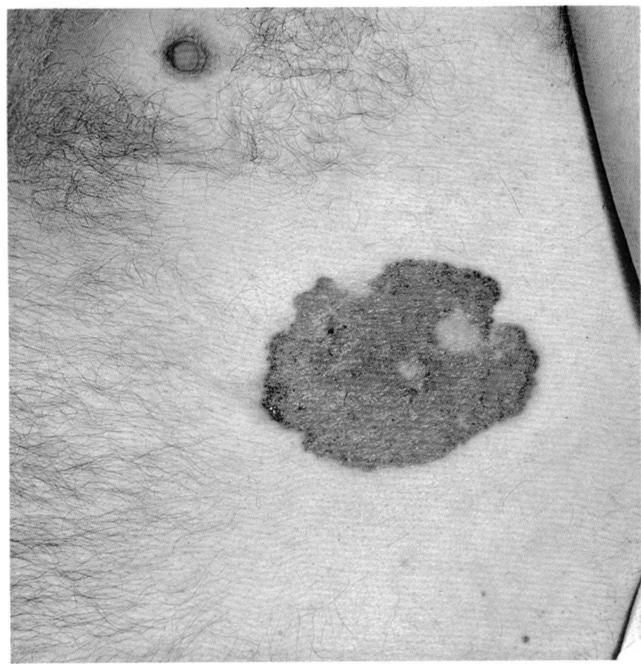

COL. FIG. 30-9. Pigmented superficial basal cell carcinomas.

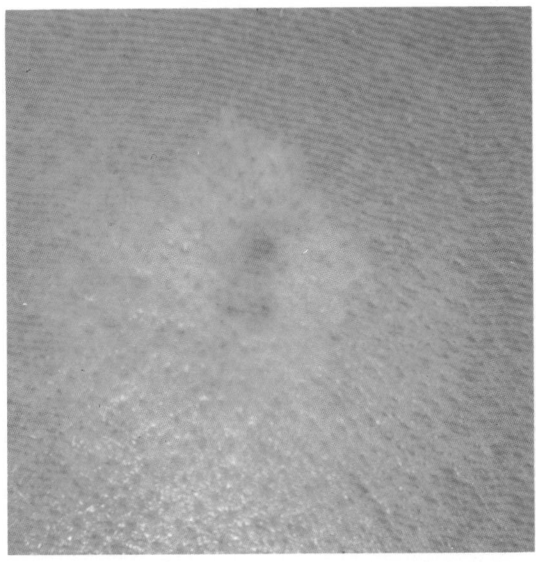

COL. FIG. 30-10. Morphea-like basal cell carcinoma. The entire pale area has been infiltrated by carcinoma; the margins are indistinct.

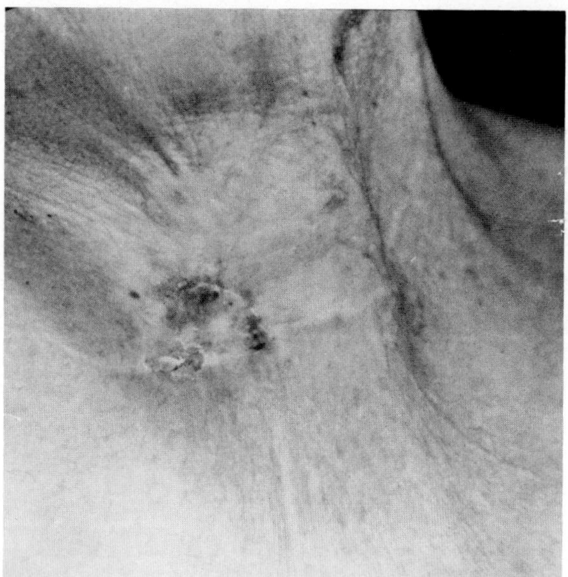

FIG. 30-1. Basal cell carcinoma arising in the periphery of a chronic radiodermatitis scar from therapy 20 years ago.

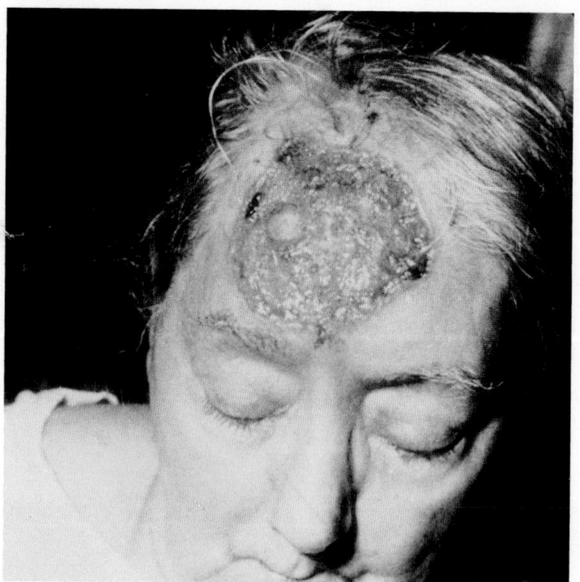

FIG. 30-2. Basal cell carcinoma, invasive into the frontal lobe.

and indirect economic costs in terms of 1971 dollars was estimated at $94.5 million. Inflation took this to $150 million in 1977 dollars.[30] While the cure rate of skin cancer exceeds 95%, the time, effort, expense, and disfigurement are of major proportions.

NATURAL HISTORY AND CLINICAL PRESENTATION

Basal Cell Carcinoma

Basal cell carcinoma is by far the most common form of skin cancer, representing at least 75% of cases in the southern U.S. and over 90% of cases in the northern U.S. Three recent publications deal with this subject in depth.[31,32,33] A nodular, or nodular ulcerative lesion, is the most frequent. It is seen most often on the skin of the head and neck, and only 10% of the time on the trunk. It is much less frequent on the upper extremities, quite uncommon on the lower extremities, rarely seen on skin that is growing, and relatively asymptomatic except for possible crusting or bleeding with minor trauma. The lesion is generally smooth, shiny, and translucent in appearance with telangiectatic vessels commonly seen just beneath the surface (see Col. Figs. 30-1 and 30-2). There is generally no tenderness or pain noted, even if ulceration occurs (see Col. Figs. 30-3 and 30-4). Generally, the overall color of the lesion is not much different from normal skin color and usually a bit lighter, except for the telangiectatic vessels. However, a certain percentage of lesions have melanin pigment within them, which appears as scattered tattoo-like dots that can become confluent to cause the whole lesion to have brown, black, or even bluish pigmentation (see Col. Figs. 30-5 and 30-6). This may cause occasional confusion with melanoma, which is readily resolved by biopsy. Patients with the basal cell nevus syndrome, also known as the nevoid basal cell carcinoma syndrome, often have nodular lesions with pigmentation that may be mistaken for pigmented nevi.

There is a variant of the nodular ulcerative lesion with some chronicity. Fibrosis occurs centrally in these lesions, with erosion being next to the fibrotic center. Outside of the area of erosion is a border of translucent shiny papules. This type of lesion may both develop to several centimeters in size and may extend, deeply injuring nerves and bone beneath (see Col. Fig. 30-7).

The next frequent type of basal cell carcinoma is the superficial type, usually found on the skin of the chest or back; in contrast to the nodular lesions, it is erythematous (see Col. Fig. 30-8). In the beginning it is a very subtle erythematous plaque, almost flat and very difficult to palpate. The surface of the lesion may be somewhat scaly with scattered fine crusting and sometimes showing an erythematous, smooth, shiny appearance. When a lesion is more mature, tiny translucent papules in a string-of-pearls-like configuration at the margin of the lesion may often be seen. It is frequent for the lesion to be mistaken as some other dermatologic problem or mild irritation. Therefore, patients with previous histories of basal cell carcinoma should have such lesions biopsied promptly. These lesions may have pigment dots scattered throughout them, but never show the reticulate, ink-blot spreading kind of pigmentation commonly seen in melanomas (see Col. Fig. 30-9).

A morphea-like or morphea-form basal cell carcinoma is an uncommon type, often masquerading as a scar (see Col. Fig. 30-10). It presents as a smooth, fibrotic patch without evident telangiectasia, ulceration, or raised, pearly papules at the edge. The margins of this kind of lesion are often quite indistinct. It may spread to great widths and depths before its true nature is recognized. Fortunately, this type of lesion is quite uncommon, occurring more often on the trunk than on the face and neck.

Uncommon types of basal cell carcinoma are those arising

in basal cell nevus syndrome, in addition to chronic radiation dermatitis from ionizing radiation, scars from vaccination, and in a variety of pre-existing genetically-determined cutaneous lesions, such as the nevus sebaceus (see Fig. 30-1).

Basal cell carcinomas of any type very rarely metastasize. However, they are capable of invading widely and deeply, extending through to the subcutaneous tissue to involve neurovascular structures and occasionally invading into bone. When located on the head they may erode through the skull and into the brain (see Fig. 30-2).

Squamous Cell Carcinoma

The clinical presentation of squamous cell carcinoma makes clinical diagnosis much more difficult than in basal cell carcinoma. Recently published material discusses this tumor in depth.[34,35,36,37] In general, the squamous cell carcinomas are erythematous lesions with varying degrees of scaling and crusting. This allows confusion with psoriasis, eczema, infections, and trauma. Squamous cell carcinomas in sun-exposed areas of the body tend to occur on the most highly-irradiated portions of skin, such as the top of the nose, forehead, tips of the helixes of the ears, lower lip, and back of the hands (see Figs. 30-3, 30-4, and 30-5). These lesions on the skin surface generally have about the same biologic malignancy as basal cell carcinomas, only rarely showing metastatic disease. An exception to this is in the case of immuno-suppressed patients who develop metastases more frequently. When squamous cell carcinoma arises on mucous membrane or mucocutaneous junction, it also tends to metastasize more frequently. The squamous cell carcinomas on skin relatively or totally not exposed to the sun have much greater biologic malignancy with a much higher frequency of metastatic disease.

As in the case of the cervix, there is an *in situ* stage of squamous cell carcinoma of the skin. In addition, there is a premalignant stage of squamous cell carcinoma known as *actinic keratosis*. These lesions are always on sun-exposed skin and present as rough, red plaques only barely raised from the skin's surface (see Fig. 30-6). If there is any accumulation of scale, this should be removed, and the residual erythematous area should not be significantly elevated. If it is, biopsy will be required to examine for possible squamous cell carcinoma. Any patient having actinic keratosis should be examined very carefuly for the presence of either basal or squamous cell carcinoma, as such patients are much more frequently affected than patients without actinic keratosis. *In situ* squamous cell carcinoma almost always looks reasonably innocuous and is a well-demarcated, slightly raised erythematous plaque with both more substance and scaling than an actinic keratosis (see Figs. 30-7 and 30-8). The type of scaling is not micaceous as in psoriasis, and the lesion is not as inflammatory appearing as eczematous dermatitis. When these lesions are present on sun-exposed skin, they are simply a stage in the development of UV-induced squamous cell carcinoma. However, when the *in situ* lesions appear on skin not exposed to the sun they are, at times, a marker for concurrent internal malignancy (5–30%), but this has been disputed.[38,39] Nodular or nodular ulcerative squamous cell carcinoma generally appears as a red, firm tumor elevated from

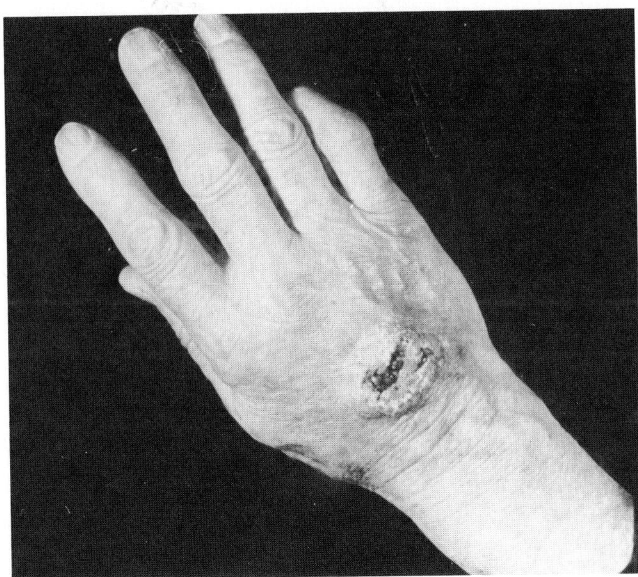

FIG. 30-3. Squamous cell carcinoma on the dorsum of the hand.

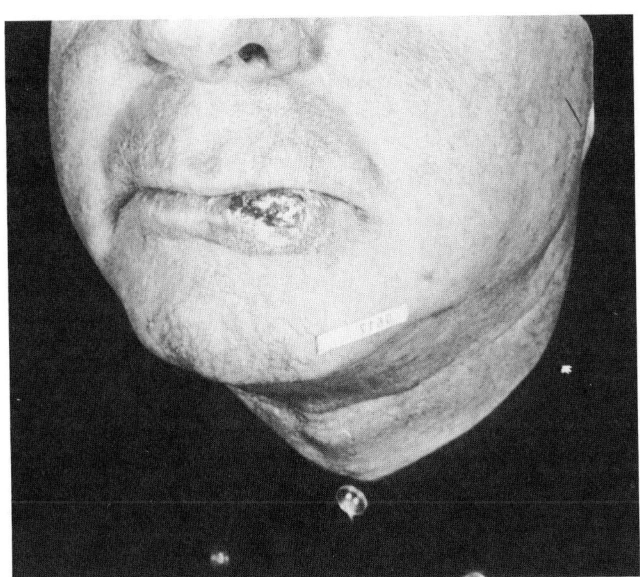

FIG. 30-4. Squamous cell carcinoma on the lower lip.

FIG. 30-5. Squamous cell carcinoma on helix.

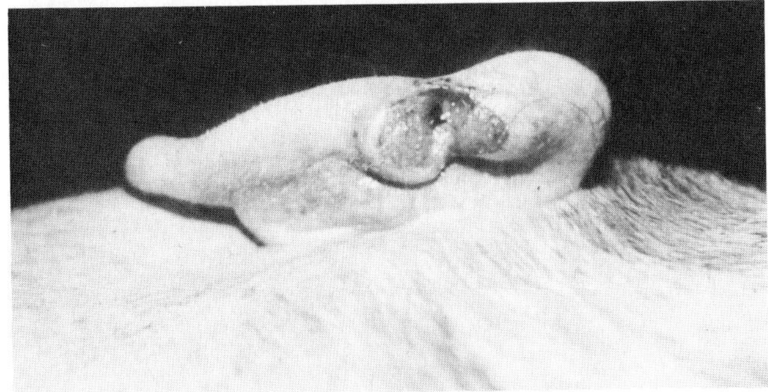

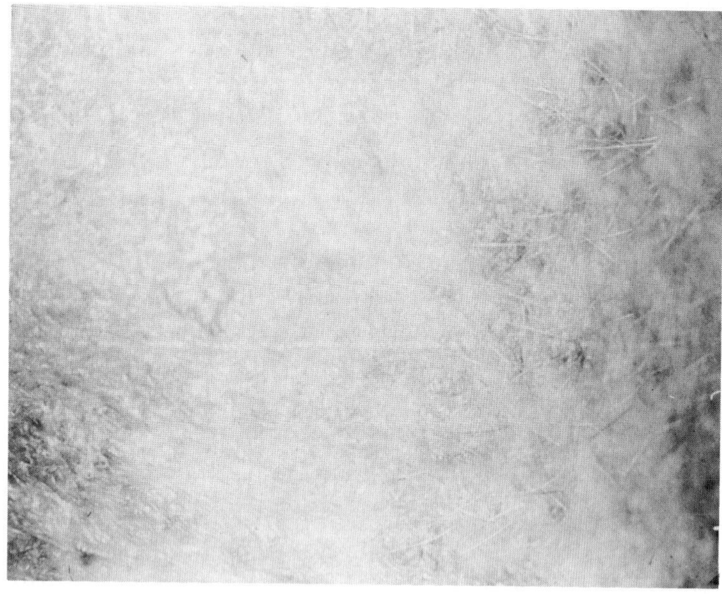

FIG. 30-6. Actinic keratosis on forehead.

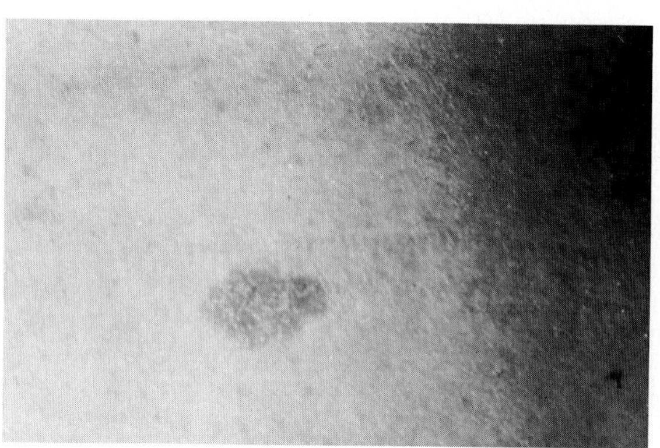

FIG. 30-7. Squamous cell carcinoma *in-situ* on the thigh.

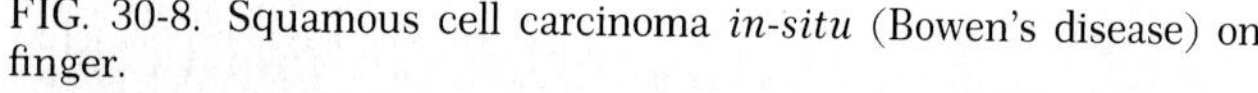

FIG. 30-8. Squamous cell carcinoma *in-situ* (Bowen's disease) on finger.

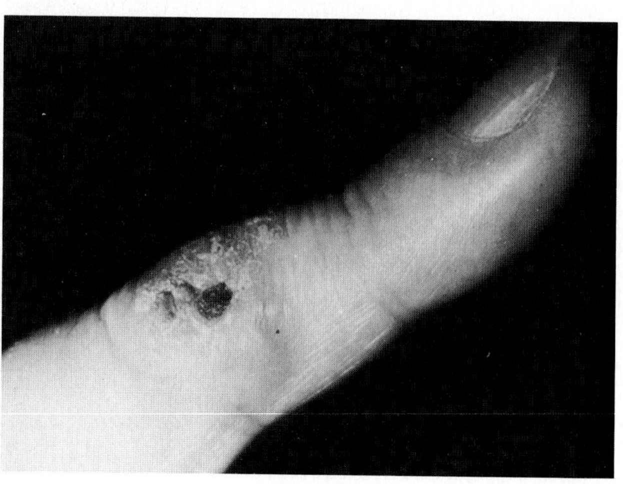

the surrounding skin with the surface consisting of scale, a cutaneous horn, or an ulceration with crusting (see Fig. 30-9). If another etiology for the lesions is not readily apparent, biopsy should be performed. On the external genitalia, erythematous plaques with weepy surfaces or verrucous nodules with ulceration are the usual presentations for squamous cell carcinoma (see Fig. 30-10). Clinically, it may be difficult to differentiate between condylomata accuminata and squamous cell carcinoma. When this clinical dilemma occurs, biopsy should be done. When cutaneous squamous cell carcinoma metastasizes it usually does so first to local lymph nodes, but hematogenous spread can appear with lung lesions being a frequent manifestation.

Bowen's Disease

This variant of *in situ* squamous cell carcinoma presents as an asymptomatic well-demarcated, slightly raised, erythematous plaque with some degree of scaling. At present, there seems little necessity to differentiate this type of squamous cell carcinoma *in situ* from other types of squamous cell carcinoma *in situ*.[39] It is not possible to distinguish these two types of squamous cell carcinoma *in situ* on clinical grounds, nor is it clear that there is any difference in therapy or prognosis in patients whose histopathologic appearance is either of the Bowen's disease or the non-Bowen's squamous cell carcinoma *in situ*. (See Figs. 30-7 and 30-8).

Keratoacanthoma

This lesion is a peculiar one and of great clinical interest. It generally appears very rapidly over a 2–3 week period on a sun-exposed site. No pre-existing lesion is present. It is a smooth, red nodule with a central keratinous plug, which at times has been avulsed. An erosion with a verrucous base may be seen in the center instead of the plug (see Figs. 30-11 and 30-12). The red rim of the tumor nodule is often a bit

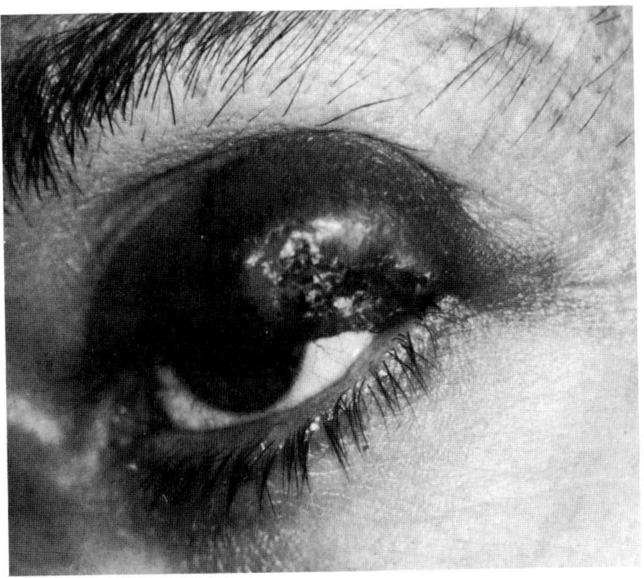

FIG. 30-9. Squamous cell carcinoma on eyelid.

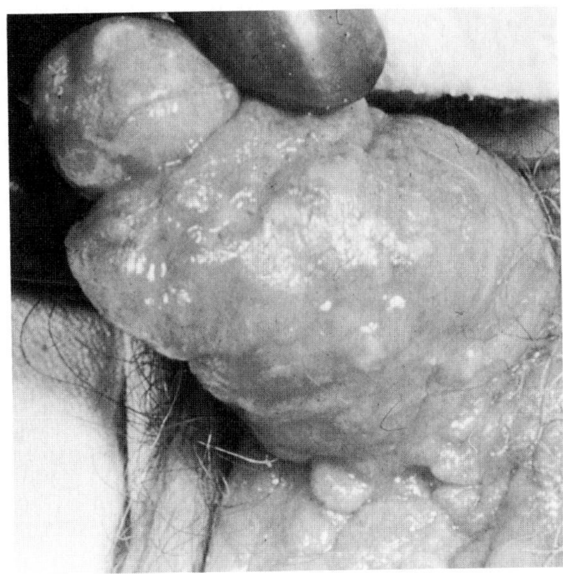

FIG. 30-10. Penile squamous cell carcinoma.

smoother than the usual squamous cell carcinoma, and telangiectatic vessels may be seen, making it difficult to differentiate from a basal cell carcinoma. The translucent characteristic of the rim of the basal cell carcinoma is absent in the keratoacanthoma. These lesions never metastasize, but the clinical problem is differentiating them from squamous cell carcinoma, which of course can metastasize. Therefore, when in doubt in an amenable location a surgical excisional biopsy should be done. In an area in which this is not feasible, a biopsy consisting of a wedge, either radially or diametrically all the way through the lesion, can be done.[40] If the histopathology confirms the diagnosis of keratoacanthoma, it is sometimes justifiable to follow the patient carefully rather than instituting surgical or radiation therapy. In a case of any questionable pathology, the lesion should be treated as though it were a squamous cell carcinoma. At times, even true keratoacanthomas may grow to substantial size, particularly on the face, producing quite a great deal of disfigurement before the tumor regresses and resulting in considerable scarring and disfigurement after the tumor regresses. Therefore, if there is any evidence of continued growth of the lesion, therapy should promptly be instituted.

Skin Appendage Carcinoma

Fortunately, carcinoma of the skin affecting the appendages is quite uncommon. This sort of carcinoma is quite aggressive and results in a high frequency of metastatic disease.[41]

There are three major types of adnexal carcinomas: pilar, sebaceous, and sweat gland carcinomas. The malignant pilar carcinomas originating from hair follicles are extremely rare and are called malignant tricholemmoma and trichochlamydocarcinoma. Apparently, these tumors tend to occur on the scalp of elderly women and may metastasize to lymph nodes.

Sebaceous carcinomas are also rare, but not as rare as the pilar carcinoma. Sebaceous carcinomas arise most often in the meibomian glands of the eyelids, and rarely in the glands of Zeis and in the sebaceous glands of the caruncle. In addition, they may occur on the nose, eyebrow, ear, lower lip, trunk, arms, and skin of the neck. These lesions tend to occur in patients over 40, and usually over 60 years of age. These tumors have no specific morphologic features that lead to a reliable clinical diagnosis, but must be diagnosed based on the histopathology. These tumors are very malignant, tend to metastasize to lymph nodes, but also to bones and other organs. A fatal outcome may occur in some 20% of the patients.

As of 1976, a review of the literature found 48 cases of metastatic sweat gland carcinoma, excluding cases of extramammary Paget's disease, carcinomas of ceruminous glands, and carcinomas of the glands of Moll.[41] These tumors are the

FIG. 30-11. Keratoacanthoma on nose.

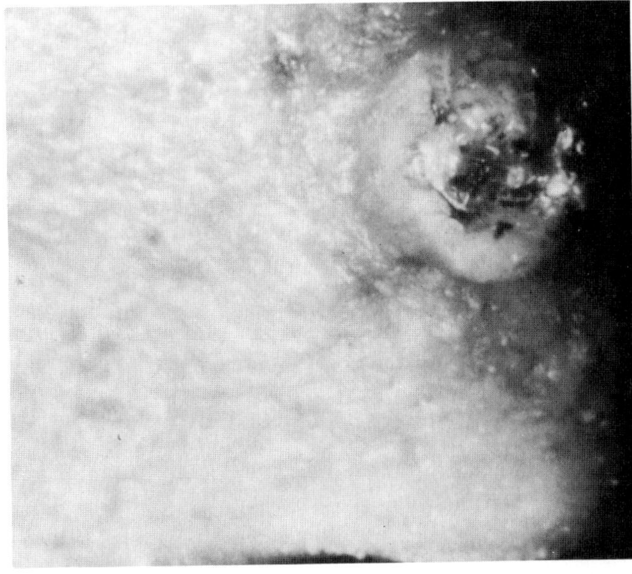

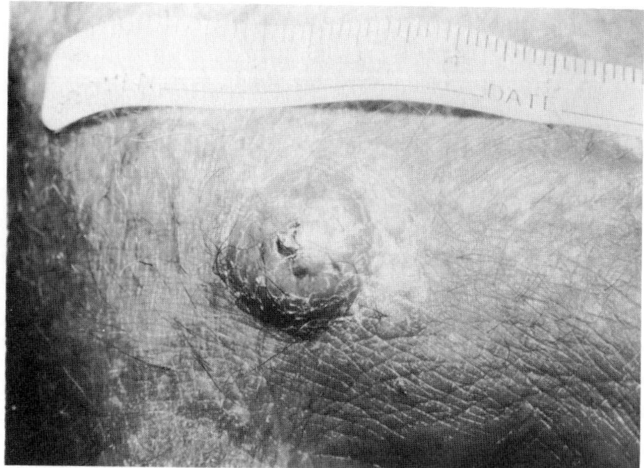

FIG. 30-12. Keratoacanthoma on dorsum of the head.

clear cell malignant hidradenoma or hidradenocarcinoma, malignant mixed tumor, and the eccrine porocarcinoma. They have no specific clinical features allowing clinical diagnosis, the appearance is generally that of a firm, nodular, hard mass, ulcerated at times, and red or purple in color. The skin of the head, particularly the scalp, is most commonly affected, but these lesions can also appear on the upper limbs, axilla, lower legs, trunk, vulva, and perianal area. The tumors grow slowly for a rather long period, then tend to suddenly increase in size and invade underlying tissues and metastasize. Metastases occur mostly to the regional lymph nodes, skin, bones, and lungs, and rarely to the brain, pelvis, and kidneys. Extramammary Paget's disease has a disputed histogenesis; some believe it to be an epidermal metastasis of an underlying ductal carcinoma, usually apocrine. Some, however, feel it is a localized epidermal de-differentiation that spreads downward to the gland ducts or the glands themselves. These lesions are generally located wherever apocrine sweat glands are found, primarily in the anogenital area, the axilla, and the areola of the breasts. The lesions are generally red plaques with flaking, scaling, and oozing that spreads to increasing size over time. Initially, these lesions may be misdiagnosed as yeast or fungal infection, eczematous dermatitis, or psoriasis. These lesions must be regarded at least as carcinoma *in situ,* and the possibility that they represent a superficial epidermal metastasis from an underlying adenocarcinoma must strongly be considered. These lesions will generally be treated by surgical extirpation. The question of depth of involvement will be answered by the histopathologic examination. It is clear that metastatic disease can occur from these lesions, although the figures on incidence are unclear.

METHODS OF DIAGNOSIS AND STAGING

In general, the principles of diagnosis and staging of the various kinds of skin cancer are similar. The diagnosis is either strongly suspected clinically, particularly for lesions such as basal and squamous cell carcinoma, or it is clinically atypical, with the diagnosis unknown until biopsy results are available. In addition, there is a lesion that was thought to be some other benign problem but failed to respond to treatment, was subsequently biopsied, and yielded the correct diagnosis. In the case of basal cell carcinoma, the most important staging is based on physical examination to determine the size of the lesion and its degree of invasion. If the lesion has invaded neurovascular bundles, bone, brain, and such, specialized complex therapy will obviously be required. Because the incidence of metastatic disease from basal cell carcinomas is so small, no work-up for this (other than a physical examination) is generally indicated unless some sign or symptom warrants further investigation. In the case of squamous cell carcinoma, it should be routine that a very careful lymph node examination is done during the physical examination; that should be adequate for most lesions arising in sun-exposed areas for which the potential of metastatic disease is rather low. In the case of squamous cell carcinoma arising on skin not exposed to the sun, (particularly in the anogenital area) gallium scans, lymphangiogram, liver-spleen scan, and chest films may be performed to investigate the possibility of metastatic disease before proceeding with therapy. Similar procedures are often indicated for chronic ulcers that have been found to be squamous cell carcinoma, or for those carcinomas arising in burn scars or in scars from radiation therapy. (These lesions tend to be more malignant than those arising on normal sun-exposed skin.) In the case of squamous cell carcinoma *in situ*, no major work-up is necessary other than removal of the lesion when it is located on sun-exposed skin. When located on skin not exposed to the sun some thought should be given as to whether there might be a concurrent internal malignancy of unrelated histology, and whether appropriate work-up should be done as indicated by screening tests after the history and physical examination. The lesion itself, however, will be cured by local removal or local ablation by cryosurgery or radiation therapy. Diagnosis of keratoacanthoma is done by clinical appearance and the histopathology; other than removal of the lesion, no staging is necessary. The skin appendage carcinomas, as mentioned previously, require diagnosis by histopathology as their clinical appearance is often atypical. Because of the frequency of metastases to local lymph nodes and bone, a careful physical examination and appropriate radiologic examination of these organs should be routine in these rare cases.

PATHOLOGY OF SKIN CANCER

The skin can be the site of origin or involvement of a substantial variety of neoplasms among which are such entities as the cutaneous T-cell lymphomas, including mycosis fungoides and Sezary's syndrome, melanoma, Kaposi's sarcoma and other dermal tumors, in addition to metastatic malignancies from a number of primary sites. However, the large majority of skin cancers are epithelial tumors arising from the epidermis and dermal appendages. The discussion of gross and microscopic pathology will be limited to these epithelial tumors, including basal cell carcinoma, squamous cell carcinoma, keratoacanthoma, the skin appendage tumors, and Bowen's disease. The reader should note that the histopathology of skin is well covered by Lever.[42]

Basal cell carcinoma is a very common form of skin cancer. It is believed by many to arise from cells in the basal layer of the epidermis, but some dispute this, regarding the cells of the dermal adenexa as the site of origin. The tumor is locally invasive but metastasizes quite rarely. Because of this feature the term *epithelioma* is preferred by some to *carcinoma*. In the rare instances of metastasis, the most common site of involvement is the regional lymph nodes; however metastases to bones, lung, and liver have been reported.[43] The large majority of basal cell carcinomas arise in regions of the body commonly exposed to the sun's rays. Between 80% and 90% of these neoplasms are found on the head and neck. Most of the remaining sites are distributed about the anterior and posterior trunk (10%) and the extremities (7%), with something under one percent appearing in the genital and perianal regions.[44]

The subclassification of basal carcinoma varies widely among authors and is generally based on either gross or histopathologic appearance. As many as ten different types have been described but the varieties most commonly encountered both in the clinic and literature include the following:

1. Nodular or nondular–ulcerative
2. Superficial
3. Pigmented
4. Cystic
5. Infiltrating or morphea-like

The nodular type is the most common form.

Histologically, basal cell carcinomas occur in a variety or patterns but the tumor cell usually has a large oval nucleus with fine chromatin and stains deeply basophilic. There is little cytoplasm and mitoses are scarce. The peripheral cells of individual tumor clusters line up in a highly characteristic palisade formation. The tumor cells form small nodular clusters, lace-like strands, and may show a glandular or cystic structure. Frequently what appears to be the point of origin in the basal layer of the epidermis is noted with nests of tumor cells extending down from this point into the dermis. In the superficial type there may be multiple such seeming points of origin with tumor cells extending into the dermis only to a depth equal to about twice the thickness of the epidermis. In infiltrating carcinoma, the stroma of the tumor predominates. It consists of dense connective tissue composed of both elastic and collagen fibers running throughout, within which are actually strands and small nests of tumor cells presenting the appearance of basal cells with oval basophilic nuclei. The appearance is reminiscent of the so-called "scirrhous" form of carcinoma of the breast.

Squamous cell carcinoma of the skin (also termed epidermoid carcinoma or prickle cell carcinoma) is second only to basal cell carcinoma in frequency in the U.S. and in other parts of the world where white populations predominate. However, among other ethnic groups squamous cell carcinoma is often the more common skin cancer.[45] The gross pathology of squamous cell carcinoma varies considerably. Often the lesions are simply ulcerated, crusted areas on the skin. At other times they may present in the early stages as an elevated nodule or plaque covered by excessive keratin. A verrucous configuration is also seen. The gross margins of these lesions tend to be less well-demarcated than that seen in basal cell carcinoma. In addition, since they tend to infiltrate more deeply, attachment to underlying structures is more common. Metastasis to lymph nodes occurs much more often than with basal cell carcinomas and in advanced stages metastasis may involve other organs, such as the lungs and liver. This is particularly true of the higher grade, less well-differentiated lesions.

Histologically, squamous cell carcinoma of the skin resembles neoplasms arising from stratified squamous eqithelium in other organ sites. In a well-differentiated tumor, the cellular appearance is similar to that seen in normal squamous epithelium with a large, polygonal outline; intercellular bridges; pale staining eosinophilic cytoplasm; and round nuclei. Keratinization of individual cells and formation of keratin pearls are common. As the tumors become less well-differentiated, keratinization and keratin pearls diminish, in higher grade tumors these changes are absent. Nuclei become more bizzare in shape and mitoses more numerous. The cells tend to lose their polygonal shape, become more elongated, and in high grade tumors they may be fusiform in appearance, resembling sarcoma cells. As might be expected, the low grade tumors tend to be relatively slow growing and show little aggressiveness toward invading other tissues. On the other hand, high grade tumors may be expected to invade relatively early, becoming readily fixed to underlying structures. Fortunately the majority of squamous cell carcinomas of the skin are of the lower grade varieties.

Keratoacanthoma is a lesion that may be easily confused with squamous cell carcinoma on clinical and histologic grounds.

Histologically, three stages are described. Initially there is marked proliferation of the epithelial cells with rapid extension into the dermis of tumor cells nests. Atypism may be noted in the advancing rim of these nests. In the second stage, a continued proliferation of the squamous cells with keratinization and formation of the characteristic keratin plug exists. In the third stage, involution occurs with dissolution of the nests; these cells are then surrounded by an inflammatory infiltrate of lymphocytes and histiocytes. The involution of the tumor cells is followed by scarring of the dermis. Many of the features (*i.e.*, cellular atypism and perforation of the basement membrane) are histologically indistinguishable from squamous cell carcinoma. In view of the marked difference in treatment of the two lesions, it is of great importance to correctly diagnose the nature of this lesion by close collaboration between the dermatologist and pathologist. The tragic results of incorrect diagnosis has been documented by Jackson, describing the development of metastatic disease from squamous cell carcinomas incorrectly diagnosed as keratoacanthomas and not removed as spontaneous involution was anticipated.[46] To provide adequate material for histopathology, an excisional biopsy or a generous wedge incisional biopsy should be done. A 3 mm or 4 mm punch biopsy is often inadequate.

Malignant tumors arising in the skin appendages are relatively rare. Sebaceous gland carcinoma usually develops on the face or scalp and its gross appearance is that of a hard yellow nodule that slowly enlarges. If left untreated it will eventually ulcerate. This lesion is capable of metastasis, generally to regional lymph nodes. Histologically, the tumor consists of sebaceous cells with large nuclei, prominent nucleoli, and foamy cytoplasm. Numerous mitotic figures are seen. Intermixed with these atypical cells may be normal-appearing sebaceous cells. Other varieties of sebaceous carcinoma include basal cell carcinoma with sebaceous differentiation and squamous cell carcinoma with sebaceous differentiation. Of the three, the pure sebaceous gland carcinoma is said to be the most malignant.[47]

Sweat gland carcinoma are so rare that the almost anecodotal case reports in the literature offer little by way of characterizing their distribution or appearance. They have been said to appear largely on the head, upper extremities, or on the trunk above the nipple line. However, Hirsh and coworkers, in a study of seven patients, could not bear this out.[48] These authors also found the gross appearance to vary considerably from the violaceous appearance previously attributed to this tumor. The tumors are usually small, very slow growing, and present as a skin nodule that can eventually ulcerate. They appear to have considerable capacity for metastasis, generally by way of the lymphatics.

Bowen's disease, frequently referred to as a premalignant lesion of the skin, is actually carcinoma *in-situ* of the skin. In contrast to basal cell carcinoma and squamous cell carcinoma, Bowen's disease often appears on unexposed areas of the skin. Characteristically, it is a minimally elevated, erythematous, plaque-like lesion with scaling or crusting. It tends to enlarge at a very slow rate and may reach considerable size before treatment is started. While some cases of Bowen's disease progress to invasive squamous cell carcinoma, many do not, even over long periods. Graham and Helwig have reported a much higher-than-normal incidence of internal organ malignancy in patients with Bowen's disease.[49]

Histologically, the appearance is that of an intact basement membrane with an orderly, normal-appearing basal layer above. However, starting just superficial to the basal layer, the cells show a loss of polarity with many large atypical nuclei and frequent mitoses. There is little evidence of cell maturation as they approach the surface. Bizzare giant cells with abnormal mitotic figures may be present.

TREATMENT

BIOPSY

The purpose of a biopsy is to obtain tissue to establish a diagnosis by microscopic analysis. It may be incisional or excisional, an incisional biopsy taking only a portion of a lesion, while an excisional biopsy is the equivalent of an excision since it removes the lesion in its entirety. To gather the most information, an incisional biopsy should have an adequate amount of tissue and come from a suspicious or characteristic part of the growth. When in doubt about arriving at a diagnosis, biopsies from more than one area should be submitted.

For some skin cancers that are small and are *not* located where primary closure may be difficult (*i.e.*, the nasal tip or tarsal plate), an excisional biopsy (excision) is usually easier for the patient. Here only one procedure is endured and the tumor is gone. An excisional biopsy has the advantage of providing the pathologist with a complete specimen, whereas an incisional biopsy may furnish an unrepresentative portion. Another disadvantage of an incisional biopsy is that after it is completed for very small lesions, it may be difficult to find the biopsy site for an adequate excision, if it is necessary.

An incisional biopsy, especially for a lesion that is large or on the face, *does* have the advantages of letting both the patient and surgeon know the precise diagnosis (if the biopsy is representative) without inflicting excessive scarring or deformity. Then the various alternative treatments can be discussed.

EXCISION

The patient must understand the purpose of excision, whether it is for a premalignant or malignant growth, at least as far as can be determined by available information. If a physician tells a patient that he has a skin cancer, the patient should receive the assurance, if justified, that almost all skin cancers (except for the very advanced) can be cured. The word "cancer" has so many frightening connotations for most patients that it is wise to differentiate between the less serious consequences of having a skin cancer (epithelioma) and a cancer of the lung, breast, or stomach. Furthermore, the surgeon can be even more optimistic if the patient's skin cancer is basal cell carcinoma.

The principal advantage of surgical excision is that it removes the lesion in one comparatively brief and usually uncomplicated procedure. It also allows a definitive assessment of the extent of the neoplasm by an examination of the margins of resection.

Any biopsy, and most excisions, of small and moderate-sized cutaneous cancers in healthy patients can be done under local anesthesia, generally on an out-patient basis. Incisional punch biopsies can easily be done in the office with the use of disposable kits. The punches are available in diameters of 2, 3, 4, and 6 mm; the 4 mm size is almost always appropriate. After skin preparation the site is infiltrated with 0.5 ml or less of lidocaine, 1% or 2%; the preparations containing epinephrine are excellent for improving hemostasis. The skin is stretched taut in the direction at right angles from the line of stress. The punch is rotated back and forth with the thumb and index finger while modest downward pressure is applied. It is usually easy to feel when the punch enters the subcutaneous fat. The biopsy specimen is then easily removed with care to avoid crushing the specimen. The biopsy site will usually assume an elliptical shape after the stretch is discontinued and can easily be closed with a single 5–0 nylon suture or left to heal by secondary intention.

A classic surgical excision can be wedge-shaped, circular, or elliptical (really lenticular since a true elipse is round at each end rather than angular).[51] Wedge excisions are usually for lesions adjacent to free margins of skin, as on the lip, nostril rim, tarsus, or ear. A circular excision of a small lesion has the advantages of sacrificing a minimal amount of normal tissue while producing a shorter scar than would result from an elliptical excision. For large lesions, closing the circular defect may create considerable tension and unwelcomed

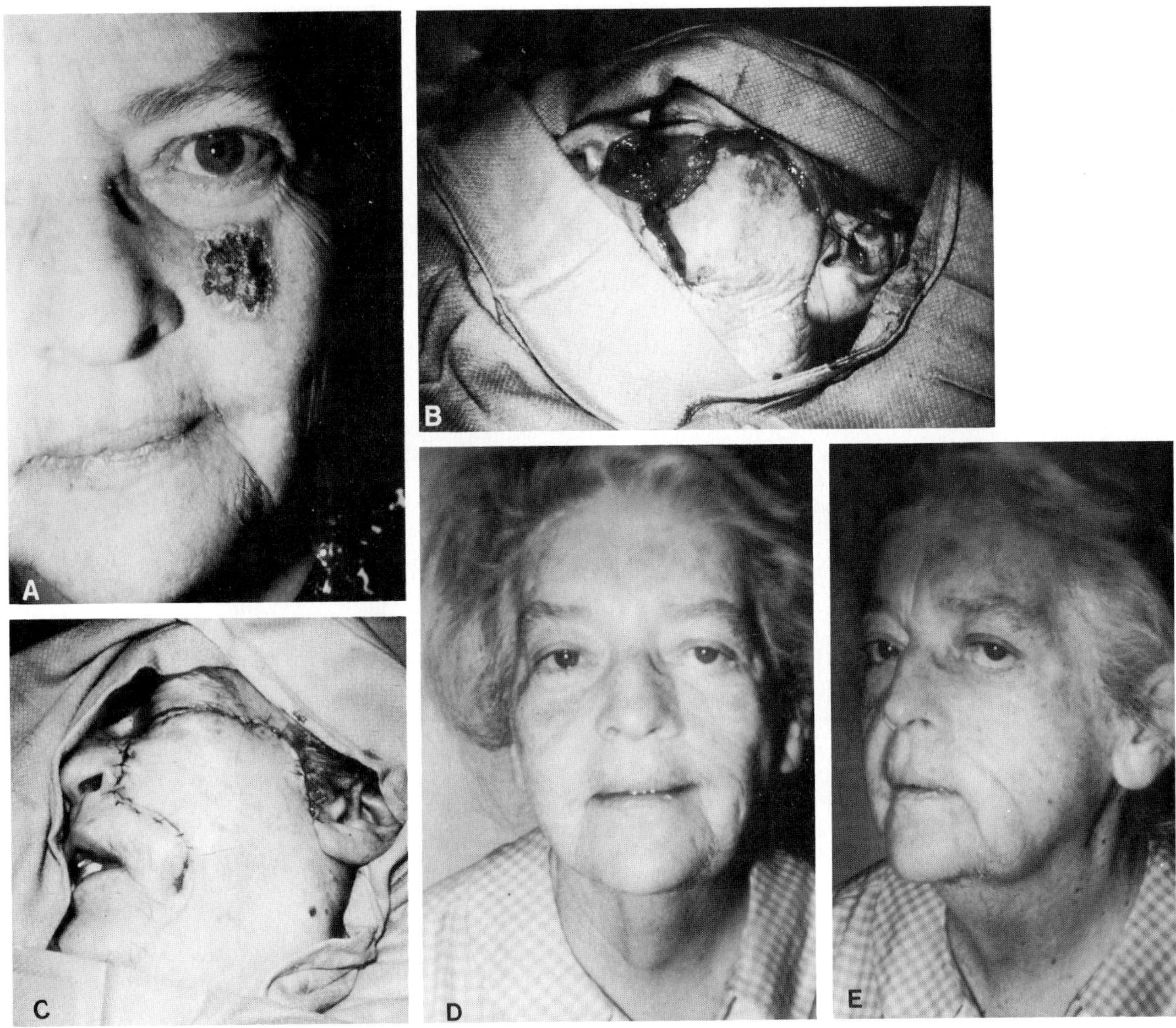

FIG. 30-13. *A*, Preoperative, 68-year-old woman with an untreated large basal cell carcinoma of left cheek. *B*, Intraoperative, following excision of basal cell carcinoma. All margins free according to multiple frozen sections. Note outline of cheek flap to be advanced into defect. *C*, Intraoperative, closure by means of advanced cheek flap. *D, E*, One year postoperative. Note normal facial nerve functioning. The patient is now 8 years without recurrence.

puckering; the final scar may be round and thick. The surgeon's elipse (elliptical excision) is the most common form of skin cancer removal and primary approximating of the skin edges is the most frequent method of closing the defect. However, if the lesion is large or located where insufficient tissue exists for primary closure without producing a deformity (*i.e.*,electropion with excision of a lesion on the lower eyelid), additional skin may be necessary in the form of a flap or graft.[52,53]

Skin Grafts

A skin flap has skin and subcutaneous tissue that is moved from one part of the body to another. However it has an attachment at its base through which it receives its nourishment and blood supply. A skin graft has no vascular pedicle; it is completely detached and easily transplanted from one area of the body to another.

A flap brings its own blood supply; a skin graft depends on the vascularity of the recipient site for its survival. For this reason, a skin graft will not take over a cavity or an avascular bed, which is commonly encountered in areas of radiation necrosis. Skin grafts also fall in the presence of infection, hematoma, or inadequate immobilization.

Flaps may be either local or distal. A local flap has the advantages of supplying ready tissue similar in color or texture to that excised. (See Figs. 30-13 through 30-20). A skin graft usually looks like a patch because of its dissimilar

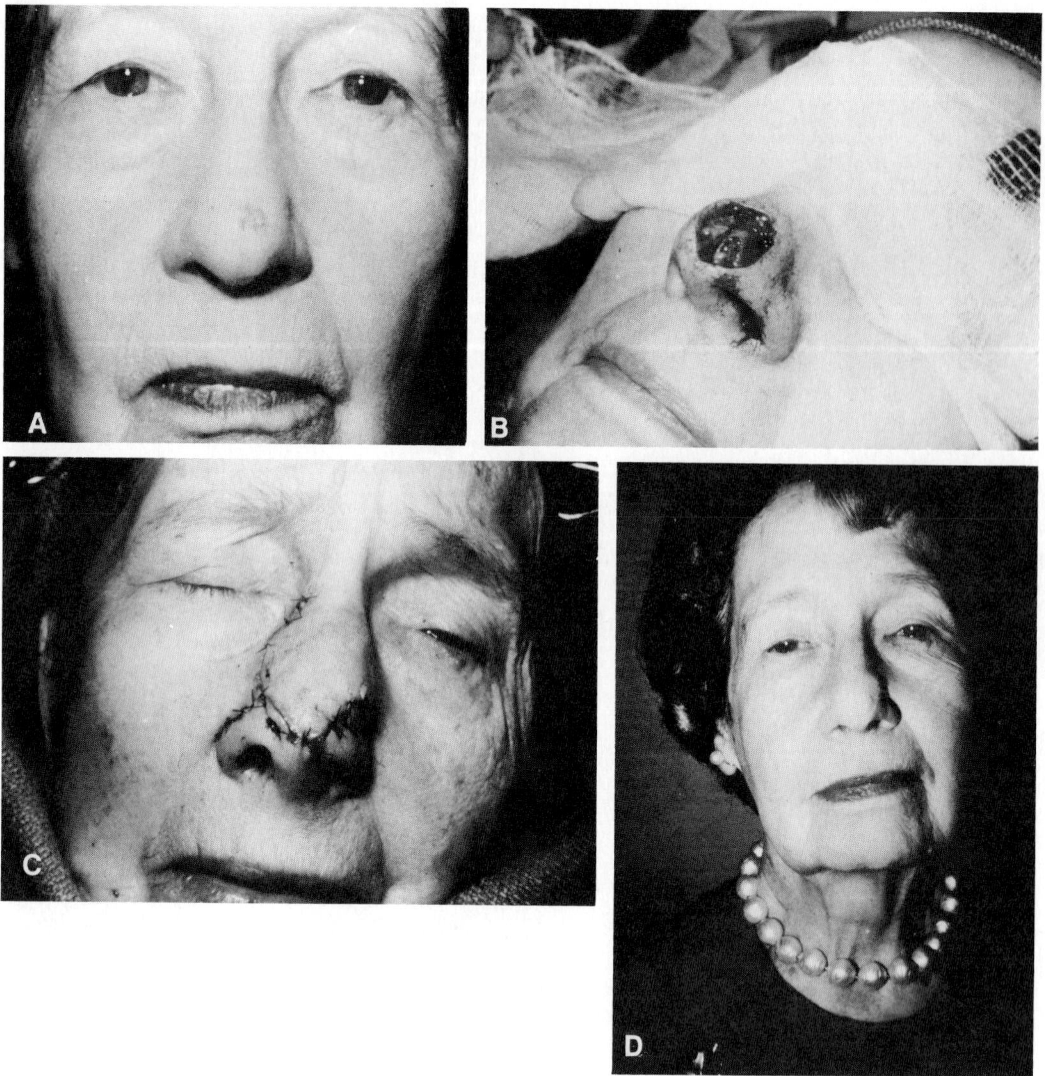

FIG. 30-14. *A,* Preoperative, 72-year-old woman with an extensive basal cell carcinoma at the tip of her nose, cartilage involved. *B,* Intraoperative defect following excision. Frozen sections of margins showed no tumor. The operation is being done under local anesthesia. *C,* Intraoperative, a large flap of nasal skin has been rotated downward to cover the defect. *D,* Postoperative, 6 years. The patient is free of tumor. The result cosmetically could be improved by a revision of the flap but the patient does not want more surgery.

thickness and hue compared to the tissue removed (see Figs. 30-21 and 30-22). Ideally, like skin should replace like skin (*i.e.,* eyelid for eyelid). This aim, however, is not always possible because many times the donor site would then have an objectionable deformity. The postauricular area is a good bank of skin. It is well hidden and closely resembles that on the face. In general, the thicker the graft, the less the subsequent contracture of the wound. A full-thickness skin graft, as from behind the ear, has all layers of skin and is preferable cosmetically to a split-thickness graft, which contains only epidermis and a segment of dermis. However, because the full-thickness graft has more tissue than a split-thickness graft, its vascular-nutritional requirements are greater. The practical consequence is that it may not take, whereas a less thick (split-thickness) skin graft will.

Factors favoring a good scar following excision and primary closure (no flap or graft) include:

Excision of the lesion in lines of facial expression.
Proper technique performed relatively atraumatically.
Inherent ability of the patient to heal well.

Some patients and their families characteristically form hypertrophic scars and keloids. Therefore, all patients should be questioned concerning their history of past healing. Age makes a difference also. Adolescents, for example, are more likely to form scars that are raised and red than are their parents and grandparents. In addition, thick oily skin with hyperactive sebaceous glands is not condusive to fine scars.

Favored Sites of Excisions

Incisions in the lower eyelids, for example, usually heal much better than those on the sternum, back, or tip of the shoulder or nose.

Uneventful Healing

A postoperative course complicated by infection and hematoma augurs poorly for eventful scarring. Removal of sutures at the proper time—not too early (dehiscence) or too late (stitch mark)—is essential.

Informing the Patient

Whether a biopsy, incisional or excisional, is done with primary closure, flap, or graft, the rationale of treatment and the realities of the procedure must be explained to the patient. This includes type of anesthesia (local or general), degree of pain, appearance of the scar. The latter factor is what often concerns the patient the most. While the physician thinks in terms of cure the patient thinks more in terms of deformity. From any excision, a patient must expect a scar. Furthermore, no surgeon can guarantee what the scar will look like. If a flap or skin graft is planned, a scar and discomfort at the donor site should be expected. The flap or a graft is necessary; it is important for the patient to understand why it is important and why one and not the other will be used. The operation can be explained by outlining the incision(s) with a marking pencil while the patient is looking in the mirror (this is done at the initial consultation). For example, most patients with a basal cell carcinoma may not understand why it is necessary to excise so far beyond what they judge to be the size of the lesion. These patients must be told that the tumor grows like an iceberg, the most visible part having the smallest diameter. If a lymph node dissection is also planned, this, of course, must also be discussed (see Fig. 30-22C).

Occasionally, a lesion that has had an incisional biopsy with a diagnosis of a basal cell carcinoma will then be excised and no tumor will be found. This is likely to happen with small lesions. The patient should be forewarned of that possibility; otherwise, he will think that he has been subjected to unnecessary surgery. Expecting more tumor but finding none can also occur with lesions that have been incompletely excised. Again, the patient must be prepared for the possibility that going back a few weeks later may not produce more cancer.

The basic objective of the excision is to totally remove the malignancy with enough margin for cure. A surgeon who skimps on the extent of the excision because he fears he cannot close the defect does the patient harm and himself little good. Some lesions that are large, in a conspicuous area such as the face, or some that will present problems in closure following adequate excision should be referred at the outset to a plastic surgeon or the equivalent. The first attempt at excision is the patient's best chance for cure. An inadequately removed tumor or one that is recurrent makes the patient undergo a more extensive operation next time, perhaps necessitating hospital admission and general anesthesia. Then, recovery will be longer, recurrence more likely, and deformity more definite.

The use of frozen sections at the time of excision is helpful when the surgeon is uncertain about the margins of the tumor. In some situations, the surgeon may choose not to use a flap for closure (even though it will give a cosmetically better result) but to employ a skin graft until either the permanent sections confirm adequacy of resection or the subsequent course for the patient indicates that he is free of malignancy, especially if the tumor is recurrent, aggressive histologically, or both.

FIG. 30-15. *A*, Preoperative, 62-year-old man with basal cell carcinoma involving tragus. *B*, Intraoperative defect produced by excision. Note outline of rotation flap. *C*, Intraoperative; flap has been rotated for closure.

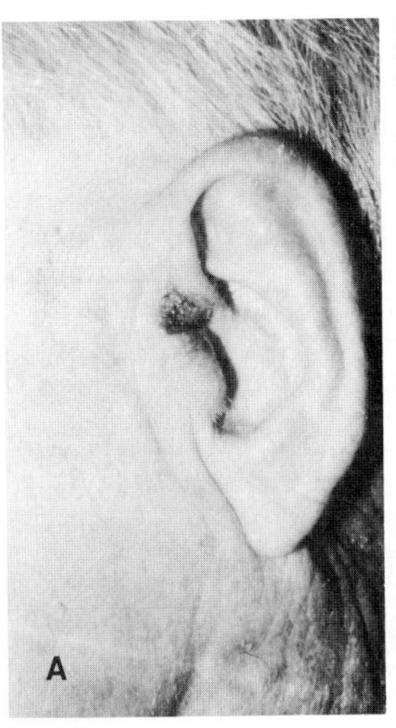

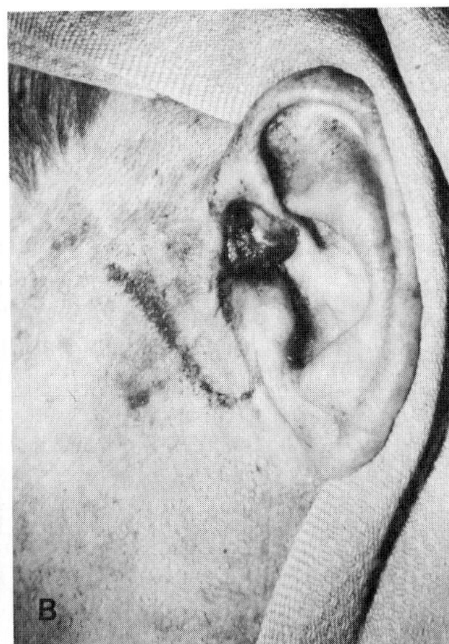

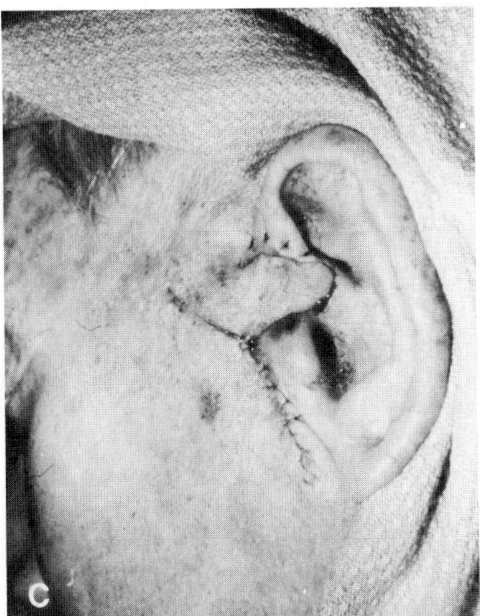

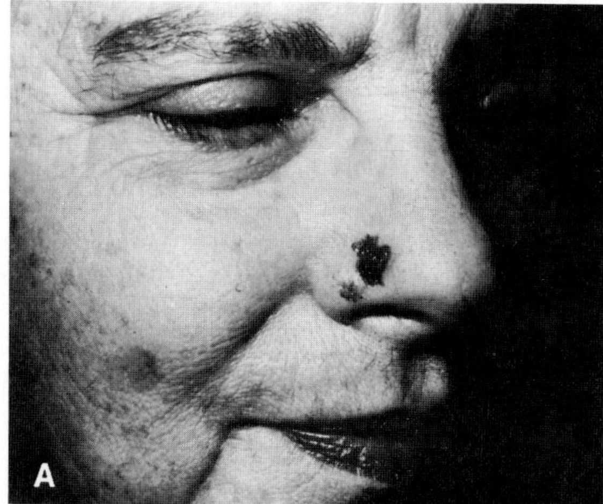

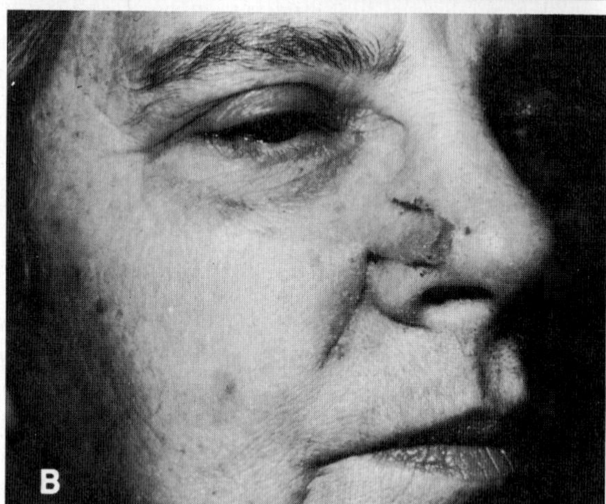

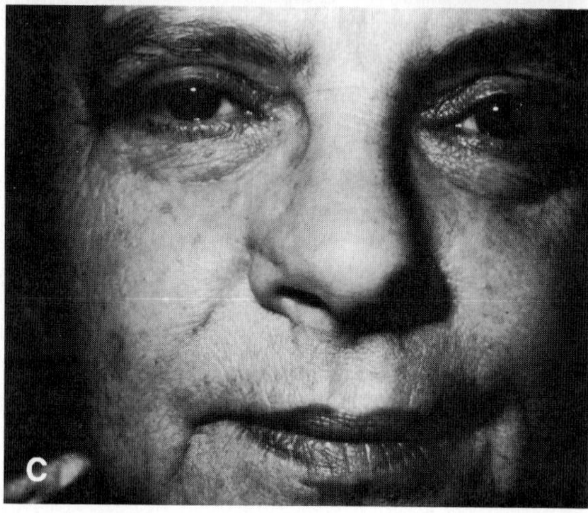

FIG. 30-16. *A*, Preoperative, 52-year-old woman with pigmented basal cell carcinoma near right nostril rim. *B*, Postoperative, 12 days following excision and rotation of nasolabial flap. *C*, Postoperative, 9 months. The patient has been free of recurrence for 12 years.

CURETTAGE

Curettage is a reasonable treatment for basal call carcinomas that are neither recurrent nor fibrotic nor extending into deep underlying tissues.[50] It is not an appropriate therapy for any other carcinomas of the skin. The technique basically involves local anesthesia with xylocaine containing epinephrine, followed by scooping out the tumor with sharp curettes, beginning with 1, 3, or 4 mm in diameter, and ending with a small curette 1 or 2 mm in diameter to search for the soft, mushy, finger-like projections of tumor that may occur at the margins. Normal dermis is quite resistant to removal by the currette; this physical property of tumor friability and normal tissue firmness constitutes the basis for the procedure. It is common to treat the base after curettage by electrodessication and perform a second curettage of the charred tissue. However, this may not be a necessary feature of the procedure. Effective, careful curettage by itself will accomplish an equal cure rate and a superior cosmetic result. The lesions are allowed to heal by secondary intention while being treated, usually with a topical antibiotic or antiseptic such as erythromycin ointment, or Silvadene cream. The cure rate is comparable to other procedures (in excess of 95%). The cosmetic result is excellent because of the wound contraction in many cases, although a smooth hypopigmented scar does result. Quite a bit of expertise in wielding the curette is necessary for an operator to be able to achieve optimal cure rates. This procedure can be used to provide tissue for biopsy diagnosis and a therapeutic procedure at one sitting. The disadvantage of this procedure is that no tissue margins are presented to the pathologist for examination or for confirmation of complete extirpation. In spite of this defect, however, statistics show it to be a reliably curative procedure in properly selected lesions.

CRYOSURGERY

Cryosurgery employing liquid nitrogen has been used in skin cancer therapy for a reasonably short time. It is only since the late 1960's that it was used in scattered academic centers in the U.S., but it has gained wide acceptance since the early 1970's. Most lesions that are suitable for curettage are also suitable for cryosurgery. In addition, lesions that are recurrent after previous therapy by x-irradiation, curettage, or by cryosurgery itself are amenable to retreatment by cryosurgery in carefully selected cases. Carcinomas having a significant component of fibrosis on a spontaneous basis are also amenable to cryosurgery, whereas they would not be able to be adequately treated by curettage. A biopsy diagnosis is necessary before cryosurgery, as the procedure does not provide tissue for examination.

There are many ways of performing cryosurgery using different techniques and equipment.[54,55,56] Most operators now employ techniques providing a liquid nitrogen spray that is directed at the tumor. In certain instances, a solid probe is applied to the tumor with liquid nitrogen circulated through it. Anesthesia is generally not necessary during the procedure as the liquid nitrogen provides a measure of its own anesthesia when the nerves are frozen. Only lesions reasonably limited to skin are appropriate for this form of therapy. The operator must carefully assess the outermost margins of the lesion by careful palpation and sidelighting with a spot source of illumination. The margins of the lesion so defined then should be marked with some form of skin marking instrument. An additional margin (usually 2–5 mm) is drawn around this to ensure complete inclusion of the lesion within the treatment area. If the liquid nitrogen spray is directed at the center of the tumor and the tumor allowed to freeze out to the treatment margin by conduction, then maintained at that area by an additional freezing for approximately 30 seconds, it will be found that the depth of freezing is appropriate for cure of the lesion. A rough rule of thumb is that the depth would equal roughly one-half the radius under these circumstances if the closest point-source, as possible, of spray is used. Generally, the depth of freezing can be adequately detected by physical examination of the ice ball while it is frozen. If any doubt exists a thermocouple needle can be inserted just deep to where the operative field of the lesion extends prior to treatment. Then, treatment can be monitored by the temperature registered by the needle. A temperature of −20°C is the ideal temperature to ensure a lethal effect on cells.

The lesion is then allowed to thaw. Slow thawing is felt to be more lethal to the tissue than rapid thawing. Rapid thawing, of course, is used in cases of frostbite to prevent as much tissue injury as possible. Another rough clinical indication of the adequacy of freezing is measuring the number of minutes it takes for the lesion to completely thaw after ceasing nitrogen application. For most small lesions on face and neck this should be at least one and a half minutes, for lesions of the skin of the back generally two or more minutes is required. It is customary to use two freeze-thaw cycles. The second freeze-thaw cycle can be adjusted to some extent to compensate for excessive or inadequate freezing on the first cycle. Even eyelid lesions can be treated with this technique if a thermal shield is placed over the globe. The cure rates from this procedure are generally between 95–97%, although most operators feel that scalp lesions have the highest recurrence rate of any site. Intraoperative pain is usually minimal, postoperative pain is generally not a problem, although in some patients, particularly when bone has been involved by the technique, there may be significant pain for a few days, which is usually relieved by aspirin-type analgesia and cool compresses. The frozen tissue develops edema within minutes of the therapy, followed within a day by purpura, and usually bulla formation. Erosion is then left after the tumor sloughs. This erosion is generally treated by a bacitracin ointment or an anti-infective, such as Silvadene cream, twice daily and allowed to be washed twice daily. Healing from the edges begins to occur after the first week, and is usually completed by 3–4 weeks for lesions on the face, but significantly longer for lesions on the back, and longer still for lesions arising within scarred areas from previous therapy, particularly from radiation therapy. Significant hemorrhage after treatment is rare. Damage to underlying nerves can occur from cryosurgery, so care must be taken to avoid treating major sensory and motor nerves in superficial locations. If accidental cryosurgery of nerves is performed, nerve function can generally be expected to return, although months may be required. The cosmetic results from cryotherapy are at least as good, and probably better, than those from curettage. A hypopigmented scar without hair growth is the result, but the scar tends to have functional qualities much like normal dermis, and often feels quite normal to the touch. The sequence of fractions to cryosurgery is shown in Fig. 30-23.

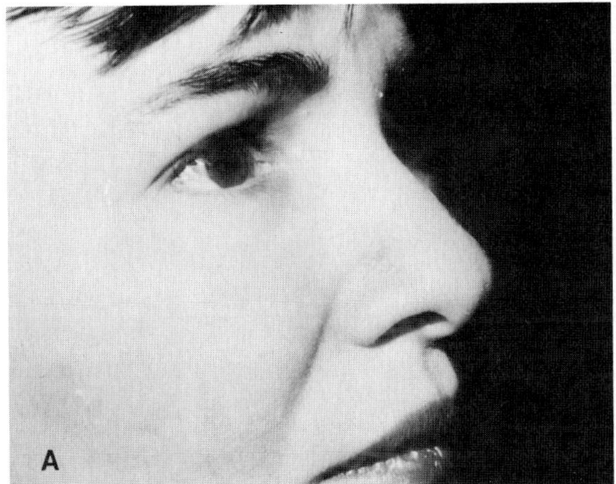

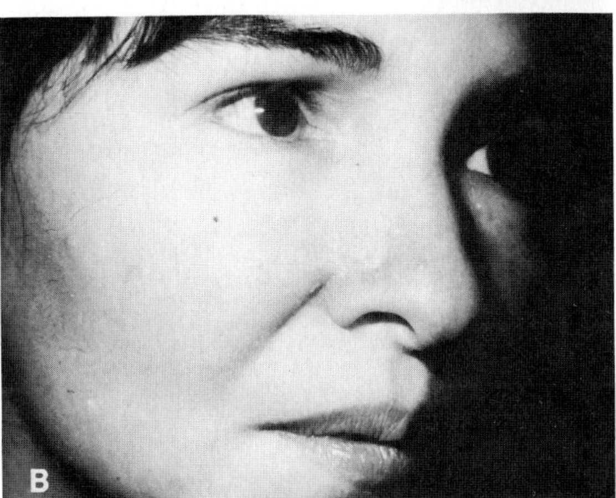

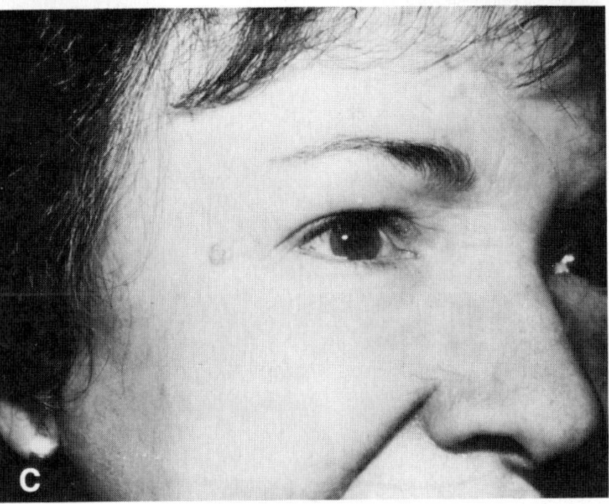

FIG. 30-17. *A*, Preoperative, 34-year-old woman with basal cell carcinoma of right nostril. *B*, Postoperative, 2 months following excision and nasolabial flap. *C*, Postoperative, 12 years with no evidence of recurrence.

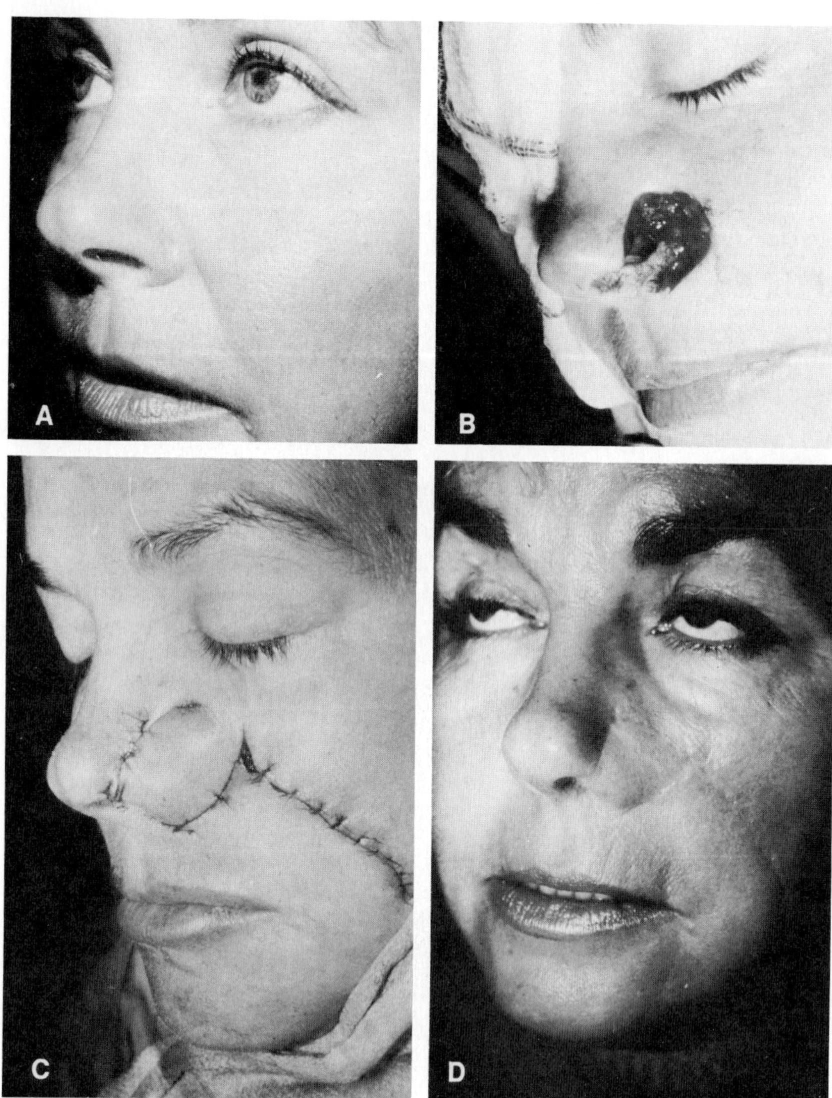

FIG. 30-18. *A,* Preoperative, 45-year-old woman with large infiltrating basal cell carcinoma of base of left nostril. *B,* Intraoperative, following wide excision. Frozen sections of margins showed no tumor. *C,* Intraoperative nasolabial flap used for coverage. *D,* Postoperative, 7 months. *E,* Postoperative, 9 months. *F, G,* Postoperative 4 years; no evidence of recurrence. (*Continues on facing page*)

This procedure is most appropriate for fair-skinned patients, who naturally form the bulk of patients with these lesions. In patients with very ruddy complexions or significant pigmentation, the resulting white scar will be cosmetically undesirable.

CHEMOSURGERY (MOHS' TECHNIQUE)

Dr. Mohs originated a microscopically controlled technique of excision of skin carcinoma called *Mohs' technique* or *chemosurgery*. The chemosurgery name came from the original form of the technique, in which the tissue to be removed was pretreated with zinc chloride paste, fixing it *in situ* before renewal. In recent years, this *in vivo* fixation is not a necessary part of the procedure; it is now commonly performed as a fresh tissue technique.[57] The technique basically employs the serial horizontal shave excision of skin carcinoma, followed by immediate careful mapping of the removed tissue so as to relate it to the wound, and frozen sections performed horizontally on the base of the excised specimen along the inferior margin of the tissue under local anesthesia. Any areas of the specimen found to contain tumor are assumed to be matched by residual tumor in the patient deep to the excision. These areas are then mapped out and re-excised, the specimens being examined in an identical fashion. This procedure continues serially until the excised specimen shows no evidence of tumor. Inasmuch as basal cell carcinomas extend by continuity, this technique allows the physician to follow the tumor wherever it leads, giving high assurance of complete removal, while allowing no removal of tissue that is not involved. The resulting ulceration is allowed to heal by secondary intention most often, with the resulting cosmetic results being much better than anticipated by looking at the extensive wound immediately after the procedure.

If necessary, cosmetic revision of the wound can be performed, either as a second stage, or in rare cases, as an

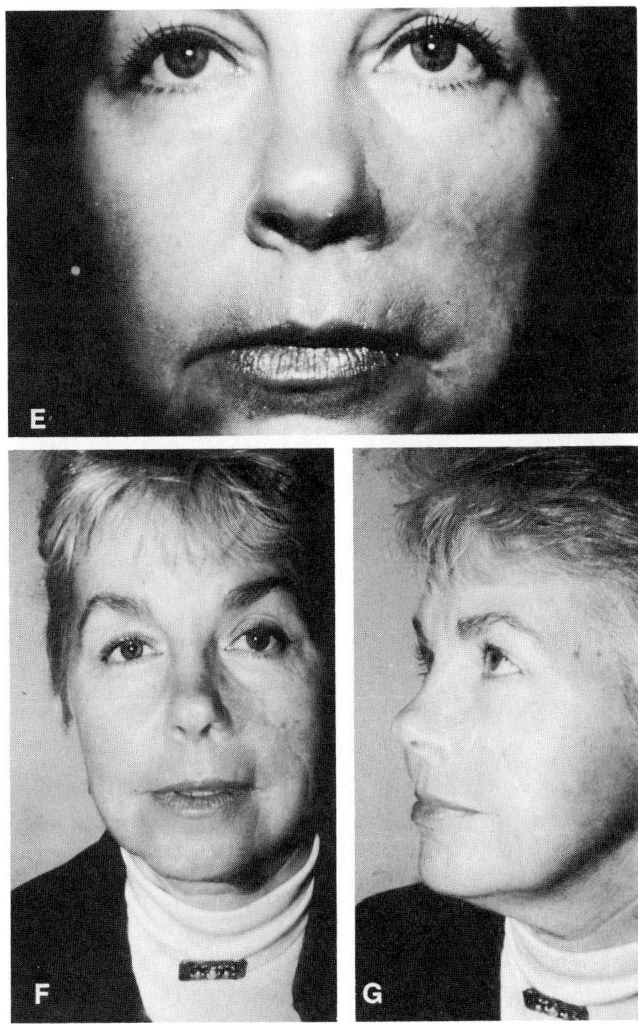

FIG. 30-18. *(Continued)*

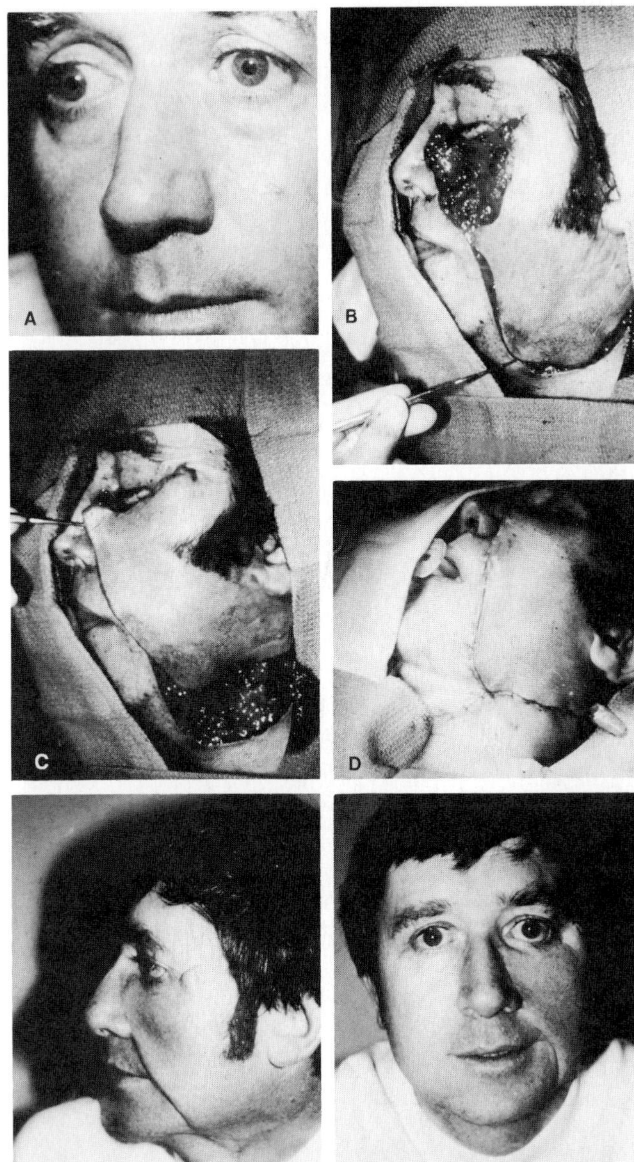

FIG. 30-19. *A*, Preoperative, 43-year-old man with sclerosing basal cell carcinoma of cheek infiltrating a much larger area than the photograph shows. *B*, Intraoperative, after excision with frozen sections to determine its adequacy. *C*, Intraoperative, cervicofacial flap used for coverage. *D*, Intraoperative, closure. *E*, *F*, Postoperative, 9 months. Patient is now 3½ years without recurrence.

immediate postoperative event. This technique has the highest cure rate for removal of skin carcinomas, being in excess of 99%. However, the operator must be highly trained and skilled in this technique for its successful implementation. There are only a few such highly and skillful operators at this time in the U.S. Therefore, patients are generally preselected for this procedure on the criteria of having lesions of unusual extent, poorly-defined margins, or recurrence after previous therapies

RADIATION THERAPY

Basal and squamous cell carcinomas of the skin are both highly curable by radiation therapy. However, certain exceptions do exist when the tumor has invaded bone. In addition, certain lesions, while treatable with radiation therapy, are better treated by other modalities because of previous damage to normal tissues in or about the tumor site. These include skin carcinomas arising in burn scars, in previously irradiated regions, and areas where the tumor itself has been deeply destructive, particularly to underlying cartilage, such as in the nose or ear.

Contrary to popular belief, there is no difference in the radiocurability of basal and squamous cell carcinoma of the skin. This point was analyzed by von Essen as part of a study of 565 skin cancers treated by irradiation.[58] He found no difference in the recurrence rate of these tumors nor that of mixed basosquamous carcinomas. It must be kept in mind, however, the potential for metastasis to lymph nodes by

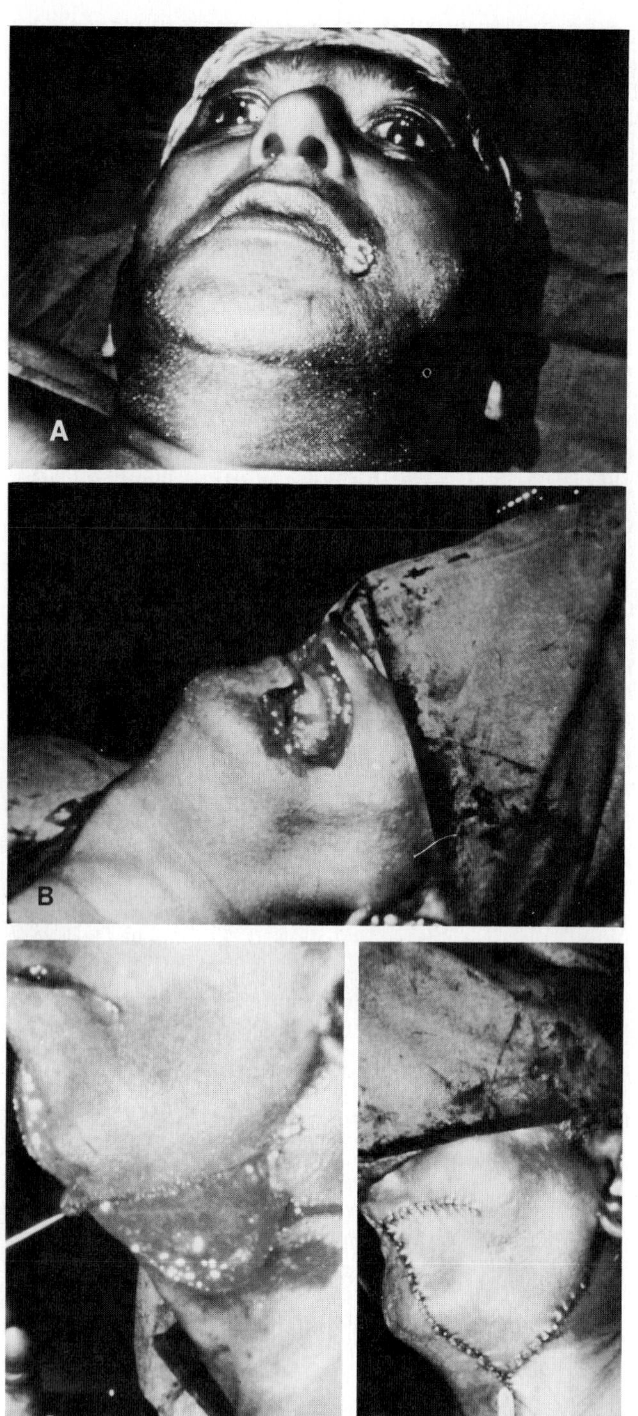

FIG. 30-20. *A,* Preoperative, 64-year-old man with squamous cell carcinoma of the left commissure and left cheek. *B,* Intraoperative, after excision. Frozen sections used to determine its adequacy. *C,* Intraoperative cervicofacial flap used for reconstruction of defect. *D,* Intraoperative, closure. Patient is now 10 years without recurrence.

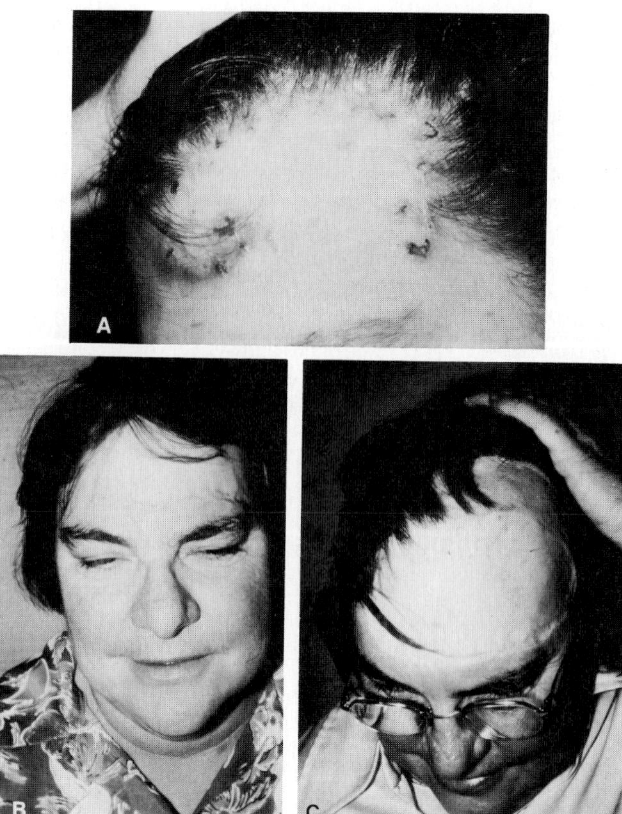

FIG. 30-21. *A,* Preoperative, 42-year-old woman treated for 8 years by cauterization, partial excision, and cryotherapy for recurrent basal cell carcinoma of forehead. *B,* Postoperative, one year, after wide excision and split thickness graft. A portion of the outer table had to be removed because of involvement by tumor. *C,* Postoperative, 2 years, no evidence of recurrence. Patient has been free of disease for 7 years.

squamous cell carcinoma, particularly those of the higher grades. This problem is almost never encountered with basal cell carcinoma.

The radiocurability of the skin appendage tumors (*i.e.*, sweat gland and sebaceous carcinomas) is less well documented. Such lesions have been successfully treated by irradiation, but since the majority are subjected to surgical excision with curative intent, the experience with radiation therapy of these tumors is limited.

Keratocanthoma is generally regarded as a self-limiting tumor. However, if allowed to run its natural course it will eventually heal. This lesion is occassionally treated by radiation therapy either because it is sited in a location where it may cause unacceptable destructive changes or because there is doubt in the minds of those responsible for treatment that it is not indeed a squamous cell carcinoma. When treated, it should be treated as a squamous cell carcinoma.

Bowen's disease is, too, a highly curable lesion with radiation therapy. In situations where large areas are involved, it may be preferable to employ irradiation to avoid grafting. The treatment, both in terms of radiation dose and fractionation, does not differ from that employed with invasive epithelial skin tumors.

In most instances, skin tumors of the above types are treated for cure. Rarely is a skin neoplasm seen of such extent and location that a palliative philosophy must be adopted. However, it is important to be sure that all other curative techniques for advanced disease have been exhausted before a decision is made to treat palliatively. Chemosurgery with Mohs paste, as previously discussed, may offer a curative approach when other modalities are at best palliative.

The site of the lesion is probably the most important single factor in deciding when radiation therapy is to be employed. While plastic surgery is capable of achieving excellent cosmetic and functional results in areas that are difficult to treat (*i.e.*, the nose, eyelid, and external ear), many lesions may be cured as effectively by irradiation at a greatly reduced expenditure of time and effort (see Figs. 30-24 through 30-27).

The vast majority of skin lesions treated by irradiation receive treatment through a single "en face" portal with the central ray at right angles to the skin surface. The volume of tissue irradiated is kept small by limiting the field size and by using radiation whose energy and penetration is in keeping with the depth and nature of the lesion. The margin of normal tissue irradiated is somewhat dependent on the nature of the neoplasm. Small nodular and superficial basal cell carcinomas can be very accurately assessed as to tumor margin with the aid of good lighting and a small magnifying glass. Epstein showed that it was possible to delineate the tumor margin with an accuracy of 1 mm in 94% of basal cell carcinomas.[59] He further demonstrated that using a 2 mm margin of apparently normal tissue gave surgical tumor-free margins in 122 of 125 basal cell carcinomas so treated. However, as tumors increase in size the margin of normal tissue irradiated must be increased. This is also true for poorly-defined lesions or those that tend to infiltrate subcutaneously. Obviously, clinical judgement based on experience must aid the physician in determining the margin of normal tissue included in the treatment portal. This may vary from 3 mm for a small, well-defined lesion to several centimeters for an extensive lesion with poorly-defined borders. When in doubt, a large field can be used to deliver the initial dose and then reduced to encompass the gross tumor when the normal skin has received a tumoricidal dose at a depth of a few millimeters. Lead sheets cut to fit the size and shape of the desired area to be irradiated should be used rather than standard cones or rectangular fields produced by collimator jaws (see Fig. 30-27). Five half-value layers of lead will reduce the transmitted dose to about 3%. The precise size and shape of the area to be treated can be reproduced in the lead cutout by marking the area on the skin. This should include a suitable margin of normal tissue and a marking on cleared x-ray film using the outline on the cleared film to transfer the desired shape to the lead sheet. A linoleum knife is an excellent tool for transfering the cutout design and for actually cutting the hole in the lead sheet, no matter how irregular it may be. The lead cutout is secured in place by tape during treatment assuring that the radiation will be delivered to the desired area.

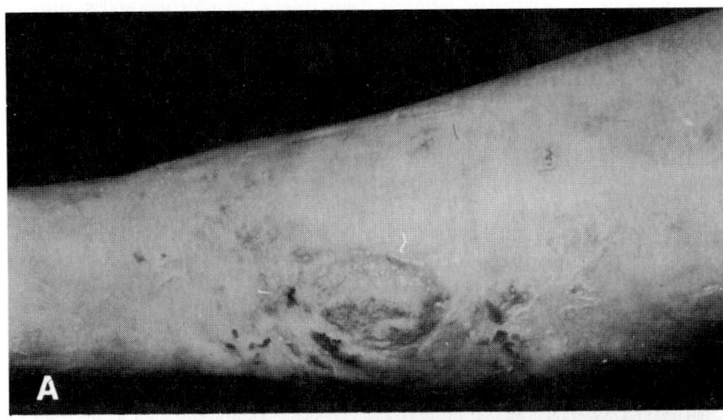

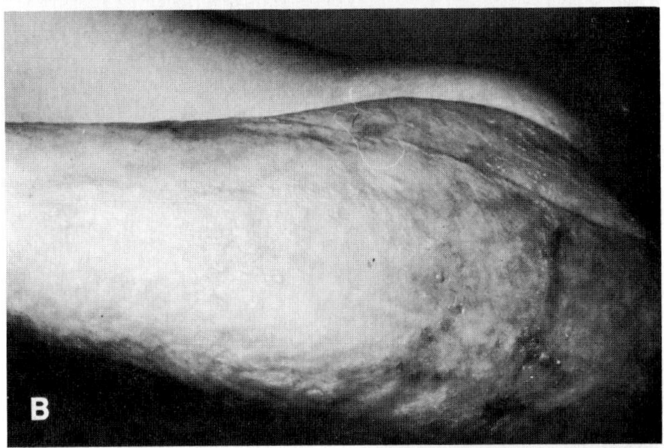

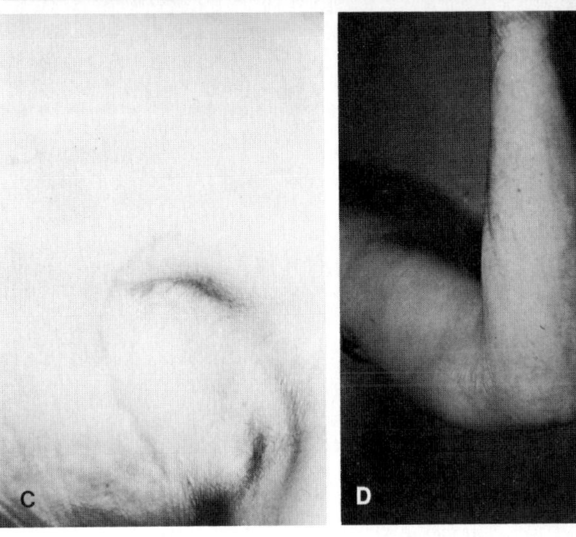

FIG. 30-22. *A*, Preoperative, 38-year-old woman with squamous cell carcinoma in burn scar sustained when she was a child. *B*, Postoperative, 5 months, following wide excision and split thickness grafts for coverage. *C*, Patient also had an axillary node dissection. No metastases were found. *D*, Postoperative, 8 years. The patient is now 16 years without recurrence.

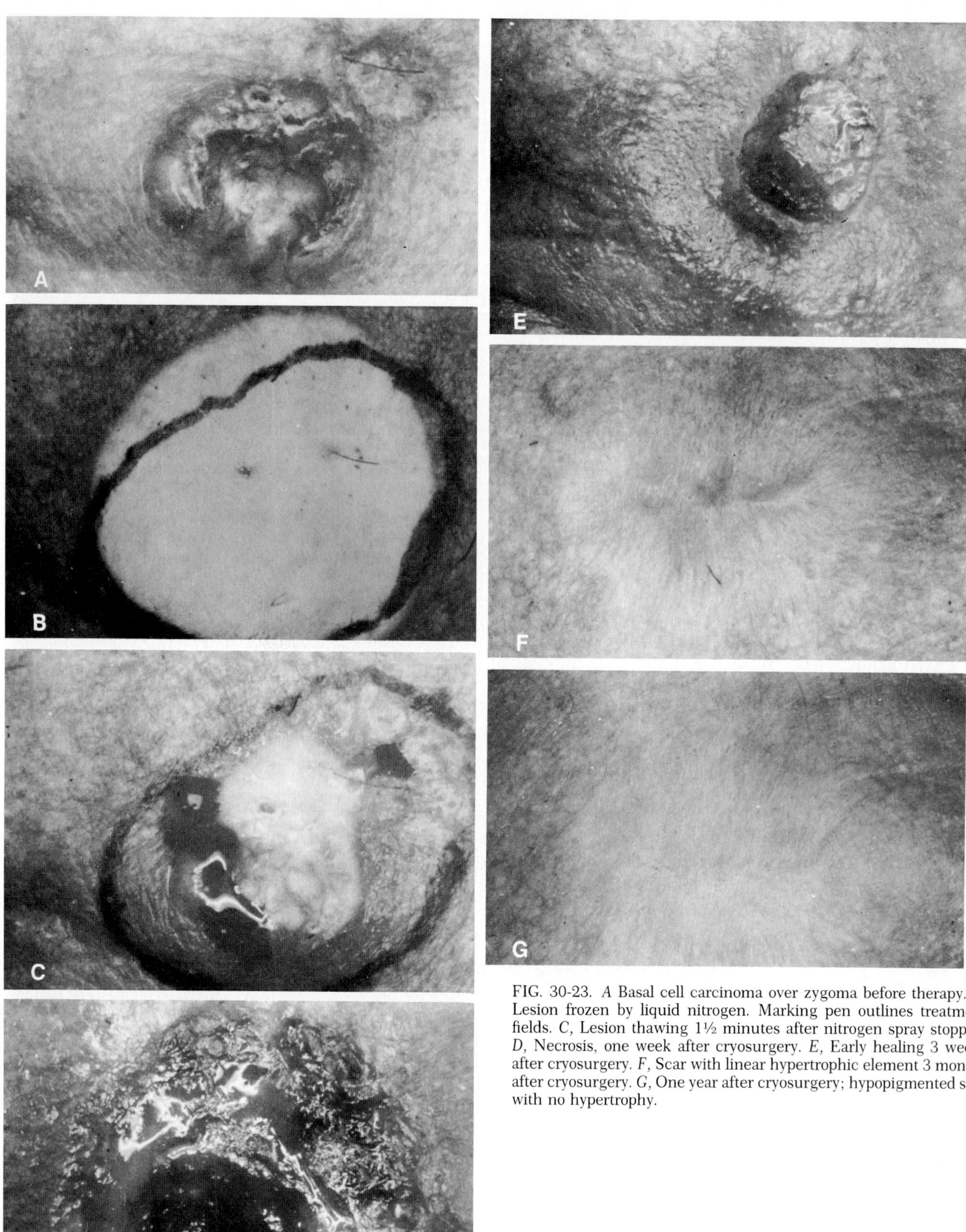

FIG. 30-23. *A* Basal cell carcinoma over zygoma before therapy. *B*, Lesion frozen by liquid nitrogen. Marking pen outlines treatment fields. *C*, Lesion thawing 1½ minutes after nitrogen spray stopped. *D*, Necrosis, one week after cryosurgery. *E*, Early healing 3 weeks after cryosurgery. *F*, Scar with linear hypertrophic element 3 months after cryosurgery. *G*, One year after cryosurgery; hypopigmented scar with no hypertrophy.

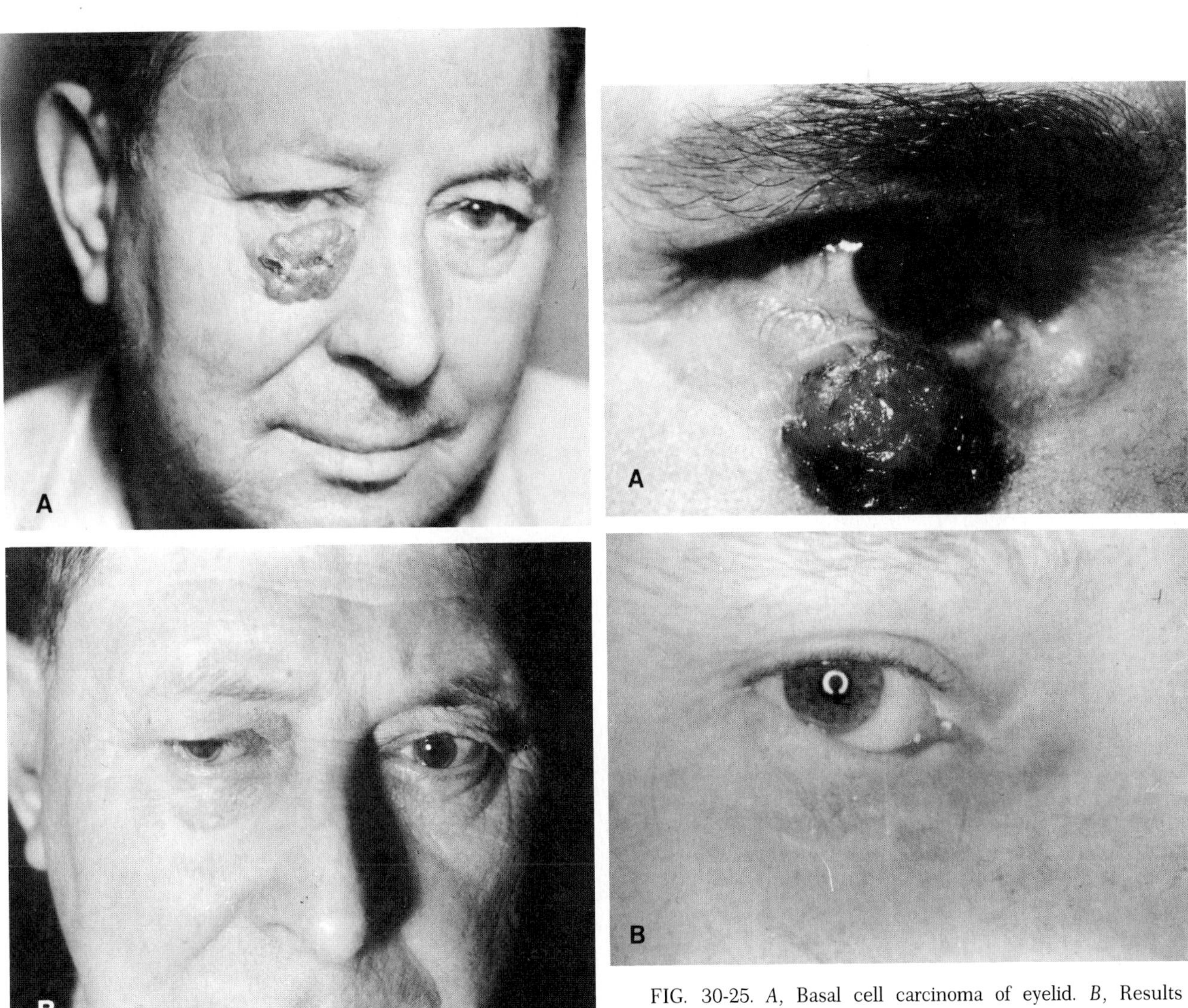

FIG. 30-24. *A*, Basal cell carcinoma, involving lower eyelid. *B*, Same patient 15 months after radiation therapy.

FIG. 30-25. *A*, Basal cell carcinoma of eyelid. *B*, Results after radiation therapy.

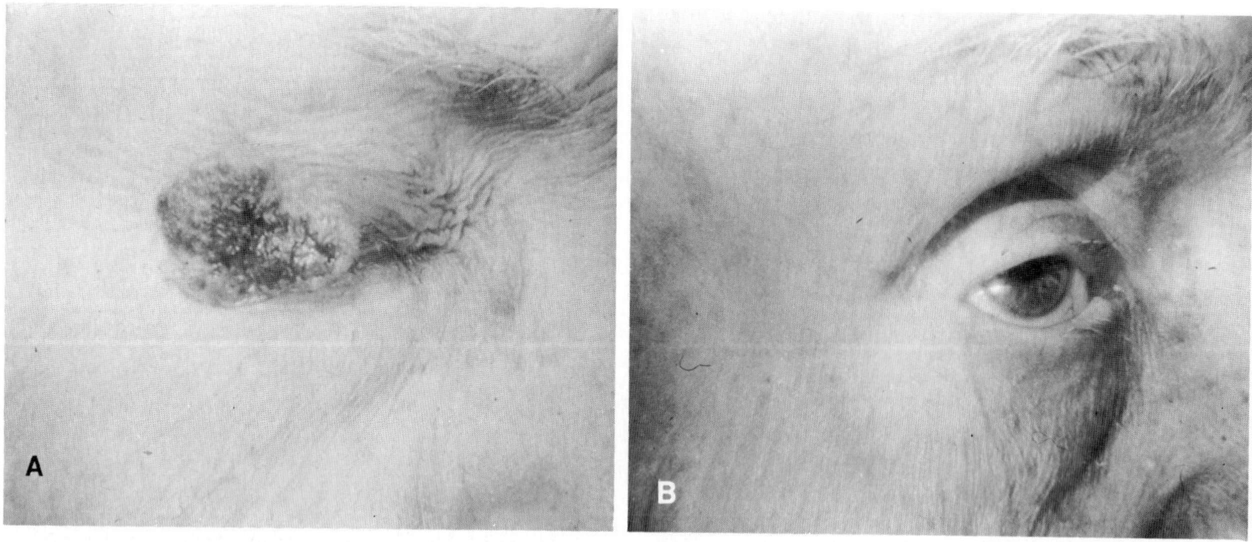

FIG. 30-26. *A*, Squamous cell carcinoma of the eyelid in an 86-year-old woman. *B*, Results 7 months after radiation therapy.

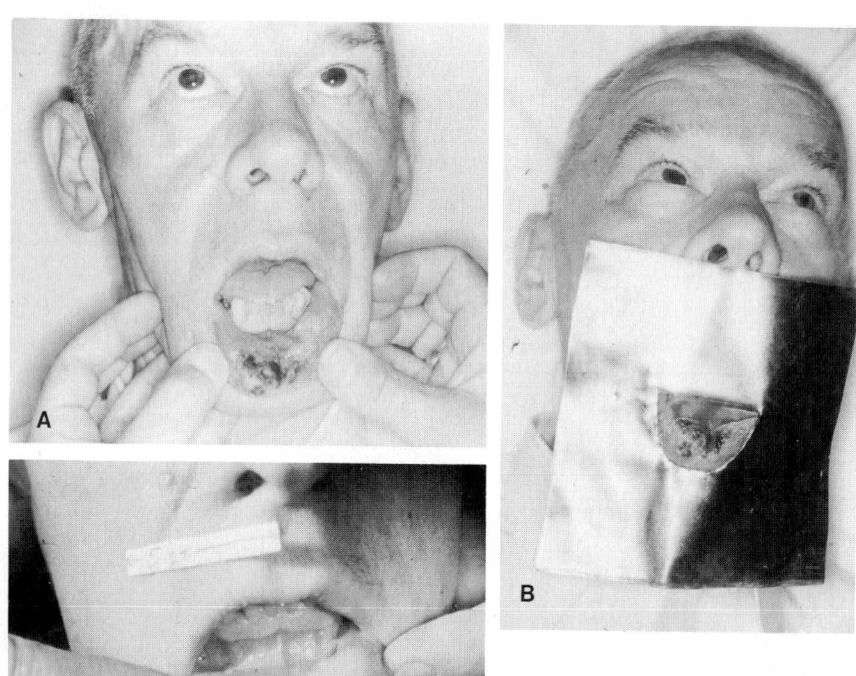

FIG. 30-27. Squamous cell carcinoma of the lower lip. *B*, Lead shield cut-out to expose the treatment field. *C*, Results after radiation therapy.

In planning treatment, it must be remembered that the skin itself is most often the dose-limiting normal tissue. Excessive doses of radiation to the skin will cause necrosis, failure to heal, atrophy, telangectasis, loss of pigmentation, and generally poor cosmetic results. The principal site of such injury is in the dermis and is largely mediated by damage to the vascular supply. Structures underlying the skin must also be considered. When treating scalp lesions brain tissue may be damaged if the radiation factors are poorly chosen. The eye, and lens in particular, must be shielded from the radiation beam if feasible. Bone and cartilage can be injured, but without gross tumor involvement, osteonecrosis and chondronecrosis due to properly performed irradiation are rare (see Figs. 30-28 and 30-29).[60]

The radiation dose required to cure basal and squamous cell carcinoma must be considered in terms of the area to be treated and the fractionation scheme employed. Very small lesions (*i.e.*, less than 1 cm), may be satisfactorily treated with a single dose of 2,200 rad, particularly if contact therapy with 50 kvp radiation is used. On the other hand, large lesions may require doses as high as 6,000 rad fractionationed over an appropriate period of time. Three factors must be determined in arriving at an optimum time-dose scheme for a given lesion. Starting with the size of the area to be irradiated, the dose to produce a cure without accompanying necrosis is determined from time-dose isoeffect curves published by von Essen.[4] These isoeffect curves maintain that the slope of the time-dose curves for tumor curability is less than that for skin necrosis. Adequate protraction of treatment will therefore allow selection of a dose within the curative range, but below that which will produce skin necrosis. An example of this is shown in Fig. 30-30. It shows the curves adopted from von Essen for a 10 cm^2 treatment area.[61] A family of parallel curves is available for areas ranging from 1 cm^2 to 100 cm^2. In Table 30-1, values are suggested for fractionation schemes for lesions of various sizes and thicknesses.

Radiation modalities to be used for the treatment of skin cancer are quite numerous. They include external beam

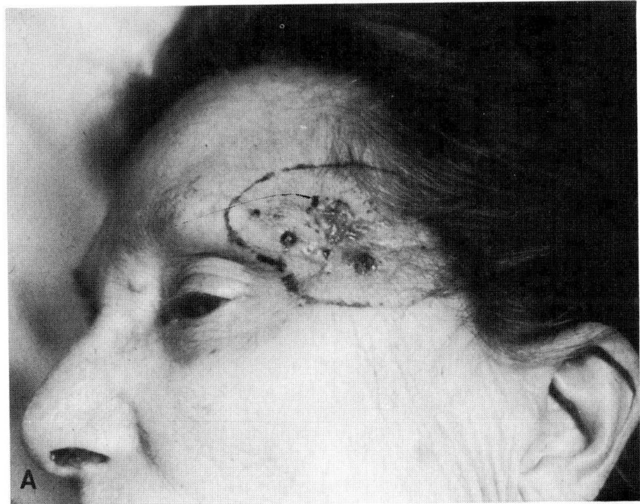

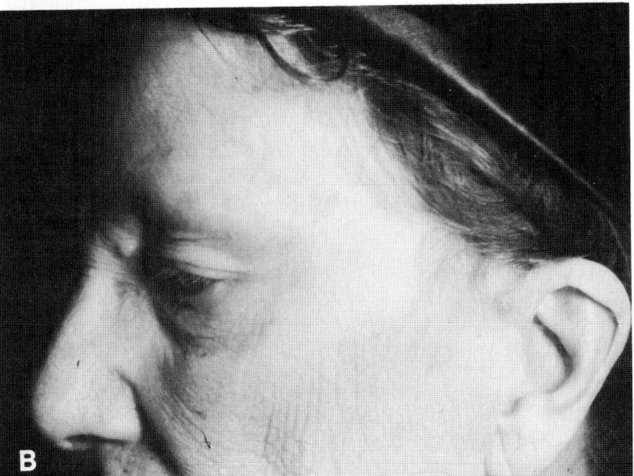

FIG. 30-28. *A*, Basal cell carcinoma. *B*, Results 6 months after radiation therapy.

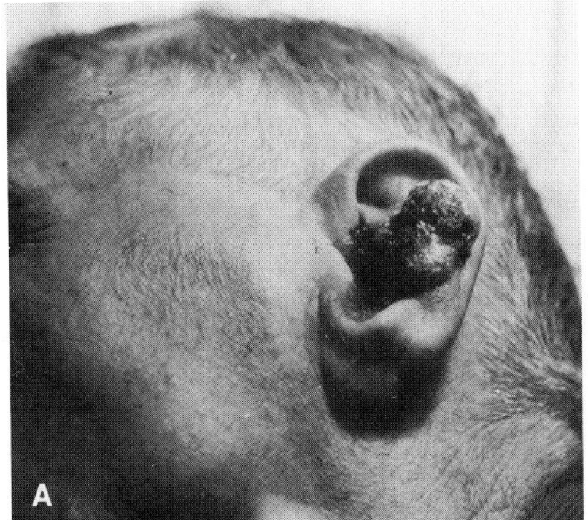

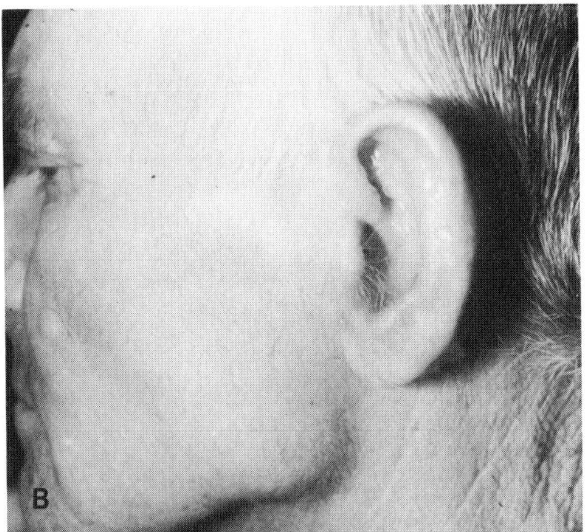

FIG. 30-29. *A*, Squamous cell carcinoma of ear. *B*, Results 2 months after radiation therapy.

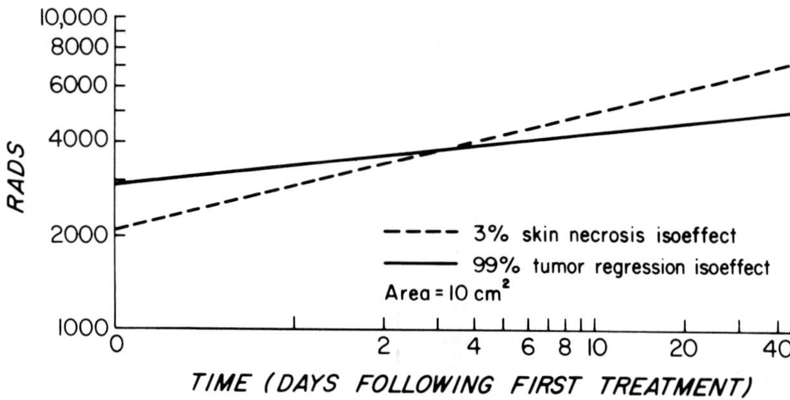

FIG. 30-30. Dose required for either 99% likelihood of tumor regression or 3% likelihood of skin necrosis as a function of the overall treatment time. (Adapted from von Essen CF: A spatial model of time-dose-area relationships in radiation therapy. Radiology 81:881–883, 1963)

irradiation with photons or electrons, interstitial implantation with radioactive source, and molds containing radioactive sources that are applied topically. The most commonly used of these modalities is external photon beam irradiation using x-ray photons of varying energies, going from about 50 kvp up to the megavoltage range. Usually lesions of small to moderate size are treated with what is termed superficial therapy (with 100 kvp radiation) whose depth-dose characteristics are determined by the amount of filtration employed. Adequate protraction of treatment is the key to good cosmetic results. While it is possible to treat small lesions with five or even fewer fractions, superior results will be obtained if 10 fractions are employed for small lesions (<2 cm diameter) and 15 or 20 fractions for larger lesions.

Superficial therapy is commonly carried out at target to skin distances (TSD) of 15–20 cm. Increasing the TSD has the effect of increasing the relative depth dose; conversely, decreasing the TSD decreases the dose in depth relative to the surface dose. In the contact therapy unit this characteristic is taken advantage of. A TSD of 2 cm is employed and the distance guide of the machine is placed in contact with the patient's skin (Fig. 30-31). This, coupled with a low energy of 50 kvp and a minimum of inherent filtration by use of a berylium window in the x-ray tube, gives a photon beam of relatively limited penetration that provides an excellent modality for treating small lesions of limited thickness. Comparison of the depth-dose characteristics of 50 kvp contact therapy and 100 kvp superficial therapy is shown in Fig. 30-32. A Philips contact therapy unit has a maximum field size of 2 cm at 2 cm TSD, but by increasing the TSD to 4 cm, lesions up to about 3.5 cm diameter can be treated with an adequate margin provided the border of the lesion can clearly be outlined. Contact therapy has the major advantage over superficial therapy of allowing treatment with a minimum of protraction without impairing cosmetic results. A dose of 3,300 rad delivered in three fractions calculated at the base of the lesion will cure basal and squamous cell carcinoma and leave little, if any, recognizable radiation changes in the skin. In general, contact therapy should not be used for lesions of greater than 5 mm thickness.

Contact therapy is of particular utility in treating lesions of the eyelid. Excellent cosmetic and functional results are attainable.[62,63] If the lesion is at the medial canthus and the punctum is involved, stenosis of the nasolacrimal duct can be prevented by inserting a metal stint or silastic tube prior to irradiation.[64,65] This is sutured in place and left in for at least

TABLE 30-1. Suggested Dose, Energy, and Fraction Number for Lesions of Different Dimensions

MAXIMUM FIELD DIAMETER (cm)	THICKNESS (cm)	HVL (mm)	MINIMUM TUMOR DOSE RADS	NUMBER OF FRACTIONS
1.5	0.3 or less	0.2 Al	2,200	1
3.0	0.35	0.2 Al	3,300	3
3.0	0.5	0.2 Al	4,000	5
3.0	0.3	1.0 Al	4,500	15
3.0	0.5	2.0 Al	4,500	15
5.0	0.5	2.0 Al	5,200	20
5.0	1.0	3.6 Al	5,500	25
5.0	1.5	0.5 Cu	5,500	25
5.0	2.0	0.5 Cu	5,800	29
8.0	0.5	1.0 Al	6,000	30
8.0	1.0	3.0 Al	6,000	30
8.0	1.5	0.5 Cu	6,000	30
8.0	2.0	0.5 Cu	6,000	30

several weeks (or longer if tolerated by the patient) after radiation therapy is completed (see Fig. 30-33). A lead eyeshield either plated with silver or dipped in melted paraffin is placed beneath the lids to protect the globe and lens.

Deeply infiltrating skin cancers, if treated by irradiation, require the use of a more penetrating photon beam. This may be in the form of orthovoltage radiation, ranging from 140 kvp to 300 kvp with appropriate filtration and TSDs, or megavoltage photons in the 4–8 MV range. When the MV beam is employed, material of approximate tissue density must be placed on the irradiated skin to overcome the skin-sparing effect of high energy photons and bring the point of maximum dose to the surface. The thickness of this bolusing material will depend on beam energy. In treatment with MV photons, it is often advantageous to use portals with an angle between them, generally ranging from 90–135 degrees, for entry. The dose distribution in the treatment volume when such a treatment plan is used must be made reasonably homogeneous by the use of wedges.

The electron beam, with energies ranging from 3–18 MV, has also proved a useful modality for irradiation of skin neoplasms. The physical characteristics of the electron beam with relatively high surface dose, rapid build-up to the maximum dose, and rapid fall-off of dose beyond a certain depth are all desirable for treatment of this type of lesion. The

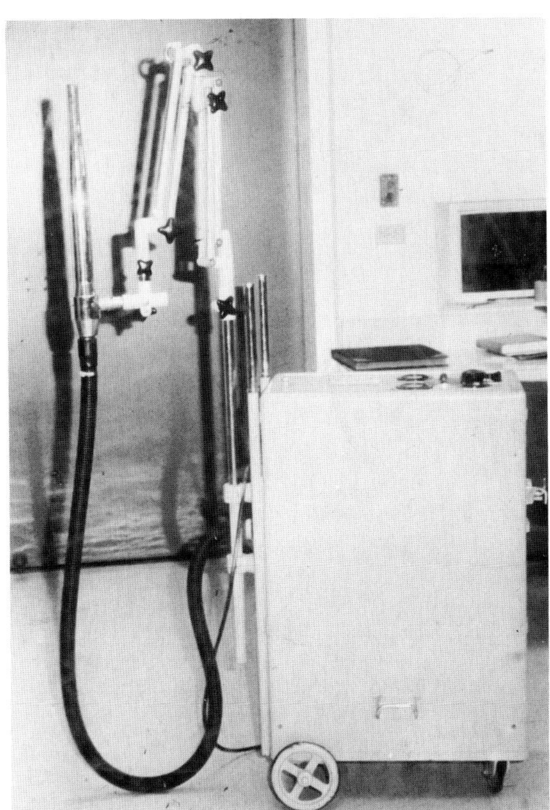

FIG. 30-31. Contact therapy unit.

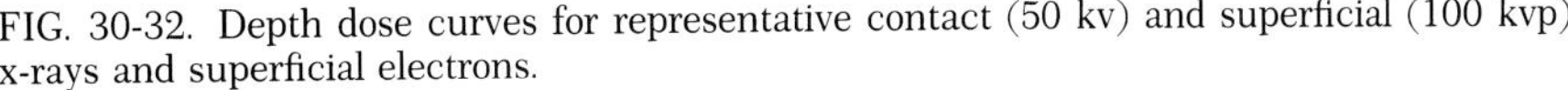

FIG. 30-32. Depth dose curves for representative contact (50 kv) and superficial (100 kvp) x-rays and superficial electrons.

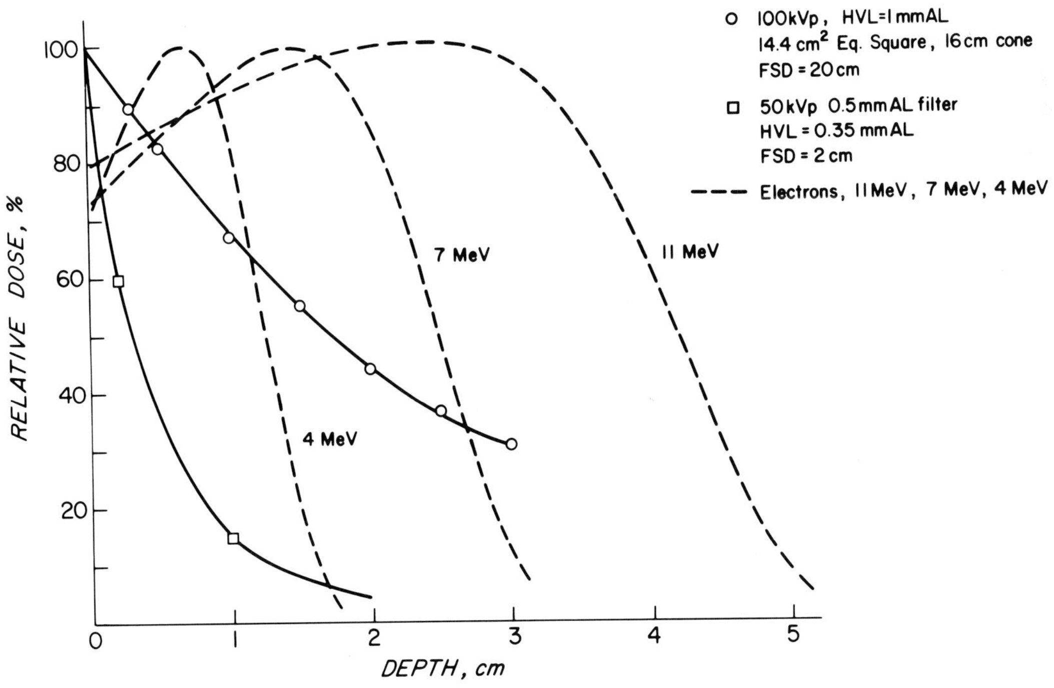

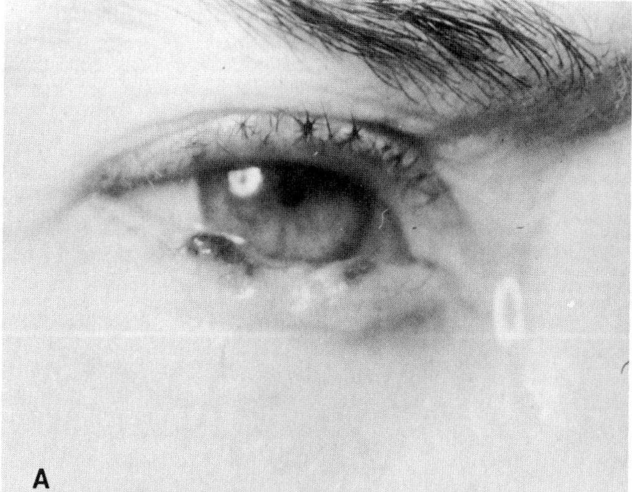

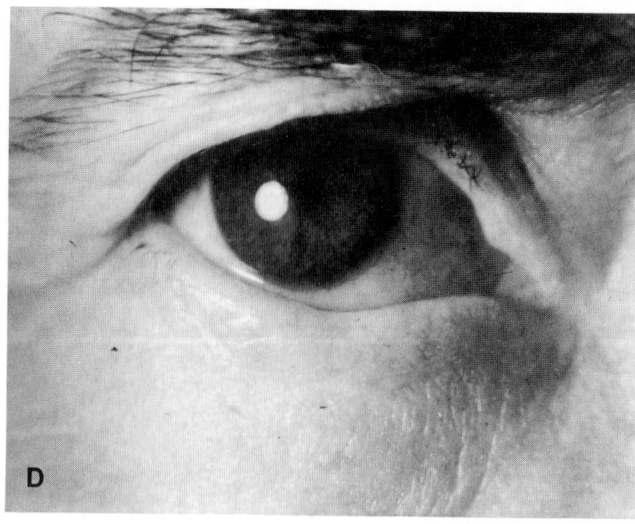

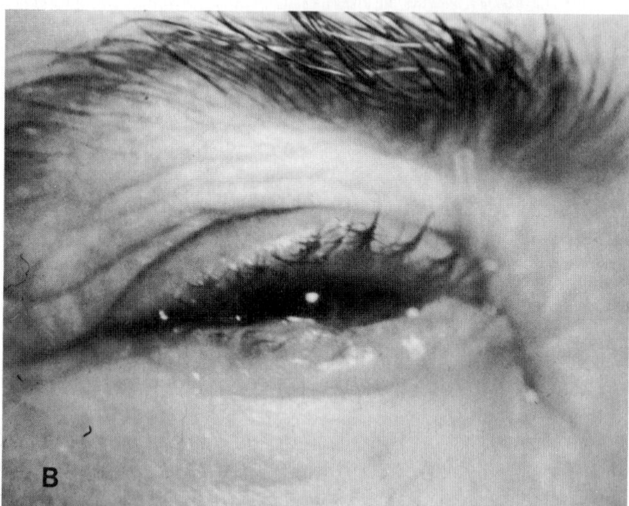

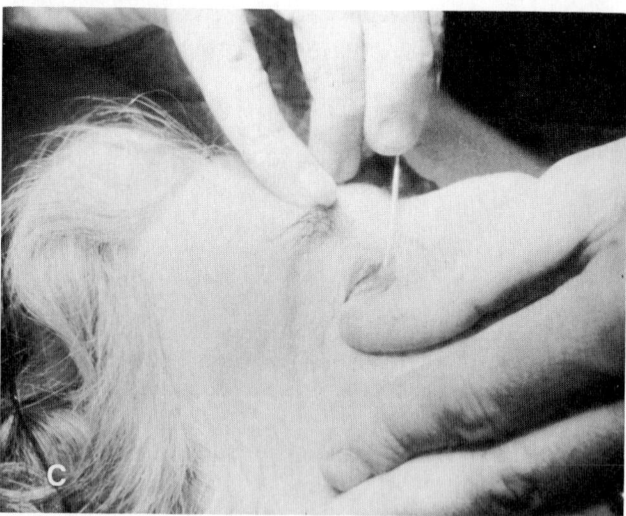

FIG. 30-33. *A*, Basal cell carcinoma of eyelid, recurrent after surgery. *B*, Probe being inserted in lacrimal duct. *C*, Tube in place in lacrimal duct. *D*, Results 4 months after radiation therapy. The lacrimal duct is patent.

exact details of these parameters are determined by the energy of the electron beam chosen. However, the surface dose is generally about 85% of the maximum dose and rises to 90% at a depth of 2 mm so that no bolusing is required. The fall-off after the 80% level is reached is extremely rapid. Some characteristic depth dose curves for various electron energies compared with superficial photon beams are shown in Fig. 30-32. Since treatment with electrons is usually more time-consuming and complex than photon irradiation, its use should be reserved for those lesions where it appears to convey some special advantage over other forms of radiation therapy. Tapley and Fletcher have found electrons particularly useful in treating large destructive lesions in the head and neck area and in multiple recurrent lesions after previous treatment with cautery, radiation, and surgery.[66]

Two other techniques of irradiating skin carcinomas involve the use of radioactive-sealed sources such as radium, cesium, iridium, or tantalum. The sources are used to implant the lesion interstitially or to load a mold made for surface application. Because of the time involved in these forms of treatment, the need for hospitalization, and, in some instances, anesthesia, neither form of therapy is in very common use. However for certain specific situations where extenal beam irradiation is difficult to administer, an interstitial implant or surface mold may occasionally be the treatment of choice.

Interstitial implantation has proved to be particularly useful in treating lesions about the nasal vestibule where the ala nasi, nasal septum, and nasolabial sulcus may be involved. The technique confines the radiation dose to the desired tumor volume and takes advantage of the benefits of low-dose rate irradiation. Wang and associates have described an afterloading technique using Angiocaths in conjunction with Ir-192 sources in plastic tubing, which is easily carried out with a minimum of exposure.[67] However, conventional radium or cesium needles can be employed. Interstitial implants are planned to deliver a dose of about 1,000 rad per day. The entire dose of 6,000–7,000 rad may be delivered over 6–7-days. However, quite often a portion of the radiation dose is given with external beam irradiation and supplemented by the interstitial technique. An example of an Angiocath—Ir—192 implant of the region between the upper lip and the nasal vestibule is shown in Fig. 30-34.

Surface molds have proved most useful for moderately large superficial lesions in close proximity to underlying bone. Molds can be constructed using dental molding materials or simply built-up layers of elastoplast. The relative depth dose can be controlled by the distance between the sources and the tumor, *i.e.*, the thickness of the mold. Distribution of the sources and the treatment distance to be employed are established by consulting the Paterson and Parker rules and tables.[68] Surface molds are designed to be worn daily during the treatment period, generally for about 6–8 hours a day or sometimes longer. As with interstitial implants, the entire dose may be given using the mold, or, the treatment can be combined with external beam irradiation.

TOPICAL CHEMOTHERAPY

Topically-applied 5-fluorouracil is excellent therapy for the premalignant precursor lesion of sun-induced squamous cell carcinoma—the actinic keratosis.[69] A 1–5% cream or solution is applied to the lesion every morning and night for 2–3 weeks. After one week erythema and possibly some erosion may develop. At the end of 2 or 3 weeks (preferably 3 weeks), the therapy is discontinued and a topical antibiotic, such as bacitracin ointment, is applied until healing has occurred. Generally, scarring does not occur. This therapy is also *suggested* for basal cell carcinoma therapy. If there are a small number of lesions that can be well-treated by one of the previously described modalities, that would be preferable. Nodular lesions do not respond well to topical chemotherapy. The most likely application for carcinoma is in the case of large or multiple superficial basal cell carcinomas. Therapy by topical 5-fluorouracil for these lesions must be continued for at least 6 weeks to attain a respectable rate of cure. Even then, this modality has a lower cure rate than surgery, cryosurgery, curettage, or Mohs' technique. Occasionally, it may be desirable to treat squamous cell carcinoma *in situ* with this approach. The risk of eventual invasive disease with possible metastatic disease exists if any tumor is not destroyed at the depth of the lesion, particularly when the epithelium of the hair follicle is affected as it extends into the dermis. Therefore, conventional therapy is preferred when possible.

IMMUNOTHERAPY

Sensitization to DNCB (dinitrochlorobenzene) or BCG followed by local application to carcinomas of the skin has been reported to cause resolution of many lesions. Sometimes this has been added to topical chemotherapy with 5-fluorouracil. At present, this form of therapy is experimental.[70,71] It is doubtful that the cure rate could exceed the 95–98% attained by conventional therapy. However, consideration may be given to experimental therapy if there are a large number of basal cell carcinomas that would be very difficult to treat by standard measures.

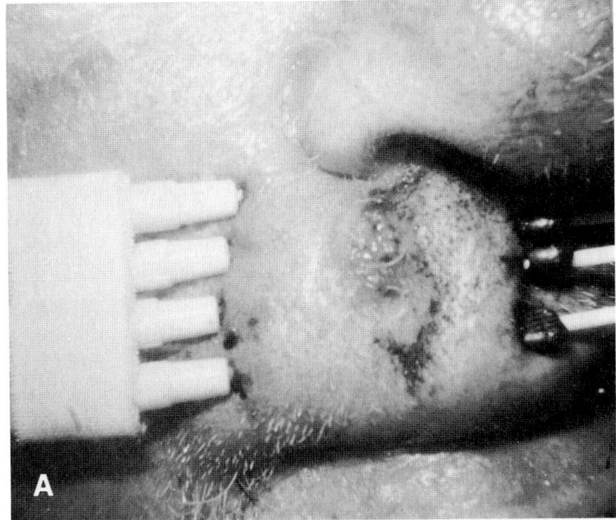

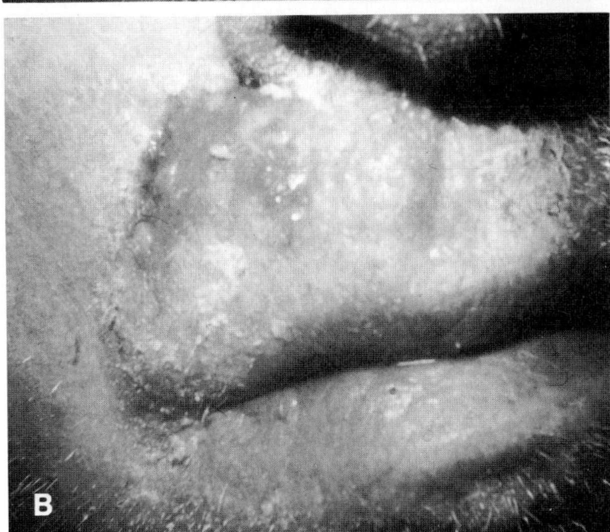

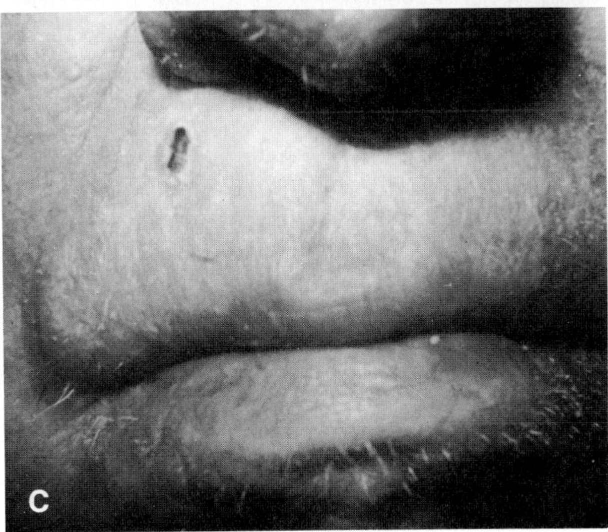

FIG. 30-34. *A*, Angiograph 1r-192 implant in place. *B*, Results one month after therapy. *C*, Results 2 months after therapy.

CHOICE OF THERAPY

It is very difficult to briefly describe the multiple factors influencing the choice of therapy for carcinomas of the skin. The pros and cons have been summarized by Helm.[72] In general, no therapy is better than surgical excision for those lesions which can be totally extirpated and closed with minimal cosmetic disfigurement. For lesions not readily treatable surgically, it is reasonable to consider locally destructive techniques. All of these leave an area of scarring rather than the linear scar from excisional surgery. Cryosurgery seems to give better cosmetic results than curettage and can be used in the presence of scarring where curettage is ineffective. Both are relatively quick office procedures with several weeks required for subsequent healing by secondary intention. Radiation therapy should generally be reserved for lesions not easily treated by surgery, curettage, or cryosurgery. As the scar from radiation therapy becomes more atrophic and fibrotic with time, younger patients will develop a worse cosmetic result after many years than older patients whose life expectancy will shorten the postradiation interval. Carcinomas invasive to bone do not respond well to radiation therapy. In the older patient, or on the eyelid at any age, excellent cosmetic results without the need for surgery can be obtained; in these cases, the authors recommend radiation therapy.

REFERENCES

1. Clayson DB: Chemical Carcinogenesis. Boston, Little, Brown & Co, 1962
2. Rous P, Kroo JG: Conditional neoplasms and subthreshold neoplastic states. J Exp Med 73:365, 1941
3. Berenblum I: The two-stage mechanism of carcinogenesis as an analytical tool. In Emmelot P, Muhlbock, O (eds): Cellular Control Mechanisms and Cancer. Amsterdam, Elsevier, 1964
4. Miller EC, Miller JA: The molecular biology of cancer, pp 377–402. New York, Academic Press, 1974
5. Slaga TJ, Sivak A, Boutwell RK (eds): Carcinogenesis, Vol. 2. Mechanisms of tumor promotion and carcinogenesis. New York, Raven Press, 1978
6. Lowe N, Verma AK, Boutwell RK: Ultraviolet light induces epidermal ornithine decarboxylase activity. J Invest Derm 71:417–418, 1978
7. Unna PG: Die Histopathologie der Hautkrenkheiten. Berlin, Hirschwald, 1894
8. Shield AM: A remarkable case of multiple growths of the skin caused by exposure to the sun. Lancet 1:22–23, 1899
9. Heuper WC: Occupational Tumors and Allied Diseases. Springfield, Illinois, Charles C Thomas, 1942
10. Hyde JN: On the influence of light in the production of cancer of the skin. Amer J Med Sci 131:1–22, 1906
11. Findlay GM: Ultraviolet light and skin cancer. Lancet 2:1070–1073, 1928
12. Blum HF: Sunlight as a causal factor in cancer of the skin of man. JNCI 9:247, 1948
13. Blum HF: Carcinogenesis by Ultraviolet Light. Princeton, Princeton University Press, 1959
14. Roffo AH: Cancer et soleil. Carcinomes et sarcomes provoques par l'action de soleil *in toto*. Bull Assoc Franc. Etude Cancer, 23:590–616, 1934
15. Macdonald, EJ: Epidemiology of skin cancer, 1975. In Neoplasms of the Skin and Malignant Melanoma, pp 27–42. Chicago, Year Book Medical Publishers, 1976
16. Scotto J, Kopf AW, Urbach F: Nonmelanoma skin cancer among Caucasians in four areas of the United States. Cancer 34:1333–1338, 1974
17. Urbach F, Epstein JH, Forbes RD: Ultraviolet carcinogenesis: experimental, global, and genetic aspects. In Fitzpatrick TB (ed): Sunlight and Man, p. 259. Tokyo, University of Tokyo Press, 1974
18. Scott EL, Bloomfield P, Cole P et al: Estimates of increases in skin cancer due to increases in ultraviolet radiation caused by reducing stratospheric ozone. In Environmental Impact of Stratospheric Flight, pp 177–221. Washington, DC, National Academy of Sciences, 1975
19. van der Leun JC, Daniels F Jr: Biologic effects of stratospheric ozone decrease: a critical review of assessments. In Grobecker AJ (ed): Impacts of Climatic Change on the Biosphere, CIAP Monograph 5, Chap 7, DOT-TST-75-55. Washington, DC, Department of Transportation, 1975
20. Protection Against Depletion of Stratospheric Ozone by Chlorofluorocarbons, National Academy of Sciences, Washington, DC, 1979
21. Cleaver, JE: Defective repair replication of DNA in xeroderma pigmentosum. Nature 218:652–656, 1968
22. Setlow RB, Regan JD, German J et al: Evidence that xeroderma pigmentosum cells do not perform the first step in the repair of ultraviolet damage to their DNA. Proc Natl Acad Sci, USA 64:1035–1041, 1969
23. Epstein JH, Fukuyama K, Read WB et al: Defect in DNA synthesis in the skin of patients with xeroderma pigmentosum demonstrated *in vivo*. Science 168:1477–1478, 1970
24. Kripke ML: Antigenicity of murine skin tumors induced by ultraviolet light. JNCI 53:1333–1336, 1974
25. Kripke ML, Fisher MS: Immunologic parameters of ultraviolet carcinogenesis. JNCI 57:211–215, 1976
26. Kripke ML: Ultraviolet radiation and tumor immunity. J Reticuloendothelial Soc 22:217, 1977
27. Toews GB, Bergstresser PR, Streilein JW: Langerhans Cells: sentinels of skin associated lympoid tissue. J Invest Derm 75:78–82, 1980
28. O'Dell BL, Jessen RT, Becker LE et al: Diminished immune response in sun-damaged skin. Arch Dermatol 116:559–561, 1980
29. Upton AC: Radiation carcinogenesis. In Bush H (ed): Methods in Cancer Research, Vol. III. New York, Academic Press, 1967
30. Anderson A, Bradley R, Haas JE et al: CIAP Monograph #6. Economic and social measures of biologic and climatic change pp 4–139. Springfield, Virginia, Natural Technical Information Service, 1975
31. Popkin GL, DeFeo CP Jr: Basal cell epithelioma. In Andrade R, Gumport SL, Popkin GL et al (eds): Cancer of the Skin, Biology—Diagnosis—Management, pp 821–844. Philadelphia, WB Saunders, 1976
32. Van Scott EJ: Basal cell carcinoma. In Fitzpatrick TB, Eisen AZ, Wolff K et al (eds): Dermatology in General Medicine, 2nd ed, pp. 377–383. New York, McGraw-Hill, 1979
33. Sanderson KV, Mackie R: Tumors of the skin. In Rook A, Wilkinson DS, Ebling FJG (eds): Textbook of Dermatology, 3rd ed, pp 2171–2179. London, Blackwell Scientific Publications, 1979
34. Stoll HL Jr: Squamous cell carcinoma. In Fitzpatrick TB, Eisen AZ, Wolff K et al (eds): Dermatology in General Medicine, 2nd ed, pp 362–377. New York, McGraw-Hill, 1979
35. Sage HH, Casson PR: Squamous cell carcinoma of the scalp, face, and neck. In Androde R, Gumport SL, Popkin, GL et al (eds): Cancer of the Skin, pp 899–915. Philadelphia, WB Saunders, 1976
36. Grier WRN: Squamous cell carcinoma of the body and extremities. In Andrade R, Gumport SL, Popkin GL et al (eds): Cancer of the Skin, pp 918–932. Philadelphia, WB Saunders, 1976
37. Sanderson KV, Mackie R: Tumors of the skin. In Rook A, Wilkinson DS, Ebling FJG (eds): Textbook of Dermatology, 3rd ed, pp 2186–2192. London Blackwell Scientific Publications, 1979
38. Andersen SLC, Nielson A, Raymann F: Relationship between Bowen's disease and internal malignant tumors. Arch Dermatol 108:367–370, 1973
39. Callen JP, Headington J: Bowen's and non-Bowen's squamous

intraepidermal neoplasia of the skin. Arch Dermatol 116:422–426, 1980
40. Kopf SW: Keratoacanthoma, clinical aspects. In Andrade R, Gumport SL, Popkin GL et al (eds): Cancer of the Skin, pp 755–781. Philadelphia, WB Saunders, 1976
41. Civatte J, Tsoitis G: Adnexal skin carcinomas. In Andrade R, Gumport SL, Popkin GL et al (eds): Cancer of the Skin, pp 1045–1068. Philadelphia, WB Saunders, 1976
42. Lever WF, Schaumberg-Lever G: Histopathology of the Skin, 5th ed. Philadelphia, JB Lippincott, 1975
43. Costanza ME, Dayal Y, Binder S et al: Metastatic basal cell carcinoma: Review, report of a case and chemotherapy. Cancer 34:230–235, 1974
44. Rahhari H, Melregan AH: Basal cell epitheliomas in usual and unusual sites. J Cutaneous Path 6:425–431, 1979
45. Freeman RG, Knox JM: Recent experience with skin cancer. Arch Derm 101:403–408, 1970
46. Jackson IT: Diagnostic problem of keratoacanthoma. Lancet 1:490–492, 1969
47. Urban FH, Winkelmann RK: Sebaceous malignancy. Arch Derm 84:63, 1961
48. Hirsh LF, Enterline HT, Rosato EF et al: Sweat gland carcinoma. Ann Surg 174:283–286, 1971
49. Graham JH, Helwig EB: Precancerous skin lesions and systemic cancer. In: Tumors of the Skin. Chicago, Year Book Medical Publishers, 1964
50. Davis TS, Graham WP III, Miller SH: The circular excision. Ann Plast Surg 4:21–24, 1980
51. Grabb WC: Basic techniques of plastic surgery. In Grabb WC, Smith JW (eds): Plastic Surgery, 3rd ed, pp 3–74. Boston, Little, Brown & Co, 1979
52. Converse JM, McCarthy JG, Brauer RO et al: Transplantation of skin: Grafts and flaps. In Converse JM (ed): Reconstructive Plastic Surgery, 2nd ed, vol 1, pp 152–239. Philadelphia, WB Saunders, 1977
53. McGregor IA: Fundamental techniques of plastic surgery, 2nd ed. Edinburgh, E&S Livingstone, 1962
54. Torre D: Cryosurgery. In Andrade R, Gumport SL, Popkin GL et al (eds): Cancer of the Skin, pp 1569–1587. Philadelphia, WB Saunders, 1976
55. Zacharian SA (ed): Cryosurgical advances in dermatology and tumors of the head and neck. Springfield, Illinois, Charles C Thomas, 1977
56. McLean DI, Haynes HA, McCarthy PL et al: Cryotherapy of basal-cell carcinoma by a simple method of standardized freeze-thaw cycles. J Dermatol Surg Oncol 4:175–177, 1978
57. Robins P: Mohs surgery in the treatment of basal cell and squamous cell carcinoma of the skin. In Andrade R, Gumport SL, Popkin GL et al (eds): Cancer of the Skin, pp 1537–1550. Philadelphia, WB Saunders, 1976
58. von Essen CF: Roentgen therapy of skin and lip carcinoma: Factors influencing success and failure. Am J Roentgenol Rad Ther Nuc Med, 83:556–570, 1960
59. Epstein E: How accurate is the visual assessment of basal cell carcinoma margins? Brit J Dermatol 89:37–43, 1973
60. Del Regato JA, Vuksanovic M: Radiotherapy of carcinomas of the skin overlying the cartilages of the nose and ear. Radiology 79:203–208, 1962
61. von Essen CF: A spatial model of time-dose-area relationships in radiation therapy. Radiology 81:881–883, 1963
62. Domonkos AN; Treatment of eyelid carcinoma. Arch Dermatol 91:364–370, 1965
63. Levene MB: Radiotherapeutic management of carcinoma of the eyelid. In Brockhurst RJ, Boruchaff SA, Hutchinson BJ et al (eds): Controversies in Ophthalmology, pp 390–397. Philadelphia, WB Saunders, 1977
64. Leventhal HH, Messer RJ: Malignant tumors of the eyelid. Am J Surg 124:522–526, 1972
65. Johnson CC: A canaliculus wire. Am J Ophthalmol 78, 1974
66. Tapley N duV, Fletcher GH: Applications of the electron beam in the treatment of cancer of the skin and lips. Radiology 109:423–428, 1973
67. Wang CC, Boyer A, Mendiondo O: Afterloading interstitial radiation therapy. Int J Radiat Oncol Biol. Phys 1:365–368, 1976
68. Meredith WJ: Radium dosage, the Manchester system. Edinburgh, E&S Livingstone, 1958
69. Stoll HL: Topical chemotherapy. In Helm F (ed): Cancer Dermatology, pp. 435–448. Philadelphia, Lea and Febiger, 1979
70. Bigazzi PE, Klein E, Helm, F: Introduction to tumor immunotherapy. In Helm F (ed): Cancer Dermatology, pp 471–480. Philadelphia, Lea and Febiger, 1979
71. Moore GE, Klein E,: Immunotherapy of skin cancer. In Andrade R, Gumport SL, Popkin GL et al (eds): Cancer of the Skin, pp 1647–1661. Philadelphia, WB Saunders, 1976
72. Helm F: Comparison of different methods of treatment. In Cancer Dermatology, pp 481–487. Philadelphia, Lea and Febiger, 1979

Michael J. Mastrangelo
Steven A. Rosenberg
Alan R. Baker
Harry R. Katz

CHAPTER 31

Cutaneous Melanoma

Cutaneous melanoma is a malignant neoplasm arising from melanocytes. Melanocytes are melanosome-containing cells that specialize in the biosynthesis and transport of melanin pigment. Historically, the earliest description of melanoma is in the writings of Hippocrates in the 5th century, B.C.; in addition, the disease was found in several Pre-Columbian Inca mummies from approximately the same era.[1] The term *melanoma* was first suggested by Carswell in 1938 in a paper describing the malignant character of the tumor.[2]

Cutaneous melanoma has been considered a rare tumor with an unpredictable behavior that varied from spontaneous regression to rapid progression and death. However, the disease is no longer rare. The rate of increase in the incidence of melanoma is greater than for any other cancer, with the exception of bronchogenic carcinoma. The cutaneous location of this tumor has allowed detailing of its evolutionary history. Important prognostic factors have been identified and criteria established for the clinical recognition of melanoma at a surgically curable stage.

Several excellent books and monographs on this subject have recently been published, if the reader desires an expanded discussion of this material.[3–7]

EMBRYOLOGY OF CUTANEOUS MELANOMA

In embryologic terms, the pigment-producing cells are neural crest derivatives that migrate during early gestation to skin, uveal tract, meninges, and ectodermal mucosa.[8] Melanocytes reside in the skin at the basal layer of the epidermis and under a variety of stimuli elaborate melanin pigment. Synthesis occurs on the melanosome, a well-defined intracellular organelle, where the amino acid tyrosine, under the catalytic influence of tyrosinase, is oxidized to dihydroxyphenylalanine (dopa) and then to dopaquinone before undergoing polymerization to melanin.[9] The melanosome-pigment package is passaged out of the melanocyte, by way of its dendritic processes, and phagocytized by surrounding keratinocytes.[10] These, in turn, migrate upward through the epidermis, conferring the phenotypic patterns and degrees of skin coloration observed.

The number of melanocytes per unit area of skin surface shows no significant correlation with the propensity to develop melanoma. Two lines of evidence support this observation. First, melanocyte density among Caucasians and Blacks is roughly the same for any skin site despite a 5-fold difference in the age-adjusted incidence of melanoma reported for these groups in the U.S. (see Table 31-1).[12] Second, melanocyte density varies by several-fold from one skin site to another with the trunk (900/mm^2) and extremities (1150/mm^2) showing the lowest concentration, while the head (2000/mm^2) and penis (2400/mm^2) have the highest.[8] Although melanoma occurs with a disproportionately high frequency on the head, it occurs commonly on the trunk and extremities as well; it is rarely seen on the penis.[13]

EPIDEMIOLOGY AND ETIOLOGY

Presently, melanoma accounts for roughly 1% of cancers in the U.S. and about the same proportion of cancer deaths. Although it represents approximately only 3% of cutaneous neoplasms, its malignant potential is more aptly reflected in the fact that it results in 65% of skin cancer deaths. Numerical data that put the problem in epidemiologic perspective are well-summarized in the results of the Third National Cancer Survey (1975).[12] The information in Table 31-1 in conjunction with other data, suggests that both environmental and genetic factors are important in the pathogenesis of this tumor.

TABLE 31-1. Melanoma-Epidemiology Data for U.S. (1975)[12]

Prevalence: 9000 cases/year	
Age-Adjusted Incidence (per 100,000 population)	
A. Overall	4.2
B. *Sex*	
Male	4.3
Female	4.1
C. *Race*	
White	4.5
Black	0.8
D. Age 0–9	0.1
10–19	0.4
20–29	2.3
30–39	5.4
40–49	7.3
50–59	7.9
60–69	8.6
70–79	11.3
80 +	16.1
E. Geographic Location	
North	*White*
Minn./St. Paul	3.5
Detroit	3.2
Pittsburgh	3.0
Iowa	3.0
Central	
San Francisco/ Oakland	5.7
Colorado	5.3
South	
Dallas/Ft. Worth	7.6
Atlanta	6.6
Birmingham	5.6

The overall incidence of melanoma in the U.S. in 1975 was 4.2 cases per 100,000 population. Of real concern is the fact that most epidemiologists report that the incidence, both here and in other countries, is rising rapidly with an apparent doubling occurring every 10–17 years (see Table 31-2).[14–18] Ressequie reported an exception to this trend in his analysis of the population of Rochester, Minnesota.[18] Here, the incidence of melanoma remained stable at about 4 per 100,000 between 1958 and 1974.

The generally observed increase in incidence does not appear to be due to more complete case reporting or an alteration in pathologic criteria for diagnostic inclusion, either of which might artifactually explain the observation. Consistent with the reported rise in melanoma incidence being real, there is a parallel increase noted in melanoma mortality. These data, summarized in Table 31-3, show a 25–267% increase for the time intervals studied, the mean increase for all locations being 83%.

Melanoma does not exhibit any overall sex predilection, the incidence among men and women being roughly equal (see Table 31-3). There are, however, striking differences in distribution of the primary lesion by skin sites, with most series showing a disproportionately larger number of lower extremity lesions in women and a similar increase in truncal lesions in men.[21]

The occurrence of metastasizing melanoma is exceedingly rare in children.[22–24] Although in most reported series the age-incidence rate increases successively by decade (see Table 31-1), the majority of patients presenting with primary lesions for treatment are between 30 and 60 years-old.[12,15,19,25]

The relatively infrequent occurrence of melanoma in people of Black and Oriental races is a genetic comment on the clearly protective roll that skin pigment plays.[17,26–34] When non-Caucasians develop melanoma, they exhibit an unusual propensity to develop lesions on the less deeply pigmented parts of the body (*i.e.*, the plantar surface of the foot, palm of

TABLE 31-2. Changes in Reported Incidence of Melanoma with Time for Different Geographic Locations

LOCATION	SEX	EARLIER TIME OF OBSERVATION	INCIDENCE PER 10[5]	LATER TIME OF OBSERVATION	INCIDENCE PER 10[5]
Connecticut[14,16]	M	1935–1939	1.37	1965–1972	4.72
	F	1935–1939	1.05	1965–1972	4.62
New York[14,16]	M	1941–1943	1.22	1966–1970	4.33
	F	1941–1943	1.77	1966–1970	3.61
*Texas[17]	M	1944–1948	2.28	1962–1966	7.32
	F	1944–1948	2.88	1962–1966	6.66
Rochester, Minn[18]	M&F	1950–1958	4.40	1967–1974	4.00
Norway[15]	M	1953–1957	2.36	1968–1972	6.60
	F	1953–1957	2.62	1968–1972	6.48
Sweden[15]	M	1953–1957	3.10	1967–1971	5.54
	F	1953–1957	3.32	1967–1971	5.94
Denmark[15]	M	1955	2.1	1970	4.6
	F	1955	2.5	1970	6.5
Finland[19]	M	1953–1957	1.36	1969–1973	3.22
	F	1953–1957	1.76	1969–1973	3.04

* Numbers represent average of incidence reported for 6 regions surveyed—Houston, El Paso, San Antonio, Laredo, Harlingen, Corpus Christie.

TABLE 31-3. Changes in Reported Mortality of Melanoma for Different Geographic Locations

LOCATION	SEX	EARLIER TIME OF OBSERVATION	MORTALITY PER 10^5	LATER TIME OF OBSERVATION	MORTALITY PER 10^5
U.S.[20]	Both	1950–1953	1.02	1964–1970	1.55
Norway[14]	M	1956–1960	1.59	1966–1970	2.68
	F	1956–1960	1.33	1966–1970	1.81
Sweden[14]	M	1956–1960	1.65	1966–1968	2.14
	F	1956–1960	1.06	1966–1968	1.48
Denmark[14]	M	1956–1960	1.59	1966–1969	2.37
	F	1956–1960	1.61	1966–1969	2.13
Finland[19]	M	1953–1960	1.0	1961–1970	1.4
	F	1953–1960	0.8	1961–1970	1.0
Australia[14]	M	1931–1940	0.98	1961–1970	3.60
	F	1931–1940	0.76	1961–1970	2.49
Canada[14]	M	1951–1955	0.71	1966–1970	1.37
	F	1951–1955	0.59	1966–1970	1.22
U.K.[14]	Both	1950	0.51	1967	1.02

the hand, or mucous membranes of the mouth, rectum, or vagina).[26,27] While lesions in these sites account for less than 10% of melanomas seen in Caucasians, they represent about two-thirds of those seen among Negroes.

Although no definitive proof causally linking any specific factor or insult to any given human tumor exists today, a fairly strong case can be made for the etiologic role that sunlight plays in melanoma. Much has been written, based largely on epidemiologic observations, on the importance of solar trauma in the pathogenesis of melanoma.[15,19,35–46]

Most compelling among the lines of evidence supporting a causal relationship is the "latitude effect" first described by Lancaster.[35] Within any given region studied, the incidence and mortality of melanoma rises significantly as you approach the equator. Data corroborating this observation have been reported for the U.S., Australia, Canada, and Norway.[12,38,42,45,46] Further implicating exposure to sunlight in the pathogenesis of melanoma are data reported from Israel.[36,37] These data emphasize the importance of duration of exposure and show that the incidence of melanoma is highest among Israeli natives of European extraction, intermediate for those European-born but long-term residents in Israel, and lowest for the newly arrived European-born immigrants.

Although a more convincing case can be made for basal and squamous cell skin cancer, the anatomic distribution of primary melanomas on the body is consistent with sun exposure as an etiologic factor. A clear excess of melanoma occurs on the head and neck region in both sexes, on the lower extremities in women, and on the trunk in men compared to the expected incidence at these sites if melanoma occurrence was directly relation to skin surface area (see Table 31-4). The latter two observations may reflect changes in dress habits and recreational activity patterns occurring over the past several decades that have led to greater sun exposure for these parts.

The most likely candidates to develop melanoma are those persons who tolerate the sun poorly; they freckle, burn easily, and tan lightly if at all.[39] Sober and coworkers noted that melanoma patients experienced a greater number of multiple sun burns than controls.[47] Williams and associates demon-

TABLE 31-4. Distribution of Melanoma by Sex and Site

SERIES	SEX	LOWER EXTREMITY	TRUNK	UPPER EXTREMITY	H&N	OTHER
Davis[52] (Queensland)	M(523)*	19% (101)	47% (246)	13% (66)	21% (110)	
	F (664)	39% (256)	19% (128)	23% (161)	18% (119)	
Knutson[53] (Ellis Fischel)	M(123)	21% (26)	22% (27)	18% (22)	39% (48)	
	F (106)	40% (42)	17% (18)	13% (14)	30% (32)	
Teppo[19] (Finland)	M(1108)	17% (184)	48% (531)	9% (94)	19% (212)	7% (87)
	F (1393)	36% (506)	28% (396)	11% (153)	19% (257)	6% (81)
Luce[21] (M.D. Anderson)	M(1225)	16% (196)	26% (319)	20% (245)	26% (318)	12% (147)
	F (1224)	36% (441)	18% (220)	20% (245)	18% (220)	8% (98)
TOTAL	M(2979)	17% (507)	38% (1123)	14% (427)	23% (688)	8% (234)
	F (3387)	37% (1245)	22% (762)	17% (573)	19% (628)	5% (179)

* ( ) = number of patients

strated an association between melanoma and school teaching, an occupation that does not usually entail protracted sun exposure.[48] These latter two observations suggest that the pattern of sun exposure (*i.e.*, brief but intense) may be as important as total duration of exposure.

Mechanical trauma was suggested as an etiologic factor in melanoma based on the disproportionately high occurrence of lesions on the sole of the foot among Bantu Africans who go barefoot.[49] More critical analysis of the information available showed that the incidence of melanoma on the sole of the foot similarly was high among urbanized Bantus who wear shoes as well as among American Blacks who wear shoes.[26,27] A causal role for mechanical trauma in melanoma is doubtful.

The role of hormonal factors in the etiology of melanoma is unclear. Although the sex ratio is about equal, women overall fare better than men with their disease, even when corrected for stage.[50,51,54] That hormonal factors may very well be of importance is further suggested by the fact that the survival advantage noted for women disappears in the postmenopausal subgroup.[54] The questions usually posed by women in regard to the importance of hormonal factors in melanoma are: Should I take oral contraceptives, and, Should I become pregnant? The paucity of available data makes it difficult to give hard answers to these questions. Beral reported a weak association between oral contraceptive use and melanoma, while Shaw noted that oral contraceptive users had a slightly better 5-year survival than non-users.[54,55] The effect of pregnancy on prognosis of melanoma has long been questioned. There have been several reports of patients experiencing spontaneous regression following termination of pregnancy.[56–58] In retrospectively analyzing the impact of pregnancy on course of disease in 251 women, Shiu reported no statistically significant difference in 5-year, disease-free intervals between nulliparous, parous nonpregnant, and pregnant women with stage I disease.[59] With stage I melanoma, pregnant women or women whose disease became reactivated with pregnancy, however, had statistically significant lower survival rates than nulliparous or other women in the parous group. However, the data from this retrospective study must be interpreted cautiously. For example, the group in which pregnancy appears to have had an adverse effect contained a greater number of patients with truncal primaries, an indicator of poor prognosis. This may have occurred as a result of pregnancy or perhaps chance alone. At present, the relationship between pregnancy and prognosis in patients with melanoma remains unresolved.

Bahn and coworkers have suggested a possible relationship between exposure to polychlorinated biphenyls and melanoma.[60] However, this brief report remains unconfirmed. Several reports suggest that levodopa may exacerbate melanoma.[61–63] However, Sober and Wick found only one patient taking levodopa among 1,099 questioned prospectively, concluding that levodopa, if a factor in the induction of melanoma, must play an inconsequential role.[64]

Parsons and associates have detected particles with RNA tumor virus-like properties in six established human melanoma cell lines. Birkmayer and associates found an RNA-instructed DNA polymerase with enzymatic activity characteristic of that of oncogenic RNA viruses.[66] It remains unclear whether these investigators have detected an etiologic agent or simply contaminating or passenger viruses.

GENETICS

In 1820, Norris was the first to describe the hereditary variant of cutaneous melanoma.[67] The next report of human familial melanoma did not appear until 1952.[68] On reviewing the literature in 1967, Anderson found 74 pedigrees demonstrating familial melanoma.[69] The subject was more recently reviewed by Greene and Fraumeni who identified 165 different kindreds with 490 persons with melanoma.[70] Their observations are summarized here.

Surveys of patients with cutaneous melanoma report a positive family history in 0.4–12.3% of patients with the higher figures being reported when intensive case-finding was employed. Using data from a population-based survey in Australia, these investigators estimate that first-degree blood relatives of melanoma patients are 1.7 times more likely to develop cutaneous melanoma than persons in the general population. Further, they estimate that 11% of melanoma may be hereditary. The sex distribution of cases of familial melanoma was similar to that for sporadic melanoma. Age at first diagnosis was approximately 10 years younger in patients with familial melanoma, but it is not certain if this is an important biologic characteristic or ascertainment bias. It is generally believed that the survival rate is better for hereditary cutaneous melanoma than it is for the sporadic type.[71] This may simply be a reflection of a greater awareness resulting in earlier diagnosis.

Multiple primary melanomas occurred in 50 of 406 familial melanoma patients (12.3%) with an average of 2.8 tumors per person. In contrast, only 2.8% of patients with sporadic melanoma developed multiple primaries. Cancers other than melanoma have been reported in close relatives of patients with familial melanoma but no consistent pattern has emerged. An association may exist between sporadic melanoma and breast cancer in females.[72,73]

Clark et al[74] recently described the familial occurrence of melanoma with an associated constellation of clinical and histologic features, which he termed the "B–K mole" syndrome. Patients with the syndrome typically have between 10 and 100 pigmented lesions, located largely over the trunk, buttocks, and lower extremities (see Fig. 31-1). Such precursor moles have been followed with serial photographs as they evolved into frank melanomas. The lesions tend to be large (about 10 mm in diameter) and histologically resemble a compound melanocytic nevus but exhibit atypical melanocytic hyperplasia, lymphocytic infiltration, and neovascularization as well.[74] The inheritance pattern for the syndrome is most often that of autosomal dominance.[75] Treatment of the B–K mole involves excisional biopsy of any such lesion that arouses suspicion followed by further surgery if the histology reveals melanoma. The importance of recognizing a patient as a member of the syndrome lies in both the need for added vigilance in the follow-up of the patient's other pigmented lesions as well as the need to screen family members to define afflicted members.

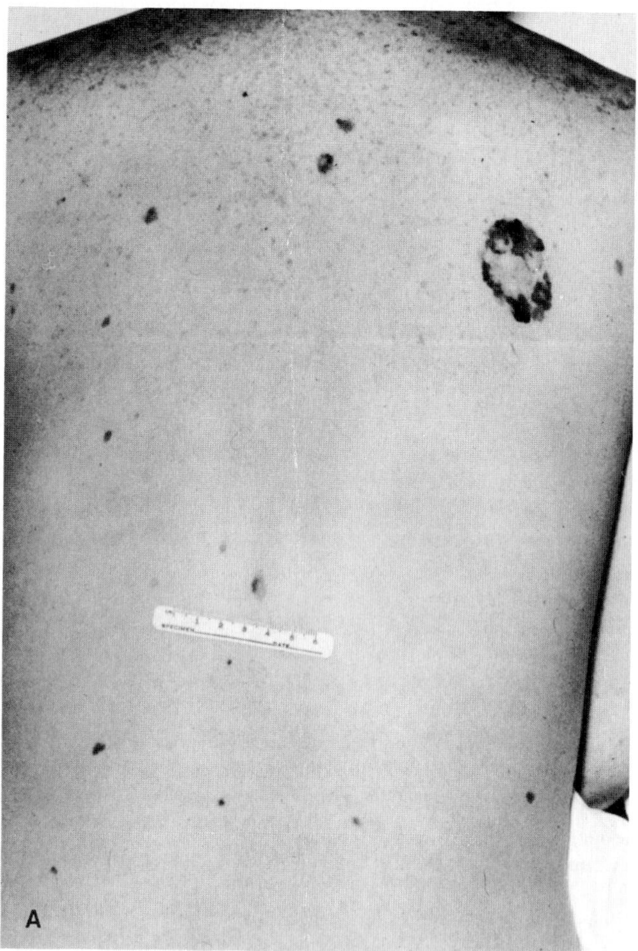

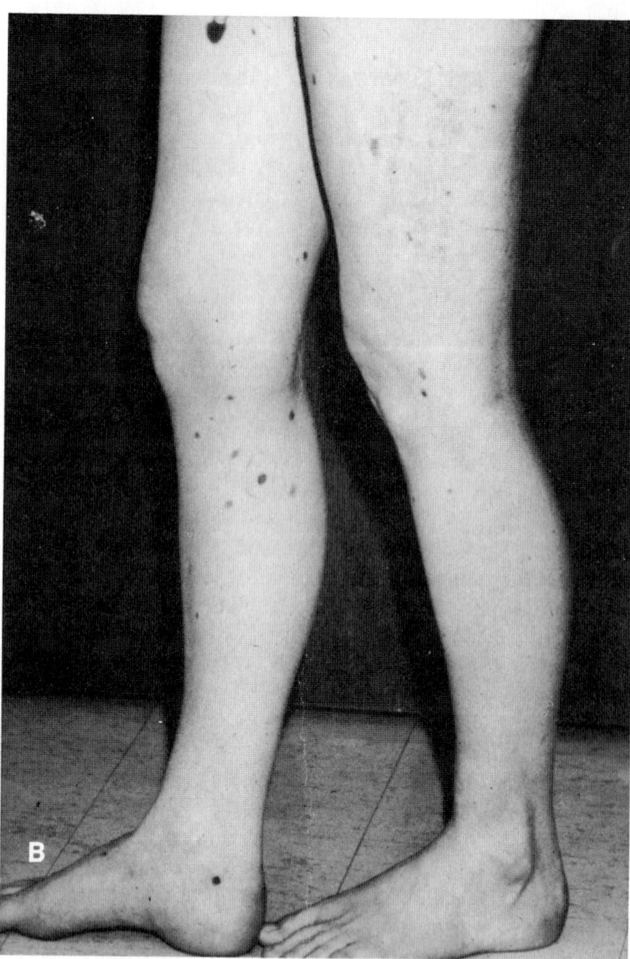

FIG. 31-1. The back (*A*) and lower extremities (*B*) of a 26-year-old Caucasian female with familial melanoma and the B-K mole syndrome. This patient had three primary cutaneous melanomas, one of which is obvious in the area of the right scapula. Two siblings also had cutaneous melanoma. The numerous B-K moles are apparent on the back and lower extremities.

CLASSIFICATION AND CLINICAL DIAGNOSIS

Clark distinguishes 11 types of extraocular melanoma on clinical and histologic grounds (see Table 31-5).[76] Of these the most common cutaneous types are lentigo maligna melanoma (LMM), superficial spreading melanoma (SSM), nodular melanoma (NM), and acral lentinginous melanoma (ALM).[77,78] The proper understanding and recognition of the four dominant types of melanoma will allow for clinical diagnosis at a developmental stage when the disease is curable. The reason for this is that three of the four common varieties of cutaneous melanoma (LMM, SSM, ALM) are characterized by indolent, peripheral enlargement of relatively flat, complex colored, primary lesions. This period of centrifugal growth generally lasts for several years and has been termed the *radial growth phase* of the primary lesion. While a melanoma is in the radial growth phase, it acquires little or no competence to metastasize and may therefore be cured by relatively simple surgical procedures.

The acquisition of competence to metastasize by a primary melanoma is associated with a focal change in the neoplasm, a change characterized by penetration into deeper cutaneous tissues. This focal, deep penetration is called the *vertical growth phase*. The extent of this second growth phase is the basis for the levels of invasion and the tumor thickness measurements that are presently the mainstays to estimate prognosis and assignment of risk immediately following surgery for the primary tumor.

Mihm and Sober and their respective associates have delineated the positive signs that suggest malignant change:

1. Variegated Color
   This is most common in SSM and LMM. The presence of red, white, or blue in a lesion that was basically brown or black suggests malignancy. Blue is most ominous, white generally denotes an area of spontaneous regression, and nodular melanomas are usually uniform in color, being blue–black or gray.
2. Irregular Border
   Notching of the border resulting from spontaneous

TABLE 31-5. Classification of Human Extra-Ocular Melanomas

1. Superficial spreading type
2. Lentigo maligna type
3. Melanoma with an unclassified radial growth phase
4. Nodular type
5. Melanoma arising in a giant hairy nevus
6. Volar-subungual melanoma (acral lentiginous melanoma)
7. Oral, vaginal, and anal mucous membrane melanoma
8. Melanoma without a demonstrable primary lesion
9. Melanoma arising in a blue nevus
10. Melanoma arising in a visceral site
11. Other melanoma such as those arising in childhood and those arising in dermal nevi

regression or segmental peripheral expansion is common in melanomas with a radial growth phase, especially SSM.

3. Irregular Surface Elevations
   Either palpable or visible.

LMM constitutes 10–15% of cutaneous melanomas and is the most benign of the four types. LMM most commonly occurs in areas heavily exposed to the sun, such as the head, neck, and dorsum of the hands. The median age at diagnosis is about 70 years, and females are probably more frequently affected. The histology of this lesion is represented schematically in Fig. 31-2. There are both radial and vertical growth phases.

The radial growth phase of LMM is characterized by abnormal melanocytes extending centrifugally in the epidermis with minimal invasion into the papillary dermis. There is minimal epidermal hyperplasia, thus the radial growth phase is only minimally elevated. When only radial growth is present, the lesion is called lentigo maligna and is not malignant melanoma.[81] Radial growth precedes the development of vertical growth by decades, and it is this slow progression to vertical growth that accounts for the relative benignity of LMM. Although the radial growth phase is relatively innocuous, the vertical growth phase is associated with metastases in about 25% of cases.

Clinically, the early LMM lesions are large, flat, and tan or brown in color (see Col. Fig. 31-1). With the development of the vertical growth phase, the lesion becomes focally elevated, but the basic tan–brown pattern of the radial growth phase persists (see Col. Fig. 31-2). The focal elevation may be darker or lighter in color than the surrounding radial growth phase. LMM is distinguished from superficial spreading melanoma by the rarity of rose and pink colors and the minimal elevation of the radial growth phase.

SSM accounts for about 70% of all cutaneous melanoma in Caucasians and is intermediate in malignancy. The tumor has its peak incidence in the fifth decade; the sexes are affected with equal frequency, with the legs more commonly affected in females. In males, the upper back is the predominant site. The histology of this lesion is represented schematically in Fig. 31-3.

As in LMM, there are both radial and vertical growth phases. The radial growth phase of SMM is characterized by melanoma cells within the epidermis (with epidermal thickening) and papillary dermis and by a host response composed of inflammatory cells, fibroplasia, and new blood vessel formation. This epidermal hyperplasia results in a radial growth phase which is more obviously elevated than is the radial growth phase of LMM. The duration of the radial growth phase is difficult to document since the lesions are small and inconspicuous; one-third are present on the back where they are not readily visible. This growth phase ranges from one to as many as a dozen years. It is associated with recurrent or metastatic disease in less than 5% of affected patients.

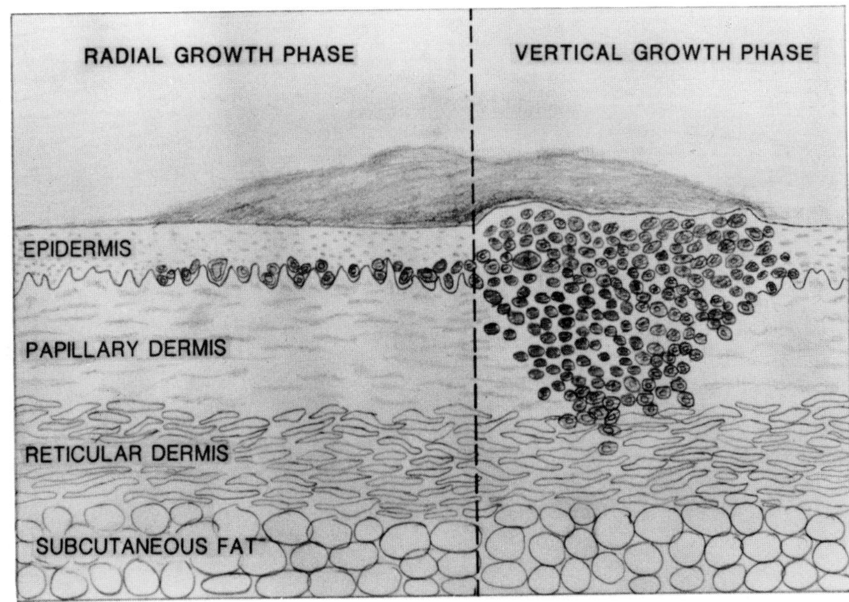

FIG. 31-2. Schematic of the cross-sectional histology of lentigo maligna melanoma. (Mastrangelo M, et al. Prog Cancer Res Ther 6:1–18, 1978)

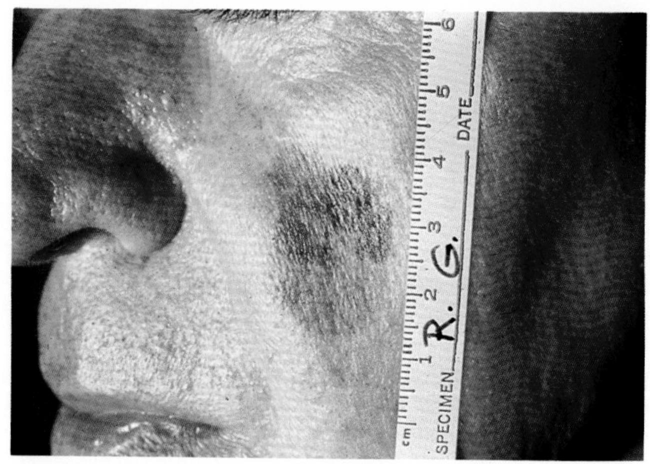

COL. FIG. 31-1. Lentigo maligna.

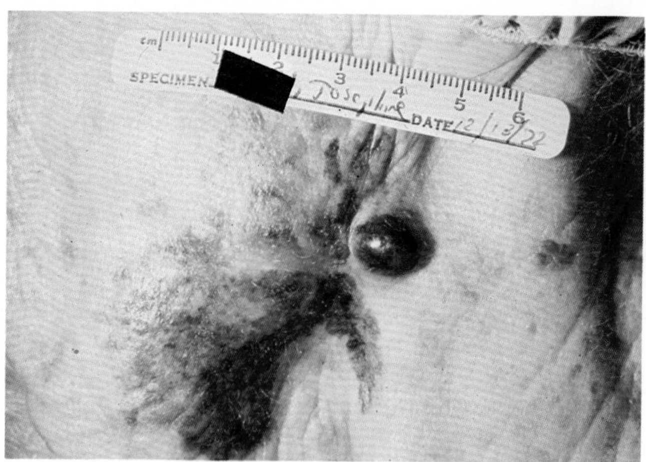

COL. FIG. 31-2. Lentigo maligna melanoma with vertical growth (nodule formation).

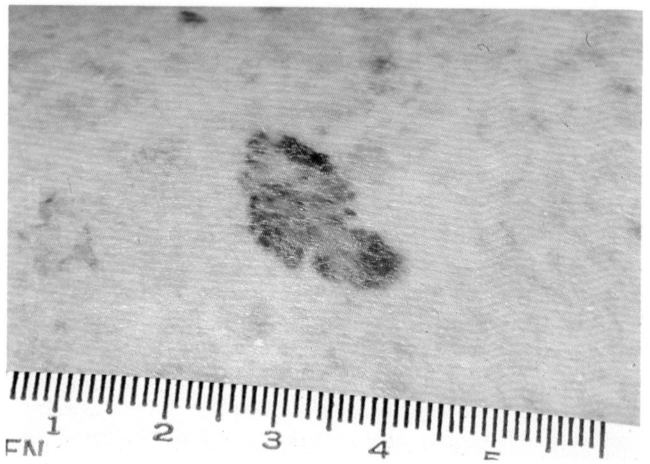

COL. FIG. 31-3. Superficial spreading melanoma in radial growth.

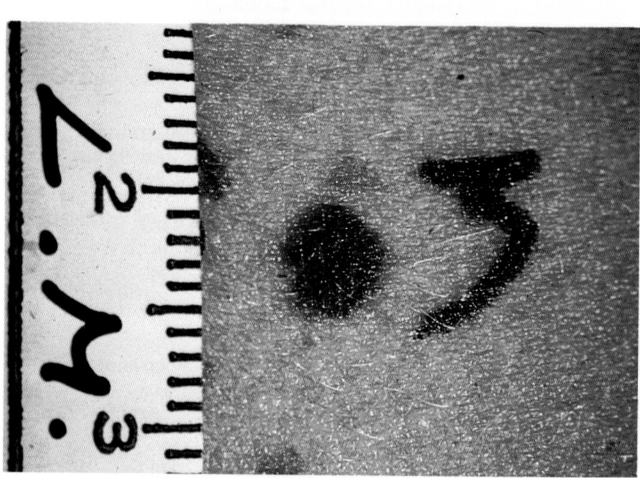

COL. FIG. 31-4. Intradermal nevus.

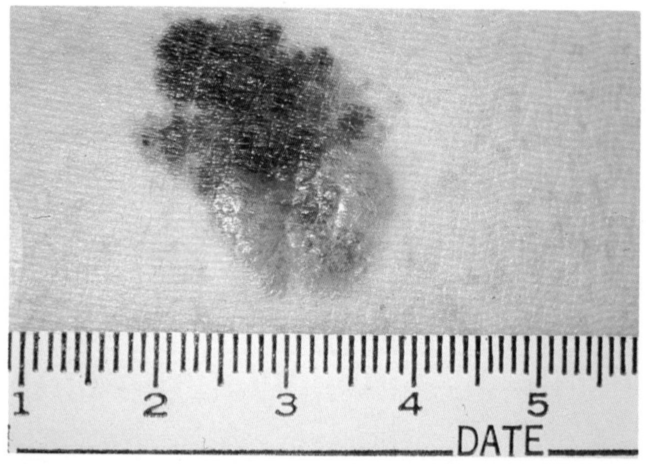

COL. FIG. 31-5. Superficial spreading melanoma with radial and early vertical growth.(Early nodule formation.)

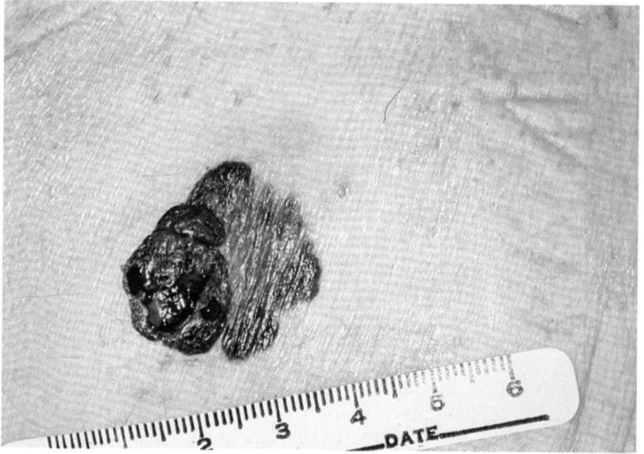

COL. FIG. 31.6. Superficial spreading melanoma with radial and advanced vertical growth. (Large nodule with bleeding.)

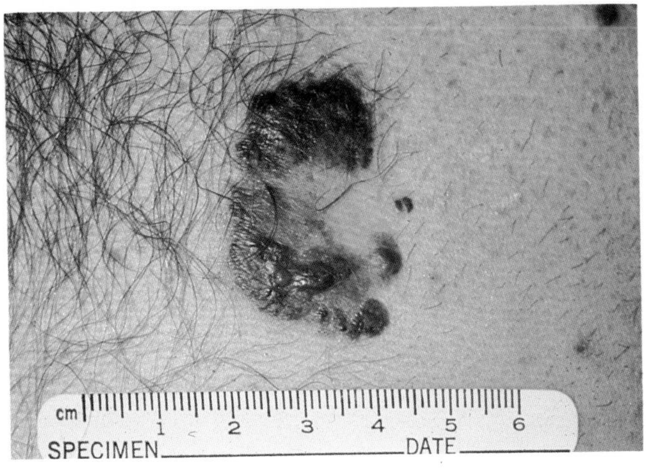

COL. FIG. 31-7. Superficial spreading melanoma with spontaneous regression of central (white) area.

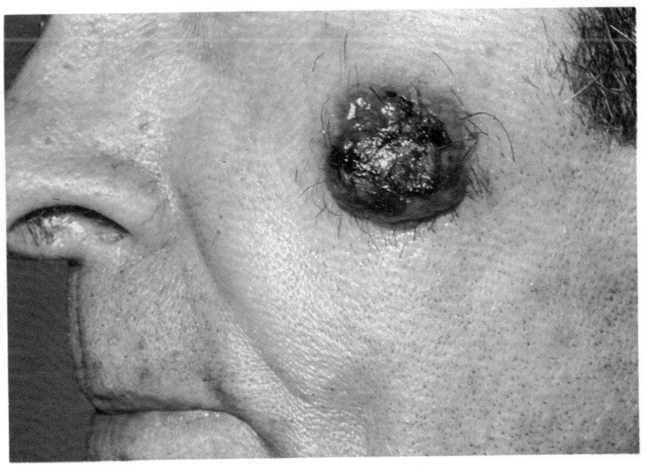

COL. FIG. 31-8. Nodular melanoma.

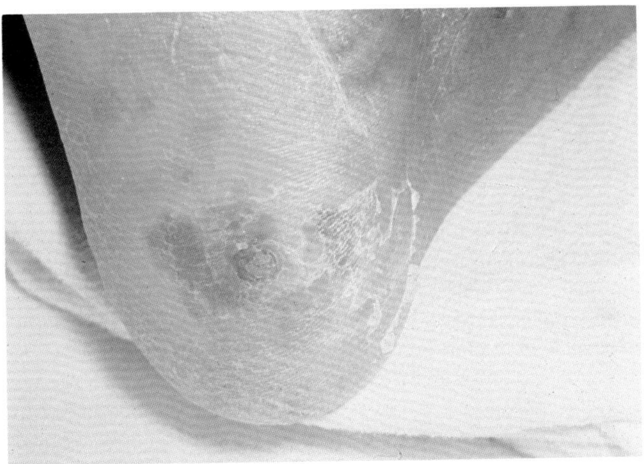

COL. FIG. 31-9. Plantar (heel) melanoma, showing typical "stain" appearance. Because of mechanical and anatomic factors, nodules infrequently develop even in deeply invasive lesions.

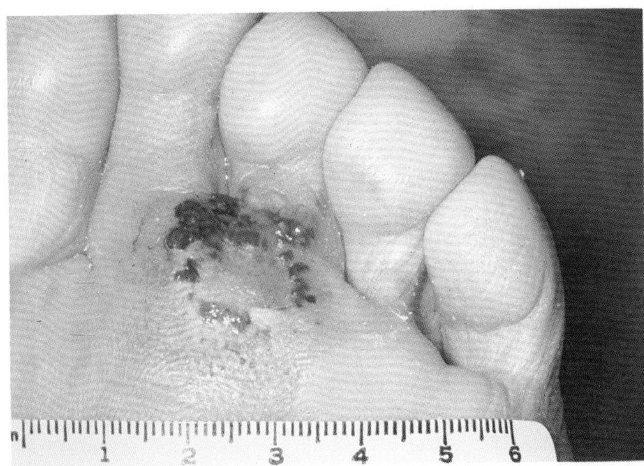

COL. FIG. 31-10. Plantar melanoma at the base of the toes. Nodule development is more common in this location.

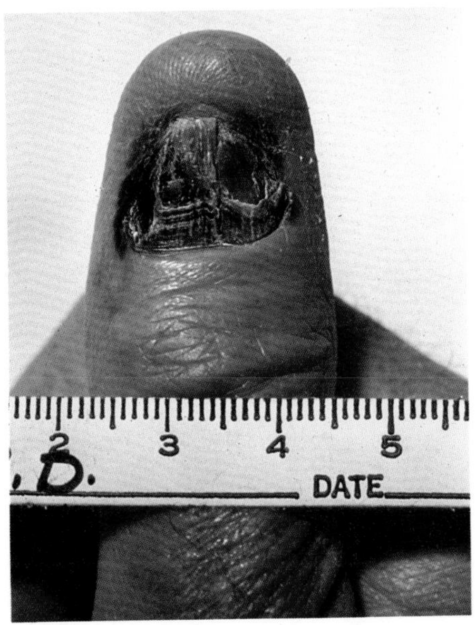

COL. FIG. 31-11. Subungual melanoma.

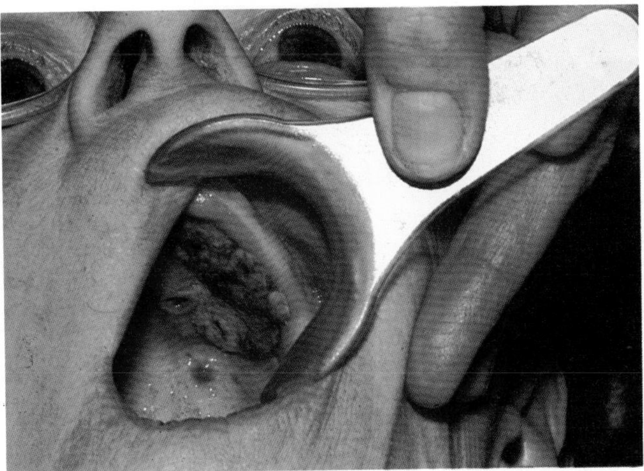

COL. FIG. 31-12. Oral mucosal melanoma.

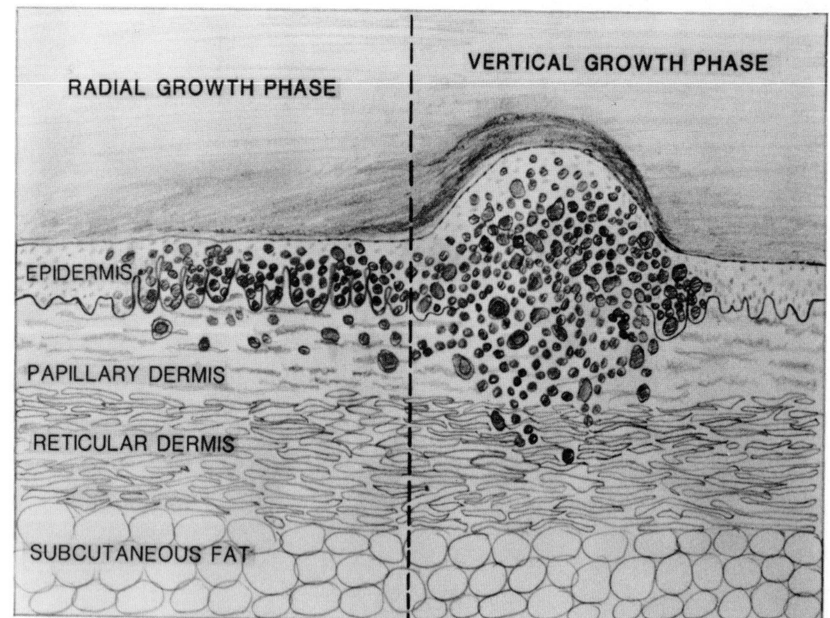

FIG. 31-3. Schematic of the cross-sectional histology of superficial spreading melanoma. (Mastrangelo M, et al. Prog Cancer Res Ther 6:1–18, 1978)

The vertical growth phase develops clinically rather rapidly, in a few weeks to a few months, and is heralded by the appearance of a nodule. Depending on the depth of invasion and other cellular parameters, vertical growth phase lesions metastasize in 35–85% of cases.

Early SSM lesions are a haphazard combination of tan, brown, blue, and black; in most lesions, shades of rose and pink are also present. Col. Fig. 31-3 illustrates an SSM entirely in radial growth. Note the marked variegation in color, marginal notching, and loss of skin creases that distinguish this lesion from the more common intra-epidermal or junctional nevus (see Col. Fig. 31-4), which, in addition, is usually considerably smaller in size (< 5 mm). More advanced lesions have the nodularity indicative of vertical growth and have a characteristic red, white, and blue appearance (see Col. Figs. 31-5 and 31-6). The white areas represent spontaneous regression (see Col. Fig. 31-7).

NM, the most malignant of the four varieties, constitutes about 12% of all cutaneous melanomas. The median age at diagnosis is 50 years. NM occurs twice as commonly in males as in females. This may account, at least in part, for the poorer prognosis of melanoma in males. The histology of NM is presented schematically in Fig. 31-4.

NM is composed exclusively of a vertical growth phase, with melanoma cells usually invading into the deeper dermis. The host cellular response is variable, but is generally less than in other forms of melanoma. Clinically, these lesions evolve quickly over several months to a year and rarely longer. Even the earliest lesions are raised and usually contain a characteristic gray appearance with pinkish hues (see Col.

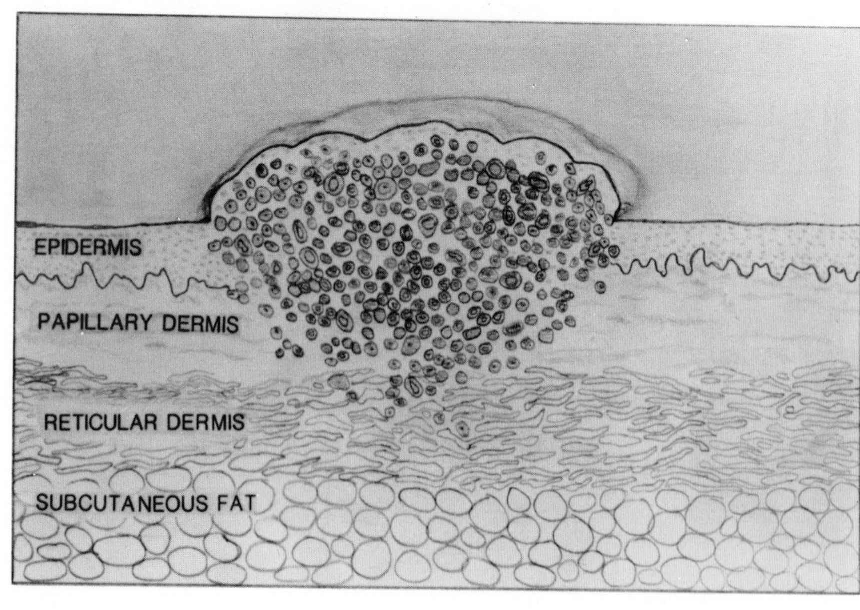

FIG. 31-4. Schematic of the cross-sectional histology of nodular melanoma. (Mastrangelo M, et al. Prog Cancer Res Ther 6:1–18, 1978)

TABLE 31-6. Comparison of Four Varieties of Melanoma

TYPE OF MELANOMA	RADIAL GROWTH	DURATION OF RADIAL GROWTH	FOCI OF REGRESSION/ PROGRESSION	PAGETOID CELLS IN EPIDERMIS	DESMOPLASIA IN VERTICAL GROWTH
Lentigo maligna	Lentiginous	Decades	Yes	No	Common
Superficial spreading	Epitheliod	1–10 years	Yes	Yes	Rare
Nodular	None	None	No	No	Rare
Acral lentiginous	Usually lentiginous	Months to years	Yes	Rarely	Very common

Fig. 31-8). As the lesion continues to grow, the dominant color changes to blue–black, giving the tumor a blueberry-like appearance (see Col. Fig. 31-8). The lack of a radial growth phase makes early diagnosis difficult.

Arrington and coworkers have documented the development and biologic characteristics of ALM. This form of melanoma occurs on the palms and soles and in subungual locations (see Col. Figs. 31-9, 31,10- and 31-11). The developmental biology is also characterized by radial and vertical growth phases. The radial growth phase is flat, the margin nonpalpable, and the color a mosaic of rich tans, browns, and black. In subungual locations, the radial growth phase may be a streak in the nail associated with an irregular tan–brown stain, diffusing proximally from the nail bed. The radial growth phase has a duration of years, but if ignored, it will be followed by the elevated nodular areas of the vertical growth phase. The exact prognostic significance of the vertical growth phase has not been determined in a large series of cases, but once it has supervened, metastases are common.

The distinguishing histologic characteristics of LMM, SSM, NM, and ALM are summarized in Table 31-6.

The key to control of cutaneous melanoma is early diagnosis. This involves an awareness of the clinical characteristics of early melanoma (described above) and a willingness to conduct thorough cutaneous examinations, especially of high-risk patients. High-risk groups include persons who have already had one cutaneous melanoma; a first-degree blood relative of patients who have had melanoma, particularly if they have had multiple primary melanomas or the BK-mole syndrome; or normal persons of Celtic ancestory. If clinical characteristics suggest melanoma, if an uncertain etiology exists, or if the patient is concerned (particularly if symptomatic conditions exists), the lesion should be biopsied. All excised lesions must be submitted for histologic examination.

DIFFERENTIAL DIAGNOSIS

Many cutaneous lesions appear pigmented and thus require differentiation from melanoma.* This discussion addresses the three most common problems confronting the clinician:

1. Distinguishing superficial spreading melanoma from common acquired nevi, pigmented seborrheic keratosis, and pigmented basal cell carcinoma
2. Differentiating nodular melanoma from a hemangioma, Spitz nevus, or dermatofibroma
3. Distinguishing subungual melanoma from hemorrhage

Common acquired nevi present in three clinical and histologic patterns—junctional, compound, and dermal.[84,85] Common acquired nevi or moles are proliferative aggregates of apparently normal melanocytes. In a junctional nevus all the melanocytes are above the basement membrane. Clinically, these lesions are flat, tan or brown in color, and tend to be circular in outline (see Col. Fig. 31-4). They can be distinguished from an SSM in radial growth (see Col. Fig. 31-3). Color is orderly rather than markedly and haphazardly variegated. Normal skin markings are usually observed. Most are less than 5 mm in diameter and almost all are less than 9 mm in longest dimension. The margin lacks the notching characteristic of SSM.

In a compound nevus melanocytes are present in both the epidermis and the dermis. In the deeper dermis, cells loose pigment and have a clear cytoplasm. Other cells have a neural appearance. These may be modified melanocytes or an ingrowth of cells of Schwann cell origin. Clinically, these begin as slightly elevated tan–brown lesions with the subsequent slow development of a nodular component in many. These lesions can be distinguished from an SSM in vertical growth in several ways. Historically, nodule development is slow in these benign lesions as opposed to the abrupt and rapid vertical growth in SSM. The flat component of a compound nevus is characterized by an orderly pattern of coloration and marginal integrity.

As its name implies, a dermal nevus has only a dermal component that is histologically similar to the dermal component of a compound nevus. These lesions are dome-shaped and usually devoid of pigment. Thus, they are generally easily distinguishable from melanoma. An entirely amelanotic primary melanoma is a rare lesion.

The pigmented seborrheic keratosis has a dull, waxy surface studded with small keratin plugs and a tan to dark brown coloration. The lesion presents a "stuck-on" appearance and indeed can be scraped from the surface. Melanomas are firmly attached to the skin.[83]

Pigmented basal cell carcinomas may display bluish, reddish–brown, and gray–white coloration. True brown or black are not present because the melanin pigment in the tumor is confined to the dermis. Careful examination with side lighting may reveal the characteristic peripheral ring of tumor nodules and telangiectasia over and between nodules. (The telangiectasia is best seen with the aide of a hand lens.[83])

* For a detailed presentation of the differential diagnosis of pigmented cutaneous lesions the reader is referred to the reports by Winkelmann and Mihm and coworkers.[82,83]

Nodular melanomas must be distinguished from hemangiomas, dermatofibromas, and Spitz nevi. The hemangioma presents as a globoid, dark blue–red or purple lesion. On occasion, the blood can be expressed from the lesion by applying pressure with a glass slide. Most often, however, the diagnosis only becomes apparent when the lesion is sectioned following excision.

The typical dermatofibroma has been described by Fitzpatrick and Gilchrest as a firm nodule less than 1 cm in diameter with a uniform moderate or dark brown pigmentation.[86] They occur most commonly on the extremities of middle-aged women. The application of lateral pressure with thumb and index finger produces dimpling. In contrast, melanomas will protrude above the skin.

The Spitz nevus presents a major problem in clinical and histologic diagnosis. The lesion was first described by Spitz in 1948 and has a variety of names, including juvenile melanoma.[87] The average age at the time of histologic diagnosis is about 10 years.[88] Typically, these are small (6–7 mm) dome-shaped, pink to red lesions that grow rapidly within a few months. A rapidly growing globoid lesion in a young patient should alert the clinician to consider a Spitz nevus. Without clinical information these lesions are often difficult to distinguish histologically from malignant melanoma.[89] Clark describes these as tumors of relatively uniform histology.[84] Cells are often fat, elongated, and contain no pigment. Multinucleated giant melanocytes are frequently present.* The treatment of choice is excision.

Subungual melanoma must be distinguished from subungual hemorrhage. The latter is usually sudden in onset and the lesion is sharply defined beneath the nail. By comparison, melanoma is gradual in onset and characterized by poorly demarcated streaks extending along the long axis of the nail. A diagnosis of hemorrhage can be confirmed by puncturing the nail and evacuating the blood. Further, with the passage of time the entire subungual hemorrhage will migrate distally with clearing of the nail bed. Subungual melanoma is a persistent lesion.[91]

The differential diagnosis of pigmented skin lesions is a difficult task for the non-specialist. If doubt exists concerning the precise etiology of a lesion, the patient should be referred to a dermatologist. All excised lesions must be examined histologically.

PROGNOSTIC FACTORS

PATIENT FACTORS

Sex

Data regarding the relationship between the sex of the patient and 5-year survival are presented in Table 31-7. Females have a clear advantage in survival after initial diagnosis. Heise, Krementz, and Bodenham note an improved survival for females irrespective of whether the stage at diagnosis was local or regional.[92,93] It is less clear whether females survive longer after first recurrence. Einhorn and coworkers reported

* For a detailed description of the histopathology, the reader is referred to the review by Paniago–Pereria and coworkers.[90]

TABLE 31-7. Five-Year Survival Related to Sex

STUDY (Reference No.)	% MALES*	% FEMALES*
Perzik & Baum (95)	43 (33/76)	63 (45/72)
Jones et al (96)	25 (12/48)	41 (26/63)
Shah & Goldsmith (50)	48 (368/766)	62 (445/717)
Mundth et al (51)	35 (63/180)	54 (92/170)
Lehman et al (97)	23 (5/22)	65 (13/20)
Nathanson et al (98)	24 (22/92)	38 (27/72)
Cochran (99)	30 (16/54)	63 (55/88)
Elias et al (100)	32 (48/148)	48 (48/100)
TOTALS	41 (567/1386)	58 (751/1302)

* $p = <0.00001$

that females survived longer than males following the start of chemotherapy despite the lack of a real difference in objective response rates. Sex appears to be an important prognostic factor in patients with operable local or regional disease. Its importance in patients with more advanced disease remains a question.

Age

Data are conflicting regarding the impact of age at initial diagnosis on subsequent survival. Several investigators have noted an improved survival for patients less than 45 years of age.[95,96,101] However, Cochran and Elias and coworkers could not demonstrate an impact of age on survival at initial diagnosis. There are few data correlating age with survival after first recurrence or dissemination.

Immunologic Status

There have been numerous attempts to correlate prognosis with various parameters of immune reactivity. The most extensively studied immune parameters include delayed-type hypersensitivity to DNCB and recall antigens, lymphocyte microcytotoxicity against autologous and allogeneic melanoma cells, lymphocyte transformation to PHA and T-cell enumeration.[102–122] Taken as a whole, these immunologic studies suggest that melanoma patients, especially those with advanced disease, are less easily sensitized to DNCB, have lower delayed hypersensitivity responses to a variety of antigens, and display impaired transformation responses to PHA and various antigens. It has not been demonstrated that any of these responses constitutes a significant independent variable in estimating the prognosis or response to treatment of melanoma patients. Attempts to measure tumor specific immunity such as the lymphocyte cytotoxicity assay are hampered by a lack of specificity.

PRIMARY LESION

Microstaging

Several workers have clearly shown that prognosis in melanoma is related to the depth of tumor invasion.[123,124] These studies were subsequently refined by the work of Clark and associates who defined five levels of microinvasion.[76,77,81,125]

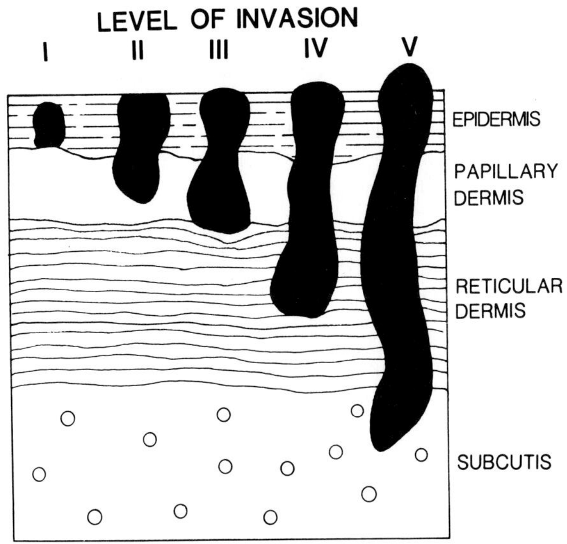

FIG. 31-5. Schematic of Clark's levels of invasion.

These are as follows:

Level I. All tumor cells confined to the epidermis with no invasion through the basement membrane (*in situ* melanoma)

Level II. Tumor cells penetrating through the basement membrane into the papillary dermis but not extending to the reticular dermis

Level III. Tumor cells filling the papillary dermis and abutting against the reticular dermis, but not invading it

Level IV. Extension of tumor cells between the bundles of collagen characteristic of the reticular dermis

Level V. Invasion into the subcutaneous tissue.

Clark levels of invasion are depicted schematically in Fig. 31-5. The correlation of level of invasion with survival is presented in Table 31-8. Survival decreases with increasing level of invasion. The correlation is most accurate in patients with pathologic stage I disease. Balch and coworkers found that Clark level of invasion did not correlate with survival in patients presenting with pathologic stage II disease.[131] The number of lymph nodes involved with tumor was an overriding factor in determining survival.

TABLE 31-9. Relationship of Tumor Thickness to Prognosis

THICKNESS (mm)	DISEASE-FREE 5 YEARS BRESLOW[129]	SURVIVAL BALCH ET AL[128]
<0.76	38/38 100%	19/20 95%
0.76–1.5	14/19 74%	32/47 68%
1.51–2.25	11/14 79%	
1.5–3.0		50/78 65%
2.26–3.0	4/9 44%	
>3.0	4/18 22%	
>4.0		9/44 20%

Breslow has correlated the thickness of the primary lesion, as measured with an ocular micrometer, with prognosis.[129] Thickness is measured by determining the vertical dimension of each melanoma from the top of the granular layer to the base of the tumor. Breslow found an inverse relationship between thickness and survival. This work was confirmed and extended by Hansen and McCarten, Wanebo and coworkers, and Balch and coworkers.[127,128,130] Because of variation in the thickness categories used to assess prognosis, these data cannot be pooled; however, data from two comparable studies are presented in Table 31-9.

Correct assessment of Clark levels and tumor thickness requires that the primary melanoma be properly sectioned. The correct procedure for this is presented in Fig. 31-6. The entire specimen is serially blocked with sections cut at about 3 mm intervals at right angles to the long axis through the entire specimen. Likewise, it is important to examine the lesions clinically and histologically for areas of regression. Of 121 thin (<0.76 mm thick) melanomas examined by Gromet and associates, 23 displayed areas of regression and 5 (22%) subsequently metastasized.[131] Only 2 of 98 thin lesions without evidence of regression metastasized.

Patients with non-ulcerated lesions have an improved prognosis when compared with patients with ulcerated primary melanomas.[95,135] Ulceration is associated with nodule formation and the onset of vertical growth. This suggests that this latter parameter alone may be adequate in assessing prognosis. Balch and coworkers noted that lesion ulceration as determined by microscopic evaluation correlated strongly with thickness. Nonetheless, ulceration was an independent var-

TABLE 31-8. Correlation of Level of Invasion of the Primary Lesion With Survival

LEVEL OF INVASION	CLARK[77]	McGOVERN[126]	% FIVE-YEAR SURVIVAL WANEBO ET AL[127]*	BALCH ET AL[128]
I	—	—	—	—
II	72	82	100	85
III	47	65	88	72
IV	32	49	65	57
V	12	29	16	28

* Clinical stage I patients with only extremity lesions.

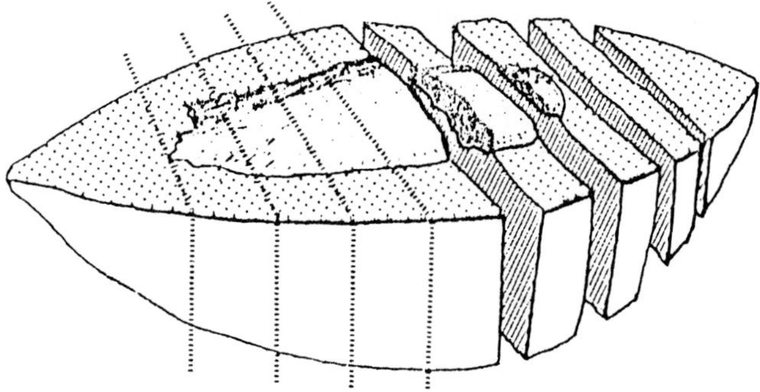

FIG. 31-6. Proper sectioning of a lesion suspected of being malignant melanoma. Many sections of all specimens suspected of being a malignant melanoma should be cut at about 3 mm intervals at right angles to the long axis. By this technique the pathologist can be certain of the actual thickness of the neoplasm and other valuable information, such as the presence of a pre-existing melanocytic nevus. (Ackerman and Su: In Malignant Melanoma, pp. 25–148. New York, Masson Publishing, 1979)

iable that influenced survival within stage of disease (I vs II) and thickness groups.

The location of the primary lesion also appears to influence survival (see Table 31-10). Extremity lesions carry the best prognosis, head and neck primaries an intermediate prognosis, and trunk lesions the poorest prognosis. For all sites, women live longer than men.[92,93,96]

Various other aspects of the primary lesion have been studied to ascertain their relationship to prognosis. These include shape, mitotic activity, vascular invasion, pigmentation, host cellular infiltrate, and surface contour.[93,96,126,128,129,136,137] These parameters have either been of little prognostic value or are related to other more widely accepted indicators.

In a direct comparison of 11 prognostic factors in patients with stage I melanoma, Balch and coworkers found that thickness was the single most important index of outcome, reflecting the biologic risks for local recurrences as well as for regional and distant metastases.[134] Clark levels were a less predictive prognostic guide because of the wide variation in thickness for each level. Ulceration of the epithelium overlying the melanoma is also an important prognostic variable that independently predicted survival in stage I disease. An ulcerative lesion indicates a worse prognosis than a non-ulcerative primary when thickness is equivalent. Anatomic location of the primary was a dominant prognostic variable only for melanomas >0.76 mm thick.

STAGE OF DISEASE

The demonstration that a primary melanoma has the biologic ability to leave the site of origin and take up residence in a regional lymph node is an ominous sign that portends a poor prognosis (see Table 31-11). Further, although the 5-year survival of patients with regional lymph node involvement is about 30%, deaths can continue to occur. McNeer and DasGupta found only 12% of stage II patients alive and free of disease at 10 years and 9% at 15 years.[138]

Correlation of prognosis with the number of histologically involved nodes is presented in Table 31-12. An inverse relationship exists between survival and the number of involved nodes.

Patients with disseminated disease are a heterogeneous group since melanoma has several metastatic patterns. Amer and associates report a median survival of 9 months from the time of dissemination.[143] Prognosis varies with metastatic site (see Table 31-13). Patients with only skin and lymph node metastases live substantially longer than patients with visceral disease. Melanoma metastases, even those in the same site, may vary widely in their growth rates. Presently, there are no clearly useful prospective indices for quantitating this phenomenon. The length of time from initial diagnosis to recurrence or dissemination may reflect, among other things, the growth pattern of the tumor. Amer and associates report that patients with disseminated disease who previously had a disease-free interval of more than 6 months had a mean survival of 7.1 months compared with 3 months ($p = 0.001$) for patients with prior disease-free intervals of less than 6 months.[143]

TABLE 31-10. Correlation of 5-Year Survival with the Location of the Primary Lesion

STUDY (Ref. No.)	H&N %(A)	ARM %(B)	LEG %(C)	TRUNK %(D)
Perzik & Baum[95]	53 (16/30)	71 (20/28)	53 (23/43)	57 (17/30)
Jones et al[96]	33 (9/21)	27 (4/15)	45 (21/47)	19 (4/21)
Franklin et al[132]	41 (21/51)	73 (22/30)	68 (59/87)	60 (47/78)
Shah & Goldsmith[50]	57 (130/228)	63 (167/265)	60 (299/498)	42 (167/397)
Mundth et al[51]*	53 (60/114)	43 (20/46)	43 (38/89)	29 (26/91)
Lehman et al[97]	45 (5/11)	50 (6/12)	66 (4/6)	0 (0/5)
McLeod[133]†	77	88	83	70
Balch et al[134]‡	68	88	70	58
TOTALS	52 (241/461)	60 (239/396)	58 (444/770)	42 (261/622)

* Survival from onset symptoms
† Total 342 patients
‡ Total 248 clinical stage I patients
H&N = head and neck
B vs. C, NS; A vs. B, P = 0.02; A vs. C, P = 0.07
D vs. A, B, or C, p < 0.00

TABLE 31-11. Correlation of 5-Year Survival with Stage of Disease

STUDY (Reference No.)	PERCENT FIVE-YEAR SURVIVAL	
	LOCAL	REGIONAL
McNeer & Das Gupta[137]	71 (255/359)	19 (56/295)
Goldsmith et al[50,139]	80 (256/321)	39 (178/456)
Cochran[99]	66 (67/102)	14 (5/36)
Fortner et al[101]	55 (47/85)	19 (21/109)
TOTALS	72 (625/867)	29 (277/950)

Clinical or histologic staging
p = <0.0001

Clinical-Diagnostic Staging

The foundation of accurate staging is a careful examination.[144] The primary lesion should be evaluated for size, color (especially areas of depigmentation), and topography (ulceration and nodularity). White areas are indicative of spontaneous regression, a phenomenon that McGovern reported to have occurred in 12.3% of 437 primary cutaneous melanomas.[145] This is an important consideration in assessing risk in patients with thin (<0.76 mm) primary tumors. Ulceration is an important independent prognostic variable and nodularity is indicative of vertical growth. The surrounding skin and subcutaneous tissue should be examined for satellites and intransit metastases. The entire body surface (including the scalp, conjunctivae, oral and genital mucosa, scrotum, and subungual and perianal areas) should be examined for additional primary melanomas and for the presence of precursors lesions. Examination of suspect lesions is facilitated by use of a 10 power hand lens.

The primary lesion is occult in one to 15% of patients.[146-148] In these cases a careful history must be obtained regarding the possible complete regression of a pigmented lesion. Further, the body surface must be carefully examined for an occult primary or areas of depigmentation, which can result following the complete regression of a primary tumor (see Fig. 31-7). Use of a Wood's light facilitates the search for depigmentation.

Laboratory studies should include a chest film, hemogram, and blood chemistry profile.[149] Liver function chemistries, particularly the lactic dehydrogenase (LDH), are helpful in detecting liver metastases.[94,150] Liver, brain, and bone scans are not useful in detecting metastases in asymptomatic patients.[151] However, they are valuable as a baseline for future studies. Lung tomography is reserved for patients with suspicious routine chest roentgenograms. The role of CT scans and lymphangiography in the pretreatment evaluation of melanoma patients requires further definition.[152-156]

Following this exercise, patients can be classified preoperatively using the staging system presented in Table 31-14.

TABLE 31-12. Correlation of Survival with the Number of Histologically Positive Regional Lymph Nodes

	NUMBER OF NODES POSITIVE		
Cohen et al[140]	1–3 nodes	4 nodes	
5-year survival	55%	26% p = <0.01	
10-year survival	55%	26% p = <0.01	
Fortner et al[141]	1 node	multiple nodes	
5-year survival	50%	15%	
10-year survival	50%	15%	
Karakousis et al[142]	1 node	2 nodes	≥3 nodes
median survival	36.1 mos	26.9 mos	20.2 mos
5-year survival NED	41%	30%	18%

TABLE 31-13. Metastatic Site and Survival in Patients with Advanced Malignant Melanoma

	INITIAL PRESENTATION			ANY TIME		
	NO. OF PATIENTS	SURVIVAL (months)		NO. OF PATIENTS	SURVIVAL (months)	
		MEAN	MEDIAN		MEAN	MEDIAN
Skin, lymph nodes	24	19.9	14	83	9.7	5
Bone and marrow	15	7.2	5	46	5.3	3
Lung	26	7.2	6	76	8.7	3
Liver	20	7.5	4	73	3.9	1
Gastrointestinal tract	10	16.8	4	29	7.9	2
Central nervous system	17	13.9	8	60	4.2	2
Multiple	28	1.3	1	109	3.4	2
TOTAL	140	9.7	5			

Amer MN, A.–Sarraf M, Vaitkevicius VK: Surg Gynecol Obstet 149:168, 1979

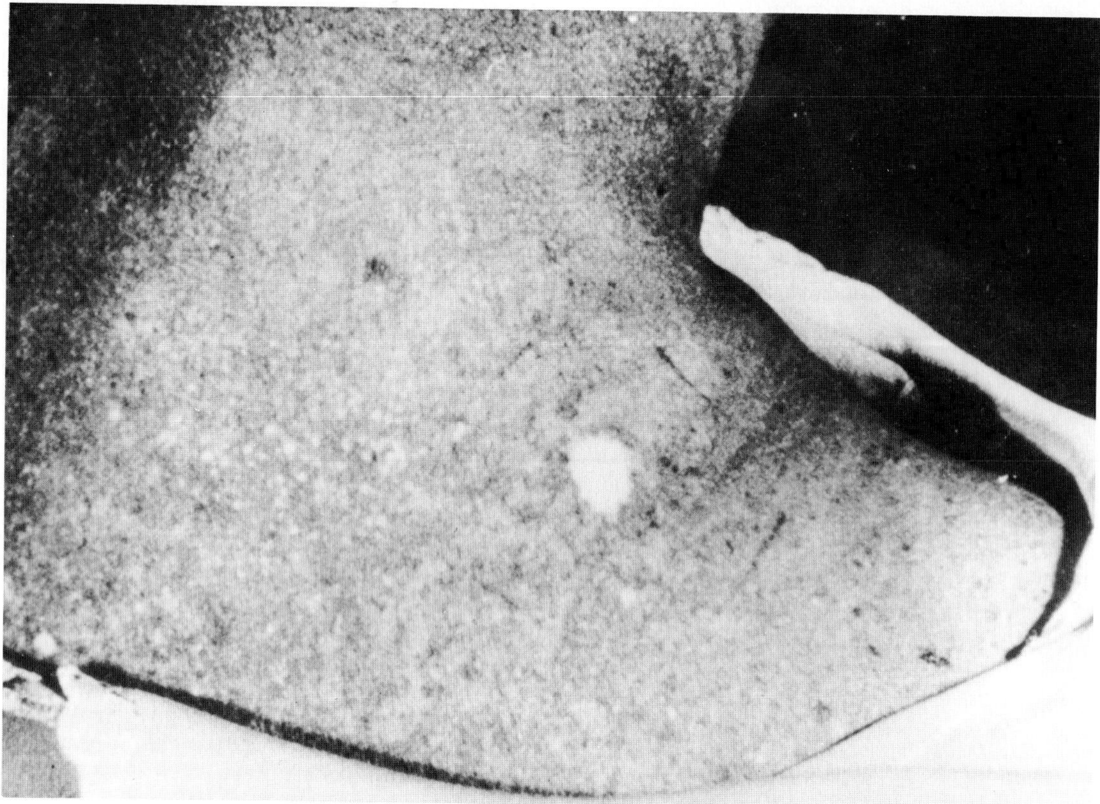

FIG. 31-7. Ultraviolet light photograph of the right posterior shoulder of a patient who presented with melanoma metastatic to the right axillary nodes. History revealed that a pigmented lesion present on the right shoulder became inflamed and regressed several years earlier. Wood's light examination demonstrated the residual patch of depigmentation.

Postsurgical Treatment and Pathologic Staging

The entire primary tumor should be examined histologically using the technique illustrated in Figure 31-6. Both thickness and Clark level should be reported. If removed, regional lymph nodes should be thoroughly evaluated; the number positive as well as the total number examined should be reported. These data can then be used to assign a TNM classification using the system presented in Table 31-15. However, because of its complexity, the TNM classification is rarely used by most clinical investigators. Rather, the staging system outlined in Table 31-14 is most frequently relied upon.

Table 31-14. Clinical Staging System

I. Local
  A. Primary lesion alone
  B. Primary and satellites within a 5 cm radius of the primary
  C. Local recurrence within a 5 cm radius of a resected primary
  D. Metastases located more than 5 cm from the primary site but within the primary lymphatic drainage area

II. Regional Nodal Disease

III. Disseminated Disease

TREATMENT OF THE PRIMARY SITE

SURGERY

Biopsy of the Primary Lesion

Any skin lesion suspected of being a malignant melanoma should be biopsied. When feasible, an excisional biopsy should be performed with a margin of several millimeters around the suspected lesion.[157,158] Some lesions may be too large for an excisional biopsy; however, the incisional or punch biopsy of these lesions should be performed. The local excision required for proper treatment of primary melanoma cannot be undertaken without proof of diagnosis by biopsy.

The biopsy should include the full thickness of skin into and including subcutaneous tissue. This will permit the pathologist to evaluate the thickness of the lesion and its depth of vertical invasion. A scalpel should be used for all biopsies. Electrocoagulation, curettage, or shave biopsies should never be performed. All skin lesions worthy of removal should be sent to the pathologist and none should be "burned off."

For lesions that cannot be excisionally biopsied, incisional biopsy is acceptable. However, care should be taken to perform this biopsy through the most clinically suspicious area of the lesion. Melanomas may arise in benign skin lesions and biopsy

TABLE 31-15. TNM Classification[144]

PRIMARY TUMOR (T)

T0	No evidence of primary tumor (unknown primary tumor or primary tumor removed and not histologically examined)
T1	Invasion of papillary dermis (L–II) or 0.75 mm thickness or less
T2	Invasion of the papillary-reticular dermal interface (L–III) or 0.76–1.5 mm thickness
T3	Invasion of the reticular dermis (L–IV) or 1.51–3.0 mm thickness
T4	Invasion of the subcutaneous tissue (L–V) or more than 3.0 mm thickness

T1a, T2a, T3a, T4a: Satellite(s) within 2 cm of the primary lesion

T1b, T2b, T3b, T4b: Regional satellites more than 2 cm from the primary lesion or intransit metastasis directed toward primary lymph node draining basin

NODAL INVOLVEMENT (N)

NX	Minimum requirements cannot be met
N0	No regional lymph node involvement
N1a	Regional lymph node involvement of first station nodes only
N1b	Regional nodes, massive or fixed
N2a	Regional lymph node involvement contralateral or bilateral or primary and secondary lymphatic basin
Ns2b	Massive or fixed lymph nodes, contralateral or both

DISTANT METASTASIS (M)

MX	Not assessed
M0	No (known) distant metastasis
M1a	Skin or subcutaneous tissue or distant lymph nodes Specify ____________
M1b	Visceral metastasis present (any structure other than skin, subcutaneous tissue or lymph nodes) Specify ____________

Specify sites according to the following notations:

Pulmonary — PUL
Osseous — OSS
Hepatic — HEP
Brain — BRA
Lymph Nodes — LYM
Bone Marrow — MAR
Pleura — PLE
Skin — SKI
Eye —EYE
Gastrointestinal — GI
Subcutaneous — SUBC
Other — OTH

of such a lesion at an inappropriate site may lead to falsely negative results. In general, incisional biopsy should be performed with a scalpel although a 5–7 mm punch biopsy, if care is taken to perform this in a full thickness fashion, can be acceptable. Local anesthesia is always used for these biopsies.

Prognosis of the patient does not appear to be adversely affected by prior biopsy. In a review of 193 cases of melanoma from the California Tumor Registry, Epstein showed that the survival rate of patients who had initial biopsies or simple excision was similar to those patients who had immediate definitive surgery.[159] In fact, at 10 years, those patients who had biopsies survived longer than those patients who had immediate primary excision (83.5% vs. 66.5% respectively, $p < 0.05$). In a study of 230 melanoma patients Knutson and coworkers, reported the same survival for patients who had previous biopsy, whether incisional or excisional, compared to those patients who did not.[53] Similarly, Jones and coworkers found the 5-year survival of patients who had incisional biopsy was similar to that of other patients.[96] However, Ames and coworkers found no significant difference in survival or local recurrence when comparing patients treated with intact primary melanomas of the head and neck to those who had had either excisional or incisional biopsy.[160] A prospective trial by the WHO Collaborating Centers for Evaluation of Methods of Diagnosis and Treatment of Melanoma showed no difference in survival between patients not previously biopsied and patients submitted to excisional biopsy within a month of definitive treatment.[161] Thus, prior biopsy, does not appear to affect ultimate prognosis in patients being treated for melanoma. Despite these studies it would seem wise to excisionally biopsy lesions when possible to minimize any chance of local spread of the tumor or any chance of tumor cells entering the blood vessels.

Surgical Excision of the Primary Melanoma

Wide surgical excision of melanomas in the skin was strongly advocated first by W. Sampson Handley in 1907, based on his pathologic studies of the frequency of centrifugal dermal lymphatic permeation into the surrounding skin.[162] No prospective studies have been performed to evaluate the exact extent of the local excision necessary for adequate primary melanoma treatment. Most surgeons advocate excision of full thickness skin with margins of 3–4 cm in all directions from the lesion.[5,162–167] While lesser resections may be acceptable in special circumstances, the surgical excision of melanomas using this rule provides excellent local control. Excision of primary melanomas in the skin with 3–5 cm margins results in a local recurrence rate of 5% or less in virtually all reported series. The results of eight typical series are shown in Table 31-16.[5,15,166,168–172] Local recurrence rates are not affected by whether a lymph node dissection is performed simultaneously; however, higher rates of local recurrence appear to occur in patients with clinical Stage II disease.[173]

The large defects created by excising skin and subcutaneous tissue (3–5 cm in all directions) from the primary melanoma almost always require a split thickness skin graft to provide adequate coverage. This technique is greatly preferred over the advancement of skin flaps because of the tendency of this

TABLE 31-16. Local Recurrence Following Wide Excision of Skin Melanomas

REFERENCE	NO. OF PATIENTS	PATIENT POPULATION	EXTENT OF LOCAL RESECTION	LOCAL RECURRENCE	COMMENTS
Olsen, 1972 (168)	211	All sites	Not stated	8 (4%)	No effect of fascial excision
Cady et al 1975 (1969)	176	All sites	Not stated	12 (7%)	Most without skin grafts
McBride et al 1975 (70)	99	Clinical stage I Trunk	Not stated	5 (5%)	
Veronesi et al 1977 (171)	395	Clinical stage I Extremity	3 cm margin	6 (2%)	No effect of lymph node dissection
Das Gupta, 1977 (164)	150	All sites Clinical Stage I and II	5 cm margin	10 (7%)	
	21	Head and neck		1 (5%)	
	41	Trunk		3 (7%)	
	54	Lower extremity		4 (7%)	
	34	Upper extremity		2 (6%)	
Milton, 1977 (5)	224	All sites	5 cm margin	4 (2%)	
Goldman, 1978 (166)	115	All sites	3–5 cm margin	0	Only 2–5 year follow-up
Balch et al 1979 (172)	287	Clinical stage I All sites	Not stated	8 (3%)	None if primary less than 0.76 mm thick

latter technique to obscure local recurrences in the excision bed when they occur. Except in very obese patients or in some areas of the trunk, split thickness skin grafts are required. As a general rule, adequate excision has probably not been performed unless a split thickness skin graft has been placed.

The exact extent of excision required to insure against local recurrence is a matter of some controversy. McNeer reported limited excisional surgery in a series of 194 patients with melanoma that resulted in a 24.7% local recurrence rate.[173] However, Breslow has recently presented evidence that very thin melanomas require far less local excision than do thicker melanomas.[174] In 62 patients with melanomas less than 0.76 mm in thickness no local recurrences were seen despite local excisions that varied from 0.5 to greater than 3 cm from the site of the local lesion. In addition, Balch has reported on 36 patients with melanomas less than 0.76 mm thick with margins of excision from less than one to 5 cm from the lesion, again with no local recurrences.[172] It thus appears that very thin melanomas (less than 0.76 mm) may not require extensive local excisions. Cady has reported no difference in local recurrence rates in 83 patients who underwent wide excision without a skin graft compared to 36 patients who underwent wide excision with a skin graft.[169] This was not a prospective study however, and it is difficult to determine how patients were selected for different local therapies. In contrast, Milton has reported a local recurrence rate of 0.5% in 185 patients undergoing wide excision with split thickness skin grafting compared to a local recurrence rate of 7.7% in 39 patients who did not undergo split thickness skin grafting.[5]

Though the exact extent of local excision necessary in melanoma patients is unknown the morbidity of wide excision (3–5 cm margins) with placement of a split thickness skin graft is minimal and advocated for virtually all patients with melanoma greater than 0.76 mm thick. This may be somewhat more than is required for some patients, but local recurrence rates will be in the range of 5% when this approach is followed.

The site of the melanoma will, of course, affect the extent of possible local excision. Compromise of margins for melanomas on the face must, of course, be taken into account. Though mastectomy has been advocated for melanoma occurring on the nipple or areola, adequate local control is most often attainable by standard wide excision.[175-178] Subungual melanomas should always be treated by amputation of the digit, generally at the metatarsal or metacarpophalangeal joint so that adequate closure can be obtained with adequate skin removal.[161,179,180] Both plantar and palmar melanomas in weight-bearing portions of the foot have lead many surgeons to use muscle transpositions, free myocutaneous rotation, or transpositional, cross-foot or cross-leg flaps.[32,180-183] In most patients, however, split thickness skin grafts will support normal weight when properly padded shoes are used. (This has been convincingly demonstrated in a recent report by Woltering and coworkers.[181]) The simple and uncomplicated nature of this latter treatment makes it the treatment of choice even in weight-bearing areas.

Technique of Wide Excision for Melanoma

The technique used for wide excision and split thickness skin grafting of primary melanoma excision sites at the National

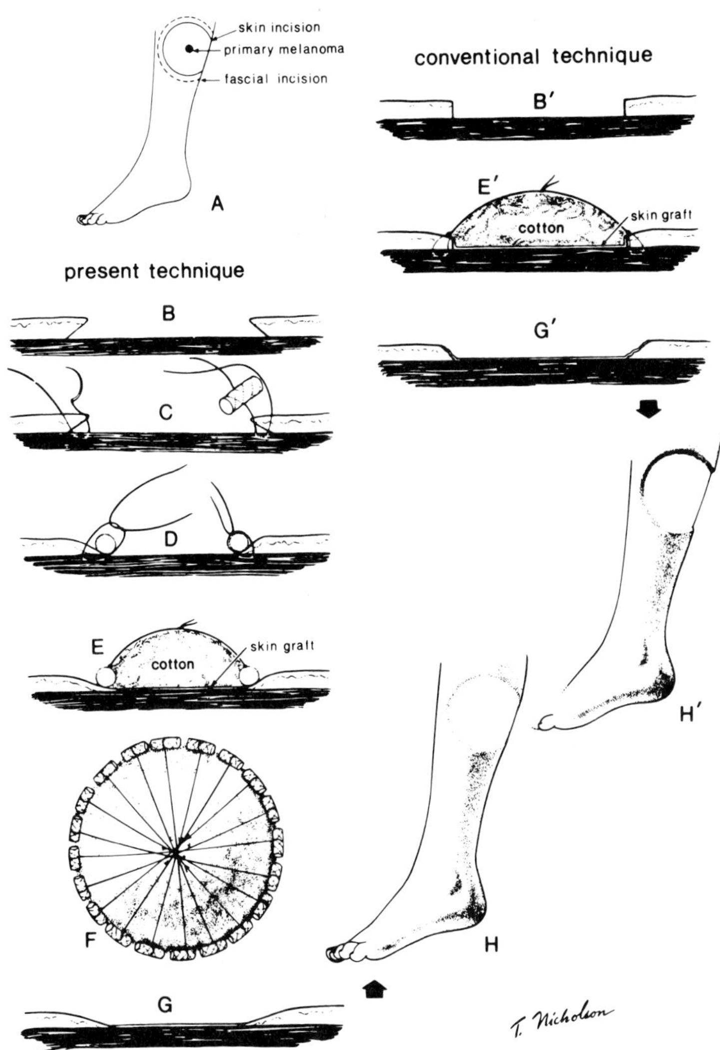

FIG. 31-8. The technique of wide excision and split-thickness skin grafting. See text for explanation. (Neifeld, JP, Chretien PB: An improved technique of excision and skin grafting for primary malignant melanomas. Surg Gynecol Obstet 143:585, 1976. By permission of Surgery, Gynecology and Obstetrics)

Cancer Institute is illustrated in Figure 31-8.[184] This technique is highly reliable and provides excellent cosmetic results. The margins of resection 4–5 cm around the melanoma in all directions are measured with a ruler and marked on the skin. As the incision is made through the skin and subcutaneous tissue, it is bevelled at an angle of 45–60°, undermining the skin (see Fig. 31-8, parts A and B). This results in a larger fascial than skin defect. Vertical mattress sutures of 2-0 nylon that extend from skin to muscle and back to skin are placed and tied over ¼ inch dental cotton rolls with the ends of the sutures left, approximately 5 inches long (see Fig. 31-8, parts C and D). These sutures serve to attach the skin edges to the muscle surface and provide a gradual transition from normal skin thickness to the depths of the excision site. The placement of these stitches also serves to advance the skin and reduce the size of the defect. A split thickness skin graft is then placed in the defect and a continuous suture of 4-0 chromic catgut is used to secure the skin graft to the skin excision margins. Soft cotton immersed in mineral oil is then packed over the skin graft. The nylon sutures are tied over the cotton to provide a bolus pressure dressing (see Fig. 31-8, parts E and F). This pressure dressing is removed after approximately 7 days, the cotton bolsters in the skin are removed after approximately two weeks. This technique prevents retraction of the incised skin margins and reduces the unsightly consequences of the sharp demarcation that occur with conventional skin excision techniques that do not involve beveling.

It is essential to avoid contamination of the skin graft donor site with melanoma. It is for this reason that the skin graft is taken prior to beginning the melanoma excision and placed in saline until needed.

It is advisable to remove the deep fascia as a part of all excisions for primary melanoma. Most melanomas have been biopsied prior to definitive surgical excision and wide excision, which includes the deep fascia and insures against entering the previous biopsy site. While contamination from biopsies can extend to the deep fascia it rarely extends below this anatomic plane. Though Olsen has reported an increased tendency to subsequent tumor dissemination when the deep fascia is excised, this observation has not been confirmed by other workers.[185]

RADIATION THERAPY

Definitive Irradiation of Primary Cutaneous Melanoma

Radiotherapy with curative intent, either alone or in combination with surgical excision for early primary cutaneous melanoma, has been described by a number of researchers.[186–199] However, many of these reports contain several flaws.[200] These include:

The proportion of unbiopsied lesions diagnosed clinically and treated as melanoma varied from 32% of the 259 patients in Hellriegel's study to 62% of the 78 patients of Pearsons' group, and 77% of the 13 patients of Koneckny's.[188,189,198] Pearson stated that most of the survivors in her group of 49 patients irradiated without biopsy confirmation probably had pigmented basal cell carcinomas.[198]

The relative effectiveness of radiotherapy, either alone or with surgery, in definitively treating primary cutaneous melanoma can only be adequately evaluated by comparison with similar surgically treated control patients. The cited reports all have this in common—a failure to provide adequate surgical controls against which the effectiveness of the radiotherapy can be compared.[186–190,193–198]

Patients in these reports were not staged according to clinicopathologic type, level of invasion, or thickness, all of which are important prognostic indicators.

The lack of uniformity of total radiation doses, individual fraction size, overall treatment times, and beam characteristics makes comparisons of the effectiveness of radiotherapy within and between series reports meaningless. Indeed, information on radiation technique is often missing, except for that given in a few illustrative cases, which may not have been representative of the treatment plans for the entire patient group.[200,201]

The only exceptions to the above flawed studies are a few recent reports on the role of local radiotherapy in the treatment of lentigo maligna and uncomplicated and previously untreated lentigo maligna melanoma, particularly in elderly patients where radiation may be used as an alternative to surgical excision.[193,196,202] For other primary melanomas, however, surgical excision is the preferred treatment.

IMMUNOTHERAPY

Several investigators have attempted pre-operative intralesional adjuvant immunotherapy (see Table 31-17). Everall injected the primary melanoma with vaccinia virus in 23 patients, 2 weeks prior to definitive surgical therapy.[203] The disease-free intervals for these patients were compared (actuarial method) to those achieved in a group of 25 patients who received standard surgical therapy. Allocation to treatment and control groups was not random. The two groups were comparable in age but the vaccinia virus treated group contained significantly more tumors of the superficial spreading type. Relapse rates are shown in Table 31-17. The data suggest that vaccinia virus treated patients may have benefited therapeutically.

Castermans–Elias and associates treated 37 clinical stage I patients with DNCB.[204] Some 23 patients presented with their primary melanoma intact (clinical diagnosis). In these patients, 2 mg of DNCB were applied to the tumor for 48 hours (repeated twice at weekly intervals). Eight to 19 days later a standard surgical excision was performed. The results after 3 years of observation are presented in Table 31-17. The

TABLE 31-17. Intralesional Pre-operative Adjuvant Immunotherapy

Everall (203)		Excision plus vaccinia	Excision only	
No. of patients		25	23	
Relapses (%): (all patients)	1 yr	5	20	NS
	2 yr	5	30	NS
	3 yr	15	35	NS
Relapses (%): (IV + V only)	2 yr	5	50	$p = 0.05$
	4 yr	20	50	$p = 0.05$
Castermans–Elias (204)				
		DNCB before surgery	DNCB after surgery	
No. of patients		23	14	
Relapses		0/23	4/14	$p = 0.05$
Deaths		0/23	0/14	NS
Rosenberg (205)				
		BCG	Control	
No. of patients		13	13	$p = <0.05$
Recurrences		5	10	
Regional nodes				
Tumor positive		0	4	

NS = not significant

statistically significant difference in relapse rates suggest an advantage for pre-operative DNCB. However, this was not a randomized trial and further, diagnosis in the treated group was on clinical grounds and microstaging was done after several applications of DNCB.

Rosenberg and coworkers randomized 26 patients to receive intralesional BCG or no treatment prior to definitive surgical excision and have noted an improvement in disease-free survival for BCG-treated patients.[205] Despite the statistical significance of this observation the number of patients is too small to allow generalization of the therapeutic benefit.

Based on the above observations and trials in animals, pre-surgical intralesional therapy warrants further investigation in the treatment of high-risk melanoma patients.

TREATMENT OF REGIONAL LYMPH NODES

SURGERY

The question of whether to prophylactically dissect the regional lymph nodes in patients with clinical stage I malignant melanoma has been an area of considerable controversy. Many reports of retrospective analyses of selected patient series argue either for or against prophylactic lymph node dissection.[124,127,139,141,142,164–166,172,206–213] Only since 1977 have two prospective randomized clinical trials been performed to help elucidate the answer to this question.[167,171]

Proponents of prophylactic lymph node dissection have argued that approximately 20% of patients with clinically normal regional lymph nodes will harbor micrometastases. If left intact, these metastases may lead to tumor dissemination. Arguments against performing prophylactic lymph node dissection have emphasized the immunologic importance of the draining regional nodes in the host response to the tumor and the unnecessary morbidity of lymph node dissection in those 80% of patients without micrometastases in draining nodes. Lymph node dissection in the 20% of patients with micrometastases can be performed without adversely affecting overall patient survival when their lymph nodes become clinically positive. A summary of the results of seven representative retrospective series concerning the efficacy of prophylactic lymph node dissection in clinical stage I melanoma patients and two prospective series is presented in Table 31-18. In each of these series, patients were selected for either wide excision alone or wide excision plus lymph node dissection based on the judgement of the surgeon or for undefined clinical criteria. The series of Cade, Goldsmith and coworkers, Fortner and coworkers, and Kapelanski and coworkers show no dramatic differences between these two treatments.[139,141,206,211] The series of Southwick and coworkers and Mehnert and coworkers exhibit an improvement in 5-year survival for those patients undergoing prophylactic lymph node dissection.[124,207] However, the Sandeman series indicates a poorer prognosis for patients undergoing prophylactic lymph node dissection.[208] Variability of the results among these seven

TABLE 31-18. Studies of the Efficacy of Prophylactic Lymph Node Dissection in Clinical Stage I Malignant Melanoma

	NO. OF PATIENTS			% 5 YR. SURVIVAL	
	TOTAL	WE	WE & LND	WE	WE & LND
Retrospective studies, reference					
Cade, 1961 (206)	176			65	69
Southwick et al 1962 (207)	96	71	25	32	80
Mehnert et al 1965 (124)	75	46	29	50	72
Sandeman et al 1965 (208)	80	40	40	57	28
Goldsmith et al 1970 (139)	707	411	296	68	78
Fortner et al 1977 (141)	404	145	259	70	76
Kapelanski et al 1979 (211)	91	65	26	55	65
Prospective studies					
Veronesi et al 1977 (171)	553	286	267	70	71
Sim et al 1978 (167)	117	63	54	85–90*	85–90

* Most patients not at 5 years.
WE = wide excision
LND = lymph node dissection

TABLE 31-19. Incidence of Regional Lymph Node Micrometastases in Patients with Clinical Stage I Malignant Melanoma

REFERENCE	NUMBER OF PATIENTS	PRIMARY SITE	% NODAL METASTASES CLARK LEVEL			
			II	III	IV	V
Wanebo et al 1975 (127, 212)	151	Extremity	4	7	25	70
Fortner et al 1977 (141)	162	Trunk and extremity	0	14	31	33
Holmes et al 1977 (214)	160	All	—	18	27	33
Cohen et al 1977 (140)	61	All	15	14	35	33
Goldman et al 1978 (166)	42	All	—	4	26	
Kapelanski et al 1979 (211)	26	All	0	18	17	
	692					
TOTAL	692	Mean	5%	14%	33%	49%

studies is characteristic of many additional reports existing in the literature. Because of the wide variation in 5-year survival in these series and the need to control the wide diversity of subgroups of melanoma patients based on prognostic factors, this question cannot be resolved by retrospective analyses.

The advent of techniques for predicting the likelihood of micrometastases in patients with clinically negative regional lymph nodes led to the hope that subgroups of patients could be identified that would benefit from prophylactic lymph node dissection. Table 31-19 presents six series demonstrating the correlation of Clark level of invasion with the incidence of nodal micrometastases in patients with clinical stage I malignant melanoma.[127,140,141,166,211,212,214] Though there is some variation from series to series, the mean percentage of patients with micrometastases is 5% for patients with Clark level II disease, 14% for level III, 33% for level IV, and 49% for level V.

The direct thickness measurement of the primary melanoma as described by Breslow is also predictive of the presence of micrometastases in regional nodes of patients with clinical stage I melanoma.[215] The results of three series reveal that patients with lesions less than 0.76 mm thick rarely have micrometastases in regional nodes; a 14% incidence is found in patients with 0.76–1.5 mm thick lesions; 37% of lymph node dissections are positive in patients with lesions of 1.5–4 mm thickness; and 51% are positive in patients with lesions thicker than 4 mm (see Table 31-20).[127,172,214]

Several clinical series in which some patients underwent wide excision alone and some underwent wide excision plus prophylactic lymph node dissection have been analyzed retrospectively by subgroups of known Clark level of invasion and thickness of the primary lesion (see Table 31-21).[127,172,211,215] These are retrospective series and the choice of treatment for any individual patient was not randomly assigned. Kapelanski and coworkers found that a statistically significant improvement in 5-year survival was obtained in patients undergoing prophylactic lymph node dissection who had Clark level IV melanoma.[211] He found no significant differences in patients with lesions of other Clark levels or in any subgroups when using the thickness of the lesion as a prognostic guide. However, Wanebo and coworkers found

TABLE 31-20. Incidence of Regional Lymph Node Metastases in Patients with Clinical Stage I Malignant Melanoma

REFERENCE	NUMBER OF PATIENTS	PRIMARY SITE	THICKNESS (approximate range in mm)			
			<0.76	0.76–1.5	1.5–4	>4
			(% with positive lymph nodes)			
Balch et al 1979 (172)	78	All	0	25	51	62
Wanebo et al 1975 (127)	151	Extremities	—	7	22	39
Holmes et al 1977 (214)	250	All	—	10	20	
TOTAL	479	Mean	0%	14%	37%	51%

TABLE 31-21. Retrospective Studies of the Efficacy of Prophylactic Lymph Node Dissection in Clinical Stage I Melanoma Patients Based on Invasion and Thickness of the Primary Lesion

	KAPELANSKI ET AL 1979 (211)		WANEBO ET AL 1975 (127)		BALCH ET AL 1979 (172)		BRESLOW 1975 (215)	
TOTAL NUMBER OF PATIENTS	91		151		134		138	
	% 5-year Survival							
	WE	WE + LND	WE	WE + LND	WE	WE + LND	WE	WE + LND
Clark Level II	80	67	100	100	—	—	—	—
III	55	59	67	93*	—	—	—	—
IV	24	80*	57	68	—	—	—	—
V	29	100	50	0	—	—	—	—
<.76 mm	75	75	—	—	100	100	100	100
0.76–1.5 mm	73	100	—	—	58	94*	70	70
>1.5 mm	33	58	—	—	37	83†	31	64*

* $p < 0.05$
$p < 0.01$
WE = wide exicision
LND = lymph node dissection

that patients with Clark level III lesions benefited from prophylactic lymph node dissection ($p < 0.05$) but no statistically significant differences were seen in analyzing other subgroups based on Clark levels.[127] Balch and associates found a statistically significant improvement in patients undergoing prophylactic dissection for those patients with lesions between 0.76 and 1.5 mm thick and for those patients with lesions greater than 1.5 mm thick.[172] Breslow, however, could find no difference in survival depending on therapy for patients with lesions between 0.76 and 1.5 mm thick. However, he did find a statistically significant improvement in patients undergoing prophylactic dissection for those patients with lesions greater than 1.5 mm thick ($p < 0.05$).[215] These studies have suggested that patients with a high likelihood of having micrometastases in draining regional nodes might benefit from prophylactic node dissection. However, difficulties in analyzing these historically controlled series and the wide variations in five-year survivals between these series cast considerable doubt on these conclusions.

Two prospective randomized series have now been performed to evaluate the efficacy of regional prophylactic lymph node dissection in patients with clinical stage I melanoma.[167,171] In both series no improvement was seen in those patients undergoing prophylactic lymph node dissection. From September 1967 to January 1974, the WHO Melanoma Group carried out a prospective randomized protocol in patients with clinical stage I melanoma of the extremities.[171] Some 267 patients were prospectively randomized to receive wide excision of the primary melanoma and immediate regional lymph node dissection. Some 286 patients were randomized

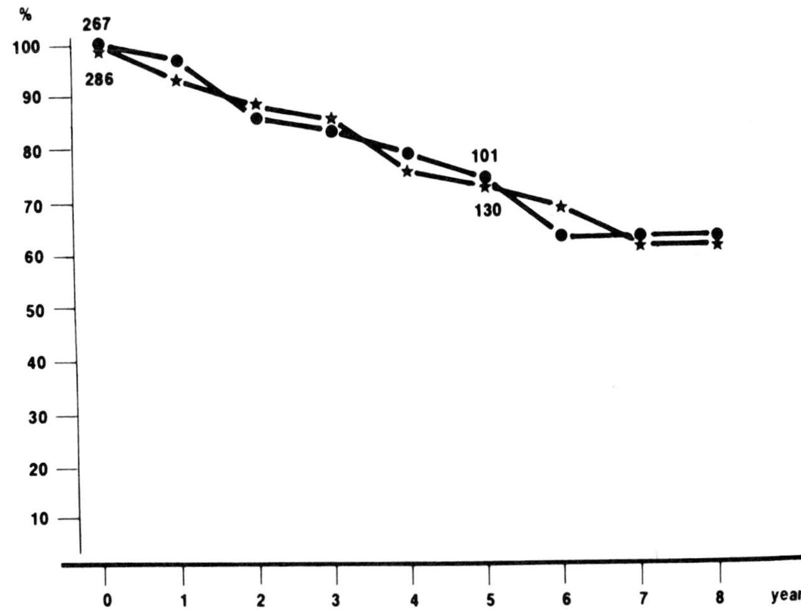

FIG. 31-9. Actuarial analysis of WHO prospective randomized study of the efficacy of prophylactic lymph node dissection in patients with melanoma of the extremities. (Veronesi U, Adams J, Bandiera DC et al: N Engl J Med 297:627, 1977)

TABLE 31-22. Analysis of WHO Study of Prophylactic Lymph Node Dissection in Clinical Stage I Melanoma: Effect of Prognostic Factors

		5-YEAR SURVIVAL*		
CRITERION	NO. OF PATIENTS	EXCISION + LYMPH NODE DISSECTION	EXCISION ONLY	P VALUE
Sex:				
M	103	64.7	55.9	
F	450	72.8	74.1	0.90
Maximum diameter (mm):				
0–10	164	73.1	85.4	
11–20	237	77.1	63.0	0.96
>21	89	48.0	60.2	
Site:				
Upper limbs	95	54.7	45.3	
Lower limbs	458	74.0	69.5	0.90
Histology findings:				
Level 3	71	75.4	82.4	
Level 4	178	70.1	58.3	0.15
Superficial spreading	124	58.8	58.1	
Nodular	120	61.3	60.0	0.85
Thickness (mm):				
≤1.5	52	81.8	90.0	
1.6–4.5	187	78.5	69.7	0.36
≥4.6	70	52.9	51.7	

* Computed from reference 171

to receive wide excision alone with regional lymph node dissection only at the time of appearance of metastases. With follow-up for the great majority of patients in excess of 5 years, no improvement in survival was seen in patients undergoing prophylatic lymph node dissection. Approximately 73% of patients were alive in both groups (see Fig. 31-9). Patient groups were balanced for sex, maximum diameter of the lesion, site of the lesion, level of invasion, histologic type, and thickness. Careful analysis was performed for a large number of subgroups of these patients and no difference in 5-year survival could be seen in subgroups separated by sex, diameter, site, Clark level of invasion, histologic morphology or thickness of the primary lesion (see Table 31-22). Of the 178 patients with level IV melanoma, the 5-year survival was 58.3% for the excision-only group and 70.1% for the excision-plus lymph node dissection group though this difference was not statistically significant. Of the 193 patients with follow-up for 5 years who, underwent prophylactic node dissection, 38 or 19.7% had regional micrometastases. In those 202 patients with similar follow-up who had undergone excision only, 49 cases (24.2%) ultimately developed palpable lymph nodes and required lymph node dissection. This trial, which represented a joint effort of 17 cancer institutions in 12 countries, clearly demonstrated no survival improvement for patients undergoing prophylactic lymph node dissection. It also suggested that vigilent follow-up coupled with therapeutic lymph node dissection for those patients whose nodes became clinically suspicious both spares 80% of node-negative patients an unnecessary operation and does nothing to compromise survival for the subgroup of node-positive patients.

The second prospective randomized study of prophylactic lymphadenectomy in clinical stage I melanoma patients was performed at the Mayo Clinic and also demonstrated no improvement in survival for patients undergoing prophylactic lymph node dissection.[167] In this study, 173 patients were randomized to receive either wide excision of the primary lesion alone (63 patients), lymphadenectomy at 3 months after wide excision (56 patients), or wide excision and immediate lymphadenectomy (54 patients). Patient groups in this study were comparable with respect to all known prognostic factors. No difference in survival was seen when comparing any of the treatment groups. Though the number of patients in this series is relatively small no difference could be seen when analyzing any subgroup based on the Clark level of the primary lesion.

The available data therefore suggest that prophylactic lymph node dissection is not of therapeutic benefit in patients with clinical stage I melanoma. Though it also appears unlikely that any subgroup will benefit from prophylactic lymph node dissection, several retrospective studies suggest a small improvement in patients with deeply invasive or thick primary melanomas.[127,172,211,215] Clark level IV patients also fared somewhat better in the WHO prospective randomized trial when prophylactic lymph node dissection was performed, though this was not statistically significant.[171] Much data exist, however, suggesting that the pathologic status of the draining lymph nodes is an important prognostic indicator and prophylactic lymph node dissection may indeed be indicated when it is necessary to identify those patients with poor prognosis for trials of adjuvant therapy.

The above discussion dealt only with patients with clinical stage I melanoma. Any patient with clinically positive regional lymph nodes or nodes suspicious of containing melanoma should undergo prompt regional lymph node dissection. Approximately 10–20% of patients with palpable disease in draining lymph nodes can be cured by lymph node dissection. Because of the short median survival of patients with metastatic disease beyond the regional nodes no lymphadenectomy is indicated in the treatment of most patients with disseminated disease except as is necessary for palliation of symptoms.

Selecting the Regional Lymph Node Group to be Dissected

The axillary and superficial inguinal lymph nodes represent the first regional drainage group (for primary melanomas of the upper and lower extremity respectively). The lymphatic drainage of the trunk, however, is less predictable. Lymphatic vessels from the upper half of the trunk generally drain into the axilla and those from the lower half of the trunk drain into the inguinal region; therefore, much variation exists.[216] Fortner and coworkers proposed the eighth rib as the line of division on the trunk that determines whether drainage will occur to the axillary or to the inguinal area, though this has proved to be unreliable.[88] A more accurate predictor of the lymphatic watershed for the groin and axillary lymph nodes is Sappey's line, which runs from 2 cm above the umbilicus curving upward to the level of the second and third lumbar vertebra.[217] This line is lower than the course of eighth rib. A series by Sugarbaker and associates appeared to more accurately predict the nodal drainage group.[217] Occasionally, melanomas of the upper trunk drain to the neck.

Sappey originally delineated the lymphatic drainage of the trunk by the injection of mercury into the skin. Fee and coworkers have attempted to localize draining lymph nodes by injecting radioactive colloidal gold into the skin and observing its migration patterns.[218] Holmes and coworkers have also used colloidal gold to predict the drainage pattern of individual melanomas.[214] Prospective studies of the efficacy of these techniques have not been performed and they do not have wide applicability. Decreasing enthusiasm for performing prophylactic lymph node dissections has lessened interest in finding methods for predicting the drainage patterns of truncal lesions when no lymph nodes are palpable.

Melanomas on the scalp and face drain to the neck though the first eschelon of nodes likely to be involved depends on the exact location of the primary. Ballantyne and Smith have carefully delineated the most likely sites of metastases from scalp and facial lesions.[219] Lesions from the anterior portion of the scalp and cheek areas drain to the superficial parotid nodes and then to the nodes of the anterior neck. Neck lymph node dissections for patients with primary lesions in this area should include superficial parotidectomy. Though standard neck dissections should be performed for most head and neck melanomas, sometimes it is possible to modify this procedure.[220] Lesions in the anterior portion of the scalp and face can sometimes be treated by dissection of the neck nodes with preservation of the spinal accessory nerve. Though little functional or physiologic disturbance accompanies division of the spinal accessory nerve some cosmetic deformity and anterior displacement of the clavical results. Similarly for posterior lesions, posterolateral neck dissections can be performed omitting dissection of the submaxillary and submental triangles.[221]

Technique of Axillary Dissection

A simple and safe technique for performing axillary dissection using an incision in the hairline of the axilla results in excellent exposure and excellent cosmetic results.[222] This technique is detailed in Fig. 31-10. The operation is performed with the patient in the supine position with the arm draped so that it is free to move in the operative field. The incision lies on a plane extending from the junction of the middle and medial thirds of the clavical to the lateral third of the latissimus dorsi muscle approximately 2 inches below its confluence with the triceps muscle and passes approximately one inch below the apex of the axilla. The incision extends from the anterior aspects of the pectoralis major muscle to the posterior aspect of the latissimus dorsi muscle (see Fig. 31-10, parts A and B). The flaps are raised to allow dissection caudad to the course of the thoracodorsal nerve inferiorly, to the pectoralis major muscle anteriorly, the latissimus dorsi muscle posteriorly, and the axillary vein superiorly. All subcutaneous fat and lymphatic tissue within this area to the apex of the axilla can easily be removed. While exposure to the apex of the axilla can most often be obtained with the pectoralis minor muscle intact, it is sometimes necessary to detach the head of this muscle from the coracoid or to remove the muscle completely to achieve adequate exposure. Either can easily be performed through this approach. Care should be taken to preserve the long thoracic and thoracodorsal nerves if they are not involved with tumor. Following removal of the specimen, suction catheters are placed and left for several days to secure adhesion of the flaps and to remove lymphatic effusions. Though temporary dysfunction of the shoulder may result following lymphatic dissection due to traction on the thoracodorso and long thoracic nerves, permanent dysfunction occurs in less than 1% of patients. Arm edema is also a very rare occurrence following axillary dissection without concomitant radiation therapy to the axilla.

Technique and Complications of Inguinal Lymph Node Dissection

Superficial inguinal lymph node dissections are best performed through a transverse incision in the inguinal crease extending from the anterior superior iliac spine to within one centimeter of the pubis, though many other incisions have been used.[214,223–226] This incision is adequate for raising skin flaps both inferiorly and superiorly, which provide good exposure to the femoral triangle. The contents of the femoral triangle bordered by the sartorius muscle laterally, the adductor magnus muscle medially, and the inguinal ligament superiorily should be excised down to the femoral artery and vein as well as the fat and lymphatic tissue beneath the upper flap cephalad to the inguinal ligament (see Fig. 31-11). The greater saphenous vein is also removed from the crossing point of the sartorius and adductor magnus muscles to its attachment to the femoral vein. Because of the potential

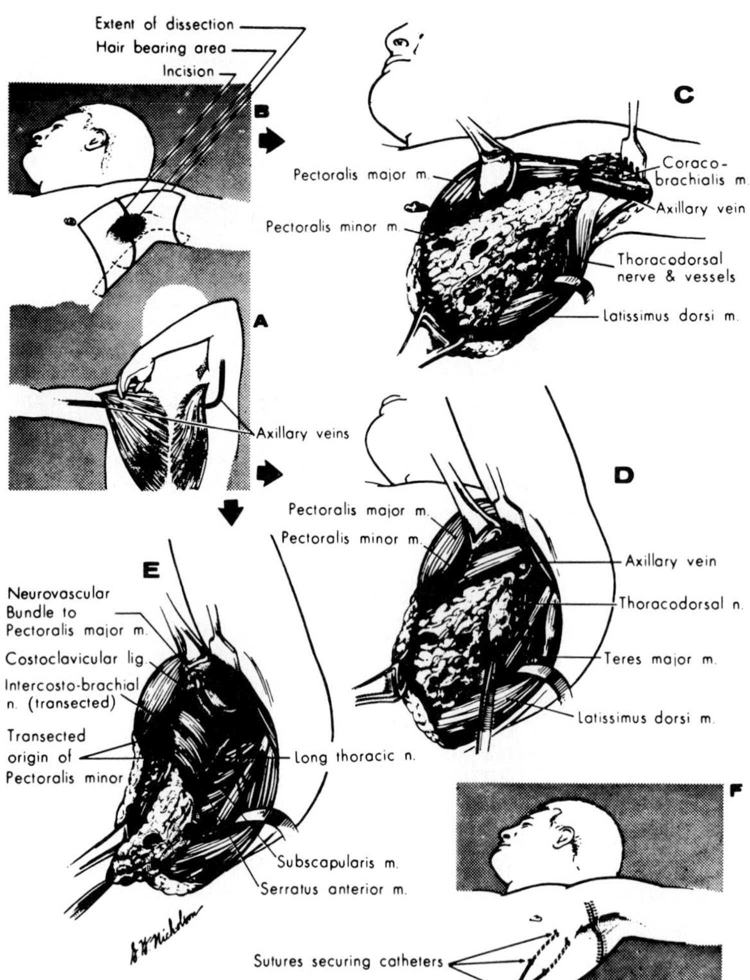

FIG. 31-10. Technique of axillary lymph node dissection. See text for details. (Chretien PB, Ketchan AS, Hoye RC et al: Ann Surg 173:554, 1971).

contamination of the skin in this area and the tenuous vascularity of the flaps, complications of superficial inguinal dissections are common. Minor flap necrosis will occur in from 5–20% of patients and edema of the lower extremity in approximately the same number.[214,223–226]

Deep inguinal lymph node dissections encompassing the iliac and obturator lymph nodes should be performed only in patients with grossly positive superficial inguinal nodes. In a series completed by Cohen and coworkers positive deep iliac and obturator lymph nodes were present only in patients with clinically positive superficial nodes.[227] The rarity of involvement of the deep inguinal nodes when the superficial nodes are either pathologically negative or contain only micrometastases do not warrant engendering the additional complications encountered by dissection of the deep iliac and obturator lymph nodes. When these deep lymph nodes are to be dissected a midline abdominal incision is preferred and will lead to a lower incidence of lower extremity and wound complications.[227] An alternate approach is the use of a long inguinal incision, dividing the inguinal ligament.[224] The iliac and obturator lymph nodes can also be dissected using a retroperitoneal approach with an incision extending superior to and parallel with the inguinal ligament and extending laterally into the flank.[226] Midline abdominal incisions have the advantage of allowing exploration of the para-aortic lymph nodes and the liver, in addition to providing excellent exposure for dissection of the deep inguinal lymph nodes.[227]

RADIOTHERAPY AS A REGIONAL SURGICAL ADJUVANT

Several reports deal with radiation therapy as a regional adjunct to surgery in clinically palpable node metastases.[228,229] The results of a randomized prospective study comparing postoperative radiotherapy to lymphadenectomy alone for patients presenting with clinically involved regional nodes was reported by Creagan and coworkers.[229] Three of 27 patients given postoperative irradition (5000 rad/28 fractions as a split course) developed recurrences within the portals, compared with one local recurrence in 29 unirradiated patients. No statistically significant differences in the disease-free intervals and overall survivals between the irradiated and surgical control groups were observed.

Radioactive endolymphatic therapy has also been employed in an effort to sterilize subclinical regional node metastases.[230–235] At present, there are insufficient data to allow a conclusion regarding the utility of this therapeutic modality.

ADJUVANT THERAPY

Pinsky and coworkers performed a prospective, randomized trial to investigate the therapeutic efficacy of BCG in poor prognosis melanoma patients with micrometastatic disease. The authors found no significant difference in disease-free interval or survival between 24 BCG-treated patients and 23 surgical controls.

Morton and coworkers found no difference in disease-free survival among patients treated with adjuvant BCG or BCG + allogeneic tumor cells when compared with control patients treated by surgery alone in a randomized prospective trial.[237]

Terry and coworkers randomized 174 evaluable stage I (level IV and V) and stage II melanoma patients following surgery to one of four arms: no further treatment, BCG, BCG and allogeneic tumor cells, or methyl-CCNU.[238] The disease-free survival was similar in all groups.

The Eastern Cooperative Oncology Group randomized stage I melanoma patients to receive either BCG or no further treatment.[239] Stage II (trunk) patients were randomized to receive BCG or DTIC. Immunotherapy showed no beneficial effect.

A WHO study compared surgery alone to BCG, DTIC or BCG + DTIC following surgery in 696 patients with stage I and II melanoma. DTIC-treated stage II patients had a prolonged disease-free interval when compared to patients treated with surgery alone (p = 0.018). No other statistically significant differences in disease-free interval or survival were noted and the magnitude of the advantage for DTIC treated patients was modest. The Central Oncology Group was unable to demonstrate a therapeutic advantage for intermittent (every 3 months), short-term (one year) DTIC treatment in a heterogeneous group (stage I, II and III) of melanoma patients when compared to an untreated randomized control.[241]

Spitler and Aggeler compared levamisole and placebo as postsurgical adjuvants in patients at high risk for recurrence following surgery.[242] With a total of 204 patients entered there were no differences in disease-free interval, time to appearance of visceral metastases, and survival.

Based on these data it does not appear that chemotherapy or immunotherapy has a role in the conventional management of patients free of disease following surgery but at high risk for recurrence (see immunotherapy chapter for further details).

REGIONAL PERFUSION

The principle of treating malignancies by regional perfusion of chemotherapeutic agents resulted from studies by Klopp and coworkers who infused small doses of nitrogen mustard into arteries supplying tumors while blocking venous return from the area to maximize exposure of tumor to the chemotherapeutic agent.[243] In 1957, Ryan, Krementz, and Creech used extracorporeal circulation using a pump oxygenator that made it possible to administer large doses of nitrogen mustard by continuous perfusion.[244,245] One of the first large reported series of patients undergoing regional perfusion was by Stehlin and coworkers who reported on 116 regional perfusions in 1960.[246] In 1967, Cavaliere used heated blood

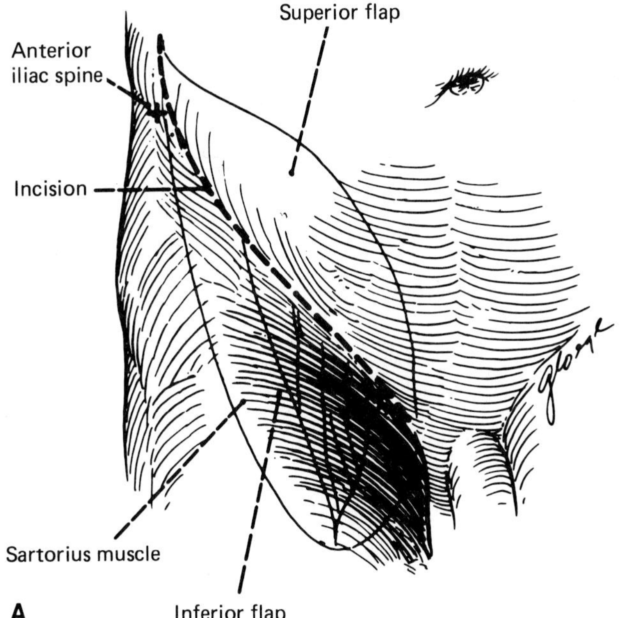

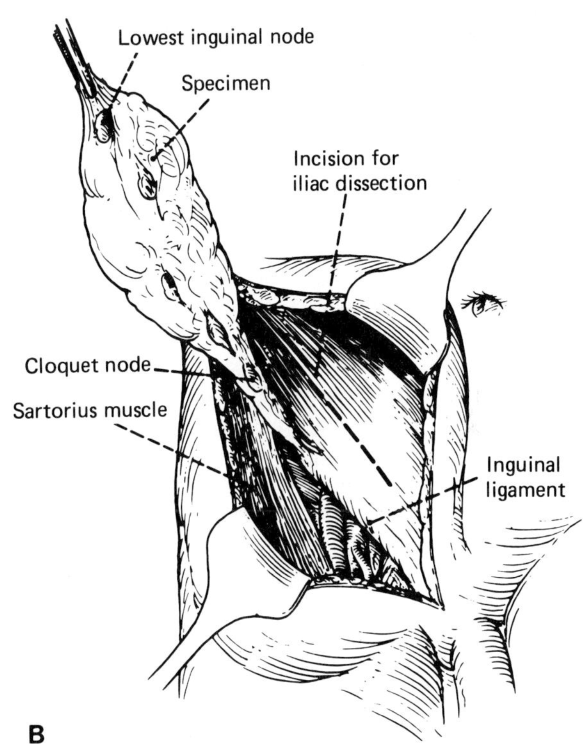

FIG. 31-11. Technique of superficial inguinal lymph node dissection. (See text for details.) (Holmes C, Moseley HS, Morton DL et al, Ann Surg 186:481, 1977)

as a perfusate in an attempt to improve the chemotherapeutic response and thus introduced the principle of heated perfusion.[247] In the last 20 years, many workers have employed isolation perfusion techniques for the treatment of the local primary melanoma, recurrent melanoma, satellitosis, in-transit metastases, or for patients with metastatic melanoma

TABLE 31-23. Chemotherapeutic Agents Used in Regional Perfusion

DRUG	REFERENCES
Melphalan	248–250, 253, 255, 256, 258–262
Mechlorethamine	250, 252
Thiotepa	251
Melphalan + thiotepa	254, 257
Melphalan + dactinomycin + mechlorethamine	263

to draining lymph nodes.[248–267] Perfusion is often combined with local surgical excision of the melanoma.

The technique of isolation perfusion is relatively simple though technically exacting. The afferent and efferent vessels supplying the extremity are isolated and connected to a low flow perfusion pump in continuity with an oxygenator and a heat exchanger. The iliac vessels are generally used for perfusion of the lower extremity and the axillary vessels are cannulated high in the axilla for upper extremity lesions. Chemotherapeutic agents are added to the perfusion circuit and the perfusion continued for approximately one hour. The drugs often used are listed in Table 31-23. Perfusion rates for lower extremity lesions are generally from 100–150 ml/min; upper extremity perfusions are approximately half this rate. Systemic heparinization is used throughout the perfusion and often reversed after perfusion is complete. Some drug leakage into the systemic circulation is inevitable and can be measured by including I^{131}-labeled albumin in the perfusate and monitoring radioactivity over the heart using a gamma detector. This provides a safeguard against excessive leakage of potentially lethal amounts of drugs into the systemic circulation and minimizes bone marrow depression. By use of this isolation perfusion technique, higher doses of chemotherapeutic agents can be administered than would be tolerated when infused into the arterial or venous systemic circulation.

Despite its application in several major cancer treatment centers the lack of critical comparative studies makes it difficult to evaluate the current role that perfusion should play in the treatment of patients with melanoma. A review of selected series is presented in Table 31-24. It has been difficult to define the exact results obtained with perfusion because many studies combine patients with a variety of different disease stages as well as perfusion with varied amounts of surgery. Most reported series involve small numbers of patients. In no instance has perfusion therapy been compared with other standard treatment for any stage patients with melanoma in a controlled fashion.

In the treatment of localized (stage I) melanoma, perfusion is often combined with local excision. As can be seen from Table 31-24, 5-year survival rates of 80–90% in clinical stage I patients are achieved. These survival rates may not be better than would be expected by wide excisional surgery alone. Detailed information concerning exact prognostic features of the primary lesion is not available in most series. Local recurrence rates following excision and perfusion therapy of local melanomas are 2% in the series by McBride, 6% in the series by Schraffordt and Koops, and 3.2% in the series by Wagner.[258,260,261] These local recurrence rates are comparable to those reported for series using wide excision alone (see Table 31-16).

Several series adequately document the regression of multiple cutaneous recurrences following perfusion therapy. While these results cannot be compared to the application of wide excisional surgery or even amputation in these patients because of unknown factors of patient selection, it does appear as if regional perfusion can play a role in the control of multiple cutaneous metastases. Recently, Stehlin and coworkers have presented evidence that hyperthermic perfusion is more effective than normothermic perfusion in the treatment of patients with in-transit metastases.[259] They reported a 76.7% 5-year survival in 30 such patients treated with hyperthermic perfusion compared to 22.2% 5-year survival

TABLE 31-24. Treatment of Malignant Melanoma by Regional Perfusion

	LOCAL DISEASE		LOCAL RECURRENCE		SATELLITES OR IN TRANSIT METASTASES	
Reference	*Number of Patients*	*5-Year Survival*	*Number of Patients*	*5-Year Survival*	*Number of Patients*	*5-Year Survival*
McBride et al 1975 (260)	92	86%	—	—	—	—
Stehlin, 1975 (259)	70	84%	8	Not stated	30	77%
Krementz et al 1975 (265)	249	85%	13	88%	62	33%
Schraffordt-Koops, 1977 (261)	31	77%	—	—	—	—
Wagner, 1976 (258)	144	93%	—	—	—	—
Rochlin et al 1972 (266)	238	92%	44	71%	142	43%
Golomb, 1972 (267)	—	—	20	35%	—	—

for 27 patients treated with normothermic perfusion. Again, problems of patient selection confuse interpretation.

A major problem with the widespread application of regional perfusion is the relatively high incidence of complications associated with its use. Stehlin reported two deaths in 165 patients, Krementz had nine deaths in 608 patients, and McBride and associates reported one death in 202 patients being perfused.[259,260,265] The local tissue necrosis resulting from the use of chemotherapeutic agents in the perfusate can also be a source of local morbidity, especially when multiple drugs are used. Occasional patients have required extensive debridement, fasciotomies, or even amputation for treatment of these complications. Krementz has reported 206 complications in 726 perfusions including mild edema, thrombophlebitis, infection, or bleeding.[265] Further complications due to the leakage of chemotherapeutic agents into the systemic circulation can occur. Most groups studying the role of perfusion in the treatment of melanoma report a decrease in the incidence of complications as increased experience in the use of these techniques accumulates.

It must be concluded that good evidence does not exist for a role for regional perfusion in the treatment of otherwise resectable melanoma of the extremities. Wide excision of local melanoma probably provides as good an overall survival with a lower incidence of complications as regional perfusion. Regional perfusion may have a role, however, in the treatment of multiple cutaneous metastases in an extremity that is otherwise not amenable to local surgery. Further studies and prospective controlled trials of regional perfusion compared to standard surgical therapy are necessary to elucidate the role of isolation perfusion in patients with melanoma.

FOLLOW-UP OF DISEASE-FREE PATIENTS

Patients rendered disease-free are followed not only to detect recurrence of the initial melanoma but also to diagnose any additional primary lesions that may develop. The frequency of follow-up is dependent upon risk of recurrence. Table 31-25 is an attempt to categorize patients into risk groups. Very high and very low risk groups are relatively easy to define. There remains however a large, less well-defined middle group. For the purpose of determining frequency of follow-up, patients are divided into two risk groups: low and intermediate/high. Low-risk patients are followed every 6 months with a history and physical examination; chest film, hemogram, and serum chemistry profile are performed yearly. Patients at intermediate or high-risk are followed every 3 months for 2 years, every 4 months for an additional year, and every 6 months thereafter. A history and physical examination, chest film, hemogram, and serum chemistry profile are performed on each visit.

Nodes at risk for regional spread must be carefully examined at each visit in those patients who have not undergone lymphadenectomy. Further, irrespective of whether or not the patient had a regional lymph node dissection, the area between the primary site and the lymph nodes must be carefully examined for intradermal and subcutaneous metastases.

When cutaneous melanoma disseminates, it has no preferential pattern of metastasis.[94,143] Serial routine chest films (with tomography for suspicious lesions) are adequate for detecting asymptomatic lung metastases. Serial liver enzyme determinations are more useful for detecting liver metastases in asymptomatic patients than are serial liver scans. The serum LDH is a sensitive indicator of hepatic and other intra-abdominal metastases.[94,150] A confirmed LDH elevation requires a liver scan and, if this is negative, ultrasonography or CT scan of the abdomen.[268] Evaluation of other sites is only undertaken if suggestive signs or symptoms exist. Persistent gastrointestinal complaints or unexplained blood in the stool should be evaluated with appropriate roentgenograms. "Bull's-eye" lesions on radioopaque studies are characteristic of melanoma metastatic to the GI tract.[269-272] Brain metastases may be the initial presentation of recurrent disease. The CT scan is the single most reliable technique for demonstrating these metastases and documenting their extent.[273] The urographic manifestations of metastatic melanoma have been reviewed.[274] Stewart and coworkers have characterized the roentgenographic evidence of skeletal metastases of melanoma. It is important to remember that melanoma can colonize virtually any anatomic site.[276] Further, in patients who have had a long disease-free interval, a second non-melanocytic primary should be considered.[73] Histologic confirmation of recurrent melanoma should be obtained whenever practical.

Yearly examination is adequate for the detection of a second primary cutaneous melanoma. In the patient with multiple large atypical pigmented lesions, follow-up is facilitated by the use of yearly close up color photographs or slides. The latter technique allows a large area to be photographed while providing magnification with projection for visible detail.

TABLE 31-25. Risk Estimate Based on Clark Levels, Thickness, and Regional Lymph Node Status

CLARK's LEVEL	THICKNESS (mm)	REGIONAL NODES		ESTIMATED 5-YEAR SURVIVAL NED	RISK
		CLINICAL	HISTOLOGIC		
I Thin II	<0.76	—	—	95–100%	Low
Thick II Thin III	0.76–1.5	—	—	50–85%	Intermediate
Thick III IV, V	>1.5	—	—	35–60%	High
Any	Any	—	+	20–35%	High
Any	Any	+	+	5–20%	High

TREATMENT OF DISSEMINATED DISEASE

SURGERY

Although surgery only plays a limited role in the management of patients with stage III disease, it should not be overlooked in treatment planning. Resection of melanoma metastases should be performed when relatively simple resections can leave the patient clinically disease-free. There is no role for the "debulking" of asymptomatic melanoma metastases.[277]

The palliative role of surgery should not be overlooked. Resection of a bleeding or partially obstructive bowel metastasis can not only afford significant palliation but at times may result in prolonged survival.[278]

The lungs are not infrequently the initial, and apparently sole, site of systemic spread.[279] Several reports have addressed the role of surgical resection in the management of pulmonary metastases from melanoma.[280,281] Mathiesen and coworkers collected data on 71 reported cases and found that 15 (21%) survived longer than 5 years.[280] Despite these few long-term survivors, the uncontrolled nature of these studies makes it difficult to determine the therapeutic potential of this approach. Of interest was the large number of benign processes or primary lung cancer and not melanoma metastases that were found in melanoma patients with radiologic evidence of pulmonary nodules.[280,281]

RADIOTHERAPY

Palliative Irradiation of Soft Tissue, Osseous, and Visceral Metastases

The publication by Hilaris and associates in 1963 marked the beginning of serious interest in this aspect of the radiotherapeutic management of melanoma.[282] Using conventional radiation fractionation and total doses of 2,000–4,000 rad in most cases, response rates were obtained ranging from 48% for skin metastases to 67% for brain metastases, averaging 57% for all sites. In the years following this publication, radiobiologic experiments suggesting a better response rate in melanoma using large individual fraction sizes prompted Habermalz and Fischer to adopt this practice.[283-285] They found a striking improvement in the response rate for skin metastases treated with individual dose fractions of 600 rad or higher. Responses were seen in 28 of 31 metastases treated with individual doses of 600 rad or more, compared with no responses in 11 lesions treated with fractions of 500 rad or less, independent of total dose. Hornsey confirmed this clinical observation in a series of patients with predominantly lymph node metastases, with a significantly better response rate of 80% in patients using fraction sizes of 400–800 rad, compared to a 54% response rate using fractions of less than 300 rad.[286] Overgaard reported similar improvements in response rates in skin and lymph node metastases with the response rates increasing from 35%, using fractions less than 400 rad, to 70%, with fractions of 400–700 rad, and 100% with fractions of 800 rad or higher.[287]

In a review of the large series of patients treated at the American Oncologic Hospital in Philadelphia, the improvement in response rates of intrathoracic and visceral melanoma metastases using fraction sizes larger than 500 rad, independent of total dose, was greater (82% vs. 44%) than the response rates using fractions of less than 500 rad.[288] In comparing the response of bone metastases, however, no improvement was observed in response rates with large fraction sizes compared with conventional palliative fraction sizes of 400 rad or less. There was a significant difference in response rates for bone metastases when comparing total doses above 3,000 rad with those of 3,000 rad or less (88% vs. 72%). The reasons for this behavior in bone metastases from that seen in soft tissue disease is not known. However, it provides an alternative to the use of large fractions for palliation of bone metastases in clinical settings where acute or late normal tissue tolerance would preclude the use of large fractions. The treatment options available for palliative irradiation of soft tissue, visceral, and bone metastases are presented in Table 31-26.

Palliative Irradiation of Central Nervous System Metastases

The published reports on the role of palliative radiotherapy for brain metastases from melanoma have claimed response rates ranging from 37% to 100% (average 68%), with the mean duration of response varying from 2 to 4.9 months (average 3.5), and mean survival following irradiation varying from 2 to 7.6 months (average 3.8 months).[282, 289-295] No one treatment regimen, either conventional palliative fractionation, large individual fraction sizes, or hyperfractionation has shown to be superior to others in improving the response rates, duration of response, or length of survival.[282,289-296] While the large majority of reported patients have been treated with corticosteroids concomitantly with irradiation, no evaluation of the relative effectiveness of each modality in relieving symptoms had been performed.[289-295] Furthermore, the relative responses to irradiation of patients with solitary versus multiple cerebral metastases (a common occurrence in melanoma) had not been studied. In a recently analyzed series of 63 patients at the American Oncologic Hospital, 73% of patients achieved symptomatic improvement with corticosteroids and irradiation. Most of the symptomatic improvement was attributable to the corticosteroid effect before irradiation and in only 42% to the effects of irradiation.[296] The mean duration of response in patients with multiple cerebral metastases was 0.9 months, compared with 1.9 months for patients with solitary metastases. Mean survivals post-irradiation were 2.2 and 3.2 months respectively. No improvement was seen in either duration of response or survival when large fraction sizes were used compared with conventional fractionation, either for solitary or multiple cerebral metastases. However, several retrospective studies show prolonged survival in patients treated with corticosteroids and irradiation over those treated with radiotherapy alone or no treatment.[289,292,293] A separately analyzed group of eight patients at American Oncologic Hospital who underwent excision of a solitary intracerebral metastasis followed by whole brain irradiation had a five-fold increase in duration of response and survival (13.5 months and 14.7 months respectively) over those patients with solitary intracerebral metastases treated only by irradiation and corticosteroids. Four of the eight

TABLE 31-26. Treatment Options for Palliative Irradiation of Melanoma Metastatic to Soft Tissue, Viscera, and Bone

	SMALL TREATMENT VOLUMES OR ACUTE/LATE NORMAL TISSUE TOLERANCE NOT CRITICAL	LARGE TREATMENT VOLUMES OR ACUTE/LATE NORMAL TISSUE TOLERANCE CRITICAL*
PERIPHERAL LYMPH NODE AND SOFT TISSUE METASTASES	Large individual fractions (≥ 500 rads) twice weekly to total dose of ~2000–4000 rads†	Same as for small volumes†
INTRATHORACIC, INTRA-ABDOMINAL, AND PELVIC NODAL AND VISCERAL METASTASES	Large individual fractions (≥ 500 rads) twice weekly to total dose of ~2000–4000 rads†	Conventional palliative fractions of 200–400 rads to total doses within normal tissue tolerance. Consideration may be given to hyperfractionation (115 rads × 2, 3–4 hours apart/daily to total dose ~3500–4500 rads)
BONE METASTASES	Large individual fractions (≥500 rads) or conventional palliative fractions of 200–400 rads (total dose in either case > 3000 rads)	Conventional palliative fractions of 200–400 rads (total dose >3000 rads)

* Esophagus, heart, small bowel, spinal cord
† Responses are not dependent on total dose (see text)

TABLE 31-27. Treatment Options for Melanoma Metastatic to the Brain

SOLITARY INTRACEREBRAL METASTASIS ON CT SCAN		MULTIPLE INTRACEREBRAL METASTASES ON CT SCAN	
Other metastases: none or stable and performance >30*	Other metastases: Rapidly progressing or performance ≤30*	Other metastases: None or stable and performance >30*	Other metastases: Rapidly progressing or performance ≤30*
Surgical excision of the metastasis and postoperative radiation†	Corticosteroids and irradiation† or corticosteroids alone if no symptomatic improvement	Corticosteroids and irradiation†	Corticosteroids and irradiation† or corticosteroids alone if no symptomatic improvement

* Karnofsky scale
† The optimum radiotherapeutic treatment regimen for each category has not been established (see text)

patients survived at least one year, compared with two of 28 patients with solitary intracerebral metastases receiving irradiation and steroids only ($p < 0.01$). This compares favorably with the 29–44% one-year survival rates in recently reported series of patients undergoing surgical excision and postoperative radiotherapy for solitary cerebral metastases from a variety of primary malignancies, including melanoma.[297-299] It suggests the value of combined surgical and radiotherapeutic treatment in selected patients, with solitary intracerebral metastases of melanoma with stable disease elsewhere, in prolonging symptom-free and absolute survival. Treatment options for brain metastases are presented in Table 31-27.

Epidural cord compression from metastatic melanoma is best managed by laminectomy, if there is a solitary blockage on myelogram and the patient has an anticipated life expectancy of at least 4 months. In the American Oncologic Hospital series, each of the four patients undergoing laminectomy had significant symptomatic improvement, while none of three patients receiving irradiation alone (either with conventional or high-dose fractionation schemes) had any symptomatic improvement.

SYSTEMIC CHEMOTHERAPY

Dimethyl-triazeno-imidazole-carboxamide (DTIC) is the most active single agent for the treatment of metastatic melanoma (see Table 31-28).[316] DTIC is the standard against which other single agents or combinations should be compared. The

TABLE 31-28. Activity of DTIC

INVESTIGATOR (Reference)	DOSE SCHEDULE	NO. EVALUABLE PTS.	CR and PR	RESPONSE RATE (%)
Wagner et al (300)	4.5 mg/kg/d × 10	393	109	28
Luce (301)	250 mg/m²/d × 5	125	20	16
Nathanson et al (302)	2 or 4.5 mg/kg/d × 10	115	32	28
Costanza et al (303)	150 mg/m²/d × 5	51	9	18
Moon et al (304)	300 mg/m²/d × 6, or 100 mg/m² q 8 h× 6	46	12	27
Van der Merwe et al (305)	100 mg/m² q 8 h × 6, or 150 mg/m²/d × 10, or 300 mg/m²/d × 6	29	8	28
Gottlieb et al (306)	150 mg/m²/d × 5 or 350–450 mg/m² biweekly	25	3	12
Burke et al (307)	4.5 mg/kg/d × 10	20	4	20
Cowan et al (308)	650–1450 mg/m²	20	4	20
Gerner et al (309)	3.5–5.5 mg/kg/d × 10	15	3	20
Vogel et al (310)	300–400 mg/m²/d × 5	12	1	8
Carter et al (311)	4.5 mg/kg/d × 10	48	8	16
Einhorn et al (94)	250 mg/m²/d × 5	113	19	17
Carter et al (312)	4.5 mg/kg/d × 10	71	15	21
Bellet et al (313)	2 mg/kg/d × 10	36	8	22
Ahmann et al (314)	275–400 mg/m²/d × 5	23	2	11
Costanzi (315)	150–250 mg/m²/d × 5	110	21	19
Costanza et al (331)	200 mg/m²/d × 5	127	9	15
	TOTALS	1379	293	21

CR and PR = complete response and partial response

overall objective response rate is 21%. Patients with subcutaneous, lymph node or pulmonary metastases respond most favorably. The median duration of response can approach one year.[301,313] Hematologic toxicity is modest with most regimens and gastrointestinal toxicity varies in severity, with 10-day regimens being best tolerated and a single infusion least well-tolerated. A 5-day course seems a reasonable compromise. The need for IV administration produces considerable inconvenience.

The nitrosoureas, of which BCNU, CCNU, and methyl-CCNU are best known, are the other single agents with well-documented activity against malignant melanoma (see Table 31-29).[317] Response rates range from 12–18%. Median response duration varies from 2–6 months. Hematologic toxicity is more severe than with DTIC but the oral nitrosoureas offer a major advantage in convenience of administration.

A large number of other single agents have demonstrated some anti-tumor activity against melanoma with response rates ranging from 3% to 35% (see Table 31-30). The reported experience with each of these drugs is small; thus, the observed response rates may not accurately reflect the true response rates. It is not necessarily true that actinomycin D with a response rate of 35% is better than cyclophosphamide with a 13% response rate.

A large number of combination regimens have been used in Phase II and controlled clinical trials. These are presented in Tables 31-31, 31-32, and 31-33. The questions to be asked regarding these trials are the following: Does any DTIC containing regimen have a better response rate than DTIC alone when compared in a randomized prospective trial? Does any regimen containing an active agent (DTIC or a nitrosourea) produce a better therapeutic effect than the components when used singly in sequence? The answers to both of these questions are no. Are combinations of marginally active drugs clinically worthwhile (see Table 31-33)? Although the reported experience with these regimens is modest, several seem promising and deserving of more extensive trials against DTIC and in DTIC-resistant patients.

DTIC is the obvious first choice for single agent conventional therapy. An oral nitrosourea is a logical second choice. It is not possible at present to select, on a rational basis, additional single agents from those with reported activity. Hopefully the development of a successful chemosensitivity assay will select those drugs which, although marginally active in general, will produce a useful anti-tumor effect in a given patient.[454] Some combinations of marginally effective agents seem promising but as yet do not appear ready for conventional application.

There is an urgent need for the development of more effective agents. Drug evaluation could be facilitated by the development of secondary pre-clinical screens (for example, human melanoma xenografted to nude mice).[455] Further research is warranted to exploit the tyrosinase-catalyzed pigment biosynthesis mechanism that is unique to normal and malignant melanocytes.[456]

HORMONAL THERAPY

Exogenous estrogen can increase melanin production in ovariectomized guinea pigs.[465] Lerner and coworkers demonstrated an increased quantity of melanocyte-stimulating substance in the urine of pregnant women. The relationship of melanoma to pregnancy and use of oral contraceptives has been discussed. These and similar observations have led some to consider melanoma an endocrine-dependent tumor.[467,468] Bodenham and Hale demonstrated an estrogen-induced increased uptake of ^{32}P by melanoma metastases.[467,468] Data indicate that melanoma tissue from some patients contain low levels of cytoplasmic estrogen, progesterone, androgen, and dexamethasone receptors.[463,464,472,474] Chaudhuri has demonstrated estrogen receptors in tissue from primary melanomas as well as from benign nevi removed from melanoma patients.[475] Beattie and associates have preliminary data suggesting that the growth of human melanoma in the nude mouse may be susceptible to hormonal control in relationship to estrogen receptors. Data on hormonal therapy are fragmentary (see Table 31-34). Responses are infrequent and where measured seem to occur without regard to hormone receptor status. Recently, Mossler and coworkers have suggested that estrogen binding in melanoma cytosol may be an artifactual function of proteins (*e.g.*, tyrosinase) other than steroid specific receptors. Considerable additional research will be required to clarify this area.

IMMUNOTHERAPY

The natural history of melanoma suggests that immunologic intervention by the host may significantly alter its growth and dissemination. Decades may separate the initial appearance of a primary lesion and its subsequent dissemination. During the radial phase of growth, with lymphocytic infiltration prominent, a melanoma may persist indolently for years, to be followed by sudden vertical growth activity, diminution of infiltrating lymphocytes, and rapidly developing metastases.[76] Further, there are well-documented cases of spontaneous regression of primary melanomas as well as metastatic disease.[145,478] Some of these regressions have been attributed to an attendant immunologic response.[479] For these and other reasons patients with cutaneous malignant melanoma have been the subject of intense immunobiologic investigation. The research dealing with melanoma-specific antigens and the host's immune response to these antigens has been extensively reviewed.[112]

Local Immunotherapy

In 1970, Morton demonstrated that the direct injection of live BCG organisms into cutaneous melanoma deposits could

TABLE 31-29. Activity of the Nitrosoureas

INVESTIGATOR AND REF. NO.	DOSE SCHEDULE	NO. OF EVALUABLE PATIENTS	RESPONSE	
			NO.	OVERALL % (CR + PR)
BCNU				
Ramirez et al. (318)	1.5 mg/kg/day × 5	99	19	19
DeVita et al (319)	150 mg/m²/day × 3	20	3	15
Lessner (320)	100 mg/m²/day × 2–3	3	0	0
		122	22	18
CCNU				
Pugh (321)	130 mg/m²q6wk	48	2	4
Cruz (322)	130 mg/m²q6wk	27	7	26
Ahmann et al (323)	130 mg/m²q6wk	19	1	5
Hoogstraten et al (324)	100 or 130 mg/m²q6wk	14	3	21
Broder et al (325)	130 mg/m²q4–6wk	4	0	0
De Conti et al (326)	130 mg/m²q6wk	4	1	25
Perloff et al (327)	130 mg/m²4–6wk	3	1	33
Hansen et al (328)	100–130 mg/m²q6wk	2	0	0
Wasserman (329)	variable	136	17	13
		257	32	12
METHYL-CCNU				
Ahmann et al (330)	225 mg/m²q6wk	28	5	18
Costanza et al (331)	200 mg/m²q6wk	119	18	15
Young et al (332)	220 mg/m²q6wk	28	6	21
Tranum et al (333)	150 or 200 mg/m²	10	0	0
Firat et al (334)	200 mg/m²q6wk	5	0	0
Wasserman (335)	variable	124	15	12
		314	44	14

Modified from Cannis RL: Cancer Treat Rep 60:165, 1976

TABLE 31-30. Activity of Single Agents

DRUG (Reference)	EVALUABLE PATIENTS	CR+PR	RESPONSE RATE (%)
ALKYLATING AGENTS			
Thiotepa (336, 337)	24	5	21
L-PAM (336, 338, 339)	24	4	17
Chlorambucil (Leukeran) (340)	22	2	9
Cyclophosphamide (336, 341–348)	32	4	13
ANTIMETABOLITES			
Methotrexate (349–351)	41	3	7
Cytarabine (Cytosine Arabinoside) (352–354)	27	3	11
5-fluorouracil (336, 355)	20	1	5
6-mercaptopurine (356–358)	29	2	7
ANTIBIOTICS			
Mitomycin C (359–361)	65	9	14
Bleomycin (362, 363)	40	1	3
Actinomycin D (387)	23	8	35
SPINDLE INHIBITORS			
Vincristine (364–368)	26	3	12
Vinblastine (369–377)	58	7	8
Vindesine (378–380)	75	13	17
Trimethyl colchicinic acid (381–383)	90	13	14
MISCELLANEOUS AGENT			
Dibromodulcitol (384–386)	43	8	18
TIC-mustard (388, 389)	26	3	12
Hydroxyurea (326, 375, 390–397)	86	7	8
Hexamethylymelamine (398)	42	2	5
Streptozotocin (399, 400)	19	2	10
cis-dichlorodiammine-platinum (II) (401)	11	3	27
Dianhydrogalactitol (402)	21	1	5
Cyclocytidine (403)	29	1	3
Estramustine phosphate (404)	26	1	4
Piperazinedione (405)	41	2	5

TABLE 31-31. Combination Chemotherapy with Regimens Containing DTIC

REGIMEN	EVALUABLE PATIENTS	CR+PR	RESPONSE RATE (%)	REFERENCES
DTIC + VA	126	22	17	406–410
DTIC + NU	212	37	17	303, 331, 415
DTIC + DDP	79	17	22	411–414
DTIC + Procarb	77	14	18	94, 410
DTIC + CTX	29	7	24	410
DTIC + Act-D	106	20	19	416–418
DTIC + Adria	27	5	19	415
DTIC + HU	28	5	19	415
DTIC + Cyclo	17	3	18	419
DTIC + VA + NU	749	177	24	94, 311, 420–428
DTIC + VA + CTX	20	5	25	429
DTIC + NU + Act-D	61	19	31	430
DTIC + NU + HU	119	30	25	311, 431
DTIC + NU + HU + VA	68	27	40	431
DTIC + NU + VA + Chl	121	27	22	432
DTIC + DDP + Procarb	13	2	15	413

Uncomon abbreviations: VA = vinca alkaloid; NU = nitrosourea; Cyclo = cyclocytidine; Chl = chlorpromazine

induce tumor regression in immunocompetent patients. Following his example, intralesional BCG therapy for metastatic malignant melanoma was adopted by a large number of investigators. The pooled data of 14 investigators reveal that in approximately 66% of patients treated by intralesional BCG there was regression of injected nodules (see Table 31-35). In 21% of patients, there was also regression of uninjected nodules (the latter were in close proximity to injected lesions). Some 27% of patients experienced complete remission of all clinically evident disease; this group was composed almost exclusively of immunocompetent patients with small tumor burdens limited to the dermis. Regression of injected and

TABLE 31-32. Combination Chemotherapy Regimens Containing A Nitrosourea (NU) as Most Active Component

REGIMEN	EVALUABLE PATIENTS	CR + PR	RESPONSE RATE (%)	REFERENCES
NU + VA	148	36	24	304, 413, 433–435
NU + CTX	40	4	10	406, 436
NU + CTX + VA + Bleo	39	7	18	437
NU + VA + Bleo	48	21	43	438, 439
NU + VA + CTX + Procarb	12	4	33	440
NU + VA + Procarb	30	18	60	441
NU + Caffeine + Chl	75	9	12	442

Unusual abbreviations: NU = nitrosourea; VA = vinca alkaloid; Chl = chlorpromazine

TABLE 31-33. Combination Chemotherapy Regimens That Do Not Contain DTIC or A Nitrosourea

REGIMEN	EVALUABLE PATIENTS	CR + PR	RESPONSE RATE (%)	REFERENCES
VA + Procarb + Act-D	53	13	24	443, 444
VA + Procarb + CTX	6	2	33	445
VA + Bleo + MTX	15	3	20	446
VA + Bleo	9	4	44	447
VA + Bleo + DDP	17	13	76	447, 448
DDP + Ifosfamid	15	8	53	449
5FU + Procarb	19	7	37	450
5FU + CTX + MTX + VA	26	4	24	451–453

Unusual abbreviation: VA = vinca alkaloid

TABLE 31-34. Hormonal Therapy

REGIMEN	EVALUABLE PATIENTS	CR + PR	RESPONSE RATE (%)	REFERENCES
Pregnanetrione	155	11	7	457, 458
Estramustine	40	5	12	404, 459
Diethylstilbestrol	18	4	22	460
Medroxyprogesterone acetate	15	1	6	461
Tamoxifen	25	4	16	462–464
Orchiectomy	2	1	50	470, 471

uninjected metastases is generally limited to patients with dermal disease. Uninjected lesions that regress are located in the same body region (usually an extremity) and in close proximity to injected lesions. On occasion, injected and uninjected subcutaneous lesions will regress. Fig. 31-12 illustrates dermal melanoma metastases and the responses to intralesional BCG of injected and uninjected lesions.

Immunostimulants other than BCG have been employed topically and intralesionally in the treatment of dermal lesions of recurrent malignant melanoma. The results are summarized in Table 31-36; the agents, in these small series of patients, have some efficacy and response rates that appear similar to those obtained with intralesional BCG. A variety of agents such as purified protein derivative (PPD), methanol-extracted residue (MER), cell wall skeleton (CWS) and P3, *C. parvum,* and dinitrochlorobenzene (DNCB) are likely to have mechanisms of action similar to BCG. An obvious advantage over BCG is that these are nonviable materials. Direct comparisons against BCG have not been attempted except for the study done by Cohen and coworkers using DNCB.[498] As that trial contained a total of only 11 patients, few definitive conclusions were possible. Once the efficacy of BCG has been detailed, it seems reasonable to undertake direct comparisons with potentially superior materials.

Systemic Immunotherapy

Several investigators have attempted active specific and nonspecific immunotherapy in patients with macrometastatic disease.[511–518] Objective remissions have been noted but these have been brief and considerably less frequent than those achieved with conventional chemotherapy. This result is to be expected based on animal tumor models demonstrating that these therapies are only effective against small tumor burdens.

The often large tumor burdens of patients receiving im-

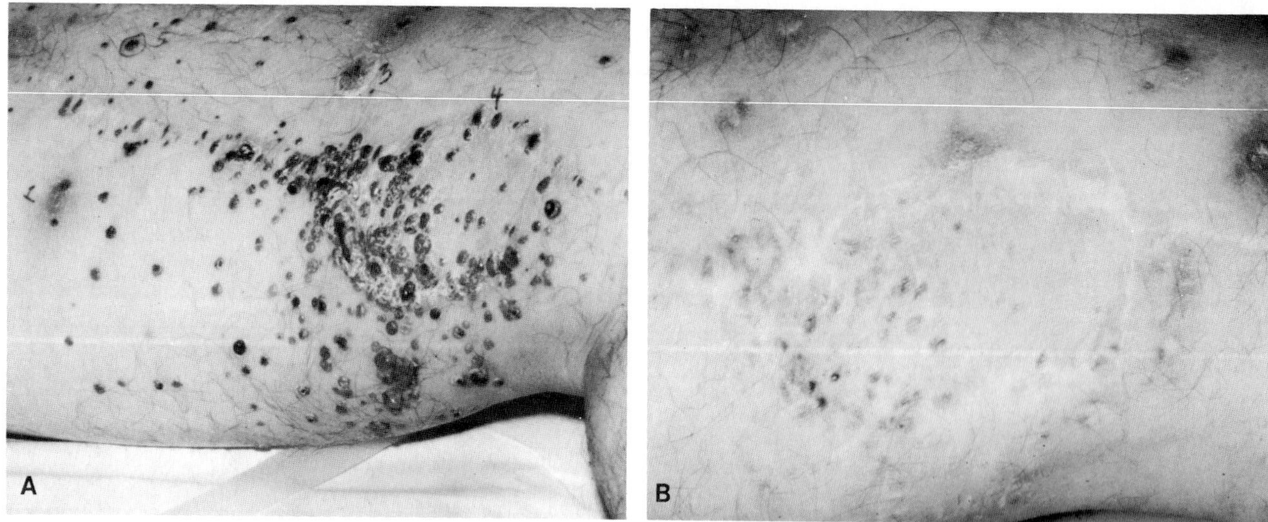

FIG. 31-12. Dermal melanoma metastases on the medical aspect of the thigh before (*A*) and after (*B*) intralesional *BCG* therapy.

munotherapy led to efforts to couple immunotherapy with tumor reductive chemotherapy regimens. The results of recent chemoimmunotherapy trials in melanoma patients with disseminated disease are summarized in Table 31-37. Gutterman and coworkers evaluated the efficacy of dimethyl-triazeno-imidazole-carboxamide (DTIC) plus Pasteur BCG by scarification in 89 patients, using a retrospective group of 111 patients treated with DTIC alone as controls.[519] Patients receiving DTIC-BCG exhibited a response rate significantly greater than patients treated with DTIC alone ($p = 0.05$). Mean survival was also greater in the chemoimmunotherapy group ($p = 0.001$). Patients with lymph node metastases and no evidence of visceral disease particularly benefited by the DTIC-BCG regimen, demonstrating a remission rate of 55% compared with 18% for controls ($p = 0.025$).

Randomized, prospective studies have yielded less encouraging results regarding an enhanced efficacy of chemoimmunotherapy regimens compared with chemotherapy alone in melanoma patients. Costanzi evaluated the contribution of BCG to a triple drug regimen (BHD) of 1,3-bis(2-chlorethyl)-1-nitrosourea (BCNU), hydroxyurea, and DTIC.[520] Addition of BCG to the BHD regimen did not result in enhanced overall response rates. Analysis by age, sex, and site of disease indicated that patients with pulmonary metastases had longer remissions and survival on BCG. Further, BCG seemed to yield longer survivals in patients over 60 years of age. These observations need confirmation in trials specifically designed to evaluate these points.

Presant and coworkers evaluated *C. parvum* added to a drug regimen of DTIC and cyclophosphamide, and observed

TABLE 31-35. Immunotherapy of Melanoma With Intralesional BCG

AUTHOR	SOURCE BCG	REGRESSION OF NODULES* INJECTED	UNINJECTED	CR
Morton (480–482)	Glaxo, Tice	25/29†	6/36	11/36
Krementz (483)	?	1/4	1/4	1/4
Nathanson (484)	Tice	7/9	2/9	2/9
Levy (485)	Glaxo	0/1	0/1	0/1
Pinsky (486)	Tice, Glaxo	15/25	2/25	2/25
Mastrangelo (487–489)	Tice, Glaxo	12/15	11/14‡	7/15
Smith (490)	Tice	3/7	1/7?	?
Minton (491)	?	2/8?	?	?
Baker (492)	Tice	1/2	0/2	?
Klein (493, 494)	Connaught	2/3	1/3	?
Liberman (495)	Tice	4/6	2/6?	3/6
Israel (496)	Pasteur	7/11?	0/11	?
Grant (497)	Glaxo	1/2	0/2	0/2
Cohen (498)	Glaxo, Tice	5/5	?	?
		85/127(66%)	26/120(21%)	26/98(27%)

CR = Complete responders; * = Number of patients showing regression of nodules/total number patients treated; † = regression on a per patient basis available on only 29 patients; ‡ = one patient had only a single nodule.

TABLE 31-36. Local Immunotherapy of Melanoma With Miscellaneous Nonspecific Immunostimulants

AUTHOR	NSI	REGRESSION OF NODULES*		CR
		INJECTED	UNIN-JECTED	
Tisman et al (499)	PPD	1/1	1/1	?
Klein et al (500)	PPD,DNCB	5/9	0/9	?
Malek–Mansour et al (501)	DNCB	1/1	?	1/1
Cohen et al (498)	DNCB	164/255†	?	?
Hunter–Craig et al (502)	Vaccinia	9/10	0/10	6/10
Milton and Brown (503)	Vaccinia	4/30?	?	3/30
Burdick (504)	Vaccinia	1/1	0/1	0/1
Burdick and Hawk (505)	Vaccinia	1/1		1/1
Milton and Belisario (506)	Vaccinia	1/1	?	1/1
Krown et al (507)	MER	12/18	?	6/18
Cunningham–Rundles et al (508)	*C. parvum*	6/14‡	0/14	3/14
Cohen (498)	*C. parvum*	31/86§	?	?
Cohen (498)	Nitrogen mustard	6/10§	?	?
Richman et al (509)	CWS + P3	11/23‡	0/23	?
Vosika et al (510)	CWS + P3	6/15	4/15	?

CWS + P3 = mycobacterium cell wall skeleton + trehalose dimycolate
NSI = Nonspecific Immunostimulants; CR = complete response
* = Number of patients showing regression of nodules/total number patients treated
† = Number of nodules showing regression in a total of 11 patients
‡ = Several patients had tumors other than melanoma
§ = Number of nodules showing regression in a total of five patients

TABLE 31-37. Chemoimmunotherapy in Disseminated Melanoma

GUTTERMAN ET AL (519)				
Treatment	DTIC–BCG (89)	DTIC (111) (HC)		
Response Rate*	27%	14.4%		
MDR (mos)	6	5	p = 0.05	
MDS (mos)	7	5	p = 0.01	
Remissisin rate at one year	20%	0		
COSTANZI (520)(R)				
Treatment	DTIC–BCG (119)	BHD–BCG (150)	BHD (82)	
Response Rate*	19%	29%	35%	NS
PRESANT ET AL (521)(R)	DTIC–C–CP (27)	DTIC–C (29)		
Response Rate*	29%	18%		NS
MDR (wks)	13	15.6		NS
MDS (mos)	5.7	6.1		NS
MASTRANGELO ET AL (552)(R)	M–V–BCG–TC(31)	M–V(31)		
Response Rate*	19%	23%		NS
MDR (mos)	8	6		NS
MS (mos)	8.0	6.5		NS

C = cyclophosphamide; CP = Corynebacterium parvum; D = DTIC; BHD = BCNU, hydroxyurea, and DTIC; M = MeCCNU; V = vincristine; TC = allogeneic tumor cells; HC = historical controls; MDR = median duration response; MDS = median duration survival; * = complete and partial responses; ( ) = number of patients in group; R = randomized study.

no difference in response or survival between treatment groups.[521] Mastrangelo and coworkers, using a regimen that included BCG and allogeneic tumor cells, failed to demonstrate a greater efficacy of the chemoimmunotherapy regimen.[522]

The addition of currently available immunotherapies to chemotherapy regimens may yield a small biologic effect but this is not of sufficient magnitude to be of clinical interest.

OCCULT MELANOMAS AND MELANOMAS ARISING IN ATYPICAL SITES

In various series of melanoma patients, the prevalence of occult primary lesions varies from 1% to 15%.[146–148,523] In about 10% of patients there is no historical or physical evidence suggesting a regressed cutaneous primary melanoma.[523] Fifty-five to 60% of those patients present with stage II disease, while the remainder have visceral metastases.[148,523] Survival is similar to that of patients with known cutaneous primaries.[523] Treatment is dependent on disease stage and is identical to that described for patients in whom the primary melanoma can be identified.

The Third National Cancer Survey determined the incidence of primary cutaneous melanoma to be 4.2/100 000 population.[12] The second most common primary site was the eye (0.56/100 000 population). (See Chapter 32) Non-cutaneous, non-ocular melanomas had an incidence of 0.15/100,000 population, largely mucosal in origin. Primary melanoma has been reported to occur in the mucosa of the respiratory, alimentary, and urogenital tracts.

The distribution of primary mucosal melanomas among 1,058 melanoma patients registered at the Cancer Control Agency of British Columbia is presented in Table 31-38.[524] The mucosa of the head and neck and the vulvo-vaginal areas are most commonly involved. However, melanoma of the female urethra constituted 7% of all malignancies at that site (see Col. Fig. 31-12). Attempts to correlate survival with the degree of invasion of the primary lesion have been hampered by their relative rarity and differences in mucosal anatomy. However, in their study of vulvar melanoma, Chung and associates found that thickness correlated with prognosis in that no patient with a tumor thickness of less than 1 mm experienced recurrence or nodal metastases.[525] Treatment of the primary lesion is often hampered by anatomic restrictions and large size, which results from the delayed diagnosis caused by their location. These primary lesions are best managed by wide excision, which may require vaginectomy, abdominoperineal resection, and so forth depending on the location of the primary lesion. No consensus exists on the merit of elective regional lymph node dissection in patients with mucosal melanomas. Treatment of stage III disease is similar to that described for melanoma of cutaneous origin. For a more detailed discussion of mucosal melanomas, the reader is referred to Iversen and Robins.[524]

Melanoma can arise in almost any location—as a desmoid cyst of the ovary, in the central nervous system, pituitary gland, pleura, and gall bladder.[526-530] These lesions are rare; therefore, surgical therapy must be guided by the general principles of surgical oncology for the particular anatomic site.

TABLE 31-38. Anatomic Distribution of Mucosal Malignant Melanomas (CCABC, 1938 to 1978)

LOCATION	NO.	PERCENT OF ALL MELANOMAS	PERCENT OF ALL MALIGNANCIES, SAME SITE
Head and neck	20	1.9	1
Vulva	14	1.3	5
Vagina	7	0.7	5
Anal canal	3	0.3	2
Female urethra	2	0.2	7
Esophagus	1	0.1	0.1
TOTAL	47	4.5	—

CCABC = Cancer Control Agency of British Columbia
Iversen K, Robins RE: Mucosal Malignant Melanomas. Am J Surg 139:660–664, 1980

REFERENCES

1. Urteaga O, Pack GT: On the antiquity of melanoma. Cancer 19:607–610, 1966
2. Carswell R: Pathological Anatomy, part 9, Melanoma. London, Longman, 1838.
3. Clark WH Jr, Goldman LI, Mastrangelo MJ (eds): Human Malignant Melanoma. New York, Grune & Stratton, 1979
4. Kopf AW, Bart RS, Rodriguez-Sains RS et al: Malignant Melanoma. New York, Masson Publishing, 1979
5. Milton GW: Malignant Melanoma of the Skin and Mucous Membranes. Edinburgh, Churchill-Livingston, 1977
6. McGovern VJ: Malignant Melanoma—Clinical and Histological Diagnosis. New York, John Wiley & Sons, 1976
7. Andrade R, Gumport SL, Popkin GL et al: Cancer of the Skin, pp 950–1044. Philadelphia, WB Saunders, 1976
8. Rawles ME: Origin of the Mammalian pigment cell and its role in the pigmentation of hair. In Gordon M (ed): Pigment Cell Growth, pp 1–15. New York, Academic Press, 1953
9. Fitzpatrick TB, Szabo G: The melanocyte-cytology and cytochemistry. J Invest Dermatol 32:197–209, 1959
10. Wolff K: Melanocyte-keratinocyte interactions in vivo: The fate of melanosomes. Yale J Biol Med 46:384–396, 1973
11. Szabo G: The number of melanocytes in the human epidermis. Br Med J 1:1016, 1954
12. Cutler SJ, Young JL Jr: Third National Cancer Survey: Incidence Data. Natl Cancer Inst Mongr 41:20–25, 1975
13. Kherzi AA, Dounis A, Roberts JBM: Primary malignant melanoma of the penis: Two cases and a review of the literature. Br J Urol 51:147–150, 1979
14. Elwood JM, Lee JAH: Recent data on the epidemiology of malignant melanoma. Semin Oncol 2:149–154, 1975
15. Magnus K: Incidence of malignant melanoma of the skin in the five Nordic countries. Significance of solar radiation. Int J Cancer 20:477–485, 1977
16. Cosman B, Heddle SB, Crikelair GF: The increasing incidence of melanoma. Plast Reconstr Surg 57:50–56, 1976
17. MacDonald EJ: Incidence and epidemiology of melanoma in Texas. In Neoplasmas of the Skin and Malignant Melanoma, pp 279–292. Chicago, Year Book Medical Publishers, 1976
18. Ressequie LJ, Marks SJ, Wenkelmann RK et al: Malignant melanoma in the resident population of Rochester, Minnesota. Mayo Clin Proc 52:191–195, 1977
19. Teppo L, Pakkanen M, Hakulinen T: Sunlight as a risk factor of malignant melanoma of the skin. Cancer 41:2018–2027, 1978
20. Lee JAH, Carter AP: Secular trends in mortality from malignant melanoma. JNCI 45:91–97, 1970
21. Luce JK, McBride CM, Frei E III: Melanoma, pp 1823–1844. In Holland JF, Frei E III (eds): Cancer Medicine. Philadelphia, Lea & Febiger, 1973
22. Lerman RI, Murray D, O'Hara JM et al: Malignant melanoma of childhood. Cancer 25:436–449, 1970
23. Skov–Jensen T, Hastrup J, Lambrethsen S: Malignant melanoma in children. Cancer 19:620–626, 1966
24. McGovern VJ, Goulston E: Malignant moles in children. Med J Aust 1:181–182, 1963
25. Lee JAH, Yongchaiyudha S: Incidence of and mortality from malignant melanoma by anatomical site. JNCI 47:253–263, 1971
26. Krementz ET, Sutherland CM, Carter RD et al: Malignant melanoma in the American Black. Ann Surg 183:533–542, 1976
27. Lewis MG: Malignant melanoma in Uganda. Br J Cancer 21:483–495, 1967
28. Fleming ID, Barnawell JR, Burlison PE et al: Skin cancer in black patients. Cancer 35:600–605, 1975

29. Hinds MW, Kolonel LN: Malignant melanoma of the skin in Hawaii, 1960–1977. Cancer 45:811–817, 1980
30. Oshumi T, Seiji M: Statistical study on malignant melanoma in Japan (1970–1976). Tohoku J Exp Med 121:355–364, 1979
31. Oluwasanmi JO, Williams AO et al: Superficial cancer in Nigeria. Br J Cancer 23:714–728, 1969
32. Higginson J, Oettle AG: Cancer incidence in the Bantu and "Cape Colored" races of South Africa: Report of a cancer survey in the Transvaal (1953–55). JNCI 24:589:671, 1960
33. Anderson WAD: Disease in the American Negro. Surgery 9:425–432, 1941
34. Morris GC Jr, Horn RC Jr: Malignant melanoma in the Negro. Surgery 29:223–230, 1951
35. Lancaster HO: Some geographical aspects on the mortality from melanoma. Med J Aust 1:1082–1087, 1956
36. Anaise D, Steinitz R, Ben Hur N: Solar radiation: A possible etiologic factor in malignant melanoma in Israel. Cancer 42:299–304, 1978
37. Movshovitz M, Modan B: Role of sun exposure in the ethiology of malignant melanoma: Epidemiologic influence. JNCI 51:777–779, 1973
38. Magnus K: Incidence of malignant melanoma of the skin in Norway 1955–1970: Variation in time and space and solar radiation. Cancer 32:1275–1286, 1973
39. Gellin GA, Kopf AW, Garfinkel L: Malignant melanoma: A controlled study of possible associated factors. Arch Dermatol 99:43–48, 1969
40. Kripke ML: Speculations on the role of ultraviolet radiation in the development of malignant melanoma. JNCI 63:541–548, 1979
41. Lee JAH, Merrill JM: Sunlight and the etiology of malignant melanomas: A synthesis. Med J Aust 2:846–851, 1970
42. Elwood JM, Lee JAH, Walters SD et al: Relationship of melanoma and other skin cancer mortality to latitude and ultraviolet radiation in the United States and Canada. Int J Epidemiol 3:325–332, 1974
43. Fears TR, Scotto J, Schneiderman M: Skin cancer, melanoma and sunlight. Am J Public Health 66:461–464, 1976
44. Viola MV, Houghton A, Munster EW: Solar cycles and malignant melanoma. Medical Hypothesis 5:153–160, 1979
45. Mason TJ, McKay FW, Hoover R et al: Atlas of cancer mortality for US countries: 1950–1969. DHEW Publ. No. (NIH) 75–78, 1975
46. Beardmore GL: The epidemiology of malignant melanoma in Australia. In McCarthy WH (ed): Melanoma and Skin Cancer, pp 40–64. Sydney, VCN Blight, 1972
47. Sober AJ, Lew RA, Fitzpatrick TB et al: Solar exposure patterns in patients with cutaneous melanoma. Clin Res 27, 536A, 1979
48. Williams RR, Stegens NL, Goldsmith JR: Association of cancer site and type with occupation and industry from the Third National Cancer Survey Interview: JNCI 59:1147–1185, 1977
49. Hewer TF: Malignant melanoma in colored races: Role of trauma in its causation. J Path Bact 41:473–477, 1935
50. Shah JP, Goldsmith HS: Prognosis of malignant melanoma in relation to clinical presentation. Am J Surg 123:286–288, 1972
51. Mundth ED, Guralnick EA, Raker JW: Malignant melanoma: A clinical study of 427 cases. Ann Surg 162:15–28, 1965
52. Davis NC: Cutaneous melanoma: The Queensland experience. Curr Prob Surg 13:1–63, 1976
53. Knutson CO, Hori JM, Spratt JS Jr: Melanoma. In Current Problems in Surgery, pp 1–55. Chicago, Year Book Medical Publisher, 1971
54. Shaw HM, Milton GW, Farago G, et al: Endocrine influences on survival from malignant melanoma. Cancer 42:669–677, 1978
55. Beral V, Ramcharan S, Faris R: Malignant melanoma and oral contraceptive use among women in California. Br J Cancer 36:804–809, 1977
56. Allen EP: Malignant melanoma—spontaneous regression after pregnancy. Br Med J 2:1067, 1955
57. Stewart H: A case of malignant melanoma and pregnancy, Br Med J 1:647, 1955
58. Summer WC: Spontaneous regression of melanoma: Case report. Cancer 6:1040–1043, 1953
59. Shiu MH, Schottenfeld D, Maclean B et al: Adverse effect of pregnancy on melanoma. Cancer 37:181–187, 1976
60. Bohn AK, Rosenwaike I, Herrmann N et al: Melanoma after exposure to PCB's. N Engl J Med 295:450, 1976
61. Lieberman AN, Shupack JL: Levodopa and melanoma. Neurology 24:340–343, 1974
62. Skibba JL, Pinckley J, Gilbert EF et al: Multiple primary melanoma following administration of levodopa. Arch Path 93:556–561, 1972
63. Robinson E, Wajsbort J, Hirshowitz B: Levodopa and malignant melanoma. Arch Path 95:213, 1973
64. Sober AJ, Wick MM: Levodopa therapy and malignant melanoma. JAMA 240:554–555, 1978
65. Parsons PG, Goss P, Pope JH: Detection in human melanoma cell lines of particles with some properties in common with RNA tumor viruses. Int J Cancer 13:606–618, 1974
66. Birkmayer GD, Balda BR, Miller F: Oncorna-viral information in human melanoma. Europ J Cancer 10:419–424, 1974
67. Norris W: A case of fungoid diseases. Edinb Med Surg J 96:562–565, 1820
68. Cawley EP: Genetic aspects of malignant melanoma. Arch Dermatol 65:440–450, 1952
69. Anderson DE, Smith JL, McBride CM: Hereditary aspects of malignant melanoma. JAMA 200:741–746, 1967
70. Greene MH, Fraumeni JF Jr: The hereditary variant of malignant melanoma. In Clark WH, Goldman LI, Mastrangelo, MJ (eds): Human Malignant Melanoma, pp 139–166. New York, Grune & Stratton, 1979
71. Anderson DE: Clinical characteristics of the genetic variety of cutaneous melanoma in man. Cancer 288:721:–725, 1977
72. Lokich JJ: Malignant melanoma and carcinoma of the breast. J Surg Oncol 7:199–204, 1975
73. Bellet RE, Vaisman I, Mastrangelo MJ et al: Multiple primary malignancies in patients with cutaneous melanoma. Cancer 40: 1974–1981, 1977
74. Clark WH Jr, Reimer RR, Greene M et al: Origin of familial melanoma from heritable melanocytic lesions—the BK mole syndrome. Arch Dermatol 114:732–738, 1978
75. Reimer RR, Clark WH Jr, Greene MH et al: Precursur lesions in familial melanoma. JAMA 239:744–746, 1978
76. Clark WH Jr, Ainsworth AM, Bernardino EA et al: The developmental biology of primary human malignant melanomas. Semin Oncol 2:83–103, 1975
77. Clark WH Jr, From L, Bernardino EA et al: The histogenesis and biologic behavior of primary human malignant melanoma of the skin. Cancer Res 29:705–727, 1969
78. Arrington JH III, Reed RJ, Ichinose H et al: Acral lentiginous melanoma: A distinctive variant of human cutaneous malignant melanoma. J Surg Path 1:131–143, 1977
79. Mihm MC Jr, Fitzpatrick TB, Lane Brown MM et al: Early detection of primary cutaneous malignant melanoma. N Engl J Med 289:989–996, 1973
80. Sober AJ, Fitzpatrick TB, Mihm MC et al: Early recognition of cutaneous melanoma. JAMA 242:2795–2799, 1979
81. Clark, WH Jr, Mihm MC: Lentigo maligna and lentigo maligna melanoma. Am J Pathol 55:39–67, 1969
82. Winkelmann RK: The differential diagnosis of melanoma. In McCarthy WH (ed): Melanoma and Skin Cancer, pp 175–184. Sydney, VCN Blight, 1972
83. Mihm MC Jr, Clark WH Jr, Reed RJ: The clinical diagnosis of malignant melanoma. Semin Oncol 2:105–118, 1975
84. Clark WH Jr, Mihm MC Jr: Moles and malignant melanoma. In Fitzpatrick TB, Arndt KA, Clark WH Jr et al: (eds): Dermatology in General Medicine, pp 491–511. New York, McGraw-Hill, 1971
85. Bhawan J: Melanocytic nevi. A review. J Cut Path 6:153–169, 1979
86. Fitzpatrick TB, Gilchrest BA: Dimple sign to differentiate benign from malignant pigmented cutaneous lesions. N. Engl J Med 296:1518, 1977

87. Spitz S: Melanomas in childhood. Amer J Path 24:591–609, 1948
88. Kopf AW, Andrade R: Benign juvenile melanoma. In: The Year Book of Dermatology, pp 7–52. Chicago, Year Book Medical Publishers, 1966
89. Okun MR: Melanoma resembling spindle and epithelioid cell nevus. Arch Dermatol 115:1416–1420, 1979
90. Paniago–Pereira C, Maize JC, Ackerman AB: Nevus of large spindle cells and/or epithelioid cells (Spitz's nevus). Arch Dermatol 114:1811–1823, 1978
91. Leppard B, Sanderson KV, Behan F: Subungual malignant melanoma: Difficulty in diagnosis. Br Med J 1:310–312, 1974
92. Heise H, Krementz ET: Survival experience of patients with malignant melanoma of the skin, 1950–1957. Natl Cancer Inst Monogr 6:69–84, 1961
93. Bodenham DC: Basic principles of surgery—Malignant melanoma. In McCarthy WH (ed): Melanoma and Skin Cancer, pp 375–383. Sydney, VCN Blight, 1972
94. Einhorn LH, Burgess MA, Vallejos C et al: Prognostic correlations and response to treatment in advanced metastatic melanoma. Cancer Res 34:1995–2004, 1974
95. Perzik SL, Baum RK: Individualization in the management of melanoma: A review of 164 consecutive cases. Am Surg 35:177–180, 1969
96. Jones WM, Williams WJ, Roberts MM el al: Malignant melanoma of the skin: Prognostic value of clinical features and the role of treatment in 111 cases. Br J Cancer 22:437–451, 1968
97. Lehman JA Jr, Cross FS, Richey DeWG: A clinical study of 49 patients with malignant melanoma. Cancer 19:611–619, 1966
98. Nathanson L, Hale TC, Vater GF et al: Melanoma as a medical problem. Arch Intern Med 119:479–492, 1967
99. Cochran AJ: Malignant melanoma: Review of 10 years experience in Glasgow, Scotland. Cancer 23:1190–1199, 1969
100. Elias EG, Didolkar MS, Goel IP et al: A clinicopathologic study of prognostic factors in cutaneous malignant melanoma. Surg Gynecol Obstet 144:327–334, 1977
101. Fortner JG, DasGupta T, McNeer G: Primary malignant melanoma of the trunk. Ann Surg 161:161–169, 1965
102. Ketcham AS, Chretien PB: Therapeutic implications of cellular immune defects in operable cancer patients revealed by dinitrochlorobenzene skin contact sensitivity. Pan Med 17:174–178, 1975
103. Ziegler JL, Lewis MG, Luyombya JBS et al: Immunologic studies on patients with malignant melanoma in Uganda. Br. J Cancer 23:729–734, 1969
104. Catalano WJ, Chretien PB: Abnormalities of quantitative dinitrochlorobenzene sensitization in cancer patients: Correlation with tumor stage and histology. Cancer 31:353–356, 1973
105. Eilber FR, Morton DL: Impaired immunologic reactivity and recurrence following cancer surgery. Cancer 25:362–367, 1970
106. Camacho ES, Pinsky CM, Wanebo HJ et al; DNCB reactivity and prognosis in 358 patients with malignant melanoma. Proc Am Assoc Cancer Res 18:226, 1977
107. Pritchard DJ, Ritts RE Jr, Taylor WF et al: A prospective study of immune responsiveness in human melanoma. Cancer 41:2165–2173, 1978
108. Roses DF, Campion JF, Harris MN et al: Malignant melanoma. Delayed hypersensitivity skin testing. Arch Surg 114:35–38, 1979
109. Seigler HF, Shingleton WW, Metzgar RS et al: Non-specific and specific immunotherapy in patients with melanoma. Surgery 72:162-174, 1972
110. Gross NJ, Eddie–Quartery AC: Monitoring of immunologic status of patients receiving BCG therapy for malignant disease. Cancer 37:2183–2193, 1976
111. Aranha GV, McKhann CF, Simmons RL et al: Recall skin-test antigens and the prognosis of Stage I melanoma. J Surg Oncol 11:13–16, 1979
112. Mastrangelo MJ, Bellet RE, Berd D: Immunology and immunotherapy of human cutaneous malignant melanoma. In Clark WH Jr, Goldman LI, Mastrongelo, MJ (eds): Human Malignant Melanoma, pp 355–416. New York, Grune & Stratton, 1979
113. Gillespie GY, Barth RF: Lymphocyte mediated reactivity against malignant melanoma detected by a microcytotoxicity assay employing technetium–99m labeled target cells. Cancer 41:2174–2182, 1978
114. Livingston PO, Shiku H, Bean MA et al: Cell-mediated cytotoxicity for cultured autologous melanoma cells. Int J Cancer 24:39–44, 1979
115. Hersey P, Edwards A, Milton GW et al: Relationship of cell-mediated cytotoxicity against melanoma cells to prognosis in melanoma patients. Br J Cancer 37:505–513, 1978
116. Golub SH, O'Connell TX, Morton DL: Correlation of *in vivo* and *in vitro* assays of immunocompetence in cancer patients. Cancer Res 34:1833–1837, 1974
117. DeGast GC, The TH, Koops HS et al: Humoral and cell-mediated immune response in patients with malignant melanoma. Cancer 36:1289–1297, 1975
118. Lui VK, Karpuchas J, Dent PB et al: Cellular immunocompetence in melanoma: Effect of extent of disease and immunotherapy. Br J Cancer 32:323–330, 1975
119. Golub SH, Rangel DM, Morton DL: *In vitro* assessment of immuno-competence in patients with malignant melanoma. Int J Cancer 20:873–880, 1977
120. Reynolds PM, Grimsley G, Dawkins RL et al: Immunologic status may predict clinical outcome in BCG treated melanoma. Aust NZ J Med 10:39–43, 1980
121. Babusikova O, Novotna L, Schnekova K et al: T and B lymphocytes in malignant melanoma patients. Neoplasm 23:635–644, 1976
122. Bertoglio J, Gerlier D, Bourgoin A et al: Increase in E. active rosette forming lymphocytes in melanoma patients treated with BCG. Eur J Cancer 13:321–323, 1977
123. Lane N, Lattes R, Malm J: Clinicopathological correlations in a series of 117 malignant melanomas of the skin of adults. Cancer 11:1025–1043, 1958
124. Mehnert JH, Heard JL: Staging of malignant melanoma by depth of invasion. Am J Surg 110:168–176, 1965
125. Clark WH Jr: A classification of malignant melanoma in man correlated with histogenesis and biologic behavior. In Montagna W, Hu F (eds): Advances in Biology of Skin and the Pigmentary System, pp 621–647. London, Pergamon Press, 1967
126. McGovern VJ: The classification of melanoma and its relationship with prognosis. Pathology 2:85–98, 1970
127. Wanebo HJ, Woodruff J, Fortner JG: Malignant melanoma of the extremities: A clinicopathologic study using levels of invasion (microstage). Cancer 35:666–676, 1975
128. Balch CM, Murad TM, Soong SJ et al: A multifactorial analysis of melanoma: Prognostic histopathological features comparing Clark's and Breslow's staging methods. Ann Surg 118:732–742, 1978
129. Breslow A: Thickness, cross-sectional area and depth of invasion in prognosis of cutaneous melanoma. Ann Surg 172:902–908, 1970
130. Hansen MG, McCarten AB: Tumor thickness and lymphocyte infiltration in malignant melanoma of the head and neck. Am J Surg 128:557–561, 1974
131. Gromet MA, Epstein WL, Blois MS: The regressing thin melanoma. A distinctive lesion with metastatic potential. Cancer 72:2282–2292, 1978
132. Franklin JD, Reynolds VH, Page DL: Cutaneous melanoma: A twenty year retrospective study with clinicopathologic correlation. Plast Reconstr Surg 56:277–285, 1975
133. McLeod GR: Factors influencing prognosis in malignant melanoma. In McCarthy WH (ed): Melanoma and Skin Cancer, pp 367–373. Sydney, VCN Blight, 1972
134. Balch CM, Soong JJ, Murad TM et al: A multifactorial analysis of melanoma. II. Prognostic factors in patients with Stage I (localized) melanoma. Surgery 86:343–351, 1979
135. Huvos AG, Mike V, Donnellan MJ et al: Prognostic factors in cutaneous melanoma of the head and neck. Am J Pathol 71:33–45, 1973
136. Little JH: Histology and prognosis in cutaneous malignant melanoma. In: McCarthy WH (ed): Melanoma and Skin Cancer, pp 109–119. Sydney, VCN Blight, 1972
137. Beardmore GL, Davis NC, McLeod R et al: Malignant melanoma in Queensland: A study of 219 deaths. Aust J Dermatol 10:158–168, 1969

138. McNeer G, DasGupta T: Prognosis in malignant melanoma. Surgery 56:512–518, 1964
139. Goldsmith HS, Shah JP, Kim DH: Prognostic significance of lymph node dissection in the treatment of malignant melanoma. Cancer 26:606–609, 1970
140. Cohen MH, Ketcham AS, Felix EL et al: Prognostic factors in patients underdoing lymphadenectomy for malignant melanoma. Ann Surg 186:635–642, 1977
141. Fortner JG, Woodruff J, Schottenfeld D et al: Biostatistical basis of elective node dissection for malignent melanoma. Ann Surg 186:101–103, 1977
142. Karakousis CP, Seddiq MK, Moore R: Prognostic value of lymph node dissection in malignant melanoma. Arch Surg 115:719–722, 1980
143. Amer MH, AL–Sarraf M, Vaitkevicius VK: Clinical presentation, natural history and prognostic factors in advanced melanoma. Surg Gynecol Obstet 149:168–192, 1979
144. American Joint Committee for Cancer Staging and End-Results Reporting: Manual for staging of cancer, 1978, pp 131–135. Whiting Press, 1978
145. McGovern VJ: Spontaneous regression of melanoma. Pathology 7:91–99, 1975.
146. Brownstein MH, Helwig EB: Patterns of cutaneous metastasis. Arch Dermatol 105:862–868, 1972
147. DasGupta T, Bowden L, Berg JW: Malignant melanoma of unknown primary origin. Surg Gynecol Obstet 117:341–345, 1963
148. Baab GH, McBride CM: Malignant melanoma. The patient with an unknown site of primary origin. Arch Surg 110:896–900, 1975
149. Meyer JE, Stolbach L: Pretreatment radiographic evaluation of patients with malignant melanoma. Cancer 42:125–126, 1978
150. Garg R, McPherson TA, Lentle B et al: Usefulness of an elevated serum lactate dehydrogenase value as a marker of hepatic metastases in malignant melanoma. Can Med Ass J 120:1114, 1979
151. Thomas JH, Panoussopoulous D, Liesmann GE et al: Scintiscans in the evaluation of patients with malignant melanoma. Surg Gynecol Obstet 149:574–576, 1979
152. deRoo T: Lymphangiographic studies in a series of 55 patients with malignant melanoma. Lymphology 6:6–12, 1973
153. Musumeci R, Acerbil L, Balzarini GP et al: Lymphographic evaluation of 116 cases of malignant melanoma. Tumori 58:1–12, 1972
154. Musumeci R, LaMonica G, Orefice S et al: Lymphographic evaluation of 250 patients with malignant melanoma. Cancer 38:1568–1573, 1976
155. Cox K, Hare WSC, Bruce PT: Lymphography in melanoma. Cancer 19:637–647, 1966
156. Edwards JM: The value of lymphography in the management of melanoma. Clin Radiol 20:444–446, 1969
157. Roses DF, Ackerman AB, Harris MN et al: Assessment of biopsy techniques and histopathologic interpretations of primary cutaneous malignant melanoma. Ann Surg 189:294–297, 1979
158. Little JH, Davis NC: Frozen section diagnosis of suspected malignant melanoma of the skin. Cancer 34:1163–1172, 1974
159. Epstein E, Bragg K, Linden G: Biopsy and prognosis of malignant melanoma. JAMA 208:1369–1371, 1969
160. Ames FC, Sugarbaker FV, Ballantyne AJ: Analysis of survival and disease control in Stage I melanoma of the head and neck. Am J Surg 132:484–491, 1976
161. Veronesi U, Cascinelli N: Surgical treatment of malignant melanoma of the skin. World J Surg 3:279–288, 1979
162. Handley WS: The pathology of melanotic growths in relation of their operative treatment. Lancet 1:927–1003, 1907
163. Rosenberg SA: Surgical treatment of malignant melanoma. Cancer Treat Rep 60:159–163, 1976
164. DasGupta TK: Results of treatment of 269 patients with primary cutaneous melanoma: A five-year prospective study. Ann Surg 186:201–209, 1977
165. Kopf AW, Bart RS, Rodriguez-Sains RS: Surgical management of malignant melanomas. J Dermatol Surg Oncol 3:41–125, 1977
166. Goldman LI: The treatment of malignant melanoma of the skin. Surg Gynecol Obstet 146:779–782, 1978
167. Sim FH, Taylor WF, Ivins JC et al: A prospective randomized study of the efficacy of routine elective lymphadenectomy in management of malignant melanoma: Preliminary results. Cancer 41:948–956, 1978
168. Olsen G: Surgical treatment of primary melanoma. Some views on the size and depth of the excision. In McCarth WH (ed): Melanoma and Skin Cancer, pp 389–398. Sidney, VCB Blight, 1972
169. Cady B, Legg MA, Redfern AB: Contemporary treatment of malignant melanoma. Am J Surg 129:472–482, 1975
170. McBride CM, Sugarbaker EV, Brown BW: Malignant melanoma of the trunk. In Neoplasms of the Skin and Malignant Melanoma, pp 363–374. Chicago, Year Book Medical Publishers, 1975
171. Veronesi U, Adamus J, Bandiera DC et al: Inefficacy of immediate node dissection in Stage I melanoma of the limbs. New Engl J Med 297:627–630, 1977
172. Balch CM, Murad TM, Soong SJ et al: Tumor thickness as a guide to surgical management of clinical Stage I melanoma patients. Cancer 43:883–888, 1979
173. McNeer G, Cantin J: Local failure in the treatment of melanoma. Am J Roentgen Rad Ther Nucl Med 99:790–808, 1967
174. Breslow A, Macht SD: Optimal size of resection margin for this cutaneous melanoma. Surg Gynecol Obstet 145:691–692, 1977
175. Roses DF, Harris MN, Stern JS et al: Cutaneous melanoma of the breast. Ann Surg 189:112–115, 1979
176. Lee YTN: Sparks FC, Morton DL: Primary melanoma of skin of the breast region. Ann Surg 185:17–22, 1977
177. Papachristou DN, Kinne D, Ashikari R et al: Melanoma of the nipple and areola. Br J Surg 66:287–288, 1979
178. Papachristou DN, Kinne DW, Rosen PP et al: Cutaneous melanoma of the breast. Surgery 85:322–328, 1979
179. Welvaart K, Koops HS: Subungual malignant melanoma: A nail in the coffin. Clin Oncol 4:309–315, 1978
180. Keyhani A: Comparison of clinical behavior of melanoma of the hands and feet. A study of 283 patients. Cancer 40:3168–3173, 1977
181. Woltering EA, Thorpe WP, Reed JK Jr et al: Split thickness skin grafting of the plantar surface of the foot after wide excision of neoplasms of the skin. Surg Gynecol Obstet 149:229–232, 1979.
182. Allen SC, Spitz S: Malignant melanoma. A clinicopathological analysis of the criteria for diagnosis and prognosis. Cancer 6:1–45, 1953
183. Cochran A: Method of assessing prognosis in patients with malignant melanoma. Lancet 2:1062–1064, 1968
184. Neifeld JP, Chretien PB: An improved technique of excision and skin grafting for primary malignant melanomas. Surg Gynecol Obstet 143:585–586, 1976
185. Olsen G: The malignant melanoma of the skin. New theories based on a study of 500 cases. Acta Chirurgica Scand Suppl 365:128–136, 1966
186. Jorgsholm B, Engdahl I: Malignant melanoma. Acta Radiol (Stockh) 44:417–433, 1955
187. Nitter L: The treatment of malignant melanoma with special reference to the possible effect of radiotherapy. Acta Radiol (Stockh) 44:547–562, 1956
188. Hellriegel W: Radiation therapy of primary and metastatic melanoma. Ann NY Acad Sci 100:131–141, 1963
189. Konevny M, Krenarova V: A contribution to the radiotherapy of malignant melanoma. Neoplasma 16:335–337, 1969
190. Weitzel G: Die Strahlenbehandlung des melanomas. Schweiz Med Wochenschr 100:982–987, 1970
191. Ghanrawi KAE, Glennie JM: The value of radiotherapy in the management of malignant melanoma of the nasal cavity. J Laryngol Otol 88:71–75, 1974
192. von Lieven H, Skopal D: Zur strahlenempfindlichkeit des malignen melanomas. Strahlentherapie 152:1–4, 1976
193. Storck H: Treatment of melanotic freckles by radiotherapy. J Dermatol Surg Oncol 3:293–294, 1977
194. Kynaston B: The radiotherapy of melanoma. Aust NZ J Surg 48:36–39, 1978

195. Proppe A: The worth of radiotherapy in malignant melanomas. J Dermat Surg Oncol 4:613–616, 1978
196. Dancuart F, Harwood AR, Fitzpatrick PJ: The radiotherapy of lentigo maligna and lentigo maligna melanoma of the head and neck. Cancer 45:2279–2283, 1980
197. Creagan ET, Woods JE, Cupps RE et al: Radiation therapy for malignant melanoma of the head and neck. Am J Surg 138:604–606, 1979
198. Pearson D: Radiotherapy in malignant melanoma. Proc Roy Soc Med 67:96–97, 1974
199. Dickson RJ: Malignant melanoma. A combined surgical and radiotherapeutic approach. Am J Roentgenol 79:1063–1070, 1958
200. Kopf AW, Bart RS, Rodriguez-Sains RS et al: Malignant melanoma, pp 197–199. New York, Masson Publishing USA, 1979
201. Cooper JS, Kopf AW, Bart RS: Present role and future prospects for radiotherapy in the management of malignant melanomas. J Dermat Surg Oncol 5:134–139, 1979
202. Harmer CL: The radiotherapy of melanoma. Clin Exp Dermatol 1:29–35, 1976
203. Everall JD, O'Doherty CJ, Ward J et al: Treatment of primary melanoma by intralesional vaccinia before excision. Lancet 2:583–586, 1975
204. Castermans–Elias S, Simar L, Vanijck R et al: Immunosurgical treatment of Stage I malignant melanoma. Cancer Immunol Immunother 2:179–187, 1977
205. Rosenberg SA, Rapp H, Terry W et al: Intralesional BCG therapy of patients with primary Stage I melanoma. Proceedings Second International Conference on Immunotherapy of Cancer, Bethesda, Maryland, April 28–30, 1980, p 8
206. Cade S: Malignant melanoma. Ann R Coll Surg, Engl 28:334–366, 1961
207. Southwick HW, Slaughter DP, Hinkamp JF et al: The role of regional node dissection in the treatment of malignant melanoma. Arch Surg 85:63–68, 1962
208. Sandeman TF: Treat or watch? An evaluation of elective treatment of clinically uninvolved nodes in malignant melanoma. Med J Aust 1:42, 1965
209. Goldsmith HS, Shah JP, Kim D: Malignant melanoma. Current concepts of lymph node dissection. Cancer 22:216–220, 1972
210. Goldsmith HS: The debate over immediate lymph node dissection in melanoma. Surg Gynecol Obstet 148:403–405, 1979
211. Kapelanski DP, Block GE, Kaufman M: Characteristics of the primary lesion of malignant melanoma as a guide to prognosis and therapy. Ann Surg 189:225–235, 1979
212. Wanebo JH, Fortner JG, Woodruff J et al: Selection of the optimum surgical treatment of Stage I melanoma by depth of microinvasion: Use of the combined microstage technique (Clark–Breslow). Ann Surg 182:302–315, 1975
213. Polk HC, Linn BS: Selective regional lymphadenectomy for melanoma: A mathematical aid to clinical judgment. Ann Surg 174:403–413, 1971
214. Holmes C, Moseley HS, Morton DL et al: A rational approach to the surgical management of melanoma. Ann Surg 186:481–490, 1977
215. Breslow A: Tumor thickness, level of invasion and node dissection in Stage I cutaneous melanoma. Ann Surg 182:572–575, 1975
216. McNeer G, DasGupta T: Routes of lymphatic spread of malignant melanoma. CA 15:168, 1965
217. Sugarbaker EV, McBride CM: Melanoma of the trunk: The results of surgical excision and anatomic guidelines for predicting nodal metastasis. Surgery 80:22–30, 1976.
218. Fee HJ, Robinson DS, Sample WF et al: The determination of lymph shed by colloidal gold scanning in patients with malignant melanoma: A preliminary study. Surgery 84:626–632, 1978
219. Ballantyne AJ: Malignant melanoma of the head and neck region. In Neoplasms of the Skin and Malignant Melanoma, pp 345–362. Chicago, Year Book Medical Publishers, 1975
220. Lore JM Jr: An Atlas of Head and Neck Surgery. Philadelphia, W B Saunders, 1973
221. Rochlin DB: Posterolateral neck dissection for malignant neoplasms. Surg Gynecol Obstet 115:369–373, 1962
222. Chretien PB, Ketcham AS, Hoye RC et al: Axillary dissection with preservation of the pectoralis major muscle. Ann Surg 173:554–560, 1971
223. Hovnanian AP: The evolution and present status of pelvic–inguinal lymphatic excision. Surg Gynecol Obstet 124:851–865, 1967
224. Harris MN, Gumport SL, Berman IR et al: Ilioinguinal lymph node dissection for melanoma. Surg Gynecol Obstet 136:33–39, 1973
225. McCarthy JG, Haagensen CD, Herter FP: The role of groin dissection in the management of melanoma of the lower extremity. Ann Surg 179:156–159, 1974
226. Wagner DE, Rochlin DB, Weber AP: A new approach to radical retroperitoneal iliac and femoral node dissection. Arch Surg 103:681–683, 1971
227. Cohen MH, Schour L, Felix EL et al: Staging laparotomy in the treatment of metastatic melanoma of the lower extremities. Ann Surg 182:710–714, 1975
228. Sandeman TF: The radical treatment of enlarged lymph nodes in malignant melanoma. Am J Roentgenol 97:967–976, 1966
229. Creagan ET, Cupps RE, Ivins JC et al: Adjuvant radiation therapy for regional nodal metastases from malignant melanoma. A randomized prospective study. Cancer 42:2206–2210, 1978
230. Jantet GH, Edwards JM, Gough MH et al: Endolymphatic therapy with radioactive gold for malignant melanoma. Br Med J 2:904–906, 1964
231. Edwards JM: Malignant melanoma: Surgical aspects of treatment. Proc Roy Soc Med 65:140–144, 1072
232. Edwards JM: Treatment of melanoma by endolymphatic therapy. Proc Roy Soc Med 67:97–99, 1974
233. Ariel IM: Malignant melanoma, its treatment by the endolymphatic administration of radioactive isotopes. Am J Roentgenol 111:310–322, 1971
234. Ariel IM: Results of treating malignant melanoma intralymphatically with radioactive isotopes. Surg Gynecol Obstet 139:726–730, 1974
235. MRC Working Party on Endolymphatic Therapy in Malignant Melanoma: A clinical trial of endolymphatic therapy in malignant melanoma: Interim report of the progress of the Medical Research Council trial. Br J Surg 66:9–13, 1979
236. Pinsky CM, Hirshaut Y, Wanebo HJ et al: Surgical adjuvant immunotherapy with BCG in patients with malignant melanoma: Results in a prospective randomized trial. In Terry WD, Windhorts D, (eds): Immunotherapy of Cancer, Current Status of Trials in Man, pp 27–33. New York, Raven Press, 1978
237. Morton DL: Adjuvant immunotherapy of malignant melanoma. Results of a randomized trial. Proceedings Second International Conference on the Immunotherapy of Cancer, Bethesda, Maryland, April 28–30, 1980, p 11
238. Terry WD, Hodes RJ, Rosenberg SA et al: Treatment of stage I + II malignant melanoma with adjuvant immunotherapy or chemotherapy: Preliminary analysis of a prospective randomized trial. Proceedings Second International Conference on the Immunotherapy of Cancer, Bethesda, Maryland, April 28–30, 1980, p 11
239. Cunningham TJ, Schoenfeld D, Nathanson L et al: A controlled ECOG study of adjuvant therapy (BCG, BCG–DTIC) in patients with Stage I and II malignant melanoma—1980. Proceedings Second International Conference on the Immunotherapy of Cancer, Bethesda, Maryland, April 28–30, 1980, p 9
240. Beretta G: Randomized study of prolonged chemotherapy, immunotherapy and chemoimmunotherapy as an adjuvant to surgery for stage I and II malignant melanoma (Trial 6). Proceedings of the Second International Conference on the Immunotherapy of Cancer, Bethesda, Maryland, April 28–30, 1980, p 8
241. Hill GJ II, Johnson RO, Melter G: Multimodal surgical adjuvant therapy for a broad spectrum of solid tumors in humans. Surg Gynecol Obstet 142:882–892, 1976
242. Spitler LE, Aggeler PM: Levamisole in melanoma. Proceedings Second International Conference on Immunotherapy of Cancer, Bethesda, Maryland, April 28–30, 1980, p 10

243. Klopp CG, Alford TC, Batemen J et al: Fractionated intra-arterial cancer chemotherapy with methyl bis amine hydrochloride: A preliminary report. Ann Surg 132:811–832, 1950
244. Ryan RF, Krementz ET, Creech O et al: Selected perfusion of isolated viscera with chemotherapeutic agents using an extracorporeal circuit. Surg Forum 8:158–161, 1957
245. Creech O Jr, Krementz ET, Ryan RF et al: Chemotherapy of cancer: Regional perfusion utilizing an extracorporeal circuit. Ann Surg 148:616–632, 1958
246. Stehlin JS Jr, Clark RI Jr, White EC et al: Regional chemotherapy for cancer: Experiences with 116 perfusions. Ann Surg 151:605–619, 1960
247. Cavaliere R, Giocatto EC, Giovanella BC et al: Selective heat sensitivity of cancer cells. Biochemical and clinical studies. Cancer 20:1351–1381, 1967
248. Rochlin DB, Smart CR: Treatment of malignant melanoma by regional perfusion. Cancer 18:1544–1550, 1965
249. Irvine WT, Luck RJ: Review of regional limb perfusion with melphalan for malignant melanoma. Br Med J 1:770–774, 1966
250. Goldman LI, Tyson RR, Rosemond GP: Isolation perfusion in malignant melanoma of the extremity. Oncology 22:61–66, 1968
251. Cox KR: Regional perfusion for peripheral melanoma. Aust NZ J Surg 36:24–32, 1966
252. Key JA: The role of perfusion therapy in malignant melanoma. Can Med Assoc J 99:11–16, 1968
253. Stehlin JS Jr: Perfusion for melanoma of the extremities: 6½ years experience with 221 cases. Proc Natl Cancer Conf 5:525–531, 1964
254. Krementz ET, Creech O Jr: Advances in the treatment of malignant melanoma. Proc Natl Cancer Conf 6:529–542, 1970
255. Alrich EM, Manwaring JL, Horsley JJ III: Isolation perfusion: An adjunct to surgical excision in the primary treatment of melanoma of the extremities. Am J Surg 121:583–585, 1971
256. Fontaine CJ, Jamieson CW: Perfusion in limb melanoma: Indications and results. Proc R Soc Med 67:99–110, 1974
257. Cox KR: Survival after regional perfusion for limb melanoma. Aust NZ J Surg 45:32–36, 1975
258. Wagner DE: A retrospective study of regional perfusion for melanoma. Arch Surg 111:410–413, 1976
259. Stehlin JS Jr, Giovanelli BC, De Ipolyi PD et al: Results of hyperthermic perfusion for melanoma of the extremities. Surg Gynecol Obstet 140:339–348, 1975
260. McBride CM, Sugarbaker EV, Hickey RC: Prophylactic isolation-perfusion as the primary therapy for invasive malignant melanoma of the limbs. Ann Surg 182:316–324, 1975
261. Schraffordt Koops H, Oldhoff J, van der Ploeg E et al: Some aspects of the treatment of primary malignant melanoma of the extremities by isolated regional perfusion. Cancer 39:27–33, 1977
262. Shingleton WM: Perfusion chemotherapy for recurrent melanoma of extremity: A progress report. Ann Surg 169:969–973, 1969
263. McBride CM: Advanced melanoma of the extremities: Treatment by isolation-perfusion with a triple drug combination. Arch Surg 101:122–126, 1970
264. Golomb FM: Perfusion. In Andrade R, Gumport SL, Popkin GL et al (eds): Cancer of the Skin, pp 1623–1636. Philadelphia, WB Saunders, 1976
265. Krementz ET, Carter RD, Sutherland CM et al: Malignant melanoma of the limbs: An evaluation of chemotherapy in regional perfusion. In Neoplasms of the Skin and Malignant Melanoma, pp. 375–400. Chicago, Year Book Medical Publishers, 1975
266. Rochlin DB, Wagner DE, Rochlin S: The therapy of malignant melanoma as treated by regional perfusion. In McCarthy WH (ed): Melanoma and Skin Cancer, pp 443–451. Sydney, VCN Blight, 1972
267. Golomb FM: Treatment of recurrent melanoma—chemotherapy. In McCarthy WH (ed): Melanoma and Skin Cancer, pp 497–502. Sydney, VCN Blight, 1972
268. Bernardino ME Goldstein HM: Gray scale ultrasonography in the evaluation of metastatic melanoma. Cancer 42:2529–2533, 1978
269. Reeder MM, Cavanagh RC: Bull's-eye lesions, solitary or multiple nodules in the gastrointestinal tract with large central ulceration. JAMA 229:825–826, 1974
270. Meyer JE: Radiographic evaluation of metastatic melanoma. Cancer 42:127–132, 1978
271. Pomerantz H, Margolin NH: Metastases to the gastrointestinal tract from malignant melanoma. Am J Rotengenol 88:712–717, 1962
272. Oddson TA Rice RP, Seigler HF et al: The spectrum of small bowel melanoma. Gastrointest Radiol 3:419–423, 1978
273. Bragg DG: Medical imaging problems in the patient with advanced cancer. JAMA 244:597–599, 1980
274. Goldstein HM, Kaminsky S, Wallace S et al: Urographic manifestations of metastatic melanoma. Am J Roentgenol Radium Ther Nucl Med 121:801–805, 1974
275. Stewart WR, Gelberman RH, Harrelson JM et al: Skeletal metastases of melanoma. J Bone Joint Surg 60–A:645–649, 1978
276. Patel JK, Didolkar MS, Pickren JW et al: Metastatic patterns of malignant melanoma. A study of 216 autopsy cases. Am J Surg 135:807–810, 1978
277. Moore GE: Debunking debulking. Surg Gynecol Obstet 150:395–396, 1980
278. Fortner JG, Strong EW, Mulcare RJ et al: The surgical treatment of recurrent melanoma. Surg Clin N Amer 54:865–870, 1974
279. Gromet MA, Ominsky SH, Epstein WL et al: The thorax as the initial site for systemic relapse in malignant melanoma. Cancer 44:776–784, 1979
280. Mathisen DJ, Flye MW, Peabody J: The role of thoracotomy in the management of pulmonary metastases from malignant melanoma. Ann Thoracic Surg 27:295–299, 1979
281. Cahan WG: Excision of melanoma metastases to lung: Problems in diagnosis and management. Ann Surg 178:703–709, 1973
282. Hilaris BS, Raben M, Calabrese AS et al: Value of radiation therapy for distant metastases from malignant melanoma. Cancer 16: 765–773, 1963
283. Dewey DL: The radiosensitivity of melanoma cells in culture. Br J Radiol 44:816–817, 1971
284. Hornsey S: The radiation response of human malignant melanoma cells *in vitro* and *in vivo*. Cancer Res 32:650–651, 1972
285. Habermalz HJ, Fischer JJ: Radiation therapy of malignant melanoma. Experience with high individual treatment doses. Cancer 38:2258–2262, 1976
286. Hornsey S: The relationship between total dose, number of fractions, and fraction size in the response of malignant melanoma in patients. Br J Radiol 51:905–909, 1978
287. Overgaard J: Radiation treatment of malignant melanoma. Int J Radiat Oncol Biol Phys 6:41–44, 1980
288. Katz HR: The results of different fractionation shemes in the palliative irradiation of metastatic melanoma. Int J Radiat Oncol Biol Phys 7, July 1981
289. Beresford HR: Melanoma of the nervous system. Neurology 19:59–65, 1965
290. Gottlieb JA, Frei E, Luce JK: An evaluation of the management of patients with cerebral metastases from malignant melanoma. Cancer 29:701–705, 1972
291. Nisce LZ, Hilaris BS, Chu FCH: A review of experience with irradiation of brain metastases. Am J Roentgenol 111:329–333, 1971
292. Withers HR, Harter D: Radiotherapy in the management of malignant melanoma. In Neoplasms of the Skin and Malignant Melanoma, pp 453–460. Chicago, Year Book Medical Publishers, 1976
293. Amer MH, Al-Sarraf M, Baker LH et al: Malignant melanoma and central nervous system metastases. Incidence, diagnosis, treatment and survival. Cancer 42:660–668, 1978
294. Cooper JS, Carella R: Radiotherapy of intracerebral metastatic malignant melanoma. Radiology 134:735–738, 1980
295. Carella RJ, Gleber R, Hendrickson F et al: Value of radiation therapy in the management of patients with cerebral metastases from malignant melanoma. Radiation Therapy Oncology Group brain metastases study I and II. Cancer 45:679–683, 1980

296. Katz HR: The relative effectiveness of radiation therapy, corticosteroids, and surgery in the management of melanoma metastatic to the central nervous system (in press)
297. Galicich JH, Sundaresan N, Arbit E et al: Surgical treatment of single brain metastasis: Factors associated with survival. Cancer 45:381–386, 1980
298. Galicich JH, Sundaresan N, Thaler HT: Surgical treatment of single brain metastasis. Evaluation of results by computerized tomography scanning. J Neurosurg 53:63–67, 1980
299. Bremer AM, West CR, Didolkar, MS: An evaluation of the surgical management of melanoma of the brain. J Surg Oncol 10:211–219, 1978
300. Wagner DE, Ramirez G, Weiss AJ et al: Combination phase I–II study of imidazole carboxamide (NSC-45388). Oncology 26:310–316, 1971
301. Luce JK: Chemotherapy of malignant melanoma. Cancer 30:1604–1616, 1972
302. Nathanson L, Wolter K, Horton J et al: Characteristics of prognosis and response to an imidazole carboxamide in malignant melanoma. Clin Pharmacol Ther 12:955–962, 1971
303. Costanza ME, Nathanson L, Lenhard R et al: Therapy of malignant melanoma with an imidazole carboxamide and bis-chloroethyl nitrosourea. Cancer 30:1457–1461, 1972
304. Moon JH, Gailani S, Cooper MR et al: Comparison of the combination of 1,3-bis (2-chloroethyl)-1-nitrosourea (BCNU) and vincristine with two dose schedules of 5-(3,5-dimethyl-1-triazeno) imidazole-4-carboxamide (DTIC) in the treatment of disseminated malignant melanoma. Cancer 35:368–371, 1975
305. Van der Merwe AM, Falkson G, van EB et al: Metastatic malignant melanoma. Imidazole carboxamide in its treatment. Med Proc 17:399–405, 1971
306. Gottlieb JA, Serpick AA: Clinical evaluation of 5-(3,3-dimethyl-1-triazeno) imidazole-4-carboxamide in malignant melanoma and other neoplasms. Comparison of twice weekly and daily administration schedules. Oncology 25:225–233, 1971
307. Burker PJ, McCarthy NWH, Milton GW: Imidazole carboxamide therapy in advanced malignant melanoma. Cancer 27:744–750, 1971
308. Cowan DH, Bergsagel DE: Intermittent treatment of metastatic malignant melanoma with high dose 5-(3,3-dimethyl-1-triazeno) imidazole-4-carboxamide (NSC-45388). Cancer Chemother Rep 55:175–181, 1971
309. Gerner RE, Moore GE: Study of 5-(3,3-dimethyl-1-triazeno) imidazole-4-carboxamide (NSC-45388) in patients with disseminated melanoma. Cancer Chemother Rep 57:83–84, 1973
310. Vogel CL, Comis RL, Ziegler JL et al: Clinical trials of 5-(3,3-dimethyl-1-triazeno) imidazole-4-carboxamide (NSC-45388) given intravenously in the treatment of malignant melanoma in Uganda. Cancer Chemother Rep 55:143–149, 1971
311. Carter RD, Krementz ET, Hill GJ II et al: DTIC (NSC-45388) and combination therapy for melanoma. I. Studies with DTIC, BCNU, CCNU, vincristine, and hydroxyurea. Cancer Treat Rep 60:601–609, 1976
312. Carter SK, Fiedman MA: 5-(3,3-dimethyl-1-triazeno) imidazole-4-carboxamide (DTIC, DIC, NSC-45388) a new anti-tumor agent with activity against malignant melanoma. Europ J Cancer 8:85–92, 1972
313. Bellet RE, Mastrangelo MJ, Laucius JF et al: Randomized prospective trial of DTIC (NSC-45388) alone versus BCNU (NSC-409962) plus vincristine (NSC-67574) in the treatment of metastatic malignant melanoma. Cancer Treat Rep 60:595–600, 1976
314. Ahmann DL, Hahn RG, Bisel HF: Clinical evaluation of 5-(3,3-dimethyl-1-triazeno) imidazole-4-carboxamide (NSC-45388), melphalan (NSC-8806) and hydroxyurea (NSC-32065) in the treatment of disseminated malignant melanoma. Cancer Chemother Rep 56:369–372, 1972
315. Costanzi JJ: DTIC (NSC-45388) studies in the Southwest Oncology Group. Cancer Treat Rep 60:189–192, 1976
316. Comis RL: DTIC (NSC-45388) in malignant melanoma: A perspective. Cancer Treat Rep 60:165–176, 1976
317. Ahmann DL: Nitrosoureas in the management of disseminated malignant melanoma. Cancer Treat Rep 60:747–751, 1976
318. Ramirez G, Wilson W, Grage T et al: Phase II evaluation of 1,3-bis(2-chloroethyl-1-nitrosourea) (BCNU; NSC-409962) in patients with solid tumors. Cancer Chemother Rep 56:787–790, 1972
319. DeVita VT, Carbone PP, Owens AH Jr et al: Clinical trials with 1,3-bis(2-chloroethyl)-1-nitrosourea, NSC-409962. Cancer Res. 25:1875–1881, 1965
320. Lessner HE: BCNU (1,3-bis(2-chloroethyl)-1-nitrosourea). Effects on advanced Hodgkin's disease and other neoplasia. Cancer 22:451–456, 1968
321. Pugh R, Jacobs E, Bateman J et al: CCNU versus CCNU + vincristine in disseminated melanoma. Proceedings of the 11th International Cancer Congress, Florence, Italy, 1974, pp. 540–541
322. Cruz AB Jr, Armstrong DM, Aust JB: Treatment of advanced malignancy with CCNU (1-(2-chloroethyl)-3-cyclohexyl-1-nitrosourea, NSC-79037). A phase II cooperative study. Proc Am Assoc Cancer Res 15:184, 1974
323. Ahmann DL, Hahn RG, Bisel HF: A comparative study of 1-(2-chloroethyl)-3-cyclohexyl-1-nitrosourea (NSC-79037) and imidazole carboxamide (NSC-45388) with vincristine (NSC-67574) in the palliation of disseminated malignant melanoma. Cancer Res 32:2432–2434, 1972
324. Hoogstraten B, Gottlieb JA, Caoili E et al: CCNU (1-(2,chloroethyl)-3-cyclohexyl-1-nitrosourea, NSC-79037) in the treatment of cancer. Phase II study. Cancer 32:38–43, 1973
325. Broder LE, Hansen HH: 1-(2-chloroethyl)-3-cyclohexyl-1-nitrosourea (CCNU, NSC-79037): A comparison of drug administration at four-week and six-week intervals. Europ J Cancer 9:147–152, 1973
326. DeConti RC, Hubbard SP, Pinch P et al: Treatment of advanced neoplastic disease with 1-(2-chloroethyl)-3-cyclohexyl-1-nitrosourea (CCNU; NSC-79037). Cancer Chemother Rep 57:201–207, 1973
327. Perloff M, Muggia FM, Ackerman C: Role of a nitrosourea CCNU, NSC-79037) in advanced nonhematologic cancer. Cancer Chemother Rep 58:421–429, 1974
328. Hansen HH, Muggia FM: Treatment of malignant brain tumors with nitrosoureas. Cancer Chemother Rep 55:99–100, 1971
329. Wasserman TH, Slavik M, Carter SK: Review of CCNU in clinical cancer therapy. Cancer Treat Rev 1:131–151, 1974
330. Ahmann DL, Hahn RG, Bisel HF: Evaluation of 1-(2-chloroethyl-3-4-methyl-cyclohexyl)-1-nitrosourea (methyl-CCNU, NSC-95441) versus combined imidazole carboxamide (NSC-45388) and vincristine (NSC-67574) in palliation of disseminated malanoma. Cancer 33:615–618, 1974
331. Costanza ME, Nathanson L, Schoenfeld D et al: Results with methyl-CCNU and DTIC in metastatic melanoma. Cancer 40:1010–1015, 1977
332. Young RC, Canellos GP, Chabner BA et al: Treatment of malignant melanoma with methyl-CCNU. Clin Pharmacol Ther 15:617–622, 1974
333. Tranum BL, Haut A, Rivkin S at al: Methyl-CCNU in Hodgkin's disease and other tumors. Proc Am Assoc Cancer Res 15:171, 1974
334. Firat D, Tekuzman G: Treatment of solid tumors and lymphomas with methyl-CCNU. Proc Am Assoc Cancer Res 15:5, 1974
335. Wasserman TH, Slavik M, Carter SK: Methyl-CCNU in clinical cancer therapy. Cancer Treat Rev 1:251–259, 1974
336. Larsen RR, Hill GJ: Improved systemic chemotherapy for malignant melanoma. Am J Surg 122:36–41, 1971
337. Gumport SL, Wright JC, Golomb FM: The treatment of advanced malignant melanoma with triethylene thiophosphoramide (Thio-TEPA or TSPA). Ann Surg 147:232–238, 1958
338. Clifford P, Clift RA, Gillmore JH: Oral melphalan therapy in advanced malignant disease. Br J Cancer 17:381–390, 1963
339. Holland JF, Regelson W: Studies on phenylalanine nitrogen mustard (CB 3025) in metastatic malignant melanoma of man. Ann NY Acad Sci 68:1122–1125, 1958
340. Moore GE, Bross IDJ, Ausman R et al: Effects of chlorambucil (NSC-3088) in 374 patients with advanced cancer. Cancer Chemother Rep 52:661–666. 1968
341. Buckner CD, Rudolph RH, Fefer A et al: High dose cyclophos-

phamide therapy for malignant disease: Toxicity tumor response and the effects of stored autologous marrow. Cancer 29:357–365, 1972

342. Bergsagel DE, Levin WC: A prelusive clinical trial of cyclophosphamide. Cancer Chemother Rep 8:120–134, 1960
343. Haar H, Marshall GJ, Bierman HR et al: The influence of cyclophosphamide upon neoplastic disease in man. Cancer Chemother Rep 6:41–51, 1960
344. Gottlieb JA, Mendelson D, Serpick AA: An evaluation of large intermittent intravenous doses of cyclophosphamide (NSC-26271) in the treatment of metastatic malignant melanoma. Cancer Chemother Rep 54:365–367, 1970
345. Korst DR, Johnson FD, Frenkel EP et al: Preliminary evaluation of the effect of cyclophosphamide on the course of human neoplasms. Cancer Chemother Rep 7:1–12, 1960
346. Shnider BI, Gold GL, Hall T et al: Preliminary studies with cyclophosphamide. Cancer Chemother Rep 8:106–111, 1960
347. Rundles RW, Laszlo J, Garrison FE et al: The anti-tumor spectrum of cyclophosphamide. Cancer Chemother Rep 16:407–411, 1962
348. Mullens GM, Colvin M: Intensive cyclophosphamide (NSC-26271) therapy for solid tumors. Cancer Chemother Rep 59:411–419, 1975
349. Sullivan RD, Muller E, Zurek WZ et al: Re-evaluation of methotrexate as an anti-cancer durg. Surg Gynecol Obstet 125:819–824, 1967
350. Vogler WR, Huguley CM, Kerr W: Toxicity and anti-tumor effect of divided doses of methotrexate. Arch Intern Med 115:285–293, 1965
351. Karakousis CP, Carlson M: High dose methotrexate in malignant melanoma. Cancer Treat Rep 63:1405–1407, 1979
352. Burke PJ, Owens AH, Colsky J et al: A clinical evaluation of a prolonged schedule of cytosine arabinoside (NSC-63878). Cancer Res 30:1512–1515, 1970
353. Frei E, Bickers JN, Hewlett JS et al: Dose schedule and antitumor studies of arabinosyl cytosine (NSC-63878). Cancer Res 29:1325–1332, 1969
354. Hart JS, Ho DH, George SL et al: Cytokinetic and molecular pharmacology studies of arabinoslcytosine in metastatic melanoma. Cancer Res 32:2711–2716, 1972
355. Moore GE, Bross IDJ, Ausman R et al: Effects of 5-fluorouracil (NSC-19893) in 389 patients with cancer. Cancer Chemother Rep 52:641–653, 1968
356. Regelson W, Holland JF, Gold GL et al: 6-Mercaptopurine (NSC-755) given intravenously at weekly intervals to patients with advanced cancer. Cancer Chemother Rep 51:277–282, 1967
357. Fink DJ, Foye LV: 6-Mercaptopurine (NSC-755) given intermittently in high doses. Phase II study. Cancer Chemother Rep 54:31–34, 1970
358. Moore GE, Bross IDJ, Ausman R et al: Effects of 6-mercaptopurine (NSC-755) in 290 patients with advanced cancer. Cancer Chemother Rep 52:655–660, 1968
359. Whittington RM, Close HP: Clinical experience with mitomycin C (NSC-26980). Cancer Chemother Rep 54:195–198, 1970
360. Godfrey TE, Wilbur DW: Clinical experience with mitomycin C in large infrequent doses. Cancer 29:1647–1652, 1972
361. Moore GE, Bross IDJ, Ausman R et al: Effects of mitomycin C (NSC-26980) in 346 patients with advanced cancer. Cancer Chemother Rep 52:675–684, 1968
362. Blum RH, Carter SK, Agre K: A clinical review of bleomycin: A new anti-neoplastic agent. Cancer 31:903–914, 1973
363. Clinical Screening Cooperative Group of the European Organization for Research on the Treatment of Cancer: Study of the clinical efficiency of bleomycin in human cancer. Br Med J 2:643–645, 1970
364. Costa G, Hreshchyshyn MM, Holland JF: Initial clinical studies with vincristine. Cancer Chemother Rep 24:39–44, 1962
365. Gubisch NJ, Norena D, Perlia CP et al: Experience with vincrisrine in solid tumors. Cancer Chemother Rep 32:19–22, 1963
366. Shaw RK, Bruner JA: Clinical evaluation of vincristine (NSC-67574). Cancer Chemother Rep 42:45–48, 1964
367. Reitmeier RJ, Moertel CG, Blackburn CM: Vincristine (NSC-67574) therapy of adult patients with solid tumors. Cancer Chemother Rep 34:21–23, 1964
368. Smart CR, Ottoman RE, Rochlin DB et al: Clinical experience with vincristine (NSC-67574) in tumors of the central nervous system and other malignant diseases. Cancer Chemother Rep 52:733–741, 1968
369. Frei E, Franzino A, Shnider BI et al: Clinical studies of vinblastine. Cancer Chemother Rep 12:125–129, 1961
370. Armstrong JG, Dyke RW, Fouts PJ et al: Hodgkin's disease, carcinoma of the breast and other tumors treated with vinblastine sulfate. Cancer Chemother Rep 18:49–71, 1962
371. Acute Leukemia Group B, Eastern Cooperative Group: Neoplastic diseases: Treatment with vinblastine. Arch Intern Med 111:846–852, 1965
372. Bond WH, Rohn RJ, Bates LH et al: Treatment of neoplastic diseases with an improved oral preparation of vinblastine sulfate. Cancer 19:213–219, 1966
373. Hodes ME, Rohn RJ, Bond WH et al: Vincaleukoblastine: A summary of two and one-half years experience in the use of vinblastine. Cancer Chemother Rep 16:401–406, 1962
374. Hill JM, Loeb E: Treatment of leukemia, lymphoma and other malignant neoplasms with vinblastine. Cancer Chemother Rep 15:41–61, 1961
375. Falkson G, Van Dyk JJ: The chemotherapy of malignant melanoma. S Afr Med J 42:89–90, 1968
376. Wright TL, Hurley J, Kurst DR et al: Vinblastine in neoplastic disease. Cancer Res 23:169–179, 1963
377. Smart CR, Rochlin DB, Nahum AM et al: Clinical experience with vinblastine sulfate (NSC-49842) in squamous cell carcinoma and other malignancies. Cancer Chemother Rep 34:31–45, 1964
378. Camacho FJ, Young CW, Wittes RE: Phase II trial of vindesine in patients with malignant melanoma. Cancer Treat Rep 64:179–181, 1980
379. Retsas S, Newton KA, Westbury G: Vindesine as a single agent in the treatment of advanced malignant melanoma. Cancer Chemother Pharmacol 2:257–260, 1979
380. Smith IE, Hedley DW, Powles TJ et al: Vindesine: A phase II study in the treatment of breast carcinoma, malignant melanoma and other solid tumors. Cancer Treat Rep 62:1427–1433, 1978
381. Johnson FD, Jacobs EM: Chemotherapy of metastatic malignant melanoma: Experience with 73 patients. Cancer 27:1306–1312, 1971
382. Stolinsky DC, Jacobs EM, Bateman JR et al: Clinical trial of trimethylcolchicinic acid, methyl ether d-tartrate (TMCA; NSC-36354) in advanced cancer. Cancer Chemother Rep 51:25–34, 1967
383. Stolinsky DC, Jacobs EM, Braunwald J et al: Further study of trimethylcolchicinic acid, methyl ether d-tartrate (TMCA; NSC-36354) in patients with malignant melanoma. Cancer Chemother Rep 56:263–265, 1972
384. Andrews NC, Weiss AJ, Ansfield FJ et al: Phase I study of dibromodulcitol (NSC-104800). Cancer Chemother Rep 55:61–65, 1971
385. Phillips RW, Brook J: Clinical experiences with dibromodulcitol (NSC-1048000) in solid tumors. Cancer Chemother Rep 55:567–573, 1971
386. Bellet RE, Catalano RB, Mastrangelo MJ et al: Positive Phase II trial of dibromodulcitol in patients with metastatic melanoma refractory to DTIC and a nitrosourea. Cancer Treat Rep 62:2095–2099, 1978
387. Hall SW, Benjamin RS, Lewinski U et al: Actinomycin D, levamisole chemoimmunotherapy of refractory malignant melanoma. Cancer 43:1195–1200, 1979
388. Falkson G, Van der Merwe AM, Falkson HC: Clinical experience with 5-3,3-bis(2-chloroethyl)-1-triazeno) imidazole-4-carboxamide (NSC-82196) in the treatment of metastatic malignant melanoma. Cancer Chemother Rep 56:671–677, 1972
389. Bagley CM, Canellos GP, Young RC et al: Clinical trials with 5-(3,3-bis(2-chloroethyl)-1-triazeno) imidazole-4-carboxamide (NSC-82196) given intravenously. Cancer Chemother Rep 56:387–391, 1972

390. Slack NH, Jones R: Single reversal trial of hydroxyurea (NSC-32065) in 91 patients with advanced cancer. Cancer Chemother Rep 54:53–63, 1970
391. Cole DR, Beckloff GL, Rousselot LM: Clinical results with hydroxyurea in cancer chemotherapy: Preliminary report. NY State J Med 65:2132–2136, 1961
392. Creasey WA, Capizzi RL, DeConti RC: Clinical and biochemical studies of high dose intermittent therapy of solid tumors with hydroxyurea (NSC-32065). Cancer Chemother Rep 54:191–194, 1970
393. Bolton BH, Kaung DT, Lawton RL et al: Hydroxyurea (NSC-32065): A Phase II Study. Cancer Chemother Rep 39:47–51, 1964
394. Cassileth PA, Hyman GA: Treatment of malignant melanoma with hydroxyurea. Cancer Res 27:1843–1845, 1967
395. Gottlieb JA, Frei E, Luce JK: Dose-schedule studies with hydroxyurea (NSC-32065) in malignant melanoma. Cancer Chemother Rep 55:277–280, 1971
396. Nathanson L, Hall TC: Phase II study of hydroxyurea (NSC-32065) in malignant melanoma. Cancer Chemother Rep 51:503–505, 1967
397. Lerner HJ, Beckloff GL, Godwin MC: Hydroxyurea (NSC-32065) intermittent therapy in malignant disease. Cancer Chemother Rep 53:385–395, 1969
398. Blum RH, Livingston RB, Carter SK: Hexamethylmelamine: A new drug with activity in solid tumors. Europ J Cancer 9:195–202, 1973
399. duPriest RW, Huntington MC, Massey WH et al: Streptozotocin therapy in 22 cancer patients. Cancer 35:358–367, 1975
400. Schein PS, O'Connell MJ, Blom J et al: Clinical antitumor activity and toxicity of streptozotocin (NSC-85998). Cancer 34:993–1000, 1974
401. Chary KK, Higby DJ, Henderson ES et al: Phase I study of high dose cis-dichlorodiammineplatinum (II) with forced diuresis. Cancer Treat Rep 61:367–370, 1977
402. Ahmann DL, Bisel HF, Edmonson JH et al: Phase II study of VP-16-213 versus dianhydrogalactitol in patients with metastatic malignant melanoma. Cancer Treat Rep 60:1681–1682, 1976
403. McKelvey EM, Hewlett JS, Thigpen T et al: Cyclocytidine chemotherapy for malignant melanoma. Cancer Treat Rep 62:469–471, 1978
404. Lopez R, Karakousis CP, Didolkar MS et al: Estramustine phosphate in the treatment of advanced malignant melanoma. Cancer Treat Rep 62:1329–1332, 1978
405. Presant CA Bartolucci AA, Ungaro P et al: Phase II trial of piperazinedione in malignant melanoma. Cancer Treat Rep 63:1367–1369, 1979
406. Ahmann DL, Hahn RG, Bisel HF et al: Comparative study of methyl-CCNU (NSC-95441) with cyclophosphamide (NSC-26271) and 5-(3,3-dimethyl-1-triazeno) imidazole-4-carboxamide (NSC-45388) with vincristine (NSC-67574) in patients with disseminated melanoma. Cancer Chemother Rep 59:451–453, 1975
407. Ahmann DL, Hahn RG, Bisel HF: A comparative study of 1-(2-chloroethyl)-3-cyclohexyl-1-nitrosourea (NSC-79037) and imidazole carboxamide (NSC-45388) with vincristine (NSC-67574) in the palliation of disseminated malignant melanoma. Cancer Res 32:2432–2434, 1972
408. Ahmann DL, Hahn RG, Bisel HF: Evaluation of 1-(2-chloroethyl)-3-(4-methylcyclohexyl)-1-nitrosourea (methyl-CCNU, NSC-95441) versus combined imidazole carboxamide (NSC-45388) and vincristine (NSC-67574) in palliation of disseminated malignant melanoma. Cancer 33:615–618, 1974
409. Chauverqne J, Clavel B, Klein T et al: Chemotherapy of malignant melanoma. Bull Cancer 65:107–109, 1978
410. Wittes RE, Wittes JT, Golbey RB: Combination chemotherapy in metastatic melanoma. Cancer 41:415–421, 1978
411. Goodnight JE Jr, Moseley HS, Eilber FR et al: Cis-dichlorodiammineplatinum (II) alone and combined with DTIC for treatment of disseminated malignant melanoma. Cancer Treat Rep 63:2005–2007, 1979
412. Friedman MA, Kaufman DA, Williams JE et al: Combined DTIC and cis-dichlorodiammineplatinum (II) therapy for patients with disseminated melanoma: A Northern California Oncology Group study. Cancer Treat Rep 63:493–495, 1979
413. Karakousis CP, Getaz EP, Bjornsson S et al: Cis-dichlorodiammineplatinum (II) and DTIC in malignant melanoma. Cancer Treat Rep 63:2009–2010, 1979
414. Ahmann DL, Edmonson JH, Frytak S et al: Phase II study of ICRF-159 vs. combination cis-dichlorodiammineplatinum (II) and DTIC in patients with disseminated melanoma. Cancer Treat Rep 62:151–153, 1978
415. Gerner RE, Moore GE, Dickey C: Combination chemotherapy in disseminated melanoma and other solid tumors in adults. Oncology 31:22–30, 1975
416. Gerner RE, Moore GE, Didolkar MS: Chemotherapy of disseminated malignant melanoma with dimethyl imidazole carboxamide and actinomycin D. Cancer 32:756–760, 1973
417. Samson MK, Baker LH, Talley RW et al: Phase I-II study of intermittent bolus administration of DTIC and actinomycin D in metastatic malignant melanoma. Cancer Treat Rep 62:1223–1225, 1978
418. Ramseur WL, Richards F II, Muss HB et al: Chemoimmunotherapy for disseminated malignant melanoma: A prospective randomized study. Cancer Treat Rep 62:1085–1087, 1978
419. Samson MK, Baker LH, Izbicki RM et al: Phase I–II study of DTIC and cyclocytidine in disseminated melanoma. Cancer Treat Rep 60:1369–1371, 1976
420. Beretta G, Bojetta E, Bonadonna G et al: Combination chemotherapy with 5-(3,3-dimethyl-1-triazeno) imidazole carboxamide (DTIC; NSC-45388), 1,3-bis(2-chloroethyl)-1-nitrosourea (BCNU; NSC-409962) and vincristine (VCR; NSC-67574) in metastatic malignant melanoma. Tumori 59:239–248, 1973
421. Cohen SM, Greenspan EM, Ratner LH et al: Combination chemotherapy of malignant melanoma with imidazole carboxamide, BCNU and vincristine. Cancer 39:41–44, 1977
422. Beretta G, Bonadonna G, Cascinelli N et al: Comparative evaluation of three combination regimens for advanced malignant melanoma: Results of an international cooperative study. Cancer Treat Rep 60:33–40, 1976
423. Luce JK, Torin LB, Price H: Combination dimethyl-triazeno-imidazole-carboxamide (NSC-45388; DIC), vincristine (NSC-67574; VCR) and 1,3 bis(2-chloroethyl)-1-nitrosourea (NSC-409962; BCNU) chemotherapy of disseminated melanoma. Proc Am Assoc Cancer Res 11:50, 1970
424. Hill GJ II, Metter GE, Krementy ET et al: DTIC and combination therapy for melanoma. II Escalating schedules of DTIC with BCNU, CCNU and vincristine. Cancer Treat Rep 1989–1992, 1979
425. Einhorn LH, Furnas B: Combination chemotherapy for disseminated malignant melanoma with DTIC, vincristine and methyl-CCNU. Cancer Treat Rep 61:881–883, 1977
426. McKelvey EM, Luce JK, Talley RW et al: Combination chemotherapy with bischloroethylnitrosourea (BCNU), vincristine and dimethyl-triazeno-imidazole-carboxamide (DTIC) in disseminated malignant melanoma. Cancer 39:1–4, 1977
427. Carmo–Pereira J, Costa FO, Pimental P: Combination cytotoxic chemotherapy for metastatic cutaneous malignant melanoma with DTIC, BCNU and vincristine. Cancer Treat Rep 60:1381–1382, 1976
428. Kleeberg UR, Schreml W: Treatment of metastasizing melanoma with a combination of cytostatic agents. Deut Med Wochen 101:890–894, 1976
429. Gardere SH, Cowan DH: Treatment of metastatic malignant melanoma with a combination of 5-(3,3-dimethyl-1-triazeno) imidazole-4-carboxamide (NSC-45388), cyclophosphamide (NSC-26271) and vincristine (NSC-67574). Cancer Chemother Rep 56:357–361, 1972
430. Beretta G. Bonadonna G, Cascinelli N et al: Comparative evaluation of three combination regimens for advanced malignant melanoma. Results of an international cooperative study. Cancer Treat Rep 60:33–40., 1976
431. Costanzi JJ, Vaitkevicius VK, Quagliana JM et al: Combination chemotherapy for disseminated malignant melanoma. Cancer 35:342–346, 1975
432. McKelvey EM, Luce JK, Vaitkevicius VK et al: Bis-chloroethyl-

nitrosourea, vincristine, dimethyltriazeno-imidazole-carboxamide and chlorpromazine combination chemotherapy in disseminated malignant melanoma. Cancer 39:5–10, 1977

433. Moon JH: Combination chemotherapy in malignant melanoma. Cancer 25:468–473, 1970
434. Marsh JC, DeConti RC, Hubbard SP: Treatment of Hodgkin's disease and other cancers with 1,3-bis (2-chloroethyl)-1-nitrosourea (BCNU, NSC-409962). Cancer Chemother Rep 55:599–606, 1971
435. Stolinsky DC, Puch RP, Bohannon RA et al: Clinical trial of BCNU combined with vincristine in disseminated gastrointestinal cancer and other neoplasms. Cancer Chemother Rep 58:947–950, 1974
436. Murphy, WK: Phase I–II study of combination chemotherapy with cyclophosphamide and methyl-CCNU. Proc Am Soc Clin Oncol 16:253, 1975
437. Livingston RB, Einhorn LH, Bodey GP et al: COMB (cyclophosphamide, oncovin, methyl-CCNU, and bleomycin): a four drug combination in solid tumors. Cancer 36:327–332, 1975
438. Dewasch G, Bernheim J, Michel J et al: Combination chemotherapy with three marginally effective agents, CCNU, vincristine, and bleomycin in the treatment of stage III melanoma. Cancer Treat Rep 60:1273–1276, 1976
439. Everall JD, Doud PM: Use of combination chemotherapy with CCNU, bleomycin and vincristine in the treatment of metastatic melanoma in patients resistent to DTIC chemotherapy. Cancer Treat Rep 63:151–155, 1979
440. Green MR, Dillman RO, Horton C: Procarbazine, vincristine, CCNU and cyclophosphamide in the treatment of metastatic melanoma. Cancer Treat Rep 64:139–142, 1980
441. Carmo–Pereira J, Costa FO, Pimentel P et al: Combination cytotoxic chemotherapy with CCNU, procarbazine and vincristine in disseminated cutaneous malignant melanoma: 3 years followup. Cancer Treat Rep 64:143–145, 1980
442. Cohen MH, Schoenfeld D, Wolter J: Randomized trial of chlorpromazine, caffeine and methyl CCNU in disseminated melanoma. Cancer Treat Rep 64:151–153, 1980
443. Perlin E, Engeler J, Reid JW et al: Treatment of malignant melanoma with vinblastine, procarbazine, and actinomycin D. Cancer Chemother Rep 59:767–768, 1975
444. Kostinas JE, Leone LA, Cuttner JA et al: Procarbazine, vinblastine and actinomycin D in stage III and IV melanoma with or without methanol extracted residue of Bacillus-Calmette-Guerin. Cancer Treat Rep 63:197–200, 1979
445. Byrne MJ: Cyclophosphamide, vincristine, and procarbazine in the treatment of malignant melanoma. Cancer 38:1922–1924, 1976
446. Porcile G, Musso M, Boccardo F et al: Combination chemotherapy with vinblastine, bleomycin and methotrexate in DTIC-resistant metastatic melanoma. Tumori 65:237–240, 1979
447. Nathanson L, Wittenberg BK: Pilot study of vinblastine and bleomycin combinations in the treatment of metastatic melanoma. Cancer Treat Rep 64:133–137, 1980
448. Nathanson L, Kaufman SD, Carey RW: Vinblastine-bleomycin-platinum: A high response rate regimen in metastatic melanoma. Proc Am Soc Clin Oncol 21:479, 1980
449. Schmidt CG, Becker R: Combination chemotherapy of metastasizing melanoblastoma using ifosfamide and cis-platinum (II)-diamminodichloride. Deut Med Wochen 104:872–875, 1979
450. Nordman EM, Mäntylä: Treatment of metastatic melanoma with combined 5-fluorouracil and procarbazine. Cancer Treat Rep 61:1709–1710, 1977
451. Coltman C Jr, Costanzi JJ, Dudley GM III et al: Further clinical studies of combination chemotherapy using cyclophosphamide, vincristine, methotrexate and 5-fluorouracil in solid tumors. Am J Med Sci 261:73–78, 1971
452. Hanham IWF, Mewton KA, Westbury G: Seventy-five cases of solid tumors treated by a modified quadruple chemotherapy regimen. Cancer 25:462–478, 1971
453. Shnider BI, Baig M, Serpic A et al: Combination therapy with 5-fluorouracil, cyclophosphamide, vincristine, and methotrexate. J Clin Pharmacol 15:69–73, 1975
454. Salmon SE, Hamburger AW, Soehnlen BJ et al: Quantitation of differential sensitivities of human tumor cells to anti-cancer drugs. N Engl J Med 298:1321–1327, 1978
455. Bellet RE, Danna V, Mastrangelo MJ et al: Evaluation of a "nude" mouse-human tumor panel as a predictive secondary screen for cancer chemotherapeutic agents. JNCI 63:1185–1188, 1979
456. Wick MM, Byers L, Frei E III: L-DOPA: Selective toxicity for melanoma cells *in vitro*. Science 197:468–469, 1977
457. Ramirez G, Weiss AJ, Rochlin DB et al: Phase II study of 6α-methylpregn-4-ene-3, 11, 20 -trione (NSC-17256). Cancer Chemother Rep 55:265–268, 1971
458. Johnson RO, Bisel HF, Andrews N et al: Phase I clinical study of 6α-methylpregn-4-ene-3, 11, 20-trione (NSC-17256). Cancer Chemother Rep 50:671–673, 1966
459. Didolkar RC, Catane R, Lopez R et al: Estramustine phosphate (estracyt) in advanced malignant melanoma. Proc Am Soc Clin Oncol 19:381, 1978
460. Fisher RI, Young RC, Lippman MC: Diethylstilbesterol therapy of surgically non-resectable malignant melanoma. Proc Am Soc Clin Oncol 19:339, 1978
461. Beretta G, Tabiadon D, Fossati P: Clinical evaluation of medroxiprogesterone acetate (MAP) in malignant melanoma. Cancer Treat Rep 63:1200, 1979
462. Meyskens FL Jr, Voakes JB: Tamoxifen in metastatic malignant melanoma. Cancer Treat Rep 64:171–173, 1980
463. Karakousis CP, Lopez R, Bhakoo HS et al: Steroid hormone receptors and tamoxifen treatment in malignant melanoma. Proc Am Soc Clin Oncol 21:345, 1980
464. Papac R, Luikhart S, Kirkwood J: High dose tamoxifen in patients with advanced renal cell cancer and malignant melanoma. Proc Am Soc Clin Oncol 21:358, 1980
465. Snell RS, Bischitz PG: The effect of large doses of estrogen and progesterone on melanin pigmentation. J Invest Derm 35:73–82, 1960
466. Lerner AB, Shizume K, Bunding I: The mechanism of endocrine control of melanin pigmentation. J Clin Endocr 14:1463–1490, 1954
467. Sadoff L, Winkley J, Tyson S: Is malignant melanoma an endocrine dependent tumor? Oncology 27:244–257, 1973
468. Rampen FHJ, Mulder JH: Malignant melanoma: An androgen dependent tumor? Lancet 1:562–565, 1980
469. Bodenham DC, Hale B: Malignant melanoma. In Stoll BA (ed): Endocrine Therapy in Malignant Disease, p 377. London, W B Saunders, 1972
470. Herbst WP: Malignant melanoma of the choroid with extenstive metastases treated by removing secreting tissue of the testicles. JAMA 122: 597, 1943
471. Howes WE: Removal of testes in treatment of melanoma. JAMA 123: 304, 1943
472. Fisher RI, Neifeld JP, Lippman ME: Estrogen receptors in human malignant melanoma. Lancet 2:337–338, 1976
473. Rumke P, Persijn JP, Korsten CB: Oestrogen and androgen receptors in melanoma. Br J Cancer 41:652–656, 1980
474. Stedman KE, Moore GE, Morgan RT: Estrogen receptor proteins in diverse human tumors. Arch Surg 115:244–248, 1980
475. Chaudhuri PK, Walker MJ, Briele HA et al: Incidence of estrogen receptor in benign nevi and human malignant melanoma. JAMA 244:791–793, 1980
476. Beattie CW, Chaudhuri PK, Walker MJ et al: Hormonal regulation of the growth and metastasis of human melanoma. Cancer Treat Rep 63:1199, 1979
477. Mossler JA, Stowers S, Lubahn D et al: Comparative analysis of sex steroid binding in human melanoma. Proc Am Soc Clin Oncol 21:476, 1980
478. Cole WH: Spontaneous regression of cancer: The metabolic triumph of the host? Ann NY Acad Sci 230:111–141, 1974
479. Bodurtha AJ: Spontaneous regression of malignant melanoma. In Clark WH, Goldman LI, Mastrangelo MJ (eds): Human Malignant Melanoma, pp 227–241. New York, Grune & Stratton, 1979
480. Morton DL: Immunological studies with human neoplasms. J Reticuloendothel Soc 10:137–160, 1971
481. Morton DL, Eilber FR, Malmgren RA et al: Immunological

factors which influence response to immunotherapy in malignant melanoma. Surgery 68: 158–164, 1970
482. Sparks FC, Silverstein MJ, Hunt JS et al: Complications of BCG immunotherapy in patients with cancer. N Engl J Med 289:827–830, 1973
483. Krementz ET, Samuels MS, Wallace JH: Clinical experience in the immunotherapy of cancer. Surg Gynecol Obstet 133:209–217, 1971
484. Nathanson L: Regression of intradermal melanoma after intralesional injection of *Mycobacterium bovis* strain BCG. Cancer Chemother Rep 56:659–665, 1972
485. Levy NL, Mahaley MS Jr, Day ED: Serum-mediated blocking of cell-mediated antitumor immunity in a melanoma patient: Association with BCG immunotherapy and clinical deterioration. Int J Cancer 10:244–248, 1972
486. Pinsky CM, Hirshaut Y, Oettgen HF: Treatment of malignant melanoma by intra-turmoral injection of BCG. Natl Cancer Inst Monogr 39:255–228, 1973
487. Mastrangelo MJ, Bellet RE, Laucius JF et al: Immunotherapy of Malignant Melanoma—A review. In Sutnick AI, Engstrom PF (eds): Oncologic Medicine, pp 71–93. Baltimore, University Park Press, 1976
488. Mastrangelo MJ, Sulit HL, Prehn LM et al: Intralesional BCG in the treatment of metastatic malignant melanoma. Cancer 37:684–692, 1976
489. Mastrangelo MJ, Bellet RE, Berkelhammer J et al: Regression of pulmonary metastatic disease associated with intralesional BCG therapy of dermal melanoma metastases. Cancer 36:1305–1308, 1975
490. Smith GV, Morse PA Jr, Deraps GD et al: Immunotherapy of patients with cancer. Surgery 74:59–68, 1973
491. Minton JR: Mumps virus and BCG vaccine in metastatic melanoma. Arch Surg 106:503–506, 1973
492. Baker MA, Taub RN: BCG in malignant melanoma. Lancet 1:1117–1118, 1973
493. Klein E, Holterman OA: Immunotherapeutic approaches to the management of neoplasm. Natl Cancer Inst Monog 35:379–402, 1972
494. Klein E, Holterman OA, Papermaster B et al: Immunologic approaches to various types of cancer with the use of BCG and purified protein derivatives. Natl Cancer Inst Monogr 39:229–239, 1973
495. Lieberman R, Wybran J, Epstein W: The immunologic and histopathologic changes in BCG-mediated tumor regression in patients with malignant melanoma. Cancer 35:756–777, 1975
496. Israel L, DePierre A, Edelstein R: Effect of intranodular BCG in 22 melanoma patients. Proceedings IV International Symposium on the Locoregional Treatment of Tumors, Turin, Italy, UICC, Sept. 19–21, 1973
497. Grant RM, Mackie R, Cochran AJ et al: Results of administering BCG to patients with melanoma. Lancet 2:1096–1098, 1974
498. Cohen MH, Felix E, Jessup J et al: Treatment of metastatic melanoma by intralesional injection of BCG, organic chemicals and *C. parvum*. In Crispen RG (ed): Neoplasm Immunity Mechanism, pp 121–134. Philadelphia, Franklin Institute Press, 1975
499. Tisman G, Wu SJG, Safire GE: Intralesional PPD in malignant melanoma. Lancet 1:161–162, 1975
500. Klein E, Holterman OA, Helm F et al: Immunologic approaches to the management of primary and secondary tumors involving the skin and soft tissues. Review of a ten year program. Transplant Proc 7:297–315, 1975
501. Malek–Mansour S, Castermans–Elias S, Lapiere CM: Regression de metastases de mélanome aprés thérapeutique immunlogique. Dermatologica 146:156–162, 1973
502. Hunter–Craig I, Newton KA, Westbury G et al: Use of vaccinia virus in the treatment of metastatic malignant melanoma. Br Med J 2:512–515, 1970
503. Milton GW, Brown MML: The limited role of attenuated smallpox virus in the management of advanced malignant melanoma. Aust NZJ Surg 35:286–290, 1966
504. Burdick KH: Malignant melanoma treated with vaccinia injections. Arch Dermatol 82:438–439, 1960
505. Burdick K, Hawk WA: Vitiligo in a case of vaccinia virus-treated melanoma. Cancer 17:708–712, 1964
506. Belisario JC, Milton GW: The experimental local therapy of cutaneous metastases of malignant melanoblastomas with cow pox vaccine or colcemid. Aust J Dermatol 6:113–118, 1961
507. Krown SE, Hilal EY, Pinsky CM et al: Intralesional injection of the methanol extraction residue of Baccilus Calmette-Guerin (MER) into cutaneous metastases of malignant melanoma. Cancer 42:2648–2660, 1978
508. Cunningham–Rundles WF, Hirshaut Y, Pinsky CM et al: Phase trial of intralesional *C. parvum*. Clin Res 26:337A, 1978
509. Richman SP, Gutterman JU, Hersh EM et al: Phase I–II study of intratumor immunotherapy with BCG cell wall skeleton plus P3. Cancer Immunol Immunother 5:41–44, 1978
510. Vosika GJ, Schmidtke JR, Goldman A et al: Intralesional immunotherapy of malignant melanoma with myobacterium smegmatis cell wall skeleton combined with trehalose dimycolate (P3). Cancer 44:495–503, 1979
511. Laucius JF, Bodurtha AJ, Mastrangelo MJ et al: A Phase II study of autologous irradiated tumor cells plus BCG in patients with metastatic melanoma. Cancer 40: 2091–2093, 1977
512. Arlen M, Hollinshead A, Scherrer J: Tumor-specific immunity in patients with malignant melanoma. Surg Forum 28:168–169, 1977
513. Orefice S, Cascinelli N, Vaglini M et al: Intravenous administration of BCG in advanced melanoma patients. Tumori 64:437–443, 1978
514. Israel L, Edelstein R, Depierre A et al: Daily intravenous infusions of *Corynebacterium parvum* in twenty patients with disseminated cancer. JNCI 55:29–33, 1975
515. Falk RE, Mann P, Largen B: Cell-mediated immunity to human tumors. Arch Surg 107:261–266, 1973
516. Wallack MK, Steplewski Z, Koprowski H et al: A new approach to specific active immunotherapy. Cancer 39:560–564, 1977
517. Murray DR, Cassel WA, Torbin AH et al: Viral oncolysate in the management of malignant melanoma. Cancer 40:680–686, 1977
518. Israel L, Edelstein R, Mannori P et al: Plasmapheresis in patients with disseminated cancer. Clinical results and correlation with changes in serum protein. Cancer 40:3146–3154, 1977
519. Gutterman JU, Mavligit G, Gottlieb JA et al: Chemoimmunotherapy of disseminated malignant melanoma with dimethyltriazeno-imidazole-carboxamide and Bacillus Calmette–Guerin. N Engl J Med 529:291–297, 1974
520. Costanzi JJ, Al-Saraf M, Dixon DO: Chemoimmunotherapy of disseminated melanoma. Proc Am Assoc Clin Oncol 19:362, 1979
521. Presant CA, Bartolucci AA, Smalley RV et al: Cyclophosphamide plus 5-(3,3-dimethyl-1-triazeno) imidazole-4-carboxamide (DTIC) with or without *Corynebacterium parvum* in metastatic malignant melanoma. Cancer 44:899–905, 1979
522. Mastrangelo MJ, Bellet RE, Berd D: A Phase II comparison of Methyl-CCNU + vincristine with or without BCG + allogeneic tumor cells in malignant melanoma. Cancer Immunol Immunother 6:231–236, 1979
523. Giuliano AE, Moseley HS, Morton DL: Clinical aspects of unknown primary melanoma. Ann Surg 191:98–104, 1980
524. Iverson K, Robins RE: Mucosal malignant melanomas. Am J Surg 139:660–664, 1980
525. Chung AF, Woodruff JM, Lewis JL: Malignant melanoma of the vulva. Obstet Gynecol 45:638–646, 1975
526. Leo S, Rorat E, Parekh M: Primary melanoma in a desmoid cyst of the ovary. Obstet Gynecol 41:205–210, 1973
527. Bergdahl L, Boquist L, Liliequist B et al: Primary malignant melanoma of the central nervous system. Acta Neurochirurgica 26:139–149, 1972
528. Scholtz CL, Siu K: Melanoma of the pituitary. J Neurosurg 45:101–103, 1976
529. Smith S, Opipari MI: Primary pleural melanoma. J Thor Cardiovasc Surg 75:827–831, 1978
530. Hatae Y, Kikuchi M, Segawa M et al: Malignant melanoma of the gallbladder. Path Res Pract 163:281–287, 1978

CHAPTER 32

Daniel M. Albert

Intraocular Melanomas

OCCURRENCE AND LOCATION OF OCULAR MELANOMAS

Intraocular melanomas constitute the most common primary ocular malignancy in Caucasians. They hold a special significance to the ophthalmologist. Whereas many eye diseases have the potential for loss of vision, ocular melanomas may result in death of the patient as well. This chapter will deal with melanomas of the uveal tract (*i.e.* the iris, ciliary body, and choroid). However melanomas may also occur on the skin of the lid, on the conjunctiva, and even within the orbit. Moreover, in addition to the uveal melanocytes (the cells probably giving rise to uveal melanomas), a second population of pigmented cells exist within the eye. These are the pigmented epithelium of the iris, ciliary body, and retina. These cells are derived from the neuroepithelium of the embryonic optic cup. The pigmented epithelium commonly undergoes non-neoplastic proliferation or reactive hyperplasia in response to a variety of stimuli and, in rare instances, undergoes neoplastic differentiation. The uveal melanocytes originate from the neural crest and possess long, dendrite-like processes emanating from the center of the cell body. They reside in the stromal components of the uvea and, as discussed below, are considered the cell of origin for most intraocular pigmented neoplasms.[1,2]

The annual age-adjusted incidence of non-skin melanoma as reported in the Third National Cancer Survey, 1969–1971, was 0.7/100,000 population in the U.S.[3] Ocular tumors comprise 79% of all the noncutaneous melanomas reported in that survey. The precise anatomic origin of ocular melanomas was unspecified in some 25%; the tumors arose within the globe, (mainly from the choroid) in 73%; and finally, 2% developed from the conjunctiva. Melanoma accounted for 70% of all eye malignancies, followed in frequency by the childhood tumor, retinoblastoma (13%). In persons over the age of 20, melanoma was the reported diagnosis for 80% of all primary ocular cancers.[3] Data from the Connecticut Tumor Registry are similar to those from the Third National Cancer Survey.[4]

The annual age-adjusted incidence of ocular melanomas is about one-eighth the rate of melanoma of skin in the U.S.[5] The risk among whites for ocular melanomas was 8-fold over blacks (compared to a risk six-times greater for skin melanomas). The overall risk of ocular melanomas did not vary by sex.[5] However, ocular and skin melanomas showed similar age patterns, with women predominating at younger ages and men later in life. The Third National Cancer Survey indicated a left-sided excess of 18% for ocular melanomas in males, contrasted with a right-sided excess in females.[5] This is consistent with a previous survey of ocular melanoma in armed service veterans, in which 65% of tumors developed in the left eye.[6]

ETIOLOGY, HISTOGENESIS, AND HISTOPATHOLOGY OF OCULAR MELANOMAS

ETIOLOGY

As is the case with other human cancers, the etiology of ocular melanomas is unknown. Some evidence based on electron microscopy of ocular melanomas and biomolecular studies suggests that there may be a viral role.[7] Viruses have been used in the induction of animal ocular melanoma models.[8]

In a recent study of a single population of chemical workers, a statistically significant and higher-than-expected incidence of ocular melanomas was found.[4] Various chemicals, including nickel subsulfide, platinum, methycholanthrene, ethionine, N-2-fluorenylacetamide, and radium have been reported to induce ocular melanomas in animals.[8-12] Exposure to sunlight is now cited as a major causative factor for melanomas of the skin and probably conjunctiva.[5,13] No comparable latitudinal gradient for eye melanomas could be demonstrated similar to that which exists for skin melanomas. This indicates that intraocular melanoma is not related to sun exposure, either directly or through activation of a "solar circulating factor."[14] Scotto and coworkers suggested a relationship between the laterality of ocular melanoma as related to sex and a possible relationship to automobile driving habits and exposure to road pollutants.[5]

Aside from rare instances of familial aggregation of ocular melanoma, little evidence for inborn susceptibility to eye melanoma exists, except in the case of certain associated conditions, such as melanomis oculi, nevus of Ota, and neurofibromatosis.[15-17]

HISTOGENESIS

In the older literature it has been stated that malignant melanomas were derived from mesenchymal (mesodermal) cells in the uvea and, consequently, the term "melanosarcoma" persisted for many years.[18] The argument as to the source or sources of this tumor has persisted over many years, with the Schwann cell, the dendritic melanocyte of neural crest origin, and the uveal nevus all having their advocates.[19-21]

HISTOPATHOLOGY

The major histopathologic types of uveal malignant melanoma have long been recognized.[18] Callender, in 1931, provided the initial data relating the histologic appearance to prognosis. The Callender classification, in somewhat modified form, remains in general use today as follows:

1. Spindle A Melanomas
   Spindle A melanomas are made up of cohesive cells with small, spindle-shaped nuclei containing a central dark strip contributed by a nuclear fold. The nucleoli are not distinct, the cytoplasm is ill-defined, and the cell borders are difficult to identify. These comprise approximately 5% of ciliary body and choroidal melanomas.
2. Spindle B and fascicular melanomas
   These melanomas are composed of cohesive cells having distinct spindle-shaped nuclei with prominent nucleoli. The cytoplasm is indistinct and the cell borders are difficult to discern by light microscopy. This cell type comprises approximately 39% of ciliary body and choroidal melanomas. The fascicular type is a subgroup of spindle B melanomas characterized by a palisading arrangement of the spindle-shaped cells termed a "fascicular pattern." These comprise approximately 6% of choroidal melanomas. As discussed below, spindle A and spindle B melanomas are the cell types seen in essentially all iris melanomas.
3. Epithelioid Melanomas
   Epithelioid melanomas are composed of poorly cohesive large cells and round nuclei with prominent nucleoli. Abundant eosinophilic cytoplasm and well-demarcated cell borders are seen. This is the rarest type of ciliary body and choroidal melanoma, occurring in only 3% of all cases.
4. Mixed cell type melanomas
   These are neoplasms showing significant spindle cells (usually spindle B) together with a predominant epithelioid population. This is the most common type of ciliary body and choroidal melanoma, accounting for 45% of these lesions.
5. Necrotic Melanoma
   This refers to a tumor so necrotic that the cell type may not be identified. An uncommon variety, it occurs in only 7% of all ciliary body and choroidal tumors.

For the sake of convenience, it is sometimes easier to consider melanomas of the uveal tract in two primary categories: the spindle cell variety (combining spindle A and spindle B types) and the epithelioid, mixed, and necrotic types, or non-spindle cell variety.

In the years following the introduction of Callender classification, numerous studies were undertaken attempting to correlate additional morphologic features with behavior of the tumor.[23-27] These studies generally confirmed that the best correlation exists between cell type and prognosis. Paul and coworkers analyzed 2,652 cases of choroidal and ciliary body melanoma accessioned at the Armed Forces Institute of Pathology (AFIP) prior to 1956. Actuarial data from that study showed that five years after enucleation 95% of the patients with spindle A tumors, 85% with spindle B tumors, 60% with mixed tumors, and 43% with epithelioid tumors were alive. At 15 years after enucleation, 85% of the patients with spindle A melanomas, 80% with spindle B tumors, 46% with mixed tumors, and 34% with epithelioid tumors were alive. Applying the "simplified classification" to these data, the authors observed that a little under 50% were of the "non-spindle" variety; approximately 35% of these patients had survived 15 years after enucleation.

In Jensen's series of 230 cases from Denmark that had been observed for a total of 15 years, 121 or 53% of the patients died of metastatic melanoma.[28,29] Less than 1% of patients with spindle A tumors died from metastatic disease; 62% with mixed tumors died; and in 81% with epithelioid tumors the cause of death was metastatic melanoma.

Other parameters have been examined as well, including tumor size and location, scleral invasion, fiber content, pigmentation, and lymphocytic infiltration. McLean and coworkers studied 217 small malignant melanomas, each with a volume less than 14 mm^3. Using a single-factor approach with 16 risk factors, they found seven that correlated well with outcome. These included cell type, pigmentation, size (largest diameter), scleral extension, mitotic activity, location of anterior tumor margin, and optic nerve extension. Using a linear discriminant function, the four best factors in combination were cell type, largest dimension, scleral extension, and mitotic activity. Four other variables (largest diameter, location of anterior margin, mitotic activity, and optic nerve invasion) that can be correlated with clinical observations were less accurate in separating fatal and nonfatal cases than cell type alone.

In another study of prognostic factors in choroidal and ciliary body melanomas carried out by Shammas and Blodi, 293 cases of choroidal and ciliary body melanoma with a follow-up period of 5 years or more were reviewed. They identified nine factors that significantly influenced prognosis: age of the patient at enucleation; location of the tumor and its anterior border; largest tumor diameter in contact with the sclera; height of the tumor; integrity of Bruch's membrane; cell type; pigmentation; and scleral infiltration by tumor cells. They stated that the largest tumor diameter is the single most important clinical and pathologic prognostic factor. The prognosis is relatively good when the diameter is 10 mm or less and becomes poor when it exceeds 10 mm.

DIAGNOSIS OF UVEAL MELANOMAS

As Zimmerman points out, tumors of the iris have several important distinguishing clinical features that contrast with tumors of the posterior uveal tract. First these tumors are located where not only the ophthalmologist can see them but also where the patient, family, and friends can see them as well. Such patients are frequently aware of a spot on the iris that has been there for many years but only recently shows growth. The ophthalmologist can examine the lesion carefully with a slit lamp biomicroscope and gonioscopy. With the aid of both serial and iris fluorescein photography, the ophthalmologist can sequentially document the size and vasculature of the tumor. Iris tumors are usually small, discrete lesions, but may be diffuse and infiltrative or even multiple. In a study of lesions mistaken for malignant melanoma of the iris, Ferry noted that conditions which caused increased pigmentation of the iris may be confused with a diffuse melanoma of the iris.[33] This includes congenital melanosis, siderosis bulbi, and heterochromia iridis. In addition, foreign bodies lodged in the iris and encapsulated by fibrous tissue, cysts or tumors of the iris pigment epithelium, leiomyomas, granulomas (as seen in sarcoid or tuberculosis), metastatic neoplasms, implantation cysts, and nevoxanthoendothelioma may be confused with iris melanomas.

Nonetheless, diagnosis of ciliary body and choroidal melanomas, although more difficult than iris melanomas, has reached a high degree of accuracy at eye centers where experienced clinicians and ancillary testing facilities are available. Probably representative of the degree of accuracy of diagnosis at major centers are the findings in a review of 876 eyes enucleated between 1954 and 1977 at the Mayo Clinic.[34] Only six of 224 eyes enucleated for clinically suspected melanoma had a mimicking lesion, a misdiagnosis rate of 2.7 percent. In addition, six melanomas that were clinically unsuspected were found. This high rate for correct clinical diagnosis is particularly impressive since only outpatient procedures (including clinical examination, ultrasound, and fluorescein angiography) were used and without biopsy, as is done for many other tumors.

The cornerstone of diagnosis in posterior uveal melanoma remains to be clinical examination and, in particular, indirect ophthalmoscopy through the dilated pupil. Fundus contact lens examination as well as the use of the three-mirror lens in the case of ciliary body melanomas can be extremely helpful. Scleral transillumination, as advocated by Reese, is also a useful aid.[35] Visual field studies are less specific, but are easily accomplished.[36] While clinical examination by an experienced observer remains far and away the most important diagnostic test in establishing the presence of an ocular melanoma, ancillary diagnostic testing can be extremely valuable.[37] The combined use of A- and B-scan ultrasound techniques has been of great value in confirming the clinical diagnosis of choroidal melanoma, especially in the presence of opaque media.[38] Small tumors elevated less than 2–3 mm above the sclera cannot be accurately evaluated with most ultrasound equipment in use. In larger tumors, ultrasound provides valuable size data for serial measurements. In addition, ultrasound has been helpful in differentiating primary choroidal tumors from metastatic lesions and choroidal hemangioma.

Fluorescein angiography has proven to be of considerable diagnostic value in some cases where it has demonstrated inherent tumor vasculature and has permitted differentiation among subretinal or choroidal hemorrhage, hemangioma, and melanoma.[39] Of particular value is the ability of fluorescein angiography to detect minute degrees of damage to the retinal pigment epithelium and neovascularization along the plane of Bruch's membrane, changes that indicate the rate of choroidal tumor growth.

The usefulness of radioactive phosphorus (^{32}P) in determining malignancy is more controversial than ultrasound or fluorescein. In addition, it probably has limited indications for use in routine cases where adequate support for a diagnosis of ocular melanoma can be obtained with less complicated procedures.[37,40]

Radiologic examinations, including the use of CT scans, are not often indicated in the clinical evaluation of ocular melanoma. Such studies, however, can be extremely valuable in some instances to confirm the presence of intraocular bone in rare simulating lesions (osseous choristoma) or to provide preoperative indication of extraocular or optic nerve extension.

The development of immunologic testing shows exciting potential for future usefulness in the diagnosis of ocular melanomas. It does not as yet, however, offer results as reliable as the other methods for confirming the presence of an ocular melanoma.[41–43]

Patients with suspected intraocular melanoma should have a physical examination. Clinical laboratory studies should be performed, including routine blood work and chest films, liver enzyme measurements, and probably radioisotope liver scanning to rule out the possibility of metastatic disease.[44]

ANTERIOR UVEAL MELANOMAS: DISTINGUISHING FEATURES AND TREATMENT

GENERAL CONSIDERATIONS

Malignant melanomas are the most common primary tumors of the iris. Their reported occurrence varies between 49% and 72.4% in a variety of series.[45-47] The occurrence of malignant melanomas of the iris is low in comparison with melanomas of the rest of the uvea, with various estimates ranging from 1:6 to 1:30.[28,48-50] A number of clinical, cytologic, histologic, and oncologic differences distinguish melanomas of the iris, with and without ciliary body involvement, from those involving the posterior uveal tract. Because of their position, iris melanomas are detected early and generally removed early. Clinically, the average age of patients operated on for iris melanomas is between 40 and 50 years.[51] Many patients give a long history of a noticeable pigmented iris lesion prior to clinical diagnosis, interpreted by many to suggest that the tumor has arisen from a pre-existing nevus.[52-54] The rate of growth of malignant melanomas of the iris is generally slower than choroidal or ciliary body melanomas. The clinical feature that Zimmerman believes to be the single most important difference between tumors of the iris and those of the posterior uveal tract is size. These are almost always invariably small lesions, usually much smaller than the tumors the physician must deal with in the posterior uveal tract.[32]

Both the older and more recent literature stress the relatively benign behavior and good prognosis of iris melanomas compared with malignant melanomas of the choroid and ciliary body. Zimmerman, reviewing the major studies of iris melanomas, found only 12 deaths reported among 258 patients followed at least 5 years after treatment with a 5-year mortality rate of about 4% for these iris tumors.[32] In a more recent study from the Institute of Ophthalmology in London, Sunba and associates reported only seven patients developing metastases out of 196 cases in their files followed for a minimum of 5 years, representing an incidence of metastasis of 3.5%.[51]

This very favorable prognosis for iris melanomas is undoubtedly closely related to the fact that these tumors are predominantly of the spindle cell type, in particular, the spindle A variety.[32,49,51] Histologically, spindle A melanomas of the iris are compact, cohesive lesions composed of small, slender cells with fusiform nuclei and little evidence of mitotic activity. The histologic features are consistent with slow growth and benign behavior. It should be noted that there is a significant incidence of errors in preoperative clinical evaluation, and that the lesions comprising the differential diagnosis of iris melanomas differ considerably from those of the ciliary body and choroid.[33]

TREATMENT

In the management of iris melanomas, if the following factors are present, surgical intervention is not necessary:

1. No clinical evidence exists that the lesion is progressing
2. Absence of pronounced neovascularization
3. The lesion is not producing any vision disturbances
4. No significant complications, such as hemorrhage into the anterior chamber, secondary glaucoma, or an obvious extension outside of the eye are evident
5. The lesion arises in the patient's better eye.[32]

On the other hand, enucleation should be carried out in the following circumstances:

1. If there is diffuse involvement of the iris
2. Circumferential extension exists along a large portion of the chamber angle, particularly if the entire chamber angle is involved
3. Tumors are too bulky to be removed by excisional procedures
4. In the presence of complications such as severe secondary glaucoma that does not respond to medical therapy
5. In the presence of extraocular extension
6. When the tumor has recurred after previous iridectomy or iridocyclectomy and is judged not suitable for further excisional treatment.[32]

However, Reese, Zimmerman, and others have noted examples of cases where the tumor has extended outside of the eye and has still been successfully removed by corneoscleroiridocyclectomy.[32,55]

Reese points out that beginning around 1958, iris melanomas, with or without ciliary body involvement, were seldom recognized to metastasize or seed and that they are malignant only in the sense that they infiltrate locally. Consequently, interest in *iridectomy, iridocyclectomy,* and *corneoscleroiridocyclectomy* with graft as alternatives to enucleation has grown.[52]

The object of excisional iridectomy is to remove the tumor entirely without permitting tumor cells to disseminate in the eye or the incision (see Fig. 32-1). The general procedure is that described by Reese in which a limbal incision is made that is large enough to permit removal of the lesion by basal iridectomy under direct observation.[52]

When the iris tumor extends not only to the root of the iris but also into the face of the ciliary body, iridectomy is an inadequate procedure for its removal. Raubitschek and Verhoeff suggested the use of iridocyclectomy many years ago for the removal of such tumors.[56,57] Until the 1960s, however, such lesions continued to be treated by enucleation. Through the pioneering efforts of Müller and Stallard, the use of iridocyclectomy for the treatment of such tumors has gained wide acceptance.[58-60] A basic technique for resecting the iris tumor together with involved ciliary body is that given by Jones (see Figure 32-2).[61]

Many cases requiring more than iridectomy for iris tumor removal also require an cperation more extensive than iridocyclectomy. Examples are eyes in which the tumor not only invades the ciliary body, but also fills the chamber angle and is adherent to the tissues in the angle or to the cornea itself. In such cases the surgeon should consider corneoscleroiridocyclectomy with or without a corneoscleral graft. An alternative method not requiring a transplant is that described by Sears.[62]

Surgical complications include intraocular hemorrhage, hypotony, subluxation of the lens, cataract, late detachment

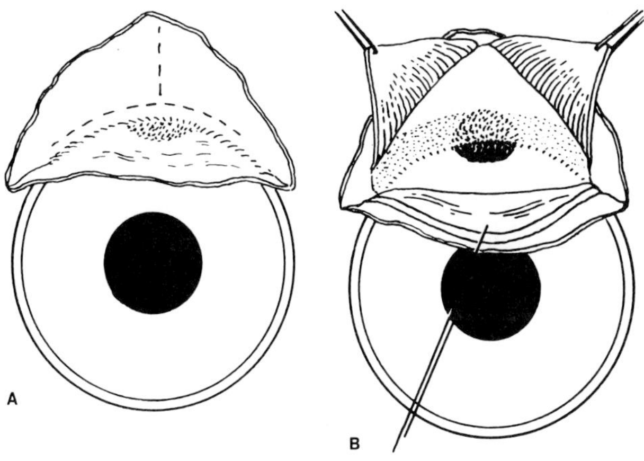

FIG. 32-1. Limbal incision with single perpendicular scleral cut. Exposure by folding back sclera. (Jones IS: Iridocyclectomy and corneoscleroiridocyclectomy. In Reese AB (ed): Tumors of the Eye, pp 240, 241. Hagerstown, Harper & Row, 1976)

of the retina, corneal edema, macular edema, and vitreous loss. If incompletely excised, the tumor may recur. If metastasis occurs following iridocyclectomy, it is difficult to assess the operative role in its causation[32]

Forrest and associates, in a study of 107 cases of ciliary body melanomas treated by iridocyclectomy, found that 6% of the patients operated on culminated in enucleation. The majority of problems relating to surgical management or to the tumors arose within 4 years of surgery.

In summary, conservative management of iris melanomas is generally advocated. Therefore, no surgical treatment should be undertaken unless there is a clear-cut indication for it. However, when surgery is indicated, every effort should be made to use excisional methods and to avoid enucleation of the eye.

THE TREATMENT OF CHOROIDAL AND CILIARY BODY MELANOMAS

In the late 19th century, enucleation became the standard and almost universally accepted treatment for all choroidal or ciliary body melanomas.[18] Even today, early enucleation continues to have its ardent advocates.[64] However, in the last few years reassessment has been made of enucleation as a conventional means of treating malignant melanomas of the choroid and ciliary body. This has resulted from the development of newer and more precise diagnostic tests now available for recognizing malignant melanomas and the serial documentation of their size; more information about clinical and pathologic features that determine survival; additional observations about the natural course of ciliary body and choroidal melanomas when untreated; and therapeutic developments other than enucleation to treat these tumors without destroying the eye. A major spur to the re-evaluation of enucleation in the treatment of ciliary body and choroidal melanomas has been the contention that the peak mortality from uveal melanomas is causally connected to the surgical procedure.[65,66]

In light of current knowledge, it is useful to consider the treatment of melanomas of the choroid, with and without involvement of the ciliary body, in terms of size:

1. Small melanomas, less than 10 mm in diameter and less than 2 mm elevated
2. Medium melanomas, between 10 and 15 mm in diameter and 2–5 mm elevated
3. Large melanomas, greater than 15 mm in diameter and greater than 5 mm elevation[37,67]

SMALL TUMORS

As with melanomas of all sizes, the choices open to the clinician in following a small choroidal melanoma include

1. Enucleate
2. Use some method of local treatment, such as radiotherapy, photocoagulation, cryotherapy or local resection
3. Immunotherapy or chemotherapy
4. Observation

There is an accumulating body of evidence indicating that the risks in observing these small tumors are low.[68–70] In cases in which patients with small melanomas are asymptomatic, appropriate work-up and subsequent observation is the treatment of choice, particularly in elderly patients. If the diagnosis is equivocal, observation is most certainly indicated. If the lesion shows progression, particularly rapid growth or an increase in size beyond 10 mm in diameter and 2 mm in elevation, or, if the lesion results in significant impairment of vision (as with a lesion of the posterior pole), treatment is indicated. In such cases, if the prospect of good vision exists, proton beam irradiation appears the treatment of choice; in the case of an only eye, such treatment should be undertaken. This modality of treatment is discussed later, together with other methods of local therapy. In the case of a young patient with a healthy second eye who shows evidence of rapid progression or growth beyond 10 mm in diameter and 2 mm in elevation, or, in patients in whom invasion of the optic nerve or extraocular extension is suspected, enucleation is advised. Should transsection of the tumor be demonstrated, subsequent exenteration must be considered.

TREATMENT OF LARGE MELANOMAS

There is general agreement that it would not presently be advisable to treat these cases other than by enucleation.[71] Possible exceptions include patients with only one seeing eye, rare patients in whom vision can be salvaged, and patients refusing enucleation.[67] Abramson and Ellsworth recommend local irradiation in such cases.[67]

Zimmerman and associates have suggested that when enucleation is carried out, the "no-touch" technique of Fraunfelder should be considered (see Fig. 32-3).[72] This method was designed to eliminate all flow of blood or fluid to and from the tumor during enucleation.

The authors claim that this technique avoids intraocular pressure elevations above 15 mm Hg before complete freezing occurs around the tumor. Subsequently, cryotherapy prevents

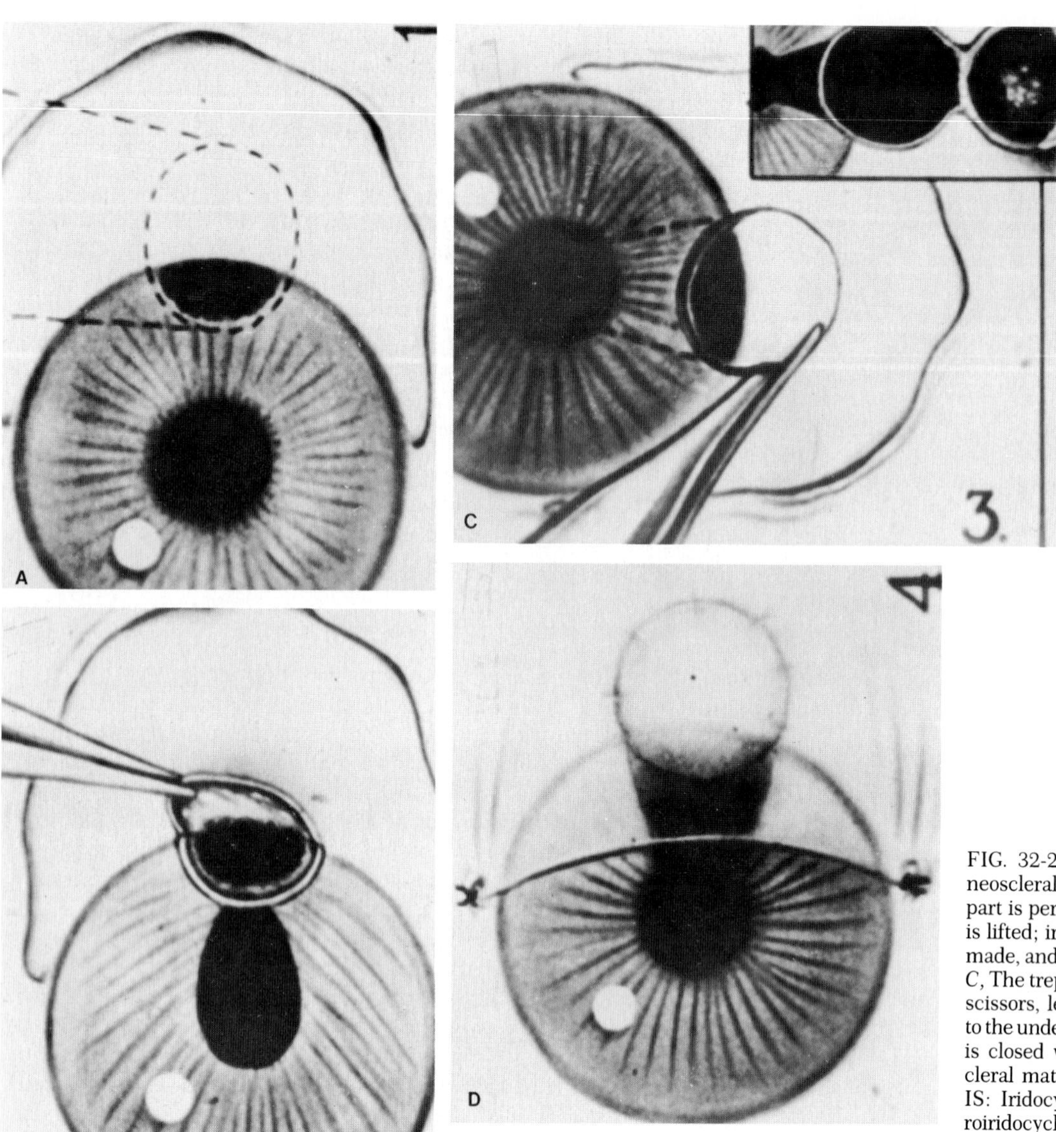

FIG. 32-2. *A,* In full-thickness corneoscleral trephination, the corneal part is perforated first. *B,* The button is lifted; iris and ciliary body cuts are made, and the vitreous is stroked free. *C,* The trephine cut is completed with scissors, leaving the button attached to the underlying tumor. *D,* The wound is closed with a corneal or corneoscleral matching button graft. (Jones IS: Iridocyclectomy and corneoscleroiridocyclectomy. In Reese AB (ed): Tumors of the Eye, pp 240, 241. Hagerstown, Harper & Row, 1976)

flow of fluid and blood to or from the tumor prior to the manipulation necessary for enucleation. While most surgeons do not use the "no-touch" technique, it is becoming increasingly recognized that enucleation be carried out by operators skilled and experienced in the procedure, and that the surgery be done with a minimum of manipulations possibly expressing tumor cells into the blood.

MEDIUM-SIZED TUMORS

Treatment of these tumors is the subject of current controversy. While general agreement exists that the observation of small melanomas carries little risk and that large melanomas should generally be treated by enucleation, there is less consensus regarding the therapy of melanomas between 10 and 15 mm in diameter and 2–5 mm in elevation.

Enucleation

Traditionally, most medium-sized melanomas have been treated by enucleation. Concern regarding enucleation as a mode of therapy, however, has been raised by Zimmerman and coworkers.[65,66] Their re-appraisal of survival data for patients with ciliary body and choroidal melanoma has led them to the conclusions that: (1) the mortality before enucleation is low (estimated at 1% per year), and, (2) the mortality rises abruptly following enucleation, reaches a peak of about 8% during the second year after enucleation, and then drops off monotonically.[65,66] They suggest that about two-thirds of fatalities following enucleation can be attributed to the dissemination of tumor emboli at surgery. These assumptions have been challenged by several investigators. Seigel and associates of the National Eye Institute pointed out that there are other ways to interpret this statistical data,

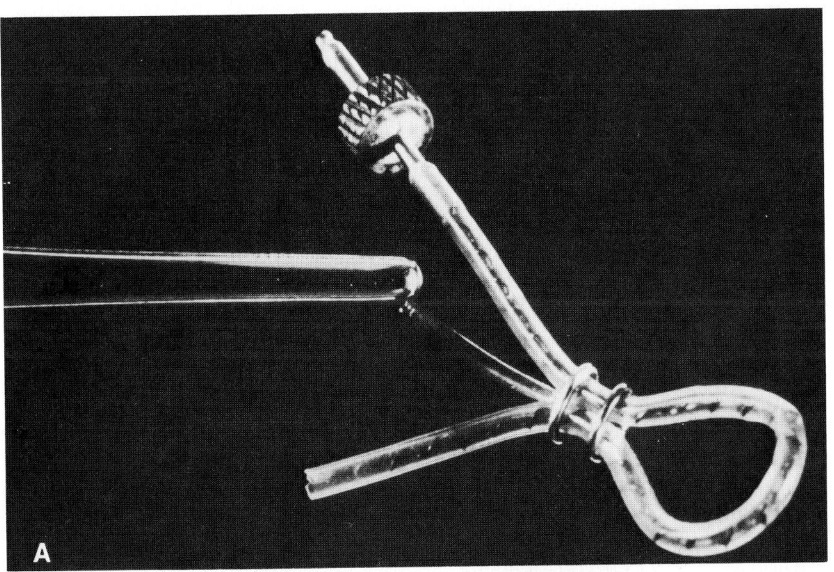

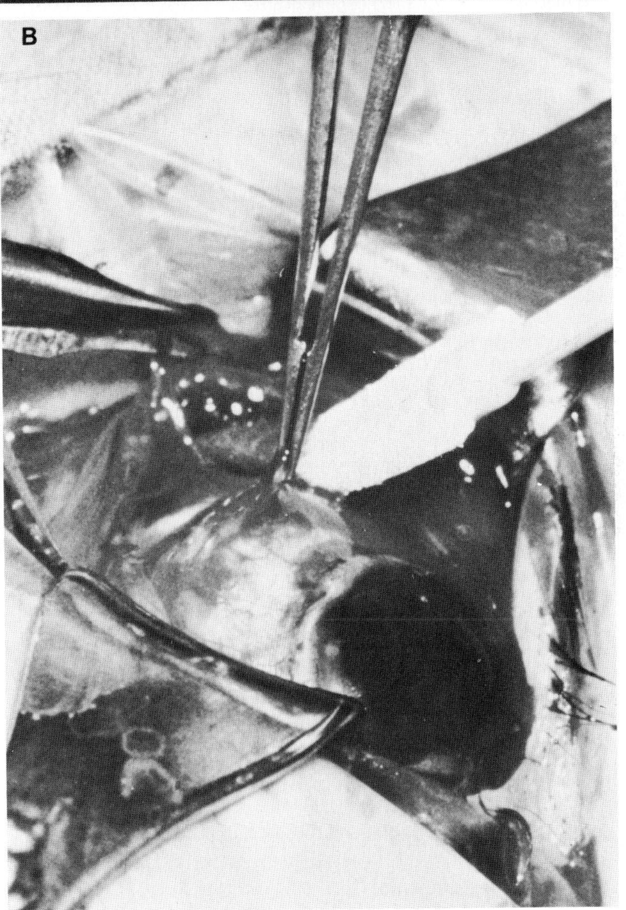

FIG. 32-3. *A*, Adjustable cryo-ring. A silastic tube with an obturator inside to prevent collapse of the tubing is held together by two metal coils. The size and shape of the loop can be varied by simply adjusting the tubing through the coils. *B*, The cryo-ring is placed on the outside of the eye to completely encircle the tumor. The sheets of styrofoam are placed between the ring and the orbit to prevent freezing of periocular tissue. A cryogen is then intermittently passed through the tubing to completely freeze the tumor area. Intermittent freezing is important since constant flow would cause the whole orbit to become frozen. (Courtesy of Fredrick T. Fraunfelder)

and concluded that there is no evidence at present to suggest that the existing pattern of treatment be altered for malignant melanoma of the uvea.[73] Another report from the Netherlands National Committee on Ocular Melanomas reached the opposite conclusions of Zimmerman and coworkers based on their study of tumor doubling time.[64] They advise immediate enucleation once the correct diagnosis has been established. Blodi believes that there is general agreement among most clinicians that it would not be advisable at present to change the type of management that is routinely recommended for patients with malignant melanoma of the uveal tract.[71] Although the "no-touch" technique has not as yet received wide acceptance, there is a greater awareness that necessary preoperative diagnostic studies and enucleation should be conducted with greater care and with no unnecessary trauma.

Radiation

The most exciting alternative to enucleation for treatment of choroidal malignant melanomas is the use of proton irradiation.[74] High-energy proton beams offer significant advantages for irradiation of ocular tumors. The high-energy, heavily charged particles have minimal scatter and a well-defined range in tissues that is both finite and energy-dependent. They can be collimated into small beams and thus deliver maximal density of ionization as they stop, resulting in the maximum dose called the Bragg peak, at the end of the beam path. According to the method developed by Gragoudas and coworkers, the proton beam can be accurately aimed at lesions within the eye.[74] Fortified tantalum rings 2 mm in diameter are sutured to the sclera at the edges of the tumor, which is localized by indirect ophthalmoscopy and transillumination. The rings are used as markers for stereotactic radiography to align the tumors precisely within the proton beam. Patients are given a total tumor dose of approximately 4700–6700 rad, delivered in five equal fractions over an 8–9 day period. Results of this treatment have been extremely impressive with regard to small tumors and show promise in the treatment of larger tumors as well.

Good results have also been reported with older techniques of local radiation, particularly ^{60}Co plaques and radon seeds.[75-77] Stallard, in his study that convincingly refuted the argument that choroidal malignant melanomas are not responsive to radiation, treated 100 eyes. In 69 eyes, the tumor completely disappeared.[75] Only six tumor deaths occurred in his group. These methods require a surgical procedure by which the plaque is sutured to the sclera directly over the base of the tumor. The dosage is calculated according to tumor size as measured with ultrasound. Once the proper amount of irradiation has been delivered, the plaque is surgically removed. Evidence of regression is seen weeks to months following treatment. Cases require careful selection and care must be taken to treat lesions peripheral enough from the optic nerve and macula so that these structures are not damaged by radiation. With regard to the ^{60}Co plaques, Abramson and Ellsworth suggest the treatment of tumors 8–10 disc diameters in size by this method, although noting they have treated melanomas filling two-thirds of an eye in rare cases.[67]

Radiation has also been coupled to enucleation, with European reports stating that postenucleation radiation therapy doubles the 5-year survival rate.[78,79]

Photocoagulation

Xenon arc photocoagulation has been advocated by several authors as a useful treatment method for eradicating small malignant melanomas of the choroid.[67,80,81] Meyer-Schwickerath and Vogel have suggested the following criteria for selecting patients with melanoma for photocoagulation treatment:

1. The diagnosis of malignant melanoma should be documented with as many modalities as possible
2. The lesion cannot be greater than 2 mm in elevation
3. The tumor should not be greater than six disc diameters in its greatest diameter
4. The lesion should not have significant subretinal fluid, which would in turn prevent adequate photocoagulation
5. The tumor should be far enough from the fovea so that vision is not significantly destroyed by treatment
6. The patient should have the technique thoroughly explained and should be informed of the possible complications and prognosis[81]

The technique involves several outpatient treatment sessions and is carried out after mydriasis and retrobulbar anesthesia. The normal retina around the tumor is treated heavily with photocoagulation forming two rows around the tumor. In about 3 weeks a second treatment is performed over the same area. Three weeks following this, the peripheral portions of the tumor are encroached upon with the photocoagulation and, in subsequent treatments, photocoagulation is carried to the center of the tumor. The hoped-for conclusion is a focal area of bare sclera with no ophthalmoscopic evidence of tumor and only residual pigment clumping in the center.

It is difficult to destroy large vessels over the tumor by this technique. Complications of photocoagulation include visual field defects, macular pucker, traction retinal detachment, and recurrence. Recurrences usually appear within 2 years of treatment. In Vogel's 10-year follow-up of photocoagulated melanomas, 18% of patients had died as a result of the tumor. The smallest tumor to cause death was 6 × 5 disc diameters in size; the mean size of the tumor causing death was 8–10 disc diameters.[81]

Cryotherapy

Cryotherapy of ocular melanomas was attempted by Lincoff and coworkers in four patients with discouraging results.[82] Although the technique has largely been abandoned, Abramson and Ellsworth have stated that additional work is going on at present to determine what role, if any, this modality has.[67]

Local Full-Thickness Eyewall Resection of Melanomas

Peyman has reported encouraging results using local sclerochorioretinal resection.[83,84] Peyman's technique involves a series of photocoagulation treatments around the tumor to create a firm chorioretinal adhesion or an area of bare sclera. Subsequently, the tumor is surgically removed together with the adjacent sclera and retina. The defect is replaced by a scleral graft. Approximately 25% of cases so treated have eventually required enucleation. Complications have included retinal detachment, vitreous hemorrhage, cataract, wound leak, and incomplete resection. This technique has not been widely adopted and must be considered experimental at this time.

Other Techniques

Immunotherapy and chemotherapy have future promise, but are not yet established as either useful principal modalities or effective adjuvant modes of therapy.[85-88]

Observation

In medium-sized melanomas, there are certain instances where careful periodic observation is warranted. Particularly in elderly patients with tumors that show little or no growth on serial examination, observation and documentation of size on a monthly or semi-monthly basis may be justified. Since prognosis is not improved by performing enucleation in older patients this course is probably supported.[89] Observation would appear particularly appropriate in an extremely old patient or in severely ill patients with a short life expectancy.

TUMORS WITH EXTRASCLERAL EXTENSION

It is generally recognized that patients with extrascleral extension have a poor prognosis. Exenteration of the orbit is probably the procedure employed most often and may yield good results, particularly when employed promptly after recognition of residual tumor in the orbit.[90] The precise technique (partial vs. complete exenteration) varies among different ophthalmic surgeons. Evaluation of data, by and large, is difficult, as it is often not clear if cases of apparent extrascleral extension truly have residual tumor in the orbit, or if the tumor extended close to the line of transsection. It seems likely that adjuvant therapy will find increasing use in these cases in upcoming years.[91]

METASTATIC DISEASE

The pattern of metastatic disease in ocular melanoma varies from that of cutaneous melanoma in that the lack of lymphatic drainage of the eye precludes the presence of lymphatic metastases prior to orbital spread. Hepatic metastases tend to predominate in ocular melanoma, but the tumor is capable of widespread metastatic dissemination. Metastatic melanoma is clearly incurable at present, and is generally treated with palliative chemotherapy and radiotherapy in a manner similar to metastatic cutaneous melanomas.[91]

REFERENCES

1. Rawles ME: Origin of pigment cells from neural crest in mouse embryo. Physiol Zool 20:248–266, 1947
2. Zimmerman LE: Melanocytes, melanocytic nevi and melanocytomas. Invest Ophthalmol 4:11–41, 1965
3. Cutler SJ, Young JL (eds): Third National Cancer Survey: Incidence Data. Natl Cancer Inst Monogr 41:1–454, 1975
4. Albert DM, Puliáfito CA, Fulton AB et al: Increased incidence of choroidal malignant melanoma occurring in a single population of chemical workers. Am J Ophthalmol 89:323–337, 1980
5. Scotto J, Fraumeni JF, Lee JAH: Melanomas of the eye and other noncutaneous sites. J Natl Cancer Inst 56:489–491, 9176
6. Keller AZ: Histology, survivorship, and related factors in the epidemiology of eye cancers. Am J Epidemiol 97:386–393, 1973
7. Albert DM: The association of viruses with uveal melanoma. Trans Am Ophthalmol Soc 77:367–421, 1980
8. Albert DM, Shadduck JA, Liu HS et al: Animal models for the study of uveal melanomas. Intl Ophthalmol Clin 20(2) (in press)
9. Evgen'eva TP: Pigmented tumors in rats induced by introduction of platinum and cellophane films into the chamber of the eye. Byulletin' Éksperimental' noi Biologii i Meditsiny 74:75–77, 1972
10. Patz A, Wulff LB, Rogers SW: Experimental production of ocular tumors. Am J Ophthalmol 48:98–111, 1959
11. Benson WR: Intraocular tumor after ethionine and N-2-fluorenyl-acetamide. Arch Pathol 73:404–406, 1962
12. Taylor GN, Dougherty TF, Mays CW et al: Radium-induced eye melanomas in dogs. Radiat Res 51:361–373, 1972
13. Elwood JM, Lee JA, Walter SD et al: Relationship of melanoma and other skin cancer mortality to latitude and ultraviolet radiation in the United States and Canada. Int J Epidemiol 3:325–332, 1972
14. Lee JA, Merrill JM: Sunlight and aetiology of malignant melanoma: a synthesis. Med J Aust 2:846–851, 1970
15. Walker JP, Weiter JJ, Albert DM et al: Uveal malignant melanoma in three generations of the same family. Am J Ophthalmol 88:723–726, 1979
16. Sang DN, Albert DM, Sober AJ et al: Nevus of Ota with contralateral cerebral melanoma. Arch Ophthalmol 95:1820–1824, 1977
17. Gartner S: Malignant melanoma of the choroid in von Recklinghausen's disease. Am J Ophthalmol 23:73–78, 1940
18. Fuchs E: Das Sarcom des Uvealtractus. Wein, Wilhelm Braumüller, 1882
19. Albert DM, Lahav M, Packer S et al: Histogenesis of malignant melanomas of the uvea: occurrence of nevus-like structures in experimental choroidal tumors. Arch Ophthalmol 92:318–328, 1974
20. Yanoff M, Zimmerman LE: Histogenesis of malignant melanoma of the uvea. II. Relationship of uveal nevi to malignant melanomas. Cancer 20:493–507, 1967
21. Yanoff M, Zimmerman LE: Histogenesis of malignant melanoma of the uvea. III. The relationship of congenital ocular melanocytosis and neurofibromatosis to uveal melanomas. Arch Ophthalmol 77:331–336, 1967
22. Callender GR: Malignant tumors of the eye: a study of histologic types in 111 cases. Trans Am Acad Ophthalmol Otolaryngol 36:131–142, 1931
23. Bierring F, Jensen OA: Electron microscopy of melanomas of the human uveal tract: the ultrastructure of four malignant melanomas of the mixed cell type. Acta Ophthalmol (Kbh) 42:665–671, 1964
24. Callender GR, Wilder HC, Ash JE: Five hundred malignant melanomas of the choroid and ciliary body followed five years or longer. Am J Ophthalmol 25:962–967, 1942
25. McLean IW, Zimmerman LE, Evans RM: Reappraisal of Callender's spindle A type of malignant melanoma of the choroid and ciliary body. Am J Ophthalmol 86:557–564, 1978
26. Wilder HC, Callender GR: Malignant melanoma of the choroid: further studies of prognosis by histologic type and fiber content. Am J Ophthalmol 22:851–855, 1939
27. Wilder HC, Paul E: Malignant melanoma of the choroid and ciliary body: a study of 2,533 cases. Milit Surg 109:370–378, 1951
28. Jensen OA: Malignant melanoma of the uvea in Denmark, 1943–1952: a clinical, histopathologic and prognostic study. Acta Ophthalmol (suppl) 75:1–220, 1963
29. Jensen OA: Malignant melanoma of the human uvea: recent follow-up of cases in Denmark, 1943–1952. Acta Ophthalmol 48:1113–1128, 1970
30. McLean IW, Foster WD, Zimmerman LE: Prognostic factors in small malignant melanomas of the choroid and ciliary body. Arch Ophthalmol 95:48–58, 1977
31. Shammas HF, Blodi FC: Prognostic factors in choroidal and ciliary body melanomas. Arch Ophthalmol 95:63–69, 1977
32. Zimmerman LE: Histologic considerations in the management of tumors of the iris and ciliary body. Ann Ist Barraquer 10:27–56, 1972
33. Ferry AP: Lesions mistaken for malignant melanoma of the iris. Arch Ophthalmol 74:9–18, 1965
34. Robertson DM, Campbell RJ: Errors in the diagnosis of malignant melanoma of the choroid. Am J Ophthalmol 87:269–275, 1979
35. Reese AB: Tumors of the Eye, 2nd ed. New York, Hoeber, 1963
36. Flindall RJ, Drance SM: Visual field studies of benign choroidal melanoma. Arch Ophthalmol 81:41–44, 1969
37. Shields JA: Current approaches to the diagnosis and management of choroidal melanomas. Surv Ophthalmol 21:443–463, 1977
38. Coleman DJ, Abramson DH, Jack RL et al: Ultrasonic diagnosis of tumors of the choroid. Am J Ophthalmol 91:344–354, 1974
39. Norton EWD, Smith JL, Curtin VT et al: Fluorescein fundus photography, an aid in the differential diagnosis of posterior ocular lesions. Trans Am Acad Ophthalmol Otolaryngol 68:755–765, 1964
40. Shields JA, McDonald PR, Leonard BC et al: The diagnosis of uveal malignant melanoma in eyes with opaque media. Am J Ophthalmol 83:95–105, 1977
41. Michelson JB, Felberg NT, Shields JA: Carcinoembryonic antigen: its role in the evaluation of intraocular malignant tumor. Arch Ophthalmol 94:414–416, 1976
42. Char DH: Inhibition of leukocyte migration with melanoma-associated antigen in choroidal tumors. Invest Ophthalmol Visual Sci 16:176–179, 1977
43. Brownstein S, Phillips TM, Lewis MG: Specificity of tumor-associated antibodies in serum of patients with uveal melanoma. Can J Ophthalmol 13:190–193, 1978
44. Char DH: Metastatic choroidal melanoma. Am J Ophthalmol 86:76–80, 1978
45. Heath P: Tumors of the iris: classification and clinical follow-up. Trans Am Ophthalmol Soc 62:51–85, 1964
46. Duke JR, Dunn SN: Primary tumors of the iris. Arch Ophthalmol 59:204–214, 1958

47. Ashton N: Primary tumors of the iris. Br J Ophthalmol 48:65–68, 1964
48. Holland G: Clinical features and pathology of pigmented tumors of the iris. Klin Monatsbl Augenheilkd 150:359–370, 1976
49. Rones B, Zimmerman LE: The prognosis of primary tumors of the iris treated by iridectomy. Arch Ophthalmol 60:193–205, 1958
50. Raivio I: Uveal melanoma in Finland. Acta Ophthalmol (suppl) (Kbh) 133:1–64, 1977
51. Sunba MN, Rahi AHS, Morgan G: Tumors of the anterior uveal tract. I. Metastasizing malignant melanoma of the iris. Arch Ophthalmol 98:82–85, 1980
52. Reese AB: Tumors of the Eye, 3rd ed, pp 229–262. Hagerstown, Maryland, Harper and Row, 1977
53. Cleasby GW: Malignant melanoma of the iris. Arch Ophthalmol 60:403–417, 1958
54. Duke-Elder WS, Stallard HH: Leukosarcoma of the iris. Br J Ophthalmol 14:158–161, 1930
55. Reese AB, Jones IS, Cooper WC: Surgery for tumors of the iris and ciliary body. Am J Ophthalmol 66:173–184, 1968
56. Raubitschek E: Über iristumoren. Klin Monatsbl Augenheilkd 52:683–694, 1914
57. Verhoeff FH: Sarcoma of the iris. Trans Am Ophthalmol Soc 31:270–271, 1933
58. Muller HK, Sollner F, Lund OE: Erfahrungen bei der Operativen Entferung von Tumoren der Iriswurzel und des Ciliarkörpers, Ber Und 63, pp 194–199. Heidelberg, Zusam Deutsch Ophthalmol Ges, 1960
59. Stallard HB: Partial cyclectomy. Br J Ophthalmol 45:797–802, 1961
60. Stallard HB: Partial iridocyclectomy and sclerectomy. Br J Opthalmol 50:656–659, 1966
61. Jones IS: Iridocyclectomy and corneoscleroiridocyclectomy. In Reese AB (ed): Tumors of the Eye, 3rd ed, pp 238–239. Hagerstown, Harper and Row, 1976
62. Sears ML: Technique for iridocyclectomy. Am J Ophthalmol 66:42–44, 1968
63. Forrest AW, Keyser RB, Spencer WH: Iridocyclectomy for melanomas of the ciliary body: a follow-up study of pathology and surgical morbidity. Trans Am Acad Ophthalmol Otolaryngol 85:1237–1250, 1978
64. Manschot WA, von Peperzeel HA: Choroidal melanoma: enucleation or observation? A new approach. Arch Ophthalmol 98:71–77, 1980
65. Zimmerman LE, McLean IW, Foster WD: Does enucleation of the eye containing a malignant melanoma prevent or accelerate the dissemination of tumor cells? Br J Ophthalmol 62:420–425, 1978
66. Zimmerman LE, McLean IW: An evaluation of enucleation in the management of uveal melanomas. Am J Ophthalmol 87:741–760, 1979
67. Abramson DH, Ellsworth RM: Treatment of choroidal melanomas. Bull NY Acad Med 54:849–854, 1978
68. Gass JDM: Problems in the differential diagnosis of choroidal nevi and malignant melanomas. Am J Ophthalmol 83:299–323, 1977
69. Barr CC, Sipperley JO, Nicholson DH: Small melanomas of the choroid. Arch Ophthalmol 96:1580–1582, 1978
70. Thomas JV, Green WR, Maumenee AE: Small choroidal melanomas: a long-term follow-up study. Arch Ophthalmol 97:861–864, 1979
71. Blodi FC: Ophthalmology. JAMA 243:2202–2203, 1980
72. Fraunfelder FT, Boozman FW III, Wilson RS et al: No-touch technique for intraocular malignant melanomas. Arch Ophthalmol 95:1616–1620, 1977
73. Seigel D, Myers M, Ferris F III et al: Survival rates after enucleation of eyes with malignant melanomas. Am J Ophthalmol 87:761–765, 1979
74. Gragoudas ES, Goitein M, Koehler AM et al: Proton irradiation of small choroidal malignant melanomas. Am J Ophthalmol 83:665–673, 1977
75. Stallard HB: Radiotherapy for malignant melanoma of the choroid. Br J Ophthalmol 50:147–155, 1966
76. Long RS, Galin MA, Rotman M: Conservative treatment of intraocular melanomas. Trans Am Acad Ophthalmol Otolaryngol 74:84–93, 1971
77. Davidorf FH, Makley TA, Lang JR: Radiotherapy of malignant melanoma of the choroid. Trans Am Acad Ophthalmol Otolaryngol 81:849–861, 1976
78. Lommatzsch P, Dietrich B: The effect of orbital radiation on the survival rate of patients with choroidal melanoma. Acta Ophthalmol 173:49–52, 1976
79. Sobanski J, Zeydler-Grzebzielewska L, Szusterowska-Martinowa E: Decreased mortality of patients with intranuclear malignant melanoma after enucleation of the eye, followed by orbit x-ray irradiation. Polish Med J 11:1512–1516, 1972
80. Shields JA: Current approaches to the management of posterior uveal melanomas. Trans Penna Acad Ophthalmol Otolaryngol 28:128–134, 1975
81. Vogel MH: Treatment of malignant choroidal melanomas with photocoagulation. Evaluation of one-year follow-up data. Am J Ophthalmol 74:1–11, 1972
82. Lincoff H, McLean J, Long R: The cryosurgical treatment of intraocular tumors. Am J Ophthalmol 63:389–390, 1977
83. Peyman GA, Ericson ES, Axelrod AJ et al: Full-thickness eyewall resection in primates. An experimental approach to the treatment of choroidal melanoma. Arch Ophthalmol 89:410–412, 1973
84. Peyman GA, Apple DJ: Local excision of a choroidal malignant melanoma. Full-thickness eyewall resection. Arch Ophthalmol 92:216–218, 1974
85. Smith GM: Ocular melanoma and immunotherapy. Ophthalmologica (Basel) 178:111–113, 1979
86. The TH, deGast GC, Huiges HA et al: Immunologic aspects of melanoma. Ophthalmologica (Basel) 175:25–27, 1977
87. Stark WJ, Rosenthal AR, Mullins GM, Green WR: Simultaneous bilateral uveal melanomas responding to BCNU therapy. Trans Am Acad Ophthalmol Otolaryngol 75:70–83, 1971
88. Liu HS, Refojo MF, Albert DM: Experimental combined systemic and local chemotherapy for intraocular malignancy. Arch Ophthalmol 98:905–908, 1980
89. Westerveld-Brandon ER, Zeeman WPC: The prognosis of melanoblastoma of the choroid. Ophthalmologica 134:20–29, 1957
90. Shammas HF, Blodi FC: Orbital exenteration of choroidal and ciliary body melanomas. Arch Ophthalmol 95:2002–2005, 1977
91. Nathanson L: National Eye Institute Ocular Melanoma Task Force Report. Am J Ophthalmol (in press)

Paul L. Kornblith
Michael D. Walker
J. Robert Cassady

CHAPTER 33

Neoplasms of the Central Nervous System

Tumors of the brain and spinal cord comprise a challenging area for clinicians as well as for research scientists. The tumors may be conveniently grouped into primary and secondary lesions. This chapter will deal with the primary or intrinsic group.

The intrinsic tumors of the central nervous system (CNS) pose particularly difficult problems. First, they rarely metastasize beyond the central nervous system pathways, yet they are often locally invasive. Second, the structures they involve are incapable of significant regeneration. Third, even tumors of benign histology may behave in a malignant fashion owing to their strategically inaccessible locations.

The modern era of brain tumor therapy began in the late 19th century. The first successful brain tumor removal was performed in 1879 by Sir William Macewen.[1] Another early craniotomy for tumor (a meningioma) was performed in 1884.[2] Other early reports of brain tumor therapy involved the work of V. Horsley and W.W. Keen.[3-4] Following Keen's report in 1898 there were additional successful tumor extirpations. It remained for Harvey Cushing to introduce a system for the successful care of brain tumor patients![5] Cushing, in a series of over 2000 brain tumor cases, described the behavior, histology, and classification of the lesions and designed successful approaches to their surgical removal and pre- and postoperative care.[6] Although Cushing's work was followed by a plethora of technical and neuropathological studies, the next major advances came from a better use of anesthesia and the introduction of neuroradiological contrast procedures, particularly the pneumoencephalogram (PEG) by Dandy, and the arteriogram by Moniz.[7-9] Following World War II, tremendous advances were seen in technical surgery and anesthetic support and it became possible to routinely remove benign, accessible brain and spinal cord tumors. Coincidentally, technical improvement in radiation therapy, especially the development of megavoltage equipment, occurred, making precisely delivered, high-dose treatment possible. Malignant lesions, frustrating to the neurosurgeon because of their invasiveness, usual unresectability, and propensity to subarachnoid spread, could now be effectively irradiated in many instances. Radiation therapy became the first measure to make a significant difference in the outcome of histologically malignant lesions, especially in children and young adults.[10] Improved skill in the use of radiotherapy has brought continued gains in therapeutic applications.

The current era of brain and spinal tumor therapy has seen a remarkable advance in microsurgical techniques for the treatment of difficult and inaccessible lesions. The treatment of histologically malignant tumors has also shown that certain chemotherapeutic agents, including the nitrosoureas, combined with surgery and irradiation, produce some improvement in therapy.[11]

In this chapter, the biological, anatomical, and pathological considerations of primary CNS neoplasms will be discussed and the clinical pictures of the tumors as a group will be described. Inasmuch as multimodal therapy is often required for each of the tumor types, the therapy discussions will include radiation and chemotherapy. The most speculative aspect, prospects for the future, will conclude the chapter.

EPIDEMIOLOGY AND INCIDENCE

EPIDEMIOLOGY

Genetics

We lack clearcut epidemiologic studies indicating any particular factors (viral, chemical, or traumatic) that cause brain tumors. Proof of a genetic predisposition for all central nervous system (CNS) tumors is not available; however, certain evidence pertains to specific tumor types which are of interest.

In human meningiomas it has been found that chromosome 22 has frequent abnormalities. These are usually in the form of dislocations and translocations.[12] Their significance is not known, but this does represent one of the few observations correlating chromosomal abnormalities in human tumors.

Neurofibromatosis clearly represents a genetic condition and is inherited as an autosomal phenomenon, evidence of hereditary predisposition. These patients develop not only cutaneous manifestations (*cafe-au-lait* and subcutaneous neurofibromas) but are likely to have bony and mesenchymal abnormalities related to the CNS and malignant glial tumors.[13] Twenty percent to over 50% of patients with optic glioma have co-existing von Recklinghausen's disease, especially patients with more anteriorly placed lesions.

Tuberous sclerosis, a disease involving CNS and cutaneous sites (Bourneville's disease), is another example of a condition with a genetic predisposition. In the intracranial tubers there may be nests of very bizarre astrocytes or neural-like cells. In addition to the acneiform facies (adenoma sebaceum) there are other cutaneous manifestations, including angiofibromas and periungual fibromas. Other intracranial tumors such as gangliogliomas are similar in histological features to those of tuberous sclerosis but merely lack the cutaneous picture. Most of the individuals afflicted with tuberous sclerosis manifest their problems early in life and mental retardation is common.[13]

In Turcot syndrome, a familial polyposis of the colon associated with malignant gliomas of the CNS, there are evidences of genetic factors.[14]

Chemical

At present there is little specific evidence linking CNS tumors to environmental carcinogens. However, many chemicals show carcinogenic activity in animals and produce CNS tumors. The most notable are those induced by ethyl- and methylnitrosourea, and those induced by anthracene derivatives.[15–17] In the ethylnitrosourea induction, exposure of the maternal animal results in a high proportion of her offspring developing nervous system lesions with the CNS predominantly involved. In methylnitrosourea treated animals, prolonged prenatal exposure leads to a virtually uniform incidence of CNS tumors with many being of a highly malignant, invasive nature.

Methylcholanthrene, anthracycline, and other anthracene derivatives have shown a propensity for CNS tumor production. In the few clinical studies done, vinyl chloride and rubber industry work have been implicated.

Viral

There is no evidence in humans for a viral etiology. The evidence deduced from animal models is, however, of interest. Using *Rous sarcoma* virus, a beagle tumor quite comparable to human malignant astrocytomas was obtained.[18] A murine astrocytoma was also produced by inoculation with purified avian sarcoma virus.[19] Perhaps the most striking evidence is recent work in which human polyoma J C virus injected into primates produced tumors compatible with human astrocytomas after an 18-month incubation period.[20] This type of "slow virus" effect may account for some of the problems in isolating viruses from human tumors.

Trauma

There is no evidence that trauma can lead to true CNS neoplasia. Trauma to the CNS, however, can result in indirect effects on tumors already present, especially hemorrhage, and thus appear to bear a causal relation.

INCIDENCE

The overall incidence of brain tumors is 10,000 cases per year and of spinal cord tumors is 4,000 cases per year. Central nervous system tumors comprise the most common group of solid tumors of the young, accounting for 20% of all pediatric neoplasms, and appear to have a second peak of incidence in later years.

The majority of brain tumors occur in two age peaks, one in childhood (3 years to 12 years); the other in later life (50 years to 70 years).[21,22] The pediatric tumors are quite different in histology and behavior from those of adult life. Nearly two-thirds of pediatric CNS lesions are infratentorial in location, whereas an equivalent proportion of adult tumors are supratentorial. Therefore, most pediatric gliomas arise in the cerebellum, brain stem, or midbrain/thalamus region. Cortical or hemispheric lesions are seen with much greater frequency in the adult population. Males are afflicted equally with females but astrocytomas are more common in males and meningiomas in females. The age and sex incidence are shown in Tables 33-1 *A,B*.

ANATOMIC CONSIDERATIONS

The anatomic location of a CNS tumor has critical implications on morbidity to be expected following surgery. These anatomical barriers to safe surgical treatment have required the development of elaborate clinical strategies to provide effective therapy. The major problem is the inability of the CNS tissues to undergo regeneration. Even minimal surgical interference may result in permanent deficits.

In this section anatomical features that need to be considered in understanding the pathophysiology of tumor evolution and in the planning of therapy will be discussed. Specific CNS areas will be considered separately and the information provided is modified from several sources of neuroanatomical correlation.[23–25] The primary emphasis will be on the surgical implications of the neuroanatomy. There are two major

TABLE 33-1*A*. Incidence of Brain Tumors According to Age

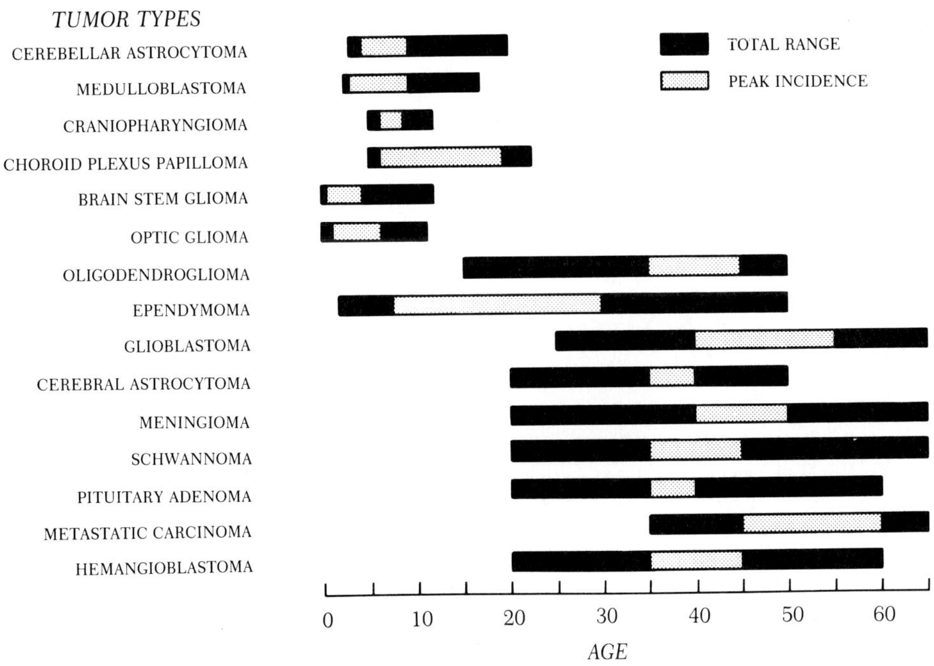

TUMOR TYPES

CEREBELLAR ASTROCYTOMA
MEDULLOBLASTOMA
CRANIOPHARYNGIOMA
CHOROID PLEXUS PAPILLOMA
BRAIN STEM GLIOMA
OPTIC GLIOMA
OLIGODENDROGLIOMA
EPENDYMOMA
GLIOBLASTOMA
CEREBRAL ASTROCYTOMA
MENINGIOMA
SCHWANNOMA
PITUITARY ADENOMA
METASTATIC CARCINOMA
HEMANGIOBLASTOMA

TOTAL RANGE
PEAK INCIDENCE

0 10 20 30 40 50 60
AGE

(Youmans JR: Neurological Surgery, vol III. Philadelphia, WB Saunders, 1973, p 1321)

intracranial compartments, the supratentorial and the infratentorial. The supratentorial includes the cerebral hemispheres and the sellar, pineal, and upper brain stem regions. The infratentorial includes the brain stem, pons, medulla, and cerebellum and leads into the upper spinal cord.

CEREBRAL HEMISPHERES

The majority of CNS tumors are situated in the cerebral hemisphere and these distinct boundaries of an anatomic and functional nature are significant. As can be seen in Fig. 33-1, the hemispheres comprise frontal, parietal, occipital, and temporal lobes as major loci. The frontal lobes are concerned with behavioral organization, planning and association; parietal lobes with motor, sensory, and complex intellectual functions; occipital lobes with vision; and temporal lobes with behavior, memory, speech, emotion, and auditory–visual pathways.

Unilateral removal of either frontal lobe can be tolerated. Deficits of intellectual function which may occur are often transient.[26] Bifrontal removal or removal of one frontal lobe in a patient whose contralateral frontal lobe is already compromised by tumor usually results in behavioral and association losses that are irreparable.[27] Unilateral occipital lobectomy results in loss of vision of a hemianoptic type but may be acceptable in certain cases in which circumscribed benign tumors are entirely confined to the occipital lobe. Bilateral occipital ablation results in total blindness, and is virtually never indicated.

Lesions in the parietal lobe pose particular problems, as removal of significant amounts of these areas produces major and often disabling deficits. The left parietal lobe in patients who are right handed controls speech as well as sensory and motor functions and should not be considered an area for normal tissue removal. The right parietal lobe, which has control of the left side of the body, is concerned with complex cognitive functions (concepts of space, music, and other abstractions) and motor–sensory control.

TABLE 33-1*B*. Incidence of Brain Tumors According to Sex

TYPE OF TUMOR	M:F RATIO	
Medulloblastomas	5:2	
Oligodendrogliomas	9:7	
Astrocytomas	3:2	
Glioblastomas	2:1	
Ependymomas	6:5	
Pinealomas	3:1	
Angioblastomas	2:1	Male preponderance
Craniopharyngiomas	2:1	
Epidermoids	5:2	
Teratomas	7:4	
Angiomas and aneurysms	2:1	
Metastases	6:5	
Meningiomas	7:6	
Neurinomas	2:1	Female preponderance

(McKeran RO, Thomas DGT: The clinical study of gliomas. In Thomas DGT, Graham DI (eds): Brain Tumours: Scientific Basis, Clinical Investigation and Current Therapy, p 197. London, Butterworths, 1980)

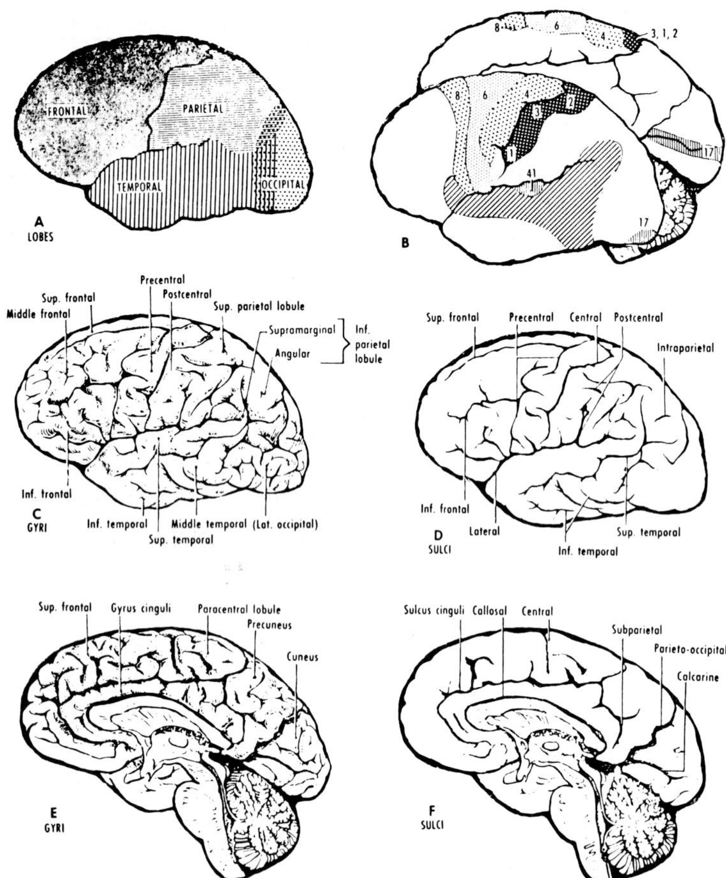

FIG. 33-1. Cerebral hemispheres, gross anatomy. The primary lobes, gyri and sulci are depicted in *A, C, D, E*, and *F*. In *B* the functional areas according to Brodmann are described. (Gardner E, Gray DJ, O'Rahilly R: Anatomy—A Regional Study of Human Structure, 4th ed. Philadelphia, WB Saunders, 1975, p 585)

Unilateral, anterior temporal lobe resections produce minimal deficits whereas bilateral surgical intervention is quite likely to result in marked behavioral and memory problems.[26,27] Posterior temporal areas are not amenable to surgical removal, as the hippocampal formation, dentate gyrus, and parahippocampal gyrus are needed for memory.

In addition to these fundamental functional anatomic limitations there are major anatomic considerations of a vascular nature. Whereas removal or encroachment upon certain vessels can be tolerated, it is crucial to determine what vessels are involved pre-operatively, so that accurate judgements can be made as to the territory supplied.

Certain specific vessels must be carefully considered anatomically in view of their essential blood supply to critical areas. For example, the middle cerebral arteries, their proximal branches, and even the small proximal penetrating vessels, which supply major motor and speech areas of the parietal lobe, are critical. The anterior and posterior communicating arteries and their small branches provide cerebral as well as brain stem vascularization. Obviously, all vessels in the brain are important for the area supplied; however, there can be a preoperative appreciation for potential cross-circulation or anastomotic channels through preoperative arteriography. A further important consideration is the role played by the extracranial circulation in supplying tumors, especially meningiomas. It is often necessary to visualize these vessels separately before surgery by selective external carotid study to determine their contributions.

An important general anatomic consideration of cerebral tumors is that they can manifest their effects through intracranial pressure increase. This increase can cause specific cranial nerve compression—such as optic nerve compression resulting in blindness, or ocular motor nerve damage resulting in ocular motility defects. Increased pressure can also indirectly cause clinical symptoms by way of ventricular compression or blockage resulting in hydrocephalus. Detection of hydrocephalus by way of CT scan is therefore a very useful pre-operative finding.

The most critical type of tumor related pressure syndromes results from effects on the major cerebral elements, such as the temporal lobes. Tumors impinging on the temporal region can result in the syndrome of uncal herniation, with compression of the uncus and the midbrain with resultant death. Because of the long pathway of the oculomotor nerve, this process of herniation results in a characteristic dilated pupil.

CEREBELLUM

The posterior fossa is an extremely confined space and even minimal increments in pressure in this space can result in death from cerebellar tonsillar herniation. On the other hand, removal of relatively large portions of the cerebellum other than the midline and deep nuclei can be tolerated after transient periods of cerebellar deficits.

Resection of either cerebellar hemisphere can be followed by ipsilateral dysmetria, dysdiadochokinesia, and intention tremor. Removal of, or injury to, the midline cerebellum (vermis) results in ataxia and gait instability, which can be in part compensated for by the patient.

The vascular supply to the cerebellum from the basilar artery and the posterior communicating vessels relates also to critical brain stem functions. Furthermore, ischemic or occlusive vascular disease in the basilar distribution can result in cerebellar infarction, swelling, and tonsilar herniation.

BRAIN STEM, PONS, MEDULLA OBLONGATA

Tumors in these areas are generally not amenable to surgical resection and even small tumor masses cause significant deficits. Occasionally a biopsy of a pontine lesion is feasible.

Although tumors involving these structures can infiltrate surrounding areas, nonsurgical treatment such as radiotherapy can be useful. The intrinsic lesions which have a predilection for this area are almost exclusively infiltrating tumors, usually of fairly primitive neuroectodermal elements; that is, medulloblastoma or pontine glioma. The anatomic relations of these structures are shown in Fig. 33-2*A*,*B*. The vascular supply depicted is essential and damage to vessels supplying these structures results in significant deficits. The syndromes associated with these areas are given in Table 33-2*A*.

Tumors in the region of the IV ventricle can produce hydrocephalus with its sequelae of increased pressure and neurological dysfunction.

CEREBELLOPONTINE ANGLE (CPA)

An area of particular anatomic import in relation to tumors is the CPA. Certain of the most treatable yet potentially devastating tumors, such as acoustic neuromas and meningiomas, reside in this region. The relation of acoustic nerve tumors to cranial nerve VIII makes hearing loss an important finding. As tumors progress the relation to nerve VII may result in facial weakness. If tumor growth continues, then the direct compression of the vital structures of the brain stem results in paralysis or death.

The vessels of this area include branches of the posterior inferior cerebellar artery (PICA). Small perforating vessels can be crucial to brain stem function. Even traction of tumors in the CPA can cause brain stem dysfunction on either a direct or a vascular basis. Until the advent of microsurgical techniques, the anatomic relations of CPA tumors precluded their surgically safe treatment. With these techniques, the PICA, the perforating vessels, and nerves VII and VIII can be so well visualized that surgical extirpation is feasible with minimal risk and a reasonable likelihood of preserving facial nerve function and, occasionally, some acoustic nerve function.

SELLA AND SUPRASELLA

This discrete anatomical region has both intrasellar and suprasellar lesions. These tumors and their corresponding

(Text continues on page 1188)

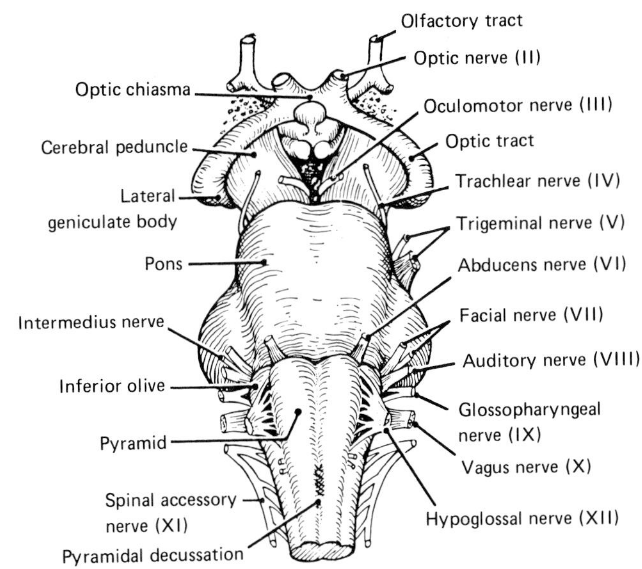

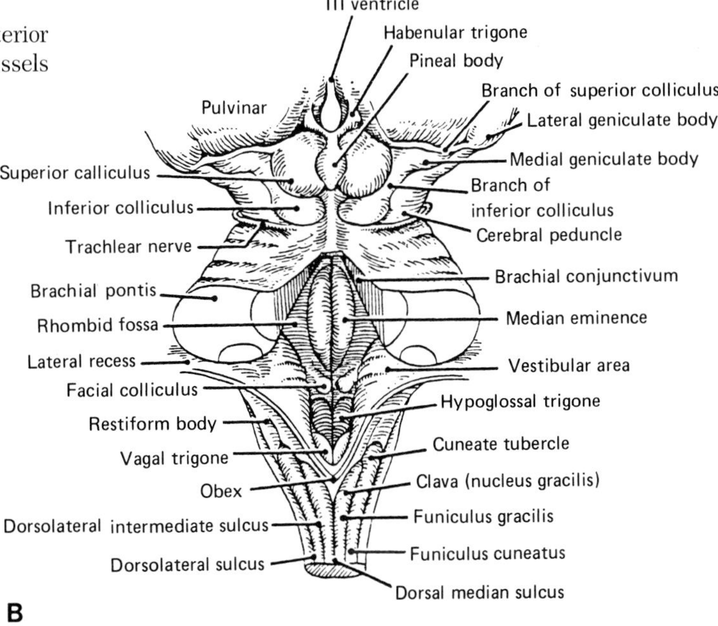

FIG. 33-2. Medulla, pons, and midbrain: (*A*) anterior view, (*B*) posterior view. (Truex RC, Carpenter MB: Strong and Elwyn's Human Neuroanatomy, 5th ed. Baltimore, Williams and Wilkins, 1964, pp 252, 253)

TABLE 33-2*A*. Clinical Syndromes Associated with Lesions of Brain Stem, Pons and Medulla Oblongata

SITE OF LESION	EPONYM	CLINICAL SYMPTOMS	ETIOLOGY
Anterior part of the base of the skull		Olfactory disturbances (uni- or bilateral anosmia), possibly psychiatric disturbances, epileptic attacks.	Tumors that have invaded the anterior part of the base of the skull from the frontal sinus or the ethmoid bone, osteomas. Malignant tumors; meningiomas of the olfactory groove.
Superior orbital fissure	Rochon–Duvigneau; syndrome of the pterygopalatine fossa (Behr) and the base of the orbit (DeJean) commencing with a lesion of the maxillary and pterygoid rami and evolving into the superior orbital fissure syndrome.	Lesions of the IIIrd, IVth, and VIth nerve and first division of the VIth nerve with ophthalmoplegia, pain and sensory disturbances in the area of V_1; often exophthalmos, some vegetative disturbances.	Tumors: meningiomas, osteomas, dermoid cysts, giant cell tumors, tumors of the orbit, nasopharyngeal tumors, more rarely optic nerve gliomas, eosinophilic granulomas, angiomas, local or neighbouring infections, trauma.
Apex of the orbit (infraclinoid syndrome of Dandy)	Jacod–Rollet (often combined with the syndrome of the superior orbital fissure).	Optic nerve symptoms with visual disturbances, central scotoma, papilloedema, optic nerve atrophy; occasional exophthalmos, chemosis.	Optic nerve glioma, infraclinoid aneurysm of the internal carotid artery (Dandy), trauma, orbital tumors, Paget's disease.
Cavernous sinus	Foix–Jefferson; syndrome of the sphenopetrosal fissure (Bonnet and Bonnet) corresponding in part to the cavernous sinus syndrome of Raeder, involving the trigeminal nerve and the sympathetic plexus–paratrigeminal syndrome.	Ophthalmoplegia due to lesions of the IIIrd, IVth, VIth, and often Vth nerves, exophthalmos, vegetative disturbances. Jefferson distinguished three symptom complexes: the anterior–superior syndrome corresponds to the superior orbital fissure syndrome. The middle one causes ophthalmoplegia and lesions of V_1 and V_2. The caudal syndrome also in addition affects the whole trigeminal nerve.	Tumors of the sellar and parasellar area, infraclinoid aneurysms of the internal carotid artery, nasopharyngeal tumors, fistulae of the sinus cavernosus and the carotid artery (traumatic), tumors of the middle cranial fossa, *e.g.*, chondromas, meningiomas, and neurinomas.
Apex of the petrous temporal bone	Gradenigo–Lannois	Lesions of the Vth and VIth nerves with neuralgia, sensory and motor disturbances, double vision.	Inflammatory processes (otitis), tumors of the pyramids such as cholesteatomas, chondromas, meningiomas, neurinomas of the gasserian ganglion and trigeminal root, primary and secondary sarcomas of the base of the skull.
Sphenoid and petrosal bones (petro–sphenoidal syndrome)	Jacod	Ophthalmoplegia due to loss of function of the IIIrd, IVth, and VIth nerves, amaurosis, trigeminal neuralgia possibly with sensory disturbances.	Tumors of the sphenoid and petrosal bone areas, the middle cranial fossa, nasopharyngeal tumors, metastases.
Jugular foramen	Vernet	Lesions of IXth, Xth, and XIth nerves with disturbance of deglutition, curtain phenomenon, sensory disturbances of the tongue, soft palate, pharynx and larynx, hoarseness, weakness of the sternocleido mastoid and the trapezius.	Tumors of the glomus jugulare. Neurinomas of VIIIth, IXth, Xth and XIth nerves, chondromas, cholesteatomas, meningiomas, nasopharyngeal and ear tumors, infections, angiomatose processes, rarely trauma.
Anterior occipital condyles	Sicard–Collet (Vernet–Sargnon)	Loss of XIIth nerve function in addition to the symptoms of the jugular foramen with loss of normal tongue mobility.	Tumors of the base of the skull, ear, the parotid, disease of the hematopoietic system, aneurysms, angiomas, and inflammations.
Retro-parotid space (retro-pharyngeal syndrome)	Villaret	Lesions of the lower group of nerves (Sicard–Collet) and Bernard–Horner syndrome with ptosis, miosis, and enophthalmos.	Tumors of the retro-parotid space (carcinomas, sarcomas), trauma, inflammations.

TABLE 33-2*A*. (Continued)

SITE OF LESION	EPONYM	CLINICAL SYMPTOMS	ETIOLOGY
Half of the base of the skull	Garcin (Guillain–Alajouanine–Garcin). This syndrome was also described by Hartmann in 1904.	Loss of function of all XII cranial nerves of one side. In many cases, isolated cranial nerves spared. Rarely signs of raised intracranial pressure or pyramidal tract symptoms.	Nasopharyngeal tumors, primary tumors of the base of the skull, disease of the hematopoietic organs, trauma, metastases.
Cerebello–pontine angle		Loss of function of VIIIth nerve (hearing loss, vertigo, nystagmus), cerebellar disturbances, lesions of the Vth, VIIth, and possibly IXth–XIIth, cranial nerves. Signs of raised intracranial pressure, brain stem symptoms.	Tumors; acoustic neurinomas (raised protein in CSF), meningiomas, cholesteatomas, metastases, cerebellar tumors, neurinomas of the caudal group of nerves and the trigeminal nerve, vascular processes such as angiomas, basilaris ektasia (own case), aneurysms.

(Bingas B: Tumours of the Base of the Skull. In Vinken PJ, Bruyn GW (eds): Handbook of Clinical Neurology: Tumours of the Brain and Skull, Part II, Vol. 17. Amsterdam, North-Holland, 1974; pp 181, 182)

TABLE 33-2*B*. Clinical Syndromes Associated with Tumors of Sellar Region

		DISORDERS OF			
LOCALIZATION	TUMOR	*Anterior Pituitary Gland*	*Hypo-thalamus*	INCIDENCE AND DEGREE	SYNDROMES
In the sella	Adenoma	+			Cushing's disease,
	Active				acromegaly, gigantism
	Inactive	+			Forbes–Albright
			(+)		syndrome, hypopituitarism
	Chondroma	+			
	Metastasis	+			
	Craniopharyngioma			Regular	
	Intrasellar	+		Clinically manifest	
	Intrasellar + suprasellar	+	+		
Close to the sella	Suprasellar craniopharyngioma		+	Regular, clinically manifest	Adiposogenital dystrophy (Fröhlich)
	Suprasellar meningioma		(+)		
	Suprasellar epidermoid				
	Optic pathway glioma		(+)	Rare	Russell's syndrome
	Hypothalamic glioma		+	Frequent	Precocious puberty
	Hypothalamic hamartoma		+	Clinically manifest	
	Pineal tumors		+	Frequent, clinically manifest	
	Tumors with aqueductal obstruction and hydrocephalus		+		Cushingoid
Remote from the sella	Cerebral hemispheres	(+)	(+)	Rare	
	Meningioma glioma			Latent	

(Fahlbusch R, Marguth F: Endocrine Disorders Associated with Intracranial tumors. In Vinken PJ, Bruyn GW (eds): Handbook of Clinical Neurology; Tumors of the Brain and Skull, Part I, Volume 16, p 345. Amsterdam, North Holland, 1974)

endocrinological disorders are depicted in Table 33-2*B*. Intrasellar lesions (pituitary adenomas) are usually confined by the bony sellar floor and the tough diaphragma sellae above with the result that their early effects cause bony erosion particularly of the clinoid processes or the floor of the sella. Slow but progressive growth may cause bone remodeling without invasion or erosion and create a so-called "double floor." As tumor growth progresses, the diaphragma can become distorted and the optic nerves immediately above the diaphragma become stretched, compressed, and compromised resulting in the typical bitemporal hemianoptic field defect. Further growth then can result in extension either into the sphenoid sinus below, by continued bony erosion, or into the temporal lobes by lateral extension. The proximity of the carotid and jugular vessels is of serious concern, as the tumor may erode or compress these structures.

Suprasellar lesions may either arise from within the sella and then extend upwards in a dumbbell-shaped fashion (pituitary adenomas, craniopharyngiomas); arise from the dura (meningiomas); or be entirely suprasellar (craniopharyngiomas). The upward extension brings these tumors in contact with the hypothalamus, possibly causing serious metabolic and behavioral dysfunction. If these tumors enlarge sufficiently they may project into the third ventricle, causing ventricular obstruction either at the foramen of Munro or at the aqueduct of Sylvius. The vascular supply of the pituitary has particular significance to its endocrine functions.[28] The detailed surgical vascular anatomy of the pituitary has been described by Rhoton.[29,30]

PINEAL AREA

Tumors of the pineal gland are in a position to encroach upon ventricle III and also impinge upon the midbrain (mesencephalus tegmentum), resulting in the typical Parinaud's syndrome (paralysis of conjugate upward movement of the eyes, pupillary arreflexia to light, and loss of convergence) associated with many pineal neoplasms.

Until relatively recently, the pineal area was considered largely inaccessible. However, as demonstrated by Stein and others pineal tumors can now be approached surgically with significant risk.[31,32]

SPINAL CORD

The major anatomic considerations of spinal cord tumors relate to the tumor location and the spinal dura. Those tumors outside the dura are usually secondary (metastatic) in nature. The intradural tumors may be in the cord itself (intradural, intramedullary) or on the nerve roots or coverings of the cord (intradural, extramedullary). The intramedullary lesions (usually astrocytomas or ependymomas) are located in the substance of the cord and present difficult problems in surgical removal. The extramedullary lesions are often removable when situated on a nerve root (neurofibroma) or associated with the coverings (meningiomas).

The intradural tumors cause compression of neural structures and vasculature. The syndromes produced vary by the level, the size, and the extent of the lesion. Partial or intermittent CSF blockage may occur initially, followed by complete block, resulting in cessation of cord function and neural transmission below the affected level. Both partial and complete blocks can be visualized on myelography with their features depending on the compartment harboring the tumor. The relations are shown in Fig. 33-3.

PATHOLOGY

The classification of brain tumors has been categorized in many different ways depending upon the concept of "cell of origin." With evolution in our understanding of the biology and embryology of the cells these concepts continue to change. In Table 33-3 are given the classifications of Bailey-Cushing and of Kernohan-Sayre.[22] The latter classification and the one used by Rubinstein are the framework for this discussion.[33]* The superb scholarship of Penfield and of Rio Hortega is crucial to our knowledge of tumor cell types and is integrated in part in this system.[35,36] The tumors are grouped by their cell of origin and described in the order of their frequency.

In assessing the malignant potential of a brain tumor it is important to understand the difference between cytologic and biologic malignancy. Cytologic malignancy is a morphologic assessment of anaplasia based upon cytologic and nuclear pleomorphism, cellularity, necrosis, mitoses, and invasiveness. Biologic malignancy is the likelihood that a tumor will kill the patient. Most cytologically malignant brain tumors are also biologically malignant despite treatment presently available. Various factors, including the brain's exquisite sensitivity to increased internal pressure, dictate that certain cytologically benign tumors are biologically malignant.

GLIOMAS

Gliomas comprise about 60% of all primary CNS tumors. Their common embryonic layer of origin is neuro–ectodermal and they constitute the bulk of the intrinsic intraparenchymal tumors of both brain and spinal cord.

There are five fairly distinct types among glial cells: astrocytes, oligodendroglia, ependymal cells, microglia, and neuroglial precursors. Each of these gives rise to tumors of different biological and anatomic characteristics. The neuroepithelial origin of microglia is in question.[37] The histiocytic lymphoma may be the neoplastic counterpart of microglia and is discussed on page 1193.

Astrocytoma

Astrocytes comprise the vast majority of the intraparenchymal cells of the brain. Their function appears to be as a supporting tissue for neurons, but the precise interrelations of astrocytes and neurons remain unclear.

From astrocytes arise a variety of tumors ranging from benign to highly malignant. The benign lesions include cystic cerebellar astrocytomas, juvenile pilocytic astrocytomas, and the fairly distinctive optic nerve glioma. The malignant forms include the graded series of astrocytomas with the ultimate

* A new classification has been developed which is going to come into common usage.[34]

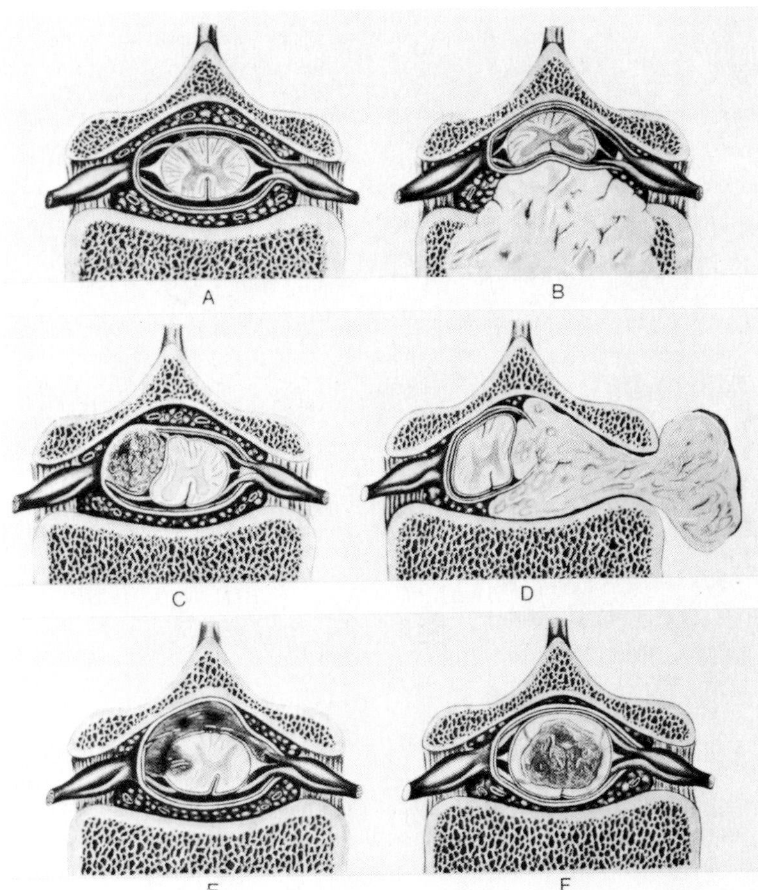

FIG. 33-3. Relationship of different types of spinal cord tumor to the spinal cord: (*A*) normal relationship; (*B*) extradural, extramedullary tumor (usually metastasis); (*C*) intradural, extramedullary tumor, *e.g.*, meningioma; (*D*) extradural and intradural tumor, *e.g.*, neurofibroma, meningioma; (*E*) intradural, extramedullary and intramedullary tumor, *e.g.*, neurofibroma; (*F*) intradural, intramedullary astrocytoma, epindymoma. (Shafer ER: Chirurgie des Gehirns und Rückenmarks im Kindes- und Jugendalter (Bushe KA, Glees P, eds). Stuttgart, Hippokrates-Verlag, 1968, p 1159)

being the highly malignant glioblastoma multiforme. A prognostically valuable system of subclassification of astrocytomas is that of Kernohan in which astrocytomas are graded from I–IV with Grade IV the most malignant and Grade I cytologically (but not necessarily biologically) benign. The features used in this classification scheme depend upon cellularity, vascularity, nuclear detail, and amount of necrosis. In the Grade I astrocytoma hypercellularity is the major feature. It is at times difficult to determine whether a Grade I is "astrocytosis" or an astrocytoma. In ascending grades (Grade II and above) there is a gradual progression of vascular proliferation and nuclear pleomorphism. Grade III astrocytomas have malignant cytologic features including mitoses and hyperchromatic nuclei. In the Grade IV neoplasm there is a significant amount of necrosis, and hemorrhage and marked variation in cell size and detail. In an attempt to define pediatric cerebellar astrocytomas more precisely, Winston and colleagues have developed a scheme utilizing clusters of histological details to determine activity.[38,39] This allows further subdivision of many of these astrocytomas (vide infra).

TABLE 33-3. Classification and Grading of Brain Tumors According to Cushing-Bailey and Kernohan.

MODIFIED BAILEY-CUSHING	KERNOHAN AND OTHERS
Astrocytoma	Astrocytoma, Grades I and II
Oligodendroglioma	Oligodendroglioma, Grades I to IV
Ependymoma	Ependymoma
Medulloblastoma	Medulloblastoma
Glioblastoma multiforme	Astrocytoma, Grades III and IV
Pinealoma (teratoma)	Pinealoma
Ganglioneuroma (ganglioglioma)	Neuroastrocytoma, Grade I
Neuroblastoma (sympathicoblastoma)	Neuroastrocytoma, Grades II to IV
Papilloma of choroid plexus	
Mixed	
Unclassified	

(Youmans JR: Neurological Surgery, vol III, Philadelphia, WB Saunders, 1973, p 1303)

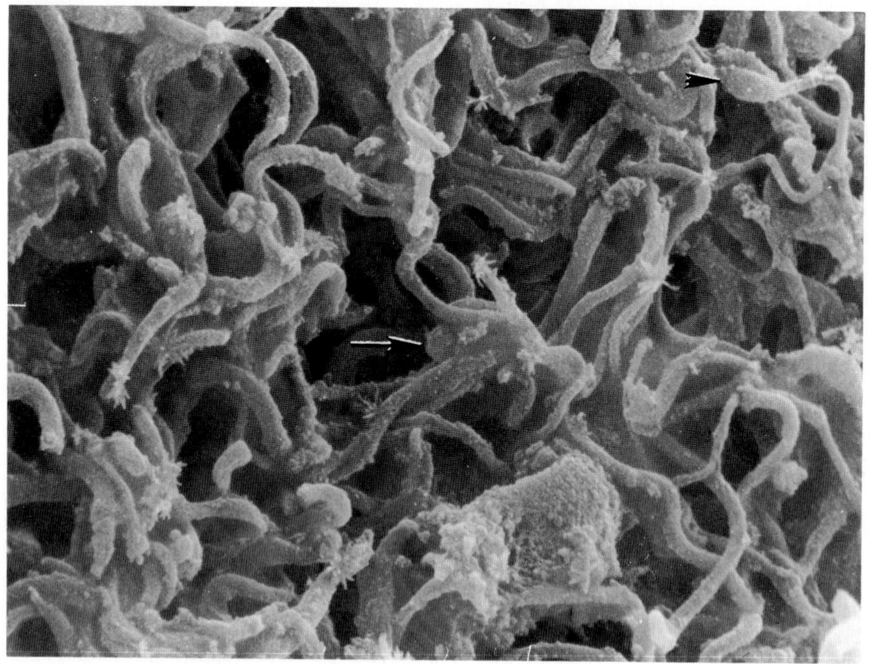

FIG. 33-4. Scanning micrograph of astrocytoma fibrils. Juvenile piloid astrocytoma seen by scanning electron microscopy. Octapoid cells (arrow) project numerous, twisted, cylindrical processes with smooth surfaces. Focally thickened processes (arrowhead) contain Rosenthal fibers; × 7700. (McKeever PE: Scanning electron microscopy in the evaluation of neurosurgical neoplasms: A review of new approaches. Neurosurgery 4:345, 1979)

As demonstrated by Rubinstein, tissue culture may also be useful in helping to characterize tumors as to their cells of origin and biological characteristics.[33] Kinetics and morphological and ultrastructural details, as well as tumorogenicity, may be refined sufficiently to help give a dynamic characterization of tumor growth potentials as described by Kornblith.[40] In the astrocytomas there is more rapid growth, tumor doubling, loss of morphological features such as processes and glial fibrils, as one progresses from benign to malignant lesions.

Certain specific subgroups of astrocytomas deserve special mention. Optic nerve glioma is an astrocytoma of childhood in which astrocytes proliferate within the optic nerve sheath. It may be accompanied by the CNS form of von Recklinghausen's neurofibromatosis (10%).[33] The appearance of the cells is often like the more malignant astrocytomas with large cells, occasionally multinucleated and quite bizarre. However, the clinical behavior of this tumor is often characterized by slow growth over a period of years and an evolution of a fairly benign lesion. Some data suggest that certain of these tumors may regress spontaneously.

Microcystic cerebellar astrocytomas of children are extremely benign tumors in which a localized tumor nodule is associated with a cystic fluid-filled mass comprising the bulk of the tumor.[36] In juvenile cortical astrocytomas and in some of the adult piloid astrocytomas there is sufficiently slow growth that the tumors develop Rosenthal fibers and gliofibrillary tangles. Scanning electron microscopy shows stellate and octapoid cells which project serpentine, cylindrical fibrils swollen in place by Rosenthal fibers (Fig. 33-4). At the other end of the histologic spectrum, semistocytic astrocytomas are populated with large "gemistocytes" swollen with eosinophilic cytoplasm and, in the glioblastoma multiforme, extremely bizarre multinucleated pleomorphic cells appear.

In adults, brain tumors have a predilection for the cerebral hemispheres whereas in children, the predilection is for the cerebellum and brain stem.

The local gross pathological behavior is determined by the degree of histologic malignancy and by the invasive nature of the lesions. Paradoxically, some benign Grade I astrocytomas may be quite extensive and indeed invasive. Even certain malignant astrocytomas may be encapsulated or pseudoencapsulated. Generally, the benign tumors tend to be more localized and the malignant tumors more invasive. A continuing problem is the apparent multifocal nature of many malignant astrocytomas in which distant tumor loci are found. It represents migration of cells from the original tumor.

Oligodendroglioma

Oligodendroglia are satellite cells which are found in proximity to neurons and are involved in the process of myelination. They may even form myelin figures when in tissue culture. The cells have a distinctive "halo" or "fried egg" appearance with a clear zone surrounding a round or ovoid nucleus and relatively scant cytoplasm.

The tumors from these cells are usually benign but may occasionally be malignant. Frequently oligodendroglial tumors have astrocytic admixtures. The presence of a significant portion of oligodendroglia in an astrocytoma is a favorable sign. Oligodendrogliomas, in particular the benign, slow growing forms, are frequently likely to have calcifications in association with the tumor mass. They tend to be fairly solid and discrete from surrounding brain. The sites of predilection are the cortex and in particular the frontal and parietal lobes.

Medulloblastoma

This tumor is primarily a pediatric age group tumor. The exact nature and location of the neuroglial precursor cell of origin of the medulloblastoma is a matter of debate. The likely candidates are the cells which populate the external granular cell layer of the fetal and neonatal cerebellum and the cells in the medullary vela.[41] Recent ultrastructural and tissue culture studies of medulloblastomas tend to support combination of astroglial and neuronal features.[42] Their cells have both glial type fibrils and synaptic type vesicles.

This tumor tends to grow aggressively and is always malignant in its histology. The tumor is invasive and not encapsualted. The cells have an elongated "carrot" shape and a field of cells are distinctively homogeneous. The cells and nuclei are very darkly staining.

The tumor originates in the cerebellum. It can spread by way of CSF pathways and secondary tumors can appear in cervical or lumbar spinal areas as well as in other areas proximate to the ventricular system. Widespread distant metastases are occasionally seen, especially with better local control and prolongation of survival.

Ependymoma

Ependymal cells line the cavities of the CNS and are distinguished by their cilia which help in CSF movement. The cells are of neuroectodermal origin and can be found in the linings of the ventricular cavities and the central canal of the spinal cord. Tumors which arise from these cells can be located either in brain or spinal cord and are deeply situated within the CNS.

Ependymomas may vary greatly in their rates of growth and certain lesions may be relatively benign, whereas others grow quite rapidly. These tumors are more common in children and comprise a major group of spinal cord intramedullary tumors.

The tumor can be identified by its angulated cells, oval nuclei with pinpoint chromatin, true ependymal rosettes, perivascular pseudorosettes, or the finding of blepharoblasts which appear to be the anchoring points for the attachment of the cilia. In true rosettes, the cells tend to form circular arrangements as if enclosing a cavity or tube and, occasionally, cilia can be seen. The more common pseudorosettes are formed by numerous tumor cell processes surrounding central vessels like spokes surrounding an axle (Fig. 33-5). Scanning electron microscopy shows long, thin, cylindrical fibrils which project from spherical cells.

These tumors are quite invasive but sometimes have an indolent growth pattern. The tumors are not encapsulated but may be fairly well demarcated from surrounding normal CNS tissues. Their texture and coloration (somewhat purplish) are helpful in distinguishing tumor from surrounding tissue.

NEURAL SERIES

Neural tumors of the CNS are extremely rare. The most common neural series tumor, the neuroblastoma, almost never occurs as a primary CNS lesion. Of the CNS neural tumors, the ganglion cell tumors, ganglioglioma, and ganglioneuroma are most representative. Tuberous sclerosis is accompanied in certain cases by CNS tubers, which are histologically similar to the ganglioglioma.[43,44]

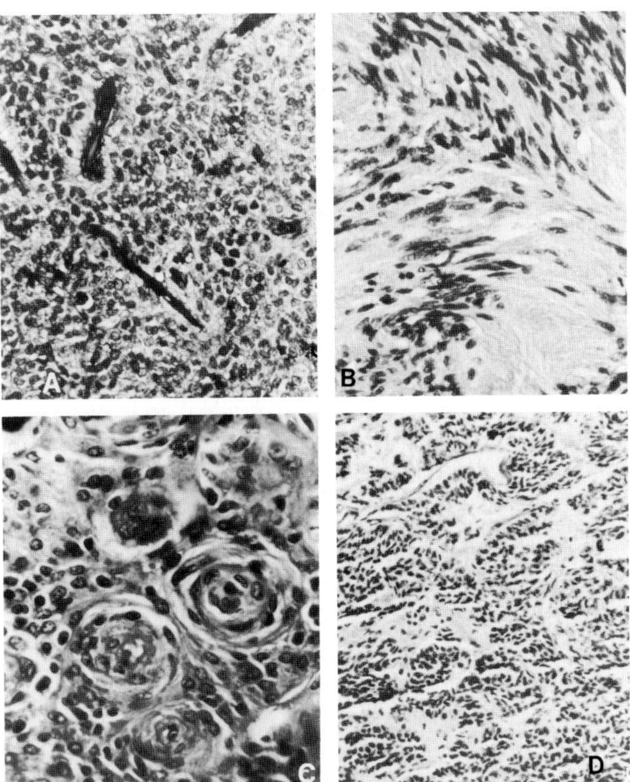

FIG. 33-5. Brain tumors stained with hematoxylin and eosin and seen by light microscopy. (*A*) Perivascular pseudorosettes of this ependymoma surround the vessels producing a gliovascular fibrillar structure. Nuclei are round to oval with punctuate chromatin; × 275. (*B*) Palisading cells with their parallel arrangement of nuclei and processes characterize this acoustic schwannoma; × 375. (*C*) Whorls of meningothelial cells are an important diagnostic feature of the meningioma; × 400. (*D*) This pituitary adenoma has a sinusoidal pattern. Each nest consists of many small cells which lack fibrils surrounded by a fibrovascular stroma; × 200. (*A, B, D,* McKeever PE, Brissie NT: Scanning electron microscopy of neoplasms removed at surgery: Surface typography and comparison of meningioma, colloid cyst, ependymoma, pituitary adenoma, schwannoma and astrocytoma. J Neuropathol Exp Neurol 36:881–883, 1977. *C,* McKeever PE: Scanning electron microscopy in the evaluation of neurosurgical neoplasms: A review of new approaches. Neurosurgery 4:347, 1979)

The ganglion cell tumors usually occur in the fronto–temporal or parietal cortex. The histology of these lesions is distinctive in the presence of numerous large ganglion cells, which are neuron-like and stain densely for Nissl substance with cresyl violet. In gangliogliomas the astrocytic component predominates and in ganglioneuromas the abnormal neurons predominate.

These tumors tend to occur in the young and cover a range from benign to malignant. Although they are clearly demarcated from normal brain tissue they are rarely encapsulated.

ACOUSTIC SCHWANNOMAS

The tumors of the Schwann sheath grow in association with several cranial nerves. The acoustic nerve is the most frequently involved. The cells are small, have scant cytoplasm and are considered responsible for myelination of peripheral nerves. The germ layer of origin of these cells has been somewhat controversial but recent studies demonstrate marked immunological and biochemical correlations with astrocytes. These tumors should be considered to be derived from neuro–ectoderm rather than mesoderm.

In histological study the tumors can be grouped into Antoni types A and B. In type A the cells form a highly distinctive palisading pattern (Fig. 33-5) whereas in type B a more reticulated pattern is found. By scanning electron microscopy the long, flat cells have a rough, beaded surface owing to the basement membranes between cells.[45] These tumors are cytologically benign and do not undergo malignant transformation. Schwannomas of peripheral nerve origin, however, may be quite malignant.

The tumors tend to be encapsulated and grow in relation to both auditory and vestibular portions of nerve VIII. Initially they are entirely in the auditory canal but gradually grow out into the area of the CPA, where they come into contact with vital brain stem centers. When small, these tumors can be considered intratemporal and only as they enlarge are they really "brain" tumors. This distinction plays a major role in surgical management.

MENINGIOMAS

Meningeal cells arise from the pia or arachnoid, which are the covering layers of the CNS. The cells are of mesodermal origin and have many features in common with the mesodermal fibroblasts which serve as the stromal cells in othei somatic tissues. The cells are prevalent throughout the CNS and tumors arising from them can be found in both intracranial and spinal regions.

As a group, meningiomas are considered relatively benign lesions but they can become malignant and several subclasses appear to be invasive from the start. Except for the invasive types, the majority of benign meningiomas are encapsulated and are well demarcated from surrounding tissues. Their sites of predilection can be seen in Table 33-4 within the intracranial region. They represent the most common group of extramedullary intradural spinal cord tumors. Sites of surgical importance include sphenoid wing, tuberculum sellae, parasagittal areas, olfactory groove, clivus, foramen magnum, and convexity. Of these lesions there are certain ones in which anatomical features make the tumors' behavior "malignant" although the histology may be benign. Sphenoid wing meningiomas in the medial portion, which can press upon the carotid and jugular vessels, represent this behavior most clearly.

A somewhat simplified classification of meningiomas is used here combining features of the schemes of Rubinstein, and Burger and Vogel.[46–47] By considering the primary cell type one can divide meningiomas into fibroblastic, syncytial (meningothelial), angioblastic, and sarcomatous varieties. There may be combinations present in any tumor. Combinations of fibroblastic and syncytial meningiomas called transitional meningiomas are particularly common (Fig. 33-5). The fibroblastic and syncytial varieties are self-descriptive and are benign, slow-growing tumors. An important diagnostic feature of most meningiomas is a circular nest of cells which tends to form a "whorl." These whorls are the probable source of "psammoma" bodies when they eventually

TABLE 33-4. Sites of Predilections of Meningiomas within the Intracranial Regions

SITE	NUMBER	PERCENT
Sagittal (attached to superior sagittal sinus)	63	9
Falx (not attached to superior sagittal sinus).	90	13
Convexity		
Prerolandic	111	16
Rolandic	116	17
Postrolandic	38	5
Sphenoid ridge–sylvian fissure	78	11
Olfactory groove–tuberculum sellae	70	10
Diaphragma sellae	19	3
Anterior fossa floor	16	2
Temporal fossa floor	11	2
Tentorium	28	4
Posterior fossa		
Cerebellar convexity	12	2
Cerebellopontine angle	7	1
Clivus	4	1
Lateral ventricle	7	1
Other (petrous, 4: cavernous sinus, 5: intraorbital, 2: torcula, 2: lateral sinus, 3: oramen magnum, 3)	19	3
TOTAL	689	100

(Youmans, JR: Neurological Surgery, Vol. III, Philadelphia, WB Saunders Co., 1973, p. 1389.)

become calcified. These bodies connote a slow-growing benign subclass called the psammomatous meningioma when present in great abundance.

The angioblastic and sarcomatous varieties are essentially malignant meningiomas. In the angiomatous type, vascular pericytial or endothelial proliferation is quite marked. In the sarcomas, the appearance is analogous to that of sarcomas elsewhere in the body.

PITUITARY TUMORS

Three types of tumors, the chromophobe, eosinophilic and basophilic adenomas which arise from the adenohypophysis have historically been included in this group. The tumors are derived from neuroectoderm. Tumors of the neuro-hypophysis are very rare. This nomenclature is based upon the staining characteristics of the tumors, with the chromophobe being the non-staining type. The chromophobe tumors are "nonfunctional" and produce their clinical effects by pressure on surrounding structures. The eosinophilic tumors secrete growth hormone (GH), resulting in acromegaly, and the basophilic adenomas secrete ACTH, resulting in Cushing's syndrome. Progress in pituitary endocrinology and some recent tissue culture studies require that this classification now be altered.

It is now clear that pituitary tumors are capable of producing a wide range of pituitary hormones and that the older classification merely describes the dominant hormonal effect. Further, prolactin-secreting adenomas have to be added to the group of pituitary hormonal tumors. The hormones, their releasing factors, and the pituitary-hypothalamic interplay need to be put in a new perspective as part of the body's ability to produce peptides.

In their gross pathological behavior the tumors can be divided into those which are purely intrasellar and those which have extended beyond the sellar margins. The intrasellar lesions tend to be the hormonally active tumors. Chromophobe adenomas have a greater likelihood of extension above the sella or into the temporal lobes. Correspondingly, the chromophobe tumors are more likely to exhibit invasive properties. The hormonally active lesions rarely become malignant and are often of small size. Indeed many prolactin secreting adenomas are really "microadenomas," fairly discrete from the rest of the gland.

The pituitary tumors are composed of small cells with relatively scant cytoplasm, no fibrils, and large round nuclei (Fig. 33-5). Scanning electron microscopy shows angulated, polyhedral cells, most of which lack fibrils. Both secretory and storage granules are often visible by light microscopy. With electron microscopy the size of the granules can be quantitated and aid in definition of hormonal products. Radioisotopic or fluorescent labelled antibodies to the peptide hormones can also be useful in characterizing endocrinologic cell types. Special staining has traditionally been very helpful and among the stains the Alcian Blue and PAS orange G are most commonly used.

On gross study, pituitary tumors may be small and well demarcated and often encapsulated, even when larger.

CRANIOPHARYNGIOMAS

The craniopharyngiomas are tumors derived from the embryologic remnants of Rathke's pouch. They are found primarily in young patients but may present later. The tumors are composed of epithelial cells which can produce a cholesterol-containing viscous fluid, very irritating to CNS tissues. The demonstration of cholesterol production has been documented in tissue culture studies in which cells from these tumors produce a saturated solution so rich in cholesterol that typical cholesterol crystals may form. Frequently, the epithelial solid tumor portion represents only a small part of the lesion, with the larger part being a fluid-filled, thinly walled cyst.

Craniopharyngiomas are benign tumors on histologic study. Their behavior can frequently be malignant, due to the strategic location or invasive potential. These tumors are located in the suprasellar region. Occasionally, a portion may be intrasellar in a dumbbell-shaped fashion. Their upper extension may press upon or adhere to hypothalamic structures. This hypothalamic relationship is therefore principal to their "location" problem. Some craniopharyngiomas appear to behave in an aggressive or "atypical" fashion. As demonstrated in tissue culture studies, these "atypical" lesions have a rapidly growing cell population, "malignant" ultrastructural features (microvilli, nuclear detail) and the ability to form cholesterol crystals. Benign or "typical" tumors do not exhibit these characteristics.

CHORDOMAS

Chordomas arise from the primitive notochord and can be found at either the caudal or cranial ends of the neuraxis. Thus they occur at either clival or sacral loci.

These tumors are benign by histological criteria and do not metastasize. They do possess an ability to invade surrounding structures, especially bone. This may reflect an enzymatic action of the tumor cells. They are not encapsulated and are always locally invasive. They are another example of a histologically benign tumor whose behavior is malignant. This tumor has large "physoliferous" cells which appear to contain lipid material in large vacuoles. The cells grow slowly and mitotic figures are infrequent.

PRIMARY LYMPHOMAS ("HISTIOCYTIC LYMPHOMAS")

Primary CNS lymphoma is a tumor of the CNS which has received increasing attention, as it occurs more frequently in patients who have received immunosuppressive therapy for transplantation. This tumor has caused some confusion as to its cell of origin. Some tumors may contain neoplastic microglial cells or macrophages which have a predilection for the perivascular space.[37] At present, evidence suggests that this is primary lymphoma of the CNS and thus of lymphoreticular origin and not neuroepithelial.[48,49] Certain cases of primary CNS lymphoma contain intracellular or surface immunoglobulin.[48,50] The tumor is composed of mononuclear cells with anaplastic nuclei which invade the neural parenchyma. These reticuloendothelial cells congregate in the Virchow–Robin space and the picture can be confused with encephalitis. This neoplasm tends to be cortical in location and contains a stroma of fibrous or reticulum network which stains with reticulum stains.

These CNS lymphomas are malignant tumors, invade locally, and may develop subarachnoid seeding. When other sites of lymphoma are found, the CNS tumor is considered as part of the systemic disease and not a primary site. These metastic tumors are usually meningeal in location and not focal within the brain. They are not encapsulated.

PINEAL AREA TUMORS

The group of tumors which cluster in the pineal gland region are unified by their common location and not by any histological similarities. They include the pineal area astrocytoma. They are often of low or intermediate grade malignancy. The pineal area teratoma is a benign, often encapsulated tumor analogous to teratomas elsewhere in the body.

Tumors distinctive to the pineal region are the dysgerminoma and pineoblastoma. The dysgerminoma has a propensity for local and CSF pathway spread and is similar to the testicular seminoma or ovarian dysgerminoma with nests of germinal large cells intermixed with lymphocytes. The pineoblastoma is derived from actual pineal glandular cells and is extremely rare. The tumor is characterized by end feet which are best seen with silver stains.

VASCULAR TUMORS

Vascular tumors include the hemangioma, hemangioblastoma, and arteriovenous malformation (AVM). The hemangioma is composed of closely packed, abnormally dilated blood vessels and the hemangioblastoma contains a peculiar mixture of capillaries and lipid-laden, large stromal cells. Both tumors are usually benign though in either intracranial or spinal locations even a modest growth, or a moderate amount of bleeding can be lethal. The arteriovenous malformation is a haphazard disordered tangle of enlarged or tortuous blood vessels and may be present as a mass lesion.

COLLOID CYSTS

The colloid cyst is an uncommon brain tumor almost exclusively located in the third ventricle.[51] Rare cysts of similar morphology have been found in the fourth ventricle.[52,53] These 0.5 cm to 4 cm diameter cysts have a fibrovascular wall with an inner lining of ciliated and microvillous columnar epithelium. The colloid is a carboxymucin mixed with a minor sulfomucin component.[54]

Recent evidence indicates that colloid cysts closely resemble tissues outside of the brain. The epithelial surface coat is endodermal.[55] The colloid has the histochemical properties of tissue outside of the CNS.[54] Certain colloid cysts contain sensory cilia like olfactory epithelium.[45,56]

Colloid cysts can cause obstructive hydrocephalus and episodic, severe headaches which may change with position of the head. They are distinctive on CT scan. When recognized and excised, they are cytologically and biologically benign.

NATURAL HISTORY

PATHOGENESIS

The development of CNS tumors can be considered in relationship to two variables; the kinetics of tumor growth and the local evolution. Distant metastases are sufficiently rare that this is not a major consideration.

Kinetics

The kinetics of each class of CNS tumor vary. There are marked variations in the growth rates of tumors within each class. The overall growth kinetics of both intracranial and spinal tumors is slow. There is a low growth fraction even in the highly malignant tumors.[57] Because of the confined nature of both intracranial and spinal regions, even a slow-growing tumor can have devastating effects. In the slow-growing lesions of the brain, gradual compression of surrounding structures allows them to adapt better to the pressure, and long histories of vague symptomatology often accompany lesions such as olfactory groove meningiomas. In tissue culture studies, the variability of growth rate of individual tumors appears to be predictive of their clinical outcome.[58]

Local Evolution

The local evolution of CNS tumor growth depends largely on the degree of tumor invasiveness. The malignant potential is measured primarily on the ability of the tumor to infiltrate normal, CNS, or bony tissues. Benign tumors cause effects primarily by pressure, whereas the malignant or invasive lesions act by both pressure and actual functional destruction.

The pressure effects of CNS tumors can be grouped as displacements, herniations, ventricular obstructions, and vascular compressions.

Displacement of normal CNS structures is the most common feature of growth and is often the finding in contrast radiography which demonstrates the presence of a mass lesion. Herniation occurs when either the cerebellar tonsils or the uncus of the temporal lobe are forced against immovable bony structures and may often result in cerebral death. Ventricular obstruction can occur with any tumor in proximity to the ventricles but is particularly common with tumors in the region of the ventricle III or IV. Such obstruction then results in the syndrome of obstructive hydrocephalus, in which continued CSF production causes increasing pressure on brain substance. Peritumoral edema may cause local venous stasis with resultant increase in edema.

PATTERNS OF SPREAD

The patterns of spread of CNS tumors are quite distinct from those of other tumors. There is no lymphatic system within the CNS. Hematogenous spread does occur but is rare. A factor often present with such hematogenous spread is operative intervention. It is not clear whether the relative infrequency of hematogenous spread is related to a relatively immunologically privileged status of the CNS or whether the short life expectancy of most patients with the highly malignant tumors merely does not allow sufficient time for systemic metastases to become manifest.

The major patterns of spread, therefore, involve local invasion and CSF seeding. These tumors, in particular the intracranial astrocytomas, have cells with the capability of invading normal brain to a remarkable degree. The cells can be found at points distant from the primary focus, even 6 cm or more distant. This distant spread has led many to question whether the lesions may have multifocal origins. Some basis for this invasiveness can be appreciated from tissue cultures of astrocytomas which show remarkable cellular motility and from a recent study by Scott, in which astrocytoma cells were able to find, penetrate, and grow through a 1 mm opening in a nucleopore filter.

The spread of tumors by seeding locally or distally by way of CSF pathways is another rather significant concern. The majority of gliomas, meningiomas, pituitary tumors, and chordomas rarely seed, whereas medulloblastomas and dysgerminomas seed extremely frequently. The seeding of these latter two occurs both by spread along the surface of the brain to local sites and by the so called "drop metastases" which fall by way of the CSF to the spinal subarachnoid space and then form secondary tumors.

This process of CSF seeding is an extremely important part of the pathogenesis of these two tumor types in that treatment must include these problems. The secondary seedings may grow on nerve roots, causing root distribution pain, or on the coverings of the spinal cord resulting in cord compression. All levels of the spinal axis can be involved but the lumbosacral area is the most frequent site.

Systemic spread by way of the hematogenous route is rare. However, specific instances of extracranial metastasis of malignant astrocytomas, ependymomas, medulloblastomas, and malignant meningiomas have been reported.[60] On rare occasion, an intracranial malignant tumor may even present first by its extracranial metastasis. In most patients with systemic metastases prior surgical intervention has occurred, but there are reports of metastases prior to any surgery.[61] With improvements in the prognosis of malignant astrocytoma patients perhaps more metastases will become manifest.

CLINICAL PRESENTATION

The clinical presentations of CNS tumors will be discussed in a general overview and then certain symptoms referable to specific ares of the CNS will be described. Symptoms and their frequency are given in Table 33-5. Brain tumors will be discussed first, followed by spinal cord tumors.

History

The history in a patient suspected of having a CNS tumor is the most crucial part of the diagnostic evaluation as it pertains to the outcome. With CNS lesions any loss of function represents an extremely difficult problem and thus early, accurate historical data are critical.

BRAIN TUMORS. In most brain tumor cases the initial presenting symptom is headache (see Table 33-5 for frequency of symptoms). The headache is often worse in the morning and lightens during the day, due to the differences in CSF drainage in the supine *versus* the recumbent position. There is often a regional correlation to the headache, especially with frontal lesions causing frontal headache and occipital or posterior fossa lesions causing occipital or posterior cervical pain. However, many patients will complain of a diffuse headache of a vertex location. The headache may be partially relieved by medication but the patient will often find it more severe and less responsive to medication than other prior headaches.

A second prominent early symptom is a seizure. This may take the form of a generalized grand mal type, or a focal Jacksonian seizure (which can be helpful in localization). Often the first seizure is a momentary loss of alertness or concentration and may be ignored by the patient. It is of great interest that the presence of a seizure as an early presenting symptom has a positive correlation in prognosis. This factor and other patient characteristics which are factors in predicting survival are given in Table 33-6.

Focal neurological symptoms usually connote a fairly well developed mass lesion. Weakness, sensory loss, or deficits in vision, hearing, or smell can occur in relation to specific tumor sites. In analyzing these focal findings it is clear that weakness or sensory symptoms denote a lesion of the cerebral fronto–parietal sensorimotor regions or their deeper pathways. Visual deficits involve the visual pathway from occipital lobe to optic nerve. Hearing loss involves the CPA, brain stem, or temporal lobes. Problems with smell (anosmia) suggest lesions of the cribriform plate, olfactory groove, temporal lobe, or other rhinencephalic connections and may also be involved in aberration in the sense of smell. Defects in mental functions may be associated with frontal, temporal, or parietal regions.

TABLE 33-5. Frequency of Symptoms of Intrinsic Brain Tumors (Gliomas)

SYMPTOM	RELATIVE FREQUENCY AS INITIAL SYMPTOM (%)	RELATIVE FREQUENCY AT ASSESSMENT AND DIAGNOSIS (%)
Epilepsy	38.3	53.9
Grand mal	15.9	20.4
Focal	14.7	22.8
Temporal lobe	7.2	8.6
Minor absence	0.5	2.1
No epilepsy	61.7	46.1
Headache	35.2	71.4
Mental change	16.5	52.2
Hemiparesis	10.3	43.3
Vomiting	7.5	31.5
Dysphasia	6.9	27.0
Impaired consciousness	4.6	24.8
Visual failure	4.3	17.9
Hemianaesthesia	3.4	13.6
Hemianopia	1.8	8.1
Cranial nerve palsy	1.8	10.9
Miscellaneous	2.3	7.0

(McKeran RO, Thomas DGT: The clinical study of gliomas. In Thomas DGT, Graham DI (eds): Brain Tumours: Scientific Basis, Clinical Investigation and Current Therapy, p 202. London, Butterworths, 1980.)

Difficulties with balance or gait suggest cerebellar vestibular or extrapyramidal involvement.

Increased intracranial pressure represents an even further advance of the tumor. By the time this appears either a significant tumor mass or corresponding amounts of cerebral edema are present. These symptoms include lethargy, drowsiness, irritability, and difficulty with ambulation. When these are present there is a real urgency to attending to the acute management of the patient in relieving the raised pressure (see chapter on acute CNS emergencies). A key element in the symptom complex of the brain tumor patient is the relentless progression of symptomatology which accompanies the evolution of an intracranial mass lesion.

SPINAL CORD TUMORS. In patients with spinal cord tumors, the prominent symptoms include pain, weakness, loss of sensation and difficulty with bowel and bladder control. There is a marked difference in the appearance of these symptoms in time. Pain may be the only early symptom. The onset of the other symptoms often connotes not just the presence of tumor but actual spinal cord compression or vascular compromise.

Pain occurs in somewhat different forms with relation to the type of tumor and its location. An intramedullary, intradural tumor can produce a deep, extremely severe pain and may, depending on the tracts involved, produce a radiating type of pain sensation. Intradural, extramedullary tumors, such as neurofibromas, may be restricted to one nerve route and thus produce a radicular pain confined to that particular root distribution. Cervical spine tumors often cause severe neck pain and patients may complain of neck stiffness at an early time.

TABLE 33-6. Correlation between Early Symptoms and Prognosis of Brain Tumors

PATIENT CHARACTERISTIC	NUMBER OF PATIENTS	NUMBER OF DEATHS	MEDIAN SURVIVAL WEEKS	P
Age, yr				
0–49	61	54	40	
50–59	76	75	29	0.005
60 and over	88	86	18	
Diagnosis				
Glioblastoma multiforme and malignant glioma	191	184	25	
Malignant astrocytoma	18	16	33	0.19
All others	16	15	36	
Sex				
Male	143	135	27	0.24
Female	82	80	25	
Location				
Cerebellum	3	3	18	
BG thalamus	2	2	14	
Frontal	72	67	25	
Occipital	15	14	43	0.15
Parietal	59	59	21	
Temporal	74	70	27	
Tumor characteristics				
Hypovascular				
No	207	199	25	0.03
Yes	18	16	40	
Invasive				
No	98	9	25	0.78
Yes	127	12	27	
Solid				
No	161	156	27	0.44
Yes	64	59	22	
Necrotic				
No	110	102	24	0.95
Yes	115	113	27	
Soft				
No	115	111	24	0.33
Yes	110	104	28	
Friable				
No	195	187	24	0.055
Yes	30	28	35	
Cystic				
No	174	165	27	0.21
Yes	51	50	25	
Hard				
No	200	191	28	0.13
Yes	25	24	14	
Vascular				
No	153	147	25	0.45
Yes	72	68	28	
Encapsulated				
No	212	203	26	0.28
Yes	13	12	26	
Symptoms				
Headache				
No	97	94	28	0.56
Yes	128	121	25	
Personality change				
No	144	137	27	0.85
Yes	81	78	25	
Motor symptoms				
No	111	105	27	0.37
Yes	114	110	26	
Seizure				
No	163	160	24	0.05
Yes	62	55	31	

TABLE 33-6. (Continued)

PATIENT CHARACTERISTIC	NUMBER OF PATIENTS	NUMBER OF DEATHS	MEDIAN SURVIVAL WEEKS	P
Speech				
No	166	157	27	0.43
Yes	59	58	25	
General complaints				
No	209	199	26	0.68
Yes	16	16	27	
Sensory				
No	194	186	27	0.70
Yes	31	29	23	
Cranial nerves II, III, IV, VI				
No	208	198	25	0.13
Yes	17	17	34	
Rapid unconsciousness				
No	212	202	26	0.82
Yes	13	13	26	
Cranial nerves other				
No	217	207	26	0.62
Yes	8	8	27	
Cerebellar				
No	222	212	27	0.77
Yes	3	3	12	
Other				
No	182	173	27	0.32
Yes	43	42	21	
Time from symptoms to operation, wk				
0–25	200	191	27	0.85
26–51	12	12	19	
52 or more	13	12	22	
Left or right				
Left	102	99	22	0.13
Right	123	116	28	
Type of operation				
Biopsy only	12	12	14	0.01
Partial or total resection	213	203	27	
All Patients	225	215	26	

(Gehan EA, Walker MD: Prognostic factors for patients with brain tumors. Natl Cancer Inst Monogr 46: 189–195, 1977)

Weakness and sensory complaints come relatively late in spinal cord tumor patients. The weakness tends to be at first noticeable in distal parts of the extremities gradually progressing proximally. With intramedullary intradural tumors, the patients may have gait difficulty as one of the first manifestations of tumor. The sensory complaints include the gamut of modalities affected by a particular tumor. Often, difficulty with proprioception manifested by a hesitant, uncertain gait will occur and be noticeable to the patient even earlier than numbness. Changes in temperature, sensitivity to hot or cold may be present.

In general, it can be stated that the rapid progression of spinal cord tumors follows a pattern of early pain and in the case of some slow-growing lesions slight weakness or numbness, followed by a relatively short period (hours, days) of rapid deterioration in motor and sensory function. By the time that bowel and bladder function has been affected, the cord can be considered to be severely, and usually irreversibly, compressed. As a corollary, rapidly progressing symptoms of spinal cord compression are frequently followed by poorer recovery in comparison with the more slowly growing lesions.

The components of the syndromes associated with spinal cord lesions are given in Tables 33-7*A*, *B*

Neurological Findings

BRAIN TUMORS. The evaluation of a patient suspected of having a brain tumor must consider the following areas; intellectual, cranial nerve, motor, sensory, reflex, and coordination functions.

Of these areas the most crucial is that of intellectual function and in particular the *"level of consciousness."* This level determines the urgency of the total evaluation process and allows one to decide whether meticulous consideration of the neurological status is in order or if one had better first deal with the relatively acute problem presented by a rapidly declining level of consciousness. Orientation to person, place, time, and promptness of response is the critical first test.

TABLE 33-7*A*. Clinical Manifestations of Spinal Cord Lesions

CLINICAL MANIFESTATIONS	SPINAL CORD LESIONS (Myelopathies)
Motor	Upper or lower motor neuron type weakness, depending on acuity and "age" of the lesion and its location in relation to cord segments Trunk and limb(s) below the lesion affected Atrophy from disuse only
Sensory	Cutaneous "sensory level" or "suspended sensory level" on trunk Sensory dissociation, if present, usually in terms of cord tracts
Reflexes	Hyperactive tendon reflexes below lesion except during "spinal shock" with acute lesions At level of lesion, if limb segments are involved, hyporeflexia or areflexia persists or both hyper- and hyporeflexia occur in same limb(s) Pathological reflexes (Babinski sign, spontaneous flexor or extensor spasms) below lesion likely Cutaneous reflexes lost below lesion
Sphincters	External urethral and anal sphincters often impaired

(Youmans JR: Neurological Surgery, vol I. Philadelphia, WB Saunders, 1973, p. 35)

The more subtle evaluation of intellectual function involves evaluation of speech, memory (recent and past), arithmetic and verbal skills, and association and coherence of logical thought. The performance of step commands, involving multiple functions, is a good general parameter of intact mental function. Simple tests of speech, including repetition of phrases, content, and appropriateness help determine whether dysphasic or aphasic defects are present. Memory can be tested by providing the patient with the names of several items to recollect and then asking for these several minutes later. Simple subtraction in series from 100 allows testing of arithmetic function.

In general, the association of intellectual functions with anatomic areas can be described, speech being involved with temporal and parietal areas, especially left parieto–temporal (in right-handed patients), memory being frontal and temporal, and mathematical skills being parietal. Association functions are primarily frontal and temporal in location. These loci and their associated functions are depicted in Fig. 33-6

Cranial nerve findings can be very important in diagnosis and those details are described in Table 33-8.

Motor functions involve pathways from the contralateral parietal motor area through the midbrain, brain stem, and spinal cord. Thus lesions at any point in the course of these tracts can result in weakness. Cerebral lesions affecting motor function tend to produce a spastic paralysis and often affect distal parts first. Fine motor functions are affected at first. Testing involves observing both active spontaneous movements, and testing of strength against resistance. Quantitation of strength should be made on a numerical scale. This is particularly important with CNS neoplastic lesions, in that the rate of evolution or the response to treatment requires measurable parameters. Motor strength is one of the easiest parameters to monitor.

Sensory functions follow a complex pathway from the sensory areas of the contralateral parietal lobes by way of the midbrain, thalamus, and medulla to the spinal cord. The various sensory modalities have very different interconnections and relationships, requiring detailed descriptions as can be found in anatomic texts.[23,62] In general, brain tumors of the parietal lobes produce sensory loss in distal parts first and testing with pin, temperature (hot and cold), vibration, and tactile discrimination are all valuable. Sensory functions can often be affected earlier than motor losses. Thus, careful and thorough sensory exams can be a great help in diagnosis.

Reflexes are hyperactive with intracranial mass lesions, becoming hypoactive only in terminal phases. Toes are often upgoing on plantar stroking (Babinski sign) and a unilateral finding of this sign is useful in localizing lesions of the contralateral hemisphere localization. Reflexes also lend themselves to quantitation and careful determination of the amplitude of the responses on a numerical scale is helpful. Coordination refers to cerebellar function and tumors of this area may cause deficits. Cerebellar deficits tend to be transient and frequently are observable only for relatively short intervals. Ataxia often suggests a midline cerebellar lesion. Dysmetria and dysdiadochocinesia reflect cerebellar hemisphere deficits usually of ipsilateral representation.

SPINAL CORD TUMORS. The neurologic examination of the patient with suspected spinal cord tumor depends on evaluation of three major modalities: motor, sensory, and reflex functions.

Motor testing may reveal a hypotonic or flaccid paralysis in advanced lesions. Spasticity may be seen both in early lesions as well as late. There may even be atrophic changes in muscles late in tumor progression. Reflexes follow a biphasic pattern with early hyperactivity and later hypoactivity.

Sensory testing is critical in that it helps determine the level of the lesion. Spinal nerves supply sensation on a dermatomal basis and thus sensory levels can determine the tumor level. Temperature, proprioception, pain and touch may all be affected. The organization of the major sensory pathways in the spinal cord is depicted in Fig. 33-7.

TABLE 33-7*B*. Frequency of Symptoms of Spinal Cord Lesions, in Order of Appearance (Gliomas)

FIRST		SECOND		THIRD		FOURTH	
Pain	60%	Motor	43%	Motor	40%	Sensory	50%
Motor	20%	Sensory	30%	Sensory	27.5%	Sphincter	40%
Sensory	16%	Pain	14%	Sphincter	27.5%	Pain	5%
Sphincter	4%	Sphincter	13%	Pain	5%	Motor	5%

(Stein WE: Localization and diagnosis of spinal cord tumors. Clin Neurosurg 25:480–494, 1978)

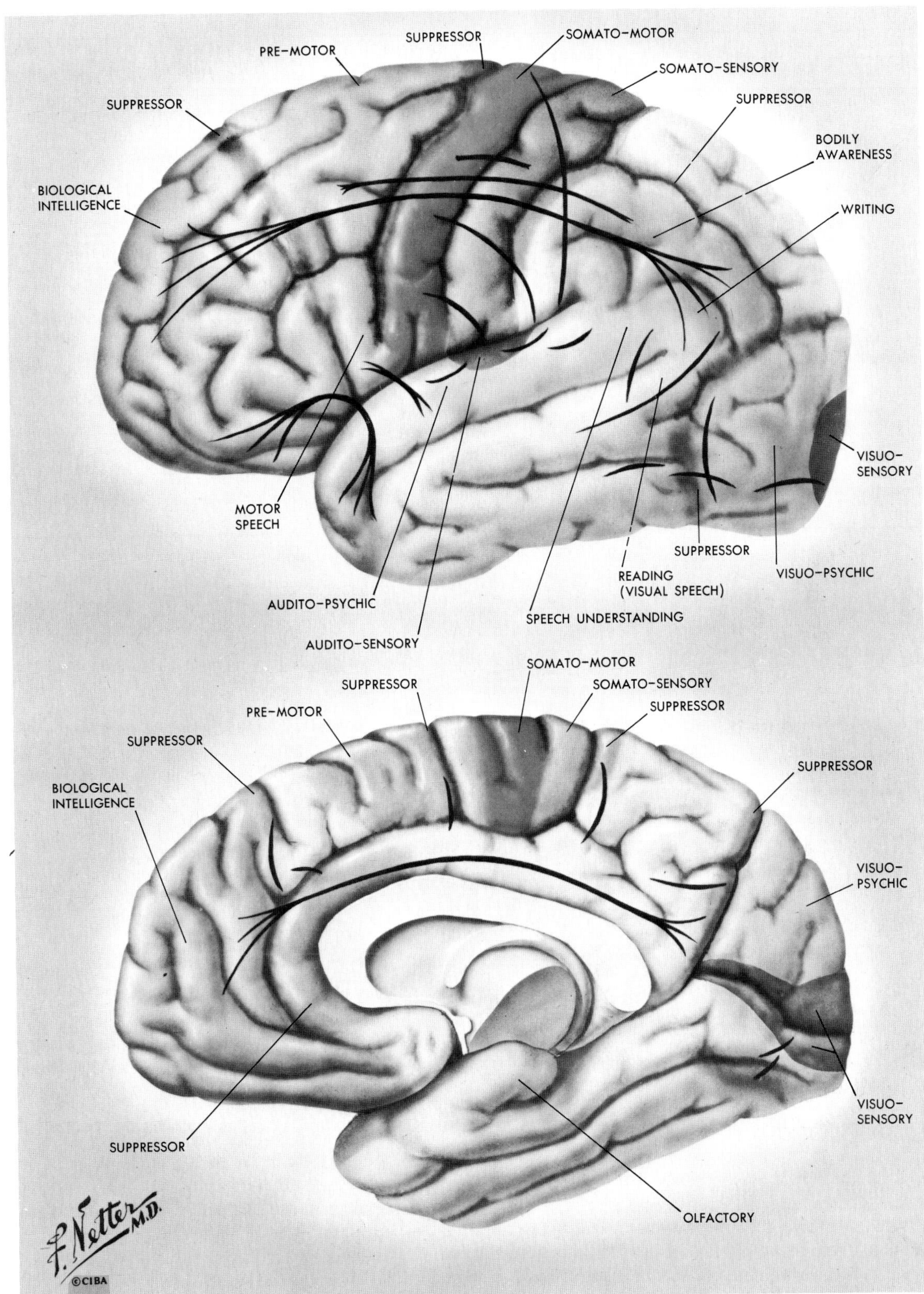

FIG. 33-6. Areas of functional localization in cerebral cortex. (Copyright 1953, 1972, CIBA Pharmaceutical Company, Division of CIBA–GEIGY Corporation. Reprinted with permission from The CIBA Collection of Medical Illustrations by Frank H. Netter, M.D. All rights reserved.)

TABLE 33-8. Clinical Symptoms Associated with Cranial Nerves

SITE	CRANIAL NERVES INVOLVED	EPONYMIC SYNDROME	USUAL CAUSE
Sphenoidal fissure	III, IV, ophthalmic V, VI		Invasive tumors of sphenoid bone, aneurysms
Lateral wall of cavernous sinus	III, IV, ophthalmic V, VI	Tolosa–Hunt	Aneurysms of cavernous sinus, cavernous sinus thrombosis, invasive tumors from sinuses and sella turcica
Petrosphenoidal space	II, III, IV, V, VI	Jacob	Large tumors of middle cranial fossa
Apex of petrous bone	V, VI	Gradenigo	Petrositis, tumors of petrous bone
Internal auditory meatus	VII, VIII		Tumors of petrous tone (dermoids, etc.), infectious processes
Pontocerebellar angle	V, VII, VIII, and sometimes IX		Acoustic neuromas, meningiomas
Jugular foramen	IX, X, XI	Vernet	Tumors and aneurysms
Posterior laterocondylar space	IX, X, XI, XII	Collet–Sicard	Tumors of parotid gland, carotid body, and secondary tumor, lymph node tumors, tuberculous adenitis
Posterior retroparotid space	IX, X, XI, XII, and Bernard–Horner syndrome	Villaret	Same as above

(Adams RD, Victor M: Principles of Neurology. New York, McGraw-Hill, 1977, p. 455)

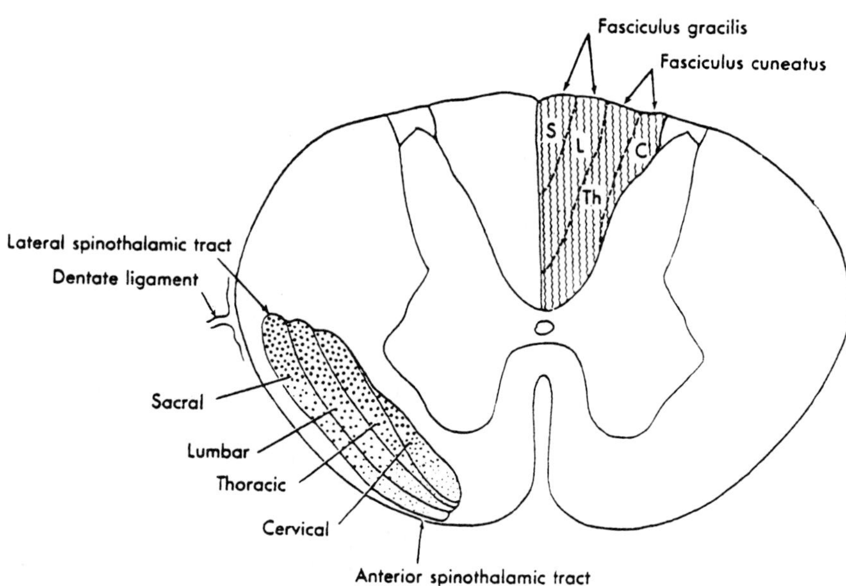

FIG. 33-7. Sensory pathways in spinal cord, indicating lamination of the posterior column, lateral corticospinal tract, and spinothalamic tracts. In the lateral spinothalamic tracts the coarse dots indicate the fibers conveying heat and cold impulses; the medium-sized dots, those carrying pain impulses; and the fine dots, those carrying tactile impulses. The lateral thalamic tract reaches dorsally to the level of the dentate ligament. *C*, cervical; *TH*, thoracic; *L*, lumbar; and *S*, sacral segments. (Haymaker W: Bing's Local Diagnosis in Neurological Diseases, 15th ed. St Louis, CV Mosby, 1969, p 8. Originally adapted from Foerster O, Gagel O: Zbl Ges Neurol Psychiatr 138:1–92, 1932; and Walker AE: Arch Neurol Psychiatr 43:284–298, 1940)

METHODS OF DIAGNOSIS

Intracranial Techniques

NEUROLOGICAL EXAMINATION AND CLINICAL HISTORY. The presumptive diagnosis of brain tumor can be made with the symptoms of headache, seizure, or focal deficit being the crucial clues. A relentless progression is helpful in differentiating evolving mass lesions from vascular lesions such as stroke.

The neurological examination enables one to determine the overall neurological status of the patient, the degree of urgency of the evaluation process and often can be helpful in localizing the lesion. In addition, as shown by Walker and Gehan it is of real help in predicting outcome.[63]

The history and neurological exam provide the framework for the entire evaluation process. The frequency of specific symptoms and signs in the diagnosis of intrinsic tumors (gliomas) is given in Table 33-9.

QUANTITATIVE TECHNIQUES ADJUNCTIVE TO THE NEUROLOGICAL EXAM. *Tangent Screen and Perimetry.* In the evaluation of visual fields the finding of deficits on confrontation requires specific confirmation. With these instruments the extent of the deficits, the margins and the degree of regularity (congruity) of the deficits can be determined. Subtle changes not found by confrontation will often become manifest. Pre- as well as postoperative exams provide another means of quantifying the effects of tumor and the results of surgery and the postoperative course on the status of the visual pathways. Visual field defects and their relationships are depicted in Fig. 33-8.

Caloric Testing. In a normal patient, cold caloric stimulation results in nystagmus with the fast component away from the site of stimulation. The test, most useful in a comatose patient, can be used to help detect brain stem or CPA mass lesions. The complete absence of caloric responses connotes brain stem death, unless nerve is destroyed, but more subtle abnormalities are of localizing value. In caloric testing, cold or warm water is sequentially placed in the external canal of each ear and the resultant tonic or nystagmoid movements of each eye are observed. If these movements are abnormal, either decreased or increased in amplitude, they suggest lesions of brain stem or CPA regions.

Electronystagmography. This technique of quantifying ocular movements, especially nystagmus, finds application in the diagnosis of CPA lesions in which abnormal nystagmus patterns can be of specific help in distinguishing brain stem from CPA type lesions. It utilizes cold water caloric testing as a stimulus and quantifies the result with an ocular motility device.[64,65]

Audiometry. With hearing deficits the detailed audiometric exam is needed. This includes evaluation of low and high tone losses, and testing of auditory discrimination ability. Whereas some high-tone loss with age is likely, a low-tone loss, especially unilaterally coupled with decreased discrimination, is suggestive of CPA tumors. The early detection of acoustic tumors, and their improved cure rate, can be traced to the widespread application of these techniques.[66] The use of brain stem evoked responses is coming into routine clinical neurophysiological use and is particularly useful in non-cooperative patients.

Muscle Testing. Various devices have been developed for quantitating grip, plantar flexion and extension, and actions of other muscle groups. They may be helpful in supplementing findings on physical examination.

LUMBAR PUNCTURE. Discussion of lumbar puncture (LP) in the diagnosis of intracranial tumors should begin with the caution that this procedure holds significant risks for certain categories of patients. Those who have elevated ICP as indicated by lethargy and perhaps the finding of papilledema are at particular risk. Patients with lesions of the temporal lobe and cerebellum are at higher risk. The danger consists of the alteration in pressure relationships that can occur when CSF is withdrawn from the lumbar space. This risk can be minimized by the use of a small-caliber needle, slow withdrawal of minimal amount of CSF, and in some cases pre-treatment with steroids or mannitol.

The pertinent parameters to measure on examination include CSF pressure dynamics, color, protein, sugar cell counts, bacterial culture and gram stain, millipore filtration, cytocentrifugation, and tissue culture for malignant cells.

The procedure is performed with the patient in the lateral position, preferably at the L4,5 interspace, using a 22-gauge spinal needle. Assurance that one is in the subarachnoid space can be made by observing the movement of CSF with respiration. Initially, the evaluation of ICP is performed using a manometer. Findings of over 150 mm of H_2O are of concern, although not always abnormal. Readings of well over 200 mm of H_2O in a fairly relaxed patient suggest true raised ICP and supports the diagnosis of mass lesion. At levels above 200 mm only minimal CSF amounts should be withdrawn and the needle removed promptly. Although there are certain instances in which relieving ICP by lumbar drainage may be therapeutic, it is not often indicated as part of the diagnostic evaluation.

The CSF dynamics can be observed by asking the patient to breathe deeply and watching the CSF excursions in the manometer. The Valsalva maneuver is not a part of the evaluation of intracranial mass lesions.

The color and appearance of the CSF can aid in determining whether bleeding, high protein, or possibly infection are present. Reddish fluid suggests recent hemorrhage. Yellowish (xanthochronic) fluid suggests old bleeding or high protein content. A viscous appearance may occur with either high protein or infection. Turbidity suggests infection.

CSF protein has classically been one of the most useful biochemical parameters indicating tumor presence. Elevation of CSF protein above 20 mg/100 ml to 40 mg/100 ml is highly suggestive of tumor. Increased protein can, however, be produced by blood in the CSF or infection, less frequently even by cerebrovascular occlusive disease. Numerous efforts have been made to characterize the CSF proteins. For example, α-fetoprotein has been found in the CSF of patients with dysgerminomas.

CSF sugar decreases below 50 mg/ml are suggestive of infectious processes such as meningitis or viral encephalitis. Tumors may lower CSF sugar, especially in leukemic meningitis.

Gram stains and bacterial culture represent two of the most important CSF diagnostic studies in differential diagnosis. Identification of organisms in the CSF and determining antibiotic sensitivity are essential for the treatment of meningitis. The presumption of meningitis and the need for CSF assays constitute the single most important indications for an LP as an early diagnostic procedure in a patient where brain tumor is being considered.

Millipore filtration, its modifications and, more recently,

TABLE 33-9. Frequency of Neurological Findings in Brain Tumor Patients at the Time of Diagnosis (Cerebral Gliomas)

SIGNS	ABSOLUTE NUMBER OF CASES	RELATIVE FREQUENCY (%)
Hemiparesis	403	61.7
Cranial nerve palsy	354	54.2
Mental deterioration	349	53.4
Papilloedema	340	52.1
Hemianaesthesia	226	34.6
Hemianopia	214	32.8
Dysphasia	183	28.0
Visual failure	139	21.3

(McKeran RO; Thomas DGT: The clinical study of gliomas. In Thomas DGT, Graham DI (eds): Brain Tumours: Scientific Basis, Clinical Investigation and Current Therapy, p 206). London, Butterworth, 1980

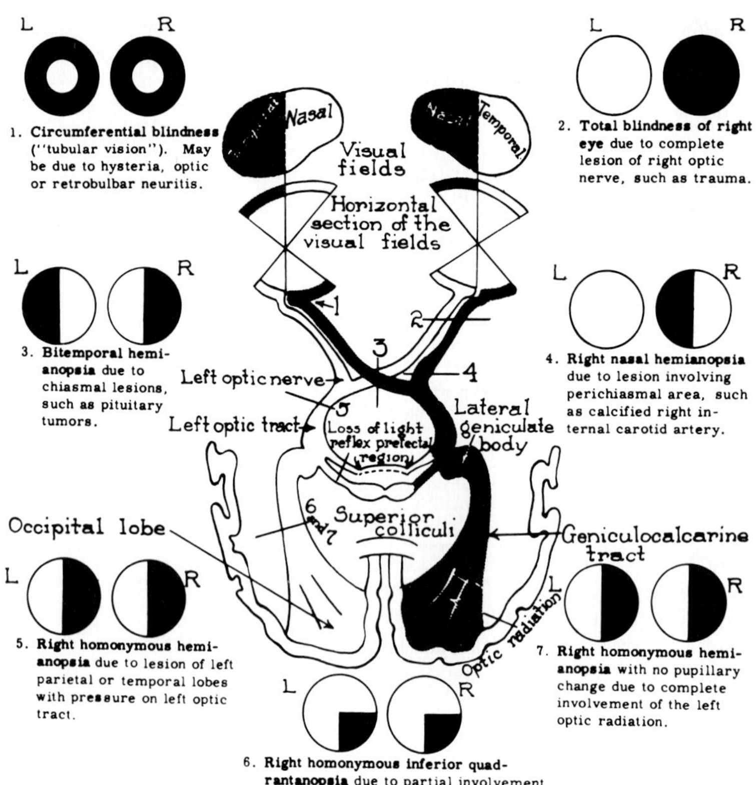

FIG. 33-8. Visual field deficits and their relationship to the optic pathways. (Chusid JG, McDonald JJ: Correlative Neuroanatomy and Functional Neurology, 13th ed. Los Altos, CA, Lange Medical Publications, 1967, p 85)

CSF tissue culture can be very useful diagnostic adjuncts. These techniques find their greatest utility in tumors with a presentation on the brain surface, such as metastatic tumors and in cases of CSF seeding, as with medulloblastoma where exfoliated tumor cells may be identified. Millipore study can describe nuclear abnormalities in some detail and thus indicate malignancy, but little if any cytoplasmic detail is evident.

CSF tissue culture can improve the ability to evaluate size, shape and cell process formation. In recent studies an almost twofold higher rate of tumor detection by CSF culture was found.[67,68] Combining Millipore and culture techniques, better results can be obtained. Fluorescent antibody testing has offered additional help in specificity.[33] The use of CSF cell identification techniques should be considered a routine adjunct in patients with tumors likely to have CSF seeding.

SKULL FILMS. Plain skull films may be useful in the diagnosis of tumors. The types of abnormalities may be classifed as calcifications, bony erosions, and hyperostoses.

Calcifications. Intracranial calcifications relevant to specific brain tumors most commonly involve gliomas, oligodendrogliomas, astrocytomas, craniopharyngiomas, and some meningiomas. Tuberous sclerosis may occasionally have calcified lesions. Although the incidence of calcification is substantially lower with astrocytomas than with oligodendrogliomas, their overall frequency more than compensates and these tumors represent the greatest number of calcifying tumors.

In oligodendrogliomas the calcifications are often large and diffuse, appearing as fluffy white patches. They occur in 50% of such tumors,[33] an example of which is shown in Fig. 33-9. Approximately 20% of astrocytomas have calcifications.[33] Although calcification is less frequent in astrocytomas, the fact that these tumors occur more frequently makes most calcified cerebral tumors astrocytomas.

In craniopharyngiomas the calcifications often follow the contours of the tumor capsule and are curvilinear and thin. They are seen in some form in 70% to 80% of these tumors,[69] an example of which is shown in Fig. 33-10. Calcification occurs with much greater frequency in pediatric patients with craniopharyngiomas than in adults.

Meningiomas vary in their tendency to form calcifications. The psammomatous varieties are most likely to calcify and small speckled flecks may be seen. Five percent to 10% of meningiomas have visible calcifications.[70]

In general, calcifications represent slow tumor growth and thus suggest a benign lesion. Many vascular lesions such as hemangiomas can also calcify. In addition to these specific abnormal calcifications, the normal calcification of the pineal gland in most patients (55%) allows a good reference point to detect shifts in intracranial structures due to tumors. Shifts of over 0.5 cm are usually significant indicators of hemispheric mass lesions.[71]

Bone Erosions. Persistent elevations in intracranial pressure can result in erosion of normally calcified structures. The clinoid processes of the sella turcica are often affected early in patients with tumors. In children, chronic pressure erosion of the inner table of the skull can lead to the

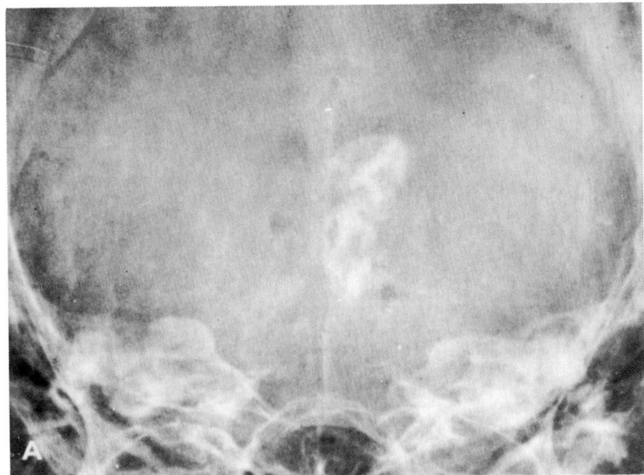

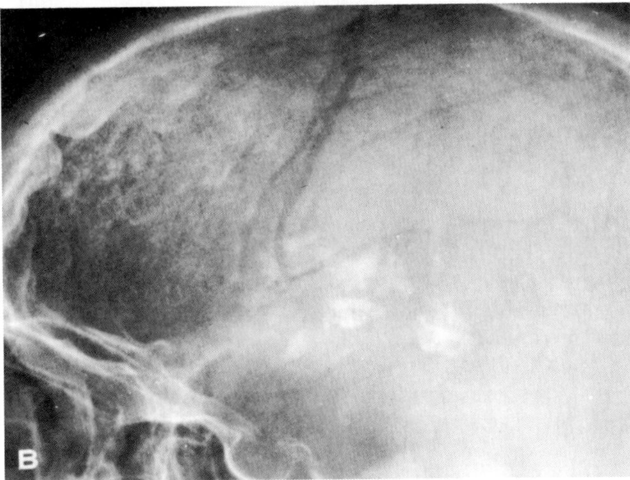

FIG. 33-9. Calcification in mixed oligodendroglioma and astrocytoma: (*A*) lateral view, (*B*) posterior view. (Taveras JM, Wood EH: Diagnostic Radiology, vol 1, 2nd ed, Baltimore, Williams and Wilkins, 1976, p 215)

"hammered metal" appearance. Occasionally, malignant tumors may erode through the dura and invade the skull with resultant erosive changes.

Hyperostosis of the Skull. Hyperostosis usually occurs in relation to the slow-growing tumor, such as a meningioma. Sphenoid wing and supraorbital meningiomas classically have significant hyperostosis attributed with their presence.

TOMOGRAPHY. This technique allows demonstration of such processes as erosion or hyperostosis in greater detail and can help differentiate subtle conditions. The "double floor" of the sella, as is shown in Fig. 33-11, in certain pituitary tumors or the localized erosion of the anterior sella in microadenomas of the pituitary are examples. This technique is most often used with a pneumoencephalogram to give better visualization of ventricular area III or IV abnormalities. The use of polytomography, as contrasted to linear tomography, markedly decreases artifacts and has major advantages especially for the evaluation and diagnosis of lesions affecting bone, such as pituitary tumors or acoustic neuromas.

Tomograms of the internal auditory canal can demonstrate the quantitative unilateral enlargement that often accompanies acoustic nerve tumors. Optic nerve gliomas may similarly widen the optic foramina and this effect can be quantitated with tomography.

EEG. The EEG allows demonstration of either increased or diminished electrical activity of the brain. In general, brain tumors produce a regional slowing of electrical activity. When there is a specific EEG focus, however, spikes or spike and wave foci can occur in relation to a tumor.

The EEG is often normal in patients with brain tumors and thus has limited value as a screening device. It is helpful in tumor localization in patients who present with seizures.

BRAIN SCAN. Brain scanning with radiolabelled isotopes, such as ^{99m}Tc, had been a very important technique in tumor

FIG. 33-10. Calcification in craniopharyngioma. (*A*) intrasellar lesion enlarging sella; (*B*) suprasellar lesion, (*C*) tomographic view. (Taveras JM, Wood EH: Diagnostic Radiology, vol 1, 2nd ed, Baltimore, Williams and Wilkins, 1976, p 197)

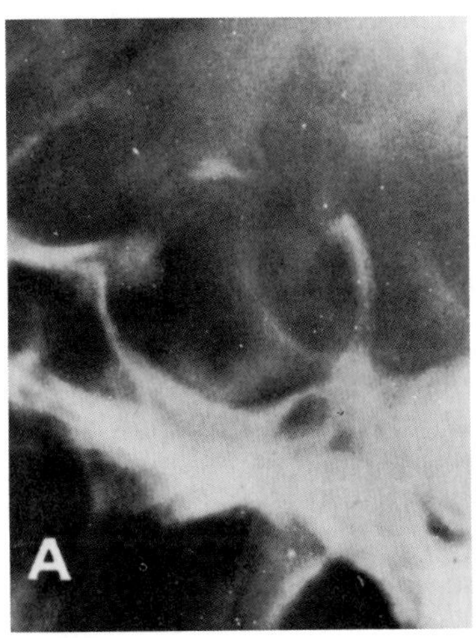

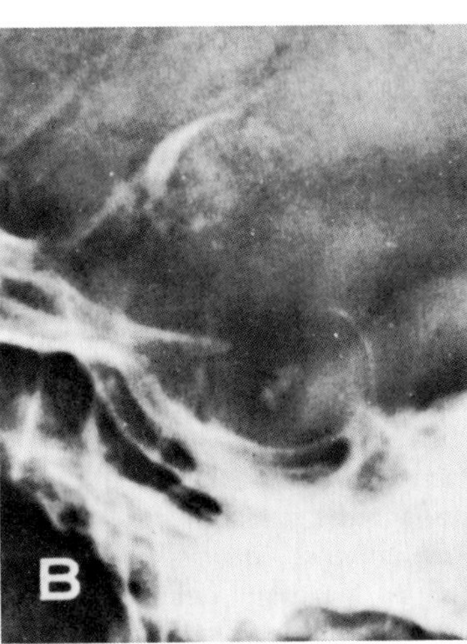

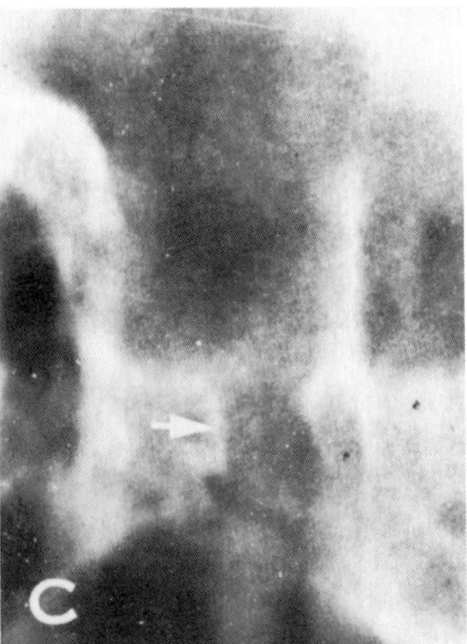

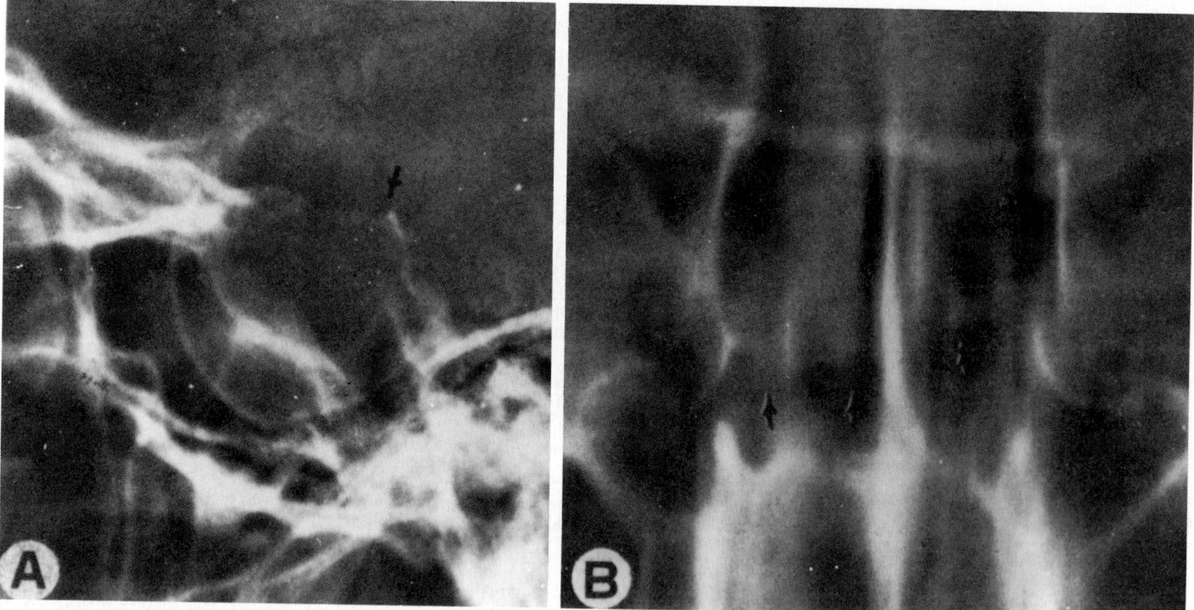

FIG. 33-11. Double floor of sella turcica in patient with pituitary adenoma. The lateral view (*A*) demonstrates a typical double contour of the sella turcica; one side is almost normal whereas the other side shows marked enlargement with undermining of the anterior clinoid process and tuberculum sellae and posterior displacement of the dorsum sellae. There is only very slight posterior displacement of the posterior clinoid process, however, because this portion of the sella is fixed by the interclinoid ligaments. A frontal laminagram (*B*) demonstrates the depression of the sella involving only one side of the pituitary fossa (arrows). There is marked increase in width of the floor of the sella turcica, which measured a total of 30 mm. (Taveras JM, Wood EH: Diagnostic Neuroradiology. Baltimore, Williams and Wilkins, 1976, p 1.109)

diagnosis. At present, the primary value of isotopic techniques lies in detecting meningiomas, and certain well-vascularized astrocytomas. It is often of great help in the three-dimensional visualization of a tumor prior to surgery. Its use, in combination with CT scan, increases the accuracy of diagnosis from 85% to 95%.

Using radioisotopically labelled, metabolically active substances is of particular promise. The development of the PET scan (positron emission tomography) may make the combination of isotopic and computerized imaging a new tool for studying the dynamic aspects of tumor biology.

CT SCAN. The CT scan has markedly changed the diagnostic approach to the patient with a possible tumor. In this technique, computerized tomographic cuts allow a detailed analysis of density changes to be made with precision. It distinguishes between CSF, blood, edema, tumor, and normal brain tissue by means of quantitative density differences.

A 90% success rate in diagnosis of presence or absence of tumors has been noted with intraparenchymal lesions.[72] Low-grade, well-differentiated astrocytomas still present a problem, with rates as low as 70% being reported. Lesions of 1 cm^3 and above can be detected. Localization in three dimensions is achievable and the patient risks are minimal. The use of contrast enhancement can often sharpen the tumor delineation and is helpful with vascularized lesions.

Cerebellar tumors are more difficult to visualize because of the surrounding dense bony structures. Intrasellar tumors require exceptionally high-resolution equipment for detection of the smaller lesions. Surgical intervention can produce artifactual changes, and the use of any metallic materials produces a scatter problem. The use of an iodinated contrast material does raise a risk of idiosyncratic or allergic reaction. Young children or hyperactive patients may require sedation or anesthesia to allow them to remain still, thus adding risk for these patients.

If the history and neurological findings are suggestive of a brain tumor, the performance of a CT scan is often the most logical next step. Examples of CT scans are given in Fig. 33-12 *A*, *B*, *C* and Fig. 33-13.

ANGIOGRAPHY. Angiography of the intracranial vasculature has been a great aid in brain tumor diagnosis. Presently, the majority of angiograms are performed by way of the retrograde femoral route using a catheter to inject opaque contrast material into either the carotid or vertebral arteries. For most injections, a transfemoral common carotid route is used but selective internal or external injections have specialized uses, such as an external carotid injection for visualizing a meningioma. Direct carotid injections are less frequently used. Angiography does carry risks, including stroke, embolism, and hemorrhage (the last two both at the local site of injection and intracerebrally). Some patients may have allergic or idiosyncratic reactions to contrast (with its

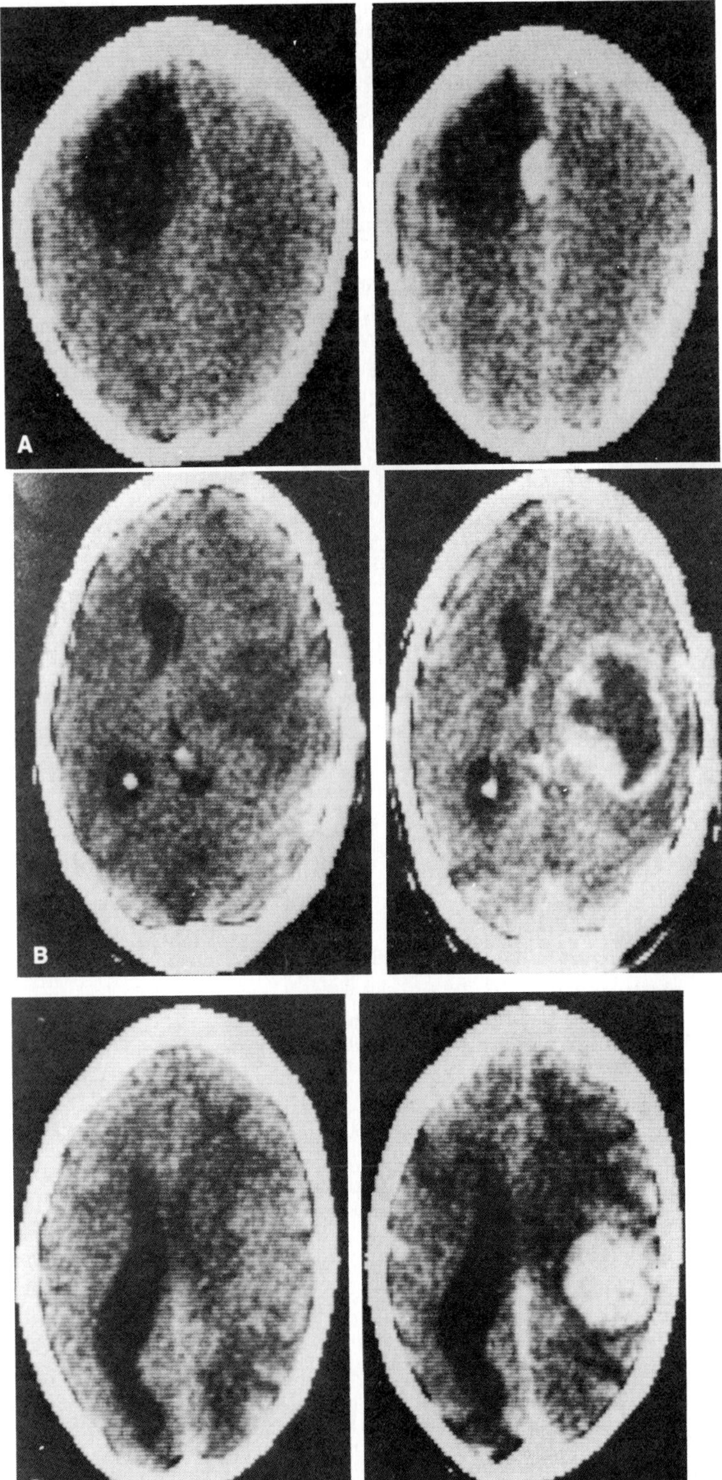

FIG. 33-12. (*A*) CT scan of low-grade glioma. *Left:* Plain CT scan. The large area of decreased density in the left frontal lobe was found at surgery to be a cystic astrocytoma. *Right:* The mural nodule is seen on the scan enhanced by contrast material. (*B*) CT of glioblastoma. *Left:* Plain CT scan shows area of decreased density in the right insula and temporal lobe, with somewhat regular margins. *Right:* On the IV–CT scan, enhancement shows a thick ring outlining the extent of the tumor. (*C*) CT of anaplastic glioma. *Left:* Plain CT scan shows extensive area of decreased density mainly due to edema. The finger-like appearance is the result of sparing of cortical layers. *Right:* On the IV–CT scan the enhancement is homogeneous, involving all the tumor and mimicking the appearance of meningiomas. (Tchang S, Scotti G, Terbrugge K et al: Computerized tomography as a possible aid to histological grading of supratentorial gliomas. J Neurosurg 46:737–738, 1977. Taylor S, Ethier R, Scotti G et al: CT evaluation of intracranial meningiomas. Presented at the International Symposium and Course on Computerized Tomography (CT), Puerto Rico, April 4–9, 1976)

iodine content). For further complications of angiography see Table 33-10.

For a period of about 20 years (1955–1975) angiography was crucial in cerebral tumor diagnosis. The CT scan has altered the use of angiography and currently angiography has as its major role outlining the detailed vascular supply of a tumor. Tumors are seen on angiography but not on CT scan in certain instances.

The findings seen in angiography which are of diagnostic importance are (see Table 33-11): blush (Fig. 33-14), displacements of vessels from their normal positions (Figs. 33-15 and 33-16), tumor "staining" due to the development of

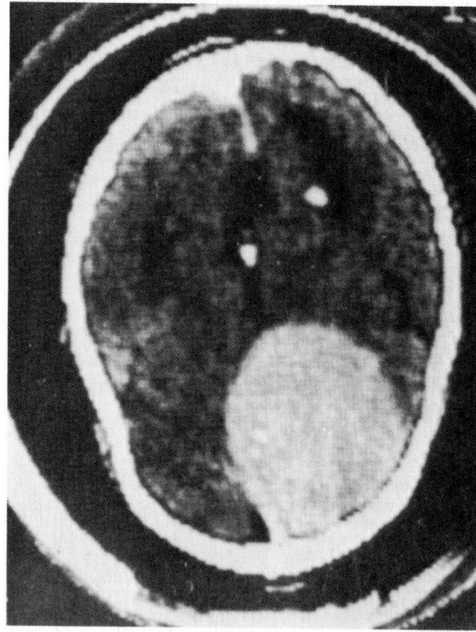
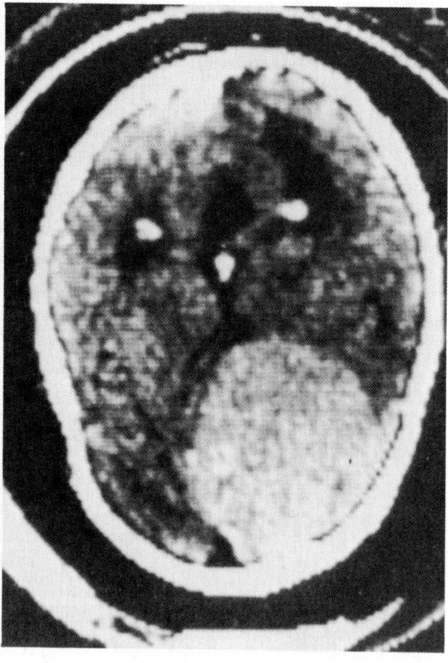

FIG. 33-13. Meningioma of the left frontal polar convexity. *Left:* The unenhanced scan shows a large, well defined "spotty" tumor containing visible calcium aggregates with minimal surrounding edema. *Right:* The contrast-enhanced scan emphasizes the marked enhancement, good definition, and "spotty" appearance. (Vassilouthis J, Ambrose J: Computerized tomography scanning appearances of intracranial meningiomas. J Neurosurg 50:325, 1979)

abnormal tumor vessels, and filling patterns of veins and arteries in a tumor area.

The displacements of vessels can often be subtle, with only minimal changes in location of a small vessel such as the anterior choroidal artery. These changes can, however, be extremely crucial. Other displacement changes can be massive, such as the shift of the anterior cerebral artery across the midline in cases of large hemispheric tumors. A classification for angiographic localization of tumors has been devised by Taveras and is described in Fig. 33-17.

TABLE 33-10. Complications of Angiography

A. Local complications
   1. Local hematoma requiring drainage
   2. Osteomyelitis of cervical spine due to infection
   3. Abscess of neck
   4. Radicular pain
   5. Aneurysm at injection site
   6. Persistent arterial spasm
   7. Pneumothorax
   8. Subcutaneous emphysema with subclavian punctures
   9. Thrombosis of femoral or brachial artery at site of entry
   10. Loss of pulse
   11. Rupture of a vein

B. Embolic complications
   1. Plugging of artery and its branches
   2. Retinal artery embolism
   3. Accidental injection of air
   4. Foreign body emboli

C. Neurologic complications
   1. Result of interference with circulation through a vessel due to
      a. Intramural injection
      b. Occasional spasm
      c. Obstruction of the vessel lumen by a catheter
      d. Embolism
   2. Hemiparesis
   3. Dysphasia
   4. Unilateral sensory disturbances
   5. Hemianopia

(Adapted from Taveras JM; Wood EH: Diagnostic Neuroradiology, 2nd ed, vol 2. Baltimore, Williams & Wilkins, 1976, pp 567–573.)

Tumor stain or blush can be very helpful in diagnosing a tumor and in distinguishing peritumoral edema from tumor. Subtraction techniques can help in highlighting tumor stains, particularly in areas of bony overlap.

Venous and arterial filling patterns are of particular help in distinguishing astrocytomas. Late or delayed venous filling is commonly seen with astrocytomas. In many cases of meningiomas, engorged venous channels develop in response to the increased vascular needs of the growing tumor and these can be visualized.

In addition to these direct diagnostic data, arteriograpy is of considerable value in planning surgical strategy. It is still appropriate to consider the arteriogram as a valuable preoperative adjunct, although it no longer represents the primary screening technique as it did prior to the CT scan.

PEG AND VENTRICULOGRAPHY. The air contrast studies as developed by Walter Dandy revolutionized the diagnostic approach.[7] Prior to their introduction, only the neurological exam and the occasional finding on the skull film were available for either tumor screening or localization.

In the ventriculogram, a burr hole is made (usually frontally) and a small quantity of CSF removed and replaced by air (or in some cases by positive contrast material). In the pneumoencephelogram, air is introduced by way of the lumbar route. In both techniques, the air is circulated through the intracranial ventricular and cisternal system by means of

TABLE 33-11. Indications for Angiography in Brain Tumor Patients

1. Preoperative evaluation of surgically relevant tumor vasculature
2. To detect possible vascular lesion producing mass effect, *i.e.*, AVM
3. To differentiate hemorrhage associated with aneurysms from that of tumor
4. To aid in diagnosis of lesions poorly visualized on CT scan, *i.e.;* posterior fossa tumors

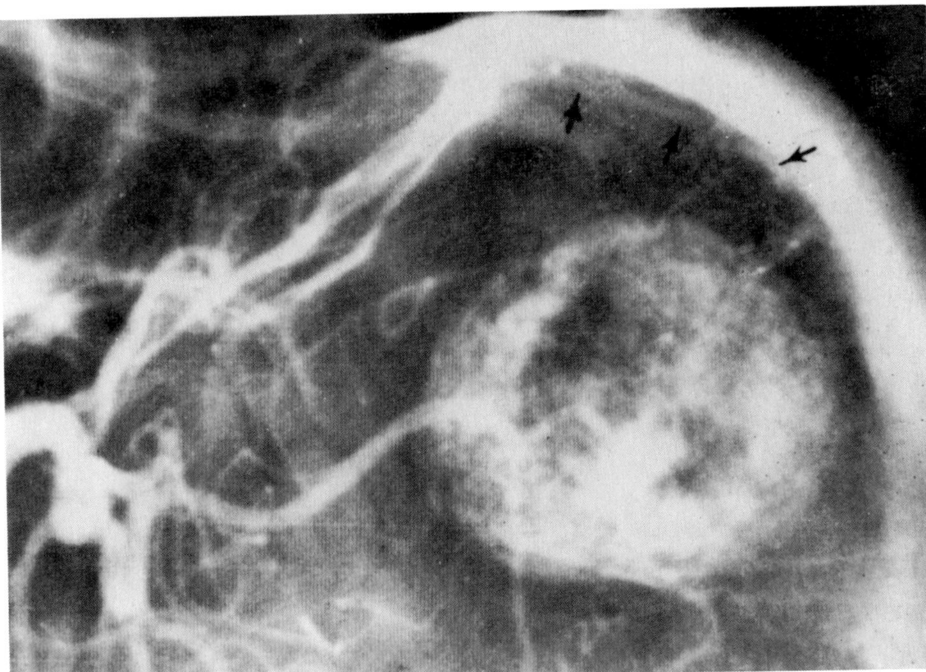

FIG. 33-14. Arteriographic demonstration of tumor blush in frontal falx meningioma. Also seen is the filling of the tumor by the anterior meningeal branch of the ophthalmic artery. (Taveras JM, Wood EH: Diagnostic Neuroradiology. Baltimore, Williams and Wilkins, 1976, p 668)

rotating and positioning the patient. These techniques allow for detection of mass lesions by visualization of displacements, blockages, or identations affecting the ventricular systems or cisterns.

These techniques involve significant risk and marked discomfort for the brain tumor patient. Rapid decrease in blood pressure often occurs, headache is severe, and the displacement of fluid by air can result in major shifts in intracranial structures and even death. The use of the CT scan has significantly decreased the need for these procedures except for deep midline lesions, particularly those of sellar, third and fourth ventricular regions and of posterior fossa. For further indications for PEG see Table 33-12.

In cases in which there is a particular risk of increased ICP the performance of the ventriculogram may be indicated. This procedure allows removal of fluid from above, decreasing the ICP and permitting decompression. It finds use when a posterior fossa or deep midline lesion blocks CSF flow resulting in obstructive hydrocephalus.

The PEG is now used primarily in patients with sellar lesions to observe whether the sellar diaphragm is elevated and there is encroachment into the area of ventricle III. It is very helpful in the "empty sella syndrome," in which pituitary tissue is largely absent from the sella, and a clinical syndrome with effects on vision can occur in the absence of an actively growing pituitary tumor.

For certain lesions, especially CPA tumor in the cerebellum, positive contrast encephalography is needed. Contrast material may be introduced from either above (ventriculogram) or

TABLE 33-12. Indications for Pneumoencephalogram

1. Detection of mass lesions by visualization of displacements, blockages or indentation affecting ventricular system or cisterns
2. Midline lesions, particularly those of sella, third, and fourth ventricular regions and of the posterior fossa
3. Extent of encroachment on cisterna magna
4. Exact site of blockage in ventricular system
5. Differentiate between pituitary tumor and "empty" sella syndrome
6. Pituitary tumors (most common use today)

FIG. 33-15. Arteriographic demonstration of "rounded" shift of anterior cerebral artery as seen in frontal masses. (Taveras JM, Wood EH: Diagnostic Neuroradiology, vol 2, 2nd ed. Baltimore, Williams and Wilkins, 1976, p 654)

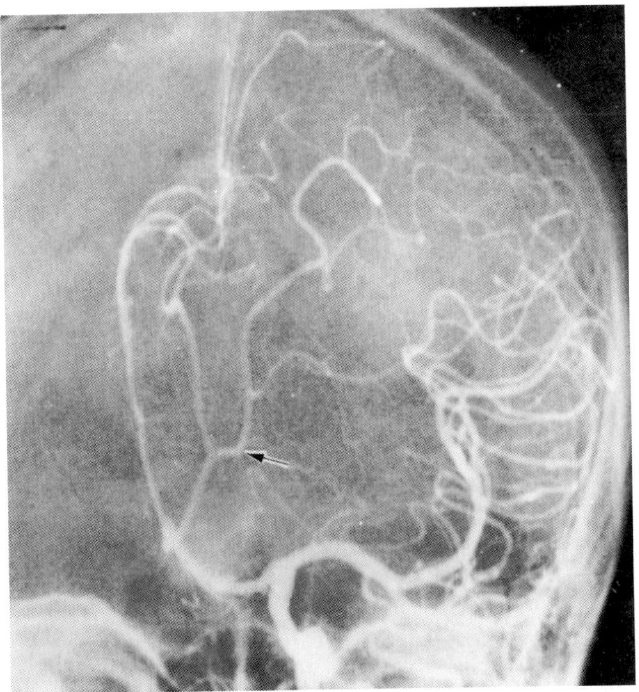

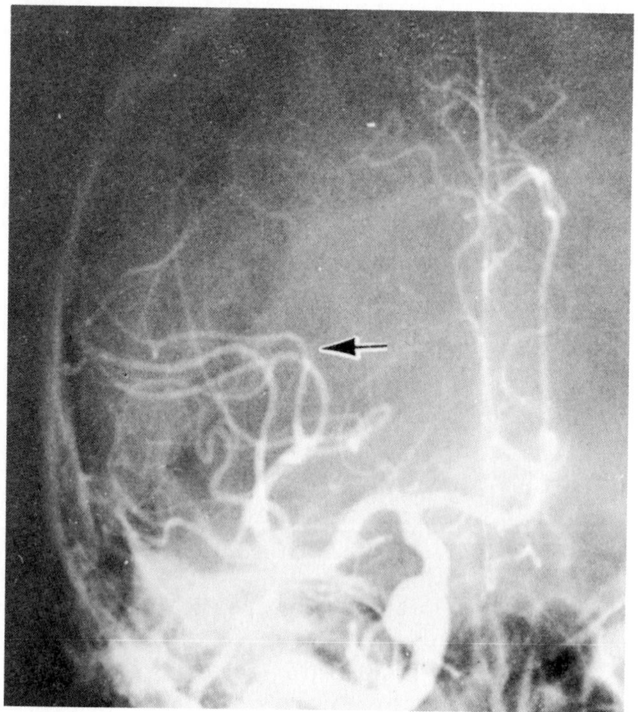

FIG. 33-16. Arteriographic demonstration of "squared" shift of anterior cerebral artery as seen in supra-sylvian tumors. (Taveras JM, Wood EH: Diagnostic Neuroradiology. vol 2, 2nd ed. Baltimore, Williams and Wilkins, 1976, p 654)

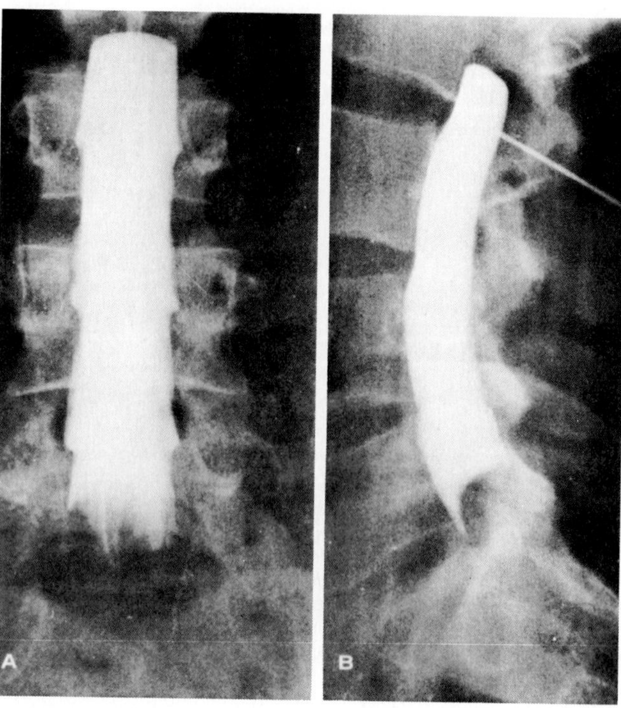

FIG. 33-18. Myelographic demonstration of complete block in flow of contrast material due to spinal tumor: (*A*) frontal view, (*B*) lateral view. (Taveras JM, Wood EH: Diagnostic Neuroradiology, vol 2, 2nd ed. Baltimore, Williams and Wilkins, 1976, p 1177)

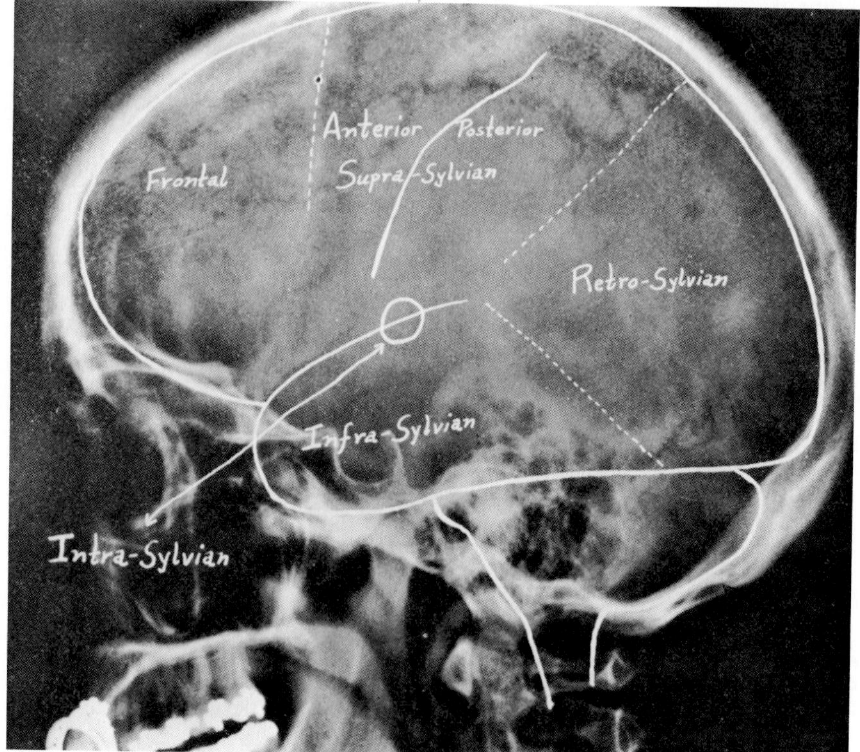

FIG. 33-17. Angiographic classification of brain tumors. (Taveras JM, Wood EH: Diagnostic Neuroradiology. Baltimore, Williams and Wilkins, 1964, p 1579)

TABLE 33-13. Sequence of Clinical Evaluation for Brain Tumor Patients

A. Clinical History (general symtpoms for intracranial tumors)	
1. Progressive course	
2. Headache	
3. Seizures	
4. Weakness or sensory loss	
5. Visual loss	blurring of field of vision
6. Hearing loss	tinnitus or decreased acuity
B. Neurological Examination	
1. Mental status	decreased alertness and decline in intellectual function with increased intracranial pressure in frontal, temporal and parietal lesions
2. Cranial nerves	
CN-I. Anosmia	suggestive of frontal lobe tumor, especially olfactory groove meningioma
CN-II. Papilledema	increased intracranial pressure
Field defects	localize lesion depending on portion of pathways affected
CN-III, IV, VI. Decreased ocular motility	due to increased pressure or tumors at base of brain
CN-V. Facial sensation loss and corneal reflex loss	tumors of cerebellopontine angle
CN-VII. Facial movement loss	tumors of carebellopontine angle
CN-VIII. Hearing loss—balance problems	tumors of cerebellopontine angle
CN-IX, X. Difficulty in swallowing	tumors at base of brain
CN-XI. Asymmetry in shoulder shrugging	tumors at base of brain
CN-XII. Aysmmetry in protruding tongue	tumors deviate tongue to side of lesion
3. Motor function	weakness of hemiplegic type with spasticity in lesions of motor cortex and descending motor pathways
4. Reflex dysfunction	hyperactive reflexes with abnormal reflexes
5. Sensory loss	corresponding to area of sensory cortex or ascending pathways involved
6. Coordination deficits	ataxia, dysmetria in cerebellar and some brain stem lesions
C. Radiological Studies	
1. Skull films	shifts in calcified structures, hyperostosis, decalcification, abnormal calcification
2. CT scan	masses, location and edema
3. Isotope scan	location and extent of masses
4. Angiography	for feeding vessels and localization as well as sequence of vessel filling
5. Pneumoencephalography	for masses in midline and posterior fossa areas
6. Ventriculogram	for deep lesions especially in posterior fossa which have caused increased intracranial pressure
D. Ancillary Studies for Diagnosis	
1. Audiometric examination	for lesions of cerebellopontine angle, temporal cortex
2. Tangent screen and perimetry	detailed visual field documentation
3. Lumbar puncture	when concerned about possibility of infectious process

below (PEG) and the course of its flow outlined. Often, sharper detail of mass lesions in the relevant areas can be obtained and a fairly small amount of material (5 cc) can offer useful data.

SPINAL CORD TECHNIQUES. *Spine Films.* Films of the lumbar, thoracic and cervical spine can be useful in tumor diagnosis. Often, however, the changes seen are those accompanying metastatic lesions (see Chapter 41) and not primary tumors.

A primary tumor which can cause spinal changes, including gross deformities such as scoliosis, is the neurofibroma.

MYELOGRAPHY. The primary radiological procedure for detecting spinal cord tumors is myelography. A radiopaque positive contrast material is introduced by way of the lumbar and occasionally by way of the lateral cervical approach. On

TABLE 33-14. Sequence of Clinical Evaluation for Spinal Cord Tumor Patients

A. History
  1. Pain
  2. Difficulty in ambulation
  3. Sensory disturbances
  4. Bladder and bowel difficulties
  5. Sensory dermatomes

B. Clinical Examination
  1. Sensory loss
    a. Distribution
    b. Levels
    c. Symmetry
  2. Motor loss
    a. Muscles involved
    b. Distribution
    c. Levels
    d. Atrophy
  3. Reflex abnormalities
    a. Hyper- or hyporeflexia
    b. Abnormal reflexes

C. Radiological Examination
  1. Spine films
  2. Myelography
    a. Contrast
    b. Air
  3. Angiography
  4. CT scan

D. Ancillary Studies
  1. Lumbar puncture and CSF examination
    a. Manometrics
    b. Protein
  2. Spinal evoked potentials
  3. EMG and nerve conductive

occasion, air can be used rather than positive contrast material and there has been recent interest in water-soluble agents for myelography.

The use of myelography in tumors can help determine the upper and lower margins of a tumor, the size of the lesion, and its location with respect to the spinal cord, in addition to aiding in the detection of the lesions themselves.

In myelography, the early detection of lesions depends upon noting either enlargement of the cord with intradural, intramedullary tumors or indentation of the contrast column by intradural, extramedullary tumors. Later in tumor progression a partial or complete blockage of contrast flow may occur. In such "blocks" an intramedullary tumor will often produce a contrast margin with crescentic borders, whereas an extramedullary tumor will produce a more irregular margin.

In cases of block (Fig. 33-18) it is often important to know the lower and upper margins of the lesion for either surgical or radiotherapeutic treatment and so lumbar myelography may need to be supplemented by cisternal injections.

Air myelography is most useful when a contrast lighter than CSF is needed and is often used to complement positive contrast myelography. Water-soluble contrast is much less viscous than the lipid-based media and can often show the intricacies of spinal lesions in greater detail.

Myelography of all types carries risks. CSF removal in itself can disrupt the balance of fluid dynamics in certain tumors and neurological findings may worsen. Infection, reaction to contrast, and arachnoiditis have been reported.[73] Spinal cord and cortical seizure activity has occurred from water-soluble agents.[74]

ANGIOGRAPHY. Spinal angiography is a highly specialized technique involving catheterization of the small arteries supplying the spinal cord. The injections are made by way of a femoral artery catheter directed into a specific vessel. This technique is of primary value in evaluating the feeding and draining vessels supplying vascular malformations and occasionally highly vascular cord tumors.[75]

SPINAL CT SCAN. This relatively new technique offers the promise of detecting mass lesions in the spine with the same proficiency as cerebral CT scans. Early developmental reports suggest excellent resolution and significant diagnostic potential.[76]

Diagnostic Workup

As indicated in Table 33-13 there is a specific sequence of the clinical evaluation for the brain tumor suspect. The sequence for the spinal cord tumor suspect is shown in Table 33-14.

There is still no substitute for the careful history and neurological exam. The general physical examination is extremely valuable in differential diagnosis and in evaluating the clinical condition regarding the patient's ability to tolerate

TABLE 33-15. Role of Diagnostic Techniques in Evaluation for Brain Tumor Patients

TECHNIQUE	INDICATIONS
History	All patients
Neurological examination	All patients
General medical and metabolic evaluation	All patients
Skull films	All patients
CT scan	Patients with history and exam suggestive of brain tumor findings
EEG	Patients with findings suggestive of seizure disorder
Isotope scan	Localization of certain tumors, *e.g.*, meningioma, *esp.* prior to surgery
Angiography	1. Preoperative evaluation of specific vascular supply 2. Differentiation of dynamics of vascular pattern, *i.e.*, early or late filling 3. Determination of general vascularization of tumor
Pneumoencephalography	1. Centrally located masses in midline, *i.e.*, pituitary tumors 2. Posterior fossa tumors
Ventriculogram	Patients with deep midline lesions who may need decompression from above prior to procedure
Lumbar puncture	1. Differentiating infection from tumor 2. Screening patients with no evidence of increased pressure 3. Follow-ups of patients with known tumors 4. Monitoring of pressure

surgery. In older patients, chest radiography to exclude primary lung carcinoma presenting because of cerebral metastases is often helpful. After these principal steps, the CT scan seems the most dependable, safest, and highest yield diagnostic approach for brain tumors.

Indications for Use of Diagnostic Techniques

Table 33-15 illustrates certain indications for the use of the major diagnostic techniques which have been described.

TREATMENT

The discussion of the treatment of CNS tumors will be divided into intracranial and spinal cord lesions. A presentation of the basic treatment modalities, their applications and then risks will be given. This will be followed by anatomically oriented descriptions of the major tumor types which occur in that area. The therapeutic plans discussed in this section will emphasize those in current general use. The last section will describe some of the newer and potentially useful approaches.

INTRACRANIAL TUMORS

General Treatment Modalities

SURGERY. Surgical procedures in the treatment of intracranial tumors can be of four types: biopsy, partial resection (decompression), tumor removal, and lobectomy. In addition, procedures for drainage of CSF (shunts) can be of value in relieving pressure.

"Biopsy" implies the removal of sufficient tissue for establishing the diagnosis without any attempt at significant tumor removal. Partial resection involves removing a portion of the tumor which is safely accessible. Tumor removal applies primarily to benign, well-demarcated lesions which often have a capsule and can be extirpated from surrounding normal tissues. Complete or partial lobectomy is applicable in certain frontal, occipital, temporal, and cerebellar lesions, usually of a malignant nature. Operative mortality is less than 1%. For complication of surgical procedures see Table 33-16. Some sites in the brain are inaccessible for surgery. These are listed in Table 33-17.

Biopsy. The techniques of biopsy include needle biopsy, open biopsy, and stereotactic biopsy. The indications for biopsy are a likely malignant tumor in a crucial location (*e.g.*, parietal astrocytoma), a deep-seated lesion (*e.g.*, thalamic glioma) and an extremely ill or elderly patient unable to tolerate a more strenuous procedure. Biopsy has been suggested as the overall surgical approach to malignant brain tumors.[77] In this view a biopsy is done for most lesions and then followed by therapy with radiation or chemotherapy. The risks of biopsy include a relatively high rate of inadequate diagnosis (30%).[78] This may be due to either too small a sample, a sample from a non-representation area, or inadequate viability of the tissue for complete study. A second risk is the danger of an uncontrollable hemorrhage in an area rendered inaccessible by either the lack of a craniotomy or the lack of adequate exposure; this occurs in about 5% of cases so treated. A third major risk of biopsy is the danger of postoperative swelling unrelieved by the decompression of surrounding tissues. The use of high dosage corticosteroids pre-operatively has diminished this problem somewhat but it still is of concern and occurs in about 20% of patients biopsied. However, biopsy may be the only technique even worth considering for those categories of patients in whom other techniques are far too dangerous.

TABLE 33-16. Complications of Intracranial Surgery for Tumor

A. Cerebral edema, postoperative
B. Cerebral vascular accidents (occlusive or hemorrhagic)
C. Hematoma (subdural or epidural)
D. Hydrocephalus (obstructive or communicating)
E. Increased incidence of thrombophlebitis and pulmonary embolism
F. Infection
G. Neurological focal deficits, transient or permanent (depending upon tumor location)

TABLE 33-17. Surgical Inaccessible Cerebral Areas

A. Brain stem
B. Corpus callosum
C. Medulla
D. Midbrain
E. Pons
F. Thalamus (except for tumors which are present on ventricular surface or extend laterally into temporal regions).

If at all possible, open biopsy is preferable to either needle or stereotactic techniques. In open biopsy, a small craniotomy or trephine is made in the area of the lesion and then, upon opening the dura, a 1 cm or smaller cortical incision is made to gain access to the tumor tissue. The gross appearance of the tissue and the location of major blood vessels can be visualized. Repeated samples can also be obtained if the initial samples do not clarify the diagnosis on frozen section.

PARTIAL RESECTION, TUMOR REMOVAL, AND LOBECTOMY. These three major operative approaches will be discussed together, inasmuch as the general techniques and risks are quite similar. The major differences in the approaches occur during the surgical procedure when a decision is made on the basis of the surgical pathology and anatomy which procedure is best suited to the specific situation.

The basic considerations for these surgical procedures involve preoperative medical preparations, intra-operative anesthesia and medical management, the surgical techniques themselves, and postoperative care.

The preoperative preparations (see Table 33-18) include a detailed diagnostic evaluation with a considerable effort to localize the main mass of tumor, the peripheral edema, and the major supplying vessels. Cardiovascular status is crucial, as many procedures involve relatively abrupt changes in blood pressure. The respiratory status, including blood gases and tidal volume, is crucial, as retained CO_2 can be extremely harmful in raising ICP and thus encouraging postoperative cerebral edema. Hyperventilation to remove CO_2 can be a technique for decreasing cerebral swelling. Renal function is important in that there is a need to restrict intra-operative

TABLE 33-18. Pre-operative Preparation of Patient

A. Neurological examination and clinical history

B. Quantitative techniques adjunctive to the neurological examination (see text)

C. Medical status of patient
   1. Cardiovascular status including abrupt changes in blood pressure and ability to tolerate these changes
   2. Respiratory status including blood gases and tidal volume
   3. Renal function tests
   4. Bladder function and status of urethra
   5. Hematological evaluation
   6. Other medical status, *i.e.*, ocular disorder, diabetes mellitus
   7. Status of airway, larynx

D. Preparation for surgery
   1. Corticosteroids, at least 2 days prior to surgery
   2. Preoperative shampoo
   3. Anticonvulsant

E. Anesthesia phase
   1. Blood pressure
   2. Ventilation
   3. Placement of padding
   4. Elastic stockings
   5. Placement of arterial catheter
   6. Urinary catheter

F. Positioning of patient

G. Cleansing of scalp

fluid intake and often a further need to "dry out" the brain with osmotic diuretics. The function of the bladder and the status of the urethra are of further specific import, since urinary drainage catheters may be necessary for long durations. Hematological factors can be critical. Any blood dyscrasia which results in a prolonged bleeding time or coagulation problems can make neurosurgery extremely dangerous. Corrections of such bleeding problems are a prerequisite for elective neurosurgical procedures. Other medical aspects to consider include whether a patient has an ocular disorder, such as glaucoma, for a long procedure may require intra-operative medications. Diabetes mellitus is a consideration, as the use of dextrose-containing solutions and corticosteroids are part of the procedures. The status of the airway, the larynx in particular, is also a factor, for the endotracheal tube may also be in place for long periods.

After diagnostic and medical considerations have been completed, the patient is ready for surgical preparation. There are at least three important measures which need to be carried out routinely. First the patient should be given corticosteroids at a dose equivalent to 4 mg to 8 mg of dexamethasone, every 6 hours beginning at least 2 days prior to surgery, preferably earlier if significant cerebral edema is present. The efficacy of this maneuver has been demonstrated in many studies.[79] For one or two nights prior to surgery the pre-operative shampoo is done, often with an agent effective in diminishing staphylococcal organisms.

A third measure, especially for supratentorial tumors, is the use of an anticonvulsant, especially diphenylhydantoin 100 mg tid, started several days before surgery, since it takes this interval to reach an effective blood level.

In the anesthesia phase of the operative procedure, there are several important facets. The blood pressure needs to be prevented from rising excessively, as this increases cerebral swelling. Care is necessary in providing optimum ventilation, as retained CO_2 is another cause of raised ICP. Inhalation agents, such as Halothane, which do not alter cerebral blood flow or systemic blood pressure to a marked degree, are commonly used for anesthesia. Padding is placed to prevent neurovascular or skin compression of arms or legs during the longer procedures. Elastic stockings decrease the risks of pulmonary embolism from venous stasis. The anesthesia induction period is often fairly lengthy, to protect the patient from too rapid changes in blood pressure and from coughing, as this serves to raise the ICP. An arterial catheter is often placed in the radial artery for precise BP control. Prior to surgery a urinary catheter is placed, the availability of cross-matched blood is checked, and all or part of the scalp hair is removed.

A good operative procedure depends upon excellent exposure and this is in part dependent on proper operative positioning. In general, the patient lies supine for frontal, temporal, and anterior parietal lesions, and in the lateral position for posterior parietal and occipital lesions. Low occipital and cerebellar access requires either the prone position or the sitting position. The sitting position poses special problems but offers significant benefits. In the sitting position, the cerebellum is more accessible surgically, and there is less arterial bleeding due to the elevation of the head. On the other hand, air embolism through open subatmospheric pressure venous channels and hypotension are more serious problems. The use of a precordial Doppler device with a large bone CVP line in the right heart allows for detection of air embolism. Careful monitoring of BP and the use of hypertensive agents (such as isoproterenol) help in preventing severe hypotension.

Once the patient has been positioned and the scalp thoroughly cleansed, a scalp flap appropriate to the tumor site is made. In general, the flap should be large enough to create good exposure but the smaller the flap the less the blood loss. A representative series of scalp flaps for the different operative areas is seen in Fig. 33-19 *A, B, C, D, E*. The crucial steps in making the scalp flap include extreme care with hemostasis and cutting the skin edges perpendicular to the skull. When the scalp flap is retracted and it has adequate continuing blood supply, the bone is removed. In supratentorial tumors, a craniotomy is usually done and in cerebellar lesions a craniectomy. In the craniotomy the bone is removed as one segment using a craniotome or Gigli saw after initial burr holes have been made. In a craniectomy the bone is totally removed, often in small pieces, using a ronguer. After waxing the bone edges to prevent bleeding or air intake, the dura is opened above the tumor site. This must be done with care not to damage pial vessels or the cortex itself, as the brain is often under increased pressure and tightly pressing on the dura. The use of I.V. mannitol about 20 minutes to 30 minutes prior to dural opening is often indicated to lessen this pressure and in some cases lumbar or ventricular CSF drainage can additionally relieve the pressure. Dural sutures, attaching the dural edges to the pericranium, prevent extradural blood loss intra-operatively and help in preventing postoperative extradural hematomas from accumulating.

Upon reflection of the dural flap, the cerebral or cerebellar

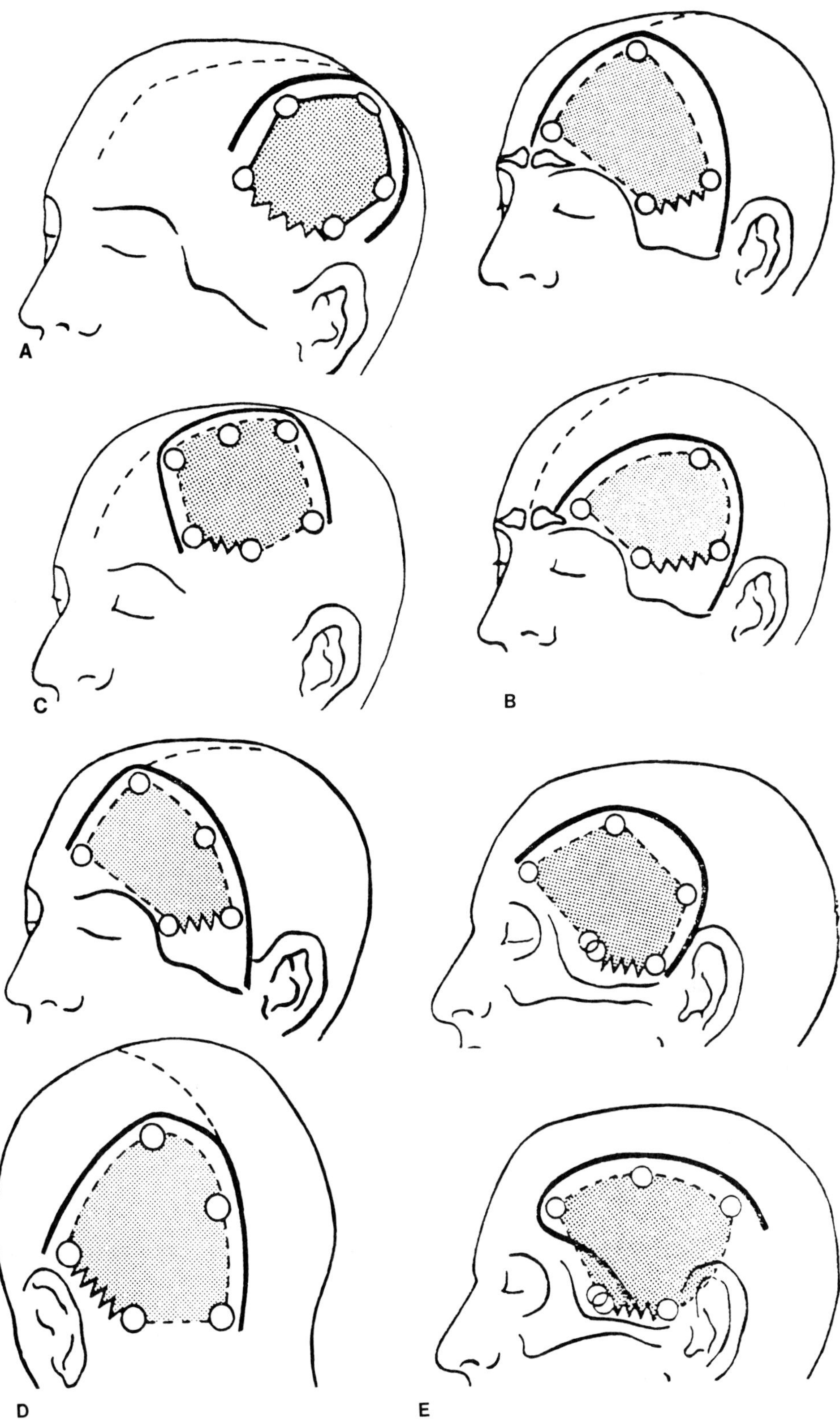

FIG. 33-19. Types of scalp incisions to expose different areas of the brain: (*A*) exposure of the surface of cerebral hemisphere (for convexity lesions); (*B, top and bottom*) exposure of the base of the brain frontally for meningiomas and pituitary adenomas; (*C*) exposure of midline region for perisagittal and falx meningiomas; (*D, top and bottom*) exposure for frontal lobectomies and occipital lobectomies such as for astrocytoma; (*E, top and bottom*) exposure for removal of temporal lobe tumors. (Illingworth RD: Craniotomy. In Rob C, Smith R (eds): Operative Surgery: Neurosurgery, 3rd ed. London, Butterworth, 1979, pp 54–56)

surface is encountered. Initially the inspection of the brain is a very useful maneuver. One can detect hyperemia, swelling, vascular engorgement, discoloration, flattening of gyri, obliteration of sulci and, in some cases, the tumor itself presenting at the surface.

Using the radiological localization data, the presence of a tumor not presenting on the surface can then be confirmed by gentle palpation if subjacent to the surface or by probing with a #16 ventricular needle if deep to the surface. A small pial area is electrocoagulated prior to needle placement. When the depth and location of the tumor have been ascertained, the lesion is approached by a cortisectomy or opening into the cortex of the brain. The techniques used involve gentle dissection of the tumor from the surrounding normal brain tissue using suction, electrocoagulation, and extremely gentle retraction. The brain is quite soft and can easily be displaced by retraction, but it is very sensitive to such retractor pressure, especially over long periods. In general, it is best to put pressure only on tumor and protect the normal brain with moist cotton patties or rubber sheets.

This general description of brain tumor surgery now diverges, based on the gross pathology of the lesion. For an encapsulated, non-infiltrating tumor, the lesion can now be removed by either *en bloc* technique, if the opening in the cortex permits, or in smaller sections if necessary. It is important to attempt to remove the capsule. If the tumor is to be partially resected then that portion to be left behind is often in close relation to normal brain and must be protected. In lobectomy, anatomic landmarks are noted and if areas susceptible to electrical stimulation are involved, the use of cortical stimulation can help mark the boundaries of safety for resection.

After the tumor has been removed and sent for pathological study, meticulous hemostasis is the next step and all vessels need to be observed, coagulated if necessary or packed with a hemostatic agent (surgical or oxycel). When the tumor has been removed, there is often a remarkable decrease in tension of the brain and the dura can usually be closed easily. If only a small area of tumor has been removed, the brain may be swollen, and dural closure, which should be watertight, may require the use of a grafted piece of pericranium.

Mention should be made of the importance of lighting, magnification, and microsurgical techniques to the safe surgical treatment of tumors. The operative microscope provides excellent light, allows the use of smaller cortical openings, and provides the magnification needed to fully visualize the minute feeding vessels which may supply a crucial brain area. Microsurgical instruments and bipolar coagulation allow extremely fine control of the operative dissection.

After dural closure the bone is wired in place, a dural tenting suture is tied, the galea and then the skin are approximated, and a suitable dressing applied.

Immediately postoperatively, the care of respiratory and blood pressure status is critical and adequate ventilation and reasonable alertness should be assured prior to extubation. Postoperatively, very frequent neurological and vital sign checks are needed. The patients are continued on fluid restriction, anticonvulsants, and corticosteroids. Any evidence of pupillary dilatation, rapid change in pulse or blood pressure, or development of new neurological deficits in the postoperative period may reflect intracranial bleeding. CT scanning is the most effective means of making this diagnosis. In most postoperative patients, some changes in neurological status can be anticipated at the second to fourth postoperative day owing to evolving cerebral edema.

If the postoperative course is satisfactory (see Table 33-19 for postoperative management of patients), the patient should be able to be out of bed in 24 hours to 48 hours, have fluids by mouth, and have the sutures removed in about 7 days. In addition to the neurological concerns in the postoperative period, thrombophlebitis and pulmonary embolism deserve special note. These patients are dehydrated, have been in one position for a long interval and are thus prime candidates for thrombotic problems. Because of the risk of intracranial bleeding, the use of anticoagulants is contraindicated in the first 2 weeks to 3 weeks postoperatively. If elevation, bed rest, and elastic or pneumatic stockings are not deemed sufficient therapy, these patients may require early vascular surgical intervention of some type (vena cava ligation or balloon catheter placements).

RADIATION THERAPY. Several critical questions face the radiation therapist evaluating a patient with a primary CNS neoplasm. Many of these will be discussed in this introductory section and several technical aspects necessary for optimal results will be briefly discussed.

Perhaps more frequently than in any other clinical setting, the therapist involved with CNS tumors must consider the necessity and desirability of surgical intervention to obtain biopsy confirmation of tumor. In addition, the extent of surgery considered optimum should be discussed by the therapeutic team *prior* to any surgical intervention.

A significant fraction of brain tumors occur in functionally critical areas, such as the brain stem, hypothalamus, thalamus, and midbrain. When the likelihood of tumor is considered to be very great following appropriate studies, the potential morbidity and mortality of operative intervention merely to obtain tissue confirmation is not warranted. Several studies have demonstrated that tumor is overwhelmingly likely and, as surgical resection beyond biopsy is clearly not possible, local control with irradiation is essential.

A second consideration is the desirability of potential complete resection when tedious and prolonged surgical intervention will be necessary to accomplish this end. In certain settings, that is, the glioma A or microcystic astrocytoma of the cerebellum in childhood, such careful attempts are nearly always warranted. However, the radiation therapist should caution against such an approach when irradiation will clearly be necessary, as with medulloblastoma.

The therapist must also decide if radiation fields with relatively restricted margins about the evident tumor will suffice, as with pituitary neoplasms, or if regionally extensive fields are desirable, as with intermediate grade gliomas. Finally, craniospinal treatment may be necessary, as with medulloblastomas. Clearly, the age, radiation dose necessary for microscopic control, and relative size of the patient, as well as the long-term risk of seeding, must be considered in arriving at a final decision, especially when temporary palliation is the goal. Unfortunately, patients most frequently requiring such craniospinal treatment are often in the younger

TABLE 33-19. Considerations of Postoperative Management of Patients Following Intracranial Surgery

A. Immediate management
   1. Respiration
   2. Pulse
   3. Blood pressure
   4. Ventilation
   5. Alertness

B. Check of neurological and vital signs

C. Medication
   1. Fluid restriction
   2. Anticonvulsants (first 2–3 days)
   3. Corticosteroids

D. Postoperative course
   1. Out of bed (24–48 hours) versus bed rest, depending upon condition
   2. Fluids by mouth
   3. Removal of sutures (day 7)
   4. Check for thrombophlebitis and pulmonary embolism
   5. Surgical intervention (vena cava ligation or balloon catheter placements)
   6. Elastic or pneumatic stockings

age group, where morbidity is greatest. The ultimate risk of craniospinal dissemination can only be accurately evaluated when a group of patients who have survived for a relatively long period with clinical primary control are considered. Studies estimating the risk of seeding based on short-term evaluation of patients dying relatively rapidly of primary progression are certain to underestimate the true risk.

The radiation dose desired, technique to be used, and the question of dose modification for the pediatric patient must be considered. No study accurately compares the risk of brain necrosis for a given treatment regimen for a child versus an adult. Numerous studies are available detailing pediatric patients who have received radiation doses in excess of 5000 rad to limited portions of the brain without an unacceptable incidence of necrosis.[80–83] Relatively few documented instances of radiation brain necrosis in patients of any age have been reported.[84] When biologically different types or regimens of irradiation have been used or when chemotherapy (especially methotrexate) has been combined with irradiation, this incidence has clearly increased.[85–87] Conversely, children, especially those under the age of 5 years, seem to be more susceptible to certain functional consequences of moderate or high dose irradiation, such as hypothalmic/pituitary hormonal dysfunction or certain types of learning disabilities. Myelinization appears to be nearly completed by 2 years to 3 years. Prior to this time, high doses of irradiation might be expected to be associated with substantially more risks. Fortunately, primary brain tumors in this age child are quite infrequent.

Choice of a radiation dose or regimen that has minimal likelihood for ultimate disease control solely because of the young age of the patient is clearly to be condemned. Selection for the pediatric patient of a regimen yielding nearly equivalent disease control but with an appropriate decrease in treatment morbidity represents a difficult clinical problem. Nearly always in such situations, use of a total radiation dose, volume, and fractionation plan which closely approximates those found to be effective in adults will usually be found to be optimum.

Development of radiation treatment plans which optimize homogeneity of radiation dose throughout the tumor volume selected and minimize high dose regions in normal brain transited by the radiation beam is always desirable. Such technique improvements represent the easiest and most certain way to improve the therapeutic ratio regardless of a patient's age. With available megavoltage equipment, such optimization is most often accomplished by use of multiple fields, rotational techniques, or radiation beam modifiers such as wedges, compensators, or individually shaped blocks to protect normal tissue.

Several representative treatment plans for tumors in specific anatomic locations are shown in Fig. 33-20 *A,B,C,D,E*. An arc wedge plan is shown in Fig. 33-20*A*. This plan is particularly useful for centrally located lesions such as pituitary neoplasms, craniopharyngiomas, or chordomas or to boost treatments for deep-seated cerebral gliomas or pineal neoplasms. A typical right angle "wedge pair" plan, useful for treatment of lesions restricted to one quadrant of the cranial cavity, is also shown (Fig. 33-20 *B*)

Figure 33-20 *C* depicts treatment details and fields necessary for treatment of the craniospinal axis to avoid areas of treatment overlap or underlap. In addition to precise field arrangements facilitated by routine use of permanent pinpoint tatoos placed at critical points, construction of an individualized immobilization device (Fig. 33-20 *D*) must be accomplished for reproducibility of day-to-day treatments. Other important questions relate to the timing of irradiation following surgery and the necessity to use graded "build-up" doses when initiating treatment.

For most patients, the clinical setting permits a period of 1 week to 2 weeks to elapse following surgical therapy prior to initiation of irradiation. During this period, considerable postoperative stabilization will occur, acute but transient complications such as diabetes insipidus may resolve and significant wound healing can take place, potentially lessening the risks of infection or dehiscence. A waiting period of this approximate duration is recommended. However, many patients will require more rapid definitive treatment (*i.e.*, the child with only partially resected medulloblastoma). Such rapid initiation of irradiation is usually well tolerated, without a major increase in the incidence of complications.

Considerable controversy exists over the value of initiating irradiation by means of small incremental increases in daily dose (*i.e.*, 25, 50, 75, 100, 150, 180 rad). Proponents feel that this type of schedule lessens the risk of treatment-associated edema and the risk of brain swelling. Others argue that tumor response to these small doses is insufficient and use of such a protracted schedule only delays adequate treatment and thus prolongs or increases the period of risk. No definitive study has been performed; however, where surgical decompression or a shunt procedure has been performed prior to irradiation, such a technique is rarely necessary. On occasion, particularly with spinal compression or with a marginally compensated undecompressed patient, use of such a protracted schedule appears to be of benefit. Often, in this setting, a patient may receive two or more fractions per day,

(Text continues on p. 1218)

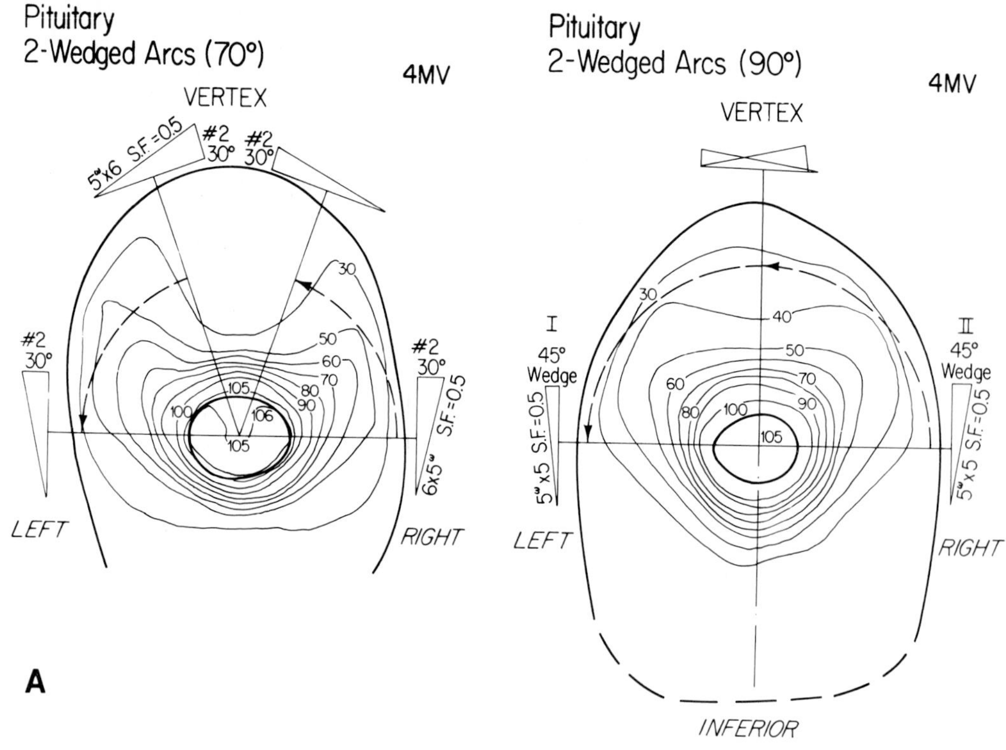

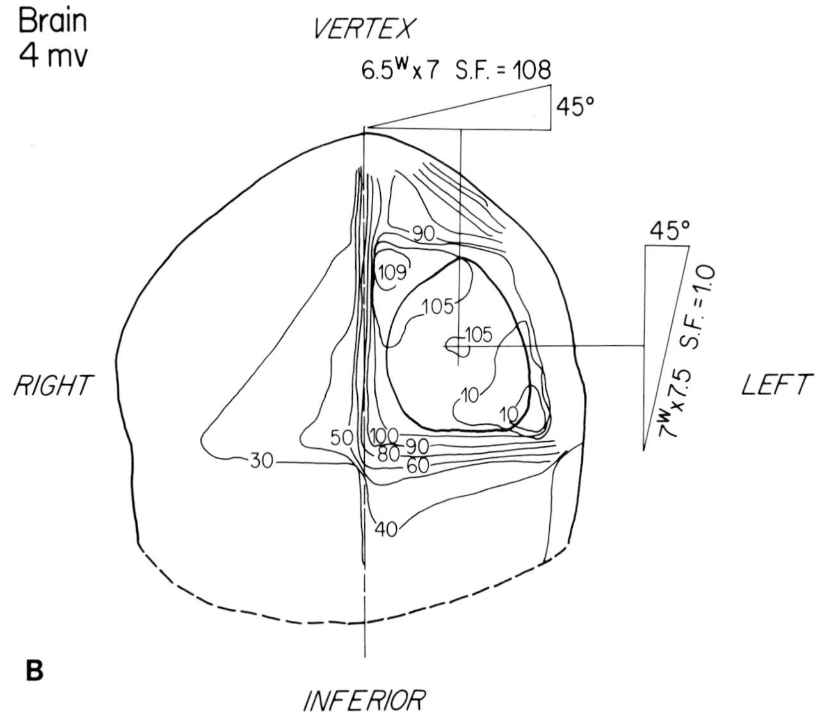

FIG. 33-20. (*A*) Isodose distributions using an arc wedge plan especially suitable for spherical or ovoid tumors in the pituitary, pineal, or third ventricular area. This treatment plan is also useful in treatment of spinal cord lesions. Note should be taken of the excellent hemogeneity throughout the tumor volume (dark line) and rapid fall-off of dose in normal brain. S.F. = scaling factor. (*B*) Isodose distribution for a right angle wedge plan particularly suitable for limited lesions in one area of the cortex such as the frontal region. This plan may be adapted to either frontal (antero–posterior or postero–anterior) and lateral beam directions or a frontal or lateral and vertex beam direction. S.F. = scaling factor. (*C*) Schematic illustration of medulloblastoma treatment technique. The left panel demonstrates approximate regions to be irradiated in dotted lines and also shows usual locations for field junctions. Multiple junction sites are utilized (usually at least three) to minimize any inhomogeneity in dose across the junction. The central illustration demonstrates the cephalic angulation of the lateral skull portal necessary to establish a parallel juncture with the posteriorly directed spine field. The inclusion of the sacral roots is also schematically shown. The panel at the right shows the field block which is individually constructed to shield the eye and nasopharynx region from irradiation and also demonstrates the orientation of the lateral skull field in relation to the posterior spine field(s). (*D*) Isodose distribution for three-field plan (anterior, posterior, and lateral) useful in treatment of extensive hemispheral tumor. The anterior and posterior fields must have a wedged beam absorber in order to achieve dose homogeneity. S.F. = scaling factor. (*E*) Isodose distribution for three-field plan (two wedged laterals and one vertex) useful for extensive centrally placed lesions such as a large tumor of the optic pathways with posterior extension. S.F. = scaling factor. (*Figure continues on opposite page*)

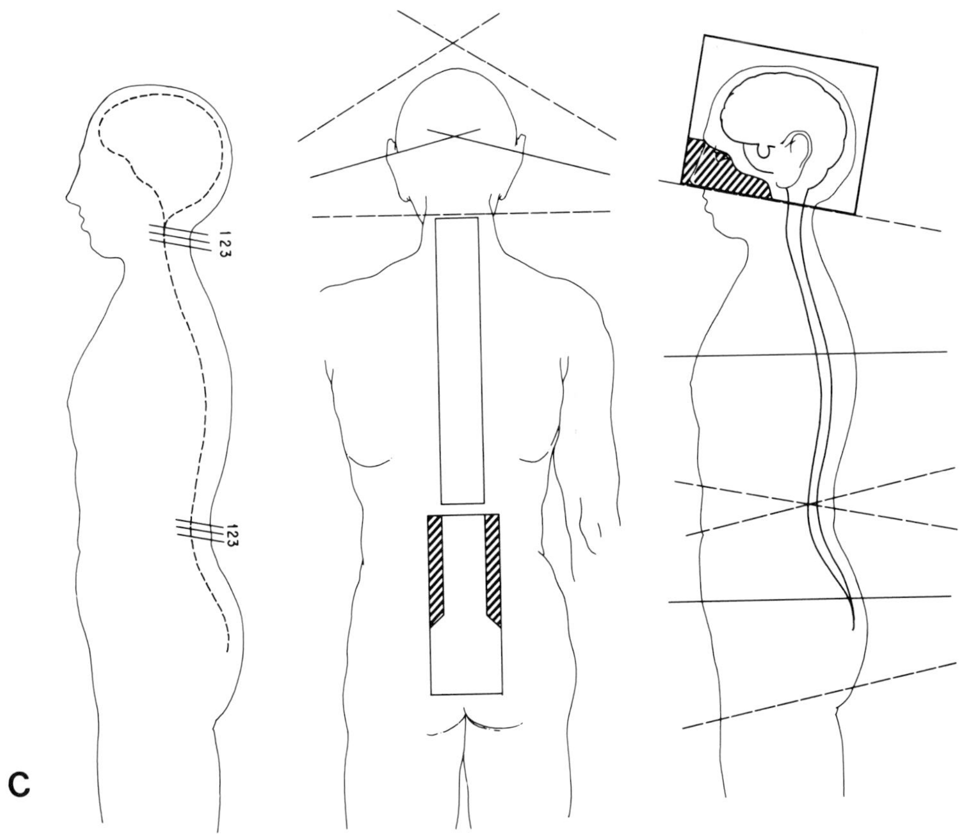
123
123
C

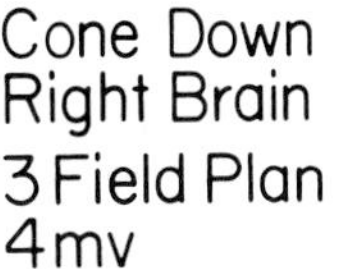
Cone Down
Right Brain
3 Field Plan
4mv

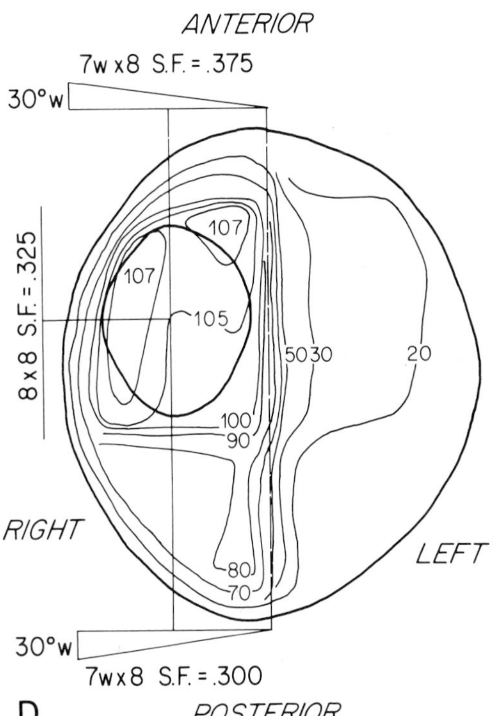
ANTERIOR
7w x 8 S.F. = .375
30°w
8 x 8 S.F. = .325
107
107
105
50
30
20
100
90
80
70
RIGHT
LEFT
30°w
7w x 8 S.F. = .300
D
POSTERIOR

Cone Down
Optic Pathways
4 mv

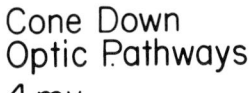

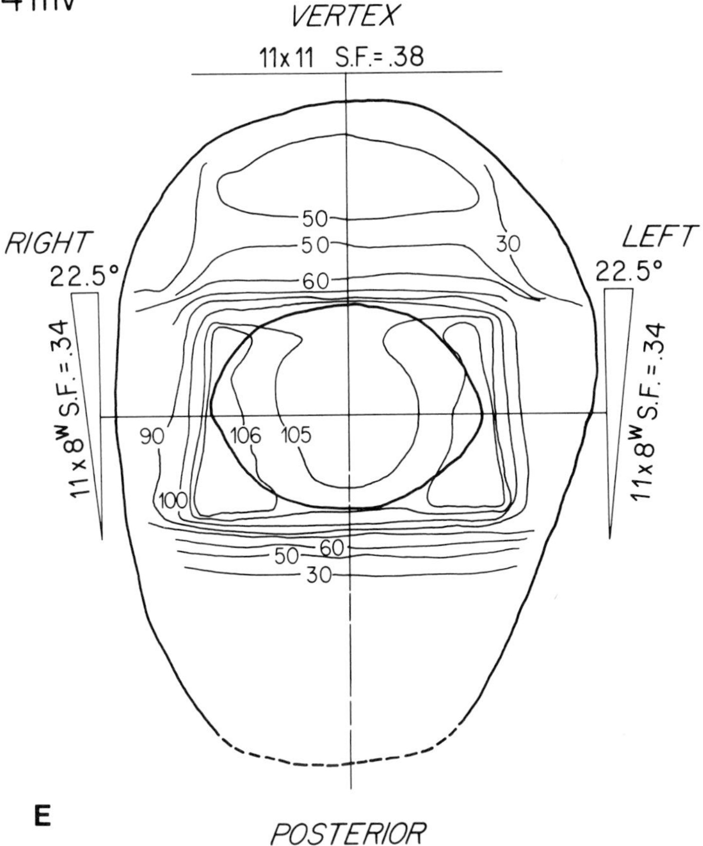
VERTEX
11x11 S.F. = .38
RIGHT
22.5°
LEFT
22.5°
50
50
60
30
11 x 8W S.F. = .34
11 x 8W S.F. = .34
90
106
105
100
50
60
30
E
POSTERIOR

thus increasing the daily dose and hastening the "build-up" period.

Several studies relate the size of the daily radiation fraction to the incidence of complications.[88,89] For this reason, a maximum daily dose greater than 200 rad is rarely recommended except when dealing with an obviously palliative situation, as in treatment of brain metastases. When a course of high dose definitive irradiation is to be given, we favor daily radiation fractions of 175 rad to 180 rad (900 rad/week).

The total radiation dose recommended may vary considerably depending on tumor type, location, size of radiation field to be used, prior treatment, or anticipated delivery of concurrent or adjuvant chemotherapeutic treatment. Specific recommendations are given in the following section devoted to individual tumor types.

CHEMOTHERAPY: GENERAL PRINCIPLES. The treatment of malignant brain tumors, until recently, has been limited to surgery followed by radiotherapy for a considerably smaller proportion of patients. Surgery is limited by virtue of the fact that these procedures can be carried out relatively infrequently owing to the trauma and hazard to the patient, as well as to the inability in many instances to fully resect the tumor. Since many brain tumors (malignant gliomas being the most common and a case in point) do not have clear demarcation from normal brain, frequently merge from frankly neoplastic tissue into edematous brain, and often have apparently separate local spread, such tumors cannot be clearly and cleanly removed. Their intrinsic involvement with vital areas of brain function frequently means "large margins" cannot be taken and often the tumor is in such a location that judicious surgery is confined to a modest subtotal resection. Because of either increased intracranial pressure caused by a mass lesion or local space-occupying effects of a tumor, surgery is usually considered as the first and most important treatment. Thus, with judicious use of the knife the surgeon can markedly control increased intracranial pressure, reduce the tumor burden present and obtain tissue for neuropathologic and biologic analysis. However, the tumor has been perturbed by surgical intervention and its kinetics in all probability altered.

Irradiation, on the other hand, has as its prime advantage the fact that it is local therapy for what is clearly a local and non-metastasizing tumor. The toxicity then is only to the immediately involved brain parenchyma, its vasculature and supporting structures. Radiotherapy has as its limitations the maximally tolerated dose that normal brain tissue can accept without the development of radiation necrosis. There is a further perturbation by the use of ionizing irradiation, usually delivered daily, 5 days a week for some 6 weeks.

The remaining modality of treatment therefore is chemotherapy, which may be applied locally or systemically. Chemotherapy almost inevitably exhibits its primary toxicity in organs other than the brain and hence it is systemic therapy which is limited by virtue of its systemic side-effects.

Chemotherapy cannot be considered independent of surgery and irradiation but must be integrated into therapeutic planning, which takes into account the biology of brain tumor. The majority of other cancers that have responded to therapeutic approaches have usually done so in relation to multimodal treatment (surgery, radiation, and chemotherapy), which has been utilized either in sequential or concomitant treatment schedules. The interrelationship of radiotherapy and chemotherapy has not clearly been elucidated.

The classic concept of phased studies in the application of chemotherapy is no place more clearly found than in the treatment of brain tumor. Phase I studies of new drugs may be carried out in patients with brain tumors, provided they have sufficient marrow reserve. In one sense they are more ideal patients for such investigations, as they rarely have systemic disease and therefore do not have hepatic, renal, or pulmonary compromise. However, it is inappropriate use of patient material to utilize patients with brain tumors for Phase I studies if there are any other treatment modalities which should be investigated that will specifically aid patients with brain tumors. From a therapeutic point of view the Phase II study of chemotherapeutic agents in patients with brain tumor is extremely important.

Drugs entering into Phase II studies are selected because they have: (1) the appropriate pharmacologic characteristics which allow them to enter into the brain; (2) evidence of efficacy in one of the various experimental brain tumor models; (3) an indication from the treatment of other malignant disease that the drug in question is one which has potential wide application; and (4) a specific biochemical mode of action that directly relates to brain tumor metabolism. The conduct of the Phase II study is one which relies primarily on the judgement of the investigator supported by some objective and statistically manipulatable measurement factors. Because of the complexity of measuring outcome in patients with malignant glioma, Phase II studies are extraordinarily difficult to analyze in a meaningful fashion. Therefore, any drug which shows a reasonable indication of value in Phase II should be subjected to more carefully controlled studies.

The Phase III study is clearly the most important and the most difficult to carry out in the treatment of malignant brain tumors. Strict selection criteria, careful documentation of pathology, randomization procedure, and the requirement for close and continuous follow-up all add severe limitations to the study of this disease. The implication of the null hypothesis expressed by the randomization procedure places the surgeon in an antithetical position. That is, his training and inherent disposition is that of decision-making on behalf of and for the benefit of his patient. When he must state that he does not know which treatment is better and therefore must revert to the randomization procedure, a discordant note is rung. Nevertheless, the Phase III control study for evaluating chemotherapeutic efficacy remains the most effective way of *proving* efficacy.

There are a number of biologic variables as related to chemotherapy of brain tumor which are either different or unique compared to other cancers. The histopathology as commonly reported is not necessarily related to the biologic events of the tumor and is therefore only one part of the equation. An examination of Fig. 33-21 indicates that there are clearcut differences between astrocytoma Grade I and astrocytoma Grade II. Malignant astrocytomas (Grade III) and glioblastoma (Grade IV) share essentially the same survival curve through the median point and are not as distinct from each other as are Grades I and II. A review of some 417 cases of intracranial astrocytoma from the Mayo Clinic (where the Kernohan Grading system originated) noted that the survival patterns for Grade I and II tumors were extremely similar and in fact combined them into what they now call "low-grade" astrocytoma. Similarly, they noted that Grade III and IV astrocytomas had no significant difference and therefore reunited them into "high-grade" astrocytomas.[90] Thus, they now propose two grades on the basis of histology. The studies of Winston and colleagues have demonstrated that very few of the histopathologic variables which are graded and described bear any significant relationship to survival.[37,38] It is evident from the above information that histopathologic classification of brain tumors is far from clear. Precisely what factors observed under the light microscope are truly significant and relate to biologic events and what factors are merely observations without known biologic significance remain to be determined.

The brain is traditionally thought to be protected by the blood brain barrier.[91] This pharmacologic–physiologic entity has been located in the endothelium of the majority of cerebral capillaries.[92] Pentalaminar fusions of endothelial cell membranes form relatively continuous zones of occlusions which obstruct the passage of substances having a molecular weight greater than 200 daltons. Drugs that have high lipid solubility and hence are capable of passing cell membranes in general are considered as not being excluded by the blood brain barrier. Finally, drugs must either not be ionized or have readily reversible ionization equations in order to pass through the blood brain barrier. Although the blood brain barrier has been traditionally cited as one of the more important factors in the choice of chemotherapeutic agents for the treatment of malignant brain tumor, it is both pharmacologically, as well as histopathologically, not intact in the midst of the tumor.[93] Capillary endothelial cells within tumor have been shown to have abnormal or discontinuous tight junctions.[93] CT and radionuclide scanning, both of which are dependent upon the entrance into the area of tumor of large protein molecules which are isotope labeled, are able to attain contrast differential between tumor and normal brain by virtue of leaks in the blood brain barrier.[94] Studies utilizing an extracellular peroxidase marker and horseradish peroxidase (44,000 daltons) in experimental tumor systems have demonstrated the discontinuous nature of the endothelium of brain tumor vasculature.[95] Thus, the role of the blood brain barrier remains obscure in human brain tumor therapy.

The kinetics of brain tumor have only been partially elucidated.[96] Of particular note is the fact that normal glia essentially does not replicate (in adults or older children). Cerebral vasculature and some of the other supporting elements do replicate, but at comparatively slow turnover times. Brain tumors, on the other hand, are in part by their very

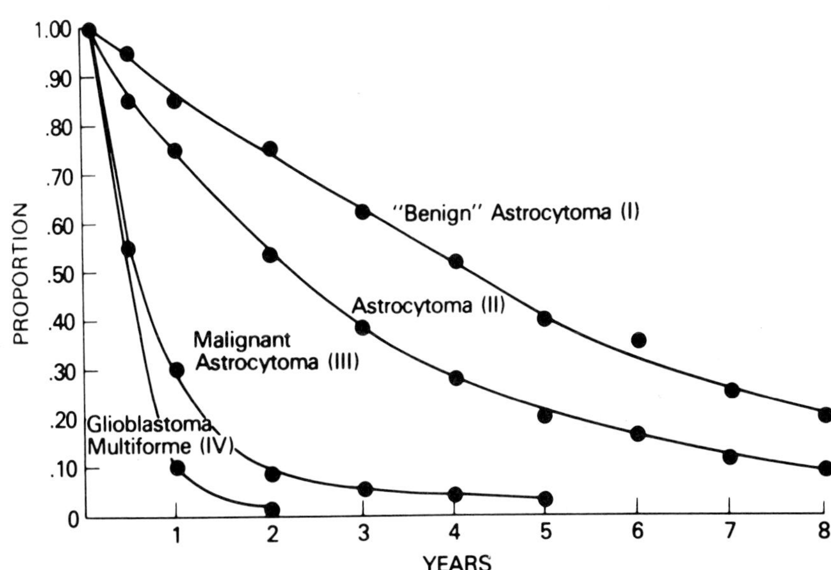

FIG. 33-21. Survival from surgery of patients with different types of astrocytoma. (Walker MD: Malignant Glioma In Wilson CB, Hoff JT (eds): Current Surgical Management of Neurologic Disease. New York, Churchill Livingstone, 1980, p 73)

nature actively going through the cell cycle. Low-grade astrocytomas have been demonstrated to have extremely few cells undergoing active proliferations, whereas high-grade gliomas appear to have a greater but nevertheless still small percentage of cells actively replicating.[97] A very wide distribution of kinetic parameters was seen in those patients who were studied. Thus, the labelling index is on the order of 0% to 10%, the S phase is approximately 7 hours to 10 hours, and the growth fraction is 0.30 and extremely variable. Birthrate of tumor cells is between 0.5% hour and 1.7% hour. The estimated turnover time is therefore between 3 days and 7 days, which is obviously not consistent with the clinical entity. If a computed cell loss factor of 85% is included, the more common clinically accepted doubling time of 6 weeks to 8 weeks can be obtained. However, this has marked implications for both the previous kinetic observations as well as chemotherapeutic considerations.[97]

Recently, the concept of the "microenvironment" of brain tumor has evolved and includes a number of factors.[98] The brain is devoid of lymphatic drainage and therefore one of the major paths of egress of drugs (and metabolites) from extracellular fluid is not available. Such lack of drainage also has implications for formation of edema as well as drainage from the extracellular space into the CSF. Second, there is frequently seen, in the histology of most brain tumors areas of necrosis in the center of the tumor, an actively proliferating edge of tumor which is well vascularized that intermingles with an outer zone, the so-called "brain adjacent to tumor" (BAT).[99] Each of these areas is felt to have a different pharmacologic environment and contains viable tumor cells, but in very different proportions, and has different kinetic considerations for the cells in each of these zones. There is increasing evidence of diverse biologic heterogeneity found in brain tumor.[100] Studies evaluating the chromosomal content, number, and karyotyping of freshly explanted serially transplanted brain tumors has provided evidence of marked changes in tumor characteristics within a matter of a few generations. Thus, what appears histopathologically as a single type of brain tumor cell, may in fact have extremely different kinetic, immunologic, and metabolic activity and response to therapy.

With the wide variety of kinetics seen and the marked heterogeneity of cell populations, the therapist is faced with an extraordinarily difficult problem in that a radio- or chemotherapeutically sensitive tumor today may be in fact replaced by its resistant variant within a short time. The development of resistant strains of bacteria to antibiotics is well known. However, it takes many generations before resistance becomes apparent and it may well not be an analogous phenomenon.

Despite the foregoing considerations, chemotherapy remains a potential avenue in which modest success has already been seen. Such drugs as the nitrosoureas and procarbazine do possess the appropriate pharmacologic characteristics for passing the blood brain barrier and have application in a wide variety of tumors. The development and investigation of new drugs is of extreme importance and requires the concerted effort of the medicinal chemist, pharmacologist, and neurooncologist in their design. Carefully controlled clinical trials of both Phase II and Phase III variety should be carried out in all appropriate drugs both to develop a backlog of information concerning the tumor and its biologic variables as well as efficacy. The use of experimental models, both *in vivo* and *in vitro*, must be expanded so as to provide the comparative data base necessary for evaluating new drugs and determining the relative meaning of the model systems themselves.

Several noteworthy attempts have been made to circumvent what might be considered the "rate limiting step" of brain tumor chemotherapy. Systemically delivered drugs are distributed throughout the body as well as to the brain. By the time one has entered the cerebral circulation its plasma concentration has been diluted to a considerable extent. Intra-arterial chemotherapy might therefore possess considerable advantage. Studies utilizing intracarotid infusion of radiolabeled modeled substances (inulin, antipyrine, and pentobarbital) in the dog produced between 1.5 and 3 times greater concentration of drug in normal brain as compared to a similar intravenous infusion.[101] Intracarotid ^{14}C-BCNU in the monkey achieved between 1.9 and 2.8 times greater brain nucleic acid-bound drug.[102] Intra-arterial BCNU has been utilized in a Phase II study of patients with malignant glioma and in a preliminary report failed to reveal marked therapeutic results.[103] In addition, there were a number of serious complications.

Since the blood brain barrier has been implicated as a major limiting factor to the egress of chemotherapeutic agents to neoplasms in the brain, attempts have been made to temporarily disrupt the blood brain barrier for the sake of increasing drug concentration.[104] Internal carotid artery infusions of 25% mannitol were shown to produce a transient reversible osmotic disruption of the blood brain barrier which resulted in several-fold higher concentrations of subsequently delivered methotrexate. Such techniques are not without hazard but are of interest in modulating the microenvironment of the brain.

The small therapeutic index possessed by BCNU limits the total amount of drug which may be delivered at any one time. The dose-limiting critical organ for the nitrosoureas is the bone marrow and thus if one could protect the marrow from the comparatively brief pharmacologic effects of BCNU, considerably higher concentrations of drug might be achieved in tumor. In a pilot study, 10 ml/kg of bone marrow was removed from patients under general anesthesia and stored frozen. Between 600 mg/m^2 to 280 mg/m^2 BCNU were delivered intravenously over the course of 2 hours divided into three daily doses. Several days later the autologous bone marrow was retransplanted into the patient. Some 55 patients with refractory malignancies have been so treated, with tumor responses seen in approximately half. However, considerable amounts of toxicity have been encountered and, although the hematapoietic system was protected, the next most significant dose-limiting organ would appear to be the liver or lungs. Such investigations need to continue to be carefully carried out in order to document this interesting approach.

Chemotherapy of brain tumor presents a unique challenge to the therapists because of the small tumor burden present, its highly localized position, its failure to metastasize, and the frustrating inability to get to it because it is inextricably intertwined within vital brain parenchyma. Thus, new drugs with highly specific activity for brain tumor, or various methods by which the dose-limiting steps of marginally effective drugs may be enhanced, must all be explored.

Cerebral Tumors

The common cerebral primary tumors are astrocytoma, meningioma, oligodendroglioma, and histocytic lymphoma. The treatments for these tumor types will be discussed separately. In general, when lesions are in the anterior frontal, occipital, and anterior temporal regions, aggressive surgical treatment is a prime therapeutic treatment modality. In other areas, surgery may serve only to aid in diagnosis or to achieve decompression in the cases of malignant tumors. Encapsulated benign tumors can often be approached, even in more restricted areas such as the parietal or posterior frontal lobes.

ASTROCYTOMAS. Cerebral astrocytomas comprise the single largest group of primary brain tumors of one histological cell type. They may be located at any site and range from low grade (Grade I) to high grade (Grade IV) in malignancy.

Low-Grade Astrocytomas (Grades I–II). For lowgrade lesions located in surgically accessible sites, surgery is the basic treatment modality and the location of the tumor and its extent determine the type of operative procedure. For Grade I lesions in the cortex of a patient in good general health, long term survival without recurrence of 10 years or more is common and, depending on the specific location and extent of tumor, there may be only minimal deficit resulting from therapy. The major anatomic features determining prognosis for surgery are whether the tumor is accessible and clearly demarcated from surrounding normal brain tissue. The surgical approaches most often used are partial or total resection in appropriate locations with biopsy for lesions in difficult areas.

The importance of the anatomic location on the type of operative procedure is again relevant to cerebral astrocytomas of low grade. Anterior frontal, occipital, and anterior temporal lesions can be resected or treated by partial lobectomy. Posterior frontal or temporal and parietal lesions are often diffuse, with infiltration of surrounding brain, even though low in histologic malignancy. Thus biopsy is the relevant surgical measure unless the tumor is well encapsulated and can be separated cleanly from surrounding brain.

Certain low-grade cerebral astrocytomas require separate discussion. These include microcystic astrocytomas, juvenile cerebellar astrocytomas, optic nerve gliomas, and the subependymal gliomas associated with tuberous sclerosis. All of these are primarily tumors of the pediatric age group. Microcystic astrocytomas have a particularly favorable prognosis and surgical removal of the mural nodule carries an excellent prognosis with relatively low rates of recurrence. These juvenile cerebellar astrocytomas may be solid, are usually well demarcated and respond well to surgery.[5,37,38]

The subependymal gliomas are usually benign, well demarcated, occur in relation to the ventricles and can be largely resected. They can undergo malignant change and then should be treated as the more invasive lesions.

Radiation Therapy of Low-Grade Astrocytoma. Radiation therapy delivered postoperatively has not been shown to increase the high survival rate of completely excised low-grade gliomas.[114] Controversy exists regarding the place of irradiation following incomplete removal of low-grade cerebral or cerebellar gliomas. No study is available comparing survival and relapse rates in patients with equivalent tumor extent who were randomly treated with irradiation or observed. However, most available studies, comparing survival in patients with incomplete removal of Grade I or II tumors who received localized irradiation with doses in excess of 5000 rad with unirradiated patients treated in the same period at the same institution, show a significant advantage for the irradiated group. This advantage increases with increasing periods of follow-up.[80–83,114–117] Leibel and colleagues were able to demonstrate 5-year and 10-year survival rates of 46% and 35% versus 19% and 11% for irradiated versus unirradiated patients.[114] Similar results have been obtained by others.[118–121] Results achieved in children have generally been superior to those in adults—60% to 80% 5-year survival versus 20% 5-year survival respectively for children versus adults.[114,120] As the grade of the lesions increases, recurrence time shortens in unirradiated patients.

Based on the highly suggestive reports cited, routine postoperative irradiation, totaling 5000 rad to 6000 rad to limited radiation fields, relying on accurate surgical and radiologic assessment of tumor extent with adequate treatment margins, is recommended. Daily tumor dose should range from 150 rad to no more than 200 rad with four or five treatments delivered each week. Care must be taken to restrict treatment volumes where possible to minimize morbidity from the high dose necessary for tumor control.

Nearly complete surgical removal of a Grade I cerebral lesion in a very young child (less than 5 years of age) may represent one clinical setting where an exception to the desirability of routine postoperative irradiation should be considered. Delay in administration of irradiation may be possible and permit further maturation of the nervous system with lessened complications. The risk to ultimate survival of such a delay is unknown. Postoperative irradiation should not be delivered to the microcystic astrocytoma of the cerebellum occurring in young children, unless exceptional circumstances are present.

Chemotherapy of Low-Grade Astrocytomas. Low-grade "benign" astrocytomas (Kernohan Grade I) have a median life span of 4 years to 5 years (See Fig. 33-21)[5,37,38,105] Immediate chemotherapy after obtaining a biopsy and establishing the diagnosis does not appear to be logical either for kinetic considerations (the long doubling times and few cells actively proliferating) or for chemotherapeutic toxicity considerations (long-term exposure and depletion of bone-marrow reserve). The usual course of events of low-grade astrocytomas is to continue in a somewhat indolent state for months to years, at which time, for unknown reasons, they appear to become more active, start to grow larger in size and frequently dedifferentiate histopathologically. At this time they are often reoperated upon and demonstrate a more aggressive, actively growing tumor. If the maximum cumulative dose of radiotherapy has already been utilized and the bone marrow had been severely compromised by several years of chemotherapy, maximum doses of both these forms of therapy at a time when they are most needed cannot be utilized. Therefore, chemotherapy should not be considered in low-grade astrocytomas until after recurrence has been demonstrated. This is particularly true of the juvenile cerebellar astrocytomas, optic nerve gliomas, and microcystic astrocytomas, all of which may be considered as cured or at least stabilized in a reasonable proportion of patients following surgery. There is a pressing need for a detailed analysis of the long-term events of patients with low-grade astrocytomas with the hope that the natural history will make more apparent the appropriate timing for both radiotherapeutic and chemotherapeutic intervention.

Low-grade gliomas (astrocytomas, Grade II) are located on the histopathology continuum of gliomas somewhere between benign astrocytomas and those which truly show malignant tendencies. To whatever extent possible, a re-review of the pathologic material, the clinical course of the patient, the surgeon's notes, and a neuroradiologic presentation of the tumor should be undertaken so as to attempt to either declare it of the low-grade astrocytic series or recognize its malignant potential. There is some question as to the indications of chemotherapy in the low-grade gliomas of either the cerebral or cerebellar hemisphere. As noted above, the value of radiotherapy is unproven but is indeed highly suggestive. However, until effective minimally toxic agents are identified, it would probably be more appropriate to wait for evidence of recurrence following radiotherapy for patients in whom the degree of anaplasia cannot be more clearly defined.

Optic Gliomas. Optic glioma represents an uncommon tumor largely occurring in children. From 20% to 60% of these patients are noted to have von Recklinghausen's disease at diagnosis.[105-107] In addition to its well-recognized unpredictable behavior, its heterogeneity in primary location, histologic grade and appearance, and variation in clinical management have clouded most clinical reports of this tumor with controversy.

In general, lesions which affect an optic nerve without reaching the optic chiasm appear to enjoy the most indolent and favorable course. Lesions with chiasmal involvement without extension into the hypothalamus or third ventricle region are more favorable than tumors where such extension is present.[106,107] Lesions with such "anterior" involvement appear to be present more often with known von Recklinghausen's disease. The histologic appearance of the anterior lesions is often that of a fibrillary pilocytic astrocytoma and almost always are of extremely low grade. The more posterior lesions tend to be of higher grade, and, in some adult cases, glioblastoma has been observed.[108] Most fatal cases have been posterior in origin or extent.

Hoyt and others have postulated that optic gliomas represent hamartomatous lesions.[109,110] Although the clinical course of many of the anterior lesions, especially those confined to one optic nerve, support this contention, pathologic examination rarely suggests a hamartoma and both clinical and pathologic features of the more posterior lesions are at variance.[111]

Numerous clinical reports confirm that optic glioma often causes morbidity (blindness) and, when posterior in location, not infrequently mortality. Several reports and personal experience document the ability of properly applied, high-dose megavoltage irradiation to cause objective tumor reduction, clinical improvement or stabilization and, often, long-term disease-free survival for lesions affecting the optic chiasm with or without affecting both nerves.[105,106,111-113] When clear evidence of objective or symptomatic progression is noted in a patient with optic glioma, we recommend an attempt at definitive radiation therapy. A tumor dose of approximately 5000 rad delivered in 6 weeks time in 180-rad fractions should be given. Care must be taken to include potential sites of extension posteriorly (optic tracts), superiorly (hypothalamus and third ventricle); and anteriorly along the optic nerve pathways.

A representative treatment plan is shown for a patient with bilateral nerve, chiasma, and hypothalamic involvement in Fig. 33-20 *E*. A high rate of local control and arrest or reversal of clinical progression has been documented in several series using megavoltage irradiation to appropriate volumes and dose.

More difficult questions are posed when an apparently isolated lesion affects one nerve only. Controversy regarding the importance and advisability of biopsy of all such lesions exists. When the often indolent and uncertain clinical course of these lesions is considered, the advisability of surgical removal of such lesions, with resultant blindness, is questioned. Data supporting the use of irradiation in verified cases exist with functional preservation in such patients.

Clear documentation of progression by appropriate clinical and radiographic means should be present prior to surgical intervention. Should surgery be necessary, evidence of tumor extension to the optic chiasma should limit surgery to a biopsy followed by irradiation. If the lesion is circumscribed and progressive and can be removed with an adequate margin, complete surgical removal is recommended.

There appears to be little reason at this juncture to subject optic nerve gliomas to chemotherapy because of the comparatively long survival of these patients and the lack of highly efficacious agents. However, an optic nerve glioma which has dedifferentiated, becomes invasive and is actively proliferating should be considered as though it were a malignant glioma and therefore aggressively treated.

High-Grade Astrocytomas (Grades III, III–IV). These astrocytomas have a spectrum of variable growth rates with the mean survival of a Grade III patient being 1 year to 2 years and a Grade IV patient only 15 weeks after surgery alone. They share, however, such a malignant growth potential that treatment is quite similar. The surgical intervention in these highly malignant lesions is unlikely to be curative and palliation by tumor removal has to be balanced against the risks of altering cerebral function and quality of life during the relatively brief lifespan. Therapeutic decisions include a detailed evaluation of the known prognostic factors and consideration of the patient's feelings, occupation, and family and social needs.[63] The application of comprehensive treatment approaches is never more relevant than in this patient group. The neurological and functional status (often measured on the Karnovsky scale) have been useful indicators of the projected response to therapy.

Despite the poor prognosis of these tumors with surgery alone, surgery for the confirmation of the nature of the tumor is indicated in most cases in which the tumor is accessible and the patient's condition permits. The same general surgical principles apply to these lesions as to the less malignant lesions with the significant difference being that total removal is an indistinct possibility. The goals of surgery are to make the diagnosis, determine the extent of the lesion and, if possible, decompress the tumor to allow for a smoother postoperative recovery and safer administration of radiation therapy and possible chemotherapy. The evidence that extensive surgical resection increases life expectancy in any statistically significant way is meager but in the individual case of a frontal or occipital lesion, extensive resection and even lobectomy may offer significant palliation. It does not appear that massive resections involving predictable major loss of neurological function have any benefits which outweigh the cost to the quality of life. Large parietal or deep-seated cerebral lesions of this degree of malignancy should at most be biopsied or if decompression is needed only noncritical tissue should be removed. It should be noted that an occasional tumor even in the parietal lobes may be sufficiently "pseudoencapsulated" that significant resections can be achieved.

A major area of controversy exists as to whether any surgery, even biopsy, should be undertaken in a patient with a neurological CT scan and angiographic demonstration of a lesion most likely to be a malignant astrocytoma. Major reasons favoring surgery whenever feasible and acceptable to the patient include: (1) a clear diagnosis allows the patient and the family to plan intelligently for whatever future exists; (2) planning of radiation fields may be more specific and precise based on information gained at the time of surgery; (3) on occasion, even the best of diagnostic workups will suggest a malignant tumor of primary nature when actually the tumor is benign (meningioma, abcess, aneurysm, AVM, cyst); (4) apparent total resection may be unexpectedly possible in certain individuals with quite good results; and (5) an uncertainty about diagnosis, while initially acceptable to the patient and family, can become a crisis in later management if nonsurgical therapies create serious complications or if there is an unexpectedly long but poor quality survival.

The arguments in favor of performing no surgery include: (1) improvements in nonsurgical diagnostic techniques make incorrect diagnosis in the adequately evaluated patients unlikely; (2) significant additional morbidity and occasional instances of mortality may occur; (3) as a significant resection is unlikely, nonsurgical therapy, especially radiation therapy, will likely be the principal treatment mode. The total dose used and volume which will be irradiated will probably vary relatively little for the varying diagnostic possibilities and the difference in morbidity between the extremes in radiation dose and volume is likely to be outweighed by the surgical morbidity; and (4) patients with a limited survival duration may spend a significant fraction of their remaining life confined to the hospital.

Should tumor tissue be removed, careful pathological assessment is necessary. Tissue culture studies may be of experimental and/or clinical interest. After a 1-2 week recovery period a decision as to further therapy must be made. Unless the patient or family declines such treatment the use of radiotherapy and/or chemotherapy is usually indicated. Whereas surgery alone for Grade IV astrocytomas carries a prognosis of only 15 weeks the use of combined modality therapy considerably improves the outlook, although "cures" or 5 year survivals in properly diagnosed Grade IV astrocytomas are extremely rare (less than 1%).

Radiotherapy of High-Grade Astrocytomas. With rare exceptions, treatment of malignant astrocytomas continues to be unsatisfactory. Several studies demonstrate that irradiation improves survival duration. A recent randomized study confirms this.[122-124] Both the extent of the radiation fields used and total dose correlate with treatment efficacy.[125-130]

Based on earlier studies, which demonstrated the inability of certain radiographic studies to precisely determine the true extent of malignant gliomas, the current practice of whole brain irradiation for a major portion of the treatment course has evolved.[125,126] Data are available demonstrating that the use of radiation fields less than 100 cm^2 for malignant glioma is associated with decreased efficacy.[127,129] Data confirming the value of whole brain treatment, as opposed to the use of wide fields with generous margins, are not available. Radiation doses of greater than 5000 rad delivered in 5 weeks to 6 weeks yield improved results over lesser doses. Recent data suggest that routine use of radiation doses in excess of 7000 rad in 7.5 weeks to 8 weeks to the area of radiographic or clinically demonstrated tumor yields improved short-term survival for adults with more malignant lesions.[129] This improvement disappears after 2 years to 3 years. The advantage of these high radiation doses for younger patients or those with less aggressive lesions is not certain. The potential longer survival for these patients makes the risk of radiation associated brain necrosis more likely and improvements in short-term survival may be more than compensated for by an increased rate of late brain necrosis.

A systematic examination of results following high dose, large volume irradiation has demonstrated the importance of tumor grade or degree of malignancy on both short and long term prognosis. Virtually no patient with Grade IV glioblastoma multiforme survives 5 years following treatment. Approximately 35% to 50% of treated patients with high grade lesions survive 1 year but less than 20% will survive 2 years (Tables 33-20*A*, *B*).

Results for patients with Grade III lesions are more encouraging. Sixty-five percent to 70% of these patients survive 1 year, 40% survive 2 years and 10–20% will survive 5 years or more.[117,118,129-132]

Young patients less than 15 years or 20 years of age fare significantly better than older patients.[118,129] This improvement includes both total survival and relative quality of life.[118]

Based on experience and results available in the literature, postoperative high dose (6000 rad–6500 rad/7 weeks–7½ weeks) megavoltage treatment is recommended. Treatment fields should be generous but the use of whole brain irradiation fields beyond a dose of 4000 rad to 4500 rad, especially for younger patients and those with less aggressive tumors (Grade III), is not advocated. Smaller radiation fields delivered only to the radiographically abnormal area should follow to a total dose of 5500 rad to 6500 rad in 6 weeks to 7½ weeks. Careful treatment planning is of importance for similar reasons. Experimental techniques currently being clinically tested for patients with malignant gliomas will be discussed in a later section.

Chemotherapy of High-Grade Astrocytomas. The greatest amount of work and the most significant effects of both radiotherapy and chemotherapy have been seen in patients with high-grade malignant gliomas. Included within this category are glioblastoma multiforme, malignant astro-

TABLE 33-20*A*. Representative Survival Figures for Patients Treated in Varying Fashions for Cerebral Gliomas

GRADE	SURGERY	XRT	AGE	SURVIVAL (%) 5 year	10 year
I & II	C*	Yes	P‡	?	?
		No	P	90+	90+
	C	Yes	M§	?	?
		No	M	90	25
	I†	Yes	P	50–80	40–70
		No	P	20–40	10–30
	I	Yes	M	40–50	30–35
		No	M	15–35	0–<15

C* = Complete
I† = Incomplete
P‡ = Pediatric
M§ = Mixed pediatric and adult

cytoma, and Kernohan Grades III and IV. The vast majority of these patients have also undergone surgical resection and a smaller portion have undergone radiotherapy. These factors must be taken into consideration when examining adjuvant chemotherapy.

Almost every drug which has been utilized for the treatment of malignancies has been applied to the treatment of brain cancer.[133] The vast majority of these studies are uncontrolled, utilizing patients with different histology who appear at different times during the course of their disease and who, by and large, are both recurrent and debilitated. Intercomparison between these studies is extremely difficult because the advertent and inadvertent selection factors which modulate the choice of patient population may often have a greater effect than some of the therapies available. Thus, controlled perspective randomized trials become extremely important, as a majority of these variables will have less impact on the results. The first multi-institutional control perspective randomized trial in the treatment of malignant glioma was carried out by the Brain Tumor Study Group (a clinical cooperative group of neurosurgeons, neurologists, radiotherapists, and neuropathologists under the aegis of the National Cancer Institute).[10] In this study, the use of mithramycin was compared to no mithramycin in patients who had a surgical resection and some radiotherapy. The importance of this study is not so much that it definitively demonstrated that mithramycin is an ineffective agent for the treatment of malignant glioma, but in that it established that controlled perspective randomized trials can be carried out in the treatment of this disease and develop meaningful results.

The nitrosoureas were among the first rationally designed chemotherapeutic agents which have the specific properties necessary in order to cross the blood brain barrier. They are highly lipid soluble, of small molecular weight, and are not ionized, therefore, they will not only penetrate normal brain tissue but they will equidistribute throughout the body. 1-3-*bis*-2-chloroethyl-1-nitrosourea (BCNU) was the first of these to be utilized clinically. Early Phase II studies demonstrated improvement in approximately 50% of patients treated with doses of 80 mg/m²/day–100 mg/m²/day on 3 successive days, delivered intravenously every 6 weeks to 8 weeks.[134,135] However, the median time to progression was brief and in the order of 12 weeks to 20 weeks.

Following these initial observations, a wide variety of trials of both controlled and uncontrolled design have been undertaken and are summarized in Table 33-21. Contained within this table are important factors, such as tumor type and the number of patients, that were both entered into the study as well as becoming part of the evaluated group. The results are reported as either median time to progression (MTP) or median survival time (MST) in weeks. One of the major deficits in most of these trials was the lack of an adequate number of patients in order to demonstrate true efficacy or to satisfy the null hypothesis. Only three of the randomized trials had over 100 patients in all groups for purposes of analysis.

The subsequent study of Brain Tumor Study Group attempted to define the quantitative (in contradistinction to the qualitative) value of radiotherapy. It clearly demonstrated that the use of 5000 rad to 6000 rad whole-head through bilateral opposing ports increased median survival by 150%, whereas the use of BCNU alone increased median survival by an insignificant 30%.[11] However, at 18 months, approximately 20% of the patients who received both BCNU and radiotherapy were still alive, while less than half as many patients who received monotherapy were still alive.

In a study utilizing radiotherapy as a control and examining the use of methyl-CCNU alone and in a combination with radiotherapy *versus* the best arm from the prior study of radiotherapy and BCNU[136] it was clearly demonstrated again that nitrosourea alone is inadequate treatment, that radiotherapy is an effective mode of treatment and that the combination of BCNU and radiotherapy is modestly better than BCNU alone.

A number of other studies have examined CCNU, as it is

TABLE 33-20*B*. Representative Survival Figures for Patients Treated in Varying Fashions for Cerebral Gliomas

GRADE	SURGERY*	XRT (>4500 rad)	SURVIVAL (%) 1 year	2 year	5 year
III	+	(−)	10–15	5–10	0
	+	(+)	40	30	15–20
IV	+	(−)	5	0	0
	+	(+)	25–50	10	0–3

*Surgery for these grades is always considered to be incomplete.

an oral nitrosourea, and therefore relatively easy to deliver. The EORTC, in a carefully controlled trial, gave CCNU immediately after surgery and radiotherapy in comparison with giving it after the patient demonstrated progression.[137] The median time to progression for both groups is exactly the same; however, a significant improvement was seen in patients following progression who then received CCNU. In a smaller study in patients with poor performance status and requiring steroids, they demonstrated that patients who received CCNU had a better median survival time than those who did not. Several other studies have been unable to demonstrate the specific value of CCNU.[138-140] Some studies in Table 33-21 of non-randomized nature have examined various forms of combination chemotherapy.[141-144] The majority of these have failed to substantiate the significance of their combination.

Egan and co-workers treated a randomized group of 42 patients with dianhydrogalactitol and found a remarkable improvement in median survival (67 wks) as compared to those who received radiotherapy alone.

Procarbazine has been reported as an effective treatment for malignant glioma and therefore has been brought forward into the current BTSG study. Following definitive surgical resection, all patients will receive 6000 rad of radiotherapy and will be randomized to procarbazine, high-dose corticosteroid, and high-dose corticosteroid plus BCNU *versus* BCNU alone. The purpose of this study is to evaluate the oncolytic effect of corticosteroids in comparison with their well-known ability to control cerebral edema, the effect which they might have in combination with BCNU, and the efficacy of procarbazine. The current trend indicates that corticosteroids have no independent oncolytic effect in the doses used and do not add to the efficacy of BCNU. Further, procarbazine appears to be an effective agent with the same approximate efficacy as BCNU. The absolute results must await the final analysis.

Several factors of significance have been derived from these controlled studies. A group of pretreatment prognostic factors which play an important role on survival rates of patients with malignant glioma have been identified.[145] Such determinants as age, performance status, the duration of symptoms, and histopathologic classification all are of considerable significance and must be accounted for in intercomparisons between studies. As the treatment of high-grade glioma becomes more prevalent and patients live longer, the complications of both chemotherapy and radiotherapy can be expected to become more apparent. Late delayed radiation necrosis was identified in four of 25 brains examined that had received between 5000 rad and 6000 rad of radiotherapy.[146] Two of the four had received BCNU, 1-dibromodulcitol and one had received other chemotherapy. The complications of prolonged nitrosourea therapy are also becoming apparent, as scattered case reports identify patients with pulmonary fibrosis, hepatic toxicity, or renal failure. Cases of second tumor in association with nitrosourea treatment are also being reported.[147]

OLIGODENDROGLIOMAS. These tumors when pure are most often benign and extremely slow-growing. They often calcify and are well demarcated from surrounding normal brain. For a *purely* oligodendroglial lesion of benign nature, surgical extirpation is usually possible with good short-term results and a favorable long-term prognosis if complete resection has been possible.

There are two major facets of this cerebral tumor which render its management more complicated. These tumors are frequently composed of both astrocytic and oligodendroglial elements and thus are rarely "pure." The second problem is represented by the relatively rare malignant oligodendroglioma.

In the case of the mixed oligo–astrocytoma the treatment plan is dependent on which cell is most prominent. The presence of oligodendroglia in the midst of an astrocytoma is a good prognostic sign but the presence of malignant astrocytes in an oligodendroglia is unfavorable. It is extremely important to sample the pathological material thoroughly to see whether foci of either type are present. These mixed tumors are therefore difficult to describe as a group because of the spectrum of malignancy which they encompass, depending on the makeup of the "mix."

The malignant "pure" oligodendroglioma behaves in much the same way as in infiltrating astrocytoma and the management is similar. However, these lesions have been noted to develop subarachnoid seeding deposits with greater regularity than astrocytomas, especially when periventricular in location or when histologically less well differentiated.[51] A peculiar diffuse involvement of the entire periventricular region has been noted with oligodendroglioma.[51,148]

Indications for use of radiation therapy, radiation dose, and techniques recommended generally parallel those for astrocytomas. However, the increased propensity for subarachnoid seeding should be considered, particularly for higher grade, periventricular lesions and these patients may benefit from craniospinal irradiation in addition to local treatment. Series comparing results achieved with postoperative irradiation to those with surgery alone show an advantage for the irradiated group.[149,150] Sheline demonstrated improvement in survival at 5 years (85% *vs.* 31%) and this continued at 10 years (55% *vs.* 25%).[130] Similar results have been achieved by Bouchard and Peirce.[82]

Oligodendroglioma account for only 1.5% of all brain tumors (3.7% of gliomas) and therefore are not seen frequently enough to be included for chemotherapy studies. However, upon recurrence and reoperation of oligodendroglioma, progressive dedifferentiation is frequently seen and the tumor takes on more of the characteristics of a malignant glioma or glioblastoma multiforme.[150] Following the demonstration of such changes the patient should promptly receive radiotherapy, and chemotherapy with a nitrosourea utilized for the treatment of malignant glioma.

MENINGIOMAS. *Surgical Treatment.* Meningiomas are generally considered as benign tumors with a favorable outlook. It is best to group these tumors into three general therapeutic groups: (1) accessible, (resectable) benign lesions, (2) inaccessible (only partially resectable) benign lesions, and (3) malignant meningiomas.

Accessible (Resectable) Meningiomas. The concept of resectability as it applies to meningioma patients depends to a large part on the anatomic location of the lesion but other factors, including the size of the lesion and the age

(Text continues on p. 1228)

TABLE 33-21. Summary of Chemotherapy Trials

AUTHOR	STUDY DESIGN	TUMOR TYPE* AND PERCENT		NUMBER (Evaluable / Entered)	PRETREATMENT CONDITIONS	TREATMENT GROUPS	RESULTS†		COMMENTS
							MTP	MST	
Levin	Randomized	GBM Non-GBM	62% 37%	99/130	Surgery	RadTh & BCNU	31 wk		Significant at $p = 0.04$
						RadTh, BCNU & Hydroxyurea	42		
Sweet	Randomized	Astrocytoma III & IV		21	Surgery & RadTh	BCNU BCNU & VM26	61 wk 94		Difference not statistically significant
Solero	Randomized	GBM	100%	102/105	Surgery Randomize in 2 wk	RadTh RadTh & BCNU RadTh & CCNU	38 wk 45 52	45 wk 52 69	RadTh & CCNU only significantly better than RadTh alone $p = 0.05$
Jellinger	Consecutive, Historic Selective	GBM MA	66% 44%	116	Surgery	Supportive Care RadTh COMP*** RadTh & COMP	16 wk 29 29 30	23 wk 46 46 58	Uncontrolled, consecutive and selected patients. Any therapy better than supportive care alone
Garrett	Randomized	GMB MA Other	68% 29% 3%	69/74	Biopsy	RadTh RadTh & CCNU		35 wk 56	Not statistically significant
Heiss	Consecutive & Historic	GMB	100%	77	Surgery Some RadTh	Control CCNU Polychemotherapy COMP‡	11 wk 15 20 39	27 wk 28 35 46	Combined retrospective and previous series. Not stratified by RadTh. COMP appeared better
EORTC-BTG (Hildebrand)	1)Randomized	GBM Astro III–IV	40% 31%	81/111	Surgery & RadTh *Good* performance status, no steroids	CCNU (after Surg) CCNU (after Prog)	34.5 wk 31	43 wk 62	} Significant $p = 0.05$
	2)Randomized	Other	29%	22/111	Surgery & RadTh *Poor* performance status, steroids required	Control CCNU		21.5 wk 31	Population stratified into two groups by performance status } Significant $p = 0.01$
Walker	Randomized	GBM MA Other	90% 9% 1%	222/303	Surgery & Randomize in 2 wk	Control BCNU RadTh BCNU & RadTh		14 wk 18.5 35.0 34.5	RadTh and RadTh & BCNU statistically significant from control $p = 0.001$
Shapiro	Randomized	Malignant glioma		33	Surgery	BCNU & VCR BCNU, VCR & RadTh		30.0 wk 44.5	No significant difference demonstrated
Reagan	Randomized	Astrocytoma Gr. III & IV		63/72	Surgery Randomize in 2 wk	RadTh CCNU RadTh & CCNU	30 wk 17 30	49 wk 28 52	Suboptimal RadTh (5000 rad) Stopped treating upon recurrence CCNU inferior to other treatments $p = 0.02$

Walker	Randomized	GBM MA Other	84% 11% 5%	358/467	Surgery Randomize in 2 wk	MeCCNU RadTh RadTh & MeCCNU RadTh & BCNU		24 wk 36 42 51	RadTh and BCNU vs RadTh, $p = 0.072$ MeCCN vs RadTh $p = 0.048$
Weir	Randomized & Crossover	Astrocytoma III & IV Other	97% 7%	40	Surgery Randomize in 2 wk	RadTh CCNU RadTh & CCNU	23 wk 14 31	27 wk 37 36	7 RadTh crossed to CCNU 10 CCNU crossed to RadTh Those who had combination treatment survived longer
Seiler	Consecutive vs Historic	GBM MA	63% 37%	52	Surgery RadTh	CCNU, Procarbazine, Bleomycin Control		56 wk 51 wk	No significant difference
Eagan	Randomized	GBM MA	71% 29%	42/43	Surgery RadTh Randomize in 2 wk	Dianhydrogalactitol Control		67 wk 35	Split course RadTh given to half the patients DAG *vs* Control $p = 0.02$

*GMB = Glioblastoma multiforme; MA = Malignant Astrocytoma

†MTP = Median time to Progression; MST = Median Survival Time

‡"COMP" = CCNU, vincristine, methotrexate, and procarbazine

(Levin VA, Wilson CB, Davis R et al: A Phase III comparison of BCNU, hydroxyurea, and radiation therapy to BCNU and radiation therapy for treatment of primary malignant gliomas. J Neurosurg 51:526–532, 1979; Sweet DL, Hendler FJ, Hanlon K et al: Treatment of Grade III and IV astrocytomas with BCNU alone and in combination with VM-26 following surgery and radiation therapy. Cancer Treat Rep 63:1707–1711, 1979; Solero CL, Monfardini S, Brambilla C et al: Controlled study with BCNU *vs* CCNU as adjuvant chemotherapy following surgery plus radiotherapy for glioblastoma multiforme. Cancer Clin Trials 2:43–48, 1979; Jellinger K, Kothbauer P, Volc D et al: Combination chemotherapy (COMP protocol) and radiotherapy of anaplastic supratentorial gliomas. Acta Neurochirurgica 51:1–13, Springer-Verlag, 1979; Garrett MJ, Hughes HJ, Freedman LS: A comparison of radiotherapy alone with radiotherapy and CCNU in cerebral glioma. Clin Oncol 4:71–76, 1978; Heiss, W-D: Chemotherapy of malignant gliomas: Comparison of the effect of polychemo- and CCNU-therapy. Acta Neurochirurgica (Wien) 42:109–115, 1978; EORTC Brain Tumor Group: Effect of CCNU on survival rate of objective remission and duration of free interval in patients with malignant brain glioma—Final evaluation. Eur J Cancer 14:851–856, 1978; Walker MD, Alexander E Jr, Hunt WE et al: An evaluation of BCNU and/or radiotherapy in the treatment of anaplastic gliomas. (A cooperative clinical trial) for the Brain Tumor Study Group. J Neurosurg 49:333–343, 1978; Shapiro WR, Young DF: Chemotherapy of malignant glioma with BCNU and vincristine. Neurology Minn 24:380, 1974; Reagan TJ, Bisel HJ, Childs DS et al: Controlled study of CCNU and radiation therapy in malignant astrocytoma. J Neurosurg 44:186–190, 1976; Walker MD, Green SB, Byar DP et al: Randomized comparisons of radiotherapy and nitrosoureas for malignant glioma after surgery. N Engl J Med, 303:1323–1329, 1980; Weir B, Band P, Urtasun R et al: Radiotherapy and CCNU in the treatment of high-grade supratentorial astrocytomas. J Neurosurg 45:129–134, 1976; Seiler RW, Greiner RH, Zimmerman A et al: Radiotherapy combined with procarbazine, bleomycin, and CCNU in the treatment of high-grade supratentorial astrocytomas. J Neurosurg 48:861–865, 1978; and Eagan RT, Childs DS Jr, Layton DD Jr et al: Dianhydrogalactitol and radiation therapy: Treatment of supratentorial glioma. JAMA 241:2046–2050, 1979)

and health of the patient, need to be taken into account. This is particularly so because even these "accessible" lesions are often difficult to resect, involve long and strenuous procedures, and carry significant morbidity. In general, meningiomas located in the convexity, in the olfactory groove region, and those intraparenchymally in the cortex can be removed in their entirety.

When these tumors are in the parasagittal region the concerns about the sagittal sinus can often lead to leaving a portion of the tumor adherent to the sinus. The risks of ligating and removing a portion of the sinus with the tumor are greatest in posterior falx lesions and less in anterior ones. On many occasions, a partial resection of the portion of the wall of the sinus with grafting or oversewing of the sinus can still allow venous flow and tumor removal can be completed. If the sinus is completely resected, especially posteriorly, cerebral swelling and venous engorgement can present serious problems.

Meningiomas of the sphenoid wing have been divided into two groups, lateral and medial. The lateral lesions are both lateral and anterior and can present with proptosis and may be first seen and managed by ophthalamic surgeons. Total removal with as much tumor as possible being resected should be planned for young, healthy patients. These lesions often, however, are in the sphenoid bone, expanding the bone itself and extensive bony removal may be difficult. These lesions may be mistaken for fibrous dysplasia and followed for years before their true neoplastic origin is clear. Special techniques for bony removal using air drills with steel and diamond burrs enable this bony removal to be accomplished.

Medial sphenoid wing lesions can involve the carotid and jugular vessels, can be extremely adherent to these structures and, although benign, are not completely resectable. Even microsurgical techniques may not permit complete removal. The use of magnifications and micro-instruments has increased significantly the amount of tumor which can be safely resected.[151]

The likelihood of local recurrence of these benign meningiomas depends on the completeness of the surgical removal. It is important to remove even the smallest points of tumor attachment if safely possible, as these foci can allow tumor recurrence.[152,153]

In the benign lesions, consideration of the age of the patient is an important factor in surgical planning. In an elderly patient with a slow-growing tumor, debulking and decompressing the tumor, or in some cases no surgery at all, may be safer than total removal. However, failure to remove tumor completely can increase the risks of postoperative bleeding. These relatively long and difficult procedures require careful medical evaluation. Significant medical contraindications, especially in the elderly, may be a strong factor against surgery.

For benign tumors which are not totally removed or for lesions which pre-operatively are thought to be unresectable, consideration should be given to radiotherapy.

Radiation Therapy. The meningiomas with malignant potential include the angioblastic and the sarcomatous types. The angioblastic tumors may be relatively circumscribed, but are extremely vascular and have a remarkable rate of recurrence. Often their diagnosis is not appreciated until pathological study is completed and the resection performed may be too modest for such a potentially aggressive tumor. Tumors which appear to be very vascular meningiomas, not clearly encapsulated, should be studied by frozen section at operation.

Incomplete removal is followed by clinical recurrence in the majority of patients. Even after apparent complete removal a small number of patients will suffer recurrence. Incomplete removal of larger tumors is particularly common in certain locations including the posterior two-thirds of the central venous sinus, olfactory groove, clivus, and Meckel's cave–middle cranial fossa region.[154] Plaque-like tumors of the inner portion of the sphenoid wing are relatively common, usually very slow growing, quite extensive, and often impossible to completely resect.[155]

Reports documenting the efficacy of irradiation for incompletely resected or recurrent meningiomas are sparse.[156] Perhaps most encouraging is the report of Wara and colleagues.[157] Of 104 patients with incompletely resected meningioma, 74% of 58 patients not receiving postoperative irradiation developed clinical recurrence as opposed to 29% of 34 patients receiving postoperative irradiation following healing of the craniotomy site. The 12 remaining patients underwent biopsy or minimal resection followed by postoperative irradiation and planned re-operation approximately 6 months following completion of irradiation. Eight of these 12 were subsequently able to undergo total resection and seven are living and well. Supporting data have been repeated by King and colleagues.[158] Similar data are available for children.[159]

Therefore a course of high-dose irradiation following attempted initial surgical resection is recommended, where minimal residual disease remains, in an attempt to delay or decrease the overall incidence of clinical recurrence. When gross residual disease remains, high-dose irradiation, followed by delayed reoperation and attempted resection, seems indicated. The delay prior to reoperation is recommended to permit maximum tumor regression to take place as it is well recognized that tumors that enlarge slowly may decrease over a protracted time following irradiation. A radiation dose in excess of 4500 rad to 5000 rad delivered in 5 weeks to 6 weeks in 150 rad to 280 rad fractions appears to be needed.

Finally, it must be emphasized that ultimate clinical control appears to require nearly complete or complete resection, as attempts to deliver radiation doses in excess of 5500 rad are often limited in deep-seated lesions by the frequent proximity and radiation tolerance of normal brain or brainstem. The necessity for careful treatment planning with multiple fields of irradiation to permit maximum tumor dose homogeneity and optimum sparing of surrounding normal brain is evident. If there is evidence of the angioblastic type lesions, then a more extensive operative procedure may be indicated, including lobectomy if the tumor is situated in an appropriate site.

Meningeal sarcomas are essentially primary malignant tumors of the brain which at times develop metastasis to the lung or other sites. These tumors are rarely resectable, but when anatomy permits, a significant tumor removal is indicated.[160] In meningiomas with malignant potential there is a role for radiation and even consideration of chemotherapy is appropriate.

Treatment techniques and general rationale discussed previously with less aggressive lesions pertain. Radiation doses should be carried to tolerance levels of the adjacent normal brain, even when only microscopic residual tumor remains. Treatment volumes must be restricted to include as little normal brain as possible within the high dose volume and careful treatment planning and simulation to accomplish this aim is mandatory. It is possible that development of newer techniques, such as intra-operative irradiation with electrons, will permit higher radiation doses and yield improved results. For most sites, radiation doses of 5500 rad to 6500 rad in 6 weeks to 7 weeks will be possible.

Although the primary treatment of meningioma is surgical, adjuvant chemotherapy should be considered in those cases where the tumor has regrown after multiple procedures and has failed to respond to radiotherapy. Under such circumstances, the tumor frequently undergoes progressive neoplastic degeneration and may take on a sarcomatous appearance. In such cases, chemotherapeutic regimens for sarcomas or adriamycin may be considered.

POSTERIOR FOSSA TUMORS. The major tumor types which occur in the posterior fossa include astrocytomas, medulloblastomas, ependymomas, hemangioblastomas, and meningiomas. Although these lesions may not be restricted to the posterior fossa, their presentation and management can be conveniently considered from this anatomic vantage point.

The tumors which reside completely in the posterior fossa can, on many occasions, be dealt with effectively by surgery, if limited. Those lesions which have involved deeper midline structures are malignant or invasive and are rarely amenable to complete surgical removal.

Astrocytomas. Astrocytomas of the posterior fossa include a variety of lesions which are most often found in childhood. These have been discussed earlier in the section on astrocytomas and include the microcystic astrocytoma (glioma A of Winston), which can nearly always be dealt with effectively by surgery alone and has an excellent prognosis. More aggressive lesions, especially these with necrosis or calcification, regularly recur following surgery and require additional treatment. These lesions may have cystic components; however, they almost never contain the microcysts associated with Rosenthal fibers, foci of oligodendroglia, or leptomeningeal deposits noted to be associated together.[38]

The more diffuse solid cerebellar astrocytomas are often of relatively low grade but the chances of invasiveness and recurrence are higher. These solid tumors may also present in older patients. These astrocytomas tend to involve the cerebellar hemispheres more than the vermis, and resection of a single cerebellar hemisphere does not carry great risk of permanent neurological deficit.

Patients with more aggressive astrocytomas of the cerebellum and posterior fossa can benefit from irradiation. For lesions which are incompletely resected but not frankly malignant, postoperative megavoltage irradiation to limited radiation fields that include the posterior fossa and immediately adjacent structures with adequate margin suffices. These lesions can extend into the brain stem, medulla–oblongata and even into the upper cervical spinal cord and, when indicated, myelography may be useful in better defining appropriate treatment volumes.

Radiation doses of 5000 rad to more than 5500 rad in 6 weeks to 6.5 weeks should be delivered utilizing three-field or rotational techniques.[161] These more complex field arrangements often follow opposing lateral fields and are useful in minimizing radiation dose inhomogeneity at the lateral aspects of the cerebellar hemispheres. Care must be taken so that vertex or posteriorly placed radiation fields do not exit through the orbits and produce later cataracts.

Malignant astrocytomas of the posterior fossa carry a much more ominous prognosis. However, high-dose irradiation is capable of achieving long-term control in some younger patients. High-grade astrocytomas of the posterior fossa in younger patients carry a substantial risk of subarachnoid seeding and this proclivity must be considered in treatment planning.

Cerebellar astrocytomas account for 38% of the infratentorial tumors of childhood. Since they are predominately a well differentiated low-grade astrocytoma, respond well to subtotal excision, frequently may not recur until years later and the median survival is in excess of 18 years for children with cerebellar astrocytomas, the employment of additional therapy should be withheld until such time as they demonstrate more malignant and aggressive characteristics. Cases have been reported to become malignant some two decades after remaining asymptomatic.[162] In such cases, or when the tumor demonstrates malignant potential at the outset, chemotherapy should be employed in the same method as treating any other malignant glioma.

Postoperative hydrocephalus is seen in approximately one-fifth of children with cerebellar astrocytoma.[163] There are indications that shunting may be of value for some patients who demonstrate progressive deterioration of mental status, or abnormal gait. The need for postoperative shunts was found more frequently in patients who had an extensive tumor resection or subtotal removal and postoperative radiotherapy.[163] However, any additional therapy in children with cerebellar astrocytomas must be carefully balanced with the fact that these children will live a long time and that the secondary effects of the brain, endocrine system, or bone marrow is not fully understood and must be seriously considered.

MEDULLOBLASTOMAS. This infiltrative malignant tumor is present most often in children and young adults and by nature of its strategic location can cause devastating neurological deficits. This tumor represents the most common malignant tumor in childhood. Although anatomically an intrinsic tumor of the medulla, its surgical approaches are by way of the posterior fossa route.

The overall treatment plan for medulloblastoma at the present time includes both surgery and radiation. The value of various chemotherapeutic regimens in improving survival is currently being tested.

Surgery of Medulloblastoma. The role of surgery has as its goals to establish the diagnosis, to relieve acute problems related to tumor pressure, and to reduce the bulk of the tumor mass. It is clear that surgery alone is not curative and can be considered only the first step in therapy.[164] The operative procedure involves a posterior fossa craniectomy with retraction of the appropriate portions of the cerebellum, giving access to the tumor. The tumor is usually grossly apparent, being often fleshy and somewhat darker in appearance than the surrounding normal tissues. The surgical techniques require magnification and the procedure is often done with the patient in the sitting position. In addition to the risks which apply generally to neurosurgical procedures, the approach to the medulloblastoma has the additional problems brought about by the close relationship of the tumor to vital medullary and brain stem control centers. Even traction or manipulation of the tumor mass can result in postoperative neurological deficits.

At present, surgery is a part of the standard approach to these tumors. A considerable surgical morbidity and mortality continues to be recorded, even with neurosurgical and anesthesial improvement. It may be possible with improved diagnostic accuracy of the CT scan to make a sufficiently definitive pre-operative diagnosis, where radiation or chemotherapy could be instituted without surgery in certain specific cases in which the patient's condition makes any surgery hazardous. The use of CSF cytology and CSF tissue culture may allow, in certain instances, in combination with the CT scan, definitive tumor location and histologic diagnosis.

It should be emphasized that medulloblastoma very commonly spreads by way of the CSF pathways intracranially as well as along the spinal neuraxis.[165] This proclivity for spread makes the definitive diagnosis of medulloblastoma a critical therapeutic issue, for with this diagnosis there is an almost absolute indication for treatment of the entire neuraxis with radiation and it may also commit the patient to adjuvant chemotherapy[166,167]

Radiation Therapy of Medulloblastoma. Following surgery and a suitable interval for recovery, radiation therapy with or without chemotherapy should begin. Like most CNS tumors in childhood, medulloblastoma tends to cause symptoms by obstruction of the ventricular system with subsequent increased intracranial pressure. Rarely a patient presents with symptoms of spinal cord compromise from a subarachnoid deposit and evaluation reveals a primary lesion in the posterior fossa. Virtually all lesions tend to arise in the cerebellum. Chang and colleagues have proposed a staging system based on primary extent and extent of subarachnoid disease (Table 33-22).[168] Histologic separation into varying subtypes with suggestive differences in prognosis has been attempted.[169]

The role of surgery, as detailed earlier in this chapter, should be to re-establish as normal CSF dynamics as possible and remove bulk tumor if this can be safely accomplished. Overly aggressive attempts to remove all evident tumor, with resultant neurologic morbidity and possible mortality, are strongly discouraged, as are shunting procedures which potentially place systemic sites, circulating system, pleura, or peritoneum at risk.

Surgical treatment alone is never sufficient therapy for this tumor, as Cushing aptly demonstrated.[166] Radiation therapy represents the only currently available modality which offers the demonstrated potential of cure. Early studies demonstrated the necessity for treatment of the entire neuraxis by irradiation and a technically demanding treatment plan must be followed to permit optimum efficacy with acceptable morbidity. Treatment techniques used at the Joint Center for Radiotherapy (JCRT) are in Fig. 33-22 and dosimetric aspects have been described by Van Dyk and colleagues.[170] Following initial treatment of the site, concurrent treatment of the entire neuraxis is essential rather than sequential treatment of separate geographic regions, to minimize the risk of cells migrating from untreated to treated areas.[171] Many studies suggest that posterior fossa primary site irradiation to doses approaching 5500 rad with 180 rad fractions in 6 weeks to 7 weeks are preferable to lower dose treatment, especially for locally more advanced or prognostically unfavorable lesions.[81,117,130,168,171,173]

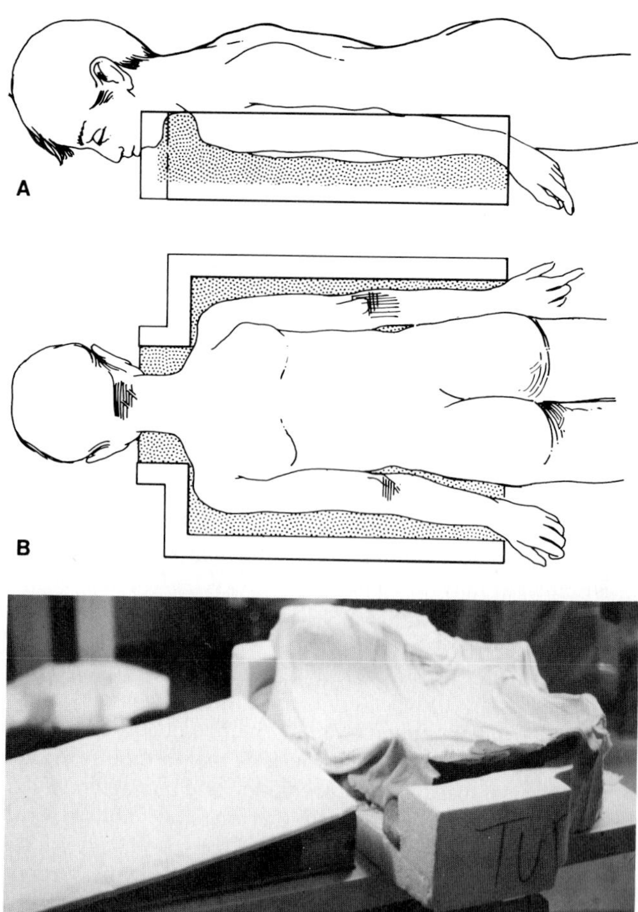

FIG. 33-22. Medulloblastoma: treatment technique at Joint Center for Radiotherapy (JCRT). (*A, B*) Schematic for individualized device for immobilization in treatment for medulloblastoma at JCRT in frontal and lateral projections. (*C*) Photograph of actual device in use at JCRT.

Although radiation doses of 3500 rad or more are usually recommended for treatment of subclinical spinal subarachnoid disease and more than 4000 rad for the remainder of the brain, data confirming these recommended dose levels are scant. Bloom and colleagues, using lower doses in the past, achieved substantial survival improvement and long-term control in approximately 25% of treated patients.[173-175] Virtually all initial failures in patients receiving neuraxis treatment were, and continue to be, at the primary, posterior fossa

TABLE 33-22. Staging System for Medulloblastoma

T_1	Tumor less than 3 cm diameter and limited to the classic midline position in the vermis, the roof of the fourth ventricle, and less frequently to the cerebellar hemispheres.
T_2	Tumor 3 cm or greater in diameter, further invading one adjacent structure or partially filling the fourth ventricle.
T_3	This stage is subdivided into T_{3a} and T_{3b}. T_{3a}: Tumor further invading two adjacent structures or completely filling the fourth ventricle with extension into the aqueduct of Sylvius, foramen of Magendie, or foramen of Luschka, thus producing marked internal hydrocephalus. T_{3b}: Tumor arising from the floor of the fourth ventricle or brain stem and filling the fourth ventricle.
T_4	Tumor further spreading through the aqueduct of Sylvius to involve the third ventricle or midbrain, or tumor extending to the upper cervical cord.
M_0	No evidence of gross subarachnoid or hematogenous metastasis.
M_1	Microscopic tumor cells found in cerebrospinal fluid.
M_2	Gross nodular seedings demonstrated in the cerebellar, cerebral subarachnoid space, or in the third or lateral ventricles.
M_3	Gross nodular seeding in spinal subarachnoid space.
M_4	Metastasis outside the cerebrospinal axis.

(Chang CH, Housepian EM, Herbert C Jr: An operative staging system and a megavoltage radiotherapeutic technic for cerebellar medulloblastomas. Radiology 93:1351–1359, 1969)

site. We are unaware of a series of patients treated with appropriate neuraxis irradiation and receiving more than 2500 rad to prophylactic sites in which the overwhelming primary relapse site has not been the posterior fossa, *not* the remainder of the neuraxis. The issue of dose to these sites of potential subclinical disease is of considerable importance, as a major portion of the radiation-related morbidity of treatment occurs outside the PF and is clearly dose related. We do not recommend use of radiocolloids to treat potential CSF disease, owing to the potential for significant arachnoiditis.[176]

In contrast to the absence of clear dose/response data for these subclinical sites, considerable evidence has accumulated demonstrating the improved local and overall control following higher posterior fossa doses in excess of 5000 rad. Harisiadis and colleagues, studying similarly staged lesions, were able to demonstrate significant control improvement with higher doses.[171] Several other recent series tend to confirm this view.

Improvements in equipment and technical aspects of treatment combined with the use of higher radiation doses to the posterior fossa have resulted in substantial improvement in results. In particular, 3-year survival has improved with more than 60% of irradiated patients living at this interval. However, although a substantial increase in the time to relapse has occurred and these late relapses decrease the overall differences at 5 years, (35%–40% vs. 20%–25%), Bloom and others have shown the value of the Collin's risk period (age at diagnosis plus 9 months) in predicting an accurate risk period for recurrence. [164,173,177] Relapse in patients with medulloblastoma beyond this period is extremely rare. In association with better local control and a longer duration of survival, a larger percentage of patients now demonstrate systemic, extra-CNS metastases, especially to bones where a characteristic diffuse blastic appearance is produced. Placement of shunts to pleural or peritoneal locations certainly increases the risk of tumor seeding to these locations. It has also been credited as increasing the risk of systemic dissemination to other sites; however, this increase is controversial and a shunt is certainly not necessary for this occurrence, as there have been several instances without prior shunting.[178]

The prognosis of older (15 years) patients with medulloblastoma has been stated to be better than that of younger children. In fact, although 3-year survival appears to be superior for older patients, at 5 years, survival for younger patients is superior and shows apparent advantage with longer followup.

Should tumor recurrence develop several years after initial treatment and be limited to the posterior fossa, a second course of limited irradiation can result in substantial aftersurvival and, on rare occasions, apparent cure.

The clinical benefit of such retreatment has clearly outweighed the increased risk of brain necrosis. The increasing frequency of appearance of late relapses has heightened interest in the combined use of systemic chemotherapy with irradiation.

Chemotherapy of Medulloblastoma. Medulloblastoma accounts for one-fourth of all pediatric age brain tumors and therefore a significant number of patients may be accrued on therapeutic trials. The advent of carefully planned maximal dose radiotherapy has resulted in a median survival of patients with medulloblastoma of some 4 years to 5 years. The majority of patients often recur at the original site of disease and therefore chemotherapeutic trials are appropriate. Most reports, unfortunately, contain less than a half dozen cases who have been treated on a comparatively *ad hoc* basis at the time when they become symptomatic.

There is a general impression that medulloblastomas are comparatively radiosensitive as well as chemosensitive. The duration of response is frequently brief or not reported. Table 33-23 contains a series of currently reported studies evaluating various modalities in the treatment of medulloblastoma. Two major prospective randomized studies are currently underway and only preliminary information is available.[179,180] Both studies require the patient to have had a surgical biopsy and then compare radiotherapy to radiotherapy plus CCNU and vincristine. In addition, the study carried out by Evans and co-workers adds prednisone.[180] A preliminary analysis of a study being carried out by the International Society of Pediatric Oncology (SIOP) indicates a slightly greater median time to progression for patients receiving radiotherapy and chemotherapy in comparison with those who receive radiotherapy alone. A study carried out by the Children's Cancer Study Group (CCSG) has not yet reached significance. It is too early to determine if the preliminary analysis will continue to show the same trend or if, in fact, selective and prognostic factors may in the long run account for differences seen. These studies will form a basis for controlled clinical trials in the treatment of children with medulloblastoma.

Although vincristine has been reported as being useful for the treatment of gliomas, it has rarely been used alone. Rosenstock reported response in three out of four patients with recurrent medulloblastomas.[181] A wide variety of other Phase II therapeutic studies in patients with recurrent or progressive tumor symptoms have added vincristine to other drugs, such as the nitrosoureas, procarbazine, nitrogen mustard, and methotrexate. Cangir had an impressive 80% re-

TABLE 33-23. Current Chemotherapy: Studies on Treatment of Medulloblastoma

AUTHOR	STUDY DESIGN	PATIENT POPULATION	NUMBER	PRETREATMENT CONDITIONS	TREATMENT GROUPS	RESULTS* MTP	RESULTS* MST	COMMENTS
Bloom (SIOP)	Randomized (Preliminary)	Postop	191	Surgery	RadTh RadTh, VCR & CCNU	2 yrs 3+ yrs		Slight benefit to chemotherapy $p = 0.408$
Evans (CCSG)	Randomized (Preliminary)	Postop Age 2–16 years	128/144	Surgery	RadTh vs RadTh, VCR, CCNU & Prednisone	69% 2 yr survival 72% 2 yr survival		No significant difference
Crafts	Phase II	Recurrent & Symptomatic	16/17	Surgery & RadTh	Procarbazine + Vincristine + CCNU	Response Stable Progression	63% 31% 6%	
Cangir	Phase II	Recurrent & Progressive	10	Surgery & RadTh	Nitrogen mustard + Vincristine + Procarbazine + Prednisone	Response = 80% No Response = 20%	11 mos 2	Moderately acceptable toxicity
Rosenstock	Phase II	Recurrent	4	Surgery & RadTh	Vincristine	Response = 75%		VCR used alone
Thomas	Phase II	(1) Recurrent (2) Early Treatment	8 9	Surgery & RadTh Surgery & RadTh	Vincristine BCNU Dexamethosone Methotrexate IV Methotrexate IT	Response = 100% MDR = 18.8 mos		IT-MTX and BCNU stopped during RadTh as very toxic when used early (4 deaths)

*MTP = Median time to Progression; MST = Median Survival Time

(Bloom HJG: Prospects for increasing survival in children with medulloblastoma: present and future studies. Multidisciplin Aspects Br Tum Ther, 1:245–259, 1979; Evans AE, Anderson J, Chang C et al: Adjuvant chemotherapy for medulloblastoma and ependymoma. Multidisciplin Aspects Br Tum Ther, 1:219–222, 1979; Crafts DC, Levin VA, Edwards MS et al: Chemotherapy of recurrent medulloblastoma with combined procarbazine, CCNU, and vincristine. J Neurosurg 49:589–592, 1978; Cangir A, van Eys J, Berry DH et al: Combination chemotherapy with MOPP in children with recurrent brain tumors. Med Ped Oncol, 4:253–261, 1978; Rosenstock JG, Evans AE, Schut L: Response to vincristine of recurrent brain tumors in children. J Neurosurg 45:135–140, 1976; Thomas PR, Duffner PK, Cohen ME et al: Multimodality therapy for medulloblastoma. Cancer 45:666–669, 1980)

sponse rate in ten patients with the median duration of response of 11 months in a group of ten patients who received MOP.[182] Thomas had 100% response rate in eight patients with recurrent symptoms of medulloblastoma whom he treated with vincristine, BNCU, dexamethosone, intravenous methotrexate, and intrathecal methotrexate. In nine patients who were treated immediately after surgery and in combination with radiotherapy, severe toxicity was seen with four early deaths.[183] The toxicity was attributed to the intrathecal methotrexate and BCNU being delivered during radiotherapy. Considerably less toxicity was seen when they were discontinued while radiotherapy was being delivered.

The design of a therapeutic study in the treatment of medulloblastoma is complicated by the long life span and therefore long therapeutic period which these patients can enjoy. Radiotherapy, chemotherapy, and the combination of both can have severe effects upon the endocrine and mental function of children and their general growth and development. All of these factors must be taken into consideration when designing therapeutic studies.

EPENDYMOMAS. *Surgical Treatment.* Ependymomas are tumors which arise from the ependymal linings of the CSF pathways. Although they can arise in any portion of the brain lined with ependyma, approximately 70% of intracranial lesions occur in the posterior fossa and they are thereby considered in the discussion of posterior fossa tumors.[184] These tumors, particularly those in the posterior fossa, are found in younger patients and cover a wide spectrum from benign to malignant and have a highly variable clinical course. The mean age at presentation in one series was 21 years.[184]

The anatomical relationship of these tumors makes total surgical removal quite difficult, regardless of the histological degree of malignancy. They are rarely encapsulated, although grossly demarcated from the surrounding normal brain. The surgical approach is therefore primarily by way of posterior fossa craniectomy with an attempt being made to remove that portion of the tumor safely. The results of surgery of ependymomas are given in Table 33-24. It is clear that surgical removal alone is applicable in only the minority of cases. Often, repeated surgical procedures are indicated. The indolent and often slow-growing nature of the tumor makes such repeated surgical resections worthwhile, particularly in the young patients whom this tumor most often afflicts. The use of CSF shunting procedures may be required when the tumor restricts flow of CSF in the fourth ventricular region. As discussed with medulloblastoma, such shunts place usually protected sites at risk for spread and should not be utilized unless clearly necessary. Initially, shunting devices, by which increased pressure can be decreased by external needle aspiration but which do not circulate CSF and possible malignant cells to areas which cannot be irradiated, are to be preferred.

The incompleteness of surgical removal results in frequent need to consider both radiation and chemotherapy.

Radiation Therapy of Ependymoma. Virtually all studies demonstrate that postoperative irradiation considerably improves survival for both children and adults with ependymoma. Mørk and Løken were able to demonstrate a 20% to 30% increase in survival at 5 years with intracranial

Table 33-24*A*. Survival from Time of Diagnosis in Treatment of Ependymomas

INFRATENTORIAL TUMORS		SUPRATENTORIAL TUMORS	
Years Surviving	*Number of Patients*	*Years Surviving*	*Number of Patients*
<1	52(7)	<1	18(6)
1–3	36	1–3	11
3–5	19	3–5	6
5–10	15	5–10	2
>10	13	>10	1

(The number of operative deaths included are noted in parentheses.)

(Kricheff II, Becker M, Schneck SA et al: Intracranial ependymomas: A study of survival in 65 cases treated by surgery and irradiation. Am J Roentgenol Radium Ther Nucl Med 91:167–175, 1964)

lesions.[185,186] Similar results have been shown by others.[184,186] Radiation doses in excess of 4500 rad have been shown to achieve improved results compared with lower doses.[187–190] Numerous studies are available which demonstrate that ependymomas have a considerable incidence of subarachnoid seeding.[188,191,192] Pathologic evaluation has demonstrated this risk to average 20% to 30% in most series. Clinically, symptomatic seeding is less frequent, although several recent papers have focused attention on this problem.[81,189,190,192] Factors which tend to increase this risk include infratentorial intracranial location, proximity to the ventricular linings, and higher grade lesions.[189,190,193] Based on this information, irradiation of the craniospinal axis is recommended for posterior fossa lesions or high-grade tumors at any site. Such treatment for supratentorial, lower grade lesions that are somewhat removed from the ventricular lining does not seem warranted.

Radiation doses in excess of 5000 rad delivered 5.5 weeks to 6 weeks are recommended for the primary lesion and, when craniospinal treatment is necessary, doses of 3000-3500 rad in 3.5 weeks to 4 weeks and more have been recommended. Radiation techniques identical to those described for the treatment of medulloblastoma should be utilized.

From 40% to 60% of patients with intracranial ependymoma survive 5 years. Histologic grade is of considerable prognostic significance, as patients with poorly differentiated tumors fare considerably less well than those with lower grade lesions. The prognostic significance of location within the cranial cavity is unclear with infratentorial lesions faring less well in some series and better in others.[185,190]

Chemotherapy of Ependymoma. Although ependymomas are highly responsive to radiotherapy and a prolonged high quality of life can be anticipated, recurrence may eventually take place. This may be either at the original site of the tumor or more distally, owing to metastasis. Chemotherapy has been carried out only occasionally in late-stage recurrent tumors. In Cangir's study utilizing MOPP, one recurrent patient was treated with no response.[182] Four out of six late-recurrent ependymomas treated with the nitrosoureas were noted to have a positive response.[194]

The major study that will provide the basic information on

TABLE 33-24*B*. 5-Year Survival from Time of Diagnosis in Treatment of Ependymomas

	NUMBER FOLLOWED	NUMBER SURVIVING	PERCENT SURVIVING
All Cases	59	17	28
All Surviving Surgery and Receiving Radiation	41	17	41
All Infratentorial Tumors	45	15	33
Infratentorial Cases Surviving Surgery and Receiving Radiation	33	15	45
All Supratentorial Tumors	14	2	14
Supratentorial Cases Surviving Surgery and Receiving Radiation	9	2	22

(Kircheff II, Becker M, Schneck SA et al: Intracranial ependymomas: A study of survival in 65 cases treated by surgery and irradiation. Am J Roentgenol Radium Ther Nucl Med 91:167–175, 1964)

the treatment of ependymoblastoma is that being carried out by the CCSG in conjunction with the previously discussed medulloblastoma study.[91] As a separate stratification, patients with ependymoblastoma will receive standard prescribed courses of radiotherapy and be randomized to no additional therapy or to receive CCNU, vincristine, and prednisone. Over 40 patients have been entered into this study, however, it is too early for results to be meaningful.

The survival curve of patients who have ependymomas is generally biphasic, in which the first half succumb rather promptly to their disease with a median survival of approximately 1 year, regardless of the supra- or infratentorial location of the tumor. After 5 years the slope of the survival curve has markedly flattened out with approximately 25% of patients alive. Clearly, these patients describe a different biologic entity than those seen in the earlier portion of the survival curve and deserve vigorous investigation as to what characteristics might account for their increased survivorship.

HEMANGIOBLASTOMA AND HEMANGIOMA. These tumors are highly vascular lesions involving the cerebellum and occurring primarily in the young. The majority are benign, but highly malignant cases have been reported. The surgical approach is by way of posterior fossa craniectomy with an attempt to remove the lesion. As they occupy primarily cerebellum, total removal is often possible. Leaving even a small portion of these tumors can lead to massive recurrence. In view of the extreme vascularity, particular care needs to be taken to have adequate sources of blood replacement, pay meticulous attention to hemostasis, and check for any potential bleeding diathesis. When total removal is accomplished, patients can usually be considered cured. The association of these tumors with other hemangiomas, particularly renal and hepatic loci, makes systemic evaluation important.[195] A frequent association with von Hippel–Lindau disease has been noted and these patients may be polycythemic. Familial aggregations with many affected members have been noted.[196]

Surgical morbidity and mortality has been appreciable with lesions that are solid rather than cystic, especially when the floor of the IV ventricle of brain stem has been affected.[197,198] For these patients, more conservative surgical procedures followed by high dose (5000 rad to 5500 rad in 5 weeks to 6 weeks) irradiation is recommended. Anecdotal experience confirms the ability of irradiation to accomplish tumor control.[199,200]

In the malignant hemangioblastoma total removal may be quite difficult as this tumor may invade deeply into midline structures. In such cases radiation therapy should be considered.

Brain Stem and Thalamus Tumors

The tumors of these basal structures are primarily intrinsic lesions of the glioma group. Because of the risk of surgical morbidity, lesions are often grouped by region rather than histology. Meningioma of the foramen magnum is a benign tumor which may occur in this region and may be amenable to surgical removal. In general, the intrinsic tumors of this region are astrocytic and range from low-grade to high-grade malignancy. A significant fraction of these lesions are of high grade, especially in the pontine and brain stem region. Other than glioma, only ependymomas and medulloblastomas are seen with any frequency. Surgery for tumors of the brain stem, pons, and midbrain is rarely indicated. Even surgical biopsy carries unacceptable risks in all but a few cases. There have been successful thalamic biopsies and subtotal resections reported. Occasional, more vigorous surgical approaches to thalamic lesions that have extended to the temporal lobes may be of value, especially for decompression of cystic lesions. The astrocytic tumors as a group in these regions are more common in young patients and tend to have a somewhat slower growth rate than their cerebral counterparts. However, the vital nature of the structures involved causes significant deficits relatively early in the clinical course. The primary treatment for these tumors involves radiation possibly supplemented by chemotherapy.

Nearly two-thirds of patients with mid-brain and thalamic tumors are children less than 15 years of age. In this age group, these lesions constitute a relatively common clinical problem and are seen with a frequency only exceeded by cerebellar gliomas and approximated by malignant posterior fossa tumors such as medulloblastoma.

Symptoms of ventricular obstruction such as headache, nausea, or vomiting predominate and cranial nerve palsies (especially CN VI or VII) or cerebellar ataxia with subtle changes in mental status are the neurologic signs seen with greatest frequency. Symptom duration is usually short, usually less than 6 months. Consultation with an experienced neuroradiologist is essential so that optimum radiographic evaluation is obtained, especially as most of these patients will not undergo biopsy or surgical exploration.

Many series demonstrate the efficacy of irradiation.[80–83,119,130,161,201–205] Following delivery of 5000 rad to 5500 rad delivered in 6 weeks to 7 weeks to volumes that include the posterior fossa, mid-brain and a sufficient margin, most patients will have significant improvement in their neurologic status and demonstrate reversal or prior neurologic deficits and show functional improvement. Attempts to improve results by delivery of higher radiation doses have not generally been successful.

Treatment results permit separation of patients with pontine and brain stem lesions from those with mid-brain or thalamic lesions.[81,83,161] From 15% to 25% of the former group will enjoy 3-year to 5-year survival following treatment whereas 40% to 60% of the patients with mid-brain lesions will survive disease-free for this period.

For brain stem lesions, radiation appears to increase survival by an average of 1 year with an occasional long term disease-free survivor. Results for the mid-brain and thalamic lesions are much more encouraging. Reasons for this difference are not known, although a higher frequency of more favorable histology in the mid-brain group has been proposed as a possible explanation.[83]

These tumors, all essentially inaccessible lesions, comprise a group wherein treatment without firm histological diagnosis is often the only recourse. Particular care needs to be given to the neurological diagnosis and the radiological findings. The use of CSF cytology and tissue culture may play an important role in tumors of this area.

By virtue of their interaxial location, tumors of the brain stem, medulla, and thalmus are among the most sensitive to therapeutic manipulation. Small changes in tumor mass within these vital areas can produce dramatic clinical responses. The brain stem is not more than a few centimeters in diameter and is in continual contact with CSF. It might therefore, be considered as the ideal tumor for intrathecal chemotherapy. However, in those few cases in which intrathecal methotrexate has been utilized, the results have been unsatisfactory.[194]

A group of patients with pontine glioma were studied by Rosen, utilizing high-dose methotrexate followed by citrovorum factor rescue.[206] Encouraging temporary symptomatic improvement, as well as a decrease in tumor volume seen on serial CT scans, has been reported. However, the therapy is difficult and requires careful monitoring and control. In addition, severe encephalomalacia with loss of white matter and brain damage has been reported following both intrathecal and high-dose intravenous methotrexate.[207]

Brain stem gliomas are relatively infrequently seen and are therefore often placed on adult brain tumor chemotherapy protocols with the hope of showing some results.[208,209]

The nitrosoureas (BCNU and CCNU) produced temporary responses in three out of 12 of a heterogeneous group of patients so studied. Symptomatic improvement was reported in one patient treated with procarbazine.[209] A complex protocol involving a six-drug combination (6-mercaptopurine, procarbazine, cyclophosphamide, methotrexate, 5-fluorouracil, vinblastine) has been tried in a small series of patients who received concurrent radiotherapy and failed to show significant results.[208]

Pineal Area Neoplasms

The area of pineal gland and region of the third ventricle gives rise to four different tumor groups, each of which differs in management approach. These tumors are usually diagnosed after either visual symptoms (such as paralysis of upward gaze) or obstructive effects (hydrocephalus syndrome). Most tumors occur within 10 years of puberty.[210] The use of the CT scan has made the detection of these tumors much easier and allowed for the development of a rational management approach as described in Fig. 33-23. Astrocytomas, dysgerminomas and teratomas are the more common pineal region tumors. Pinealomas and pinealoblastomas are extremely rare.

Clinical symptoms at presentation may be extremely helpful in reaching a likely diagnosis even in the absence of histology.[211] The presence of diabetes insipidus in a teenage patient with delayed or absent development of secondary sexual characteristics, other evidence of pituitary dysfunction and visual symptoms nearly always indicates a germinoma. Precocious puberty may be noted. Often, two distinct separated lesions are identified, one located in the suprasellar (floor of ventricle III) region and the other in the pineal region. Involvement of the hypothalamus, midbrain, and brain stem may produce striking symptoms of memory loss, emotional lability, or marked fluctuation in temperature control or regulation of other vital functions. Surgical intervention, even for biopsy only, does not appear warranted.

Patients with these signs and any patient thought clinically to have a dysgerminoma is best treated with radiation therapy (*vide infra*). Response to treatment is often extremely rapid and a repeat CT scan taken after delivery of 2000 rad to 3000 rad may show striking reduction in tumor size.[212–214]

More aggressive germ cell tumors may also be seen including embryonal carcinoma, teratoma, and teratocarcinoma and the so-called Teilum tumor more frequently seen in the ovary in adolescent girls or testis in young males. HCG determination, including measurement of the B-subunit of CSF, may be helpful and, as with medulloblastoma and ependymoma, CSF cytology following cytocentrifugation should always be performed.[215]

The surgical approach to the pineal area has recently undergone considerable evaluation. The work of Stein and others has indicated that with careful microsurgical technique, surgery can be carried out with acceptable risks.[31] It has been suggested that surgery be considered as a primary treatment modality.[216] The pineal region can be approached either by the posterior fossa or from above through the ventricle. The early management of many pineal tumors requires the placement of a ventricular shunt in one or both ventricles prior to radiation. If the tumor is believed to be a germinoma likely to respond quickly to irradiation, then early irradiation with careful monitoring may eliminate this requirement. Certainly, if the tumor is felt to be of a germ cell

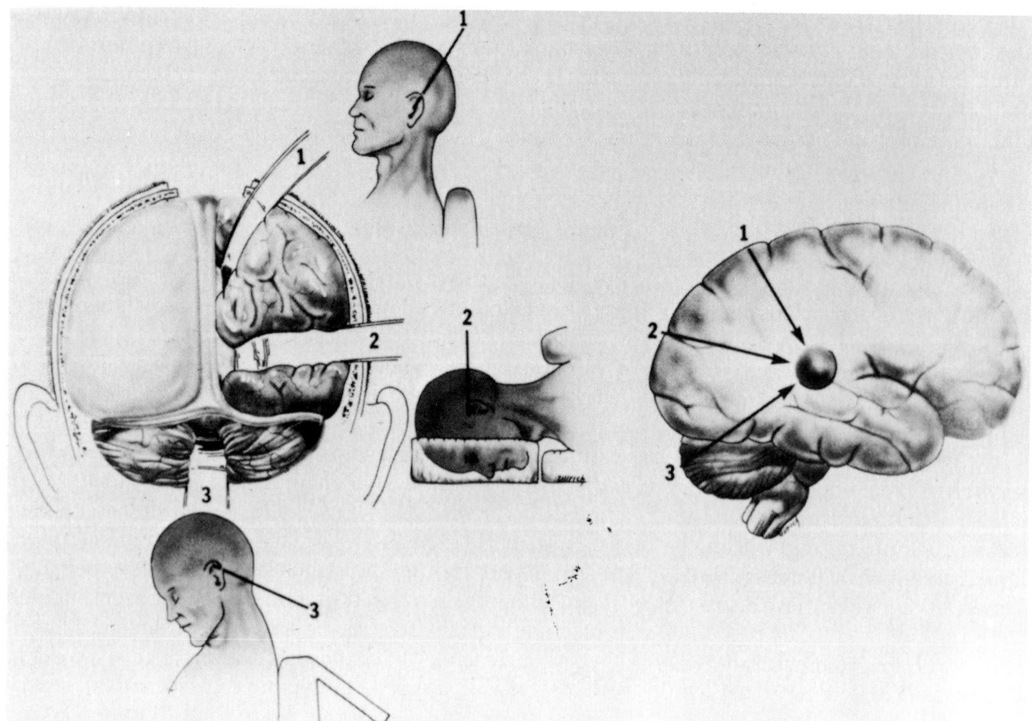

FIG. 33-23. Surgical exposures for neoplasms of pineal area, showing the three basic routes to the pineal area. The supracerebellar–infratentorial approach used by Stein is shown as 3. (Stein BM: Supracerebellar–infratentorial approach to pineal tumors. Surg Neurol 11:331–337, 1979)

nature, shunts to areas untreatable by irradiation should be rigorously avoided, (see discussion earlier on "closed" tappable shunts) as these tumors seed regularly and frequently.[81,212]

Should none of the characteristic clinical symptoms (especially diabetes insipidus) be present and radiographic studies suggest a mature or differentiated teratoma, surgery may be appropriate. Its use, other than for possible biopsy, for the other histologic types, is either not appropriate (germ cell tumor, pinealoblastoma) or debatable (astrocytoma).

Most patients with long term disease-free survival following treatment for pineal area neoplasms have either had a benign teratoma or have received relatively high-dose, large volume radiation therapy.[81,210–214,217,218] Most authors agree on the necessity of relatively high dose (approximately 5000 rad/5.5 weeks–6 weeks) megavoltage treatment to the primary lesion. Current reports also agree on the desirability for treatment of relatively wide margins around the primary lesions. However, considerable disagreement is present on the necessity for craniospinal treatment for these patients. Virtually all series of any size include several examples of subarachnoid seeding either within the cranial cortex and/or the spinal axis. Most series suffer in that the cumulative risk of seeding is not described.[217] Therefore, the relatively few examples of seeding become the numerator and the entire group with pineal neoplasms become the denominator and craniospinal treatment is rejected.[217]

The only series which describes the cumulative risk of seeding has described a 37% likelihood for "suprasellar ectopic pinealoma," a 10% risk for any pineal lesion and a greater than 50% for biopsy-proven germinoma.[213] Based on these data, we strongly urge craniospinal treatment for patients with clinical characteristics of dysgerminoma (*i.e.*, diabetes insipidus—*vide supra*). In other unbiopsied patients with pineal neoplasms, serial CT scans should be performed during the period of irradiation. The demonstration of significant response after a relatively modest dose of irradiation (2000 rad to 3000 rad) is sufficiently common with the group of tumors that regularly seed and rare with the other possibilities (teratoma; astrocytoma). We feel these patients should also receive prophylactic craniospinal treatment.[81,213] When necessary, doses of 2000 rad to 3000 rad have been effective in eliminating the risk of subarachnoid spread. Radiation techniques described earlier for treatment of medulloblastoma should be used. Attempts to achieve long term salvage for patients initially treated to local fields who develop subarachnoid spread, by subsequent irradiation are almost never successful.

Nearly 60% of patients with midline pineal tumors will survive 5 years following treatment with irradiation and an even higher proportion of these with "ectopic pinealoma" will survive for this period.[81,213,214,217,218] To maintain this level of disease-free survival beyond 3 years to 5 years appears to require initial craniospinal treatment.[213] The results of surgical treatment of pineal area neoplasms are shown on Table 33-25.

Pineal tumors, because of their heterogeneity of cell type, rarity, and complications noted above, have not been frequently subjected to chemotherapy. A case report of an adult

TABLE 33-25. Results of Treatment of Pineal Area Neoplasms

CASE NUMBER	HISTOLOGICAL DIAGNOSIS	SHUNT	OCCIPITAL TRANSTENTORIAL CRANIOTOMY	RADIATION	CHEMOTHERAPY	OUTCOME
1	germinoma	VP	subtotal decompression	none	–	alive & well; receiving Laetrile
2	dysgerminoma	VP	–	craniospinal	+	alive & well; tumor-free after 3 yrs
3	dysgerminoma	VP	subtotal decompression	craniospinal	–	alive & well; tumor-free after 3 yrs
4	pineoblastoma	VP	–	cranial only	–	died of spinal metastases
5	pineoblastoma	VP	complete excision	craniospinal	–	alive & well; tumor-free after 6 mos
6	pineocytoma	VP	complete excision	craniospinal	–	alive & well; undergoing irradiation
7	pineocytoma	VP	complete excision	craniocervical	–	alive & well; tumor-free after 2 yrs
8	malignant ependymoma	VP	complete excision	cranial only	–	alive & well; tumor-free after 6 yrs

(Neuwelt EA, Glasberg M, Frenkel E et al: Malignant pineal region tumors. J Neurosurg 51:597–607, 1979)

with pinealoma diagnosed on CT scan and CSF cytology was treated with adriamycin and vincristine upon recurrence of symptoms after a brief period of radiotherapeutic control. The tumor was noted to markedly decrease in size on subsequent CT scans.[219] The rationale for choice of adriamycin was that germinoma is the most frequently encountered histology in pineal tumors and adriamycin has been shown to be effective in germ cell tumors.

Glomus Jugulare Tumors

These tumors, which arise from glomus bodies in the adventitia of the jugular bulb or nearby are often clinically detected because of slowly progressive aural (deafness, tinitis, vertigo, external canal bleeding) or neurologic (swallowing or phonation difficulties) symptoms or both. Histologically, they have been grouped with the other nonchromaffin paragangiomas or chemodectomas, such as carotid body tumors. Females are most commonly affected. One study has attempted to separate lesions histologically into three groups: predominantly vascular, cellular, and mixed types. Although lymph node and, rarely, distant metastases have been noted, they are most commonly locally progressive. A definite familial and bilateral group has been defined.

Because of their vascular nature and location, surgical management is often accompanied by major blood loss and major morbidity and mortality. Complete extirpation, despite these complications, is rarely possible.[220–223] In view of this, radical radiation therapy following biopsy or attempted removal has been increasingly recommended.

These lesions were formerly considered to be "radioresistant." This mistaken surmise was probably due to lower maximum tumor doses possible using only orthovoltage equipment as well as the protracted regression commonly seen following irradiation of slowly progressive lesions. With newer megavoltage techniques, several recent reports document the efficacy of irradiation in control of glomus tumors.[220,224] A tumor dose of approximately 5000–5500 rad in 6–7 weeks time has produced superior results when compared to results achieved with lower doses.[220,224–227] Chemotherapy has not been utilized in tumors of the glomus jugulare.

Cerebellopontine Angle (CPA) Tumors

The primary tumor of the cerebellopontine angle (CPA) is the acoustic schwannoma. Less frequently, meningiomas arise in this area. Perhaps no other intracranial tumor group has so changed in its outlook in the last 10 years. The development of sophisticated audiometric and neuroradiologic techniques has allowed early diagnosis and microsurgical technique has found a major application.[228] Whereas Harvey Cushing had a 40% mortality in his series, today mortality rates are less than 1% for all but those with either very large tumors or poor preoperative neurological status.[229–231] When these tumors are diagnosed very early, that is, when still completely within the auditory canal, total removal with sparing of the seventh nerve and possibly even the auditory portion of the eighth nerve is possible in the majority of cases.[232]

The surgical approach may be either a one-stage or two-stage procedure. The first stage involves a translabyrinthine attack through the temporal bone, carefully drilling away the bone until the tumor is reached in the auditory canal. Intracanalicular tumors can be completely removed by this route. When the tumors extend medially, they come to press upon the brain stem, causing serious neurological sequelae. This CPA portion of the tumor usually requires a second-stage approach by way of the posterior fossa. In those cases requiring two stages, surgery may be performed all at one time consecutively or on two separate days. The procedures are coordinated so that the acoustic nerve and the seventh nerve are identified during the translabyrinthine approach and can be better protected during the posterior fossa stage. The translabyrinthine is most useful in attempting to preserve the seventh nerve function and, occasionally, some degree of eighth nerve function. The vestibular nerve can rarely be preserved. In cases in which seventh and eighth nerve destruction is unlikely to be reversed by surgery, a single stage posterior fossa operation may suffice. The proximity and

TABLE 33-26. Results of Surgery for Acoustic Neuroma (Microsurgical Suboccipital Operation)

SIZE (cm)	NUMBER OF CASES	RESULTS*			
		Good	*Fair*	*Poor*	*Died*
<2 cm (small)	8	8	–	–	–
2–3 cm (medium)	21	20	1	–	–
>3 cm (large)	74	60	7	5	2
Total	103	88	8	5	2

*Good = returned to full activity; fair = able to return to most of previous activity with mild impairment; poor = significant residual disability. Facial and auditory nerve function are not included in the assessment of disability.

(Ojemann RG, Crowell RC: Acoustic neuromas treated by microsurgical suboccipital operations. Prog Neurol Surg 9:337–373, 1978)

adherence of these tumors to the brain stem makes their removal an extremely delicate task. It is often safest to use a type of anesthesia which permits spontaneous respiration. Thus slight alterations in the respiratory pattern signal potential danger resulting from traction or manipulation of the tumor mass which affects brain stem function. These tumors are virtually always benign and if completely removed do not recur. In patients with neurofibromatosis they may be bilateral. The results of surgery and the possible complications are given in Table 33-26.

Meningiomas of this region rarely have an intracanalicular portion and can be dealt with by the posterior fossa approach. Surgical removal involves the same factors as for the schwannomas. At the current juncture there is little indication for either radiotherapy or chemotherapy in the treatment of CPA tumors.

Sellar and Suprasellar Tumors

The tumors of the sellar region include the intrinsic tumors of the pituitary gland, which are largely intrasellar tumors, and these of the suprasellar region which are primarily craniopharyngiomas and ectopic pinealomas. Tumors of the clivus will also be discussed in this area, with the primary tumors being clivus chordomas and meningiomas.

Pituitary tumors are comprised of both hormonally active and hormonally inactive lesions. The hormonally active tumors are primarily the eosinophilic (GH) and basophilic adenomas (ACTH) and the prolactin (PRL) secreting adenomas. These three hormone-producing tumors are often of relatively small size and infrequently protrude outside the sella. The nonhormonally active chromophobe adenomas are often larger in size, may protrude outside of the sella and are more likely to exhibit invasive characteristics. The treatment of these tumors will be described under two categories, active and inactive. In the eosinophilic and basophilic adenomas the major problems from a clinical standpoint usually lie in the hormonal effects of the tumor rather than the mass effect of the tumor on surrounding brain or nervous system structures. The management plan, therefore, is directed at eliminating their secretory functions. This can be accomplished by surgery, radiation therapy, or both. The prolactin secreting tumors represent a special type of clinical problem in that prolactin secretion can be suppressed by the use of a medical regime based upon bromocryptine.[233] This agent allows a medical regime to be followed which can significantly diminish the production of excessive prolactin and markedly ameliorate the clinical symptomatology. Surgical or radiotherapeutic management of these lesions is necessary when the tumors protrude from the sella or have suprasellar extension with neurological deficits.[234] However, surgical intervention carries sufficiently small risks that intervention transsphenoidally can be considered as an early treatment measure.

Prolactin secreting tumors have a particular propensity for growing as small so-called microadenomas. These microadenomas are often anterior and inferior in the sella and can be approached from the transphenoidal route with ease and removed with minimal neurologic interference.[235]

A further indication for surgery for a hormonally active tumor, especially eosinophilic adenoma, is the need for rapid cessation in hormonal function. This occurs when the effects of the excessive hormonal production have produced serious sequelae, such as extreme hypertension in the eosinophilic adenoma.

Radiation therapy, principally in the form of external megavoltage photon treatment, but including heavy particle proton or α-particle irradiation, has been utilized with considerable success.

In one of the few studies to evaluate the necessity of treatment of clinically evident but apparently inactive pituitary adenomas, it was noted that 87% of untreated but followed patients eventually required definitive treatment. Of more significance, 50% of these patients developed permanent damage which earlier treatment could have prevented.[236,237]

Patients who present with clinical symptoms of headache and visual symptoms as well as the clinical facial changes of an eosinophilic adenoma in whom no urgent reason for surgical decompression exists may be treated by primary irradiation without biopsy. In virtually all other settings, surgical decompression and biopsy appear to be of value. Rapid determination in visual signs and symptoms should be managed by initial rapid surgical decompressions.

The efficacy of relatively small doses of irradiation in rapidly reversing the clinical symptoms of pituitary tumors is well recognized. Several studies document the superiority of an initial definitive course of high dose irradiation delivering 4500 rad or more when compared to smaller multiple repeated courses. In particular, the poor results and increased morbidity

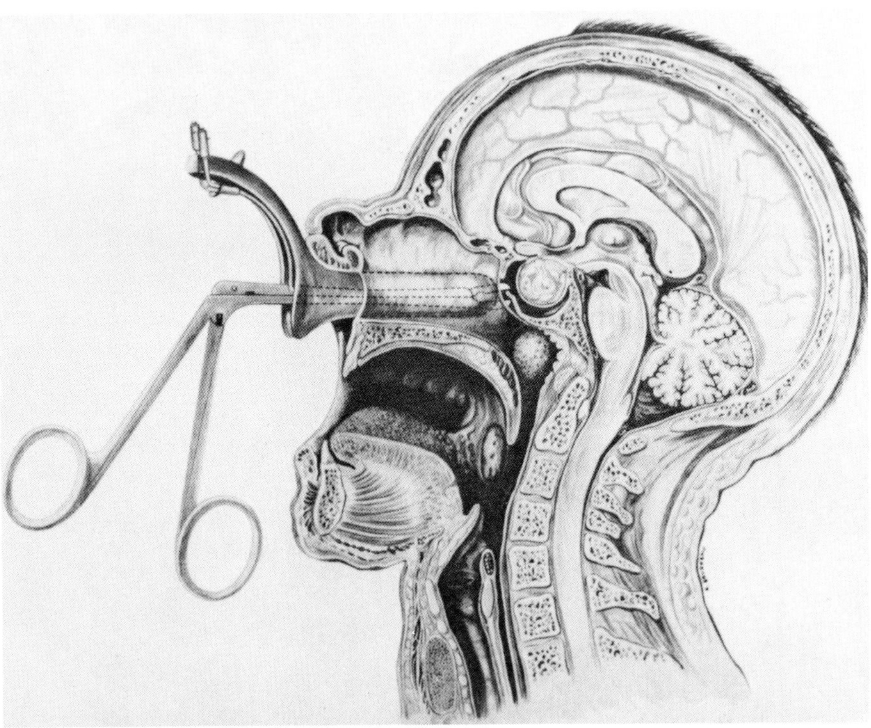

FIG. 33-24. Anatomic root for transsphenoidal hypophysectomy. (Hardy J, Wigser SM: Trans-sphenoidal surgery of pituitary fossa tumors with televised radiofluoroscopic control. J Neurosurg 23:613, 1965)

associated with repeated courses of treatment averaging 1000 rad to 1500 rad is clear.[238]

More than 75% of irradiated patients with acromegaly can be clinically controlled as measured by reversal of chemical abnormalities and arrest or reversal of soft tissue changes.[236-240] Many of these patients have extensive disease with suprasellar extension and therefore are not eligible for control by transsphenoidal hypophysectomy alone. Following development of the growth hormone assay, it was noted by several investigators that levels in the normal range were present in the minority.[241,242] More recent studies evaluating patients treated several years earlier demonstrate regular decrease in GH levels in the majority. This decrease may take up to two years for levels to reach normal limits.[237-240, 243] In one study, 84% of treated patients ultimately had growth hormone levels within normal limits following treatment.[243]

A significant advantage of radiation therapy without hypophysectomy is the retention of normal pituitary hormone secretion. In one study, 17 of 22 treated patients required no replacement following treatment.

A dose of 4500 rad to 5000 rad in 5 weeks or more using 180 rad daily fractions is recommended. Three-field, five-field, or rotational techniques are strongly recommended. Chemotherapy has not been employed in tumors in the sellar region.

Pituitary Tumors

CHROMOPHOBE ADENOMAS. The chromophobe adenomas are often larger and more vigorous in their growth and require treatment with surgery or radiation or both. They represent the most common pituitary tumor. The likelihood of compression of the optic nerves by extension beyond the sella is much more likely.

There are three surgical approaches available for the treatment of pituitary tumors. The first is the transfrontal approach. This procedure, popularized by Bronson Ray, involves a transfrontal craniotomy with elevation of the frontal lobe on the appropriate side.[244] The right side represents the safest general approach, but if visual effects have been more pronounced on the left then a left-sided approach is more appropriate. The pituitary gland and the tumor with suprasellar extension are then visualized and the tumor removed, often with the use of microsurgical techniques. This approach carries with it an excellent chance for complete pituitary gland removal and a lower risk of recurrence of hormonal activity if the suprasellar extension is minimal. It carries, however, a risk of craniotomy and of potential compression of the frontal lobes during the surgical procedure. It is the most rigorous and riskiest of the surgical approaches to the pituitary gland.

A second surgical approach is that of the transsphenoidal or, occasionally, transethenoidal removal. This approach was initially described and popularized by Harvey Cushing.[245] It fell into disuse until revived by Guiot and Hardy in the past decade.[246,247] The transsphenoidal approach allows direct access to the pituitary gland without having to disturb or disrupt the CNS structures. In this procedure (see Fig. 33-24) a nasal speculum is used to expose the sphenoid. The sphenoid is then entered and the pituitary gland approached by way of the sellar floor. The bony floor of the sella is opened and the tumor removed from beneath. The use of microsurgical technique and image intensification fluoroscopy made this procedure extremely safe with relatively minimal morbidity.

TABLE 33-27. Results of Treatment of Pituitary Tumors

AUTHOR	TYPE OF PROCEDURE	TYPE OF DISEASE	NUMBER OF PATIENTS	NUMBER OF OPERATIONS	PERCENT SUCCESS	PERCENT MORTALITY	PERCENT RECURRENCE	PERCENT VISUAL IMPROVEMENT
A. Ray	Transfrontal craniotomy	Chromophobe						
		Adenoma	63	68				
		Acromegaly	14	14				
		Cushing's Syndrome	3	3				
		TOTAL	80	85	100	0	8-10	75
B. Laws	Transseptal–Trans-phenoidal	Pituitary Adenoma		408	99.02	0.98		
		Functioning	265					
		Non-Functioning	135					
		Other	89	97				
		TOTAL	489	505	98.61	1.39		95.3 (81 of 85 studied)
C. Wilson	Transsphenoidal Microsurgical	Cushing's Disease						
		Basophilic Adenoma	1					
		Chromophobe						
		Adenoma	10					
		Mixed	3					
		Insufficient Tissue	3					
		Total Hypophysectomy	1					
		No specimen	2					
		TOTAL	20	20	100	0		
D. Hardy	Transsphenoidal	Pituitary Adenoma						
		Cromophobe	8					
		Recurrent						
		Chromophobe	3					
		Mixed	4					
		Eosinophilic	1					
		Craniopharyngioma	2					
		Reticulosarcoma	1					
		Chondrosarcoma	1					
		TOTAL	20	20	100	0		90

(Adapted from Ray BS, Patterson RH: Symposium on pituitary tumors: I, Surgical treatment of pituitary adenomas. J Neurosurg 19:1–8, 1962; Kern EB, Pearson BW, McDonald TJ et al: The transseptal approach to lesions of the pituitary and parasellar regions. Laryngoscope 89, Suppl 15:1–34, 1979; Tyrell JB, Brooks RM, Fitzgerald PA et al: Cushing's Disease: Selective Trans-sphenoidal resection of pituitary microadenomas. N Engl J Med 298:753–758, 1978,* and Hardy J, Wigser SM: Trans-sphenoidal surgery of pituitary fossa tumors with televised radiofluoroscopic control. J Neurosurg 23:612–619, 1965)

*Reprinted by permission of The New England Journal of Medicine.

Mortality for this procedure is extremely low and the neurological sequelae rare.[248] The problems of infection and CSF rhinorrhea which earlier complicated this procedure are now less common because of the availability of antibiotics for the occasional infection and meticulous placement of materials such as fascia lata or fat to plug the opening in the sphenoid sinus. These procedures have the additional advantage of not requiring access through the calivarium and the postoperative course is less stressful. Aside from the need for general anesthesia and the placement of nasal packs following surgery, the procedure is well tolerated. A variation of this approach is that of Zervas, in which an electrical coagulation of the intrasellar material is carried out stereotatically by the transsphenoidal route.[249] In this procedure an electrode is introduced by the same transsphenoidal approach through a small hole in the sellar floor and, by carefully manipulating the electrode tip into all the regions of the sellar tissue, the electrocoagulation is accomplished. This allows for relatively rapid destruction of pituitary tissue, has an extremely low morbidity, and minimal mortality. It is not as easy to obtain large amounts of pituitary tissue for careful pathological analysis by this technique but enough tissue can be obtained for evaluation of tumor type. All three approaches and their relative successes and risks are given in Table 33-27. All these approaches, particularly the transsphenoidal versions, now have to be given serious consideration as relatively safe procedures.

Transsphenoidal decompression prior to irradiation has three potential advantages. It achieves diagnostic confirmation, thereby ruling out the possibility of craniopharyngioma, which requires a higher dose for control. It also eliminates cystic spaces which potentially can cause radiation failure. Further, it decompresses the visual system, providing rapid relief from tumor impression.

Prior to 1950, utilizing orthovoltage techniques with tumor doses of less than 2500 roentgens, less than one-third of treated patients maintained useful vision or showed improvement. Following introduction of megavoltage techniques delivering more than 4000 rad, significant improvement occurred. In one series, only eight of 66 patients so treated required subsequent surgery and the majority showed improvement. In most large reported series, 75% to 80% of patients will be controlled by the initial course of irradiation. Although suggested in some series, no clear evidence is available confirming the advantage of initial surgery in lowering recurrence rates following irradiation.[250,251]

Although treatment response in the absence of visual signs may be difficult to gauge, especially following initial decompressive surgery, bone changes with restoration of a more normal sella turcica may be approximated in many patients 12–18 months following irradiation.[252] However, hormonal replacement, if needed prior to irradiation, will generally continue to be required.

CUSHING'S DISEASE. Basophilic or chromophobe adenoma of the pituitary has been associated with a syndrome of hypertension, obesity, plethora, striae, diabetes mellitus, and virilism or feminization. When the possibility of an adrenal tumor has been satisfactorily excluded, primary radiation therapy has proved to be effective therapy in many patients, especially children.[89,253–256] More than 4000 rad, delivered in 4 weeks to 5 weeks has generally been required to achieve a satisfactory response rate. Although success rates achieved in the treatment of children mimic results using irradiation seen in other pituitary tumors, control rates in adults tend to be lower, with most studies showing 50% or less of treated patients to be controlled.

Heavy Particle Irradiation (Protons and α-Particles). Although limited in general availability, considerable success has been achieved using either high energy α-particles or protons derived from a cyclotron. One or a very few large fractions (*i.e.*, 6,000–10,000 rad/1 fraction) of irradiation can be delivered by stereotactic or similarly precise localization techniques. Charged particles deposit rapidly increasing amounts of energy per unit path length as their velocity slows near the termination of their path in tissue. This "Bragg peak" portion of the proton beam's path can be used and permits a greater deposition of energy in the tumor than in intervening normal brain, especially when multiple beams are used which converge at the tumor site. From 80% to 90% of patients with a variety of pituitary lesions can be controlled by these specialized techniques.[257–263] However, large lesions, especially those with suprasellar extension, are not suitable and significant complications, especially visual field abnormalities, have ensued when attempts were made to treat such patients with heavy particles.[86,257,258]

Craniopharyngiomas

Craniopharyngiomas are tumors which arise from remnants of Rathke's pouch. They are usually principally suprasellar in location, but may have sellar involvement. They are often adherent to the hypothalamus and may compress ventricular pathways. It is often necessary to treat these patients with a shunting procedure prior to a definitive surgical or radiation treatment. These tumors are for the most part benign. Their strategic location makes the treatment of these tumors by surgical means a very high-risk procedure.[264] Matson was able to demonstrate that by careful extirpation of these lesions cures were obtainable in many patients.[265] Katz has recently updated and summarized this series.[51,263] Of 40 children originally operated on by Matson, six (15%) had incomplete resection.[263] Of 34 with apparent complete surgical removal, six (15%) additional patients were shown to have residual tumor within 1 month of surgery and three others (7½%) recurred later. Three patients died of hypothalamic and hypophyseal dysfunction. Only 22 (55%) were continuously disease-free and living for substantial periods after initial surgery. Seven of these 22 (32%) have been noted to have only a fair to poor quality of survival. The dangers involved in this procedure, in terms of hypothalamic function following surgery and of potential loss of neurological and neuro–endocrine function, have given impetus to the use of a combined approach wherein radiation is the primary therapeutic modality and surgery is used to biopsy and decompress the lesion if it is cystic. The surgical portion of this combined approach to the treatment of craniopharyngioma can often be accomplished by the transsphenoidal route but may involve a direct transfrontal procedure.

Because of the considerable surgical morbidity and mortality, especially prior to the availability of corticosteroids, Kramer initiated an attempt at the Royal Marsden Hospital to control this lesion with irradiation following conservative surgery.[266-268]

Initially using radiation doses of 6000 rad to 7000 rad in 7 weeks to 8 weeks by a multiple field or rotational technique almost uniform control was obtained. A recent update of this series, with radiation dose reduction to 5500 rad in 6 weeks shows 5-year and 10-year survival rates of 85% and 72%, respectively.[81,117] Thirty-eight patients receiving uniform 6 MEV megavoltage treatment have a five-year survival rate in excess of 90%. Similar results have been obtained in a series of patients treated at the Jefferson Medical School by Kramer and by the group at the Joint Center for Radiotherapy.[266,267] Virtually uniform local control has been obtained in children treated with conservative surgery followed by multiple field or rotational megavoltage irradiation totaling 5500 rad in 6 weeks using 180 rad daily fractions. Similar results, especially with children, have recently been reported by Onoyama and others.[269-272]

Although results continue to be superior to radical surgery, overall disease-free survival is reduced when adult patients have been treated or lower doses of radiation have been used.

For recurrent craniopharyngiomas which have already been operated upon, radiation is the primary treatment modality as surgical morbidity and mortality are unacceptable. Results following attempted radiation salvage of recurrence following apparent complete surgical resection are not as uniformly successful as when irradiation immediately follows conservative surgery. Although occasional recurrences are seen, even in children, overall survival and reduced morbidity and mortality make this the only reasonable therapy. Appropriate initial therapy should considerably reduce the incidence of this problem.

Lesions of the Clivus

The primary clivus lesion is the chordoma. This notochordal remnant tumor has a tendency to dissolve the bony structures of the clivus and, although benign in nature, is extremely difficult to remove in its entirety. Attempted surgical resection carries significant morbidity. The so-called Stevenson approach by way of the cervical region is a rather indirect and long route to the clivus.[273] The transtemporal route involves significant retraction and disruption of brain tissue. Both of these approaches have significant risks. The tumor can also be approached by the transsphenoidal route and, when possible, this is a safer approach to the clivus, allowing removal of significant amounts of tissue of the tumor without disturbing the normal brain. There are virtually no patients who have survived with this tumor for periods in excess of 10 years.

Lesions of the clivus represent somewhat less than half the reported cases of chordoma, the others arising in the sacrococcygeal region or rarely, at another vertebral site. There is a male predominance of 2:1 or 3:1 in most series. Most patients are in the third to fifth decade of life. Although metastases occur the tumor usually causes death by progressive local extension with ultimate compromise of vital structures.[272] Soft tissue extension is nearly always greater than bony abnormalities would suggest.[274] Symptom duration prior to diagnosis can be quite long owing to the relatively slow growth rate and average doubling time of nearly 1 year for clivus lesions. Headache and/or visual symptoms predominate. A variety of radiographic studies may be helpful, especially CT scans and polytomography. Myelography or positive contrast studies using water soluble media may be informative.

All reported series demonstrate the importance of surgery as primary therapy. Extensive and, when necessary, repeated surgical removal may be of great benefit. Rarely, however, is surgery totally successful and the overwhelming majority of tumors recur. Location of these lesions and their extensive and insidious growth is primarily responsible for local failure.

Radiation therapy regularly produces tumor regression and this response may persist for years. However, very high radiation doses in excess of 5000 rad in 5 weeks are necessary to produce a significant duration of response and local failure nearly always occurs. Suit and colleagues currently recommend radiation doses in excess of 6000 rad with supplementation by proton beam therapy for an additional 1000 rad or more.[275] Data from Pearlman and Friedman demonstrate that the incidence of 5-year survival increases considerably with doses above 6000 rad.[276] Based on the almost routine development of local failure following surgery, postoperative radiation therapy is recommended for virtually all patients.[274-278]

SPINAL CORD TUMORS

Primary tumors of the spinal cord present one of the major neuro-oncologic emergencies. Frequently, warning signs and symptoms have been experienced for many weeks prior to the precipitation of events leading to severe disability and hospitalization. Spinal cord tumors contain a comparatively small tumor burden, as the cord with its extra and intradural compartments is contained within the rigid vertebral canal. Small masses therefore can have profound effects, with local ischemia and irreversible dysfunction the result.

The role of corticosteroids in the treatment of spinal cord tumor is not clear. Clearly, there is local edema secondary to the effects of tumor which potentially may be reversed by the utilization of corticosteroids. However, if the mass is too large or the effect has been too prolonged, the control of small amounts of edema will be of no avail. While the patient is undergoing diagnostic workup, preparation for surgery, or radiotherapy, high-dose corticosteroid might be considered as a comparatively benign adjunct to control any additional edema which may develop.

Chemotherapy has not been employed in the treatment of spinal cord tumors except on individual basis utilizing therapeutic regimes available for the same histologic type elsewhere.

Extradural Tumors

These tumors are primarily of metastatic origin and are considered in the chapter on metastatic disease. One tumor, however, is primary to the CNS and may involve the spinal canal, namely, the spinal chordoma. This tumor occurs in the lumbosacral region, erodes bone and soft tissue extensively, and is difficult to remove in its entirety, even though benign in histology. Multiple operative procedures are usually necessary and of value. Long term survival is more frequent with these lesions and higher doses of irradiation can be given by techniques that minimize bowel irradiation. When the lesion is inferior to the spinal cord, the risk of central nervous system damage is eliminated. When disease extent permits, radiation dose of 7000 rad in $7\frac{1}{2}$ weeks to 8 weeks delivered by suitably directed fields is suggested.[278]

Intradural Extramedullary Tumors

The two primary tumors in this compartment are the neurofibroma and the meningioma. Neurofibromas are usually found connected to nerve roots and are primarily unilateral lesions with radicular and myelopathic neurological sequelae. The treatment of these lesions is primarily surgical. They are virtually always benign and with the use of microsurgical techniques can be totally removed. An appropriate-sized laminectomy is performed, the dura opened, and the tumor identified and then carefully dissected. The encapsulated nature of these tumors makes much of the surgical procedure straightforward. The major surgical problem involves the intimate relation of these tumors to the nerve roots and spinal cord. It is often not possible to separate the tumors completely from the roots. A decision thus has to be made whether the root can be sacrificed safely. If only a single root is involved, as is usually the case, then removing the tumor with the nerve root attachment is advisable. When totally removed these tumors rarely recur. In cases of neurofibromatosis, however, multiple tumors may be present and removal of all the lesions may not be feasible. The basic risks of surgery for these lesions are those of the laminectomy itself, coupled with possible neural or vascular compromise of the spinal cord as the tumor is manipulated during its removal. The use of microsurgical techniques minimizes these dangers.

Meningiomas may occur anywhere within the intradural compartment, arising from the covering layers of the cord. These are most often benign and can be removed surgically. A major concern is their close attachment to the cord and, after prolonged compression, a moderate to large sized spinal meningioma can have compromised and compressed the cord to such a degree that the remaining structure is quite fragile. If complete removal can be accomplished, including all attachments of the tumor to dura and the cord, recurrence is rare. It is particularly important to remove any dura involved by tumor and replace the resultant dural defect with a watertight dural graft. Should total removal be limited, consideration should be given to the use of radiation therapy. However, experience with radiation treatment is virtually non-existent with spinal cord meningiomas. Isolated case reports have documented response and long-term control of aggressive neurofibromas at several sites following radiation therapy. However, these reports and those previously discussed for meningioma have usually involved radiation doses at or beyond spinal cord tolerance. Should a lesion of this type be considered initially unresectable, radiation therapy given prior to planned second-look surgery might prove beneficial, as it has for meningiomas elsewhere.[157]

Intradural Intermedullary Tumors

The primary tumors in this category are astrocytomas, ependymomas and vascular malformations.

ASTROCYTOMAS. Astrocytomas of the spinal cord vary considerably in their histologic differentiation. The determining factor in their surgical treatment is the degree of infiltration of the surrounding cord by the tumor. Where the tumor is both histologically benign and well demarcated from the cord, surgical removal provides successful treatment. Benign lesions that have invaded the cord structure may not be totally removable. Malignant invasive tumors can rarely be removed surgically and require postoperative radiation therapy. Results of treatment of spinal cord astrocytomas are given in Table 33-28 *A*, *B*. The basic treatment plan for these tumors involves maximal safe tumor resection followed by radiotherapy.

Owing to the relative rarity of these tumors, few reports are available detailing results following radiation therapy of spinal cord tumors. More than half of the treated patients with adequate follow-up survive 3 years to 5 years or more following irradiation. Most of these patients are disease-free; however, a significant number suffer local recurrence, but continue to survive for protracted periods. Radiation therapy produces improvement or reversal of symptoms in most patients and substantially improves the symptom-free interval even in patients who are not cured. A tumor dose of approximately 5000 rad, delivered in 150 rad to 180 rad fractions over 6+ weeks appears safe and relatively effective.[279,280,281] Substantially higher radiation doses given for spinal cord tumors have produced a significant incidence of radiation myelitis.[282] Three of 15 patients treated with a mean dose of 5700 rad (range 5000 rad–6700 rad) developed late complications.[280] It would appear that the optimum dose range lies between 4500 rad and 5500 rad, delivered in a relatively protracted fashion.

EPENDYMOMAS. These intrinsic tumors rise from the ependymomal lining cells of the central canal at almost any point in the spinal cord. Histopathologically, many of the lesions, especially at the filum terminale are of the myxopapillary type. Although often benign histologically, their central location makes removal difficult without serious neurological risk. It is sometimes possible with smaller tumors, to achieve complete surgical removal; however, unless margins or resection is adequate, local recurrence is likely.[283] When complete removal is not possible, or when margins are questionable, radiotherapy should be delivered. Any patient presenting with such a lesion should have careful and thorough assessment of the brain, especially posterior fossa, ensuring that the patient is not presenting with a "drop" metastasis from a primary tumor in the brain.

Somewhat greater experience is available for ependymomas of the spinal cord compared with astrocytomas, detailing results of irradiation. Almost all reports attest to the considerable efficacy of such treatment, with the great majority of patients surviving for protracted time periods without evidence of recurrent disease when adequate radiation doses and fields have been used. Surprisingly low radiation doses have been reported to result in long-term symptom control when gross

TABLE 33-28*A* Results of Treatment of Intrinsic Spinal Cord Tumors in Children

PATHOLOGY	TYPE OF SURGERY				RADIO-THERAPY	DIED POSTOP	LIVING			MEAN FOLLOW-UP PERIOD (YEARS)
	Number of Cases	*Total Removal*	*Subtotal Removal*	*Biopsy*			*Normal*	*Improved*	*Not Walking*	
Astrocytomas	11	0	0	11	5	4	4	2	1	13
Ependymomas	7	2	5	3	6	1	5	0	1	6
Lipomas	8	3	3	2	0	0	3	4	0	13
Neurinomas	9	6	2	1	0	1	5	2	1	5
Epidermoid & dermoid cysts	8	6	2	0	0	1	4	2	0	8
Sarcomas	11	0	6	4	11	10(1)	0	1	0	2
Neuroblastomas	6	1	4	2	6	2(1)	1	1	0	12
Teratomas	6	4	2	0	1	2	4	0	0	3
Meningiomas	3	2	1	0	2	1	1	1	0	10
Granulomas	4	3	1	0	0	0	3	0	0	8
Others	8	1	3	3	6	3	0	3	1	10

* There were six patients who were lost to follow-up review (lipoma, dermoid cyst, granuloma, aneurysmal bone cyst, two neuroblastomas)
(DeSousa AL, Kalsbeck JE, Mealey J Jr, et al: Intraspinal tumors in children. J Neurosurg 51:437–445, 1979)

TABLE 33-28*B* Results of Treatment of Intrinsic Spinal Cord Tumors in Adults and Children

PATIENT NUMBER	AGE (YEARS)	LOCATION	HISTOLOGY	PRIOR SURGERY	REMOVAL	PREOPERATIVE NEUROLOGICAL DEFECTS	RESULT	FOLLOW-UP
1	40	Conus	Epend	0	T	1+	Improved	6 mo
2	24	Conus	Epend	0	T	2+	Improved	6 mo
3	49	C	Epend	+	T	3+	Improved	2 yr
4	28	C-D	Epend	+	T	4+	Static	2 yr
5	38	C	Epend	+	T	3+	Static	2 yr
6	17	D	Teratoma	+	T	4+	Improved	2 yr
7	13	Conus	Dermoid	0	T	2+	Improved	8 yr
8	4 mo	Conus	Epidermoid	0	T	2+	Improved	7 yr
9	60	D-C	Astroc	+	90%	4+	Static	4 yr
10	13	D-L	Astroc	+	T	2+	Static	18 mo
11	3	C-D	Astroc	0	95%	1+	Improved	18 mo
12	48	C	Astroc	0	T	1+/pain	Improved	2 yr
13	38	C	Astroc	+	T	2+	Improved	3 yr

D, dorsal; C, cervical; T, total; 1+, mild defect; 2+, paresis; 3+, moderate deficit; 4+ para-quadriplegia.
(Stein BM: Surgery of intramedullary spinal cord tumors. Clin Neurosurg 26: 529–542, 1979)

residual disease has been irradiated.[284] The myxopapillary type of ependymoma appears to often be limited and responsive. Thus Schwade, and colleagues have reported control in 12 of 12 patients with spinal cord ependymoma followed for 2.5 years or more (maximum 17 years).[281] Similar results have been obtained by Bouchard and Wood.[82,279] A radiation dose of approximately 5000 rad delivered in 150 rad to 180 rad fractions in 6 weeks has been well tolerated and effective. Radiation fields for ependymomas and astrocytomas should have generous superior and inferior margins of at least 2 cm to 3 cm around known disease or the radiographic abnormality.

VASCULAR LESIONS. A variety of vascular tumors form intrinsic lesions of the spinal cord. These include hemangiomas and arteriovenous malformations (AVM) as the most common types. The use of microsurgery has made direct removal of these lesions possible. Hemangiomas of relatively small size can be completely removed. Larger lesions may have vascular supplies crucial to spinal cord function, limiting total removal.

Should these hemangiomas be the infantile type noted in the first 6 months to 9 months of life, steroid therapy can often produce substantial regression. If steroids are ineffective or only partially successful, and the secondary neurologic disability from progression of the hemangioma serious, then low doses of radiation therapy (450 rad–900 rad in 3–6 fractions) will almost uniformly cause substantial response. The efficacy of both steroids and irradiation for treatment of the hemangiomas and AVMs occurring in older patients is much less likely or predictable. Considerably larger radiation doses (2000 rad–3000 rad in 15 fractions in 3 or more weeks) are necessary and have produced occasional significant clinical regression.

Arteriovenous malformations can often be extensive lesions involving multiple levels of the spinal cord. The entire length of the cord may be at least partially involved in certain cases. The treatment of AVMs involves microsurgical removal of as much of the lesion as possible. Attempts at merely coagulating feeding vessels may result in temporary shrinkage of the lesion, but eventually revascularization takes place. Embolization by catheter may be useful if surgery is contraindicated or to diminish the size of a lesion prior to surgery. Removal of these lesions in their entirety depends upon their being posteriorly located and not having feeding vessels which cannot be sacrificed. Since these conditions do not always exist, total removal is difficult.[285] Re-operation or postoperative radiation therapy may be necessary.

There are other intrinsic tumors of the spinal cord that are less common and less distinctive. The management of these tumors follows the general principles which have been just discussed.

FUTURE CONSIDERATIONS

LIMITATIONS OF PRESENT TECHNIQUES FOR MALIGNANT TUMORS

Although much progress has been made in the area of improved surgical technique for the treatment of benign intracranial and spinal cord tumors, it is obvious that there is a tremendous need for improvement in the therapy of malignant CNS tumors. The malignant tumors of the CNS have not greatly changed in their prognosis in the last 10 years, despite advances in surgical technique, radiation therapy approaches and the recent development of useful chemotherapeutic agents. Even with the best of therapeutic modalities currently available, a prognosis of under 1-year survival, as for glioblastoma multiforme, seems quite grim.[11] The major problem in CNS malignant tumors involves the invasive nature of the lesions and the fact that the surrounding normal brain invaded by the tumors cannot be resected without significant deficit. The removal of normal central nervous system tissue and the inability of CNS tissue to regenerate is a clear limitation to the effective use of surgery. The relatively thin margin between the sensitivity of tumor and the sensitivity of normal brain is a limitation to the effectiveness of conventional modality of radiation therapy. Further, the relatively small growth fraction of malignant brain tumors gives less opportunity for effective chemotherapy.[57,286] Chemotherapy has advanced in recent decades and offers tremendous hope for improvement in outlook of patients with CNS malignancies. A major current limitation is that only one agent or group of agents, the nitrosoureas, has been proven to be consistently effective and then only to a small degree.[11] The development of further effective agents, differing in their mechanisms of action, would significantly change the treatment of human CNS malignancies. The challenge is clear to those involved in neurooncology to develop new approaches for the diagnosis and treatment of human brain and spinal cord neoplasms.

ROLE OF EARLY DIAGNOSIS

The diagnosis of CNS neoplasms of the brain has been marked by a tremendous improvement due to the use of the computerized tomographic technique.[70] This technique, which allows detection of even extremely small, relatively early tumors, has certain discrete limitations. Tumors which are not well vascularized, tumors whose density does not differ greatly from that of surrounding brain, and tumors with diffuse infiltration are not as easily detected by CT scan. There is difficulty in considering the CT scan as a simple primary diagnostic technique. Therefore, there are two levels at which earlier diagnosis needs to be improved. The first level is that of screening: the second level is that of improved specific pre-operative diagnosis.

In the area of screening, perhaps the most important single measure is increased awareness of the originally consulted physician. All too often a patient with a brain tumor will present to a physician and be followed for headache or for occasional drowsiness or for some fairly indistinct symptoms only peripherally referable to the neoplasm before the diagnosis becomes strongly suspected. In addition, it is necessary for the physicians caring for brain tumor patients or brain tumor suspect patients to have an increased hope for the outlook of these patients. This is particularly important in moving aggressively to make a diagnosis as early as possible and thereby allow the tumor to have as minimal effect as possible on cerebral or spinal cord function.

The concept of screening diagnosis for brain tumors has

been augmented by the development of techniques which allow a simple, safe, outpatient diagnostic adjunct. These techniques include the development of immunological assays, using allogeneic humoral responses and cultured human brain tumor cells.[287] Such techniques are still in the developmental stage, but show evidence of differentiating between the patient who has a brain tumor *versus* the normal patient. Approximately 90% of patients with astrocytomas will have a positive humoral immune response against a common target cell line.[288] Only 9% of normal patients exhibit such a response. In the lower grades of astrocytomas, this percentage of response approaches 100% detection. It is precisely these low-grade astrocytomas in which early detection is both important and also difficult. This humoral immune response is extremely promising.

The second aspect of improved diagnosis involves the development of more sophisticated technology for differential diagnosis of human brain tumors. The most interesting new technological development is the so-called PET scan or positron emission tomogram.[289] This device incorporates the localizing ability of computerized tomography with the ability of isotopically labelled agents to concentrate in specific lesions. It is likely that this technique may be useful for differentiating between different types of CNS lesions, be they neoplasm, infections, or degenerative states. The PET scan offers the clinician a potential of differential metabolic and functional diagnosis to add to that of anatomical diagnostic approaches currently in use. This technique is still in its early stages of development and will in the next several years become an interesting but selectively used technique in differential diagnosis.

There has been great interest throughout the years in the development of further diagnostic approaches using the cerebral CSF which surrounds the tumors. The area of using CSF study for tumor diagnosis has certain clear limitations. Patients with brain or spinal cord tumors are at risk when a spinal puncture is done and there is increased intracranial or spinal pressure due to an expanding tumor. For this reason, the use of early diagnostic approaches involving CSF sampling must be done on an extremely selective basis. In those instances where increased pressure is not a problem, the use of CSF study can be of value. Numerous biochemical substances are found to increase in CSF of patients with brain tumors. In addition to the overall increase in protein, certain of these specific proteins, lipids, and other biochemical substances can be detected even in small quantities.[290] Further, the use of CSF tissue culture and use of immunofluorescent labelling as an adjunct to millipore filtration offers hope of increased accuracy and frequency of diagnosis of tumors which seed the CSF pathways.[67]

SURGICAL TREATMENT

The major new development of brain tumor surgery which will continue to bear fruit involves microsurgical techniques. These techniques have grown considerably in the last decade and are still under development. Part of the impact of these microsurgical techniques will be felt when the majority of neurosurgeons performing brain tumor operations are able to use them fully. Microsurgical technology for the future may include such approaches and the use of the laser, which already has been tried in preliminary fashion, and the development of new instrumentation, new lighting devices, and new intra-operative monitoring techniques to determine the direct effects of surgery during the procedure. This last possibility, particularly the use of the evoked potential technique, may permit intra-operative determination of the effects on the normal brain or spinal cord that extirpation of tumor or normal tissue may have. This may allow more vigorous approaches to tumors without destruction of CNS function.

RADIATION THERAPY

A number of experimental approaches have been tested or are currently undergoing investigation in an attempt to improve the efficacy and local control of irradiation for patients with malignant glioma.

Shaw and colleagues have utilized 700 rad to 1800 rad of fractionated 8MV fast neutron irradiation in the treatment of 34 patients with glioblastoma multiforme.[85] Patients who received lower doses of neutron treatment received supplemental, fractionated photon irradiation (3000 rad–3600 rad). The median survival for these patients was 5 months from completion of treatment, not different from results achieved with photon treatment alone. However, postmortem examination performed on 13 patients demonstrated a marked coagulative necrosis as well as considerable decrease in apparent tumor. The cause of death appeared to be related to treatment effects on the brain in most cases. Virtually identical results have recently been reported by Catterall and colleagues, using 7.5 MeV fast neutrons in 30 patients with glioblastoma.[291]

A different approach has been examined by Douglas.[292] Photon irradiation, using superfractionation with three fractions per day of 100 rad separated by 3 hours to 3½ hours, was tested. Forty-five to 60 fractions of 100 rad were delivered to the entire brain with a 1000 rad boost in five daily fractions to a restricted volume at the completion of treatment. Using historical controls for comparison, improved results appear to have been achieved, although median survival (~50 weeks) is not substantially different from results achieved by the Brain Tumor Study Group using conventional irradiation following surgery. Very few of these patients had been followed for periods beyond 60 weeks to 70 weeks, so that longer terms results are unknown.

Three different types of radiosensitizers have been used in combination with irradiation.[293] Sano and Hoshino have utilized the halogenated thymidine analog, 5-bromo-deoxy uridine (BUDR) given by intra-arterial infusion.[294] This compound has been shown to be a radiosensitizer and only is incorporated by actively dividing cells (*i.e.*, tumor) and not by resting or non-dividing cells (*i.e.*, normal brain). A 3-year survival of 21% was accomplished in "moderately" malignant tumors and a 7% 3-year survival for "highly" malignant lesions when 5000 rad to 6000 rad of irradiation was combined with BUDR.

Chang[295] has shown a modest improvement in 1- and 2-year survival (40% *vs.* 28% and 12% *vs.* 0%, respectively) when irradiation was combined with hyperbaric oxygenation at 3 atmospheres of pressure. These differences were not statistically significant.

Finally, the hypoxic cell sensitizer metronidazole, combined with nine fractions of 300 rad photon irradiation, had been shown by Urtasun to significantly improve results over x-ray treatment alone.[296,297] Unfortunately, toxic side effects, principally gastrointestinal, of this agent precluded giving it in combination with irradiation for a larger number of fractions. Overall survival results in the study group are not significantly better than results achieved by larger total doses of irradiation, so that the overall treatment effect by addition of this compound is still in question. Studies to evaluate the efficacy of these compounds in combination with more conventional doses of irradiation are currently in progress.

Combination of photon irradiation with lipophylic chemotherapy agents such as the nitrosoureas (BCNU, CCNU, methyl-CCNU) has also been tested in a randomized fashion by the Brain Tumor Study Group. Although prolonged survival was achieved, the gain was modest and median improvement was measured in weeks.[122-124] More recently, a trial of two fractions of very high dose CCNU (600 mg/M^2) sandwiched around conventional, high-dose radiation therapy is being tested by Takvorian.[298] Because of the potential of prolonged and severe myelosuppression with this regimen, bone marrow removal and storage for possible autologous marrow transfusion precedes this therapeutic attempt. This trial has been initiated too recently for any meaningful data to be available.

Thus, although a variety of experimental approaches have been tested using radiation therapy with and without other agents, glioblastoma has thus far proven remarkably resistant to further improvement in therapy.

CHEMOTHERAPY

Advances in chemotherapy of CNS tumors are likely to include the development of new agents with greater specificity for such tumors as well as a means of designing individualized therapy. The new agents being sought would be those with a greater ability to penetrate the blood brain barrier, a better tumoricidal effect, and a diminished toxicity for normal organs. In addition to new agents, the use of a combination of the existing agents may prove valuable. Higher dosages to tumor may be achievable using bone marrow transplantation to reconstitute marrow after higher dose chemotherapy.

A major new approach for the therapy of human CNS tumors involves the concept of using tissue cultures of human tumors for prediction of clinical response. Human CNS neoplasms lend themselves extremely well to this technique. In a study of 2000 human brain tumors about 90% of these were successfully grown in tissue culture.[38] This high percentage of success allows the use of chemotherapeutic approaches in the majority of human brain tumor patients. Several different techniques have been used including the microtiter plate technique and the clonogenic assay.[299-301] From both of these approaches the same types of information are being derived. It appears at this time that approximately 60% of patients who will respond to a nitrosourea clinically will have an *in vitro* positive response by either technique. Similarly between 90% and 100% of patients who will be unresponsive to the nitrosoureas can be predicted from the *in vitro* data.[301] This ability to correlate clinical and tissue culture information holds great promise. The effectivensss of this technique will be multiplied immeasurably should other chemotherapeutic agents be proven to be of consistent effectiveness in the treatment of such tumors. The development of an understanding of the resistance of cell lines may also be helpful in gaining insight as to why certain tumors are more resistant to treatment than others.

IMMUNOTHERAPY

Immunotherapy for brain tumor has been attempted in a variety of ways. Presently, there have been reports of the use of BCG, C parvum, levamisole and cellular preparations in the treatment of human brain tumors.[114,302] Although extremely interesting data have been generated, no significant influence on survival has been achieved. There is a study by Bloom on the effect of cellular preparations from culture on human medulloblastoma patients showing some evidence of altered survival.[117] The great number of different approaches to immunotherapy makes it apparent that only through a marked improvement of our understanding of the entire concept of the immune response in patients can we hope to utilize this tool effectively. It is not likely that an empirical approach to immunotherapy will greatly alter the survival of brain tumor patients. It, however, is extremely intriguing that these tumors do metastasize so infrequently and there does appear to be a relatively immunologically privileged site in the brain which could be expected to respond quite differently than other parts of the body to immune manipulation. Attempts to manipulate the humoral and cellular immune responses in patients as well as to alter the status of the target tumor cells may prove to be an effective approach to the introduction of immunotherapy into the clinical armamentarium for brain tumor patients. The ability to grow tissue cultures from most of the patients with CNS tumors allows us also to have optimism regarding the development of information as to the antigenic components of human CNS malignancies.

SUMMARY

In summary, the future of the treatment of human CNS neoplasms offers a tremendous challenge to all of those concerned with the treatment of these patients. We need to have a positive and vigorous outlook and yet one tempered by extreme care and conservatism in our approach to the individual patient. It will be necessary to introduce new modalities of radiation, chemotherapy, and immunotherapy, perhaps singly or in combination in order to develop a sound treatment approach. It may well be that the customizing of therapy based on the use of individual cells from patients may be one of the most effective means of improving survival.

REFERENCES

1. Bucy P: Research on Brain Tumors. In Paoletti P, Walker MD, Butte G et al (eds): Multidisciplinary Aspects of Brain Tumor Therapy. Amsterdam, Elsevier North-Holland Biomedical Press, 1979, pp 3–6
2. Durante F: Trattato di tatologia e terapie chirurgica generale e speciale. Alighieve D. (ed): Roma Societa 3:227–233, 1898
3. Horsely V, Krause F: The Treatment of Tumors of the Brain and Indications for Operation. Trans Int Cong Med, London, sec 2, Pt 1, pp 161–257, 1913
4. Gurdjian ES, Thomas LM: Operative Neurosurgery. Baltimore, Williams and Wilkins, 1970.
5. Cushing H: Experiences with cerebellar astrocytomas—A critical review of 76 cases. Surg Gynecol Obstet 52:129–204, 1931
6. Cushing H: Intracranial Tumors. Notes upon a series of two thousand verified cases with surgical-mortality percentages pertaining thereto. Springfield, Ill, Charles C Thomas, 1932
7. Dandy WE: Ventriculography following the injection of air into the cerebral ventricles. Ann Surg 68:5–11, 1918
8. Dandy WE: Röentgenography of the brain after injection of air into the spinal canal. Ann Surg 70:397–403, 1919
9. Moniz E: L'Angiographie Cerebrale: Ses applications et résultats en anatomie, physiologie, et clinique. Paris, Mason 1934
10. Walker MD, Alexander E Jr, Hunt WE et al: Evaluation of mithramycin in the treatment of anaplastic gliomas. J Neurosurg 44:655–667, 1976
11. Walker MD, Alexander E Jr, Hunt WE et al: Evaluation of BCNU and/or radiotherapy in the treatment of anaplastic gliomas. A Cooperative clinical trial. J Neurosurg 49:333–343, 1978
12. Zankl H, Zang KD: Cytological and cytogenetical studies on brain tumors. IV. Identification of the missing G chromosome in human meningiomas as no 22 by fluorescence technique. Humangenetik 14:167–169, 1972
13. Adams RD, Victor M: Principles of Neurology. New York, McGraw-Hill, 1977
14. Dorland WAN: Illustrated Medical Dictionary. 25th ed, Philadelphia, WB Saunders, 1974
15. Wechsler W, Kleihues P, Matsumoto S et al: Pathology of experimental neurogenic tumors chemically induced during prenatal and postnatal life. Ann NY Acad Sci 159:360–408, 1969
16. Benda P, Someda K, Messer J et al: Morphological and immunochemical studies of rat glial tumors and clonal strains propagated in culture. J Neurosurg 34:310–323, 1971
17. Zimmerman HM: Brain tumors: Their incidence and classification in man and their experimental production. Ann NY Acad Sci 159:337–359, 1969
18. Wodinski I, Kensler CJ, Rall DP: The induction and transplantation of brain tumors in neonate beagles. Proceedings of American Association for Cancer Research, San Francisco, March 1969, Abs #394, p 99
19. Copeland DD, Bigner DD: Glial–mesenchymal tropism of *in vivo* avian sarcoma virus neuro–oncogenesis in rats. Acta Neuropathol (Berl) 41:23–25, 1978
20. London WT, Houff SA, Madden DL et al: Brain tumors in owl monkeys inoculated with a human polyoma virus (JC Virus). Science 201:1246–1249, 1978
21. Farwell JR, Dohrmann GJ, Flannery JT: Central nervous system tumors in children. Cancer 40:3123–3132, 1977
22. Youmans JR: Neurological Surgery, vol. III. Philadelphia, WB Saunders, 1973
23. Carpenter MB: Human Neuroanatomy, 7th ed. Baltimore, Williams & Wilkins, 1976, 741 pp
24. Crosby EC, Humphrey T, Lauer EW: Correlative Anatomy of the Nervous System. New York, Macmillan, 1962
25. Haymaker WE: Bing's Local Diagnosis in Neurological Diseases, 15th ed. St. Louis, CV Mosby, 1969
26. Scoville WB, Milner B: Loss of recent memory after bilateral hippocampal lesions. J Neurol Neurosurg Psychiat 20:11–21, 1957
27. Penfield W, Milner B: Memory deficit produced by bilateral lesions in the hippocampal zone. Arch Neurol Psychiat 79:475–497, 1958
28. Bergland R, Ray BS: The arterial supply of the human optic chiasm. J Neurosurg 31:327–334, 1969
29. Rhoton AL Jr, Hardy DG, Chambers JM: Microsurgical anatomy and dissection of the sphenoid bone, cavernous sinus and sellar region. Surg Neurol 12:63–104, 1979
30. Saeki N, Rhoton AL: Microsurgical anatomy of the upper basilar artery and the posterior circle of Willis. J Neurosurg 46:563–578, 1977
31. Stein BM: Supracerebellar–infratentorial approach to pineal tumors. Surg Neurol 11:331–337, 1979
32. Reid WS, Clark WK: Comparison of the infratentorial and transtentorial approaches to the pineal region. Neurosurgery 3:1–8, 1978
33. Russell DS, Rubinstein LJ: Pathology of Tumours of the Nervous System, 4th ed, Baltimore, Williams & Wilkins, 1977
34. Zulch DJ: Principles of the New World Health Organization (WHO) Classification of Brain Tumors. Neuroradiology 19:59–66, 1980
35. Penfield W: Cytology and Cellular Pathology of the Nervous System, vol. 3, New York, Hoeber, 1932
36. del Rio Hortega P: The Microscopic Anatomy of Tumors of the Central and Peripheral Nervous System. Springfield, Ill, Charles C Thomas, 1962
37. McKeever PE, Balentine JD: Macrophage migration through the brain parenchyma to the perivascular space following particle ingestion. Am J Path 93:153–164, 1978
38. Gilles FH, Winston K, Fulchiero A et al: Histologic features and observational variation in cerebellar gliomas in children. J Natl Cancer Inst 58:175–181, 1977
39. Winston K, Gilles FH, Leviton A et al: Cerebellar gliomas in children. J Natl Cancer Inst. 58:833–838, 1977
40. Kornblith PL: Role of tissue culture in prediction of malignancy. Clin Neurosurg 25:346–376, 1978
41. Kadin ME, Rubinstein LJ, Nelson JS: Neonatal cerebellar medulloblastoma originating from the fetal external granular layer. J Neuropath Exp Neurol 29:583–600, 1970
42. Cole M, Nauta WJH: Retrograde atrophy of axons of the lemniscus of the cat. An experimental study. J Neuropath Exp Neurol 29:354–369, 1970
43. Jervis GA: Spongioneuroblastoma and tuberous sclerosis. J Neuropath Exp Neurol 13:105–116, 1954
44. Davis RL, Nelson E: Unilateral ganglioglioma in a tuberosclerotic brain. J Neuropath Exp Neurol 20:571–581, 1961
45. McKeever PE: Scanning electron microscopy in the evaluation of neurosurgical neoplasms: A review of new approaches. Neurosurgery 4:343–352, 1979
46. Rubinstein LJ: Tumors of the Central Nervous System. Atlas of Tumor Pathology, Fasc 6. Washington, DC, Armed Forces Institute of Pathology, 1972
47. Burger PC, Vogel FS: Surgical Pathology of the Nervous System and Its Coverings. New York, John Wiley and Sons, 1976
48. Garvin AJ, Spicer SS, McKeever PE: The cytochemical demonstration of intracellular immunoglobulin in neoplasms of lymphoreticular tissue. Am J Path 82:457–478, 1976
49. Henry JM, Heffner RR, Dillard SH et al: Primary malignant lymphomas of the central nervous system. Cancer 34:1293–1302, 1974
50. Varadachari C, Palutke M, Climie ARW et al: Immunoblastic sarcoma (histiocytic lymphoma) of the brain with B cell markers. Case report, J Neurosurg 49:887–892, 1978
51. Russell DS, Rubinstein J: Pathology of Tumours of the Nervous System, 3rd ed. Baltimore, Williams and Wilkins, 1971
52. Parkinson D, Childe AE: Colloid cyst of the fourth ventricle. Report of a case of two colloid cysts of the fourth ventricle. J Neurosurg 9:404–409, 1952
53. Hoenig EM, Ghatak NR, Hirano A et al: Multiloculated cystic tumor of the choroid plexus of the fourth ventricle. Case report, J Neurosurg 27:574–579, 1967
54. McKeever PE, Hall BJ, Spicer SS: The origin of colloid cysts of the third ventricle. J Neuropath Exp Neurol 29:658 (#232), 1978

55. Hirano A,, Ghatak NR: The fine structure of colloid cysts of the third ventricle. J Neuropath Exp Neurol 33:333–341, 1974
56. McKeever PE, Brissie NT: Scanning electron microscopy of neoplasms removed at surgery: Surface topography and comparison of meningioma, colloid cyst, ependymoma, pituitary adenoma, schwanoma and astrocytoma. J Neuropath Exp Neurol 36:875–896, 1977
57. Hoshino T, Barker M, Wilson CB: The kinetics of cultured human glioma cells. Acta Neuropath (Berl) 32:235–244, 1975
58. Brooks BR, Hochberg F, Kornblith PL et al: Morphologic and kinetic analysis of explant cultures of 100 CNS biopsy specimens. J Neuropath Exp Neurol 34:112 (Abs. #122), 1975
59. Scott RM, Liszczak TM, Kornblith PL: "Invasiveness" in tissue culture: A technique for study of gliomas. Surg Forum 29:531–533, 1978
60. Shuangshoti S, Hongsaprabhas C, Netsky MG: Metastasizing meningioma. Cancer 26:832–841, 1970
61. Labitzke HG: Glioblastoma multiforme with remote extracranial metastases. Arch Pathol 73:223–229, 1962
62. Gray H, Goss CM (eds): Anatomy of the Human Body, 28th ed. Philadelphia, Lea and Febiger, 1970
63. Gehan EA, Walker MD: Prognostic factors for patients with brain tumors. Natl Cancer Inst Monogr 46:189–195, 1977
64. Linthicum FH, Churchill D: Vestibular test results in acoustic neuroma cases. Arch Otolaryngol 88:604–607, 1968
65. Nelson JR: The minimal ice water caloric test. Neurology 19:577–585, 1969
66. Ojemann R, Montgomery W, Weiss L: Evaluation and surgical treatment of acoustic neuroma. N Engl J Med 287:895–899, 1972
67. Black PM, Callahan LV, Kornblith PL: Tissue cultures from cerebrospinal fluid specimens in the study of human brain tumors. J Neurosurg 49:697–704, 1978
68. Kajikawa H, Ohta T, Ohshiro H et al: Cerebrospinal fluid cytology in patients with brain tumours; A simple method using the cell culture technique. Acta Cytol 21:162–167, 1977
69. duBoulay GH, Trickey SE: Case reports. Calcification in chromophobe adenoma. Br J Radiol 35:793–795, 1962
70. Taveras JM, Wood EH: Diagnostic Neuroradiology, 2nd ed, vols 1 & 2. Baltimore, Williams & Wilkins, 1976
71. Chambers AA, Lukin R, Tsunekawa N: Calcification in a chromophobe adenoma. Case Report. J Neurosurg 44:623–625, 1976
72. Greitz T: Computer tomography for diagnosis of intracranial tumors compared with other neuroradiological procedures. In Lindgren (ed): Computer Tomography of Brain Lesions. Acta Radiol (supp. 346):14–20, 1975
73. Shipiro R: Myelography, 3rd ed. Chicago, Year Book Medical Publishers, 1975
74. Picard L, Vespignani H, Vieux-Rochat P et al: Serious neurological complications of metrizamide myelography: Report of eight cases. J Neuroradiol 6:3–14, 1979
75. Di Chiro G, Doppman H, Ommaya AK: Selective arteriography of arteriovenous aneurysms of the spinal cord. Radiology 88:1065–1077, 1967
76. Di Chiro G, Schellinger D: Computed tomography of spinal cord after lumbar intrathecal introduction of metrizamide (computer-assisted myelography). Radiology 120:101–104, 1976
77. Jelsma R, Bucy PC: Glioblastoma multiforme. Its treatment and some factors effecting its survival. Arch Neurol 20:161–171, 1969
78. Rossi GR, Feoli F, Fernandez E et al: The role of surgery in the treatment of supratentorial brain gliomas. In Paoletti P, Walker MD, Butte G et al: (eds): Multidisciplinary Aspects of Brain Tumor Therapy. Amsterdam, Elsevier North-Holland Biomedical Press, 1979, pp 155–163
79. Marshall LF, King J, Langfitt TW: The complications of high-dose corticosteroid therapy in neurosurgical patients: A prospective study. Ann Neurol 1:201–203, 1977
80. Sheline GE: Radiation therapy of tumors of the central nervous system in childhood. Cancer 35:957–964, 1975
81. Bloom HJG, Walsh LS: Tumors of the central nervous system. In Bloom HJG, Lemerle J, Neidhardt MK (eds): Cancer in Chidlren, Clinical Management, pp 93–119. New York, Springer Verlag, 1975
82. Bouchard J, Peirce CB: Radiation therapy in the management of neoplasms of the central nervous system, with a special note in regard to children: 20 years experience (1939–1958). Am J Roentgenol Radium Ther Nucl Med 84:610–628, 1960
83. Marsa GW, Profert JC, Rubinstein LC et al: Radiation therapy in the treatment of childhood astrocytic gliomas. Cancer 32:646–654, 1973
84. Kramer S, Southard ME, Mansfield CM: Radiation effect and tolerance of the central nervous system. Front Rad Ther Oncol. Baltimore, Karger, Basel & University Park Press, 6:332–345, 1972
85. Shaw CM, Sumi SM, Alvord EC et al: Fast neutron irradiation of glioblastoma multiforme. J Neurosurg 49:1–12, 1978
86. Dawson DM, Dingman JF: Hazards of proton-beam pituitary irradiation. N Engl J Med 282:1434, 1970
87. Aur R, Hustu HO, Simone J: Leukoencephalopathy in children with acute lymphocytic leukemia receiving preventive central nervous system therapy. Proc Am Soc Clin Oncol 17:97, 1976
88. Harno JR, Levene MB: Visual complications following irradiation for pituitary adenomas and craniopharyngiomas. Radiology 120:167–171, 1976
89. Aristizibal S, Caldwell WL, Avila J et al: Relationship of time dose factors to tumor control and complications in the treatment of Cushing's disease by irradiation. Int J Radiat Oncol Biol Phys 2:47–54, 1977
90. Scanlon PW, Taylor WF: Radiotherapy of intracranial astrocytomas: Analysis of 417 cases treated from 1960 through 1969. Neurosurgery 5: 301–308, 1979
91. Rall DP, Zubrod CG: Mechanism of drug absorption and excretion. Passage of drugs in and out of the central nervous system. Annu Rev Pharmacol 2:109–128, 1962
92. Reese TS, Karnofsky J: Fine structural localization of a blood-brain barrier to exogenous peroxidase. J Cell Biol 34:207–217, 1967
93. Long DM: Capillary ultrastructure and the blood-brain barrier in human malignant brain tumors. J Neurosurg 32:127–144, 1970
94. Oldendorf WH: Blood–brain barrier permeability to drugs. Annu Rev Pharmacol 14:239–248, 1974
95. Vick NA, Khandekar JD, Bigner DD: Chemotherapy of Brain Tumors (editorial). Arch Neurol 34:523–526, 1977
96. Hoshino T, Wilson CB, Rosenblum MD et al: Chemotherapeutic implications of growth fraction and cell cycle time in glioblastomas. J Neurosurg 43:127–135, 1975
97. Hoshino T: Therapeutic implications of brain tumor cell kinetics. Modern Concepts in Brain Tumor Therapy: Laboratory and Clinical Investigations. NCI Monograph 46, DHEW, 1977, pp 29–36
98. Levin VA: A pharmacologic basis for brain tumor chemotherapy. Semin Oncol 2:57–61, 1975
99 Levin VA, Freeman MA, Landahl HD: The permeability characteristics of the edematous brain adjacent to intracerebral rat brain tumors. Arch Neurol 32:785–791, 1975
100. Shapiro WR, Yung WA, Basler GA, et al.: Heterogeneous response to chemotherapy of human gliomas grown in nude mice and as clones *in vitro*. Cancer Treat Rep 65 (Suppl 2):55–59, 1981
101. Walker MD, Goldware SI, Rockswold GL et al: Regional infusion chemotherapy of head and neck in dogs. Fed Proc 29:681, 1970
102. Levin VA, Kabra PM, Freeman-Dove MA: Pharmacokinetics of intracarotid artery C-BCNU in the squirrel monkey. J Neurosurg 48:587–593, 1978
103. West CR, Avellanosa AM, Barua NR et al: Phase II study on malignant gliomas of the brain treated with intra-arterial BCNU in combination with vincristine and procarbazine. Proceedings, AACR. 21:482, 1980
104. Neuwelt E, Frenkel E, Bartnett P et al: Methotrexate (MTX) pharmacokinetics after osmotic blood brain barrier (BBB) disruption. Proceedings, AACR, 21:286, 1980
105. Danoff BF, Kramer S, Thompson N: The radiotherapeutic management of optic nerve gliomas in children. Int J Radiat Oncol Biol Phys 6:45–50, 1980

106. Miller NR, Iliff WJ, Green WR: Evaluation and management of gliomas of the anterior visual pathways. Brain 97:743–754, 1974
107. Myles ST, Murphy SB: Gliomas of the optic nerve and chiasm. Can J Ophthalmol 8:508–514, 1973
108. Hoyt WF, Meshel LG, Lessell S et al: Malignant optic glioma of adulthood. Brain 96:121–132, 1973
109. Hoyt WF, Baghdassarian SA: Optic glioma of childhood. Br J Ophthal 53:793–798, 1969
110. Bynke H, Kagstrom E, Jernstrom K: Aspects on the treatment of gliomas of the anterior visual pathway. Acta Ophthal 55:269–280, 1971
111. Montgomery AB, Griffin T, Parker RG et al: Optic nerve glioma: The role of radiation therapy. Cancer 40:2079–2080, 1977
112. Chang CH, Wood EH: The value of radiation therapy for gliomas of anterior visual pathway. In Brockhurst R, Boruchoff S, Hutchinson B et al (eds): Controversy in Ophthalmology. Philadelphia, WB Saunders, 1977, pp 878–886
113. Dosoretz DE, Blitzer PH, Wang CC et al: Management of glioma of the optic nerve and/or chiasm: An analysis of 20 cases. Cancer 45:1467–1471, 1980
114. Leibel SA, Sheline GE, Wara WM et al: The role of radiation therapy in the treatment of astrocytomas. Cancer 35:1551–1557, 1975
115. Griffin TW, Beaufait D, Blasko JC: Cystic cerebellar astrocytomas in childhood. Cancer 44:276–280, 1979
116. Fagekas JT: Treatment of Grades I and II brain astrocytomas. The role of radiotherapy. Int J Radiat Oncol Biol Phys 2:661–666, 1977
117. Bloom HJG: Combined modality therapy for intracranial tumors. Cancer 35:111–120, 1975
118. Stage W, Stein J: Treatment of malignant astrocytomas. Am J Roentgenol Radium Ther Nucl Med 120:7–18, 1974
119. Kramer S: Cancer of the central nervous system—Radiation therapy in the management of malignant gliomas. IN: Seventh Natl Cancer Conf Proc, Philadelphia, JB Lippincott, 1973, pp 823–826
120. Gol A: Cerebral astrocytomas in childhood: A clinical study. J Neurosurg 19:577–582, 1962
121. Dibden FA: Radiotherapy of brain tumors. J Coll Radiol Aus 6:122–129, 1962
122. Walker MD: Chemotherapy: adjuvant to surgery and radiation therapy. Semin Oncol 2:69–72, 1975
123. Walker MD: Nitrosoureas in central nervous system tumors. Cancer Chemo Reg 4:21–26, 1973
124. Walker MD, Gehan E: An evaluation of 1,3 *bis*(2-chloroethyl)-1-nitrosourea (BCNU) alone and irradiation alone and in combination for the treatment of malignant glioma (abstract). Proc Am Assoc Cancer Res 15:67, 1972
125. Concannon JP, Kramer S, Beny R: The extent of intracranial gliomata at autopsy and its relationship to techniques used in radiation therapy of brain tumors. Am J Roentgenol Radium Ther Nucl Med 84:99–107, 1960
126. Kramer S: Tumor extent as a determining factor in radiotherapy of glioblastomas. Acta Radiol (Ther) 8:111–117, 1969
127. Aristizibal SA, Caldwell WL: Time–Dose–Volume relationships in the treatment of glioblastoma multiforme. Radiology 101:201–202, 1971
128. Todd IDH: Choice of volume in the x-ray treatment of supratentorial gliomas. Br J Radiol 36:645–649, 1963
129. Salazar OM, Rubin P, McDonald JV et al: High dose radiation therapy in the treatment of glioblastoma multiforme: a preliminary report. Int J Radiat Oncol Biol Phys 1:717–727, 1976
130. Sheline GE: Radiation therapy of primary tumors. Semin Oncol 2:29–42, 1975
131. Sheline GE: The importance of distinguishing tumor grade in malignant gliomas: treatment and prognosis. Int J Radiat Oncol Biol Phys 1:781–786, 1976
132. Walsh JM, Cassady JR, Frei E III et al: Recent advances in the treatment of primary brain tumors. Arch Surg 110:696–702, 1975
133. Walker MD: Brain Tumors. In Holland JF, Frei E III (eds): Cancer Medicine. Philadelphia, Lea & Febiger, 1973, pp 1385–1407
134. Walker MD, Hurwitz BS: BCNU 1,3-*bis*(2-chloroethyl)-1-nitrosourea (NSC 409962) in the treatment of malignant brain tumor—a preliminary report, Cancer Chemother Rep 54:263–271, 1970
135. Wilson CB, Boldrey EB, Enot KJ: 1,3-*bis*(2-chloroethyl)-1-nitrosourea (NSC-409962) in the treatment of brain tumors. Cancer Chemother Rep 54:273–281, 1970
136. Walker MD, Green SB, Byar DP. et al: Randomized comparisons of radiotherapy and nitrosoureas for malignant glioma after surgery. N Engl J Med, 303:1323–1329, 1980
137. EORTC Brain Tumor Group: Effect of CCNU on survival rate of objective remission and duration of free interval in patients with malignant brain glioma—Final evaluation. Eur J Cancer 14:851–856, 1978
138. Garrett MJ, Hughes HJ, Freedman LS: A comparison of radiotherapy alone with radiotherapy and CCNU in cerebral glioma. Clinical Oncol 4:71–76, 1978
139. Reagan TJ, Bisel HF, Childs DS et al: Controlled study of CCNU and radiation therapy in malignant astrocytoma. J Neurosurg 44:186–190, 1976
140. Weir B, Band P, Urtasun R et al: Radiotherapy and CCNU in the treatment of high-grade supratentorial astrocytomas. J Neurosurg 45:129–134, 1976
141. Jellinger K, Kothbauer P, Volc D et al: Combination Chemotherapy (COMP Protocol) and Radiotherapy of Anaplastic Supratentorial Gliomas. Acta Neurochir 51:1–13, 1979
142. Heiss W-D: Chemotherapy of malignant gliomas: Comparison of the effect of polychemo- and CCNU-therapy. Acta Neurochir (Wien) 42:109–115, 1978
143. Shapiro WR, Young DF: Chemotherapy of malignant glioma with BCNU and vincristine. Neurology (Minneapolis) 24:380, 1974
144. Seiler RW, Greiner RH, Zimmerman A et al: Radiotherapy combined with procarbazine, bleomycin, and CCNU in the treatment of high-grade supratentorial astrocytomas. J Neurosurg 48:861–865, 1978
145. Gehan EA, Walker MD: Prognostic factors for patients with brain tumors. Natl Cancer Inst Monogr 46:189–195, 1977
146. Burger PC, Mahaley MS Jr, Dudka L et al: The morphologic effects of radiation administered therapeutically for intracranial gliomas. Cancer 44:1256–1272, 1979
147. Cohen RJ, Wiernik PH, Walker MD: Acute nonlymphocytic leukemia associated with nitrosourea chemotherapy: Report of two cases. Cancer Treat Rep 60, no 9, September 1976
148. Beck DJK, Russell DS: Oligodendrogliomatosis of the cerebro–spinal pathway. Brain 65:352–372, 1942
149. Chui HW, Hazel JJ, Kim TH et al: Oligodendrogliomas. Cancer 45:1458–1466, 1980
150. Roberts M, German WJ: A long term study of patients with oligodendrogliomas. Follow-up of 50 cases, including Dr. Harvey Cushing's series. J Neurosurg 24:697–700, 1966
151. Konovalov AN, Fedorov SN, Faller TO et al: Current problems in the surgical management of parasellar meningiomas. Zentralbl Neurochir 39:273–284, 1978
152. Simpson D: Recurrence of intracranial meningiomas after surgical treatment. J Neurol Neurosurg Psych 20:22–39, 1957
153. Earle KM, Richany SF: Meningiomas: a study of the histology, incidence and biologic behavior of 243 cases from the Frazier–Grant collection of brain tumors. Med Ann DC 38:353–358, 1969
154. Quest DO: Meningiomas, an update. Neurosurgery 3:219–225, 1978
155. Castellano F, Guidetti B, Olivecrona H: Pterional meningiomas "*en plaque.*" J Neurosurg 9:188–196, 1952
156. Friedman M: Irradiation of meningioma: a prototype circumscribed tumor for planning high-dose irradiation of the brain. Int J Radiat Oncol Biol Phys 2:949–958, 1977
157. Wara WM, Sheline GE, Newman H et al: Radiation therapy of meningiomas. Am J Roentgenol Radium Ther Nucl Med 123:453–458, 1975
158. King DL, Chang CH, Pool JL: Radiotherapy in the management of meningiomas. Acta Radiol (Ther) 5:26–33, 1966
159. Leibel SA, Wara WM, Sheline GE et al: Treatment of meningiomas in childhood. Cancer 37:2709–2712, 1976
160. Ludwin SK, Rubinstein LJ, Russell DS: Papillary meningioma:

a malignant variant of meningioma. Cancer 36:1363–1373, 1975
161. Greenberger JS, Cassady JR, Levene MB: Radiation therapy of thalamic, midbrain, and brainstem gliomas. Radiology 122:463–468, 1977
162. Gjerris, F, Klinken L: Long-term prognosis in children with benign cerebellar astrocytoma. J Neurosurg 49:179–184, 1978
163. Stein BM, Tenner MS, Fraser AR: Hydrocephalus following removal of cerebellar astrocytomas in children. J Neurosurg 36:763, 1972
164. Quest DO, Brisman R, Antunes JL et al: Period of risk for recurrence in medulloblastoma. J Neurosurg 48:159–163, 1978
165. Deutsch M, Reigel DH: Value of myelography in the management of childhood medulloblastoma. Cancer 45:2194–2197, 1980
166. Cushing H: Experiences with cerebellar medulloblastomas; a critical review. Acta Pathol Microbiol Scand 7:1–86, 1930
167. Bryan P: CSF seeding of intra-cranial tumors: a study of 96 cases. Clin Radiol 25:355–360, 1974
168. Chang CH, Housepian EM, Herbert C Jr: An operative staging system and a megavoltage radiotherapeutic technic for cerebellar medulloblastomas. Radiology 93:1351–1359, 1969
169. Berger EC, Elvidge AR: Medulloblastomas and cerebellar sarcomas: A clinical survey. J Neurosurg 10:139–144, 1963
170. VanDyk J, Jenkin RD, Lering PMK et al: Medulloblastoma: treatment technique and radiation dosimetry. Int J Radiat Oncol Biol Phys 2:993–1005, 1977
171. Harisiadis L, Chang CH: Medulloblastoma in children: a correlation between staging and results of treatment. Int J Radiat Oncol Biol Phys 2:833–841, 1977
172. Smith CE, Long DM, Jones TK et al: Experiences in treating medulloblastoma at the University of Minnesota Hospitals. Radiology 109:179–182, 1973
173. Bloom HJG, Wallace EWK, Henk JM: The treatment and prognosis of medulloblastoma in children. A study of 82 verified cases. Am J Roentgenol Radium Ther Nucl Med 105:43–62, 1969
174. Hope-Stone HF: Results of treatment of medulloblastomas. J Neurosurg 32:83–88, 1970
175. Aron BS: Twenty years' experience with radiation therapy of medulloblastoma. Am J Roentgenol Radium Ther Nucl Med 105:37–42, 1969
176. D'Angio GJ, French LA, Stadlam EM et al: Intrathecal radioisotopes for the treatment of brain tumors. Clin Neurosurg 15:288–299, 1968
177. Wilson CB: Medulloblastoma: Current views regarding the tumor and its treatment. Oncology 24:273–290, 1970
178. Black SPW, Keats TE: Generalized osteosclerosis secondary to metastatic medulloblastoma of the cerebellum. Radiology 82:395–399, 1964
179. Bloom HJG: Prospects for increasing survival in children with medulloblastoma: Present and future studies. Multidisciplin Aspects Br Tum Ther, 1:245–259, 1979
180. Evans AE, Anderson J, Chang C et al: Adjuvant chemotherapy for medulloblastoma and ependymoma. Multidisciplin Aspects Br Tum Ther 1:219–222, 1979
181. Rosenstock JG, Evans AE, Schut L: Response to vincristine of recurrent brain tumors in children. J Neurosurg 45:135–140, 1976
182. Cangir A, Eys J, Berry DH et al: Combination chemotherapy with MOPP in children with recurrent brain tumors. Med Ped Oncol 4:253–261, 1978
183. Thomas PR, Duffner PK, Cohen ME et al: Multimodality therapy for medulloblastoma. Cancer 45:666–669, 1980
184. Fokes EC, Earle KM: Ependymomas: Clinical and pathological aspects. J Neurosurg 30:585–594, 1969
185. Mørk SJ, Løken AC: Ependymoma: A follow-up study of 101 cases. Cancer 40:907–915, 1977
186. Barone BM, Elridge AR: Ependymomas: A clinical survey. J Neurosurg 33:428–438, 1970
187. Phillips TL, Sheline GE, Boldrey E: Therapeutic considerations in tumors affecting the central nervous system: Ependymomas. Radiology 33:98–105, 1964
188. Shuman RM, Alvord EC, Leech RW: The biology of childhood ependymomas. Arch Neurol 32:731–739, 1975
189. Salazar OM, Rubin P, Bassano D et al: Improved survival of patients with intracranial ependymomas by irradiation: Dose selection and field extension. Cancer 35:1563–1573, 1975
190. Kim YH, Fayos J: Intracranial ependymomas. Radiology 124:805–808, 1977
191. Kricheff II, Becker M, Schneck SA et al: Intracranial ependymomas: A study of survival in 65 patients treated by surgery and irradiation. Am J Roentgenol Radium Ther Nucl Med 91:167–175, 1964 (cited p 172)
192. Sagerman RH, Bagshaw MA, Hanberg J: Considerations in the treatment of ependymomas. Radiology 84:401–408, 1965
193. Dohrmann GJ, Farwell JR, Flannery JT: Ependymomas and ependymoblastomas in children. J Neurosurg 45:273–283, 1976
194. Shapiro WR: Chemotherapy of primary malignant brain tumors in children. Cancer 35:975, 1975
195. Wohlwill FJ, Yakovlev PI: Histopathology of meningiofacial angiomatosis (Sturge–Weber's disease). J Neuropathol Exp Neurol 16:341–364, 1957
196. Horton WA: Genetics of central nervous system tumors. Birth Defects 12:91–97, 1976
197. Okawara SH: Solid cerebellar hemangioblastoma. J Neurosurg 39:514–518, 1973
198. Ulkowski M, Kaczmarczyk Z: Post-operative x-ray therapy of malignant brain tumors: Results and analysis of vital adaptation of patients after treatment. Pol Przesl Radiol 42:481–485, 1978
199. Belli JA: Personal communication.
200. Richardson RG, Griffin TW, Parker RG: Intramedullary hemangioblastoma of the spinal cord. Cancer 45:49–50, 1980
201. Shin KH, Fisher G, Webster JH: Brain stem tumors in children. J Can Assoc Radiol 30:77–78, 1979
202. Kim TH, Chin HW, Pollan S et al: Radiotherapy of primary brain stem tumors. Int J Radiat Oncol Biol Phys 6:51–57, 1980
203. Sheline GE, Phillips TL, Boldrey E: The therapy of brain stem tumors. Radiology 93:664–670, 1965
204. Urtasun RC: ^{60}Co radiation treatment of pontine gliomas. Radiology 104:385–387, 1972
205. Whyte TR, Colby MY, Layton DD: Radiation therapy of brain stem tumors. Radiology 93:413–421, 1969
206. Rosen G, Ghavimi F, Vanucci R et al: Pontine glioma: High-dose methotrexate and leucovorin rescue. JAMA, 230:1149–1152, 1974
207. Smith B: Brain damage after intrathecal methotrexate. J Neurol Neurosurg Psych 38:810–815, 1975
208. Zaunbauer F, Pichler E, Fodor M: Experiences with radiotherapy and chemotherapy in the treatment of tumors involving the caudal brain stem. Mod Probl Paediat 18:80–83, 1977
209. Vansantha Kumar AR, Renaudin J, Wilson CB et al: Procarbazine hydrochloride in the treatment of brain tumors—Phase 2 study. J Neurosurg 40:365–371, 1974
210. El-Mahdi AM, Phillips E, Lott S: The role of radiation therapy in pinealoma. Radiology 103:407–412, 1972
211. Swischuk LE, Bryan RN: Double midline intracranial atypical teratomas. Am J Roentgenol Radium Ther Nucl Med 122:517–524, 1974
212. Bradfield J, Perez CA: Pineal tumors and ectopic pinealomas. Analysis of treatment and failures. Radiology 103:399–406, 1972
213. Sung DI, Harisiadis L, Chang CH: Midline pineal tumors and suprasellar germinomas: highly curable by irradiation. Radiology 128:745–751, 1978
214. Rubin P, Kramer S: Ectopic pinealoma: radiocurable neuro–endocrinologic entity. Radiology 85:512–523, 1965
215. Jordan RM, Kendall JW, McClung M et al: Concentration of human chorionic gonadotroph in the cerebrospinal fluid of patients with germinal cell hypothalamic tumors. Pediatrics 65:121–124, 1980
216. Obrador S, Soto M, Gutierrez-Diaz JA: Surgical management of tumours of the pineal region. Acta Neurochir (Wien) 34:159–171, 1976
217. Wara WM, Jenkin RDT, Evans A et al: Tumors of the pineal and suprasellar region: Children's cancer study group treatment results 1960–1975. Cancer 43:698–701, 1979

218. Jenkin RDT, Simpson JK, Keen CW: Pineal and suprasellar germinomas. J Neurosurg 48:99–107, 1978
219. de Tribolet N, Barrelet L: Successful chemotherapy of pinealoma (letter). Lancet 2:1228–1229, 1977
220. Newman H, Rowe JF, Phillips T: Radiation therapy of the gliomas jugulare tumor. Am J Roentgenol Radium Ther Nucl Med 118:663–669, 1973
221. Hawkins TD: Glomus jugulare and carotid body tumours. Clin Radiol 12:199–213, 1961
222. Bradley WH, Maxwell JH: Neoplasms of middle ear and mastoid: Report of 54 cases. Laryngoscope 64:533–556, 1954
223. Rosenwasser H: Glomus jugularis tumor of middle ear. Laryngoscope 62:623–633, 1952
224. VanMiert PJ: The treatment of chemodectomas by radiotherapy. Proc Roy Soc Med 57:1964
225. Grubb WB Jr, Lampe I: Role of radiation therapy in treatment of chemodectomas of glomus jugulare. Laryngoscope 75:1861–1871, 1965
226. Hudgins PT: Radiotherapy for extensive glomus jugulare tumors. Radiology 103:427–429, 1972
227. Maruyama Y, Gold LHA, Kieffer SA: Clinical and angiographic evaluation of radiotherapeutic response of glomus jugulare tumors. Radiology 101:397–399, 1971
228. Ojemann RG: Microsurgical suboccipital approach to cerebello–pontine angle tumors. Clin Neurosurg 25:461–479, 1978
229. Cushing HW: Tumors of the Nervus Acusticus and the Syndrome of the Cerebellopontine Angle. Philadelphia, WB Saunders, 1917
230. Ojemann RG, Crowell RM: Acoustic neuromas treated by microsurgical suboccipital operations. Prog Neurol Surg 9:337–373, 1978
231. Drake CG: Surgical treatment of acoustic neuroma with preservation or reconstitution of the facial nerve. J Neurosurg 26:459–464, 1967
232. Hitselberger WE, House WF: Combined approach to cerebellopontine angle. Suboccipitalpetrosal approach. Arch Otolaryng 84:267–285, 1966
233. George SR, Burrow GN, Zinman B et al: Regression of pituitary tumors, a possible effect of bromergocryptine. Am J Med 66:697–702, 1979
234. Hardy J, Vezina JL: Transsphenoidal neurosurgery of intracranial neoplasm. Adv Neurol 15:261–273, 1976
235. Nielson KD, Watts C, Clark K: Transsphenoidal microsurgery for selective removal of functional pituitary microadenomas. World J Surg 1:79–84, 1977
236. Sheline GE: Untreated and recurrent chromophobe adenomas of the pituitary. Am J Roentgenol Radium Ther Nucl Med 112:768–773, 1971
237. Sheline GE: Treatment of chromophobe adenomas of the pituitary gland and acromegaly. In Kohler PO, Ross GT (eds): Diagnosis and Treatment of Pituitary Tumors. Amsterdam, Exerpta Med, 1973, pp 201–216
238. Chang CH, Pool JL: The radiotherapy of pituitary chromophobe adenomas. Radiology 89:1005–1016, 1967
239. Kramer S: Indications for, and results of, treatment of pituitary tumors by external radiation. In Kohler PO, Ross GT (eds): Diagnosis and Treatment of Pituitary Tumors. New York, Elsevier, Exerpta Med, 1973, pp 217–229
240. Levene MB: Radiotherapy and pituitary tumors. In Deeley TJ (ed): Modern Radiotherapy and Oncology Central Nervous System Tumors. London, Butterworths, 1974, pp 224–241
241. Christy NP: Anterior pituitary. In Beeson PB, McDermott W (eds): Textbook of Medicine, 11th ed. Philadelphia, WB Saunders, 1963, pp 1342–1364
242. Daughaday WH: The adenohypophysis. In William RH (ed): Textbook of Endocrinology, 3rd ed. Philadelphia, WB Saunders, 1962, pp 11–79
243. Lawrence AM, Pinsky SM, Goldfine ID: Conventional radiation therapy in acromegaly: A review and reassessment. Arch Intern Med 128:369–377, 1971
244. Ray BS, Patterson RH: Symposium on pituitary tumors. I. Surgical treatment of pituitary adenomas. J Neurosurg 19:1–8, 1962
245. Cushing H: Disorders of the pituitary gland: Retrospective and prophetic. JAMA 76:1721–1726, 1921
246. Guiot G: Indications for the transsphenoidal approach of the hypophyseal fossa. Rhinology 11:137–152, 1973
247. Hardy J: Transsphenoidal hypophysectomy. J Neurosurg 34:582–594, 1971
248. Wilson CB, Dempsey LC: Transsphenoidal microsurgical removal of 250 pituitary adenomas. J Neurosurg 48:13–22, 1978
249. Zervas NT: Stereotaxic thermal surgery of the pituitary. In Linfoot JA (ed): Recent Advances in the Diagnosis and Treatment of Pituitary Tumors. New York, Raven Press, 1979, pp 407–417
250. Pistenma DH, Goffinet DR, Bagshaw MA et al: Treatment of acromegaly with megavoltage radiation therapy. Int J Radiat Oncol Biol Phys 1:885–893, 1976
251. Hayes TP, Davis RA, Raventos A: The treatment of pituitary chromophobe adenomas. Radiology 98:140–153, 1971
252. Lewtes NA: Symposium on pituitary tumors. Radiology in diagnosis and management. Clin Radiol 17:149–153, 1966
253. Orth DN, Liddle GW: Results of treatment in 108 patients with Cushing's syndrome. N Engl J Med 285:243–247, 1971
254. Jennings AS, Liddle G, Orth DN: Results of treating childhood Cushing's disease with pituitary irradiation. N Engl J Med 297:957–962, 1977
255. Edmonds MW, Simpson WJK, Meakin JW: External irradiation of the hypophysis for Cushing's disease. Can Med Assoc J 107:860–862, 1972
256. Heuschele R, Lampe I: Pituitary irradiation for Cushing's syndrome. Radiol Clin Biol 36:27–31, 1967
257. Kjellberg RN, Kliman B: Proton beam therapy. N Engl J Med 284:333, 1971
258. Lawrence JH, Born JL, Linfoot JA et al: Heavy particle radiation treatment of pituitary tumors. JAMA 214:2061, 1970
259. Kjellberg RN, Shintani A, Freintz AG et al: Proton-beam therapy in acromegaly. N Engl J Med 278:689–695, 1968
260. Lawrence JH, Tobias GA, Linfoot JA et al: Successful treatment of acromegaly: metabolic and clinical studies in 145 patients. J Clin Endo Metab 31:180–198, 1970
261. Kjellberg RN, Kliman B: A system for therapy of pituitary tumors. In Kohler PO, Ross GT (eds): Diagnosis and Treatment of Pituitary Tumors, Amsterdam, Excerpta Med, 1973, pp 234–252
262. Lawrence JH, Chong CY, Lyman JT et al: Treatment of pituitary tumors with heavy particles. In Kohler PO, Ross GT (eds): Diagnosis and Treatment of Pituitary Tumors, New York. Elsevier, 1973, pp 253–262
263. Katz EL: Late results of radical excision of craniopharyngiomas in children. J Neurosurg 42:86–90, 1975
264. Sweet WH: Radical Surgical Treatment of Craniopharyngioma. In Schmidek HH, Sweet WH (eds): Current Techniques in Operative Neurosurgery. New York, Grune & Stratton, 1977, pp 199–221
265. Matson DD, Crigler JF Jr: Management of craniopharyngioma in childhood. J Neurosurg 30:377–390, 1969
266. Kramer S, McKissock W, Concannon J: Craniopharyngiomas, treatment by combined surgery and radiation therapy. J Neurosurg 18:217–226, 1961
267. Kramer S, Southard M, Mansfield C: Radiotherapy in the management of craniopharyngiomas. Am J Roentgenol Radium Ther Nucl Med 103:44–52, 1968
268. Kramer S: Radiation therapy in the management of brain tumors in children. Ann NY Acad Med 159:571–584, 1969
269. Onoyama Y, Ono K, Yabumoto E et al: Radiation therapy of craniopharyngioma. Radiology 125:799–803, 1977
270. Lichter AS, Wara WM, Sheline GE et al: The treatment of craniopharyngioma. Int J Radiat Oncol Biol Phys 2:675–683, 1977
271. Bartlett JR: Craniopharyngiomas—A summary of 85 cases. J Neurol Neurosurg Psychiat 34:37–41, 1971
272. Wang CC, James AE: Chordoma: Brief review of the literature and report of a case with wide spread metastases. Cancer 22:162–167, 1968
273. Stevenson GC, Stoney RJ, Perkins RK et al: A transcervical

approach to the ventral surface of the brain stem for removal of a clivus chordoma. J Neurosurg 24:544–551, 1960

274. Tewjik HH, McGinnis WL, Nordstrom DG et al: Chordoma, evaluation of clinical behavior and treatment modalities. Int J Radiat Oncol Biol Phys 2:959–962, 1977
275. Suit H, Rich T: Personal communication.
276. Pearlman AW, Friedman M: Radical radiation therapy of chordoma. Am J Roentgenol Radium Ther Nucl Med 108:333–341, 1970
277. Phillips TL, Newman H: Chordoma. In Deeley TJ (ed): Modern Radiotherapy and Oncology: Central Nervous System Tumours. London, Butterworths, 1974, pp 184–203
278. Steckler RM, Martin RG: Sacrococcygeal chordoma. Ann Surg 40:579–581, 1974
279. Wood EH, Berne AS, Traveras JM: The value of radiation therapy in the management of intrinsic tumours of the spinal cord. Radiology 63:11–22, 1954
280. Marsa GW, Goffinet DR, Rubinstein LR et al: Megavoltage irradiation in the treatment of gliomas of the brain and spinal cord. Cancer 36:1681–1689, 1975
281. Schwade JG, Wara WM, Sheline GE et al: Management of primary spinal cord tumors. Int J Radiat Oncol Biol Phys 4:389–393, 1978
282. Wara WM, Phillips TL, Sheline GE et al: Radiation tolerance of the spinal cord. Cancer 35:1558–1562, 1975
283. Coulon RA, Till K: Intracranial ependymomas in children: A review of 43 cases. Childs Brain 3:154–168, 1977
284. Scott M: Infiltrating ependymomas of the cauda equina. Treatment by conservative surgery plus radiotherapy. J Neurosurg 41:446–448, 1974
285. Luessenhop AJ, Presper JH: Surgical embolization of cerebral arteriovenous malformations through internal carotid and vertebral arteries: Long term results. J Neurosurg 42:443–451, 1975
286. Hoshino T, Barker M, Wilson CB et al: Cell kinetics of human gliomas. J Neurosurg 37:15–26, 1972
287. Kornblith PL, Dohan FC Jr, Wood WC et al: Human astrocytoma: serum-mediated immunologic response. Cancer 33:1512–1519, 1974
288. Kornblith PL, Pollock LA, Coakham HB et al: Cytotoxic antibody responses in astrocytoma patients: an improved allogeneic assay. J Neurosurg 51:47–52, 1979
289. Phelps ME, Huang SC, Hoffman EJ et al: Tomographic measurement of local cerebral glucose metabolic rate in humans with (F-18)2-fluoro-2-deoxy-D-glucose: Validation of method. Ann Neurol 6:371–388, 1979
290. Grossi-Paoletti E, Paoletti P, Fumagalli R: Lipids in brain tumors. J Neurosurg 34:454–455, 1971
291. Catterall M, Bloom HJG, Ash DV et al: Fast neutrons compared with megavoltage x-rays in the treatment of patients with supratentorial glioblastomas: A controlled pilot study. Int J Radiat Oncol Biol Phys 6:261–266, 1980
292. Douglas BG: Preliminary results using superfractionation in the treatment of glioblastoma multiforme. J Can Assoc Radiol 28:106–110, 1977
293. Hatanaka H, Takakura K, Nagai M: Irradiation plus drugs aids brain tumor patients (Medical News). JAMA 220:1289–1290, 1972
294. Sano K, Hoshino T, Nagai M: Radiosensitization of brain tumor cells with thymidine analaogue (biomoundine). J Neurosurg 28:530–538, 1968
295. Chang CH, Housepian EM, Sciana D et al: Hyperbaric oxygen for radiation therapy for malignant gliomas. In Seydel HG (ed): Tumors of the Nervous System. New York, John Wiley & Sons, pp 71–76, 1975
296. Urtasun R, Band P, Chapman JD et al: Radiation and high-dose metronidazole in supratentorial glioblastoma. N Engl J Med 294:1364–1367, 1976
297. Urtasun RC, Band PR, Chapman JD et al: Radiation plus metronidazole for glioblastoma. N Engl J Med 296:757, 1977
298. Takvorian R: Personal communication, 1980.
299. Kornblith PL, Szypko PE: Variations in response of human brain tumors to BCNU *in vitro*. J Neurosurg 48:580–586, 1978
300. Thomas DGT, Darling JL, Freshney RI et al: *In vitro* chemosensitivity assay of human gliomas by scintillation autofluorography. In Paoletti P, Walker MD, Butte G et al (eds): Multidisciplinary Aspects of Brain Tumor Therapy. Amsterdam, Elsevier North-Holland Biomedical Press, 1979, pp 19–34
301. Rosenblum ML, Vasquez DA, Hoshino T et al: Development of a clonogenic cell assay for human brain tumors. Cancer 41:2305–2314, 1978
302. Young HF, Sakalas R, Kaplan AM: Inhibition of cell mediated immunity in patients with brain tumors. Surg Neurol 5:19–23, 1976

Joseph V. Simone
J. Robert Cassady
Robert M. Filler

CHAPTER 34

Cancers of Childhood

Childhood cancer has provided unique opportunities for the advancement of our understanding and therapeutic success in the treatment of cancer as a whole. Malignancies in children are predominantly of embryonic or blastemic origin or take on the characteristics of such tissue. Consequently, the spectrum of responsiveness to various therapeutic agents differs from the predominant carcinomas seen in adults. In general, the childhood cancers are more responsive to current therapeutic methods. This has been borne out by remarkable success in the treatment of Wilms' tumor, acute lymphocytic leukemia, retinoblastoma, and lymphoma. Childhood leukemia has been an especially fruitful testing ground for general hypotheses of cancer therapy generated in animal systems. Because the child is a growing and developing organism, therapeutic success has also been associated with a magnification of the complication rate due to the effects of chemotherapy, radiation, and surgery. When a malignancy is almost universally fatal, there is little concern about the consequences of therapy except that it be effective. Once effective, then modifications of therapy are required to minimize the late effects, physical and psychosocial.

Childhood cancer, because of its appearance chronologically closer to the etiologic event, has provided an opportunity to understand associations and potential etiological factors. A number of associations of childhood cancer with predisposing genetic and chromosomal abnormalities have been described. This is especially evident in tumors such as retinoblastoma, Wilms' tumor, and a small proportion of patients with leukemia. Although direct causative factors have not been defined, complex schema of etiology are emerging which, in some cases, apparently require two or more events for cancer to develop. This hypothesis has been developed by Knudson, using as a prototype the difference in frequency of retinoblastoma when it occurs sporadically and in families.[1] He postulates that it requires two events for malignant transformation to occur. In patients with familial retinoblastoma who frequently develop bilateral disease, the first event is the genetic predisposition of the retinal tissue to transformation. The second event, which probably occurs relatively frequently to the population at large, finds fertile soil for conversion in the patients with familial disease. In the general population with no genetic predisposition, the two "hits" of the cell or tissue is a much less likely statistical probability.

The association of Down's syndrome with a high frequency of leukemia has long been observed.[2] It is likely that the trisomy is associated with general aberration in hematopoietic control mechanisms because of the occurrence of a pseudoleukemia syndrome in some of these patients shortly after birth.[3]

Thus, although childhood cancer accounts for only 3% of all cancers, the impact that the study of childhood cancer and its treatment has had on the field as a whole has been proportionately greater. There is a great deal to learn from the study of childhood cancer and the purpose of this chapter is to provide a basis for understanding each of the tumor types and developing a rational therapeutic approach.

CHEMOTHERAPY PRINCIPLES IN PEDIATRIC ONCOLOGY

The introduction and clinical trial of a new agent usually develops in a systematic fashion. A new agent that showed promise in animal systems is first used in Phase I (toxicity and dose-finding) studies. Phase I studies determine dose tolerance and simultaneously permit assessment of the degree of responsiveness of a broad variety of tumors. If the toxicity is found tolerable and there is demonstrable antitumor activity, the agent is then evaluated in Phase II studies, in which the agent is given in the previously determined dosage, but this time for a specific tumor with the primary intention of observing the degree and duration of antitumor effect. The patients entered in Phase II studies usually have had conventional treatment and their tumors have become refractory. It is not anticipated that a Phase II study will result in permanent cures. Once an agent demonstrates a significant antitumor effect, either by inducing remissions or preventing progression for a significant period of time, it is moved up to the Phase III study, in which the objective is a realistic attempt at permanent cure. Phase III studies almost always involve the use of combinations of agents and modalities. However, even when an agent is found effective throughout the three phases of development it is still possible that the optimal method of application may not be known. A good example is methotrexate, which has been available as an effective agent for over 30 years, yet is still the object of intense study to find the optimal dosage and route of administration for the different disease categories.

An agent which is found to be ineffective in a Phase II trial is unlikely to become effective when used in combination with other agents. However, agents which are moderately effective when used alone in Phase II studies may have a sufficient additive effect when combined with other agents to form a potent combination. Examples of this are mercaptopurine and methotrexate for acute lymphocytic leukemia, doxorubicin (Adriamycin), and cyclophosphamide for neuroblastoma and the MOPP therapy for Hodgkin's disease. However, there has been a trend to the belief that "more is better," that is, the untested addition of many agents with potential effectiveness unproven in combination. This may lead to more toxicity without more efficacy because of redundancy, drug antagonism, or inappropriate drug schedules for the combination.[4] Combinations of drugs become difficult to modify or take apart to determine the essential facets unless they are put together systematically at the very outset.

Chemotherapy is given in prescribed doses but it becomes readily apparent that not all patients will tolerate the same dosage at all times. Whereas fixed doses are frequently employed in adult oncology, the range of body size and fluid pools in children is enormous. The most useful standard by which chemotherapy dosage is calculated is based on body surface area. Although this method works well most of the time, there are major exceptions. First, a particular agent may require an upper dosage limit because of excessive toxicity at a given dosage per square meter in larger patients, as with vincristine. The common dosage of 1.5 mg/mm^2 or 2 mg/mm^2 may be given at all childhood ages, but in adolescents and young adults, repetitive dosages of more than 2 mg/mm^2 often causes severe neuropathy. Many treatment regimens establish an upper limit of 2 mg/mm^2. A second circumstance requiring modification of dosage is the innate variability of a particular patient's tolerance. The dosages prescribed in a well-established protocol may be tolerated without modification by a large minority of patients, perhaps one-third to one-half. Another minority of patients may tolerate the prescribed dosage most of the time but will have intermittent periods of intolerance that may be associated with infections or other complications. Finally, some patients are never able to tolerate the full dosage and always receive chemotherapy in lower dosage or less frequently.

The principle to be employed is not that one must make each patient conform to a predetermined dosage level, but that one must determine the maximum dosage that the patient may receive without life-threatening or chronically debilitating toxicity. Tumor cell-kill is clearly dose-related, so one should strive to give the maximum tolerable dosage. What is maximum tolerable? Transient neutropenia is not sufficient to permanently modify chemotherapy or radiation therapy dosage, but recurring sepsis, pneumonia, and progressive weight loss are. Chemotherapy dosage may be modified in a variety of ways. The two most common are to continue chemotherapy at the prescribed intervals but at reduced dosage, or to omit a dose or series of doses until the toxic effect is largely resolved and then to resume at full dosage. It is not clear which is the better approach for optimal antitumor activity. One might choose to reduce dosage rather than lengthen the interval on the assumption that the tumor cells and hemopoietic cells are equally sensitive and the latter serves as an accurate barometer of tumoricidal dosage. The reduced tolerance is blamed on the patient's peculiar metabolism. This approach is often used when drugs are given daily or weekly, because titration to tolerance is relatively easy. The alternative approach—prolong the interval but maintain the dosage—is often employed in regimens using several agents intensively during 1 week of every 3 weeks or 4 weeks.

The administration of chemotherapy to its maximum effectiveness depends on a variety of factors. In many cases, individual agents and combinations have been given empirically and because of success have not been modified appreciably. However, it has become clear from investigations of pharmacology and cell kinetics that the application of certain principles may enhance the effectiveness of agents.[5-7] That the product of drug concentration and time is an indicator of antitumor effectiveness is a concept that has evolved in recent years.[8] This concept states that it is not only drug dosage and tumor cell concentration that is important, but also the duration of effective concentrations. For example, one might achieve a superior result using a smaller dose maintained over a protracted period of time rather than a much higher peak level which disappears rapidly. The reason for this may be that cells are not equally sensitive to the effects of chemotherapy at all times in their life cycle and maintaining an effective dose level for a more prolonged period of time may be more likely to affect the entire cell population. Furthermore, it is well known that some chemotherapeutic agents are most effective in only one phase of the cell cycle. Cytosine arabinoside is effective during DNA synthesis, but is relatively ineffective at other times. Because of rapid plasma clearance, therefore, cytosine arabinoside must be given in multiple doses or by continuous infusion to maintain effective blood and tissue levels for a sufficient period of time to attack a majority of cells at a susceptible time.

Children and adults may experience unique and different side-effects with the same agents, either because of differences in tissue tolerance, such as in the gonads, or in available body space for distribution of the drug, as in the case of intrathecal therapy. The risk of side-effects from brain irradiation with intrathecal or systemic methotrexate appears to be greater in preschool children than in older children and adults.[9] Pediatricians wonder what the cardiac late effects of "safe" doses of doxorubicin will be in children who survive their tumor. The relatively acute toxicity resulting in congestive heart failure may be only one end of a spectrum of potential effects. Long-term follow-up studies are difficult and often done poorly or not at all, but they are essential if we are to maximize the quality of life of children cured of cancer.

SURGERY IN PEDIATRIC ONCOLOGY

The role of the surgeon in the management of children with cancer has many facets. For most solid tumors, surgery provides the best definitive treatment of the primary tumor and, in some cases, metastatic deposits as well. With malignancies that are better treated by radiation or chemotherapy, the surgeon's role may be to obtain tissue for accurate diagnosis. For other tumors, such as Hodgkin's lymphoma, surgery is needed for definitive staging of the tumor so that nonsurgical therapy is delivered appropriately. Complications of treatment, such as peptic ulcer disease, intestinal obstruction, or pneumothorax, often require surgical intervention. More recently, the surgeon's involvement in the supportive care of the child with cancer has expanded because of his or her skills in providing total parenteral nutrition, which is often necessary when gastrointestinal complications of anticancer therapy seriously affect the child's nutritional status or threaten to interrupt therapy.

In contrast to the adult who requires surgery for cancer, the child rarely has underlying cardiovascular, respiratory, renal, or nervous system disease and special pre-operative preparation usually is not necessary. The complications seen are directly related to the operative procedure and problems such as pulmonary embolus and myocardial infarction do not occur.

The major problem encountered during surgery for childhood cancer is excessive blood loss, because the common tumors encountered are large and vascular. They often originate in vascular organs (*e.g.*, hepatoma) or, as in the case of Wilms' tumor and neuroblastoma, they tend to surround major vascular structures such as the vena cava and aorta. Successful removal of these lesions requires meticulous attention to the details of monitoring for blood loss and management of blood replacement during and after surgery. One or two intravenous cannulas (with a sufficiently large internal diameter) are necessary. In preparation for surgery to remove an abdominal tumor, these cannulas should be placed in the upper extremity and not the leg, so that transfused blood will reach the heart in the event that the inferior vena cava is opened or clamped. As a guide to proper transfusion, accurate measurement of blood lost in sponges and by suction in the operating room is necessary. Monitoring of intra-arterial blood pressure, central venous pressure and urine output is essential during the removal of a large tumor. When rapid transfusion is necessary, the blood should be warmed to 37°C and its pH buffered to pH 7.4 to avoid the likelihood of cardiac arrest, which often occurs when large volumes of cold, acid, bank blood (10°C, pH 7.0) are administered to the small child. The surgeon and anesthetist must be aware that what is considered insignificant blood loss in an adult might be life-threatening in a small child with a small circulating blood volume. For example, in an 1 year old, loss of 400 ml of blood represents half of the child's blood volume. Similarly, dangerous overtransfusion can occur with administration as little as 100 ml.

One of the most important differences between the adult and the child is that loss of body heat is greater in the young because of the child's relatively large body surface area, especially under general anesthesia. The small subject tends to become hypothermic, and hypothermia increases cardiac irritability and may cause metabolic acidosis and disturbance in blood clotting. To avoid these problems, normal body temperature should be maintained during surgery by providing a warm operating room environment (as high as 80°F), by using a warming blanket, and by avoiding the infusion of cold intravenous fluids and blood.

A special philosophy of care has developed among pediatric surgeons who treat children with cancer. With rare exception, no child is considered to have disease which is so far advanced that treatment for cure can be ruled out. Therefore, the child with extremely large lesions in difficult to reach locations, and those with metastatic disease are considered operable. At surgery, every attempt is made to remove the entire tumor, but when this is not possible other options are usually exercised. For certain tumors, such as neuroblastoma, subtotal or partial resection is performed because a decrease in tumor volume can improve the results of chemotherapy and radiation. For other tumors, such as rhabdomyosarcoma, a plan which includes biopsy of the tumor, chemotherapy and radiotherapy, and a "second look" operation to remove residual tumor is indicated.

While there is no hesitation to perform a radical procedure for cure, every attempt is made to minimize disability and deformity. Recent advances in chemotherapy and radiotherapy have reduced the need for radical resection in children with certain tumors. For example, in the past, pelvic exenteration and urinary or fecal diversion or both were necessary to cure rhabdomyosarcoma of pelvic organs. It now appears that pre-operative anticancer treatment can reduce tumor size sufficiently so that exenteration and diversion can be avoided in most cases. Similarly, current chemotherapy of osteogenic sarcoma has allowed surgeons to resect the primary tumor and preserve the involved limb without decreasing the cure rate.

An aggressive positive approach is always indicated for the child with cancer because so many potential years of life lie ahead. The otherwise healthy child can tolerate surgical procedures of great magnitude and the ability of young people to adjust to long-term disabilities is truly remarkable.

RADIOTHERAPY IN PEDIATRIC ONCOLOGY

Many differences between children and adults have led to the distinct subspecialty of pediatric radiation therapy. These differences include distinctive histologic types of malignancy with unique clinical features, as well as radiation toxicities seen only in children (*i.e.* growth retardation). Toxic effects such as second tumors may also be more likely in children owing to developing tissues and longer life. Another essential difference is the difficulty in immobilization posed by an uncooperative child who often requires the use of deep sedation or anesthesia to accomplish technically acceptable irradiation. Unlike current adult practice, most children with malignancy undergo surgery, irradiation, and chemotherapy, rather than treatment with only one or two of these modalities. This requires close collaboration in pretreatment planning.

Immobilization is a problem primarily in children 18 months to 25 months of age. It is, fortunately, uncommon for children younger than this age to require irradiation, and when necessary, appropriate restraint and sedation usually suffice to permit adequate treatment. Children older than 3 years can usually be reasoned with and convinced to cooperate by experienced and patient personnel. It is often useful to show a child the treatment room and equipment, introduce him to personnel, and have him observe, by closed-circuit television, another child being treated, to gain his confidence prior to actual treatment. Nonetheless, the 18 month to 36 month old child is often difficult to sedate properly to accomplish the rigorous immobilization demanded: the strength of these children is prodigious and they are able to move about in every restraint device tested. When a protracted series of treatments are required, as for retinoblastoma, the use of ketamine anesthesia offers advantages: optimal immobilization, none of the respiratory depression seen with most sedative and anesthetic agents, and a very short period of anesthesia, sufficient to accomplish treatment but not so prolonged as to risk weight loss from inability to eat or orthostatic pneumonia from prolonged bed rest.

The acute tolerance of radiation therapy by children is at least equal to and, we believe, superior to that of adults, in many respects. Acute gastrointestinal tolerance to wide-field abdominal irradiation at equivalent or larger daily radiation fractions appears to be superior in the child, and recovery of normal tissues, such as the gastrointestinal mucosa, oral mucosa, skin, and bone marrow, appears to be more prompt in the child. For these reasons, we see no point in significantly decreasing the daily radiation fraction size in the child (*i.e.* to <150 rad/fx/day) as advocated by some.[10]

A number of schedules have been published advocating variable radiation doses for specific tumors depending on age at the time of irradiation. Modifications of radiation schedule may be justified by major age-related changes of CNS neurons in normal tissue. For example, incomplete myelinization in the infant has led to a dose reduction of CNS prophylaxis from 2400 rad to 1500 rad or 2000 rad for infants less than 24 months of age with acute lymphoblastic leukemia. The risk of a somewhat lower control rate is justified by the presumably lower risk of functional impairment of successfully treated patients. However, to date no data are available documenting such a functional improvement at the lower doses, and the steep dose–response curve of most human tumors must be considered. Apparently, minor changes in radiation can translate into major differences in control rates. We cannot, however, support the use of schedules that permit variations in dose of more than 100%, such as that advocated by the National Wilms' Tumor Study.[11] No data are available demonstrating a marked difference in radiation sensitivity of Wilms' tumor according to the age of the child at the time of irradiation, and therefore such published schedules almost certainly significantly underdose or overdose the majority of patients. For the National Wilms' Tumor Study, comparison with other published series with nearly uniform control suggests that most children have received higher-than-necessary radiation doses.[12,13]

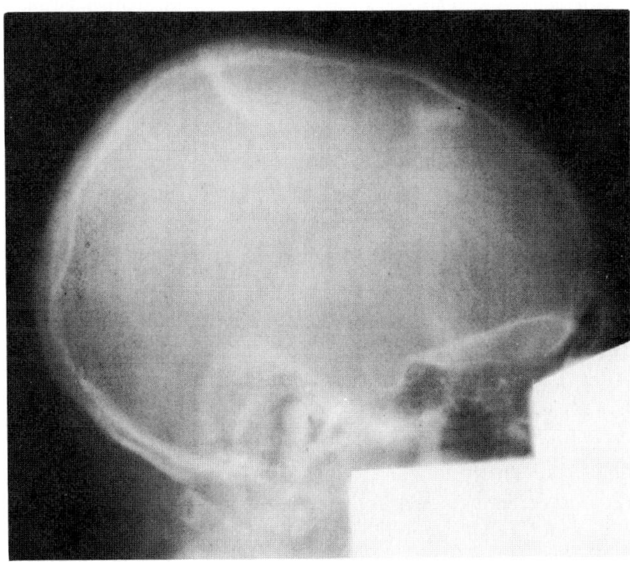

FIG. 34-1. Port film for cranial irradiation. The entire brain and cranial meninges are included. The port includes the first two cervical vertebrae, the retro-orbital spaces and extends beyond the scalp.

Optimum radiation therapy requires precision and reproducibility in daily treatment and appropriate volumes. Also, what may be appropriate treatment for an adult may be inadequate for the pediatric patient. An example of this is represented by "whole brain" irradiation. Principally used for palliative treatment of metastatic disease to brain parenchyma in adults, these fields, when employed for radical treatment of meningeal leukemia, are not appropriate. Technically inadequate fields have been responsible for most instances of primary CNS relapse in irradiated patients referred to our institutions (see Fig. 34-1). This figure illustrates an appropriate field for childhood CNS lymphoma or leukemia, compared with typical adult "whole brain" field.

Several points deserve emphasis. Growth retardation or arrest as a consequence of irradiation represents one of the most noticeable differences between pediatric and adult radiation therapy. Asymmetry created by growth retardation represents a striking consequence of decreased growth. The experienced pediatric therapist will, therefore, plan treatment fields with an attempt to create symmetry wherever possible, especially in visible areas such as the head and neck, or where asymmetry will have major future consequences, as in the spine. Figure 34-16 in the Wilms' tumor section demonstrates the significant dose heterogeneity that will occur when the radiation field is directed so as to just include the edge of the spine. With a radiation dose that is somewhat above the threshold for significant bone growth arrest (2000 rad to 2500 rad), such heterogeneity can lead to major differences in growth across a vertebral body and resultant structural scoliosis despite inclusion of the spine in the treatment field.

Differences in growth rate across a bone may not become evident until the child enters a growth phase.[14]

In addition to growth arrest in bones, a variety of other tissues may fail to develop normally following irradiation. Soft tissue and muscle bulk is often noticeably decreased within a prior radiation field, and this relative asymmetry (especially in muscle strength) may also produce a secondary or acquired scoliosis. Other tissues which may not develop fully include the breast or, less commonly, a major artery or bowel viscus.[15–17]

As the majority of children receiving radiation therapy are also being treated with a variety of chemotherapeutic agents, the potential interaction of these drugs with irradiation must be recognized. Perhaps the most striking and well-recognized of these is the so-called "recall" phenomenon, whereby a child, previously irradiated, with complete disappearance of radiation effects, is administered actinomycin-D, with striking and rapid redevelopment of the prior radiation reaction.[18] Such "recall" has now been described for other agents in addition to actinomycin-D.[19,20] The endothelial vasculitis which appears to be responsible for the overt findings may occur in a variety of other sites including the lung, kidney, and liver.[21,22] A rapid and fulminant pneumonitis or hepatitis may develop which requires intensive therapy, principally with prednisone, to combat it.[23]

A second way in which radiation may interact with drugs is by altering their metabolism, thereby heightening or prolonging the effect of a "safe" dose. An example of this has been described in the treatment of Wilms' tumor, where hepatic irradiation has been shown to enhance the neurotoxicity of vincristine which is metabolized by that organ.[24]

Finally, irradiation toxicity may simply combine in an additive way with toxicity of chemotherapeutic agents. Possible examples of this might include enhanced vincristine neurotoxicity in an irradiated peripheral nerve, or the enhanced cardiotoxicity of doxorubicin when administered to a patient who has received substantial prior irradiation.[25,26]

Perhaps the most tragic complication of treatment is a second malignancy appearing years later in a cured patient. Evidence suggests that tumor incidence is related to site and age treated, use of and technique of irradiation, chemotherapy, or combined treatment, and duration of follow-up[27–34] In addition, mounting evidence suggests that a genetic predisposition for tumor development may significantly enhance risk.[35]

Thus children appear to be more susceptible than adults, and certain organs, such as the thyroid gland, are particularly prone.[29,30,32] The enhanced risk of acute myelogenous leukemia and non-Hodgkin's lymphoma in patients with Hodgkin's disease receiving both irradiation and chemotherapy is well recognized.

Most second tumor data in children have been accumulated in children receiving orthovoltage treatment.[27] Current reports suggest that this incidence may be considerably reduced by the improved technique (and decrease in bone dose) possible with megavoltage.[34] Finally, children with certain conditions, especially retinoblastoma, appear to be particularly prone to the development of second tumors, suggesting a strong genetic association between tumor development, both spontaneous and induced.[35] Based on these findings, Knudsen has postulated a two-hit model for carcinogenesis in these patients.[8]

CHILDHOOD LEUKEMIAS

Leukemia is a neoplastic disease of the hematopoietic and lymphoid tissues which is always disseminated at the time of diagnosis. Leukemia may involve any tissue of the body, but because of its universal involvement of the bone marrow and its greatest concentration there even in the earliest cases, bone marrow involvement is the *sine qua non* of the disease. The types of leukemia seen in children are acute lymphocytic leukemia, acute nonlymphocytic leukemia and chronic myelocytic leukemia. Chronic lymphocytic leukemia, if it occurs at all in children, is extremely rare and will not be discussed further. Acute lymphocytic leukemia (ALL) is the most common variety, accounting for 75% to 80% of all leukemias in childhood. Acute nonlymphocytic leukemia (ANLL), including all of its cytological subtypes (*e.g.* myeloblastic-AML, monoblastic-AMOL, promyelocytic-APML, and so forth) accounts for approximately 20% of all leukemias in children.[36] The remaining 2% to 5% is made up of the two forms of chronic myelocytic leukemia: the adult type, usually with a Philadelphia chromosome, and the juvenile type, which differs in clinical features and course from the adult variety.[37]

EPIDEMIOLOGY AND GENETICS

The etiology of leukemia is unknown. There remains a strong suspicion that leukemia and lymphoma are virus-induced in humans, as they are in several animal species. However, at this time there is no concrete evidence for a human leukemia or lymphoma virus. Clues to etiology come from unusual circumstances in which the frequency of leukemia is greater than in the population at large. Exposure to ionizing radiation or to chemicals such as benzene is associated with an increased frequency of leukemia.[38] The risk of developing leukemia is about 15 times greater in children with Down's syndrome.[39] This real incidence of leukemia (primarily ALL) should not be confused with a self-limited leukemoid reaction sometimes seen in newborns with Down's syndrome.[40] The latter mimics ANLL but disappears without chemotherapy. The occurrence of this phenomenon in a phenotypically normal child with mosaicism for trisomy-21 indicates the need for routine karotyping of all neonates with apparent acute leukemia.[41]

Bloom syndrome, ataxia–telangiectasia, and Fanconi anemia are all autosomal recessive disorders with an increased risk of leukemia.[42] These conditions have in common a defect in DNA repair mechanisms which predisposes to chromosomal instability and resultant malignant degeneration. Such observations are consistent with Knudson's hypothesis that individuals bearing certain germinal cell mutations are at high risk for malignancy after subsequent exposure to poorly defined leukemogenic stimuli.[43] Of particular interest in this regard is the increased occurrence of leukemia in phenotypically normal people who are heterozygotes for Fanconi anemia. Leukemia in childhood is much more likely to occur in an identical twin of an index case than in other siblings.[44] Should acute leukemia develop in one of a pair of twins, the risk of the disease developing in the other is as high as 20% if the first case occurs prior to age 5 years. Most reported cases of leukemia in twins have borne a temporal relationship to each other, with both being diagnosed within a year or two. All of these associations account for only a small fraction of all the childhood leukemia cases but provide potentially important clues in the search for etiology.

One of the contributing factors to the hypothesis that childhood leukemia, and particularly ALL, is caused by a virus is the peak-age frequency between 2 years and 6 years. This is precisely the age at which children are subject to a wide range of viral infections and often develop hyperplasia of such lymphoid organs as tonsils and adenoids as well as lymph nodes. Unlike ALL, there is no peak age incidence during the childhood years for ANLL and the frequency is also similar in both black and white children. In ALL the frequency among blacks is approximately one-half that seen in white children.[45] The significance of this difference is unknown. The chronic leukemias are equally rare in blacks and whites. The juvenile form tends to occur in younger children during the preschool age period, whereas the Philadelphia chromosome-positive variety may occur at any age, but usually in school-age children.[37]

CELLULAR TYPES

The predominant cell type in acute leukemia determines the diagnosis. Most of the time it is not difficult to distinguish ALL from the various types of ANLL using Wright or Romanovsky stains of the bone marrow aspirate. Lymphoblasts are usually relatively small and uniform with scanty cytoplasm showing around the relatively large nucleus. Myeloblasts and monoblasts have more abundant cytoplasm, with cytoplasmic organelles often visible. The presence of an Auer rod is diagnostic of ANLL but is present in the cells of only about 20% to 25% of patients. A cytological subclassification has been developed by a French–American–British group (FAB classification).[46] In ALL three morphologic subtypes are recognized: L-1 (most common), with small cell predominance, scanty cytoplasm and dense homogeneous chromatin; L-2, with a heterogenous cell population, the majority being larger cells having greater amounts of cytoplasm; and L-3 (very rare), with a large uniform basophilic cell population, round nuclei, and dense granular chromatin with one or more prominent nucleoli. Recent evidence suggests that the best prognosis is associated with the L-1 cases. Additional heterogeneity is recognized with the application of cell marker studies (see below). Most cases with L-3 morphology have markers of B-cell differentiation. Otherwise, the appearance of the lymphoblasts does not correlate with the presence of T-cell or other markers. In ANLL, the subtypes are grouped as follows: M-1, poorly differentiated with myeloblasts predominant; M-2, AML with maturation in which bizarre myeloid differentiation is seen; M-3, hypergranular promyelocytic leukemia; M-4, myelomonocytic leukemia; M-5, pure monocytic leukemia; and M-6, erythroleukemia. In 5% or fewer cases of acute childhood leukemia, cytochemical stains are required to establish the specific diagnosis. The problems in morphologic distinction are among L-2 ALL, M-1 AML, and M-5 AMOL. The following stains are helpful when positive: periodic acid Schiff in ALL, sudan black B and peroxidase in AML, and nonspecific esterase in AMOL. When all stains are negative, most hematologists consider such undifferentiated leukemias to be ALL for treatment purposes. This is supported by the fact that many such patients do indeed respond to ALL therapy and that at least half will have surface antigens indicative of lymphoid origin (see below). In addition, the great majority of acute lymphocytic leukemias will have readily detectable nuclear terminal deoxynucleotidyl transferase activity, in contrast to the rarity of this enzyme in acute nonlymphocytic leukemia.[47]

The classification of functional subtypes of acute leukemia has assumed increasing importance in recent years because of differences in prognosis. There are now subtypes of ALL which are antigenically similar to normal T-lymphocytes, normal B-cells, or lymphoid stem cells at various stages of differentiation. In general, patients whose leukemia cells are T-like or B-like do not respond to therapy as well as those who have neither characteristic.[48,49] Subdivisions of even these varieties are also being elucidated, but their prognostic value is not yet established.[50] The use of monoclonal antibodies is enlarging the capacity for biological correlation enormously and also increasing the demonstrable heterogeneity of these diseases.[51] It is possible that direct clinical, etiological, or pharmacological correlations may be made in the future because of the power of distinguishing subclasses of leukemia.

Studies of chromosomes and G-6-PD variants support the hypothesis that the leukemia cell line is a clone.[52,53] This suggests that the leukemogenic event occurs in a single cell and that the conditions for growth and perpetuation of that cell line prevail. It is presumed that most leukemias begin in the bone marrow because of the universal involvement of this tissue and because the marrow is the largest hematopoietic organ. However, the lymphoid malignancies may originate in another tissue and rapidly find extremely fertile soil in the bone marrow to give the clinical features observed at the time of diagnosis.

CLINICAL FEATURES

The chief complaint of children who present with leukemia is often related to the suppression of hematopoietic activity (Table 34-1). Thus, they may present with a minor or major infection, pallor or bruising. Other common complaints are bone pain, which is sometimes misdiagnosed as "growing pains," rheumatic fever, or rheumatoid arthritis.[54] Less common chief complains include enlarged lymph nodes, enlarged abdomen due to hepatosplenomegaly, unexplained fever, and lassitude. Leukemia cells are capable of invading any tissue in the body and, consequently, can cause a wide variety of manifestations, either at the time of clinical presentation or later during the course of the disease. The duration of symptoms may vary from a few days to several months. Often the children with the briefest histories are those with the most fulminant rapidly growing leukemic cell populations.

TABLE 34-1. Clinical Features of Acute Leukemia in Children

Anemia	Pallor, weakness, fatigue
Neutropenia	Infection
Thrombocytopenia	Bleeding tendency
Infiltration of bony cortex and periosteum	Bone swelling and pain
Infiltration of synovial membranes	Arthralgia, sometimes migratory
Splenomegaly	Abdominal protuberance and pain; shortened red cell survival
Hepatomegaly	Abdominal protuberance, loss of appetite, clotting disorders
Lymphadenopathy	Cervical, axillary, inguinal masses, mediastinal widening, abdominal pain
Thymus enlargement (10% of cases)	Superior vena cava syndrome, dyspnea, cough
Hyperplasia of submucosal lymphatic tissue	Abdominal pain, intussusception, G.I. ulceration and bleeding, bowel obstruction
Nephromegaly	Renal failure and/or hypertension
Pericardial effusion (very rare)	Dyspnea, narrow pulse pressure, EKG changes, pericardial friction rub, cardiomegaly
Cranial nerve infiltration (very rare)	Cranial nerve palsies

METHODS OF DIAGNOSIS

The diagnosis may be suspected by the history, by physical findings such as hepatosplenomegaly, pallor, and petechiae and, finally, by the blood count that reveals neutropenia, thrombocytopenia, or anemia, with or without blast cells. A majority of patients with acute leukemia and most patients with chronic leukemia have an elevated leukocyte count. In acute leukemia, a varying proportion of these cells may be blasts, the higher leukocyte count usually associated with a higher proportion of blasts. Patients may present with pancytopenia and have few or no identifiable blasts circulating. In acute nonlymphocytic leukemia and chronic leukemia, the circulating leukemia cells usually reflect the distribution of cells in the bone marrow. However, examination of a carefully prepared bone marrow aspirate is essential for the specific diagnosis of acute leukemia and the cell type of origin. Bone marrow biopsy is not usually required except in very rare cases in which an insufficient quantity of material can be aspirated.

The cerebrospinal fluid should be examined at diagnosis; some defer this examination for a few days. To diagnose central nervous system leukemia, it is not sufficient only to enumerate cells in a counting chamber. Careful examination of a Wright-stained centrifugate is essential to identify small numbers of blast cells in the fluid.

The standard workup for a patient with leukemia should also include a careful history with special attention to questions of exposure to radiation or chemicals and of genetic abnormalities in the family. Blood counts, serum uric acid, electrolytes, and liver and kidney function tests should be obtained. All patients should have a chest roentgenogram in search of thymic enlargement or infectious infiltrate. A serum uric acid and urea nitrogen are mandatory requirements, because they may be elevated at the outset or may become elevated after treatment is begun should there be rapid lysis of leukemia cells.[55] Hypercalcemia is a very rare presenting feature in acute leukemia but needs to be ruled out, as it may contribute to renal dysfunction and hypertension.[56]

The two types of CML must be distinguished from each other and from leukemoid reactions. Helpful points are the presence in "adult" type CML of a Philadelphia chromosome (90% of cases), a low leukocyte alkaline phosphatase, a very high myeloid–erythroid ratio in the marrow, and thrombocytosis. In juvenile CML, the white blood count is not as high as in the adult type (rarely above 70,000/mm^3), anemia and thrombocytopenia are prominent, and the hemoglobin F is elevated.

PROGNOSTIC FACTORS

In children with ALL there are clinical features which are associated with a poor prognosis. An elevated leukocyte count is by far the most important of all clinical prognostic features.[57,58] The prognosis seems to be inversely related to the height of the leukocyte count. Factors of less influence associated with a poor prognosis include central nervous system involvement at diagnosis, massive enlargement of the liver or spleen, age below 2 years or above 10 years of age, and thymic enlargement.[57] The significance of the latter as an independent prognostic feature has been disputed; however, the strong association of the T-cell variant of ALL with mediastinal enlargement and an elevated leukocyte count suggests that they are influential if not independent prognostic features.[59]

Although not completely developed, surface markers, identifying leukemic cells as having B- or T-cell features appear to have prognostic significance.[48,49] The degree of independence of the influence of these variables (discussed further below) is not yet known. For example, patients with T-cell leukemia often have elevated leukocyte counts and therefore have a poor prognosis. Only a small number of patients with T-cell leukemia are in the favorable age range and have leukocyte counts below 10,000/mm^3 with no other poor prognostic features. Until a sufficient number of these patients is followed for a long period of time, it will not be clear whether the biological implications of a T-cell leukemia are independent of the extent of tumor mass.

The most important prognostic feature is often overlooked in discussions of the subject—it is the treatment. Suboptimal or poorly administered treatment has a greater negative impact on the outcome of the disease than any single clinical prognostic feature.

Prognostic features are not well developed for acute nonlymphocytic leukemia and the chronic leukemias because treatment has not been as effective in these types and clinical features are not as readily segregated as a consequence. Among patients with ANLL, those with APML generally have a longer remission and survival duration if one can support the patient past the dangerous initial period of therapy when fatal hemorrhage is a major risk.[60] Such hemorrhage is a consequence of disseminated intravascular coagulation (DIC) triggered by the release of thromboplastic substances from the granules of the malignant cells.[61] DIC also occurs frequently in AMOL and rarely in ALL.[62,63] Patients who present with serious systemic infections are less likely to attain remission and have a shorter duration of survival than those who do not present with such infections. In general, patients with ANLL who present with very high leukocyte counts do not do as well as those who present with normal or low leukocyte counts.[36] In the pediatric age group there are no other major clinical prognostic factors among patients with ANLL. However, recent observations suggest that cytogenetic abnormalities may be an indicator of prognosis.[64]

In the chronic leukemias the Philadelphia chromosome-positive or adult type behaves in children in the same way it does in adults and the prognosis is similar.[37] The median survival is approximately 3 years and the accelerated or blastic phase is the signal for a relatively short subsequent survival. Juvenile chronic myelocytic leukemia, which some have called subacute monocytic leukemia, has a median survival of approximately 1 year and there are no known features at the time of diagnosis which help one to predict the outcome in a given patient or group of patients.[37]

TREATMENT

The strategy for treatment of leukemia is relatively simple and uniform. First, reduce the tumor burden with chemotherapy to the point that normal hematopoietic and metabolic function returns. During this phase of remission-induction therapy, infectious and metabolic complications that either pre-exist or develop during the initial phases of chemotherapy must be managed vigorously. The intensity of chemotherapy must be sufficiently aggressive to induce remission as rapidly as possible and yet not so toxic as to delay substantially the return of normal hematopoietic function. The rationale for more aggressive treatment during this phase is based on the supposition that leukemia cells are most sensitive during the initial period of treatment and that one should take maximum advantage of this opportunity to reduce the leukemia cell mass even lower than that which is required to induce remission. However, one must balance the risk of increased morbidity and mortality of the initial treatment.

The second phase of therapy, which begins after the patient has attained remission, entails the continued destruction of residual leukemia cells that are known to be present, despite the fact that they are undetectable by the usual clinical means. This is the most difficult phase, because treatment must be administered with no visible enemy and one is tempted to give as little treatment as possible to avoid toxic side effects. This phase of therapy would be scientifically enhanced immeasurably should a method become available for detecting extremely small concentrations of leukemia cells in the bone marrow and blood. These principles of treatment may be applied to any form of leukemia, or indeed, any form of cancer.[65] Although the strategy is the same for all forms of leukemia, the tactics differ because of differences in sensitivity to therapy of the major subtypes of leukemia.

Once the diagnosis of acute leukemia is made, treatment should begin promptly, though it is often preferable to invest a day or two in improving the patient's general condition prior to beginning specific therapy.

Supportive Measures

During the initial days of treatment, transfusions of washed packed red blood cells are given to relieve the anemia which is almost invariably present. These must be initiated cautiously in those cases presenting with profound anemia (Hb less than 4 gm/dl) in order to avoid volume overload and heart failure. Platelet concentrates are used to control bleeding due to thrombocytopenia. However, they need not be given simply because the platelet count is low. Many patients, especially during remission induction, experience no significant bleeding despite platelet counts below 20,000/mm^3. The rapid progression of cutaneous bleeding, mucosal bleeding, or suspicion of bleeding into a vital organ are indications for platelet transfusion. Bacterial sepsis should also be suspected in such patients. Despite intensive combination therapy, patients receiving induction therapy for ALL require relatively few platelet transfusions. The major usage of platelet transfusion at many institutions is for patients in relapse, often infected and receiving experimental chemotherapy. In addition, the risk of severe spontaneous bleeding is greater for children with ANLL which justifies a more liberal approach to platelet transfusion in these cases. Depletion of coagulation factors is also more likely for certain subtypes of ANLL (see above). The value of anticoagulation with heparin in patients with DIC due to leukemia is controversial and should not be undertaken prior to an attempt at providing adequate replacement with platelets and fresh plasma. The use of heparin in low dosage as prophylaxis against DIC has been recommended prior to chemotherapy for patients with APML who do not already have an established coagulopathy.[66]

Fluid and electrolytes by intravenous infusion are given mainly during periods of potential hyperuricemia. Potassium-containing solutions should be avoided during maximum cell lysis (first 3 days to 7 days of remission induction therapy). If the leukocyte count is elevated or there is splenomegaly, nephromegaly, thymus enlargement or initial hyperuricemia, sodium bicarbonate and allopurinol are given.

Except for the seriously ill, many children with ALL may be managed as outpatients. Children with ANLL usually require admission in order to manage the complications of the more aggressive chemotherapy they receive. A minimum of hospitalization is desirable for obvious reasons including the comfort of the child and parents, reduced exposure to infectious agents, and reduced cost. Hospital-acquired infections represent a hazard to the leukemic child. The major effort in prevention of infections is directed to diligent attention to simple means such as hand washing, personal hygiene, and education of the patients, their parents, and hospital personnel to these precautions. Routine prophylactic administration of antibiotics is not recommended because it may produce changes in the host's nasopharyngeal and intestinal flora predisposing to the development of antibiotic-resistant organisms. When clinical signs suggest infection, efforts are directed at the identification of the causative infectious agents and their sensitivities to antibiotics. Bactericidal antibiotics are given by the intravenous route and in dosages often greater than used for treating children without underlying diseases. For undiagnosed or suspected sepsis, antibiotic coverage should be directed against both gram-positive and gram-negative organisms.[67]

Life-threatening septicemia during initial induction therapy usually responds to appropriate antibiotic therapy. Rarely, when the causative agents are resistant gram-negative enteric bacteria or when there is deep tissue or intra-abdominal localization, additional support in the form of daily granulocyte transfusions is required until normal hematopoiesis recovers.

Therapy of ALL

As a drug-responsive neoplasm ALL has been a testing ground for the development of concepts in cancer therapy that have broad potential application. In fact, the modern era of cancer chemotherapy was heralded in 1948 by Dr. Sidney Farber's demonstration of the responsiveness of childhood ALL to aminopterin.[68] In the 1950s the disease was seen to respond to several drugs, often to disappear completely, entering a period of remission, only to return and pursue a fatal course within weeks or months. Since then progress has been dramatic.

From studies in the early 1960s which had curative intent has come a framework for leukemia treatment upon which all current programs are built. The first step is to induce remission, making all evidence of leukemia disappear and permitting restoration of normal marrow function and apparent health. The next step is to eradicate the residual, undetectable disease that would otherwise grow again, causing relapse and the eventual death of the patient. This continued therapy during remission aims at leukemia in the bone marrow, the apparent site of origin and most likely site of relapse, but also at leukemia in extramedullary sites such as the meninges of the central nervous system (CNS) where leukemia cells enjoy an environment relatively protected from chemotherapy and multiply unless specific measures are taken. The phases of treatment—remission induction, CNS preventive therapy, and systemic continuation therapy—are discussed individually but it must be emphasized that they are interdependent; the effectiveness as well as the toxicity of one phase has a bearing on that of the others.

REMISSION INDUCTION. Since leukemia is by definition disseminated at clinical presentation, systemic therapy is required throughout the treatment period. A number of drugs such as prednisone, vincristine, or mercaptopurine used as single agents will induce remissions, but none is more than 50% effective. The additive effect of certain combinations of agents demonstrated the superiority of combination chemotherapy over single agents, especially when drugs with different mechanisms of action were employed. For example, the relatively non-toxic combination of prednisone and vincristine could induce remissions with 1 month in 90% of patients, and thus became standard therapy by the late 1960s. The addition of a third drug, such as daunomycin or asparaginase gave marginally superior results and initially was not recommended due to the risk of extra toxicity. However, as indicated earlier, the effectiveness of one phase of therapy may influence the success of another. In particular, the intensity of initial remission induction therapy may affect a patient's chances for leukemia-free survival. An analysis was performed of studies in which the major variable was the nature of the remission induction therapy; the treatment that followed was very similar for all patients.[69] Only 38% of those receiving the two drugs for induction were still in continuous complete remission after 30 months compared to 50% to 60% of those receiving three drugs. Because of these findings the inclusion of three remission-inducing agents has been standard therapy since 1975.

THERAPY DURING REMISSION. Following the attainment of remission one does not continue giving the same drug combination. The toxicity would become intolerable, but more importantly, this approach rapidly selects drug-resistant cells, leading to relapse. By the mid-1960s a number of drugs were known to prolong remissions when given singly. The most active of these were methotrexate, mercaptopurine, and cyclophosphamide in that order. Once again, combinations of these and other agents proved superior and increasing numbers of patients began to experience remissions of 2 years or 3 years duration—in fact, about 15% of patients so treated survive free of leukemia to this day, as long as 12 years after stopping all chemotherapy.

With the use of multiple agent therapy and inevitable toxicity, an important issue was how aggressively one needed to use these drug combinations during remission maintenance. Consequently, a randomized trial was performed in which one group of patients received therapy in maximum tolerated dosages designed to produce a continuous state of leukopenia between 2000 WBC/mm^3 and 3500 WBC/mm^3. A second group received the same treatment schedule but with only one-half the same total daily and weekly doses. Though patient numbers were small in this early study, the results were clear. Nearly one-half of the full dose group were still in remission 3 years later, while the majority of the one-half dose group had relapsed.[70]

With these superior results attainable and fewer patients dying early from uncontrolled leukemia in the bone marrow, proliferation of leukemic cells in the meninges began to assume a greater importance. A CNS relapse became a frequent occurrence for patients still in their first bone marrow remission. Though such a relapse could usually be controlled, it was often followed by neurological morbidity and bone marrow relapses as well, and usually precluded long survival. The pathogenesis of these meningeal proliferations of leukemic cells was uncertain. It did not seem sensible that they could be ongoing metastases from a bone marrow in remission as they occurred so often in the same site while the disease was quiescent elsewhere. Dr. Donald Pinkel proposed the hypothesis that the presence of leukemic cells in the meninges was due to bloodborne seeding *before any therapy* had been given. Conceivably, the CNS was a pharmacological sanctuary wherein lymphoblasts were protected and uninhibited from growth by the same drugs that kept the marrow in remission.

In his early "Total Therapy Studies," the first attempts were made to prevent CNS leukemia with craniospinal irradiation following remission induction. In the low doses of 500 rad to 1200 rad there was still a *primary* CNS relapse rate of 40%. These results were not significantly better than in Study IV in which CNS preventive therapy was temporarily abandoned. A major breakthrough came with Studies V and VI conducted from 1967 to 1971.[71,72] Both employed aggressive combination induction and continuation chemotherapy. Study V was designed to test prophylactic irradiation in a higher dosage for prevention of CNS leukemia. All patients received 2400 rad cranial irradiation combined with intrathecal methotrexate shortly after attaining complete remission. The results were dramatic; CNS leukemia terminated remission in only three patients (10%). Eighteen of the original 31 patients remain in remission and have been off all therapy now for 9 years and are presumed cured. Study VI was a larger randomized clinical trial designed *before* the results of Study V were known. One-half of the patients received 2400 rad craniospinal radiation and one-half no preventive therapy. The irradiated patients had a markedly superior outcome; primary CNS relapse occurred in only two patients of 45, compared to 33 patients of 49 unirradiated. In the subsequent study, the two effective modalities, 2400 rad craniospinal and 2400 rad cranial plus intrathecal methotrexate, were compared prospectively and found to be equally effective.[73] Due to its lower toxicity, the latter was adopted in 1972 as the preferred method of CNS preventive therapy. Its 90% to 95% effectiveness makes it still the standard against which all others must be judged. It is important that the opposing lateral ports include all the meninges and retro-orbital spaces to avoid inadequate therapy (Fig. 34-1).

However, the new found success was not without its price. The intensive treatment program delivered over a period of 3 years was immunosuppressive and left the patient vulnerable to opportunistic infection. As a result an unfortunate 5% to 10% of children tragically died while in remission.

In Study VIII the possibility that more therapy might not be better was explored for the first time.[74] The variable in question was the number of drugs used in combination to maintain remission. Control of leukemia was just as good with maximum tolerated dosages of the two-drug combination methotrexate plus mercaptopurine as with these two plus a third, cyclophosphamide, or a fourth agent, cytosine arabinoside. Two-thirds of the patients on the two-drug regimen were able to have their therapy stopped after 30 months CCR and 80% of those stopping therapy have continued leukemia-free. In fact, the multiple drug regimens were clearly inferior owing to their associated higher risk of infection. The two major culprits were *Pneumocystis carinii* pneumonia and disseminated varicella-zoster, each of which produced marked morbidity and a significant mortality.[75,76] Other toxic manifestations required consideration, but the two-drug program is the basic therapy around which other modifications are tested.[77,78]

The sequential studies of the Cancer and Leukemia Group B (CALGB) demonstrated the progressive improvement of the outcome of treatment for children with ALL using the basic regimen of a three-drug induction including asparaginase, central nervous system prophylaxis and two-drug maintenance with mercaptopurine and methotrexate with periodic pulses of vincristine and prednisone.[79,80] Holland and Glidewell demonstrated that over the years, the complete remission duration progressively improved, reaching an approximately 50% long-term complete remission with the best arms of the series of protocols. The same group also demonstrated that the addition of asparaginase to vincristine and prednisone was more effective when given after prednisone and vincristine had been started. The series of studies from the CALGB and other studies reported by the Children's Cancer Study Group and the Southwest Oncology Group demonstrated that many of the advances in treatment were transferable on a broad scale to a large number of institutions participating in the cooperative group movement, despite the inherent difficulty of attempting to follow protocols in multiple institutions. The effort of these groups was instrumental in raising the overall level of medical care for children with leukemia by establishing standards for treatment and for responsiveness. In institutions where treatment would otherwise be given on an *ad hoc* basis according to the personal whim of the specialist, the existence of a thoughtful protocol from the cooperative group helped to standardize treatment. Many problems were avoided because information was disseminated more rapidly to the participants providing cautions for toxic side effects much earlier than would be noted in an individual's experience. In more recent years, the cooperative groups have employed individual institutions to perform major pilot studies which later became effective groupwide studies. For example, the promising study of Freeman and colleagues employing moderate dose methotrexate, has been transferred to a groupwide study of the CALGB and early reports show similar promise for that treatment approach.[84]

To summarize to this point, a series of studies have established that 30% to 60% long-term leukemia-free survival is attained with treatment for childhood ALL using three drugs for remission induction, CNS preventive therapy with cranial irradiation and intrathecal methotrexate, and the two-drug combination for continuation therapy. Numerous other regimens yielding similar results have been studied including multiple drugs in rotations and intermittent high dose "pulse" therapy.[81,82] Even better results, though with shorter follow-up, have been reported using regimens that give very aggressive multiple agent therapy during the first 2 months and traditional therapy thereafter, and regimens employing infusions of intermediate dose methotrexate.[83-85]

TREATMENT TOXICITY. Most of the short-range toxicity induced by therapy is predictable, self-limited, and can be handled with the supportive measures described above. Following the attainment of complete remission and the delivery of CNS preventive therapy, the majority of children can resume fairly normal lifestyles—continuation therapy does not render them chronic invalids. Opportunistic infections, of which *Pneumocystic carinii* pneumonia was paramount in some centers, are now less frequent. *Pneumocystis carinii* pneumonia has recently been shown to be 100% preventable with the regular administration of oral trimethoprim–sulfamethoxazole.[75,76] Varicella–zoster remains a dangerous infection for these children.

The most significant and disturbing area of toxicity is to the central nervous system. Leukoencephalopathy is a progressive degenerative condition of central white matter which leads to ataxia, spasticity, dementia, and often death. Several cases were observed in the early 1970s when attempts were made to deliver higher than usual doses of intravenous methotrexate during continuation therapy.[74,77] Cranial irradiation seemed to have an adverse effect on the blood–brain barrier, predisposing to the entry of methotrexate into the cerebral substance where it is a potent neurotoxin. As a result, it is now necessary to limit the individual dosage of intravenous methotrexate *following radiation* to avoid this complication.[74] Leukoencephalopathy is rarely seen anymore and is usually restricted to patients who develop recurrent or refractory CNS leukemia in spite of preventive therapy.

The possibility of more subtle long-range CNS toxicity in survivors of ALL is a subject which is lately receiving increased attention. Computerized axial tomography brain scans show some evidence of vertricular dilatation and cerebral calcifications in as many as 50% of patients receiving cranial irradiation, most of whom are asymptomatic.[78] Neuropsychological testing demonstrates gross intellectual function to be satisfactory in most patients but certain abnormalities are becoming apparent. Studies at St. Jude show that one-third to one-half of these children have a shortened attention span, poor short-term memory, and specific learning disabilities particularly in the development of mathematical skills. Those irradiated before the age of 8 years seem to be especially at risk for this complication and should be examined prospectively so that appropriate remedial measures can be taken. Most investigators believe that cranial irradiation is responsible for these problems but to keep things in perspective it must be mentioned that this is just one of a number of medical and social factors which may have a bearing on the school performance of a child treated for a malignant disease. Controlled studies are in progress to define the role of cranial irradiation in contributing to these learning disabilites.

In the meantime, alternative methods of CNS preventive therapy are being explored. The nature of the systemic therapy may have an influence on the risk of CNS leukemia. At Memorial Sloan–Kettering Cancer Center, an aggressive multiple drug program lacking irradiation but utilizing periodic intrathecal methotrexate has been effective in preventing CNS leukemia but the drug schedule has more acute toxicity and is inconvenient to administer.[81] The use of intrathecal methotrexate alone with the more conventional two-drug systemic therapy may be adequate for an as yet undefined subgroup of patients. However, the distribution in the cerebrospinal fluid of drug administered by way of the lumbar route is erratic and unpredictable and may not eradicate leukemic blasts that reside in the meninges over the cerebral convexities or deep within the cortical sulci. Prolonged intravenous infusions of methotrexate in higher than conventional doses may overcome the relatively high CNS threshold and allow a more even distribution of therapeutic concentrations there.[84] This approach is currently under study and seems effective and does not predispose to leukoencephalopathy in patients not previously irradiated. It is also attractive in view of the prospect that higher doses might also favorably influence control of disease in the marrow and other extramedullary sites, a concept presently being tested. Finally, doses of irradiation lower than 2400 rad merit further exploration. Though 1200 rad was not effective in the early studies, it may be possible to define a subgroup of patients for whom 1800 rad is adequate.[86] Long-term prospective studies are underway to determine if these latter two methods are as effective and, at the same time, less toxic than the standard regimen.

TREATMENT FAILURE—"HIGH RISK" ALL. Though toxicity is an important consideration, the most disturbing problem the leukemia therapist faces is failure to control the primary disease. In spite of best efforts, one-half of the patients still relapse in the bone marrow and, though further remissions may be induced, most of these cases have a fatal outcome. Most of the relapses occur early, that is during the 2 years to 3 years that the patient is receiving continuation therapy, and indicate the ominous development of drug resistant disease. An area of active current research involves studies seeking a better understanding of patients at high risk for treatment failure and designing imaginative new programs for them from the outset.

In the early 1970s, when a substantial number of patients were beginning to experience longer remissions, it was recognized that some were much less likely to do well than others. Prognosis was inversely related to the initial leukocyte count. Children with thymic enlargement and those wih massive tumor burdens also had a relatively poor response to therapy. A major breakthrough in the understanding of leukemia cell biology came with the demonstration of the E-rosette-forming lymphoblast.[87] It had earlier been shown that the major subpopulation of normal circulating lymphocytes bears surface receptors which generate rosettes when incubated with sheep erythrocytes. These cells are now well-known as T-lymphocytes, because processing in the thymus is required for them to reach functional maturity. The demonstration that there was a corresponding leukemic T-lymphoblast was the first evidence for variation in the cell lineage of ALL. We now know that patients with T-cell leukemia as defined by E-rosette formation are at high risk for treatment failure. Subpopulations of T-cell leukemia are now being defined using monoclonal antibody techniques. Laboratory and clinical high-risk features overlap each other to some extent, and though a patient may express only one, it is more common to have two or more together. For example, two-thirds of all E-positive patients have a high leukocyte count, a thymic mass, or CNS leukemia at diagnosis. Conversely, not all patients with high risk clinical features have E-rosette positive leukemic cells. What binds the high risk group together is a 20% or worse chance of remaining in complete remission for 2½ years. The initial complete remission rate is 80%, not as good as for the remaining patients, but the main reason for treatment failure is early relapse—the median duration of complete remission is 6 months to 12 months. In view of consistently unfavorable results, it is justifiable to explore radically new directions in treatment for such patients. The likelihood of drug resistance in these patients is so high that new chemotherapeutic agents are needed. Recent investigations suggest a possible future role for the epipodophyllotoxin derivative VM-26 in treatment of "high risk" cases.[88]

The remaining majority of patients, presently designated

"standard risk," are not homogeneous. Though their prognosis is better, and drastic departures from previous treatment design are harder to justify, 30% to 60% will fail conventional therapy. Studies in progress will determine whether further application of lymphoid cell marker studies will refine the ability to assign prognosis and in so doing elucidate additional functional heterogeneity within the ALL population. Surface markers indicative of different phases of lymphoid differentiation are being applied systematically to the study of blast cells from all new patients and a new tentative classification system of ALL is beginning to take shape. We now recognize an expanded concept of T-cell ALL (about 20% of all patients) in which not all are E-rosette forming but in which some express only a T-antigen, evidence of definite but more primitive T-cell origin.[89] Differentiation of the lymphoblast along the B-cell axis to the level of surface immunoglobulin expression is very rare, at most 2% of childhood cases.[49] However, these are important to recognize in view of their remarkably aggressive clinical behavior and apparent identity with non-edemic Burkitt's lymphoma in a leukemic phase. B-cell ALL is also unique in having L-3 morphology (FAB classification).[46,49] The remaining 75% to 80% of cases, until recently labeled null-cell ALL, can be further subdivided. The majority are now referred to as common ALL by virtue of their expression of a common lymphoid stem cell antigen first described by Greaves and known as the ALL antigen.[90] These leukemias are fixed at an earlier stage of differentiation than their T- or B-cell counterparts. In some of these common ALL cases, evidence of differentiation potential along the T or B lines has been described following the recognition of thymic antigens ("pre-T") or cytoplasmic immunoglobulin ("pre-B") respectively.[91] Finally, there is a totally undifferentiated group—about 15% of cases, which fail to express any of the above markers.

It is of interest to see how patients classified according to this compare with respect to presenting clinical features (Table 34-2). With the expanding concept of T-ALL, the majority of clinically high risk patients may be accounted for.[92] On the other hand, high leukocyte counts and other adverse features are unusual in the common ALL group. A preliminary analysis of outcome (average follow-up 20 months) of a group of patients receiving the same therapy shows that induction failures and early relapses are more frequent among T-cell patients (Table 34-3). The great majority of children with common ALL do well. An interesting observation of as yet uncertain significance is a high early failure rate among the patients with undifferentiated blasts that express neither common nor T-cell markers. Perhaps the common ALL antigen is indeed a marker of good prognosis which in the future may contribute to treatment planning.

TABLE 34-2. Clinical Features and Leukemia Cell Surface Markers

	COMMON	T	UNDIFFERENTIATED
WBC > 50,000/mm³	13	19	4
Mediastinal Mass	1	17	0
Early CNS Leukemia	2	5	1
TOTAL	126	33	16

TABLE 34-3. Preliminary Outcome Correlation With Surface Markers

	COMMON	T	UNDIFFERENTIATED
Induction Failure	3	4	4
Relapse	13	8	3
Remission	58	13	5
TOTAL	74	25	12

TREATMENT OF RELAPSE. The management of relapse in ALL differs considerably depending on the site of relapse. Focal relapses in the testes or central nervous system must be treated aggressively since it is still possible that the child may be cured despite the relapse.[93] In either case, it has been our practice to treat focal relapse with irradiation and additional chemotherapy. In the case of CNS relapse, control is usually achieved with periodic intrathecal methotrexate. Following a 1-year period of intrathecal chemotherapy, craniospinal irradiation is given if the patient remains in remission because intrathecal therapy has never permanently eradicated CNS leukemia once it has become clinically active.[88] With this approach one-third of patients with CNS relapse may still enjoy long-term disease-free survival.

Testicular relapse is usually suspected following discovery of painless enlargement of one testicle. The diagnosis should be established by biopsy of both testes; an examination of bone marrow and spinal fluid must be done to establish the focal nature of relapse. Affected testes are irradiated with a dose of at least 2000 rad. In some institutions both testes are irradiated even if only one is shown to be positive on biopsy. It is recommended that a course of systemic remission induction therapy be given on the chance that any leukemia cells that have metastasized from the testes might be destroyed while they are still few in number. Unlike CNS relapse, testicular relapse during the course of continuation therapy is usually accompanied or shortly followed by bone marrow relapse. In fact, it is believed by some that the testes are an entirely different type of focal relapse than CNS because of this accompaniment and that testicular relapse may simply be a harbinger of impending systemic relapse in most cases.

The management of bone marrow relapse is not satisfactory because, with rare exceptions, the child who has had a bone marrow relapse ultimately dies of his disease. Reinduction of remission can be achieved in the majority of cases with conventional agents. The problem is that there are no effective drugs remaining for maintaining remission and further relapses ensue, with the patient becoming totally refractory to therapy within months or at most, a year or two. When promising agents are discovered they are moved to primary therapy since the objective is to attempt to cure the patient with the first remission rather than to allow relapses to occur and to save therapy for that eventuality. However, studies are underway which attempt to improve results for relapsing patients and the development of new agents such as the epipodophyllotoxins and 2′-deoxycoformycin holds promise.

CESSATION OF THERAPY AND THE RISK OF LATE RELAPSE. No one knows the optimal duration of therapy for the child with ALL in continuous complete remission. While the object of continuation therapy is the eradication of all leukemia (or at least leukemic potential), we have no way of knowing whether this has happened when the disease is in remission and below the threshold of detectability. We do know, however, that the drugs used have cumulative toxicities which make it undesirable to continue them indefinitely. It is common practice to electively stop treatment for all patients who have remained in continuous complete remission for 30 months. This length of remission is not synonymous with cure, however, for there is a small but significant risk of late relapse after stopping therapy—16% in the first year after cessation, and thereafter 3% or less.[94] Relapse is extremely rare 4 years or more after cessation of therapy. Cooperative groups currently have ongoing comparative studies of duration of therapy. However, longer therapy with the same agents is unlikely to be more effective and alternative strategies are needed. The pathogenesis of such relapses is not clear at this time. In some patients, late relapse merely represents delayed reappearance of drug resistant cells. The speculation that late relapse is due to a brand new clone, that is, a fresh leukemogenic event in a susceptible host, is tantalizing but cannot be established at present. Though the prognosis has generally been poor, relapses after cessation of therapy tend to be more responsive to treatment than do earlier ones. We now have had the experience in a few cases of delivering a second complete, though slightly different, 30-month course of treatment and of taking patients off therapy a second time.[95]

Some off-therapy relapses may represent persistent leukemia in sites that are protected from the full effects of drugs administered during continuation therapy. Of interest in this regard is that the off-therapy relapse rate is greater in boys than in girls by a factor of 2:1. This is partly explained by the fact that 40% of the late relapses in boys involve the testes, either alone or combined with marrow involvement. The testes may be a protected environment for leukemic cells to persist, inhibited from growth, but not eradicated. In an effort to prevent these late marrow relapses many centers now routinely obtain testicular biopsies prior to stopping therapy in all boys. In these centers so far, subclinical leukemic infiltration is found in about 10%. Testicular radiation therapy (and a 1-year course of chemotherapy) for this selected group may decrease the frequency of relapse after cessation of therapy. However, focal testicular relapse after cessation of therapy is not as unfavorable a sign as it is during therapy. Radiation therapy and additional chemotherapy are effective and the majority of such patients do not go on to relapse in the marrow.

THERAPY FOR ACUTE NONLYMPHOCYTIC LEUKEMIA (ANLL). The treatment of ANLL is not nearly as satisfactory as it is for ALL although significant advances have been made. It is now possible to achieve remission in three of every four patients with acute nonlymphocytic leukemias but the durations of remissions are usually short, averaging only a year or so.[36,96] ANLL in children is substantially the same disease biologically as seen in adults except for a slight therapeutic advantage of youth.

A wide variety of remission induction therapies has been employed.[36,96–99] The two most effective agents are cytosine arabinoside and anthracyclines (daunomycin or adriamycin).[97–99] The most successful regimens have included three days of daunomycin and 5 to 16 days of cytosine arabinoside, the latter by constant infusion. This therapy and all forms of remission induction treatment for ANLL are more toxic than the treatment employed for ALL because of the much narrower therapeutic index. Hypoplasia or aplasia of the marrow is achieved in both types of leukemia. The difference between the two is that lymphoblasts are much more sensitive to chemotherapy and disappear more quickly, allowing rapid recovery of the normal marrow; myeloblasts are more resistant, requiring more aggressive chemotherapy, which has a deleterious effect on normal stem cells. Therefore, the duration of hematopoietic suppression is longer. Most patients will attain remission following one or two courses of aggressive chemotherapy. However, 14 days to 21 days of severe granulocytopenia is to be anticipated and predisposes to a greater risk of early death from sepsis than is the case for ALL patients.

There is no specific form of therapy during remission that can be recommended. In many regimens, the same therapy used for remission induction is employed in a less aggressive scheme throughout the course of remission. Others have taken the approach of giving an intensive consolidation phase of therapy but not subsequent maintenance therapy. Unfortunately, the majority of ANLL patients have drug-resistant cells which lead ultimately to relapse. The most promising chemotherapeutic strategy described has been the use of repetitive intensive treatment resulting in recurrent episodes of marrow aplasia.[93] This approach may indeed provide better control of leukemia but is fraught with complications and can be undertaken only in specialized referral centers.

The frequency of CNS leukemia at the time of diagnosis is higher in ANLL than ALL and the attack rate of CNS relapse is about the same when adjusted for period of time at risk.[36,100] Preventive CNS therapy is effective, but is not a major issue because bone marrow relapse cannot be controlled for sufficiently long periods of time to permit CNS relapse to be a major factor limiting complete remission duration.[101] Nonetheless, modest preventive CNS therapy, such as periodic intrathecal injections of methotrexate, should be given as much to avoid the nuisance of CNS relapse as to prolong remission.

The optimal duration of therapy for those children with AML who remain in complete remission is unknown. Treatment periods ranging from 4 months to indefinitely have been proposed.[96–99] However, the data are insufficient to draw firm conclusions concerning the relative efficacy of each.

CHRONIC MYELOCYTIC LEUKEMIA IN CHILDREN. The treatment of CML is completely unsatisfactory. The adult or Philadelphia chromosome positive (Ph′-positive) type of CML is generally treated in the same way in children as it is in adults. A conventional approach is to administer busulphan to lower the leukocyte count and reduce the size of the enlarged abdominal organs. This results in a variable period of symptom-free disease control, but is not a remission in the true sense as the circulating blood cells remain Ph′-positive. Chemotherapy has not resulted in cure and, in fact, the median duration of survival has not changed appreciably over the past 30 years. A more aggressive approach has been tried in which an attempt is made to eradicate the Philadelphia chromosome.[102] This is based on the premise that there remains a non-Philadelphia chromosome-bearing clone of normal cells that has been overwhelmed by the malignant clone. Aggressive chemotherapy has successfully eliminated the Philadelphia chromosome, at least temporarily, in some patients, but this method requires further study. Bone marrow transplantation also shows promise for this disease.[103] The natural history of Ph′-positive CML is to remain in a stable phase for months to years when the leukemic cells lose their capacity to differentiate resulting in the accumulation of primitive cells and bone marrow failure (a "blast crisis").

In 60% of these cases the crisis then resembles ANLL but is extremely refractory to attempts at remission induction with a complete response rate below 10% and subsequent survival rarely exceeding 2 months. The remaining 40% have an acute phase in which the blast cells are indistinguishable morphologically from those of ALL. In addition, they are usually positive for terminal deoxynucleotidyl transferase and the common ALL antigen.[104] Patients with lymphoid blast crisis frequently attain complete remission with prednisone and vincristine though relapse can be expected within a few months.[105] Occasionally, the blast crisis of CML has a mixed lymphoid/myeloid character and differential sensitivity to chemotherapeutic agents can be seen in the two leukemic populations. These divergent courses in the evolution of Ph′-positive CML should not be interpreted to mean that more than one leukemic clone is present. In fact, the Ph′ chromosome is found in all the leukemic cells. Instead, these observations suggest that CML begins in a very primitive stem cell with the potential to differentiate along one or more lines. More recently, the Philadelphia chromosome has been found in cases of ALL occurring with no antecedent chronic phase.[106] A few of those reported have gone on to manifest typical CML while in apparent complete remission of ALL.[107] Most likely the spectrum of Ph′-positive disease will enlarge as more systematic studies are done of bone marrow chromosomes in leukemic patients.

Juvenile CML is a strange disorder which has many features in common with but is easily distinguished from the adult form of CML.[37] It tends to occur in younger children, to have a lesser degree of myeloid hyperplasia, and a greater degree of thrombocytopenia. The malignant cells frequently have a monocytic appearance and tend to form monocyte colonies *in vitro*.[108] There is no specific chromosomal marker and true blast crisis does not occur. However, the disease may have an accelerated phase in which the proportion of primitive cells increases and thrombocytopenia worsens. There is no satisfactory form of treatment for this disorder. The median survival is approximately one year and this course has not been significantly modified by chemotherapy. Splenectomy has been proposed as a treatment in the past, but this form of therapy would appear to be effective in only a peculiar subgroup of juvenile CML.[37] Apparent cure of juvenile CML has been reported following marrow transplantation.[109]

BONE MARROW TRANSPLANTATION FOR LEUKEMIA. This approach is one of the more exciting developments in leukemia therapy. It is still under development and considered a research effort rather than a definitive treatment, but progress for the treatment of all forms of leukemia has been most impressive. Results are especially good for the acute leukemias when the patient receives a transplant during remission rather than while in relapse and infected and bleeding.[110,111]

The sequence of events for a bone marrow transplantation are the following: the patient who has an HLA-matched donor, usually a sibling, is given total body irradiation or aggressive chemotherapy or both in an attempt to eradicate all residual leukemia cells. In addition, of course, this should eradicate normal bone marrow stem cells. The donor's marrow is infused into the patient and engraftment occurs readily in this population. The problems that are encountered subsequently include serious infection, graft *versus* host disease and relapse of leukemia despite the treatment. However, whereas only 10% to 15% of patients were survivors in the initial studies, it appears that a higher proportion of long-term survivors will result from more recent studies in which patients are given the transplant during clinical remission of leukemia.

It is impossible to make detailed recommendations of who should receive a bone marrow transplant because the procedure remains investigative and facilities are limited. As a rule, however, it would appear that the risk and difficulties of bone marrow transplantation would be worthwhile when no effective alternative therapy is available. Since only one-third of patients have an acceptable donor, however, for the time being it is unlikely that this will become a therapeutic substitute for conventional therapy.

CONCLUSIONS

Current therapy for childhood ALL is good and certainly much better than what was available as little as 10 years ago. Depending on the study, between 40% and 60% of children with ALL are now long-term survivors, even after therapy has been discontinued for several years. However, results are not nearly as good in patients who have identifiable poor risk features and no modification of therapy has significantly changed the outcome of this population of patients. There is good evidence that the answer is not "more is better," since a variety of aggressive multiagent regimens has failed to modify the course of this population of patients.

The hope for the future lies in the development of new agents such as the epipodophyllotoxins and 2-deoxycoformycin, the more effective use of current agents such as methotrexate and the anthracyclines, the more strategic combining of agents to take advantage of therapeutic synergism, and the identification through biological studies of potential areas in which a therapeutic advantage may be identified. The identification of subclasses of leukemia by immunological probes may provide leverage in this direction. Though progress has been less dramatic for the non-lymphocytic leukemias, based upon recent results, there is reason to be optimistic about the future.

Among those who are already long-term survivors of leukemia therapy, the quality of life is generally good. For some, however, the cumulative effects of combination chemotherapy and radiation therapy have resulted in undesirable disturbances of neuropsychological and endocrine function, and of growth. The possibility of second malignancy is of concern but so far has been very rare. Obviously, with considerable progress being made toward the cure of childhood leukemias, the issue of late effects assumes increasing importance. The next generation of treatment studies, in addition to further attempts at improving the proportion of survivors, will need to develop strategies aimed at clearly defining and minimizing these late sequelae.

NON-HODGKIN'S LYMPHOMA

All malignant lymphomas not considered to represent Hodgkin's disease have been designated as non-Hodgkin's lymphoma (NHL).[112] The use of this negative terminology has brought little clarification and considerable confusion to understanding with the implication that NHL is a single entity. In fact, it represents a varied and heterogenous collection of diseases with differing clinical presentation, behavior, pathology, and prognosis. Therapeutic strategies must also differ if optimum results are to be achieved. Unlike Hodgkin's disease, where relatively minor differences in natural history exist between the pediatric and adult populations, the group of NHL malignancies differ in many respects from their adult counterparts. Using the Rappaport classification, the pediatric tumors are virtually always diffuse rather than nodular, tend to present in different primary locations (terminal ileum, gastrointestinal tract, mediastinum), develop more frequent "conversion" to a leukemic picture and also develop more frequent primary central nervous system (CNS) relapse.[113–117] Cell surface markers carry different prognostic implications, with B-cell tumors in children usually causing rapid demise, while in adults, tumors with these markers often have a more indolent course.[116–118] Finally, 2-year disease-free survival in children usually constitutes cure while continuing relapse is seen even after 10 years in adults, especially those with certain nodular lymphomas.[117,119]

Another difficulty in classification is posed by the separation between childhood NHL and acute leukemia. To date, this separation has been arbitrary and based on the presence or absence of circulating malignant cells or extent of involvement of the bone marrow rather than on any proven biological difference. Thus, at St. Jude Children's Research Hospital (SJCRH), children must have greater than 25% marrow involvement with blasts to be considered leukemic. Eleven of 69 children with NHL seen from 1975 to 1978 at SJCRH had greater than 5% and equal to or less than 25% blasts in the bone marrow.[120] In contrast, at Memorial Hospital in New York, any confirmed marrow involvement in a child with NHL does not currently categorize a child as leukemic, while at the Children's Hospital Medical Center (CHMC), the Joint Center for Radiotherapy (JCRT), and the Sidney Farber Cancer Institute (SFCI), children with greater than 5% blasts in their initial marrow aspirate are considered to have leukemia.[116] These differing definitions create obvious differences in the homogeneity of patient mix from one institution to another. This relative heterogeneity makes intercomparison of treatment efficacy between institutions difficult. The most cogent criticism of the arbitrary nature of the separations between leukemia and NHL has been well summarized by Magrath and Zeigler.[121] They state that

> the terms leukemia and lymphoma can be seen to have definite limitations in their usefulness. They have evolved as descriptive terms . . . but they do not accurately represent major subdivisions of lymphoid malignancy. In particular, arbitrary designations of lymphoid malignancy . . . on the basis of the percentage of tumor cells in the bone marrow is probably of little or no value. Apart from the inaccuracy of such quantitation . . . the basing of therapeutic decisions on this type of information is hazardous.[121]

INCIDENCE AND EPIDEMIOLOGY

NHL is approximately 1.5 times as common as Hodgkin's disease in childhood and collectively these tumors represent the third most frequent category of childhood malignancy.[116,122] As annual incidence rate of approximately 7 cases per million children less than 15 years old has been reported. A striking male predominence of 2.5:1 to 3:1 has been regularly observed.[117,123] The peak incidence occurs from the age of 7 years to 11 years. Involvement before 3 years of age is uncommon.[124]

A greater than expected risk of development of NHL has been reported in a variety of conditions, including the Wiskott–Aldrich syndrome, ataxia–telangectasia, X-linked agammaglobulinemia, Chediak–Higashi syndrome, and a number of other diseases with associated abnormalities in immune function.[125,126] A specific immuno deficiency to Epstein–Barr virus may account for the increased risk of NHL, especially Burkitt lymphoma, observed in a syndrome recently reported by Purtilo and colleagues.[127,128]

Patients receiving chronic immunosuppressive therapy following organ transplantation have been shown to carry a heightened risk of developing NHL, especially of the brain.[129]

Both Epstein–Barr virus and malaria have been implicated in the development of Burkitt's lymphoma in African children.[121,130–132] Nearly all African Burkitt children have been noted to have the genome for EB virus incorporated in their DNA. Similar associations do not appear to be present in most children developing American Burkitt lymphoma.[133–135]

Chronic treatment with hydantoid drugs including phenytoin (Dilantin) has been associated with development of both pseudolymphomas and true malignant lymphomas, including both Hodgkin's disease and NHL.[136]

Despite circumstantial evidence implicating both abnormalities in immune function and chronic immune stimulation, principally related to the Epstein–Barr virus, the precise etiology of NHL remains unknown.

CLINICAL PRESENTATION

The variety of sites containing lymphoid tissue, including lymph nodes, Peyer's patches, Waldeyer's ring, thymus, and bone marrow, creates considerable heterogeneity in clinical presentation. However, a few typical symptom aggregations account for the majority of case presentations.

More than one-third of affected children present with gastrointestinal involvement.[114,116,117,124] Symptoms for this group range from right-lower quadrant pain and other symptoms, including nausea and vomiting typical of intussusception seen in children with ileo-caecal and appendiceal tumors, to rapid onset of diffuse abdominal pain, ascites, fatigue, malaise, and weight loss, seen most often in children with diffuse, undifferentiated tumors, especially of the Burkitt type.[137,138]

Approximately one-quarter of children with NHL present with mediastinal involvement, especially in the anterior compartment. These tumors are typically of the diffuse lymphoblastic type with T-cell surface markers.[139,140] These children are characteristically pre-teen or early teen-age males who present because of respiratory difficulty, cervical or supraclavicular lymphadenopathy, or on occasion, with the superior vena caval syndrome.

Less commonly, children present with regionally limited disease affecting the tonsil, nasopharynx or other portions of Waldeyer's ring, or adenopathy involving the neck. Other regional sites include the bone, usually monostotic but occasionally multiple and very rarely contiguous (*i.e.*, pelvis, femur, and sacrum) bones, skin, gonad, or central nervous system. Systemic symptoms, including unexplained fevers, often of an erratic and widely fluctuating nature, night sweats, often drenching in character, and weight loss are relatively common, particularly in children with more advanced disease. The importance of these symptoms as independent prognostic factors is not known in view of their frequent association with extensive disease.[117,141]

The typical presentation of African Burkitt's lymphoma with often massive tumors of the maxilla or mandible, with or without orbital involvement, is rarely seen in the United States, even in patients with Burkitt histology.[142–144] The overwhelming majority of children with American Burkitt tumors present with massive abdominal disease, occasionally combined with central nervous system or bone marrow involvement at presentation.[138] Only 30% to 50% of African children present with this advanced disease. Involvement of the pleura, pericardium, and kidneys is noted quite frequently in American cases (see below). As noted above, the histologic subtype and immunologic surface characteristics, as well as the likely natural history can often be predicted by the mode of clinical presentation.

These tumors are rapidly growing and clinical symptoms and signs are usually of short duration, rarely extending more than 6 weeks to 8 weeks.

PRETREATMENT EVALUATION

A rapid and expeditious assessment of disease extent is mandatory to permit treatment to commence with as little delay as possible. The child who presents with probable lymphoma should be rapidly evaluated with a thorough history and physical examination. A complete blood and platelet count should be obtained as well as a careful differential looking for circulating blasts. A postero–anterior and lateral chest roentgenogram should be obtained to assess mediastinal, hilar, pericardial or pleural involvement, in addition to evaluating the trachea and bronchi for patency and displacement.

In the child suspected of having NHL, especially when the mediastinum is involved, a bone marrow aspirate may establish the diagnosis and obviate the necessity for surgical intervention.[145]

In general, the role of surgery will be limited to lymph node biopsy or, perhaps, incisional or excisional biopsy of a mass. In view of the relative frequency of abdominal presentations, laparotomy will be necessary for biopsy or therapy in many children. In those children with regionally limited disease affecting the terminal ileum and caecum with or without mesenteric nodes, an ileo–transverse colectomy and anastamosis will be both diagnostic and therapeutic. In the more frequently seen child with massive abdominal involvement with or without malignant ascites, surgery will usually be limited to biopsy although some investigators have suggested that more aggressive attempts at removal of bulk abdominal tumor in patients with Burkitt's tumor has yielded improved results.[146]

Should abdominal exploration be necessary, the surgeon should take this opportunity to biopsy the liver and regional lymph nodes, including the para-aortic nodes, as well as any other suspicious areas to evaluate their status. Splenectomy for staging is not recommended, as it will almost never influence therapeutic management decisions. Similarly, for those children in whom it is not essential for establishment of the diagnosis, laparotomy is not recommended for staging purposes. It is important that tissue at the time of biopsy be made available not only for histopathologic study including imprints, but also for immunologic surface typing, as management decisions may differ considerably, depending on immunologic characteristics (see below).

Mandatory and optional staging procedures for the child in whom a diagnosis of NHL has been confirmed are shown in Table 34-4.

TABLE 34-4. Staging Procedures for NHL

MANDATORY
1. CBC, Platelet count, differential
2. Chest PA and lateral
3. Bone marrow aspirate and biopsy
4. Lumbar puncture with millipore or cytocentrifuge exam of CSF
5. Liver function tests
6. BUN and creatinine
7. Uric acid level

OPTIONAL (depending on clinical circumstances)
1. Bone scan ± skeletal survey
2. Intravenous urogram
3. Barium studies of the GI tract
4. Myelography
5. Tomography
6. Lymphangiography*
7. Serum electrolyte levels

*rarely indicated

Histopathology and Immunologic Classifications

As noted earlier, nearly all children with NHL have a diffuse pattern on conventional histologic examination of affected tissue. Rare examples of true nodular NHL in childhood have been reported, however, most examples will, in fact, constitute benign conditions or the lymphocyte predominant subtype of Hodgkin's disease.[116,147] Diffuse, well-differentiated lymphocytic lymphoma is not seen in childhood.

Most pediatric NHL can histologically be grouped in one of four categories if the Rappaport classification is used with suitable modifications.[148,149] Most common is the diffuse lymphoblastic type encountered most frequently in patients with supradiaphragmatic disease especially with anterior mediastinal involvement.[139] Seen with approximately equal frequency are histiocytic, undifferentiated Burkitt type and undifferentiated non-Burkitt lesions. The latter two categories are seen most often in children with primary gastrointestinal disease, while the histiocytic lesions may occur at a variety of sites, including Waldeyer's ring, bone and, on occasion, with axial nodal disease. Of 49 consecutive children seen at CHMC/SFCI, 23 had lymphoblastic, seven had histiocytic and 13 had undifferentiated lesions (six, Burkitt, and seven, non-Burkitt). Six patients' lesions were unclassified.[116,120]

A number of other systems have been proposed for classification of NHL. Of these, the system of Lukes and Collins has gained the most widespread use.[150] In this system, the lymphoblastic (convoluted) lesion is equated with "convoluted lymphocytic" while the remainder of lesions seen in children are "follicular center cell" lesions, except for the rare immunoblastic sarcoma and true histiocytic lesions.[116]

The surface characteristics of the lymphoblastic lesions are similar to T-lymphocytes and form rosettes with sheep erythrocytes or react with human antithymocyte sera.[139,151] Burkitt lymphoma cells react immunologically as B-lymphocytes and can be shown to have surface immunoglobulins.[121,152,153] The remainder of the lesions seen in NHL react in a heterogeneous way and many react as null cells with no definite T- or B-cell surface antigens.[154-156] The development of monoclonal antibodies may improve the analysis of surface markers considerably and improve the subclassification of these lesions.[157-158]

STAGING SYSTEMS

Although used in the past and shown to have some prognostic significance when treatment was largely limited to the local modalities of surgery and irradiation, the Ann Arbor Classification, devised for Hodgkin's disease, has numerous deficiencies when applied to childhood NHL.[159] These deficiencies have been discussed at length and will only be briefly summarized here.[117,120,160-162] Unlike Hodgkin's disease, NHL in the child is not orderly or predictable in its relapse pattern. In addition, prognosis is not readily determined by the number of sites affected. As an example, solitary mediastinal involvement carries a grave prognosis in most reported series. The indistinct separation between NHL and leukemia also makes a system which relies primarily on anatomic extent of lymph node disease of doubtful significance. Finally, many pediatric lymphomas do *not* arise in a lymph node or node groups which further complicates the use of the Ann Arbor system.

Murphy and Wollner have proposed systems which answer many of these problems and are clearly superior to the Ann Arbor system:[141,160,161] Murphy's system is shown in Table 34-5. As can be seen, any patient with thoracic disease and patients with extensive abdominal disease are assigned advanced stages. Certain problems remain, however, even with this improved system. Any patient with bone marrow involvement is considered to have Stage IV disease and it is conceivable that certain of these children, considered to have leukemia in other institutions, are overstaged. Children with extensive abdominal disease, who account for the majority of treatment failures in most recent series where routine aggressive multiagent chemotherapy combined with surgery and irradiation has been used, are grouped as Stage III and may thus be understaged, especially should this system be used for Burkitt lymphoma. No system to date has incorporated

TABLE 34-5. SJCRH Staging System for Childhood NHL

STAGE I

A single tumor (extranodal) or single anatomic area (nodal), with the exclusion of mediastinum or abdomen.

STAGE II

A single tumor (extranodal) with regional node involvement.
Two or more nodal areas on the same side of the diaphragm.
Two single (extranodal) tumors with or without regional node involvement on the same side of the diaphragm.
A primary gastrointestinal tract tumor, usually in the ileocaecal area, with or without involvement of associated mesenteric nodes only.

STAGE III

Two single tumors (extranodal) on opposite sides of the diaphragm.
Two or more nodal areas above and below the diaphragm.
All the primary intrathoracic tumors (mediastinal, pleural, thymic).
All extensive primary intraabdominal disease.

STAGE IV

Any of the above with initial CNS and/or bone marrow involvement.

(Murphy SB, Childhood non-Hodgkin's lymphoma. N Engl J Med 299:1446—1448, 1978; Murphy SB: Prognostic factors and obstacles to cure of childhood non-Hodgkin's lymphoma. Sem Oncol 4:265–271, 1977)

TABLE 34-6. Burkitt Tumor Clinical Staging System

A.	A single extra-abdominal tumor
B.	Multiple extra-abdominal tumors
C.	Intra-abdominal tumor ± a single jaw tumor
D.	Intra-abdominal tumor with extra-abdominal sites
AR.	Patients in whom all intra-abdominal tumor has been resected*

(Magrath IT, Lwanga S, Carswell W et al: Surgical reduction of tumor bulk in management of abdominal Burkitt's lymphoma. Br Med J: 308–312, 1974; Ziegler JL, Magrath IT: Burkitt's lymphoma. In Ioachim HL, (ed): Pathobiology Annual. New York, Appleton-Century Crofts, 1974, pp 129–142; Magrath IT, Lee YJ, Anderson T et al: Prognostic factors in Burkitt's lymphoma. Cancer 45:1507–1515, 1980)

*Patients who have had more than 90% of tumor removed may also be considered 2 in this category in some studies.

immunologic marker information. In view of its relatively different natural history, a separate staging system has been proposed for patients with Burkitt lymphoma.[146,162] This system, which appears to have prognostic value for this variant of lymphoma, is shown in Table 34-6.

TREATMENT

Optimum therapy for the child with NHL is a matter of considerable controversy. However, certain principles of treatment are agreed upon by most investigators and will be enumerated here followed by more detailed and potentially controversial recommendations for individual presentation sites.

1. Multiagent systemic chemotherapy should be utilized in all patients with childhood NHL, regardless of initial stage. Despite a substantial and well-documented fraction of survivors following aggressive local treatment (principally irradiation) for early stage disease in certain sites, results, even for favorable patients, can usually be significantly enhanced by the routine use of systemic therapy. Survival of 30% to 60% of patients with early stage disease was reported in the past, using aggressive local treatment with or without single agent systemic treatment.[114,164,165] Results for these favorable patients have been considerably improved by addition of more aggressive systemic treatment and 70% to 90% of these patients appear to be controlled currently with multidisciplinary treatment. This observation, coupled with the infrequent salvage of patients with relapsed NHL, makes optimum initial treatment essential.[116,117,120,141,168]

2. With the exception of patients who present with limited mediastinal, skin, or Burkitt tumors, the incidence of primary CNS relapse is sufficiently low in patients with regional disease limited to a single site that specific therapy directed against potential CNS disease ("prophylaxis") does not appear to be indicated. Conversely, patients who present with primary mediastinal disease have a substantial risk of CNS relapse and appear to benefit from CNS prophylaxis, as do patients with more advanced disease.[117,120,140,166–168]

3. Although several systemic regimens have yielded impressive results for the majority of children with NHL, to date no single multiagent regimen is appropriate for all patients. Thus, regimens omitting doxorubicin have been less effective for patients with mediastinal T-cell disease and doxorubicin regimens omitting cyclophosphamide have not been successful in treatment of Burkitt lymphoma.[116,117,120,168]

4. Involved field high-dose irradiation delivered to patients with limited disease (excluding mediastinum) combined with one of a number of multiagent systemic regimens has achieved a high level of local control and overall success. This successful multidisciplinary approach for these patients is favored as optimum therapy by most investigators. Table 34-7 details several systemic regimens that have been successfully utilized for both this group and those with more extensive disease.[117,120,165–170]

5. Supplemental irradiation delivered to all known disease sites or prior "bulk disease" sites for patients with advanced disease that is not regionally limited has not been shown to improve results over those achieved with systemic therapy alone (excluding CNS disease) and is associated with increased acute and potential long-term morbidity. It is not, therefore, generally recommended.[117,120]

THERAPEUTIC RECOMMENDATIONS FOR SPECIFIC SITES OF PRESENTATION AND HISTOLOGY

Undifferentiated Non-Burkitt Tumors of the Terminal Ileum, Cecum, and Appendiceal Region

Surgical resection of all gross disease should be performed if possible. Usually, this can be accomplished by ileo–transverse colectomy in patients with limited disease.[137,171] In addition to removal of the appropriate regional mesentery, biopsy of liver and para-aortic nodes should be routinely accomplished. Should no additional therapy be delivered, local recurrence and relapse occur regularly even in children with limited disease.[170]

Routine administration of whole abdomen irradiation to 2400 rad to 3000 rad will markedly improve both local control and survival for children with disease limited to the bowel with or without mesenteric node involvement.[137,170,171] This is one of the few clinical settings where withholding systemic therapy can be proposed for a child with NHL with justification. However, because relapse is still a potential risk, routine administration of systemic therapy in addition to surgery and irradiation is favored.[117]

More recently, the administration of systemic chemotherapy following surgery without irradiation has been proposed and accomplished in selected patients.[172] To date, a rigorous trial of the possible therapeutic options (radiation plus chemotherapy, radiation without chemotherapy, chemotherapy without irradiation) has not occurred, and such a trial, assessing

TABLE 34-7. Several Chemotherapy Regimens in use for Childhood Non-Hodgkins Lymphoma*

REGIMEN (REFERENCE NUMBER)	REMISSION INDUCTION	CONSOLIDATION	MAINTENANCE
LSA_2/L_2 (141,165)	Cyclophosphamide Prednisone Vincristine Daunomycin Methotrexate (I.T.) ± Radiotherapy	Cytosine Arabinoside Thioguanine Asparaginase BCNU Methotrexate (I.T.)	Thioguanine Cyclophosphamide Hydroxyurea Daunomycin Methotrexate BCNU Cytosine Arabinoside Vincristine Methotrexate (I.T.)
APO (140)	Adriamycin Prednisone Vincristine ± Radiotherapy	Adriamycin Prednisone Vincristine Mercaptopurine Asparaginase Methotrexate (I.T.) Cranial Radiation	Adriamycin Prednisone Vincristine Mercaptopurine Methotrexate
SJCRH (120)	Cyclophosphamide Prednisone Vincristine ± Adriamycin ± Radiotherapy	± Cranial Radiation Methotrexate (I.T.)	Mercaptopurine Methotrexate
COMP (167)	Cyclophosphamide Prednisone Vincristine Methotrexate (I.V. + I.T.) Radiotherapy	) Repeated monthly	

*See Reference 168 for other regimens.

both relative disease control and late treatment consequences, is necessary prior to endorsing therapy other than the currently recommended approach.

Children with more advanced disease (*i.e.*, with para-aortic nodes) or with an unresectable primary lesion are more difficult to manage and carry a much more ominous prognosis. Multiagent chemotherapy should take therapeutic precedence for several cycles, perhaps followed by a second laparotomy with primary site resection with or without irradiation. Routine CNS prophylaxis for children with advanced disease is recommended.

T-Cell Lymphoblastic Lymphoma of the Mediastinum

Aggressive multiagent chemotherapy with an anthracycline-containing regimen is the mainstay of treatment for these children. Emergency irradiation for tumor-related compromise or superior vena caval syndrome may be necessary, but such irradiation should be stopped as soon as the acute problem has improved. Although an occasional patient will show persistent or recurrent mediastinal disease, the substantial morbidity (esophagus, heart and lung) of adding mediastinal irradiation to effective chemotherapy makes routine irradiation inadvisable. Should persistence or recurrence develop, localized irradiation of 3500 rad to 4000 rad in 3.5 weeks to 4.5 weeks, combined with an alternate chemotherapy regimen, may be effective.[116,117,140]

In addition to "leukemic conversion," these patients have a substantial risk for primary CNS relapse, which may occur prior to development of bone marrow disease or a leukemic state.[167] Routine prophylaxis with craniocervical irradiation or intrathecal methotrexate or both as recommended for acute lymphoblastic leukemia is advised[116,117,165]

The best results to date have occurred when either the LSA_2/L_2 regimen, utilized at New York Memorial Hospital, or the APO regimen (JCRT, CHMC, SFCI) has been used. A recent randomized trial conducted by the CCSG also verifies the efficacy of the LSA_2/L_2 regimen for this clinical setting, as contrasted to a regimen containing cyclophosphamide, vincristine, prednisone, and methotrexate. Using these regimens, more than 65% to 70% of these patients have been disease-free at more than 3 years.[116,117,165,167,169]

Some patients treated with the APO regimen have developed late testicular relapse, which further supports the close relationship of this disease with T-cell leukemia.[173] At present, the advisability and place of routine testicular "prophylaxis" for such patients is not known.

Despite many similarities between lymphoblastic lymphoma and T-cell leukemia, the difference in response to similar therapy is striking. The excellent results using the APO regimen for children with no detectable marrow involvement have been cited. Using a very similar regimen for children with bone marrow involvement, results were poor, with relapse-free survival of much less than 20% at 2 years.[175]

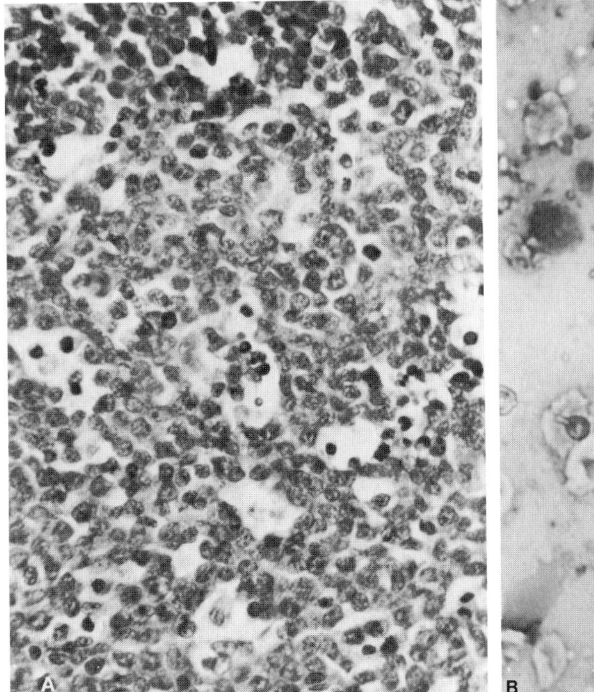

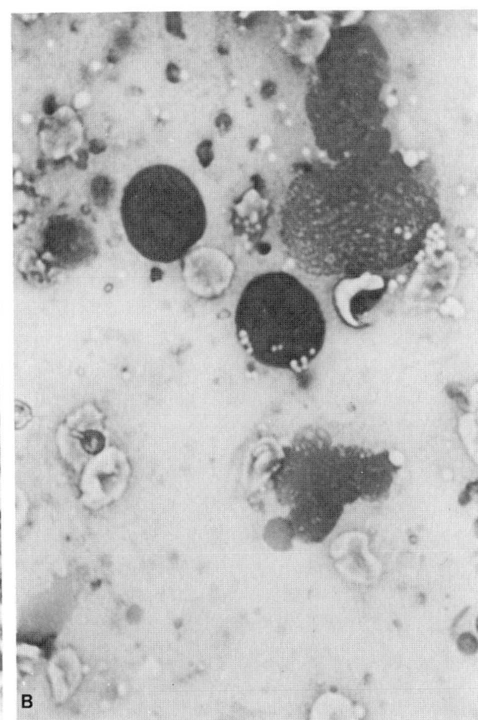

FIG. 34-2. Photomicrographs of Burkitt lymphoma. Typical "starry-sky" appearance is seen on left (*A*) with interspersed macrophages with ingested lipid, nuclear, and cytoplasmic debris in presence of undifferentiated Burkitt cells. Panel on right (*B*) demonstrates magnified appearance of Burkitt cells with vacuoles.

Perhaps a difference in tumor cell biology or tumor burden explains these disparate results.

Burkitt Lymphoma

Originally described as "a sarcoma involving the jaws of African children" by Burkitt, this lymphoma continues to represent both a chemotherapeutic success story and a continuing challenge, as it currently represents the subset of pediatric NHL accounting for most treatment failure.[131,143,144,176–178]

It has been noted to be monoclonal in origin and has characteristics of B lymphocytes, with surface immunoglobulin present.[179,180,182,183] Several differences are apparent between African children and North American children affected with the tumor. Epstein–Barr virus DNA is nearly always noted in tumor cells of African children but is rare in American cases.[133–135] American children have been noted to have a high incidence of abnormalities on chromosome I, although both African and non-African children have been noted to carry cells with the t(8:14) translocation.[180] Perhaps the most readily apparent difference is in the clinical presentation, with African children having a very high proportion of primary jaw lesions and American children presenting nearly always with abdominal disease (Table 34-8).[121]

As B-cell tumors containing surface immunoglobulins are not invariably Burkitt tumors, a certain degree of subjectivity may be present in deciding when a histologic preparation represents Burkitt tumor as opposed to an undifferentiated lymphoma, non-Burkitt type.[121] For this reason, in 1969, under the auspices of the World Health Organization, a pamphlet titled "Histopathologic Definition of Burkitt's Tumor" was published.[181] The authors noted "predominantly undifferentiated lymphoreticular cells" with a diffuse pattern and a characteristic appearance. In addition, the presence of macrophages containing lipid and cellular debris dispersed intermittently throughout gives a characteristic "starry-sky" appearance (Fig. 34-2). Other undifferentiated tumors, including diffuse histiocytic lymphoma, immunoblastic sarcoma, and undifferentiated lymphoma, non-Burkitt type, may pose diagnostic difficulties. It is felt that the differences between African and non-African patients (including the relationship with EB virus and malaria in the former) may merely be due to differences in racial or epidemiological factors or might, in fact, indicate that they are different pathologic entities.[121]

Limited early stage disease presenting as a mandibular or maxillary mass is rare in the United States. Most children tend to present with primary abdominal disease, and in most of these patients, resection of a significant portion of the intra-abdominal tumor is rarely possible at initial presentation.

TABLE 34-8. Common Sites of Presentation in African and Non-African Children with Burkitt's Lymphoma

SITE	PERCENT (%) OF CHILDREN WITH SITE INVOLVEMENT	
	African	*Non-African*
Abdomen	58	78
Pleura	3	22
Jaw	58	4
CNS	19	10
Bone Marrow	7	18
Peripheral Nodes	4	18

(Magrath IT, Ziegler JL: Bone marrow involvement in Burkitt's lymphoma and its relationship to acute B-cell leukemia. Leuk Res 4:33–59, 1979.)

The tumor in these patients is usually exquisitely responsive to cyclophosphamide; however, rapid reappearance of tumor in a period of weeks to months occurs very frequently. Initial treatment of these patients requires expert pediatric medical care, as compromise of renal function, occasionally combined with actual renal infiltration with tumor, is often present initially. The rapid lysis of tumor cells often creates an elevation in serum uric acid to a very high level and a combination of pretreatment renal compromise and acute uric acid nephropathy occurs in a substantial number of patients. A variety of techniques, including temporary periods of dialysis, are often required to overcome these problems. A major effort must be made to provide optimal hydration, alkalinization, and appropriate treatment with allopurinol, to minimize the possibility of these renal difficulties.[138,142–144,146] Other acute medical problems that may occur include hyperkalemia, hyperphosphatemia, and hypocalcemia.[182,183] These problems also appear to relate to rapid cell destruction due to the extreme responsiveness of large volumes of tumor tells to chemotherapeutic agents, particularly cyclophosphamide.

Using, in African children, one or two doses of cyclophosphamide (40 mg/kg I.V. with 2-week interval between doses), six doses (same concentration as above) given at 2-week intervals, or a cyclic sequential regimen, consisting of cyclophosphamide, vincristine, methotrexate, and cytosine arabinoside, for patients with advanced disease, a complete response of 95% was obtained.[184] Fourteen percent of patients (all with advanced disease) died within the first 2 weeks of treatment, of complications primarily of the medical type discussed previously. Sixty-one percent (58 of 95 patients) of complete responders relapsed (39% of early stage patients and nearly 70% of late stage patients). The relapse frequency was similar in the three therapy groups and nearly half of the relapsed patients could be salvaged. Only 30% of patients who relapsed within the first 10 weeks could be salvaged, contrasted to 64% of "late" relapsers. Many of the relapsing patients developed CNS disease which could be controlled in a surprisingly large number by intrathecal chemotherapy. Overall nearly 50% of all patients were long-term survivors (more than 2 years)—Stages I and II, 74%; Stage II, 50%) Stage IV, 44%.[144] More recent data from Uganda are not so encouraging, with less than 20% of advanced stage patients surviving more than 2 years, although more than 85% of early stage (A and B) patients survive.[177]

American children tend to present with advanced disease and less than 35 percent of all children achieve long-term disease-free survival in most published reports. Obstacles to more effective treatment include tumor bulk and frequent development of CNS disease which has not been able to be eradicated with frequency equal to that achieved in African children. Magrath has suggested the value of aggressive surgical reduction of tumor bulk in improving therapy in patients with abdominal disease.[146] However, such tumor reduction is frequently not ultimately successful.[184]

Although hyperfractionation of radiation doses has resulted in an improved response rate and duration of response, hyperfractionated craniospinal irradiation (2000 rad to 2400 rad in 10 treatment days with three fractions of 70 rad to 75 rad delivered each day) was ineffective in preventing CNS relapse.[185,186] A similar lack of efficacy has been reported for intrathecal methotrexate, cytosine arabinoside, combinations of these two agents, and hydroxyurea or CCNU taken by mouth.[187] More recently, high dose systemic methotrexate with citrovorum rescue has been utilized with coordinated intrathecal therapy with success reported in a small number of treated patients. However, CNS relapses continue to occur even with these regimens.[188]

The addition of whole abdominal irradiation to intensive chemotherapy in an effort to reduce the high incidence of local recurrence in children with unresectable abdominal tumors has not yielded substantially better results.[184] Therefore, although success has often been striking, children with Burkitt tumor, especially those with massive unresectable abdominal tumors, continue to frequently develop relapse despite progressively more aggressive treatment.

Non-Hodgkin's Lymphoma of Bone

Although uncommon, this represents a distinct and, with appropriate therapy, favorable clinical group. Most children present because of symptoms referable to the affected bone with localized pain, limp, or on occasion, pathologic fracture after minor trauma. Radiographically, the lesions simulate Ewing's tumor or other round cell tumors of bone, with a permeative appearance often affecting the diaphysis of a long bone or involving a flat bone such as the pelvis or spine. A mixed lytic and blastic appearance is seen more commonly than with Ewing's tumor. Histologically, biopsy may show a picture compatible with a diffuse histiocytic tumor or, less commonly, a diffuse, poorly differentiated lymphocytic or lymphoblastic picture. Regional nodal involvement is seen on occasion and, more commonly, involvement of another bone, so that a bone scan should be routinely obtained. Treatment for monostotic or regionally limited disease should be with irradiation and systemic chemotherapy. Radiation techniques utilized for patients with Ewing's tumor, including treatment of the entire bone and affected soft tissue, sparing of an adequate strip of unirradiated tissue, use of compensators, and so forth, should be used.[116,117,165] We have utilized a dose of 4000 rad in 4 weeks to the entire affected bone and then, using a shrinking field technique, have delivered an additional 1000 rad to the radiographically abnormal area (total, 5000 rad in 5 weeks) in combination with systemic chemotherapy. Unlike Ewing's tumor, local recurrence following appropriate treatment is virtually unheard of. CNS prophylaxis has been reserved for children with more than simple monostotic involvement. Using the APO regimen with irradiation as described, all patients seen to date have achieved local control and continuing disease-free survival.[116,117] Less optimistic results have been reported when the LSA_2/L_2 regimen has been utilized.[141,165]

RESULTS

Disease-free survival of more than 2 years in 70% to 80% or more of all patients, exclusive of those with Burkitt tumor, is now being reported by several centers. In general, these results have been achieved with combinations of intensive multiagent chemotherapy, supplemental irradiation, especially in patients with regionally limited disease, and some form of CNS prophylaxis delivered soon after achievement of a clinical complete response, as in patients with leukemia.[116,117,120,141,165,166]

COMPLICATIONS

The several renal and metabolic problems possible following massive rapid cell lysis after initiation of therapy have been previously discussed. In addition to the usual acute risks of aggressive multiagent systemic chemotherapy, such as myelosuppression, infection, risk of bleeding, and a variety of gastrointestinal complications, the potential for sterility and, in girls, failure of secondary sexual characteristics to develop, must be considered, especially in regimens containing cyclophosphamide. Doxorubicin cardiomyopathy is by now a well-recognized complication that is usually related to total dose administered.

Radiation complications include acute problems such as mucositis, nausea, vomiting, and diarrhea. Two complications seen in these children when irradiation is administered with doxorubicin, are a striking esophagitis following radiation doses of less than 1000 rad delivered for acute relief of respiratory or vascular compromise related to mediastinal tumor, and the phenomenon of "recall" of a prior radiation reaction occasioned by administration of doxorubicin.[172]

Compromise in growth of an irradiated body part or extremity may occur if treatment must be delivered prior to achievement of total growth.

FUTURE PROSPECTS

In marked contrast to clinical reports prior to 1970, the great majority of children with NHL are now long-term disease-free survivors. For this group of children, future studies should be directed towards minimizing the complications of therapy without sacrificing efficacy. Such questions as the necessity of irradiation when intensive chemotherapy is to be delivered and the possibility of combining irradiation with *less* intensive chemotherapy for children with regional, favorable site disease to minimize overall complications need to be investigated. The desirability of routine CNS prophylaxis for certain high risk presentations is becoming apparent from current studies.[116,117,120,140] Ways to deliver this CNS therapy earlier, prior to the development of overt disease need to be considered and the optimum combination of efficacy with least morbidity should be developed. Finally, improved therapy for the high-risk children with widespread, undifferentiated tumors of the abdomen needs to be discovered.

NEUROBLASTOMA

Neuroblastoma is a malignant tumor of neural crest origin which may arise at any location containing sympathetic nervous system tissue, but is found most often in or around the adrenal glands. It is the most common extracranial malignant solid tumor of childhood and represents approximately 10% of childhood malignancies. First described by Virchow, neuroblastoma remains one of the most studied tumors of childhood; however, many aspects of its clinical behavior continue to be poorly understood.[189] Despite progressively more aggressive therapy by surgeons, radiation therapists, and pediatric oncologists, only minor improvements in ultimate survival have been achieved in the past two decades, although some prolongation of median survival has been achieved.[190,191]

EPIDEMIOLOGY AND GENETICS

Epidemiological studies have not been helpful. An association of neuroblastoma with von Recklinghausen's disease has been reported.[192] Infants dying of congenital heart disease have been noted to have an excessive number of occult primary neuroblastomas ("neuroblastoma *in situ*"); however, the latter association may well represent a selection bias, with congenital heart disease representing one of the major causes of infant mortality permitting complete *post mortem* study.[193,194] No convincing evidence is available relating these pathologic findings to clinically overt neuroblastoma.

Familial associations of neuroblastoma have been noted. However, these reports are rare and no easily recognized or numerically significant genetic association has been recognized.[195,196] Recently, an association of neuroblastoma with familial nisidioblastosis has been reported.[198] Studies with pathologically assessed infant adrenals show a substantially greater incidence of *in situ* neuroblastoma than is recognized clinically.[193,194] Presumably, spontaneous regression or maturation occurs to account for this discrepancy. This is one of the more intriguing aspects of neuroblastoma.

Although neuroblastoma is one of the more frequent pediatric solid tumors, fewer than 500 new cases are seen in the United States in a year. The incidence is slightly lower in black children (7.0 per million) than whites (9.6 per million).[197] Neuroblastoma accounts for one-quarter to one-half of all neonatal malignancies (under 30 months of age).[199] Approximately 25% of children with this tumor are diagnosed in the first year of life. However,, 50% to 60% present after the age of 2 years and these older children, unfortunately, tend to have an increased frequency of advanced disease.[199,200]

ANATOMIC CONSIDERATIONS

Analysis of several collected series reveals that 60% to 70% of children present with primary abdominal disease.[199-201] Approximately half of these have adrenal lesions, while the remainder have lesions occurring in the perirenal, paraspinal, or celiac regions. About 5% have pelvic primary lesions (*i.e.*, organ of Zuckerkandl), while 15% to 20% of lesions arise in the cervico–thoracic region. No definite primary site can be identified in the significant remaining fraction of patients. The frequency of a site of primary involvement is related to age at diagnosis (Fig. 34-3).

Most neuroblastomas are not resectable at the time of presentation. This is due to the high frequency of both disseminated and locally advanced disease, but even small tumors are often located in areas that do not permit complete excision. Diffuse soft tissue involvement and invasion along tissue planes around major vascular structures, such as the aorta, superior mesenteric artery, and vena cava, tend to make surgical excision difficult or impossible.

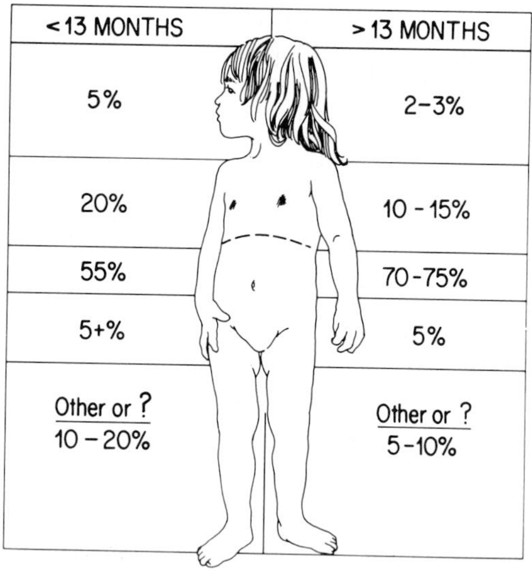

FIG. 34-3. This schematic illustration demonstrates the different distribution of primary tumor sites seen in the infant compared with the child more than 13 months of age. Note greater percentage of adrenal and peri-adrenal disease in older child.

PATHOLOGY

A variety of histologic patterns have been noted in patients with neuroblastoma, ranging from a monotonous collection of densely packed round cells (neuroblastoma) to a primary aggregation of mature or nearly mature ganglion cells with occasional interspersed neuroblasts (ganglioneuroblastoma) (Fig. 34-4).[202–209] Careful pathologic analysis of all parts of a tumor must be performed prior to making a diagnosis of benign ganglioneuroma, as marked variation from one region to another is common. Mature ganglioneuroma should not be considered with neuroblastoma, as the natural history and prognosis are quite different. Although controversial, lesions in infants and in extra-adrenal sites tend to demonstrate a somewhat higher proportion of more differentiated ganglioneuroblastoma than adrenal lesions. Histology as an independent variable has not been convincingly shown to correlate with ultimate prognosis. However, survival duration appears to be slightly longer in patients with more differentiated tumors.[201,203–207] Reports that demonstrate correlations between tumor grade and survival have attempted to correct for other factors, but generally fail to adjust simultaneously for all significant prognostic variables: age, stage, and site.[208,209]

NATURAL HISTORY

The initial diagnostic feature in most children with neuroblastoma is an abdominal mass discovered by a parent or by a physician as part of a routine visit or in response to vague, nonspecific complaints. However, a variety of presenting signs and symptoms deserve comment because of their characteristic association with this tumor. These include opsoclonus and polymyoclonus, paresis or paralysis due to extension of paraspinous lesions through neural foramina, Horner's syndrome and heterochromia iridis seen with cervicothoracic primaries and, quite commonly, periorbital ecchymosis in the absence of trauma, with or without proptosis.[211,216,238] Bone pain related to metastatic disease, especially of the spine, pelvis, or femur, is common. Chronic diarrhea and malabsorption is an important and often overlooked complaint, which may only be elicited by careful questioning.[217] Coagulation abnormalities have been noted in association with widespread disease, and marked change in temperament and increased irritability, presumably related to disease-related inanition or diffuse metastases, are seen on occasion.[210]

Table 34-9 illustrates stage as a function of age at presentation and demonstrates that more than 60% of children over 2 years of age have Stage IV disease at presentation. The Evans–D'Angio staging system is widely accepted for this condition (Table 34-10).[212] However, dissatisfaction exists, especially with the designation of midline primary lesions, presumably Stage III by this system, but with a widely recognized favorable prognosis. The prognostic significance of the Stage IVS designation in contradistinction to the well-recognized import of age at diagnosis has also been questioned.[207] From published data, it is unclear what the prognostic significance of regional lymph node disease is. The development and routine use of TNM system would permit a more accurate designation of midline lesions and it would also facilitate analysis of the relative prognostic importance of primary size, lymph node extent, and so forth, within a given age group and primary site.

TABLE 34-9. Neuroblastoma: Stage (extent) of disease as a Function of Age

STAGE	AGE		
	< 13 Mo.	*13–24 Mo.*	*> 24 Mo.*
I	20%	20%	12½%
II	20%	12½%	12½%
III	5%	12½%	10%
IV	25%	50%	60%
IVS	30%	5%	5%

TABLE 34-10. A Staging System for Neuroblastoma

Stage I:	Tumor confined to the organ structure of origin
Stage II:	Tumors extending in continuity beyond the organ or structure of origin but not crossing the midline. Regional lymph nodes on the homolateral side may be involved.
Stage III:	Tumors extending in continuity beyond the midline. Regional lymph nodes may be involved bilaterally.
Stage IV:	Remote disease involving skeleton, soft tissues, distant lymph node groups, etc.
Stage IVS:	Patients with local Stage I or II disease but who have remote disease confined to one or more of the following: liver, skin, and bone marrow (without radiographic evidence of bone metastases on complete skeletal survey)

(Evans A, D'Angio GJ, Randolph JA: A proposed staging for children with neuroblastoma. Cancer 27:347, 1971.)

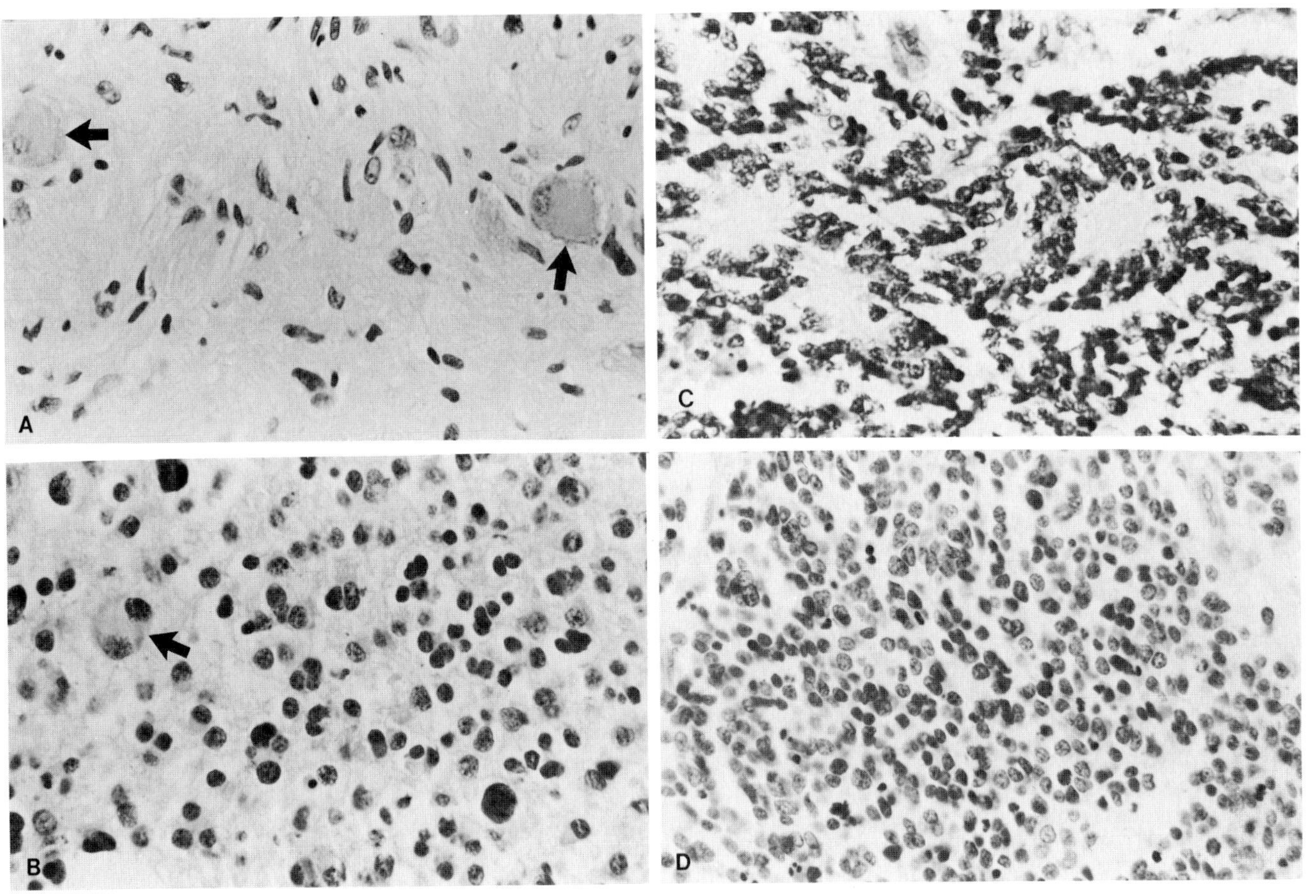

FIG. 34-4. Histological features of ganglioneuroma and neuroblastoma (400×). (*A*) Benign ganglioneuroma. Arrow demonstrates a mature ganglion cell. No areas of immaturity or neuroblastoma. Nissl substance is noted in the periphery of the cytoplasm. (*B*) Ganglioneuroblastoma. Arrow illustrates binucleate immature malignant ganglion cell. Admixture of densely staining neuroblasts is seen. (*C*) Neuroblastoma. Homer Wright rosette in presence of numerous neuroblasts with virtually no more mature elements. (*D*) Typical neuroblastoma.

Finally, the extent to which completeness of surgical excision should be considered in clinical/anatomic staging is questionable. The potential for inter-institutional variability, depending on the skill and aggressiveness of the surgeon, is clear and introduces obvious potential bias in treatment comparisons. At the time of surgical exploration for diagnosis or therapy, thorough assessment of primary size and extent, lymph node sampling and, when possible, liver biopsy, should be performed.

Widespread metastatic disease is common. Frequent sites of involvement include regional and distant lymph node sites, bone marrow, bone, liver, skin, and subcutaneous tissue. Pulmonary nodules, common with Wilms' tumor, are rarely seen and involvement of the lung generally occurs by extension from pleural sites, which in turn have developed following extension from ribs or lymph nodes. We have recently noted that children who are beyond 10 years of age at diagnosis have developed clinically evident pulmonary nodules with greater frequency than younger children.[213]

The poor therapeutic results are explained partly by the high frequency of wide local extension and metastatic disease. Even though neuroblastoma is recognized as having the highest incidence of spontaneous regression of any tumor, this is rare and virtually limited to young infants.[214]

INITIAL EVALUATION

In addition to a careful history, the initial examination should include blood pressure analysis and careful evaluation of the periorbital regions, entire skin and subcutaneous tissue, lymph node regions including both supraclavicular fossae, and thorough abdominal examination. Careful neurologic evaluation is also of importance,

Routine radiographic studies must include evaluation of the chest with particular attention to the paraspinous region posterior to the heart, a region commonly abnormal in neuroblastoma patients, owing to paravertebral lymph node involvement with pleural displacement (Fig. 34-5). Other essential radiographic studies include intravenous urography (Fig. 34-6), isotopic bone scan, and abdominal ultrasonography (Fig. 34-7). Depending on clinical history, primary site, and results of other studies, radiographic assessment of neural foramina, myelography, computerized tomography, angiog-

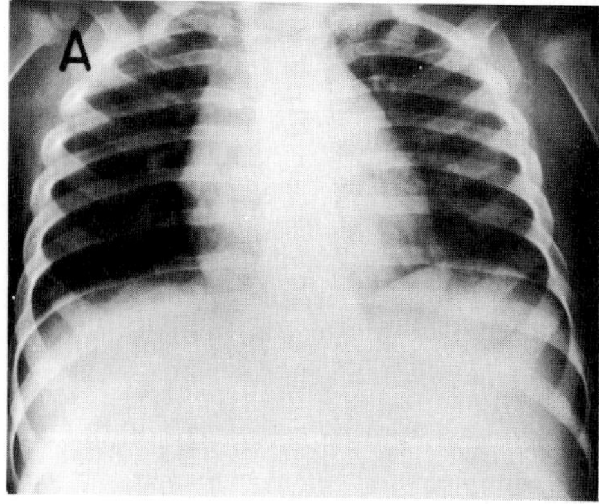

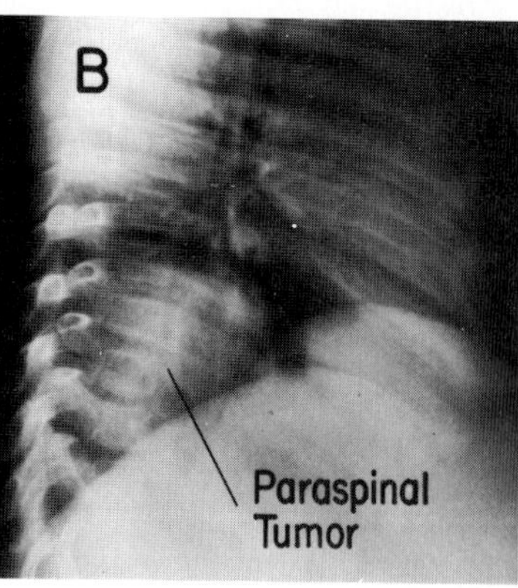

FIG. 34-5. Chest roentgenograph in frontal (*A*) and lateral (*B*) projections demonstrating paravertebral pleural displacement. Size of the thoracic component can be appreciated on the lateral projection.

raphy (Fig. 34-8), or radiographs of individual bones may be necessary.

Levels of vanilylmandelic acid (VMA) and homovanillic acid (HVA) are useful for diagnosis when elevated.[218,219] Apparent elevations of VMA may occur when diet has not been appropriately controlled and a nonspecific "spot-test" is performed, especially when foods such as chocolate, bananas, and vanilla are not eliminated. However, when VMA, HVA, total metanephrines, cystathionine and creatinine are measured in a prolonged urine collection (usually 24 hours) and results expressed as catechol excretion per mg creatinine no dietary restriction is necessary. However, no medications containing catecholamines should be given concurrent with the collection. Normal values include total metanephrines less than 1.6 mcg/mg creatinine, VMA less than 20 mcg/mg creatinine, and HVA less than 40 mcg/mg creatinine. When properly performed, more than 50% of patients will have an elevated VMA and up to 90% of patients will have elevation of either VMA or HVA. The LaBross VMA spot test is a much less reliable study and many patients with abnormal quantitative VMA results will have intermediate or negative VMA spot test results.[220] Cytathionine excretion has also been shown to be elevated in some patients with neuroblastoma, but these patients also have VMA elevations.[221] Routine hematologic and serum studies should be obtained in all patients.

Bone marrow examination is essential. If positive in an appropriate clinical setting, laparotomy can be precluded with its attendant risks and the delay in systemic treatment.

In the absence of a diagnosis by bone marrow analysis, tissue documentation is essential. With limited disease, complete excision of all evident tumor may be possible with acceptable morbidity. If resection is not possible, biopsy of an abnormal lymph node, hepatic nodule, or incisional biopsy of the primary lesion may confirm the diagnosis. At the time of surgery, the radiation therapist should be present to assess tumor extent and instruct the surgeon in judicious placement of clips potentially useful in treatment planning. Potential interference of metallic clips with computed tomography must, however, be considered. Regardless of the resectability of the primary, regional lymph node biopsy should be performed for more accurate surgical staging.

IMMUNOLOGIC RESPONSE

In part because of its known tendency for spontaneous regression and maturation, a number of *in vitro* immunologic

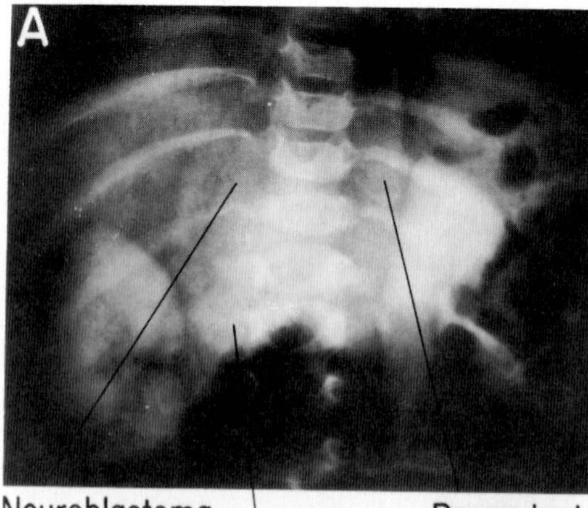

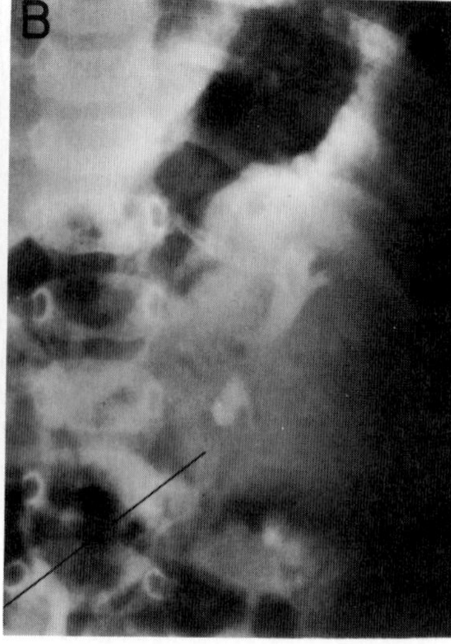

FIG. 34-6. Intravenous urogram demonstrating typical findings in child with neuroblastoma and Wilms' tumor. Note the outward and downward displacement of the right kidney ("drooping lily") in the child with neuroblastoma (*A*) as well as the faint calcification (*arrow*). Presence of para-aortic nodal involvement is shown by displacement of the left kidney and abnormal paravertebral stripe (see Fig. 24-5). The kidney with Wilms' tumor (*B*) has a typical intra-renal mass with calyceal distortion and displacement but little change in axis of the kidney.

studies have been performed on lymphocytes and serum of patients with neuroblastoma and on their family members. Lymphocytes from patients with neuroblastoma will produce a positive colony inhibition test as demonstrated by the Hellströms.[222] Lymphocytes from matched controls failed to produce similar inhibition; however, lymphocytes from the patients' mothers demonstrated activity.[223,224] Serum from patients with active neuroblastoma blocked the colony inhibition, although serum from cured patients demonstrated no blocking effect. This so-called "blocking" antibody requires the presence of tumor. After tumor removal, blocking antibody quickly disappears.[225] Serum of patients and family members also contains cytotoxic antibodies against tumor cells. Serum complement is necessary for a positive result.[222] Despite this accumulated evidence of immunologic activity, no clinically useful therapeutic application has yet been found.

TREATMENT

Prognosis in neuroblastoma is dependent on age at diagnosis, stage, and, to a lesser degree, primary site. With the exception of complete surgical removal, the influence of therapy on prognosis is controversial. As suggested earlier, the necessity and desirability of partial surgical removal when complete excision is not possible for children with regional disease, and the usefulness of attempted surgical treatment of the primary for children with metastatic disease is controversial. No data exist to support such an attempt in children with a known poor prognosis.[199,201,203,207,212,236,237]

Surgery is indicated as initial therapy for all children with Stage I and Stage II neuroblastoma and for those with Stage III tumors that originate in the mediastinum. In more advanced neuroblastoma, excision of the primary tumor is delayed until distant metastatic disease has been controlled and the size of the primary mass has been reduced by chemotherapy, with or without irradiation.

The principles of surgical care which are employed for removal of an abdominal neuroblastoma are similar to those used in the treatment of any large intraabdominal neoplasm. Hemorrhage is the most significant problem, mainly because neuroblastoma encases major vascular structures as it grows. As a rule, one must be prepared to transfuse as much as one or two blood volumes, and if this much blood is actually used, fresh blood should be available. As already noted, bank blood should be warmed to 37°C and buffered to pH 7.4, and upper extremity veins should be used for intravenous cannulas.

A long abdominal or thoraco–abdominal incision is recommended to provide adequate exposure for removal of the tumor. In the past 4 years, we have had success with a somewhat different operative approach in 10 children with large neuroblastomas (Fig. 34-9). The technique which is demonstrated is similar to that which is currently used to expose the spine for anterior spinal fusion. The retroperitoneum is approached extraperitoneally through a vertical lateral abdominal incision, which is extended into the chest to expose the lower thoracic and upper abdominal aorta after circumferential detachment of the diaphragm. In contrast to transperitoneal operations in which the anterior approach to the upper abdominal aorta encased by tumor is often unsatisfactory, the lateral retroperitoneal exposure provides access to these vessels, so that a safe and more complete dissection can be accomplished. A movie demonstrating this technique is available in the film library of the American College of Surgeons.*

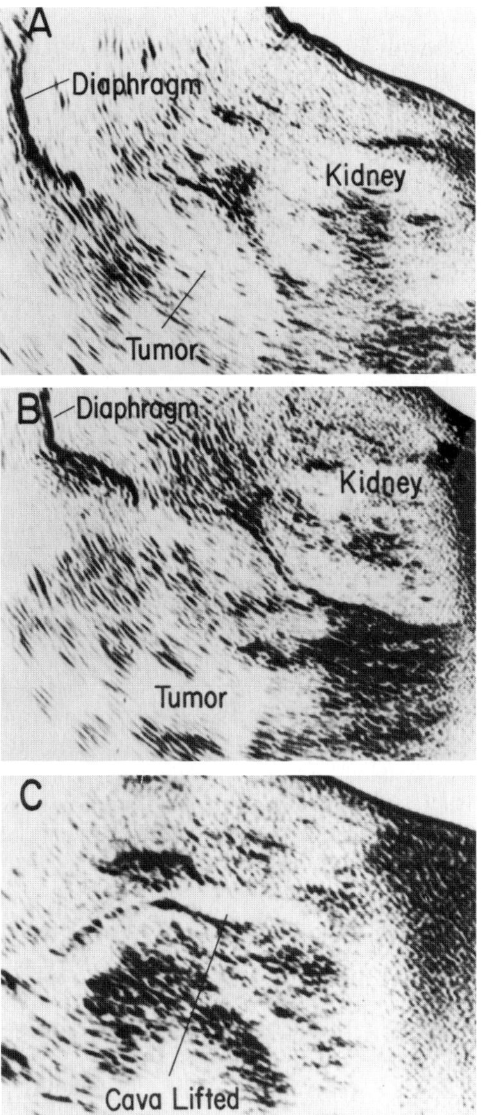

FIG. 34-7. Abdominal ultrasound demonstrating striking displacement forward of the inferior vena cava (*C*), forward and downward displacement of the kidney (*B*, *C*), and transdiaphragmatic extension of tumor in lymph nodes (*B*).

A variety of chemotherapy regimens is shown in Table 34-11. The single most effective agent for neuroblastoma is cyclophosphamide followed by doxorubicin. Platinum compounds and the epipodophyllotoxin VM-26 also show significant activity.[240]

Children with primary extraadrenal disease, especially in the mediastinum and paraspinal regions, have a surprisingly

* Filler RM: New Thoracolumbar Approach for Excision of Neuroblastoma. American College of Surgeons Film Library, 55 East Eric Street, Chicago, IL 60611.

favorable outlook.[203,237,238] Thus, 85% of all patients with primary mediastinal and neck disease survived over 2 years and 47% of those with spinal canal disease were cured in two reported series.[238] This is in contrast to an expected overall cure rate of 30% to 35%. In part, however, these results can be related to favorable selection by age and stage. Table 34-12 shows approximate survival by stage and age at presentation. It should be noted that with increasing efficacy of chemotherapy, median survivals are increasing and 2-year survival is no longer reliable as an index of cure. In the following section, therapeutic recommendations will be given for different age groups as a function of stage or primary site.

Infants Under 12 Months of Age

Children with Stage I or limited Stage II disease in this age group are currently best treated by surgical excision without postoperative radiation therapy or chemotherapy, regardless of primary site. The only exceptions would include those children with locally extensive Stage II disease with gross residual disease or with disease in the spinal canal not amenable to surgical removal, especially if neurologic signs are present.

The role of chemotherapy in this clinical setting is more controversial.[226,227] We do not recommend single agent treatment (*i.e.*, with cyclophosphamide or vincristine) or combination of these two agents alone, as the benefit of this therapy has not been demonstrated when tested in a somewhat similar setting.[226] Although numbers are small, mortality has been

TABLE 34-11. Chemotherapy Regimens for Neuroblastoma

	"MADDOC" PROGRAM	
	Course 1,3,5, . . .	*Course 2,4,6 . . .*
Nitrogen Mustard	4 mg/m² I.V.	3 mg/m²
Adriamycin	40 mg/m² I.V.	30 mg/m²
DD Cis-platinum II*	45 mg/m² I.V.	45 mg/m²
DTIC	750 mg/m² I.V.	–
Oncovin	2 mg/m² I.V.	2 mg/m²
Cyclophosphamide	750 mg/m² I.V.	600 mg/m²

Therapy courses are given at 21 day intervals, and doses are modified depending on degree of myelosuppression.

	CCSG-331
Cyclophosphamide	750 mg/m² × 1 on day 1
DTIC	250 mg/m²/day × 5 on days 1–5
Vincristine	1.5 mg/m² × 1 on day 5

Cycles are repeated every 22 days.

	ST. JUDE PROGRAM
Cyclophosphamide	150 mg/m²/day for 7 days
Adriamycin	35 mg/m² on day 8

Cycles repeated every 21 days

*5% Mannitol—750 cc/m² over 3 hours

(Frantz C: Personal communication; Finklestein JZ, Klemper MF, Evans A et al: Multiagent chemotherapy for children with metastatic neuroblastoma: A report from CCSG. Med Ped Oncol 6:179–188, 1979. Hayes FA, Green AA, Mauer AM: The correlation of cell kinetic and clinical response to chemotherapy in disseminated neuroblastoma. Cancer Res 37:3766–3770, 1977)

FIG. 34-8. Angiogram in child with neuroblastoma showing typical neovascularity and extra renal appearance of tumor. Note displaced vena cava.

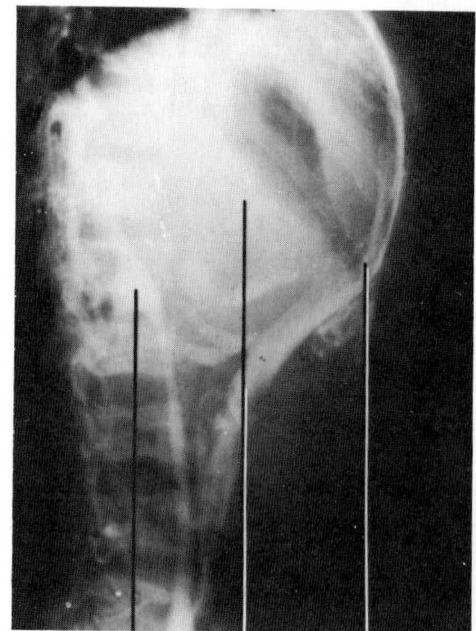

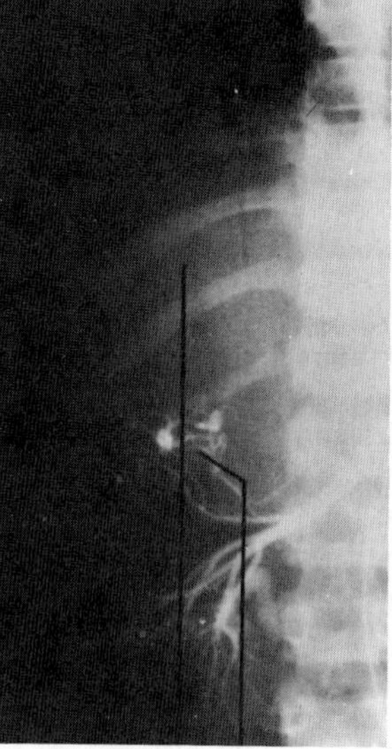

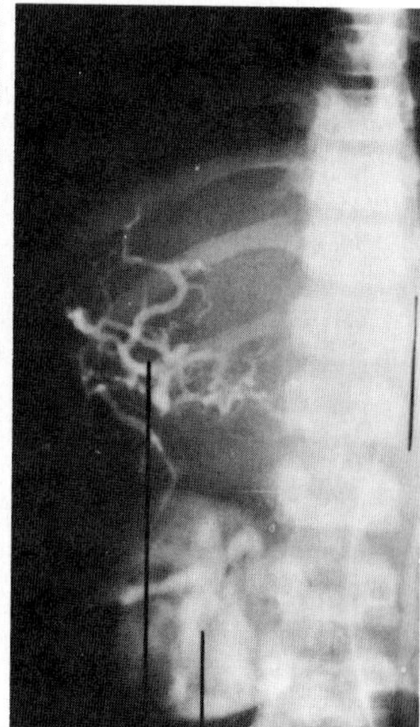

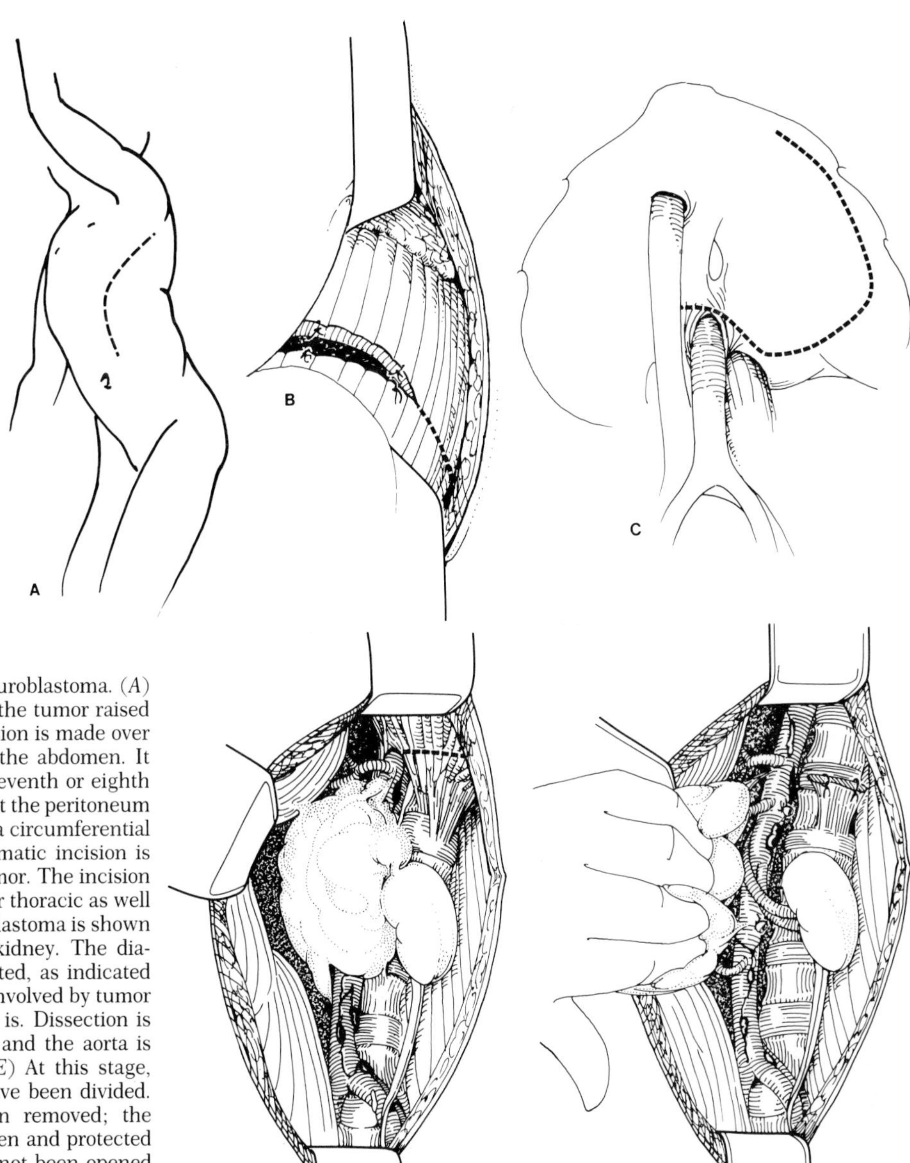

FIG. 34-9. Thoracolumbar excision of neuroblastoma. (*A*) The patient is positioned with the side of the tumor raised approximately 45° from the table. An incision is made over the lateral edge of the rectus muscle in the abdomen. It extends across the costal margin in the seventh or eighth interspace. The pleural cavity is opened but the peritoneum is not. (*B*) The diaphragm is opened with a circumferential incision. (*C*) The extent of the diaphragmatic incision is shown for this patient with a left-sided tumor. The incision opens the aortic hiatus, exposing the lower thoracic as well as upper abdominal aorta. (*D*) The neuroblastoma is shown encasing the aorta and depressing the kidney. The diaphragmatic incision is just being completed, as indicated by the dotted lines. The celiac axis is not involved by tumor in this case, but the superior mesenteric is. Dissection is begun at the periphery of the neoplasm and the aorta is exposed as tumor is removed from it. (*E*) At this stage, most of the attachments of the tumor have been divided. The tumor has almost completely been removed; the branches of the abdominal aorta easily seen and protected with this approach. The peritoneum has not been opened during the procedure, so that the intestines do not block the view of the surgical field nor is there prolonged ileus from retracting them.

significant in infants with Stage III disease and an argument can be made for use of an aggressive multiagent regimen following irradiation. More effective multiagent chemotherapy programs in current use at several institutions are shown in Table 34-11. The optimal multiagent regimen of those currently in clinical use is not known.

Infants with Stage IV disease require aggressive, multiagent chemotherapy. Such an approach has recently been shown to significantly improve survival in this group of patients, one of the few instances where aggressive, combination chemotherapy has been demonstrated to increase the number of surviving patients rather than simply prolonging survival (Fig. 34-10).[190,229] Therapy for infants with Stage IVS disease is more controversial. These infants have a relatively favorable outcome, considering initial disease extent.[230] Although hepatic and skin involvement have been recognized as not conferring an unduly poor prognosis upon these children, documented bone marrow involvement is much more controversial and requires further study. Therapeutic intervention has improved survival, by permitting children to survive the organ dysfunction (*i.e.*, hepatic or pulmonary failure) created by tumor growth for a sufficient period of time to permit regression or maturation to take place. The mechanism whereby spontaneous regression occurs is unknown. When therapy has been unwisely withheld in all children, regardless of clinical status, children have died of organ dysfunction and pulmonary–hepatic–metabolic consequences. Some therapy, in addition to biopsy confirmation, will be required in a substantial majority of these patients. At present, we feel that these children should be carefully observed following biopsy

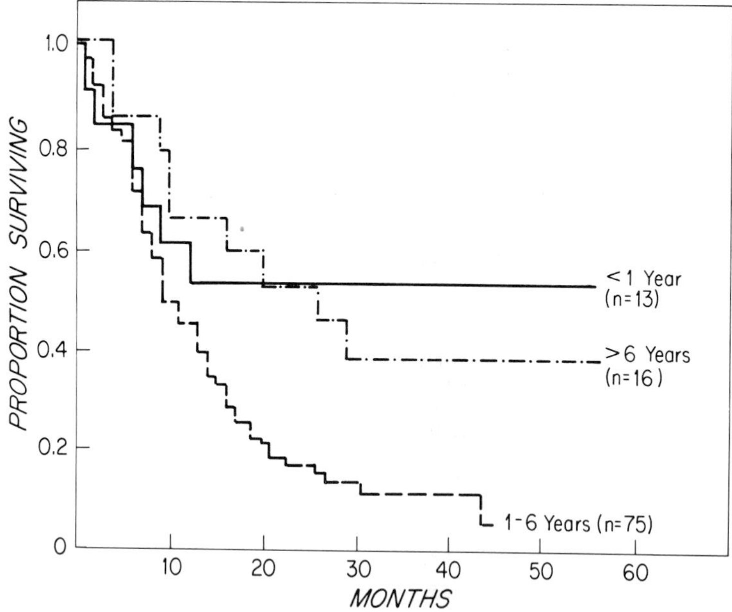

FIG. 34-10. Survival curves of children with Stage IV neuroblastoma treated with a three-drug (CCG-331, vincristine, cyclophosphamide, cytosine arabinoside) or four-drug (CCG-334, same drugs plus adriamycin) regimens in combination with surgery with and without irradiation. Note improved prognosis for children less than one year or greater than 6 years. (Finklestein JZ, Klemperer MR, Evans AE et al: Chemotherapy for metastatic neuroblastoma. Med Ped Onc 6:179–188, 1979)

confirmation. Routine use of single agent cyclophosphamide therapy following diagnosis is recommended by some pediatric oncologists but is controversial.

Any significant progression of disease causing increased organ dysfunction mandates therapy. Choice of treatment in such patients must be made by considering the potential long-term sequelae of the modalities available, especially as the known tendency of this tumor in this age child is to ultimately undergo regression. In the absence of adequate long-term data, current recommendations generally include less aggressive chemotherapeutic (*i.e.*, vincristine/cyclophosphamide) intervention with reservation of irradiation for persistent problems. When required, modest doses of irradiation are effective in causing response and rarely should exceed 1000 rad to 1500 rad.

Children Aged 12 Months to 24 Months

This age group in the most difficult for which to choose an appropriate regimen. The prognosis and tendency to progressive growth is not so uniformly bad as with the patient more than 2 years of age, nor is the prospect of a favorable natural history and regression as high as with the younger infant. Clearly, the age in months within this group is important, and survival of children greater than 18 months of age closely resembles that of the older child.

Stage I. Complete surgical excision is recommended. No data is known suggesting an improvement in survival by addition of irradiation or chemothrapy, although overall survival is significantly inferior to that in the younger child.

Stage II. This stage and age pose the most problems, and choice of treatment should be based on considerations of adequacy of surgical removal and age of child. Any child under the age of 18 months with known residual disease and any child greater than 18 months with positive margins of resection should receive local irradiation. Dose necessary is a controversial matter but probably need not exceed 2000 rad in the younger group and 2500 rad in the older. The desirability of chemotherapy is even more controversial. Cyclophosphamide has been tested and shown to influence neither the time to recurrence nor the incidence of relapse.[226]

Stage III. Prognosis is substantially poorer for this group and aggressive treatment is indicated. In view of the greater likelihood of rapid dissemination, children with tumors of the adrenal or abdomen not in the pelvis or midline (*i.e.*, paraspinous or "dumbbell") should receive aggressive multiagent systemic chemotherapy for a suitable period (3 months to 6 months) and, should resection of an initially unresectable mass then be possible, "second-look" surgery performed. Irradiation should then be delivered to appropriate volumes with doses of approximately 2500 rad or more in 3 weeks, depending on the extent of residual disease.

Stages IV and IVS. Both these groups should be approached with aggressive chemotherapy as detailed above for the younger child with Stage IV disease. The role of surgical resection and radiation therapy is highly questionable, with

TABLE 34-12. Prognosis of Neuroblastoma by Age and Stage at Presentation Representative 3-Year Disease-Free Survival

STAGE	<12 MONTHS	12–24 MONTHS	>24 MONTHS	TOTAL
I			60%	80–85%
	85%	50–60%		
II				60–65%
			15%	
III	50%	50%		30%
IVS	75%	25%	25%	75%
IV	20–50%	3–10%	3–5%	5–10%
ALL STAGES	70–75%	25–30%	10–15%	30–35%

*The higher figure reflects best current results with aggressive systemic therapy.

irradiation currently being studied as either a local agent (JCRT) or as a whole body treatment used as a systemic agent.[231,232]

Children Aged More Than 24 Months

Limited disease is rare and complete resection of all evident tumor even less common.

Stages I and II. As in the younger patient, surgical resection is desirable. Regional lymph nodes should be biopsied. Any patient with Stage I disease in whom adequacy of local excision is questionable, and virtually all Stage II patients should receive postoperative irradiation. Areas of potential microscopic disease should receive 2500 rad to 3000 rad, while regions of residual bulk disease should be treated more aggressively (~3500 rad). In the absence of clear information, aggressive systemic therapy is probably indicated for most patients, especially those with adrenal and abdominal tumors.

Stages III, IV, and IVS. Aggressive combination therapy of all patients is indicated with systemic treatment receiving priority. Use of surgery and extensive irradiation interdigitated with chemotherapy clearly appears beneficial in the rare child with Stage III disease, or with those who are Stage IV solely by virtue of extensive nodal disease (*i.e.*, mediastinum and/or supraclavicular regions). Improvement in prognosis for this group of children has clearly been noted in recent years by virtue of such aggressive treatment.[190,233] Three of five such children treated at the JCRT/SFCI/CHMC are currently surviving 2 years without evidence of tumor.[234]

Except for children over 6 years of age, who may have unusual features (*e.g.*, pulmonary metastases) and an indolent course, treatment in the great majority of these children clearly remains suboptimal and has primarily accomplished prolongation of survival rather than successful eradication of disease.[190,199,233,234]

FOLLOW-UP

As most children will be receiving chemotherapy, follow-up exams will be frequently performed for this group during this period. Table 34-13 lists appropriate follow-up studies and their frequency assuming no untoward symptoms for children with this disease.

TABLE 34-13. Follow-up Studies Following Treatment Cessation for Neuroblastoma

1. Physical examination every 1–2 months for first year then every 2–3 months for second year then every four to six months for an additional 2–3 years, every 6 months or yearly thereafter.
2. Radiographic studies.
   - A. Chest x-ray film every 3–4 months in first 2 years then every 6 months.
   - B. Ultrasonography every 4–6 months in first 2 years.
   - C. Intravenous urography every 6 months—one year in first two years.
   - D. Bone scan every 3–6 months in first year, every 6 months in second year.
3. Bone marrow study every 3–4 months in first year. Every 6–12 months in next year.
4. VMA collection every 3–6 months in first 2 years.
5. Appropriate visits for cardiac, renal or orthopedic problems as needed.

COMPLICATIONS AND FUTURE CONSIDERATION

Complications of treatment include a wide range of structural, growth, and organ dysfunctions necessitated by major surgical resection, variable doses and fields of irradiation, and use of cytotoxic chemotherapy as considered elsewhere in this chapter. These effects are of special importance in neuroblastoma, both because of the young age of most patients, and because of the unpredictable nature of the tumor in younger patients.

These considerations should weigh heavily in future therapeutic studies. Of principal importance is the development of more effective systemic treatment capable of producing more than temporary arrest and modest prolongation in survival for the majority of children with metastatic disease. Table 34-9 and Fig. 34-3 demonstrate the unfortunate fact that most patients with neuroblastoma are more than 18 months to 24 months of age at presentation and therefore do not enjoy the favorable natural history of the younger patient. The tables also show that the great majority of all patients have metastatic disease at presentation. Current therapy permits long-term survival in only 25% to 35% of affected children. Progressively more aggressive combinations of chemotherapeutic modalities have, to date, proved disappointing in altering the eventual outcome of this disease.

Future studies should be designed to answer the many questions regarding the necessity and advantages of therapy in patients with more favorable prognoses. Blanket recommendations for no treatment in infants with Stage IVS disease result in an unacceptably high mortality rate. Even recommendations advocating early intervention for this group only when worrisome clinical progression has occurred result in many patients ultimately succumbing to overwhelming metastatic disease. Carefully performed studies are necessary to determine if current aggressive systemic treatment can further improve the prognosis for these relatively favorable patients, as it has for younger children with a poor prognosis.[190,233]

The necessity of adding radiation therapy to surgery in younger children with only microscopic residual disease or of adding chemotherapy to any patient with Stage I or Stage II disease needs to be demonstrated in similarly controlled studies, and these questions may ultimately prove to be more amenable to study than attempts to control tumor in older patients with metastatic disease have been to date.

Studies of growth kinetics and relationship to clinical responsiveness to chemotherapy may provide a scientific basis for developing more effective systemic therapy for disseminated disease.[239]

WILMS' TUMOR

Wilms' tumor or nephroblastoma is the most common primary renal tumor in children and accounts for about 10% of the malignant tumors seen in this age group.[241] About 500 new cases are seen in the United States each year.[242] Although previous workers had described the same tumor, the 1899 paper by Max Wilms has become the classical monograph and the eponym "Wilms' tumor" persists.[243] In 1938, a survey of 383 cases recorded a cure rate of 5.7%.[244] Ladd showed that improved surgical technique increased survival to 20%, and in 1950 Gross and Neuhauser indicated that the use of postoperative radiotherapy raised the cure rate to 50%.[245,246] With the addition of actinomycin-D to the antitumor regimen, combined with more aggressive treatment of metastatic disease, and improved radiotherapy techniques, Farber reported that 81% of children survived for 2 years or longer.[247] Recent modifications in therapy protocols have not substantially increased survival. However, they have reduced toxicity, by eliminating flank radiation in selected cases, and they have decreased the number of children requiring treatment of metastatic disease in the lungs, since the incidence of pulmonary relapse has been reduced.

EPIDEMIOLOGY

Wilms' tumor is often associated with patterns of congenital anomalies suggesting a relationship between oncogenesis and teratogenesis.[248] Among the more common anomalies seen in conjunction with Wilms' tumor are genitourinary anomalies, aniridia, and hemihypertrophy. Pendergrass reviewed 547 patients with Wilms' tumor and found that 24 had genitourinary anomalies.[249] The most common types were hypospadias, cryptorchidism, and fusion anomalies of the kidney. Six children in this series had aniridia (absence or a hypoplasia of the iris stroma), and 16 had hemihypertrophy. The incidence of these anomalies seems to be more frequent in children with bilateral disease.

Children with Wilms' tumor and aniridia are more likely to have genitourinary anomalies and other anomalies than those without aniridia, although histology of the nephroblastoma and its outlook in these cases are no different.[250] Adrenal and liver tumors, as well as renal tumors, have been reported in those children with hemihypertrophy.[251] The Wilms' tumor does not always develop on the hypertrophic side.

Familial incidence of Wilms' tumor is rare, although it has been noted.[252] Knudson and Strong have suggested germinal mutation may be present in all cases of bilateral tumors and one-third of the cases of unilateral tumors.[253] The rare occurrence of Wilms' tumor in successive family generations supports their concept that gene mutation predisposing to Wilms' tumor may exist as a nonlethal dominant character.

ANATOMIC CONSIDERATIONS

The tumor may arise from any portion of either kidney but the upper pole is the most common location. Because development of symptoms is usually delayed, tumors grow to large size before discovery. Despite the teaching that Wilms' tumor does not cross the midline as does neuroblastoma, the mass in many cases is so large that it can be felt on both sides of the abdomen.[254] In treating such large masses, the surgeon must be thoroughly prepared to deal with the likelihood of massive hemorrhage or capsular rupture. Furthermore, the necessity for inferior vena cava and right atrial exploration to remove neoplasm must be anticipated, because extension into the renal veins is common and in some cases gross tumor reaches the chambers of the heart and even the pulmonary artery. In about 10% of children with Wilms' tumor, both kidneys are involved so that proper examination of the contralateral kidney before and during surgery is always necessary.

In contrast to neuroblastoma, which usually has no capsule and which grows along tissue planes in the retroperitoneum to encase major blood vessels, Wilms' tumor usually remains as a single expansile mass so that complete resection is possible in most cases.

PATHOLOGY

Recent electron microscopic studies and organ culture studies support the theory of derivation of Wilms' tumor from the metanephric blastema.[255–258] Since the cells comprising the metanephric blastema disappear 4 weeks to 6 weeks prior to term in a normal human gestation, the prevailing concept is that all Wilms' tumors arise during intra-uterine life. However, Bove and McAdams have questioned the theory that all Wilms' tumors are present at birth, because of the rarity of congenital Wilms' tumor and the increasing incidence of these lesions to age 3 years or 4 years.[259] In a careful histologic review of 69 cases, they showed that one or more independent foci of malformation or benign neoplasia accompanied at least one-third of the cases of Wilms' tumor. These authors postulate that classic Wilms' tumor arises in a hamartomatous metanephric precursor which persists in a stable state for months or years prior to the carcinogenic event that results in Wilms' tumor. They also believe that many foci disappear spontaneously.

Grossly, a Wilms' tumor is surrounded by a fibrous external capsule with dilated blood vessels on its surface. The surface is usually smooth, as compared to the irregularity and nodularity seen with neuroblastoma. The cut surface usually has a grey-yellow appearance and areas of liquefaction necrosis, hemorrhage, and cystic degeneration are common. A pseudocapsule usually separates the tumor from the remaining compressed renal parenchyma.

Microscopically, an embryonic type of malignant stroma containing undifferentiated spindle-shaped cells surrounds epithelial cells arranged as tubules of various shapes and sizes, or as abortive glomeruli. A mixture of smooth and striated muscle, myxomatous tissue, and occasionally fat, bone, or cartilage may be found. Many histologic variations exist and several histologic classifications have been proposed. However, the recent classification described by Beckwith and Palmer seems to have the most merit, because these workers were able to correlate histologic type with response to treatment and outcome.[260] This classification placed tumors into one of four categories, according to the predominance of each cell type in a representative section of tumor: epithelial predominant, blastema predominant, stromal predominant, and mixed (no one element predominant). Within each histologic type the cells are also graded for the degree of anaplasia, or the presence of sarcoma in the stromal type. Studies reveal that tumors with marked anaplasia and those with stromal predominant type composed mainly of sarcomatous cells are associated with an unfavorable outcome using current therapeutic approaches. Three sarcomatous patterns

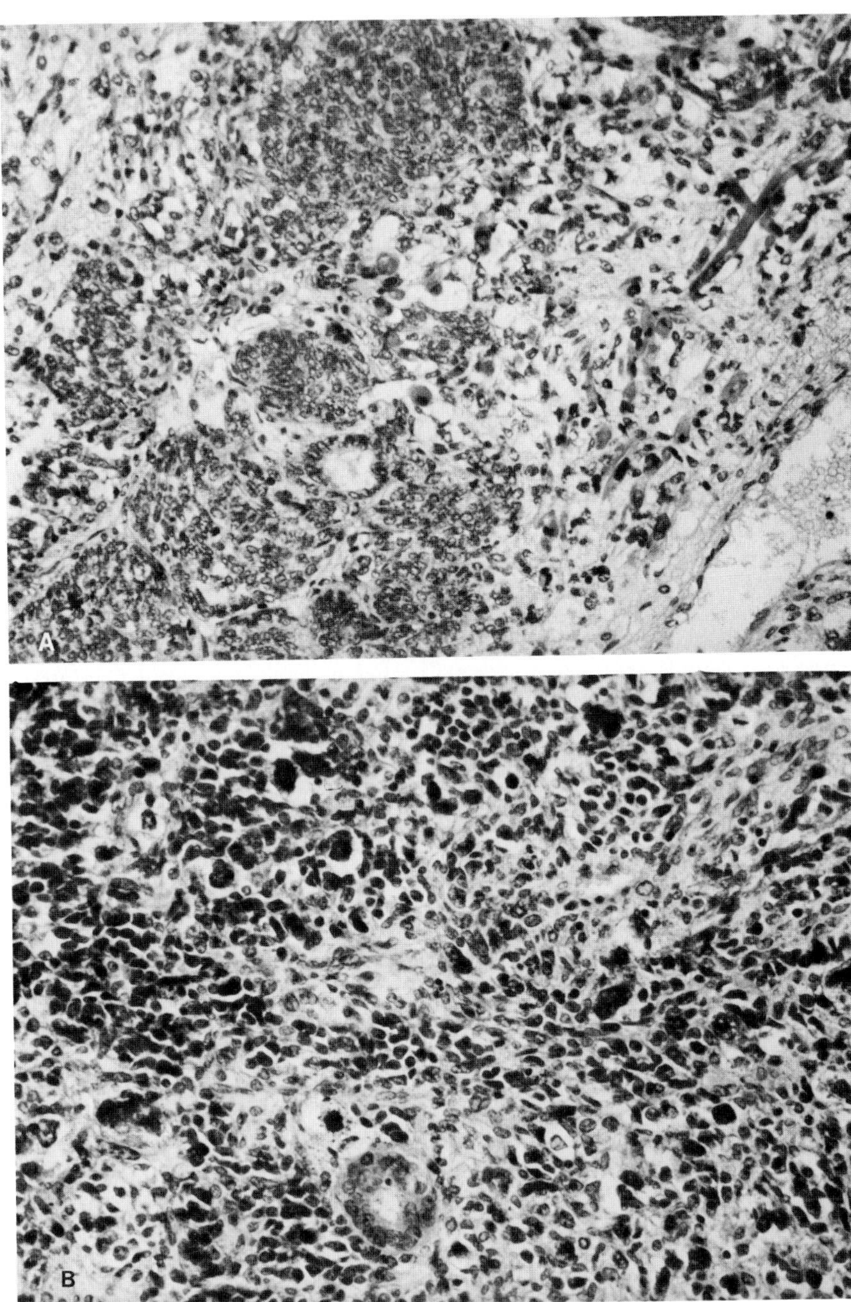

FIG. 34-11. (*A*) Wilms' tumor, showing blastema (undifferentiated spindle cells), epithelial differentiation (tubules) and stromal differentiation on the right hand side of the photograph (striated muscle fibers). The tumor lacks anaplasia. (*B*) Wilms' tumor, showing anaplasia, nuclei varying in diameter by a factor greater than three. As well as blastema, some epithelial differentiation is apparent. Hematoxylin and eosin, magnification.

are recognized, one of which, designated "clear cell sarcoma," has a predilection for bony metastases.[260] An example of a tumor with favorable histology and one with unfavorable histology is shown in Fig. 34-11.

NATURAL HISTORY

Approximately 30% of children are less than 1 year of age and 70% are less than 4 years of age at diagnosis. Presentation with Wilms' tumor after the age of 7 years is rare. The usual presenting finding is an asymptomatic flank mass discovered by the parents or by routine physical examination. Wilms' tumors often appear to reach great size suddenly, either because of recent growth, hemorrhage within the tumor, or cystic degeneration. In a series of 164 patients, 68% presented with an abdominal mass, 29% with pain, 26% with hematuria, 18% with fever, and 14% with anorexia.[262] Although gross hematuria is rare in Wilms' tumor as compared to renal cell carcinoma in older patients, about one-third of children with Wilms' tumor have microscopic hematuria. Other less common symptoms include malaise, weight loss, anemia, dysuria, and frequency.

Hypertension, usually mild but sometimes severe, is more commonly found in children with Wilm's tumor than is

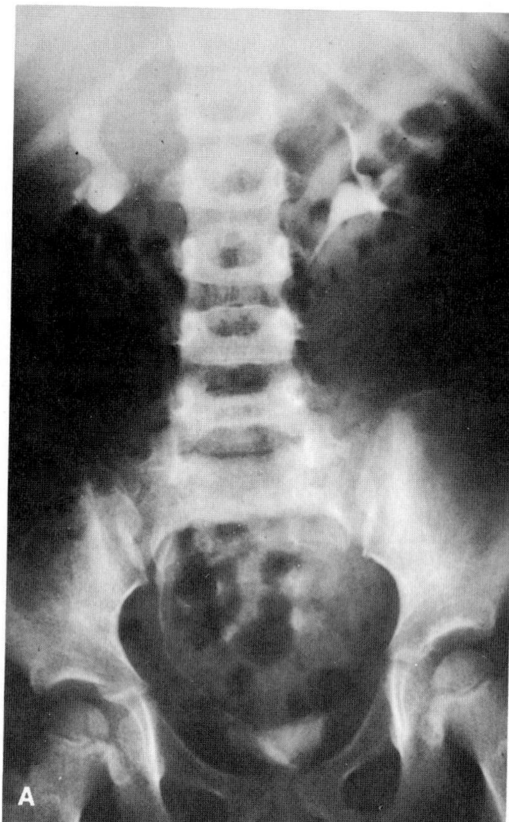

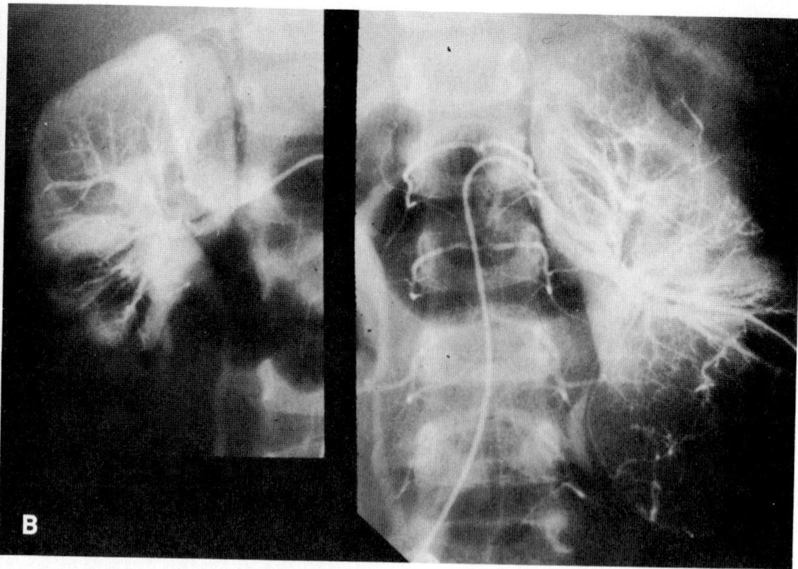

FIG. 34-12. (*A*) Intravenous pyelogram in 3-year-old with bilateral Wilms' tumor. The major mass is in the lower pole of the left kidney end and the stretched out lower pole calyx is evident. The mass in the right is not obvious. (*B*) Selective renal angiogram of each kidney demonstrates intrarenal mass in upper pole of right kidney and larger mass at lower pole of left kidney.

generally appreciated. Dibbins and Wiener have described an incidence as high as 75% to 90%.[263] Elevated plasma renin levels have been found to be associated with hypertension in many cases, presumably due to renin production by neoplastic cells, or from normal renal parenchyma whose blood flow is diminished by the surrounding neoplasm.[264,265]

Metastases are noted at initial presentation in about 15% of patients. An additional 30% develop metastases subsequently, 90% of these within 24 months of diagnosis.[262] The lungs are the most common site of tumor spread and the lesions may be single or multiple. Tumor is present in hilar or periaortic lymph nodes in about 25% of cases.[266] Hepatic metastases are not common and they are usually associated with lesions elsewhere. The presence of urothelial spread is well documented and indicates the need for extensive ureterectomy at the time of resection of the primary tumor.[267] Bone metastasis occurs in less than 5% of cases.

DIAGNOSIS

The initial investigation of a child with suspected Wilms' tumor includes complete blood count, urinalysis, blood urea nitrogen, serum creatinine, intravenous pyelography, and chest roentgenography.

The diagnosis is suspected from the characteristics of the mass as seen by pyelography, which usually shows intrinsic distortion of the collecting system with compression or elongation of the calyces (Fig. 34-12). Calcification is noted in about 10% of cases. Occasionally, the affected kidney shows no excretion of dye because of renal vein obstruction by tumor, but a nonfunctioning kidney is more often due to hydronephrosis. The contralateral kidney should be studied carefully for evidence of bilateral involvement, although a normal pyelogram does not exclude this possibility.

Ultrasonography is now used routinely to evaluate children with abdominal masses (Fig. 34-13). While this test can differentiate between solid and cystic areas, it is rarely sufficiently specific in children with suspected Wilms' tumor to provide a definitive diagnosis. However, in many cases this study is useful in detecting the presence of tumor in the inferior vena cava. If ultrasonography is inconclusive in this regard, then inferior vena cavagram is necessary to identify those cases with involvement of the vena cava, so that the surgeon is aware of the possible need for vascular control above the diaphragm or cardiotomy to remove the intravascular neoplasm. Ruling out caval extension is particularly important for left-sided lesions for the usual operative approach to these tumors does not allow easy access to the region of the right atrium.

Arteriography may be used to confirm the diagnosis and is particularly useful in those cases in which the pyelographic findings are not clearcut, and in those in which there is a suspicion of tumor in the contralateral kidney (Fig. 34-12).

Standard chest roentgenographs are used to determine the presence of pulmonary metastases, the most common site of spread. Computer tomography (CT scan) is capable of detecting smaller lesions than chest roentgenography, and will undoubtedly complement the latter procedure as its availa-

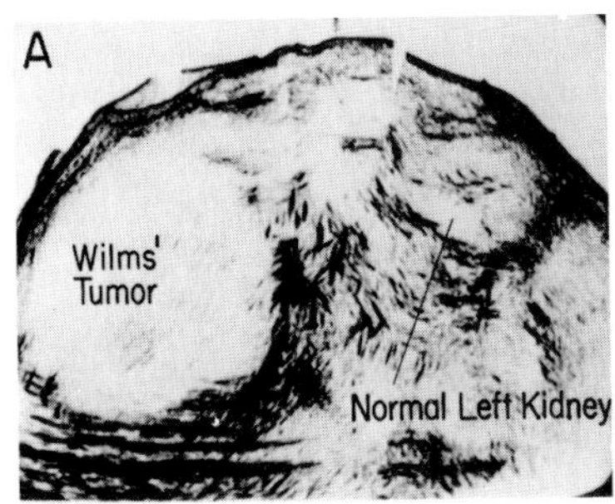

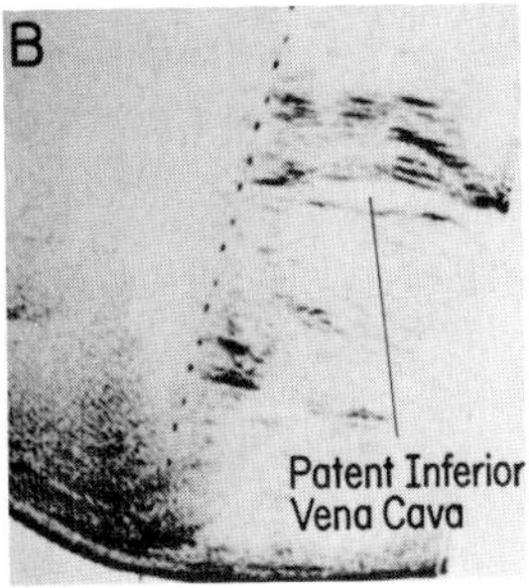

FIG. 34-13. Ultrasound study of patient with right Wilms' tumor: (*A*) Large right renal mass and normal left kidney; (*B*) Patent inferior vena cava.

bility increases and its expense decreases. Skeletal survey, bone scan, and liver scan may reveal the rare metastatic bone or liver lesion. Bone marrow examination and urine studies for VMA excretion are indicated mainly to exclude neuroblastoma.

STAGING

The extent of disease is staged according to the findings at surgery (confirmed by the pathologist) and the presence of distant metastatic disease. The staging system (grouping) used in the National Wilms' Tumor Study (NWTS) is given in Table 34-14. This system is used in most institutions in the United States and has been found to be of benefit in evaluating effects of different therapy protocols.[268]

However, despite its widespread use, this staging system has some shortcomings. To a degree, staging of disease is treatment related, and as a result the stage may vary with the skill of the surgeon rather than with a characteristic of the tumor. NWTS staging does not separate certain features known to affect prognosis. For example, the stage is not related to the size of the primary tumor, although tumor size clearly influences the result of treatment.[262,269] A modified staging system based on anatomic extent such as that proposed by Cassady and associates might be better suited for evaluation of data from different institutions.[262] Any new system of staging would also have to take into account tumor histology since this feature of Wilms' tumor is so closely related to outcome.[260]

TREATMENT OF WILMS' TUMOR

The evolution of treatment of Wilms' tumor is one of the most remarkable stories in cancer therapy. A major revolution took place in each of the effective modalities of therapy: surgery, radiotherapy, and chemotherapy. However, the advances made in each of these modalities were subsequently brought together and developed as one of the first unified multimodal approaches to the treatment of a solid tumor. This multimodal approach was highly effective, resulting in a high proportion of cures. Subsequently, Wilms' tumor was one of the first in which it was recognized that less therapy might be just as effective and might avoid some of the adverse consequences. This is best demonstrated by the National Wilms' Tumor Studies[268,269]

For many years, the surgical approach was through flank incisions, which did not permit accurate visualization of the affected kidney and no opportunity to explore the opposite kidney or the para-aortic lymph nodes. Although the transabdominal approach was first tried in the 1930s it was not widely employed until the 1950s. This was an essential step for the subsequent staging systems that were employed to assess the effectiveness of treatment. Postoperative irradiation of the tumor bed was introduced by Gross and Neuhauser and reported in 1950.[270] Subsequently, postoperative irradiation became an almost routine part of treatment and it was only many years later that it was learned this was no. necessary for every patient. Nonetheless, the second of the three modalities had been introduced, contributing to an improved overall outcome. In 1956, Dr. Sidney Farber and his colleagues reported that actinomycin-D was active against Wilms' tumor and was added to the armamentarium.[271] Subsequently, vincristine was also found to be effective and the basic components of therapy were later combined in many studies showing progressive improvement in the outcome of these patients, even those with extensive disease[272-274] Wilms' tumor remains one of the few tumors which can be cured in patients with multiple pulmonary metastases.[274] A wide variety

TABLE 34-14. Clinical Grouping; National Wilms' Tumor Studies 1 and 2

The patient's group is decided by the surgeon in the operating room, and is confirmed by the pathologist. If the histological diagnosis and grouping will take more than 48 hours, the surgical grouping stands, the patient is registered and started on treatment.

Group I—Tumor limited to kidney and completely resected.
The surface of the renal capsule is intact. The tumor was not ruptured before or during removal. There is no residual tumor apparent beyond the margins of resection.

Group II—Tumor extends beyond the kidney but is completely resected.
There is local extension of the tumor; *i.e.*, penetration beyond the pseudocapsule into the peri-renal soft tissues, or peri-aortic lymph node involvement. The renal vessels outside the kidney substances are infiltrated or contain tumor thrombus. There is no residual tumor apparent beyond the margins of resection.

Group III—Residual nonhematogenous tumor confined to abdomen.
Any one or more of the following occur: (1) The tumor has been biopsied or ruptured before or during surgery; (2) there are implants on peritoneal surfaces; (3) there are involved lymph nodes beyond the abdominal peri-aortic chains; (4) the tumor is not completely resectable because of local infiltration into vital structures.

Group IV—Hematogenous metastases.
Deposits beyond Group III; *e.g.*, lung, liver, bone and brain.

Group V—Bilateral renal involvement either initially or subsequently.

(D'Angio GJ, Evans AE, Breslow N et al: The treatment of Wilms' tumor: Results of the National Wilms' Tumor Study. Cancer 38:633–646, 1976)

*For National Wilms' Tumor Study 3, this system has been slightly modified. Groups I–V are now called Stages I–V. However, the following changes should be noted: (1) All patients with biopsy-proven positive lymph nodes are Stage III; (2) Children with biopsy of tumor or localized tumor "spills" are Stage II. (Children with gross tumor "spills" are still Stage III.)

of approaches, including surgery, radiotherapy, and chemotherapy, has been reported, however, an up-to-date review of the National Wilms' Tumor Studies has been reported recently by D'Angio and colleagues.[275–286] The National Wilms' Tumor Studies have been most effective in identifying subpopulations of patients who require less therapy and those who require considerably more therapy or different therapy because of a poor outcome, such as those with anaplastic histology.[274,286]

The history of the treatment of Wilms' tumor has a great deal to teach us about the effectiveness of multimodal therapy, the role of single institution and multi-institutional studies, and a necessary concern for the adverse late effects of therapy and definitive studies attempting to avoid those effects. Below are listed some specific aspects of each of the treatment modalities.

SURGERY

The initial goal of therapy is to remove the primary tumor even if distant metastases are present. The need for emergency operation in all cases is no longer advocated. However, there should be no unnecessary delay, and in most cases diagnostic studies can be completed within 48 hours, so that an operation can be performed within 3 days of admission. In about 5% of cases, pre-operative irradiation or primary chemotherapy is instituted because of the extent of the primary and its presumed inoperability, or because of the child's poor clinical status.[275] In these cases, surgery is delayed 2 weeks to 3 weeks, when the size of the tumor is much reduced.

In children with gross hematuria, cystoscopy preceding excision is employed to determine if the tumor has extended into the bladder. In the rare case in which the lower urinary tract is involved, the entire ureter and the involved portion of the bladder must be included with the resection.

At surgery, a generous transabdominal incision, extending into the chest if necessary, is used for proper exposure. If possible, the renal vein is occluded before extensive dissection to prevent further dissemination of tumor. During dissection, care must be taken to avoid rupture of the tumor. Tumors which invade the liver capsule usually do not penetrate deeply into the liver substance and they can be removed *in toto* by a superficial excision of the liver involved. The greatest hazard in removing the Wilms' tumor is injury to the inferior vena cava. It must be isolated above and below the tumor in all cases to be certain that an opening into it can be controlled.

After the primary is removed with a long segment of ureter, para-aortic nodes are inspected, and all enlarged or suspicious nodes are removed if possible. Biopsy of grossly negative nodes is essential for staging. Some surgeons perform retroperitoneal node dissection in all cases of Wilms' tumor, but data from NWTS do not indicate increased survival from this procedure.[266,269] In fact, when the surgeon has been confident that lymph nodes are negative, biopsy has indicated a correct appraisal in 96% of cases.[269]

Some of the details of the operation are shown in Fig. 34-14. Tumor which extends into the vena cava usually is not adherent to the wall of the vein. Therefore, it can be removed relatively easily after venotomy and control of vena cava above and below by gentle traction with a forceps. Occasionally, a blunt dissector can be passed between the vein wall and the tumor to facilitate this dislodgement. If the tumor embolus extends into the heart, removal can be aided by inserting a finger into an opening in the right atrial appendage while the tumor embolus is withdrawn from below. Cardiopulmonary bypass usually is not needed.

The contralateral kidney is carefully examined after it is mobilized and its capsule opened. If a small easily resectable tumor is found on this side, and if renal function will not be compromised, then the nodule and a small portion of normal kidney should be removed. Otherwise, the tumor should be biopsied, marked with radiopaque clips and treated as outlined below.

The liver and remainder of the abdomen are inspected for metastases. The tumor bed or areas of extension or residual disease are outlined with metallic clips where appropriate, as a guide for the radiotherapist. Leape, Breslow, and Bishop have recently reviewed the surgical treatment of Wilms' tumor from NWTS data.[269] Their study was capable of analyzing certain aspects of surgical technique. Their findings indicated that operative spill was a serious mishap, for it resulted in twice the frequency of abdominal recurrence, which led to a significantly higher mortality rate (22.8%). Possibly this incidence was related to difficulties with radiation technique because we have not observed this problem when all peritoneal surfaces have been irradiated after spill.[262] Operative spill was not more common with either a vertical, transverse, or thoraco–abdominal incision, but it is clear that good exposure and careful handling of the tumor are necessary to avoid this problem.

Relapse-free survival was not affected by ligation of the renal vein prior to resection. Similarly, leaving small amounts of visible tumor in the abdomen did not affect outcome. This finding supports the thesis that heroic or destructive efforts to remove the last vestige of tumor are not warranted or beneficial.

Children who present with, or develop, one or more pulmonary metastases usually are treated first with systemic chemotherapy and irradiation (1500 rad/10 Fx/2 wks) to both lung fields, because of the likelihood of multiple foci of gross and microscopic tumor deposits in the lung. However, surgical resection of pulmonary metastases is indicated for treatment failures or relapses, provided that the extent of disease is sufficiently limited to allow resection without severe compromise of pulmonary function. Wedge pulmonary resection, which minimizes the loss of lung, appears to be as effective as lobectomy for Wilms' tumor metastases.[275] Resection has been used to eradicate resistant metastases in the liver and in the brain.[276] Unfortunately, resection for metastases in these regions has not been successful as for those in the lung.[262]

CHEMOTHERAPY

Both actinomycin-D (ACD) and vincristine (VCR) have been widely used alone and in combination for chemotherapy of Wilms' tumor. Data from the National Wilms' Tumor Study indicate that the combination of these agents is better than either alone. Recently doxorubicin has been shown to be effective, but because of its potential cardiac toxicity, its routine use in several institutions has been reserved for

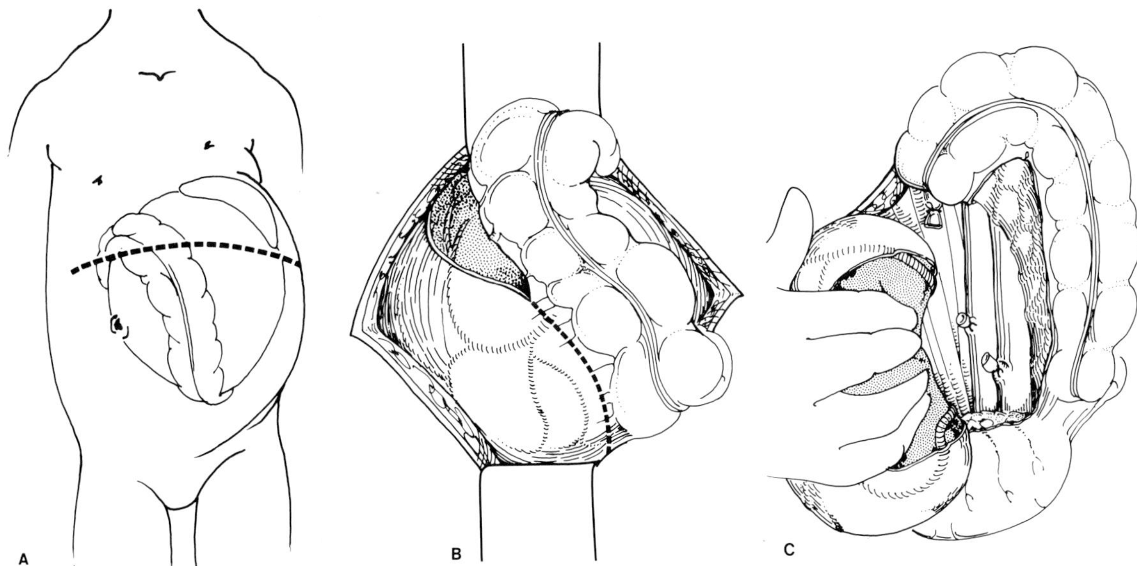

FIG. 34-14. Operative excision of Wilms' tumor of the left kidney. (*A*) Position of the bulging mass and the long transverse abdominal incision. (*B*) The colon is displaced downward and medially by the tumor. The peritoneum will be cut to mobilize the colon and expose the neoplasm. (*C*) The colon is pulled medially and the renal pedicle is divided. It does not seem to matter if the vein is tied before the artery or not. The tumor is being removed from the renal fossa. The ureter is seen at the lower end of the operative field, where it has been ligated. The colon will be replaced into the raw space left by the neoplasm.

patients with resistant or recurrent disease and for those whose tumor displays an unfavorable histology.[247,262,277–280]

Many slightly different therapy protocols have been designed.[262,268,281] At the Sidney Farber Cancer Center in Boston, actinomycin D, 10 mcg/kg I.V. (maximum dose 400 mcg), is initiated at surgery and continued for the next 6 days for a total dose of 70 mcg/kg. Vincristine, 2 mg/m^2 I.V. (maximum dose 2 mg), is begun when normal gastrointestinal motility is established following a nephrectomy. Vincristine is continued weekly for 12 courses if well tolerated, while actinomycin-D is repeated at 6 week to 8 week intervals for 24 months.[281]

RADIOTHERAPY

The routine use of radiotherapy to the flank or abdomen has been advocated for Wilms' tumor since 1938.[245] Recommended dose, dose–time relationships, and ports have varied considerably. However, no evidence is available supporting radiation doses greater than 2400 rad to 2600 rad in 2½ weeks to 3 weeks for treatment of potential microscopic residual disease, regardless of patient age at the time of treatment. Larger doses should be used for treatment of gross residual disease.[282,283] Renal fossa treatment suffices in most patients. Indications for treatment of the entire peritoneal cavity ("whole abdomen") are controversial. A standardized radiation scheme is shown in Figs. 34-15 through 34-17. Examination of this scheme, which is based on anatomic extent of tumor, demonstrates that routine use of irradiation for all patients is not necessary or desirable (see below). Figure 34-16 shows a simulation film for a typical renal fossa field. The heterogeneity in dose across the vertebral body that may occur if the medial border of the radiation field is too close to the vertebra is graphically shown in Fig. 34-16. Figures 34-17A and 34-17B show simulation and portal films for treatment of the entire abdomen, including all peritoneal surfaces and used when timer spill or rupture has occurred or overt residual disease remains in the abdomen.

TREATMENT ACCORDING TO STAGE OF DISEASE

In the past, when new effective therapy for Wilms' tumor was discovered, all children regardless of stage of disease were given the benefit of the new development. In the past 15 years, a more scientific approach has been taken, and individual institutional and cooperative group studies have been conducted to determine optimal therapy according to anatomic extent of disease. The aim of such studies has been to increase survival while decreasing the toxicity associated with therapy.[242,262,268] On the basis of these studies, it is now apparent that certain modifications in original therapy protocols are indicated in certain cases.

NWTS Group I patients less than 2 years of age did not benefit by routine postoperative irradiation. A significant improvement in survival and better local control and disease-free survival were demonstrated in irradiated Group I patients more than 2 years of age.[268] From this study, and other retrospective data, routine irradiation is not indicated in Group I children less than 2 years of age or any age child with anatomic T_1N_0, Stage I disease.[262,268]

NWTS I also demonstrated a superior disease-free survival in children with Group II or Group III disease who received both actinomycin-D and vincristine, as opposed to either agent singly. However, to date, overall survival has not increased because aggressive surgery, whole lung irradiation, and chemotherapy have salvaged patients who relapsed.

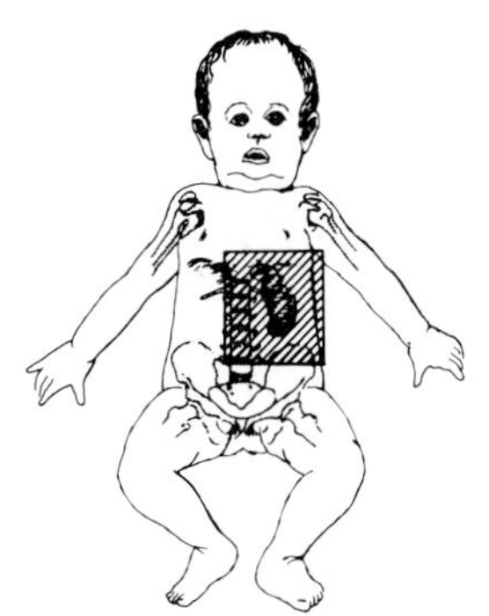
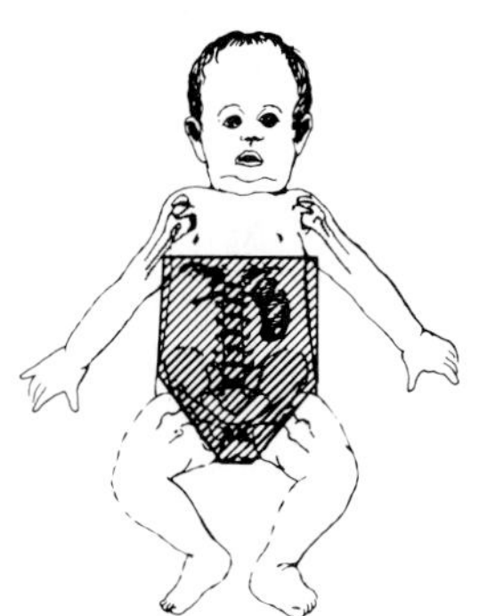
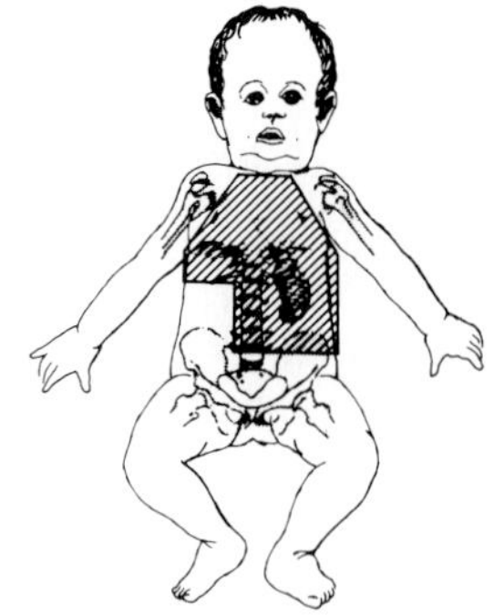

RENAL LESION ± LOCAL LYMPH NODES
• No surgical spill or other abdominal disease.
• No pulmonary metastases.
THERAPY
2500–3000 RAD/3 weeks to renal fossa.
AMD
• Surgical tumor spill ± other abdominal disease.
• No pulmonary metastases
THERAPY
2000 RAD/2½ weeks whole abdominal contents with normal kidney shielded at 1200 RAD.
+ Additional 750–1000 RAD/1 week to renal fossa.
AMD ± VCR
• No surgical spill or other abdominal disease.
• Pulmonary metastases.
THERAPY
1650 RAD/2 weeks to entire thorax and renal fossa.
Additional 1000–1500 RAD/1½ week to renal fossa.
AMD + VCR

FIG. 34-15. Diagrammatic treatment plan of radiotherapeutic fields in relation to extent of disease. (Cassady JR, Tefft M, Filler RM et al: Considerations in the radiation therapy of Wilms' tumor. Cancer 32:598, 1973)

NWTS II attempted to assess the efficacy of actinomycin-D and vincristine in all children with Group I disease without irradiation, regardless of age, since NWTS I Group I children had received only actinomycin-D. Excellent and equivalent disease-free survival was shown whether drugs were administered for 6 months or 15 months.[268] However, the radiotherapy question was left unanswered, as Group I children with unfavorable features (age more than 2 years, those with large tumors, or those with suspicious capsular involvement) were arbitrarily treated with irradiation at the discretion of the individual therapist.[282] NWTS II showed superior disease-free survival in children with Group II and Group III disease who received actinomycin-D, vincristine, and doxorubicin as opposed to actinomycin-D, and vincristine only. The two-drug schedule used in this study differed from that used in previous studies, as the course of actinomycin-D administered 6 weeks to 8 weeks following surgery was eliminated. The necessity and desirability of routine doxorubicin administration remains controversial. However, most oncologists feel that doxorubicin should be used definitively in those patients with tumors that have adverse histology.

For children with Group II and Group III disease, routine flank or abdominal irradiation or both appears indicated, although the necessity and optimum radiation dose and fields continue to be controversial. Because of the findings of Beckwith and Palmer, studies are now underway to determine if a more extensive therapy protocol will improve the survival in those children whose tumors have unfavorable histopathology.[260] To date, treatment of bilateral Wilms' tumor (Group V) has been individualized, and in most series, better than 50% survival has been noted with various methods.[262,284] Bilateral Wilms' tumor does not appear to be extremely aggressive and a conservative approach, preserving as much renal parenchyma as possible, seems indicated. In cases with a dominant mass on one side and a relatively small lesion on the other, most oncologists would recommend nephrectomy and heminephrectomy followed by standard chemotherapy and radiotherapy to both sides, but not more than 1500 rad/10 Fx/2 weeks to the remaining kidney parenchyma. If there is extensive bilateral involvement, then combined radiotherapy and chemotherapy, with or without subsequent surgery to remove residual tumor, can be curative. Approaches using chemotherapy followed by bilateral heminephrectomy or "tumorectomy" have also been described.[284] The place of bilateral nephrectomy and renal transplantation in these cases has been reviewed by DeMaria and associates.[285] They noted that only five of 17 patients were alive without metastasis at the time of their report, whereas nine of 17 died of overwhelming sepsis and another three died of metastatic tumor. At present, it would appear that bilateral nephrectomy and transplantation should be considered only as the last resort.

RESULTS OF TREATMENT

Most current studies indicate an overall cure of about 80% in children with Wilms' tumor, using the treatment plan outlined above (Fig. 34-18).[268,283] When the results are analyzed by clinical group, 2-year survival for those in Group I is about 95%, whereas salvage is about 30% for those who develop pulmonary metastases.[262] Those with metastases in liver, bone, or brain do not do as well, but only a few patients fall into this category.

As noted, relapse occurs in about 50% of children who initially present without metastases. Metastasis in the lung

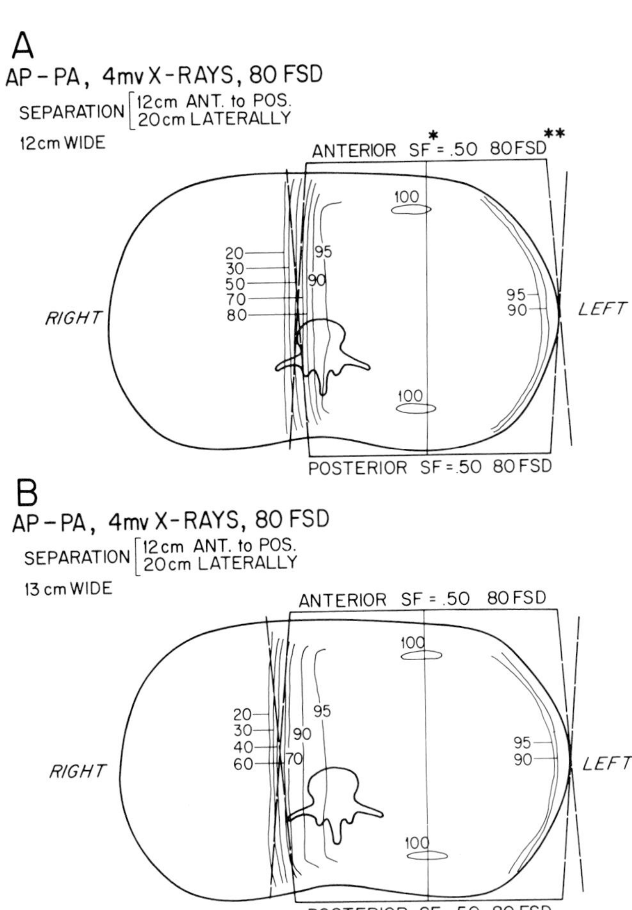

FIG. 34-16. Simulation field for radiation therapy of Wilms' tumor.

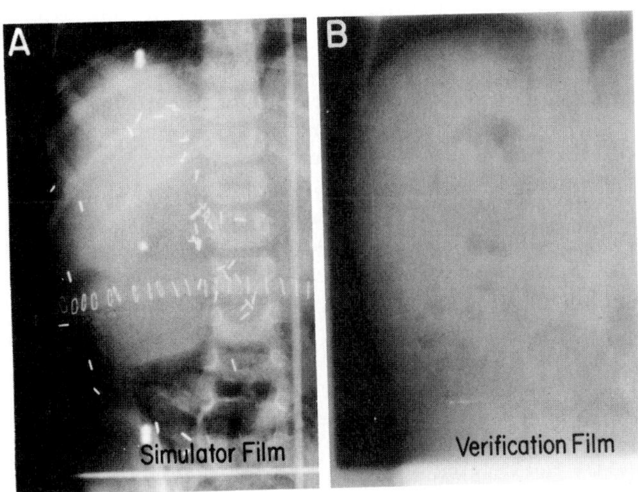

FIG. 34-17. (*A*) Simulation field for whole abdominal radiation. (*B*) Portal film for whole abdominal radiation.

accounts for about two-thirds of the relapses. Control of these metastases is possible in at least half of the cases by aggressive treatment, primarily with irradiation and chemotherapy, while reserving surgical excision for lesions which do not respond, or recur at a later date.[262]

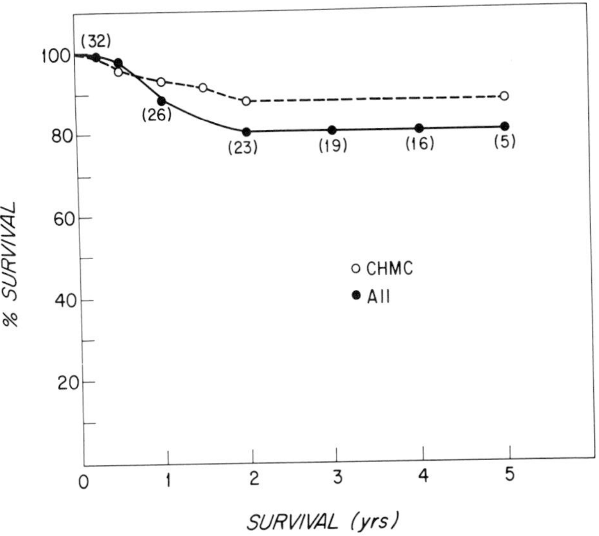

FIG. 34-18. Actuarial survival in Wilms' tumor. (Cassady JR, Jaffe N, Filler RM: The increasing importance of radiation therapy in the improved prognosis of children with Wilms' tumor. Cancer 39:825, 1977)

When the abdomen, retroperitoneum, or pelvis is the site of relapse, subsequent salvage is much less likely. However, local recurrences have been shown to be primarily related to radiation technique.[262] When tumor spill or local extension is not properly irradiated, relapse rates will be high.

Beckwith and Palmer's study related the prognosis to histopathology. Of 427 cases of Wilms' tumor treated by standard methods in the National Wilms' Tumor Study, 49 had unfavorable histology by their criteria and 28 (57.1%) of these children died of tumor.[260] Of the 378 cases with favorable histology, only 26 (6.9%) died of tumor. Seven of the 10 deaths due to tumor in patients diagnosed before 2 years of age were associated with sarcomatous histology.

FUTURE CONSIDERATIONS

Efforts to further modify therapy by the stage of disease must continue. Now that it has been shown that unfavorable results can be correlated to histopathology, trials to evaluate more aggressive therapy in these cases have already started. The results of studies in progress may also indicate that therapy can be further reduced in those with favorable histology.

RHABDOMYOSARCOMA

Rhabdomyosarcoma (RMS) is a highly malignant tumor thought to be derived from unsegmented, undifferentiated mesodermal tissue. This tumor, although numerically uncommon, represents a relatively frequent pediatric problem and, in fact, accounts for 5% to 10% of solid tumors and the majority of soft tissue sarcomas occurring in the pediatric age group.[287,288] Early therapeutic attempts focused on radical extirpative surgical procedures, which were often locally unsuccessful, both by virtue of local invasiveness and prox-

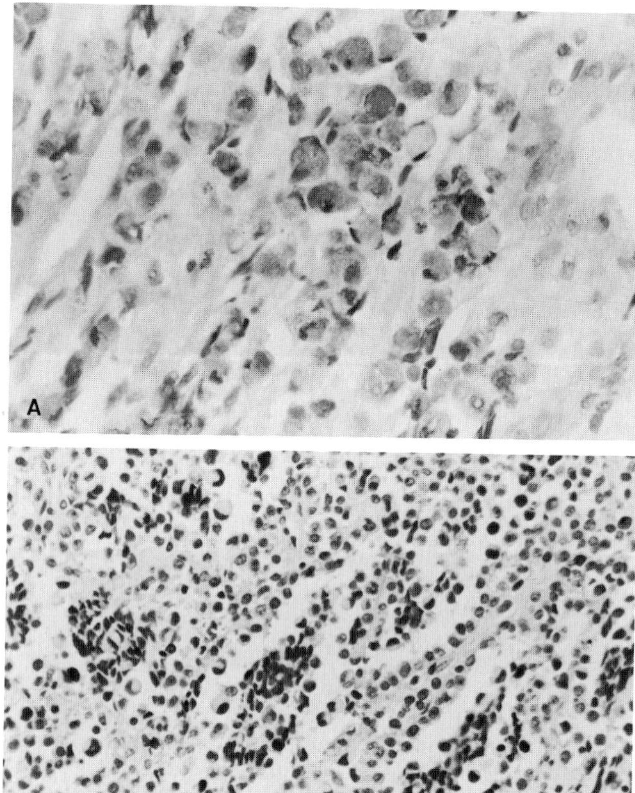

FIG. 34-19. (*A*) Typical embryonal rhabdomyosarcoma. Numerous rhabdoymyoblasts are interspersed throughout the section. (*B*) Alveolar rhabdomyosarcoma. Alveolar appearance resembling lung tissue is suggested by the cytologic arrangement of cells.

imity of vital normal structures. Even when local disease was successfully removed, the frequent and rapid appearance of metastatic disease often resulted in the patient's death. Following development of megavoltage radiation devices, permitting high-dose, large volume treatment, the ability of properly applied irradiation to routinely accomplish local control, with or without prior major surgery, was recognized. Almost simultaneously, the introduction of routine adjuvant systemic treatment permitted significant reduction in the incidence of metastatic disease and further improved overall control rates. Most recently, therapeutic approaches designed to minimize functional, cosmetic, and other long-term sequelae of treatment, without sacrificing overall control, have received increasing attention.

EPIDEMIOLOGY AND GENETICS

The etiology of RMS is not known. An association of RMS with breast cancer has been suggested; however, no definite genetic or familial associations are recognized. The relevance of murine sarcoma studies to human RMS is highly speculative.[289-292]

Two definite age peaks are recognized; one occurring between the ages 2 years and 6 years, the other in the early or mid-teens. Although numerous exceptions occur, tumors in the young tend to be embryonal in type and occur in the head and neck or genitourinary region, while tumors in older patients tend to arise on the trunk or extremities and be alveolar or undifferentiated in histology.[293]

ANATOMIC CONSIDERATIONS

Nearly 40% of all tumors occur in the head and neck region, with the orbit being the most frequently affected regional and general primary location. Other head and neck sites include the paranasal sinuses, oro- and nasopharynx, and tempero–parotid regions. One-third occur in the genitourinary region, while the remainder of tumors occur on the trunk and extremities.[291,294,295] As noted earlier, tumor location frequently precludes definitive surgical resection and, even when feasible (*i.e.*, genito–urinary sites), such resections produce significant disability.

PATHOLOGY

Formerly considered under a variety of histologic designations, current concepts of the true nature of many poorly differentiated pediatric soft tissue tumors changed approximately 20 years ago, when most of these lesions were reconsidered and designated as RMS.[296,297] Subsequently, they have been grouped into three major subtypes: embryonal, alveolar, and pleomorphic, or undifferentiated. Cross-striations are seen with frequency only in the pleomorphic variety. Specimens from fewer than 20% of patients with the embryonal type have cross-striations. Sarcoma botryoides ("grape-like") is a gross morphologic characterization of the embryonal type when it occurs in a submucosal location adjacent to a hollow viscus. Alveolar soft part sarcoma and the so-called "soft tissue Ewing's tumor" should be considered separately, although the latter lesion appears to have a similar prognosis and behaves like more typical RMS (Fig. 34-19).[298-300]

Embryonal RMS, the most frequent variety, is characterized by a mixture of round cells and cells with enlargement about an eccentric nucleus, so-called "tadpole" or "tennis racquet" cells. Alveolar RMS is characterized by connective tissue latticework, with cells arranged about this supporting structure, giving an overall appearance of lung alveoli with spaces between the cells. Pleomorphic RMS consists principally of spindle cells with considerable pleomorphism and, occasionally, strap-like cells that may contain cross-striations.[291,296]

Following diastase digestion, PAS stains with demonstration of glycogen in the cytoplasm may be helpful in diagnosis. Electron microscopic demonstration of cytoplasmic myofilaments or Z-band material may suggest or confirm the diagnosis. These specialized techniques may be of special value in the lesion without clear cross-striations, where lack of differentiation makes a specific diagnosis by light microscopy difficult or impossible.[301]

NATURAL HISTORY

RMS most frequently presents as an asymptomatic mass and has been noted in virtually every part of the body. The orbital tumors often present as tumors of the eyelid with or without associated proptosis or restriction of extraocular motion. RMS

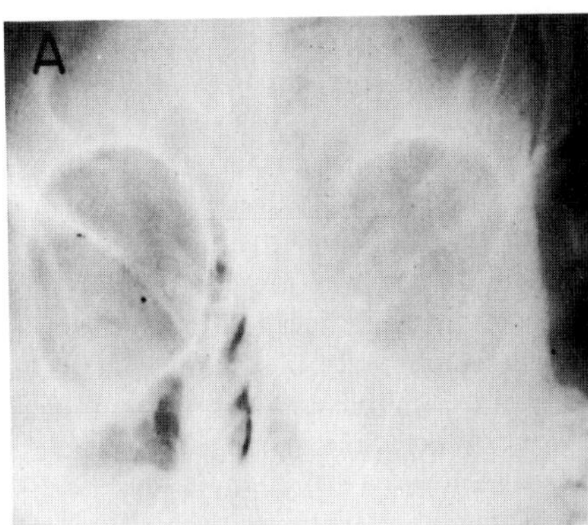

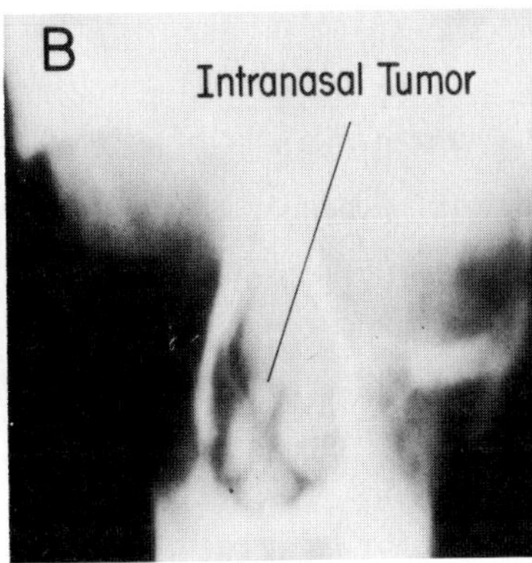

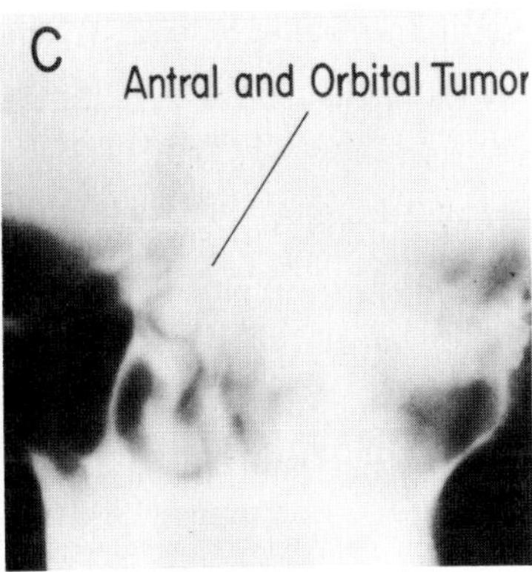

FIG. 34-20. Hypocloidal polytomography to show extent of tumor intransasally (*B*) and into antrum and orbit (*C*).

in other head and neck sites may present with such typical symptoms as ear pain, nasal stuffiness or discharge, trismus, or epistaxis. Genitourinary (GU) lesions may present with urinary retention or hematuria, vaginal discharge, or a scrotal mass. Pain, associated with the primary lesion or its metastases, may be the presenting complaint.

RMS spreads by three basic routes. Locally, wide regional soft tissue extension along fascial or muscle planes or direct invasion is the rule, and any reasonable therapeutic plan must consider this characteristic.[296] Metastatic extension to regional and distant node sites in an orderly fashion is common. Hematogenous metastases are found at presentation in about 20% of patients, especially those with trunk and extremity sites.[291] The disease tends to remain localized for a longer period of time in certain sites such as the orbit, bladder, and female genital tract, and this tendency explains the relative success obtained with tumors of these sites using only local treatment techniques in the past.[302]

Clinical lymph node metastases are rare at the time of presentation with orbital tumors, and the Intergroup RMS Study noted them to be uncommon in other head and neck sites.[295,303,304,308] Conflicting data exist on this point, and we have been struck by the frequency of clinically or pathologically involved lymph nodes in virtually every site except orbit.[305,306] Pathologic node involvement is relatively common with GU (especially paratesticular lesions) or lower extremity primaries.[306–308] Pathologic sampling of regional lymph nodes following confirmation of primary disease should be routine. One recent review compiling the overall incidence of involved lymph nodes by anatomic location of several large series demonstrated involvement of nodes in 0 of 19 (0%) orbital, 14 of 93 (15%) other head and neck, 13 of 55 (24%) genitourinary, 6 of 36 (17%) trunk and retroperitoneum, and 9 of 50 (18%) extremity primary sites.[301] The low incidence of node involvement in all head and neck sites reported by the Intergroup RMS Study may relate to the necessity for surgical confirmation for a node or node group to be considered to be affected and the frequent treatment of head and neck rhabdomyosarcoma by primary radiation therapy and more conservative surgical techniques. Routine lymph node sampling has not been required as necessary pretreatment evaluation in any large published series.

The necessity for a careful physical examination, history, and the usual laboratory tests (*i.e.*, CBC, urinalysis, and liver function studies) is evident. In addition to clinical and pathologic assessment of lymph node status, initial evaluation should include careful assessment of primary extent by a variety of radiographic techniques, including appropriate plain films, tomography (both conventional and computerized), ultrasonography, intravenous urography, angiography, and myelography when indicated. Hypocycloidal polytomography is essential for accurate assessment of head and neck primary extent into adjacent bony structures (Fig. 34-20).

Other workup should include isotopic bone scanning as well as analysis of the chest by plain films and tomography. Bone marrow aspiration and biopsy should be performed in all patients. Complete evaluation should be completed within 1 week of diagnosis, so that treatment can be initiated as soon as possible.

STAGING

No currently utilized staging system is entirely satisfactory. Systems developed and utilized by the Intergroup RMS Study (Table 34-15*A*) or Memorial Sloan Kettering Cancer Center are most commonly used.[308,309] Both place primary emphasis on surgical resection and therefore are heavily dependent on the skill and aggressiveness of the individual surgeon. Both also presume the superiority of primary surgical treatment, as unresected lesions are accorded higher stage, regardless of initial size. Intercomparison of data, a principal function of staging, is therefore difficult or impossible, and lesions of similar extent may be assigned widely varying stages.

The clinical TNM system of Jones and Campbell eliminates many of these problems; however, the artibrary size criteria (Table 34-15*B*) utilized may be inappropriate for very small children or critical locations.[310] As an example, a 10 cm orbital tumor with bone invasion in 2-year-old child is a massive tumor, although only Stage II in the TNM system depicted. A more recent, and more complicated, TNM system that incorporates grade has been recently proposed but suffers from many of the same problems for the pediatric patient.[311]

An anatomic staging system that considers the differences in site (*i.e.*, head and neck, genitourinary, and extremities)

TABLE 34-15*A*. Staging System, Intergroup Rhabdomyosarcoma Study

Group I:	Localized disease, completely resected Regional nodes not involved a. Confined to muscle or organ of origin b. Contiguous involvement—infiltration outside the muscle or organ of origin, as through fascial planes
Group II:	Regional disease a. Grossly resected tumor with microscopic residual disease. No evidence of gross residual tumor. No clinical or microscopic evidence of regional node involvement b. Regional disease, completely resected (regional nodes involved completely resected with no microscopic residual) c. Regional disease with involved nodes, grossly resected, but with evidence of microscopic residual
Group III:	Incomplete resection or biopsy with gross residual disease
Group IV:	Metastatic disease present at onset

TABLE 34-15*B*. Jones and Campbell Staging System

T_1:	Tumor less than 1 cm. in maximum dimension, no radiographic evidence of bone involvement by tumor
T_2:	Tumor 5-10 cm. in maximum diameter and/or radiographic evidence of bone invasion by tumor
T_3:	Tumor with contamination of the contiguous serosal cavity or greater than 10 cm. in maximum diameter
N_0:	No lymph node metastases
N_1:	Histologically involved lymph nodes in the first draining lymph node group
N_2:	Histologically or radiographically involved lymph nodes in the second draining lymph node group
M_0:	No extranodal metastases
M_1:	Pulmonary metastases
M_2:	Extrapulmonary metastases (bone, liver, bone marrow, etc.)

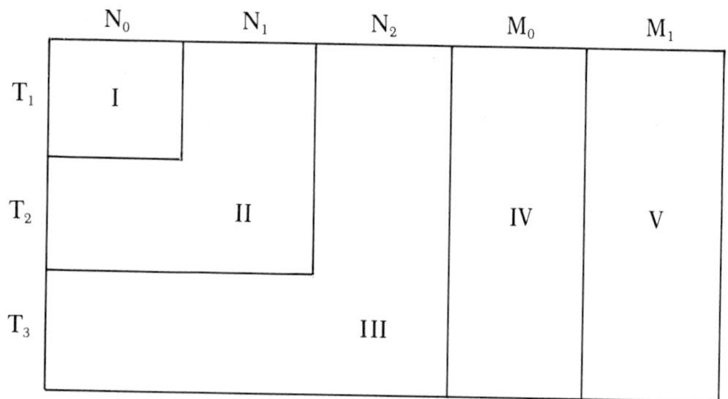

and considers variation of size with age and in which variation in surgical techniques is not important, is essential.

TREATMENT

The anatomic location of many of these tumors is such that aggressive surgical or radiotherapeutic treatment techniques may have far-reaching cosmetic as well as functional results. These considerations, in combination with surgical feasibility, will have the major influence on choice of the treatment plan for the primary lesion. Certain sites, such as the orbit, nasopharynx, or prostate, are nearly always best managed following biopsy confirmation by primary irradiation and adjuvant chemotherapy. Conversely, the primary management in limited trunk or extremity lesions or paratesticular primaries will usually include excisional removal of all gross disease, reserving irradiation for situations where its use permits less functionally destructive surgery (*i.e.*, amputation), improved local control (*i.e.*, close surgical margins) or regional control (*i.e.*, clinical or pathologic evidence of regional node involvement).

The goal of the therapeutic team should always be to achieve the best possible functional results as well as optimum survival.

Treatment for the child with RMS clearly requires close collaboration between the disciplines of radiation therapy, medical oncology, and surgery. General considerations for each discipline will be covered briefly, followed by a section discussing recommended treatment approaches for certain more common primary sites.

SURGICAL CONSIDERATIONS

The efficacy of radiation therapy and chemotherapy for rhabdomyosarcoma has had a major impact on the surgical procedures recommended for this tumor. Formerly, radical operations were the only means to affect a cure, although even with extensive and often disabling surgery, local recurrence rates were high and cure rates were low.[312] At present, more conservative, function-preserving operations are possible in a "total" treatment plan that utilizes the tumoricidal effects of modern chemotherapy and radiation therapy.

The exact role of surgery varies with the location, size, and extent of the tumor at presentation. Treatment of rhabdomyosarcoma initially by surgery is indicated when excision of the primary tumor imposes no major functional disability, especially if removal of the primary tumor will permit elimination or a significant dose reduction of irradiation. When only partial removal of the tumor is likely, and particularly when such attempts will result in significant long-term disability, initial surgery should be limited to biopsy, sampling of regional nodes, and placement of radiopaque markers, which can be used to plan radiation fields. After the size of the mass has been reduced by other therapeutic modalities, residual tumor can be removed at a second operation by a much less extensive procedure. When reduction of the tumor mass has been accomplished by multiagent chemotherapy only, irradiation is used after second-look surgery, because of the likelihood of residual microscopic tumor at sites outside of the surgical field that were originally occupied by the neoplasm. Some rhabdomyosarcomas, such as those involving the orbit, can be treated successfully by a combination of chemotherapy and radiotherapy. In these children, further surgery is necessary only for the rare patient who develops a solitary local recurrence. Utilizing these principles, amputation, orbital and pelvic exenteration, radical node dissection, and other similar procedures can be avoided and local tumor control, functional survival, and cure rates improved.[307,313-316]

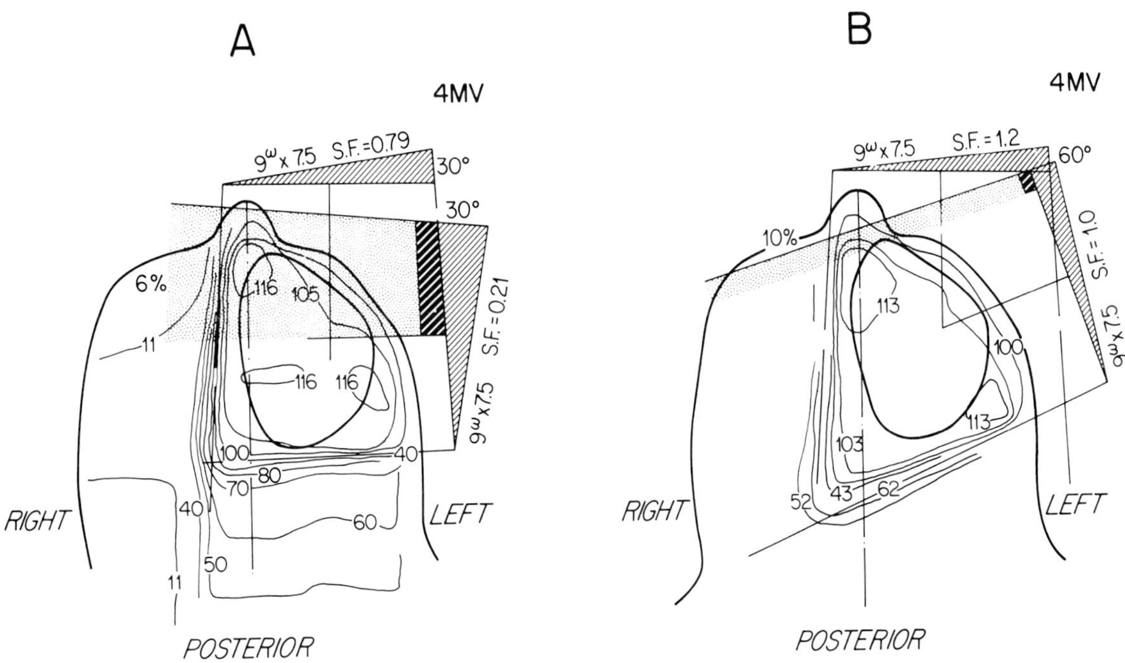

FIG. 34-21. Isodose contours for an extensive tumor of the paranasal sinus region with regional nodal involvement. Contours at the eye, palate, and neck level are shown and demonstrate the technical complexity essential for appropriate homogeneous treatment. Use of individually contoured blocks, appropriate scaling of the radiation beam, and level of homogeneity within tumor volume achieved are shown in the face of very dramatic changes in contour.

RADIATION THERAPY

The majority of patients with RMS will require irradiation for control of primary or regional disease. On rare occasions, control of limited metastatic disease utilizing combinations of chemotherapy, irradiation, and surgery will permit resultant long-term disease-free survival.

The multiplicity of potential primary sites precludes detailed descriptions of radiation fields; however, general principles include:

1. The importance of using radiation fields which are relatively large for the apparent clinical extent of gross tumor. RMS is insidiously invasive and experience has shown that use of such *large* fields results in improved local control.[317]

2. Local control of gross or macroscopic RMS in a high percentage of patients requires doses of 5500 rad to 6000 rad using conventional fractionation in combination with multiagent chemotherapy.[302,308,329] Presence of extensive bony invasion, seen more often in patients with RMS in the head and neck region, is worrisome and may require higher radiation doses for equivalent control rates.[302,318–321]

3. Control of microscopic or presumed subclinical disease may be accomplished with lower radiation doses of 4500 rad to 5000 rad. Although controversial, when primary control is to be achieved with irradiation, treatment of one tier of lymph nodes beyond those clinically involved appears to result in improved local–regional control.[291,307,329]

4. Judicious and extensive treatment planning, utilizing simulation with rotational or multiple field techniques and using individually constructed blocks and beam-shaping devices to minimize normal tissue damage is mandatory (Fig. 34-21).

Simple two-field treatment plans will usually result in excessive morbidity and a poor therapeutic result, and when technical aspects of radiation therapy are omitted or performed incompletely, treatment failure from both local tumor recurrence and poor function often results.

CHEMOTHERAPY

A number of series, using historical controls for comparison, have demonstrated progressive improvement in overall and disease-free survival following the introduction of routine adjuvant chemotherapy. In part, these results were clouded by the fact that concurrent improvements were obtained with radiation techniques, especially with respect to both field size and total dose. However, Jenkin and Sonley, comparing results at the Princess Margaret Hospital using similar radiation techniques and doses, with or without adjuvant chemotherapy (historical), showed an overall improvement in 5-year survival (all stages) from 32% to 43% by the introduction of routine chemotherapy. Of greater significance, the study of Heyn and associates, a randomized, prospective clinical trial, demonstrated an improvement in disease-free survival from 47% (7 of 15 cases) to 82% (14 of 17 cases) in patients with limited disease receiving routine adjuvant actinomycin-D and vincristine, rather than local treatment alone.[291,295,309,320,326,327,335,336]

Several classes of agents have been shown to have activity against this tumor. Alkylating agents, including cyclophos-

TABLE 34-16. Representative Combination Drug Schedules in Clinical Use (Duration 18-24 Months)

REFERENCE NUMBER	VINCRISTINE	ACTINOMYCIN-D	CYCLOPHOSPHAMIDE	ADRIAMYCIN
(291)	1. ⊕, 1.5 mg/m² IV weekly × 6, then every other week	⊕, 0.4 mg/m² IV weekly × 6 every 12 weeks	⊕, 300 mg/m² weekly × 6, then every other week	(−)
(309)	2. ⊕, 0.075 mg/Kg IV weekly × 4 every 12 weeks	⊕, 0.015 mg/Kg IV q day × 5 every 12 weeks	⊕, 10 mg/Kg by mouth every day × 10 every 12 weeks	(−)
(326)	3. ⊕, 2 mg/m² IV weekly × 12, then weekly as tolerated	⊕, 0.32 mg/m² IV every day × 7 every 12 weeks	⊕, 300 mg/m² IV every day × 7 every 6 weeks	(−)
(327)	4. ⊕, 2 mg/m² IV weekly × 4 every 13 weeks	⊕, 0.45 mg/m² IV q day × 5 every 13 weeks	⊕, 1200 mg/m² IV every other week × 2 every 13 weeks	⊕, 20 mg/m² IV every day × 3, × 2 course, × 13 weeks
(325)	5. ⊕, 2 mg/m² IV weekly × 12	⊕, 0.015 mg/Kg IV q day × 5 every 3 months	⊕, 2.5 mg/Kg by mouth every day × 2 years	(−)

phamide and nitrogen mustard, vinca alkaloids, especially vincristine, and antibiotics, principally actinomycin-D and doxorubicin, have all been extensively utilized in treatment. Response rates to these agents utilized alone range from 25% to 30% with complete responses noted rather infrequently.[291,322-324] Surprisingly, combinations of three or more agents have not been demonstrated to be more effective than the combination of vincristine and actinomycin-D. Thus, the Intergroup RMS Study and Children's Cancer Study Group have tested the efficacy of VAC (actinomycin-D) compared to VA for patients with Stage II disease and shown no significant difference.[308,325] Similarly, disease-free survival and response rates with doxorubicin added to VAC have not been shown to be significantly different.[308] The possibility remains that more optimum drug schedules for the three-drug or four-drug regimens would have yielded substantially different qualitative and quantitative results. A number of representative drug combinations and schedules currently in clinical use are shown in Table 34-16. A brief perusal of this table is sufficient to indicate the considerable variation in drug schedules and intensity possible using primarily the same agents.

INTEGRATION OF THERAPEUTIC TECHNIQUES

Combining surgery, radiation therapy, and chemotherapy to produce maximum efficacy of each treatment mode within tolerable limits of morbidity represents one of the greatest challenges in treatment of these children.

For children who present with widespread metastatic disease, it is clear that initial aggressive systemic treatment, with integration of local treatment modes considerably later in the therapy course, is appropriate. Conversely, children with limited early stage disease, especially in favorable sites, fare well when systemic treatment follows or, when appropriate, is utilized concurrently with appropriate local modalities. The Intergroup RMS Study has shown that for children with intermediate disease extent, pretreatment with chemotherapy for periods up to 6 weeks following diagnosis does not adversely affect results.[328]

Suitable modification of one treatment mode so as to not compromise another is equally important. Therefore, in the treatment of pelvic RMS, temporary use of nitrogen mustard rather than cyclophosphamide during irradiation to prevent unacceptable cystitis is clearly useful and does not appear to compromise results. When large areas of mucosa must be irradiated, suitable modification in chemotherapeutic schedules during the period of irradiation to prevent extremely disabling mucositis is also helpful and no therapeutic compromise has been demonstrated. Conversely, split courses of irradiation permitting interdigitation of chemotherapy during local treatment so as to not interfere with effective drug scheduling is often necessary. It is apparent that frequent and close collaboration between physicians must occur to achieve optimal results.

RESULTS

Most current series report disease control in more than 60% of children with RMS. Overall success is clearly related to disease extent and primary site. Cure is likely in more than 80% of all patients with limited or regional orbital tumor and tumors in most patients with regionally limited genitourinary lesions are currently controlled by aggressive interdisciplinary treatment.[291,295,307,309,317,319,320,327,329]

Patients with regionally limited head and neck RMS have a similarly favorable outlook, although extensive bone destruction or extensive regional nodal disease is worrisome.[327] Patients with trunk or extremity lesions, even when localized, have a less favorable outlook in our experience, while cure in the patient who presents with distant metastatic disease is extremely unlikely.[330] Using optimal surgery and irradiation combined with systemic chemotherapy, primary local control should be possible in more than 90% of all patients[302,307,320,329]

FUTURE CONSIDERATIONS

The obvious necessity for a more appropriate staging system is clear and has been noted earlier. As with many other pediatric solid tumors, better systemic therapy to permit more effective treatment for patients who present with metastatic disease is necessary. In addition, patients with certain disease sites, especially trunk and extremity lesions, continue to fare poorly in most reports, even when apparently limited at presentation, and would clearly benefit from more effective systemic treatment.

Local control rates in more than 90% of all patients utilizing integrated, definitive surgery, irradiation and chemotherapy are currently achieved at several institutions.[302,307,320,329] Current and future studies are needed to confirm the necessity for use of all treatment modes in all patients. Surgical treatment, utilized alone in certain highly selected patients with early stage disease, seems sufficient and local control rates of approximately 90% have been achieved with this approach. Thus, the Intergroup RMS Study has demonstrated no significant advantage when irradiation was added to complete excision followed by multiagent chemotherapy (actinomycin-D and vincristine, with or without cyclophosphamide) in patients with Group I tumors. Two of 24 patients without irradiation relapsed locally as opposed to none of the 13 who received postoperative irradiation. The incidence of distant metastases was equivalent in the two groups. Of note, only 16% of all patients were Group I in this study and a disproportionate number (39 of 50 patients, or 78%) had primary lesions of the extremities or genitourinary region, sites more amenable to extirpative surgery. Similarly, no clear benefit in local control has been achieved when surgery has been added to optimum irradiation for tumors of the orbit, other head and neck sites, and genitourinary sites.[289,307,319,327]

ORBIT

Following biopsy confirmation, primary irradiation is recommended in combination with systemic chemotherapy. For limited tumors at this favorable site, we recommend initial irradiation with delay in chemotherapy until approximately 2500 rad to 3000 rad has been administered, following which completion of irradiation should be accomplished. It is very important that the eye be open for a major portion of radiation treatment, if possible, as treatment for the entire course with eyelid closed is associated with a significantly greater likelihood of subsequent chronic keratoconjunctivitis, dryness, phthisis, and painful eye, presumably related to elimination of the relative sparing of conjunctival dose made possible with megavoltage equipment. A two-field or three-field plan with wedges is recommended with irradiation of the preauricular and upper cervical lymph nodes if clinically negative, although the necessity of including node groups for this site is controversial (Fig. 34-22).

OTHER HEAD AND NECK SITES

Surgical resection with sufficiently wide margins to permit elimination of irradiation will rarely be possible without unacceptable cosmetic or functional consequences. Therefore, radiation therapy in combination with judicious surgery will constitute the principal mode of primary treatment for most of these patients.[327] Careful attention to common routes of tumor spread and technical details of irradiation is necessary. Although parameningeal RMS has been noted to have a high rate of meningeal relapse in the Intergroup RMS Study, virtually all of these patients had one or more major alterations in recommended irradiation treatment plans and we and others have not observed a similar rate of relapse when radiation parameters were carefully controlled.[329,331–333] Patients with extensive bone involvement account for virtually all local failures in our series and radiation doses should approach a minimum of 6000 rad in virtually all of these patients.[329,334] Chemotherapy should either precede irradiation by a brief period or be given concurrently.

TRUNK

A higher proportion of tumors at this site tend to be of the alveolar or pleomorphic type. Surgical resection of bulk disease should be possible in many of these patients without unacceptable consequences. If margins are widely adequate, no postoperative irradiation appears necessary at this time, so long as aggressive systemic chemotherapy is administered.[304] If margins are inadequate, irradiation is necessary. If microscopic residual (*i.e.*, close margin) is to be treated, a dose of 5000 rad will suffice. Use of electron beam irradiation, interstitial techniques, and creative and judicious use of photon irradiation to minimize normal tissue damage are essential.

EXTREMITY

Many of the comments made for truncal RMS are also appropriate for extremity lesions. Wide surgical resection should be accomplished where feasible without resultant major functional defect. Amputation is rarely appropriate and, when surgically necessary, should be considered only when growth discrepancies following irradiation will be functionally unacceptable. Even in this latter setting, initial radiation treatment with reservation of surgical amputation only when functionally mandatory has many advantages. As a group, these patients fare poorly, owing to failure in control of distant rather than local disease. As relapse usually occurs within 2 years of initial treatment, many children will be thereby spared unnecessary amputation. Unlike osteosarcoma, where a similar treatment philosophy was espoused earlier, control of RMS with irradiation is regularly accomplished and doses necessary to this high control probability can be delivered with excellent resultant function.[329] Amputation for upper extremity lesions is virtually never recommended. Lymph node involvement is often seen with these lesions and lymph node sampling (NOT dissection) is especially recommended.

GENITOURINARY

Most patients with a morphologic appearance of sarcoma botryoides have lesions of this location and, as noted earlier, most are of the embryonal type. Patients tend to be younger and lymph node involvement is common.[304,307,312–315] The dual goals of function and tumor control require careful interposition of all major modalities. Radical anterior, posterior, or combined exenterations should not be performed, and complications, including ejaculatory impotence, should discourage radical node dissections.[301] Similarly, careful and precise

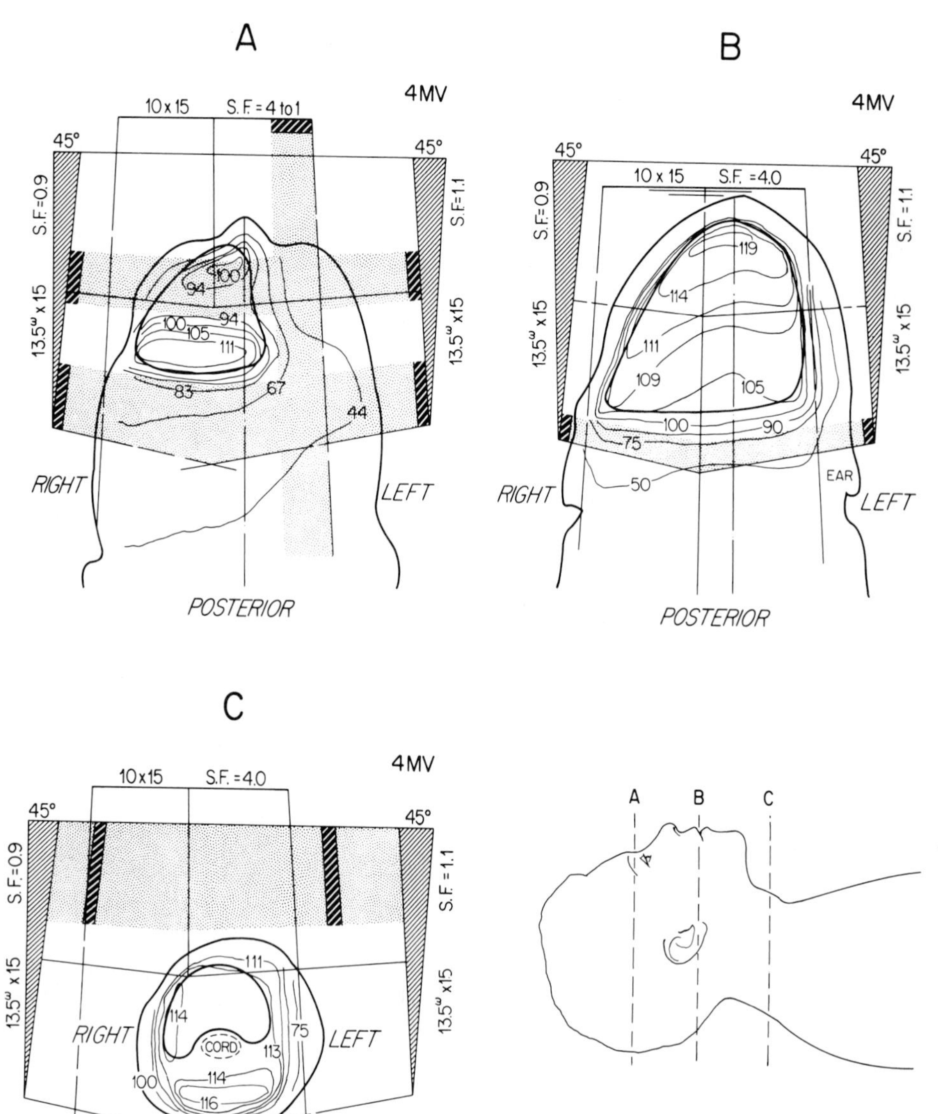

FIG. 34-22. Isodose contours of two treatment plans for orbital rhabdomyosarcoma. *A* includes a greater contribution from the anterior field with a resultant contralateral lens dose of approximately 6%. We have not observed this dose delivered in multiple small increments to lead to cataract formation. Cataract formation in the treated eye is routine and is generally noted about 1½ years following treatment. *B* demonstrates that the lateral field is angled posteriorly with an appropriated placed lens block for the contralateral eye. Use of a block placed at the central portion of the lateral field, thereby avoiding divergency, is shown in *A*.

radiation treatment planning and use of rotational and multiple field techniques are necessary to prevent an unacceptable incidence of bowel and other complications. Fortunately, the majority of these children can be cured even when they present with extensive disease.

EWING'S SARCOMA

Ewing's sarcoma is a highly malignant round cell tumor of bone which represents the second most common primary bone tumor in children and young adults.[328–330] First distinguished by Ewing in 1921 by virtue of its composition with small round cells rather than the spindle cells of osteosarcoma, and its characteristic diaphyseal tumor location, this tumor continues to defy easy histopathologic separation from other small round cell tumors affecting bones in children.[331]

Major diagnostic and therapeutic advances occurring in the past decades involving this highly malignant tumor of bone have created a number of new questions and controversy for the pediatric oncology team. Paradoxically, improved survival, local control, and a significant increase in the number of cured patients, developments which have occurred by virtue of markedly improved radiation therapy techniques in association with the introduction and routine use of progressively more effective systemic therapy, have created new questions about optimum local treatment, especially the place of radiation therapy, because of the potential of late complications.

Local treatment with either surgical procedures or moderate dose (4000 rad or less) orthovoltage irradiation, produces long-term survival in less than 10% of all patients.[330] More recently, the introduction of more effective systemic treatment, combined with improved local treatment techniques principally using megavoltage irradiation, has produced striking improvement in local control of the primary lesion and significant improvement in disease-free survival for patients with no metastases at presentation.[332–336] Although survival has been substantially extended for patients who present with metastases, most such patients ultimately develop additional sites of tumor and die.

Current questions concern the optimum treatment of the primary lesion to accomplish local control, good function, and a minimum of late morbidity, and the best choice of several available systemic approaches to improve therapy for the large number of patients who present with axial primary lesions or with metastatic disease and regularly relapse currently.

EPIDEMIOLOGY AND GENETICS

The etiology of this highly malignant tumor is not known. The tumor is seen most frequently in the second decade of life and is rare before the age of 5 years and after the age of 30 years. Males predominate with a usual sex ratio of 1.5:1 to 2:1.[328,329,332,337,338]

As are patients with osteosarcoma, those with Ewing's sarcoma are taller as a group than their peers without bone tumors.[328] In addition, Ewing's tumor is exceptionally rare in blacks.[328,337] The significance of these findings is not known, although they certainly suggest an important genetic element in the development of this tumor.

FIG. 34-23. Frequency of primary involvement in patients with Ewing's tumor. Note relative frequency of femur and pelvis involvement.

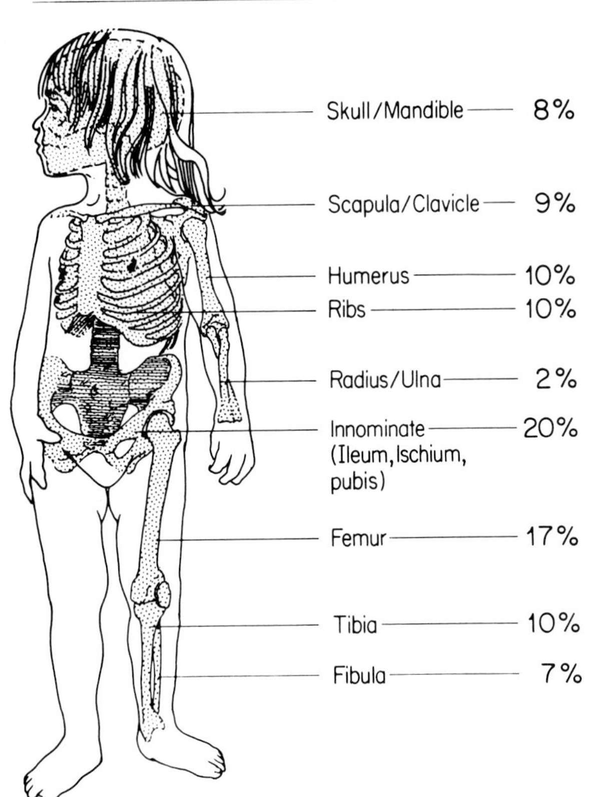

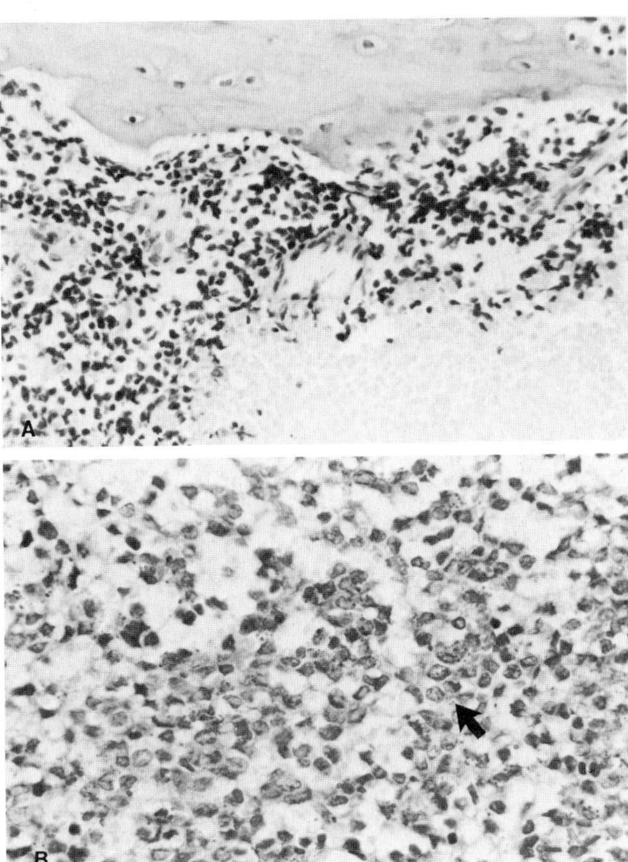

FIG. 34-24. Histopathology of Ewing's sarcoma. (*A*) Relatively uniform Ewing's tumor cells present in medullary cavity of bone with adjacent, relatively normal, bone. No osteoid formation by tumor evident. (*B*) PAS (periodic acid Schiff) stain of Ewing's sarcoma. Arrow illustrates PAS granule in cytoplasm.

ANATOMICAL CONSIDERATIONS

As in osteosarcoma, the femur is among the most frequently affected primary sites of involvement.[339] However, unlike osteosarcoma, the flat bones, especially those constituting the innominate bone, are frequently affected and collectively represent the most frequently affected sites in many series.[329] Frequency by site in two large collected series is shown in Fig. 34-23.[329,340] More than half of the lesions in these series originate in the axial skeleton.

PATHOLOGY

The lesion is composed of large numbers of round cells, usually rather small in size and quite anaplastic (Fig. 34-24). Ewing noted frequent vascular invasion in this tumor and postulated that the cell of origin was a primitive endothelial cell, hence "diffuse endothelioma of bone."[331]

Non-Hodgkin's lymphoma of bone, metastatic neuroblastoma, and embryonal rhabdomyosarcoma, either metastatic or invading from a soft tissue primary into bone, all constitute potential *differential problems*. Generally, other clinical findings enable the physician to differentiate neuroblastoma and

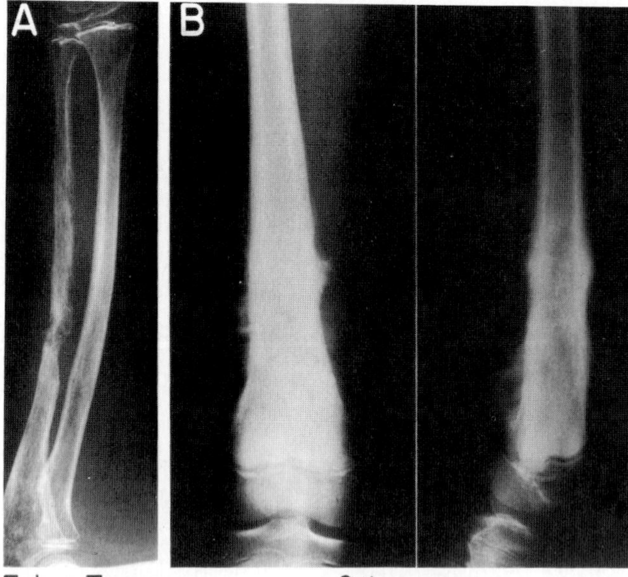

FIG. 34-25. Radiographs of "typical" osteosarcoma and Ewing's tumor. (*A*) Ewing's tumor of ulna. Note diaphyseal involvement with no tumor-related new bone and extensive permeative appearance. (*B*) Classic osteosarcoma of femur in frontal and lateral projections. Typical metaphyseal location with new bone formation, lack of permeation, Codman's triangle, and spiculation are evident.

rhabdomyosarcoma from the other two lesions. In particular, the presence of an elevated catecholamine level will serve to distinguish neuroblastoma.

More recent studies, utilizing cytochemistry, tissue culture, and electron microscopy in addition to light microscopy, have suggested that the cell of origin of Ewing's tumor is a primitive myeloid element with the capacity for further differentiation.[341]

The presence of glycogen-rich cytoplasm has been suggested as a principal differential point between Ewing's tumor and non-Hodgkin's lymphoma of bone.[342] However, the utility of this finding in all instances has been questioned in more recent reports.[341] Newer developments in cell surface typing and analysis combined with regular use of electron microscopy should serve to distinguish many patients with non-Hodgkin's lymphoma from those with Ewing's tumor and probably represent the greatest hope for future improvement in this confusing area.

In summary, although advances in the ability of the pathologist to distinguish Ewing's tumor from other lesions have occured, Stout's lack of a "clear and definitive mental picture, which on the basis of histopathology alone, enables me to differentiate this neoplasm from others involving bone" seems to be shared by many pathologists and continues to represent a major clinical problem.[341,343]

NATURAL HISTORY

Most patients present because of pain and swelling of the affected region. Often the duration of clinical symptoms, especially with axial lesions, can be prolonged and extended over many months. Fever, weight loss, and generalized fatigue are frequently present, and more than one-half of all patients have a mass evident at the time of presentation.[344] On occasion, the presence of metastases (*i.e.*, lung) may cause symptoms that cause the patient to seek initial medical attention.

PATTERNS OF SPREAD

Ewing's tumor tends to affect the diaphysis of long bones and, less frequently, the metaphysis.[338,340,345] Involvement of the epiphysis is rare. The entire medullary cavity of affected bones should be considered to be affected for treatment purposes.

Extension through the bony cortex and into the soft tissues is regularly present and, as noted previously, a large soft tissue component is common. On occasion, especially with axial lesions, the soft tissue mass may, in fact, be larger than the intraosseous component. Fig. 34-25*A*, *B* compares radiographs of a "classic" osteosarcoma with those of a "classic" Ewing's tumor. However, these "typical" changes must be viewed with caution, as numerous exceptions occur (Table 34-17).

Lymph node involvement is said to be uncommon, although reports suggesting more frequent involvement are available.[346] In fact, no study is known in which routine pathologic sampling of appropriate regional nodes has been accomplished. Certain patients in the current Intergroup Ewing's Tumor Study are undergoing node sampling.[347] For the present, however, the true incidence of nodal involvement remains an unanswered question.

Hematogenous spread to the lungs is well recognized, and this probably represents the most frequent site of metastatic disease at presentation or as a site of initial relapse.

Although recognized clinically for some time, the introduction of radioisotopic bone scanning has emphasized the relative frequency of bony involvement at sites other than the presenting location.[348] Although generally considered to be sites of hematogenous metastases, the possibility that these may represent sites of multifocal origin has been raised.[341] If they do represent metastatic disease, a "soil" factor making bone a preferential site for growth of metastases should be considered. Bone marrow involvement, either focal or diffuse, is not uncommon, especially in patients with pelvic primary lesions.

With the advent of routine systemic adjuvant treatment with various chemotherapeutic agents or combinations, central nervous system and meningeal involvement similar to that recognized as "sanctuary site" relapse in leukemia and pediatric non-Hodgkin's lymphoma was described and recommendations were made for treatment including cranio–spinal irradiation.[349,350] Recent experience and review of numerous reported studies fails to confirm the frequency of this finding.[335–337,351] No patient seen at the JCRT/CHMC/SFCI has developed initial meningeal or central nervous system relapse despite routine adjuvant systemic treatment with no attempt at CNS prophylaxis. CNS involvement, is, however, commonly seen in patients with advanced metastatic disease, usually as a consequence of prior bony metastatic disease with subsequent soft tissue extension and compromise of adjacent CNS structures (*i.e.*, vertebral body involvement with extradural spinal cord disturbance).[350]

TABLE 34-17. Typical Radiographic Characteristics

FEATURE	OSTEOSARCOMA	EWING'S TUMOR
Location in bone	Metaphyseal	Diaphyseal
Involvement of long bones	Yes	Yes
Involvement of flat bones	Rare	Yes
Diffuse medullary cavity involvement	Rare	Common ("moth-eaten" or permeative involvement)
New bone formation	Yes	No—only as secondary phenomenon
Periosteal reaction	Yes ("Codman Triangle") or spiculation	Yes ("onionskin" appearance)
Soft tissue mass	Not prominent but may be present	Yes

The frequency of overt metastatic disease at presentation in appropriately staged patients has been surprising. Approximately half of the patients seen at our institutions in the last decade have been shown to have metastases at presentation.

DIAGNOSIS AND STAGING

A careful history and physical examination must be performed in addition to radiographic assessment of the primary lesion using tomography where appropriate. Several other studies are necessary for optimum evaluation prior to institution of therapy. They are listed in Table 34-18.

The diagnosis of Ewing's tumor must be confirmed by biopsy; however, it is critically important that the biopsy site and approach be discussed in advance by the surgeon and radiation therapist, as a poorly placed biopsy incision may make optimum irradiation technically more difficult or impossible by eliminating the possibility of sparing an adequate strip of subcutaneous and lymphatic tissue.

The extent of biopsy should be just sufficient to enable pathologic diagnosis. As noted earlier, many patients have a considerable soft tissue mass, which can be biopsied without actual intra-osseous biopsy. Further weakening of bony integrity, already compromised by tumor extent in many patients, especially those with lesions of weight-bearing bones, can thereby be avoided. Large intraosseous biopsies that are poorly placed are to be decried and substantially increase the patient's morbidity (especially pathologic fracture), to no purpose.

STAGING

No generally accepted staging system has been adopted for Ewing's tumor. Features of prognostic importance include primary site, with distal extremity lesions being less serious than proximal lesions. Axial lesions are distinctly unfavorable, especially lesions of the pelvis. Significant elevation of the serum LDH appears to be an indicator of poor prognosis as, to a lesser degree, are fever and leukocytosis. The presence of metastases or multifocal bone involvement almost invariably represents an incurable situation. Based on current clinical results, separation of patients into the several categories shown in Table 34-19 would appear to be prognostically significant and, therefore, may represent a potentially useful staging system.

TREATMENT

The striking propensity for this tumor to develop distant metastatic disease makes aggressive systemic treatment essential, as compilations of survival results prior to routine use of systemic treatment demonstrated control in less than 10% of all patients.[330] Assumptions based on patients treated in the past must be made with great caution, however, as patients treated currently are much more accurately staged (therefore current "nonmetastatic" patients are more favorably selected). In addition, radiation techniques used historically have generally been inadequate, both with respect to dose used and field adequacy (see below).

Two forms of systemic treatment have been utilized. Phy-

TABLE 34-18. Pre-Therapy Studies for Ewing's Sarcoma

1. Radiographic studies
   a. Plain films of primary lesion with tomography where indicated
   b. Radioisotope bone scan
   c. Computer-assisted tomography, essential in axial lesions
   d. Full lung tomography or CT study of lungs
   e. Angiography and/or intravenous pyelography and/or myelography where indicated
2. Blood and serum studies
   a. CBC and platelet count
   b. Serum BUN, LDH, SGOT, and alkaline phosphatase
3. Bone marrow aspiration and biopsy
4. Urinalysis and urine VMA and HVA

TABLE 34-19. Potential Staging System—Ewing's Tumor

Stage I—Any extremity lesion in a patient with no evidence of distant metastases.*
- a. Distal extremity lesion
- b. Proximal extremity lesion

Stage II—Any axial lesion in a patient with no evidence of distant metastases.
- a. Extrapelvic lesion
- b. Innominate bone lesion

Stage III Any lesion, axial or appendicular, in a patient with distant metastatic disease.

*Following evaluation

sicians at the Princess Margaret Hospital and Hospital for Sick Children initially used a single dose of 300 rad of whole body irradiation in addition to conventional irradiation of the primary site, and demonstrated apparent improvement in both disease-free and total survival.[351,352] Of note was the control of two patients who had metastatic disease at presentation with this approach.

However, this approach has been largely superceded by the introduction of multiagent chemotherapy. Several classes of agents have shown activity with Ewing's tumor, including the vinca alkaloids (vincristine), alkylating agents (cyclophosphamide), antibiotics (actinomycin-D and doxorubicin), and a variety of other agents, including BCNU and mithramycin. Many adjuvant chemotherapy regimens have been utilized without clear superiority for any particular regimen, although multiagent regimens containing doxorubicin are felt by many to be preferable.[332,333,335–337,344,353–356]

Doxorubicin, actinomycin-D, Cytoxan, and vincristine are currently the most active and effective agents, and the VAC and VACA regimens represent two of the combinations utilized most often currently (Table 34-20).[332,335,336] In addition to a variety of different drug combinations, many different schedules of certain of these combinations exist (*i.e.*, VAC). The current Intergroup Ewing's study shows clear superiority in disease-free survival for the VACA regimen or for a VAC regimen combined with pulmonary irradiation when compared with VAC alone. However, the schedule and doses of VAC used are different than those used by others reporting a higher level of success with this regimen.[332] No data exist, however, to suggest that actinomycin-D is a more active agent than doxorubicin for this tumor.

In addition to improved survival, optimum function should be a principal goal of the therapeutic team. This consideration should be of paramount importance in the choice of local treatment. Most often, irradiation of the primary lesion and adjacent soft tissue will represent the most appropriate therapy for both tumor control and function. The necessity for meticulous radiation technique is clear when analyzing functional consequences of treatment.[357] However, when care is directed to irradiaion details, functional consequences will generally be excellent. Necessary technical details include megavoltage apparatus, appropriate cast or other immobilization device for daily reproducibility, and use of beam-modifying devices, including compensators, wedge filters, and individually constructed blocks. In addition, appropriate treatment of the entire bone with preservation of an unirradiated strip of skin and subcutaneous tissue must be accomplished to prevent late lymphedema and contractures (Fig. 34-26).[358–360] Currently, using modern, megavoltage techniques in combination with systemic chemotherapy, in excess of 80% to 90% of all unselected primary lesions will be controlled by irradiation, with doses of approximately 6000 rad delivered in 6 weeks to 8 weeks utilizing 180 rad to 200 rad fractions.[335,360]

Suit and colleagues demonstrated that radiation doses of 4000 rad, although producing prompt symptomatic relief and complete clinical regression of tumor, regularly resulted in local failure, if the patient survived for a sufficient period of time.[358,359] In response, progressively higher radiation doses were utilized, often resulting in poor functional results and not always achieving local control.[357] More recently, with combined multiagent chemotherapy and radiation protocols, delivery of 4000 rad to 5000 rad to the entire affected bone followed by an additional 1000 rad to 1500 rad to successively smaller "cone down" radiation fields has resulted in excellent local control and good-to-excellent functional results in most patients.[360]

Certain primary sites and clinical settings clearly require primary surgical treatment. Lesions of the rib, clavicle, foot and, when limited, fibula, are often best managed by surgical excision, often with the addition of postoperative irradiation. Distal lower extremity lesions in very young patients (less than 6 years to 8 years of age), if treated with primary irradiation, will result in substantial growth discrepancy, and primary surgical management will usually result in ultimately superior functional results in these patients. However, should major functional loss result from surgical management that could be avoided by irradiation (*i.e.*, sacrifice of the peroneal nerve in resection of a fibular lesion in a teenager), then irradiation is to be preferred.

Although currently being utilized in several patients, the long-term functional and disease control consequences of partial bone resection combined with lower dose irradiation for certain primary sites remains unknown. Early or delayed resection of the clinically and radiographically evident lesion

TABLE 34-20. Multiagent Chemotherapy Regimens

INSTITUTION	VINCRISTINE Dose	VINCRISTINE Schedule	CYCLOPHOSPHAMIDE Dose	CYCLOPHOSPHAMIDE Schedule	ACTINOMYCIN D Dose	ACTINOMYCIN D Schedule
Intergroup Ewing's VAC	1.5 mg/M² (Single dose 2 mg)	Weekly × 6, then 2 weeks break, then weekly × 5	500 mg/M²	Weekly	0.015 mg/Kg (Single dose 0.5 mg)	Daily × 5 every 12 weeks
JCRT/CHMC/SFCI VAC	2.0 mg/M² (Single dose 2.0 mg)	Weekly × 12, then weekly as tolerated	300 mg/M²	Daily × 7–10 days every 6 weeks	225 mcg/M²	Daily × 7 every 12 weeks
Memorial-SKI VACA*	2.0 mg/M² (Single dose 2 mg)	Weekly × 4 every 13 weeks	1200 mg/M²	Every other week × 2 every 13 weeks	0.45 mg/M²	Daily × 5 every 13 weeks

*VACA includes adriamycin as well as the other three agents.

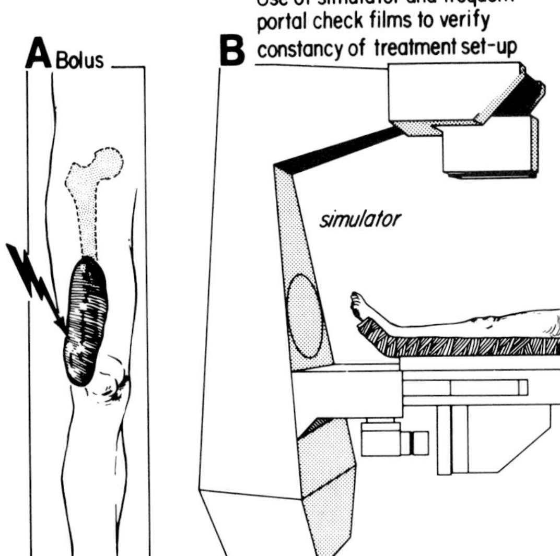

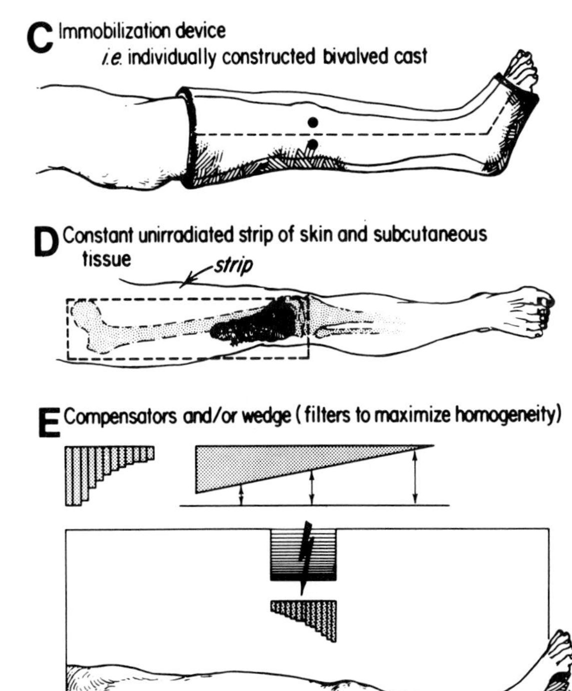

FIG. 34-26. Composite figure demonstrating some of the technically essential features for optimum results. Included are sparing of an adequate strip of skin and subcutaneous tissue to avoid late constrictive fibrosis and edema, use of appropriate treatment simulation and portal verification, appropriate immobilization during treatment, and use of wedges and compensators for homogeneity of treatment.

without other local treatment of the entire bone and appropriate initially affected soft tissues clearly represents inadequate therapy. A study by Pritchard and associates has been the basis for recent recommendations for surgery as primary treatment for a larger proportion of patients with this disease.[365] In this study, patients without initial metastases at the Mayo Clinic who received surgical removal of the affected bone fared better than patients treated with primary irradiation. Unfortunately, this study spanned several decades and no information was available regarding possible selection bias, as treatment was not randomized. Most importantly, no information was supplied regarding radiation technique. In fact, most patients were irradiated by techniques and doses considered inadequate today. Many doses, for example, were specified in "erythema dose" units.[366]

RESULTS

Utilizing current treatment, more than 60% of patients with initially nonmetastatic disease can be controlled. Thus, approximately 70% of Rosen's patients treated adjuvantly with VACA chemotherapy survived disease-free, with similar results reported by Jaffe and colleagues and others. Somewhat less optimistic results have been reported by Johnson and Pomeroy, with a 53% 5-year survival rate and, more recently, by Cham and associates. Late recurrence or metastases continue to be seen by all investigators. However, most patients who present with or subsequently develop metastases succumb eventually to their tumor. Even though no metastases may be evident following evaluation, patients with axial lesions, especially of the pelvis, as noted earlier, have a poorer prognosis.[332,335,336,360–363]

Most treatment regimes extend for 18 months to 24 months following diagnosis, and patients will be seen frequently (every 3 weeks to 6 weeks) during this time period. Particular care should be directed to ensure that excellent function is maintained during this interval, as general morbidity produced by vigorous systemic therapy may cause the patient to ignore or inadequately perform local exercise and physiotherapy of the affected extremity. The requirement for an active program of physical therapy for these patients is clear. The severe contracture resulting from neglect of the program may not be fully correctable.

Regular evaluation of the primary lesion, lungs, and other bones should be performed. Chest radiographs should be performed at 1-month to 2-month intervals, and radiographs of the primary lesion (if present) at 2-month to 3-month intervals. In the first 4 weeks to 6 weeks following irradiation, films may suggest extension of the bony destruction, despite objective and subjective evidence of improvement. This radiographic "extension" should not be regarded as "resistant" tumor, as it virtually always represents radiographically evidence of demineralization and not tumor extension.[360] Healing, often delayed by continuing systemic therapy, ultimately occurs. Serial bone scans at approximately 6-month intervals, and, when appropriate, repeat chest tomography or CT scanning, also represent important follow-up measures.

COMPLICATIONS AND FUTURE PROSPECTS

Substantial improvement has occurred in treatment results in the past 15 years. However, the majority of patients who develop this tumor continue to die of it. Better systemic therapy is clearly necessary if further improvements are to be made. Although occasional patients continue to develop isolated primary relapse, development of distant relapse or inability to control widespread metastatic disease represents the most frequent cause of failure.

Although better scheduling of currently available chemotherapeutic agents may result in significant improvements, it is likely that substantial progress will require introduction and use of new agents or techniques. One possible example of this is the use of whole body irradiation following a planned course of chemotherapy—currently being subjected to trial by the Toronto group.[364]

Three major categories of complications are seen most frequently. Acute problems associated with aggressive systemic therapy including fever, neutropenia, mucositis, nausea, vomiting, and diarrhea, are regularly observed. In addition to erythema (or "recall") within the irradiation field, these acute difficulties are often significantly enhanced by irradiation, depending on location and size of radiation fields. Subacute and late changes of edema, fibrosis, contractures, and growth arrest have been previously discussed and can often be avoided or minimized by use of optimum technique. More recently, osteosarcoma arising in bones previously treated successfully with irradiation and chemotherapy for Ewing's tumor has been reported.[336] Megavoltage-treated patients experiencing this complication have generally been treated with radiation doses in excess of 6000 rad to 6500 rad. In patients receiving doxorubicin, both acute and late cardiac damage represent an obvious potential complication. Sterility and related endocrine dysfunction may follow cyclophosphamide administration or pelvic irradiation. Combinations of cyclophosphamide and significant pelvic irradiation may also result in a significantly increased risk of hemorrhagic cystitis. Potential development of these complications clearly indicates the necessity for indefinite, continuing follow-up. Choice of primary therapy considered optimum may require revision, should the ultimate incidence of second tumors observed be extremely high, even in patients irradiated with somewhat lower doses. At present, this complication has been reported principally in patients treated with very high radiation doses delivered with megavoltage equipment or in patients treated with orthovoltage apparatus. It is to be hoped that continued refinement in radiation technique will minimize this complication, as function consequences of radiation treatment have been improved through more judicious techniques.

HEPATIC TUMORS

A variety of malignant and benign tumors of the liver are seen in childhood. Hepatic tumors are the eighth most common cause of cancer mortality in children less than 15 years of age in the United States.[367] Most liver tumors pose a significant challenge for the surgeon because they reach a very large size before discovery and as a rule major hepatic resection is necessary for cure.

TABLE 34-21. Anomalies and Conditions Associated with Hepatoblastoma and Hepatocellular Carcinoma

Hemihypertrophy
Osteoporosis
Lipid Storage Disease
Glycogen Storage Disease
DeToni–Fanconi Syndrome
Virilization in Males
Retarded Sexual Development in Males

EPIDEMIOLOGY

A number of diseases and congenital malformations have been reported in association with childhood primary epithelial neoplasms of the liver. Some appear to be coincidental. Those that have been reported on more than one occasion are listed in Table 34-21. Virilization in young males has been reported in at least eight cases, most of whom had hepatoblastoma.[368] In these cases, urinary gonadotropin levels are elevated and testicular histology shows Leydig cell hyperplasia without spermatogenesis. Most authors suggest that the hepatic neoplasm is the source of gonadotropin; however, pituitary abnormalities in some cases indicate that the liver may not always be the site of abnormal gonadotropin production.[369] The association of hemihypertrophy and hepatoblastoma suggests an etiologic relationship with Wilms' tumor and adrenal cortical neoplasms, which also occur in children with hemihypertrophy.

ANATOMIC CONSIDERATIONS

Like the lung, the liver can be divided into lobes and segments according to its vascular supply. From a surgical standpoint, these anatomic divisions indicate the proper sites for liver resection (Fig. 34-27).

The right lobe of the liver contains about 70% of the total liver mass and each segment of the left lobe represents an additional 15%. Because of the liver's remarkable ability to regenerate rapidly, it is possible to remove as much as 85% of the total liver at one time and expect complete regeneration of liver cell mass.

Thus, tumors which are contained in one lobe of the liver and those that arise in the right lobe but do not extend beyond the medial segment of the left lobe are amenable to surgical resection.

PATHOLOGY

A comprehensive list of liver tumors occurring in childhood and their relative frequency has been compiled from a recent survey of member of the Surgical Section of the American Academy of Pediatrics.[370] A total of 375 tumors, 252 malignant, and 123 benign, were reported. The types of lesions seen over a 10 year span are noted in Table 34-22.

Hepatoblastoma and hepatocellular carcinoma are the most

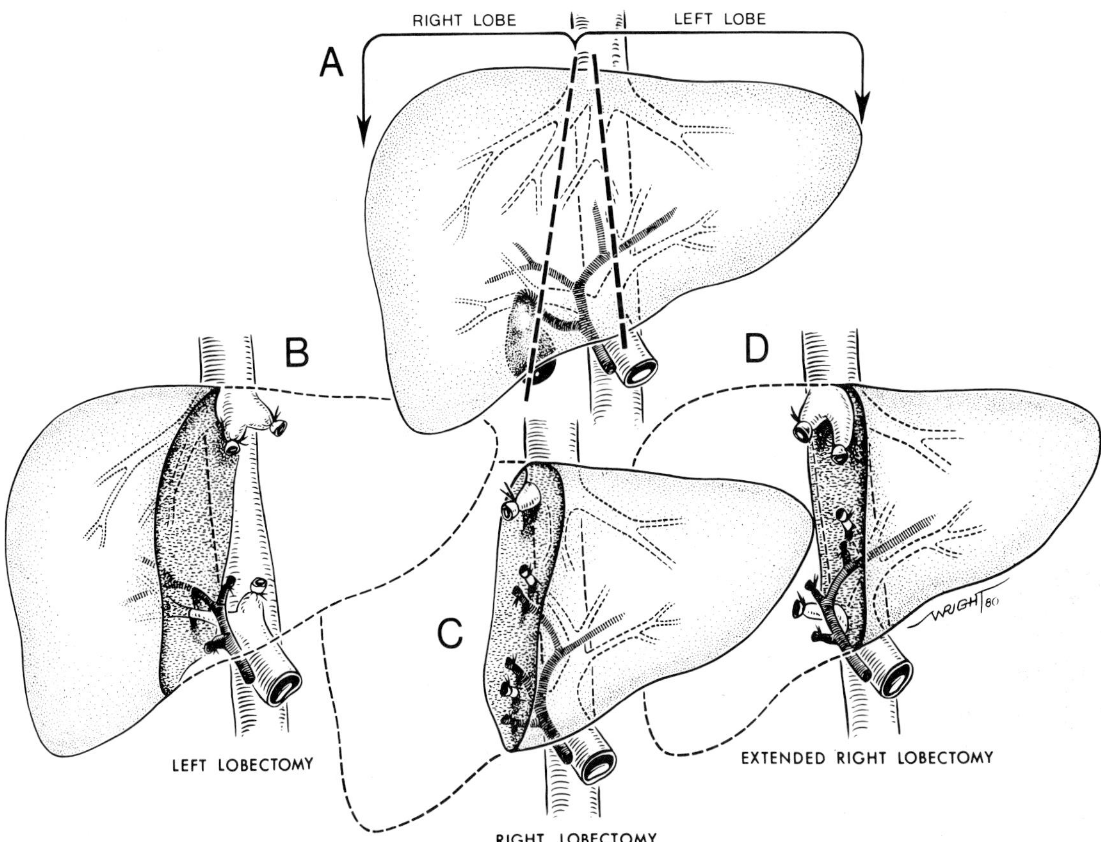

FIG. 34-27. (*A*) The lobar anatomy of the liver and possible plans of surgical resection. (*B*) Left lobectomy, (*C*) right lobectomy. The right and left lobes of the liver are separated by a vertical plane located to the right of the midline which extends from the bed of the gallbladder to the dome of the liver at the point where the inferior vena cava traverses the diaphragm. The left lobe of the liver is subdivided into medial and lateral segments. The medial segment begins at the interlobar plane to the right of the midline and extends to the falciform ligament (midline). The lateral segment comprises all the hepatic tissue to the left of the midline. (*D*) An extended right hepatic lobectomy removes about 85% of the liver, the maximum resection compatible with survival.

common malignant tumors. These epithelial neoplasms represent about 2% of all malignancies seen in childhood. Most workers recognized two morphologic types of hepatoblastoma.[368] The epithelial type is composed of fetal or immature hepatic epithelial cells, and the mixed epithelial and mesenchymal type contains tissues of mesenchymal derivation in addition to the epithelial element. Hepatoblastoma occurs in infants and almost all cases are below 3 years of age.[368,370] Hepatocellular carcinoma in childhood is histologically identical to hepatoma seen in the adult. Hepatocellular carcinoma is rare under 3 years of age and most cases occur in children over 5 years old.

Rhabdomyosarcoma is the most common sarcoma seen. Its histologic appearance and clinical characteristics are similar to rhabdomyosarcoma at other sites.

Vascular neoplasms are the commonest benign liver tumors in children. Although these tumors are reported in adults, in the pediatric age group about 90% are discovered before the age of 6 months. Two types have been identified. The hemangioendothelioma is composed of many small vascular channels lined by one or more layers of endothelial cells and appears identical to skin and subcutaneous lesions similarly named. Although generally thought of as a benign tumor, some observers believe that the presence of hemangioendothelioma at multiple sites indicates that this tumor can metastasize. However, death from metastatic disease is exceedingly rare. Cavernous hemangioma in the liver is composed of various sized vascular spaces, lined by a single layer of flat endothelial cells. The vascular spaces are often partially occluded with recent or old thrombi. This lesion also resembles cavernous hemangioma seen at other sites in the body. Some authors make a clear distinction between hemangioendothelioma and hemangioma while it is clear that others use the term hemangioma for both types.[371,372] An excellent review of the characteristics of the less common benign hepatic neoplasms can be found in a publication by Ishak and Rabin.[371]

NATURAL HISTORY

Regardless of exact histology, hepatic epithelial malignancies most frequently involve the right lobe. Metastases to other parts of the liver occur by direct extension or by way of

TABLE 34-22. Types of Hepatic Tumors Seen in 375 Children

MALIGNANT TUMORS		BENIGN TUMORS	
Pathology	*Number of Cases*	*Pathology*	*Number of Cases*
Hepatoblastoma	138	Hemangioma	54
Hepatocellular Carcinoma	98	Hamartoma	37
Sarcomas	13	Miscellaneous	
		Cysts	16
Other	3	Adenoma	7
		Other	9
TOTAL	252	TOTAL	123

(Exelby PR, Filler RM, Grosfeld JL: Liver tumors in children in the particular reference to hepatoblastoma in hepatocellular carcinoma. American Academy of Pediatric Surgical Section Survey, 1974. J Ped Surg 10:329–337, 1975)

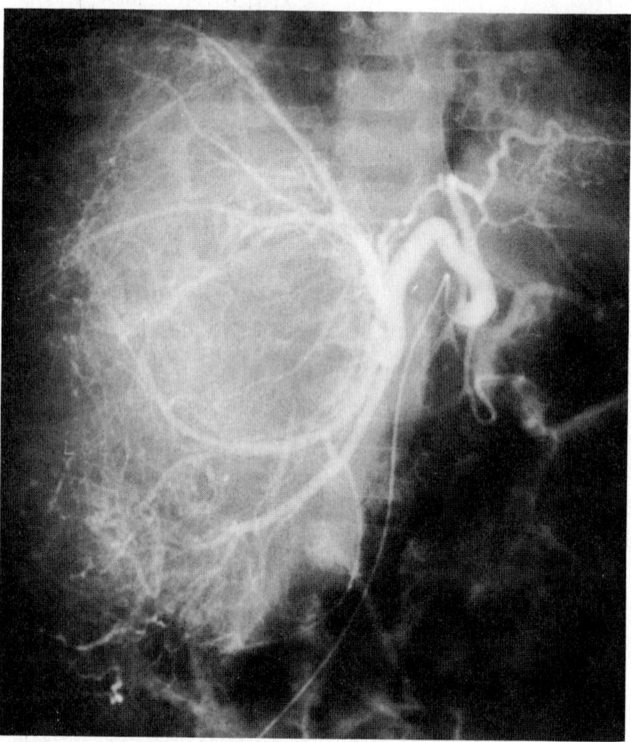

FIG. 34-28. Celiac arteriogram in 1½-year-old boy with abdominal distention for 3 months. Celiac axis is displaced to the left by a large vascular mass containing many tumor vessels and involving inferior portion of right lobe of liver. A second mass can be seen in the left lobe. At surgery both lobes were involved by hepatoblastoma and resection was not possible.

intrahepatic vascular or lymphatic channels. Extrahepatic spread of tumor is usually to regional lymph nodes in the porta hepatis and the lung.

Most children with hepatic tumors present with an asymptomatic abdominal mass. Abdominal pain, weight loss, and irritability are signs of advanced malignancy and are present in less than 25% of cases.[368,373] Children with hemangioendothelioma and cavernous hemangioma may present in cardiac failure due to arteriovenous shunting. In addition, some children with vascular neoplasms present with petechial hemorrhage due to thrombocytopenia. Occasionally, shock due to rupture of a malignant or benign vascular tumor is the first indication of a hepatic neoplasm. Rarely, precocious puberty will be the presenting complaint in a child with cancer of the liver. Approximately 25% of children with malignant epithelial tumors have diffuse hepatic involvement or pulmonary metastases at diagnosis.[370,373]

DIAGNOSIS

Routine laboratory studies are often normal. Anemia and thrombocytopenia have been noted with hepatoma and benign vascular tumors. In most children with a hepatic mass, serum bilirubin is normal. SGOT and alkaline phosphatase may be normal or slightly elevated. α-Fetoprotein is a normal α-globulin that is produced by embryonic hepatocytes. It is present in the fetus and may be found in the serum of two-thirds of the children with malignant hepatic epithelial neoplasms.[374] This marker is useful for diagnosis and, when positive, serial determinations can be used to follow the child's progress after treatment. α-Fetoprotein also can be found in the serum of children with embryonal carcinoma of the testis and in others with teratoma. Cystothionuria has been reported in children with hepatoblastoma.[375]

Radiographic examination of the child with an abdominal mass begins with plain films of the abdomen and chest. An intravenous pyelogram is essential, since most abdominal masses in childhood originate in a kidney, adrenal gland, or retroperitoneum. More precise evaluation of a liver mass is obtained by radionuclide liver scanning, ultrasound, computerized axial tomography (CT scan), and arteriography.[376] Hepatic imaging by radionuclide scans and CT scans are useful in delineating the distribution of tumor within the liver substance. Ultrasonography and CT scan can differentiate solid from cystic tumor masses. These studies also can be used after surgery to estimate the degree of liver regeneration and recurrence of neoplasia after resection.

Of all the diagnostic tests, selective celiac arteriography gives the most useful information (Figs. 34-27, 34-28). This study usually demonstrates the extent of the tumor and allows one to predict whether complete resection is possible. The differentiation of one type tumor from another is often possible, since many tumors have a characteristic vascular pattern. In addition, the abnormal anatomy of the hepatic vasculature displayed by angiograms aids in planning the hepatic resection. However, except in the case of a typical hepatic hemangioma, angiography rarely obviates the need for surgery. Surgical exploration is still necessary to provide a definitive tissue diagnosis and to avoid errors in interpretation such as those which may occur when a large but resectable mass causes sufficient vascular distortion to produce an angiogram in which the tumor appears to be too extensive for removal.

TREATMENT

Hepatic Resection

Despite advances in cancer treatment, current data indicate that the cure of children with malignant hepatic tumors is not possible without complete resection of the primary tumor.

Anatomic hepatic lobectomy is usually necessary for complete excision of these tumors.

Improvements in anesthetic and surgical techniques and proper attention to details of management before, during, and after surgery have minimized the hazards of hepatic resection.[373,377,378] As much as 85% of the liver can be removed safely. A significant portion of the hepatic cell mass will regenerate in 1 month and liver regeneration will be complete in 3 months. Therefore, in the absence of distant metastases, resection for cure is possible for tumors of the right hepatic lobe that do not extend beyond the medial segment of the left lobe and for tumors confined to the left lobe.

The operative technique recommended for hepatic resection in children is similar to that recommended by others for adults (Fig. 34-29).[379-381] A thoracoabdominal approach is preferred because it offers excellent exposure and precludes the development of negative intrathoracic pressure, which may cause the aspiration of air into an open venous system. This approach also provides excellent visualization of the entire supradiaphragmatic inferior vena cava, into which an internal venous shunt can be placed so that liver blood flow can be isolated in the event of catastrophic hemorrhage.[382]

Once the porta hepatis is dissected, the vessels and ducts to the lobe to be excised are ligated and divided. The liver is mobilized by dividing the diaphragmatic attachments and the diaphragm divided radially to the vena cava. Tapes are passed around the vena cava above and below the liver to ensure control if excessive bleeding should occur. Before the hepatic veins are isolated, the liver capsule is incised along a lobar or segmental division and the liver substance is divided bluntly. Bridging vessels and bile ducts are ligated as they are encountered. Because of the very short extrahepatic length of the hepatic veins in a child, they are approached by dissection through the liver substance rather than at their exit from the liver. By this technique, inadvertent venous injury, which results in difficult to control bleeding, can be minimized. After resection is completed, hemostasis and bile drainage are controlled with mattress sutures to the raw surface of the liver. Sump and Penrose drains are placed in the liver bed and the incision is closed. T-tube drainage of the common duct has not been used because of the potential risk of stricture in the small bile duct of an infant.

Recently, Theman et al have excised massive intra-abdominal tumors with total circulatory arrest.[383] We have applied this technique to hepatectomy. Prior to division of the liver, cardiopulmonary bypass is instituted and hypothermia is induced. With the child's body temperature at 20°C, the circulation can be stopped for as long as 60 minutes and resection and repair of vascular structures can be performed in a bloodless operative field. Similarly, Offenstadt and colleagues have described the use of normothermic isolated hepatic circulatory arrest as an adjunct to hepatic resection.[384] These surgeons clamped the lower thoracic aorta, porta hepatis, and the vena cava above or below the liver and thereby effectively stopped liver circulation. These techniques should be considered for all children with very large hepatic tumors.

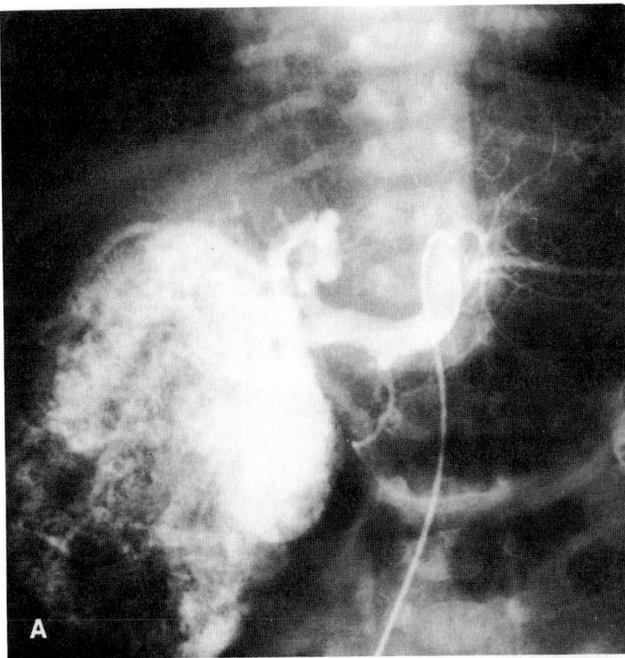

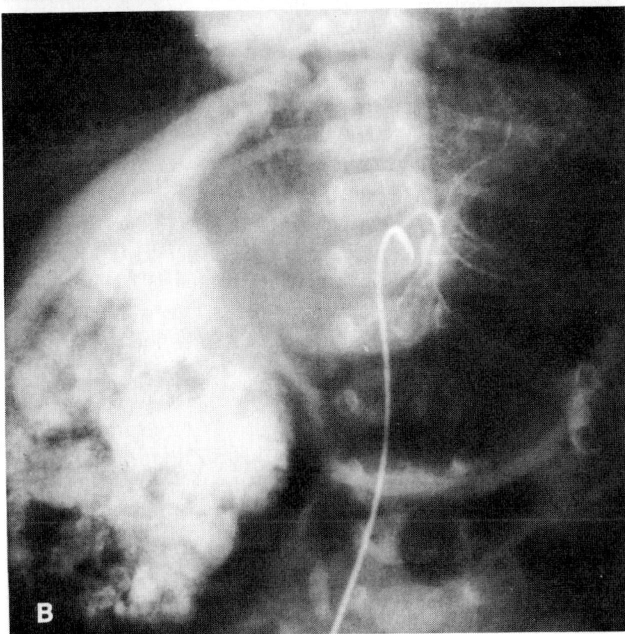

FIG. 34-29. Hepatic arteriogram in 1-month-old boy who presented with heart failure and an abdominal mass. Note how the vascular pattern in this child differs from that in Fig. 24-27. (*A*) Early phase of hepatic arteriogram shows an extremely large hepatic artery filling or hemangioma in right lobe of the liver. The blood flow to the remainder of the normal liver is decreased. (*B*) Later phase of angiogram shows pooling of blood in portions of the tumor and rapid filling of hepatic veins and vena cava through arteriovenous shunts. Heart failure was controlled by digitalis and diuretics and the lesion has regressed spontaneously.

INTRA-OPERATIVE MANAGEMENT. The most frequent and serious intra-operative problem is hemorrhage. Even in the absence of uncontrolled bleeding, the loss of one blood volume (800 ml in a 10 kg child) is not unusual. As a guide to proper replacement, accurate measurement of blood lost in sponges and by suction, and monitoring of intra-arterial blood pressure, central venous pressure, and urine output are necessary. Since hypothermia tends to cause cardiac irritability, metabolic acidosis, and disturbed blood clotting mechanisms, blood which is administered at surgery should be warmed to 37°C. In addition, the child's normal body temperature should be maintained by providing a warm operating room temperature and by the use of a warming blanket. Adjusting the pH of bank blood (pH 7.0) to pH 7.4 will also decrease the incidence of cardiac arrest, which can be triggered by the rapid infusion of large volumes of cold, acid blood.

POSTOPERATIVE MANAGEMENT. Blood loss is the most immediate concern and must be managed judiciously. A single blood-stained dressing may represent a significant loss in the infant and yet, overreplacement may result in pulmonary edema. Continual monitoring of the central venous pressure and urine output is mandatory.

Hepatic resection is likely to cause several metabolic derangements.[385] However, problems usually can be avoided by simple prophylactic measures. Ten percent dextrose solution should be administered intravenously during the first few days to avoid hypoglycemia due to the removal of hepatic glycogen stores. The daily infusion of albumin (25 g to 50 g) for the first postoperative week avoids hypoalbuminemia and vitamin K administration for 7 days to 10 days after surgery ensures adequate prothrombin levels.

Chemotherapy and Radiation

The use of chemotherapy and radiation in the treatment of hepatic epithelial neoplasms is currently under study. Although no cures have been reported without surgical resection, many reports now indicate that a marked reduction in the size of both primary and secondary tumor deposits can be achieved by radiation and the administration of a variety of chemotherapeutic agents, including doxorubicin, vincristine, cyclophosphamide, and carmustine (BCNU).[386–390] In these reports, a combination of radiation and drugs were used in children whose hepatic tumors were deemed inoperable because of their great size, unfavorable position or the presence of intrahepatic or pulmonary metastases. In most of these children, tumor regression was such that resection for cure was possible. Doxorubicin seemed to be the most effective drug in total dose between 400 mg/m^2 and 500 mg/m^2. When radiation has been added, tumor dose of 1200 rad to 2000 rad has been used.

Clinical trials which are now underway may indicate that adjunctive chemotherapy or radiation or both may have a place in the management of all children with malignant hepatic tumors. However, the timing of such therapy will be critical, for clinical and laboratory studies have indicated that the cytotoxic agents can inhibit normal liver regeneration and that the toxicity from radiation and drugs is enhanced in the recently hepatectomized individual.[391]

RESULTS

Despite advances in techniques, surgical mortality and morbidity are still significant. In some series, operative mortality from hepatic resection has been as high as 25%. Exelby and colleagues recorded 25 operative and postoperative deaths in 223 operations for malignant hepatic tumors.[370]

TABLE 34-23. Results of Hepatic Resection in the Treatment of Hepatoblastoma (129 Cases) and Hepatocellular Carcinoma (92 Cases)

TYPE OF RESECTION	NUMBER OF PATIENTS	NUMBER ALIVE	PERCENT SURVIVAL
Left lobectomy	31	14	45
Right lobectomy	56	25	45
Extended Right lobectomy	30	16	53
Wedge Resection	5	2	40
Biopsy Only	99	0	0
TOTAL	221	57	25

(Exelby PR, Filler RM, Grosfeld JL: Liver tumors in children in the particular reference to hepatoblastoma in hepatocellular carcinoma. American Academy of Pediatric Surgical Section Survey, 1974. J Ped Surg 10:329–337, 1975)

Excessive blood loss is the most common complication during and immediately after operation. Other relatively frequent postoperative complications of hepatic lobectomy include subphrenic abscess, wound infection, biliary fistula, small bowel obstruction, and biliary obstruction. However, most of these problems can be managed without mortality.

Approximately one-fourth of children with malignant epithelial tumors have diffuse hepatic involvement or pulmonary metastases at diagnosis, so that only biopsy of the tumor can be performed. As already mentioned, none of these children have been salvaged to date. For those in whom the entire tumor can be resected, the outlook is much brighter, for approximately 50% of these children can be cured (Table 34-23).[370,373,377,378] The results of surgery are somewhat better for children with hepatoblastoma than for those with hepatocellular carcinoma. Approximately 90% of the deaths from metastatic cancer occur in the first year after diagnosis.

FUTURE

It now appears that the operability of hepatic tumors can be increased by chemotherapy and radiation, which suggests that significant improvement in cure rates can be obtained by adding these modalities to a standard treatment protocol. Improved surgical techniques over the years have led to a decrease in operative mortality, but significant problems remain. Preoperative chemotherapy and radiation, which reduce tumor size, may reduce surgical risk but this will need further study. Recent innovations that also may prove to reduce surgical risk include liver resection during hypothermic total circulatory arrest and resection during normothermic hepatic circulatory arrest.[383,384]

RETINOBLASTOMA

Retinoblastoma (RB) represents the commonest primary tumor of the eye in children.[392] Although accounting for 1% or less of all childhood malignancies and 5% of childhood blindness, it has received an inordinate amount of attention, owing to its genetic features and the known predisposition of bilaterally affected children to develop other malignancies.[393-395] It also represents one of the earliest instances of the interdisciplinary use of irradiation for achieving functional preservation as well as improved survival in a childhood tumor.

ETIOLOGY AND DEMOGRAPHIC FEATURES

Retinoblastoma is inherited as an autosomal dominant with nearly complete penetrance from an affected parent.[396] However, such cases represent less than 10% of all affected patients.[397] Much more commonly, retinoblastoma develops as an apparently spontaneous event: one in 15,000 to 30,000 children is so affected.[398] It has been suggested that the condition is increasing in frequency.[399-401] The overwhelming majority of children with a known family history have bilateral disease. However, only 20% to 30% of children with no known family history are bilaterally affected.[397] It is presumed that the timing of the mutational event in embryological development determines whether the entire retinal anlage or only that of one eye is at risk. Less than one-third of all bilaterally affected children have a known family history. Other than this known genetic association, the etiology of retinoblastoma is not known. A deletion of the long arm of chromosome 13 (13q) has been noted in a very small percentage of all patients.[402,403] It has been postulated that a small deletion, not detectable with current techniques, may in fact be present in all patients and perhaps be responsible for tumor induction.[404] Fibroblasts from patients with hereditary RB, especially those with the recognized chromosomal defect, have been shown to have enhanced radiation sensitivity and have been postulated to have a defect in repair of sublethal radiation damage.[405-407]

There is approximately a 1% likelihood that apparently normal parents who have a child with retinoblastoma will have another similarly affected child. However, should the child have bilateral disease, this risk will significantly increase.[397]

PRESENTATION

In the absence of a known family history, most children with RB are diagnosed following detection of leukokoria (white or "cat's eye" reflex).[408,409] Other common presenting signs or symptoms include unexplained strabismus or "squint." Any child developing strabismus requires careful ophthalmologic examination to rule out causes of blindness, especially RB, rather than ascribing such symptoms to "lazy" or "weak" muscles. Other, much rarer, reasons for presentation include blindness, proptosis, a painful inflamed eye, cervical lymphadenopathy, or other evidence of metastatic disease.[409] In other areas of the world, exophthalmos is the most common presenting sign.[410]

The mean age at presentation is 17 months, with a range from birth to 62 years.[397] Presentation after age 5 years to 6 years is quite rare.[411] Children with a known family history, or with bilateral disease, present at a significantly younger age than spontaneously affected children.[397,411,412] Any child with a known family history should be examined at birth and at regular intervals thereafter.

Therapy for a patient with retinoblastoma may need to be performed without biopsy, to achieve maximal functional preservation. Several other ophthalmologic conditions may pose differential problems. These include visceral larval migrans (toxocara granuloma), Coats' disease, retrolental fibroplasia, persistent hyperplastic primary vitreous, and a variety of other rare ophthalmologic conditions.[395,397,408,413] An experienced ophthalmologist rarely has difficulty in distinguishing these conditions from retinoblastoma. The presence of either flocculent "cottage cheese" calcification with the lesion or vitreous seeding usually confirms the diagnosis of RB.[413,414]

EVALUATION

A thorough history and physical examination, especially of the orbits and head and neck region, is essential. Careful questioning for a history of eye disease in the family is obviously important. Careful ophthalmologic examination of both parents and any siblings should also be routinely performed, in view of genetic considerations and several recognized instances of spontaneous regression.

Careful and complete examination of both retinas by direct and indirect ophthalmaloscopy under anesthesia must be performed. Numerous unexpected instances of bilateral involvement have been discovered by this means. Mapping of all known or suspicious lesions on appropriate diagrams is necessary. Other studies should include a bone marrow aspirate, with or without biopsy, and lumbar puncture with millipore or cytocentrifuge evaluation of spinal fluid to exclude meningeal involvement.[415] Special ultrasound evaluation of affected eyes can be helpful in excluding involvement of the optic nerve head, which may have been suggested by routine ophthalmoscopic examination. Exophytic lesions, extending over the appropriate location of the nerve head, may otherwise pose significant problems.

Computerized axial tomography (CT) may be of considerable assistance in combination with polytomography in better defining local orbital extension in more severely affected patients. Routine use of these studies for children with limited retinal disease does not appear to be warranted. Similarly, although a chest roentgenograph is warranted in all patients, a routine skeletal survey or bone scan should not be obtained unless clinically warranted by extensive local involvement.

STAGING

Reese and Ellsworth have developed a widely adopted grouping system to assess the likelihood of tumor control with vision following radiation therapy.[397,413] This classification is reproduced in Table 34-24 and demonstrates that size, number of lesions, vitreous seeding, and anterior location are apparent adverse prognostic factors. Recent data would suggest, however, that anterior location may have been unfavorable because of the radiation technique utilized.[414-416] Irradiated patients were treated entirely by lateral fields which, based on the low incidence of subsequent cataract formation, almost certainly underdosed the anterior retina and ora serrata region.[417] As noted earlier, the Reese–Ellsworth system predicts local control with vision, but *not* survival. Only Group V patients in the Reese–Ellsworth system have any appreciable mortality.[414]

A more conventional staging system predicting prognosis is necessary. One recently proposed system is shown in Table 34-25*A*, and a simplified version in Table 34-25*B*.[415,418,419]

TABLE 34-24. Staging Classification for Retinoblastoma (Reese)

Group I: Very favorable
1. Solitary tumor, less than 4 disc diameters in size, at or beyond equator.
2. Multiple tumors, none over 4 disc diameters in size, all at or behind equator.

Group II: Favorable
1. Solitary tumor, 4 to 10 disc diameters in size, at or behind equator.
2. Multiple tumors, 4 to 10 disc diameters in size, at or behind equator.

Group III: Doubtful
1. Any lesion anterior to equator.
2. Solitary tumors larger than 10 disc diameters behind equator.

Group IV: Unfavorable
1. Multiple tumors, some larger than 10 disc diameters.
2. Any lesion extending anteriorly to ora serrata.

Group V: Very unfavorable.
1. Massive tumors involving over half the retina.
2. Vitreous seeding.

(Reese AB: Tumors of the Eye, 2nd ed, pp 1–593. New York, Harper & Row, 1963.)

PATHOLOGY

The cell of origin of retinoblastoma appears to be a cell of outer layer of the retina with photoreceptor elements. On microscopic examination the tumor is seen to be composed of numerous small round cells with scanty cytoplasm and a chromatin-rich nucleus. These cells aggregate about blood vessels and the tumor demonstrates true Flexner–Wintersteiner rosettes.[397,413,420–423]

LOCAL AND METASTATIC SPREAD

Two forms of local extension are recognized: endophytic and exophytic.[397] The endophytic tumors grow into the vitreous cavity. Should cells or fragments separate from the main tumor mass, they may form vitreous seeds. Exophytic tumors grow into the subretinal space with resultant detachment of the retina.

Progressive growth of tumor is associated with extension into the choroid or sclera. Gross extension into either of these two sites has unfavorable prognostic significance, although microscopic choroid involvement is relatively common and does not carry the same adverse significance.[397,424–426]

Extension into the optic nerve head and subsequent growth along the optic nerve permits tumor to gain access to the cranial meninges, with the subsequent possibility of gross meningeal involvement.[415] This route of spread has been recognized for some time from pathologic and autopsy examination and has considerable therapeutic significance.[420]

Distant metastases are uncommon and occur most often to bones, bone marrow and, especially with local orbital disease, to cervical lymph nodes.[397,425]

TREATMENT

The great majority of patients with retinoblastoma have multifocal disease of one or both retinas. Eighty-four percent of the patients at Columbia-Presbyterian Institute of Ophthalmology had two or more tumors, with an average of four to five per patient.[397] This multifocal involvement has considerable therapeutic implication for radiation therapy planning. Thirty percent to 35% of all patients have bilateral disease at initial presentation.

The technique offering the highest likelihood of local control for retinoblastoma limited to the globe is surgical enucleation. Functional preservation, including restoration or preservation of vision, represents the principal indication for irradiation. Therefore, any eye with permanent loss of vision should be treated by surgical enucleation with removal of the longest possible section of optic nerve to remove any tumor which may have infiltrated this structure. Because of possible risk to survival posed by uncontrolled but clinically inapparent disease in the optic nerve following radiation therapy, enucleation is also recommended for eyes with optic nerve head involvment.

Most children with spontaneous unilateral disease have far-advanced local disease, often with little or no sight in the affected eye at presentation. Enucleation also seems appropriate for these patients, as even if sight is still present, the likelihood of tumor control with vision retention is less than 15% to 30% in advanced disease.[414,417] When the potential morbidity of irradiation is considered for a child who has vision in the other, apparently normal, eye, enucleation is generally preferred as local therapy. Children with unilateral disease that is early or intermediate in extent have a significantly greater likelihood (more than 70%) of tumor eradication with visual preservation, and radiation therapy should be seriously considered. Should tumor extent be quite limited in one eye (unifocal and less than 4 dd*), other local techniques

* 1 dd = 1.6 mm

TABLE 34-25*A*. Prognostic Staging System for Retinoblastoma (Pratt)

I. Tumor (unifocal or multifocal) confined to retina
 A. occupying 1 quadrant or less
 B. occupying 2 quadrants or less
 C. occupying more than 50% of retinal surface

II. Tumor (unifocal or multifocal) confined to globe
 A. with vitreous seeding
 B. extending to optic nerve head
 C. extending to choroid
 D. extending to choroid and optic nerve head
 E. extending to emissaries

III. Extraocular extension of tumor (regional)
 A. extending beyond cut end of optic nerve (including subarachnoid extension)
 B. extending through sclera into orbital contents
 C. extending to choroid and beyond cut end of optic nerve (including subarachnoid extension)
 D. extending through sclera into orbital contents and beyond cut end of optic nerve (including subarachnoid extension)

IV. Distant metastases
 A. extending through optic nerve to brain
 B. blood-borne metastases to soft tissue and bone
 C. Bone marrow metastases

(Pratt CB: Management of malignant solid tumors in children. Ped Clin N Am 19:1141–1155, 1972.)

TABLE 34-25*B*. Simplified Staging System for Retinoblastoma

Stage I
a. Tumor limited to less than one-half of the retina, no evidence of optic nerve involvement, no vitreous seeding.
b. Involvement of more than one-half of the retina and/ or presence of vitreous seeding.

Stage II
Tumor limited to the globe. There is evidence of optic nerve invasion and/or massive choroidal involvement.

Stage III
Extension of tumor beyond the globe into the orbital contents. No evidence of distant metastases.

Stage IV
Evidence of metastatic spread to bones, bone marrow, or lymph nodes; or meningeal involvement.

such as photocoagulation by the technique of Meyer–Schwickerath, or cryotherapy by the freeze–thaw method of Lincoff and Rubin, may offer a preferable alternative to either enucleation or external beam photon irradiation.[394,415,427,428]

As noted earlier, nearly all children with a known family history have or develop bilateral disease. Irradiation for these children and those with spontaneous bilateral disease offers the possibility of tumor control with preservation of sight and should be utilized, unless sight is absent in both eyes. Children with bilateral disease who have one eye with no sight or with worrisome local features such as a suggestion of optic nerve involvement should have enucleation of the blind eye and irradiation of the less affected one. However, should sight be present in both eyes and no features requiring enucleation be present, both eyes should be irradiated. The oft-repeated treatment plan of enculeation of the more severely affected eye is not to be recommended if sight remains in both. It is impossible to predict with certainty which eye will be successfully treated with retention of vision and therefore quite possible that the only eye with vision following treatment will be the initially more severely affected one. Should one eye be blind at presentation and minimal disease be present in the other, then enucleation of the blind eye and photocoagulation or cryotherapy of the minimal (unifocal) disease may be attempted, thereby avoiding the use of photon irradiation. Unfortunately, this is rarely possible (see below).

RADIATION TECHNIQUE

The overwhelming majority of patients with retinoblastoma have multiple tumors in one or both eyes. In patients with bilateral disease, the entire retinal anlage is at risk for multicentric tumor development. Radiation fields therefore must include the entire geographic extent of the retina, the anterior border of which is the ora serrata. Two other observations make inclusion of the ora of importance. Ellsworth has noted that cells shed from more posterior regions of the retina are channeled to this area.[397,414] In addition, this anterior portion is the last to develop embryologically and therefore tumor formation in this region is more likely to be less advanced and clinically less apparent, although present.

It is technically not possible using lateral fields to treat the ora serrata without irradiation of the posterior lens with subsequent cataract formation. Therefore anterior irradiation with lens protection, combined with lateral field irradiation, is necessary. This technique depicted graphically in Fig. 34-30 has been described previously.[416,419] General anesthesia utilizing ketamine is necessary for the immobilization required for this demanding procedure. The immobilization achieved when only sedation and restraint are used is not satisfactory in our experience.

A radiation dose of 3500 rad to 5000 rad delivered in 20 to 25 fractions in 4 to 5 weeks is recommended.[417,419] If the maximal retinal dose is kept below 5000 rad to 5500 rad, the function results achieved will be quite satisfactory. The pattern and rapidity of tumor regression following irradiation does not correlate with the results ultimately achieved.[397,414]

Techniques treating localized portions of the retina are very useful in salvage of localized relapse following external beam irradiation. Thus, cryotherapy and photocoagulation used for this purpose have been quite successful.[417] However, the utility of these techniques for primary treatment is quite limited. New tumors developed in more than 60% of 43 patients treated with localized ^{60}Co plaques by Stallard.[429,430] This finding, emphasizing the multicentricity of retinoblastoma, combined with the relative rarity of patients presenting with solitary lesions, demonstrates the unfortunate limitations of such localized techniques.

Residual orbital disease or tumor at the cut end of the optic nerve should be treated by postoperative irradiation. The entire orbit and course of the optic nerve should be treated. Radiation doses in excess of 5000 rad to 5500 rad should be used, delivered in 200 rad fractions over a 5 week to 6 week period.[417]

CHEMOTHERAPY

Triethylene melanine has been administered by oral, intramuscular, and intra-arterial means, combined with irradiation, in an attempt to increase local control. Although no randomized trial exists, no apparent advantage was evident in patients who received chemotherapy.[417]

Only patients with gross choroidal extension or regionally extensive disease have any appreciable likelihood for metastatic disease. A variety of agents including nitrogen mustard, cyclophosphamide, and vincristine have been utilized in an attempt to reduce the incidence of metastatic disease for these patients without definite evidence of improvement.[417,431–433] One report, utilizing cyclophosphamide and vincristine supplemented, where appropriate, by intrathecal methotrexate, claims improved survival for the patients reported; however, overall survival was not significantly different from that of several current series.[414,415,417,434,435]

Currently, randomized trials are in progress testing the efficacy of vincristine, cyclophosphamide, and methotrexate or doxorubicin or both in prevention of metastatic disease.[436] It is important in assessing the results of these studies to realize that interinstitutional differences in survival for retinoblastoma may equal the total mortality present at centers with broad experience in treatment and follow-up of this disease.[394]

FIG. 34-30. A schematic representation of the relationship of the retina to the lens and externally evident landmarks is shown on the left. Use of an anterior field with a divergent lens block positioned close to the anesthetized patient is shown on the right. When the level of ketamine anesthesia is satisfactory, the eyes maintain an "eyes front" position.

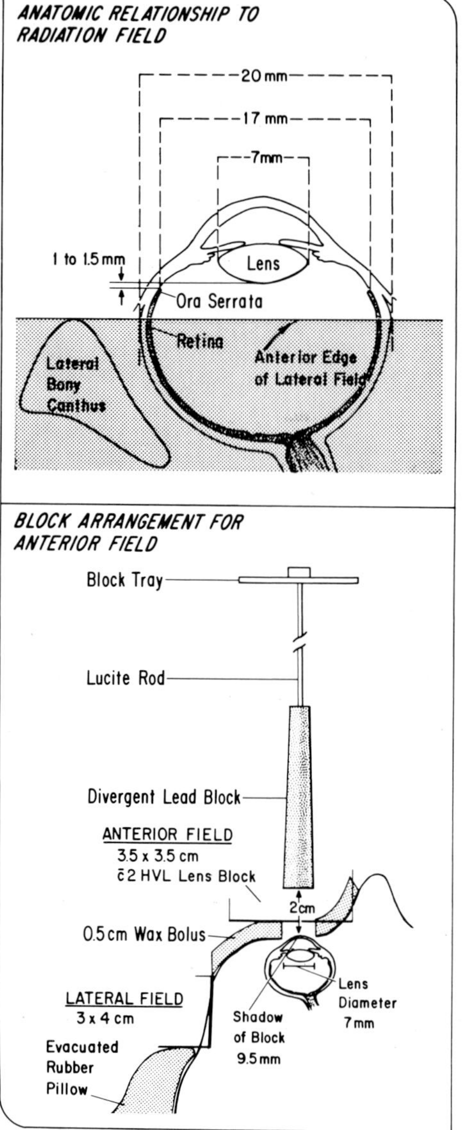

RESULTS

More than 85% of patients with retinoblastoma survive following therapy. No apparent increased mortality is evident in patients with unilateral or bilateral disease who receive irradiation in an attempt to preserve vision.[397,415,417,434,435]

Nearly one-half of the patients with extensive optic nerve infiltration or residual orbital disease succumb to metastatic tumor (Table 34-25A).[417] Despite numerous instances of response to chemotherapeutic agents, no patient with metastatic disease has been cured. In contrast, virtually all patients with Ellsworth Group I through IV disease survive following treatment, when managed by an experienced team.[414] Local control with vision for patients with Group I–V disease is shown in Table 34-26.

A second course of external beam irradiation is rarely indicated in patients who develop multiple foci of retinal relapse after an initial course of irradiation. Tumor control is rarely achieved and useful vision is even less frequent because of retinal complications which often ensue after two courses of irradiation. An increased incidence of metastatic disease (and therefore death) also is present in patients subjected to multiple courses of irradiation.[417,419]

Treatment with cranial or craniospinal irradiation and intrathecally administered chemotherapeutic agents (principally intrathecal methotrexate) has been suggested for children with any evidence of optic nerve involvement beyond the surgical cut end, with known subarachnoid invasion or intracranial tumor, or malignant CSF pleocytosis.[415] Aside from the extreme technical problems posed by craniospinal treatment of an infant, there is no definite evidence that this approach improves control probability in the child with disease and no evidence that the child with overt meningeal disease can have disease control achieved by such treatment.

COMPLICATIONS, FOLLOW-UP, AND FUTURE PROSPECTS

Patients with retinoblastoma may suffer a wide range of complications. It is evident that surgical enucleation of the affected eye in patients with unilateral disease results in permanent monocular, non-stereoscopic vision. Radiation therapy may result in a variety of local orbital, ocular, and dental complications.[417,437] Included among these are cataract formation, mild to moderate orbital or temporal fossa bony hypoplasia, failure of tooth eruption and, most tragically, second or induced tumors within the radiation field.[438–440] It has been proposed that patients with hereditary RB have one of two mutations postulated to be necessary for tumor induc-

TABLE 34-26. Likelihood of tumor control with vision*

GROUP	PERCENT
I	95
II	85
III	69
IV	67
V	35

*Based on results achieved in several series.

tion within all their cells.[441] Patients have therefore been presumed to be more susceptible to second tumors following radiation, chemotherapy, or other mutagens, as compared to children treated for other conditions. With the exception of one report, little data are available to support this contention.[442] The second tumor incidence in irradiated RB patients treated with current doses and megavoltage techniques has been 1% to 2%.[438] These patients nearly all have bilateral disease and therefore hereditary disease as defined by geneticists. However, this second tumor incidence is, in fact, significantly less than found in other series of children irradiated for malignant disease.[443] These latter series almost exclusively utilized orthovoltage treatment techniques, which may account for their high incidence figures. The incidence in megavoltage-treated patients is substantially lower.[444]

Patients with hereditary retinoblastoma also have a strikingly increased risk of second tumors unrelated to radiation therapy. Most of these tumors have been osteosarcomas, although other lesions, including Wilms' tumor, have occurred.[393] They therefore appear to be genetically at risk for a wide range of neoplasms other than RB. These features make regular and continuous follow-up care, including complete physical examination in addition to ocular examination, essential.

Regular and careful retinal examination under anesthesia should be performed following irradiation of the intact eye. Initially, following irradiation, these exams should be at 4-week to 6-week intervals with prolongation to 2-month to 3-month intervals after stability is apparent following the first several exams.

Fortunately, few children with RB in this country present with regionally far advanced or metastatic disease. Survival rates are therefore good. Unfortunately, although temporary palliation is possible, no child with metastatic or overt meningeal disease has a realistic possibility for cure at this time. Even children with regionally advanced but not metastatic disease have a substantial risk of death from metastatic disease. For this reason, improved systemic regimens are essential in order to improve current survival for this unfavorable group.

Systematic and regular use of improved radiotherapeutic techniques should result in improved function in survivors. Finally, genetic counseling and a better understanding of the nature of the genetic lesion that leads to RB formation should lead to a reduction in incidence and, it is to be hoped, to prevention of this disease.

GERM CELL TUMORS

Germ cell tumors are those which arise from the pluripotential cells of the embryonic primitive streak and primitive knot. These cells ordinarily populate the gonads, but on occasion some are left behind during migration from yolk sac to gonad. In childhood, germ cell tumors develop in the sacrococcygeal region, the testis, ovary, retroperitoneum and mediastinum. Tumors classified as pure teratoma are usually benign. The common malignant germ cell neoplasms in childhood are malignant sacrococcygeal teratoma and yolk sac tumor of the testis. In this section, only germ cell tumors in these sites will be discussed.

SACROCOCCYGEAL TERATOMA

Sacrococcygeal teratomas are the most frequent germ cell tumors encountered in infants and children. Approximately 75% occur in girls. Altman and colleagues compiled a comprehensive review of a 10-year experience of 405 clinical cases among the membership of the Surgical Section of the American Academy of Pediatrics.[445]

All sacrococcygeal teratomas have a malignant potential, regardless of location or size. The overall rate of malignancy varies between 15% and 40%.[445,446] The tendency for malignant degeneration is appreciably greater in the male and in the older child. When the diagnosis is made before 2 months of age, the incidence of malignancy is about 10%. When the diagnosis is established at an older age, about two-thirds of the males and approximately one-half of the females have malignant tumors.[445]

Anatomic Considerations

Sacrococcygeal teratomas appear to arise at the coccyx, and this structure must be removed at the time of surgery. Many sacrococcygeal teratomas grow inferiorly and away from the pelvis, so that the bulk of the tumor presents as an external mass posterior to the anus. Others have a significant presacral component, and some grow only in the presacral space, so that no evidence of a mass is seen externally.

Those that grow predominantly externally are detected at an earlier age, are less likely to be malignant, and can be removed more readily than those with a large pelvic component.

Pathology

Lesions may be solid or cystic. Solid teratomas are more likely to contain malignant elements. There appears to be no direct correlation between size and malignancy. The tissues most commonly found include epidermis, brain, glial tissue, intestinal and respiratory mucosa, mesenchymal tissues, fat, cartilage, bone, connective tissue, and muscle.

Histologically, teratomas may be composed of a mixture of mature, immature (embryonic), or unequivocably malignant tissues.[446–448] Hence, for proper evaluation of a given tumor, multiple histologic sections are necessary. Neoplasms containing only mature and immature elements are generally considered to be benign, whereas those with areas of malignant cells are more likely to recur or spread. The most common malignant histology is yolk sac tumor. Theoretically, other malignant germ cell tumors, such as choriocarcinoma, seminoma, and embryonal carcinoma can occur.

Natural History

About 75% of teratomas are detected on the first day of life, because they present with an obvious external mass at the coccyx.[449] Occasionally, a sacrococcygeal tumor is so large that a cesarean section is necessary for delivery. Death due to uncontrolled hemorrhage has been reported upon rupture of the tumor during vaginal delivery. Some teratomas have been found by routine rectal examination shortly after birth when suspicion was aroused by asymmetry of the intergluteal fold.

In children with presacral teratomas that do not protrude externally, diagnosis is often delayed for several months or years. These children usually present with bowel or bladder dysfunction due to pressure from the tumor mass or destruction of the presacral nerves. Lower extremity paralysis and pain may be noted if the tumor invades the lumbosacral plexus or spinal canal. As many as 20% of these children have pulmonary metastasis at diagnosis.[445]

Diagnosis

The diagnosis is usually made by physical examination. The principal differential diagnostic considerations are meningocele, chordoma, duplication of the rectum, neurogenic tumors, lipoma, hemangioma, vestigial tail, and other lesions which cause urinary or rectal obstruction. Radiographic examination of the pelvis may demonstrate calcification in the mass or destruction or aplasia of the sacrum. Barium enema and intravenous pyelography may be helpful in evaluating the extent of tumor and the degree of impairment of urinary function. Chest film is necessary to evaluate the possibility of pulmonary metastases.

Elevation of α-fetoprotein in the serum should be looked for in these children, so that serial determinations can be used in those with high serum levels to monitor the effect of therapy.

Treatment and Results

The treatment of sacrococcygeal teratoma is principally surgical, regardless of the size of the mass or the age of the patient. The surgical approach has been outlined in a number of communications.[449,450] Lesions which are predominantly extrapelvic are usually removed in a one-stage procedure by a posterior sacral approach.[449] The coccyx must be removed with the tumor to minimize the chance of recurrence. For lesions extending high in the sacral region, it is usually necessary to enter the abdomen through a separate anterior approach so that the superior extent of tumor can be completely and safely removed. The major surgical complication has been excessive bleeding. In most children anal and urinary sphincter function is not interrupted.

No additional therapy is recommended for patients whose tumors are benign except for those with local recurrence. In these cases, excision of the recurrence is indicated. The coccyx should be excised if this important step has been previously omitted.

Because of the poor prognosis, patients with malignant teratomas should be given additional therapy postoperatively. Adjunctive vincristine, actinomycin-D, and cyclophosphamide is given to patients whose malignant teratoma has been completely removed.[451] Because of its effect on the bladder, pelvis, and rectum, "prophylactic" high-dose radiation therapy to sterilize the tumor bed is not recommended. However, with incomplete removal or in those patients in whom local recurrence of malignant tumors has occurred, radiation therapy should be employed. Radiation dose and volume will vary depending on clinical extent of tumor but doses greater than 3500 rad to 4000 rad are often necessary when irradiation is required.

The outcome of treatment correlates most closely with the histology of the primary tumor. With few exceptions, all patients with benign tumors have survived.[445,452] In contrast, very few children with tumors containing a malignant component have been cured. In a collected series, only 12 of 114 survived.[445,452–454]

GERM CELL TUMORS OF THE TESTIS

Pathology

Testicular tumors are the seventh most common pediatric neoplasm and most are of germinal origin.[455]

Teratomas of the testis in childhood are invariably benign. The yolk sac tumor is the most common type malignant germ cell neoplasm. In the past, a number of different names have been applied to this tumor including embryonal carcinoma, Teilum's tumor, endodermal sinus tumor, clear cell adenocarcinoma, and orchioblastoma. Theories on the histogenesis of yolk sac tumor have been discussed by Young and his associates.[456] Although sometimes called embryonal carcinoma, the histology and clinical behavior of the yolk sac tumor of the testis in the child is quite different from the embryonal carcinoma of the testis seen in the adult.

The relative frequency of the different types of testicular tumors seen in childhood at two large pediatric institutions is shown in Table 34-27.[457,458] Seminomas are exceedingly rare in patients under 16 years of age. Rhabdomyosarcoma is the commonest sarcoma seen.

Natural History

Most boys with a testicular tumor present with a painless mass that has been present for one to several months. Most of the children affected are less than 6 years of age and those with yolk sac tumor are usually under the age of 3 years. Physical examination usually reveals a hard, painless, testic-

TABLE 34-27. Frequency of Types of Testicular Tumor Seen in Two Large Series of Children

	HOPKINS	FILLER
TUMORS OF GERMINAL ORIGIN		
Yolk sac tumor	20	21
Teratocarcinoma	3	2
Chorio carcinoma	1	1
Teratoma	6	11
TUMORS OF NON-GERMINAL ORIGIN		
Sarcomas	7	8
Interstitial Cell Tumor	2	1
Sertoli Cell Tumor	0	1

(Hopkins TB, Jaffe N, Colodny A et al: The management of testicular tumors in children. J Urol 120:96–102, 1978; Filler RM, Hardy B: Testicular tumors in children. World J Surg 4:63–70, 1980.)

ular mass, 2 cm or more in diameter, not involving the scrotal wall or spermatic cord. Transillumination may be misleading, because translucency may be noted in cystic teratomas and in yolk sac tumor when hydrocele is associated with tumor. Metastatic spread is to retroperitoneal and supraclavicular lymph nodes, and to lung.

Diagnosis and Staging

Initial diagnosis is suggested by the presence of a testicular mass. To evaluate the extent of disease, sites of lymphatic and blood-borne metastases must be examined. The presence of tumor in retroperitoneal lymph nodes has been evaluated traditionally by intravenous pyelography. However, more recently ultrasound and CT scan have been used for assessment of the retroperitoneum. Lymphangiogram is technically difficult in the young child and it has not been widely used in children with testicular tumors. Chest roentgenographs will identify most metastases, but lung tomograms or CT scans are needed to detect pulmonary lesions less than 0.5 cm in diameter.

The beta sub-unit of human chorionic gonadotropin (HCG) and α-fetoprotein (AFP) have been found in the serum of children with germ cell tumors of the testis. In recent studies, as many as 90% of patients of all ages with nonseminomatous testicular tumors were found to have elevated levels of HCG, AFP, or both. Since active tumor growth is necessary to produce elevations in the blood, serial determinations are useful to follow the progress of a patient whose tumor produces these markers. Some workers have suggested the use of these studies as an aid in staging.[459]

The most widely accepted staging system for testicular tumors is that proposed by Boden and Gibb.[460] In Stage A disease, tumor is confined to the scrotum. Stage B signifies that tumor has spread to retroperitoneal nodes, Stage C indicates that tumor is present above the diaphragm. In the evaluation of reports from different centers treating patients of all ages, the distinction between clinical staging (evaluation by all diagnostic techniques except retroperitoneal node dissection) and pathologic staging must be recognized. However, as noted in Table 34-28 retroperitoneal node dissection is rarely positive in childhood yolk sac tumor. Therefore pathologic stage and clinical stage are nearly always the same in children with this tumor in contradistinction to the findings in adults.

Treatment of Yolk Sac Tumor of the Testis

ORCHIECTOMY. It is generally agreed that the initial modality of treatment for all malignant tumors of the testis should be radical orchiectomy with high ligation of the spermatic cord. In any child with a scrotal mass an inguinal incision should be made to establish the diagnosis before orchiectomy. Needle biopsy for diagnosis is contraindicated, because contamination of the scrotal contents is likely. If at exploration the diagnosis is uncertain, the testis is walled off with sponges and an incisional biopsy performed. Frozen section diagnosis is used to determine further treatment. Node dissection is not done at the same sitting but when indicated it is performed 3 days to 7 days later. According to

TABLE 34-28. Yolk Sac Tumor of the Testis: Results of Lymphadenectomy in Children with Clinical Stage A Disease

SERIES (REFERENCE NUMBER)	NUMBER OF PATIENTS HAVING LYMPHAD-ENECTOMY	NUMBER OF PATIENTS WITH POSITIVE NODES
McCullough (462)	14	2
Hopkins (457)	11	0
Young (456)	8	0
Filler (458)	6	0
TOTAL	39	2

reports in the literature 50% survival can be expected with orchiectomy alone (Table 34-29). However, in Filler's report, all 12 boys treated only by radical orchiectomy were cured and similarly five of 6 boys in Young's series were long-term survivors.[456,458]

RETROPERITONEAL NODE DISSECTION. The need for retroperitoneal node dissection in the management of testicular tumors is a point of controversy. In addition, there is argument as to whether unilateral or bilateral dissection is preferable.

In the adult experience, node dissections have been recommended for accurate pathologic staging of germinal tumors.[461] However, the experience from many pediatric centers noted in Table 34-28 indicates the presence of positive nodes in only two of 39 children with yolk sac tumors undergoing node dissection.[456,458,462] Therefore, the need for node dissection in the evaluation and treatment of germ cell testicular tumors in young boys is debatable. If most dissections are negative, then one would expect that orchiectomy would cure as many patients with Stage A disease as orchiectomy plus retroperitoneal node dissection. Data from some institutions indicate that this is indeed the case (Table 34-29).[458] However, reports from other centers indicate that orchiectomy and node dissection result in more survivors at 1 year than orchiectomy alone.[463] A good reason for these discrepancies is not apparent. Perhaps undetectable tumor deposits are present in the histologically negative lymph nodes. Since published reports do not accurately describe the distribution of disease in those who relapse after orchiectomy, it is difficult to be certain if omission of node dissection was responsible.

In view of these findings, our current policy is to perform node dissection for staging purposes after the diagnosis is confirmed. On the basis of data which indicate that contralateral nodes are rarely affected when ipsilateral nodes are negative, only a unilateral node dissection is performed when nodes are clinically negative.[464–466] When ipsilateral nodes are grossly positive, then modified bilateral lymphadenectomy is performed.

RADIATION AND CHEMOTHERAPY. The indication for radiation and chemotherapy in clinical Stage A disease is also open to debate. The report of Matsumoto and colleagues indicates that all 19 boys treated by orchiectomy and retro-

TABLE 34-29. Yolk Sac Tumor of the Testis. Results of Orchiectomy *versus* Orchiectomy plus Node Dissection for the Treatment of Stage A Disease

	ORCHIECTOMY		ORCHIECTOMY & NODE DISSECTION	
SERIES (REFERENCE NUMBER)	*Number of Patients*	*Number of 1-Year Disease-free Survivors*	*Number of Patients*	*Number of 1-Year Disease-free Survivors*
Sabio (463)	52	25	25	21
Filler (458)	12	12	6	5
TOTAL	64	37	31	26
	58% Survival		84% Survival	

peritoneal radiation (2000 rad to 3000 rad in 4 weeks to 7 weeks) were alive and well 1 year to 5 years later.[467]

Seven boys treated with lymphadenectomy, radiotherapy, and chemotherapy, after orchiectomy by Tefft and colleagues were long-term survivors, although two developed pulmonary metastases which required further therapy.[468] Four additional children treated at the same institution were treated similarly, except that radiation was omitted in two and all have survived more than 2 years. In ten of these 11 boys, repeated courses of actinomycin-D have been given over 2 years and, in the most recent cases, vincristine and cylophosphamide have been added to the regimen. Sabio's review of the literature uncovered four other children who were treated by orchiectomy and chemotherapy, with or without radiotherapy, all of whom survived over a year.[463]

Despite these favorable results, most workers feel that retroperitoneal radiation is not indicated for those with negative retroperitoneal nodes, because the risks of oncogenesis and skeletal growth retardation outweigh the possible benefits. On the other hand, the use of adjunctive chemotherapy appears to be indicated. Data from collected series indicate that at least 80% of children with testicular embryonal carcinoma have Stage A disease. Yet orchiectomy cures 50% to 60% and most die with tumor in the lung with no disease in the retroperitoneum. Fatal pulmonary metastases also occur in about 15% to 20% of those who have had a negative retroperitoneal node dissection. These treatment failures suggest that micrometastases are often present in the lung at the time of initial treatment. Since actinomycin-D appears to be active against embryonal carcinoma, there is a reasonable chance that adjunctive chemotherapy with this agent will eradicate micrometastases and improve overall survival.

Most oncologists recognize the importance of chemotherapy and radiation for the treatment of those who present with Stage B and Stage C disease and those who develop metastases. Tefft and associates salvaged two children with pulmonary metastases with whole lung radiation and actinomycin-D.[468] Other survivors with metastatic disease treated similarly were noted by Sabio and colleagues and by Young and colleagues.[456,463] A summary of recommendations for the treatment of yolk sac tumors of the testis in childhood is given in Table 34-30.

HISTIOCYTOSIS X

The collection of clinical disorders which have been termed "histiocytosis X" represents a widely varied group. Initially, these entities were described as separate clinical syndromes, most notably Hand–Schuller–Christian and Letterer–Siwe syndromes and solitary eosinophilic granuloma of bone, without consideration of pathologic appearance.[469–471] In particular,

TABLE 34-30. Yolk Sac Tumor of the Testis: Recommendations for Treatment

STAGE OF DISEASE	RADICAL ORCHIECTOMY	UNILATERAL RETROPERITONEAL NODE DISSECTION	MODIFIED BILATERAL RETROPERITONEAL NODE DISSECTION	CHEMOTHERAPY	RADIATION
A	Yes	For Staging	No	Adjunctive Actinomycin D	No
B	Yes	Yes	When ipsilateral nodes grossly positive	Actinomycin D Vincristine Cyclophosphamide	Yes
C	Yes	No	No	Actinomycin D Vincristine Cyclophosphamide	Yes

the Hand–Schuller–Christian syndrome was initally considered to represent a primary disorder of lipid metabolism or primary xanthomatosis.[472]

Subsequently, a number of investigators, in particular, Wallgren, Lichtenstein, and Green and Farber, recognized pathologic similarities between the three syndromes and suggested that they were linked disorders.[473–475] Observed clinical variations were felt to represent differences in host response and disease severity. Recently, an increasing number of investigators describe apparently reproducible pathologic differences between the clinically fulminant disease, with substantial mortality affecting children under the age of 2 years (roughly corresponding to the Letterer–Siwe syndrome as originally described), and the clinically indolent but heterogeneous entities broadly equated with eosinophilic granuloma and Hand–Schuller–Christian disease.[476–478] In these reports, the clinically aggressive disease is thought to represent a form of relatively differentiated histiocytic lymphoma affecting children.[476–479]

ETIOLOGY AND DEMOGRAPHIC FEATURES

There is a predominance of males in most series. The age at presentation averages approximately 3 years to 3½ years, with children with limited disease tending to be significantly older than those with generalized disease.[480–481]

Although a variety of agents and disease processes have been considered to be causally responsible, ranging from tuberculosis to a disorder in lipid metabolism, no recognized etiology is apparent. Many investigators currently consider the Letterer–Siwe syndrome to be malignant (see above), while controversy continues regarding the true nature of the less aggressive entities.[478]

Recently, it has been theorized that most, if not all, of these disorders are related to an immunologic abnormality.[482] Similarity between typical clinical features of histiocytosis X, including skin, liver, and lung involvement, and chronic graft-*versus*-host disease has been suggested.[483,484]

Thymic pathology has been abnormal in many of these patients at autopsy and, in some patients, when sampled soon after presentation.[483] Nearly two-thirds of one group of patients with histiocytosis X have been found to have immunologic abnormalities; either spontaneous lymphocyte cytotoxicity to cultured fibroblasts, or an antibody to autologous erythrocytes.[482] More typical immunological function tests have usually been unremarkable.[482,484] Based on these findings as well as a demonstrated deficiency in surface receptors for histamine (H_2 locus) on T-cells, a deficiency in suppressor T-cells has been suggested as the principal lesion. Patients with more severe and rapidly progressive disease (Letterer–Siwe type) have not shown these findings and have failed to respond to attempts at therapeutic manipulation of immune function.[482]

Many cases have recently been described which suggest at least a partial hereditary basis.[485–487] When the family members of five siblings of affected patients were assessed, 19 of 43 children were reported to have histiocytosis.[485] Twin studies also suggest a genetic predisposition.[488,489] In five twins where each member was affected, monozygosity was likely in at least three.[485] Taken together, these studies suggest that a sibling of an affected child has a substantially elevated risk of also developing histiocytosis X.[477] Finally, a recent review of the Boston Children's Hospital patient material suggests a possible association between histiocytosis X and mental retardation.[490]

EVALUATION

The necessary evaluation for a child with histiocytosis is controversial. A careful physical examination must be performed with particular attention to the skin, especially of the scalp and groin regions. A scaling, eczematoid rash is typical, especially at these locations.

Careful evaluation of the skull (raised areas suggesting calvarial involvement), mastoids, and external ear canals (chronic otitis and middle ear disease representing two of the commonest types of involvement), eyes and orbits (proptosis), and teeth and gums (floating teeth) should be performed. Involvement of lymph nodes, liver, and spleen must also be ruled out. Radiographic evaluation should include a chest roentgenograph (excluding pulmonary involvement with so-called "honeycomb lung") and skeletal survey, as histiocytosis represents one of the few conditions where conventional radiographs are more accurate and sensitive than radioisotopic bone scan. In addition to conventional serum and blood studies, more controversial studies include bone marrow aspiration and biopsy, routine dental evaluation with panorex films of the mandible and maxilla, and a wide range of immunologic evaluations. Urine specific gravity should be assessed and, when indicated, careful water deprivation test performed to rule out diabetes insipidus.

STAGING

No widely recognized staging system is available (Table 34-31). The first prognostically useful system was devised by Lahey, who assigned points for involvement of various organ systems, including the skin, liver, spleen, lung, pituitary, skeleton, and bone marrow (anemia or thrombocytopenia).[492] Modification of this system into a two-stage classification (with or without organ dysfunction), although helpful in distinguishing a favorable group (without organ involvement), fails to adequately subdivide patients with organ involvement into prognostically useful groups. More recently, the overriding importance of age as a prognostic variable has become apparent, and Greenberger and colleagues, after retrospective review of a large group of patients, have devised a system which utilizes both age and disease extent.[481,490] A somewhat simpler, four-stage system has been suggested by Osband and associates.[482]

The failure to use some clinico–anatomic system for staging makes most reports claiming therapetutic efficacy for one or more agents or regimens difficult to assess, and use of such a system is an obvious necessity.

PATHOLOGY

Accumulations of macrophages, occasionally with a foamy appearance and admixed with plasma cells, lymphocytes, and eosinophils histologically characterize the lesions of Hand–Schuller–Christian disease. With increased clinical activity, lesions contain a greater cellular infiltrate with

TABLE 34-31. Staging Systems for Histiocytosis

I. Lahey System (reference 491)

Points are assigned for involvement of each of the following:

a. skin
b. liver
c. spleen
d. lung
e. pituitary (diabetes insipidus)
f. skeleton
g. anemia
h. leucopenia or thrombocytopenia
i. lymph nodes

II. Greenberger et al (reference 481)

Stage I	a. Single monostotic bone lesion b. Multiple lesions in (one bone or multiple bones)
Stage II	a. ≥24 months of age at diagnosis and: having one or more of the following organ systems involved: diabetes insipidus; teeth and gingivae; lymph nodes; skin; seborrhea, any site; "mild lung involvement" (*i.e.*, infiltrates seen on chest x-ray without pulmonary symptoms or gross consolidation); bone marrow focally positive.
Stage III	a. age < 24 months at diagnosis with any of the systems involved in above II or: b. age ≥24months with involvement of liver and/or spleen; massive nodal involvement (nodes >5 × 5 × 5 cm in several sites above or below the diaphragm); "honeycomb lung" (major lung involvement in all areas with apparent fibrosis); bone marrow packed.
Stage IV	spleen >6 cm palpable below costal margin and fever >1 month with or without any or all of the above systems involved.
Stage V	"special" -monocytosis in peripheral blood >20% of differential cell count, in addition to Stage III or Stage IV findings.

(The categories (a) and (b) do not indicate differences in prognosis within the particular stage. The node size 5 × 5 × 5 in Stage III is intended to indicate massive adenopathy.)

III. Osband et al (reference 482)

Factor	*Points*
Age at Presentation	
<2	0
>2	1
Number of Organs Involved	
<4	0
>4	1
Presence of Organ Dysfunction*	
No	0
Yes	1

Stage	*Total Points*
I	0
II	1
III	2
IV	3

(Patients are staged according to the three prognostic variables derived by Lahey: age, number of organs involved and presence of organ dysfunction. A patient received one point for being in the 'poorer risk' group in each variable: age under 2 years; more than four organs involved and the presence of organ dysfunction. The points were then added and the stage determined.)

*Either hepatic, pulmonary or hemopoietic, as defined by Lahey.

variable eosinophilic infiltration. When inactive, more fibrosis is noted, with the presence of lipid-laden macrophages or "foam cells."[473–477]

Letterer–Siwe disease is characterized by a proliferation of moderately differentiated histiocytes. Newton and Hamondi feel that lesions can be separated into two types: Type 1 and Type 2.[476] In a clinicopatholgoic review of 51 patients, patients with Type 2 lesions were characterized by sheets of histiocytes with a mixture of eosinophils and giant cells. Histiocytic cells formed a somewhat syncytial appearance with areas of fibrosis, necrosis, and occasional hemorrhage. This pattern was associated with a favorable outcome; 42 of 44 patients who demonstrated it survived.

Type 1 lesions were characterized by a diffuse infiltration of the reticulo–endothelial system by individual histiocytes with preservation of architecture. Histiocytes were large with pale cytoplasm and distinct cell membranes. No eosinophils, giant cells, necrosis, or fibrosis was seen. Seven of nine patients with this histology succumbed, usually very rapidly.[476] The reproducibility of such systems has not been reported by all authors.[492]

CLINICAL BEHAVIOR

Nearly all patients with limited or generalized disease will have one or more bony sites affected, most commonly a flat or membranous one. Of those with generalized disease, 25% to 50% will develop diabetes insipidus at some time in their course, and in approximately half, the lungs will be affected to some degree. Skin and node involvement is more common, whereas splenic and bone marrow involvement is distinctly less common.[477,480,481,490]

A wide range of clinical symptoms may be responsible for patient presentation. Isolated bone pain, proptosis, chronic otitis, and floating teeth may all signal the presence of lesions in bone. The triad of geographic skull lesion, diabetes insipidus, and exophthalmos, supposedly typical of the HSC syndrome is, in fact, rare and noted in only 10% of patients with this entity. An apparently isolated site at presentation may be followed, with great variation in disease tempo, by one or more sites of disease in the same or different organ systems.

Involvement of a vertebral body, producing so-called "vertebra plana," occurs with relative frequency and may result in complete recovery and restoration of vertebral height (usually with treatment) or may, on occasion, result in severe neurologic disability through spinal cord injury, if not treated appropriately.

Diabetes insipidus is relatively common and rarely is associated with radiographic abnormalities of the sella turcica. Early treatment with irradiation is necessary if this clinical entity is to be reversed in a substantial fraction of treated patients.[481]

Skin involvement may precede more widespread disease in some patients. As noted, early age is commonly associated with a more fulminant disease course, and an all-too-frequent clinical setting is represented by the 4 month old to 12 month old infant with massive hepatosplenomegaly, widespread skin involvement, anemia or thrombocytopenia, and a variable degree of bone, lung, or nodal involvement. Disease tempo in these younger children is often fulminant and death within weeks is not uncommon.[476]

TREATMENT

A striking variety in treatment, including surgery, irradiation, corticosteroids, cytotoxic chemotherapy, and immunotherapy has been used for histiocytosis X. A substantial number of patients, especially in earlier years, have also been simply observed or received only symptomatic therapy with substantial survival. Controversy surrounds almost all analyses of efficacy of treatment for varying stages of disease, because of the frequent occurrence of spontaneous regression and the unpredictable course of this disease. In addition, clinical staging is rarely reported.

Isolated, monostotic bone involvement most commonly occurs in children aged 4 years to 9 years and is best treated by surgical curettage or low dose megavoltage irradiation (450 rad to 1200 rad in three to six fractions) or both.[481,492] Routine use of postoperative irradiation following thorough curettage of lesions is not recommended. Instead, careful observation should occur and, only when clinical or radiographic evidence of recurrence or progression develops should irradiation be used. A possible exception is represented by lesions at sites where early local recurrence may be difficult to clinically appreciate and may pose a serious threat to the patient (*i.e.*, pathologic fracture of a weight-bearing bone). Incompletely curetted lesions or surgically less accessible sites (*i.e.*, vertebral body) should receive treatment with irradiation. Cases of spinal cord injury caused by extradural compression from untreated histiocytosis in this site have been reported.[494]

Systemic treatment for patients with multisystem disease, but with an indolent course, is controversial but appears to improve survival, especially for patients less than 2 years of age.[495] Observation, steroid treatment, single-agent chemotherapy (i.e., vinblastine or chlorambucil), thymic extract therapy, and multiagent chemotherapy have all been utilized and advocated.[495–497] Although acute leukemia has been suggested as an appropriate model and multiagent combinations recommended, evidence supporting this suggestion for older patients or those with HSC disease is lacking.[477] The optimum agent(s) and schedule(s) of cytoxic drugs are not known.

Single agent treatment with chlorambucil, vinblastine or methotrexate, with or without prednisone, yields response rates (both complete and partial) of 40% to 60% or more.[495–498] Factors which decrease the likelihood of response include age (more than 2 years more favorable than less than 2 years and less than 2 years more favorable than less than 1 year), organ involvement, and stage.[495–499] Overall response rates to combinations of more than two agents do not yield definitely superior results, although one study suggested that the effect of one such regimen on children aged 1 year to 2 years with more extensive disease was superior.[499] Clearly, however, more aggressive chemotherapeutic regimens have a greater acute and possibly late morbidity.[495,499–501]

The presence of chronic disease exacerbations combined with chronic treatment may result in a number of sequelae. 67% of two series of patients had significant late problems, including diabetes insipidus, pulmonary fibrosis, or bone abnormality.[495,500] 27% of patients had short stature (less than third percentile).[495] Treatment with thymic humoral factor has been associated with response rates equivalent to those obtained with cytotoxic chemotherapeutic agents.[482]

In general, the therapeutic goal should be to prevent both excessive disease-associated morbidity and, of equal importance, iatrogenic morbidity, especially in later life. Intensive treatment at the time of initial presentation is not, therefore, usually appropriate, as would be the case with a true malignancy, and initial recommended therapy should probably constitute prednisone plus single-agent therapy, or thymic extract treatment. Progression of disease will clearly require more aggressive systemic forms of treatment. Histiocytosis X is rapidly responsive to irradiation and surprisingly low total doses of irradiation are very effective in obtaining local control.[481,493] Specific clinical settings, such as diabetes insipidus treated soon after initial symptoms, progressive destruction of a weight-bearing bone, extensive and progressive mandibular involvement with floating teeth, mastoid involvement, or progressive proptosis, can often be rapidly and most effectively treated by a short course of localized irradiation.[481]

Should all conventional chemotherapy techniques prove ineffective, low-dose whole or half body irradiation, similar to treatment used in adults with nodular non-Hodgkin's lymphomas has been helpful in isolated cases.[502,503]

Unfortunately, treatment has been much less effective for the child of less than 2 years of age with widespread involvement at presentation who suffers rapid disease progression. Despite intensive treatment with single-agent therapy or multiagent-systemic treatment, many of these patients succumb rapidly. For these prognostically unfavorable infants, improved techniques of therapy are clearly necessary. The addition and use of wide field or whole body irradiation should be performed only in the setting of a carefully controlled study.

RESULTS

Virtually all patients with early stage monostotic bone involvement survive and frequently suffer no additional signs or symptoms of the disease. Although disease-related death may occur in the older child with multisystem, intermediate stage disease, the frequency is rare and more than 80% of these children should survive with adequate supportive treatment, aggressive use of antibiotic treatment, and judicious use of all currently available modalities of therapy. It is with this group of children that survival has been significantly improved in recent years, due in part at least to better supportive management as well as systemic treatment of their disease.

Using the staging system of Greenberger and colleagues, 80% of all patients with Stage I through Stage III disease survive. No patient of 15 with Stage IV disease survived, and 38% of those in a special group of patients with Stage III or IV disease but with a greater than 20% peripheral monocytosis (Stage V) survive.

Infants with widespread, progressive disease continue to prove resistant to most therapies and constitute the principal therapeutic challenge.

FUTURE GOALS

Better characterization of the primary nature or natures of histiocytosis X and a better understanding of its pathophysiology should constitute the major goal of future investigations. It will be of importance to ascertain if, in fact, two separate conditions with somewhat similar clinical signs and symptoms, only one of which constitutes a true neoplasm, have been incorrectly considered as one entity. Routine use of clinical staging is essential in clinical reports. Finally, further attempts to improve current therapy for the "typical" child, while minimizing morbidity of therapy will continue to command attention.

REFERENCES

1. Knudson AG Jr: Mutation and cancer: statistical study of retinoblastoma. Proc Natl Acad Sci 68:820–823, 1971
2. Krivit W, Good RA: The simultaneous occurrence of leukemia and mongolism; report of 4 cases. AMA J Dis Child 91:218–222, 1956
3. Ross JD, Maloney WC, Desforges JF: Ineffective regulation of granulopoiesis masquerading as congenital leukemia in a mongoloid child. J Ped 61:1–5, 1963
4. Aur RJA, Simone, JV, Verzosa MS et al: Childhood acute lymphocytic leukemia Study VIII. Cancer 42:2123–2134, 1978
5. DeVita VT Jr, Young RC, Canellos GP: Combination *versus* single agent chemotherapy: A review of the basis for selection of drug treatment of cancer. Cancer 35:98–110, 1975
6. Razek A, Vietti T, Valeriote F: Optimum time sequence for the administration of vincristine and cyclophosphamide *in vivo*. Cancer Res 34:1857–1861, 1974
7. Bertino JR: Toward improved selectivity in cancer chemotheapy: The Richard and Hinda Rosenthal foundation award lecture. Cancer Res 39:293–304, 1979
8. Bleyer, WA, Poplack, DG, Simon RM: "Concentration X time" methotrexate *via* a subcutaneous reservoir: a less toxic regimen for intraventricular chemotherapy of central nervous system neoplasms. Blood 51:835–842, 1978
9. Eiser C, Lansdown R: Retrospective study of intellectual development in children treated for acute lymphoblastic leukemia. Arch Dis Child 52:525–529, 1977
10. Williams IG, Price BS: Tumours of Childhood. New York, Appleton-Century-Crofts, 1973
11. D'Angio GJ, Evans AE, Breslow N et al: The treatment of Wilms' tumor. Results of the National Wilms' Tumor Study. Cancer 38:633–646, 1976
12. Neal PN, Jenkin RJT: Abdominal irradiation in the treatment of Wilms' tumor. Int J Radiat Oncol Biol Phys 6:655–661, 1980
13. Cassady JR, Jaffe N, Filler RM: The increasing importance of radiation therapy in the treatment of Wilms' tumor. Cancer 39:825–829, 1977
14. Probert JC, Parker BR, Kaplan HS: Growth retardation in children after megavoltage irradiation of the spine. Cancer 32:634–639, 1973
15. Littman PS, D'Angio GJ: Growth considerations in the radiation therapy of children with cancer. Ann Rev Med (in press)
16. Painter MJ, Chutorian AM, Hilal SK; Cerebrovasculopathy following irradiation in childhood. Neurology 25:189–194, 1975
17. Rubin P, Duthie RB, Young LW: Significance of scoliosis in postirradiated Wilms' tumor and neuroblastoma. Radiology 79:539–559, 1962
18. D'Angio GJ: Clinical and biologic studies of Actinomycin D and roentgen irradiation. Am J Roent 87:106–109, 1962
19. Jaffe N, Farber S, Traggis D et al: Favorable response of metastatic osteogenic sarcoma to pulse high-dose methotrexate

with citrovorum rescue and radiation therapy. Cancer 31:1367–1373, 1973
20. Cassady JR, Richter M, Piro AJ et al: Radiation–Adriamycin interactions: preliminary clinical observations. Cancer 36: 946–949, 1975
21. Phillips TL, Fu KK: Acute and late effects of multimodal therapy on normal tissues. Cancer 40:489–494, 1977
22. Glatstein E, Fajardo LF, Brown JM: Radiation injury in the mouse kidney. I. Sequential light microscopic study. Int J Radiat Oncol Biol Phys 2:933–943, 1977
23. Phillips TL: Effects on lung of combined chemotherapy and radiotherapy. Front Rad Ther Onc 13:133–135, Karger, Basel, 1979
24. Cassady JR, Carabell, S, Jaffe N: Chemotherapy-irradiation related hepatic dysfunction in patients with Wilms' tumor. Front Rad Ther Onc 13:147–160, Basel, Karger, 1979
25. Gilladoga AC, Manuel C, Tan CTC et al: The cardiotoxicity of adriamycin and daunorubicin in children. Cancer 37:1070–1078, 1976
26. Tonnesen GL, Cassady JR, Sallan SE et al: Augmentation of vincristine neurotoxicity by irradiation of peripheral nerves. Cancer Treat Rep 64:963–965, 1980
27. Li FP, Cassady JR, Jaffe N: Risk of second tumors in survivors of childhood cancer. Cancer 35:1230–1235, 1975
28. Arseneau JC, Sponzo RW, Levin DL et al: Non-lymphomatous malignant tumors complicating Hodgkin's disease. N Engl J Med 287:1119–1122, 1972
29. Hutchinson GB: Late neoplastic changes following medical irradiation. Radiology 105:645–652, 1972
30. Hempelmann LH: Risk of thyroid neoplasms after irradiation in childhood. Science 160:159–163, 1968
31. Mole RH: Ionizing radiation as a carcinogen: practical questions and academic pursuits. Br J Radiol 48:157–169, 1975
32. Upton AC: The dose–response relation in radiation-induced cancer. Cancer Res 21:717–729, 1961
33. Sagerman RH, Cassady JR, Tretter P et al: Radiation induced neoplasia following external-beam therapy for children with retinoblastoma. Am J Roentgenol 105:529–535, 1969
34. Haselow RE, Nesbit M, Kehner LP et al: Second neoplasms following megavoltage radiation in a pediatric population. Cancer 42:1185–1191, 1978
35. Kitchin FD, Ellsworth RM: Pleiotropic effects of the gene for retinoblastoma. J Med Genetics 11:244–246, 1974
36. Choi SI, Simone JV: Acute nonlymphocytic leukemia in 171 children. Med Ped Oncol 2:119–146, 1976
37. Smith KL, Johnson W: Classification of chronic myelocytic leukemia in children. Cancer 34:670–679, 1974
38. Roath S: Observations on the aetiology of acute leukemia. Clinics Haematol 1:23–47, 1972
39. Miller RW: Persons with exceptionally high risk of leukemia. Cancer Res 27:2420–2423, 1967
40. Ross JD, Maloney WC, Desforges JF: Ineffective regulation of granulopoiesis masquerading as congenital leukemia in a mongoloid child. J Ped 61:1–5, 1963
41. Brodeur GM, Dahl GV, Williams DL et al: Transient leukemoid reaction and trisomy 21 mosaicism in a phenotypically normal newborn. Blood 55:691–693, 1980
42. Hecht F, McCaw BK: Chromosome instability syndromes. Genetics of Human Cancer. New York, Raven Press, 1977, pp 105–123
43. Knudson AG, Jr: Mutation and cancer: statistical study of retinoblastoma. Proc Natl Acad Sci 68:820–823, 1971
44. Falletta JM, Starling KA, Fernbach DJ: Leukemia in twins. Pediatrics 52:846–849, 1973
45. Young JL, Miller RW: Incidence of malignant tumors in U.S. children. J Ped 86:254–258, 1975
46. Bennett JM, Catovsky D, Daniel MT et al: Proposals for the classification of the acute leukaemias. Br J Haematol 33:451–458, 1976
47. Bollum FJ: Terminal deoxynucleotidyl transferase as a hematopoietic cell marker. Blood 54:1203–1215, 1979
48. Chessells JM, Hardisty RM, Rapson NT: Acute lymphoblastic leukaemia in children: classification and prognosis. Lancet 2:1307–1309, 1977
49. Flandrin G, Brouet JC, Daniel MT et al: Acute leukemia with Burkitt's tumor cells: a study of six cases with special reference to lymphocyte surface markers. Blood 45:183–188, 1975
50. Reinherz EL, Nadler LM, Sallan SE et al: Subset derivation of T-cell acute lymphoblastic leukemia in man. J Clin Invest 64:392–397, 1979
51. Reinherz EL, Schlossman SF: Regulation of the immune response—inducer and suppressor T-lymphocyte subsets in human beings. N Engl J Med 303:370–374, 1980
52. Zuelzer WW, Inoue S, Thompson RI et al: Long-term cytogenetic studies in acute leukemia of children, the nature of relapse. Am J Hemat 1:143–190, 1976
53. Fialkow PJ: Clonal origin of human tumors. Biochem Biophys Acta 458: 283–321, 1976
54. Schaller J: Arthritis as a presenting manifestation of malignancy in children. J Ped 81:793–797, 1972
55. Yolken RH, Miller DR: Hyperuricemia and renal failure—presenting manifestations of occult hematologic malignancies. J Ped 89:775–778, 1976
56. Jayaraman J, David R: Hypercalcemia as a presenting manifestation of leukemia: Evidence of excessive PTH secretion. J Ped 90:609–610, 1977
57. Simone JV, Verzosa MS, Rudy JA: Initial features and prognosis in 363 children with acute lymphocytic leukemia. Cancer 36:2099–2108, 1975
58. Robison LL, Nesbit ME, Sather HN et al: Assessment of the interrelationship of prognostic factors in childhood acute lymphoblastic leukemia. Am J Ped Hem Oncol 2:5–13, 1980
59. Dow, LW, Borella L, Sen L et al: Initial prognostic factors and lymphoblast-erythrocyte rosette formation in 109 children with acute lymphocytic leukemia. Blood 50:671–682, 1977
60. Bernard J, Weil M, Boiron M et al: Acute promyelocytic leukemia: results of treatment by daunorubicin. Blood 41:489–496, 1973
61. Jones ME, Saleem A: Acute promyelocytic leukemia. Am J Med 65:673–677, 1978
62. McKenna RW, Bloomfield CD, Dick F et al: Acute monoblastic leukemia: diagnosis and treatment of ten cases. Blood 46:481–494, 1975
63. Champion LAA, Luddy RE, Schwartz AD: Disseminated intravascular coagulation in childhood acute lymphocytic leukemia with poor prognostic features. Cancer 41:1642–1646, 1978
64. Golomb HM, Vardiman JW, Rowley JD et al: Correlation of clinical findings with quinacrine-banded chromosomes in 90 adults with acute nonlymphocytic leukemia. N Engl J Med 299:613–619, 1978
65. Simone JV: Childhood leukemia as a model for cancer research: The Richard and Hinda Rosenthal foundation award lecture. Cancer Res 39:4301–4307, 1979
66. Gralnick HR, Sultan C: Acute promyelocytic leukaemia: haemorrhagic manifestations and morphologic criteria. Br J Haematol 29:373–376, 1975
67. Hughes WT, Smith DR: Infection during induction of remission in acute lymphocytic leukemia. Cancer 31:1008–1014, 1973
68. Farber S, Diamond L, Mercer R et al: Temporary remission in acute leukemia in children produced by folic acid antagonist, 4-aminopteryl glutamic acid (Aminopterin). N Engl J Med 238:787–782, 1948
69. Simone JV: Factors that influence haematological remission duration in acute lymphocytic leukaemia. Br J Haematol 32:465–472, 1976
70. Pinkel D, Hernandez K, Borella L et al: Drug dosage and remission duration in childhood lymphocytic leukemia. Cancer 27:247–256, 1971
71. Aur RJA, Simone J, Hustu HO et al: Central nervous system therapy and combination chemotherapy of childhood lymphocytic leukemia. Blood 37:272–281, 1971
72. Aur RJA, Simone JV, Hustu HO et al: A comparative study of

central nervous system irradiation and intensive chemotheapy early in remission of childhood acute lymphocytic leukemia. Cancer 29:381–391, 1972

73. Aur RJA, Hustu HO, Verzosa MS et al: Comparison of two methods of preventing central nervous system leukemia. Blood 42:349–357, 1973
74. Aur RJA, Simone JV, Verzosa MS et al: Childhood acute lymphocytic leukemia. Study VIII. Cancer 42:2123–2134, 1978
75. Hughes WT, Kuhn S, Chaudhary S et al: Successful chemoprophylaxis for *Pneumocystis carinii* pneumonitis. N Engl J Med 297:1419–1426, 1977
76. Wilber RB, Feldman S, Malone WJ et al: Chemoprophylaxis for *Pneumocystis carinii* pneumonitis. Am J Dis Child 134:643–648, 1980
77. Price RA, Jamieson PA: The central nervous system in childhood leukemia. I Subacute leukoencephalopathy. Cancer 35:306–318, 1975
78. Peylan-Ramu N, Poplack DG, Pizzo PA et al: Abnormal CT scans of the brain in asymptomatic children with acute lymphocytic leukemia after prophylactic treatment of the central nervous system with radiation and intrathecal chemotherapy. N Engl J Med 298:815–818, 1978
79. Holland JF, Glidewell O: Chemotherapy of acute lymphocytic leukemia of childhood. Cancer 1480–1487, 1970
80. Jones B, Holland JF, Glidewell O et al: Optimal use of l-asparaginase (NSC-109229) in acute lymphocytic leukemia: Med Ped Oncol 3:387–400, 1977
81. Haghbin M, Murphy ML, Tan CC et al: A long-term clinical follow-up of children with acute lymphoblastic leukemia treated with intensive chemotherapy regimens. Cancer 46:241–252, 1980
82. Sallan SE, Camitta BM, Cassady JR et al: Intermittent combination chemotherapy with adriamycin for childhood acute lymphoblastic leukemia: clinical results. Blood 51:425–433, 1978
83. Riehm H, Gadner H, Welte K: Die West-Berliner studie zur behandlung der akuten lymphoblastischen leukämie des kindes—erfahrungsbericht nach 6 jahren. Klin pädiat 189:89–102, 1977
84. Freeman AI, Wang JJ, Sinks LF: High-dose methotrexate in acute lymphocytic leukemia. Cancer Treat Rep 61:727–731, 1977
85. Moe PJ, Seip M: High dose methotrexate in acute lymphocytic leukemia in childhood. Acta Paediatr Scand 67:265–268, 1978
86. Henze G, Langermann HJ, Lampert F et al: Die studie zur behandlung der akuten lymphoblastischen leukamie 1971–1974 der deutschen arbeitsgemeinschaft fur leukamieforschung und behandlung im kindesalter e.V. Analyse der prognostischen bedeutung von initialbefunden und therapievarianten. Klin Padiat 191:114–126, 1979
87. Sen L, Borella L: Clinical importance of lymphoblasts with T markers in childhood acute leukaemia. N Engl J Med 292:828–832, 1975
88. Rivera G, Dahl GV, Bowman WP et al: VM-26 and cytosine arabinoside combination chemotherapy for initial induction failures in childhood lymphocytic leukemia. Cancer 46:1727–1730, 1980
89. Thiel E, Rodt H, Netzel B et al: T-Zell-Antigen positive, E-Rosetten negative akute lymphoblastenleukämie. Blut 36:363–369, 1978
90. Roberts M, Greaves M, Janossy G et al: Acute lymphoblastic leukaemia (ALL) associated antigen-I. expression in different haematopoietic malignancies. Leuk Res 2:105–114, 1978
91. Vogler LB, Crist WM, Bockman DE et al: Pre-B-cell leukemia: a new phenotype of childhood lymphoblastic leukemia. N Engl J Med 298:872, 1978
92. Sallan SE, Ritz J, Pesando J et al: Cell surface antigens: Prognostic implications in childhood acute lymphoblastic leukemia. Blood 55:395–402, 1980
93. Hustu HO, Aur RJA: Extramedullary leukemia. Clin Haematol 7:313–337, 1978
94. George SL, Aur RJA, Mauer AM et al: A reappraisal of the results of stopping therapy in childhood leukemia. N Engl J Med 300:269–273, 1979
95. Rivera G, Aur RJA, Dahl GV et al: Second cessation of therapy in childhood lymphocytic leukemia. Blood 53:1114–1120, 1979
96. Gale RP: Advances in the treatment of acute myelogenous leukemia. N Engl J Med 300:1189–1199, 1979
97. Vaughan WP, Karp JE, Burke PJ: Long chemotherapy-free remissions after single-cycle timed-sequential chemotherapy for acute myelocytic leukemia. Cancer 45:859–865, 1980
98. Priesler HD, Rustum Y, Henderson ES et al: Treatment of acute nonlymphocytic leukemia: use of anthracycline–cytosine arabinoside induction therapy and comparison of two maintenance regimens. Blood 53:455–464, 1979
99. Weinstein HJ, Mayer RJ, Rosenthal DS et al: Treatment of acute myelogenous leukemia in children and adults. N Engl J Med 303:473–478, 1980
100. Kay HEM: Development of CNS leukaemia in acute myeloid leukaemia in childhood. Arch Dis Child 51:73–74, 1976
101. Dahl GV, Simone JV, Hustu HO et al: Preventive central nervous system irradiation in children with acute nonlymphocytic leukemia. Cancer 42:2187–2192, 1978
102. Cunningham I, Gee T, Dowling M et al: Results of treatment of PH'+ chronic myelogenous leukemia with an intensive treatment regimen (L-5 protocol). Blood 53:375–395, 1979
103. Fefer A, Cheever MA, Thomas ED et al: Disappearance of Ph^1-positive cells in four patients with chronic granulocytic leukemia after chemotherapy, irradiation and marrow transplantation from an identical twin. N Engl J Med 300:333–337, 1979
104. Janossy G, Greaves MF, Revesz T et al: Blast crisis of chronic myeloid leukaemia (CML). II. Cell surface marker analysis of 'lymphoid' and myeloid cases. Br J Haematol 34:179–192, 1976
105. Marks SM, Baltimore D, McCaffrey R: Terminal transferase as a predictor of initial responsiveness to vincristine and prednisone in blastic chronic myelogenous leukemia. N Engl J Med 298:812–814, 1978
106. Priest JR, Robison LL, McKenna RW et al: Philadelphia chromosome positive childhood acute lymphoblastic leukemia. Blood 56:15–22, 1980
107. Kelsen DP, Gee TS, Chaganti RSK: Philadelphia chromosome positive chronic myelogenous leukemia developing in a patient with acute lymphoblastic leukemia. Cancer 43:1782–1787, 1979
108. Altman AJ, Baehner RL: In vitro colony-forming characteristics of chronic granulocytic leukemia in childhood. J Pediatr 86:221–224, 1975
109. Sanders JE, Buckner CD, Stewart P et al: Successful treatment of juvenile chronic granulocytic leukemia with marrow transplantation. Pediatrics 63:44–46, 1979
110. Thomas ED, Sanders JE, Flournoy N et al: Marrow transplantation for patients with acute lymphoblastic leukemia in remission. Blood 54:468–476, 1979
111. Thomas ED, Buckner CD, Clift RA et al: Marrow transplantation for acute nonlymphoblastic leukemia in first remission. N Engl J Med 301:597–599, 1979
112. Pinkel D, Johnson W, Aur RJA: Non-Hodgkin's lymphoma in children. Br J Cancer 31 (Suppl II):298–323, 1975
113. Murphy SB, Frizzera G, Evans AE: A study of childhood non-Hodgkin's lymphoma. Cancer 36:2121–2131, 1975
114. Jenkin RDT, Sonley MJ; The management of malignant lymphoma in childhood. In: Neoplasia in Childhood. Chicago, Year Book: 1969, pp 305–319
115. Jones B, Klingberg WG: Lymphosarcoma in children. A report of 43 cases and review of the recent literature. J Ped 63:11–20, 1963
116. Weinstein HJ, Link MP: Non-Hodgkin's lymphoma in childhood. Clin Haematol 8, 699–716, 1979
117. Carabell S, Cassady JR, Weinstein H et al: The role of radiation therapy in the treatment of pediatric non-Hodgkin's lymphomas. Cancer 42:2193–2205, 1978
118. Murphy S: The lymphomas, lymphadenopathy and histiocytoses. In Nathan DG, Oski FA (eds): Hematology in Infancy and Childhood, 2nd ed. Philadelphia, WB Saunders 1980

119. Qazi R, Aisenberg AC, Long JC: The natural history of nodular lymphoma. Cancer 37:1923–1927, 1976
120. Murphy S, Hustu H: A randomized trial of combined modality therapy in childhood non-Hodgkin's lymphoma. Cancer 45: 630–637, 1980
121. Magrath IT, Ziegler JL: Bone marrow involvement in Burkitt's lymphoma and its relationship to acute B-cell leukemia. Leuk Res 4: 33–59, 1979
122. Young JL, Miller RW: Incidence of malignant tumors in U.S. children. J Pediatrics 86:254–258, 1975
123. Rosenberg SA, Diamond HD, Jaslowitz B et al: Lymphosarcoma: A review of 1269 cases. Medicine 40:31, 1960
124. Jenkin RDT, Morris-Jones P: In Bloom HJG, Lemerle J, Neidhardt MK et al (eds): Malignant lymphomas In Cancer in Children. Berlin, Heidelberg, New York, Springer-Verlag, 1975, pp 162–179
125. Grundy GW, Creagan ET, Fraumeni JF: Non-Hodgkin's lymphoma in childhood: Epidemiologic features. JNCI 51: 767–776, 1973
126. Kersey JH, Spector BD, Good RA: Immunodeficiency diseases and cancer: the immuno deficiency—cancer registry. Int J Cancer 12:333–347, 1973
127. Purtilo DT; Opportunistic non-Hodgkin's lymphoma in X-linked recessive immunodeficiency and lymphoproliferative syndromes. Sem Oncol 4, 335–343, 1977
128. Purtilo DT, DeFlorio D, Hutt LM et al: Variable phenotypic expressions of an X-linked recessive lymphoproliferative syndrome. NEJM 297:1077–1081, 1977
129. Hoover R, Fraumeni JF: Risk of Cancer in renal transplant recipients. Lancet II: 55–57, 1973
130. Epstein MA, Achong BG, Barr YM: Virus particles in cultured lymphoblasts from Burkitt's lymphoma. Lancet I: 702, 1964
131. Burkitt DP: The trail to a virus. In Biggs PM, DeThe G, Payne LN (eds): Oncogenesis and Herpes viruses. Lyon, France, International Agency for Research in Cancer, 1972, pp. 345–348
132. O'Conor GT: Persistant immunologic stimulation as a factor in oncogenesis with special reference to Burkitt's tumor. Am J Med 48:279–285, 1970
133. Pagano JS, Huang CH, Levine PH: Absence of Epstein-Barr viral DNA in American Burkitt's Lymphoma. N Engl J Med 289:1395–1399, 1973
134. DeThe G: Is Burkitt's lymphoma related to perinatal infection by Epstein-Barr virus? Lancet I: 335, 1977
135. Anderson M, Klein G et al: Association of Epstein-Barr viral genomes with American Burkitt lymphoma. Nature 260:357, 1976
136. Li FP, Willard DR, Goodman R et al: Malignant lymphoma after diphenylhydantoin (Dilantin) therapy. Cancer 36:1359–1362, 1975
137. Nelson DF, Cassady JR, Traggis D et al: The role of radiation therapy in localized, resectable intestinal non-Hodgkin's lymphoma in children. Cancer 39:89–97, 1977
138. Arseneau JC, Canellos GP, Banks PM et al: American Burkitt's lymphoma: A clinicopathiologic study of 30 cases. Am J Med 58, 314–321, 1975
139. Nathwani BN, Kim H, Rappaport H: Malignant lymphoma, lymphoblastic. Cancer 38:964–983, 1976
140. Weinstein H, Vance Z, Jaffe N et al: Improved prognosis for patients with mediastinal lymphoblastic lymphoma. Blood 53:687–694, 1979
141. Wollner N, Burchenal JH, Lieberman O et al: Non-Hodgkin's lymphoma in children, a comparative study of two modalities of therapy. Cancer 37:123–134, 1976
142. Ziegler JL, Monow RH, Fass L et al: Treatment of Burkitt's tumor with cyclophosphamide. Cancer 26:474–484, 1970
143. Ziegler JL, Magrath IT, Olweny CLM: Cure of Burkitt's lymphoma. Lancet II:936–938, 1979
144. Ziegler JL: Chemotherapy of Burkitt's lymphoma. Cancer 30:1534–1540, 1972
145. Pasmantier M, Coleman M, Silver RT: Value of biopsy in diagnosis of primary lymphosarcoma of marrow. Arch Int Med: 137, 52–54, 1977
146. Magrath IT, Lwanga S, Carswell W et al: Surgical reduction of tumor bulk in management of abdominal Burkitt's lymphoma. Br Med J II: 308–312, 1974
147. Frizzera G, Murphy S: Follicular (nodular) lymphoma in childhood: A rare clinical-pathological entity: Report of eight cases from four cancer centers. Cancer 44:2218–2235, 1979
148. Byrne GE: Rappaport classification of non-Hodgkin's lymphoma: Histologic features and clinical significance. Cancer Treat Rep 61:935, 1977
149. Nathwani BN, Kim H, Rappaport H et al: Non-Hodgkin's lymphoma—a clinicopathologic study comparing two classifications. Cancer 41:303–325, 1978
150. Lukes R, Collins RD; Immunologic characterization of human malignant lymphomas. Cancer 34: 1488–1503, 1972
151. Siegal FP, Filippa DA, Koziner B: Surface markers in leukemias and lymphomas. Am J Pathol 90:451–460, 1978
152. Fialkow PJ, Klein E, Klein G et al: Immunoglobulin and glucose-6-phosphate dehydrogenase as markers of cellular origin in Burkitt's lymphoma. J Exp Med 138:89–95, 1973
153. Mann RB, Jaffe ES, Braylan RC et al: Non-endemic Burkitt's lymphoma: A B-cell tumor related to germinal centers. N Engl J Med 295:685–670, 1976
154. Lukes RJ, Taylor CR, Parker JW et al: A morphologic and immunologic surface marker study of 299 cases of non-Hodgkin's lymphomas and related leukemias. Am J Pathol 90: 461–486, 1978
155. Sen L, Borella L: Clinical importance of lymphoblasts with T markers in childhood acute leukemia. N Engl Med 292: 828–832, 1975
156. Bloomfield C, Kersey J, Brunning R et al: Prognostic significance of lymphocyte surface markers in adult non-Hodgkin's lymphoma. Lancet II:1330–1333, 1976
157. Reinherz EL, Nadler LM, Sallan SE et al: Subset derivation of T-cell acute lymphoblastic leukemia in man. J Clin Invest 64:392–397, 1979
158. Carbone PP, Kaplan HS, Musshoff K et al: Report of the Committee on Hodgkin's Disease staging classification. Cancer Res 31:1860–1861, 1971
159. Murphy SB, Childhood non-Hodgkin's lymphoma. N Engl J Med 299:1446–1448, 1978
160. Murphy SB: Prognostic factors and obstacles to cure of childhood non-Hodgkin's lymphoma. Sem Oncol 4:265–271, 1977
161. Rosenberg SA: Validity of the Ann Arbor staging classification for the non-Hodgkin's lymphomas. Cancer Treat Rep 61:1023, 1977
162. Ziegler JL, Magrath IT: Burkitt's lymphoma. In Ioachim HL (ed): Pathobiology Annual. New York, Appleton-Century Crofts, 1974, pp 129–142
163. Glatstein E, Kim H, Donaldson SS, et al: Non-Hodgkin's lymphomas: VI. Results of treatment in childhood. Cancer 34:204–211, 1974
164. Lemerle M, Gerard-Marchant R, Sanazin D et al: Lymphosarcoma and reticulum cell sarcoma in children: A retrospective study of 172 cases. Cancer 32:1499–1507, 1973
165. Wollner N, Exelby PR, Lieberman PH: Non-Hodgkin's lymphoma in children: A progress report on the original patients treated with the LSA_2L_2 protocol. Cancer 44:1990–1999, 1979
166. Hutter JJ, Favara B, Nelsen M et al: Non-Hodgkin's lymphoma in children. Cancer 36:2132–2137, 1975
167. Jenkin R, Anderson J, Chilcote R et al: Grossly localized childhood non-Hodgkin's lymphoma (NHL). Response to irradiation and elective 4 or 10 drug combination chemotherapy (abstr). Proc Am Soc Clin Oncol 20:354, 1979
168. Murphy SB: Management of childhood non-Hodgkin's lymphoma. Cancer Treat Rep 61:1161–1173, 1977
169. Meadows A, Jenkin R, Chilcote R, et al: Remission induction in childhood non-Hodgkin's lymphoma (NHL) with cyclophosphamide (CPM), vincristine (VCR), prednisone, and intravenous methotrexate (MTX) (abstr). Proc Am Soc Clin Oncol 19:365, 1978
170. Jenkin RDT, Sonley MJ, Stephens CA et al: Primary gastrointestinal tract lymphoma in childhood. Radiology 92:763, 1969

171. Zea JM, Exelby P, Wollner N; Abdominal non-Hodgkin's lymphoma in childhood. J Ped Surg 11:363–369, 1976
172. Newburger P, Cassady JR, Jaffe N: Esophagitis due to adriamycin and radiation therapy for childhood malignancy. Center 42:417–423, 1978
173. Weinstein HJ, Cassady JR, Nadler LM et al: Prolonged remissions in patients with mediastinal lymphoblastic lymphoma (MLL) (abstract C-452). Proc Am Soc Clin Oncol 21:433, 1980
174. Frei EF III, Sallan SA: Acute lymphoblastic leukemia: treatment. Cancer 42:828–838, 1978
175. Burkitt D: A sarcoma involving the jaws of African children. Br J Surg 46:218, 1958.
176. Appelbaum FR, Deisseroth AB, Graw RG et al: Prolonged complete remission following high dose chemotherapy of Burkitt's lymphoma in relapse. Cancer 41:1059–1063, 1978
177. Magrath IT, Lee YJ, Anderson T et al: Prognostic factors in Burkitt's lymphoma. Cancer 45:1507–1515, 1980
178. Fialkow PJ, Klein G, Gartler SM et al: Clonal origin for individual Burkitt tumors. Lancet, Feb 21, 1970, 384–386
179. Editorial: Lancet, Feb 21, 1970, 400–401
180. Douglass EC, Magrath IT, Lee EC et al: Cytogenetic studies in Non-African Burkitt lymphoma. Blood 55:148–155, 1980
181. Berard C, O'Conor GT, Thomas LB: Histopathological definition of Burkitt's tumor. Bull WHO 40:601, 1969
182. Arseneau JC, Bagley CM, Anderson T et al: Hyperkalemia, a sequel to chemotherapy of Burkitt's lymphoma. Lancet I:10–14, 1973
183. Cadman EC, Lundberg WB, Bertino JR: Hyperphosphatemia and hypocalcemia accompanying rapid cell lysis in a patient with Burkitt's lymphoma and Burkitt cell leukemia. Am J Med 62:283–290, 1977
184. Ziegler JL, DeVita VT, Graw R-G et al: Combined modality treatment of American Burkitt's lymphoma. Cancer 38: 2225–2231, 1976
185. Norin T, Onyango J: Radiotherapy in Burkitt's lymphoma. Int J Rad Oncol Biol Phys 2:399–406, 1977
186. Olweny CLM, Atine I, Kaddu-Mukasa A et al: Cerebrospinal irradiation of Burkitt's lymphoma. Acta Radiol Ther 16:225–231, 1977
187. Ziegler JL, Bluming AZ: Intrathecal chemotherapy in Burkitt lymphoma. Br Med J 3:508–512, 1971
188. Ramirez I, Sullivan MP, Wang Y et al: Effective therapy for Burkitt's lymphoma: High dose cyclophosphamide + high dose methotrexate with coordinated intrathecal therapy. Cancer Chemother Pharm 3:103–109, 1979
189. Virchow R: Die krankhaften Geschwülste, vol II. Berlin, A Hirschwald, 1864, p 149
190. Finklestein JZ, Klemperer MR, Evans AE et al: Chemotherapy for metastatic neuroblastoma. Med Ped Oncol 6:179–188, 1979
191. Leikin S, Evans A, Heyn R et al: The impact of chemotherapy on advanced neuroblastoma: Survival of patients diagnosed in 1956, 1962 and 1966–68 in Children's Cancer Study Group A. J Ped 84:131, 1974
192. Bolande RP, Towler WF: Possible relationship of neuroblastoma to Von Recklinghausen's disease. Cancer 26:162–174, 1970
193. Beckwith JB, Perrin EV: *In situ* neuroblastomas. A contribution to the natural history of neural crest tumors. Am J Path 43:1089, 1963
194. Guin GH, Gilbert EF, Jones B: Incidental neuroblastoma in infants. Am J Clin Path 51:126–136, 1968
195. Chatten J, Voorkess ML: Familial neuroblastoma. N Eng J Med 277:1230, 1967
196. Wagget J, Aherne G: Familial neuroblastoma. Arch Dis Child 48:63, 1973
197. Young J, Miller RW: Incidence of malignant tumors in U.S. children. J Pediatr 86:254, 1975
198. Grotting JC, Kassel S, Dehner L: Nesidioblastosis and congenital neuroblastoma. Arch Path Lab Med 103:642–646, 1979
199. Jaffe N: Neuroblastoma: Review of the literature and an examination of factors contributing to its enigmatic character. Cancer Treat Rev 3:61–82, 1976
200. deLorimer AA, Bragg KU, Linden G: Neuroblastoma in Childhood. Am J Dis Child 118:441–450, 1969
201. Breslow N, McCann B: Statistical estimation of prognosis for children with neuroblastoma. Cancer Res 31:2098–2103, 1971
202. Gross RE, Farber S, Martin LW: Neuroblastoma sympatheticum: A study and report of 217 cases. Pediatrics 23:1179–1191, 1959
203. Young LW, Rubin P, Hanson RE: The extra-adrenal neuroblastoma: High curability and diagnostic accuracy. Am J Roent 108:75–91, 1969
204. Fortner J, Nicastri A, Murphy ML: Neuroblastoma: Natural history and results of treating 133 cases. Ann Surg 167:132–142, 1968
205. Bailey BJ, Barton S: Olfactory neuroblastoma. Arch Otolaryngol 101:1–5, 1975
206. Gerson JM, Koop CE: Neuroblastoma. Sem Oncol 1:35–46, 1974
207. Hayes FA, Green A: Neuroblastoma: Practice of Pediatrics, vol 3, chap 77. Hagerstown Md, Harper and Row, pp 1–6
208. Mäkinen J: Microscopic patterns as a guide to prognosis of neuroblastoma in childhood. Cancer 29:1637–1646, 1972
209. Hughes M, Marsden HB, Palmer MK: Histologic patterns of neuroblastoma related to prognosis and clinical staging. Cancer 34:1706–1711, 1974
210. McMillan CW, Gaudry CL, Holemans R: Coagulation defects and metastatic neuroblastoma. J Pediatr 72:347–250, 1968
211. Alfano J: Ophthalmological aspects of neuroblastomatosis: A study of 53 verified cases. Trans Am Acad Ophth Otol 72:830–848, 1968
212. Evans A, D'Angio GJ, Randolph JA: A proposed staging for children with neuroblastoma. Cancer 27:347, 1971
213. Kushner D, Parker B: Personal communication, 1980
214. Everson TC: Spontaneous regression of cancer. Ann NY Acad Sci 114:721, 1964
215. Bill AH: The regression of neuroblastoma. J Ped Surg 3:103, 196
216. Solomon GE, Chutorian AM: Opsoclonus and occult neuroblastoma. N Engl J Med 279:475, 1968
217. Rosenstein BJ Engelman K: Diarrhea in a child with catecholamine-secreting ganglioneuroma. J Pediatr 63:217, 1963
218. Voorhess M, Gardner LI: Studies of catecholamine excretion by children with neural tumors. J Clin Endocrinol 22:126, 1962
219. Williams CM, Green M: Homovanillic acid and vanilmandelic acid in the diagnosis of neuroblastoma. JAMA 183:836, 1963
220. Ong M, Dupont CL: The LaBrosse spot test revisted. J Pediatr 86:238, 1975
221. Geiser CF, Efron ML: Cystathioninuria in patients with neuroblastoma or ganglioneuroblastoma. Cancer 22:856, 1968
222. Hellstrom I, Hellstrom KE, Pierce GE et al: Demonstration of cell-bound and humoral immunity against neuroblastoma cells. PNAS 60:1231–1238, 1968
223. Hellstrom KE, Hellstrom I: Immunity to neuroblastoma and melanomas. Ann Rev Med 23:191, 1972
224. Hellstrom I, Hellstrom KE, Bell AH et al: Studies on cellular immunity to human neuroblastoma cells. Int J Cancer 6:172, 1970
225. Bill AH: Immune aspects of neuroblastoma. Am J Surg 122:142–147, 1971
226. Evans AE, Albo V, D'Angio GJ et al: Cyclophosphamide treatment of patients with localized and regional neuroblastoma: a randomized study. Cancer 36:655–660, 1976
227. Evans AE, Albo V, D'Angio GJ et al: Factors influencing survival of children with nonmetastatic neuroblastoma. Cancer 38:661–666, 1976
228. Frantz C: Personal communication, 1981
229. Finklestein JZ, Klemperer MF, Evans A et al: Multiagent chemotherapy for children with metastatic neuroblastoma: A report from CCSG. Med Ped Oncol 6:179–188, 1979
230. D'Angio GJ, Evans AE, Koop CE et al: Special pattern of widespread neuroblastoma with a favorable prognosis. Lancet 1:1946, 1971
231. Kun L, Camitta B: Personal communication, 1981
232. D'Angio GJ: Personal communication, 1981
233. Grosfeld JL, Schatzlein M, Ballantine TV et al: Metastatic

neuroblastoma: Factors influencing survival. J Ped Surg 13: 59–65, 1978
234. Frantz C: Personal communication, 1981
235. Kinnier-Witson LM, Draper GJ: Neuroblastoma, natural history and prognosis: A study of 487 cases. Br Med J 3:301, 1974
236. Knudsen AG Jr, Amronin GD: Neuroblastoma and ganglioneuroma in a child with multiple neurofibromatosis. Cancer 19: 1032, 1966
237. Filler RM, Traggis DG, Jaffe N et al: Favorable outlook for children with mediastinal neuroblastoma. J Ped Surg 7:136–143, 1972
238. Traggis DG, Filler RM, Druckman H et al: Prognosis for children with neuroblastoma presenting with paralysis. J Ped Surg 12:419–425, 1977
239. Hayes FA, Green AA, Mauer AM: The correlation of cell kinetic and clinical response to chemotherapy in disseminated neuroblastoma. Cancer Res 37:3766–3770, 1977
240. Rivera G, Green A, Hayes A et al: Epipodophyllotoxin VM-26 in the treatment of childhood neuroblastoma. Cancer Treat Rep 61:1243–1248, 1977
241. Aron B: Wilms' tumor—a clinical study of eighty-one children. Cancer 33:637–646, 1974
242. D'Angio GJ (chairman): Childhood cancer: The national Wilms' tumor study: a progress report. Urology 3:798–806, 1974
243. Wilms M: Die Mischgeschwülste der Nieren. Leipzig, Arthur Georgi, 1899, pp. 1–90
244. McNeill WH Jr, Chilko AJ: Status of surgical and irradiation treatment of Wilms' tumor and report of 2 cases. J Urol 39:287–302, 1938
245. Ladd WE: Embryoma of the kidney (Wilms' tumor). Ann Surg 108:885–902, 1938
246. Gross RE, Neuhauser EBD: Treatment of mixed tumors of kidney in childhood. Pediatrics 6:843–852, 1950
247. Farber S: Chemotherapy in the treatment of leukemia and Wilms' tumor. JAMA 198:826–836, 1966
248. Meadows AT, Lichtenfeld JL, Koop EC: Wilms' tumor in three children of a woman with congenital hemihypertrophy. N Engl J Med 291:23–24, 1974
249. Pendergrass TW: Congenital anomalies in children with Wilms' tumor, a new survey. Cancer 37:403–408, 1976
250. Haicken BN, Miller DR: Simultaneous occurrence of congenital aniridia, hamartoma, and Wilms' tumor. J Ped 78:497–502, 1971
251. Fraumeni JF Jr, Geiser CF, Manning MD: Wilms' tumor and congenital hemihypertrophy: Report of five new cases and review of literature. Pediatrics, 40:886–899, 1967
252. Brown WT, Puranik SR, Altman DH, Hardin HC Jr: Wilms' tumor in three successive generations. Surgery 72:756–761, 1972
253. Knudson AG, Strong LC: Mutation and cancer: A model for Wilms' tumor of the kidney. J Natl Cancer Inst 48:313, 1972
254. Snyder WH Jr, Hastings TN, Pollock WF: Retroperitoneal tumors. In Mustard WT, Ravitch MM, Snyder WH Jr et al (eds): Pediatric Surgery, 2nd ed. Chicago, Year Book Publishers, 1969, p 1020
255. Balsaver AM, Gibley CW Jr, Tessmer CF: Ultrastructural studies in Wilms' tumor. Cancer 22:417–427, 1968
256. Tremblay M: Ultrastructure of a Wilms' tumour and myogenesis. J Pathol 105:269–277, 1971
257. Williams AO, Ajayi OO: Ultrastructure of Wilms' tumor (nephroblastoma). Exp Mol Pathol 24:35–47, 1976
258. Rousseau MF, Nabarra B, Nezelof C: Behaviour of Wilms' tumour and normal metanephros in organ culture. Eur J Cancer 10:461–466, 1974
259. Bove KE, McAdams AJ: The nephroblastomatosis complex and its relationship to Wilms' tumor: A clinicopathologic treatise. In Rosenberg HS, Bolande RP (eds): Perspectives in Pediatric Pathology, vol. 3. Chicago, Year Book Medical Publishers, 1976, pp 185–223
260. Beckwith JB, Palmer NF: Histopathology and prognosis of Wilms' tumor: Results from the First National Wilms' Tumor Study. Cancer 41:1937–1948, 1978
261. Chatten J: Epithelial differentiation in Wilms' tumor: A clinicopathologic appraisal. In Rosenberg HS, Bolande RP (eds): Perspectives in Pediatric Pathology, vol. 3. Chicago, Year Book Medical Publishers, 1976, pp 225–254
262. Cassady JR, Tefft M, Filler RM et al: Considerations in the radiation therapy of Wilms' tumor. Cancer 32:598–608, 1973
263. Dibbins AW, Wiener ES: Retroperitoneal tumors in children. In: Current Problems in Surgery, pp 1–70. Chicago, Year Book Medical Publishers, October, 1973
264. Sukarochana K, Tolentino W, Kiesewetter WB: Wilms' tumor and hypertension. J Ped Surg 7:573–576, 1972
265. Ganguly A, Gribble J, Tune B et al: Renin-secreting Wilms' tumor with severe hypertension: Report of a case and brief review of renin-secreting tumors. Ann Intern Med 79:835–837, 1973
266. Martin LW, Schaffner DP, Cox JA et al: Retroperitoneal lymph node dissection for Wilms' tumor. J Ped Surg 14:704–707, 1979
267. Stevens PS, Eckstein HB: Ureteral metastasis from Wilms' tumor. J Urol 115:467–468, 1976
268. D'Angio GJ, Evans AE, Breslow N et al: The treatment of Wilms' tumor: Results of the National Wilms' Tumor Study. Cancer 38:633–646, 1976
269. Leape LL, Breslow NE, Bishop HC: The surgical treatment of Wilms' tumor: Results of the National Wilms' Tumor Study. Ann Surg 187:351, 1978
270. Gross RA, Neuhauser EBD: Treatment of mixed tumors of the kidney in childhood. Pediatrics 6:843–852, 1950
271. Farber S, Toch R, Sears EM et al: Advances in chemotherapy of cancer in man. Adv Cancer Res 4:1–71, 1956
272. Wolff JA, D'Angio G, Hartmann J et al: Long-term evaluation of single *versus* multiple courses of actinomycin D therapy of Wilms' tumor. N Engl J Med 290:84–86, 1974
273. Lemerle J, Voute PA, Tournade MF et al: Preoperative versus postoperative radiotherapy, single *versus* multiple courses of actinomycin D., in the treatment of Wilms' tumor. Cancer 38:647–654, 1976
274. Breslow NE, Palmer NF, Hill LR et al: Wilms' tumor: prognostic factors for patients without metastases at diagnosis. Cancer 41:1577–1589, 1978
275. Ballantine TVN, Wiseman NE, Filler RM: Assessment of pulmonary wedge resection for the treatment of lung metastases. J Ped Surg 10:329–337, 1975
276. Filler RM, Tefft M, Vawter GF et al: Hepatic lobectomy in childhood: Effects of x-ray and chemotherapy. J Ped Surg 4:31–41, 1969
277. Sullivan MP, Sutow WW: Successful therapy for Wilms' tumor. Tex Med 65:46, 1969
278. Wolff JA, D'Angio G, Hartmann J et al: Long-term evaluation of single versus multiple courses of actinomycin D therapy of Wilms' tumor. N Engl J Med 290:84–86, 1974
279. Sutow WW: Proceedings: Chemotherapy in Wilms' tumor: An appraisal. Cancer 32:1150–1153, 1973
280. Wolff JA: Advances in the treatment of Wilms' tumor. Cancer 35:901–904, 1975
281. Sieber WK, Dibbins AW, Wiener ES: Retroperitoneal tumors. In Ravitch MM, Benson CD (eds): Pediatric Surgery, vol 2, 3rd ed. Chicago, Year Book Medical Publishers, 1979, p 1082
282. Jeal PN, Jenkin RDT: Abdominal irradiation in the treatment of Wilms' tumor. Int J Rad Oncol Biol Phys 6:655–661, 1980
283. Cassady JR, Jaffe N, Filler RM: The increasing importance of radiation therapy in the improved prognosis of children with Wilms' tumor. Cancer 39:825–829, 1977
284. Bishop HC, Tefft M, Evans AE et al: Survival in bilateral Wilms' tumor—Review of 30 National Wilms' Tumor Study Cases. J Ped Surg 12:631–638, 1977
285. DeMaria JE, Hardy BE, Brezinski A et al: Wilms' tumors, nephromas, and urogenital tumors. J Ped Surg 14:577–579, 1979
286. D'Angio GJ, Beckwith JB, Breslow NE et al: Wilm's tumor: An update. Cancer 45:1791–1798, 1980.
287. Mahour GH, Soule EH, Mills SD et al: Rhabdomyosarcoma in infants and children: A clinico-pathologic study of 75 cases. J Ped Surg 2:402–409, 1967

288. Enziger FM, Shiraki M: Alveolar rhabdomyosarcoma: An analysis of 110 cases. Cancer 24:18–31, 1969
289. Li FP, Fraumeni JF: Letter. Ann Int Med 83:833, 1975
290. Lynch HT, Krush AJ, Harlan WL et al: Association of soft tissue sarcoma, leukemia, and brain tumors in families affected with breast cancer. Am Surgeon 39:199–206, 1973
291. Green DM, Jaffe N: Progress and controversy in the treatment of childhood rhabdomyosarcoma. Cancer Treat Rev 5:7–27, 1978
292. Li FP, Fraumeni JP: Rhabdomyosarcoma in children: epidemiologic study and identification of a familial cancer syndrome. J Nat Cancer Inst 43:1365–1373, 1969
293. Young J, Miller RW: Incidence of malignant tumors in U.S. children. J Ped 86:254–258, 1975
294. D'Angio GJ, Evans A: Soft tissue sarcomas. In Bloom HJG, Lemerle J, Neihardt M et al (eds): Cancer in Childhood. Berlin, Springer-Verlag, 1975, pp 217–241
295. Heyn RM, Hollan R, Newton WA et al: The role of combined chemotherapy in the treatment of rhabdomyosarcoma in children. Cancer 34:2128–2142, 1974
296. Horn RC, Enterline HT: Rhabdomyosarcoma: a clinicopathological study and classification of 39 cases. Cancer 11:181–199, 1958
297. Soule EH, Mahour GH, Mills SD et al: Soft tissue sarcomas in infants and children: a clinico–pathologic study of 135 cases. Mayo Clin Proc 43:313–326, 1968
298. Lieberman PB: Alveolar soft-part sarcoma. JAMA 198: 1047–1051, 1966
299. Christopherson WM, Foote FW, Stewart FW: Alveolar soft-part sarcomas: structurally characteristic tumors of uncertain histogenesis. Cancer 5:100–111, 1952
300. Soule EH, Newton W, Moone TE et al: Extraskeletal Ewing's sarcoma: A preliminary review of 26 cases controlled in the Intergroup Rhabdomyosarcoma Study. Cancer 42:259–264, 1978
301. Donaldson S: Rhabdomyosarcoma. In Carter SK, Glatstein E, Livingston RB (eds): Principles in Cancer Treatment. New York, Blakiston (in press)
302. Cassady JR, Sagerman RH, Tretter P et al: Radiation therapy for rhabdomyosarcoma. Radiology 91:116–120, 1968
303. Lawrence W, Hays DM, Moon TE: Lymphatic metastases with childhood rhabdomyosarcoma. Cancer 39:556–559, 1977
304. Masson JK, Soule EH: Embryonal rhabdomyosarcoma of the head and neck: Report on 88 cases. Am J Surg 110:585–591, 1965
305. Soule EH, Geitz M, Henderson ED: Embryonal rhabdomyosarcoma of the limbs and limb-girdle. Cancer 23:1336–1346, 1969
306. Raney B, Hays D, Lawrence W et al: Paratesticular rhabdomyosarcoma in childhood (asbstract C-30). Proc ASCO 18:274, 1977
307. Weichselbaum RR, Cassady JR, Jaffe N et al: The evolution of combination therapy of genitourinary rhabdomyosarcoma in children: A preliminary report. Int J Rad Oncol Biol Phys 2:267–272, 1977
308. Maurer HM, Moon TE, Donaldson M et al: The Intergroup Rhabdomyosarcoma Study. Cancer 40:2015–2026, 1977
309. Ghavimi F, Exelby PR, D'Angio GH et al: Multidisciplinary treatment of embryonal rhabdomyosarcoma in children. Cancer 35:677–686, 1975
310. Jones PG: Tumors of Infancy and Childhood. In Jones PG, Campbell PE (eds): Oxford, Blackwell Scientific Publications, 1976, pp 20–24
311. Russell WO, Cohen J, Enzinger F et al: A clinical and pathological staging system for soft tissue sarcomas. Cancer 40:1362–1370, 1977
312. Tefft M, Jaffe N: Sarcoma of the bladder and prostate in childhood. Cancer 32:1161–1177, 1973
313. Exelby PR, Ghavimi F, Jereb B: Genitourinary rhabdomyosarcoma in childhood. J Ped Surg 13:746–752, 1978
314. Rivard G, Ortega J, Hittle R et al: Intensive chemotherapy as primary treatment for rhabdomyosarcoma of the pelvis. Cancer 36:1593–1597, 1975
315. Kumar APM, Wrenn EL, Fleming ID et al: Combined therapy to prevent complete exenteration for rhabdomyosarcoma of the vagina and uterus. Cancer 37:118–122, 1976
316. Johnson DG: Trends in surgery for childhood rhabdomyosarcoma. Cancer 35:916–920, 1975
317. Jenkin RDT: Rhabdomyosarcoma of childhood III. In Vuksanovic MM (ed): Clinical Pediatric Oncology. Mt. Kisco, NY, Futura Publishing, 1972
318. Jereb B, Cham W, LaHin P et al: Local control of embryonal rhabdomyosarcoma in children by radiation therapy when combined with concomitant chemotherapy. Int J Rad Oncol Biol Phys 1:217–225, 1976
319. Sagerman, RH, Tretter P, Ellsworth RM: Orbital rhabdomyosarcoma in children. Trans Am Acad Ophthalmol Otol 78:602–605, 1974
320. Fernandez CH, Sutow WW, Merino OR et al: Childhood rhabdomyosarcoma: Analysis of coordinated therapy and results. Am J Roent Rad Ther Nucl Med 123:588–597, 1975
321. Flamant F: Therapeuic trial on rhabdomyosarcoma with low-regional extension. International Soc Ped Oncol, SIOP #3, Protocol UICC–76004, 1977
322. Sweency MJ, Tuttle AH, Etteldorf JN et al: Cyclophosphamide in the treatment of common neoplastic diseases of childhood. J Ped 61:702–708, 1962
323. Tan CTC, Aduna NS: Preliminary clinical experience with leucocristine in children (abstract 271). Proc Am Assoc Cancer Res 3:367, 1962
324. Tan CTC, Golbey RB, Yap CL et al: Clinical experiences with actinomycin D, KS_2, and F_1 (KS_4). Ann NY Acad Sci 89:426–444, 1960
324. Tan CTC, Rosen G, Ghavimi F et al: Adriamycin (NSC-123127) in pediatric malignancy. Cancer Chemother Rep 6(3):259–366, 1975
325. Heyn R, Holland R, Joo P et al: Treatment of rhabdomyosarcoma in children with surgery, radiotherapy, and chemotherapy. Med Ped Oncol 3:21–32, 1977
326. Pratt CB, Hustu HP, Pinkel D: Coordinated treatment of childhood rhabdomyosarcoma. Prog Clin Cancer 6:87–94, 1975
327. Donaldson SS, Castro JR, Wilbur JR et al: Rhabdomyosarcoma of the head and neck in children: Combination treatment by surgery, irradiation, and chemotherapy. Cancer 31:26–35, 1973
328. Tefft M, Fernandez CH, Moon TE et al: Rhabdomyosarcoma: Response to chemotherapy prior to radiation in patients with gross residual disease. Cancer 39:665–670, 1977
329. Dritschilo A, Weichselbaum R, Cassady JR et al: The role of radiation therapy in the treatment of soft tissue sarcomas of childhood. Cancer 42:1192–1203, 1978
330. Okamura J, Sutow W, Moon T et al: Prognosis in children with metastatic rhabdomyosarcoma. Med Ped Oncol 3:243–251, 1977
331. Tefft M, Fernandez C, Donaldson M et al: Incidence of meningeal involvement by rhabdomyosarcoma of the head and neck in children. Cancer 42:253–258, 1978
332. Gerson JM, Jaffe N, Donaldson M et al: Meningeal seeding from rhabdomyosarcoma of the head and neck with base of skull invasion. Med Ped Onc 5:137–144, 1978
333. Chan RC, Sutow WW, Lindberg R: Parameningeal rhabdomyosarcoma. Radiology 131:211–214, 1979
334. Healy GB, Jaffe M, Cassady JR: Rhabdomyosarcoma of the head and neck: Diagnosis and management. Head Neck Surg 1:334–339, 1979
335. Kilman JW, Clatworthy HW Jr, Newton WA et al: Reasonable surgery for rhabdomyosarcoma: A study of 67 cases. Ann Surg 178:346–351, 1973
336. Jaffe N, Murray J, Traggis D et al: Multidisciplinary treatment for childhood sarcoma. Am J Surg 133:405–413, 1977
337. Jenkin D, Sonley M: Soft tissue sarcomas in the young. Cancer (in press)
328. Glass AG, Fraumeni JF Jr: Epidemiology of bone cancer in children. J Natl Can Insti 44:187–199, 1970
329. Falk S, Alpert M: The clinical and roentgen aspects of Ewing's sarcoma. Am J Med Sci 250:492–508, 1965

330. Falk S, Alpert M: Five year survival of patients with Ewing's sarcoma. Surg Gynecol Obstret 124:319–324, 1967
331. Ewing J: Diffuse endothelioma of bone. Proc NY Pathol Soc 21:17–24, 1921
332. Jaffe N, Traggis D, Sallan S et al: Improved outlook for Ewing's sarcoma with combination chemotherapy and radiation therapy. Cancer 38:1925–1930, 1976
333. Rosen G, Wollner N, Tan C et al: Disease-free survival in children with Ewing's sarcoma treated with radiation therapy and adjuvant four-drug sequential chemotherapy. Cancer 33:384–393, 1974
334. Chabora B, Rosen G, Cham W et al: Radiotherapy of Ewing's sarcoma. Radiology 120:667–671, 1976
335. Rosen G: Primary Ewing's sarcoma: The multidisciplinary lesion. Int J Radiat Onc Biol Phys 4:527–532, 1978
336. Chan RC, Sutow WW, Lindberg RD et al: Management and results of localized Ewing's sarcoma. Cancer 43:1001–1006, 1979
337. Hustu HO, Pinkel D, Pratt CB: Treatment of clinically localized Ewing's sarcoma with radiotherapy and combination chemotherapy. Cancer 30:1522–1527, 1972
338. Dahlin D, Coventry M, Scanlon P: Ewing's sarcoma: A critical analysis of 165 cases. J Bone Joint Surg 43A:185–192, 1961
339. Rosen G: Management of malignant bone tumors of children and adolescents. Ped Clin N A 23:183–213, 1976
340. Vohre VG: Roentgen manifestations in Ewing's sarcoma. Cancer 20:727–733, 1967
341. Kadin ME, Bensch KG: On the origin of Ewing's tumor. Cancer 27:257–272, 1971
342. Schajowicz F: Ewing's sarcoma and reticulum cell sarcoma of bone. J Bone Joint Surg 41A:349, 1959
343. Stout AP: Discussion of the pathology and histogenesis of Ewing's tumor of bone marrow. Am J Roent 50:334, 1943
344. Pomeroy TC, Johnson RE: Prognostic factors for survival in Ewing's sarcoma. Am J Roent Rad Ther Nuc Med 123:598–606, 1975
345. Sherman RS, Soong KY: Ewing's sarcoma—its roentgen classification and diagnosis. Radiology 66:529–539, 1956
346. Tallroth K: Lymphatic dissemination of bone and soft tissue sarcomas. Acta Radiologica (supplement) 549:38–65, 1976
347. Tefft M, Razek A, Perez C et al: Local control and survival related to radiation dose and volume and to chemotherapy in non-metastatic Ewing's sarcoma of pelvic bones. Int J Radiat Oncol Biol Phys 4:367–372, 1978
348. Frankel RS, Jones AE, Cohen JA et al: Clinical correlations of ^{67}Ga and skeletal whole body radionuclide studies with radiography in Ewings' sarcoma. Radiology 110:597–603, 1974
349. Marsa GW, Johnson RE: Altered pattern of metastases following treatment of Ewing's sarcoma with radiation and adjuvant chemotheapy. Cancer 27:1051–1054, 1971
350. Mehta Y, Hendrickson FR: CNS involvement in Ewing's sarcoma. Cancer 33:859–862, 1974
351. Jenkin RDT, Rider WD, Sonley MJ: Ewing's sarcoma. Int J Radiat Onc Biol Phys 1:407–413, 1976
352. Jenkin RDT: Radiation treatment of Ewing's sarcoma and osteogenic sarcoma. Canad J Surg 20:530–536, 1977
353. Fernandez CH, Lindberg RD, Sutow WW et al: Localized Ewing's sarcoma, treatment and results. Cancer 34:143–148, 1974
354. Haggard ME: Cyclophosphamide (NSC-26271) in the treatment of children with malignant neoplasms. Cancer Chemo Rep 51:403–405, 1967
355. DeVita VT, Carbone PP, Owens AH Jr et al: Clinical trials with 1, 3-*bis* (2-chlorethyl)-1-nitrosourea (NSC 409962). Cancer Res 25:1876–1881, 1965
356. Kofman S, Perlia CP, Economou SG: Mithramycin in the treatment of Ewing's sarcoma with radiation therapy and adjuvant chemotherapy. Cancer 27:1051–1054, 1971
357. Lewis RJ, Marcove RC, Rosen G: Ewing's sarcoma: functional effects of radiation therapy. J Bone Joint Surg (Am) 59A:325–331, 1977
358. Suit HD: Ewing's sarcoma: Treatment by radiation therapy. In: Tumors of Bone and Soft Tissue: A Collection of Papers Presented at the Eighth Annual Clinical Conference on Cancer, 1963, at The Univ of Texas M. D. Anderson Hospital and Tumor Institute, Houston, Tx. Chicago, Year Book Medical Publishers, 1965, pp 191–200
359. Sutow WW, Suit HD, Martin RG: Bone tumors. In Bloom HJG, Lemerle J, Neidhardt MK et al (eds): Cancer in Children, Clinical Management, pp 200–216. Berlin, Heidelberg, New York, Springer-Verlag, 1975
360. Cassady JR: Ewing's sarcoma—the place of radiation therapy. In Jaffe N (ed): Bone Tumors in Children. Littleton, MA, PSG Publishers, 1979
361. Johnson RE, Pomeroy TC: Evaluation of therapeutic results in Ewing's sarcoma. Am J Roentgen 123:583–587, 1975
362. Graham-Pole J: Ewing's sarcoma: Treatment with high dose radiation and adjuvant chemotherapy. Med Ped Oncol 7:1–8, 1979
363. Tefft M, Razek A, Perez C et al: Local control and survival related to radiation dose and volume and to chemotherapy in non-metastatic Ewing's sarcoma of the pelvic bones. Int J Radiat Onc Biol Phys 4:367–372, 1978
364. Jenkin RDT: Personal communication, 1981
365. Pritchard DJ, Dahlin D, Dauphine R et al: Ewing's sarcoma. J Bone and Joint Surg 57A:10–16, 1975
366. Bruckman J: Personal communication, 1981
367. Fraumeni JF Jr, Miller RW, Hill SA: Primary carcinoma of the liver in childhood: An epidemiologic study. J Natl Cancer Inst 40:1087–1099, 1968
368. Ishak KG, Glunz PR: Hepatoblastoma and hapatocarcinoma in infancy and childhood. Report of 47 cases. Cancer 20:396–422, 1967
369. Reeves RL, Tesluk H, Harrison CE: Precocious puberty associated with hepatoma. J Clin Endocrinol 19:1651–1660, 1959
370. Exelby PR, Filler RM, Grosfeld JL: Liver tumors in children in the particular reference to hepatoblastoma in hepatocellular carcinoma. American Academy of Pediatric Surgical Section Survey 1974. J Ped Surg 10:329–337, 1975
371. Ishak KG, Rabin L: Benign tumors of the liver. Med Clin N Am 59:995–1013, 1975
372. Matolo NM, Johnson DG: Surgical treatment of hepatic hemangioma in the newborn. Arch Surg 106:725–727, 1973
373. Randolph JG, Altman RP, Arensman RM et al: Liver resection in children with hepatic neoplasms. Ann Surg 187:599–605, 1978
374. Alpert ME, Seeler RA: Alpha-fetoprotein in embryonal hepatoblastoma. J Pediatr 77:1058–1060, 1970
375. Geiser CF, Baez A, Schindler AM et al: Epithelial hepatoblastoma associated with congenital hemihypertrophy and cystathioninuria: Presentation of a case. Pediatrics 46:66–73, 1970
376. Nebesar RA, Tefft M, Filler RM: Correlation of angiography and isotope scanning in abdominal diseases of children. Am J Roentgenol Rad Ther & Nucl Med 153:365–385, 1970
377. Taylor PH, Filler RM, Nebesar RA et al: Experience with hepatic resection in childhood. Am J Surg 117:435–441, 1969
378. Clatworthy HW Jr, Schiller M, Grosfeld, JL: Primary liver tumors in infancy and childhood: 41 cases variously treated. Arch Surg 109:143–147, 1974
379. Pack GT, Islami AH: Surgical treatment of hepatic tumors. In Popper H, Schaffner F (eds): Progress in Liver Diseases, ch 29. vol 2. New York, Grune & Stratton, 1965, pp 499–511
380. Longmire WP: Hepatic surgery: Trauma, tumors, and cysts. Ann Surg, 161:1–14, 1965
381. Wilson H, Wolf RY: Hepatic lobectomy: Indications, technique, and results. Surgery 59:472–482, 1966
382. Blaisdell FW, Lim RC: Liver resection. In Madding GF, Kennedy PA (eds): Major Problems in Clinical Surgery. Philadelphia, WB Saunders, 1971, pp 131–145
383. Theman T, Williams WG, Simpson JS et al: Tumor invasion of the upper inferior vena cava: The use of profound hypothermia and circulation arrest as a surgical adjunct. J Pediatr Surg 13:331–334, 1978
384. Offenstadt G, Huguet C, Gallot D et al: Hemodynamic moni-

toring during complete vascular exclusion for extensive hepatectomy. Surg Gyn Obstet 146:709–713, 1978
385. McDermott WV Jr, Greenberger VJ, Isselbacher KJ et al: Major hepatic resection: Diagnostic techniques and metabolic problems. Surgery 54:56, 1963
386. Ikeda K, Suita S, Nakagawara A, Takabayashi K: Preoperative chemotherapy for initially unresectable hepatoblastoma in children. Survival in two cases. Arch Surg 114:203–207, 1979
387. Hermann RE, Lonsdale D: Chemotherapy, radiotherapy, and hepatic lobectomy for hepatoblastoma in an infant: Report of a survival. Surgery 68:383–388, 1970
388. Shafer AD, Selinkoff PM: Preoperative irradiation and chemotherapy for initially unresectable hepatoblastoma. J Pediatr Surg 12:1001–1007, 1977
389. Siegel MM, Siegel SE, Andrassy RJ et al: Primary chemotherapeutic management of metastatic and unresectable hepatoblastoma of childhood (abstract). Proc Am Assoc Cancer Res 20:342 (C-212), 1979
390. Senzer NN, Terrell W, Pratt CB: Evaluation of a chemotherapeutic regimen for primary liver cancer in children. Cancer Treat Rep 62:1403–1404, 1978
391. Filler RM, Tefft M, Vawter GF et al: Hepatic lobectomy in childhood: Effects of x-ray and chemotherapy. J Ped Surg 4:31–41, 1969
392. Howard RO, Berg WR, Albert DM et al: Retinoblastoma and chromosome abnormality. Arch Ophthalmol 92:490–493, 1974
393. Jensen RD, Miller RW: Retinoblastoma: epidemiologic characteristics. N Engl J Med 283:307–311, 1971
394. Lennox EL, Draper GJ, Sanders BM: Retinoblastoma: a study of natural history and prognosis of 268 cases. Br Med J 3:731–734, 1975
395. Fraser GR, Friedman AI: The causes of Blindness in Children. Baltimore, John Hopkins Press, 1967
396. Falls HF, Neel JV: Genetics of retinoblastoma. Arch Ophthalmol 46:367–389, 1951
397. Ellsworth R: In Duane TD (ed): Clinical Ophthalmology, chap 35, vol 3. New York, Harper & Row, 1976, pp 1–18
398. Macklin MT: A study of retinoblastoma in Ohio. Am J Human Gen 12:1–43, 1960
399. Tarkkanen A, Tuovinen E: Retinoblastoma in Finland, 1912–1964. Acta Ophthalmol 49:293–300, 1971
400. Schappert-Kimmijser J, Hemmes GD, Nijland R: The heredity of retinoblastoma. Ophthalmologica 151:197–213, 1966
401. Francois J: Heredity of malignant tumors of the eye. Symposium on surgery and medical management of congenital anomalies of the eye. St. Louis, CV Mosby, 1968, pp 199–246
402. Knudson AG, Meadows AT, Nichols WW, et al: Chromosomal deletion and retinoblastoma. N Engl J Med 295:1120–1123, 1976
403. Francke U: Retinoblastoma and Chromosome 13. Cytogenet Cell Genet 16:131–134, 1976
404. Yunis J, Ramsey N: Retinoblastoma and subband deletion of chromosome 13. Am J Dis Child 132:161–163, 1978
405. Weichselbaum RR, Nove J, Little JB; Skin fibroblasts from a D-deletion type retinoblastoma patient are abnormally sensitive. Nature 266: 726–727, 1977
406. Weichselbaum RR, Nove J, Little JB: X-ray sensitivity of diploid fibroblasts from patients with hereditary or sporadic retinoblastoma. Proc Natl Acad Sci USA 75:3962–3964, 1978
407. Nove J, Little JB, Weichselbaum RR et al: Retinoblastoma, chromosome 13, and *in vitro* cellular radiosensitivity. Cytogen Cell Gene 24:176–184, 1979
408. Tapley N, Du V, Tretter P: Retinoblastoma. In Sutow W (ed). Clinical Pediatric Oncology. St. Louis, CV Mosby, 1978, pp 411–430
409. Bedford MA, Bedotto C, MacFaul PA: Retinoblastoma, a study of 139 cases. Br J Ophthalmol 55:19–27, 1971
410. Kodilinye HC: Retinoblastoma in Nigeria: problems of treatment. Am J Ophthal 63:469–481, 1967
411. Lennox EL, Draper GF, Sanders BM: Retinoblastoma: A study of natural history and prognosis of 268 cases. Br Med J 3:731–734, 1975
412. Devesa SS: The incidence of retinoblastoma. Am J Ophthalmol 80:263–265, 1975
413. Reese AB: Tumors of the Eye, 2nd ed. New York, Harper & Row, 1963
414. Ellsworth RM: Retinoblastoma. Modern Prob Ophthalmol 18:94–100, 1977
415. Howarth C, Meyer D, Hustu HO et al: Stage related combined modality treatment of retinoblastoma. Cancer 45:851–858, 1980
416. Weiss DR, Cassady JR, Petersen R: Retinoblastoma: A modification in radiation therapy technique. Radiology 114:705–708, 1975
417. Cassady JR, Sagerman RH, Tretter P et al: Radiation therapy in retinoblastoma. Radiology 93:405–409, 1969
418. Pratt CB: Management of malignant solid tumors in children. Ped Clin NAM 19:1141–1155, 1972
419. Cassady JR: Retinoblastoma: Questions in management. In Carter SB, Glatstein E, Livingstone RB (eds): Principals of Cancer Treatment. New York, Blakiston (in press)
420. Merriam GR: Retinoblastoma, an analysis of 17 autopsies. Arch Ophthalmol 44:71–108, 1950
421. Zimmerman LE: Retinoblastoma including a report of illustrative cases. Med Ann DC 38:366–374, 1969
422. Ts'o MO, Fine BS, Zimmerman LE et al: Photoreceptor elements in retinoblastoma. Arch Ophthalmol 82:57–59, 1969
423. Ts'o MO, Zimmerman LE, Fine BS et al: A cause of radioresistence in retinoblastoma: Photoreceptor differentiation. Trans Am Acad Ophth Otol 74:959–969, 1970
424. Carbajal UM: Observations on retinoblastoma. Am J Ophthalmol 45:391–402, 1958
425. Carbajal UM: Metastases in retinoblastoma. Am J Ophthalmol 48: 47–69, 1959
426. Redler LD, Ellsworth RM: Prognostic importance ot choroidal invasion in retinoblastoma. Arch Ophthalmol 90:294–296, 1973
427. Hopping W, Meyer-Schwickerath, RG: Indications and limitations of light coagulation of the retina. Trans Am Acad Ophthalmol 63:725–738, 1959
428. Lincoff H, McLean JM, Long R: The cryosurgical treatment of intraocular tumors. Am J Ophthalmol 63:389–399, 1967
429. Stallard HB: Multiple islands of retinoblastoma: Incidence rate and time span of appearance. Br J Ophthalmol 39:241–243, 1955
430. Stallard HB: The conservative treatment of retinoblastoma. Trans Ophthalmol Soc UK 82:473, 1962
431. Kupfer C: Retinoblastoma treated with intravenous nitrogen mustard. Am J Ophthalmol 36:1721, 1953
432. Wolff J, Pratt CB, Sitarz A: Chemotherapy of metastatic retinoblastoma. Cancer Chemo Rep 16:437, 1962
433. Lonsdale D, Berry DH, Holcomb TM et al: Chemotherapeutic trials in patients with metastatic retinoblastoma, Cancer Chemo Rep 52:634, 1968
434. Thompson RW, Small RC, Stein JJ: Treatment of retinoblastoma. Am J Roentgenol 114:16–23, 1972
435. Bagshaw M, Kaplan HS: Supervoltage linear accelerator radiation therapy: VIII. Retinoblastoma. Radiology 86:242–246, 1966
436. Wolff J: Personal communication, 1981
437. Doline S, Needleman H, Petersen RA et al: The effect of radiotherapy in the treatment of retinoblastoma upon the developing dentition. J Ped Ophthalmology (in press)
438. Sagerman RH, Cassady JR, Tretter P et al: Radiation-induced neoplasia following external beam therapy for children with retinoblastoma. Am J Roentgenol 105:529–535, 1969
439. Soloway HB: Radiation-induced neoplasms following curative therapy for retinoblastoma. Cancer 19:1984–1988, 1966
440. Tefft M, Vawter GF, Mitus A: Second primary neoplasms in children. Am J Roentgenol 103:800–822, 1968
441. Knudson AG Jr: Mutation and cancer: statistical study of retinoblastoma. Proc Natl Acad Sci USA 68:820–823, 1971
442. Meadows A, Strong LC, Li FP et al: Bone sarcoma as second malignant neoplasm (SMN) in children: influence of radiation (RT) and predisposition (abstract 508). Proc Am Assoc Cancer Res, 1979
443. Li F, Cassady JR, Jaffe N: Risk of second tumors in survivors of childhood cancer. Cancer 35:1230–1235, 1975

444. Haselow RE, Nesbit M, Dehner LP et al: Second neoplasms following megavoltage radiation in a pediatric population. Cancer 42:1185–1191, 1978
445. Altman RP, Randolph JG, Lilly JR: Sacrococcygeal teratoma: American Academy of Pediatrics Surgical Section Survey—1973. J Ped Surg 9:389–398, 1974
446. Mahour GH, Woolley MM, Trivedi SN et al: Teratomas in infancy and childhood: Experience with 81 cases. Surgery 76:309–318, 1974
447. Berry CL, Keeling J, Hilton C: Teratoma in infancy and childhood: A review of 91 cases. J Pathol 98:241–252, 1969
448. Carney JA, Thompson DP, Johnson CL et al: Teratomas in children: Clinical and pathologic aspects. J Ped Surg 7:271–282, 1972
449. Gross RE, Clatworthy HW Jr, Meeker IA Jr: Sacrococcygeal teratomas in infants and children: A report of 40 cases. Surg Gynecol Obstet 92:341–354, 1951
450. Hendren WH, Henderson BM: The surgical management of sacrococcygeal teratomas with intrapelvic extension. Ann Surg 171:77–84, 1970
451. Jaffe N, Murray J, Traggis D et al: Multidisciplinary treatment for childhood sarcoma. Am J Surg 133:405–413, 1977
452. Filler RM, Jaffe N: Teratomas in infants and children. In Holland JF, Frei E III (eds): Cancer Medicine, vol 2. Philadelphia, Lea & Febiger (in press)
453. Donnellan WA, Swenson O: Benign and malignant sacrococcygeal teratomas. Surgery 64:834–846, 1968
454. Mahour GH, Wooliey MM, Trivedi SN et al: Sacrococcygeal teratoma: A 33-year experience. J Ped Surg 10:183–188, 1975
455. The Third National Cancer Study: Advanced 3 Year Report 1969–1971 Incidence, DHEW Publication No (NIH) 74-637
456. Young PG, Mount BM, Foote FW Jr et al: Embryonal adenocarcinoma in the prepubertal testis. A clinicopathologic study of 18 cases. Cancer 26:1065–1075, 1970
457. Hopkins TB, Jaffe N, Colodny A et al: The management of testicular tumors in children. J Urol 120:96–102, 1978
458. Filler RM, Hardy B: Testicular tumors in children. World J Surg 4:63–70, 1980
459. Javadpour N, Bergman S: Recent advances in testicular cancer. Curr Prob Surg 15(2):1–64, Feb 1978
460. Boden G, Gibb R: Radiotherapy and testicular neoplasms. Lancet 2:1195–1197, 1951
461. Whitmore WF Jr: Cancer Management. The Treatment of Germinal Tumors of the Testis. Special Graduate Course on Cancer sponsored by The American Cancer Society. Philadelphia, JB Lippincott, 1966 pp 347–355
462. McCullough DL, Carlton CE, Seybold HM: Testicular tumors in infants and children: Report of 5 cases and evaluation of different modes of therapy. J Urol 105:140–148, 1971
463. Sabio H, Burgert EO Jr, Farrow GM et al: Embryonal carcinoma of the testis in childhood. Cancer 34:2118–2121, 1974
464. Ray B, Hajdu SI, Whitmore WF Jr: Distribution of retroperitoneal lymph node metastases in testicular germinal tumors. Cancer 33:340–348, 1974
465. Skinner DG, Leadbetter WF: The surgical management of testis tumors. J Urol 106:84–93, 1971
466. Maier JG, Van Buskirk KE, Sulak MH et al: An evaluation of lymphadenectomy in the treatment of malignant testicular germ cell neoplasms. Trans Am Assoc Genitourin Surg 60:71–74, 1968
467. Matsumoto K, Nakauchi K, Fujita K: Radiation therapy for the embryonal carcinoma of testis in childhood. J Urol 104:778–780, 1970
468. Tefft M, Vawter GF, Mitus A: Radiotherapeutic management of testicular neoplasms in children. Radiology 88:457–465, 1967
469. Hand A: Defects of membranous bone, exopthalmos and polyuria in childhood: Is it dispituitarism: Am J Med Sci 162:509, 1921
470. Abt AF, Denholz EJ: Letterer-Siwe's disease; splenomepatomegaly associated with widespread hyperplasia of non-lipid storing macrophages: discussion of so-called reticuloendotheliose s. Am J Dis Children 51:499, 1936
471. Lichtenstein L, Jaffe HL: Eosinophilic granuloma of bone. Am J Path 16:595, 1940
472. Roland RS: Xanthomatosis and the reticuloendothelial system. Arch Intern Med 42:611, 1928
473. Wallgren A: Systemic reticuloendothelial granuloma; non lipid reticulo-endotheliosis and Schüller-Christian disease. Am J Dis Child 60:471, 1940
474. Lichtenstein L: Histiocytosis X. Integration of eosinophilic granuloma of bone, "Letterer-Siwe disease," and Schüller-Christian disease as related manifestations of a single nosologic entity. Arch Path (Chicao) 56:84, 1953
475. Green WT, Farber S: "Eosinophilic or solitary granuloma" of bone. J Bone Joint Surg (Am) 24:499, 1942
476. Newton WA Jr, Hamondi AB: Histiocytosis: a histologic classification with clinical correlation. In: Rosenberg H, Bolande RF (eds): Perspectives in Pediatric Pathology, vol 1. Chicago, Yearbook Medical Publishers, 1973, pp 251–283
477. Vogel JM, Vogel P: Idiopathic histiocytosis: A discussion of eosinophilic granuloma, the Hand–Schüller–Christian syndrome, and the Letterer–Siwe syndrome. Sem Hematol 9:349–369, 1972
478. Cline MJ, Golde DW: A review of reevaluation of the histiocytic disorders. Am J Med 53:49–60, 1973
479. Frederiksen P, Thommesen P: Histiocytosis X, II. Histologic appearance correlated to progress and extent of disease. Acta Rad Oncol 17:10–16, 1978
480. Nesbit ME Jr, Krivit W: Histiocytosis. In Bloom HJG, Lemerle J, Neidhardt MK et al (eds): Cancer in Children, Ch 16. Berlin, Springer-Verlag, 1975, pp 193–199
481. Greenberger J, Cassady JR, Jaffe N et al: Radiation therapy in patients with histiocytosis: management of diabetes insipidus and bone lesions. Int J Rad Oncol Biol Phys 5:1749–1755, 1979
482. Osband M, Lipton J, Larvin P et al: Histiocytosis X: Demonstration of abnormal immunity, T-cell histamine H_{2x} receptor deficiency and successful treatment with thymic extract. N Engl J Med (in press)
483. Vawter GF: Does Letterer–Siwe disease exist? Or, who's not afraid of infantile histiocytosis: In Vuksanvik MM (ed): Clinical Pediatric Oncology: Research, Diagnosis, Treatment and Prognosis of Malignant Tumors. Mt. Kisco, NY, Futura Publishing, 1972, pp 165–169
484. Gotoff SP, Esterly NB: Histiocytosis. J Ped 85:592, 1974
485. Miller DR: Familial reticuloendotheliosis: Concurrence of disease in five siblings. Pediatrics 38:986, 1966
486. Rogers DL, Benson TE: Familial Letterer–Siwe disease: Report of a case. J Ped 60:550, 1962
487. Reese AJM, Levy E: Familial incidence of non-lipoid reticuloendotheliosis (Letterer–Siwe disease). Arch Dis Child 26:573, 1951
488. Juberg RC, Kloepfer HW, Oberman HA: Genetic determination of acute disseminated histiocytosis X (letterer–Siwe Syndrome). Pediatrics 45:753, 1970
489. Glass AG, Miller RW: U.S. mortality from Letterer–Siwe disease, 1960–1964. Pediatrics 42:364, 1968
490. Greenberger JS, Crocker AC, Jaffe N et al: Treatment and end result in 139 patients with histiocytosis. Proc Am Soc Clin Oncol 19, 1978 (abstract C 371), p 399
491. Lahey ME: Prognosis in reticuloendotheliosis in children. J Ped 60:664, 1962
492. Nezelof C, Frileux-Herbert F, Cronier-Sachot J: Disseminated histiocytosis X, Cancer 44, 1824–1838, 1979
493. Smith DG, Nesbit ME, D'Angio GJ et al: Histiocytosis-X: role of radiation therapy in management with special reference to dose levels employed. Radiology 106:419–422, 1973
494. Loos D: Hokes Querschmitts-Syndrom durch eosinophiles granulom. Med Monatssehr 10:681–683, 1956
495. Lahey ME: Histiocytosis X—comparison of three treatment regimens. J Ped 87:179–183, 1975
496. Starling KA, Donaldson MH, Haggard ME et al: Therapy of histiocytosis X with vincristine, vinblastine and cyclophosphamide. Am J Dis Child 123:105–110, 1972
497. Jones B, Kung K, Chevalier L et al: Chemotherapy of reticuloendotheliosis. Cancer 34:1011–1017, 1974

498. Starling KA, Iyer R, Silva-Sosa M et al: Chlorambucil in histiocytosis X: A southwest oncology group study. J Ped 96, 266–268, 1980
499. Komp DM, Viehi TJ, Berry DH et al: Combination chemotherapoy in histiocytosis-X, Med. and Ped. Oncology 3, 267–273, 1977
500. Komp DM, El-Mahdi A, Starling KA et al: Quality of survival in histiocytosis X, Ped Res 10:455, 1976
501. Komp DM, Trueworthy R, Hvizdala E et al: Prednisone, methotrexate and 6-mercapto-purine in the treatment of histiocytosis X, Cancer Treat Rep 63:2125–2126, 1979
502. West G: Personal communication
503. Griffin TW: The treatment of advanced histiocytosis-X with sequential hemibody irradiation. Cancer 39:2435–2436, 1977

Vincent T. DeVita, Jr.
Samuel Hellman

CHAPTER 35

Hodgkin's Disease and the Non-Hodgkin's Lymphomas

ETIOLOGY AND EPIDEMIOLOGY

The lymphomas are the seventh commonest causes of death from cancer in the United States.[1] About 30,000 new cases of lymphoma occurred in 1980. Twenty-four percent have Hodgkin's disease. Because of young average age of the lymphoma population (32 years for Hodgkin's disease and 42 years for the other adult lymphomas), the toll in person-years of life lost each year ranks the lymphomas fourth in terms of economic impact among cancers in the United States. For unexplained reasons, the incidence of lymphomas appears to be increasing each year.[2,3] Studies on the epidemiology of lymphomas have been hampered in the past by the lack of a worldwide standard histopathologic classifications of the disease.

There is a bimodal incidence curve of Hodgkin's disease in economically developed countries. Correa and O'Connor recognized that in economically underdeveloped countries there is a lower incidence of Hodgkin's disease but the incidence prior to the age of 15 years is higher than in developed countries, with only a modest increase throughout adolescence and young adulthood.[5] An increased incidence of histologic subtypes less common in young people in developed countries (mixed cellularity and lymphocyte depleted) accompanies the increased incidences below the age of 15 years in poorly developed countries. One exception to the increased incidence of Hodgkin's disease in young adults in economically developed countries is that of Japan where the first peak in the western bimodal curve is absent. The reason for this is of considerable interest, but is as yet unexplained.

In the United States there is a steady increase in the incidence of the non-Hodgkin's lymphomas from childhood through age 80 years and in the United States, non-Hodgkin's lymphoma is more common in males (8.1:100,000) than in females (5.7:100,000).[6–8] The incidence rates for non-Hodgkin's lymphomas also show marked variations from country to country ranging from 1/100,000 in rural Poland to 9.1/100,000 in the non-Jewish population of Israel.[9] Non-Hodgkin's lymphoma appears with a greater frequency in earlier ages in Egypt than in America or European countries. In Africa and New Guinea, Burkitt's lymphoma is very common, while in the United States, Great Britain, and tropical Latin America, Burkitt's lymphoma is rare.

The etiology of the lymphomas is unknown. McMahon has postulated that the dual peak incidence of Hodgkin's disease is compatible with the hypothesis that Hodgkin's disease is a result of two etiologic processes: a biologic agent of low infectivity which causes the disease in young adults, and a mechanism similar to other lymphomas in the older age groups.[2] An alternative explanation is that these data are a reflection of a variation in host response to a single etiologic mechanism. There is an increased risk of Hodgkin's disease with increasing educational level. The relative risk varies from 0.7 to 1.8, depending on the level. The reason for this is unknown.

The potential infectious nature of Hodgkin's disease has

been a topic of discussion since its earliest description. Mycobacterium tuberculosis was early suspected to be the etiologic organism because of the high incidence of tuberculosis in patients with this disease. The idea was first seriously advanced by Sternberg in 1898, and by others since.[10–14] Since that time there has been considerable other epidemiologic evidence which suggests an infectious etiology, particularly a virus (see below). There have been a number of studies addressing the question of the increased risk of Hodgkin's disease in infectious mononucleosis.[15–18] A small but consistent increase in the incidence of lymphomas has been noted after infectious mononucleosis after long followup in patients compared to controls. These data are summarized in Table 35-1. This etiologic relationship has been enhanced by the identification of Sternberg–Reed cells in the lymph node biopsies of patients with infectious mononucleosis. The known etiologic relationship between the Epstein Barr virus (EBV) and infectious mononucleosis prompted a number of investigators to examine patients with Hodgkin's disease for elevated EBV antibody titers. No significant differences between patient and control populations have been identified, although mean antibody titers are significantly more elevated in the patients with Hodgkin's disease than in control patients. Tumor specimens from Hodgkin's disease patients have been examined for the presence of the DNA of the Epstein–Barr virus in their genome and no evidence of the virus has been found.[20] Thus, the etiologic association between Hodgkin's disease and Epstein-Barr virus has not been confirmed.[20]

There are certain similarities between Hodgkin's disease and graft host disease which led Kaplan and Smithers to speculate that the disease process might include an interaction between normal lymphocytes and antigenically different neoplastic cells.[21] Order and Hellman carried this further suggesting that T-lymphocytes may be infected by a single or by a number of viruses which alter their antigenicity.[22] Uninvolved T-cells react against these altered cells, resulting in an anti-immune response similar to graft vs host disease. Swartz and Beldotti have shown in mice that chronic graft versus host disease often results in lymphoma and the hypothesis suggests a similar consequence in humans.[23] DeVita modified the hypothesis suggesting an active role for B-cells engaged in a "lymphocyte civil war."[24] Whatever the pathogenesis, Hodgkin's disease has a number of unusual characteristics that require explanation. These include: axial distribution of lymph node disease, large numbers of nonmalignant lymphocytes and eosinophils intermixed with the malignant cells, frequent lymphoid hyperplasia either preceding or adjacent to the disease, and early derangement of cell mediated immunity.

There is convincing evidence that viruses are a cause of other types of lymphomas in rodents, birds, cats and cows.[25–28] Marek's disease, a lymphoma of chickens, is caused by a herpes-like DNA virus, and can now be prevented by vaccines.[29] A horizontally transmitted type C retrovirus of cows is a highly infectious cause of bovine lymphosarcoma.[30] Inbreeding appears to play an important role in the viral etiology of these animal cancers. In humans, there is a strong association between the Epstein–Barr virus and the lymphoma described by Burkitt in East Africa (anti-EBV antibodies have been identified in the serum of patients and complementary viral DNA in the DNA of Burkitt cells), but the association is less strong for Burkitt's lymphoma diagnosed in the United States.[31] Cells cultured from patients with Hodgkin's disease and some patients with diffuse non-Hodgkin's lymphoma have been shown to express type C RNA virus particles and appear to contain viral information such as protein coat antigens and viral reverse transcriptase.[32,33] All these observations lend credence to a viral etiology of human lymphomas but do not yet provide definitive proof. At the moment, it is not possible to distinguish among the three possible alternatives: a true etiologic relationship, contamination of tissue cultures by ubiquitous viruses, or, the most likely explanation, infection by virus *in vivo* or expression of a virogene after the cell has been altered by malignant transformation.

A cluster of Hodgkin's disease has been reported by Vianna and associates.[34,35] The infectious relationship of the cluster implied by the authors has been questioned because of the nature of the selection of contacts to the patients. Population based studies, using the cancer registries of Connecticut and California, have made a rather convincing argument that the reported cluster of Hodgkin's disease occurred by chance alone.[36,37] A study repeating the methodology of Vianna in a different location failed to confirm the findings.[38] Medical personnel who specialize in the care of patients with lymphomas do not seem to have a higher incidence of these diseases than others of the same socioeconomic level. Recently, there has been additional epidemiologic evidence suggesting an infectious etiology of Hodgkin's disease that is more convincing.[39] These authors investigated the association of Hodgkin's disease with childhood factors that influence age of exposure to infectious agents. They found that the risk of Hodgkin's disease was positively associated with a set of factors (fewer siblings, single family houses, early birth order, fewer playmates, and the rate of mononucleosis) that tend to decrease or delay early exposure to infections and suggest the association can be best explained by a viral origin with age at infection the major modifier of risk. There have been other interesting and as yet unexplained observations such

TABLE 35-1. The Risk of Developing Hodgkin's Disease After Infectious Mononucleosis

SOURCE	SIZE OF POPULATION AT RISK	OBSERVED	EXPECTED	YEARS OF FOLLOW-UP	REFERENCE NUMBER
U.S soldiers	2,437	2	1	22	(15)
Connecticut	4,529	5	1	16	(16)
Denmark	17,000	17	6	–	(17)

as the increased risk of acquiring Hodgkin's disease among wood workers; the relationship between the development of Hodgkin's disease and tonsillectomy and appendectomy; and the association of Hodgkin's disease with certain HLA antigens.[40-45]

A hereditary influence on the incidence of lymphomas is suggested by their higher incidences in patients with inherited immunologic deficiency diseases and by a small increase in the incidence in families of patients with immunologic disorders.[46] In one study, a significant increase in the incidence of Hodgkin's disease was noted in siblings of the index case, particularly in siblings of the same sex.[47] A slight increase in the incidence of lymphomas has been noted in large series of patients with collagen vascular diseases, as compared with the general population adjusted for age.[48] This increased incidence approached 10% in patients with long-standing Sjögren's syndrome who tend to develop diffuse lymphomas or immunoblastic sarcomas.[49-51]

Lymphoma-like syndromes associated with lymphadenopathy have been found in patients who take phenytoin to control seizeures.[52] Although in most cases the disease regresses when the patient stops taking phenytoin, a small fraction proceed to develop malignant lymphoma of several different varieties, including Hodgkin's disease. Such observations suggest that the drug is acting on patients within an inherited tendency to develop the disease. Patients who are chronically immunosuppressed by drugs, particularly those who have received renal transplants, have a higher incidence of diffuse histiocytic lymphoma and immunoblastic sarcomas, often in the brain.[53,54] Except for the higher incidence of Hodgkin's disease in siblings and the influence of phenytoin on the development on lymphomas, it is difficult to separate the influence of inheritance, *per se*, from immunosuppression, which may be of etiologic importance without an inherited background.

Although it appears that ionizing radiation can cause malignant lymphoma in humans, the mechanism of neoplastic transformation and the condition under which it occurs have yet to be clearly delineated. An increased prevalence of lymphocytic and histiocytic lymphoma has been demonstrated in survivors of the atomic bomb in Hiroshima who were exposed to 100 rad or more.[55,56] An increased incidence of lymphoma has been demonstrated in patients irradiated for ankylosing spondylitis.[57] In both groups, the ratio of observed to expected cases of lymphoma was 2:1.

Investigations of the association of histocompatibility antigens with lymphoma report an association of nodular lymphomas with HLA-B-12 antigen.[58,59] Klinefelter's syndrome has been associated with reticulum cell sarcoma and Chediak–Higashi syndrome has been associated with an increased risk of lymphoreticular malignancy.[60,61]

The development of the technique of chromosome banding in 1970 has revolutionized the field of human cytogenetics.[62] Using quinacrine and Giemsa metaphase banding techniques, patients with both African and American Burkitt's lymphoma have been found to have an abnormally long arm of chromosome 14.[63] Changes in chromosome 14 have also been reported in a number of other types of malignant lymphomas.[64] The diseases that have been shown to predispose to the development of lymphomas are listed in Table 35-2.

TABLE 35-2. Diseases with a Predisposition to Develop Lymphomas

Klinefelter's syndrome
Chediak-Higashi syndrome
Ataxia telangiectasia syndrome
Wiscott-Aldrich syndrome
Swiss-type agammaglobulinemia
Common variable immunodeficiency disease
Acquired hypogammaglobulinemia
Renal transplant recipients
Sjögren's syndrome
Rheumatoid arthritis and systemic lupus erythematosus

THE MICROSCOPIC ANATOMY OF NORMAL LYMPHOID TISSUE

The reticulo–endothelial system can be divided into (1) hematopoietic and (2) lymphoreticular components.[65-69] Lymphoreticular cells are widely distributed throughout the body, both singly and in centers of aggregation. The centers of aggregation include lymph nodes, white pulp of the spleen, Waldeyer's ring (tonsils and adenoids), thymus gland, and lymphoid aggregates in the lamina propria and submucosa of the respiratory and gastrointestinal tracts, where they are referred to in the latter location as Peyer's patches. Lymphoreticular cells also populate the bone marrow, as cohabitants of the more numerous hematopoietic elements. In addition to these major sites of aggregation and proliferation, lymphoreticular cells are distributed as normally inconspicuous interstitial elements in essentially all tissues except the central nervous system.

The various cells of the lymphoreticular system are conceived of as including reticular supporting cells, lymphoid cells, and cells of monocyte–macrophage series. The reticular cells provide the basic three-dimensional matrix of lymph nodes by virtue of their long cytoplasmic processes joined by tight junctions or desmosomes. Within this matrix, the functional cells of the lymphoid and monocyte–macrophage series migrate, proliferate, and serve as the primary arm of the host immunologic defense apparatus. The lymphoreticular system is thus the anatomical basis of cellular and humoral immunity. Because lymphoreticular cells differ from hematopoietic cells in complexities of anatomical distribution and function, their neoplastic proliferation is distinguishable from that of common hematopoietic malignancies. Depending on the primary site of proliferation, the lymphoreticular cancers may initially become manifested either in the bone marrow and peripheral blood or in one of the centers of aggregation, most commonly lymph nodes. When the bone marrow is a major site of the involvement of the lymphorecticular neoplasms, the disease is classified as acute or chronic lymphocytic or, less frequently, monocytic leukemia. When they present as extramedullary tumor fractions, rising primarily in lymph nodes or other sites, solid lymphoreticular tumors are collectively referred to as malignant lymphomas. Among the most common forms of malignant lymphomas is Hodgkin's disease. Malignant lymphomas other than Hodgkin's disease can be conveniently viewed as the spectrum of diseases we, unfortunately, term the non-Hodgkin's lymphoma. Since the lymphoreticular system is the anatomical basis of the immune system, the the non-Hodgkin's lymphomas can be most easily understood as tumors of the immune system.[70]

In contrast to lymphoreticular components, hematopoietic elements of the reticulo–endothelial system are postnatally normally confined to the bone marrow and responsible for the production of red blood cells, granulocytes and platelets. Abnormal proliferations of these elements are usually manifested in the marrow and peripheral blood as myeloproliferative syndromes (polycythemia vera, agnogenic myeloid metaplasia, idiopathic thrombocythemia, megakaryocytic myelosis, erythremic myelosis, and erthroleukemia) or the more common acute and chronic granulocytic leukemias. Extramedullary infiltration of hematopoietic elements does occur but is an unusual manifestation of leukemias (see Chapters 34 and 36).

Normally both the lymphoid and monocytic cells of the lymphoreticular system originate in the bone marrow and from there migrate by way of the blood and lymphatic vessels to populate other lymphoreticular tissues.[65–69] The lymphocytes processed through the thymus gland are referred to as thymus-dependent T-cells. Other lymphocytes are thymus-independent and are processed through an as yet unknown equivalent of the avian bursa of Fabricius. They are termed B-cells, based on the avian system. T-cells and B-cells comprise the two major components of lymphocytic series, but there are smaller populations of other lymphocytes that are as yet less well understood and characterized. Monocytes also originate in the bone marrow and, like lymphocytes, circulate and eventually populate extramedullary tissues as cells of the monocyte–histiocytic series.[71] These three populations of lymphoreticular cells (T-cells, B-cells, and monocyte–macrophages) subserve different functions in the system and are to some degree compartmentalized anatomically.[72–75]

LYMPHORETICULAR CELL SURFACE MARKERS

Different normal cells of the lymphoreticular system can be identified by characteristic surface markers. The markers commonly used to identify B- and T-lymphocytes and mononuclear phagocytes are listed in Table 35-1.[67,68] Surface membrane-bound immunoglobulin (SIg) is the hallmark of B-lymphocytes. The surface immunoglobulin must be produced by the cell and consist of a heavy chain and only one type of light chain per lymphocyte in a given time. Immunofluorescence is the most widely used technique for detecting SIg. Monospecific antiserum prepared against individual light and heavy chains is essential to evaluate clonicity of normal and abnormal lymphoid populations. The presence of an immunoglobulin on the surface of a mononuclear cell, however, is not adequate evidence to identify it as a B-lymphocyte. Other cells may have immunoglobulins on their surface which are nonspecifically bound by way of the Fc fragment to complement receptors. These cells do not produce the surface immunoglobulins and they are usually not monoclonal in origin when examined with monospecific antisera. Most B-lymphocytes bear receptors for the third component of complement (C_3). A rosette technique employing erythrocytes (E) coated with IgM antibody (A) and complement (C) is most commonly used to identify these receptors (referred to as EAC in Table 35-3). B-lymphocytes will bind this EAC reagent in suspension and in frozen tissue sections. B-lymphocytes and monocytes also bear receptors for the Fc portion IgG immunoglobulin. The Fc receptors of monocytes have a stronger affinity for antigen–antibody complexes than those of B-lymphocytes and are easily identified by rosetting techniques employing erythrocytes (E) coated with IgG antibody (A), (EA in Table 35-3). Using conventional methods, this reagent does not readily adhere to Fc receptors of B-lymphocytes.

Live, human T-lymphocytes form rosettes with unsensitized sheep erythrocytes (E).[76] The rosettes may be strengthened by incubation in the cold, in the presence of serum, or by pretreatment of the sheep erythrocytes with either neuraminidase or 2-aminethyliso-thiuronium bromide (AET). The mechanism of binding of erythrocytes to human T-lymphocytes is not clear but a charge phenomeon has been suggested.

The ability to phagocytize particular material is a hallmark of macrophages and monocytes. These cells will ingest latex particles and neutral red and iron fillings. They will also phagocytize the adherent red cells used in EA or EAC rosette assays. In contrast, B-lymphocytes, which bear some of the same receptors as monocyte–macrophages will not perform phagocytosis. Thus, a phagocytic assay can be extremely helpful in differentiating B-lymphocytes from monocytes and histiocytes.

The demonstration of various hydrolytic enzymes by cytochemical and histochemical techniques has been useful in identifying certain cells of the lymphoreticular system. The most helpful hydrolytic enzymes are acid phosphatase (AP) and tartrate-resistant acid phosphatase (T-AP). The former can be used to identify lymphoid elements as T-lymphocytes and the latter is characteristic of the cells of the disorder

TABLE 35-3. Markers of Normal Human Mononuclear Cells

CELL TYPE	SIg	EAC	EA	E	PHAGOCYTOSIS	HTLA	HBLA
T-lymphocyte	−	−	+/−	+	−	+	−
B-lymphocyte	+	+	+	−	−	−	+
Monocyte/Histiocyte	−	+	++	−	+	−	+

SIg = Cell-sensitized membrane-immunoglobulin
EAC = Rosette formation with erythrocyte-IgM antibody-complements complexes
EA = Rosette formation with erythrocyte-IgG antibody complexes
E = Rosette formation with unsensitized sheep erythrocyte
HTLA = Human T-lymphocyte-associated antigens
HBLA = Human B-lymphocyte-associated antigens

TABLE 35-4. Immunologic Characterization of Cells of Origin of Lymphomas

LYMPHORETICULAR NEOPLASMS OF B-CELL ORIGIN	LYMPHORETICULAR NEOPLASMS OF T-CELL ORIGIN	LYMPHORETICULAR NEOPLASMS OF HISTIOCYTES	NULL-CELL NEOPLASMS
Chronic lymphocytic leukemia Cells in Richter's syndrome*	Acute lymphatic leukemia of childhood with mediastinal adenopathy and convoluted cells	Hodgkin's disease 10% of patients with "diffuse histiocytic lymphoma"	Most patients with childhood acute lymphatic leukemia
Diffuse-well differentiated lymphocytic lymphomas	Sézary syndrome, mycosis fungoides Chronic lymphatic leukemia (some cases)	Histiocytic medullary reticulosis	40% of patients with diffuse "histiocytic" lymphoma of Rappaport
Nodular poorly differentiated lymphocytic lymphomas	Diffuse "histiocytic" lymphoma of Rappaport (some cases)	Monocytic leukemia	
Nodular mixed lymphoma			
Nodular "histiocytic" lymphomas			
Diffuse poorly differentiated lymphocytic lymphomas			
Most patients with diffuse-"histiocytic" lymphoma			
Burkitt's lymphoma			
5% of children with acute lymphatic leukemia			
Poorly differentiated lymphoblastic lymphoma of children			
Immunoblastic lymphadenopathy			
Immunoblastic sarcoma			

* Local overgrowth of lymphoid tumor in patients with chronic lymphatic leukemia often designated as reticulum-cell sarcomas in the past classification schemes

called leukemic reticuloendotheliosis (hairy cell leukemia). Terminal deoxynucleotidyl transfersase (TdT) is a DNA polymerase which catalyses the addition of deoxyribonucleoside triphosphates to the 3'-hydroxy end of single-stranded poly- or oligodeoxyribonucleotide primers.[77] This enzyme has been found to be present in thymic-committed lymphocytes and in uncommitted blast cells. The enzyme is found in low levels in normal bone marrow. Mature peripheral blood B- and T-lymphocytes, and PHA-stimulated lymphocytes do not contain detectable TdT. This enzyme has been identified in the cells of nearly all patients with acute lymphoblastic leukemia, in certain forms of lymphoblastic lymphoma, and in the cells of some cases of blastic crisis of chronic myelogenous leukemia. TdT determinations may be performed on fresh or frozen tissues in cell suspension.

THE CELLULAR ORIGIN OF THE LYMPHOMAS

The lymphomas can now, in most cases, be classified by their cell of origin.[65–70] The majority of the non-Hodgkin's lymphomas (NHL) appear either to derive from a monoclonal population of B-cells or to have no distinctive cell markers (Table 35-4). The origin of tumors of the lymphoreticular system related to the anatomy of the lymph node is shown in Fig. 35-1. Only a few lymphomas appear to be true derivatives of tissue monocyte–macrophages (histiocytic lymphomas), despite the morphologic similarity of the large cell lymphomas to histiocytes. Even those histologic types of lymphomas characterized by mixtures of different morphologic cell types in the same node (mixed lymphomas of Rappaport, see below) have been shown by cell surface markers to derive from a monoclonal B-cell line. While identification of immunologically homogenous clinico–pathological entities may ultimately have prognostic and therapeutic implications, great variations in behavior can occur within each major immunologic classification of lymphomas. For example, those B-cell lymphomas which grow in a nodular pattern usually tend to have an indolent natural history with relapses and recurrences spread over 5 years to 10 years or more. In contrast, B-cell lymphomas with cells resembling histiocytes (termed "histiocytic" by Rappaport) without nodule formation usually have a more aggressive clinical course, but when responsive to treatment, are more susceptible to permanent control by drugs.

The cell of origin of Hodgkin's disease is still uncertain but it may be derived from either a T-lymphocyte or a macrophage line.[22,24,65–69] Cells from patients with Hodgkin's disease have now been grown in tissue culture.[78–81]* These cells are often

*Since preparation of this chapter, the cell lines referred to by the authors of references 78 and 81 have, in all but one instance, been found to be derived from the owl monkey. The single human line was derived from spleen not involved with tumor.

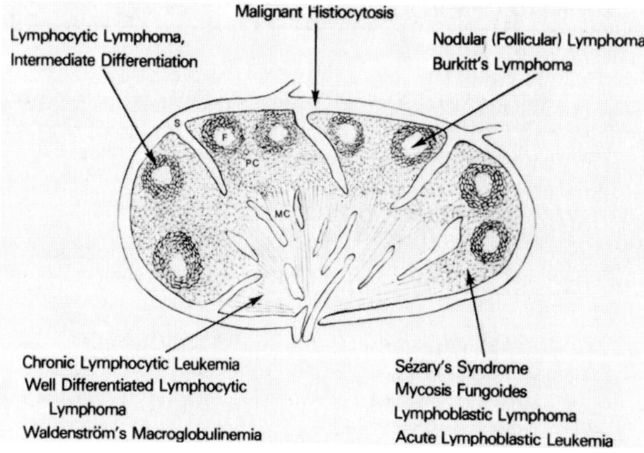

FIG. 35-1. Normal lymph node showing compartments of the immune system, relating the malignant lymphomas to each compartment as shown. *S* = sinuses; *F* = follicles; *PC* = paracortex; *MC* = medullary cords. (Adapted from Berard CW, Gallo RC, Jaffe ES et al: Current concepts of leukemia and lymphoma: Etiology, pathogenesis and therapy. Ann Intern Med 85:351–366, 1976)

binucleate and resemble the Sternberg–Reed cell characteristic of Hodgkin's disease. In culture they are often surrounded in rosette fashion by T-lymphocytes. They are aneuploid, a characteristic of malignancy.[79,80,82] When implanted into immune-deprived mice, they produce tumors.[79,80] They also have been to shown to phagocytize and possess surface receptors for Fc fragment of immunoglobulins and complement (C3b). All these findings are more characteristic of cells derived from the monocyte-histiocyte series than from T-lymphocytes and lend strong support to the thesis that Hodgkin's disease is a true histiocytic lymphoma.

THE PATHOLOGY OF LYMPHOMAS

The beginnings of the pathologic description of lymphomas can be traced to the description of tumors of the lymph glands by Thomas Hodgkin in 1832. The historical evolution of the pathology of the lymphomas is shown in Table 35-5 and 35-6.[83,86,88,89,91–95,107–118]

The diagnosis and classification of lymphoma can only be made by biopsy and histopathologic examination under a light microscope. Needle aspirations of lymph nodes may suggest a diagnosis, but do not yield sufficient tissue to classify lymphomas accurately, and the error rate is high. A careful study of a large number of cases accrued to a clinical cooperative group treatment protocol has shown that even experienced pathologists, using fixed sections of lymph nodes, disagree on subclassification of lymphoma in up to 25% of cases and also disagree on whether the resected tissues show evidence of malignancy in as many as 6% of cases.[84] Frozen section material should not be used when lymphoma is suspected, because slightly crushed normal lymphoid tissue in frozen sections mimics malignancy of other kinds. Some patients diagnosed by frozen section as having carcinoma of the head or neck regions have actually had lymphoma or benign reactive hyperplasia, and have undergone neck dissection unnecessarily.

HODGKIN'S DISEASE

Hodgkin's disease is unique among cancers because the tumor palpated by the physician largely contains normal lymphocytes, plasma cells, and fibrous stroma of the lymph node and only a scattering of the characteristic malignant cell of Hodgkin's disease, the Sternberg–Reed cell. The diagnosis of Hodgkin's disease should rarely be made in the absence of Sternberg–Reed cells, although the presence of such a cell by itself is not pathognomonic of the disease. Cells simulating the Sternberg–Reed cells have been found in tissue of patients with infectious mononucleosis and breast cancer.[19,85] Since the detailed descriptions by Sternberg and Reed, Hodgkin's disease has been recognized as a form of lymphoreticular malignancy with distinctive clinical and pathologic features.[10,86] Histologically, one sees a polymorphous admixture of cytologic abnormal cells (Sternberg–Reed cells and their mononuclear variants) and a variety of apparently normal reactive elements. The Sternberg–Reed cell is a large cell with two or more mirror-image nuclei, each containing a single prominent nucleolus (Fig. 35-2). In the first clinically useful subclassification of Hodgkin's disease, developed by Jackson and Parker, their cases were divided in three groups: paragranuloma, granuloma, and sarcoma.[87] This classification identified the 9 to 10% of cases with the most favorable and least favorable prognoses (paragranuloma and sarcoma, respectively), but approximately 90% of cases remained in the category of granuloma. A major advance occurred when Lukes, Hicks, and Butler proposed a new histiologic classification in 1966, which appeared to correlate well with clinical stage and aggressiveness of the disease.[88] This scheme was later simplified into the Rye subclassification, which is now widely accepted and employed by both pathologists and clinicians. These two classifications are compared in Table 35-7. In the Rye classification, Hodgkin's disease is divided into four categories: lymphocyte predominant, mixed cellularity, lymphocyte depleted, and nodular sclerosis. The first three categories differ primarily in the relative proportions of neoplastic mononuclear and Sternberg–Reed cells to reactive elements, especially lymphocytes. An indolent natural history and prolonged survival appear to be directly related to the ratio of lymphocytes to abnormal cells in diagnostic biopsies. The fourth subcategory, nodular sclerosis, has distinctive clinical and morphologic features which were first hinted at by Greenfield in 1878, but more clearly described by Lukes and colleagues in 1963, and are shown in Fig. 35-3.[89,90]

In lymphocyte predominant Hodgkin's disease, the lymph node architecture may be completely or partially destroyed. The cellular proliferation is composed of benign appearing lymphocytes with or without benign histiocytes. It is often necessary to examine multiple sections to identify diagnostic Sternberg–Reed cells. Fibrosis is usually not seen. This subtype is more common in males than in females and often occurs in the younger age groups (less than 35 years of age). The majority of patients have clinically localized disease, and are asymptomatic, and the prognosis is usually favorable.

The mixed cellularity type occupies an intermediate position between lymphocyte predominant and lymphocyte depleted Hodgkin's disease with respect to both proportion of neoplastic cells and prognosis. In this type, Sternberg–Reed cells and

TABLE 35-5. Landmarks in the Description of Hodgkin's Disease

AUTHOR (Reference Number)	YEAR	OBSERVATION
Hodgkin (83)	1832	"On some morbid appearances of the absorbent glands and spleen"
Wilks (91)	1865	"Cases of the enlargement of the lymph glands and spleen (or Hodgkin's disease)"
Langhans (92) Greenfield (89)	1872 1878	First description of histologic features of Hodgkin's disease, including a description of giant cells and intense fibrous bands
Pel & Epstein (94)	1887	Described cyclical fever in Hodgkin's disease
Sternberg (10) Reed (7)	1898	First definitive description of Hodgkin's disease and clear illustrations of the cells bearing their names
Parker & Jackson Fitzhugh & Speis (93)	1932 1934	Described the absence of response to tuberculin in the presence of tuberculosis in Hodgkin's disease
Jackson (95)	1937	First histopathologic classification of Hodgkin's disease
Lukes, Butler, & Hicks (88)	1963	Described the current histopathologic classification of Hodgkin's disease

TABLE 35-6. Landmarks in the Description of the Other Lymphomas

AUTHOR	YEAR	OBSERVATION
Craigie (107), Bennett (108) Virchow (109)	1845	Described the first cases of leukemia
Virchow (109)	1845	Distinguished lymphosarcoma from leukemia. Included cases described by Hodgkin in the lymphosarcoma group
Bilroth (110)	1871	Coined phrase "malignant lymphomas"
Dreshfield (111) Kundradt (112)	1892 1893	Developed histiologic criteria for diagnosing lymphosarcoma
Brill, Bearh (96), & Rosenthal (113) Symmers (114)	1925 1927	Described giant follicular lymphoma and considered it a benign disease "Brill–Symmers disease"
Roulet (115)	1930	Developed histologic criteria for diagnosing reticulum cell sarcoma. Considered it a malignancy of the supporting cells of the lymph node.
Gall & Mallory (116)	1942	Developed criteria for distinguishing benign hyperplasia from malignant follicular lymphoma
Rappaport, Winter & Hicks (117)	1956	Described different cell types within follicular lymphomas and termed them "nodular lymphomas"
Burkitt (118)	1958	Described lymphoma of the jaw, which bears his name, in Africa

their variants are usually quite plentiful (5–15 per high power field and easily identified). The lymph node is usually diffusely effaced, but occasionally, focal involvement is observed. Broad bands of fibrosis are not seen. Focal necrosis may be present but is usually not marked. This type of Hodgkin's disease is slightly more common in males than in females and is often associated with systemic symptoms. It occurs in all clinical stages.

In lymphocyte depleted Hodgkin's disease, in contrast to the other types, there is a predominance of abnormal cells and Sternberg–Reed cells (usually more than 15 per high power field) with a relative paucity of lymphocytes. Fibrosis and necrosis are common but are diffuse and not of the broad band type seen in the nodular sclerosis type. The majority of patients are older and symptomatic and the disease is usually disseminated at the time of diagnosis.

The nodular sclerosis category is distinctive both morphologically and clinically. From the histologic standpoint there are two features that distinguish this form of Hodgkin's disease from all other types. The first is the presence of a particular variant of the Sternberg–Reed cell, the so-called lacunar cell.[96,97] In formalin-fixed tissue the cytoplasm often

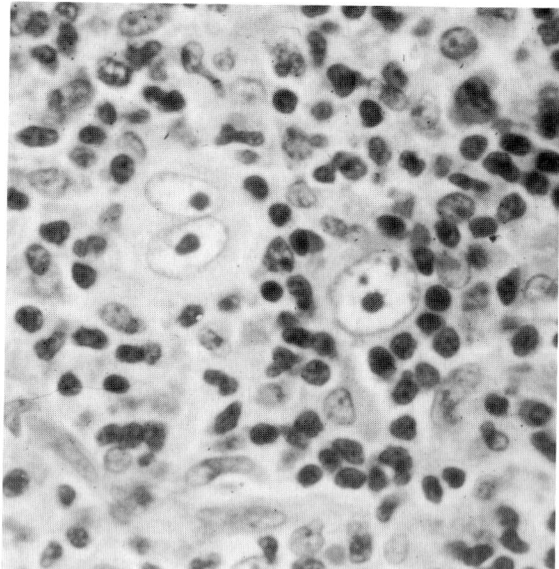

FIG. 35-2. Characteristic Sternberg-Reed cell and mononuclear variant of Hodgkin's disease. (Hematoxylin and eosin × 400)

artifactually retracts and gives the appearance of cells in a space. The second feature seen in most, but not all cases, is a thickened capsule with a proliferation of orderly collagenous bands which divide the lymphoid tissue into circumscribed nodules (Fig. 35-3). In some cases the sclerosis and nodularity are either absent or minimal, but the presence of numerous lacunar cells, often in focal aggregates, has led some investigators to refer to this as the "cellular phase" of nodular sclerosis. Strum and Rappaport have observed progression from the cellular phase to classic nodular sclerosis with fibrous bands in sequential biopsies in five patients.[98] Necrosis, often accompanied by numerous inflammatory cells, may be striking in the center of some nodules. Nodular sclerosis is the only form of Hodgkin's disease that is more common in females than in males. It most frequently occurs in adolescents and young adults and is unusual in patients over 50 years of age. The process has a striking propensity to involve lower cervical, supraclavicular, and mediastinal lymph nodes. Patients with nodular sclerosis, particularly those with localized tumors, usually have a good prognosis. The category of

TABLE 35-7. Histologic Classification of Hodgkin's Disease Comparing the Jackson and Parker Classification to That of Lukes and Butler

JACKSON AND PARKER (1944)	LUKES AND BUTLER (1966)
Paragranuloma (10%)*	Lymphocytic predominant (16%)
Granuloma (80%)	Nodular sclerosis (35%) Mixed cellularity (33%) Lymphocyte depletion (16%) 1. Diffuse fibrosis 2. Reticular type
Sarcoma (10%)	

* The figures in parenthesis indicate percentage of patients in various subcategories in the National Cancer Institute population.

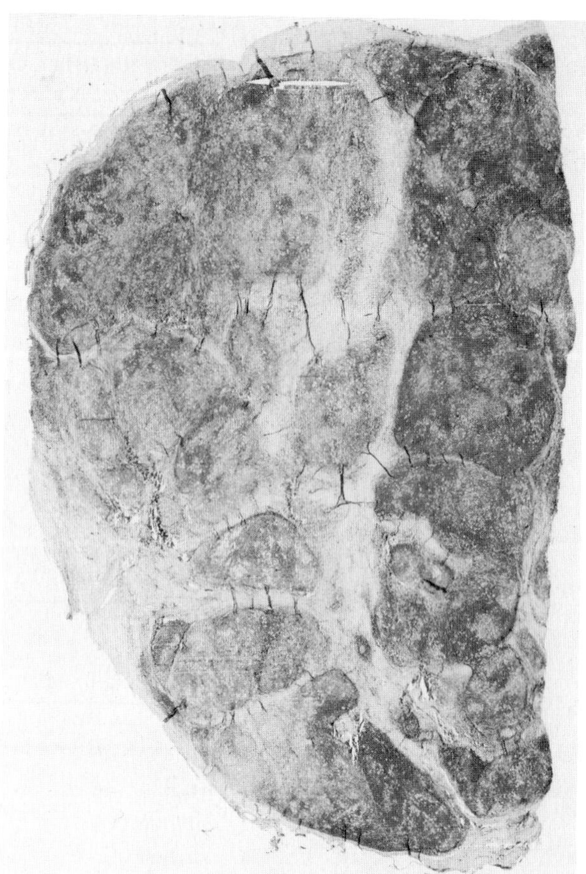

FIG. 35-3. Characteristic fibrous bands in nodular sclerosing Hodgkin's disease. (Hematoxylin and eosin × 8)

nodular sclerosing Hodgkin's disease can be further subclassified into lymphocyte depleted or mixed cellularity. A multivariant analysis of a population of patients so subclassified at the National Cancer Institute indicated that this subclassification also has prognostic importance.[99] The subclassification lymphocyte depleted nodular sclerosis had the worst prognosis. Venous invasion has been described in Hodgkin's disease and reported to be associated with a poor prognosis.[100] The malignant cells of Hodgkin's disease appear to home into the regions of the lymph nodes populated by T-cells, such as the paracortical region.

PATHOLOGY OF THE NON-HODGKIN'S LYMPHOMA

At least five different pathologic classifications for malignant lymphoma are in use throughout the world.[101–106] One classification of lymphomas is based entirely on the immunologic derivation of the lymphoreticular system.[70] While this is of great interest, the best classification for clinical purposes is the one which is easiest to use by pathologists, which has clinical relevance in designing therapeutic plans, and which accurately predicts response to treatment and prognosis. The classification of malignant lymphomas currently most widely used and established as valuable for clinical-pathologic studies is the one proposed by Rappaport, and will be described in detail below and used in this text.[101,107]

The use of five different pathologic classifications for non-Hodgkin's lymphomas throughout the world obviously makes the international analysis and comparison of clinical trials extremely difficult. The Rappaport classification has been criticized because some of the terminology and concepts are now known to be inaccurate. A new classification system has been proposed, based on an international study comparing the five major systems and is shown in Table 35-8.[103] Designation of tumor types using the new system appears in parentheses next to the Rappaport diagnosis in the text. The other classification schemes are compared in Table 35-9.

In the Rappaport scheme, the non-Hodgkin's lymphomas are divided into two major groups, those with nodular (follicular), pattern of growth, and those with a diffuse pattern of growth.

Nodular Lymphomas

Nodular lymphomas are those in which the neoplastic cells form circumscribed aggregates morphologically resembling germinal centers. The nodular pattern may be present throughout the tumor or may be manifested in only a portion of the lymphoma, which elsewhere is composed of diffuse cellular proliferation. Nodular lymphomas can be distinguished from reactive hyperplasia of normal nodes by the disordered appearance of nodules throughout the medullary cords and the cortex of the lymph nodes (Fig. 35-4) as opposed to the regular progression of nodules from large to small in the cortex to the medulla of normal lymph node, shown diagrammatically in Fig. 35-1. In areas of the nodules, the neoplastic cells may be either within or between the nodules, or confined to the nodules, with normal-appearing cells in the internodular tissue. In the latter situation, these neoplasms may be mistaken for benign follicular hyperplasia, unless careful scrutiny is given to the cells comprising the nodules. Whereas normal germinal centers are composed of cytologically heterogeneous populations representing the entire spectrum of proliferating B-cells, neoplastic nodules appear more homogeneous and "clonal." It has now been definitely proven that nodular lymphomas are neoplasms of follicular B-cells.

Using the Rappaport histopathologic classification the cells of nodular lymphomas can be either *poorly differentiated lymphocytic* (small cleaved cell), *mixed lymphocytic–histiocytic* (mixed large and small cell) or *histiocytic* (large cell). The term histiocytic was originally used to denote large cells resembling histiocytes seen amidst the small indented and cleaved neoplastic lymphocytes. These cells were interpreted as histiocytes because of their overall size, abundant cytoplasm, and large nucleoli which, at the time this system was developed, were not conceived of as features possible within the lymphoid series. It is now appreciated that proliferating lymphocytes, whether B- or T-cells, can undergo transformation to large cells previously described morphologically as histiocytes or "reticulum cells." In the B-cell series, this transformation is a known process within germinal centers and the nodular lymphomas represent neoplastic expressions of this same phenomenon. The term "histiocytic" is thus a misnomer, since both the large and small cells of these tumors are of follicular origins. The larger cells appear to be the

TABLE 35-8. A Working Formulation of Non-Hodgkin's Lymphoma for Clinical Usage: Recommendations of an Expert International Panel; Comparisons to the Rappaport Scheme

WORKING FORMULATION	RAPPAPORT TERMINOLOGY
LOW GRADE	
A. Malignant lymphocytic Small lymphocytic consistent with chronic lymphocytic leukemia plasmacytoid	Diffuse well-differentiated lymphocytic
B. Malignant lymphoma, follicular, predominantly small cleaved cell diffuse areas sclerosis	Nodular poorly differentiated lymphocytic
C. Malignant lymphoma, follicular mixed, small cleaved and large cell diffuse areas sclerosis	Nodular mixed lymphocytic histiocytic
INTERMEDIATE GRADE	
D. Malignant lymphoma, follicular Predominantly large cell diffuse areas sclerosis	Nodular histiocytic
E. Malignant lymphoma, diffuse small cleaved cell	Diffuse poorly differentiated lymphocytic
F. Malignant lymphoma, diffuse mixed, small and large cell sclerosis epithelioid cell component	Diffuse mixed lymphocytic-histiocytic
G. Malignant lymphoma, diffuse large cell cleaved cell non-cleaved cell sclerosis	Diffuse histiocytic
HIGH GRADE	
H. Malignant lymphoma large cell, immunoblastic plasmacytoid clear cell polymorphous epithelioid cell component	Diffuse histiocytic
I. Malignant lymphoma lymphoblastic convoluted cell non-convoluted cell	Diffuse lymphoblastic
J. Malignant lymphoma small non-cleaved cell Burkitt's follicular areas	Diffuse undifferentiated

replicative component of the process wherein the smaller lymphoid cells are relatively indolent, but perhaps more motile. These observations also shed light on the clinical behavior of these lymphomas.

In the most common type of nodular lymphoma, the *nodular poorly differentiated lymphocytic* variety (NPDL) (malignant lymphoma, follicular, predominantly small cleaved cell), the vast majority of neoplastic cells are small cleaved, indented lymphocytes, with only occasional large cells. (Fig. 35-5) Mitotic figures are few. Recent studies have demonstrated that monoclonal populations of lymphocytes, identical to those

TABLE 35-9. A Comparison of Classifications of Non-Hodgkin's Lymphomas

POPULAR TERMINOLOGY	RAPPAPORT (1966)	DORFMAN (1974)	BENNETT ET AL (1974)		"KIEL CLASSIFICATION" (1974)	LUKES AND COLLINS (1974)
	Nodular Lymphomas	*Follicular Lymphomas*	*Follicular Lymphomas*		*Low-Grade Malignancy*	*Undefined Cell Type*
	(b-F)* Lymphocytic, poorly differentiated	Small lymphoid	Follicle cell, predominantly small		(a)* Lymphocytic (a) Lymphoplasmacytoid	*T Cell Types* (b) Convoluted lymphocytic
GIANT FOLLICLE LYMPHOMA	(c-F) Mixed lymphocytic-histiocytic	Mixed small and large lymphoid	Follicle cell, mixed small and large		(b) Centrocytic	(e) Immunoblastic sarcoma (T cell)
	(e-F) Histiocytic	Large lymphoid	Follicle cell, predominantly large		(c) Centroblastic-centrocytic follicular (b-,c-,e-,F) follicular and diffuse diffuse	*B Cell Types*
	Diffuse Lymphomas	*Diffuse Lymphomas*	*Diffuse Lymphomas*	Grade 1		(a) Small lymphocytic (a) Plasmacytoid lymphocytic
LYMPHOSARCOMA	(a) Lymphocytic, well-differentiated	Small lymphocytic (± plasmacytic (differentiation)	Lymphocytic, well differentiated Lymphocytic, intermediate differentiation		*High-Grade Malignancy* (e) Centroblastic	Follicular center cell (follicular, follicular and diffuse, diffuse , sclerotic):
	(b) Lymphocytic, poorly differentiated	Atypical small lymphocytic Convoluted lymphocytic (thymic)	Lymphocytic, poorly differentiated		Lymphoblastic (q) Burkitt's type (b) Convoluted cell type	(b) Small cleaved (e) Large cleaved
	(c) Mixed lymphocytic-histiocytic	Mixed small and large lymphoid	Mixed small lymphoid and undifferentiated large cell		(e) Immunoblastic	(q) Small non-cleaved (e) Large non-cleaved (e) Immunoblastic sarcoma (B cell)
RETICULUM CELL SARCOMA	(d) Histiocytic, well-differentiated	Histiocytic	True histiocytic	Grade 2		*Histiocytic* (d)
	(e) Histiocytic, poorly differentiated	Large lymphoid (pyroninophilic)	Undifferentiated large cell			*Unclassifiable*
	(f) Undifferentiated, pleomorphic	Undefined (undifferentiated)	Lymphocytic poorly differentiated (lymphoblastic)			
BURKITT'S TUMOR	(g) Undifferentiated, Burkitt's type	Burkitt's lymphoma	Burkitt's tumor			

* Small case letters in parentheses allow comparison of entities in recently proposed systems to those in the modified Rappaport system.

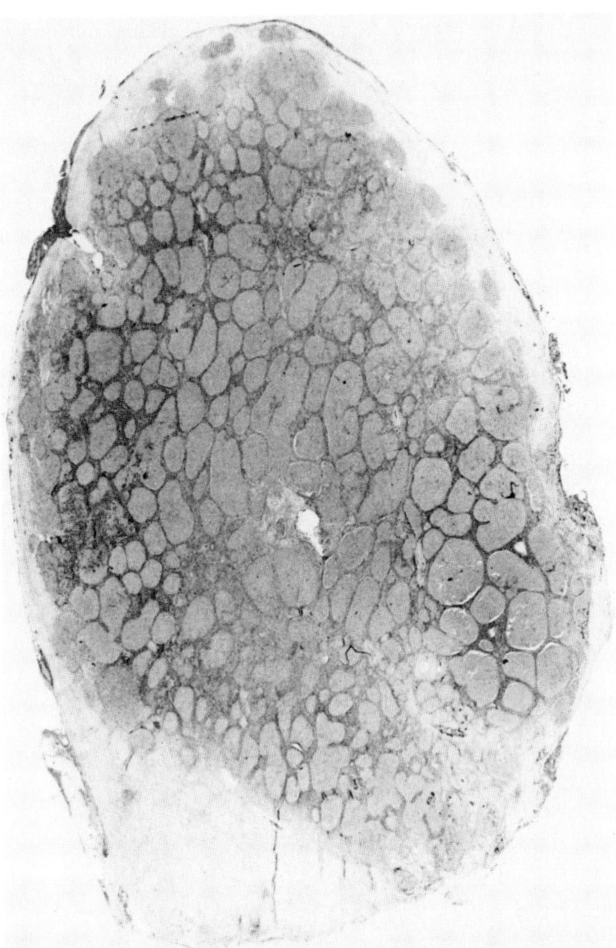

FIG. 35-4. Chaotic nodule formation in nodular lymphoma. Compare to orderly nodularity of normal node shown schematically in Fig. 35-1. (Hematoxylin and eosin × 10)

found in lymph nodes involved with tumor, are present in the peripheral blood of many patients with nodular lymphomas who do not otherwide have morphologic evidence of leukemia. When leukemia does appear, the lymphoid cells in the peripheral blood exhibit notches in the nucleus ("buttock cells" to some hematologists) and the process has been referred to as lymphosarcoma cell leukemia.

Nodular Mixed Lymphomas (Malignant Lymphoma, Follicular, Mixed Small Cleaved and Large Cells)

In nodular lymphomas with a mixture of lymphocytes and histiocytic appearing cells, the large nucleolated cells are more abundant, numbering more than 5 per high powered field and, in some cases, appearing to be admixed in almost equal numbers with smaller lymphoid cells. These patients usually have easily detected disseminated disease at presentation but it is not uncommon to find only the smaller lymphoid cells in sites distant from the nodes of origin, such as liver or bone marrow. This observation underscores the belief that the smaller cells are the migratory component of the normal and malignant lymphoreticular system and the larger cells are the replicative forms.

Nodular Histiocytic Lymphoma (Malignant Lymphoma, Follicular, Predominantly Large Cell)

This is the least common form of nodular lymphoma. The motile small lymphoid cells, seen in appreciable numbers in the other nodular lymphomas, are few in these tumors and the patients often appear to have localized tumors. Despite their earlier clinical stage at diagnosis, they nevertheless have had, until recently, the least favorable prognosis of all nodular lymphomas because their localized appearance is deceptive and frequent recurrences and progression to diffuse large cell tumors occur.

Diffuse Lymphomas

WELL-DIFFERENTIATED DIFFUSE LYMPHOMAS (malignant lymphoma, small lymphocytic). Diffuse lymphocytic lymphomas with well-differentiated small lymphocytes are the solid tumor counterpart of chronic lymphocytic leukemia (CLL). If patients with the usual peripheral blood manifestations of CLL are excluded, these neoplasms comprise approximately 5% of all non-Hodgkin's lymphomas. The patients, even when aleukemic or subleukemic, often have focal involvement of the bone marrow, liver and other visceral sites at presentation. With time, the natural history of this disease seems to be a progression to CLL. In the vast majority of patients the malignant cells are B-lymphocytes, analogous to the normal small B-cells of the medullary cords of lymph nodes (Fig. 35-1) which are in free exchange with the B-cells of peripheral blood. These B-cells are at a different stage of maturation than follicular B-cells and are no longer follicle associated. These considerations are reflected in the fact that these tumors have a diffuse pattern of growth, are usually disseminated at diagnosis, and in most cases are, or become, leukemic. These neoplastic cells, like normal medullary cord B-lymphocytes, may exhibit some functional differentiation toward the plasma cells and become immunosecretory in addition to bearing monoclonal membrane-bound immuno-

FIG. 35-5. Malignant lymphocytes in nodular, poorly-differentiated lymphoma (predominantly small cleaved cell). (Hematoxylin and eosin × 1000)

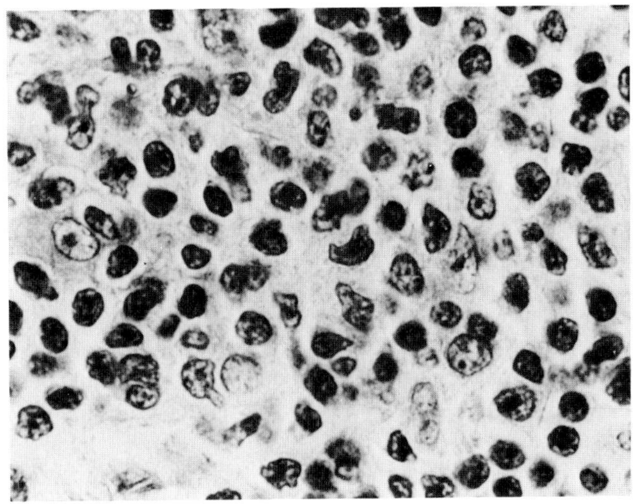

globulin. Approximately 15% of these patients have monoclonal protein spikes detected by immuno-electrophoretic studies.[67] The monoclonal protein secreted may be of any heavy chain class, including Fc fragments of IgG or IgM, but the gammopathy is most commonly monoclonal IgM of the kappa light chain type.

WALDENSTROM'S MACROGLOBULINEMIA. The disorder known as Waldenstrom's macroglobulinemia, can be most helpfully viewed as a form of well-differentiated lymphocytic neoplasia with immunoglobulin secretion as its *sine qua non* (see chapter on plasma cell neoplasms).[119,120] The cells of Waldenstrom's tumor are intermediate between lymphocytes and plasma cells, often exhibiting a spectrum, even in the same patients. Clinically, the disease also presents a spectrum from CLL-like features to a form characterized predominately by lymphadenopathy and hepatosplenomegaly. In both CLL and Waldenstrom's macroglobulinemia, a small percentage of patients (less than 1%) may at some time in their clinical course manifest a large cell lymphoma, initially reported as pleomorphic reticulum cell sarcoma by Richter, and thenceforth referred to as "Richter's syndrome."[121] Immunologic studies have now shown these large cells to bear the same surface determinants as the small lymphoid cells of the original disease.[122] Heavy-chain diseases corresponding to the three most plentiful classes of immunoglobulins are discussed in the chapter on plasma cell neoplasms.

INTERMEDIATE TYPES OF DIFFUSE LYMPHOMAS. Closely related to the above tumors, and included within the same class by many observers, are diffuse malignant lymphomas of intermediate lymphocyte type. Cytologically they differ only in that they are composed of an admixture of small round lymphocytes and less numerous small cleaved and indented lymphoid cells. The latter cells are identical to the small lymphoid cells of nodular lymphomas and these tumors can be conceived of as emanating from the interface of follicles and small medullary B-lymphocytes. (Fig. 35-1) While they are usually diffuse in growth pattern, their prognosis and natural history are suggestive of NPDL. Their recognition is important because inclusion of such cases in studies of diffuse lymphomas can improve and distort interpretations of the therapeutic results. These neoplasms, like NPDL, frequently involve the bone marrow and peripheral blood.

DIFFUSE, POORLY DIFFERENTIATED LYMPHOCYTIC LYMPHOMAS (Malignant lymphoma, diffuse small cleaved cell). Diffuse malignant lymphomas of poorly differentiated *lymphocytic* type are morphologically, clinically and immunologically not a homogeneous group. Two variants account for most of the cases. One occurs characteristically in adults with an age range similar to that of patients with nodular lymphomas. The neoplastic cells are cleaved and indented lymphocytes, identical to those of nodular lymphomas, and are often admixed, as in the latter, with occasional large nucleated cells. These tumors may have originally been nodular but have undergone progression to a diffuse pattern by the time of diagnostic biopsy. B-cell markers identical to those of nodular lymphomas may be demonstrable on the cells and additional biopsies may reveal nodular growth patterns in other anatomic sites.

The second common type of diffuse, poorly differentiated lymphocytic lymphomas is most common in adolescents and young adults. The neoplastic cells appear blastic with finely distributed nuclear chromatin, small nucleoli, scant cytoplasm and numerous mitotic figures. The nuclei in some cases are round to oval, while in others a variable percentage of these cells have nuclei with marked lobulations and convolutions. Many of these patients have mediastinal masses and a relationship to the thymus gland that was suggested on clinical grounds long before the discovery of T- and B-cell systems. Progression to acute lymphoblastic leukemia is a frequent phenomenon in these patients. While the malignant cells of some of these cases have no demonstrable surface markers, those with markers have exhibited features consistent with neoplastic T-cells. The enzyme terminal deoxynucleotydyl transferase has been found in all cases so far. In organs partially involved by tumors, these cells also selectively infiltrate T-cell zones, such as the paracortical regions of the lymph node and peri-arterial lymphoid sheaths of the spleen. Clinically, cytologically, and immunogically, these patients are closely related to the 20% to 30% of patients with acute lymphoblastic leukemia whose cells bear T-cell markers (see chapter on pediatric oncology). Even those patients presenting with solid forms of these tumors, a careful workup will often reveal occult marrow involvement. There is also a high risk of infiltration of the leptomeninges, with neoplastic cells demonstrable in the cerebrospinal fluid. Although the disease may appear circumscribed at the time of diagnosis, progression to systemic disease is such a common feature that these patients are now treated in most centers with regimens similar to those for acute lymphoblastic leukemia of childhood.

DIFFUSE MALIGNANT LYMPHOMAS OF MIXED LYMPHOCYTIC-HISTIOCYTIC TYPES (Malignant lymphoma, diffuse, mixed small and large cell). In most cases, the neoplastic cells of diffuse mixed lymphomas are cytologically identical to those of nodular mixed lymphomas and it is likely that the tumors are diffuse outgrowths of formally nodular proliferations. B-cell markers with the same features as the cells of nodular lymphomas may be demonstrable on the cells of these diffuse tumors and the term "histiocytic" is again an apparent misnomer for the large nucleated transformed B-cell. Adequate biopsy sampling may even reveal focal residual nodularity. These patients have an age distribution similar to those with nodular lymphomas and the disease is often of advanced clinical stage at the time of diagnosis, with occult disease in the liver, bone marrow, and extranodal sites.

In a few diffuse lymphomas of mixed cell type, the cells do not resemble those of nodular lymphomas but appear instead to be a pleomorphic mixture of large and small completely round cells. The small cells are immature and atypical but distinctively lymphoid, whereas the larger cells have very prominent central nuclei and pyroninophilic cytoplasm. Binucleated forms of larger cells may simulate Sternberg–Reed cells, and these cases may be misdiagnosed as lymphocyte predominate Hodgkin's disease if the fact that the small lymphoid cells also have a neoplastic appearance, in contrast to Hodgkin's disease, is not recognized. In a few cases, the malignant cells have been known to bear T-cell markers.

DIFFUSE LARGE CELL LYMPHOMAS. Diffuse histiocytic and pleomorphic lymphomas are best discussed as one group since they are not sharply separable on either histopathological or clinical grounds. They occur in all ages and present in both nodal and extranodal sites. These tumors tend to disseminate rapidly and their prognosis is distinctly unfavorable unless modern intensive chemotherapeutic regimens can induce a sustained, complete remission.

In the *undifferentiated pleomorphic group* (malignant lymphoma, large non-cleaved cell) the cells have features similar to those of Burkitt's tumor, with sharp nuclear membranes, one to four distinct basophilic nucleoli, coarsely reticulated chromatin and pyroninophilic cytoplasm. They differ from Burkitt cells predominately in the variation of their nuclear size and shape. While Burkitt tumor cells have uniformly round–oval nuclei and a size of 10 μ to 25 μ, the cells of undifferentiated pleomorphic lymphomas range from 10 μ to 45 μ and include forms with nuclear indentations, lobulations, binucleation and even multinucleation. Mitotic figures are usually numerous and are often associated with a starry sky pattern, the cytologically benign tingible-body macrophages admixed with neoplastic cells.

Diffuse histiocytic lymphomas (DHL) (malignant lymphoma, diffuse, large cell) differ from the undifferentiated pleomorphic types principally on the basis of overall cell size, nuclear size, and prominence of nucleoli. The nuclei of DHL cells are characteristically large and vesicular with marginated chromatin and from one to three distinct nucleoli (Fig. 35-6). The nucleoli may be either central or eccentric and apparently in juxtaposition to the nuclear membrane. The larger nucleoli tend to be eosinophilic and the neoplastic cells may resemble those of Hodgkin's disease. When multinucleated giant cells are present, the histiologic appearance may be indistinguishable from that of Hodgkin's disease with extreme lymphocyte depletion. Such cases should, however, be interpreted as pleomorphic histiocytic lymphomas, unless unequivocal Hodgkin's disease can be found in previous biopsies of that or another anatomic site.

In some histiocytic lymphomas the cells have large reniform and clefted nuclei and are readily distinguishable from Hodgkin's disease. In these tumors, there is, in some cases, a minor admixture of small cleaved lymphoid cells resembling those of nodular follicular lymphomas, and it is likely that such cases were formerly nodular. They may have numerous mitotic figures and a starry sky pattern and their apparent rapid growth rate could readily have effaced any previous follicular pattern. There is, in fact, considerable evidence that many of these large cells are neoplasms of transformed lymphoid cells, most commonly of B-cell type, although occasionally with T-cell characteristics. However, 40% of all diffuse histiocytic lymphomas have no characteristic surface markers. A consistent observation has been the retention of B-cell markers in diffuse histiocytic lymphomas supervening on chronic lymphoid disorders.[123] In those patients with diffuse histiocytic lymphomas within B-cell markers, but no evidence of a previous or underlying lymphoid disorder, it is supposed that transformation of the lymphoid cells occurred with loss of nodules. In the newly proposed classification, the lymphoid nature of most of the tumors referred to as histiocytic in the Rappaport scheme is reflected in the substitution of terms such as large lymphoid, undifferentiated large cell, central blastic, large cleaved and non-cleaved, or immunoblastic for histiocytic. Most of the schemes still retain a category of true histiocytic lymphoma, but it is generally conceded that malignant lymphomas composed of cells probably related to the monocyte-macrophage system must be very rare.

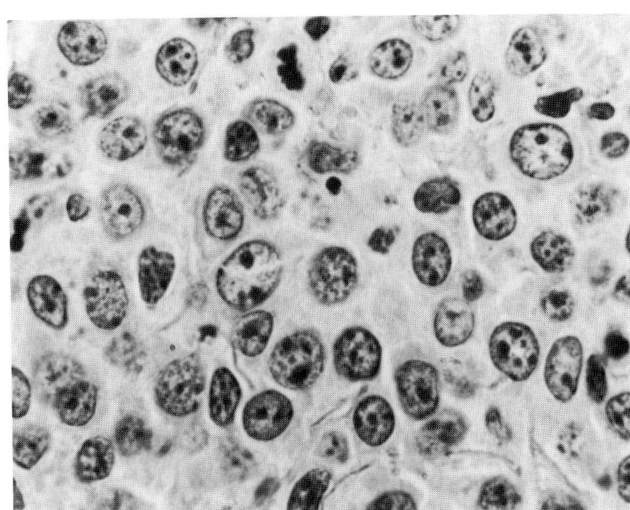

FIG. 35-6. Cells of diffuse histiocytic lymphoma (malignant lymphoma, diffuse large cell). Note comparison of size at similar magnification with cells in Fig. 35-5. (Hematoxylin and eosin × 1000)

Malignant Histiocytosis (Histiocytic Medullary Reticulosis, HMR)

Within the entire spectrum of lymphoreticular malignancies, the only tumor conclusively proven to be composed of neoplastic histiocytes is the usually fulminant systemic disease known as histiocytic medullary reticulosis or malignant histiocytosis.[124]

This is a rare, usually rapidly progressive systemic disease characterized by abrupt onset, fever, progressive pancytopenia, hepato–splenomegaly and mild lymphadenopathy.[67,125] In all lymph nodes there is a systemic proliferation of morphologically atypical histiocytes with a distinctive distribution. They characteristically proliferate within the sinusoids of the splenic red pulp, lymph nodes, liver, and bone marrow, and occasionally infiltrate the skin and other organs. The malignant cells exhibit phagocytic activity of erythrocytes and leukocytes. When erythrophagocytosis is prominent, patients usually demonstrate fulminant and progressive pancytopenia and jaundice. The neoplastic cells have strong Fc receptors, a feature of normal histiocytes.[126] In this true histiocytic malignancy the neoplastic cells preferentially proliferate in sites occupied normally by histiocytes such as the subcapsular and medullary sinuses of lymph nodes and the sinusoids of the spleen and liver. Although not much has been written on the treatment of this disease, the authors have observed long-term disease-free survival in patients treated with high intermittent large doses of cyclophosphamide.

Angio-immunoblastic Lymphadenopathy

A new histopathologic entity was described in 1975 by Lukes and Tindle and by Fizzera, Moran and Rappaport and termed angio-immunoblastic lymphadenopathy.[127,128] It is a distinct hyperimmune disorder apparently of B-cell origin that can be mistaken for Hodgkin's disease. In 24 patients described by Fizzera and colleagues, the median age was 68 years. The disease had an acute onset with generalized lymphadenopathy. Hepatosplenomegaly and constitutional symptoms occurred in almost all cases (20 of 24). Skin rashes, constitutional symptoms and a positive Coombs' test were commonly found. A polyclonal hypergammaglobulinemia was found in 17 of 22 patients. Similar results were reported in the series of Lukes and Tindle. A characteristic morphologic triad has been noted: (1) proliferation of arborizing small blood vessels, (2) immunoblastic proliferation of normal-appearing lymphocytes, and (3) amorphous acidophilic interstitial material. The cellular infiltrate consists of rounded or slightly indented small lymphocytes, plasma cells, and numerous immunoblasts. Occasional multi-indented cells have been noted. At autopsy, all lymph node areas tend to be involved. Although the disease is progressive and often fatal (median survival, 15 months), the cells are not morphologically malignant. The clinical and laboratory findings are consistent with an autoimmune disorder in which a deficiency of T-cell regulatory functions probably predisposes to an abnormal proliferative and aggressive reaction of B-cell system. To date, cytotoxic treatment has proven ineffective. Corticosteroid therapy in small doses appears to provide temporary control of the disease in some cases.

THE NATURAL HISTORY OF THE LYMPHOMAS

SUPERFICIAL LYMPH NODE PRESENTATIONS

Eighty percent or more of adult patients with lymphomas present to their physicians with superficial adenopathy. The contrasting clinical features of Hodgkin's disease and the non-Hodgkin's lymphomas are shown in Table 35-10. Lymph node enlargement is usually painless, rubbery, discrete, and located in the neck region. It may have been detected by the patient or found as a result of a physical examination for another purpose.

Most patients are asymptomatic, although 20% of patients with the non-Hodgkin's lymphomas and as many as 40% of patients with Hodgkin's disease may have some combination of fever, night sweats, weight loss, or pruritus, with fever being the commonest associated symptom.[129,130] Often patients will give a history of waxing and waning adenopathy over periods extending from months to years prior to diagnosis with an average duration of 5 months. Isolated axillary or inguinal lymph node presentations occur but are less common then cervical node presentations. It is not possible to make accurate distinctions among the various lymphomas by the size, shape, or feel of the lymph nodes. The distribution of peripheral adenopathy can, however, yield diagnostic information. Involvement of Waldeyer's ring occurs in less than 1% of patients with Hodgkin's disease, but is identified in 15% to 33% of patients with the non-Hodgkin's lymphomas.[129-131] The higher figure has been found in a series where lymphatic tissue of Waldeyer's ring is routinely biopsied. Epitrochlear node involvement is unusual in Hodgkin's disease but relatively common in patients with the nodular lymphomas. When obtaining the patient's medical history, care should be taken to document the presence or absence of night sweats before the diagnosis is made, since anxious patients can have night sweats on the basis of anxiety alone. The duration of signs and symptoms, unexplained weight loss,

TABLE 35-10. Clinical Features of the Lymphomas

HODGKIN'S DISEASE	NON-HODGKIN'S LYMPHOMA
Lymph node disease "centripetal", tends to be in axial lymph nodes	Lymph nodes disease "centrifugal" noncontiguous
Epitrochlear nodes, Waldeyer's ring, testicular and gastrointestinal sites uncommon	More common involvement of epitrochlear nodes, Waldeyer's ring, testes and gastrointestinal tract
Mediastinal presentation in 50% of patients	Mediastinal presentation less common (~20%) Distinct syndrome of T cell lymphoma with mediastinal presentation most commonly in 2nd or 3rd decades
Abdominal nodal involvement uncommon in asymptomatic but common in older patients and/or when fever or night sweats present	Abdominal lymph node involvement common
Commonly localized; contiguous nodal disease	Rarely localized nodal disease (<10%)
Bone marrow involvement uncommon	Bone marrow involvement common
Liver involvement uncommon; when present spleen is usually involved, rare without fever or night sweats	Liver commonly involved in nodular lymphoma rare in diffuse lymphoma

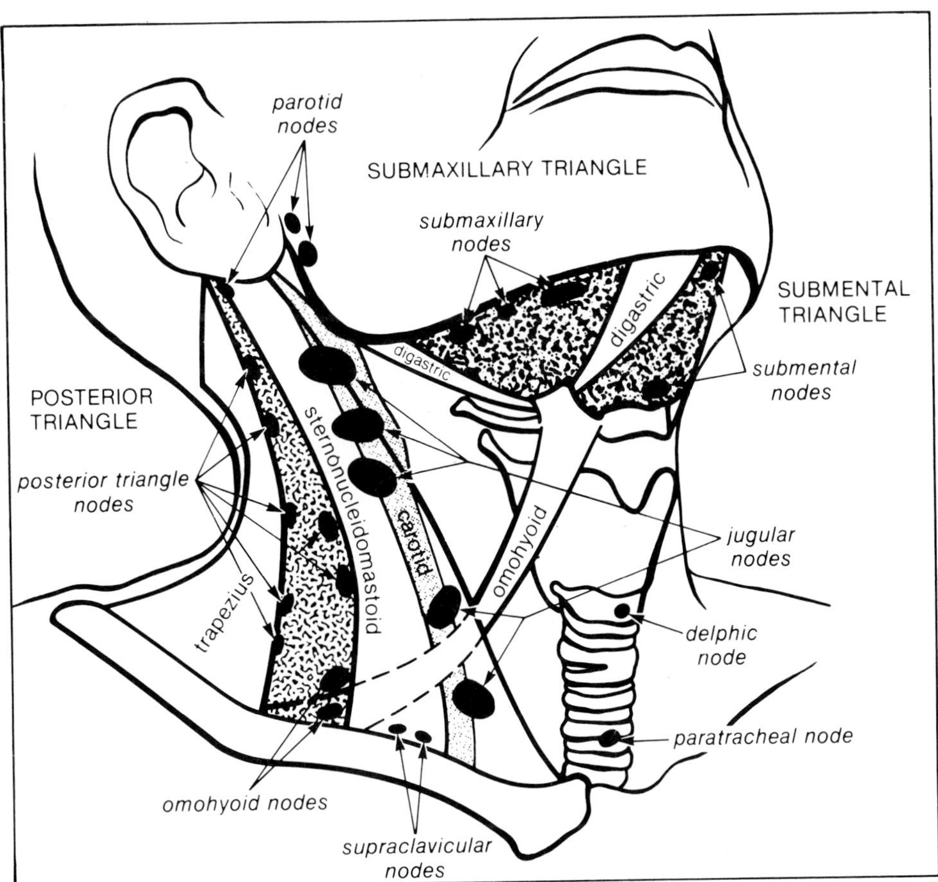

FIG. 35-7. Anatomic subdivisions of the neck depicting lymph node areas. (Adapted from Sage HH: Palpable cervical lymph nodes. JAMA 168:496, 1958)

particularly that in excess of 10% of body weight, and a family history of similar or related illnesses such as mononucleosis and immunologic disorders, should be noted. During the physical examination the status of lymph nodes in all peripheral sites including the spleen should be determined and each site recorded separately.

DIFFERENTIAL DIAGNOSIS OF SUPERFICIAL LYMPHADENOPATHY

The differential diagnosis of adenopathy depends on the age of the patient, the size, shape, and feel of lymph nodes as well as the location of the adenopathy. Palpable lymph nodes are commonly found in normal individuals on careful examination, particularly in the neck region. A display of the lymph node areas of the head and neck region is shown in Fig. 35-7. Soft, flat, eliptical submandibular nodes of 0.5 cm to 1 cm are commonly palpable in the submandibular and submental regions while soft eliptical nodes of about 0.5 cm are found with careful examination in as many as 50% of normal people in the superficial jugular and/or posterior cervical chain.[132] In young patients, superficial adenopathy in the head and neck region is most often related to acute infectious illnesses of the mouth or pharynx. Mononucleosis is a common cause of cervical adenopathy and although often associated with pharyngitis, adenopathy can occur without pharyngeal symptoms. Toxoplasmosis can mimic mononucleosis as well; these disorders can be easily diagnosed by standard methods if suspected. Adenopathy due to infection usually causes firm, sometimes tender, spherical enlargement of nodes which can easily be confused with lymphomas if they are nontender. A reasonable rule of thumb is that a spherical lymph node greater than 1 cm in diameter, thought to be due to an infectious process, that does not diminish in size over a 4 week to 8 week period of observation after resolution of the acute process, should be biopsied. Discrete hard lymph nodes, particularly if fixed or matted, are more worrisome and should be promptly biopsied for diagnosis, particularly in older people. Hard lymph nodes in the submandibular or submental region in older people are more likely related to tumors of the floor of the mouth or larynx. Nasopharyngeal cancers often drain to, and present as, posterior cervical lymph node enlargements. Thyroid carcinoma can mimic lymphoma although the lymph nodes involved with thyroid cancer are generally firmer and often found in the submental, and superficial jugular region, an area less commonly involved in isolation by lymphomas.

Since supraclavicular lymph nodes drain regions of the lung and retroperitoneal space, they can reflect either lymphoma or tumors and infectious processes originating in these areas. Isolated axillary lymph node enlargement can be related to local phenomena in the hands or arms, such as infections, trauma, or insect bites. A young male adult with a tumor in an axillary lymph node is most likely to have a lymphoma or a malignant melanoma. In the female, the same two tumors plus breast cancer are the most likely diagnoses. Isolated inguinal adenopathy is often difficult to separate from the normal 0.5 cm to 1 cm elliptical lymph nodes found in the region of the inguinal ligament, which are also influenced by disorders occurring on the legs and feet. Concomitant enlargement of nodes in the femoral triangle or adenopathy along the external iliac chain should make inguinal adenopathy more suspicious and decrease the threshold for biopsy.

THORACIC PRESENTATIONS

Thoracic adenopathy is relatively common in patients with lymphomas. It may be detected by routine roentgenogram or films taken for another purpose such as the workup after the discovery of peripheral adenopathy, or because the patient has had a chronic dry, nonproductive cough with or without fever. The overall frequency of mediastinal adenopathy in Hodgkin's disease is 50%. The highest frequency of mediastinal adenopathy occurs in young women with Hodgkin's disease (70%).[129] The mediastinum is involved in less than 20% of patients with the other lymphomas.[133] Mediastinal adenopathy is a common presenting problem in adolescents with T-cell lymphoblastic lymphoma.[134,135] Involvement of hilar or mediastinal nodes in patients with lymphoma is usually unilateral.

The differential diagnosis of mediastinal and hilar adenopathy includes primary lung disorders and some systemic illnesses that characteristically involve hilar or mediastinal nodes. In the young, mediastinal adenopathy occurs commonly in patients with infectious mononucleosis and sarcoidosis which in both cases is usually panhilar. In endemic regions, histoplasmosis can cause unilateral paratracheal node enlargement which mimics lymphoma but is usually associated with the node calcification and esophageal symptoms. Unilateral tuberculous adenopathy is not often confused with lymphoma because of the associated Ghon complex. Primary lung cancer is an important part of the differential diagnosis in older people, especially smokers, and can usually be distinguished from lymphomas by the presence of a parenchymal lesion.

The argument over involvement of a thymus gland with Hodgkin's disease seems to be settled. The entity, granulomatous thymoma, in all carefully studied series, appears to invariably represent involvement of the thymus gland with Hodgkin's disease. It is, however, difficult to determine how often the thymus is involved, when the mediastinal lymph nodes are involved, without surgical examination, which is rarely done for this purpose.

ABDOMINAL PRESENTATIONS

Hodgkin's disease and the common non-Hodgkin's lymphomas frequently involve either retroperitoneal lymph nodes or the primary lymphatic tissue of the gut and its mesenteric drainage sites. Patients who present with abdominal lymphoma usually have either a painless mass discovered on physical examination, or pain associated with a palpable mass. Some patients present only with splenomegaly and most often have one of the non-Hodgkin's lymphomas, not uncommonly leukemic reticuloendotheliosis (hairy cell leukemia).[136] This is discussed further in Chapter 37. Rarely, previously untreated patients may present with perforation of a viscus through tumor, or hemorrhage from the upper or lower gastrointestinal tract. Previously unsuspected abdominal lymphomas are much more commonly found after the staging workup is completed in patients who have superficial lymph node presentations. Patients whose abdominal disease alone prompts their visit to their physician most often have one of the non-Hodgkin's lymphomas. It is distinctly unusual to be able to palpate significant abdominal adenopathy in patients with Hodgkin's disease. Hodgkin's disease may rarely make its appearance associated with idiopathic thrombocytopenic purpura and splenomegaly, but only a few of those patients with such a presentation have been described.[137]

The commonest clinical constellation of symptoms and signs in patients with Hodgkin's disease who have ultimately abdominal tumor only is that of fever and weight loss. The diagnosis of Hodgkin's disease is made at laparotomy performed as part of a diagnostic evaluation for fever of undetermined origin. Such patients usually have involvement of the retroperitoneal lymph nodes and the histologic subtype is likely to be lymphocyte depleted Hodgkin's disease. The so-called "Mediterranean lymphoma" often presents with disease in the abdomen. Pathologically, these tumors resemble diffuse plasma cell tumors and are often associated with aberrant production of immunoglobulin heavy chains and malabsorption.[138] They are discussed in the chapter on plasma cell neoplasms. Abdominal presentations of lymphoma may also mimic any type of intraabdominal disease.

OTHER CLINICAL PRESENTATIONS

Lymphomas should be included in the differential diagnosis of superior vena cava syndrome (most often Hodgkin's disease or diffuse histiocytic lymphoma), acute spinal cord compression, isolated tumor nodules of the skin, bone tumors, and unexplained anemias. While these manifestations occur with considerable frequency in patients with widespread advancing tumor, they are uncommon as initial presentations of the disease.

DISEASE EVOLUTION

With the advent of modern treatment, patients with lymphoma are rarely left untreated and the natural history is interrupted, often successfully, by treatment.

THE CLINICAL EVOLUTION OF HODGKIN'S DISEASE

Hodgkin's disease was first suspected to spread by contiguity by the Swiss radiotherapist, Gilbert.[139,140] His work was expanded by Peters and Kaplan, who tested the value of prophylactic radiotherapy to nodes adjacent to those involved with the disease.[141–144] Two relatively recent diagnostic procedures have greatly increased our knowledge of the natural history of Hodgkin's disease. The development of the bipedal lymphogram or lymphangiogram, in the early 1960s, provided the first diagnostic tool delineating the status of the retroperitoneal lymph nodes, and the use of routine staging laparotomy, introduced by the Stanford group, detected tumors in previously unsuspected sites by all other tests.[145-147]

Hodgkin's disease is now believed by most to be unifocal in origin and to spread by involving adjacent lymph nodes structures first. With unchecked tumor growth, either direct extension into adjacent visceral organs occurs or blood vessel invasion occurs with dissemination of the disease to the spleen, bone marrow, liver, bone, and other organs, in a fashion similar to metastases from epithelial cancers. The two commonest lymph nodes groups involved with tumor are in the cervical and retroperitoneal regions.[148] Left cervical lymph node involvement is more common than right and more often associated with retroperitoneal lymph node invasion, not rarely (15%) in the absence of mediastinal tumor. This skipping of a contiguous lymph node site initially led to the suggestion that on some occasions Hodgkin's disease did not spread by continuity. Laparotomy studies have shown that left cervical node involvement also occurs in the absence of abdominal tumor, leaving Kaplan to postulate that when the site of primary tumor is in the left cervical region, retroperitoneal lymph node disease occurs as a result of retrograde spready by way of the thoracic duct. This hypothesis has been questioned by some on physiologic grounds as the pressure required to create a complete block of lymph flow is in excess of what can be achieved by involvement of lymph nodes with tumor. An important finding from all laparotomy studies is that the spleen is often involved with tumor when otherwise normal by physical examination and all other tests (± 30%).[149-153] The spleen has also been shown to be involved with Hodgkin's disease, on occasion, in the absence of retroperitoneal lymph nodes. This observation, and the known absence of afferent splenic lymphatics strongly suggests that hematogenous dissemination to the spleen from the primary tumor site occurs commonly, and early in the course of the disease, with subsequent spread to the splenic hilar and retroperitoneal nodes and the liver. Finally, it is possible that retroperitoneal lymph nodes are the commonest site of primary tumor but are not detected early because of the inaccessibility of the retroperitoneum to clinical examination. The disease could then spread anterograde through the thoracic duct, physiologically, to involve cervical lymph nodes and from there disseminate to the spleen through vascular channels. None of the hypotheses completely explains the evolution of the disease. The single most important fact for the physician to remember is that Hodgkin's disease appears to be a unifocal process that most often spreads by contiguity. These two facts influence both staging and selection of treatment.

The histologic subtype as depicted in the Lukes–Butler classification also has a bearing on the natural history of Hodgkin's disease. Patients with nodular sclerosing Hodgkin's disease tend to have larger lymph nodes most often located in the upper thorax and their disease tends to remain localized longer than those with the mixed cellularity or lymphocyte depleted varieties.[154] Although patterns of presentation differ, the natural history of lymphocyte predominant disease is in many ways similar to that of nodular sclerosing. Isolated high right neck presentations are common in the lymphocyte predominant variety and, when clinically localized, distant disease is rarely found at laparotomy. On the other hand, patients who present with apparently localized *lymphocyte depleted* histology usually develop noncontiguous recurrences, if treated with local therapy only, suggesting that the tumor cells in the worse histologic subtypes proceed to invade blood vessels early and spread widely.[155]

Current data suggest that histologic evolution occurs with progressive loss of lymphocytes. Hodgkin's disease probably begins as either lymphocyte predominant or the cellular phase of nodular sclerosing disease. Evolution of the histologic appearance within the nodular sclerosing variety has been shown to occur with progressive depletion of lymphocytes, and increases in the number of malignant cells.[156] This appears to occur at varying rates of speed in different patients under the influence of unknown host factors. Even with extreme lymphocyte depletion, however, the fibrous characteristic of nodular sclerosing Hodgkin's disease is usually manifest in lymph node structures in autopsy material. Patients who present with lymphocyte predominant Hodgkin's disease have been shown to evolve to mixed cellularity and, subsequently, to lymphocyte depletion as the tumor advances from stage to stage. It is, for example, unusual for any patient to have primarily lymphocyte predominant histology at autopsy. It seems likely that patients who present with lymphocyte depleted Hodgkin's disease have very rapidly progressive disease with essentially no clinical phase of lymphocyte predominant disease. This probably occurs in patients who present with fever, weight loss, and retroperitoneal lymph node involvement and lymphocyte depleted Hodgkin's disease. Retrogressive histologic evolution has also been shown to occur after successful therapy. Patients with lymphocyte depleted or mixed cellularity disease who have been induced into remission for long periods of time with chemotherapy, and then relapse, have had lymphocyte predominant disease on rebiopsy, suggesting a restoration of histology to a more favorable type.

Since histology is correlated with stage (lymphocyte predominant and nodular sclerosing disease more commonly Stages I and II) and propensity for vascular invasion, and stage is correlated with immune function, a probable evolution of Hodgkin's disease can be constructed as follows.[129,157,158] Hodgkin's disease most likely begins as a unifocal involvement of a lymph node in the cervical or retroperitoneal areas in response to an as yet unknown stimulus but perhaps exposure to an infecious agent. The malignant cells, the Sternberg-Reed cell or its mononuclear variant, are in the minority, and are generally surrounded by normal lymphocytes, macrophages, and plasma cells, or in the case of nodular sclerosing disease, by a more intense fibrous inflammatory reaction. The major early increase in mass of the lymph node is due to reactive hyperplasia of the normal cells and overgrowth of fibrous tissue. Spread occurs to adjacent lymph nodes through normal lymphatic channels. The rate of spread is determined by host factors yet unknown, and is accompanied at varying rates of speed by effacement of the lymph node architecture, gradual depletion of lymphocytes, and as the ratio of the number of tumor cells to normal cells increases, symptoms of fever, sweats, pruritus, weight loss and a tendency for vascular invasion by the malignant cells. At some point, the tumor mass becomes visible or palpable and offers the prospect of diagnosis. Depending on where the process is interrupted, patients may appear to the physician as having early disease with favorable histology, no symptoms, a relatively intact immune system, or present with advanced disease and the reverse of all of the above. It is now possible to interrupt the progression of the disease at all stages of clinical, histologic, and immunologic evolution with either local treatment with radiotherapy or chemotherapy or both and reverse all the abnormalities mentioned above. If treatment fails, however, progressive involvement of other lymph nodes and organ systems occurs. Symptoms become more common and are associated with cachexia, which is often out of proportion to the visible volume of tumor. Immunologic function deteriorates and peripheral lymphocytopenia becomes common. The patient becomes vulnerable to infections, either as a consequence of the disease or because of the negative impact of treatment on bone marrow and organ function, and usually dies as a consequence of infection. A single series of untreated patients reported by Craft in 1941 leads us to believe that the course of patients with Hodgkin's disease left untreated, regardless of the stage, is brief, measured in 1 year to 2 years.[159] In that series the median survival was less than 1 year and most patients were dead by 2 years with fewer than 5% alive at 5 years.

THE CLINICAL EVOLUTION OF THE NON-HODGKIN'S LYMPHOMAS

The natural history of the other lymphomas is quite different from Hodgkin's disease. Predictability of spread is less certain, although some tendency toward contiguity of spread has been demonstrated in a series from Stanford.[160] The disease may be unifocal in origin, but, if so, it remains localized so briefly that widespread disease is the rule at the time of diagnosis rather than the exception. A reasonable estimate of the percentage of patients with truly localized non-Hodgkin's lymphomas is 10%, compared to the 50% or so of patients who present with localized Hodgkin's disease. Now that it is apparent that the majority of the common types of the non-Hodgkin's lymphomas in adults originate from a monoclonal population of B-cells, and the anatomic compartmentalization of these cells in lymph nodes is more clearly understood, certain generalizations can be made relating the type of disease to the clinical course of patients with non-Hodgkin's lymphomas.

The commonest histologic subgroup of patients with the non-Hodgkin's lymphoma are those with nodular (follicular) patterns in the lymph node. These patients make up almost half of all cases in most series. When patients with nodular lymphomas present with apparently localized adenopathy, it is usually easy to demonstrate generalized adenopathy with few additional examinations. This propensity to have widespread disease matches the normal tendency of the small untransformed follicular B-cell to migrate in the circulation. Nonetheless, in spite of wide dissemination, the NPDL variety of lymphoma is often clinically indolent. An as-yet-undetermined fraction of such patients can be left untreated and will evidence waxing and waning adenopathy for months to years before unsightly or painful lymph node enlargement, or compression of a vital organ, requires treatment.[161] Involvement of the bone marrow and liver, frequently easily demonstrated at initial diagnostic evaluation, does not impart the same adverse prognosis as involvement of these organs by Hodgkin's disease. Several studies have now clearly indicated there is no difference in survival in patients with widespread disease confined to lymph nodes (Stage III) and those with involvement of lymph nodes, bone marrow, and liver.[162,163]

Patients with diffuse non-Hodgkin's lymphomas, although these also most often of B-cell origin, have a vastly different natural history than patients with nodular lymphomas. In keeping with the lack of motility of transformed follicular B-cells, the diffuse large cell lymphomas (pleomorphic undifferentiated or histiocytic of Rappaport), the second most common type, more often appear to be clinically localized, although the recurrence rate after local treatment indicates otherwise. In contrast to patients with NPDL, when tumor is identified in organs like the bone marrow, liver, and bone, patients with diffuse large cell lymphomas have aggressive, rapidly fatal illnesses unless treated successfully.

There is now also evidence for a link between NPDL (follicular small cleaved cell lymphomas) and the diffuse large cell lymphomas of B-cell origin. At the National Cancer Institute, a series of 515 patients with non-Hodgkin's lymphomas has been analyzed for frequency of histologic evolution.[164,165] The clinical course of 114 of these patients had led to a repeat biopsy more than 3 months after the initial diagnostic biopsy. Among patients with nodular types of lymphoma at diagnosis, repeat biopsies revealed histologic progression in 41%. These data indicate that a substantial number of patients with nodular lymphomas will evolve to a diffuse variety as part of the natural history of their disease.

A likely evolution of the non-Hodgkin's lymphoma can be constructed as follows. The follicle associated cells of B-cell lymphomas (Fig. 35-1) that initially retain the characteristic of forming nodules are close to normal tissue in their growth characteristics and migrate easily while minimally dedifferentiated. This accounts for the ease of detectability of these cells in other organs and yet the indolent natural history. Their growth rate and invasive potential, for unknown reasons, remains low. In time, the malignant B-cell dedifferentiates to take on the morphologic characteristics of transformed lymphocytes or histiocytes. This transformation may occur slowly over several years, or so rapidly that the evolution antedates diagnosis. These transformed cells are less motile, which accounts for the difficulty in detecting them outside the site of origin (dedifferentiation) with normal staging procedures, but they are more invasive and produce a rapidly fatal disease if growth is unchecked. In the past, these histologic types were called reticulum cell sarcomas, and in the more recent Rappaport classification, diffuse histiocytic lymphoma. It also seems likely that NPDL subtype evolves to nodular mixed (NM) and nodular histiocytic (NH) lymphomas of Rappaport as the percentage of large cells increases until, finally, effacement of the lymph node occurs and a pathologic picture of diffuse large cell lymphoma is observed under the microscope. As with the evolution of the histologic effacement of a lymph node in Hodgkin's disease, the reasons for the varying rate of transformation from nodule-forming indolent lymphocytes to large transformed cells are unknown. Lymphomas of diffuse small cells disseminate widely at an early stage but have an indolent course in keeping with their benign histologic appearance. They evolve to large cell B-neoplasms much less frequently and usually kill patients by causing bone marrow failure, with hypogammaglobulinemia leading to fatal infections.

DIAGNOSIS AND STAGING OF LYMPHOMAS

HODGKIN'S DISEASE

The diagnosis of Hodgkin's disease is made by biopsy of an enlarged lymph node. Occasionally, multiple biopsies are necessary for proper diagnosis, because reactive hyperplasia of nodes adjacent to those involved by tumor may lead to biopsy of an easily accessible but uninvolved node.[166] Needle aspiration biopsy of lymph nodes is never adequate for initial diagnosis since it is impossible to subclassify the disease with such limited amounts of biopsy material it provides. The Lukes–Butler classification of Hodgkin's disease is currently used to classify the disease.[88] In Table 35-7 it is compared to the distribution of case material at the National Cancer Institute under the old Jackson–Parker classification.[95]

The first useful staging classification for Hodgkin's disease was developed by Peters and colleagues.[167] It divided patients into three categories indicated by Roman numerals. Stages I and II included patients with localized tumor easily treated with radiotherapy. Stage III included patients with both extensive nodal disease and tumor involving organ systems. This classification system was modified in the early 1960s to delineate the patients who are most suitable for radiation therapy treatment.[129] The modification included a category, Stage IV, for patients who had disease disseminated outside the lymph node system. This staging system has been accepted and widely used since its adoption at the Rye staging conference in 1965.[168] A subsequent modification was developed at the Ann Arbor Staging Conferences in 1970 and is shown in Table 35-11.[169] The Ann Arbor version modifies the previous classification in two major ways. First, based on therapeutic data provided by Musshoff, patients whose disease has spread by contiguity from lymph nodes to adjacent organs are not considered as Stage IV; they are staged by the extent of lymph node involvement followed by the subscript "E" which denotes direct extension.[170] Second, involvement of the spleen is indicated by the subscript "S." In all systems, patients are further classified as either "A" or "B" on the basis of the absence or presence of constitutional symptoms, such as fever higher than 38°C (100.4°F) for three consecutive days, night sweats, or unexplained loss of more than 10% of body weight. As a result of the Ann Arbor deliberations, pruritis, previously considered an important systemic symptom, is no longer considered sufficient to include a patient in category B when it occurs alone.

Recommendations for proper staging procedures made at the Ann Arbor symposium are shown in Tables 35-12 and 35-13.[171] A detailed history and physical are necessary to determine the presence or absence of systemic symptoms, to note symptoms or signs suggesting extranodal involvement and to properly characterize the extent of lymph node involvement. Equivocally abnormal adenopathy that would change the patient's stage should be biopsied. In addition, a chest roentgenogram and bipedal lymphangiography are always necessary for proper staging unless medically contraindicated. When bone marrow examination is indicated, bone marrow biopsy, not aspiration, is required. Bone marrow biopsy is particularly important in symptomatic patients and in those with bone lesions, bone pain, hypercalcemia, or an elevated serum alkaline phosphatase. Whole chest tomography should be performed if mediastinal disease or any suspicious abnormality is present on a conventional chest roentgenogram.[172] Isotope scanning of the liver, spleen, and bone may be helpful in defining possible sites of additional disease, but a positive or negative study cannot be thought of as definitive for diagnosis without biopsy confirmation. It is particularly important that suspicious extranodal sites be biopsied because the finding of visceral disease markedly alters the therapeutic approach and obviates the need for further staging procedures.

Recently, computerized axial tomography (CT) scanning has been introduced as a supplement to staging in lymphomas.[172–174] Good correlation has been found between the results of CT scanning and lymphangiography. Clear visualization of the para-aortic lymph nodes is possible and can supplement lymphangiography. It is not uncommon for lymphangiograms to fail to visualize nodes in the upper abdominal lymph node regions and it is not possible to visualize mesenteric nodes using lymphangiography. CT has been shown to have a high degree of accuracy identifying enlarged mesenteric lymph nodes and upper abdominal nodes not

TABLE 35-11. Ann Arbor Staging Classification for Hodgkin's Disease

STAGE I	Involvement of a single lymph node region (I) or a single extralymphatic organ or site (I_E)
STAGE II	Involvement of 2 or more lymph node regions on the same side of the diaphragm (II) or localized involvement of an extralymphatic organ or site (II_E)
STAGE III	Involvement of lymph node regions on both sides of the diaphragm (III) or localized involvement of an extralymphatic organ or site (III_E) or spleen (III_S) or both (III_{SE})
STAGE IV	Diffuse or disseminated involvement of 1 or more extralymphatic organs with or without associated lymph node involvement. The organ(s) involved should be identified by a symbol: A = Asymptomatic B = Fever, sweats, weight loss >10% of body weight

TABLE 35-12. Staging Hodgkin's and Non-Hodgkin's Lymphomas: Required Evaluation Procedures

1. Adequate surgical biopsy, reviewed by an experienced hematologist
2. A detailed history recording the presence or absence of and duration of fever, unexplained sweating and its severity, unexplained pruritus and unexplained weight loss
3. A careful and detailed physical examination; special attention to all node-bearing areas, including Waldeyer's ring, and determination of size of liver and spleen
4. Necessary laboratory procedures:
   a. Complete blood count, including an erythrocytic sedimentation rate
   b. Serum alkaline phosphatase
   c. Evaluation of renal function
   d. Evaluation of liver function
5. Radiologic studies include:
   a. Chest roentgenogram (PA and lateral)
   b. Intravenous pyelogram
   c. Bilateral lower extremity lymphogram
   d. Views of skeletal system to include thoracic and lumbar vertebrae, the pelvis, proximal extremities and any areas of bone tenderness

TABLE 35-13. Staging Hodgkin's Disease and Non-Hodgkin's Lymphomas: Procedures Required Under Certain Circumstances

1. Whole-chest tomography if any abnormality is noted or suspected on the routine chest roentgenogram
2. Abdominal CAT scan, ultrasonogram, inferior cavography or pyelogram to supplement lymphographic findings
3. Bone marrow *biopsy* (needle or open) in the presence of:
   a. An elevated alkaline phosphatase
   b. Unexplained anemia or other blood count depression
   c. Other evidence of bone disease (scan or x-ray)
   d. Generalized disease of Stage III or greater
4. Exploratory laparotomy and splenectomy, if management decision will depend on the identification of abdominal procedures

Useful Ancillary Procedures Not Required for Staging

1. Skeletal scintigrams*
2. Hepatic and spleen scintigrams*
3. Serum chemistries to include serum calcium and uric acid for overall management of patient
4. Estimates of the patient's delayed hypersensitivity of the tuberculin type
5. Gallium whole-body scans*

* Cannot be used as evidence of Hodgkin's disease without biopsy confirmation

visualized by lymphangiography. CT scanning, however, has not been shown to provide sufficient information over normal roentgenographic procedures used to diagnose thoracic disease, and in some cases may be too sensitive. Ultrasonography has also been investigated as a means of diagnosing intra-abdominal masses.[175,176] Sonograms of lymph nodes involved with lymphoma appear as lucent areas. It has not been noted that detection of an abnormality of a lymph node is not entirely related to size using sonography. Normal size lymph nodes involved with tumor show sonolucency when compared to uninvolved lymph nodes. Also, large hyperplastic normal lymph nodes do not have the same sonolucent pattern as nodes involved with lymphoma. This adds an additional distinctive feature to the use of sonography. The correlation between the presence of an abnormal sonogram and the finding of positive lymph nodes at time of surgery is in excess of 85% and correlates well with what can be achieved using other methods such as lymphangiography.

STAGING LAPAROTOMY

Staging laparotomy initially was developed to study the pattern of spread and frequency of involvement of various abdominal sites and was utilized as a research tool.[147] Treatment was not initially reduced as a result of the negative findings at laparotomy. As a research tool, it has provided an enormous amount of information about the patterns of involvement of Hodgkin's disease, the accuracy of lymphangiography and other tests, such as CT scanning and sonography, and the accuracy of clinical evaluations of the liver and spleen. In order to be complete and accurate, and to justify its application in the staging of Hodgkin's disease, it should only be carried out routinely by investigators skilled in the technique who will use the data obtained to advance our knowledge of the natural history of the disease. The decision to use laparotomy in staging is closely linked to the therapeutic approach.[177] Physicians who first perform laparotomy and then inquire about therapy have done their patients a disservice. The Committee on Hodgkin's Disease Staging Procedures at Ann Arbor recommended that laparotomy and splenectomy should be performed only if management decisions depend on identification of abdominal disease (Table 35-13).[169] The so-called staging laparotomy, in which the spleen is removed and sectioned only a few times, or the para-aortic nodes are palpated, felt to be normal, and either biopsied once or not biopsied at all, is to be condemned as inadequate. The procedure is not justified unless extreme care to ensure that the patient is staged completely.[178–180] Laparotomy should include detailed inspection of the abdomen and splenectomy. The spleen should be sectioned in 1 cm slices. Examination of the liver should include an ample wedge biopsy of the right lobe as well as three needle biopsies of both the right and left lobes, and a biopsy of any grossly abnormal hepatic lesions. After inspection and palpation of the nodal groups, a biopsy should be taken of the right and left para-aortic and iliac nodes, *regardless* of their character on palpation or appearance on lymphangiography. In addition, lymph nodes should be removed from the splenic hilar, celiac, porta hepatis, mesenteric, and iliac regions and clips should be placed at all biopsy sites. Oophoropexy should be performed in female patients who wish to avoid sterilization during radiotherapy. In patients with positive lymphangiograms it is vitally important to be certain that the suspicious nodes have actually been removed. In many instances it may be necessary to clip areas adjacent to nodes removed, and perform diagnostic abdominal roentgenograms during surgery to ensure the appropriate nodes have been biopsied. Iliac bone wedge biopsy should be performed at the time of operation. As should be apparent from this description, a complete staging laparotomy is a major surgical procedure and requires considerable skill, time, and effort on the part of the surgeon. Its risks should be constantly weighed against its benefits.

The most significant finding gained from exploratory laporatory and splenectomy has concerned the frequency and character of splenic involvement. Data from laparotomy studies have clearly established that clinical evaluation of the spleen is incapable of accurately assessing the frequency of splenic disease. Only about 50% to 60% of patients believed to have splenic disease on clinical evaluation actually have proved to have such involvement.[181] More importantly, about 25% of patients with normal sized spleens without any clinical evidence of splenic abnormalities will be found to have histologically proven Hodgkin's disease of the spleen when it is removed. In addition, the spleen may be the only site of involvement by tumor below the diaphragm. Another important finding in laparotomy studies is that the liver is virtually never involved with Hodgkin's disease in the absence of splenic involvement. In contrast to the frequent finding of splenic involvement, the liver is uncommonly found to be involved by tumor at routine laparotomy. It was involved in only three patients of the Stanford series of 100 unselected patients.[147,181] Of 406 liver biopsies in a collected series reported by Desser and colleagues, 47 (12%) were positive for Hodgkin's disease.[182] In this series, the majority of the positives occurred in patients with advanced symptomatic disease (Stage IIB or greater) or in patients who were not evaluated with any other biopsy procedures prior to laparotomy. It is important to note that staging laparotomy studies have revealed that the usual clinical determination of liver size and liver function (including liver scans) correlates poorly, if at all, with the presence of Hodgkin's disease in the liver, although completely negative evaluations are generally confirmed. Since the finding of liver involvement by Hodgkin's disease necessitates a marked change in the treatment plan, it is extremely important to ensure accurate assessment of the liver before a treatment plan is initiated. It is not necessary to perform routine laparotomy in all patients in order to properly evaluate the liver. First, clinical information indicates that patients found to have liver involvement usually have one or all of the following characteristics: (1) high para-aortic nodes positive on lymphangiogram, (2) splenomegaly, and (3) poor risk histology (lymphocyte depleted or mixed cellularity).[171] Such patients should have evaluation of their liver by biopsy. Percutaneous biopsy will yield some positives and should be performed prior to more aggressive staging. Peritoneoscopy, with multiple liver biopsies under direct visualization, is associated with lower morbidity than laparotomy, and leads to the diagnosis of liver involvement in a frequency similar to that at laparotomy.[183,184] Recently, a study of the use of peritoneoscopy followed by laparotomy has been reported.[185] Only two of 110 patients with negative peritoneoscopy were found to have liver involvement at laparotomy. All patients should have this procedure performed, if possible, before undergoing laparotomy.

Ordinarily, the nodes found to be positive at the time of laparotomy are those in the para-aortic, iliac, or splenic hilar areas, and these would be expected to be incorporated into a conventional radiation field. Of considerable interest are those nodes outside such fields that would not be treated. Fortunately, in Hodgkin's disease, such involvement is unusual, but disease sometimes is found in the portal and even more uncommonly, in the mesenteric nodes. In a recent study, where laparotomy was performed in 99 patients, two of 54 patients with clinical Stages I and II (4%) were found to have occult disease in the porta hepatis.[186] Even this low incidence is higher than that reported in most other series. Seven patients in the entire series of 99 had unexpected findings of either nodal disease outside traditional radiation ports or liver disease. However, if the criteria for laparotomy and laparoscopy set forth above had been used, only two patients would not have had disease incorporated in an appropriate radiation port. Thus, although disease outside traditional nodal areas is occasionally found at staging laparotomy, it generally is in patients who are otherwise candidates for staging laparotomy. Furthermore, disease is most often found in the porta hepatis region, which can be be included in an upper abdominal radiation field by extending the para-aortic port 2 cm laterally from the eleventh thoracic vertebra to the first lumbar vertebra. Whether routine laparotomy is justified to discover the 2% of patients with nodal disease outside traditional ports is conjectural, since those patients who relapse from radiation therapy may do well with subsequent chemotherapy.

A number of studies have been done to determine the frequency of therapeutic alteration on the basis of laparotomy findings. At institutions where therapy is tailored by stage, this can be important. In 114 successive laparotomies performed at the Joint Center for Radiation Therapy between April, 1969, and December, 1971, there were 33 patients whose stage was changed, 18 who were downstaged, while 15 were found to have more extensive disease than was suspected. Using the treatment regimens felt appropriate at that time, 40 of the 114 patients (35%) had the therapeutic plan altered: 18 received radiation to a reduced volume, 10 to a greater volume, two received radiation instead of chemotherapy, four received chemotherapy instead of radiation; four received both.[190,191] When reviewing therapeutic approaches later in this chapter, physicians should note that changes in stage as a result of findings at laparotomy often do not result in a change in treatment plan, especially if chemotherapy is planned for part of the treatment. A thorough knowledge of treatment alternatives will often obviate the need for staging by laparotomy. Thus, as treatment alternatives change, and other diagnostic tools become available, the place of laparotomy must be reevaluated. For example, Sweet and colleagues have proposed that the accuracy of assessment of the retroperitoneal lymph nodes using CT scans and sonography in conjunction with lymphangiography is sufficiently good to replace surgical biopsy and obviate the need for laparotomy.[192]

Current practice requires that after staging is completed, patients be assigned to a clinical stage (CS) based on preoperative assessment and a pathologic stage (PS) based on the findings at the time of laparotomy or other invasive procedure such as laparoscopy. Because staging laparotomy alters the clinical stage frequently, a significant number of changes often will occur between the CS and the PS. Examples of the use of this staging classification are shown in Table 35-14.

Recently, a further subclassification of the Ann Arbor staging system has been proposed by Desser and associates.[187,188] They analyzed their patients with Stage III disease to determine where the location of involved abdominal sites had influence on survival. They found that patients with disease limited to the spleen, or splenic, celiac or portal nodes (anatomic Substage III_1) had a significantly more favorable 5-year survival (93%) than did patients with involvement of para-aortic, iliac, or mesenteric nodes (anatomic Substage III_2) whose 5-year survival was 57%. Hoppe and colleagues, however, found no difference in their series between III_1 and III_2 but, rather, an influence of total number of sites of involvement on ultimate survival.[189]

Complications of Staging Laparotomy

Staging laparotomy is a major surgical procedure with established morbidity and mortality. Institutions with the most extensive experience report mortality statistics as low as 0.5%.[193] Nevertheless, one study of a cooperative hospital experience reported a 27% morbidity and an unacceptable 6.6% mortality.[194] More recently a study of the experience of other institutions, including university hospitals, has reported a significant morbidity (16%) in patients with Hodgkin's disease undergoing routine laparotomy under non-study circumstances.[195] Morbidity included wound infections, subphrenic abscesses, pulmonary emboli, stress ulcers with gastrointestinal bleeding, pulmonary infections, and wound dehiscence. Tabulation of some of the available information on complications of laparotomy is presented in Table 35-15. Categories in Table 35-15 are mutually exclusive, so that the overall significant complication rate is 69 of 555 (12.8%).[171] In this analysis, less significant complications such as atelectasis and postoperative fever were deleted, even though mentioned by the authors. The resulting figures, 0.7% mortality and 12.8% morbidity, therefore, are likely to be minimal estimates.

TABLE 35-14. Staging Classification (CS and PS): Typical Examples

PATIENT	EXPLANATION
1. CS IB PS $IIIB_{S-H-N+M-}$	Patient has clinical Stage I disease with systematic symptoms and at laparotomy was found to have positive para-aortic nodes. Spleen, liver and bone marrow biopsies were negative.
2. CS IIA PS $IIIA_{S+H-N-M}$	Patient 2 had clinical Stage II disease without systemic symptoms. The spleen was positive at laparotomy. Liver, node and bone marrow biopsies were negative.
3. CS IIIB PS $IVB_{S+H+N+M-}$	Patient 3 had clinical Stage III disease with systemic symptoms. The spleen, liver and nodes were positive at laparotomy. The marrow biopsy was negative.
4. CS IIA PS $IA_{S-,H-,N-,M-}$	Patient 4 had positive cervical node biopsy and an enlarged spleen. At laparotomy, the spleen, liver, nodes and marrow were negative.

CS = clinical staging; PS = pathologic staging; N = lymph nodes (other than primary); H = liver; L = lung; P = pleura; S = spleen; M = marrow; O = osseous; D = skin

TABLE 35-15. Complications of Staging Laparotomy for Hodgkin's Disease

PATIENT NUMBER	MORTALITY	MORBIDITY			TOTAL COMPLICATIONS
		Significant	*Severe*	*Contributed to death*	
99	0	21 (21%)	1 (1%)	2 (2%)	24 (24%)
291	0	23 (8%)	6 (2%)	1 (0.3%)	30 (10%)
30	2 (6.6%)	2 (6.6%)	4 (13.3%)	–	8 (27)%
81	1 (1.3%)	–	1 (1.3%)	–	2 (2.6%)
54	1 (1.9%)	4 (7.4%)	–	–	5 (9.3%)
TOTAL 555	4 (0.7%)	50 (9%)	12 (2.2%)	3 (0.5%)	69 (12.8%)*

Significant morbidity—includes significant infectious complications, wound dehiscence, axilliary thrombophlebitis

Severe morbidity—(life threatening) includes pulmonary emboli, complications requiring re-exploration, ulcers with gastrointestinal hemorrhage

Contributed to death—as stated by authors

* Not considered in morbidity figures are complications such as atelectasis and postoperative fever

(Adapted from Young, RC, Anderson T, DeVita VT: The treatment of Hodgkin's disease: emphasizing programs at the Clinical Center, National Institutes of Health. Curr Probl Cancer 1(7):1–29, 1977)

Staging Laparotomy and Splenectomy in Children

Staging laparotomy and splenectomy in children has been advocated by some investigators because of the increased need for accurate staging to avoid the deleterious effects of extensive radiation therapy or prolonged chemotherapy. Recent studies of the procedure, performed in the pediatric age group, indicate a nonlethal complication rate of 8%, similar to that observed in the adult population.[196] Of great concern, however, is the increased incidence of severe, sudden, overwhelming infection seen in children after staging laparotomy and splenectomy. Studies indicate an incidence of 10% to 20% for this late and often catastrophic complication.[197,198] The risk of developing these complications increases as the age decreases below 10 years. Until the results of ongoing studies demonstrate that knowledge resulting from staging laparotomy in children improves survival, it seems prudent to be very selective in the use of such a procedure for individual patients in the pediatric age group.

Staging Laparotomy and the Effect on Subsequent Radiotherapy and Chemotherapy

Laparotomy with splenectomy has been advocated because it has been suggested that removal of the spleen will enable the patient to tolerate radiotherapy or chemotherapy more easily. It has been suggested further that such increased tolerance to therapy might be expected to improve response to therapy and survival. Data on these points are not yet conclusive. Begent and Wiltshaw found minimal effects of splenectomy on the tolerance to 3400 rad to 4300 rad administered to a mantle field.[199] In contrast, Salzman and Kaplan found that splenectomy led to improved peripheral blood counts, shortened the time of treatment, and improved ability to complete a projected course of 4400 rad of total nodal radiation.[200] However, even in that report, appropriate therapy was completed finally in all patients, regardless of the whether the spleen had been removed or not. Panettiere and Coltman suggested that splenectomy enabled administration of greater amounts of combination chemotherapy in a shorter period of time with resultant higher blood counts.[201] At first they postulated that this effect might result in an enhanced response rate. A recent reanalysis of these data indicates that there is no improvement in response rate or survival between the group undergoing splenectomy and those who did not have the operation.[202] Studies at the National Cancer Institute on the effect of splenectomy on the tolerance to combination chemotherapy also indicate that the total dose of drugs, the time required to complete six cycles of treatment, and the portion of patients entering and remaining in complete remission are not significantly different between patients who underwent splenectomy and those who did not, although peripheral leukocyte and platelet counts were higher prior to each cycle of drug treatment in patients whose spleen had been removed.[203] At present there appears to be no evidence that splenectomy *per se* in patients without hypersplenism, improves the ability to administer chemotherapy, increases the response rate, or alters the survival rate.[171] Laparotomy does, however, treat the involved spleen. The reduction on the radiation field may avoid irradiation of a significant portion of the stomach, intestine, and left kidney.

Patterns of Anatomic Distribution

Figure 35-8 illustrates the frequency of sites of involvement by Hodgkin's disease in 285 unselected, consecutive cases from Stanford University who underwent routine laparotomy.[181] Only three patients had mesenteric lymph node involvement at the time of laparotomy, in striking contrast to the frequency with which nearby lumbar para-aortic nodes are involved with disease. The rarity of epitrochlear and popliteal lymph node involvement in Hodgkin's disease compared to the other lymphomas has been mentioned previously. Hilar lymph nodes were involved in about 20% of the cases in which mediastinal lymphadenopathy was present. The spleen was the most common site of intra-abdominal involvement and often was undetected on clinical examination.

A remarkably low frequency of involvement of the tonsil and Waldeyer's ring occurs in Hodgkin's disease, in contrast to the other lymphomas. The lungs are rarely involved with Hodgkin's disease, *per se,* without involvement of the hilar lymph nodes first, which is a consequence of involvement of

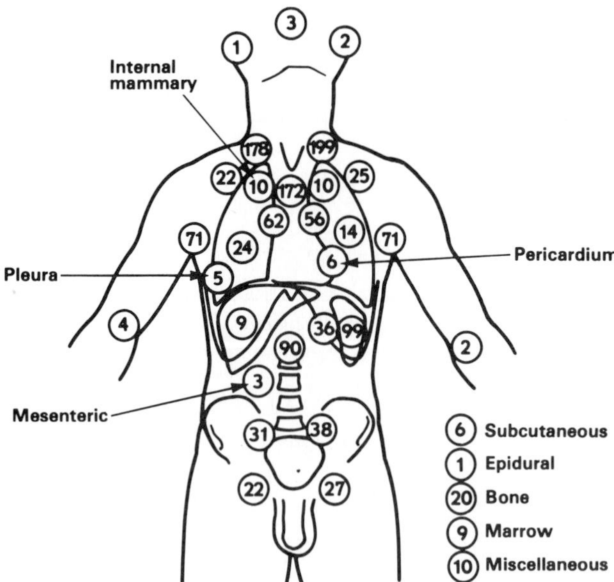

FIG. 35-8. Hodgkin's disease showing the anatomic distribution of sites of involvement in 285 consecutive, unselected, previously untreated cases. (Adapted from Kaplan HS, Dorfman RF, Nelson TS et al: Staging laparotomy and splenectomy in Hodgkin's disease: Analysis of indications and patterns of involvement in 285 consecutive, unselected patients. Natl Cancer Inst Monogr 36:291, 1973)

the mediastinal lymph nodes.[129] When mediastinal or hilar adenopathy is evident, whole chest tomography will, on occasion (±3.5%), demonstrate involvement of pulmonary parenchyma undetected by routine chest roentgenograms. Invasion of the pleura by Hodgkin's disease may occur with or without pulmonary parenchymal involvement, but is almost invariably associated with prior or concomitant mediastinal lymphadenopathy. It is difficult to diagnose Hodgkin's disease in pleural fluid. Pleural effusions with low specific gravity, and low protein content are usually simple transudates. Neither these, nor exudative pleural effusions, can be regarded as indicative of pleural invasion by Hodgkin's disease. It is imperative to obtain histologic confirmation either with the Cope pleural biopsy needle or by open thoracotomy and biopsy. Involvement of the pericardium occurs as a result of direct invasion from mediastinal adenopathy.

The liver is rarely involved with Hodgkin's disease in the absence of splenic invasion. The risk of liver involvement increases to 28% as the size of the involved spleen increases. Liver involvement is unusual in patients who have normal size spleens, even if they are involved with Hodgkin's disease (<0.5%).[129,171]

Bone marrow involvement with Hodgkin's disease is associated with extensive tumor and usually with systemic symptoms.[204,205] It is not often associated with leukopenia, anemia, or thrombocytopenia. An elevated serum alkaline phosphatase may give some hint of the involvement of the bone marrow. It has been conclusively demonstrated that it is necessary to biopsy the bone marrow either by an open surgical technique or by the use of a Westerman–Jensen cutting needle. Bone marrow involvement may be associated with diffuse fibrosis of the marrow or may be evidenced by focal involvement. The diagnosis can be made in the absence of characteristics of Sternberg–Reed cells by identification of the mononuclear variant of these cells.

The bones are often involved when patients have advancing systemic disease but, on occasion, local invasion of bone adjacent to massive adenopathy may be seen. Osteolytic lesions are the commonest manifestation, but a diffuse osteoblastic increase in bone density is more characteristic of Hodgkin's disease, although less frequent than osteolytic lesions. Radioisotopic bone scans may reveal focal areas of increased uptake when conventional radiographs are normal.[206] Involvement of bone should not be equated with involvement of bone marrow unless there is evidence of widely disseminated disease. Mussoff and colleagues have pointed out that there are well-documented cases of long disease-free survivals in patients with isolated bone lesions when treated appropriately with radiotherapy.[207]

Involvement of the skin, subcutaneous tissue, and breast with Hodgkin's disease can occur as a result of advancing systemic disease.[208] It is most often noted in conjunction with massive involvement of the lymph nodes draining the region.

Hodgkin's disease may rarely invade the central nervous system.[209] Invasion of the epidural space can occur by extension through the intervertebral foramina from para-aortic lymph node masses, usually in the dorsal or lumbar spine regions, although direct invasion can occur from involved vertebra or compression of nutrient blood vessels. The process is usually clinically silent until significant compression of either nerve roots or spinal cord itself becomes evident. Pain is usually the prominent feature but often it is accompanied by numbness and paresthesias.[210]

Unlike other malignant lymphomas, Hodgkin's disease rarely arises in the gastrointestinal tract. In the series reported from Stanford, there were no instances of involvement of the gastrointestinal tract at the time of initial diagnosis.[129] Nonetheless, there are well-documented instances of Hodgkin's disease involving the esophagus, stomach, and small intestine. Likewise, involvement of the genitourinary tract is seldom clinically evident during the course of the disease. Compression of the urinary drainage tracts may occur as a result of lymph node enlargement, and nephrotic syndrome has been reported as a result of compression of the renal blood supply.

An unusual complication of Hodgkin's disease is lipoid nephrosis, which may occur at a time when no other clinical manifestations or persistence of recurrence of lymphoma can be detected.[211,212]

STAGING OF THE NON-HODGKIN'S LYMPHOMAS

In contrast to Hodgkin's disease, patients with the other lymphomas do not commonly have localized disease.[213] This realization has influenced the approach to staging. This information has actually been available from therapeutic data for some time. Table 35-16 illustrates the results of treatment reported in several old series.[214] Patients in the studies referred to were staged without lymphangiograms, CT scans, ultrasound and laparotomy, or laparoscopy. The major point illustrated in Table 35-16 is that only 20% of the total number of patients seen at the institutions shown had localized disease, even with the crude staging techniques available at

TABLE 35-16. Survival of Patients with Non-Hodgkin's Lymphoma—Crude Survival Rates (Percent)

	CLINICALLY LOCALIZED (Stage I)				ALL STAGES	
AUTHOR	*Total Number of Cases*	*5 Year*	*10 Year*	*15 Year*	*Total Number of Cases*	*5 Year*
Craver	–	–	–	–	239	26
Rosenburg	245	47	–	–	1269	28
Peters	102	51	43	36	415	26
Easson	194	48	43	43	716	30

TABLE 35-17. Change in Patient Stage During Sequential Work-up; 170 Consecutively Staged, Previously Untreated Patients with Non-Hodgkin's Lymphoma—Percent of Patients Each Stage After Indicated Procedure

	STAGE I	STAGE II	STAGE III	STAGE IV
Clinical stage on referral	13	21	42	24
After lymphogram	8	15	54	24
After bone marrow	7	13	33	48
After closed liver biopsies	6	11	25	58
After laparotomy	6	8	21	65

(Adapted from Chabner BA, Johnson RE, Young RC et al: Sequential nonsurgical and surgical staging of non-Hodgkin's lymphoma. Ann Intern Med 85:149–154, 1976)

the time. Long-term followup, after only local treatment, indicated that, at best, half of those 20% had prolonged disease free survival. This led to the conclusion that 10% or less of patients had truly localized tumors, regardless of the histologic subtype.

Because of the divergent clinical features of patients with non-Hodgkin's lymphoma, no rigid or routine staging plan is appropriate for all patients. The staging classifications and staging procedures used in Hodgkin's disease are used for the non-Hodgkin's lymphomas, although they are less applicable because of the high incidence of extra nodal sites of origin in patients with non-Hodgkin's lymphoma (Tables 35-12 and 35-13). In particular, the role of staging laparotomy, a morbid and expensive procedure, requires even more careful consideration in the staging of the non-Hodgkin's lymphoma. The technique of staging laparotomy is similar to that described previously for the patients with Hodgkin's disease, except that greater care must be taken to inspect the mesentary, porta hepatis, and splenic pedicle, since lymph tissues in these areas are much more frequently involved in patients with non-Hodgkin's lymphomas.[215,217] The abdominal cavity should be washed with saline and samples obtained for cytologic evaluation as this may be the only site of intra-abdominal disease.

While the Ann Arbor staging scheme is extremely useful in defining the patient composition in clinical trials (Table 35-11) there exists considerable uncertainty at present as to whether the distinction between the various stages in patients with non-Hodgkin's lymphoma is as prognostically important in certain histologic groups as it is for Hodgkin's disease. For example, the distinction between Stage III and Stage IV non-Hodgkin's lymphoma is of little importance in determining therapy since Stage III disease is rarely curable with total nodal radiotherapy as it is in Hodgkin's disease.[218] Certain other factors, not explicitly recognized by the Ann Arbor classification, such as the bulk of the tumor and the specific sites of organ involvement in certain histologic subtypes may have a more profound influence on the prognosis than does the distinction between Stage III and Stage IV disease.

The results of a study of 170 consecutively staged and previously untreated patients with non-Hodgkin's lymphoma at the National Cancer Institute, are shown in Table 35-17.[213] Of particular importance is that 34% of patients were Stage I or II at the time of referral to the National Cancer Institute. Lymphangiography decreased this number to 23%, bone marrow biopsy further decreased it to 20%, and liver biopsies and laparotomy decreased it to 14%, leaving as Stage I and II only five of 81 patients (6.3%) with nodular lymphoma and 12 of 40 (30%) with diffuse histiocytic lymphoma. Thus, rigorous staging even before laparotomy placed virtually all patients with nodular lymphoma in advanced categories of disease (Stage III or IV). A substantial number of patients with limited disease was found only in those with histiocytic lymphoma. The frequency of liver involvement in patients undergoing a sequential liver biopsy protocol was 63 of 98, or 64%. In the complete series of 170 patients, liver involvement was documented in 73, or 43%. The sequence of tests was abbreviated in 72 patients. Liver was the only site of organ disease in 30 patients (18%) while bone marrow was the only site in 22 patients (13%).

CLINICAL STAGING

Clinical staging should be performed on all patients with non-Hodgkin's lymphoma and should include careful history, physical examination, blood counts and chemistries, and radiologic studies as indicated for Hodgkin's disease in Tables

TABLE 35-18. Yield of Non-Surgical Procedures in Staging Non-Hodgkin's Lymphoma*

	LYMPHOGRAM		BONE MARROW BIOPSY		PERCUTANEOUS LIVER BIOPSY		PERITONEOSCOPY LIVER BIOPSY	
	No. + /no.tested	*Percent*	*No. + /no. tested*	*Percent*	*No. + /no. tested*	*Percent*	*No. + /no. tested*	*Percent*
Nodular								
PDL	38/42	90	19/48	40	14/45	31	6/28	21
Mixed	18/20	90	11/24	46	4/21	21	7/17	41
Hist	6/7	86	1/7	14	0/6	0	3/6	50
TOTAL	62/69	90	31/79	39	18/72	25	16/51	32
Diffuse								
WDL	5/5	100	6/6	100	2/4	50	0/1	0
PDL	10/16	63	15/28	54	5/15	33	5/7	71
Mixed	6/7	86	2/6	33	1/4	25	2/5	40
Hist	21/37	57	6/39	15	2/33	5	3/26	12
Stem	3/3	100	4/7	57	0/3	0	0/1	0
TOTAL	45/68	66	33/86	38	10/59	17	10/40	25

* WDL = well-differentiated lymphocytic; PDL = poorly differentiated lymphocyctic; Mixed = mixed lymphocyctic-histiocytic; Hist = histiocytic; Stem = pleomorphic or stem cell lymphoma

35-12 and 35-13.[219] Patients should be questioned about the date that the lymph node enlargement was first noted and the rate of subsequent tumor growth, as this information may influence the choice of therapy and, indeed, even the decision to institute treatment in patients with NPDL (follicular small cleaved cell) of Rappaport. As with Hodgkin's disease, the recording of all the sites of involvement of lymph nodes should be meticulous. In contrast to Hodgkin's disease, however, certain clinical correlations must be made during the physical examination. Preauricular nodal enlargement is often associated with disease in the Waldeyer's ring area, which is uncommon in Hodgkin's disease. Indirect laryngoscopy is an absolute requirement of the staging workup. Primary lesions in extranodal sites such as bone or skin are frequently associated with involvement of regional nodes. Patients with skin lesions that occur as primary or secondary lesions often have multiple cutaneous lesions which may be remote from one another. Thus, a careful inspection of the skin and biopsy of suspicious lesions is necessary, especially in patients with diffuse lymphomas.

The correlation between peripheral blood counts and marrow involvement by lymphoma is poor. Some abnormality in blood counts is found in only 37% of patients with bone marrow infiltration by lymphoma.[220] Approximately one-half of patients with abnormal blood counts will not even have bone marrow involvement on biopsy. Examination of the peripheral smear in patients with non-Hodgkin's lymphoma may yield evidence of malignant cells in approximately 15% of patients, primarily those with poorly differentiated lymphocytic lymphomas (nodular or diffuse). Chest roentgenograms yield positive information in 26% of patients. The most frequent abnormalities are hilar or mediastinal adenopathies, which occur in only 18% of patients (pleural effusions 8% and parenchymal lesions 4%). Parenchymal lesions and pleural effusions require pathologic verification. A chylous or transudative effusion which lacks malignant cells does not change the pathologic stage of the patient. As in Hodgkin's disease, pulmonary parenchymal lesions are usually associated with concurrent hilar lymph node involvement and, if they involve only one hemithorax, they are considered to be an extension from the lymph nodes and do not necessarily change the patient's stage. Full lung tomograms are usually not needed in the search for parenchymal nodes in the presence of a completely normal chest roentgen film in view of the infrequency of parenchymal disease in these patients (<2%) but should be done on any patient with extensive mediastinal or hilar adenopathy. Routine roentgenographic studies of bone have largely been replaced by bone scanning, a technique with greater sensitivity. Bone lesions are particularly common in patients with diffuse histiocytic lymphoma. In a recent series from the National Cancer Institute, ten of 40 patients, or 25%, with this diagnosis had bone lesions detected radiologically.[213,221,222] All ten of these lesions were seen on bone scan, while bone films showed the lesions in only eight patients. Thus, as an initial procedure it is unnecessary to do both bone roentgen films and scans. A positive bone scan should be confirmed by plain films and biopsied if possible.

Bipedal lymphangiography is a particularly valuable procedure in the staging of non-Hodgkin's lymphoma. Filling defects, or absence of filling, with collateral lymphatic drainage are signs of malignant disease, although less specific for lymphoma. An accurate assessment of abdominal lymph nodes has been reported in 83% to 90% of patients studied in three large series in which the roentgenographic interpretations were verified by laparotomy.[223-226] In patients with a negative study, 20% to 30% had involvement with tumor at laparotomy. A striking feature of the non-Hodgkin's lymphoma is that the frequency of retroperitoneal nodal involvement as demonstrated by lymphangiography varies sharply with histiologic type and ranges from about 90% for patients with nodular types of disease to 57% of those with diffuse histiocytic lymphoma (Table 35-18).[213] Most patients with positive lymphograms also have generalized palpable adenopathy, so that an advance in stage only occurs in 10% of the patients as a result of a positive lymphangiogram.

The lymphangiogram is also an accurate predictor of the chances of finding intra-abdominal lymphoma in extranodal sites, or in splenic, portal, or mesenteric lymph nodes. In the National Cancer Institute series, 81% of patients with a positive lymphangiogram had disease in liver or in lymph nodes outside the para-aortic chain or in ascites fluid.[213] Only 18% of patients with negative lymphangiograms had similar findings at laparotomy. The group at Stanford has shown a similar positive correlation between lymphangiogram and mesenteric lymph node involvement.

These findings have important implications for staging and treatment. There appears to be little reason, aside from research considerations, for undertaking routine staging laparotomy in patients with non-Hodgkin's lymphoma with positive lymphograms, in view of the high likelihood of disease in sites outside traditional radiation ports. Since widespread clinical disease often is present, and lymphangiography only changes the clinical stage in 10% of patients, consideration should even be given to using other modes of diagnosing tumor involvement of retroperitoneal lymph nodes, such as the CT scan or sonography, particularly in patients who have significant pulmonary disease or who are elderly.

^{67}Ga scanning is of some value in patients with histiocytic lymphomas, in whom 60% to 80% of involved nodal sites can be visualized.[227-229] In the better differentiated lymphocytic lymphomas, this test is quite unreliable, with less than 50% of nodal sites known to be involved by tumor detected by the scan. Lesions in or near the liver may be obscured by the normal accumulation of ^{67}Ga in the bowel. Iliac lymph nodes are difficult to interpret because of the usual accumulation of ^{67}Ga in the cecum and sigmoid colon. Thus ^{67}Ga scans are a poor substitute for lymphangiography or other tests such as the CT scan and sonography.

In the largest comparative series using the CT scan published to date, Best and colleagues found that only nine of 45 patients with a negative CT scan and a negative lymphangiogram had positive abdominal nodes at laparotomy.[230,231] Two patients with a positive CT scan but with negative lymphangiography had positive lymph nodes at surgery. In addition, CT scans appear to provide a true estimate of the size of the involved nodes which are often underestimated by lymphangiography. CT scans detect abnormal nodes in the mesentery, porta hepatis, and splenic hilum, areas that are commonly involved in patients with non-Hodgkin's lymphoma. Thus, the CT scan may be an acceptable substitute for lymphangiography when the latter procedure cannot be obtained, although like lymphangiography, CT scanning has a considerable false-negative rate.

BONE MARROW EVALUATION

One of the major findings of exhaustive staging studies, and indeed an important reason for the decline of interest in staging laporatoy in non-Hodgkin's lymphoma, is the approximately 50% incidence of bone marrow and hepatic involvement.[213] The incidence of bone marrow metastasis in lymphoma is highest in patients with the lymphocytic lymphomas, nodular or diffuse, (40%–100%, depending on the specific type, Table 35-18) and lowest in those with diffuse histiocytic lymphoma (5%–15%). Each subtype of disease tends to have a identifiable pattern of bone marrow involvement.[219] Patients with NPDL had a predominance of para-trabecular location of tumor while in patients with diffuse poorly differentiated tumors involvement assumes a more diffuse pattern. Bone marrow metastases in patients with diffuse histiocytic and diffuse mixed lymphoma also occur in a diffuse pattern and may be associated with focal or diffuse myelofibrosis. While bone marrow involvement is less frequent in diffuse histiocyte lymphoma, its detection is important because of its strong correlation with later spread of disease to the central nervous system.[232] Cytologic examination of the spinal fluid should be performed in all patients with diffuse types of lymphoma with bone marrow involvement, since prophylactic therapy of the CNS is indicated in such patients.[233] As with Hodgkin's disease, aspiration of the bone marrow is inadequate for staging purposes. In view of the clinical importance of bone marrow evaluation, and the focal nature of metastases, more than one biopsy should be obtained for evaluation. For patients having two biopsies, between 10% and 20% will have positive findings in only one biopsy. Assuming an even chance of obtaining the positive biopsy on the first attempt, a second biopsy should increase the number of positives by 5% to 10%. Overall, bone marrow biopsy can be expected to advance the stage in approximately 25% of patients to Stage IV, since some of those with marrow disease will have previously been classified as Stage IV on the basis of other extranodal sites. The shift to Stage IV occurs predominantly in patients with Stage III disease and in those with NPDL and DWDL lymphomas. In these patients, it is then unnecessary to proceed with further staging unless documentation of liver involvement will influence the choice of therapy. In most clinical situations this is not the case.

Intensive efforts to identify hepatic metastases in non-Hodgkin's lymphoma have led to the recognition of a surprisingly high incidence of involvement in some categories of disease. This is also illustrated in Table 35-18.[213,219] The yield increases as the size and number of biopsy specimens increase. Percutaneous biopsy reveals disease in approximately 30% of patients with NPDL or DPDL, but in only 6% of patients with diffuse histiocytic lymphoma. Peritoneoscopy directed biopsies add an additional 30% after a negative percutaneous biopsy. Laparotomy in patients having a negative biopsy by a nonsurgical technique (percutaneous biopsy or biopsy at time of peritoneoscopy) reveals an additional 20% positive liver biopsies, primarily in patients with NPDL who have a positive lymphangiogram prior to biopsy. By all biopsy techniques patients with diffuse histiocytic lymphoma have a much lower incidence of liver metastases than the other major categories of disease.

In view of the above results, the discussion of staging laparotomy in the non-Hodgkin's lymphoma takes on an entirely different meaning. While as in Hodgkin's disease, it has enhanced our understanding of the behavior of the non-Hodgkin's lymphoma, it should never be performed in general practice as a routine staging procedure. Because patient's with non-Hodgkin's lymphoma generally are older than those with Hodgkin's disease, postoperative complications are more common. While surgical mortality is approximately 0.5%, significant morbidity, primarily pneumonia, pulmonary embolism, pancreatitis, subdiaphragmatic abscesses, or gastrointestinal bleeding has been reported in 11% to 40% of patients in three larger series.[223–226]

Thus, the primary factor which accounts for the limited need for laparotomy in non-Hodgkin's lymphoma is the high yield of less morbid procedures and the recognition that precise definition of involvement probably has limited importance in treatment planning for most patients. Since most patients have easily demonstrated Stage III and IV disease, and these patients are treated with chemotherapy in most centers, routine staging laparotomy is obviously not indicated. Staging laparotomy could be considered for the 20% of patients who remain in clinical Stage I or II, after sequential staging tests, but only if they are to be subsequently treated with radiotherapy alone rather than systemic treatment. The procedure has its greatest usefulness in patients with diffuse histiocytic lymphoma, since fully one-third of this group remain in Stage I or Stage II after a complete sequence of staging procedures, including laparotomy, and may be candidates for local radiotherapy.

IMMUNOLOGIC ABNORMALITIES IN PATIENTS WITH LYMPHOMA

HODGKIN'S DISEASE

The history of the immunologic abnormalities in Hodgkin's disease is linked closely to tuberculosis. In 1928, Ewing, observing an incidence of tuberculosis of around 20% in patients with Hodgkin's disease, commented that "In New York State, where the disease is very common, tuberculosis follows Hodgkin's disease like a shadow."[233] That this heightened susceptibility might be related to an immunologic problem in Hodgkin's disease was independently noted by Parker and colleagues (1932) and Steiner (1934).[93,104] Parker noted that in contrast to the high reactivity of the general population at the time to tuberculin testing, 27 of 33 patients with Hodgkin's disease studied exhibited no cutaneous reaction to either human or avian tuberculosis antigen and 20 of 28 patients remained unresponsive despite a tenfold increase in the dose of tuberculin protein. Both investigators noted that the tuberculin test was not infrequently negative, even in the presence of active tuberculosis. These observations were confirmed by Dubin in 1947, who reported on positive tuberculin tests in only one of 38 patients with Hodgkin's disease in an area where skin test postivity in the general population was 52%.[234]

The first systematic studies of the capacity of patients with Hodgkin's disease to react to battery of antigens were reported in 1956 by Scheir and his associates.[235] These investigators studied a series of 43 patients with Hodgkin's disease and 79 normal and disease controls. They reported that delayed reactivity to purified tuberculin, *Trichophyton gypseum, candida albicans,* and mumps skin test antigens were severely depressed in patients with Hodgkin's disease. They reported no correlation with skin test response and severity of disease or type of treatment. Similar studies were reported by Lamb and associates, who, in addition, first suggested that the absence of response to tuberculin skin testing in patients in good condition might indicate that anergy was related to the primary disease process itself.[236]

The first definitive study of the question of the relationship of anergy to the stage of the disease awaited the modern era of staging and was reported by Brown and associates from the National Cancer Institute in 1967.[237] They reported a series of 50 previously untreated patients staged with the aid of lymphangiography and other modern diagnostic tests. They compared the skin test response to a battery of antigens in these patients to 17 healthy individuals and found that 28 of 50 patients (56%) gave a positive response to one or more antigens while all controls responded. They noted, however, that the response to two or more antigens in patients in Stage I disease (five of eight, or 63%) was similar to controls (17 of 25, or 68%) and responsiveness decreased with increasing stage. The same relationship was noted in seven of eight Stage I patients tested with dinitrochlorobenzene (DNCB), a chemical allergen. Brown and associates reasoned, in contrast to the data reported by Sokal and Primikiros, that anergy was the consequence of progressive Hodgkin's disease.[238] A conflict arose when data reported by Aisenberg, and later by the Stanford group, indicated a lack of responsiveness to skin tests even in patients with early stage disease.[239,240] This dispute was later settled when the technique of skin sensitization with DNCB was standardized and only previously untreated patients were studied. The main reason for the differences in the reported data was related to the fact that patients reported by Aisenberg, and from Stanford, had received radiation to the lymph node areas draining the skin test sites. Since then, experimental induction of anergy by local radiotherapy of axillary lymph nodes draining the sensitized limb has been convincingly demonstrated in rodents in 1970 by Eltringham and Weissman. Recently, the Stanford group has shown that responsiveness to DNCB in patients with early stage disease is not an "all or none" phenomenon.[242] At lower doses that sensitized all normal individuals, less than half of the previously untreated patients with Stage I disease responded.

The studies at the National Cancer Institute have been extended by Young and colleagues and reported in 1972.[243] These authors confirm the findings of Brown and associates.[237] The most significant additional observation from the latter study of 103 patients is that cutaneous anergy did not influence prognosis as measured by response to treatment, relapse rate, and survival within a given stage. These authors also reported that patients who were anergic prior to treatment regained skin test sensitivity while in remission to recall antigens to which they previously failed to respond, providing further fuel for the argument that anergy was a secondary and reversible aspect of Hodgkin's disease. King and colleagues subsequently reported that patients in remission after chemotherapy and radiotherapy react normally to recall antigens, but not to neoantigens, such as keyhole limpet hemocyanin (KLH) and DNCB.[244,245] Both King and colleagues and Fuks and colleagues have reported an increased tendency to respond to neoantigens with time (1 year to 3 years) after either chemotherapy or radiotherapy.[246] Sokal and colleagues have attempted to convert PPD-negative patients to positivity by vaccination with BCG and have succeeded in some cases.[247] They reported a striking difference in survival in favor of patients who converted. Since these patients were not treated with the more effective modern programs, however, these good results seem more likely related to the variable clinical condition of the patients in the study group. Others have reported that the delayed homograft rejection is a manifestation of anergy in patients with Hodgkin's disease.[248-250]

Lymphocytopenia is a common concomitant of Hodgkin's disease. It was first described by Bunting in 1914 and his observation was extended by Wisman and Rosenthal in 1936.[251-253] In 1965, Aisenberg analyzed lymphocyte counts in 50 consecutive fatal cases of Hodgkin's disease, both at the onset of the disease and during the last 6 months of their lives.[254] Only two of the near-terminal patients had lymphocyte counts in the normal range (1500/mm^3 to 3000/mm^3). The study by Brown and associates reported lymphocytopenia in 19 of their 50 patients (38%).[237] In general, there was a relationship between advancing stage and decreased skin test reactivity with more severe lymphocytopenia. This question was examined more definitively at NCI in the 1972 report on 103 previously untreated patients.[243] This study showed significant differences in peripheral lymphocyte counts between Stage I and Stages III and IV; and Stage II and Stage IV. Anergic patients had significantly lower lymphocyte counts than those in whom the reactions to all major skin test antigens were positive. This was particularly significant in reference to reactions to mumps and DNCB. The NCI workers also showed that the histologic subtype was important. Those patients with nodular sclerosing Hodgkin's disease had significantly higher lymphocyte counts than those with lymphocyte depleted disease.

Further information on the status of delayed hypersensitivity of patients with Hodgkin's disease has been provided by analyzing the response of patients' lymphocytes *in vitro* to phytohemagglutinin (PHA), pokeweed antigen, or antigens such as tuberculin and vaccinia. The first definitive studies in Hodgkin's disease were those of Hersh and Oppenheim in 1965.[255] They showed a striking impairment in the capacity of peripheral blood lymphocytes from patients with Hodgkin's disease to undergo lymphoblastic transformation after *in vitro* incubation with tuberculin or vaccinia. The study of Brown and colleagues correlated the lymphocyte transformation response to clinical stage and anergy.[237] Once again, lymphocyte transformation was normal in patients with Stage I disease. The poorest response was in patients with Stage IV disease. Brown and collegues did not observe any correlation between the capacity of lymphocytes to transform and the peripheral lymphocyte count.

Refinement of the technique has since revealed unambiguous abnormalities of PHA stimulation response, even in patients with the earliest stages of disease. Matchett and associates noted good initial *in vitro* lymphocyte response in the first 2 days in patients with localized disease, but these responses were not sustained after 4 days to 5 days.[256] These authors concluded that impaired lymphocyte function is inherent to Hodgkin's disease, even in its earliest stages.

Levy and Kaplan have reported similar results, using the uptake of tritiated leucine into stimulated lymphocytes.[247] These authors demonstrated a concentration dependent defect in *in vitro* lymphocyte response to DNCB. These results have since been confirmed by others.[257,258]

The capacity to form spontaneous E-rosettes with uncoated sheep erythrocytes, a property of T-lymphocytes, was observed by Bobrove and colleagues, to be impaired in 13 of 15 patients with untreated Hodgkin's disease, relative to the percentage of T-lymphocytes detected by another assay using cytotoxic antibody.[259] The mean percentage of E-rosette-forming cells was only 43 ± 3.9% whereas the percentage of T-lymphocytes scored by the cytotoxic assay was 63 ± 2.9%. Thus, T-lymphocytopenia cannot account for the observed defect in cell mediated immunity.

Since cells capable of inhibition or suppression of immune responses exist in the lymphoid system, investigators have searched for such an effect in Hodgkin's disease. Twomey and colleagues observed that *in vitro* stimulation of lymphocytes was increased when mononuclear cells of patients were removed by passage through glass wool.[260] Goodwin and colleagues found that the inhibitory activity of glass adherent cells in culture could be inhibited by adding indomethacin, a known prostaglandin inhibitor to cultures, leading to the suggestion that production of prostaglandin E_2 by suppression cells could be responsible for lymphocyte hyporesponsiveness.[261] Suppressor responses have now been reported by other investigators.[262,263] Other studies have demonstrated that a subpopulation of lymphocytes in patients with Hodgkin's disease appears to have membrane alterations reflected in enhanced lectin agglutinability and diminished cap formation, but no direct link has been established between these defects and impairment of cell mediated immunity. A major observation was made by Fuks and associates when they discovered that impaired E-rosette formation by lymphocytes from patients with Hodgkin's disease could be consistently restored to normal levels by short incubation in fetal calf serum and such incubation could restore lymphocyte transformation in response to PHA to normal as well.[264] Later, Fuks, Stokes, and Kaplan were able to show that depression of E-rosette formation could be produced by an extract from the spleen of patients with Hodgkin's disease.[265] The actual material proved to be a glycolipid, which is still incompletely characterized. Later, Moroz and colleagues demonstrated the presence of a blocking protein that could be released from the cell surface by incubation with levamisole, the antihelminthic drug.[266] The blocking protein appears to be apoferritin. After release by levamisole, E-rosette response of peripheral blood lymphocytes returned to normal.

Others have now had the opportunity to restudy lymphocyte responsiveness in patients with Hodgkin's disease who have been successfully treated with either radiotherapy or chemotherapy while in remission. At the National Cancer Institute, Fisher et al have shown that although the total number of circulating lymphocytes in patients who have been in remission for anywhere from 1.3 years to 12.8 years (mean, 6.5 years) was not different than normals, the percent of E-rosetting cells was significantly reduced (60.4% in controls, compared to 45.2% in disease-free Hodgkin's patients.)[267] The responses to conconavalin A and PHA were also significantly depressed when compared to normals. Even those patients whose T-cell numbers, as measured by the percent of rosetting cells, were in the normal range had depressed *in vitro* response to antigens. This decrease in E-rosetting is shown in Fig. 35-9. It can be seen that even some very long disease-free survivors had diminished E-rosetting. Fisher and colleagues found no decrease in the number of lymphocytes in the peripheral blood with easily detectable surface immunoglobulins (B-cells). Thirty-nine of 47 patients also had measurement of their serum immunoglobulins and there was no significant difference when compared to normal individuals.

To examine the question as to whether the persistent defect in T-cell function was related to the disease or type of chemotherapy the patients received, Fisher and colleagues studied a group of 16 patients with a diagnosis of diffuse histiocytic lymphoma who had been in continuous complete remission after treatment with the same chemotherapy used for the treatment of Hodgkin's disease. While the percentage of E-rosetting cells was reduced in patients with diffuse histiocytic lymphoma, their lymphocyte responsiveness to both PHA and conconavalin A was similar to normal controls. These results have led the authors to conclude that the defect in lymphocyte responsiveness in Hodgkin's disease is inherent to the disease process itself, and not a sequela of treatment. Fuks and associates reported that lymphocytopenia induced by radiotherapy returned to normal from 12 months to 111 months after the cessation of radiation treatment.[246] In their patients, however, there was a striking T-cell lymphocytopenia and a reactive B-cell lymphocytosis. They, like the NCI workers, also reported, little or no recovery of *in vitro* responsiveness of their patients' lymphocytes to either PHA or conconavalin A. They also studied mixed lymphocyte reactivity and found it markedly impaired in the first 2 years after treatment and partially restored in the next 3 years.

Similar results have been reported by Case and associates in 20 patients treated with roentgen therapy and studied while in remission from 5 years to 25 years.[268] In their study, the absolute number and percentage of T- and B-cells, as measured by surface immunoglobulins and E-rosetting, was normal but the cellular response to PHA was also significantly decreased. Identical results in a small group of successfully treated patients have been reported by King and colleagues.[245]

Taken *in toto*, the studies on delayed hypersensitivity, as measured by skin test responsiveness to recall and neoantigens, lymphocyte counts, and *in vitro* lymphocyte responsiveness to PHA and conconavalin A, as well as spontaneous E-rosetting and surface changes of lymphocytes, leave little doubt that a functional defect in T-lymphocytes occurs simultaneously with the appearance of the disease itself. This

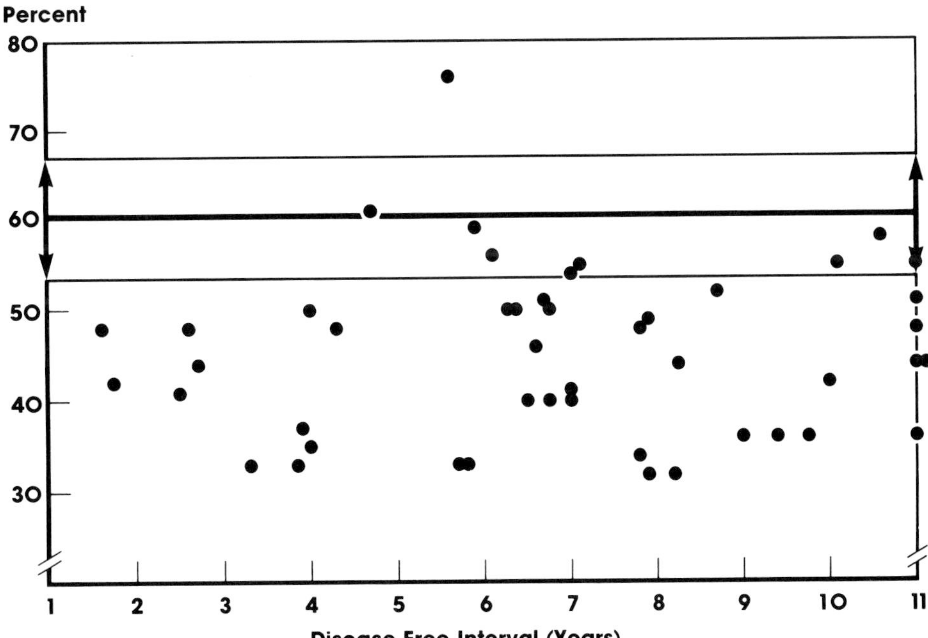

FIG. 35-9. Percent of E-rosetting cells in the peripheral blood of patients with Hodgkin's disease in remission from 1.3 to 12 years after treatment with MOPP chemotherapy.

defect in T-cell number and function appears to be aggravated by treatment, particularly radiotherapy, and persists in a variable time-dependent way with recovery. Humoral inhibition in the sera of patients with Hodgkin's disease and suppressor cell effects may be involved in the underlying mechanism of these impaired responses. This defect in T-cell function has now been shown to persist for as long as 10 years to 12 years after cessation of successful treatment. Despite this defect, skin test reactivity returns to normal after successful treatment, which may reflect a minimum number of T-cells required for skin test reactivity and dose–response relationships with antigen and lymphocyte counts. The data from the National Cancer Institute comparing results in successfullly treated DHL patients to those with Hodgkin's disease seem to provide further evidence that the defect is more disease- than treatment-related.

In contrast to the defects in delayed hypersensitivity, most studies show that antibody response and B-cell number are normal in all but the patient with most advanced Hodgkin's disease, although B-cell function is affected by therapy. In the 1956 study by Scheir, it was reported that there was a normal antibody response to mumps vaccine in 12 patients, and Kelly reported similar results in 1958.[235,258] Aisenberg and Leskowitz studied antibody response to pneumococcal polysaccharide types 1 and 2 in a series of patients with active Hodgkin's disease who were known to be unresponsive to DNCB.[269] They observed normal responses in 13 of 19 patients. The remaining six patients were considered terminal and all died within 6 months. They did note, however, that there was an abnormally rapid decline of the antibody titers in eight of the patients who had responded normally. In the study by Brown and colleagues, a normal antibody response to tuleremia antigen was noted, even though there was no evidence of delayed hypersensitivity to the tuleremia skin test.[237] As in the studies of delayed hypersensitivity, many of the older studies on antibody response in Hodgkin's disease, except that of Brown and colleagues, reported results in patients who were heavily pretreated with either radiation or drugs. Nonetheless, the data taken *in toto* suggests that B-cell function is normal in untreated patients with Hodgkin's disease. Followup studies of successfully treated patients have shown no decrease in B-cell number and in fact, in some cases, a relative B-cell lymphocytosis.[246] All these studies have shown normal quantitative immunoglobulins.

Weitzman and colleagues measured antibody response to hemophilious influenza type B in patients after splenectomy who had received radiation therapy, chemotherapy, or combinations of both.[270] Antibody titers were significantly reduced in patients receiving combined radiotherapy and chemotherapy but not significantly reduced in those who received either chemotherapy or radiotherapy alone. Untreated patients, and those studied after splenectomy, but before treatment, had normal values. Immunoglobulin levels likewise were normal in untreated patients, but chemotherapy significantly reduced levels of IgM, an effect that was potentiated in the group undergoing splenectomy. Minor and colleagues examined the response of 41 successfully treated patients, all of whom had undergone splenectomy, to pneumococcal vaccine.[271] Postimmunization antibody level was significantly lower for ten of 12 serotypes measured. Antibody recovery was time-dependent from the end of treatment, with several patients in remission for more than 3 years having normal responses. Studies by Walzer and associates have also shown significant decreases in IgM levels post splenectomy, radiotherapy, and chemotherapy which have persisted for longer than 36 months.[272]

In summary, B-cell function appears normal in untreated patients with Hodgkin's disease. Splenectomy by itself does not alter their function, but the combination of splenectomy and chemotherapy or splenectomy, chemotherapy, and radiotherapy diminishes B-cell function, as measured by antibody response to several bacterial antigens. Vaccination with pneumococcal antigen is therefore not likely to be useful in this infection prone population. In fact in the study by Minor and colleagues, pneumococcal sepsis, in one case, and meningitis in another, were reported after vaccination. These data give explanation to the high risk of sepsis in patients who are treated with aggressive combination treatment with radiotherapy and chemotherapy after undergoing staging laparotomy.

NON-HODGKIN'S LYMPHOMAS

Since the early studies of delayed hypersensitivity in lymphoma patients did not reveal distinct abnormalities in patients with non-Hodgkin's lymphomas, there have been fewer studies in these patients and data are surprisingly scarce. Interpretation of results of available studies needs to be qualifed as well since, in general, investigators have not allowed for differences among the various histologic subtypes of non-Hodgkin's lymphoma, and staging.

In 1977, Jones and colleagues studied the first group of previously untreated patients with non-Hodgkin's lymphoma, uniformly staged and classified according to the Rappaport scheme.[273] They measured peripheral lymphocyte number, serum immunoglobulins, and delayed hypersensitivity to six recall antigens. The major abnormality noted was in the group of 38 patients classified as having diffuse histiocytic lymphoma. This group exhibited marked impairments in reaction to five of the six recall antigens as well as lymphocytopenia and reduced levels of serum IgA. They also noted that within this group of patients, response to antigens was significantly improved in patients who had localized disease and no constitutional symptoms. This was the first evidence of decreased immunologic function, of the delayed hypersensitivity type, in patients with a non-Hodgkin's lymphoma. In their study of 33 patients with NPDL, they showed an impairment in response to only two specific antigens (streptokinase–streptodornase, and mumps). Reactivity to the other three antigens was normal. In spite of the B-cell origin of these lymphomas, there is not apparent consistent defect in antibody production in patients with the non-Hodgkin's lymphoma, except for the reports of decreased levels of immunoglobulins, usually of the IgM type, concomitant with the production of a monoclonal antibody spike in some patients with diffuse lymphomas.

A recent study by Avdani and associates confirms the data of Jones and colleagues.[274] They studied 101 uniformly staged patients using the Rappaport histologic classification, measuring skin test response to DNCB, PPD, candida, mumps, and streptokinase–streptodornase antigens. The reactions of DNCB and six recall antigens were found to be significantly diminished in patients with non-Hodgkin's lymphomas as compared to normal controls. Loss of skin test reactivity was greater in histiocytic types and in patients with generalized disease. IgG levels tended to be elevated. They studied eight cases of angio-immunoblastic lymphadenopathy as well and found anergy in seven of eight patients.

CLINICAL IMMUNOLOGIC DISORDERS IN LYMPHOMA PATIENTS

The commonest immunologic disorder in patients with lymphomas is a monoclonal gammopathy which has been shown by Moore and colleagues to occur in 6% to 8% of patients with diffuse lymphomas, but only 1% or less of patients with the nodular lymphomas.[278] These incidence figures reflect the origin of the former cells from the immunoglobulin-producing cells of the medullary cords (Fig. 35-1). This region is thought to be the site of origin of the cells of Waldenstrom's macroglobulinemia as well as the chronic variety of lymphocytic leukemia and diffuse, well-differentiated lymphocytic lymphomas. A monoclonal protein spike is less common in Hodgkin's disease.

In a study by Ko and Pruzansky of 1246 patients identified in a screening process to have M components in their serum, 62 were found to have lymphomas (0.05%).[276] Thirty-three of these patients had an elevated level of IgM, 20 had elevated IgG levels, five had elevated IgA levels, and one had a Bence-Jones protein spike. Fifty-four of 67 patients had diffuse lymphomas and only 13 had evidence of nodularity. Nine patients had Hodgkin's disease. An associated decrease in the normal serum globulin levels was noted in 20 patients (IgM, 16; IgG, four). Seven patients had cryoglobulinemia, five with IgM and two with IgG. Six patients had cold agglutinins identified of IgM type with anti-I specificity.

In a report by Jones in 1973, focusing on immune disorders in lymphoma patients, nine patients with Coomb's positive autoimmune hemolytic anemia (AIHA) (an incidence of 1.7%) and four cases of idiopathic thrombocytopenia purpura (ITP) (0.4%) were identifed.[277] He analyzed four additional cases of Hodgkin's disease with immune disorders previously known to him, two each with AIHA and ITP. In only two patients did the autoimmune disorder precede the diagnosis. Autoimmune hemolytic anemia was associated with splenomegaly, systemic symptoms, and, in eight of nine patients with non-Hodgkin's lymphoma of the diffuse histiocytic or lymphoblastic variety, widely disseminated disease. No patient in their series died of the autoimmune disorder, which could usually be controlled with the drugs used to treat the underlying lymphoma.

In a recent study of 71 patients with Hodgkin's disease, unexplained positive Coomb's tests were identified in seven male patients.[278] All had extensive disease (Stages III and IV) and six had constitutional symptoms. Four patients had mixed cellularity and three had nodular sclerosing Hodgkin's disease. The Coomb's test was positive at initial diagnosis in three and at the time of relapse in four. Only three patients in this group had overt hemolysis. The authors emphasized that when autoimmune hemolytic anemia occurs in lymphoma patients, it is associated with advanced stages. In their series, the antibody was characterized in three patients and all of them fulfilled the criteria for an IgG with anti-I^t specificity, as described by Booth and colleagues in 1966.[279] This antibody may be a unique antibody for Coomb's positive hemolytic anemia associated with Hodgkin's disease.

Another review of ITP associated with Hodgkin's disease added two new cases to the literature. Waddel and Cimo were able to locate only a total of 30 cases in the English literature, including those previously discussed by Jones.[280] In seven cases, no further analysis was done, as the data reported was not sufficient to characterize the syndrome. In three of the cases, the diagnosis of ITP antedated the diagnosis of lymphoma. In the remaining 23 patients, ITP always occurred either at the time or subsequent to the diagnosis. The authors pointed out several characteristic features of ITP associated with Hodgkin's disease. (1) While ITP occurs predominately in females, ITP associated with Hodgkin's disease is more common in males (15 males to eight females). (2) ITP associated with Hodgkin's disease appeared to be more severe and resistant to treatment than ITP when it occurs alone or in association with other illnesses. Only six of 23 patients responded to steroids, although six of nine patients who underwent splenectomy specifically for ITP appeared to have a good and durable response. (3) Autoimmune hemolytic anemia, a frequent concomitant of ITP occurring in other disorders, was present in only three of 23 patients in their series. (4) They also noted that ITP occurred after splenectomy had been performed for staging purposes in 11 reviewed patients including their own two patients. This indicates that the antibody responsible for thrombocytopenia can be produced in sites other than the spleen. (5) All the patients with a recorded histology had either nodular sclerosing or mixed cellularity Hodgkin's disease. (6) The majority of patients developed ITP while in remission after successful radiotherapy or chemotherapy and the occurrence of ITP did not necessarily indicate relapse. Since most reported cases occurred after splenectomy, a combination of corticosteroids and immunosuppressive drugs is required for treatment. Five of their patients were treated this way and three had an excellent response; the two remaining patients had useful responses.

RADIATION THERAPY OF HODGKIN'S DISEASE

The extreme radiation responsiveness of the lymphomas was noted shortly after the discovery of x-rays. Pusey, in 1902, reported a series of patients with Hodgkin's disease treated with radiation.[281] In the early part of the century, therapists were limited by the equipment available to them. The machines had poor depth–dose characteristics and caused extensive skin reactions, limiting their utility. Despite this, there was a great deal of interest in using radiation on this tumor. Teschendorf, Voorhoeve, and Kruchen all described therapy for such patients.[282–284] It was Gilbert who laid the foundation for the principles for modern radiation therapy.[139,140] Despite the availability of only orthovoltage radiation, Gilbert recognized the importance of treating all involved disease to the maximum dose possible if cure was to be the treatment goal. He suggested that, to the extent to which it was possible, one should treat adjacent sites, because of the frequency of adjacent recurrence. These are the principles of radiotherapy today. Gilbert's technique was followed in Toronto and reported by Peters in 1950.[141] Subsequently, she described patients as long as 20 years after treatment, indicating that patients could be cured with radiation, as there were no recurrences in those patients who were disease-free 10 years after treatment.[142] Peters also first described the staging system for the disease described earlier in this chapter. The dose to the involved areas in these reports depended on the site and extent of the disease, with higher doses given when the disease was relatively localized. The concept of irradiation of adjacent nodal groups with lower doses of radiation was utilized by Peters.[143] Easson and Russell in 1963 published a paper entitled "The Cure of Hodgkin's Disease."[285] This reported the long-term results of local treatment of both Hodgkin's disease and localized non-Hodgkin's lymphomas. The title and emphasis of the paper were that Hodgkin's disease could be cured. There were others who also reported in the early 1950s and 1960s the results of localized radiation; however, it was Henry Kaplan and his group at Stanford who systematically studied the place of radiation therapy in the treatment of Hodgkin's disease and devised new techniques using supervoltage radiation to treat the disease.[117,239–243,105] It is these pioneering studies that form the basis of much of what we know today of the curability of Hodgkin's disease. Figure 35-10 is redrawn from Kaplan to indicate that although low doses of radiation cause tumors to disappear, high doses are required to ablate them permanently.[244] Hodgkin's disease, like all other tumors, has a dose-response curve. This was a very important concept, because the prevailing attitude at the time was that, since the disease was so responsive to radiation but, of course, incurable, one should give low doses and make local nodal masses regress while "saving" the radiation tolerance for the required subsequent therapies when the disease reappeared. Such a philosophy of treatment confirmed the self-fulfilling prophecy of the incurability of Hodgkin's disease. As can be seen from the figure, when high doses were given,

FIG. 35-10. Risk of recurrence in the treatment field after radiotherapy related to dose.

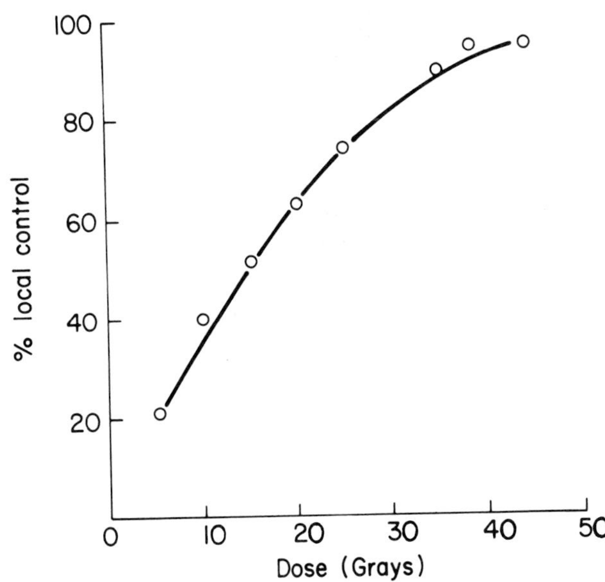

local recurrence was very uncommon. While suspected by Gilbert and Peters, the Stanford group gave evidence of the orderliness and continuity of the initial presentation of Hodgkin's disease, as well as its subsequent extension.[254] The adaptation of modern supervoltage techniques for the treatment of Hodgkin's disease for the first time allowed high doses of radiation to be given to extensive volumes, and careful beam direction and shielding allowed such treatment to be tolerated by normal tissues.

It is generally recommended that local tumor masses receive "boost therapy" to a minimum dose of 4000 rad to 4400 rad, while apparently uninvolved areas treated for subclinical disease appear to be adequately controlled with doses of 3000 rad to 3500 rad. The dose–time relationship for Hodgkin's disease is less well known. Because of normal tissue tolerance, patient acceptance, and tumor control, tumor doses of between 150 rad and 220 rad per day given five times a week appear to be most appropriate. When there is a significant interruption in the treatment then it appears that larger doses should be given.[293] Supervoltage radiation must be used in order to deliver the wide field radiation required. This has the advantages of (1) skin sparing, (2) increased depth dose, and (3) sharp beam edges with reduced lateral scatter. A basic tool for the treatment of patients with Hodgkin's disease is the modern linear accelerator providing x-ray beams in the 4 MeV to 8 MeV range. Although cobalt units can be used, conventionally available cobalt units have significant limitations. When used at distances of less than 80 cm, they tend to have poor depth–dose characteristics. They often have far less well defined beam edges, owing to the large source and short treatment distances. This latter factor causes significantly greater irradiation to adjacent and apparently shielded tissues.

Hodgkin's disease treatment may be divided into three volumes to be irradiated: the mantle, para-aortic area, and pelvis.[294] The mantle technique has been well described by the Stanford group. It is an attempt to treat in continuity the lymph nodes of the neck, axilla, and mediastinum, including the occipital and preauricular lymph nodes, in one contiguous treatment volume. In order to do this, a wide field is placed upon the patient and individually made blocks are fashioned to shield the normal tissues not under treatment. In order for this to be done accurately, not only is the supervoltage linear accelerator required but a treatment planning simulator or localizer must be available as well, which will allow the duplication of therapy fields using diagnostic quality radiation so that detailed x-rays can be made for the fabrication of the blocks. Such a simulator film is shown in Fig. 35-11 with the appropriate block outlines. The check films are made on the supervoltage machine; however, because of the radiation energy, this film, while useful for check purpose, is much less satisfactory than the simulator films. In our institution and others, these blocks conform to the divergent x-ray beam so that the edge of the field can be as sharp as possible. The mantle treatment irradiates a large volume of normal tissues and therefore care must be taken to limit the unnecessary normal tissue irradiation while at the same time assure adequate irradiation of the tumor volume. This requires careful evaluation and planning using diagnostic roentgen films, simulation, and dosimetric calculations and measurements. The normal tissue tolerance of the lung and heart have been evaluated in the course of treatment of Hodgkin's disease.[295-297] Such whole lung irradiation is used frequently when the ipsilateral hilum is involved with tumor. The whole heart should not be treated, unless there is evidence of pericardial involvement. Under normal circumstances, a significant portion of the cardiac silhouette can be shielded. Of vital importance is to be sure that the "matchline" between the mantle and the para-aortic area does not allow overlap of a portion of the spinal cord. If this is the case, the dose received can cause significant neurological damage. The treatment of the para-aortic nodes and pelvis are frequently done together as described by the Stanford group.[298,299] It is our experience that this treatment is better tolerated when divided into a para-aortic field and a separate pelvic field. Perhaps this latter is the case because the midline pelvic block used to shield the ovaries is much smaller in our case than that described by Stanford. In either circumstance the para-aortic field must be wide enough to include the para-aortic lymph nodes as demonstrated on the lymphangiogram. Most modern radiotherapeutic technique has been influenced by the results of laparotomy. As discussed earlier, laparotomy is only of value if the results may alter therapy. It allows removal of the spleen and the placement of radiopaque clips on the splenic pedicle, so that the radiotherapy field may be tailored accurately to this volume. The normal right side of the para-aortic field as shown in Fig. 35-12 does not treat the porta hepatis, and if this is to be treated, then this field must be extended laterally. The same considerations for field overlap apply between the para-aortic and pelvic field; however, these are less critical, as this overlap is placed below the level of the spinal cord. Considerations for the pelvic field include the treatment of the lymph nodes with as little radiation as possible to important sacral and pelvic bone marrow. The marrow irradiated may be greatly reduced by careful blocking and the use of linear accelerators rather than cobalt units. Adequate covering of the inguinal and femoral lymph nodes

FIG. 35-11. Simulated film for radiation treatment fields in a patient with mediastinal Hodgkin's disease. *Dark lines* indicate shielding blocks.

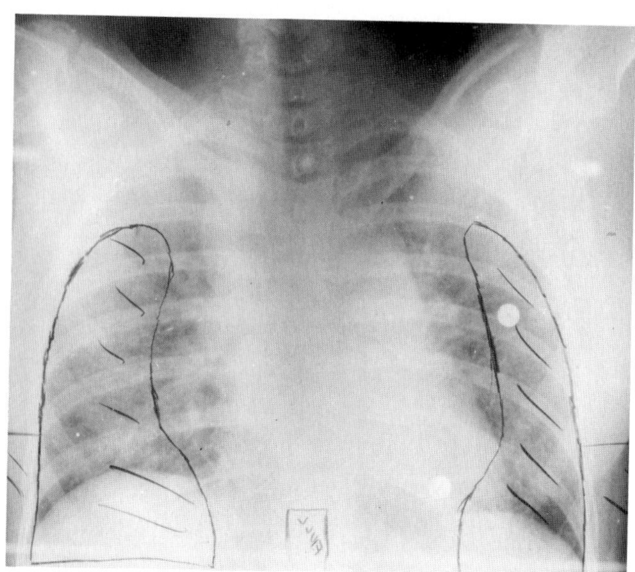

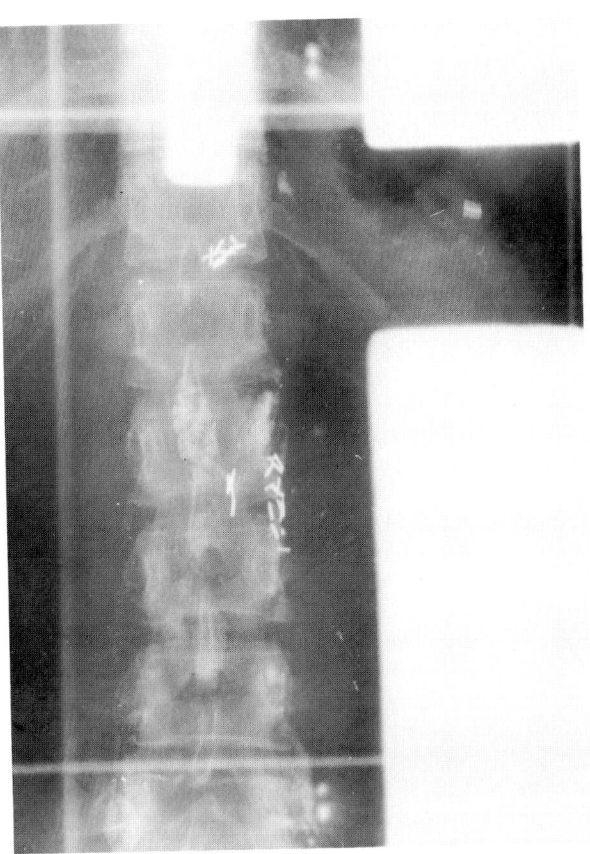

FIG. 35-12. Normal para-aortic field in treating a patient with Hodgkin's disease below the diaphragm. Field for porta hepatic nodes not involved.

must be assured and the testes should be shielded. In the case of the female, a central block can be placed and the ovaries moved to the midline by being tacked either in front or in back of the uterus. This can allow total nodal irradiation with the continuation of the menses in many patients. This technique, first described by Trueblood, is used in many institutions.[300] While individual preference in technique may have a role, most important are the general principles of careful beam definition, detailed patient positioning, use of simulators, individually constructed shielding techniques, and, finally, verification of dose, usually using thermo-luminescent dosimetry. Small technical considerations, such as the positions of the arm, can greatly influence the amount of normal tissue treated and thus must be carefully considered. While further details of radiotherapy of Hodgkin's disease are beyond the scope of this chapter, it must be emphasized that with Hodgkin's disease as with other malignancies, maximum cure with minimal complications can occur only when all the technical aspects of radiotherapy are carefully considered.

RESULTS OF RADIATION THERAPY

With the results of radiation therapy reported by Peters and associates and Easson and Russell, the question of whether or not uninvolved areas ought to be irradiated becomes an important one.[141,142,285] In 1966, Peters carefully analyzed her data in an attempt to answer this.[143] Review of these data make it difficult to prove that irradiation of the uninvolved lymph nodes in Stage I or Stage IIA disease affect the outcome. In order to study this point further, the Stanford group did a randomized prospective clinical trial (LI) which compared local irradiation to extended field irradiation in Stage I and Stage II disease.[129] This study showed no significant difference between involved field and extended field irradiation with respect to either survival or freedom from relapse. A similar national collaborative study also failed to show significant differences.[301] Both of these studies preceded, in part, the use of staging laparotomy and also failed to consider the para-aortic area as a contiguous site for supraclavicular node disease. A new trial was introduced at Stanford (HI), in which the alternatives for Stage I and Stage IIA disease involved field irradiation and total nodal irradiation (TNI). This study was started 1 year before the introduction of laparotomy at Stanford, therefore most of the patients in this study had staging laparotomy. Results of this study showed a highly significant difference in relapse-free survival in favor of TNI, although overall survival was not affected. Total nodal irradiation is far more extensive than the intended irradiation of subclinical contiguous disease in Stage I and Stage IIA patients. Surely, for supradiaphragmatic disease, pelvic irradiation might be eliminated. This would be important, as it would greatly reduce the amount of bone marrow irradiated and would limit the dose to the gonads. Such a technique for supradiaphragmatic Stage I and Stage IIA patients has been a treatment recommended at the Joint

FIG. 35-13. Survival and relapse-free survival of stage IA patients treated to the pelvic brim. Recent results from the Joint Center for Radiation Therapy, Harvard University.

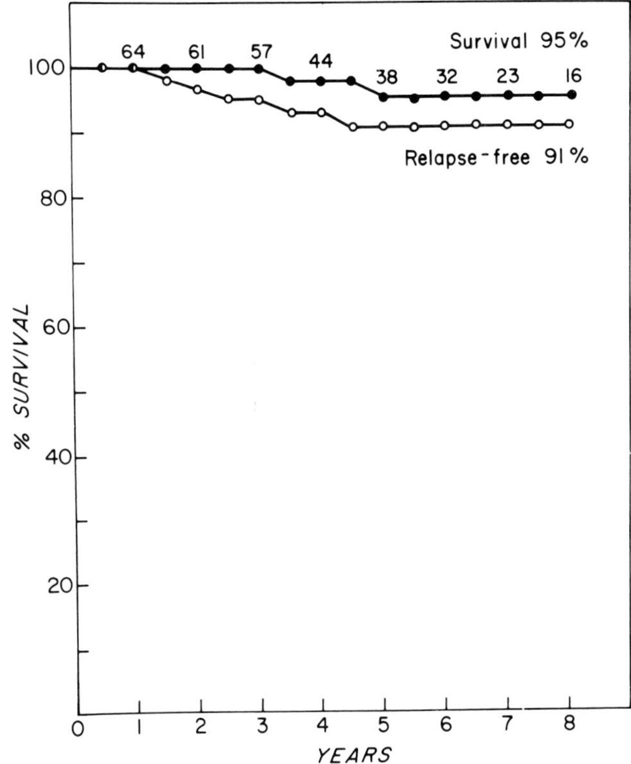

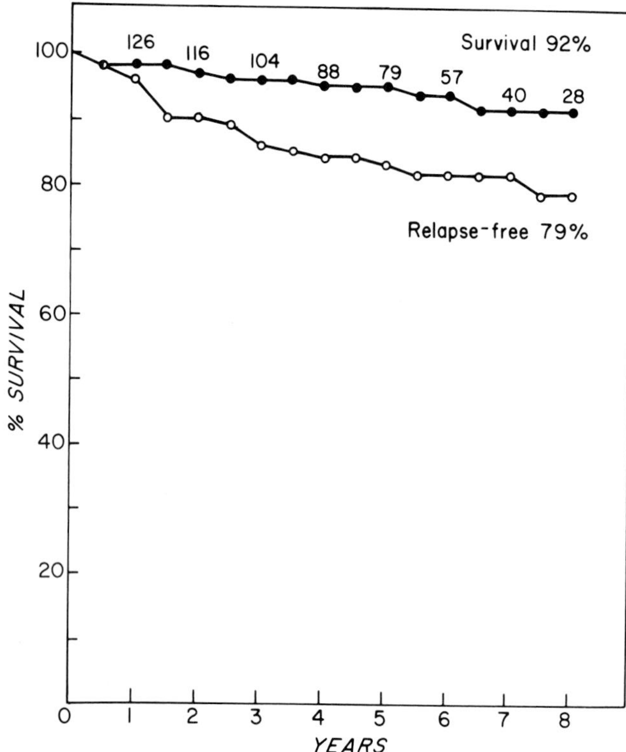

FIG. 35-14. Survival and relapse-free survival of stage IIA patients treated with irradiation to the pelvic brim. Recent results of Joint Center for Radiation Therapy, Harvard University.

Center for Radiation Therapy.[302] The results of such treatment are shown in Fig. 35-13 and 35-14. Relapse-free and overall survivals for Stage IA are 91% and 95%, respectively, and for Stage IIA are 79% and 92%, respectively. The most recent review of the 169 patients treated in this manner with a median followup of 68 months reveals only four (2%) pelvic nodal recurrences.[303] This would seem to indicate that the pelvis can be spared irradiation, while the patient still derives the value of extended field irradiation. The importance of pelvic sparing, even in those patients who eventually fail and require chemotherapy, will be discussed later. It is important to emphasize that these studies were done in laparotomy staged patients in whom the spleen had been removed.

There appears to be a separate subgroup of Stage I and IIA patients who have a higher likelihood for relapse. These are patients with large mediastinal masses. Review of such patients at the Joint Center for Radiation Therapy revealed that of 111 Stage I and IIA patients, there were 18 who had mediastinal masses greater than one-third of the total chest diameter (Table 35-19).[304] Patients relapsed both within the initial treatment volume as well as in adjacent untreated lymph nodes and extranodal relapse is primarily in the lung. These patients are more likely to recur even at involved sites separate from the mediastinum. This analysis is shown in Table 35-20. Despite the high failure rate, subsequent treatment of these patients largely with chemotherapy has resulted in excellent survival. These results have been confirmed by others.[305,306] The majority of patients with Stage I and Stage IIA disease have no, or little, mediastinal involvement. For them, the relapse-free survival is 92% and the overall survival is 97%, using a technique which spares the pelvis from irradiation.[304]

Extensive mediastinal involvement causes a number of additional problems. Such patients appear to be anesthesia risks with difficulty occurring during extubation and the risk–benefit ratios of laparotomy increases. Such risk can be greatly reduced by irradiating the mass before exploratory laparotomy, if laparotomy is essential.[307] Irradiation of these large mediastinal masses is in itself a real problem, as it may require extensive irradiation of lung or heart. Therefore, it appears that Stage I and Stage IIA disease with large mediastinal masses ought best to be considered separately.[308] Laparotomy in this group carries an increased risk, radiation treatment is more difficult to apply with normal tissue sparing more difficult to obtain, and, finally, treatment of such patients results in a higher proportion of failure than in those patients without mediastinal disease. Appropriate management of such patients will be discussed later.

While the data for subdiaphragmatic presentation Stage I and Stage IIA disease are far more limited, the results of extended field treatment appear equally satisfactory. In the Joint Center experience there were 12 such patients, with two recurrences.[303] The question of the importance of histology is not certain. In general, it is felt that mixed cellularity and lymphocyte depleted disease more likely present with higher stage disease when carefully evaluated. Within each stage, however, there may be some greater likelihood for failure with these histologies than with lymphocyte predominance or nodular sclerosis. The most recent Joint Center for Radiation Therapy results are shown in Table 35-21.

The first curative attempt at treatment of Stage III disease was presented in the Stanford (L2) protocol. This compared low dose irradiation as was the convention, since this disease was considered incurable and thus should receive palliative therapy, with radical irradiation to all lymph node bearing areas, including the spleen. Relapses occurred earlier and more frequently in the palliatively treated groups; however, their ultimate survival was not statistically significantly lower, presumably because of the success of salvage therapy. This was the first demonstration that these patients could, in fact, be cured.[129]

Figure 35-15 reveals the actuarial survival and relapse-free survival for laparotomy Stage IIIA patients from the Joint Center for Radiation Therapy.[309] In spite of the increased accuracy of staging, over 50% of the patients so treated will relapse. A majority of these can be salvaged by subsequent combination chemotherapy.[303,309,310] Total lymphoid irradiation in the hands of Stanford has been associated with a better relapse-free survival (67%) in surgically staged patients.[311]

TABLE 35-19. Influence of Mediastinal Hodgkin's Disease on Relapse

	PATIENTS	RELAPSE
No mediastinal disease	51	1
Mediastinal disease		
<⅓ chest diameter	33	4
>⅓ chest diameter	18	9

TABLE 35-20. Relapse Frequency with and without Mediastinal Disease

	INITIAL SITES	RELAPSES	PERCENT RELAPSE
No mediastinal disease	85	1	1.1
Mediastinal disease <⅓ all sites	124	4	3.2
mediastinal sites alone	50	1	2.0
non-mediastinal sites	74	3	4.1
Mediastinal disease >⅓ all sites	92	16	17.4
mediastinal sites alone	25	10	40.0
non-mediastinal sites	67	6	9.0

These data are better than those from Yale and the Joint Center.[303,309,312] Possible reasons for the difference include a larger proportion of nodular sclerosis patients seen at Stanford, and perhaps because, in those patients with splenic involvement, the Stanford group routinely irradiated the liver.[129]

Treatment of Stage IIB and Stage IIIB Hodgkin's disease with radiation alone can result in some long-term relapse-free survival (approximately 30% in the Stanford L1 and L2 protocols using total nodal irradiation). While there is general agreement that, for Stage IIIB disease, radiation therapy alone is unsatisfactory treatment, the data suggest that in surgically staged Stage IIB disease, irradiation alone may have the same results as combined modality treatment.[129,311,313] The Joint Center for Radiation Therapy had six recurrences in 18 patients treated with radiation alone; three of the failures have been successfully salvaged with chemotherapy.[303]

COMPLICATIONS OF RADIATION TREATMENT

Complications of treatment are related to the technique employed, dose administered, and irradiated volume. Most of the complications associated with irradiation are seen in the mantle field.[314] Following such irradiation there are usually no immediate changes on the chest roentgenogram or clinical function. With time, a paramediastinal pulmonary density which outlines the irradiated field may be seen on roentgen film. These are usually without symptoms, although occasionally the patients may develop dry cough or dyspnea on exertion. A more important potential complication is acute radiation pneumonitis. This depends very much on the volume of lung irradiated and the total dose given. Some changes in pulmonary function after irradiation can be seen if looked for carefully; however, symptomatic radiation pneumonitis is much less common if one is careful to restrict the pulmonary volume irradiated. When whole lung irradiation is required, the dose should be restricted to less than 1650 rad. For example, of 209 mantle patients at the Joint Center for Radiation Therapy, there were only four who developed symptomatic radiation pneumonitis.[314] Symptoms associated with this are shortness of breath, cough, and occasional fever. If a large volume of lung had been irradiated to high doses, then these changes may become progressive and sometimes fatal. In an attempt to reduce pulmonary complications, a variety of techniques have been used. Radiation therapy has been given to large pulmonary masses and interrupted at approximately 1500 rad to allow time for the mass to shrink and then the radiation continued after a 2 week or 3 week hiatus using smaller fields. Similarly, whole lung irradiation has been given to patients with hilar lymph node involvement, using either transmission blocks that allow only a portion of the dose to reach the lungs or using fields that include the whole lungs but only to tolerable doses.[129] Both of these techniques have allowed pulmonary irradiation without complications.

TABLE 35-21. Influence of Histology on Prognosis for Stage I and IIA Hodgkin's Disease

HISTOLOGY	PATIENTS	RELAPSE	DEAD
Lymphocyte predominant	22	1 (5%)	0
Nodular sclerosis	102	10 (10%)	2
Mixed cellularity	68	15 (22%)	7

FIG. 35-15. Survival and relapse-free survival of patients with stage IIIA Hodgkin's disease staged by laparotomy and treated with total nodal irradiation.

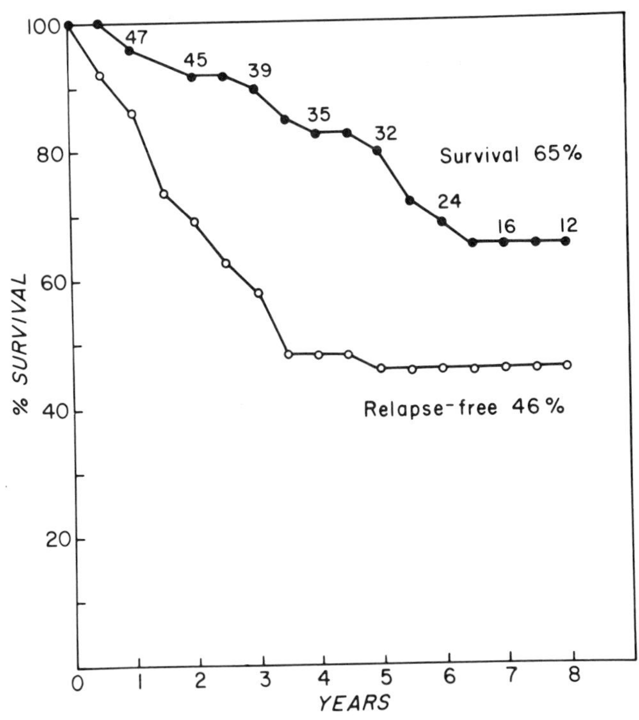

Cardiac complications of radiation therapy in Hodgkin's disease were first reported by the Stanford group.[297] With attention to limiting the volume of pericardium irradiated, keeping the radiation fraction less than 250 rad, and limiting the total dose, this had become a very uncommon complication. When the whole heart is irradiated to doses of greater than 3000 rad, then as many as 50% of the patients will develop pericardial complications.[295] It is quite important to avoid treating the whole pericardium, but if whole pericardium irradiation is required, the dose must be limited. The symptom complex seen is largely that of pericarditis and, in some patients, continued pericardial fluid causing tamponade or eventual pericardial fibrosis. Both of these can be treated surgically. There appears to be some evidence that early coronary artery disease may be a consequence of mediastinal irradiation. This is currently being reviewed. Thus far, in a large epidemiologic study, there appears to be no significant increase in cardiac-related deaths in Hodgkin's disease patients.*

The most common neurologic complication seen with irradiation is Lhermitte's syndrome. This transient complication of radiation therapy consists of numbness, tingling, or "electric" sensations, which are produced or exacerbated by head flexion. Carmel and Kaplan reported an incidence of 15% in their patients treated with mantle fields.[295] These symptoms are transitory and are not associated with permanent sequelae. The pathogenesis is unknown. Significant spinal cord transection can occur when a portion of the spinal cord is included in both the mantle and para-aortic fields. If overlap is avoided, this complication does not occur at the doses of 3600 rad to 4000 rad used. Radiation fibrosis in the brachial plexus has been rarely seen. This usually occurs when high doses of radiation are given to large neck and axillary tumor masses. When these large doses are given, patients have been recorded with progressive motor and sensory loss. Rare malignant tumors of nerve sheath origin have been reported long after radiation therapy.[315] These are usually associated with both radiation and chemotherapy.

Complications related to para-aortic fields are quite uncommon and if the doses and fields are as described, gastrointestinal complications are almost unheard of. In 216 para-aortic field irradiation patients, there have been no reported complications at the Joint Center for Radiation Therapy.[314] Pelvis treatment alone similarly causes persistent thrombocytopenia or leukopenia. This is quite rare with current techniques using well-collimated linear accelerators and judicious blocks. Infectious complications of treatment are seen when total nodal irradiation and splenectomy are used.

CHEMOTHERAPY OF LYMPHOMAS

Mention of the chemotherapy of lymphomas with Fowler's solution is made in 1892 in the first edition of Osler's textbook of medicine.[316] Because Osler recognized that waxing and waning adenopathy frequently occurs in lymphomas, he was uncertain as to the impact of this arsenic-containing material on the natural history of the disease. The modern era of lymphoma chemotherapy began in the early 1940s when mustard gases were first submitted for study to Goodman and Gilman at Yale and were found to produce profound effects on lymphatic and hemopoietic tissue in rodents. A derivative, nitrogen mustard, was first used in the treatment of a group of six patients with neoplastic diseases, including Hodgkin's disease and lymphosarcoma at Yale University in 1943. Because of the secrecy surrounding the war gas program, the results were not published until 1946.[317] It was obvious from the results that dissolution of tumor masses occurred in Hodgkin's disease and lymphosarcoma following intermittent dosing with nitrogen mustard. Subsequent studies by Alpert and Peterson and by Dameshek and colleagues confirmed these effects.[318,319] These early studies were the source of both great excitement and disappointment. Never before had such marked regression of tumor masses occurred in humans as a result of drug treatment and the possibility of curing cancer with drugs was first realistically entertained. However, with rapid regrowth of the tumor masses and death of these patients, the long debate began as to whether drugs provided any significant benefit, let alone cure, to patients with these diseases.

While the identification of the antitumor activity of the antifols in the 1950s had no immediate bearing on the treatment of lymphomas, it did lead to the development of the National Cancer Institute's Drug Development Program, which would add other agents to the therapeutic armamentarium (see Chapter 8).[320] In the 1950s, corticosteroids provided an additional therapeutic tool for physicians to use with alkylating agents, but even in combination, these agents did not provide durable benefit for patients with lymphomas. Thus, during the 1950s, investigators compared the effects of a variety of alkylating agents, evaluating various routes and schedules of administration and debating their effects on survival.

The first attempt to elucidate the effect of an induction treatment *versus* continued maintenance treatment in a comparative study was published by Scott in 1963.[321] Eighty-nine patients with advanced Hodgkin's disease received a conventional induction course of nitrogen mustard (0.4 mg/kg), of which 40 patients with "satisfactory response" were randomized to receive either no further treatment or continuous treatment with chlorambucil. In the 16 patients who received chlorambucil, time to relapse averaged 35 weeks (range 4 weeks to 84 weeks) compared to 11.7 weeks (range 4 weeks to 51 weeks) without further treatment. This highly significant difference in the duration of a "satisfactory remission" provided the first useful information on alternatives in the management of patients with Hodgkin's disease. No mention was made in this study, however, as to whether any survival benefit accrued to the patients maintained on chlorambucil. Subsequent studies comparing remission induction with nitrogen mustard and maintenance with chlorambucil to induction and maintenance with oral cyclophosphamide revealed no significant differences in either the response rate or remission duration. In a report by Jacobs and colleagues, one of the first survival curves published in the modern chemotherapy era was presented.[322] It indicated that drug treatment in patients with advanced lymphomas was associ-

* Boivin J: Personal communication, 1981

ated with a median survival of less than 2 years with only 5% to 10% living beyond 4 years (Fig. 35-16). While these results were slightly superior to the untreated series reported by Croft in 1942, they did not provide convincing data that chemotherapy was improving survival.[159]

The next major advance in the chemotherapy of the lymphomas came with the identification of the vinca alkaloids.[323] The availability of two apparently non-cross-resistant classes of antitumor agents and the conceptual separation of induction and maintenance therapy gave impetus to a large study initiated through the combined effort of two clinical cooperative groups supported by the National Cancer Institute (Acute Leukemia Group B and the Eastern Solid Tumor Group).[324] This study provided the foundation for future studies on combination chemotherapy, which were to prove so effective.

Three hundred and forty-two patients were randomized by disease and prior therapy to remission induction with cyclophosphamide, or one of the vinca alkaloids. Vinblastine was used in Hodgkin's disease and vincristine in non-Hodgkin's lymphomas, known then as lymphosarcoma and reticulum cell sarcoma. The objectives of this study were to compare the effectiveness of the two vinca alkaloids to cyclophosphamide in remission induction in lymphoma. These investigators also studied the duration of response when patients received either cyclophosphamide or placebo to maintain the remission, and compared the effectiveness of continuous therapy *versus* intermittent reinduction with cyclophosphamide. The results of this study established the superiority of vinblastine over cyclophosphamide for remission induction in patients with advanced Hodgkin's disease. In the non-Hodgkin's lymphomas, cyclophosphamide proved superior to the vinca alkaloid, vincristine. In all disease categories, the average duration of placebo-maintained remission was a remarkably short, 4 weeks to 6 weeks, irrespective of the drug used to induce the remission. Daily oral cyclophosphamide significantly prolonged remission duration when compared to placebo, confirming the observation of Scott.[321] Remission duration with drug maintenance treatment varied by tumor type, with a range from 11 weeks in reticulum cell sarcoma to 32 weeks in Hodgkin's disease. There were two other features of this study that were not initially emphasized. First, patients were separated by whether they had partial or complete remissions, a practice not generally employed at that time. Response duration was always significantly longer for patients who achieved complete remission. Second, regardless of the approach to treatment, overall survival in the various subgroups in each disease category was almost identical. These data indicated that, while maintenance drug treatment did prolong remission duration and provided a smooth way to manage patients in the normal practice of medicine, survival was not compromised by a decision to induce remissions and leave patients untreated until relapse. The value of obtaining a complete remission and the failure of the maintenance treatment to prolong survival allowed physicians who subsequently developed the drug combination programs to set as their major initial goal achieving a high complete remission rate. It was possible to assess the quality of these complete remissions by observing their duration with no further therapy, without imposing an ethical dilemma.

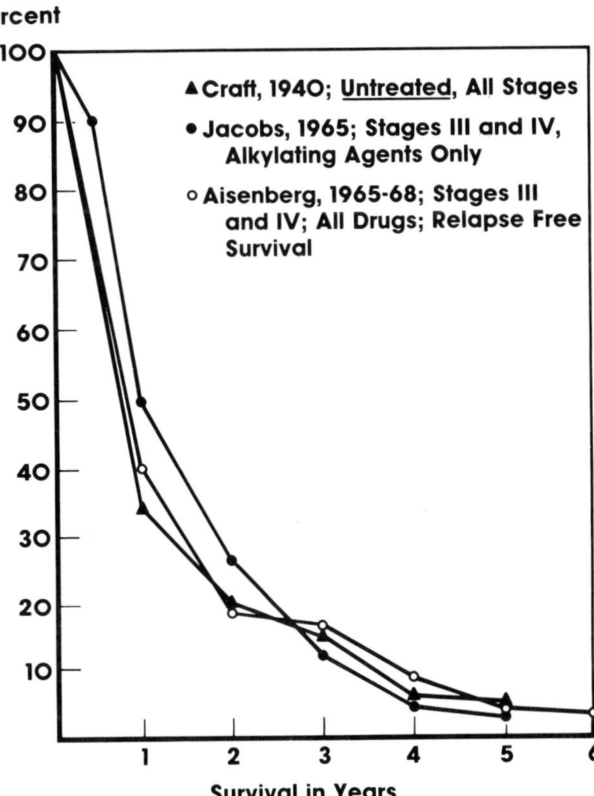

FIG. 35-16. Three survival curves of patients with advanced Hodgkin's disease treated with single agent chemotherapy compared to a group left untreated. (From DeVita VT Jr: Consequences of the chemotherapy of Hodgkin's disease. Cancer 47:1, 1981)

The appearance of vinca alkaloids was followed shortly by the discovery of the antitumor activity of the methylhydrazine derivative, procarbazine, then called ibenzamethyzin in Hodgkin's disease by Bollag and Grunberg, and Mathe and colleagues, in Europe, and by DeVita and colleagues, in the United States.[325–329] These studies and others indicated that procarbazine was almost exclusively useful in Hodgkin's disease and in occasional patients with reticulum cell sarcoma.

As the influx of anti-cancer drugs accelerated, other drugs have since been identified with activity against patients with lymphomas. These are shown in Tables 35-22 and 35-23. The availability of numerous drugs allowed investigators to approach the problem of exploring their use in combination.

THE USE OF SINGLE AGENT CHEMOTHERAPY TO MANAGE HODGKIN'S DISEASE

The use of single drugs has no important role as initial treatment in most patients with advanced Hodgkin's disease. Single agents have been compared in controlled clinical trials to drug combinations, and proven inferior.[332] A fixed sequential use of five active single agents has also proven inferior to the combination programs.[333] Similarly, since maintenance treatment has not proven beneficial, single agents are no longer

TABLE 35-22. Single Agents in Advanced Hodgkin's Disease

DRUG	DOSE AND SCHEDULE	NUMBER OF STUDIES	EVALUATED	NUMBER OF PATIENTS	PERCENT RESPONSE
Mechlorethamine	0.4 mg/kg q3-4 wk I.V.	5	106	67	63
Cyclophosphamide	15 mg/kg/wk I.V.	3	91	50	55
Vincristine	0.025–0.075 mg/kg qwk I.V.	4	38	24	63
Vinblastine	0.1–0.3 mg/kg/wk I.V.	2	57	82	70
Procarbazine	100 mg/m² qD continous p.o.	1	33	22	67
Adriamycin	75 mg/m² q3 wk I.V.	2	33	13	39
Bleomycin	10 units/m² 2 × wk I.V./I.M.	3	100	29	29
Dacarbazine	250 mg/m² qD × 5 q3-4 wks I.V.	1	18	10	56
BCNU	200 mg/m² q6 wk I.V.	3	83	38	46
CCNU	100–130 mg/m² q6 wk p.o.	2	38	20	53
MeCCNU	125–200 mg/m² q6 wk p.o.	1	16	9	56
VP 16-213	45 mg/m² qD × 5 q3 wk I.V.	1	17	3	18
VM 26	100 mg/m² qwk q3 wk I.V.	1	9	2	22
Methyl GAG	200 mg qD × 7	1	8	5	63
Thiotepa	0.8 mg/kg q3 wk I.V.	2	14	31	45

(Adapted from Coltman CA: Chemotherapy of advanced Hodgkin's disease. Serv Onc 7:155–173, 1980)

used in this setting. There are two clinical circumstances when single drug rather than combination therapy may be useful. The first is when medical infirmity caused by associated illnesses or age makes combination chemotherapy too risky to be used, and the second is in the patient who has failed after treatment with drug combinations.

Previously untreated patients ill from other diseases, with a life expectancy to from 1 year to 3 years, may best be managed by single agents. To date, the best and easiest drug to use is vinblastine, given on a weekly schedule for the duration of the patient's illness (Table 35-22). Vinblastine may also be combined with chlorambucil. Such an approach may produce a smooth remission of useful quality in as many as 40% of patients, and these remissions may be maintained from 1 year to 2 years.[334] The likelihood of cure, nonetheless, is remote. Induction of remission with an alkylating agent, with or without continuous maintenance treatment, is the second choice therapy that might be selected in very elderly patients who are less able to tolerate the constipating effects of the vinca alkaloids. With relapse, procarbazine, adriamycin, one of the nitrosoureas, dacarbazine, or one of the newer agents shown in Table 35-22 may be used in sequence. Since each of these drugs has unique toxicities (see Chapter 47; a Practical Guide for Physicians and Oncology Nurses), their selection should be based on the clinical circumstances in each case.

The second circumstance where single agents are sometimes useful is in the treatment of patients who fail after combination chemotherapy. They should first be treated with a second non-cross-resistant drug combination in an attempt to induce a second durable complete remission. If the patient fails to respond satisfactorily the second time, attempts to use more than a two-drug combination should generally be abandoned. Newer drugs should be used and selected on the basis of the degree of morbidity associated with their use. If new drugs fail, or are unavailable, then a drug should be selected from a class of agents that has produced a response in the patient since there is evidence that patients may respond to a different chemical structure in a given class. This is particularly true of alkylating agents and may be due to differences in drug distribution or transport into the cells (see Chapter 8). Sometimes drugs used in combination are used in abbreviated schedules. An example is the use of the methylhydrazine derivative, procarbazine, in the MOPP program. When used alone, it is given continuously and in larger doses than when used in combination. It has been the author's experience that some patients who have failed combination chemotherapy with MOPP will respond to procarbazine when used alone continuously at doses of 100 mg/m²/day to 200 mg/m²/day. This phenomenon, often referred to as schedule resistance, may be exploited using different alkylating agents as well.

In Hodgkin's disease, vinblastine is thought to be superior to vincristine but the published data do not speak firmly on this point. Experimental data in rodents also show little evidence of cross resistance between vincristine and vinblastine. Patients exposed to one or the other agent in a drug combination may then be treated with the alternate compound as a single agent. Occasionally, drugs not commonly used in Hodgkin's disease, such as methotrexate and 5-fluorouracil, may produce benefit and these drugs can be used with minimal side effects in failing patients. Nonetheless, the prognosis for these patients is poor. Remissions are usually incomplete and of short duration; complications of the disease commonly supervene and death is the outcome.

THE USE OF SINGLE AGENT CHEMOTHERAPY TO MANAGE PATIENTS WITH NON-HODGKIN'S LYMPHOMA

There are more similarities than differences in the spectrum of response of patients with non-Hodgkin's lymphoma to single agent chemotherapy when compared to Hodgkin's disease. Some of the differences in drug activity are important to note and are highlighted in Table 35-23.

The data suggested that vincristine is superior to vinblastine when used as a single agent, and presumably in combination.[324] Comparative studies have shown that the vinca alkaloids are inferior to alkylating agents as remission-inducing drugs for patients with non-Hodgkin's lymphoma.[335] Procarbazine has no real role in the management of patients with

TABLE 35-23. Single Agents in Advanced Non-Hodgkin's Lymphomas

DRUGS	AND DOSE SCHEDULE	HISTIOCYTIC LYMPHOMAS				LYMPHOCYTIC LYMPHOMAS			
				(Response)				*(Response)*	
		Number of studies	*Patients evaluated*	*Number of patients*	*Percent*	*Number of studies*	*Patients evaluated*	*Number of patients*	*Percent*
Mechlorethamine	0.4 mg/kg q 4 wk I.V.	2	11	2	18	4	70	42	60
Cyclophosphamide	3-4 mg/kg q D × 5 I.V. P.O.	5	158	90	57	2	77	52	67
Vincristine	0.025-0.75 mg/kg q wk I.V.	3	100	65	65	1	47	18	38
Vinblastine	0.1-0.15 mg/kg q wk I.V.	3	40	11	28	2	21	4	19
Procarbazine	2-3 mg/kg q D continuous P.O.	3	15	4	27	–	–	–	–
Adriamycin	45-75 mg/m² q 3 wks I.V.	2	63	31	49	2	60	21	35
Bleomycin	10-15 m/m² BIW I.V. or I.M.	2	42	17	40	2	34	15	44
BCNU	200-250 mg/m² q 6 wks I.V.	1	24	8	33	2	70	14	20
Dacarbazine	250 mg/m² q D × 5 q 3-4 wks I.V.	1	13	–	–	1	15	4	27
VP 16-213	60 mg/m² q D × 5 q 3 wks I.V.	1	22	8	36	1	12	7	58
VM-26	30 mg/m² q D × 5 q 3 wks I.V.	1	21	4	19	1	7	2	28
Methotrexate (high dose)	30 mg/kg + Citrovorum factor rescue	2	43	30	70	–	–	–	–

(Bender RA, DeVita VT: Non-Hodgkin's lymphoma. In Staquet MJ (ed): Randomized Clinical Trials in Cancer: A Critical Review by Sites. New York, Raven Press, 1978, pp 77–102)

nodular lymphomas but has been reported to have some consistent effect in some patients with diffuse histiocytic and lymphoblastic lymphomas.

No distinction can be made in responses of patients with non-Hodgkin's lymphoma to a variety of alkylating agents. The nitrosoureas are more effective in Hodgkin's disease than in the various non-Hodgkin's lymphomas.[336,337] The only agent that is useful in non-Hodgkin's lymphomas but not in Hodgkin's disease is the enzyme, L-asparaginase. Response rates as high as 60% are observed in patients with the more indolent non-Hodgkin's lymphomas, although the response duration is usually brief. This appears to be the only malignant disease, other than acute lymphocytic leukemia, that responds to L-asparaginase.[338] There are differences and some considerable controversy in the use of single agent chemotherapy for the heterogeneous group of patients with non-Hodgkin's lymphomas.

Diffuse well-differentiated lymphocytic lymphomas (DWDL) have a natural history similar to patients with chronic lymphocytic leukemia (CLL). Although the response rate of patients with this disease to combination chemotherapy is reported to be high, the duration of these responses is very short. Neither the response rate nor the duration of the response has been shown to have much impact on survival which averages in excess of 6 years with any approach to management.[339,340] Therefore, patients with diffuse well-differentiated lymphocytic lymphomas are best treated by conservative approaches, usually sequential use of single agents when clinically necessary. Usually an oral alkylating agent coupled with intermittent administration of corticosteroids is sufficient.

The situation is quite different for patients with diffuse poorly differentiated, lymphocytic, mixed or histiocytic lymphomas. These diseases are clinically aggressive. There are no data indicating that use of single agent chemotherapy provides a sufficient number of complete or durable remissions to warrant its use.[331] Data to be reviewed below indicate that long-term survival is possible only after the use of aggressive combination chemotherapy.[342] Even in the studies of Carbone and associates and Jones and associates, the quality of response to alkylating and vinca alkaloids had an influence on survival.[324,339] Patients who attained complete remissions lived longer than those who did not respond. Survival beyond 2 years was consistently noted only in the minority of patients who had complete tumor disappearance. To date, no study using single agents for patients with advanced diffuse histiocytic, diffuse undifferentiated, or diffuse lymphoblastic lymphomas has reported a significant fraction of long-term disease-free survivors.

The situation with the nodular lymphomas is more complex. The series of Jones and colleagues from Stanford and the older literature, indicate that the average survival for patients with NPDL is 6 years, even when the treatment used is regional radiotherapy, or radiotherapy followed by single agent chemotherapy, usually chlorambucil.[331,339] Although in the Stanford series there were some differences in survival between patients with NPDL or NM or NH lymphoma, all nodular lymphomas fared better than patients with diffuse lymphomas. Average survival, curiously, is not affected by infiltration of organs such as the bone marrow and liver by lymphoma cells in nodular lymphomas. Results of radiotherapy of localized NHL offer some additional insights into the natural history of these diseases. Data from Stanford indicates that diffuse lymphomas have a tendency to relapse early and frequently, with almost all relapses occurring within the first 2 years.[342] In patients with localized NPDL, on the other hand, the pressure of relapse is constant and continuous at 10% to 15% per year, even beyond the sixth year of followup. The paradox of the "good prognosis" lymphomas is that although NPDL is an indolent illness, all patients ultimately succumb to their disease. Anderson and associates reported a similar continuous pattern of relapse in patients with advanced disease who achieve a complete remission after combination chemotherapy.[343] There is no convincing evidence that combinations of drugs can cure patients with advanced stages of NPDL.

In a randomized clinical trial, conducted at Stanford University, patients were assigned to receive either a single oral alkylating agent or the combination of cyclophosphamide, vincristine, and prednisone (CVP) (see below) or CVP combined with total lymph node irradiation.[344] Although the complete response rate after the first 6 months of treatment was higher in the CVP group, by 4 years the single agent complete response rate was equivalent, and survival was not significantly different in any group at 5 years.

This has led the Stanford group to advance the proposition of no initial therapy for such patients. Surprisingly, the literature is relatively silent on this point. Portlock and Rosenberg reported on a highly selected group of 44 patients with favorable histologic types given no initial therapy.[345] Twenty-nine patients had nodular lymphomas, eight had diffuse well-differentiated lymphomas, and seven had diffuse lymphocytic poorly differentiated lymphomas. All were either Stage III or Stage IV. The median time required before therapy was needed was 31 months, and at the time of the report, 19 patients had not yet required therapy for periods ranging from 3 months to 104 months. At 4 years, the actuarial survival of the 44 patients who had received no initial treatment was 77.3% compared to 83.2% for 112 retrospectively matched control patients treated on a routine protocol at Stanford. The difference was not significant. The defects of such a retrospective analysis are obvious. This group of 44 patients was selected out of a group of over 1000 such patients seen at Stanford since 1963, and they represent a highly selected group of patients. The true fraction of patients who can be followed without treatment remains unknown. The very old literature collected in 1919 by Yates, when no chemotherapy was available, suggests that most patients require some form of therapy within 1 year to 2 years.[346,347] Nonetheless, these data suggest that some patients can be followed for significant periods of time without therapy. Are there any advantages for such an approach?[348] Many patients do not care for the constant and visible enlargement of lymph nodes which are an everpresent reminder of their illness, and the uncertainties associated with no therapy. This approach, on the other hand, spares the patients the long-term, toxic effects of drugs on bone marrow, which can be particularly severe with continuous exposure to chlorambucil, and the disruption associated with continued therapy, especially since cure of patients with NPDL by chemotherapy does not yet seem possible.

Recently, the National Cancer Institute workers have reported three observations that may influence the approach to the management of patients with NPDL. First, there is clearcut evidence that NPDL evolves to DHL, probably by evolving through NM and NH lymphoma first.[163,349] Second, there is evidence, in contrast to NPDL, that patients with NM may be curable by combination chemotherapy but not by the use of single agents.[343] Third, patients with nodular histiocytic lymphomas are curable by combination chemotherapy, as well.[350]

These data highlight the paradox facing the physician. For patients with advanced NPDL, there is, at present, no curative chemotherapy. When the disease evolves, the only therapy that offers the potential for long-term disease-free survival are the more aggressive drug combination programs that do not work in NPDL. The commonly used drug, chlorambucil, cannot cure patients with NPDL, but can compromise the patient's ability to respond to drug combinations later. The same can be said for using non-curative combination therapy during the indolent phase of NPDL as well. Taken *in toto,* these data make a reasonable case for management of patients with NPDL on an expectant basis unless the clinical situation dictates treatment. In most cases, small field local radiotherapy should be used for dangerous or unsightly lymph node masses. When drug treatment is required because of evolution to a more aggressive histiologic type, one of the programs used for DHL, described below, is the treatment of choice. Thus, the role of single agent chemotherapy as initial treatment for NPDL seems limited, as in Hodgkin's disease, to those patients who failed drug combinations and have advancing disease, and the same principles presented for Hodgkin's disease apply.

EXPERIMENTAL SINGLE AGENT THERAPY

Some of the drugs listed in Tables 35-22 and 35-23 are not marketed. The cancer drug development process and distribution of experimental anticancer drugs is detailed in Chapter 8. Results of phase I and II clinical trials of newer antitumor agents are also detailed in references 351 through 357. Recently, biological materials have been evaluated as antitumor agents. Interferon, a protein normally produced by cells in response to viral infections has been tested in patients with two types of B-cell lymphomas by Merigan and colleagues and Gutterman and colleagues.[358,359] While partial responses were seen in previously untreated patients with NPDL, those with DHL failed to respond. Large scale trials of interferon have been initiated by the Division of Cancer Treatment of the NCI, to evaluate interferon further in a variety of cancers including lymphomas. Two groups have evaluated anti T-cell antibody in patients with T-cell lymphomas with evidence of regressions, but considerable side effects.[360,361] As pure nonclonal antibody becomes available using hybridoma technology, this approach may prove to have some merit.

COMBINATION CHEMOTHERAPY OF HODGKIN'S DISEASE

Seventeen years after the initiation of the first studies on the combination chemotherapy of Hodgkin's disease it is now possible to say with some confidence that such programs can cure a significant fraction of patients with advanced disease.[350-365] The development of a variety of these programs will be discussed here. The application of combination chemotherapy to the various stages of Hodgkin's disease will be discussed below. The details of the principles of the use of curative combination chemotherapy using the lymphomas as the human example are discussed in detail in Chapter 8.

The first studies on combination chemotherapy followed the identification of the multiple, independently active, chemotherapeutic agents discussed above. In 1964, Skipper and associates published data on the curability of L-1210 leukemia in rodents and established some principles which have proven to be of fundamental importance to chemotherapy programs since that time.[350,366] The first intensive drug combination program designed to exploit these principles in Hodgkin's disease utilized the combination of vincristine, methotrexate, cyclophosphamide, and prednisone (MOMP) given for 2½ months.[350,367] The goal of this pilot protocol was to test the safety of such an approach in advanced Hodgkin's disease. Only 14 patients were studied, but the data showed the approach to be safe and a high complete remission rate (80%) was attained. In 1965, Lacher and Durant reported that the administration of low dose vinblastine and chlorambucil in combination achieved a complete remission rate of approximately 40%.[334] However, this difference was not a significant improvement in the response rate achieved with vinblastine alone and no further reports have been published on these patients. As experience accrued, with procarbazine, then a new drug, the MOMP program was modified in several ways in 1964. The duration of treatment was increased to 6 months and procarbazine was substituted for the antifol, methotrexate. This program, named MOPP, has proven to be a standard drug combination for the treatment of patients with advanced Hodgkin's disease and for use in combination with radiotherapy in patients with earlier stages.[363] In 1967, when the results of the use of MOPP in the first 43 patients were reported, an 80% complete remission rate was noted, a fourfold increase over results achieved with the best use of single agents. Other studies have confirmed the results of the MOPP program either in controlled or uncontrolled studies (Table 35-24).[363,369-375] Studies comparing MOPP to other regimens are shown in Table 35-25.[332,333,376-381] Hugeley and associates compared the use of MOPP chemotherapy to intensive use of the single agent, nitrogen mustard. Although the complete remission rate for the MOPP program (48%) was less than that reported by the National Cancer Institute, there was a statistically significant difference between the ability of MOPP and nitrogen mustard to induce complete remissions; nitrogen mustard induced complete remissions in only three of 23 patients (13%).

Numerous investigators attempted to modify the MOPP program. These data are illustrated in Table 35-26.[382-390] Nicholson and colleagues reported on modification of the MOPP program that substituted vinblastine for vincristine, and was able to achieve a 42% complete remission rate. A complete remission rate comparable to that at the National Cancer Institute was reported by the group from Stanford and Frei and colleagues in a large study from the Southwest Oncology Group, with remission rates ranging from 66% to 74% (Table 35-24).[363,373] Several prognostic factors influencing remission rates emerged from these studies. Patients previously treated with chemotherapy responded less well to MOPP

TABLE 35-24. MOPP as Primary Treatment

AUTHOR (Reference Number)	YEAR	PRIOR THERAPY	TOTAL PATIENTS	PERCENT CR	DFS(%/yr)	SURVIVAL(%/yr)
DeVita et al (363)	1970	Local RT	43	81	50/3.5	63/4
Ziegler et al (369)	1972	–	24	100	–	–
Canellos et al (370)	1972	RT only	21	76	50/1 +	75/3
Frei et al (371)	1973	CT & RT	178	66	75/4*	80/4
Coltman et al (372)	1973	CT & RT	206	62	46/4†	59/3
Moore et al (373)	1973	–	81	74	50/1,5	–
Focan et al (374)	1975	–	34	41	50/2	–
Olweny et al (375)	1978	–	48	88	74/10	67/10
DeVita et al (365)	1980	Local RT	198	80	63/10	54/10

Abbreviations: CR = Complete Response; DFS = Disease Free Survival; RT = Radiotherapy
*18 months maintenance therapy
†No maintenance
‡3 different maintenance programs
(Adopted from Coltman CA: Chemotherapy of advanced Hodgkin's disease. Sem Onc 7:155–173, 1980)

TABLE 35-25. Randomized Studies Comparing MOPP with Other Regimens as Primary Treatment

AUTHOR (Reference Number)	REGIMEN*	YEAR	PRIOR THERAPY	TOTAL PATIENTS	PERCENT CR	DFS (%/yr)	OS (%/yr)
Huguley et al (332)	MOPP *vs*	1975	Yes	61	48	40/3	55/3
	HN_2			47	13	23/3	35/3
Nissen et al (333)	MOPP *vs*	1973	Yes	81	61	50/2	–
	VPBCPr† vs			89	61	25/2	–
	VPBCPr‡			77	49	20/2	–
British National Investigation (376)	MOPP *vs*	1975	Yes	49	80	–	No significant difference
	MOPr			41	44	–	
Bonadonna et al (377)	MOPP *vs*	1975	RT only	25	76	–	
	ABVD			20	75	–	
Bennett et al (378)	MOPP	1976	Yes	115	69		
	BCVPP			115	68		
Coltman et al (379)	MOPP *vs*	1978	Yes	44	70	62/3	62/3
	MOPP LDB *vs*			118	84	64/3	78/3
	MOPP HDB *vs*			38	76	53/3	65/3
	MOPP CPF			28	64	60/3	58/3
Cooper et al (380)	MVPP *vs*	1975	Yes		59–66		
	COPPr§ *vs*						
	CVPPr						
	MOPP *vs*						
Nissen et al (381)	MOPP *vs*	1979	Yes	104	62	62/4	71/4
	BOP *vs*			107	40	30/4	46/4
	OPP *vs*			112	42	50/5	72/4
	BOPPr			103	67	54/4	70/4

Abbreviations: CR = Complete Response; DFS = Disease Free Survival; OS = Overall Survival
†Simultaneous administration
‡Sequential administration
§CCNU
*For drug designation see Abbreviations and Acronyms—Table 35-39
(Adopted from Coltman CA: Chemotherapy of advanced Hodgkin's disease. Sem Onc 7:155–173, 1980)

chemotherapy than previously untreated patients as reported by Lowenbraun and colleagues.[391] Exposure to prior radiotherapy did not seem to compromise the patient's ability to respond to chemotherapy.[364,365,370] There seemed to be a significant difference in the overall response rate in the initial reports between those patients who were asymptomatic and those who had constitutional symptoms (category B).

In a recent update of the NCI experience, DeVita and associates reported on the 17-year results of treatment of 198 patients with MOPP program as their primary treatment.[365] One-hundred-fifty-nine of 198 patients, or 80%, achieved a complete remission. These patients required a median number of three cycles to attain remission. The only characteristic significantly associated with a greater probability of attaining a complete remission in this population was the absence of fever, night sweats, and weight loss (B-symptoms). For example, all 23 patients without symptoms attained complete remission, compared to 78% of the symptomatic patients. This difference was highly significant. Of the 32 patients who had received local radiotherapy, before MOPP treatment, all

TABLE 35-26. MOPP Modifications as Primary Treatment

AUTHOR (Reference Number)	REGIMEN*	PRIOR THERAPY	TOTAL PATIENTS	PERCENT CR	DFS (%/yr)
Nicholson et al (382)	MVPP	Yes	52	42	–
Durant et al (383)	BCVPPr	Yes	324	68-73	70/4
Bloomfield et al (384)	CVPP	Yes	38	74	–
Diggs et al (385)	CVPP	Yes	50	62	–
Harrison et al (386)	BVPP	Yes	12	75	–
McElwain et al (387)	ChlVPP	Yes	70	76	–
Suttcliffe et al (388)	MVPP	Yes	133	59	46/70/4
Morgenfeld et al (389)	CVPP *vs*	Yes	157	71	50/3
	CCVPP		141	78	64/3
Eckhardt et al (390)	VM-26 PP	Yes	50	40	–

Abbreviations: CR = Complete Response; DFS = Disease Free Survival
*For drug designations see Abbreviations and Acronyms—Table 35-39
(Adapted from Coltman CA: Chemotherapy of advanced Hodgkin's disease. Semi Onc 7:155–173,1980)

but two (94%) attained complete remission, compared to 78% of the unirradiated patients. While this difference was not significant, the *p*-value was 0.065. The authors report the survival results in terms of tumor mortality since treatments were not compared in the MOPP study. Sixty-three and one-half percent of patients achieving complete remission, who are at risk for longer than 5 years, have remained disease free. Because 80% of the entire treated population achieved a complete remission, the proportion of all treated patients who remained free of relapse at 5 years was 54.6%. Although most relapses tended to occur with 42 months after cessation of the therapy, three relapses occurred at 77, 82, and 92 months, respectively. The relapse-free survival curve of patients with Hodgkin's disease who achieved a complete remission is illustrated in Fig. 35-17. The NCI authors further reported that two factors had an influence on the durability of the remissions. The first was, again, the absence of systemic symptoms. Only one of the 23 asymptomatic patients relapsed. The second was the histologic subtype of the disease. A significantly worse prognosis was noted in patients with nodular sclerosing Hodgkin's disease. When this group was further analyzed, the poor prognosis was related to patients with nodular sclerosing disease which had progressed to lymphocyte depletion. The overall survival of the population is shown in Fig. 35-18. Patients who died without evidence of disease were considered alive and lost to followup at the time of death. There were 98 recorded deaths, 23 (24%) of which represented patients who died without evidence of Hodgkin's disease. Autopsies were done in 15 of these patients and no Hodgkin's disease were detected in 14, further supporting the contention that in patients who appear to be in clinical remission, the disease was eradicated by chemotherapy.

While 80% of patients treated with MOPP or variants of MOPP enter complete remission, anywhere from 36% to 50% of patients relapse by the fifth year of followup.

The next question posed by a number of investigators was whether maintenance drug therapy would be beneficial after achieving a complete remission. These data are shown in Table 35-27. The first such study was conducted at the National Cancer Institute. Patients were randomly allocated after achieving complete remission to intermittent cycles of carmustine (the nitrosourea BCNU) or no therapy, or intermittent cycles of MOPP. Maintenance treatment was given for 15 months. When the results of this study were reported in 1973, and when reanalyzed in 1980, there was no significant advantage for either continued intermittent MOPP or intermittent carmustine therapy.[365,392] The toxicity in the two chemotherapeutic arms was significantly greater than in the no maintenance treatment arm, and the trial has been discontinued. At the same time the Southwest Oncology Group made a comparison study between the use of intermittent MOPP, given as two cycles every 3 months, and no further therapy after the initial six cycles of MOPP. While these authors initially reported a prolongation of remission duration with MOPP maintenance this difference has been

FIG. 35-17. Relapse-free survival curve of patients with advanced Hodgkin's disease who attained a complete remission after MOPP treatment.

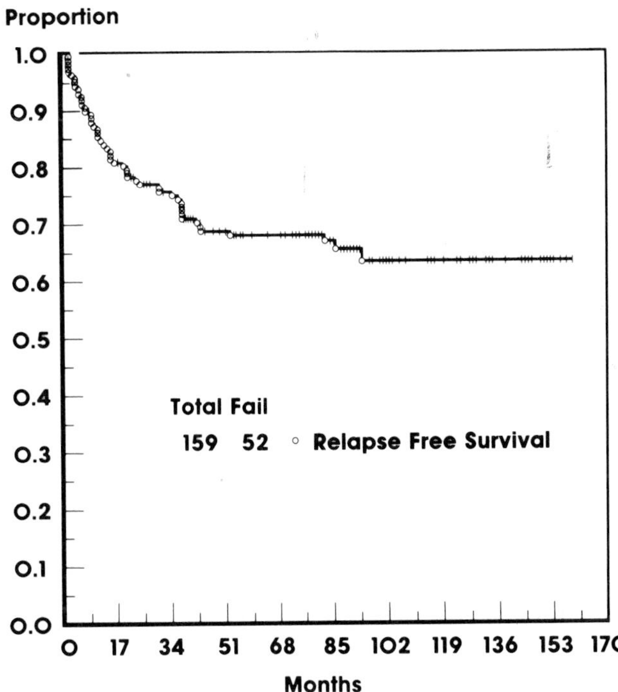

TABLE 35-27. Studies Which Fail to Show Significant Benefit From Maintenance Drug Therapy on Remission Duration and Survival

REGIMEN*	YEAR	AUTHOR (Reference Number)
MOPP *vs* BCNU *vs* No Therapy	1973	Young et al (392)
MOPP q2 mo. × 9 *vs* No Therapy	1973	Frei et al (371)
Actinomycin D *vs* Methotrexate *vs* Vinblastine	1973	Coltman et al (372)
Chlorambucil *vs* Chlorambucil and reinforcements *vs* Vinblastine	1973	Nissen et al (333)
MOPP *vs* BCVPP *vs* No Therapy	1975	Durant et al (383)
CCNU + Vinblastine *vs* No Therapy	1976	Bennet et al (378)
MOPP q2 mo. × 9 *vs* RT + MOPP q2 mo × 9 *vs* MOPP q1m8 × 18	1977	Coltman et al (379)
Vinblastine and Procarbazine MVPP	1978	Suttcliffe et al (388)
CVPP *vs* CCVPP	1979	Morgenfeld et al (389)
MOPP q2 mo. × 9 *vs* No Therapy	1976	Coltman et al (393)

*For drug designation see Abbreviations and Acronyms—Table 35-39

lost by the seventh year of followup and there is now no survival advantage for the use of maintenance therapy. Eight other studies have addressed the same question of using a variety of maintenance treatments, and to date, none of these programs has shown a positive effect (Table 35-27). These data make an impressive case for discontinuation of therapy after it has been carefully documented that a remission has been achieved. These data also provide further indirect evidence that a substantial number of patients who achieve a complete remission are indeed cured of their disease. It might be expected that continuation of therapy, in the form of maintenance, would have no benefit in cured patients. The initial advantage in the relapse-free survival curve reported by Frei and colleagues can be explained by the effect of drug maintenance on patients who failed to achieve a true complete remission and, therefore, profited by temporary suppression of tumor regrowth. Physicians are advised not to treat patients with further chemotherapy after documentation of complete remission.

Patients who attain a complete remission and relapse can be successfully retreated under certain circumstances. Fifty-nine percent of 32 patients who relapsed after treatment with MOPP at the NCI achieved a second complete remission when retreated with MOPP and intermittent maintenance with two cycles every three months for two years.[394] As with primary MOPP therapy, no disease variable seemed to affect the second response rate. However, only five out of 17 patients whose initial complete remission was less than 1 year in duration achieved a second complete remission (29%) compared to 14 out of 15 patients whose initial complete remission

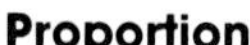

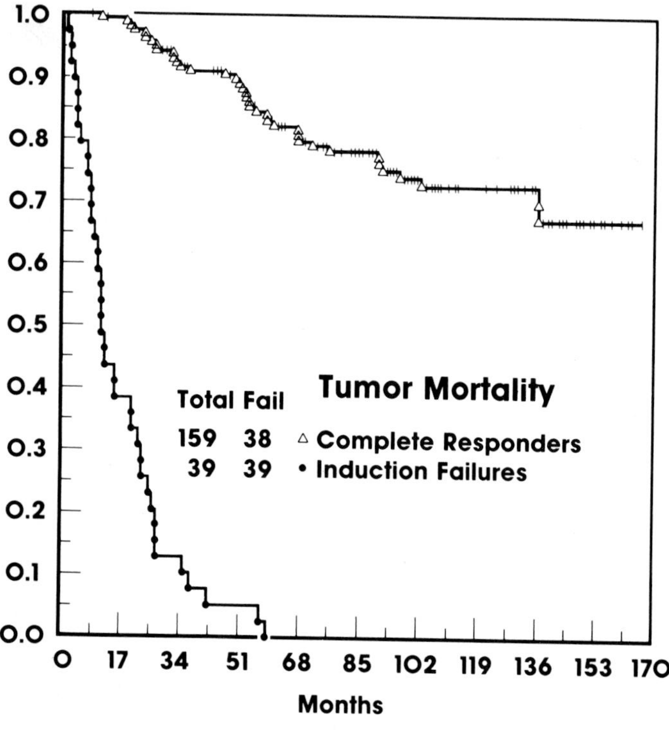

FIG. 35-18. Tumor mortality of patients treated with MOPP at the National Cancer Institute. Note that patients who died of other causes without evidence of disease [23 patients] are considered alive and lost to followup at the time of their death for purposes of evaluating the impact of MOPP therapy.

was a year or longer (93%), a statistically significant difference ($p = 0.001$). The duration of the second remission was also longer in patients whose initial complete remission exceeded 1 year than in those whose initial remission was less than 1 year. Overall survival is significantly improved in those patients who achieve second remissions over those who do not achieve a second remission ($p = 0.005$, Fig. 35-19). Thus, the duration of an initial complete remission attained with MOPP represents an important variable that must be taken into consideration in the management of patients who relapse. The duration of first complete remission is also an important variable that should influence the interpretation of any new treatment program evaluated in patients with Hodgkin's disease who relapse after combination chemotherapy.

Data on the importance of the initial remission duration and data that demonstrated that maintenance therapy in complete responders does not improve relapse-free survival have led to several conclusions.[365] Patients who are truly cured during remission induction cannot experience beneficial effects from maintenance therapy. Long initial remissions and retained sensitivity to MOPP in patients who stay in remission in excess of 1 year probably indicate that patients were almost cured by the intensive induction program. This is suggested by the fact that 14 out of 15 patients who relapsed one year or more after the end of therapy achieved a durable second remission. These data suggest that the initial remission induction treatment was not continued long enough. The failure of maintenance program to prevent relapse is therefore probably related to dose reduction and less intensive schedules of administration that are ineffective in eradicating occult residual tumor (see Chapter 8). The relative insensitivity of the tumor of patients who experience short remissions (<12 months) suggests that the primary cause of treatment failure in this group is the presence and overgrowth of cells resistant to the drugs in the MOPP program.

The studies tabulated in Table 35-26 evaluated the effect of drug combinations substituting drugs from the same general class as in the MOPP program in an attempt to alter its toxicity. The British group substituted vinblastine for vincristine. The study by Durant and associates added the nitrosourea BCNU and changed the alkylating agent to Cytoxan, substituted vinblastine for vincristine, and changed the schedule of the MOPP administration. Other programs removed nitrogen mustard and substituted a nitrosourea, and substituted vinblastine for vincristine. To date, none of these studies has reported a significant difference in the ability to induce durable complete remissions in patients with previously untreated Hodgkin's disease and toxicity has been substantial with all programs.

The randomized clinical trials conducted to compare various programs are shown in Table 35-25. The study by Hugeley and colleagues has been previously discussed. A study by the Acute Leukemia Group B comparing MOPP to a five-drug combination and the same five drugs used in sequence, showed that while the complete remission of MOPP and the 5-drug combination were similar, relapse-free survival was significantly better for the MOPP program. Most importantly, the same five drugs used in sequence were no better than the five-drug combination, which proved inferior to MOPP. This result indicates caution is necessary in evaluating programs solely on the basis of their capacity to induce complete remissions. Remission durability with no further treatment must be assessed as well. The British attempted to make a comparison of the use of MOPP with and without prednisone and found that the complete remission rate was significancly better using prednisone. The Eastern Cooperative Oncology Group compared the Durant regimen to the MOPP program. This study is still in progress, but intermittent reports do not show any significant advantage for the BCVPP over MOPP. The most instructive studies have been those of the Southwest Oncology Group, recently reviewed by Coltman (Table 35-25). In this series of studies, MOPP has been compared to MOPP plus bleomycin given in high and low doses. Interestingly, MOPP–high-dose bleomycin proved to be less effective than MOPP–low-dose bleomycin, and more toxic. While MOPP–low-dose bleomycin initially appeared superior to MOPP alone, there is now no difference in relapse-free survival amongst the various groups. No program listed in Table 35-25 has proven superior to MOPP as measured by complete remission rate, remission duration, or degree of toxicity.

In the early 1970s, other drugs with significant activity in Hodgkin's disease began to appear on the scene, as shown in Table 35-22. The most useful have been adriamycin, bleo-

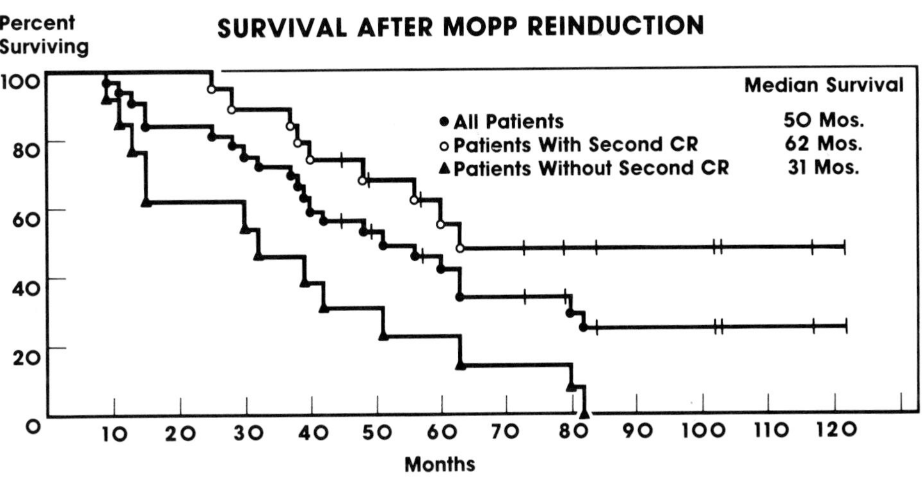

FIG. 35-19. Survival of patients with Hodgkin's disease retreated with MOPP after relapsing from their remission.

mycin, and the imidazole derivative dacarbazine. The availability of these drugs led to the development of non-cross-resistant combinations for the treatment of patients who fail MOPP chemotherapy. The results with the use of these regimens are shown in Table 35-28.[394–402] Of the greatest interest is the combination reported by Santoro and colleagues, using adriamycin, bleomycin, vinblastine, and dacarbazine, (ABVD) and a variant of this regimen (B-DOPA) reported by Lokich and associates.[395,396] Although the number of patients in their initial reports is small, the complete remission rate is approximately the same as can be achieved in a previously untreated population. In addition, the B-DOPA, ABVD, B-CAVE, and SCAB combinations are reported to be effective in patients who failed primary treatment with MOPP, a particularly difficult group of patients to treat.

A number of studies have emphasized that the site of relapse in patients who achieve complete remission is usually in areas previously involved with tumor, particularly in those with nodular sclerosis histology.[403] These data have led to the exploration of the use of chemotherapy and radiotherapy in combination with chemotherapy in patients with advanced disease. These studies fall in two general categories: the use of full doses of chemotherapy with full dose radiotherapy, and the more recent studies exploring chemotherapy interspersed with low dose radiotherapy to sites previously known to have been involved with tumor. (These are detailed in Table 35-29, and references 379 and 404–409.) In the first category, Kun et al reported the only study using MOPP preceding total nodal radiation therapy.[405] In that study of patients with stage IIIB disease, 96% of patients achieved a complete remission, but the toxicity of the combined approach used this way proved to be prohibitive and this approach is not to be recommended. Rosenberg and associates, as part of a larger randomized control trial from Stanford, compared use of MOPP alone in Stage IV disease to MOPP plus full dose radiotherapy to sites involved with tumor.[406] They also compared MOPP plus radiotherapy to radiotherapy alone in patients with Stage IIIB disease. In the latter arm of the study, MOPP plus radiotherapy proved superior to radiotherapy alone. In the former arm, the addition of radiotherapy to MOPP chemotherapy did not improve relapse-free or overall survival when compared to the use of MOPP alone. Their more recent study using a modification of the MOPP program, referred to as PAVe, shows similar results.[408] Two studies, those of Strauss and colleagues and Prosnitz and colleagues, illustrated in Table 35-29 deserve special mention.[407] In the Strauss study, the MOPP program is alternated with a version of the combination reported by Bonadonna, referred to as ABDV, and *low dose* radiotherapy is given to sites involved with tumor between cycles of chemotherapy. In addition, levamisole, the immunostimulant compound that enhances lymphocyte reactivity *in vitro* in Hodgkin's disease, is given to a random half of the study group. In the update of this report, complete remission rates were 80% for previously untreated, 65% for patients with prior or minimal radiotherapy or chemotherapy, and 50% for heavily pretreated patients, which is in the range reported for other studies including those using chemotherapy alone. Among 49 previously untreated patients there have, however, been no primary treatment failures. The estimated 2-year relapse rate for the entire group who achieved complete remission was 9%. Prosnitz and colleagues reported the use of a new drug combination, alternating it with low dose radiotherapy.[407] In their report, a total of 80 patients were treated and 75% of patients achieved a complete remission, a rate similar to drugs used alone. Disease-free survival at 5 years was 68%, with overall survival of 73% at 5 years. These data, again, are not significantly different from other studies. Since no random comparison is made to standard programs, it is difficult to draw any firm conclusions from these data. Similar results have been reported in small studies by Hoppe and associates, Bonadonna and associates and Goodman and associates.[408–410] To date, the use of combination of drugs and irradiation for patients with advanced Hodgkin's disease should not be considered routine until results are further evaluated. A major consideration is the added carcinogenic burden imposed on successfully treated patients by the addition of radiotherapy to the chemotherapy (see below).

A more recent approach to improving the results of chemotherapy of patients with advanced Hodgkin's disease has been

TABLE 35-28. Salvage Treatment of MOPP Failures

AUTHOR (Reference Number)	REGIMEN*	PRIOR THERAPY	TOTAL PATIENTS	PERCENT CR	MEDIAN DFS (months)	MEDIAN SURVIVAL (months)
Fisher et al (394)	MOPP	MOPP	32	59	21	50
Santoro et al (395)	ABVD	MOPP	21	62	70%/36	73%/36
Lokich et al (396)	B-DOPA	MOPP	15	60	–	–
Levi et al (397)	SCAB	CVPP or MOPP	17	35	8+	16+
Goldman et al (398)	CVB	MOPP or MVPP	39	26	–	–
Vinciguerra et al (399)	BVDS	MOPP	10	30	–	–
Case et al (400)	ABVD	MOPP	24	29		
Porzig et al (401)	B-CAVe	MOPP	22	50		17
Krikorian et al (402)	ABVD	MOPP	27	22		

Abbreviations: CR = Complete remission; DFS = Disease free survival; OS = Overall survival
*For abbreviations and definitions of acronyms see Table 35-39

TABLE 35-29. Value of Radiotherapy in Addition to Chemotherapy in Advanced Hodgkin's Disease

AUTHOR (Reference Number)	YEAR	REGIMEN*	PRIOR THERAPY	TOTAL PATIENTS	PERCENT CR	DISEASE FREE SURVIVAL (%/month)	OVERALL SURVIVAL (%month)
Straus et al (404)	1980	MOP alternating with ABDV +	–	49	80		
		RT + BDV alternating with	RT	18	50		
		MOP +/– levamisole between cycles	RT+CT	17	65		
Kun et al (405)	1976	MOPP + TNI	–	28	96		
Coltman et al (379)	1978	MOPP × 6 + RT + MOPP q2mo × 4	Yes				
Rosenberg et al (406)	1978	MOP(P) × 6 + TNI	–	18		67/82	59/82
		vs MOP(P)	–	15		58/82	43/82
Prosnitz et al (407)	1978	MVVPP × 3 + Low dose RT + MVVPP × 2	RT	124	84	74/60	80/60
Hoppe et al (375)	1979	MOPP/PAVe Alternating with RT	Yes	25	88	79/42	84/42
Bonadonna et al (407)	1979	MOPP + RT vs ABVD	–	29	93	95/48	
		+ RT		26	96	93/48	

*For abbreviations and definitions of acronyms see Table 35-39.

to use two non-cross-resistant combinations in alternating cycles. The first data on such an approach were reported by Santoro and colleagues, who alternated cycles of MOPP and ABVD and compared the results to MOPP alone.[411] In their most recent report, a total of 61 patients completed 12 cycles of chemotherapy and the authors were able to give results at 3 years of followup. Complete remission rate achieved with MOPP was 63%, compared with 87% for MOPP and alternating cycles of ABVD. The difference is almost entirely due to the better results with symptomatic patients. In symptomatic patients, a complete remission was noted in 59% for MOPP, compared to 86% for MOPP plus ABDV. At the time of their report, relapse-free survival was not significantly different between the two programs, although the difference in patients with symptomatic disease (61.5% *versus* 100%) is approaching statistical significance. The authors report that myelosuppression was not increased by MOPP plus ABDV. Cardiomyopathy or lung fibrosis was not yet observed to be a problem. A similar study is in progress at the National Cancer Institute, comparing the use of MOPP alone to alternating cycles of MOPP and the drug combination of streptozotocin, cyclohexylnitrosourea, adriamycin, and bleomycin.[397] This approach offers the possibility of improving both response rate and relapse-free survival of patients with advanced disease, without adding the additional burden of radiotherapy and the consequent risks in their combined use.

A controversy exists over the treatment of Stage IIIA Hodgkin's disease.[412–414] Results of radiotherapy alone, previously discussed, indicate relapse-free survivals of approximately 50%. The best results of radiotherapy, from Stanford, show relapse-free survival of 75%. Chemotherapy alone in small groups of asymptomatic patients is yielding relapse-free survival of near 100%. Similar results can be achieved by adding chemotherapy to radiotherapy, but with the increased risk of second cancers. A single randomized trial comparing TNI to MOPP showed equivalent results in clinical Stage IIIA patients and an advantage for TNI over MOPP in patients staged by laparotomy (PS IIIA). With current information, radiotherapy seems the treatment of choice for Stage PS IIIA patients and CS IIIA with nodular sclerosing disease, while chemotherapy is the treatment of choice for all other CS IIIA patients.

In summary, the MOPP chemotherapy program is the standard program for use in patients with Stage III and Stage IV Hodgkin's disease. To date, none of the studies comparing MOPP to other programs has provided a superior drug combination. Attempts to improve the complete response rate and remission duration by the addition of radiotherapy has yielded interesting but as yet indefinite results. The most promising new approach to the management of patients with advanced disease is the use of alternating cycles of non-cross-resistant combinations (MOPP and ABVD), now possible because of the recent addition of newer drugs to the therapeutic armamentarium.

THE ADMINISTRATION OF MOPP CHEMOTHERAPY

The MOPP program is illustrated in Table 35-30 along with a sliding scale for modification of drug doses. Details of some of the more commonly used alternatives to MOPP are shown in Tables 35-31 and 35-32. Because of the variability of speed of response among patients it is necessary to establish guidelines to adjust the total dose and duration of treatment to the speed of the response of individual patients. Unless chemotherapy is contraindicated for medical reasons, all patients treated with MOPP and other combinations should be given a minimum of six cycles or as many cycles as needed to achieve a complete remission, plus two additional cycles to consolidate the remission. Cycles should be given in a way to assure consistency and to preserve the integrity of the combination of drugs.

They are generally given every 28 days with the doses of myelosuppressive drugs, adjusted according to a sliding scale

TABLE 35-30. MOPP Regimen with Sliding Scale for Dose Modification

Nitrogen mustard	6 mg/m² IV	day 1 and 8
Vincristine (Oncovin)	1.4 mg/m² IV	day 1 and 8
Procarbazine	100 mg/m² PO	day 1 through 14
Prednisone*	40 mg/m² PO	day 1 through 14, cycles 1 & 4 only

Repeat cycle every 4 weeks

6 cycles minimum

Complete remission to be documented before discontinuing therapy

WBC COUNT	PLATELET COUNT	DOSE ADJUSTMENT
>4000/mm³	>100,000/mm³	100% all drugs
3000–4000/mm³	>100,000/mm³	100% vincristine, 50% nitrogen mustard and procarbazine
2000–3000/mm³	50,000–100,000/mm³	100% vincristine, 25% nitrogen mustard and procarbazine
1000–2000/mm³	>50,000/mm³	50% vincristine, 25% nitrogen mustard and procarbazine
<1000/mm³	<50,000/mm³	No therapy

*No dosage adjustment required.

based on the peripheral blood counts, as shown in Table 35-30. If the blood counts do not return to normal by day 28 of the previous cycle, but more than 50% of the myelotoxic drugs (procarbazine and nitrogen mustard) can be given according to the sliding scale, physicians are urged to proceed with the next cycle at reduced doses to preserve the timing of sequential cycles, while still giving some of all of the drugs. If the peripheral blood counts on day 28 are reduced to a level that required dose reduction of more than 50% of the myelosuppressive drugs, or omission of a drug from the combination would be required, an additional week is generally allowed between cycles to allow further recovery of the blood counts. MOPP chemotherapy is then reinstituted, if necessary at reduced doses. Generally, it has been advisable not to allow more than an extra week of waiting time between cycles of chemotherapy. Experience with patients who present with bone marrow involvement with Hodgkin's tumor, including those with pancytopenia, indicates that full doses of chemotherapy are necessary in order to achieve maximum effect. Dissolution of the tumor in the bone marrow usually results in rapid return of the blood counts. Full dose chemotherapy is, therefore, recommended in all these patients. Analyzing the results of the patients with proven bone marrow involvement indicates that this approach leads to complete response rates and relapse-free survivals equivalent to patients with tumor in other visceral sites.

TABLE 35-31. Alternatives to MOPP: Minor Variations

B-MOPP (LOW-DOSE BLEOMYCIN)
Bleomycin 2 U/m² day 1 and 8
Nitrogen Mustard 6 mg/m² day 1 and 8
Vincristine (Oncovin®) 1.4 mg/m² day 1 and 8
Procarbazine 100 mg/m² day 1 thru 10
Prednisone 50 mg/m² day 1 thru 10 (Cycles 1 and 4 only)
Repeat every 28 days

BVCPP
BCNU 100 mg/m² day 1
Vinblastine 5 mg/m² day 1
Cyclophosphamide 600 mg/m² day 1
Procarbazine 100 mg/m² day 1 thru 10
Prednisone 60 mg/m² day 1 thru 10
Repeat every 28 days

MVPP
Nitrogen Mustard 6 mg/m² day 1 and 8
Vinblastine 10 mg day 1, 8, and 15
Procarbazine 100 mg/m² day 1 thru 15
Prednisolone 40 mg day 1 thru 15
Repeat every 28 days

CVPP
Cyclophosphamide 300 mg/m² day 1 and 8
Vinblastine 10 mg day 1, 8, and 15
Procarbazine 100 mg/m² day 1 thru 15
Prednisone 40 mg/m² day 1 thru 15 (Cycles 1 and 4 only)
Repeat every 28 days

CVPP-CCNU
Cyclophosphamide 600 mg/m² day 1
Vinblastine 6 mg/m² day 1
Procarbazine 100 mg/m² day 1 thru 14
Prednisone 40 mg/m² 1 thru 14
CCNU 75 mg/m² day 1 (on alternative cycles)
Repeat every 28 days

MVVPP
Nitrogen Mustard 0.4 mg/kg day 1
Vincristine 1.4 mg/m² days 1, 8, 15
Vinblastine 6 mg/m² days 22, 29, 36
Prednisone 40 mg/m² day 1 thru 22 then taper 14 days
Procarbazine 100 mg (total) days 22 thru 43
Repeat every 57 days

TABLE 35-32. Alternatives to MOPP: Non-Cross Resistant

ABVD Doxorubicin (Adriamycin) 25 mg/m² day 1 and 15 Bleomycin 10 U/m² day 1 and 15 Vinblastine 6 mg/m² day 1 and 15 Dacarbazine 375 mg/m² day 1 and 15 Repeat every 28 days	B-CAVe Bleomycin 2.5 U/m² day 1, 28, and 35 CCNU 100 mg/m² day 1 Doxorubicin (Adriamycin) 60 mg/m² day 1 Vinblastine (Velban®) 5 mg/m² day 1 Repeat every 42 days
B-DOPA Bleomycin 4 U/m² day 2 and 5 Dacarbazine 150 mg/m² day 1 thru 5 Vincristine (Oncovin®) 1.5 mg/m² day 1 and 5 Prednisone 40 mg/m² day 1 thru 6 Doxorubicin (Adriamycin) 60 mg/m² day 1 Repeat every 21 days	BVDS Bleomycin 5 U/m² day 1 and 15 Vinblastine 6 mg/m² day 1 and 15 Doxorubicin 30 mg/m² day 1 Streptozotocin 1500 mg/m² day 1 and 15 Repeat every 28 days
SCAB Streptozotocin 500 mg/m² day 1 thru 5 CCNU 100 mg/m² day 1 Doxorubicin (Adriamycin) 45 mg/m² day 1 Bleomycin 15 U/m² day 1 and 8 Repeat every 28 days	CVB CCNU 100 mg/m² day 1 Vinblastine 6 mg/m² day 1 and 8 Bleomycin 15 units day 1 and 8 Repeat every 28 days
ABDV Doxorubicin (Adriamycin) 25 mg/m² days 1 and 15 Bleomycin 2 mg (total) days 4 thru 12, and 18 thru 26 Dacarbazine 250 mg/m² days 1 and 15 Vinblastine (Velban®) 6 mg/m² day 1 Repeat every 28 days	

In order to determine whether further treatment after six cycles is required, it is necessary to ascertain whether a patient has achieved a complete remission. Since maintenance chemotherapy has not improved the prognosis of patients with Hodgkin's disease, this becomes a critical point of management. Patients should be restaged 1 month after the sixth cycle of treatment, at a time when blood counts have returned to normal, or 1 month after the last cycle of therapy needed to consolidate the complete remission. Restaging is accomplished by repeating all previous positive tests, such as tomography and lymphangiography, and repeating biopsies of both liver and bone marrow if these organs were previously involved by tumor. Lymphangiograms should be repeated if insufficient dye remains in the retroperitoneal lymph nodes to judge their size. If previously enlarged lymph nodes have returned to normal size, they are considered normal even if residual morphologic abnormalities are present, since these defects cannot be refilled with dye unless the lymphogram is repeated. If no evidence of tumor is found, no further therapy is given and patients can be followed at monthly intervals for the first year, two-monthly intervals for the second year and every 4 months to 6 months for the next 2 years. Annual restaging, short of repeating biopsies is useful for the first 4 years.

COMBINED RADIATION AND CHEMOTHERAPY IN HODGKIN'S DISEASE, STAGES I, II AND III

Chemotherapy has been used with radiation in a number of centers. Most of the older studies used single drugs and radiation therapy techniques which would not be acceptable today. Since the advent of MOPP combination chemotherapy, a number of attempts at combined modality therapy have been described. The systematic studies by Stanford to compare combined modality therapy *versus* radiation therapy alone appear to indicate that MOPP chemotherapy does reduce relapse in those patients in whom relapse with radiation alone appears likely.[311] In those groups in which radiation treatment appears to be associated with a significant recurrence rate, combined modality treatment appears attractive. Unfortunately, this treatment can be associated with considerable complications. Wide field irradiation with chemotherapy has been associated with a significant increase in leukemia and non-Hodgkin's lymphoma, with a cumulative likelihood of such tumors predicted to be about 5% at 10 years (see Chapter 45 on Secondary Cancers).[416–418] This appears to be true whether the radiation and chemotherapy are given in the initial treatment or whether the chemotherapy is given at the time of radiation failure. Combined modality treatment can also result in fatal infectious complications.[419] Deaths due to both of these appear to be reduced when the irradiated volume is less than total nodal irradiation.[420] Table 35-33 shows the results from the Joint Center comparing the likelihood of fatal complications, either leukemia or infection, when total nodal irradiation and chemotherapy are given as compared to subtotal nodal irradiation. Because of these results it is important to analyze the consequences of a treatment philosophy that would restrict combined modality therapy and add chemotherapy to only those patients who fail initial radiation. Such an approach represents a radical change in our current treatment principles, which try to assure the highest likelihood of relapse-free survival. This philosophy suggests that the lower relapse-free survival after radiotherapy alone may be acceptable because failing patients could subsequently be salvaged by chemotherapy. To analyze whether this is the case requires analysis of the outcome of treatment of the patients who have failed radiation. A review by Mauch and colleagues of the Joint Center for Radiation Therapy experi-

TABLE 35-33. Fatal Complications of Combined Modality Treatment

	XRT + MOPP	XRT RELAPSE MOPP	TOTAL
M-PA	0/48	0/31	0/79
TNI	3/33 (2 leukemia) (1 disseminated herpes)	3/26 (1 leukemia) (1 herpes) (1 non-Hodgkin's lymphoma)	6/59

ence has indicated that the most important prognostic factor for patients with relapsing Hodgkin's disease was their initial pathological stage.[310] They could identify two groups, those patients with initial early stage disease including Stage IA, IIA, IIB, or IIIA (spleen only). The cumulative survival at 4 years following relapse in this group is 81%, while in those patients who initially had IIIA disease with lymph node involvement or IIIB disease it was 42%. The difference between these two groups was almost completely due to the proportion of patients who achieved a complete response with chemotherapy; this being 86% in the favorable group and 56% in the unfavorable group. These data suggest that early stage patients can be treated with radiation alone, with chemotherapy being reserved for only those patients who fail. In these patients, such salvage therapy is quite effective. However, those with Stage III disease with lymph node involvement or systemic systems are not salvaged well and should be treated with initial chemotherapy, either alone or in combination with radiation.

The techniques of combining radiation and chemotherapy vary. Some studies administer all the radiation, then all of the chemotherapy. Others divide the chemotherapy, after two or three cycles give the radiation, then finally complete the chemotherapy. Still others interspace cycles of chemotherapy after completion of each radiation volume. It is uncertain which is preferable and this may depend on the clinical circumstances. One must be careful not to compromise both the chemotherapy and the radiation in programs of combined modality therapy. The one technique associated with the greatest toxicity is full course chemotherapy followed by total nodal irradiation, and this is not recommended.

CURRENT RECOMMENDATIONS FOR TREATMENT OF HODGKIN'S DISEASE BY STAGE

Based on the previous data, the following recommendations for treatment appear appropriate:

Clinical and pathologic Stage I and Stage IIA supradiaphragmatic disease without large mediastinal masses should be treated with mantle and para-aortic field radiation, except for those with lymphocyte depleted histology, who should receive at least TNI and, in some centers, chemotherapy as well. Such treatment is associated with very high relapse-free survival and ultimate survival and without significant major complications.

Clinical and pathologic Stage I and Stage IIA disease with large mediastinal masses currently represent a clinical quandry. An acceptable treatment alternative appears to be combination chemotherapy initially, with radiation to areas of previous bulk disease (mediastinum). Such a treatment technique means that, in patients presenting initially with large mediastinal masses, laparotomy is not indicated since it will not significantly alter therapy and does have an anesthesia risk. Full course chemotherapy should be given with the radiation volume restricted. The total dose of radiation under such circumstances is uncertain. A second alternative is to use radiation as in the other Stage I and Stage II patients, but using techniques of dividing the mantle radiation into two courses to allow the mass to shrink and thus reduce the volume irradiated in the second course. Such treatment will be associated with approximately a 50% failure rate; however, thus far most of these patients can be salvaged with subsequent chemotherapy. A third alternative is to treat such patients with chemotherapy only. Data on this approach is incomplete and studies are in progress to evaluate it. Since nodular sclerosing Hodgkin's disease, so common in patients with mediastinal tumors, appears to be the worst prognostic group for chemotherapy-treated patients this approach is not recommended in practice. Subdiaphagmatic CS and PS I and IIA disease should be treated with para-aortic and pelvic irradiation for pelvic or inguinal presentation and with TNI for para-aortic presentations.

Stage PS IIB disease can be treated with subtotal nodal radiation. It does not appear that combined modality therapy should be used in such patients unless they have very large mediastinal disease. Patients with CS IIB disease should received TNI or TNI plus MOPP chemotherapy. It is possible that this group should be treated with chemotherapy only, although there has not been a significant experience with this technique.

Stage PS IIIA patients are best subdivided into favorable, called either IIIA (spleen only) or PS $IIIA_1$, and unfavorable, called either PS IIIA (nodal) or $IIIA_2$. It is our current recommendation that combination of TNI and MOPP should be avoided because of the high risk of secondary malignancies and fatal infections. Therefore, for PS $IIIA_1$, we would treat with TNI. If the patient fails this treatment then we would treat with combination chemotherapy. Clinical Stage IIIA patients and Stage IIIB patients would be treated with combination chemotherapy either alone or in combination with limited volume irradiation to sites of bulky disease (in patients with nodular sclerosing Hodgkin's disease). Stage IVA and Stage IVB patients should be treated with combination chemotherapy.

Exceptions to these general recommendations must be applied to very young children. Such children have a greater risk of infectious complications after splenectomy making surgical staging less desirable. Radiation therapy in the dose ranges used in Hodgkin's disease results in significant retardation of growth in the treated volume. This volume must be limited and care taken to attempt symmetrical irradiation in order to limit the deformity produced as a consequence of unilateral asymmetric bone growth. Some authors have suggested low-dose radiation be used with chemotherapy in such patients, while others favor using localized radiation for early stage disease with combination chemotherapy reserved for those patients who fail initial therapy. Finally, some groups recommend chemotherapy as initial therapy for most if not all patients in order to avoid these irradiation complications.

THE PLACE OF RADIATION IN THE TREATMENT OF NON-HODGKIN'S LYMPHOMA

The curative role of radiation therapy in the treatment of non-Hodgkin's lymphoma is quite different from that in Hodgkin's disease. While non-Hodgkin's lymphoma is quite responsive to radiation, only a small proportion of patients are amenable to cure with local or regional radiation. In addition to histologic variants, the term "non-Hodgkin's lymphoma" includes a variety of clinical constellations. For example, lymphoma of bone, mediastinal lymphoma of childhood and adolescence, and lymphoma in Waldeyer's ring are all quite different and may require different therapeutic approaches. Such approaches range from local field irradiation to whole body irradiation, from single agent chemotherapy to aggressive multi-drug treatment protocols and finally to a combination of radiation and chemotherapy. In the study of all of these approaches, it should be remembered that it is extraordinarily easy to make many lymph nodes in patients with non-Hodgkin's lymphomas regress; however, it is not always clear how frequently one alters the natural history of these diseases with treatment for some disease categories. In order to understand this, one must be careful to separate survival from freedom from first relapse. Since, as described earlier, the nodular lymphomas may have a more indolent course, but with a consistent force of relapse and mortality, fixed time survival such as the commonly used 5-year survival may in fact be misleading. The survival curves may still be continuing downward.

Radiation therapy has its major role in the treatment of localized lymphomas. Unfortunately these Stage I and Stage II nodal lymphomas are quite uncommon presentations on non-Hodgkin's lymphoma. Of the 338 consecutive patients seen at the Peter Bent Brigham Hospital, only 11% were thought to have local or regional non-Hodgkin's lymphoma.[421] Older and similar data are shown in Table 35-16. Evaluation of these patients did not include staging laparotomy and thus the proportion with localized lymphoma would in fact have been less. Using similar criteria at the Princess Margaret Hospital, about 20% of the patients were found to have localized disease.[422] The sequential staging of 100 non-Hodgkin's lymphoma patients at the University of Chicago revealed 12 patients to have Stage I or Stage II disease and similar results have been already discussed from the staging study reported from the National Cancer Institute.[213,219,423] Review of the experience at the Joint Center for Radiation Therapy shows that while radiation achieves both reasonable survival and relapse-free survival for Stage I disease, this is not true for Stage II.[421] Stage II disease has been subdivided and it appears that contiguous Stage II disease may behave like Stage I while noncontiguous Stage II disease behaves as though it is generalized disease.[422,424,425] Thus, like Stage I disease, contiguous Stage II disease seems to be amenable to localized treatment. This appears to be true for both nodular and diffuse disease; however, it is more difficult to evaluate nodular disease because of the indolent nature of the disease.

There have been a large number of studies reporting the results of localized radiation therapy for non-Hodgkin's lymphoma.[342,394,395,421,422,424–432] Unfortunately many of these were reported before or do not use current histopathologic classifications and vary in the extent of pretreatment evaluation. A careful, representative review is that from the Princess Margaret Hospital, which indicates that there is about 55% cure rate in localized lymphoma treated with localized radiation therapy. In general, histiocytic lymphoma tends to recur early with few if any late relapses. As this is not true with lymphocytic disease, it is of interest that in the Princess Margaret Hospital series the curve for lymphocytic disease, like that for histiocytic, became parallel with the age-adjusted peer population, indicating cure in both groups.

The technique of radiation therapy should be different from that used with Hodgkin's disease. There are no data to suggest that adjuvant wide field irradiation to clinically uninvolved contiguous locations is of value.[342] There are good dose–response relationships for all the Rappaport subtypes of non-Hodgkin's lymphoma except diffuse histiocytic.[422,433] In general, the doses used are approximately 3500 rad in $3\frac{1}{2}$ weeks for localized non-Hodgkin's lymphoma, except for the histiocytic variety. For this it is suggested that the dose be 4500 rad to 5000 rad given in 200-rad fractions, 5 days a week.

Attempts to combine chemotherapy with radiation depend on the combination chemotherapy used. The Stanford study comparing total nodal radiotherapy and three-drug combination chemotherapy showed no advantage for the addition of drugs to radiation therapy.[434] In contrast, the Milan group, using local or regional radiation with or without CVP, report a significant increase in freedom from relapse for patients with diffuse histology, either lymphocytic or nodular, Stage I or II, nodal or extranodal disease.[435]

Total body irradiation (TBI) has been used in cancer treatment since early in this century. Advanced non-Hodgkin's lymphoma was first treated by TBI by Heublein at Memorial Hospital in the 1930s.[436] Medinger and Craver, using his methods, reported a doubling in the average survival time for patients with disseminated non-Hodgkin's lymphoma.[437] With the development of systemic chemotherapeutic agents, there was a diminished interest in TBI until Johnson and associates suggested a new role for this treatment.[438] The technique is to give 5 rad to 15 rad, three to five times a week to the whole body to a total dose of between 100 rad to 250 rad. The initial treatment of nodular lymphoma using this technique showed good results at the NIH and at the Joint Center for Radiation Therapy, equal to those with CVP.[439–441] The exact mechanism of action of the treatment technique is unknown, although in mice, low doses of whole body irradiation is selectively lethal to elements of the immune system that may regulate growth. Marked bone marrow depression can be seen with this treatment, especially in a prolonged and protracted thrombocytopenia. If this technique is to be used, we recommend that 15 rad twice a week be given with an interruption after 75 rad or so. Routine white blood cell and platelet counts should be done before each treatment. These must be plotted and watched carefully for the appearance of thrombocytopenia. Using such a technique in nodular lymphomas the 5-year survival for Stage II and Stage IV patients at the Joint Center for Radiation Therapy was 60%, while the relapse-free survival was 25%. There is no evidence of a plateau on these curves and thus the treatment is considered to be palliative.[441] The diffuse lymphomas may achieve a remission with such treatment but it is of shorter duration. In this study the median time to relapse was 24 months for nodular lymphoma while only 12 months for diffuse lymphoma.

Primary extranodal tumor may present initially as local or regional disease. If, on evaluation, the presence of distant disease can be eliminated, most of these presentations respond to radiation and are treated similarly to Stage I and localized Stage II nodal disease.[442,443] Occurrence of tumors in a number of extranodal sites is quite common and has been reported separately. Primary lymphoma of bone may spread to regional lymph nodes and still be amenable to local treatment. It is often called "reticulum sarcoma of bone," however, lymphoma of bone is more accurate.[444] The pelvis, femur, humerus and ribs, and tibia are involved most frequently. When treated with radiation, care must be taken to treat the entire medullary cavity. With local treatment, 5-year survivals are in the 40% to 50% range.[444–446] There have been some who have suggested a role for Coley's toxins as an adjuvant to radiation therapy in management of this tumor.[447] Waldeyer's ring is another frequent site of involvement usually with diffuse lymphoma.[448] Stage I and contiguous Stage II disease have a 50% to 70% cure rate with local or regional treatment.[442,448–450] One series reports an association of gastrointestinal involvement either initially or as a site of recurrent disease in 10% of patients with a Waldeyer's ring presentation.[450] Primary gastrointestinal lymphoma may arise in the stomach or small intestine.[451] When it is of the former, it is often a diffuse histiocytic histology. There are frequent ulcer-like symptoms and regional node involvement. Small intestine involvement is usually multifocal and thus local resection is not adequate. This is usually of a lymphocytic cell type. This disease is more common in the Middle East and may be associated with malabsorption of the α-chain IgA in the peripheral blood.[452,453] Treatment reviews emphasize resection of the gastric lesion if possible to avoid possible bleeding or perforation due to tumor necrosis following radiation of chemotherapy. Current series emphasize the role of combined modality management of intestinal lymphoma.[454]

COMBINATION CHEMOTHERAPY OF THE NON-HODGKIN'S LYMPHOMA

The results of combination chemotherapy of the non-Hodgkin's lymphoma need to be sharply separated into two groups of patients: those with nodular and diffuse lymphomas. The controversy over the proper approach to treat NPDL in routine practice has been discussed. In contrast to treatment of NPDL, unequivocal progress has been made in the development of successful drug programs for treatment of the non-Hodgkin's lymphoma of the diffuse, undifferentiated, lymphoblastic, and histiocytic varieties in the Rappaport scheme.[342] There is now also data that indicate differences in response rate among some of the different types of nodular lymphomas.[343,349] Long-term disease-free survivals appear to be increasingly possible as the fraction of undifferentiated cells in the lymph node increases. Thus, patients with NM or NH lymphomas have been reported to have complete response rates and relapse-free survivals equal or superior to those of patients with diffuse lymphoma. Combination chemotherapy is now indicated for all patients with diffuse large cell lymphomas, and appears superior to a single agent therapy in patients with NML and NHL. The treatment of Burkitt's lymphoma is reviewed in Chapter 34.

The era of combination chemotherapy of the non-Hodgkin's lymphomas began simultaneously with that of Hodgkin's disease. The MOPP program was initially used to treat patients with the non-Hodgkin's lymphoma in 1964 as part of the original Hodgkin's disease study. Patients at NCI were then classified using the older terminology, lymphosarcoma (LSA) and reticulum cell sarcoma (RCS). In the initial study of 15 patients with LSA and eight with RCS, it was reported that seven of 15 LSA patients had complete remissions, while three of 8 RCS patients had a complete response.[455] At the time of that report, all but the two of the LSA patients had relapsed but all three of the RCS patients who responded to MOPP remained disease free. Although the number of patients was small, durable complete remission after drug therapy had not previously been reported for patients with advanced reticulum cell sarcoma. The results in LSA were initially disappointing compared with Hodgkin's disease and the use of MOPP program for NHL was discontinued in favor of the CVP combination (see below).[456] By this time, the Rappaport classification was coming into general use and NCI investigators used it to redefine the patients in this population. Further patients with diffuse histiocytic lymphoma were added to the study and the results in 27 patients with advanced DHL treated with the MOPP program (or C-MOPP Cytoxan substituted for nitrogen mustard) revealed a 41% complete response rate with only one of the 11 complete responding patients relapsing up to 10 years after therapy had been discontinued.[457] The three patients of the original series, were still in remission in 1975.[455] Interestingly enough, the relapse curve for patients with advanced disease was similar to that reported by Jones and colleagues in patients with early disease treated with radiotherapy. All relapses tended to occur after the first 2 years off treatment. The difference between the survival curves in patients with advanced and localized disease was only in the median survival, which was 6 months for patients with advanced disease and about a year for patients with localized disease. Only one patient who achieved complete remission in the NCI study relapsed at 5 months and died at 23.5 months.

Levitt and associates in a study of a four-drug combination of cyclophosphamide, vincristine, arabinosyl cytosine, and methotrexate, with citrovorum factor rescue, reported preliminary results in 15 patients with lymphomas also described by the older terminology.[458] They reported that nine of 15 patients had complete remissions and six patients remained in remission at the time of that report. No histologic subtype analysis was given in that report. A later re-analysis of these data, using the Rappaport classification was made in 1975 by Berd.[459] Of the 17 patients reported in that study, eight were found to have DHL and six of the eight patients had complete remissions. At that time, only one patient had relapsed, at seven months. The other five remained in complete remission up to 65 months. These two small series gave impetus to the idea that patients with this aggressive tumor in its advanced stages, could be successfully treated, and started a concerted effort to develop better programs for the treatment of DHL. With the demonstration that adriamycin was an active antitumor drug in patients with DHL, newer drug programs exploited its use in combination. Procarbazine was not usually used in newer combination programs because of its low individual activity in patients with non-Hodgkin's lymphoma. One of these regimens, the BACOP program, reported from the NCI, produced 48% complete response rate in patients with far advanced disease.[460] Again, while failure to achieve a complete remission was associated with rapid demise, if a complete remission was attained, few patients relapsed. The survival of the population of 56 MOPP and BACOP patients treated at NCI is shown in Fig. 35-20.[461] Only four of 26 patients who attained complete remission have relapsed, and 84% of patients who achieved a complete remission remain disease-free beyond 2 years. It should be noted that all patients with partial or no responses died by 24 months. Of all treated patients, approximately 40% remained disease-free beyond 2 years and are probably cured of their disease. Sweet and colleagues reported the results of their attempt to use the drug program reported by Levitt and colleagues and Berd and colleagues.[458,459,461] The response rate was similar: Pooled results of the Yale and Chicago groups allowed an analysis of the results in a total of 45 patients. A complete remission rate of 58% and long disease-free survival were noted.

A summary of the data from these and other studies is shown in Table 35-34.[341,459,462–471] The Southwest Oncology Group has reported complete response rates of 68% and 66% in patients with advanced diffuse histiocytic lymphoma treated with the adriamycin-containing combinations, CHOP and HOP, respectively.[472] The true impact of these programs is, however, difficult to define, because all patients received some form of maintenance treatment after discontinuation of therapy.

In order to determine the relative importance of the various pathologic features that influence the survival of patients with diffuse lymphomas, investigators at the NCI have analyzed the clinical course of 151 such patients seen over a decade at the NCI.[461] The stage and response to treatment are shown in Table 35-35. Combination chemotherapy was the initial treatment (C-MOPP or BACOP) in 91 patients (60%). Localized radiotherapy was the initial therapy in 29 patients with Stage I disease. Only those patients who achieved a complete remission had a long disease-free survival. Fifty-four percent of patients had a complete remission and their median survival has not been reached with 76% of complete responders alive at 70 months. Eight clinical factors were identified that appeared to adversely affect the capacity to attain a complete

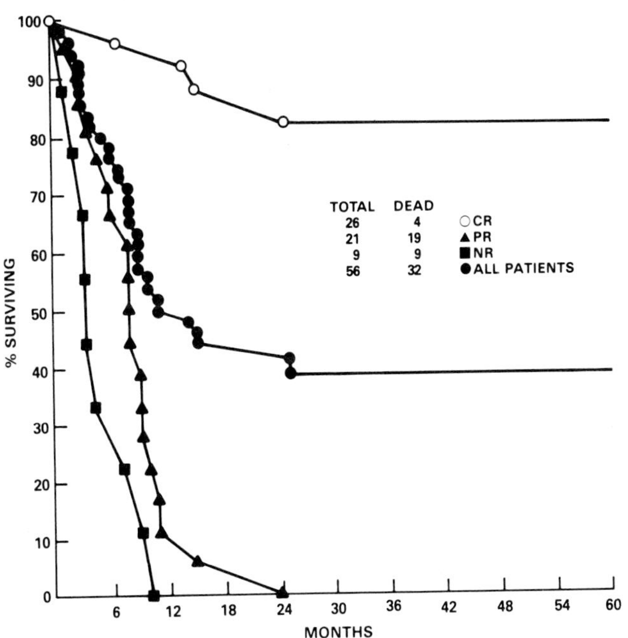

FIG. 35-20. Survival of patients with stage III and IV treated at NCI with MOPP, C-MOPP, or BACOP.

remission. All save one tend to reflect a large volume of tumor cells. The only exception is sex, a characteristic that significantly influenced survival without affecting the complete remission rate. Advanced stage, the presence of constitutional symptoms, bone marrow involvement, large gastrointestinal masses greater than 10 cm in diameter, liver involvement, a hemoglobin of less than 12 gm%, and a level of the serum lactate dihydrogenase greater than 250 units/ml, all negatively influenced response rate (Table 35-36). In the latter case, the LDH level appeared to reflect tumor volume. Patients with an LDH less than 250 units/ml had a complete remission rate of 74%, compared to a complete response rate of 39% for those with serum level of greater than 250 units/ml. A multifactorial analysis to delineate the relative strength of these primary prognostic factors identified four of the variables as the best predictors of the patient's course: bone marrow involvement, large gastrointestinal masses greater than 10 cm in diameter, symptoms, and sex. These factors influence survival because fewer patients achieved complete remissions; survival of patients with poor prognostic factors, however, was not compromised if a complete remission was achieved.

Complete response rates for the numerous treatment programs in the literature vary from 13% to 69% (Table 35-34). There is also considerable variability in the fraction of patients free of any recurrence of disease at the critical 2-year point. It seems likely, but is not discernible in the data from most reported studies, that much of the variability is accounted for by a different mix of sites of involvement, size of primary tumor masses, and histologic subtypes. The four best programs for treating DHL are the MOPP (or C-MOPP), COMLA, CHOP (or HOP) and BACOP.

The use of chemotherapy alone or in combination may also be effective in patients with early stage DHL. In a recent report by Miller and Jones, the use of chemotherapy in patients

TABLE 35-34. Primary Chemotherapy of Advanced Diffuse Histiocytic Lymphoma

AUTHOR	YEAR	REGIMEN	TOTAL PATIENTS	NUMBER OF PATIENTS WITH CR	CR PERCENT	PERCENT DFS AT 2 YEARS	COMMENTS
DeVita (342)	1977	MOPP, CMOPP or BACOP	56	32	46	41	DFS at 5 yr = 39%
Skarin et al (463)	1977	BACOP (Farber)	18	10	56	N.A.	Still in remission - 33%
Berd et al (459)	1975	COMA	8	6	75	63	Still in remission - 63%
McKelvey et al (464)	1976	$CHOP_{(a)}$	35*	22*	63*	–	Maintenance CXT
McKelvey et al (464)	1976	HOP	29*	22*	76*	–	Maintenance CXT
Luce et al (465)	1973	BCVP	16	10	66	–	Maintenance CXT
Durant et al (466)	1975	BCCP	28	14	50	21	Still in remission-21%
Bonadonna et al (467)	1974	MABOP	26*	14*	54	N.A.	
Rodriquez et al (468)	1977	CHOP-Bleo	26	18	69	58	
Elias et al (469)	1978	$CHOP_{(b)}$	23	9	39	30	Includes 2 patients with Stage I
Sweet et al (462)	1980	COMLA	42	23	55	48	3 relapses—all achieved 2nd CR
Fisher et al (470)	1980	ProMACE/MOPP	22*	11*	50	N.A.	
Stein et al (471)	1974	COPP	6	1	16	16	

*Date modified to exclude other histologic categories and early stages of disease.
For drug names and definitions of acronyms see Table 35-39.

TABLE 35-35. Influence of Stage on Complete Response Rate and Survival of Patients with Diffuse Histiocytic Lymphoma Treated with Involved Field Radiation (Stage I Only) or Combination Chemotherapy with CVP, C-MOPP, or BACOP

	PERCENT TOTAL PATIENTS	COMPLETE RESPONDERS	MEDIAN SURVIVAL (MONTHS)
Stage I	13%	100%	N.R.*
Stage II	23%	56%	33
Stage III	14%	66%	71
Stage IV	50%	38%	11

*Not reached
(Fisher RI, Hubbard S, DeVita VT et al: Factors predicting long term survival in diffuse mixed, histiocytic, or undifferentiated lymphoma. Blood 58:45–51, 1981)

with localized DHL has been examined.[473] Of 22 patients with localized (Stage I or II), 14 patients received chemotherapy as their only treatment and eight received chemotherapy plus local radiation. Adriamycin-containing combinations were used in all but two of these patients. All 22 patients achieved a complete remission and all were alive at the time of the report. Only one patient has relapsed. The group from Milan, Italy, has also reported a randomized clinical trial using CVP chemotherapy plus radiotherapy to radiotherapy alone.[435] They reported a highly significant advantage for the use of a combined program in patients with diffuse histology.

Of recent concern has been the development of the central nervous system involvement in patients with diffuse large cell lymphomas. This has been particularly notable in patients with bone marrow involvement. The development of CNS disease, as the only site of relapse in patients in remission, is reminiscent of the pattern of relapse in children with lymphoblastic leukemia. These results reported by Bunn and associates have led to the recommendation that patients with diffuse large cell lymphomas, with bone marrow involvement, should have prophylactic central nervous system therapy with intrathecal methotrexate.

SPECIAL CONSIDERATIONS IN THE TREATMENT OF PATIENTS WITH ADVANCED DIFFUSE LARGE CELL LYMPHOMAS

There are several important points to consider when charged with the welfare of patients with one of the diffuse large cell lymphomas. First, diffuse large cell lymphomas (mostly reticulum cell sarcomas in the older terminology) are curable

TABLE 35-36. Prognostic Factors Influencing Complete Remission Rate in Patients with Diffuse Lymphoma

FACTOR	FRACTION OF PATIENTS WITH FACTOR (%)	CR RATE AND MEDIAN SURVIVAL OF PATIENTS WITH FACTOR		CR RATE (%) AND MEDIAN SURVIVAL OF PATIENTS WITHOUT FACTOR		p VALUE
Liver involvement	12	25%	6 mo	59%	51 mo	$p < 0.002$
"B" symptoms	45	38%	10 mo	67%	N.R.	$p = 0.002$
Bone marrow involvement	15	9%	6 mo	62%	51 mo	$p < 0.002$
Hgb < 12 gms%	39	41%	10 mo	63%	71 mo	$p < 0.002$
LDH >250	62	39%	13 mo	74%	N.R.	$p = 0.003$
Gastrointestinal mass <10 cm in diameter	10	7%	6 mo	60%	51 mo	$p < 0.002$

(Fisher RI, Hubbard S, DeVita VT et al: Factors predicting long term survival in diffuse mixed, histiocytic, or undifferentiated lymphoma. Blood 58:45–51, 1981)

illnesses, even when the patient has widespread tumor. Second, unlike patients with nodular lymphomas, a decision not to treat the patient is not a viable option. Left untreated, this type of lymphoma is clinically and biologically aggressive and death supervenes in less than 2 years in almost all cases. Since complete tumor disappearance is uncommon with single agent chemotherapy and long survival is not possible without achieving a complete remission, single drugs are not good choices for first treatment. Third, all the potentially curative treatments listed in Table 35-34 are difficult to administer. Side effects are severe and the schedule of administration must be rigidly adhered to in order to achieve the best results. For example, prolongation of the interval between cycles of treatment, even by a week or so, can be associated with a rapid regrowth of tumor between cycles. Regrowth is almost always followed shortly by death. This reason for treatment failure has led to the redesign of some of the programs. Physicians are advised, therefore, to consult with other investigators studying ways of improving these treatments before treating a patient and should attempt to participate in such clinical trials.

The initial goal of treatment for diffuse large cell lymphomas is to produce a complete remission. The quality of these remissions can be judged by the fraction of patients who remain free of disease 2 years after all therapy is discontinued. Selection of a therapy, new or old, should be based on both these points. A therapy less than 2 years old is unlikely to be the best first choice in routine practice. A number of treatment programs listed in Table 35-34 are less than ideal because the high complete remission rates have been offset by a low relapse-free survival at 2 years. In many cases, these data are complicated by the fact that drug maintenance treatment is given continuously after remission is achieved. In other reported programs, the initial high complete remission rates are related to the selection of patients with an excellent prognosis, such as those with only skin or soft tissue involvement. In such patients the complete and durable remissions occur in greater than 85% of cases.

Recently, the NCI group has developed a treatment program called ProMACE-flexi-therapy (Table 35-34).[437] The overall complete remission rate for this program is 68% and there have been few relapses. Several parts of this regime have been modified to match the clinical evolution of diffuse lymphomas. It includes alternating cycles of two non-cross-resistant drug combinations, MOPP and ProMACE. The schedules of this and other combinations of drugs to treat NHL are detailed in Table 35-37.

The decision to switch from the initial drug combination to the second combination is not a fixed point but made at the bedside at the first evidence of a change in the slope of the clinical response curve of measurable lesions (the concept of flexi-therapy). Such an approach attempts to use the patient's response to treatment as an indicator of the magnitude of the antitumor effect. Experimental evidence in rodents shows that when the slope of the response diminishes it is usually due to two things: a decreased cell kill and regrowth of drug resistant cells (see Chapter 8). Switching to the second non-cross-resistant combination at this point is designed to maximize the initial chances to achieve a complete remission. ProMACE-flexi-therapy also includes the use of high dose methotrexate, and citrovorum factor rescue, to bridge the interval between cycles of treatment to prevent tumor regrowth while the bone marrow is recovering. The study was initially combined with a randomization of half the patients to intravenous hyperalimentation to test the hypothesis that nutritional support during remission induction might improve the overall results. This phase of the study has been discontinued owing to lack of good effect and highly significant toxicity associated with intravenous hyperalimentation.

NODULAR MIXED AND NODULAR HISTIOCYTIC LYMPHOMAS

Nodular mixed and nodular histiocytic lymphomas differ from NPDL in the size of the fraction of large undifferentiated cells resembling histiocytes. A diagnosis of nodular mixed lym-

TABLE 35-37. Drug Combinations in Clinical Use for the Primary Treatment of Non-Hodgkin's Lymphoma

BACOP (NATIONAL CANCER INSTITUTE)
Bleomycin 5 U/m^2 day 15 and 22
Adriamycin 25 mg/m^2 day 1 and 8
Cyclophosphamide 650 mg/m^2 day 1 and 8
Vincristine (Oncovin) 1.4 mg/m^2 day 1 and 8
Prednisone 60 mg/m^2 day 15 through 28
Repeat every 28 days

BACOP
(Sidney Farber Cancer Center)
Bleomycin 4 U/m^2 day 1,5,8,12,15,19
Adriamycin 45 mg/m^2 day 1
Cyclophosphamide 600 mg/m^2 day 1
Vincristine (Oncovin) 1.2 mg/m^2 day 1,8,15
Prednisone 40 mg/m^2 day 1 through 21, then taper
Repeat every 21 days

CMOPP
Cyclophosphamide 650 mg/m^2 day 1 and 8
Vincristine (Oncovin) 1.4 mg/m^2 day 1 and 8
Procarbazine 100 mg/m^2 day 1 through 10
Prednisone 40 mg/m^2 day 1 through 14
Repeat every 28 days

CVP (NCI)
Cyclophosphamide 400 mg/m^2 po day 1 through 5
Vincristine 1.4 mg/m^2 day 1
Prednisone 100 mg/m^2 day 1 through 5
Repeat every 21 days

COMLA
Cyclophosphamide 1500 mg/m^2 day 1
Vincristine (Oncovin) 1.4 mg/m^2 day 1,8,15
Methotrexate 120 mg/m^2 day 22,29,36,43,50,57,64,71
Leucovorin 25 mg/m^2 po Q 6 hr × 4 doses, start 24 hours after methotrexate
Cytarabin (Ara-C) 300 mg/m^2 day 22,29,36,43,50,57,64,71
Repeat every 91 days

BCVP
Bleomycin 10 U/m^2 day 1 through 4
Cyclophosphamide 125 mg/m^2 day 1 through 4
VCR 1.4 mg/m^2 day 1 and 8
Prednisone 60 mg/m^2 Q D d through 5

CHOP A
Cyclophosphamide 750 mg/m^2 day 1
Adriamycin (Hydroxyldaunomycin/doxorubicin) 50 mg/m^2 day 1
Vincristine (Oncovin) 1.4 mg/m^2 day 1
Prednisone 100 mg day 1 through 5
Repeat every 21 to 28 days

CHOP B (STANFORD CHOP = PRED 50 MG/M^2 1–5)

HOP
Adriamycin (Hydroxyldaunomycin/doxorubicin) 80 mg/m^2 day 1
Vincristine (Oncovin) 1.4 mg/m^2 day 1
Prednisone 100 mg day 1 through 5
Repeat every 21 days

BCOP
BCNU 100 mg/m^2 day 1
Cyclophosphamide 600 mg/m^2 day 1
Vincristine (Oncovin) 1 mg/m^2 day 1 and 14
Prednisone 40 mg/m^2 day 1 through 7
Repeat every 28 days

CHOP-BLEO
Cyclophosphamide 750 mg/m^2 day 1
Adriamycin (Hydroxyldaunomycin/doxorubicin) 50 mg/m^2 day 1
Vincristine (Oncovin) 2 mg day 1 and 5
Prednisone 100 mg day 1 through 5
Bleomycin 15 U day 1 and 5
Repeat every 21 or 28 days

MEV
Methotrexate 20 mg/m^2 day 3
Cyclophosphamide (Endoxan) 800 mg/m^2 day 1
Vincristine 2 mg/m^2 day 2

ProMACE-MOPP
Prednisone 60 mg/m^2 day 1 through 14
Methotrexate 1500 mg/m^2 day 15 + leucovorin rescue
Adriamycin 25 mg/m^2 day 1 and 8
Cyclophosphamide 650 mg/m^2 day 1 and 8
VP-16 120 mg/m^2 day 1 and 8

MOPP
Nitrogen Mustard 6 mg/m^2 I.V. day 1 through 8
Vincristine (Oncovin) 1.4 mg/m^2 day 1 through 8
Procarbazine 100 mg/m^2 po day 1 through 14
Prednisone 40 mg/m^2 P.O. po day 1 through 14

MABOP
Nitrogen Mustard 6 mg/m^2 day 1 and 8
Adriamycin 25 mg/m^2 day 1 and 8
Bleomycin 30 U/m^2 day 1 and 8
Vincristine (Oncovin) 1.2 mg/m^2 day 1 and 8
Prednisone 40 mg/m^2 day 1 through 14

COP (ROESER)[163]
Cyclophosphamide 800 mg day 1
Vincristine (Oncovin) 2 mg/m^2 day 1
Prednisone 100 mg/m^2 day 1 through 5

COP (HOOGSTRATEN)
Cyclophosphamide 350 mg/m^2 q wkly
Vincristine 1.0 mg/m^2 q wkly
Prednisone 40 mg/m^2 po Q D
Then MTX maintenance or nothing

COP (LUCE)
Cyclophosphamide 800 mg day 1
Vincristine 2 mg/m^2 day 1
Prednisone 100 mg/m^2 day 1 through 5

phoma can be made by pathologists with as little as 5% of such cells present per high powered field. In tissue specimens, nodular histiocytic lymphomas retain nodularity but the lymph node is totally replaced by these large undifferentiated histiocytic appearing cells. Since nodular mixed and nodular histiocytic lymphomas are known to be monoclonal population of B-cells, they most likely almost always are examples of dedifferentiation of NPDL. Eventual effacement of the lymph node architecture, with loss of nodularity produces the morphologic appearance of diffuse large cell lymphomas (DHL, DUL, DILL).

Since patients with NM and NH may be DHL in evolution, workers at NCI examined the results of treatment of such patients separately. The first large series of patients with non-Hodgkin's lymphoma, classified with the Rappaport scheme, and treated with single agent chemotherapy by a single group of investigators was reported by Jones and colleagues.[339] One-hundred-and-ten patients with non-Hodgkin's lymphomas were treated with orally administered alkylating agents. Jones and colleagues reported that the complete remission rates were higher in nodular lymphomas than in diffuse (48% *versus* 5%) and that although there were slight differences in the response duration in the various subcategories of nodular lymphomas, the response rate and duration of response of all nodular lymphomas were similar. In contrast, in the NCI series, 31 patients with nodular mixed lymphomas were identified. Twenty-four of these 31 patients (77%) achieved a complete remission with the CVP or MOPP program (see Tables 35-37 and 35-38).[343] Only four patients have relapsed and the median duration of remission or survival has not been reached, with 79% of the patients still in their first remission and 91% of the patients still alive. No treatment was given to these patients beyond the initial remission induction. Partial responders or those who did not respond to therapy fared poorly, with a median survival of only 13 months (range, 4 months to 32 months). These results have now been confirmed by Ezdinli and colleagues in a retrospective analysis of patients from Eastern Cooperative Oncology Group studies in which results of therapy of 80 patients with NML were compared to 249 patients with NPDL.[474] While overall, the prognosis for long-term survival decreased with increasing mixtures of large lymphoma cells, those patients with NML who attained a complete remission have remained in remission significantly longer than those with NPDL.

Patients with nodular histiocytic lymphomas are even less common than those with nodular mixed varieties. What happens with these patients is, however, pivotal to the evaluation of the hypothesis that cell dedifferentiation leads to greater vunerability to the cell killing effects of chemotherapy. A recent report from the NCI gave the results of treatment in 16 patients with nodular histiocytic lymphoma (3.4% of 473 patients with non-Hodgkin's lymphoma).[349] Thirteen of 16 patients had Stage III or Stage IV disease, and 11 of these patients were treated with variants of the MOPP program. Eight of 11 patients achieved a complete remission and only one has since relapsed after therapy was discontinued. The other seven patients remain in complete remission off therapy with a minimal followup of 4.5 years. These data support the use of aggressive combination chemotherapy of the types shown in Tables 35-34 and 35-37 used for DHL, in patients with nodular lymphomas with a significant mixture of large histiocytic appearing cells.

RESULTS OF TREATMENT OF NODULAR POORLY DIFFERENTIATED LYMPHOCYTIC LYMPHOMA

Interpretation of results of the use of combination chemotherapy in the late 1960s is complicated by the failure of most investigators to use consistent criteria for pathologic classification, staging and response to treatment. For example, a report by Hoogstratten and associates, in 1969, randomized patients then designated as having lymphosarcoma or reticulum cell sarcoma, to single agents, or a combination of cyclophosphamide, vincristine, and prednisone given either as a high or low dose combination.[475] Neither form of the combination was given in substantial doses. Also, a fixed 42-day interval was used for induction treatment. A significantly better overall remission rate (but not complete remission rate) was noted for both forms of the combination regimen when compared to the single agents. No comments were made on the response rate by the presence or absence of nodularity. Bagley and colleagues reported the first aggressive use of a combination chemotherapy in patients with NPDL using cyclophosphamide, vincristine and prednisone (CVP, Tables 35-37 and 35-38).[456] These subsequent studies are listed in Table 35-38. In the early Bagley study of 35 patients with advanced NPDL, 57% of patients attained a complete remission in a median time of 2 months, with 89% of complete responders remaining in complete remission at the first year of followup. A more recent re-analysis of these data reported by Anderson in 1977 (Table 35-38), showed that although complete remission rates in patients treated with CVP have consistently remained higher than previous reports using single agents, a consistent pressure of relapse has always been noted.[343] These relapse rates for patients with advanced NPDL are similar to that reported from Stanford in patients with localized forms of NPDL treated only with radiotherapy.[342] Although a tendency was noted for the relapse-free survival curve to plateau by the fifth year of followup, the numbers of patients at that time were too small to speak with any confidence about our capacity to achieve long-term disease-free survival after combination chemotherapy. An analysis of the sites of relapse in those patients who achieved a complete remission by the NCI group revealed that lymph nodes and bone marrow previously involved with tumor were almost always the site of relapse.[476] The persistent tendency of NPDL patients to relapse after chemotherapy and the findings by Johnson and colleagues that total body irradiation (TBI) could also induce complete remissions, led to a random comparison of CVP to TBI, and later a comparison of TBI plus CVP to CVP alone.[438,439] TBI proved equal to CVP in remission induction and relapse-free survival in the early phase of the study

TABLE 35-38. Combination Chemotherapy of Advanced Nodular Lymphomas

AUTHOR (Reference Number)	YEAR	REGIMEN	TOTAL PATIENTS	PERCENT CR	MEDIAN SURVIVAL (MO)	SURVIVAL 5 YEARS
Jones et al (339)	1972	Cytoxan or Chlorambucil	49	31–48	24	–
Anderson (343)	1977	CVP (NCI), (CMOPP)	46	67	30+	>67%
Portlock et al (344)	1976	CVP (Stanford)	–	–	–	–
Roeser (163)	1975	COP	35	49	>60	55%
McKelvey (348)	1976	HOP	98	59	12+	–
McKelvey (348)	1976	CHOP	98	69	12+	–
Bonadonna (481)	1975	MABOP	57	53	–	81% (at 2 years)

but beyond 4 years, late relapses after TBI and a high complication rate, including the development of variants of acute leukemia, made the use of TBI less attractive as a first line treatment. Adding TBI to CVP also provided no advantage over CVP alone.

CVP, as reported by the NCI group, has been used at Stanford with similar results.[477] However, when a prospective comparison of CVP to CVP plus interspersed total lymphoid irradiation, with continuous single agent therapy (chlorambucil or cyclophosphamide) in patients with favorable histology (mostly NPDL), the complete remission rate was 78.3%, 65%, and 55%, respectively, for the three treatment programs.[344] These results are not significantly different. The authors reported that continuous treatment with single agents, furthermore, would produce complete remission rates in up to 80% of patients, if one allowed the time of assessment to be extended as long as 40 months. At the time of last analysis there was also no significant difference among the three groups in disease-free or overall survival. These data led the authors to conclude that single agent therapy was as good as combination chemotherapy. In reality, the study proved that neither therapy was sufficiently good to justify its continued routine use. These data have, unfortunately, led many physicians to manage NPDL patients conservatively with single agents, usually chlorambucil. Another comparison of CVP to the same three drugs used in sequence in patients with NPDL has been made by Kennedy and associates.[478] They noted that 81% of patients achieved complete remission with CVP compared with 46% with the same drugs used in sequence. CVP proved no more effective than single agents in patients with diffuse lymphomas as in the Stanford Study. Monfardine and colleagues used CVP alternately with a combination of adriamycin, bleomycin, and prednisone in 31 patients with NPDL.[479] Although 74% of patients attained a complete remission, relapse-free survival at 4 years (44.2%) does not appear to be significantly different from results reported with single agent or CVP alone. Another controlled trial by Lister and associates compared CVP with to the use of chlorambucil in patients with favorable histology lymphoma.[480] The CVP program produced a higher complete remission rate than chlorambucil but overall survival appeared no different. NCI authors and Lister and associates have reported, however, that patients who achieve a complete remission live longer than those who do not. If this observation is confirmed, the CVP regimen may eventually improve survival when compared to single drug treatment. It is likely that due to the indolent nature of NPDL, followup time in most studies has been too short to make this distinction. Other regimens have been compared to single agents and although the complete remission rates are consistently higher than single agents, the overall results are not superior to the results reported using CVP at Stanford and NCI.

In all studies testing drug maintenance treatment as a way to prevent relapse, continuous drug maintenance therapy prolongs remission duration but produces no overall impact on survival. A case in point is the large Southwest Oncology Group study of patients with non-Hodgkin's lymphoma using CHOP or HOP (Table 35-38).[464] Of 73 patients treated with CHOP in this study, 78% attained a complete remission, while 67% of 75 patients with NPDL treated with HOP did so. These results were not significantly different. Unfortunately, all patients in this study were placed on maintenance regimens of either cyclophosphamide, prednisone and vincristine, or arabinosyl cytosine, vincristine, and prednisone. While relapse-free survival appears excellent, reflecting the impact of maintenance therapy, overall survival at the time of the report did not appear significantly different than that reported from other programs not using maintenance treatment. Recently, the Southwest Oncology Group has evaluated the use of BCG scarification in conjunction with CHOP chemotherapy to maintain drug induced remissions. Preliminary analysis reveals some positive effect on relapse-free survival. Given the ultimate disappointment of other similar observations, this approach requires further evaluation before it becomes widely used.[482-417]

A study that is in progress at the Clinical Center of the NCI is comparing two alternate ways of managing patients with advanced nodular lymphomas.[164] Half of all patients are randomly allocated to a new treatment program designed to be more intensive than those used in the past. This arm will test the hypothesis that the reason for the inability of drug combination programs to produce a significant fraction of NPDL patients who remain relapse-free is due to the failure in dose escalation. The other half of the patients are randomized to a "watch and wait" treatment arm and followed closely to determine two pieces of important information, the fraction of patients with nodular lymphomas who can be followed without drug treatment, and the number that evolve to NM, NH, and DHL over time. Clinically aggressive tumor masses are biopsied at intervals to determine the histologic subtype. If therapy is required, and the histology is still NPDL, low-dose small-field radiotherapy is used as long as possible. If chemotherapy is required, the use of chlorambucil is prohibited. When histologic evolution to NM, NH or diffuse lymphoma occurs in the "watch and wait" arm, treatment with a more aggressive combination chemotherapy program (ProMACE-flexi-therapy, Tables 35-36 and 35-37) is used. The data on the evolution of NPDL to a more vulnerable histologic subtype is an important conceptual advance in this disease. In the NCI retrospective analysis of the evolution of nodular lymphomas patients whose histology progressed to less nodularity and greater numbers of undifferentiated cells had a median survival of 46 months when compared to those whose histologic subtype remained the same.[349] In both groups, the average duration of illness prior to biopsy was not significantly different. Following progression from nodular to diffuse pathologic types; however, some patients may have been cured by combination chemotherapy, although the response rate is lower than in previously untreated patients. Twenty-two were treated with drug combinations and seven achieved complete remission (32%). All seven remain free of disease. The 16 patients who progressed to diffuse lymphomas who did not attain a complete remission had a median survival of 28 months, significantly shorter than those attaining a complete remission ($p < 0.004$).

The study by the Italian group that tested CVP as an adjuvant to irradiation of localized NHL in all histologic subtypes reported no significant difference in relapse-free and overall survival for the addition of chemotherapy to radiotherapy in patients with NPDL.

TABLE 35-39. Abbreviations and Acronyms

ABVD	: adriamycin, bleomycin, vinblastine, and DTIC
ABDV	: Same as above but different schedule
AC	: adriamycin and CCNU
ADBC	: adriamycin, DTIC, bleomycin, and CCNU
B-CAVe	: bleomycin, CCNU, adriamycin, and velban
BCNU	: 1,3-*bis*(2-chloroethyl)-1-nitrosourea
BCVPP	: BCNU, cyclophosphamide, velban, procarbazine, and prednisone
B-DOPA	: bleomycin, DTIC, vincristine, prednisone, and adriamycin
BOAP	: bleomycin, vincristine, adriamycin, and prednisone
BOP	: BCNU, vincristine, and prednisone
BOPP	: BCNU, vincristine, procarbazine, and prednisone
BVDS	: bleomycin, velban, adriamycin, and streptozotocin
BVPP	: BNCU, vincristine, procarbazine, and prednisone
CCNU	: (1-(2-chloroethyl)-3-cyclohexyl-1-nitrosourea)
CCVPP	: CCNU, cyclophosphamide, velban, procarbazine, and prednisone
CH_3CCNU	: methyl CCNU
Ch1VPP.	: chlorambucil, vinblastine, procarbazine, and prednisone
COPP	: CCNU, vincristine, procarbazine, and prednisone
CVB	: CCNU, velban, and bleomycin
CVPP	: cyclophosphamide, velban, procarbazine, and prednisone
DTIC	: 5-(3,3-dimethyl-1-triazino) imidazole-4-carboxamide
HN_2	: nitrogen mustard
MABOP	: nitrogen mustard, adriamycin, bleomycin, vincristine, and prednisone
Methyl GAG	: methylglyoxal bis (guanylhydrazone)dihidro-chloride
MOP	: nitrogen mustard, vincristine, and prednisone
MOPr	: nitrogen mustard, vincristine, and procarbazine
MOPP	: nitrogen mustard, vincristine, procarbazine, and prednisone
MOPPCPF	: nitrogen mustard, vincristine, procarbazine, and prednisone for patients with compromised pulmonary functions
MOPPHDB	: nitrogen mustard, vincristine, procarbazine, prednisone, and high-dose bleomycin
MOPPLDB	: nitrogen mustard, vincristine, procarbazine, prednisone, and low-dose bleomycin
MVVPP	: nitrogen mustard, vincristine, vinblastine, procarbazine, and prednisone
MVPP	: nitrogen mustard, vinblastine, procarbazine, and prednisone
OPP	: vincristine, procarbazine, and prednisone
PAVe	: procarbazine, phenylalanine mustard, and velban
SCAB	: streptozotocin, CCNU, adriamycin, and bleomycin
VP-16-213	: 4′ dimethyl-epipodophyllotoxin 9-(4,6-0-ethylidene-β-D-glucopyranoside)
VM-26	: 4′ dimethyl-epipodophyllotoxin-β-D-thenyliden glucoside
VM-26PP	: VM-26, procarbazine, and prednisone
VPBCPr	: vincristine, prednisone, vinblastine, chlorambocil, and procarbazine

RECOMMENDATIONS FOR TREATMENT BY STAGE: NODULAR LYMPHOMA

Stage I and contiguous Stage II nodular poorly differentiated lymphocytic (NPDL) lymphoma should be treated with localized radiation therapy alone. This may afford cure in some patients. At present, there are no other satisfactory curative alternatives. Care must be taken to limit the radiation field so that there is not significant bone marrow compromise.

Stage III and Stage IV NPDL should be entered on clinical trials or treated symptomatically as there appear to be no curative therapies presently available. We recommend limited local radiation as the best of such symptomatic palliative therapies. Care should be taken again to preserve bone marrow function and tumors should be rebiopsied if the disease changes *in tempo* as it may have progressed to a more aggressive lymphoma. Should the latter occur then it should be treated as such.

Nodular mixed and nodular histiocytic lymphoma should be treated with radiation for Stage I and contiguous Stage II disease. For any disease more advanced than this (Stages III and IV), combination chemotherapy of the types listed in Tables 35-34 and 35-37 should be given with or without regional irradiation to the area of involvement.

TREATMENT RECOMMENDATIONS BY STAGE: DIFFUSE LYMPHOMA

Stage I and contiguous Stage II diffuse lymphoma should be treated with local radiation with doses of 4500 rad to 5000 rad. Preliminary results suggest that the use of combination chemotherapy serves as a useful adjuvant. Although there are reports of the successful use of combination chemotherapy alone for patients with Stage I and II disease, this approach is not recommended at present. All other patients should be treated with combination chemotherapy of the type shown in

Tables 35-37 and 35-38. Table 35-39 lists abbreviations and acronyms of commonly used drug combinations.

Complications of Chemotherapy

The major long-term complications of chemotherapy of lymphomas are sterility and the risk of second cancers. These subjects are covered in detail elsewhere in this text (see Chapter 45). Acute and chronic side effects of individual drugs are discussed in the Chapters 43 and 47.

CONCLUSION

Two decades ago the lymphomas were considered incurable cancers. Now 70% of all patients with Hodgkin's disease and half of all patient with the non-Hodgkin's lymphomas are curable. National mortality from cancer below the age of 50 years, when most lymphomas occur, has fallen precipitously as a result of the widespread applications of treatment results (see Chapter 8, Principles of Chemotherapy). There is still a good distance to go to improve the cure rate for lymphoma patients and make the current morbid treatment programs more acceptable and easy to use. The progress achieved thus far has been the result of vigorous clinical trials. The lymphomas serve as an example of what can be done to improve the lot of patients with cancer.

REFERENCES

1. Cancer Facts and Figures 1980. New York, American Cancer Society 1980, p 9
2. Cole P, MacMahon B, Aisenberg A: Mortality from Hodgkin's disease in the United States. Evidence for the multiple etiology hypothesis. Lancet 2:1371–1376, 1968
3. MacMahon B: Epidemiology of Hodgkin's disease. Cancer Res 26:1189–1200, 1966
4. MacMahon B: Epidemiological evidence of the nature of Hodgkin's disease. Cancer 10:1045–1054, 1957
5. Correa P, O'Conor GT, Berard CW et al: International comparability and reproducibility in histologic subclassification of Hodgkin's disease. J Nat Cancer Inst 50:1429–1435, 1973
6. Cantor KP, Frameni JF: Distribution of Non-Hodgkin's Lymphoma in the United States between 1950 & 1975. Cancer Res 40:2645–2652, 1980
7. Third National Cancer Survey, 1969 Incidence. Preliminary Report. Department of Health, Education and Welfare, Publ No (NIH) 71-128, 1971
8. Higginson J, Muir CS: Epidemiology. In Holland JF, Frei E (eds): Cancer Medicine. Philadelphia, Lea and Febiger, 1973, pp 241–306
9. Anderson RE, Ishida K, Li Y, et al: Geographic aspects of malignant lymphoma and multiple myeloma. Amer J Pathol 61:85, 1970
10. Sternberg C: Uber eine eigenartige unter dem Bilde der Pseudoleukamie verlaufende Tuberculose des lymphatichon Apparates. Ztschr Heilk, 19:21–90, 1898
11. Steiner PE: Hodgkin's disease: search for infective agent and attempts at experimental reproduction. Arch Path 17:749–763, 1934
12. L Esperance ES: Experimental innoculation of chickens with Hodgkin's nodes. J Immunol 16:37–60, 1929
13. Van Rooyea CE: Etiology of Hodgkin's disease with special reference to B. Tuberculosis avis. Brit Med J 1:50–51, 1933
14. Van Rooyan CE: Recent Experimental work on the etiology of Hodgkin's disease. Brit Med J 2:519–524, 1934
15. Miller RW, Beebe: Infectious mononucleosis and the empirical risk of cancer. J Nat Cancer Inst 50:315–321, 1973
16. Connolly RR, Chistene BW: A cohort study of cancer following infectious mononucleosis. Cancer Res 34:1172–1178, 1974
17. Rosdahl N, Larsen SO, Clemmensen J: Hodgkin's disease in patients with previous mononucleosis, 30 years experience. Br Med J 2:253–256, 1974
18. Munoz N, Davidson RJ, Witthoff B et al: Infectious mononucleosis and Hodgkin's disease. Internat J Cancer 22:10–13, 1978
19. Lukes RJ, Tindle BH, Parker JW: Reed–Sternberg-like cells in infectious mononucleosis. Lancet 2:1000–1004, 1969
20. Nonoyama M, Kawai Y, Huang CH et al: Epstein Barr virus DNA in Hodgkin's disease, American Burkitts lymphoma and other human tumors. Cancer Res 34:1228–1231. 1974
21. Kaplan HS, Smithers DW: Auto-immunity and homologous disease in mice in relation to the malignant lymphomas. Lancet 2:1–4, 1959
22. Order SE, Hellman S: Pathologenesis of Hodgkin's disease. Lancet 1:571–573, 1972
23. Schwartz RS, Beldotti L: Malignant lymphomas following allogenic disease: transition from an immunological to a neoplastic disorder. Science 149:1511–1514, 1965
24. DeVita VT: Lymphocyte reactivity in Hodgkin's disease: a lymphocyte civil war. New Engl J Med 289:801–802, 1973
25. Kaplan HS: Etiology of Lymphomas and Leukemia: Role of C-type RNA viruses. Leukemia Res 2:253–271
26. Dmochowski L: Viral studies in human leukemia and lymphoma. In Zarafonetis CJD (ed): Proceedings of the International Conference on Leukemia–Lymphoma. Philadelphia, Lea and Febiger, 1968, pp 97–113
27. Kawakami TG, Theilan GH, Dungworth DL et al: "C" type viral particles in plasma of cats with feline leukemia. Science 158:1049–1050, 1967
28. Kawakami TG, Hull SD, Buckley DM et al: C-Type virus associated with Gibbon Lymphosarcoma. Nature New Biol 235:170–171, 1972
29. Rapp F: Viruses as an etiologic factor in cancer. Sem Onc 3:49–53, 1976
30. Van der Maaten MJ, Miller JM, Booth AD: Replicating Type-C virus particles in monolayer cell cultures from cattle with lymphosarcoma. J Nat Cancer Inst 52:491–497, 1974
31. Reedman BM, Klein G: Cellular localization of an Epstein–Barr virus (EBV)—associated complement fixing antigen in producer and non producer lymphoblastoid cell lines. Int J Cancer 11:499–520, 1973
32. Kaplan HS, Goodenow RS, Gartner BA et al: Biology and virology of the human malignant lymphomas. Cancer 43:1–24, 1979
33. Epstein AL, Kaplan HS: Biology of the human malignant lymphomas. I. Establishment in continuous culture and heterotransplantation of diffuse Histocytic Lymphomas. Cancer 34:1851–1872, 1974
34. Vianna NJ, Greenwald P, Davies JNP: Extended epidemic of Hodgkin's disease in high school students. Lancet 1:1209–1210, 1971
35. Vianna JH, Polan AK: Epidemiological evidence for transmission of Hodgkin's disease. N Engl J Med 289:499–502, 1973
36. Smith PG, Pike MC, Kinlam LJ, et al: Contacts between young patients with Hodgkin's disease: a case control study. Lancet 2:59–62, 1977
37. Zack MM, Heath CW, Jr, Andrews MD, et al: High school contact among persons with leukemia and lymphoma. J Nat Cancer Inst 59:1343–1349, 1977
38. Gutterman S, Cole P, Levitan TR: Evidence against transmission of Hodgkin's disease in high schools. New Engl J Med 300:1000–1011, 1979
39. Gutensohn N, Cole P: Childhood social environment and Hodgkin's disease. New Engl J Med (in press)
40. Milham S Jr, Hesser J: Hodgkin's disease in woodworkers. Lancet 2:136–137, 1967

41. Vianna NJ, Greenwald P, Davies JNP: Tonsillectomy and Hodgkin's disease: the lymphoid tissue barrier. Lancet 1:431–432, 1971
42. Bierman HR: Human appendix and neoplasia. Cancer 21:109–118, 1968
43. Hyams L, Wynder EL: Appendectomy and cancer risk: an epidemiological evaluation. J Chronic Disease 21:319–415, 1968
44. Lilly F, Pincus T: Genetic control of murine viral leukemogenesis In Klein G and Weinhouse S (eds): Advances in Cancer Research, Vol 17. New York, Academic Press, 1977, pp 231–277
45. Graff KS, Simons RM, Yankee RA et al: HL-A antigens in Hodgkin's disease: Histopathologic and clinical correlations. J Nat Cancer Inst 52(4):1087–1090, 1974
46. Vianna NJ, Davies JNP, Polan AK et al: Familial Hodgkin's disease: an environmental and Genetic disorder. Lancet 854–857, Oct 12, 1974
47. Grufferman S, Cole P, Smith PG et al: Hodgkin's disease in siblings. New Engl J Med 296:248–250, 1977
48. Miller DG: The association of immune disease and malignant lymphoma. Ann Int Med 66:507–521, 1967
49. Zulman J, Jaffe R, Talal N: Evidence that the malignant lymphoma of Sjogrens syndrome is a monoclonal B-Cell neoplasm. New Engl J Med 299:1215–1220, 1978
50. Talal N, Sokoloff L, Barth W: Extra salivary Lymphoid Abnormalities in Sjogrens Syndrome (Reticulum Cell Sarcoma, "Pseudolymphoma," Macroglobulinemia). Am J Med 43:50–65, 1967
51. Kassan JS, Thomas TL, Montsopoulos HM et al: Increased risk of lymphoma in Sicca syndrome. Ann of Int Med 89:888–892, 1978
52. Hyman G, Sommers S: The development of Hodgkin's disease and other lymphomas during anticonvulsant therapy. Blood 28:416–427, 1966
53. Penn I: The incidence of malignancies in transplant recipients. Tranplant Proc 7:323, 1975
54. Matas AJ, Hertel BF, Rosai J, et al: Post-transplant malignant lymphoma. Distinctive morphologic features related to its pathogenesis. Am J Med 61:716, 1976
55. Anderson RE, Nishiyama H, Yohei I, Kenzo T, Nobukazo O: Pathogenesis of radiation related leukemia and lymphoma. Speculations based primarily on experience of Hiroshima and Nagasaki. Lancet 1:1060–1062, 1972
56. Miller RW: Delayed radiation effects in atomic bomb survivors. Science 166:569–574, 1969
57. Court Brown WM, Doll R: Leukemia and aplastic anemia in patients irradiated for ankylosing spondylitis. Med Res Council Spec Rep Ser (Lond), No 295, Her Majesty's Stationary Office, 1957
58. Kissmeyer-Nielsen F, Bjorn-Jensen K, Femara RB et al: HLA phenotypes in Hodgkin's disease: preliminary report. Transplantation Proceedings, Vol III #3, 1287–1289, 1971
59. Dick FR, Fortuny I, Theologides A, et al: HL-A and lymphoid tumors. Cancer Res 32:2608, 1972
60. MacSween RNM: Reticulum cell sarcoma and rheumatoid arthritis in a patient with XY/XXY/XXX/Y Klinefelter's syndrome and normal intellignece. Lancet 1:460, 1965
61. Tan C, Etcubanas E, Lieberman P et al: Chediak–Higashi syndrome in a child with Hodgkin's disease. Am J Dis Child 121:135–139, 1971
62. Caspersson T, Zech L, Johansson C, et al: Identification of human chromosomes by DNA-binding fluorescent agents. Chromosoma 30:215, 1970
63. Manolov G, Manolova Y: Marker band in one chromosome 14 from Burkitt lymphomas. Nature 237:33, 1972
64. Fukuhara S, Rowley JD, Variakojiis D et al: Banding studies on chromosomes in diffuse histiocytic lymphoma: correlation of 14Q+ marker chromosome with cytology. Blood 52, 989–1002, 1978
65. Berard CW, Gallo RC, Jaffee ES et al: Current concepts of leukemia and lymphoma: Etiology, pathogenesis and therapy. Ann Int Med 85:351–366, 1976
66. Braylan RC, Jaffee ES, Berard CW: Malignant lymphomas: Current classification and new observations. In Sommers SC (ed): Pathology Annual, pp 213–270, Appleton Century-Crofts, New York, New York, 1975
67. Mann RB, Jaffe ES, Berard CW: Malignant lymphomas—a conceptual understanding of morphologic diversity. A review. Am J Pathol 94(1):105–191, 1979
68. Berard CW: Reticuloendothelial system. An overview of neoplasia. In The Reticuloendothelial System. Baltimore, Williams & Wilkins, 1975, pp 310–317
69. DeVita VT, Fisher RI, Johnson R et al: Non-Hodgkin's lymphoma. Cancer Med (in press)
70. Lukes RJ, Collin RD: Immunologic characterization of human malignant lymphomas. Cancer 34:1488, 1974
71. Golde D, Cline MJ: A review and reevaluation of the histiocytic disorders. Amer J Med 55:49–60, 1973
72. Gupta S, Good RA: Markers of human lymphocyte subpopulations in primary immunodeficiency and lymphoproliferative disorders. Sem in Hematol 17:1–29, 1980
73. Jaffe ES, Shevach EM, Frank MM et al: Nodular lymphoma: Evidence for origin from follicular B lymphocytes. New Engl J Med 290:813, 1974
74. Ross GD: Identification of human lymphocyte subpopulations by surface marker analysis. Blood 53:799–811, 1979
75. Seligmann M, Brouet JC, Preud'homme JL: The immunological diagnosis of human leukemias and lymphomas: An overview. In Thierfelder S and Rudt H (eds): Immunological Diagnosis of Leukemias and Lymphomas, Springer-Verlag, Berlin, 1977
76. Jaffe ES, Shevach EM, Sussman EH et al: Membrane receptor sites for the identification of lymphoreticular cells in benign and malignant conditions. Brit J Cancer 31(II) 107, 1975
77. Kung PC, Long JC, McCaffrey RP, Ratliff RL, Harrison TA, Baltimore D: Terminal deoxynucleotidyl transferase in the diagnosis of leukemia and malignant lymphoma. Am J Med 64(5):788–794, 1978
78. Long JC, Zamecnik PC, Aisenberg AC et al: Tissue culture studies in Hodgkin's disease: Morphologic, cytogenetic, cell surface, and enzymatic properties of cultures derived from splenic tumors. J Exp Med 145(6):1484–1500, 1977
79. Kadin ME, Stites DP, Levy R et al: Exogenous immunoglobulin and the macrophage origin of Reed-Sternberg cells in Hodgkin's disease. New Engl J Med 299(22):1208–1214, 1978
80. Kaplan HS, Gartner S: "Sternberg-Reed" giant cells of Hodgkin's disease: Cultivation in vitro, heterotransplantation, and characterization as neoplastic macrophages. Int J Cancer 19:511–525, 1977
81. Zamecnik PC, Long JC: Growth of cultured cells from patients with Hodgkin's disease and transplantation into *nude* mice. Proc Natl Acad Sci 74:754–758, 1977
82. Seif GSF, Spriggs AI: Chromosome changes in Hodgkin's disease. J Nat Cancer Inst 39:557–570, 1967
83. Hodgkin T: On some morbid appearances of the absorbent glands and spleen. Med-Chir Trans 17:68–114, 1832
84. Jones SE, Butler JJ, Byrne GE Jr et al: Histopathologic review of lymphoma cases from the Southwest Oncology Group. Cancer 39(3):1071–1076, 1977
85. Strum SB, Dark JK, Rappaport H: Observations of cells resembling Sternberg-Reed cells in conditions other than Hodgkin's disease. Cancer 26:176–190, 1970
86. Reed DM: On the pathological changes in Hodgkin's disease with especial reference to its relationship to tuberculosis. Johns Hopkins Hospital Rev 10:133–196, 1902
87. Jackson H Jr, Parker F Jr: Hodgkin's disease. II Pathology. New Engl J Med 231:35–44, 1944
88. Lukes RJ, Butler JJ, Hicks ED: Natural history of Hodgkin's disease as related to its pathologic picture. Cancer 19:317–344, 1966
89. Greenfield WS: Specimens illustrative of the pathology of lymphadenoma and leucocythemia. Trans Path Soc London 29:272–304, 1878
90. Lukes RJ: Relationship of histiologic features to clinical stages in Hodgkin's disease. Am J Roentgenol 90:944–955, 1963
91. Wilks Sir S: Cases of enlargement of lymphatic glands and spleen, (or Hodgkin's disease), with remarks. Guy's Hosp Rep 11:56–67, 1865

92. Langhans T: Das Maligne Lymphosarkom (Pseuddukamie). Virchow's Arch f path Anat 54:509–537, 1872
93. Parker F Jr, Jackson H Jr, Fitzhugh G et al: Studies of diseases of the lymphoid and myeloid tissues. IV. Skin reactions to human and avian tuberculin. J Immunol 22:277–282, 1932
94. Pell PK: Zur Symptomatologie der sogenannten Pseudoleukamie II. Pseudoleukamie oder chronisches Ruckfallsfieber? Berlin Klin Wchnschr 24:644–646, 1887
95. Jackson H Jr: Classification and prognosis of Hodgkin's disease and allied disorders. Surg Gynec Obst 64:465–467, 1937
96. Anagnostou D, Parker JW, Taylor CR et al: Lacunar cells of nodular sclerosing Hodgkin's disease. An ultrastructural and immunohistologic study. Cancer 39:1032–1043, 1977
97. Kadin ME, Glatstein E, Dorfman RF: Clinicopathologic study of 117 untreated patients subjected to laparotomy for the staging of Hodgkin's disease. Cancer 27:1277–1294, 1971
98. Strum SB, Rappaport H: Interrelations of the histologic types of Hodgkin's disease. Arch Path 91:127–134, 1971
99. Axtel LM, Myers MH, Thomas LB et al: Prognostic indications in Hodgkin's disease. Cancer 29:1481–1488, 1972
100. Rappaport H, Strum SB, Hutchison G et al: Clincial and biological significance of vascular invasion in Hodgkin's disease. Cancer Res 31:1794–1798, 1971
101. Rappaport H, Winter WJ, Hicks EB: Follicular lymphoma—A re-evaluation of its position is the scheme of malignant lymphoma, based on a survey of 253 cases. Cancer 9:792, 1956
102. Rappaport H: Tumors of the hematopoietic system. In Atlas of Tumor Pathology, Sec III, Fasc 8. Washington, DC, Armed Forces Institute of Pathology, 1966
103. Berard CW: Personal communication, 1980
104. Bennett MH, Farrer-Brown G, Henry K et al: Classification of non-Hodgkin's lymphomas. Lancet ii:405, 1974
105. Dorfman RF: Classification of non-Hodgkin's lymphomas. Lancet i:1295, 1974
106. Lennert K, Stein H, Kaiserling E: Cytological and functional criteria for the classification of malignant lymphomata. Br J Cancer 31(II):29, 1975
107. Craigie D: Case of disease of the spleen, in which death took place in consequence in the presence of purulent matter in the blood. Edinburgh Med Surg J 64:400–413, 1845
108. Bennett JH: Case of hypertrophy of the spleen and liver in which death tool place from suppuration of the blood. Edinburgh Med Surg J 64:413–423, 1845
109. Virchow R: Weisses blut. Neue Notizen aus den Geb der Natur- und Heilkunde. (Froriep's neue Notizen) 36:151–156, 1845
110. Bilroth T: Multiple lymphome. Erfolgreiche Behandling mit arsenik. Wien Med Wochengchie 21:1066–1067, 1871
111. Dreschfeld J: Clinical lecture on acute Hodgkin's (or Pseudo-leucocythermia). Brit Med J I: 893–896, 1892
112. Kundrat H: Uber. Lympho-sarkomatosis. Wien klin Wchnschr 6:211–234, 1893
113. Brill NE, Baehr G, Rosenthal N: Generalized giant lymph-follicle hyperplasia of lymph nodes and spleen, a hitherto undescribed type. JAMA 84:668–671, 1925
114. Symmers D: Follicular lymphodenopathy with splenomegaly. A newly recognized disease of lymphatic system. Arch Path Lab Med 3:816–820, 1927
115. Roulet F: Dasprinare Retothelsarkom der Lymphkonten. Virchows Arch path anat 277:15–47, 1930
116. Gall EA, Mallory TB: Malignant lymphoma. A clinical pathologic survey of 618 cases. Am J Path 18:381–429, 1942
117. Rappaport H, Winter WJ, Hicks EB: Follicular lymphoma. A reevaluation of its position in the scheme of malignant lymphomas, based on a survey of 253 cases. Cancer 9:792–821, 1956
118. Burkitt D: A sarcoma involving the jaws in African children. Brit J Surg 46:218–223, 1958
119. Harrison CV: The morphology of the lymph node in the macroglobulinaemia of Waldenstrom. J Clin Path 25:12–16, 1972
120. Dutcher TF, Fahey JL: The histopathology of the macroglobulinaemia of Waldenstrom. JNCI 22:887–917, 1959
121. Richter MN: Generalized reticular cell sarcoma of lymph nodes associated with lymphatic leukemia. Am J Pathol 4:285, 1928
122. Trump DL, Mann RB, Phelps R, Roberts HUW et al: Richter's syndrome: Diffuse histiocytic lymphoma in patients with chronic lymphocytic lymphoma. A report of 5 cases and review of the literature. Am J Med 68:539–548, 1980
123. Woda BA, Knowles DM: Nodular lymphocytic lymphoma eventuating into diffuse histiocytic lymphoma: Immunoperoxidase demonstration of monoclonicity. Cancer 43:303–307, 1979
124. Scott RB, Robb-Smith ANT: Histiocytic medullary reticulosis. Lancet 2:194–198, 1939
125. Warnke RA, Kim H, Dorfman RF: Malignant histiocytosis (histiocytic medullary reticulosis) I. Clinicopathologic study of 29 cases. Cancer 35:215–230, 1975
126. Jaffe ES, Shevach EM, Sussman EH et al: Membrane receptor sites for the identification of lymphoreticular cells in benign and malignant conditions. Br J Cancer (Suppl; 2):107–120, 1975
127. Lukes RJ, Tindle BH: Immunoblastic lymphadenopathy. A hyper-immune entity resembling Hodgkin's disease. N Engl J Med 292:1–12, 1975
128. Frizzera G, Moran EM, Rappaport H: Angioblastic lymphadenopathy: Diagnosis and clinical course. Am J Med 59:803–819, 1975
129. Kaplan HS: Hodgkin's Disease. 2nd ed Cambridge, Harvard University Press, 1980
130. Rosenberg SA, Diamond HD, Jaslowitz B et al: Lymphosarcoma: A review of 1269 cases. Medicine 40:31, 1961
131. Banfe A, Bonadonna G, Riece SB et al: Malignant lymphomas of Waldeyer's ring—Natural history and survival after radiotherapy. Br Med J 2:140–143, 1972
132. Sage HH: Palpable cervical lymph nodes. JAMA 168:496–498, 1958
133. Filly R, Blank N, Castellino RA: Radiographic distribution of intrathoracic disease in previously untreated patients with Hodgkin's disease and non-Hodgkin's lymphoma. Radiology 120:277–281, 1976
134. Simone JV, Verzosa MS, Rudy JA: Initial features and prognosis in 363 children with acute lymphoblastic leukemia. Cancer 36:2099, 1975
135. Nathwami BN, Kim H, Rappaport H: Malignant lymphoma, lymphoblastic. Cancer 38:964, 1976
136. Golumb H: "Hairy" cell leukemia: an unusual lymphoproliferative disease. Cancer 42:946–956, 1958
137. Rudders RA, Aisenberg AC, Schiller AL: Hodgkin's disease presenting as "idiopathic" thrombocytopenic purpura. Cancer 30:220–230, 1972
138. Rappaport H, Ramot B, Hulu N et al: The pathology of so-called mediterranean abdominal lymphoma with malabsorption. Cancer 29:1502–1511, 1972
139. Gilbert R: La roentgentherapie de la granulomatose maligne. J Radiol electrol 9:509–514, 1925
140. Gilbert R: Radiotherapy in Hodgkin's disease (Malignant granulomatosis): anatomic and clinical foundations: governing principles: results. Am J Roentgenol 41:198–241, 1939
141. Peters MV: A study of survival in Hodgkin's disease treated radiologically. Am J Roentgenol 63:299–311, 1950
142. Peters MV, Middlemiss KCH: A study of Hodgkin's disease treated by irradiation. Am J Roentgenol 79:114–121, 1958
143. Peters MV: Prophylactic treatment of adjacent areas in Hodgkin's disease. Cancer Res 26:1232–1243, 1966
144. Kaplan HS: The radical radiotherapy of regionally localized Hodgkin's disease. Radiology 78:553–561, 1962
145. Kinmonth JB, Taylor GW, Harper, RK: Lymphography: A technique for its clinical use in the lower limbs. Brit Med J 1:940–942, 1955
146. Lee BJ, Nelson JH, Schwarz G: Evaluation of lymphangiography, inferior venocavography and intravenouse pyelography in the clinical staging and management of Hodgkin's disease and lymphosarcoma. New Engl J Med 271:327–337, 1964
147. Glatstein E, Guernsey JM, Rosenberg SA et al: The value of laparotomy and splenectomy in the staging of Hodgkin's disease. Cancer 24:709–718, 1969
148. Kaplan HS: On the natural history, treatment and prognosis of Hodgkin's disease. Harvey Lectures, 1968–1969. New York, Academic Press, 1970, pp 215–259
149. Glatstein E, Trueblood HW, Enright LP et al: Surgical staging

of abdominal involvement in unselected patients with Hodgkin's disease. Radiology 97:425, 1970
150. Desser RK, Moran EM, Ultmann JE: Staging of Hodgkin's disease and lymphoma. Med Clin N Am 57:479, 1973
151. Rosenberg SA: A critique of the value of laparotomy and splenectomy in the evaluation of patients with Hodgkin's disease. Cancer Res 31:1737, 1971
152. Piro AJ, Hellman S, Moloney WC: The influence of laparotomy on management decisions in Hodgkin's disease. Arch Intern Med 130:844, 1972
153. DeVita VT: The role of staging laparotomy in combined modality therapy of Hodgkin's disease. World J of Surg 2(1):105–107, 1978
154. Peters MV, Alison RE, Buch RS: Natural history of Hodgkin's disease as related to staging. Cancer 19:308–346, 1966
155. Johnson RE, Thomas LB, Chretien P: Correlationa between clinico-histologic staging and extranodal relapse in Hodgkin's disease. Cancer 25:1071–1075, 1970
156. Strum SB, Rappaport H: Interrelationships of the histologic types of Hodgkin's disease. Arch Path 91:127–134, 1971
157. Corder MP, Young RC, DeVita VT: Delayed hypersensitivity in patients with cancer. New Engl J Med 285:522–524, 1971
158. Corder MP, Young RC, Brown RS et al: Phytohemagglutinin induced lymphocyte transformation: The relationship to prognosis of Hodgkin's disease. Blood 39(5):595–602, 1972
159. Craft CB: Results with roentgen ray therapy in Hodgkin's disease. Bull Staff Meet Univ Mim Hosp 11:391–409, 1940
160. Jones SE, Fuks Z, Bull M, Kadin ME, Dorfman RF, Kaplan HS, Rosenberg SA, Kim H: Non-Hodgkin's lymphomas: IV. Clinicopathologic correlation in 405 cases. Cancer 31:806–823, 1973
161. Portlock CS, Rosenberg SA: No initial therapy for stage III and IV non-Hodgkin's lymphomas of favorable histologic types. Ann Int Med 90:10–13, 1979
162. Rosenberg SA, Kaplan HS: Clinical trials in the non-Hodgkin's lymphomata at Stanford University: Experimental design and preliminary results. Br J Cancer 31(Suppl II):456–464, 1975
163. Roeser HP, Hocker GK, Kynaston B et al: Advanced non-Hodgkin's lymphomas: Response to treatment with combination chemotherapy and factors influencing prognosis. Br J Haem 30:323–327, 1975
164. DeVita VT: Human models of human disease: Breast cancer and the lymphomas. Intl J Rad Onc Biol Phys. 5:1855–1867, 1979
165. Jones R, Hubbard SM, Osborne C et al: Histologic conversions in non-Hodgkin's lymphoma: Evolution of nodular lymphomas to diffuse lymphomas. Clin Res 26:437, 1978
166. Slaughter DP, Economou SG, Southwick HW: The surgical management of Hodgkin's disease. Ann Surg 148:705–710, 1958
167. Peters MV, Hasselbach R, Brown TC: The natural history of the lymphomas related to the clinical classification. In Zarafonetis CJD (ed): Proceedings of the International Conference on Leukemia-Lymphoma. Philadelphia, Lea and Febiger, 1968, pp 357–370
168. Lukes RJ, Craver LF, Hall TC et al: Report of the nomenclature committee. Cancer Res 26:311, 1966
169. Carbone PP, Kaplan HS, Musshoff K et al: Report of the committee on Hodgkin's disease staging. Cancer Res 31:1860–1861, 1971
170. Musshoff K, Ronemann H, Bourlis L et al: Die extranodulare lymphogranulomatose. Diagnose, therapie und prognose bei zwei unterschiedlichen formen des organ befalls, Ein Beitrag zur Stadienein teilung des morbus Hodgkin Fortschr. Geb Roentgenstr 109:776–786, 1968
171. Young RC, Anderson T, DeVita VT: The treatment of Hodgkin's disease: emphasizing programs at the Clinical Center, National Institutes of Health. Curr Probl Cancer 1(7):1–29, 1977
172. Redman HC, Glatstein E, Castellino RA et al: Computed tomography as an adjunct in the staging of Hodgkin's disease and non-Hodgkin's lymphomas. Radiology 124(2):381–385, 1977
173. Breeman RS, Castellino RA, Harell GS et al: CT-Pathologic correlations in Hodgkin's disease and non-Hodgkin's lymphoma. Radiology 126:159–166, 1978
174. Jones SE, Tobias DA, Waldman RS: Complete tomographic scanning in patients with lymphoma. Cancer 41:480–486, 1978
175. Rochester D, Bowie JD, Kunzmann A et al: Ultrasound in the staging of lymphoma. Radiology 124(2):483–487, 1977
176. Filly R, Marglin S, Castellino RA: The ultra sonographic spectrum of abdominal and pelvic Hodgkin's disease and non-Hodgkin's lymphoma. Cancer 38:2143–2148, 1976
177. Johnson RE: Is staging laparotomy routinely indicated in Hodgkin's disease? Ann Intern Med 75:459, 1971
178. Enright LP, Trueblood HW, Nelson TS: The surgical diagnosis of abdominal Hodgkin's disease. Surg Gynec Obst 130:853–858, 1970
179. Ferguson DJ, Allen LW, Griem ML, Moran ME, Rappaport H, Ultmann J: Surgical experience with staging laparotomy in 125 patients with lymphoma. Arch Int Med 131:356–361, 1973
180. Cannon NB, Nelson TS: Staging of Hodgkin's disease: a surgical perspective. Am J Surg 132:224–230, 1976
181. Kaplan HS, Dorfman RF, Nelson TS et al: Staging laparotomy and splenectomy in Hodgkin's disease: Analysis of indications and patterns of involvement in 285 consecutive, unselected patients. Nat Cancer Inst Mono No 36:291–301, 1973
182. Desser RK, Moran EM, Ultmann JE: Staging of Hodgkin's disease and lymphoma. Diagnostic procedures including staging laparotomy and splenectomy. Med Clin N Am 57:479–498, 1973
183. DeVita VT, Bagley CM, Goodell B et al: Peritoneoscopy in the staging of Hodgkin's disease. Cancer Res 31:1746–1750, 1971
184. Bagley CM, Roth JA, Thomas LB et al: Liver biopsy in Hodgkin's disease. Clinicopathologic correlations in 127 patients. Ann Intern Med 76(2):219–225, 1972
185. Berretta G, Spinelli P, Rilke F et al: Sequential laparoscopy and laparotomy combined with bone marrow biopsy in staging Hodgkin's disease (in press)
186. Levi JA, Wiernik PH: The therapeutic implications of splenic involvement in stage III Hodgkin's disease. Cancer 39:2158–2165, 1977
187. Desser RK, Golomb HM, Ultmann JE et al: Prognostic classification of Hodgkin's disease in pathologic stage III, based on anatomic considerations. Blood 49(6):883–893, 1977
188. Stein RS, Golumb HM, Diggs CH et al: Anatomic substages of Stage III-A Hodgkin's disease. Ann Int Med 92:159–165, 1980
189. Hoppe RT, Rosenberg SA, Kaplan HS et al: Prognostic factors in pathologic Stage IIIA Hodgkin's disease. Cancer 46:1240–1246, 1980
190. Piro AJ, Hellman S: Laparotomy alters treatment in Hodgkin's disease. Nat Cancer Inst Mono 36:307–311, 1973
191. Hellman S: Current studies in Hodgkin's disease: What laparotomy has wrought. New Engl J Med 290:894–898, 1974
192. Sweet DL Jr, Kinnealey A, Ultmann JE: Hodgkin's disease: Problems of staging. Cancer 42(2):957–970, 1978
193. Desser RL, Ultmann JE: Risk of severe infection in patients with Hodgkin's disease of lymphoma after diagnostic laparotomy and splenectomy. Ann Int Med 77:143–147, 1972
194. Meeker WR, Richardson JD, West W et al: Critical evaluation of laparotomy and splenectomy in Hodgkin's disease. Arch Surg 105:222, 1972
195. Brogadir S, Fialk MA, Coleman M, Vinciguerra VP, Degnan T, Pasmantier M, Silver RT: Morbidity of staging laparotomy in Hodgkin's disease. Am J Med 64(3):429–433, 1978
196. Jenkin RRT, Berry MP: Hodgkin's disease in children. Sem Onc 7:202–211, 1980
197. Chilcote RR, Baehner RH, Hammond D: Septicemia and meningitis in children splenectomized for Hodgkin's disease. New Engl J Med 295:798–800, 1976
198. Slaven R, Nelson TS: Complications from staging laparotomy for Hodgkin's disease. Nat Cancer Inst Monogr 36:457, 1973
199. Begent RHJ, Wiltshaw E: The effect of splenectomy in the haematological response to radiotherapy in Hodgkin's disease. Br J Haematol 27:331–336, 1974
200. Salzman JR, Kaplan HS: Effect of splenectomy on hematologic tolerance during total lymphoid radiotherapy of patients with Hodgkin's disease. Cancer 27:471–478, 1971

201. Panattiere FJ, Coltman CA: Splenectomy effects on chemotherapy in Hodgkin's disease. Arch Int Med 131:363–366, 1973
202. Panattiere FJ, Coltman CA, Delaney FC: Splenectomy, chemotherapy, and survival in Hodgkin's disease. Arch Int Med 137:341–343, 1977
203. Ihde DC, DeVita VT, Cannelos GP et al: Effect of splenectomy on tolerance to combination chemotherapy in patients with lymphoma. Blood 47(2):211–222, 1976
204. Myers CE, Chabner BA, DeVita VT et al: Bone marrow involvement in Hodgkin's disease: Pathology and response to MOPP chemotherapy. Blood 44(2):197–204, 1974
205. Rosenberg SA: Hodgkin's disease of the bone marrow. Cancer Res 31:1733–1736, 1971
206. Ferraut A, Rodhain JL, Michaux L et al: Detection of skeletal involvement in Hodgkin's disease: A comparison of radiography bone scanning and bone marrow biopsy in 38 patients. Cancer 35:1346–1353, 1975
207. Musshoff K, Boutis L: Therapy results in Hodgkin's disease. Freiburg i Br 1948–1966. Cancer 21:1100–1113, 1968
208. Rubins J: Cutaneous Hodgkin's disease: Indolent causes and control with chemotherapy. Cancer 42: 1219–1221, 1978
209. Valtysson G, Fisher-Beckfield P, Carbone PP: Cerebellar degeneration with Hodgkin's disease. Cancer 29(4):246–249, 1979
210. Young RC, Howser DM, Anderson T et al: Central nervous system comnplications of non-Hodgkin's lymphoma. The potential role for prophylactic therapy. Am J Med 66(3):435–443, 1979
211. Moorthy AV, Zimmerman SW, Burkholder: Nephrotic syndrome in Hodgkin's disease: Evidence for pathogenesis alternative to immune complex deposition. Am J Med 61:471–477, 1976
212. Yum MN, Edwards JL, Kleit S: Glomerular lesions in Hodgkin's disease. Arch Path 99:645–649, 1975
213. Chabner BA, Johnson RE, Young RC et al: Sequential nonsurgical and surgical staging of non-Hodgkin's lymphoma. Ann Int Med 85(2):149–154, 1976
214. DeVita VT, Canellos GP: Treatment of the lymphomas. Semin Hematol 9(2):193–209, 1972
215. Veronesi U, Musumeci R, Pizzetti F et al: The value of staging laparotomy in non-Hodgkin's lymphomas (with emphasis on the histioctyic type). Cancer 33:446–469, 1974
216. Goffinet, DR, Castellino RA, Kim H et al: Staging laparotomies in unselected previously untreated patients with non-Hodgkin's lymphomas. Cancer 32:672–681, 1973
217. Lotz MJ, Chabner B, DeVita VT et al: Surgical staging of 100 consecutive untreated patients with non-Hodgkin's lymphomas: Extramedullary sites of disease. Cancer 37:266–270, 1976
218. Glatstein E, Fuks Z, Goffinet DR et al: Non-Hodgkin's lymphoma of stage III extent: Is total lymphoid irradiation appropriate treatment? Cancer 37:2806, 1976
219. Chabner BA, Fisher RI, Young RC et al: Staging of non-Hodgkin's lymphoma. Semin Onc 7(3):285–291, 1980
220. McKenna RW, Bloomfield CD, Brunning RD: Nodular lymphoma: Bone marrow and blood manifestations. Cancer 36:428, 1975
221. Reimer RR, Chabner BA, Young RC et al: Lymphoma presenting in bone: results of histopathology, staging and therapy. Ann Intern Med 87(1):50–55, 1977
222. Shoji H, Miller T: Primary reticulum cell sarcoma of bone. Significance of clinical features upon prognosis. Cancer 28:1234–1244, 1971
223. Castellino RA, Goffinett DR, Blank N et al: The role of radiography in the staging of non-Hodgkin's lymphoma with laparotomy correlation. Radiology 110:329–338, 1974
224. Dunnick NR, Fuks Z, Castellino RA: Repeat lymphography in non-Hodgkin's lymphoma. Radiology 115:349–354, 1975
225. Bitran JD, Golomb HM, Ultmann JE et al: Non-Hodgkin's lymphoma, poorly differentiated lymphocytic and mixed cell types: results of sequential staging procedures, response to therapy, and survival of 100 patients. Cancer 42(1), 88–95, 1978
226. Herman TS, Jones SE: Systematic re-staging in the management of non-Hodgkin's lymphoma. Cancer Treat Rep 61:1009–1015, 1977
227. Longo DL, Schilsky RL, Blei L et al: Gallium-67 scanning has limited usefulness in staging patients with non-Hodgkin's lymphoma. Am J Med 68:695–700, 1980
228. Moran EJ, Ultmann JE, Ferguson DJ: Staging laparotomy on non-Hodgkin's lymphoma. Br J Cancer 31(Suppl II):228–237, 1975
229. Turner DA, Fordham EW, Amjad A et al: Gallium-67 imaging in the management of Hodgkin's disease and other malignant lymphomas. Semin Nucl Med 8:205–218, 1978
230. Best JJK, Blackledge G, Forbes WS et al: Computed tomography of abdomen in staging and clinical management of lymphoma. Br Med J 2:1675–1677, 1978
231. Schaner EG, Head GL, Doppman JL et al: Computed tomography in the diagnosis, staging, and management of abdominal lymphoma. J Compu Assist Tomography 1:176–180, 1977
232. Bunn PA Jr, Schein PS, Banks PM et al: Central nervous system complications in patients with diffuse histiocytic and undifferentiated lymphoma: Leukemia revisited. Blood 47(1):3–10, 1976
233. Ewing J: Neoplastic diseases. Philadelphia, WB Saunders, 1928
234. Dubin IN: The poverty of the immunologic mechanism in patients with Hodgkin's disease. Ann Int Med 27:898–913, 1947
235. Schier WW, Roth A, Ostroff J: Hodgkin's disease and immunity. Am J Med 20:94–99, 1954
236. Lamb D, Pilney F, Kelly WD et al: A comparative study of the incidence of anergy in patients with carcinoma, leukemia, Hodgkin's disease, and other lymphomas. J Immunol 89:555–558, 1962
237. Brown RS, Haynes HA, Foley HJ et al: Hodgkin's disease. Immunological, clinical and histologic features of 50 untreated patients. Ann Int Med 67:291–302, 1967
238. Sokol JE, Primikirios M: The delayed skin test response in Hodgkin's disease and lymphosarcoma. Cancer 14:597–607, 1961
239. Aisenberg AC: Immunologic status of Hodgkin's disease. Cancer 19:385–394, 1966
240. Eltringham JR, Kaplan HS: Impaired delayed hypersensitivity responses in 154 patients with untreated Hodgkin's disease. Nat Cancer Inst Monog 36 107–115, 1973
241. Eltringham JR, Weissmand A: Regional lymph node irradiation effect on immune responses. Radiology 94:438–441, 1970
242. Levy RA, Kaplan HS: Impaired lymphocyte function in untreated Hodgkin's disease. New Engl J Med 290:181–186, 1974
243. Young RC, Corder MP, Haynes HA et al: Delayed hypersensitivity in Hodgkin's disease: A study of 103 patients. Am J Med 52:63–71, 1972
244. King GW, Yanes B, Hurtubise PE et al: Immune function of successfully treated lymphoma patients. J Clin Invest 57:1451–1460, 1976
245. King GW, Grozea PC, Eyre HG et al: Neoantigen response in patients successfully treated for lymphoma. Ann Int Med 90:892–895, 1979
246. Fuks Z, Strober S, Bobrove AM et al: Longterm effects of radiation on T and B lymphocytes in peripheral blood of patients with Hodgkin's disease. J Clin Invest 58:803–814, 1976
247. Sokol JE, Aungst CW: Response to BCG vaccination and survival in advanced Hodgkin's disease. Cancer 24:128–134, 1969
248. Kelly WD, Good RA, Varco RL et al: The altered response to skin homographs and to delayed allergens in Hodgkin's disease. Surg Forum 9: 785–789, 1958
249. Green I, Corso P: Experiences with skin homografting in patients with lymphoma. Transp Bull 5:427–428, 1958
250. Green I, Inkelas, Allen LB: Hodgkin's disease: a maternal-to-foetal lymphocyte chimera? Lancet 1:30–32, 1960
251. Bunting CH: The blood picture in Hodgkin's disease. Bull Johns Hopkins Hosp 25:173–177, 1914.
252. Wiseman BK: Blood picture in primary disease of lymphatic system: their character and significance. JAMA 107:2016–2022, 1936
253. Rosenthal SR: Significance of tissue lymphocytes in the prognosis of lymphogranulomatosis. Arch Path 21:628–646, 1936

254. Aisenberg AC: Lymphocytopenia in Hodgkin's disease. Blood 25:1037–1042, 1965
255. Hersh EM, Oppenheim JJ: Impaired lymphocyte transformation in Hodgkin's disease. New Engl J Med 273:1006–1012, 1965
256. Matchett KM, Huang AT, Kremer WB: Impaired lymphocyte transformation in Hodgkin's disease. Evidence for depletion or circulating T-lymphocytes. J Clin Invest 52:1908–1917, 1973
257. Ziegler JB, Hansen P, Penny R: Intrinsic lymphocyte defect in Hodgkin's disease: Analysis of the phytohemagglutinen dose-response. Cell Immunol Immunopath 3:451–460, 1975
258. Faquet GB: Quantitatation of immunocompetence in Hodgkin's disease. J Clin Invest 56: 951–957, 1957
259. Bobrove AM, Fuks Z, Strober S et al: Quantitation of T and B lymphocytes and cellular immune function in Hodgkin's disease. Cancer 36:169–179, 1975
260. Twomey JJ, Laughter AH et al: Hodgkin's disease. An immunodepleting and immunosuppressive disorder. J Clin Invest 56:467–475 1975
261. Goodwin JS, Messner RP, Barkhurst AD et al: Prostaglandin-producing suppressor cells in Hodgkin's disease. New Engl J Med 297:963–968, 1977
267. Engleman EG, Hoppe R, Kaplan HS et al: Surpressor cells of a mixed lymphocyte reaction in healthy subjects and patients with Hodgkin's disease and sarcoidosis. Clin Res 20:513A, 1978
263. Hillinger SM, Herzig GP: Impaired cell-mediated immunity in Hodgkin's disease mediated by suppressor lymphocytes and monocytes. J Clin Invest 61:1620–1627, 1978
264. Fuks Z, Strober W, King DP et al: Reversal of cell surface abnormalities of T lymphocytes in Hodgkin's disease after *in vitro* incubation in fetal sera. J Immunol 117:1331–1335, 1976
265. Fuks Z, Strober S, Kaplan HS: Interaction between serum factors and T-lymphocytes in Hodgkin's disease. New Engl J Med 295:1273–1278, 1976
266. Moroz C, Labat M, Biniaminov M et al: Ferritin on the surface of lymphocytes in Hodgkin's disease patients. A possible blocking substance removed by levamisole. Clin Exp Immunol 29:30–35, 1977
267. Fisher RI, DeVita VT, Bostick F et al: Persistent immunologic abnormalities in long-term survivors of advanced Hodgkin's disease. Ann Int Med 92(5):595–599, 1980
268. Case DC, Hansen JA, Corrales E et al: Depressed in vitro lymphocyte responses to PHA in patients with Hodgkin's disease in continuous long remissions. Blood 49:771–778, 1977
269. Aisenberg AC, Leskowitz S: Antibody formation in Hodgkin's disease. New Engl J Med 268: 1269–1272, 1963
270. Weitzman SA, Aisenberg AC, Siber GR et al: Impaired humoral immunity in treated Hodgkin's disease. New Engl J Med 297(5):245–248, 1977
271. Minor DR, Schiffman G, McIntosh LS: Response of patients with Hodgkin's disease to pneumococcal vaccine. Ann Int Med 90:887–892, 1979
272. Walzer PD, Armstrong D, Weisman P et al: Serum immunoglobulin levels in childhood Hodgkin's disease: Effect of splenectomy and long-term followup. Cancer 45:2084–2089, 1980
273. Jones SE, Griffith K, Dombrowski P et al: Immunodeficiency in patients with non-Hodgkin's lymphomas. Blood 49: 335–344, 1977
274. Avdani SH, Dinshaw KA, Nair CN, et al: Immune dysfunction in non-Hodgkin's lymphoma. Cancer 45:2843–2848, 1980
275. Moore DF, Migliore PH, Shullenberger CC et al: Monoclonal macroglobulinemia in malignant lymphoma. Ann Int Med 72:43, 1970
276. Ko HS, Pruzanski W: M components associated with lymphoma: A review of 62 cases. Amer J Med Sci 272:175–183, 1976
277. Jones SE: Autoimmune disorders and malignant lymphoma. Cancer 31:1092–1098, 1973
278. Levine AM, Thorton P, Forman SJ et al: Positive Coombs test in Hodgkin's disease: Significance and implications. Blood 55:607–611, 1980
279. Booth PB, Jenkins WJ, Marsh WL: Anti-It; a new antibody of the I blood group system occuring in certain Melanesian sera. Br J Haemat 12:341–344, 1966
280. Waddell CC, Cimo PL: Idiopathic thrombocytopenic purpura occuring in Hodgkin's disease after splenectomy. A report of two cases and review of the literature. Am J Hematol 7:381–387, 1979
281. Pusey WA: Cases of sarcoma and of Hodgkin's disease treated by exposures to x-rays: a preliminary report. JAMA 38:166–170, 1902
282. Teschendorf W: Veber bestrahlung der ganzen menschluchen korpers bel blutkrankheiten. Struhlenther 26:720–729, 1927
283. Voorhoeve N: La lymphogranulomatose maligne. Acta Radiol 4:567–589, 1925
284. Kruchen C: Beitrag zur Rontgentherapie der lymphogranulomatose mit besonder berucksichtigung der neuren klinischen ergelnisse. Strahlenther 31:623–670, 1929
285. Easson EC, Russell MH: The cure of Hodgkin's disease. Brit Med J 1:1704, 1963
286. Kaplan HS: Long-term results of palliative and radical radiotherapy of Hodgkin's disease. Cancer Res 26:1250–1252, 1966
287. Kaplan HS: Role of intensive radiotherapy in the management of Hodgkin's disease. Cancer 19:356–367, 1966
288. Kaplan HS, Rosenberg SA: The treatment of Hodgkin's disease. Med Clin North Amer 50:1591–1610, 1966
289. Kaplan HS: Clinical evaluation and radiotherapeutic management of Hodgkin's disease and the malignant lymphomas. New Engl J Med 278:892–899, 1968
290. Kaplan HS: On the natural history, treatment and prognosis of Hodgkin's disease. Harvey lectues 1968–1969. New York, Academic Press. 215–259, 1970
291. Kaplan HS: Evidence for a tumorocidal dose level in the radiotherapy of Hodgkin's disease. Cancer Res 26:1221–1224, 1966
292. Rosenberg SA, Kaplan HS: Evidence for an orderly progression in the spread of Hodgkin's disease. Cancer Res 26:1225–1231, 1966
293. Landberg T, Liden K, Forslo H: Split-course radiation therapy of mediastinal Hodgkin's disease. TSD and CRE concepts Acta Radiol 12:33–39, 1973
294. Page V, Gardner A, Karsmark CJ: Physical and dosimetric aspects of the radiotherapy of the malignant lymphomas. I The mantle technique. Radiol 96:609–618, 1970
295. Carmel RJ, Kaplan HS: Mantle irradiation in Hodgkin's disease. An analysis of technique, tumor irradiation, and complications. Cancer 37:2812–2825, 1976
296. Kaplan HS, Stewart: Complications of intensive magavoltage radiotherapy for Hodgkin's disease. Nat Cancer Inst Monograph 36:439–444, 1973
297. Stewart HR, Cohn KE, Fajardo LF et al: Radiation-induced heart disease; a study of twenty-five patients. Radiology 89:302–310, 1967
298. Page V, Gardner A, Karsmark CJ: Physical and dosimetric aspects of the radiotherapy of malignant lymphoma. II. The inverted Y technique. Radiology 96:619–626, 1970
299. Lutz WR, Larsen RD: Technique to match mantle and paraaortic fields. Int J Rad Oncol Biol Phys 5 (Supple 2):159, 1979
300. Trueblood HW, Enright LP, Roy GR et al: Preservation of ovarian function in pelvic irradiation for Hodgkin's disease. Arch Surg 100:236–237, 1970
301. Collaborative Study. Survival and complications of radiotherapy following involved and extended field therapy of Hodgkin's disease, stage I and II—a collaborative study. Cancer 38:288–305, 1976
302. Goodman RL, Piro AJ, Hellman S: Can pelvic irradiation be omitted in patients with pathologic stages IA and IIA Hodgkin's disease. Cancer 37:2834–2839, 1976
303. Mauch P, Lewin A, Hellman S: Role of radiation therapy in the treatment of early stage Hodgkin's disease (in press)
304. Mauch P, Goodman R, Hellman S: The significance of mediastinal involvement in early stage Hodgkin's disease. Cancer 42:1039–1045, 1978
305. Thar TL, Million RR, Hausner RJ et al: Hodgkin's disease stage I and II: Relationship of recurrence to size of disease, radiation dose and number of sites involved. Cancer 43:1101–1105, 1979
306. Hoppe RT, Coleman CN, Kaplan HS et al: Hodgkin's disease, pathological stage I and II, the prognostic importance of initial sites of disease and extent of mediastinal involvement. Proc Amer Soc Clin Oncol 21:471, 1980

307. Piro AJ, Weiss DR, Hellman S: Mediastinal Hodgkin's disease: a possible danger for intubation anasthesia. Internat J Radiat Oncol Biol Phys 1:415–419, 1976
308. Mauch P, Hellman S: Supradiaphragmatic Hodgkin's disease: Is there a role for MOPP chemotherapy in patients with bulky mediastinal disease? Internat J Radiat Oncol Biol Phys 6:947–949, 1980
309. Hellman S: An evaluation of total nodal irradiation as treatment for stage IIIA Hodgkin's disease. Cancer 43:1255–1261, 1979
310. Mauch P. Ryback ME, Rosenthal D et al: The influence of initial pathological stage on the survival of patients who relapse from Hodgkin's disease. Blood (in press)
311. Rosenberg SA, Kaplan HS, Glatstein EJ et al: Combined modality therapy of Hodgkin's disease. A report of the Stanford trials. Cancer 42:991–1000, 1978
312. Prosnitz LR, Montalvo RI, Fischer DB et al: Treatment of stage IIIA Hodgkin's disease. Is radiotherapy alone adequate? Internat J Radiat Oncol Biol Phys 4:481–489
313. Goodman R, Mauch P, Piro A et al: Cancer 40:84–89, 1977
314. Hellman S, Mauch P, Goodman RL et al: The place of radiation therapy in the treatment of Hodgkin's disease. Cancer 42:971–978, 1978
315. Foley KM, Woodruff J, Ellis F et al: Radiation induced malignant and atypical schwannomas. Ann Neurology 7:311–318, 1979
316. Osler W: The Principles and Practice of Medicine. New York, D Appleton & Company, 1892
317. Goodman LS, Wintrobe MM, Dameshek W et al: Nitrogen mustard therapy. Use of methy *bis* (B-chloreothyl) amine hydrochloride and *tris* (B-chloroethy) amine hydrochloride for Hodgkin's disease lymphosarcoma, leukemia, certain allied and miscellaneous disorders. JAMA 132:126–132, 1946
318. Alpert LK, Petersen SK: The use of nitrogen mustard in the treatment of lymphomata. Bulletin of the US Army Medical Dept 7:187–194, 1947
319. Damesheck W, Weisfuse L, Stein T: Nitrogen mustard therapy in Hodgkin's disease. Analysis of 50 consecutive cases. Blood 4:338–379, 1949
320. Farber S, Diamond LK, Mercer RD et al: Temporary remission in acute leukemia in children produced by folic acid antagonist, 4-amino-pteroyl glutamic acid Aminopterin. New Engl J Med 238:787, 1948
321. Scott JL: The effect of nitrogen mustard and maintenance chlorambucil in the treatment of advanced Hodgkin's disease. Cancer Chemother Rep 27:27–32, 1963
322. Jacobs EM, Peters FC, Luce JK et al: Mechlorethamine HCL and cyclophosphamide in the treatment of Hodgkin's disease and the lymphomas. JAMA 203:392–398, 1969
323. Johnson IS, Armstrong JG, Gorman M et al: The vinca alkaloids: A new class of oncolytic agents. Cancer Res 23:1390, 1963
324. Carbone PP, Spurr C, Schneiderman M et al: Management of patients with malignant lymphoma: a comparative study with cyclophosphamide and vinca alkaloids. Cancer Res 28:811–822, 1968
325. Bollag, Grunberg E: Tumor inhibitory effects of a new class of cytotoxic agents: methyl hydrazine derivatives. Experientia 19:751, 1963
326. Mathe G, Schweisguth O, Schnieder M et al: Methylhydrazine in treatment of Hodgkin's disease Lancet 2: 1077, 1963
327. Martz G, D'Alessandri A, Keel HJ et al: Preliminary clinical results with a new anti-tumor agent RO 4-6467 (NSC 77213). Cancer Chemother Rep 33:5–14, 1963
328. Falkson G, de Villieb PC, Falkson HC: N-Isopropyl-(2-methyl-hydrazine)-p-toluamide hydrochloride (NSC 77213). Cancer Chemother Rep 39:77–79, 1964
329. DeVita VT, Hahn MA, Oliverio VT: Monoamine oxidase inhibition by a new carcinostatic agent, N-isopropyl-a-(2-methyl-hydrazine)-p-toluamide (MIH). Proc Soc Exp Biol Med 120:561–565, 1965
330. Coltman CA: Chemotherapy of advanced Hodgkin's disease. Sem Onc 7:155–173, 1980
331. Bender RA, DeVita VT: Non-Hodgkin's lymphoma. In Staquet MJ (ed): Randomized Clinical Trials in Cancer: A Critical Review By Sites. New York, Raven Press, 1978; pp 77–102.
332. Huguley CM Jr, Durant JR, Moores RR et al: Comparisons of nitrogen mustard, vincristine, procarbazine and prednisone (MOPP) *vs* nitrogen mustard in advanced Hodgkin's disease. Cancer 36:1227–1240, 1975
333. Nissen NI, Stutzman L, Holland JF et al: Chemotherapy of Hodgkin's disease in studies by Acute Leukemia Group B. Arch Intern Med 13:396–401, 1973
334. Lacher MJ, Durant JR: Combined vinblastine and chlorambucil therapy of Hodgkin's disease. Ann Int Med 62:468–476, 1965
335. Stutzman L, Ezdinli EZ, Stutzman MA: Vinblastine sulfate vs. cyclophosphamide in the therapy for lymphoma. JAMA 195:111–116, 1965
336. Selawey OS, Hansen H: Superiority of CCNU (1-[2-chloroethyl]-3-cyclohexyl)-1-nitrosourea; NSC 409962) in treatment of advanced Hodgkin's disease. Proc AACR 13:46, 1972
337. Lessner HE: BCNU (NSC 409962) in the treatment of advanced Hodgkin's disease and other neoplasia. Cancer 22:451–456, 1968
338. Haskell CM, Canellos GP, Leventhal BG et al: L-asparaginase therapeutic and toxic effects in patients with neoplastic disease. New Engl J Med 281:1028, 1969
339. Jones SE, Rosenberg SA, Kaplan HS et al: Non-Hodgkin's lymphoma II: single agent chemotherapy. Cancer 30:31–38, 1972
340. Schein PS, Chabner BA, Canellos GP et al: Potential for prolonged disease-free survival following combination chemotherapy of non-Hodgkin's lymphoma. Blood 43(2):181–189, 1974
341. DeVita VT, Fisher RI, Young RC: Treatment of diffuse histiocytic lymphomas: New opportunities for the future. In Staquet MJ, Tagnon HJ (eds): Recent Advances in Cancer Treatment. New York, Raven Press, 1977, pp 39–54
342. Jones SE, Fuks Z, Kaplan HS et al: Non-Hodgkin's lymphomas. Results of radiotherapy. Cancer 32:682–691, 1973
343. Anderson T, Bender RA, Fisher RI et al: Combination chemotherapy in non-Hodgkin's lymphoma: results of long-term followup. Cancer Treat Rep 61(6):1057–1066, 1977
344. Portlock CS, Rosenberg SA, Glatstein E et al: Treatment of advanced non-Hodgkin's lymphomas with favorable histologies. Preliminary results of a prospective trial. Blood 47:747–756, 1976
345. Portlock CS, Rosenberg SA: No initial therapy for stage III and IV non-Hodgkin's lymphomas of favorable histologic types. Ann Intern Med 90(1):10–13, 1979
346. Yates JL, Bunting CH: The rational treatment of Hodgkin's disease. JAMA 64:1953, 1915
347. Yates JL: The proper treatment of chronic malignant diseases of the superficial lymph glands. Arch Surg 5:65, 1922
348. Chabner BA: Nodular non-Hodgkin's lymphoma: the case for watchful waiting. Ann Intern Med 90(1):115–117, 1979
349. Osborne CK, Norton L, Young RC et al: Nodular histiocytic lymphoma: An aggressive nodular lymphoma with potential for prolonged disease-free survival. Blood 56(1):98–103, 1980
350. DeVita VT, Moxley JH, Brace K et al: Intensive combination chemotherapy and x-irradiation in the treatment of Hodgkin's disease. Proc Am Assoc Cancer Res 6:15, 1965
351. Corder MP, Elliott TE, Maguire LC, et al: Phase II study of cis-dischlorodiamminepoatinum(II) in stage IVB Hodgkin's disease. Cancer Treat Rep 63(5):763–766, 1979
352. Bender RA, Anderson T, Fisher RI et al: Activcity of the epipodophyllotoxin VP-16 in the treatment of combination chemotherapy-resistant non-Hodgkin's lymphoma. Am J Hematol 5(3):203–209, 1978
353. Sklaroff RB, Straus D, Young C: Phase II trial of vindesine in patients with malignant lymphoma. Cancer Treat Rep 63(5):793–794, 1979
354. Radice PA, Bunn PA Jr, Ihde DC: Therapeutic trials with VP-16-213 and VM-26: active agents in small cell lung cancer, non-Hodgkin's lymphomas, and other malignancies. Cancer Treat Rep 63(8):1231–1239, 1979
355. Bodey GP, Rodriguez V, Cabanillas F et al: Protected environment-prophylactic antibiotic program for malignant lymphoma.

Randomized trial during chemotherapy to induce remission. Am J Med 66(1):74–81, 1979
356. Turman S, Coleman M, Silver RT et al: High dose methotrexate with citrovorum factor in adult resistant lymphoma. Cancer 40(6):2823–2828, 1977
357. Appelbaum FR, Herzig GP, Ziegler JL et al: Successful engraftment of cryopreserved autologous bone marrow in patients with malignant lymphoma. Blood 521(1):85–95, 1978
358. Merigan TC, Sikora K, Breeden JH et al: Preliminary observations on the effect of human leukocyte interferon in non-Hodgkin's lymphoma. New Engl J Med 299(26):1449–1453, 1978
359. Gutterman JU, Yap Y, Buzdar A et al: Leukocyte interferon-induced tumor regression in human metastatic breast cancer, multiple myeloma, and malignant lymphoma. Ann Intes Med 93:399–406, 1980
360. Edelson RL, Raafat J, Berger CL Antithymocyte globulin in the management of cutaneous T cell lymphoma. Cancer Treat Rep 63(4):675–680, 1979
361. Fisher RI, Kubota TT, Mandell GL et al: Regression of a T-cell lymphoma after administration of antithymocyte globulin. Ann Intern Med 88(6):799–80, 1978
367. DeVita VT, Serpick A: Combination chemotherapy in the treatment of advanced Hodgkin's disease. Proc Am Assoc Cancer Res 8:13, 1967
363. DeVita VT, Serpick AA, Carbone PP: Combination chemotherapy in the treatment of advanced Hodgkin's disease. Ann Intern Med 73:891–895, 1970
364. DeVita VT Jr: Consequences of the chemotherapy of Hodgkin's disease. Cancer 47:1–13, 1981
365. DeVita VT, Simon RM, Hubbard SM et al: Curability of advanced Hodgkin's disease with chemotherapy: Long-term follow up of MOPP treated patients at NCI. Ann Int Med 92(5):587–595, 1980
366. Skipper HE, Shabel FM, Wilcox WS: Experimental evaluation of potential anti-cancer agents. XIII. On the criteria and kinetics associated with "curability" of experimental leukemia. Cancer Chemother Rep 35:1–11, 1964
367. Skipper HE (ed): Cancer Chemotherapy, vol I: Reasons for success and failure in treatment of murine leukemia with the drugs now employed in treating human leukemias. Ann Arbor, University Microfilms International, 1978
368. Moxley JH III, DeVita VT, Brace K et al: Intensive combination chemotherapy and x-irradiation in Hodgkin's disease. Cancer Res 27:1258–1263, 1967
369. Zeigler JL, Bluming AZ, Fass L et al: Chemotherapy of childhood Hodgkin's disease in Uganda. Lancet 2:679–680, 1972
370. Canellos GP, Young RC, DeVita VT: Combination chemotherapy for advanced Hodgkin's disease in relapse following extensive radiotherapy. Clin Pharmacol Ther 13:750–754, 1972
371. Frei E III, Luce JK, Gamble JE et al: Combination chemotherapy in advanced Hodgkin's disease: Induction and maintenance of remission. Ann Intern Med 79:376–382, 1973
372. Coltman CA, Frei E, Delaney FC: Effectiveness of actinomycin (a), methotrexate (MTX) and vinblastine (V) in prolonging the duration of combination chemotherapy (MOPP) induced remission in advanced Hodgkin's disease. Proc ASCO 9:78, 1973
373. Moore MR, Jones SE, Bull JM et al: MOPP chemotherapy for advanced Hodgkin's disease. Prognostic factors in 81 patients. Cancer 32:52–60, 1973
374. Focan C, Bricteux N, Lemaire M et al: MOPP chemotherapy for Hodgkin's disease at advanced stages. Acta Clin Belg 4:298–309, 1975
375. Olweny CLM, Katon Gole Mbidde E, Kiire CL et al: Childhood Hodgkin's disease in Uganda: a ten year experience. Cancer 42:787–792, 1978
376. British National Lymphoma Investigation: Value of prednisone in combination chemotherapy of Stage IV Hodgkin's disease. Br J Med 3:413–414, 1975
377. Bonadonna G, Zucali R, Monfardini S et al: Combination chemotherapy of Hodgkin's disease with adriamycin, bleomycin, vinblastine, and imidazole carboximide versus MOPP. Cancer 36:252–259, 1975
378. Bennett JM, Bakemeier RF, Carbone PP et al: Clinical trials with BCNU (NSC 409962) in malignant lymphomas by ECOG. Cancer Treat Rev 60:737–745, 1976
379. Coltman CA, Jones SE, Grozea PN et al: Bleomycin in combination with MOPP for the management of Hodgkin's disease. SWOG experience. In Carter SK, Crooke ST, Umezawa H (eds): Bleomycins—Current status and new developments. New York, Academic Press, 1978. pp 227–242
380. Cooper MR, Spurr CL, Glidewell O et al: The superiority of a nitrosourea (CCNU) containing four drug combination over MOPP in the treatment of stage III and IV Hodgkin's disease. Proc Am Soc Haematol 18:60, 1976
381. Nissen NI, Pajak TF, Glidewell O et al: A comparative study of a BCNU containing 4-drug program versus MOPP *versus* 3-drug combinations in advanced Hodgkin's disease: A cooperative study by the Cancer and Leukemia Group B. Cancer 43:31–40, 1979
382. Nicholson WM, Beard MEJ, Crowther D et al: Combination chemotherapy in generalized Hodgkin's disease. Br Med J 3:7–10, 1970
383. Durant JR, Gams RA, Velez-Garcia E et al: BCNU, velban, cyclosphosphamide, procarbazine, and prednisone (BVCPP) in advanced Hodgkin's disease. Cancer 42(5):2101–2110, 1978
384. Bloomfield CD, Weiss RB, Fortuney I et al: Combined chemotherapy with cyclophosphamide, vinblastine, procarbazine, and prednisone (CVPP) for patients with advanced Hodgkin's disease: an alternative program to MOPP. Cancer 38: 42–48, 1976
385. Diggs CH, Wiernik PH, Levi JA ed al: Cyclophosphamide, vinblastine, procarbazine and prednisone with CCNU and vinblastine maintenance for advanced Hodgkin's disease. Cancer 39(5):1949–1954, 1977
386. Harrison DT, Neiman PE: Primary treatment of disseminated Hodgkin's disease with BCNU alone and in combination with vincristine, procarbazine and prednisone. Cancer Treat Rep 61:789–795, 1977
387. McElwain TJ, Toy J, Smith E et al: A combination of chlorambucil, vinblastine, procarbazine and prednisolone for treatment of Hodgkin's disease. Br J Cancer 36(2): 276–280, 1977
388. Sutcliffe SB, Wrigley RF, Peto J et al: MVPP chemotherapy regimen for advanced Hodgkin's disease. Br Med J 1(6114): 679–683, 1978
389. Morgenfeld M, Somoza N, Magnasco J et al: Combined chemotherapy with cyclophosphamide, vinblastine, procarbazine, and prednisone (CVPP) *vs* CVPP plus CCNU (CCVPP) in Hodgkin's disease. Cancer 43:1579–1586, 1979
390. Eckhardt S, Dobrensy E, Bodrogi I: Results obtained with combination chemotherapy of VM26, natulan and prednisolone in generalized Hodgkin's disease. Chemotherapy 21:248–254, 1975
391. Lowenbraun S, DeVita VT, Serpick AA: Combination chemotherapy with nitrogen mustard, vincristine, procarbazine, and prednisone in previously treated patients with Hodgkin's disease. Blood 36(6): 704–717, 1970
392. Young RC, Canellos GP, Chabner BA et al: Maintenance chemotherapy for advanced Hodgkin's disease in remission. Lancet 1:1339–1343, 1973
393. Coltman CA Jr, Frei E, Moon TE: MOPP maintenance (MM) *vs* (VMR) for MOPP induced complete remission (CR) of advanced Hodgkin's disease. Proc ASCO 17:300, 1976
394. Fisher RI, DeVita VT, Hubbard SP et al: Prolonged disease-free survival in Hodgkin's disease with MOPP reinduction after first relapse. Ann Int Med 90(5):761–763, 1979
395. Santoro, A, Bonadonna G: Prolonged disease-free survival in MOPP-resistant Hodgkin's disease after treatment with adriamycin, bleomycin, vinblastine and dacarbazine (ABVD). Cancer Chemother Pharmacol 2:101–105, 1979
396. Lokich JJ, Frei E III, Jaffee N et al: New multiple agent chemotherapy (B-DOPA) for advanced Hodgkin's disease. Cancer 38:667–671, 1976
397. Levi JA, Wiernik PH, Diggs CH: Combination chemotherapy of advanced previously treated Hodgkin's disease with streptozotocin, CCNU, adriamycin and bleomycin. Med Pediatr Oncol 3(1):33–40, 1977

398. Goldman JM, Dawson AA: Combination therapy for advanced Hodgkin's disease. Lancet 11:1224–1227, 1975
399. Vinciguerra V, Coleman M, Iarowski CI et al: A new combination chemotherapy for resistant Hodgkin's disease. JAMA 33:237, 1977
400. Case DC, Young CW, Lee BJ: Combination chemotherapy of MOPP-resistant Hodgkin's disease with adriamycin, bleomycin, dacarbazine and vinblastine (ABDV). Cancer 39(4):1382–1386, 1977
401. Porzig KJ, Portlock CS, Robertson A et al: Treatment of advanced Hodgkin's disease with B-CAVE following MOPP failure. Cancer 41(5):1670:1675, 1978
402. Krikorian JG, Portlock CS, Rosenberg SA: Treatment of advanced Hodgkin's disease with adriamycin, bleomycin, vinblastine, and imidazole carboxamide (ABVD) after failure of MOPP therapy. Cancer 41(6):2107–2111, 1978
403. Young RC, Canellos GP, Chabner BA et al: Patterns of relapse in advanced Hodgkin's disease treated with combination chemotherapy. Cancer 42(2):1001–1007, 1978
404. Strauss DJ, Myers J, Passe S et al: The eight drug/radiation therapy program (MOPP/ABDV/RT) for advanced Hodgkin's disease: a followup report. Cancer 46:233–240, 1980
405. Kun LE, DeVita VT, Young RC et al: Treatment of Hodgkin's disease using intensive chemotherapy followed by radiotherapy. Int J Rad Onc Biol Phys 1:619–626, 1976
406. Rosenberg SA, Kaplan HS, Portlock CS et al: Combined modality therapy of Hodgkin's disease: a report on the Stanford trials. Cancer 42(Suppl 2):991–1000, 1978
407. Farber LR, Prosnitz LR, Cadman EC et al: Curative potential of combined modality therapy for advanced Hodgkin's disease. Cancer 46:1509–1517, 1980
408. Hoppe RT, Portlock CS, Glatstein E et al: Alternating chemotherapy and irradiation in the treatment of advanced Hodgkin's disease. Cancer 43(2):472–481, 1979
409. Bonadonna G, Santoro A, Zucali R et al: Improved five-year survival in advanced Hodgkin's disease. Cancer Clin Trials 2:217–226, 1979
410. Goodman R, Mauch P, Piro A et al: Stages IIB and IIIB Hodgkin's disease: Results of combined modality treatment. Cancer 40:84–89, 1977
411. Santoro A, Bonadonna G, Bonfante V et al: Non-cross resistant regimens (MOPP and ABVD versus MOPP alone) in stage IV Hodgkin's disease. Proc ASCO 16:470, 1980
412. DeVita VT Jr, Lewis BJ, Rozencweig M et al: The chemotherapy of Hodgkin's disease: past experiences and future directions. Cancer 42(2):979–990, 1978
413. Glick JH: The treatment of stage IIIA Hodgkin's disease: what is the role of combined modality therapy? Int J Radiat Oncol Biol Phys 4(9–10):909–911, 1978
414. Prosnitz LR, Montalvo RL, Fischer DB: Treatment of stage IIIA Hodgkin's disease: is radiotherapy alone adequate? Int J Radiat Oncol Biol Phys 4(9–10):781–787, 1978
415. British National Lymphoma Investigation: Initial treatment of stage IIIA Hodgkin's disease. Lancet 2:991–995, 1976
416. Canellos GP, Arseneau JC, DeVita VT et al: Second malignancies complicating Hodgkin's disease in remission. Lancet 1:947–949, 1975.
417. Coleman CN, Williams CJ, Flint A et al: Hematological neoplasia in patients treated for Hodgkin's disease. New Engl J Med 300:452–458, 1979
418. Krikorian JG, Burke JS, Rosenberg SA et al: The occurrence of non-Hodgkin's lymphoma following therapy for Hodgkin's disease. New Engl J Med 300:452–458, 1979
419. Reboul R, Donaldson SS, Kaplan HS: Herpes zoster and varicella infections in children with Hodgkin's disease. Cancer 41:95–99, 1978
420. Mauch P, Rosenthal D, Canellos G et al: Reduction of fatal complications from combined modality therapy in Hodgkin's disease (in preparation)
421. Hellman S, Chaffey JT, Rosenthal DS et al: The place of radiation therapy in the treatment of non-Hodgkin's lymphomas. Cancer 39:843–851, 1977
422. Bush RS, Gaspodarowicz M, Sturgeon J et al: Radiation therapy of localized non-Hodgkin's lymphoma. Cancer Treat Rep 61:1129–1136, 1977.
423. Bitran JD, Golomb HM, Ultmann JE et al: Non-Hodgkin's lymphoma, poorly differentiated and mized cell types. Cancer 42:88–95, 1978
424. Peters MV, Bush RS, Brown TC et al: The place of radiotherapy in the control of non-Hodgkin's lymphoma. Br J Cancer 31(Suppl II):386–401, 1975
425. Banfi A, Bonadonna G, Buraggi G et al: Clinical staging and treatment of lymphosarcoma and reticulum cell sarcoma. Tumori 51:153–178, 1965
426. Tubiana M, Pouillart P, Hayat M et al: Results of radiotherapy of stages I and II non-Hodgkin's lymphoma. Br J Cancer 31(Suppl II): 402–412, 1975
427. Hansen HS: Reticulum cell sarcoma treated by radiotherapy. Significance of clinical features upon prognosis. Acta Radiol (ther) 8:439, 1969
428. Lipton A, Lee BJ: Prognosis of stage I lymphosarcoma and reticulum cell sarcoma. New Engl J Med 284:230–233, 1971
429. Peters MV: The contribution of radiation therapy in the control of early lymphomas. Am J Roentgenol 90:956, 1963
430. Prosnitz LR, Hellman S, Von Essen CF et al: The clinical course of Hodgkin's disease and other malignant lymphomas treated with radical radiation therapy. Am J Roentgenol 105:618–628, 1969
431. Robinson T, Fischer JJ, Vera R: Reticulum cell sarcoma treated by radiation. Radiology 99:669, 1971
432. Reddy S, Saxena VS, Pellettiere EU et al: Early nodal and extranodal non-Hodgkin's lymphomas. Cancer 40:98–104, 1977
433. Fuks Z, Kaplan HS: Recurrence rates following radiation therapy of nodular and diffuse malignant lymphomas. Radiology 108:675–684, 1973
434. Glatstein E, Donaldson SS, Rosenberg SA et al: Combined modality therapy in malignant lymphomas. Cancer Treat Rep 61:1199–1207, 1977
435. Bonadonna G, Lattuada A, Manfardina S et al: Combined radiotherapy—chemotherapy in localized non-Hodgkin's lymphomas: 5 year results of a randomized study. In Jones SE, Salmon SE (eds): Adjuvant Therapy of Cancer, 2nd ed, New York, Grune & Stratton, pp 145–153
436. Heublein SC: Preliminary report on continuous irradiation of the entire body. Radiology 18:1051–1062, 1932
437. Medinger FG, Craver LF: Total body irradiation. Am J Roentgenol 48:651–671, 1942
438. Johnson RE, O'Conor GT, Levin D: Primary management of advanced lymphosarcoma with radiotherapy. Cancer 25:787–791, 1970
439. Young RC, Johnson RE, Canellos GP et al: Advanced lymphocytic lymphoma: Randomized comparisons of chemotherapy and radiotherapy alone or in combination. Cancer Treat Rep 61:1153–1159, 1977
440. Chaffey JT, Hellman S, Rosenthal DS et al: Total body irradiation in the treatment of lymphocytic lymphoma. Cancer Treat Rep 61:1149–1152, 1977
441. Carabell SC, Chaffey JT, Rosenthal DS et al: Results of total body irradiation in the treatment of advanced non-Hodgkin's lymphomas. Cancer 43:994–1000, 1979
442. Peckham MJ, Guay JP, Hamlin ME et al: Survival in localized nodal and extranodal non-Hodgkin's lymphoma. Br J Cancer 31 (Suppl II):413–424, 1975
443. Musshoff K, Schmidt-Vollmer H: Prognostic significance of primary site after radiotherapy of non-Hodgkin's lymphoma. Br J Cancer 31 (Suppl II):425–434, 1975
444. Boston HC, Dahlin DC, Ivins JC et al: Malignant lymphoma (so called reticulum cell sarcoma) of bone. Cancer 34:1131–1137, 1974
445. Wang CC, Fleichli DJ: Primary reticulum cell sarcoma of bone. Cancer 22:994–998, 1968
446. Newall J, Friedman M: Reticulum cell sarcoma part III prognosis. Radiology 97:99–102, 1970
447. Miller TR, Nicholson JT: End results in reticulum cell sarcoma of bone treated by bacterial toxin therapy alone or combined

with surgery and/or radiotherapy or with concurrent infection. Cancer 27:524–548, 1971
448. Wang CC: Malignant lymphoma of Waldeyer's ring. Radiology 92:1335–1339, 1969
449. Hoppe RT, Burke JS, Glatstein E et al: Non-Hodgkin's lymphoma: Involvement of Waldeyer's ring. Cancer 42:1096–1104, 1978
450. Banfi A, Bonadonna G, Ricci et al: Malignant lymphomas of Waldeyer's ring. Natural history and survival after radiotherapy. Br Med J 3:140, 1972
451. Freeman C, Berg JW, Cutler SJ: Occurrence and prognosis of extra-nodal lymphomas. Cancer 29:252
452. Novis BH, Bank S, Marks S et al: Abdominal lymphoma presenting with malabsorption. Q J Med 40:521–540, 1971
453. Seligmann M, Danon F, Hurez B et al: Alpha chain disease: A new immunoglobulin abnormality. Science 162:1396
454. Vawter GF, Jaffe N, Filler RM: The role of radiation therapy in localized resectable intestinal non-Hodgkin's lymphoma in children. Cancer 39:89–97, 1977
455. Lowenbraun S, DeVita VT, Serpick AA: Combination chemotherapy with nitrogen mustard, vincristine, procarbazine, and prednisone in lymphosarcoma and reticulum cell sarcoma. Cancer 25(5):1018–1025, 1970
456. Bagley CM, DeVita VT, Berard CW et al: Advanced lymphosarcoma: Intensive cyclical combination chemotherapy with cyclophosphamide, vincristine, and prednisone. Ann Intern Med 76(2):227–234, 1972
457. DeVita VT, Canellos GP, Chabner B et al: Advanced diffuse histiocytic lymphoma, a potentially curable disease. Results with combination chemotherapy. Lancet 1:248–250, 1975
458. Levitt M, Marsh JC, DeConti RC et al: Combination sequential chemotherapy in advanced reticulum cell sarcoma. Cancer 29:630–636, 1972
459. Berd D, Cornog J, DeConti RC et al: Long-term remission in diffuse histiocytic lymphoma treated with combination sequential chemotherapy. Cancer 35:1050–1054, 1975
460. Schein PS, DeVita VT, Hubbard S et al: Bleomycin, adriamycin, cyclophosphamide, vincristine, and prednisone (BACOP): Combination chemotherapy in the treatment of advanced diffuse histiocytic lymphoma. Ann Int Med 85(4):417–422, 1976
461. Fisher RI, DeVita VT, Johnson BL et al: Prognostic factors for advanced diffuse histiocytic lymphoma following treatment with combination chemotherapy. Am J Med 63(2):177–182, 1977
467. Sweet DL, Golomb HM, Ultmann JE et al: Cyclophosphamide, vincristine, methotrexate with leucovorin rescue, and cytosine arabinoside (COMLA) combination sequential chemotherapy in the treatment of advanced diffuse histiocytic lymphoma. Ann Intern Med 92:785–790, 1980
463. Skarin AT, Rosenthal DS, Moloney WC et al: Combination chemotherapy of advanced non-Hodgkin's lymphoma with bleomycin, adriamycin, cyclophosphamide, vincristine, and prednisone (BACOP). Blood 49:759–770, 1977
464. McKelvey EM, Gottlieb JA, Wilson HE: Hydroxydaunomycin (Adriamycin) combination chemotherapy in malignant lymphoma. Cancer 38:1481–1493, 1976
465. Luce JK, Delaney FC, Gehan EA: Remission induction chemotherapy of malignant lymphoma with combination bleomycin, cyclophosphamide, vincristine, and prednisone. Proc Am Assoc Cancer Res 14:66, 1973
466. Durant JR, Loeb V Jr, Dorfman R et al: 1,3-bis(2-chloroethyl-1-nitrosourea (BCNU), cyclophosphamide, vincristine, and prednisone (BCOP). A new therapeutic regimen for diffuse histiocytic lymphoma. Cancer 36:1936–1944, 1975
467. Bonadonna G, Beretta G, Tancini G et al: Adriamycin in combination and in combined treatment modalities. Tumori 60:393–416, 1974
468. Rodriguez V, Cabanillas F, Burgess MA et al: Combination chemotherapy ("CHOP-Bleo") in advanced (non-Hodgkin) malignant lymphoma. Blood 49:325–333, 1977
469. Elias L, Portlock CS, Rosenberg SA: Combination chemotherapy of diffuse histiocytic lymphoma with cyclophosphamide, adriamycin, vincristine, and predisone (CHOP). Cancer 42:1705–1710, 1978
470. Fisher RI, DeVita VT Jr, Hubbard SM et al: Pro-MACE-MOPP combination chemotherapy: Treatment of diffuse lymphomas. Proc ASCO 16:468, 1980
471. Stein RS, Moran EM, Desser RK et al: Combination chemotherapy of lymphomas other than Hodgkin's disease. Ann Intern Med 81:601–609, 1974
472. Coltman CA, Luce JK, McKelvey EM et al: Chemotherapy of non-Hodgkin's lymphomas: 10 years experience in the Southwest Oncology Group. Cancer Treat Rep 61:1067–1078, 1977.
473. Miller TP, Jones SE: Chemotherapy of localized histiocytic lymphoma. Lancet 1(8112):358–360, 1979
474. Ezdinli EZ, Costello WG, Icli F et al: Nodular mixed lymphocytic-histiocytic lymphoma (NM). Response and survival. Cancer 45:261–267, 1980
475. Hoogstraten B, Owens AH, Lenhard RE et al: Combination chemotherapy in lymphosarcoma and reticulum cell sarcoma. Blood 33:370–378, 1978
476. Schein PS, Chabner BA, Canellos GP et al: Non-Hodgkin's lymphoma: Patterns of relapse from complete remission after combination chemotherapy. Cancer 35:354–357, 1975
477. Portlock CS, Rosenberg SA: Combination chemotherapy with cyclophosphamide, vincristine and prednisone in advanced non-Hodgkin's lymphoma. Cancer 37:1275–1282, 1976
478. Kennedy BJ, Bloomfield CD, Kiang DT et al: Combination versus successive single agent chemotherapy in lymphocytic lymphoma. Cancer 41:23–28, 1978
479. Monfardini S, Tancini G, DeLena M et al: Cyclophosphamide, vincristine, and prednisone (CVP) versus adriamycin, bleomycin, and prednisone (ABP) in stage IV non-Hodgkin's lymphomas. Med Pediatr Oncol 3(1):67–74, 1977
480. Lister TA, Cullen MH, Beard ME et al: Comparison of combined and single-agent chemotherapy in non-Hodgkin's lymphoma of favourable histological type. Br Med J 1(6112):533–537, 1978
481. Bonadonna G, DeLena M, Lattuada A et al: Combination chemotherapy and radiotherapy in non-Hodgkin's lymphomata. Br J Cancer 31(Suppl 2):481–488, 1975
482. Jones SE, Salmon SE: Adjuvant immunotherapy with BCG in lymphoma. In Salmon SE, Jones SE (eds): Adjuvant Therapy of Cancer. Amsterdam, North–Holland, 1977, pp 549–556
483. Jones SE: Chemoimmunotherapy versus chemotherapy for remission induction in patients with non-Hodgkin's lymphoma: progress report of a Southwest Oncology Group study. Recent Results Cancer Res 65:164–169, 1978
484. Hoerni B, Durand M, Richaud P et al: Successful maintenance immunotherapy by BCG of non-Hodgkin's malignant lymphomas: results of a controlled trial. Br J Haematol 42(4):507:514, 1979.

CHAPTER 36

Peter H. Wiernik

Acute Leukemias of Adults

Acute leukemia, untreated, is a rapidly fatal disease that is characterized by a proliferation of abnormal immature blood cell progenitors in the bone marrow and other tissues. The progressive disappearance of normal cells from the blood—erythrocytes, granulocytes, and platelets—leads to progressively more severe fatigue, infection, and hemorrhage during the course of the disease. Disease control in adults requires more intensive treatment than in children. Intensive chemotherapy and radiotherapy along with substantial supportive care, which includes infection prevention and treatment measures and granulocyte, platelet, and red cell transfusions, are required to affect favorably the course of the disease. This treatment must be administered by a team of trained health care professionals thoroughly knowledgeable in the disease, its treatment, and the complications of both if optimal results are to be obtained. Because of the difficulty and expense of administering proper care to the leukemia patient, the patient's interests are usually best served by referral immediately upon diagnosis to a facility that specializes in leukemia treatment.

Patients with signs and symptoms of anemia, granulocytopenia, and thrombocytopenia, associated with splenomegaly or lymphadenopathy have been reported since the time of Hippocrates. However, it was not until the mid-19th century that leukemia was recognized as a distinct disease entity, after Donne made meticulous microscopic studies of the blood of patients and Virchow recorded clinical and autopsy data.[1] The disease was called leukemia by Virchow, who observed that the blood of some patients had a whitish color. The development of cellular stains by Ehrlich in 1877 when he was a medical student allowed him to recognize lymphocytic, myelocytic, and blastic forms of the disease. Naegeli in 1900 described the myeloblast and divided the blastic leukemias into myelocytic and lymphocytic varieties. Reschad and Schilling-Torgau a decade later described the monocytic variety of blastic leukemia.

Radiation therapy was shown to offer palliation to many patients with chronic leukemia in the second decade of this century. The startling observation that drugs could favorably affect the course of a malignant disease was made in the immediate post World War II period when nitrogen mustard was shown to have anti-lymphomic activity. Soon thereafter, Farber and others demonstrated the antileukemic activity of glucocorticoids and folic acid antagonists in children with acute lymphocytic leukemia.[2] These landmark observations represent the seeds from which modern day medical oncology has grown.

More recently, treatments from which the majority of patients with acute leukemia substantially benefit have been developed. Current treatment research has been directed primarily at reducing the toxicity of and prolonging the response to treatment. Today it is clear that a small fraction, perhaps 15% to 20%, of treated adults with acute leukemia is actually cured with drug treatment.

ETIOLOGY

Although factors leading to the development of acute leukemia in the vast majority of patients have not been identified, some rare predisposing causes as well as some potential leukemogens have been defined.

GENETIC FACTORS

The observations that children with Down syndrome have a 20-fold increased incidence of acute leukemia and that the risk of Down syndrome is increased among siblings of children with acute leukemia suggest that alterations or reorganization of the information on chromosome 21 can lead to the development of acute lymphocytic or myelocytic leukemia.[3] This suspicion is strengthened by the fact that the Philadelphia chromosome, the hallmark of chronic myelocytic leukemia which terminates as an acute leukemia, results from a translocation of some information from chromosome 21 to some other chromosome.[4] It has been recognized recently that some patients with acute leukemia who have no history or evidence of chronic myelocytic leukemia also have the Philadelphia chromosome. In most cases the survival of such patients and their response to therapy is somewhat poorer than expected for the type of acute leukemia with which they present, that is, acute lymphocytic or acute myelocytic leukemia, but better than expected for blast crisis of chronic myelocytic leukemia.[5]

A number of new, specific chromosomal aberrations have been recently reported in patients with acute leukemia. C-group trisomy has been reported in patients with ANLL.[6] A patient who, after treatment for acute lymphocytic leukemia (ALL), developed ANLL coincident with the emergence of a monosomy-7 marrow clone has also been reported.[7] ANLL patients with monosomy-7 have been described with increasing frequency lately.[8] The fact that the T-antigen genome of SV40 virus has been demonstrated on human chromosome 7 after transformation of human cell lines *in vitro* by that virus makes that observation especially intriguing.[9]

A number of congenital disorders that have in common an inherited tendency for chromosomal fragility or an association with unstable chromosome patterns such as aneuploidy are associated with an increased incidence of ANLL. The list of such diseases is rather long and includes congenital agranulocytosis, Ellis–van Creveld syndrome, celiac disease, Bloom's syndrome, Fanconi's anemia, Wiskott–Aldrich syndrome, Kleinfelter's syndrome, D^1-trisomy syndrome, and von Recklinghausen's neurofibromatosis.[10–18]

Environmental factors known to cause acquired chromosomal breaks, such as ionizing radiation, and some chemicals such as benzene and drugs such as some used for cancer treatment or more benign conditions, are associated with an increased incidence of acute leukemia, especially ANLL.[19–23]

VIRUSES

Certain viruses are known to cause acute leukemia in many species of subhuman vertebrates. They may be leukemogenic to the host in which they are inoculated or may be carried by germ cell or milk to a future generation in which the disease becomes manifest.[24] Whether or not the innoculated virus leads to the development of acute leukemia apparently depends on a myriad of modulating factors such as age, sex, and strain of the host; quantity of the innoculum; immunologic factors; and the presence or absence of certain environmental cocarcinogens such as chemicals or ionizing irradiation.[25,26]

There is no conclusive evidence that human leukemia is a viral disease. However, several molecular biological bits of evidence have nurtured speculation in this regard. RNA-dependent DNA polymerase (reverse transcriptase) has been detected in human leukemic blood cells but not in normal blood cells. This enzyme is known to be present primarily only in oncogenic viruses such as C-type viruses, a group of RNA viruses that can cause leukemia in animals, including primates other than man.[27] This enzyme allows the virus to synthesize genetic material that can be incorporated into the infected cell's genome. Viral genetic information can then be passed on through replication of the infected host cell.[28]

Electron microscopic and other classical virologic studies have failed to yield evidence of intact C-type viral particles in human leukemia cells. However, the study of two pairs of identical twins, each with one member afflicted with leukemia, revealed that DNA from the patient contained specific polynucleotide sequences not found in the DNA of the healthy twin[29] These data suggest that acquired genetic information may be related to the development of leukemia in humans.

These data together with the suspicion that, under certain circumstances some sort of human-to-human transmission of leukemia may occur, have served to intensify research in the area of viral oncogenesis.[30]

CHEMICALS AND DRUGS

Chronic exposure to a variety of substances has been associated with an increased incidence of acute leukemia, especially ANLL. Turkish cobblers who are chronically exposed to benzene during their work are an example. Drugs that can cause aplastic anemia such as chloramphenicol and phenylbutazone, and anticancer alkylating agents such as melphalan and chlorambucil have resulted in a 1% to 17% incidence of ANLL within 5 years after initiation of treatment. The incidence of leukemia varies with the primary disease and the intensity and duration of treatment with these drugs.[22,23] These drugs are known to cause chromosomal breaks in a large proportion of patients who receive them.

RADIATION EXPOSURE

Ionizing radiation is the external factor most clearly leukemogenic in both animals and man. Both ANLL and CML occur with increased frequency after exposure to such radiation and dose-response curves have been established for man and animals.[31,32] The increased incidence of ALL in man after exposure to irradiation is minimal, and not detected in all studies. Radiologists experienced a ten-fold increase in incidence of leukemia prior to the recognition of the need to protect them from exposure.[33] Japanese atomic bomb survivors sustained up to a greater than 20-fold increased incidence of ANLL and CML, depending on their distance from the hypocenter of the explosion. The peak incidence of leukemia occurred 5 years to 7 years after the explosion and the incidence of new cases continued above the expected rate for 20 years after the exposure.[34] Similarly, a 14-fold increased incidence of ANLL has been observed in patients with the benign disease ankylosing spondylitis who were treated with at least 2000 rads irradiation compared with patients with the disease who were not irradiated.[35] Similar data are available for patients therapeutically irradiated for malignant disease.[36]

Recent evidence suggests that as many as 6% of patients who receive radiation and alkylating agents as therapy for a malignant disease develop acute leukemia within 5 years of treatment.[37] This is especially true if many months or years separate the two modalities of treatment. It must be remembered, however, that the number of patients who develop acute leukemia after therapy for another malignant disease is tiny compared to patients who benefit from the treatment.

SPONTANEOUS REGRESSION

Rarely, babies born with widespread marrow, blood, and organ infiltration with myeloblast experience a spontaneous complete regression of the disease which is transient or permanent.[38,39] Transient spontaneous regression of ANLL in older patients has rarely been observed and is usually associated with a pyogenic bacterial infection.[40] The mechanism of these phenomena is not known. Careful study of such patients may provide insight into control mechanisms that regulate myeloblast differentiation and their aberrations in ANLL.

MORPHOLOGIC AND ANATOMIC CONSIDERATIONS

Acute leukemia is subclassified as lymphocytic or nonlymphocytic according to the morphology of the marrow and blood leukemic cells. Acute nonlymphocytic leukemia (ANLL) is further subclassified as acute myelocytic (granulocytic), promyelocytic (progranulocytic), monocytic, myelomonocytic, erythroleukemia, and other rarer varieties on the same grounds. The major morphologic distinction to be made is between ALL and ANLL, however. This distinction is important for two reasons. First, the response to therapy and prognosis are often better in ALL and, secondly, different treatments are usually prescribed for the two diseases. Distinction among the various subtypes of ANLL is more difficult but is possible with greater precision lately due to the development of new histochemical stains (Table 36-1). Identification of the many varieties of ANLL is becoming increasingly more important since several new drugs appear to have

TABLE 36-1. Interpretation of Histochemical Stains in Acute Leukemia

CYTOCHEMICAL REACTION	DISCRIMINATION	INTERPRETATION	ACUTE MYELOCYTIC LEUKEMIA	ACUTE MYELOMONOCYTIC LEUKEMIA	ACUTE MONOCYTIC LEUKEMIA	ACUTE LYMPHOCYTIC LEUKEMIA
PEROXIDASE & SUDAN BLACK	Lymphoid *vs* Non-lymphoid	Positive = dark granular cytoplasmic reaction = Non-lymphoid process (granulocytic–monocytic)	Positive	Positive	Usually positive	Negative
SPECIFIC ESTERASE (Chloracetate esterase)	Granulocytes *vs* Monocytes	Positive = pink cytoplasmic reaction = Granulocytic differentiation	Usually Positive	Usually Positive	Negative	Negative
NONSPECIFIC ESTERASE (α-naphthyl butyrate)	Granulocytes *vs* Monocytes	Positive = Brown cytoplasmic reaction = Monocytic–histiocytic differentiation	Negative	By FAB criteria 30% of leukemia cells positive	Positive (inhibited by Fluoride)	Negative
		Exceptions: May see weak rxns in Megs, plasma cells etc. Also "Block" positivity in "T" lymphs				
PAS (with & without diastase)	In some cases may discriminate lymphoid *vs* nonlymphoid; usually not of value	Block Positivity—diastase digestible, *i.e.*, glycogen = Lymphoid process.				
		Other rxns—granular positivity & diastase resistant products are NONSPECIFIC	May see granular positivity	May see granular positivity	Often see granular positivity	Ideally see Block positivity
ACID PHOSPHATASE	May be of value in discriminating "T" from Null ALL; otherwise nondiscriminatory	Block Positivity = "T" cell process				
		Tartrate-resistant granular positivity found in hairy cell leukemia	Often granular positivity	Often granular positivity	Often strong granular positivity	"T" cell ALL Block positivity; other ALL—may show granular positivity

significant activity against some varieties and essentially none against others. In addition, several characteristic features of the pathogenesis of some of the variants have been documented since the advent of more accurate classification techniques.

ACUTE LYMPHOCYTIC LEUKEMIA (ALL)

The blast cells that always infiltrate the bone marrow and often the blood of patients with this disease have several important cytologic features. They are round cells with usually only a scant rim of cytoplasm. Granules are almost never present in the cytoplasm, although an occasional azurophilic tiny granule may be seen. The nucleus is usually round and contains finely reticulated, homogeneous, open chromatin. The nucleus may contain one or two small nucleoli, which are often inconspicuous and difficult to see. These cells appear to be essentially undifferentiated. The morphologic variation from cell to cell in a given patient is minimal, although more variation is usually noted in adults than in children. Certain histochemical stain reactions are characteristic of the blast cells in ALL. Stains for lysosomal granules, such as the myeloperoxidase and Sudan black stains must give negative reactions to support the diagnosis of ALL. The periodic acid–Schiff (PAS) reagent will result in clumpy reddish positivity in the cytoplasm of most cells in more than half the patients. Various esterase stains yield negative results. The blast cells of more than 95% of patients with ALL contain the enzyme deoxynucleotidyl terminal transferase (TdT). This enzyme may be demonstrated by biochemical assay of a marrow aspirate, or by an immunofluorescent stain of a marrow or blood smear.[41] With the latter technique the vast majority of leukemic lymphoblasts will demonstrate nuclear fluorescene with a fluorescent microscope. Although low levels of TdT activity can rarely be detected biochemically in the marrow aspirate of a patient with ANLL, the fluorescent stain technique will identify only an occasional cell as positive in such a patient. Some patients with the blast crisis of chronic myelocytic leukemia (CML) will demonstrate significant TdT activity with either technique.[41] The patient usually has had the typical clinical course of CML, however. Thus, the demonstration of TdT activity in the leukemic cells of a patient with newly diagnosted acute leukemia is very convincing evidence that the leukemia is ALL.

Acute lymphocytic leukemia is primarily a disease of the marrow and blood. However, at least 80% of patients will have lymphadenopathy, primarily of the neck, and/or splenomegaly at the time of diagnosis due to infiltration of those organs with leukemic cells. In addition, the liver will be barely palpable in half of adults with ALL.

ACUTE NONLYMPHOCYTIC LEUKEMIA (ANLL)

The blast cells in the marrow and blood of patients with this disease are usually larger than lymphoblasts, and their variation in size and shape is much greater. Leukemic cells in ANLL have more abundant cytoplasm and cytoplasmic granulation is usually, but not always, evident. Auer rods, which are reddish-staining abnormal lysosomal granules with Wright's stain are present in the cytoplasm of at least some cells in approximately 10% of patients with ANLL (Fig. 36-1). The cell nucleus is relatively large and usually slightly or greatly irregular in shape. Usually, some evidence of nuclear or cytoplasmic differentiation is evident. The nuclear chromatin pattern is more heavily reticulated than in the blast cells of ALL and multiple nucleoli are usually seen within each nucleus. The nucleoli often vary greatly in size within the same nucleus and from cell to cell. Occasionally they are relatively large. Nucleolar staining characteristics are also quite variable. Occasionally the nucleoli are amphophilic, sometimes they are pale blue, but more often they are lightly eosinophilic.

ACUTE MYELOCYTIC LEUKEMIA

The leukemic cells in this variant of ANLL are the most uniform of all ANLL variants, although variation in size and shape is still evident. The cytoplasm usually contains fine azurophilic granules, especially in the perinuclear area. The nucleus is generally round. Lysosomal granule stains such as myeloperoxidase and Sudan black are almost always positive. Sometimes, however, the granules are so small that they are evident only on electron-microscopy. The PAS stain is almost always negative.

ACUTE PROMYELOCYTIC LEUKEMIA

The leukemic cells in this disease are almost always heavily granulated, although sometimes electron microscopy is necessary to demonstrate them (microgranular variant).[42] Often the granules stain very basophilic with Wright's stain. Curiously, the nucleus of the leukemic cell is often lobulated, folded, or highly irregular and suggests a monocytoid morphology. Sometimes, although heavy and bizarre granulation is evident with Wright's stain, the usual lysosomal granule stains give negative reactions.

ACUTE MONOCYTIC LEUKEMIA

The leukemic cells are large with abundant sparsely or ungranulated cytoplasm. Cytoplasmic buds that look like

FIG. 36-1. A Wright's stained bone marrow aspirate from a patient with acute myelocytic leukemia. Many of the blasts have auer bodies in the cytoplasm.

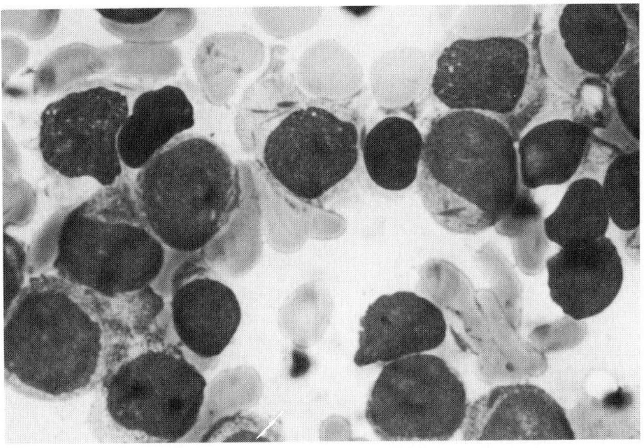

pseudopodia may be evident. The nucleus is large and convoluted, or folded. Great morphologic variation from cell to cell is evident. The peroxidase and Sudan black stains may show light, punctate positivity in some cells and occasionally do so in most cells. Some cells also show punctate PAS positivity, but never the "clumpy" positivity of lymphoblasts. Certain esterase stains are usually positive, and sodium fluoride inhibiton of esterase activity is characteristic of the cells of acute monocytic leukemia.[43]

ACUTE MYELOMONOCYTIC LEUKEMIA

In this variant, cells characteristic of acute myelocytic and acute monocytic leukemia are seen in various ratios. In both acute monocytic and myelomonocytic leukemia, muramidase (lysozyme) activity is evident in the leukemic cells.[43] Intramedullary destruction of leukemic cells in these two variants often leads to greatly elevated levels of that enzyme in the blood and urine which can be detected and quantitated with a simple turbidimetric technique.[44] Patients with acute monocytic or myelomonocytic leukemia often have evidence of significant extramedullary leukemic infiltration of tissues. Thus, gingival hypertrophy, leukemia cutis, and meningeal leukemia are more common in these variants of ANLL than any other. This observation may be related to the greater ability of leukemic cells in these ANLL variants to migrate to skin windows.[45]

ERYTHROLEUKEMIA

This ANLL variant was first described by DiGuglielmo and is often referred to as the acute DiGuglielmo syndrome. A more chronic variant, called by some the chronic DiGuglielmo syndrome, is characterized by less morphologic immaturity initially and may, at first glance, appear to be a refractory anemia with ineffective erythropoiesis. The chronic DiGuglielmo syndrome becomes indistinguishable from the acute syndrome with time. It, therefore, seems appropriate to refer to this ANLL variant as erythroleukemia, a term suggested by DiGuglielmo himself.

The predominant proliferating cell in the bone marrow is an abnormal erythroblast. Usually the morphology of most of the marrow cells is such that the erythrocytic derivation is obvious. Often, many bizzare, abnormal erythrocyte forms are present, and occasionally they may be the dominating element. In such cases, multinucleated red cells are usually found, and often cells as young as proerythroblasts with three or more nuclei are seen in clumps. The red cell precursors are usually megaloblastic and show obvious nuclear–cytoplasmic maturation dissociation. This abnormality is usually represented by relatively mature red cell precursors with little or no hemoglobinization of the cytoplasm which, in such cases, stains intensely basophilic with Wright's stain. An iron stain will usually reveal rare or abundant ringed sideroblasts in erythroleukemia and the PAS stain will usually demonstrate blocks of positivity in cytoplasm of many abnormal erythrocytes. Erythrocyte PAS positivity does not occur in any other malignant disease or anemia except, perhaps, extremely rarely in thalassemia major. In many patients the abnormal erythroblasts can be shown to have esterase activity by histochemical staining.[46] Normal erythroblasts contain no such activity. Ringed sideroblasts may be found on occasion in other variants of ANLL, especially when the leukemia can be related to previous alkylating agent therapy for another malignancy such as multiple myeloma.[47] As erythroleukemia progresses, the erythroid element becomes less obvious and a morphologic picture more characteristic of acute myelocytic or myelomonocytic leukemia emerges.

Some erythroleukemia patients have a peculiar rheumatic disorder that responds to aspirin but not antileukemic treatment. In addition, about a quarter of patients have a positive Coombs' test and one-third have rheumatoid factor demonstrable.[48] The significance of these findings is unclear.

HAIRY CELL LEUKEMIA

There is disagreement in the literature concerning the origin of the leukemic cell in this rare variety of acute leukemia. It is very important to recognize the entity, however, because the early course may mimic that of chronic lymphocytic leukemia and require little treatment. The latest information suggests that hairy cells are distinctive and contain properties of both monocytes and B lymphocytes.[49] Others, however, have reported hairy cell leukemia with cells that have T-cell properties.[50]

Peripheral blood cytopenia is common in this disorder and marrow hypoplasia may be so severe that the diagnosis of aplastic anemia is incorrectly entertained.[51] The classic hairy cell looks, at first glance, like a somewhat immature lymphocyte. The nucleus is large and round, and nucleoli are rarely seen. The agranular cytoplasm is usually very lightly stained. Closer scrutiny reveals multiple fine hair-like clear cytoplasmic projections around the perimeter of the cell. A peculiar acid phosphatase that is tartrate resistant can be histochemically demonstrated in the cytoplasm of hairy cells and, indeed, its demonstration is necessary for the diagnosis.[52] Unlike hairy cells, the acid phosphatase activity in T-lymphoblasts is eradicated upon incubation with tartrate. The results of other histochemical tests are variable. Confusion with monocytic leukemia may arise from the fact that many hairy cell leukemia patients have α-naphthylesterase-positive leukemic cells, and the esterase activity is almost always inhibited by sodium fluoride.[53]

Of special interest is the fact that hairy cell leukemia cells do not have reverse transcriptase activity, a feature which distinguishes them from all other leukemia cells.[54]

Patients with hairy cell leukemia are often young males who are surprisingly asymptomatic. The most significant finding on physical examination is a moderately or greatly enlarged spleen. Lymphadenopathy is absent or minimal.

PATHOLOGY

The acute leukemias may be responsible for dysfunction of various organs due to either direct invasion with leukemic cells or compression of a vital conduit by enlarged lymph nodes or other tissues, or as a consequence of the release of a variety of substances from leukemic cells. These manifestations of acute leukemia will be reviewed according to organ site.

BONE MARROW

An increased number of blast cells in the bone marrow is necessary to diagnose acute leukemia. It is said that the blast count in a normal marrow may be as high as 5%. However, blasts are usually very difficult to find in a normal marrow. Therefore a patient whose marrow contains even a low percentage of blasts should have another examination in a month or so. The marrow may be completely replaced by leukemic cells or such cells may account for a large minority of marrow nucleated cells at the time of diagnosis of acute leukemia. Very early in the disease, especially in patients with ALL, marrow infiltration with leukemic cells may vary in degree from site to site. Thus, it may be possible for a marrow aspirate from one iliac crest to be nondiagnostic while the aspirate from the other is frankly leukemic.

The marrow is usually hypercellular due to infiltration with leukemic cells. The number of nucleated cells is usually increased, and the amount of fat is decreased. However, in many patients whose leukemia is considered secondary to prior radiotherapy or chemotherapy for another disease the marrow aspirate may appear hypocellular and sometimes essentially aplastic. Some ANLL patients, especially elderly ones, who are leukopenic at the time leukemia is diagnosed also have hypocellular bone marrows. It should be remembered that marrow cellularity cannot be properly assessed by reviewing an aspirate. A marrow biopsy must be studied in order to determine the true cellularity of the area sampled.

The number of normal elements in a leukemic marrow is almost always reduced. There is a fairly good inverse relationship between the number of normal elements and the number of leukemic cells. In ALL the normal elements of the marrow have essentially normal morphology. In ANLL, however, distinct morphologic abnormalities of the normal elements are often discernible. In such patients cytoplasmic granulation of granulocytes beyond the myelocyte stage may be reduced or absent.[55] Rarely, an acquired Pelger–Huet anomaly, principally characterized by a reduction of nuclear segments to two or less in mature neutrophils, may be evident. Abnormalities may be evident in the red cell series also. There may be erythroid hyperplasia with or without megaloblastoid maturation and immaturity of the red cell series may be striking. Megakaryocyte abnormalities, in the form of decreased budding or nuclear morphologic abnormalities may be seen. These erythroid and megakaryocytic abnormalities are quite common in acute myelomonocytic leukemia. Thus, the marrow picture in ANLL may often be best described as that of a panmyelosis.

A radioisotope marrow scan will usually show peripheral extension of the active marrow into areas that are largely replaced by fat in the adult, such as distal long bones. Thus isotope uptake in the distal tibia may be as great as in the pelvic bones.

BONES AND JOINTS

The most commonly appreciated radiologic finding in bone in adult acute leukemia is thinning of the cortex of long bones due to the expansion of the marrow cavity. Osteolytic lesions very rarely occur and the metaphyseal lines commonly seen in children with ALL do not occur in adults. These lines represent functional impairment of the metaphyseal growth centers in the child and, since these centers are inactive in adults, they are not affected by the expanding marrow cavity. Arthritis secondary to infiltration of synovium by leukemic cells occasionally occurs in children but not in adults. However, patients with acute leukemia of all ages may experience a migratory polyarthritis secondary to hyperuricemia. This is especially true of patients with an unusually large leukemic cell mass as evidenced by an extremely high white blood cell count and hypercellular marrow, or by bulky lymphadenopathy or splenomegaly. In addition, migratory polyarthritis may occur after the administration of a xanthine oxidase inhibitor such as allopurinol given to reduce the blood uric acid level.

SKIN AND SOFT TISSUE

The most common skin lesions in patients with acute leukemia are petechiae resulting from capillary hemorrhage. They tend to occcur on dependent or traumatized areas of the body. Leukemic infiltration of skin may be found in patients who present with high white counts, or in patients with far advanced disease no longer responsive to therapy. Such infiltration usually results in small (2 mm to 5 mm) raised, pinkish nodules that are painless, nontender, and not pruritic. These lesions are most common on the extremities or trunk. Occasionally they may involve the face and other areas of the body, and rarely they may be massive (1 cm to 5 cm) in size (Fig. 36-2). These lesions usually occur when the bone marrow and blood are actively involved in the leukemic process. However, on occasion, the appearance or reappearance of these lesions in a patient in hematologic remission may be the first harbinger of relapse. These lesions, like all extramedullary leukemic lesions, are more common in patients with acute monocytic or myelomonocytic leukemia. The leukemic cells in these variants of ANLL have been shown to have the greatest potential for migration to soft tissue.[45]

Ecchymoses, characteristic of bleeding secondary to clotting factor deficiencies, may be found in the skin of any acute leukemia patient after local trauma. They most frequently occur in patients with acute promyelocytic leukemia and may appear even in the absence of trauma. Patients with this variant of ANLL very often have a disseminated intravascular coagulopathy which can lead to clotting factor depletion. Procoagulant released from the abnormal granules of the leukemic cells in this variant triggers the intravascular clotting.[56]

Chloromas, or granulocytic sarcomas are focal soft-tissue masses of leukemic cells.[57] They rarely, if ever, occur in ALL and arise in only a small minority of ANLL patients. The term chloroma derives from the fact that some of these lesions have a greenish color from the high myeloperoxidase content of the leukemic cells. However, most such lesions are not green, and the term granulocytic sarcoma seems more appropriate. Chloromas often arise from the subperiosteal area of bone and grow into soft tissue. They usually occur in association with bones of the orbit, ribs, or sternum. However lesions unassociated with bone have been observed on the face (Fig. 36-3), and in ovary, breast and other tissues,

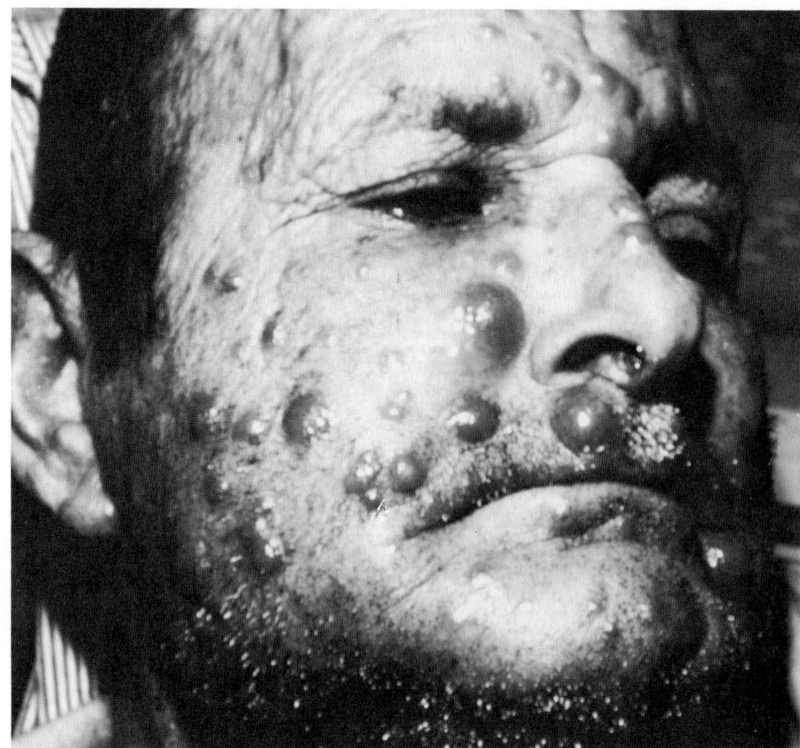

FIG. 36-2. Large cutaneous leukemic infiltrates of a patient with acute myelomonocytic leukemia.

FIG. 36-3. A patient with acute myelocytic leukemia complicated by facial granulocytic sarcomas (chloromas). The lesions were dull light green.

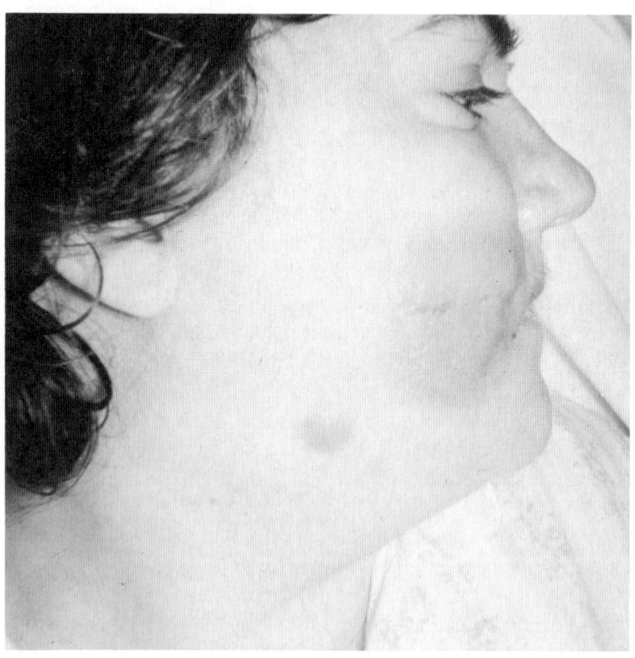

including the dura (Fig. 36-4). Most patients with granulocytic sarcomas have only one or two such lesions.

Granulocytic sarcomas are usually composed primarily of immature leukemic cells. The true character of the lesion may not be appreciated with routine surgical pathology sections stained with hematoxylin and eosin. Such a preparation may be misinterpreted as anaplastic carcinoma, diffuse histiocytic lymphoma, plasmacytoma, or other lesions. This is particularly true when a granulocytic sarcoma is the first sign of malignant disease. Whenever a suspected granulocytic sarcoma is biopsied, touch preparations stained with Wright's stain should be made and the pathologist should be alerted to the possible diagnosis.

Rarely, a nonspecific exfoliative dermatitis may occur any time during the course of ANLL, and a febrile neutrophilic dermatosis of unknown etiology which responds to steroids has also been reported.[58,59]

LESIONS OF THE HEAD AND NECK

The most frequent manifestation of acute leukemia in this area is cervical lymphadenopathy in the patient with ALL. Oropharyngeal infections are common in acute leukemia patients prior to or during therapy. Periodontal infections are particularly common, and should be treated if possible prior to the institution of antileukemic therapy in order to prevent subsequent septicemia. Each acute leukemia patient should be examined by a dentist shortly after diagnosis.[60]

Antileukemic drugs frequently cause oral mucosal ulcerations that are usually minimal but can be extensive. Such lesions tend to become infected particularly with *Candida albicans* when the patient is granulocytopenic. The vast majority of such infections can be prevented with prophylactic oral antifungal drug administration.

Ocular involvement with ANLL may produce protean complications. There may be retinal hemorrhages due to leukemic infiltration or thrombocytopenia. Fundic lesions secondary to leukemic infiltration are usually associated with Roth-like

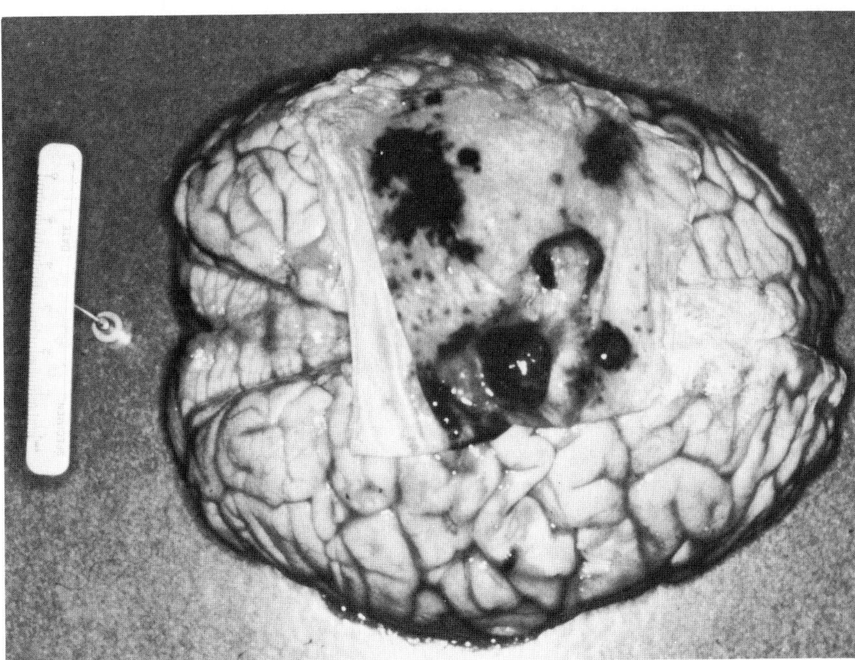

FIG. 36-4. Dural granulocytic sarcomas at the base of the brain of a patient with acute myelomonocytic leukemia. The dark lesions gradually faded upon exposure to air.

spots, whereas thrombocytopenia usually results in fundic hemorrhage alone (Fig. 36-5). Fundic leukemic infiltration is often associated with other evidence of CNS leukemia. It is important to recognize it because low-dose irradiation may save the vision in the involved eye.

Gingival hypertrophy (Fig. 36-6), sometimes marked, is common in patients with acute myelomonocytic or monocytic leukemia. The hypertrophy is due to massive infiltration of the gingiva with leukemic cells. The gingiva often become necrotic and superinfected. The degree of gingival hypertrophy usually parallels the activity of the disease in marrow and blood.

CARDIOPULMONARY MANIFESTATIONS

The most common pulmonary lesion in a patient with acute leukemia is pneumonia, which can occur whenever the patient is granulocytopenic because of the disease or its treatment. The pneumonia is most often due to gram negative bacteria, but after prolonged antibacterial treatment fungal pneumonias are common. Fungal penumonias tend to occur in relapsed patients with advanced disease. The incidence of fungal and bacterial pneumonia may be sharply reduced by conducting therapy in a laminar air flow room or any other essentially sterile environment (see below).

It should be remembered that the usual signs and symptoms of pneumonia in a granulocytopenic leukemia patient may be absent due to the lack of granulocytes. Thus, sputum production, cough, and roentgenographic changes may be minimal.[61] Therefore, fever may be the only clue to a life-threatening infection in such a patient.

Some patients with longstanding acute leukemia in relapse may have evidence of impaired respiration due to capillary plugging with leukemic cells in the lung. This is especially true of acute monocytic and myelomonocytic leukemia patients with very high white counts. Such a patient may occasionally present with an asthma-like attack of sudden onset and histologic examination of the lung will often show capillaries and alveoli engorged with leukemic cells.

Cardiovascular abnormalities due to leukemic infiltration are rarely clinically important. However, conduction defects, murmurs, pericarditis, and congestive heart failure have rarely been observed owing to leukemic infiltration of the bundle of His, cardiac valves, pericardium, or myocardium, respectively.[62]

FIG. 36-5. Roth spots in the optic fundus of a patient with acute monocytic leukemia. The clearer central areas of the hemorrhages are due to leukemic infiltration.

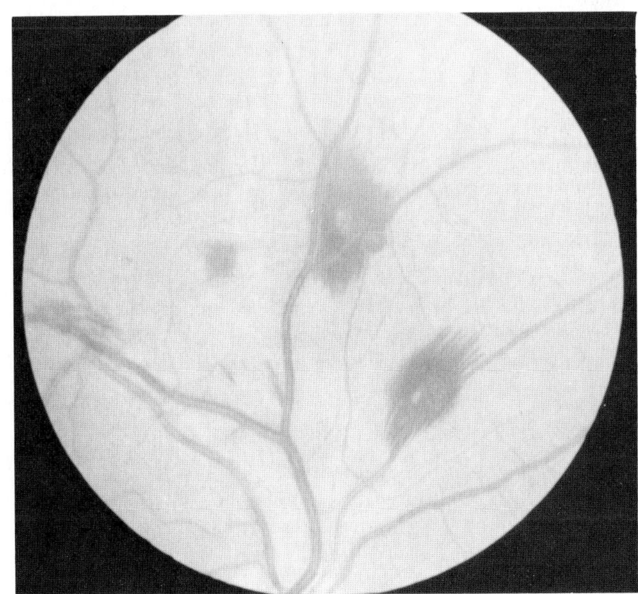

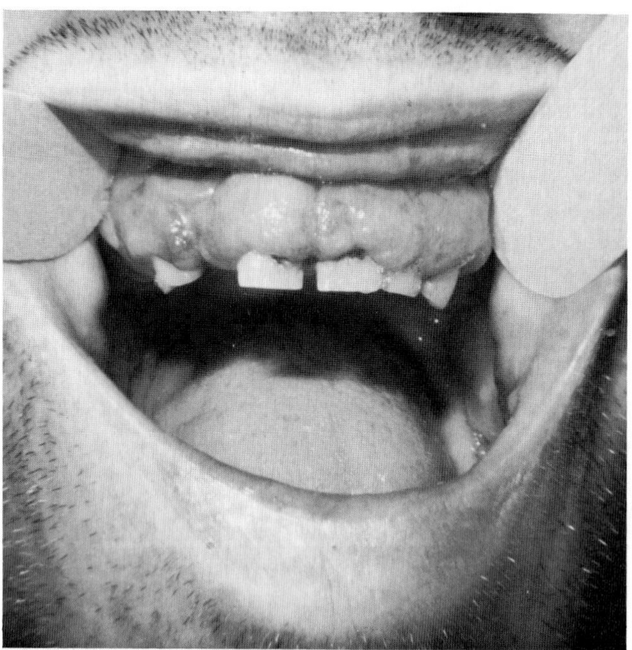

FIG. 36-6. Marked gingival hypertrophy due to leukemic infiltration in a patient with acute monocytic leukemia.

GASTROINTESTINAL MANIFESTATIONS

Dysphagia is common in acute leukemia patients. It may be due to hypopharyngeal infection, especially Candidiasis, or to mucosal ulceration secondary to chemotherapy, or both. Rarely, leukemic infiltration of the tonsils or uvula is the cause of dysphagia (Fig. 36-7).[63] Substernal burning and dysphagia are clues to esophagitis due to Candida or gram negative organisms. The classic radiographic findings of Candida esophagitis are also seen with bacterial esophagitis. Occasionally these lesions are caused by instrumentation of the granulocotopenic patient with unsterile equipment prepared for routine use.[64]

Thrombocytopenic leukemia patients may have significant gastrointestinal bleeding. However, this has become rare since the general acceptance of prophylactic platelet transfusion. Occasionally hematemesis in a far advanced, relapsed patient is due to leukemic infiltration of the stomach. If the patient has become refractory to platelet transfusion, irradiation of the stomach may be useful in stopping the bleeding. Usually a total dose of 1000 rad given in 200 rad daily fractions will be successful.

Small bowel granulocytic sarcoma has rarely been reported to cause obstruction in the adult with acute leukemia.[65] Although such lesions are often complications of advanced

FIG. 36-7. Massive leukemia infiltration of the uvula in a patient with acute myelomonocytic leukemia. Irradiation was necessary to relieve the patient's dysphagia.

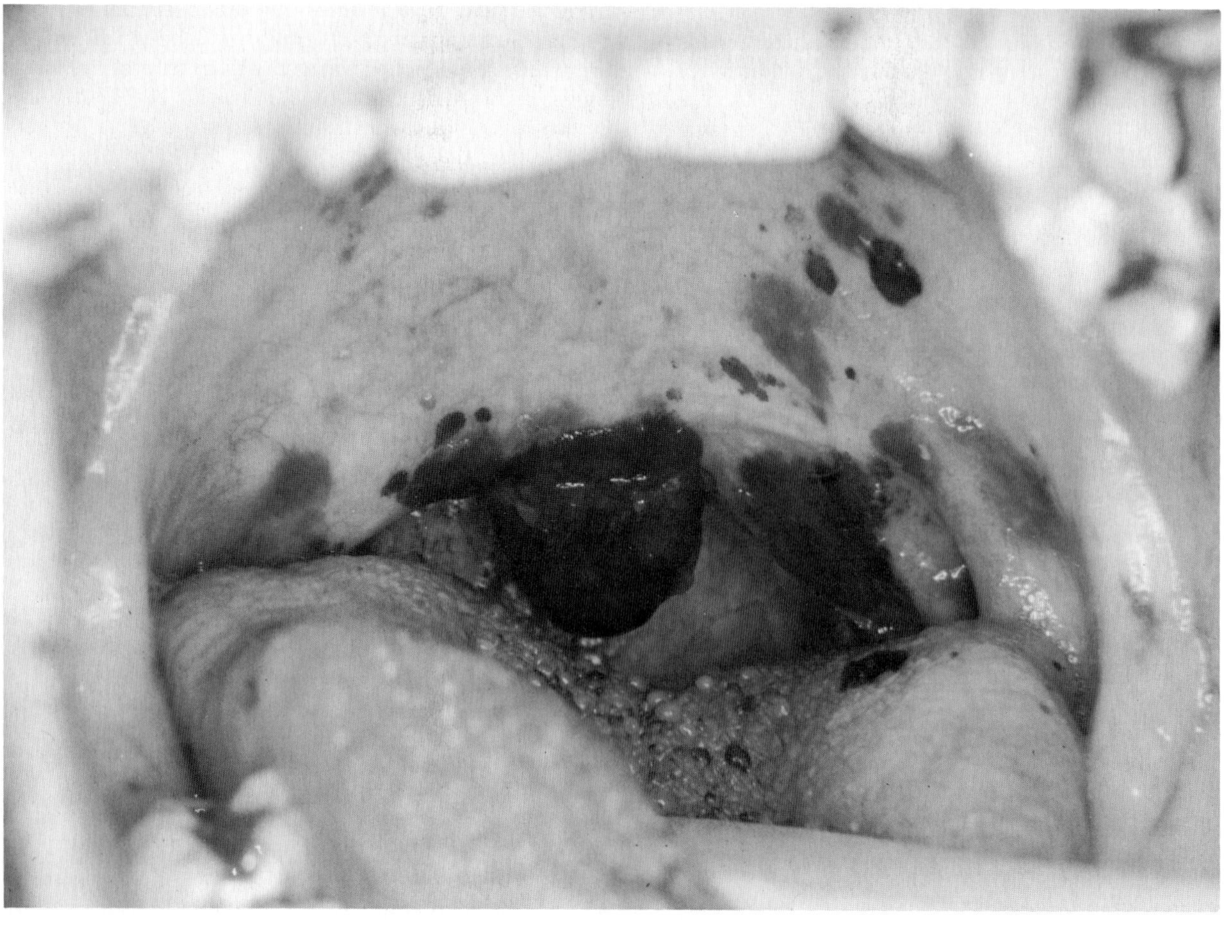

disease, they may rarely be the first manifestation of leukemia.

Perirectal abscess is relatively common in patients with acute monocytic or myelomonocytic leukemia who have not undergone bowel decontamination procedures. The only signs of the lesion may be a small mucosal tear and fever and the only symptom may be pain on defecation if the patient is severely granulocytopenic.[66] It is important to recognize these lesions, which are due to gram negative bacterial infection, because they may rapidly progress to septicemia if not treated. Typhlitis, or fulminant necrotizing colitis, occurs rarely in acute leukemia patients and may be related to granulocytopenia, cytotoxic therapy, or both. The majority of reported cases have been recognized only at autopsy. When recognized clinically, surgical intervention may be lifesaving.[67]

GENITOURINARY MANIFESTATIONS

Clinically important leukemic infiltration of the kidney is rare. However, the kidneys may be diffusely enlarged due to infiltration in a small fraction of patients. In such cases the renal cortex is usually more heavily infiltrated than the medulla, and both kidneys are involved.

Occasionally, a patient with acute leukemia presents with some evidence of renal failure or may even be anuric. Uric acid nephropathy accounts for the majority of such cases. This compromise of renal function usually occurs in patients with high white counts (>1000,000/d1) who have been untreated for a period of time. The high turnover of leukemic cells in such patients leads to more uric acid production than can be solubilized in the normally acid urine. Consequently, urate crystals precipitate in the renal tubules when the urine is acidified and mechanically impede the urine flow.

Urine flow may rarely be obstructed in a male patient by acute prostatism secondary to massive leukemic infiltration of the prostate.[68]

Patients with acute myelomonocytic or monocytic leukemia may have evidence of proximal renal tubular dysfunction secondary to the toxic effects of muramidase on the renal tubular epithelium. The major clinically important manifestation of this problem is potassium wasting, which may lead to severe hypokalemia.[44]

NERVOUS SYSTEM MANIFESTATIONS

Meningeal leukemia is much more common in ALL than in ANLL. In both diseases, it is less common in adults than children. Prophylactic meningeal leukemia treatment of children and adults with ALL has become a standard component of therapy. Patients who receive it subsequently experience an incidence of meningeal leukemia that is one-half or less that of ALL patients who did not have such prophylaxis. Prophylactic meningeal leukemia treatment has not been clearly shown to be of value in ANLL. Such prophylaxis in ALL not only reduces the incidence of meningeal leukemia but reduces the incidence of systemic relapse as well. Despite widespread acceptance of prophylactic meningeal leukemia treatment, however, approximately 20% of adults with ALL and 10% of those with ANLL will either present with or develop meningeal leukemia sometime during their course.[69] The incidence is higher in acute monocytic and myelomonocytic leukemia than in other variants of ANLL. Headache, due to increased intracranial pressure, is the most frequent complaint. Since the elevated pressure is evenly distributed within the cranium, a lumbar puncture may be safely performed. Examination of the CSF will reveal elevated pressure and protein with normal sugar. The routine cell count on the CSF may reveal increased numbers of cells. The cytocentrifuge (Fig. 36-8) or millipore filter techniques for examining the CSF will allow stained preparations of concentrated specimens to be examined.[70] This is important for accurate and early diagnosis.

Cranial nerve palsies may suddenly appear in an acute leukemia patient secondary to leukemic infiltration of the nerve sheath. Cranial nerves VI and VII are most often affected. The palsy may occur without other evidence of CNS leukemia and the CSF examination may be negative. The course of the affected nerve must be irradiated within 24 hours of onset of the palsy if as much function as possible is to be restored.

METABOLIC PATHOLOGY

A number of important derangements of metabolism can occur in the acute leukemia patient as a consequence of the disease, its treatment or both. Two important biochemical causes of renal functional impairment, urate nephropathy and muramidasuria, have already been discussed above.

Lactic acidosis has been rarely observed in patients with acute leukemia.[71] Often the morphology of the leukemic cells in such patients is unusual and cytoplasmic vacuolization has been a prominent feature of such cells. Most acute leukemia patients with lactic acidosis have had poorly controlled leukemia with only brief remissions. Many have had evidence of an unusually large body burden of tumor as estimated by the presence of very high white counts, massive organomegaly or other masses, and extremely hypercellular bone marrows. Some reported patients have, however, been leukopenic. The etiology of lactic acidosis in acute leukemia is unclear. The acidosis may be profound, and arterial lactate concentrations as high as 36 mEq/l have been recorded. The acidosis has

FIG. 36-8. A Wright's stained cytocentrifuge preparation of cerebrospinal fluid from an acute lymphocytic leukemia patient. The diagnosis of meningeal leukemia was easily made although the routine cell count on the fluid was only two cells/mm^3.

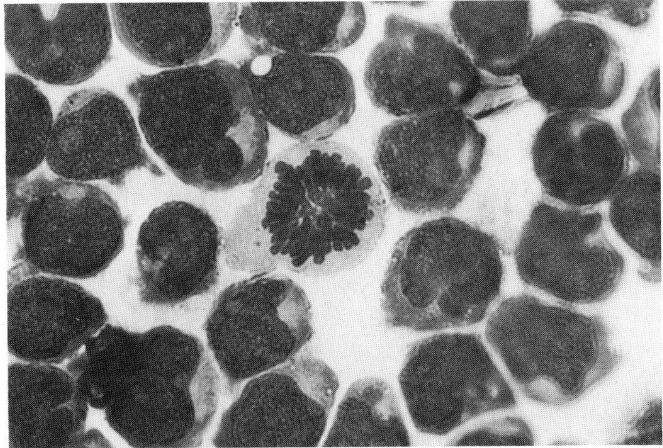

been at least partially corrected by bringing the leukemia under control in all cases in which chemotherapy resulted in a remission, and the degree of acidosis roughly paralleled disease activity in such cases.

Hypercalcemia secondary to ectopic parathyroid hormone production by leukemic cells has been observed on occasion in both ANLL and ALL.[72] The blood calcium level usually parallels disease activity in such cases. Hypocalcemia also occurs in patients with acute leukemia, and may be more common than hypercalcemia. Hypocalcemia is most common in patients with greatly elevated leukemic cell counts in the peripheral blood and some degree of renal failure. It is usually associated with hyperphosphatemia and hyperphosphaturia. The hypocalcemia in such patients is most likely secondary to the increased endogenous phosphorus load that results from the destruction of leukemic cells either as a result of ineffective leukopoiesis or chemotherapy or both. Often, septicemia is present in the hypocalcemic leukemia patient.[74]

Hypercalcemia may result from the rapid destruction of large numbers of leukemic cells just as hyperphosphatemia may. The sudden elevation of blood potassium levels has caused cardiac arrest in at least one patient.[75] On occasion, the hyperkalemia is spurious.[76] Potassium release from large numbers of leukemic cells during clotting *in vitro* results in the misinformation. It is important, therefore, to repeat serum electrolyte studies by examining anticoagulated blood immediately after venipuncture when elevated blood potassium levels are reported for a leukemia patient and hyperkalemic effects are not seen on the electrocardiogram.

PATHOLOGY OF THE IMMUNE SYSTEM

Impairment of cell-mediated immunity measured by reaction to a variety of intradermal tests of delayed hypersensitivity has been observed in 10% to 45% of acute leukemia patients in various studies. The significance of this finding is unclear. Some investigators believe that the immunoincompetence is a direct effect of the leukemia on the immune system, while others consider it a nonspecific manifestation of cachexia which may accompany advanced leukemia. In some, but not all, studies anergy prior to treatment had a poor prognosis, while intact cell mediated immunity—or conversion to it during therapy—had a very favorable prognosis.[77,78]

Abnormalities of the humoral immune system in acute leukemia patients were observed in some studies. In a large minority of patients decreased IgG and increased IgM and IgA levels were measured prior to therapy. These abnormalities usually normalized during the initial phase of chemotherapy, and their significance is unclear. Rarely, an abnormal paraprotein is present in the serum prior to therapy and disappears with successful treatment. Such paraproteins have been more frequently reported with acute monocytic or myelomonocytic leukemia than with other varieties of acute leukemia.[79]

At least two-thirds of ANLL patients have a relatively normal ability to develop a secondary antibody response as measured by the development of lymphocytotoxic or anti-red blood cell (ABO) antibodies or both after multiple ABO-incompatible platelet transfusions. The ability to develop such antibodies does not correlate with pretreatment blood immunoglobulin levels or skin test reactivity, nor with subsequent response to therapy or ultimate prognosis.[80]

Significant elevations of whole complement and C5, C8, and C9 were observed in acute leukemia patients in one study but the significance of these observations is unclear.[81] It is interesting that one mouse model of spontaneously arising acute leukemia, the AKR mouse, is deficient in C5.[82]

NATURAL HISTORY

PATHOGENESIS

Acute leukemia patients, in general, suffer from the lack of normal numbers of normal blood cells more so than from the presence of leukemic cells. Thus, infection and hemorrhage due to decreased number of circulating granulocytes and platelets, respectively, are the most serious threats to the well-being and life of a patient with acute leukemia. Decreased production of granulocytes, platelets, and red cells by the leukemic marrow has classically been attributed to a "crowding" phenomenon in which it is held that the normal marrow stem cell clone is physically crowded out by the unchecked proliferation of the leukemic clone. However, the mechanism by which proliferation and maturation of normal blood cell precursors is reduced may be more complicated than that simple mechanical explanation implies. Some recent evidence suggests that leukemic cells may produce certain chalones which inhibit proliferation and differentiation of normal marrow stem cells.[83]

When a patient with acute leukemia achieves a complete remission of his disease after therapy the bone marrow and peripheral blood cells become relatively normal in appearance and the proportions of the various cells within each compartment become normal. The explanation for this observation has been that the therapy successfully reduces the body burden of leukemic cells to a point that it cannot be observed by clinically employed techniques, and derivatives of the normal stem cell clone, now relatively unopposed, have repopulated marrow and blood. This explanation is consistent with the widely accepted theory that acute leukemia is a disease that begins with the development of a single malignant clone of cells. Some evidence against this theory has been collected over the past few years, however. Rare patients who achieve complete remission after chemotherapy for ANLL have been observed to have Auer rods in their otherwise morphologically normal mature polymorphonuclear leukocytes.[84] In addition, some patients have been noted to lose the normal granulation of their mature polymorphonuclear leukocytes as the first evidence of impending relapse with ANLL.[51] The granulation becomes normal if another remission is subsequently achieved. The buffy coats of some patients in complete remission after treatment for ANLL have been shown to contain significant reverse transcriptase activity even though the peripheral white blood cells appear to be morphologically normal.[85] These data suggest that in some patients with ANLL the morphologically normal leukocytes in marrow and blood may be derived from the abnormal leukemic cells. Thus, it is possible that, in some ANLL patients at least, there is no normal marrow stem cell and that remission results from differentiation and maturation of leukemic cells induced in some unknown manner by the treatment. In fact, some naturally occurring leukemic cell differentiation-inducing proteins have been described, such as protein MGI of Sachs.[86]

This section began with the statement that, in most patients, the presence of leukemic cells was less dangerous than the relative absence of normal cells. There are exceptions to this general statement. As stated above, patients with acute promyelocytic leukemia often experience a disseminated intravascular coagulopathy triggered by the release of procoagulant from leukemic cells, and significant renal tubular dysfunction may result from muraminadasuria in patients with acute myelomonocytic and monocytic leukemia. Acute leukemia patients with high peripheral blood blast counts, especially those with ALL, may present with urate nephropathy severe enough to cause anuria. Rare patients with acute leukemia may present with lactic acidosis or other metabolic abnormalities which sometimes can be attributed to ectopic production of a bioactive substance by leukemic cells, as discussed above.

There is one organ system, the central nervous system, in which the presence of leukemic cells can be life-threatening. ANLL patients with a very high peripheral blood blast count (>150,000 blasts/dl) have at least a 25% risk of fatal intracerebral hemorrhage within 24 hours to 48 hours if not treated.[87] The viscosity of blood with such a high concentration of large, sticky cells is increased and sludging tends to occur at the venous end of the capillary bed. Plugging of the low pressure side of the capillary network may be caused by these blast cells and the capillary may rupture. The resultant bleeding will go undetected if it occurs in a tissue such as muscle, but it may be fatal if it occurs in brain. Therefore the presentation of an ANLL patient with a greatly elevated blood blast count is a medical emergency requiring immediate treatment as discussed below. Patients with ALL who have extreme leukocytosis do not appear to have the same risk because the more rigid lymphoblast does not alter blood viscosity as greatly as the blasts in ANLL do. However, some increased risk of intracerebral hemorrhage may exist. Patients with chronic leukemia, except patients with blast crisis of chronic myelocytic leukemia, are not at risk for this complication.

Another manifestation of central nervous system leukemia is meningeal leukemia. Patients rarely present with this complication but can develop it months or years after treatment while in hematologic complete remission especially if prophylactic treatment for this complication was not part of the initial treatment program (see below).

The pathogenesis of meningeal leukemia has been explained by some as follows. At the time of presentation, the acute leukemia patient has a marrow cavity packed with leukemic cells, including areas of marrow that are usually inactive in the adult such as the marrow of the skull bones. Leukemic cells from skull marrow may rupture through the periosteum and infiltrate the dura. The cells may then migrate down the adventitia of vessels that traverse the potential space between the dura and pia-arachnoid and then infiltrate that membrane. Systemic chemotherapy usually will not cross the so-called blood–brain barrier. This is true because most cancer chemotherapeutic agents are lipid insoluble. Capillary endothelial cells of the brain, unlike other such cells elsewhere in the body, restrict passage of drugs bound to plasma protein and also limit diffusion of drugs in general and lipid insoluble drugs in particular. Entry of drugs into the brain from cerebrospinal fluid is limited by choroid plexus cells in a similar fashion. Therefore systemic chemotherapy might eradicate leukemic cells on the blood side of that barrier (dura) but not kill cells on the brain side (pia-arachnoid). Leukemic cells in the pia-arachnoid will divide and, with time, block the flow of cerebrospinal fluid between the dura and pia-arachnoid. Hydrocephalus will result and the patient will present with signs and symptoms of increased intracranial pressure.[88] Examination of the cerebrospinal fluid will reveal leukemic cells and establish the diagnosis.[89]

A simpler, alternative explanation for this phenomenon has been offered.[90] Leukemic meningitis occurs more frequently in ALL patients who present with high blast counts (>20,000/μl) and low platelet counts (<20,000/μl). It has been suggested that, in such a patient, petechial hemorrhage in the pia-arachnoid may deposit leukemic cells in that membrane and thereby set up a focus of leukemic cells in a relative pharmacologic sanctuary with respect to systemic antileukemic therapy. Whatever the true pathogenesis of this lesion, prophylactic treatment greatly reduces its clinical incidence and effective palliative therapy exists for most patients who develop it (see below).

PATTERNS OF SPREAD

Leukemia, at the time of diagnosis, is a widespread disseminated systemic disease. It is difficult to, therefore, discuss patterns of spread in the way that we do with more common tumors such as those of lung, colon, or breast. Certain useful, general statements can be made, however. Parenchymal organ dysfunction secondary to leukemic cell infiltration is not common in ALL or ANLL. When it does occur, it usually occurs late in the course of a patient who has had relapsed, poorly controlled disease for months. In addition, extramedullary relapses in both diseases are more common than extramedullary presentations. A notable exception to this statement is gingival infiltration in a patient with acute monocytic or myelomonocytic leukemia, which is commonly present at the time of diagnosis.

CLINICAL PRESENTATION

Acute Lymphocytic Leukemia (ALL)

Most adults with ALL are young adults in the third or fourth decade of life. The disease is less frequently observed in succeeding decades. The patient usually gives a history of lassitude for several weeks or more. Moderate signs and symptoms of anemia are present at the time of diagnosis, and some evidence of minor bleeding is elicited from the history or detected by physical examination in one-third of patients. The patient is usually not infected at the time of diagnosis. Perhaps 10% of patients are entirely well at the time a diagnosis is made by routine examination. The physical examination reveals generalized minimal or moderate lymphadenopathy, especially of the cervical region and minimal or moderate splenomegaly. The white blood cell count is normal or elevated in at least 85% of patients, while 15% of patients are leukopenic. Approximately 25% of adults with ALL present with a WBC >50,000/μl. The differential white blood cell count reveals at least some lymphoblasts in almost every patient and at least 50% of the white cells are lymphoblasts in approximately two-thirds of patients. The platelet count is reduced in most patients, but below 50,000/μl in only one-third of patients. Moderate decreases in hematocrit to 30% to 35% are noted initially in approximately three-quarters of patients. The bone marrow biopsy is hypercellular in virtually all patients and a smear of the marrow aspirate reveals decreased numbers of erythrocyte and granulocyte precursors, and megakaryocytes. The normal cells present generally have normal morphology. At least half of the marrow nucleated elements are lymphoblasts in three-quarters of patients.

Serum uric acid is elevated in almost all patients and the degree of elevation roughly parallels the degree of marrow infiltration with lymphoblasts. Serum and urinary muramidase are normal or reduced.

In an untreated patient the blood and marrow blast count will rise almost daily and the granulocyte and platelet count will fall roughly in parallel. The rise is usually gradual but at times can be alarming. Patients with ALL rarely have a spontaneous stabilization of disease. Therefore "preleukemia" and "smouldering leukemia" are terms that rarely, if ever, apply to ALL. It is important to initiate therapy as soon after diagnosis as possible in order to prevent infection and hemorrhage from complicating the management of the patient.

Acute Nonlymphocytic Leukemia (ANLL)

This disease is much more common in adulthood than ALL and can occur at any age. In most series the bulk of patients are 30 years to 60 years old. Patients with ANLL give a history similar to the ALL patient, but the history may be very brief with only a week or two of symptoms prior to diagnosis. Significant evidence of hemorrhage is more likely to be found in the patient with ANLL than the patient with ALL. Approximately one-third of ANLL patients have had a serious orificial bleed or have noted major petechial rashes that may be confluent in some areas. Patients with acute promyelocytic leukemia commonly present with moderately severe hemorrhage and large areas of cutaneous ecchymoses. Approximately one-third of ANLL patients present with a serious or even life-threatening infection such as a pyogenic abscess or septicemia. Rarely the patient will be entirely asymptomatic and will be diagnosed after a routine examination. The physical examination is entirely normal except for evidence of intracutaneous bleeding in three-quarters of patients. Lymphadenopathy is unusual and splenomegaly is found in less than one-quarter of patients. Gingival hypertrophy may be prominent in patients with a monocytic component of the disease and may be the problem for which the patient initially seeks help. The white blood cell count is low in one-third, normal in one-third, and elevated in one-third of patients at the time of diagnosis. The white blood cell count is less than 50,000/μl in approximately a quarter of newly diagnosed patients. It is much less common today for a patient to present with an extremely high white count (>300,000/μl) than it was only several years ago. This may be so because of earlier diagnosis now than previously for a variety of reasons. The differential white blood cell count reveals some blast forms in most patients, but in approximately 10% of patients no blasts are seen in the peripheral blood. The platelet count is almost always reduced sharply, and platelet counts of less than 20,000/μl are common. Almost all patients have a moderate reduction of hematocrit to at least 30% to 35%. The peripheral blood granulocyte count is reduced in virtually all patients and is below 1000/μl in at least half of patients when first diagnosed.

The bone marrow biopsy is hypercellular in the majority of patients but may be hypocellular in patients who have developed ANLL after another hematologic disorder such as aplastic anemia or paroxysmal nocturnal hemoglobinuria, or after treatment with radiotherapy, chemotherapy, or both for another malignant disease.[91] Leukemic cells comprise at least 50% of the marrow nucleated elements in most patients at the time of diagnosis. Striking changes may be evident in other marrow elements. There may be erythroid hyperplasia or bizarre granulation of more mature granulocytes.

The serum uric acid is elevated in approximately half of patients, but is usually only 1 mg% to 2 mg% above normal. Serum lactic dehydrogenase is elevated in many patients, but less so than in patients with ALL. Serum and urine muramidase may be greatly elevated in acute monocytic leukemia and moderately so in acute myelomonocytic leukemia.[44]

This disease is rapidly progressive in most patients if not treated. It is imperative to begin treatment before the blood granulocyte count falls below 1500/μl to 1000/μl if at all possible, because ANLL patients who have a serious infection have less than half the chance of obtaining a complete remission after treatment than has an uninfected patient.[92]

Approximately 10% of patients who eventually are diagnosed as ANLL present with a hematologic disorder that cannot be completely characterized. Such patients are often elderly and present with complaints referable to anemia or thrombocytopenia. Anemia, leukopenia, and thrombocytopenia may be present in any combination. An occasional blast may be seen on the blood smear, and there may be a monocytosis. The bone marrow may be normocellular, hypercellular, or hypocellular. An increased number of sideroblasts (often ringed) may be present, and a maturation arrest at the myelocyte level of white cell maturation may be observed together with an excess number of blasts (perhaps 9–15% of marrow nucleated elements).[93] The terms "refractory sideroblastic anemia with excess blasts," or "pre-leukemia" have been applied to these patients. Many patients presenting in this manner, with time (months to years), progress to unequivocal ANLL, especially acute myelomonocytic leukemia. One-third to one-half of patients with this syndrome will have an abnormal chromosome pattern with aneuploidy or a marker chromosome being noted. Progression to frank leukemia occurs in the majority of patients with abnormal cytogenetics but in only a small minority of patients with normal karyotypes.[94]

A variation of the preleukemic syndrome called "smoldering leukemia" includes patients with frank ANLL, usually acute myelomonocytic leukemia, whose disease may remain stable for weeks or many months without treatment.[95] The patient demonstrates stable peripheral granulocyte and platelet counts above dangerous levels (>1500 granulocytes/µl and >20,000 platelets/µl) and a marrow blast count of less than 30% to 50% of marrow nucleated elements. It is not clear why the disease does not progress, but it is important to realize that treatment may be withheld until progression is evident from serial blood and marrow examinations.

METHODS OF DIAGNOSIS

The work-up for patients with acute leukemia is demonstrated in Table 36-2. Acute leukemia may be diagnosed from a peripheral blood smear in the majority of cases. In a minority of patients with acute myelomonocytic leukemia only a few immature cells will appear on the blood smear and a marrow aspirate examination will be necessary to make the diagnosis.

TABLE 36-2. Work-up for Patient with Acute Leukemia

I. Complete history, including:
   a. Family history
   b. Work history
   c. Past medical history
   d. Radiation and chemical exposure history

II. Complete physical examination, with special atttention to:
   a. Temperature
   b. Lymph node-bearing areas and splenic area
   c. Optic fundi and cranial nerves
   d. Potential sites of infection
      1. Skin, including axillae
      2. Oropharynx, including gingivae
      3. Lungs
      4. Perianal area

III. Peripheral blood studies
   a. Hematocrit, white blood cell count, platelet count
   b. White cell differential count.

IV. Bone marrow examination
   a. Biopsy to determine cellularity
   b. Aspirate smears stained with Wright's, Sudan Black, and esterase stains; Periodic acid-Schiff reagent; Prussian blue iron stain; and immunofluorescent stain for terminal transferase.
   c. Aspirate for karyotyping

V. Blood chemistries and other studies
   a. Serum electrolytes, uric acid, BUN and muramidase
   b. Coagulation profile, including fibrinogen level, prothrombin time and partial thromboplastin time

VI. Cerebrospinal fluid
   Examine Wright's-stained spun sediment

VII. Radiographs
   Chest PA and lateral x-ray films

VIII. Transfusion work-up
   a. Determine blood type and HLA type if patient has circulating lymphocytes
   b. Do same for family members who are willing to serve as platelet or granulocyte donors for patient

SPECIAL WORK-UP OF PATIENT WITH ACUTE LYMPHOCYTIC LEUKEMIA

I. Peripheral blood
   a. Determination of B- and T-cell surface markers. If not possible, do acid phosphatase stain of blood smear
   b. Do tartrate-resistant acid phosphatase stain of blood smear to exclude hairy cell leukemia

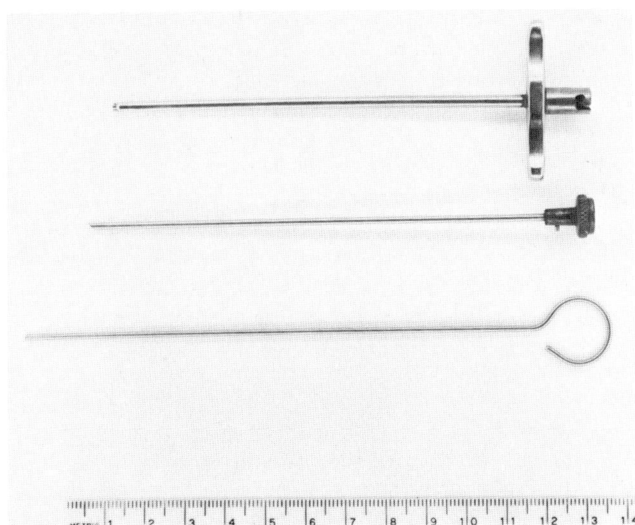

FIG. 36-9. The Jamshidi adult needle for posterior iliac crest marrow aspiration and biopsy. The patient is placed on his abdomen and the posterior superior iliac spine is located and marked with an indelible pen. The operator then dons sterile gloves, swabs the operative site with antiseptic, and covers surrounding areas with surgical drapes. Local anesthetic is then infiltrated into the operative site down to and including the periosteum. (A particularly anxious or frightened patient may require nitrous oxide inhalation instead.) The operator then makes a skin incision a few millimeters in length over the marked area with a scalpel. The operator then introduces the needle (top of figure) with the stylet locked in place (middle of figure) through the incision and with a gentle rotating motion advances the needle through soft tissue to the periosteal surface. The instrument should come in contact with the posterior iliac spine at such an angle that it is aimed at the ipsilateral anterior superior iliac spine. The instrument is then advanced with firmer pressure and a rotating counterclockwise–clockwise motion until entrance into the marrow cavity is perceived by sudden decreased resistance or "give." The stylet is then removed and a 10 cc syringe is attached to the hub of the needle. Negative pressure is briskly applied to the syringe and a few cc's of marrow are aspirated into the syringe. The syringe is quickly removed from the needle and the stylet is replaced. One small drop of marrow is quickly placed on each of five specially cleaned cover slips. Each cover slip is covered with a dry cover slip placed so that the corners of each pair form a six-pointed star. The weight of the dry cover slip, without other pressure, is allowed to spread the drop of marrow aspirate over the surface of both cover slips. The pair of cover slips are briskly pulled apart, making ten thin coverslip marrow aspirate preparations for staining. If a biopsy is also to be performed, the needle with stylet in place is withdrawn from the marrow cavity and repositioned through the same skin incision into a slightly different place in the marrow cavity. The stylet is then removed and the needle is advanced approximately 5 mm into the marrow cavity. A core of marrow will enter the needle. The needle is then pulled back a few millimeters and its tip is then advanced at a slightly different angle for a few millimeters. This maneuver ensures that the specimen is severed from the marrow. The needle is then briskly rotated several times along its long axis in one direction and then in the other. The needle is then removed. The probe (bottom of figure) is introduced into the distal end of the needle and the biopsy specimen is pushed out through the hub of the needle into a specimen bottle containing formalin and sent to the laboratory. A small gauze dressing is taped to the operative site unless the patient is thrombocytopenic, in which case a pressure dressing is applied. The patient is instructed to keep the area dry for 24 hours.

The marrow should always be examined in a newly diagnosed acute leukemia patient, since in many cases proper subclassification of the diagnosis will be facilitated and cellularity can be assessed.

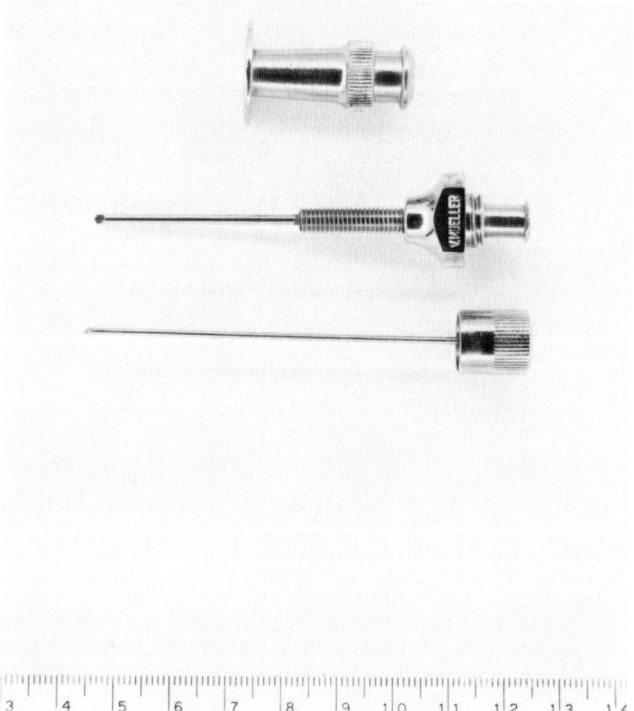

FIG. 36-10. The Illinois needle for sternal marrow aspiration. The patient is supine and the sternal angle is identified. The operative site is prepared and locally anesthetized as described in Fig. 36-9. The guard (top of figure) is screwed onto the needle and adjusted so that no more than 1 cm of the needle will enter the marrow cavity. The stylet (bottom of figure) is put into the needle and locked in place. A small incision is made with a scalpel in the skin just under the ridge of the sternal angle, midpoint from each side of the sternum. The marrow aspiration needle is introduced through the incision at a 45° angle just under the sternal angle in a cephalad direction. When the periosteum is reached, gentle pressure is applied as the needle is rotated clockwise–counterclockwise until a sudden "give" indicates that the marrow cavity has been entered. The stylet is then withdrawn, a syringe is attached to the needle, marrow is aspirated, and slides are prepared as described in Fig. 36-9. The needle is withdrawn with the stylet in place and the patient is dressed as described in Fig. 36-9. Sternal marrow aspiration should be attempted only when posterior iliac crest aspiration is not possible because damage to vital intrathoracic structure may occur if the posterior sternum is accidentally penetrated.

The most important subclassification of acute leukemia to be made is to distinguish between ALL and ANLL since the treatment is different. The distinction is made by proper interpretation of morphology and histochemical stains as discussed above. Determination of terminal transferase activity by biochemical or immunofluorescent techniques is extremely helpful since it is virtually impossible to make a diagnosis of ALL if terminal transferase is not present in the leukemic cells.

It is important to perform cell surface marker studies on the blast cells of a patient with ALL.[96] A small minority of ALL patients will have T-cell markers on the blast cells. These are usually male patients with mediastinal masses. Although the likelihood of such a patient achieving a complete response to therapy is equal to that of a patient with the much more common null cell ALL, patients with T-cell ALL have shorter remission durations and a much poorer overall survival than null-cell ALL patients. If cell surface marker determinations are not available an acid phosphatase stain of the patient's blasts should be performed since acid phosphatase positive lymphoblasts are usually T-lymphoblasts.[43]

Cell surface marker studies are not as helpful in ANLL as in ALL. However, some clinically useful information is slowly evolving from certain studies. Monocytoid cells in acute monocytic or myelomonocytic leukemia usually have Fc-receptors and membrane-bound IgG. Myeloblasts are characteristically Fc-receptor negative.[96] Thus cell surface marker studies in ANLL may facilitate subclassification.

The usual site chosen for marrow aspiration and biopsy is the posterior iliac crest. In a very obese patient it may be difficult to perform the procedure at this site. An alternative site for marrow *aspiration* is the sternum. Great care should be taken in performing a sternal marrow aspirate since retrosternal bleeding could cause serious problems and even be life-threatening. Of course, the sternal marrow is never biopsied (Figs. 36-9, 36-10).

A careful lumbar puncture with a small needle should be performed on a newly diagnosed acute leukemia patient since an occasional patient will have meningeal leukemia at the time of diagnosis. The CFS spun sediment should be smeared on a slide and stained with Wright's stain prior to examination. The platelet count should be 20,000/μl at the time of the procedure. The procedure should be performed, therefore, after platelet transfusion if the patient presents with a lower count.

ASSESSING PROGNOSIS PRIOR TO THERAPY

A number of characteristics of the acute leukemia patient at the time of diagnosis have prognostic import. Age is the most consistent such factor. Patients over the age of 70 years are less likely to survive the rigors of treatment and achieve a complete response. This is particularly true of patients with ANLL because the chemotherapy is more toxic than that usually given to patients with ALL. Thus, every possible means of supportive care must be given to the elderly patient if treatment is to be successful. It should be remembered that, once the elderly patient achieves complete remission, his subsequent survival and remission duration can be expected to be as long as younger patients.[97]

As discussed earlier in this chapter several poor prognostic factors for ALL patients have been identified. These include high white blood cell count, the presence of meningeal leukemia at diagnosis, infection at that time, the presence of the Philadelphia chromosome in lymphoblasts, and T-cell markers on lymphoblasts. None of these characteristics, except infection, impairs the patient's chance of obtaining a complete response to chemotherapy. They are all associated with a propensity for early relapse, however, and therefore overall survival can be expected to be reduced in patients with one or more of these characteristics.

The factors that have been identified as prognostically important in ANLL affect the likelihood of a complete response to chemotherapy, rather than remission duration. Perhaps the single most important negative prognostic factor in ANLL is prior treatment with radiation or chemotherapy. Patients with therapy-related "secondary leukemia" have a notoriously poor response to chemotherapy and less than 10% of such patients achieve complete remission.[98] It is not clear why the leukemic cell is so resistant to chemotherapy in these patients.

As discussed earlier, the presence of a serious infection at the time of diagnosis reduces by one-half the patient's chances of achieving complete remission. Although the leukemic cell is as sensitive to chemotherapy as in an uninfected patient, death from uncontrolled infection during chemotherapy is, unfortunately, common. However, if an infected patient achieves complete remission his subsequent prognosis is similar to other patients.[97]

The percent labeling index of bone marrow leukemic cells had prognostic importance with respect to probability of complete remission in one study of ANLL patients.[99] Young patients with high labeling indices had the highest complete response rate in that study. Interestingly, in the same study, marrow percent labeling index had no prognostic significance in ALL.

The presence of an abnormal karyotype in a patient with ANLL may impair response to chemotherapy. In one study none of 43 patients with an initially abnormal karyotype achieved a complete response with chemotherapy in contrast to 37 patients with a normal karyotype who had a complete response rate of 69%.[100] This important observation needs confirmation from other laboratories.

The prognostic values of colony forming and colony stimulating capacities of bone marrow cells from patients with ANLL have been studied.[101] The number of colonies and clusters in both *in vitro* soft agar marrow and blood cultures was significantly lower at presentation in patients who later entered remission than in those who did not. Thus, growth pattern of both bone marrow and circulating colony forming units may be of value in predicting response to chemotherapy.

A recent attempt to correlate therapeutic response to morphologic subclass of ANLL failed.[102] However, some data suggest a poorer prognosis for acute monocytic leukemia because of brief remission duration often due to extramedullary relapse.[103]

As the therapy for a given disease improves, the importance of previously recognized prognostic factors diminishes. There is some evidence that such may be the case for patients with ANLL.[104]

TREATMENT

It is very important to remember that some patients with ANLL do not require specific immediate treatment. A minority of patients, as discussed above, present with a "smouldering" disease that does not appear to be progressive. Such patients are usually elderly and are either entirely well clinically or have only signs and symptoms of anemia that can be corrected with blood transfusion. Although variable degrees of thrombocytopenia or granulocytopenia may be present, platelet and granulocyte counts are above danger levels. Bone marrow examination is diagnostic of ANLL but adequate granulocyte and platelet production is evident. This quiescent status may persist for only a few weeks or, occasionally, for months or years. Weekly blood counts should be performed in order to determine when the disease becomes progressive so that treatment may be instituted while the patient is still clinically well. Initiation of treatment is indicated when serial studies reveal (a) progressive thrombocytopenia with platelet counts falling to the 30,000/μl to 50,000/μl range, or (b) progressive granulocytopenia with the granulocyte count falling below 1500/μl, or (c) progressive marrow infiltration with leukemic cells to the point that they account for more than 50% of marrow hematopoietic cells.

An ALL patient should begin treatment as soon as the diagnosis is firmly established since that disease almost always steadily progresses. Moreover, there is compelling evidence that prognosis is directly related to the body burden of tumor in the patient with ALL.

Adult acute leukemia patients should almost always undergo treatment in a facility that has essentially unlimited supportive care capabilities, including access to sufficient quantities of platelets and granulocytes for transfusion, and, above all, a multidisciplinary team of physicians, nurses, and pharmacists thoroughly experienced in the management of such patients. Obvious exceptions to this recommendation include patients who refuse the intensive chemotherapy necessary for optimal results, and patients who refuse transfusion of blood products. In addition, patients over the age of 70 years are much less likely to respond favorably to treatment than are younger patients and are therefore often candidates for largely symptomatic care which can be delivered by any competent physician. All other patients should be strongly advised to accept treatment at the nearest facility specializing in the management of acute leukemia patients.

MANAGEMENT OF EMERGENCIES

Some readily treatable emergencies may exist at the time acute leukemia is diagnosed. Their recognition and proper management will preclude early death in many patients and allow them to survive long enough to receive an adequate trial of chemotherapy to which the majority of adult acute leukemia patients will respond.

HEMORRHAGE

Bleeding in a setting of thrombocytopenia and normal clotting factor studies is most likely the result of the thrombocytopenia. In such cases the platelet count is usually well below 20,000/μl. However, if the platelet count has been falling rapidly, serious hemorrhage may occur with higher platelet counts. Platelet concentrate transfusion will almost always stop the bleeding, although the platelets from 10 or more units of fresh whole blood may be required to do so (see Chapter 43, Supportive Care of the Cancer Patient). Such hemorrhage can almost always be prevented by the prophylactic transfusion of fewer platelets (3 units to 5 units) every 2 days to 3 days when the platelet count is below 20,000/μl.

Disseminated intravascular coagulation may result in life-threatening bleeding, as discussed above. The use of heparin is controversial in this coagulopathy *except* when it occurs in association with acute leukemia. It is clear that bleeding in acute leukemia patients that is secondary to disseminated intravascular coagulation can be prevented or stopped with low doses of heparin (50 units/kg) given intravenously every 6 hours.[105] Heparin should be administered prophylactically in that dose and schedule before bleeding starts in an acute leukemia patient with laboratory evidence of this syndrome. Such evidence includes a falling plasma fibrinogen concentration below 100 mg%, and elevated and rising titers of fibrin degradation products. If the blood fibrinogen concentration does not rise within 24 hours or the concentration of fibrin degradation products does not fall in that period of time, the dose of heparin should be doubled. If the platelet count is below 20,000/μ, as is often the case, platelet concentrate transfusions should also be given, but only after heparin therapy is well underway. Otherwise, the coagulopathy may be exacerbated. Heparin therapy may be successful in active bleeding secondary to disseminated intravascular coagulation, but prevention is more successful than treatment.

INFECTION

A febrile granulocytic leukemia patient must be considered to be infected until proven otherwise. Treatment with empiric broad-spectrum parenteral antibiotics should be instituted immediately after the patient is examined and cultured.[106] Intravenous carbenicillin, 5 grams every 4 hours and gentamicin 80 mg intravenously every 6 hours is a commonly used empiric antibiotic regimen for this situation. Appropriate antibiotic changes are made when pre-therapy culture results identify a specific organism. When those cultures yield no growth, the patient's clinical response to the therapy must serve as a guide to continue, discontinue, or change it. It is important to remember that resolution of fever may be the only clue that an infection was successfully treated by the empiric therapy. Since the infected patient is less likely to have a favorable outcome after antileukemia treatment than an uninfected patient, it is necessary to bring the infection under as much control as possible before beginning chemotherapy. It is essential to withold chemotherapy in an infected ANLL patient who has circulating granulocytes, since the marrow suppressive drugs used in the treatment of leukemia may reduce the circulating granulocyte count to zero and impair the patient's chances of surviving the infection (see Chapter 43, Supportive Care of the Cancer Patient).

INTRACEREBRAL LEUKOSTASIS

The likelihood of fatal intracerebral hemorrhage associated with a greatly elevated blood blast count in a patient with ANLL can virtually be eliminated by (a) immediately delivering cranial irradiation, 600 R in one dose, and (b) placing the patient on hydroxyurea, 3 grams per square meter of body surface area daily orally for 2 days.[107] The irradiation will destroy intracerebral foci of leukemic cells that already may be established, and the drug will cause a rapid fall in the blood blast count over 24 hours to 48 hours and prevent the reaccumulation of potentially lethal intracerebral lesions.

URATE NEPHROPATHY

Patients with acute leukemia, especially ALL, who have a high white blood cell count will occasionally present with anuria and uremia associated with a greatly elevated serum uric acid concentration. Urine alkalinization, reduction of uric acid production, and even renal dialysis may be necessary to reverse urate nephropathy. The xanthine oxidase inhibitor, allopurinol, should be given three or four times daily in a dose of 300 mg or 400 mg in such cases. Pyrazinamide, a potent inhibitor of tubular secretion of urate may be very helpful for patients with serum uric acid levels greater than 20 mg% if given at a dose of 1 gram every 8 hours for several days. Acetazolamide, 500 mg at bedtime, will keep the urine alkaline overnight and should be given to the patient until the serum uric acid is within the normal range. Dialysis should be strongly considered when the BUN is in the 100 mg% to 150 mg% range and rising. These potentially lifesaving emergency measures must be undertaken, when indicated, by the referring physician prior to transfer to another facility if they are to be successful.

ADDITIONAL PREPARATION FOR DEFINITIVE TREATMENT

Chemotherapy designed to induce complete remission of acute leukemia will have the greatest chance of success if the patient is brought into stable condition prior to its initiation. Hemorrhage and infection must be brought under control as discussed above before chemotherapy is begun if at all possible. Even if urate nephropathy were not present at the time of diagnosis, it might be precipitated by the rapid destruction of leukemic cells by chemotherapy. Therefore, allopurinol, 100 mg to 200 mg orally three times daily should be administered for at least 24 hours prior to beginning chemotherapy. The higher dose is usually only necessary for patients with ALL. If the patient has significant extramedullary leukemic infiltration, such as a mediastinal mass, the higher dose of allopurinol should be given for at least 48 hours prior to chemotherapy if at all possible. Allopurinol should be continued in all patients until chemotherapy results in leukopenia and marrow hypocellularity, at which time it may safely be discontinued.

All patients with ANLL and some with ALL are likely to undergo a prolonged period of severe granulocytopenia after chemotherapy and therefore infection prevention methods are of paramount importance. After several showers with topical disinfectants, the patient is placed in strict reverse isolation in a specially cleaned private room. Some physicians prefer to use a special laminar air flow room equipped with a high efficiency particulate air filter for reverse isolation of acute leukemia patients.[108] These rooms are expensive to build and to operate, but available data indicate that ANLL patients treated in them sustain fewer infections and fewer fatal infections during chemotherapy. Patients so treated experience one-third to one-half the incidence of bacterial pneumonias and virtually no fungal pneumonias compared to patients undergoing leukemia treatment without mechanical and chemical protection from organisms in their internal and external environments. This is especially true if the patient is also placed on a gut sterilization regimen consisting of several oral nonabsorbable antibiotics. A typical regimen consists of gentamicin liquid, 200 mg, vancomycin liquid, 500 mg, nystatin tablets, 4 million units, and nystatin liquid, 1 million units. All drugs are given every 4 hours around the clock beginning 24 hours prior to the first chemotherapy dose and continued through the chemotherapy treatment until the patient is no longer granulocytopenic. This regimen is highly successful in preventing such serious infections as esophageal candidiasis, and perirectal abscess and septicemia. The regimen is very expensive and most patients find it foul-tasting and nauseating. Therefore, many physicians choose to use trimethoprim and sulfamethoxazole tablets instead of gentamicin and vancomycin.[109] This new regimen given in a dose of 150 mg/m²/day to 170 mg/m²/day PO is quite inexpensive and palatable. Recent studies indicate that this regimen may be as efficacious as the older treatment, but this impression needs to be confirmed by larger trials before it can be generally accepted. Since infection during chemotherapy is less likely in patients with ALL than ANLL, the trimethoprim–sulfamethoxazole regimen will almost always suffice as infection prophylaxis for ALL patients. (See Chapter 44, Management of Infections of the Cancer Patient.)

SPECIFIC THERAPY FOR ALL

The treatment of ALL in children has characteristically been delivered in 4 phases: (1) initial or remission induction therapy, (2) consolidation therapy, (3) maintenance therapy, and (4) meningeal prophylactic therapy. These phases of treatment also comprise most programs for treatment of adult ALL. Therapy in the remission induction phase is designed to result in complete remission as soon as possible. Complete remission is defined as a post-treatment state in which it is impossible to make the diagnosis of leukemia. All signs and symptoms of the disease are absent once complete remission has been achieved, and all blood counts are normal. The bone marrow biopsy and aspirate are nondiagnostic and essentially normal also.

Remission induction therapy for adult ALL, usually begun in the hospital, may result in dramatic improvement in hematologic parameters and physical examination in days or 1 week to 2 weeks. Complete remission will usually not be achieved until 3 weeks or more of treatment have been given, however. Clinical improvement in many patients may be sufficient enough in several days to allow the treatment to be completed in the clinic.

The cornerstone of remission induction treatment for adult ALL is vincristine and prednisone. More than 60% of adults will achieve complete remission with these drugs alone.[110] The complete response rate can be increased to 80% or more by adding an anthracycline such as adriamycin or daunorubicin to that basic regimen.[110,111] Equally impressive results may be obtained by adding L-asparaginase instead of an anthracycline to the basic vincristine and prednisone treatment with less bone marrow and other potentially serious toxicity.[112] Thus, with multidrug combinations, the rate of complete response in adults with ALL currently approaches that of children with the disease.

Once complete remission is achieved, several additional courses of the initially successful drugs are usually given in an attempt to reduce the now clinically undetectable leukemic cell mass as much as possible (consolidation therapy). In some studies different drugs are used for this purpose. The drugs are delivered in doses designed to result in toxicity similar to induction therapy and the schedule of drug administration is such that the courses of treatment are delivered as quickly as hematologic recovery from the preceding course will allow.

Prophylactic meningeal leukemia therapy is usually delivered immediately before or after consolidation therapy. In one recent study patients who received meningeal prophylaxis subsequently had an 11% incidence of meningeal leukemia compared to a 32% incidence in the control group which did not receive it.[111] Thus meningeal leukemia prophylaxis, which has been eminently successful in children, has also been shown to be of significant value in adults with ALL. Cranial irradiation and intrathecal methotrexate are usually used for meningeal prophylaxis, but in some studies intrathecal methotrexate alone has been equally as effective.[111,113,114] Until confirmation of the simpler treatment is reported, however, combined modality prophylaxis is recommended.

The maintenance phase of treatment begins after the consolidation phase has been completed and the patient has fully recovered. It is usually carried out in the clinic with doses and schedules of drugs that are not associated with significant acute toxicity. Usually drugs not previously used in the patient's treatment comprise all or at least part of the maintenance regimen. It is not known whether maintenance therapy can be safely discontinued in an adult with ALL who has been in long-term continuous complete remission. At present it is highly recommended that maintenance therapy be continued for at least 3 years. A recommended treatment for adult ALL is given in Table 36-3.

TABLE 36-3. An Accepted Treatment for Adult ALL

A. Induction therapy
   1. Vincristine 2.0 mg I.V. weekly for 3 doses beginning on day 1.
   2. Prednisone 40 mg/M² P.O. daily for 3 weeks beginning on day 1 followed by dosage reductions to zero for an additional week
   3. Daunorubicin 45 mg/M² I.V. daily on each of the first 3 days of treatment
   4. L-asparaginase 500 I.U./kg/day daily for 10 days beginning on day 22

B. Prophylactic meningeal leukemia therapy
   (Start after complete remission is achieved and full hematologic recovery is evident)
   1. Cranial irradiation, 2400 R over 16 treatments
   2. Intrathecal methotrexate, 15 mg, is given weekly for 6 doses beginning on the first day of cranial irradiation

C. Maintenance therapy
   (Start 1 week after cranial irradiation is begun and continue to relapse or for at least 3 years of continuous complete remission)
   1. 6-mercaptopurine 200 mg/M² daily P.O. for 5 days every other week
   2. Methotrexate 7.5 mg/M² daily P.O. each day that 6-mercaptopurine is given. Omit an oral methotrexate dose if intrathecal methotrexate is to be given on the same day.
   3. After every third course of methotrexate and 6-mercaptopurine omit a course and substitute the following:
      a. Vincristine, 2 mg I.V., weekly for 2 doses beginning 1 week after the last doses of methotrexate and 6-mercaptopurine.
      b. Prednisone 40 mg/M² P.O. daily for 2 weeks beginning with first vincristine dose, then taper to zero over several days.

(Modified from Gottlieb AJ, Weinberg V: Efficacy of daunorubicin in induction therapy of adult acute lymphocytic leukemia (ALL): A controlled Phase III study (abs 496). (CALGB 7612) Blood (suppl) 54:188a, 1979. Maintenance doses must be modified according to tolerance.)

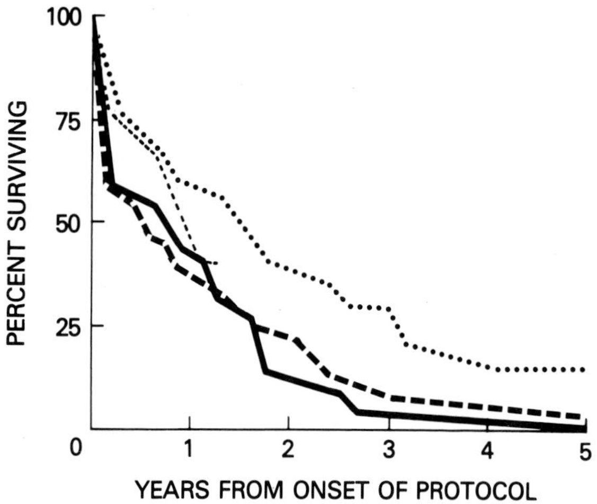

FIG. 36-11. Survival curves for all adult ALL patients treated on sequential Cancer and Leukemia Group protocols since 1967. The studies with the poorest median survivals and the least number of long-term survivors employed various doses and schedules of vincristine, prednisone, methotrexate and 6-mercaptopurine. The two studies with the better results employed vincristine, prednisone, L-asparaginase and, in most patients, daunorubicin. In addition, most patients in those two studies received meningeal leukemia prophylaxis. The shortest curve represents the latest study which, at the time the curve was drawn, had accrued only a small number of patients. The curves show that L-asparaginase and daunorubicin are important new drugs for the treatment of this disease. When they are used in conjunction with vincristine, prednisone, and meningeal leukemia prophylaxis, a significant additional fraction of adults survive 5 years after the diagnosis of ALL.

Although the rate of complete response in adult ALL now approaches that of childhood ALL in many studies, the long-term results are poorer in adults. Current therapeutic programs are associated with median remission durations of only 15 months to 21 months and median survivals of slightly more than 2 years.[111-114] However, in most recent studies, approximately one-third of patients appear to be long-term disease-free survivors judging from 4 years to 5 years of follow-up (Fig. 36-11).[111-114]

A multitude of therapeutic regimens are capable of inducing a second complete response in relapsed adults with ALL almost as frequently as first remissions are obtained.[115] Newer drugs such as AMSA may be useful in this regard, although this agent seems more useful in ANLL thus far (see below)[116] The duration of second remission is directly related to the duration of first remission.[115]

Several investigators have attempted to treat ALL patients with transplantation of normal marrow from a histocompatible donor. Thomas and colleagues treated 22 ALL patients in second or subsequent remission and 26 ALL patients in relapse with marrow obtained from an HLA identical sibling.[117] Transplantation during remission was generally more successful than transplantation during relapse. The projected post-transplanation survival curve for the patients transplanted during remission is flat at 50% survival from approximately 1 year to 3 years. More than half of the patients on that plateau have survived less than 2 years to date, however, and at least two of them have relapsed. Therefore, the final survival curve for these transplanted patients is likely to be inferior to the projected one. The same remarks apply to the remission duration curve for these patients, which is currently projected to plateau at 50% from approximately 9 to 24 months. Thus, although these data are very encouraging, bone marrow transplantation for adults with ALL must still be considered an experimental procedure.

Many agents with immunotherapeutic potential have been tested in ALL. Results to date have not shown useful activity of any of these treatments, however.

TREATMENT OF HAIRY CELL LEUKEMIA

The treatment of this disease has not been as well worked out as treatment for other leukemias. This may be because the entity is uncommon and has only recently been relatively precisely defined from a clinical point of view. Some recent data have contributed to the management of the disorder, however. Splenectomy is the most generally accepted initial treatment for hairy cell leukemia, and it often produces longlasting improvement of many months or even several years duration.[118] This procedure almost never results in complete remission. Instead, improvement in white cell and platelet counts, and reduction in the requirement for red cell transfusion usually occur. These changes are associated with an improved sense of well-being on the part of the patient.

Although irradiation has been said to be ineffective in this disorder, it is occasionally very useful as are low dose alkylating agents when the disease recurs after splenectomy.[119,120] Some early data also suggest that anthracycline drugs such as adriamycin and rubidazone may also be useful.[121,122] Although such intensive treatment is probably never justified as initial therapy, these new observations do pave the way for additional therapeutic research in this disorder.

SPECIFIC THERAPY FOR ANLL

The phases of treatment of ANLL are patterned after those of ALL, but many variations on the theme are commonly employed. This is testimony to the fact that, except for remission induction therapy, no one philosophy of management has emerged as clearly superior to another. Thus, controversy exists concerning the value of consolidation and maintenance therapy, and prophylactic meningeal leukemia treatment of patients with ANLL as discussed below.

Remission induction therapy for ANLL differs from that of ALL in several important ways. The treatment for ANLL is much more toxic primarily because of the toxicity associated with the most useful drugs, but also because of the more greatly impaired normal marrow reserve in the ANLL patient. Thus, while few ALL patients will be required to receive most of their induction therapy in the hospital, most ANLL patients will need to remain hospitalized for the majority of the treatment time. This is so because of the moderate to severe nausea and vomiting usually experienced during the first week of continuous intravenous drug administration, the great susceptibility to infection and bleeding that exists during the subsequent 2 weeks or 3 weeks of drug-induced marrow hypoplasia and resultant pancytopenia, and the frequent laboratory testing necessary to properly assess the results of therapy.

The most successful remission induction therapy for ANLL

consists of the anthracycline daunorubicin given in conjunction with cytosine arabinoside.[123,124] Daunorubicin treatment alone will result in a 40% to 50% complete response rate and cytosine arabinoside as a single agent is productive of a complete response in approximately a quarter of patients. Combination treatment with both drugs given simultaneously gives better results, with complete responses occurring in 65% or more of adult ANLL patients so treated irrespective of ANLL subgroup.[125] The drugs have been combined in a variety of ways with approximately equal success. A popular daunorubicin–cytosine arabinoside remission induction regimen for ANLL is outlined in Table 36-4. Some recent studies suggest that the addition of thioguanine to such a regimen augments the response rate, but major augmentation has not been observed in all such studies.[98,126,127] A three-drug treatment plan is outlined in Table 36-5.

The patient will experience profound marrow hypoplasia and pancytopenia after remission induction therapy. Some evidence of marrow recovery will usually be noted in 2 weeks to 3 weeks after the completion of therapy, and 80% of patients who will ultimately achieve a complete remission will do so within 1 month after finishing the first induction therapy course. The vast majority of the remainder of patients destined to completely respond to treatment will do so after the second course. When the marrow becomes repopulated after the first course of treatment, a decision about further induction therapy will have to be made. If the marrow shows evidence of normal megakaryocytic and myeloid regeneration, the marrow should be reassessed in several days. If, at that time, more evidence of normal marrow regeneration is obtained, and leukemic blast cells are difficult to find, the patient's blood counts should be followed until they have become normal. At that time the marrow should be re-examined to confirm complete remission or recurrent leukemia. If the first marrow examined after initial induction therapy appears predominantly leukemic, retreatment should be withheld until the need for it is confirmed by another marrow examination several days later. This is recommended because a regenerating *normal* marrow after anthracycline drug administration may look frankly leukemic due to the large number of megaloblastoid normal myeloblasts present that are destined to mature.

TABLE 36-4. An Accepted Treatment Plan for ANLL

A. Induction therapy
   1. Daunorubicin 45 mg/M² I.V. is given daily on each of the first 3 days of treatment.
   2. Cytosine arabinoside is given as a continuous I.V. infusion for 7 days beginning on the day of the first daunorubicin dose, at the rate of 100/mg/M²/day

B. Maintenance therapy
   (Start as soon as complete remission is achieved and full hematologic recovery is evident. Continue until relapse or for at least 3 years of continuous complete remission.)
   1. Cytosine arabinoside 100 mg/M² subcutaneously every 12 hrs for a total of 10 doses
   2. 6-thioguanine 100 mg/M² P.O. every 12 hrs for a total of 10 doses beginning on the same day that cytosine arabinoside is started.
   Begin subsequent cytosine arabinoside and 6-thioguanine courses 8 weeks after the first day of the last course.

(Modified from Yates JW, Glidewell O, Wiernik P et al: A CALGB study of adriamycin vs daunorubicin induction and a four vs eight week maintenance in acute myelocytic leukemia. (CALGB 7721) Proc Am Soc Clin Oncol (in press). Maintenance doses must be modified according to tolerance.)

TABLE 36-5. A More Intensive Treatment Plan for ANLL

A. Induction therapy
   1. Daunorubicin 45 mg/m² daily I.V.² for 3 days starting on day 1
   2. Cytosine arabinoside, 100 mg/m² is given I.V. every 12 hours for 5 days (total of 10 doses) starting on day 1.
   3. 6-Thioguanine is given orally in the same dose and schedule as cytosine arabinoside

B. Maintenance therapy
   (This phase of treatment consists of 4 different regimens given sequentially. Each regimen is given 4 times at monthly intervals. Maintenance therapy is discontinued after the fourth course of the fourth regimen, which usually occurs approximately 15 months after beginning treatment.)
   Regimen 1: Daunorubicin 30 mg/m² I.V. day 1 and cytosine arabinoside 200 mg/m²/day is given as a continuous I.V. infusion for 5 days beginning on day 1.
   Regimen 2: The same dose of daunorubicin is given I.V. day 1 and azacytidine, 150 mg/m²/day is given as a continuous infusion for 5 days beginning day 1.
   Regimen 3: Each of the following drugs is given as a daily I.V. bolus for 5 days: Methylprednisolone 800 mg/m², 6-mercaptopurine 500 mg/m², and methotrexate 7.5 mg/m², vincristine, 2 mg. total dose is given on day 1, I.V.
   Regimen 4: Cytosine arabinoside 200 mg/m²/day as a continuous I.V. infusion for 5 days.

(Modified from Wiernik PH, Schimpff SC, Schiffer CA et al: A randomized comparison of daunorubicin alone with a combination of daunorubicin, cytosine arabinoside, thioguanine, and pyrimethamine for the treatment of acute nonlymphocytic leukemia. Cancer Treat Rep 60:41, 1976 and from Weinstein HJ, Mayer RJ, Rosenthal DS et al: Treatment of acute myelogenous leukemia in children and adults. N Eng J Med 303:473, 1980)

Several clues may be taken from peripheral blood studies after induction treatment that may serve as early signals of response or the lack of it. The earliest clue of success is a gradual and steady daily rise in the platelet count which may begin 5 days or more before a rise in the granulocyte count. A transient rise in platelet count is usually a sign of incomplete response to induction therapy, a suspicion that must be confirmed by marrow examination.

Differences of opinion exist as to whether consolidation therapy should be administered to the ANLL patient who has just achieved a complete response, and conflicting data concerning the value of maintenance therapy have been reported. It seems reasonably clear that both consolidation *and* maintenance therapy are rarely necessary, so most treatment programs incorporate one or the other. When consolidation therapy is given, the same drugs used during induction are commonly used. Different drugs than those initially employed are usually recommended for maintenance therapy (see Tables 36-4 and 36-5). Many authors have suggested that a reasonably well-tolerated 5 day course of several active drugs given monthly prolongs complete remission duration, but other studies have cast doubt on this assumption.[128,129] At least one study has suggested that the intensity of remission induction therapy is a more powerful determinant of remission duration than is maintenance ther-

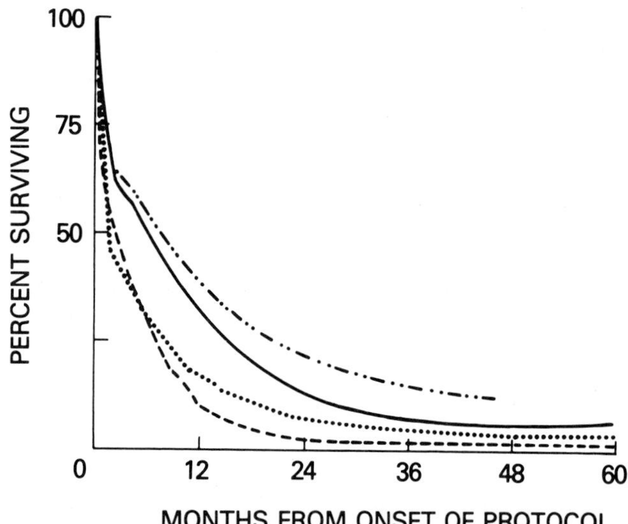

FIG. 36-12. Survival curve for all ANLL patients treated on sequential Cancer and Leukemia Group B protocols since 1967. --- Patients treated with daunorubicin alone in several different schedules. ... Patients treated with 1 hour infusions of cytosine arabinoside and oral 6-thioguanine at a high and a low dose level on an open-ended schedule. - Patients treated with 5 day courses of cytosine arabinoside given in conjunction with 6-thioguanine, CCNU, cyclophosphamide, or daunorubicin. -..- Patients treated with two or three daily doses of daunorubicin in conjunction with a continuous infusion of cytosine arabinoside of 5 or 7 days' duration. Improvement in median duration of survival of all treated patients is noted only after the use of daunorubicin-cytosine arabinoside combinations, in addition to when the proportion of long-term survivors directly correlates with the intensity of treatment.

apy.[130] On the other hand some studies employing intensive maintenance therapy have yielded very impressive remission duration results.[131,132] Some current studies conducted by large cooperative study groups are likely to resolve some of these questions in the near future.

The role of meningeal leukemia prophylaxis in ANLL is also controversial. Meningeal leukemia is more common in children than adults with ANLL. Therefore many pediatric oncologists routinely employ meningeal leukemia prophylaxis in childhood ANLL similar to that routinely used in ALL. No study has been performed to date that clearly shows the need for such therapy, however. Meningeal leukemia is so uncommon in adults with ANLL that prospective studies designed to show the value, if any, for meningeal prophylaxis are rare and usually provide inconclusive results.[133] On the other hand, meningeal leukemia incidence in ANLL appears to have decreased even further since the popularization of treatments employing continuous intravenous infusions of cytosine arabinoside. The reduced incidence may be related to the fact that the large parenteral infusions of the drug result in therapeutic drug levels in the cerebrospinal fluid.[134] Thus, current induction treatment may also be delivering effective meningeal leukemia prophylaxis.

It may be more important from a therapeutic standpoint to precisely subclassify ANLL in the future. Some recent data suggest that some drug specificity with respect to the various subgroups may be emerging. Acute progranulocytic leukemia appears to be highly sensitive to daunorubicin and acute monocytic leukemia appears to be the only ANLL variant sensitive to the experimental epipodophyllotoxin derivative known as VP16-213.[135,136] The dose of this new drug has not yet been completely worked out, but doses in the range of 60 mg/m^2/day to 100 mg/m^2/day for 5 days have yielded the best results to date.

While the results of current day treatment of ANLL leave much to be desired, results are infinitely better than only a few years ago. With treatments such as that outlined in Tables 36-4 and 36-5, approximately 65% of all treated patients and 70% or more of patients less than 50 years of age will achieve a complete response. The median remission duration for complete responders of all ages is approximately 1 year to 1½ years. More importantly, in many recent studies, approximately 25% of all complete responders appear to be long-term disease-free survivors who are well 4 to 5 years after initial treatment (Fig. 36-12).

The feasibility of treating ANLL with bone marrow transplantation has been studied by Thomas and colleagues.[137] The post-transplant median survival for 19 young patients already in complete remission after chemotherapy at the time of the transplantation (from an HLA-identical sibling) will be at least 18 months. The projected survival curve for all surviving patients in that study has a plateau at 60% survival ranging from 1 year to 3 years. Much more time will be needed to determine the true shape of this curve and the relative merits of treatment of ANLL with chemotherapy alone or chemotherapy followed by transplantation. It is clear already, however, that in some studies utilizing chemotherapy alone, results have been at least as encouraging as the most successful transplantation studies.[138-141]

Immunotherapy with a variety of agents derived from bacteria given with or without allogeneic irradiated leukemic cells has been extensively studied in ANLL patients. These studies were based on successful studies in mice with leukemia L1210 in which treatment with BCG and irradiated leukemic cells yielded some cures in animals with a minimum body burden of tumor cells.[142] The human experiments presume the existence of a human leukemia-specific antigen or antigens for which there is no conclusive proof to date.[143] Most human trials were conducted with patients in chemotherapy induced remission to mimic the state of disease in animals that has been most successfully treated with immunotherapy. Results of early human trials with BCG were initially encouraging but enthusiasm for this treatment has recently waned, since larger, controlled trials in this country and abroad have now shown no statistically significant effect on remission rate or duration, or survival for patients treated with various BCG preparations.[143] The same results have been obtained with other similar agents such as *Corynebacterium parvum*[144] In some small studies, however, modest improvement of post-relapse survival seems to have resulted from immunotherapy for unclear reasons.[143,145] In one study in which neuraminidase-treated allogeneic cells were used as immunotherapy, enhanced remission duration and survival resulted from treatment.[146] This approach must be confirmed by others before it can be generally recommended.

TREATMENT OF RELAPSED PATIENTS WITH ANLL

The treatment of relapsed ANLL patients is unrewarding, for the most part. In general, irrespective of treatment, complete responses are obtained in a small minority of patients, are more frequent in patients who previously obtained a complete remission, and are usually of brief duration.[147,148] Recently, AMSA has been shown to have significant activity in relapsed ANLL patients. In one study in which the drug was given in a dose of 75 mg/m² to 90 mg/m² daily for 7 days, nine of 30 patients responded with a complete remission.[149] Most of these patients were refractory to anthracyclines and cytosine arabinoside. AMSA, therefore, deserves further study in ANLL, especially in combination with other active drugs. This investigational drug is supplied by the National Cancer Institute for approved studies.

TREATMENT OF PRELEUKEMIA

Most patients with preleukemia need only careful observation and periodic blood transfusion. However, with time, blood transfusion requirements increase and platelet transfusions may also be necessary. Induction chemotherapy for ANLL will ultimately be required by most preleukemia patients but, in some, the requirement for intensive treatment may be put off for variable periods of time by the administration of corticosteroids alone.[150] This is especially true if cortisol enhances *in vitro* colony formation from the patient's bone marrow cells. Preleukemia patients whose *in vitro* marrow colony forming activity is not enhanced by cortisol are unlikely to respond to it clinically and should, therefore, go directly to more intensive therapy when therapy is required.

TREATMENT OF ACUTE LEUKEMIA DURING PREGNANCY

The delivery of normal children by mothers receiving antileukemic therapy has been amply documented although no long-term follow-up of children born of such mothers has been reported.[151,152] Treatment of women in the second or third trimester of pregnancy appears to be safe for the fetus. There is little information on treatment of women with earlier pregnancies, however.

MONITORING RESPONSE TO ACUTE LEUKEMIA TREATMENT

The bone marrow must be examined serially in order to properly assess the results of chemotherapy as discussed above. However, a wealth of laboratory evidence strongly suggests that a significant number of leukemic cells may still be present in the patient when the marrow examination gives normal results. Thus, the marrow examination is a relatively crude method of monitoring disease activity. For that reason, much effort has gone into the search for a tumor-specific biomarker of disease activity such as an antigen or an enzyme, the blood level of which might be a more sensitive indicator of residual disease. Recently, plasma levels of an 2-L-fucosyltransferase specified by the human blood group H gene has been shown to correlate with disease activity in acute leukemia patients.[153] Perhaps in the future, serial determinations of biomarkers in the blood will prove to be a more accurate and less painful means of following response to therapy than serial bone marrow aspiration.

Other methods of predicting relapse earlier are under investigation. Principal among these is a method utilizing premature chromosome condensation which allows for the determination of the relative number of bone marrow cells in early versus late G1 phase of the cell cycle.[154] Since normal cells appear to come to rest in early G1 and malignant cells seem to do so in late G1 of the cell cycle, determining the fraction of all G1-phase cells of a population that are in late G1 may reveal a repopulation of the marrow with leukemic cells before generally applied morphologic studies will do so. This potentially useful test is difficult to perform and has been done in only one laboratory on a small number of patients to date.[154]

TREATMENT CONSIDERATIONS FOR THE FUTURE

Present day treatment of adult acute leukemia is difficult to deliver properly, and quite toxic to the patient. There are reasons to believe that therapy will become more specific and less toxic in the near future as second-generation treatments such as chalones, other differentiation-inducing substances, and less toxic analogs of useful drugs such as aclacinomycin begin to emerge from the laboratory.[155–158] If these new experimental treatments prove useful in the clinic, major benefit to the patient may accrue.

REFERENCES

1. Rundles RW: Myeloproliferative disorders: General considerations. In Williams WJ, Buetler E, Erslev AJ, Rundles RW (eds): Hematology, pp 673–679. New York: McGraw-Hill, 1972
2. Farber S, Diamond LK, Mercer RD et al: Temporary remissions in acute leukemia in children produced by folic acid antagonist, 4-aminopteroyl-glutamic acid (Aminopterin). N Engl J Med 238:787, 1948
3. Rosner F, Lee SL: Down's syndrome and acute leukemia: Myeloblastic or lymphoblastic? Am J Med 53:203, 1972
4. Nowell PC, Hungerford DA: Chromosome studies in human leukemia. II. Chronic granulocytic leukemia. J Natl Cancer Inst 27:1013, 1961
5. Catovsky D: Ph¹-positive acute leukaemia and chronic granulocytic leukaemia: One or two diseases? Br J Haematol 42:493, 1979
6. Hilton HB, Lewis IC, Trowell HF: C-group trisomy in identical twins with acute leukemia. Blood 35:222, 1970
7. Walker LMS, Sandler RM: Acute myeloid leukemia with monosomy-7 follows acute lymphoblastic leukaemia. Br J Haematol 38:359, 1978
8. Kaufmann U, Loffler H, Foerster W et al: Fehlendes chromosom nr. 7 in der praleukamischen phase einer myeloblastenleukose bei einem kind. Blut 29:50, 1974
9. Croce CM, Girardi AJ, Kaprowski H: Assignment of the T-antigen gene of simian virus to human chromosome C-7. Proc Natl Acad Sci (USA) 70:3617, 1973
10. Gilman PA, Jackson DP, Guild HG: Congenital agranulocytosis: prolonged survival and terminal acute leukemia. Blood 36:576, 1970
11. Miller DR, Newstead GJ, Young LW: Perinatal leukemia with a possible variant of the Ellis-van Creveld syndrome. J Pediatri 74:300, 1969
12. Gupte SP, Perkash A, Mahajan CM et al: Acute myeloid leukemia in a girl with celiac disease. Am J Dig Dis 16:939, 1971
13. Sawitsky A, Bloom D, German J: Chromosomal breakage and acute leukemia in congenital talangiectasia erythema and stunted growth. Ann Intern Med 65:487, 1966
14. Bloom GE, Warner S, Gerald PS et al: Chromosomal abnormalities in constitutional aplastic anemia. N Engl J Med 274:8, 1966

15. Zuelzer WW, Cox DE: Genetic aspects of leukemia. Semin Hematol 6:228, 1969
16. Jackson LG: Chromosomes and cancer: Current aspects. Semin Oncol 5:3, 1978
17. Schade H, Schoeller L, Schultze KWD: D-Trisomie (Patau) mit kongenitaler myeloischer leukaemie. Med Welt 50:2690, 1966
18. Reich SC, Wiernik PH: Von Recklinghausen neurofibromatosis and acute leukemia. Am J Dis Child 130:888, 1976
19. Conard RA: Acute myelogenous leukemia following fallout radiation exposure. JAMA 232:1356, 1975
20. Karchmer RK, Caldwell GG, Chin TDY: Acute leukemia following localized irradiation for carcinoma of the larynx. Blood 43:721, 1974
21. Aksoy M, Erdem S: Follow-up study on the mortality and the development of leukemia in 44 pancytopenic patients with chronic exposure to benzene. Blood 52:285, 1978
22. Casciato DA, Scott JL: Acute leukemia following prolonged cytotoxic agent therapy. Medicine 58:32, 1979
23. Brauer MJ, Dameshek W: Hypoplastic anemia and myeloblastic leukemia following chloramphenicol therapy. N Engl J Med 277:1003, 1967
24. Jarrett WFH: Viruses and leukaemia. Br J Haematol 25:287, 1973
25. Rowe WP, Hartley JW, Landes MR et al: Noninfectious AKR mouse embryo cell lines in which each cell has the capacity to product infectious murine leukemia virus. Virology 46:866, 1971
26. Weiss RA, Fris RR, Katz E et al: Induction of avian tumor viruses in normal cells by physical and chemical carcinogens. Virology 46:920, 1971
27. Gallo RC, Miller N, Saxinger W et al: Primate RNA tumor virus-like DNA synthesized endogenously by RNA-dependent DNA polymerase in virus-like particles from fresh human acute leukemic blood cells. Proc Natl Acad Sci USA 70:3219, 1973
28. Baltimore D: Viral-dependent NDA polymerase in virions of RNA tumor viruses. Nature 226:1209, 1970
29. Baxt W, Yates JW, Wallace HJ Jr: Leukemia-specific DNA sequences in leukocytes of the leukemic members of identical twins. Proc Natl Acad Sci USA 70:2629, 1973
30. Schimpff SC, Brager DM, Schimpff CR et al: Leukemia and lymphoma patients linked by prior social contact. Evaluation using a case-control approach. Ann Intern Med 84:547, 1976
31. Brill AB, Tomonaga M, Heyssell RM: Leukemia in man following exposure to ionizing radiation: Summary of finds in Hiroshima and Nagasaki and comparison with other human experience. Ann Intern Med 56:590, 1962
32. Kaplan HS: The role of irradiation in experimental leukemogenesis. Natl Cancer Inst Monogr 14:207, 1964
33. March HC: Leukemia in radiologists, ten years later: With review of pertinent evidence for radiation leukemia. Am J Med Sci 242:137, 1961
34. Bizzozero OJ, Johnson KG, Ciocco A: Leukemia in Hiroshima and Nagasaki. N. Engl J Med 274:1095, 1966
35. Court-Brown WM, Doll R: Leukemia and aplastic anemia in patients irradiated for ankylosing spondylitis. Med Res Council Spec Rep Ser No. 295, London, Her Majesty's Stationery Office, 1957
36. O'Donnell JF, Brereton HD, Greco FA et al: Acute nonlymphocytic leukemia and acute myeloproliferative syndrome following radiation therapy for non-Hodgkin's lymphoma and chronic lymphocytic leukemia: Clinical studies. Cancer 44:1930, 1979
37. Coleman CN, Williams CJ, Flint A et al: Hematologic neoplasia in patients treated for Hodgkin's disease. N Engl J Med 297:1249, 1977
38. van Eys J, Flexner JM: Transient spontaneous remission in a case of untreated congenital leukemia. Am J Dis Child 118:507, 1979
39. Zussman WV, Khan A, Shayesteh P: Congenital leukemia. Cancer 20:1227, 1967
40. Wiernik PH: Spontaneous regression of hematologic cancers. Natl Cancer Inst Monogr 44:35, 1976
41. Bollum FJ: Terminal deoxynucleotidyl transferase as a hematopoietic cell marker. Blood 54:1203, 1979
42. Golomb HM, Rowley JD, Vardiman JW et al: "Microgranular" acute promyelocytic leukemia: A distinct clinical, ultrastructural, and cytogenetic entity. Blood 55:253, 1980
43. Bennett JM, Catovsky D, Daniel MT et al: Proposals for the classification of the acute leukaemias. Br J Haematol 33:451, 1976
44. Wiernik PH, Serpick AA: Clinical significance of serum and urinary muramidase activity in leukemia and other hematologic malignancies. Am J Med 46:330, 1979
45. Schiffer CA, Sanel FT, Stechmiller BK et al: Functional and morphologic characteristics of the leukemia cells of a patient with acute monocytic leukemia: Correlation with clinical features. Blood 46:17, 1975
46. Kass L: Esterase activity in erythroleukemia. Am J Clin Pathol 67:368, 1977
47. Foucar K, McKenna RW, Bloomfield CD et al: Therapyrelated leukemia. A panmyelosis. Cancer 43:1285, 1979
48. Hetzel P, Gee TS: A new observation in the clinical spectrums of erythroleukemia. A report of 46 cases. Am J Med 64:765, 1978
49. Davey FR, Dock NL, Terzian J et al: Immunological studies in hairy cell leukemia. Arch Pathol Lab Med 103:433, 1979
50. Saxon A, Stevens RH, Golde DW: T-lymphocyte variant of hairy-cell leukemia. Ann Itern Med 88:323, 1978
51. Brearley RL, Chapman RM, Brozovic B: Hairy-cell leukemia presenting as aplastic anemia. Ann Intern Med 91:228, 1979
52. Yam LT, Li CY, Lam KW: Tartrate-resistant acid phosphatase isoenzyme in the reticulum cells of leukemic reticuloendotheliosis. N Engl J Med 284:357, 1971
53. Variakojis D, Vardiman JW, Golomb HM: Cytochemistry of hairy cells. Cancer 45:72, 1980
54. van Muijen GNP, de Velde J, den Ottolander GJ et al: On the presence of reverse transcriptase in myelo- and lymphoproliferative disorders. Cancer 43:1682, 1979
55. Davis AT, Brunning RD, Quie PG: Polymorphonuclear leukocyte myeloperoxidase deficiency in a patient with myelomonocytic leukemia. N Engl J Med 285:789, 1971
56. Sultan C, Heilmann-Gouault M, Tulliez M: Relationship between blast cell morphology and occurrence of a syndrome of disseminated intravascular coagulation. Br J Haematol 24:155, 1973
57. Wiernik P, Serpick AA: Granulocytic sarcoma (chloroma). Blood 35:361, 1970
58. Nicolis GD, Helwig EB: Exfoliative dermatitis. Arch Dermatol 108:788, 1973
59. Klock JC, Oken RL: Febrile neutrophilic dermatosis in acute myelogenous leukemia. Cancer 37:922, 1976
60. Peterson DE, Overholser CD Jr: Dental management of leukemia patients. Oral Surg 47:40, 1979
61. Sickles EA, Young VM, Greene WH et al: Pneumonia in acute leukemia. Ann Intern Med 79:528, 1973
62. Wiernik PH, Sutherland JC, Stechmiller BK et al: Clinically significant cardiac infiltration in acute leukemia, lymphocytic lymphoma, and plasma cell myeloma. Med Pediatr Oncol 2:75, 1976
63. Sklansky BD, Jafek BW, Wiernik PH: Otolaryngologic manifestations of acute leukemia. Laryngoscope 84:210, 1974
64. Greene WH, Moody, M, Hartley R et al: Esophagoscopy as a source of Pseudomonas aeruginosa sepsis in patients with acute leukemia: The need for sterilization of endoscopes. Gastroenterol 67:912, 1974
65. Brugo EA, Marshall RB, Riberi AM et al: Preleukemic granulocytic sarcomas of the gastrointestinal tract. Am J Clin Pathol 68:616, 1977
66. Schimpff SC, Wiernik PH, Block JB: Rectal abscesses in cancer patients. Lancet 2:844, 1972
67. Varki AP, Armitage JO, Feagler JR: Typhlitis in acute leukemia. Successful treatment by early surgical intervention. Cancer 43:695, 1979
68. Rader ES: Leukemic infiltration of the prostate. Urology 3:779, 1974
69. Lister TA, Whitehouse JMA, Beard MEJ et al: Early central

nervous system involvement in adults with acute non-myelogenous leukaemia. Br J Cancer 35:479, 1977
70. Woodruff KH: Cerebrospinal fluid cytomorphology using cytocentrifugation. Am J Clin Pathol 60:621, 1973
71. Wainer RA, Wiernik PH, Thompson WL: Metabolic and therapeutic studies of a patient with acute leukemia and severe lactic acidosis of prolonged duration. Am J Med 55:255, 1973
72. Zidar BL, Shadduck RK, Winkelstein A et al: Acute myeloblastic leukemia and hypercalcemia. A case of probable ectopic parathyroid hormone production. N Engl J Med 295:692, 1976
73. Zussman J, Brown DJ, Nesbit ME: Hyperphosphatemia, hyperphosphaturia and hypocalcemia in acute lymphoblastic leukemia. N Engl J Med 289:1335, 1973
74. Alberts DS, Serpick AA, Thompson WL: Hypocalcemia complicating acute leukemia. Med Pediatric Oncol 1:289, 1975
75. Wilson D, Stewart A, Szwed J et al: Cardiac arrest due to hyperkalemia following therapy for acute lymphoblastic leukemia. Cancer 39:2290, 1977
76. Salomon J: Spurious hypoglycemia and hyperkalemia in myelomonocytic leukemia. Am J Med Sci 267:359, 1974
77. Hersh EM, Whitecar JP McCredie KB et al: Chemotherapy, immunocompetence, immunosuppression and prognosis in acute leukemia. N Engl J Med 285:1211, 1971
78. Greene WH, Schimpff SC, Wiernik PH: Cell-mediated immunity in acute nonlymphocytic leukemia: Relationship to host factors, therapy and prognosis. Blood 43:1, 1974
79. Van Camp B, Reynaerts Ph, Naets JP et al: Transient IgA_1—paraproteinemia during treatment of acute myelomonocytic leukemia. Blood 55:21, 1980
80. Schiffer CA, Lichtenfeld JL, Wiernik PH et al: Antibody response in patients with acute nonlymphocytic leukemia. Cancer 37:2177, 1976
81. Lichtenfeld JL Wiernik PH, Mardiney MR Jr et al: Abnormalities of complement and its components in patients with acute leukemia, Hodgkin's disease, and sarcoma. Cancer Res 36:3678, 1976
82. Hartveit F: The complement content of the serum of normal as opposed to tumour bearing mice. Br J Cancer 18:714, 1964
83. Boll ITM, Sterry K, Maurer HR: Evidence ofr a rat granulocyte chalone effect on the proliferation on normal human bone marrow and of myeloid leukemias. Acta Haematol 61:130, 1979
84. Davies AR: Auer bodies in mature neutrophils. J Am Med Assoc 202:895, 1968
85. Viola MV, Frazier M, Wiernik PH et al: Reverse transcriptase in leukocytes of leukemic patients in remission. N Engl J Med 294:75, 1976
86. Sachs L: The differentiation of myeloid leukaemia cells: New possibilities for therapy. Br J Haematol 40:509, 1978
87. Fritz RD, Forkner CD Jr, Freireich EJ: The association of fatal intracranial hemorrhage and "blastic crisis" in patients with acute leukemia. N Engl J Med 261:59, 1959
88. Law IP, Blom J: Adult central nervous system leukemia. South Med J 69:1054, 1976
89. Dawson DM, Rosenthal DS, Moloney WC: Neurological complications of acute leukemia in adults: changing note. Ann Intern Med 79:541, 1973
90. West RJ, Graham-Pole J, Hardisty RM et al: Factors in pathogenesis of central nervous system leukaemia. Br Med J 2:311, 1972
91. Jenkins DE Jr, Hartmann RC: Paroxysmal nocturnal hemoglobinuria terminating in acute myeloblastic leukemia. Blood 33:274, 1969
92. Kansal V, Omura GA, Soong S-J: Prognosis in adult acute myelogenous leukemia related to performance status and other factors. Cancer 38:329, 1976
93. Koeffler HP, Golde DW: Human preleukemia. Ann Intern Med 93:347, 1980
94. Heath CW Jr, Bennet JM, Whang-Peng J et al: Cytogenetic findings in erythroleukemia. Blood 32:453, 1979
95. Rheingold JJ: Acute leukemia. Its smouldering phase, or leukemia never starts on Thursday. J Am Med Assoc 230:985, 1974
96. Gordon DS, Hubbard M: Surface membrane characteristics and cytochemistry of the abnormal cells in adult acute leukemia. Blood 51:681, 1978
97. Wiernik PH, Glidewell OJ, Hogland HC et al: A comparative trial of daunorubicin, cytosine arabinoside and thioguanine, and a combination of the three agents for the treatment of acute myelocytic leukemia. Med Pediatr Oncol 6:261, 1979
98. Reiner RR, Hoover R, Fraumeni JF Jr et al: Acute leukemia after alkylating-agent therapy of ovarian cancer. N Engl J Med 297:17, 1977
99. Hart JS, George SL, Frei III E et al: Prognostic significance of pretreatment proliferative activity in adult acute leukemia. Cancer 39:1603, 1977
100. Golomb HM, Vardiman JW, Rowley JD et al: Correlation of clinical findings with quinacrine-banded chromosomes in 90 adults with acute nonlymphocytic leukemia. N Engl J Med 299:613, 1978
101. Beran M, Reizenstein P, Uden AM: Response to treatment in acute nonlymphatic leukaemia: Prognostic value of colony forming and colony stimulating capacities of bone marrow and blood cells compared to other parameters. Br J Haematol 44:39, 1980
102. Foon KA, Naiem F, Yale C et al: Acute myelogenous leukemia: morphologic classification and response to therapy. Leukemia Res 3:171, 1979
103. Tobelem G, Jacquillat C, Chastang C et al: Acute monoblastic leukemia. A clinical and biologic study of 74 cases. Blood 55:71, 1980
104. Brandman J, Bukowski RM, Greenstreet R et al: Prognostic factors affecting remission, remission duration, and survival in adult acute nonlymphocytic leukemia. Cancer 44:1062, 1979
105. Gralnick HK, Bagley J, Abrel E: Heparin treatment for the hemorrhagic diathesis of acute promyelocytic leukemia. Am J Med 52:167, 1972
106. Schimpff SC, Landesman S, Hahn DM et al: Ticarcillin in combination with cephalothin or gentamicin as empiric antibiotic therapy in granulocytopenic cancer patients. Antimicrob Agents Chemother 10:837, 1976
107. Grund FM, Armitage JO Burns CP: Hydroxyurea in the prevention of the effects of leukostasis in acute leukemia. Arch Intern Med 137:1246, 1977
108. Schimpff SC, Greene WH, Young VM et al: Infection prevention in acute nonlymphocytic leukemia. Ann Intern Med 82:351, 1975
109. Gurwith MJ, Brunton JL, Lank BA et al: A prospective controlled investigation of prophylactic trimethoprim/sulfamethoxazole in hospitalized granulocytopenic patients. Am J Med 66:248, 1979
110. Woodruff R: The management of adult acute lymphoblastic leukemia. Cancer Treat Rev 5:95, 1978
111. Omura GA, Moffitt S, Vogler WF et al: Combination chemotherapy of adult acute lymphoblastic leukemia with randomized central nervous system prophylaxis. Blood 55:199, 1980
112. Polli EE: A cooperative study on the therapy of acute lymphoblastic leukemia. Haematologica 64:119, 1979
113. Armitage JO, Burns CP: Remission maintenance of adult lymphoblastic leukemia. Med Pediatri Oncol 3:53, 1977
114. Willemze R, Hillen H, den Ottolander GJ et al: Acute lymfatische leukemie bij adolescenten envolwassenen: behandelings-resullaten bij 75 patienten in de periode 1970–1977. Ned T Geneesk 123:1782, 1979
115. Woodruff RK, Lister TA, Paxton AM et al: Combination chemotherapy for haematological relapse in adult acute lymphoblastic leukaemia (ALL). Am J Hematol 4:173, 1978
116. Tan C, Haghbin M, Rosen G et al: Acridinylamino anisidine in children with advanced cancer. Proc Am Assoc Cancer Res 20:154, 1979
117. Thomas ED, Sanders JE, Flournoy N et al: Marrow transplantation for patients with acute lymphoblastic leukemia in remission. Blood 54:468, 1979
118. Turner A, Kjeldaberg CR: Hairy cell leukemia: A review. Medicine 57:477, 1978
119. Ooyirilangkumaran T: Hairy cell leukaemia. Medicine 71:604, 1978
120. Golomb HM, Mintz U: Treatment of hairy cell leukemia (Leu-

kemic reticuloendotheliosis) II. Chlorambucil therapy in post-splenectomy patients with progressive disease. Blood 54:305, 1979

121. McCarthy D, Catovsky D: Response to doxorubicin in hairy cell leukaemia. Scand J Haematol 21:445, 1978
122. Stewart DJ, Benjamin RS, McCredie KB et al: The effectiveness of rubidazone in hairy cell leukemia (Leukemic reticuloendotheliosis). Blood 54:298, 1979
123. Wiernik PH, Serpick AA: A randomized trial of daunorubicin and a combination of prednisone, vincristine, 6-mercaptopurine, and methotrexate in adult acute nonlymphocytic leukemia. Cancer Res 32:2023, 1972
124. Ellison RR, Holland JF, Weil M et al: Arabinosyl cytosine: a useful agent in the treatment of acute leukemia in adults. Blood 32:507, 1978
125. Casaileth PA, Katz ME: Chemotherapy of adult acute nonlymphocytic leukemia with daunorubicin and cytosine arabinoside. Cancer Treat Rep 61:1441, 1977
126. Gale RP, Cline MJ: High remission–induction rate in acute myeloid leukaemia. Lancet 1:497, 1977
127. Rees JKH, Sandler RM, Challener J et al: Treatment of acute myeloid leukaemia with a triple cytotoxic regime: DAT. Br J Cancer 36:770, 1977
128. Embury SH, Elias L, Heller PH et al: Remission maintenance therapy in acute myelogenous leukemia. West J Med 126:267, 1977
129. Omura GA, Vogler WR, Lynn MJ: A controlled trial of chemotherapy vs BCG immunotherapy vs. no further therapy in remission maintenance of acute myelogenous leukemia (AML). Proc Am Assoc Cancer Res 18:272, 1977
130. Burke PJ, Karp JE, Braine HG et al: Timed sequential therapy of human leukemia based upon the response of leukemic cells to humoral growth factors. Cancer Res 37:2138, 1977
131. Bodey GP, Frerieich EJ, McCredie KB et al: Late intensification (LI) chemoimmunotherapy in adult acute leukemia. Proc Am Soc Clin Oncol 20:400, 1979
132. Weinstein HJ, Mayer RJ, Rosenthal DS et al: Treatment of acute myelogenous leukemia in children and adults. N Engl J Med 303:473, 1980
133. Wiernik PH, Schimpff SC, Schiffer CA et al: A randomized comparison of adunorubicin alone with a combination of daunorubicin, cytosine arabinoside, thioguanine, and pyrimethamine for the treatment of acute nonlymphocytic leukemia. Cancer Treat Rep 60:41, 1976
134. van Prooijen R, van der Kleijn E, Haanen C: Pharmacokinetics of cytosine arabinoside in acute myeloid leukemia. Clin Pharmacol Ther 21:744, 1977
135. Bernard J, Weil M, Boiron M et al: Acute promyelocytic leukemia: results of treatment by daunorubicin. Blood 41:489, 1973
136. Chard RL Jr, Hammond D: 4'-Demethyl-epipodophyllotoxin- -D-ethylidene glucoside (VP16-213). Phase II study for refractory acute leukemias of childhood. Proc Am Soc Clin Oncol 18:354, 1977
137. Thomas ED, Buckner CD, Clift RA et al: Marrow transplantation for acute nonlymphoblastic leukemia in first remission. N Engl J Med 301:597, 1979
138. Durie BGM: Marrow transplantation for acute nonlymphoblastic leukemia. N Engl J Med 302:408, 1980
139. Begg CG, Bennett JM, Cassileth PA: Marrow transplantation for acute nonlymphoblastic leukemia. N Engl J Med 302:408, 1980
140. Glucksberg H, Cheever M, Bowman W et al: Intensification therapy in adult acute non-lymphocytic leukemia (ANL). Proc Am Soc Clin Oncol 20:381, 1979
141. Peterson BA, Bloomfield CD: Prolonged disease-free survival in adult acute non-lymphocytic leukemia. Proc Am Soc Clin Oncol 20:441, 1979
142. Mathé G, Pouillart P, Lapeyraque F: Active immunotherapy of L1210 leukaemia applied after the graft of tumour cells. Br J Cancer 23:814, 1969
143. Whittaker JA: Immunotherapy in the treatment of acute leukaemia. Br J Haematol 45:187, 1980
144. Eppinger-Helft M, Pavlovsky S, Hidalgo G et al: Chemoimmunotherapy with *Corynebacterium parvum* in acute myelocytic leukemia. Cancer 45:280, 1980
145. Powles RL, Russell J, Lister TA et al: Immunotherapy for acute myelogenous leukemia: A controlled clinical study $2\frac{1}{2}$ years after entry of the last patient. Br. J Cancer 35:265, 1977
146. Holland JF, Bekesi JG, Cuttner J et al: Chemoimmunotherapy in acute myelocytic leukemia. Israel J Med Sci 13:694, 1977
147. Omura GA, Vogler WR, Bartolucci A et al: Treatment of refractory adult acute leukemia with 5-azacytidine plus 2-deoxythioguanosine. Cancer Treat Rep 63:209, 1979
148. Elias L, Shaw MT, Raab SO: Reinduction therapy for adult acute leukemia with adriamycin, vincristine, and prednisone. Cancer Treat Rep 63:1413, 1979
149. Tegha SS, Keating MJ, Zander AR et al: 4′-(9-acridinylamino) Methanesulfon-*m*-Ansidide (AMSA): A new drug effective in the treatment of adult acute leukemia. Ann Intern Med 93:17, 1980
150. Bagby CG Jr, Gabourel JD, Linman JW: Glucocorticoid therapy in the preleukemic syndrome (hemopoietic dysplasia). Ann Intern Med 92:55, 1980
151. Doney KC, Kraemer KG, Shepard TH: Combination chemotherapy for acute myelocytic leukemia during pregnancy. Cancer Treat Rep 63:369, 1979
152. Hamer JW, Beard MEJ, Duff GB: Pregnancy complicated by acute myeloid leukemia. N Z Med J 89:212, 1979
153. Khilanani P, Chou TH, Lomen PL et al: Variation of levels of plasma guanosine diphosphate 1-fucose: -d-galactosyl- -2-La1 fucosyltransferase in acute adult leukemia. Cancer Res 37:2557, 1977
154. Hittelman WN, Broussard LC, Dosik G et al: Predicting relapse of human leukemia by means of premature chromosome condensation. N Engl J Med 303:479, 1980
155. Rytomaa T, Vilpo JA, Levanto A et al: Effect of granulocytic chalone on acute myeloid leukaemia in man. Lancet 1:771, 1977
156. Huberman E: Induction of terminal differentiation in human myeloid leukemia cells by tumor-promoting agents. Proc Am Assoc Cancer Res 20:281, 1979
157. Brennan JK, DePersio JF, Abboud CN et al: The exceptional responsiveness of certain myeloid leukemia cells to colony-stimulating activity. Blood 54:1230, 1979
158. Suzuki H: Aclacinomycin A in acute leukemias and lymphomas. Lancet 2:310, 1979
159. Gottlieb AJ, Weinberg V: Efficacy of daunorubicin in induction therapy of adult acute lymphocytic leukemia (ALL): A controlled Phase III study (abstr 496) (CALGB 7612) Blood (suppl) 54:188a, 1979
160. Yates JW, Glidewell O, Wiernik P et al: A study of daunorubicin vs adriamycin induction and monthly vs bimonthly maintenance in acute myelotic leukemia from CALGB. Proc Am Soc Clin Oncol 22:487, 1981

CHAPTER 37

George P. Canellos

Chronic Leukemias

CHRONIC LYMPHOCYTIC LEUKEMIA

INTRODUCTION

Chronic lymphocytic leukemia (CLL) is a diagnosis that encompasses a variety of closely related chronic lymphoproliferative leukemic disorders characterized by the excessive accumulation of neoplastic lymphocytes. The grades of differentiation vary from small mature-appearing cells to larger cells of varying degrees of intermediate lymphoid maturation. These disorders are usually characterized by lymphadenopathy, peripheral lymphocytosis, bone marrow infiltration, and eventual interference with normal hematopoiesis. The extent of organ involvement, immunologic abnormalities, and subsequent prognosis are generally determined by the duration of disease prior to diagnosis.

The vast majority involve clonal proliferation of neoplastic lymphocytes of B-lymphocytic derivation, although a minority have been clearly defined as T-cell in origin. These disorders are usually easily distinguishable from acute lymphoblastic leukemia in adults. As they occur generally in adults above the age of 30 years (median age 60 years), it is sometimes difficult to consider them biologically different disorders from certain lymphocytic lymphomas of well differentiated lymphocytes or those lymphocytic lymphomas which may eventuate into a leukemic picture.

Generally, an absolute lymphocytosis of at least 15,000/dl with at least 40% lymphocytosis in the bone marrow is the minimal criteria required for diagnosis. The chronic lymphocytic leukemias include common B-cell CLL, rare T-cell CLL, lymphosarcoma cell leukemia, and prolymphocytic leukemia B- or T-cell type. Leukemic reticuloendotheliosis or hairy cell leukemia might also be considered in the above categories.

Clinical and Hematologic Characteristics

The diagnosis of CLL is based on a triad of peripheral lymphocytosis, lymphadenopathy, and splenomegaly. Most series have less than 20% of cases diagnosed with only lymphocytosis.[1,2]

Lymphadenopathy is usually generalized, with 75% of patients having splenomegaly. Depending upon the duration of undetected disease, normal hematopoiesis can be affected. About 35% of cases will be anemic with a hemoglobin less than 12.0 g%. Less than 25% of cases will be thrombocytopenic (less than 100,000/dl). Initial symptoms are usually related to lymph node enlargement or anemia. Patients with CLL have a median age of 60 years and are predominantly male (75% of cases).

Bone marrow aspiration or biopsy will often show a monotonous replacement by small lymphocytes with increased cellularity despite normal hemoglobin and platelets.

The lymph node biopsy will often have extensive effacement with mature-appearing lymphocytes but one-third will have varying degrees of immaturity that can be confused with poorly differentiated diffuse lymphocytic lymphoma (Rappaport).[3] The moderate degree of immaturity does not appear to influence the prognosis. A useful clinical staging system (Rai) based on extent of tissue involvement and compromise of bone marrow function has permitted a definition of patients with a poor prognosis (Tables 37-1, 37-2).[4] In the absence of anemia or thrombocytopenia, the median survival can exceed 70 months, although the expected median survival will be less than 2 years in patients with anemia, thrombocytopenia, lymphadenopathy, and splenomegaly.

The prognosis has also been predicted on the basis of the cytology of the peripheral cells. There is still controversy as

TABLE 37-1. Chronic Lymphocytic Leukemia

STAGING

Stage	*Absolute Lymphocytosis > 15,000/mm³*	*Enlarged nodes*	*Herpato- and/or Splenomegaly*	*Anemia <11 gm%*	*Thrombocyto-penia (11,000/dl)*
0	+	–	–	–	–
I	+	+	–	–	–
II	+	±	+	–	–
III	+	±	±	+	–
IV	+	±	±	±	+

SURVIVAL (MONTHS)

Stage	*Rai* NO. OF PATIENTS	*Rai* MEDIAN	*Boggs* NO. OF PATIENTS	*Boggs* MEDIAN	*Phillips* NO. OF PATIENTS	*Phillips* MEDIAN
0	22	>150	3	–	11	150
I	29	101	7	130	25	84
II	39	71	41	108	60	48
III	21	19	13	9	29	24
IV	14	19	20	42	32	24

TABLE 37-2. Intensive Chemotherapy: Chronic Phase of CGL

TRIAL	NUMBER OF PATIENTS	NUMBER CONVERTED TO 100% PH'NEG.	DURATION	REFERENCE NUMBER
1. MSKI (L-5) Splenectomy Ara-C, 6-thioguanine Asparaginase	37	7	1–43 months	(90)
2. SEG (Smalley et al) Ara-C, 6-thioguanine	12	2	1–5 months	(91)
3. (Sharp et al) Ara-C, 6-thioguanine Adriamycin, Vincristine	12	1	few weeks	(92)

to the significance of large lymphoid cells in the peripheral blood of CLL. It has been proposed that when there are benign appearing atypical lymphocytes present in excess of 35%, the prognosis is better.[5] This has not been confirmed by others.[6]

Prolymphocytic Leukemia

A rare variant of CLL called prolymphocytic leukemia has been defined in which the characteristic cell is a large lymphoid cell with large vesicular nucleoli and well-condensed chromatin with abundant cytoplasm. This is in contradistinction to the small lymphocyte of classic CLL with a dense chromatin and scant rim of cytoplasm. Prolymphocytic leukemia usually has massive splenomegaly, insignificant lymphadenopathy, and a uniformly poor prognosis.[7,8]

Lymphosarcoma Cell Leukemia

There rarely has been general agreement as to the application of this diagnostic term. The appearance of larger lymphoid cells with or without cleaved lymphocytes such as might be seen in touch preparations of lymphomatous nodes can occur in over one-half of the cases of CLL. Some have been inclined to refer to this as lymphosarcoma cell leukemia. If all of the other features are typical of CLL, the survival of these patients is said to be somewhat worse than classic CLL.[9] Others would reserve this term for patients with histologically defined lymphoma in the nodes and secondary leukemic manifestations. The usual setting is that of a diffuse poorly differentiated lymphocytic lymphoma (Rappaport) with bone marrow involvement which subsequently has abnormal cells in the peripheral blood in increasing quantities.[10] It can occur in nodular lymphomas as well. These variants may have a worse prognosis than classic CLL.

The Malignant Lymphocyte

The neoplastic cells of CLL are abundant and have been extensively studied. They have been shown to bear surface immunoglobulin of single light and heavy isotypes, usually IGM and, rarely, IgG.[11,12] The immunofluorescent staining is usually fainter than that seen in the B-cell lymphomas. The technique, however, of surface marker analysis allows for the distinction of early CLL from benign lymphocytosis.[13] Bone marrow derived B-lymphocytes have surface immunoglobulin as well as complement receptors. In CLL there is a loss of sensitivity for complement binding.[14] Plant lectins transform CLL lymphocytes poorly, and do not transform well in mixed lymphocyte cultures.[16] The normal T-cell lymphocyte in CLL is decreased proportionally but not in absolute terms.[17]

Immunologic Abnormalities

CLL frequently has abnormalities in B-cell function with hypogammaglobulinemia (50% of cases) or presence of monoclonal immunoglobulin, usually IgM, in small amounts in the serum (less than 10% of cases).[2] In addition, auto-immune hemolytic anemia (Coombs' test positive) and immune thrombocytopenia with platelet membrane bound IgG have been described.[2,18] These can occur at any time in the natural history of the disease. The impaired immunity, especially in antibody production, can be hazardous, not only because of the increased risk of fungal and pyogenic infection, but also viral infections. Dissemination of vaccinia following vaccination has been reported such that vaccination should be discouraged. Patients with CLL may also experience exaggerated hypersensitivity responses to insect bites.[19] Other autoimmune phenomena reported with CLL include pure red cell aplasia and bullous pemphigoid.[20,21]

Complications of CLL

The most common fatal complication is infection. The end stage of the disease can evolve to a refractory state of anemia, progressive splenomegaly, leukemic cell replacement of the bone marrow, and profound hypogammaglobulinemia, which usually terminates with a fatal septicemia.

Rarely, patients with CLL can develop tumors in lymph nodes or extranodal sites which, following biopsy, have all of the histologic characteristics of large cell lymphoma or diffuse histiocytic lymphoma. This has been called Richter's Syndrome and usually represents a refractory terminal condition, since by this time these patients have been exposed and become resistant to chemotherapy.[22] Patients will complain of fever, weight loss, increasing lymphadenopathy, and abdominal pain. These lymphomas are often in retroperitoneal nodes, but can occur in the gastrointestinal tract as well. The length of survival is usually a few months after the diagnosis.

A blastic leukemic transformation as a terminal event is extremely rare in the course of CLL occurring in two of 340 cases in one series.[23] Rarely, CLL can terminate with a progressive increase in immature-appearing cells which resemble prolymphocytes. Prolymphocytic transformation retains the surface marker characteristics of the original CLL.[24] The risk of developing other cancers is somewhat increased, including a higher incidence of melanoma, skin cancer, sarcoma, and lung cancer.[25]

T-Cell CLL

A distinct but rare variant of CLL has been noted to be of T-cell origin. Its incidence is increased in Japan, where B-cell CLL is rare. The cells lack surface immunoglobulin and form rosettes with sheep red blood cells, possess T-cell surface antigens and mark as mature T-lymphocytes.[26,27] Patients have hepatosplenomegaly without lymphadenopathy, neutropenia, and skin infiltration. The cells can have an abnormal karyotype with a pattern of 45 chromosomes.[28] T-cell CLL is quite refractory to treatment with agents effective in B-cell CLL and has a survival less than 1 year.

LEUKEMIC RETICULOENDOTHELIOSIS (HAIRY CELL LEUKEMIA)

Hairy cell leukemia, also referred to as leukemic reticuloendotheliosis, is an uncommon lymphoproliferative disorder characterized by massive splenomegaly, leukocytosis, and bone marrow replacement by an atypical cell with prominent cytoplasmic projections ("hairy cells"). There is an uncertainty as to the lineage of the malignant cell. There are characteristics of a B-lymphocytic, as well as monocytic features. The cells contain the tartrate resistant isoenzyme 5 of acid phosphatase. Like monocytes, they adhere to glass and plastic surfaces as well as ingesting latex or zymosan particles.[29,30] They do ingest sensitized erythrocytes. The lymphocytic characteristics include Fc receptors, synthesis of surface monoclonal immunoglobulin, and lectin (concanavalin A) induced cap formation.[31]

The clinical features of the disease that distinguish it from other chronic lymphoproliferative diseases include the morphology of the cells, absence of lymphadenopathy, and general refractoriness to chemotherapy. There is often dramatic benefit from splenectomy in the presence of hypersplenism, and this remains the only effective therapy for the majority of patients. Splenic irradiation and corticosteroids have been of little and only temporary benefit.[32]

Progressive bone marrow replacement with pancytopenia refractory to treatment can occur at any time over a period of years. Chemotherapy with other single agent alkylating agents or combination therapy can reduce elevated blood counts and extent of bone marrow involvement. However, complete hematologic remissions are distinctly rare.[33] Splenectomy in asymptomatic patients without evidence of hypersplenism does not prolong survival.

TREATMENT OF CLL

Because of the indolent nature of the disease in many patients, as well as their relatively advanced age, intensive therapy is rarely applied. It is clear that progression of CLL can lead to symptomatic lymph node enlargement, hepatosplenomegaly, involvement of extralymphatic tissue, hypermetabolism, and infection. The prognosis is worse and the urgency for therapy greater when bone marrow function is compromised.

Symptomatic, isolated lymph node tumors in CLL can be effectively treated by involved field radiation therapy. Relatively low doses of radiation will effect an excellent response lasting months to years. Splenic irradiation is rarely employed, since splenomegaly in the absence of other manifestations of disease is rare in CLL. Splenic irradiation, at a dose ranging from 300 rad to 450 rad, can result in reduction in size and relief of symptoms with improvement in blood counts in a minority of patients.[34]

Systemic therapy for CLL has centered on the use of

steroids and alkylating agents. The indications for therapy have not been well defined prior to the introduction of staging classifications which defined poor prognosis patients on the basis of anemia or thrombocytopenia (Table 37-1). The latter group of patients has a median survival of 19 months.[4] In addition to compromise of bone marrow function, systemic therapy will relieve constitutional symptoms due to expanded lymphocytic mass. The best evaluated systemic agent is *chlorambucil,* which given in any one of a number of schedules will control the symptoms and result in hematologic involvement in 40% to 50% of patients.

The daily oral dose is 0.1 mg/kg to 0.2 mg/kg, resulting in a dose of 6 mg to 12 mg (see chs. 9, 47). At this dose level, the elevated blood count will begin to fall within a week. The extent and rate of response is usually related to the dose. Reduction in lymph node size and splenomegaly will follow the drop in white count, usually in the second or third week of treatment. At this dose level, the white count will reach 15,000/dl to 20,000/dl after 4 weeks to 8 weeks, depending on the height of the initial count. The drug should be stopped at this point. An alternate schedule would employ continuous daily oral therapy at lower dose levels with a slower and less complete response. The daily oral treatment (0.1 mg/kg–0.2 mg/kg) has been compared to an intermittent single monthly dose of 0.4 mg/kg to 0.8 mg/kg without an advantage to either schedule.[35]

Yet another schedule gives chlorambucil 0.4 mg/kg as a single dose every 2 weeks with increases of 0.1 mg/kg to toxicity or response.[36] The overall response was 58% but did not result in superior results.

Corticosteroids are lymphocytolytic and have a major role in the systemic control of CLL, especially the autoimmune complications, which can be severe. Autoimmune hemolytic anemia requires high doses of steroids and rarely splenectomy to relieve the extreme hemolysis.[37] Corticosteroids (prednisone) in doses of 0.8 mg/kg/day given orally over 6 weeks with tapering doses will effect a hematologic remission in about 15% of patients. Most often they are combined with alkylating agents in patients with compromised blood counts.[38] Antitumor activity of chlorambucil combined with predinsone is better than the chlorambucil alone.[39,40] When the bone marrow is heavily infiltrated with CLL cells and neutropenia, thrombocytopenia (platelet counts <100,000/dl) and anemia can occur. It is often referred to as the packed marrow syndrome. More aggressive use of an alkylating agent, usually the platelet sparing drug cyclophosphamide, in combination with corticosteroids, in doses and schedules used to treat patients with lymphocytic lymphomas, can reverse progression of the disease. Generally, advanced stages of CLL refractory to alkylating agents and radiation are treated with steroids with little benefit and often with steroid toxicity, adding to the compromised defenses against infection.

The treatment of CLL is primarily palliative, with rare complete remissions and then only in patients with minimal disease. It is rare to improve the depressed levels of immunoglobulin.

Alternate radiotherapeutic techniques have been employed, including fractionated total body radiation (TBI) and thymic radiation.[41] TBI, given in weekly or semiweekly 10 rad doses to 150 rad, can improve many of the features of CLL, even to the point of a clinical complete remission with improvement to normal or depressed immunoglobulin.[42] Patients with early stage disease had the more striking responses. As a systemic treatment, TBI seems to be equivalent to systemic chemotherapy. Intensive leukopheresis has been studied in small numbers of patients with removal of 3×10^{10} to 18×10^{10} lymphocytes.[43,44] The lymphocyte counts and organomegaly can be reduced with a decrease of the median lymphocyte counts from 70,000/dl to 20,000/dl. The median doubling time of the peripheral blood counts was 71 days. Hemoglobin and platelet counts are less dramatically improved.

Extracorporeal irradiation was employed in the past with an analogous goal of lymphocyte destruction without systemic toxicity. The benefits were mainly limited to reduction of lymphocytosis.[45] The technique is now rarely used. There has been limited experience with combination chemotherapy. Regimens designed for lymphoma and myeloma have been tried with a high initial response rate but show no clear advantage over conventional therapy.[46]

The therapy for CLL should be gauged according to the stage and activity of the disease. In most instances, it provides excellent palliation. Many early stage cases of CLL clearly do not require treatment for extended periods of time.

CHRONIC GRANULOCYTIC LEUKEMIA

INTRODUCTION

Chronic granulocytic leukemia has been regarded as one of a group of myeloproliferative syndromes which include polycythemia vera, agnogenic myeloid metaplasia, essential thrombocytosis, and erythroleukemia. Recent investigation has cast some doubt on the exclusively myeloid character of the disease. It is basically considered a disorder of bone marrow stem cell proliferation. The initial phase is represented by excessive production of mature elements derived from the myeloid stem cell. The terminal phase of the disease is a progression to a less differentiated or blastic phase. The majority of cases have a characteristic cytogenetic abnormality, the Philadelphia (Ph^1) chromosome, which was the first characteristic marker chromosome in all of human malignant disease.[47]

At any time in the natural history of the disease, the characteristics of the other myeloproliferative disorders can occur. In the vast majority of cases, initial symptoms are related to the excessive production of mature myeloid cells and platelets. As opposed to the other chronic myeloproliferative disorders, almost all patients with CGL have a terminal phase which resembles acute leukemia or an otherwise definable acute myeloproliferative disorder.

No specific etiologic mechanism has been defined for the Ph^1 chromosome and the disease. Although exposure to ionizing radiation has been associated with a higher incidence of acute and chronic granulocytic leukemia, especially at Hiroshima and Nagasaki, in almost all patients with CGL an etiologic factor cannot be identified.

Clonal Origin of CGL

Ph[1] chromosome-bearing cells of a patient with CGL are the progeny of a single cell which acquired the defect. The evidence for this is derived from the fact that the Ph[1] chromosome has not been identified without a hematologic abnormality. Studies in CGL patients who have sex chromosome mosaicism show the skin, blood, and marrow to contain cells which are XY or XYY or XXY. The Ph[1] chromosome is associated with the XY only and, in the evolution to the blastic phase, aneuploidy is confined solely to the line bearing the Ph[1] chromosome.[48]

In vitro cultures of bone marrow cells from such patients showed a preferential growth of leukemic cells with the chromosomal abnormality in colonies confined to cells derived from these colonies. A more direct line of evidence involves the study of glucose-6 phosphate dehydrogenase isoenzymes in females with CGL who are heterozygous for this X-chromosome–linked enzyme. A single female cell can only have one X-chromosome dominant. Thus female heterozygote normal tissues have cells with A or B bands in approximately equal proportion. A variety of hematologic malignancies, including acute leukemia, agnogenic myeloid metaplasia, polycythemia vera, and CGL, have been studied.[49,50] In all instances the malignant cells show only a single enzyme type. This has also been shown in cells obtained directly or grown in *in vitro* colonies.[51] Thus, peripheral blood and bone marrow cells have a single enzyme type, while skin fibroblasts have both types of enzyme. If one of a pair of identical twins has Ph[1] positive CGL, the normal twin has normal cytogenetics.[52]

THE PHILADELPHIA CHROMOSOME. Approximately 90% of patients with the clinical and hematologic features of CGL will have the Philadelphia chromosome (Ph[1]) abnormality in their bone marrow and peripheral blood cells. This was first described by Nowell and Hungerford.[47] It consists of a shortening of the long arms of the number 22 (G group) chromosome, due to a translocation of chromosomal material to the long arms of the number 9(9:22).[53]

The classic pattern occurs in most cases. However, translocation from the number 22 to chromosomes other than the number 9 have been reported to occur with numbers 2, 6, 11, 13, 14, 15, 16, 17, 19, 21, and 22 chromosomes and these X chromosomes.[54] These usual translocations have been reported with classic CGL and in the setting of an acute myeloproliferative disorder.[55] The Ph[1] chromosome has been identified in the erythroid and megakaryocytic elements as well as myeloid cells.[56,57] It has not been seen in the normal-appearing lymphocytes transformed with phytohemagglutinin or otherwise purified from peripheral blood.[58] Skin and bone marrow-derived fibroblasts lack the Ph[1] abnormality, but it has been identified in macrophages derived from *in vitro* colonies growth from bone marrow cells placed in semi-solid medium.[59]

No specific biochemical abnormality or specific surface antigen has been related to the Ph[1] chromosome. The majority of patients will have 100% Ph[1] positive metaphases from bone marrow specimens; however, chromosome mosaicism has been described. It is felt that an improved prognosis occurs when normal karyotypes occur in the marrow of CGL patients at the time of diagnosis.[60] A similar mosaicism may occasionally follow treatment of the chronic phase with busulfan resulting in extremely long remissions, often with hypoplasia.[61]

Ph[1] CHROMOSOME AND THE COURSE OF CGL. The vast majority of cases will present with the well-recognized hematologic characteristics of CGL of granulocytic hyperplasia in the bone marrow, peripheral myeloid leukocytosis with or without splenomegaly, thrombocytosis, anemia, and basophilia, depending on the point in the natural history of the disease. The usual cytogenetic picture consists of 46XX or 46XY Ph[1] positive. The Ph[1] abnormality will remain throughout the course of the illness, although other aberrations may occur such as additional chromosomes or deletions (aneuploidy).[62,63] The single most common form of aneuploidy is reduplication of the Ph[1] chromosome. Progression of the disease through to its accelerated myeloproliferative or blastic phase will be associated with aneuploidy in about 50% of cases—usually hyperdiploidy involving extra chromosomes in numbers 8, 17, 19. Abnormalities of the number 17 as an isochromosome of the long arm represent one of the more frequent abnormalities together with trisomy of chromosome number 8.[64] Less than 10% of male cases with Ph[1] positive CGL appear to lose the Y chromosome (X0) in marrow cells during the chronic phase but this does not influence the prognosis.[65] The detection of new aneuploid cell lines usually connotes an imminent change in the course of the illness, regardless of the hematologic picture. Rarely, extramedullary myeloblastic tumors (granulocytic sarcoma), such as lymph node enlargement due to blast cell infiltration, without other features of the blastic phase will show aneuploidy in the cells of the tumors.[66] Serial cytogenetic studies during the course of the blastic phase can demonstrate progressive cytogenetic abnormalities showing clonal evolution of new cell lines usually with progressively increasing number of chromosomes.

The Ph[1] chromosome has been definitely identified in a variety of myeloproliferative disorders which at the time of diagnosis had the clinical and hematologic features of agnogenic myeloid metaplasia, erythroleukemia, eosinophilic leukemia, and chronic myelodysplastic syndrome (preleukemia).[67,68]

PHILADELPHIA CHROMOSOME NEGATIVE CGL. About 12% of adults with the hematologic characteristics of CGL lack the Ph[1] chromosome.[69,70] There is usually no other characteristic karyotypic abnormality. The median age is between 60 years and 65 years, which is considerably higher than the 40 years to 45 years of classic Ph[1] positive CGL. These patients characteristically do poorly with therapy and have a median survival in the range of 14 months to 19 months, whereas the median survival of Ph[1] positive patients is 36 months to 44 months.

CHRONIC PHASE

The Chronic Phase of CGL

The majority of patients with CGL will develop symptoms owing to the expansion of the granulocytic mass. The accompanying thrombocytosis in some instances can result in hemorrhagic manifestations. Approximately 10% of cases will have asymptomatic leukocytosis.

CLINICAL AND HEMATOLOGIC CHARACTERISTICS. Granulocytic leukocytosis is the fundamental abnormality, averaging 200,000/dl, with a wide range from 15,000/dl to 600,000/dl. The peripheral blood film will have the spectrum of myeloid maturation. The neutrophils are usually 50% with 22% myelocytes and usually less than 10% blasts and promyelocytes. The eosinophils and basophils are less than 5% at diagnosis.[71] Thrombocytosis above 450,000/dl occurs in about half of the cases and thrombocytopenia less than 100,000/dl is distinctly rare.[72] The bone marrow is hypercellular with granulocytic hyperplasia and, often, increased megakaryocytes. The bone marrow and spleen may occasionally contain lipid-laden histiocytes which resemble Gaucher cells and have been described as sea-blue histiocytes. Unlike the true hereditary Gaucher's disease, glucocerebrosidase in the leukocytes of CGL is elevated.[73]

The mature neutrophils of CGL prior to therapy appear to function normally as to rate of phagocytosis, oxygen consumption, and bacteriocidal capacity against yeast and *Escherichia coli*.[74] These and other subtle metabolic parameters tend to become abnormal during the course of the disease. The neutrophil alkaline phosphatase has been used to distinguish CGL from other myeloproliferative disorders, since the levels are low or undetectable in almost all cases of CGL in relapse, as opposed to elevated levels in myeloid metaplasia and polycythemia vera.[75,76] All studies show a decrease in enzyme content, which can increase in a remission of the chronic phase or during the blastic phase. CGL granulocytes transfused into a leukopenic recipient will show a rise of neutrophil alkaline phosphatase.[77]

The anemia is normocytic normochromic with an average hemoglobin level of 9 g% to 10 g%. Patients with early CGL will usually have a normal hemoglobin, leukocytosis less than 100,000/dl and absent splenomegaly. Splenomegaly is noted in most cases, however, but massive splenic enlargement is a late finding.

Similarly, slight hepatomegaly associated with an expanded granulocytic mass is a common finding. Lymphadenopathy is distinctly uncommon in the chronic phase and its *de novo* appearance should alert the physician to an extramedullary myeloblastoma and impending blastic transformation.

The platelets in CGL are abnormal but hemorrhagic problems are rare, except in extreme leukocytosis with an associated thrombocytosis. Morphologically, there are often giant forms, paucity of granulation, and scarcity of microtubules by electron microscopy. The platelets have a decreased content of ADP and serotonin (storage pool deficiency), but synthesize prostaglandin and thromboxanes normally in response to adrenaline and arachidonic acid.[78] A variety of functional defects have been described, but an abnormality in the second wave of aggregation with adrenaline is the most frequent. Rarely, there will occur periodic or cyclic oscillation of leukocyte and platelet counts with wide fluctuations over a period of 55 days to 70 days.[79]

Patients with myeloproliferative disorders have increased serum B_{12} content and unsaturated B_{12} binding capacity.[80] The levels are the highest in CGL and tend to be proportional to the granulocytic level.[81] They reflect an increased serum B_{12} binding protein, transobalamin I, which is derived from granulocytes and represents a circulating storage protein with no abnormalities in B_{12} delivery to tissues.[82]

The blood histamine can be elevated in circumstances of increased basophilia resulting in histamine excess symptoms such as pruritis, cold urticaria, and gastroduodenal ulceration.[83] These can be effectively treated with histamine H-2 receptor inhibition by cimetidine.[84]

TREATMENT OF THE CHRONIC PHASE. Patients rarely die in the chronic or stable phase because the granulocytic hyperplasia can be controlled without undue toxicity to the patient. Splenic irradiation was an early form of effective therapy that was shown to be inferior to cytotoxic chemotherapy with busulphan.[85] The latter is the most extensively studied cytotoxic agent in the chronic phase of CGL. Busulphan is given orally at doses of 0.1 mg/kg to 0.2 mg/kg or 4 mg to 10 mg per day continuously with weekly determination of blood count. Treatment is interrupted when the white count reaches 10,000/dl. In most cases there is no urgent need to lower the blood counts, so the more gradual approach reduces the risk of busulphan-induced aplasia. The latter occurs in about 10% of cases and reflects an inordinate sensitivity of the marrow stem cell to the drug. Busulphan induced aplasia can be severe and last from a few months to several years. Depending on the dose, the rate of decline of the white blood count proceeds over 2 weeks to 6 weeks. A "complete" remission can be achieved with disappearance of all stigmata of the disease, including return of serum B_{12} and leukocyte alkaline phosphatase to normal. A safe practice includes reducing the dose by one-half as the total white count is reduced by one-half.[86] A clinical and hematologic remission is achieved in most instances without a change in the percentage of Ph^1-positive metaphases. The remission can endure without further therapy from several months up to 2 years and, rarely, longer.[87] Other oral alkylating agents such as cyclophosphamide and L-phenylalanine mustard (L-PAM) have been used but are not superior to busulphan. Oral antimetabolic therapy with hydroxyurea in daily oral doses of 0.5 g to 2.0 g per day can control the white count, often with worsening of the anemia. Long term remissions without therapy have not been seen with hydroxyurea.[88] The long-term complications of busulphan are rare and include dryness of mucous membranes, pulmonary fibrosis, subtle lens changes, and alterations in exfoliative cytology.[89]

Previous experience with the chemotherapy in the chronic phase demonstrated that remissions could be readily achieved with a variety of antineoplastic agents. However, as mentioned above, in almost all instances, the Philadelphia chromosome remained in 100% of the metaphases, even in the presence of normal bone marrow and peripheral counts. Thus, true remissions with reconstitution of a normal stem cell had not been achieved. In rare instances, severe aplasia of the bone marrow following busulphan therapy was associated with the disappearance of the Philadelphia chromosome and return of cells of normal karyotype.[61]

In order to explore the possibility that the Philadelphia chromosome stem cell may be relatively more vulnerable to cytotoxic agents, three trials have explored the application of acute leukemia-type chemotherapy in the chronic phase of CGL in order to reduce or eradicate the Philadelphia chromosome (Table 37-2, p. 1428). Chemotherapy included cytosine arabinoside, 6-thioguanine, vincristine and prednisone, and in addition, in one trial, anthracycline antibiotic.[90–92] The Memorial–Sloan Kettering Group preceded the intensive chemotherapy with splenic irradiation and splenectomy followed by a maintenance chemotherapy program.[90] Karyotypic conversion was rare (10 of 61 cases) and of short duration. The Philadelphia chromosome-bearing stem line could not be eradicated by the cell cycle active chemotherapy that characterizes the treatment of acute leukemia.

It is noteworthy that the intensive regimen used to prepare patients for bone marrow transplantation including total body irradiation, intravenous cyclophosphamide, and dimethylmyleran was successful in eradicating the Ph^1 chromosome in the majority of cases of identical twin transplants (*vide infra*). It is unknown whether total ablation of the bone marrow stem cell or whether a more intensive regimen without a transplant might exert a selective effect on the Philadelphia-positive stem cell. Even conversion of the marrow to 100% normal metaphases may fail to detect residual Ph^1-positive stem cells. Techniques for the *in vitro* eradication of residual Ph^1-positive cells may be required in marrow cells that can be used for autologous transplantation.

SPLENECTOMY. Splenectomy during the chronic phase as an elective procedure will not change the incidence of blastic transformation and thus, the overall survival.[93] The procedure should be reserved for those instances of hypersplenism during the chronic phase or when experimental bone marrow transplantation might be considered.[94] In rare instances, the removal of a symptomatic enlarged spleen can palliate a patient in the blastic phase. The period of benefit is brief, and this procedure is not without risk in that phase. Intensive leukopheresis has been attempted in the chronic phase but rarely results in long term benefit, and often makes the anemia worse despite lowering of the white count.[95]

DURATION OF CHRONIC PHASE. The chronic or stable phase can be measured from a few months to years. The median survival from diagnosis varies from 36 months to 44 months. The majority of time is spent in the chronic phase since the median duration of the blastic phase is only 2 months to 3 months.[96]

There is a gradual tendency to refractoriness to stable phase therapy and shortening of the doubling time of the leukocyte count as the chronic phase of the disease progresses. Failure of previously effective therapy to control the disease usually heralds the terminal phase.

THE TERMINAL PHASE OF CGL

The terminal phase of CGL can occur at any time in the natural history of the disease. It can vary in duration from weeks to many months depending on the mode of presentation. The clinical and hematologic presentation of the terminal phase can present either as an (1) accelerated phase or (2) blastic phase.

The Accelerated Myeloproliferative Phase

The majority of patients (75%) will evolve a hematologic state which can be indistinguishable from the accelerated phase of any chronic myeloproliferative disorder.[97] This "myeloproliferative acceleration" can appear gradually over several months and usually includes progressive leukocytosis with an increase in intermediate myeloid precursors, including blast cells. The elevated blood count and splenomegaly become more refractory to control by busulphan or previously effective therapy. Thrombocytosis with large, bizarre platelets may occur, but more often the platelet count will tend to fall as increasing doses of chemotherapy are given.

Myelofibrosis, especially reticulin fibrosis, will occur in this setting in approximately one-third of cases.[98] "Basophilic leukemia," or increased basophils, is another characteristic of the myeloproliferative acceleration. The morphology of the peripheral red cells can be abnormal, especially in splenectomized patients, with marked anisopoikilocytosis, leukoerythroblastosis, and basophilic stippling of erythroid cells. Symptoms of this phase include weight loss, weakness due to progressive anemia, and pain due to splenomegaly.[99]

The proliferative component can be treated with hydroxyurea in doses of 0.5 g to 4.0 g by mouth per day.[88] It is advisable to discontinue busulphan and refrain from conventional splenic irradiation, since the latter will usually exacerbate thrombocytopenia with only minimal regression of an enlarged spleen. The myeloproliferative acceleration can be controlled for about 4 months to 6 months, but in patients with elevated platelet counts control may be even longer. The course of the accelerated phase may deteriorate with rapidly increasing blast cell count, bleeding, sepsis, and extramedullary blast cell tumors.

The Blastic Phase

Blastic transformation or metamorphosis has been synonymous with the terminal phase. Rarely is there a blastic "crisis." The blastic phase usually has 30% to 40% of marrow cells as blasts or promyelocytes, although anemia and thrombocytopenia are usually required to support the diagnosis.[99] The "crisis" occurs when the blast cell count rises rapidly, exceeding 100,000/dl. In that circumstance leukostatic lesions can develop in the microvasculature of the central nervous system, or even in the lungs.[100] Therapy is urgent and should include high doses of hydroxyurea 75 mg/kg by mouth daily or intravenous cyclophosphamide 20 mg/kg to 30 mg/kg as a single dose. Any regimen which rapidly lowers the blast cell count would suffice. The blastic phase can evolve so rapidly that significant anemia and splenomegaly may not be present. The majority of patients have a myeloblastic transformation, but 20% to 30% will have the morphologic features of lymphoblasts.[101] Rarely, an erythroblastic or even megakaryoblastic component will predominate. The majority eventuate to a state where the blast cells can be described as myeloblastic or undifferentiated.

Extramedullary Blastic Tumors

Extramedullary blastic tumors (myeloblastomas, granulocytic sarcoma) are usually a late manifestation but can, rarely,

TABLE 37-3. Chemotherapy of Blastic Transformation of Chronic Granulocytic Leukemia

REGIMEN	NUMBER OF PATIENTS	COMPLETE REMISSIONS	PARTIAL REMISSIONS	REFERENCE NUMBER
Vincristine and prednisone	38	18	18	103, 124
Vincristine and prednisone	24	9	–	118
Vincristine and prednisone	4	1	–	119
Prednisone, vincristine, methotrexate and 6-MP[b] (POMP)	13	1	2	120
Cytosine arabinoside and BCNU[a]	47	3	5	121
Cytosine arabinoside, BCNU, vincristine and prednisone	39	1	4	121
Multiple regimens (M.D. Anderson Hospital)	39	4	6	122
Trampco (L) (Hammersmith, London)	9	4	1	123
Cytosine arabinoside and 6-thioguanine	13	1	3	124
Hydroxyurea, 6-MP and dexamethasone, vincristine	60	8	7	125
Hydroxyurea, 6-MP, dexamethasone, vincristine	64	7	16	125
Vincristine, prednisolone, thioguanine, L-asparaginase, cytosine arabinose	24	8	8	126
TOTAL	485	55 (11.5%)	8	126

[a]BCNU = 1,3-*bis* (2-chloroethyl-l-nitrosourea)
[b]6-MP = 6-mercaptopurine

precede the systemic manifestations of the blastic phase. This occurs most commonly as lymph node enlargement. They have been reported in the meninges, skin, breast, bone, or intestinal tract.[99,102] Biopsies of such tumors stained with hematoxylin–eosin are often confused with histiocytic lymphoma (reticulum cell sarcoma). "Touch preps" of fresh biopsies will make the diagnosis as well as cytogenetics with detection of aneuploid Ph^1-positive cells.

THERAPY OF THE BLASTIC PHASE

The blastic phase occurring abruptly *de novo* or evolving from a myeloproliferative acceleration requires intensive acute leukemia-type therapy. The wide variety of regimens used in the treatment of acute myeloblastic leukemia and variant adaptations for blastic CGL have had disappointing results, with improvement noted in less than 20% of cases, and with complete hematologic remission an extremely rare event.[89] Most regimens include cytosine arabinoside, 6-thioguanine, and an anthracycline. These are summarized in Table 37-3.

In patients with lymphoblastic transformation, vincristine–prednisone may also be included, since the relatively non-toxic combination can effect a remission and a return to chronic phase morphology in 20% to 30% of patients entering the blastic phase. The usual dose is 1.4 mg/m^2 of vincristine, given intravenously as a weekly dose. Prednisone is given at 60 mg/m^2 per day by mouth over 5 days to 7 days with tapering over the subsequent 7 days to 14 days. Antileukemic response should be seen with the first dose.[103] If no response occurs after two weekly doses another regimen should be used. Maintenance with oral hydroxyurea or twice-weekly methotrexate should accompany intermittent monthly reinduction courses of vincristine–prednisone. The response can be correlated with the lymphoid biochemical and morphologic characteristics of the blast cells. Resistance to vincristine–prednisone is usually accompanied by blastic cells that have lost the lymphoid features. The median survival of patients in the blastic phase is 2 months but is longer (6 months to 8 months) in those who achieve a remission.

Alternative treatments recently introduced include cryopreservation of chronic phase bone marrow or buffy count peripheral blood cells for subsequent autologous transfusion into blastic phase patients treated with intensive chemotherapy or radiation. Although this technique has theoretic appeal, it has been extremely difficult to eradicate the blastic leukemia.[104] The transfused cells appear to have grafted successfully. This experimental treatment may be improved by better techniques of leukemic cell ablation.

Treatment of the blastic phase by allogeneic and even isogeneic transplantation has been disappointing for a number of reasons, including refractory leukemia, relatively advanced age of patients, myelofibrosis, and infection (Table 37-4).[105,106] There has been an interesting report of successful isogeneic transplantation in four cases of CGL in the chronic phase from their normal identical twins.[107] Intravenous cyclophosphamide 120 mg/kg and dimethyl myleran 5 mg/kg followed by total body irradiation (920 rad) were used to prepare the patients. All four had disappearance of the Ph^1 chromosome for 30, 43 plus, 46 plus and 51 plus months.* The success of this approach would support the concept of early transplantation for CGL patients with normal identical twins. Broad application of allogeneic transplantation is limited by the toxicity of the preparation; age of patients since CGL has a median of 45 years; and the problem of graft *versus* host disease still exists.

LYMPHOBLASTIC TRANSFORMATION OF CGL

Approximately 20% to 30% of cases of the blastic phase have cells bearing lymphoid morphologic and surface marker char-

*Fefer A: personal communication.

TABLE 37-4. Transplantation in Chronic Granulocytic Leukemia Transplantation

	NO OF PATIENTS	ENGRAFTMENTS	DURATION	REFERENCE NUMBER
BLASTIC PHASE				
A. Cryopreserved autologous graft				
1. Seattle (Buckner et al) 1978 (marrow cells)	7	2	72,120 days	(106)
2. Hammersmith (Goldman et al) 1980 (buffy coat)	9	8	5 cases—13 wks. 3 cases:26,32,74	(104)
B. Allogeneic				
1. Seattle (Doney et al) 1978	14	10	median 43 days survival	(105)
CHRONIC PHASE				
A. Isogeneic				
1. Seattle (Fefer et al) 1979	12	12	11/12 alive 7+–51+ months 10/12 no evidence of Ph[1] (personal communication)	(107)

acteristics.[108] This is more likely to occur in Ph[1]-positive acute leukemias. The incidence of Ph[1] positivity in acute lymphoblastic leukemia (ALL) of childhood is less than 10%.[109] Adult ALL appears to have a higher frequency of Ph[1] chromosome, in some series approaching 25%.[110] Ph[1]-positive acute lymphoblastic leukemias, whether appearing *de novo* or as a terminal phase or preceding CGL, have shown many of the phenotypic characteristics of common ALL of childhood (Table 37–5). The cells react with a non-B, non-T common ALL antiserum; anti-Ia antiserum and show high levels of the enzyme terminal deoxynucleotidyl transferase (TdT).[111] The presence of this enzyme, as well as the other characteristics, can be used to predict a response to vincristine–prednisone.[112]

Terminal deoxynucleotidyl transferase is a DNA-synthetic enzyme that is measurable in 75% of cases of childhood ALL. It is not present in the chronic phase of CGL or CLL, and only rarely in acute myeloblastic leukemia.[113] A few patients with Ph[1]-positive lymphoid blastic leukemia whose cells are reactive with anti-ALL antiserum and TdT will show cytoplasmic IgM, indicating a "pre-B" phenotype.[114] These findings suggest that at least some, and perhaps all, cases of CGL are diseases of the pluripotent stem that is a precursor to both myeloid and lymphoid cells.[115] To date the Ph[1] chromosome has not been demonstrated in true B- or T-cells. The pluripotential stem cell hypothesis rests on the assumption that the ALL phenotype is unique to lymphoid cells and that this phenotype can occur in the pluripotent stem cell itself.

JUVENILE CHRONIC GRANULOCYTIC LEUKEMIA

CGL in children is rare, occurring in 1% to 3% of cases of childhood leukemia.[116] Childhood CGL consists of two main types. The Ph[1]-chromosome-positive "adult" disease and the juvenile Ph[1]-negative type. The latter occurs almost exclusively in children under 6 years of age and is characterized by skin rash, splenomegaly, thrombocytopenia, elevated fetal hemoglobin, and resistance to chemotherapy. The median

TABLE 37-5. Philadelphia Chromosome Positive Leukemia Surface Marker and Enzymatic Characteristics

	Ia	ALL ANTIGEN	TdT*	E†	SmIg‡
1. Chronic phase	–	–	–	–	–
2. Blastic phase (myeloid)	+	–	–	–	–
3. Blastic phase (lymphoid)	+	+	+	–	–
4. Ph[1]-positive acute lymphoblastic leukemia	+	+	+	–	–

	RESPONSE TO VINCRISTINE–PREDNISONE	
TdT+	8/13 patients	(ref. 112)
ALL+	14/15 patients	(ref. 108)

*terminal deoxynucleotidyl transferase
†sheep red cell rosettes
‡surface membrane immunoglobulin
(Marks SM, Baltimore D, McCaffrey R: Terminal transferase as a predictor of initial responsiveness to vincristine and prednisone in blastic chronic myelogenous leukemia. New Eng J Med 298:812–814, 1978)

white count is usually 50,000/mm³. The majority of patients have no consistent cytogenetic abnormality, although a few have marker chromosomes providing evidence for clonal proliferation.[117]

REFERENCES

1. Boggs DR, Sofferman SA, Wintrobe et al: Factors influencing the duration of survival of patients with chronic lymphocytic leukemia. 40:243–254, 1966
2. Sweet DL, Golomb HM, Ultmann JE; Clin Hematol 6:185–202, 1977
3. Dick FR, Maca RD; The lymph node in chronic lymphocytic leukemia. Cancer 41:283–292, 1978
4. Rai KR, Sawitsky A, Cronkite EP, et al: Clinical staging of chronic lymphocytic leukemia. Blood 46:219–234, 1975
5. Knospe WH, Gregory SA, Trobaugh FE Jr et al: Chronic lymphocytic leukemia: Correlation of clinical course and therapeutic response with in vitro testing and morphology of lymphocytes. Am J Hematol 2:73–101, 1977
6. Peterson LC, Bloomfield CD, Brunning RD: Relationship of clinical staging and lymphocyte morphology to survival in chronic lymphocytic leukaemia. Br J Haematol 45:563–567, 1980
7. Galton DAG, Goldman JM, Wiltshaw E et al: Prolymphocytic leukaemia. Br J Haematol 27:7–23, 1973
8. Bearman RM, Pangalis GA, Rappaport H: Prolymphocytic leukemia: Clinical, histopathological, and cytochemical observations. Cancer 42:2360–2372, 1978
9. Zacharski LR, Linman JW: Chronic lymphocytic leukemia versus chronic lymphosarcoma cell leukemia: Analysis of 496 cases. Am J Med 47:75–81, 1969
10. Schnitzer B, Loesel LS, Reed RE: Lymphosarcoma cell leukemia. Cancer 26:1082–1096, 1970
11. Preud'home JL, Seligmann M: Surface bound immunoglobulins as a cell marker in human lymphoproliferative diseases. Blood 40:777–794, 1972
12. Aisenberg AC, Bloch KJ, Long JC: Cell-surface immunoglobulins in chronic lymphocytic leukemia and allied disorders. Am J Med 55:184–198, 1973
13. Rudders RA, Howard JP: Clinical and cell surface marker characterization of the early phase of chronic lymphocytic leukemia. Blood 52:25–35, 1978
14. Logue GL, Cohen HJ: Human lymphocyte complement receptors. J Clin Invest 60:1159–1164, 1977
15. Speckart SF, Boldt DH, MacDermott RP: Chronic lymphatic leukemia (CLL): Cell surface changes detected by lectin binding and their relation to altered glycosyltransferase activity. Blood 52:681–695, 1978
16. Halper JP, Fu SM, Gottlieb AB et al: Poor mixed lymphocyte reaction stimulatory capacity of leukemic B-cells of chronic lymphocytic leukemia patients despite the presence of Ia antigens. J Clin Invest 64:1141–1148, 1979
17. Davis S: The variable pattern of circulating lymphocyte subpopulations in chronic lymphocytic leukemia. New Eng J Med 21:1150–1153, 1976
18. Kaden BR, Rosse WF, Hauch TW: Immune thrombocytopenia in lymphoproliferative diseases. Blood 53:545–551, 1979
19. Weed RI: Exaggerated delayed hypersensitivity to mosquito bites in chronic lymphocytic leukemia. Blood 26:257–268, 1965
20. Abeloff MD, Waterbury L: Pure red blood cell aplasia and chronic lymphocytic leukemia. Arch Int Med 134:721–724, 1974
21. Cuni LJ, Grunwald H, Rosner F: Bullous pemphigoid in chronic lymphocytic leukemia with the demonstration of antibasement membrane antibodies. Am J Med 57:987–992, 1974
22. Trump DL, Mann RB, Phelps R et al: Richter's syndrome: Diffuse histiocytic lymphoma in patients with chronic lymphocytic leukemia. A report of five cases and review of the literature. Am J Med 68:539–548, 1980
23. McPhedran P, Heath CW Jr: Acute leukemia occurring during chronic lymphocytic leukemia. J Hematol 35:7–11, 1970
24. Catovsky ED, O'Brien M, Cherchi M et al: 'Prolymphocytoid' transformation of chronic lymphocytic leukaemia. Br J Haematol 41:9–18, 1979
25. Greene MH, Hoover RN, Fraumeni JF: Subsequent cancer in patients with chronic lymphocytic leukemia—A possible immunologic mechanism. J Nat Canc Inst 61:337–340, 1978
26. Brouet J, Sasportes M, Flandrin G et al: Chronic lymphocytic leukemia of T-cell origin. Immunological and clinical evaluation in eleven patients. Lancet I:890–893, 1975
27. Marks SM, Yanovich S, Rosenthal DS et al: Multimarker analysis of T-cell chronic lymphocytic leukemia. Blood 51:435–443, 1978
28. Nowell P, Jensen J, Winger L et al: T-cell variant of chronic lymphocytic leukaemia with chromosome abnormality and defective response to mitogens. Br J Haematol 33:459–468, 1976
29. Cohen HJ, George ER, Kremer WB: Hairy cell leukemia: Cellular characteristics including surface immunoglobulin dynamics and biosythesis. Blood 53:764–775, 1979
30. Utsinger P, Yount WJ, Fuller CR et al: Hairy cell leukemia: B-lymphocyte and phagocytic properties. Blood 49:19–27, 1977
31. Golomb HM, Mitz U, Vardiman J et al: Surface immunoglobulin, lectin-induced cap formation, and phagocytic function in five patients with the leukemic phase of hairy cell leukemia. Cancer 46:50–55, 1980
32. Bouroncle BA: Leukemic reticuloendotheliosis (Hairy cell leukemia). Blood 53:412–436, 1979
33. Golomb HM, Mintz U: Treatment of hairy cell leukemia (leukemic reticuloendotheliosis) II. Chlorambucil therapy in postksplenectomy patients with progressive disease. Blood 54:305–309, 1979
34. Byhardt RW, Brace KD, Wiernik PH: The role of splenic irradiation in chronic lymphocytic leukemia. Cancer 35:1621–1625, 1975
35. Silver RT: The treatment of chronic lymphocytic leukemia. Sem Hematol 6:344–356, 1969
36. Knospe WH, Loeb V, Huguley CM: Bi-weekly chlorambucil treatment of chronic lymphocytic leukemia. Cancer 33:555–562, 1974
37. Freymann JG, Vander JB, Marler EA et al: Prolonged corticosteroid therapy of chronic lymphocytic leukaemia and the closely allied malignant lymphomas. Br J Haematol 6:303–323, 1960
38. Sawitsky A, Rai DR, Glidewell O et al: Comparison of daily versus intermittent chlorambucil and prednisone therapy in the treatment of patients with chronic lymphocytic leukemia. Blood 50:1049–1059, 1977
39. Han T, Ezdinli EZ, Shimaoka K et al: Chlorambucil versus combined chlorambucil–corticosteroid therapy in chronic lymphocytic leukemia. Cancer 31:502–508, 1973
40. Galton DAG, Szur WL, Dacie JV: The use of chlorambucil and steroids in the treatment of chronic lymphocytic leukemia. Br J Haematol 7:73–98, 1961
41. Sawitsky A, Rai KR, Aral I et al: Mediastinal irradiation for chronic lymphocytic leukemia. Am J Med 61:892–896, 1976
42. Johnson RE, Ruhl U: Treatment of chronic lymphocytic leukemia with emphasis on total body irradiation. Int J Rad Oncol Biol Phys 1:387–397, 1976
43. Cooper IA, Ding JC, Adams PB et al: Intensive leukapheresis in the management of cytopenias in patients with chronic lymphocytic leukaemia (CLL) and lymphocytic lymphoma. Am J Hematol 6:387–398, 1979
44. Curtis JE, Hersh EM, Freireich EJ: Leukapheresis therapy of chronic lymphocytic leukemia. Blood 39:163–174, 1972
45. Storb R, Epstein RB, Buckner CD et al: Treatment of chronic lymphocytic leukemia by extrancorporeal irradiation. Blood 31:490–502, 1968
46. Phillips EA, Kempin S, Passe et al: Prognostic factors in chronic lymphocytic leukaemia and their implications for therapy. Clin Haematol 6:203–222, 1977
47. Nowell PC, Hungerford DA: A minute chromosome in human chronic granulocytic leukemia. Science 132:1497, 1960
48. Fitzgerald PH, Pickering AF, Eiby JR: Clonal origin of the

Philadelphia chromosome and chronic myeloid leukaemia: Evidence from a sex chromosome mosaic. Br J Haematol 21:473–480, 1971

49. Fialkow PJ, Gartler SM, Yoshida A: Clonal origin of chronic myelocytic leukemia in man. Proc Nat Acad Sci 58:1468–1471, 1967
50. Fialkow PJ, Jacobson RJ, Papayannopoulou T: Chronic myeloctic leukemia: Clonal origin in a stem cell common to the granulocyte, erythrocyte, platelet and monocyte/marcophage. Am J Med 63:125–130, 1977
51. Singer JW, Fialkow PJ, Steinmann L et al: Chronic myelocytic leukemia (CML): Failure to detect residual normal committed stem cells in vitro. Blood 53:264–268, 1979
52. Bauke J: Chronic myelocytic leukemia. Cancer 24:643–648, 1969
53. Rowley JD: A new consistent chromosomal abnormality in chronic myelogenous leukaemia identified by quinacrine fluorescence and giemsa staining. Nature 243:290–293, 1973
54. Sonta S, Sandberg AA: Chromosomes and causation of human cancer and leukemia. XXIV. Unusual and complex Ph^1 translocations and their clinical significance. Blood 50:691–697, 1977
55. Oshimura M, Sandberg AA: Chromosomes and causation of human cancer and leukemia. XXV. Significance of the Ph_1 (including unusual translocations) in various acute leukemias. Cancer 40:1149–1160, 1977
56. Clein GP, Flemans RJ: Involvement of the erythroid series in blastic crisis of chronic myeloid leukaemia. Further evidence for the presence of Philadelphia chromosome in erythroblasts. Br J Haematol 12:754–758, 1966
57. Golde DW, Burgaleta C, Sparkes RS et al: The Philadelphia chromosome in human macrophages. Blood 49:367–370, 1977
58. Fialkow PJ, Denman AM, Jacobson RJ et al: Chronic myelocytic leukemia. Origin of some lymphocytes from leukemic stem cells. J Clin Invest 62:815–823, 1978
59. Greenberg BR, Wilson FD, Woo L et al: Cytogenetics of fibroblastic colonies in Ph^1-positive chronic myelogenous leukemia. Blood 51:1039–1044, 1978
60. Sakurai M, Hayata I, Sandberg AA: Prognostic value of chromosomal findings in Ph^1-positive chronic myelocytic leukemia. Cancer Res 36:313–318, 1976
61. Finney R, McDonald GA, Baikie AG et al: Chronic granulocytic leukaemia with Ph^1-negative cells in bone marrow and a ten year remission after busulphan hypoplasia. Br J Haematol 23:283–288, 1972
62. Whang-Peng J, Canellos GP, Carbone PP et al: Clinical implications of cytogenetic variants in chronic myelocytic leukemia (CML). Blood 32:755–766, 1968
63. Sonta S, Sandberg AA: Chromosomes and causation of human cancer and leukemia. XXIX. Further studies on karyotypic progression in CML. Cancer 41:153–163, 1978
64. Lyall JM, Garson OM: Non-random chromosome changes in the blastic transformation stage of Ph^1-positive chronic granulocytic leukaemia. Leuk Res 2:213–222, 1978
65. Lawler SD, Lobb DS, Wiltshaw E: Philadelphia-chromosome positive bone-marrow cells showing loss of the Y in males with chronic myeloid leukaemia. Br J Haematol 27:247–252, 1974
66. Stoll C, Oberling F, Flori E: Chromosome analysis of spleen and/or lymph nodes of patients with chronic myeloid leukemia (CML). Blood 52:828–838, 1978
67. Krauss S: Chronic myelocytic leukemia with features simulating myelofibrosis with myeloid metaplasia. Cancer 19:1321–1332, 1966
68. Roth DG, Richman CM, Rowley JD: Chronic myelodysplastic syndrome (Preleukemia) with the Philadelphia chromosome. Blood 56:262–264, 1980
69. Canellos GP, Whang-Peng J, DeVita VT: Chronic granulocytic leukemia without the Philadelphia chromosome. Am J Clin Pathol 65:467–470, 1976
70. Kohno S, Abe S, Sandberg AA: The chromosomes and causation of human cancer and leukemia: XXXVII. Cytogenetic experience in Ph^1-negative chronic myelocytic leukemia (CML). Am J Hematol 7:281–291, 1979
71. Spiers ASD, Bain BJ, Turner JE: The peripheral blood in chronic granulocytic leukaemia. Study of 50 untreated Philadelphia-positive cases. Scand J Haematol 18:25–38, 1977
72. Mason JE Jr, DeVita VT, Canellos GP: Thrombocytosis in chronic granulocytic leukemia: Incidence and clinical significance. Blood 44:483–487, 1974
73. Kattlove HE, Williams JC, Gaynor E et al: Gaucher cells in chronic myelocytic leukemia: An acquired abnormality. Blood 33:379–390, 1969
74. Cramer E, Auclair C, Hakim J et al: Metabolic activity of phagocytosing granulocytes in chronic granulocytic leukemia: Ultrastructural observation of a degranulation defect. Blood 50:93–106, 1977
75. Rosner F, Schreiber ZR, Parise F: Leukocyte alkaline phosphatase. Fluctuations with disease status in chronic granulocytic leukemia. Arch Int Med 130:892–894, 1972
76. Rosenblum D, Petzold SJ: Neutrophil alkaline phosphatase: Comparison of enzymes from normal subjects and patients with polycythemia vera and chronic myelogenous leukemia. Blood 45:335–343, 1975
77. Schiffer CA, Aisner J, Daly PA et al: Increased leukocyte alkaline phosphatase activity following transfusion of leukocytes from a patient with chronic myelogenous leukemia. Am J Med 66:519–522, 1979
78. Gerrard JM, Stoddard SF, Shapiro RS et al: Platelet storage pool deficiency and prostaglandin synthesis in chronic granulocytic leukaemia. Br J Haematol 40:597–607, 1978
79. Chikkappa G, Borner G, Burlington H et al: Periodic oscillation of blood leukocytes, platelets and reticulocytes in a patient with chronic myelocytic leukemia. Blood 47:1023–1030, 1976
80. Gilbert HS, Krauss S, Pasternack B et al: Serum vitamin B_{12} content and unsaturated vitamin B_{12}-binding capacity in myeloproliferative disease. Value in differential diagnosis and as indicators of disease activity. Ann Int Med 71:719–729, 1969
81. Chikkappa G, Corcino J, Greenberg ML et al: Correlation between various blood white cell pools and the serum B_{12}-binding capacities. Blood 37:142–151, 1971
82. Corcino J, Krauss S, Waxman S et al: Release of vitamin B_{12}-binding protein by human leukocytes in vitro. J Clin Invest 49:2250–2255, 1970
83. Youman JD, Taddeini L, Cooper T: Histamine excess symptoms in basophilic chronic granulocytic leukemia. Arch Int Med 131:560–562, 1973
84. Swisher RW, Mueller JM, Halloran LG: Basophilic leukemia presenting as gastroduodenal ulceration effect of H-2-receptor blockade. Dig Dis 23:952–955, 1978
85. Witts LJ: Chronic granulocytic leukaemia: Comparison of radiotherapy and busulphan therapy. Report of the medical research council's working party for therapeutic trials in leukaemia. Br Med J 1:201–208, 1968
86. Galton DAG: Chemotherapy of chronic myelocytic leukemia. Sem Hematol 6:323–343, 1969
87. Canellos GP, Young RC, Nieman PE et al: Dibromomannitol in the treatment of chronic granulocytic leukemia: A prospective randomized comparison with busulfan. Blood 45:197–203, 1975
88. Schwartz JH, Canellos GP: Hydroxyurea in the management of the hematologic complications of chronic granulocytic leukemia. Blood 46:11–16, 1975
89. Canellos GP: The treatment of chronic granulocytic leukaemia. Clin Haematol 6:113–128, 1977
90. Cunningham I, Gee T, Dowling M et al: Results of treatment of Ph′ + chronic myelogenous leukemia with an intensive treatment regimen (L-5 protocol). Blood 53:375–395, 1979
91. Smalley RV, Vogel J, Huguley CM Jr et al: Chronic granulocytic leukemia: Cytogenetic conversion of the bone marrow with cycle-specific chemotherapy. Blood 50:107–113, 1977
92. Sharp JC, Wayne AW, Crofts M et al: Karyotpic conversion in Ph^1-positive chronic myeloid leukaemia with combination chemotherapy. Lancet I:1370–1372, 1979
93. Ihde DC, Canellos GP, Schwartz JH et al: Splenectomy in the chronic phase of chronic granulocytic leukemia. Effects in 12 patients. Ann Int Med 84:17–21, 1976

94. Wolf DJ, Silver RT, Coleman M: Splenectomy in chronic myeloid leukemia. Ann Int Med 89:684–689, 1978
95. Lowenthal RM, Buskard NA, Goldman JM et al: Intensive leukapheresis as initial therapy for chronic granulocytic leukemia. Blood 46:835–844, 1975
96. Monfardini S, Gee T, Fried J et al: Survival in chronic myelogenous leukemia: Influence of treatment and extent of disease at diagnosis. Cancer 31:492–501, 1973
97. Spiers ASD: Annotation, Metamorphosis of chronic granulocytic leukaemia: Diagnosis; classification of management. Br J Haematol 41:1–7, 1979
98. Clough V, Geary CG, Hashmi K et al: Myelofibrosis in chronic granulocytic leukaemia. Br J Haematol 42:515–526, 1978
99. Rosenthal S, Canellos GP, DeVita VT Jr et al: Characteristics of blast crisis in chronic granulocytic leukemia. Blood 49:705–714, 1977
100. Freireich EJ, Thomas LB, Frei E III et al: A distinctive type of intracerebral hemorrhage associated with "blastic crisis" in patients with leukemia. Cancer 13:146–154, 1960
101. Rosenthal S, Canellos GP, Whang-Pheng J et al: Blast crisis of chronic granulocytic leukemia. Morphologic variants and therapeutic implications. Am J Med 63:542–547, 1977
102. Chabner BA, Haskell CM, Canellos GP: Destructive bone lesions in chronic granulocytic leukemia. Medicine 48:401–410, 1969
103. Canellos GP, DeVita VT, Whang-Peng J et al: Hematologic and cytogenetic remission of blastic transformation in chronic granulocytic leukemia. 38:671–679, 1971
104. Goldman JM, Johnson SA, Islam A et al: Haematologic reconstitution after autografting for chronic granulocytic leukaemia in transformation: the influence of previous splenectomy. Br J Haematol 45:223–231, 1980
105. Doney K, Buckner CD, Sale GE et al: Treatment of chronic granulocytic leukemia by chemotherapy, total body irradiation and allogeneic bone marrow transplantation. Exp Hemat 6:738–747, 1978
106. Buckner CD, Stewart P, Clift RA et al: Treatment of blastic transformation of chronic granulocytic leukemia by chemotherapy, total body irradiation and infusion of cryopreserved autologous marrow. Exp. Hemat 6:96–109, 1978
107. Fefer A, Cheever MA, Thomas ED et al: Disappearance of Ph[1]-positive cells in four patients with chronic granulocytic leukemia after chemotherapy, irradiation and marrow transplantation from an identical twin. New Engl J Med 300:333–337, 1979
108. Janossy G, Woodruff RK, Pippard MJ et al: Relation of "lymphoid" phenotype and response to chemotherapy incorporating vincristine–prednisolone in the acute phase of Ph[1] positive leukemia. Cancer 43:426–434, 1979
109. Priest JR, Roberts M, Oreaucs MR et al: Philadelphia chromosome positive childhood acute lymphoblastic leukemia. Blood 56:15–22, 1980
110. Bloomfield CD, Peterson LC, Yunis JJ et al: The Philadelphia chromosome (Ph[1]) in adults presenting with acute leukaemia: a comparison of Ph[1] and Ph[1]-patients. Br J Haematol 36:347–358, 1977
111. Janossy G, Woodruff RK, Paxton A et al: Membrane marker and cell separation studies in Ph[1]-positive leukemia. Blood 51:861–877, 1978
112. Marks SM, Baltimore D, McCaffrey R: Terminal transferase as a predictor of initial responsiveness to vincristine and prednisone in blastic chronic myelogenous leukemia. New Eng J Med 298:812–814, 1978
113. Marks SM, McCaffrey R: The significance of terminal transferase in normal and neoplastic hematopoietic cells. Contemp Hematol Oncol 1:277–296, 1980
114. Greaves MF, Verbi W, Reeves BR et al: "Pre-B" phenotypes in blast crisis of Ph[1] positive CML: Evidence for a pluripotential stem cell "target." Leuk Res 3:181–191, 1979
115. Boggs DR: Hematopoietic stem cell theory in relation to possible lymphoblastic conversion of chronic myeloid leukemia. Blood 44:449–453, 1974
116. Smith KL, Johnson W: Classification of chronic myelocytic leukemia in children. Cancer 34:670–679, 1974
117. Brodeur GM, Dow LW, Williams DL: Cytogenetic features of juvenile chronic myelogenous leukemia. Blood 53:812–819, 1979
118. Marmont AM, Damasio EE: The treatment of terminal metamorphosis of chronic granulocytic leukaemia with corticosteroids and vincristine. Acta Haematol 50:1–8, 1973
119. Shaw MT, Bottomley RH, Grozea PN et al: Heterogeneity of morphological, cytochemical, and cytogenetic features in the blastic phase of chronic granulocytic leukemia. Cancer 35:199–207, 1975
120. Foley HT, Bennett JM, Carbone PP: Combination chemotherapy in accelerated phase of chronic granulocytic leukemia. Arch Int Med 123:166–170, 1969
121. Hayes DM, Ellison RR, Glidewell O et al: Chemotherapy for the terminal phase of chronic myelocytic leukemia. Canc Chemother Rep 4:233–247, 1974
122. Vallejos CS, Trujillo JM, Cork A et al: Blastic crisis in chronic granulocytic leukemia: Experience in 39 patients. Cancer 34:1806–1812, 1974
123. Spiers ADS, Costello C, Catovsky D et al: Chronic granulocytic leukaemia: Multiple-drug chemotherapy for acute transformation. Br Med J 13:77–80, 1974
124. Canellos GP, DeVita VT, Whang-Peng J et al: Chemotherapy of the blastic phase of chronic granulocytic leukemia: Hypodiploidy and response to therapy. Blood 47:1003–1009, 1976
125. Coleman M, Silver RT, Pajak TF et al: Combination chemotherapy for terminal-phase chronic granulocytic leukemia: Cancer and leukemia Group B studies. Blood 55:29–36, 1980
126. Beard M, Gauci C, Sikora E et al: Blast crisis of chronic myeloid leukaemia: The effect of intensive chemotherapy. Scand J Haematol 16:258–262, 1976

Daniel E. Bergsagel
Walter D. Rider

CHAPTER 38

Plasma Cell Neoplasms

DEFINITION

Plasma cell neoplasms arise when a cell of the B-lymphocyte lineage proliferates to form a large population of similar cells. This population is belived to be monoclonal, that is, derived from a single cell, because the cells produce a homogeneous immunoglobulin composed of a single class of heavy chain and one type of light chain, or fragments of these components. Each clone produces a unique protein, with an ideotypic marker determined by identical variable regions in the heavy and light chains, which distinguishes it from all other immunoglobulins.

The appearance of a homogeneous M-protein (M for monoclonal) in a serum electrophoresis pattern provides evidence that the population of cells producing the M-protein has reached a size of at least 5×10^9 cells, and is producing enough protein to be recognized as an "M-spike' (more than 0.5 g/dl). A classification of the diseases associated with the appearance of an M-protein is shown in Table 38-1.

The proliferation of the monoclone appears to be controlled and regulated in the disorders listed under Section A in Table 38-1. The stable status of the monoclone in patients with benign monoclonal gammopathy (BMG) and the chronic cold agglutination syndrome will be discussed later (see page 1455). In some patients, the M-protein may be transient, disappearing after recovery from an infection, a reaction to a drug, or some other illness.[1-3] In addition, some patients with α–heavy-chain disease may have a "controlled proliferation" because the M-protein has been noted to disappear either spontaneously, or after treatment with antibiotics alone.[4]

Uncontrolled expansion (neoplasia) of an M-protein–producing clone is distinguished by continuing growth that results in an exponential increase in the serum M-protein concentration, the formation of tumors composed of lymphoplasmacytic cells, the appearance of lytic skeletal lesions, and other manifestations of the underlying diseases listed under Section B in Table 38-1.

HISTORY

Many of the important clinical features of plasma cell myeloma were described in a series of five papers by John Dalrymple, Henry Bence Jones, and William MacIntyre, between 1846 and 1850. The patient investigated by these physicians has been identified as Thomas Alexander McBean, as a result of the inventive sleuthing of John Clamp.[5] Clamp also analysed the contributions of the three physicians, and concludes that the unique heat-coagulation properties of McBean's urinary protein were discovered by MacIntyre, and not by Bence Jones.

Rustizky, working independently, described a similar patient in 1873, and introduced the term *multiple myeloma* to emphasize the fact that multiple bone tumors are important features of the disease.[6] The work of Kahler, who published a detailed review of multiple myeloma in 1889, aroused considerable interest in Europe, where the disease is still often referred to as *Kahler's disease*.[7] The elevated serum protein and increased erythrocyte sedimentation rate in multiple myeloma were noted by Ellinger in 1899, and in 1900, Wright recognized the close relationship of myeloma cells and plasma cells.[8,9] The diagnosis, however, remained difficult and uncertain until the 1930s, when marrow aspiration and

TABLE 38-1. Classification of Diseases Associated with M-Proteins

A. Controlled proliferation of an M-protein-producing clone
 1. Benign monoclonal gammopathy
 2. Chronic cold agglutinin syndrome
 3. Transient M-proteins
 4. Some patients with α heavy-chain disease

B. Uncontrolled proliferation (neoplasia) of an M-protein-producing clone
 1. Plasma cell myeloma—plasma cell neoplasms producing γ, α, δ, or ϵ heavy chains plus κ or λ light chains, or light chains only (κ or λ).
 2. Plasma cell neoplasms associated with dermatologic lesions.
  i. Papular mucinosis
  ii. Pyoderma gangrenosum
 2. Waldenström's macroglobulinemia—a lympho–plasmacytic neoplasm producing M heavy chains and κ or λ light chains.
 4. Immunoglobulin-related amyloidosis—plasma cell neoplasms producing free κ or λ light chains (and possibly a heavy chain) which becomes incorporated into tissue deposits of amyloid.
 5. Heavy-chain diseases—lympho–plasmacytic neoplasms producing γ, α, or μ heavy chains (or fragments) and no light chains.
 6. Chronic lymphocytic leukemia and diffuse, poorly differentiated lymphocytic lymphomas—these are B-lymphocyte neoplasms which produce usually μ ± δ and, occasionally, γ or α heavy chains, plus κ or α light chains.

studies of serum proteins by ultracentrifugation and electrophoresis were introduced. Magnus-Levy described amyloidosis as an important complication, occurring in 15% of myeloma patients, long before the relationship of amyloid fibrils to light-chain proteins provided evidence that immunoglobulins are involved in the pathogenesis of amyloidosis.[10,11]

Treatment was almost totally ineffective until 1947, when Alwall reported dramatic improvement in one of two patients treated with stilbamadine and urethane.[12] Further study showed that the anti-myeloma effect was produced by urethane. This drug, however, did not prove to be very useful, for it caused considerable nausea and vomiting, and objective improvement occurred in less than 15% of patients.[13] Many other agents, including pentamidine, nitrogen mustard, 6-mercaptopurine, and 5-fluorouracil, were tried without success.[14] In 1958, Blokhin and colleages reported to the New York Academy of Sciences that D L-phenylalanine mustard (Sarcolysin) produced significant improvement in three of six myeloma patients, including healing of skull lesions in one. Because of this report, the Southwestern Cancer Chemotherapy Study Group tested the effectiveness of the L-isomer (L-phenylalanine mustard, melphalan), and found that objective improvement occurred in one-third of patients.[16] Cyclophosphamide was soon shown to be equally effective, and the value of adrenocortical steroids demonstrated.[17,18]

INCIDENCE

The commonest cause of a serum M-protein is BMG. Axelsson and co-workers screened the serum of 6995 asymptomatic Swedish adults over the age of 25 for the presence of an M-protein by serum electrophoresis.[19] This sample represented about 70% of the adult population of four parishes in the district of Värmland. An M-protein was found in 64 sera. The initial investigation demonstrated plasma cell myeloma in one serum, and chronic lymphocytic leukemia (CLL) in another. An evaluation of the causes of death and the status of the surving patients 11 years later showed that the original myeloma patient had died of the disease, the patient thought to have CLL had progressed and died with plasma cell myeloma, while another had died with a malignant lymphoma.[20] Thus, in this series of 64 asymptomatic patients with M-proteins followed for 11 years, a B-lymphocyte neoplasm was diagnosed in only three patients, and the remaining 61 are thought to have BMG. The incidence of BMG increases with age to 2.0% in the eighth decade and 5.7% in the ninth decade.[19] Hällén found M-proteins in the sera of nine of 294 patients (3.1%) over the age of 70 years.[21] Using a more sensitive technique, Englišová et al found M-proteins in the sera of 11.7% of 51 octogenerians, and a surprising 19% of 26 nonagenerians.[22] As judged from the results of the Swedish screening study, the *prevalence* of BMG in asymptomatic adults is 61:6995 (0.872%), or 872 per 100,000 persons over the age of 25.[19]

Most subjects with symptomatic disease did not have blood drawn for electrophoresis in the Swedish screening study. However, inquiry at local hospitals and interviews with doctors who knew the population revealed two additional patients with plasma cell myeloma.[19] Thus, at least three patients with myeloma were identified in four parishes with an adult population of about 10,000, suggesting that prevalence of myeloma is about 30 per 100,000 persons over the age of 25 years.

It should be noted that the above figures represent the numbers of patients found to have BMG or plasma cell myeloma at a certain point in time. Because patients with BMG survive for prolonged periods, while patients with plasma cell myeloma have a median survival of about 30 months, the numbers of patients with BMG tend to accumulate and greatly exceed the numbers of surviving myeloma patients at any point in time. The annual incidence of BMG has not been reported.

The annual incidence of plasma cell myeloma per 100,000 population has been estimated to be 2.6 in England, 3.1 in Olmstead County, Minnesota, and 3.3 for Sweden.[23–25] The increased incidence in blacks reported from Brooklyn and Jamaica has been confirmed by a complete survey of the incidence of plasma cell myeloma in Atlanta, Georgia, where rates per 100,000 were 4.0 in blacks and 2.1 in whites.[26–28]

The incidence of myeloma increases progressively with age, with the highest rates being observed in men over the age of 80 years, and in women over 70 years of age. The mean age at diagnosis was 64 years in a recent large series.[29] Less than 2% of patients are under 40 years at diagnosis, but the disease has been reported in young adults and children.[30]

Plasma cell myeloma occurs slightly more frequently in males than in females. An analysis of 2844 cases reported in recent large studies revealed that 55.1% were male, in contrast to earlier studies in which males appeared to be more commonly affected than this.[14,23,28,29,31–37]

PATHOGENESIS

Spontaneous plasma cell tumors, or lymphomas producing immunoglobulins, have been reported in dogs, cats, hamsters, rats, and mice.[38–49] These tumors tend to develop in older animals, but an identifiable etiologic agent has not been found for any species. The plasma cell tumors of inbred mouse strains have been studied extensively, for they have proven to be useful models for the study of plasma cell neoplasms in humans.

MOUSE PLASMA CELL TUMORS

Plasma cell tumors are induced in 60% to 70% of BALB/c mice by the intraperitoneal (but not by subcutaneous) implantation of plastics or mineral oil. Hormonal factors may play a role, for plasmacytomas develop more frequently in males, and simultaneous cortisol reduces the incidence.[50] The plasmacytomas develop within peritoneal and mesenteric oil granulomas. Each plasmacytoma appears to represent a clone of plasma cells producing a unique M-protein.

Intraperitoneal pristane leads to the appearance of a growth factor in the ascitic fluid that facilitates the sustained proliferation of plasma cells and also causes local immunosuppression.[51,52] In cell cultures, irradiated myeloma-infiltrated spleen cells stimulate colony formation by mouse myeloma cells in soft agar.[53] In this system, ascorbic acid is required for the progressive growth of myeloma colonies.[54] Ascitic fluid from pristane-treated mice also stimulates the growth of human myeloma cells.[55] A variety of other cells produces growth factors for mouse myeloma cells, and serum from mice injected with Freunds adjuvant, endotoxin, or bacterial antigens contain increased amounts of a growth factor for myeloma colonies which is non-dialyzable, heat-labile, and migrates as a β-globulin.[56–58]

Antigenic stimulation by the normal bacterial flora appears to play a role in the induction of plasmacytomas in BALB/c mice, for the incidence of plasmacytomas is greatly reduced in germ-free mice treated with pristane.[59] Genetic factors are also important; pristane induces plasmacytomas only in BALB/c or NZB mice. These strains appear to be unique in possessing specific genes involved in the pathogenesis of plasma cell tumors; at least one gene is recessive.[49,60,61]

The role of viruses in the induction of mouse plasmacytomas is not clear. The infectious MLV-A virus accelerates the induction of plasmacytomas in pristane-treated BALB/c mice, and the rapidity with which these tumors develop suggests that they are derived from cells transformed by MLV-A.[62]

PREDISPOSING FACTORS IN HUMANS

There is an increased incidence of myeloma in first-degree relatives. At the Mayo Clinic, myeloma was found in the siblings of eight among 440 myeloma patients seen over a 6-year period.[63] This is far in excess of the anticipated incidence of myeloma in the general population. Familial myeloma has been reported in at least 14 additional families.[63] Furthermore, there are many reports of BMG occurring in family members of patients with myeloma and macroglobulinemia, and the familial occurrence of macroglobulinemia and BMG has been recognized.[63] This striking familial association of myeloma, macroglobulinemia, and BMG, the finding that the 4c complex of HL-A antigens occurs more frequently in myeloma patients than in the general population, and the increased incidence of myeloma in blacks strongly suggest that genetic factors play a role in determining susceptibility to this disease in humans.[26–28,64,65] Although myeloma has been reported in at least five husband-and-wife pairs in the United States, the frequency in spouses is less than expected, and does not favor the hypothesis of horizontal transmission.[66,67]

An important association between high-dose radiation exposure and plasma cell myeloma has been observed in a cohort of approximately 100,000 controls and survivors of the atomic bombs in Hiroshima and Nagasaki for the period 1950 to 1976.[68] The standardized relative risk for persons with an estimated air-dose exposure of more than 100 rads was about 4.7 times greater than controls. The excess risks for myeloma in the high-exposure group became apparent about 20 years after exposure. An association between low-dose radiation and the development of myeloma has not been firmly established.[68]

Chronic antigenic stimulation, for example, in cholecystitis, osteomyelitis, hyposensitization with repeated allergen injections, rheumatoid arthritis, hereditary spherocytosis and Gaucher's disease, has been proposed as a factor predisposing to the development of plasma cell neoplasms in humans.[1,69–81] The association of a plasma cell neoplasm with many of these conditions is difficult to establish with certainty. The incidence of myeloma in Finnish patients with rheumatoid arthritis does appear to be more than twice as common as in the general population, and the occurrence of an M-protein in ten patients with Gaucher's disease (7 BMG, 3 myeloma) and the occurrence of two BMG in patients with hereditary spherocytosis does suggest an association between these uncommon disorders.[76–81]

The occurrence of four patients with myeloma, one with macroglobulinemia, and one with chronic lymphocytic leukemia in a group of 61 patients with asbestosis raises the question of whether this carcinogen may be involved in the initiation of B-lymphocyte neoplasms.[82,83] Much further work will be required to establish this association.

Aleutian disease of mink is a viral illness characterized by excessive plasmacytosis and hyperglobulinemia. A small proportion of infected mink develop a homogeneous M-spike and light chain proteinurea.[84] The Aleutian disease virus (ADV) appears to be transmissible to humans, for half of the individuals handling high concentrations of ADV developed ADV antibodies, although none developed illness.[84] Two cases thought to be Aleutian disease in humans have been described.[85,86] Confirmation of the diagnosis by the demonstration of ADV antibodies could not be done, as the cases were described before the antibody assay was developed. The report of myeloma in a mink handler following exposure to Aleutian disease is of interest, but there is no clear evidence that ADV was involved, since no antibody to ADV could be detected in the patient's serum.[87]

The natural history of BMG has been investigated at the Mayo Clinic by following 241 patients for at least 7 years.[88]

During this period there was no significant increase in the serum M-protein of 137 patients (57%), 55 (23%) died with no known change, and 27 (11%) progressed so that a diagnosis of plasma cell myeloma was made in 18, macroglobulinemia in four, amyloidosis in four, and chronic lymphocytic leukemia in one. In addition, there was a more than 50% increase in the serum M-protein concentration, or the appearance of a urinary light chain, in 22 patients (9%). A progressive increase in the serum M-protein suggests an expanding plasma cell population, and the appearance of light chains in the urine is also thought to be an unfavorable sign. However, the patients in the latter group will have to be followed for a longer period before the diagnosis of a B-lymphocyte neoplasm is established. Thus, at least 11% of these BMG patients progressed to develop plasma cell neoplasms or chronic lymphocytic leukemia, and an additional 9% showed a progressive increase in a serum or urinary M-protein.

ANATOMIC CONSIDERATIONS

Plasma cells are produced mainly in hematopoietic marrow, lymph nodes, spleen, the submucosa of the upper air passages, and the gastrointestinal tract. Plasma cell tumors can develop in any of these, as well as in other sites. Most of the plasma cell neoplasms, producing immunoglobulins of class G, A, D, or E or only light chains, originate in hematopoietic marrow, and progress to cause typical "punched out" lytic lesions, fractures, or osteoporosis in 79% of patients at the time of diagnosis.[34] About 5% of these patients will present with lymphadenopathy or splenomegaly. In contrast, the majority of patients with plasma cell tumors producing IgM will have lymphadenopathy and splenomegaly and only about 14% will have osteolytic bone lesions.[89]

Most plasma cell neoplasms form multiple tumors in bone, and cause a generalized increase in marrow plasma cells. These neoplasms rarely present as solitary tumors in bone or in extramedullary sites (see Table 38-2 and definitions on p. 1447).

Plasma cell tumors originating in extramedullary sites usually develop in the upper air passages. Less commonly, they present in the spleen or lymph nodes, the skin, and in the gastrointestinal tract. Occasionally, plasma cell tumors can arise in almost any organ, such as the vagina, breast, pancreas, parotid, thyroid, and testes (Table 38-3).

Extramedullary plasmacytomas have many features that differ markedly from other plasma cell neoplasms (Table 38-4). They occur in a broader age group, including children and young adults, and long-term control can often be achieved with local treatment (radiation therapy and salvage surgery) directed at the primary site (Fig. 38-1). The observation that a serum M-protein will often persist following irradiation of a nasopharyngeal plasmacytoma, with long-term disappearance following surgical removal of tonsils and adenoids, indicates that some of the myeloma cells survive tumor doses of 3000 to 4500 rad, and also that the tumor tends to remain localized, in contrast to both solitary and multiple plasma cell tumors of bone.[91]

A serum or urinary M-protein has been reported in less than 30% of patients with extramedullary plasmacytomas, or solitary plasmacytomas of bone, in contrast with 98% of patients with multiple myeloma. This probably indicates that the plasma cell tumor mass is smaller in the former two diseases, however, the number of patients tested is rather small.

Solitary plasmacytomas of bone and extramedullary plasmacytomas differ markedly from multiple myeloma in that the incidence in males is 72% and 73%, respectively, in the former diseases and 55% in multiple myeloma.

Solitary plasmacytomas of bone appear to be an uncommon, early stage of myeloma. The median age at diagnosis is about 11 years younger than for multiple myeloma, survival from the recognition of the solitary lesion is much longer than the survival of patients who present with multiple myeloma, progression to multiple myeloma is common, and survival after progression is similar to that of patients who present with multiple myeloma.

Although the overall survival of patients presenting with extramedullary plasmacytomas and solitary plasmacytomas

TABLE 38-2. Plasma Cell Tumors Originating in Skeletal (Multiple and Solitary) or Extramedullary Sites

	NUMBER	PERCENT
Plasma cell tumors of bone		
multiple	856	93.2
solitary	26	2.8
Extramedullary plasma cell tumors	37	4.0
TOTALS	919	100.0

(Adapted from Crowin J, Lindberg RD: Solitary plasmacytoma of bone *vs* extramedullary plasmacytoma and their relationship to multiple myeloma. Cancer 43:1007–1013, 1979 and from Knowling M, Harwood A, Bergsagel DE: A comparison of extramedullary plasmacytomas with multiple and solitary plasma cell tumors of bone. (in press))

TABLE 38-3. Sites of Extramedullary Plasma Cell Tumors

	NUMBER	PERCENT
Upper air passages (tonsil, palate, nasal sinuses, nasopharynx, nose, orbit)	248	76
Lymph nodes and spleen	18	6
Bronchi and lung	13	4
Skin and subcutaneous	12	3.5
Gastrointestinal tract	10	3
Thyroid	9	3
Testes	3	1
Other	12	3.5
TOTALS	325	100

(Adapted from Crowin J, Lindberg RD: Solitary plasmacytoma of bone *vs* extramedullary plasmacytoma and their relationship to multiple myeloma. Cancer 43:1007–1013, 1979, Knowling M, Harwood A, Bergsagel DE: A comparison of extramedullary plasmacytomas with multiple and solitary plasma cell tumors of bone (in press), Wiltshaw E: The natural history of extramedullary plasmacytoma and its relation to solitary myeloma of bone and myelomatosis. Medicine 55:217–238, 1976, and from Woodruff RK, Whittle JM, Malpas JS: Solitary plasmacytoma. I: Extramedullary soft tissue plasmactyoma. Cancer 43:2340–2343, 1979)

of bone is long (Table 38-4), it is easy to demonstrate the difference between the two conditions by plotting progression-free survival (Fig. 38-1). It will be noted that progression does not occur in 80% of extramedullary plasmacytomas treated by local measures. In contrast, progression continues exponentially following local treatment of solitary plasmacytomas, and the majority of these patients progress to multiple myeloma. Progression to multiple myeloma occurs rarely with extramedullary plasmacytomas, unless the tumor invades adjacent bone.[91] The overall survival of extramedullary and solitary plasmacytomas of bone is similar because the former tumor occurs in an older age group, and deaths result from unrelated causes.

PATHOLOGY

Plasma cell tumors have a relatively uniform appearance in histologic sections, imprints, or in spreads of marrow and tissue aspirates. These preparations show sheets or lobules of plasma cells within a fine reticular framework and with a generous supply of small blood vessels. The plasma cell population often varies from small, mature cells, to larger cells with more cytoplasm, to more immature cells with a distinct nucleolus and multinucleated cells. In Wright-stained films, the plasma cell is round or oval, with an eccentric nucleus composed of coarsely clumped chromatin, a densely basophilic cytoplasm, and a perinuclear clear zone (hof) containing the Golgi apparatus. Plasma cells producing IgA often have a diffuse reddish tinge throughout the cytoplasm, and are known as "flaming" plasma cells (see Fig. 38-2).[95] Intranuclear inclusions, which stain positively with PAS and the

FIG. 38-1. Progression-free survival of patients with extramedullary plasmacytomas or solitary plasmacytomas of bone from date of first treatment. Patients who died from unrelated causes without any evidence of progression were withdrawn at the time of death, being progression-free. The patients reported in references 90, 91, 93, and 94 were combined for these progression-free survival curves.

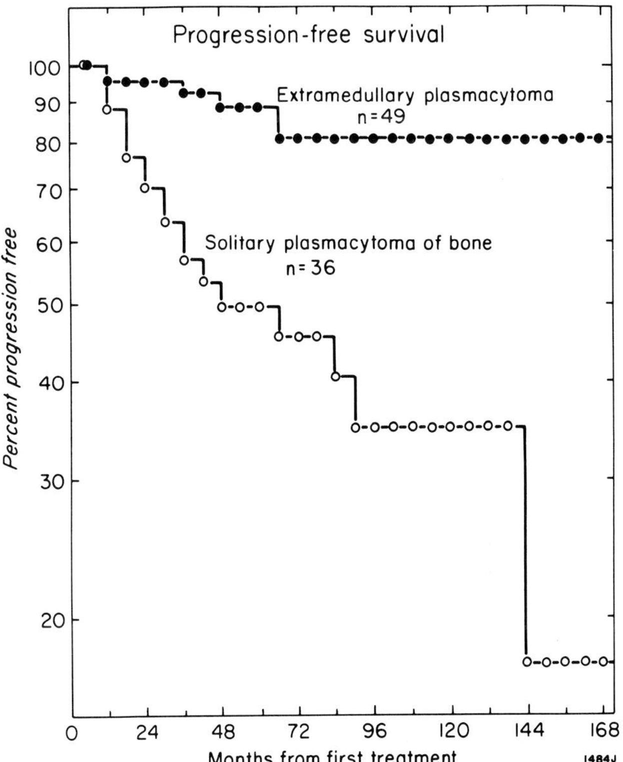

TABLE 38-4. Comparison of Plasma Cell Tumors Originating in Skeletal (Multiple and Solitary) and Extramedullary Sites

	SOLITARY BONE PLASMACYTOMA	MULTIPLE MYELOMA*	EXTRAMEDULLARY PLASMACYTOMAS
Number	114	290	325
Age (years)			
median	53	64	62
range	14–72	29–93	10–87
Percent males	72	55	73
M-protein in serum or urine	10/38	–	8/29
M-protein/tested	26%	98%	28%
Median survival (months)	114	30	192

(Adapted from Crowin J, Lindberg RD: Solitary plasmacytoma of bone *vs* extramedullary plasmacytoma and their relationship to multiple myeloma. Cancer 43:1007–1013, 1979, Knowling M, Harwood A, Bergsagel DE: A comparison of extramedullary plasmacytomas with multiple and solitary plasma cell tumors of bone (in press), Wiltshaw E: The natural history of extramedullary plasmacytoma and its relation to solitary myeloma of bone and myelomatosis. Medicine 55:217–238, 1976, Woodruff RK, Whittle JM, Malpas JS: Solitary plasmacytoma. I: Extramedullary soft tissue plasmactyoma. Cancer 43: 2340–2343, 1979, and from Woodruff RK, Malpas JS, White FE: Solitary plasmacytoma. II: Solitary plasmacytoma of bone. Cancer 43:2344–2347, 1979)

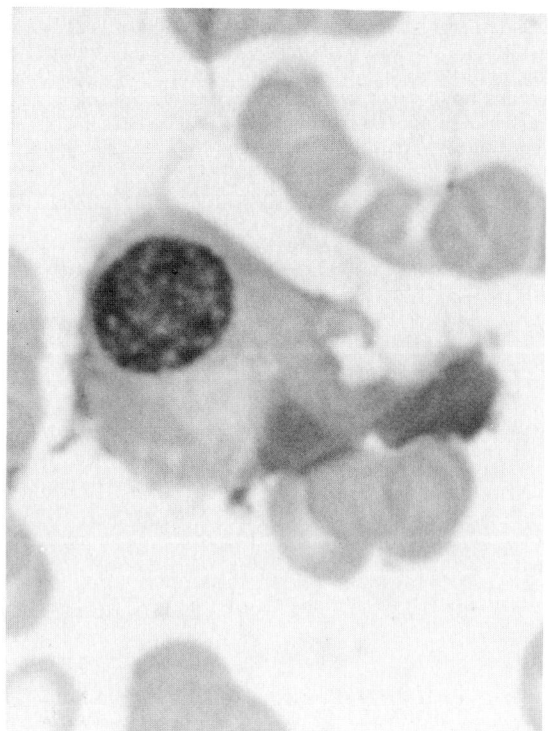

FIG. 38-2. "Flaming" plasma cell from the marrow of a patient with IgA/κ myeloma. Similar cells may also be seen in plasma cell tumors producing IgM.

Schiff method, are often found in plasma cells producing IgM.[31] The various types of cytoplasmic granules found in plasma cells, known as Mott cells, cells with Russell bodies, grape cells, and morula cells, all appear to result from collections of proteins in dilated cisterns of the rough endoplasmic reticulum.[31,96] Although these cytological features of plasma cells are interesting, and it appears to be possible to distinguish most cells producing IgA from other types of plasma cell, it is usually not possible to relate cytological features to the course of the disease.[31] Indeed, there are no cytological features that clearly distinguish benign from malignant plasma cells.

In multiple myeloma, the collections of cords of plasma cells within an open reticular framework are usually separated from an increased number of multinucleated osteoclasts in resorption lacunae lining the surface of bone by a thin fibrous membrane (Fig. 38-3).

Local amyloid deposits have been found in biopsies of the primary lesion from several patients with extra medullary plasmacytomas.[91,92] Tumors heavily infiltrated with amyloid frequently do not regress completely following local radiation therapy.

NATURAL HISTORY

The disease manifestations of plasma cell neoplasms are exceedingly variable. These tumors can appear in almost any site, and to the symptoms and signs caused by the tumor must be added those resulting from the M-protein produced

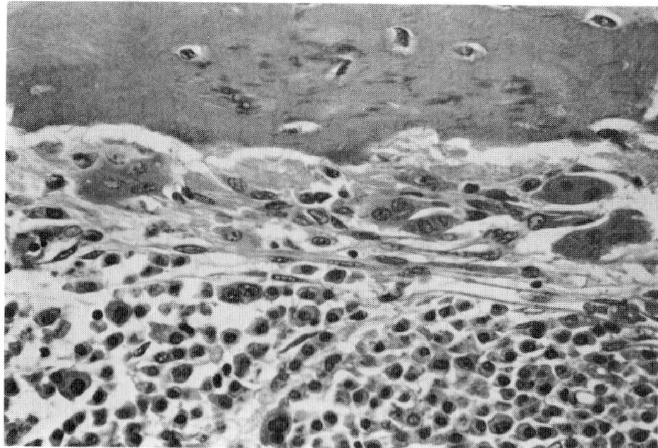

FIG. 38-3. Histologic section through a rib invaded by plasma cell myeloma. The lower portion, packed with plasma cells, is separated from the osteoclast layer by a thin, fibrous membrane. Note the numerous multinucleated osteoclasts in the resorption lacunae along the edge of the bone matrix.

by the neoplasm, such as hypervolemia, hyperviscosity, and renal failure.

At least 68% of patients present with bone pain, which usually affects the back and ribs and, less often, the extremities.[34] The pain is usually precipated by movement and does not occur at night except with a change in position. This is in contrast with the pain of metastatic carcinoma which is frequently worse at night. Persistant or localized pain in a myeloma patient usually indicates a pathological fracture. Other manifestations of acute or advanced disease include

TABLE 38-5. Investigation of Patients with Plasma Cell Neoplasms

1. Hematology: Hgb, WBC, platelets, differential
   marrow aspiration
2. Biopsy: solitary lytic lesion
   extramedullary plasmacytoma
   skin nodules
   enlarged lymph nodes
3. Biochemistry: calcium, BUN or creatinine, uric acid, alkaline phosphatase, total serum protein
4. Serum proteins: electrophoresis, measure (g/dl) M-protein and albumin
   identify M-protein by immunoelectrophoresis
   quantative immunoglobulin assay
5. Urine: measure 24 hour urine protein and creatinine
   calculate creatinine clearance (ml/min)
   electrophoresis of concentrated urine to determine the relative amounts of light chain, albumin, and other serum proteins being excreted
   identify the type of light and/or heavy chain by immunoelectrophoresis
6. Complete skeletal survey, including skull and long bones
7. Myelogram, if there is a paraspinal mass or neurological signs and symptoms of spinal cord or nerve root compression.
   Send CSF for cytospin, cell count, protein, glucose & chloride
8. Special: serum viscosity
   check for cryoglobulins
   plasma volume
   Congo red, rectal biopsy—search for amyloid
   check joint effusions for amyloid

weakness, weight loss, intermittent or sustained fever without infection, dehydration, confusion, and uremia.

Since plasma cell neoplasms are now recognized at earlier, relatively asymptomatic stages, minor diagnostic clues have become important. These include susceptibility to infection, an unexplained elevated erythrocyte sedimentation rate, rouleau formation, anemia, a reduced anion gap, transient skeletal pain, diffuse skeletal demineralization, and proteinurea without hypertension or an abnormal urinary sediment.

The diagnosis is established, using the tests outlined in Table 38-5. Thereafter, the course of plasma cell myeloma is far from natural. Many forms of treatment are available to relieve symptoms and prolong survival.

The course of plasma cell myeloma during treatment shows many similarities to chronic granulocytic leukemia. During the chronic phase, both diseases usually respond well to treatment with an alkylating agent, achieving remissions with a 1-log to 2-log cell-kill. The regrowth rate during relapse, as measured by the M-protein doubling time or the leukocyte doubling time, shortens progressively with each relapse (Fig. 38-4), until the terminal acute phase is reached. The acute blast phase of chronic granulocytic leukemia, and the acute terminal phase of plasma cell myeloma are both marked by marrow failure. This is shown in chronic granulocytic leukemia by anemia, thrombocytopenia, a falling proportion of neutrophils, and increasing blast cells. Myeloma patients develop anemia, neutropenia, thrombocytopenia, and a cellular marrow containing immature plasma cells. There is also an increased risk of a terminal acute leukemia.[29]

DIAGNOSIS, INVESTIGATION, AND STAGING

The diagnosis of a plasma cell neoplasm requires the demonstration of *uncontrolled* growth of a plasma cell clone. Evidence of uncontrolled growth is provided by the invasion of normal tissues by plasma cells causing osteolytic bone lesions, or plasmacytomas in extraskeletal sites. A progressive increase in the amount of a serum M-protein or light chain proteinurea provides additional evidence of uncontrolled growth. The criteria for diagnosis are:

1. Plasma Cell Myeloma. The classical diagnostic triad is

FIG. 38-4. A progressive shortening of the M-protein doubling time is shown for 3 IgA and 3 IgG myeloma patients during successive relapses. The ratio of the M-protein serum concentration at the indicated times divided by the initial M-protein concentration is plotted vs. time in days. The numbers associated with each curve indicate the doubling time of the M-protein in days. (Bergsagel DE: Assessment of the response of mouse and human myeloma to chemotherapy and radiotherapy. In Drewinko B, Humphreys RM (eds): Growth Kinetics and Biochemical Regulation of Normal and Malignant Cells. University of Texas Cancer Center, M. D. Anderson Hospital and Tumor Institute, 29th Annual Symposium on Fundamental Cancer Research, pp 705–717. Baltimore, Williams & Wilkins, 1977)

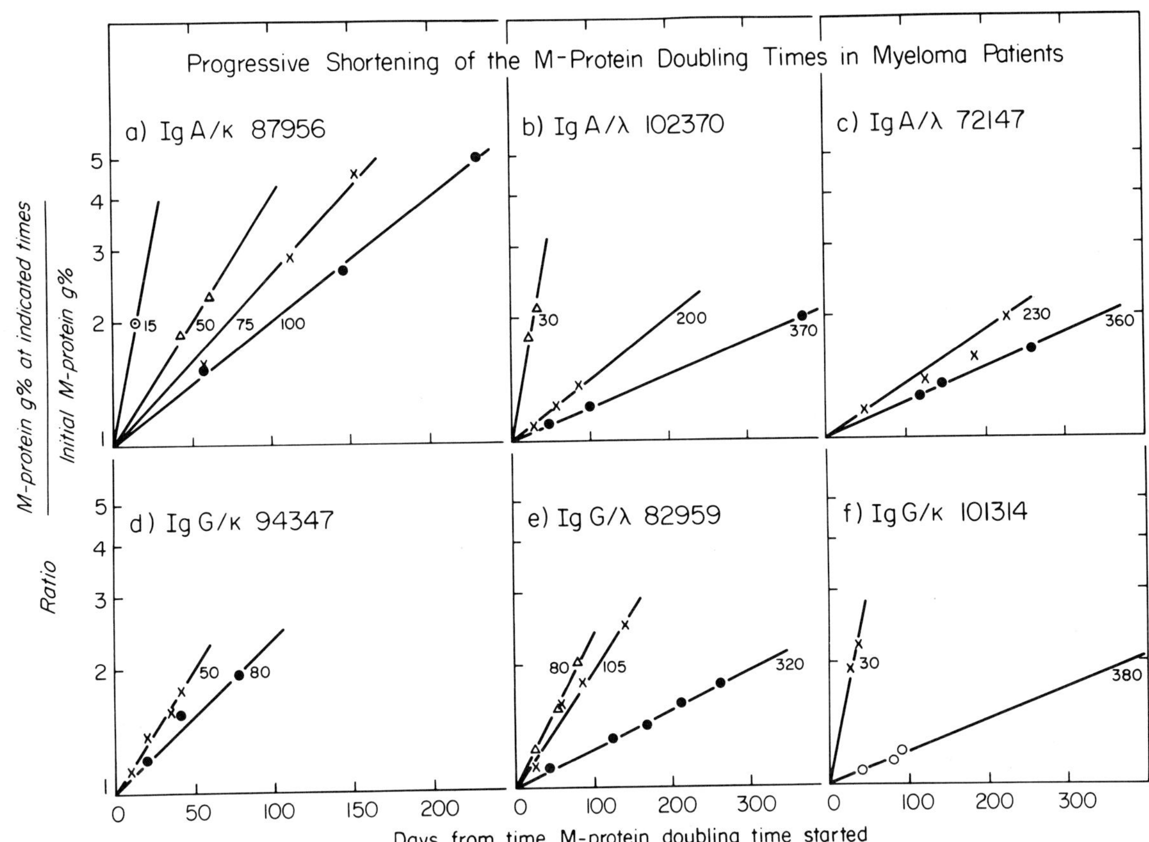

the association of marrow plasmacytosis of at least 10%, osteolytic bone lesions, and a serum or urinary M-protein. In the absence of osteolytic lesions, the diagnosis is also established if marrow plasmacytosis is associated with a progressive increase in the M-protein, or the formation of extramedullary plasmacytomas.

2. Solitary Osseous Plasmacytoma. A diagnosis is suspected when a *solitary* lytic lesion is discovered on a skeletal survey. The diagnosis is confirmed by a biopsy showing that the lytic lesion is composed of plasma cells, and a marrow aspiration containing less than 5% plasma cells. If an M-protein is found in the serum or urine, it should disappear following radiation therapy to the lytic lesion.

3. Extramedullary Plasmacytomas. These appear as tumors, most commonly in the submucosal lymphoid tissue of the nasopharynx and paranasal sinuses. Biopsy shows the tumors to be composed of plasma cells. Skeletal radiographs are usually normal, but direct invasion may occur into bones adjacent to the tumor. Marrow aspirations usually contain less than 5% plasma cells.

The clinical investigation of patients with plasma cell neoplasms is outlined in Table 38-5. With these tests it is possible to stage patients, using the criteria outlined in Table 38-6. This staging system was developed by correlating estimates of total body myeloma cell mass with certain clinical manifestations of the disease.[102] Patients with a high myeloma cell mass manifested one or more of the findings shown for Stage III, those with low numbers of myeloma cells satisfied all of the criteria listed for Stage I, while those with intermediate tumor cell numbers had intermediate values. Renal function is an important factor influencing prognosis, which is independent of myeloma cell mass. The influence of clinical stage and renal function on survival is illustrated in Fig. 38-5.

Serum uric acid levels have been suggested as another independent prognostic variable.[317] However, in this study only patients who had all of the 23 variables measured were included. Many of the patients who died early did not have all of the variables measured, and were excluded. As a result the overall survival of this group was unusually long, and the conventional prognostic factors shown in Table 38-6 did not appear to be important. Further study will be required before the significance of serum uric acid as an independent prognostic factor in an unselected population of myeloma patients can be assessed.

SCREENING

Sera from large numbers of asymptomatic adults, and from patients with a variety of chronic diseases, have been screened for the presence of an M-protein (Table 38-7).

The incidence of serum M-proteins is not elevated in patients with cancer, Hodgkin's disease or the nodular malignant lymphomas, but is increased in patients with diffuse malignant lymphomas and those with chronic lymphocytic leukemia. In the latter two diseases the M-protein is frequently IgM, and there is good evidence that it is produced by the neoplastic B-cell responsible for the lymphoma.

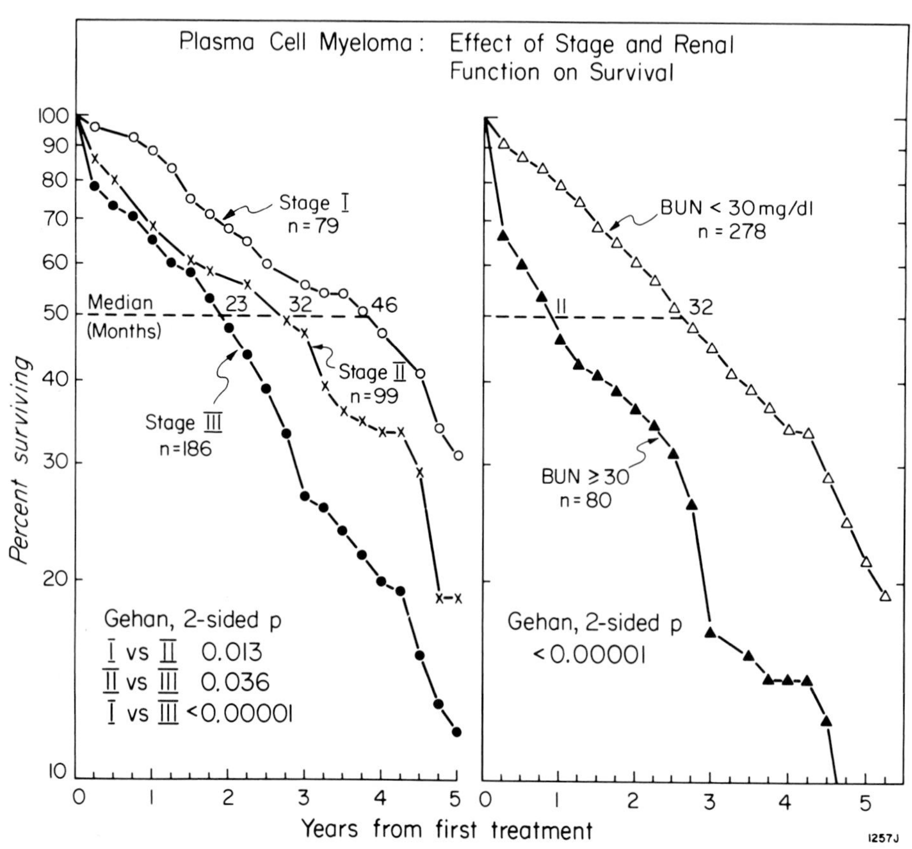

FIG. 38-5. Influence of clinical stage and renal function on the survival of patients with plasma cell myeloma. Survival is plotted from the time of first treatment. (Bergsagel DE, Bailey AJ, Langley GR et al: The chemotherapy of plasma-cell myeloma and the incidence of acute leukemia. N Engl J Med 301:743–748, 1979)

TABLE 38-6. Criteria for Staging Plasma Cell Myeloma Patients

STAGE	CRITERIA	MYELOMA CELL MASS (cells × $10^{12}/M^2$)
I	All of the following: 1. Hemoglobin >10 g/dl 2. Normal serum calcium 3. Normal bone structure, or solitary bone plasmacytoma 4. Low M-protein production rates: a. IgG < 5.0 g/dl b. IgA < 3.0 g/dl c. Urinary κ or λ < 4 g/24 hr	<0.6 (low)
II	Fitting neither Stage I or III	0.6–1.2 (intermediate)
III	One or more of the following: 1. Hemoglobin < 8.5 g/dl 2. Serum calcium > 12.0 mg/dl 3. More than 3 lytic bone lesions 4. High M-protein production rates: a. IgG > 7.0 g/dl b. IgA > 5.0 g/dl c. Urinary κ or λ > 12.0 g/24 hr	>1.2 (high)
SUBCLASSIFICATION		
	A. BUN < 30 mg/dl, creatinine < 2.0 mg/dl	
	B. BUN ≥ 30 mg/dl, creatinine ≥ 2.0 mg/dl	

(Adapted from Durie BGM, Salmon SE: A clinical staging system for multiple myeloma. Correlation of measured myeloma cell mass with presenting clinical features, response to treatment and survival. Cancer 36:842–854, 1975)

TABLE 38-7. Serum Electrophoresis Screening for M-Proteins

DIAGNOSIS	M-PROTEIN DETECTED	TOTAL TESTED	PERCENT
Asymptomatic adults			
Sweden > 25 years (19)*	65	6995	0.9
Minnesota > 50 years (103)	15	1200	1.25
Sweden > 70 years (21)	9	294	3.1
Cancer (104)	32	5043	0.6
Hodgkin's disease (105)	1	218	0.5
Nodular lymphomas (105)	4	292	1.4
Diffuse lymphomas (105)	27	374	7.2
Chronic lymphocytic leukemia (105)	17	266	6.4

*The figures in brackets refer to references.

The detection of an M-protein requires a careful investigation to rule out the presence of plasma cell myeloma, macroglobulinemia, amyloidosis, a malignant lymphoma, and chronic lymphocytic leukemia. However, it is uncommon to find an associated disease to explain the presence of an M-protein detected in screening studies.

The incidence of B-cell neoplasms in patients with M-proteins varies with the type of patient screened. B-cell neoplasms were found in 11 of 123 patients (8.9%) discovered to have an M-protein in five large series of asymptomatic adults.[20,21,100–103] In active treatment hospitals, where serum electrophoresis is often done because the presence of an M-protein is suspected, it is more common to find a B-cell neoplasm. The diagnoses associated with the presence of an M-protein in 1244 sera studied in one immunodiagnostic laboratory are shown in Table 38-8.

Most patients with BMG are not treated, and there is no evidence that starting treatment early for asymptomatic myeloma is better than withholding it until progressive disease is

TABLE 38-8. Diagnosis in 1244 Patients with M-Protein

	NUMBER	PERCENT
M-proteins with B-cell neoplasms	795	63.9
Plasma cell myeloma	632	50.8
Macroglobulinemia	45	3.6
Primary amyloidosis	31	2.5
Malignant lymphoma, diffuse	53	4.3
Chronic lymphocytic leukemia	34	2.7
M-proteins of unknown significance, with	449	36.1
Hodgkin's disease	11	0.9
Other leukemias	12	1.0
Cancers	72	5.8
Collagen diseases	53	4.3
Other benign diseases (including BMG)	301	24.2
	1244	100.0

(Adapted from Ameis A, Ko HS, Pruzanski W: M-components—A review of 1242 cases. Can Med Assoc J 114:889–895, 1976)

clearly evident. Thus, there is no known therapeutic benefit for M-protein screening studies designed to detect early B-cell neoplasms. These screening studies have produced a great deal of interesting information, but it must be recognized that the discovery of a BMG means a prolonged period of uncertainty for the patient and the physician who struggle to determine its significance.

DIFFERENTIAL DIAGNOSIS

The combination of osteolytic skeletal lesions, marrow plasmacytosis, and a serum or urinary M-protein almost always indicates the presence of a plasma cell neoplasm. However, each of these manifestations can be caused by several diseases, and there may be some difficulty in establishing a diagnosis when they occur singly.

Marrow plasmacytosis occurs in association with certain infections (especially chronic granulomatous infections such as tuberculosis or syphilis), cirrhosis, metastatic cancer, collagen diseases, and hypersensitivity reactions. In these conditions the marrow plasmacytosis usually does not exceed 20%, but there are exceptions. A reactive plasmacytosis is usually distinguished from a plasma cell neoplasm by examining the serum immunoglobulins. The occurrence of polyclonal hyperglobulinemia virtually rules out a plasma cell neoplasm, and favors a reactive plasmacytosis.

FIG. 38-6. Bony lesions in plasma cell myeloma. *A*, Typical "punched-out" osteolytic skull lesions, which healed after treatment with R-48 for 8 months. *B*, Myeloma patient with severe, diffuse osteoporosis and compression collapse of several vertebrae, especially L-5. *C*, Typical "punched-out" osteolytic myeloma lesions in a femur. *D*, Metastatic breast cancer in a femur showing a diffuse, poorly-defined osteolytic lesion and an osteoblastic reaction in the upper portion.

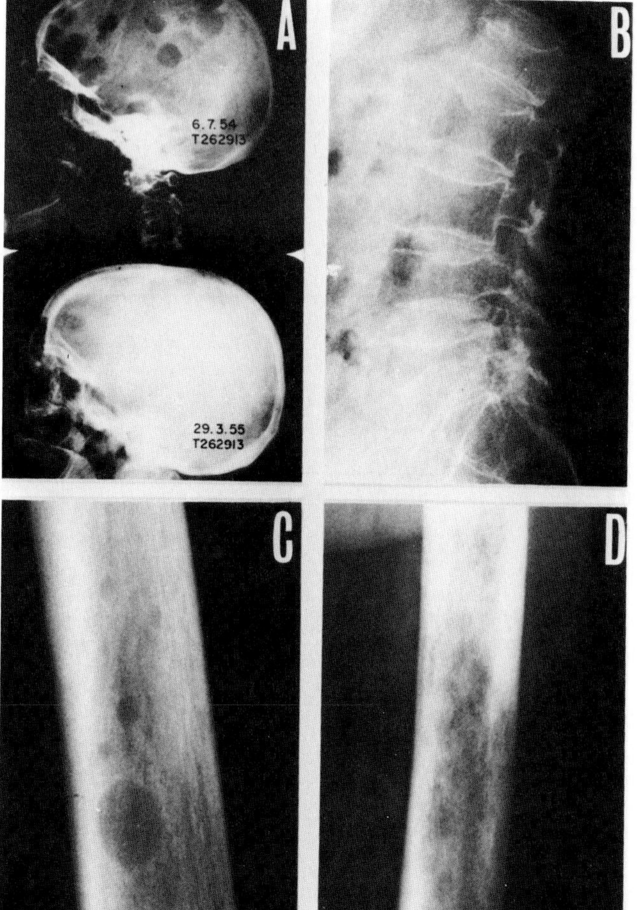

The occurrence of an osteoblastic reaction around the rim of an osteolytic bone lesion should immediately raise the suspicion that the lesion is caused by metastatic carcinoma, for plasma cell neoplasms usually cause purely lytic "punched out" lesions (Fig. 38-6).

Many diseases are associated with an M-protein (Table 38-8). BMG is difficult to distinguish from plasma cell myeloma and macroglobulinemia, because the differences between the benign and the neoplastic disorder are quantitative rather than qualitative. The major distinguishing feature of BMG is that the M-protein level remains constant.

Extensive proliferation is required to expand a clone of cells producing a homogeneous immunoglobulin to a population of 5×10^9 cells, capable of producing enough M-protein to be detected readily as a "spike" (approximately 0.5 g/dl) by serum electrophoresis. In patients with BMG, the proliferation of this monoclonal population appears to be controlled by some unexplained mechanism, because the monoclone expands to between 5×10^9 and 5×10^{11} cells, and then remains constant. It has been suggested that a serum M-protein greater than 3.0 g/dl, the occurrence of Bence Jones proteinurea, depressed normal serum immunoglobulins, or an increase in marrow plasma cells (especially when atypical multinucleated plasma cells are present) favors a diagnosis of plasma cell myeloma or macroglobulinemia over BMG.[109] However, alone, none of these features are sufficient to establish a diagnosis of a plasma cell neoplasm. In the absence of osteolytic lesions and plasma cell infiltrations causing soft tissue tumors, lymphadenopathy, or splenomegaly, it is usually necessary to follow the M-protein in the serum and urine of an asymptomatic patient for at least a year in order to differentiate BMG from a neoplastic disorder. If the M-protein remains stable for a year, the working diagnosis is BMG.[110] Thereafter the M-protein should be measured at least at yearly intervals in BMG patients, for at least 11%, and possibly as many as 20%, progress to develop a B-cell neoplasm.[88]

TREATMENT

GENERAL PRINCIPLES

The chronic phase of plasma cell neoplasms may last from 1 year to more than 10 years. During this phase most patients respond well to chemotherapy and derive considerable benefit from radiotherapy, supportive care, and encouragement. The acute terminal phase is usually short, and unresponsive to treatment.

An important initial objective is to relieve pain so that patients can be ambulated. Skeletal roentgenographic films are a useful guide in the choice of appropriate treatment, that is, whether to radiate lytic lesions or use chemotherapy for diffuse osteoporosis.

All patients should be encouraged to be as active as possible in order to avoid further demineralization and weakening of the bone structure. Simple lumbar corsets often help to relieve back pain by stabilizing the spine and preventing rapid rotational movements, which may precipitate microfractures and muscle spasms. Lumbar and cervical supports are required only until the back pain is relieved by radiotherapy or chemotherapy.

Pathologic fractures should be prevented by irradiation of large lytic lesions before the fracture occurs. If a fracture of a long bone does occur, it should be stabilized with an intramedullary pin and then irradiated.

Throughout the course of the disease patients must be encouraged to drink 2000 ml to 3000 ml of fluid daily to maintain the increased urinary output required for the excretion of light chains, calcium, uric acid, and other metabolites. All infections must be investigated and treated promptly.

EVALUATING THE RESPONSE TO TREATMENT

The tests outlined in Table 38-9 are used to follow the response to treatment. The most useful primary indices of response and relapse are measurements of the serum and urinary M-protein.

It is important to maintain a flow sheet (Fig. 38-7) throughout the course of the disease, recording systematically all relevant hematologic and treatment data, indices of the response to treatment and the clinical status of the patient. It is impossible to evaluate the response of plasma cell neoplasms to treatment, the status of the remission, or the onset of relapse without a quantitative chronological record of changes in the M-protein.

THE ONTARIO CANCER INSTITUTE
SUMMARY FLOW SHEET

white male, age 69
IgG/λ + λ in urine

Ht. 185.5 cm 2.14 m²

DATE d/mo./yr.	Wt kg.	Temp °C / P.S.	Hb g%	Poly & Bands / Wbc × 10³	Plat × 10³	M / alb (urine)	Prot. (urine)	Ca / BUN		SYMPTOMS AND SIGNS	Therapy XRT, Chemotherapy, Blood, Supportive
						g/dl	g/24	mg/dl		5x4cm Ⓡ clav. plasmacytoma. multiple lytic lesions skull, ribs, pelvis, vertebrae	
19 Aug 77	90.5	36.5/60	13.4	57%/8.2	360	6.2/2.5	2.0	10.4/32		Marrow - 45% P.C; Ccr · 28 ml/min. ①	Melphalan 18 mg × 4; Prednisone 100 mg × 4
26 Aug			12.3	67/6.6	330	4.7/2.3	3.7	8.8/61			
2 Sept			9.4	41/2.2	64						
9 Sept			8.9	52/1.6	80						
16 Sept	90.0	36/70	10.2	54/3.7	380	2.9/4.2	0.7	8.5/20		plasmacytoma not palpable ②	M - 18 mg/d × 4; P - 100 mg/d × 4
14 Oct	90.3	36.8/70	9.2	49/4.7	300	1.8/3.1	0.4	8.7/14		no pain ③	—"—
11 Nov	90.7	36.9/80	10.9	55/3.0	350	2.3/3.2	0.3	9.5/12		feels well ④	—"—
09 Dec	93.1	36.8/90	12.5	55/3.7	260	1.7/3.5	0.10	9.5/12		Ccr - 60 ml/min. ⑤	—"—
06 Jan '78	94.6	36.8/90	12.5	66/2.5	250	1.5/3.0	0.20	9.5/18		⑥	—"—
03 Feb	94.7	36/90	11.9	61/3.7	260	1.5/3.2	0.22	8.9/18		⑦	—"—
03 Mar	94.5	36.8/90	12.3	55/3.8	300	1.4/3.6	0.26	9.1/17		electroph. conc. urine - Albumin only. ⑧	—"—
31 Mar			12.5	68/3.0	174					in Florida ⑨	—"—
28 Apr	94.0	36.4/90	12.3	57/3.7	260	1.9/3.7	0.25	9.6/19		Skull - good healing of lytic l.	RANDOMIZED TO NO MAINTENANCE THERAPY
23 June	93.0	36.2/90	14.1	80/4.5	330	1.7/4.0	0.28	9.4/18			0
18 Aug	93.0	36.2/90	15.4	62/5.0	350	1.5/4.3	0.24	9.8/17			0

Diagnosis Plasma cell myeloma Clinical Stage III B
Initial sign or symptom, and date of onset back pain Apr. '77 Date of Biopsy 10 Aug 77
Other Significant Medical Problems:

75-44-69-R77

FIG. 38-7. Summary flow sheet for recording clinical, laboratory, and treatment information chronologically on myeloma patients. The synthetic index calculated for the serum M-protein concentrations have been graphed in Fig. 38-7 for the estimated myeloma cell-kill.

TABLE 38-9. Evaluating the Response to Treatment

1. Physical examination: record weight, temperature, performance status, symptoms, and signs.
2. Hemoglobin, leukocytes, platelets and differential—once weekly until an acceptable pattern of toxicity is established, then repeat only before each treatment.
3. Measure the M-protein regularly, every 1 month to 2 months.
   a. Serum M-protein—serum electrophoresis is more reliable than immunoglobulin assays if an M-peak is visible.
   b. Urine protein—grams per 24 hours. Measurement of the total protein excreted per 24 hours is usually sufficient, with occasional checks of the electrophoresis pattern to determine the fraction of urinary light chains.
4. Serum calcium and BUN (or creatinine) should be checked regularly, with a frequency determined by the status of the patient. Check the serum calcium whenever the patient mentions nausea, vomiting, polydipsia, somnolence or confusion.
5. If the initial creatinine clearance was decreased, this test should be repeated to evaluate the response to treatment.
6. Bone roentgen films should be repeated to investigate the cause of new painful sites. Skull roentgen films, at 6 month to 12 month intervals, help to assess skeletal healing.
7. Look for evidence of paraspinal mass whenever the patient complains of back pain. If a paraspinal mass is suspected, a myelogram should be done. Do a cytospin on the CSF and look for myeloma cells.
8. A marrow aspiration and biopsy should be done to evaluate the onset of pancytopenia. A hypocellular marrow suggests that the pancytopenia may be caused by treatment. However, if the marrow is cellular, pancytopenia indicates the onset of the acute terminal phase. Look for ring sideroblasts (a pre-leukemic sign), or an increase in blasts indicating the development of acute leukemia.

TABLE 38-10. SWOG Myeloma Response Criteria

A. Responsive patients who satisfy *all* of the following criteria are considered to have achieved definite objective improvement.
   1. A sustained decrease in the synthesis index of serum M-protein to 25% or less of the pretreatment value, and to less than 2.5 g/dl on at least two measurements separated by 4 weeks. For IgA and IgG_3 M-proteins, the synthetic index is the same as the serum concentration. For IgG M-proteins of subclasses 1, 2, and 4, the synthetic index must be estimated using the nomogram shown in Fig 38-7.
   2. A sustained decrease in 24 hour urine globulin to 10%, or less, of the pretreatment value, and to less than 0.2 g/24 hr on at least two occasions separated by 4 weeks.
   3. In all responsive patients the size and number of lytic skull lesions must not increase, and the serum calcium must remain normal. Correction of anemia (hematocrit >27 vol. %) and hypoalbuminemia (>3.0 g/dl) is required if they are considered to be secondary to myeloma.

   With equivocal data (e.g. non-secretors, or L-chain producers for whom the pretreatment urine collection was lost), the following support the conclusion that an objective repsonse has occurred.
   4. Recalcification of lytic skull lesions.
   5. Significant increments in depressed normal immunoglobulins, e.g. increments >20 mg/dl for IgM, >40 mg/dl IgA, and >400 mg/dl IgG.

B. Improved patients show a decline in the serum M-protein synthesis rate to less than 50%, but not less than 25% of the pretreatment value.

C. Unresponsive patients fail to satisfy the criteria for responsive or improved patients.

(Alexanian R, Bonnet J, Gehan E et al: Combination chemotherapy for multiple myeloma. Cancer 30:382–389, 1972)

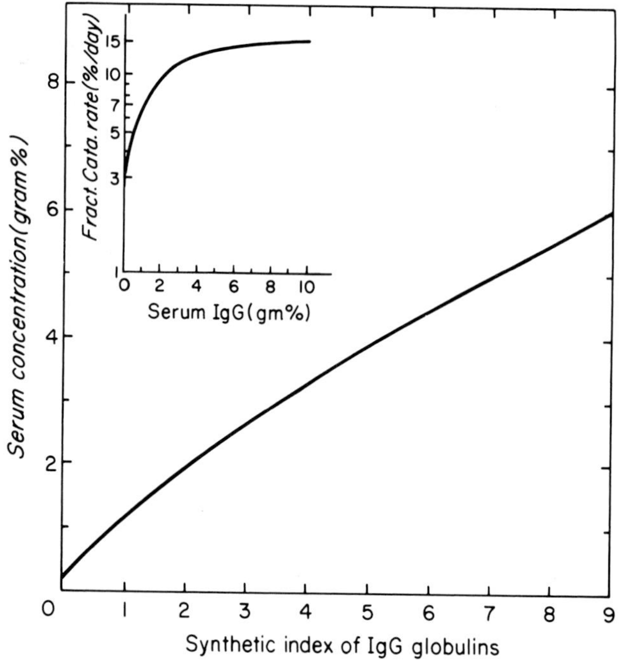

FIG. 38-8. Nomogram for deriving a synthesis index for IgG M-proteins of subclasses 1, 2, and 4 from the serum M-protein concentration. The nomogram corrects for concentration-dependent changes in the fractional catabolic rate of these subclasses of IgG and provides a better means of assessing changes in M-protein synthesis (and myeloma cell number). *Inset*—Relation of serum IgG concentration to the fractional catabolic rate. (Salmon SE: Immunoglobulin synthesis and tumor kinetics of multiple myeloma. Semin Hematol 10:135–147, 1973)

CRITERIA OF RESPONSE

An adequate definition of response is required to guide treatment and assess prognosis. The definition of response should include all patients with actual tumor regression, and exclude those who show non-specific improvement in symptoms, or indirect manifestations of the disease.

The Southwest Oncology Group (SWOG) have developed the excellent response criteria shown in Table 38-10.[111] In order to use these criteria, the serum concentration of some IgG M-proteins must be converted to a "synthetic index," using the nomogram shown in Fig. 38-8.[112] This is done because the fractional catabolic rate of IgG_1, IgG_2, and IgG_4 are strongly concentration-dependent. The fractional catabolic rate of these M-proteins increases from about 6% per day with a serum IgG concentration of 1 g/dl, to almost 15% when the IgG rises to 6 g/dl. Thus, as the IgG M-protein concentration falls, the fractional catabolic rate also decreases. As a result, the serum M-protein concentration does not fall as far as would be predicted if the fractional catabolic rate remained constant. For this reason Salmon recommends that when serial data for IgG myeloma patients are analyzed, corrections should be made for this concentration–catabolism effect.[112] If this is not done, changes in the total body synthesis rate for the M-protein (and tumor cell number) will be underestimated. This is an important phenomenom because IgG myelomas comprise about 50% of plasma cell tumors. These corrections are not required for IgG_3, IgA, IgD, or IgM because these immunoglobulins have fixed fractional catabolic rates which do not vary with serum concentration.

The SWOG has shown that the improvement in survival is related to the reduction in the M-protein synthesis rate.[111] Patients with M-protein synthesis rates suppressed to less than 10% survived longer than those with rates reduced to 10% to 24%, while these in turn survived longer than those with rates suppressed to 25% to 49%. A reduction of less than 50% in the M-protein synthesis rate was not associated with improved survival. It was also noted that the prognosis for patients who show a sustained rise in hemoglobin and albumin, and a fall in BUN, is better than for those in whom these abnormalities fail to improve. With these refinements it is possible to describe several degrees of response, with improved survival for the patients who satisfy the more restricted criteria. Patients classified as "improved" or "responsive" will also have an improvement in their performance status, gain weight, and have a marked reduction in pain.

ANTINEOPLASTIC THERAPY

Alkylating agents, radiotherapy, and prednisone are the mainstays of treatment. Many other chemotherapeutic agents have been evaluated in the treatment of plasma cell neoplasms, but most of them have not proven to be sufficiently effective to be used regularly. Successful chemotherapy relieves bone pain, causes weight gain, reduces the myeloma cell mass by 1 log to 2 logs, occasionally initiates skeletal healing, and improves survival. However, there is no evidence that the neoplastic plasma cells can be eliminated by the chemotherapy currently available. Thus, the treatment of plasma cell neoplasms is largely palliative, being directed at controlling the disease during the chronic phase and preventing death from complications such as infections, hypercalcemia, hyperviscosity, renal failure, and so forth.

ALKYLATING AGENTS

Many alkylating agents, including melphalan, cyclophosphamide, chlorambucil, and carmustine (BCNU), have been reported to produce objective improvement in 30% to 50% of patients with plasma cell neoplasms.

Most alkylating agents are equally toxic for resting and proliferating cells. In this respect, cyclophosphamide is unique, for regenerating mouse marrow cells are much more sensitive to this agent than are resting marrow cells.[113] Cyclophosphamide is schedule-dependent, producing greater anti-tumor effects when given intermittently than when given daily at doses that produce the same toxicity. This schedule-dependency may be partly explained by the fact that the drug becomes increasingly toxic for hematopoietic cells during daily administration as resting stem cells are drawn into cycle to replace injured cells. For these reasons, many chemotherapists favor administering cyclophosphamide in large doses intermittently, allowing marrow function to recover before the dose is repeated. However, there has been no clinical trial to determine the superiority of high-dose intermittent cyclophosphamide in the treatment of plasma cell neoplasms.

The dosage schedules commonly used for these alkylating agents are shown in Table 38-11. Although melphalan and carmustine are not schedule-dependent, the intermittent administration of these agents permits the patient to be seen at 4 week to 6 week intervals for blood counts, measurement of the M-protein, and a repeat course of therapy. Alternatively,

TABLE 38-11. Dosage Schedules for Alkylating Agents

DRUG	INTERMITTENT	CONTINUOUS
	The full dose is given for 1 day to 4 days, and repeated at regular intervals	After a *loading dose*, the drug is stopped until the leukocyte count rises to 4000/μl. *Daily* therapy is then started and adjusted to maintain the count between 2000–3500/μl.
1. Cyclophosphamide		
IV	1000 mg/M² (27 mg/kg) q 3 wk	
Oral	250 mg/M²/d × 4 q 3 wk	*Loading*: 10 mg/kd/d × 7–10 *Daily*: 1–3 mg/kg/d
2. Melphalan		
IV	Start 9 mg/M² (0.25 mg/kg) q 4 wk. Increase by 3 mg/M² until hematologic toxicity results.	
Oral	9 mg/M²/d × 4 q 4 wk. Increase until hematologic toxicity results.	*Loading*: 10 mg/d × 7–10 *Daily*: 1–3 mg/d
3. Carmustine (BCNU)	150 mg/M² IV q 4–6 wk	
4. Chlorambucil		*Loading*: 0.2 mg/kg/d orally × 21 to 42 *Daily*: 1–3 mg/d

daily therapy with small doses of the alkylating agent may be used.[114] Such maintenance therapy may require more frequent visits for blood counts. However, the same proportion of objective responses and the same prolongation of survival is achieved with low-dose continuous melphalan therapy as with the high-dose intermittent regimen.

When intermittent doses of melphalan or carmustine are used, patients should have blood counts done at weekly intervals after the first course. If the granulocyte count does not fall below 500/dl; or platelets below 70,000/dl, and granulocytes have increased to more than 1000/dl and platelets to more than 100,000/dl by the fourth to sixth week, the original dose should be repeated. The dose should be reduced if granulocytopenia or thrombocytopenia is more marked or prolonged. If the counts are too low for therapy to be repeated by the fourth week, the second course of the drug should be delayed for 2 weeks or more, until recovery occurs. The appropriate dose, causing only moderate granulocytopenia or thrombocytopenia with recovery, should be repeated regularly at 4-week to 6-week intervals.

The absorption of melphalan from the gastrointestinal tract has been shown to be erratic.[115,116] A dose of 0.25 mg/kg/day for 4 days usually causes some degree of neutropenia and/or thrombocytopenia. However, for occasional patients the total dose may need to be increased to 1.5 mg/kg to 2.0 mg/kg, or more, in order to cause marrow toxicity. The dose of melphalan should be increased until there is evidence of a response or hematologic toxicity. If there is no response or toxicity with doses of 0.5 mg/kg/day for 4 days administered orally, consideration should be given to using the intravenous form of melphalan. Intravenous melphalan is more toxic than oral melphalan. The initial intravenous dose should be reduced to a total of 0.25 mg/kg, and increased subsequently until moderate toxicity is observed.

Once the dose that causes moderate toxicity or a response has been established, it is usually adequate to check blood counts only prior to repeating the drug treatment, to be sure that cumulative toxicity is not developing. Some patients will develop a progressive fall in leukocytes and platelets following repeated courses of melphalan or carmustine. When this happens, treatment should be stopped until the blood counts return to pre-treatment levels, and then be restarted using longer intervals between courses of treatment.

Following a 1000 mg/m^2 dose of cyclophosphamide intravenously, the leukocyte count falls to a nadir at 10 days to 12 days, with recovery by 17 days to 21 days.[117] Blood counts should be obtained on days 10, 12, and 21 after a course of cyclophosphamide. If the granulocyte nadir is above 500/μl, and the count is near pre-treatment levels by day 21, the same dose is repeated. The dose should be reduced if the granulocytopenia is more severe than this. When the appropriate dose is determined, it should be repeated regularly at 3-week to 4-week intervals, with blood counts before each treatment. Cumulative toxicity usually does not occur with cyclophosphamide. The drug should be given in the morning so that most of the drug is excreted before the patient goes to sleep. Patients are instructed to take 2500 ml to 3000 ml of fluids to ensure the prompt excretion of the drug and its metabolites, and to minimize contact with the bladder mucosa. Patients who become so nauseated that they cannot drink adequate amounts of fluid should be hospitalized and given intravenous fluids. These measures are necessary to reduce the chance of developing cyclophosphamide-induced hemorrhagic cystitis.

The frequency of objective improvement following the treatment of groups of patients with plasma cell neoplasms is probably very similar for melphalan, cyclophosphamide, carmustine, and chlorambucil. Melphalan and cyclophosphamide are the most commonly used drugs, however.

The sensitivity of a plasma cell neoplasm to different alkylating agents may vary considerably. A mouse plasma cell tumor has been described which is highly resistant to carmustine, moderately resistant to melphalan, and very sensitive to cyclophosphamide.[118] It would appear that intrinsic cellular factors determine whether a cell will be sensitive to an alkylating agent, rather than the proliferative state of the cell or the alkylating function of the agent. Patients who have been found to be resistant to melphalan have achieved an objective response with high-dose intermittent cyclophosphamide therapy.[119]

Cyclophosphamide is recommended for the treatment of patients who present with platelet counts of less than 100,000 μl, or for those who develop thrombocytopenia during treatment with another alkylating agent. Cyclophosphamide is less toxic to thrombopoiesis than other alkylating agents, and thrombocytopenic patients are usually able to tolerate this drug better than other alkylating agents.

PREDNISONE

Treatment of patients with plasma cell myeloma with corticosteroids corrects hypercalcemia by blocking the activation of osteoclasts by osteoclast activating factor, and thus reduces bone resorption.[120] Treatment also causes a fall in serum protein concentrations, including that of the M-protein and albumin, decreases proteinurea, and produces a substantial rise in the hematocrit of some patients. The persistence of marrow plasmacytosis suggests that the fall in the M-protein associated with prednisone therapy may not be due to a direct, injurious effect on myeloma cells, but instead to the induction of hypercatabolism of proteins, resulting in a negative nitrogen balance and lowered serum protein concentrations.[121] Prednisone therapy alone, however, has been observed to decrease the size of a plasmacytoma in at least one patient, suggesting that this drug may have a direct antineoplastic action in some patients.[122]

OTHER AGENTS

Procarbazine has been shown to lower the M-protein concentration, and to lengthen the median survival of mice bearing the ascitic plasma cell tumor LPC-1.[123] In clinical trials, a lowering of the serum M-protein concentration to less than 50% of the pre-treatment value was observed in five of 36 patients previously treated with melphalan, but this improvement was not associated with a significant change in marrow plasmacytosis.[124,125] This observation suggests that procarbazine may have some activity against plasma cell neoplasms.

Adriamycin reduced short objective remissions in six of 32 patients who were resistant to other forms of treatment.[126,127]

The mechanism of action of this drug is markedly different from that of alkylating agents, and it has been tested extensively in various combinations explored by the SWOG. The results of these trials will be reviewed later.

Cis-platinum appears to be an effective agent in the treatment of mouse myeloma to date.[128,129]

Interferons are potent antiviral glycoproteins which have been shown to inhibit the proliferation of tumor cells in experimental systems. Interferon has been shown to inhibit the growth of neoplastic human cell lines in culture, and has induced objective improvement in at least 11 of 15 myeloma patients.[130-132] Excellent, long-lasting remissions have been achieved, with a fall in serum M-protein, improvement in bone pain, and weight gain. The major toxicity is fever, which has been attributed to impurities in the human leukocyte interferon. Other toxic effects, which may be caused by the inhibition of growth and differentiation by interferon, include leukopenia, thrombocytopenia, and hair loss. The biological mechanisms underlying the anti-tumor properties of interferon are unknown, but are of great interest because this substance is produced by normal cells. The effectiveness of human leukocyte interferon in the treatment of plasma cell myeloma is being compared to melphalan in a Swedish trial.

DRUG COMBINATIONS

The effectiveness of drug combinations in the treatment of plasma cell myeloma is shown in Table 38-12. The treatment results in this table are restricted to the reports of groups that use the SWOG criteria of response.

The addition of prednisone (P) to intermittent courses of melphalan (M) doubles the response rate but has little influence on survival. Combining procarbazine with M and P appeared to increase the response rate, but again, had little effect on survival. Further experience suggests that procarbazine contributes little in the management of myeloma, and it has been dropped from subsequent SWOG myeloma trials. The non-specific effects of prednisone, however, are so useful that it is now included in most therapeutic drug trials for myeloma. The addition of adriamycin (A) to MP or cyclophosphamide (C) and P, did not improve the response rate or survival.

The discovery that mouse and human plasma cell tumors, which are resistant to one alkylating agent, may still respond to another drug of this class indicated that different alkylating agents are not necessarily cross-resistant.[118,119] Furthermore, combinations of alkylating agents have been shown to be synergistic in the treatment of two murine tumors.[136,137] These observations stimulated clinical trials of combinations of alkylating agents in the treatment of plasma cell myeloma. The SWOG found that combinations containing MC, or MC and carumustine (B), did not significantly change the response rate or survival. Similarly, the National Cancer Institute of Canada (NCI-C) Clinical Trials Group found no advantage for the MCBP combination, administered either alternately or concurrently, over MP alone. In contrast, the Cancer and Acute Leukemia Group B (CALGB) found that MCBP significantly improved the response rate in several parameters over that obtained with MP alone, but did not improve the survival of patients.[138] The CALGB study of MCBP differs from those of the SWOG and NCI-C in that all of the alkylating agents in the combination were administered intravenously; the results were compared with the oral administration of M to the MP group. Since the absorption of M may be erratic, the improved response rate could be the result of the intravenous administration of M to the MCBP group in this study.[115,116]

Studies of the labelling index of myeloma marrow plasma cells before and after treatment demonstrated a marked temporary increase in the index after treatment with alkylating

TABLE 38-12. Combination Chemotherapy for Plasma Cell Myeloma

DRUGS*	GROUP (Reference Number)	NO. RESPONSIVE† / NO. EVALUABLE	RESPONSE RATE (%)	SURVIVAL‡ MEDIAN, (Months)
M	SWOG (111)	13/54	24	18
MP	SWOG (111)	67/139	48	21
	NCI-C (29)	40/100	40	28
MP + Proc	SWOG (111)	120/205	59	23
MAP	SWOG (133)	31/67	46	21–26
CAP	SWOG (133)	23/59	39	21–26
MCP	SWOG (133)	35/74	47	21–26
MCBP	SWOG (133)	34/70	49	~34
	NCI-C (29)			
	alternating	28/91	31	31
	concurrent	39/83	47	31
VMP + Proc	SWOG (133, 134)	64/127	50	34
VMCP	SWOG (133)	48/77	62	~34
VCAP	SWOG (133)	42/74	57	~34
VCMP–VCAP	SWOG (135)	–	–	$p = 0.05$
VMCP–VBAP	SWOG (135)	–	–	
MP	SWOG (135)	–	–	$p = 0.02$

* Abbreviations used are: A = adriamycin, B = carmustine, C = cyclophosphamide, M = melphalan, P = prednisone, Proc = procarbazine, V = vincristine.

† Responsive as defined by SWOG, i.e., ≥75% regression.

‡ Survival from the onset of treatment.

agents.[139,140] This observation led to the suggestion that an increase in growth fraction after treatment maintained the myeloma cell mass constant after an initial reduction of one to two orders of magnitude. Trials of cycle-specific agents were initiated in an attempt to destroy the increased fraction of proliferating myeloma cells occurring after treatment with an alkylating agent. In a preliminary trial, vincristine (V), caused a modest further decrease in myeloma cell number, and was selected for further study in drug combinations.[141] The SWOG was encouraged by a modest improvement in response rate and survival of patients treated with combinations containing V. However, as noted in Table 38-12, combinations that do not contain V have been reported to produce similar high response rates (e.g., MP plus procarbazine) and survival (e.g., MCBP).

A recent SWOG study allocates patients at random to one of three arms: (1) VMCP alternating with VCAP; (2) VMCP for 3 cycles alternating with VBAP for 3 cycles, and (3) MP. The doses of these drugs were adjusted so that they could be repeated at 3-week intervals (Table 38-13). At 2 years the response rates on the three arms are similar. The survival at 2 years for all patients receiving arm 1 ($p = 0.02$) or arm 2 ($p = 0.05$) is superior to MP. The superiority of VMCP–VBAP over MP was marked for Stage III patients ($p = 0.01$), but was also seen in patients with a hemoglobin greater than 10 g/dl ($p = 0.03$). For patients with an elevated creatinine, the survival of patients treated with VMCP–VCAP was superior to the survival with MP ($p = 0.02$). These combinations appear to improve survival by reducing the numbers of early deaths. It has been suggested that combination therapy may provide more uniform drug delivery, perhaps because oral M is known to have variable absorption which may reduce its toxicity and response. The results of this study are interesting, but longer follow-up will be required to confirm the early results.

The M-2 protocol for myeloma patients employed at Memorial Hospital in New York combines VMCBP; this combination reportedly produces a higher response rate and longer survival than MP.[142] However, certain factors make it difficult to evaluate the relative merit of the M-2 protocol. Patients treated with M-2 were compared with an historical control group treated with MP, and it is always difficult to know whether the historical control group is truly comparable. Furthermore, it is the practice at Memorial Hospital to follow asymptomatic myeloma patients without treatment until evidence of progressive disease develops. Myeloma patients called "asymptomatic," "stable," or "indolent" may not require treatment for intervals varying from a few months to more than 8 years.[143] In the M-2 study, survival was measured from time of diagnosis. The admission of a cohort of untreated, asymptomatic myeloma patients to the M-2 study would improve the early part of a survival curve measured from diagnosis. The size of this cohort has not been reported, but it is possible that it is large enough to account for the improved survival reported in this study. It is not possible to compare the results of the M-2 protocol directly with other studies in which survival is measured from the onset of treatment.

TUMOR CELL-KILL ACHIEVED BY CHEMOTHERAPY

The amount of M-protein produced by a mouse plasma cell tumor correlated directly with the tumor mass.[144] In humans, it is possible to evaluate the effectiveness of chemotherapy by following changes in the concentration of the serum M-protein. One method of estimating myeloma cell-kill is illustrated in Fig. 38-9. It is also useful to measure the amount of light-chain protein excreted in the urine per 24 hours to follow the effectiveness of treatment in a qualitative way, but it is difficult to use this measurement to estimate cell-kill quantitatively, because an unknown fraction of light-chain protein is catabolized by the kidney.[145]

A more sophisticated method for estimating changes in the total myeloma cell number is based on measuring the amount of M-protein produced per myeloma cell, the total amount of M-protein in the plasma volume, and the catabolic rate of the M-protein.[146]

Estimates by both of these methods suggest that the maximum tumor cell-kill achieved by chemotherapy is between 90% and 99% and this is followed by a plateau in which continued treatment does not reduce the tumor cell mass further.

If the improved survival of myeloma patients who respond to treatment results from the effect of that treatment on myeloma cells, one would expect to find a correlation between the estimated cell-kill and survival. The estimated myeloma cell-kill following treatment varied from $10^{-0.3}$ to $10^{-6.4}$, with survivals ranging from 3 months to more than 10 years. No correlation was found between cell-kill and survival.[98]

The results of treating a patient with total body irradiation are also consistent with the view that the duration of response

TABLE 38-13. Dosage Schedules for VMCP, VCAP and VBAP

DRUGS	VMCP	VCAP	VBAP
V-vincristine, IV	1.0 mg total	same	same
M-melphalan, PO	5 mg/M²/d × 4* (6)	–	–
C-cyclophosphamide, PO	100 mg/M²/d × 4 (125)	100 mg/M²/d × 4 (125)	
A-adriamycin, IV	–	30 mg/M²/d.1 (40)	30 mg/M²/d.1 (40)
B-carmustine (BCNU) IV	–	–	30 mg/M²/d.1 (40)
P-prednisone, PO	60 mg/M²/d × 4	same	same

* The recommended initial doses are shown. If these are well tolerated, subsequent doses are increased to those shown in parentheses.

is not determined by the cell-kill.[98] The radiation sensitivity of myeloma cells suggests that a dose of 225 rad would reduce the myeloma cell number by 1 log, and result in a remission of about 3 years. The administration of this dose to one patient caused the serum M-protein to disappear, and lytic skeletal lesions to heal; this excellent remission has now persisted for more than 9 years. It is not possible to explain the duration of this remission on the basis of the myeloma cell-kill expected from the dose of irradiation that was used. In addition, we have observed an unmaintained remission of 5 years in an IgG κ myeloma, and a remission in a Stage III λ light-chain patient which continues 7 years after melphalan was discontinued. Moreover, at least one long remission of more than 5 years has been reported following one course of melphalan in a κ light-chain myeloma patient.[147] It is difficult to attribute these long remissions to the myeloma cell-kill achieved with melphalan. The failure of maintenance therapy to prolong the duration of remission or survival provides additional evidence that these myeloma-response parameters are not determined by the myeloma cell-kill.[134]

The myeloma growth rate, as reflected by the M-protein doubling time, has been measured repeatedly on myeloma patients in unmaintained remissions.[98] A progressive shortening in the M-protein doubling time was observed. Most of the patients who progressed to an M-protein doubling time of less than 30 days also developed marrow failure.[97,148] This marrow failure apparently did not result from treatment, because the marrow remained cellular and the pancytopenia persisted after all therapy was stopped. About one-third of myeloma patients progress to develop marrow failure and die during the "acute terminal phase" of the disease.[29] The M-protein doubling time during relapse correlates strongly with subsequent survival; short M-protein doubling times predict brief survival.[98] The survival of myeloma patients appears to be determined largely by the time required for a progressive loss of myeloma growth control and marrow failure to occur.

MYELOMA REMISSIONS RESEMBLE BENIGN MONOCLONAL GAMMOPATHY (BMG)

In some ways the status of patients during the treatment-induced remissions resembles that of patients with BMG. The M-protein level falls progressively during remission-induction to reach a plateau, and then remains stable throughout the remission. The duration of this stable phase is not prolonged by maintenance therapy. Some of these remissions persist for unusually long periods. The persistence of a M-protein throughout the remissions and the demonstration that 12 of 24 remission marrows contained myeloma stem cells capable of forming colonies of plasma cells indicate that the myeloma clone persists but is controlled during remissions.[55]

In both BMG and myeloma remissions there are large monoclonal populations of plasma cells (greater than 10^{10} cells) that remain stable for prolonged periods. Myeloma stem cells capable of forming colonies of plasma cells are present in both BMG and remission marrows. Unmaintained myeloma remissions last for variable periods, from a few months to many years, with a median duration of 11 months.[149] A recurrence of progressive, uncontrolled growth of myeloma cells ends the remission in most myeloma patients. In contrast,

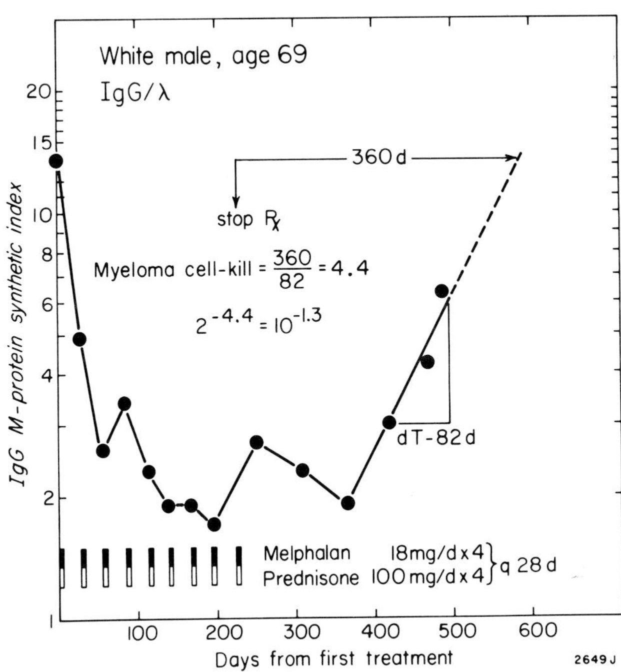

FIG. 38-9. Estimated myeloma cell-kill. The IgG synthetic index for the M-protein serum concentrations shown on the flow sheet in Fig. 38-5 are plotted against time on semi-logarithmic graph paper. The myeloma cell-kill is estimated by dividing the interval after treatment is stopped until the M-protein synthetic index returns to pre-treatment values (this is obtained by extrapolation of the early relapse rate) by the M-protein double time (dT). This indicates that nine courses of treatment inhibited myeloma growth by the equivalent of 4.4 doublings, or $10^{-1.3}$.

progression from the stable monoclone in BMG occurs definitely in only 11% and possibly in as many as 20%.[88]

RADIOTHERAPY

X-ray (roentgen) therapy (XRT) is very useful in the palliative treatment of patients who present with localized lesions, such as fractures, large osteolytic lesions in the long bones which may fracture, extraskeletal plasmacytomas, osteolytic vertebral lesions, and plasma cell tumors causing spinal cord or nerve root compression. The field used for irradiating localized lesions must be planned carefully so that all of the lesion is treated. Generous margins should be used in the treatment of osteolytic lesions of the long bones.

Tumor doses of more than 2000 rad in 5 days are rarely required to treat paraspinal masses or large lytic lesions. Smaller lesions in the ribs, vertebrae, or subcutaneous tumors are often effectively treated with a single dose of 800 rad. Solitary plasmacytomas in a bone, or in the naso–oropharynx should be treated more aggressively, with fields and doses designed to be curative. Tumor doses of about 3500 rad in 3 weeks are suggested.

Total body irradiation has been used successfully in the treatment of at least one patient, but is rarely practical.[147] The maximally tolerated dose of total body irradiation in one dose (225 rad–250 rad) would reduce the tumor cell number about tenfold. This is justified only if the patient is resistant to all alkylating agents, and has a slowly growing tumor, with an M-protein doubling time of greater than 3 months. If the doubling time is shorter than this, a tenfold tumor cell-kill would produce a remission of less than 9 months. We have observed only one good objective remission among five myeloma patients treated with total body irradiation.*

Wide-field irradiation can be administered in many different ways. Dr. Rider and his colleagues found that much larger doses of irradiation are tolerated if a period of 4 weeks to 6 weeks was allowed for marrow recovery between irradiation of the upper and the lower half-body.[150–152] The upper half-body can tolerate doses as high as 600 rad in one dose; irradiation pneumonitis is the limiting toxic effect, and becomes common with a single dose of 600 rad or more. The lower half-body will tolerate doses of 800 rad to 1000 rad in one dose. This wide-field irradiation can also be given in multiple fractions, using approximately 100 rad per day. We have treated four previously untreated myeloma patients with 300 rad to the upper and lower half-body, with a 6-week interval between each dose of irradiation. These doses were well tolerated with no significant hematologic toxicity. Bone pain was improved in all patients, but in none was there a significant change in the serum or urinary M-protein. All four patients subsequently responded to melphalan and prednisone with a significant decrease in the M-protein and additional improvement in bone pain. We have not used half-body irradiation as the initial treatment for subsequent myeloma patients, since the response was inferior to that achieved with melphalan and prednisone. Wide-field irradiation, however, remains a useful form of treatment for bone pain in patients who are unresponsive to alkylating agents, and have adequate marrow function. Half-body irradiation probably should not be used in the treatment of patients who have entered the acute terminal phase with pancytopenia.

Others have tested the value of half-body irradiation, and also report good pain relief.[153,154] In a study of ten patients treated with a single dose of 800 rad mid-plane to each half, nine patients experienced significant pain relief, and three demonstrated regression of the M-protein to less than 50% of the pre-study value.[153] In one of these patients, the M-protein disappeared and marrow plasmacytosis decreased to less than 5%. This excellent response persisted for 10 months, when the patient died of an interstitial pneumonitis, presumably radiation-related.

A TREATMENT PLAN

For most patients the initial objective is to relieve pain. Localized osteolytic lesions, paraspinal masses, and spinal cord or nerve root compression should be irradiated. However, pain associated with diffuse osteoporosis probably responds better to chemotherapy than to radiotherapy. If the serum calcium is elevated, intravenous fluids should be used to hydrate the patient.

Patients with platelet counts greater than 100,000/dl are started on intermittent courses of melphalan (0.25 mg/kg day for 4 days) and prednisone (100 mg/day for 4 days). If the patient is hypercalcemic, prednisone may need to be continued for a few extra days until the serum calcium returns to normal. Blood counts are done weekly, and therapy is repeated at 4-week intervals. The dose of melphalan should be increased until there is clear evidence that enough of the drug is absorbed to cause mild neutropenia or thrombocytopenia or the patient shows clear evidence of a response. Therapy is continued as long as the M-protein continues to decrease. It may be possible to suspend therapy after a satisfactory remission has been induced.[134] Patients who respond satisfactorily with a drop in the M-protein may show progression of the bone disease. For this reason, any new painful bony site should be examined radiologically, and treated with radiation if a lytic lesion is discovered.

If a patient treated with intermittent melphalan has, or develops, thrombocytopenia, or shows no sign of improvement after three courses of treatment, or relapses after demonstrating a response, therapy is changed to intermittent courses of cyclophosphamide and prednisone. Patients who still fail to respond, or who relapse on intermittent cyclophosphamide–prednisone regimens may respond to other alkylating agents such as chlorambucil or carmustine.

Patients are permitted to walk as soon as adequate pain relief is achieved, and are encouraged to exercise regularly. They are instructed to maintain a good fluid intake, and warned against vaccination.

*Unpublished data.

SPECIAL PROBLEMS

When should treatment be started? Asymptomatic patients with M-proteins should be investigated and followed carefully. No treatment should be given unless progressive plasma cell myeloma is confirmed as being responsible for the M-protein.

HYPERCALCEMIA

Hypercalcemia is present at diagnosis in approximately one-third of patients, and develops in an additional third during the course of the disease. The serum calcium should be measured in any patient who complains of nausea, vomiting, polyuria, polydipsia, constipation, or mental confusion. The hypercalcemia develops as a result of increased bone resorption stimulated by the release of an osteoclast-activating factor (OAF) produced by the myeloma cells.[155] Hypercalcemic patients are usually dehydrated, and fluid replacement should be started immediately, using intravenous saline. Prednisone blocks the activation of osteoclasts by OAF, and this hormone should be started immediately using doses of 40 mg to 100 mg per day.[120] Antineoplastic therapy with an alkylating agent, or other drugs, should also be started immediately to reduce the myeloma cell mass, and the amount of OAF produced by these cells. Prednisone should be continued until the serum calcium returns to normal, which usually occurs within 7 days to 10 days. The hypercalcemia associated with plasma cell neoplasms usually responds promptly to this treatment. Dichloromethane diphosphonate also inhibits osteoclast activity and reduces bone resorption in myeloma patients.[156] This agent may prove to be useful in the long term management of myeloma patients. (Additional measures to be used in the treatment of resistant cases are described in another chapter.)

The occasional serum M-protein binds calcium firmly.[157–159] These patients do not manifest the symptoms or signs of hypercalcemia, for although the total serum calcium is chronically elevated, there is no increase in free, ionized calcium. The occurrence of an elevated serum calcium in an asymptomatic patient should initiate investigations to determine whether ionized calcium is increased.

SKELETON

The increased bone resorption, described above, leads to two major types of bony changes: generalized osteoporosis, and more localized purely osteolytic, "punched out" lesions, with no evidence of osteoblastic bone repair at the margins.

The effects of generalized osteoporosis are usually seen best in the spine. The vertebrae lose much of their density, and compression collapse of the vertebral plates leads to the development of "fish mouth" deformity. With extensive demineralization, most patients complain of spasms of back pain, initiated by movement, and probably caused by microfractures of the weak bone structure. Treatment with an alkylating agent and prednisone often results in improvement in the back pain within 2 weeks to 3 weeks. Osteolytic vertebral lesions may be discovered by finding that a pedicle is missing (the "winking owl" sign).[160] Osteolytic lesions are more common than pure diffuse osteoporosis. Lytic lesions should be irradiated if they cause pain.

Strengthening of the skeleton is enhanced by ambulating the patient as soon as bone pain is controlled. Treatment with fluorides, calcium, and vitamin D have been used in an attempt to strengthen the skeleton. Extensive recalcification of bone has been reported in a patient treated for 22 months with 90 mg of sodium fluoride and 3.5 g calcium lactate daily.[161] However, a prospective clinical trial of the effect of sodium fluoride alone on the clinical course of plasma cell myeloma failed to demonstrate any beneficial effect.[162]

The administration of fluoride stimulates osteoblasts, but the new bone is poorly mineralized and osteomalacia, a fall in serum calcium, and secondary hyperparathyroidism occur.[163] The addition of calcium and vitamin D prevents the appearance of poorly mineralized bone in rats. Myeloma patients have been randomized to receive sodium fluoride (50 mg, twice daily) plus calcium carbonate (1 g, 4 times daily), or placebo, in addition to melphalan and prednisone.[164] After 1 year of treatment, microradiographic and video–densitometry studies of bone biopsies showed significant increases in bone formation and bone mass in the fluoride–calcium group. These changes could not be detected by technetium bone scans or roentgenographic films. The addition of 50,000 units of vitamin D twice weekly reduced the incidence of hypocalcemia.[165] It has also been suggested that the addition of androgens is required for maximal strengthening of the skeleton.[166]

SOLITARY PLASMACYTOMAS

If a solitary lytic lesion is found on a complete skeletal survey, and a marrow aspirate contains less than 5% plasma cells, the solitary lesion should be treated with irradiation. If the irradiated lesion is truly solitary, the M-protein should disappear from the serum and urine. The persistance or reappearance of an M-protein, or the development of marrow plasmacytosis following irradiation of an apparently solitary plasmacytoma, is an indication that the disease is more extensive, and that chemotherapy is required. Truly solitary plasmacytomas are uncommon, and most progress eventually to develop generalized disease; however, the survival of these patients is considerably better than the survival of patients who present with generalized disease (Table 38-4).

EXTRAMEDULLARY PLASMACYTOMAS

Three-quarters of these tumors appear in the tonsils, nasopharnyx and the paranasal sinuses. These patients should be investigated carefully with a complete skeletal survey, and special attention to the local involvement of bones in the area of the plasmacytoma. Marrow involvement is rare. Extramedullary plasmacytomas should be treated aggressively with irradiation, using fields and doses that are designed to be curative, and tumor doses of about 3500 rad in 3 weeks. The majority of these tumors are well controlled with local irradiation alone. In some patients the plasmacytoma regresses slowly. We have treated a patient with large plasmacytomas involving both tonsils and adenoids with 3000 rad in 14 fractions to the nasopharynx. The nasopharyngeal masses decreased for about 6 months and then remained stable. An IgG λ-M-protein decreased from 2.5 g/dl before therapy to 1.8 g/dl at the end of 1 year, and then remained stable. Two courses of melphalan and prednisone did not cause further shrinkage of the tumor masses, or any further decrease in the M-protein. Surgical removal of the tonsilar and adenoidal masses 20 months after the completion of radiotherapy resulted in the disappearance of the serum M-protein within 1 month, and the patient has remained free of recurrence on no further therapy for the past 6 years.

We have treated 25 patients with extramedullary plasmacytomas using radiation doses of 3000 rad to 4500 rad. Extramedullary plasmacytomas have recurred locally in two patients at 16 months and 17 months and in multiple extramedullary sites in one patient at 47 months after radiation was completed. Four patients have progressed to develop solitary, at 15 months, or multiple osteolytic lesions, at 24 months, 24 months, and 30 months; two of these patients were unusual in that there was local extension into adjacent bone prior to the initial radiation therapy. There has been no recurrence in the remaining patients. There have been 7 deaths, but in only three of these was death associated with a progressive plasma cell neoplasm. Thus, the prognosis for extramedullary plasmacytomas is good following radiation therapy, especially if there is no invasion of adjacent bone.

RENAL FAILURE

A unique form of renal disease, not associated with hypertension or notable abnormalities in the urinary sediment, occurs in approximately 50% of patients with plasma cell myeloma. Urinary tract infections and glomerular deposits of amyloid occur in a few cases, but the major cause of renal failure in myeloma patients is the tubular damage associated with the excretion of light chains.

The primary histopathologic changes appear in the renal tubules. DeFronzo and colleagues found marked tubular atrophy and degeneration in seven of eight myeloma patients with light chain proteinurea and creatinine clearance (C_{cr}) less than 50 ml/min.[167] Light chains are filtered and then reabsorbed and catabolized by the renal tubular cells.[168-170] The finding of positive κ and λ immunofluorescent staining within renal tubular cells and the frequent demonstration of protein-like inclusion droplets within tubular cells are consistent with this observation.[171-176] It is possible that the renal tubular cells are damaged during the process of reabsorption and catabolism of light chains, either by the release of lysozomal enzymes or by the direct nephrotoxic effect of the light chain. Renal tubular cell injury is manifested early by defects in the ability of the kidney to acidify and concentrate urine.[167] The incubation of renal cortical slices with light chain proteins inhibits a variety of tubular functions, including para-aminohippuric acid and organic ion transport, gluconeogenesis, and ammoniagenesis.[177,178] In some patients this tubular cell injury may cause specific defects in tubular reabsorption so that there is an increased loss of amino acids, glucose, phosphates, potassium, and other electrolytes in the urine (adult Fanconi syndrome). This syndrome may develop long before plasma cell myeloma is recognized, and has been found mainly in patients who excrete κ-type light chain proteins.[97,179] One of the striking features of the "myeloma kidney" at autopsy is the presence of tubular casts. These casts contain precipitated albumin, other plasma proteins, and complete immunoglobulin molecules, or only light chains.[172,180] Tubular casts were found in four of the 15 kidneys of myeloma patients biopsied by DeFronzo and colleagues.[167] Cast formation appears to be an end stage of chronic, progressive renal impairment. The glomerular filtration rate decreases progressively if tumor growth continues unabated. The increased load of free light chains must be excreted by fewer nephrons, and an increased intratubular light-chain protein concentration favors its precipitation with resultant cast formation.

Light-chain proteins can be detected in the blood of patients with marked renal impairment ($C_{cr} < 12$ ml/min).[167] These patients also excrete more than 1 g of light-chain protein per 24 hours. This high rate of light chain proteinuria may in part reflect reduced tubular catabolism secondary to progressive renal damage.

Renal tubular acidosis has been infrequently reported in patients with myeloma, but acidification defects are not often looked for. DeFronzo and co-workers found acidification defects in 14 of 35 patients.[167] This was attributed to light-chain proteinuria in 13, and to hypercalcemia in one. The renal tubular acidosis of one patient, who excreted λ light chains (with a normal serum calcium and normal creatinine clearance), resolved completely, as effective chemotherapy caused the light-chain proteinuria to disappear.[181] These observations suggest that renal tubular acidosis develops in myeloma patients as a result of a specific tubular defect caused by the excretion of light chains.

However, not all light chains are nephrotoxic. It is well known that some patients may excrete large amounts of light chains in the urine for many years without developing evidence of renal disease. In a series of myeloma patients excreting more than 1 g light-chain protein per 24 hours, eight had severely impaired renal function ($C_{cr}8 \pm 2$ ml/min) while the other three had well-preserved function.[167] Although the differences were not significant, patients excreting λ light chains tended to be at greater risk of developing renal insufficiency than those excreting κ light chains. These findings suggest that the nephrotoxic potential of light chains is variable and related in some way to the structure of the protein, and it is of interest that patients excreting only κ light chains survive significantly longer than those producing only λ light chains.[182]

When the primary lesion is in the distal and collecting tubules the proteinuria consists primarily of light chains, with albumin as a minor component. Glomeruli are usually not affected in myeloma, except in patients with an associated glomerulonephritis and in those with glomerular deposits of amyloid.[167] With glomerular lesions the proteinuria is nonselective, large amounts of albumin are excreted and the electrophoresis pattern of the urinary protein resembles that of the serum.

Other factors which may impair renal function include hyperuricosuria, hypercalciuria, and hypercalcemia with parenchymal calcium deposits, all of which occur frequently in myeloma. Dehydration is particularly hazardous in patients with severe disease and as a rule should be avoided in preparing patients for diagnostic procedures. Myeloma patients are susceptible to infections, and pylonephritis may occur. In late stages of the disease, plasma cell infiltration of the kidney may be severe enough to interfere with renal function. The plasma cells reported in the urinary sediment of 11 of 18 patients may have been derived from the circulating blood or from plasma cell infiltration of the urinary tract.[183]

Preventive measures are the best way to reduce the frequency of renal failure. All patients should be encouraged to maintain a high fluid intake to help excrete light-chain proteins, calcium, uric acid, and other metabolites. Urinary tract infections should be treated promptly, and antineoplastic therapy should be started as soon as possible. If the amount of protein excreted in the urine can be reduced, renal function will often improve.

When myeloma patients develop acute renal failure, as a result of an inability to excrete excessive amounts of light chains, there is an urgent need to reduce the load of light chains presented to the kidneys. Plasmapheresis is ten times more effective than peritoneal dialysis in removing light chains, and appears to be the most effective method for treating this acute complication.[184-186] Chemotherapy should be started immediately to reduce the production of light chains by the myeloma cells. If this treatment is successful, plasmapheresis will be required for a short period and renal function will be improved for as long as the growth of myeloma cells can be controlled. Successful renal transplantation has been reported for a patient with chronic renal failure that did not improve after effective chemotherapy; however, the indications for renal transplantation in patients with a lethal disease have been questioned.[187,188]

The clearance of alkylating agents from the plasma of patients with renal insufficiency has not been examined directly. In practice we have not found that it is necessary to reduce the dose of melphalan administered to uremic myeloma patients. This alkylating agent is not schedule-dependent, and repeat courses of the drug are given at 4-week intervals. Thus, even if the clearance of melphalan is delayed in patients with renal impairment, excessive toxicity is not observed. Cyclophosphamide, on the other hand, is schedule-dependent, and it has been our practice to reduce the dose of this drug until there is evidence that renal function is adequate to clear the drug and prevent toxic levels of the active form of cyclophosphamide from circulating for prolonged periods.

HYPERVOLEMIA AND THE HYPERVISCOSITY SYNDROME

There is a positive correlation between serum gammaglobulin concentration and plasma volume in plasma cell myeloma patients.[189] As the plasma volume expands, the hematocrit falls, and simultaneous measurements of the total red cell mass have shown that the apparent anemia is due to dilution.[190] In some patients the plasma volume expands to such an extent that congestive heart failure results.

The hyperviscosity syndrome develops when the size, shape, and concentration of a serum M-protein, or M-protein aggregate, causes a marked increase in serum viscosity. About 50% of patients with macroglobulinemia develop symptoms of hyperviscosity.[191-196] In addition, 2% to 4% of patients with IgA and IgG myeloma form unusual protein aggregates that cause the syndrome.[191,197-202] Symptoms usually do not develop unless the serum viscosity (relative to water) rises above 4.

The Sia water dilution test is a simple test for recognizing the presence of euglobulins. A drop of serum is added to a cylinder of distilled water, and if a filmy white precipitate appears, the test is read as positive. The majority of IgM proteins are Sia-positive.[203] In a series of 238 IgG myeloma patients, 29 (12%) had a positive Sia test, and of these, eight (27%) had elevated serum viscosity.[200] A positive Sia test is thus an indication for determining the serum viscosity.

Monoclonal IgG_3 proteins tend to form concentration- and temperature-dependent aggregates that are not encountered with other IgG subclasses, and to produce hyperviscosity at lower serum concentrations than IgG_1 M-proteins.[199,200]

The clinical hyperviscosity syndrome includes: (1) a bleeding diathesis marked by bruising, purpura, epistaxis, and bleeding from mucosal surfaces; (2) retinopathy with dilation and segmentation of the retinal and conjunctival veins (link-sausage appearance), retinal hemorrhages, and papilledema; (3) neurologic symptoms including weakness, fatigue, headache, anorexia, vertigo, nystagmus, transient paresis, and coma; and (4) hypervolemia, distention of peripheral blood vessels, increased vascular resistance, and cardiac failure.

Patients who develop the hyperviscosity syndrome require plasmapheresis; 4 units to 6 units of plasma should be removed daily until the relative serum viscosity falls to less than 4. Chemotherapy with an alkylating agent (melphalan, cyclophosphamide, or chlorambucil) and prednisone will often control the underlying disease, and should be given in an effort to reduce the production of the M-protein responsible for the hyperviscosity.

CRYOGLOBULINS

In patients with purpura that is precipitated or aggravated by cold weather, Raynaud's phenomenon, or cold urticaria, tests for cryoglobulins may be informative. Blood should be collected with a prewarmed syringe and allowed to clot at 37°C. The serum is cooled to 4°C to 10°C for several hours or days. Cryoglobulins settle out as a white precipitate or a thick, viscous gel on cooling, but redissolve completely on warming. Cryoglobulins are usually IgM or IgG proteins, but IgA M-proteins and light chains have also been reported to form cryoglobulin precipitates.[201-205]

Plasmapheresis may be useful to reduce symptoms of hyperviscosity, or to control excessive bleeding. Treatment with an alykylating agent and prednisone should be started immediately to reduce the production of the cryoglobulin.

DISORDERS OF HEMOSTASIS

A bleeding tendency occurs commonly in patients with macroglobulinemia and cryoglobulinemia, and occasionally in patients producing other types of M-proteins. These patients have bruising, purpura, retinal hemorrhages, epistaxis, and bleeding from mucosal surfaces. The platelet count is usually normal, but abnormalities of platelet function appear to be important causes of bleeding in these patients. Evidence of impaired platelet function includes: prolonged bleeding time, positive tourniquet test, impaired clot retraction, defective prothrombin consumption, poor thromboplastin generation with the patient's platelets, and defective platelet aggregation *in vivo* and adhesiveness *in vitro*.[206-208] Impairment of platelet aggregation and the release of platelet factor 3 appears to result from the coating of platelets with M-protein.[208-210]

Other abnormalities of the coagulation mechanism can be detected in some patients.[211] Some IgM proteins may interact with coagulation factors to inhibit coagulation.[212] The coagulation defect detected most frequently is prolongation of the thrombin time. This defect appears to result from the binding of the Fab sites of some M-proteins to fibrin during clotting and polymerization, thereby inhibiting fibrin monomer polymerization.[213] This results in a bulky, gelatinous, transparent clot with narrow fibrin strands and impaired or absent clot retraction. The inhibition of fibrin monomer aggregation does not necessarily produce a bleeding diathesis, however, unless there is a concomitant impairment of platelet function. Inhibitors of coagulation factors have been reported for a variety of M-proteins.[212] These include inhibitors of factor VIII (nonspecific inhibitors usually detected with the thromboplastin generation test), inhibitors of the prothrombin complex, factor V and factor VII, and factor X deficiency due to inactivation *in vivo* in patients with amyloidosis.

In addition, there are a number of patients who have reduced levels of one, or more, coagulation factors. Factors II, V, VII, VIII, and X and fibrinogen have all been affected. A clear explanation for the depression of these factors is not apparent. It has been proposed that the M-protein complexes with or coprecipitates labile coagulation factors.[214] With the exception of fibrinogen, the *in vitro* formation of these complexes has not been confirmed.[209,210,216] The formation of coagulation factor complexes in cryoglobulinemia could not be demonstrated.[211]

THE ANION GAP

The anion gap is usually calculated by subtracting the sum of serum chloride and bicarbonate concentrations from that of the serum sodium.[217] The anion gap was found to be reduced to 9.2 ± 0.4 mEq/l in 50 myeloma patients, a value that is significantly less than the 12.2 ± 0.4 mEq/l found in hospitalized controls.[218] The mean difference in the anion gaps of these two groups of patients was not great, but one-third of the anion gaps of myeloma patients were 6 mEq/l or less, whereas only two of 105 controls had such low values. An inverse correlation between the amount of M-protein and the anion gap has been observed.[218]

The anion gap is reduced in many myeloma patients because the M-proteins have a net positive charge, that is, they are cationic. The accumulation of these "unmeasured cations" results in the retention of chloride and bicarbonate to offset their charge. In addition, the serum sodium concentration is often reduced in myeloma patients.[219] The hyponatremia has been attributed to the displacement of sodium-containing water from serum by the non-sodium containing M-proteins. As a result, each liter of serum contains more solute (protein) and less water, thereby reducing the amount of sodium contained in a liter. The retention of chloride and bicarbonate, without a concomitant increase in sodium, results in a reduced anion gap.

Reduced anion gaps have also been reported in patients with benign monoclonal gammopathy.[220]

It is important to recognize the mechanism responsible for the low anion gap in patients with serum M-proteins. In our day of automated procedures for the routine determination of serum electrolytes, the discovery of a low anion gap should lead to the ordering of a serum electrophoresis, which may uncover an unsuspected M-protein. Myeloma patients with hyponatremia usually have no neurologic or psychiatric symptoms attributable to this finding, and no sodium replacement therapy should be instituted, for this could lead to fluid overload.

ANEMIA

The initial hemoglobin value was found to be less than 12.0 g/dl in 62% of 869 patients.[34] This anemia is usually secondary to myeloma, and the severity of the anemia is related to the total body myeloma cell mass.[102] The initial hemoglobin is an important prognostic factor.

As pointed out above, the low hematocrit may be the result of hemodilution. Other causes of anemia, such as increased blood loss, hemolysis, folic acid deficiency, and vitamin B_{12} deficiency should be considered. Folate deficiency is the commonest cause of megaloblastic changes, and appears to result from excess folate utilization by the plasma cell neoplasm.[221] The incidence of pernicious anemia in myeloma patients is much higher than would be predicted from the chance occurrence of two uncommon diseases. Between 1950 and 1960, pernicious anemia was present in 4.3% of all newly diagnosed cases of myeloma in Mälmo, Sweden.[222] Pernicious anemia has also been discovered in four of 22 newly diagnosed myeloma patients during a 6-year period in Bridgeport, Connecticut.[223]

Anemia may persist in some myeloma patients who are otherwise improved by treatment with an alkylating agent and prednisone. If the anemia is symptomatic and thought to be due to marrow failure associated with myeloma, a trial of androgen therapy is indicated. Treatment with fluoxymesterone, 15 mg to 30 mg daily by mouth, will raise the hemoglobin level in many of these patients. The response of the anemia to fluoxymesterone therapy is slow, and may not be detected until treatment has continued for 3 months to 6 months.

SUSCEPTIBILITY TO INFECTIONS

Infections occur commonly in patients with plasma cell neoplasms.[224–228] The increased susceptibility occurs early, and may lead to the discovery of a plasma cell tumor. Infections also complicate the course of treatment, and are the commonest cause of deaths.[29,34]

Patients with plasma cell neoplasms are especially susceptible to infections with organisms, such as *Streptococcus pneumoniae,* in which antibodies have a protective role. These patients usually fail to develop durable immunity to these organisms, so that repeated infections with the same strain of S. *pneumoniae* are common. Some patients are able to mount an acute, specific antibody response, but these antibodies appear to decay rapidly. Two or more episodes of herpes zoster infection have also been observed, and smallpox vaccination is dangerous because of the risk of generalized vaccinia. The incidence of infections with gram-negative organisms is also increased, but these are usually non-life-threatening urinary tract infections. The most serious infections in patients with plasma cell neoplasms (*i.e.*, pneumonias, septicemias) are usually caused by gram-positive bacteria.[224–229]

Multiple factors contribute to the vulnerability of patients with plasma cell neoplasms to infection; the most important is a defective primary antibody response. Secondary antibody responses and cellular immunity are usually well preserved in untreated patients.[225,230]

The mechanisms responsible for the failure of the primary immune response are complex, and probably multifactorial. The ability of peripheral blood lymphocytes from myeloma patients to respond to pokeweed mutogen (PWM) stimulation with the production of normal immunoglobulins is greatly impaired. Circulating mononuclear cells capable of suppressing the response of co-cultured normal lymphocytes to PWM were found in the blood of three of six myeloma patients, and the removal of these cells enhanced the normal immunoglobulin synthesis response of lymphocytes from myeloma patients.[231] The inhibitory effects may be mediated by a low molecular weight immunosuppressive factor produced by the suppressor macrophages.[232]

Another interesting mechanism has been investigated by Heller and his colleagues.[233] They found that lymphocytes, bearing surface immunoglobulin (S Ig) with the ideotype of the myeloma protein, appeared in the peripheral blood of BALB/c mice 72 hours after the subcutaneous implantation of a plasma cell tumor. The population of monoclonal lymphocytes increased rapidly to reach a plateau at 7 days to 10 days. The possibilities that passive absorption or binding of the M-protein to Fc receptors on the lymphocytes were excluded by showing that the same S Ig was synthesized by the lymphocyte after the original S Ig was removed with trypsin. It was possible to extract and purify RNA from mouse plasmacytomas which induced normal mouse lymphocytes to produce S Ig with the same ideotype as the M-protein of the plasmacytoma ("S Ig conversion"). Furthermore, a cold phenol extract of the plasma of several myeloma patients has been shown to have an RNA-containing factor which is capable of converting the S Ig of normal human lymphocytes to S Ig with the M-protein ideotype.[234] The hypothesis is that an RNA-containing factor is released from plasma cell tumors, perhaps during cell turnover, which impairs the immunologic effectiveness of lymphocytes by causing "S Ig conversion." The same factor may stimulate suppressor macrophages to inhibit normal antibody production.

Defective neutrophil function may also play a role in making patients with plasma cell neoplasms susceptible to infections. Neutropenia occurs as a result of disease-related and treatment-induced causes. Impaired neutrophil function, demonstrated by defective neutrophil adherence to nylon fibers, and the delayed appearance of neutrophils in skin windows in myeloma patients, may be important.[235,236] Impaired neutrophil adherence in myeloma patients appears to be caused by a plasma factor which is not the M-protein, for it is present in plasma and absent from serum.[236] The significance of this abnormal leukocyte function is not clear since patients with poor neutrophil adherence did not have an increased incidence of infection.[236]

An important aspect of treatment is the prompt and urgent investigation and treatment of every febrile episode. Cultures should be obtained from the blood, sputum, urine, skin lesions, and other possible sites of infection. Since the risk of septicemia is great, treatment is usually started before the culture results are available. Serious infections should be treated with a combination of cephalosporin and an aminoglycoside, to cover infections with penicillin-sensitive and -resistant bacteria and gram-negative organisms, with appropriate attention to renal function and nephrotoxicity. Prophylactic long-acting penicillin (benzanthine penicillin G) should be considered for pneumococcal, meningeococcal, and gonococcal infections, because repeated infections with these organisms tend to occur. Prophylactic gammaglobulin, given in conventional doses IM to a random group of myeloma patients, did not reduce the frequency, or severity, of infections.[237]

Patients with plasma cell neoplasms should not be vaccinated with a live organism (*e.g.*, vaccinia), because of the danger of a generalized viral infection. Although many patients have defective primary antibody responses, some are capable of mounting an acute, and possibly temporary response, to meningeococcal and pneumococcal infections.[229] This observation suggests that the role of vaccination against pneumococcal and other bacterial pathogens should be explored in patients with plasma cell neoplasms.

AMYLOIDOSIS

Immunoglobulin-related (primary) amyloidosis has been recognized with increasing frequency in patients with plasma cell neoplasms because of wider use of tissue biopsies and the intensive search for an M-protein in the serum and urine of patients with primary amyloidosis. The majority of patients who present with primary amyloidosis, and no evidence of a plasma cell neoplasm will have one, or more, of the following recognized, if they are followed long enough: a light chain protein in the urine, a serum M-protein, or marrow plasmacytosis.[238]

Most amyloid fibrils are composed of two major types of protein, occurring singly or in combination.[239] In the amyloid associated with plasma cell neoplasms, the major, and often the only protein consists of fragments of immunoglobulin light chains. This heterogeneous group of proteins are now called AL (amyloid L-chain) protein. All light chains do not form amyloid, and the special properties and circumstances required for the formation of amyloid have not been described yet. However, lambda light chains are more likely to form amyloid than kappa light chains. The κ:λ ratio in M-proteins associated with amyloidosis approaches 3:5, in striking contrast to the 3:2 ratio for M-proteins not associated with amyloid.[240] Amyloid fibrils from patients with secondary amyloidosis and certain familial forms, such as familial Mediterranean fever, consist primarily of another protein known as the AA (amyloid A) protein. This protein is not related to any known immunoglobulin. AA protein is believed to be derived from a larger, antigenically-related protein known as SAA (serum amyloid A) protein.

The evidence that AL protein is derived from light chains is based on three types of studies. The first, and clearest evidence, was the demonstration of sequence homologies between amyloid fibrils and light chains.[11] Second, proteolytic digestion of some, but not all, light-chain proteins results in the formation of fibrils that resemble amyloid fibrils.[241,242] Thirdly, there is the observation that antisera to amyloid subunits cross-react with κ- or λ-light chains.[243]

Immunoglobulin-related amyloidosis generally involves the tongue, heart, skeletal muscle, skin, ligaments, and gastrointestinal tract. Other organs, typically affected in secondary amyloidosis, are also frequently infiltrated with immunoglobulin-related amyloid. Thus, the kidney, spleen, liver, and endocrine glands are often involved.

These patients often present with macroglossia, carpal tunnel syndrome with median nerve compression, an arthropathy caused by periarticular or synovial amyloid, a sensorimotor peripheral neuropathy, occasionally autonomic nerve dysfunction, and generalized lymphadenopathy.[238,244–247] Amyloid can infiltrate all sections of the gastrointestinal tract, resulting in obstruction, hemorrhage, diarrhea, malabsorption, protein-losing enteropathy, or simply disturbances in motility.[248] Gastrointestinal blood loss appears to be caused by amyloid infiltrates in the walls of blood vessels, with erosion and bleeding.[244,249] Impaired gastrointestinal motility may be due to patchy amyloid infiltrates in smooth muscle, but impaired autonomic nerve function as a result of amyloid infiltration of these nerves, or infiltrates in the blood vessels supplying the nerves are also important.[250] Pulmonary amyloidosis can produce three forms: a mass simulating a tumor, nodular deposits throughout the tracheo–bronchial tree, and a diffuse reticulonodular parenchymal infiltrate involving the alveolar septa. In the last form, the amyloid is deposited in the walls of blood vessels and may extend into the interstitial spaces.[251] Amyloidosis of the heart may cause conduction defects and arrythmias, coronary insufficiency, and murmurs as a result of stiffening of the myocardium. Cardiomegaly, associated with cardiac failure, often results. The stiff, enlarged, poorly contractile heart physiologically resembles constrictive pericarditis. Treatment with digitalis may result in serious arrythmias, and is usually of little help in improving cardiac contractility.[238,244,252–254]

Renal involvement is seen with deposits of amyloid in the blood vessels of the glomerulus, which leads to damage to the glomerular basement membrane and non-selective proteinurea. The occurrence of the nephrotic syndrome and non-selective proteinuria in a patient with a plasma cell neoplasm should trigger a search for amyloidosis. It should be noted that liver biopsies in patients with amyloidosis are frequently complicated by excessive bleeding, and should not be attempted, while percutaneous needle biopsy of the kidney is not considered to be hazardous.[255]

The treatment of immunoglobulin-related amyloidosis should be directed against the underlying plasma cell neoplasm. If this treatment causes tumor regression, the growth of amyloid deposits will at least be slowed and, in some, clinical improvement may occur. A review of 16 cases treated with melphalan with, or without, added prednisone or penicillamine or both, showed that 12 achieved a partial remission. There was a marked reduction in proteinuria in 11, and regression of amyloid-containing lymph nodes in one.[265–263] In addition to reduced proteinuria, one patient had regression of amyloid infiltrates of the skin and gastrointestinal mucosa and improvement in a peripheral neuropathy, and another had improvement in hepatic and cardiac function.[261,263] However, most of these remissions are only partial, for amyloid deposits usually do not disappear completely.

NEUROLOGIC SYNDROMES

A variety of neurologic signs and symptoms can develop in patients with plasma cell neoplasms (Table 38-14). Hypercalcemia is common, and should be suspected whenever a patient mentions polyuria, polydipsia, nausea, vomiting, or constipation. Lethargy and mental obtundation occur in most patients, but progression to coma is rare. Patients with the hyperviscosity syndrome complain of fatigue, headache, and visual disturbances. These patients often think and respond sluggishly. A history of epistaxis, and the finding of cardiomegaly, distended veins, or retinopathy, should trigger the measurement of serum viscosity and appropriate treatment. Although "coma paraproteinemicum" has been described, it must be rare now that the symptoms of severe hyperviscosity can be relieved promptly by plasmapheresis.[264]

Spinal cord and nerve root compression is common. In 1963 it was reported to occur in about one-third of myeloma patients, but in recent years the incidence appears to have decreased to about 10%, possibly as a result of earlier diagnosis, more effective treatment of the underlying disease, and an increased awareness of potential neurologic involvement.[265,266] The plasma cell tumor often originates in a rib, or vertebra, forming a tumor which invades the spinal canal through an intervertebral foramina and causes extradural compression. The detection of a paraspinal mass is an early warning sign that a patient is at risk of developing cord compression (Fig. 38-10). Roentgenograms of the total spinal column should be obtained as part of the initial evaluation of all patients with plasma cell neoplasms and checked specifically for the presence of a paraspinal mass and destructive lesions of vertebrae. A myelogram should be done if a paraspinal mass is seen, for it is frequently possible to detect myelogram defects in these patients before any neurologic symptoms or signs become manifest. The ideal time to treat these patients with radiation therapy is before neurologic complications develop.

Early recognition of spinal cord compression is the key to successful treatment (see Chapter 42). Remember that sensory and motor loss, loss of sphincter control, and paraplegia are late signs. Radicular pain, usually well localized to a dermatome, and aggravated by coughing, sneezing, or straining, is a common early sign.

TABLE 38-14. Neurologic Manifestations Associated with Plasma Cell Neoplasms

1. Hypercalcemia	Lethargy, severe muscle weakness, anxiety, depression, mental obtundation, coma
2. Hyperviscosity	Headache, fatigue, visual disturbances, retinopathy, mental obtundation, coma.
3. Spinal cord and/or nerve root compression	Paraspinal mass, radicular pain, sensory loss, muscle weakness, loss of bladder control, paraplegia. Level determined by sensory loss and myelogram. Cranial nerves may be involved by tumors at base of skull.
4. Myelomatous meningitis	CSF contains plasma cells and increased protein. May also have spinal cord and nerve root compression.
5. Peripheral neuropathies	a. Amyloid-related (1) Carpal tunnel syndrome, with compression of the median nerve. (ii) Diffuse sensorimotor polyneuropathy caused by amyloid deposits in nerve fibers or perineural blood vessels. b. Diffuse sensorimotor polyneuropathy with increased CSF protein.
6. Cerebral plasmacytomas	Direct invasion of CNS rare, but may cause seizures and focal signs.
7. Viral infections	a. Herpes zoster b. Multifocal leukoencephalopathy

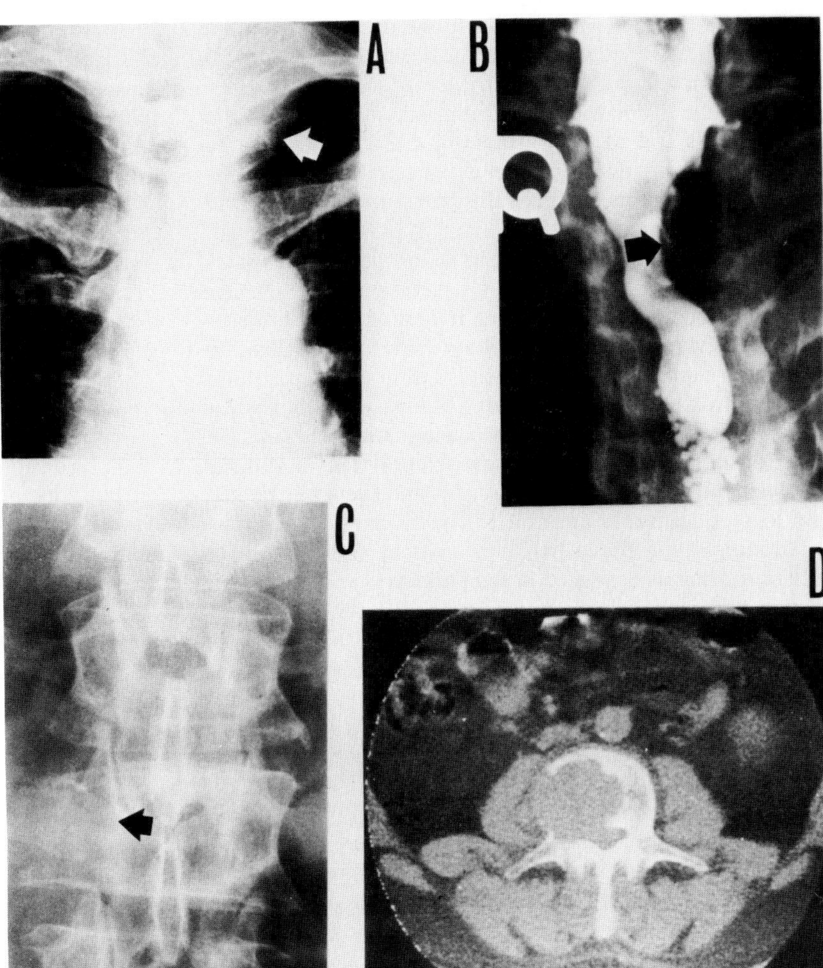

FIG. 38-10. Spinal cord compression in patients with plasma cell myeloma. *A*, A destructive plasma cell tumor in a rib has caused the formation of a paraspinal mass, visible just above the left clavicle on a chest radiograph. *B*, A myelogram shows that this plasma cell tumor has invaded the spinal canal through an intervertebral foramen and is causing extradural spinal cord compression. *C*, Lumbar vertebrae showing loss of the right pedicle of L-5, as indicated by a *black arrow* (the "winking-owl" sign). *D*, CT of L-2 shows destruction of the body of L-2 and invasion of the spinal canal.

Patients suspected of having spinal cord compression should have a myelogram done immediately to confirm the diagnosis, to demonstrate the extent of involvement if there is only partial obstruction, or to show the lower border, if the obstruction is complete. The radiopaque dye should be left in the subarachnoid space, so that follow-up studies can be done to check the response to treatment, and to make sure that the upper margin of the tumor was covered by the radiation field.

The CSF should be examined. A cytospin preparation will often contain plasma cells, but the total cell count is usually low (Fig. 38-11). The plasma cells should disappear from the CSF following radiation therapy. The CSF protein may be elevated, and frequently contains the M-protein. The presence of the M-protein in the CSF is difficult to explain when there are no plasma cells in the subarachnoid space (how does the M-protein cross the blood: CSF barrier?), but has little clinical significance. An M-protein was demonstrated by immunoelectrophoresis in the CSF of 16 of 20 unselected myeloma patients with a serum M-protein but no signs of spinal cord or nerve root compression.[267]

Plasma cell neoplasms usually regress promptly following radiation therapy. Decompression laminectomy is required only if the diagnosis is in doubt. Patients should be started on high-dose corticosteroids (*e.g.*, prednisone 100 mg/day), to reduce the risk of having post-irradiation edema cause further

FIG. 38-11. Plasma cells in a cytospin of a cerebrospinal fluid containing eight nucleated cells per μl from a patient with plasma cell myeloma.

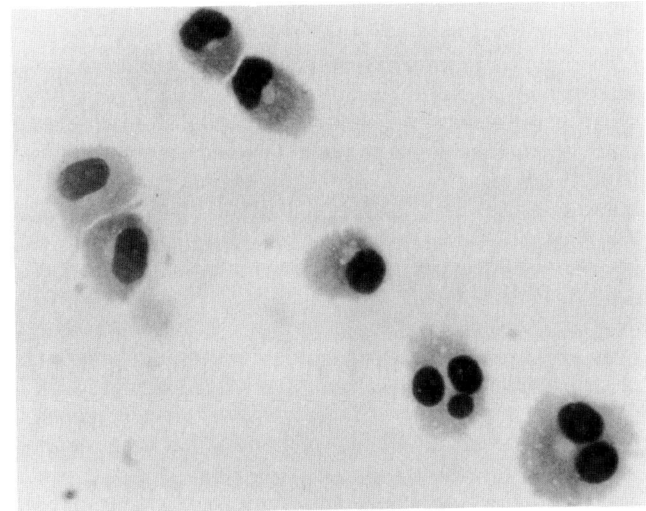

devitalization of the spinal cord. A tumor dose of 2000 rad in 5 days is usually adequate for the local control of plasma cell tumors causing spinal cord compression.

Some patients develop extensive plasma cell infiltration of the meninges and a CSF plasmacytosis (Fig. 38-11). Myelomatous meningitis usually develops during a period of rapid growth late in the course of the disease in patients with aggressive myeloma.[268,269]

The deposition of amyloid in the flexor retinaculum of the wrist frequently entraps the median nerve causing the "carpal tunnel syndrome." This is the commonest type of neuropathy associated with amyloidosis. The median nerve itself is not infiltrated with amyloid, and excision of the retinaculum usually gives lasting relief. Other patients with amyloidosis may develop diffuse sensorimotor neuropathy, with involvement of both upper and lower extremities. This neurologic involvement may ascend progressively and eventually lead to the loss of sphincter control. Nerve biopsies have shown infiltration of the nerve fibers by amyloid in some, and in others, amyloid is deposited in the perineural vessels without evidence of axonal degeneration.[246]

Somewhat less than 1% of patients with plasma cell neoplasms develop a distal sensorimotor polyneuropathy that is not caused by infiltration of the nerves with amyloid or plasma cells. This neuropathy appears to occur as a "remote effect" of the plasma cell tumor, because it often improves following radiation of solitary plasmacytomas, or treatment with melphalan and prednisone for generalized disease.[270,271]

The peripheral neuropathy begins insiduously in the feet, and progresses gradually to involve the legs and hands. Both sensory and motor functions are impaired. In some patients, the distal loss of sensation predominates, while in others, the major effect is loss of motor function. Pain and dysesthesia may be more disabling than the motor or sensory loss. These painful symptoms are uncommon in peripheral neuropathies due to other causes, but are found in the majority of patients with plasma cell neoplasms who develop peripheral neuropathies. The CSF protein was found to be elevated above 50 mg/dl in 36 of 40 (90%) myeloma patients with this sensorimotor neuropathy.[271]

Patients with plasma cell neoplasms who develop a diffuse sensorimotor polyneuropathy appear to be a recognizable subgroup, with several distinctive characteristics that distinguish them from patients without a neuropathy.[271] These patients are recognized at a younger age (mean, 50.8 years), than those with other plasma cell tumors (mean, 64 years). The polyneuropathy is recognized before the plasma cell neoplasm in 80%, and this may account in part for the earlier age at diagnosis. The polyneuropathy occurs more commonly in males, with a male:female ratio of 4:1, as compared to a ratio of 3:2 for all plasma cell tumors. Solitary osseous plasmacytomas account for only 2.8% of all plasmacytomas (Table 38-2), but 25% of those developing polyneuropathy had solitary lesions.[271] The polyneuropathy has been reported most often with tumors producing G heavy chains, but has also occurred with tumors producing A heavy chains, or only λ light chains; a surprising finding has been that the light chain has been lambda in all of the patients tested to date. The serum M-protein is usually low, and rarely exceeds 2.0 g/dl. While osteosclerotic bone lesions occur in much less than 1% of all patients with plasma cell neoplasms, sclerotic lesions have been found in 22% of patients with this type of polyneuropathy. The fact that the polyneuropathy has improved following treatment of the plasma cell tumor in 20 of the 33 (61%) reported cases strongly suggests that the neuropathy is a "remote effect" of the tumor.[271]

Plasma cell tumors in the vault of the skull rarely cause any symptoms, because these tumors tend to grow outward rather than inward. Tumors involving the base of the skull, however, can compress cranial nerves and cause palsies. Orbital lesions can cause proptosis. Plasma cell tumors rarely invade the central nervous system, but examples have been reported, including apparently solitary intracerebral plasma cell tumors.[272-274]

Herpes zoster was recorded in 2% of 869 patients seen at the Mayo Clinic.[34] We have the impression that the incidence of this infection is higher in the group of patients we have followed throughout the full course of the disease. The immune response of myeloma patients to this infection is weak and repeated infections in the same, or in different, dermatomes have been observed.

Multifocal leukoencephalopathy is a devastating, and currently untreatable, viral infection that may complicate the course of patients with plasma cell neoplasms.[275]

OSTEOSCLEROTIC MYELOMA

As noted earlier, osteosclerotic bone lesions occur in much less than 1% of all patients with plasma cell tumors, but have been found in 22% of those who develop a diffuse sensorimotor polyneuropathy.[271] This observation, and the report from Japan of a new association of osteosclerotic myeloma, polyneuropathy, certain endocrine disturbances (diabetes, hypertrichosis, and gynecomastia), and skin changes (hyperpigmentation, hyperhidrosis, and skin thickening) raises the question of whether this combination of findings represents a new syndrome.[276] All of these changes could occur as a spectrum of "remote effects" caused by a factor or factors produced by the plasma cell neoplasm. Indeed, the finding of elevated serum calcitonin in a patient with osteosclerotic myeloma is in keeping with this view, although there is not direct evidence that the neoplastic plasma cells produced this hormone.[277] The demonstration that the IgA M-protein in this patient was bound specifically on the peripheral myelinated nerve fibers, whereas IgG and IgM were not, suggests that the M-protein may have an etiologic role in producing the neuropathy.[277]

EXTRASKELETAL PLASMA CELL INFILTRATES

Almost every tissue in the body may be infiltrated with plasma cells in patients with plasma cell neoplasms. This is not surprising, since these neoplastic cells are frequently found in the peripheral blood and are consequently widely distributed throughout the body. We have already considered the occurrence of plasma cell infiltrates in the marrow, lymph nodes, the meninges, and brain. Skin infiltrations occur in advanced stages of the disease. Although infiltration of the spleen and liver is common, jaundice is rarely caused by plasma cell infiltration of the liver or as a result of lymph node or other infiltrates causing bile duct obstruction.[278-281] In one series, the commonest cause of jaundice in myeloma patients was cholestasis secondary to oxymetholone treatment.[281] Heavy infiltration of the portal tracts with plasma cells can cause intrahepatic presinusoidal portal hypertension and bleeding esophageal varicies.[282] Widespread plasma cell infiltration of the gastrointestinal mucosa also occurs. This can lead to anorexia, diarrhea, weight loss, obstruction, a protein-losing enteropathy, and excessive bleeding. Multiple gastrointestinal polyps may also be formed.[283]

SKIN DISEASES ASSOCIATED WITH A SERUM M-PROTEIN

M-proteins have been discovered in association with two dermatologic conditions. Papular mucinosis (lichen myxedematosus) is characterized by deposition in the skin of mucinous material which forms papules and plaques. Serum electrophoresis reveals a serum M-protein, characteristic of the disease, that is usually basic and has a slower mobility than most other gammaglobulins. The M-protein is usually IgG, but patients with IgA and IgM have also been reported. The ratio of κ:λ light chains is 1:2.5 in the patients with papular mucinosis who have had the light chain typed, in striking contrast to the 3:2 ratio of plasma cell neoplasms in general. In this entity, marrow plasmacytosis, osteolytic bone lesions, and light-chain proteinurea occur rarely.[284] The excellent response of two patients to melphalan therapy supports the view that papular mucinosis is an unusual variety of plasma cell neoplasm.[285,286] This disease usually follows a prolonged, benign course, but deaths do occur from unusual causes that may be related to the plasma cell neoplasm. Pyoderma gangrenosum is another skin disease in which M-proteins of the IgG, IgA, and IgM classes have been reported.[287]

ACUTE TERMINAL PHASE AND ACUTE LEUKEMIA

During the chronic phase of plasma cell myeloma there is an increase in the tumor growth rate during tumor relapses, which has been demonstrated by a progressive shortening of the M-protein doubling time (Fig. 38-4). Most of the patients who progressed to an M-protein doubling time of less than 30 days also developed marrow failure.[97] This marrow failure apparently does not result from treatment, because the marrow remains cellular, and the pancytopenia persists after all treatment is stopped. The development of pancytopenia, with a cellular marrow, marks the onset of the acute terminal phase of the disease. In addition to rapid progression of the disease, an unexplained fever may develop.[97] The marrow is usually infiltrated with immature plasma cells; dyserythropoiesis and ring sideroblasts may be noted. During this phase, plasma cell infiltrates in tissues such as the meninges, gastrointestinal tract, skin, liver, and so forth, may be recognized. Treatment during this phase is usually only of transient benefit, but the authors have observed one remission of long duration in a patient treated with a combination of lomustine, vincristine, and prednisone. Survival is usually brief after the onset of the acute terminal phase, ranging from 1 month to 9 months with a median of 3 months in one series.[97]

A high incidence of acute leukemia has been observed in patients with plasma cell myeloma (Fig. 38-12). In one large study the actuarial risk of developing acute leukemia reached 19.6% at 50 months after the onset of treatment.[29] It is not possible to decide whether treatment with leukemogenic agents (x-irradiation and alkylating agents) increases the risk of developing acute leukemia, because we do not know what the incidence is in untreated patients. The occurrence of acute leukemia in at least 17 patients with myeloma, five with macroglobulinemia, and five with benign monoclonal gammopathy, including an unpublished case from our hospital, before any treatment was started, suggests that there is an increased risk of acute leukemia in patients with plasma cell neoplasms in the absence of treatment and that acute leukemia may occur as part of the natural history of this disease.[288–295]

The acute leukemia that occurs in patients with plasma cell neoplasms may be part of the course of the disease, as it is in chronic granulocytic leukemia, polycythemia rubra vera, and myelofibrosis.

SURVIVAL AND CAUSES OF DEATH

The overall survival of 364 patients with plasma cell myeloma treated with alkylating agents and prednisone is shown in Fig. 38-13. It will be noted that 15% die within the first 3 months; thereafter deaths occur at a constant rate. Throughout the course of this study to date, deaths have occurred at an increased rate, and the survival curve for myeloma patients never parallels the survival of an age and sex-matched normal control population. Thus, there is no evidence that any of these patients are cured of the disease.

The causes of death are shown in Table 38-15. Most patients died during the chronic phase of the disease with adequate

FIG. 38-12. Actuarial risk of developing acute leukemia in myeloma patients treated with alkylating agents and prednisone. This figure has been updated to include the 15th patient who has developed acute leukemia in the NCI-C study reported. (Bergsagel DE, Bailey AJ, Langley GR et al: The chemotherapy of plasma-cell myeloma and the incidence of acute leukemia. N Engl J Med 301:743–748, 1979)

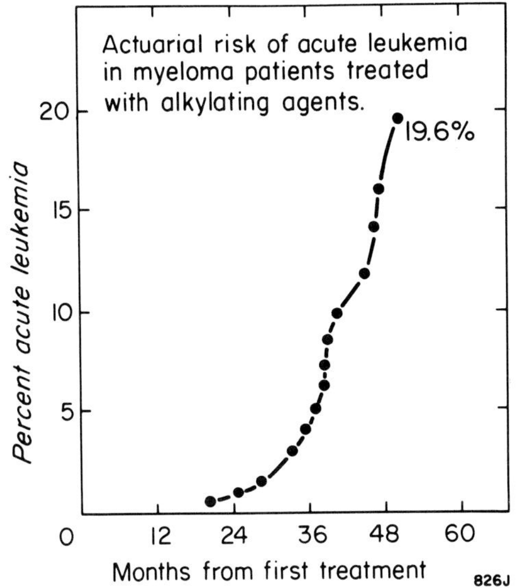

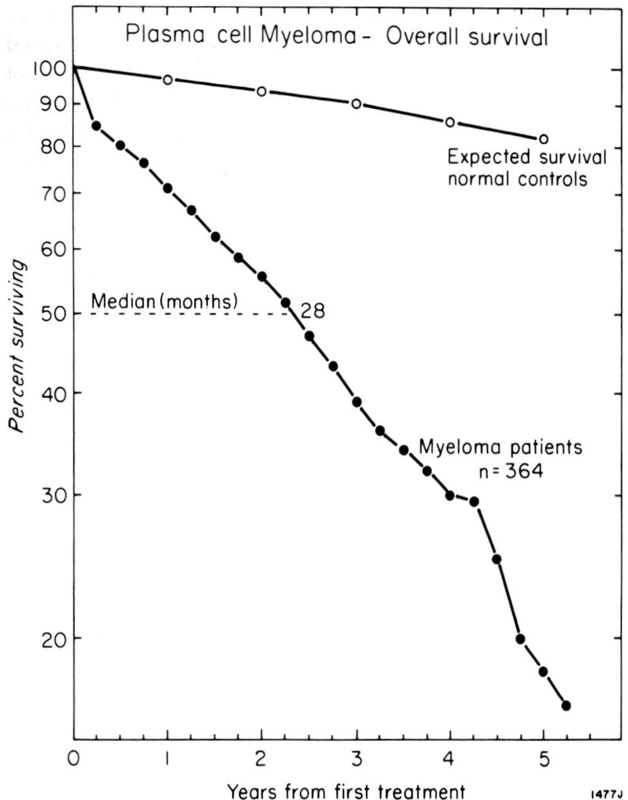

FIG. 38-13. Overall survival of all patients treated with alkylating agents and prednisone in the NCI-C clinical trials group study reported. The expected survival of age- and sex-matched normals is shown in the upper curve. (Bergsagel DE, Bailey AJ, Langley GR et al: The chemotherapy of plasma-cell myeloma and the incidence of acute leukemia. N Engl J Med 301:743–748, 1979)

marrow function and progressive myeloma plus renal failure, sepsis, or both. Those listed as dying during the acute terminal phase developed pancytopenia with a cellular marrow. These patients had evidence of rapidly progressing myeloma with short M-protein doubling times or increasing numbers of plasma cells in the blood. In addition, ring sideroblasts, a presumed pre-leukemic change were reported in 18 patients.[296] Acute leukemia has developed in nine of the patients with sideroblasts, and in six others. The acute leukemias were classified as myeloblastic in 11, monoblastic in two, and erythroleukemic in two. Other serious illnesses, such as myocardial infarctions, chronic obstructive pulmonary disease, and strokes caused deaths in 20%, and the direct cause of death is unknown for 7%.

SPECIAL SYNDROMES

MACROGLOBULINEMIA

Several disorders are associated with the appearance of a monoclonal macroglobulin M-spike in the serum electrophoresis pattern (Table 38-16).

The lymphoplasmacytic neoplasms form a spectrum of closely related disease. The separation of the three diseases is difficult, arbitrary, and of little prognostic value. Plasma cell tumors arising in an extramedullary site without involving the bone marrow are classified as extramedullary plasmacytomas. Patients with Waldenström's macroglobulinemia usually have hepatosplenomegaly and lymphadenopathy, but osteolytic bone lesions are rare. When osteolytic bone lesions are found, patients tend to be labelled as having IgM myeloma. It is not possible to differentiate Waldenström's syndrome

TABLE 38-15. Plasma Cell Myeloma: Causes of Death

PHASE AND CAUSE	NUMBER (Percent)
A. During the chronic phase	
Progressive myeloma	38
plus renal failure	24
plus sepsis	33
plus both	16
	111 (46)
B. During the acute terminal phase	
Progressive myeloma	31
plus renal failure	4
plus sepsis	22
plus both	5
	62 (26)
Acute leukemia	12 (5)
C. Other causes	48 (20)
D. Unknown	7 (3)
TOTAL	240 (100)

(Bergsagel DE, Bailey AJ, Langley GR et al: The chemotherapy of plasma-cell myeloma and the incidence of acute leukemia. N Engl J Med 301:743–748, 1979)

TABLE 38-16. Diseases Associated With a Serum IgM M-Protein

	NUMBER	PER-CENT
A. Lymphoplasmacytic neoplasms		
1. Waldenstroms macroglobulinemia	112	
2. IgM myeloma	14	
3. Extramedullary plasmacytoma	7	
	133	31
B. Controlled monoclone		
1. Cold agglutinin syndrome	9	
2. Benign macroglobulinemia	117	
	126	30
C. B-lymphocyte neoplasms		
1. Chronic lymphocytic leukemia	31	
2. Diffuse lymphomas	133	
	164	39
TOTALS	423	100

(Adapted from Carter P, Koval JJ, Hobbs JR: The relation of clinical and laboratory findings to the survival of patients with macroglobulinaemia. Clin Exp Immunol 28:241–249, 1977; Ameis A, Ko HS, Pruzanski W: M-components—A review of 1242 cases. Can Med Assoc J 114:889–895, 1976; Stein RS, Ellman L, Bloch KJ: The clinical correlates of IgM M-components: an analysis of thirty-four patients. Am J Med Sc 269:209–216, 1975) from IgM myeloma on the basis of marrow cytology. The predominant cell tends to be lymphoid in the former and plasmacytoid in the latter, but there is so much variation and overlap that clear distinctions cannot be made. Patients with Waldenström's syndrome and IgM myeloma tend to have higher serum IgM values and to develop the symptoms associated with hyperviscosity.

The IgM level tends to remain constant in patients with the cold hemagglutin syndrome, and the disease runs a benign course, similar to the course of the disease in patients with benign macroglobulinemia, in whom the significance of the M-protein is unknown.

It is relatively easy to differentiate the B-lymphocyte neoplasms associated with an IgM protein, for these patients have other features diagnostic of chronic lymphocytic leukemia or diffuse lymphocytic lymphomas. These patients rarely have a serum M-protein concentration greater than 2.5 g/dl, and complications such as hyperviscosity or cryoglobulinemia are uncommon. The course of the disease in patients with a B-lymphocyte neoplasm and an M-protein is similar to the course in patients with a normal serum electrophoresis pattern, and treatment should be appropriate for chronic lymphocytic leukemia or a malignant lymphoma.

The mean age at diagnosis of patients with macroglobulinemia associated with a lympho–plasmacytic neoplasm is 64 years. In earlier studies, 66% of the patients were males, but in three recent series the proportion of males has dropped to 50%.[89,297–300]

Guidelines for the treatment of these patients are very much the same as for plasma cell myeloma. Patients with lympho–plasmacytic tumors producing IgM usually respond well to an alkylating agent and prednisone, using the dosage schedules described in Table 38-11. This treatment should be continued until the serum IgM declines to reach a pleateau. At this point, treatment can be discontinued until the M-protein begins to increase. Patients must be observed carefully for evidence of the hyperviscosity syndrome, and treated with plasmapheresis when prompt relief from this syndrome is required. These opinions regarding the treatment of lympho-plasmacytic neoplasms producing IgM are based on personal observations and series reported in the literature. No systematic studies of different approaches to treatment have been conducted, so that it is not possible to state that one alkylating agent, one dosage schedule, or a particular drug combination is better than another. Until well-designed studies of macroglobulinemia uncover unique features of this disease that require special approaches, it is probably best to apply the same principles of treatment to this disease as have been developed for the management of patients with plasma cell myeloma.

THE HEAVY CHAIN DISEASES

Heavy chain diseases are lympho–plasmacytic diseases characterized by the proliferation of cells which synthesize and secrete a defective heavy chain with an intact F_c portion and a major deletion in the F_d region. Three of the possible five types of heavy-chain disease (γ, α, and μ) have been recognized since 1963.[301–304] Detailed studies of the heavy chain, especially those produced by patients with γ-heavy chain disease, have provided some clues as to the genetic control of immunoglobulin structure, synthesis and assembly.[304] The deletion of the amino-terminal end of the heavy chain (F_d portion) probably results from an abnormality affecting the gene or genes that control the synthesis of this part of the molecule. However, it is difficult to explain the absence of light chain synthesis by the neoplastic cells in patients with γ and α heavy-chain disease, since the synthesis of heavy and light chains is under the control of separate, non-linked genes. It is therefore necessary to postulate either a second, separate mutational event, or the existence of a regulator which controls the expression of two non-linked genes.

The heavy-chain diseases are uncommon, and while the condition may be suspected in patients who manifest the clinical syndromes described below, an accurate diagnosis requires detailed immunochemical investigations.

γ *Heavy-Chain Disease (γ-HCD)*

This disease has been recognized in North America, Europe, and Japan, and the major factor influencing the geographic incidence of γ-HCD may be the availability of a competent immunochemist.[300] The age of patients has ranged from 9 years to 76 years; most were elderly, but six were under the age of 30 years.[304,305]

The usual clinical manifestations consist of lymphadenopathy, anemia, and fever, often accompanied by malaise, weakness, and hepato- or splenomegaly. Initially, a granulomatous disease, such as toxoplasmosis, histoplasmosis, or Hodgkin's disease, has been suspected. Lymphadenopathy may wax and wane, but persistent generalized lymph node enlargement usually develops eventually. Palatal edema and erythema may result from involvement of the lymphatic tissue of Waldeyer's ring and give rise to respiratory difficulties. Bony lesions are uncommon. All patients have mild to moderate anemia, often associated with leukopenia, eosinophilia, thrombocytopenia, and the presence of atypical lymphocytes or plasma cells in the blood. A few patients have developed plasma cell leukemia terminally. The bone marrow may be normal, but usually there is an increased proportion of plasma cells or lymphocytes or both, often accompanied by eosinophilia. The bone marrow findings are rarely diagnostic.

None of the histologic changes found in tissues are diagnostic, and they often suggest other conditions such as Hodgkin's disease or a granulomatous infection. At least two patients have shown extensive amyloid infiltration at *post mortem* examination, an incongruous finding in view of the assumed relation of light chains to the formation of amyloid.

The diagnosis is usually established by the demonstration of a protein in the serum or urine which on immunoelectrophoresis reacts with anti-sera to γ chains, but not to light chains. Most of the anomalous proteins have been of the γ_1 subclass, but patients with γ_2, γ_3, and γ_4 heavy chains have been reported. In the serum electrophoresis pattern the abnormal protein usually appears to be a broad, heterogeneous compound. In 50% of patients the concentration of the anomalous protein is greater than 2.0 g/dl and marked hypogammaglobulinemia is present. About half of the patients excrete the abnormal protein in the urine in amounts ranging from 0.5 g/24 hr to 20 g/24 hr.

A satisfactory form of treatment has not been established. Limited trials of alkylating agents and steroids have produced no obvious improvement. Splenic irradiation may result in temporary hematologic improvement and irradiation of the nasopharynx may be helpful in relieving palatal edema and respiratory distress.

The course of the disease is variable, with survival ranging from a few months to more than 5 years from the onset of symptoms. Infections and progression of the disease are the usual causes of death.

α Heavy Chain Disease (α-HCD)

α-HCD was first described in 1968, and appears to be the most common form of heavy chain disease. In striking contrast to plasma cell myeloma and macroglobulinemia, the disease affects patients under the age of 50 years, with a peak of incidence in the second and third decades. The ratio of males to females is 3:2, similar to plasma cell myeloma. The geographic distribution of the enteric form of the disease reveals a high incidence in areas where intestinal infection with parasites, bacteria, and viruses is common (*e.g.*, Mediterranean, Asian, and South American countries). Patients reported from the Netherlands and the United States have had a respiratory form of α-HCD, with a lymphoplasmacytic infiltrate limited to the respiratory tract.[4,302,304,306–310]

Patients usually present with chronic diarrhea and a severe malabsorption syndrome with marked weight loss, steatorrhea, hypocalcemia, and excessive fecal losses of water and electrolytes. Abdominal masses may be palpable, and abdominal pain is often a major symptom. Clubbing of the fingers has been noted in many patients. Radiologic studies of the intestine and mucosal biopsies have shown diffuse and massive lympho–plasmacytic infiltration of the mucosa. Villous atrophy and sparsity of crypts have been found in all patients. Mesenteric lymph nodes have shown a similar plasmacytic infiltration, as have rectal biopsies. At a late stage, tumors may develop and cause intestinal obstruction.

Enlarged retroperitoneal nodes have been demonstrated by lymphography, but enlargement of peripheral lymph nodes is uncommon. Lympho–plasmacytic infiltrates have been found in the portal tracts of the liver, and in the spleen.[308] Abnormal lymphoid or plasma cells may be found in the blood of terminal patients, and although it is difficult to demonstrate an increased number of plasma cells in marrow aspirates with Wright's stain, abnormal plasma cells producing α heavy chain can be demonstrated by immunofluorescence studies.

The diagnosis of α-HCD requires the demonstration of an α_1 heavy chain in the serum. The serum electrophoresis pattern usually reveals a reduced albumin level, a moderate to marked hypogammaglobulinemia, and a broad abnormal band in the α_2- to β-globulin region. The anomalous protein usually does not produce a sharp peak on electrophoresis. The abnormal protein reacts with anti-sera to IgA, but fails to react with antisera to κ or λ light chains. The failure of light-chain anti-sera to precipitate the abnormal protein is not sufficient evidence to establish a diagnosis, since some IgA M-proteins (usually with λ chains) may not be precipitated with these anti-sera. In doubtful cases, the abnormal protein should be purified and the absence of light chains demonstrated by urea–acid–starch gel electrophoresis, or gel filtration of the reduced and alkylated protein in dissociating solutions.[4] In all of the reported cases, the abnormal protein belongs to the α_1 rather than the α_2 subtype of IgA. Light chain proteinurea has not been found, but in most patients the abnormal heavy chain protein can be demonstrated in concentrated urine. The anomalous protein is also found in large amounts in the jejunal fluid, but not in the parotid saliva.

The course of the disease is usually progressive and fatal. However, complete clinical remission has been reported, with disappearance of the abnormal protein from the serum and jejunal fluid, and disappearance of the lymphoplasmacytic infiltrate from the intestinal mucosa.[4] In some of these patients, remissions were achieved with chemotherapy for a malignant lymphoma, while in others, antibiotics alone were employed. The occurrence of complete remissions with antibiotic treatment alone makes the neoplastic nature of the disease questionable. It should also be noted that at least two patients have developed second plasma cell neoplasms while in an apparent complete remission from α-HCD.[311,312]

μ Heavy-Chain Disease (μ-HCD)

Patients with μ-HCD range in age from 39 years to 79 years, and nearly all have chronic lymphocytic leukemia (CLL).[313,314] The patients differ from the usual CLL in 3 ways: (1) enlarged lymph nodes are infrequent; (2) unusual vacuolated plasma cells are present in the marrow of the majority of patients; and (3) most of the patients excrete large amounts of κ light chains in the urine. Occasional patients excrete the anomalous μ chain as well.[315] μ-HCD is rare in CLL, for careful study of at least 180 CLL patients failed to uncover more than the index case.[313]

The diagnosis requires a high index of suspicion. Serum protein electrophoresis is usually normal, or shows only hypogammaglobulinemia, but a small M-protein may be found in some cases.[313,314] The diagnosis requires the demonstration by immunoelectrophoresis of a rapidly migrating component which precipitates with anti-sera to μ chains, but not with anti-sera to light chains. It is usually necessary to document the diagnosis further by ultracentrifugation or gel filtration, since some intact macroglobulins may not react with κ or λ anti-sera.

The patient should be treated for the underlying disease, usually CLL (see Chapter 37).

FUTURE CONSIDERATIONS

Studies during the past 2 decades have clarified the tumor biology of plasma cell neoplasms, identified the prognostic factors, and established a useful clinical staging system. The response rates and survival of myeloma patients treated with new agents and drug combinations are only minimally better than those achieved with melphalan and prednisone. The failure of more intensive treatment to improve survival and the lack of a correlation between myeloma cell-kill and survival suggests that the beneficial results of treatment may not be due to an effect of therapy on the myeloma cell mass.

Alternate hypotheses are required to explain the effect of treatment on plasma cell neoplasms. One alternate hypothesis holds that treatment reduces a population of regulator cells in myeloma patients, and allows a growth control mechanism to be re-established. This growth control mechanism maintains the myeloma cell number stable until the regulator cells regenerate sufficiently to allow the monoclone to grow again.[148,316] If research provides further support for a growth control abnormality in patients with plasma cell neoplasms, therapeutic research should be aimed at correcting the faulty control mechanisms, rather than trying to reduce the myeloma cell number.

REFERENCES

1. Osserman EF, Takatsuki K: Considerations regarding the pathogenesis of the plasmacytic dyscrasias. Series Hemat 4:28–49, 1965
2. Hällén J: Discrete gammaglobulin (M-) components in serum. Clinical study of 150 subjects without myelomatosis. Acta Med Scand Suppl 462:1–127, 1966
3. Shimm DS, Cohen HJ: Transient monoclonal immunoglobulin G with anti-dextran activity. Acta Haemat 59:99–103, 1978
4. Seligmann M: Immunochemical, clinical, and pathological features of α-heavy chain disease. Arch Intern Med 135:78–82, 1975
5. Clamp JR: Some aspects of the first recorded case of multiple myeloma. Lancet 2:1354–1356, 1967
6. Rustizky J: Multiple myeloma. Deutsch Z Chir 3:162–172, 1873
7. Kahler O: Zur symptomatologie des multiplen myeloma; Beobachtung von albumosurie. Prog Med Wochnschr 14:33, 45, 1889
8. Ellinger A: Das vorkommen des Bence-Jones's schen Körpers im harn bei tumoren des knochenmarks und seine diagnostische Bedeutang. Deutsch Arch Klin Med 62:255–278, 1899
9. Wright JH: A case of multiple myeloma. Trans Assoc Am Physicians 15:137–145, 1900
10. Magnus-Levy A: Multiple myeloma. Acta Med Scand 95:217–280, 1938
11. Glenner GG, Terry W, Harada M et al: Amyloid fibril proteins: proof of homology with immunoglobulin light chains by sequence analysis. Science 172:1150–1151, 1971
12. Alwall N: Urethane and stilbamidine in multiple myeloma: Report on 2 cases. Lancet 2:388–389, 1947
13. Holland JF, Hosley H, Scharlau C et al: A controlled trial of urethane treatment in myeloma. Blood 27:328–342, 1966
14. Bergsagel DE, Griffith KM, Haut A et al: The treatment of plasma cell myeloma. Adv Cancer Res 10:311–359, 1967
15. Blokhin N, Larionov L, Perevodchikova N et al: Clinical experiences with sarcolysin in neoplastic diseases. Ann NY Acad Sci 68:1128–1132, 1958
16. Bergsagel DE, Sprague CC, Austin C et al: Evaluation of new chemotherapeutic agents in the treatment of multiple myeloma. IV. L-phenylalanine mustard (NSC-8806). Cancer Chemother Rep 21:87–99, 1962
17. Korst DR, Clifford GO, Fowler WM et al: Multiple myeloma. II. Analysis of cyclophosphamide in 165 patients. JAMA 189:758–762, 1964
18. Alexanian R, Haut A, Khan AU et al: Treatment for multiple myeloma: Combination chemotherapy with different melphalan dose regimens. JAMA 208:1680–1685, 1969
19. Axelsson U, Bachmann R, Hällén J: Frequency of pathological proteins (M-components) in 6995 sera from an adult population. Acta Med Scand 179:235–247, 1966
20. Axelsson U: An eleven-year follow-up on 64 subjects with M-components. Acta Med Scand 201:173–175, 1977
21. Hällén J: Frequency of "abnormal" serum globulins (M-components) in the aged. Acta Med Scand 173:737–744, 1963
22. Englišová M, Engliš M, Kyral V et al: Changes of immunoglobulin synthesis in old people. Exp Geront 3:125–127, 1968
23. Martin NH: The incidence of myelomatosis. Lancet 1:237–239, 1961
24. Kyle RA, Nobrega FT, Kurland LT: Multiple myeloma in Olmstead County, Minnesota, 1945–64. Blood 33:739–745, 1969
25. Malignant neoplasms of lymphatic and haematopoietic tissues: Multiple myeloma (203). WHO Epidemiol Vital Statist Rep 18:414–415, 1965
26. MacMahon B, Clark DW: Incidence of multiple myeloma. J Chronic Dis 4:508–515, 1956
27. McFarlane H: Multiple myeloma in Jamaica: A study of 40 cases with special reference to the incidence and laboratory diagnosis. J Clin Pathol 19:268–271, 1966
28. McPhedran P, Heath CW Jr, Garcia J: Multiple myeloma incidence in metropolitan Atlanta, Georgia: Racial and seasonal variations. Blood 39:866–873, 1972
29. Bergsagel DE, Bailey AJ, Langley GR et al: The chemotherapy of plasma-cell myeloma and the incidence of acute leukemia. N Engl J Med 301:743–748, 1979
30. Hewell GM, Alexanian R: Myeloma in young persons. Ann Intern Med 84:441–443, 1976
31. Waldenström J: Diagnosis and treatment of multiple myeloma. p 230. New York, Grune & Stratton, 1970
32. MRC working party for therapeutic trials in leukemia: Report on the first myelomatosis trial. Part I. Analysis of presenting features of prognostic significance. Brit J Haemat 24:123–139, 1973
33. Fine JM, Lambin P: Distribution of heavy chain classes and light chain types in 757 cases of monoclonal gammopathies. Biomedicine 23:323–327, 1975
34. Kyle RA: Multiple myeloma. Review of 869 cases. Mayo Clinic Proc 50:29–40, 1975
35. Alexanian R, Balcerzak S, Bonnet JD et al: Prognostic factors in multiple myeloma. Cancer 36:1192–1201, 1975
36. Atkinson FRB: Multiple myelomata. M Press 195:312, 327, 1937
37. Snapper I, Turner LB, Moscovitz HL: Multiple Myeloma. p 168. New York, Grune & Stratton, 1953
38. Osborne CA, Perman V, Sautter JH et al: Multiple myeloma in the dog. J Am Vet Assoc 153:1300–1319, 1968
39. Hurvitz AI: Animal model for human disease: Canine monoclonal gammopathies/immunoglobulins. Comp Pathol Bull 3:4, 1971
40. Farrow BRH, Penny R: Multiple myeloma in a cat. J Am Vet Assoc 158:606–611, 1971
41. Kehoe JM, Hurvitz AI, Capra JD: Characterization of three feline paraproteins. J Immunol 109:511–516, 1972
42. Cotran RS, Fortner JG: Serum-protein abnormality in a transplantable plasmacytoma of the Syrian golden hamster. J Natl Cancer Inst 28:1193–1205, 1962
43. Bazin H, Deckers C, Beckers A et al: Transplantable immunoglobulin-secreting tumors in rats. I. General features of Lou/Wsl strain rat immunocytomas and their monoclonal proteins. Int J Cancer 10:568–580, 1972
44. Bazin H, Beckers A, Deckers C et al: Transplantable imnmunoglobulin-secreting tumors in rats. V. Monoclonal immunoglobulins secreted by 250 ileocecal immunocytomas in Lou/Wsl rats. J Natl Cancer Inst 51:1359–1361, 1973
45. Dunn TB: Normal and pathologic anatomy of the reticular tissue in laboratory mice, with a classification and discussion of neoplasms. J Natl Cancer Inst 14:1281–1433, 1954
46. Dunn TB: Plasma-cell neoplasms beginning in the ileocecal area in strain C3H mice. J Natl Cancer Inst 19:371–391, 1957
47. Pilgrim HI: The relationship of chronic ulceration of the ileocecal function to the development of reticuloendothelial tumors in C3H mice. Cancer Res 25:53–65, 1965
48. Mellors RC: Autoimmune and immunoproliferative diseases of NZB/Bl mice and hybrids. Int Rev Exp Pathol 5:217–252, 1966
49. Potter M: Immunoglobulin producing tumors and myeloma proteins of mice. Physiol Rev 52:631–719, 1972
50. Hollander VP, Takakura K, Yamada H: Endocrine factors in the pathogenesis of plasma cell tumors. Recent Prog Horm Res 24:81–137, 1968

51. Potter M, Pumphrey JG, Walters JL: Brief communication: Growth of primary plasmacytomas in the mineral oil-conditioned environment. J Natl Cancer Inst 49:305–308, 1972
52. Potter M, Walters JL: Effect of intraperitoneal pristane on established immunity to the Adj-PC-5 plasmacytoma. J Natl Cancer Inst 51:875–881, 1973
53. Park CH, Bergsagel DE, McCulloch EA: Mouse myeloma tumor stem cells: A primary cell culture assay. J Natl Cancer Inst 46:411–422, 1971
54. Park CH, Bergsagel DE, McCulloch EA: Ascorbic acid: A culture requirement for mouse plasmacytoma cells. Science 174:720–722, 1971
55. Hamburger A, Salmon SE: Primary bioassay of human myeloma stem cells. J Clin Invest 50:846–854, 1977
56. Namba Y, Hanaoka M: Immunocytology of cultured IgM-forming cells of mouse. I. Requirement of phagocytic cell factor for the growth of IgM-forming tumor cells in tissue culture. J Immunol 109:1193–1200, 1972
57. Metcalf D: Colony formation in agar by murine plasmacytoma cells: Potentiation by hemopoietic cells and serum. J Cell Physiol 81:397–410, 1973
58. Metcalf D: The serum factor stimulating colony formation *in vitro* by murine plasmacytoma cells: Response to antigens and mineral oil. J Immunol 113:235–243, 1974
59. McIntire KR, Princler GL: Prolonged adjuvant stimulation in germfree BALB/c mice: Development of plasma cell neoplasia. Immunology 17:481–487, 1969
60. Warner NL, Potter M, Metcalf D: Multiple myeloma and related immunoglobulin-producing neoplasms. UICC Technical Report Series, Vol 13. Geneva, International Union Against Cancer, 1974
61. Warner NL: Autoimmunity and the pathogenesis of plasma cell tumor induction in NZB inbred and hybrid mice. UICC Technical Report Series, Vol 13, p 60. Geneva, International Union Against Cancer, 1974
62. Potter M, Sklar MD, Rowe WP: Rapid viral induction of plasmacytomas in pristane-primed BALB/c mice. Science 182:592–594, 1973
63. Maldonado JE, Kyle RA: Familial myeloma. Report of eight families and a study of serum proteins in their relatives. Am J Med 57:875–884, 1974
64. Bertrams J, Kuwert E, Böhme U et al: HL-A antigens in Hodgkin's Disease and multiple myeloma. Tissue Antigens 2:41–46, 1972
65. Smith G, Walford RL, Fishkin B et al: HL-A phenotypes, immunoglobulins, and K and L chains in multiple myeloma. Tissue Antigens 4:374–377, 1974
66. Kyle RA, Heath CW Jr, Carbone P: Multiple myeloma in spouses. Arch Intern Med 127:944–946, 1971
67. Pietruszka M, Rabin BS, Srodes G: Multiple myeloma in husband and wife. Lancet 1:314, 1976
68. Ichimaru M, Ishimaru T, Mikami M et al: Multiple myeloma among atomic bomb survivors, Hiroshima and Nagasaki, 1950–1976. Radiation Effects Research Foundation Technical Report No 9-79. Hiroshima, Radiation Effects Research Foundation, 1979
69. Isobe T, Osserman EF: Pathologic conditions associated with plasma cell dyscrasias: A study of 806 cases. Ann NY Acad Sci 90:507–518, 1971
70. Schafer AI, Miller JB: Association of IgA multiple myeloma with pre-existing disease. Br J Haematol 41:19–24, 1979
71. Wohlenberg H: Osteomyelitis and plasmacytoma. N Engl J Med 283:822–823, 1970
72. Penny R, Hughes S: Repeated stimulation of the reticuloendothelial system and the development of plasma cell dyscrasias. Lancet 1:77–78, 1970
73. Rosenblatt J, Hall CA: Plasma-cell dyscrasia following prolonged stimulation of reticuloendothelial system. Lancet 1:301–302, 1970
74. Goldenberg GJ, Paraskevas F, Israels LG: The association of rheumatoid arthritis with plasma cell and lymphocytic neoplasms. Arthrit Rheum 12:569–579, 1969
75. Wegelius O, Skrifvars B: Rheumatoid arthritis terminating in plasmacytoma. Acta Med Scand 187:133–138, 1970
76. Isomäki HA, Hakulmen T, Joutsenlahti U: Excess risk of lymphomas, leukemias and myelomas in patients with rheumatoid arthritis. J Chron Dis 31:691–699, 1978
77. Schafer AI, Miller JB, Lester EP et al: Monoclonal gammopathy in hereditary spherocytosis: A possible pathogenetic relation. Ann Intern Med 88:45–46, 1978
78. Pratt PW, Estren S, Kochwa S: Immunoglobulin abnormalities in Gaucher's Disease: Report of 16 cases. Blood 31:633–640, 1968
79. Wolf P: Monoclonal gammopathy in Gaucher's Disease. Lab Med 4:28–29, 1973
80. Turesson I, Rausing A: Gaucher's Disease and benign monoclonal gammopathy. Acta Med Scand 197:507–512, 1975
81. MacDonald M, McCathie M, Faed MJW et al: Gaucher's Disease with biclonal gammopathy. J Clin Path 28:757, 1975
82. Gerber MA: Asbestosis and neoplastic disorders of the hematopoietic system. Am J Clin Path 53:204–208, 1970
83. Kagan E, Jacobson RJ, Yeung K-Y et al: Asbestosis-associated neoplasms of B cell lineage. Am J Med 67:325–330, 1979
84. Porter DD, Dixon FJ, Larsen AE: The development of a myeloma-like condition in mink with Aleutian disease. Blood 25:736–742, 1965
85. Chapman I, Jimenez FA: Aleutian mink disease in man. N Engl J Med 269:1171–1174, 1963
86. Helmboldt CF, Kenyon AJ, Dessel BH: The comparative aspects of Aleutian mink disease. In NINDB Monograph #2: Slow, latent, and temperate virus infections. pp 315–319, 1964
87. Henry LW: Multiple myeloma in a mink handler following exposure to Aleutian disease. Cancer 44:273–275, 1979
88. Kyle RA: Monoclonal gammopathy of undetermined significance. Am J Med 64:814–825, 1978
89. Carter P, Koval JJ, Hobbs JR: The relation of clinical and laboratory findings to the survival of patients with macroglobulinanemia. Clin Exp Immunol 28:241–249, 1977
90. Crowin J, Lindberg RD: Solitary plasmacytoma of bone *vs.* extramedullary plasmacytoma and their relationship to multiple myeloma. Cancer 43:1007–1013, 1979
91. Knowling M, Harwood A, Bergsagel DE: A comparison of extramedullary plasmacytomas with multiple and solitary plasma cell tumors of bone. (in press)
92. Wiltshaw E: The natural history of extramedullary plasmacytoma and its relation to solitary myeloma of bone and myelomatosis. Medicine 55:217–238, 1976
93. Woodruff RK, Whittle JM, Malpaş JS: Solitary plasmacytoma. I: Extramedullary soft tissue plasmacytoma. Cancer 43:2340–2343, 1979
94. Woodruff RK, Malpas JS, White FE: Solitary plasmacytoma. II: Solitary plasmacytoma of bone. Cancer 43:2344–2347, 1979
95. Paraskevas F, Heremans J, Waldenström J: Cytology and electrophoretic pattern in γ_1A (B_2A) myeloma. Acta Med Scand 170:575–589, 1961
96. Maldonado JE, Brown AL, Bayrd ED et al: Cytoplasmic and intranuclear electron-dense bodies in the myeloma cell. Arch Pathol 81:484–500, 1966
97. Bergsagel DE, Pruzanski W: Treatment of plasma cell myeloma with cytotoxic agents. Arch Intern Med 135:172–176, 1975
98. Bergsagel DE: Assessment of the response of mouse and human myeloma to chemotherapy and radiotherapy. In Drewinko B, Humphreys RM (eds): Growth Kinetics and Biochemical Regulation of Normal and Malignant Cells. University of Texas Cancer Center, M.D. Anderson Hospital and Tumor Institute, 29th Annual Symposium on Fundamental Cancer Research, pp 705–717. Baltimore, Williams & Wilkins, 1977
99. Bergsagel DE: The treatment of plasma cell myeloma. Br J Haematol 33:443–449, 1976
100. Fine JM, Lambin P, Muller JY: The evolution of asymptomatic monoclonal gammopathies. A follow-up of 20 cases over 3–14 years. Acta Med Scand 205:339–341, 1979
101. Zawadzki ZA, Edwards GA: Non myelomatous monoclonal immunoglobulinemia. Prog Clin Immunol 1:105–156, 1972

102. Durie BGM, Salmon SE: A clinical staging system for multiple myeloma. Correlation of measured myeloma cell mass with presenting clinical features, response to treatment and survival. Cancer 36:842–854, 1975
103. Kyle RA, Finkelstein S, Elveback LR et al: Incidence of monoclonal proteins in a Minnesota community with a cluster of multiple myeloma. Blood 40:719–724, 1972
104. Migliore P, Alexanian R: Monoclonal gammopathy in human neoplasia. Cancer 21:1127–1131, 1968
105. Alexanian R: Monoclonal gammopathy in lymphoma. Arch Intern Med 135:62–66, 1975
106. Ameis A, Ko HS, Pruzanski W: M-components—A review of 1242 cases. Can Med Assoc J 114:889–895, 1976
107. Čejka J, Bollinger R, Schuit HRE et al: Macroglobulinemia in a child with acute leukemia. Blood 43:191–199, 1974
108. Shohet SB, Mohler WC: *In vitro* growth of peripheral blood cells from a patient with chronic myelogenous leukemia. Proc AACR 4:61, 1963
109. Hobbs JR: Paraproteins, benign or malignant? Br Med J 3:699–704, 1967
110. Lindström FD, Dahlström U: Multiple myeloma or benign monoclonal gammopathy? A study of differential diagnostic criteria in 44 cases. Clin Immun Immunopath 10:168–174, 1978
111. Alexanian R, Bonnet J, Gehan E et al: Combination chemotherapy for multiple myeloma. Cancer 30:382–389, 1972
112. Salmon SE: Immunoglobulin synthesis and tumor kinetics of multiple myeloma. Semin Hematol 10:135–147, 1973
113. Ogawa M, Bergsagel DE, McCulloch EA: Chemotherapy of mouse myeloma: Quantitative cell cultures predictive of response *in vitro*. Blood 41:7–15, 1973
114. McArthur JR, Athens JW, Wintrobe MM et al: Melphalan and myeloma: Experience with a low dose, continuous regimen. Ann Intern Med 72:665–670, 1970
115. Tattersall MHN, Jarman M, Newlands ES et al: Pharmacokinetics of melphalan following oral or intravenous administration in patients with malignant disease. Eur J Cancer 14:507–513, 1978
116. Alberts DS, Chang SY, Chen H-S et al: Variability of melphalan absorption in man. Proc AACR-ASCO 19:334, 1978
117. Bergsagel DE, Robertson GL, Hasselback R: Effect of cyclophosphamide on advanced lung cancer and the hematological toxicity of large, intermittent intravenous doses. Can Med Assoc J 98:532–538, 1968
118. Bergsagel DE, Ogawa M, Librach SL: Mouse myeloma. A model for studies of cell kinetics. Arch Intern Med 135:109–113, 1975
119. Bergsagel DE, Cowan DH, Hasselback R: Plasma cell myeloma: response of melphalan-resistant patients to high-dose, intermittent cyclophosphamide. Can Med Assoc J 107:851–855, 1972
120. Raisz LG, Luben RA, Mundy GR et al: Effect of osteoclast activating factor from human leukocytes on bone metabolism. J Clin Invest 56:408–413, 1975
121. Bergsagel DE: Plasma cell myeloma: An interpretive review. Cancer 30:1588–1594, 1972
122. Salmon SE, Shadduck RK, Schilling A: Intermittent high-dose prednisone (NSC-10023) therapy for multiple myeloma. Cancer Chemother Rep 51:179–187, 1967
123. Abraham D, Carbone PP, Venditti JM et al: Evaluation of chemical agents against the plasma cell tumor LPC-1 in mice. Biochem Pharmacol 16:665–673, 1967
124. Moon JH, Edmonson JH: Procarbazine (NSC-77213) and multiple myeloma. Cancer Chemother Rep (Pt 1) 54:245–248, 1970
125. Samuels ML, Leary WV, Alexanian R et al: Clinical trials with *N*-isopropyl-x-(methylhydrazino)-*p*-toluamide in malignant lymphoma and other disseminated neoplasia. Cancer 20:1187–1194, 1967
126. O'Bryan RM, Luce JK, Talley RW et al: Phase II evaluation of adriamycin in human neoplasia. Cancer 32:1–17, 1973
127. Alberts DE, Salmon SE: Adriamycin (NSC-123127) in the treatment of alkylator-resistant multiple myeloma: A pilot study. Cancer Chemother Rep (Pt 1) 59:345–350, 1975
128. Ghanta VK, Jones MT, Woodard DA et al: Cisdichlorodiammine platinum (II) chemotherapy in experimental murine myeloma MOPC 104E. Cancer Res 37:771–774, 1977
129. Ogawa M, Gale GR, Meischan SJ et aL: Effects of dinitrato (1,2-diaminocyclohexane) platinum (NSC-239851) on murine myeloma and hemopoietic precursor cells. Cancer Res 36:3185–3188, 1976
130. Mellstedt H, Björkholm M, Johansson B et al: Interferon therapy in myelomatosis. Lancet 1:245–247, 1979
131. Idestrōm K, Cantell K, Killander D et al: Interferon therapy in multiple myeloma. Acta Med Scand 205:149–154, 1979
132. Cover story: The big IF in cancer. Time Magazine, 31 March, 1980
133. Alexanian R, Salmon S, Bonnet J et al: Combination chemotherapy for multiple myeloma. Cancer 40:2765–2771, 1977
134. Southwest Oncology Group: Remission maintenance therapy for multiple myeloma. Arch Intern Med 135:147–152, 1975
135. Salmon SE, Alexanian R, Dixon D: Non-cross resistant combination chemotherapy improves survival in multiple myeloma. Blood 54 (Suppl 1): 207a, 1979 (Abs 552)
136. Valeriote F, Bruce WR, Meeker BE: Synergistic action of cyclophosphamide and 1,3 *bis*-(2-chloroethyl)-1-nitrosourea on a transplanted murine lymphoma. J Natl Cancer Inst 40:935–944, 1968
137. Lin H, Bruce WR: Chemotherapy of the transplanted KHT fibrosarcoma in mice. Ser Haematol 5:89–104, 1972
138. Harley JP, Pajak TF, McIntyre OR et al: Improved survival of increased-risk myeloma patients on combined triple-alkylating agent therapy: A study of the CALGB. Blood 54:13–21, 1979
139. Alberts DS, Golde DW: Perterbation of DNA synthesis in multiple myeloma cells following cell-cycle-nonspecific chemotherapy. Cancer Res 34:2911–2914, 1974
140. Drewinko B, Brown BW, Humphrey R et al: Effect of chemotherapy on the labeling index of myeloma cells. Cancer 34:526–531, 1974
141. Salmon SE: Expansion of the growth fraction in multiple myeloma with alkylating agents. Blood 145:119–129, 1975
142. Case DC Jr, Lee BJ III, Clarkson BD: Improved survival times in multiple myeloma treated with melphalan, prednisone, cyclophosphamide, vincristine, and BCNU: M-2 protocol. Am J Med 63:897–903, 1977
143. Conklin R, Alexanian R: Clinical classification of plasma cell myeloma. Arch Intern Med 135:;139–145, 1975
144. Nathaus D, Fahey JL, Potter M: The formation of myeloma protein by a mouse plasma cell tumor. J Exp Med 108:121–130, 1958
145. Harrison JF, Blainey JD, Hardwicke J et al: Proteinuria in multiple myeloma. Clin Sci 31:95–110, 1966
146. Sullivan PW, Salmon SE: Kinetics of tumor growth and regression in IgG multiple myeloma. J Clin Invest 51:1697–1708, 1972
147. Von Schéele C: Light chain myeloma with features of adult Fanconi syndrome. Six years remission with one course of melphalan. Acta Med Scand 199:533–537, 1976
148. Bergsagel DE: Treatment of plasma cell myeloma. Ann Rev Med 30:431–443, 1979
149. Alexanian R, Gehan E, Haut A et al: Unmaintained remissions in multiple myeloma. Blood 51:1005–1011, 1978
150. Fitzpatrick PJ, Rider WD: Half body radiotherapy. Int J Rad Onc Biol Phys 1:197–207, 1976
151. Prato FS, Kurdyak R, Saibil EA et al: The incidence of radiation pneumonitis as a result of single fraction upper half body irradiation. Cancer 39:71–78, 1976
152. Rider WD: Half body radiotherapy. An update. Int J Rad Oncol Biol Phys (Suppl 2) 4:69–70, 1978
153. Jaffe JP, Bosch A, Raich PC: Sequential hemi-body radiotherapy in advanced multiple myeloma. Cancer 43:124–128, 1979
154. Qasim MM: Techniques and results of half body irradiation (HBI) in metastatic carcinoma and myelomas. Clin Onc 5:65–68, 1979
155. Mundy GR, Raisz LG, Cooper RA et al: Evidence for the secretion of an osteoclast stimulating factor in myeloma. N Engl J Med 291:1041–1046, 1974

156. Siris ES, Sherman WH, Baquiran DC et al: Effects of clichloromethylene diphosphonate on skeletal mobilization of calcium in multiple myeloma. N Engl J Med 302:310–315, 1980
157. Lindgärde F, Zettervall O: Hypercalcemia and normal ionized serum calcium in a case of myelomatosis. Ann Intern Med 78:396–399, 1973
158. Soria J, Soria C, Dao C: Immunoglobulin bound calcium and ultrafilterable serum calcium in myeloma. Br J Haematol 34:343–344, 1976
159. Jaffe JP, Mosher DF: Calcium binding by a myeloma protein. Ann J Med 67:343–346, 1979
160. Livingston KE, Perrin RG: The neurosurgical management of spinal metastases causing cord and cauda equina compression. J Neurosurg 49:839–843, 1978
161. Cohen P, Gardner FH: Induction of subacute skeletal fluorosis in a case of multiple myeloma. N Engl J Med 271:1129–1133, 1964
162. Harley JB, Schilling A, Glidwell O: Ineffectiveness of fluoride therapy in multiple myeloma. N Engl J Med 286:1283–1288, 1972
163. Jowsey J, Schenk RK, Reutter FW: Some results of the effect of fluoride on bone tissue in osteoporosis. J Clin Endocrinol Metab 28:869–874, 1968
164. Kyle RA, Joswey J, Kelly PJ et al: Multiple-myeloma bone disease. The comparative effect of sodium fluoride and calcium carbonate or placebo. N Engl J Med 293:1334–1338, 1975
165. Kyle RA, Jowsey J: Effect of sodium fluoride, calcium carbonate, and Vitamin D on the skeleton in multiple myeloma. Cancer (in press)
166. Gardner FH: Fluorides for multiple myeloma. N Engl J Med 287:1252–1253, 1972
167. DeFronzo RA, Cooke CR, Wright JR et al: Renal function in patients with multiple myeloma. Medicine 57:;151–166, 1978
168. Solomon A, Waldmann TA, Fahey JL et al: Metabolism of Bence Jones proteins. J Clin Invest 43:103–117, 1964
169. Waldmann TA, Strober W, Mogielnicki RP: The renal handling of low molecular weight proteins. II Disorders of serum protein catabolism in patients with tubular proteinuria, the nephrotic syndrome, or uremia. J Clin Invest 51:2162–2174, 1972
170. Wochner RD, Strober W, Waldmann TA: The role of kidney in the catabolism of Bence Jones proteins and immunoglobulin fragments. J Exp Med 126:207–221, 1967
171. Clyne DH, Brendstrup L, First MR et al: Renal effects of intraperitoneal kappa chain infection. Induction of crystals in renal tubular cells. Lab Invest 31:131–142, 1974
172. Levi DF, Williams RC Jr, Lindstrom FD: Immunofluorescent studies of the myeloma kidney with special reference to light chain disease. Am J Med 44:922–933, 1968
173. Costanza DJ, Smoller M: Multiple myeloma with the Fanconi syndrome. Study of a case, with electron microscopy of the kidney. Am J Med 34:125–133, 1963
174. Engle RL Jr, Wallis LA: Multiple myeloma and the adult Fanconi syndrome. I Report of a case with crystal-like deposits in the tumor cells and in the epithelial cells of the kidney. Am J Med 22:5–12, 1957
175. Finkel PN, Kronenberg K, Pesce AJ et al: Adult Fanconi syndrome, amyloidosis, and marked kappa light chain proteinuria. Nephron 10:1–24, 1973
176. Sirtoa JH, Hamerman D: Renal function studies in an adult subject with the Fanconi syndrome. Am J Med 16:138–152, 1954
177. Preuss HG, Hammack WJ, Murdaugh HV: The effect of Bence-Jones protein on the *in vitro* function of rabbit renal cortex. Nephron 5:210–216, 1967
178. Preuss HG, Weiss FR, Iammarino RM et al: Effect on rat kidney slice function *in vitro* of proteins from the urines of patients with myelomatosis and nephrosis. Clin Sci Mol Med 46:283–294, 1974
179. Maldonado JE, Velosa JA, Kyle RA et al: Fanconi syndrome in adults. A manifestation of a latent form of myeloma. Am J Med 58:354–364, 1975
180. Pruzanski W, Ogryzlo MA: Abnormal proteinuria in malignant diseases. Adv Clin Chem 13:335–382, 1970
181. Salmon SE: "Paraneoplastic" syndrome associated with monoclonal lymphocyte and plasma cell proliferation. Ann N Y Acad Sci 230:228–239, 1974
182. Shustik C, Bergsagel DE, Pruzanski W: κ and λ light chain disease: survival rates and clinical manifestations. Blood 48:41–51, 1976
183. Pringle JP, Graham RC, Bernier GM: Detection of myeloma cells in the urine sediment. Blood 43:137–143, 1974
184. Russell JA, Fitzharris BM, Corringham R et al: Plasma exchange v peritoneal dialysis for removing Bence-Jones protein. Br J Med 2:1397, 1978
185. Feest TG, Burge PS, Cohen SL: Successful treatment of myeloma kidney by diuresis and plasmapheresis. Br J Med 1:503–4, 1976
186. Misiani R, Remuzzi G, Bertani T et al: Plasmapheresis in the treatment of acute renal failure in multiple myeloma. Am J Med 66:684–688, 1979
187. Humphrey RL, Wright JR, Zachary JB et al: Renal transplantation in multiple myeloma. A case report. Ann Intern Med 83:651–653, 1975
188. Trivedi H, Kumar S: Renal transplantation in lethal disease (letter). Ann Intern Med 85:132, 1976
189. Bjørneboe M, Jensen KB: Plasma volume, colloid-osmotic pressure and gamma globulin in multiple myeloma. Acta Med Scand 186:475–478, 1969
190. Kopp WL, MacKinney AA Jr, Wasson G: Blood volume and hematocrit value in macroglobulinemia and myeloma. Arch Intern Med 123:394–396, 1969
191. Somer T: Hyperviscosity syndrome in plasma cell dyscrasias. Adv Microcirc 6:1–55, 1975
192. Fahey JL: Serum protein disorders causing clinical symptoms in malignant neoplastic disease. J Chron Dis 16:703–712, 1963
193. Fahey JL, Barth WF, Solomon A: Serum hyperviscosity syndrome. JAMA 192:464–467, 1965
194. Bloch KJ, Maki DG: Hyperviscosity syndromes associated with immunoglobulin abnormalities. Sem Hematol 10:113–124, 1973
195. McGrath MA, Penny R: Paraproteinemia: Blood hyperviscosity and clinical manifestations. J Clin Invest 58:1155–1162, 1976
196. MacKenzie MR, Lee TK: Blood viscosity in Waldenström macroglobulinemia. Blood 49:507–510, 1977
197. Smith E, Kochwa S, Wasserman LR: Aggregation of IgG globulin *in vivo*. I The hyperviscosity syndrome in multiple myeloma. Am J Med 39:35–48, 1965
198. MacKenzie MR, Fudenberg HH, O'Reilly RA: The hyperviscosity syndrome. I. In IgG myeloma. The role of protein concentration and molecular shape. J Clin Invest 49:15–20, 1970
199. Capra JD, Kunkel HG: Aggregation of γG_3 proteins: Relevance to the hyperviscosity syndrome. J Clin Invest 49:610–621, 1970
200. Pruzanski W, Watt JG: Serum viscosity and hyperviscosity syndrome in IgG multiple myeloma. Ann Intern Med 77:853–860, 1972
201. Whittaker JA, Tuddenham EGD, Bradley J: Hyperviscosity syndrome in IgA multiple myeloma. Lancet 2:572, 1973
202. Pruzanski W, Jancelewicz Z, Underdown B: Immunological and physiochemical studies of IgAL (λ) cryogelglobulinemia. Clin Exp Immunol 15:181–191, 1973
203. Meltzer M, Franklin EC: Cryoglobulinemia: A study of twenty-nine patients. I. IgG and IgM cryoglobulins and factors affecting cryoprecipitability. Am J Med 40:828–836, 1966
204. MacKay IR, Eriksen N, Motulsky AG et al: Cryo- and macroglobulinemia: Electrophoretic, ultracentrifugal, and clinical studies. Am J Med 20:564–587, 1956
205. Liss M, Fudenberg HH, Kritzman J: A Bence Jones cryoglobulin: Clinical, physical, and immunological properties. Clin Exp Immunol 2:467–475, 1967
206. Godal HC, Borchgrevink CF: The effect of plasmapheresis on the hemostatic function in patients with macroblobulinemia Waldenström and multiple myeloma. Scand J Clin Lab Invest 17 (Suppl 84): 133–137, 1965
207. Doumenc J, Prost RJ, Samama M et al: Anomalie de l'agrégation plaquettaire au cours de la maladie de Waldenström (à propos de 3 cas). Nouv Rev Fr Hematol 6:734–738, 1966

208. Penny R, Castaldi PA, Whitsed HM: Inflammation and hemostasis in paraproteinemias. Br J Haematol 20:35–44, 1971
209. Pachter MR, Johnson SA, Neblett TR et al: Bleeding, platelets, and macroglobulinemia. Am J Clin Pathol 31:467–482, 1959
210. Pachter MR, Johnson SA, Basinski DH: The effect of macroglobulins and their dissociation units on release of platelet factor 3. Thromb Diath Haemorrh 3:501–509, 1959
211. Perkins HA, MacKenzie MR, Fudenberg HH: Hemostatic defects in dysproteinemias. Blood 35:695–707, 1970
212. Lackner H: Hemostatic abnormalities associated with dysproteinemias. Semin Hematol 10:125–133, 1973
213. Coleman M, Vigliano EM, Weksler ME et al: Inhibition of fibrin monomer polymerization by lambda myeloma globulins. Blood 39:210–223, 1972
214. Henstell HH, Kligerman M: A new theory of interference with the clotting mechanism: The complexing of euglobulin with factor V, factor VII, and prothrombin. Ann Intern Med 49:371–387, 1958
215. Brzoza H, Lahav M: Interaction between macroglobulin and fibrinogen with partial dissociation of macroglobulin after coagulation. Isr J Exp Med 11:165–173, 1964
216. Ménaché D: Action des macroglobulines de la malade de Waldenström sur la coagulation étude *in vitro*. Ann Biol Clin 20:169–196, 1962
217. Emmett ME, Narins RG: Clinical use of the anion gap. Medicine 56:38–54, 1977
218. Murray T, Long W, Narins RG: Multiple myeloma and the anion gap. N Engl J Med 292:574–575, 1975
219. Bloth B, Christensson T, Mellstedt H: Extreme hyponatremia in patients with myelomatosis. An effect of cationic paraproteins. Acta Med Scand. 203:273–275, 1978
220. Schnur MJ, Appel GB, Karp G et al: The anion gap in asymptomatic plasma cell dyscrasia. Ann Intern Med 86:304–305, 1977
221. Hoffbrand AV, Hobbs JR, Kremenchuzky S et al: Incidence and pathogenesis of megaloblastic erythropoiesis in multiple myeloma. J Clin Path 20:699–705, 1967
222. Larsson SO: Myeloma and pernicious anemia. Acta Med Scand 172:195–205, 1962
223. Perillie PE: Myeloma and pernicious anemia. Am J Med Sci 275:93–98, 1978
224. Zinneman HH, Hall WH: Recurrent pneumonia in multiple myeloma and some observations on immunologic response. Ann Intern Med 41:1152–1163, 1954
225. Fahey JR, Scoggins R, Utz JP et al: Infections, antibody response and γ globulin components in multiple myeloma and macroglobulinemia. Am J Med 35:698–707, 1963
226. Meyers BR, Hirschman SZ, Axelrod JA: Current patterns of infection in multiple myeloma. Am J Med 52:87–92, 1972
227. Twomey JJ: Infections complicating multiple myeloma and chronic lymphocytic leukemia. Arch Intern Med 132:562–565, 1973
228. Norden CW: Editorial. Arch Intern Med, 1980 (in press)
229. Nolan CM, Baxley PJ, Frasch CE: Antibody response to infection in multiple myeloma. Implications for vaccination. Am J Med 67:331–334, 1979
230. Cone L, Uhr JW: Immunological deficiency disorders associated with chronic lymphocytic leukemia and multiple myeloma. J Clin Invest 43:2241–2248, 1964
231. Broder S, Humphrey R, Durm M et al: Impaired synthesis of polyclonal (nonparaprotein) immunoglobulins by circulating lymphocytes from patients with multiple myeloma. Role of suppressor cells. N Engl J Med 293:887–892, 1975
232. Krakauer RS, Strober W, Waldmann TA: Hypogammaglobulinemia in experimental myeloma: The role of suppressor factors from mononuclear phagocytes. J Immunol 118:1385–1390, 1977
233. Heller P: The mechanism of the immunologic deficiency in myeloma of man and mouse. Blut 37:65–68, 1978
234. Chen Y, Bhoopalam N, Yakulis V et al: Changes in lymphocyte surface immunoglobulin in myeloma and the effect of an RNA-containing plasma factor. Ann Intern Med 83:625–631, 1975
235. Zieger JB, Hansen PJ, Penny R: Leukocyte function in paraproteinemia. Aust NZ J Med 5:39–43, 1975
236. MacGregor RR, Negendank WG, Schrieber AD: Impaired granulocyte adherence in multiple myeloma: Relationship to complement system, granulocyte delivery and infection. Blood 51:591–599, 1978
237. Salmon SE, Samal BA, Hayes DM et al: Role of gamma globulin for immunoprophylaxis in multiple myeloma. N Engl J Med 277:1336–1340, 1967
238. Isobe T, Osserman E: Patterns of amyloidosis and their association with plasma cell dyscrasias, monoclonal immunoglobulins and Bence-Jones proteins. N Engl J Med 290:473–477, 1974
239. Glenner GG, Terry WD: Amyloidosis: Its nature and pathogenesis. Sem Hematol 10:65–86, 1973
240. Cathcart ES, Ritchie RF, Cohen AS et al: Immunoglobulins and amyloidosis. An immunologic study of sixty-two patients with biopsy-proved disease. Am J Med 52:93–101, 1972
241. Glenner GG, Ein D, Eanes ED et al: The creation of "amyloid" fibrils from Bence-Jones proteins *in vitro*. Science 174:712–714, 1971
242. Linke R, Tischendorf FW, Zweker-Franklin D et al: The formation of amyloid-like fibrils *in virto* from Bence-Jones proteins of the Vλ1 subclass. J Immunol 111:24–26, 1972
243. Isersky C, Ein D, Page DL et al: Immunochemical cross-reaction of human amyloid proteins with immunoglobulin light chains. J Immunol 108:486–493, 1973
244. Cohen AS: Amyloidosis. N Engl J Med 277:522–530, 1967
245. Gordon DA, Pruzanski W, Ogryzlo MA et al: Amyloid arthritis simulating rheumatoid disease in five patients with multiple myeloma. Am J Med 55:142–154, 1973
246. Benson MD, Brandt KD, Cohen AS et al: Neuropathy, M components and amyloid. Lancet 1:10–12, 1975
247. Pruzanski W: Editorial. Amyloidogenesis—theories and facts. J Rheumatol 4:219–222, 1977
248. Jarnum S: Gastrointestinal hemorrhage and protein loss in primary amyloidosis. Gut 6:14–18, 1965
249. Schroeder FM, Miller FJ Jr, Nelson JA et al: Gastrointestinal angiographic findings in systemic amyloidosis. Am J Roentgenol 131:143–146, 1978
250. Battle WM, Rubin MR, Cohen S et al: Gastrointestinal-motility dysfunction in amyloidosis. N Engl J Med 301:24–25, 1979
251. Melato M, Bianchi C: Pulmonary amyloidosis with unusual pathological features. Morphol Embryol 24:133–135, 1978
252. Cassidy JT: Cardiac amyloidosis: Two cases with digitalis sensitivity. Ann Intern Med 55:989–994, 1961
253. Barth WF, Glenner GG, Waldmann TA et al: Primary amyloidosis: combined staff conference. Ann Intern Med 69:787–805, 1968
254. Brandt K, Cathcart ES, Cohen AS: A clinical analysis of the course and prognosis of 42 patients with amyloidosis. Am J Med 44:955–969, 1968
255. Case records of the Massachusetts General Hospital (Case 5-1980). N Engl J Med 302:336–344, 1980
256. Barth WF, Willerson JT, Waldmann TA et al: Primary amyloidosis. Clinical, immunological and immunoglobulin metabolism studies in fifteen patients. Ann Intern Med 47:259–273, 1975
257. Kyle RA, Bayrd ED: Amyloidosis: Review of 236 cases. Medicine 54:271–299, 1975
258. Cohen HJ, Lessin LS, Hallal J et al: Resolution of primary amyloidosis during chemotherapy. Studies in a patient with nephrotic syndrome. Ann Intern Med 82:466–473, 1975
259. Jones NF: Renal amyloidosis: Pathogenesis and therapy. Clin Nephrology 6:459–464, 1976
260. Kaufman BM: Primary amyloidosis, paraproteinaemia and neuropathy. Proc Roy Soc Med 69:707–708, 1976
261. Bradstock K, Clancy R, Uther J et al: The successful treatment of primary amyloidosis with intermittent chemotherapy. Aust NZ J Med 8:176–179, 1978
262. Mehta AD: Regression of amyloidosis in multiple myeloma. Br J Clin Prac 32:358–361, 1978
263. Corkery J, Bern MM, Tullis JL: Resolution of amyloidosis and plasma-cell discrasia with combination chemotherapy. Lancet 2:425–426, 1978
264. Wuhrmann F: Ober das coma paraproteinaemieum bei mye-

lomen und macroglobulinaemien. Schweiz med Wschr 2:623–625, 1956
265. Silverstein A, Doniger DF: Neurologic complications of myelomatosis. Arch Neurol 9:534–544, 1963
266. Cohen HJ, Rundles RW: Managing the complications of plasma cell myeloma. Arch Intern Med 135:177–184, 1975
267. Frantzen E, Hertz H, Matzke J et al: Protein studies on cerebrospinal fluid and neurological symptoms in myelomatosis. Acta Neurol Scand 45:1–17, 1969
268. Maldonado JE, Kyle RA, Ludwig J et al: Meningeal myeloma. Arch Intern Med 126:660–663, 1970
269. Durie BGM, Salmon SE, Moon TE: Pretreatment tumor mass, cell kinetics, and prognosis in multiple myeloma. Blood 55:364–372, 1980
270. Davis LE, Drachman DB: Myeloma neuropathy. Successful treatment of two patients and review of cases. Arch Neurol 27:507–511, 1972
271. Drieger H, Pruzanski W: Plasma cell neoplasia with peripheral neuropathy. A study of five cases and a review of the literature. Medicine, 1980 (in press)
272. Weiner LP, Anderson PN, Allen JC: Cerebral plasmacytoma with myeloma protein in the cerebrospinal fluid. Neurology 16:615–618, 1966
273. Somersen A, Osgood CP Jr, Brylski J: Solitary posterior fossa plasmacytoma. J Neurosurg 35:223–228, 1971
274. McCarthy J, Proctor SJ: Cerebral involvement in multiple myeloma: case report. J Clin Path 31:259–264, 1978
275. Bethlem J, van Gool J, den Hartog Jager WA: Progressive multifocal leukoencephalopathy associated with multiple myeloma. Acta Neuropathol 3:525–528, 1964
276. Takatsuki K, Uchiyama T, Sagawa K et al: Plasma cell dyscrasia with polyneuritis and endocrine disorder: Review of 32 patients. Exerpta Medica, International Congress Series No 415. Topics in Haematology. Proc 16th Internat Congr Hematol, 5–11 Sept, p 454, Kyoto, 1976
277. Rousseau JJ, Franck G, Grisar T et al: Osteosclerotic myeloma with polyneuropathy and ectopic secretion of calcitonin. Eur J Cancer 14:133–140, 1978
278. Shapiro HD, Watson RJ: Splenic aspirations in multiple myeloma. Blood 8:755–759, 1953
279. Thomas FB, Clausen KP, Greenberger NJ: Liver disease in multiple myeloma. Arch Intern Med 132:195–202, 1973
280. Simon TL, Rughani IK, Pierson DJ et al: Multiple plasma cytomas with thoracic and biliary involvement. Arch Intern Med 138:1165–1167, 1978
281. Young GP, Bhathal PD, Wall AJ et al: Jaundice in multiple myeloma: The role of oxymetholone. Aust NZ J Med 8:14–22, 1978
282. Brooks AP: Portal hypertension in Waldenström's macroglobulinemia. Br J Med 1:689–690, 1976
283. Goeggel-Lamping C, Kahn SB: Gastrointestinal polyposis in multiple myeloma. JAMA 239:1786–1787, 1978
284. Danby FW, Danby CWE, Pruzanski W: Papular mucinosis with IgG (κ) M-component. CMAJ 114:920–922, 1976
285. Feldman P, Shapiro L, Pick AI et al: Scleromyxedema. A dramatic response to melphalan. Arch Dermatol 99:51–56, 1969
286. Degos R, Civatte J, Clauvel JP et al: Anomalies globulinigues dans les mucinoses cutanées. Bull Soc Franc Dermatol Syphiligr 77:579–591, 1970
287. Cream JJ: Pyoderma gangrenosum with a monoclonal IgM red cell agglomerating factor. Br J Dermatol 84:223–226, 1971
288. Rosner F, Grunwald H: Multiple myeloma terminating in acute leukemia: Report of 12 cases and review of the literature. Am J Med 57:927–939, 1974
289. Cleary B, Binder RA, Kales AN et al: Simultaneous presentation of acute myelomonocytic leukemia and multiple myeloma. Cancer 41:1381–1386, 1978
290. Tursz T, Flandrin G, Brouet J-C et al: Simultaneous occurrence of acute myeloblastic leukemia and multiple myeloma, without previous chemotherapy. Br Med J 1:642–643, 1974
291. Salberg D, Kurtides ES, McKeever WP: Myelomonocytic leukemia in an untreated case of Waldenström's macroglobulinemia. Arch Intern Med 137:514–516, 1977
292. Ligorsky RD, Axelrod AR, Mandell GH et al: Acute myelomonocytic leukemia in a patient with macroglobulinemia and malignant lymphoma. Cancer 39:1156–1162, 1977
293. Osserman EF: The association between plasmacytic and monocytic dyscrasias in man: Clinical and biochemical studies. In Killander J (ed): Gamma Globulins—Structure and Control Biosynthesis, 3rd Nobel Symposium held in Stockholm, June 12–17, pp 573–583. New York, Interscience Publishers, 1967
294. Poulik MD, Berman L, Prasad AS: "Myeloma protein" in a patient with monocytic leukemia. Blood 33:746–758, 1969
295. Barnard DL, Burns GF, Gordon J et al: Chronic myelomonocytic leukemia with paraproteinemia but no detectable plasmacytosis. Cancer 44:927–936, 1979
296. Khaleeli M, Keane WM, Lee GR: Sideroblastic anemia in multiple myeloma: A preleukemic change. Blood 41:17–25, 1973
297. Stein RS, Ellman L, Bloch KJ: The clinical correlates of IgM M-components: an analysis of thirty-four patients. Am J Med Sc 269:209–216, 1975
298. McCallister BD, Bayrd ED, Harrison EG Jr et al: Primary macroglobulinemia. Review with a report on thirty-one cases and notes on the value of continuous chlorambucil therapy. Am J Med 43:394–434, 1967
299. MacKenzie MR, Fudenberg HH: Macroglobulinemia: An analysis of forty patients. Blood 39:874–889, 1972
300. Krajny M, Pruzanski W: Waldenström's macroglobulinemia: Review of 45 cases. Canad Med Assoc J 114:899–905, 1976
301. Franklin EC, Lowenstein J, Bigelow B et al: Heavy chain disease: A new disorder of serum γ-globulins. Report of the first case. Am J Med 37:332–350, 1964
302. Seligmann M, Mihaesco E, Hurez D et al: Immunochemical studies in four cases of alpha-chain disease. J Clin Invest 48:2374–2389, 1969
303. Forte FA, Prelli F, Yount WJ et al: Heavy-chain disease of the μ(γM) type: Report of the first case. Blood 36:137–144, 1970
304. Frangione B, Franklin EC: Heavy-chain diseases: Clinical features and molecular significance of the disordered immunoglobulin structure. Sem Hematol 10:53–64, 1973
305. Pruzanski W, Parr DM, Prychal J et al: γ_3-Heavy-chain disease (γ_3-HCD) in a young patient with Down Syndrome. Study of peripheral blood lymphocytes and of susceptibility to infection. Clin Immunol Immunopathol 12:253–262, 1979
306. Seligmann M, Danon F, Hurez D et al: Alpha-chain disease: A new immunoglobulin abnormality. Science 162:1396–1397, 1968
307. Tabbane S, Tabbane F, Cammoun M et al: Mediterranean lymphomas with alpha heavy chain monoclonal gammopathy. Cancer 38:1989–1996, 1976
308. Galian A, Lecestre M-J, Scotto J et al: Pathological study of alpha-chain disease, with special emphasis on evolution. Cancer 39:2081–2101, 1977
309. Stoop JW, Ballieux RE, Higmans W et al: Alpha-chain disease with involvement of the respiratory tract in a Dutch child. Clin Exp Immunol 9:625–635, 1971
310. Faux JA, Crain JD, Rosen FS et al: An alpha-chain abnormality in a child with hypogammaglobulinemia. Clin Immunol Immunopathol 1:282–290, 1973
311. Manousos ON, Economidou JC: Localized plasmacytoma in a patient with α-chain disease in remission. Br Med J 2:758, 1975
312. Guardia J, Rubiés-Prat J, Gallart MT et al: The evolution of alpha hevay-chain disease. Am J Med 60:596–602, 1976
313. Franklin EC: μ-Chain disease. Arch Intern Med 135:71–72, 1975
314. Jønsson V, Videbaek A, Axelsen NH et al: μ-Chain disease in a case of chronic lymphocytic leukaemia and malignant histiocytoma. I Clinical aspects. Scand J Hematol 16:209–217, 1976
315. Bonhomme J, Seligmann M, Mihaesco C et al: MV-Chain disease in an African patient. Blood 43:485–492, 1974

316. Bergsagel DE: The duration of myeloma remissions survival cannot be explained by the myeloma cell-kill achieved. In Fox BW (ed): Advances in Medical Oncology, Research, and Education. Vol 5, Basis for Cancer Therapy 1. pp 137–143. Oxford & New York, Pergamon Press, 1979
317. Cox EB: Prognosis in myeloma: key role of uric acid in azotemia. Proc AACR-ASCO 21:483, 1980
318. Waldmann TA, Strober W: Metabolism of immunoglobulins. Prog Allergy 13:1–110, 1969
319. Rider WD, Warwick OH: Clinical experience with the use of R48 (NN-di-2′-chloroethyl-2′-naphthylamine). Ann NY Acad Sci 68:1116–1121, 1958

John D. Minna
Paul A. Bunn, Jr.

CHAPTER 39

Paraneoplastic Syndromes

Tumors produce signs and symptoms in the patient by invasion, obstruction, and bulk mass at the primary tumor site, and in regional and distant deposits. In addition, tumors can produce signs and symptoms at a distance from the tumor or its metastases. These are collectively referred to as "Paraneoplastic Syndromes" or "remote effects" of malignancy.[1-4] By definition, these syndromes should not be produced as a direct effect of the tumor or its metastases. The best characterized paraneoplastic syndromes are those produced by tumors secreting a polypeptide hormone (*e.g.*, adrenocorticotrophin, ACTH, or parathormone, PTH), which is distributed by the circulation and acts on target organ(s) at a distance from the tumor. In these instances it can be expected that the course of the paraneoplastic syndrome will run parallel to the course of the underlying malignancy since removal or destruction of the tumor will halt production of the hormone. There are many organ associated syndromes that have been reported in conjunction with malignancy for which there is no known etiology (*e.g.*, cerebellar degeneration, Eaton–Lambert syndrome). In some instances, the course of these syndromes runs parallel to the course of the underlying malignancy, suggesting a true paraneoplastic etiology with a syndrome produced by an as yet undefined tumor product or hormone. In other instances, the paraneoplastic syndrome and tumor run independent courses. In some of these cases a tumor product may have caused irreversible damage to an organ system, while in others the syndrome is not related to the tumor but to other factors (*e.g.*, treatment or opportunistic infection). For example, progressive multifocal leukoencephalopathy (PML) was initially described as a neurologic paraneoplastic syndrome.[5] More recently, it has been appreciated that PML is caused by a virus and while patients with malignancy may be prone to develop this viral syndrome, the PML is not truly "paraneoplastic."[6]

Endocrine tumors can also be functional and their hormonal products (polypeptide, catecholamines, iodothyronine, or steroidal) give symptoms at a distance from the primary tumor (and thus are "paraneoplastic"). However, for practical purposes, this chapter will deal only with syndromes produced by tumors arising in sites other than the pituitary, adrenal glands, endocrine pancreas, endocrine cells of the GI tract, and endocrine cells of the ovaries and testes, as well as all forms of the carcinoid syndrome. These are covered in detail in other chapters.

Although not rare, paraneoplastic syndrome develop in a minority of cancer patients. Their exact frequency is difficult to determine for a variety of reasons including: varying definitions, unknown etiologies, and most importantly, lack of systematic case-controlled studies. For example, in an uncontrolled study, Croft and Wilkinson reported that 7% of cancer patients have neurologic paraneoplastic syndromes while in a case controlled study, Brody found no difference in the frequency of neurologic syndromes in patients with lung cancer and controls with benign chronic lung disease.[7,8] The frequency figures given in this chapter are, in nearly all cases, from uncontrolled studies.

The importance of the paraneoplastic syndromes (including hormones detected by immunoassay) and elucidating their mechanisms are manyfold:

1. Their appearance may be the first sign of a malignancy, which allows its early detection in a curable state

2. They may simulate metastatic disease and thus prevent patients from having curative therapy
3. Conversely, treatable complications of malignancy (metastatic disease, infection) may be ascribed to a paraneoplastic syndrome leading to withholding appropriate therapy
4. They can be used as tumor markers in previously treated patients to detect early recurrence, or in patients undergoing adjuvant therapy to guide further therapy
5. In patients with metastatic disease their syndromes can be disabling and appropriate treatment of the paraneoplasia may be the best means of palliating patients
6. It is possible that the hormones released by tumors are required for tumor growth (*i.e.*, the tumor may produce its own growth factors and "autostimulate"); thus, appropriate identification of such hormones may allow a new rationale therapeutic approach to treatment of the neoplasms as well[9]

Because of their importance, numerous articles describing paraneoplastic syndromes have been published in the past 20 years. For the interested reader, excellent detailed reviews are available.[1–4,10,11]

ETIOLOGY AND PATHOGENESIS OF PARANEOPLASTIC SYNDROMES

Paraneoplastic syndromes can arise by:

1. Tumor-produced biologically active proteins or polypeptides, including peptide hormones, their precursors, prostaglandins, fetal proteins such as carcinoembryonic antigen (CEA), or alpha fetal protein (AFP), other proteins such as immunoglobulins, and enzymes produced and released by tumors
2. Autoimmunity or immune complex production and immune suppression
3. "Ectopic receptor" production or a competitive blockade of normal hormone action by tumor-produced biologically inactive hormones
4. "Forbidden contact" where there is release of enzymes (*e.g.*, placental alkaline phosphatase) or other products that normally are not circulated but which takes place because of abnormal tumor vasculature or disrupted basement membranes allowing antigenic reactions, inappropriate initiation of normal physiologic functions, and other toxic manifestations to occur
5. By unknown causes

Some syndromes of uncertain etiology may be mediated by circulating substances produced by tumors such as CNS degeneration, myopathies, myasthenic syndrome, dermatologic manifestations, hematologic syndromes, (including anemia, leukocytosis, vasculidities-thrombophlebitis), fever, and anorexia.[10,11] In other instances, the syndromes may not be paraneoplastic and infectious or other causes may be found.

DIFFERENTIAL DIAGNOSIS

The importance and frequency of paraneoplastic syndromes make it imperative that the appropriate diagnosis be established. In instances where the etiology of the paraneoplastic syndrome is unknown, this may mean excluding all other known causes of the syndrome. Each section of this chapter includes a listing of the differential diagnosis because of its central importance. In general, paraneoplastic syndromes must be distinguished from:

1. Direct invasion by the primary tumor or its metastases
2. Obstruction caused by tumor or tumor products
3. Vascular abnormalities
4. Infections
5. Fluid and electrolyte abnormalities
6. Toxicity of cancer therapy including cytotoxic chemotherapy, radiation therapy, immunotherapy or antibiotic therapy

ENDOCRINOLOGIC MANIFESTATIONS OF MALIGNANCY

Paraneoplastic syndromes caused by the production of polypeptide hormones are the most frequent and best understood paraneoplastic syndromes and consequently will be considered in the most detail. To establish a paraneoplastic etiology for alterations in hormone production, conclusive evidence that the hormone is produced by the tumor must be established. The differential diagnosis of endocrinologic abnormalities in the cancer patient is shown in Table 39-1.

The laboratory evaluation begins after a complete history and physical examination. Abnormal levels of the hormone in question should be documented, usually by radioimmunoassay. Concomitant measurements of other hormones in the feedback control of the hormones can be measured before and after stimulatory and inhibitory hormones are administered. Paraneoplastic hormone production will usually be independent of the normal regulatory mechanisms. Besides elevated hormone levels, independent of the normal control mechanisms, other direct evidence that a tumor produces a hormone or a paraneoplastic syndrome includes:

1. Fall in hormone levels after removal or treatment of the tumor
2. Maintenance of elevated hormone levels following extirpation of the "normal" gland of origin of the hormone
3. Demonstration of an arteriovenous gradient of hormone levels across the tumor
4. Demonstration of synthesis and secretion of the hormone by tumor tissue *in vitro*

TABLE 39-1. Endocrinologic Manifestations of Malignancy: Differential Diagnosis

1. Hormone production by benign cells (*e.g.*, parathyroid adenema)
2. Hormone production by a malignancy of an endocrine organ (*e.g.*, MEA)
3. Alterations in hormone production as a direct result of infiltration of an endocrine gland by a primary tumor or its metastases
4. Alterations in hormone production by therapy
5. Alteration in hormone production by infection
6. Paraneoplastic

5. Ultimately, demonstration of such synthesis and secretion by *in vitro,* clonal tissue culture isolates of the tumor cells

The endocrine paraneoplastic syndromes, the responsible hormone, the most frequently associated tumor types, and incidence are shown in Table 39-2.[12,13] With the development of radioimmunoassays and screening of cancer patients, it was found that hormone production in cancer patients (and presumably from their tumors) was much more frequent than previously realized.[3,12] Table 39-3 lists screening studies of lung cancer patients or tumor extracts for the presence of various hormones using radioimmunoassays.[14–16] It must be stressed that these frequencies are much higher than the clinically recognized paraneoplastic syndromes related to these hormones because the large molecular weight hormone precursors, fragments, or subunits secreted by tumors are often biologically inactive. Other factors that also obscure the true incidence of hormone secretion by tumors include inadequate clinical follow-up (*e.g.*, spot checks of patients rather than observation throughout the clinical course); production of a hormone that does not have easily recognizable clinical effect (such as development of the acromegalic effects of growth hormone (GH), which may take years to become manifest); operation of normal physiologic feedback mechanisms, which suppress normal hormone production; secretion of multiple hormones (*e.g.*, secretion of ACTH obscuring the clinical effect of simultaneous arginine vasopressin (AVP) secretion); and finally, investigator and available laboratory facility bias.

ACTH/CUSHING'S SYNDROME

Evidence[17–19] from analysis of cultured tumor cells, pituitary extracts, and recombination DNA work demonstrates that the prohormone ("stem hormone") molecule of ACTH contains in sequence from the C-terminal to the N-terminal end:

1. A putative signal peptide (amino acid position −141 to −110)
2. A region with unknown function (position −110 to −53)
3. Gamma −MSH (position −53 to −48)
4. A region with unknown function (position −48 to −1)
5. ACTH (position 1 to 39) = "classic" ACTH, which contains within it alpha-MSH (position 1 to 13) and corticotrophin-like intermediate lobe peptide, CLIP (position 18 to 39)

TABLE 39-2. Endocrine Paraneoplastic Syndromes[12,13]

SYNDROME	HORMONE	TUMOR	INCIDENCE (percent)
Cushing's syndrome	ACTH	Lung cancer-all types	0–2.0%
		Small-cell lung cancer	2.8,7,22
Inappropriate antidiuresis	AVP	Lung cancer-all types	0.9–2.0
		Small-cell lung cancer	8,12,35,53
Non-metastatic hypercalcemia	PTH	Lung cancer-all types	1.0–7.5
		Squamous cell lung cancer	15
		Other tumors	14
Gynecomastia		Lung cancer-all types	0.5–0.9
		Small-cell lung cancer	2.0
Hyperthyroidism		Lung Cancer	0–1.4
Calcitonin		Medullary carcinoma of the thyroid	
		Small-cell lung cancer	
		Other lung cancer types	
		Breast cancer	0–70

TABLE 39-3. Frequency of Peptide Hormone Elevation in the Blood of 110 Lung Cancer Patients*[14,15,16]

	% OF PATIENTS WITH SIGNIFICANTLY ELEVATED LEVELS			
HORMONE	SMALL-CELL	EPIDERMOID	ADENOCARCINOMA	LARGE-CELL
	(N = 149)	(N = 64)	(N = 17)	(N = 19)
ACTH	30–69	0–80	17–75	26
LPH	54	33	20	not done
Calcitonin	48–64	9	0	11
ADH	32	—	—	—
PTH	27	32	0	17
B-HCG	1–32	19	17	26
GH	0	3	0	0

* Not all studies were done in all patients.
See references for details.

6. Beta-lipotropin, beta-LPH (position 42 to 134), which contains within it gamma-LPH (position 42 to 101) and beta-MSH (position 84 to 101)
7. Met-enkephalin (position 104 to 108)
8. Beta-endorphin (position 104 to 134).

The prohormone molecule has been called "big ACTH" or pro-opiocortin and contains four repetitive sequences based on the ACTH/MSH core, with these sequences separated by paired basic residues. The importance of the promolecule is that it can be split up into many biologically active fragments. These activities include adrenal gland stimulation to make corticosteroids and androgens (*e.g.*, by ACTH); melanocyte stimulation-hyperpigmentation activity (by MSH containing peptides); and opiate-like activity (beta-LPH, beta-endorphin, and met-enkephalin). There has been an explosion of knowledge concerning the biologic activity of fragments of this molecule, particularly the opiod peptides (beta-LPH, beta-LPH, B-endorphin, met-enkephalin), which mimic morphine in their action.[20–22] The paired basic residues flank the biologically active sequences. At these sites proteolytic processing takes place which determines the biologic activity (and thus the paraneoplastic syndrome) seen in humans. Thus, the regulation of cleavage of the promolecule in neoplastic states is important. The cleavage patterns change during development and may be different in tumors than adult pituitary tissue.[22] In addition, pro-opiocortin is a glycosylated peptide and glycosylation may play an important role in proteolysis, packaging, and storage. While classically, ectopic ACTH production is thought to be unregulated, some tumor tissues studied *in vitro* continue to show some control over ACTH secretion by way of a cyclic AMP dependent mechanism.[23]

Clinical Features of "ectopic" pro-opiocortin (ACTH/LPH) excess

As discussed previously, the promolecule may circulate wih no clinically evident effect because it is biologically inactive and unable to bind to receptors. The clinical features of the ectopic ACTH syndrome include hypokalemia, hyperglycemia, edema, muscle weakness or atrophy, hypertension, and weight loss. The other features seen in pituitary Cushing's disease or exogenous corticosteroid excess (centripedal obesity, cutaneous striae, moon facies, buffalo hump, and pigmentation) are uncommonly seen but are said to be more frequent in the more indolent carcinoids, thymomas, and pheochromocytomas. While the cases first reported involved men, with the increased incidence of lung cancer in women, hirsutism may start to be a paraneoplastic syndrome feature and was seen in Brown's original case.[24]

While Cushing's syndrome is a well-recognized clinical effect of ectopic ACTH it is almost certain that other clinical states will be related to other fragments in the promolecule. Thus, neurologic syndromes, aberrant mental behavior, decreased activity, catatonia, cachexia–anorexia, inappropriate analgesia, and other states associated with the endogenous opioids should be found.

FREQUENCY OF ECTOPIC PRO-OPIOCORTIN (ACTH) PRODUCTION BY TUMORS. The major clinical association of ectopic ACTH production is with lung cancer, particularly of the small-cell carcinoma histologic type.[3,12,19] Lung cancer represents over 50% of the clinically obvious cases while bronchial carcinoids and neural crest lesions (pheochromocytomas, neuroblastomas, medullary carcinomas of the thyroid) amount to 15% each, and bronchial carcinoid and thymomas represent 10% each. Table 39-4 gives the frequency of finding significantly elevated levels of ACTH by RIA in the blood and tumor extracts of lung cancer patients. A wide range of 20–90% positivity is found in the reported series for elevations of plasma ACTH.[33] Clinically apparent Cushing's syndrome is found in 0.4–2% of patients with lung cancer of all histologic types.[34,35] However, 25% of patients with small-cell lung cancer have either Cushing's syndrome or significantly increased cortisol levels associated with ectopic ACTH, while 49% of small-cell cancer patients have AM plasma cortisol elevations not suppressed by 8 mg of dexamethasone taken the night before.[12,15,27,33,36,37] Nearly all ex-

TABLE 39-4. Frequency of ACTH Elevation in Blood and Tumor Extracts as Detected by RIA in Lung Cancer Patients Without Clinically Evident Ectopic ACTH Syndrome

SOURCE OF MATERIAL TUMOR TYPE	# PATIENTS	% POSITIVE	REFERENCES
PATIENT'S BLOOD			
All histologic types	290	19,41,42,88	25,26,27,28
Epidermoid	88	0–50	25,27
Adenocarcinoma	25	17–26	25,27
Large-cell carcinoma	28	26–49	25,27
Small-cell carcinoma	25	29–30	15,27
Chronic obstructive pulmonary disease	101	25*	26,28
TUMOR EXTRACTS (SURGICAL SPECIMENS)			
All histologic types	127	31,58,93,100	25,26,29,30
Epidermoid	49	41	25
Adenocarcinoma	17	6	25
Large-cell carcinoma	8	25	25
Small-cell carcinoma-carcinoid	12	100	31,32

* 8/48 patients with elevated ACTH levels were subsequently shown to develop lung cancer within 2 years.[26,28]

tracts of small-cell lung cancer tumors have increased levels of ACTH and LPH detected by RIA. The other histologic types vary in positivity between 6 and 40%. While non-small-cell lung cancer types have increased cortisol levels, the mechanism of this is not known.[11,12,27] Likewise, the frequency of ectopic ACTH-associated clinical syndromes and adrenal function are not well described for other tumor types.[19]

HISTOLOGY OF ACTH-PRODUCING TUMORS. Azzopardi and Williams reviewed the world's literature on Cushing's syndrome and found that 112 of 130 cases arose in the lung, pancreas, or thymus.[38] The most frequent histology was a small cell cancer of the lung-like pattern followed by a carcinoid morphology. Other tumors included pheochromocytomas, related tumors, and certain ovarian tumors. Ten years later, Skrabanek and Powell continued the literature review of cases with ectopic ACTH and Cushing's syndrome and found that all such tumors with clinically apparent ACTH excess could be grouped into a carcinoid-oat cell (small-cell) group and a pheochromocytoma–neuroblastoma class based on histology.[39] They felt that tumors found in other organs besides the lung (*e.g.*, thymus, all thymic carcinoids rather than epithelial thymoma), thyroid (medullary carcinoma), esophagus, stomach, pancreas, small intestine, appendix, salivary gland, ovary, testis, uterine cervix, and prostate had either a carcinoid or small-cell lung cancer-like histology when histology was available for review.[40,41] They and others postulated that these tumors arose only where normal Kulchitsky-type cells occur and thus could potentially have a common origin.

Whether or not ectopic ACTH production is even seen in tumor types of diverse histology and embryologic derivation or is restricted to certain classes of cells is under investigation. However, for clinical purposes, the presence of Cushing's syndrome or very high levels of ACTH is found in the large majority of cases with pituitary tumors, primary adrenal disease, small-cell lung cancer, small-cell-like cancers of other organs, carcinoids, or the pheochromocytoma–neuroblastoma group. Whenever it is suggested that another histology besides one of these is present (*e.g.*, adenocarcinoma), this should be viewed with skepticism and carefully documented. The histologic material should be reviewed and more obtained, if necessary. At present, the extrapulmonary cancers with small-cell-like histology should be treated as if they were small cell carcinoma of the lung, while those with carcinoid histology should be dealt with as carcinoids (see Chapter 14).[42,43] In the future, it will be important to obtain more studies on the efficacy of chemotherapy on tumors producing ACTH that do not have typical small-cell or carcinoid histology.

DIAGNOSIS OF ECTOPIC PRO-OPIOCORTICOID SYNDROME. Some 40% of patients presenting with overt Cushing's syndrome have pituitary Cushing's with an obvious tumor, 28% have pituitary Cushing's syndrome without tumors (and both of these usually occur in women of child-bearing age), 17% have adrenal Cushing's (usually presenting in children), while 15% have the ectopic Cushing's syndrome (which usually presents in adult men). While the production of pro-opoicorticoid molecule may have hitherto unrecognized clinical effects, the diagnosis of clinically significant ectopic ACTH excess begins with thinking about the possibility in the appropriate clinical setting, such as an older man with small-cell lung cancer or a patient with unexplained hypokalemic alkylosis, particularly if it is accompanied by edema, hypertension, profound muscular weakness or atrophy, mental changes, or glucose intolerance. Patients with ectopic ACTH from thymic tumors and bronchial carcinoids are usually younger and present with more of the other features of Cushing's syndrome, primarily because of the more indolent course of the neoplasms. When classic clinical features are present, a plasma ACTH of over 200 pg/ml is highly suggestive of ectopic ACTH production. The simplest biochemical approach is to obtain an 8 AM and a 6 PM cortisol level (in ectopic ACTH these are usually over 40 μg% showing the loss of diurnal variation with the ectopic ACTH syndrome) followed by an 8 AM cortisol and ACTH level after 2 mg of dexamethasone given every 6 hours for 8 doses (48 hours). In 95% of ectopic hormone cases, the ACTH and cortisol level will not suppress (reduction in cortisol, ACTH levels by at least 40% of the prior values); this lack of suppression is virtually diagnostic of ectopic ACTH production. The same tests can be applied if the patient presents with Cushing's syndrome without an obvious tumor. If the results are consistent with ectopic ACTH secretion, then a careful evaluation for occult tumor should proceed and be rigorously continued until the source of the ACTH is identified. With adrenal hyperplasia or carcinoma, the ACTH levels will be low (suppression of normal pituitary ACTH) even if the cortisol levels do not suppress with dexamethasone. Most pituitary tumors will suppress with the high-dose dexamethasone and the ACTH levels are usually much higher in the ectopic ACTH syndrome. Reportedly, half of patients with ectopic ACTH produced by carcinoids may suppress and occasionally a tumor may secrete in a cyclic fashion.[44,45] In difficult cases (*e.g.*, distinguishing a small pulmonary carcinoid that suppresses with dexamethasone vs a pituitary lesion), the question can be resolved by selective venous catheterization with ACTH determinations.[46] Other sources of difficulty in initial recognition can occur in the simultaneous production of two hormones (such as ACTH and AVP) or of a peptide hormone and amine product.[12,47] However, the very occurrence of multiple hormone secretion indicates the presence of a non-pituitary tumor. Other cases of dexamethasone suppression of ectopic ACTH production have been postulated to be related to secretion of a corticotropin-releasing hormone (CRF) by the tumor.[48,49] The CRF is postulated to act either on the pituitary to stimulate pituitary ACTH release or at the tumor level to stimulate tumor cell ACTH production. However, until either the normal or paraneoplastic "CRF" activity can be isolated, characterized, and actually proven to exist, the CRF paraneoplastic syndrome is in limbo.

Treatment of Ectopic ACTH and Related Syndromes

The treatment of ectopic opiocorticoid syndromes should primarily be directed at the tumor. In the case of carcinoids this can involve surgery; with thymomas, surgery or radiotherapy. With appropriate therapy, the syndrome is apparently cured and high levels of ACTH reduced in a fraction of these patients.[50] While prior reviews have stated that a bad prognosis of less than 4 months is expected for the ectopic ACTH syndrome with small-cell lung cancer, these were before the substantial gains in treatment and potential cure of some patients with small-cell carcinoma had been made. (The principles of the treatment of small-cell lung carcinomas with combination chemotherapy is discussed in detail in Chapter 14.) If the histology of any mediastinal or extrathoracic tumor is compatible with a small-cell tumor, the authors would favor treating this patient as though he had small-cell lung cancer. The data on response to therapy of Cushing's syndrome in small-cell cancer patients are anectodal but reports of fall in ACTH levels with combination chemotherapy with or without radiotherapy have appeared.[14,19] If treatment of the tumor fails, drugs that inhibit adrenal corticoid production may be used such as aminoglutethimide metyrapone or o'p'DDD.[46,51,52,53] (The reader should review appropriate endocrinology sources for directions in using these adrenal suppressants.) Obviously, after such drug treatment, patients would have to be treated with supplemental steroids to avoid hypoadrenalism. Because of the increasing use of aminoglutethimide in breast cancer patients, this drug is probably the first choice. Another possibility includes combining aminoglutethimide and metyrapone to lower the dose-related toxicity of both agents along with dexamethasone and fludrocortisone.[54] In rare cases, with chronic ectopic ACTH excess and indolent tumors, bilateral adrenalectomy can be considered.

Use of proACTH/LPH for Early Cancer Detection

Odell and coworkers have found significant blood elevations of proACTH/LPH in 92% of pancreatic cancers, 72% of lung cancers, 54% of gastric or esophagus cancers, 41% of breast cancers, and 27% of colon cancers, while corresponding values for elevated LPH were 25%, 36%, 14%, 0%, and 10%, respectively for these tumor types.[16] In general, the quantitative levels of proACTH/ACTH and LPH were correlated. Some 20% of patients with chronic obstructive pulmonary disease (COPD) had blood elevations of proACTH while 13% had elevations of LPH. Other studies have also found proACTH elevations in chronic lung disease, suggesting the lung may produce or bind proACTH or LPH in response to injury.[28,30] Some of the patients (5/20) with elevated proACTH in COPD went on to develop lung cancer while only 2/81 COPD patients with normal plasma levels of ACTH developed lung cancer.[26]

When ACTH, calcitonin, and hCG were done simultaneously, significant elevated levels were found in 65% of 109 lung cancer patients and 78% of small-cell cancer patients, suggesting use of several markers in concert to detect lung cancer.[15] More studies are needed to know whether the proACTH-LPH or other peptide hormone assays are predictors of the development of lung cancer, and whether they will be useful in following the course of the disease. Extracts of other tumors besides lung cancer showed significant elevations (over 1 ng/gm tissue) of proACTH or LPH, 6/16 colon cancers, 3/4 breasts, and 22/31 with miscellaneous tumors and metastatic lesions. However, while elevated levels of immunoreactive material were found, there is no direct evidence that the tumors themselves produced the peptides. It is possible that many tumors make the pre-opiocorticoid but only some have the ability to cleave it appropriately into biologically active forms. Thus, the expression of the syndromes may depend more on the procession of the promolecule rather than the presence of the ectopic prohormone itself.[2]

With the development and use of RIAs for measuring lipotropin, beta endorphin and receptor assays for measuring endogenous opiate peptides in human cerebrospinal fluid and plasma, it may become possible to relate unusual neurologic syndromes and mental behavior directly to fragments derived from the pro-opiocorticoid molecule.[16,20,55] It is certainly reasonable at present to start applying these assays to patients with such symptoms and appropriate tumor settings (such as lung cancer). Recently, circulating immune complexes of ACTH and human immunoglobulins have been reported.[56] Thus, it is possible that ACTH will also be involved in an immune complex paraneoplastic syndrome. A portion of the ACTH promolecule undergoes, with opioid activity, a striking increase in the pituitary of the newborn monkeys. It has been speculated that this increase in endogenous opioid helps the fetus withstand the stress of parturition.[22] Likewise, it is not unreasonable to speculate that tumor production of an analgesic-like material such as beta-endorphin may allow the cancer patient a measure of relief from tumor-related symptoms. Further work quantitating the amount and nature of such endogenous analgesics is necessary.

SYNDROME OF "INAPPROPRIATE" SECRETION OF ANTIDIURETIC HORMONE (SIADH)

The association of hyponatremia and lung cancer was noted in 1938; the syndrome of "inappropriate secretion" of antidiuretic hormone (ADH, arginine vasopressin, AVP) was postulated by Schwartz and coworkers in 1957 to be caused by stimulation of the posterior pituitary to secrete AVP by presence of the thoracic tumor.[57,58] It was then demonstrated by Amatruda and coworkers in 1963 to be related to tumor production of AVP.[59] AVP, oxytocin, and neurophysins have been found by RIA in tumors and the AVP is bioactive as well as immunoreactive.[12,60] The neurophysins are normally synthesized, stored, and secreted in parallel with AVP and oxytocin.[61] These polypeptides function as binding proteins for AVP and oxytocin; there are different neurophysins for AVP and oxytocin.[62] Whether AVP and oxytocin actually form a promolecule with their respective neurophysins is under investigation.[12] At present there are no recognized syndromes related to tumor production of neurophysins or oxytocin while tumor production of AVP results in hyponatremia.

Clinical Findings and Pathophysiology of SIADH

Continuous tumor production, exogenous administration, or posterior pituitary production of AVP all result in a syndrome of hyponatremia, hyperglycemia, urine inappropriately higher in osmolality than the plasma, and high urinary sodium concentrations in the face of serum hyponatremia.[2,3,12] This is felt to result from the action of AVP on the renal tubule with resultant water retention. The hyponatremia comes from both renal sodium loss and dilution by water retention. The mechanism of the natriuresis is not defined but could include an increased filtered sodium load, decrease in aldosterone secretion, or a decrease in tubular reabsorption of sodium. The major clinical symptomatology comes from water intoxication (hypo-osmolality and hyponatremia), and is manifested by altered mental status, confusion, lethargy, psychotic behavior, seizures, coma, and occasionally death.[2,3,12,63] Focal neurologic findings can be associated with water intoxication from SIADH alone without brain metastases.[63] Because of the predominant occurrence of SIADH with small-cell lung cancer and the frequent presence of brain metastases in this cancer, all patients with neurologic syndromes in small-cell lung cancer should have serum sodium checked for the presence of hyponatremia, and all small-cell cancer patients with hyponatremia and neurologic syndromes should also be evaluated for brain metastases.

Diagnosis of Ectopic AVP Production and the IADH Syndrome

Hyponatremia is the usual mode of presentation of SIADH because of the routine use of serum electrolytes in patient evaluation (see Table 39-5). Occasionally patients will present with neurologic symptoms. The first major problem is to differentiate SIADH from the multiple other causes of hyponatremia (such as diuretic usage, cardiac, hepatic and renal failure, dilutional causes, and diminished function of adrenals, anterior pituitary or thyroid gland). In addition, there are a variety of drugs that can impair free water excretion either by acting on the renal tubule or inducing pituitary AVP, including chlorpropamide, thiazide diuretics, and most importantly, for cancer patients, cyclophosphamide, vincristine, and morphine.[64,65,66] To separate out these causes of hyponatremia from SIADH it is mandatory to demonstrate:

1. Hypo-osmolality (usually less than 280 mOsm/kg)
2. Urinary osmolality greater than the plasma (usually in the range of 500 mOsm/kg or higher)
3. Continued urinary excretion of sodium (usually over 20 mEq/L) off of any diuretics
4. Absence of signs of volume depletion
5. Normal renal function
6. Normal adrenal and thyroid function (these are not routinely tested unless there are other signs suggesting hypofunction of these organs)

Fichman and Bethune studied 86 patients with SIADH and found serum sodiums of 88–126 mEq/L, urine sodiums of 35–175 mEq/24 hours, serum osmolalities of 190–273 mOsm/kg, and urine osmolalities of 332–780 mOsm/kg.[66] The most common mistake in diagnosis of SIADH is failing to notice the prior administration of a diuretic or occult volume depletion with resulting dilutional hyponatremia. Usually, repeat clinical examination can exclude these causes. While AVP can be measured by RIA, this is not routinely available and many conditions can be associated with both the "appropriate" and "inappropriate" secretion of AVP.

The most common disorders associated with SIADH besides small-cell lung cancer include CNS diseases (*e.g.*, CNS infection, head trauma, intracranial space-occupying lesions, subarachnoid hemorrhage, acute intermittent prophyria, pain, and emotional stress) and pulmonary infections (see Table 39-5). Clearly, if any of these factors are present in patients with SIADH and malignant disease (including small-cell cancer), they should be treated in an effort to control the SIADH. Water loading can elicit clinically occult SIADH but it can be very dangerous in the patient with hyponatremia and probably should not be done if the serum sodium is 125 mEq/L or less.[64]

In studies of lung cancer patients with SIADH and high levels of AVP by RIA, fluid restriction further increased the already elevated AVP level. This probably resulted from stimulation of the pituitary to release AVP.[67] The other causes of SIADH (particularly drugs), could account for some of the SIADH seen in tumor patients without small-cell lung cancer

TABLE 39-5. Differential Diagnosis in the Syndrome of "Inappropriate" Secretion of Antidiuretic Hormone

1. Tumors
   - Small-cell lung cancer
   - Other types
2. Pulmonary, chest conditions
   - Infection (tuberculosis, abscess, pneumonia—viral or bacterial), mitral stenosis (s/p surgical correction)
3. Central Nervous System
   - Trauma (skull fracture, subdural, concussion, subarachnoid hemorrhage, thrombosis)
   - Intracranial space-occupying lesions (primary and metastatic tumors)
   - Infections (meningitis, encephalitis, lues)
   - Vasculitis (lupus)
   - Guillian–Barré
   - Acute intermittent porphyria
   - Pain and emotional stress
4. Drugs
   - Chlorpropamide
   - Morphine
   - Nicotine
   - Ethanol
   - Cyclophosphamide
5. "Idiopathic"

or carcinoid histology and stress the need for biosynthetic studies of AVP by cultured tumor cells to prove the source of the AVP. In any event, these other complications (*e.g.*, pneumonia) usually occur because of the cancer and the development of SIADH from them represents a "secondary" paraneoplastic syndrome. For example, cyclophosphamide and vincristine are both used in the treatment of small-cell lung cancer. When cyclophosphamide is given in high doses and the patient hydrated to prevent cystitis, the combined effect of cyclophosphamide to decrease free water clearance and the water load can lead to the SIADH.[66,68,69] Whether this represents release of pituitary AVP or a direct effect of cyclophosphamide metabolites on the renal tubules is not known.[68]

If the histology of the tumor associated with SIADH is small-cell cancer, the cancer will be treated along with any other causes and correlation can be made between the tumor response and the SIADH. If the tumor histology is other than small cell or carcinoid one should be skeptical about tumor production of AVP until the cause of the SIADH and other etiologies are sought. If no other etiologies of SIADH are apparent, thought should be given to obtaining more tumor tissue as a component of small-cell carcinoma may be present. This would dictate a more aggressive chemo-radiotherapy approach than that taken for an "unresponsive" non small-cell tumor type.

If a patient presents with "idiopathic" SIADH, a careful search and follow-up for small-cell tumor must be maintained and while cases like this are uncommon, the work-up probably should include a full staging evaluation for small-cell cancer including fiberoptic bronchoscopy and CT scans of the chest and abdomen to locate small tumor masses. The tumor should declare itself within a few months. In comparing tumor-related SIADH and SIADH resulting from other causes, serum and urinary sodium, osmolality, blood urea nitrogen, plasma AVP, or renin levels all failed to distinguish neoplastic from non-neoplastic causes.[68] The speed of rise in serum sodium with water restriction is supposedly faster (occurring in 3 days compared to 7–10 days) in non-neoplastic causes compared to neoplastic causes of SIADH.[70] However, this is probably not a clear enough distinction to be clinically useful.

Frequency and Tumor Types

The vast majority of the tumors producing AVP are small-cell carcinomas of the lung[2,3,12,13] However, the SIADH has been seen with other tumor types including carcinomas of the prostate, adrenal cortex, esophagus, pancreas, duodenum, colon, bronchial carcinoids, thymomas, head and neck, Hodgkin's disease, and non-Hodgkin's lymphomas.[2,3,12] At least some of these may have had a non-pulmonary small-cell or carcinoid histology. Small-cell lung cancer lines grown in tissue culture make immunologically detectable AVP.[71,72] However, there have been no clear biosynthetic studies by cultured tumor cells of other histologic types.

Approximately 8–10% of small-cell lung cancer patients have clinically evident SIADH with hyponatremia.[12] However, AVP by RIA was significantly elevated in the blood of 32% of small-cell cancer patients and when 80 patients from two studies with small-cell cancer were water-loaded, 53% had subclinical but evocable SIADH.[15] Odell and coworkers found 41% of lung cancer patients of all histologic types and 43% of colon cancer patients to have significantly elevated blood AVP levels without clinically evident SIADH.[2] North's group has studied neurophysins in 72 small cell cancer patients and found significantly elevated levels of either one or both (AVP or oxytocin) neurophysins in 65%.[62]

Treatment of SIADH

The fundamental principle of the treatment of tumor-associated SIADH involves successful treatment of the underlying cancer. Since nearly all cases involved lung cancer, and small-cell cancer in particular, the reader is referred to Chapter 14 for tumor treatment principles. If chemotherapy is not effective then radiotherapy of bulk tumor mass, or in selected cases of non-small cell lung cancer limited to the chest, surgical removal of the tumor may be considered. The major decisions following those of antitumor treatment involve:

1. The problem of water restriction and high-dose chemotherapy
2. Management of severly symptomatic hyponatremia
3. The problem of distinguishing SIADH developing during treatment from other causes and true tumor relapse
4. Treatment of recurrent SIADH with tumor progression on primary therapy.

For symptomatic hyponatremia and serum sodium less than 130 mEq/L, fluid restriction to less than 500 ml/24 hours will allow patients to slowly increase their plasma osmolality over 7–10 days. If chemotherapy requires hydration, and the chemotherapy could induce more hyponatremia (cyclophosphamide in high doses being an example of both), this can usually be handled by careful monitoring of body weight, input and output, daily or more frequent serum sodiums, and urine sodium and potassium while giving normal saline with furosemide diuretics and electrolyte replacement[69,73,74] If the patient is severely hyponatremic or symptomatic (*e.g.* serum sodium less than 125 mEq/L) correction of this over several days may be required before instituting chemotherapy. Correlation of response to chemo-radiotherapy of SIADH has only been made in a few small-cell tumor patients. The NCI group reported correction of SIADH in 7/7 newly diagnosed small-cell cancer patients after treatment with chemotherapy and fluid restriction.[74] North and coworkers studied 18 patients with elevated neurophysins by RIA (some of which represent elevated AVP) and found complete agreement between tumor and neurophysin levels and response to chemotherapy (reduction of neurophysin levels in 12 patients with complete or partial remissions and rise in six patients with progressive tumor).[75] Since these latter markers are present in 65% of small-cell cancer patients initially, the neurophysins may prove to be excellent tumor markers.

When a patient presents severely symptomatic from SIADH (*e.g.* comatose) more acute measures are needed. The procedure of Hantman and coworkers involves using 3% hypertonic saline and IV furosemide to increase the net free water clearance.[76] Furosemide (1 mg/kg body weight) is given IV and subsequent doses are given as needed to obtain the desired negative fluid balance. Besides routine vital signs, urinary losses of sodium and potassium are measured hourly and replaced by an infusion of appropriate amounts of hypertonic sodium chloride solution to which appropriate amounts of potassium chloride are added. Using an estimated total body water content of 60% of body weight in females and 70% of body weight in males, the negative fluid balance necessary to raise the plasma osmolality to 270 mOsmols/kg water is calculated for an individual patient by the formula: Desired negative water balance in liters = Total body water (TBW = weight in kg x 0.6 or 0.7) minus $\frac{\text{TBW x plasma osmolality}}{270}$.[76] This approach resulted in the serum sodium concentrations rising from 120 to 133 mEq/L in 6–8 hours.[76] While none of these patients had small-cell carcinoma, the Johns Hopkins group has used this regime successfully in small-cell cancer.[63] This procedure could also be used to prepare patients for chemotherapy.

Sometimes during maintenance chemotherapy SIADH will reappear. If this is coincident with other signs of objective tumor progression there is no problem and the antitumor therapy should be changed. If other signs are not present it is reasonable at present to re-examine the patient for other causes of SIADH, correct any of these, and observe the effect of the SIADH before changing chemotherapy. If no causes are found, follow the patient until other signs of objective tumor progression are noted because several cases have been noted where transient hyponatremia and SIADH occurred without tumor progression. Obviously the recurrence of SIADH in a patient who had this syndrome initially is ominous.

In the patient who has relapsed and has recurrent SIADH with no or only minimal effective chemotherapy available, therapy with demeclocycline or urea can be tried. Demeclocycline has been shown to be more effective in the treatment of SIADH than lithium carbonate, another agent previously used in the treatment of SIADH.[77–79] Demeclocycline blocks AVP action at the level of the renal tubule (by inhibiting AVP induced cyclic-AMP formation and blocking the effect of any cyclic-AMP generated) with more reproducibility than lithium carbonate. Recently, a positive correlation between serum sodium and blood urea was noted in patients with SIADH. This suggested the use of urea therapy to correct SIADH. Urea given in doses of 30 g/day corrected the salt-losing tendency of SIADH in two patients with small-cell cancer and normal individuals given exogenous AVP.[80] Because it induces an osmotic diuresis, urea therapy allows a normal daily intake of water despite continued SIADH. Urea (99% pure crystalline material), 30 g is dissolved in 100 ml water with 15 grams of magnesium and aluminum hydroxide (maalox) and is taken at noon; this has been maintained for up to 11 weeks without water restriction.[80] The urea is taken orally because of good GI absorption and because cells are freely permeable to urea. There is no risk of cardiac failure from rapid shifts of water as is possible in a mannitol-induced diuresis. Usually water intake and electrolytes are monitored for the first 2 weeks until the patient has stabilized. The only risk is from hypernatremic dehydration and this is rare if the thirst center is intact and water is available.[80] Thirty grams of urea should provide an obligatory diuresis of approximately 1500 ml/day if the urine osmality is 800 mOsm/kg.[80] Urea begins working immediately and does not have the problems of potential nephrotoxicity or bacterial overgrowth that the tetracycline derivative demeclocycline has.

While hyponatremia and the SIADH are the classic presenting features of tumor secretion of AVP, other paraneoplastic syndromes are possible. The primary effect of AVP is on the renal tubule, but at much higher concentrations it acts on the cardiovascular system and other smooth muscles throughout the body.[65] AVP acts to constrict smooth muscle through the vascular system causing increase in blood pressure (hence the derivation of the name arginine vasopressin), decrease in skin and gut circulation, vasoconstriction of coronary (with myocardial ischemia) and pulmonary arterial vessels (with pulmonary hypertension). While very large amounts of AVP are required for these effects in normal persons, when baroreceptor reflexes are depressed by anesthesia, ganglionic blocking agents, or other defects in sympathetic outflow, are present. Patients can become very sensitive to the pressor effects of AVP. Myocardial ischemia, increased bowel motility, and uterine smooth muscle contractions are thus the most likely new syndromes that could be seen. While paraneoplastic syndromes with these symptoms have not been reported in the past 10 years, these features may have been overlooked or ascribed to other causes and should be considered in patients with SIADH who have such features.

HYPERCALCEMIA

Hypercalcemia is common in cancer patients; about 10% of patients with cancer will have hypercalcemia, and 10% to 15% of these will not have associated bony metastases.[81,82] The most common tumor types associated with hypercalcemia are breast cancer (15% of cases but usually associated with bony metastases), lung cancer (10%), and multiple myeloma (> 50% but usually associated with bony involvement).There are several documented mechanisms of hypercalcemia in cancer patients, including bony metastases, the simultaneous occurrence of primary hyperparathyroidism, ectopic-tumor-produced parathormone (PTH), tumor-produced prostaglandins (PGE_1,PGE_2), tumor-produced osteoblast activating factor, and potentially other produced osteolytic factors.[2,3,12,81,84–86] In normal humans, calcium is maintained by a series of control mechanisms governing bone resorption and osteolysis, which are stimulated by PGE, PTH, OAF, thyrotoxin (T4), and a monocyte derived osteolytic factor and inhibited by calcitonin and estrogen. Absorption of calcium from the gastrointestinal and renal tubular tracts is stimulated by PTH, growth hormone, and vitamin D.[81] Thus, production by tumors of any of these materials could cause hypercalcemia. In addition, whereas paraneoplastic syndromes are usually considered to be those humorally mediated at a distance from the primary tumor or its metastases, in the case of hypercalcemia the mediators released by the tumor cells may act locally (as with PGE and OAF). All of the mechanisms of hypercalcemia should be considered in the cancer patient, and determining the cause of the hypercalcemia is important because of the therapeutic implications. The pathophysiology, clinical manifestations, and treatment are covered in Chapter 42.

HYPOCALCEMIA

In patients with bony metastases hypocalcemia occurs in 16% while hypercalcemia only occurs in 9%.[116–119] Not infrequently this is with osteoblastic metastases of the breast, prostate, and lung.[117,120] Only very rarely is tetanic hypocalcemia seen with these osteoblastic metastases.[88] However, it is possible with more refined studies of nerve, muscle, or other physiologic function testing that the hypocalcemia be found to impair a patient's neuromuscular function. It is possible that hypocalcemia can be mediated by way of tumor-secreted calcitonin although there is not direct evidence for this at present. No specific therapy is indicated except in the rare case of tetany where calcium can be given.

HYPOPHOSPHATEMIC OSTEOMALACIA ASSOCIATED WITH BENIGN MESENCHYMAL TUMORS ("TUMORAL OSTEOMALACIA" OR "ONCOGENIC OSTEOMALACIA")

An acquired, adult-onset, vitamin-D resistant rickets with bone pain, severe phosphaturia, renal glycosuria, hypophasphatemia, normo-calcemia, and increased alkaline phosphatase is seen in association with benign mesenchymal tumors which occur in soft tissues or bone.[121–123] They are also called ossifying mesenchymal tumors, giant-cell tumors of bone, sclerosing hemangioma, cavernous hemangioma, or reparative giant-cell granuloma.[124] Often the syndrome precedes the discovery of the tumor by several years.[12] The basis of treatment is resection of the mesenchymal tumor, which results in resolution of the syndrome.[121,122,125] Otherwise, treatment requires large doses of vitamin D and phosphate. The mechanism behind the paraneoplastic syndrome is unknown and could include production of a vitamin D antagonist, abberant vitamin D metabolism, or an effect on the renal tubule to produce phosphaturia. The importance of recognizing this syndrome is its cure with surgical resection. Sometimes multiple osteolytic lesions, or osteoblastic-like lesions, are seen in sclerosing hemangiomas of bone. These require treatment with oral phosphate and vitamin D and give relief of bone pain and weakness.[123] These bony lesions can look like diffuse metastases on roentgenogram and so careful pathologic examination is required.

CALCITONIN PRODUCTION BY TUMORS

The polypeptide hormone calcitonin is normally produced by the C-cells of the thyroid. It causes calcium release from bone and an increase in renal excretion of calcium, sodium, and phosphate.[126] However, there are no described clinical syndromes associated with tumor production of calcitonin at present, although one small-cell cancer patient with high calcitonin levels had hypocalcemia.[14] The major clinical use of calcitonin assay is in monitoring patients with medullary carcinoma of the thyroid. This tumor produces large amounts of calcitonin without clinical signs or symptoms.[126] Calcitonin is an extremely sensitive indicator of residual tumor following surgery.[63] It is also useful in identifying patients with multiple endocrine neoplasia, type II, a familial disorder involving an association of medullary carcinoma of the thyroid, pheochromocytoma, and parathyroid adenomas. These are described in detail in the Chapter 28. Because of the excellent clinical correlation of calcitonin with medullary thyroid cancer, the hormone has been studied in other tumor types.

Elevated plasma calcitonin levels have been consistently found in 48–64% of patients with small-cell lung cancer and in variable frequency with the other lung cancer cell types.[11,14,15,127] Urine calcitonin is elevated in 75% of lung cancer patients (53% of epidermoid, 45% of adenocarcinomas, 20% of large-cell cancers, but surprisingly only 17% of small cell cancers).[128] When antiserum detecting both the C-terminal and midportion of the calcitonin molecule was used on both serum and urine samples, over 90% of lung cancer patients had abnormal values.[128] Calcitonin levels mirrored clinical tumor status 67% of the time in lung cancer patients, but selective venous sampling showed both tumoral and thyroidal production of the elevated calcitonin levels.[127] Thus its utility as a marker of lung cancer is not yet established. Other tumor types associated with increased plasma calcitonin include carcinoids, breast cancer (in some studies up to 100%), colon cancer (24%), and gastric cancer (38%). High calcitonin levels do not correlate with bony metastases.[127] However, there are a variety of non-neoplastic conditions associated with elevated calcitonin levels including hypercalcemia, chronic renal failure, pregnancy, pernicious anemia, Zollinger–Ellison syndrome, and pancreatitis.[11,127] Thus, its use as a screen for the early detection of cancer is problematic.

Because of the several possible sources of calcitonin, biosynthetic studies would be very useful. Immunoreactive calcitonin has been found in many tumor extracts including small-cell cancer, pheochromocytomas, malignant carcinoids, other types of lung cancer, breast, melanoma, colon, gastric, esophagus, and pancreatic cancer.[71,129,130] These studies failed to show that calcitonin and ACTH were on a common precursor molecule as predicted by some but did show a high molecular weight form of calcitonin.[131,132] The nature of the calcitonin precursor molecule is unknown. In summary, calcitonin is a polypeptide hormone apparently produced by many cancers waiting for definition of a clinically evident paraneoplastic syndrome and prospective documentation as a marker of response to therapy.

HUMAN PLACENTAL AND PITUITARY GLYCOPROTEIN HORMONES AND THEIR SUBUNITS PRODUCED BY TUMORS

Gonadotropins

Precocious puberty in children, gynecomastia in men, and oligomenorrhea in premenopausal women can result from excessive gonadotropin production by tumors.[2,3,12,133] In addition, very high levels of gonadotropin secretion can result in thyroid stimulation and hyperthyroidism.[134,135] Gonadroptropin secretion can occur in pituitary tumors, gestational trophoblastic tumors (choriocarcinoma and hydatidiform mole), germ cell tumors of testis and ovary, germ cell tumors arising or presenting in extragonadal primary sites, and less commonly as tumors in other sites, including hepatoblastomas in children, and large-cell and adenocarcinoma of the lung in adults.[2,3,12,133,136,137]

The tumors arising in gestational tissue, testis, ovaries and endocrine organs are covered in other chapters where the great value of gonadotropin measurement as a marker in the treatment of gestational trophoblastic tumors and testicular cancer is discussed.[138,139] Their usefulness as a marker in these tumors stimulated intense study of gonadotropin expression in other tumors to see if they could be used as markers for early diagnosis or monitoring of subsequent treatment.[140]

The human hormones with gonadotrophic properties are follicle stimulating hormone (FSH), luteinizing hormone (LH), and human chorionic gonadotropin (hCG).[133] FSH, LH, and hCG are composed of two polypeptide chains, an alpha and a beta subunit. The alpha subunit is common to all the hormones while the beta subunit confers immunologic and biologic specificity. However, both subunits together are required for bioactivity.[133] Radioimmunoassay allows distinction between the various types of beta subunits.[133] In normal persons, FSH and LH are produced by the pituitary and are normally present in serum, while biologically active hCG is produced by the placenta and thus is usually found only in pregnant women. Since levels of FSH and LH vary widely under normal physiologic conditions, the assay for β-hCG is theoretically the best to use for following patients with suspected paraneoplastic production of gonadotropin excess. Recently an hCG-like material has been found in extracts of all normal tissue by RIA and radioreceptor assay calling into question the use of hCG in cancer patients. However, this hCG is carbohydrate-free, while that produced by the placenta and many tumors contains carbohydrate. Carbohydrate-free hCG is cleared rapidly from the circulation and has marked loss of bioactivity.[133,141]

TABLE 39-6. Elevations of Human Chorionic Gonadotropin (hCG), the Beta Subunit of hCG, (CG-beta) or the Alpha Subunit of Placental and Pituitary Glycoprotein Hormones in Various Tumors*

TUMOR TYPE	% ELEVATED	
	hCG OR CG-BETA	ALPHA
Lung†	0–12	3–30
Colorectal	0–20	20–26
Breast	7–50	30
Pancreatic adenocarcinoma	11–50	
Gastric carcinoma	0–24	
Prostate cancer	1	0
Islet cell carcinoma	22–50	52
Carcinoid of gut and lung		16
Small intestine	13	
Hepatoma	17–20	
Non-malignant lung disease	7	
Non-malignant GI disease	9	
Non-malignant breast disease	4	

* References for the multiple studies—57 and 76

† Within lung there were: 32% epidermoid cancers; 27% small-cell lung cancers; 13% large-cell lung cancers; 11% adenocarcinoma; and 17% miscellaneous and undetermined histologic malignant diseases. Within GI cancer there were 13% pancreatic adenocarcinomas; 8% gastric cancers; 4% hepatomas; 10% other types of upper GI cancer; and 65% lower GI cancer. Carcinoid lesions included 80% of GI origin; Malignant islet cell neoplasms included 28% insulinomas, and 40% gastrinomas. Normal controls included: 299 healthy subjects; 123 patients with chronic lung disease; 110 with benign GI disease; and 47 with benign endocrine diseases.

Many studies have looked at "elevations" of hCG, the beta subunit of hCG (CG-beta), and the common alpha subunit (see Table 39-6). Of great interest, many of the common tumors (*e.g.*, lung, colorectal, and breast) had frequent elevations of these markers. However, 5–10% of patients with non-malignant chronic disease also had hormone elevations calling the specificity of the findings in tumor patients into doubt. In pursuing this, Blackman and coworkers have conducted a detailed study of human placental and pituitary glycopeptide hormones and their subunits in the sera of patients with lung cancer, GI cancer, malignant carcinoid, and malignant islet cell tumors and compared their results to 579 appropriately matched controls (see Table 39-7).[140] Values for the alpha subunit and the beta subunit of chorionic gonadotropin (CG-beta) were significantly higher in the cancer patients while elevations of FSH-beta, TSH-beta, and LH-beta were not observed. In addition, the sensitivity of detection of cancer patients increased by combining the results from the two tests. They and others also found differences in the ratio of alpha/CG-beta positivity between sexes and among cancer groups, a finding which is unexplained.

Because of the frequency of elevation in common tumors, such as lung and GI, and because of the correlation with response in trophoblastic disease and testicular tumors, it will be of great importance to prospectively test the role of alpha and CG beta in monitoring the therapy of common tumors. In some non-trophoblastic tumors these markers have proved of value in monitoring therapy.[142,143,144,145,146] However, these reports are still anectodal. For example, Broder and coworkers reported on a patient with prostatic cancer and elevation of hCG whose serum hCG levels mirrored the clinical course more reliably than concomitant acid phosphatase levels.[145] Muggia and coworkers reported on four patients with metastatic cancer and in seven of nine episodes, clinical remission was associated with marker decrease or exacerbation associated with marker increase.[142] Metz and coworkers reported on a patient with an hCG-secreting large-cell carcinoma of the lung with painful gynecomastia and testicular atrophy.[146] Investigation revealed elevated levels of CG-beta, and alpha subunits, normal estradiol levels, low normal testosterone levels, and abnormal (delayed) pituitary response to LHRH. These abnormal findings reverted to normal after surgical resection of the tumor (shown to contain high levels of hCG), recurred with tumor regrowth, and then regressed again with the addition of combination chemotherapy which obtained a complete clinical remission of the tumor and the biochemical parameters.[146] The CG-beta level was more sensitive than gynecomastia in predicting recurrence. This was an important case because it demonstrated the usefulness of the CG-beta marker in a common solid tumor to monitor therapy and achieve potential cure with the use of chemotherapy in a semi-adjuvant setting.

Studies of tumor lines *in vitro* agree with these studies of serum samples. CG-beta and alpha subunit have been shown to be produced by human tumor cell lines *in vitro*.[140,147,148] Unbalanced synthesis of alpha and beta subunits is seen

TABLE 39-7. Elevations of the Beta Unit of Chorionic Gonadotropin (CG-B) or the Alpha Subunit of Glycoprotein Hormones in Patients with Lung and Gastrointestinal Cancer*

	% OF TUMOR PATIENTS WITH HORMONE ELEVATIONS OVER 95TH PERCENTILE OF NORMAL CONTROLS			
TUMOR TYPE†	# PATIENTS	ALPHA	CG BETA	ALPHA OR CG BETA
Lung Cancer				
Men	269	11	41	45
Women	31	16	16	29
GI Cancer				
Men	92	32	28	48
Women	71	18	34	41
Carcinoid				
Men	25	50	0	50
Women		13	50	50
Malignant Islet Cell				
Men	40	61	6	61
Women		38	19	43

* Data summarized from Blackman and colleagues (Reference 140).
† Within lung cancer there were 32% epidermoid.

while no evidence of production of FSH-beta, TSH-beta and only rarely (and at low levels) of LH-beta were found.

While tumor produced alpha subunit and CG-beta are found frequently there are no definitive reports of tumor produced FSH, TSH, or LH.[3,12] Thus, any potential patients with suspected tumor production of these hormones should be carefully documented and reported. It should be noted that some elevations of LH and FSH can occur in cancer patients probably as the result of gonadal failure related to age, stress, chronic illness, or treatment.[140] Obviously, other causes of elevated hormones, such as those seen in physiologic causes of hypergonadotropinemia, hyperthyrotropinemia, pituitary adenomas, pregnancy, and uremia, have to be exluded.[140]

DIFFERENTIAL DIAGNOSIS. The exact frequency of symptoms associated with tumor-produced gonadotropin is not known, although both intact hormone (both subunits) and appropriate host (child for precocious puberty, man for gynecomastia, premenopausal women for oligomenorrhea) are simultaneously required for clinical expression. A detailed discussion of the differential diagnosis of these conditions is beyond the scope of this chapter. However, the most common problem is a male patient presenting with unexplained gynecomastia. In this situation, a CG-beta determination should be performed as well as a careful examination of the testes, and radiographic examination of the chest and mediastinum. It is important to use a RIA since routine urinary pregnancy tests are not sensitive enough to detect many hCG secretory neoplasms.[146] Germ cell tumors of the testis or extragonadal sites and lung cancers are the most frequent cause of the combination of gynecomastia and hCG elevation and such men should then be persistently and thoroughly evaluated since this syndrome can present before a clinical evident cancer is found.[149]

In fact, other tumors associated with biologically active hCG (*e.g.*, gynecomastia and precocious puberty) are rather rare. Skrabanek and associates found only 44 extragonadal cases in the world's literature and these involved the lung, adrenal gland, liver, GI tract, and non-gonadal portions of the genitourinary tract.[150] Analysis of the histologies revealed that all contained syncytial giant cells or frankly choriocarcinomatous elements similar to classic trophoblastic germ cell tumors. Greco and coworkers found that 40% of patients with extragonadal germ cell tumors "masquerading" as poorly-differentiated carcinomas had immunochemical tumor staining for CG beta and AFP without serum elevations of the markers.[151] Many patients responded to combination chemotherapy. These results suggest that in poorly no-differentiated midline carcinomas in young adults, immunohistochemistry and a chemotherapy approach similar to that for histologically classic germ cell tumors is at present warranted in these potentially curable lesions.

Precocious puberty has been found in children with hepatoma or hepatoblastomas. In these children, secondary sexual characteristics were prematurely developed, along with advanced skeletal maturation and hyperplasia of prostatic and testicular interstitial cells.[12,152,153]

Abnormal endocrine manifestations consisting of precocious puberty, irregular bleeding, amenorrhea, and hirsutism were present in 9/15 patients (60%) with tumors of the ovary and stained immunohistochemically for hCG (in syncytiotrophoblast-like cells) and for alpha fetoprotein (in embryonal carcinoma cells).[154]

TUMOR-PRODUCED HUMAN PLACENTAL LACTOGEN (HPL), GROWTH HORMONE (GH), PROLACTIN, AND THYROTROPIC SUBSTANCE

HPL was detected in the sera of 5–8% of patients with non-trophoblastic non-gonadal tumors.[155,156] Many of these patients with elevated HPL also had elevated levels of estrogens and gynecomastia. Apparently, some of these patients also have elevated hCG levels. When HPL is found in non-pregnant women, it is a very specific indication of malignancy.[156]

Growth hormone levels that are elevated have been reported in patients with lung cancer and gastric cancer but may be uncommon. While patients may not live long enough with these neoplasms to develop acromegaly, it has been speculated that GH may cause hypertrophic pulmonary osteoarthropathy and the syndrome has been reversed by resection of lung tumors.[158] However, a study of patients with and without osteoarthropathy failed to reveal any relationship between the syndrome and elevated plasma growth hormone levels and none were acromegalic.[159] Of interest, two patients have been described whose acromegaly was cured by removal of a bronchial carcinoid tumor.[159] These tumors appeared to secrete a growth hormone-releasing substance and the authors suggest that some other cases of "polyglandular syndromes" may be secondary to small bronchial carcinoids that produce as yet unidentified substances that can stimlulate other endocrine tissue.

Only three patients with elevated prolactin levels have been found (undifferentiated lung cancer, small-cell lung cancer, and hypernephroma), only one of which had associated galactorrhea.[3,12] Resection or irradiation resulted in the fall of prolactin in all cases. Thus, cases of non-pituitary prolactin secreting tumors are rare, and any suspected cases should be carefully distinguished from pituitary lesions and reported.

Cancer patients frequently have a "hypermetabolic state" that may resemble hyperthyroidism and 1.4% of lung cancer patients are reportedly hyperthyroid, but documentation of tumor caused syndromes is uncommon.[160] Four potential substances that could stimulate the thyroid gland are pituitary-like TSH, chorionic thyrotropin, hCG, and long-activating thyroid stimulating substances (LATS). Documented examples of hyperthyroidism produced by TSH, LATS, and chorionic thyrotropin probably do not exist. Isolated reports of tumor-associated TSH without thyrotoxicosis have been made.[161] However, a definite association is found between hyperthyroidism and gestational trophoblastic disease (choriocarcinoma and hydatidiform mole) where 8% of cases can have biochemical evidence of hyperthyroidism. This is also seen in testicular tumors.[12,162] In all such cases, the relationship seems to be between trophoblastic tumors and very high levels of hCG where the thyroid stimulating substance has been shown in some cases to be hCG.[134,135,163]

HYPOGLYCEMIA

Hypoglycemia is frequently caused by insulinomas. Hypoglycemia associated with non-islet cell tumors is an uncommon and not well-characterized paraneoplastic syndrome. The other types of neoplasms associated with hypoglycemia are:

1. Mesenchymal in 64% (including mesothelioma, fibrosarcoma, neurofibrosarcoma, hemangiopericytoma)
2. Hepatoma in 21%
3. Adrenal carcinomas in 6%
4. Gastrointestinal in 5%
5. Miscellaneous in 5% (including anaplastic carcinomas of unknown primary, pseudomyxoma, hypernephromas, lymphomas, pheochromocytomas)[2,3,52,164]

'he tumors are usually quite large (1–10 kg with an average eight of 2.4 kg), often invade the liver, and often have protracted courses over many years.[2,3] However, hypoglycemia as the presenting symptom of a tumor can also occur.[2] Mesotheliomas are the most common cause of hypoglycemia and about 50% of these occur in the abdomen, the remainder in the chest. The signs and symptoms are those of hypoglycemia with neurologic findings (stupor, coma, and occasionally focal findings and agitated behavior), predominating until the hypoglycemia is discovered.[63]

There are multiple potential ways tumors could cause hypoglycemia including:

1. Ectopic insulin production
2. Production of insulin-like activity (NSILA)
3. Over-utilization of glucose by the tumor
4. Tumor production of a material stimulating eutopic insulin release
5. Massive infiltration of the liver by tumor or tumor production of an inhibitor of hepatic glucose output.

However, only the second mechanism appears a good candidate at present. Tumor utilization of glucose to a degree to cause hypoglycemia has not yet been substantiated and only rarely is liver infiltration by tumor massive enough to cause hypoglycemia.[2,3,165] There are rare reports of insulin production by non-islet cell tumors, but there are no definitive biosynthetic studies to prove this.[166] A massive thoracic mesothelioma associated with hypoglycemia and very low glucagon levels was postulated to make a factor suppressing glucagon secretion.[167] Artifactual hypoglycemia can occur in acute leukemia when the high number of circulating leukemia cells metabolize the plasma glucose while standing in the collection tube.[168]

Currently, the most likely, although far from established mechanism, is tumor production of somatomedins, also called NSILA.[2,3,63] Somatomedins are a family of peptide hormones normally produced by the liver under growth hormone regulation.[169] By current definitions, substances with identical bioassay properties of insulin (in the rat diaphragm or epididymal fat pad) and which also react in insulin radioreceptor assays (RRA) but do not react in insulin radioimmunoassays are "somatomedins." Approximately half of the 200 μU of biologically active insulin and insulin-like activity in normal human serum is related to NSILA-somatomedin activity.[170] However, further purification using receptor assays and characterization is required, and it is possible that several molecules with these characteristics exist. Hypoglycemia associated with cancer generally occurs after fasting and physical exertion, while reactive postprandial hypoglycemia is usually not part of the paraneoplastic syndrome.[63] Thus, cancer hypoglycemia behaves like NSILA. Some cancer patients with hypoglycemia have elevated tumor extract levels of biologically active insulin-like activity that is not suppressed or reactive with anti-insulin antibodies, but is reactive in the RRA.[170,171] These patients appear to have tumors producing NSILA and it will be important to study tissue culture lines of tumors from such patients to see if they produce the NSILA. At present, the evaluation of such patients is experimental after the common causes of severe hypoglycemia (exogenous insulin or sulfomylureas, insulinoma, islet cell tumor, adrenal or pituitary insufficiency, ethanol abuse and poor nutrition) have been excluded.

Initially, the treatment of paraneoplastic hypoglycemia involves glucose infusion to control the acute symptoms. Reduction of tumor bulk usually by surgical resection should then be carried out, if possible. However, there are no good data on the long-term effectiveness of any surgical, radiotherapy, or chemotherapy treatment approach. If tumor treatment is not possible or inadequate, other possibilities include the use of glucagon (intermittent subcutaneous or long-acting glucagon given IM) or high-dose corticosteorids.[63] However, there are little data on the long-term effectiveness of these agents in controlling the hypoglycemia.

NEUROLOGIC MANIFESTATIONS OF MALIGNANCY

Neurologic problems occur frequently in patients with cancer. In the experiences of Dr. Posner and coworkers at Memorial Hospital, 17% of all admissions have neurologic symptoms and signs requiring neurologic consultation.[172] In patients with established cancer, true paraneoplastic syndromes account for a minority of neurologic problems and the diagnosis of paraneoplastic syndrome can only be established after other diagnoses are excluded. The differential diagnosis of the cancer patient with neurologic signs and symptoms is provided in Table 39-8. Most frequently, neurologic complications are caused directly by the tumor or its metastases. For example, 40%–65% of lung cancers metastasize to the brain, and overall Posner and Chernick reported that intracranial metastases were found in 24% of autopsies at Memorial Sloan-Kettering Cancer Center.[173–175]

Neurologic syndromes due to endocrine and fluid and electrolyte abnormalities are the second most common cause of neurologic symptoms and signs in cancer patients. Hepatic encephalopathy and hypercalcemia are the most frequent of these. Cerebral and spinal vascular disease are common in the cancer patient and are found in 13% of autopsied cancer patients.[172] The etiologies of the vascular problems in these autopsied patients are shown in Table 39-9. It is clear that the causes of stroke in these patients are strikingly dissimilar from those in the general population. Marantic and septic emboli, disseminated intravascular coagulation, tumor related hemorrhage, superior sagittal sinus occlusion, and many of the cases of subarachnoid hemorrhage were directly tumor related and account for well over 50% of strokes.[175–178] Risk factors for the general population, including hypertension, atherosclerotic heart disease, and diabetes, are less important in the cancer patient. Several associations of cancer and neurologic vascular disease are noteworthy. Marantic endocarditis with emboli (nonbacterial thrombotic endocarditis) occurs predominantly in patients with adenocarcinoma, especially of the lung, and may present neurologically as multifocal abnormalities, focal abnormalities, or progressive encephalopathy without any focal deficits.[176] Hemorrhage is most often seen in the leukemias, especially acute nonlymphocytic leukemia.[177] Fungi are the most frequent cause of septic emboli.

Paraneoplastic syndromes or "remote effects" of tumors on the CNS are uncommon although the incidence varies considerably in different reports. For example, Croft and Wilkinson found neuromyopathies in 7% of 1,476 cancer patients; lung cancers were the most frequent.[7] Brody, however, found no difference in the frequency of neurologic syndromes between patients with lung cancer and controls with chronic lung disease.[8] There are clearly some specific neurologic syndromes that occur exclusively or with much higher frequency in cancer patients. The patient with no known cancer developing one of these syndromes should lead to a high suspicion of an occult cancer and a full evaluation for cancer is warranted. These syndromes include subacute cerebellar degeneration, subacute motor neuropathy, dermatomyositis in older males, Eaton-Lambert syndrome, and dorsal root ganglionitis. If a patient not known to have cancer develops a neurologic syndrome less often associated with malignancy a careful history and physical examination should be performed but an exhaustive laboratory and radiologic search for tumor is not indicated (see Table 39-10). In these instances and in instances with a highly suspect syndrome with negative evaluation, careful patient follow-up is required.

Most paraneoplastic syndromes run a course parallel to the underlying tumor. This is less often the case in neurologic paraneoplastic syndrome where the course of the neurologic

TABLE 39-8. Differential Diagnosis of Neurologic Syndromes

Syndromes due to effects of primary or metastatic tumor
Syndromes due to endocrine or metabolic tumor products (*e.g.*, ADH, calcium, glucose, electrolytes)
Syndromes due to cerebral and spinal vascular disease
Syndromes due to toxicity of primary treatment (chemotherapy, radiotherapy)
Syndromes due to CNS infections
Paraneoplastic syndromes associated with malignancy with unknown mechanisms

TABLE 39-9. Etiology of Stroke in Cancer Patients

ETIOLOGY	FREQUENCY	(%)
1. Embolic infarction	27	
Septic		13
Marantic		12
Tumor		2
2. Thrombotic infarction	19	
Atherosclerotic		10
Disseminated intravascular coagulation		9
3. Miscellaneous infarction	6	
4. Intraparenchymal hemorrhage	32.5	
Spontaneous		13
Tumor related		13
Hypertension		5
Unknown		1.5
5. Subdural hemorrhage	8.5	
6. Subarachnoid hemorrhage	3	
7. Superior saggital sinus occlusion	4	
Total	100	

From Studies by Allen, Rosen, Collins, and Sigsbee

TABLE 39-10. Paraneoplastic Syndromes of the Nervous System

SITE	SYNDROME	REFERENCE	CLINICAL FEATURES	ASSOCIATED NEOPLASMS	COMMENTS
I. Cerebral	Subacute Cerebellar Degeneration*	Brain (182) Paone (183) Victor (184)	Subacute, progressive bilateral, symmetric, cerebellar failure often with dementia, dysarthria, CSF lymphocytosis, and elevated protein	Lung Prostate Colorectal Ovary Cervix Other	Some reports of improvements with removal of primary tumor; no other known treatment
	Dementia	Shapiro (185) Dorfman (186)	Variable presentation, acute to slowly progressive. Often associated with abnormalities in other areas of the neuraxis. EEG shows slowing. CSF pleocytois sometimes seen.	Lung	Relatively common (30–40%)
	Limbic Encephalitis	Corsellis (187) Dorfman (186)	Dementia with degenerative changes in the hippocampus and amygdaloid nuclei. Often associated with inflammatory and degenerative lesions in other areas of the neuraxis.	Lung Other	May not improve with removal of primary tumor
	Optic Neuritis	Sawyer (188)	Sometimes decrease in vision and papilledema; unilateral or bilateral		Rare
	Progressive Multifocal Leukoencephalopathy	Padgett (189) Richardson (5) Weiner (6)	Dementia, paralysis, aphasia, ataxia, dysarthria, visual field defects, blindness, coma, seizures. Demyelination of white matter. CSF often normal. Death usually rapid.	Leukemias, lymphomas, sarcomas, other	Due to papova viruses of 2 types: JC virus or SV-40 like virus
II. Spinal Cord	Amyotropic Lateral Sclerosis (ALS)	Norris and Engel (190)	Upper and lower motoneuron disease with spasticity, extensor plantar responses, wasting and fasiculations.		Syndrome similar to that in patients without cancer but sometimes progresses more slowly. Cancer found in 10% of ALS patients in one report but others find cancer less frequently.
	Subacute Necrotic Myelopathy	Mancall (191)	Rapid ascending motor and sensory paralysis to thoracic level. Elevated CSF protein.	Lung	Severe tissue destruction of grey and white matter.
	Subacute Motor Neuropathy*	Walton (192)	Slowly developing lower motoneuron weakness without sensory changes. Most often in irradiated patients with lymphoma.	Lymphoma	No known treatment; occasional spontaneous recovery; ? viral origin.
III. Peripheral Nerves	Sensory Neuropathy*	Horwich (194) Henson (195)	Subacute onset of sensory loss including deep tendon reflexes, with normal strength and normal motor conduction velocity. Elevated CSF protein.	Lung, other	Uncommon
	Sensorimotor Peripheral Neuropathy	Craft (196) Dayan (197) Newman (198) Victor (199)	Distal weakness and wasting, areflexia, distal sensory loss. Elevated CSF protein.	Lung, GI, breast, other	Quite common. Recovery rare even with removal of primary tumor.

TABLE 39-10. (Continued)

SITE	SYNDROME	REFERENCE	CLINICAL FEATURES	ASSOCIATED NEOPLASMS	COMMENTS
	Ascending Acute Polyneuropathy (Guillain–Barré)	Lisak (202)	Bilateral usually symmetric weakness (flaccid), usually beginning in lower extremities and ascending. Sensory symptoms and signs usually develop as well. Elevated CSF protein.	Lymphoma	Association not definite.
	Myasthenia Gravis	Tyler (193)	Weakness with predilection for ocular and cranial muscles, tendency for fluctuation, and partial reversibility by administration of cholinergic drugs.	Thymoma, lymphomas, breast, other	Except for thymoma, association not proven.
IV. Muscle and Neuromuscular Junction	Dermatomyositis and Polymyositis*	DeVere (204) Barnes (205) Williams (206)	Progressive muscle weakness developing gradually over weeks to months (proximal > distal). Usually not disabling. Elevated muscle enzymes and sedimentation rate.	Lung Stomach Ovary Other	Stringent association in older males; less frequent in colorectal tumors.
	Myasthenic Syndrome* (Eaton–Lambert Syndrome)	Lambert (207, 208) Cherrington (210) Jenkyn (209)	Weakness and fatigability of proximal muscles, especially pelvic girdle and thigh. Dryness of mouth, dysphagia, dysarthria, and peripheral paresthesias common. EMGs show a facilitated response in active muscles.	Lung (small cell) Stomach Ovary Other	Poor response to tensilon. Should respond to therapy of primary tumor. Guanidine may also be useful.
	Myasthenia Gravis	Tyler (193)	Weakness with predilection for ocular and cranial muscles, tendency for fluctuation and partial reversibility by cholinergic drugs.	Thymoma Lymphomas Breast Other	Except for thymoma, association not proven.

*These syndromes are so strongly associated with malignancy that a thorough investigation for malignancy is indicated when they develop in patients not known to have cancer.

abnormalities is frequently independent of the underlying tumor. In many instances, this can be attributed to the inability of the nervous tissue to divide and repair damage. In some instances, such as the myasthenic syndrome and polymyositis, however, cases of a parallel course of tumor and syndrome have been documented.

Numerous neurologic syndromes have been described. For convenience they are listed in Table 39-10, which is divided by area within the nervous system.

"REMOTE EFFECTS" ON THE CEREBRUM AND CRANIAL NERVES

Remote paraneoplastic syndromes involving the brain and cranial nerves are less common than those involving other areas of the neuraxis. In one large series involving 1,476 cancer patients only 162 had neurologic abnormalities and of these, only 15 had lesions of the brain.[7] These 15 all had subacute cerebellar degeneration, which is one of the syndromes with a strong association with malignancy.

Subacute cerebellar degeneration occurs most commonly in association with lung cancer but many other tumor types have been described. It is characterized by a subacute and progressive, bilateral, symmetric cerebellar failure with ataxia, dysarthria, hypotonia, and pendular reflexes. Dementia may occur. There is frequently a cerebrospinal fluid (CSF) lymphocytosis and elevated protein levels. Pathologically, there is atrophy with loss of Purkinje cells. The etiology is unknown and there is no effective treatment except removal of the primary tumor, which may be associated with improvement in the syndrome.

Dementia is probably the most frequent cerebral abnormality in cancer patients. Since it is also frequent in the general population, its association with malignancy is less strong. Dementia is often associated with abnormalities in other areas of the nervous system. The EEG shows generalized slowing and a CSF pleocytosis is sometimes present.

Limbic encephalitis is characterized by a progressive dementia associated with degenerative changes in the hippocampus and amygdaloid nuclei. Pathologically, there are inflammatory as well as degenerative changes. The CSF may be normal or show a pleocytosis. The syndrome does not appear to improve with removal of the primary tumor. The etiology is unknown although a viral etiology has been postulated.

Optic neuritis is characterized by scotomas, decreased vision, and papilledema, which may be unilaterral or bilateral. Pathologically, demyelination is found.

Progressive multifocal leukoencephalopathy is included in this section even though multiple areas of the neuraxis are involved and it is not a true paraneoplastic syndrome since a viral etiology has been quite well established in recent years. The syndrome is characterized by dementia, paralysis, aphasia, ataxia, dysarthria, visual field defects, blindness, and sometimes coma or seizures. It is usually rapidly progressive with death occurring within 6 months. The CSF is usually normal. It occurs most often in malignancies associated with impaired immunity (leukemias and lymphomas), but also occurs in many benign conditions with altered immunity (sarcoidosis or steroid therapy). Pathologically, demyelination of white matter is found throughout the nervous system. Recent evidence suggests the illness is caused by one or two types of papova virus.[6,189]

REMOTE EFFECTS INVOLVING THE SPINAL CORD

In the large series of Croft and Wilkinson, paraneoplastic syndromes primarily involving the spinal cord accounted for only 9% of all nervous system syndromes.[7] From a different perspective Norris and Engel, reported that 10% of 130 patients with amyotrophic lateral sclerosis had an underlying malignancy.[190]

Amyotrophic lateral sclerosis (ALS) is characterized by widespread lower motor neuron muscle weakness, atrophy, spasticity, hyperreflexia, extensor plantar responses, and fasiculations. When associated with cancer, the sex distribution is predominantly male, and the age is older. The course of ALS may progress more slowly in cancer patients. Despite the report of Norris and Engel, many observers feel that far less than 10% of ALS patients have an underlying cancer.[190]

Subacute necrotic myelopathy is characterized by a rapid ascending motor and sensory paralysis, which is most severe in the thoracic region. It usually terminates in death in a matter of days or weeks. There are often degenerative lesions in other areas of gray and white matter as well. The CSF protein level is usually elevated. The syndrome is most often reported in association with lung cancer, but other tumors have been reported as well.

Subacute motor neuropathy has a strong association with malignancy, particularly with the lymphomas. It is characterized by slowly developing but progressive lower motor weakness without sensory changes. It occurs most often in irradiated patients. While the course often progresses slowly, it may wax and wane and there may be spontaneous recovery. A viral etiology has been speculated.

REMOTE EFFECTS ON THE PERIPHERAL NERVOUS SYSTEM

Paraneoplastic syndromes involving the peripheral nerves are the most frequent site in the nervous system. The association was first reported in the late 1800's and a number of reports appeared in the late 1940's and early 1950's. A large series were reported by Croft and Wilkinson in 1965 who divided these neuropathies into symmetrical sensory peripheral neuropathy late in the course of the neoplasm.[7] The second group developed an acute or subacute severe sensory motor neuropathy, which often progressed to paralysis often before other signs of malignancy. The CSF protein is often elevated in these syndromes. The neurologic abnormalities may wax and wane and steroids are occasionally associated with clinical improvement. However, surgical removal of the tumor rarely leads to improvement. The syndrome has been reported with a wide variety of neoplasms, most commonly lung cancer.[193]

Pure sensory neuropathy associated with degeneration of dorsal root ganglia (dorsal root ganglionitis) is strongly associated with malignancy. In most instances, the tumor is located in the chest (lung cancer, thymoma, lymphomas, involving the mediastinum, laryngeal or esophageal carcinomas). The syndrome is characterized by the subacute development of distal sensory loss, especially proprioception, and loss of deep tendon reflexes with normal muscle strength. Motor nerve conduction velocities are normal. The CSF protein is often elevated. The illness usually precedes the development of cancer, leaves the patient severely disabled and rarely improves. An immunologic mechanism has been postulated for these sensory neuropathies since organ-specific anti-brain antibodies have been reported in sera and CSF[200]. In one patient with a plasma cell dyscrasia and peripheral neuropathy, pathologic and immunologic studies indicated an IgM kappa antibody directed against peripheral nerve myelin produced the neuropathy.[201]

Ascending acute polyneuropathy (Guillain–Barré syndrome) has been reported in some patients with malignancy, particularly Hodgkin's disease and malignant lymphomas.[202] The syndrome has been clinically similar to that found in patients without malignancy. Since both are relatively common and since parallel clinical courses have not been demonstrated, the association may be coincidental.

Peripheral nerve abnormalities may also be found as a result of other phenomena associated with the cancer. For example, patients with multiple myeloma may have neuropathies secondary to amyloid deposition. Johnson and coworkers reported three patients who developed peripheral neuropathy (mononeuritis multiplex) as a result of tumor-related vasculitis limited to the peripheral nervous system.[203] Neuropathies secondary to hemorrhage into the nerves have also been reported in leukemic patients.

REMOTE EFFECTS ON MUSCLE AND NEUROMUSCULAR FUNCTION

Dermatomyositis and Polymyositis

In large series, 7–34% of patients with dermatomyositis or polymyositis have been reported to have cancer. Thus, the patients with these disorders have five to seven times the incidence of malignancy as the general population.[204,205,206] These estimates are based on compilations of uncontrolled single institution studies lacking strict comparisons with the general population. In addition, a parallel clinical course has been reported in only a minority of patients.[205] It does appear from these retrospective series that the association is most striking in males over 50 where more than 70% have developed cancer.

Clinically, the syndrome is characterized by gradually progressive muscle weakness over a period of weeks to months. The weakness eventually stabilizes and is usually not disabling. The weakness involves the proximal musculature. Reflexes are usually present but diminished. Muscle enzymes and sedimentation rate are usually elevated. The EMG is abnormal and muscle biopsies show muscle fiber necrosis with minimal inflammatory changes.

In most instances, the myopathy and cancer present within one year of one another. There have been no long-term follow-up studies to determine whether patients with dermatomyositis who do not develop cancer within one year continue at high risk for developing cancer. Most reported cases do not relate the temporal cause of the tumor and the dermatomyositis. Barnes was able to find 29 reports of improvement in both tumor and dermatomyositis and seven reports of worsening of both in a review of 258 cases.[205] Steroids have been reported to be useful by some observers although this is controversial and there are no well-controlled therapeutic studies.

MYASTHENIC (EATON–LAMBERT) SYNDROME

This syndrome is uncommon but strongly associated with small-cell undifferentiated bronchogenic carcinoma. The syndrome is characterized by muscle weakness and fatigue, which are most pronounced in the pelvic girdle and thigh making it difficult to climb stairs or get out of a chair. Other features including dryness of mouth, dysarthria, dysphagia, blurred vision or diplopia, ptosis, paresthesias, and muscle pain. In contrast to true myasthenia gravis, muscle strength improves with exercise and there is poor response to tensilon. The EMG confirms the increase in muscle action potential with repeated nerve stimulation at rates greater than 10 per second. The majority of cases have lung cancer, particularly small-cell lung cancer. Lambert and coworkers reported that less than 1% of all lung cancer patients but 6% of all small-cell lung cancer patients have this syndrome.[207,208] In the authors' experience, these syndromes are infrequent in lung cancer patients. There are a few reports of the relationship between response to antitumor therapy and improvement in the syndrome.[209] Recovery of the syndrome has been noted in patients with small-cell lung cancer treated with combination chemotherapy. Since more than 90% of patients with small-cell lung cancer respond to combination chemotherapy, this should be tried as a first measure. For patients failing chemotherapy or having no improvement in muscle strength with response to chemotherapy, guanidine has been reported to be useful.[210]

MYASTHENIA GRAVIS

The association of myasthenia gravis and thymoma is well established. A number of tumors including lymphomas, pancreas, breast, prostate, ovary, thyroid, cervix, kidney, rectum, and palate have been reported in association with myasthenia gravis but many authors conclude the incidence is not greater than expected in the normal poulation.[193]

HEMATOLOGIC MANIFESTATIONS OF MALIGNANCY

Abnormalities in all the hematopoietic cell lines as well as in the clotting proteins have been reported in cancer patients. As with the other paraneoplastic syndromes these abnormalities are most often produced as a direct result of marrow infiltration by the tumor or its metastases. Infection and toxicity from cancer therapies are also more common than true paraneoplastic effects. As our understanding of hormones and protein factors regulating hematopoiesis has increased in recent years with newer *in vitro* cell culture techniques, the mechanisms for hematologic paraneoplastic syndromes, particularly increases in cell numbers, are better understood.

ERYTHROCYTOSIS

Tumor-associated erythrocytosis is well documented in the literature. In a review of 340 cases of tumor-associated erythrocytosis, 35% were hypernephromas, 14% were benign renal problems (cystic kidneys or hydronephrosis), 3% were other tumors involving the kidney (Wilm's, hemangioma, adenomas and sarcomas), 19% were hepatomas, 15% were cerebellar hemangioblastomas, 7% were uterine fibroids (often aldosterone secreting adenomas), 3% were adrenal (often aldosterone-secreting adenomas) tumors and pheochromocytomas, and 3% were miscellaneous tumors (ovary, lung, thymus).[211] Overall, 53% of cases had some renal involvement. It is estimated that 1–5% of patients with renal tumors and 9–20% of patients with cerebellar hemangioblastomas have erythrocytosis.[212] The erythrocytosis usually regresses with removal of the primary tumor and recurs with tumor progression.[211] Increased erythropoietin levels were found in 64% of the tumor extracts or cystic fluids tested, but no erythropoietin was detected in normal tissues. Elevated serum erythropoietin levels were found in 53% of patients. While Wilm's tumor is usually not associated with erythrocytosis, elevated plasma erythropoietin levels have been found in patients without erythrocytosis, but the exact frequency of this is unknown.[211] All of this is very suggestive that about half of certain tumors associated with erythrocytosis make erythropoietin.[211]

Erythropoietin is normally produced by the kidney but also may be produced by the liver in anephric individuals.[12] Thus, it is not surprising that certain renal and liver tumors may produce erythropoietin. However, erythropoietin has not yet been purified, bioassays remain difficult, and biosynthetic studies of cloned tumor cells do not exist.[12] This is important because there are a variety of mechanisms by which tumors could cause elevated erythropoietin levels including:

1. Tumor production of erythropoietin
2. Induction of either local kidney or systemic hypoxia by tumor mass effect, vascular obstruction, or hypoxia
3. Secretion by the tumor of a factor that stimulates the release of eutopic erythropoietin
4. Change in the metabolism of erythropoietin by the tumor.[211]

In the cases of renal cysts, local renal hypoxia is a likely cause.[211]

Other Mechanisms Generating Erythrocytosis in Cancer Patients

Since not all cancer patients with erythrocytosis had elevated tumor levels of erythropoietin, other mechanisms causing erythrocytosis must exist. Adrenal cortical tumors and virilizing ovarian tumors can produce androgenic hormones with erythropoietic effects.[12] This may be the mechanism of erythrocytosis associated with Cushing's syndrome. While pheochromocytomas and aldosterone-producing adrenal adenomas may also cause erythrocytosis by this mechanism, the exact hormonal basis is not yet defined.[211]

Another possible mechanism would be by way of tumor-produced prostaglandins since prostaglandins will enhance the effects of erythropoietin on erythroid differentiation.[12] This is likely since the demonstration of elevated prostaglandin levels associated with hypercalcemia were usually found in patients with renal tumors.[106,107] Because of this it would be extremely interesting to consider a trial of indomethacin in cancer-associated erythrocytosis in patients without elevated erythropoietin levels.

By convention, erythrocytosis is diagnosed when there is increased red cell mass, usually associated with a hematocrit over 55% for a man and over 50% for a woman.[213] Obviously, elevated but lower hematocrits in the setting of appropriate tumors (*e.g.*, hypernephromas, hepatomas, or CNS tumors) should alert clinical suspicion of a paraneoplastic syndrome. The differential diagnosis of erythrocytosis is between the panmyelosis (all blood elements) and splenomegaly of polycythemia vera, stress polycythemia, arterial unsaturation from many causes, a hemoglobinopathy with aberrent oxygen binding features, and dehydration with hemoconcentration.[213] A physical examination, arterial pO_2 determination, a hemoglobin electrophoresis, and family history will resolve most of these. Demonstration of elevated erythropoietin in the blood would confirm the diagnosis, but is usually not performed because of the difficult in bioassay. If a tumor is evident it is still probably wise to rule out other causes of erythrocytosis and an IVP (looking for cysts or other benign abnormalities), careful pelvic examination (looking for fibroids), and neurologic examination for cerebellar signs should be performed in all cases.

The erythrocytosis *per se* usually does not need treatment and phlebotomy is rarely used.[211] Tumor resection is successful in controlling the erythrocytosis in over 97% of resectable cases; this should be the primary approach.[211] There are no good data on the response of erythrocytosis to chemotherapy (*e.g.*, of a hepatoma). Since only half of the patients with resectable tumors had increased serum or tumor extract erythropoietin levels before surgery, and the erythrocytosis corrected with resection, it is clear that non-erythropoietin-mediated tumor erythrocytosis also should be primarily treated with resection, if possible.

ANEMIA ASSOCIATED WITH CANCER

Anemia occurs frequently in cancer patients and there are a variety of mechanisms postulated to explain the anemias including the anemia of "chronic disease"; bone marrow invasion; blood loss; marrow suppression by chemo-radiotherapy; hypersplenism; immune hemolysis of both the warm and cold antibody types; megaloblastic anemia; vitamin and iron deficiency; microangiopathic hemolytic anemia; and "pure red cell aplasia."[214–232] The reader is referred to other general hematologic sources for the general evaluation of anemia in the cancer patient. However, the mechanisms of anemia associated with cancer in most cases have not been elucidated.[214,215] For example, anemia found in leukemias is probably not explained by "crowding out" of normal marrow.[214] In many patients a good explanation of anemia cannot be found and the diagnosis of anemia of "chronic disease" is given. While this is easy to treat with transfusions, the cause is unknown and probably represents a remote effect of the tumor on bone marrow function, red cell metabolism, or kinetics. The anemia of "chronic malignancy" has no associated cancer types, and is usually normocytic, and normochromic or hypochromic, with normal iron stores (but low serum iron, and low total iron binding capacity), normal reticulocyte count, normal red cell maturation, moderately increased erythropoiesis, and slightly shorter red cell survival.[214,216,217] New approaches to finding the mechanisms would include study of red cell production in nude mice bearing human tumors associated with malignancy, or cocultivation of *in vitro* erythropoiesis systems with human tumor cells.

Pure red cell aplasia with a severe anemia is found in association with thymomas.[218] A selective absence of marrow erythropoiesis occurs, and hypogammaglobulinemia may occur.[218,219] Many cases with and without thymomas have responded to cyclophosphamide therapy and it is possible the mechanism of the aplasia is through some T-lymphocyte mediated system.

Megaloblastic anemia without folate or B_{12} deficiency is seen in the bone marrows of cancer patients before chemotherapy; these are unexplained. A macrocytic anemia of unknown etiology is occasionally seen in association with multiple myeloma. The marrow is megaloblastic, the serum B_{12} levels low, but the patients fail to respond to B_{12}.[220]

Hypersplenic anemia with shortened red cell survival is probably not a paraneoplastic syndrome, as it nearly always occurs with myelofibrosis or rarely with a chronic granulocytic leukemia.[213] However, it is possible that the cause of the fibrosis in the marrow and the spleen is by way of a humoral factor.

Autoimmune hemolytic anemias (AHA) associated with tumors are usually found with B-cell lympho-proliferative neoplasms.[221,222,223] The mechanisms by which the B-cell neoplasms upset the normal immuno-regulatory circuits remains to be identified. However, the monoclonal immunoglobulins produced by the B-cell neoplasms on their surface membranes are probably not themselves responsible for the hemolysis.

Rarely, autoimmune hemolytic anemia is found associated with solid tumors.[224,225,226] In a review of a large series of AHA, only 2% of patients had associated solid tumors.[227,228] In these cases the mean age is 10 years older than patients presenting with idiopathic AHA.[226] Thus, when AHA presents in the elderly it is important to consider the possibility of an underlying carcinoma. A wide variety of tumor types are reported associated with AHA, including lung cancer of all histologic types, ovarian cancer, hypernephromas, breast cancer, stomach, uterine cervix, colon, cecal cancer, and seminoma.

In tumor-associated AHA, anemia is often the presenting symptom, with mean hemoglobin levels of 7.4 g/dl and frequent reticulocytosis. Splenomegaly is also common. Response to corticosteroids is infrequent in contrast to the high response seen in idiopathic AHA. However, successful treatment of the primary tumor with resection, radiation therapy, or chemotherapy usually leads to improvement or cure of the AHA.[226,229] In some cases, recurrent tumor was associated with recurrent AHA. Thus, definitive tumor treatment should be the first approach rather than corticosteroids or splenectomy. If this fails, splenectomy can be tried and works in some patients. While the etiology is not known, the two most likely causes are immune response to antigens shared by the tumor with erythrocytes (but exposed on the erythrocyte in a non-stimulating form) or attachment of immune complexes to red cells.

Microangiopathic hemolytic anemia (MAHA) has been reported in association with 55 cancer patients in a comprehensive review.[230] By definition, the peripheral blood smear in MAHA contains fragmented red blood cell (RBC) forms.[231] Severe MAHA is rare in cancer patients, in one series occurring in only eight of 3,200 patients.[232] However, Antman and associates postulate that a careful search of the peripheral blood film for signs of microangiopathy (schistocytosis) may uncover many more cases of a milder nature.[230] In the reported MAHA cases, the hemolysis was abrupt and severe requiring several units of transfused blood daily to maintain a 20% hematocrit. The mean hemoglobin level was 7 g/dl, the mean number of nucleated red blood cells was 30%, elevated bilirubin was found in 93%, and a leukoerythroblastic blood film was found in 35% of patients. The mean number of days from diagnosis of MAHA to death was 21 (range of 2–90 days) and thus MAHA rapidly led to a patient's demise. The Coombs' test was always negative. Associated laboratory findings of disseminated intravascular coagulation (DIC) were found in 50–60% and some of the patients had migratory thrombophlebitis. However, some of the patients with MAHA did not have signs of DIC.

Most of the tumors were mucin-producing adenocarcinomas; 55% were gastric cancer, 10% were of unknown primary (possibly gastric), and breast and lung accounted for 13% and 7% each. The remainder were divided between prostate, ovary, pancreatic, colon, hepatoma, cholangiocarcinoma, and seminal vesicle.[230] Of interest, several of the gastric primaries were occult and found only at autopsy.

MAHA is easily diagnosed by the presence of a severe hemolytic anemia, with fragmented RBC forms on the peripheral blood smear and a negative Coombs' test. The causes of the MAHA syndrome represent various diseases associated with lesions of small blood vessels including thrombotic thrombocytopenic purpura (TTP); congenital vascular abnormalities such as the Kasabach–Merritt syndrome; hemolytic-uremic syndrome; DIC; malfunction at an aortic valve prosthesis; and neoplastic disease. The differential diagnosis of MAHA due to neoplastic diseases from TTP or DIC may be impossible since TTP and DIC have been reported in association with malignancy.[233,234] The renal function of patients with the MAHA associated with malignancy was not indicated, but supposedly was not unusual.

While heparin has been used to treat other causes of MAHA, particularly the hemolytic uremic syndrome, it appears ineffective when given alone in the MAHA of neoplastic disease. In contrast, in 7/9 patients, the MAHA syndrome responded to hormonal anti-cancer therapy (for breast and prostate cancer) or chemotherapy.[230] However, if DIC is associated with MAHA, it would appear reasonable to treat with heparin to control the immediate DIC problem while instituting appropriate anti-cancer therapy as is done in acute promyelocytic leukemia.[234]

The pathophysiology of MAHA associated with cancer may represent various causes of RBC shearing including fibrin strands from DIC; pulmonary intraluminal tumor emboli (found in 31% of MAHA patients); and narrowing of pulmonary arterioles by intraluminal proliferation of pulmonary arterioles due to tumor emboli or a side effect of chemotherapy.[230] The presence of tumor emboli diffusely involving pulmonary arterioles occurs in about 1% of cancer patients.[230] Association of MAHA with gastric cancer may be explained by its tendency for widespread vascular metastasis and mucin production. Mucin can act as a procoagulant and potentially cause DIC. The occurrence of intimal proliferation is postulated to give pulmonary hypertension and increase the shearing force on the RBC.[230]

GRANULOCYTOSIS ASSOCIATED WITH NON-HEMATOLOGIC MALIGNANCIES

Elevation in the peripheral granulocyte count to over 20,000/μl without overt infection or leukemia occurs in association with several neoplasms.[213,235,236,237,238] Similarly, monocyte elevation also may be seen.[239] Neoplasms associated with a granulocytosis syndrome are gastric, lung, pancreas, melanoma, brain tumors, Hodgkin's disease, and diffuse histiocytic lymphoma ("reticulum cell sarcoma").[213,240] The exact frequency in each histologic type is not known, but many cases have been reported over the past 50 years.[213] The granulocytosis is usually asymptomatic and consists of mature neutrophils.[215]

While there are many potential causes of neutrophilia in cancer patients (including infection, inflammatory disorders, drugs, metabolic disorders, physical and emotional stimuli) the major differential diagnostic problem for a persistently high neutrophil count is to distinguish it from co-existent chronic myelogenous leukemia (CML).[213] The major features distinguishing a paraneoplastic "leukemoid reaction" in the cancer patient from CML are a white blood count less than 100,000/μl; no left shift to blast or progranulocytic forms; normal platelet and basophil levels; absent splenomegaly; elevated leukocyte alkaline phosphatase; normal serum B_{12} levels; and, of course, an absent Philadelphia chromosome.[215] Once other disorders and co-existent CML are ruled out in the cancer patient a paraneoplastic granulocytosis is likely. The mechanism(s) behind this granulocytosis is not fully understood but does not seem in most cases to reflect marrow involvement with tumor.[235]

When specific bone marrow progenitor cells of granulocyte and macrophages are cultured in semi-solid agar medium they will grow to form colonies of differentiated granulocytes and macrophages.[241,242] This proliferation requires the presence of a colony stimulatory factor (CSF, CSA).[241] The human sources include urine; conditioned media of peripheral leukocyte cultures; spleen; placenta; embryonic kidney; and embryonic lung.[241,243,244] A transplantable mouse mammary tumor produces a factor like CSF that can induce granulocyte counts above 100,000/μl.[245] Following this lead, Robinson tested the serum and urine of 12 patients with cancer and unexplained, sustained granulocytosis for CFS activity using *in vitro* bone marrow culture assays.[235] Of interest, in his series there were five lung cancers (type unspecified), two melanomas, and two adrenal cancers, as well as an unknown primary, hepatoma, and multiple myeloma. He found elevated CSF levels in all these patients, and the levels correlated with the degree of elevation of the peripheral neutrophil count. The two adrenal tumors did not make CSF in culture, while the other tumors were not tested. Recently, several laboratories have reported on establishing human tumor tissue culture cell lines of lung cancer (squamous),[245] oral cavity (squamous),[243] and fibrous histiocytoma,[244] which produce large amounts of a CSF-like factor. The activity can be demonstrated in marrow cultures *in vitro*, and, interestingly, when the human tumors are heterotransplanted they cause neutrophilia in athymic nude mice.[243,245] Thus, the most likely cause of granulocytosis in most of the cancer patients is production of a CSF by the tumor. Because normal human tissues (such as embryonic and fetal lung) can produce CSF, it is not unexpected that tumors of these organs will also be found to produce CSF. However, as Robinson points out, there probably will be heterogeneity in the cause of the syndrome with different tumors, and tumors may produce factors that induce the secretion of eutopic CSF, or other mechanisms may be involved.[235] There is no specific therapy for the granulocytosis other than to treat the underlying malignancy.[215]

GRANULOCYTOPENIA AS A PARANEOPLASTIC SYNDROME

Granulocytopenia associated with cancer is usually the result of chemotherapy, radiotherapy, other drugs, or severe infection.[240] Granulocytosis rarely has been reported with thymomas and may have the same immunologic basis as pure red cell aplasia.[240] Neutropenia alone may develop with marrow involvement by carcinoma, lymphoma, myeloma, or leukemia, but a pancytopenia is more common.[240] With the exception of leukemia, the neutropenia is usually not life-threatening. Despite the frequent involvement of the bone marrow with cancer, significant granulocytopenia unrelated to therapy must be uncommon in cancer patients. However, recent experimental evidence suggests that a paraneoplastic syndrome involving granulopoiesis may exist. When 10^5 normal bone marrow cells are plated in semisolid medium with CSF, 20–100 hematopoietic colonies (containing 40 or more cells) and 5–10 times that number of "cluster" (aggregates of 3–40 cells) are found.[246] In contrast, when marrow from patients with acute leukemia, preleukemic states, and CML in blast transformation are plated, mainly clusters and only rare colonies are found, suggesting the leukemic process may inhibit the activity of the exogenously-added CSF in some unknown way. Similar findings also occur with solid tumors. McCarthy and coworkers studied nine small-cell lung cancer patients for bone marrow colony formation with CSF.[246] Two of these patients (one with and one without small-cell cancer marrow involvement) were not able to form colonies in agar but had large numbers of clusters with or without CSF. Of interest, the patient with marrow involvement had neutrophilia, while the one without had neutropenia.[246] Thus, it is likely that some tumors may suppress granulopoiesis by interfering with the action of CSF on marrow progenitor cells.

EOSINOPHILIA AND BASOPHILIA ASSOCIATED WITH NEOPLASMS

Eosinophilia is also associated with non-leukemic neoplasms, particularly Hodgkin's disease (in up to 20% of cases) and mycosis fungoides, but it has also been found with other lymphomas, melanoma, brain tumors, and other cancer. The exact frequency in these tumors is not documented.[213,240,247]

It is possible that the eosinophilia itself could be symptomatic if the count were sufficiently high and an allergic or Leoffler's-like syndrome (fleeting nodular pulmonary infiltrates with eosinophilia, the PIE syndrome, with mild cough, lassitude and low grade fever) were produced in cancer patients. A small peptide that acts as an eosinophilopoietin has recently been described and it is possible the tumor cells are producing or stimulating the secretion of this factor.[249] Therapy should be directed against the tumor, particularly in cases of the malignant lymphomas which are potentially curable. If this does not work or if pulmonary symptoms are troublesome, a trial of corticosteroids could be given as this sometimes gives dramatic results in other forms of the PIE syndrome, but data in cancer patients are lacking.[247]

Eosinopenia as a tertiary result of tumor secretion of ACTH or other hormones is possible but should give no clinical symptoms. Basophilia is commonly associated with CML, myelofibrosis, and polycythemia vera but is not reported with other malignancies and currently there is no recognized basophilic paraneoplastic syndrome.[213]

THROMBOCYTOSIS ASSOCIATED WITH CANCER

Thrombocytosis (platelet count over 400,000/μl) is said to occur in up to 30–40% of cancer patients.[249,250,251] The differential diagnosis of thrombocytosis in the cancer patient includes myeloproliferative disorders (which may represent a paraneoplastic syndrome); acute and chronic inflammatory disorders; acute hemorrhage; iron deficiency; hemolytic anemias; post-splenectomy and other surgical procedures; and as a response to vincristine or epinephrine.[249] Thrombocytosis has been seen with carcinomas, leukemias, Hodgkin's disease, and non-Hodgkin's disease; a fall in the platelet count is associated with a response to therapy.[215] Although not characterized yet there is a "thrombopoietin" which regulates normal megakaryocyte production and maturation.[252] Thus, patients with neoplasms and thrombocytosis will have to have serum and tumor levels of thrombopoietin assayed. While platelet counts over 1,000,000/μl can lead to thrombosis or hemorrhage, these are rarely seen associated with malignancy and such symptoms do not appear to occur with any regularity with the thrombocytosis of malignancy. As of now, no specific treatment of the thrombocytosis is indicated except to treat the underlying malignancy.

UNEXPLAINED THROMBOCYTOPENIA IN CANCER PATIENTS

Thrombocytopenia is commonly seen in cancer patients and is usually related to chemotherapy, radiotherapy, acute leukemia, or DIC. A syndrome resembling idiopathic thrombocytopenic purpura (ITP) is occasionally seen associated with malignancy.[253] This association is uncommon and in one series of ITP represented 4% of 381 patients with otherwise unexplained thrombocytopenia; all of these cases had lymphomas.[254] In another series of ITP, 9/52 had cancer.[253]

The diagnosis of an "ITP-like" syndrome is made by finding thrombocytopenia without anemia and with normal or increased numbers of normal red cells on peripheral smear; no evidence of DIC; and no evidence of a drug-induced thrombocytopenia.[253] The type of neoplasms reported in the literature associated with this syndrome are Hodgkin's disease; chronic lymphocytic leukemia; non-Hodgkin's lymphoma; acute lymphoblastic leukemia; immunoblastic sarcomas; and carcinomas of the lung, breast, rectum, gallbladder, and testis.[253,254] The association with CLL and Hodgkin's disease is widely known and the syndrome occurs in approximately 30% of patients with immunoblastic lymphadenopathy.[255–257] However, the association with other tumors is less widely recognized. The mean age of patients is older (54 years) than the age of patients with ITP alone. Some 80% of patients are symptomatic with bleeding, petechiae, or purpura. Most have platelet counts under 30,000/μl.[253] Response of platelet counts to high-dose (60 mg/day) prednisone is common but transient. However, 6/10 had a complete and apparently permanent response to splenectomy.[253]

The syndrome is called "ITP-like" because the course is very much like classic ITP but an immune mechanism has not been demonstrated. In the future, studies of antiplatelet antibodies will have to be done, as well as test of antibody crossreactivity with tumor cells. Nearly all patients have been treated with splenectomy, in addition to various antineoplastic therapies, so the effect of tumor treatment alone on the thrombocytopenia is currently unknown.[253] Obviously, other causes of thrombocytopenia need to be excluded; particularly the use of thiazide diuretics and quinidine, or the presence of DIC or severe infection. In thrombocytopenic patients receiving antineoplastic therapy, ITP-like syndromes should be considered. The clues are thrombocytopenia out of proportion to granulocytopenia, normal or increased numbers of marrow megakaryocytes, and a rapid fall in transfused platelets. This diagnosis should be particularly remembered in lymphoproliferative disorders. Therapy will consist of platelet transfusions, initial corticosteroids, then splenectomy. At present, because of the poor response to steroids and inconsistent response to treatment of the underlying malignancy, a reasonable approach is to take the patient directly to splenectomy after other causes of thrombocytopenia have been excluded.

Abnormalities of platelet function are sometimes seen associated with plasma cell dyscrasias and are felt to result from the interference of the monoclonal protein with platelet function.[223]

DISSEMINATED INTRAVASCULAR COAGULATION (DIC) ASSOCIATED WITH CANCER

Hemorrhagic and thrombotic complications occur frequently in cancer patients and can arise from various mechanisms, including thrombocytopenia, local tissue disruption from tumor or therapy, vitamin deficiency, circulating anticoagulants, liver disease, and DIC.[233,234,258] After therapy-induced changes in platelet count, DIC is probably the most common and important cause. Armand Trousseau first noted the clinical association between cancer and thrombophlebitis.[259] In 1949, Marder and colleagues reported afibrinogenemia in metastatic prostate cancer.[260] After these publications, many reports of DIC and malignancy appeared.[261] Disseminated intravascular coagulation can present as a chronic coagulation disorder, usually of a thrombotic nature, and as acute acquired hemorrhagic diathesis, or as a coagulation abnormality only detected by laboratory tests (Table 39-11).[233,234,258–269] The diagnosis, clinical manifestations, and pathophysiology of DIC are covered in detail in Chapter 42.

Another cause of thrombotic or hemorrhagic complications, nonbacterial thrombotic endocarditis (NBTE), can occur with or without DIC and is characterized by the presence of sterile verrucous, bland, fibrin-platelet lesions in the left-side heart valves.[176,233,270,271,272] Clinically, patients often present with emboli to the brain as well as to other organs. The brain emboli can have either an abrupt or gradual onset of neurologic symptoms with development of either focal neurologic deficits, or diffuse abnormalities such as confusion, disorientation, generalized seizure, or disturbances in consciousness. Only one-third or less of patients have heart murmurs, usually

TABLE 39-11. Frequency of Different Cancer Types Associated with DIC in Various Series*

TUMOR TYPE	CHRONIC DIC (N=213) (233)	% OF TUMORS MAKING UP VARIOUS DIC SERIES	
		BLEEDING DISORDER (N=134) (234)	COAGULATION ABNORMALITY (N=86) (234a)
Pancreas	24	2	0
Lung	20	1.5	12
Prostate	13	18	8
Stomach	12	4	0
Acute Leukemia	9	64	19
Colon	5	0.7	6
Unknown Primary	5	0	0
Ovary	4	0.7	1
Gallbladder (Cholangiocarcinoma)	4	0.7	2
Lymphomas	1	1.5	16
Breast	0.5	0	10
Melanomas	0.5	0	3
Miscellaneous others	3	3	10

*Some of the cases in reference 233 and 234 may overlap. The data in reference 233 were obtained by way of a literature review from 1960–1970 looking for the association of malignancy and thrombophlebitis, hemorrhagic diathesis, DIC, arterial embolism, or nonbacterial thrombotic endocarditis. The data in reference 234 are based on a literature review to find cases of permit a tentative diagnosis of DIC. The data in reference 234 come from review of the coagulation laboratory and medical records from 1971–1974 at the Memorial Sloan-Kettering Cancer Center looking for laboratory evidence of DIC.

systolic. Patients are usually afebrile, however, all patients should have blood cultures if emboli are suspected. Echocardiography may be of diagnostic use but no large series are yet reported. Arterial emboli can go to the CNS, heart, spleen, kidneys, and peripheral sites. Occlusion of both large and small vessels is seen pathologically in the brain. Myocardial infarction can result from emboli to coronary arteries.[270,271] It is important to note that paraneoplastic endocarditis can present with early malignancy as well as at later stages and thus does not mean incurability.[272] In Goodnight's review of NBTE, bleeding was frequently found in the skin (77–100%), CNS (22–49%), genitourinary tract (38–42%), eye, ear, nose, mouth (31–47%), and GI (24–56%) and respiratory tracts (20–31%) in leukemias and solid tumor patients respectively.[261] Of both the leukemias and solid tumor patients 37% had autopsy evidence of fibrin thrombi but only 1% had evidence of NBTE.

In cancer patients suspected of DIC, NBTE, or other thrombotic or hemorrhagic phenomena, Sack and coworkers stressed the need for sequential monitoring of coagulation tests, and the striking decreases that occurred in fibrinogen and platelet levels associated with the acute vascular events.[233] They postulated this was due to a shift from a "compensated" to a "decompensated" coagulation status engendered by the tumor.[233] While the thrombotic events of chronic DIC are clearly related to the coagulation disorder, the relationship is not so clear for the multiple organ system dysfunction seen in acute (often hemorrhagic) DIC.[234] The situations that appear most related to DIC are the adult respiratory distress syndrome; oliguric renal insufficiency with gram-negative sepsis and the hemolytic-uremic syndrome; neurologic syndromes related to intracranial bleeding and thrombosis; pulmonary hemorrhage syndrome; and the infarcted skin of purpura fulminans.[234] In any event, autopsy studies show DIC usually contributes strongly to patient morbidity, and mortality particularly with thrombosis or bleeding in the lung, CNS, or gastrointestinal tract.[234]

MANAGEMENT OF DIC IN MALIGNANCY

There is universal agreement that identification and treatment of all precipitating factors is the keystone to DIC management.[234,262] This should include not only treatment of cancer, but evaluation of patients with DIC for other precipitating factors (*e.g.*, sepsis, volume deficit, hypotension, hypoxemia, acidosis, fungus infection, transfusion reactions, and vessel manipulation). In addition, identification and correction of other hemostatic deficits should take place. A response of the malignancy to tumor treatment is often associated with response of the DIC and thus the long-term goal is appropriate anti-neoplastic therapy.[233,273]

A major controversy is whether or not heparin should be used.[234,262] There is a tendency to use heparin more in DIC with thrombotic, thromboembolic, or necrotizing complications as is often seen in the chronic DIC of malignancy.[234,235] However, randomized trials of heparin therapy in the DIC of malignancy have not been conducted. Gralnick and associates reported on three patients with acute promyelocytic leukemia (APL) who were treated with induction chemotherapy and developed DIC.[263] The patients were treated with heparin and had prompt (over 2–4 day) improvement in their bleeding and coagulation abnormalities. Drapkin and associates, in a

TABLE 39-12. Treatment of Chronic DIC Malignancy*

Treatment Given: Anti-Neoplastic	Anti-Coagulant†	# Patients	% Response	
			Short-Term	Long-Term
+	+	27	52	15
+	−	22	55	18
−	+	48	60	10
+	+	12‡	75	?

*Data from reference 233. Response is defined as cessation of signs and/or symptoms of thrombophlebitis, hemorrhage, or arterial emboli. Long term indicates for over 250 days or until death.

†In nearly all cases the anticoagulant therapy was heparin (81/87 patients reported for anticoagulant response received heparin)

‡Patients with recurrent DIC after stopping heparin were restarted on heparin.

non-randomized trial, compared 15 patients with APL treated between 1970–1975 with chemotherapy alone with nine patients treated between 1975–1976, with chemotherapy and prophylactic heparin therapy.[268] Heparin was given before the development of DIC based on the premise that chemotherapy of APL with tumor cell lysis would initiate the DIC with a high frequency. In the heparin-treated group there was a decreased incidence of fatal hemorrhage and a resulting increased incidence of remission induction. They used 5–10 units/kg/hr of heparin over 24 hours for 5-14 days and increased the dose of heparin to 10–20 units/kg/hr if clinical or laboratory indices of DIC developed.

Sack and associates,[233] in their literature review of chronic DIC in malignancy, found positive responses to anticoagulant therapy (defined as cessation of signs or symptoms of thrombophlebitis, hemorrhage, or arterial emboli) in 65% of 55 patients treated with heparin initially and 33% of 26 patients treated with heparin after failing warfarin therapy. In contrast, only 19% of 32 patients treated with warfarin alone responded. In addition, 53% of 36 patients had symptoms of the thrombotic-hemorrhage disorder recur when the heparin was stopped suggesting a therapeutic role of heparin in control of the DIC. Table 39-12 summarizes the results of anticoagulant and antineoplastic therapy in the treatment of the chronic DIC of malignancy. Clearly, all combinations of antineoplastic and anticoagulant therapy were associated with response of the DIC symptoms in over half of the cases but only 10–20% of patients had long-term control, presumably reflecting the lack of control of the underlying tumor. While in many cases, the temporal correlation of heparin therapy with cessation of DIC is persuasive, spontaneous remission of DIC occurring with persistent cancer has been reported.[274]

At present, once a diagnosis of DIC associated with malignancy is made and other factors corrected, it is wise to establish the tempo of the DIC. If the DIC is acute and symptoms life-threatening (*e.g.*, uncontrolled bleeding), or if it is chronic and the symptoms debilitating (*e.g.*, recurrent thromboembolic lesions), a trial of heparin therapy can be given. The doses used in the literature range from 300–600 units/kg/24 hr. Because continuous heparin infusion appears to have fewer bleeding complications than pulse doses of heparin, continuous infusion is recommended. Care must be used if liver or renal insufficiency are present since herapin retention is seen in these conditions. Once heparin therapy has begun, the repletion of coagulation factors with platelets, cryoprecipitates, and whole blood can be used, particularly in highly symptomatic, hemorrhagic, acute DIC.[234] It should be re-emphasized that while heparin treatment may be maintained for weeks, it is only a temporary measure and control of the underlying malignancy will afford the only long-term control of chronic DIC.

RENAL MANIFESTATIONS OF MALIGNANCY

There are numerous problems involving the kidneys that develop in patients with malignancies. The etiology of these complications are listed in Table 39-13. The table demonstrates that in most instances the renal abnormalities are not paraneoplastic in orgin. Only the glomerular lesions and obstruction by tumor products can be considered to be true paraneoplastic syndromes.

GLOMERULAR LESIONS OF INDIRECT CAUSE

Massive proteinuria with the nephrotic syndrome is the major consequence of these paraneoplastic glomerular lesions, although renal failure may later develop. In patients with malignancy the nephrotic syndrome may develop as a result of neoplastic infiltration of the kidneys, renal vein thrombosis, or amyloid infiltration. Besides the above-established causes for the nephrotic syndrome, there does seem to be a true paraneoplastic syndrome. Until 1966, there were only a few scattered case reports of an association between idiopathic

TABLE 39-13. Differential Diagnosis of Renal Abnormalities in Patients with Malignancy

1. Direct infiltration of the kidney by tumor
2. Obstruction of the urinary tract by tumor
3. Electrolyte imbalances, many of which are caused by the tumor or its treatment (*e.g.*, calcium, uric acid, potassium)
4. Fluid imbalances induced by the tumor or its treatment (pre-renal)
5. Infection
6. Toxicity of therapy (chemotherapy, radiotherapy, immunotherapy, antibiotics)
7. Glomerular lesions of uncertain etiology (usually associated with nephrotic syndrome), paraneoplastic
8. Obstruction by tumor products

nephrotic syndrome and malignancy. In 1966, Lee and associates reported that among 101 patients with the nephrotic syndrome of unknown etiology, 11 were found to have cancer.[275] The neoplastic syndrome preceded discovery of the cancer in seven of these 11 patients who were all over the age of 40. Since that time, the nephrotic syndrome has been reported in association with a wide variety of cancers.

Clinical and immunologic evidence supports the true paraneoplastic nature of this syndrome.[275,276,277,278,279,280,281] The nephrotic syndrome may precede the development of neoplastic disease.[277] Surgical removal of tumor or response to radiotherapy or chemotherapy is usually associated with dramatic diminution in proteinuria, whereas recurrence of the neoplasm is followed by increased proteinuria.[276,278,279] Tumor-specific antigens and antibodies and carcinoembryonic antigen have been found in the glomeruli of some patients.[280,281,282]

The most frequently reported associated neoplasm has been Hodgkin's disease.[276,277,279,283,284,285] In patients with Hodgkin's disease the most common renal lesion is lipoid nephrosis (minimal glomerular changes), which occurs in about 80% of cases.[286,287] In most of these instances, the renal findings have been similar to those seen in idiopathic lipoid nephrosis including an absence of electron dense deposits on electron microscopy and an absence of immunoglobulin deposits.[283] In the remaining 20% of cases, lesions typical of membranous glomerulopathy, focal sclerosis, or a membranoproliferative glomerulonephritis have been observed.[276,279,284]

In the non-Hodgkin's lymphomas (Burkitt's lymphomas, lymphocytic, and histiocytic lymphoma) the incidence of the nephrotic syndrome appears to be lower than in Hodgkin's disease and some other carcinomas, although there are numerous case reports.[288,289,290] In several of the patients with non-Hodgkin's lymphomas, immunoglobulin deposits have been identified, suggesting an immune complex etiology of the syndrome.[289,290]

There is a striking difference in the type of renal lesions described in patients with carcinomas when compared to Hodgkin's disease. The most frequently observed glomerular lesion in patients with carcinomas is membranous glomerulonephritis.[287,288,291,292] Membranous glomerulonephritis is characterized by subepithelial electron dense deposits and granular peripheral capillary deposits of IgG with or without C3.[276] It is present in 80–90% of patients with carcinoma and nephrotic syndrome. The remaining patients have lipoid nephrosis or proliferative glomerulonephritis.[276,287,288] When considering all patients with membranous glomerulonephritis, patients with neoplasia have accounted for 5–10% of cases.[293,294]

There is a similarity between the immunopathologic features of the membranous glomerulonephritis associated with carcinomas and experimentally-induced immune complex nephritis in animals. The suggestion has been made that there is a common pathophysiologic mechanism with glomerular deposition of circulating antigen–antibody complexes.[276,288] Tumor specific antibodies have been eluted from the kidneys of two patients with lung cancer and the nephrotic syndrome and a tumor-specific antigen was demonstrated in the glomeruli of a patient with colonic carcinoma.[276,281,288] In another patient with colon cancer, carcinoembryonic antigen–antibody complexes were found in the glomeruli.[282]

The pathogenesis of lipoid nephrosis, in patients with Hodgkin's disease, seems to have a different mechanism. There is some evidence that lipoid nephrosis may be a result of deficient T-cell function and abnormalities of T-cell function are common in Hodgkin's disease.[295]

Other renal abnormalities caused directly or indirectly by tumor products include renal dysfunction in patients with multiple myeloma amyloidosis; renal potassium wasting and hypocalcemia related to lysozyme in acute monocytic or myelomonocytic leukemia; intrarenal obstruction by mucoprotein in pancreatic carcinoma; and nephrogenic diabetes insipidus with leiomyosarcoma.[296–314]

The renal problems of myeloma are discussed in Chapter 42.

PARANEOPLASTIC LESIONS INVOLVING THE SKIN

There is a long list of fascinating cutaneous syndromes that have been reported with malignancies. The salient features of these syndromes are outlined in Tables 39-14 through 39-19. There is a great variation in the relationships between the cutaneous lesions and the malignancy. In some instances (*e.g.*, acanthosis nigricans and erythema gryratum repens) the cutaneous syndrome is uncommon but almost always associated with cancer. In other instances the cutaneous lesions may be common (*e.g.*, bullous lesions, exfoliative dermatitis, erythema multiforme) and have an association with various benign disorders as well as cancers. In some instances (*e.g.*, bullous lesions pemphygoid), the association of the skin lesion and cancer may not be proven. The cutaneous syndrome may always be associated with a particular tumor (*e.g.*, esophageal cancer and tylosis), while in others the cutaneous lesions may be associated with a variety of neoplasms (*e.g.*, dermatomyositis). The etiology of the cutaneous lesion is well-known in some instances (*e.g.*, hirsutism in adrenal or ovarian tumors or flushing in carcinoid tumors), while in most the mechanism is unknown. Excellent reviews of the association between skin cancers and internal malignancies are available.[315–317]

EVALUATION OF PATIENTS WITH SUSPECTED PARANEOPLASTIC SKIN LESIONS

The evaluation of cutaneous lesions suspected of being paraneoplastic in origin begins with the clinical history, with particular emphasis on drug and other exposures, associated medical conditions, and family history. An evaluation for an underlying cancer should be undertaken only if there is no evidence of drug exposure. Many of the cutaneous syndromes are hereditary. The onset of symptoms in the paraneoplastic cutaneous lesions is often more rapid than in other benign conditions (*e.g.*, dermatomyositis, malignant down, or erythema gyratum repens). The physical examination is also of

TABLE 39-14. Pigmented Lesions—Keratoses

DISORDER	REFERENCE	DESCRIPTION	PREDOM. MALIGNANCY	ETIOLOGY	COMMENTS
Acanthosis Nigricans*	Brown (320) Curth (321)	Hyperkeratosis and pigmentation especially of axillae, neck, flexures, and anogenital region.	Gastric 60%; abdominal 90%; other	Unknown	Most important to distinguish benign forms present from birth and benign forms associated with various syndromes.
Leser–Trelat*	Dantzig (324) Ronchese (323) Snedden (322)	Sudden showing of large numbers of seborrheic (wart-like) keratoses.	NHL, miscellaneous GI adenocarcinomas	Unknown	Must be distinguished from multiple seborrheic keratoses, which are common and may not be associated with malignancy. Occasionally associated with acanthosis nigricans.
Bowen's Disease	Graham (325) Anderson (326)	A persistent progressive non-elevated red, scaly, or crusted plaque due to an intra-epidermal neoplasm.	Lung, GI, GU, skin	Generally unknown. Arsenic exposure in some cases.	¼ developed systemic cancers an average of 5 years after initial skin lesions but significance of association has been questioned.
Chronic arsenism	Minkowsky (327)	A corn-like, punctate keratosis more profuse on the extremities and characteristically affecting the palms and feet.	Lung, miscellaneous	Chronic exposure to arsenic.	Not a true paraneoplastic lesion.
Generalized melanosis	Fitzpatrick (328) Helm (316)	A diffuse darkening of the skin with a ruddy gray color secondary to chronic liver disease. Generalized blue-gray appearance.	Lymphoma, hepatoma, metastatic liver tumors, melanoma	Melanin deposits in dermis.	Also seen in a variety of benign conditions. May be rapid at onset.
Paget's disease	Ashikari (329)	Erythematous keratotic patch over areola, nipple, or accessory breast tissue.	Breast	Paget cells are either migrants from the carcinoma or Langerhan's cells.	Occurs in less than 3% of breast cancers.
Bazex's disease	Braverman (317)	Erythema hyperkeratosis with scales and pruritis predominantly on palms and soles.	Head and neck, GI, lung	Unknown	Males only.

*True paraneoplastic syndromes.

critical importance. For example, while *cafe au lait* spots are not always associated with Von Recklingausen's disease, the finding of six or more *cafe au lait* spots greater than 1.5 cm in diameter or the presence of axillary freckling are diagnostic aids for the earlier recognition of neurofibromatosis.[318]

Laboratory evaluations are most helpful for cutaneous lesions suspected of being metabolic in nature (*e.g.*, hyperpigmentation in Cushing's and Addison's disease). Skin biopsy is the most important procedure for establishing the correct diagnosis and should be performed in most instances and may provide important information. For example, exfoliative dermatitis in a patient with mycosis fungoides may be associated with infiltration of the skin as in the Sézary syndrome, but may occur in patients with uninvolved skin areas. It may also occur in these patients as a result of treatment with chemotherapy or electron beam radiotherapy.

The differential diagnosis for cutaneous lesions of possible paraneoplastic origin includes benign, non-related skin conditions, cutaneous lesions resulting from a primary tumor or its metastases, cutaneous infections, and toxicity from anticancer therapy (particularly cytotoxic chemotherapy or radiotherapy). Numerous cytotoxic chemotherapeutic agents have mucocutaneous toxicities. While a detailed discussion is beyond the scope of this chapter, excellent reviews are available.[319]

Pigmented Lesions

Of special interest is acanthosis nigricans. This skin lesion is characterized by the presence of symmetric brown areas of hyperpigmentation with hyperkeratosis, exaggerated skin markings, and warty lesions, particularly in the intertriginous

TABLE 39-15. Erythemas

DISORDER	REFERENCE	DESCRIPTION	PREDOMINANT MALIGNANCY	ETIOLOGY	COMMENTS
Erythema gyratum repens*	Purdy (331) Gammell (330) Summerly (332)	Rapidly changing and advancing gyri with scaling and pruritis.	Breast, lung, other.	Unknown	Almost always associated with malignancy.
Erythema annulare centrifugum	Lazar (333)	Slowly migrating annular and configurate erythematous lesions.	Prostate, myeloma, other.	Unknown	Occurs also with infections and other disorders.
Necrolytic migratory erythema (Glucogonoma)*	Wilkinson (334) Church (335)	Circinate and gyrate areas of blistering and erosive erythema on limbs; stomatitis.	Islet cell on pancreas.	Glucoganoma or other metabolic product.	See chapter on islet cell tumors.
Flushing*	Sjoerdsma (336) Mason (337)	Episodic flushing of face and neck.	Carcinoids. Medullary carcinoma of thyroid.	Serotonin or other vasoactive peptides.	See chapter on carcinoids.
Exfoliative Dermatis*	Abrahams (338) Nicolis (339) Helm (316)	Progressive erythema followed by scaling.	Cutaneous T-cell lymphomas, NHL, Hodgkin's disease, non-Hodgkin's lymphoma.	Unknown	Account for 10–20% of all exfoliative dermatitis.
Erythema Multiforme	Elias (340)	Distinctive target lesions in symmetric distribution sometimes with plaques or bullae.			

* True paraneoplastic syndrome
† True neoplastic syndrome only in some instances

TABLE 39-16. Endocrine and Metabolic Lesions

DISORDER	REFERENCE	DESCRIPTION	PREDOMINANT MALIGNANCY	ETIOLOGY	COMMENTS
Systemic nodular panniculitis* (nodular relapsing fat necrosis) (Weber–Christian disease)*	Fitzpatrick (341)	Recurrent crops of tender erythematous subcutaneous nodules. May be accompanied by abdominal pain, fat necrosis in bone marrow, lungs and other organs.	Adenocarcinoma pancreas	Effect of pancreatic enzymes released into circulation on fatty tissues.	Usually associated with pancreatic disease but may be benign pancreatic disease.
Porphyria cutanea tarda*	Weddington (342) Thompson (343)	Photosensitive skin lesions, often painful, or pruritic.	Liver	Increased porphyrins in skin tissues.	Rare.
Cushing's syndrome		Broad purple striae, atrophy, hyperpigmentation (uncommon), plethora, telangiectasis, mild hirsutism.	Ectopic-lung (small cell), thyroid, testes, ovary, adrenal tumors. Pancreatic islet cell, pituitary, other	Increased ACTH.	
Addison's syndrome		Generalized hyperpigmentation especially scars, pressure points, points of friction.	Adrenal gland invasion, lymphomas or carcinomas.	Decreased glucocorticoids.	Rarely caused by tumors invading the adrenal.
Hirsutism		Increased amounts of hair.	Adrenal tumors, ovarian tumors.	Increased glucocorticoid. Increased testosterone.	Associated with virilism.

* True paraneoplastic syndrome

and flexural areas such as the axilla, neck, anogenital region, umbilicus, and areola. The salient features are shown in Table 39-14. The lesions of Leser–Trelat with multiple seborrheic keratoses have also been described in patients with acanthosis nigricans (see Table 39-14).[322] There is a strong association between acanthosis nigricans and malignancy with more than half of all reported cases having cancer. However, the acanthosis nigricans may precede, occur simultaneous with, or occur after the diagnosis of malignancy is made. While the etiology of the disorder is unknown it does appear to be a true paraneoplastic syndrome since there are documented cases of regression following surgical tumor removal. The most

TABLE 39-17. Bullous and Urticarial Lesions

DISORDERS	REFERENCE	DESCRIPTION	PREDOMINANT MALIGNANCY	ETIOLOGY	COMMENTS
Pemphigoid	Stone (344)	Large tense bullae with histologically absent acantholysis.	Miscellaneous	Unknown	While the clinical association of bullous pemphigoid and malignancy was once accepted, recent age-matched studies have failed to support the association.
Dermatitis herpitformis	Tobias (345) Helm (316)	Phemorphic symmetric subepidermal bullae particularly with scarring.	Lymphomas, miscellaneous.	Related to autoantibodies.	

TABLE 39-18. Miscellaneous Lesions

DISORDER	REFERENCE	DESCRIPTION	PREDOMINANT MALIGNANCY	ETIOLOGY	COMMENTS
Dermatomyositis*	Williams (206) Arundell (346) DeVere (204) Barnes (205)	Purplish pink erythema especially of eyelids, neck, and hands.	Miscellaneous	Unknown	Malignant disease reported in 7–50%. Precedes carcinoma by days-years with an average of 6 months.
Hypertrichosis languginosa* (malignant down)	Lyell (347) Hegedus (348)	Rapid development of fine long silky hair especially on ears, forehead and may involve the entire body.	Lung, colon, bladder, uterus, gall bladder.	Unknown	High association with cancer.
Acquired icthyosis*	VanDijk (349) Flint (350)	Generalized dry crackling skin, hyperkeratotic palms and soles, rhomboidal scales.	Hodgkin's disease, other lymphomas, multiple myeloma, other.	Unknown	Should be distinguished from hereditary form which occurs before age 20.
Pachydermoperiostosis*	Vogl (351)	Thickening of skin and creation of new folds. Thickened lips, ears, and lids. Macroglossia. Thick forehead and scalp. Clubbing. Excessive sweating.	Lung, (uterus)	Unknown	Occurs also in lung abscess and benign tumors.
Pruritus*	Rajka (352) Cormia (353)	Failure to determine an overt or covert cutaneous cause of generalized pruritus necessitates evaluation for a possible underlying systemic disease.	Lymphomas, leukemias, multiple myelomas, CNS tumors, abdominal tumors.	Unknown	Also associated with many benign diseases.
Amyloid deposits		Macroglossia, pinch purpura, superficial waxy yellow and pink elevated nodules.	Multiple myeloma, Waldenstrom's macroglobulinemia	Amyloid deposition in blood vessels and dermis.	Also associated with primary systemic amyloid and other benign conditions.
Herpes zoster	Schimpff (354) Dolin (355) Huberman (356)	Vesicular eruption in a dermatomal distribution.	Hodgkin's disease, non-Hodgkin's lymphomas, chronic lymphocytic leukemia, small cell lung cancer.	Immunosuppression	Increased incidence in cancers associated with immunosuppression and following severely immunosuppressive therapy.
Caput medusa					
Thrombophlebitis					
Gynecomastia					

frequent association is with adenocarcinomas of the GI tract (92%), particularly the stomach (50–60%). However, the lesions have been reported in a variety of other tumors, including breast cancer, lymphomas, and squamous carcinomas.[320,321]

The most important part of the differential diagnosis is to distinguish between true acanthosis nigricans associated with malignancy, benign acanthosis, and pseudoacanthosis. Benign acanthosis is a nevoid condition present at birth or beginning in childhood and associated with a number of benign syndromes. Pseudoacanthosis occurs in obese persons, especially those of dark complexion. It may occur in patients

TABLE 39-19. Hereditary Disorders

DISORDERS	REFERENCE	DESCRIPTION	PREDOMINANT MALIGNANCY	HEREDITY	COMMENTS
Gardner's syndrome	Gardner (357) Bussey (358) Jones (359)	Epidermal cysts, sebaceous cysts, dermoid tumors, lipomas, fibromas.	Adenocarcinoma of large or small bowel.	Autosomal dominant	Associated with polyposis of colon and bony exostoses.
Peutz–Jeghers syndrome	Jeghers (360) Riley (361)	Pigmentation of lips, face, oral mucosa, and digits.	GI adenocarcinomas	Autosomal dominant	Low (2–3%) incidence
Tylosis (palmaris and plantaris)	Howel–Evans (362)	Hyperkeratosis of palms and soles after age 10.	Esophageal carcinoma	Autosomal dominant	95% incidence of carcinoma by age 65.
Multiple mucosal neuromas	Williams (363)	Neuromas of eyelids, lips, tongue, and oral mucosa.	Pheochromocytoma, medullary carcinoma of thyroid (MEA II)	Autosomal dominant	Parathyroid adenomas, hypertension common.
Cowden's disease—multiple hamartoma syndrome	Lloyd (364)	Fibromas of oral mucosa, acral venucous papulas, trichilemmomas face.	Thyroid, breast carcinomas	Autosomal dominant	Associated with multiple hamartomas, lipomas, neuromas, hemangiomas, thyroid adenomas.
Multiple basal cell neuromas syndrome	Solomon (365)	Multiple basal cell carcinomas, pits on soles and palms.	Medulloblastoma fibrosarcoma (jaw)	Autosomal dominant	Infrequent association with internal malignancy.
PHAKOMATOSES					
Neurofibromatosis (von Recklinghausen)	Crowe (318)	Neurofibromas, cafe au lait.	Pheochromocytoma	Autosomal dominant	Malignancies develop in a minority of patients.
Tuberous sclerosis (Bourneville)	Butterworth (366)	Lipopigmented macules, adenomas, fibromas.	Neurologic malignancies	Autosomol dominant	Malignancies develop in a minority of patients.
Cerebelloretinal hemangioblastoma (von Hippel-Lindau)	Christoferson (367)	Retinal malformation, papilledema	Neurologic malignancies	Autosomol dominant	Malignancies develop in a minority of patients.
Encephalotrigeminal syndrome (Sturge–Weber)	Doll (368)	Capillary or cavernous hemangiomas within the cutaneous distribution of the trigeminal nerve.	Neurologic malignancies	Autosomol dominant	Malignancies develop in a minority of patients.
Ataxia telangiectasia	Doll (368) Frizzera (370)	Telangiectasias	Lymphomas, leukemias.	Autosomal recessive	IgA ± IgE deficiency. Sinopulmonary infections, tumors in < 10%.
Bloom's syndrome	Helm (318)	Photosensitivity, telangiectasias, erythema of face.	Leukemia	Autosomol recessive.	Stunted growth, high incidence.
Fanconi's anemia	Helm (316)	Patchy hyperpigmentation.	Leukemias.	Autosomal recessive.	High incidence
Chédiak–Higashi syndrome	Doll (367)	Recurrent pyoderma, giant melanosomes, dilution of skin and hair color.	Lymphomas	Autosomol recessive.	High incidence.
Werner's syndrome (Adult progeria)	Epstein (369)	Scleroderma-like changes, premature aging, leg ulcers, short stature.	Sarcomas, meningiomas, others.	Autosomal recessive.	Cancers in about 10%.
Wiskott–Aldrich syndrome	Doll (368) Frizzeria (370)	Eczematous dermatitis, pyroderma.	Lymphomas.	Sex-linked, (males)	> 10% incidence.
Bruton's sex-linked agammaglobulinemia	Helm (316)	Recurrent infections.	Lymphoma, leukemias.	Sex-linked.	> 5% incidence.

with gigantism, acromegaly, Stein–Leventhal syndrome, or diabetes mellitus. It may also develop after prolonged administration of corticosteroids, diethylstilbestrol (DES) or nicotinic acid. Because of the strong association of acanthosis and cancer, patients developing true acanthosis nigricans after the age of 40 should be evaluated for malignancy including a thorough evaluation of the GI tract, lymph nodes, and breasts.

Although more rare than acanthosis nigricans, the sudden development and rapid increase in size of seborrheic keratoses (sign of Leser–Trelat) are strongly associated with malignancy, particularly of the GI tract.[322-324] As with many cutaneous paraneoplastic syndromes, the most important feature is the rapid change since multiple seborrheic keratoses may be common, especially in older age groups. Salient features of other pigmented lesions are summarized in Table 39-14.

Erythemas

The major features of erythemas associated with malignancy are summarized in Table 39-15. Of note, erythema gyratum repens is nearly always associated with malignancy and necrolytic migratory erythema is pathognomonic of glucagonoma. Exfoliative dermatitis can be caused by a variety of malignancies, drug reactions, or unknown causes.[316,338,339] In various series, 10–20% of cases may be associated with malignancy, particularly lymphomas. In some instances, the skin lesions are not paraneoplastic since cutaneous infiltration of the skin can be documented by skin biopsy. In some instances, there is no demonstrable cutaneous tumor and the condition may improve following therapy. In these instances the skin condition appears to be a true paraneoplastic syndrome. Although the mechanism in these cases is unknown some have speculated that there is an immunologic response to some antigenic material derived from the tumor.[316]

Endocrine and Metabolic Lesions (Table 39-16) and Bullous and Urticarial Lesions

Important skin lesions associated with endocrine and metabolic tumors are systemic nodular panniculitus with adenocarcinoma of the pancreas and porphyria cutanea tarda with hepatomas. The associations of malignancy with bullous and urticarial lesions are as yet unproved (Table 39-17).

Miscellaneous Lesions (Table 39-18)

The cutaneous lesions in dermatomyositis are characterized by purplish-pink heliotrope erythema of the face with edema of the eyelids with spread to the neck and arms. Erythematous purplish papules and plaques over the knuckles and interphalangeal joints (Grotton's sign) may be characteristic but usually occur late. All types of malignancies have been reported.[204,205,206,346] Overall, cancers are reported in 7-52% of patients with dermatomyositis. There are reports of dramatic improvement in dermatomyositis after antitumor therapy, supporting the concept of a true paraneoplastic syndrome.[206,346]

Acquired Ichthyosis

An important feature of paraneoplastic acquired ichthyosis is also the rapid development of the lesions that are characterized by generalized dry cracking skin with hyperkeratotic palms and soles. The acquired forms are most often associated with Hodgkin's disease and other malignant lymphomas, although associations with other solid tumors have been reported.[349,350] The acquired forms can be distinguished from genetic forms by the fact the latter almost always arise before the age of 20. A parallel course of the malignant lymphoma and acquired ichthyosis has been reported in many patients.[350]

Hereditary Disorders

A large number of hereditary disorders associated with malignant disease and skin lesions of presumed paraneoplastic nature are summarized in Table 39-19.

GASTROINTESTINAL PARANEOPLASTIC SYNDROMES

The Zollinger–Ellison, carcinoid, and other syndromes resulting from hormone-producing endocrine tumors are covered in Chapter 28.

PROTEIN-LOSING ENTEROPATHIES ASSOCIATED WITH MALIGNANCY

Cancer patients have a low serum albumin in over 90% of cases.[371] Metabolic studies show that this can be due to decreased albumin synthesis; abnormal distribution of albumin in effusions; or increased loss of protein into the GI tract (protein-losing enteropathy).[371] The most common mechanism is decreased albumin synthesis but the mechanism(s) for this are not known.[371] While patients usually present with other signs of malignancy, unexplained edema and hypoproteinemia were the initial manifestations of malignancy in a few patients. The mechanisms of protein-losing enteropathy include inflammation and ulceration of the GI mucosa and exudative loss of proteins; disorders of the intestinal lymphatic channels from neoplastic obstruction (seen with lymphomas); or congestive failure (seen in patients with carcinoid or pericardial constriction) with resultant loss of protein and lymphocytes rich in lymph into the GI lumen; and a group of undefined mechanisms. The resulting hypoalbuminemia leads to edema, and the lymphopenia gives decreased cellular immunity with impaired skin test reactivity.[371] While these syndromes may not fulfill all of the criteria for paraneoplastic (that is, acting at a distance from the tumor), anecdotal case reports indicate that protein-losing enteropathy can be reversed by appropriate treatment of the underlying tumor. Profuse watery diarrhea, hypokalemia, and hypochlorhydria are usually associated with pancreatic non-beta islet cell tumors, or villous adenomas of the rectum. In addition, this syndrome can be found in patients with lung cancer; however, the mechanism is unknown.[372]

Malabsorption

Malabsorption syndromes for several or specific substances can occur by a variety of mechanisms in cancer patients including side effects of surgery, radiation, and chemotherapy. Malabsorption is often associated with lymphoma involving the small bowel or with gastric, hepatic, or biliary tract tumors, particularly if biliary obstruction is present. These examples are not "remote effects" of the tumor. However, some malabsorption syndromes may be paraneoplastic in nature as suggested by finding histologic abnormalities of the small bowel in up to 62% of various cancers in some series.[373–375] While the exact incidence for various histologic types is unknown, the histologic abnormalities include "flat" mucosa with simple or partial villous atrophy. Subtotal villous atrophy is less common. However, the severity of associated malabsorption does not correlate with the severity of the small bowel histologic changes.[373] The tumors associated with small bowel abnormalities have been colon, lung, prostate, pancreas, lymphomas, as well as other tumors. The mechanisms behind the loss of villous height is unknown. Treatment should be directed at the underlying tumor, plus administration of exogenous nutrients, and vitamins to bypass the malabsorption.

HEPATOPATHY AS A PARANEOPLASTIC SYNDROME

Elevated hepatic alkaline phosphatase has occurred with a malignant schwannoma and disappeared with surgical resection.[376] This can also be seen in hypernephroma where there can be reversible abnormalities of liver function that are not associated with liver metastases.[377–379] Decreased albumin synthesis will rise to normal after resection of the renal tumor. Biochemical abnormalities, such as elevated alkaline phosphatase or hyperglobulinemia, hypocholesterolemia, prolonged prothrombin time, as well as hepatosplenomegaly, have regressed after primary tumor removal in 4/6 patients.[377,379] The mechanisms for the hepatopathy associated with hypernephroma are unknown but may include hepatic amyloid or be related to either the generalized hepatic hypervascularity seen on angiography or the nonspecific focal periportal inflammation seen on biopsy.[377,378,380] The importance of recognizing the hepatopathy syndrome is so as not to confuse these signs with metastases to the liver. Thus, biopsy confirmation of liver metastases from renal carcinoma is highly desirable if this metastatic site alone would preclude resection of the primary renal tumor for cure.

ANOREXIA, CACHEXIA, AND TASTE ABNORMALITIES AS PARANEOPLASTIC MANIFESTATIONS

Problems with anorexia, taste, weight loss and cachexia are common in cancer patients.[381–385] One third or more of cancer patients are in negative nitrogen balance; they can even be in positive nitrogen balance and still maintain a caloric deficit.[383] The syndrome consists of anorexia, cachexia, asthenia, loss of body tissue, inability to conserve normal regulatory functions of metabolism, and bears no correlation to the amount, type, or site of neoplastic tissue.[384] It can occur as an early symptom of disease, or appear in the presence of bulk neoplasms. The best evidence of the paraneoplastic nature of the anorexia-cachexia syndrome comes when it appears before the malignancy is discovered and disappears with the resection of control of the tumor.[383] Obviously, cancer patients can have these symptoms as a result of therapy toxicity, gross invasion, or obstruction of structures by tumor. Cachexia can result from decreased caloric intake, malabsorption, loss of material from the body (*e.g.*, from effusions, hemorrhage, ulcers) or a change in the body metabolism. Anorexia and taste changes can result in decreased caloric intake. However, a variety of experimental evidence suggests that malnutrition alone cannot explain the cachexia of malignancy.[383] Thus, in malignancy and cachexia, the caloric expenditure remains high, the basal metabolic rate is increased despite the reduced dietary intake, indicating a profound systemic derangement of host metabolism.[383] These findings are in contrast to the lower metabolic rates and adaptation that normal subjects make following starvation.[384] In normal subjects with starvation, the caloric expenditure is lowered, amino acids cease being used for gluconeogenesis, and exogenous glucose is readily oxidized whereas it is not in malignancy. In addition, protein synthesis is maintained in malignancy rather than reduced as in starvation.

A whole set of normal physiologic stimuli are set in motion after a taste sensation occurs; these can be upset if the taste sensation is deranged. Aversion to meats and other protein-containing food frequently occurs in cancer patients. DeWys found 16/50 cancer patients of various types had an aversion to meat; this was correlated with a lowered threshhold for bitter taste (urea).[382] In addition, these patients had elevated thresholds for sweet (sucrose) substances. The taste abnormalities were correlated with a patient's body burden of tumor and then normalized after response to treatment.[382]

In addition to taste, the regulation of hunger and satiety is complex and involves a CNS "satiety" center in the ventromedial nuclei of the hypothalmus and a "feeding" center in the lateral hypothalamic nuclei.[383] Also, alimentary tract regulation, glucostatic, lipostatic, thermostatic, osmotic regulation, hormone regulation by insulin, growth hormone, glucagon, enterogastrone, adrenal corticosteroids, amino acids levels, and as yet unidentified anorexigenic pituitary polypeptides take place.[383] Thus, it appears likely that mechanism(s) underlying the paraneoplastic anorexia-cachexia syndrome involve molecules produced by the tumor which then impinge on one or more of the regulatory mechanisms of hunger, satiety, metabolism, or taste and cause the organism to falsy disrupt these patterns and thus enter into a metabolic "chaotic" state.[383] The treatment of the underlying tumor appears to be the best general approach to reversing the state of cancer cachexia.

MISCELLANEOUS PARANEOPLASTIC SYNDROMES

FEVER AS A PARANEOPLASTIC SYNDROME

Fever occurs frequently in cancer patients and is usually caused by infection. While other non-infectious causes (such as drug toxicity and adrenal insufficiency) exist, certain tumors are associated with fever.[386] In 351 cancer patients, Petersdorf found 30% developed fever and 5% had fever that could only be related to their cancer.[387] The major associations are with Hodgkin's disease, myxomas, hypernephromas, osteogenic sarcomas, and a variety of other tumors have also been reported to be associated with fever.[387,388] Tumor-associated fever is usually defined as unexplained fever that coincides with tumor growth, disappears promptly on tumor removal or control, and reappears with tumor regrowth. Alternatively, when the fever persists with uncontrolled tumor without any other reasonable cause, the tumor is a likely etiology of the fever.[386] In Hodgkin's disease, fever as a systemic symptom suggests a worse prognosis stage-by-stage, and its disappearance is required to document remission of tumor and subsequent cure (see Chapter 35). There are no data about the influence on prognosis of fever associated with other tumors.

The etiology of the tumor-associated fever could come from release of pyrogen from tumor cells, normal leukocytes, or a variety of other normal cells that have been demonstrated to have "endogenous" pyrogen. For example, the Kupffer cells of the liver contain endogenous pyrogen which could cause fever with hepatoma, or with metastases to the liver from other tumors.[389] The pyrogen acts upon the hypothalamus to cause some reset of temperature regulation. Tumor cells can produce pyrogen as well. Bodel showed that five of six hypernephromas placed *in vitro* released pyrogen into the supernatent medium (detected by injection into a rabbit).[386] Similarly, spleen and lymph node tissue from Hodgkin's disease patients produced pyrogen when cultured into the medium *in vitro*. However, pyrogen production, while correlated with lymph node involvement, did not correlate with histologic involvement of the spleen or with fever in the patient.[386] It is still unknown whether tumor cells themselves or other normal cells mixed in the incubated specimens produce the pyrogen. Treatment should be directed at the underlying tumor, and the most dramatic remissions of paraneoplastic fever come in successfully treated patients with Hodgkin's disease or hypernephroma.

LACTIC ACIDOSIS

Lactic acidosis is usually associated with acute lymphatic or myelogenous leukemia, Hodgkin's disease, and other lymphomas and responds in parallel with tumor regression to therapy.[390–392] Often bicarbonate therapy is also needed.

HYPERLIPIDEMIA

Hyperlipidemia is frequently seen in lymphoma-bearing hamsters and normalizes after tumor treatment.[389] Hyperlipidemias have also been seen in multiple myeloma, hepatoma, and colon cancer.[393,394,395] Total lipids of 2.0 g/dl, cholesterol over 500 mg/dl, and triglycerides of 580 mg/dl have been found. However, no associated vascular abnormalities have been reported. In the case of myeloma, the monoclonal proteins have sometimes reacted with alpha or beta lipoproteins or with lipolytic enzymes. The mechanism in the other tumor types is obscure but could involve invasion by tumor.

HYPERTENSION–HYPOTENSION

Malignant hypertension and hypokalemia associated with apparent tumor production of renin have been reported with lung cancer, hypernephroma, and Wilm's tumor.[396–399] The hypertension recedes with control of the tumor.

An antihypertension syndrome has been seen with a prostaglandin-A secreting renal-cell tumor, and abnormally low baroreceptor pressure responses have been seen with intrathoracic carcinomas.[400,401] The latter syndrome appears related to interference of transmission of impulses from intrathoracic stretch receptors resulting in orthostatic hypotension and abnormalities of sodium excretion.

AMYLASE ELEVATION

Synthesis and secretion of amylase by tumors is uncommon; the tumors have all been lung cancer usually of the adenocarcinoma variety.[402] These tumors make the salivary type of amylase, which allows distinction from a pancreatic source of the amylase elevation. The amylase itself apparently does not cause symptoms, but can lead to great concern and medical evaluation about the presence of pancreatitis or various types of pancreatic fistulas when in reality the amylase is produced by the tumor cells.[402]

HYPERTROPHIC PULMONARY OSTEOARTHROPATHY

Hypertrophic pulmonary osteoarthropathy (HPO) is a paraneoplastic syndrome consisting of clubbing of the fingers and toes, periostitis of the long bones, and sometimes a polyarthritis resembling rheumatoid arthritis.[403–406] Periostitis-arthritis produces joint pains in the knees, wrists, and ankles with pain, tenderness, and swelling of the affected bones. Involved bones include usually the distal ends of the tibia, fibula, humerus, radius, or ulna. Hyperemia of the affected joints or hands and feet are also seen.[403] HPO may precede the discovery of the neoplasm by several months and usually has a fairly defined onset. Often, patients do not present with clubbing, but appear with joint pain or polyarthritis, and in adult patients presenting with unexplained polyarthritis or joint pain, the HPO syndrome should be kept in mind.[403] Pathologic examination of the joints can show pannus formation; however, most only show hyperemia.[403] If polyarthritis is present, joint effusions, particularly of the knees, with non-inflammatory synovial fluid and good mucin clot are present. Ossifying periostitis is seen on roentgenogram at the distal end of the shafts of long bones as a thin opaque line of new bone formation, separated from the underlying denser cortex by a narrow radiolucent band. Radionuclide bone scans are often positive over the bones involved with periostitis before the other radiologic changes appear.[407] In advanced cases, other bones (e.g., the ribs, clavicle, iliac crests, and vertebral column) can be involved.

HPO is most frequently encountered in lung cancer occurring in 12% of patients with adenocarcinoma, and less frequently in the other cell types; HPO is almost non-existent in small-cell lung cancer.[408,409] Of interest, the HPO syndrome often occurs with benign mesothelioma and the rare neurolemmomas of the diaphragm, while malignant mesotheliomas are said never to produce HPO.[403] Other tumors metastatic to the chest can cause HPO including metastases from renal cancer, thymoma, leiomyoma of the esophagus, intrathoracic Hodgkin's disease, osteogenic sarcoma, fibrosarcoma, and undifferentiated nasopharyngeal tumors of young people when they metastasize to mediastinal lymph nodes.[410–416]

The diagnosis is made by the physical findings, radionuclide bone scan, and radiographic appearance of the bones. While benign causes have to be considered, the bone changes of hyperparathyroidism can simulate HPO and should be ruled out although it is possible for HPO and ectopic PTH to coexist. The etiology is unknown, although estrogens, circulatory factors, neurogenic factors, and growth hormone, have been postulated to play a role.[406,417–419]

AMYLOIDOSIS (PARANEOPLASTIC B-FIBRILLOSES)

Amyloid deposition is a pathologic process whose manifestations are dependent on the formation of a specific and unique protein conformation—the twisted B-pleated sheet fibril.[420] Histochemically, these fibrils have green polarization color after Congo red staining. This structure is not normally found in mammalian tissues and can occur with a variety of proteins produced by several different pathogenic mechanisms. Immunoglobulin fragments produced by plasma cell dyscrasias are the most common neoplastic mechanism. Because of the B-pleated structure, the fibrils are very resistant to normal proteolytic digestion under physiologic conditions and thus accumulate as inert fibrils in tissues. This results in pressure atrophy, morbidity, and death from interference of normal physiologic processes of the affected vital organs (heart, kidneys, nerve, joints).

While amyloidosis can have several non-malignant causes, 15% of cases occur with malignant disease including multiple myeloma, lymphomas, and carcinomas.[420–422] Amyloid occurs in 6–15% of multiple myeloma and Waldenstrom's macroglobulinemia, in 4% of Hodgkin's disease, and 1% of other lymphomas, and probably all B-cell lymphomas can give rise to amyloidosis. Carcinomas associated with amyloidosis are hypernephromas, bladder and renal pelvic cancer, uterine cervix, and biliary tract cancer.[421] Hypernephroma is reported to represent over 25% of all tumors associated with amyloidosis, but the nature of the protein in the amyloid deposit of hypernephromas is unknown.[420,421]

The "amyloidogenic" protein can be monoclonal light chains (designated AL), or other proteins (designated AA).[420] Amyloid fibrils from medullary carcinoma of the thyroid contain part of the calcitonin molecule; thus, it is possible that peptides produced by several tumors, if they contain sequences capable of forming B-pleated sheets, could cause amyloid.[420] In amyloidosis with multiple myeloma, usually Bence-Jones proteinuria is present, and the occurrence is higher in free light chain myeloma.[420]

The signs and symptoms of amyloidosis of malignancy, particularly with myeloma are a peripheral neuropathy (painful stocking-glove), autonomic nervous symptoms of sexual impotence, GI motility disturbances, orthostatic hypotension, and dyshidrosis.[420] Motor function is impaired from median nerve entrapment and weight loss is frequent. A restrictive cardiomyopathy, with signs and symptoms of right heart failure with only minimal radiographic evidence of cardiomegaly, occurs. ECG changes of low voltage, arrhythmias, conduction disturbances, and ECG pattern simulating myocardial infarction can occur. The patients are extremely sensitive to digitalis and several toxic deaths from this have been reported. Pinch purpura, periorbital purpura after procedures, macroglossia, waxy cutaneous papules, subcutaneous nodules, alopecia, and scleroderma-like skin infiltration can occur. Joint infiltration often gives painless limitation of range of motion. The large joints are affected in amyloid arthropathy, and the "shoulder pad" sign develops with massive infiltration of the glenohumeral articulation. Carpal and tarsal tunnel syndromes occur with infiltration of these regions.

The diagnosis of amyloid is made by the demonstration of the characteristic emerald-green bi-refringence of tissue specimens stained for Congo red and examined by polarization microscopy.[420] Biopsies of infiltrated lesions, gingiva, skin, bone marrow, or rectum can be used. The prognosis of clinically evident amyloidosis with malignancy is poor and in myeloma, median survival from diagnosis is 14 months or less.[420] There is not good evidence that treatment of myeloma or other neoplastic disorders will reverse the amyloid already deposited but it will probably halt amyloid progression. Supportive care problems abound as the congestive heart failure from amyloid does not respond to digitalis (and it is said that all amyloid patients when being started on digitalis should be hospitalized because of potential toxicity). Diuretics can cause dehydration and cardiovascular collapse because of concurrent renal damage, postural hypotension, adrenal insufficiency, autonomic neuropathy, and low-cardiac output. Mineralocorticoids, elastic stockings, broad spectrum antibiotics for bacterial overgrowth in bowel with disturbed motility, gastrostomy and tracheostomy for macroglossia, hemodialysis, and surgical decompression of carpal tunnel syndrome have all been used.[420]

ARTHRITIS, POLYMYALGIA RHEUMATICA, SYSTEMIC LUPUS ERYTHEMATOSIS

Rheumatoid arthritis, or an asymmetric polyarthritis, can occur with malignancy or may be related by chance.[4,423–425] Joint manifestations are said to regress on removal or control of the underlying malignancy in 48% of patients. Some 80% of female patients with asymmetric polyarthritis and malignancy had breast cancer. Some 83% of patients with polymyalgia rheumatica are said to develop a malignancy within 3 months, and it is possible some of these cases represent arterial emboli to muscle from nonbacterial thrombotic endocarditis. Lymphomas may be associated with systemic rheumatic disease.[425,426] In Sjogren's syndrome, a spectrum of benign to malignant lymphoproliferation can be seen but whether this is "at a distance from the tumor" remains to be determined.[427] It is also important to remember that metastases to joints can simulate rheumatoid arthritis and cytology should be done on joint effusions in cancer patients.[428,429] Systemic lupus erythematosis (SLE) is associated with lymphomas, lymphoblastic leukemia, thymomas, testicular and ovarian tumors, and lung cancer, and remission of the SLE is said to occur with tumor treatment.[4,427,430]

REFERENCES

1. Hall TC (ed): Paraneoplastic Syndromes. Ann NY Acad Sci 230:1–577, 1974
2. Odell WD, Wolfsen AR: Humoral syndromes associated with cancer. Ann Rev Med 29:379–406, 1978
3. Blackman MR, Rosen SW, Weintraub BD: Ectopic hormones. Adv Intern Med 23:85–113, 1978
4. Shneider BS, Manalo A: Paraneoplastic syndromes. Unusual manifestations of malignant disease. Disease a Month:1–60, February, 1979
5. Richardson EP: Progressive multifocal leukoencephalopathy. In Vinken PJ Bruryn GW (eds): Handbook of Clinical Neurology, pp 485–499. North-Holland, Amsterdam, 1970
6. Wiener LP, Hernden RM, Narayan O, Johnson RT, Shaw K, Rubinstein J, Prezicse TJ, Conley FK: Virus related to SV40 in patients with progressive multifocal leukoencephalopathy. N Engl J Med 286:385–390, 1972
7. Croft P, Wilkinson M: The incidence of carcinomatous neuromyopathy in patients with various types of carcinoma. Brain 88:427–434, 1965
8. Wilner EC, Brody JA: An evaluation of the remote effects of cancer on the nervous system. Neurology 18:1120–1124, 1967
9. DeLarco JE, Todaro GJ: Growth factors from murine sarcoma virus-transformed cells. Proc Natl Acad Sci (USA) 75:4001–4005, 1978
10. Waldenstrom JG: Paraneoplasia, Biological Signals in Diagnosis of Cancer. New York, John Wiley & Sons, 1978
11. Odell WD, Wolfsen AR: Hormones from Tumors: Are they ubiquitous? Am J Med 68:317–318, 1980
12. Lees LH: The biosynthesis of hormones by nonendocrine tumours—a review. J Endocrinol 67:143–175, 1975
13. Richardson RL, Greco FA, Oldham RK, Liddle GW: Tumor products and potential markers in small cell lung cancer. Semin Oncol 5:253–262, 1978
14. Gropp C, Havemann K, Scheuer A: Ectopic hormones in lung cancer patients at diagnosis and during therapy. Cancer 46:347–354, 1980
15. Hansen M, Hansen HH, Hirsch FR, Arends J, Christensen JD, Christensen JM, U Hummer L, Kuhl C: Hormonal polypeptides and amine metabolites in small cell carcinoma of the lung, with special reference to stage and subtypes. Cancer 345:1432–1437, 1980
16. Odell WD: Wolfsen AR, Bachelot I, Hirose FM: Ectopic production of lipotropin by cancer. Am J Med 66:631–638, 1979
17. Nakanishi S, Inoue A, Kita T, Nakamura M, Chang ACY, Cohen SN, Numa S: Nucleotide sequence of cloned cDNA for bovine corticotropin-B-lipotropin precursor. Nature 278:423–427, 1979
18. Bertagna XY, Nicholson WE, Pettengill OS, Sorenson GD, Mount CD, Orth DN: Corticotropin, lipotropin, and B-endophin production by a human nonpituitary tumor in culture: evidence for a common precursor. Proc Natl Acad Sci (USA) 75:5160–5164, 1978
19. Jeffcoate WJ, Rees LH: Adrenocorticotropin and related peptides in nonendocrine tumors. Curr Top Exp Endocrinol 3:57–74, 1978
20. Guillemin R: Endorphins, brain peptides that act like opiates. N Engl J Med 296:226–228, 1977
21. Huges J: Opioid peptides and their relatives. Nature 278:394–395, 1979
22. Silman RE, Holland D, Chard T, Lowry PJ, Hope J, Robinson JS, Thorburn GD: The ACTH "family tree" of the rheusus monkey changes with development. Nature 276:526–528, 1978
23. Hirata Y, Yamamoto H, Matsukura S, Imura H: In vitro release and biosynthesis of tumor ACTH in ectopic ACTH producing tumors. J Clin Endocrinol Metab 41:106–114, 1975
24. Brown WH: A case of pluriglandular syndrome: Diabetes of bearded women. Lancet 2:1022–1023, 1928
25. Yallow RS, Eastridge CE, Higgins G Jr, Wolf J: Plasma and tumor ACTH in carcinoma of the lung. Cancer 44:1789–1792, 1979
26. Wolfsen AR, Odell WD: ProACTH: Use for early detection of lung cancer. Am J Med 66:765–772, 1979
27. Liddle GW, Island D, Meador CK: Normal and abnormal regulation of corticotropin secretion in man. Recent Prog Horm Res 18:125–166, 1962
28. Ayvazian LF, Schneider B, Gewirtz G, Yalow RS: Ectopic production of big ACTH in carcinoma of the lung. Its clinical usefulness as a biologic marker. Am Rev Respir Dis III:279–287, 1975
29. Ratcliff JG, Knight RA, Besser GM: Tumour and plasma ACTH concentrations in patients with and without the ectopic ACTH syndrome. Clin Endocrinol 1:27–44, 1972
30. Gewirtz G, Yalow RS: Ectopic ACTH production in carcinoma of the lung. J Clin Invest 53:1022–1032, 1974
31. Abe K, Adachi I, Miyakawa S, Tanaka M, Yamaguchi K, Tanaka N, Kameya T, Shimosato Y: Production of calcitonin, adrenocorticotropic hormone, and B-melanocyte stimulating hormone in tumors derived from amine precursors uptake and decarboxylation cells. Cancer Res 37:4100–4194, 1977
32. Bloomfield GA, Holdaway IM, Corrin B, Ratcliffe JG, Rees GM, Ellison M, Rees LH: Lung tumours and ACTH production. Clin Endocrinol (Oxf) 6:95–104, 1977
33. Gilby ED, Rees LH, Bondy PK: Ectopic hormones as markers of response to therapy in cancer. In: Proceedings of the Sixth International Symposium of Biological Characterization of Human Tumors, pp 132–138. Amsterdam, American Elsevier Publishing Co, 1976
34. Rassam JW, Anderson G: Incidence of paramalignant disorders in bronchogenic carcinoma. Thorax 30:86–90, 1975
35. Ross EJ: Endocrine syndromes of non-endocrine origin. Cancer and the adrenal cortex. Proc R Soc Med 59:335–338, 1966
36. Amatruda TT, Upton GV: Hyperadrenocorticism and ACTH-releasing factor. Ann NY Acad Sci 230:168–180, 1974
37. Eagan RT, Maurer LH, Forcier RJ, Tulloh M: Small cell carcinoma of the lung: Staging, paraneoplastic syndromes, treatment and survival. Cancer 33:527–532, 1974
38. Azzopardi JG, Williams ED: Pathology of "nonendocrine" tumors associated with Cushing's syndrome. Cancer 22:274–286, 1968
39. Skrabanek P, Powell D: Unifying concept of non-pituitary ACTH secreting tumors. Evidence of common origin of neural-crest tumors, carcinoids, and oat-cell carcinomas. Cancer 42:1263–1269, 1978
40. Lojek MA, Fer MF, Kasselberg AG, Glick AD, Burnett LS, Julian CG, Greco FA, Oldham RK: Cushing's syndrome with small cell carcinoma of the uterine cervix. Am J Med 69:140–144, 1980
41. Matsuyama M, Inoue T, Ariyoshi Y, Doi M, Suchi T, Sato T, Tashiro K, Chihara T: Argyrophil cell carcinoma of the uterine cervix with ectopic production of ACTH, B-MSH, serotonin, histamine, and amylase. Cancer 44:1813–1823, 1979
42. Levenson RM, Ihde DC, Matthews MJ, Cohen MH, Bunn PA, Minna JD: Small cell carcinoma arising in extrapulmonary sites: Response to chemotherapy. Proc AACR-ASCO 21:143, 1980
43. Fer MF, Oldham RK, Richardson RL, Hande KR, Greco FA: Extrapulmonary small cell carcinoma. Proc AACR-ASCO 21:475, 1980
44. Rees LH, Ratcliffe JG: Ectopic hormone production by non-endocrine tumors. Clin Endocrinol 3:263–299, 1974
45. Bailey RE: Periodic "hormonogenesis"—a new phenomenon. Periodicity in function of a hormone-producing tumor in man. Clin Endocrinol 32:317–327, 1971
46. Gold EM: The Cushing Syndromes: Changing views of diagnosis and treatment. Ann Intern Med 90:829–844, 1979
47. Hattori M, Imura H, Matsukura S, Yoshimoto Y, Sekita K, Tomomatsu T, Kyogoku M, Kameya T: Multiple hormone-producing lung carcinoma. Cancer 43:2429–2437, 1979
48. Mason AMS, Ratcliffe JA, Buckly RM, Mason AS: ACTH secretion by bronchial carcinoid tumors. Clin Endocrinol 1:3–25, 1972
49. Imura H, Matsukura S, Yamamoto H, Hirata Y, Nakai Y: Studies on ectopic ACTH-producing tumors. II. Clinical and biochemical features of 30 cases. Cancer 35:1430–1437, 1975

50. Orth DN, Liddle GW: Results of treatment of 108 patients with Cushing's syndrome. N EnglJ Med 285:243–247, 1971
51. Gordon P, Becker CE, Levey GS, Roth J: Efficacy of amianoglutethimide in the ectopic ACTH syndrome. J Clin Endocrinol Metab 28:921–923, 1968
52. Carey RM, Orth DN, Hartmann WH: Malignant melanoma with ectopic production of adrenocorticotrophic hormone: Palliative treatment with inhibitors of adrenal steroid biosynthesis. J Clin Endocrinol Metab 36:482–487, 1973
53. Vaughn CB, Pearson S, Chapman J, Chinn B, Banks D: The treatment of ACTH paraneoplastic syndrome with aminoglutethimide. J Natl Med Assoc 71:21–23, 1979
54. Child DF, Burke CW, Burley DM, Rees LH, Fraser TR: Drug control of Cushing's syndrome. Combined aminoglutethamide and metapyrone therapy. Acta Endocrinol (KBH) 82:330–341, 1976
55. Naber D, Pickar D, Dionne RA, Bowie DC, Ewels BA, Moody TW, Soble MG, Pert CG: Assay of endogenous opiate receptor ligands in human CSF and plasma. Substance Alcohol Actions Misuse, 1:83–91, 1980
56. Gropp C, Havemann K, Scharfe T, Ax W: Incidence of circulating immune complexes in patients with lung cancer and their effect on antibody dependent cytotoxicity. Oncology 37:71–76, 1980
57. Winkler WA, Crankshaw OF: Chloride depletion in conditions other than Addison's disease. J Clin Invest 17:1–6, 1938
58. Schwartz WDF, Bennett W, Curelop S, Bartter F: A syndrome of reanl sodium loss and hyponatremia probably resulting from inappropriate secretion of antidiuretic hormone. Am J Med 23:529–542, 1957
59. Amatruda TT, Mulrow PJ, Gallagher JC, Sawyer WH: Carcinoma of the lung with inappropriate antidiuresis. N Engl J Med 269:544–549, 1963
60. Hamilton BPM, Upton GV, Amatruda TT: Evidence for the presence of neurophysins in tumors producing the syndrome of inappropriate antidiuresis. J Clin Endocrinol Metab 35:764–767, 1972
61. Cheng KW, Friesen HG: Physiological factors regulating secretion of neurophysin. Metabolism 19:876–890, 1970
62. Kennedy SS, Maurer LH, O'Donnell JF, North WG: Human neurophysins in small cell cancer of the lung. Proc AACR-ASCO 21:324, 1980
63. Trump DL, Baylin SB: Ectopic Hormone Syndromes. In Abeloff MD (ed): Complications of Cancer: Diagnosis and Mangement, pp 211–241. Baltimore and London, Johns Hopkins University Press, 1979
64. Moses AM, Miller M, Streeten DHP: Pathophysiologic and pharmacologic alteratiaons in the release and action of ADH. Metabolism 25:697–721, 1976
65. Goodman LS, Gilman A, Gilman AG, Koelle GB: The Pharmacological Basis Of Therapeutics, 5th ed. New York, Toronto, London, Macmillan, 1975
66. Fichman M, Bethune J: Effects of neoplasms on renal electrolyte function. Ann NY Acad Sci 230:448–472, 1974
67. Padfield PL, Morton JJ, Brown JJ, Lever AF, Robertson JIS, Wood M, Fox R: Plasma arginine vasopressin in the syndrome of antidiuretic hormone excess associated with bronchogenic carcinoma. A J Med 61:825–831, 1976
68. Harlow PJ, DeClerck YA, Shore NA, Ortega JA, Carranza A, Heuser E: A fatal case of inappropriate ADH secretion induced by cyclophosphamide therapy. Cancer 44:896–898, 1979
69. DeFronzo RA, Braine H, Colvin OM, Davis PJ: Water intoxication in man after cyclophosphamide therapy. Time course and relation to drug activation. Ann Intern Med 78:861–869, 1973
70. Thomas TH, Morgan DB, Swaminathan R, Ball SG, Lee MR: Severe hypoatremia. Lancet 1:621–624, 1978
71. Radice PA, Dermody WC: Clonal heterogeneity of hormone produce by continuous cultures of small cell carcinoma of the lung. Proc AACR-ASCO 21:41, 1980
72. Pettengill OS, Caulkner CS, Wurster-Hill DH, Maurer LH, Sorenson GD, Robinson AG, Zimmerman EA: Isolation and characterization of a hormone-producing cell line from human small cell anaplastic carcinoma of the lung. J Natl Cancer Inst 58:511–518, 1977
73. Munro AHG, Crompton GK: Inappropriate antidiuretic hormone secretion in oat cell carcinoma of bronchus: Aggravation of hyponatremia by intravenous cyclophosphamide. Thorax 27:640–642, 1972
74. Cohen MH, Bunn PA Jr, Ihde DC, Fossieck BE Jr, Minna JD: Chemotherapy rather than demeclocycline for inappropriate secretion of antidiuretic hormone. N Engl J Med 298:1423, 1978
75. North WG, Maurer H, O'Donnell JF: Human neurophysins and small cell carcinoma. Clin Res 27:390A, 1979
76. Hantman D, Rossier B, Zohlman R, Schrier R: Rapid correction of hyponatremia in the syndrome of inappropriate secretion of antidiuretic hormone. An alternative treatment to hypertonic saline. Ann Intern Med 78:870–875, 1973
77. Forrest JN Jr, Cox M, Hong C, Morrison G, Bia M, Singer I: Superiority of demeclocycline over lithium in the treatment of chronic syndrome of inappropriate secretion of antidiuretic hormone. N Engl J Med 298:173–177, 1978
78. DeTroyer A: Demeclocycline treatment for syndrome of inappropriate antidiuretic hormone secretion. J Am Med Assoc 237:2823–2826, 1977
79. White MG, Fetner DC: Treatment of the syndrome of inappropriate secretion of antidiuretic hormone with lithium carbonate. N Engl J Med 292:390–392, 1975
80. Decaux G, Brimioulle S, Genette F, Mockel J: Treatment of the syndrome of inappropriate secretion of antidiuretic hormone by urea. Am J Med 69:99–106, 1980
81. Trump DL: Abnormalities of bone and mineral metabolism. In: Complications of Cancer. Ableoff MD (ed): Diagnosis and Management, pp 263–281. Baltimore and London, Johns Hopkins University Press, 1979
82. Myers WPL: Differential diagnosis of hypercalcemia and cancer. CA 27:258–272, 1977
83. Holtz G, Johnson TR Jr, Schrock ME: Paraneoplastic hypercalcemia in ovarian tumors. Obstet Gynecol 54:483–487, 1979
84. Cryer PE, Kissane JM: Clinicopathologic conference. Malignant hypercalcemia. Am J Med 65:486–494, 1979
85. Tashjian AH, Voelkel EF, Levine L: Evidence that the bone resorption-stimulating factor produced by mouse fibrosarcoma cells is prostaglandin E2: A new model for the hypercalcemia of cancer. J Exp Med 135:1329–1343, 1972
86. Voelkel EF, Tashjian AH Jr, Franklin R, Wasserman E, Levine L: Hypercalcemia and tumor-prostaglandins: The VX2 carcinoma model in the rabbit. Metabolism 24:973–986, 1975
87. Albright F: Case records of Massachusetts General Hospital #27461. N Engl J Med 225:789–794, 1941
88. Gordon GS: Hyper- and hypocalcemia: Pathogenesis and treatments. Ann NY Acad Sci 230:181–186, 1974
89. Habener JF, Kronenberg HM: Parathyroid hormone biosynthesis: Structure and function of biosynthetic precursors. Fed Proc 37:2561–2566, 1978
90. Benson RC Jr, Riggs BL, Pickard BM, Arnaud CD: Radioimmunoassay of parathyroid hormone in hypercalcemic patients with malignant disease. Am J Med 56:821–826, 1974
91. Powell D, Singer FR, Murray TM, Minkin C, Potts JT Jr: Nonparathyroid humoral hypercalcemia in patients with neoplastic diseases. N Engl J Med 289:176–181, 1973
92. Sherwood LM, O'Riordan JLH, Aurbach GD, Potts JT Jr: Production of parathyroid hormone by nonparathyroid tumors. J Clin Endocrinol Metab 27:140–146, 1967
93. Grajower M, Barzel US: Ectopic hyperparathyroidism (pseudohyperparathyroidism) in esophageal malignancy. Report of a case and a review of the literature. Am J Med 61:134–135, 1976
94. Kumar GK, Naidu VG, Razzaque MA: Esophageal carcinoma with pseudohyperparathyroidism and hypercorticism. Am J Gastroenterol 65:222–225, 1976
95. Terz JJ, Estep H, Bright R, Lawrence W Jr, Curutchet HP, Kay S: Primary oropharyngeal cancer and hypercalcemia. Cancer 33:334–339, 1974
96. Hoeg JM, Slatopolsky E: Cervical carcinoma and ectopic hyperparathyroidism. Arch Intern Med 140:569–571, 1980

97. Malakoff AF, Schmidt JD: Metastatic carcinoma of penis complicated by hypercalcemia. Urology 5:510–513, 1975
98. Goldman JW, Becker FO: Ectopic parathyroid hormone syndrome. Occurrence in a case of undifferentiated lymphoma with bone marrow involvement. Arch Intern Med 138:1290–1291, 1978
99. Libnoch JA, Ajhlouoni K, Millman WL, Guansing AR, Theil GB: Acute myelofibrosis and malignant hypercalcemia. Am J Med 62:432–438, 1977
100. Raisz LG, Yajnik CH, Bockman RS, Bower BF: Comparison of commercially available parathyroid hormone immunoassays in the differential diagnosis of hypercalcemia due to primary hyperparathyroidism or malignancy. Ann Intern Med 91:739–740, 1979
101. Drezner MK, Lebovitz HE: Primary hyperparathyroidism in paraneoplastic hypercalcemia. Lancet 1:1004–1006, 1978
102. Shaw JW, Oldham SB, Rosoff L, Bethune JE, Fichman MP: Urinary cyclic AMP analyzed as a function of the serum calcium and parathyroid hormone in a differential diagnosis of hypercalcemia. J Clin Invest 59:14–21, 1977
103. Ackerman NB, Winer N: The differentiation of primary hyperparathyroidism from the hypercalcemia of malignancy. Ann Surg 181:226–231, 1975
104. Farr HW, Fahey TJ Jr, Nash AG, Farr CM: Primary hyperparathyroidism and cancer. Am J Surg 126:539–543, 1973
105. Seyberth HW: Prostaglandin-mediated hypercalcemia: A paraneoplastic syndrome. Klin Wochenscher 56:373–387, 1978
106. Brereton HD, Halushka PV, Alexander RW, Mason DM, Keiser HR, DeVita VT Jr: Indomethacin-responsive hypercalcemia in a patient with renal-cell adenocarcinoma. N Engl J Med 29:83–85, 1975
107. Robertson RP, Baylink DJ, Marini JJ, Adkison HW: Elevated prostaglandins and suppressed parathyroid hormone associated with hypercalcemia and renal cell carcinoma. J Clin Endocrinol Metab 41:164–167, 1975
108. Ito H, Sanada T, Katayama T, Shimazaki J: Indomethacin-responsive hypercalcemia. N Engl J Med 293:558–559, 1975
109. Seyberth HW, Segre GV, Morgan JL, Swettman BJ, Potts JT, Oates JA: Prostaglandins as mediators of hypercalcemia associated with certain types of cancer. N Engl J Med 293:1278–1283, 1975
110. Tashjian AH Jr: Prostaglandins, hypercalcemia and cancer. N Engl J Med 293:1317–1318, 1975
111. Horton JE, Raisz LG, Simmons HA, Oppenheim JJ, Mergenhagen SE: Bone resorbing activity in supernatant fluid from cultured human peripheral blood leukocytes. Science 177:793–795, 1972
112. Luben RA, Mundy GR, Trummel CL, Raisz LG: Partial purification of osteoclast-activating factor from phytohemagglutinin-stimulated human leukocytes. J Clin Invest 53:1473–1480, 1974
113. Mundy GR, Raisz LG, Cooper RA, Schechter GP, Salmon SE: Evidence for the secretion of an osteoclast stimulating factor in myeloma. N Engl J Med 291:1041–1046, 1974
114. Elion G, Mundy GR: Direct resorption of bone by human breast cancer cells in vitro. Nature 276:726–728, 1978
115. Koeffler HP, Mundy GR, Golde DW, Cline MJ: Production of bone-resorbing activity in poorly differentiated monocytic malignancy. Cancer 41:2438–2443, 1978
116. Raskin P, McClain CJ, Medsger TA: Hypocalcemia associated with metastatic bone disease. Arch Intern Med 132:539–543, 1973
117. Sackner MA, Spivak AP, Balian LJ: Hypocalcemia in the presence of osteoblastic metastases. N Engl J Med 262:173–176, 1960
118. Hall TC, Griffiths CT, Petranek JR: Hypocalcemia: An unusual metabolic complications of breast cancer. N Engl J Med 275:1474–1477, 1966
119. Jackson HJ, Taylor FHL: Calcium, potassium, and inorganic phosphate content of the serum in cancer patients. Effect of roentgen ray radiation on the level of these substances in the blood of cancer patients. Am J Cancer 19:379–388, 1933
120. Ehrlich M, Goldsten M, Heinemann HO: Hypocalcemia, hypoparathyroidism and osteoblastic metastases. Metabolism 12:516–526, 1963
121. Salassa RM, Jowsey J, Arnaud C: Hypophosphatemia osteomalacia associated with "nonendocrine" tumors. N Engl J Med 283:65–69, 1970
122. Stanbury W: Tumor-associated hypophosphatemia, osteomalacia and rickets. Clin Endocrinol Metabol 1:256–259, 1972
123. Daniels RA, Weisenfeld I: Tumorous phosphaturic osteomalacia. Report of a case associated with multiple hemangiomas of bone. Am J Med 67:155–159, 1979
124. Olefsky J, Compson R, Jones H, Reaven G: "Tertiary" hyperparathyroidism, and apparent "cure" of vitamin D resistant rickets after removal of an ossifying mesenchymal tumor of the pharynx. N Engl J Med 286:740–746, 1972
125. Evans DJ, Azzopardi JG: Distinctive tumours of bone and soft tissue causing acquired vitamin-D-resistant osteomalacia. Lancet 1:353–354, 1972
126. Tashjian AH, Wolfe HJ, Voelkel EF: Human calcitonin: Immunologic assay, cytologic localization and studies of medullary thyroid carcinoma. Am J Med 56:840–849, 1974
127. Silva OL, Broder LE, Doppman JL, Snider RH, Moore CF, Cohen MH, Becker KL: Citcitanin as a marker for bronchogenic cancer. A prospective study. Cancer 44:680–684, 1979
128. Becker KL, Nash DR, Silva OL, Snider RH, Moore CF: Urine calcitonin levels in patients with bronchogenic carcinoma. J Am Med Assoc 243:670–672, 1980
129. Ellison M, Woodhouse D, Hillyard C, Dowsett M, Coombes RC, Gilby ED, Greenberg PB, Neville AM: Immunoreactive calcitonin production by human lung carcinoma cells in culture. Br J Cancer 32:373–379, 1975
130. Bertagna XY, Nicholson WE, Pettengill OS, Sorenson GD, Mount CD, Orth DN: Ectopic production of high molecular weight calcitonin and corticotropin by human small cell carcinoma cells in tissue culture: Evidence for separate precursors. J Clin Endocrinol Metab 47:1390–1393, 1978
131. Lips CJ, Vander Sluys V, Van Der Donk JA, Van Dam RH: Common precursor molecule as origin for the ectopic-hormone-producing tumor syndrome. Lancet 1:16–18, 1978
132. Hillyard V, Coombes RC, Greenberg PB, Galante LS, MacIntyre I: Calcitonin in breast and lung cancer. Clin Endocrinol 5:1–8, 1976
133. Vaitukaitis JL, Ross GT, Braunstein GD, Rayford PL: Gonadotropins and their subunits: Basic and clinical studies. Recent Prog Horm Res 32:289–321, 1976
134. Kenimer JG, Hershman JM, Higgins HP: The thyrotropin in hydatidiform moles is human chorionic gonadotropin. J Clin Endocrinol Metab 40:481–491, 1975
135. Nisula BC, Ketelslegers JM: Thyroid-stimulating activity and chorionic gonadotropin. J Clin Invest 54:494–499, 1974
136. Faiman C, Colwell JA, Ryan RJ, Hershman M, Shields TW: Gonadotropin secretion from a bronchogenic carcinoma. N Engl J Med 277:1395–1399, 1967
137. Fusco FD, Rosen SW: Gonadotropin-producing anaplastic large-cell carcinomas of the lung. N Engl J Med 275:507–515, 1966
138. Anderson T, Waldmann TA, Javadpour N, Glatstein E: Testicular germ-cell neoplasms: Recent advances in diagnosis and therapy. Ann Intern Med 90:373–385, 1979
139. Lewis JL: Chemotherapy of gestational choriocarcinoma. Cancer 30:1517–1521, 1972
140. Blackman MR, Weintraub BD, Rosen SW, Kourides IA, Steinwascher K, Gail MH: Human placental and pituitary glycoprotein hormones and their subunits as tumor markers: A quantitative assessment. J Natl Cancer Inst 65:81–93, 1980
141. Tsuruhara T, Dufau ML, Hickman J, Catt KJ: Biological properties of hCG after removal of terminal sialic acid and galactose residues. Endocrinol 91:296–301, 1972
142. Muggia Fm, Rosen SW, Weintraub BD, Hansen HH: Ectopic placental proteins in nontrophoblastic tumors: Serial measurements following chemotherapy. Cancer 36:1327–1337, 1975
143. Kahn CR, Rosen SW, Weintraub BD, Fajans SS, Gorden P: Ectopic production of chorionic gonadotropin and its subunits by islet cell tumors: A specific marker for malignancy. N Engl J Med 297:565–569, 1977

144. Bender RA, Weintraub BD, Rosen SW: Prospective evaluation of two tumor-associated proteins in pancreatic adenocarcinoma. Cancer 43:591–595, 1979
145. Broder LE, Weintraub BD, Rosen SW, Cohen MH, Tejada F: Placental proteins and their subunits as tumor markers in prostatic carcinoma. Cancer 40:211–216, 1977
146. Metz SA, Weintraub B, Rosen SW, Singer J, Robertson RP: Ectopic secretion of chorionic gonadotropin by a lung carcinoma. Pituitary gonadotropin and subunit secretion and prolonged chemotherapeutic remission. Am J Med 65:325–333, 1978
147. Tashijian AH Jr, Weintraub BD, Barowsky NJ, Rabson AS, Rosen SW: Subunits of human chorionic gonadotropin: Unbalanced synthesis and secretion by clonal cell strains derived from a bronchogenic carcinoma. Proc Natl Acad Sci (USA) 70:1419–1422, 1973
148. Rosen SW, Weintraub BD, Aaronson SA: Nonrandom ectopic protein production by malignant cells: Direct evidence in vitro. J Clin Endocrinol Metab 50:834–841, 1980
149. Rudnick P, Odell WD: In search of a cancer. N Engl J Med 284:405–408, 1971
150. Skrabanek P, Kirrane J, Powell D: A unifying concept of chorionic gonadotropin production in malignancy. Invest Cell Pathol 2:75–85, 1979
151. Greco FA, Fer MF, Oldham RK, Schoumacher RA, Forbes JT: Intracytoplasmic localization of ectopic B-human chorionic gonadotropin and A-fetoprotein in suspected extragonadal germ cell cancers by immunohistochemical methods. Clin Res 28:415A, 1980
152. Root, AW, Bongiovanni AM, Eberlein WR: A testicular-interstitial-cell stimulating gonadotropin in a child with hepatoblastoma and sexual precocity. J Clin Endocrin Metab 28:1317–1322, 1968
153. McArthur J, Toll GD, Russfield AB, Reiss AM, Quinby WC, Baker WH: Sexual precocity attributable to ectopic gonadotropin secretion by hepatoblastoma. Am J Med 54:390–403, 1973
154. Kurman RJ, Norris HJ: Embryonal carcinoma of the ovary: A clinicopathologic entity distinct from endodermal sinus tumor resembling embryonal carcinoma of the adult testis. Cancer 38:2420–2433, 1976
155. Weintraub BD, Rosen SW: Ectopic production of human chorionic somatomammotrophin by nontrophoblastic cancers. J Clin Endocrin Metab 32:94–101, 1971
156. Rosen SW, Weintraub BD, Vaitukaitis JL, Sussman HH, Hershman JH, Muggia FM: Placental proteins and their subunits as tumor markers. Ann Intern Med 82:71–83, 1975
157. Steiner H, Dahlback O, Waldenstrom J: Ectopic growth-hormone production and osteoartropathy in carcinoma of the bronchus. Lancet 1:783–785, 1968
158. Ennis CG, Cameron DP, Burger HG: On the etiology of hypertrophic pulmonary osteoarthropathy in bronchogenic carcinoma: Lack of relationship to elevated growth hormone levels. Aust NZ J Med 3:157–161, 1973
159. Sonksen PH, Ayres AB, Braimbridge M, Corrin B, Davies DR, Jeremiah GM, Oaten SW, Lowy C, West TE: Acromegaly caused by pulmonary carcinoid tumors. Clin Endocrinol (Oxf) 5:505–513, 1976
160. Anderson G: The incidence of paramalignant syndromes. In: Paramalignant Syndromes in Lung Cancer, Anderson G (ed), p 4. London, William Heinemann, 1973
161 Hennen G: Characterization of a thyroid-stimulating factor in human cancer tissue. J Clin Endocrin Metab 27:610–614, 1967
162. Odell WD, Bates RW, Rivlin RS, Lipsett MB, Hertz R: Increased thyroid function without clinical hyperthyroidism in patients with choriocarcinoma. J Clin Endocrinol Metab 23:658–668, 1963
163. Cave WT Jr, Dunn JT: Choriocarcinoma with hyperthyroidism: Probably identify of the thyrotropin with human chorionic gonadotropin. Ann Intern Med 85:60–63, 1976
164. Bommer G, Altenahr E, Kuhnau J Jr, Kloppel G: Ultrastructure of hemangiopericytoma associated with paraneoplastic hypoglycemia. Z Krebsforsh 85:231–241, 1976
165. Younus S, Soterakis J, Sossi AJ, Chawlask, LoPresti PA: Hypoglycemia secondary to metastases to the liver. A case report and review of the literature. Gastroenterology 72:334–337, 1977
166. Kiang DT, Bauer GE, Kennedy BJ: Immunoassayable insulin in carcinoma of the cervix associated with hypoglycemia. Cancer 31:801–805, 1973
167. Silvert CK, Rossini AA, Ghazvinian S, Widrich WC, Marks LJ, Sawin CT: Tumor hypoglycemia: Deficient splanchnic glucose output and deficient glucagon secretion. Diabetes 25:202–206, 1976
168. Solomon J: Case report: Spurious hypoglycemia and hyperkalemia in myelomonocytic leukemia. Am J Med Sci 267:359–363, 1974
169. VanWyk JJ, Underwood LE, Hintz RL, Clemmons OR, Voina SJ, Weaver RP: The somatomedins: A family of insulin-like hormones under growth hormone control. Recent Prog Horm Res 30:259–318, 1974
170. Chandalia HB, Boshell BR: Hypoglycemia associated with extrapancreatic tumors. Arch Intern Med 129:447–456, 1972
171. Megyesi K, Kahn CR, Roth J, Gordon P: Hypoglycemia in association with extrapancreatic tumors: Demonstration of elevated plasma NSILA-S by a new radioreceptor assay. J Clin Endocrinol Metab 38:931–934, 1974
172. Allen JC, Deck MDF, Foley KM, Galicich JH, Holland JCB, Horten B, Pasternak JB, Posner JB, Price RW, Rottenberg DA, Shapiro WR, Young DF: Neuro-oncology. II. Dept. of Neurology, Memorial Sloan-Kettering Cancer Center, NY, 1979
173. Newman SJ, Hansen HH: Frequency, diagnosis, and treatment of brain metastases in 247 consecutive patients with bronchogenic carcinoma. Cancer 33:492–496, 1974
174. Nugent JL, Bunn PA Jr., Matthews MJ, Ihde DC, Cohen MH, Gazdar A, Minna JD: CNS metastases in small cell bronchogenic carcinoma. Increasing frequency and changing pattern with lengthening survival. Cancer 44:1855–1893, 1979
175. Posner, JB, Chernik NL: Intracranial metastasis from systemic cancer. Adv Neurol 19:575–587, 1978
176. Rosen P, Armstrong D: Nonbacterial thrombotic endocarditis in patients with malignant neoplastic disease. Am J Med 54:23–29, 1973
177. Collins RC, Al-mondhiry, H, Chernik NL, Posner JB: Neurologic manifestations of intravascular coagulation in patients with cancer. A clinical-pathological analysis of 12 cases. Neurology 25:795–806, 1975
178. Sigsbee B, Deck MDF, Posner JB: Non-metastatic superior sagital sinus thrombosis complicating systemic cancer. Neurology 29:139–146, 1979
179. Weiss HD, Walker MD, Wiernik PH: Neurotoxicity of commonly used antineoplastic agents. N Engl J Med 291:75–80, 127–133, 1974
180. Chernik NL, Armstrong D, Posner JB: Central nervous system infections in patients with cancer: Medicine 52:563–581, 1973
181. Chernik NL, Armstrong D, Posner JB: Central nervous system infections in patients with cancer: Changing patterns. Cancer 40:268–274, 1977
182. Brain WR, Wilkinson M: Subacute cerebellar degeneration associated with neoplasms. Brain 88:465, 1965
183. Paone JF, Jeyasingham K: Remission of cerebellar dysfunction after penumonectomy for bronchogenic carcinoma. N Engl J Med 302:156–157, 1980
184. Victor M, Adams RD, Mancall EL: A restricted form of cerebellar cortical degeneration occurring in alcoholic patients. Arch Neurol 1:579–688, 1959
185. Shapiro WR: Remote effects of neoplasm on the central nervous system: encephalopathy. Adv Neurol 15:101–117, 1976
186. Dorfman, LH, Forno LS: Paraneoplastic encephalomyelitis. Acta Neurol Scand 48:556–574, 1972
187. Corsellis JAN, Goldberg GJ, Norton AR; "Limbic encephalitis" and its association with carcinoma. Brain 91:481–497, 1968
188. Sawyer, RA: Blindness caused by photoreceptor degeneration as a remote effect of cancer. Am J Ophthalmol 81:606–613, 1976
189. Padgett BL: JC papovavirus in progressive multifocal leukoencephalopathy. J Infect Dis 133:686–690, 1976
190. Norris FH Jr, Engel WK: Carcinomatous amyotrophic lateral

sclerosis. In Brain WR, Norris FH Jr (eds): The Remote Effects of Cancer on the Nervous System. NY, Grune and Stratton, 1965
191. Mancall EL, Rosales RK: Necrotizing myelopathy associated with visceral carcinoma. Brain 87:636–639, 1964
192. Walton JN, Tomlinson BE, Pearce GW: Subacute "polyiomyelitis" and Hodgkin's disease. J Neurol Sci 6:435–445, 1968
193. Tyler HR: Paraneoplastic syndromes of nerve, muscle, and neuromuscular junction. Ann NY Acad Sci 230:348–357, 1974
194. Horwich MS, Cho L, Porro RS, Posner JB: Subacute sensory neuropathy: A remote effect of carcinoma. Ann Neurol 1:7–19, 1977
195. Henson, RA, Hoffman HL, Urich H: Encephalomyelitis with carcinoma. Brain 88:449–464, 1965
196. Croft PB, Urich H, Wilkinson M: Peripoheral neuropathy of sensorimotor type associated with malignant disease. Brain 90:31–66, 1967
197. Dayan AD, Croft PB, Wilkinson M: Association of carcinomatous neuromyopathy with different histological types of carcinoma of the lung. Brain 88:435–448, 1965
198. Newman MK, Gugino RJ: Neuropathies and myopathies associated with occult malignancies. JAMA 190:575–577, 1964
199. Victor M, Banker BQ, Adams RD: The neuropathy of multiple myeloma. J Neurol Neurosurg Psychiati 21:73–88, 1958
200. Croft PB, Henson RA, Ulrich H, Wilkinson PC: Sensory neuropathy with bronchial carcinoma: a study of 4 cases showing serologic abnormalities. Brain 88:501–514, 1965
201. Latov N, Sherman WH, Nemni R, Galassi G, Shyong JS, Penn AS, Chess L, Olarte MR, Rowland LP, Osserman EF: Plasma cell dyscrasia and peripheral neuropathy with a monoclonal antibody to peripheral-nerve myelin. N Engl J Med 303:618–621, 1980
202. Lisak RP: Guillain-Barre syndrome and Hodgkin's disease. Three cases with immunological studies. Ann Neurol 1:72–78, 1977
203. Johnson PC, Rolak LA, Hamilton RH, Laguna JF: Paraneoplastic vasculitis of nerve: A remote effect of cancer. Ann Neurol 5:437–444, 1979
204. DeVere R, Bradley WG: Polymyositis: Its presentation, morbility and mortality. Brain 98:637–666, 1976
205. Barnes BE: Dermatomyositis and malignancy. A review of the literature. Ann Intern Med 84:68–76, 1976
206. Williams RC Jr: Dermatomyositis and malignancy: A review of the literature. Ann Intern Med 50:1174–1181, 1959
207. Lambert EH, Eaton LM, Rooke ED: Defect of neuromuscular conduction associated with malignant neoplasms. Am J Physiol 187:612, 1956
208. Lambert EH, Rooke ED: Myasthenic state and lung cancer. In Brain WR, Norris FH Jr (eds): The Remote Effects of Cancer on the Nervous System, pp 67–80. N. Y., Grune and Stratton, 1965
209. Jenkyn LR, Brooks PL, Forcier RJ, Maurer LH, Ochoa J: Remission of the Lambert-Eaton syndrome and small cell anaplastic carcinoma of the lung induced by chemotherapy and radiotherapy. Cancer 46:1123–1127, 1980
210. Cherington M: Guanidine and germine in Eaton-Lambert syndrome. Neurology 26:944–946, 1976
211. Hammond D, Winnick S: Paraneoplastic erythrocytosis and ectopic erythropoietins. Ann NY Acad Sci 230:219–227, 1974
212. Valentine WN, Hennessy TG, Lang E, Longmire R, McMillan R, Odell W, Ross JF, Scott JL, Simmons DH, Tanaka KR: Polycythemia: Erythrocytosis and erythremia. Ann Intern Med 69:587–606, 1968
213. Williams WJ, Beutler E, Erslev AJ, Rundles RW: Hematology, 2nd ed. New York, McGraw-Hill, 1977
214. Berlin NI: Anemia of Cancer. Ann NY Acad Sci 230:209–211, 1974
215. Waterbury L: Hematologic problems. in Complications of Cancer. Diagnosis and Mangement pp 121–145. Abeloff MD (ed): Baltimore and London, Johns Hopkins Press, 1979
216. Cartwright GE, Lee GR: The anemia of chronic disorders. Br J Haematol 21:147–152, 1971
217. Crowthers D, Bateman CJT: Hematological aspects of systemic disease-malignant disease. Clin Haematol 1:447–455, 1972
218. Jacobs EM, Hutter RVP, Pool JL, Ley AB: Benign thymoma and selective erthyroid aplasia of the bone marrow. Cancer 12:47–57, 1959
219. Vasavada PJ, Bournigal LJ, Reynolds RW: Thymoma associated with pure red cell aplasia and hyogammaglobulinemias. Postgrad Med 54(6):93–98, 1973
220. Hoffbrand AV, Hobbs JR, Kremenchuzky S, Mallin DL: Incidence and pathogenesis of megaloblastic erythropoiesis in multiple myeloma. J Clin Pathol 20:699–705, 1967
221. Pirofsky B: Clinical aspects of autoimmune hemolytic anemia. Semin Hematol 13:251–265, 1976
222. Ludwin D, Sacks P, Lynch S, Jacobs P, Bezwoda W, Bothwell TH: Autoimmune hematological complications occurring during the treatment of malignant lymphoproliferative diseases. S Afr Med J 48:2143–2145, 1974
223. Lackner H: Hemostatic abnormalities associated with dysproteinemias. Semin Hematol 10:125–133, 1973
224. Burkert L, Becker G, Pisciotta AV: Ovarian malignancy and hemolytic anemia. Ann Intern Med 73:91–93, 1970
225. Dawson MA, Tolbert W, Yarbro JW: Hemolytic anemia associated with an ovarian tumor. Am J Med 50:552–556, 1971
226. Spira MA, Lynch EC: Autoimmune hemolytic anemia and carcinoma: An unusual association. Am J Med 67:753–758, 1979
227. Dacie JV: The Hemolytic Anemias: Congenital and Acquired. Part III. Secondary and Symptomatic Hemolytic Anemias New York, Grune & Stratton, 1967
228. Pirofsky B: Autoimmunization and the Autoimmune Hemolytic Anemias. Baltimore, Williams & Wilkins, 1968
229. Barry KG, Crosby WH: Autoimmune hemolytic anemia arrested by removal of an ovarian teratoma. Review of the literature and report of a case. Ann Intern Med 47:1002–1007, 1957
230. Antman KH, Skarin AT, Mayer RJ, Hargreaves HK, Canellos GP: Microangiopathic hemolytic anemia and cancer: A review. Medicine 58:377–384, 1979
231. Brain MC, Dacie JV, Hourihane OB: Microangiopathic hemolytic anemia: The possible role of vascular lesions in pathogenesis. Br J Haematol 8:358–374, 1962
232. Lohrmann HP, Adam W, Heymer B, Kubanek B: Microangiopathic hemolytic anemia in metastatic carcinoma. Report of eight cases. Ann Intern Med 79:368–375, 1973
233. Sack GH, Levin J, Bell WR: Trousseau's syndrome and other manifestations of chronic disseminated coagulopathy in patients with neoplasms. Medicine 56:1–37, 1977
234. Colman RW, Robboy SJ, Minna JD: Disseminated intravascular coagulation: a reappraisal. Ann Rev Med 30:359–374, 1979
234a. Al-Mondhiry H: Disseminated intravascular coagulation: Experience in a major cancer center. Thrombos Diathes Haemorrh (Stuttgart) 34:181–193, 1975
235. Robinson WA: Granulocytosis in neoplasia. Ann NY Acad Sci 230:212–218, 1974
236. Meyer LM, Rotter SD: Leukemoid reaction (Hyperleukocytosis) in malignancy. Am J Clin Pathol 12:218–222, 1942
237. Fahey RJ: Unusual leukocyte response in primary carcinoma of the lung. Cancer 4:930–935, 1951
238. Hughes WF, Highley CS: Marked leukocytosis resulting from carcinomatosis. Ann Intern Med 37:1095–1088, 1952
239. Barrett O Jr: Monocytosis in malignant disease. Ann Intern Med 73:991–992, 1970
240. Finch SC: Granulocytopenia and granulocytosis. In Williams WJ, Beutler E, Erslev AJ, Rundles RW (eds): Hematology 2nd ed New York, McGraw Hill, 1977
241. Metcalf D: Haemopoietic Colonies. Berlin, Springer-Verlag, 1977
242. Pike BL, Robinson WA: Human bone marrow colony growth in agar-gel. J Cell Physiol 76:77–84, 1970
243. Okabe T, Sato N, Kondo Y, Asano S, Ohsawa N, Kosaka K, Ueyama Y: Establishment and characterization of a human cancer cell line that produces human colony-stimulating factor. Cancer Res 38:3910–3917, 1978
244. DiPersio JF, Brennan JK, Lichtman MA, Speiser BL: Human

cell lines that elaborate colony-stimulating activity for the marrow cells of man and other species. Blood 51:507–519, 1978
245. Asano S, Urabe A, Okabe T, Sato N, Kondo Y, Ueyama Y, Chiba S, Ohsawa N, Kosaka K: Demonstration of granulopoietic factor(s) in the plasma of nude mice transplanted with a human lung cancer and in the tumor tissue. Blood 49:845–852, 1977
246. McCarthy JH, Sullivan JR, Ungar B, Metcalf D: Two cases of carcinoma of the lung characterized by a bone marrow agar culture pattern resembling acute myeloid leukemia. Blood 54:530–533, 1979
247. Knowles JH: Miscellaneous disorders of the lung. In Harrison TR, Adams RD, Bennett IL et al: Harrison's Principles of Internal Medicine. New York, McGraw-Hill, 5th edition pp 955–957, 1966
248. Liddle GW, Nicholson WE, Island DP, Orth DN, Abe K, Lowder SC: Clinical and laboratory studies of ecotopic humoral syndromes. Recent Prog Horm Res 25:283–314, 1969
249. Williams WJ: Thrombocytosis. In Hematology, 2nd ed, Williams WJ, Beutler E, Erslev AJ, Rundles RW New York, McGraw-Hill, 1977
250. Levin J, Conley CL: Thrombocytosis associated with malignant disease. Arch Intern Med 114:497–500, 1964
251. Davis RB, Theologides A, Kennedy BJ: Comparative studies of blood coagulation and platelet aggregation in patients with cancer and nonmalignant disease. Ann Intern Med 71:67–80, 1967
252. Aster RH: Control of platelet production. In Williams WJ, Beutler E, Erslev AJ, Rundles RW (eds): Hematology, 2nd ed. New York, McGraw-Hill, 1977
253. Kim HD, Boggs DR: A syndrome resembling idiopathic thrombocytopenic purpura in 10 patients with diverse forms of cancer. Am J Med 67:371–377, 1979
254. Doan C, Bouroncle BA, Wiseman BK: Idiopathic and secondary thrombocytopenic purpura. Clincial study and evlauation of 381 cases over a period of 28 years. Ann Intern Med 53:861–876, 1960
255. Carey RW, McGinnis O, Jacobson BM, Carvalho A: Idiopathic thrombocytopenic purpura complicating chronic lymphocytic leukemia. Arch Intern Med 136:62–66, 1976
256. Khilanani P, Al-Sarraf M: The association of autoimmune thrombocytopenia and Hodgkin's disease. Oncology 28:238–245, 1973
257. Jones SE: Autoimmune disorders and malignant lymphoma. Cancer 31:1092–1098, 1973
258. Bowie EJW, Owen CA Jr: Hemostatic failure in clinical medicine. Semin Hematol 14:341–364, 1977
259. Trousseau A: Phlegmasia alba dolens. Clinique medicale de l'Hotel-Dieu de Paris. London, The New Sydenham Society 3:94, 1865
260. Marder M, Weiner M, Shulman P, Shapiro S: Afribinogenemia occurring in a case of malignancy of the prostate with bone metastases. NY State J Med 49:1197–1198, 1949
261. Goodnight SH Jr: Bleeding and intravascular clotting in malignancy: A review. Ann NY Acad Sci 230:271–288, 1974
262. Sharp AA: Diagnosis and management of disseminated intravascular coagulation. Br Med Bull 33:265–272, 1977
263. Gralnick HR, Abrell E: Studies of the procagulant and fibroinolytic activity of promyelocytes in acute promyelocytic leukemia. Br J Hematol 24:59–99, 1973
264. Colman RW, Robby SJ, Minna JD: Disseminated intravascular coagulation (DIC): An approach. Am J Med 52:679–689, 1972
265. Siegal T, Seligsohn U, Aghai E, Modan M: Clinical and laboratory aspects of disseminated intravascular coagulation (DIC): A study of 118 cases. Thrombos Haemostas 39:122–134, 1978
266. Merskey C, Johnson AJ, Kleiner GJ, Wohl H: The defibrination syndrome: Clinical features and laboratory diagnosis. Br J Haematol 13:528–549, 1967
267. Owen CA Jr, Bowie EJ: Chronic intravascular coagulation syndromes. A summary. Mayo Clin Proc 49:673–679, 1974
268. Drapkin RL, Gee TS, Dowling MD, Arlin Z, McKenzie S, Kempin S, Clarkson B: Prophylactic heparin therapy in acute promyelocytic leukemia. Cancer 41:2484–2490, 1978
269. Gralnick HR, Sultan C: Acute prolmyelocytic leukemia: Haemorrhagic manifestation and morphologic criteria. Br J Haematol 29:333–336, 1975
270. Fayemi AO, Deppisch LM: Nonbacterial thrombotic endocarditis and myocardial infarction. Am Heart J 97:405–406, 1979
271. MacDonald RA, Robbins SL: The significance of nonbacterial thrombotic endocarditis. Autopsy and clinical study of 78 patients. Ann Intern Med 46:255–273, 1957
272. Studdy P, Wiloughby JMT: Non-bacterial thrombotic endocarditis in early cancer. Br J Med 1:752, 1976
273. Susens GP, Hendrickson C, Barto Da, Sams BJ: Disseminated intravascular coagulation syndrome with metastatic melanoma: Remission after treatment with 5-(3,3-dimethyl-l-triazeno) imidazole-4-carboxamide (DTIC). Ann Intern Med 84:175, 1976
274. Alving BM, Abeloff MD, Bell W: Spontaneous remission of recurring disseminated intravascular coagulation associated with prostatic carcinoma. Cancer 37:928–930, 1976
275. Lee JC, Yamuchi H, Hopper J Jr: The association of cancer and the nephrotic syndrome. Ann Intern Med 64:41–51, 1966
276. Glassock RJ, Friedler RM, Massry SG: Kidney and electrolyte disturbances in neoplastic diseases. Contrib Nephrol 7:2–41, 1977
277. Ghosh L, Meuhrhe RC: The nephrotic syndrome: A prodrome to lymphoma. Ann Intern Med 72:379–382, 1970
278. Cantrell EG: Nephrotic syndrome cured by removal of gastric carcinoma. Br Med J 2:739, 1969
279. Plager J, Stutzman L: Acute nephrotic syndrome as a manifestation of active Hodgkin's disease. Am J Med 50:56–66, 1971
280. Lewis MG, Loughridge LW, Phillips TM: Immunological studies in nephrotic syndrome associated with extrarenal malignant disease. Lancet II:134–185, 1971
281. Couser WG, Wagonfeld JB, Spargo BH, Lewis EJ: Glomerular deposition of tumor antigen in membranous nephropathy associated with colonic carcinoma. Am J Med 57:962–970, 1974
282. Costanza ME, Perin V, Schwartz RS, Nathansen L: Carcinoembryonic antigen–antibody complexes in a patient with colonic carcinoma and nephrotic syndrome. N Engl J Med 289:520–522, 1973
283. Sherman RL, Susin M, Weksler ME, Becker EL: Lipoid nephrosis in Hodgkin's disease. Am J Med 52:699–706, 1972
284. Lokich JJ, Galvanek EG, Moloney WC: Nephrosis of Hodgkin's disease. Arch Intern Med 132:597–600, 1973
285. Moorthy AV, Zimmerman SW, Burkholder PM: Nephrotic syndrome in Hodgkin's disease. Am J Med 61:471–477, 1976
286. Carpenter CB: Case records of the Massachusetts General Hospital. N Engl J Med 289:1241–1247, 1973
287. Richard-Mendes da Costa C, Dupont E, Hamers R, Hooghe R, Dupuis F, Potuliege R: Rephrotic syndrome in bronchogenic carcinoma: Report of two cases with immunochemical studies. Clin Nephrol 2:245–251, 1974
288. Gagliano RG, Costanzi JJ, Beathard GA, Sarles HE, Bell JD: The nephrotic syndrome associated with neoplasia: An unusual paraneoplastic syndrome. Report of a case and review of the literature. Am J Med 60:1026–1031, 1976
289. Cameron JS: Nephrotic syndrome in chronic lymphatic leukemia. Br Med J 4:164–167, 1974
290. Hyman LR, Burkholder PM, Joo PA, Segar WE: Malignant lymphoma and the nephrotic syndrome. A clinicopathologic analysis with light immunofluorescence and electron microscopy of the renal lesions. J Pediatr 82:207–217, 1973
291. Higgins MR, Randall RE, Still WJS: Nephrotic syndrome with oat-cell carcinoma. Br Med J 3:450, 1974
292. Karpen HO, Bhat JG, Feiner HD, Baldwin DS: Membranous nephropathy associated with renal cell carcinoma. Evidence against a role of renal tubular or tumor antibodies in pathogenesis. Am J Med 64:864–867, 1978
293. Hopper JH Jr: Tumor related renal lesions. Ann Intern Med 81:550–551, 1974
294. Row PG, Cameron JS, Turner DR, Evans DJ, White RHR, Ogg CS, Chantler C, Brown B: Membranous mephropathy. Long-term followup and association with neoplasia. Quart J Med 44:207–239, 1975
295. Shalhoub RJ: Pathogenesis of lipoid nephrosis: A disorder of T-cell function. Lancet 2:556–558, 1974

296. Osserman EF, Lawlor DP: Serum and urinary lysozyme (muramidase) in monocyte and monomyelocytic leukemia. J Exp Med 124:921–951, 1966
297. Pruzanki W, Platts MF: Serum and urinary proteins, lysozyme (muramidase) and renal dysfunction in mono- and myelomonocytic leukemia. J Clin Invest 49:1694–1707, 1970
298. Hobbs JR, Evans DJ, Wrong OM: Renal tubular obstruction by mucoprotein from adenocarcinoma of pancreas. Br Med J 2:87–89, 1974
299. Freibusch J, Barbosa-Saldivar JL, Bernstein RS, Robertson GL: Tumor-associated nephrogenic diabetes insipides. Ann Intern Med 92:797–798, 1980
300. Kyle RA: Multiple myeloma. Review of 869 cases. Mayo Clin Proc 50:29–40, 1975
301. DeFronzo RA, Cooke CR, Wright JR, Humphrey RL: Renal function in patients with multiple myeloma. Medicine 57:151–161, 1978
302. Zlotnick A, Rosemann E: Renal pathologic findings associated with monoclonal gammopathies. Arch Intern Med 135:40–45, 1975
303. Schubert GE, Veigel J, Lennert K: Structure and function of the kidney in multiple myeloma. Virchow Arch Abt A Pathol Anat 355:135–137, 1972
304. Brown Ww, Herbert LA, Piering WF, Piscotta AV, Lemann J Jr, Garancis JC: Reversal of chronic end stage renal failure due to myeloma kidney. Ann Intern Med 90:793–794, 1979
305. Leech SH, Polesky HF, Shapiro FL: Chronic hemodialysis in myelomatosis. Ann Intern Med 77:239–242, 1972
306. Richmond J, Sherman RS, Diamond HD, Craver LF: Renal lesions associated with malignant lymphomas. Am J Med 32:184–207, 1962
307. Martinez-Maldonado M, Ramirez de Arellano GA: Renal involvement in malignant lymphomas: A survey of 49 cases. J Urol 95:485–488, 1966
308. Matthews MJ: Problems in morphology and behavior of monchopulmonary malignant disease. In L Israel, P Chanimian (eds): Lung Cancer, Facts, Problems and Perspectives, pp 23–62. New York, Academic Press, 1976
309. Brin EN, Schiff M Jr, Weiss RM: Palliative urinary diversion for malignancy. J Urol 113:619–622, 1975
310. Fichman M, Bethune J: Effects of neoplasms on renal electrolyte function in paraneoplastic syndromes. Ann NY Acad Sci 230:448–472, 1974
311. Garnic MB, Mayer RJ: Acute renal failure associated with neoplastic disease and its treatment. Semin Oncol 5:155–165, 1978
312. Keane WF, Crosson JT, Staley NA, Anderson WR, Shapiro FL: Radiation-induced renal disease. A clinicopathologic study. Am J Med 60:127–137, 1967
313. Dosik GM, Gutterman JE, Hersh EM, Akhtar M, Senoda T, Horn RG: Nephrotoxicity from cancer immunotherapy. Ann Intern Med 89:41–46, 1978
314. Bennett WM, Muther RS, Parker RA, Feig P, Morrison G, Golper TA, Singer I: Drug therapy in renal failure: Dosing guidelines for adults. Ann Intern Med 93:286–325, 1980
315. Kierland RR: Cutaneous signs of internal malignancy. South Med J 65:563–568, 1972
316. Helm F, Helm J: Cutaneous markers of internal malignancies. In Helm F (ed): *Cancer Dermatology*, pp 247–283. Philadelphia, Lea and Febiger, 1979
317. Braverman IM: Skin signs of systemic disease. Philadelphia, WB Saunders, 1970
318. Crowe FW: Axillary freckling as a diagnostic aid in neurofibromatosis. Ann Intern Med 61:1142–1143, 1964
319. Levine N, Greenwald ES: Mucocutaneous side effects of cancer chemotherapy. Cancer Treat Rev 5:67–84, 1978
320. Brown J, Winkelmann RK: Acanthosis nigricans: A study of 90 cases. Medicine 47:33–51, 1968
321. Curth HO: Classification of acanthosis nigricans. Int J Dermatol 15:592, 1976
322. Sneddon IB, Roberts JBM: An incomplete form of acanthosis nigricans. Gut 3:269–272, 1962
323. Ronchese F: Keratoses, cancer and "The Sign of Leser-Trelat." Cancer 18:1003–1006, 1965
324. Dantzig PI: Sign of Leser-Trelat. Arch Dermatol 108:700–701, 1973
325. Graham JH, Helwig EB: Bowen's disease and its relationship to systemic cancer. Arch Dermatol 83:738–758, 1961
326. Anderson SL, Nielsen A, Reymann F: Relationship between Bowen's disease and internal malignancy. Arch Dermatol 108:367–370, 1973
327. Minkowsky S: Multiple carcinomata following the ingestion of medicinal arsenic. Ann Intern Med 61:296–299, 1964
328. Fitzpatrick TB, Montgomery H, Lerner AB: Pathogenesis of generalized dermal pigmentation secondary to malignant melanoma and melanuria. J Invest Dermatol 22:163–172, 1954
329. Ashikari R, Park K, Huvos AG, Urban JA: Paget's disease of the breast. Cancer 26:680–685, 1970
330. Gammel JA: Erythema gyratum repens. Skin manifestations of patients with carcinoma of breast. Arch Dermatol 66:494–505, 1952
331. Purdy MJ: Erythema gyratum repens. Report of a case. Arch Dermatol 80:590–591, 1959
332. Summerly R: The figurate erythemas and neoplasia. Br J Dermatol 76:370–373, 1964
333. Lazar P: Cancer, erythema annulare centrifugum and autoimmunity. Arch Dermatol 87:246–253, 1963
334. Wilkinson DS: Necrolytic migrating erythema with pancreatic carcinoma. Proc R Soc Med 64:1197–1198, 1971
335. Church RE, Crane WAJ: A cutaneous syndrome associated with islet cell carcinoma of the pancreas. Br J Dermatol 79:284–286, 1967
336. Sjoerdsma A, Weissbach H, Udenfriend S: A clinical, physiologic, and biochemical study of patients with malignant carcinoid (argentaffinoma). Am J Med 21:520–532, 1956
337. Mason DT, Melmon KL: New understanding of the mechanism of the carcinoid flush. Ann Intern Med 65:1334–1339, 1966
338. Abrahams F, McCarthy JT, Sanders SL: 101 cases of exfoliative dermatitis. Arch Dermatol 87:96–103, 1963
339. Nicolis GD, Helwig EB: Exfoliative dermatitis: A clinicopathologic study of 135 cases. Arch Dermatol 108:788–979, 1973
340. Elias PM, Fritsch PO: Erythema multiforme. In Fitzpatrick TB, Eisen AZ, Wolf K, Freedberg IM, Austen FF (eds): Dermatology in General Medicine, 2nd ed, pp 295–303. New York, McGraw-Hill, 1979
341. Fitzpatrick TB, Clark WH Jr: Recurrent attacks of abdominal pain and cutaneous lesions. N Engl J Med 270:1248–1251, 1964
342. Waddington RT: A case of primary liver tumor associated with porphyria. Br J Surg 59:653–654, 1972
343. Thompson RPH, Nicholson DC, Farman T, Whitmore DN, Williams R: Cutaneous prophyria due to a malignant primary hepatoma. Gastroenterology 59:779–783, 1970
344. Stone SP, Schroeder AL: Bullous pemphigoid and associated malignant neoplasms. Arch Dermatol 111:991–994, 1975
345. Tobias N: Dermatitis herpetiformis associated with visceral malignancy. Urol Cutan Rev 55:352, 1951
346. Arundell FD, Wilkinson RD, Haserick Jr: Dermatomyositis and malignant neoplasms in adults. Arch Dermatol 82:772–775, 1960
347. Lyell A, Whittle CH: Hypertrichosis languginosa acquired type. Br J Dermatol 63:411–413, 1951
348. Hegedus SI, Schorr WF: Acquired hypertrichosis languginosa and malignancy. Arch Dermatol 106:84–88, 1972
349. Van Dijk E: Ichthyosiform atrophy of the skin with internal malignant diseases. Dermatologica 127:413–428, 1963
350. Flint GL, Flam M, Soter NA: Acquired ichthyosis. Arch Dermatol 111:1446–1447, 1975
351. Vogl A, Goldfischer S: Pachydermoperiostosis. Primary or idiopathic hypertrophic osteoarthopathy. Am J Med 33:166–187, 1962
352. Rajka G: Investigation of patients suffering from generalized pruritus, with special references to systemic diseases. Acta Dermatol Venereal (Stock) 46:190–194, 1966
353. Cormia FE: Pruritus, an uncommon but important symptom of systemic cancer. Arch Dermatol 92:36–39, 1965
354. Schimpff S, Serpick A, Stoler B, Rumack B, Mellin H. Joseph

JM, Block J: Varicella-zoster infection in patients with cancer. Ann Intern Med 76:241–254, 1972
355. Dolin R, Reichman RC, Mazur MH, Whitley RJ: Herpes zoster-varicella infections in immunosuppressed patients. Ann Intern Med 89:375–388, 1978
356. Huberman M. Fossieck BE Jr, Bunn PA Jr, Cohen MH, Ihde DC, Minna JD: Herpes zoster and small cell bronchogenic carcinoma. Am J Med 68:214–218, 1980
357. Gardner EJ: Follow-up study of a family group exhibiting dominant inheritance for a syndrome including intestinal polyps, osteomas, fibromas, and epidermal cysts. Am J Hum Genet 16:376–390, 1962
358. Bussey HJR: Gastrointestinal polyposis. Gut 11:970–978, 1970
359. Jones EL, Cornell WP: Gardner's syndrome. Review of the literature and report on a family. Arch Surg 92:287–300, 1966
360. Jeghers H, McKusick VA, Katz KH: Generalized intestinal polyposis and melanin spots of the oral mucosa, lips and digits. A syndrome of diagnostic significance. N Engl J Med 241:933–1005, 1031–1036, 1949
361. Riley E, Swift M: A family with Pentz-Jeghers syndrome and bilateral breast cancer. Cancer 46:815–817, 1980
362. Howel-Evans W, McConnell RR, Clarke CA, Sheppard PM: Carcinoma of the esophagus with keratosis palmaris et plantaris (tylosis). Quart J Med 27:413–429, 1958
363. Williams ED, Pollock DJ: Multiple mucosal neuromatoa with endocrine tumors: A syndrome allied to Von Recklinghausen's disease. J Pathol Bacteriol 91:71–80, 1966
364. Lloyd KM, Dennis M: Cowden's disease, a possible new symptom complex with multiple system involvement. Ann Intern Med 58:136–142, 1963
365. Solomon LM, Fretzin DF, Dewald RL: The epidermal nevus syndrome. Arch Dermatol 97:273–285, 1968
366. Butterworth T, Wilson M Jr: Dermatologic aspects of tuberous sclerosis. Arch Dermatol Syphilol 43:1–41, 1941
367. Christoferson LA, Gustafson MB, Petersen AG: Von Hippel-Lindau's disease. JAMA 178:280–282, 1961
368. Doll R, Kinlen L: Immunosurveillance and cancer: Epidemiologic evidence. Br Med J 4:420–422, 1970
369. Epstein CJ, Martin GM, Schultz AL, Motulsky AG: Werner's syndrome. A review of the symptomatology, natural history, pathologic features, genetics, and relationship to the natural aging process. Medicine 45:177–221, 1966
370. Frizzera G, Rosai J, Dehner LP, Spector BD, Kersey JH: Lymphoreticular disorders in primary immunodeficiencies: New findings based on an up-to-date histologic classification of 35 cases. Cancer 46:692–699, 1980
371. Waldman TA, Broder S, Strober W: Protein-losing enteropathies in malignancy. Ann NY Acad Sci 230:306–317, 1974
372. Watery diarrhoea (WDHA) syndrome associated with carcinoma of the lung. Aust NZ J Med 6:490–491, 1976
373. Troncale FJ: Distant manifestations of colonic carcinoma. Ann NY Acad Sci 230:332–347, 1974
374. Klipstein FA, Smorth G: Intestinal structure and function in neoplastic disease. Am J Dig Dis 14:887–899, 1969
375. Gilat T, Fischel B, Danon J, Lowewnthal M: Morphology of small bowel mucosa and malignancy. Digestion 12:147–155, 1972
376. Henderson AR, Grace DM: Liver-originating isoenzymes of alkaline phosphatase in the serum: A paraneoplastic manifestation of a malignant schwannoma of the sciatic nerve. J Clin Pathol 29:237–240, 1976
377. Walsh PN, Kissane JM: Nonmetastatic hypernephroma with reversible hepatic dysfunction. Arch Intern Med 122:214–222, 1968
378. Utz, DC, Warren MM, Gregg JA, Ludwig J, Kelalis PP: Reversible hepatic dysfunction associated with hypernephroma. Mayo Clin Proc 45:161–169, 1970
379. Cronin RE, Kaehny WD, Miller PD, Stables DP, Gabow PA, Ostroy PR, Schrier RW: Renal cell carcinoma: Unusual systemic manifestations. Medicine 55:291–311, 1976
380. Mena E, Bull FE, Bookstein JJ, Goldstein HM, Neiman MD, Thornbury, JR, Lim CO: Angiography of the nephrogenic hepatic dysfunction syndrome. Radiology 111:65–68, 1974
381. DeWys WD: Working conference on anorexia and achexia of neoplastic disease. Cancer Res 30:2816–2818, 1970
382. DeWys WD: Abnormalities of taste as a remote effect of a neoplasm. Ann NY Acad Sci 230:427–434, 1974
383. Theologides A: The anorexia–cachexia syndrome: A new hypothesis. Ann NY Acad Sci 230:14–22, 1974
384. Waterhouse C: How tumors affect host metabolism. Ann NY Acad Sci 230:86–93, 1974
385. Gold J: Cancer Cachexia and gluconeogenesis. Ann NY Acad Sci 230:103–110, 1974
386. Bodel P: Tumors and fever. Ann NY Acad Sci 230:6–13, 1974
387. Petersdorf RG: Fever and cancer. Hosp Med 1:2–10, 1965
388. Lobell M, Boggs DR, Wintrobe MM: The clinical significance of fever in Hodgkin's disease. Arch Intern Med 117:335–342, 1966
389. Gluckman JB, Turner MD: Systemic manifestations of tumors of the small gut and liver. Ann NY Acad Sci 230:318–331, 1974
390. Block JB: Lactic acidosis in malignancy and observations on its possible pathogenesis. Ann NY Acad Sci 230:94–102, 1974
391. Nadiminti Y, Wang JC, Chou S, Pineles E, Tobin MS: Lactic acidosis associated with Hodgkin's disease. Response of chemotherapy. N Engl J Med 303:15–17, 1980
392. Spechler SJ, Esposito AL, Koff RS, Hong WK: Lactic acidosis in oat cell carcinoma with extensive hepatic metastases. Arch Intern Med 138:1663–1664, 1978
393. Eridani S, Burdick L, Periti M, Arosio A, Libretti A: Primary carcinoma of the colon and hyperlipemia: A paraneoplastic syndrome. Biomedicine 25:324–326, 1976
394. Glueck HL, MacKenzie M, Glueck CJ: Crystalline IgG protein in multiple myeloma: Identification of effects on coagulation and on lipoprotein metabolism. J Lab Clin Med 79:731–744, 1972
395. Santer MA, Waldmann TA, Fallon HJ: Erythrocytosis and hyperlipemia as manifestations of hepatic carcinoma. Arch Intern Med 120:735–739, 1967
396. Gangulu A, Gribble J, Tune B, Kempson RL, Luetscher JA: Renin-secreting Wilms' tumor with severe hypertension. Report of a case and brief review of renin-secreting tumors. Ann Intern Med 79:835–837, 1973
397. Genest J, Rojo-Ortega JM, Kuchel O, Boucher R, Nowaczynski W, Lefebvre R, Chretien M, Cantin J, Granger P: Malignant hypertension with hypokalemia in a patient with renin-producing pulmonary carcinoma. Trans Assoc Am Phys 88:192–201, 1975
398. Aurell M, Rudin A, Tisell LE, Kindblom LG, Sandberg G: Captopril effect on hypertension in patient with renin-producing tumor. Lancet 2:149–150, 1979
399. Hollifield JW, Page DL, Smith C, Michelakis AM, Staab E, Rhamy R: Reinin-secreting clear cell carcinoma of the kidney. Arch Intern Med 135:859–864, 1975
400. Zusman RM, Snider JJ, Cline A, Caldwell BV, Speroff L: Antihypertensive function of renal-cell carcinoma. Evidence for a prostaglandin A secreting tumor. N Engl J Med 290:43–845, 1974
401. Boasberg PD, Henry JP, Rosenbloom AA, Hall TC, Rose M, Fisher DA: Case reports and studies of paraneoplastic hypotension: Abnormal low pressure baroreceptor responses. Med Pediatr Oncol 3:59–66, 1977
402. Braganza JM, Butler EB, Fox H, Hunter PM, Qureshi MSA, Samarji W, Vallon AG: Ectopic production of salivary type amylase by a pseudomesotheliomatous carcinoma of the lung. Cancer 41:1522–1525, 1978
403. Mills JA: A spectrum of organ systems that respond to cancer: The joints and connective tissue. Ann NY Acad Sci 230: 443–447, 1974
404. Greenfield GB, Schorsch HA, Shkolnik A: The various roentgen appearance of pulmonary hypertrophic osteoarthropathy. Am J Roentgenol Radium Ther Nucl Med 101:927–931, 1967
405. LeRoux BT: Bronchial carcinoma with hypertrophic pulmonary osteoarthropathy. S Afr Med J 42:1074–1075, 1968
406. Jao JY, Barlow JJ, Krant MKJ: Pulmonary hypertrophic osteoarthropathy, spider angiomata and estrogen hypersecretion in neoplasms. Ann Intern Med 70:580–584, 1969

407. Donnelly B, Johnson PM: Detection of hypertrophic pulmonary osteoarthropathy by skeletal imaging with ^{99m}Tc-labeled diphosphonate. Radiology 114:389–391, 1975
408. Green N, Kurohara SS, George FW III, Crews QE Jr: The biologic behavior of lung cancer according to histologic type. Radiol Clin Biol 41:160–170, 1972
409. Yesner R: Spectrum of lung cancer and ectopic hormones. In Sommers SC, Rosen PP (eds): Pathology Annual, Vol 12 (part I), pp 217–240. New York, Appleton-Century Crofts, 1978
410. Goldstraw P, Walbraun PR: Hypertrophic pulmonary osteoarthropathy and its occurrence with pulmonary metastases from renal carcinoma. Thorax 31:205–211, 1976
411. Miller ER: Carcinoma of the thymus with marked pulmonary osteoarthropathy. Radiology 32:651–660, 1939
412. Ullal SR: Hypertrophic osteoarthropathy and leiomyoma of the oesophagus. Am J Surg 123:356–358, 1972
413. Shapiro RF, Zvaifler NJ: Concurrent intrathoracic Hodgkin's disease and hypertrophic osteoarthropathy. Chest 63:912–916, 1973
414. Howard CP, Telander RL, Hoffman AD, Burgert EO Jr: Hypertrophic osteoarthropathy in association with pulmonary metastasis from osteogenic sarcoma. Mayo Clin Proc 53:538–541, 1978
415. Papavasiliou C, Pavlatou M, Pappas J: Nasopharyngeal cancer in patients under the age of thirty years. Cancer 40:2312–2316, 1977
416. Ellouz R, Cammoun M, Attia RB, Bahi J: Clinical aspects Nasopharyngeal carcinoma in children and adolescents in Tunisia: Clinical aspects and the paraneoplastic syndrome. Iarc Sci Pub 20:115–129, 1978
417. Cudkowicz, L, Armstrong JB: Finger clubbing and changes in the bronchial circulation: Arterio-venous shunts in hypertrophic pulmonary osteoarthropathy. Br J Tuberc 47:227–232, 1953
418. Carroll KB, Doyle L: A common factor in hypertrophic osteoarthropathy. Thorax 29:262–264, 1974
419. Riyami AM, Anderson EG: Hypertrophic pulmonary osteoarthropathy: A clinical and biochemical study. Br J Dis Chest 68:193–196, 1974
420. Glenner GG: Amyloid deposits and amyloidosis. The B-fibrilloses. N Engl J Med 303:1283–1292, 1333–1347, 1980
421. Azzopardi JG, Lehner T: Systemic amyloidosis and malignant disease. J Clin Pathol 19:539–548, 1966
422. Kyle RA, Bayrd ED; Amyloidosis: Review of 236 cases. Medicine 54:271–547, 1975
423. Mills JA: Connective tissue disease associated with malignant neoplastic disease. J Chronic Dis 16:797–811, 1963
424. Calabro J: Cancer and arthritis. Arthritis and Rheu 10:553–567, 1967
425. Cammarata R, Rodnan GP, Jensen WM: Systemic rheumatic disease and malignant lymphoma. Arch Intern Med 111: 112–119, 1963
426. Miller D: The association of immune disease and malignant lymphoma. Ann Intern Med 66:507–521, 1967
427. Anderson LG, Talal N: The spectrum of benign to malignant lymphoproliferation in Sjogrens syndrome. Clin Exp Immunol 9:199–221, 1971
428. Murray GC, Persellin RH: Metastatic carcinoma presenting as monarticular arthritis: A case report and review of the literature. Arthritis Rheum 23:95–100, 1980
429. Karten I, Bartfield H: Bronchogenic carcinoma simulating early rheumatoid arthritis. JAMA 179:160–161, 1962
430. Tumulty PA: Systemic lupus erythematosus. In Winthrobe, Thorn, Adams, Bennett, Braunwald, Isselbacher, Petersdorf (eds): Harrison's Principles of Internal Medicine, 6th ed, pp 1962–1967. New York, McGraw-Hill, 1971

CHAPTER 40

John E. Ultmann
Theodore L. Phillips

Management of the Patient with Cancer of Unknown Primary Site

The patient with metastatic cancer with no obvious primary site presents a difficult, but not uncommon problem for the practicing physician. Between 0.5% and 7% of cancer patients have an occult primary site depending on the thoroughness of the investigation undertaken to find the primary site and the population studied. Two questions are foremost in the mind of the clinician treating the patient with an unknown primary site:

1. Which diagnostic studies should be undertaken to locate the primary site?
2. What treatment, if any, is indicated when the primary site is not found after an appropriate investigation?

This chapter will discuss these questions in detail and provide a guide for patient management.

A critical analysis of the literature concerning the patient with cancer of unknown origin is difficult. All studies have been retrospective. Comparisons between individual series are not usually valid because the patient populations studied differ and the criteria used to define the patient with an unknown primary site vary. Patient cohorts may involve all patients in a hospital tumor registry or only those patients referred to a special oncology unit. Some physicians consider a patient to have an unknown primary site if the history, physical examination, and chest films are unrevealing; others require the patient to have undergone more extensive testing, which includes biopsies. A few physicians exclude any patient for whom the diagnosis was suspected during life or eventually known, no matter how late during the clinical course it occurred. A further point of variation among studies concerns the evidence required to establish the primary site. Is one radiologic study adequate? Should two positive clinical tests be required? Is a biopsy of the suspected primary site necessary? In spite of these difficulties, sufficient clinical information is now available to form a rational basis for the management of these patients, provided physicians precisely define the patient population of interest.

OCCULT PRIMARY MALIGNANCY

For clarity of discussion, a patient will be said to have an *occult primary malignancy* (OPM) if: 1. he has a biopsy proven malignancy, and, 2. a history, physical examination, chest film, complete blood count, urinalysis, and stool test for blood are not indicative of a primary site. The histology of the biopsy must demonstrate unequivocal malignancy and must be inconsistent with a primary tumor at the biopsy site. In most cancer patients, the localization of the primary site is not difficult. If, after all clues from history, physical examination, and the above screening laboratory studies have been investigated, the primary site is not found, it is concluded that the patient has an OPM. For example, the patient presenting with squamous cell carcinoma in a high cervical node is not classified as having an OPM until he has received a meticulous ENT examination by a specialist and biopsies of any suspicious oral or pharyngeal areas are negative.

CLINICALLY UNDETECTABLE PRIMARY MALIGNANCY

In the event a primary site is eventually identified, the reader will have an entry point into patient management and can consult the chapter of this book that discusses the diagnosis, staging, and treatment of that primary malignancy.

A patient who has gone through the indicated additional diagnostic studies and the primary site is still not apparent is said to have a *clinically undetectable primary malignancy* (CUPM).

DIAGNOSTIC EVALUATION IN OCCULT PRIMARY MALIGNANCY

In many hospitals, patients with an OPM undergo extensive diagnostic studies based on the belief that optimal manage-

TABLE 40-1. The Value of Diagnostic Studies in Occult Primary Malignancy

STUDY	DESCRIPTION OF POPULATION	ANATOMIC EXCLUSIONS	HISTOLOGIC EXCLUSIONS	MINIMUM WORK-UP REQUIRED BEFORE PRIMARY SITE CONSIDERED UNKNOWN	WORK-UP TO FIND PRIMARY
Nystrom et al[1]	Referred with diagnosis of adeno- or undifferentiated carcinoma to Medical Oncology Division—University of Southern California	—	Adeno- or undifferentiated carcinoma only	Variable, referred with diagnosis of unknown primary site	History and physical, proctoscopy, upper and lower level GI contrast films, skeletal survey IV pyelogram, multiphase chemistry profile, urinalysis, mammography
Osteen et al[2]	Registered with Tumor Board of Peter Bent Brigham Hospital as unknown primary	Excluded patients with upper cervical nodes	—	History, physical examination, chest film, hematocrit, WBC, urinalysis	Minimum work-up based on symptoms followed by more extensive workup.
Stewart et al[3]	All patients referred to medical oncology unit—Royal Prince Alfred Hospital	—	—	History and physical, chest film	—

STUDY	FRACTION OF ALL SIMILAR CANCER PATIENTS WITH UNKNOWN PRIMARY	FRACTION OF PATIENTS WITH PRIMARY SITE FOUND DURING LIFE	AUTOPSY RATE	FRACTION OF AUTOPSIES DISCLOSING PRIMARY	MEDIAN SURVIVAL	NUMBER OF PATIENTS WITH HIGHLY TREATABLE MALIGNANCIES
Nystrom et al[1]	—	30/266	130/266	107/130	—	14/266 3-breast, 2-thyroid, 4-ovary, 4-prostate, 1-adrenal (including one found at post-mortem)
Osteen et al[2]	—	38/67	22/61	20/22	3 mos	16/67 5-ovary, 4-lymphoma, 4-prostate, 3-breast
Stewart et al[3]	87/1300 (6.7%)	8/87-diagnostic work-up, 2/87-exploratory laparotomy, 13/87-clinical follow-up; 23/87 total	16/63	14/16	13–14 weeks (4½ mos)	12/87 Diagnosis by noninvasive studies 2-prostate, diagnosis by laparotomy and prolonged follow-up, 4-ovary 2-germ cell, 2 thyroid, post mortem-Hodgkin's disease, histiocytic lymphoma

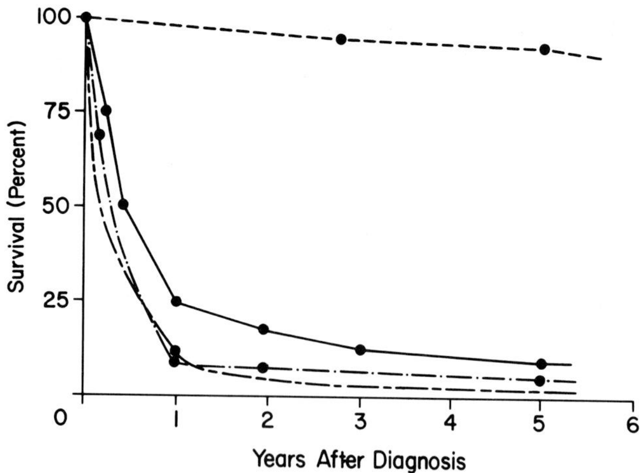

FIG. 40-1. Survival curve of patients with metastatic cancer with an unknown primary site. (●——●Smith PE, Krementz ET, Chapman W: Metastatic cancer without a detectable primary site. J Surg 113:633–637, 1967;●-·-●Holmes FF, Fouts TL: Metastatic cancer of unknown primary site. Cancer 26:816–820, 1970; ●-—● Richardson RG, Parker RG: Metastases from undetected primary cancers—Clinical experience at a radiation oncology center (Medical Information). West J Med 123:337–339, 1975); ●----● Survival of age-adjusted normal controls.

ment depends on identification of the primary site. The utility of such an approach has been questioned by investigators in three recent studies summarized in Table 40-1.[1,2,3] Median survival for OPM patients is poor, usually only 3–4 months. Survival curves from three publications show that less than 25% of patients are alive at one year and less than 10% at 5-year follow-up (see Fig. 40-1).[4,5,6] As a group, patient survival is unchanged by treatment. Hence, the cost and discomfort of elaborate diagnostic studies (which may consume a significant part of a patient's life expectancy) need to be weighed carefully. In most OPM patients a primary site will not be located during life. Even after post-mortem, the primary site will not be identified in 15% of these patients. Chemotherapy of OPM patients, prior to the advent of doxorubicin (adriamycin), was also uniformly unsuccessful with a response rate of 15% or less.

Table 40-2 lists the primary sites identified by Nystrom and coworkers either during life or at autopsy.[7] The distribution of primary sites eventually found in OPM patients is quite different from the overall incidence of primary cancers reported in the literature or reports of the End Results Group. Lung was the most common primary site in patients with supradiaphragmatic metastases, while pancreas was the most common primary site in patients with subdiaphragmatic metastases. The value of systemic therapy for most primary sites ultimately detected is in question.

The search for a primary site is difficult since the pattern of metastases may be atypical when compared to the metastatic spread of a clinically obvious primary site presenting in the traditional manner.[7] Table 40-3 compares the pattern of metastatic involvement in patients with an OPM in whom a primary site was eventually proven with literature values for patterns of metastases of patients with obvious primary sites. For example, 30–50% of patients with metastatic lung cancer can be expected to have bony involvement, but only 4% of patients with an OPM, later proven to be lung cancer, had bony metastases. The normal relative incidence of metastases from known primary sites is therefore not useful in making

TABLE 40-2. Distribution of Primary Cancer Sites: Comparison with Literature and End Results Group

PRIMARY SITE	PRESENT SERIES N	PRESENT SERIES %	LITERATURE %	END RESULTS GROUP %
Above diaphragm:				
Lung	28	17	17	10
Breast	3	2	3	26
Thyroid	2	1	5	1
Parotid	1	<1	—	<1
Subtotal	34			
Below diaphragm:				
Pancreas	30	20	21	1.5
Liver	16	11	10	1.5
Colorectal	15	10	7	14
Gastric	12	8	10	5
Renal	9	7	3	2
Ovary	4	4	2	5
Prostate	4	3	3	17
Adrenal	1	<1	2	—
Subtotal	91			
Other	4	2	—	—
Not classified	23	15	15	—
Total	152			

Nystrom JS, Weiner JM, Heffelfinger-Juttner J et al: Metastatic and histologic presentations in unknown primary cancer. Semin Oncol 4(1):53–58, 1977

TABLE 40-3. Pattern of Metastatic Involvement: Comparison of Clinically Overt Primaries (B) and Primaries Presenting as OPM (A)

PRIMARY SITE	PERCENT METASTATIC INVOLVEMENT							
	Bone		*Lung*		*Liver*		*Brain*	
	A	*B*	*A*	*B*	*A*	*B*	*A*	*B*
Lung	4	30–50	90	34	36	30–50	21	15–30
Breast	33	50–85	66	60	66	45–60	33	15–25
Thyroid	0	39	100	65	50	60	0	1
Pancreas	28	5–10	31	25–40	72	50–70	3	1–4
Liver	31	8	19	20	100	—	6	0
Colorectal	13	5–10	40	25–40	87	71	0	1
Gastric	9	5–10	18	20–30	36	35–50	9	1–4
Renal	66	30–50	77	50–75	33	35–40	0	7–8
Ovary	0	2–6	25	10	25	10–15	0	1
Prostate	25	50–75	75	13–53	50	13	25	2

Nystrom JS, Weiner JM, Heffelfinger-Juttner J et al: Metastatic and histologic presentations in unknown primary cancer. Semin Oncol 4(1):53–58, 1977

a diagnosis. Several common tumors, such as breast and prostate, are easily detectable by simple means and thus rarely present as OPM.

Patients with OPM present with a different pattern of metastatic spread as well as a different frequency of ultimately proven primary sites when compared with patients with metastatic malignancies and obvious primary sites. The statistics cited in Tables 40-2 and 40-3 describe the distribution of primary cancer sites and the patterns of metastatic involvement. The biological reasons for these observations have not yet been elucidated; however, Holmes and Foults have cited four reasons for metastatic cancer remaining undiagnosed as to the primary origin:

1. Present clinical tools are inadequate
2. The primary may remain inapparent despite autopsy because standard sampling and lack of serial sections may not constitute a sufficient search
3. The primary may have been removed by excision or fulguration (*e.g.*, melanoma), by dilatation and curettage (*e.g.*, endometrial cancer), or by sloughing the necrotic tumor from skin or the GI tract
4. A spontaneous regression of the primary may have occurred[5]

When primary sites are ultimately detected, they are smaller than tumors whose metastases have occurred from easily detectable sites. Often, the histology of the metastasis, or of the later-discovered primary, is undifferentiated or a poorly differentiated carcinoma, lymphoma, or sarcoma. Apparently, these tumors metastasize early and the metastases have a tendency to proliferate more rapidly than the primary tumor. The response to therapy and survival is poor.

Further difficulty arises since clinical studies are often incorrect, with both false-postive and false-negative results. Even chest roentgenographic patterns normally considered diagnostic of primary lung tumors may be erroneous when metastatic disease is present (see Table 40-4).[1] The sensitivity and selectivity of upper GI films, barium enemas, and intravenous pyelograms (IVP) in patients with an OPM are shown in Table 40-5.[1,2,3] Tentative diagnoses are often not confirmed at autopsy. One clinical study alone should not be considered diagnostic.

Although the above data would seem to suggest that no evaluation is justified for the patient with OPM, this is not the case. About 10% or 15% of patients with an OPM will ultimately be shown with tumors for which *effective systemic therapy* is available, though unfortunately, not all of these patients will be identifiable before death. For example, a group of female patients present with axillary lymph node and distant metastases. They are found to have breast cancer effectively controllable by combination chemotherapy. A search for these primary tumors is indicated, for their identification will select those patients who will benefit greatly from specific therapy. A list of these tumors appears in Table 40-6 and includes tumors for which there is: highly effective therapy; moderately effective, but quite specific therapy; or therapy with no toxicity. Table 40-6 lists the number and types of potentially treatable malignancies found in patients with OPM.

A second reason for diagnostic studies is the prevention of local catastrophes. For example, if searching for an OPM of a poorly-differentiated adenocarcinoma leads to the detection of a primary in the colon, local resection of the primary colon

TABLE 40-4. Comparison of Chest Roentgenogram Patterns of Verified Primary and Metastatic Nonsquamous Cell Cancer of the Lung

	LUNG PCS*	METASTATIC PCS
Single mass	6	6
Malignant effusion	8	11
Multiple nodules	2	8
Nodal disease	10	6
Infiltrates	1	6
Total	27	37

* PCS represents primary cancer site

Nystrom JS, Weiner JM, Wolf RN et al: Identifying the primary site in metastatic cancer of unknown origin. Inadequacy of roentgenographic procedures. JAMA 241:381–383, 1979

TABLE 40-5. Sensitivity and Selectivity of Contrast Roentgenography in Patients with Occult Primary Malignancies

	UPPER GI ROENTGENOGRAM				BARIUM ENEMA				IV PYELOGRAM			
RESULTS OF STUDIES	N*	O†	S‡	TOTAL	N	O	S	TOTAL	N	O	S	TOTAL
Total studies	218	—	24	242	198	—	27	225	187	43	35	265
Positive for carcinoma	14	—	4	18	17	—	7	24	16	0	2	18
True positive	8	—	1	9	9	—	4	13	5	0	0	5
False positive	6	—	3	9	8	—	3	11	11	0	2	13
False negative	4	—	1	5	8	—	0	8	4	2	1	7
Sensitivity§				64%				62%				41%
Selectivity‖				50%				54%				27%

* Nystrom et al[1]
† Osteen et al[2]
‡ Stewart et al[3]
§ true positives/total tumors
‖ true positives/total positive

carcinoma may be justified to prevent an impending bowel obstruction.

ORGANIZATION OF THE DIAGNOSTIC EVALUATION

As described previously, the diagnostic evaluation of the patient with an OPM has two goals: the identification of any tumor for which effective or at least specific therapy is available, and, the identification of any imminent local complication for which local therapy is required. These are best pursued using a systematic operational approach. Only those studies which result in data that would potentially alter therapy are useful (see Fig. 40-2). For example, the measurement of acid phosphatase, which may lead to the diagnosis of prostate carcinoma, is useful because there is specific therapy available for the tumor. However, the measurement of a carcinoembryonic antigen level, which is elevated in many tumors and non-malignant states, is useless. To distinguish between primary tumors for which there is only minimally effective systemic therapy is of no value because the patient's management will be unchanged. Therefore, before any diagnostic test is ordered, the physician should ask: "Will the results affect patient management?" If the answer is no, the tests should not be ordered.

TABLE 40-6. Tumors for Which Effective Systemic Treatment is Available

I. CURE POSSIBLE
   1. Germ cell tumors
   2. Hodgkin's disease
   3. Non-Hodgkin's lymphoma
   4. Trophoblastic tumors

II. "NON-TOXIC" HORMONAL TREATMENT
   1. Breast cancer
   2. Prostatic cancer
   3. Endometrial cancer

III. HIGHLY EFFECTIVE CHEMOTHERAPY (Response ≥ 50%)
   1. Breast cancer
   2. Ovarian cancer
   3. Oat cell carcinoma of lung

IV. SPECIFIC, MODERATELY EFFECTIVE CHEMOTHERAPY (Response ≥ 20%)
   1. Adrenal carcinoma

V. CHEMOTHERAPY EFFECTIVE AS AN ADJUVANT AFTER SURGICAL DEBULKING
   1. Osteogenic sarcoma

It is essential that diagnostic studies be carefully selected to insure that the most information is obtained at the least cost to the patient in terms of money, time, and discomfort and at the lowest risk of morbidity or mortality. Studies directed by signs or symptoms are more likely to be fruitful than those that are not. Careful attention must be directed to evaluating biopsy material for precise histologic classification. The presenting anatomic site must be analyzed for clues as to the origin of the OPM. A repeat history and physical examination may yield clues that were missed earlier. In addition, careful attention must be paid to smoking history, pains (particularly in the epigastrium), change in bowel habits or voiding pattern, vaginal or other bleeding, and pelvic discomfort. The examination must include a pelvic and rectal. Specific studies should be undertaken to systematically search for those primary sites for which therapeutic options are available and useful.

Fig. 40-2 illustrates the optimal sequence of steps when evaluating the patient with an OPM. Note that this differs from the traditional order of inquiry (history, physical examination, laboratory studies) used to delineate other clinical problems. The biopsy material should be reviewed first since a prior history and physical examination are usually unrevealing. Clues the biopsy specimen provides will facilitate a directed history and physical with emphasis on specific areas of interest.

Data from Biopsy Specimens

The first step in the evaluation of the patient with an OPM is to review the biopsy material with an experienced pathologist. Subtle features in the histology may well give an indication of likely primary sites. If there is any question regarding the adequacy of the original biopsy material and if an easily accessible site is available, a second biopsy should be done. Note that careful planning is necessary to insure

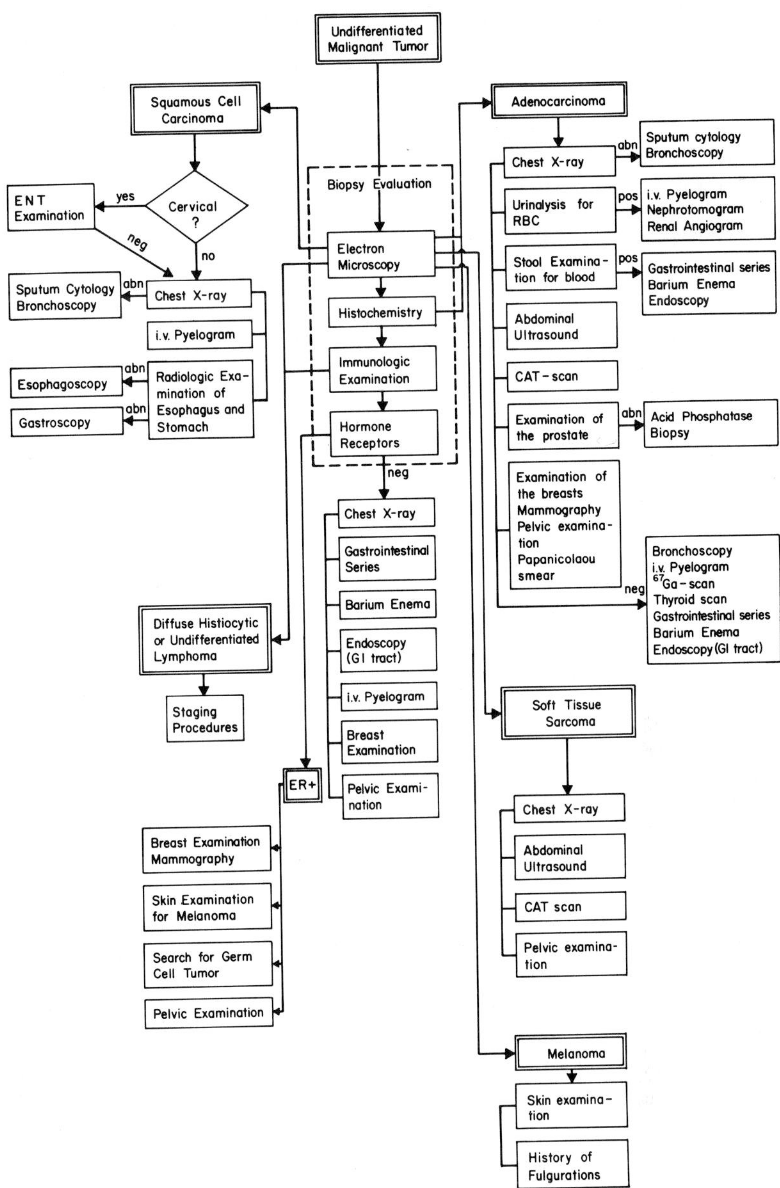

FIG. 40-2. Schematic representation of diagnostic strategy for work-up of patients with occult primary malignancy (OPM).

that the surgical specimen is properly divided for any desired special studies *before* it is put into a routine fixative.

Sometimes special stains are useful. Some tumors appear totally undifferentiated on hematoxylin-and-eosin stained sections. In the adult, the most common of these are poorly-undifferentiated squamous cell carcinoma, poorly-differentiated adenocarcinoma, diffuse histiocytic or undifferentiated lymphoma, poorly-differentiated sarcoma, amelanotic melanoma, and undifferentiated germ cell cancer (see Table 40-7). Intracellular mucin detected with a mucicarmine stain would identify an adenocarcinoma; diastase-resistant periodic acid Schiff (PAS) positivity of such an adenocarcinoma would point to a gastric carcinoma. However, electron microscopy is often much more useful (see Fig. 40-3). For example, premelanosomes are diagnostic of melanomas, while desmosomes identify poorly-differentiated carcinomas. In a female, the measurement of estrogen receptors is helpful. These are classically found in breast carcinoma, but may also be present in ovarian and endometrial carcinomas and melanomas. An axillary metastasis in a woman with a positive estrogen receptor should be considered diagnostic of breast carcinoma in spite of a negative physical examination of the breast and negative mammography.

Data From Anatomic Location

For practical purposes, patients with OPM can be divided into two major categories according to anatomic presentation—those with disease above the diaphgram and those with disease below the diaphragm. In addition, those patients with

TABLE 40-7. Usefulness of Electron Microscopy, Histochemistry, Immunologic Surface Markers, and Hormone Receptors in the Classification of OPM

	ELECTRON MICROSCOPY	HISTOCHEMISTRY	IMMUNE MARKERS	HORMONE RECEPTORS
Poorly differentiated squamous cell carcinoma	Intercellular bridges, tonofilaments, desmosomes	Anti-keratin antibodies	–	–
Poorly differentiated adenocarcinoma	Junctional complex, tight junction, intermediate junction, desmosome	Mucicarmin, diastase-resistant PAS	–	Estrogen receptor, progesterone receptor
Diffuse histiocytic or undifferentiated lymphoma	Polyribosomes, absence of junctions	PAS MGP	EAC rosettes, E rosettes, surface IG	Steroid receptor
Poorly differentiated sarcoma	Myofibrils, dilated rough endoplasmic reticulum, or extracellular osteroid	Anti-smooth muscle antibodies	–	–
Amelanotic melanoma	Premelanosomes	Fontana-Mason argyrophil stain	–	Estrogen receptor
Undifferentiated germ cell carcinoma	–	Alpha fetoprotein antibodies, β-fragment HCG antibodies	–	Estrogen receptor

involvement of only the cervical nodes or axillary nodes deserve special consideration (see Table 40-8).

CERVICAL LYMPH NODES. Despite the dismal prognosis for patients with OPM, those with OPM manifest only in cervical nodes are greatly benefited by local and regional therapy. As shown in Table 40-9, the 3-year survival after radical radiation, radical surgery, or both ranges from 35% to 59%.[8,9,10,11,12] An OPM in a cervical node is most often due to regional spread from a clinically inapparent primary in the head and neck (see Table 40-10).[8,9,11] Some 78% of the primary sites that became apparent after therapy were, in fact, in the head and neck. High cervical nodes are more likely to have a head and neck primary site in Waldeyer's ring than low cervical nodes. Consequently, high cervical nodes have a better prognosis.

An appropriate radiation port can be designed to cover most potential head and neck primary sites at the same time the cervical nodes are irradiated. Generally, ports typical for the nasopharynx, base of tongue, and tonsils are used for nodes along the jugular vein in the mid- or posterior neck region. Nodes in the submaxillary or subdigastric areas require oral cavity irradiation. Treatment of patients with radical neck dissection rather than radiation results in a higher incidence of primary site relapses. However, it has not been fully established if these relapses can be successfully salvaged by additional local resection and radiotherapy.[8,10,11] Well-differentiated squamous cell carcinoma in anterior nodes is surgically treatable; lower nodes should receive radiation. For patients with tumors of the head and neck, squamous and anaplastic carcinoma have the best prognosis. Long-term survivors with adenocarcinoma are rare. Long-term survival in patients with primary sites below the clavicle is also unusual.

Patients with OPM in the supraclavicular nodes have a much poorer prognosis. This most often represents widely metastatic disease from a distant primary. On the right side, the most likely primary sites are lung and breast. On the left side, spread from intra-abdominal malignancies by way of the thoracic duct is probable and still needs to be considered (*i.e.*, Virchow's node). The small number of long-term survivors with radical radiation (12%) are most likely due to primaries in the head and neck (see Table 40-8).

AXILLARY LYMPH NODES. Among patients with OPM above the diaphragm, those presenting with an isolated axillary node have unique clinical features. The prognosis for patients presenting with an isolated axillary node is somewhat better than for OPM in general. In the series from M.D. Anderson Hospital, 18 of 37 females presenting with a malignant axillary node and a negative breast examination were ultimately shown to have breast carcinoma.[13] Mammography was negative in nine of the 17 patients in whom the study was performed. Thus, a negative physical examination and mammography do not completely rule out breast carcinoma. In addition, nine of 60 patients in another series from the M.D. Anderson Hospital remained disease-free for 2–10 years after diagnosis. Therapy consisted only of local excision or axillary dissection. Two patients who died of other causes had no evidence of malignancy at post-mortem examination. No primary site was identified in any of these patients. Feigenberg and coworkers reported eight patients with axillary lymph node metastases. The primary growth in three of these patients was ultimately found in the ipsilateral breast.[14] The investigators advocated conservative sector mastectomy of the upper outer quadrant as a diagnostic procedure, radiotherapy to the affected axilla and, if breast cancer is proven, to the breast as well.

The ready availability of estrogen (ER) and progesterone (PR) receptor tests changes the strategy of the work-up of an isolated axillary mass. Therefore, the initial biopsy in all female patients should be processed for receptor activity. Carcinoma of the breast can be presumed to be the primary (even if no primary lesion is demonstrable) if an ER+ or PR+ adenocarcinoma is found in axillary lymph nodes. If an

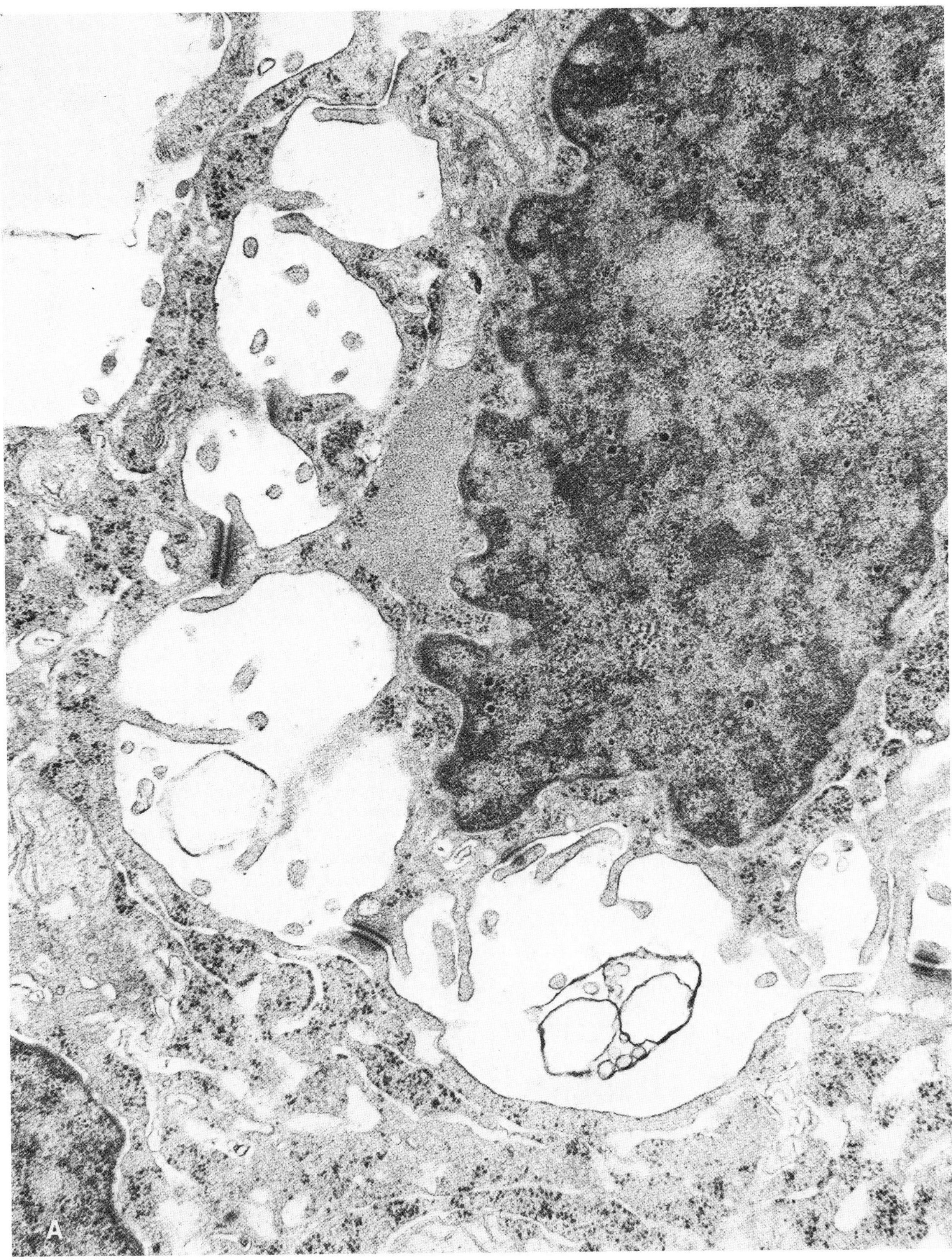

FIG. 40-3. *A*, Electron micrograph showing a portion of a cell with tonofilaments and two intracellular bridges (desmosomes). This finding is compatible with poorly-differentiated squamous cell carcinoma. (Original magnification × 17,500.) (Courtesy Dr. J. Ringus) *(Fig. 40-3 continues on pages 1526–1528)*

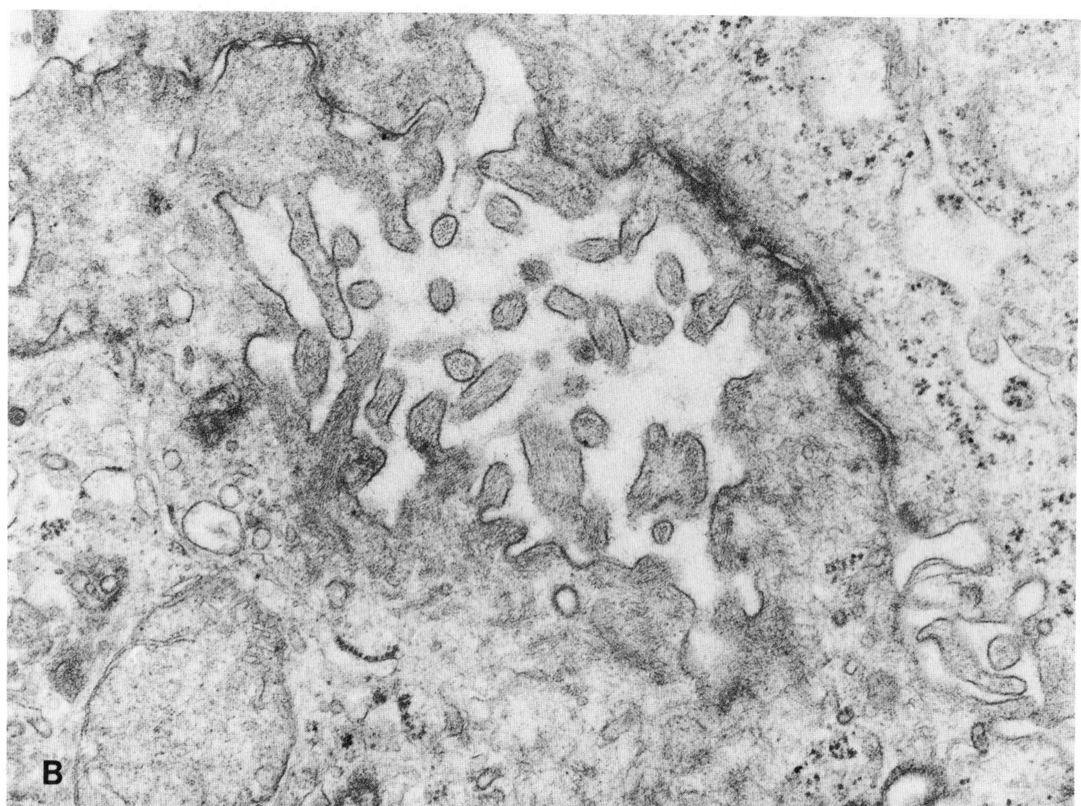

FIG. 40-3. *B,* A portion of a cell from an electron micrograph showing junctional complex and microvilli compatible with poorly differentiated adenocarcinoma. (Original magnification × 17,500.) (Courtesy Dr. J. Ringus) (*Fig. 40-3 continues on pages 1527–1528*)

ER and PR were negative or not obtained, it is best to treat the most treatable cancer for the particular region. Thus, if the patient is a 48-year-old female who has axillary involvement and no primary is found, the best way to manage her would be to treat as if she had carcinoma of the breast. This should be done whether estrogen receptor sites are found or not.

With the exceptions already discussed (*i.e.,* high cervical, axillary, and left supraclavicular lymph node presentations), lung cancer remains the most common primary site for OPM presenting *above* the diaphragm.[7]

In analyses of OPM presenting as metastases *below* the diaphragm, carcinoma of the pancreas is the most common primary site ultimately detected.[7] However, two other areas

TABLE 40-8. Anatomic Analysis of OPM

ANATOMIC LOCATION	PRIMARY SOURCE TO BE CONSIDERED
Above Diaphragm	
High cervical lymph nodes	Head and neck Thyroid Lungs
Low cervical/supraclavicular lymph nodes	Head and neck Thyroid Left or right lung Left > right gastrointestinal
Axillary lymph nodes	Breast Left or right lung Left > right gastrointestinal
All presentations above diaphragm	Lung
Below Diaphragm	
Umbilical mass (Sister Mary Joseph's Nodule)	Gastrointestinal (stomach > others) Ovarian Uterine
Groin mass/lymph nodes	Anus and rectum Prostate Vulva Testicle (after testicular biopsy or repair of hernia)
All presentations below diaphragm	Pancreas

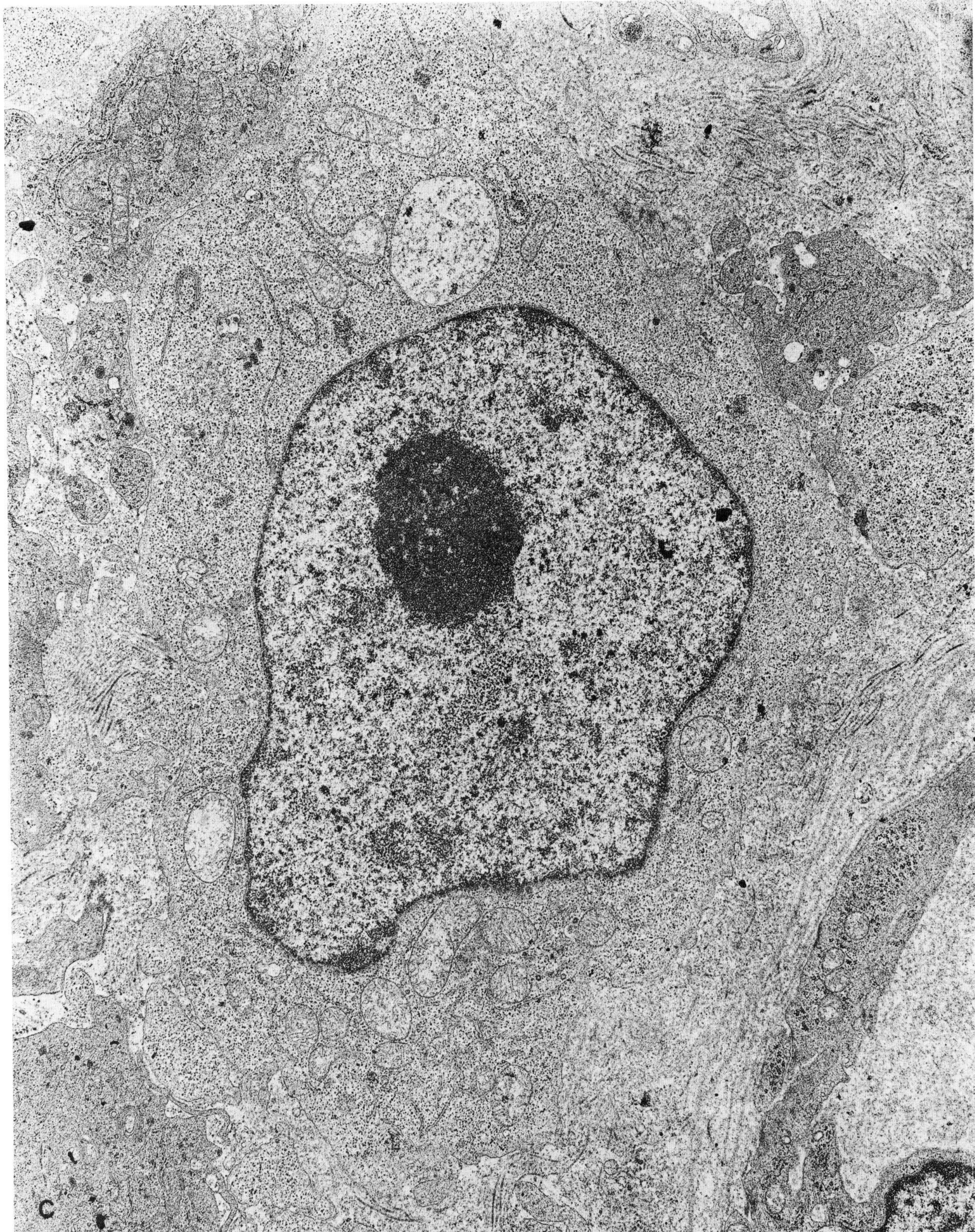

FIG. 40-3. *C,* Electron micrograph of a cell with cytoplasm packed with ribosomes in absence of junctions diagnostic of diffuse histiocytic lymphoma. (Original magnification × 17,500.) (Courtesy Dr. J. Ringus) (*Fig. 40-3 continues on page 1528*)

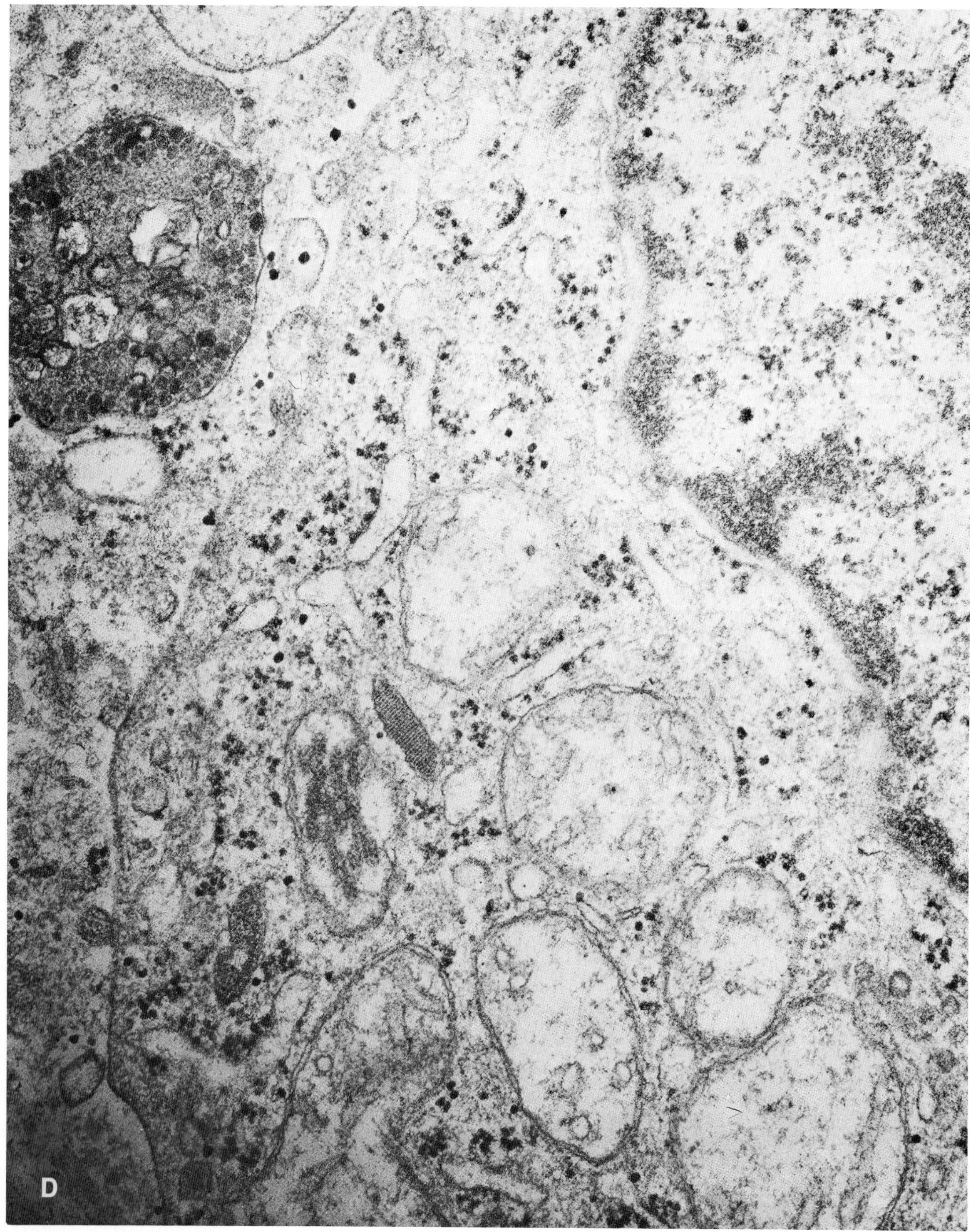

FIG. 40-3. *D*, Electron micrograph showing a single, premelanosome structure diagnostic of amelanotic melanoma. (Original magnification × 75,000.) (Courtsey Dr. J. Ringus)

TABLE 40-9. Survival in OPM Confined to Cervical Nodes

STUDY	TREATMENT	THREE-YEAR SURVIVAL (percent)	THREE-YEAR SURVIVAL WHEN PRIMARY SITE IS NEVER APPARENT (percent)	THREE-YEAR SURVIVAL WITH PRIMARY SITE EVENTUALLY APPARENT ABOVE DIAPHRAGM (percent)	THREE-YEAR SURVIVAL WITH PRIMARY SITE EVENTUALLY APPARENT BELOW DIAPHRAGM (percent)	THREE-YEAR SURVIVAL OF SIMILAR PATIENTS WITH SUPRACLAVICULAR NODE POSITIVE (percent)
Jesse et al[8]	Radical neck dissection,* RT (5000 rad), or both	53 (disease-free)	58	31	0	12
Barrie et al[9]	Radical neck dissection:- RT for a few patients	35	–	–	–	–
Fried et al[10]	RT (6000–7000 rad) followed by radical neck dissection or RT alone or RT (3000 rad) followed by dissection	39	–	–	–	–
Coker et al[11]	Radical neck dissection*	51‡	60	37	–	–
Fitzpatrick et al[12]	RT† > 4500 rad	59	–	–	–	12

*Includes additional local resection as required
†Ports to nasopharynx, tonsil and base of tongue, areas boosted as necessary
‡Squamous and anaplastic histology only
RT = radiotherapy

TABLE 40-10. Primary Sites Detected After Treatment of OPM Confined to Cervical Nodes

	JESSE ET AL[8]	BARRIE ET AL[9]	COKER ET AL[11]	TOTAL	PERCENT OF ALL PRIMARY SITES
HEAD AND NECK PRIMARIES	28/184	31/123	12/56	71/363	78%
Hypopharynx	8	9			
Tonsil or faucial arch	5	9	1		
Base of tongue or vallecula	4	5	2		
Oral cavity or salivary gland	4	1	1		
Nasopharynx	2	8	1		
Maxillary antrum	1				
A–E folds, epiglottis	2		2		
Cervical esophagus	1				
Thyroid	1				
Nasal cavity		2			
Pharyngeal wall (including pyriform sinus)		2			
True vocal cord			1		
Skin			1		
Lymphoma			3		
BELOW CLAVICLE	9/184	7/123	4/56	20/363	22%
Not specified	9				
Stomach		2			
Lung		2	3		
Pancreas		1			
Ovary		1	1		
Colon		1			

deserve special consideration—an umbilical mass and a groin mass or lymph nodes.

UMBILICAL MASS. Primary carcinoma of the umbilicus is rare and usually epidermoid in nature. Adenocarcinomas detected in the umbilicus are likely to be metastatic (35 of 36 cases) and the most common primary source is carcinoma of the stomach. Occasionally, carcinomas of the gall bladder, colon, appendix, ovary, or uterus are the primary site. In 18 of 40 patients with umbilical masses, the umbilical site was the only reason for seeking medical attention. Finding the mass (referred to as Sister Mary Joseph's nodule) initiated the appropriate work-up for the OPM.[15,16,17,18,19]

GROIN MASS. Groin masses or lymph nodes showing metastatic cancer most commonly point to a primary site in the lower extremities, the vulva, anorectal region, or prostate. Infrequently, ovarian or testicular cancers will metastasize to this region. In the latter case, this may occur following biopsy of the testis or following hernia repair when the lymphatics are interrupted.

SKIN. When an OMP is detected in the skin, consideration must be given to malignant tumors that spread by the hematogenous route; among these are melanomas and carcinomas of the lung, breast, kidney, and ovary. A previous history of skin fulguration may point to a metastasis from a melanoma. If no distant primary is detectable, further consideration must be given to the primary in the skin or its appendages. Occasionally, lymphoma, particularly diffuse histiocytic lymphoma, arises in the skin. Then the OPM may, in fact, represent the primary lesion.

LUNG. Major mass lesions detected on chest roentgenograms are most likely lung cancers. Weber and associates reported that 18 of 94 patients with confirmed carcinoma of the pancreas were initially diagnosed as having primary carcinoma of the bronchus based on clinical signs, results of radiologic examinations, lung scannning, and bronchoscopy with histologic or cytologic examination.[20] Other metastatic tumors may also mimic mass lesions of primary lung cancer.

When a single, atypical lesion is seen in chest roentgenogram, the most likely diagnosis is primary lung cancer. If the lesion is a metastasis, it is still most likely to originate from a primary lesion in the lung, particularly if the histology shows a squamous cell carcinoma. If an adenocarcinoma is demonstrated, the source may be lung, pancreas and other sites in the GI tract, or breast. Solitary nodules in the lung frequently arise from kidney or primary liver cancer. In addition, undifferentiated tumors may originate from occult sarcoma or amelanotic melanoma.

LIVER. The suspicion of an OPM in the liver arises in cases presenting with cachexia, fever, or jaundice, with or without hepatomegaly. Serum alkaline phosphatase (hepatic isozyme) is usually elevated and a liver scan may be abnormal. If stool is positive for blood, a work-up of the GI tract is indicated and a search for a primary is likely to be rewarding.

If a diagnosis is not achieved, a liver biopsy is indicated; it is preferable to perform such a procedure by laparoscopy or laparotomy rather than by closed needle biopsy since hemorrhage from a vascular tumor is a real risk. In addition to the GI tract (including pancreas), the lung or breast may be the primary site of metastases. In some cases, it is difficult to separate poorly-differentiated hepatocellular carcinomas and biliary carcinomas from OPM in the liver.

BONE. Patients presenting with pain in a bone or an unexplained fracture may have an OPM. If a fracture is present, open reduction will yield tissue that may give clues to tumor origin. Often serum alkaline phosphatase (bone isozyme) is elevated. A serum protein electrophoresis can establish the diagnosis of multiple myeloma. An elevated serum acid phosphatase can point to prostatic carcinoma, which is also characterized by purely blastic lesions on radiologic examination of the skeleton. Blastic lesions may also be seen in ovarian cancer, carcinoid, and Hodgkin's disease, and very infrequently in oat cell cancer. A mixed blastic and lytic picture is often seen in breast cancer, whereas punched-out, purely lytic lesions are characteristic of multiple myeloma. In addition to lung, breast, prostate, and ovarian cancer, cancer of the kidney and GI tract must be considered when evaluating OPM in bone.

HEMATOLOGIC ABNORMALITIES. Unexplained increases or decreases in the formed elements of the blood may suggest that a work-up be initiated; hence, lead to the discovery of an OPM. Erythrocytosis resulting from excess erythropoietin is usually associated with kidney tumors but may also occur in infratentorial hemangioblastoma and hepatic carcinoma. Thrombocytosis, without other hematologic abnormalities, has been described in a number of tumors including ovarian, lung, and pancreatic carcinoma, and Hodgkin's disease. Anemia, leukopenia, and thrombocytopenia should suggest a hematologic work-up, including a bone marrow aspiration and bone core biopsy that could reveal a tumor. Almost any primary tumor may be the source of these metastases, but the lung, breast, GI tract, and pancreas are the most common sources. A characteristic hematologic picture referred to as leukoerythroblastic anemia is seen most frequently in association with widespread bone marrow invasion from breast cancer; other primary sources, including lung, may also be found.

BRAIN. Although the routine preoperative work-up for a brain tumor includes search for OPM with emphasis on lung, breast, and prostate, it is not uncommon at craniotomy to find an unsuspected metastatic tumor. For all practical purposes, carcinomas of the lung, breast, prostate, and pancreas, and melanomas are the commonest sources of OPM. In these cases, surgical resection and postoperative radiotherapy are indicated. However, surgical resection is not required if other metastases are demonstrated. The type of radiotherapy (whole-brain vs. whole brain with local boost) will depend on the preoperative findings, including computerized axial tomography scan, as well as the operative findings. If the primary can be detected, appropriate chemotherapy can be selected.

SPINAL CORD. The dramatic events suggesting impending cord compression often lead to surgical intervention, which results in decompression and the diagnosis of an OPM. High (thoracic) spinal cord lesions most commonly originate from cancer of the lung or breast, whereas low (thoracolumbar) spinal cord lesions can usually be traced to retroperitoneal lymphomas or prostatic cancer. In any event, vigorous postoperative management with radiotherapy, chemotherapy, or both is indicated.

MALIGNANT EFFUSIONS. Infrequently, the first sign and symptom of a malignant tumor is pleural effusion or ascites. The demonstration of malignant cells not only proves the nature of the effusion but could also give clues as to the origin of the tumor. Both cytologic analysis and study of cell blocks should be undertaken. Malignant pleural effusions with positive cytology most frequently originate in the lung, breast, ovary, GI tract, or pancreas; malignant ascites originate most frequently in the ovary, pancreas, stomach, or colon.

PAIN. Pain may be the first sign of a primary cancer as well as of a tumor presenting as an OPM. Obvious examples are bone pain leading to the discovery of a bone metastasis and long tract signs leading to the detection of an intrathecal tumor. Occasionally, the pain problem is related to nerve or nerve root involvement as in Pancoast tumors, pancreatic cancer, or mesothelioma.

MIGRATORY THROMBOPHLEBITIS. Recurrent episodes of thrombophlebitis in multiple locations (migratory thrombophlebitis) that are not readily explained by the usual antecedent factors are likely to be associated with an OPM. Without trauma, an episode of thrombophlebitis in the upper extremity suggests cancer. Cancer of the pancreas is the most common primary site associated with migratory thrombophlebitis, but lung cancer, GI cancers, and other malignancies have been described.

HISTORICAL APPROACH

The discovery of an OPM should prompt a thorough, historic review to detect clues about the origin of the metastatic tumor. In general, this approach is less rewarding than the histologic and anatomic approaches already discussed. Most importantly, patients should be questioned about fulgurations or biopsies of "harmless" skin lesions, removal of benign polyps of the colon, dilatation and curettage (or conization) procedures that revealed "no cancer," biopsies of the prostate that showed "only prostatic hypertrophy," and any other surgical procedures in which tissue was removed. Occasionally, this line of questioning reveals that the tissue which was removed and considered benign, may well have been the location of the primary malignancy that now is manifest as a metastasis. The opportunity to perform a second biopsy permits the pathologist to perform "directed" procedures to support a diagnosis suspected from history.

The family history is rarely helpful since most familial and hereditary cancers are obvious as to primary site. However, the geographic or racial history may occasionally offer clues, since it is known that in certain regions particular cancers have a high incidence (*e.g.*, the prevalence of skin cancer in sunbelt residents, stomach cancer in Japanese, or nasopharyngeal cancer in Chinese populations).

Knowledge of age and sex differences in cancer incidence may be of some help in planning the strategy for the OPM patient work-up. Risk factors, including knowledge of occupational exposure, may offer subtle clues that assist in planning a directed search for the primary tumor.

BASIC SCREENING STUDIES

In the strategy for evaluating an OPM the laboratory and radiologic studies must be selected carefully based on data obtained from various clues.

Re-examination of Fig. 40-2 emphasizes the usefulness of the radiologic examination of the chest, urinalysis for detection of blood, and stool examination for blood. In addition, serum chemistries with particular emphasis on calcium, uric acid, and liver functions should be performed. In most instances, these tests are done on admission to the hospital and should pass scrutiny. However, a re-examination of these simple tests is in order to detect abnormalities that might have major impact on the strategy of further work-up.

SPECIFIC STUDIES

Kennedy and Luedke have outlined a strategy for undertaking the work-up of an OPM:

> If no clues are forthcoming from the basic screening studies, the physician faces the challenging question of how far to proceed with a low-yield diagnostic workup on a patient with a short life expectancy. The benefits of an established diagnosis must outweigh the expense, time, and risk to the patient involved in making the diagnosis. Ultimately, the extent of disease; the organ involvement; and the age, social situation, and performance level of the patient should dictate the extent of the diagnostic workup. A critically ill patient with rapidly progressive tumor requires therapeutic intervention rather than an extensive diagnostic evaluation. However, in patients able to undergo additional studies, strong consideration should be given to systematic assessment of the sites of common primary tumors which metastasize widely (lung, breast, pancreas, kidney) and of those that are most amenable to treatment (breast, prostate, ovary).[21]

Table 40-11 summarizes the cost in time and money required to perform 15 common tests to detect the primary site from which an OPM may have originated. The armamentarium available for the diagnostic work-up of an OPM spans the entire repertoire of radiologic, radioisotopic, chemical, and immunologic tests. Some tests are simple, atraumatic for the patient, and require little justification (*i.e.*, mammogram, ultrasound, bone scan, upper GI series); others are more complex and may be very expensive (*i.e.*, CAT scan, PTH-assay, ^{67}Ga scans); still other tests are complex, expensive, and may cause significant complications, thus requiring the physician to carefully weigh the cost-benefit ratio (*i.e.*, bronchoscopy, ERCP, arteriography). The guiding rule should be selectivity, keeping effectiveness in mind in terms of therapeutic decision-making, complication rate, cost, and time. Some costly tests may actually save time and money. For example, a CAT scan of the abdomen can, in many instances, replace upper GI series, IVP, barium enema, and liver scan.

TABLE 40-11. Economics of Finding the Primary Site

EXAMINATION	COST ($)*	TIME REQUIRED FOR EXAMINATION (Hours)
Chest film	32	0.5
Upper GI series	150	1.0
Barium enema	125	1.0
CAT scan of chest and abdomen	403	2.0
CAT scan of brain	392	1.0
Lymphangiogram (LAG)	619	6.0
IV pyelogram (IVP)	144	2.0
Inferior venacavagram (IVC)	712	12.0
Mammogram	90	0.5
Bone scan	230	3.0
^{67}Ga scan	300	4.0
Liver/spleen scan	200	2.0
Gastroscopy	225	1.0
Colonoscopy	250	2.0
Fiberoptic bronchoscopy	375	2.0
(One hospital day)	241	

*1980 prices
CAT stands for Computerized Axial Tomography

TREATMENT

When selective work-up reveals the primary site with a high degree of certainty, appropriate specific therapy is initiated. For squamous cell cancers presenting with high cervical lymph nodes, an aggressive approach, similar to that used in proven head and neck cancers and using radiation therapy or surgery, is indicated even if a primary site cannot be determined. Data have already been summarized that demonstrate 3-year survival in up to 60% of cases using this approach (see Table 40-9).

In general, the authors feel that treatment should only be applied when a patient becomes symptomatic, except under the unusual circumstance when the presumed treatable lesion is one that is known to be curable. For the tumors listed in Table 40-6, specific and effective systemic therapy is available and should be initiated with intent to offer cure or maximal palliation.

In a significant number of patients, a clinically undetectable primary malignancy (CUPM) will remain. Two reports offer little help concerning useful approaches in selecting combinations of agents likely to be effective in such situations.[21,22] The response rate to chemotherapy of cancer of the lung (other than oat cell), pancreas, stomach, colon, and kidney; of amelanotic melanoma; or of undifferentiated sarcoma may be as high as 40–60%, but these responses are generally short and survival is not extended. Table 40-12 lists agents or groups of agents shown to be effective in the management of disseminated cancers of known primary origin.

TABLE 40-12. Effectiveness of Chemotherapeutic Agents used Singly to Treat Various Cancers

	BREAST	CERVIX	COLON	HEAD + NECK	KIDNEY	LUNG	OVARY	PANCREAS	STOMACH	MELANOMA	*DHL/UNDIFF. LYMPHOMA	SARCOMA
Alkylating agent	+ +	+ +		+	+	+	+ +			+	+ +	+
Methotrexate	+ +	+		+		+					+ +	
5-Fluorouracil	+	+	+				+	+	+			
Vincristine	+	+	+		+	+			+		+ +	+
Cis dichlorodiammine platinum (II)	+			+			+					
Doxorubicin	+ +			+		+	+ +	+	+		+ +	+ +
Mitomycin	+	+						+	+			

*Diffuse histiocytic lymphoma
+ Moderately effective
+ + Effective

Only one published report on the management of patients with a CUPM describes the use of doxorubicin (adriamycin). Woods and coworkers describe a randomized treatment study of symptomatic patients with metastatic adenocarcinomas of unknown primary origin using two combination chemotherapy regimens.[23] One regimen combined doxorubicin and mitomycin C while the other consisted of cyclophosphamide, methotrexate, and 5-fluorouracil. While both regimens demonstrated a wide range of anti-tumor activity, the regimen containing doxorubicin and mitomycin C was found to be superior. The spectrum of usefulness of doxorubicin, alone or in combination should lead to a reassessment of treatment programs for patients with a CUPM.[23] This authors' current approach takes this into account and our program for patients with CUPM includes doxorubicin, cyclophosphamide, vincristine, and methotrexate with or without leucovorin rescue. Clearly, further studies are necessary to develop data demonstrating that such an aggressive approach for patients with a CUPM is useful. Of course, various local treatments for particular symptomatic metastatic sites should be employed as described throughout the text.

REFERENCES

1. Nystrom JS, Weiner JM, Wolf RM et al: Identifying the primary site in metastatic cancer of unknown origin. Inadequacy of roentgenographic procedures. JAMA 241:381–383, 1979
2. Osteen RT, Kopf G, Wilson RE: In pursuit of the unknown primary. Am J Surg 135:494–498, 1978
3. Stewart JF, Tattersall MHN, Woods RL et al: Unknown primary adenocarcinoma: Incidence of overinvestigation and natural history. Br Med J 1:1530–1533, 1979
4. Smith PE, Krementz ET, Chapman W: Metastatic cancer without a detectable primary site. J Surg 113:633–637, 1967
5. Holmes FF, Fouts TL: Metastatic cancer of unknown primary site. Cancer 26:816–820, 1970
6. Richardson RG, Parker RG: Metastases from undetected primary cancers—Clinical experience at a radiation oncology center (Medical Information). West J Med 123:337–339, 1975
7. Nystrom JS, Weiner JM, Heffelfinger-Juttner J et al: Metastatic and histologic presentations in unknown primary cancer. Semin Oncol 4(1):53–58, 1977
8. Jesse RH, Perez CA, Fletcher GH: Cervical lymph node metastasis: Unknown primary cancer. Cancer 31:854–859, 1973
9. Barrie JR, Knapper WH, Strong EW: Cervical nodal metastases of unknown origin. Am J Surg 120:466–470, 1970
10. Fried MP, Diehl WH Jr, Brownson RJ et al: Cervical metastasis from an unknown primary. Ann Otol Rhinol Laryngol 84:152–156, 1975
11. Coker DD, Casterline PF, Chamber RG et al: Metastases to lymph nodes of the head and neck from an unknown primary site. Am J Surg 134:517–522, 1977
12. Fitzpatrick PJ, Kotalik JF: Cervical metastases from an unknown primary tumor. Radiology 110:659–663, 1974
13. Copeland EM, McBride CM: Axillary metastases from unknown primary sites. Ann Surg 178:25–27, 1973
14. Feigenberg Z, Zer M, Dintsman M: Axillary metastases from an unknown primary source: A diagnostic and therapeutic approach. Isr J Med Sci 12:1153–1158, 1976
15. Key JD, Shephard DAE, Walters W: Sister Mary Joseph's nodule and its relationship to diagnosis of carcinoma of the umbilicus. Minn Med 59:561, 1976
16. Samitz MH: Umbilical metastasis from carcinoma of the stomach: Sister Joseph's nodule. Arch Dermatol 111:1478–1479, 1975
17. Scarpa FJ, Dineen JP, Boltax RS: Visceral neoplasia presenting at the umbilicus. J Surg Oncol 11:351–359, 1979
18. Jager RM, Max MH: Umbilical metastasis as the presenting symptom of cecal carcinoma. J Surg Oncol 12:41–45, 1979
19. Steck WD, Helwig EB: Tumors of the umbilicus. Cancer 18:907–915, 1965
20. Weber P, Troger J, Ernst H: Das pankreaskarzinom klinisch als zentrales Brouchuskarzinom maskiert. Deutsche Med Wochenschrift 98:1389–1391, 1973
21. Kennedy PS, Luedke DW: Adenocarcinoma of unknown origin: A rational approach to a diagnostic puzzle. Postgrad Med 65:151–160, 1979
22. Lleander VC, Goldstein G, Horsley JS III: Chemotherapy in the management of metastatic cancer of unknown primary site. Oncology 26:265–270, 1972
23. Woods RL, Fox RM, Tattersall MHN et al: Metastatic adenocarcinomas of unknown primary site: A randomized study of two combination chemotherapy regimens. N Engl J Med 303(2): 87–89, 1980

CHAPTER 41

John E. Ultmann
Theodore L. Phillips

Treatment of Metastatic Cancer

Considerations in the Treatment of Metastatic Cancer

The management of metastatic disease represents the largest problem in clinical oncology. Although most attention focuses on the treatment of primary disease, it is metastatic disease that afflicts the majority of patients. Sixty percent to 70% of all patients with cancer will at some time develop distant metastases. Although the management of these metastases has often played a Cinderella role, it is clear that aggressive management of metastases can contribute extensively not only to the prolongation of useful life, but also to long-term survival.

The proclivity to develop metastases by lymphatic or bloodborne routes is one of the salient features of all malignancy. It is unclear at which point in the life history of a tumor metastasis begins, but there is general agreement that tumors over 2 cm in diameter generally begin to have increasing risk of distant metastatic disease. Although there is some correlation between the degree of anaplasia in the tumor and its distant metastasis rate, clearly many other factors in the cell surface makeup of the tumor and in the biology of the periphery of the tumor influence the proclivity to metastasize. In many malignancies, circulating tumor cells may be found in the blood, as originally described by Fisher and Turnbull.* It was recognized by these authors, and subsequently by others, that not all patients demonstrating circulating tumor cells developed metastatic disease. It then became clear that tumor emboli *per se* did not mean that successful metastasis would occur and that many tumor emboli and circulating tumor cells were killed through host interaction.

The risk of metastasis is particularly high in certain specific organs that may be characteristic of a given tissue origin and cell type. Obviously certain organs are favorite sites of metastasis because they are the initial capillary bed through which the blood is filtered after leaving the primary site. Most tumors drain into the general venous circulation, which first reaches the lung after passing through the heart; therefore, lung metastases are the most common. The high blood flow to the brain makes it a likely trapping point for cells surviving passage through the lungs, and obviously the liver is the primary drainage site for gastrointestinal malignancies. Such blood flow explanations do not adequately explain the high proclivity of cells that develop clinical metastases in the bones, on the pleura, or in the adrenals.

More recently, it has become evident through the work of Fidler** and others that tumor cells have specific attractions for given capillary beds. Tumor cells may have surface receptors that lead to their preferential adherence to certain capillary beds. Experimental animal tumor cell lines have

* (Fisher ER, Turnbull RB: Cytologic demonstration and significance of tumor cells in the mesenteric venous blood in patients with colo-rectal carcinoma. Surg Gynecol Obstet 100:102–108, 1955)

** (Fidler IJ: Selections of successive tumor. Lines for metastasis. Nature New Biol 242:148–149, 1973)

been developed that have a high probability of metastasizing to one specific organ after intravenous injection despite the blood flow pattern that may precede such a cell's reaching the target organ. Clearly the outcome of cancer metastasis is dependent upon the interaction of tumor cells with their host. Not only the biological behavior of the tumor cells themselves but also the host nonspecific and perhaps specific immune response will determine the fate of potential metastases.

GENERAL APPROACH TO THE PATIENT WITH METASTATIC DISEASE

Although obviously patients with generalized metastases may benefit from effective systemic chemotherapy because of its ability to reach most portions of the body, in many situations more localized treatment may add to the patient's well-being or survival. The subsequent sections of this chapter will focus on those organs that may contain solitary metastases or that may be the only site of metastasis for a specific tumor. In those situations in which solitary metastases or single organ metastasis exists, a more aggressive, potentially curative approach may be taken using surgery or radiation or combinations of radiation and chemotherapy or surgery, radiation, and chemotherapy.

The general approach involves determining those situations in which the probability is high that only a specific organ is involved or the probability that a metastasis is indeed solitary. Based on this determination, an approach is then devised that will resect the solitary lesion or irradiate the entire organ with additional radiation to gross metastatic foci. Chemotherapy may be added to this regimen to sterilize cells at other locations and to aid the radiation and sterilization of cells within the target organ. The effect of cytotoxic chemotherapy on the tolerance of organs for radiation must be taken into account and radiation dose fractionation schedules adjusted according to the best knowledge as to organ tolerance with chemotherapy. Clearly a more aggressive approach combining the major modalities and with particular emphasis on surgical treatment of limited metastases will yield not only improved palliation, but also significant gains in survival in selected patients.

Treatment of Metastatic Cancer to Brain

with PAUL L. KORNBLITH
MICHAEL D. WALKER
J. ROBERT CASSADY

Metastases to the brain constitute a major problem in the management of patients with malignancies. Although most primary tumors sometimes give rise to brain metastases, there is a predilection for such spread among a number of specific tumors. The most common lesions that give rise to metastases to the brain are carcinomas of the lung and breast (see Table 41-1). In the surgical series of Vieth and coworkers reported in 1965, lung is the most common metastatic site (28%); a significant number of metastases from breast cancer, cancer of unknown primary, and melanoma also exist.[1] In the radiotherapy series from the Radiation Therapy Oncology Group (RTOG) recently reported by Borgelt and coworkers metastases from lung cancer represent almost 60% of all cases, with breast cancer second, and miscellaneous sites making up about 20% of cases.[2] This difference in relative incidence is probably due to the rapid increase in incidence of lung cancer over the past 20 years.

Improved management of patients with generalized metastases has recently led to longer survival and a greater incidence of brain metastases. The use of multi-agent chemotherapy, in particular, has contributed to this trend because of its ability to retard metastases in other sites; in addition, multi-agent chemotherapy fails to cross the blood-brain barrier which affects cerebral metastases. Thus, the combination of an increasing incidence of lung cancer, with its predilection for brain metastases, and patients developing metastases while on systemic chemotherapy has led to a large influx of this disease.

Brain metastasis may be the only symptomatic lesion that a particular patient faces. It is a devastating event. Correction of the neurologic deficit and return of the patient to a normal neurologic condition can markedly improve the quality of survival and, in some cases, the length of survival. Management by radiotherapy alone and the combination of surgery and radiation therapy, and the prospects for chemical modification of radiation will be discussed here. However, chemo-

TABLE 41-1. Primary Sites of Tumors Metastatic to Brain

CARCINOMAS	VIETH AND COWORKERS (1965) NO. OF CASES (%)	BORGELT AND COWORKERS (1980) NO. OF CASES (%)
Lung	86 (28)	1067 (59)
Breast	51 (16)	312 (17)
Melanoma	49 (16)	60 (3)
Unknown	44 (14)	
GU Tract	22 (7)	
Colon	16 (5)	
Skin and Sinuses	14 (4)	
Sarcoma	8 (3)	
Other	23 (7)	373 (21)
TOTAL CASES	313	1812

Vieth R, Odom GL: Intracranial metastases and their neurosurgical treatment. J Neurosurg 23:375–383, 1965

Borgelt B, Gelber R, Kramer S et al: The palliation of brain metastases: Final results of the first two studies by the Radiation Therapy Oncology Group. Int J Radiat Oncol Biol Phys 6:1–9, 1980

therapy in the management of brain metastases will only be discussed briefly.

SITES OF BRAIN METASTASES

Metastasis to the brain usually involves the cerebrum; the frontal lobe is the most common site.[1] Other common sites include the temporal, parietal, and occipital lobes. Combinations of fronto-parietal, temporo-parietal, and occipito-parietal are also common lesions (see Table 41-2). Metastases to the cerebellum are less frequent, and those to the brain stem are the least frequent. Most reports indicate that approximately one-third of patients may exhibit solitary metastases, although this number is decreasing as the accuracy of computerized tomography (CT) steadily increases. Autopsy studies suggest that the incidence of solitary metastases is less than 30%.

DIAGNOSTIC EVALUATION OF BRAIN METASTASES

The diagnosis of metastatic disease to the brain involves a combination of careful historic, neurologic and neuroradiologic evaluations. A history of headache, seizures, and focal neurologic deficits may be elicited. Among these symptoms, the most prevalent are headache, loss of motor function, and impaired mentation with lethargy. Seizures, sensory loss, and cerebellar dysfunction are also common.

Focal neurologic findings on examination may occur in relation to the site of the lesion within the brain. Initially, development of the nuclear scan, and more recently, development of CT scan has altered the diagnostic approach to the patient suspected of having brain metastasis. The most recent generation of CT scanners is more accurate in depicting the size and multiplicity of brain metastases than prior tests, including nuclear scans, arteriography, and pneumoencephalography. It is now exceedingly rare for CT not to find and delineate a brain metastasis. In certain situations, meningeal metastasis rather than focal brain lesions may be present. In that situation, the use of cerebrospinal fluid (CSF) cytology may be helpful. The elevation of CSF pressure, protein, and the discovery of malignant cells on cytologic examination are the most relevant findings. Millipore analysis of the fluid permits detection of a small number of tumor cells.

TABLE 41-2. Location of Metastases Within the Brain (Patients with Single Sites)

LOCATION	NO. OF CASES (%)
Frontal lobe	36 (27)
Temporal lobe	19 (14)
Parietal lobe	19 (14)
Occipital lobe	19 (14)
Occipito-parietal region	15 (11)
Cerebellum	11 (8)
Fronto-parietal region	6 (5)
Temporo-parietal region	6 (5)
Brain stem	2 (2)
TOTAL PATIENTS	133

Vieth RG, Odom GL: Intracranial metastases and their neurosurgical treatment. J Neurosurg 23:375–383, 1965

The presence of even vague CNS symptoms in a patient with lung cancer suggests the need for a CT scan. Most diseases do not have enough incidence of brain metastases at initial diagnosis to warrant CT scanning as a part of the original staging evaluation, but it would appear indicated in all lung cancers, particularly in small-cell carcinoma of the lung.

GENERAL APPROACH TO TREATMENT

Many factors should be considered when determining appropriate therapy for the patient with brain metastasis. The initial decision should concern the appropriateness of any treatment other than analgesia or symptomatic relief. No therapy is often the best choice for the patient with widespread, painful, metastatic disease outside of the brain that is not responding well to systemic treatment. Since the treatment of most patients with brain metastases will be palliative, the quality of life prolonged by specific therapy to the brain must be considered. Should the patient's general condition appear to indicate treatment of CNS lesions, the following factors will help to determine the type of local treatment to be employed; namely, surgery, radiation, chemotherapy, or a combination of these:

1. Number of lesions
2. Location of lesions
3. Primary site
4. Patient age and general functional condition
5. Status of other metastatic disease and the primary
6. Relative radioresponsiveness and radiocontrollability
7. Interval between treatment of the primary lesion and development of brain metastases

In general, radiotherapy will be the principal and often sole treatment in most patients. Surgery may be considered for the patient without systemic disease who is relatively young, has a solitary metastasis in a silent area, and, in particular, has a primary of the breast or other site outside the lung. For surgery, the primary site should not be of a histologic type showing extreme sensitivity to radiation (*i.e.*, lymphomas). Even for apparently solitary disease, the interval between primary therapy and development of metastases should be considered. If the interval is greater than 12 months, the duration of benefit from an aggressive surgical approach is more likely to benefit the patient. These considerations will limit patients treated surgically to the healthy, younger patient with a primary lesion such as osteosarcoma, renal cell carcinoma, or melanoma, which are generally solitary. Surgery is often appropriate for the patient with an apparently metastatic CNS lesion without evidence of primary site for diagnostic purposes. Prior to neurosurgical intervention, careful radiographic evaluation of the head, neck, nasopharynx, and lungs is mandatory since carcinoma of the lung is the primary site in 60% of patients developing brain metastases. Dexamethasone in doses of 8–60 mg/day may be very valuable in reducing symptoms while other treatment is being considered or given.

RADIATION THERAPY

The value of radiation therapy for the treatment of metastatic carcinoma to the brain was first reported by Chao and coworkers in 1954.[3] Subsequent publications include those of Chu and Hilaris; Nisce, Hilaris, and Chu; Horton and associates; Montana and associates; and, more recently, by Hendrickson and others advocating large fraction irradiation.[4–11] Order and associates demonstrated the superiority of radiation over surgery for most patients, in particular, those with primary sites originating in the lung.[12] They evaluated the functional improvement accomplished by radiation and showed that a high palliative index could be achieved by radiotherapy of brain metastases. With increasing duration of survival, the functional improvement as a fraction of survival time (palliative index) decreased and was only 31% for patients surviving one year after treatment. This suggested that supplemental irradiation to a small volume containing gross disease might be needed in patients with a longer prognosis.

In two large studies totaling 1,800 patients, RTOG evaluated various radiation fractionation schemes ranging from 2,000 rad in one week to 4,000 rad in 4 weeks for their relative efficacy employing whole brain irradiation.[2] Carcinoma of the lung was the most common source of metastases (60%), while breast was second most common (17%). More than 75% of patients improved in at least one functional category, regardless of the fractionation scheme. Those receiving the larger fraction sizes and shorter courses demonstrated more prompt improvement. Median survival varied between 15 and 18 weeks before the two portions of the study; the palliative index was equal in all dose groups.

The patients were divided into four classes of neurologic function ranging from ability to work and perform normal activities (I) to severe impairment of activities requiring hospitalization and constant nursing care (IV). Improvement in neurologic function from one class to another was, of course, not measurable in class I patients and was rare in class IV patients. Among class II and III patients, improvement occurred in 38% in the first study and in 34% in the second study. With patients in neurologic function class III (*i.e.*, requiring nursing care or hospitalization and with serious limitations on performance), improvement was shown in 60% in the first study and 69% in the second. Some 16% and 23%, respectively, improved from class III to class I. The improvement in neurologic function was related to a number of covariates. Improvement was greater in patients who were ambulatory, who had brain as the only site of metastasis, and in whom the primary was absent (Table 41-3).[2]

Specific symptoms were relieved in a higher percentage of patients since movement from one neurologic category to another required greater improvement than relief of a particular symptom. As shown in Table 41-4, complete relief of symptoms ranged from 52% of 500 patients with headache to 32% of 454 patients with motor loss.[2] These refer to complete responses; overall responses (complete and partial) were 82% and 74%, respectively. Some 80% of patients who showed improved Karnofsky performance status also improved in neurologic status; thus, the results of performance status were similar to those for neurologic function.

Overall median survival was 18 weeks in the first RTOG study and 15 weeks in the second RTOG study, with no significant difference among treatment schedules. Ambulatory patients survived longer (21 week median) than nonambulatory patients (12 week median). The breast cancer patients, as a group, survived longer (21 week median) than lung cancer patients (16 week median). Lung cancer patients

TABLE 41-3. Percent of Patients Showing Improvement in Neurologic Function and Other Covariates According to Initial Neurologic Function Class

	INITIAL NEUROLOGIC FUNCTION CLASS II		INITIAL NEUROLOGIC FUNCTION CLASS III	
COVARIATE	*First Study*	*Second Study*	*First Study*	*Second Study*
Lung	38 (259)*	37 (197)	62 (195)	72 (196)
Breast	38 (80)	32 (53)	66 (50)	66 (67)
Ambulatory (performance 1 and 2)	42 (335)	39 (244)	76 (41)	88 (40)
Nonambulatory (performance 3–5)	22 (87)	23 (109)	56 (278)	67 (319)
Brain only site of metastases	40 (250)	41 (153)	64 (171)	73 (148)
Brain with other metastases	35 (172)	29 (200)	56 (148)	66 (211)
Primary absent	42 (222)	37 (150)	63 (142)	72 (134)
Primary present	33 (200)	33 (181)	58 (177)	68 (206)
Chemotherapy	26 (76)	29 (66)	65 (49)	70 (83)
No chemotherapy	41 (336)	38 (238)	52 (251)	70 (232)

*Number in parenthesis is total number of patients.

Borgelt B, Gelber R, Kramer S et al: The palliation of brain metastases: Final results of the first two studies by the Radiation Therapy Oncology Group. Int J Radiat Oncol Biol Phys 6:1–9, 1980

TABLE 41-4. Relief of Specific Neurologic Symptoms

	FIRST RTOG STUDY		
	Number of Patients	*Complete Response (%)*	*Overall Response (%)*
Headache	500	52	82
Motor Loss	454	32	74
Impaired Mentation	355	34	71
Cerebellar Dysfunction	218	39	75
Cranial Nerve	215	40	71
Increased Intracranial			
Pressure	165	57	83
General	108	66	86
Convulsions	85	48	76
Focal			
Sensory Loss	175	41	77
Lethargy	237	39	69

Borgelt B, Gelber R, Kramer S et al: The palliation of brain metastases: Final results of the first two studies by the Radiation Therapy Oncology Group. Int J Radiat. Oncol Biol Phys 6:1–9, 1980

with brain as the only site of metastasis and the primary absent in the second study (who received 4,000 rad) survived significantly longer than the other groups (47 week median). Brain metastasis as a cause of death was reported in 49% of patients in the first study and 31% in the second study. Thus, in spite of radiotherapy, up to half of the patients will eventually develop recurrence of their brain lesions prior to death due to other metastases.

The palliative index, as originally proposed by Order and coworkers, was also evaluated in this study.[12] For all patients in this study, 75–80% of remaining life was spent in either an improved or stable neurologic state.

A study reported by West and Maor revealed that a schedule of 2,000 rad in one week or 3,000 rad in 2 weeks was as effective as more protracted schedules, findings identical to those of the randomized RTOG study.[13] Thus, the radiation therapy technique to be recommended for most patients is 3,000 rad to the whole brain in 2 weeks. The RTOG study does suggest, however, that the ambulatory patient with brain metastases as the only site of active disease may benefit from increased doses, particularly to one or a small number of easily localized lesions that would be amenable to a higher radiation dose in a boost field. The study by West and Maor also indicates that adenocarcinoma of the lung has a significantly longer survival than other histologies with a one-year survival of approximately 50% and a 2-year survival of close to 30%. Thus, patients with adenocarcinoma of the lung who meet the above-listed criteria may also benefit from increased dosage.

FUTURE DIRECTIONS

It is possible that radiotherapy of metastatic disease to the brain may be improved through using chemical modifiers of radiation effect and improved use of CT. Previous studies of radiation therapy on brain metastases relied primarily on neurologic function and general functional status to evaluate response. With these endpoints, it has been possible to show a significant difference between radiation doses ranging from 2,000 rad in one week to 5,000 rad in 4 weeks. It is possible that this failure is due not to the fact that the higher doses were not more effective, but to the non-specificity of the crude functional endpoints. The routine use of serial CT scans may allow evaluation not only of response rates but also of delayed regrowth for brain metastases and the incidence of permanent control. It will also allow better evaluation of symptoms due to radiation effect rather than recurrent tumor. From these observations, hopefully the value of higher doses and higher dose boosts, in particular, will be forthcoming. Such evaluation may also allow the employment of biologically more effective radiation modalities, such as neutrons or heavy charged particles in treatment.

Of particular interest in treatment is the application of hypoxic cell sensitizers. Most brain metastases show necrotic centers at CT scanning or surgery and obviously contain significant hypoxic cell zones. The RTOG is currently evaluating the effect of misonidazole on treatment of brain metastases. In a Phase II study, the RTOG treated 40 patients with misonidazole (2 g/m^2) twice per week for 3 weeks, with doses of 600 rad. Using this scheme, eight of nine patients with serial CT scans showed significant improvement in the size of the lesions; 23 of 34 patients showed clinical improvement. The time to progression was 3.7 months and the mean survival 4.2 months. The study suggested in this group of patients (all of whom had other metastases as well), a representative poor risk group, that response may have been increased. A Phase III randomized trial is now underway comparing 300 rad × 10, and 500 rad × 6 with and without misonidazole to determine whether this sensitizer may improve the response to radiation in cerebral radiation.

SURGERY IN THE MANAGEMENT OF CEREBRAL METASTASIS

In most patients noted with clear indications for surgery, the task is obviously to remove the lesion in its totality, if possible, without compromising cerebral function. Although metastatic lesions are highly malignant, they are often well demarcated from surrounding normal brain and can be totally removed. The surgical techniques are essentially the same as for primary tumors with the exception that resection of surrounding normal brain, such as lobectomy, is rarely indicated. Results of a selected number of surgical treatment reports are given in Table 41-5. Highly selected patients studied by Galicich and coworkers, who had only solitary lesions and who received postoperative irradiation in most cases, did quite well.[14] Although there was a 12% operative mortality, there was a 44% one-year survival and an 8 month median survival. These are both greater than in series with radiation therapy alone, although exactly comparable cases with solitary lesions are not available. The series of Winston and coworkers showed median survivals and one-year survivals not different from radiation therapy alone, but this study was not limited to solitary lesions.[15] The series of Vieth and coworkers suffers from a higher surgical mortality and much poorer diagnostic methods. Many of these patients had multiple lesions therefore, a very poor one-year survival was obtained.

TABLE 41-5. Results of Surgical Treatment of Brain Metastases

AUTHOR	NO. OF CASES	OPERATIVE MORTALITY	MEDIAN SURVIVAL	1 YEAR SURVIVAL
Galicich et al	33*	12%	8 Mo.	44%
Winston et al	79	10%	5 Mo.	22%
Vieth et al	155	15%	N.A.	14%

*Solitary lesions only

Galicich JH, Sundaresan N, Thaler HT: Surgical treatment of single brain metastases. J Neurosurg 53:63–67, 1980

Winston KR, Walsh JW, Fischer EG: Results of operative treatment of intracranial metastatic tumors. Cancer 45:2639–2645, 1980

Vieth RG Odom GL: Intracranial metastases and their neurological treatment. J Neurosurg 23:375–383, 1965

The recent report by Winston and coworkers emphasizes that 53% of neurologically impaired patients who survived at least one month after surgery were improved in condition, while only 5% were made worse.[15] They point out the influence of primary site on survival at one year in many cases drawn from the literature. Their best estimates of survival at one year after craniotomy are 48% for breast cancer and 34% for unknown primary (see Table 41-6). They also point out that survival has markedly increased in reports published since 1965 and that half of their patients who survived for more than one year had not been irradiated, indicating that surgery alone is capable of prolonged survival of limited intracranial metastases.

Galicich and coworkers reported on 33 patients who were treated surgically for solitary brain metastases, then received postoperative irradiation.[14] In this group, median survival was 8 months; one-year survival 44%, while one-year survival was 81% in those who had no evidence of other metastases at craniotomy. Only three patients died of recurrent disease in the CNS. The data indicate that recurrence in the CNS following surgery combined with radiation is far lower than with radiation alone. Therefore, patients who might benefit from such prolonged suppression of symptoms should have surgery.

TABLE 41-6. Influence of Site of Origin on Survival after Craniotomy

Breast	48%
Unknown Primary	34%
Melanoma	32%
Renal Cell	27%
Lung	19%

Winston KR, Walsh JW, Fischer CG: Results of operative treatment of intracranial metastatic tumors. Cancer 45:2639–2645, 1980

Review of the pertinent publications suggests that there is a definite subset of patients who could benefit from resection of cerebral metastases followed by radiotherapy. These include patients who are ambulatory; have no evidence of active disease in the primary site or other metastatic foci outside the brain; whose brain metastases are solitary; and whose lesions are in accessible, silent portions of the brain, resection of which will not increase neurologic deficit. Patients meeting these criteria should be offered resection followed by radiotherapy.

Treatment of Metastatic Cancer to Lung

with M. WAYNE FLYE

Approximately 30% of patients with malignant disease will have pulmonary metastases at some time during the clinical course of their disease. Almost 20% of patients dying with pulmonary metastases have no other foci of disease detectable at autopsy.[15a] Pulmonary metastases represent the major and often the only site of recurrence in a number of childhood tumors, including Wilms' tumor and Ewing's sarcoma. In addition, pulmonary metastases may represent the only site of failure in testicular tumors, as well as bone and soft tissue sarcomas. The extensive use of aggressive adjuvant combination chemotherapy has reduced the incidence of pulmonary metastases as a clinical problem in most childhood solid tumors and in certain adult tumors, with particular success achieved recently with carcinomas of the testis. In spite of these successes, chemotherapy has not eliminated the occurrence of such metastases completely. Therefore, they continue to be a major problem.

Current approaches to the management of lung metastases include chemotherapy for tumors sensitive to drugs, radiotherapy to augment chemotherapy, and pulmonary resection of focal discrete lesions. Although tolerance to radiation of the thoracic area is limited, it may be effective in sterilizing microscopic disease in combination with small field boost irradiation of gross nodules visible on chest film. The largest experience with radiotherapy in the treatment of pulmonary metastases has been in the childhood solid tumors, testicular tumors, Hodgkin's disease, and in soft tissue and bone sarcomas. The results of such treatment with radiation alone have been marginal, but they have been markedly augmented by the combination of radiotherapy and chemotherapy. While

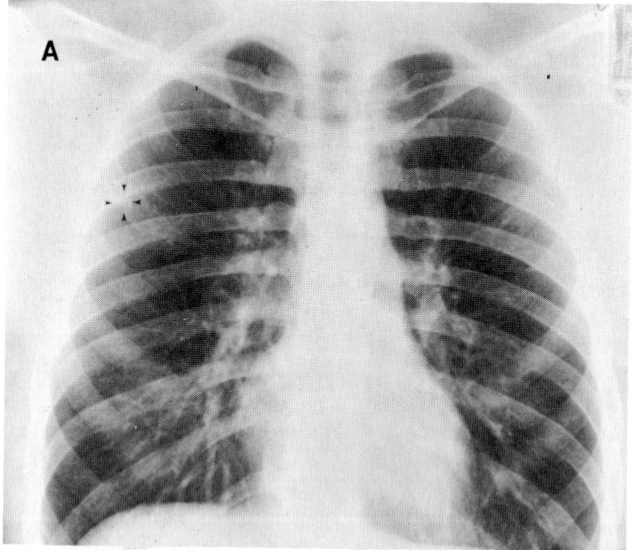

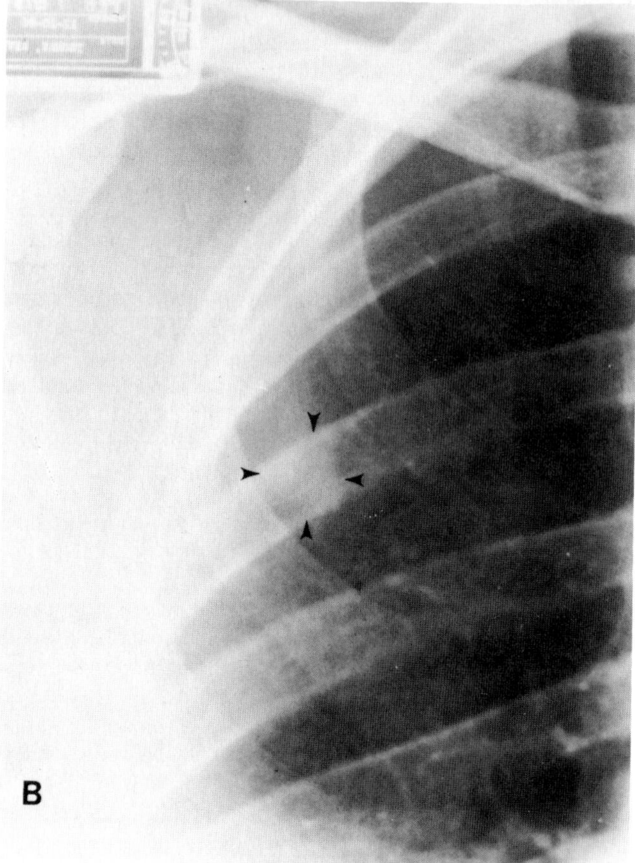

FIG. 41-1. *A,* Poorly defined metastasis in the right upper lobe of a PA chest roentgenogram, 22 months after below knee amputation for an undifferentiated neurofibrosarcoma of the ankle in a 20-year-old Caucasian male. *B,* A spot film allows better definition of right upper lobe lesion in Fig. 41-1*A*.

surgery is generally a modality best suited for the treatment of focal discrete lesions, pulmonary resection in cases where the systemic spread of a malignancy is limited to the lungs offers a significant chance for cure or prolonged survival.

PATHOGENESIS OF LUNG METASTASES

In humans, most sarcomas and some carcinomas tend to metastasize by the hematogenous route while most carcinomas spread by way of the lymphatics. While lymphogenous metastases begin with a regional lymph node and progressively spread along the lymphatic chains, hematogenous metastases to the lung or liver occur relatively early in the course of the disease.[16] The likelihood of metastatic development is thought to rest on the state of differentiation and the anatomic extent of the primary tumor. Generally, the more undifferentiated cancer is more invasive, and the degree of mitosis and pleomorphism is an index of its aggressiveness and metastatic potential. These characteristics usually are translated into tumor grading. The correlation between survival and grade supports the view that metastases occur with increasing frequency as cancer cells shift from a well-differentiated type to an anaplastic variety.[15] Blood borne dissemination to the lungs and liver is due to the peculiar anatomic relationship of these organs, which serve as filters for the systemic and portal circulations, respectively.

Hematogenous spread of most tumors is to the lung since the venous blood return of most organs is to the right side of the heart and from there to the pulmonary capillary bed. This includes tumors of the head and neck, lungs, kidney, testis, melanoma originating from skin, osteochondrosarcomas, liver, and endocrine tumors.[17] Organs drained by the systemic venous system give rise to 84% of solitary metastases. Except for rare occurrences, it is not possible for a tumor to gain access to the arterial circulation without first establishing a pulmonary metastasis. However, blood borne metastases originating from the GI tract drain into the portal circulation and are first filtered by the liver so that it is unusual for the lungs to contain the only metastases; however, they usually serve as a second relay area of metastases. In addition to hematogenous metastases, tumor cells may enter the venous circulation from the lymphatics, by way of the thoracic duct.

DIAGNOSIS

In an attempt to detect pulmonary metastases as early as possible, frequent chest roentgenograms should be obtained following primary tumor resection.[18] Conventional linear x-ray tomography has also been useful in detecting additional pulmonary nodules in 30–35% of cases (see Fig. 41-1).[19] While this modality has also been shown to be a sensitive screening study for detection of metastatic disease in the presence of a normal chest film, it underestimates the number of pulmonary metastases found at surgery in 30–50% of cases. The new technique of computed tomography (CT) is more sensitive than conventional tomography in detecting small pulmonary nodules. CT detects 78% of all nodules greater

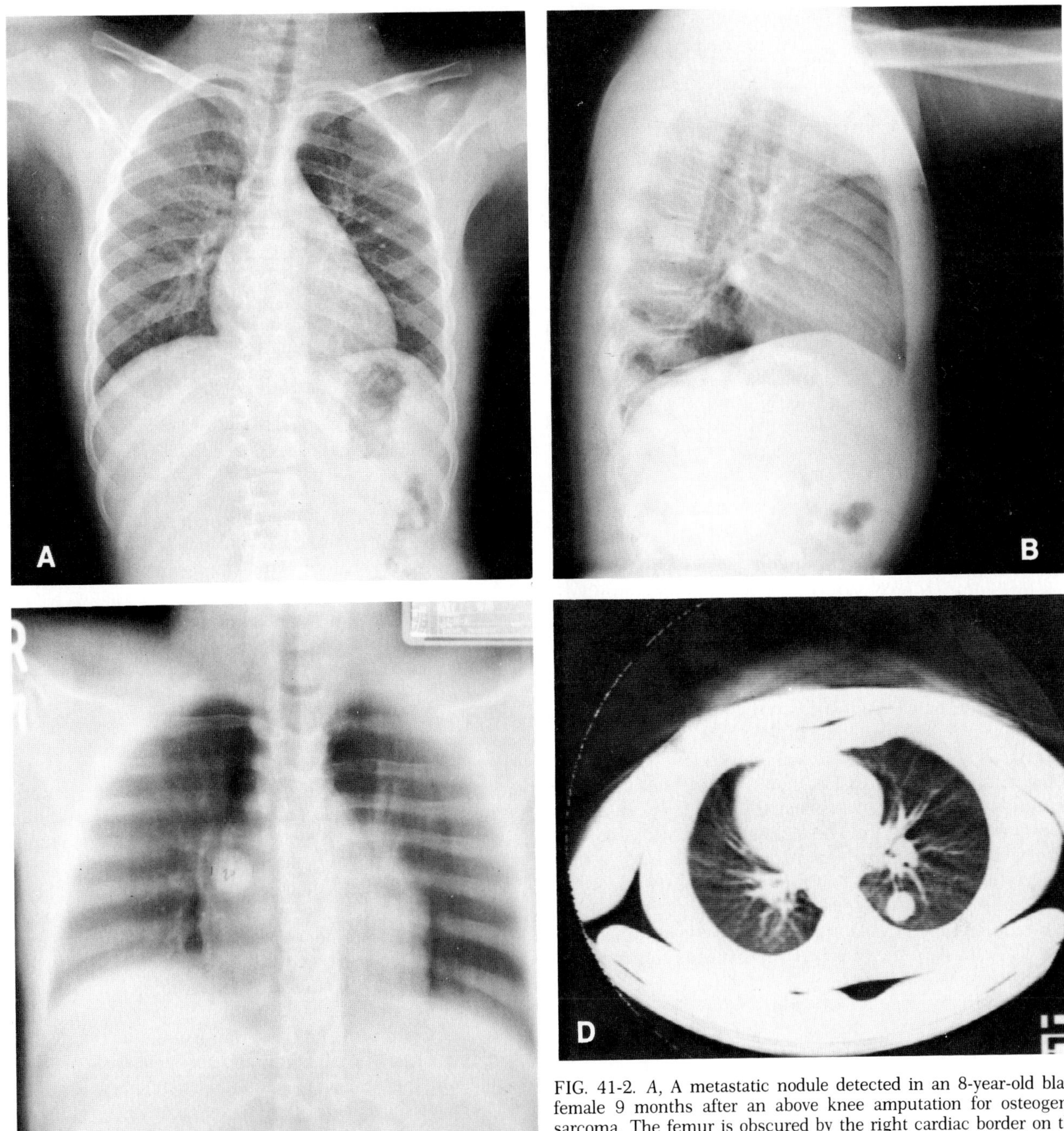

FIG. 41-2. *A*, A metastatic nodule detected in an 8-year-old black female 9 months after an above knee amputation for osteogenic sarcoma. The femur is obscured by the right cardiac border on the PA chest roentgenogram. *B*, The metastasis is seen overlying the thoracic spine on a lateral chest roentgenogram. *C*, A full lung tomogram clearly shows the metastatic deposit posterior to the right hilum. *D*, Computerized axial tomography also shows the single metastasis in the right posterior lung.

than 3 mm in diameter subsequently removed at thoracotomy, compared to 59% for conventional tomography (see Fig. 41-2).[19] However, 60% of the additional nodules are benign, thus diminishing the specificity for identifying metastatic nodules (see Table 41-7).

In contrast to patients with primary bronchogenic carcinoma where 90% have some symptoms at diagnosis, only about one-third of patients with isolated pulmonary metastases have symptoms.[20] Although seldom directly related to the metastases, these may include cough, hemoptysis, chest pain, shortness of breath, fatigue, and wheezing. Also, unlike the primary bronchogenic tumors, sputum cytology reveals malignant cells in only 5% of patients and bronchoscopy provided significant findings in only 10% of patients examined.[17] Lack of positive bronchoscopic findings and symptoms, as well as the negative cytologic results of sputum and bronchial aspi-

TABLE 41-7. Results of Preoperative Chest Film (CXR), Conventional Tomography (CLT), and Computed Axial Tomography (CAT)

	CXR	CLT*	CAT†
Nodules visible	21	38	69
Nodules found at operation‡	21 (100%)	32 (84%)	47 (68%)
Nodules proved metastatic	19 (90%)	25 (66%)	31 (45%)
Percent of total metastatic nodules found§	36%	47%	58%

*Includes all nodules visible on CXR.
†Includes all nodules visible on CLT.
‡Percentage based on nodules visible.
§53 metastatic nodules resected.
Chang AE, Schaner EG, Conkle DM et al: Evaluation of computed tomography in the detection of pulmonary metastases. Cancer 43:913, 1979

rate, reflect the usual peripheral location of the metastatic lesions and the infrequent involvement of the bronchus.

In patients who have multiple lung lesions and a known cancer outside the lung, lesions are likely to be metastatic. The appearance of a solitary pulmonary lesion in patients with a known extrapulmonary primary raises three possibilities: a new and separate cancer of the lung; metastases from the known cancer; or a benign lesion. While there is less than a 1% chance of a solitary nodule being a metastasis if there is no previous history of cancer, this increases to 81% for the group with a previous malignancy.[15] However, this varies according to the type of previous cancer. If the previous primary was of the head and neck, prostate, trachea, stomach, or breast, a solitary pulmonary nodule is most likely a new primary cancer of the lung. If the initial primary was of GI or genitourinary origin, it has an equal chance of being a metastatic or new primary cancer of the lung. It is much more likely to be a metastasis if the previous tumor was a sarcoma or melanoma.[17]

SURGICAL TREATMENT OF PULMONARY METASTASES

Prior to 1927, metastatic lung disease was not treated by pulmonary resection. This reflects the state of intrathoracic surgery at that time. Divis, of Germany, performed the first successful resection of a pulmonary metastasis. Four years later in the U.S., Torek was the first to successfully resect a pulmonary metastasis, although preoperatively it had been considered to be a primary tumor.[17] The stimulus for surgical efforts to cure patients with pulmonary metastases was provided by a report by Barney and Churchill in 1939 whose patient died of coronary artery disease 23 years after wedge resection of a solitary pulmonary metastasis from an adenocarcinoma of the kidney.[21]

Initially, the acceptance of surgery in the treatment of pulmonary metastases was slow and very selective. Resection was undertaken only in rare instances when the primary tumor site remained under control, with a long disease-free interval and with the metastatic disease solitary or limited to one lung. In 1947, Alexander and Haight reported apparent cures in three of six patients following metastatic resection.[22] Surprisingly, in 1965, Thomford and coworkers reported almost identical postoperative survival rates between unilateral solitary and multiple carcinoma and sarcoma lung metastases.[21] Martini and coworkers and Morton and coworkers later found that the survival rates after surgical resection of multiple metastatic lesions, even when they were bilateral, were comparable to those after resection of solitary lung lesions.[22,23]

For surgical resection of pulmonary metastases to offer hope for cure there must be a high probability that this represents the only site of residual tumor. Because of the tumor's contrast with the surrounding aerated lung on radiograph, detection of early metastases to the lung is easier than to other locations. It is often difficult to determine whether a single nodule seen on chest film is truly a solitary lesion or the first sign of wide dissemination. Now it is well appreciated that it is uncommon for patients with malignancy of the abdominal viscera to present solely with pulmonary metastases and that an exhaustive search for tumor in other organs must be made before pulmonary resection should be performed.[24] It is not unusual, however, for patients with sarcoma, melanoma, or extra-abdominal carcinoma to develop pulmonary nodules as the only clinically evident disease.

PRETREATMENT EVALUATION

Preoperative evaluation differs according to primary tumor type because the pattern of metastatic spread changes according to the histological type. As with primary bronchopulmonary cancers, if a metastasis is diagnosed at a time that it is giving rise to symptoms, the results of resection are much less favorable than when it is resected at its asymptomatic stage. Therefore, the usefulness of periodic radiographic examinations of former cancer patients is obvious. Sarcomas generally metastasize first to lung in preference to other sites. Carcinomas, on the other hand, tend to metastasize to more than one distant site, usually including the liver, and therefore a more careful screening program is required to select those patients whose lungs contain the only detectable metastases. Malignant melanoma can simultaneously spread to any organ system and the cause of death is frequently due to metastases to the CNS. Since the chance of having the disease confined to lung is small, these patients must fulfill the most stringent clinical criteria for resection of pulmonary metastases. In contrast, the clinical course of a hypernephroma is often characterized by long intervals between control of the primary tumor and development of metastases, which are frequently confined to the lung.[25]

Except in the case of chemoresponsive primary testicular cancers, the following are accepted as the minimal criteria for the operability of pulmonary metastases: the primary tumor should be completely controlled or controllable; no extrapulmonary metastatic sites should be demonstrable; and all metastases must be resectable. The Sloan-Kettering Memorial Hospital (Memorial Hospital) group also uses the criterion that no other therapy be available.[26,27]

CRITERIA FOR PATIENT SELECTION AND INFLUENCE ON RESULTS: THE DISEASE-FREE INTERVAL FROM CONTROL OF THE PRIMARY TUMOR TO METASTASES

In general, the longer the disease-free interval between primary and metastatic treatment, the more favorable the prognosis. In a mixed group of 140 patients with carcinomas or sarcomas undergoing 161 pulmonary resections for metastases, Wilkins found that the 5-year survival was 34%, regardless of whether the disease-free interval was less than or more than two years.[20] However, for 18 patients, the removal of metastases before or synchronous with the primary resulted in a 5-year survival of 15.1%; this was considered one of the few contraindications to surgical resection. Ramming and coworkers found that the median survival time of 91 patients who underwent resection of pulmonary metastases from carcinoma or sarcoma was 9 months when the disease interval was 6 months or less.[25] This increased to greater than 2.6 years when the disease-free interval was 12 months or more.

The Roswell Park group reported that the 5-year survival of patients who had resection of solitary pulmonary metastases of all types was 29.6% if the disease-free interval was less than one year, 37% for 1–4 years, and 50.6% if the interval was more than 4 years. When all patients were compared, regardless of the number of metastatic nodules removed, the median survival of 86 patients with a disease-free interval of 12 months or less was 19.7 months compared to 27.3 months for those disease-free for more than 12 months.[28]

Using a 3 year follow-up interval, Thomford and coworkers reported survivals of 26.6%, 42.6%, and 40.6% for disease-free intervals of less than one year, 1–4 years, and more than 4 years, respectively.[21] The Memorial Hospital group, on the other hand, has found that neither the number and size of metastases nor the disease-free interval is a primary factor in survival but that the site of origin of the primary tumor influences survival the most.[26,29]

Number of Metastatic Nodules

Prior to this last decade, pulmonary metastases were not resected unless they were solitary. Recently, an increasingly aggressive approach has been taken regardless of the number of metastases. At Roswell Park the median survival of 18.3 months for multiple metastases was not significantly less than 24.7 months for solitary metastases.[30] For 585 patients at Memorial Hospital with all types of metastases the 5-year survival rate was 15% for multiple lesions and 25% when metastases were solitary.[31]

Thomford and coworkers reported that 34% of 221 pulmonary resections for all types of metastases revealed multicentricity.[21] Whereas the one year survival was 66.7 for multiple lesions and 81.3 for solitary lesions, the 5-year survivals of 30% and 31%, respectively, were not different.

The origin of the pulmonary metastases particularly influences the results of resection. Multiple nodules from Ewing's sarcoma or malignant melanoma are considered a contraindication to surgery by some authors and are indicators of a poor prognosis for patients with colon or breast cancer.[25] In contrast, for patients with osteogenic or fibrosarcomas and carcinomas from the head, neck, and testis, the results with multiple metastases are similar to those for single lesions.[32]

Unilateral vs. Bilateral Pulmonary Metastases

The results of metastatic treatment from a primary carcinoma or sarcoma to both lungs are comparable to those for multiple unilateral lesions except for testicular metastases.[25] The poorer results for the bilateral testicular metastases probably reflect the delay in treatment of a rapidly dividing tumor when staged bilateral thoracotomies are used. When a median sternotomy is used to approach both lungs simultaneously the results are similar for unilateral and bilateral involvement.[28]

Tumor Doubling Time

A number of biological systems grow exponentially at first. However, later, when the number of cells increases and there is competition for nutrition, the growth curve flattens. The growth of solid tumors is also characterized by retardation, which increases with time. This retardation is caused by immunologic suppression, limitation of nutrition, and, most importantly, decrease in blood supply, evident microscopically as tumor necrosis. These factors cause a longer generation time of cancer cells with a resulting increase in the mean generation and doubling times. This tumor growth is best expressed by the Gompertzian equation, which expressed exponential growth when the tumor is small and contains a retarding factor; this increases exponentially with time to fit the decreasing growth rate when the tumor is large.[32]

The growth of lung metastases in humans appears to be closer to an exponential rate than tumors in other locations. This may be because the lung tissue provides a particularly favorable environment. Actually, the interval between 10 mm in diameter, when a metastasis is regularly visible on roentgenogram, and 100 mm, when the host is near death, is such a short and selected segment relative to the total life history of the neoplasm that arguments over whether the growth is logarithmic, Gompertzian, linear, or other are impossible to resolve. Growth during this interval may be interpreted as a straight line when a lesion is measured at two points in time.

Collins, when pioneering in this work, used such measurements. Tumor growth kinetics have since been examined to determine their prognostic value.[33] The tumor doubling times (TDT) of pulmonary metastases or primary lung tumors have been studied most frequently because of the ease of precisely measuring a nodule, denser than the surrounding aerated lung, on at least two chest roentgenograms taken under identical conditions and separated by a suitable time interval. The changing diameters of each nodule are plotted on semilogarithmic paper along the ventrical axis against time (in days) between determinations on the horizontal axis.[16] The slope of the line between the points represents the tumor growth rate and the horizontal distance between any two doubling points represents the TDT in days (see Fig. 41-3).

It is agreed that for all human tumors in which the TDT has been measured there is a relationship between growth rate and prognosis. In general, the shorter the TDT, the shorter the patient survival. This is most dramatically demonstrated by the study performed by Joseph and coworkers

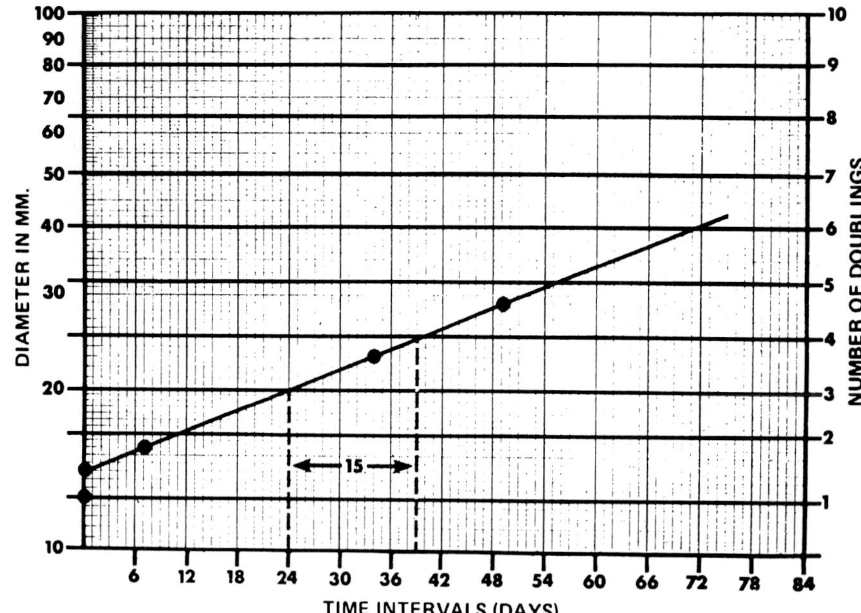

FIG. 41-3. Tumor doubling time (TDT) is estimated by plotting the changing diameters of metastatic pulmonary nodules on semilogarithmic paper (Joseph WL, Morton DL, Adkins PC: J Thor Cardiovasc Surg 61:23, 1971)

of 113 patients with pulmonary metastases from sarcomas and carcinomas.[34] Some 89 patients who had no further treatment after the onset of metastatic lung lesions were grouped according to TDT of 20 days and less, 21–40 days, and more than 40 days. The 1-year survivals of these groups were 11%, 45%, and 86%, respectively. None of the untreated patients survived 2 years. Of the 17 patients with TDTs of less than 20 days who were treated by resection of pulmonary metastases, all were dead within 18 months (see Fig. 41-4). There were no survivors beyond 30 months in the group of 17 patients with TDTs of 20–40 days treated surgically. Surprisingly, 97% of patients with TDTs greater than 40 days undergoing surgical resection were alive at 2 years and 63% at 5 years. Of the 26 patients in this third group 14 had undergone resection of bilateral pulmonary metastases.[23]

The results reported by Takita and coworkers were not as striking.[30] When the survival of 67 patients undergoing resection of lung metastases was determined for TDTs of less than 75 days and more than 75 days, the 5-year survival was 30% and 60%, respectively.

In 12 patients with metastatic osteogenic sarcoma, Giritsky reported that the TDT averaged 22 days when the patients were receiving no chemotherapy or radiation.[35] When the patients were receiving multi-drug chemotherapy during three different periods the average TDT was 74 days. This suggests that for those metastases responsive to irradiation or chemotherapy, the biological character of the tumor might be modified so that improved results can be obtained by surgical resection.

There is also a correlation between the TDT and the interval between resection of the primary lesion and the onset of pulmonary metastases. Generally, the longer the disease-free interval before detection of metastatic disease, the longer the TDT. That there is a link between tumor growth rate and prognosis seems firmly established not only as deducted from the observations on pulmonary metastases but also those made on breast and bronchogenic tumors.[15,36] This raises the question of whether there is a link between tumor growth and its tendency to metastasize since the cure rate is higher in slow growing tumors. There is no evidence thus far to indicate that even though metastases appear earlier in fast growing tumors, that they appear more often than in slow growing tumors.[15]

Histologic Type of the Primary Tumor

In spite of location and accessibility of pathways of spread, the character of the malignant tumor itself often decides its potential to disseminate as well as the eventual site of metastases. It is obvious that any generalizations about metastases, especially pulmonary metastases, that do not take into consideration the unique behavior of the various malignant tumors are idle speculations.

TECHNIQUE OF SURGICAL RESECTION

Many metastatic lesions are located peripherally and subpleurally, making them accessible to palpation and removal with wedge excisions. Resection is predicated on the findings that spread from a pulmonary metastasis is hematogenous and not lymphatic, as is the case with primary bronchogenic carcinoma. The latter lesion is usually resected by an anatomic lobectomy or pneumonectomy to encompass possible lymph node involvement. It is generally accepted that a margin of 1–2 cm of healthy pulmonary tissue around the metastasis should be removed, but with maximal conservation of lung tissue. Seldom are metastases positioned so that a lobectomy or pneumonectomy is required for complete removal.[26] Patients found to have only unilateral pulmonary metastases after a complete work-up may be explored through an anterolateral thoracotomy to minimize the greater pain associated with a muscle dividing the posterolateral incision. The appropriate rib interspace is divided and a small segment of rib is removed posteriorly to allow easier rib retraction. If lesions are present bilaterally, a median sternotomy allows resection of lesions in both lungs simultaneously. However, if the patient has adhesions from previous thoracotomies (*i.e.*, emphysema, which would make collapse of the lung difficult, or medially based lesions, which might make adequate resection difficult), bilateral staged thoracotomy is usually preferred. The left ventricle also makes it more difficult to approach the lower lobe.

After opening the thorax, the mediastinum and hilum of the lung are inspected for enlarged lymph nodes. If present, they are examined by frozen section while the pulmonary parenchyma is carefully examined to identify any nodular lesions. By careful palpation between thumb and fingers, nodules less than 1 mm in diameter can be identified. All nodules must be resected, even though there is a high proportion that are benign, since some do represent metastatic disease. Each lesion should be identified and marked prior to excision because resection invariably changes the configuration of the surrounding lung, making it difficult to identify new nodules.

For the peripheral lesions, a Pennington clamp can be placed on either side of the nodule and lifted outward while an automatic stapling device is placed across the base (see Fig. 41-5). This instrument comes in 30, 55, and 90 mm sizes. For lesions deeper in the parenchyma the GIA stapler, which staples and cuts simultaneously, may be used (see Fig. 41-6). This prevents the forceful traction sometimes needed for the TA stapler to be used and minimizes the chance of an inadequate margin of resection.

The mortality following surgical treatment of pulmonary metastases is low and ranges, in larger series, from 0–4%.[21,26] The few deaths reported have occurred in patients with respiratory compromise due to previous radiation or chemotherapy. Concomitant chemotherapy can contribute to morbidity, which is primarily related to incisional pain, infection, and atelectasis. In general, morbidity and mortality are lower than for resection of primary bronchogenic lung tumors because the patient population with metastatic disease is younger.

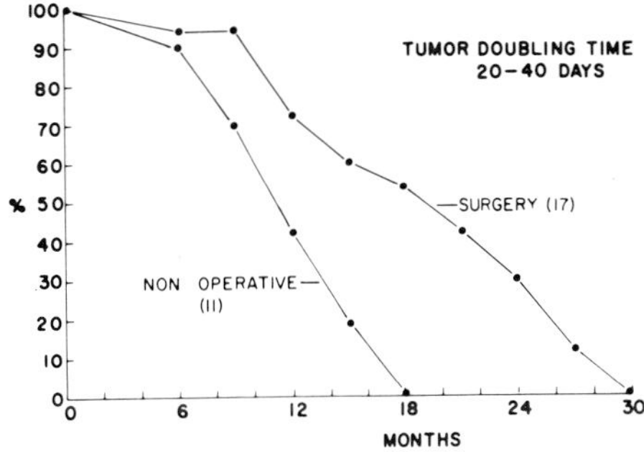

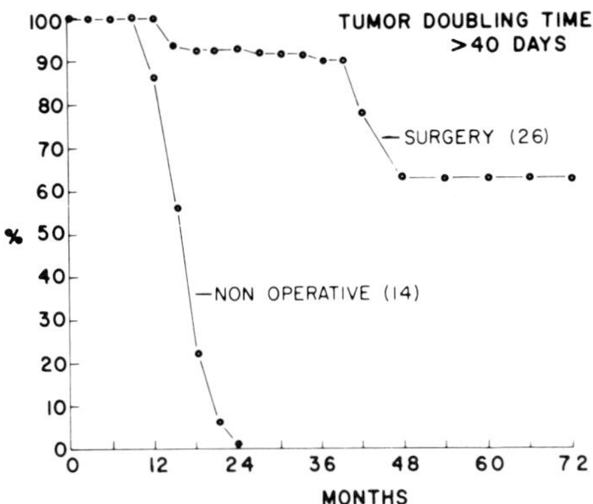

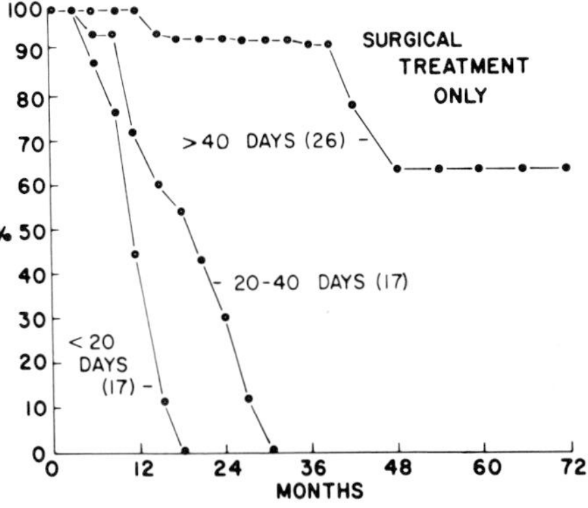

FIG. 41-4. Cumulative survival of patients after resection of pulmonary metastases grouped according to tumor doubling times of less than 20 days, 20–40 days, and more than 40 days. Number of patients in each group in parentheses. (Morton DL, Joseph WL, Ketcham AS et al: Ann Surg 178:360, 1973)

RESULTS OF SURGICAL RESECTION OF PULMONARY METASTASES

CHILDHOOD TUMORS

Although the lung is the principal site of metastasis, for most of the childhood tumors (*e.g.*, nephroblastoma or Wilms' tumor, hepatoma, hepatoblastoma, osteogenic sarcoma, Ewing's sarcoma, and rhabdomyosarcoma), lung seldom is the only site of metastases and, therefore, is rarely amenable to resection.[35] Osteogenic sarcoma represents an important exception to this pattern and is discussed with the adult tumors. The other tumors are also quite sensitive to radiotherapy and chemotherapy. Neuroblastoma, on the other hand, metastasizes principally to sites other than the lung and pulmonary involvement does not develop until after liver or bone lesions are present.

For nephroblastoma, the lungs are not only the most common metastatic site, but also the most frequent initial site of metastasis. Romansky and Landing reported that of 26 patients with a nephroblastoma, 6 had only pulmonary metastases.[36] Of these patients 5 died from massive bilateral pulmonary metastases and one from radiation pneumonitis.

The principal site of metastases for both hepatoma and hepatoblastoma is the lung, which is not surprising considering the venous drainage of the hepatic site of the primary. However, only two of 12 patients with hepatoblastoma and four of seven with hepatoma had metastases continued to the lung. The causes of death in these patients were often directly or indirectly associated with the pulmonary metastases which were not isolated.[36]

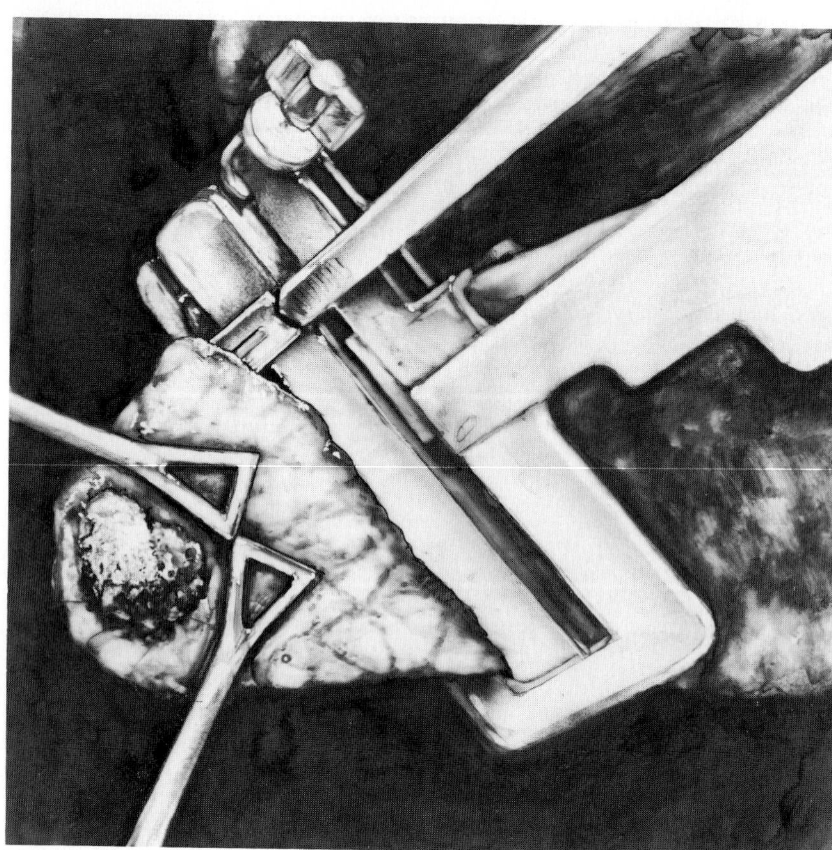

FIG. 41-5. For wedge resection of pulmonary metastases, two Pennington clamps are used to elevate the lesion and the automatic stapling device seals the lung tissue prior to transection with a scalpel.

FIG. 41-6. An alternative technique, especially for resection of deeper pulmonary lesions, is by the use of the GIA stapler which staples and divides simultaneously when the knife is advanced (*arrow*).

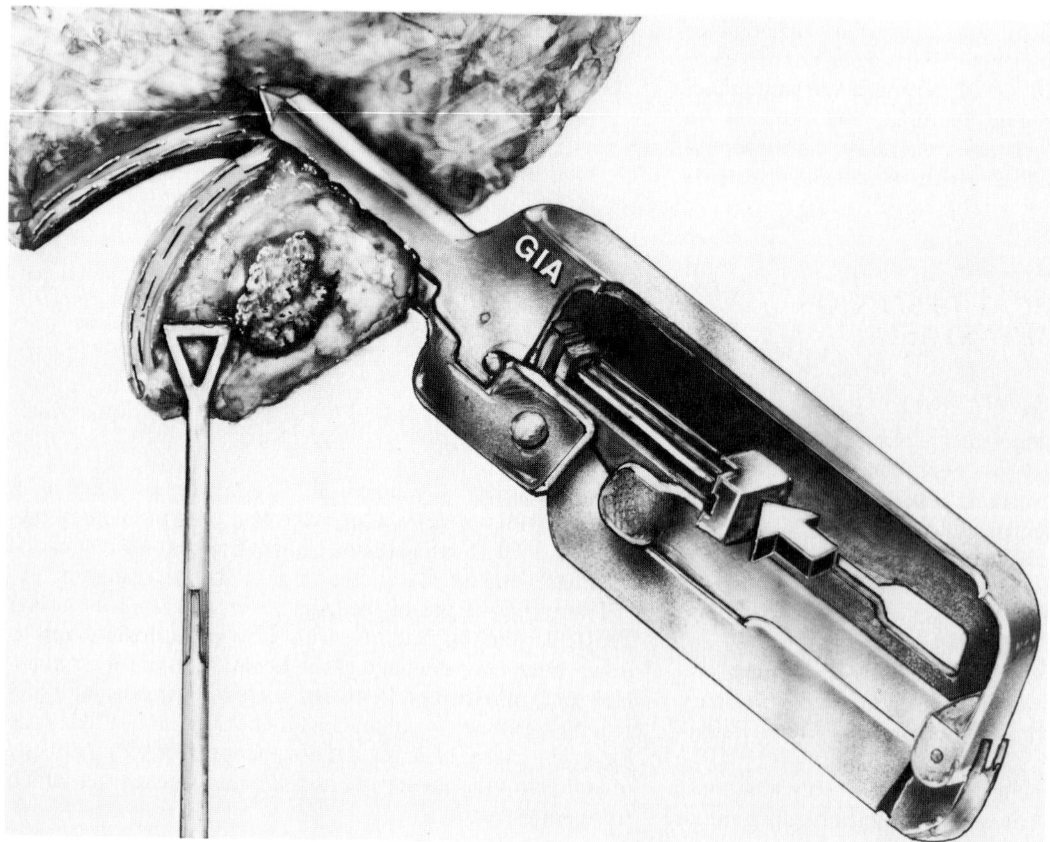

Rhabdomyosarcoma metastasis may present itself in many different sites. While the lung is the initial metastatic site for 20% of the entire group, no single anatomic primary site is peculiarly liable to produce only pulmonary metastases. Some 82% of patients with Ewing's sarcoma die from pulmonary metastases, but few have metastases confined only to the lung.[36]

Of the childhood tumors, osteogenic sarcoma metastases have been most amenable to surgical resection because, although they are relatively resistant to other therapy, they tend to metastasize primarily to the lung.[37,38] These patients often die from respiratory insufficiency if the metastases are not removed. While patients with sarcoma contribute to less than 1% of all deaths from cancer, they represent greater than 15% of the reported solitary pulmonary metastases and can be surgically resected with a 5-year survival of approximately 30% (see Table 41-8).[39]

ADULT TUMORS

In adults, the types of tumors differ from those in the pediatric group in that the metastases of many of the sarcomas and carcinomas are initially limited to the lungs. Except for trophoblastic choriocarcinoma and seminoma, most authorities feel there is currently no satisfactory mode of treatment other than surgical removal.[40]

Despite the variable routes by which a carcinoma may spread to the lungs (compared to the direct hematogenous spread of osteogenic and soft tissue sarcomas) the 5-year survival rates after resection of pulmonary metastases from carcinoma and sarcoma are comparable—approximately 30%.[3] When survival for patients with carcinoma was stratified

TABLE 41-8. Reported Survival after Resection of Pulmonary Metastases According to Site of Primary*

SITE OF PRIMARY	NO. OF PATIENTS	5-YEAR SURVIVAL (%)
Sarcoma		
Osteogenic	99	27–31
Soft Tissue†	149	20–35
	248	
Carcinoma		
Head and Neck	83	22–44
Bladder	36	33–50
Kidney	62	20–62
Uterine-Cervix	73	19–40
Colon	131	0–30
Rectum	7	52–57
Testicle	93	31–50
Breast	80	13–52
Melanoma	73	0–33
Salivary Glands	5	20
	643	

*See references 17,25,26,33,37, and 48.

†Includes fibrosarcoma; liposarcoma; undifferentiated, malignant fibrous histiocytoma; leiomyosarcoma; synoviosarcoma; angiosarcoma; neurofibrosarcoma; malignant mesenchymoma; myosarcoma; chondrosarcoma; myxosarcoma; giant cell sarcoma; rhabdomyosarcoma; hemangiopericytoma; Ewing's sarcoma.

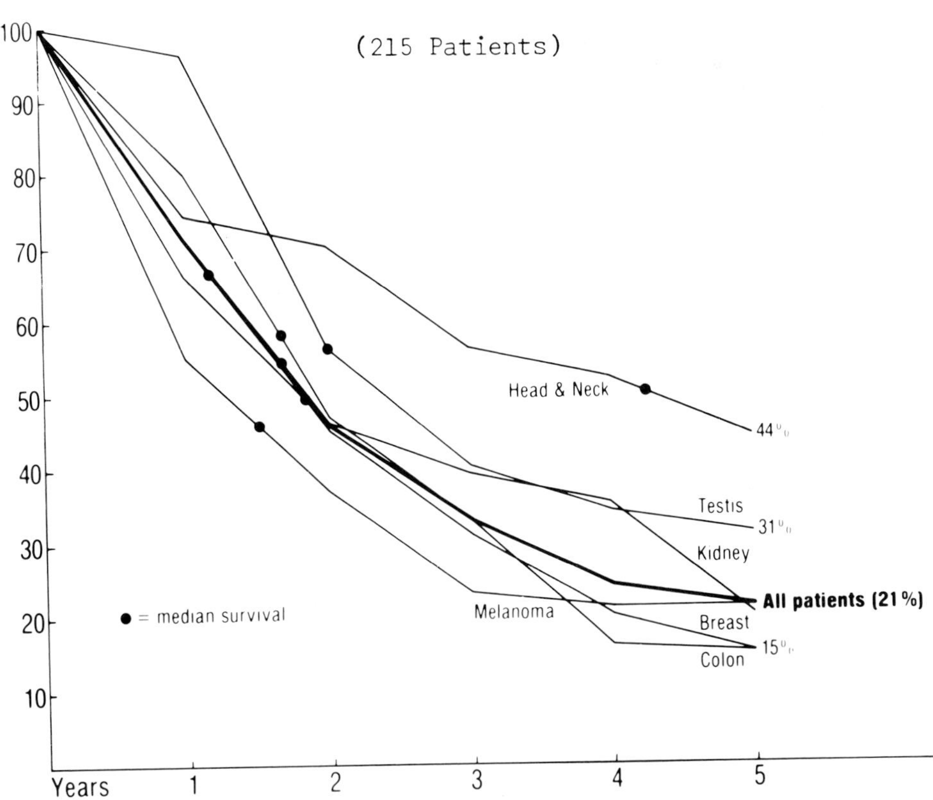

FIG. 41-7. Cumulative survival of patients after resection of pulmonary metastases from primary carcinomas (McCormack P: Surgical treatment of pulmonary metastases: The Memorial Hospital experience. In Weiss L, Gilvert HA, (eds): Pulmonary Metastasis, pp 260–270. Boston, GK Hall, 1978)

by morphology, the best prognosis was for tumors other than epidermoid carcinoma or adenocarcinoma (41% survived 5 years). The poorest prognosis was observed for patients with epidermoid carcinoma who had a 5-year survival rate of 18%.[44] The primary site of the carcinoma involvement is an important determinant of survival rates. Mountain and coworkers found that the highest 5-year survival rates were for tumors of the urinary tract (50%), male genital tract (37%), head and neck (30%), and colon-rectum (28%).[45] Similarly, McCormack and associates reported the best 5-year survival rates with tumors of the head and neck (43%) and testicle (32%).[28] In contrast, the lowest rates of survival were with carcinoma of the breast (15%) and melanoma (21%) at 5 years (see Figure 41-7, p. 1547).

Modes of Spread—Primarily Pulmonary

The mode of spread of solid tumors from the primary cancer throughout the body determines the possibility of surgical treatment. This is determined by the seeding pattern of key disseminating organs.[24] The most favorable pattern of spread for potential surgical resection is directly to the lungs from which further metastases would have to disseminate. Tumors in this group include osteogenic and soft tissue sarcomas, tumors of the head and neck, genitourinary carcinomas, testicular tumors, carcinomas of the endocrine system, and skin melanoma.

OSTEOGENIC SARCOMA. Aggressive resection of pulmonary metastases from osteogenic sarcoma was not advocated until 1970 when Marcove and coworkers reported the dismal survival results in patients treated by amputation alone at Memorial Hospital.[41] Only 17% were disease-free after 5 years. Six months after amputation of the primary tumor, 50% of the 145 patients had developed pulmonary metastases and by 12 months, this was approximately 80%. Of those that developed pulmonary metastases, 50% died within the first year, 88% within 2 years, 95% within 3 years, and none were alive at 5 years. At that time there was no effective radiation or chemotherapy.

Subsequently, when all grossly palpable pulmonary osteogenic sarcoma metastases were resected, 27% of patients were alive after 5 years. However, the other 73% of patients had relapsed and died of their disease since microscopic disease could not be detected at surgery.[22] The introduction of chemotherapy, especially high-dose methotrexate with citrovorum factor rescue, doxorubicin (adriamycin), and cyclophosphamide, appears to effectively control very small lesions before they become clinically significant and thus appears to improve surgical results.[42,43] When a regimen of "adjuvant" chemotherapy was used after the initial thoracotomy, survival was increased to 70% in 14 patients (see Fig. 41-8).

When Rosenberg and associates used adjuvant, high-dose methotrexate with leucovorin rescue, the recurrence rate for 39 patients with osteogenic sarcoma was 56.4%.[44] Of 18 patients who underwent thoracotomy for possible curative resection, 11 had all known disease resected. Although four of these 11 patients required further pulmonary resection, all were disease-free for more than 12 months (eight patients) to less than 24 months (four patients) from the time of the first recurrence. Therefore, for the entire group of 39 patients, 76.9% were alive and 71.8% had no evidence of disease with a median follow-up of 27 months. This improved survival may have been due to the high-dose methotrexate chemotherapy or to closer screening for pulmonary metastases by chest roentgenograms every 3 weeks after amputation.

SOFT TISSUE SARCOMA. The results of surgical resection of isolated pulmonary metastases from other types of sarcoma have been similar to those for osteogenic sarcoma. Of 102 patients operated on at Memorial Hospital, disease was too extensive to permit resection of all visible tumor in only 16 patients. In those patients where complete resection was possible, 26% were alive after 5 years and 17% were completely disease-free.[31] Feldman and coworkers reported better survival for soft tissue sarcomas (40%) than for osteogenic sarcoma (15%) for a group of 40 patients.[45] As for osteogenic sarcomas, the number of lesions does not appear to adversely affect the results as long as all tumor can be resected.[28]

HEAD AND NECK. Head and neck cancers, with the exception of cancers of the lip, tonsil, and adenoid, first spread to the lungs and from there to the liver, CNS, and endocrine system. Of 428 patients with primary cancers of the nose, nasopharynx, larynx, mouth, lip, tongue, salivary glands, oropharynx, tonsils, and combined head and neck, 105 had

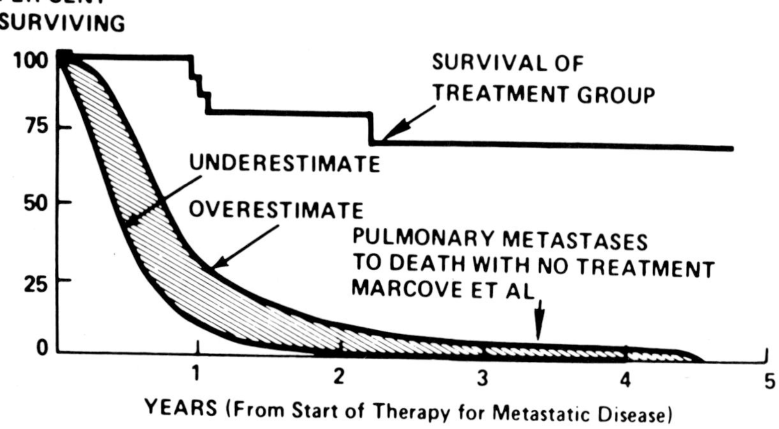

FIG. 41-8. Survival of 14 patients with pulmonary metastatic osteogenic sarcoma completely removed followed by adjuvant chemotherapy of high-dose methotrexate with citrovorum factor rescue, vincristine, doxorubicin (adriamycin), and cyclophosphamide. Their survival is compared to that of 121 patients reported by Marcove who received no treatment for the pulmonary metastases. Since there was a delay in detecting pulmonary metastases of up to 6 months the survival curve was plotted for underestimating or overestimating by 6 months. (Rosen G, Huvos AG, Mosende C et al: Cancer 41:841, 1978)

only lung metastases while 16 patients had isolated liver metastases.[24] This emphasizes that their pattern of initial spread is primarily to the lungs. The 5-year survival rate of 22–44% indicates that the results for these tumors are quite favorable (see Table 41-8). It should be kept in mind that there is also a high incidence of independently arising second primary lung tumors.

URINARY TRACT. Pulmonary metastases from genitourinary carcinomas have been one of the lesions most favorable to treatment using resection. Vincent and coworkers reported a 5-year survival of 62.5% following resection of solitary pulmonary metastases from cancers of the urinary bladder.[17] Wilkins and associates reported a 44.2% survival for 28 patients with the kidney as the primary site; Mountain and coworkers reported a 5-year survival of 50% for the urinary tract.[23,32] However, a lower 5-year survival of 20% was reported from Memorial Hospital.[26]

TESTICULAR. Testicular tumor pulmonary metastases result from hematogenous dissemination that is almost always secondary to primary lymphatic involvement. When pulmonary metastases are seen, retroperitoneal, abdominal, and often mediastinal involvement are usually also present. Therefore, the management of pulmonary metastases cannot be separated from the treatment of these other involved areas. While surgical excision for pulmonary metastases from other tumors is predicated on the absence of effective therapy by other means, the germ cell tumors of the testis are known to be sensitive to chemotherapy; in fact, chemotherapy is the primary form of therapy. Although 85% develop pulmonary metastases, surgery is recommended only when there is no response or continued progression of disease in the face of active chemotherapy or when there is partial or total response followed by prompt recurrence while on chemotherapy.[44] In these situations, thoracotomy is indicated to ascertain the histologic nature of the metastases and to determine if there has been a benign transformation as sometimes occurs in teratomas. During the thoracotomy, all palpable tumor should also be resected with minimal sacrifice of surrounding lung tissue. McCormack reported a 5-year survival of 31%; Vincent and coworkers reported that 50% of those patients who had a solitary metastasis resected survived 10 years (see Table 41-8).[17,26] In view of these results, Merrin and associates have aggressively treated patients with massive metastases using tumor reductive surgery combined with chemotherapy.[47,48] The purpose of simultaneous excision of metastases in the chest and abdomen was to reduce the tumor mass in an attempt to improve the efficiency of chemotherapy. This approach appears to be effective in producing a high percentage of complete clinical remissions in these patients.

ENDOCRINE TUMORS. The adverse effects of endocrine tumors initially resulted from inappropriate hormone production, and not until later from the mass effect of the tumor. Therefore, when their hormonal effects cannot be controlled by other measures on occasion, resection of pulmonary metastases may make the disease easier to control. This has been temporarily effective for the hypercalcemia of metastatic parathyroid carcinoma.

MELANOMA. Although malignant melanoma spreads initially to lungs after leaving its primary site or regional lymph nodes, it enjoys a reputation as an extraordinarily unpredictable disease. Although a 5-year survival of 40% can be obtained by surgical excision of the primary if regional lymphatics are involved, blood borne spread is usually an ominous sign.[51] Mathisen and coworkers found that for 22 patients operated on for isolated pulmonary metastases, no significant difference existed in mean survival between those rendered disease-free (12 months) and those deemed unresectable (10.5 months).[52] Other authors also report poor results usually with no long-term survivors. Cahan, on the other hand, reported a 33% 5-year survival for 12 patients undergoing pulmonary resection.[51]

Thoracotomy is especially useful for staging purposes in the patient with melanoma. Approximately one-third of the patients reported by Mathisen and coworkers had no metastases and, therefore, could be placed in a group with a much better prognosis.[52]

Modes of Spread—Portal Drainage

The second group of tumors are located in the abdomen or pelvis and their venous blood drains into the portal vein. Only some 9% of these tumors have pulmonary metastases without hepatic metastases. Of this group, only rectal adenocarcinoma is an exception to the pattern of spread of metastases from primary tumor to liver and then to the lungs. Adenocarcinomas located in the lower third of the rectum probably convey metastases directly to the lungs by way of the inferior hemorrhoidal veins and the inferior vena cava, whereas tumors of the upper two-thirds of the rectum metastasize by way of the portal vein to the liver.[24] The colon drains only into the portal vein and hence directly to the liver.

COLON-RECTUM. The difference between the results of resection of pulmonary metastases from the rectum and colon is well illustrated by a 52% 5-year survival for solitary metastases from a rectal primary but no 5-year survival when the colon was the primary site (see Table 41-8).[17] Other authors have not separated their results for rectal and colonic primaries and have reported combined 5-year survivals of 15–30%.[26,47,53,54]

OVARY. Ovarian adenocarcinomas are also an exception for intra-abdominal organs in that although they do not drain to the portal venous system, lymph-borne metastases originating in the pelvis and abdominal lymph nodes primarily spread to the liver. Very occasionally, metastatic disease will be isolated to the lungs and long-term survivors have been reported following resection. Every effort should be made to detect other metastases before resecting pulmonary lesions.

Modes of Spread—Independent

A third group of tumors may metastasize to the lungs and liver by independent routes. Cancer of the upper two-thirds of the esophagus is likely to spread to the lungs by way of the azygos veins and superior vena cava, but metastases otherwise go directly to the liver by way of the gastric and portal veins.

Gynecologic cancers (cervix uteri and corpus uteri) seed both the liver and lungs independently, but only the lungs are responsible for disseminating distant blood-borne metastases to the brain. The frequency of drainage directly into the vena cava explains the tendency to produce pulmonary metastases without any hepatic metastases. For these tumors the possibility of pelvic and abdominal lymph-borne metastases that may also spread to liver or lung makes it difficult to conclude that a pulmonary metastasis represents the only residual disease.

ESOPHAGUS. Because of the difficulty of adequately resecting the primary tumor and because of the high local recurrence rate, any pulmonary metastases are generally considered part of systemic disease; no attempt is made at resection.

UTERINE-CERVIX. The results of resection of isolated metastases from uterine-cervix primaries are favorable. Five-year survival ranges from 19% to 40% (see Table 41-8).[17,53] Characteristically, these tumors grow slowly and are slow to metastasize. Favorable results were achieved with both squamous and glandular carcinomas of uterine origin.

Adenocarcinoma of the breast represents a fourth complex pattern with spread independently to the lungs, vertebrae, or liver. Metastases to the liver may arise by way of the lymphatics of the rectus abdominis muscle or to the vertebrae by way of the intercostal veins and paravertebral plexuses (Batson's plexus) without lung involvement. However, the lung may be the first site of metastasis from the breast and from which subsequent metastases can disseminate to the liver and bones without vertebral involvement.[24]

BREAST. Despite the large number of women with breast cancer, there are relatively few reported cases of resection of metastatic breast pulmonary nodules. This reflects the difficulty of determining whether metastatic breast cancer is truly limited to the lungs. The 5-year survival results reported after resection are lower than for other tumors but do range from 13% to 52.7% (see Table 41-8).[17,47,53] However, the survival of 52.7% reported by Wilkins represents a total of only nine patients. The effects of chemotherapy may be particularly important in the treatment of micrometastases of breast carcinoma and, therefore, may affect resection results of pulmonary metastases.

TREATMENT OF PULMONARY METASTASES USING RADIOTHERAPY

The treatment of pulmonary metastases with radiotherapy has recently undergone re-assessment. Understanding the pathogenesis of pulmonary metastases has permitted tumor identification of those prone to spread to the lungs. Appreciation of the usefulness of adjuvant therapy for certain tumors has led to a solid rationale for the combined use of radiotherapy to the lungs and systemic chemotherapy. Finally, a better knowledge of the changes of normal lung following radiation has resulted in the development of treatment strategies permitting optimal therapeutic effect with lung radiation.

BIOLOGIC CONSIDERATIONS

Experimental studies of pulmonary metastases in the mouse have been carried out by Brown.[55] These investigations demonstrated that irradiation of the entire lung or lungs and the whole body prior to injection of tumor cells IV leads to a significantly higher incidence of pulmonary metastases resulting from a higher number of retained tumor cells in the lungs. This may be due to an increase in the capture of cells in the lung and an increased success rate of growth. Experimental studies in the dog by Owen and Bostock using both IV injected osteosarcoma cells and spontaneous osteosarcomas, melanomas, adenocarcinomas, and squamous cell carcinomas indicate that whole lung irradiation after tumor cell injection or ablation of the primary tumor reduces the volume and number of pulmonary metastases in the irradiated lung.[55] If the irradiation is given prior to IV osteosarcoma injection or prior to surgical ablation of the primary tumor, the number and volume of the metastases are increased in most dogs. Thus, both the dog and mouse experiments suggest that pulmonary irradiation for metastatic disease should not be carried out prior to ablation of the primary tumor and other gross tumor sites that might give rise to metastatic disease.

The experiments of Fu and coworkers proved that small lung tumors measuring 0.5–2.0 mm in diameter are more radiosensitive as assayed by single cell survival in culture following irradiation *in situ* than are large tumors growing in the flank of the mouse.[57] Both the width of the shoulder on the radiation response curve and the slope of dose response curves are steeper in these tumors; the hypoxic fraction is markedly lower than for larger flank masses. All of this work indicates that small, undetectable, microscopic pulmonary metastases will be far more amenable to sterilization by radiation than large deposits.

The use of prophylactic pulmonary irradiation is thus attractive and has been advocated by a number of authors, including Fernandez and coworkers, Cassady and coworkers, and Caldwell.[58–60] It is currently a part of a number of trials in the U.S. and Europe, some of which have shown encouraging results. Such prophylactic irradiation may be indicated, at least as an experimental technique, in Ewing's sarcoma and osteosarcoma, but only after removing the primary lesion.

The potential appears real for enhancing tumor cures with a combination of radiotherapy and chemotherapy in tumors with pulmonary metastases as the primary site of failure. The routine, aggressive treatment of such metastases, combining whole lung irradiation and high-dose local boost therapy, as well as the careful introduction of prophylactic irradiation and chemotherapy into clinical trials, may lead to improved cure rates in certain tumor sites. The success of such combinations will be limited, however, by the tolerance of the lung to radiation. Methods to increase this tolerance must be sought including the development of appropriate radioprotectors for pulmonary tissue.

Radiotherapeutic Approaches to Pulmonary Metastases

In general, the patient with pulmonary metastases should be considered to have multiple microscopic foci, as well as the grossly visible lesions seen on chest film or tomograms. Whole lung tomograms or CT are helpful in delineating the location of gross metastases for treatment. The treatment plan should include concomitant chemotherapy or sequential chemotherapy with effective agents. Since it appears that chemotherapy, even within several weeks of irradiation, enhances lung response to radiation, there would appear to be no gain in avoiding simultaneous combinations, which may be likely to cause greater tumor killing than separate administration of radiation and chemotherapy.

The radiotherapeutic approach should generally involve the use of megavoltage beams because of sharper collimation and better penetration. The decreased absorption of high energy radiation by the lung must be taken into account in calculating doses, although most experience with lung tolerance is based on uncorrected radiation doses. The initial treatment should generally include irradiation of the entire lung volume.

Although Caldwell has disputed the exact levels, the findings of Wara and coworkers suggest that whole lung irradiation administered at the same or approximately the same time as chemotherapy must be limited to between 1,350 and 1,500 rads at 150 rad/fraction.[60,61] These are doses uncorrected for transmission. If chemotherapy is not administered, has not been administered in the prior 3 months, and is not to be administered in the subsequent 3 months, these total doses may be increased to between 2,000 rad in 10 fractions and 3,000 rad in 20 fractions.

Following whole lung irradiation, additional radiation is given to the involved gross tumor areas. It is essential that these areas are carefully localized and that the volume of lung surrounding these nodules is limited severely. Since any additional dosage will lead to radiation pneumonitis and fibrosis in the target volume, this volume must be kept small. Because pneumonitis is inevitable, however, the doses to limited regions may be taken quite high, (*i.e.*, to between 4,000–6,000 rad) depending on the nature of the treated tumor. It is recommended that in all tumors, boost irradiation be used with the maximum dose limited to 3,000 rad in Wilms' tumor and between 5,000–6,000 rad in other histologic types.

TREATMENT OF PULMONARY METASTASES USING RADIOTHERAPY ALONE

Through the 1950's and early 1960's, the major experience in radiotherapy of pulmonary metastases was confined to childhood tumors. As seen in Table 41-9, a number of reports emphasize the small but definite complete response rate and prolonged survival seen in Ewing's sarcoma and Wilms' tumor. Combining this experience it can be seen that three of 14 patients treated for Ewing's sarcoma, and 11 of 98 treated for Wilms' tumor, survived longer than 2 years. In none of these reports was fatal radiation pneumonitis observed; a few patients did achieve long-term survival.

The value of whole lung irradiation alone in tumors originating from other sites is less clear, with most survivals over 2 years representing patients with Hodgkin's disease. Thus, it would appear that treatment of metastatic disease to the lung with radiotherapy alone yields only moderate success and is quite limited in terms of long-term survival. Failure in these cases occurred because of recurrence in the treated lung and the appearance of distant metastases in sites other than the lungs.

EXPERIENCE WITH COMBINED RADIOTHERAPY AND CHEMOTHERAPY FOR PULMONARY METASTASES

With the advent of effective multi-drug chemotherapy in the mid-1960's, the combination of radiotherapy and chemotherapy was extensively explored. A number of the available publications are summarized in Table 41-10. In addition to exploring the use of radiation with chemotherapy in Wilms' tumor and Ewing's sarcoma, this approach was applied to patients with testicular tumors and to patients with bone and soft tissue sarcomas.

The use of combined whole lung irradiation, with boosts to gross disease and chemotherapy, raised the cure rate of patients with Wilms' tumor metastatic to the lung from 10–20% to almost 50%. In the collected literature reviewed here, 100 of 226 patients lived beyond 2 years following treatment (see Table 41-9). Combined radiation and chemotherapy has also been successful in the treatment of Ewing's sarcoma and testicular tumors, with approximately 30–40% of such patients achieving long-term survival following combined treatment. The success rate with bone and soft tissue sarcomas is more modest, but in spite of the inherent lower radiosensitivity of these tumors, five of 22 patients achieved survival over 2 years.

These gains in survival have not been achieved without a price in terms of morbidity and mortality. Particularly early

TABLE 41-9. Survival of Patients Treated by Radiotherapy Alone for Pulmonary Metastases

AUTHOR	TUMOR TYPE	2-YEAR SURVIVAL NO. TREATED	%	NUMBER FATAL COMPLICATIONS
Margolis and	Ewing's	2/7	29	0
Phillips[23]	Miscellaneous	1/8	13	0
Wara et al[61]	Wilms'	0/4	0	0
Newton and	Testis	3/11	27	0
Spittle[63]	Sarcoma	0/6	0	0
	Ewing's	1/7	15	0
	Wilms'	1/4	25	0
	Hodgkin's	2/2	100	0
Hussey et al[62]	Wilms'	0/1	0	0
Monson et al[17]	Wilms'	10/89	11	No data

TABLE 41-10. Survival of Patients Treated by Combined Radiotherapy and Chemotherapy for Pulmonary Metastases

AUTHOR	TUMOR TYPE	2-YEAR SURVIVAL/ NO. TREATED	%	NUMBER FATAL PNEU-MONITIS
Wara et al[15]	Wilms'	8/13	62	1
Cassady et al[59]	Wilms'	20/42	48	4
Monson et al[63a]	Wilms'	70/168	42	No Data
Wharam et al[63b]	Testis	3/7	43	1
	Sarcoma	2/7	28	0
Cox et al[63c]	Testis	1/8	13	No Data
van der Werf-Messing[63d]	Testis	8/22	36	2
Caldwell[60]	Osteosarcoma	1/3	33	0
	Ewing's	3/4	75	0
	Sarcoma	2/8		1
	Wilms'	2/3		0
Baeza[63e]	Wilms'	4/9		3
	Ewing's	1/5		0
	Rhabdomyo-sarcoma	0/4		0
	Other	2/18		0

in combined radiation and chemotherapy, a significant number of deaths occurred due to acute radiation pneumonitis. Following the recognition that certain chemotherapeutic agents, in particular actinomycin-D and cyclophosphamide, reduced the tolerance of the lung to radiation by enhancement of the radiation effect, reductions in radiation dosage were carried out that have decreased the incidence of symptomatic and fatal reactions.[61]

Aggressive treatment of patients with apparently solitary pulmonary metastases is indicated by surgery. When these lesions are multiple and the patient is not considered a good surgical candidate, the use of whole lung irradiation and chemotherapy is indicated. The results available to date indicate that the patients most suitable for attempts to control pulmonary metastases that are not amenable to surgical resection are those with Wilms' tumor, testicular tumors, and soft tissue sarcomas, as well as selected patients with osteogenic sarcoma and Ewing's sarcoma. The combination of radiation therapy and effective chemotherapy is probably more successful than radiation alone because of chemosterilization of disease outside the irradiated fields and the effect of chemotherapy on cells within the irradiated volume augmenting the cell killing achievable by radiation.

The value of radiotherapy in patients with carcinomas metastatic to the lung is less clear. These lesions tend to be widespread and multiple, less radioresponsive, and they require a higher dose for control. Such patients usually have metastatic disease in other sites in addition to the lungs. The very limited tolerance of the lung to radiation, particularly when combined with chemotherapy, continues to be a major stumbling block in the greater exploitation of radiotherapy in the treatment of pulmonary metastases.

CHEMOTHERAPY

The treatment of pulmonary metastases with systemic chemotherapy alone will have to be considered in most patients for whom the surgical and radiotherapeutic approaches described in this chapter are not applicable. The appropriate hormonal management of the appropriate combination of chemotherapeutic agents will depend on the primary tumor that has metastasized to the lungs. The applicable protocols are described in the individual chapters according to site.

Treatment of Metastatic Cancer to Liver

with JAMES H. FOSTER

Liver metastases are considered by most doctors to be incurable. The work of Jaffe and others suggests that metastatic disease of the liver is often the component of the malignant process that most directly leads to death.[64] At least two decades of experience with systemic and intra-arterial chemotherapy and radiotherapy have shown that neither has much to offer most patients with liver metastases.

Resection of metastases in selected patients has developed some support in the last 10 years as operations on the liver have become safer and as the long-term survival results of resection have become known. However, the localized occurrence of metastatic disease in the liver suitable for resection is a rare event.[65] Most reports of success with chemotherapy or resection do not include simultaneous control patients and there is no well-documented prospective study that clearly and unequivocally demonstrates that any form of active therapy specifically directed at liver metastases provides more comfortable days at home than are provided by no therapy at all. Given these limitations, what evidence *is* available to recommend the use of any treatment for a patient who has proven metastatic disease in the liver?

NATURAL HISTORY WITHOUT TREATMENT

The first factor to consider in recommending therapy is the natural history of untreated disease progression. The extent of liver involvement is also important in determining prognosis in that those patients with a solitary metastasis or otherwise limited metastases do better no matter what treatment is employed.[64,66–68] Wood reports 60% one-year survival for patients with solitary, untreated metastases from colon and rectal carcinomas and only 5.7% survival when both lobes of the liver contain widespread disease. The mean survival was 16.7 months for patients with minimal disease in the liver and only 3.1 months for those with widespread disease.[68] When the two clinical indices of hepatomegaly and increased serum alkaline phosphatase were used to categorize the extent of metastases by Pettavel and Morgenthaler, the mean survival of 27 patients with neither criterion was 16 months, while 30 patients with both a palpable increase in liver size and increased serum alkaline phosphatase lived an average of only 1.4 months.[67] Table 41-11 uses retrospective data from a variety of sources to establish figures for mean survival of untreated patients with liver metastases from various primary tumors. (Median survival figures are almost always lower than mean survival figures.) Most patients who develop liver metastases have them at the time of diagnosis, and resection of their primary tumor, or within 2 years thereafter.

DIAGNOSIS AND RECOGNITION OF LIVER METASTASES

In the preoperative evaluation of the patient with an extrahepatic primary malignancy, decisions about therapy must be contingent on knowledge concerning spread of disease to the liver. Of the common biochemical tests of liver function, the alkaline phosphatase, serum glutamic-oxaloacetic transaminase (SGOT), and Bromsulphalein (BSP) retention are probably the most sensitive for liver metastases. However, they are often normal when the extent of the liver metastasis is small. They may be elevated in patients without liver metastasis so that such abnormalities should never be used as the sole basis of decisions about subsequent liver-directed anticancer therapy.

Radionuclide scans, particularly those using technitium 99M sulfur colloid, have been extensively used but have significantly high rates of false positive and false negative results when compared with operative findings. They seldom pick up lesions less than 2 cm in diameter. Cedermark and

TABLE 41-11. Natural History (Survival) of Patients with Untreated Hepatic Metastases

PRIMARY TUMOR	REFERENCE	NUMBER OF PATIENTS	EXTENT OF DISEASE	MEAN SURVIVAL (MOS)
Colon and rectum	Jaffe et al[64]	177	All stages	5
	Flanagan et al[109a]	43	All stages	8
	Pestana et al[109b]	353	All stages	9
	Pettavel et al[109c]	12	Solitary or minimal	21.5
		41	Moderate	6.9
		30	Widespread	1.4
	Wood et al[68]	15	Solitary	16.7
		11	Localized	10.6
		87	Widespread	3.1
Stomach	Bengmark et al[66]	23	All stages	6
Pancreas	Bengmark et al[66]	68	All stages	2.4
Breast	Foster et al[65]	54	All stages	6

coworkers report that when less than 25% of the liver is replaced by tumor there is only a random correlation of scan to operative findings.[69] Selective hepatic arteriography can demonstrate large metastatic lesions (which, with the exception of melanomas, leiomyosarcomas and metastatic endocrine tumors are usually hypovascular), but it cannot be depended upon to determine the presence and number of smaller deposits.

The role of ultrasound and CT in detecting liver metastases has yet to be clarified. However, an important point should be made about all of these preoperative examinations. If laparotomy will eventually be required to diagnose or treat a primary intra-abdominal tumor, the presence and degree of liver metastasis can be most accurately determined by the surgeon's hands. Two hands placed on opposite surfaces of both the right and left liver lobes will detect the vast majority of small and large liver metastases. Therefore, costly and time-consuming preoperative liver evaluation tests may not be indicated and should be avoided unless they will contribute directly to a decision against laparotomy. Biopsy confirmation is essential, however, since there are several benign liver tumors and other conditions that may simulate metastases.

Detection of liver metastases after resection of an extrahepatic primary tumor has prognostic significance, but is important therapeutically only if there are effective therapies available for controlling their growth once they are detected. Serial carcinoembryonic antigen determinations, usually at 1–2 month intervals, are recommended by some.[70,71] Most oncologists will include the standard liver function biochemical tests and an occasional radionuclide scan in their routine follow-up examination. Hepatomegaly denotes massive liver involvement and liver pain is usually a sign of late and extensive disease.

TREATMENT OPTIONS

Treatment can be given before there is any evidence of persistent or recurrent disease and, in this instance, will be called "prophylactic" treatment. Once the diagnosis of a definite liver metastasis is established by detection and histologic confirmation (whether at treatment of the primary tumor or at some interval thereafter), either palliative or curative therapy must then be considered. "Palliative" therapy would include radiotherapy, systemic or regional chemotherapy, interruption of tumor blood supply, immunotherapy, noncurative resection, or any combination. "Curative" therapy is limited to resection for patients with liver metastasis from the more common solid primary tumors since there is no evidence of permanent or even long-term "cure" with the other modalities at present. Chemotherapy and radiation therapy, with or without resection of liver secondaries, may occasionally be curative in those patients with rare tumors (*e.g.*, Wilms' tumor), which are unusually sensitive to the presently available techniques of radiotherapy or chemotherapy.

PROPHYLACTIC TREATMENT

Most prospective studies about adjuvant chemotherapy have failed to show significant protection of the clinically uninvolved liver against subsequent tumor deposits. However, a few recently reported ongoing trials have suggested otherwise and the favorable results are approaching statistical significance.[72] Also, a well controlled but small series of adjuvant 5-fluorouracil infusions through the portal vein reported by Taylor and coworkers suggests that liver metastases may be preventable in certain circumstances.[73] The transient protection of the liver from implantation of tumor cells dislodged from the primary site into the portal venous system by operative manipulation is theoretically sound, but should not be routinely recommended until further proof is available that adjuvant chemotherapy will do more good than harm.

PALLIATIVE THERAPY

Radiotherapy

Hepatic metastases represent a very common problem, which until recently has been ignored as subject to useful palliation by radiotherapy. When recognized at autopsy that 60–70% of patients with metastatic large bowel cancer have hepatic metastases, it can be predicted that at least 20,000 patients will suffer from this problem alone. In addition, when considering the other GI primary sites and other distant sites that lead to symptomatic hepatic metastases, it is recognized that the potential for significant palliation by radiotherapy exists. This finding is further emphasized by the fact that many hepatic metastases are solitary or exist in patients with no other evidence of distant spread. Thus, the adequate treatment of hepatic disease has the potential for inducing long-term survival and is recommended for suitable patients using a palliative course of 300 rad daily for seven treatments.

TOLERANCE OF THE LIVER TO IRRADIATION. One of the major considerations when selecting treatment techniques for the radiotherapy of hepatic metastases is the limited tolerance of the liver to radiation. The liver is a very radiosensitive organ. Doses of more than 3,000 rad given at a rate of 1,000 rad per week may produce radiation hepatitis. In 1965, Ingold and coworkers described 40 patients irradiated to the entire liver for carcinoma of the ovary employing doses between 1,300–5,100 rad.[74] The authors were able to correlate the incidence of radiation hepatitis with total dose. One of eight patients receiving doses of 3000–3450 rad developed radiation hepatitis, while five of nine patients receiving 3500–3950 rad developed this complication. The overall incidence of radiation hepatitis in this series was 13 of 40. A summary of these cases from the series by Ingold and coworkers and also from an earlier series reported by Phillips and coworkers in 1954 is shown in Table 41-12.[75] Kraut and coworkers described two cases of mild, asymptomatic, reversible radiation hepatitis occurring at doses between 2500–3000 rad.[76] From this and other information, most investigators feel that whole liver irradiation tolerance is approximately 1800–2400 rad at 300 rads/fraction, 2500 rad at 250 rad/fraction, and 3000 rad at 150–180 rad/fraction. If these doses are exceeded, the classic signs of radiation hepatitis ensue, generally within 1–3 months following irradiation.[77] Radiation hepatitis is accompanied by ascites and a Budd-Chiari-like syndrome associated with injury to the central vein region of the liver lobule, leading to obstruction

TABLE 41-12. Radiation Hepatitis—Incidence as a Function of Dose

RADS	NO. OF PATIENTS INGOLD SERIES*	PHILLIPS SERIES†	FATAL	PERSISTENT DAMAGE	TOTAL RECOVERY	INADEQUATE FOLLOW-UP
3000	1/9	0/19	0	0	0	1
3000–3500	2/9	1/11	0	0	1	1
3500–4000	7/18	0/6	1	2	3	1
4000+	3/4	—	2	0	1	0
TOTALS	13/40	1/36	3	2	5	3

* Ingold JA, et al.: Radiation hepatitis. Am J Roentgenol 93:200–208, 1965
† Phillips R et al.: Roentgen therapy of hepatic metastases. Am J Roentgenol Radiat Ther Nucl Med 71:826–834, 1954

and portal hypertension. This limitation on liver tolerance restricts radiation dosage to the entire organ to palliative levels, although such doses may be compatible with sterilization of micrometastases when used in prophylactic fashion. Most metastatic lesions are not sensitive to less than 3000 rad, but an occasional patient with radiosensitive and symptomatic liver metastasis will be symptomatically benefitted by external radiation.[78]

RADIOTHERAPY ALONE FOR HEPATIC METASTASES. The use of hepatic irradiation for patients with metastatic disease to the liver was first reported by Case and Warth in 1924.[79] Subsequently, Phillips and coworkers reported a series of 36 patients treated with doses between 2000–3750 rad in fractions of generally 250 rad over 8–22 days.[75] Of the patients treated 72% showed symptomatic improvement and 47% of patients showed improvement in liver function. Only one patient demonstrated evidence of radiation damage to the liver. That patient had received 3500 rad to the entire liver. The second patient died of radiation nephritis secondary to irradiation of both kidneys. Turek-Maischeider and Kazem employed doses between 1600 rad in two weeks and 2500 rad in three weeks for palliation of hepatic metastases.[15] Although the number of patients treated was small, eight of 11 had complete relief of symptoms and two others had moderate pain relief. These results were obtained at dose levels of 1800 rad or more; no evidence of radiation hepatitis was found at autopsy.

Prasad and associates, using doses averaging 2500 rad in 3–3½ weeks, reported symptomatic improvement in 19 of 27 patients (70%).[80] If the analysis was restricted to patients completing therapy, 19 of 20 (95%) were symptomatically improved. The authors reported improvement in bilirubin levels in two of seven patients and improvement in ascites in four of eight. The average survival was 4 months and no significant change was noted over nontreated patients.

More recently, Sherman and coworkers at the Joint Center at Harvard reviewed the experience of the New England Deaconess Hospital, where 55 patients underwent palliative irradiation for liver metastases with radiation alone or radiation combined with chemotherapy.[81] Some 64% had massive liver involvement and 92% were metastatic from adenocarcinomas. Most patients received 2100–2400 rad in 2 weeks in increments of 300 rad/fraction. Some 89% of patients showed response, with 44% showing excellent response. Of those patients having pain 90% experienced pain relief, decreased liver size, and improvement in liver function tests. Some 31 patients received concomitant chemotherapy and 14 were previous chemotherapy failures. No correlation could be found between palliative response and prior or concomitant chemotherapy administration. Radiation hepatitis was not observed. The entire group exhibited a median survival of 4.5 months with a median survival of 9 months for those showing excellent response; survival at one year was 21%. Palliation of pain and other symptoms generally lasted for the duration of the patient's survival, thus the palliative index was high. The major morbidity in the whole liver irradiation series was nausea and vomiting.

RTOG carried out a pilot study of irradiation for palliation of hepatic metastases using several fractionation schemes over 1–4 weeks. In this study, 55% of patients experienced subjective improvement in abdominal pain.[82]

EXPERIENCE WITH COMBINED RADIOTHERAPY AND CHEMOTHERAPY. Because of the liver's limited tolerance to radiotherapy, attempts have recently been made to enhance response through the addition of cytotoxic chemotherapy through both the intra-arterial and IV route. Friedman and coworkers studied 22 patients using intra-arterial 5-fluorouracil and doxorubicin with concomitant radiation therapy at levels between 1500 and 2100 rad with 300 rad fractions.[83] Of the patients 43% showed improvement in liver size with a median duration of response greater than 3.5 months. Almost all patients with pain or impaired function experienced relief of pain and improvement in liver function tests. The response rate was 55% in patients with colorectal primaries. Toxicity was acceptable, with the major side effect being nausea and fever during treatment and moderate suppression of white blood cell and platelet counts. No definite hepatotoxicity from the combined modality therapy was noted. Webber and coworkers employed radiation therapy and intrahepatic 5-FUdR; they observed a 44% response rate with a median survival of 13 months in the responders and 4.5 months in the nonresponders.[84] The Northern California Oncology Group is currently conducting a trial randomizing patients between radiation alone, radiation plus intra-arterial chemotherapy, and radiation plus systemic chemotherapy.

HYPOXIC CELL SENSITIZERS FOR HEPATIC METASTASES. RTOG has recently completed a Phase II study of the use of the hypoxic cell sensitizer, misonidazole, with radiation in the treatment of liver metastases. Patients were given 2100 rad in seven fractions to the entire liver with daily misonidazole doses of 1.5 g/m^2.[85] Of the patients 76%

experienced pain relief and there was an overall median survival of 22 weeks. There was no significant additional morbidity from the sensitizer and no evidence of radiation-induced hepatic damage. The responses of various types of symptoms in this series are shown in Table 41-13. Additional factors measured in this RTOG study included the Karnofsky status, which improved in 58% of patients, the alkaline phosphatase, which improved in 42% of patients, and the bilirubin, which was reduced when elevated in 60% of patients. Hepatic size was reduced in 32% of patients. The palliation index was 88% in patients with minimal symptoms and 72% in patients with more marked symptoms, indicating that the relief lasted most of the patient's remaining life span.

INTRA-ARTERIAL ISOTOPIC THERAPY. To increase the radiation dose to tumors within the liver and remain within organ tolerance, a number of attempts have been made to use intra-arterial and IV radioisotopic therapy. For radiosensitive diseases such as lymphomas, Kraut, Kaplan, and Bagshaw proposed fractionated radioisotopic and external irradiation of the liver in patients with Hodgkin's disease.[86] This technique employed IV injected radioactive colloidal gold, which tends to localize in the portal triad regions, regions now showing damage following external irradiation. Although this technique appeared successful in some patients with lymphoma, there were problems with bone marrow suppression due to colloidal gold uptake in the marrow. The technique has been replaced by more effective multi-drug chemotherapy.

Ariel and Padula and Grady have reported on the use of intra-arterial yttrium-90 microspheres through the cannulated hepatic artery or through the remote catheter cannulization of the hepatic artery.[87,88] These authors have combined bolus injection of radioactive microspheres with subsequent infusion of 5-fluorouracil through the hepatic artery, in addition to external beam irradiation, and systemic chemotherapy. Ariel and Padula reported on 25 patients with metastatic carcinoma. Some 35% demonstrated an objective response of 3 months or more to this combined treatment; 65% of the patients showed subjective improvement.[87]

This technique involves use of radiolabeled microspheres approximately 15 microns in diameter and preferentially trapped within tumor vessels. The concomitant use of vasoconstrictive agents can further increase the differential uptake in tumor compared to the remainder of the liver. One problem with this technique is the shunting of isotope through the liver and delivery of isotopic microspheres to portions of the stomach and duodenum with certain catheter positions. However, these problems can be avoided through pre-injection with microspheres labeled with tracer doses of technitium 199M, especially in conjunction with other treatment modalities.

The role of radiotherapy in the treatment of hepatic metastases is growing rapidly. The liver represents an excellent model system for the study of tumor treatment in a radiosensitive bed. In addition, it offers the opportunity to combine systemic irradiation with intra-arterial irradiation, systemic with intra-arterial chemotherapy, and in some situations, with surgery. Optimum combination of radiation, microspheres, sensitizers, and chemotherapy may eventually lead to the control of hepatic metastases. There is certainly a place for such approaches in the prophylactic treatment of the liver in patients at high risk for hepatic metastases.

TABLE 41-13. Summary of Changes in Signs/Symptoms—Pre-Treatment Versus Fourth Week Assessment (Numbers in Parenthesis are Number Improved/Total Number)

	INITIALLY PRESENT							INITIALLY ABSENT	
SIGNS/ SYMPTOMS	TOTAL NUMBER WITH SYMPTOMS AT PRESENTATION	PERCENT IMPROVED	INITIAL MILD	SEVERITY VS. MODERATE	IMPROVEMENT SEVERE	PERCENT COMPLETELY IMPROVED	PERCENT WORSENED	TOTAL NUMBER	PERCENT WORSENED
Abdominal Pain	23	74% (17/23)	69% (9/13)	75% (6/8)	100% (2/2)	65% (15/23)	8%	18	11%
Nausea/ Vomiting	10	60% (6/10)	50% (3/6)	75% (3/4)	— —	60% (6/10)	15%	31	16%
Anorexia	22	36% (8/22)	35% (6/17)	40% (2/5)	— —	36% (8/22)	15%	19	21%
Weakness/ Fatigue	23	35% (8/23)	50% (5/10)	43% (3/7)	— —	30% (7/23)	32%	18	39%
Abdominal Distension	15	53% (8/15)	42% (5/12)	100% (3/3)	—	40% (6/15)	10%	26	6%
Fever/ Night Sweats	6	83% (5/6)	66% (2/3)	100% (3/3)	—	83% (5/6)	12%	35	14%
Jaundice	6	17% (1/6)	(0/2)	50% (1/4)	—	17% (1/6)	15%	35	13%
Ascites	5	60% (3/5)	60% (3/5)	—	—	60% (3/5)	12%	36	14%

Chemotherapy

After two decades of extensive experience with chemotherapy for liver metastases, it is still difficult to define its role in the treatment of patients with known disease. For solid carcinomas of GI origin, most would agree that the systemic use of 5-fluorouracil for hepatic metastases will usually be followed by an objective response of 3 months or more duration in about 15%, but that such therapy will not prolong survival. Disappointment with these results led Sullivan, Watkins, Ansfield, and others to recommend regional arterial infusion, at first through catheters placed at laparotomy into major feeding arteries of the liver, and more recently through catheters placed percutaneously through the axilla or groin.[89–91] Hospital morbidity and mortality have been reduced in recent years, but a high rate of catheter displacement or sepsis, GI hemorrhage, and other complications related to the infusion techniques remain. The development of small, portable infusion pumps has allowed continuance of infusion therapy for ambulatory patients in a home setting. The technical details of catheter placement and the management of long-term infusion are discussed by Watkins and others.[92–94]

The efficacy of these methods is difficult to determine even after careful review of the frequently published results. Response is usually measured in terms of 2 or 3 months. The effects in "responders" are compared with those of "nonresponders," a practice without significance or other merit. Patient results in those with minimal liver disease are often lumped together with those with extensive disease, and, more often than not, the hepatic artery infusion of chemotherapeutic agents is combined with systemic chemotherapy, hepatic artery interruption, or some other treatment. The most important deficiency of most published results relates to the almost universal absence of untreated control patients in any of these studies and to the almost equally universal comparison of achieved results with "historic" controls carefully chosen to emphasize the beneficial effects of active treatment.

In spite of the favorable prejudice introduced by all of these "unscientific" biases, the data presented is still discouraging and has led many to abandon the use of infusion for the treatment of common solid cancers until more effective chemotherapeutic agents are found. Ansfield and Ramirez reported at least 2 months of improvement in 55% of 369 patients with liver metastases treated with intra-arterial 5-fluorouracil, but their mean survival was only 9 months after the initiation of therapy in the overall group.[89] Watkins and coworkers reported objective response of 3 months or greater in 56% of 108 patients with colorectal secondaries and median survival of 15 months from the onset of symptoms (not of treatment).[91] Sullivan reported 58% response in 102 patients with colorectal metastases for 3 months or more following initiation of hepatic artery infusion, but does not list overall median or mean survival rates.[90] Petrek and Minton reported an objective response at 5–8 weeks after the start of hepatic artery infusion therapy in 12 of 24 patients with colorectal secondaries and in 11 of 27 patients with other primary tumors. In addition, a median survival of patients with colorectal carcinoma of 9 months following the start of infusion therapy, a therapy which lasted a median of 8 months resulted. Thus, the median patient survived one month after cessation of intra-arterial infusion in this series. The patients with noncolorectal primaries lived an average of 5 months after the initiation of hepatic artery infusion therapy.[95] A Swedish report noted median survival of 9 months and a mean survival of 11.5 months in 15 patients following the onset of hepatic artery infusion with 5-fluorouracil for patients with colon and rectal metastases.[96] A Swiss report, which included an attempt at staging the degree of liver involvement, presents a more optimistic picture of what hepatic artery infusion may accomplish.[67] However, in general, a picture of mean survival of less than a year exists, a result that must be compared with the natural history of the disease. It has also become clear that the infusion must be prolonged over several months rather than weeks to be effective even in the most favorable "responders." Almost all authors report more discouraging results with liver secondaries from the stomach, pancreas, breast, and lung than with those from colorectal primaries.

Patt and coworkers have reported the combination of intra-arterial infusion of chemotherapeutic agents with *Corynebacterium parvum* in 28 patients with metastatic carcinoma in the liver. This combination of immunotherapy with chemotherapy is interesting, but the results achieved in terms of survival and objective remission were quite poor in this small series and the toxicity introduced by the *C. parvum* was impressive.[97]

One can only conclude from this data that the case for regional infusion therapy remains unproven. The cost in terms of dollars, discomfort, and iatrogenic morbidity and mortality is difficult to measure. The striking similarity in the length of overall survival with or without chemotherapy in the total groups reported should give pause to any physician who is considering treatment for a patient with asymptomatic liver metastases. It is to be hoped that most treated patients will become part of carefully controlled prospective trials in the future, and that those trials will include untreated controls.

Vessel Ligation

First suggested by Markowitz in 1952, hepatic artery ligation has a sound theoretical basis in that the great majority of primary and secondary cancers of the liver derive their nourishment from branches of the hepatic artery, even though initial seeding of the liver may have been through the portal vein. For years, ligation of the hepatic artery was thought to be a dangerous procedure. However, more recent evidence suggests that it can be safely done in most patients who do not have portal vein thrombosis or cirrhosis. In fact, the real problem with arterial ligation turns out to be that it is almost impossible to permanently exclude arterial blood from the liver. Although transient, dramatic shrinkage of hepatic metastasis has been reported by many authors after hepatic artery ligation, follow-up angiography has demonstrated rapid reestablishment of arterial flow through collateral channels and regrowth of tumor that parallels this increase in circulation. More extensive dearterialization procedures were developed but were equally unsuccessful in preventing eventual collateral development and tumor regrowth.[98,99] Hepatic artery ligation has been combined with intra-arterial infusion of chemotherapeutic agents by many investigators. El-Domeiri and Mojab have recently reported a technique for intermittent occlusion of the hepatic artery on the theoretical grounds that limited periods of warm ischemia might preferentially adversely affect the tumor cells, while reestablishment of arterial circulation might allow better distribution of cytotoxic agents to the tumor cells while protecting the normal liver cells.[100] Unfortunately, no clear advantage of any of these techniques involving permanent or transient hepatic artery ligation has yet been shown.

Honjo and coworkers have advocated ligation of one of the main branches of the portal vein on the grounds that the subsequent atrophy of that liver lobe would reduce tumor growth.[101] They report a few impressive anecdotal cases, but their results have not been reproduced elsewhere.

CURATIVE THERAPY

Resection of Liver Metastases

The final method to be discussed for the management of liver metastases is surgical resection. Advocates for resection of metastatic disease to the lung in selected patients have been successful in establishing that significant palliation and even cure may be achieved in a significant number of highly selected cases. The thesis of the authors, based on evidence that will be developed, is that curative resection of certain localized and apparently solitary liver metastases from common solid tumors should also be attempted in highly selected patients. On the other hand, palliative resection where gross tumor is left is seldom, if ever, justified except in an attempt to control disabling symptoms from a slow-growing endocrine tumor. Debulking of liver metastases may have a place in the future when more effective chemotherapeutic agents with which to treat residual disease are available. However, for the present, debulking procedures cannot be recommended. Thus, the discussion of the results and techniques of liver resection for secondary disease has been placed on the general heading of curative therapy.

Improvements in operative techniques, anesthesia, and experience with liver resection for trauma and benign disease over the last 20 years have allowed resection of up to 75–80% of non-cirrhotic livers with acceptable operative mortality rates. Pack, Wangensteen, and others were resecting liver metastases in the 1950s, but their operative mortality rates were high indeed, and the reported survivors usually succumbed to recurrent disease shortly after resection.[102,103] Orthotopic transplantation after total hepatectomy is another possibility. Although success has been achieved for many benign conditions by Starzl and others, experience with patients with primary liver tumors has been less fortunate, and no significant experience with transplantation after hepatectomy for metastatic disease has yet been reported.[99,104]

More recent reviews justify a cautious optimism about partial liver resection for cure in selected patients with limited metastatic disease of the liver. Adson and coworkers have reported the largest single institutional experience with hepatic resection for metastatic disease.[105,106] In addition, Foster has reviewed the reports of others and combined these figures with a nationwide review of collected cases to provide some firm data about the mortality of the operation and the duration of postoperative survival.[65,99] An overall generalization that might summarize their conclusions is that liver resection is indicated:

1. In selected patients with primary colon and rectal tumors who have localized liver deposits as their only manifestation of recurrent or persistent cancer
2. In even more highly selected patients with disabling symptoms from liver deposits of endocrine tumors with slow tumor growth rates
3. In children with tumors responsive to chemotherapy and radiotherapy where liver resection might remove a large focus of disease, allowing for control of smaller amounts of residual disease elsewhere by other therapeutic modalities

Current survival data after liver resection for patients with carcinoma metastatic from pancreas, stomach, lung, breast, and melanoma do not justify liver resection for these and for most other solid tumors at the present time.[65]

In adults, then, what is to be achieved by resection of liver secondaries from primary carcinomas of the colon and rectum? First, 10–30% of patients with primary colon and rectal tumors will have liver metastases at the time of resection of their primary tumor.[99] Raven studied 818 patients from the Royal Marsden Hospital with carcinoma of the stomach, colon, and rectum. Of these patients 23% had liver metastases at laparotomy for treatment of their primary tumor; 5% had limited liver disease judged to be resectable.[107] Bengmark and Hafstrom found resectable disease in nine of 156 patients undergoing laparotomy for primary tumors of the colon and rectum.[66] Pettavel and Morgenthaler also found 23% liver metastases in patients with colon and rectum primaries and, of these, only 15 patients (4.5%) had clearly resectable conditions.[67] Adson and Van Heerden also reported a 5% resectability rate for isolated liver disease in all patients undergoing resection of primary colon and rectum tumors. Thus, a surgeon resecting 100 patients with primary tumors of the colon and rectum will find a resectable focus of residual disease in the liver as the only remaining manifestation of cancer in about five patients, but in that small and selected group of patients, what should be recommended?

Wilson and Adson reported 42% five-year survival and 28% ten-year survival after resection of apparently solitary colon and rectum metastases in 40 patients. Most of these metastases were removed by wedge resection and there was no operative mortality in that report.[106] In a more recent paper, Adson and Van Heerden reviewed 34 major hepatic resections done for larger deposits of metastatic colon and rectum carcinoma, some in patients with known metastatic disease elsewhere. There were two postoperative deaths in this group and minimal postoperative morbidity. The early survival figures parallel those achieved after the "lesser" resections. Of the 24 patients operated on more than 2 years prior to reporting, 14 lived at least 2 years, although at least five of those patients had evidence of recurrent disease.[105] Fortner and coworkers reported a 72% actuarial 3-year survival after 17 "curative" liver resections for metastatic colon and rectal tumors. However, only two patients had actually survived beyond 3 years in that series and no patient in that series lived as long as 2 years after "palliative" liver resection for metastatic disease.[108]

TABLE 41-14. Survival After Liver Resection for Metastatic Cancer

PRIMARY TUMOR	NO. OF PATIENTS	SURVIVAL 2-YR	SURVIVAL 5-YR	DECEASED AFTER 5 YEARS OF RECURRENCE
Colon and rectum	259	84/192	46/206	12
Wilms' Tumor	13	8/11	4/7	0
Melanoma	12	2/10	1/10	1
Leiomyosarcoma	11	4/8	1/8	1
Pancreas	7	2/7	1/6	1
Uterus and cervix	8	1/7	0/7	—
Stomach	7	0/7	0/7	—
Kidney	5	2/5	1/5	0
Breast	5	0/4	0/4	—
Other	17	6/13	3/20	—

Table 41-14 lists the results collected by Foster and Table 41-15 describes the outcome achieved in that group of patients with primary tumors of the colon and rectum.[65,99] Careful analysis of the experience with resected cases suggests that the size and number of metastases relate directly to curability by liver resection, but that eventual survival does not correlate with the status of the mesenteric lymph nodes at primary colon tumor resection, with the amount of liver resection, or even with the interval between the primary tumor resection and the resection of the metastases (see Tables 41-15 through 41-18).[99] The late death (more than 5 years after liver resection) of 12 patients suggests a favorable natural history in some of these cases, but it is very hard to document even a 1% five-year survival rate for untreated patients with histologically proven liver metastases from tumors of the colon and rectum. Thus, about one-fourth of highly selected patients will be cured by liver resection of metastatic disease.

The selection process should be considered next. First, what should be recommended if a resectable metastasis is found at laparotomy for resection of a primary tumor of the colon or rectum? The number, location, and size of the metastatic lesion(s) should be carefully noted and histologic confirmation obtained. If the patient's condition, the location of the incision, and the surgeon's experience and vigor allow easy wedge excision of a solitary peripheral metastasis, this should be done at the time of bowel resection. In most circumstances, however, it will be better to delay a decision about liver resection until another day. This will allow careful study of the primary tumor and careful search for other metastatic disease by lung tomography and other tests. It will also allow preparation of the patient and the surgeon for liver resection. Hepatic angiography should precede any major liver resection. Although there are no figures to defend this thesis, it seems reasonable to expect that a delay of 1–4 months might allow those tumors with an aggressive nature to declare themselves by rapid growth and other metastases. Yet, such a short delay should not defeat the goal of resecting a solitary liver focus. If spread or rapid growth is not apparent and if other conditions permit it, liver resection for resectable disease should be recommended as the patient's only chance for permanent cure.

If no liver disease is apparent at resection of a primary bowel tumor, routine follow-up studies should include a baseline liver scan and liver function tests. These tests should

TABLE 41-15. Survival After Liver Resection for Metastatic Colorectal Cancer*

OPERATIVE MORTALITY	5%
OPERATIVE SURVIVORS	259 patients
2-Year Survival	84/192 (44%)
5-Year Survival	46/206 (22%)
DEAD WITH RECURRENT CANCER MORE THAN 5 YEARS AFTER LIVER RESECTION	12 patients

* Foster JH: Survival after liver resection for secondary tumors. Am J Surg 135:389, 1978

TABLE 41-16. Liver Resection for Metastatic Colorectal Cancer: Solitary versus Multiple Nodules

	SOLITARY	MULTIPLE
Patients at risk	108	54
Operative deaths	1	7
5-Year Survivors	33 (30%)	7 (13%)

TABLE 41-17. Liver Resection for Metastatic Colorectal Cancer: Operation versus Survival*

	LOBECTOMY	SEGMENTAL RESECTION	WEDGE
Patients	46	25	97
Operative deaths	5	0	3
5-year survivors	6/45 (13%)	5/24 (21%)	22/93 (24%)

*Foster JH: Survival after liver resection for secondary tumors. Am J Surg 135:389, 1978

TABLE 41-18. Colon and Rectum Primary: Interval between Bowel and Liver Resection

	SYNCHRONOUS	METACHRONOUS LESS THAN 2 YEARS	METACHRONOUS MORE THAN 2 YEARS
No. of Patients	111	60	69
Mean Survival (mos)*	27	26	34
2-Year Survival*	43/88(49%)	25/50(50%)	19/56(34%)
5-Year Survival*	15/81(19%)	12/47(26%)	10/51(20%)

*After liver resection; excludes operative death.

be repeated reasonably often during the first 2 or 3 years following bowel resection since metastasis is most common during this interval. Liver metastasis is probably more common than bowel recurrence, which is often routinely searched for by barium enema and sigmoidoscopy during the follow-up period). Also, if liver involvement is found early, the situation may still be amenable to cure or palliation. Clinical evidence of liver recurrence (*i.e.*, hepatomegaly, right upper quadrant pain, weight loss, etc.) are bad prognostic signs, but occasionally resectable situations will be found even in the symptomatic patient.

ENDOCRINE TUMORS. There have been at least 44 reported instances of liver resection to control disabling symptoms from a malignant carcinoid tumor.[99] Most often, liver metastases will be diffuse and preclude resection, since at least 95% of liver disease must be removed to achieve palliation from the hormone-mediated symptoms. However, when the geography of the metastases allows total or subtotal resection, good palliation can be expected when the rate of tumor growth is slow. Palliation of endocrine symptoms from insulinomas, glucagonomas, and other endocrine tumors can also be achieved in rare instances by liver resection when medical measures have failed and when the tumor deposits are localized.

PEDIATRIC TUMORS. At least 15 cases of liver resection for metastatic Wilms' tumors have been reported and at least nine of these children were alive and apparently disease-free from 18 months to 7 years after hepatectomy. Most of these children had a combination of resection with radiation and chemotherapy; a few also had resection of pulmonary metastases.[65]

FIG. 41-9. Mattress suture wedge excision. Usually, interlocking mattress sutures of heavy absorbable materials are placed prior to sharp wedge excision of a peripheral tumor, but they may also be placed after tumor excision if required by hemostasis. (Foster JH, Berman MM: Solid liver tumors. In Major Problems in Clinical Surgery, Vol 23. Philadelphia, WB Saunders, 1977)

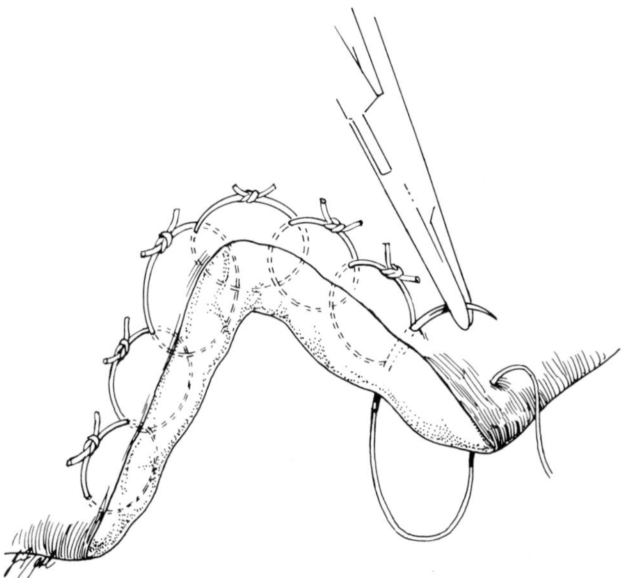

TECHNIQUE OF LIVER RESECTION FOR METASTATIC DISEASE. The collected data show clearly that results achieved do not correlate with the amount of liver resected or with the width of the resected margin of normal liver surrounding the metastases. Wedge resection with a narrow margin of normal liver is apparently as likely to cure as major lobectomy, so that resection should be planned on the basis of patient safety. With larger metastases, lobectomy, even if not required by the geography of the tumor, may be less bloody and therefore safer than "anatomic" segmental resections of liver. There are few serious metabolic problems associated with either right or left lobectomy, and the noncirrhotic liver quickly resumes its preoperative volume and weight by a process of hypertrophy and hyperplasia.

Fig. 41-9 shows a useful technique for the wedge resection of a small tumor at the free edge of the liver. Although large mattress sutures through the center of the liver should not be used because they cause necrosis and are associated with an increased risk of postoperative infection, their use as illustrated is usually well tolerated. Because catgut slides more easily, and thus tension on the knots can be more accurately adjusted, it is preferred over the synthetic absorbable sutures for a liver mattress technique in spite of its increased tissue reactivity. The larger wedge excisions illustrated in Fig. 41-10 are better performed with the blunt section technique described below.

For larger and more central lesions, some type of formal hepatectomy will be needed. Several principles are important. The surgeon must be familiar with the normal anatomy of the vascular and biliary compartments and should have specific information about his patient's arterial supply. This is often anomalous, and therefore preoperative selective arteriography should be done whenever possible. Also, hilar identification and distal dissection of the components of the portal triad should precede any major resection. This dissection can almost always be carried out to the proposed line of transection without dividing any liver substance. One can go well beyond the bifurcation of portal vein and hepatic artery and the confluence of the right and left hepatic ducts without entering Glisson's capsule. The liver substance should be divided by blunt technique, not by a cold knife or electrocautery. When possible, all vessels and ducts encountered, however small, should be controlled with clips and ties before they are transected. Metal clips are most useful for all but the largest vessels. There are no bloodless planes in the human liver. Lastly, the outflow vessels (*i.e.*, the hepatic veins) should be controlled last in most patients. They are thin-walled, large, and friable, and their junctions with the inferior vena cava are almost always largely intrahepatic. The technique preferred at the University of Connecticut Health Center for most major liver resections involves several steps:

1. Adequate exposure is obtained by mobilization of the lobe to be resected by transection of the falciform and triangular ligaments where appropriate and, for right lobectomy, by incision of the peritoneal fold between

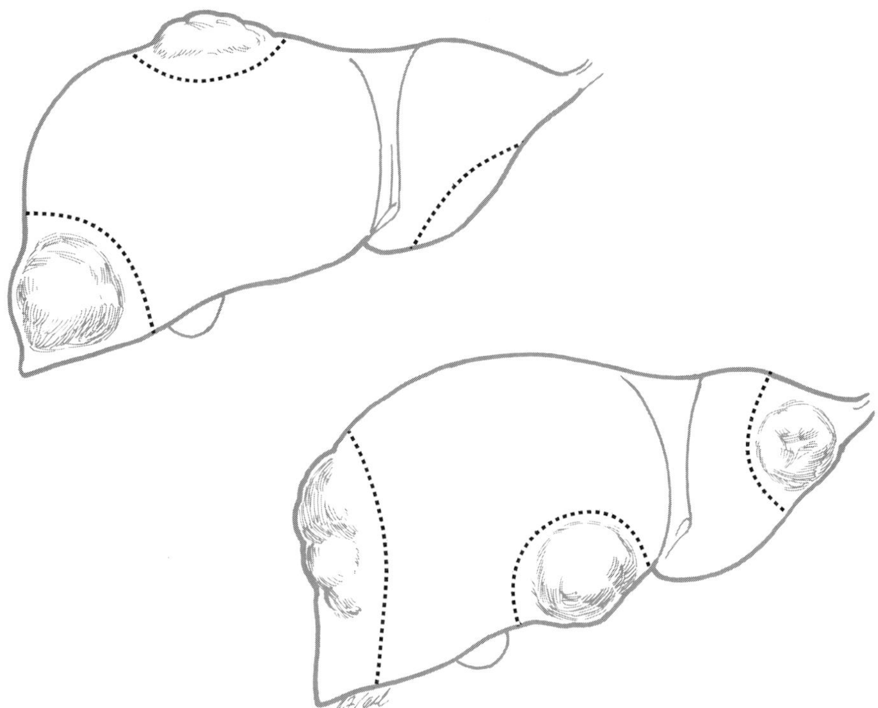

FIG. 41-10. Wedge excisions. Although wedge excision is most useful for small tumors along the free edge of the liver, it also may be done for more bulky disease. Typical large wedge excisions are illustrated. Individual circumstances will dictate whether preliminary hilar control is necessary. The upper diagram illustrates the type of peripheral excision of the lower part of the left lateral segment often done to satisfy the "en bloc" principle in removing a large gastric carcinoma that has invaded adjacent liver. (Foster JH, Berman MM: Solid liver tumors. In Major Problems in Clinical Surgery, Vol 23. Philadelphia, WB Saunders, 1977)

the inferior vena cava and the back of the right lobe of the liver. Right lobectomy and extended right lobectomy will require thoracic extension of the incision either by median sternotomy or right thoracotomy. Most left lobe tumors, all tumors in children, and some large but low lying right-sided tumors can be resected entirely through an abdominal incision.

2. Hilar dissection and control of the arterial, portal venous, and biliary radicals feeding and draining the segment to be resected should next be accomplished.
3. Careful capsular incision with blunt elevation and then sharp transection of a centimeter or so of capsule to the tumor side of the proposed line of resection should be done circumferentially around the serosa-covered surfaces of the liver (see Fig. 41-11). This will aid orientation as the transaction of the liver substance proceeds rapidly.
4. Rapid transection of liver substance using blunt technique is the most important step in the operation. Use of the abdominal sucker tip, as illustrated in Fig. 41-12, is preferred. Controlling the tumor with the non-dominant hand, the surgeon exposes all the vessels and ducts with the sucker tip held in the dominant hand. An assistant clips and then cuts all small vessels or ties in continuity all larger vessels as they are encountered (see Fig. 41-13). An extra scrub assistant should pass the clips during this transection.

   Finger fracture is another acceptable technique but will leave the surface more liable to ooze blood and bile. Various liver clamps have been used to reduce blood loss, but they are often difficult to apply for major lobar resection. When hilar control is accurate, the surgical team is practiced, the surgeon's non-dominant hand adequately controls back-bleeding from the tumor site, and when this step of the operation is done rapidly, major lobectomy can be done with minimal blood loss. However the anesthesiologist must be prepared to transfuse rapidly should the tempo of the operation slack off.
5. After removal of the tumor and adjacent liver, gentle compression of the transected surface for several minutes will result in permanent control of all but a few vessels. Any remaining bleeding points are best handled by suture ligation with fine stitches. Clamps and clips are not as effective for vessels partially retracted into the liver substance.
6. The raw surface does not need to be covered with omentum or adjacent bowel. However, hemostasis is often aided by the gentle compression afforded by sutures that bring together the two free edges of the transected liver capsule.
7. After elective liver resection, drainage may not be required at all. Certainly a T-tube is not needed for biliary decompression unless a major bile duct has been injured. When minor oozing of blood persists, it is often wiser to close the abdominal wound and to use suction drainage for a day or two than to pick away at the bleeding surface. The prolonged use of either sump or soft drains probably does more harm than good after most elective liver resections.

A more detailed discussion and illustration of the techniques of liver resection are described by Foster.[99]

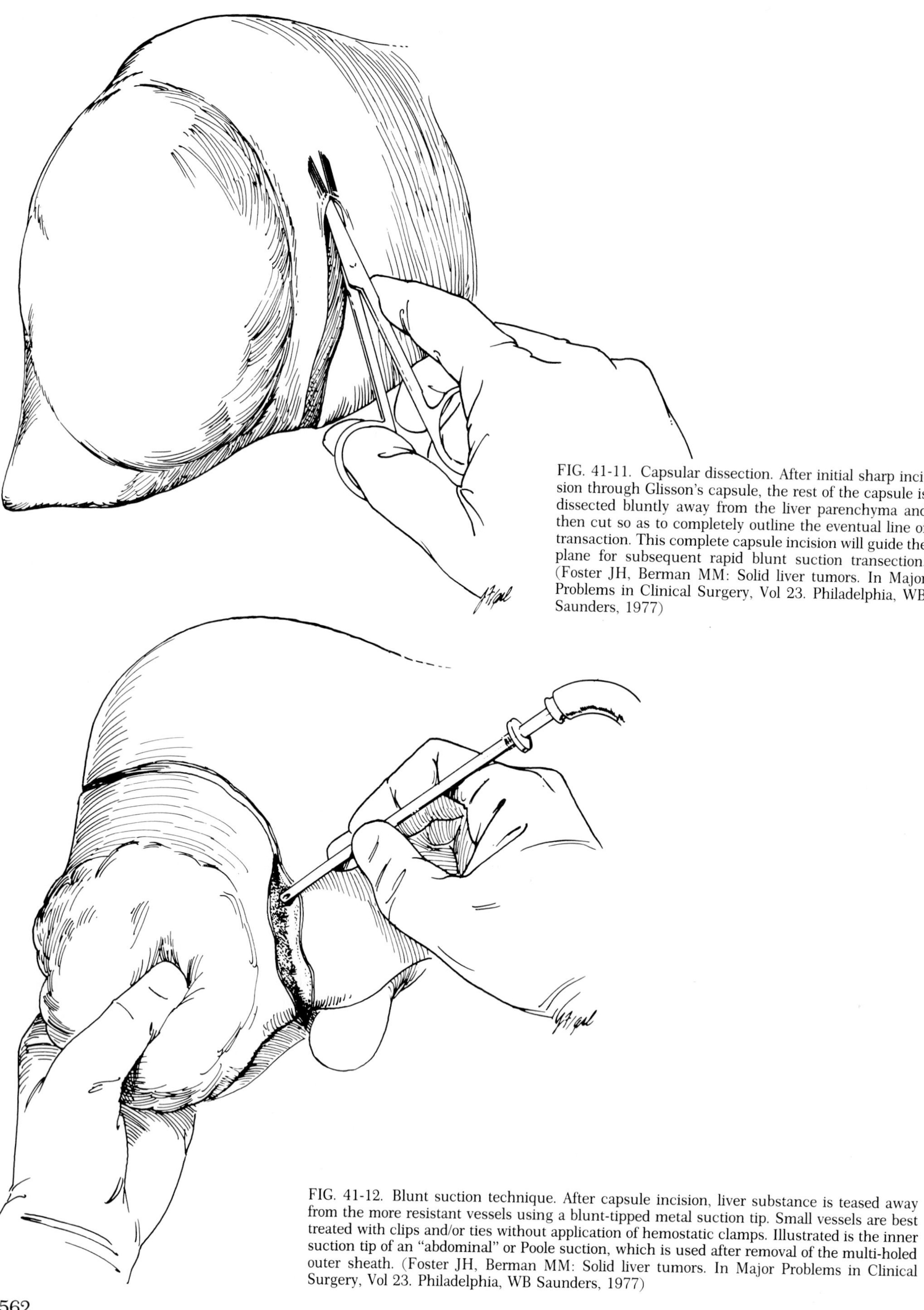

FIG. 41-11. Capsular dissection. After initial sharp incision through Glisson's capsule, the rest of the capsule is dissected bluntly away from the liver parenchyma and then cut so as to completely outline the eventual line of transaction. This complete capsule incision will guide the plane for subsequent rapid blunt suction transection. (Foster JH, Berman MM: Solid liver tumors. In Major Problems in Clinical Surgery, Vol 23. Philadelphia, WB Saunders, 1977)

FIG. 41-12. Blunt suction technique. After capsule incision, liver substance is teased away from the more resistant vessels using a blunt-tipped metal suction tip. Small vessels are best treated with clips and/or ties without application of hemostatic clamps. Illustrated is the inner suction tip of an "abdominal" or Poole suction, which is used after removal of the multi-holed outer sheath. (Foster JH, Berman MM: Solid liver tumors. In Major Problems in Clinical Surgery, Vol 23. Philadelphia, WB Saunders, 1977)

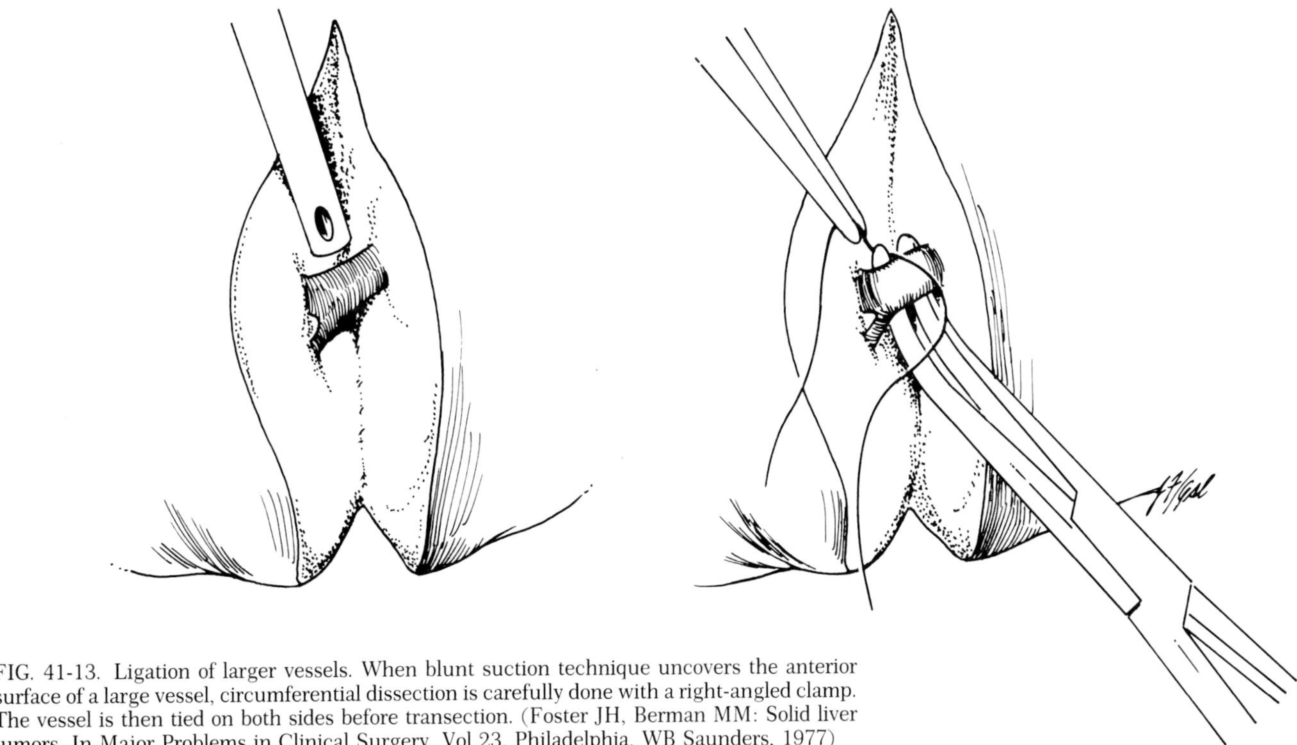

FIG. 41-13. Ligation of larger vessels. When blunt suction technique uncovers the anterior surface of a large vessel, circumferential dissection is carefully done with a right-angled clamp. The vessel is then tied on both sides before transection. (Foster JH, Berman MM: Solid liver tumors. In Major Problems in Clinical Surgery, Vol 23. Philadelphia, WB Saunders, 1977)

SUMMARY

Metastatic disease in the liver is usually a very bad prognostic sign and few patients with metastases from most of the common solid tumor will derive benefit from modern therapy in terms of significant increase in comfortable days at home. The cost/benefit ratio for systemic or regional chemotherapy, radiation therapy, vessel ligation, and of combination therapies, both in terms of dollars and of human suffering remains unclear. Chemotherapy has a clear role to play when liver metastases occur from certain rare primary tumors, where experience has shown good sensitivity to specific agents. Hormone manipulation may play a palliative role for patients with endocrine-sensitive disease. Operative resection of liver metastases is rarely indicated but should be considered for carefully selected patients with certain tumors.

The model of the pediatric tumor provides us with our brightest prospects for the future. Imaginative combinations of new, more effective chemotherapeutic agents with resection and radiation may prevent liver metastases when primary lesions are being treated and may also allow for cure even after liver metastasis has been established. The role of tumor markers in the discovery of early recurrence and the therapeutic benefits of immunotherapy, hyperthermia, and other experimental methods may also augment future effectiveness.

For the present, when unresectable liver metastases are recognized but produce no symptoms, should the patient receive any treatment at all? Two principles apply to that difficult question. First, there is a need to keep searching for effective treatment, so that some patients should be included in well-controlled prospective trials of treatment regimens that do not rob the patient of comfortable days at home. Second, it must be remembered that the first law of therapeutics, which is to do no harm (primum non nocere) and Hoerr's rule (*i.e.,* "It is difficult to make the asymptomatic feel better") concludes that for many asymptomatic patients, a recommendation should be made to withold treatment specifically aimed at their liver disease.[109]

When symptoms can be related to liver metastases from these tumors for which there is little or no effective therapy, the choice of what to offer the patient is more in the realm of art than science. Fortunately, liver disease is often asymptomatic until very close to the end, and among the routes of exodus for the cancer patient, liver failure is not the worst.

Treatment of Metastatic Cancer to Bone

with PETER M. MAUCH

The development of a bone metastasis is a common and often catastrophic event for the cancer patient. The pain, pathological fractures, frequent neurologic deficits, and forced immobility caused by bone metastases significantly decrease the quality of life for the cancer patient. Over 80% of all patients who develop bone metastases have tumors originating in the breast, lung, or prostate. Nearly 50% of all patients who present with breast, lung, or prostate carcinoma will eventually develop bone metastases. Bone metastases are also seen in patients with carcinoma of the kidney, thyroid, bladder, cervix, endometrium, pancreas, and in other tumors, but collectively these represent less than 20% of patients who develop bone metastasis.[110,111]

The most frequent symptom associated with bone metastases is pain, which characteristically develops gradually over weeks or months and becomes progressively more severe. This pain is usually localized and is classically more severe at night.[110] Percussion tenderness at the site of involvement is a highly reliable clinical sign. Stretching of the periosteum of the involved bone by either direct tumor pressure or by weakening of the bone with mechanical stress at the tumor site precipitates pain in some of these patients. In patients with multiple sites of bony metastases, the initial site of pain is often brought on by weight bearing. In this situation radiographs must be obtained to rule out a pathologic fracture. The pain will often be positional in nature, and can be temporarily relieved by shifting weight from the involved area. Bone involvement may also cause pain by nerve entrapment, which results from tumor expansion and pressure on the nerve or by direct destruction of bone with collapse. This pain is most often seen with metastases to the vertebral bodies or sacrum and is characterized by its radicular nature. Careful neurologic evaluation of the patient with back pain is essential as vertebral body destruction is often associated with extradural spine disease, which contributes a high risk of spinal cord compression. The patient with back pain and neurologic signs should undergo a myelogram. Early treatment of a partial or complete spinal cord block may prevent the almost certain tragic neurologic sequelae of motor paresis and sensory loss.

Metastatic bone cancer is rarely life threatening and occasionally patients live for years following the discovery of bone metastases. Treatment goals should center on relieving pain, reducing requirements for narcotic medication, and increasing ambulation. If possible, prolonged hospitalization and an excessive number of outpatient appointments should be avoided. With longer survival, retreatment or orthopaedic stabilization may be needed and these should be considered in the initial management plans.

EPIDEMIOLOGY AND ANATOMIC LOCATION

Bone metastases occur as the primary tumor spreads through lymph or blood vessels to circulate to a site permissive for new tumor growth. Tumor cells may gain access to the circulation by the direct invasion of blood vessels or by neovascularization, although the relationship of circulating tumor cells to development of metastases is complicated.[112] Often the pattern of metastases is related to the specific vascular area invaded. For example, the frequent metastases to the skull from adrenal neuroblastomas and to the shoulder girdle and pelvis from cancer of the prostate can be attributed to tumor invasion of the vertebral vein system.[113] The arterial system, in contrast, is very resistant to neoplastic invasion and this may explain the infrequent involvement of the hands, feet, forearms, and distal legs with bone metastases in the patient with systemic disease.

A solitary metastasis to bone by tumor is unusual and radiographic detection of a single lesion predicts the eventual development of other metastatic disease; most frequently involved are the vertebral bodies, pelvic bones, and ribs. With widespread metastases, lesions in the humerus, femur, scapula, sternum, skull, or clavicle may also be seen. Although involvement of the distal extremities is uncommon, unusual sites of metastases are occasionally seen.[114] One report noted initial metastatic sites that included the maxilla, metatarsal-phalangeal joint, mandible, and antecubital fossa.[115] Occasionally, bony metastases have a soft tissue tumor component, which may make it difficult to distinguish hematogenous metastases from an expanding soft tissue mass eroding into the bone. Soft tissue masses are seen with vertebral body or sternal destruction. Patients with soft tissue metastases to the scalp from breast cancer may have underlying bone destruction as well. Metastases to the ribs or clavicles may also be present as expanding tumor masses.

PATHOLOGY AND RADIOGRAPHIC APPEARANCE

Bone metastases can take on different radiographic appearances. Osteolytic lesions begin in the medullary canal and can infiltrate the entire length of the bone so that treatment localized to the radiographic lesion may often fail due to spreading of the disease beyond the initial radiation portal. As the tumor grows it eventually involves the cortex, thus predisposing to pathologic fracture. The lytic-appearing lesions have ragged margins; when the margins are sharp or smooth a benign process should be considered (see Fig. 41-14*A*). In some instances only a granular, mottled-appearing area is seen. There is usually no periosteal reaction or sclerosis around the margin of the malignant lesion. Breast, kidney, and thyroid carcinomas most commonly produce lytic lesions. In the spine, the vertebral bodies as well as the pedicles may be involved, such that the loss of the outline of one or more pedicle may be the earliest sign of tumor involvement. In the sacrum, loss of the detailed radiographic laminar appearance may help distinguish bone metastasis from bowel gas. In the patient with multiple bone lesions and no known primary,

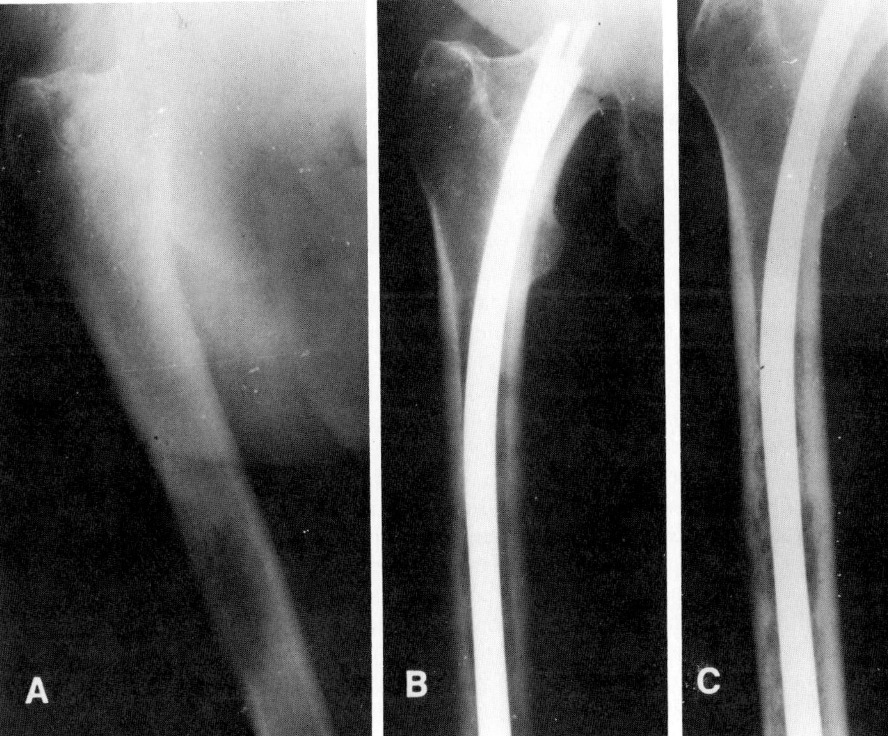

FIG. 41-14. *A*, 57-year-old female with metastatic breast carcinoma. Her first site of bone involvement was this lytic area in the right mid-femoral shaft. *B*, A radiograph taken 6 months after intramedullary fixation of the right femur and systemic therapy with doxorubicin (adriamycin) and cyclophosphamide. Significant bone reformation and recalcification has taken place. *C*, A radiograph taken 18 months after intramedullary fixation. There is now progressive disease with increased destruction in the original area. Radiation therapy was planned.

multiple myeloma must be considered and its radiographic appearance at times cannot be differentiated from metastatic tumor. In the spine, myeloma is less likely to involve the pedicles, and an associated soft tissue mass is more common than in metastatic disease. In the skull, lesions of myeloma are more sharply defined.[116]

Osteoblastic lesions are sclerotic metastatic foci characterized by increased radiographic density. They may occur as isolated rounded foci or as a diffuse sclerosis involving a large area in the bone. Within the involved region the normal bony architecture is lost (see Fig. 41-15). Most patients with osteoblastic lesions have metastatic breast or prostatic carcinoma.[116] Occasionally, metastatic lesions have mixed sclerotic and lytic patterns. Radiographically they appear mottled with intermixed areas of decreased and increased density. Following radiation therapy and occasionally chemotherapy, these destructive lesions often develop some degree of sclerosis, sometimes with complete recalcification of the area.[116,117]

The development of vertebral body collapse in the cancer patient who has diffuse osteoporosis but no known metastatic disease may present a difficult diagnostic problem. Occasionally, laminograms or magnification views of the bone will be useful. With osteoporosis, the cortex of the bone may still be intact while metastatic disease should cause cortical destruction. A syndrome of hypercalcemia and osteoporosis has been associated with certain tumors. Possible mechanisms include parathyroid hormone-like polypeptide production by tumor tissue, and chronic immobilization of patients. Tumor production of vitamin-D-like steroids and prostaglandins has also been implicated.[118,119] The development of osteoporosis due to tumor-accelerated skeletal resorption and calcium release is

FIG. 41-15. Osteoblastic metastases to the fourth lumbar vertebral body and to the sacrum of a patient with prostatic carcinoma. Note the loss of structural detail in the vertebral body.

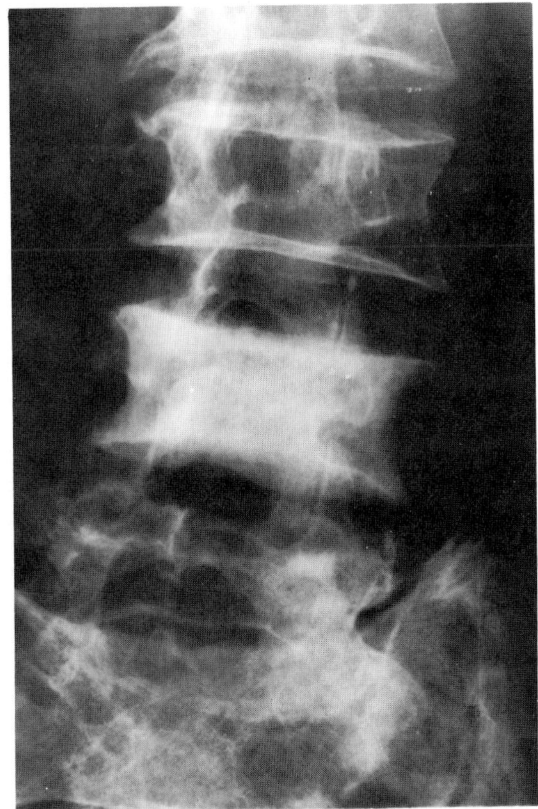

more frequently seen with multiple myeloma than with other tumors.[116]

NATURAL HISTORY

Although the presence of bone metastases almost always predicts eventual progressive disease, the time to progression and development of additional metastases varies tremendously and depends on several factors including host resistance, tumor histology, tumor doubling time, and tumor responsiveness to systemic treatment. Once malignant melanoma has spread to bone the median survival is only 3½ months.[120] In patients with colon cancer metastatic to bone the median survival is 13 months.[121] In metastatic carcinoma of the cervix 96% of patients die within 18 months.[122] However, patients with bony metastases from carcinoma of the breast may occasionally have a prolonged survival as combination chemotherapy or hormonal therapy can produce gratifying responses. Similarly, patients with Hodgkin's disease metastatic to bone may have long survivals following response to therapy with combination chemotherapy.[123] The extent of disease at diagnosis may vary tremendously and the patient with a solitary, asymptomatic lesion on bone scan may have a longer survival than the patient presenting with pain and widespread metastasis. When effective chemotherapy or hormonal therapy is available, progression of bone disease may be delayed. With tumors that respond poorly to systemic management local irradiation may provide significant pain relief but is unlikely to prevent eventual metastases in other sites, even when there is initially only one site recognized.

DIAGNOSIS AND EVALUATION

The physical examination is one of the most important elements in the evaluation of the patient with osseous metastases. Patients with severe pain are often heavily medicated and precise localization requires interviewing and examining the patient just before the next dose of medication is required. Pain localization requires patient cooperation. In the patient who is confused or heavily sedated, precise localization may not be possible. In patients with extensive bony metastases multiple areas of pain are often noted. In this situation, treating the area that is "most painful" is likely to be frustrating and unrewarding for both physician and patient.

Before changes in density can be appreciated on routine radiographs changes of 30–50% must occur in bone mineralization. Even with these changes lesions smaller than 1 cm will often go undetected.[124,125] Initial attempts to devise a more sensitive test by radioactive scanning with calcium-47 were not completely successful due to lack of a photon emission satisfactory for external detection.[124] A great many radiopharmaceuticals, including barium-139, strontium-85, strontium-87 M, fluorine-18, and gallium-68 have subsequently been used in bone scanning. Most recently, technetium polyphosphate-99M has been employed. In a compilation by Charkes of 14 reported series using earlier scanning techniques, scans were positive in 14–34% of patients with metastatic cancer without skeletal radiographic abnormalities.[126] Other nonspecific chemical markers have been used to screen for bone metastasis. These include serum alkaline phosphatase and urine hydroxyproline excretion and serum acid phosphatase in patients with carcinoma of the prostate. These tests are not specific enough to be reliable in the diagnosis of bone metastasis.[127] In one study, 39% of patients with known bone metastases from carcinoma of the prostate had normal acid phosphase levels; 23% had normal alkaline phosphatase levels.[128] A localized area of increased activity identified on a bone scan is not specific for skeletal malignancies. Abnormal scans have been observed in a variety of benign tumors and non-neoplastic skeletal lesions. When the bone scan is positive and radiographs are negative in a patient with a known primary malignancy, bone biopsy may be the only means of immediately confirming or ruling out osseous metastasis. A history of previous trauma or evidence of arthritis may rule in favor of benign disease, especially if the increased uptake is in the area of the previous benign process. A lesion outside the joint or the presence of multiple lesions may favor metastatic disease. Solitary abnormalities are seen in approximately 15% of all positive bone scans. On further investigation in one study, 64% were due to metastatic disease and 36% due to benign processes.[129] In another study, 40% of women with breast cancer who had positive bone scans and negative roentgenograms survived 8 years without evidence of any metastatic disease, emphasizing the importance of histologic or radiographic confirmation in these patients if therapy is to be based on the scan results.[130]

Both the bone scan and the radiograph are important in the management of the cancer patient and they often complement each other. In 2–8% of patients who have destructive radiographic lesions the bone scan is negative.[131] This is especially true with multiple myeloma. Radiographs can help confirm the bone scan abnormalities and can define the structural integrity of the bone and the potential risk for fracture. Pathologic fractures may be seen in the pelvis, the head of the femur, the head of the humerus, and in the vertebral bodies. Their presence may decrease likelihood of relief with radiation therapy alone and increase the need for orthopaedic intervention. With radiography, one may be able to distinguish between a benign and malignant process, both of which are positive on the bone scan. Often tomograms can distinguish the cortical destruction seen with metastases from benign changes that leave the bone cortex intact. The image detail available in magnification radiographs is far superior to the bone scan for assessing progressive changes over time. Sequential scans may show progression by demonstrating additional lesions, but scans are not useful in following disease progression once a specific lesion has been noted. However, the bone scan can be helpful in planning treatment even with local pain and a positive radiograph present. Asymptomatic involvement demonstrated by bone scan adjacent to a symptomatic area may allow alteration of the radiation field used.

Occasionally, patients develop pain without bone scan or radiographic evidence of bony involvement in the symptomatic area. If other bony disease is present, a trial of localized therapy could be initiated. However, if there is no previous evidence of metastatic disease, additional diagnostic studies including biopsy may be needed. In these situations the recent clinical history may be very important. For example, a long history of constant radicular low back pain in a patient who recently developed cancer makes tumor involvement of the low lumbar area less likely than in the patient whose back pain has recently increased in intensity even though the pain is characteristic of either benign or malignant disease.

TREATMENT

Bone metastases require treatment to palliate pain and to prevent fracture of weight-bearing bones. With few exceptions, a radical curative approach to the treatment of bone metastases is unrealistic and its attempt will only risk treatment complications in the patient with incurable disease.[132,133] Patients with bone metastases often have severe pain which limits ambulation. The use of narcotic medication risks oversedation and constipation. Various modalities are available as potentially effective methods of treating bone pain and proper selection and administration of these requires careful evaluation of tumor type, extent of disease, degree of symptomatology, and physical status of the patient.

Localized radiation therapy is a highly effective modality in the treatment of bone pain offering partial or complete relief in 73–96% of patients treated.[133–136] The probability of relief appears slightly better with metastatic breast cancer than with carcinoma of the kidney or prostate and occasionally higher doses are needed for the latter. Treatments can often be given on an outpatient basis and with megavoltage equipment treatments are usually well-tolerated with little morbidity. There continues to be considerable controversy regarding the total dose and number of treatments required for treating bone metastases. Several studies have retrospectively demonstrated that low dose, short fraction irradiation (500–2000 rad in 1–5 fractions) appears as effective and durable in relieving pain as more protracted irradiation (3000–4500 rad in 2½–4½ weeks).[136–139] In these studies a greater portion of patients who received protracted irradiation had relief by the end of therapy than patients with shorter course treatment, but within one month following treatment, the results of therapy were equivalent for the two groups. The duration of palliation was difficult to assess in these studies, as the median survival was often short (4 months in one study).[138] For this reason, some have advocated higher dose or more protracted irradiation in those patients who have a prolonged survival potential (*e.g.*, the patient with early metastatic breast cancer or the patient with a solitary metastasis).[134] The daily planned fractionation also depends on the field size and on acute and long-term normal tissue tolerance. Daily fractionation greater than 300–400 rad should not be employed in treating vertebral body metastasis or in treating large fields that may include portions of the small or large bowel. In this fashion, time dose recommendations for the treatment of bone metastases can vary tremendously. Rib metastases can be treated with a single fraction of 1000 rad. Bone pain from lesions in the humerus or femur is relieved with 2000–2400 rad in 4–6 daily fractions. A solitary bone metastasis, in an otherwise healthy patient, should receive 3000–4000 rad in 2½–4 weeks if long-term control is desired. Cervical or thoracic vertebral body metastases should receive similar doses as treatment with a lower dose makes recurrent symptoms more likely while spinal cord tolerance limits retreatment. The selection of the field size in the patient with metastatic disease is often difficult. Neurologic dysfunction may require more extensive treatment of vertebral body disease than would be indicated by radiographic evaluation. Asymptomatic bone lesions detected radiographically near a painful lesion may allow for inclusion of both lesions in the treatment field. Some have advocated treatment of the entire vertebral spine in patients with metastatic breast carcinoma on the theory that future potential overlap difficulties could be avoided.[140] In contrast, one may want to restrict the size of the radiation field if systemic therapy is to be given. Multiple radiation fields may treat extensive areas of bone marrow making it more difficult to deliver adequate chemotherapy.

Other radiation modalities have been used in the treatment of bone pain. The administration of radioactive I-131 may provide pain relief in certain patients with well-differentiated carcinoma of the thyroid.[141] Testosterone or parathyroid hormone-potentiated radiophosphorus (P32) administration has resulted in substantial palliation of bone pain in 50% of patients with breast cancer and over in 86–93% of patients with cancer of the prostate.[142,143] Strontium-89 has also been effective as a systemic agent in palliating bone pain in patients with carcinoma of the prostate.[143]

HEMIBODY RADIATION

Hemibody irradiation has been an effective treatment modality in selected patients with extensive metastases. In one series, patients with carcinoma of the breast received 600–800 rad half-body irradiation as a single dose. In 12 of 21 patients, complete pain relief was observed within 48 hours.[144] In another study of 84 patients receiving half-body irradiation with cobalt-60 or 35 MeV electrons, dramatic pain relief was noted in many patients.[145] Treatment to the lower half of the body resulted in few or no side effects, while upper half-body irradiation was followed by moderately severe retching, nausea, vomiting, and diarrhea.

Systemic treatment may effectively relieve bone pain from some tumors and may be preferable to localized irradiation in the patient with rapidly progressive bone metastases. Hormonal therapy with estrogens, tamoxifen, or surgical ablation has provided relief from pain in 25–50% of patients with carcinoma of the breast metastatic to bone.[146–148] Similarly, diethylstilbestrol (DES) provides at least temporary pain relief in 75% of patients with metastatic prostatic carcinoma, although serial radiographs rarely demonstrated bone healing.[148] Improvement in serial bone scans has been seen in patients with prostate carcinoma treated with DES.[149] Systemic treatment with 5-fluorouracil improved bone pain in 30% of patients with metastatic breast carcinoma reported in one large series.[150] Results with a five drug chemotherapy regime has produced partial or complete relief in greater than 50% of patients with skeletal metastases from breast cancer.[151] In some of these patients there is bone healing (see Fig. 41-14*A*, *B*, *C*). The use of systemic therapy in patients with renal or lung carcinoma has not been as gratifying and these patients are not as likely to have significant pain relief with combination chemotherapy.[146]

Lytic lesions in weight-bearing bones require special attention. A pathologic fracture can be a catastrophic occurrence for the cancer patient and can increase the risk of early death. Severe pain often will not allow full weight bearing until the area is treated, thus making the bone especially vulnerable to fracture following relief with radiation therapy. Internal fixation followed by radiation therapy should be considered in patients who have lytic lesions in weight-bearing bones to reduce the risk of pathologic fracture. A variety of means for internal fixation are available. In general, intramedullary devices or prosthetic replacement are preferred to external plating in the treatment of pathologic fractures or impending fractures. An endoprosthesis can be used to replace the femoral neck and head. The Zickel intramedullary nail has been commonly used to stabilize the femoral shaft in the patient who has subtrochanteric lesions. A large variety of other external and internal fixation devices are available (see Fig. 41-14*B*).[152–154] Methylmethacrylate may be necessary to help stabilize the internal fixation when there is extensive bony destruction.[47,48] Methylmethacrylate may also produce tumor cell killing as in mixing; the polymerization generates temperatures between 106–110°C, which drop to room temperature in 12–25 minutes.[157] Patients should receive post-operative irradiation following the internal fixation as continued growth and bone destruction by tumor will eventually weaken the bone in spite of the fixation (see Fig. 41-14*C*). Once a fracture occurs, patients who undergo internal fixation have relief of pain 80% of the time and satisfactory healing and excellent functional results 75% of the time. With external fixation these occur only 40% and 33% of the time, respectively.[158,159]

The patient with metastatic bone disease often presents a therapeutic and diagnostic challenge. Many treatment techniques are available allowing for individualization. Aggressive local radiation therapy with orthopaedic stabilization, if necessary, may be appropriate in the patient with a significant life expectancy. Combination chemotherapy or hemibody radiation therapy may provide pain relief and allow treatment of additional systemic disease in patients with progressive or widespread disease. For the critically ill patient, analgesic medication may provide sufficient pain relief, although this is a poor long-term solution. Further advances in the treatment of bone metastasis will come only with earlier detection of disease and with development of more effective adjuvant chemotherapy.

Treatment of Malignant Pleural Effusions

with PETER M. MAUCH

Many cancer patients develop pleural effusions during the course of their disease. Malignant effusions are most commonly associated with carcinomas of the lung and breast, or with lymphomas (see Table 41-19).[160] The survival of patients who develop pleural effusions varies widely and reflects the ability of systemic therapy to control specific types of tumor. Median survivals following diagnosis of malignant effusions have varied from 3.1 months in one study to greater than 19 months in other series.[160,161] Many alternative methods have been developed over the last 20 years to treat pleural effusions.

TABLE 41-19. Site of Primary Tumor Most Frequently Causing Malignant Effusions*

PRIMARY TUMOR	INCIDENCE IN SERIES (%)
Breast	26–49
Lung	10–24
Ovary	6–17
Lymphoma	13–24
Non-Hodgkin's Lymphoma	13–15
Hodgkin's Disease	7–9

* Principles of Internal Medicine, 9th ed. p. 1267, 1979

Each form of treatment has its own set of potential advantages and disadvantages; effective treatment of malignant effusions depends on understanding and evaluating them. Patients with pleural effusions commonly present with dyspnea, cough, or chest pain and only 23% of patients are asymptomatic at presentation.[160] The successful treatment of malignant pleural effusions may allow months or years of productive life. Without treatment, the patient faces repeated thoracenteses and prolonged hospitalization may be required. Pleural effusions cause respiratory embarrassment by mechanical impairment of lung expansion and the resultant reduction in lung volume may predispose to atelectasis and recurrent infection. Thus, effective treatment of pleural effusions may prevent repeated hospitalization, respiratory compromise, and allow for an improved quality of survival.[162]

PATHOGENESIS

The pleural space is formed by a continuous serosal lining that encases the lung on one side (visceral pleura) and the muscles and cartilage of the thoracic cavity (parietal pleura) on the other. In the normal, healthy state, the pleural cavity contains a few milliliters of fluid. The formation and removal of pleural fluid is governed by the relations in the Starling equation in which fluid movement is dependent on four factors: the capillary hydrostatic pressure, the interstitial hydrostatic pressure, the plasma protein osmotic pressure, and the interstitial protein osmotic pressure. The parietal pleural capillary bed, supplied by the branches of the intercostal arteries, has a higher hydrostatic pressure than the visceral pleural capillaries supplied by the pulmonary circulation. Under normal circumstances, fluid is continuously filtered from the parietal pleural surface because of this pressure differential and is about 80–90% reabsorbed through the visceral pleura.[162,163] The remaining 10–20% including large molecular substances is reabsorbed through lymphatic channels lying just beneath the serosal membrane. An imbalance of this equilibrium may result from changes in hydrostatic or osmotic pressure or from an increase in capillary permeability. Intrathoracic malignancies can affect these factors in several ways. Direct involvement of the pleural surface by tumor and the associated inflammation may produce increased capillary permeability. Obstruction of lung or pleural lymphatic channels impairs reabsorption of fluid and protein. Obstruction of the pulmonary veins by tumor increases the capillary hydrostatic pressure thus reducing gradient between the parietal and visceral pleura. This may occur in patients with endobronchial obstruction, with atelectasis, or with postobstructive pneumonitis. Severe hypoproteinemia may also impair the reabsorptive process.[160,164] True chylous pleural effusion arises from central impairment due to obstruction and damage of the thoracic duct by tumor.

DIAGNOSIS

Pleural effusions have been associated with many different malignant and non-malignant diseases. In one review of 436 patients with pleural effusions from the Mayo Clinic, 53% were associated with malignant disease, 10% were associated with congestive heart failure, 8% were related to infection, 12% were from other miscellaneous causes, and in 17% the cause was never determined.[165] In another review, malignancy-caused effusions were seen in 39% of cases.[166] Of the neoplastic pleural effusions, carcinomas of the lung, breast, and the lymphomas and leukemias were the cause in more than 85% of cases. Cardiac-related effusions were most commonly due to chronic rheumatic heart disease, hypertensive heart disease, or calcific aortic stenosis. The most common cause of infection-related effusions was tuberculosis.[165] Other causes of pleural effusions included pulmonary infarction, cirrhosis of the liver, renal disease, and lupus erythematosus. Pleural effusions have also been reported following routine abdominal surgery.[167]

The initial separation of effusions into transudates and exudates has been a useful concept that can be helpful in determining the cause of pleural effusions. With transudates, an increase in the amount of pleural fluid is due primarily to an increased leakage of water. Diseases that result in an imbalance of sodium and water often have associated transudative effusions. Cirrhosis, nephrosis, and congestive heart failure should be strongly suspected in patients with transudative effusions. Changes that affect the capillary or interstitial hydrostatic pressure (such as obstruction by mediastinal nodes) may also result in a transudative effusion. Patients with lymphoma or Hodgkin's disease may have significant mediastinal adenopathy with an associated transudative effusion that should not be interpreted as pleural involvement by the lymphoma. One study analyzed patients with primary bronchogenic carcinoma who had associated pleural effusions that were cytologically negative. Most patients were eventually found to have metastatic disease but in five of these patients long-term survival was achieved following local resection. Thus, cytologic evidence of direct pleural involvement must be made in patients with primary tumors who have pleural effusions but no other known metastatic disease.[168]

Exudates represent an abnormal accumulation of protein in the pleural space. Malignancy is the most frequent cause of exudative effusions but they can also be associated with tuberculosis, pneumonia, pulmonary embolism, collagen vascular disease, and trauma. There has been no general agreement on the diagnostic criteria needed for separation of transudate and exudates. However, one classic study frequently cited identifies three criteria that are highly useful in the diagnostic evaluation of pleural effusions: a ratio of pleural fluid protein to serum protein greater than 0.5; a ratio of pleural fluid LDH to serum LDH greater than 0.6, and a LDH value greater than 200 mg/dl usually indicate exudative effusions.[169]

Various methods have been used to diagnose malignant pleural effusions. The most common is routine thoracentesis. Following thoracentesis, fluid should be sent for culture to rule out tuberculosis or other infection. Cytologic examination of the fluid as well as examination of the cell block after fixation and sectioning should be carried out. Several chemical tests can be performed on the fluid. Pleural fluid glucose levels have been reported to be low in both tuberculosis and in neoplastic effusions. Pleural fluid amylase determinations have been elevated in patients with pancreatitis and with pancreatic tumors. These two tests are not specific enough, however, to result in a definitive diagnosis.[170] Thirty-four to 55% of patients with malignant effusions will have pleural fluid carcinoembryonic antigen (CEA) levels greater than 12 ng/ml.[171–173] Similar results have been reported with beta$_2$ microglobulin levels in the pleural fluid. Elevated CEA levels are rarely associated with benign effusions. Thus, elevated CEA levels above 12 ng/ml are pathognomonic of malignant effusions. Cell counts should be made on the pleural effusion and cytologic examination performed. Through thoracentesis a cytologic diagnosis of malignancy can be made in as many as 65–67% of patients who are eventually found to have malignant effusions. Cytogenic techniques identifying hyperdiploid cells or cells containing abnormal chromosomes can aid in making a diagnosis of malignancy.[174–176] If diagnosis cannot be made by thoracentesis then a thoracostomy directed biopsy may be necessary. Using these two techniques, 94–96% of patients with malignant effusions can be diagnosed without further study.[177] An absolute cell count in malignant effusions may help determine the pathogenesis. With an acellular effusion, obstruction of small vessels and lymphatics is most likely.[161] In this situation systemic therapy and perhaps mediastinal irradiation can be most useful. When there is tumor implantation on the serosal surface, usually fewer than 1000 cells/mm^3 are seen. With the tumor implantation clumps of cells, often well-differentiated, will be seen in the effusion. Intracavitary chemotherapy may be therapeutic by pleural irritation. At times the tumor may be free-growing in the effusion. Morphologically, these cells would be less differentiated, often single cells, and 1000–4000 cells/mm^3 would be seen. Intracavitary chemotherapy in this situation may act as both a cytotoxic agent and as a pleural irritant. Milky-appearing fluid may indicate a chylothorax. Therefore, fluid should be sent for staining with Sudan III to microscopically demonstrate the presence of fat. The fat may be removed by acidification of the fluid followed by extraction with ether. Other conditions called pseudochylous effusions may be associated with a cloudy or milky-appearing pleural fluid. The turbid appearance of the fluid is usually due to protein and desquamated cells and the turbidity will not be removed with ether.

TREATMENT

Thoracentesis alone, even when the pleural space is completely evacuated, does not prevent reaccumulation of fluid in metastatic malignant effusions.[178] Similarly, a small number of patients treated with tube thoracostomy may remain fluid free, but most patients will have recurrence of pleural effusion within a short period.[174] Nonetheless, one or more thoracenteses should be performed both for obtaining initial diagnostic material and for establishing the recurrent nature of the effusion. Rapidly reaccumulating effusions that cause respiratory symptoms require treatment and a choice of therapy must then be made. Patients with effusions from breast cancer or lymphoma may respond to systemic therapy and avoid the need for intrathoracic manipulation.

The primary goal for treatment of malignant pleural effusions is relief of symptoms. Obliteration of the pleural space prevents reaccumulation of fluid and thus the effectiveness of an intracavitary agent depends primarily on its ability to produce mesothelial fibrosis and pleural sclerosis rather than its specific antineoplastic activity. There is some evidence to suggest that instillation of an alkylating agent or antibiotic following tube thoracostomy is superior to results obtained with the instillation of these agents through thoracentesis. Various agents have been instilled intrapleurally in an attempt to diminish the incidence of recurrent pleural effusion. Intrapleural instillation of nitrogen mustard reduced or prevented pleural fluid reaccumulation in 64% of patients reported in one study.[166] However, in another study only 25% of patients had beneficial results.[180] Median patient survival may influence reported statistics as in one study where 57% of patients who were treated with tube thoracostomy and instillation of nitrogen mustard were free of effusion 3 months after therapy, but only 29% were free of effusion 6 months following treatment.[174] The use of other agents has resulted in a 38% benefit from instillation of intracavitary 5-fluorouracil, an improvement in 37–57% of patients treated with intracavitary thiotepa, and improvement in 63% of patients given intrapleural bleomycin.[161,183] Intracavitary chemotherapy is administered at doses similar to that administered systemically. For nitrogen mustard, 10–40 mg, for thiotepa, 30–45 mg, for 5-fluorouracil, 2–3 g, and for bleomycin, 15–240 mg. Toxicity commonly has included nausea and vomiting, with chest pain, fever and leukopenia occurring less frequently.

Both quinacrine, an antimalarial agent, and tetracycline have been administered intrapleurally for the treatment of malignant pleural effusions with good to excellent results. The mode of action of these agents is solely by means of their sclerosing properties. The intrapleural administration of quinacrine has resulted in reduction of effusions in 67–70% of patients studied.[184–186] Pain and fever are commonly reported side effects with quinacrine administration although hypotension, oliguria, and skin discoloration have also been noted.[186,187]. Tetracycline is also an effective intrapleural agent with over 80% of patients requiring no additional therapy following administration.[188,189] Pleuritic pain is the only significant side effect reported with the use of tetracycline.

External beam irradiation of the hemithorax or mediastinum has been used to control pleural effusions in some patients. In one study seven of 10 patients required no additional treatment following 1400–2600 rad external beam irradiation to the hemithorax for lymphoma.[190] In another study, out of 14 evaluable patients given 1800 rad over 3 weeks duration ten demonstrated no reaccumulation or improvement of their pleural effusions.[191] Radioactive colloidal gold (Au^{198}) and

FIG. 41-16. Treatment of malignant pleural effusions.

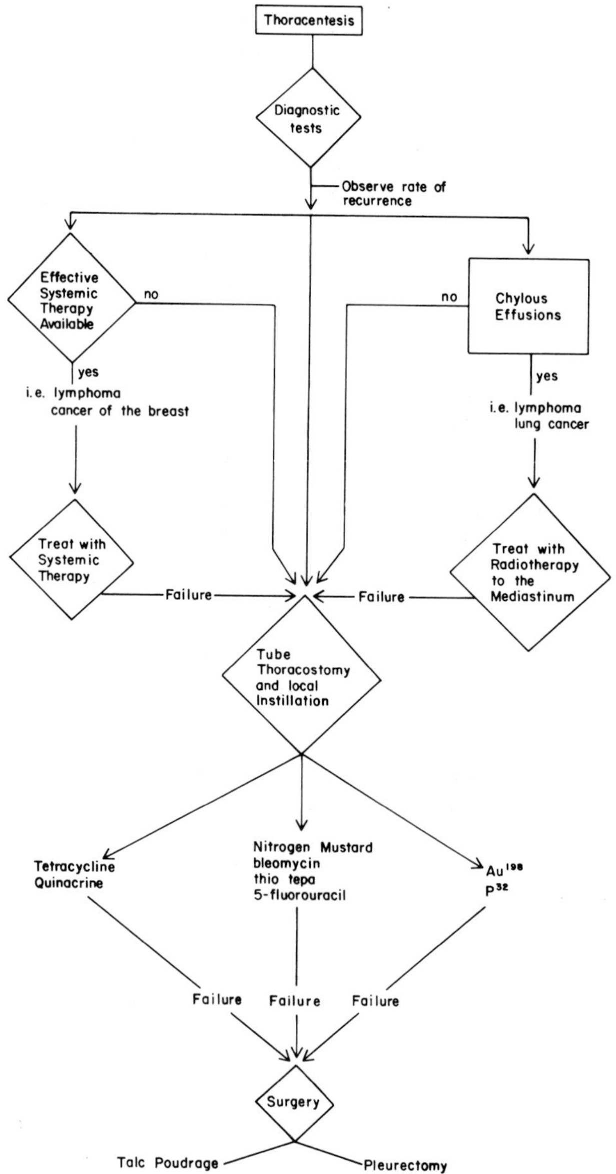

radioactive colloidal phosphorus (P^{32}) have been used intrapleurally in the treatment of malignant effusions. Several studies have reported a marked decrease or absence of pleural fluid reaccumulation in approximately 50% of patients receiving radioactive gold or colloid chromic phosphate.[192–195] Mild anemia and leukopenia have been seen following Au^{198} 50–100 mCi administration. Other difficulties with the use of radioisotopes include the lack of homogeneous distribution in some patients, and the need for specialized personnel and facilities to prevent radiation contamination.

Surgical techniques have been used in the treatment of malignant effusions with varying degrees of risk and effectiveness. Talc poudrage uses a silicate that is closely related chemically to asbestos and produces a chronic granulomatous reaction in the lung when inhaled. The installation of talc into the pleural space causes an intense pleuritis and subsequent obliteration of the pleural space.[196–198] In one study, 90% of patients treated with talc pleurodesis required no additional treatment.[197] Intrapleural talc administration is painful and is often done under general anesthesia. One study reported an improvement in 37% of patients treated with closed drainage thoracostomy alone.[199] The average hospital stay for patients receiving tube drainage alone was 8 days versus 11 days for patients receiving both thoracostomy drainage and instillation therapy. In another study, however, all patients treated with thoracostomy drainage alone recurred within one month.[174]

Pleurectomy has been shown to be highly effective treatment for patients with malignant pleural effusions[174,184]. In one series, none of the 146 patients who underwent pleurectomies have had recurrence of their effusion following surgical treatment.[199] The median survival after pleurectomy was 16 months. Complications, however, are high and persistent pneumonia and empyema complicate the course in more than 20% of patients postoperatively. Mortality from the procedure is about 10%.[199]

External beam irradiation to the mediastinal nodes can completely control a chylothorax due to thoracic duct obstruction. In other instances, aspiration or continuous catheter drainage may allow relief although instillation of a sclerosing agent will often be necessary. A diet, low in fatty acids, may provide temporary relief by decreasing the flow of chyle.

Many modalities for the treatment of pleural effusions have been described or reported in the literature. These include repeated thoracentesis, use of diuretics, systemic chemotherapy, instillation of chemotherapy intrapleurally, instillation of antibiotics, thoracostomy drainage alone, intracavitary radioactive colloid administration, external beam irradiation, thoracostomy with talc administration, and pleurectomy. Effectiveness of these various treatments varies widely as do their potential side effects. In Fig. 41-16 one treatment approach is outlined. Drainage alone is associated with a high recurrence rate and aggressive surgical treatment may have a high associated mortality such that other treatments should be initially considered. Patients with malignant effusions have a limited life expectancy and treatment goals should include relieving symptoms and avoiding repeated hospitalizations. In many patients, intrapleural chemotherapy or antibiotic administration through a thoracostomy tube can provide significant palliation without significant morbidity.

Treatment of Malignant Pericardial Effusions

with PETER M. MAUCH

The development of metastatic pericardial disease often goes undiagnosed in the cancer patient. The formation of a pericardial effusion may be gradual and the associated symptoms, which include dyspnea, cough, hepatomegaly, pain, orthopnea, cyanosis, venous distension, leg edema, and cardiac enlargement may all be attributed to the overall systemic effects of carcinomatosis unless there are reasons to suspect pericardial involvement.[200,201] Left unattended the rapid development of a pericardial effusion can lead to cardiac tamponade sudden death; in one series, 36% of patients with pericardial disease died as a direct result of the pericardial involvement.[200] However, if cardiac tamponade can be avoided the mean survival of the patient with a pericardial effusion is quite satisfactory and is 9–13 months, respectively, in two studies.[202,203]

A variety of tumors have been reported to metastasize to the pericardium. The ones most commonly reported include lung cancer, breast cancer, leukemia, Hodgkin's disease, non-Hodgkin's lymphoma, melanoma, GI tumors, and sarcomas.[204–208] Occasionally, cardiac tamponade may be the first manifestation of metastatic tumor or leukemia.[209] Certain primary tumors of the heart may cause pericardial effusions; these include mesothelioma and sarcoma.[210,211] Metastatic involvement of the pericardium may occur from either direct invasion by an adjacent primary tumor or by lymphatic or hematogenous spread.

PATHOGENESIS

Metastasis can involve the pericardium in a variety of ways. By direct extension, tumor can involve the pericardium with or without involvement of the heart. With hematogenous or lymphatic spread there can be studding of the pericardium with diffuse tumor nodules or diffuse infiltration by tumor and thickening of the pericardium. Extension to the epicardium or myocardium may also be present. Constrictive pericarditis occurs when a thickened fibrous pericardium hampers the diastolic filling of the ventricles. If the constriction is significant enough cardiac tamponade can occur even without fluid accumulation.[212]

Cardiac tamponade is caused by the accumulation of fluid in the pericardium in an amount sufficient to cause serious obstruction to the inflow of blood to the ventricle. The amount of fluid necessary to produce this critical state may be as small as 250 ml when fluid develops rapidly or it may be well over 1000 ml with a slowly developing effusion where the pericardium has had the opportunity to stretch and adapt to the increasing volume of fluid.[213]

Clinically, the progressive elevation of intrapericardial pressure interferes with ventricular expansion and results in a decrease in the cardiac volume. There is a rapid rise in the ventricular diastolic pressure followed subsequently by a rise in the mean left atrial, the pulmonary venous, the pulmonary atrial, the right atrial, and the vena caval pressure. In an effort to maintain the normal cardiac output various compensatory mechanisms come into play. The heart rate increases and peripheral vasoconstriction occurs in an attempt to maintain arterial pressure and venous return. There is decreased renal blood flow which results in increased sodium and water retention and an increase in blood volume. With a rapidly increasing intrapericardial pressure these compensatory methods may not be able to counterbalance the rise in ventricular diastolic pressure; total circulatory collapse and death can occur. With a more gradual increase the pericardium has time to stretch and the intrapericardial pressure does not rise to such high levels allowing compensatory mechanisms to be able to effectively maintain the cardiac output.[201]

DIAGNOSIS

Many of the signs and symptoms of neoplastic pericardial effusions result from a decrease in ventricular stroke volume and an increase in ventricular diastolic pressure and include dyspnea, hepatomegaly, venous distension, orthopnea, and occasionally cyanosis. Other signs include hiccups, cough, and pain.[200] With constrictive pericarditis, atrial arrhythmias, an early diastolic sound, and a pericardial friction rub may also be seen.[214]

Similarly, the symptoms of cardiac tamponade are due to a falling cardiac output and systemic venous congestion. Most frequently, tamponade develops slowly and symptoms resemble those of heart failure: orthopnea, tachycardia, and hepatic engorgement. Bilateral pleural effusions may be present. Palpation of the precordium may reveal weakness or absence of the cardiac impulse. Percussion may reveal a marked increase in precordial dullness. On auscultation there may be tachycardia and arrhythmias. Heart sounds may be weak and distant except when there is excessive tumor involvement or constrictive pericarditis present during which sounds can remain loud. One important clue in the diagnosis of cardiac tamponade is the presence of a greater-than-normal respiratory decrease in the systolic atrial pressure; if severe this may be detected by palpating the arterial pulse during inspiration. Concomitant inspiratory swelling of the neck veins may be seen during respiration. This respiratory fall in the systolic pressure when greater than 10 mm Hg is known as pulsus paradoxus and can occasionally occur from other causes—severe myocardial failure, hemorrhagic shock, chronic obstructive airway disease, and severe bronchial asthma.[200,201] Finally, when cardiovascular collapse is imminent more severe symptoms may be seen including facial plethora, profuse perspiration, confused or impaired consciousness, rapid and shallow breathing, and peripheral cyanosis.

The radiographic changes seen with neoplastic pericarditis include cardiomegaly if there is significant pericardial effusion present. The heart may have a globular or water bottle appearance and, in some instances, even nodular appearances to the normal cardiac contour can be seen. Mediastinal widening and hilar adenopathy are frequently seen. Fluoroscopic examination may reveal a striking absence of pulsations of the cardiac border but a vigorous aortic pulsation.[201] Radioactive-labeled I^{131} human serum albumin injected IV can measure by photoscanning the size of the intraventricular volume. When compared to a chest radiograph, differences in the transverse diameter can be seen if pericardial effusion is present. Echocardiographic changes are best seen by studying the posterior wall where normally single echo is seen moving synchronously with the heartbeat. In the presence of a pericardial effusion two distinct echoes are observed—one from the pericardium and one from the posterior heart border. With impending cardiac tamponade abnormalities in the anterior mitral leaflet motion may also be seen on echocardiography.[215,216]

The EKG changes seen with neoplastic pericarditis are often minimal. Reported changes include cyanosis, tachycardia, premature contraction, low QRS voltage, and non-specific ST and T wave changes.[200] If constrictive pericarditis is present a flattened or inverted T wave may be seen.[214] However, pathognomonic of cardiac tamponade is the presence of total electrical alternans involving both atrial and ventricular complexes. This is seen electrocardiographically as alternation of the P wave as well as the QRS complex and is an especially unfavorable prognostic finding even if it resolves following pericardiocentesis. Ventricular alternation (QRS only) may occur with cardiac tamponade but is a less specific sign. Pulsus alternans, an indication of serious myocardial weakness, is rarely seen with cardiac tamponade.[217–219]

In evaluation of the patient with known malignancy and pericardial effusion other potential diagnoses should be considered. Pericarditis and pericardial effusions can be caused by a large number of diseases including tuberculosis, rheumatic fever, trauma, uremia, collagen vascular disease, myxedema, severe chronic anemia, previous irradiation, and by some drugs including procainamide and hydralazine.[213] Examination of the fluid following pericardiocentesis may be helpful. Malignant cells can occasionally be seen although even in the presence of neoplastic pericarditis a high percentage of false negative cytologic results are seen.[220] Fluid should also be sent for culture and stained for acid fast organisms. Pericardial effusions are almost always exudative in nature. Bloody fluid is commonly due to tuberculosis or tumor but may be seen with administration of anticoagulants or with uremia.[213] The presence of regional tumor or adenopathy may add circumstantial evidence for the diagnosis of neoplastic pericarditis when other such evidence is not available.

Pericardial injury is a well-known complication of modern radiation therapy. One study estimated that approximtely

4000 rad of fractionated radiation therapy to a considerable volume of heart is required for radiation injury to occur to normal cardiac structures.[221] The injury to the pericardium may manifest itself as an acute pericarditis during the course of the treatment, weeks or months after completion, or as a chronic form up to 20 years after treatment. Acute radiation pericarditis is frequently self-limited and often subsides without residual constriction. Chronic radiation pericarditis may lead to constriction, tamponade, and eventual death. The differential diagnosis between radiation-induced pericarditis and progressive malignant disease with pericardial metastasis is often difficult to make in a patient who has had prior radiation therapy. The findings from the pericardial fluid may not be helpful, as in both instances the fluid may be bloody and cytology is often negative even when neoplastic pericarditis is present. A careful understanding of the volume of heart irradiated and the total dose delivered may help to determine whether radiation pericarditis is a likely possibility or not.

TREATMENT

The diagnosis of malignant pericardial effusion and cardiac tamponade should always be considered in the patient with metastatic cancer. In the presence of a pericardial effusion, arterial and venous pressures and heart rate should be monitored and serial radiographs obtained. With cardiac tamponade sudden death may occur. If there are symptoms of cyanosis, dyspnea, shock, impairment of consciousness, falling pulse pressure, or a rising venous pressure, pericardiocentesis should be performed as soon as possible.[215] Other supportive measures may be needed at the same time. These include IV fluids, pressor agents, and nasal oxygen. As much fluid should be removed as possible at pericardiocentesis. The procedure itself has some risk including induction of cardiac arrhythmias and hemorrhage from an injured coronary vessel, and the puncture should be done under EKG and blood pressure monitoring. With removal of the first 50–100 cc of fluid, disappearance of some of the signs may occur.[215,222] Following relief of cardiac tamponade there may be rapid fluid reaccumulation. For more prolonged palliation some recommend formation of a pericardial pleural window. This is a successful procedure which is well-tolerated surgically and is limited mainly by rapid reformation of adhesions, which sometimes block the window. Technically, the procedure is difficult to perform when the tumor encases the heart and pericardium.[223,224] Others have favored insertion of an indwelling pericardial catheter by way of chest intubation. Talc can then be inserted to cause pericardial irritation, subsequent fibrosis, and obliteration of the pericardial space.[225] Pericardiectomy is a highly effective treatment for cardiac tamponade but it involves a more extensive surgical approach, usually a left thoracotomy, has a higher morbidity, and thus is rarely justified. However, in patients with chronic constrictive pericarditis, either from tumor or from radiation therapy, it may be the only effective treatment available.[226]

Various agents have been injected into the pericardial cavity either following pericardiocentesis or catheter placement in an attempt to control recurrent pericardial effusion. These include the use of intrapericardial tetracycline and quinacrine.[202,227,228] Antineoplastic agents have also been used intrapericardially and include nitrogen mustard, thiotepa, and 5-fluorouracil.[229–232] Although the number of patients treated with these agents is too small for individual comparison, collective intrapericardial instillation of these drugs provides for approximately a 50% likelihood of significant decrease in pericardial fluid production. This is presumably due to sclerosis of the pericardial membrane and obliteration of the pericardial sac. Side effects include nausea, mild chest pain, and transient fever. If effective systemic chemotherapy or hormonal therapy is available to the patient with widespread metastatic disease, this may be attempted prior to the administration of intrapericardial agents. With a slowly developing pericardial effusion, systemic agents may have time to effect tumor regression and decrease fluid production.

Radioactive gold and colloidal chromic phosphate have also been used intrapericardially in an attempt to control malignant effusions.[203,233] In one study 28 patients were treated with pericardiocentesis and colloidal chromic phosphate instillation intraperitoneally. Only eight patients in this study had further difficulty with effusion. External beam radiation therapy has also been effective in treating pericardial effusions in some patients.[234–236] In one study, 11 of 16 patients with pericardial effusions from breast cancer and two of seven patients with lung cancer had significant improvement following a 2500–3500 rad cardiac irradiation. Furthermore, with significantly lower doses, six of seven patients with lymphoma or leukemia had relief of their effusion.[234]

The symptoms of pericardial effusion and cardiac tamponade may mimic the symptoms of generalized carcinomatosis; if not part of the routine evaluation, this diagnosis may be missed. Initial conservative therapy in most patients is warranted. This includes repeated pericardiocentesis, hormonal or systemic chemotherapy, and perhaps intrapericardial administration of antibiotics, radioactive colloid, or antineoplastic agents. Neoplastic cardiac tamponade is one of the emergencies of clinical oncology. It may appear abruptly and cause death in a patient who has a potentially controllable disease and otherwise good short-term life expectancy. In patients who have impending cardiac tamponade formation, a pericardial pleural window may be indicated. When constrictive pericarditis or extensive tumor involvement is present a more extensive pericardiectomy may be the only way to relieve symptoms. This procedure has a higher morbidity and should be used only under carefully selected circumstances. As outlined, the treatment of pericardial effusions should proceed in a stepwise fashion and these patients should have a mean life expectancy of 9–13 months if tamponade does not occur. Even with cardiac tamponade, long-term survivals have been reported.[235]

Treatment of Malignant Ascites

with PETER M. MAUCH

Abdominal distension, weight gain, and general discomfort are presenting signs of ascites. The increased intra-abdominal pressure associated with ascites may result in indigestion or heartburn. Localized pain is unusual unless liver or splenic congestion or peritonitis is present. Dyspnea, orthopnea, or tachypnea may result from elevation of the diaphragm. Leakage of ascitic fluid through diaphragmatic lymphatic channels may produce a coexistent pleural effusion and cause additional respiratory embarrassment. Decreased bowel motility from abdominal carcinomatosis and ascites may lead to obstruction of the small bowel. Ascites is diagnosed by physical examination. A tensely distended abdomen with tightly stretched skin and bulging flanks is characteristic. Auscultation may reveal a high-pitched rushing sound of early intestinal obstruction or a succussion sound due to increased fluid and gas in a dilated hollow viscus. Fluid wave and flank dullness that shifts with changes in the patient's position are important signs that indicate the presence of peritoneal fluid.[238]

There are multiple causes of ascites, both neoplastic and non-neoplastic, and in the patient with a primary malignancy other causes of ascites must be ruled out. The major non-malignant causes of ascites include cirrhosis of the liver, tuberculosis, peritonitis, pyogenic peritonitis, congestive heart failure, nephrosis, and pancreatitis.[238] A variety of factors play a role in ascites formation. Increased capillary permeability due to damaged capillary endothelium occurs with bacterial infection or with widespread peritoneal carcinomatosis. Increased venous pressure from congestive heart failure or from a local obstructive process results in elevation of microcirculatory vessel pressure and decreased reabsorption of fluid from the abdomen. The plasma oncotic pressure may be reduced from the hypoalbuminemia seen with malignant tumors, liver disease, or loss of protein from other causes. In this circumstance, the ascitic fluid protein is greater than the serum protein and additional fluid is drawn into the abdominal cavity. With peritoneal seeding from a malignant tumor perhaps the most common cause of ascites is obstruction of the diaphragmatic lymphatics. One study in a murine ovarian tumor model has demonstrated that the egress of ^{51}Cr-labeled erythrocytes through the diaphragmatic lymphatic channels becomes blocked prior to ascites development and may in fact predict this development.[239]

A careful clinical history and physical examination can help determine the cause of ascites. The presence of congestive heart failure or nephrosis can usually be diagnosed non-invasively. Diagnostic paracentesis is an important test in the routine evaluation of ascites. Turbid or purulent ascites would favor pyogenic peritonitis. Culturing the ascites fluid may help rule out tuberculosis; protein determination may also be important. Cirrhosis and nephrosis rarely cause ascitic protein values greater than 2.5 g/100 ml fluid. In contrast, in neoplastic effusions approximately 75% of patients have ascitic fluid protein greater than 2.5 g/100 ml. Cytologic and cell block examination may disclose an otherwise unsuspected carcinoma or may help confirm metastatic cancer in a patient with a known primary malignancy. Careful cytogenetic analysis of cells from peritoneal fluid may reveal hyperdiploid cells or cells with an abnormal number of chromosomes.[240] One study has indicated that measurement of the carcinoembryonic-antigen (CEA) level in the peritoneal fluid is helpful in testing for malignant disease.[241] Approximately 50% of patients who have malignant ascites have CEA levels greater than 12 ng/ml. None of the patients with non-malignant peritoneal effusions had CEA levels greater than this value. Chylous ascites refers to a turbid milky or creamy fluid due to presence of thoracic duct or intestinal lymph. The causes of chylous peritonitis include trauma with mechanical damage to the lymphatic system, intestinal obstruction with rupture of a major lymphatic channel, and malignant disease or tuberculosis infection obstructing the intestinal lymphatics. Lymphangiography may be of value in determining the location of the leak or site of obstruction to the lymphatic channels.[238] Chylous ascites has also been described in patients who have undergone retroperitoneal lymphadenectomy and in patients who have had lymphatic injury during intra-abdominal surgery.[242,243]

Radiographs, ultrasonography, and CT may be helpful in evaluation of the patient with ascites. Routine abdominal radiographs can evaluate areas of potential small bowel obstruction. Ultrasonography has been of some help in evaluating the retroperitoneum; however, distended loops of bowel often interfere with the quality of this study. For this reason, CT is more accurate in evaluating the liver, spleen, and retroperitoneum.[244]

Malignant ascites has been associated with a number of different tumors. In order of decreasing frequency, ovarian, endometrial, breast, colonic, gastric, and pancreatic carcinomas make up more than 80% of the tumors associated with intra-abdominal seeding and ascites formation.[245–248] There have been rare cases of ascites associated with multiple myeloma and malignant melanoma.[249–251]

Several major therapeutic modalities have been used in the treatment of malignant ascites: systemic chemotherapy; radioactive colloidal chromic phosphate or radioactive gold; chemotherapeutic agents administered intra-abdominally; and surgical techniques that shunt peritoneal fluid back into the general circulation. Repeated paracentesis of abdominal fluid has not been effective in reducing ascites and only results in protein loss and risks fluid deprivation. If effective chemotherapy is available it should be tried initially as a gratifying response that will treat both the ascites and the disease itself.

Intraperitoneal administration of Au^{198} has been a common treatment for malignant ascites. In a review of 566 patients treated with Au^{198} over a 10-year interval, 47% of patients responded with a decrease in the production of peritoneal fluid.[252] Doses of 125–150 millicuries of intraperitoneal Au^{198} resulted in complete cessation of fluid formation in many patients. Late effects included mild anemia and leukopenia but treatments were well tolerated. Autopsy findings have revealed that gold particles are deposited on the serous surfaces as relatively large aggregates and subsequently undergo partial phagocytosis.[253] The major hazard in the use of radioactive gold is the risk of leakage or spillage. The material must be handled by specialized personnel in an approved facility. The short half-life of radioactive gold somewhat reduces this risk of contamination. Colloidal chromic phosphate (P^{32}) has also been used in the treatment of malignant ascites and in one series, 31% of patients had complete cessation of their effusion.[254]

Various chemotherapeutic agents have been used intra-abdominally in the treatment of malignant ascites. The major toxicity of these agents has been mild leukopenia and occasional fever. Reduction or complete cessation of the production of peritoneal fluid has been reported in 35% of patients treated with 5-fluorouracil, 36% with the use of bleomycin, 32% with administration of thiotepa, and 53% in one report with the use of nitrogen mustard.[255-258] Reported doses include bleomycin (60–120 mg), 5-fluorouracil (2–3 g), and nitrogen mustard (10–40 mg). Intracavitary treatment may be more effective if the tumor has been responsive to systemic therapy; this is most likely in patients who have metastases from ovarian or breast cancer. Intracavitary treatment has little cytotoxic effect on peritoneal implants and its main effect is in inducing fibrosis of the peritoneal membrane. However, in the ascites tumor model, with single undifferentiated cells (1000–4000/mm^3), there may be tumor growth within the ascites fluid itself and some cytotoxic effect may be seen.

Intra-abdominal chemotherapy is unlikely to be effective in patients with chylous ascites. Tumor-causing lymphatic dysfunction may be sensitive to systemic chemotherapy. A median chain triglyceride diet may be of some help in reducing production of chyle. If leakage of lymphatic vessels is demonstrated, conservative measures including diet and paracentesis should be attempted reserving laparotomy as a last resort. LeVeen shunt placement has been effective in some patients with chylous ascites.[242,259]

Several different surgical methods for the relief of ascites have been reported. One is to devise a peritoneal vessicle catheter such that ascitic fluid will drain into the bladder and can be voided per urethrum.[260] A more popular technique has been the use of the peritoneal venous shunt. This has been popularized by Leveen and has been described in various reports.[246,261-263] The shunt drains fluid from the abdominal cavity into the superior vena cava. The effectiveness of the shunt is due to a pressure sensitive one-way valve that permits flow when intraperitoneal pressure exceeds the central venous pressure by 3–5 cm of water pressure. In this fashion, back-up of blood from the venous system into the peritoneum is prevented. The initial shunt was devised for non-malignant ascites and was initially successful in 28 of 37 patients into whom it was implanted.[264] A more recent study has evaluated the shunt in patients with malignant ascites. Out of 37 patients 27 (73%) treated with peritoneal venous shunting for malignant ascites achieved long-term palliation longer than 3 months duration or until death of their underlying

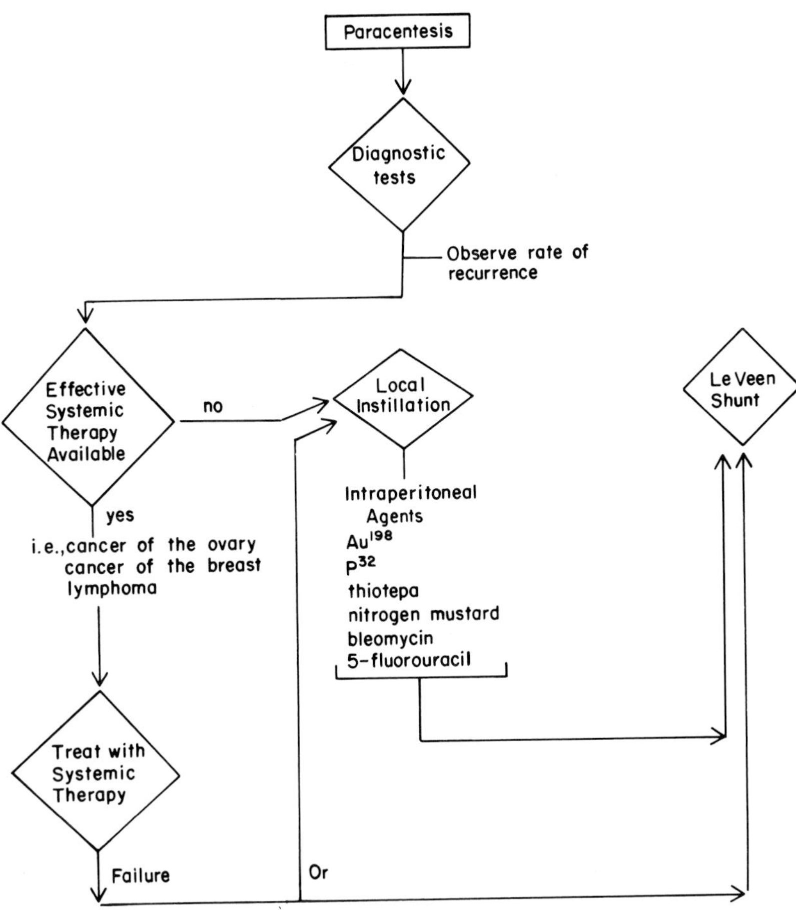

FIG. 41-17. Management of malignant ascites.

disease. In the 31 patients in whom initial shunt function was established, the mean duration of shunt function was 10.6 weeks and the mean survival from time of shunt placement was 11.6 weeks.[246] Most patients who had shunt failures had bloody ascites at the time of shunt placement. One of eight patients with bloody ascites had normal shunt function and presumably clotting of the valve was responsible for the lack of function. The shunt placement is usually well tolerated. Patients may have a febrile response for 2–4 days following placement of the shunt which spontaneously resolves. Shunt-related infections are rare. Shunt placement is a relatively simple procedure rarely lasting longer than 45 minutes and is usually carried out under local infiltration anesthesia plus sedation with diazepam.[264]

SUMMARY

Malignant ascites and its often associated nausea, distension, and shortness of breath can provide an uncomfortable existence for patients with metastatic disease. Various methods of treating malignant ascites have been reported. (Some of these are outlined in Fig. 41-17.) The use of diuretics or repeated paracentesis is ineffective. In 30–50% of patients intraperitoneal administration of radioactive colloid or antineoplastic chemotherapy can reduce peritoneal fluid formation. Peritoneal venous shunting has been an effective alternative method to the instillation of these agents and can provide relief in a very high percentage of patients. Side effects are minimal for all three major modalities and the proper choice of treatment must in part depend on the experience of the physician and institution to administer such therapy.

REFERENCES

1. Vieth RG, Odom GL: Intracranial metastases and their neurosurgical treatment. J Neurosurg 23:375–383, 1965
2. Borgelt B, Gelber R, Kramer S et al: The palliation of brain metastases: Final results of the first two studies by the Radiation Therapy Oncology Group. Int J Radiat Oncol Biol Phys 6:1–9, 1980
3. Chao JH, Phillips R, Nickson JJ: Roentgen-ray therapy of cerebral metastases. Cancer 7:682–689, 1954
4. Chu FCH, Hilaris BS: Value of radiation therapy in the management of intracranial metastases. Cancer 14:577–581, 1961
5. Nisce LZ, Hilaris BS, Chu FCH: A review of experience with irradiation of brain metastasis. Am J Roentgenol Radium Ther Nucl Med 111:329–333, 1971
6. Horton J, Baxter DH, Olson KB: The management of metastases to the brain by irradiation and corticosteroids. Am J Roentgenol Radium Ther Nucl Med 111:334–336, 1971
7. Montana GS, Meacham WF, Caldwell WL: Brain irradiation for metastatic disease of lung origin. Cancer 29:1477–1480, 1972
8. Hendrickson FR: The optimum schedule for palliative radiotherapy for metastatic brain cancer. Int J Radiat Oncol Biol Phys 2:165–168, 1977
9. Hindo WA, DeTrana III, FA, Lee MS et al: Large dose increment irradiation in treatment of cerebral metastases. Cancer 26:138–141, 1970
10. Kramer, S, Hendrickson F, Zelen M et al: Therapeutic trials in the management of metastatic brain tumors by different time/dose fractionation schemes of radiation therapy. Natl Cancer Inst Monogr 46:213–221, 1977
11. Shehata WM, Hendrickson FR, Hindo WA: Rapid fractionation technique and re-treatment of cerebral metastases by irradiation. Cancer 34:257–261, 1974
12. Order SE, Hellman S, Von Essen CF et al: Improvement in quality of survival following whole-brain irradiation for brain metastases. Radiology 91:149–153, 1968
13. West J, Maor M: Intracranial metastases: Behavioral patterns related to primary site and results of treatment by whole brain irradiation. Int J Radiat Oncol Biol Phys 6:11–15, 1980
14. Galicich JH, Sundaresan N, Thaler HT: Surgical treatment of single brain metastases. J Neurosurg 53:63–67, 1980
15. Winston KR, Walsh JW, Fischer EG: Results of operative treatment of intracranial metastatic tumors. Cancer 45:2639–2645, 1980

15a. Malaise EP, Chavaudra N, Courdi A et al: Tumor Growth Rate and Pulmonary Metastases. In Weiss L, Gilbert HA (eds): Pulmonary Metastasis. Boston, GK Hall & Co, 1978

16. Edlich RF, Shea MA, Foker JE et al: A review of 26 years' experience with pulmonary resection for metastatic cancer. Dis Chest 49:587–594, 1966
17. Vincent RG, Choksi LB, Takita H et al: Surgical Resection of the Solitary Pulmonary Metastasis. In Weiss L, Gilbert HA (eds): Pulmonary Metastasis. Boston, GK Hall & Co, 1978
18. Neifield JP, Michaelis LL, Doppman JL: Suspected pulmonary metastases: Correlation of chest x-rays, whole lung tomograms and operative findings. Cancer 39:383–387, 1977
19. Chang AE, Schaner EC, Conkle DM et al: Evaluation of computed tomography in the detection of pulmonary metastases: A prospective study. Cancer 43:913–916, 1979
20. Wilkins EW Jr: The Status of Pulmonary Resection of Metastases: Experience at Massachusetts General Hospital. In Weiss L and Gilbert HA (eds): Pulmonary Metastasis. Boston, GK Hall & Co, 1978
21. Thomford NR, Woolner LB, Clagett OT: The surgical treatment of metastatic tumors in the lungs. J Thorac Cardiovasc Surg 49:357–363, 1965
22. Martini N, Huvos AG, Mike V et al: Multiple pulmonary resections in the treatment of osteogenic sarcoma. Ann Thorac Surg 12:271–280, 1971
23. Morton DL, Joseph WL, Ketcham AS et al: Surgical resection and adjunctive immunotherapy for selected patients with multiple pulmonary metastases. Ann Surg 178:360–365, 1973
24. Viadana E, Brass IDJ, Pickren JW: Cascade Spread of Blood-borne Metastases in Solid and Non-solid Cancers of Humans. In Weiss L and Gilbert HA (eds): Pulmonary Metastasis. Boston, GK Hall & Co, 1978
25. Ramming KP, Holmes EC, Skinner DG et al: Surgery for Pulmonary Metastases: The UCLA Approach. In Weiss L and Gilbert HA (eds): Pulmonary Metastases. Boston, GK Hall & Co, 1978
26. McCormack P: Surgical Treatment of Pulmonary Metastases: Memorial Hospital Experience. In Weiss L and Gilbert HA (eds): Pulmonary Metastases. Boston, GK Hall & Co, 1978
27. McCormack PM, Martini N: The changing role of surgery for pulmonary metastases. Ann Thorac Surg 28:138–145, 1979
28. Takita H, Merrin C, Didolkar MS et al: The surgical management of multiple lung metastases. Ann Thorac Surg 24:359–363, 1977
29. McCormack P, Bains MS, Beattie EJ Jr et al: Pulmonary resection in metastatic carcinoma. Chest 73:163–166, 1978
30. Takita H, Edgerton F, Vincent RG et al: Surgical Management of Lung Metastases. In Weiss L and Gilbert HA (eds): Pulmonary Metastasis. Boston, GK Hall & Co, 1978
31. Martini N, McCormack PM, Bains MS et al: Surgery for solitary and multiple pulmonary metastasis. NY State J Med 78:1711–1713, 1978
32. Turney SZ, Haight C: Pulmonary resection for metastatic neoplasms. J Thorac Cardiovasc Surg 61:784–794, 1971
33. Collins VP, Loeffler RK, Tivey H: Observations on growth rates of human tumors. Am J Roentgenol 76:988–1000, 1956
34. Joseph WL, Morton DL, Adkins PC: Prognostic significance of tumor doubling time in evaluating operability in pulmonary metastatic disease. J Thorac Cardiovasc Surg 61:23–32, 1971

35. Giritsky AS, Etcubanas E, Mark JBD: Pulmonary resection in children with metastatic osteogenic sarcoma. J Thorac Cardiovasc Surg 75:354–362, 1978
36. Romansky SG, Landing BH: Metastatic Patterns in Childhood Tumors. In Weiss L and Gilbert HA (eds): Pulmonary Metastases. Boston, GK Hall & Co, 1978
37. Telander RL, Pairolero PC, Pritchard DJ et al: Resection of pulmonary metastatic osteogenic sarcoma in children. Surgery 84:335–341, 1978
38. Beattie EJ, Martini N, Rosen G: The management of pulmonary metastases in children with osteogenic sarcoma with surgical resection combined with chemotherapy. Cancer 35:118–121, 1975
39. Turnbuss AD, Pool JL, Arthur K et al: The role of radiotherapy and chemotherapy in the surgical management of metastases. Am J Roentgenol Rad Ther Nucl Med 114:99–105, 1971
40. Van Dongen JA, Van Slooten EA: The surgical treatment of pulmonary metastases. Cancer Treat Rev 5:29–48, 1978
41. Marcove RC, Mike V, Hajek JV et al: Osteogenic sarcoma under the age of 21: A review of 145 operative cases. J Bone Joint Surg 52A:411–421, 1970
42. Rosen G, Huvos AG, Mosende C et al: Chemotherapy and thoracotomy for metastatic osteogenic sarcoma: A model for adjuvant chemotherapy and rationale for the timing of thoracic surgery. Cancer 41:841–849, 1978.
43. Huth JF, Holmes EC, Vernon SE et al: Pulmonary resection for metastatic sarcoma. Am J Surg 140:9–16, 1980
44. Rosenberg SA, Flye MW, Conkle D et al: Treatment of osteogenic sarcoma. II. Aggressive resection of pulmonary metastases. Cancer Treat Rep 63:753–756, 1979
45. Feldman PS, Kyriakos M: Pulmonary resection for metastatic sarcoma. J Thorac Cardiovasc Surg 64:784–799, 1972
46. Wilkins EW, Head JM, Burke JF: Pulmonary resection for metastatic neoplasms of the lung. Am J Surg 135:480–482, 1978
47. Bains MS, McCormack PM, Coitkovic E et al: Results of combined chemo-surgical therapy for pulmonary metastases from testicular carcinoma. Cancer 41:850–853, 1978
48. Mountain CF, Khalh KG, Hermes KE et al: The contribution of surgery to the management of carcinomatous pulmonary metastases. Cancer 41:833–840, 1978
49. Merrin C, Takita H, Beckley S et al: Treatment of recurrent and widespread testicular tumor by radical reductive surgery and multiple sequential chemotherapy. J Urol 177:291–301, 1977.
50. Merrin CE: Combined Surgical and Chemotherapeutic Approach to Metastases from Testicular Tumors. In Weiss L and Gilbert HA (eds): Pulmonary Metastasis. Boston, GK Hall & Co, 1978
51. Cahan WG: Excision of melanoma metastases to lung: Problems in diagnosis and management. Ann Surg 178:703–709, 1973
52. Mathisen DJ, Flye MW, Peabody J: The role of thoracotomy in the management of pulmonary metastases from malignant melanoma. Ann Thorac Surg 27:295–299, 1979
53. Mountain CF: The basis for surgical resection of pulmonary metastasis. Int J Radiat Oncol Rad Ther 1:749–755, 1976
54. Cahan WG, Castro EB, Hajdu SI: Therapeutic pulmonary resection of colonic carcinoma metastatic to lung. Dis Colon Rectum 17:302–309, 1974
55. Brown JM: The effect of lung irradiation on the incidence of pulmonary metastases in mice. Br J Radiol 46:613–618, 1973
56. Owen LN, Bostock DE: Prophylactic X-irradiation of the lung in canine tumors with particular reference to osteosarcoma. Eur J Cancer 9:747–752, 1973
57. Fu KK, Phillips TL, Wharam MD et al: The influence of growth and irradiation conditions on the radiation response of the EMT6 tumor. Sixth L.H. Gray Conference Proceedings, pp 251–258. London, Institute of Physics, 1975
58. Fernandez CH, Lindberg RD, Sutow WW et al: Localized Ewing's sarcoma—treatment and results. Cancer 34:143–148, 1974
59. Cassady JR, Tefft M, Filler RM et al: Considerations in the radiation therapy of Wilms' tumor. Cancer 32:598–608, 1973
60. Caldwell WL: Elective whole lung irradiation. Radiology 120:659–666, 1976
61. Wara WM, Phillips TL, Margolis LW et al: Radiation pneumonitis: A new approach to the derivation of time-dose factors. Cancer 32:547–552, 1973
62. Hussey DH, Castro JR, Sullivan MP et al: Radiation therapy in the management of Wilms' tumor. Radiology 101:663–668, 1971
63. Newton KA, Spittle MF: An analysis of 40 cases treated by total thoracic irradiation. Clin Radiol 20:19–22, 1969
63a. Monson KJ, Brand WN, Boggs JD: Results of a small-field irradiation of apparent solitary metastasis from Wilms' tumor. Radiology 104:157–160, 1972
63b. Wharam MD, Phillips TL, Jacobs EM: Combination chemotherapy and whole lung irradiation for pulmonary metastases from sarcomas and germinal cell tumors of the testes. Cancer 34:136–143, 1974
63c. Cox JD, Gingerelli F, Ream NW et al: Total pulmonary irradiation for metastases from testicular carcinoma. Radiology 105:163–167, 1972
63d. van der Werf–Messing B: The treatment of pulmonary metastases of malignant teratoma of the testes. Clin Radiol 24:121–123, 1973
63e. Baeza MR, Barkley HT, Fernandez C: Total lung irradiation in the treatment of pulmonary metastases. Radiology 116:151–154, 1975
64. Jaffe BM et al: Factors influencing survival in patients with untreated hepatic metastases. Surg Gynecol Obstet 127:1, 1968
65. Foster JH: Survival after liver resection for secondary tumors. Am J Surg 135:389, 1978
66. Bengmark S, Hafstrom L: The natural course for liver cancer. Prog Clin Cancer 7:195, 1978
67. Pettavel J, Morgenthaler F: Protracted arterial chemotherapy of liver tumors: An experience of 107 cases over a 12-year period. Prog Clin Cancer 7:217, 1978.
68. Wood CB, Gillis CR, Blumgart LH: A retrospective study of the natural history of patients with liver metastases from colorectal cancer. Clin Oncol 2:285, 1976.
69. Cedermark BJ et al: The value of liver scan in the follow-up study of patients with adenocarcinoma of the colon and rectum. Surg Gynecol Obstet 144:745, 1977
70. Evans JT et al: Pre- and postoperative uses of CEA. Cancer (Suppl): 42:1419, 1978
71. Martin EW Jr et al.: A retrospective and prospective study of serial CEA determinations in the early detection of recurrent colon cancer. Am J Surg 137:167, 1979
72. Woolley PV, Higgins GA, Schein PS: Ongoing trials in surgical adjuvant management of colorectal cancer. Recent Results Cancer Res 68:231, 1978
73. Taylor I, Brooman P, Rowling JT: Adjuvant liver perfusion in colorectal cancer: Initial results of a clinical trial. Br Med J 2:1320, 1977
74. Ingold JA et al: Radiation hepatitis. Am J Roentgenol 93:200–208, 1965
75. Phillips R et al: Roentgen therapy of hepatic metastases. Am J Roentgenol Radium Ther Nucl Med 71:826–834, 1954
76. Kraut J et al: Hepatic effects of irradiation. In Vaeth JV (ed): Frontiers in Radiation Therapy and Oncology, Vol 1, p 18. Baltimore, University Park Press, 1972
77. Rubin P (ed): Radiation Hepatopathy in Set Radiation Therapy. I. In: Radiation Oncology–Radiation Biology and Radiation Biology Syllabus, pp 59–75. Chicago, Waverly Press, 1975
78. Turek-Maischeider M, Kazein I: Palliative irradiation for liver metastases. JAMA 232:625, 1975
79. Case TJ, Worthen AS: The occurrence of hepatic lesions in patients treated by intensive deep roentgen irradiation. Am J Roentgenol 12:27–46, 1924
80. Prasad B et al: Irradiation of hepatic metastases. Int J Radiat Oncol Biol Phys 2:129–132, 1977
81. Sherman DM et al: Palliation of hepatic metastases. Cancer 41:2013–2017, 1978
82. Gelber RD et al: Technical report no. 60R—Analysis of RTOG

protocol 76–05. Pilot protocol for palliation of hepatic metastases, pp 1–24, 1979
83. Friedman M et al: Combined modality theory of hepatic metastases. Cancer 44:906–913, 1979
84. Webber BM et al: A combined treatment approach to management of hepatic metastases. Cancer 42:1087–1095, 1978
85. Leibel SA, Order SE: Unpublished data, 1980
86. Kraut JW, Kaplan HS, Bagshaw MA: Combined fractionated isotopic and external irradiation of the liver in Hodgkin's disease—a study of 21 patients. Cancer 30:39–46, 1972
87. Ariel IM, Padula G: Treatment of symptomatic metastatic cancer to the liver from primary colon and rectal cancer by the intra-arterial administration of chemotherapy and radioactive isotopes. Prog Clin Cancer 7:247, 1978
88. Grady ED: Internal radiation therapy of hepatic cancer. Dis Colon Rectum 22:371, 1979
89. Ansfield FJ, Ramirez C: The clinical results of 5-fluorouracil intrahepatic arterial infusion in 528 patients with metastatic cancer to the liver. Prog Clin Cancer 7:201, 1978
90. Sullivan RD: Systemic and arterial infusion chemotherapy for metastatic liver cancer. Int J Radiat Oncol Biol Phys 1:973, 1976
91. Watkins E, Oberfield RA, Cady B et al: Arterial infusion chemotherapy of diffuse hepatic malignancies. Prog Clin Cancer 7:235, 1978
92. Ramming KP et al: Management of hepatic metastases. Semin Oncol 4:71, 1977
93. Watkins E Jr et al: Surgical basis for arterial infusion chemotherapy of disseminated carcinoma of the liver. Surg Gynecol Obstet 130:581, 1970
94. Sullivan RD, Zurek WZ: Chemotherapy for liver cancer by protracted ambulatory infusion. JAMA 194:481, 1965
95. Petrek JA, Minton JP: Treatment of hepatic metastases by percutaneous hepatic arterial infusion. Cancer 43:2182, 1979
96. Sundquist K et al: Treatment of liver cancer with regional intra-arterial 5-FU infusion. Am J Surg 136:328, 1978
97. Patt YZ et al: Hepatic arterial infusion of corynebacterium parvum and chemotherapy. Surg Gynecol Obstet 147:897, 1978
98. Bala Segaram M: Complete hepatic de-arterialization for primary carcinoma of the liver. Am J Surg 124:340, 1972
99. Foster JH, Berman MM: Solid liver tumors. In Major Problems in Clinical Surgery, Vol 23. Philadelphia, WB Saunders, 1977
100. El-Domeiri AA, Mojab K: Intermittent occlusion of the hepatic artery and infusion chemotherapy for carcinoma of the liver. Am J Surg 135:771, 1978
101. Honjo I et al: Ligation of a branch of the portal vein for carcinoma of the liver. Am J Surg 130:296, 1975
102. Gans H, Koh SK, Aust JB: Hepatic resection. Arch Surg 93:553, 1966
103. Pack GT, Brasfield RD: Metastatic carcinoma of the liver: Clinical problems and its management. Am J Surg 90:704, 1955
104. Starzl TF, Koep LJ: Surgical approaches for primary and metastatic liver neoplasms, including total hepatectomy and orthotopic liver transplantation. Prog Clin Cancer 7:181, 1978
105. Adson MA, Van Heerden JA: Major hepatic resections for metastatic colorectal cancer. Ann Surg 191:576–583, 1980
106. Wilson SM, Adson MA: Surgical treatment of hepatic metastases from colorectal cancers. Arch Surg 111:330, 1976
107. Raven RW: Hepatectomy. XVI Congress de la Societe Internationale de Chirurgie, Copenhagen, p 1099. Brussels, Imprimerie Medicale et Scientifique, 1955
108. Fortner JG et al: Major hepatic resection for neoplasia. Ann Surg 188:363, 1978
109. Hoerr SO: Hoerr's law. Am J Surg 103:411, 1962
109a. Flanager LH, Foster JH: Hepatic resection for metastatic cancer. Am J Surg 113:551–557, 1967
109b. Pestana C, Reitemeier RJ, Moertic CG, et al: The natural history of carcinoma of the colon and rectum. Am J Surg 108:826–829, 1964
109c. Pettavel J, Morgenthaler F: Protracted arterial chemotherapy of liver tumors; on experience of 107 cases over a 12-year period. Prog Clin Cancer 7:217–233, 1978
110. Hendrickson FR, Sheinkop MB: Management of osseous metastasis. Semin Oncol 2:399, 1975
111. Johnson AD: Pathology of metastatic tumors in bone. Clin Orthop 73:8, 1970
112. Sugarbaker EV, Ketcham AS: Mechanisms and prevention of cancer dissemination: An overview. Semin Oncol 4:19, 1977
113. Batson OV: The function of the vertebral veins and their role in the spread of metastasis. Ann Surg 112:138, 1940
114. Gall RJ, Sim FH, Pritchard DJ: Metastatic tumors to the bones of the foot. Cancer 37:1492, 1976
115. Brady LW, O'Neill EA, Farber SH: Unusual sites of metastasis. Semin Oncol 4:59, 1977
116. Paul LW, Juhl JH: Essentials of Roentgen Interpretation, pp 214–216. Hagerstown, Harper & Row, 1972
117. Unger JD, Chiang LC, Unger GF: Apparent reformation of the base of the skull following radiotherapy for nasopharyngeal carcinoma. Radiology 126:779, 1978
118. Besarab A, Caro JF: Mechanisms of hypercalcemia in malignancy. Cancer 41:2276, 1978
119. Muggia FM, Heinemann HO: Hypercalcemia associated with neoplastic disease. Ann Intern Med 73:281, 1970
120. Stewart WR, Gelberman RH, Harrelson JM et al: Skeletal metastasis of melanoma. J Bone Joint Surg 60-A:645, 1978
121. Besbeas S, Stearns MW Jr.: Osseous metastasis from carcinoma of the colon and rectum. Dis Colon Rectum 21(4):266, 1978
122. Blythe JG, Ptacek JJ, Buchsbaum HJ et al: Bone metastases from carcinoma of the cervix. Cancer 36:475, 1975
123. Mauch P, Ryback MG, Rosenthal D et al: The influence of initial pathological stage on the survival of patients who relapse from Hodgkin's disease. Blood 56:892, 1980
124. Maynard CD: Clinical Nuclear Medicine, pp 255–267. Philadelphia, Lea & Febeiger, 1970
125. Borah J: Relationship between clinical and roentgenological findings in bone metastases. Surg Gynecol Obstet 75:599, 1942
126. Charkes ND: Radioisotope scanning of roentgeno-graphically occult disorders of bone. AEC Symposium Series, Clin Uses of Radionuclides 27:101, 1972
127. Bishop MC, Fellows GJ: Urine hydroxypyroline excretion—a marker of bone metastases in prostatic carcinoma. Br J Urol 49:711, 1977
128. Schaffer DL, Pendergrass HP: Comparison of enzyme, clinical, radiographic and radionuclide methods of detecting bone metastases from carcinoma of the prostate. Radiology 121:431, 1976
129. Corcoran RJ, Thrall JH, Kyle RW et al: Solitary abnormalities in bone scans of patients with extraosseous malignancies. Radiology 121:663, 1976
130. Sklaroff RB, Sklaroff DM: Bone metastases from breast cancer at the time of radical mastectomy as detected by bone scan. Cancer 38:107, 1976
131. Blair RJ, McAfee JG: Radiological detection of skeletal metastasis: Radiographs versus scans. Int J Radiat Oncol Biol Phys 1:1201, 1976
132. Grabstald H: Is there a surgical role in managing bone metastasis? Int J Radiat Oncol Biol Phys 1:1207, 1976
133. Delclos L: New and old concepts in radiotherapeutic treatment. Int J Radiat Oncol Biol Phys 1:1217, 1976
134. Garmatis CJ, Chu FCH: The effectiveness of radiation therapy in the treatment of bone metastasis from breast cancer. Radiology 126:235, 1978
135. Gilbert HA, Kagan AR, Nussbaum H et al: Evaluation of radiation therapy for bone metastases: Pain relief and quality of life. Am J Roentgenol 129:1095, 1977
136. Hendrickson FR, Shehata WM, Kirchner HB: Radiation therapy for osseous metastasis. Int J Radiat Oncol Biol Phys 1:275, 1976
137. Allen KL, Johnson TW, Hibbs GG: Effective bone palliation as related to various treatment regimens. Cancer 37:984, 1976
138. Jensen NH, Roesdahl K: Single dose irradiation of bone metastasis. Acta Radiol Ther Phys Biol 15:337, 1976
139. Penn CRH: Single dose and fractionated palliative irradiation for osseous metastasis. Clin Radiol 27:405, 1976

140. Bagshaw MA: Presumptive palliative irradiation in metastatic carcinoma of the breast. Cancer 28:1692, 1971
141. Harkness JR, Thompson NW, Sisson JC et al: Differentiated thyroid carcinomas. Arch Surg 108:410, 1974
142. Cheung A, Driedger AA: Evaluation of radioactive phosphorus in the palliation of metastatic bone lesions from carcinoma of the breast and prostate. Radiology 134:209, 1980
143. Firusian N, Mellin P, Schmidt CG: Results of **89 Strontium therapy in patients with carcinoma of the prostate and incurable pain from bone metastasis. J Urol 116:764, 1976.
144. Bartelink H, Battermann J, Hart G: Half body irradiation. Int J Radiat Oncol Biol Phys 6:87, 1980
145. Fitzpatrick PJ, Rider WD: Half body radiotherapy. Int J Radiat Oncol Biol Phys 1:197, 1976
146. Cadman E, Bertino JR: Chemotherapy of skeletal metastasis. Int J Radiat Oncol Biol Phys 1:121, 1976
147. Kennedy BJ: Hormonal therapies in breast cancer. Semin Oncol 1:119, 1974
148. Mellette SJ: Management of malignant disease metastatic to bone by hormonal alterations. Clin Orthop 73:73, 1970
149. Antar MA, Remblish R, Waserman I et al: Serial bone scan for prostatic bony metastasis during diethylstilberstol therapy. Invest Radiol 13:389, 1978
150. Ansfield FJ, Ramirez G, Mackman S et al: A 10-year study of 5-fluorouracil in disseminated breast cancer with clinical results and survival times. Cancer Res 2:1062, 1969
151. Kaufman S, Goldstein M: Combination chemotherapy in disseminated carcinoma of the breast. Surg Gynecol Obstet 136:83, 1973
152. Douglas HO, Skukla SK, Mindell E: Treatment of pathological fractures of lung bones excluding those due to brest cancer. J Bone Joint Surg 58A:1055, 1976
153. Ryan JR, Rowe DE, Salcicciolì GG: Prophylactic internal fixation of the femur for neoplastic lesions. J Bone Joint Surg 58A:1071, 1976
154. Zickel RE, Mouradian WH: Intramedullary fixation of pathological fractures and lesions of the subtrochanteric region of the femur. J Bone Joint Surg 58A:1061, 1976
155. Harrington KD, Johnston JO, Turner RH et al: The use of methylmethacrylate as an adjuvant in the internal fixation of malignant neoplastic fractures. J Bone Joint Surg 54-A:1665, 1972
156. Harrington KD, Sim FH, Enos JF et al: Methylmethacrylate as an adjunct in internal fixation of pathological fractures. J Bone Joint Surg 58A:1047, 1976
157. Chan PY, Norman A: Hyperthermia (HT) effects of methyl methacrylate (MM) in bone metastases (BM). Proc Am Assoc Cancer Res 20:299, 1979
158. MacAusland WR Jr, Wyman ET: Management of metastatic pathological fractures. Clin Orthop 73:39, 1970
159. Perez CA, Bradfield JS, Morgan HC: Management of pathological fractures. Cancer 29:684, 1972
160. Chernow B, Sahn SA: Carcinomatous involvement of the pleura. Am J Med 63:695, 1977
161. Rosato FE, Wallach MW, Rosato GF: The management of malignant effusions from breast cancer. J Surg Oncol 6:441, 1974
162. Leff A, Hopewell PC, Costello: Pleural effusion from malignancy. Ann Intern Med 88:532, 1978
163. Leininger BJ, Barker WL, Langston HT: A simplified method for management of malignant pleural effusion. J Thorac Cardiovasc Surg 58:758, 1969
164. Tisi GM: Neoplasms of the Lung. In Isselbacher KJ, et al (eds): Principles of Internal Medicine, 9th ed, p. 1267. New York, McGraw Hill, 1979
165. Levallen EC, Carr DT: Pleural effusion: A statistical study of 436 patients. N Engl J Med 252:250, 1955
166. Hirsch A, Ruffie P, Nebut M et al: Pleural effusion: Laboratory tests in 300 cases. Thorax 34L:106, 1979
167. Light RW, George RB: Incidence and significance of pleural effusions after abdominal surgery. Chest 69:621, 1976
168. Decker DA, Dines DE, Payne WS et al: The significance of a cytologically negative pleural effusion in bronchogenic carcinoma. Chest 74:640, 1978
169. Light RW, MacGregor I, Luchsinger PC et al: Pleural effusions: The diagnostic separation of transients and exudates. Ann Intern Med 77:507, 1972
170. Light RW, Ball WC: Glucose and amylase in pleural effusions. JAMA 255:257, 1973
171. Vladutiu AO, Adler RH, Brason FW: Diagnostic value of biochemical analysis of pleural effusions. Carcinoembryonic antigen and beta[2] microglobulin. Am J Clin Pathol 71:210, 1979
172. Vladutiu AO: Carcinoembryonic antigen in pleural effusions. Lancet 2:423, 1978
173. Rittgers RA, Lowenstein MS, Feinerman AE et al: Carcinoembryonic antigen levels in benign and malignant pleural effusions. Ann Intern Med 88:631, 1978
174. Anderson CB, Philpott GW, Ferguson TB: The treatment of malignant pleural effusions. Cancer 33:916, 1974
175. Dewald G, Dines DE, Weiland LH et al: Usefulness of chromosome examination in the diagnosis of malignant pleural effusions. N Engl J Med 295:1494, 1976
176. Fraisse J, Brizard CP, Emonot A et al: Diagnosis of malignancy by cytogenetic means in effusions (202 pleural, 300 ascites). Methods and results. Clin Genet 14:288, 1978
177. Loddenkemper R, Mai J, Scheffler N et al: Diagnostic yield of blind needle biopsy and of thorascopy in pleural effusion—an intraindividual comparison. Endoscopy 10:143, 1978
178. Lambert CJ, Shah HH, Urschel HC et al: The treatment of malignant pleural effusions by closed tricor tube drainage. Ann Thorac Surg 3:1, 1967
179. Weisberger AS: Direct instillation of nitrogen mustard in the management of malignant effusions. Ann NY Acad Sci 68:1091, 1961
180. Fracchia AA, Knopper WH, Carey JT et al: Intrapleural chemotherapy for effusion from metastatic breast carcinoma. Cancer 26:626, 1970
181. Suhrland LG, Weisberger AS: Intracavitary 5-fluorouracil in malignant effusions. Arch Int Med 116:431, 1965
182. Anderson AP, Brincker H: Intracavitary thiotepa in malignant pleural and peritoneal effusions. Acta Radiol (Stockholm) 7:369, 1968
183. Paladine W, Cunningham TJ, Sponzo R et al: Intracavitary bleomycin in the management of malignant effusions. Cancer 38:1903, 1976
184. Borja ER, Pugh RP: Single dose quinacrine (atabrine) and thoracostomy in the control of pleural effusions in patients with neoplastic diseases. Cancer 31:899, 1973
185. Dollenger MR, Krahoff JH, Karnofsky DA: Quinacrine (atabrine) in the treatment of neoplastic effusion. Ann Intern Med 66:249, 1967
186. Hickman JA, Jones MC: Treatment of neoplastic pleural effusions with local instillations of quinacrine (mepacrine) hydrochloride. Thorax 25:226, 1970
187. Rocklin DB, Smart CR, Wagner DE et al: Control of recurrent malignant effusions using quinacrine hydrochloride. Surg Gynecol Obstet 118:991, 1964
188. Bayly TC, Kisner DL, Sybert A et al: Tetracycline and quinacrine in the control of malignant pleural effusions. A randomized trial. Cancer 41:1188, 1978
189. Wallach HW: Intrapleural tetracycline for malignant pleural effusions. Chest 68:510, 1975
190. Austin EH, Flye W: The treatment of recurrent malignant pleural effusion. Ann Thorac Surg 28:190, 1979
191. Strober SJ, Klotz E, Kuperman A et al: Malignant pleural disease. JAMA 266:296, 1973
192. Ariel IM, Oropeza R, Pack GT: Intracavitary administration of radioactive isotopes in the control of effusions due to cancer. Cancer 19:1096, 1966
193. Bateman JC, Moulton B, Larson WJ: Control of neoplastic effusion by phosphoramide chemotherapy. Arch Int Med 95:713, 1955
194. El-Mahdi A, Levene A, Lott S: Observations and management of malignant pleural effusions in breast carcinoma. Johns Hopkins Med J 132:44, 1973
195. Izbicki R, Weyhing BT, Baker L et al: Pleural effusion in cancer patients. A prospective randomized study of pleural drainage

with the addition of radioactive phosphorus to the pleural space vs. pleural drainage alone. Cancer 36:1151, 1975
196. Adler RH, Sayek I: Treatment of malignant pleural effusion: A method using tube thoracostomy and talc. Ann Ther Surg 22:8, 1976.
197. Jones GR: Treatment of recurrent malignant pleural effusion by iodized talc pleurodesis. Thorax 24:69, 1969
198. Shedbalkar AR, Head JM, Head LR et al: Evaluation of talc pleural symphysis in the management of malignant pleural effusion. J Thorac Cardiovasc Surg 61:492, 1971
199. Martini N, Bains MS, Beattie EJ: Indications for pleurectomy in malignant effusion. Cancer 35:734, 1975
200. Thurber DL, Edwards JE, Achor RWP: Secondary malignant tumors of the pericardium. Circulation 26:228, 1962
201. Theologides A: Neoplastic cardiac tamponade. Semin Oncol 5:181, 1978
202. Smith FE, Lane M, Hudgins PT: Conservative management of malignant pericardial effusion. Cancer 33:47, 1974
203. Martini N, Freeman AH, Watson RC et al: Intrapericardial instillation of radioactive chromic phosphate in malignant pericardial effusion. AJR 128:639, 1977
204. DeLoach JF, Haynes JW: Secondary tumors of heart and pericardium: Review of the subject and report of one hundred thirty-seven cases. Arch Intern Med 91:224, 1953
205. Terry LN Jr, Kligerman MM: Pericardial and myocardial involvement by lymphomas and leukemias: The role of radiotherapy. Cancer 25:1003, 1970
206. Biran S, Hachman A, Levij IS et al: Clinical diagnosis of secondary tumors of the heart and pericardium. Dis Chest 55:202, 1969
207. Goudie RB: Secondary tumors of the heart and pericardium. Br Heart J 17:183, 1955
208. Gassman HS, Meadows R Jr, Baker LA: Metastatic tumors of the heart. Am J Med 19:357, 1955
209. Chia BL, DaCosta JL, Ransome GA: Cardiac tamponade due to leukaemic pericardial effusion. Thorax 28:658, 1973
210. Sytman AL, MacAlpin RN: Primary pericardial mesothelioma: Report of two cases and review of the literature. Am Heart J 81:760, 1971
211. Poole-Wilson PA, Farnsworth A, Braimbridge MV et al: Angiosarcoma of pericardium: Problems in diagnosis and management. Br Heart J 38–240, 1976
212. Williams C, Soutter L: Pericardial tamponade: Diagnosis and treatment. Arch Intern Med 94:571, 1954
213. Wintrobe MM, Thorn GW, Adams RD, et al: Principles of Internal Medicine 7th edition, McGraw-Hill, 1974, p 1211
214. Hancock EW: Constrictive pericarditis: Clinical clues to diagnosis. JAMA 232:176, 1975
215. Spodick DH: Acute cardiac tamponade: Pathologic physiology, diagnosis and management. Prog Cardiovasc Dis 10:64, 1967
216. D'Cruz IA, Cohen HC, Prabhu R et al: Diagnosis of cardiac tamponade by echocardiography: Changes in mitral valve motion and ventricular dimensions with special reference to paradoxical pulse. Circulation 52:460, 1975
217. Spodick DH: Electric alternation of the heart: Its relation to the kinetics and physiology of the heart during cardiac tamponade. Am J Cardiol 10:155, 1962
218. Lawrence LT, Cronin JF: Electrical alternans and pericardial tamponade. Arch Intern Med 112:415, 1963
219. Niarchos AP: Electrical alternans in cardiac tamponade. Thorax 30:228, 1975
220. Zipf RE Jr, Johnston WW: The role of cytology in the evaluation of pericardial effusions. Chest 62:593, 1972
221. Stewart JR, Cohen KE, Fajardo LF et al: Radiation-induced heart disease: A study of twenty-five patients. Radiology 89:302, 1967
222. Cassell P, Dullum P: The management of cardiac tamponade: Drainage of pericardial effusions. Br J Surg 54:620, 1967
223. Hill GJ II, Cohen BI: Pleural pericardial window for palliation of cardiac tamponade due to cancer. Cancer 26:81, 1970
224. Fredriksen RT, Cohen LS, Mullins CB: Pericardial windows or pericardiocentesis for pericardial effusions. Am Heart J 82:158, 1971
225. Flannery EP, Gregoratos G, Corder MP: Pericardial effusions in patients with malignant diseases. Arch Intern Med 135:976, 1975
226. Moorton DL, Kagan AR, Roberts WC et al: Pericardiectomy for radiation-induced pericarditis with effusion. Ann Thorac Surg 8:195, 1969
227. Rubinson RM, Bolooki H: Intrapleural tetracycline for control of malignant pleural effusion: A preliminary report. South Med J 65:847, 1972
228. Davis A, Sharma SM, Blumberg ED et al: Intraperitoneal tetracycline for the management of cardiac tamponade secondary to malignant pericardial effusions. NEJM 299:1113, 1978
229. Weisberger AS, Levine B, Storaasli JP: Use of nitrogen mustard in treatment of serous effusions of neoplastic origin. JAMA 159:1704, 1955
230. Suhrland LG, Weisberger AS: Intracavitary 5-fluorouracil in malignant effusions. Arch Intern Med 116:431, 1965
231. Terpenning M, Orringer M, Wheeler R et al: Interapericardial nitrogen mustard with catheter drainage for the treatment of malignant effusions. Proc Am Assoc Cancer Res 20:286, 1979
232. Biran S, Brufman G, Klein E et al: The management of pericardial effusion in cancer patients. Chest 71:182–186, 1977
233. Clarke TH: Radioactive colloidal gold Au^{198} in the treatment of neoplastic effusions. Northwest U Med School Q Bull 26:98–104, 1952
234. Cham WC, Freiman AH, Carstens PHB et al: Radiation therapy of cardiac and pericardial metastases. Ther Radiol 114:701–704, 1975
235. Jaffe N, Traggis DG, Tefft M: Acute leukemia presenting with pericardial tamponade. Pediatrics 45:461–465, 1970.
236. Kaetz HW, Selsky LM: X-ray therapy in the treatment of cardiac tamponade in chronic myelocytic leukemia. Conn Med 32:523–524, 1968
237. Kusnoor VS, D'Souza RS, Bhandarkar SD et al: Malignant pericardial effusions: Report of two cases. J Assoc Phys India 21:101–104, 1973
238. Isselbacher KJ, Adams RD, Braunwald E et al: Principles of Internal Medicine, 9th ed, McGraw-Hill, 1979
239. Feldman GB, Knapp RO, Order SE et al: The role of lymphatic obstruction in the formation of ascites in a murine ovarian carcinoma. Can Res 32:1663, 1972
240. Fraisse J, Brizard CP, Emonot A et al: Diagnosis of malignancy by cytogenetic means in effusions (202 pleural, 300 ascites). Methods and results. Clin Genet 14:228, 1978.
241. Lowenstein MS, Rittgers RA, Feinerman AE et al: Carcinoembryonic antigen assay of ascites and detection of malignancy. Ann Intern Med 88:635, 1978
242. Herz J, Shapiro SR, Konrad P et al: Chylous ascites following retroperitoneal lymphadenectomy. Report of two cases with guidelines for diagnosis and treatment. Cancer 42:349, 1978
243. Lewis JW, Storer EH: The management of iatrogenic chylous ascites. Henry Ford Hosp Med J 27:140, 1979
244. Callen PW, Marks WM, Filly RA: Computed tomography and ultrasonography in the elevation of the retroperitoneum in patients with malignant ascites. J Comp Assist Tomogr 3:581, 1979
245. Osborne MP, Copeland BE: Intracavitary administration of radioactive colloidal gold (Au^{198}) for the treatment of malignant effusions. N Engl J Med 255:1122, 1956
246. Straus AK, Roseman DL, Shapiro TM: Peritoneovenous shunting in the management of malignant ascites. Arch Surg 114:489, 1977
247. Wilbanks GD, Straus AK, Roseman DL et al: Peritoneo-venous shunting in the management of refractory ascites from gynecologic malignancy. Proc Am Assoc Can Res 20:364, 1979
248. Wolff JP, Vignier M, Goldfarb E et al: Ascites in cancer of the ovary. Gynecologie 28:517, 1977
249. Koeffler HP, Cline MJ: Multiple myeloma presenting as ascites. West J Med 127:248, 1977
250. Nutting NG, McPherson TA: Ascites in malignant melanoma after oral BCG immunotherapy. N Engl J Med 295:395, 1976
251. Poth JL, George RP: Hemorrhagis ascites: An unusual complication of multiple myeloma. Calif Med 115:61, 1971

252. Dybecki J, Balchum OJ, Meneely GR: Treatment of pleural and peritoneal effusion with intracavitary colloidal radiogold (Au^{198}). Arch Int Med 104:802, 1959
253. Kniseley RM, Andrews GA: Pathological changes following intracavitary therapy with coloidal Au^{198}. Cancer 6:303, 1953
254. Jacobs ML: Radioactive colloidal chromic phosphate to control pleural effusion and ascites. JAMA 166:597, 1958
255. Suhrland LG, Wiesberger AS: Intracavitary 5-flourouracil in malignant effusions. Arch Intern Med 116:431, 1965
256. Paladine W, Cunningham TJ, Sponzo R et al: Intracavitary bleomycin in the management of malignant effusions. Can 38:1903, 1976.
257. Anderson AP, Brincker H: Intracavitary thiotepa in malignant pleural and peritoneal effusions. Acta Radiol Ther Phys Biol 7:369, 1968
258. Weisberger AS: Direct instillation of nitrogen mustard in the management of malignant effusions. Ann NY Acad Sci 60:1091
259. Miedema EB, Bissada NB, Finkbeiner AE et al: Chylous ascites complicating retroperitoneal lymphadenectomy for testis tumors: Management with peritoneovenous shunting. J Urol 120:377, 1978
260. Mulvany D: Vesico-coelomic drainage. Lancet 2:748, 1955
261. Leveen HH, Christoudias G, Moon IP et al: Ann Surg 180:580, 1974
262. Leveen HH, Wapneck S, Grosbey S et al: Further experience with peritoneo-venous shunt for ascites. Ann Surg 184:574, 1976
263. Reinhardt GF, Stanley MM: Peretoneovenous shunting for ascites, Surg Gynecol Obstet 145:419, 1977
264. Leveen HH, Wapnick S: Operative details of continuous peritoneo-venous shunt for ascites. Bull Soc Int Chir 34:579, 1975

CHAPTER 42

Oncologic Emergencies

Superior Vena Caval Syndrome

STEVEN C. CARABELL
ROBERT L. GOODMAN

Superior vena caval (SVC) syndrome is an acute or subacute oncologic emergency with typical clinical features that require prompt action. The incidence of SVC syndrome has been reported to vary from 3% to 8% in patients with carcinoma of the lung and malignant lymphoma.[1,2] It was first described as a clinical entity by William Hunter in 1757 in a patient with a syphilitic saccular aortic aneurysm.[3]

The syndrome usually has an insidious onset, and progresses to develop characteristic signs and symptoms. In a large recent review of 84 patients with SVC syndrome from the Mallinckrodt Institute of Radiology in St. Louis, the most common presenting symptom was shortness of breath, which was seen in more than half their patients.[1] Facial swelling was observed in 43% of patients, and swelling of the trunk or upper extremities was almost as frequent (40%). Chest pain, cough, and dysphagia were less frequently reported (each in about 20% of patients).

The physical findings and signs in the carefully analyzed group of 84 patients are listed in Table 42-1. The most frequent finding was thoracic and neck vein distention, seen in 67% and 59%, respectively. Facial edema (56%) and tachypnea (40%) were also common signs.

The pathophysiology of the syndrome is related to obstruction of venous drainage in the upper part of the thorax, with increased venous pressure leading to superficial venous dilatation of collateral veins, facial plethora, conjunctival edema, with or without proptosis, and various CNS symptoms, such as headache, visual disturbances, and altered states of consciousness.[4] The effect on the CNS can be ascribed to increased intracranial pressure secondary to the SVC obstruction. The review of Roswit and coworkers provides a thorough understanding of the anatomic and pathophysiologic features of the syndrome.[5]

The superior vena cava is the major venous channel for return of blood to the right of the heart from the head, neck upper extremities, and upper thorax (see Fig. 42-1). The vulnerability of the superior vena cava to obstruction is related to the thinness of the vessel walls and to the low venous pressure. The SVC is locked in a tight compartment of the right anterior-superior mediastinum behind the rigid sternum, adjacent to the right mainstem bronchus, and completely encircled by chains of lymph nodes that drain all the structures of the right thoracic cavity and the lower part of the left. Anterior to the SVC lie the right anterior mediastinal nodes, and posterior to it lie the right lateral or paratracheal nodes. The main auxiliary vessel, the azygos vein, is also threatened by enlarged paratracheal nodes. Without appropriate therapeutic intervention in this anatomic setting the symptoms may progress, and prolonged SVC obstruction may lead to irreversible thrombosis, CNS damage, or pulmonary complications.

An interesting anatomic feature is the occasional association of SVC syndrome and spinal cord compression, which occurs because of the proximity of these structures. The venous occlusion usually precedes the spinal cord compression, which is usually localized to the low cervical or upper thoracic spinal cord. Rubin and Hicks reported five patients with these two syndromes secondary to lymphoma or carcinoma, and recommended myelography as part of the diagnostic evaluation of a patient with venous obstruction and back pain.[6]

In current practice, by far the most common cause of superior vena caval obstruction is malignant disease. Benign conditions formerly were more common, but with effective antibiotic therapy, aneurysm secondary to syphilis, and tuberculous mediastinitis are rare. The report of Schechter in 1954 indicated that 40% of 274 cases were related to syphilis or tuberculosis, but now cancer accounts for approximately 97% of all cases of superior vena cava syndrome.[4,7] The most frequent non-malignant cause of SVC syndrome is thyroid goiter.[8] Other benign causes include primary superior vena cava thrombosis, pericardial constriction, and idiopathic sclerosing mediastinitis. Carcinoma of the lung and lymphoma are the two most common malignant causes for the syndrome, accounting for the vast majority of cases. In a combined series, 75% were due to bronchogenic carcinoma, 15% to lymphomas, and 7% from metastatic disease.[7]

The analysis of Perez and coworkers revealed that the most frequent histologic type of lung carcinoma was small cell undifferentiated, found in 46% of patients.[1] Epidermoid carcinoma was the pathologic diagnosis in 25% of the lung

TABLE 42-1. Superior Vena Caval Syndrome: Physical Findings

FINDING	NUMBER	PERCENT
Thorax vein distention	56	67
Neck Vein Distention	49	59
Edema of Face	47	56
Tachypnea	34	40
Plethora of Face	16	19
Cyanosis	13	15
Edema of Upper Extremities	8	9.5
Paralyzed True Vocal Cord	3	3.5
Horner's Syndrome	2	2.3

(Perez CA, Presant CA, Amburg AL: Management of Superior Vena Cava Syndrome. Sem Oncol 5:123–134, 1978)

cancers resulting in superior vena caval syndrome. The preponderance of small cell tumors resulting in SVC syndrome is predictable from the known tendency of these tumors to occur in central and perihilar locations in the lung. Of the 14 patients with malignant lymphoma in their series, there was an equal distribution of histologic types with five cases classified as lymphocytic, four as histiocytic, three as mixed, and two as unclassified (see Table 42-2).

The obstruction resulting in SVC syndrome may result from extrinsic compression of the SVC by nodal metastases or tumor, or the vessel wall may be directly involved with

FIG. 42-1. Schematic representation of the frontal (*left*) and sagittal (*right*) sections of the thorax showing the relationship of azygos vein to superior vena cava (SVC), coalescence of innominates to form SVC at the right second rib, and the encasement of the SVC by nodal structures. *Shaded area* indicates classical site of obstruction.

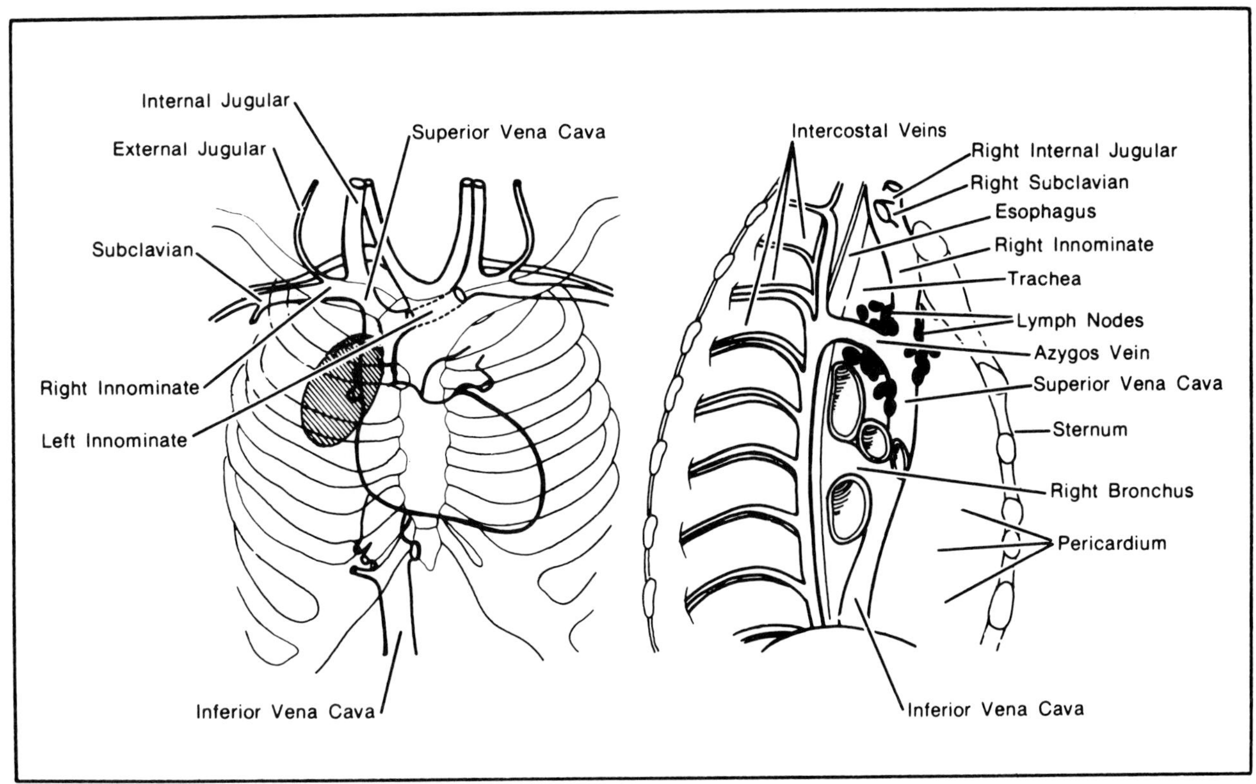

TABLE 42-2. Superior Vena Caval Syndrome: Primary Pathologic Diagnosis

DIAGNOSIS	# OF PATIENTS	TOTAL
BRONCHOGENIC CARCINOMA		67
Small Cell Undifferentiated	31	
Epidermoid	17	
Large Cell Undifferentiated	10	
Adenocarcinoma	8	
Malignant	1	
MALIGNANT LYMPHOMA		14
Lymphocytic	5	
Histiocytic	4	
Mixed	3	
Unclassified	2	
OTHER		
Kaposi's Sarcoma (Heart)	1	
Adenocarcinoma (Breast)	1	
Metastatic Seminoma (Testicle)	1	
TOTAL		84

(Perez CA, Presant CA, Amburg AL: Management of Superior Vena Cava Syndrome. Sem Oncol 5:123–134, 1978)

TABLE 42-3. Superior Vena Caval Syndrome: Methods of Diagnosis

METHODS	TOTAL NUMBER OF PATIENTS	POSITIVE DIAGNOSIS ESTABLISHED	
		NUMBER OF PATIENTS	PERCENT
Thoracotomy and biopsy	19	19	100
Mediastinoscopy and biopsy	11	9	81
Bronchoscopy and biopsy	45	28	62
Lymph node biopsy scalene	22	11	50
Supraclavicular (palpable)	19	16	84
Cytology sputum	24	15	63
Bronchial washings	12	6	50
Pleural effusion	4	4	100

(Perez CA. Present CA. Amburg AL: Management of Superior Vena Cava Syndrome. Sem Oncol 5:123–134, 1978)

tumor.[9] Associated thrombosis within the SVC is found in post-mortem examination in ½ to ⅓ of patients with SVC syndrome.[7] The failure of response to promptly instituted therapy is often a sign of thrombotic obstruction of the superior vena cava. In a recent series of 35 patients, two failures were documented at autopsy to be from large thrombi of the superior vena cava.[10]

The clinical diagnosis is usually apparent without extensive diagnostic tests. The chest film shows a mass in almost all patients, usually in the superior mediastinum (75% on the right side). This is combined with pulmonary lesions or hilar adenopathy in about 50% of patients. Mediastinal tomograms, though they may further delineate the mass and show obstruction of the tracheo-bronchial tree, should not be pursued at the expense of prompt treatment of the condition. Approximately 20–25% of patients have an associated pleural effusion, usually in the right hemithorax.

Venograms are relatively contraindicated, since interruption of the integrity of the vessel wall in the presence of increased intraluminal pressures may result in excessive bleeding from puncture sites. The clinical features with venous distention, frequently an obvious finding, make imaging procedures such as superior venacavograms unnecessary.

Invasive diagnostic procedures such as bronchoscopy, esophagoscopy, mediastinoscopy, scalene node biopsy, or exploratory thoracotomy are frequently used to establish a histopathologic diagnosis and the extent of disease. Such investigation should be pursued if there is abnormal tissue that is superficial and readily accessible or if the syndrome is stable, slowly progressive, or relatively early in clinical stage. However, since superior vena caval syndrome often represents an oncologic emergency requiring immediate therapy to alleviate the symptoms, attempts to obtain a tissue diagnosis should be deferred in favor of immediate therapeutic intervention. In addition, the increased venous pressure adds an increased risk of excessive bleeding during such procedures. In fulminant cases, surgical manipulations, such as scalene node biopsy or mediastinoscopy would be fraught with difficulty.

Since future therapy and prognosis are influenced by the histologic nature and anatomic site of the primary tumor, a definitive diagnosis is, nevertheless, important. Once appropriate therapeutic management is underway diagnostic biopsy procedures can be pursued. It is unlikely that the histologic pattern of the malignancy is substantially altered immediately following the institution of therapy. Sputum cytology and bronchoscopy, bronchial washings, and biopsy of palpable supraclavicular nodes will yield the correct diagnosis in about 70% of patients.[1] Thoracotomy is almost always successful in obtaining a tissue diagnosis, but this should be done only in patients in good general condition once the acute stage of the syndrome has subsided, and if the diagnosis has not been established by less invasive procedures. The efficacy of the various biopsy procedures in establishing a histologic diagnosis is described in Table 42-3 from the Mallinckrodt series.[1]

The modalities available for treatment of the syndrome include radiation therapy, chemotherapy, surgery, and medical measures, including anticoagulation. The primary therapeutic modality is usually radiation therapy, although chemotherapy has been reported as the sole modality used (*vide infra*). The fractionation schedule of radiation usually includes 2–4 large initial fractions of 300–400 rad, followed by additional daily doses of 180–200 rad to complete the total of 3000–3500 rad tumor dose. The fear of producing additional compromise of the superior vena cava by radiation-induced edema after large fractions appears to be unfounded.[11] Patients treated with high-dose irradiation showed slightly faster symptomatic improvement in comparison to patients receiving conventional dose radiation (180–200 rad/day).[8] Improvement within 14 days was observed in 70% of patients treated with initial high-dose fractions in contrast to 50% of patients treated conventionally, although this difference was not statistically significant.

The total dose of radiation is determined by the type and extent of the underlying malignancy. Lymphomas are more responsive to radiation than are carcinomas. Lower doses of from 2000–4000 rad are sufficient depending on the stage of disease and the additional therapy contemplated. Epithelial tumors, including squamous cell carcinoma of the lung, or adenocarcinomas in general require higher doses of from 5000–6000 rad to achieve local control. If the disease is extensive, with extrathoracic tumor spread, then radiation to relieve superior vena caval syndrome is considered palliative in intent, and a lower total dose is warranted. If the disease can be encompassed by the radiation portal, then a higher dose of radical, potentially curative radiation is appropriate. Nevertheless, even with the lower total doses used for lymphomas, the likelihood of achieving local control is greater. In the St. Louis series, five of 14 patients with malignant lymphomas showed no evidence of recurrence in the mediastinum, whereas all but two of the patients with bronchogenic carcinoma eventually relapsed in the primary site.[8] Persistent or recurrent superior vena caval syndrome occurred in 19% of patients with small cell carcinoma of the lung and 10% of the patients with other histologic types of lung carcinoma. No patients with lymphoma developed recurrent superior vena caval syndrome after irradiation.

The portal of irradiation is designed to encompass the mediastinal, hilar, and any adjacent pulmonary parenchymal lesions. For lymphomas, the field is generally extended to include adjacent node-bearing areas, including the cervical, mediastinal, and axillary areas (almost a "mantle" field, as used in the treatment of Hodgkin's disease). If there is an upper lobe lung lesion or superior mediastinal adenopathy, then the supraclavicular nodes should probably be included in the radiation portal. Such supraclavicular irradiation prevented supraclavicular recurrence in all except five of 57 patients (87%), in contrast to two of six patients (33%) who recurred in the supraclavicular area after these nodes were not irradiated.[1]

The response to irradiation is usually prompt, with complete symptomatic relief (resolution of dyspnea, facial edema, and neck vein distention) achieved more often in patients with malignant lymphoma (75%) than in bronchogenic carcinoma (20%). However, most patients with lung cancer do respond to irradiation with only about 15% showing no significant response to treatment. The time to response in a large series of patients treated with radiation therapy is noted in Table 42-4, with 27 of 35 patients (77%) subjectively responding in 3–4 days.[10] By the end of 7 days, subjective response had been achieved in 91% of patients.

If the clinical syndrome does not respond to irradiation, this may indicate that thrombosis has occurred. Indeed, in a recent series, one of 19 patients did not respond and was found at autopsy to have a large thrombus arising from a stricture in the superior vena cava extending up the interval jugular veins to the base of the skull.[12]

Survival after treatment is better for patients with lymphoma than bronchogenic carcinoma. In the St. Louis series, 45% of lymphoma patients survived 30 months, in comparison to only 10% of patients with lung tumors.[1] The overall survival of their entire series was approximately 25% at one year and 10% at 30 months following initial therapy. The survival of patients with carcinoma of the lung treated with radiation therapy alone was the same as those receiving concomitant radiation therapy and chemotherapy.

TABLE 42-4. Subjective and Objective Response of Superior Vena Caval Obstruction to Radiation Therapy

	RESPONSE OF SVC SYNDROME		
	PATIENTS	DAYS	PERCENT
SUBJECTIVE	27/35	3–4	77%
	32/35	7	91%
OBJECTIVE	23/35	7	66%
	31/35	14	89%

(Davenport D, Ferree C, Blake D et al: Radiation Therapy in the treatment of Superior Vena Cava Obstruction. Cancer 42:2600–2603, 1978)

Chemotherapy has usually been used in conjunction with radiation therapy, although in cases in which radiation tolerance of the mediastinum has been reached, it has been employed as the primary therapeutic modality. Lymphomas may respond as quickly to chemotherapy as to irradiation. There are clinical circumstances in the treatment of SVC produced by lymphoma in which there are advantages to starting treatment with chemotherapy. If the mediastinal mass is so large that a large volume of lung must be irradiated to encompass the tumor, then it would be reasonable to start treatment with chemotherapy. If the tumor responds to chemotherapy and shrinks in size, the subsequent portals of irradiation could be smaller, thus sparing more normal lung tissue. Chemotherapy can also be used as the primary modality of treatment for superior vena caval syndrome due to Hodgkin's disease, diffuse histiocytic lymphoma and small cell anaplastic lung carcinoma, which are known to be quite responsive to combinations of drugs.[13,14]

In a randomized study of 26 patients with SVC syndrome, Levitt reported 13 patients treated with radiation therapy alone using 150–200 rad fractions to a total dose of 4000–5000 rad in 4–5 weeks, and 13 patients who received radiation therapy plus conservative use of nitrogen mustard 0.4 mg/kg body weight prior to the institution of radiation therapy.[15] Approximately the same number of patients with carcinoma of the lung was present in both groups, although there were two lymphomas in the radiation-only group. The time to relief of symptoms (5–6 days) and the median survival (7.5 months) were about the same in both groups. These results showing no advantage to nitrogen mustard therapy in the management of SVC syndrome were confirmed by the retrospective study of Perez and coworkers.[1]

In treating SVC resulting from small cell carcinoma of the lung (often considered a systemic disease even at presentation), there is a rationale for primary chemotherapeutic management as the sole form of treatment. Also, since normal tissue tolerance may be compromised by combined treatment, the case for chemotherapy alone is stronger. In a series of 26 such patients, radiation and combination chemotherapy (cyclophosphamide, methotrexate, and CCNU, occasionally with vincristine) were used in the initial four patients, and chemotherapy alone in the following 22.[13] All of the latter group had resolution of the SVC syndrome within 7 days. Another report describes seven patients treated with a combination regimen (lomustine, cyclophosphamide, and methotrexate) who similarly attained complete resolution of symptoms by 7 days. This rapid improvement of SVC syndrome secondary to small cell carcinoma of the lung is consistent with the growth kinetics and responsiveness of this tumor to combinations of active chemotherapeutic agents.[16] Current chemotherapeutic regimens are thus effective in relieving SVC syndrome caused by small cell carcinoma of the lung. Since all patients may not respond to chemotherapy alone, however, an alternative approach would be to begin combined modality treatment and terminate the radiation after only a modest dose of 1000–2000 rad.

When chemotherapy is to be administered, injection into arm veins, especially on the right side, should be avoided. Slow blood flow can lead to slow drug distribution, and local irritation with resultant thrombosis or phlebitis. Venous access procedures should be limited and employ venous tributaries in the lower extremities.

Direct surgical intervention with a bypass graft of superior vena caval obstruction has been employed with limited success and high attendant morbidity. The advantage of surgery is the rapid removal of obstruction, and the possible ancillary benefit of a tissue diagnosis. The mortality of surgical treatment is considerable, and there is a high incidence of complication, including hemorrhage.[17] To provide a good bypass, the graft should have a surface that is nonthrombogenic, the lumen should be rigid enough to resist external pressure, the suture line should be large enough to prevent stricture at the anastomotic site, and good flow rate and pressure should be achieved to maintain graft patency. Partial excision of the superior vena cava has been reported by Lome and Bush.[18] Various sites have been proposed for distal anastomosis to bypass the region of obstruction (*e.g.*, azygos vein, right atrial appendage, inferior vena cava, and femoral vein). The use of the right atrial appendage was first suggested by McIntire and Sykes and later successfully adopted by others.[19] This recipient site for distal anastomosis is convenient, easily accessible, and has a large diameter. Successful bypass of an obstructed superior vena cava with a Dacron prosthesis between the left innominate vein and the right atrial appendage has been reported with rapid palliation and minimal morbidity.[20] Surgical intervention should be considered only after other therapeutic maneuvers with radiation and chemotheraphy have been exhausted.

Other measures not studied in controlled fashion include medical measures involving anticoagulation in rapidly progressive causes. Fibrinolytic drugs in addition to radiotherapy have been used by Salsali and Cliffton, who showed more rapid clinical improvement and prolonged survival with such therapy.[22] Because of thrombosis occurring as a result of decreased flow through the obstructed vessel, anticoagulants such as heparin and warfarin (Coumadin) have been used. A prospective study comparing irradiation and chemotherapy with anticoagulants with irradiation or chemotherapy showed a relatively better course with shorter hospitalization, but no significant difference in survival.[21] Diuretic therapy can be used for symptomatic relief of edema and may be quickly, though temporarily, effective.

Steroids are of limited effectiveness, and are possibly useful in the presence of respiratory compromise. Steroids may improve obstruction by decreasing inflammatory reactions associated with tumor. However, Green and coworkers have demonstrated the lack of inflammatory reaction and edema following irradiation for SVC syndrome.[22]

SVC syndrome is a relatively uncommon oncologic emergency, occurring in 3–4% of patients with carcinomas of the lung or with lymphoma. Radiation therapy is the mainstay of clinical management, and is particularly effective in relieving SVC obstruction secondary to lymphoma. The response and prognosis for carcinoma of the lung causing SVC syndrome is less favorable. For small cell carcinoma of the lung the primary treatment involves combination chemotherapy, since this disease is properly considered a systemic problem. If early SVC syndrome develops, chemotherapy alone is a reasonable form of management. If the syndrome is advancing rapidly in a patient with small cell carcinoma of the lung, however, then combined modality treatment with radiation and chemotherapy is probably indicated to reverse the symptoms as rapidly as possible. For other types of tumors, chemotherapy has not significantly enhanced the rapidity of response or long-term survival when added to radiotherapy.

Increased Intracranial Pressure

PAUL L. KORNBLITH

The mechanism of acute decompensation in brain tumor patients involves changes in the intracranial pressure (ICP). These changes can cause neurologic damage in themselves or can cause indirect effects by way of herniation of the cerebellar tonsil or uncus, or by secondary vascular compromise.

It is essential that prompt management be instituted inasmuch as losses in cerebral function become rapidly irreversible.

DIAGNOSIS

The diagnosis of ICP increases depends on the history, neurologic findings, and, in some cases, neuroradiologic study. The use of the lumbar puncture as a tool for diagnosis is to be discouraged although it is useful in monitoring.

The key features in the history are deterioration in mental status, lethargy, somnolence and confusion, all of which suggest ICP increases. The background of the patient is of course crucial and a history of tumor is obviously important. A sudden rise in ICP may be heralded by a seizure, which further serves to compromise the situation by decreasing oxygenation and increasing cerebral swelling.

Changes in pulse (decrease) and blood pressure (increase) often accompany increases in ICP. Cerebellar masses may, however, have the reverse picture. Pupillary changes, especially dilation of one or both pupils, suggest rapid and significant ICP changes. Focal neurologic deficits, hyperreflexia, and abnormal reflexes (Babinski sign) may be found. The major finding, and the most crucial one in early diagnosis, is *alteration in states of consciousness*.

Papilledema is a particularly important finding in the diagnosis of increased intracranial pressure. The dilitation and venous engorgement that results as the pressure increases may cause either unilateral or bilateral swelling of the optic disk. This finding suggests that the pressure has reached a dangerous level and constitutes an indication for consideration of radical therapy, even in a patient who is otherwise alert. The site of papilledema is also a contraindication for the performance of a lumbar puncture.

When there are changes suggestive of an elevated ICP and time permits, CT scan can be very helpful. In many cases there is not time for any delay in management. Either medical or surgical measures should be initiated prior to detailed radiologic study.

The CT scan has now become the easiest and safest diagnostic technique and offers a wide range of data useful in management. The information obtained from it includes:

1. Size and location of tumor mass or masses
2. Amount of peri-tumoral edema
3. Shifts in intracranial structures
4. Ventricular size

These findings can greatly influence clinical management. Finding a tumor in the temporal or cerebellar regions on CT scan in association with changes in vital signs and decline in level of consciousness indicates a need for rapid action. Similarly, even a small tumor with extensive peritumoral edema causing a marked shift in intracranial structures is cause for action. Ventricular enlargement, representing hydrocephalus, suggests a need for ventricular drainage, whereas small ventricles suggest a generalized increase in intracranial pressure and a situation that would not be greatly aided by ventricular drainage.

It is important to distinguish solid metastases from tumors, whether they be single or multiple, from the diffuse infiltrative processes that may occur as a cause of increased intracranial pressure. Leukemic meningitis and diffuse leukemic infiltration can give a generalized picture of increased intracranial pressure without the focal neurologic or radiographic findings found in primary or secondary brain tumors. In the diffuse process, intracranial pressure increases without concomitant findings will be the only effects of clinical CNS involvement. Radiographically, some generalized increase in cerebral density, decreases of ventricular size, and loss of normal gyral and sulcal patterns may be noted. In solid tumors, the neurologic findings may be more focal and the CT scan is more likely to reveal a specific mass lesion.

MEDICAL MANAGEMENT

Once a probable diagnosis of intracranial mass lesion has been made, with evidence of increased ICP, a decision must be made as to the management plan. In earlier eras surgical measures were the only option. However, today certain medical approaches can often preclude the need for acute surgical intervention, although surgery needs to be done on a more elective basis later in the course of care.

The first measure of value is the use of corticosteroids such as dexamethasone (Decadron) and methylprednisolone (Medrol) given IV in large doses. Fluid restriction is an essential concomitant measure and one must be extremely careful not to give the "routine IV" approach in the emergency management of a patient suspected of having raised ICP. Dehydration is the appropriate course and IV fluids must be strictly restricted. Whereas steroids and fluid restriction are sufficient for the patient with only mild evidence of ICP increase the use of more vigorous dehydrating agents (mannitol or urea) may be needed to reverse an acute decompensation. Diuretics such as furosemide (Lasix) may also be useful. In cases where such vigorous measures are needed, surgical intervention on an acute basis is more frequently required.

With early detection of increased CIP the medical measures described will be sufficient to provide time for either further clinical evaluation or at least better preparation for surgery. The dosages and routes of these primary agents are given in Table 42-5. It should be also noted that the use of a non-CNS depressing anticonvulsant such as phenytoin (Dilantin) should be an early treatment measure.

TABLE 42-5. Plan of Management of Acute Intracranial Pressure from Tumors

EVALUATION OF PATIENT
1. Evaluation of state of consciousness
2. Basic neurological examination
3. Determination of parameters of intracranial pressure
   1. pulse
   2. blood pressure
   3. respiration
   4. state of consciousness
   5. papilledema
   6. hyperreflexia
   7. abnormal reflexes
   8. gait impairment

MEDICAL MEASURES IN MANAGEMENT
1. Maintenance of airway
2. Administration of corticosteroids (dexamethasone, 8 ml IV)
3. Start IV
4. Mannitol, 50 g IV either in bolus or in 20% solution

RADIATION THERAPY

SURGICAL MEASURES IN MANAGEMENT (In extreme cases)
1. Ventricular tap through twist drill or burr hole
2. Acute decompression

The use of mannitol and urea should be reserved for those cases in which either surgery is contemplated in a short time or wherein the status of the patient is quite poor. These agents produce their effects in 15–30 minutes, but after 4–6 hours there is not only a decrease in their effects but a tendency to rebound with some increase in ICP. The use of steroids in patients with history of ulcers, bleeding disorders, or diabetes needs to be carefully evaluated.

RADIATION THERAPY

In many of the cases of raised intracranial pressure due to intracranial tumors the primary treatment is radiotherapy rather than surgery. This is particularly true when the increased intracranial pressure is due to a diffuse infiltration process such as leukemic meningitis, or to multiple metastatic tumors. If the primary diagnosis is known, or other sites of metastases have already been confirmed, the urgent use of radiation therapy can be considered as an acute management measure. In those instances in which a primary or unknown secondary tumor present as an acute increase in intracranial pressure, surgery should be carried out to confirm the diagnosis. There are, however, instances where either due to location of the tumor or the condition of the patient, surgery is contraindicated even with a primary tumor. Radiation therapy may be a consideration in an acute situation.

SURGICAL MANAGEMENT

In most patients who present with an increased ICP due to tumor the medical regime is sufficient to deal with the acute problem. Certain patients, however, require rapid surgical treatment. These groups include those with massive hydrocephalus due to ventricular obstruction (*e.g.*, pineal tumors, pituitary tumors, tumors of the area of the IV ventricle). This group will not be treated adequately without direct drainage of CSF either by ventricular needle or by shunting. A second group includes those patients with temporal or cerebellar masses who have decompensated and are not rapidly improved by dehydration. This second group may require acute surgical tumor decompression.

The basic emergency techniques are:

1. Needle drainage of ventricles
2. Shunting procedures
3. Bony decompression
4. Tumor resection and decompression

Needle drainage involves the use of a #16 ventricular needle or a Scott cannula with stylette introduced by way of a frontal or occipital burr hole. Rarely, if ever, is a twist drill hole used. The burr hole need be only 1 cm in diameter and the dura can be entered avoiding any surface vessels. The needle or cannula is then directed towards the medial canthus of the ipsilateral eye. The location of the burr holes are 2 cm from midline and 9 cm from nasion frontally and 2 cm from midline and 7 cm from the external occipital protuberance posteriorly. The ventricles are about 4 cm beneath the inner table. Establishing drainage is a prompt and effective technique for temporary decompression. On occasion a sterile drainage system can be attached to the catheter but a shunting procedure is preferred due to the lowered risk of infection.

Shunting procedures may be either ventriculo-atrial (VA) or ventriculo-peritoneal (VP) shunts with the VP now preferred. The procedure intracranially is similar to the needle drainage but silastic catheters are used at the ventricular end by way of silastic tubing passed subcutaneously to the peritoneal cavity. These procedures have low initial risks but require 1–2 hours and do have a longer term risk of blockage or infection.

Decompression of bone involves removing either the temporal or frontal bone to relieve tumor pressure. This procedure is now a rarely used temporary expedient. Leaving the bone off in a patient with an expanding tumor is not an indicated approach and getting it back in place without intracranial tumor removal is very difficult. Thus, at present, bone removal alone is viewed only as a short-term measure used prior to more definitive surgery.

Surgical tumor decompression is useful in cases where lifesaving measures are needed. The acute intervention into an edematous vascular tumor in a sick patient is a very high-risk procedure and should be reserved for those patients in whom medical measures are failing or those patients with specific temporal or cerebellar masses requiring rapid decompression to save the patient's life. The actual procedure is that of the craniotomy or craniectomy described in Chapter 33 with the major change being that tumor margins are rarely identifiable in infiltrating lesions and decompression rather than formal resection is the goal. Often, after successful acute decompression a second, more definitive procedure is needed.

MONITORING

For a patient who has either had surgery or vigorous medical measures for ICP increases, the monitoring process is of importance. Again, the level of consciousness, vital signs, and pupillary findings are of paramount import. Continuation of steroid, anti-convulsant, and dehydration is required. Rarely should repeated use of mannitol or urea be indicated.

The quantitation of the ICP can be done either by lumbar puncture (LP) or a pressure measuring device. LP should be used only when adequate decompression has been accomplished and not in the presence of a temporal or cerebellar mass lesion. A small needle, minimal CSF removal and a rapid measurement should be the extent of the procedure.

ICP monitoring devices are many and allow continuous or intermittent monitoring of pressure intracranially. Their placement requires an operative procedure and their use has not as yet become routine.

SUMMARY

The general plan of management is given in Table 42-5. The keys are early diagnosis, prompt institution of medical measures, or CSF drainage when indicated. LP and hydration should be avoided. It should be possible to manage most patients with steroids and dehydration prior to *elective* surgery. This is far preferable to acute surgical intervention. Acute surgical decompression should be reserved for extreme cases and those of temporal or cerebellar sites.

Spinal Cord Compression

STEVEN C. CARABELL
ROBERT L. GOODMAN

Most malignant lesions affecting the spinal cord are metastases from various types of primary tumors. Indeed, extradural spinal cord compression is one of the most frequent neurologic complications of systemic malignancy. It has been estimated that 5% of all patients with systemic cancer who are autopsied have pathologic evidence of a tumor invading the extradural spaces.[27] Metastatic intramedullary spinal cord tumors are relatively rare; more than 95% of spinal cord metastases were found to be extramedullary in a review of spinal cord metastases from a large cancer center.[28,29] Spinal cord compression from malignant tumor metastatic to the epidural space will inevitably result in permanent neurologic damage unless emergency measures are taken. Prompt diagnosis, evaluation, and treatment are necessary to achieve reversal of existing neurologic deficits and to prolong active and functional survival.

It should be noted that epidural lesions below the L1–2 region can result in compression of the cauda equina, rather than the spinal cord itself. Treatment of these more distal lesions are similar, and no differences in outcome between spinal cord and cauda equina compression have been reported.[29] Therefore, those remarks and guidelines may be applied to all cases of epidural compression of the spinal cord and cauda.

CLINICAL PRESENTATION

Early recognition and treatment are required for successful therapy of spinal cord compression, and all oncologists must maintain a high index of suspicion for the problem. The diagnosis is easy once there are extensive neurologic deficits, such as paraplegia or loss of bladder or bowel sphincter control. Early presentations are less obvious and should be detected by appropriate screening before irreversible damage has occurred.

The interval between first diagnosis of cancer and the development of spinal cord compression can be quite long. In a recent large series of 130 patients, the time varied from 0–19 years after initial diagnosis.[29] The long intervals involved may lull the clinician's suspicion, but the clinical presentation of spinal cord compression is surprisingly similar, regardless of the primary tumor.

A recent review described four symptoms that characterized the presenting clinical picture: pain, weakness, autonomic dysfunction, and sensory loss, including ataxia.[29,30] Symptoms were present for 5 days to 2 years (median, 2 months) before the diagnosis was established by myelography. Pain was the initial symptom in 96% of patients, and this finding of central back pain with or without radicular pain has been described in other series as well.[29,31,32]

The pain can be either local or radicular, and the site of vertebral involvement is usually responsible for the former. Radiographs of the spine often reveal bony abnormalities at the painful site of suspected compression.[33,34] Radicular pain may vary with the location of the tumor, and is more common in the cervical and lumbosacral regions than in the thoracic area.[29] In the thoracic area, radicular pain is almost always bilateral, and when it is present, such pain can localize the lesion within one or two vertebral segments. However, radicular pain can be mistaken for non-malignant visceral disorders such as pleurisy, pancreatitis, or cholecystitis.

Another diagnostic possibility for local back pain is, of course, herniated intervertebral disc. However, the quality of pain described for epidural tumors is usually different from that arising from a herniated intervertebral disc.[35] The pain of epidural tumor is frequently worse when the patient is lying down, and many patients are awakened from sleep several times during the night, finding relief while sleeping in a sitting position.[29]

Weakness is rarely the presenting complaint. By diagnosis, however, about 75% of all patients complain of weakness; neurologic evaluation reveals weakness in even more patients, 87% in a large series.[29] The diagnosis of spinal cord compression is probably being made at earlier stages in more recent series because of greater awareness of the problem by oncologists. In the more recent Memorial Hospital experience, a greater proportion of patients were ambulatory with only slight weakness at diagnosis.

Sensory loss and autonomic dysfunction are not usually presenting complaints, but by the time of diagnosis, numbness or paresthesias are common complaints (51%).[29] Bowel and bladder dysfunction are present in about half of the patients at diagnosis. This type of autonomic dysfunction is a relatively unfavorable prognostic sign. Two-thirds of patients with urinary incontinence or retention at the time of diagnosis became non-ambulatory, whereas less than 50% of patients without autonomic dysfunction became non-ambulatory.[29]

CAUSES

Tumors that arise in or metastasize to bone are those that commonly cause spinal cord compression. Carcinoma of the lung, breast, prostate, and lymphoma are the most common primary tumors responsible for epidural metastases resulting in spinal cord compression. The incidence of spinal cord compression by site of primary tumor has been evaluated in several series and there is general agreement. A recent review of this problem surveyed many reported series and found the totals as noted in Table 42-6, which lists the incidence of spinal cord compression by sites of primary tumor.[36]

Most of the epidural tumors resulting in spinal cord compression arise in a vertebral body, and there are several interesting anatomic features.[27,32,37] These tumors usually invade the epidural space, and remain largely anterior to the spinal cord. The vertebral body at the level of the cord compression is often destroyed, or at least extensively involved with tumor. However, a posterior surgical approach to the tumor is the usual route when surgery is used (*vide infra*). There is considerable limitation imposed on the surgeon in

TABLE 42-6. Incidence of Spinal Cord Compression by Site of Tumor

	LUNG	BREAST	UNKNOWN PRIMARY	LYMPHOMA	MYELOMA	SARCOMA	PROSTATE	KIDNEY	GI	THYROID	MISC.	TOTAL
Number of Patients	129	94	91	86	68	65	52	44	34	24	116	803
Percent	16	12	11	11	9	8	7	6	4	3	15	100%

TABLE 42-7. Site of Spinal Cord Compression by Primary Tumor in Recent Series

PRIMARY TUMOR	CERVICAL		THORACIC		LUMBOSACRAL		TOTAL
	NO.	%	NO.	%	NO.	%	NO.
Breast	4	14	22	79	2	7	28
Lung	8	38	12	57	1	5	21
Prostate	2	14	10	71	2	14	14
Kidney	1	8	9	75	2	17	12
Lymphoma	1	13	5	63	2	25	8
Myeloma	1	13	5	63	2	25	8
Melanoma	1	14	4	57	2	29	7
GI	0	0	2	40	3	60	5
Others	2	7	20	74	5	19	27
No. of Patients	20	15	89	68	21	16	130

(Gilbert RW, Kim JH, Posner JB: Epidural spinal cord compression from metastatic tumor: Diagnosis and treatment. Ann Neurol 3:40–51, 1978)

removing a mass anterior to the spinal cord through a posterior approach. Damage to the spinal cord itself and an unstable spine may result, since the posterior elements of the spine are removed at laminectomy and the anterior supporting elements may have already been destroyed by tumor.

Another relevant anatomic feature is the known unusual and tenuous vascular supply of the upper thoracic spinal cord.[38] Compression of the cord eventually results in spinal cord infarction, usually within white matter.[35] With the watershed vascular zone, any vascular embarrassment would be expected to have more serious consequences. Indeed, the results of treatment are more favorable for lesions in the lower as compared to the upper thoracic spine.

The site of the epidural tumor is also related to the type of primary cancer. The overall incidence in the various regions was 15% cervical, 68% thoracic, and 16% lumbosacral in the Memorial Hospital series.[29] Cancers arising in the GI tract metastasize more frequently to the lumbosacral spine, a fact that is explicable by their anatomic location and the presacral venous plexus draining the pelvis (see Table 42-7). Cancers of the breast and lung generally result in thoracic spinal cord compression, which is again understandable based on anatomic considerations.[28] Breast cancer has a known pattern of axial osseous metastases, with distal skeletal metastases seen less often. Venous blood draining a breast lesion can flow in a retrograde manner through Batson's paravertebral venous plexus, and metastases may lodge in the spine and axial skeleton in this manner. The thoracic predilection of epidural metastases from thoracic primary tumors such as breast and lung is thus understandable.

Spinal cord compression resulting from lymphomas probably arises from direct extension of tumor from involved paraspinous retroperitoneal and mediastinal nodes through the intervertebral foramina. Interestingly, lymphomas were less frequently seen as the sources of spinal cord compression in the more recent of the two Memorial Hospital series, possibly because of the increased use of total nodal irradiation (including the spine) at that institution as the initial treatment.[29,39] Myeloma is a relatively frequent cause of spinal cord compression because of the high incidence of vertebral body involvement in this disease.

INVESTIGATIONS

Myelography is indicated in all cases of suspected spinal cord compression to determine the upper and lower extent of the lesion, and to ascertain if there is more than one lesion. If complete block is found upon lumbar myelography, then cisternal myelography is required to identify the upper end of the block.

The contrast medium that was most widely used was the oily organic iodine compound, iodophenylundecylic acid (Pantopaque). This substance does not mix with CSF and, being more dense, sinks downward through it. Water soluble contrast agents are less viscous and mix with CSF, thereby spreading more easily in the subarachnoid and ventricular spaces. Until recently, the water soluble agents were limited in their use because of irritant side effects. However, the newer agent metrizamide (Amipaque) has been widely used without such difficulty and is becoming more popular.

Contrast agent left in the subarachnoid space can be used for repeat films to assess the results of treatment. Plain films of the spine occasionally reveal a paraspinous mass, or even loss of a transverse pedicle, producing the "winking owl sign." If the dense vertebral end-plate is disrupted, an infectious etiology must be suspected, tuberculosis or Pott's disease, for example. Bony involvement of the spine is usually seen at the site of epidural tumor demonstrated by myelography, although no bony involvement was noted at the site of epidural block in 15% of patients in the recent Memorial Hospital series.[29]

CT scanning is not the first diagnostic procedure that should be tried, although if myelography cannot be performed or is contraindicated, contrast-enhanced CT scanning reveals useful information.

TREATMENT

The choice of treatment for epidural spinal cord compression must be made arbitrarily, since there are no randomized, prospective studies that evaluate the efficacy of the three treatment options: surgery only, radiation therapy only, surgery followed by radiation. Decision as to therapy must be made depending on the type of tumor, the level of block, the rapidity of onset or duration of symptoms, and the available clinical experience.

As described above, laminectomy can achieve prompt decompression of the spinal cord, but can rarely remove all tumor. The surgical morbidity and mortality must be considered also, since some of these patients do not have a long life expectancy. Indeed, in early neurosurgical experience the prognosis after laminectomy for decompression of epidural tumor was so poor that laminectomy was even considered contraindicated.[40,41] More recent advances in surgical technique have improved this bleak outlook, and the operative mortality for laminectomy ranges from 3–13%.[29,32,42] Even in the latest modern Memorial Hospital series, however, surgical treatment resulted in one death in 31 patients. Surgical morbidity is still an imporitant factor; there are several series that report 10–33% of operated patients to be worse following surgery.[43,44]

Analysis of many series shows that 50% or less of patients treated with surgery only, or surgery and postoperative irradiation, are improved with ambulation as the end-point. Since most of the tumor remains following decompression, postoperative irradiation should be administered to prevent regrowth of tumor and to relieve pain. The value of postoperative irradiation is noted in several series comparing surgery vs. surgery and postoperative irradiation. In a study of 45 cases, 44% of patients treated with surgery and postoperative irradiation became ambulatory, as opposed to 26% treated with surgery alone.[33] Another retrospective analysis of a group of patients with moderately severe paraparesis showed that eight of 17 treated with postoperative irradiation became ambulatory, compared to three of 21 treated with surgery alone.[34]

The best reported results are contained in the report of Brady and coworkers who achieved a response rate of 61% in 90 patients treated with laminectomy and postoperative irradiation.[30] This was markedly better than the rate of 29% in their 24 patients treated with surgery only, and 47% in 19 patients receiving radiation therapy alone. The improved result for surgery and radiation may have been influenced by patient selection, since the patients who were treated surgically may have been in better condition.

There are several series that have evaluated the treatment of spinal cord compression by irradiation only. An early report from Memorial Hospital in 1966 found a response rate of 34% in 41 patients treated with radiation therapy.[45] Khan and coworkers reported a 42% response rate among 82 patients, 58 of whom had either breast carcinoma or lymphoma.[31] The recent Memorial Hospital experience compared the results of radiation therapy alone in 170 patients with surgical decompression followed by irradiation in 65 patients.[29] No differences were found in the percentage of ambulatory patients, as 46% of the patients operated on walked, compared with 49% of those who had irradiation. Those patients who were ambulatory at the onset of treatment had the best outcome, whether treated by surgery or radiation therapy. Paraplegia at the onset of treatment was an adverse prognostic feature, regardless of the type of treatment, as only two of 39 paraplegic patients (<5%) became ambulatory. Even when the patients in this series were stratified by the severity of neurologic symptoms or the radiation responsiveness of the primary tumors there were no significant differences between the two treatment groups. Tumors that were generally considered highly responsive to radiation therapy, such as seminoma, lymphoma, myeloma, and Ewing's sarcoma, had a better response whether treatment was surgery followed by radiation therapy or radiation therapy alone. Patients whose tumors were considerd less responsive to radiation therapy (carcinomas, melanomas, soft tissue sarcomas) had a poorer outcome than the former more responsive group, regardless of the treatment.

The nature of the primary tumor is more important with respect to prognosis and potential for response to therapy than the nature of the treatment itself. The results of treatment for spinal cord compression from various primary tumors are shown in Table 42-8, which pools data from several series.[39,42,44,46,47] Satisfactory results imply sphincter control and ambulation for greater than three months. This shows the results to be most satisfactory for lymphoma and myeloma, where 50% of patients are improved. The response rate for breast and prostate metastases is about one-third.

Comparison of the response rate for various primary tumors treated with either surgery and radiation therapy or radiation therapy alone shows that these treatments achieve equivalent results. Table 42-9 is from the recent Memorial Hospital series, and in that institution at least, radiation therapy was as effective as surgery plus radiation therapy.[29]

The total dose of irradiation can affect the result of treatment. Appropriate doses are in the range of 3000–4000 rad

TABLE 42-8. Treatment Outcome and Primary Tumors

PRIMARY TUMORS	NUMBER OF PATIENTS	SATIS-FACTORY	PER-CENTAGE
Lymphoma	147	76	52
Multiple Myeloma	40	20	50
Breast	79	26	33
Prostate	35	11	31
Lung	101	14	14
Kidney	21	2	10

(Bruckman JE, Bloomer WD: Management of Spinal Cord Compression. Semin Oncol 5:135–140, 1978)

TABLE 42-9. Initial Response to Treatment by Tumor Type

	SURGERY PLUS RT			RT ALONE		
TUMOR	NUMBER OF PATIENTS	NUMBER AMBULATORY	% IMPROVED	NUMBER OF PATIENTS	NUMBER AMBULATORY	% IMPROVED
Myeloma	3	3	100	5	3	60
Lymphoma	3	2	67	5	4	80
Breast	1	1	100	26	17	65
Kidney	2	0	0	10	6	60
Lung	5	1	20	16	8	50
Prostate	5	1	20	8	2	25
Melanoma	2	0	0	5	1	20

(Gilbert RW, Kim JH, Posner JB: Epidural spinal cord compression from metastatic tumor: Diagnosis and treatment. Ann Neurol 3:40–51, 1978)

delivered over 2–4 weeks, depending on the fractionation schedule. Earlier studies were unable to demonstrate the expected dose response relationship, but Friedman noted a 71% complete response in lymphomas treated with greater than 2500 rad compared to 34% in patients treated with lower doses.[31,40,48] The radiation portal should encompass the site of block, extending two vertebral bodies above and below the block. Generally, a single posterior field is used, and the tumor dose is calculated to a depth of 6–8 cm. More sophisticated treatment plans have been described for this problem, such as a posterior wedge pair using two oblique posterior portals, but since the treatment has palliative intent, the simpler and effective *en face* posterior, single field arrangement is generally used.[49]

The technique of irradiation can be altered according to the anatomic region of involvement. Since the lumbar vertebrae are almost midline structures, treatment of metastatic lesions in this area can be delivered with parallel opposed anterior–posterior portals. This would deliver a more homogeneous dose of irradiation to the tumor volume than a single posterior field. For treatment of the cervical spine, the oblique wedge pair arrangement described above, or opposed lateral portals can be used to avoid irradiation of the pharynx and resulting mucositis.

The first dose of irradiation should be given immediately after diagnosis (30 minutes to 2 hours), following myelographic demonstration of the lesion. The optimum fractionation schedule is unknown, but some schedules appear superior in experimental studies.[50,51] In the model of epidural spinal cord compression produced in rats by injection of a suspension of tumor cells anterior to the thoracic spine, the best fractionation schedule was 500 rad every other day for three doses, compared to 200 rad daily for eight doses or a single dose of 1000 rad.[52] Additional experimental and clinical experience also supports the use of high initial doses of irradiation.[50,53] The clinical advantage of high initial fractions of radiation therapy is that rapid reduction in tumor volume is required, and greater cell kill is to be expected with higher doses of irradiation. Rapid tumor cell destruction and cytolysis could also lead to improved vascular supply and reoxygenation of tumor that would help eliminate the relatively radioresistant hypoxic component of solid tumors.

There has been much discussion among radiotherapists about the initial use of multiple small fractions of irradiation, presumably to avoid inducing edema in an already confined space. However, because of the routine use of corticosteroids in the management of spinal cord compression, this issue seems to be unimportant. Steroids can prevent and promote transient resolution of edema, and may have an oncolytic as well as anti-edema effect.[44,51,54]

There are no systemic data on the use of steroids only for spinal cord compression, since this neurologic emergency is usually treated vigorously with radiation, surgery, or both, in addition to steroids. The dose of steroids is not established, although high doses are generally used. The earlier Memorial Hospital series used 60 mg of prednisone daily, and the later series 16 mg of dexamethasone daily.[29,55] Since the optimal daily dose is not established and there is some evidence from the treatment of brain tumors that higher doses may be more effective than lower doses, these authors recommend a high initial dose of 100 mg of dexamethasone daily for 3 days with rapid tapering as tolerated.[56] Though this dose is well-tolerated, the question of whether this schedule is better than standard dosage is unanswered.

The role of chemotherapy in the treatment of spinal cord compression is that of adjuvant rather than primary treatment. For lymphomas, alkylating agents have been used alone or in combination with radiation therapy in the successful treatment of spinal cord compression.[48,57] However, Khan found no benefit from chemotherapy.[42] In the rat model of spinal cord compression using the Walker 256 carcinoma that is known to be exquisitely sensitive to cyclophosphamide, this drug was very effective.[52] This responsiveness to chemotherapy suggests a similarity to Hodgkin's disease, also known to respond rapidly to chemotherapy as well as radiation therapy. Indeed, there is a report of three cases of spinal cord compression caused by Hodgkin's disease treated by chemotherapy with nitrogen mustard or cyclophosphamide with dramatic improvement of neurologic dysfunction.[58] Chemotherapy alone is not generally used as the primary mode of therapy, however, and this animal tumor model should not be extrapolated to humans.

PROGNOSIS

The best prognostic index for eventual recovery of function is the pretreatment status. Not surprisingly, 60% of patients

TABLE 42-10. Comparison of Preoperative Motor Status with that Attained Postoperatively

PREOPERATIVE STATUS	NUMBER OF PATIENTS	POSTOPERATIVE STATUS		
		AMBULATORY	PARAPARETIC	PARAPLEGIC
Ambulatory	48	29(60%)	13(27%)	6(13%)
Paraparetic	204	71(35%)	88(43%)	45(22%)
Paraplegic	60	4(7%)	8(13%)	48(80%)

(Bruckman JE, Bloomer WD: Management of Spinal Cord Compression. Semin Oncol 5:135–140, 1978)

who are ambulatory at diagnosis remain so postoperatively, while only 7% of patients with paraplegia at diagnosis are ambulatory after treatment (see Table 42-10).

The rapidity of onset of neurologic dysfunction is an important prognostic feature as well. Slowly progressive neurologic symptoms are associated with a better outcome than rapidly progressing dysfunction (less than 48–72 hours).[29,42] There is particular controversy regarding the optimum approach to the frightening clinical picture of rapidly progressing dysfunction.

Many neurosurgeons regard this as an indication for surgical intervention, agreeing with the recommendation of Wild and Porter that "immediate surgical decompression is indicated in cases with progressing paresis."[33] However, there are little supportive data as described by Gilbert and coworkers.[29] Their recent Memorial Hospital series showed that none of nine patients with rapidly progressing weakness who were treated surgically improved, while seven of 13 such patients treated with radiation therapy alone improved. They concluded that patients with rapidly progressing symptoms respond best to radiation therapy rather than to surgical decompression.

Another adverse prognostic feature is loss of sphincter control, especially of long duration.[31,42] Also, the results of treatment are better for distal rather than proximal thoracic spinal lesions, as mentioned above. Wild noted that 43% of patients with T5 to T12 lesions recovered, compared to 24% with T1 to T4 lesions.[57] Similarly, White reported that two-thirds of patients with T5 to T12 lesions recovered function, while only half the patients with T1 to T4 lesions improved.[44]

CONCLUSIONS

Spinal cord compression must be managed promptly. A high index of suspicion is required to allow early detection of cases, and thereby improve the results of treatment. Myelography should be performed to demonstrate the block, its limits, and possible extension, and corticosteroids should be instituted. The issue of the best form of treatment, radiation therapy or surgery followed by radiation therapy, is unsettled. However, a large recent study has described radiation therapy as the treatment of choice for most patients with extradural spinal cord compression.[29] Even in cases of rapidly progressing neurologic dysfunction, there are little data to support immediate surgical intervention. However, in such rapidly evolving clinical situations in which the primary is known to be particularly unresponsive to irradiation (*e.g.*, melanoma), it would be reasonable to advocate immediate surgical decompression followed by postoperative irradiation. Surgical laminectomy is more clearly indicated when the nature of the primary tumor is not known or the diagnosis is in doubt; relapse occurs after radiation therapy, and additional radiation therapy is contraindicated because of the risk of exceeding spinal cord tolerance to irradiation; and progression of symptoms occurs during radiation therapy after several fractions have been administered. If surgery is performed, then radiation therapy should be added postoperatively if spinal cord tolerance had not been exceeded from previous irradiation. Laminectomy cannot achieve complete removal of tumor, and postoperative irradiation should be used. For most patients surgical decompression may not be necessary or desirable as the initial form of treatment. Even in the controversial area of rapidly progressing symptoms, early surgical intervention appears to offer no advantage. Adjuvant chemotherapy may be beneficial in patients whose tumors are known to be responsive to particular agents. Whatever the modality, early diagnosis is required to achieve better results, since the outcome is clearly more favorable in patients treated with early neurologic dysfunction.

Metabolic Emergencies

ANTHONY L.A. FIELDS
ROBERT G. JOSSE
DANIEL E. BERGSAGEL

A wide variety of symptoms due to neoplasia are not caused solely by the anatomic distortion and functional impairment of organs and tissue that result from the invasive properties of enlarging tumors. These systemic manifestations frequently include endocrine and metabolic abnormalities, the most important of which are discussed in this section (see Table 42–11). The production of humoral mediators (ectopic hormone secretion) responsible for some of these metabolic disturbances is assumed, and in many cases has now been proven.

TABLE 42-11. Acute Metabolic Problems in Oncology

I. RELATED TO TUMOR
Hypercalcemia
Hypoglycemia
Lactic acidosis
Hypokalemic metabolic alkalosis
Hyperuricemia
Hyponatremia
II. RELATED TO TREATMENT
Hyperuricemia
Hyponatremia

TABLE 42-12. Causes of Hypercalcemia

Cancer
with bone metastases
without bone metastases
a) with ectopic PTH secretion
b) without ectopic PTH secretion
Primary hyperparathyroidism
Thyrotoxicosis
Renal Disease
Secondary hyperparathyroidism
Post-transplantation
Acute renal failure
Drugs
Thiazides
Calcium carbonate (e.g., in antacids)
Lithium
Hypervitaminosis
D
A
Granulomatous diseases
Sarcoidosis
Tuberculosis
Coccidioidomycosis
Adrenal Insufficiency
Immobilization
Paget's disease
Fractures
Paraplegia

*Rarer still are factitious hypercalcemia, idiopathic hypercalcemia of infancy (with elfin facies), milk-alkali syndrome, familial hypocalciuric hypercalcemia, and hypercalcemia due to pheochromocytoma or periostitis.

Hypercalcemia is probably the most frequently encountered of the acute medical problems in oncology. Prominent among the mechanisms responsible for this complication is the production of humoral mediators. Other conditions thought to be simlarly mediated include hyponatremia due to inappropriate secretion of antidiuretic hormone (ADH), hypokalemic metabolic alkalosis due to ectopic ACTH secretion, and tumor-induced hypoglycemia.

However, not all acute metabolic disturbances seen with cancer are due to ectopic production of known or as yet unidentified substances. Some, such as hyperuricemia and lactic acidosis, may be due to metabolism of the tumor itself or to the effects of this metabolism on the host. Still others may be of iatrogenic causation or precipitation.

The acute metabolic abnormalities associated with cancer, requiring urgent treatment, may be important causes of debilitating symptoms and substantial morbidity, and may constitute a more immediate threat to life than the cancer itself. These disturbances could, on occasion, lead the clinician to falsely believe that the tumor has progressed irretrievably. However, treatment of the complication may render the patient salvageable, and other appropriate cancer therapy may be undertaken. It is also important to direct attention to the prevention of the metabolic emergencies that may be precipitated by the therapeutic management of cancer patients.

HYPERCALCEMIA

The precision of calcium homeostasis is a reflection of the vital role of calcium ions in a variety of physiologic functions. Normally the ionized serum calcium is maintained within narrow and constant limits that depend on sensitive regulatory mechanisms involving primarily the coordinated secretion of parathyroid hormone, the active metabolites of vitamin D, and calcitonin.[64] Failure of these homeostatic mechanisms is accompanied by serious disease states in man. Hypercalcemia will ensue if the entry of calcium into the extracellular fluid, which in cancer is mainly due to increased bone resorption, is greater than the ability of the kidney to clear this calcium load.

Neoplastic disease is the commonest cause of hypercalcemia (see Table 42–12). About 10–20% of cancer patients will develop hypercalcemia at some stage of their disease. Three major subgroups of patients can be identified.

CLINICAL GROUPS

Patients With Solid Tumors and Bone Metastases

These comprise the major group. The severity of hypercalcemia is not necessarily correlated with the extent of metastatic bone destruction.[65]. Metastases to bone occur with advanced solid tumors, but are less common in patients with sarcomas than carcinomas.[66] The solid tumors most commonly associated with hypercalcemia and metastatic bone involvement include carcinomas of the breast, lung, kidney, and to a lesser extent, thyroid, ovary, colon and epidermoid tumors of the head, neck, and esophagus.[64–74] With breast cancer the frequency of hypercalcemia may range as high as 40–50%.[67,75,76] In this context it is important to mention that breast cancer patients with metastatic disease treated with hormone preparations occasionally experience rapid progression of hypercalcemia presumably due to hormonal stimulation of the tumor.[69,77–79]

Patients With Solid Tumors Without Bone Metastases

Solid tumors without clinically demonstrable skeletal metastases account for 15–20% of cases of hypercalcemia associated with neoplasia.[80–81] In this situation, it is thought that metabolically active substances produced by the tumor cells (or by normal cells responding to the presence of tumors) circulate in the bloodstream and stimulate bone resorption.

The tumors that most frequently cause hypercalcemia in the absence of bone involvement are carcinomas of the lung and kidney.[82] In a review of 200 consecutive untreated patients with lung cancer, Bender and Hansen found that 12.5% of patients developed hypercalcemia at some stage of their disease.[70] This complication was found predominantly with epidermoid and large cell anaplastic carcinoma, but was uncommon with adenocarcinoma and oat cell carcinoma, the two cell types most frequently associated with skeletal metastases.

Patients With Hematologic Malignancies

In multiple myeloma, hypercalcemia is particularly frequent, occurring in over 50% of patients during the course of their disease (see Chapter 38).[83,84] The hypercalcemia is associated with clinical features of skeletal involvement such as widespread osteolytic bone lesions. Patients with other lymphoproliferative disorders such as lymphosarcoma, Burkitt's lymphoma, and acute lymphoblastic leukemia also occasionally develop bone lesions and hypercalcemia.[66] In these lymphocyte and plasma cell neoplasms increased osteoclastic activity causes accelerated bone resorption.

MAJOR CLINICAL MANIFESTATIONS OF HYPERCALCEMIA

These have been summarized in Table 42–13. For any given degree of hypercalcemia the clinical manifestations may vary from person to person. In general their severity is proportional to the rate of development and the degree of hypercalcemia, modified by factors such as age, associated electrolyte or metabolic disturbances, and underlying primary disorders.[74]

Protein-bound and ionized calcium are present in roughly equal proportions in serum or plasma, but it is the ionized calcium that is clinically important. Since the measurement of ionized serum calcium is complex, the total serum calcium level is often adjusted for variations in serum albumin to detect significant changes. The formula is as follows: adjusted serum calcium = calcium-albumin + 4.0, where reports are in mg/dl for calcium and g/dl for albumin. For Sl units the equation for adjusted calcium = calcium − (0.025 × albumin) + 1.0, where reports are in mmol/l for calcium and g/l for albumin.[85] In one laboratory the 95% confidence limits for adjusted calcium were 9.0 − 10.4 mg/dl.[86–88]

Severe hypercalcemia suggests non-parathyroid causes, usually malignant conditions. Table 42–14 lists some features

TABLE 42-13. Symptoms, Signs, and Complications of Hypercalcemia

GENERAL
Soft tissue calcification, vascular calcification, itching

NEUROLOGIC
Fatigue, muscle weakness, hyporeflexia, lethargy apathy, disturbance of perception and behavior, stupor, coma

RENAL
Polyuria, polydipsia, renal insufficiency
Late: Nephrocalcinosis, renal calculi

GASTROINTESTINAL
Anorexia, nausea, vomiting, constipation, abdominal pain, peptic ulcer, pancreatitis

CARDIOVASCULAR
Hypertension, arrythmias, digitalis sensitivity

OCULAR
Conjunctivitis, corneal calcification (band keratopathy)

TABLE 42-14. Differentiation of Hypercalcemia of Cancer and Primary Hyperparthyroidism

FEATURE	HYPERCALCEMIA OF CANCER	PRIMARY HYPERPARATHYROIDISM
History	Short, rapidly progressive	Long fluctuating, slowly progressive
Major symptoms of diagnostic value	Moderate to severe weight loss, no renal calculi, pancreatitis rare.	Minimal weight loss, renal calculi, pancreatitis and peptic ulcer common
Serum calcium concentration	Usually high (14 mg/dl in 75% of cases)	Variable (14 mg/dl in 25% of cases)
Serum phosphate concentration	Increased, normal or decreased	Normal or decreased
Serum alkaline phosphatase concentration	Elevated in more than 50% of cases	Significantly elevated only in patients with gross bone disease
Serum chloride concentration	Low (usually <102 mmol/L)	High (usually >102 mmol/L)
Chloride/phosphate ratio	<30 in 50% of cases	>30
Serum bicarbonate concentration	Elevated or normal	Normal or low
Erythrocyte sedimentation rate	Usually elevated	Normal
Roentgenograms	Normal or show metastatic disease	May show subperiosteal erosions in hands
Steroid suppression	Serum calcium concentration is often decreased	Serum calcium concentration is rarely decreased

that may be helpful in differentiating the hypercalcemia of malignant diseases from that of primary hyperparathyroidism.

While the effects of an elevated serum calcium concentration are legion they are particularly evident in the GI, neuromuscular, renal, and cardiovascular systems.

Gastrointestinal

Typically these occur early and are non-specific. Anorexia, nausea, vomiting, constipation, and vague abdominal pain are very common. Increased gastric acid secretion may occur with hypercalcemia from any cause and is possibly responsible for the reported increased prevalence of peptic ulcer disease, especially in primary hyperparathyroidism. Pancreatitis, the most serious GI complication of hypercalcemia, is also more commonly reported in association with primary hyperparathyroidism than with the hypercalcemia of malignant disease.[89–91] Ileus and obstipation, when they occur, are usually late in the course of the hypercalcemia.

Neuromuscular

The protean symptoms are detailed in Table 42-13. Most commonly one sees apathy, depression, fatigue, lethargy, and clouding of consciousness.[92,93] Profound muscle weakness, usually with severe hypercalcemia, may be misinterpreted as one of the neurologic paraneoplastic syndromes.[94] Stupor and coma are typically late features; the serum calcium is often very high and the electroencephalogram may show diffuse slow wave changes and other characteristic abnormalities.[95,96]

Renal

Early symptoms of hypercalcemia are polyuria and nocturia caused by a reversible renal tubular defect in urine concentrating ability leading to a syndrome resembling nephrogenic or vasopressin-resistant diabetes insipidus.[97,98] This tubular defect further aggravates the extracellular fluid volume contraction initiated by vomiting and poor fluid intake. The stage is set for the vicious cycle of decreased glomerular filtration increasing the hypercalcemia leading to further renal impairment with subsequent nitrogen retention, acidosis and eventually, renal failure.

Other renal tubular defects produced by hypercalcemia include renal tubular acidosis, glycosuria, aminoaciduria, increased electrolyte loss, phosphaturia and excretion of small molecular weight proteins including lysozymes.[99,100] Reversible hyperuricemia, due to diminished renal urate excretion may also be seen.[101] Renal calculi are not usually a feature of the hypercalcemia of malignant disease, although nephrocalcinosis may occur in patients with prolonged hypercalcemia and azotemia.[72]

TABLE 42-15. Hypercalcemia in Cancer: Putative Chemical Mediators

1. Parathyroid hormone (ectopic) PTH
2. Osteoclast activating factor (OAF)
3. Prostaglandins (PGE_2 ± metabolites)
4. Peptides
5. Vitamin D-like sterols
6. Local osteolytic factors from metastases
7. Other osteolytic factors

Cardiovascular

Calcium ions play a critical role in neurotransmission as well as in determining the contractility of cardiac, smooth, and skeletal muscle. In acute hypercalcemia ventricular systole is shortened and the heart rate is slowed.[102] With moderate hypercalcemia the QT interval is shortened, but with calcium levels above 16 mg/dl apparent lengthening of the QT interval occurs due to widening of the T wave.[103] Of more diagnostic utility than the T wave change is the characteristic configuration of the ST junction and T waves which assume a "cove-like" appearance.[72] Hypercalcemia can also prolong the PR interval and occasionally causes significant arrhythmia.[104,105] The pharmacologic effects of digitalis are partly mediated by alteration of the membrane-bound calcium. This drug must be used with caution in patients with hypercalcemia, as its toxic effects may be potentiated. Acute hypercalcemia may cause hypertension, probably as a direct effect of the calcium ion on the smooth muscle of blood vessels.[106] Chronic hypercalcemia, particularly when due to primary hyperparathyroidism may be associated with hypertension in 20–50% of patients.[107–109]

PATHOGENETIC MECHANISMS IN THE HYPERCALCEMIA OF MALIGNANT DISEASE

In patients with neoplasms, hypercalcemia is usually caused by increased bone resorption which may occur in the presence or absence of bone metastases (see Table 42-15). Theoretically, the increased bone resorption could result from increased osteoclast activity stimulated by the tumor, or from the direct invasion of bone by tumor cells.

Although increased calcium absorption from the gut is a potential cause of hypercalcemia, available data suggest this is unlikely as the intestinal absorption of calcium is low or low-normal in the majority of hypercalcemic cancer patients.[110,111] Decreased renal function may contribute to the hypercalcemia of malignancy, for the final serum calcium of any patient with increased bone resorption is dependent on the renal capacity for calcium clearance. Increased renal tubular reabsorption of calcium does not occur in most hypercalcemic patients (Josse and Murray, unpublished data). However, renal mechanisms may be contributory in certain subgroups, such as persons with tumors that produce ectopic parathyroid hormone, breast cancer, metabolic alkalosis, or salt depletion.[112]

Morphologic data from both animal and human studies have provided evidence that osteoclast number and activity are increased in many hypercalcemic cancer patients.[66] It is postulated that the tumor cells secrete a mediator which causes osteoclast stimulation, resulting in bone resorption. *In vitro* production of bone resorbing activity has been described with many tumors.[113–119]

Recent investigation into the mechanisms of tumor-associated hypercalcemia has concentrated on three putative mediators: parathyroid hormone (PTH), prostaglandin E_2 (PGE_2) and osteoclast activating factor (OAF).

Parathyroid Hormone (PTH)

Many cases have been reported in which immunoreactive PTH has been extracted in relatively high concentrations from tumors of hypercalcemic cancer patients. Sherwood and colleagues demonstrated that this hormone possessed some immunochemical properties similar to those of pure bovine PTH.[120] In these patients, the biochemical changes simulate those of hyperparathyroidism, with hypercalcemia, hypophosphatemia, and sometimes elevated serum values of alkaline phosphatase (pseudohyperparathyroidism). In a few cases, immunoreactive PTH has been demonstrated in the venous effluent of the tumors. However, there is no general agreement as to the exact chemical nature of the PTH-like substance released, or to the frequency of this syndrome.[121,122] Sherwood and colleagues have claimed that the immunoreactivity of the hormone extracted from tumors is identical to that of pure bovine PTH, although Buckle found slight differences.[120,121] Also, Benson and associates found immunochemical differences between PTH in the plasma of the hypercalcemic cancer patients and PTH in the plasma of patients with primary hyperparathyroidism.[123] This may be because of the release of hormonal precursors such as pro-PTH or pre-pro-PTH from the tumor, as suggested by recent *in vitro* and *in vivo* studies.[123–125] The differences might also be explained by the release of C-terminal fragments of PTH from the parathyroid glands during hypercalcemia, as Mayer and colleagues showed for hypercalcemic calves.[126]

Many tumors have been shown to produce PTH; squamous carcinoma of the lung and renal cell carcinoma account for more than 50% of these cases.[99] While strong evidence for PTH secretion by some non-endocrine tumors has been presented, it does not seem likely that PTH secretion explains the hypercalcemia in most cancer patients. In addition, tumors from some hypercalcemic patients produce hormonal mediators that induce osteolysis *in vitro,* but are not immunochemically related to PTH.[127] The finding of elevated values of plasma PTH by radioimmunassay is not sufficient evidence for the diagnosis of ectopic PTH secretion, since cancer patients with coexistent primary hyperparathyroidism may also have elevated values. Coincidential primary hyperparathyroidism is not infrequent in patients with cancer. Heath noted 118 cases of such coexistence in a recent review.[128] Definitive proof of the diagnosis of "ectopic hyperparathyroidism" requires at least one (and preferably more) of the following: demonstration of an arteriovenous difference in plasma PTH across the tumor bed, temporal correlation of plasma PTH and serum calcium concentrations with tumor growth or tumor therapy, extraction of large amounts of immunoreactive PTH from the tumor, absence of a plasma PTH gradient in parathyroid venous effluent, and observation of normal or atrophic parathyroid glands at surgery or autopsy. In most hypercalcemic cancer patients with elevated PTH values such evidence has been lacking. Nevertheless ectopic PTH production still appears to be one of the important mechanisms of hypercalcemia in cancer.

Prostaglandins

Prostaglandin production by tumors is now strongly implicated in the hypercalcemia of cancer. The initial evidence was provided by two animal models, the $HSDM_1$ fibrosarcoma in mice and the VX_2 tumor in rabbits.[129,130] Prostaglandins are potent bone-resorbing substances *in vitro*. PGE_2 was initially correlated with hypercalcemia in the animal models, but more recently the prostaglandin metabolite 15-keto-13,14-dihydro-PGE_2 has been detected in much greater amounts.[131,132] However, the exact structure of the prostaglandin responsible for the hypercalcemia is still not certain.

Recent studies in humans with cancer and hypercalcemia have implicated prostaglandins pathogenetically. Plasma prostaglandin concentrations are higher in some hypercalcemia than in normocalcemic cancer patients.[133,134] Also, a metabolite of PGE_2, 7-B-hydroxy-5,11-diketotetranorprostane-1,16-dioate (PGE-M), has recently been found in elevated concentrations in the urine of 14 hypercalcemic patients with solid tumors (mainly bronchogenic carcinomas).[135] However, the association of prostaglandin production with hypercalcemia is not always observed.

Another observation supporting the thesis that prostaglandins cause hypercalcemia in some cancer patients is that inhibition of prostaglandin synthesis by indomethacin may reduce or correct the hypercalcemia. Indomethacin has corrected the associated hypercalcemia in some patients.[136] Acetylsalicylic acid has inhibited tumor-induced osteolysis *in vitro*.[137] Glucocorticoids, long known to be effective in treating some types of hypercalcemia associated with cancer, have recently been shown to reduce prostaglandin synthesis in animal models.[138,139] Inhibitors of prostaglandin synthesis, however, have not been very effective in treating patients.[139,140] The failure of such therapy may be explained by insufficient dosage, or the presence of widespread tumor. On the other hand, it may simply be that hypercalcemia is not related to prostaglandin production in all patients. Indomethacin appears to be less effective in the presence of skeletal metastases.[136]

While the evidence linking prostaglandin production with hypercalcemia in animal models is convincing, the data from human studies are less strong at present. Prostaglandins are ubiquitous substances and it is possible in some situations that the prostaglandin system may not have a direct role, but merely reflect the amount of tumor present in a specific individual.[82] Although the association seems valid on the basis of currently available data, further studies are needed to establish more definitely the relationship between prostaglandin production and tumor hypercalcemia.

Osteoclast Activating Factor

Horton and coworkers reported that supernatants from cultures of human peripheral leukocytes caused bone resorption in organ cultures of fetal rat bones when these leukocytes were stimulated by phytohemagglutinin, or by antigenic material from human dental plaque.[141] Results of subsequent experiments suggested that supernatants from a variety of cultured lymphoid cell lines from patients with multiple myeloma, Burkitt's lymphoma or malignant lymphoma spontaneously produced a similar factor that also caused bone resorption *in vitro*.[113] In addition, such factors have been identified in media from cultures of myeloma cells and lymphosarcoma cell leukemia.[114,115] The factor responsible for these effects has been named osteoclast activating factor (OAF). It is possible that OAF is produced by other tumor cells, and it may also be elaborated by normal cells as part of the cell-mediated immune response to a tumor, and could cause or enhance bone resorption in patients with solid tumors.[66]

OAF is a peptide, but its detailed chemical structure is not yet known. OAF may exist in two interconvertible forms with molecular weights of approximately 14,000 and 2000 Daltons (big and little OAF respectively).[142] OAF-stimulated osteoclasts increase in number, become more active and release lysosomal enzymes and collagenase.[143] The activation of osteoclasts by OAF is inhibited by glucocorticoids, and this distinguishes OAF from PTH.[144] This may in part explain the beneficial effects of steroids used to treat the hypercalcemia of hematologic neoplasms (*e.g.*, multiple myeloma, lymphoma).

Although OAF is strongly implicated as a mediator of hypercalcemia in some types of malignant disease in humans, the extent of its importance will not be known until there is a more satisfactory assay for its activity.

Other Mechanisms

Other substances may also be implicated in the pathogenesis of the hypercalcemia of cancer, although evidence for their existence is much less strong. One example is suggested by recent findings in some cancer patients in whom hypercalcemia has been associated with elevated urinary concentrations of adenosine 3′5′-cyclic monophosphate and elevated plasma concentrations of chloride, but no detectable PTH in the plasma and, in one study, normal urinary PGE-M concentrations.[136,145] These findings may be explained by the action of a compound chemically different from PTH but with the same biologic actions, perhaps interacting with the same receptor as PTH.

TABLE 42-16. Summary of Treatment of Hypercalcemia in Cancer Patients

GENERAL MEASURES (OF SOME VALUE IN ALL CASES)
Rehydration and fluid replacement with normal saline
Diuretics (furosemide or ethacrynic acid, not thiazides)
Avoidance of protracted immobilization when possible
Hemodialysis or peritoneal dialysis
MEASURES DIRECTED AGAINST HYPERCALCEMIA AND INCREASED BONE RESORPTION
Phosphate (oral and IV)
Corticosteroids
Mithramycin
Calcitonin
Diphosphonates
Indomethacin
SPECIFIC MEASURES AGAINST TUMOR (PREFERRED WHENEVER POSSIBLE)
Removal of tumor
Endocrine manipulation (either surgically or with drugs)
Chemotherapy
Radiation therapy

Gordan and associates presented evidence for the production of osteolytic vitamin-D-like phytosterols by breast tumors.[146,147] However, it is now known that phytosterols may be found in plasma from healthy lactating and nonlactating women, in breast cancer tissue from persons with or without hypercalcemia.[148] Thus, the significance of these substances in tumor-associated hypercalcemia has been seriously questioned. Also of importance may be cellular mechanisms that, in contrast to those previously discussed, do not involve the normal process of osteoclastic bone resorption. It is possible that some tumor cells are capable of resorbing bone directly. Mundy and coworkers found that cultured cells can release factors that directly cause resorption of dead bone, a situation in which there could be no contribution by osteoclastic mechanisms since the bone is devitalized.[149,150] The molecular mechanisms by which tumors cells resorb bone directly are unknown.

TREATMENT OF HYPERCALCEMIA

Treatment is directed at reducing calcium resorption from bone, augmentation of renal calcium excretion and perhaps a decrease in oral calcium intake. The urgency required in the treatment of hypercalcemia depends on the clinical situation. A summary of the various treatment modalities are listed in Table 42-16.

General Measures

The clinical features common to all forms of hypercalcemia, namely anorexia, nausea, vomiting, polyuria, and electrolyte disturbances result in extracellular fluid volume contraction. Therefore, the first principle of treatment is the restoration of intravascular volume, which improves the general condition of the patient while increasing glomerular filtration and thus augmenting urinary calcium excretion. Any medications that might increase the serum calcium should be discontinued. These will include thiazide diuretics, vitamins A and D and, in some circumstances, hormonal agents in patients with breast cancer. The dosage of any drug whose action is influenced by the serum calcium concentration, such as digoxin, should be adjusted appropriately. Protracted immobilization should be avoided if possible.

Saline and Calciuretic Agents

Physiologic maneuvers that increase the renal clearance of sodium also increase the clearance of calcium. Over a wide range of sodium clearance rates the excretion of ionized calcium is nearly equal to that of sodium.[146,147] The relationship between sodium and calcium excretion is independent of GFR since when the GFR is increased by means other than sodium infusion there is only a slight increase in calcium clearance.[153]

Once adequate volume repletion has been achieved, certain diuretics can be used to enhance calcium excretion. Furosemide and ethacrynic acid promote calciuresis by decreasing the renal tubular reabsorption of sodium and calcium. Mild hypercalcemia (<12 mg/dl) can usually be managed adequately by rehydration with normal saline and small doses of furosemide or ethacrynic acid. Severe sustained hypercalcemia (>14 m/dl) requires more aggressive measures. Forced diuresis with furosemide may be undertaken if the clinical condition of the patient allows. Suki and coworkers suggested treatment with 80–100 mg of furosemide every 1–2 hours.[154] Combined with very careful fluid and electrolyte replacement, urinary calcium excretions exceeding 1000 mg/day are possible and the serum calcium may decrease by 2–4 mg/dl in 24 hours. Severe potassium and magnesium losses are inevitable unless careful replacement is given. This form of therapy should probably not be undertaken unless facilities for careful monitoring are available.

Glucocorticoids

Pharmacologic doses of glucocorticoids increase urinary calcium excretion, decrease intestinal absorption and, in the long term, cause a negative skeletal calcium balance.[155–159] Glucocorticoids are most useful in the hematologic malignancies such as the leukemias, the lymphomas, and multiple myeloma.[160] Hypercalcemia associated with breast cancer also responds to this therapy (particularly when the hypercalcemia is precipitated by the administration of hormonal agents), at least in the early stages of disease.[68,72,161] However, with other solid tumors the effectiveness of glucocorticoid treatment is unpredictable. The mechanism of action is poorly defined but is probably related in part to a direct effect of these agents on both tumor and bone.[160,161,175] Recent *in vitro* studies have shown that glucocorticoids block the activation of osteoclasts by OAF, the mediator thought to be involved in the hypercalcemia of hematologic malignancies.[144] This *in vitro* response may in some situations (*e.g.*, multiple myeloma) explain the *in vivo* effectiveness of glucocorticoid drugs.

The hypocalcemic effect of glucocorticoids takes several days to develop. Large doses of glucocorticoids are usually administered (40–100 mg of prednisone, or its equivalent) in divided doses. The side–effects are well-known and require no elaboration.

Mithramycin

This cytotoxic antibiotic has proved to be particularly useful in the management of acute hypercalcemia unresponsive to other measures. It acts by directly inhibiting bone resorption (it probably has a toxic effect on osteoclasts) and is equally effective in the presence or absence of bone metastases.[66,162–166] It exerts its effect at the molecular level by inhibiting DNA-directed RNA synthesis.[167] It decreases excessive skeletal turnover as mirrored by a reduction in serum calcium and alkaline phosphatase, plus a fall in urine calcium and hydroxyproline, not only in malignant disease but in such conditions as Paget's disease, and also in normal persons.[168]

Mithramycin is administered IV at a dose of 25 μg/Kg body weight either as a rapid infusion or over 4–24 hours. Its effect is usually evident within 24–48 hours.[164,165] The duration of action is variable and may be for a week or more. The dose may be repeated if no detectable calcium lowering effect is seen within 48 hours. One or two doses per week are usually sufficient. Treatment should not be repeated until the hypercalcemia recurs.

Mithramycin has significant side effects that are directly related to the frequency of treatment and the total dosage given.[169] It causes nausea and vomiting fairly frequently but the major toxic effects are thrombocytopenia, bleeding diathesis, postural hypotension, hepatocellular necrosis, and renal damage with azotemia and proteinuria.[164,165,170] Hypocalcemia and tetany can also occur.[163] In addition, the injudicious administration of mithramycin may limit the dose, or restrict the use of other cytotoxic agents to be used for specific cancer chemotherapy.

Despite these potential problems, mithramycin is a major therapeutic agent in the treatment of hypercalcemia.

Phosphate

The IV administration of inorganic phosphate is one of the fastest and most effective methods for decreasing the blood calcium.[171–174] However, its use can cause serious side effects and there are some who express reservations regarding its administration, while others deplore its use altogether.[175]

The administration of inorganic phosphate is associated with a reduction in urinary calcium excretion, no significant change in intestinal calcium loss, and a positive calcium balance.[174] The decline in serum calcium, therefore, reflects a redistribution of calcium within the body. The results of strontium and calcium kinetic studies suggest that the calcium lowering effect of phosphate occurs primarily by the acute precipitation of some calcium phosphate salt, which is presumably sequestered principally in bone.[176] This appears to result from the supersaturation of the body fluids with calcium and phosphate, since the decrease in serum calcium concentration is directly proportional to the mean ion product of calcium and phosphate.[177] However, the effect of phosphate is probably not limited solely to the mechanisms cited above, because *in vitro* bone culture studies have shown that increasing phosphate concentration in the medium not only increases the rate of bone formation but also decreases the rate of resorption.[178]

The sequestration of calcium, however, is not limited to bone. Calcification in extraskeletal tissues has been reported with both IV and oral phosphate therapy.[172,179–182] Extraskeletal calcifications have been observed in the heart, kidneys, lens, and other soft tissues.[182,183] Although hypercalcemia alone can cause soft tissue calcification, there is evidence to indicate that phosphate administration can initiate, as well as accelerate, the process of metastatic calcification.[184–186]

The other major complications of inorganic phosphate therapy include hypocalcemia, hypotension, renal failure, and death.[174,181,183,187] These problems are largely related to the dose and rate of administration.[188] The incidence of side effects is reduced if the dose of inorganic phosphate (mono and dibasic anhydrous potassium phosphate) is limited to 1.5 g (50 mMol) infused over 6–8 hours.[187] The fall in calcium is dependent on the amount of phosphate used. In patients with renal impairment and hyperphosphatemia it is best to avoid IV phosphate altogether. If IV phosphate is used, only one dose should be given in a 24-hour period and generally no more than two doses are necessary. Serum calcium may fall within minutes, but the maximum decline may be delayed for up to five days after cessation of the infusion.[74]

Oral phosphate therapy, although less rapid in action, is very useful particularly for the chronic treatment of hypercalcemia. The usual dose is between 1 and 3 gms of sodium acid phosphate daily; the maximum effect is seen after several days. This therapy is not complicated by hypocalcemia or hypotension, although GI upset and diarrhea may limit the quantities that can be used. The mechanism of action is essentially the same as for IV phosphate, although in addition, oral phosphate may bind calcium in the gut and prevent its absorption. Phosphate enemas can be used as an alternative to the oral route in patients with nausea and vomiting.

Diphosphonates

These are a class of compounds capable of selectively inhibiting the action of osteoclasts on bone.[189,190] They are stable analogs of inorganic pyrophosphate, a naturally occurring inhibitor of hydroxy-apatite crystal growth and dissolution, an action seen *in vivo* by their ability to suppress both mineralization and bone resorption. The two diphosphonates that have been studied most extensively are ethane-l-hydroxy-l-diphosphonate (EHDP) and dichloromethylene diphosphonate (Cl_2MDP). EHDP has been used successfully to treat Paget's disease, but its ability to inhibit mineralization results in its major side effect, the occurrence of dose-dependent osteomalacia.[191] Cl_2MDP appears to be a more potent inhibitor of osteoclastic bone resorption, but it does not cause osteomalacia. A third diphosphonate under active study is aminohydroxypropylidene diphosphonate (APD). Preliminary studies have recently been reported using the diphosphonates to treat hypercalcemia and the osteocytic bone disease of cancer (metastatic breast cancer and multiple myeloma).[192,193] The results are encouraging and further therapeutic trials to assess their long-term efficacy and safety will be awaited with interest.

Prostaglandin Synthesis Inhibitors

It is axiomatic that prostaglandin synthesis inhibitors, such as indomethacin or aspirin, will only be of therapeutic benefit in situations where excess prostaglandin production is implicated in the pathogenesis of the hypercalcemia. Because methods for prostaglandin measurement are not widely available, the usual practice is to perform a therapeutic trial with either aspirin (to produce a serum salicylate level of 20–30 mg/dl) or indomethacin (25 mg every 6 hours). Sometimes these drugs do alleviate the hypercalcemia. In general, however, the use of prostaglandin synthesis inhibitors in hypercalcemia associated with neoplasia has been rather disappointing, particularly in patients with osteolytic metastases, even if excessive prostaglandin production has been demonstrated.[135,139]

Calcitonin

Calcitonin is a polypeptide secreted by the parafollicular cells of the thyroid gland. Its hypocalcemic effect is principally due to an inhibition of bone resorption.[194,195] Salmon calcitonin is the most potent of the available preparations (porcine, human, and salmon) and has the longest duration of action.[196–197] It is only moderately effective in the treatment of tumor-associated hypercalcemia. Subjects with the most rapid bone turnover show the greatest fall in serum calcium. Calcitonin is administered IV (3–6 MRC units/kg of body weight/day), intramuscularly (25–50 units every 6–8 hours), or sometimes subcutaneously (2 units/kg every 4 hours). When given IV plastic equipment should be used as this peptide adsorbs to glass.

The hypocalcemic effect of calcitonin is manifest within a few hours and the expected fall in serum calcium is 1-4 mg/dl. However, after several days' administration (and sometimes earlier) escape from the metabolic effects of calcitonin occurs in patients and animals.[198,199] This problem seriously limits its therapeutic effectiveness. There is some suggestion that this resistance may be attenuated by the concomitant administration of phosphate or prednisone.[200,201] This putative synergism deserves further evaluation. Calcitonin is not regarded as an agent of first choice. However, because of its virtual freedom from toxicity and relatively rapid action, it may be useful as an adjunctive therapy, sometimes allowing a reduction in dose of the more potent but toxic alternative agents.

Dialysis

Both peritoneal and hemodialysis have proved equally effective in managing acute hypercalcemia, particularly when it is severe and complicated by renal failure.[202–204] The dialysance of ultrafiltrable calcium approaches and may even exceed that of urea. Large quantities of phosphate may be lost during dialysis and as phosphate depletion aggravates hypercalcemia, appropriate phosphate supplementation may be necessary.[205,206] Table 42-16 offers a summary of the treatment of hypercalcemia.

HYPERURICEMIA

Hyperuricemia is a well-recognized complication of certain malignant disorders. This condition is common in the lymphoproliferative and myeloproliferative disorders, including lymphoma acute and chronic myelogenous leukemia, polycythemia vera, and myelofibrosis with myeloid metaplasia.[207,208] Additionally, hyperuricemia may be seen in association with multiple myeloma and occasionally with disseminated metastatic carcinoma.[209,210]

Although the presence of a high concentration of uric acid in the blood does not by itself produce symptoms, the sparing solubility of this compound in urine and in tissue fluids may lead to its precipitation within the kidney, the joints, or extra-articular tissues, giving rise to renal complications, gouty arthritis, or tophus formation. Patients with leukemia or lymphoma are particularly susceptible to severe hyperuricemia, which may occur spontaneously, but more commonly follows the rapid destruction of neoplastic cells induced by aggressive chemotherapy or radiotherapy.[211–213] Under these conditions, acute renal failure due to the hyperuricemia may develop. This life-threatening complication is the most important aspect of hyperuricemia in the neoplastic disorders, and the physician contemplating treatment of leukemia or lymphoma must take steps to prevent it.

PATHOGENESIS

In humans, uric acid is the major product of purine catabolism, and serves no specific function besides its role in the elimination of purines from the body. Most of the uric acid produced daily is excreted by the kidney. The remainder is degraded within the body by uricolytic processes, mainly effected by intestinal bacteria. Hyperuricemia may result from increased production or decreased excretion of uric acid or both.[207,208,214] The derivation, metabolism, and excretion of purines in health and disease is shown schematically in Fig. 42–2. In primary gout, increased *de novo* purine synthesis without increased turnover of tissue nucleic acids is responsible for the increase in the uric acid pool. In the lymphoproliferative and myeloproliferative disorders, increased cell turnover in the neoplastic tissue involves increased synthesis and degradation of nucleic acids. The lysis of malignant cells by cytotoxic therapy releases quantities of nucleic acids whose degradation leads to further uric acid production.

Serum uric acid is frequently elevated in patients with renal failure, even of modest degree, due to impaired excretion. This mechanism is largely responsible for the hyperuricemia that is often encountered in patients with multiple myeloma, although increased cell turnover probably also contributes. Similarly, patients with disseminated carcinoma and hyperuricemia often have coexistent renal impairment. In Ultmann's series, hypercalcemia was a common association and may have contributed to the renal insufficiency.[209] Lastly, in the assessment of the hyperuricemic patient it must be borne in mind that chronic administration of certain drugs may lead to elevation of the serum uric acid. Various diuretics, including thiazides, furosemide, and ethacrynic acid, are important examples.[207,208]

RENAL COMPLICATIONS

Three types of renal disease are attributable to hyperuricemia: acute hyperuricemic nephropathy, uric acid nephrolithiasis, and gouty nephropathy.[215]

Acute Hyperuricemic Nephropathy

This is the most important complication of the hyperuricemia of leukemia and lymphoma. Patients with bulky disease are at risk for this complication, and this risk is greatly enhanced by the institution of cytotoxic therapy. Clinically there is the generally sudden onset of acute renal failure with oliguria or anuria. In the oliguric patient crystals of uric acid are usually present in the urine and there may be microscopic or gross hematuria. Flank pain, suggesting ureteral obstruction, sometimes occurs. Unless recovery is rapid, the symptoms, signs, and complications of uremia may develop. Recovery is heralded by the onset of diuresis.[211–213,215]

The mechanism of acute hyperuricemic nephropathy is precipitation of uric acid crystals in the distal nephron, principally in the collecting ducts, resulting in obstruction.[215–218] Obstruction of the ureters by clumps of uric acid crystals is also reported, particularly in the older literature.[219] The factors contributing to precipitation of uric acid are the increased uric acid excretion and the acidity of the urine. In acid urine (*e.g.*, pH 5), uric acid (pK 5.4) exists predominantly as the less soluble, un-ionized form, in contrast to the situation in the blood (pH 7.4), where the dominant species is the monovalent urate ion.[215] Urine concentration tends to be maximal in the collecting duct, making this the most likely site for crystallization of the uric acid.

The diagnosis of acute hyperuricemic nephropathy should

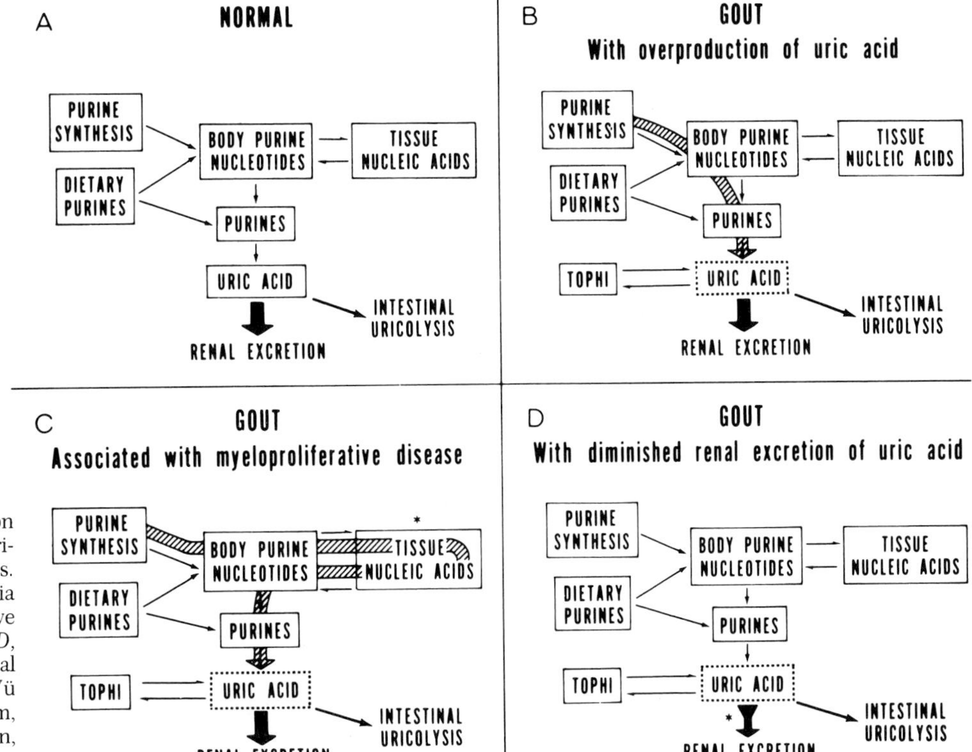

FIG. 42-2. Formation and excretion of uric acid in normal and hyperuricemic subjects. *A*, Normal subjects. *B*, Primary gout. *C*, Hyperuricemia associated with myeloproliferative or lymphoproliferative disorders. *D*, Hyperuricemia due to diminished renal excretion of uric acid. (Talbott JH, Yü TF: Gout and Uric Acid Metabolism, p 41. New York, Grune & Stratton, 1976)

be considered in any patient with leukemia or lymphoma and renal failure associated with elevated serum uric acid. However, the elevation of uric acid that may accompany renal failure of any etiology must be borne in mind in this situation. The finding of uric acid crystals in the urine is strong evidence for the diagnosis of hyperuricemic nephropathy. These may be absent, however. Under these circumstances, a value of serum uric acid that is elevated disproportionately in relation to the BUN is suggestive of the diagnosis.[220] Also, the ratio of urinary uric acid to urinary creatinine is generally greater than one in patients with acute hyperuricemic nephropathy and less than one in renal failure of other cause.[221]

Prophylactic measures against the development of acute hyperuricemic nephropathy are mandatory when cytotoxic therapy is to be undertaken in patients with leukemia in relapse or with lymphoma with bulky disease. Dehydration, if present, must be corrected. Establishing an alkaline diuresis is valuable for two reasons: it tends to lessen the concentration of uric acid in the renal tubules and it promotes conversion to the more soluble urate ion. Alkaline diuresis may be achieved by IV administration of 5% dextrose in water containing 50–100 mEq of sodium bicarbonate per liter as required to maintain a urine pH of seven or greater. The patient must be monitored carefully for the development of fluid overload.

The carbonic anhydrase inhibitor, acetazolamide, is effective in alkalinizing the urine and also has diuretic properties. However, increased clearance of uric acid is not consistently observed when this drug is administered.[216]

Allopurinol, an inhibitor of the enzyme xanthine oxidase, is effective in lowering the uric acid concentration in hyperuricemic subjects, and in attenuating the expected rise in uric acid following cytotoxic therapy of patients with leukemia and lymphoma. Thus it is effective in preventing acute hyperuricemic nephropathy.[222,223] However, this complication occasionally occurs when allopurinol alone is used as a preventative measure.[224] For this reason, alkaline diuresis should be instituted in addition to the administration of allopurinol in patients at high risk.

Doses of allopurinol ranging from 300–800 mg daily have been recommended in the prophylaxis of hyperuricemia. The most common side effects are skin rashes and GI upset. Drug fever, vasculitis, and blood dyscrasias occur infrequently. The incidence of skin rash is much higher when ampicillin is used concomitantly. Allopurinol may potentiate the effects of 6-mercaptopurine and azathioprine, and the doses of these drugs should therefore be reduced in patients taking allopurinol.[225] The formation of xanthine stones in the urine is a rare complication of therapy with allopurinol.[226]

When acute hyperuricemic nephropathy is diagnosed, treatment should involve administration of allopurinol and an attempt to institute alkaline diuresis. Optimal hydration of the patient should be achieved and cautious fluid challenge with sodium bicarbonate should be tried. The administration of mannitol has been successful on occasion in starting a diuresis when fluid challenge has failed. When these measures fail to initiate diuresis, hemodialysis has proven effective in lowering serum uric acid levels and improving azotemia.[224] Peritoneal dialysis is less effective than hemodialysis in clearing uric acid from the blood.[224] The use of hemodialysis may contribute to the good prognosis of established hyperuricemic nephropathy in the collected series of Kjellstrand and coworkers (1974), as compared with the 47% mortality rate reported by Lilje (1970).[224,227]

Cystoscopy with cannulation and alkaline lavage of the ureters has been advocated in the management of acute hyperuricemic nephropathy. Current practice is to reserve this procedure for cases in which there is evidence of ureteral obstruction.[224] When this situation is suspected, (*e.g.*, when flank pain is present) non-invasive investigative measures that may be useful include radionuclide renography and high-dose IV pyelography.

Uric Acid Nephrolithiasis

This condition is seen in cases of long-standing hyperuricemia, including patients with lymphoproliferative and myeloproliferative disorders and patients with primary gout.[215,228–230] This disorder results from precipitation of uric acid in the renal pelvis to form the nidus of the stone, which progressively enlarges. The clinical hallmark of this complication is flank pain when a stone obstructs the ureter. Patients may pass small stones or "sand" with a reddish color.[229] IV pyelography may reveal the presence of radiolucent calculi within the pelvis or ureters. Pyelonephritis is a common complication, and, when chronic, may lead to renal insufficiency.[228,229] Rarely, renal failure may result from bilateral pelvic or ureteral obstruction.[229]

Treatment consists of prolonged administration of allopurinol to suppress uric acid formation. Forced oral fluids and oral administration of sodium bicarbonate may be useful adjuncts in dissolution of stones. Occasionally, surgical removal of a stone may be necessary.[224,228–230]

Gouty Nephropathy

This is a slowly progressive condition with mild renal insufficiency, which typically occurs in the setting of the prolonged hyperuricemia of primary gout. Pathologically it is marked by deposition of crystals of monosodium urate within the renal parenchyma.[215]

Gouty Arthritis

Arthritis, clinically indistinguishable from that of primary gout, is well recognized in association with the lymphoproliferative and myeloproliferative disorders.[207,208] It is a common feature of polycythemia vera and of myeloid metaplasia. It is uncommon in patients with leukemia and lymphoma. Tophus formation is more frequent in patients with secondary gout than in patients with primary gout.[207]

The principles of diagnosis and management of secondary gout are the same as for primary gout. The interested reader is directed to a monograph on gout.[207,231]

LACTIC ACIDOSIS

Lactic acidosis is best defined as a metabolic acidosis due to the accumulation of lactic acid in the blood.[232] This disorder is a potentially lethal complication of a number of diseases. In general, two major subcategories of lactic acidosis are recognized: cases in which oxygen delivery is insufficient for tissue demands (Type A lactic acidosis), and cases in which a reduced oxygen supply is not primarily involved in the pathogenesis (Type B lactic acidosis; see Table 42-17).

In any cancer patient, lactic acidosis may occur as a result of impaired tissue oxygen delivery, a situation most commonly due to shock. In such cases, the lactic acidosis is attributable to the tumor only to the extent that the latter is responsible for the underlying tissue hypoxia.

Lactic acidosis associated with neoplasia without clinical evidence of circulatory insufficiency or hypoxemia is rare. Most reported cases have been in patients with leukemia or lymphoma, but a few cases associated with solid tumors have also been documented.[233-242c]

CLINICAL FEATURES

When lactic acidosis is due to a catastrophic complication such as shock, the symptoms and signs of the latter may dominate the clinical picture (see Table 42-18). This type of lactic acidosis typically runs a fulminant course with profound circulatory collapse, increasing acidemia, and a mortality rate of over 90%.[232,242d]

In cases of lactic acidosis in which tissue hypoxia is not the cause, the clinical manifestations are more clearly attributable to the metabolic disorder. The symptoms, listed in Table 42-18, are non-specific and variable. The most characteristic sign is hyperpnea. This type of lactic acidosis may run a progressive course, in which case circulatory collapse and death may supervene. On the other hand, a chronic, stable acidosis with a relatively good prognosis may be seen.[236,237,242a,242c]

DIAGNOSIS

The diagnosis of lactic acidosis can be established with certainty only by measurement of the blood lactate. In resting subjects, this value is normally less than 2 mmol. To exclude cases in which minor elevations may be secondary to other processes, it has been proposed that the diagnosis of lactic acidosis be reserved for cases in which the blood lactate exceeds an arbitrary value of 4 mmol or 5 mmol.[232,242d]

The major laboratory clue to the presence of lactic acidosis is widening of the "anion gap" of the serum electrolytes. When uremia, ketonemia, and the ingestion of certain toxins (methanol, ethylene glycol, paraldehyde, salicylates) have been ruled out as the cause of an increased anion gap, the latter is most likely due to lactic acidosis.[242e] These criteria are adequate for a working diagnosis in the appropriate clinical setting when facilities for rapid determination of blood lactate are not available.

Although the blood pH is typically low in patients with lactic acidosis, it may be normal or even high, particularly in the early stages of this disorder, due to the coexistence of a second acid/base disturbance. Coexistent respiratory alkalosis is not uncommon.[232] Thus, the diagnosis of lactic acidosis cannot be ruled out by the presence of a normal blood pH.

PATHOGENESIS

When tissue oxygenation is inadequate, the major biochemical pathway for ATP synthesis is glycolysis, the final metabolic product of which, under these anaerobic conditions, is lactate. Lactate removal, principally effected by liver and kidney, is severely compromised when these organs are hypoxic. Thus, net lactate accumulation results from both increased production and decreased utilization. Further details of the biochemistry of lactic acidosis are to be found in several excellent recent reviews.[232,242c,242d,242f,242g]

The pathogenesis of lactic acidosis associated with malignancy without clinical evidence of tissue hypoxia is not clearly defined. It is possible that increased glycolysis in tumor tissue, resulting in excessive production of lactate, may be a cause of this acid/base disturbance.[235,242h] However, the capacity of the normal liver for metabolizing lactate is large, and this makes it unlikely that increased lactate production alone is responsible for this disorder.[242c,242i] In virtually all reported cases of lactic acidosis associated with lymphomas and solid tumors, extensive neoplastic involvement of the liver was evident. Compromised lactate removal by the diseased liver in these cases was probably the major factor in the pathogenesis of the lactic acidosis. A similar metabolic picture is occasionally seen in severe liver disease of other etiology.[242j,242k]

TREATMENT

Type A lactic acidosis is typically a fulminant disorder that is fatal unless the underlying tissue hypoxia can be corrected. Treatment involves the restoration of adequate oxygenation and perfusion, and the IV administration of sodium bicarbonate to correct life-threatening acidemia. In spite of heroic measures, the mortality rate remains high.[242c]

The management of Type B lactic acidosis caused by

TABLE 42-17. Classification of Lactic Acidosis*

Type A
- Due to tissue hypoxia

Type B
1. Associated with various common disorders: Diabetes, renal failure, liver disease, infection, malignancy, pancreatitis
2. Due to drugs or toxins: Biguanides, ethanol, fructose, methanol, ethylene glycol
3. Hereditary forms

Modified from Cohen RD, Woods HF: Clinical and Biochemical Aspects of Lactic Acidosis. Oxford, Blackwell Scientific Publications, 1976

TABLE 42-18. Symptoms and Signs of Lactic Acidosis

DUE TO CIRCULATORY COLLAPSE	DUE TO ACIDOSIS
Hypotension	Hyperpnea
Tachycardia	Malaise
Pallor	Weakness
Peripheral cyanosis	Anorexia
Oliguria	Nausea, vomiting
	Clouding of consciousness

malignancy is less well defined. The available evidence suggests that successful treatment of the malignant disorder results in correction of the lactic acidosis. For example, in two patients with leukemia and lactic acidosis of prolonged duration, partial remission of the leukemia was accompanied by improvement of the acid/base status.[236,237]

Oral or IV sodium bicarbonate has been used to treat the acidemia in these cases. As with Type A lactic acidosis, it is reasonable to use sodium bicarbonate to correct acidemia when it is life-threatening. When the acid/base disturbance is less severe, the potential risks of alkali therapy should be weighed against the benefits.[242a,242d] This form of treatment may enhance lactate production, so that the overall impact on the acid/base status of the patient may be small, at the cost of a large administered sodium load. Under these circumstances, as sodium bicarbonate is infused, sodium lactate may be excreted in the urine in almost stoichiometrically equivalent quantities. The lactate so excreted is necessarily derived from glucose or glucose precursors, the loss of which may be detrimental to the patient with poor dietary intake.[242a]

Other approaches to the treatment of lactic acidosis have included the administration of dichloroacetate or insulin and glucose. Dichloroacetate activates the enzyme pyruvate dehydrogenase. Lactate removal by way of conversion to pyruvate and oxidation of the latter through the pyruvate dehydrogenase pathway is thus promoted.[254l] Administration of insulin and glucose infusions has been successful in the management of phenformin-induced lactic acidosis.[242m] However, the efficacy of these approaches in the therapy of lactic acidosis associated with malignancy remains to be proven.

Surgical Emergencies

RICHARD E. WILSON

Abdominal complications of an acute nature are frequent in patients with malignant disease. They may be the result of the primary tumor, per se, or may occur during or after treatment of the malignancy. This section will define the problems in both general and specific terms and discuss the appropriate methods of management.

GENERAL ASPECTS OF SURGICAL EMERGENCIES

DEFINITIONS

The primary decision required in treating abdominal problems is whether or not surgical intervention is necessary.[243] The acute nature of the problem relates to the timing of the decision and potential intervention. The frequency of observation of the patient and the continuous balance between the decision for intervention vs. non-intervention is the critical judgement factor. This decision is most difficult in patients with malignant disease and its complications because the usual responses and criteria for decision making are altered and specific expertise is necessary.

SYMPTOMS

Pain remains the most important indicator of acute abdominal disease, even in the patients with muted responses. The complaints of oncologic patients must be even *more* carefully evaluated and investigated because they frequently seem less significant to the inexperienced physician. Important aspects of the definition of pain are location, timing, radiation, description, relationship to normal functions (such as eating, defecation, and urination), and what makes it better or worse.

The presence of nausea or vomiting may also be an important complaint, but along with diarrhea and constipation, represents abnormalities of GI function so frequently a complication of treatment of malignancy has to be especially confounding. The presence or absence of blood in the stool or vomitus, the timing of the complaints, and their relationship to other signs and symptoms are particularly critical. Other abdominal complaints, such as distention, cramps, lack of passage of flatus, or anorexia should also be identified. Chills and fever are important constitutional symptoms that may be the only markers of acute abdominal disease in these patients. The timing of fever—particularly when patients are receiving chemotherapy—is important. Previous history, presence or absence of positive blood cultures or accompanying findings such as jaundice, localized pain or physical signs may be needed to place the complaint in proper perspective.

SIGNS

Nowhere in the body is the use of the four hallmarks of physical diagnosis—inspection, percussion, palpation, and auscultation—more valuable than for the acute abdomen. The physician must look for abnormalities of skin color and tone, distention, abdominal venous patterns, disproportionate swelling or edema, and how the patient tries to protect himself from discomfort. Percussion performed in a most gentle manner can localize pain without alarming or hurting the patient. A cooperative patient is essential for accurate physical examination. Absence of liver dullness may indicate free abdominal air, while a resonant epigastric region may define acute gastric dilation. The identification of acute urinary retention and shifting dullness also depends on accurate percussion. Palpation should define localized muscle spasm, organomegaly, abdominal masses, and areas of specific point tenderness. It, like percussion, should be gentle, otherwise false impressions of pain will be assumed or masses can be missed. Auscultation should be directed at identifying the presence and quality of bowel sounds, a succussion splash in the dilated stomach or unusual bruits. The pelvic and rectal examination should be a direct part of the abdominal exam, not to be deferred or delayed. They provide the most critical information of all for lower abdominal complaints Not only can masses or tumor nodules be palpated, but also evidence of peritoneal irritation, dilated bowel loops, pelvic wall disproportions, evidence of fistulous drainage, and insidious abscesses in the peri-rectal tissues can be found. Great care must be taken with proper comfort and positioning of the patient. Rectal examination should always be performed in the lithotomy position with patients of both sexes to maximize the definition of pelvic disease. Examination of the pelvis often requires both right- and left-handed examination to accurately palpate each side. Careful anal and peri-rectal examination will require having the patient turn in to the lateral position as well. Anoscopy and sigmoidoscopy should be almost a routine accompaniment of the rectal examination, even without prior bowel preparation. Anoscopy is best performed in the lateral position, while sigmoidoscopy is best accomplished in the knee-chest position. If inadequate information is obtained, they can be repeated after an enema, but frequently this is unnecessary. Important observations include the presence or absence of fissures, fistulas, and peri-anal abscesses, the status of the intestinal mucosa, the level of positive guaiac stool, and the identification of rectal lesions as being either intra- or extraluminal. Gastric aspiration can also be an important extension of the physical examination of the abdomen as is catheterization of the bladder or paracentesis if a pelvic mass is difficult to define.

LABORATORY AIDS

In the patient with malignancy where complex problems are frequent, the use of more sophisticated laboratory studies may be critical in defining and following acute abdominal problems. They cannot, however, supplant a careful physical examination and history. Rather, as in all other aspects of medicine, these basic elements lead the physician to the appropriate studies. In addition to routine complete blood counts and the SMA-20 examinations, consideration of standard enzyme determination such as the serum amylase or unique enzyme measurements and serial determination of special tumor markers such as hormone and CEA assays may be particularly important.[244] Frequent blood cultures are essential in febrile patients as well as the determination of antibiotic and other drug levels in the serum. Radiologic examinations have grown in sophistication and value and include routine plain films of the abdomen, nuclide scans, ultrasound evaluation, contrast studies of the GI tract, urinary tract, pancreatico-biliary ducts, and fistulae. Ultrasound-guided biopsies and contrast studies are now also available.[245] Angiography to define vascular anatomy may be particularly useful for the surgeon once he has decided that operative intervention is necessary. CT scan has opened up whole new areas of non-invasive evaluation, particularly of the liver, pelvis, and retroperitoneum. The specific roles of these various techniques will be discussed as individual problems are reviewed.

COMPLICATING FEATURES OF ONCOLOGIC PATIENTS

Because the malignant disease and its treatment may confuse and confound the acute abdominal problem, it is *essential* that the examiner obtain the most complete history possible. This may require questioning the family and other involved physicians, as well the patient. A thorough understanding of previous operative procedures, forms of radiation and chemotherapy, and previous abnormal findings is necessary for the correct management of acute abdominal complaints. The patient's symptoms such as pain and fever may be suppressed by corticosteroids or opiates, while ongoing radiation or chemotherapy can cause nausea, vomiting, or diarrhea. Jaundice, GI mucosal bleeding, or anemia may be drug or disease induced. Generalized serositis with its full gamut of acute peritoneal signs may result from drug therapy, diffuse tumor infiltrates, or local perforative lesions. Pneumonia or pulmonary embolism, both so frequent in cancer patients, may present to the physician as an acute abdominal condition. Immunologic anergy is well-known in Hodgkin's disease and in patients with advanced malignancy.[246,247] Their normal immune responses, including those of inflammation, can be lacking. In addition, pancytopenia may be the result of drug or radiation therapy or from marrow involvement with tumor itself.[248] The lack of white blood cell response to acute disease may be misleading in some cancer patients.

If marrow response is blunted, the expected leukocytosis will not occur to indicate a complicating infectious process. On the other hand, collections of pus may not develop and abscesses cannot form in the usual sense. This is particularly true in extraperitoneal invasive sepsis of the perineum or abdominal wall. Ubiquitous infections with viral or fungal organisms in immunosuppressed patients may induce lymphocytosis rather than leukocytosis, further confusing diagnostic decisions. Bleeding and clotting factors may be totally disturbed; bleeding from mucosal surfaces into the retroperitoneum or into a necrotic tumorous lesion is common and may be the cause of abdominal complaints. Febrile reactions may be the result of host-tumor interactions or a new complicating illness. Frequent transfusions requirements, daily alteration in bone marrow function, and infection with unique bacteria, viruses, and fungi complete the picture of diagnostic and therapeutic confusion.[249] This is why the need for a multidisciplinary approach to all problems of cancer patients is so essential.

SURGICAL PROCEDURES AND LOGISTICS

The armamentarium of surgical procedures for dealing with acute abdominal problems is broad, but in cancer patients, certain special considerations are necessary. Because of the many complicating features mentioned above, the diagnosis may be unusually obscure, even when laparotomy is performed! Previous abdominal surgery and abnormal wound repair make the surgical decisions especially critical. Staging of operative procedures may become necessary when that is not the usual practice. Poor host "reserve" may make earlier surgical intervention essential, even though apparent risks are greater and diagnosis may be less certain.

Modern techniques permit better preparation of patients with leukopenia and thrombocytopenia for surgical procedures. In general, white cell transfusions are not necessary prior to surgical exploration for drainage of a septic process. Identification of the offending organism, appropriate antibiotics, and adequate drainage usually suffice. Frequently, white blood cells will spontaneously rise if successful drainage occurs. If no operable focus can be identified or if the predicted response is not achieved, then white blood cell transfusions are indicated. On the other hand, platelet transfusions can be critical for a successful operative procedure. Usually, 6–12 units of platelets are given during induction of anesthesia. The surgeon must take special pains to control every possible bleeding point and then platelet transfusions, six units at a time, can be administered postoperatively only if bleeding is a problem.

The use of peritoneal tap and lavage may be useful, combined with laparoscopy for more accurate diagnosis.[250] Surgeons dealing with cancer patients should become expert in this latter technique. Exploratory laparotomy may be the only way to be certain of the abdominal status of a given patient, despite the lack of more specific operative indications. The simplest operative concepts of diversion, drainage, and decompression may be the only procedures to be performed; complicated resectional or anastomotic operations may be doomed to failure by the underlying nature of the disease or the patient's status.

INFLAMMATORY LESIONS

Inflammatory lesions causing acute abdominal disease may be divided into non-perforative problems. Obviously, many of the non-perforative lesions may progress to perforation and this must be considered in their management. For this reason, non-perforative lesions will be discussed first.

NON-PERFORATIVE LESIONS

Inflammatory lesions can involve the entire GI tract and its accessory organs, as well as the genitourinary system. They are, by far, the most frequent cause of acute abdominal complaints in oncologic cancer patients. Their identification and differentiation from those lesions that require acute surgical intervention are often particularly hard in this patient population.

Esophagitis

This can occur from prolonged nasogastric intubation, specific drug therapy, radiation, or bacterial, fungal, or candidal infection. Intra-oral ulceration may often accompany it and aid in the diagnosis. Perforation is rare but transmural penetration with mediastinitis may occur. Endoscopy is the best technique for diagnosis; acute abdominal pain may be the primary complaint as well as dysphagia. Treatment must be based on the diagnosis of the specific cause of the esophagitis. Very rarely, prolonged vomiting and retching may lead to spontaneous perforation of the esophagus which occurs in the distal third just above the hiatus.[251]

Gastritis and Duodenitis

Epigastric pain, nausea and vomiting, hematemesis, gastric dilation and discreet or diffuse ulceration may be present. Again, endoscopic examination is the best diagnostic tool, although upper gastrointestinal series can sometimes be helpful, particulary for identifying discrete ulcers or obstruction. Bleeding points are also best seen by endoscopy or angiography. Treatment of choice is the combination of decompression and the removal of the offending agents, where possible. Antacid drip therapy is useful in acid-peptic gastritis and steroid induced ulcerations. Conservative management is best except for complications of the gastritis.

Cholecystitis

Localized right upper quadrant pain, jaundice and the identification of gallstones classically define cholecystitis. However, unexplained fever may be the only finding in cancer patients. Ultrasound examinations for gallstones or CT may be useful in the acute situation where an oral cholecystogram would fail to provide critical information.[252] A previous history of stones and fatty food intolerance is most valuable. Treatment will depend on the status of the patients; cholecystostomy under local anesthesia or cholecystectomy under general anesthesia can both provide definitive management if the attack fails to subside. The need for common duct exploration in the presence of jaundice and sepsis may be essential, regardless of the cholangiographic findings or the status of the common duct at surgical inspection.

Pancreatitis

Pancreatitis can be an insidious lesion in patients with other abdominal disease.[253] It can produce pain out of all proportion to the abdominal findings and may be associated with sudden development of generalized ileus, nausea and vomiting and unexplained fever. Any sudden plasma volume deficit as indicated by a rising hematocrit, reduced urine output, hypovolemia or hypotension may be the clue to this diagnosis. Serum or urine amylase elevation, falling serum calcium level, serum lipase elevation or urinary amylast/creatinine ratio measurements confirm the diagnosis. Treatment is conservative, directed toward suppression of pancreatic secretions, since this is primarily an obstructive disease. Both cholangitis and pancreatitis are more common in patients that have fasted and then begun to eat, a pattern frequently seen in cancer patients particularly on chemotherapy. Operative intervention in pancreatitis is for its complications only, either persistent pseudocyst, fistula, or abscess. Common duct obstruction can result from recurrent pancreatitis and may be impossible to differentiate from primary or metastatic carcinoma.[254] Ultrasound examination of the pancreas as well as CT scanning can be extremely useful but not always accurate. Endoscopic retrograde dye-studies of the common and pancreatic ducts may also be valuable.

Enterocolitis

This may frequently be the result of radiation therapy to the abdomen or chemotherapy. In the latter case, it can usually be temporally related to the treatment pattern, frequently occurring right after treatment when reflex diarrhea or vomiting ensue, or at the time of the white cell nadir, when mucosal damage to the bowel is associated with local inflammation. Antibiotic therapy can also produce muscosal inflammation, vasculitis, and pseudomembranous colitis.[255] Mucosal bleeding with intramural hemorrhage can occur in these patients as well. Radiation effects tend to be later, usually 2–10 years after treatment, although early edematous and inflammatory reaction may produce acute symptomatology.

Appendicitis

The localizing symptoms of acute appendicitis are frequently more difficult to identify in debilitated patients. Constipation and other alterations of acute illness probably make appendicitis a greater risk, since this disease starts as an obstructive phenomenon in the appendiceal lumen. Smoldering local sepsis, with eventual abscess formation is a serious risk. The surgeon must look for reproducible localizing abdominal signs in patients with abdominal pain, as the best index of appendicitis. Laboratory studies are unreliable, with fever and leukocytosis often not apparent. Newer studies with ultrasound and CT scans in this patient population may be particularly useful. Operative treatment remains the same, appendectomy, with drainage only if there is a localized abscess. As with other surgical procedures in this patient population, prophylactic antibodies during the acute operative period in short, high dose courses are definitely indicated.

Diverticulitis

Diverticular disease is much more frequent in patients with chronic illness, inactivity, dehydration, constipation and poor immune responses. Instead of a walled off inflammation of the diverticular microabscess, which normally produces some crampy pain, low grade fever and a tender sigmoid, with or without a mass, diveriticulitis in this patient group has a high incidence of free perforation, fecal peritonitis, and death.[256] This often occurs with the most minimal signs and symptoms, sometimes acute left lower quadrant abdominal pain, groin pain, diarrhea, or fever. Early diagnosis, rapid operation and sigmoid resection with double-end colostomies are the steps needed for salvage. We have learned to obtain limited emergency barium or Gastrograffin enema examinations in these patients at the least provocation. This has been a highly successful method of effective diagnosis and treatment.

Proctitis and Perirectal Inflammation

Proctitis is a common consequence of pelvic radiation; pain, tenderness, rectal bleeding and mucosal discharge are the most common findings. Proctitis can also result from chemotherapy, especially if diarrhea is present as well. It must be distinguished from perirectal abscess, fistula-in-ano, cryptitis, and situlas. The perirectal and perianal lesions are more localized and may require surgical treatment. They can occur with proctitis, however, and careful anoscopic and sigmoidoscopic examination is necessary. Local pain may be so great that anesthesia is required for adequate evaluation of the area. With severe neutropenia, perirectal abscess may be devoid of pus and instead appear as an area of dense and painful cellulitis. High dose antibiotics for gram negative bowel organisms, covering both aerobes and anaerobes, as well as sitz baths, stool softeners, and bed rest, should precede any plans for surgical drainage. As white blood cells return, the local condition often improves; white blood cell or platelet transfusions may be very helpful, since some of these lesions start as intramural hematomas related to constipation. Careful and frequent examination is necessary for the proper decision, especially if fever and septicemia are present. If drainage is necessary in the patient with pancytopenia, small incisions with packs sewn into the cavity will reduce bleeding and local pain.

Prostatitis and Pyelonephritis

Male patients requiring prolonged or frequent urinary catheterization are at high risk for these complicating infections. Fever, urinary retention, deep pelvic pain, and a boggy, tender prostate on rectal examination is the way prostatitis presents. Appropriate high dose antibiotics followed by chronic suppressive therapy is the treatment of choice, with urinary catheterization to be used only for retention. Pyelonephritis, particularly if there is a previous history, is a risk when pancytopenia is present. This can be another source of septicemia in a debilitated patient population; urinary cultures will frequently define the organism and its sensitivity. Abdominal and flank pain with fever, sometimes associated with reflex nausea and vomiting, will lead to the diagnosis.

PERFORATIVE LESIONS

Although some of the potentially perforative lesions, such as appendicitis and diverticulitis, have been referred to in the section above, there are some circumstances that particularly present as gastrointestinal perforations. Many of these are related to the primary malignancy itself.

Gastro-duodenal

Gastric carcinoma frequently can present with perforation as the initial complaint, as can acid-peptic gastric and duodenal ulcers. Acute upper abdominal pain, muscle rigidity and free air in the abdomen on plain abdominal upright films represent the most common triad of findings. The presence of anemia, guaiac positive stool or a history of weight loss and obstructive symptoms will frequently provide a suggestion that the lesion is malignant rather than benign. Early laparotomy is the treatment of choice. If the perforation is beyond the pylorus, simple plication remains the best treatment, unless the patient has a long and definite history of peptic ulcer disease.[257] For lesions in the stomach, frozen section is essential to be certain that one is not dealing with a perforated carcinoma. With local inflammation and edema, it is not always possible to identify a gastric carcinoma by palpation, and the frozen section may be difficult as well. That is why the history and complete physical examination are important. Existence of cancer throughout the gastric wall may be accomplished by supraclavicular (Virchow) nodes, rectal shelf, celiac lymph node involvement or liver metastases, and the surgeon should look for these. Gastric resection is the treatment of choice—routine or extended subtotal gastrectomy with omentectomy. This should be done even in the presence of proven distant metastases, since the best possible palliation and opportunity for chemotherapy will result. If uncertain about the benign or malignant nature of a gastric ulcer, gastric resection should be performed since that is the most efficient treatment for benign gastric ulcer as well.[258]

Small Intestine

Small bowel perforation is rare. It results from strangulating obstruction, vasculitis, tumor perforation or sometimes during treatment of intestinal lymphomas. The treatment is always surgical and is difficult to differentiate from gastro-duodenal perforation, unless there is known enteric disease. It is most unusual for small intestinal obstruction secondary to extrinsic tumors to strangulate, but obstruction in cancer patients can be on a benign basis. Tumor of the small intestine usually presents with obstruction rather than perforation. Vasculitis from drugs or in collagen disease is on the anti-mesenteric surface and can be mimicked by intraluminal hemorrhage and necrosis in the thrombocytopenic patient. The signs and symptoms of small bowel perforation are those of diffuse peritonitis; usually of sudden onset, with pain, rigidity, absent bowel sounds and free abdominal air. Immediate laparotomy is indicated and resection of the perforation should be performed. If there is extensive soilage so that primary enteric anastomosis is deemed unwise, temporary end-enterostomy and mucous fistula for the divided bowel loops is far safer.

Appendix and Colon

Although the diagnostic criteria for acute appendicitis in the patient population have been discussed, it should be stressed that perforation, particularly with free peritonitis, is far more frequent, thus, early decision for operation is required, usually with less diagnostic findings.

Colonic perforations are usually either at or just proximal to the obstructing tumor or at the cecum.[259] Encircling colonic tumors in the recto-sigmoid region can produce local perforation and abscess formation, but far more frequently are responsible for colonic obstruction in a closed loop limited by the ileocecal valve. The cecum is the most distensible portion of the colon and likewise has the thinnest wall. Free perforation and varying degrees of necrosis of the cecal wall are the usual consequences of colonic obstruction. Generalized peritonitis results with dangerous fecal soilage. Obstructive symptoms will be discussed below, but they may be amazingly minimum. A history of progressive constipation, some cramps and fullness and sometimes blood in the stool can usually be elicited. The simplest diagnostic work-up is usually all that is necessary or justified. CBC shows an elevated hematocrit and a leucocytosis. The hematocrit rise is associated with plasma loss and outpouring of peritoneal fluid. The acute onset of the perforation is rarely associated with any other serum abnormality and the abdominal plain films confirm the clinical diagnosis.

Immediate operation with resection of the right colon, temporary end-ileostomy, and mucous fistula for the transverse colon is the treatment of choice. Extensive irrigation, wide drainage and aggressive antibiotic therapy are usually successful, although septic shock and death can occur. Subsequent resection of the primary cancer and closure of the diverted limbs of bowel provide colonic continuity. Local perforation of the tumor is best treated by primary resection of the lesion, drainage of the abscess, if such is present and either direct or delayed colonic anastomosis, depending on the state of the bowel and the surrounding peritoneal surfaces. Diversion and drainage alone are not the preferred treatment. If the lesion is too low in the pelvis to permit distal mucous fistula, then a Hartmann turn-in at the pelvic floor can be used with a proximal end-sigmoid colostomy. Although the cancer prognosis in patients with colonic perforation is usually not as good as it is for nonperforated lesions, aggressive surgical management is clearly justified because the end results are surprisingly good.[259]

OBSTRUCTIVE DISEASE

Obstruction of the gastrointestinal tract constitutes a common and serious abdominal problem in cancer patients. Essentially, there are two types of obstructive situations: those due to malignant tumor and those resulting from benign lesions that accompany some form of malignant process. Even in patients with known previous cancer, it cannot be assumed that all obstruction results from tumor recurrence nor need be treated by operative intervention.

Since intestinal obstruction results in a severe metabolic deficit, it is important that prompt replacement of extra-renal fluid and electrolyte losses be initiated promptly. In addition, nutritional support in the form of either peripheral or central hyperalimentation can proceed while either operative or non-operative treatment is considered.[260] High intestinal obstruction results in greater risk for metabolic alkalosis because of the relatively high levels of gastric fluid losses and its disproportionate hydrogen ion concentration. Vomiting and distention are the key features for all sites of intestinal obstruction. Crampy abdominal pain, particularly coming in waves, associated with high-pitched peristalsis, absence of flatus, and the lack of any specific site of tenderness is the typical finding of lower small bowel or large intestinal obstruction. When large bowel obstruction is associated with an incompetent ileocecal valve, then it is more difficult to distinguish from small bowel obstruction (see Fig. 42-3). The closed loop form of colonic obstruction, as mentioned earlier, is far more likely to rupture the cecum.

FIG. 42-3. Formation of uric acid.

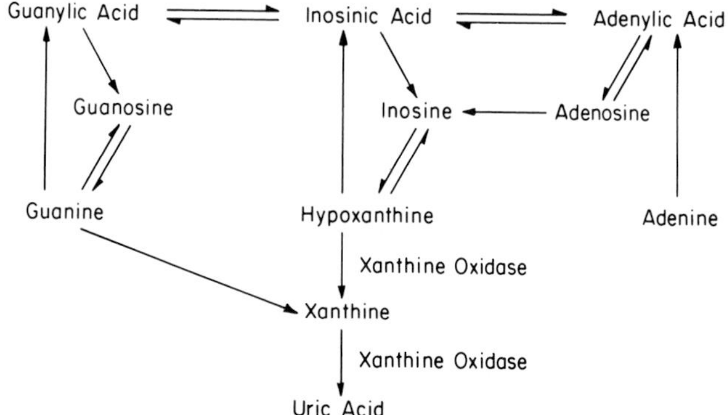

The initial investigation of all forms of intestinal obstruction should be the flat and upright plain films of the abdomen. Serial examinations will serve to document progression or improvement of obstruction if conservative treatment is chosen. The barium enema is a valuable and very safe examination and can identify unrecognized colonic obstruction; upper GI series is contraindicated, except for esophageal or gastric lesions. In general, the treatment of all forms of mechanical intestinal obstructions should be surgical. Early postoperative obstruction, associated with new adhesive bands and partially functioning small bowel loops, can respond to nasogastric or small intestinal intubation and decompression. Experience at the Peter Bent Brigham Hospital with intestinal obstruction in cancer patients reveals that one-third had a benign cause.[261] Obstruction was more likely to be due to a malignant process if the patient had known metastatic carcinoma, the primary was in advanced stage, colorectal cancer had been the primary lesion, or the free interval from the time of initial treatment was short. Relief of obstruction with nasogastric suction alone occurred in 24% of the episodes in these patients and always was seen within 3 days of admission. Of those patients achieving relief by conservative means, however, 41% eventually were readmitted and required surgical decompression. Specific aspects of obstructive lesions at different locations in the intestinal tract will be discussed from the standpoint of diagnosis and treatment.

ESOPHAGUS

Esophageal obstruction as a result of tumor, inflammatory reaction related to infection, radiation, or ulceration secondary to chemotherapy rarely presents as an acute complaint. The symptoms of dysphagia and local pain are usually progressive. However, perforation can occur, with acute epigastric complaints, and the acute pain of an obstructing ulcer can be severe. The diagnosis is best made with endoscopy so that biopsy can be obtained. Treatment is expectant and symptomatic.

GASTRIC

Gastric outlet obstruction is either the result of a benign peptic ulcer in the duodenum or pyloric channel or a gastric carcinoma of the antrum. It is rare for duodenal ulcers to obstruct without a significant history. Acute ulcers often perforate or bleed, but rarely obstruct. Hydrogen ion concentration is always high so that a metabolic alkalosis is usually present by the time the diagnosis is made.[262] Pyloric channel ulcers most frequently obstruct, even when they heal. Duodenal ulcer disease can develop or be aggravated as a result of corticosteroid therapy, operative procedures, and the general anxiety state surrounding cancer management. Although conservative treatment with gastric decompression and fluid and electrolyte replacement is necessary as the initial therapy, obstructing duodenal ulcer almost uniformly requires operative therapy. Pyloroplasty and vagotomy is the treatment of choice. This is a particularly safe operation for patients with a debilitating disease such as malignancy or during the course of chemotherapy because there is no circumferential anastomosis and tissue healing is excellent.

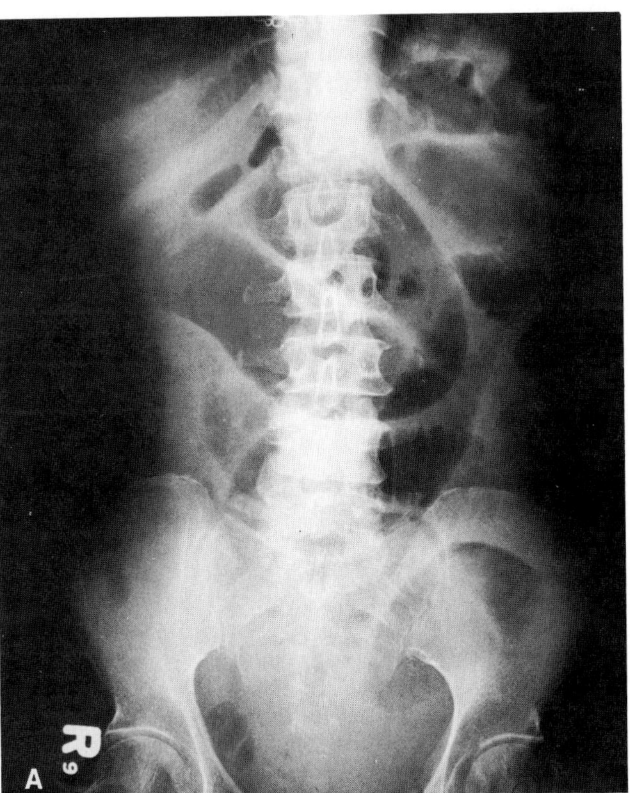

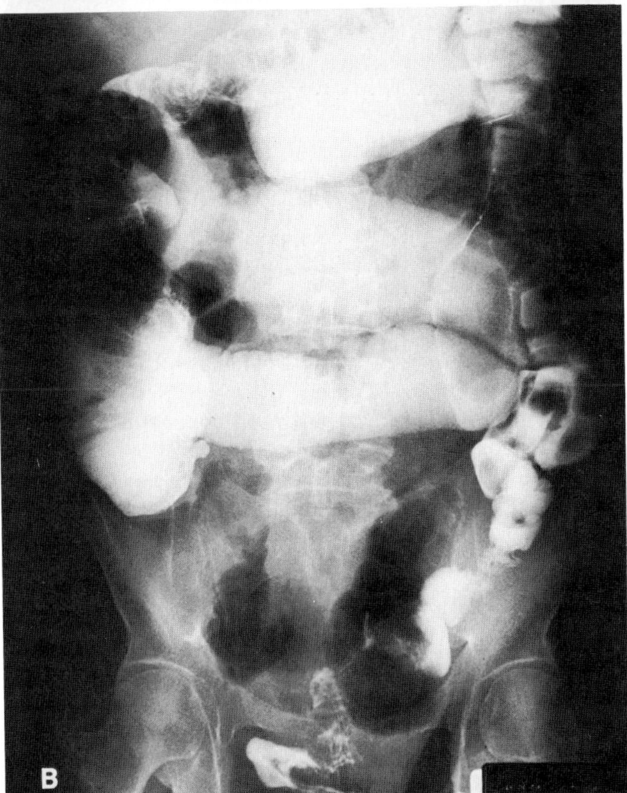

FIG. 42-4. Mechanical small bowel obstruction secondary to right colon carcinoma. *A*, Plain film of the abdomen shows small bowel obstructive pattern involving the entire jejunum and ileum. *B*, Barium enema demonstrates the responsible lesion—an annular carcinoma of the ascending colon. Barium enema is the diagnostic study of choice for patients with small bowel obstruction.

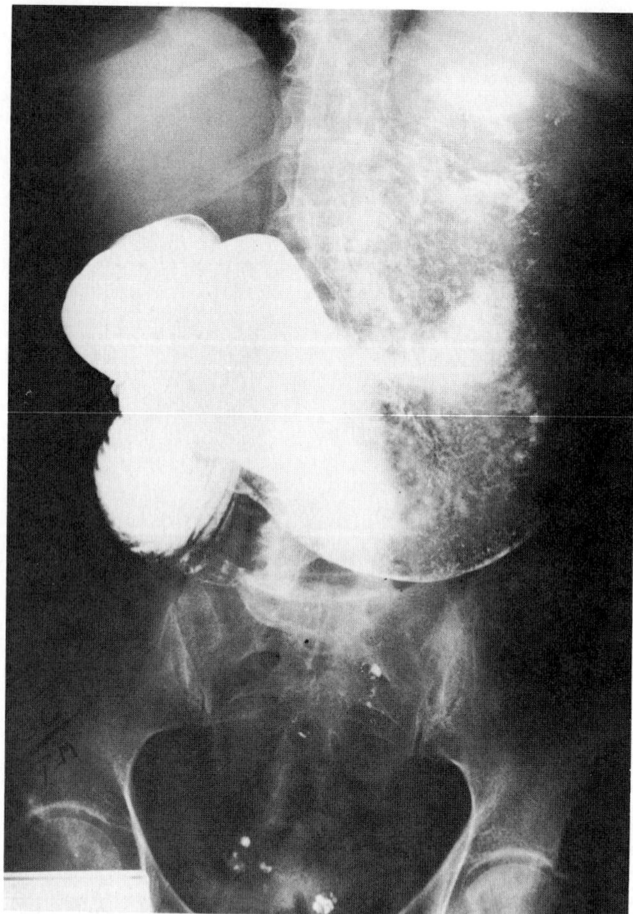

FIG. 42-5. Gastric outlet obstruction. This upper GI series demonstrates massive gastric dilatation with duodenal obstruction. The obstruction was produced by metastatic carcinoma of the breast involving the retroperitoneum in the vicinity of the duodenum and the ligaments of Trietz.

Obstructing gastric carcinoma or obstruction of the gastric outlet by extension of pancreatic carcinoma or other metastatic malignancy requires a different approach (see Fig. 42-4). Obstruction by gastric carcinoma need not be a late stage or an antral carcinoma, thus, a radical subtotal gastrectomy is indicated if operative findings warrant it. Even if there is evidence of metastatic disease to the liver, celiac nodes, or pelvis, palliation is best achieved by a gastric resection, albeit more limited. Obstruction of the stomach by a diffuse gastric carcinoma, such as linitis plastica, which extends from esophagus to duodenum, and is spread to local lymph nodes, carries a much more grave prognosis and the decision as to whether a total gastrectomy should be performed in such a patient depends on the age and general status of the patient as well as the availability of radiation and chemotherapy programs to follow.

Gastric outlet obstruction by extension of pancreatic or biliary tract carcinoma, or as a result of metastatic lesions such as carcinoma of the cervix, colon, ovary and the like, is best treated by gastrojejunostomy (side-to-side). Retro-colic posterior gastroenterostomy is sometimes easier if there is extensive omental involvement with tumor, making access to

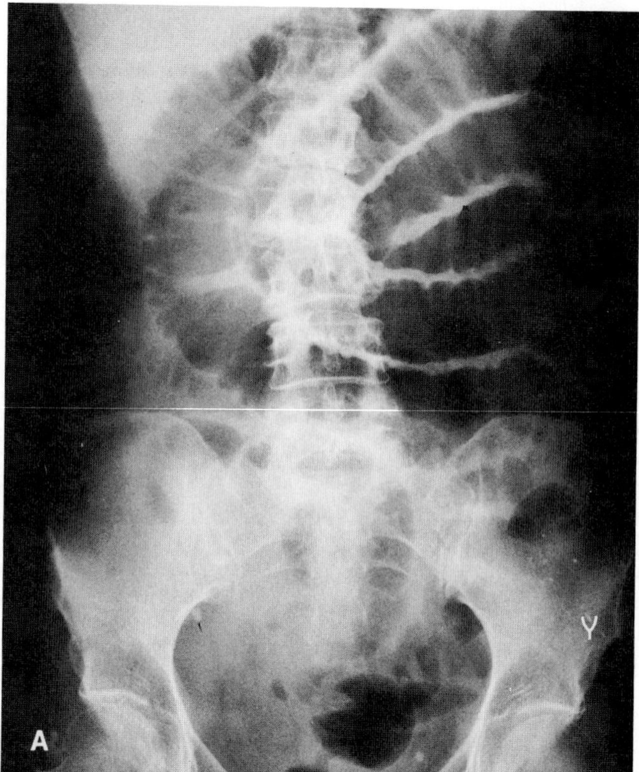

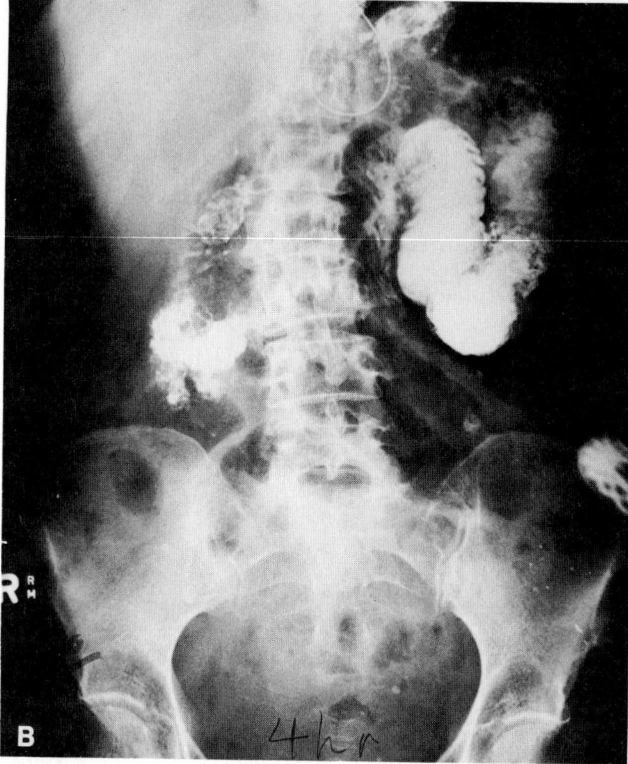

FIG. 42-6. Small bowel obstruction due to post-irradiation enteritis and metastatic endometrial carcinoma. *A*, The plain film of the abdomen shows small bowel dilatation, thickened intestinal wall, and some air in the distal colon. *B*, History was that of intermittent obstruction, confirmed by upper GI series which demonstrated moderate dilatation and poor motility. Upper GI series is indicated in this type of patient where the obstructive pattern is much less clear.

the anterior gastric surface difficult. It is essential to anastomose the jejunum to uninvolved stomach, otherwise peristalic activity will be ineffective and the procedure will fail to provide gastric emptying.

SMALL INTESTINE

As mentioned above, most small bowel obstruction in cancer patients with previous abdominal malignancy is the result of neoplastic implants. Since many of these patients have multiple foci of involvement and the obstruction may not be complete, conservative management with intubation is appropriate as the initial step, as a general rule (see Figs. 42-5 and 42-6). This is particularly true if previous operation for malignant obstruction has taken place. It is rare for multiple surgical attempts to be successful when treating intestinal obstruction due to malignant bowel involvement. An initial operative procedure is always justified if decompression fails to reverse the situation. Sometimes, preoperative passage of a Miller-Abbott, or other long intestinal tube, will permit better identification of both the site of obstruction and the proximal and distal limbs of obstructive bowel. These features may be completely obscured by extensive peritoneal carcinomatosis, the most frequent type of metastatic disease producing obstruction. Pancreatic, ovarian, colonic, and gastric carcinomas are the most common offenders. No aggressive attempts at freeing up loops of involved bowel or resection should be made; it is preferable to perform the simplest side-to-side bypass anastomosis possible. Frequently, transverse colon is the most identifiable distal bowel. The second choice is the terminal ileum. The risk of small bowel fistula is very high if dissection of tumor-involved bowel is attempted, and that is a dire complication. If the intestinal lumen is accidentally opened where tumor is present, it is wise to either resect or bypass that site. Abdominal cavity drainage and enterostomy catheters should be avoided because of the high incidence of tumor growth along the tracts.

If the cancer patient presenting with small bowel obstruction is fortunate enough to have a benign cause, such as adhesive bands, internal hernia, and the like, standard treatment should be used. More attention should be paid to wound management and to early nutritional support, since the patient may be significantly depleted of calories and protein even before the onset of the obstruction. The diagnosis may be somewhat obscured in patients receiving chemotherapy or radiation, because of the high incidence of GI symptoms associated with these treatments. It is therefore important to be certain that patients with persistent vomiting on chemotherapy do not also have crampy abdominal pain or lack passage of flatus!

COLONIC

Presentation of the problem of colonic obstruction has been partially discussed in the section on colonic perforation. The symptoms may be insidious or very acute. The end result, however, is dilated bowel, vomiting, crampy pain and absence of flatus or stool passage (see Fig. 42-7). It is rare for the right colon to be obstructed by tumor but, in the rest of the colon, except the rectum, it is not an uncommon occurrence.

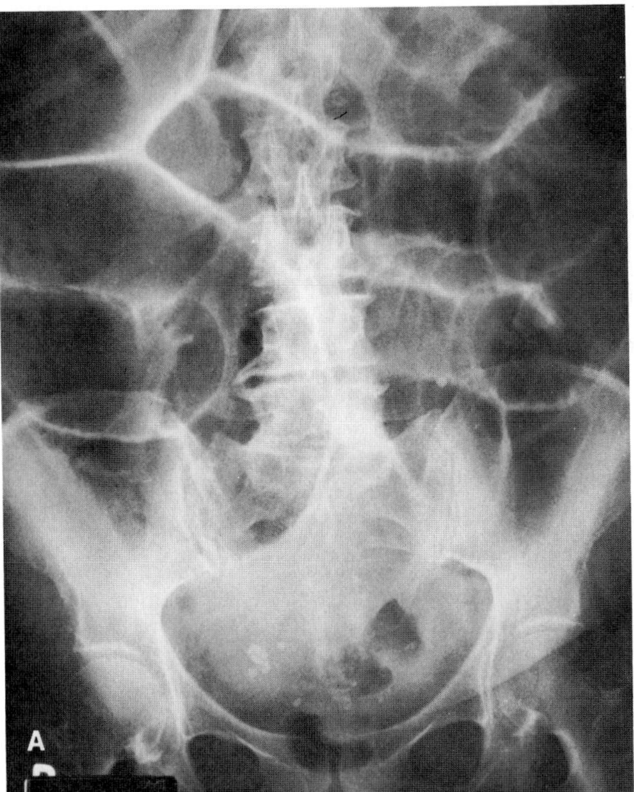

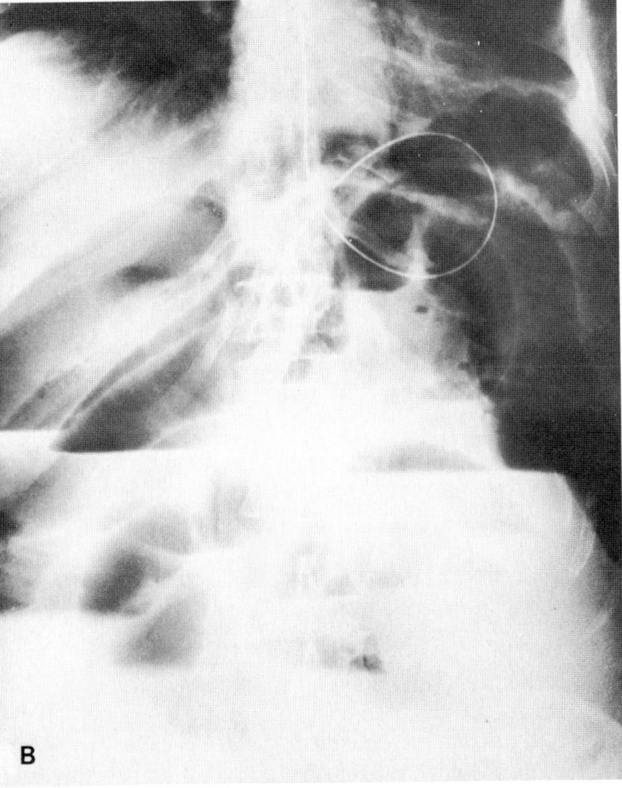

FIG. 42-7. Mechanical small bowel obstruction secondary to metastatic carcinoma of the cervix. *A*, Obstruction is complete and acute with thin bowel wall, large air-fluid filled loops of bowel and minimal large intestinal gas. *B*, The upright film shows the air-fluid levels most dramatically. The site of obstruction was in the terminal ileum.

Prompt treatment is required to avoid perforation. No attempts should be made to resect the obstructing lesion in unprepared colon. It is far safer to perform a diverting colostomy, usually right transverse, or, if necessary, an end-ileostomy or cecostomy for hepatic flexure lesions. This diverting procedure can usually be performed under local anesthesia, with or without intercostal block, and the dangers of using a general anesthetic in a sick, distended, depleted and frequently uncompensated patient can be avoided. Rapid restoration of homeostasis and thorough work-up usually can be followed by a safe, elective bowel resection in 10–14 days. Barium enema is the x-ray study of choice, once the plain films have defined the problem. No preparation is necessary and minimal pressure should be used by the radiologist.

Rectal cancers that obstruct are rare and generally are locally advanced lesions. Rectal exam will usually reveal a large fungating tumor with extension to the adjacent organs of the pelvis or the pelvic wall. Most patients with this form of obstructing rectal carcinoma will require radiation therapy, with a diverting colostomy, before an attempt is made to resect the primary. Resection should be performed, however, because radiation alone can rarely achieve good palliation. With no evidence of distant metastases, after a thorough evaluation particularly of the liver, exenterative procedures are justified for locally extensive rectal cancer.

STRATEGIES FOR MANAGING INTESTINAL OBSTRUCTION

This is a practical summary for the management of various forms of intestinal obstruction.

1. The diagnosis of the site of obstruction is critical for treatment.
2. Plain films of the abdomen may rapidly separate gastric, small bowel or large bowel obstruction.
3. Upper GI series should only be obtained in patients with gastric or duodenal obstruction.
4. Barium enema should be performed for patients with large or small bowel obstructions.
5. Patients with incomplete small bowel obstruction may require a small bowel series by mouth or through a tube to define the site of disease.
6. All patients with intestinal obstruction should be initially treated with a naso-gastric tube. For most patients this will suffice until a diagnosis is made and surgical treatment carried out.
7. A long intestinal tube is of value only in treating patients with early postoperative small bowel obstruction or those with incomplete obstruction. In either of these two situations, the obstruction may be reversible, which is the prime indication for small bowel intubation.
8. Large bowel obstruction requires early surgical decompression, particularly if the ileo-cecal valve is competent. Right transverse colostomy is the treatment of choice because it can usually be performed under local anesthesia and doesn't interfere with subsequent cancer resection.
9. Gastric obstruction and small bowel obstruction should be surgically treated unless a brief period of decompression reverses the situation. Non-operative management is particularly justified if no obstructing lesion can be identified or if acute gastric dilatation or ileus is presumed to be the cause of GI malfunction.

HEMORRHAGE

Hemorrhagic complications in the abdomen are particularly prevalent in patients with malignancy, because of the high risk for mucosal damage, combined with pancytopenia, in patients being treated with aggressive multi-modal therapy for a variety of tumors. While the majority of hemorrhagic complications are intraluminal, extraluminal bleeding can likewise occur. Prompt diagnosis as to the site of bleeding is even more critical in this patient population, because treatment decisions may be particularly complex. The critical factor is always whether or not bleeding is sufficiently massive that emergency operation is necessary. This decision is often difficult, even in people without malignant disease or complicating treatment plans. Three important considerations include the causes of bleeding correctable, short of surgery, how effectively can a surgical procedure control the bleeding, and how disabling is the surgery? The final decision for or against a surgical procedure must include the answers to these questions.

INTRALUMINAL BLEEDING

Esophagus

Esophageal varices can be a complication of primary hepatic tumors, liver metastases or myeloproliferative disorders with either liver involvement or intrahepatic hematopoiesis. Obviously, the degree of portal hypertension and associated trauma or ulceration will be responsible for variceal bleeding. Emergency porto-caval shunt may be required for such variceal bleeding if it becomes exsanguinating and cannot be controlled by either Sengstaaken tube or vasopressin. All patients with variceal bleeding may be treated initially with IV vasopressin but should this fail, then intra-arterial vasopressin should be administered through the superior mesentery artery. The dose for intra-arterial vasopressin is between 0.2 and 0.4 units per minute. If the patient is relatively stable and not bleeding too vigorously, then 0.2 units per minute would be the starting dosage. Rapid bleeding requires initiation of the dose at 0.4 units per minute. Dosages above that level usually are not any more effective and do have a greater complication rate from systemic effect of vasopressin. Older patients will even have complications, particularly in the form of arrhythmias even at the 0.2 to 0.4 unit per minute level. The usual length of intra-arterial vasopressin therapy is 12 hours. If successful cessation of bleeding occurs, then the dosage should be tapered, with reduction at the rate of 0.1 unit per 12 hours. The catheter is left in place for 12 hours after vasopressin therapy has been discontinued before it is removed. As with treatment of GI bleeding in other sites, failure of response to vasopressin would indicate the possibility of using autogenous embolization to the varices, and then if that fails, surgical treatment would be the choice.

Patients with hiatus hernia and reflux esophagitis can develop significant GI bleeding with ulceration, particularly during corticosteroid therapy or if vomiting is prolonged. Usually, antacid therapy with dietary management is sufficient for control, but on occasion an anti-reflux procedure, such as the Nissen fundoplication, is required.[263]

Stomach

Massive life-threatening bleeding can occur from gastritis, benign ulcers, or gastric carcinoma. Gastritis is common in patients with malignancy; pain medications, so frequently taken, are often irritating to the gastric muscosa. Likewise, specific forms of chemotherapy may either damage the gastric mucosa or certainly be associated with gastric irritation, dilatation, and vomiting. Septic episodes may invoke gastritis and shallow gastric ulcers, as may corticosteroid ingestion. Thrombocytopenia, uremia, and hepatic dysfunction will aggravate the problem. The diagnosis is best made by endoscopy but selective angiography may be effective not only in defining the bleeding point but in permitting control with either vasopressin or autogenous clots. Bleeding must be sufficiently vigorous from a site in the GI tract to identify the bleeding point by this technique, so it has limited usefulness. Treatment of gastritis, induced bleeding should be conservative at first; gastric decompression, lavage with cold saline to reduce mucosal flow, irrigation with antacids for acid blockage, and cimetidine therapy should all be attempted. If, after adequate blood replacement, correction of clotting and bleeding abnormalities and sufficient vasopressin administration by intra-arterial infusion (see schedule above) the bleeding persists, then surgical control will be required.[264] The surgical treatment of choice is a radical subtotal gastrectomy. Even though the entire mucosa appears to be the source of bleeding, it is rarely necessary to perform a total gastric resection for gastritis. Even preserving a small gastric cuff, reduced the incidence of anastomotic disruption and postoperative difficulties.

Benign gastric ulcers rarely result in major bleeding. Pain or perforation is more common. However, occasionally, they will bleed massively, so that emergency gastric resection is required. Upper GI series or endoscopy is the method of diagnosis. It is difficult to distinguish benign ulcer from carcinoma particularly when bleeding. Persistent gastric ulcers which do not heal promptly require surgical resection, anyway, so that subtotal gastrectomy produces the most effective treatment. Older patients with arteriosclerotic vessels and those with abnormal clotting factors will bleed more persistently and more prompt resection will be required. As stated above, in the emergency treatment of gastric carcinoma, whether it is perforated, obstructing, or bleeding, radical subtotal gastrectomy is the treatment of choice. Extensive carcinomas of the entire gastric lumen will require total gastrectomy for bleeding control, contrary to the experience with diffuse gastritis.

Other malignant lesions that may produce major gastric bleeding are leiomyosarcoma of the stomach, carcinoid tumors of the stomach, gastric lymphoma and metastatic tumor, particularly melanoma. The latter, on GI series, produces a typical "donut" ulcer in the stomach, a metastatic focus with a necrotic center that bleeds. Leiomyosarcomas of the stomach commonly present with bleeding when the mucosa over the tumor becomes eroded. The treatment of choice for all these lesions is gastric resection, attempting to leave some normal proximal or distal stomach. Any proximal resection should be accompanied by a pyloroplasty, because of vagal nerve resection and gastric atony.

Small Intestine

The most common bleeding point in the small intestine is in the duodenum. Acute duodenal ulcer with bleeding can occur after any surgical operation, after major injury, as a complication of corticosteroid or other drug therapy or following major septic episodes. A prior history of duodenal ulcer makes it more likely and bleeding will be more frequent in the pancytopenic patient. Treatment should be conservative at the start, with cimetidine or other histamine H_2-receptor antagonists, antacids, decompression if vomiting is present, and correction of bleeding problems. Bleeding from duodenal and some gastric ulcers may be successfully controlled by embolization of the artery from which the bleeding is identified by angiography. Embolization, rather than intra-arterial vasopressin, is the treatment of choice for specific ulcers in either duodenum or the stomach.[265] If bleeding cannot be controlled, prompt surgical attack should be made before problems of coagulation and pneumonia develop. Pyloroplasty, suture ligation of the bleeding point with non-absorbable material, and vagotomy is the treatment of choice. Massive hemorrhage will not usually occur from a duodenal ulcer unless the gastroduodenal artery or one of its branches is eroded. Duodenitis will not produce that lesion.

Major bleeding is rare from metastases to the small intestine. Ovarian metastases may not even extend through the serosa but most other tumors can invade into the mucosa and produce hemorrhage. Likewise, effective treatment of lymphomatous nodules in the small intestine can produce tumor necrosis and bleeding. Lymphoma and large mesenteric lymph nodes can extend into the intestinal wall, and produce bleeding when necrosis ensues. Intestinal fistula from neoplastic growth may also bleed extensively. The diagnosis of these lesions is usually made by small intestinal barium study, but sometimes not until laparotomy is performed. The treatment of small intestinal tumors is important because loss of enteric continuity in a cancer patient results in severe nutritional consequences, the large intestine serves no digestive function and can always be partially or totally bypassed.

Colo-rectum

Major bleeding from the colon and the rectum is not common in patients with malignant disease, unless there are serious bleeding abnormalities. Primary tumors usually bleed slowly and insidiously. Polypoid tumors, particularly of the rectum, may bleed sufficiently so that rectal bleeding is the cause for presentation of the patient to the physician. Any other causes of major colonic bleeding, such as diverticular disease, colitis or proctitis can be treated expectantly, assuming attempts are made to correct any defects and clotting factors. Angiographic identification and arterial infusion of vasopressin are most

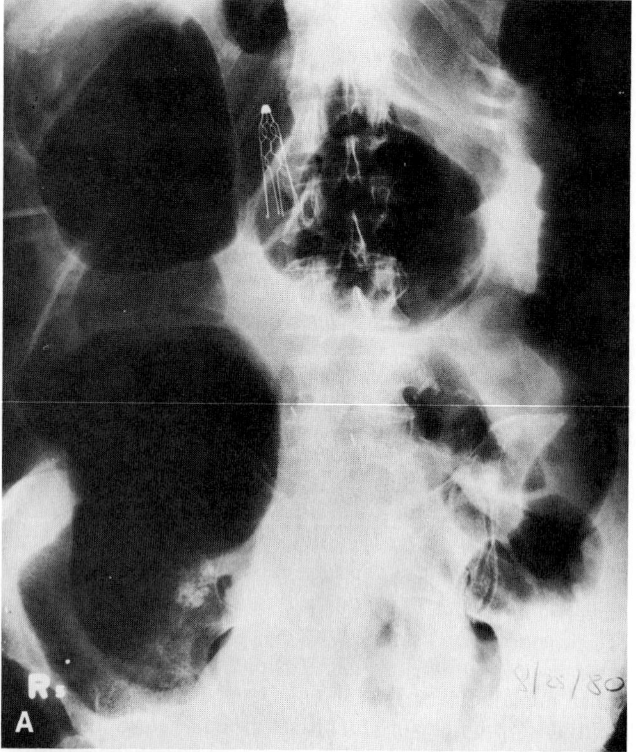

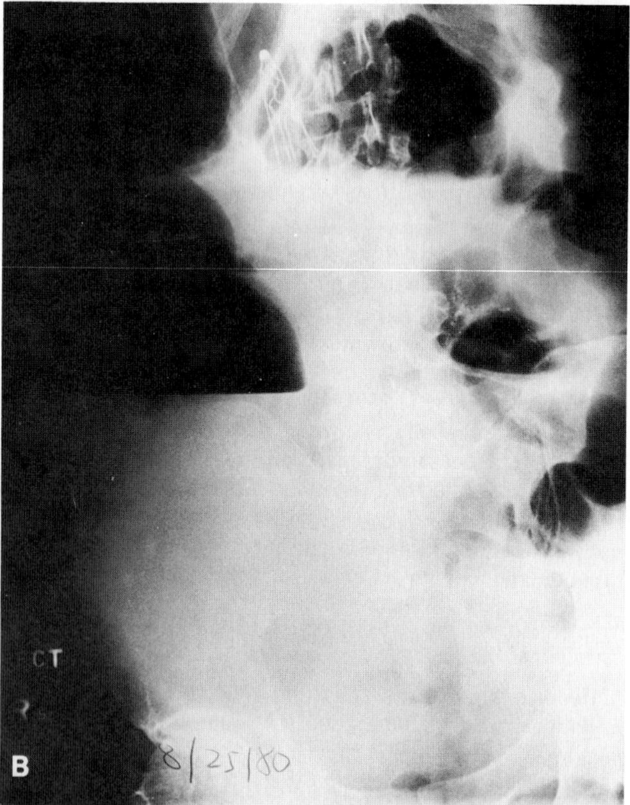

FIG. 42-8. Colonic obstruction with competent ileo-cecal valve produced by an intra-abdominal sarcoma. *A*, Obstruction was at the level of the sigmoid colon where the gas pattern ends. *B*, The cecum is critically dilated requiring emergency transverse colostomy. No small bowel dilatation is seen, as evidence of the close loop obstruction. A caval umbrella is present in the right upper quadrant.

effective for colonic bleeding and should be attempted before any surgical attack is considered (see Fig. 42-8).[266] Large villous adenomas in the rectum can be directly fulgerated or excised transrectally to control bleeding.[267] As with all chronically ill patients, stool softeners and adequate hydration will minimize the risk of ano-rectal bleeding and other complications.

EXTRALUMINAL BLEEDING

Abdominal bleeding outside the intestinal lumen most frequently is in the retroperitoneum and mesentery or in other abnormal organs. The diagnosis of bleeding is rarely made as early or as accurately as it is with intraluminal bleeding and the treatment is more varied.

Retroperitoneal bleeding is usually the result of thrombocytopenia or some other coagulopathy. It is for the most part spontaneous and is controlled by restoration of the clotting defect and retransfusion. Surgery should not be considered for this problem. Extension of bleeding into the mesentery is common and likewise should be treated conservatively. The diagnosis is usually made when bulging of the flanks of the abdomen is identified, frequently with ecchymosis and sometimes accompanied by tenderness. Hypovolemia, falling hematocrit, and unexplained hypotension without evidence for intraluminal bleeding are the usual observations.

Bleeding can occur suddenly into the spleen which is enlarged, usually from either infarct or trauma. There are numerous forms of malignancy that are associated with splenomegaly and such spleens are at greater risk to rupture as well, usually with subscapular tears but sometimes with free perforations and rapid hypovolemic shock. Pain, either referred to the left shoulder or the left flank, is the most common specific complaint. In the case of trauma, the history of the type and direction of injury is valuable. The presence of fractured ribs in the left lower rib cage is also important evidence leading to a diagnosis. Plain films showing shift of the gastric air bubble and the splenic flexure on either nuclide or CT scan are helpful in showing splenic infarcts or fracture. Angiogram with placement of autogenous clots in the splenic artery can occasionally prevent emergency splenectomy in selected patients, where this is contraindicated. When free perforation has occurred, peritoneal tap will demonstrate free blood. Splenectomy is the treatment of choice for splenic bleeding and can usually be performed safely.

Hepatic bleeding most frequently results from primary hepatomas, liver cell adenoma, or focal nodular hyperplasia. It is a rare finding for patients with focal nodular hyperplasia but is very commonly seen in primary hepatomas and liver cell adenoma patients. This is particularly true for liver cell adenomas where aside from the presence of a mass, retroperitoneal bleeding is the most common method of presentation.[268] Bleeding from both hepatoma and liver cell adenomas can be massive and exsanguinating. Evaluation of hepatic lesions with angiography, CT and ultrasound scans, as well as nuclide scans, should provide useful evidence of the location and the resectability of primary hepatic tumors but generally, laparotomy is necessary for the ultimate decision. Metastatic hepatic tumors rarely produce bleeding.

In the female patient, significant menorrhagia can occur

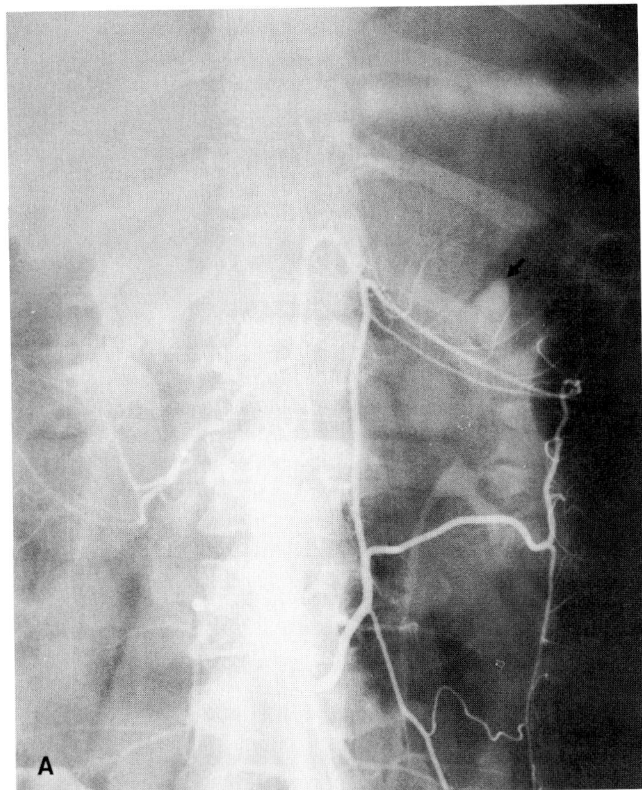

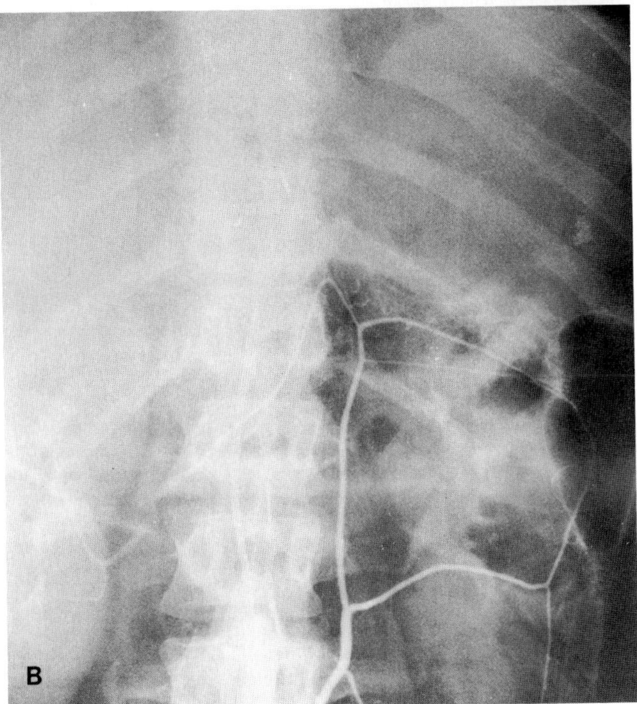

FIG. 42-9. Angiographic technique for controlling GI bleeding. *A*, Intraluminal bleeding point identified in transverse colon (*arrow*) by infusion of middle colic artery with contrast. *B*, Bleeding controlled by infusion of vasopressin at 0.3 units/minute by way of *both* superior mesenteric and inferior mesenteric arteries. Infusion of either artery alone failed to control the bleeding. No surgical treatment was required for this patient.

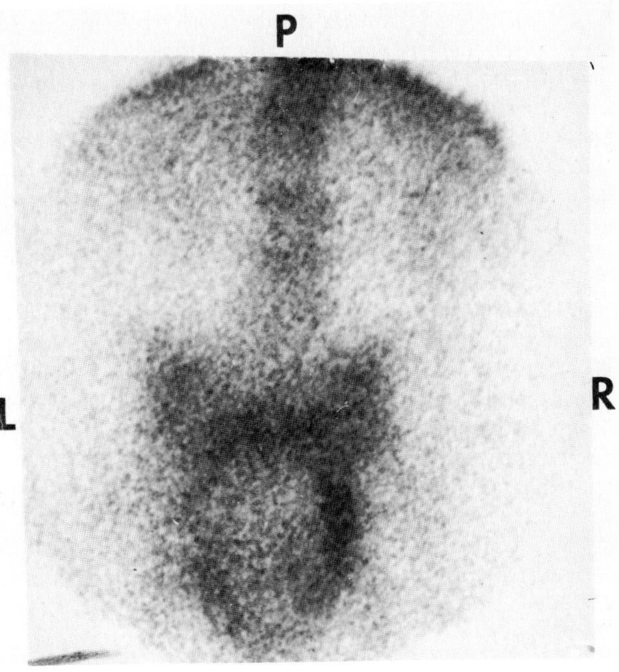

FIG. 42-10. Pelvic abscess defined by gallium[67] citrate imaging. This is a posterior view of the abdomen and pelvis in a 77-year-old female with fever one week after an anterior resection with Hartmann turn-in of the distal sigmoid colon. A large extraperitoneal pelvic abscess was defined by this scan. There is a prominent ring-shaped accumulation of the isotope in the abscess cavity around the rectum.

with thrombocytopenia. It may be necessary to suppress menstrual cycles with hormone therapy or, even rarely, perform hysterectomy to control this.

Another important cause of extraluminal bleeding is from abdominal aortic aneurysms. Although this would be considered only a coincidental problem in cancer patients, they can coexist. Since this is such a treatable condition, it must be considered in the differential diagnosis of any major abdominal catastrophy, even in patients with malignant disease.

SPECIAL ABDOMINAL PROBLEMS IN POSTOPERATIVE PATIENTS

Certain acute abdominal conditions can occur after major surgical procedures in any part of the body. These include acute pancreatitis, acute cholecystitis, mesenteric vascular accident, and pulmonary embolism with infarction on the diaphragmatic surface. Following abdominal surgery, there are a variety of complications that can present as acute abdominal problems including bleeding, anastomotic leak, abscess formation, and diffuse peritonitis. Most patients with malignant disease are more prone to develop problems of tissue healing and control of sepsis, so much a part of the normal recovery process after surgery.

Because of usual problems after major surgery, such as incisional pain, tachycardia, low grade fever, and the like, acute abdominal complications are often more difficult to diagnose than they might be in their usual setting. The nutritionally-depleted patient with extensive abdominal surgery, which often characterizes the cancer patients, makes concern for the type and form of anastomosis critical and consideration of diversion and staging of procedures important. The surgeon must be alert to the postoperative circumstances of unexplained, prolonged ileus, pleural effusion, jaundice, unusual pain, tachycardia, and hypotension. These findings may be the only indicators that the patient's course is not proceeding normally after surgery. Frequent observation and the possibility of re-exploration must always be considered if these findings persist.

Ultrasound examination can be particularly useful in identifying postoperative abscess, biliary stones in acutely jaundiced patients, and evidence of pancreatitis. Intra-abdominal abscess formation may be particularly insidious and difficult to define. Recently, McNeil and coworkers reported a prospective study comparing CT, ultrasound, and gallium-67 citrate imaging in patients suspected of having a focal source of sepsis (see Fig. 42-9).[269-271] These authors found that if any two of these three examinations were used and if either examination was abnormal, the sensitivity of the evaluation increased from 60% to nearly 90% but the false positive rate increased from 15% to 25%. On the other hand, if focal sepsis was diagnosed only when two examinations were abnormal, the false positive rate dropped to near zero but the sensitivity dropped to under 40%. They concluded that all three modalities appeared similar in their ability to detect focal sources of sepsis and that it was more advisable to use multiple methods of evaluation rather than a single study. One of the disadvantages of gallium citrate imaging is the 48 to 72 hour delay necessary for the most favorable type of study whereas ultrasound and computerized tomography can provide immediate information.

Contrast studies will identify anastomotic leaks, usually with Gastrograffin to minimize barium staining. Wound dehiscence will often result from sepsis, pancreatitis, or anastomotic leakage, depending on the time of occurrence after operation. The surgeon caring for patients with malignant disease must use special diagnostic and therapeutic expertise to reduce the risk of complications and achieve the best possible results.

Urologic Emergencies

NASSER JAVADPOUR

The clinical features of genitourinary emergencies in the cancer patient are those related to hemorrhage, obstructive uropathy, sepsis, and uremia. The urologic presentation includes disturbance of urination, hematuria, fever, pain, pyuria, and oliguria. Diagnosis and management of genitourinary emergencies in the cancer patient require a meticulous history and physical examination, as well as radiologic, laboratory, endoscopic, operative, and histopathologic examinations. This section will briefly discuss the diagnosis and management of these urologic emergencies in the cancer patient (see Table 42-19).

HEMATURIA

Hematuria may be classified as initial, total or terminal. Bleeding from the distal urethra often manifests as initial hematuria whereas terminal hematuria often originates from the proximal urethra or base of the bladder. Total hematuria often originates from the ureter, renal pelvis or kidney.

In the diagnosis and management of patients with hematuria it is important to realize that the causes of hematuria are numerous and usually vary with age and sex (see Table 42-20). However, in a known cancer patient hematuria is usually due to chemotherapy, pelvic radiotherapy, coagulation disturbances or the presence of tumor in the genitourinary tract.[272]

The diagnosis of hematuria in a cancer patient includes a careful urologic history, examination, excretory urogram, and endoscopic examination preferably during active bleeding to localize the source.

Although neoplastic diseases of the genitourinary tract may be the cause of acute bleeding in a cancer patient, the cause of bleeding is usually secondary to systemic or localized lesions of the urinary tract induced by chemotherapy or radiotherapy. Perhaps the most frequent emergency pertaining to bleeding from the urinary tract in cancer patients is secondary to cyclophosphamide induced hemorrhagic cystitis. This form of panmural cystopathy deserves a detailed discussion because of its seriousness and yet encouraging response to the appropriate local therapy.

TABLE 42-19. Urologic Emergencies in the Cancer Patient

1. Hematuria
   Cyclophosphamide-induced cystitis
   Radiation-induced cystitis
   Tumors and metastases of the urinary tract
   disseminated intravascular coagulation and other coagulation disturbances
2. Obstructive Uropathy With or Without Uremia
   Ureters: Pelvic and retroperitoneal tumors
   Trigone and urethra: Cancer of the cervix and prostate
3. Abscesses of the Urinary Tract
   Renal and perirenal area
   Perivesical and prostatic area
   Periurethral, epididymal, and scrotal structures
4. Miscellaneous
   Priapism: Acute leukemia
   Acute phimosis and paraphimosis

TABLE 42-20. Causes of Hematuria in Various Age Groups (1–60 Years of Age)

MALE AND FEMALE				MALE		FEMALE		
1–5	*5–10*	*11–30*	*31–40*	*41–50*	*51–60*	*31–40*	*41–50*	*51–60*
Infection Nephritis	Nephritis Infection	Infection Calculus Bladder tumor	Infection Bladder tumor Calculus	Bladder tumor Calculus Infection	Bladder tumor BPH Calculus Infection	Infection Calculus Bladder tumor	Infection Calculus Bladder tumor	Bladder tumor Infection Calculus

HEMORRHAGIC CYSTITIS INDUCED BY CYCLOPHOSPHAMIDE

Cyclophosphamide is a cytotoxic alkylating agent widely used in the treatment of leukemia, lymphoma, and certain solid tumors. It is unique among chemotherapeutic agents in causing urinary bladder injuries. The side-effects of cyclophosphamide on the bladder include mucosal edema, hemorrhage, mucosal ulceration, subendothelial telangiectasia, and fibrosis of detrusor muscles leading to a permanently contracted bladder.[272–277]

Bladder toxicity is caused by the metabolites of cyclophosphamide. Metabolites including chlorethyl aziridine and acrolein are activated by liver microsomes and excreted in the urine. These metabolites react with the bladder wall including its urothelium. Since the urine accumulates in the bladder the pathologic changes are mostly seen in this organ. These changes have also been seen in obstructed ureters after administration of high doses of cyclophosphamide. Although direct contact with these metabolites appears to be the cause of bladder toxicity, dogs with ileal conduits receiving IV cyclophosphamide exhibit a small amount of bladder toxicity. This finding indicates that the hematogenous route is also responsible for a part of cyclophosphamide induced bladder toxicity.

Massive telangiectasia and ulceration may cause severe life-threatening bleeding from the bladder requiring emergency treatment. Most series report urinary tract complications in about 25% of cases with approximately 7–12% having acute hemorrhagic cystitis. The histopathologic changes in acute cyclophosphamide-induced hemorrhagic cystitis have been well established. Grossly, the mucosa appears edematous and hyperemic with multiple punctate hemorrhagic areas and a diffuse capillary ooze. The mucosa may slough and erosions may extend almost through the bladder wall. Microscopically, granulation tissue and reactive fibroblasts, many of which are multinuclear, may be found beneath the mucosal surface. Hemorrhagic cystitis has also been a major problem in patients receiving radiochemotherapy with bone marrow ablation and marrow transplantation in acute leukemia. Long-term cyclophosphamide therapy may produce either an acute hemorrhagic cystitis or chronic bladder fibrosis. Hemorrhagic cystitis and bladder fibrosis have also been reported in patients with MOPP therapy for Hodgkin's disese.[278] Atypical epithelial cell hyperplasia and carcinoma of the bladder have been reported in patients receiving cyclophosphamide. Experimental and clinical experience indicate that atypical cellular changes are reversible and it is not clear whether carcinoma of the bladder is a consequence of cyclophosphamide or merely a coincidental finding in reported cases.

The treatment of cyclophosphamide bladder injuries should be divided into emergency treatment to control bleeding and elective therapy to expand the bladder capacity of a contracted bladder caused by fibrosis of detrusor muscles. A number of modalities of treatment, varying according to the severity of the hemorrhage, have been recommended. These include searing the telangiectatic capillaries in the bladder with electrocautery using a ball tip electrode and a light coagulation current, ligation of the hypogastric arteries, and urinary diversion with or without cystectomy.

The recent introduction of refined formaldehyde instillation into the bladder has made an important contribution to controlling hemorrhagic cystis.[272,274,279] The instillation of 4% formaldehyde solution is performed after cystoscopy and bladder biopsy in the following manner: The patient is sedated or anesthetized; a number 24 urethral catheter is inserted through the urethra; a cystogram is performed to rule out possible perforation or bladder fistulas which can cause leakage of formaldehyde solution into the peritoneal cavity with subsequent fixation of the bowel, the retroperitoneal space, or vagina; in a female the vagina is packed to prevent leakage of formaldehyde solution around the catheter into the vagina, which could cause severe irritation and burning sensations; the bladder is well irrigated to remove all blood clots; and a 4% formaldehyde solution (150–300 cc) is instilled into the bladder under gravity using an Asepto syringe and drained out after ten minutes. The Asepto syringe is kept at the level of the pubic symphysis during the period so that if the patient's bladder contracts or if the patient tries to urinate, the formaldehyde solution can drain out. Clamping of the catheter should be avoided, because if the patient tries to urinate while the catheter is clamped, the formaldehyde solution may enter into the circulatory system via the dilated bleeding capillaries, due to increased intravesical pressure. It is also important to note that formaldehyde cannot be used in the presence of vesicoureteral reflux due to its deleterious effect on renal papillae causing papillary necrosis. We have encountered a number of patients with vesicoureteral reflux and intractable hematuria induced by cyclophosphamide. The formaldehyde instillation has been performed in these patients after the ureters have been occluded with Fogarty catheters.[280]

Postoperatively a urethral catheter is left in the bladder for 24–72 hours to drain the urine and clots. Copious amounts of fluid intake and irrigation of the urethral catheter and discontinuance of cyclophosphamide are also advisable to these patients.

TABLE 42-21. Results of Therapy with Formaldehyde Instillation Into the Bladder For Cyclophosphamide-Induced Cystitis

	PATIENTS	PATIENTS SUCCESSFULLY TREATED
First Instillation	106	91 (86%)
Second Instillation	23	19 (83%)

In 106 cases of hemorrhagic cystitis treated by formaldehyde, 91 (86%) were successful in controlling the hemorrhage, and in 23 cases of recurrent bleeding, a second instillation of formaldehyde was successful in controlling the hemorrhage in 19 cases (83%) (see Table 42-21).[281] In addition to instillation of 4% formaldehyde in the bladder, we suggest discontinuance of cyclophosphamide, vigorous hydration with concomitant diuretic therapy in an attempt to dilute toxic metabolites in the urine. A urethral catheter is inserted to allow the bladder to remain contracted and for irrigation of clots. Antispasmodics and prophylactic antibiotics are also administered. Contracted bladder with fibrosis and subsequent hydronephrosis may require a suprapubic vesical diversion such as ileal or sigmoid conduits. Although the utilization of N-acetylcysteine has been reported in experimental animals to reduce cystitis it has not helped to reduce the toxicity of cyclophosphamide in patients in terms of panmural cystitis.[282]

FIG. 42-11. A retrograde urethrogram in a patient with urinary retention secondary to a large cystic adenocarcinoma of the right seminal vesicle (*arrow*). Note the narrowing and elongation of posterior urethra (*arrowheads*).

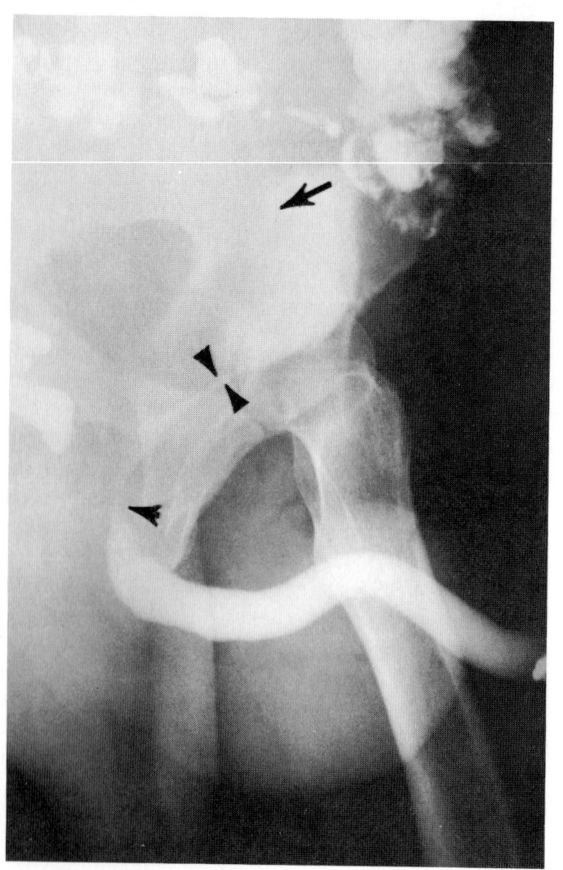

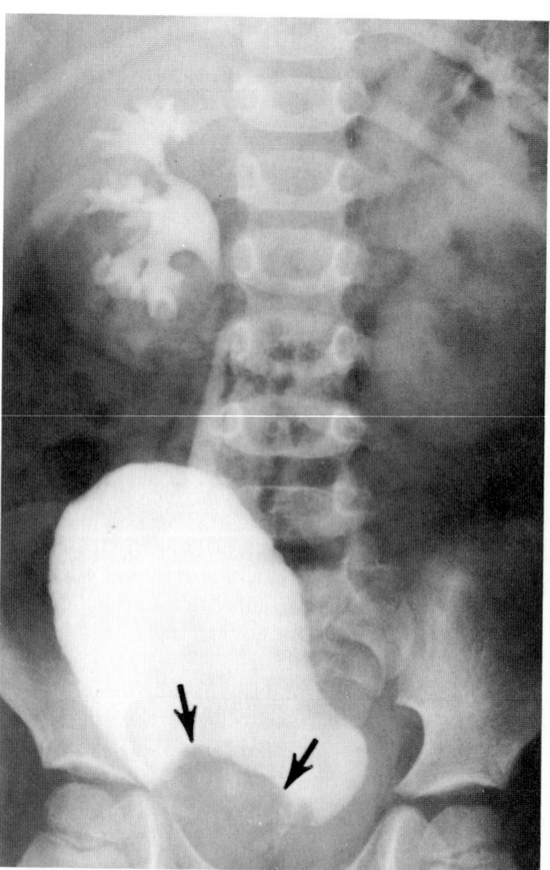

FIG. 42-12. Infusion IVP of a child with prostatic embryonal rhabdomyosarcoma. Note the filling defect at the base of the bladder (*arrows*) and a nonfunctioning left kidney proven to be caused by obstruction of the left ureterovesical junction.

In a randomized clinical trial of 20 patients receiving cyclophosphamide with prophylactic administration of mesnum (sodium-2-mercap-toethane sulfonate), Scheef and coworkers have reported a lower incidence of hematuria.[283] These investigators have indicated that administration of mesnum did not decrease the efficacy of cyclophosphamide. The mechanism of action of mesnum is inactivating the urinary metabolites of cyclophosphamide apparently being responsible for the bladder injury.

ACUTE OBSTRUCTIVE UROPATHY

Acute obstruction to the free flow of urine may result in stasis, infection, calculus formation, and eventually destruction of the portion of the urinary tract above the obstructive site. The end result of acute obstructive uropathy is hydronephrotic atrophy of the kidney, renal insufficiency and uremia. The sequence of events following an obstruction are hemorrhagic areas proximal to the obstruction, hydroureter, hydronephrosis, and caliectasis leading to loss of the functioning

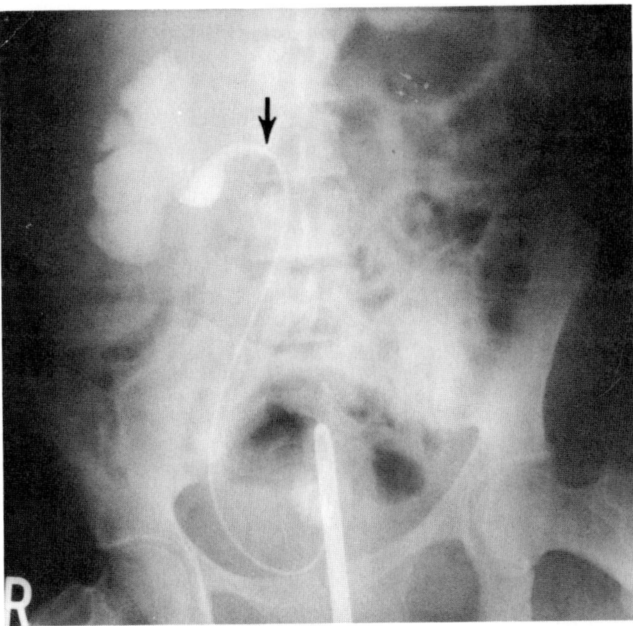

FIG. 42-13. A right retrograde pyelogram in a patient with nonfunctioning right kidney due to lymphoma involving the retroperitoneal area. Note upward deviation of the proximal ureter and renal pelvis (*arrow*).

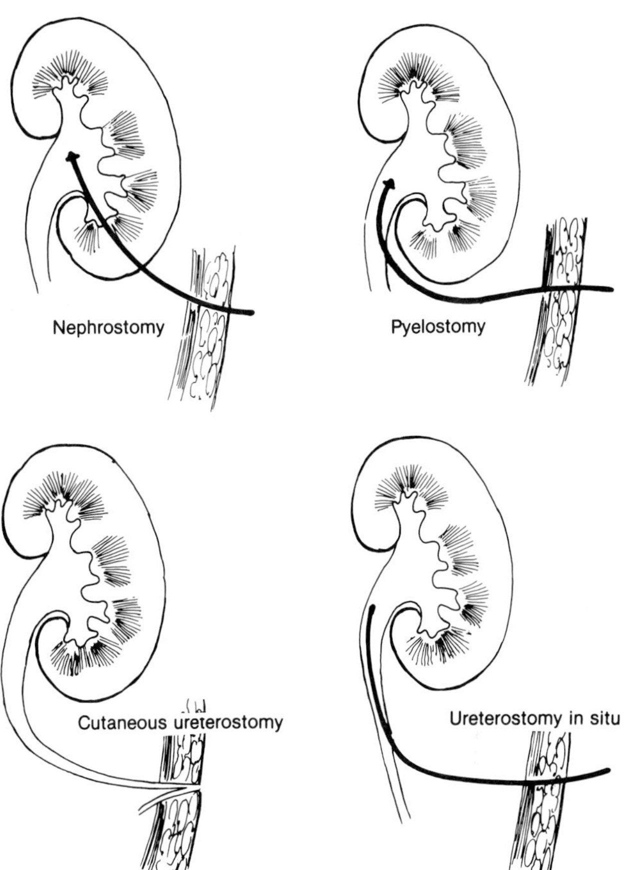

FIG. 42-15. Methods of supravesicular urinary diversions for relieving the obstruction of the upper urinary tract.

nephrons. The clinical features of acute obstruction are urinary retention, acute flank pain, hematuria (resulting from calculus, infection or tumor), chills, and fever. The significant physical findings are those of urethral lesions, prostatic neoplasms, and abdominal or flank masses. The inability to catheterize the urethra usually indicates urethral stricture, prostatic neoplasm or urethral tumor. Urethrogram and endoscopy is essential to localize the exact size and nature of an obstruction (see Fig. 42-11). Obstruction of the upper urinary tract may be diagnosed by an infusion excretory urogram with delay films (see Fig. 42-12). If the ureters are not visualized a retrograde pyelogram and occasionally brushing of ureteral lesions may be necessary to locate and diagnose the cause of obstruction (see Fig. 42-13). CT, ultrasound, and angiograms are occasionally needed for diagnosis and localizing the site of obstruction. The laboratory findings of obstruction may be hematuria, pyuria, proteinuria, leukocytosis, elevated blood urea nitrogen, creatinine, serum phosphorous, and serum potassium. These laboratory findings raise the possibility of an obstruction leading to renal failure but do not assist in precise diagnosis. The diagnosis of acute obstruction is made by demonstration of abnormal retention of urine by way of catheterization of the bladder, by urethrocystogram, excretory urogram, retrograde pyelogram, and radioisotopic renogram. The most common primary tumors causing ureteral obstruction are from cancer of the cervix, bladder, prostate, ovary, and rectum. Although the immediate release of obstruction is essential, the intactness of the urinary tract and complete recovery from the obstruction is dependent on definitive treatment of the cancer. The immediate treatment of obstructive uropathy is relief of obstruction and control of infection. The obstruction in the lower urinary tract may be temporarily controlled by passage of an indwelling urethral catheter. If passage of a urethral catheter is not possible, suprapubic cystostomy or cutaneous vesicostomy may be necessary (see Fig. 42-14). Suprapubic cystostomy has major advantages over the indwelling catheter. These advantages include the following: fewer infections, because exposure to urethral and perianal pathogenic bacteria is avoided; greater comfort for the patient; fewer occurrences of epididymitis in the male with avoidance of trauma to the ejaculatory ducts; ability to assess voiding capability without

FIG. 42-14. Methods of urinary diversion from the bladder with or without tubes.

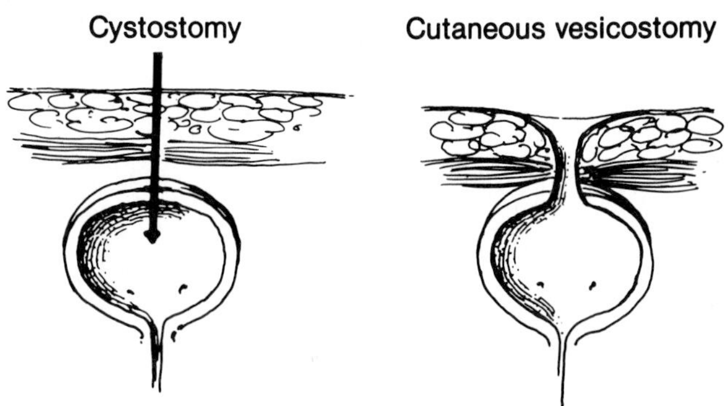

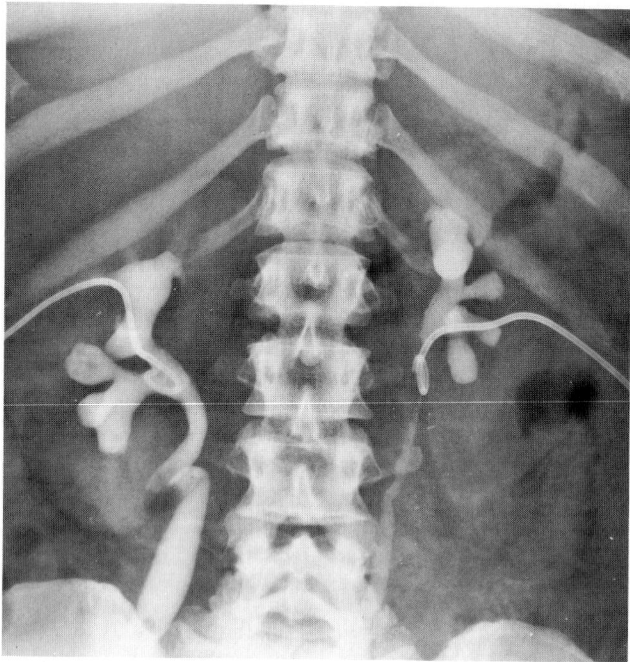

FIG. 42-16. Bilateral percutaneous nephrostomies in a patient with pelvic malignant sarcoma causing bilateral hydronephrosis. Note two No. 8 "pigtail" catheters in both renal pelves.

removing the catheter and risking recatheterization of the urethra in the event of inability to void satisfactorily; and less discomfort to the male patient than that caused by urethral catheterization provided percutaneous suprapubic cystostomy is performed with adequate local anesthesia in skilled hands. It should also be noted that, in acute urinary retention caused by prostatic obstruction, suprapubic cystostomy avoids the prostatic edema which accompanies urethral catheterization and thus, the patient is more likely to resume satisfactory voiding 24 to 48 hours after decompressing the bladder suprapubically than when retention is relieved by an indwelling urethral catheter. In lower urinary obstruction, a tubeless cystostomy can be used especially in children (see Fig. 42-14). In upper urinary tract obstruction, a cutaneous ureterostomy or ureterostomy *in situ* may relieve the obstruction. However, in practice a majority of the upper urinary tract obstructions requiring urinary diversion may be controlled by nephrostomies (see Fig. 42-15).[284-288] The advent of unilateral or bilateral cutaneous nephrostomies under fluoroscopic control has made important contributions in immediate control of the obstruction.[289,290] This technique may save an already sick patient the morbidity of anesthesia and surgical intervention (see Fig. 42-16).

The indications for permanent urinary diversion and bladder augmentation are pelvic malignancies and fibrotic contracted bladder secondary to radiochemotherapy. In our experience utilization of ileum is satisfactory to augment a contracted fibrotic bladder with small capacity. Also, in patients with high dose preoperative radiation necessitating permanent urinary diversion, we prefer a jejunal loop or transverse colon for interposition.[291]

ACUTE INFLAMMATORY DISEASES

Acute infection and abscess formation of the genitourinary tract are generally manifested as disturbance in urination, hematuria, chills, fever, GI, and abdominal manifestations. The factors contributing to the infections are generally stasis, obstruction, presence of foreign body such as a stone, and compromised host defense due to cancer or radiochemotherapy. The most common invaders are the gram negative bacteria, particularly *E. coli* followed by *A. aerogens, P. vulgaris* and *P. mirabilis, P. aeroginosa*, and occasional gram-positive cocci such as staphylococci and streptococci.[292] The main pathways of entry into the urinary tract are ascending, hematogenous, lymphogenous, and direct extension. The acute infections of the genitourinary tract requiring emergency surgical interventions are generally renal, perirenal, and prostatic abscesses. The diagnosis of these abscesses requires a careful history and physical examination. Laboratory findings are generally leukocytosis and elevated sedimentation rates in patients with uncompromised host defense mechanisms. The diagnosis of renal and perirenal abscesses is made by excretory urogram and gallium scan with clinical features of localized infection. The plain film of an excretory urogram may disclose evidence of a mass in the flank. The renal and psoas shadows are obliterated. Excretory urogram may show nonfunctioning kidney or evidence of a renal or perirenal mass (see Fig. 42-17*A*). Ultrasound, CT, and renal angiogram may reveal the mass to be cystic in nature (see Fig. 42-17*B*,*C*). The clinical findings of sepsis together with these radiologic findings including gallium scan will usually make a diagnosis of a renal or perirenal abscess. The immediate management is adequate drainage of the abscess and administration of proper antibiotic based on sensitivity of the cultured purulent material.[293] Antibiotics alone will not eradicate the infection in the presence of obstruction or abscess.[294]

Acute epididymo-orchitis may be caused by hematogenous, ascending, or descending infection along the urethra. The

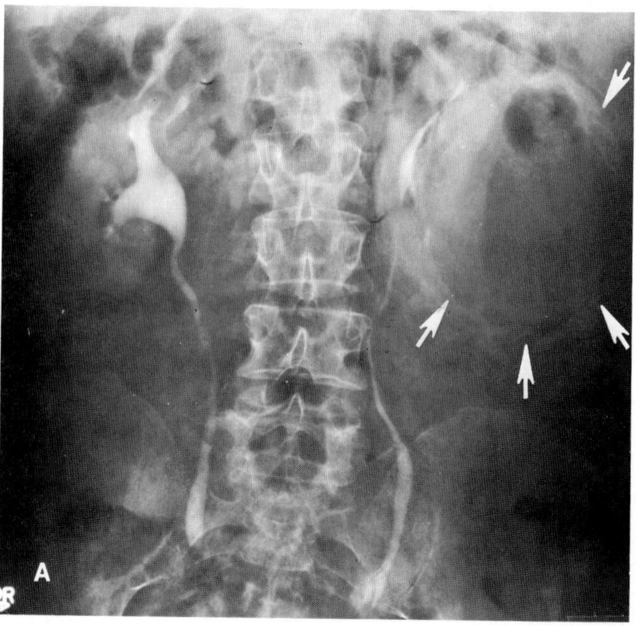

[Legend for Fig. 42-17A is on p. 1621.]

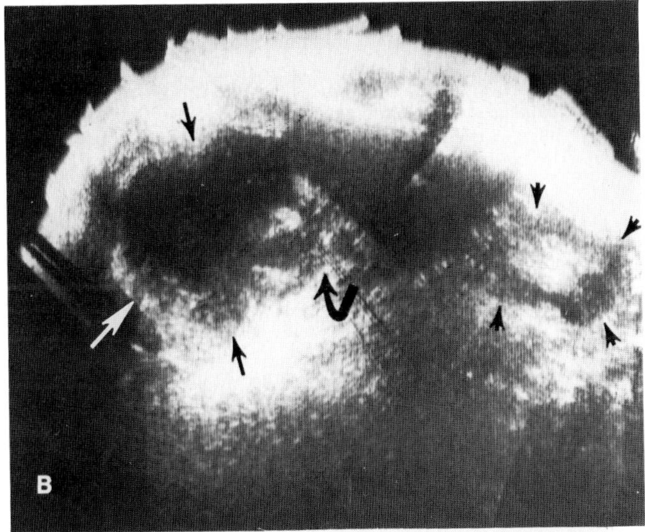

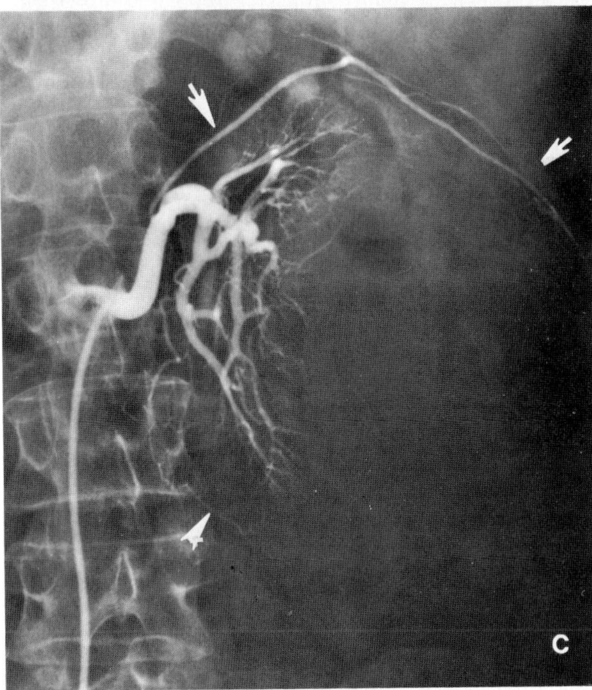

◀FIG. 42-17. *A,* Excretory urogram of a patient on immunosuppressive chemotherapy who developed chills, fever, and left flank mass. Note a large mass displacing the calyceal system medially, proven to be a staphylococal abscess of the left kidney. *B,* A transverse ultrasound of the same patient in prone position revealed a normal right kidney (*arrowheads*) with central dense collecting system echoes. The left kidney has been displayed by a large, poorly marginated fluid containing mass (*arrows*). Note the remaining portion of left kidney (*curved arrows*). *C,* A selective arteriogram of the left kidney in the same patient revealed a large avascular mass compressing the renal parenchyma. Note the capsular vessel and the remaining kidney being displaced (*arrows*).

symptoms are sudden pain, swelling of the testicle, fever and edematous scrotum. Appropriate antibiotic, bed rest, and drainage of the abscess are the immediate treatment and the underlying cause such as urethral stricture or recurrent urinary tract infection should be also treated after the acute infection is under control.

OTHER UROLOGIC EMERGENCIES IN CANCER PATIENTS

The management of iatrogenic injuries to the urinary tract during abdominal surgery for cancer requires immediate recognition and repair of the injuries. If these urinary tract injuries are not recognized during surgery, they generally manifest as obstructive uropathy or sepsis during the postoperative period.

Acute phimosis and paraphimosis also are not uncommon in patients receiving radiochemotherapy or local pelvic lymphatic obstruction due to cancer. These need immediate circumcision or urinary drainage by way of a urethral or suprapubic catheter.

Priapism defined as acute prolonged and painful erection may occur in patients with leukemia, lymphoma, and polycythemia. The treatment of priapism should be directed toward the eradication or control of these underlying cancers. In refractory cases anastomosis of saphenous veins to the ipsilateral corpus cavernosum may be necessary to relieve the patient from pain and lessen the incidence of impotence.

REFERENCES

1. Perez CA, Presant CA, Amburg AL: Management of superior vena cava syndrome. Semin Oncol 5:123–134, 1978
2. Salsali M, Cliffton EE: Superior vena caval obstruction with carcinoma of the lung. Surg Gynecol Obstet 121:783–788, 1965
3. Hunter W: History of aneurysm of the aorta with some remarks on aneurysm in general. M Obser Inq (London) 1:323, 1757
4. Schechter MM: The superior vena cava syndrome. Am J Med Sci 227:46–56, 1954
5. Roswit B, Kaplan G, Jacobson HG: The superior vena cava obstruction in bronchogenic carcinoma. Radiology 61:722–737, 1953
6. Rubin P, Hicks GL: Biassociation of superior vena caval obstruction and spinal-cord compression. NY State J Med 73:2176–2182, 1973
7. Lokich JJ, Goodman RL: Superior vena cava syndrome. JAMA 231:58–61, 1975
8. Silverstein GE, Burke G, Goldberg D et al: Superior vena caval system obstruction caused by benign endothoracic goiter. Dis Chest 56:519–523, 1969
9. Failor HJ, Edwards JE, Hodgson CH: Etiologic factors in obstruction of the superior vena cava: A pathologic study. Staff Meetings Mayo Clin 33:671–678, 1958
10. Davenport D, Ferree C, Blake D et al: Radiation therapy in the treatment of superior vena cava obstruction. Cancer 42: 2600–2603, 1978
11. Rubin P, Green J, Holzwasser G et al: Superior vena cava syndrome. Radiology 81:388–401, 1963
12. Davenport D, Ferree C, Blake D et al: Response of superior vena cava syndrome to radiation therapy. Cancer 38:1577–1580, 1976
13. Dombernowsky P, Hansen HH: Combination chemotherapy in the management of superior cava canal obstruction in small-cell anaplastic carcinoma of the lung. Acta Med Scand 204:513–516, 1978
14. Kane RC, Cohen MH, Broder LE et al: Superior vena caval obstruction due to small-cell anaplastic lung carcinoma: response to chemotherapy. JAMA 235: 1717–1719, 1976
15. Levitt SH, Jones TK, Kilpatrick SJ et al: Treatment of malignant superior vena caval obstruction. Cancer 24:447–451, 1969
16. Eagan RT, Maurer LH, Forcier RJ et al: Small cell carcinoma of the lung: Staging, paraneoplatic syndromes, treatment and survival. Cancer 33:527–532, 1974
17. Effeney DJ, Windsor HM, Shanahan MX: Superior vena cava

obstruction: Resection and bypass for malignant lesions. Aust NZ J Surg 42:231–237, 1973
18. Lome LG, Bush IM: Resection of vena cava for renal cell carcinoma. An experimental study. J Urol 107:717–719, 1972
19. McIntire FT, Sykes EM: Obstruction of the superior vena cava: a review of the literature and report of two personal cases. Ann Intern Med 30:925–960, 1949
20. Avasthi RB, Moghissi K: Malignant obstruction of the superior vena cava and its palliation. J Thorac Cardiovasc Surg 74: 244–248, 1977
21. Ghosh BC, Cliffton EE: Malignant tumors with superior vena cava obstruction. NY State J Med 73:283–289, 1973
22. Green J, Rubin P, Holzwasser G: The experimental production of superior vena cava obstruction. Radiology 81:400–414, 1963
23. Muggia FM, Krezoski SK, Hansen HH: Cell kinetic studies in patients with small cell carcinoma of the lung. Cancer 34:1683–1690, 1974
24. Nixon DW, Carey RW, Suit HD et al: Combination chemotherapy in oat cell carcinoma of the lung. Cancer 36:867–872, 1975
25. Roswit B, Patno ME, Rapp R et al: The survival of patients with inoperable lung cancer: A large-scale randomized study of radiation therapy versus placebo. Radiology 90:688–697, 1968
27. Barron KD et al: Experiences with metastatic neoplasms involving the spinal cord. Neurology (Minneap) 8:91–106, 1959
28. Del Regato J: Pathways of Metastatic Spread of Malignant Tumors. Semin Oncol 4:33–38, 1977
29. Gilbert RW, Kim JH, Posner JB: Epidural spinal cord compression from metastatic tumor: Diagnosis and treatment. Ann Neurol 3:40–51, 1978
30. Brady LW et al: The Treatment of metastatic disease of the nervous system by radiation therapy. In Seydel, HD (ed): Tumors of the Nervous System, pp 177–188. New York, John Wiley & Sons, 1975
31. Khan FR, Glickman AS, Chu FCH et al: Treatment by radiotherapy of spinal cord compression due to extradural metastasis. Radiol 89:495:500, 1967
32. Törmä T: Malignant tumors of the spine and the spinal extradural space. A study based on 250 histologically verified cases. Acta Chir Scand (suppl) 255:1–138, 1957
33. Wild WO, Porter RW: Metastatic epidural tumor of the spine. A study of 45 cases. Arch Surg 87:137–142, 1963
34. Wright RL: Malignant tumors in the spinal epidural space: Results of surgical treatment. Ann Surg 227–231, 1963
35. Love JG: The differential diagnosis of intraspinal tumors and protruded intervertebral discs and their surgical treatment. J Neurosurg 1:275–290, 1944
36. Bruckman JE, Bloomer WD: Management of Spinal Cord Compression. Semin Oncol 5:135–140, 1978
37. Arseni CN, Simionescu MD, Horwath: Tumors of the spine. Acta Psychiatr Neurol Scand 34:398–410, 1959
38. Carpenter MB: Human Neuroanatomy, 7th ed, pp 600–603. Baltimore, Williams & Wilkins, 1976
39. Friedman M, Kim TH, Panahon AM: Spinal cord compression in malignant lymphoma. Cancer 37:1485–1491, 1976
40. Elsberg CA: Surgical Disease of the Spinal Cord, Membranes and Nerve Roots, pp 499–502. New York, Paul B Hoeber, 1941
41. Shenkin HA, Horn RC, Grant FC: Lesions of spinal epidural space producing cord compression. Arch Surg 51:125–146, 1945
42. Brice J, McKissock W: Surgical treatment of malignant extradural spinal tumors. Br Med J 2:1341–1344, 1965
43. Mullan J, Evans JP: Neoplastic disease of the spinal extradural space. Arch Surg 74:900–907, 1957
44. White WA, Patterson RH, Bergland RM: Role of surgery in the treatment of spinal cord compression by metastatic neoplasm. Cancer 27:558–561, 1971
45. Mones RJ, Dozier D, Berrett A: Analysis of medical treatment of spinal cord compression by metastatic neoplasm. Cancer 19:1842–1853, 1966
46. Hall AJ, Mackay NNS: The results of laminectomy for compression of the cord and cauda equina by extradural malignant tumor. J Bone Joint Surg 55B:497–505, 1973
47. Mullins GM, Flynn MB, El-Mahdi AM et al: Malignant lymphoma of the spinal epidural space. Ann Intern Med 74:416–423, 1971
48. Murphy WT, Bilge N: Compression of the spinal cord in patients with malignant lymphoma. Radiology 82:495–500, 1964
49. Milburn L, Hibbs GG, Hendrickson FR: Treatment of spinal cord compression from metastatic carcinoma. Cancer 21:447–452, 1968
50. Rubun P: Extradural spinal cord compression by tumor. Part I: Experimental production and treatment trials. Radiology 93:1243–1248, 1969
51. Ushio Y, Posner R, Kim JH, et al: Treatment of experimental spinal cord compression caused by extradural neoplasms. J Neurosurg 37:380–390, 1977
52. Ushio Y, Posner R, Posner JB, et al: Experimental spinal cord compression by epidural neoplasms. Neurology 27:422–429, 1977
53. Rubin P, Mayer E, Poulter C: Extradural spinal cord compression by tumor. Part I: High daily dose experience without laminectomy. Radiology 93:1248–1260, 1969
54. Posner JB, Howieson J, Cvitkovic E: "Disappearing" spinal cord compression: oncolytic effect of glucocorticoids (and other chemotherapeutic agents) on epidural metastatses. Ann Neurol 2:409–413, 1977
55. Raichle ME, Posner JB: The treatment of extradural spinal compression. Neurology (Minneap)20:391, 1970
56. Renaudin J, et al: Dose dependence of Decadron in patients with partially excised brain tumors. J Neurosurg 39:302–305, 1973
57. Williams HM, Diamond HD, Craver LF et al: Neurological Complications of Lymphomas and Leukemias, pp 33–34. Springfield, Ill, Charles C Thomas, 1959
58. Silverberg IJ, Jacobs EM: Treatment of spinal cord compression in Hodgkin's disease. Cancer 27:308–313, 1971
59. Bansal S, Brady LW, Olsen A et al: The Treatment of metastatic spinal cord tumors. JAMA 202:686–688, 1967
60. Cobb CA, Leavens ME, Eckles N: Indications for nonoperative treatment of spinal cord compression due to breast cancer. J Neurosurg 47:653–658, 1977
61. Edelman RN, Deck MDF, Posner JB: Intramedullary spinal cord metastases: clinical and radiographic findings in 9 cases. Neurology (Minneap) 22:1222–1231, 1972
62. Irvine RA, Robertson WB: Spinal cord compression in the malignant lymphomas. Br Med J 1:1354–1356, 1964
63. McAlhany HJ, Netsky MG: Compression of the spinal cord by extramedullary neoplasms. J Neuropathol Exp Neurol 14: 276–287, 1955
64. Schneider AB, Sherwood LM: Calcium homeostasis and the pathogenesis and management of hypercalcemic disorders. Metabolism 23(10:975–1007, 1974
65. Lafferty FW: Pseudohyperparathyroidism. Medicine 45: 247–260, 1966
66. Mundy GR: Calcium and Cancer. Life Sci 23:1735–1744, 1978
67. Jessiman AG, Emerson K Jr, Shah RL et al: Hypercalcemia in carcinoma of the breast. Ann Surg 157:377–393, 1963
68. Mannheimer IH: Hypercalcemia of breast cancer. Cancer 18:679–691, 1965
69. Davis HL Jr, Wiseley AN, Ramirez G et al: Hypercalcemia complicating breast cancer. Clinical features and management. Oncology 28:126–137, 1973
70. Bender RA, Hanson H: Hypercalcemia in bronchogenic carcinoma. A prospective study of 200 patients. Ann Intern Med 80:205–208, 1974
71. Myers WP: Hypercalcemia in neoplastic disease. Arch Surg 80:308–318, 1960
72. Muggia FM, Heinemann HO: Hypercalcemia associated with neoplastic disease. Arch Intern Med 73:281–290, 1970
73. Stephens RL, Hansen HH, Muggia FM: Hypercalcemia in epidermoid tumors of the head and neck and esophagus. Cancer 31:1487–1491, 1973
74. Lee DBN, Zawada ET, Kleeman CR: The pathophysiology and clinical aspects of hypercalcemic disorders. West J Med 129:278–320, 1978

75. Thomas AN, Loben HF, Gordan GS et al: Hypercalcemia of metastatic breast cancer. Surg Forum 11:70–71, 1960
76. Gardner B, Graham WP, Gordan GS et al: Calcium and phosphate metabolism in patients with disseminated breast cancer. Effect of androgens and of prednisone. J Clin Endocrinol 23:1115–1124, 1963
77. Kennedy BJ, Tibbetts DM, Nathanson IT et al: Hypercalcemia, a complication of hormone therapy of advanced breast cancer. Cancer Res 13:445–459, 1953
78. Kauffman RJ, Rothschild EO, Escher GL et al: Hypercalcemia in mammary carcinoma following administration of a progestational agent. J Clin Endocrinol Metab 24:1235–1243, 1964
79. Cornbleet M, Bondy PK, Powler TJ: Total irreversible hypercalcemia in breast cancer. Br Med J 1:145, 1977
80. Murray TM, Josse RG, Heersche JNM: Hypercalcemia and cancer: An update. Can Med Assoc J 119:915–920, 1978
81. Chopra D, Clerkin EP: Hypercalcemia and malignant disease. Med Clin North Am 59:441–447, 1975
82. Besarab A, Caro JF: Mechanisms of hypercalcemia in malignancy. Cancer 41:2276–2285, 1978
83. Gutman AB, Tyson TL, Gutman EB: Serum calcium, inorganic phosphorus and phosphatase activity in hyperparathyroidism, Paget's disease, multiple myeloma and neoplastic disease of the bones. Arch Intern Med 57:379–413, 1936
84. Kyle RA, Bayrd EA: The Monoclonal Gammopathies, 1st ed. Springfield, Charles C thomas, 1976
85. Waldenström J: Diagnosis and Treatment of Multiple Myeloma, 1st ed, pp 196–203. New York, Grune & Stratton, 1970
86. Berry EM, Guta MM, Turner SJ et al: Variation in plasma calcium with induced changes in plasma specific gravity, total protein and albumin. Br Med J 4:640–643, 1973
87. Payne RB, Little AJ, Williams RB et al: Interpretation of serum calcium in patients with abnormal serum proteins. Br Med J 4:643–646, 1973
88. Husdan H, Rapoport A, Locke S et al: Effect of venous occlusion of the arm on the concentration of calcium in serum, and methods for its compensation. Clin Chem 20:529–532, 1974
89. Barreras RF, Donaldson RM Jr: Effects of induced hypercalcemia on human gastric secretion. Gastroenterology 52:670–675, 1967
90. Barreras RF: Calcium and gastric secretion. Gastroenterology 64:1168–1184, 1973
91. Mixter CG Jr, Klynes WM, Chir M et al: Further experience with pancreatitis as a diagnostic clue to hyperparathyroidism. N Engl J Med 266:265–272, 1962
92. Petersen P: Psychiatric disorders in primary hyperparathyroidism. J Clin Endocrinol 28:1491–1495, 1968
93. Lehrer GM, Levitt MF: Neuropsychiatric presentation of hypercalcemia. J Mt Sinai Hosp 27:10–18, 1960
94. Henson RA: The neurological aspects of hypercalcemia: with special reference to primary hyperparathyroidism. J R Coll Physicians Lond 1:41–50, 1966
95. Allen EM, Singer FR, Melamed D: Electroencephalographic abnormalities in hypercalcemia. Neurology 20:15–22, 1970
96. Moure JMB: The electroencephalogram in hypercalcemia. Arch Neurol 17:34–51, 1967
97. Zeffen JL, Heinemann HO: Reversible defect in renal concentrating mechanism in patients with hypercalcemia. Am J Med 33:54–63, 1962
98. Epstein FM: Calcium and the kidney. Am J Med 45:700–714, 1968
99. Mazzaferri EL, O'Dorisio TM, LoBuglio AF: Treatment of hypercalcemia associated with malignancy. Semin Oncol 5(2):141–153, 1978
100. Greenwald RA: Lysozyme and calcium. Ann Intern Med 85:261, 1976
101. Ultmann JE: Hyperuricemia in disseminated neoplastic disease other than lymphomas and leukemias. Cancer 15:122–129, 1962
102. Shiner PT, Harris WS, Weissler AM: Effects of acute changes in serum calcium levels on the systolic time intervals in man. Am J Cardiol 24:42–48, 1969
103. Bronsky D, Dubin A, Waldstein SS et al: Calcium and the electrocardiogram: II. The elctrocardiographic manifestations of hyperparathyroidism and of marked hypercalcemia from various etiologies. Am J Cardiol 7:833–839, 1961
104. Bronsky D, Dubin A, Kushner DS et al: Calcium and the electrocardiogram: III. The relationship of the intervals of the electrocardiogram to the level of the serum calcium. Am J Cardiol 7:840–843, 1961
105. Voss DM, Drake EH: Cardiac manifestations of hyperparathyroidism, with presenation of a previously unreported arrhythmia. Am Heart J 73:235–239, 1967
106. Earll JM, Kurtzman NA, Moser RH: Hypercalcemia and hypertension. Ann Intern Med 64:378–381, 1966
107. Hellström J, Birbe G, Edwall CA: Hypertension in hyperparathyroidism. BR J Urol 30:13–24, 1958
108. Rosenthal FD, Roy S: Hypertension and hyperparathyroidism. Br Med J 4:396–397, 1972
109. Brinton JS, Jubiz W, Lagerquist LD: Hypertension in primary hyperparathyroidism. The role of the renin–angiotensin system. J Clin Endocrinol Metab 41:1025–1029, 1975
110. Myers WPL: Hypercalcemia associated with malignant disease. In Endocrine and Nonendocrine Hormone-producing Tumors, pp 147–171. Chicago, Year Book Medical Publishers, 1973
111. Coombes RC, Ward MK, Greenberg PB et al: Calcium metabolism in cancer. Studies using calcium isotopes and immunoassays for parathyroid hormone and calci tonin. Cancer 38:2111–2120, 1976
112. Nordin BEC, Peacock M: The role of the kidney in serum calcium homeostasis In Taylor S, Foster G (eds): Calcitonin 1969 International Symposium Proceedings, pp 472–482. London, Heinemann, 1970
113. Mundy GR, Luben RA, Raisz LG et al: Bone-resorbing activity in supernatants from lymphoid cell lines. N Engl J Med 290:867–871, 1974
114. Mundy GR, Raisz LG, Cooper RA et al: Evidence for the secretion of an osteoclast stimulating factor in myeloma. N Engl J Med 291:1041–1046, 1974
115. Mundy GR, Rick ME, Turcotte R et al: Pathogenesis of hypercalcemia in lymphosarcoma cell leukemia. Am J Med 65:600–606, 1978
116. Tashjian AH, Voelkel EF, Levine L et al: Evidence that the bone resorption stimulating factor produced by mouse fibrosarcoma cells is prostaglandin E2. J Exp Med 136:1329–1343, 1972
117. Hough a Jr, Seyberth H, Oates J et al: Changes in bone and bone marrow of rabbits bearing the VX2 carcinoma. Am J Pathol 87:537–552, 1977
118. Rice BF, Ponthier RL Jr, Miller MC III: Hypercalcemia and neoplasia: A model system. Endocrinology 88:1210–1216, 1971
119. Hilgard P, Schmitt W, Minne H et al: Acute hypercalcemia due to Walker carcinosarcoma 256 in the rat. Horm Metab Res 2:255–256, 1970
120. Sherwood LM, O'Riordan JLH, Aurback GD et al: Production of parathyroid hormone by non-parathyroid tumor. J Clin Endocrinol Metab 27:140–146, 1967
121. Buckle R: Ectopic PTH syndrome, pseudohyperparathyroidism: hypercalcemia of malignancy. Clin Endocrinol Metab 3:237–251, 1974
122. Samaan NA, Hickey RC, Sethi MR et al: Hypercalcemia in patients with known malignant disease. Surgery 80:382–389, 1976
123. Benson RC Jr, Riggs BL, Pickard BM et al: Radioimmunoassay of parathyroid hormone in hypercalcemic patients with malignant disease. Am J Med 56:821–826, 1974
124. Martin TJ, Greenberg PB, Beck C et al: Synthesis of peptide hormones by human tumours in cell culture. In Scow RO, Ebling FJG, Henderson IW (eds): Endocrinology Proceedings of the 4th International Congress of Endocrinology, pp 1198–1204. Amsterdam, Excerpta Medica, 1973
125. Greenberg PB, Martin TJ, Sutcliffe HS: Synthesis and release of parathyroid hormone by a renal carcinoma in cell culture. Clin Sci Mol Med 42:183–191, 1973
126. Mayer GP, Keaton JA, Hwist JG et al: Effects of plasma calcium concentration on the relative proportion of hormone and carboxyl

fragments in parathyroid venous blood. Endocrinology 104:1778–1784, 1979
127. Powell D, Singer FR, Murray TM et al: Non-parathyroid humoral hypercalcemia in patients with neoplastic diseases. N Engl J Med 289:176–181, 1973
128. Heath DA: Hypercalcemia and malignancy. An Clin Biochem 13:555–560, 1976
129. Tashjian AH Jr, Voelkel EF, Goldhaber P et al: Prostaglandins, calcium metabolism and cancer. Fed Proc 33:81–86, 1974
130. Voelkel EF, Tashjian AH Jr, Franklin R et al: Hypercalcemia and tumor–prostaglandins: The VX2 carcinoma model in the rabbit. Metabolism 24:973–986, 1975
131. Seyberth HW, Hubbard WC, Oelz O et al: Prostaglandin-mediated hypercalcemia in the VX2 carcinoma bearing rabbit. Prostaglandins 14:319–331, 1977
132. Tashjian AH Jr, Voelkel EF, Levine L: Effects of hydrocortisone on the hypercalcemia and plasma levels of 13,14-dihydro-15-ketoprostaglandin E_2 in mice bearing the $HSDM_1$ fibrosarcoma. Biochem Biophys Res Commun 74:199–207, 1977
133. Robertson RP, Baylink DJ, Metz SA et al: Plasma prostaglandin-E in patients with cancer with and without hypercalcemia. J Clin Endocrinol Metab 43:1330–1335, 1976
134. Demers LM, Allegra JC, Harvey HA et al: Plasma prostaglandins in hypercalcemic patients with neoplastic disease. Cancer 39:1559–1562, 1977
135. Seyberth HW, Segre GV, Morgan JL et al: Prostaglandins as mediators of hypercalcemia associated with certain types of cancer. N Engl J Med 293:1278–1283, 1975
136. Seyberth HW, Segre GV, Hamet P et al: Characterization of the group of patients with the hypercalcemia of cancer who respond to treatment with prostaglandin synthesis inhibitors. Trans Assoc Am Physicians 89:92–104, 1976
137. Powles TJ, Dowsett M, Easty GC et al: Breast cancer osteolysis, bone metastases and anti-osteolytic effect of aspirin. Lancet 1:608–610, 1976
138. Tashjian AH Jr, Voelkel EF, McDonough J et al: Hydrocortisone inhibits prostaglandin production by mouse fibrosarcoma cells. Nature 258:739–741, 1975
139. Tashjian AH Jr: Prostaglandins, Hypercalcemia and cancer. N Engl J Med 293:1317–1318, 1975
140. Coombes RC, Powles TJ, Joplin GF: Calcium metabolism in breast cancer. Proc R Soc Med 70:195–199, 1977
141. Horton JE, Raisz LG, Simmons HA et al: Bone resorbing activity in supernatant fluid from cultured human peripheral blood leukocytes. Science 177:793–795, 1972
142. Mundy GR, Raisz LG: Big and little forms of osteoclast activating factor. J Clin Invest 60:122–128, 1977
143. Eilon G, Raisz LG: Comparison of the effects of stimulators and inhibitors of resorption on the release of lysosomal enzymes and radioactive calcium from fetal bone in organ culture. Endocrinology 103:1969–1975, 1978
144. Raisz LG, Luben RA, Mundy GR et al: Effect of osteoclast activating factor from human leukocytes on bone metabolism. J Clin Invest 56:408–413, 1975
145. Rude RK, Sharp CF Jr, Oldham SB et al: Plasma cyclic AMP, urinary cyclic AMP, and nephrogenic cyclic AMP in the hypercalcemia of malignancy. (abstr). Clin Res 26:427A, 1978
146. Gordan GS, Cantino TJ, Erhardt L et al: Osteolytic sterol in human breast cancer. Science 151:1226–1228, 1966
147. Gordan GS, Fitzpatrick ME, Lubich W: Identification of osteolytic sterols in human breast cancer. Trans Assoc Am Physicians 80:183–189, 1967
148. Haddad JG Jr, Couranz SJ, Avioli LV: Circulating phytosterols in normal females, lactating mothers and breast cancer patients. J Cin Endocrinol Metab 30:174–180, 1970
149. Mundy GR, Eilon G, Altman AJ: Direct resorption of bone by cultured exogenous cells. In: Endocrinology of Calcium Metabolism: Proceedings of the 6th Parathyroid Conference, Vancouver, p 374. Amsterdam, Exerpta Medica, 1978
150. Mundy GR, Altman AJ, Gondek MD et al: Direct resorption of bone by human monocytes. Science 196:1109–1111, 1977
151. Walser M: Calcium clearance as a function of sodium clearance in the dog. Am J Physiol 200:1099–1104, 1961
152. Massry SG, Friedler Rm, Coburn JW: Excretion of phosphate and calcium: Physiology of their renal handling and relation to clinical medicine. Arch Intern Med 131:828–859, 1973
153. Massry SG, Kleeman CR: Calcium and magnesium excretion during acute rise in glomerular filtration rate. J Lab Clin Med 80:654–664, 1972
154. Suki WN, Yium JJ, Von Minden M et al: Acute treatment of hypercalcemia with furosemide. N Engl J Med 283:836–840, 1970
155. Pechet MM, Bowers B, Bartter FC: Metabolic studies with a new series of 1,4-diene steroids. II. Effects in normal subjects of prednisone, prednisolone, and 9-a-fluoroprednisilone. J Clin Invst 38:691–701, 1959
156. Kimberg DV, Baerg RD,Gershon E et al: Effect of cortisone treatment on the active transport of calcium by the small intestine. J Clin Invest 50:1309–1321, 1971
157. Laake H: The action of corticosteroids in the renal absorption of calcium. Acta Endocrinol 34:60–64, 1960
158. Jowsey J: Quantitave microradiography. A new approach in the evaluation of metabolic bone disease. Am J Med 40: 485–491, 1966
159. Storey E: Cortisone-induced bone resorption in the rabbit. Endocrinology 68:533–542, 1961
160. Lazor MZ, Rosenberg LE: Mechanisms of adrenal–steroid reversal of hypercalcemia in multiple myeloma. N Engl J Med 270:749–755, 1964
161. Myers WPL: Cortisone in the treatment of hypercalcemia in neoplastic disease. Cancer 11:83–88, 1958
162. Kennedy BJ, Sandberg-Wollheim M, Loken M et al: Studies with tritiated mithrammycin in C_3H mice. Cancer Res 27: 1534–1538, 1967
163. Parsons V, Baum M, Self M: Effect of mithramycin on calcium and hydroxyproline metabolism in patients with malignant disease. Br Med J 1:474–477, 1967
164. Perlia CP, Gubisch NJ, Wolter J et al: Mithramycin treatment of hypercalcemia. Cancer 25:389–394, 1970
165. Elias EG, Evans JT: hypercalcemic crisis in neoplastic diseases. management with mithramycin. Surgery 71:631–635, 1972
166. Godfrey TE: Mithramycin for hypercalcemia of malignant disease. Calif Med 115:1–4, 1971
167. Varbro JW, Kennedy BJ, Barnum CP: Mithramycin inhibition of ribonucleic acid synthesis. Cancer Res 26:36–39, 1966
168. Ryan WG, Schwartz TB, Perlia CP: Effects of Mithramycin on Paget's disease of bone. Ann Intern Med 70:549–557, 1969
169. Brown JH, Kennedy BJ: Mithramycin in the treatment of disseminated testicular neoplasms. N Engl J Med 272:111–118, 1965
170. Kennedy BJ: Metabolic and toxic effects of mithramycin during tumor therapy. Am J Med 49:494–503, 1970
171. Albright F, Bauer W, Claflin D et al: Studies in parathyroid physiology: Effect of phosphate ingestion in clinical hyperparathyroidism. J Clin Invest 11:411–435, 1932
172. Goldsmith RS, Ingbar SH: Inorganic phosphate treatment of hypercalcemia of diverse etiologies. N Engl J Med 274:1–7, 1966
173. Massry SG, Mueller E, Silverman AG et al: Inorganic phosphate treatment of hypercalcemia. Arch Intern Med 121:307–312, 1968
174. Fulmer DH, Dimich AB, Rothschild EO et al: Treatment of hypercalcemia: Comparison of intravenously administered phosphate, sulphate, and hydrocortisone. Arch Intern Med 129:923–930, 1972
175. Walser M: Treatment of hypercalcemias. Mod Treat 7:662–674, 1970
176. Eisenberg E: Effect of intravenous phosphate serum strontium and calcium. N Engl J Med 282:889–892, 1970
177. Herbert LA, Lemann J Jr, Petersen JR et al: Studies of the mechanism by which phosphate infusion lowers serum calcium concentration. J Clin Invest 45:1886–1894, 1966
178. Raisz LG, Niemann I: Effect of phosphate, calcium and magnesium on bone resorption and hormonal responses in tissue culture. Endocrinology 85:446–452, 1969

179. Dent CE: Some problems of hyperparathyroidism. Br Med J 2:1495–1500, 1962
180. Shackney S, Hasson J: Precipitous fall in serum calcium, hypotension, and acute renal failure after intravenous phosphate therapy for hypercalcemia. Report of two cases. Ann Intern Med 66:906–916, 1967
181. Breuer RI, LeBauer J: Caution in the use of phosphates in the treatment of severe hypercalcemia. J Clin Endocrinol Metab 27:695–698, 1967
182. Carey RW, Schmitt GW, Kopald HH et al: Massive extraskeletal calcification during phosphate treatment of hypercalcemia. Arch Intern Med 122:150–155, 1968
183. Dudley FJ, Blackburn CRB: Extraskeletal calcification complicating oral neutral-phosphate therapy. Lancet 2:628–630, 1970
184. Scheeberger EE, Morrison AB: Increased susceptibility of magnesium-deficient rats to a phosphate-induced nephropathy. Am J Pathol 50:549–558, 1967
185. Spaullding SW, Walser M: Treatment of experimental hypercalcemia with oral phosphate. J Clin Endocrinol Metab 31:531–538, 1970
186. Jowsey J, Balasubramaniam P: Effect of phosphate supplements on soft tissue calcification and bone turnover. Clin Sci 42:289–299, 1972
187. Goldsmith RS, Ingbar SH: Phosphate, sulphate, and hypercalcemia. Ann Intern Med 67:463–464, 1967
188. Goldsmith RS, Ingbar SH: Hyper- to hypocalcemia. N Engl J Med 274:284, 1966
189. Schenk R, Merz WA, Mihlbauer R et al: Effect of ethane-1-hydroxy-1, diphosphonate (EHDP) and dichloromethylene diphosphonate (Cl_2MDP) on the calcification and resorption of cartilage and bone in the tibial epiphysis and metaphysis of rats. Calcif Tissue Res 11:196–214, 1973
190. Miller SC, Jee WS: The comparative effects of dichloromethylene diphosphonate (Cl_2MDP) and ethane-1-hydroxy-1,1-diphosphonate (EHDP) on growth and modeling of the rat tibia. Calcif Tissue Res 23:207–214, 1977
191. Canfield R, Rosner W, Skinner J et al: Diphosphonate therapy of Paget's disease of bone. J Clin Endocrinol Metab 44:96–106, 1977
192. Van Breukelen FJM, Bijvoet OLM, Van Oosterom AT: Inhibition of osteolytic bone lesions by (3-amino-1-hydroxypropylidene)-1,1-diphosphonate (ADP). Lancet 1:803–805, 1979
193. Siris ES, Sherman WH, Baguiran DC et al: Effects of dichloromethylene diphosphonate on skeletal mobilization of calcium in multiple myeloma. N Engl J Med 302:310–315, 1980
194. Krane SM, Harris ED Jr, Singer FR et al: Acute effects of calcitonin on bone formation in man. Metabolism 22:51–58, 1973
195. Vaughn CB, Vaitkevicius K: The effects of calcitonin in hypercalcemia in patients with malignancy. Cancer 34: 1268–1271, 1974
196. Potts JT Jr, Deftos LJ: Parathyroid hormone, calcitonin, vitamin D, bone and bone mineral metabolism. In Bondy PK, Rosenberg LE (eds): Duncan's Diseases of Metabolism, 7th ed. pp 1224–1430. Philadelphia, Saunders, 1974
197. Habener JR, Singer FR, Deltos LJ, Potts JT Jr: Immunological stability of calcitonin in plasma. Endocrinology 90:952–960, 1972
198. Neer R, Singer F, Habener J, Peacock M, Murray T: Escape from calcitonin (CT) during therapy of hypercalcemia. Clin Res 18:676, 1970
199. Sorensen OH, Hindberg I: Calcitonin and bone. Lancet 1:1061–1062, 1970
200. Brautbar N, Luboshitzky R: Combined calcitonin and oral phosphate treatment for hypercalcemia in multiple myeloma. Arch Intern Med 137:914–916, 1977
201. Au WYN: Calcitonin treatment of hypercalcemia due to parathyroid carcinomasynergistic effect of prednisone on long-term treatment of hypercalcemia. Arch Intern Med 135:1594–1597, 1975
202. Miach PJ, Dawborn JK, Martin TJ, Moon WJ: Management of the hypercalcemia of malignancy by peritoneal dialysis. Med J Aust 1:782–784, 1975
203. Nolph KD, Stoltz M, Maher JF: Calcium free peritoneal dialysis. Treatment of vitamin D intoxication. Arch Intern Med 128:809–814, 1971
204. Eisenberg E, Gotch FA: Normocalcemic hyperparathyroidism culminating in hypercalcemic crisis. Treatment with hemodialysis. Arch Intern Med 122:258–264, 1968
205. Wolf AV, Remp DG, Kiley JE, Currie GD: Artificial kidney function: Kinetics of hemodialysis. J Clin Invest 30:1062–1070, 1951
206. Stoltz ML, Nolph KD, Maher JF: Factors affecting calcium removal with calcium-free peritoneal dialysis. J Lab Clin Med 78:389–398, 1971
207. Talbott JH, Yü T-F: Gout and Uric Acid Metabolism. New York, Grune & Stratton, 1976
208. Boss GR, Seegmiller JE: Hyperuricemia and gout: Classification, complications and management. N Engl J Med 300:1459–1468, 1979
209. Ultmann JE: Hyperuricemia in disseminated neoplastic disease other than lymphomas and leukemias. Cancer 15: 122–129, 1962
210. Crittenden DR, Ackerman GL: Hyperuricemic acute renal failure in disseminated carcinoma. Arch Intern Med 137: 97–99, 1977
211. Robinson RR, Yarger WE: Acute uric acid nephropathy. Arch Intern Med 137:839–840, 1977
212. Frei E, Bentzel CJ, Rieselbach R et al: Renal complications of neoplastic disease. J Chronic Dis 16:757–776, 1963
213. Pochedly C: Hyperuricemia in leukemia and lymphoma. Postgrad Med 55:93–99, 1974
214. Seegmiller JE, Laster L, Howell RR: Biochemistry of uric acid and its relationship to gout. N Engl J Med 268:712–716, 1963
215. Klinenberg JR, Kippen I, Bluestone R: Hyperuricemic nephropathy: Pathologic features and factors influencing urate deposition. Nephron 14:88–98, 1975
216. Rieselbach RE, Bentzel CJ, Cotlove E et al: Uric acid excretion and renal function in the acute hyperuricemia of leukemia. Am J Med 37:872–884, 1964
217. Smith JF, Lee YC: Experimental uric acid nephritis in the rabbit. J Exp Med 105:615–622, 1957
218. Spencer HW, Yarger WE, Robinson RR: Alterations of renal function during dietary-induced hyperuricemia in the rat. Kidney Int 9:489–500, 1976
219. Bedrna J, Polcak J: Akuter Harnleiterverschluss nach Bestrahlung chronischer Leukämien mit Röntgenstrahlen. Med Klin 25:1700–1701, 1929
220. Warren DJ, Leitch AG, Leggett RJE: Hyperuricemic acute renal failure after epileptic seizures. Lancet 2:385–387, 1975
221. Kelton J, Kelley WN, Holmes EW: A rapid method for the diagnosis of acute uric acid nephropathy. Arch Intern Med 138:612–615, 1978
222. Deconti RC, Calabresi P: Use of allopurinol for prevention and control of hyperuricemia in patients with neoplastic disease. N Engl J Med 274:481–486, 1966
223. Krakoff IH, Meyer RL: Prevention of hyperuricemia in leukemia and lymphoma: Use of allopurinol, a xanthine oxidase inhibitor. JAMA 193:1–6, 1965
224. Kjellstrand CM, Campbell DC, Von Hartitzsch et al: Hyperuricemic acute renal failure. Arch Intern Med 133:349–359, 1974
225. Woodbury DM, Fingl E: Analgesic-antipyretics, anti-inflammatory agents and drugs employed in the therapy of gout. In Goodman LS, Gilman A (eds): The Pharmacological Basis of Therapeutics, pp 325–358. New York, Macmillan, 1964
226. Band PR, Silverberg DS, Henderson JF et al: Xanthine nephropathy in a patient with lymphosarcoma treated with allopurinol. N Engl J Med 283:354–357, 1970
227. Lilje AE: Hyperurikaemi og akut nyreinsufficiens. Ugeskr Laeg 132:12–14, 1970
228. Yü T-F, Gutman AB: Uric acid nephrolithiasis in gout. Predisposing factors. Ann Intern Med 67:1133–1148, 1967
229. Atsmon A, De Vries A, Frank M: Uric Acid Lithiasis. New York, Elsevier, 1964
230. Pyrah LN: Renal Calculus. New York, Springer-Verlag, 1979

231. Wyngaarden JB, Kelley WN: Gout and Hyperuricemia. New York, Grune & Stratton, 1976
232. Relman AS: Lactic acidosis. In Brenner BM, Stein JH (eds): Acid–Base and Potassium Homeostasis, pp 65–100. New York, Churchill Livingstone, 1978
233. Scheerer PP, Pierre RV, Schwartz DL et al: Reed–Sternberg-cell leukemia and lactic acidosis. N Engl J Med 270:274–278, 1964
234. Block JB, Bronson WR, Bell WR: Metabolic abnormalities of lactic acid in Burkitt-type lymphoma with malignant effusions. Ann Intern Med 65:101–108, 1966
235. Field M, Block JB, Levin R et al: Significance of blood lactate elevations among patients with acute leukemia and other neoplastic proliferative disorders. Am J Med 40:528–547, 1966
236. Roth GJ, Porte D: Chronic lactic acidosis and acute leukemia. Arch Intern Med 125:317–321, 1970
237. Wainer RA, Wiernik PH, Thompson WL: Metabolic and therapeutic studies of a patient with acute leukemia and severe lactic acidosis of prolonged duration. Am J Med 55:255–260, 1973
238. Block JB: Lactic acidosis in malignancy and observations on its possible pathogenesis. Ann NY Acad Sci 230:94–102, 1974
239. Kachel RG: Metastatic reticulum cell sarcoma and lactic acidosis. Cancer 36:2056–2059, 1975
240. Mintz U, Sweet DL, Bitran J et al: Lactic acidosis and diffuse histiocytic lymphoma (DHL). Am J Hematol 4:359–365, 1978
241. Nadiminti Y, Wang JC, Chou S-Y et al: Lactic acidosis associated with Hodgkin's disease: Response to chemotherapy. N Engl J Med 303;15–17, 1980
242. Spechler SJ, Esposito AL, Koff RS et al: Lactic acidosis in oat cell carcinoma with extensive hepatic metastases. Arch Intern Med 138:1663–1664, 1978
242a. Fields ALA, Wolman SL, Halperin ML: Chronic lactic acidosis: Therapy and metabolic consequences, Cancer 47:2626–2029, 1981
242b. Goodgame JT, Pizzo P, Brennan MF: Iatrogenic lactic acidosis in association with hypertonic glucose administration in a patient with cancer. Cancer 42:800–803, 1978
242c. Cohen RD, Woods HF: Clinical and Biochemical Aspects of Lactic Acidosis. Oxford, blackwell Scientific Publications, 1976
242d. Park R, Arieff AI: Lactic acidosis. Adv Intern Med 25:33–68, 1980
242e. Emmett M, Nairns RG: Clinical use of the anion gap. Medicine 56:38–54, 1977
242f. Halperin ML: Lactic acidosis and ketoacidosis: Biochemical and clinical implications. Can Med Assoc J 116:1034–1038, 1977
242g. Kreisberg RA: Lactic homeostasis and lactic acidosis. Ann Intern Med 92(1):227–237, 1980
242h. Warburg O: Metabolism of Tumors. New York, Smith, 1931
242i. Berry NM: The liver and lactic acidosis. Proc R Soc Med 60:1260–1262, 1967
242j. Mulhausen R, Eichenholz A, Bumentals A: Acid–base disturbances in patients with cirrhosis of the liver. Medicine 46:185–189, 1967
242k. Record CO, Iles RA, Cohen RD et al: Acid–base and metabolic disturbances in fulminant hepatic failure. Gut 16:144–149, 1975
242l. Stacpoole PW, Moore GW, Kornhauser DM: Metabolic effects of dichloroacetate in patients with diabetes mellitus and hyperlipoproteinemia. N Engl J Med 298:526–530, 1978
242m. Dembo AJ, Marliss EB, Halperin ML: Insulin therapy in phenformin-associated lactic acidosis. Diabetes 24:28–35, 1975
243. Botsford RW and Wilson RE: The Acute Abdomen. An Approach to Diagnosis and Management, 2nd ed. Philadelphia, WB Saunders, 1977
244. Steele G Jr, Sonis S, Stelos P et al: Circulating immune complexes in patients following clinically curative resection of colorectal cancer. Surgery 83:648–654, 1978
245. Rainer P, Deyhle P: Guided puncture under real-time sonograhic control. Radiology 134:784–785, 1980
246. Kelly WD, Good RA: Immunologic deficiency in Hodgkin's disease. In Good RA, Bergsma D (eds): Immunologic Deficiency Diseases in Man, Birth Defects Original Article Series, Vol IV, pp 349–356. New York, National Foundation Press, 1968
247. Rosenberg SA: Cancer immunology. In Munster AM (ed): Surgical Immunology, pp 231–281. New York, Grune & Stratton, 1976
248. Sugarbaker PH, Skarin AT, Wilson RE: Thrombocytopenia from metastatic carcinoma of the breast. Effective managements of patients with this complication. Arch Surg 107:523–527, 1973
249. Gantz NM, Myerowitz RL, Medeiros AA et al: Listeriosis in immunosuppressed patients. A cluster of eight cases. Am J Med 58:637–643, 1975
250. Sugarbaker PH, Wilson RE: Using celioscopy to determine stages of intra-abdominal malignant neoplasms. Arch Surg 111:41–44, 1976
251. Rosoff L, White EJ: Perforation of the esophagus. Am J Surg 128:207–218, 1974
252. McIntosh DMF, Penney HF: Gray-scale ultrasonography as a screening procedure in the detection of gallbladder disease. Radiology 136:725–727, 1980
253. Peterson LM, Collins JJ Jr, Wilson RE: Acute pancreatitis occurring after operation. Surg Gynecol Obstet 127:23–28, 1968
254. Sidel VW, Wilson RE, Shipp JC: Pseudocyst formation in chronic pancreatitis. A cause of obstructive jaundice. AMA Arch Surg 77:933–937, 1958
255. Bartlett JG, Chang TW, Gurwith M et al: Antibiotic associated pseudomembranous colitis due to toxin-producing Clostridia. N Eng J Med 298:531–534, 1978
256. Misra MK, Pinkus GS, Birtch AG et al: Major colonic diseases complicating renal transplantation. Surgery 73:942–948, 1973
257. Sawyers JL, Herrington JL Jr, Mulherin JO et al: Acute perforated duodenal ulcer. An evaluation of surgical management. Arch Surg 110:527–536, 1975
258. Grossman MI: Resume and comment. In The Veterans Administration Cooperative Study on Gastric Ulcer. Gastroenterology 61:635–638, 1971
259. Miller LD, Boruchow IB, Fitts WT Jr: An analysis of 284 patients with perforative carcinoma of the colon. Surg Gynecol Obstet 123:1212–1218, 1966
260. Dudrick SJ, Wilmore DW, Vars HM et al: Can intravenous feeding as the sole means of nutrition support growth in the child and restore weight loss in an adult? An affirmative answer. Ann Surg 169:974–984, 1969
261. Osteen RT, Guyton S, Steele G et al: Malignant intestinal obstruction. Surgery 87:611–615, 1980
262. Harken AH, Gabel RA, Fencl V et al: Hydrochloric acid in the correction of metabolic alkalosis. Arch Surg 110:819–821, 1975
263. Demeester TR, Johnson LF, Kent AH: Evaluation of current operations for the prevention of gastroesophageal reflux. Ann Surg 180:511–525, 1974
264. Athanasoulis CA, Baum S, Waltman AC et al: Control of acute gastric mucosal hemorrhage: Intra-arterial infusion of posterior pituitary extracts. N Engl J Med 290:597–603, 1974
265. Rosch J, Dotter CT, Brown MJ: Selective arterial embolization. A new method for control of acute gastrointestinal bleeding. Radiology 102:303–306, 1972
266. Baum S, Athanasoulis CA, Waltman AC et al: Angiographic diagnosis and control of gastrointestinal bleeding. In Welch C (ed): Advances in Surgery, Vol 7, pp 149–198. Chicago, Year Book Medical Publishers, 1973
267. Welch CE: Practical consideration in treatment of polypoid lesions of colon and rectum. In Dunphy JE (ed): Polypoid Lesions of the Gastrointestinal Tract, pp 98–122. Philadelphia, WB Saunders, 1964
268. Foster JH, Berman MM: The benign lesions: Adenoma and focal nodular hyperplsia. In Ebert PA (ed): Solid Liver Tumors, pp 138–178. Philadelphia, WB Saunders, 1977
269. McNeil BJ, Sanders R, Alderson PO et al: A prospective study of computed tomography ultrasound, and gallium imaging in patients with fever. Radiology (in press)
270. Kumar B, Alderson PO, Geisse G: The role of Ga-67 citrate imaging and diagnostic ultrasound in patients with suspected abdominal abscesses. J Nucl Med 18:534–537, 1977
271. Levitt RG, Biello DR, Sagel SS et al: Computed tomography and ^{67}Ga citrated radionuclide imagery for evaluating suspected abdominal abscess. Am J Roentgenol 132:529–534, 1979

272. Javadpour N, Barakat HA: Bladder toxicity due to cyclophosphamide. Urology 2:634, 1973
273. Johnson WW, Meadows DC: Urinary–bladder fibrosis and telangiectasia associated with long-term cyclophosphamide therapy. N Engl J Med 284:290, 1971
274. Duckett JW Jr, Peters PC, Donaldson MH: Severe cyclophosphamide hemorrhagic cystitis controlled with phenol. J Pediatr Surg 8:55, 1973
275. Blue KG et al: Bone-marrow ablation and allogeneic marrow transplantation in acute leukemia. N Engl J Med 302: 1041–1046, 1980
276. Ershler WB, Gilchrist KW, Citrin DL: Adriamycin enhancement of cyclophosphamide-induced bladder injury. J Urol 123:121, 1980
277. Bischel MD: Cyclophosphamide hemorrhagic cystitis following prolonged low dose therapy. JAMA 20:238, 1979
278. Royal JE, Seeler RA: Hemorrhagic cystitis with MOPP therapy. Cancer 41:1261–1264, 1978
279. Whittaker JR, Freed SZ: Effects of formalin on bladder urothelium. J Urol 114:866, 1975
280. Bergman S, Javadpour N: Massive intractable hematuria secondary to cyclophosphamide—Intravesical instillation of formaldehyde in patients with vesicoureteral reflux. Urology 10:256, 1977
281. Sharon SH et al: Formalin treatment for intractable hemorrhagic cystitis—A review of the literature with 16 additional cases. Cancer 38:1785–1789, 1976
282. Levy L, Harris R: Effect of N-acetylcysteine on some aspects of cyclophosphamide-induced toxicity and immunosuppression. Biochem Pharmacol 26:1015–1020, 1977
283. Scheef W, Klein HO, Brock N et al: Controlled clinical studies with an antidote against urotoxicity of oxazaphosphorines: Preliminary results. Cancer Treat Rep 63:501–505, 1979
284. Grayback JT: The urinary system. In Davis-Christopher (ed): Textbook of Surgery, p 1509. Philadelphia, Saliston-Saunders, 1972
285. Kohler JP, Lyon ES, Schoenberg HW: Reassessment of circle tube nephrostomy in advanced malignancy. J Urol 123:17, 1980
286. Loening S, Carson CC, Faxon DP, et al: Ureteral obstruction associated with Hodgkin's disease. J Urol 111:345, 1974
287. Michigan S, Catalona WJ: Ureteral obstruction from prostatic carcinoma: Response to endocrine and radiation therapy. J Urol 118:733, 1977
288. Brin EN, Schiff M, Weiss RM: Palliative urinary diversion for pelvic malignancy. J Urol 113:619, 1975
289. Barbaric ZL: Interventional uroradiology. Radiol Clin North Am 17:413, 1979
290. Pfister RC, Newhouse JH: Interventional percutaneous pyeloureteral techniques—Percutaneous nephrostomy and other procedures. Radiol Clin North Am 17:351, 1979
291. Norton JA, Javadpour N: Jejunal loop interposition in patients with ileal loop conduit failure after pelvic exenteration. Am J Surg 134:404, 1977
292. Pizzo PA,, Ladsich SL, Robichand K: Treatment of gram-positive septicemia in cancer patients. Cancer 45:206–207, 1980
293. Howard RJ: Host defense against infection; Part I. Current Probl Surg 15:272, 1980
294. Grahstald H: Life-threatening complications in cancer patients. Part II. Curr Probl Cancer 6:27, 1980

CHAPTER 43

Supportive Care of the Cancer Patient

Section 1

Nutritional Support

MURRAY F. BRENNAN

The association of malnutrition and the presence of cancer is so common as to lead one to believe that the two are causally related. The demonstration that weight loss is not only common, but a factor in prediction of therapeutic response and survival has been emphasized in a number of disease entities. This observation has led to aggressive attempts at restoring the nutritional status of the patient, sometimes independent of anti-neoplastic therapy.

ETIOLOGY OF MALNUTRITION IN CANCER PATIENTS

The commonest attributed cause of malnutrition in cancer patients is anorexia. The etiology of the anorexia associated with cancer has been variously debated.[1] Although abnormalities in the central control of food intake have been incriminated there is minimal evidence that the central control of feeding by the hypothalamic centers is disturbed in the cancer patient.[2] Possible mechanisms for diminished intake in the cancer patient have been extensively examined. That cancer patients have diminished intake when compared to proportionately malnourished controls has been questioned.[3] Specific malfunctions of the GI tract that occur as a consequence of either local effects of malignancy or side effects of therapy are easily recognized.[4] These observations cannot, however, explain the anorexia and diminished intake of patients with tumors remote from the GI tract.

Abnormalities of taste have been incriminated and linked to diminished intake.[5] If, however, taste abnormalities and diminished intake were the solitary cause of malnutrition in cancer patients, this would either easily be overcome by conventional methods of enteral nutritional support (which bypass the oropharynx) or by the use of IV feeding. The latter technique would further circumvent any abnormalities of digestion or absorption that may or may not contribute to the syndrome of advanced malnutrition associated with cancer cachexia. Certainly, total parenteral nutrition (TPN) can support growth and development of newborn man and animals, indicating that the technique is an effective form of reversing malnutrition.[6,7,8]

The extrapolation from the studies in normal and growing humans to the cancer patient is dependent upon the ability to demonstrate that total parenteral nutrition or enteral nutritional support can reverse malnutrition in the cancer patient. This, by implication, requires that whatever the etiology of cancer cachexia, it can be reversed by nutritional support or supplementation. The fact that cancer cachexia is not solely due to diminished intake makes this assumption unreasonable until proven.[9]

Evidence to support mild to moderate increases in energy demands and failure to adapt energy expenditure to available intake does exist, but seems insufficient to be incriminated as a sole etiology.[2,10–15]

Various other causes for cancer cachexia have been suggested. Evidence to support, in part, all of the causes listed

TABLE 43-1. Etiology of Cancer Cachexia

1°	2°	3°
Diminished nutrient intake	Anorexia	• Taste, smell abnormality • Malaise, weakness • Loss of central anticipatory stimuli
	Malfunction of gastrointestinal tract	• Nausea, vomiting, diarrhea • Obstruction, ileus • Mucositis, esophagitis
	Increased nutrient demand	• Catabolic consequences of therapy, including fever.
Tumor consumption of nutrient	Metabolic "activity" of the tumor	
Remote metabolic effects of tumor on the host	Hormonal production by the tumor	• Tumor hypoglycemia • Diarrheal syndromes
	Inability of host to adapt to diminished intake	• Failure to adapt to fat utilization for energy • Loss of substrate-hormonal feedback
	Increase in host lean tissue dissolution	• Gluconeogenesis for tumor consumption
	Utilization of wasteful energy cycles	• Increase in recycling of lactate.

on Table 43-1 is available, with the most likely explanation being a combination of the factors listed. It is possible to calculate substrate consumption by a human tumor. The arterial-venous difference for glucose across the human brain is 9.9±2.39 (x̄ ± s.d) mg/100 ml. Normal human cerebral blood flow is 64.7±12.1 ml/min/100 g brain. The glucose consumption by the human brain is 6.2±1.41 mg/min/100 g, and a 1400 g brain would consume 125 g of glucose per day.[16] This number is similar to the 140 g commonly quoted.[17]

A large (1.4 kg) metabolically active tumor with consumption equal to that of brain, could consume the equivalent of 140 g of glucose. This is 44% of the energy intake of a group of hospitalized cancer patients, and approximates the 61% excess of expenditure over intake seen in the same group of patients.[13] A 1.4 kg tumor approximates to 2% of the body weight and is uncommon in man.

An alternative method yields similar results. The *in vivo* utilization of glucose by a rat tumor is 40 mmol/min/100 g.[18,19] A 1.4 kg tumor can therefore consume 143 g of glucose per day. Calculations can then be made as to what percentage of caloric intake goes to tumor consumption (see Table 43-2). By examination of human tumor-bearing limbs *in vivo*, the limb with the largest tumor can be shown to consume as much as 500 g of glucose![20] It is clear that for tumors greater than 1 kg, the amount of substrate consumed by the tumor begins to be a significant percentage of total caloric intake.

NUTRITIONAL CONSEQUENCES OF THE CANCER-BEARING STATE

A great deal is known of normal body composition and the consequences of injury and starvation.[11,17] Body energy reserves in normal man are retained mainly as fat (see Fig. 43-1).[21] The limiting factors in survival in the absence of food intake are the protein reserves. Under simple fasting, there is a progressive adaptation by the obligatory glucose users, such as brain, to the use of the products of fat breakdown, the ketone bodies, especially acetoacetate and βOH butyrate.[11,17,21] As a consequence of the well-dissected response of nitrogen and protein metabolism under the influence of starvation, it is possible to calculate what amounts of the lean tissue reserve are "saved" by these processes. The signal for this adaptation to a fat-free economy is unknown; various

TABLE 43-2. Potential Tumor Consumption as a Percent of Daily Intake

TUMOR SIZE	TUMOR SIZE AS % BODY WEIGHT*	GLUCOSE CONSUMPTION G/DAY	% OF DAILY CALORIC INTAKE A	B
1 g	0.001%	0.1	0.03	0.01
100 g	0.1%	10.2	3.4	1.45
500 g	0.8%	51.0	17	7.3
1 kg	1.6%	102	34	14.5
1.5 kg	2.5%	153	51	21.9
2.0 kg	3.3%	204	67	28.7

*Body weight = 60 kgm
A Intake = 1200 cal/day
B Intake = 2800 cal/day

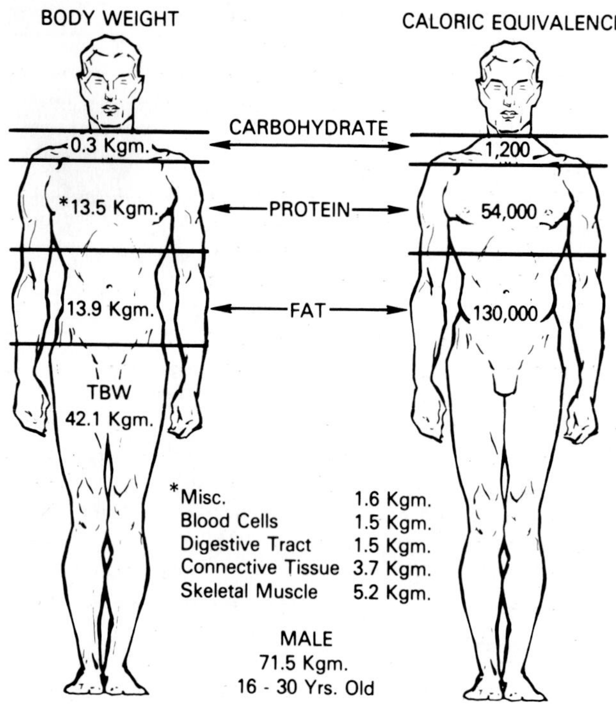

FIG. 43-1. Body Composition of a healthy, well-developed young male, expressed as caloric equivalence. (Brennan MF: Metabolic response to surgery in the cancer patient. Consequences of aggressive multimodality therapy. Cancer 43:2053–2064, 1979)

suggestions have been made involving the direct effect of hyperketonemia on muscle amino acid release[23] or the local alterations in mitochondrial and cytosol redox potential.[24,25]

Unfortunately, rarely is the cancer-bearing host in an uncomplicated semi-starved state. The presence of the neoplasm, or the use of aggressive antineoplastic therapy, which is often associated with episodes of infection and sepsis, produces a much more "hypercatabolic" state than simple starvation.

Under these circumstances, crude calculations can be made as to the time it would take to lose 50% of the body cell mass (see Table 43-3). It is clear that many patients with cancer, who enter hospital malnourished, have protein reserves such that the effects of aggressive therapy, or treatment-related complications, will translate into death from malnutrition within a month unless some nutritional support is provided. It should be abundantly clear that the best nutritional support is a full and complete response to cancer therapy, such that normal substrate intake and body composition restoration can take place. The challenge for those interested in maximizing nutritional support during therapy is to overcome the host dissolution, even when the response to anti-cancer therapy is poor.[26]

INDICATIONS FOR NUTRITIONAL SUPPORT

These would seem to be easy to document, despite a lack of significant, meaningful studies as to the significance of such indications in the cancer-bearing host (see Table 43-4).

Certainly, weight loss is a known prognostic factor in disease outcome,[27,28] so that aggressive attempts at nutritional support are widely advocated. Any patient whose in-hospital stay is expected to exceed 15 days and who is unable to ingest at least 1,000 calories a day is a candidate for some form of nutritional support. The question of the availability of effective antineoplastic therapy as a criterion for nutritional support is addressed later. Clinical and biochemical indices that are thought to support the use of, or need for, nutritional support are: a weight loss in excess of 10% of pre-illness weight; decreases in serum albumin (<3.5 g%); abnormality in anthropometric indices, diminished transferrin; plasma vitamin and trace mineral deficiencies; creatinine-height ratio less than 80% of predicted, and demonstrated immune incompetence (see Table 43-4).[3,30–34] Unfortunately, these data are imprecise in the individual patient and are altered by a large number of variables, including the degree of hydration of the patient. Indeed, these determinants have been questioned as to whether they have any value.[35] Given an awareness that the patient is receiving an intake that is less than his energy expenditure, nutritional support can be considered (see Table 43-5). The options are divided into two forms of support: enteral and parenteral. When the patient is able to eat and ingest normally with a functional GI tract, then the sensible approach to manipulating food according to patient choice can be effective. It is hard to underemphasize the amount of time and effort that this takes to be successful, often requiring the active cooperation of family members.

Unfortunately, as a consequence of the neoplasm or of therapy, the oral ingestion of adequate nutrient for host support is often impossible. As it has been shown that patients with cancers remote from the GI tract rarely have abnormal-

TABLE 43-3. Body Substrate Reserves: Depletion Times for Varying Catabolic Rates

	NITROGEN LOSS EACH DAY (g)	EQUIVALENT LEAN TISSUE LOSS (g)	DAYS TO LOSE 50% OF BCM
Acute Fasting	10	280	69
Chronic Fasting	3	84	232
Major Infection or Injury	20	560	34
Month Prior Starvation and Sepsis	15	420	35

BCM = Body cell mass

TABLE 43-4. Indications for Nutritional Support in the Cancer Patient

1°	2°	3°
Aggressive, nutritionally morbid, but therapeutically effect anti-cancer therapy	Weight loss ≥ 6% of preillness body weight	Demonstrated deficiency states
Weight loss ≥ 15% of pre-illness body weight	Therapy planned	Host functional deficits (anergy, impaired wound healing)

TABLE 43-5. Options for Nutritional Support in the Cancer Patient

1°	2°	3°
Enteral	• Increased oral feeding • Specific digestive problems	Involve the family Liquid supplements Patient preferences Multiple small meals Pancreatic enzymes Elemental diets Liquid formulae
	• Tube feeding	Soft small bore weighted feeding tube
Parenteral	• Central TPN	Non-functional GI tract High energy and protein demand
	• Peripheral IV nutritional support	Poorly functional GI tract Low caloric need

ities of absorption, and if ileus is not present, then we prefer the use of a small pediatric feeding tube. Suitable types are the Dobbhoff with a small weighted end which allows passage without difficulty, the Keofeed, or the Bardic. Some considerable success has been obtained with the use of a 24-inch 16 gauge polyethylene tube (marketed as a central venous catheter) used as a nasogastric tube.[36] If the tube is placed in the stomach then complete non-processed liquid formulae can be administered. One development is the movement away from liquid formulae based on large quantities of whole milk or milk products because of the relative inadequacy, in the adult, of sufficient lactase to permit adequate digestion of large quantities of lactose. Numerous nutritionally complete liquid diets are now available. There are however, virtually no significant comparative studies to assess the effectiveness of the various commercially available preparations in the nutritional support of the cancer patient. A most helpful summary of such formulae has recently been provided.[37] With the use of liquid-defined formula diets, patients require about 1,500–2,000 cc of fluid to meet recommended daily requirements of protein, fat, carbohydrates, vitamins, and minerals. In the majority of patients, progressive increments up to 3,000 Cal is the aim. It is not essential that the patient receive all nutrient by such means, they can be used as support for standard fare. The more chemically defined formulae containing hydrolyzed protein (as soybean or MCT oil) and carbohydrate (as oligo saccharides) are also efficacious. The absolute indications for the use of these are quite restrictive. They are required only when pancreatic exocrine insufficiency, small intestinal disease or limited surface area (short bowel) exists. The unfortunate side effect of the elemental or chemically defined diets is the high osmolality induced,

TABLE 43-6. Options for Enteral Support

TYPE	EXAMPLE	SOURCE
I. Supplementary feedings	Ca-Sec Liprotein Hi-Den Nutr	Mead-Johnson Upjohn Control Drugs
II. A. Complete formula defined (with milk, moderate residue)	Instant breakfast Compleat B Formula 2 Vitaneed	Carnation Doyle Cutter Organon
B. Intact protein (with milk, low residue)	Meritene Nutri-1000 Sustacal	Doyle Cutter Mead-Johnson
C. Intact protein (Low lactose, low milk)	Ensure Isocal Magnacal Mull-Soy Nutri-1000 Osmolite Precision	Ross Mead-Johnson Organon Syntex Cutter Ross Doyle
III. Complete formula defined (Protein Hydrolysates)	Flexical Nutramigen Vital Vivonex	Mead-Johnson Mead-Johnson Ross Eaton
IV. Defined formulae:		
Renal failure	Amin Aid	McGaw
Hepatic failure	Hepatic Aid	McGaw
Phenylketonuria	Lofenalac	Mead-Johnson

TABLE 43-7. Options for Enterel Feeding

OPTION	ROUTE	COMMENTS
Supplementary feeding	Oral	Multiple small feedings.
Complete formula defined	Oral or nasogastric tube	Multiple small feedings
	Gastrostomy	Use small bore 8F pediatric feeding tube, continuous infusion
Complete formula	Nasogastric tube	Start slowly with dilute solutions
Protein hydrolysates	Jejunal or gastrostomy tube, occasionally oral	Multiple small feedings or continuous infusion
Defined formulae for organ failure	Nasogastric tube	Of only occasional value due to other organ failure

nausea and diarrhea. These problems can be overcome by slow introduction of dilute solutions used continuously throughout 24 hours or over the awake hours (see Tables 43-6, 43-7).[4,36] Except in experienced units many problems arise from tube feeding. Persistence and diligence are required to overcome patient objection and physician resistance. The only absolute contraindications are repetitive aspiration or failure of the GI tract to function. If patient intolerance to a nasogastric tube is a major feature then a surgically placed gastrostomy or jejunostomy can be inserted. The jejunostomy kit can be used.[37]

INDICATIONS FOR TOTAL PARENTERAL NUTRITION (TPN) IN THE CANCER PATIENT

Unfortunately, the cancer patient is commonly unable to ingest, digest or absorb via the gastro-intestinal tract. When a small tube is no longer acceptable, the choice is either a surgical procedure to implant a jejunal or gastric tube or TPN. Even with a functional GI tract many physicians prefer to move directly to the IV route. If the GI tract is not functional, then IV feeding is the only alternative.

PRACTICAL ASPECTS

Numerous IV mixtures are now available. What is required is a standard amino acid source, preferably of the synthetic type so as to avoid amino nitrogen loss as polypeptides, and a caloric source. In the U.S., glucose is the preferred solitary energy source, whereas physicians involved in TPN in other parts of the world prefer a more balanced mixture containing a high percentage of IV fat as part of the caloric source. Recent animal studies would support this higher fat containing regimen[38] in the cancer-bearing animal, but as yet no data exist for humans. Alternative substrates, such as sucrose, xylitol, sorbitol, are mentioned only to be avoided. Where glucose is used as a solitary caloric source then an essential fatty acid source needs to be given, (1,000 cc a week of a 10% solution) to prevent essential fatty acid deficiency.[39,40] All solutions should contain daily requirements of essential electrolytes. At the Clinical Center, NIH, a "Three Solution System" designed for maximum flexibility without incompatibility is employed (see Table 43-8). The daily requirements of all essential nutrients are provided in the first two bottles each day, with a third bottle available, to allow administration of increased calories and nitrogen and the repletion of excess electrolyte losses. Our choice of 40% dextrose is deliberate and based on known need for adequate calorie to nitrogen ratio, but with the intended avoidance of the problems

TABLE 43-8. Suggested Daily TPN Solution Orders with Maximal Flexibility without Incompatibility for Cancer Patients

BOTTLE A	
Synthetic Amino Acid (5–10%)	500ml
Dextrose (40%)	500ml
NaCl	____meq
Na Acetate	____meq
K Cl	____meq
Ca gluconate	5meq
Iron dextran*	0.25ml
Vitamin Vial 1 & 2†	5ml
Vitamin K	0.1mg
Trace Metal Solution‡	1.0ml
Insulin	____units
Albumin	____(12.5 g)
BOTTLE B	
Synthetic Amino Acids (5–10%)	500ml
Dextrose (40%)	500ml
NaCl	____meq
NaAc	____meq
K Cl	____meq
K Phosphate	____meq
$MgSO_4$	10meq
Insulin	____units
Albumin	____(12.5 gm)
BOTTLE C	
Synthetic Amino Acids (5–10%)	500ml
Dextrose (40%)	500ml
NaCl	____meq
Na Acetate	____meq
K Cl	____meq
$MgSO_4$ or	____meq
K Phosphate or	____meq
Ca gluconate	____meq
Insulin	____units
Albumin	____(12.5 g)

*Imferon, Merrell National Laboratories.
†Vial 1 and Vial 2 = MV1–12, USV Laboratories.
‡See Table 43-9.

TABLE 43-9. Current Trace Metal and Daily Vitamin Supplementation

TRACE METAL SOLUTION		
Zinc	4.99	mg/ml
Copper	1.43	mg/ml
Manganese	0.49	mg/ml
Iodine	0.056	mg/ml
Chromium	0.016	mg/ml
VITAMINS: Vial 1 (MVI-MAINTENANCE)*		
A	3300	I.U.
D	200	I.U.
E	10	I.U.
C	100	mg
B_1 Thiamine	3	mg
B_2 Riboflavin	3.6	mg
B_3 Dexpanthenol	15.0	mg
B_5 Niacin	40	mg
B_6 Pyridoxine	4	mg
Vial 2 (*Biofol-12*)*		
B_7 Biotin	60	μg
B_{12}	5	μg
Folate (B_9)	0.4	mg

*Vial 1 and Vial 2 = MVI-12, USV Laboratories.

associated with excess glucose in the cancer patient.[41-44] Although the value of adding albumin to the patient's regimen is entirely unproven, it can be safely added to the bottle, and in situations where insulin is being used, will diminish insulin binding to the container.

The trace metals, zinc, copper, selenium and chromium, are now being increasingly employed to prevent trace metal deficiency. The trace metal solution that the authors use is listed in Table 43-9.[45,46] The question of the need for selenium and cadmium is only now being evaluated.[47,48] Vitamin deficiencies are not uncommon on vitamin-free TPN and a suggested regimen that will maintain vitamin levels in the plasma is given in Tables 43-8 and 43-9. It should be emphasized that, many vitamin preparations are currently undergoing evaluation in an effort to define a more adequate formula for use with TPN. Certainly, the concern for use of plasma levels of vitamins as reflective of adequate tissue levels remains under investigation. Given the present status of our own and other studies, one might predict that the regimen suggested, based on maintenance of plasma levels, will be low in vitamins C and D, and possibly low in vitamins B_1 and B_{12}; hence, it is these deficiencies that should be looked for.[49-51] Prior concerns about the use of IV iron dextran are undergoing re-evaluation and it seem not unreasonable to add small quantities of IV iron to parenteral nutrition formulas.[52] Choline, not previously thought essential, is currently being evaluated because plasma deficiencies of choline during TPN, have been identified. Insulin can be added directly to the mixture to correct glucose intolerance. The authors prefer to try to avoid the early glucose intolerance that accompanies rapid escalation of TPN solution volume at the start of nutritional support, preferring a slow (two- to three-day) increase to the 3–4 liters per day required. With this approach, insulin is only occasionally required, except in those patients undergoing rigorous therapy with corticosteroids, where insulin is almost invariably needed.

TECHNICAL CONSIDERATIONS

Venous Access

Venous access remains a problem in all cancer patients, as a consequence of the repetitive venesection required for the administration of vein-sclerosing drugs and for the frequent monitoring of hematologic toxicity. For TPN, a central site of infusion is essential because of the high osmolality of the solution and the subclavian route is the most common approach (see Table 43-10). Two primary alternatives exist. The standard percutaneous transneedle catheter bedside insertion or the surgically placed, tunnelled Broviac or Hickman silastic catheter with a Teflon cuff (see Figs. 43-2 and 43-3).[8,35,51,53,57] The use of the latter catheters is based on the assumption that they are less irritating than the conventional, widely-used, polyvinyl chloride catheters and that a high incidence of superior vena-caval thrombosis occurs when polyvinyl catheters are employed.[58,59] Prospective studies are not available comparing the two types of catheter in patients with cancer as to their freedom from complications. The ease of insertion and replacement of the conventional subclavian catheter make this approach the most widely acceptable. Comparative costs are significant with the percutaneous standard catheter $1–2, the percutaneous silicone catheter $8–10, and the indwelling Hickman type $35–40. On occa-

TABLE 43-10. Options in the Administration of TPN

ROUTE	CATHETER TYPE	COMMENTS
Percutaneous subclavian or jugular puncture	Polyvinylchloride-intracath*	Preferred approach.
	Silicone-Centrasil†	Undergoing evaluation but occasionally migrates.
Peripheral insertion to superior vena cava	Silicone-Intrasil†	Peripheral access is often not available and phlebitis incidence is high.
Surgically placed tunelled, cuffed catheter	Silicone-Hickman or Broviac type‡	Used extensively for home TPN, and long-term venous access.

*Becton Dickinson, #3162, Sandy, Utah.
†Vicra, Travenol Laboratories, Inc., Dallas, Texas.
‡Evermed, Medina, Washington.

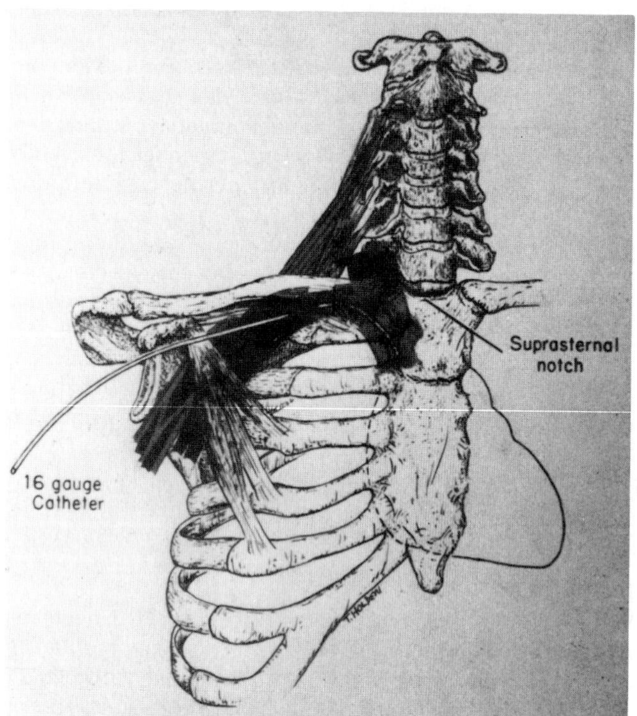

FIG. 43-2. Surgical anatomy of access site to the subclavian vein.

sions, the percutaneous subclavian route is unavailable because of prior use or difficulty in placement. The authors have found that in the patient with extensive mediastinal radiation, this may be a problem. Our preferred alternative is to use the supraclavicular approach between the two heads of the sternomastoid muscle. This ensures direct catheterization at or just above the confluence of the internal jugular and subclavian vein. The theoretical risk to the lymphatic duct has not been a problem in our experience. One potential disadvantage to this approach is the difficulty in placing a dressing over the site of exit. This latter problem is solved by making a percutaneous tunnel under the skin, such that the catheter exit site is again over the upper anterior chest wall. This tunnel can be readily created with the use of the large bore needle through which the catheter was initially inserted into the vein. A similar procedure can be used to move the exit site away from a tracheostomy site (see Fig. 43-4). In passing a catheter subcutaneously, it is necessary to remove the hub of the catheter. This can be replaced by a number of alternative "stubby needles." It is preferred, however, to use a scored needle to guarantee that the catheter hub connection cannot come apart (see Fig. 43-5).[60] In some cancer patients, with difficult access, rather than remove a catheter and replace it when it is malfunctioning, exchange the catheter for a new one over a guide wire. The series 7008, flexible tip, tapered cone guide wire which is 70 cm long with a 0.5 mm diameter is available in any x-ray department. If any difficulty is encountered, either at primary insertion or during an exchange, then fluoroscopic control can be employed to great advantage.

On the assumption that subclavian vein thrombosis may be due to the high osmolality of the infused solution, the role of catheter composition has been given less emphasis than it deserves. The high incidence of fibrin sheath formation with any intravascular catheter might suggest that attempts to decrease the thrombogenicity of such catheters by anticoagulant impregnation may be an area of fruitful research.[61] The true incidence of superior venacaval thrombosis is not known.[62,63] In an autopsy study, it was as high as 25%.[58] More recently, a review of the controlled studies supported by the Diet Nutrition and Cancer Program of the National Cancer Institute suggested a clinically detectable incidence of ap-

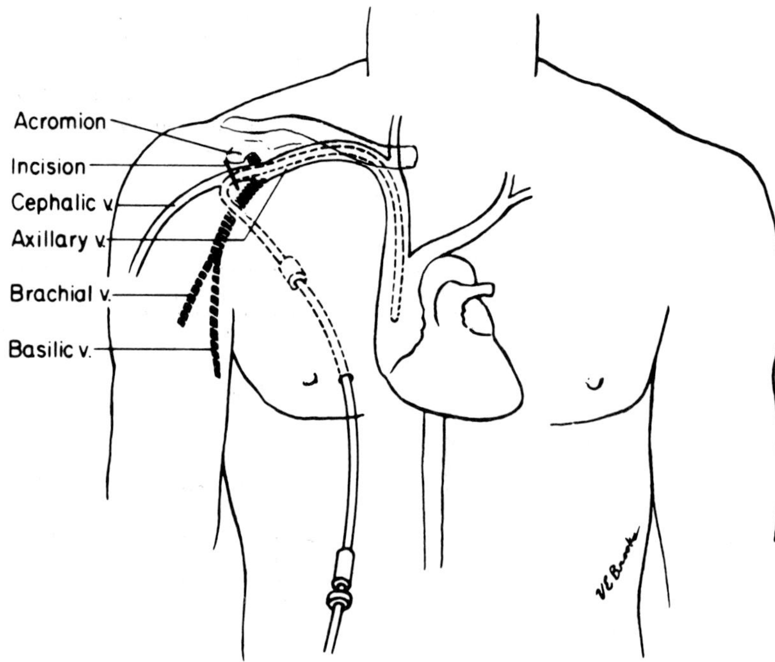

FIG. 43-3. The position and placement of the cuffed silicon rubber catheter suitable for long-term parenteral nutrition. (Riella MC, Scribner BH: Five year's experience with a right atrial catheter for prolonged parenteral nutrition at home. Surg Gynecol Obstet 143:205–208, 1976. By permission of Surgery, Gynecology and Obstetrics)

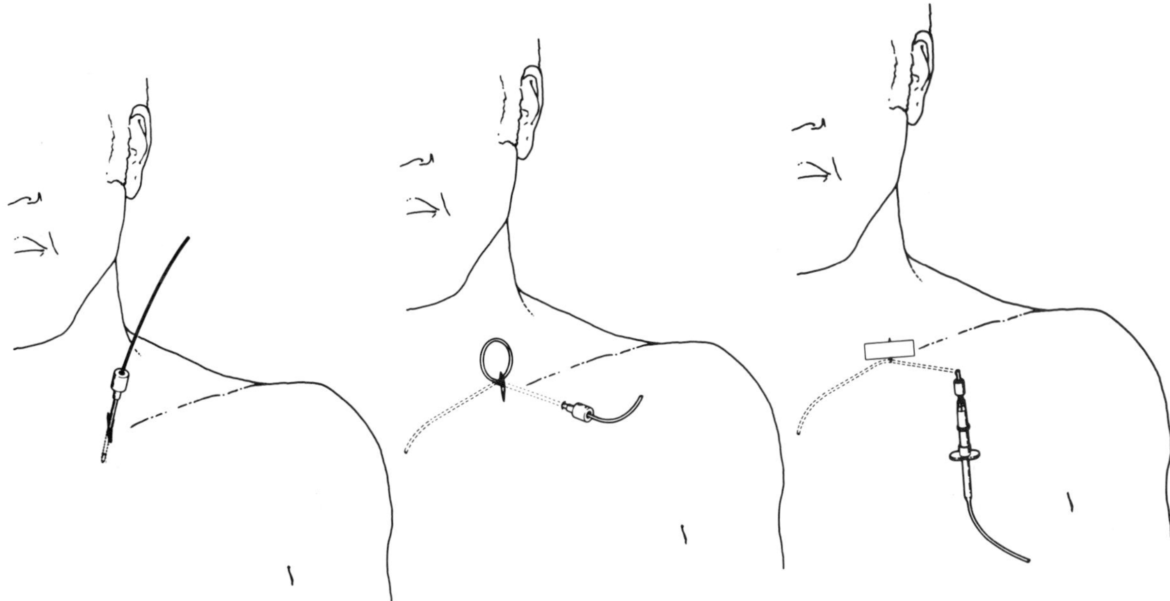

FIG. 43-4. Schematic of tunnelling a catheter placed in the internal jugular percutaneously above the clavicle, so as to have an anterior chest wall exit site remote from a tracheostomy.

proximately 5%.[64] However, an incidence of 10% of subclavian vein thrombosis in 33 patients undergoing aggressive chemotherapy and nutritional support for oat cell lung cancer has also been documented.[65] In this latter study, there was an additional 33% incidence of phlebitis with eight of 13 requiring catheter removal. These and other data would suggest that the actual incidence of clinically undetected subclavian vein thrombosis is much closer to that of the autopsy series. Regardless of the frequency with which such thrombosis occurs, it may not be important as venous collaterals develop readily. The problem is then only manifest when the patient requires repetitive venous access by the subclavian or internal jugular route, or if such thrombosis is shown to be the cause of further complications such as pulmonary emboli.

Fever

Fever is a common accompaniment to aggressive anti-neoplastic therapy and is specifically addressed elsewhere in this text. In the patient who is immunosuppressed, with a white blood count below 500 mm³, fever is almost invariable. This is complicated when a central venous catheter is in place for the use of parenteral nutrition. It is tempting to attribute fever to the presence of the catheter, but most studies have failed to confirm this. The authors have become more conservative about leaving catheters in place during periods of fever in the immunosuppressed patient. The patient often has a central line as his only source of access and indiscriminant removal would create major access problems. Consequently, in the absence of positive blood cultures or the development of new glucose intolerance, we have been willing to exchange the catheter over a wire, culturing the tip and then not removing the new catheter unless the patient has frank sepsis or hemodynamic instability. It should be emphasized that in patients in whom other sites of access are readily available, then unexplained fever is more satisfactorily treated by the removal of the catheter. The catheter can then be replaced subsequently, once fever has resolved or an explanation for the source of the fever identified.

Metabolic Complications

The techniques of total parenteral nutrition are now at a sufficient stage of development that metabolic complications due to TPN should be prevented or readily recognized and

FIG. 43-5. Modified needle adaptor for connection to a central venous catheter. (Maher MM, Bowers WG, Thomas GM et al: An improved needle adaptor for central venous catheters. J Parent Ent Nutr 3:77–78, 1979)

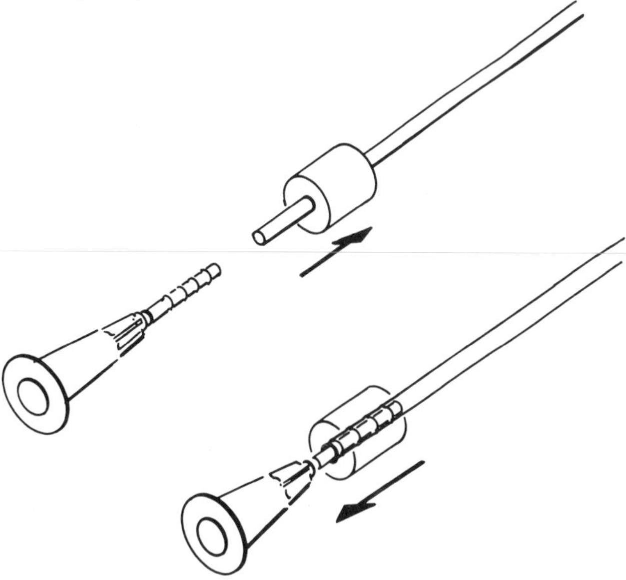

treated. Most clinical deficiency states should no longer occur and as better understanding of electrolyte requirements are identified, problems such as the long-term bone disease should occur less frequently.[66,67] In a recent comparative study of the complications occurring in patients undergoing cancer treatment, metabolic complications were no more frequent in patients on than off TPN.[64]

TUMOR STIMULATION BY NUTRITIONAL SUPPORT

A common concern is that the nutritional support of the patient with cancer may cause nutritional stimulation of tumor growth. This has been suggested by some short-term animal studies, but not by others.[68-70] The question is, in some aspects, moot as most nutritional support studies in animals are either short-term or are performed in the absence of anti-neoplastic therapy. There is little doubt that in long-term total parenteral nutrition of an animal, the tumor will be much larger than in the anorectic, non-nutritionally supported control animal.[71] This matter becomes only an issue when one considers that on occasions this "experiment" is performed in man. Patients who are receiving nutritional support at a time when they receive anti-neoplastic therapy, which is either ineffective or subsequently shown to be of no benefit, have the potential for having tumor progression induced. In a recent prospective randomized study, patients receiving total parenteral nutrition in conjunction with 5 FU-Methyl CCNU chemotherapy for advanced GI adenocarcinoma died earlier than the controls not receiving TPN. While tumor progression was not identified as a cause of death and many objections were raised as to the study design, such observations merit emphasis and concern.[72]

JUSTIFICATION FOR NUTRITIONAL SUPPORT OF CANCER PATIENTS

For nutritional support to be advocated, it must be able to be shown that the metabolic and nutritional defects of the cancer-bearing host are amenable to reversal by nutritional support.

RESTORATION OF WEIGHT LOSS

Numerous studies have shown that weight gain can be achieved with nutritional support by enteral or parenteral routes.[29-31,36,73-76] Concern has been expressed, however, that the weight gain may reflect greater fat accretion than lean tissue restoration.[77] The authors and others have certainly shown that in some patients, who have responded to anti-neoplastic therapy, lean tissue can be restored, as measured by total body potassium determinations or by nitrogen balance and nitrogen flux studies.[78]

PROVISION OF EXCESS ENERGY NEEDS OF THE CANCER-BEARING PATIENT

Increased energy requirements by the cancer patient have been invoked as a cause of cancer cachexia. The data to support this are somewhat confusing. It would certainly appear that patients who have cancer have a relative inability to adjust energy expenditure to meet energy intake.[13-15] Where energy needs are increased, then nutritional support by enteral or parenteral routes can readily match such increased need.[12] Fluid limitations then become the only limiting factor in the provision of adequate calories. However, it should be emphasized that the use of excess calories far in excess of energy requirements can only be associated with increased deposition of fat, and may result in an increased metabolic cost due to increased quantitative, but not relative, recycling rates.[79,80]

DEFICIENCY STATES

As mentioned above, the vast majority of the deficiency states should be readily reversed by either oral or IV nutrition. Certainly, deficiencies of trace metals and electrolytes once thought to be a cause of cancer or cancer progression should no longer be seen.

SUPPRESSION OF GLUCONEOGENESIS

The cancer-bearing host is, like other patients who are in a semi-starved state, endogenously producing glucose by gluconeogenesis or glycogenolysis in an effort to provide glucose for the obligatory glucose using tissues. This continuous obligatory gluconeogenesis can result in rapid lean tissue mass dissolution and subsequent death from starvation. The use of nutritional support has been shown to suppress such gluconeogenesis from amino acids in the cancer-bearing host, although at a cost of increased glucose recycling in some.[78,81-83]

IMMUNE DEFICIENCIES

The cancer-bearing host is commonly immunosuppressed. This immunosuppression may be due to the disease state, the therapy the patient is receiving, or to associated diseases. Impressive claims have been made for the reversion of this immunosuppression by IV nutritional support.[30] It is, however, difficult to tell whether the concomitant reversal of the patient's relative anergy is a function of the nutritional support the patient received or to his response to anti-neoplastic therapy. Animal data would suggest an active role for nutritional support in the reversal of anergy in patients responding to anti-neoplastic therapy.[32]

THERAPEUTIC TRIALS OF EFFICACY

The use of total parenteral nutrition in the malnourished cancer patient undergoing effective anti-neoplastic therapy can be one of the more gratifying supportive measures. Such patients can demonstrate major changes in well-being, regrowth and restoration of multiple nutritional deficits, and functional ability to withstand further non-neoplastic injury. A large number of publications have supported this approach.[29-32,74,84-86] The metabolic defects that can and have been shown to be reversed in ideal circumstances are listed in Table 43-11. It should be emphasized that the majority of

TABLE 43-11. Metabolic Consequences of TPN in the Cancer Patient

- Weight gain
- Improved serum albumin
- Improved nitrogen retention (Nitrogen balance)
- Restoration of deficiency states (vitamins, trace metals)
- Increase in subcutaneous fat (anthropometrics)
- Increased lean tissue (K^{40})
- Increase in whole body protein synthesis (^{15}N glycine)
- Suppression of gluconeogenesis from alanine (^{14}C-Alanine)
- Increase in quantitative glucose recycling (^{3}H-glucose, ^{14}C-glucose)

these studies, although not all, have been performed in situations where the patient has responded to the anti-neoplastic therapy and the analogy of regrowing a normal malnourished adult is much more appropriate.

The use of nutritional support, either enteral or parenteral, as a generalized, indiscriminantly applied adjunct to antineoplastic therapy, rests on less secure ground. Prospective randomized trials are now being performed and reported.

Studies have been reported in both heterogenous and defined populations, and in all the numbers have been small. The majority of studies have not stratified for disease stage or degree of preceding malnutrition and, as has been repetitively emphasized, malnutrition at the time of presentation is a bad prognostic sign.[1,3,27,34,87]

The studies employing enteral nutritional support have examined the efficacy of giving a supplemental high nitrogen elemental diet to patients receiving radiation therapy for locally advanced radiation therapy.[88] No difference in survival was demonstrated, 24% for the standard diet, and 38% for the supplemental high nitrogen diet. As the total group studied was 30 patients, there would have had to have been a 55% difference from control for a significant difference to be identified in such a small cohort.[89] This would be an unlikely event in patients receiving radiation therapy for advanced pancreatic, gastric, or colorectal cancer. This study, and similar studies of nutritional supplementation versus self-selected diets, emphasize the difficulty of showing any effect from a nutritional adjunct if the primary therapy is relatively ineffective.[75]

Such a comment can be similarly addressed to the studies of the use of TPN as an adjunct in advanced, low response therapies (see Table 43-12).

It would seem most unlikely that any impact of nutritional support would be identified when advanced abdominal, pelvic, colorectal carcinomas or squamous cell cancer of the lung are the diseases being examined. Unfortunately, the antineoplastic therapies for these low-response, low-cure rate, advanced malignancies are sufficiently ineffective to prevent any meaningful improvement in survival to be demonstrated.

It would seem that to examine the effects of nutritional support as an adjunct to cancer therapy, either tolerance to therapy in low response tumors, or improvement in tumor response rates in high response tumors, must be examined.

This has been examined in a random fashion in diffuse histiocytic lymphoma, where an attempt was made to determine if the percent administered of a planned course of

TABLE 43-12. Results of Prospective Randomized Trials in the Use of TPN as an Adjunct to Cancer Therapy

AUTHOR, REF.	TOTAL # OF PATIENTS	CANCER	STAGE	THERAPY	EFFECT OF TPN VS CONTROL
Holter (92, 93)	56	GI	All	Surgery	No difference in operative mortality Slight improvement in operative morbidity with TPN Improved serum albumin with TPN Decreased weight loss with TPN
Valerio (95)	20	Pelvic and abdominal	Advanced	RT	No significant difference in response, tolerance
Issell (40)	27	Squamous cell of the lung	All	Chemoimmunotherapy	Decrease in WBC and platelet nadir with TPN No difference in response
Solassol (96)	40	Abdominal-pelvic	Advanced	RT	Improved survival by TPN
Solassol (96)	81	Ovarian	Advanced	RT	No difference in survival
Heatley (94)	74	Esophogeal and gastric	Localized	Surgery	Post-operative death in TPN 15%, control 22% Complications less in TPN
Popp (87)	33	Diffuse histiocytic lymphoma	II, III, IV	Chemotherapy	No improvement in % planned dose with TPN No improvement in tolerance with TPN
Nixon (72)	45	Colorectal	IV	Chemotherapy	Decrease in survival with TPN
Valdivieso (65)	30	Oat cell lung	All	Chemotherapy	Improved complete response rate with TPN
Lanzotti (91)	33	Non-oat cell lung	All	Chemotherapy	No difference in median survival or response rate with TPN

RT = Radiation therapy

chemotherapy could be increased by the use of TPN.[87] The tolerance to chemotherapy was not significantly improved by TPN, as measured by white blood cell and platelet nadirs. In addition, these authors did not demonstrate an improvement in serum albumin by TPN. They did suggest that the chance of responding to therapy was diminished if, at the time of entry into therapy, the patient was already malnourished. This study could be criticized for the relative lack of the predicted toxicity and nutritional morbidity in the control group. However, when the data were examined to compare only those patients who were initially malnourished, no increase in percent of planned dose administered, response rate, or decrease in nutritional morbidity was seen in the group receiving TPN.

In randomized studies examining high response, low cure rate malignancies there has been a suggestion of an improved response rate in the TPN group.[65,97] This has yet to reach statistical significance. In two of these studies, subclavian vein thrombosis was higher than the conventionally accepted 5%.[65,87]

In the low-response, low-cure rate malignancy, some improvement in chemotherapeutic toxicity has been seen in one study, but no difference in another.[90,91]

Perhaps the patients most likely to benefit are the patients undergoing resectional surgery for GI malignancy. In randomized studies, improvement in nutritional indices have been seen postoperatively, with some small but real diminuition in operative morbidity and mortality in patients receiving perioperative TPN.[92-94] Again, in one of the studies, the "cross over" for nutritional "failure" postoperatively makes the data less easily interpreted.[94]

Finally, in the situation where anti-neoplastic therapy is ineffective, then routine TPN cannot be advocated and indeed, in the patient without weight loss, may decrease survival.[72]

Nutritional support of the patient undergoing rigorous anti-neoplastic therapy is now an accepted fact. There seems no reason for patients who are expected to undergo effective anti-neoplastic therapy to suffer the nutritional ravages that may accompany such therapy. The GI tract continues to be the preferred route of nutritional support. In circumstances where this is unavailable, total parenteral nutrition can now be recommended as a safe source of nutrient and micronutrient replenishment. Like other forms of patient support discussed in this chapter, the exact role of nutritional support continues to be defined.

REFERENCES

1. DeWys WD: Anorexia as a general effect of cancer. Cancer 43:2013–2019, 1979
2. Morrison SD: Limited capacity for motor activity as a cause for declining food intake in cancer. J Natl Cancer Inst 51:1535–1539, 1973
3. Nixon DW, Heymsfield SB, Cohen AE et al: Protein-calorie under nutrition in hospitalized cancer patients. Am J Med 68:683–690, 1980
4. Shils ME: Nutritional problems associated with gastrointestinal and genito urinary cancer. Cancer Res 37:2366–2372, 1977
5. DeWys WD: Changes in taste sensation and feeding behavior in cancer patients. A review. J Hum Nutr 32:447–453, 1978
6. Dudrick SJ, Wilmore DW, Vars HM et al: Long term total parenteral nutrition with growth, development and positive nitrogen balance. Surgery 64:134–142, 1968
7. Dudrick SJ, Wilmore DW, Vars HM et al: Can intravenous feeding as the sole means of nutrition support growth in the child and restore weight loss in an adult. An affirmative answer. Ann Surg 169:974–984, 1969
8. Wilmore DW, Dudrick SJ: Safe long term venous catheterization. Arch Surg 98:256–258, 1969
9. Terepka AR, Waterhouse C: Metabolic observations during forced feeding of patients with cancer. Am J Med 20:225–238, 1956
10. Bozzetti F, Pagnoni AM, Delvecchio M: Excessive caloric expenditure as a cause of malnutrition in patients with cancer. Surg Gynecol & Obstet 150:229–234, 1980
11. Brennan MF: Uncomplicated starvation versus cancer cachexia. Cancer Res 37:2359–2364, 1977
12. Steinberg JL, Crosby LO, Feurer ID et al: Indirect calorimetry and cancer patients (abstr). Am Soc Clin Oncol C–229, 1980
13. Warnold I, Falkheden T, Hulten B et al: Energy intake and expenditure in selected groups of hospital patients. Am J Clin Nutr 31:742–749, 1978
14. Warnold I, Lundholm K, Schersten T: Energy balance and body composition in cancer patients. Cancer Res 38:1801, 1978
15. Young VR: Energy metabolism and requirements in the cancer patient. Cancer Res 37:2336–2347, 1977
16. Scheinberg P, Stead EA: The cerebral blood flow in male subjects as measured by the nitrous oxide technique. Normal values for blood flow oxygen utilization, glucose utilization, and peripheral resistance with observations on the effect of tilting and anxiety. J Clin Invest 28:1163–1171, 1949
17. Cahill GF: Starvation in man. N Engl J Med 282:668–675, 1970
18. Burt ME, Lowry SF, Gorschboth C et al: Metabolic alterations in a non-cachetic animal tumor system. Cancer 47:2138–2146, 1981
19. Gullino P, Granthham FH, Courtney AH et al: Relationship between oxygen and glucose consumption by transplanted tumors in vivo. Cancer Res 27:1041–1052, 1967
20. Norton JA, Burt ME, Brennan MF: In vivo utilization of substrate by human sarcoma bearing limbs. Cancer 45: 2934–2939, 1980
21. Brennan MF: Metabolic response to surgery in the cancer patient. Consequences of aggressive multimodality therapy. Cancer 43:2053–2064, 1979
22. Owen OE, Morgan AP, Kemp HG et al: Brain metabolism during fasting. J Clin Invest 46:1589–1595, 1967
23. Fery F, Balasse EO: Differential effects of sodium acetate and acetoacetic acid infusions on alanine and glutamine metabolism in man. J Clin Invest 66:323–331, 1980
24. Aoki TT, Toews CJ, Rossini AA et al: Glucogenic substrate levels in fasting man. Adv Enzyme Regul 13:329–336, 1975
25. Buse MG, Weigand DA, Peeler D et al: The effect of diabetes and the redox potential on amino acid content and release by isolated rat diaphragms. Metabolism 29:605–616, 1980
26. Michallet M, Hollard D, Guignier HM et al: Parenteral nutrition in patients with leukemia and non-Hodgkin's malignant lymphoma under chemotherapy. JPEN 3:247–254, 1979
27. DeWys WD, Begg C, Lavin PT et al: Prognostic effect of weight loss prior to chemotherapy in cancer patients. Am J Med 69:491–497, 1980
28. Studley HO: Percentage of weight loss, a basic indicator of surgical risk. JAMA 106:458–460, 1936
29. Copeland EM, MacFadyen BV, Lanzotti V et al: Intravenous hyperalimentation as an adjunct to cancer chemotherapy. Am J Surg 129:167–170, 1975
30. Copeland EM, MacFadyen BV, Dudrick SJ: Effect of intravenous hyperalimentation on established delayed hypersensitivity in the cancer patient. Ann Surg 184:60–64, 1976
31. Copeland EM, Daly JM, Dudrick SJ: Nutrition as an adjunct to cancer treatment in the adult. Cancer Res 37:2451–2456, 1977
32. Daly JM, Copeland EM, Dudrick SJ: Effect of intravenous nutrition on tumor growth and host immunocompetence in malnourished animals. Surgery 84:655–658, 1978

33. Harvey KB, Bothe A, Blackburn GL: Nutritional assessment and patient outcome during oncological therapy. Cancer 43:2065–2069, 1979
34. Hickman DA, Miller RA, Rombeau JL et al: Serum albumin and body weight as predictors of postoperative course in colorectal cancer. JPEN 4:314–316, 1980
35. Forse RA, Shizgal HM: The assessment of malnutrition. Surgery 88:17–24, 1980
36. Bethel RA, Jansen RD, Heymsfield SB et al: Nasogastric hyperalimentation through a polyethylene catheter: an alternative to central venous hyperalimentation. Am J Clin Nutr 32:1112–1120, 1979
37. Shils ME, Block AS, Chernoff R: Liquid formulas for oral and tube feeding, 2nd ed. New York, Memorial Sloan–Kettering Cancer Center, 1979
38. Buzby GP, Mullen JL, Stein TP et al: Host–tumor interaction and nutrient supply. Cancer 45:2940–2948, 1980
39. Goodgame JT, Lowry SF, Brennan MF: Essential fatty acid deficiency intotal parenteral nutrition: Time course of devlopment and suggestions for therapy. Surgery 84:271–277, 1978
40. McCarthy DM, May RJ, Maher M et al: Trace metal and essential fatty acid deficiency during total parenteral nutrition. Am J Dig Dis 23:1009–1016, 1978
41. Peters C, Fischer JE: Studies on calorie to nitrogen ratio for parenteral nutrition. Surg Gynecol Obstet 151:1–8, 1980
42. Askanazi J, Elwyn DH, Silverberg PA et al: Respiratory distress secondary to a high carbohydrate load: A case report. Surgery 87:596–598, 1980
43. Goodgame JT, Pizzo P, Brennan MF: Iatrogenic lactic acidosis: Association with hypertonic glucose administration in a patient with cancer. Cancer 42:800–803, 1978
44. Lowry SF, Brennan MF: Abdominal liver function during parenteral nutrition correlation with infusion excess. J Surg Res 26:300–307, 1979
45. Lowry SF, Goodgame JT, Smith JC et al: Abnormalities of zinc and copper during total parenteral nutrition. Ann Surg 189:120–128, 1979
46. Lowry SF, Smith J, Brennan MF: Zinc and copper replacement during total parenteral nutrition. Am J Clin Nutr (in press)
47. Jacobson S, Webster PO: Balance study of twenty trace elements during total parenteral nutrition in man. Br J Nutr 37:107–126, 1977
48. Smith JL, Goos SM: Selenium nutriture in total parenteral nutrition: Intake levels. J Parent Ent Nutr 4:23–26, 1980
49. Jeejeebhoy KN, Langer B, Tsallas G et al: Total parenteral nutrition at home: studies in patients surviving four months to five years. Gastroenterology 71:943–953, 1976
50. Lowry SF, Goodgame JT, Maher MM et al: Parenteral vitamin requirements during intravenous feeding. Am J Clin Nutr 31:2149–2158, 1978
50A. Burt ME, Hanin I, Brennan MF: Choline deficiency associated with total parenteral nutrition. Lancet 11:638–639, 1980
51. Nichoalds GE, Meng HC, Caldwell MD: Vitamin requirements in patients receiving total parenteral nutrition. Arch Surg 112:1061–1064, 1977
52. Hamstra RD, Block MH, Schocket AC: Intravenous iron dextran in clinical medicine. JAMA 243:1724–1731, 1980
53. Abrahm J, Mullen JL, Jacobson N et al: Chronic central venous access in patients with leukemia. Cancer Treat Rep (in press)
54. Broviac JW, Cole JJ, Scribner BH: A silicone rubber atrial catheter for prolonged parenteral alimentation. Surg Gynecol Obstet 136:602, 1974
55. Hickman RD, Buckner CD, Clift RA et al: A modified right atrial catheter for access to the venous system in marrow transplant recipients. Surg Gynecol Obstet 148:872–875, 1979
56. Miller DG, Ivey M, Ivey T et al: Experience with an indwelling right atrial catheter for home parenteral nutrition. Surg Gynecol Obstet 151:108–110, 1980
57. Riella MC,Scribner BH: Five years experience with a right atrial catheter for prolonged parenteral nutrition at home. Surg Gynecol Obstet 143:205–208, 1976
58. Ryan JA, Abel RM, Abbott WM et al: Catheter complications of total parenteral nutrition. N Engl J Med 290:757–761, 1974
59. Welch GW, McKeel DW, Silverstein P et al: The role of catheter composition in the development of thrombophlebitis. Surg Gynecol Obstet 138:421–424, 1974
60. Maher MM, Bowers WG, Thomas GM et al: An improved needle adaptor for central venous catheters. JPEN 3:77–78, 1979
61. Hoshal VL, Ause EG, Hoskins FA: Fibrin sleeve formation on indwelling subclavian central venous catheters. Arch Surg 102:353–358, 1971
62. Peters WR, Bush WH, McIntyre RD et al: The development of fibrin sheath on indwelling venous catheters. Surg Gynecol Obstet 137:3–7, 1973
63. Pruitt BA, McManus WF, Kim SH et al: Diagnosis and treatment of cannula-related intravenous sepsis in burn patients. Ann Surg 191:546–553, 1980
64. Mullen JL: Complications of total parenteral nutrition in cancer patients. Cancer Treat Rep (in press).
65. Valdivieso M, Bodey GP, Benjamin RS et al: Role of intravenous hyperalimentation as an adjunct to intensive therapy for small cell bronchogenic carcinoma: Preliminary observations. Cancer Treat Rep (in press)
66. Shike M, Harrison JE, Sturtridge WC et al: Metabolic bone disease in patients receiving long term total parenteral nutrition. Ann Intern Med 92:343–350, 1980
67. Blackburn GL, Maini BS, Bistrian BR et al: The effect of cancer on nitrogen, electrolyte and mineral metabolism. Cancer Res 37:2348–2353, 1977
68. Goodgame JT, Lowry SF, Brennan MF: Nutritional manipulations and tumor growth. II. The effects of intravenous feeding. Am J Clin Nutr 32:2285–2294, 1979
69. Lowry SF, Goodgame JT, Norton JA et al: Effect of chronic protein malnutrition on host–tumor composition and growth. J Surg Res 26:79–86, 1979
70. Steiger E, Oram-Smith J, Miller E et al: Effects of nutrition on tumor growth and tolerance to chemotherapy. J Surg Res 18:455–461, 1975
71. Popp MB, Morrison SD, Brennan MF: Total parenteral nutrition in a methyl cholanthrene induced rat sarcoma model. Cancer Treat Rep (in press)
72. Nixon D, Kutmer MH, Ansley J et al: Survival with and without hyperalimentation. Cancer Treat Rep (in press)
73. Collins JP, Oxby CB, Hill GL: Intravenous amino acids and intravenous hyperalimentation as protein-sparing therapy after major surgery. Lancet i:788–791, 1978
74. Dietl M, Vasic V, Alexander MD: Specialized nutritional support in the cancer patient. Cancer 41:2359–2363, 1978
75. Elkort RJ, Baler FL, Vitale JT et al: Optional enteral nutritional support as an adjunct to breast cancer chemotherapy. J Parent Ent Nutr 2:676–686, 1978
76. Moghissi K, Hornshaw J, Teasdale PR et al: Parenteral nutrition in carcinoma of the eosophagus treated by surgery: Nitrogen balance and clinical studies. Br J Surg 64:125–128, 1977
77. Nixon D, Rudman D, Heymsfield S et al: Response to nutritional support in cachetic patients (abstr). Am Assoc for Cancer Res #698, 1978
78. Brennan MF, Burt ME: Nitrogen metabolism in cancer. Cancer Treat Rep (in press)
79. Holyroyde CP, Myers RN, Smink RD et al: Metabolic response to total parenteral nutrition in cancer patients. Cancer Res 37:3109–3114, 1977
80. Holyroyde CP, Reichard GA: Carbohydrate metabolism in cancer cachexia. Cancer Treat Rep (in press)
81. Waterhouse C, Kemperman JH: Carbohydrate metabolism in subjects with cancer. Cancer Res 31:1273–1278, 1971
82. Waterhouse C, Jeanpetre N, Keilson J: Gluconeogenesis from alanine in patients with progressive malignant disease. Cancer Res 39:1968–1972, 1979
83. Waterhouse C: Oxidation and metabolic interconversions in malignant cachexia. Cancer Treat Rep (in press)
84. Ericksson B, Douglass HO: Intravenous hyperalimentation: An adjunct to treatment of malignant disease of upper gastrointestinal tract. JAMA 243:2049–2052, 1980
85. Ford JH, Dudan RC, Bennett JS et al: Parenteral hyperalimentation in gynecologic oncology patients. Gynecol Oncol 1:70–75, 1972

86. Lanzotti VC, Copeland EM, George SL et al: Cancer chemotherapeutic response and intravenous hyperalimentation. Cancer Chemotherapy Rep 59:437–439, 1975
87. Popp MB, Fisher RI, Simon RM et al: A prospective randomized study of adjuvant parenteral nutrition in the treatment of diffuse lymphoma: I. Effect on drug tolerance. Cancer Treat Rep (in press)
88. Douglass HO, Milliron S, Nava H et al: Elemental diet as an adjuvant for patients with locally advanced gastrointestinal cancer receiving radiation therapy. A prospectively randomized study. J. Parent Ent Nutr 2:682–686, 1978
89. Behan EA, Schneiderman MA: Experimental design of clinical trials in cancer medicine. In Cancer Medicine, Holland JF, Frei EM (eds): Philadelphia, Lea and Febiger, pp 513–514, 1973
90. Issell BF, Valdivieso M, Zaren HA et al: Protection against chemotherapy toxicity by IV hyperalimentation. Cancer Treat Rep 59:437–439, 1978
91. Lanzotti V, Copeland EM, Bhuchar V et al: A randomized trial of total parenteral nutrition (TPN) with chemotherapy for non-oat cell cancer (NOCLC) (abstr). Am Soc Clin Oncol C–277, 1980
92. Holter AR, Rosen HM, Fischer JE: The effects of hyperalimentation on major surgery in patients with malignant disease a prospective study. Acta Chir Scand (suppl) 466:86–87, 1976
93. Holter AR, Fischer JE: The effects of perioperative hyperalimentation on complications in patients with carcinoma and weight loss. J Surg Res 23:31–34, 1977
94. Heatley RV, Williams RHP, Lewis MH: Preoperative intravenous feeding—a controlled trial. Post-graduate Med J, 55:541–545, 1979
95. Valerio D, Overett MT, Malcolm A et al: Nutritional support for cancer patients receiving abdominal and pelvic radiotherapy: A randomized prospective, clinical experiment of intravenous vs oral feeding. Surg Forum 29:145–148, 1978
96. Solassol C, Joyeuz H, DuBois JB: Total parenteral nutrition (TPN) with complete nutritive mixtures. An artificial gut in cancer patients. Nutr and Cancer 1:13–18, 1979.
97. Serrou B, Cupissol D: Adjunct effect of parenteral intravenous nutrition (PIVN) depends on the tumor sensitivity to chemotherapy (abstr). Am Soc Clin Oncol C–157, 1980

Section 2

The Use of Blood and Blood Products

ROSS A. ABRAMS
ALBERT DEISSEROTH

Cancer patients frequently require hematopoietic supportive care in the form of red cell, platelet, or granulocyte transfusions. Alternatively, pheresis procedures may be required to remove from the bloodstream abnormal and excessive accumulations of either cells or proteins, when the extent of such accumulations threatens normal blood and tissue function. Finally, under circumstances where recovery of endogenous hematopoietic function has been compromised by intensive or ablative levels of antineoplastic therapy, the use of hematopoietic stem cell transfusions may be required to expeditiously restore hematopoietic function.

A rational utilization of these therapeutic options, as in all other areas of medicine, can best proceed through an understanding of their current indications, potential benefits, and possible risks. Decisions regarding the specific, clinical application of these techniques will frequently be complex, requiring both careful consideration of each of the patient's problems and consultation with other physicians. In this chapter current uses of blood component therapy, "pheresis" procedures, and hematopoietic reconstitution in the management of patients with cancer are discussed.

TRANSFUSION THERAPY

A detailed discussion of blood collection, handling, storage, cross-matching, and processing is beyond the scope of this discussion. In the discussions that follow the availability of physician-specialists trained in the complexities of blood center hematology is presumed.

In cancer management the transfusion of whole blood is rarely indicated; careful use of appropriately selected blood components is preferred in most situations.

The transfusion of any blood product may produce an undesired reaction. As summarized in Table 43-13, these reactions may take several forms and may be either "immediate" in onset, occurring within a few minutes or hours of the initiation of transfusion, or they may be delayed. As summarized by Masouredis, immediate reactions include hemolytic transfusion reactions (usually from A, B, O incompatibility), febrile reactions, allergic reactions, sepsis or septic shock due to bacterial contamination by organisms able to grow in the cold (*e.g.*, Pseudomonads or colo-aerogenes), and circulatory overload.[1] A brief summary of symptoms and physical findings associated with these reactions and an outline of management principles are summarized in Tables 43-14 and 43-15 respectively. An example of a delayed reaction is hemolysis occurring from 4 to 14 days after transfusion, involving an anamnestic response to prior recipient sensitization from an earlier transfusion or pregnancy. In these situations, a low level of antibody at the time of initial cross-matching may be undetected. When antibody titers rise in an anamnestic response to transfused red cells containing offending antigen, such red cells become antibody coated and destroyed. This phenomenon may be associated with mild levels of jaundice and a positive direct Coombs' test (direct antiglobulin test).

Thus, in this situation, the mixture of the red cells in the blood of the patient with a heterologous IgM antihuman gammaglobulin serum will show that some of the red cells in the bloodstream of the patient are coated with IgG immunoglobulin molecules, as is the case in autoimmune hemolytic anemia, with which this problem may be confused. If an indirect Coombs' test is performed (exposure of test red cells to a test serum before exposure to the heterologous IgM antihuman gammaglobulin serum), the test will be positive

TABLE 43-13. Possible Untoward Events That May Be Associated With Transfusion of Blood or Blood Components*

1. Intravascular volume overload
2. Major antibody-mediated hemolytic reactions including disseminated intravascular coagulation, bleeding, and renal compromise.
3. Hemolysis due to overwarming or rapid infusion under pressure through small bore needles.
4. Leukagglutinin reactions including fever, pulmonary infiltrates, or pulmonary distress.
5. Anaphylactic and anaphylactoid reactions involving anti-IgA antibodies in IgA deficient persons.
6. Sepsis, endotoxemia, or death from transfusion of blood components heavily contaminated with bacteria or bacterial products.
7. Transmission of viral hepatitis, malaria, syphilis, cytomegalovirus, Brucellosis, toxoplasmosis, infectious mononucleosis.
8. Air embolism, phlebitis, embolism of intravenous catheters, and other complications associated with maintaining an IV infusion.
9. Graft versus host disease (in immunocompromised recipients).
10. Complications associated with massive transfusion including potassium-citrate toxicity, dilution of platelet numbers and coagulation factors, and pulmonary accumulation of platelet-fibrin microaggregates.

*Modified from Data in Masouredis (1) and in Mollison (2). See Tables 43-14 and 43-15.

TABLE 43-14. Clinical Events Associated With Immediate Transfusion Reactions*

1. Hemolytic Transfusion Reaction—fever, low back and flank pain, nausea, chest discomfort, headache, anxiety, restlessness, flushing cyanosis, hypotension; bleeding; oliguria. Usually associated with A, B, O incompatibility and signs of intravascular hemolysis (hemoglobinemia, hemoglobinuria).
2. Febrile Reactions—fever (may occur without chills or rigor). No signs or symptoms of hemolysis associated with reactions to leukocyte or platelet antigens.
3. Allergic Reactions
   a. Urticaria (Hives), pruritis (rarely bronchospasm, angioneurotic edema, axaphylaxis)—thought to be due to sensitivity to protein components in transfused plasma.
   b. Anaphylaxis following transfusion of IgA-containing plasma to IgA deficient recipient with anti-IgA antibody (approximately one person in 500 to 1000)—dyspnea, nausea, cramps, chills, diarrhea, hypotension.
4. Transfusion of blood contaminated with bacteria—rigor, fever, hypotension, disseminated intravascular coagulation, septic shock.
5. Circulatory Overload—dyspnea, increased venous pressure, rales, other evidence of congestive heart failure.
6. Air embolism—cough, chest pain, acute onset of dyspnea. Usually not seen with current use of plastic transfusion equipment (systems are closed to external air).
7. Complications of Massive Transfusion
   a. Potassium Toxicity—EKG changes (peaked T waves, depressed S-T segments, decreased R waves, widened QRS complexes), arrhythmias, cardiac arrest.
   b. Citrate Toxicity-tremor, prolongation of Q-T interval on EKG. (Note: Potassium toxicity and citrate toxicity may reinforce each other. However, in the absence of pre-existing renal or hepatic compromise, potassium and citrate toxicity are uncommon).
   c. Hypothermia from rapid transfusion of cold blood—may increase chances of cardiac arrhythmia.

*Modified from Masouredis (1), Mollison (2), and Hickman (3).

TABLE 43-15. Outline for Managing Immediate Transfusion Reaction*

REACTION CONSIDERED	ACTION
1. Hemolytic reaction or bacterial contamination	a. Stop transfusion; maintain intravenous line. b. Save remaining donor blood—repeat cross-match; examine for gross hemolysis; culture; obtain gram stain on plasma. c. Obtain venous blood from recipient to be used for repeat cross-match and culture. d. Examine recipient plasma and urine for free hemoglobulin. e. Maintain blood pressure with intravenous fluids. Avoid blood products if cross-matching error suspected until source of error identified. If possible, avoid use of vasopressors to minimize renal damage. f. Try to maintain urine output at 100 cc/hr with intravenous fluids. If needed, use mannitol (not to exceed more than 100 gm mannitol per 24 hours). Initial mannitol dose: 25 gm intravenously over 5 minutes. g. Monitor for evidence of acute renal failure. h. If bacterial contamination present—support aggressively. Treat for septic shock. Administer broad spectrum antibiotics with emphasis on covering gram negative organisms (e.g. gentamycin or tobramycin *plus* carbenicillin or ticarcillin *plus* a cephalosporin).
2. Allergic reaction *without* anaphylaxis or bronchospasm	Consider use of antihistamine. For future transfusions, consider use of washed or resuspended blood products.
3. Febrile reaction—no evidence of hemolysis or bacterial contamination	Administer an antipyretic (caution: do not use aspirin in thrombocytopenic patients). Consider use of leukocyte-poor red cell or resedimented platelet preparations.
4. Vascular overload	Treat for pulmonary edema (diuretics, morphine, digitalis, etc). Administer only packed cells to nonbleeding patients with cardiac compromise.
5. Anaphylactic reactions and severe pulmonary reaction to leukagglutinins	Oxygen, epinephrine, fluids, antihistamines, and steroids as needed. Check for IgA deficiency in recipient. Test for leukagglutinins. Eliminate offending plasma or leukcyte antigens from future transfusions by using washed or sedimented blood components.
6. Air embolism	a. Clamp IV tubing b. Place patient on left side with head down and legs elevated (this will lift air in the right ventricle away from the pulmonary outflow tract).

*Modified from Masouredis (1), Mollison (2), and Hickman (3).

if the cells from the appropriate donor to which the patient is sensitized are incubated with the serum of the patient, but will be negative if the serum of the patient is mixed with red cells which are identical to those of the patient with respect to red cell antigens. Other delayed reactions include manifestations of disease transmitted by transfusion (hepatitis, malaria, toxoplasmosis, etc.) and the risk of iron overload in multiply transfused patients with chronic, severe anemias (secondary hemochromatosis).

Of special concern in patients undergoing intensive therapy for the management of malignant disease is the risk of developing an engraftment syndrome (graft versus host disease) following the transfusion of blood products containing viable lymphocytes into severely immunocompromised recipients. This debilitating syndrome, which presents with erythematous and exfoliative skin rashes, diarrhea, and evidence of hepatic dysfunction, may be severe or even fatal.[4] Initially reported to occur following the transfusion of blood products (especially leukocytes) from donors with chronic granulocytic leukemia, graft vs. host disease has now been observed following transfusions of platelets and granulocytes from normal donors.[5-8] Consequently, it is strongly suggested that patients undergoing intensive cytoreductive therapy (*e.g.*, induction therapy for acute leukemia, total body irradiation, and intensive levels of combined modality therapy) receive blood products that have been exposed to irradiation so as to prevent proliferation of donor lymphoid cells in the recipient after they have been transfused. The precise dose of irradiation required is unknown, but as Cohen and coworkers have indicated, radiation doses in the range of 1500–7500 rads are severely inhibitory of lymphocyte proliferation *in vitro*.[8] To stay well above the minimal dose known to be inhibitory, our practice has been to use 2500 rads to irradiate all blood products at the NCI on the clinical oncology wards. Radiation doses in this range are not known to damage the function of transfused red cells, platelets, or granulocytes. Current practice at the National Cancer Institute is to administer 2500 rads from a commercially available Cesium source to all blood products intended for patients on the in-patient cancer treatment services, outpatients recovering from intensive or ablative levels of therapy, and patients with inherent immune defects (*e.g.*, patients with Wiskott-Aldrich syndrome).

TABLE 43-16. Common Causes of Anemia in Patients With Malignancy

1. Hemorrhage—may be acute or chronic
   Common underlying factors include surgery, disruption of vascular and mucosal integrity, and thrombocytopenia.
2. Decreased red cell production—may be related to cytotoxic therapy, nutritional deficiencies, myelophthesis and impaired iron utilization (anemia of chronic illness).
3. Hemolysis—nonimmunologic mechanisms include G6PD deficiency, hypersplenism, microangiopathic destruction, and Clostridial sepsis.
   —Immunologic mechanisms may be noted in association with lymphoreticular malignancy or nonhematopoietic malignancy; occasionally following viral, mycoplasma, or bacterial infection; after the use of numerous drugs.

RED CELL TRANSFUSION

Indications

The physiologic role of the red cell is to provide oxygen (O_2) transport from the lung to body tissues. Oxygen is only minimally soluble in plasma water (0.3 ml of oxygen will dissolve in 100 ml of plasma) and the ability of blood to transport O_2 is directly dependent upon the presence of red cell hemoglobin. At normal arterial O_2 pressures (PaO_2) of 95–100 mm Hg each gram of hemoglobin is capable of reversibly binding about 1.34 ml of O_2 so that in a normal person, each 100 ml of blood is capable of carrying roughly 20 ml of O_2 of which only 1–2% is directly dissolved in plasma water.

Although hemoglobin content is critical in determining the amount of O_2 available in the blood for transport, numerous other factors are essential in determining the balance between oxygen availability and oxygen need. These include cardiac and pulmonary function for providing adequate circulation and opportunity for gaseous exchange, basal oxygen requirements, and the presence or absence of additional clinical demands for tissue oxygen including fever, sepsis, or surgery.

In practice these factors may be difficult to quantify, but the following observations can be made. Due to the well-known sigmoid shape of the oxygen-hemoglobin dissociation curve, the O_2 saturation of hemoglobin does not fall appreciably until PaO_2 levels are below 70 mm Hg. At a PaO_2 of 70 mm Hg O_2 saturation is approximately 90% and at a PaO_2 of 50 mm Hg oxygen saturation is about 80%. However, below PaO_2 levels of 50 mm Hg, O_2 saturation rapidly decreases. Second, the ability of cardiac output to increase blood flow in response to increased tissue demand for O_2, or decreased tissue availability of O_2, is limited by virtue of the heart's own oxygen needs, and the increased O_2 need imposed by tachycardia and increased stroke volume.[9] Third, major surgery, fever, and sepsis have been estimated to increase tissue demand for O_2 by 20–50% above the basal resting levels of about 250 ml/minute.[10] And, fourth, in the chronic state at least one compensatory mechanism exists within the red blood cell for increasing tissue O_2 availability. By means of increasing red cell levels of diphosphoglycerate, the hemoglobin-O_2 dissociation curve is "shifted" to the right, favoring the release of more O_2 at any given level of PaO_2.

In deciding whether to transfuse a patient these considerations should be integrated with the overall clinical setting to determine whether underlying cardiac, pulmonary, or other intercurrent conditions that might impair tolerance to anemia are present. Obviously, the etiology of the anemia should also be considered. Among the causes of anemia frequently encountered on in-patient cancer services, decreased red cell production secondary to myelosuppressive therapy and the primary disease process are usually prominent (see Table 43-16). Such patients typically receive multiple cycles of antineoplastic therapy, are regularly phlebotomized for numerous laboratory analyses, frequently become febrile, and are subject to acute and chronic blood loss in association with thrombocytopenia and mucosal disruption. Consequently, it is common practice to maintain hemoglobin levels in such patients at 10 g/100 ml, using packed red cells as necessary, in order to allow them the fullest level of function and activity permitted by their disease and its treatment.

The signs and symptoms of anemia are well known and may be either systemic (malaise, fatigueability) or organ-related (tachycardia, dyspnea, headache). However, such signs and symptoms are highly nonspecific and may exist as a consequence of numerous etiologies. When managing cancer patients such findings should not be ascribed to anemia unless other causes have been excluded and the severity of the anemia is consistent with the appearance of such symptoms (typically, hemoglobin levels of 8–9 g/100 ml or less).

The currently available red cell preparations include whole blood, packed red cells, saline washed red cells, leukocyte and platelet poor red cells, buffy coat rich cells, genotyped cells, and frozen reconstituted cells.[11] Autologous cells may also be collected in advance of anticipated need, but this approach is unlikely to be applicable to many patients with advanced hematologic or systemic malignancy.[12]

Whole blood and packed red cells are uniformly available in all blood banks. Packed red cells are obtained by separating donor plasma from the donor cells by differential centrifugation. Saline washed cells are also available in most blood banks and are generated by rinsing the packed red cells with normal saline following concentration from the donor plasma. This product is useful in patients with impaired hepatic function or frequent reactions. Buffy coat rich cells provide a mixture of platelets, leukocytes and red cells but are infrequently used due to obvious problems of interpreting any reaction which may occur to them. Buffy coat poor red cells can be obtained in most blood banks by centrifugation of the unit of whole blood in the inverted position, and expressing out of the bottom of the bag only the lower portion of the red cells, leaving the buffy coat and the platelets behind. Genotyped cells, most frequently needed in oncology in situations in which an autoantibody or alloantibody has emerged, can be obtained from larger centers if not available in the local blood bank. Frozen washed cells, indicated for use in patients whom an allograft or long-term support is anticipated, or for patients with such a rare type that donors are available from larger centers where such units are stockpiled in frozen form, are available by consultation with such larger centers.

For chronic anemias associated with malignancy, transfusion needs will generally be most appropriately met through the use of packed cells. As summarized by Becker and Aster, packed cell preparations have distinct advantages over whole blood; namely, they provide more oxygen carrying capacity at smaller transfusion volumes and are associated with decreased infusion of anticoagulant and decreased patient exposure to plasma proteins, white cells, and platelets.[13] Those patients demonstrating allergic or leukoagglutinin reactions, especially after multiple transfusions, may benefit from the use of leukocyte and platelet poor preparations, just as patients demonstrating sensitivity to plasma components may benefit from the use of washed red cells. In general, the use of whole blood should be limited, with acute, massive hemorrhage being the most common indication in patients with malignancy. However, even this use might be considered controversial by some.[11]

At present, one interesting experimental use for red cell transfusions in the setting of malignant disease seems noteworthy. In 1978 Toogood and coworkers reported their results with hypertransfusion in a small group of patients undergoing induction therapy for childhood acute lymphocytic leukemia.[14] This study was prompted by animal data suggesting that "hypertransfusion" with red cells would allow accelerated myeloid recovery by shifting hematopoietic stem cell differentiation toward myelopoiesis. By transfusing one group of patients to a median hemoglobin level of 15.1 g/100 ml, small differences in granulocyte levels were observed at 7 and 10 days after chemotherapy. However, after 14 days these differences were not significant. This concept, though interesting, requires further investigation in clinical settings and cannot at present be recommended for routine use in patients receiving systemic chemotherapy.

One final indication for red cell transfusion in the presence of "asymptomatic" anemia should be noted. Rubenstein and coworkers reported that when significant thrombocytopenia is present, severe anemia (8 g/100 ml or less) increases the likelihood of developing retinal hemorrhages.[15] Since the retina represents an extension of the CNS, retinal hemorrhages occurring in the presence of thrombocytopenia are generally felt to be an indication for platelet transfusion (*vide infra*). However, Rubenstein's data suggest that patients with retinal hemorrhages, thrombocytopenia, and substantial (8 g/100 ml), but otherwise asymptomatic, anemia might well be considered candidates for red cell, as well as platelet, transfusion.

PLATELET TRANSFUSIONS

Background

Like anemia, thrombocytopenia is a common occurrence among cancer patients, especially among those with extensive marrow replacement by malignant cells and among those receiving systemic chemotherapy or large field radiotherapy. Thus, the usual cause of thrombocytopenia in the setting of malignancy derives from underproduction of platelets (amegakaryocytic thrombocytopenia). However, the possible etiologies are diverse and important to delineate since the implications for risk of bleeding and for management vary considerably with the etiology, as well as the severity, of thrombocytopenia (see Table 43-17).[18,19]

In 1962, Gaydos, Freireich, and Mantel documented that a quantitative relationship existed between platelet count levels and the occurrence of hemorrhage in patients with acute leukemia (see Fig. 43-6).[20] In these patients the incidence of hemorrhage of any kind, as well as the incidence of gross hemorrhage rose dramatically as platelet counts declined, especially to levels less than 20,000/mm^3. They also observed that bleeding episodes occurring in association with thrombocytopenia are frequently heralded by a decline in platelet count, especially in cases where bleeding occurred at

TABLE 43-17. Causes of Thrombocytopenia in Adults

1. Acute thrombocytopenia due to increased platelet depletion (utilization, sequestration or destruction)
   a. Massive blood replacement
   b. Cardiac surgery
   c. Splenomegaly
2. Immune destruction of platelets
   a. Self-limited acute idiopathic thrombocytopenic purpura (ITP)
   b. Post-transfusion purpura
   c. Drug purpura
   d. Chronic idiopathic thrombocytopenic purpura
3. Consumptive thrombocytopenia
4. Hereditary defects
5. Thrombocytopenia with decreased platelet production
   a. Aplastic anemia
   b. Acute leukemia
   c. Idiopathic megakaryocytic aplasia
   d. Marrow infiltration—
      1. Malignant
      2. Non-malignant—Gaucher's disease, granulomatous diseases
   e. Following radiation or myelosuppressive drugs
   f. Drugs producing specific suppression of platelet production (e.g., thiazides, ethanol, estrogens)
   g. Nutritional deficiency—megaloblastic anemia, severe iron deficiency (rare)
   h. Viral infections
   i. Paroxysmal nocturnal hemoglobinuria

*Adapted from References 16 and 17.

platelet counts higher than 5000/mm³. In addition, they reported that of eight cases of intracranial hemorrhage unassociated with high blast counts and intracerebral leukostasis seven patients had platelet counts of less than 5000/mm³. No intracranial bleeding was observed at a platelet count of 10,000/mm³ or more.

These observations prompted further studies incorporating platelet transfusion in the management of leukemia. Subsequently the value of platelet transfusions for controlling thrombocytopenic hemorrhage, for preventing thrombocytopenic hemorrhage, and for preventing death from hemorrhage were all well documented.[21–24]

The risk of hemorrhage in leukemic patients supported on a regimen of four units of single donor platelets is a function of the type of leukemia and the regimen used for its treatment. In good risk childhood acute lymphocytic leukemia, the risk of hemorrhage from the disease or its treatment is low. However, thrombocytopenia requiring intensive platelet support is almost a universal concomitant of standard induction regimens for acute myelogenous leukemia. In the hypergranular form of acute promyelocytic leukemia, in which disseminated intravascular coagulation, consumptive thrombopathy and hemorrhage occur, management may involve heparin in addition to fresh frozen plasma and transfusions of platelets. Following the infusion of a single donor four unit transfusion in a patient in whom thrombocytopenia arises not only from decreased production but also from increased peripheral destruction, one should obviously not expect a post-transfusion increment of 23,000/mm³/unit/M² or 13,000/mm³/unit M² which one would ideally predict in a normal person at one or 24 hours, respectively. Even in a patient whose platelets are not being consumed at an accelerated rate, one-third of the infused platelets do not appear in the peripheral blood but are sequestered in the spleen.

The clinical correlates of thrombocytopenia are well known. In the presence of otherwise normal platelet function thrombocytopenia is usually not clinically evident until platelet counts of less than 50,000/mm³ are observed, when petechiae and ecchymoses may begin to appear spontaneously especially in dependent areas such as the lower legs in ambulatory patients and the buttocks and back in bed-ridden patients.

The bleeding time may be slightly prolonged at platelet counts below 100,000/mm³ but begins to be significantly prolonged below 60,000/mm³. The Ivy bleeding time is a means of establishing the existence of clinically significant

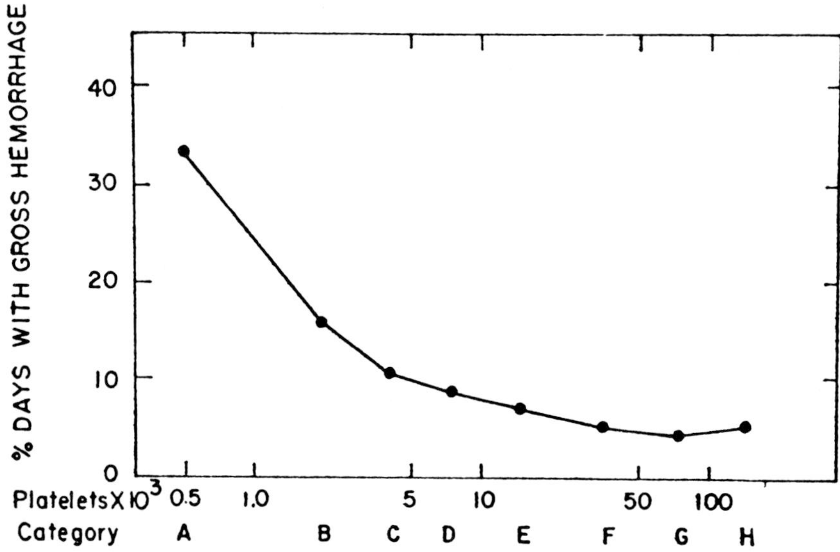

FIG. 43-6. Relationship between platelet count and the number of days spent by a patient with grossly visible hemorrhage. Capital letters along the abscissa refer to the following categories of platelet counts: *A* = less than 1,000/mm³, *B* = 1,000–3,000/mm³, *C* = 3,000–5,000/mm³, *D* = 5,000–10,000/mm³, *E* = 10,000–20,000/mm³, *F* = 20,000–50,000/mm³, *G* = 50,000–100,000/mm³, and *H* = greater than 100,000/mm³.

qualitative or quantitative defects of platelet function. (A spring lancet is applied to the volar surface of the arm to produce three small wounds, 3 mm deep. The time to achieve hemostasis is measured, by blotting excess blood from each incision, but never touching the clot forming at the incision itself. A normal bleeding time is from 1–9 minutes.) Epistaxis may also be observed at this time, and occasionally these findings will be observed with platelet counts between 50,000 and 100,000 mm^3. As platelet counts continue to decline below 50,000/mm^3 the incidence of nasal and dermal bleeding and bleeding from mucosal surfaces (gastrointestinal, genitourinary, pulmonary) also increases. Although as elegantly demonstrated by Slichter and Harker, otherwise stable patients (no fever, taking no drugs) with chronic thrombocytopenia may tolerate extremely low platelet counts (5,000–10,000/mm^3) without incidence of increased blood loss from the GI tract as compared to normals; the use of prednisone or semisynthetic penicillins substantially increases blood loss into the stool when such levels of thrombocytopenia are present.[18]

For many years clinicians were confused by an apparent lack of correlation between the level of thrombocytopenia and severity of bleeding when groups of patients with thrombocytopenias of diverse etiologies were observed. It is now well established that hemostatic effectiveness is a function of platelet age, with younger platelets being more efficient than older platelets in promoting hemostatic effectiveness.[25] Younger platelets are morphologically distinguishable from senescent platelets by size (they are larger) and by other structural and biochemical characteristics.[25,26] The single best measure of overall platelet function is generally agreed to be the standardized Ivy bleeding time when rigorously performed in a systematic way.[27] Using this test, Harker and Slichter convincingly demonstrated that between platelet counts of 10,000 and 100,000/mm^3 bleeding time increases in a strictly linear fashion as platelet counts decrease because of platelet underproduction (in contrast to increased destruction) and that at platelet counts below 10,000/mm^3 bleeding times are invariably in excess of 30 minutes (normal 4.5 ± 1.5 minutes in their hands). These data agree well with the earlier observations made by Gaydos and coworkers regarding clinical bleeding and thrombocytopenia. Their data also demonstrated that at any given level of thrombocytopenia, patients with immune thrombocytopenic purpura (ITP) and patients in the early phase of bone marrow recovery from chemotherapy have substantially shorter bleeding times than patients with ongoing thrombocytopenia from underproduction. This observation further supports the concept of improved hemostatic efficiency of younger platelets, since in ITP there is rapid destruction of circulating platelets and increased platelet turnover, and by definition platelet age is decreased as platelet counts are rising during recovery from chemotherapy-induced bone marrow suppression.

Platelet transfusion differs from red cell transfusion in several important respects. Under normal circumstances red cells have a mean survival of 120 days, whereas platelets survive only 9–10 days.[28] Aside from the well-known, numerous red cell antigens that form the basis for defining crossmatching criteria, red cells apparently do not contain other tissue antigens. In contrast, platelets do contain these antigens on their surfaces and recipients who are not immunosuppressed may quickly become alloimmunized to these antigens, of which the HLA antigens are perhaps the best known.[29] Once alloimmunization has occurred, platelet survival is seriously diminished and patients may become "refractory" to the beneficial effects of further platelet transfusions, unless proper identification and matching for known HLA antigens are carried out.[30–32] Under normal circumstances red cells are not significantly sequestered in the spleen and in the absence of disseminated intravascular coagulation (consumption coagulopathy) (DIC) their survival is not usually compromised by the presence of fever or sepsis. In contrast, even normal sized spleens routinely sequester 20–30% of both endogenous and transfused platelets, especially younger platelets and platelet survival is strikingly decreased in the presence of fever.[31,33–35] Finally, whereas red cells may be stored for up to 21 days after collection, platelets can be routinely stored for only 2–3 days even when maintained at 22°.[36]

Although much controversy has surrounded the way in which platelets are stored, most authorities now feel that the optimal manner in which to store platelets is at 22°C on a rocking platform rather than at 4°C.[36] With the former method, the post transfusion increments are higher than when platelets are stored at 4°C. Poor post-transfusion increments frequently accompany clinical settings which include fever, sepsis, disseminated intravascular coagulation, or splenomegaly. When efforts to control fever, sepsis, or disseminated intravascular coagulation are successfully undertaken, post-transfusion platelet increments will frequently improve. The occurrence of thrombocytopenia in a setting which includes clinical splenomegaly and poor post-transfusion platelet increments raises two questions: namely, the extent to which the splenomegaly is contributing to the thrombocytopenia as well as the extent to which the splenomegaly is impairing response to platelet transfusion therapy. In such settings, careful assessment must be undertaken before rational management can occur. Careful review of the patient's recent management (*e.g.*, underlying diseases, recent exposure to chemotherapy) and assessment of megakaryocyte numbers by bone marrow aspirate or biopsy will be helpful in differentiating platelet underproduction from platelet sequestration and destruction in the spleen. Valuable clinical information may also be achieved through empiric trials of leukocyte-poor platelets or HLA-matched platelets. In some cases, platelet sequestration studies, measurement of surface bound platelet immunoglobulin, and determination of one hour and 24-hour post transfusion increments may also be of help. Splenomegaly due to infiltration of these organs by neoplastic cells is usually approached through the conventional use of chemotherapy or radiation therapy. Splenectomy is reserved for the rare patient in whom profound thrombocytopenia is life threatening, in whom the thrombocytopenia has been shown to be due in large part to that organ and no other, who is unresponsive to HLA matched platelets, and in whom the irradiation and chemotherapy have been shown to be ineffective in managing the splenomegaly or in whom its use is contraindicated by the splenomegaly.

A unit of platelets is defined as the number of platelets routinely harvested from a unit of fresh whole blood.[37] Initially, this was an operational definition since platelets for transfusion could only be prepared by generating platelet rich plasma from whole blood using standard phlebotomy and centrifugation techniques. Harvesting platelets in this manner from single unit donations of whole blood usually yields about 0.7 $\times 10^{11}$ platelets per unit and initial studies on the efficacy of platelet transfusion were performed by pooling the platelets harvested from single unit donations from several donors for each transfusion.[21–23]

Platelet donation requires only 2–3 hours to complete, and involves the insertion of one or two venous needles, and thus is tolerated well by most donors.

Studies exploring the possibility of removing multiple units of platelets from individual donors at a single donation have been undertaken.[35,38] These efforts were prompted by recognition of the rapid allosensitization that occurred from exposing patient-recipients to the tissue antigens from multiple donors with each pooled platelet transfusion and of the increased risk for transmission of hepatitis when pooled products are used.[38] These studies demonstrated that several units of platelets can be safely removed from individual donors at a single sitting providing donor platelet counts are monitored. Using this approach, donors are serially phlebotomized of several units of whole blood, one at a time. Platelet rich plasma is generated by a "gentle" centrifugation (800 rpm/10 minutes) and the platelets are then concentrated by a "harder" centrifugation (2700 rpm/10 minutes) of the platelet rich plasma. The red cells and plasma are returned to the donor and the process repeated. This methodology usually provides a minimum of 0.5-0.6 $\times 10^{11}$ platelets per unit of whole blood processed, and 3–4 units are usually processed in a single sitting.[38]

Currently available blood cell separators are also used extensively for collecting multiple units of platelets from individual donors.[39,40] These instruments provide direct connection between the donor and the centrifuge used to separate the blood into its components. In these systems blood flow between the donor and the instrument is either continuous throughout the donation period (Aminco, IBM instruments) or semicontinuous (Haemonetics). The platelet product obtained using the Haemonetics model 30 separator has been directly compared to platelets obtained by multiunit platelet pheresis of single donors and no advantage observed in terms of post-transfusion increments, even though the efficiency of collection was somewhat better with the cell separator.[41]

The optimal collection, preparation, and storage of platelet concentrates have been subjects of intensive study.[36] Numerous factors have been identified as important in promoting optimal platelet collection, yield, viability, and post-transfusion increment. These include the type of anticoagulant, type of plastic collection bag, temperature of storage, agitation during storage, and amount of residual plasma remaining with the concentrated platelets.[36] In general, platelet viability declines rapidly during storage, and platelets more than 72 hours old are currently not felt to be satisfactory for clinical use. Platelets stored at 4°C have been shown to produce substantially lower transfusion increments than platelets stored at 22°C, and to have a shorter half-life in the recipient's circulation.[36]

RATIONAL USE OF PLATELET THERAPY

Rational platelet therapy seeks to optimize the balance among three factors: risk to the patient from thrombocytopenic bleeding, risk to the patient from transfusion, and scarcity of platelets as a support commodity. In the setting of thrombocytopenia from marrow failure (underproduction of platelets) previously cited data suggest that risk of spontaneous, serious hemorrhage begins to have clinical significance at platelet counts below 20,000/mm^3 and in the absence of leukostasis the risk of spontaneous intracranial bleeding appears to be substantially increased at platelet counts of 10,000/mm^3 or less.[20] Although stable, afebrile patients with thrombocytopenia from underproduction may tolerate levels of thrombocytopenia of 5,000–10,000/mm^3 very well, patients with malignancy and thrombocytopenia are clearly at risk of spontaneous serious hemorrhage when platelet counts fall below 20,000/mm^3. Such patients are susceptible to numerous problems which may compromise platelet function including fever, sepsis, the use of medications that interfere with platelet function, and disruption of normal vascular and mucosal integrity by the presence of neoplastic tissue. Consequently, most authors choose to use platelet transfusions prophylactically in nonbleeding cancer patients at counts in the range of 20,000–30,000/mm^3.[22,23,37,39] The prophylactic use of platelets in doses in the range of 2–5 units per transfusion given as needed up to once every 24 hours to maintain platelet counts in excess of 25,000/mm^3 or given 2–3 times per week have been demonstrated to decrease all bleeding episodes by 86% in one study and 53% in another.[22,23] In these same studies the incidences of serious bleeding were decreased by 70 to 90%, respectively.[22,23] Although the results of Roy and coworkers involved the use of an historic control group, the results reported by Higby and coworkers were obtained in a prospective randomized fashion.[22,23] In the study of Roy and coworkers three groups of leukemic children were studied, One in which prophylactic transfusions were not used and two in which different doses of platelets were used. In both transfusion groups, the incidence of serious bleeding episodes was less than 4% while that of the non-transfused group was 11.8%. This study was not prospectively randomized; rather both transfused groups were compared with a "historic control" group which was not supported prophylactically. In the study of Higby and coworkers, 18 patients with thrombocytopenia were prospectively randomized in a double blind manner between two groups: one in which each patient received one 4 unit transfusion of platelets/day and another group in which no platelet transfusions were used.[23] Serious hemorrhage occurred in 3/12 patients in the transfused group while 6/9 patients in the non-transfused group had serious hemorrhage. The total incidence of bleeding episodes in the transfused and non-transfused groups was 5/12 and 8/9 respectively, in this study which showed no difference in the daily platelet pre-transfusion platelet counts in the two groups of patients.[23]

In the presence of established serious hemorrhage in association with thrombocytopenia from underproduction of platelets, exact criteria for platelet transfusion therapy are less well defined. Djerassi and coworkers achieved hemostasis using 0.08 to 0.10 units of platelet concentrate per pound of recipient and Han and coworkers also reported good results in controlling hemorrhage using a similar dose of 0.2 units/kg.[21,37] In the latter study, platelet transfusions were given daily in the presence of fresh hemorrhage or fever or as infrequently as 3–4 times weekly if platelet counts of 50,000/mm³ were achieved or bleeding controlled with this less intensive support.

Although the theoretically expected increment in platelet count from the transfusion of a unit of platelets is about 10,000–12,000/mm³, increments of this magnitude are seldom, if ever, achieved in bleeding, febrile patients especially if there is associated sepsis, splenomegaly, or an extensive history of prior transfusions.[32] Management of thrombocytopenic bleeding in such cases can be extremely difficult and transfusion decisions must be predicated on platelet availability, the expected overall prognosis of the patient's clinical situation, and the patient's bleeding status after transfusion. In those circumstances where minimal increments in platelet count are observed, platelet survival is usually shortened to substantially less than 24 hours. Under these circumstances the authors have used frequent, small doses of platelets (*e.g.*, two units every 4–6 hours). Whether this approach has any significant advantage over giving a similar total dose as a single bolus every 24 hours is to our knowledge not documented.

In the presence of hemorrhage and less severe thrombocytopenia (platelet counts between 20,000 and 50,000/mm³) the authors usually recommend platelet transfusion up to a count of 50,000/mm³ in addition to whatever definitive local measures are necessary. This approach is based in part on the bleeding time observations of Harker and Slichter previously cited and the surgical impression that platelet counts of 50,000/mm³ will permit adequate hemostasis during operation.[27,42] With platelet counts in excess of 50,000/mm³ the authors are reluctant to recommend platelet transfusions as the only therapy for hemorrhage unless factors such as surgically correctable lesions, thrombocytopathy or concomitant use of drugs known to interfere with platelet function have been ruled out.

REFRACTORINESS TO PLATELET TRANSFUSION

Yankee and colleagues have demonstrated that patients with protracted thrombocytopenia in association with marrow failure states such as aplastic anemia will, in time, become refractory to platelet transfusions from randomly selected donors when such patients are repetitively transfused with platelets.[29–32] This "refractory state" was shown to be "reversible" through the use of platelet transfusions selected from donors matched at HLA A a and B loci. Unfortunately, the HLA system is extremely polymorphic involving approximately 60 antigens. Since each person may harbor up to four antigens, the chances of a random donor matching any given recipient are vanishingly small. In addition, there appears to be substantial variability in the rate at which refractoriness will develop. Refractoriness due to HLA alloimmunization should not be confused with the previously cited, nonspecific factors of fever, sepsis, and splenomegaly. Also, refractoriness due to leukoagglutinin reactions directed at non-HLA leukocyte antigens can be distinguished from HLA refractoriness. Such leukoagglutinin reactions, which may also be associated with transient exacerbations of leukopenia, can be ameliorated by decreasing leukocyte contamination of platelet concentrates.[43,44] Both platelets obtained by simple platelet pheresis and platelets collected using cell separators contain substantial numbers of leukocytes (primarily mononuclear leukocytes) usually in ratio of 1:100 with the platelets.[44,45] Herzig and coworkers demonstrated that a "gentle" centrifugation at 178 xg for 3 minutes at room temperature would allow separation of 96% of these contaminating leukocytes with 79% recovery of platelet numbers.[44] These leukocyte-poor platelet concentrates were associated with improved platelet increments and diminished incidence of transfusion reactions.

In thinking about which patients will eventually require HLA matched platelet support, one should consider the following: most patients with acute leukemia undergoing induction therapy will require platelet support for two or more weeks, while only 30% of solid tumor patients will develop sufficient thrombocytopenia to require platelet support. Only 16% of the total number of patients on an oncology service in whom intensive therapy is used will ultimately develop a pattern which is suggestive of sensitization to non-HLA matched platelets. Thus, the oncologist will find it necessary to procure an HLA phenotyping only in those solid tumor patients in whom the probability of relapse is significant and for whom intensive therapeutic protocols exist. In addition, all acute leukemia patients and their siblings should be HLA typed for future platelet support as well as the investigation of the family for potential allograft donors. A 15 cc tube of venous blood with preservative free heparin is adequate for most typing centers.

Recent advances in the use of "selective" HLA mismatching have been reported by Duquesnoy and coworkers and reviewed by Schiffer.[40,46,47] However, as Schiffer points out, in the immunosuppressed host alloimmunization appears to require a minimum of 4–6 weeks before refractoriness to random platelets will occur.[40] Although this time period may be approached by the periods of aplasia seen during intensive therapy of leukemia and other selected neoplasms, the importance of HLA matching for patients needing infrequent, occasional platelet transfusions during the course of cyclic chemotherapy is completely unclear. In fact, according to Schiffer, even the importance of single donor platelets in such settings is not well established and should remain a subject of continued investigation.[40]

Non-Transfusion Considerations in the Management of Thrombocytopenia

In the presence of thrombocytopenia, IM injections are to be avoided in an effort to minimize the development of painful, intramuscular hematomas. In the presence of granulocytopenia such hematomas may be sites of infection. When administering pharmacologic agents to such patients, if parenteral administration is required, the IV route should be selected whenever possible. Physicians should also bear in mind that numerous drugs impact adversely both on platelet function as measured *in vitro* and on bleeding time measurement *in vivo*.[48,49] This has been most clearly demonstrated for acetylsalicylic acid (aspirin) but apparently is true for the other nonsteroidal anti-inflammatory agents as well, including indomethacin, phenylbutazone, and meclofenamic acid.[49] Plasma expanders such as dextran and hydroxyethyl starch are associated with prolonged bleeding times and other drugs have been shown *in vitro* to impair platelet function, although the *in vivo* significance of these observations is less well documented.[49] Agents in this category include tricyclic antidepressants, antihistamines, phenothiazines, and some penicillin-derived antibiotics.[48,49]

Drugs affecting platelet function listed in the 1974 edition of Clinical Hematology by Wintrobe include anti-inflammatory drugs (aspirin, phenylbutazone, sulfinpyrazone, indomethacin), antidepressants (chlorpromazine, promethazine, reserpine, imipramine, and amitryptyline), andrenergic blocking agents (phentolamine and dihydroergotomine), and several in a miscellaneous category (ethanol, clofibrate, dipyridamole, diphenhydramine, papevarine, and carbenicillin). In addition, platelet function is impaired in various clinical settings including uremia and possibly liver disease, some cases of dysproteinemia, and in association with various hematologic disorders, especially the myeloproliferative syndromes. In women with thrombocytopenia, uterine hemorrhage of substantial degree may be associated with the menses. If necessary, this can be suppressed by using progestational agents. One such regimen suggested by Gardner uses an initial parenteral dose of 300 mg of medroxyprogesterone acetate followed by daily oral doses of 20 mg of the same agent.[19] Women receiving chemotherapy that does not result in profound depression of the platelet count (below 20,000/mm^3) or in whom a single episode of intensive induction is therapy followed by less intensive maintenance therapy may not require suppression of menses. The decision to suppress menses must be individualized to the patient, the schedule and intensity of the regimen, and the patient's response to the treatment. It must also be remembered that continuous suppression of menses eventually leads to breakthrough bleeding and significant uterine bleeding. Thus, in patients requiring suppression for prolonged periods, it is prudent to suppress them for this period, but to then withdraw suppressive therapy during periods of high platelet count, so as to avoid the occurrence of breakthrough bleeding during periods of low platelet count.

COMPLICATIONS OF PLATELET TRANSFUSIONS

Although any of the known complications of transfusion therapy may be associated with the use of platelets, a few are worthy of additional emphasis. The amount of red cell contamination present in platelet concentrates varies from unit to unit and with the method of preparation. Although, in general, platelets may be transfused across incompatibilities for the major red cell antigens (A,B,0), this practice should probably be avoided when gross red cell contamination is present.[22,47] There is a definite, though small, risk of bacterial contamination in platelet units stored at 22°C. In the presence of febrile reactions to platelets, many of which will be due to leukoagglutinin reactions, the possibility of bacterial contamination should be considered. Among patients with concomitant granulocytopenia the prompt institution of broad spectrum antibiotics directed at gram-negative organisms (especially pseudomonads and colon-aerogenes groups) and the obtaining of cultures of both the platelet concentrate and patient's blood should be undertaken whenever bacterial contamination is strongly suspected.

As previously cited, the risk of graft versus host disease from the large number of allogeneic lymphocytes present in platelet concentrates is present when dealing with severely immunosuppressed recipients and in these settings platelet concentrates should be irradiated prior to transfusion.[8] A dose of 2500 rads would appear to be adequate.[4,50]

GRANULOCYTE TRANSFUSION

The two most frequent causes of death among cancer patients are infection and bleeding, together accounting for consistently greater than 90% of mortality.[24,51] With the development and availability of platelet transfusions for controlling episodes of thrombocytopenic hemorrhage infection has remained as a frequent cause of death.[51,52] In 1966, Bodey and coworkers demonstrated the relationship of increasingly severe granulocytopenia to increased incidence and severity of infection. Their data also suggested that among patients with acute leukemia and granulocytopenia a relationship exists between granulocyte response to infection and the probability of mortality from the infectious episode. As shown in Table 43-18, both the percent of days with infection and the number of severe infections per 1000 patient days increased as granulocyte counts declined below a level of 1000/mm^3 with the highest rates of infection being observed below granulocyte counts of 100/mm^3. In the same paper these authors also demonstrated that a decline in granulocyte counts to levels below 1000, 500, or 100/mm^3 were associated with increasing frequency of severe infectious episodes (10%, 19%, and 28% respectively); that 100% of patients with granulocyte counts below 100/mm^3 and 50–60% of patients with granulocytes below 1000/mm^3 would be infected by 3 weeks and that among these same patient groups 100% and 70% would be afflicted with severe infection by 6 weeks. Severe infection was defined as urinary tract infection, pneumonia, septicemia, or evidence

TABLE 43-18. Relationship Between Granulocytopenia and Infections

Granulocyte Level (cells/mm^3)	<100	100–500	500–1000	1000–1500	>1500
% of Patient Days with Infection	53	38	20	10	11
Number of Severe Infections Per 1000 Patient Days	43	20	12	5	5

*Modified from Bodey et al (53).

of systemic fungal dissemination. Finally, their data demonstrated that for patients with less than 1000 granulocytes/mm^3, failure of granulocyte counts to rise above a level of 1000 mm^3 within one week of developing severe infection was associated with a mortality rate of 40%. If the granulocyte count did not rise at all or, instead fell, the mortality rate was about 60%. In spite of the improvements in antibacterial chemotherapy that have occurred since 1966, the validity of these observations regarding infection, granulocyte count, and response of granulocyte count to infection persists as demonstrated by recent data summarized by Gaya.[54] He observed that among patients being managed with two drug combinations of potent antibiotics (carbenicillin, gentamycin, and cephalothin) favorable outcome of infectious episodes still depended on the initial granulocyte count at the time of infection and the response of the granulocyte count during infection.

In essence, the data of Bodey and coworkers for granulocytes were analogous to the data of Gaydos and coworkers, cited above, for platelets.[20] Just as Gaydos and coworkers had established a relationship between thrombocytopenia and bleeding and a level of thrombocytopenia above which risk of serious hemorrhage appeared reduced, Bodey and coworkers had established qualitative and quantitative correlations between granulocytopenia and infection.

Logically, these data would suggest that patients with granulocytopenia should receive transfusions at granulocytes adequate to sustain granulocyte counts at levels of 1000/mm^3 until endogenous granulocyte recovery occurs.

Unfortunately, as a practical matter, this is virtually impossible. In contrast to red cells and even platelets, granulocytes are more difficult to collect, occupy several body space "compartments" in addition to the intravascular space, and have a normal half-life in the circulation measured in hours rather than days or weeks.

Golde and Cline have summarized relevant data regarding granulocyte kinetics and compartments.[55] It appears that granulocytes move in essentially a unidirectional manner from the bone marrow to the blood, and eventually into tissue spaces where they expire. The total blood granulocyte pool can be shown to consist of two components, namely those granulocytes actually in the circulating blood and an approximately equivalent number apparently marginated along the endothelium of small vessels. This marginated granulocyte pool is considered part of the total blood pool because under appropriate circumstances (exercise, stress, or epinephrine injection) the cells of the marginated pool enter the circulating blood stream. The mean size of the total blood granulocyte pool and the mean blood clearance of circulating granulocytes have been reported as 7.0×10^8 granulocyte per kilogram and 6.7 hours respectively, suggesting a mean granulocyte turnover rate of 1.6×10^9/kg/day.[56] Thus, for a normal 70 kg man the total blood granulocyte pool should be about 4.9×10^{10} and the number of granulocytes produced per day about 1.1×10^{11}.

In contrast, the number of granulocytes that may be collected from a single unit of blood from a normal donor is only about 5×10^8, or about 1% of a normal total blood granulocyte pool.[57] Following development of blood cell separators using either continuous or intermittent blood flow, collection capabilities were increased to about $1.1–1.4 \times 10^9$ granulocytes/hour and the incorporation of Rouleauxing agents such as hydroxyethyl starch further increased collection capabilities to about $2.7–4.6 \times 10^9$ cells/hour.[57] Based on early experience using patients with chronic myelogenous leukemia as donors of granulocytes for neutropenic patients, it was known that neutrophilia increased the ease with which granulocytes could be collected from blood and that there was a dose response between infection control and increasing the number of granulocytes transfused.[58] Thus, efforts were undertaken to induce granulocytosis in normal donors by administering steroids such as dexamethasone or etiocholanolone.[59,60]

It was also observed that granulocytes could be collected in large numbers by perfusing nylon filters with donor blood, allowing the granulocytes to adhere to the nylon surfaces while returning the blood to the donor, and then washing the granulocytes from the filter for transfusion. This procedure was observed to yield about 1.1×10^{10} granulocytes per hour.[61,62]

Thus, granulocyte collections containing roughly $1.0–2.0 \times 10^{10}$ granulocytes could be obtained over 2–4 hours by these improved methodologies.[57] Even so, such collections represent only 10–20% of the estimated granulocyte turnover per day for an adult and can be expected to survive in the circulation for only brief periods of time based on the known half-life of 6.7 hours for circulating granulocytes. Using DF^{32}P labeling techniques one can also demonstrate that about half of all transfused granulocytes marginate.[63]

These factors make substantial increments in granulocyte counts difficult to obtain by transfusion, and the logistics and expense of collection (including donor, nurse, physician, hematology, and blood banking technical efforts) make the use of multiple daily collections pragmatically unattractive. Moreover, at the present time granulocytes cannot be routinely stored for periods in excess of 24 hours, although efforts at both liquid and frozen preservation are being studied.[64–67]

A substantial body of data, based on *in vitro* measurement of granulocyte functions and dose studies of granulocytes required to protect neutropenic animals from experimentally induced infection, suggest that granulocytes collected by filtration leukapheresis may suffer functional impairment as compared to granulocytes collected by flow leukapheresis.[68–70] However, there is no question that both filtration leukapheresis and flow leukapheresis yield granulocyte collections, which have been shown to be clinically efficacious, and it is possible that the increased numbers of granulocytes obtained by filtration techniques compensate for any qualitative deficit they may harbor.[71–73] Recent improvements in the technology of continuous flow equipment have been shown to substantially increase granulocyte collection efficacy.[74] Since filtration leukapheresis collections and transfusions are associated with substantially more adverse donor and recipient reactions (side effects), such improved technology may further encourage the use of flow collection techniques over filtration techniques.

Based on several clinical trials of granulocyte transfusion that have been reported, the patient who is most likely to benefit from granulocyte transfusion would appear to be defined by the following characteristics: granulocyte count of less than 1000/mm^3 or perhaps even less than 500/mm^3;

documented or very probable source of gram negative bacterial infection (in contrast to unexplained fever); bone marrow recovery not expected earlier than 10 days following the beginning of the septic episode.[71-73,75] In such patient populations granulocyte transfusions have been consistently shown to be associated with statistically significant increases in survival (see Table 43-19).

Based on these data we are inclined to offer granulocyte support under the following circumstances: granulocyte count less than 500/mm³; documented gram (−) sepsis (+ blood culture) or strong clinical evidence of gram negative bacterial pneumonia or other specific site of gram negative bacterial infection; early bone marrow recovery not expected; failure to show clinical improvement within 24 hours of instituting appropriate, broad spectrum antibiotic coverage; overall clinical setting and prognosis warranting the use of aggressive clinical supportive measures. Since there is no foolproof way with which to predict in any given cycle of therapy the precise time course of hematopoietic recovery (hematopoietic recovery times seen during several sequential cycles of therapy may abruptly change when sepsis or other complications supervene), we recommend initiation of granulocyte transfusions on a daily basis in all patients documented to have gram negative sepsis, fever and a granulocyte count below 500/mm³ without waiting to see how rapidly the granulocyte count will return to levels above 500/mm³.

These criteria are consistent with those recently suggested by Higby and Bennett, but should only be viewed as guidelines to be applied during a careful risk-benefit analysis of any particular clinical situation under consideration.[76]

In an excellent, detailed review of the entire field of leukapheresis and granulocyte transfusion, McCullough has summarized the various reactions reported for donors and recipients of granulocytes.[77]

During both flow and filtration procedures donors have reported anxiety, chills, vasovagal reactions, nausea, arm pain, fever, menorrhagia, and possible heparin allergy.

In the case of granulocytes collected by nylon wool filtration leukapheresis sequestration of granulocytes in the pulmonary capillary bed due to the presence of activated fragments of complement is very frequent, but this complication is rare in granulocytes collected by continuous flow centrifugation. Almost every Red Cross center as well as most university blood banks will have the equipment necessary for such support. Small hospitals, or hospitals in which such support is not available can procure granulocytes for their patients by consultation with larger centers. Blood banks in hospitals in which intensive therapy is not routine have no need to become involved with granulocyte transfusions. Obviously, centers without adequate hematologic support capabilities should not be engaged in treatment regimens known to result in significant frequency of complications requiring such support.

Recipient reactions also occur, and are substantially more frequent when filtration cells are infused. Pulmonary reactions may be particularly severe and Wright has recently suggested an association between pulmonary reactions of a severe degree and the concomitant use of amphotericin among patients receiving granulocyte transfusions.[78] In such patients the concomitant use of amphotericin and granulocyte transfusions was associated with dyspnea, arterial hypoxemia, and pulmonary infiltrates, which were shown to be associated with pulmonary hemorrhage on a microscopic level. This picture was observed by Wright and coworkers in 33% of patients in whom amphotericin had been initiated following the initiation of granulocytes. Patients in whom amphotericin is started a week in advance of granulocyte transfusions, do not exhibit the high frequency of pulmonary reactions. Higby and Bennett have suggested five mechanisms for pulmonary reactions associated with granulocyte transfusion including congestive heart failure, granulocyte sequestration in infected pulmonary lesions, interaction of transfused granulocytes with circulating endotoxins, intravascular aggregation of leukocytes by circulating leukoagglutinins, and administration of aggregated leukocytes.[76] Their management suggestions include the usual intervention in cases of suspected congestive heart failure and for other causes the administration of 100–200 mg of hydrocortisone, discontinuing the transfusion, and providing other supportive care as indicated.

Beyond cross-matching for ABO and Rh compatibility, (granulocyte collections are invariably "contaminated" with obvious and measurable numbers of red cells, essentially about 30–100 cc of red cells per collection), the role of other immunologic matching (*e.g.*, for HLA-antigens or leukoagglutinins) remains substantially more controversial.[56,76] Matching of these other two parameters has been shown to be associated with higher post-transfusion increments, but leukoagglutinins apparently do not predict for transfusion reactions, and neither HLA antigens nor leukoagglutinins have been documented to be of importance in promoting the efficacy of granulocyte transfusion.[51,79]

The role of prophylactic granulocyte transfusions remains experimental. Such studies are difficult to design and execute.

TABLE 43-19. Granulocyte Transfusion Clinical Trials Survival—Survival

STUDY	REF.	TRANSFUSED WITH GRANULOCYTES	CONTROLS	P
Herzig, 1977[a]	71	8/12	0/8	<0.005
Alvai, 1977[b]	72	6/8	2/10	0.03
Vogler, 1977[c]	75	6/9	0/8	0.01

[a]Patients with documented sepsis; delayed marrow recovery, granulocytes less than 1000/mm³

[b]Patients with documented infection, delayed marrow recovery, granulocytes less than 250/mm³

[c]Patients with documented infection, granulocytes less than 300/mm³, no response to 72 hours of appropriate antibiotics

In the setting of bone marrow transplantation, Clift has demonstrated decreased incidence of infection but no difference in mortality using predominantly HLA matched granulocytes from each recipient's bone marrow donor.[80] The importance of prophylactic granulocytes in less rigorous settings is even less clearly defined.

Among infected patients in whom granulocyte support has been initiated, granulocyte transfusions should be continued daily until endogenous bone marrow recovery occurs, the infection is completely controlled, or the overall prognosis is irreversibly altered by deterioration apparently unrelated to the infectious process.

SURGICAL EMERGENCIES IN PATIENTS WITH NEUTROPENIA OR THROMBOCYTOPENIA

The availability of platelet concentrates and granulocyte transfusions, as discussed above, has had a substantial impact on the management of thrombocytopenic hemorrhage and serious infection in the presence of profound neutropenia. In addition, there has been increasing recognition that judicious utilization of these support modalities may permit surgical intervention for abdominal catastrophes (*e.g.*, perforated viscus, peritonitis, typhlitis) which, if left unoperated, would likely lead to mortality in patients with severe thrombocytopenia or neutropenia.[81-84] Although the difficulties of correct preoperative diagnosis in such patient populations are substantial, the use of platelet concentrates to maintain platelet counts above 50,000/mm³ has been associated with effective surgical hemostasis.[81] Similarly, there would appear to be a role for the use of granulocyte support in these settings along with appropriate broad spectrum antibiotics.[84] Surgical decisions involving patients with severe hematopoietic compromise remain difficult. Clinical settings requiring such decisions are clearly ominous, and mortality will undoubtedly remain significant.[82,83] However, it does appear that adequate platelet and granulocyte support can make *necessary* emergency surgery in cytopenic patients at least technically feasible by helping to control both hemorrhagic and infectious sequelae.

PHERESIS PROCEDURES IN THE MANAGEMENT OF MALIGNANT DISEASE

Currently available blood cell separators have substantial versatility for selectively extracting blood components from patients as well as donors. Although this methodology has been used experimentally in a number of chronic settings, for example lymphocyte removal in chronic lymphocytic leukemia, Sezary syndrome, leukemic reticuloendotheliosis, and chronic phase chronic myelocytic leukemia, there are several acute situations where selective pheresis would appear to be of definite clinical value in controlling and preventing the sequelae of unrestrained proliferation of immature leukocytes (blasts), platelets, and immunoglobulin into the blood.[85-87] Specifically, the risks of intracerebral and intrapulmonary leukostasis associated with circulating leukemic blast counts in excess of 50,000/mm³, of bleeding or thrombosis in association with platelet counts in excess of 1,000,000/mm³ due to myeloproliferative disease, and the hyperviscosity syndromes associated with Waldenstrom's macroglobulinemia and, less frequently, with myeloma can all be acutely benefited by selective removal of offending blasts, platelets, or immunoglobulins by using appropriate pheresis procedures.[88-94]

Plasma exchange for hyperviscosity merely involves use of the continuous flow centrifuge to separate the patients whole blood into cellular elements, which are returned to the patient, while plasma is removed in a collection bag. A plasma substitute like 5% human albumin or commercial preparations of plasma substitutes, supplemented so as to contain 4 mEq KCl/liter and 4.6 mEq of calcium gluconate/liter are returned to the patient at a rate that equals the rate of removal of the patient's plasma. This is carried on until 6 liters of the patients plasma has been exchanged (in a 70 kg person), which will result in reduction of circulating levels of plasma substances to 33% of the pretreatment values. In our center, patients with platelet counts below 20,000/mm³ are anticoagulated with acid citrate dextrose, while those with higher platelet counts may require a combination of acid citrate dextrose and heparin. Such intervention will lack sustained benefit without more definitive intervention (usually chemotherapy), but may nevertheless, provide substantial immediate relief of emergent or life-threatening symptoms including those involving the CNS.

Finally, animal studies have shown that tumor regressions may occur in cases of canine mammary carcinoma following perfusion of plasma through extravascular chambers containing immunoadsorbents.[95] Clinical use of this technique in association with continuous flow centrifugation methodology has been reported to yield responses in cases of human cancer.[96] Such responses have been attributed to the removal by the immunoadsorbents of immunologic blocking factors that act to inhibit antitumor immunity in the patient. This work, though fascinating, remains in the early stages of its development, and additional studies will be required to define the import and significance of these concepts.

HEMATOPOIETIC RECONSTITUTION IN SUPPORT OF PATIENTS RECEIVING INTENSIVE AND ABLATIVE LEVELS OF ANTINEOPLASTIC THERAPY

At present there are many tumors against which the appropriate use of standard therapeutic regimens will consistently eventuate in significant clinical responses.[97] In some cases these clinical responses will be "complete", that is on careful clinical and histologic examination using currently available non-invasive and invasive (bronchoscopy, peritoneoscopy, bone marrow biopsy, etc.) techniques no residual evidence of tumor presence will be identified.[99-105] In other cases, the responses observed, although real and measurable, will be of lesser degree and residual tumor will be identified.[106-108]

Moreover, following initial treatment, tumors that have shown complete response may relapse, even during the use of maintenance therapy, and they are then usually substantially more resistant to therapeutic intervention at standard levels of intensity.

Finally, there are many tumor types including numerous examples of frequently occurring neoplasms such as non-oat cell carcinomas of the lung, carcinoma of the colon, pancreas, and stomach, carcinoma of the prostate, and melanoma for which, following tumor dissemination, current therapeutic regimens are substantially less effective in producing complete clinical responses, even though they may result in significant clinical palliation.

Having achieved these gains new problems arise. What can be done to improve survival and control tumor following relapse? What can be done to increase both the rate of complete response and disease free interval among patients with disseminated neoplasms that have high rates of incomplete response? What can be done to prolong duration of complete response among patients with disseminated neoplasms that have a high rate of complete response followed by eventual relapse?

One approach to these questions has been to examine the effect of intensifying treatment to the point of maximally tolerated toxicity either at time of relapse or earlier in the course of management.

An additional approach involves improving hematopoietic tolerance to intensive therapy by effecting reconstitution of hematopoietic function through the use of transfused hematopoietic stem cells that have not been exposed to the cytotoxic effects of the intensive therapy used. This approach should then remove hematopoietic toxicity as the dose-limiting organ toxicity for anti-neoplastic treatment.

A substantial amount of success has been achieved with this approach using autologous (self), isogeneic (identical twin), and allogeneic (non-identical) marrow. Bone marrow for reconstitution purposes must be collected in "bulk" amounts (10 ml/kg) under anesthesia using sterile technique.

Each marrow source has associated advantages and disadvantages. Isogeneic marrow is rarely available, but, when available, combines the dual advantages of genetic identity and lack of tumor contamination. Autologous marrow is more commonly available, but requires that the patient be able to tolerate anesthesia to undergo bulk bone marrow collection and that the bony pelvis, the most easily accessible source of large amounts of marrow, be uncompromised by tumor or prior radiation therapy. In most cases autologous marrow must also be cryopreserved prior to use, a procedure associated with risk of lost viability. Allogeneic marrow from HLA matched sibling donors is available for about one patient in four and is free of tumor, but may be associated with both failure to engraft and graft versus host disease (GVHD). In GVHD the skin, liver, and GI tract may be severely damaged and the presence of GVHD is also associated with a high rate of interstitial pulmonary disease, impaired immunity, and active cytomegalovirus infection.

Graft versus host disease is the reaction which occurs when immunocompetent donor cells that are capable of recognizing and responding to recipient cellular antigens are infused and transplanted into an immunologically compromised host unable to reject the infused donor cells. Patients with acute post-transplantation graft versus host disease may have an exfoliative dermatitis with induration and a pink to purple discoloration of the skin, diarrhea with concomitant fluid and electrolyte loss, and elevation of serum levels of transaminases, alkaline phosphatase, and conjugated bilirubin.

A substantial experience involving hematopoietic reconstitution with allogeneic marrow from sibling donors found to be identical at HLA antigen loci A, B, and D has been accumulated. Using combined modality therapy consisting of total body irradiation at levels that would be hematopoietically lethal (800–1000 rads) in combination with large doses of cyclophosphamide (60 mg/kg × 2) and sometimes other agents. Thomas and colleagues have been able to observe long-term survivors among relapsed patients with acute leukemia who were clearly resistant to management with more conventional forms of therapy.[109] In 1977, they reported that 13 of 100 such patients were long-term disease-free-survivors and that hematopoietic recovery was extremely reliable. They encountered substantial morbidity and mortality in their study including deaths from graft versus host disease and interstitial pulmonary disease. However, all of these patients would otherwise have been expected to die from their refractory acute leukemia, and the demonstration that responses and even some cures could be achieved in this patient population indicated that this therapeutic resistance was relative rather than absolute.

These observations, and the fact that good clinical condition at the time of ablative therapy correlated with survival and a decreased incidence and severity of complications, suggested that patients with acute leukemia should undergo ablative therapy and allogeneic bone marrow transplantation earlier in their courses. For patients with acute nonlymphocytic leukemia (ANLL) this would logically imply ablative intervention shortly after achieving a first complete response, since the frequency of long-term disease-free remission in adults with acute non-lymphocytic leukemia is 10–20%, with standard maintenance therapy. For patients with acute lymphocytic leukemia (ALL) ablative therapy should be delayed until the first relapse followed by reinduction of complete response, since as many as 50% of ALL patients in first complete response may in fact be long-term disease-free survivors without ablative therapy. These studies have been undertaken, and results reported to date indicate that about 60% of patients with ANLL treated with ablative therapy after first complete remission will have long-term disease-free survival (off therapy) and that about 50% of patients with ALL in remission following first relapse will be long-term disease-free survivors following ablative therapy and allogeneic bone marrow transplantation.[110,112] Allogeneic transplantation in these patients in new trials has shown decreases in both the incidence of GVHD (from 70% to 40%) and interstitial pneumonia (from 60% to 20%). Both of these studies have confirmed that this early intervention with ablative therapy is associated with decreased acute morbidity and mortality.

Thus, for patients who are in a physiologic condition that permits them to tolerate the administration of intensive therapy and for whom an HLA matched sibling bone marrow donor is available, referral to an allogeneic bone marrow transplantation center is indicated. Thomas has reported that among 533 patients with at least one sibling, who were candidates for bone marrow transplantation, 233 (48%) had an HLA matched compatible donor.[4] For the time being, allogeneic bone marrow transplantation should be restricted to patients who have an HLA matched sibling donor although studies are currently underway to try to extend this support modality to non-sibling donors.

These workers have also reported successful results using isogeneic marrow after ablative therapy in the setting of various hematopoietic neoplasms including acute leukemia and lymphoma[112] and chronic phase, chronic myelogenous leukemia.[112,113]

Studies have also been carried out using autologous cryopreserved marrow. Initial studies were aimed at demonstrating both that such marrow preparations actually effected hematopoietic recovery and that the increased therapeutic intensity eventuated in increased tumor response. The techniques for procuring marrow from the pelvic bones in man as well as the procedure used in the cryopreservation of autologous marrow cells have been reviewed in detail in previous publications.[4,114,115] Both results were suggested by work at the National Cancer Institute in a study involving patients with relapsed Burkitt's lymphoma refractory to standard therapy and by subsequent reports of hematopoietic recovery and transient tumor responses in patients with relapsed hematopoietic malignancy and relapsed small cell carcinoma of the lung.[116–118] More recent studies at the National Cancer Institute involving patients with Ewing's sarcoma have suggested that autologous marrow can effectively accelerate marrow recovery after intermediate levels of intensive therapy and that accelerated marrow recovery may be associated with improved ability to tolerate subsequent maintenance therapy.[119]

Studies in a preclinical canine model have shown that the rate at which restoration of normal hematopoietic function occurs following marrow ablation is dependent on the dose of nucleated marrow cell used in the original aspirate. Although the absolute rate of hematopoietic recovery induced by infusion of cryopreserved autologous stem cells in dogs is more rapid than in man, we recommend on the basis of this canine data that all populations of human cryopreserved marrow used for reconstitution contain at least four times the dose of nucleated marrow cells in the original suspension which was found in animal models to be associated with 100% recovery (one should collect at least 2×10^8/kg of nucleated marrow cells).

Efforts using autologous marrow in the setting of acute leukemia have been less encouraging, undoubtedly reflecting the continued persistence of contaminating tumor cells in the stored marrow specimens as well as the substantial nonhematopoietic toxicity encountered.[120] In fact, it should be noted that nonhematopoietic toxicity including cardiac, pulmonary, and gastrointestinal effects has been substantial in a number of these trials.[120,121] A review of the published trials using intensive combination chemotherapy or combined modality therapy supported by autologous marrow infusion in relapsed patients with disease resistant to conventional dose therapy has shown a 30% complete response frequency and 16% long-term unmaintained remissions.[122]

The majority of patients exhibiting complete remissions following systemic high-dose chemotherapy or combined modality were those with undifferentiated lymphoma of childhood, although one patient with diffuse histiocytic lymphoma, one patient with testicular cancer, one patient with soft tissue sarcoma and one patient with neuroblastoma, exhibited complete responses for prolonged periods of time as well.

Nonhematopoietic toxicity has also led to treatment deaths in 16% of the patients. Nevertheless, this significant number of apparent cures has indicated that:

1. Marrow cells collected from solid tumor patients in complete remission can restore hematopoietic function after ablative levels of total body irradiation and chemotherapy.
2. Infusion of engrafting doses of hematopoietic cells are not necessarily associated with clinically significant levels of tumor cells since long-term unmaintained complete remissions have been achieved.
3. Autologous hematopoietic reconstitution has permitted the testing of intensive combination therapy as well as intensive use of single agents.
4. Autologous marrow infusions may increase hematopoietic tolerance to conventional doses of subsequent maintenance chemotherapy.

Preliminary studies of intensive therapy with autologous marrow rescue for neoplasms generally regarded as poorly responsive to standard chemotherapeutic regimens, (*e.g.*, intracranial gliomas, disseminated melanoma, and disseminated colon cancer) have been undertaken.[123,124] Although results have been observed in the form of unsustained responses, the role and value of this approach for such tumors remain to be defined.

POTENTIAL AREAS OF FUTURE INVESTIGATION

In the realm of allogeneic bone marrow transplantation, efforts are underway to further understand and control GVHD and to transplant across potential genetic barriers.[125,126] Treatment of the engrafting marrow with anti-lymphocyte or anti-T cell serum *in vitro* before infusion, has been reported by Thierfelder et al to have reduced the incidence of GVHD in allograft recipients in animal models and in man.[127,128] Total nodal irradiation (not total body irradiation) of the allograft recipient before transplantation has been reported to alter the course of graft rejection in organ transplants in man and has decreased the severity of GVHD, in the absence of infection, in animal models.[129] However, no clear picture of the mechanism exists and no convincing data in man have been published to establish that irradiation of nodal areas in the marrow allograft recipient before transplantation will alter the course of graft versus host disease. Finally, the use of cyclosporin A in one published series has reduced the incidence and severity of acute graft versus host disease in marrow allograft recipients and this remains the most exciting area for future development in this field.[130]

At some point, trials involving allogeneic bone marrow transplantation for patients with selected nonhematopoietic malignancies will be undertaken, especially in settings where bone marrow involvement precludes the use of autologous marrow. In autologous settings efforts are currently ongoing to remove contaminating tumor cells using physical and immunologic means including cytotoxic heteroantisera directed at the malignant cells.[120] Billings and coworkers have reported the development of heteroantisera which exhibit complement dependent cytotoxicity for leukemia cells without undermining the levels of normal hematopoietic precursor cells.[132] Engraftment in man has been achieved after treatment by autologous marrow with such reagents, but studies in animal models will be necessary to determine if such *in vitro* immunotherapy can remove all contaminating leukemia cells. Obviously, such a strategy, if successful, would permit the use of autologous remission marrow preparations for the support of the intensive therapy for AML patients in first remission or ALL patients after first relapse.

For patients in whom regional radiation therapy, tumor distribution, or physiological status precludes the collection of an engrafting dose of autologous cells from the marrow space, collection of autologous stem cells from the peripheral blood through the use of continuous flow centrifugation would be of use. In the setting of chronic myelogenous leukemia studies have been undertaken utilizing stem cells collected from the peripheral blood. This is possible in chronic myelogenous leukemia due to the unusual stem cell expansion into the peripheral blood associated with this disease in the untreated chronic state.[133] Whether such studies might also be undertaken in man in non-chronic myelogenous leukemia settings seems possible based on canine studies and recent observations in man regarding the behavior of circulating stem cells following chemotherapy.[134] Studies of autologous stem cells from the peripheral blood in animal models have shown complete reconstitution following 900 rad of total body irradiation but attempts in man to reconstitute patients with peripheral blood cells have suggested that amplification of the levels of circulating stem cells may be a prerequisite for the use of this technique. Studies at the National Cancer Institute have shown that hematopoietic recovery following conventional dose cyclical chemotherapy is associated with amplification in CFU_c levels.[125] (CFU_c is the term for the granulocytemacrophage precursor cell.) During the recovery of normal peripheral blood white cell counts following chemotherapy induced depression of white cells, a 5–10 fold increase in the circulating levels of the CFU_c occurs in man. Since animal studies suggest that this amplification of CFU_c is accompanied by pluripotent stem cell amplification, it may be possible to collect an engrafting dose of stem cells from the peripheral blood of patients undergoing cyclical conventional dose therapy, and thus use the peripheral blood as a source of stem cells for the support of intensive therapy of the solid tumor patient.[137]

Until such time as the use of peripheral blood mononuclear cells is established to be associated with hematopoietic recovery in a carefully controlled trial, marrow cells should be used exclusively for the support of patients undergoing intensive therapy.

Our current guidelines for transfusing red cells, platelets, and granulocytes are summarized in Table 43-20. It should be emphasized that such guidelines are by no means absolute or definitive, and may not be adequate for all contingencies. The role of hematopoietic reconstitution in the management of hematopoietic and nonhematopoietic malignancies will undoubtedly increase and expand as experience and methodologies improve. Patients with identical twins, in particular, and HLA identical siblings in general, should be given every opportunity for early management at transplant centers when clinical settings involve acute non-lymphocytic leukemia and relapsed acute lymphocytic leukemia. The increased success seen in the current trials of intensive therapy for AML in first remission and ALL in second remission followed by allograft, suggests an increasing role for these strategies in the treatment of resistant hematopoietic neoplasms, and the results of ongoing trials will hopefully define the ultimate value of this approach. Determining the exact role of hematopoietic reconstitution in association with intensive and ablative therapies for selected patients with other advanced stage hematopoietic and nonhematopoietic neoplasms (especially nonseminomatous testicular neoplasms, small cell carcinoma of the lung, epithelial ovarian neoplasms, and various soft tissue

TABLE 43-20. Transfusion Guidelines for Some Commonly Encountered Hematologic Problems

1. Chronic Anemia
   a. No significant cardiopulmonary compromise; stable patient
      —no absolute indication for transfusion when hemoglobin is above 6–7 g/100 ml
      —consider transfusion in the presence of otherwise unexplained lassitude, malaise, tachycardia, dyspnea in association with hemoglobin less than 9–10 g/100 ml
   b. Cardiopulmonary disease; fever; surgery
      —maintain hemoglobin level at 10 g/100 ml
   c. If management protracted (years), monitor for evidence of iron overload (secondary hemochromatosis)
2. Thrombocytopenia Due to Failure of Platelet Production
   a. Platelet count $\geq$20,000/mm^3; stable patient without retinal hemorrhages—platelet transfusion probably not necessary
   b. Platelet count less than 20,000/mm^3; patient not bleeding—provide prophylactic platelet transfusion once daily.
   c. Platelet count $\leq$50,000/mm^3; patient clinically bleeding or surgery anticipated—use local measures to control bleeding; look for defects in coagulation pathways; maintain platelet counts at 50,000/mm^3 or above with transfusion q 12–24 hours as available.
   d. Platelet count less than 20,000/mm^3; patient refractory to random platelet transfusion—consider transfusion for evidence of bleeding, when retinal hemorrhages noted, or when platelet count is less than 10,000/mm^3; consider use of leukocyte poor or HLA matched platelets.
3. Granulocytopenia—Patient Candidate for Aggressive Supportive Care
   a. Granulocytes less than 1000/mm^3; afebrile, stable patient—no established indication for granulocyte transfusion.
   b. Granulocytes less than 1000/mm^3; patient febrile, but cultures negative and no clinical evidence of infected area or tissue—no established indication for granulocyte transfusion.
   c. Gram negative sepsis, fever, granulocytes less than 500/mm^3, and poor response to antibiotics—granulocytes indicated.
   d. Local infection, thought to be due to gram negative organisms, not responsive to appropriate antibiotic therapy occurring in a patient with a granulocyte count below 500/mm^3—granulocytes probably indicated.

sarcomas) will require further studies, and should remain an area of active investigation.

Patients will likely continue to benefit from the clinical application of advances in cell separator technology.[96] In particular, the use of the cell separator to perfuse plasma through extracorporeal chambers containing substances which may enhance the immune response of the cancer patient against neoplastic cells may provide the means to alter the otherwise poor response patterns of resistant neoplasms.

REFERENCES

1. Masouredis SP: Preservation and clinical use of erythrocytes and whole blood. In Williams WJ, Rundles N, Beutler E (eds): Hematology, 2nd ed, pp 1539–1544. New York, McGraw-Hill, 1977
2. Mollison PL: Blood Transfusion in Clinical Medicine, 5th ed, pp 538–616. Oxford, Blackwell Scientific, 1972
3. Hickman SG: Anemia. In Costrini NV, Thomas WM (eds): Manual of Medical Therapeutics, 22nd ed, pp 252–256. Boston, Little, Brown & Co, 1977
4. Thomas ED, Storb R, Clift RA et al: Bone marrow transplantation (2 parts). N Engl J Med 292:832–843, 895–902, 1975
5. Graw RG Jr, Buckner CD, Whang-Peng J et al: Complications of bone marrow transplantation. Graft host disease resulting from chronic-myelogenous-leukaemia leukocyte transfusions. Lancet ii:338–341, 1970
6. Ford JM, Lucey JJ, Cullen MH et al: Fatal graft versus host disease following transfusion of granulocytes from normal donors. Lancet ii:1167–1169, 1976
7. Rosen RC, Huestis DW, Corrigan JJ: Acute leukemia and granulocyte transfusion: Fatal graft-versus-host reaction following transfusion of cells obtained from normal donors. J Pediatr 93:268–270, 1978
8. Cohen D, Weinstein H, Mihm M et al: Nonfatal graft-versus-host disease occurring after transfusion with leukocytes and platelets obtained from normal donors. Blood 53:1053–1057, 1979
9. Erslev AJ: General effects of anemia. In Williams WJ et al (eds): Hematology, 2nd ed, pp 251–255. New York, McGraw-Hill, 1977
10. Kinney JM: Ventilation and ventilatory failure. In Kinney JM et al (eds): Manual of Preoperative and Postoperative Care, pp 172–194. Philadelphia, WB Saunders, 1971
11. Mitchell R: Red cell transfusion. In Cash JD (ed): Blood Transfusion and Blood Products. Clinics in Haematol, Vol 5, no 1, pp 33–52. London, WB Saunders, 1976
12. Brzica SM, Pineda A, Taswell HF: Autologous blood transfusion. CRC Critical Reviews in Clinical Laboratory Sciences, Vol 10, pp 31–56. January, 1979
13. Becker GA, Aster RH: Red blood cell transfusion. Transfusion 13:109–111, 1973
14. Toogood IRG, Ekert H, Smith PJ, et al: Controlled study of hypertransfusion during remission induction in childhood acute lymphocytic leukemia. Lancet ii:862–864, 1978
15. Rubenstein RA, Yanoff M, Albert DM: Thrombocytopenia, anemia, and retinal hemorrhage. Am J Opthalmol 65:435–549, 1968
16. Gardner FH: Annotation: Use of platelet transfusions. Br J Haematol 27:537–542, 1974
17. Aster RH: Thrombocytopenia due to diminished or defective platelet production. In Williams WJ et al (eds): Hematology, 2nd ed, pp 1317–1325. New York, McGraw-Hill, 1977
18. Slichter SJ, Harker LA: Thrombocytopenia: Mechanisms and management of defects in platelet production. In Thomas ED (ed): Aplastic Anemia. Clin Hematol 7:523:539, 1978
19. Gardner FG: Preservation and clinical use of platelets. In Williams WF et al (eds): Hematology, 2nd ed, pp 1553–1560. New York, McGraw-Hill, 1977
20. Gaydos LS, Freireich EJ, Mantel N: The quantitative relation between platelet count and hemorrhage in patents with acute leukemia. N Engl J Med 266:905–909, 1962
21. Han T, Stutzman L, Cohen E et al: Effect of platelet transfusion on hemorrhage in patients with acute leukemia—an autopsy study. Cancer 19:1937–1942, 1966
22. Roy AJ, Jaffe N, Djerassi I: Prophylactic platelet transfusions in children with acute leukemia: A dose response study. Transfusion 13:282–290, 1973
23. Higby DJ, Cohen E, Holland JF et al: The prophylactic treatment of thrombocytopenic leukemia patients with platelets: A double blind study. Transfusion 14:440–446, 1974
24. Hersh EM, Bodey GP, Nies BA et al: Causes of death in acute leukemia. JAMA 193:99–103, 1965
25. George JN, Morgan RK: Platelet behavior and aging in the circulation. In Greenwalt TJ, Jamieson GA (eds): Progress in Clinical and Biological Reserach, Vol 28, pp 39–64. New York, Alan R. Liss, 1978
26. Corash LM: Platelet heterogeneity: Relationship between density and age. In Greenwalt TJ, Jamieson GA (eds): Progress in Clinical and Biological Research, Vol 28, pp 79–82. New York, Alan R. Liss, 1978
27. Harker LA, Slichter SJ: The bleeding time as a screening test for evaluation of platelet function. N Engl J Med 287:155–159, 1972
28. Tessier C, Steiner M, Baldini MG: Measurement of platelet kinetics using ^{51}CR. In Baldini MG, Ebbe S (eds): Platelets: Production, Function, Transfusion, and Storage, pp 327–337. New York, Grune & Stratton, 1974
29. Yankee RA: HL-A antigens and platelet therapy. In Baldini MG, Ebbe S (eds): Platelets: Production, Function, Transfusion, and Storage, pp 313–326. New York, Grune & Stratton, 1974
30. Yankee, RA, Grumet FC, Rogentine GN: Platelet transfusion therapy—The selection of comparable platelet donors for refractory patients by HL-A typing. N Engl J Med 281:1208–1212, 1968
31. Grumet FC, Yankee RA: Long-term platelet support of patients with aplastic anemia—Effect of splenectomy and steroid therapy. Ann Intern Med 78:1–7, 1970
32. Lohrmann HP, Bull MI, Decter JA et al: Efficacy of platelet transfusions from HL-A compatible unrelated donors to alloimmunized patients. Ann Intern Med 80:9–14, 1974
33. Harker LA, Finch CA: Thrombokinetics in man. J Clin Invest 48:963–974, 1969
34. Aster RH: Pooling of platelets in the spleen: Role in the pathogenesis of "hypersplenic" thrombocytopenia. J Clin Invest 45:645–657, 1965
35. Freireich EJ, Kliman A, Gaydos LA et al: Response to repeated platelet transfusion from the same donor. Ann Intern Med 59:277–287, 1963
36. Slichter SJ: Preservation of platelet viability and function during storage of concentrates. In Greenwalt TJ, Jamieson GA (eds): Progress in Clinical and Biological Research. The Blood Platelet in Transfusion Therapy, Vol 28, pp 83–100. New York, Alan R. Liss, 1978
37. Djerassi I, Farber S, Evans AE: Transfusion of fresh platelet concentrates to patients with secondary thrombocytopenia. N Engl J Med 268:221–226, 1963
38. Schiffer CA, Buchholz DH, Wiernik PH: Intensive multiunit platelet pheresis of normal donors. Transfusion 14:383–394, 1974
39. Hoak JC, Koepke JA: Blood transfusion and blood products. In Cash JD (ed): Clinics in Haematology, Vol 5, pp 69–79. Philadelphia, WB Saunders, 1976
40. Shiffer CA: Annotation: Some aspects of recent advances in the use of blood cell components. Br J Haematol 39:289–294, 1978
41. Daly PA, Schiffer CA, Aisner J et al: A comparison of platelets prepared by the Haemonetics Model 30 and multiunit bag platelet pheresis. Transfusion 19:778–781, 1979
42. Troup SB, Schwartz SI: Hemostasis, surgical bleeding, and transfusion. In Schwartz SI et al (eds): Principles of Surgery, pp 84–118. New York, McGraw-Hill, 1969
43. Herzig RH, Poplack DG, Yankee RA: Prolonged granulocyto-

penia from incompatible platelet transfusions. N Engl J Med 290:1220–1223, 1974
44. Herzig RH, Herzig GP, Bull MI et al: Correction of poor platelet transfusion responses with leukocyte-poor HL-A matched platelet concentrates. Blood 46:743–750, 1975
45. Aisner J, Schiffer CA, Wolff JH et al: A standardized technique for efficient platelet and leukocyte collection using the Model 30 Blood Processor. Transfusion 16:437–445, 1976
46. Duqesnoy RJ, Filip DJ, Aster RH: Influence of HLA-A2 on the effectiveness of platelet transfusions in alloimmunized thrombocytopenic patients. Blood 50:407–412, 1977
47. Duqesnoy RJ: Donor selection in platelet transfusion therapy of alloimmunized thrombocytopenic patients. In Greenwalt TJ, Jamieson GA (eds): Progress in Clinical and Biological Research: The Blood Platelet in Transfusion Therapy, Vol 28, pp 229–243. New York, Alan R. Liss, 1978
48. Packham MA, Mustard JF: Drug-induced alteration of platelet function. In Baldini MG, Ebbe S (eds): Platelets: Production, Function, Transfusion, and Storage, pp 265–275. New York, Grune & Stratton, 1974
49. Weiss HJ: Acquired qualitative platelet disorders. In Williams WJ et al (eds): Hematology, 2nd ed, pp 1377–1384. New York, McGraw-Hill, 1974
50. Buskard NA, Kaur J, Goldman JM et al: Engraftment with chronic granulocytic leukemia cells in acute myeloid leukemia. Transfusion 19:317–320, 1979
51. Graw RG, Herzig G, Perry S et al: Normal granulocyte transfusion therapy—Treatment of septicemia due to gram negative bacteria. N Engl J Med 287:367–371, 1972
52. Bodey GP: Infections in cancer patients. Cancer Treat Rev 2: 89–138, 1975
53. Bodey GP, Buckley M, Sathe YS et al: Quantitative relationships between circulating leukocytes and infection in patients with acute leukemia. Ann Intern Med 64:328–340, 1966
54. Gaya H: Empirical therapy in febrile granulocytopenic patients. Eur J Cancer 15:51–58, 1979
55. Golde DG, Cline MJ: Production, distribution, and fate of granulocytes. In Williams WJ et al (eds): Hematology, 2nd ed, pp 699–706. New York, McGraw-Hill, 1977
56. Athens JW, Haab OP, Raab SO et al: Leukokinetic studies IV. The total blood, circulating and marginal granulocyte pools and the granulocyte turnover rate in normal subjects. J Clin Invest 40:989–995, 1961
57. Herzig GP, Graw RG Jr: Granulocyte transfusions for bacterial infections. Prog Hematol 9:207–228, 1975
58. McCredie KB, Hester JP: White blood cell transfusions in the management of infections in neutropenic patients. In Bodey GP (ed): Infectious Complications in Haematological Diseases. Clinics In Hematology, Vol 5, No 2. Philadelphia, WB Saunders, 1976
59. McCredie KB, Freireich EJ, Hester JP et al: Increased granulocyte collection with the blood cell separator and the addition of etiocholanolone and hydroxyethyl starch. Transfusion 14:357–364, 1974
60. Mishler JM, Higby DJ, Rhomberg W et al: Leukapheresis: Increased efficiency of collection by the use of hydroxyethyl starch and dexamethasone. In Goldman JM, Lowenthal RM (eds): Leucocytes: Separation, Collection, and Transfusion, pp 61–75. New York, Academic Press, 1975
61. Djerassi I, Kim JS, Mitrakaul C et al: Filtration leukapheresis for separation and concentration of tranfusable amounts of normal human granulocytes. J Med (Basel) 1:358–364, 1970
62. Herzig GP, Root RK, Graw RG Jr: Granulocyte collection by continuous flow filtration leukapheresis. Blood 39:554–567, 1972
63. McCullough J, Weiben B, Deinard AR et al: In vitro function and post-transfusion survival of granulocytes collected by continuous flow centrifugation and by filtration leukapheresis. Blood 48:315–326, 1976
64. Lane TA, Windle B: Granulocyte concentrate function during preservation: Effect of temperature. Blood 54:216–225, 1979
65. Glasser L: Effect of storage on normal neutrophils collected by discontinuous-flow centrifugation leukapheresis. Blood 50: 1145–1150, 1977
66. McCullough J: Granulocyte function during short term liquid storage. Exp Hematol (Suppl) 7, 5:95–104, 1979
67. French JE, Jemionek JF, Contreras TJ: Cryopreservation of dog polymorphonuclear leukocytes for transfusion (abstr). Exp Hematol (Suppl) 6, 3:107, 1978
68. Glasser L: Functional consideration of granulocyte concentrates used for clinical transfusions. Transfusion 19:1–6, 1979
69. Appelbaum FR, Norton L, Graw RG Jr: Migration of transfused granulocytes in leukopenic dogs. Blood 49:483–488, 1977
70. Appelbaum FR, Bowles CA, Makuch RW et al: Granulocyte transfusion therapy of experimental pseudomonas septicemia: Study of cell dose and collection technique. Blood 52:323–331, 1978
71. Herzig RH, Herzig GP, Graw RG Jr et al: Successful granulocyte transfusion therapy for gram-negative septicemia. N Engl J Med 296:701–705, 1977
72. Alavi JB, Root RK, Djerassi I et al: A randomized clinical trial of granulocyte transfusions for infection in acute leukemia. N Engl J Med 296:706–711, 1977
73. Aisner J, Schiffer CA, Wiernik PH: Granulocyte transfusions: Evaluation of factors influencing results and a comparison of filtration and intermittent centrifugation leukapheresis. Br J Haematol 38:121–129, 1978
74. Hester JP, Kellog RM, Mulzet AP et al: Principles of blood separation and component extraction in a disposable continuous-flow single-stage channel. Blood 54:254–268, 1979
75. Vogler WR, Winton EF: A controlled study of the efficacy of granulocyte transfusions in patients with neutropenia. Am J Med 63:548–555, 1977
76. Higby DJ, Burnett D: Granulocyte transfusions: Current status. Blood 55:2–8, 1980
77. McCullough J: Leukapheresis and granulocyte transfusion. CRC Crit Rev Clin Lab Sci 10:275–327, 1979
78. Wright DG, Robichaud KJ, Pizzo PA et al: Lethal pulmonary reactions associated with the combined use of amphotericin B and leukocyte transfusions (abstr). Blood (Suppl) 54, 1:130a, 1979
79. Ungerleider RS, Appelbaum FR, Trapani RJ et al: Lack of predictive value of antileukocyte antibody screening in granulocyte transfusion therapy. Transfusion 19:90–94, 1979
80. Clift RA, Saunders JE, Thomas ED et al: Granulocyte transfusions for the prevention of infection in patients receiving bone marrow transplants. N Engl J Med 298:1052–1057, 1978
81. Spier ASD: Surgery in management of patients with leukemia. Br Med J 3:528–532, 1973
82. Bjornsson S, Yates JW, Mittelman A et al: Major surgery in acute leukemia. Cancer 34:1272–1275, 1974
83. Rasmussen BL, Freeman JS: Major surgery in leukemia. Am J Surg 130:647–651, 1975
84. Varki AP, Armitage JO, Feagler JR: Typhlitis in acute leukemia. Cancer 43:695–697, 1979
85. Lowenthal RM: Chronic leukaemias: Treatment by leukapheresis. Exp Hematol (Suppl) 5:73–84, 1977
86. Edelson R, Facktor M, Andrews A et al: Successful management of the Sezary Syndrome. Mobilization and removal of extravascular neoplastic T cells by leukapheresis. N Engl J Med 291:293–294, 1974
87. Fay JW, Moore JO, Logue GL et al: Leukapheresis therapy of leukemic reticuloendotheliosis (Hairy Cell Leukemia). Blood 54:747–749, 1979
88. McKee LC Jr, Collins RD: Intravascular leukocyte thrombi and aggregates as a cause of morbidity and mortality in leukemia. Medicine 53:463–478, 1974
89. Eisenstaedt RS, Berkman EM: Rapid cytroreduction in acute leukemia. Management of cerebral leukostasis by cell pheresis. Transfusion 18:113–115, 1978
90. Carpentieri U, Patten EV, Chamberlin PA et al: Leukapheresis in a 3 year old child with lymphoma in leukemic transformation. J Pediatr 94:919–921, 1979
91. Panlilio AL, Reiss RF: Therapeutic platelet pheresis in thrombocythemia. Transfusion 19:147–152, 1979
92. Taft EG, Babcock RD, Scharfman WB et al: Platelet-pheresis in the management of thrombocytosis. Blood 50:927–933, 1977

93. Goldfinger D, Thompson R, Lowe C et al: Long-term platelet pheresis in the management of primary thrombocytosis. Transfusion 19:336–338, 1979
94. Russell JA, Toy JL, Powles RL: Plasma exchange in malignant paraproteinemias. Exp Hematol (Suppl) 5:105–116, 1977
95. Terman D, Yamamoto T, Mattioli M et al: Extensive necrosis of spontaneous canine mammary adenocarcinoma after extracorporeal perfusion over Staph A. I. J Immunol 124:795–805, 1980
96. Bansal SC, Bansal BR, Thomas HC et al. Ex vivo removal of serum IgG in a patient with colon carcinoma. Cancer 42:1, 1978
97. Zubrod CG: Contributions of chemotherapy to the control of cancer. In Zubrod CG (ed): Cancer Chemotherapy—Fundamental Concepts and Recent Advances, pp 7–17. Chicago, Year Book Medical Publishers, 1975
98. Hammond CB, Borchert LG, Tyrey L et al: Treatment of metastatic trophoblastic disease: Good and poor prognosis. Am J Obstet Gynecol 115:451–457, 1973
99. Maller AM: Treatment of acute leukemia in children. In Simone JV (ed): Clinics in Haematology, Vol 7: Acute Leukemia, pp 245–248. Philadelphia, WB Saunders, 1978
100. Gale RP: Advances in the treatment of acute myelogenous leukemia. N Engl J Med 300:1189–1199, 1979
101. DeVita VT Jr, Serpick A, Carbone PP: Combination chemotherapy in the treatment of advanced Hodgkin's disease. Ann Intern Med 73:881–895, 1970
102. Ziegler JL, Deisseroth AB, Appelbaum FR et al: Burkitt's lymphoma—A model for intensive chemotherapy. Semin Oncol 4:317–324, 1977
103. Schein PS, DeVita VT, Hubbard S et al: Bleomycin, adriamycin, cyclophosphamide, vincristine, and prednisone (BACOP) combination chemotherapy in the treatment of advanced diffuse histiocytic lymphoma. Ann Intern Med 85:417–422, 1976
104. Cohen MH, Creaven PJ, Fossieck BE Jr et al: Intensive chemotherapy of small cell bronchogenic carcinoma. Cancer Treat Rep 61:349–354, 1977
105. Anderson T, Waldmann TA, Javadpour N et al: Testicular germ cell neoplasms: Recent advances in diagnosis and therapy. Ann Intern Med 90:373–385, 1979
106. Rozencweig M, Henson JC, Von Hoff DD et al: Breast Cancer. In Staquet MJ (ed): Randomized Trials in Cancer: A Critical Review by Sites, pp 231–272. New York, Raven Press, 1978
107. Young RC, Chabner BA, Hubbard SP et al: Advanced ovarian adenocarcinoma: A prospective clinical trial of melphalan (L-PAM) vs combination chemotherapy (Hexa-CAF). N Engl J Med 299:1261–1266, 1978
108. Benjamin RS, Baker LH, O'Bryan RM et al: Advances in the chemotherapy of soft tissue sarcomas. Med Clin North Am 6115): 1039–1044, 1977.
109. Thomas ED, Buckner CD, Fefer A et al: Marrow transplantation in the treatment of acute leukemia. In Klein G, Weinhouse S (eds): Advances in Cancer Research, Vol 27, pp 269–279. New York, Academic Press, 1978
110. Thomas ED, Buckner CD, Clift RA et al: Marrow transplantation for acute nonlymphoblastic leukemia in first remission. N Engl J Med 301:597–599, 1979
111. Thomas ED, Sanders JE, Flournoy N et al: Marrow transplantation for patients with acute lymphoblastic leukemia in remission. Blood 54:468–476, 1979
112. Fefer A, Buckner CD, Thomas ED et al: Cure of hematologic neoplasia with transplantation of marrow from identical twins. N Engl J Med 297:146–148, 1977
113. Fefer A, Cheever MA, Thomas ED et al: Disappearance of Ph[1]-positive cells in four patients with chronic granulocytic leukemia after chemotherapy, irradiation, and marrow transplantation from an identical twin. N Engl J Med 300:333–337, 1979
114. Appelbaum R, Herzig G, Zeigler J et al: Successful engraftment of cryopreserved autologous bone marrow in patients with malignant lymphoma. Blood 52:85–95, 1978
115. Thomas ED, Storb R: Technique for human marrow grafting. Blood 36:507–515, 1970
116. Appelbaum FR, Deisseroth AB, Graw RG Jr et al: Prolonged complete remission following high dose chemotherapy of Burkitt's lymphoma in relapse. Cancer 41:1059–1063, 1978
117. Kaizer H, Wharam MD, Munoz LL et al: Autologous bone marrow transplantation in the treatment of selected human malignancies. The Johns Hopkins Oncology Center Program. Exp Hematol (Suppl) 7, 5:309–320, 1979
118. Graze PR, Wells JR, Ho W et al: Successful engraftment of cryopreserved autologous bone marrow stem cells in man. Transplantation 27:142–145, 1979
119. Abrams RA, Glaubiger D, Lichter A et al: Haemopoietic recovery in Ewing's sarcoma after intensive combination therapy and autologous marrow infusion. Lancet II:385–389, 1980
119a. Appelbaum FR, Herzig GP, Graw Jr et al: Study of cell dose and storage times on engraftment of cryopreserved autologous bone marrow in a canine model. Transplantation 26:245–248, 1978
120. Dicke KA, Spitzer G, Peters L et al: Autologous bone marrow transplantation in relapsed adult acute leukemia. Lancet i:514–517, 1979
121. Gale RP, Graze PR, Wells J et al: Autologous bone marrow transplantation in patients with cancer. Exp Hematol (Suppl) 7, 5:351–359, 1979
122. Deisseroth A, Abrams R, Bode U et al: Current status of autologous bone marrow transplantation. In Gale RP, Fox CF (eds): Biology of Bone Marrow Transplantation, ICN-UCLA Symposium on Molecular and Cellular Biology, Vol XVII. New York, Academic Press, 1980
123. Phillips GL, Fay JW, Herzig GP et al: Intensive 1,3-bis (2-chloroethyl)-1-nitrosourea (BCNU)—Autologous bone marrow transplantation therapy of refractory cancer: A Preliminary Report. Exp Hematol (Suppl) 7, 5:389–397, 1979
124. McElwain TJ, Hedley DW, Burton G et al: Marrow autotransplantation accelerates haematological recovery in patients with malignant melanoma treated with high dose melphalan. Br J Cancer 40:72–80, 1979
125. Storb R, Weiden PL, Deeg HJ et al: Rejection of marrow from DLA-identical canine littermates given transfusions before grafting. Blood 54:477–484, 1979
126. Opelz G, Gale RP, Feig SA et al: Significance of HLA and non-HLA and non-HLA antigens in bone marrow transplantation. Transplant Proc 10:43–46, 1978
127. Thierfelder S, Rodt H, Kolb H et al: Prevention and treatment of GVHD by anti-thymocyte globulin. J Supramol Struct (Suppl) 4: 7, 1980
128. Rodt H, et al: Experimental Hematology Today, p 197. Springer-Verlag, 1979
129. Slavin S, Weiss L, Morecki S et al: Specific transplantation tolerance to bone marrow allografts in dogs using total lymphoid irradiation. J Supramolec Struct (Suppl) 4: p 8, 1980
130. Powles RL, Clink H, Spence D et al: Reduction of graft versus host disease by Cyclosporin A. Lancet 1:327–329, 1980
131. Clince JG: The frontiers of leukemia research. In Cline MJ (Moderator): Acute Leukemia: Biology and Treatment, pp 769–770. Ann Intern Med 91:758–773, 1979
132. Billing R, Minowada J, Cline J et al: Acute lymphocytic leukemia-associated cell membrane antigen. J Natl Cancer Inst 61:423–429, 1978
133. Goldman JM: Modern approaches to the management of chronic granulocytic leukemia. Semin Hematol 15:420–430, 1978
134. Nothdurft W, Brudh C, Fliedner TM et al: Studies on the regeneration of the CFU-c population in blood and bone marrow of lethally irradiated dogs after autologous transfusion of cryopreserved mononuclear blood cells. Scand J Haematol 19: 470–481, 1977
135. Abrams RA, Johnston-Early A, Kramer C et al: Amplification of circulating myeloid-macrophage stem cells (CFUc) numbers following chemotherapy in patients with extensive small cell carcinoma of the lung. Cancer Res (in press)
136. Hershko C, Ho WG, Gale RP et al: Cure of aplastic anaemia in paroxysmal noctural haemoglobinuria by marrow transfusion from identical twin: Failure of peripheral leukocyte transfusion to correct marrow aplasia. Lancet i: 945–947, 1979
137. Abrams R, McCormack K, Bowles C et al: Significance of cyclophosphamide induced expansion of peripheral blood granulocyte-macrophage precursor cell for hematopoietic reconstitution (abstr). Clin Res 28:524A, 1980

Section 3

Management of Pain

Pharmacologic Approaches

BRIAN J. LEWIS

Most people strongly associate pain with cancer and regard it as an inevitable and dread aspect of malignant illness. Definitive, population-based incidence figures on the frequency and severity of cancer pain are not available, but it appears from the data at hand that a significant fraction of cancer patients do experience pain related to their disease and at some point require pain control, most often in the form of analgesics.[1-3]

Unfortunately, medical personnel too infrequently make optimal use of analgesics, largely because of misinformation and misapprehension about their pharmacology. This is particularly true of the narcotic analgesics.[1,4,5] For example, a survey of inpatients in a teaching hospital indicated that 32% of 37 patients continued to experience severe distress, while 41% were in moderate distress after being prescribed narcotic analgesic therapy. Analysis of hospital records suggested significant undertreatment in terms of prescribed doses and schedules of drug. Questioning of the house staff revealed that many were greatly misinformed about the pharmacology of the narcotic analgesics. In particular, those who overestimated the danger of drug addiction were more likely to undertreat patients, even those with terminal cancer.[4]

Such observations support the conclusion that there has been a failure to give sufficient priority to the principles of supportive care in initial medical education, in continuing medical education programs, and in daily practice habits.[1] Most importantly, there is a lack of understanding that the fear of abandonment to a condition of unrelieved suffering is an intense and often frequent concern of cancer patients; that anxiety about availability of adequate pain control is one concrete expression of this fear; and that an important antidote is a physician's reassurance that he or she will stand by the patient, whatever the outcome of antitumor therapy, and knowledgeably and effectively relieve pain.

GENERAL CONSIDERATIONS

It is useful to consider briefly counterproductive attitudes sometimes brought to bear in the approach to cancer patients in pain, attitudes which diminish health personnel as historians, diagnosticians and therapists. In particular, there can be a nihilism towards cancer patients which arises out of the despair and frustration encountered in trying to manage chronic disease states, especially terminal ones, which we cannot "fix," once and for all. They can make us weary and apprehensive, make us feel inadequate, and make us act less than willing to take an active approach toward supportive care (as we more gladly do in trying to *cure* cancer). Accordingly, history-taking becomes more automatic, less individualized (a complex patient has become a simple cancer); the physical examination superficial, less probing (after all, it is just another wasted or swollen body); the differential diagnosis stunted, less comprehensive (the vague notion of "cancer pain" heads a list of one rather than being more properly a "rule out" diagnosis at the end of a range of specific possibilities); and the therapeutic plan routinized, less individualized (often irrelevant to the needs of the patient at hand). And through the whole process, there may be neglect of what the cancer in general and the pain in particular mean to the patient; of what are his or her concomitant emotional states (*e.g.*, anxiety, depression); and of what is the cost of severe, unrelieved pain (*i.e.*, loss of sleep, *increased* sensitivity to discomfort, despair, inanition, incapacitation, loss of independence, isolation from family and friends, and an inability to concentrate on anything other than the pain).[1]

INITIAL MANAGEMENT

While analgesic drugs are an important component of the overall management of cancer pain, discussion of their use and practice should come only after the prior consideration of other important elements.

ASSESSMENT OF THE PATIENT

The goal here is the identification of the cause of the pain and the documentation and specific therapy of responsive lesions. Examples pertinent to clinical oncology are listed in Table 43-21.[6] Causative factors include the cancer itself, complications of therapy, and concomitants of debilitation. Early in a patient's course, the likelihood is greater than in the terminal stages of illness that therapy directed at the cancer itself will be associated with relief of pain. At any time during a patient's course it may be necessary to intervene with local palliative measures such as radiotherapy for painful bone lesions, surgery to relieve an obstructed viscus, or mechanical stabilization for threatened long bones. Such measures should not be shunned simply because they are not curative, for they are often critical to keeping a patient out of bed, independent, and free from additional and potentially burdensome therapies such as analgesics or neurosurgical interventions.

GENERAL PRINCIPLES OF ANALGESIC USE

The selection of analgesics rests upon matching a drug with the severity of the patient's pain. Traditionally, analgesics have been classified according to their use for the treatment of either moderate or severe pain. Bonica has estimated, after reviewing data from several surveys of small groups of patients,

TABLE 43-21. Causes of Pain in Cancer Patients Amenable to Corrective Therapy

CAUSE	MANIFESTATION	LOCAL THERAPY	SYSTEMIC THERAPY
malignant growth	bone metastasis	radiotherapy, mechanical stabilization	drugs, hormones, radiotherapy
	infiltration or compression of nerves, vessels, or lymphatics	radiotherapy, surgery	drugs, hormones, radiotherapy
	compartmental swelling	radiotherapy, surgery, intracavitary therapy	drugs, hormones, radiotherapy
	destruction of epithelial surfaces	radiotherapy, local care	drugs, hormones, radiotherapy
	obstruction of a viscus	surgery, radiotherapy	drugs, hormones, radiotherapy
complications of antitumor therapy	mucositis	local care	
	chemical phlebitis, local tissue reactions to drugs	local care	anti-inflammatory agents
	radiation enteritis	surgery, ? local steroids	
debilitated state	decubitus ulcers	local care, positioning, physical therapy	
	hypercalcemia, osteoporosis fractures	try to maximize physical activity prophylactically	

Bonica JJ: Introduction to management of pain of advanced cancer. International Symposium on Pain of Advanced Cancer. In Bonica JJ et al (eds): Advances in Pain Research and Therapy, vol 2, pp 115–130. New York, Raven Press, 1979

that moderate to severe pain will occur in about one-third of cancer patients with intermediate stages of disease and in 60–80% of patients with advanced disease.[1] Drugs commonly employed singly or in combination for mild pain include aspirin, acetaminophen, propoxyphene, codeine,and pentazocene. Drugs used for severe pain are the narcotic analgesics such as morphine, meperidine, and hydromorphone.

The number of available analgesics is quite large, and as with other areas of pharmaceutical redundancy among classes of drugs (*e.g.*, diuretics and minor tranquilizers) it is best to select a few agents, learn their characteristics in detail, and employ them in a sequence according to their potency, formulation, onset and duration of effect, and adverse reaction potential. It is important to know how well a patient has responded in the past to a given drug and whether there have been any untoward reactions. It is also necessary to have a therapeutic end-point in mind for each drug, dose and schedule, so that the drug can be maintained at a given level or else augmented or replaced in the event of failure. On occasion, it may be beneficial to add non-analgesic drugs such as tranquilizers, stimulants, or anti-depressants, depending upon the patient's emotional state. However, these types of agents have never been shown to specifically enhance an analgesic's effect. Rather, they have independent properties and are used additively, not synergistically.[5,8,9] Examples of their use are outlined in Table 43-28 and discussed in a later section.

The dose and schedule of narcotic analgesics require particular mention. Traditionally and inappropriately, physicians have prescribed these drugs, especially for inpatients, in inadequate doses and on a demand schedule. Illogically, this practice requires that patients must experience pain in order to ask for their next PRN dose. Even when the drug does come, too low a dose may render it ineffective or only partially effective. In contrast, with proper recognition of a drug's half-life and potency, physicians should be able to establish a dose and a fixed schedule which provides continuous pain relief. Additionally, this approach should decrease the likelihood of the development of pain-centered behavior, it may well decrease the total analgesic requirement over time, and most importantly, it will do what analgesics are supposed to do, relieve pain.[10]

To critically evaluate the literature on analgesia, especially as it relates to cancer patients, we need to consider the problems listed in Table 43-22, which are inherent in studies on pain.[7] Where pain research has involved short-term observation of patients with postoperative or post-partum pain, it is obviously difficult to make inferences from these data about the long-term administration of analgesics in cancer patients with chronic pain. Likewise, there is a problem in using estimates of side-effect potential and addiction liability made in the types of patients just mentioned who have acute pain states or who are post-addicts.

On the other hand, investigators such as Houde have conducted careful studies of analgesics in cancer patients. Their efforts have yielded valuable principles of analgesic usage and should serve to dispel popular misconceptions about various agents, especially narcotic analgesics. Well-controlled trials have shown that patients' objective reports

TABLE 43-22. Shortcomings in Studies of Analgesics

a. Failure to construct a dose-response curve
b. Failure to vary schedule and route of administration
c. Failure to use uniform reporting of data to permit interstudy comparisons
d. Failure to address differences between acute and chronic drug administration
e. Difficulty in controlling for population differences (age, diagnosis, performance status, source of pain) and in extrapolating from a study of one type of subject (*e.g.*, normal volunteer, postoperative patient) to another (*e.g.*, cancer patient)

Lasanga L: The clinical evaluation of morphine and its substitutes as analgesics. Pharmacol Rev 16:47–83, 1964

give reliable indications of the relative potency and relative usefulness of analgesics.[8] At the same time, differences between patients have also been recognized to be important in clinical practice. Variations in responses to analgesics have been related to: the type of illness itself; the physical setting (home *versus* hospital); the ability to tolerate pain based on past experience and attitudes; the concomitant use of other drugs; and variations between individuals in the pharmacokinetics of a given drug.[8] Other important factors include the site of pain production (bone *versus* viscus *verses* nerve root); the type of noxious stimulus (erosion *versus* inflammation *versus* compression), and the baseline status of the patient (well rested *versus* fatigued; active *versus* bed-ridden).

Inferences to be drawn from these observations are that patients should be carefully listened to and questioned about the quality of their responses, that their overall situation should be considered in planning therapy and judging responses, and that one should be flexible in setting and adjusting the level of therapy, not hide-bound by the published "standard" doses and schedules. In addition, since the degree of a response to a narcotic analgesic relates to the logarithm of the dose, any attempt to increase the degree of analgesia will require more than a fractional increase in dose (See Fig. 43-7).[8]

The placebo effect is also an important element in analgesic usage. Houde has emphasized that a placebo reaction has been inherent in every patient population studied.[8] However, it is ironic that physicians have tended to regard response to placebo as evidence that a patient is malingering rather than as an indication that his or her confidence in the doctor is such as to permit a high degree of suggestibility. The point is that the context surrounding drug administration, a positive, supportive, hopeful attitude by the medical staff, in itself has a measure of therapeutic effect, independent of drug action, and should be part of the armamentarium.

FIG. 43-7. Hypothetical plot of a clinical test of the analgesic effect of two narcotics, curve *A* and curve *B*.[8,11] Note that dose is on a log scale. Over the dose range studied, neither drug A nor drug B shows a ceiling effect, that is, the shape of the log-dose response curve remains linear, implying that a continued increase in dose will be matched by an increase in analgesic effect (in reality, however, adverse side effects set dose limits). The dashed curve *C* shows the leveling off in analgesic effect that would occur if drug *B* had a ceiling effect. The interval *D* is a measure of the relative potency of drug *A* vs drug *B*, *A* being more potent than *B*. The development of drug tolerance would shift the curves to the right.

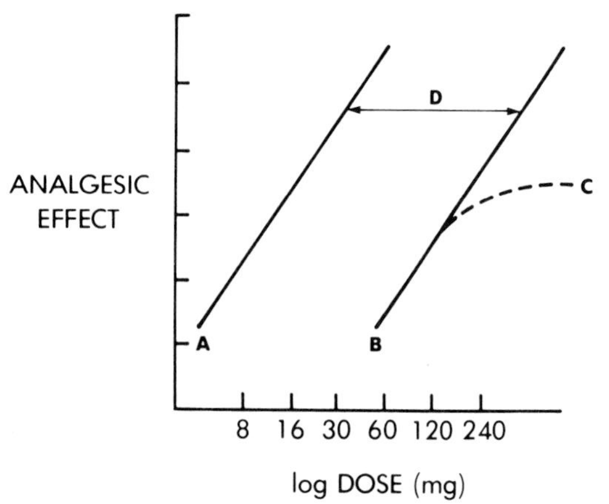

On the other hand, extensive concern for the addiction potential of narcotic analgesics should be avoided in treating pain in cancer patients.[1] It takes two weeks of parenteral administration of morphine at a dose of 60 mg or more per day for physical dependence to develop.[8] Even if it should develop in a patient with a limited life span, it is at that point one of the least worrisome items in the patient's management. In addition, Twycross, in summarizing a large experience in narcotic usage in advanced cancer patients, noted that physical dependence was rarely a significant problem, and that psychological addiction, the compulsion to experience a drug's psychological effects, did not occur when pain control was part of a pattern of total care.[12,13] Unfortunately, experience indicates that physicians tend to underuse narcotics because of an exaggerated fear of addicting their patients.[4] This is not to say, however, that the administration of narcotics does not require careful management and supervision of patients. The opposite tack of indiscriminately "snowing" cancer patients in pain or in terminal stages, is as inappropriate or harmful as undertreatment with narcotics.[3]

Tolerance to narcotic analgesics potentially poses more of a practical problem in cancer patients than does physical dependence. Tolerance has been well-documented and occurs at roughly the same pace as physical dependence.[8] It means that after several weeks, the duration of analgesic action may decrease and the dose of a narcotic may have to be increased several-fold to obtain the same analgesic effect. Fortunately, tolerance to the CNS side effects develops at a similar rate, and there is only a small risk of an increase in serious toxicity such as respiratory depression if the dose is escalated over time.[8]

Tolerance is less of a problem with drugs in the narcotic agonist-antagonist class such as pentazocine and with the "weak" narcotic codeine. It has not been reported with analgesic–antipyretic drugs such as aspirin and acetaminophen.[8] There is thus a rationale for continuing or introducing these latter two drugs, for whatever additive value they have, when placing the patient on the more potent narcotic analgesics.

SELECTION OF ANALGESIC DRUGS

AGENTS FOR MODERATE PAIN

General Considerations

Beaver, in a detailed review of the clinical pharmacology of the mild analgesics, defined this heterogenous group of agents by contrasting their properties with the more potent, narcotic analgesics.[14,15] Firstly, the mild analgesics, even in large doses, are less potent than narcotics in relieving most types of pain and are considered by many to have ceiling effects. Secondly, the mild analgesics are usually given orally, infrequently produce severe side-effects (especially considering the frequency of their use), have almost no addiction liability, and are more commonly used for chronic or mild pain in either the inpatient or outpatient setting. Thirdly, these agents probably relieve pain by diverse mechanisms, including direct effects on the cause of the pain, in contrast to the narcotics which are thought to act through CNS pathways. Whereas the narcotic analgesics have qualitatively similar pharmacologic properties, the mild analgesics as a group have dissimilar pharmacologic characteristics.

For convenience, mild analgesics may be classified into three groups: antipyretic-antiinflammatory agents; "weak" narcotics and chemically-related non-narcotics; and a host of chemically-unrelated agents, to date, of limited demonstrable value in the setting of cancer patients in pain.

Among the anti-inflammatory–antipyretic analgesics, aspirin and acetaminophen are of most interest from the standpoint of frequency of usage and limited side effect liability. Salicylates other than aspirin are uncommonly employed, have no advantage over aspirin, and are often less effective. The other types of drugs in the first group above are phenacetin, indomethacin, phenylbutazone, and the newer class of nonsteroidal anti-inflammatory agents.[16] Since phenacetin is metabolized to acetaminophen and is associated with renal damage after chronic use, it would seem to have little merit. There are no reports of extensive use of indomethacin or phenylbutazone for cancer-related pain, and these two drugs have relatively high adverse side-effect potentials. Indomethacin, however, because of its inhibition of prostaglandin systhesis, may have a specific role when pain is causally linked to prostaglandin production.[17] The same may be true for the phenylproprionic acid derivatives such as ibuprofen (Motrin), likewise inhibitors of prostaglandin synthesis. Definition of their general utility as mild analgesics in oncology practice awaits further study, though a controlled study suggests that one compound, indoprofen, is more potent than aspirin as an analgesic in cancer patients.[18]

The group of "weak" narcotics and related compounds includes codeine, dextropropoxyphene, ethoheptazine, and pentazocine. Codeine and pentazocine are the most important drugs here because of their establised analgesic potential. Dextropropoxyphene and ethoheptazine have been shown to be inferior to aspirin and would seem to have little value.[19]

The third group of drugs includes agents such as muscle relaxants, hypnotics, stimulants, and the like. The interested reader can consult Beaver's review for more details about these compounds.[15] Suffice it to say that their analgesic action is not established and that their use may be more likely to create unwanted side effects than relief of pain.

Pharmacology—Aspirin *and* Acetaminophen

Aspirin and acetaminophen are administered orally at a customary dose of 600 mg every four hours. For aspirin, at least, there is some question whether it has a ceiling effect and whether graded increases in dose will augment the degree of analgesia (see Fig. 43-7, curve c).[14] Beaver referred to data indicating that 400, 600, and 900 mg produced progressively greater pain relief in cancer patients.[14] Nine hundred mg produced greater "total relief" (a function of both intensity and duration of analgesia) of pain than 600 mg, but the peak level of relief was not significantly different between the two doses. As mentioned before, there are no data to suggest that patients develop tolerance to this class of agents.

In terms of side effects, aspirin at standard doses most commonly causes dyspepsia. It has the potential to cause occult or even frank GI bleeding and there appears to be no association between the frequency of dyspepsia and bleeding.[14] Its antiplatelet properties are well known, and it may cause allergic reactions, especially in patients with nasal polyps. In larger doses, it can prolong the prothrombin time and can cause hyperventilation and tinnitus. It has been associated with hepatic toxicity in patients with systemic lupus erythematosis and even in normal volunteers.[20]

Acetaminophen can cause dyspepsia, but it is not associated with GI bleeding or with clotting dysfunction. Acetaminophen does not exhibit cross-sensitivity in patients allergic to aspirin, and it has rarely been associated with agranulocytosis.[14] Unlike phenacetin, it produces little or no methemoglobin, is not a cause of hemolytic anemia, and its chronic use at standard doses has not yet been linked to renal toxicity. Overdoses of the drug produce a serious hepatotoxicity, however, and it has yet to be seen whether prolonged frequent administration of standard doses will produce similar damage.

In cancer patients, especially those undergoing antitumor treatement, the use of steroids (which carry a risk for peptic ulcer disease in their own right), agents lowering the platelet count, or anticoagulants, make aspirin more hazardous. Likewise, there is a theoretically greater risk of hemorrhage in patients with GI mucosal involvement with tumor who receive aspirin. Accordingly, acetaminophen will generally be a safer choice than aspirin. On the other hand, since acetaminophen has minimal anti-inflammatory activity, aspirin (or other nonsteroidal anti-inflammatory agents) would be potentially more useful in instances where inflammation contributes to a patient's discomfort.

Pharmacology—Codeine *and* Pentazocine

Codeine, along with aspirin, has been widely employed as a mild analgesic. It is effective orally over a dosage of 30–120 mg every 4–6 hours. It probably does not have a ceiling effect, tolerance to standard doses is not a practical problem, and its appearance as a drug of abuse is rare, a feature also especially striking in view of its frequent use as an analgesic and antitussive. There have been occasional instances of primary codeine addiction noted in the literature; the drug has some potential to support a preexisting physical dependence; but in fact there appears to be little risk of the development of drug dependence on standard doses given under medical supervision.[14] Codeine also has a very favorable oral:parenteral potency ratio of 0.68 (compared to 0.17 for morphine).

Pentazocine, a benzomorphan-derivative, is a weak morphine antagonist with demonstrated analgesic potential. However, the original claims that it would be free of addiction liability have turned out to be incorrect, at least for a parenterally administered drug.[21] It is effective orally at doses of 50–100 mg every 4–6 hours and parenterally at 30–60 mg (thus its oral:parenteral potency ratio is about 0.3). Compared to morphine, its onset of action is more rapid, and it is shorter acting (see Table 43-23).[5]

In terms of side effects, codeine is potentially capable of producing the adverse reactions characteristic of narcotics in general (see below and Table 43-26), but at standard doses,

TABLE 43-23. Commonly Used Narcotic Analgesics*

ANALGESIC	DOSE EQUIANALGESIC TO 10 MG IM MORPHINE		ORAL: PARENTERAL POTENCY RATIO	TIME TO ONSET (MIN)	DURATION OF ACTION (HR)	COMPARISON TO MORPHINE
	IM	PO				
oxymorphone (Numorphan)®	1	6	0.17	10–15 IM	3–6	more rapid onset; rectal suppository available
hydromorphone (Dilaudid)®	1.5	7.5	0.2	15–30 PO or IM	4–5	shorter acting
levorphanol (Levodromoran)®	2	4	0.5	60–90 PO or IM	6–8	high PO to IM potency; longer acting
methadone (Dolophine)®	10	20	0.5	30–60 PO	4–6	high PO to IM potency
morphine	10	60	0.17	30–60 IM	up to 7	—
oxycodone (in Percodan®, Percoset)®	15	30	0.5	10–15 PO	3–6	high PO to IM potency; shorter acting
anileridine (Leritine)®	30	50	0.6	15 PO or IM	2–3	high PO to IM potency; more rapid onset; shorter acting
alphaprodine (Nisentil)®	45	—	—	1–2 IV	½–1	more rapid onset; shorter acting
pentazocine (Talwin)®	60	180	0.3	20 IM	3	partial antagonist; shorter acting; more adverse CNS effects
meperidine (Demerol)®	75	300	0.25	30–50 IM	2–4	shorter acting
codeine	130	200	0.65	15–30 PO or IM	4–6	high PO to IM potency

See references 3 and 10.

serious side effects are rare. Respiratory depression, while measurable, is of little clinical significance, but constipation can be a troublesome problem after repeated doses. In addition, nausea, vomiting, sedation, dizziness, and allergic reactions all are occassionally seen.

At doses equianalgesic with morphine, pentazocine has similar side effects. It also has a troublesome frequency of associated CNS reactions including mood changes, vertigo, and hallucinations.[5,10,22] Because pentazocine has antagonist properties, it should not be used in combination with other narcotics, and it should not be given to a patient who has developed physical dependence upon a narcotic, since it can precipitate withdrawal symptoms.[3]

Management Considerations

It has been noted that in spite of the enormous popularity of the mild analgesics, there are comparatively few well-controlled studies of their use.[14] This paucity of inquiry is particularly striking when one considers the widespread prescription of "analgesic" mixtures such as aspirin, phenacetin, and caffeine, whereas certain components such as caffeine and propoxyphene have no well-established analgesic effect or where others such as aspirin and phenacetin lack any evidence of a special intermingling of effects which would justify their combination.[9,15]

On the other hand, since the relatively flat slopes of the log-dose response curves of these analgesics imply that multiples of doses of a drug will produce only modest increments of analgesia, and since two disparate drugs such as aspirin and codeine presumably act by different mechanisms and should be additive in producing analgesia, there is a rationale for forming certain drug combinations.[15] To this point, Moertel and coworkers studied aspirin in combination with a variety of other mild analgesics in cancer patients and showed that drugs approaching the potency of aspirin in an earlier drug study were additive in analgesic effect when combined with aspirin (see Tables 43-24 and 43-25).[9,19]

Thus, for the treatment of mild pain in cancer patients, one would begin with acetaminophen or aspirin (however, if their antipyretic properties posed a hazard in patients for whom fever is a critical sign—*i.e.*, those who are immunosuppressed or leukopenic—then this class of agents would be bypassed). For aspirin, there may be some rationale in pushing the dose upwards to 900 mg if the standard 600 mg dose is ineffective and if the risk and incidence of side effects is acceptable at

TABLE 43-24. Comparison of Single Analgesics

DRUGS BETTER THAN PLACEBO (DOSE IN MG)	DRUGS INFERIOR TO ASPIRIN (DOSE IN MG)
Aspirin (650)	Propoxyphene (65)
Mefenamic acid (250)	Ethoheptazine (75)
Phenacetin (650)	Promazine (25)
Acetaminophen (650)	Placebo
Codeine (65)	
Pentazocine (50)	

Moertel CG, Ahmann DL, Taylor WF et al: A comparative evaluation of marketed analgesic drugs. N Engl J Med 286:813–815, 1972

TABLE 43-25. Comparison of Analgesic Combinations

COMBINATIONS BETTER THAN ASPIRIN ALONE (DOSE IN MG)	COMBINATIONS NO BETTER THAN ASPIRIN ALONE
Codeine (65) + Aspirin (650)	Propoxyphene Napsylate (100) + Aspirin (650)
Oxycodone (9.75) + Aspirin (650)	Promazine HCl (25) + Aspirin (650)
Pentazocine (25) + Aspirin (650)	Pentabarbital (32) + Aspirin (650) Caffeine (65) + Aspirin (650) Ethoheptazine (75)+ Aspirin (650)

Moertel CG, Ahmann DL, Taylor WF et al: Relief of pain by oral medications: A controlled evaluation of analgesic combinations. JAMA 229:55–59, 1974

the higher level. The next step would be to add codeine or pentazocine, though the latter has the disadvantage of adverse CNS effects and higher cost. Codeine would be titrated over the range of 30–120 mg per dose until effective or until adverse side effects become limiting, and the next step would be to move to the stronger analgesics.

AGENTS FOR SEVERE PAIN

General Considerations

The narcotic analgesics most commonly prescribed for severe pain are listed in Table 43-23. In general, their therapeutic and pharmacologic similarities overshadow differences in analgesic potential, antitussive action, sedative effect, emetic properties, respiratory depression, constipating effect, and addiction liability.

Because clinicians tend to forget that "geometric progressions in dose are required to achieve equal increments in analgesic effect," there is the mistaken belief that these drugs have ceiling effects (see Fig. 43-6).[8] In addition, the relative potencies of the agents are often misconstrued as indicating, for example, that a drug such as meperidine is less effective than morphine (in a qualitative sense), because it takes 75 mg of meperidine IM to be equally analgesic with only 10 mg of morphine IM. The point is that even though investigators have been able to determine in clinical studies the relative doses of the different agents required to produce a given analgesic effect, each dose is simply that, a number of milligrams, and says nothing about what makes one drug better than another.

The factors which do allow for discrimination and for selection of a given narcotic include its optimal route of administration, rapidity of onset of action, and duration of action. Individual differences between patients are also important, requiring a degree of empiricism and trial and error in choosing an agent, a dose, and a schedule for each situation.

Pharmacology

The commonly used narcotic analgesics in Table 43-23 are listed according to an IM or oral dose equianalgesic to 10 mg of IM morphine. Also included are the oral:parenteral potency ratios and estimates of the time course of clinical analgesic effects for each drug. It is helpful to keep in mind that in the comparative testing of narcotic analgesics, equianalgesic doses reflect either the peaks of the time curves (peak effect) or the areas under the curves (total effect). In treating an individual patient, however, the actual effectiveness of a narcotic will relate to the clinical situation—a rapid acting or short acting drug will be more useful for the relief of acute, short-lived pain, while a long acting drug would better treat continuous pain. Thus, while the rapid acting drug may have a higher peak effect and lower total effect, or the longer acting drug a lower peak effect and greater total effect, neither parameter confers an absolute value on one drug as opposed to the other.[8,10] Older patients require smaller doses to achieve a given analgesic effect and the narcotics are generally better at relieving dull, continuous pain rather than colicky pain.[20,23]

Note that five drugs have oral:parenteral ratios of 0.5 or better (levorphanol, methadone, oxycodone, anilerdine, and codeine) and that one agent, oxymorphone, is available as a rectal suppository. There is considerable variation in time to onset of analgesia, ranging from 1–2 minutes for IV alphaprodine to 60–90 minutes for oral or IM levorphanol. Likewise, some agents are short-lived in effect (one-half to one hour for alphaprodine, 2–3 hours for anileridene, and 2–4 hours for meperidine); others have a relatively long duration of action (up to 7 hours for morphine, 6-8 hours for levorphanol); and the rest give an intermediate length of analgesia (3–6 hours for oxycodone, 4–5 hours for hydromorphone, 4–6 hours for methadone). Again, these figures are only guidelines. They will vary from patient to patient, with past duration of drug exposure, and with the degree of tolerance which has developed.

The non-analgesic effects of the narcotics are important to know and to anticipate. Table 43-26 summarizes the major reactions. Those marked with an asterisk have the greatest frequency or practical significance.

Euphoria is a frequent and desired side effect, but some patients do experience dysphoria. Nausea, vomiting, and depression of consciousness are not infrequent at the beginning of therapy and may improve with continued administration or may require a change in dose or frequency or a switch to another agent. Antiemetics such as the phenothiozines can be useful in blocking the first two side effects during the initiation of treatment. Depression of respiration, while almost always measurable and occasionally significant, has now been reported as a severe side effect in debilitated patients receiving methadone. In this instance, too rapid a build-up of dose

TABLE 43-26. Side Effects of Narcotic Analgesics

A. Central Nervous System
 *euphoria (dysphoria)
 *sedation
 lowering of seizure threshold
 *central depression of respiration, cough reflex
 *nausea, vomiting

B. GI Tract
 *decreased secretions
 *constipation
 increased smooth muscle tone in biliary tract

C. Genitourinary System
 *urinary retention

D. Circulatory System
 postural hypotension

E. Miscellaneous
 anaphylactoid reaction
 autonomic reactions
 (diaphoresis, hyperglycemia, miosis, dry mouth)
 antidiuresis
 adverse interaction with monoamineoxidase inhibitors
 (esp. meperidine)

*Those side effects more common in the treatment of cancer pain. (Catalano RB: The medical approach to management of pain caused by cancer. Semin Oncol 2:379–392, 1975)

occurred and metabolites accumulated which presumably were non-analgesic but were still able to depress the medullary respiratory centers. The effects were reversed with a narcotic antagonist.[24] In addition, in a patient with pre-existent respiratory insufficiency, the ability of the narcotics to diminish the sensitivity of the respiratory chemoreceptors may precipitate coma because of further carbon dioxide retention. This could be an especial hazard in patients with increased cranial blood flow produced by hypercarbia.[5] Suppression of the cough reflex may be beneficial in patients with an irritative cough, but harmful where any depression of the capacity to expectorate cannot be tolerated. While infrequently of clinical significance, the ability of narcotics to lower the seizure threshold may be a problem in patients with a history of seizures or with cerebral metastases.[10]

Of the GI side effects, constipation represents a major difficulty. Patients who take narcotics chronically, especially older people, frequently become constipated and require strict monitoring of bowel frequency and the administration of laxatives, stool softeners, and adequate fluid intake to avoid the obstipation which can lead to frank bowel obstruction. Urinary retention (secondary to increased vesical sphincter and detrusor tone) is more common in older patients, particularly men with prostatic enlargement. As one would expect, postural hypotension, when seen, usually occurs in ambulatory patients and is more of a risk in older patients or in those with a lowered blood volume.[5] Finally, there are several other phenomena associated with narcotic analgesic use, such as an anaphylactoid reaction and various autonomic reactions (see Table 43-26).[10]

Physical dependence upon narcotics develops over time and can be unmasked by sudden withdrawal of the analgesic. In general, a short course of therapy, one or two weeks long, will not produce clinically significant withdrawal symptoms upon cessation of the analgesic. Narcotic antagonists can precipitate severe withdrawal symptoms in dependent patients and should be used only in cases of drug overdose.

Management Considerations

The literature gives few details on sequentially selecting or changing narcotic analgesics for cancer patients with severe pain. Most of the underlying principles one uses to approach this problem have already been mentioned: the employment of a fixed rather than a demand dose schedule; the selection of a drug and the titration of the dose and schedule according to the patient and the clinical situation at hand; the recognition and treatment of untoward side effects; the avoidance of excessive concern for drug addiction or of indifference towards the hazards of narcotic use; and the awareness of the possibility of drug tolerance and of the log/dose response relationship for narcotic analgesics.

There should be a commitment to maintain a patient on oral medication for as long as possible. Unfortunately, there seems to be a tendency to link strong analgesics to only the parenteral route of administration. Extensive experience in England has shown it is possible to maintain the majority of advanced cancer patients on oral narcotics until the last few days of their lives.[12] Adverse effects such as sedation tended to disappear early on in the course of therapy, and many patients remained ambulatory and able to maintain a degree of independence and self-care.

Finally, each physician should develop his or her own cascade for the sequential use of narcotics in cancer patients. Although one narcotic can produce cross-tolerance to another, the cross-tolerance is not usually complete.[3] For example, in addition to the concomitant use of aspirin or acetaminophen mentioned earlier, this writer generally starts with oral drugs, first codeine, and later turns to oxycodone, hydromorphone, and then levorphanol or methadone. The starting dose employed for a drug as it replaces a previous one will be higher than if narcotics were being used *de novo,* and the success of each agent will depend upon the frequency of the pain and its severity in relation to the schedule and pharmacokinetics of the drug. It should be borne in mind that while drug absorption is more erratic by the oral route, and the peak effect tends to be blunted, the period of drug effect is usually more extended than with parenteral administration.[8] The favorable oral:parenteral potency ratio and long duration of action of levorphanol in particular may allow for less frequent dosaging and smoother control of pain. Empirically, methadone appears to have similar clinical usefulness. For patients

TABLE 43-27. Brompton's Solution

Morphine hydrochloride (15 mg)
Cocaine hydrochloride (10 mg)
Alcohol 90% (2 ml)
Syrup (4 ml)
Chloroform water to 15 ml

Anonymous: The Brompton Cocktail. Lancet 1:1220–1221, 1979

unable to take oral medications, oxymorphone suppositories can provide effective analgesia in doses of 10–20 mg.

A particularly successful approach to the chronic administration of narcotic analgesics has been Brompton's solution.[13,25-27] An example of its components appears in Table 43-27. As originally constituted, it contained heroin, cocaine (to counteract the sedative effect of the opiate), alcohol, and chloroform water (both elements to solubilize the heroin and cocaine), and flavoring.[26,27] A phenothiozine such as prochlorperazine (Compazine) has been given concomitantly to diminish opiate-induced nausea and vomiting.[26]

Subsequent observation has shown morphine to be equal to or better than heroin, and there has been the suggestion that the cocaine and alcohol are unnecessary (however, the alcohol does serve to prevent bacterial contamination).[28,29] A comparative study of a morphine elixir with and without cocaine showed no difference between patients with regard to sedation and ability to concentrate.[29] More important than the number of components is that the use of the solution has permitted the ready titration of oral drug doses by the patient or the physician in a manner which usually leaves the patients with a maximum degree of comfort and independence.[12] Patients began with a set dose given every four hours, say 20 mg of morphine, and the dose was increased until a satisfactory level of analgesia was reached. Initial side effects such as sedation abated relatively quickly, and nausea was blocked by a phenothiozine as mentioned above (also with titration of the dose of this drug as needed). After a stable narcotic dose had been maintained for several days, it was often possible to lower the amount of opiate required (perhaps in part because of the loss of the anxiety associated with the dread of pain). Physical dependence did not interfere with the downward adjustment of dose, and observation of a large number of patients in England did not show tolerance and physical dependence to be clinical problems.[12]

For parenteral administration of narcotics, morphine, at a starting dose of 10 mg every 4–6 hours, has been the standard. Alphaprodine would be used when a very rapid analgesic effect would be required, but its short duration of action would necessitate following up with a longer acting drug such as morphine to subsequently maintain pain relief. In this regard, meperidine's short duration of action would also tend to dictate more frequent administration, thus making intervening periods of pain more likely if subsequent doses were delayed to any extent. Other drugs to consider for parenteral use are oxymorphone, hydromorphone, levorphanol, and methadone. It may also be useful to combine oral and parenteral drugs. Differences and overlap in their time course of action may provide more complete and lasting relief.[8]

Table 43-28 contains a list of other classes of drugs which, according to anecdote or studies in groups of patients with conditions other than cancer and chronic pain (*e.g.*, postoperative and post-partum patients), have been said to augment the analgesic potential of narcotics. Recent reports have suggested that hydroxyzine and dextroamphetamine potentiate morphine analgesia in postoperative patients with acute pain.[30,31] There are reports that phenothiozines or tricyclic antidepressants have analgesic potential alone in disease states such as headache or diabetic neuropathy.[32] However, it is extremely difficult to extrapolate from these types of experience to the situation of a cancer patient with chronic pain. Certainly the agents in Table 43-28 can be used as concomitants of standard analgesics to take advantage of their independent properties, but there are as yet no convincing data that they interact in a synergistic fashion. In addition, drugs such as the phenothiozines have the potential for adding to the sedation and respiratory depression produced by narcotic analgesics, and in their own right have the liability of inducing characteristic adverse reactions, in particular, extrapyramidal side effects.[33]

TABLE 43-28. Examples of Drugs Considered for Use with Narcotic Analgesics

Stimulants
Methylphenidate (Ritalin)
Dextroamphetamine (Dexedrine)
Tricyclic Antidepressants
Imipramine (Tofranil)
Amitriptyline (Elavil)
Major Tranquilizers
Chlorpromazine (Thorazine)
Haloperidol (Haldol)
Ataractics
Hydroxyzine (Vistaril)

NEW DEVELOPMENTS IN PHARMACOLOGIC CONTROL OF PAIN

Of most immediate importance for future progress in pain control with drugs is the appearance and proliferation of multispecialty pain clinics and hospice facilities.[1] In themselves, they provide a hopeful sign as they symbolize wider efforts to comprehensively and more compassionately tackle the problems posed by chronic pain, cancer, and terminal illness. They also provide a context in which clinical research can proceed more rationally and deliberately to discover better ways to dose and schedule analgesics, to find other modes of pain control, and to test different forms of supportive care.

The discovery of the opiate receptor and of endogenous opioid polypeptides (the endorphins) within the CNS has opened fertile lines of research into how pain is produced and how it might be controlled at a more fundamental level.[34,35] Pilot studies in a limited number of patients have demonstrated that beta-endorphins given intraventricularly or intrathecally-administered morphine or beta-endorphin, can rapidly provide profound and long-lasting analgesia.[36-38] Adverse side effects in these reports were relatively minor and may turn out to be far less severe than seen with equianalgesic doses of systemically administered opiates. Comparative clinical testing will be needed to confirm these results. Direct and repeated instillations of these agents into the cerebrospinal fluid is possible now with an Ommaya reservoir, and the future development of less troublesome delivery systems or of an endorphin-like agent effective orally or parenterally may allow pain relief with fewer complications than exist with currently available methodolgies.

Neurosurgical Approaches

EUGENE A. QUINDLEN

Excluding stimulation of the central and peripheral nervous system, all other neurosurgical procedures presently designed to relieve pain are destructive procedures. In each case the surgeon attempts to interrupt specific pain pathways which carry "pain impulses" to the level of consciousness. These procedures have evolved as our understanding of neuroanatomy and neurophysiology has evolved. The basic neuroanatomy involved is that of the lateral spinothalamic tract.[39] Painful sensations are recorded by free nerve endings, nocioceptors, and transmitted over small unmyelinated axons that arise from the dorsal root ganglion cells. These synapse on a second neuron situated in the dorsal aspect of the spinal cord in an area called the substantia gelatinosa. These neurons have axons that cross in the anterior commissure and ascend to the posterior ventrolateral nucleus of the thalamus by traveling in the ventral quadrant of the spinal cord. Neurons in the thalamus project to the somatosensory cortex in the post-central gyrus of the cerebrum (see Fig. 43-8). Clinical and experimental evidence suggest that pain impulses must reach the level of the thalamus before pain can be consciously appreciated as pain.

There have been neurosurgical procedures performed to interrupt these pain pathways at every level of the nervous system. In general, the success and risk of these procedures are proportional to the level of the nervous system at which the pain pathways are interrupted. Those pain syndromes which are localized to the caudal extent of the body and unilateral are more likely to be relieved; for example, by dorsal rhizotomy, or anterolateral cordotomy. However, diffuse bilateral pain extending up to the cervical region is much more difficult to relieve and entails higher risks for the patient. Table 43-29 lists some of the neurosurgical procedures frequently used to relieve cancer pain and the results reported in representative surgical series.

PAIN

It is important to characterize fully the nature, location, and extent of the patient's pain. Clues as to a particular lesion which may be the predominant cause of the patient's pain may often be elicited on history and physical examination. This information is vital in determining the subsequent treatment. For instance, bilateral sacral pain would be better

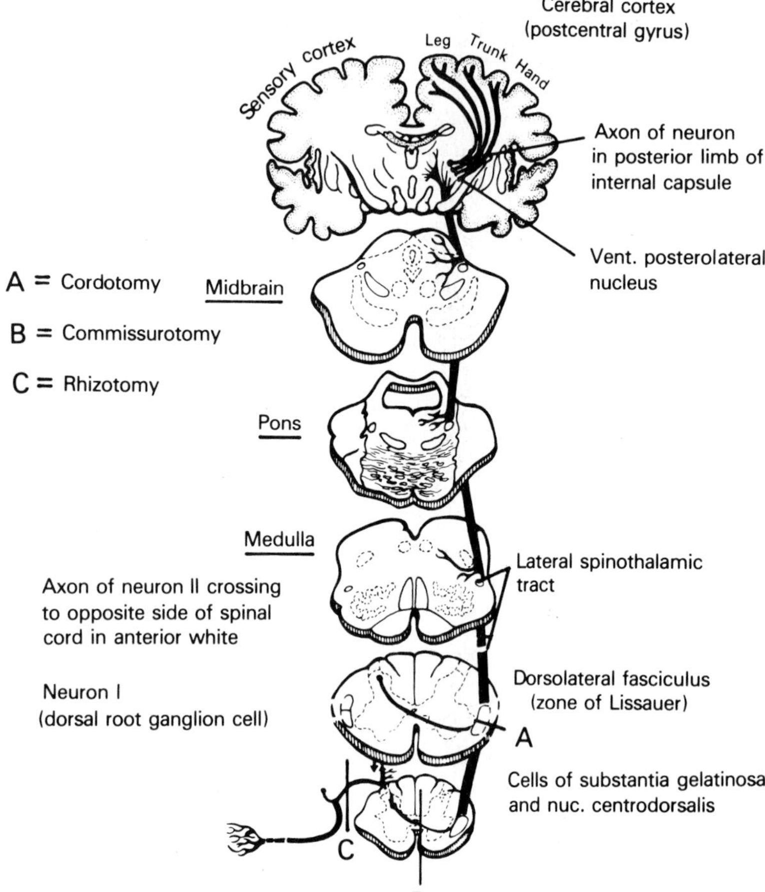

FIG. 43-8. Diagram illustrating the course of the lateral spinothalamic tract and the level of interruption of its course by three different neurosurgical procedures. (Carpenter MB: Human Neuroanatomy, p 245. Baltimore, Williams & Wilkins, 1979)

TABLE 43-29. Results of Various Surgical Procedures for Cancer Pain

OPERATION	TYPE OF PAIN	PERCENT RELIEVED OF PAIN	PERCENT SERIOUS MORBIDITY	PERCENT MORTALITY
open unilateral thoracic cordotomy (ref.)	lower trunk lower extremity with unilateral predominance	72	13	6.5
open bilateral thoracic cordotomy (ref.)	bilateral trunk lower extremity	81	42	13.0
percutaneous cervical cordotomy including bilateral (ref)	trunk and lower extremity	87	8	1.4
commissurectomy (ref)	bilateral trunk and lower limbs	87	0	0
transphenoidal hypophysectomy (ref)	diffuse bone pain from prostate carcinoma	91	0	7.5

treated with a sacral rhizotomy or a commissurotomy rather than a unilateral or bilateral cordotomy. By the same token pain localized to a single dermatome or a few dermatomes or originating in a peripheral nerve might be better treated with an appropriate posterior rhizotomy.

The physician must have a clear idea of whether the patient's pain is localized or diffuse. Furthermore, he must be able to distinguish as much as possible between discrete physical pain and suffering.[40] The distinction is difficult especially in the setting of chronic unrelieved pain, but is paramount in determining the likelihood of success in obtaining relief with a neurosurgical procedure. The aspect of suffering includes not only the aspect of pain but the psychological effects of pain and illness. Successful treatment of the patient as a whole will require the expertise of the psychiatrist, the nurse and perhaps the use of psychotropic medications.

PATIENT SELECTION

The neurosurgeon's expertise should be sought in those patients whose pain can not be controlled by more conservative measures including narcotic analgesics, endocrine manipulation, or radiation therapy. Many patients can be controlled with narcotics on a carefully regulated regimen which provides relief of pain and minimal amount of disturbed sensorium. Some patients will experience objectionable side effects of narcotic analgesia and may wish to return home free of drug effect if they can obtain relief of pain. These patients should be offered a neurosurgical procedure for control of their pain.

Patients who are considered for a pain relieving procedure should be expected to survive at least three months to justify the normal recuperative post operative period and operative risk for these procedures. However, considerable individual judgement must be exercised in this regard since many procedures are justified to make the last days of the patient more comfortable.

DORSAL RHIZOTOMY

Sectioning of the sensory roots to interrupt afferent pain fibers has several advantages and disadvantages. It is most useful when the pain is well localized to the trunk or neck and not usually practical when pain is limited to an otherwise functioning extremity since complete deafferentation of a limb renders it useless. However, partial selective rhizotomy involving the upper or lower limb has been helpful in some patients.[41] In patients with severe pain where tumor is invading the brachial plexus, (breast or Pancoast lung tumors) high cervical cordotomy may have to be performed. Since all incoming sensory fibers serving a given dermatome are cut, the patient is left with anesthesia as well as analgesia and the former effect may be disagreeable to some patients. Rarely is any effect noted from the division of a single dorsal root so that in general several dorsal roots above and below the segmental level of the pain must be divided. When analgesia is obtained, however, it is usually much more lasting than cordotomy. The operative procedure involves a laminectomy, identification, and sectioning of the appropriate dorsal roots under local anesthesia or general anesthesia. Paravertebral injection of local anesthesia into the intervertebral foramen is a very useful maneuver to determine the exact level and extent of the required rhizotomy.

Dorsal rhizotomy has been commonly used to alleviate pain in the chest or abdominal wall and pain arising in the sacral and perineal area. Sacral rhizotomy has been helpful in relieving pain caused by carcinoma of the rectum, vulva, and cervix. Bilateral sacral rhizotomies can be performed provided the sacral roots of S_2 and S_3 are preserved at least on one side to reduce the risk of urinary incontinence and impotence in the male. Failure of adequate dorsal rhizotomy to relieve pain within the dermatome involved has been attributed to sensory axons entering the cord through the ventral roots. Indeed, such axons have been found in ventral roots in recent experimental studies.[42]

Often when a decompressive laminectomy is performed for

epidural metastasis the neurosurgeon can perform extradural root section, which can relieve pain due to tumor invasion of bone and nerves at the same level of the metastasis.

COMMISSURAL MYELOTOMY

This procedure is useful in relieving bilateral sacral and lower extremity pain. After laminectomy and exposure of the lower spinal cord, a midline myelotomy is performed from the L_1 to sacral segments of the cord dividing both the dorsal and anterior commissures. The operating microscope is often used to perform the procedure to ensure adequate division of the crossing fibers and safety of the vessels of the spinal cord.

Recently, midline myelotomies have been performed at higher levels of the cord including the cervical region to relieve bilateral or midline pain in the chest wall and neck.[43] It has been observed that the pain can be relieved in areas outside of the demonstrable areas of analgesia, suggesting that simple interruption of the spinalthalamic tract crossing fibers may not be the only mechanism involved.

Mortality from this procedure has been less than 3% and the morbidity is less than cordotomy. Patients will often have uncomfortable dysesthesiae and posterior column tract deficits immediately following the procedure but these usually resolve within two weeks. Unlike cordotomy, urinary incontinence is rarely seen and motor weakness is rare. The long-term success in cancer patients in one recent series was 80% with a low operative mortality and morbidity. This operation should become an increasingly useful procedure for patients with bilateral and midline pain.[44]

ANTEROLATERAL CORDOTOMY

Cordotomy has been practiced by neurosurgeons in this country since its introduction by Frazier in 1920.[45] It is the most frequently used neurosurgical procedure for the relief of pain in cancer patients. Its aim is to cut the spinothalamic tract fibers in the anterolateral quadrant of the spinal cord at a level well above the patient's pain. Since this tract is a crossed tract, the incision in the spinal cord is made on the side opposite the patient's pain.

The operation is most effective when the patient's pain is unilateral but is also useful in reducing the discomfort of bilateral pain. When pain is worse on one side, a cordotomy can be performed on both sides of the cord at different levels of the cord at a single operation but the risk of a serious neurological complication such as paralysis or urinary incontinence is higher in bilateral cordotomy. Nonetheless, in a bedridden patient with serious pain it may give excellent relief of pain.

Two types of operations are currently employed: an open cordotomy (cervical or thoracic) and a closed cordotomy or percutaneous cervical cordotomy. The latter is a stereotactic procedure performed under fluoroscopic control and is generally replacing the older open cordotomy in most medical centers in the country.

An open cordotomy can be performed in the high thoracic region (T_2–T_4) for pain below the level of the umbilicus or in the high cervical region for pain in the chest and upper abdomen. The operation should be done at the lowest level possible consistent with adequate relief of pain since the complications at a high level of the cord can be disastrous. The operation is performed by performing a standard laminectomy, opening the dura and identifying the dentate ligament attaching the equator of the cord to the dura. The dentate ligament is then grasped with a hemostat. A knife blade is inserted 4 mm into the antereolateral quadrant of the cord, parallel to equator of the cord and swept ventral, exiting 2 mm from the midline of the cord. A blunt hook is used to insure division of all of the fibers. The operation can be performed under general or local anesthesia. Under local anesthesia the surgeon has the obvious advantage of being able to test the patient during the procedure to ensure adequate analgesia.

An open thoracic cordotomy is successful in relieving pain in over 75% of patients with a 4–5% mortality risk in most reported series.[46] Morbidity is as high as 25% and includes such complications as hemiparesis, urinary retention, sexual impotence, and skin breakdown.

If carefully examined, many post-cordotomy patients can be found to have a mild hemiparesis which becomes undetectable 2–3 weeks following the procedure. About 5% of patients will remain with a permanently detectable or long-lasting weakness on the side of the cordotomy.[47]

When pain is higher as in the chest and upper abdomen it will best be relieved by a cervical cordotomy. If this is performed by an open operation the mortality is higher than the thoracic procedure but the chance for relief of pain much better. One complication which is seen in both open and closed cervical cordotomy is respiratory depression with sleep apnea. This complication resulted in deaths early in Rosomoff's series of patients with closed cervical cordotomy so that he recommends constant observation of these patients for the first 3 days postoperatively.[48]

The percutaneous cervical cordotomy introduced by Mullan in 1963 has largely supplanted the open cordotomy technique.[49] The technique was refined by Rosomoff who built a stereotactic needle electrode holder that can precisely advance an electrode into the cord.[48] The operation is performed with the patient supine on a fluoroscopic table with the patient's head held still with a special head holding device. After local anesthesia, a standard lateral C_1–C_2 puncture is performed under fluoroscopic control with an 18 gauge spinal needle. Through this needle air or contrast material is introduced into the subarachnoid space so that the outline of the cord and the dentate ligament can be seen. When the anterior half of the spinal cord can be visualized a wire electrode insulated except at the tip is introduced through the needle into the CSF and into the anterolateral quadrant of the spinal cord. At the point at which the electrode enters the cord there is an increase in impedance across the electrode compared to an indifferent electrode. After the electrode is in place, stimulation of the anterior quadrant of the cord can verify if the electrode is in the correct position if the patient reports a warm feeling, tingling, or even pain in the contralateral body. After stimulation, a series of heat lesions are made with controlled radiofrequency current. After each lesion, the patient is tested for any sensory or motor neurological deficit. The lesions are continued until the desired level of analgesia without motor deficit is produced.

The entire procedure rarely takes longer than an hour and it affords great flexibility to the surgeon since one can persist with lesions to eradicate the pain or terminate the procedure quickly if necessary. Most series have reported success in relief of pain in over 85% of patients with a mortality rate less than 3%.[50–53] The closed cervical cordotomy carries less risk than an open procedure at the same level. However, patients must still be observed closely for signs of respiratory depression in the immediate postoperative period. Cordotomies at the cervical level can and will relieve visceral pain, which originates predominantly on one side of the abdomen (gallbladder, spleen, liver).

If bilateral cordotomies are necessary it is probably best to carry out one at a cervical level and the other at the thoracic level, since bilateral cervical cordotomies often carry a very high risk of respiratory depression.

TRANSSPHENOID HYPOPHYSECTOMY

Hypophysectomy was first used to obtain palliative remissions in premenopausal women with breast cancer who had previously responded to adrenalectomy or estrogens.[54] These patients often have a dramatic reduction in skeletal pain sometimes within hours of the operation. This technique has also been applied to patients with metastatic prostate carcinoma with gratifying results.[55,56] As tumors were investigated for the presence of estrogen receptors it was observed that some patients had relief of pain even though they had no estrogen receptors present on the tumor. This has led several neurosurgeons to perform transsphenoidal hypophysectomy in many different types of tumors with some success.[57] This would indicate that there might be some more general mechanism operating to relieve bone pain than just hormonal specificity for the tumor. In fact, a recent study of hypophysectomized women with breast cancer found that all of the women had relief of bone pain despite endocrinologic evaluation indicating incomplete hormonal ablation of the pituitary.[58]

Recently, Moricca has introduced chemical hypophysectomy which he performs by the injection of alcohol into the sella.[59] He reports dramatic relief of pain in the majority of patients with many different types of cancer. These patients do not often develop endocrinological deficits despite their good therapeutic response to the procedure. In a recent study, when contrast material was injected prior to alcohol it was found to track along the pituitary stalk and entered the third ventricle implying that this procedure may be exerting its effect on central pain pathways in the hypothalamus.[60]

At the present time in this country, transsphenoidal hypophysectomy is indicated in patients with breast or prostate carcinoma and diffuse bone pain unrelieved by standard medical measures. The operative mortality is less than 2% in most series and the complication rate 4% and includes, CSF rhinorrhea, intrasellar hematoma, sinusitis, abscess, and rarely meningitis. The operation is performed by a sublabial submucous elevation of the nasal mucosa, opening the sphenoid sinus and the anterior inferior wall of the sella. After opening of the pituitary dura the gland is mobilized and the stalk sectioned and the gland removed. The sella is packed with fat and nasal cartilage and the nasal mucosa repositioned and held in place with nasal packs. The entire procedure is performed using the operating microscope and aided by fluoroscopic control.

RHIZOTOMY OF THE CRANIAL NERVES

Patients with head and neck cancer present one of the most difficult pain problems for the physician. Some of these patients can have their pain alleviated by sectioning of the appropriate cranial nerves carrying sensory fiber from the head, ear, pharynx, or larynx. This usually involves sectioning the V, IX, X and the nervus intermidius, which travels with the facial nerve and in some cases the upper cervical roots C_1–C_3.

The operation is performed by performing a suboccipital craniectomy just behind the mastoid bone on the side of the pain. After opening of the dura and gentle retraction on the lateral cerebellum the lower cranial nerves can be found in the cerebellopontine angle. The operating microscope is an invaluable tool in the proper identification of the neuroanatomic structures in this region.

The postoperative management of these patients can be difficult, since the IX and X cranial nerves are sectioned the patient will be hoarse and normal swallowing and protective gag reflex may be absent thus making aspiration more likely. If the patient has been previously tracheotomized or has had a laryngectomy these concerns are not relevant.

Other procedures for the relief of head and neck pain have been less frequently tried. These include trigeminal tractotomy, and mesencephalic section of the spinothalamic tract.[61,62]

In those patients with a malignant process and pain involving the face, maxilla, or mouth, rhizotomy confined to the trigeminal rootlets may be sufficient for relief. In this regard, percutaneous differential thermal rhizotomy of the rootlets as performed by Sweet is the procedure of choice.[63] Like a percutaneous cordotomy, this procedure is performed under local anesthesia with a needle electrode to conduct controlled radiofrequency current. This allows controlled thermocoagulation of the trigeminal rootlets and continuous monitoring of the patient for the desired level of analgesia. Since the small unmyelinated pain fibers are more sensitive to the destructive effects of heat, these fibers can be destroyed preferentially while sparing touch sensation. Although first developed for the treatment of trigeminal neuralgia, this procedure should be used more often in malignant facial pain because of its zero mortality and low morbidity.

The operation is performed by inserting a needle electrode through the skin of the cheek and into the foramen of ovale under x-ray of fluoroscopic control. During the insertion of the needle and subsequent lesions the patient is given small doses of ultrashort-acting barbiturate IV. The effects of this type of agent last only minutes and allow testing of the patient between lesions. The electrode is connected to a stimulator and when low threshold paresthesiae are produced in the appropriate division of the trigeminal nerve, the proper location of the electrode is found. Next, staged amounts of current are applied to the electrode using a radiofrequency generator. The patient is tested between each increasing lesion to determine the level and extent of analgesia produced. The entire lesion-making process is best controlled by an electrode, which contains a built-in thermocouple which records the temperature of each lesion.

SUBARACHNOID INJECTION OF PHENOL

Since this technique was first described by Meyer it has been increasingly used by neurosurgeons and anesthesiologists to produce pain relief in the trunk and lower extremities. Sweet has estimated that the use of this procedure has reduced the need for cordotomy in 50% of his patients.[64] However, with the advent of the low risk percutaneous cordotomy it is often preferable to proceed directly with cordotomy.

The analgesic effect produced by a phenol block is highly variable and may last only 2 weeks or as long as many months. However, it usually produces relief for 3–6 months. The procedure is performed by injecting 5% phenol in pantopaque or a glycerol solution through a lumbar needle that has been placed into the subarachnoid space. Since these solutions are hyperbaric the patient is placed in the decubitus position with the side of the pain down. The table is tilted downward slightly at the caudal end. Small increments of the solution are injected and the patient examined between each injection. The use of phenol in pantopaque allows direct visualization of the solution puddle on a fluoroscopic unit. However, phenol in glycerol may be more effective. The extent of analgesia is difficult to control exactly and care must be taken not to allow the solution to extend above the mid-dorsal area and subsequently into the cervical region since respiratory paralysis may result. Deaths, although rare, have been reported because of this latter complication. If too many injections are made too quickly and insufficient time is allowed to lapse to determine the full effect of the phenol, extensive root damage can occur resulting in bladder and bowel incontinence.

When performed by an experienced person, however, this procedure can afford rapid and uncomplicated pain relief for several months.

Neurostimulation

CHARLES V. BURTON
CHARLES D. RAY

Neuroaugmentation refers to the use of external and implanted electronic devices designed to augment the function of the intact nervous system. Presently, the practical uses of these devices are essentially limited in the treatment of disease to either improving body function or relieving pain. Neuroaugmentive surgery pertains to the implantation of electronic neurostimulators. The first-generation medical devices now in use function relatively passively; second-generation devices, reflecting more advanced technology, will permit function via biofeedback mechanisms in which sensors placed in the body will monitor pathophysiologic changes and then allow the implanted devices to influence body function positively. For example, an artificial pancreas delivers insulin based on blood sugar monitoring.

In oncology, neuroaugmentive devices are presently limited to nonpharmacologic, nondestructive means of producing pain relief. When prudently applied by experienced professionals in adequately equipped medical centers, these devices are capable of producing significant improvement in the quality of life for cancer patients whose life expectancy is reasonably long.

The purpose of this chapter is to provide the oncologist with adequate information about the realistic expectation of potential benefits and limitations of such devices in the treatment of pain.

BACKGROUND

Neuroaugmentive devices owe their existence to the development of cardiac pacemaker technology. Actually, the cardiac pacemaker *is* a neuroaugmentive device acting on the myoneural system within the heart. The first modern, radio frequency-coupled, implanted, neuroaugmentive device designed for human use was developed in 1964 by Szekley, Henny, and Zanes at the Temple University Department of Physics in Philadelphia. It was intended by Spiegel and Wycis to be used for brain implantation to control tremor.[65] In 1967 Shealy inaugurated practical clinical use of implanted neuroroaugmentive devices.[66,67] His first two patients had pain from metastatic carcinoma and underwent implantation of spinal dorsal column stimulators. Both patients experienced relief. The first patient died a short time (10 days) after implantation owing to complications of lung carcinoma with liver and pleural metastases. The second, having endometrial carcinoma, was doing well 2 years after surgery.

The commercial sale of neuroaugmentive devices for pain relief began in 1970 and focused on the use of dorsal cord neurostimulators (DCN) for pain relief in patients previously screened with transcutaneous electrical nerve stimulators (TENS).

Initial enthusiasm for the use of DCN in neurosurgery was markedly diminished when the many limitations of instrumentation and clinical applications became evident. Because of this, clinical efficacy was not as high as originally predicted.[68] A major initial problem with DCN was placement of the stimulating electrode in the subarachnoid space close to the spinal cord. The significant incidence of spinal cord compression, spinal fluid leak, meningitis, and progressive collagen deposition around the stimulating electrode (pro-

TABLE 43-30. Neuromodulation: Use and Estimated Improvement

PAIN CONTROL DEVICE	ESTIMATED NUMBER WORLDWIDE	ESTIMATED SIGNIFICANT IMPROVEMENT* SHORT-TERM %	LONG-TERM %
Transcutaneous electrical nerve stimulator (TENS)	100,000	80	35
Percutaneous epidural neurostimulaor (PENS), acute and chronic	1,200	80	†
Dorsal cord neurostimulator (DCN)	7,500	80	35
Peripheral nerve neurostimulator (PNS)	500	80	50
Depth brain neurostimulator (DBS)	100	90	70

*Significant improvement = 50% or more (moderate to marked) improvement in pretreatment pain. Criteria are variable and depend on patient population, clinical pain problem, selection criteria, device used, and method of use. Long-term improvement averages over 2 years in patients who continue to use the device

†Thought to be about 50–60%

ducing gradual decrease in current transfer) were primary factors in early failures. In 1972, the development of a technique which placed the stimulating electrode within the microsurgically defined layers of the dura (endodural) alleviated the previously mentioned problems, allowing study of the basic limitations of the devices themselves.[69] These included insulation breakdown, lead wire breakage, and component failure. As a result of study of these difficulties over the past 8 years, actual device efficacy can now be appreciated.

A major disadvantage of the DCN is that there was no reliable means of screening the patient to determine the effectiveness of electrical stimulation prior to surgical placement of the device. A battery-operated TENS device called the "Electreat" was initially used for this screening. At various times, this rather crude electrical device, manufactured in the United States since 1918, had been touted as a cure for most of the ailments of mankind (including pain relief). It soon became evident that more reliable solid-state devices were required; the development of these has resulted in approximately 50 TENS manufacturers in this country alone. Recent improvements in TENS skin electrode systems have greatly added to TENS' use. Although effective in its own right for pain control, TENS is no longer regarded as a valid tool for screening patients for pain relief by implanted neuroaugmentive devices.

In 1973, Hoppenstein first reported on the use of percutaneously inserted, epidural neurostimulating electrodes (PENS) which could be left in place over a period of time to evaluate relief of pain.[70] The PENS system has proven to be a reliable indicator of pain relief and has also served, in many cases, as the definitive treatment. Because of ease and the low risk of application, PENS has progressively gained acceptance while use of the DCN has declined, remaining as a means of treatment in patients who have had good initial results with PENS (in whom PENS ceased to function because of electrode movement, lead migration, or other device malfunction).

The placement of subcortical recording and stimulating electrodes is a well-known neurophysiologic technique. In humans, the specific application to mask intractable pain is relatively new. It appears that Mazars was the first to employ chronic electrode stimulation of the nucleus ventralis posterialis for pain relief in 1961.[71] Since 1973, implanted depth brain neurostimulators (DBN) have been developed. These devices are now considered the most effective means known of controlling the most intractable chronic pain.

In 1977, Ray reviewed the approximate number of patients in whom neuromodulation had been used worldwide and estimated significant improvement (see Table 43-30).[72] The efficacy figures given for pain control devices still appear to be accurate, although with better screening, the long-term significant improvement with TENS is now about 45%; the figure for PENS is probably 50 to 60%.

THEORIES OF PAIN

With the publication of their "Gate Theory" in 1965, Melzak and Wall opened the "gate" on a new era of investigation on pain mechanisms.[73] In simplified terms, their theory implied that pain-gating mechanisms existed in the spinal cord. If an induced stimulation exceeded the level of pain, the brain would experience only that induced input. Based on this premise, the dorsal column stimulator was developed. By inducing activity of the large-diameter, afferent fibers in the posterior columns of the spinal cord, the "pain" input mediated by the smaller-diameter afferent fibers could be controlled. Although some element of this theory no doubt applies, the situation is much more complex.

Humans appear to have been equipped with two basic pain appreciating systems. Phylogenetically, the paleo–spinal–thalamic pathway is the oldest. It is a nonspecific system, typified by dull, aching discomfort designed to keep the organism informed that the body part is injured to avoid use and reinjury.

The newer system is the neo–spinal–thalamic system which represents a well-localized system of sharp, intense pain designed for fast reflex removal of the affected body part from insult. When a bone is fractured, the latter pain is experienced followed later by the aching of the paleo–spinal–thalamic residual. Peripheral and spinal neurostimulation is of little value in modulating neo–spinal–thalamic type pain and of maximal value in alleviating that due to the paleo–spinal–thalamic system. Fortunately, most pain resulting from cancer is of the dull, aching, paleo–spinal–thalamic type.

The biochemical aspect of pain is perhaps one of the most exciting areas of contemporary medical activity. The discovery, in the early 1970s, of opiate receptors (specific CNS sites where morphine and other narcotics act) and the apparent similarity to analgesia produced by brain stimulation or by morphine, led to the suggestion that stimulation triggered the release of an endogenous opiate-like (endorphan) material. This was further supported by the observed tendency of naloxone (a specific inhibitor of both endogenous and exogenous opiate action) to block the analgesic effects of such stimulation. Reports of analgesia produced by stimulating the periaqueductal (aqueduct of Sylvius) area in animals has been confirmed in humans. Periaqueductal and periventrical (both rich in endorphans) gray matter stimulation has now become standard neuroaugmentive procedures to relieve intractable pain (see Fig. 43-9). It is of interest that the intraventricular administration of human beta-endorphan in humans produces a prolonged state of analgesia and that periaqueductal gray stimulation is accompanied by increases in the beta-endorphan concentrations of ventricular cerebrospinal fluid. This suggests that future neurostimulators might function based on CSF neurotransmitter monitoring sensors.

Since the regions of the brain most effective for stimulation-induced analgesia are not directly involved in the pain signal transmission pathways, it seems likely that they are part of an analgesia system which actively modulates pain transmission. This system appears to extend down the spinal cord by way of neurotransmitter (serotonin) projection pathways located in the dorsolateral funiculus (Fig. 43-10). This system probably acts where the electrical phenomena, "gate" mechanisms, and neurotransmitters interact to a high degree. According to recent evidence, endorphin-activated neurons exist in the dorsal horn of the spinal cord.

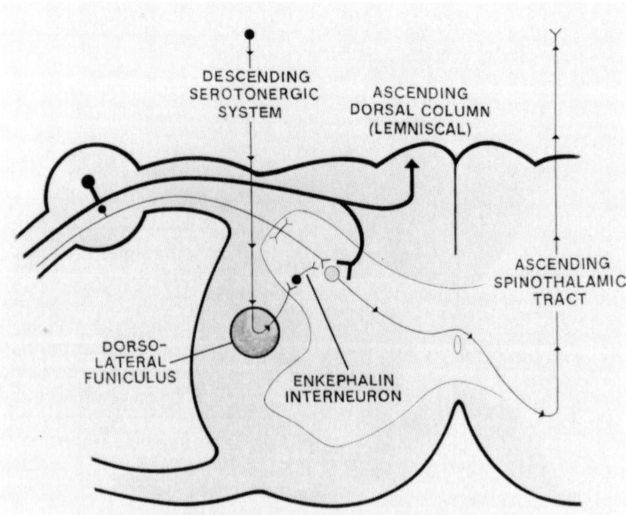

FIG. 43-10. When the periaqueductal and periventricular (meso-diencephalic) system is activated by neurostimulation, the descending intrinsic analgesic system set into operation appears to involve excitation of neurons in the nucleus raphe magnus and adjacent magnocellular reticular formation. The descending serotonergic neurons from these nuclei project to the dorsolateral funiculus of the spinal cord where they interact with pain-transmitting neurons in the dorsal horn. The presence of enkephalin interneurons in the dorsal horn suggest a close relationship of the intrinsic analgesic system to entering pain impulses. (Sister Kenny Institute, 1979).

FIG. 43-9. The largest amount of opiate binding has been found in the limbic system of the brain outlined in this drawing. The electrical stimulation of its central periventricular and periaqueductal portion has induced the highest degree of pain relief. (Sister Kenny Institute, 1979)

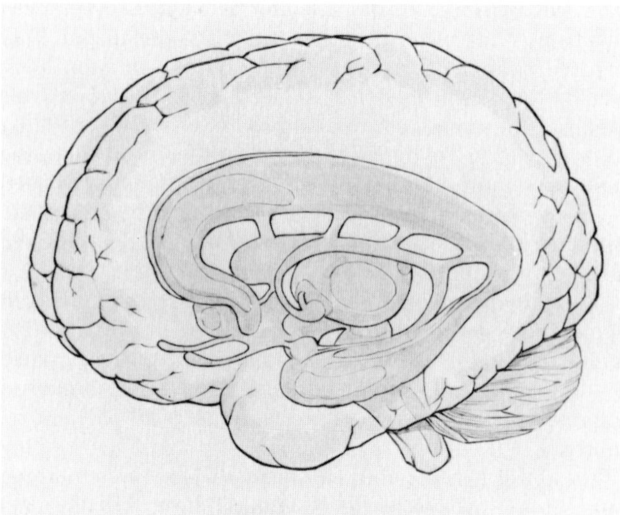

As with most medical devices, a definite placebo effect has been documented with the use of neurostimulators. This placebo effect has been associated with activation of the intrinsic analgesic system producing endorphin release. The placebo effect can also be blocked by naloxone. The intimate relationship between thought and analgesia can be better appreciated when we consider that beta-endorphin (which is found in all mammals and produces both analgesic and behavioral effects) seems to derive from a large prohormone precursor molecule (called "31 k") which can be broken down to beta-lipotropin, adrenocorticotropic hormone (ACTH), beta-lipotropin, and a number of other peptide substances that can affect behavior.

TRANSCUTANEOUS ELECTRICAL NERVE STIMULATION

The modern effort to treat pain with TENS began in 1967 with Wall's and Sweets' work on infraorbital nerve stimulation.[74] The field has grown rapidly, not only for pain relief but also for treatment of postoperative ileus and muscle pacing for many purposes including prevention of thrombophlebitis, sports medicine, and postpartum uterine contraction. The

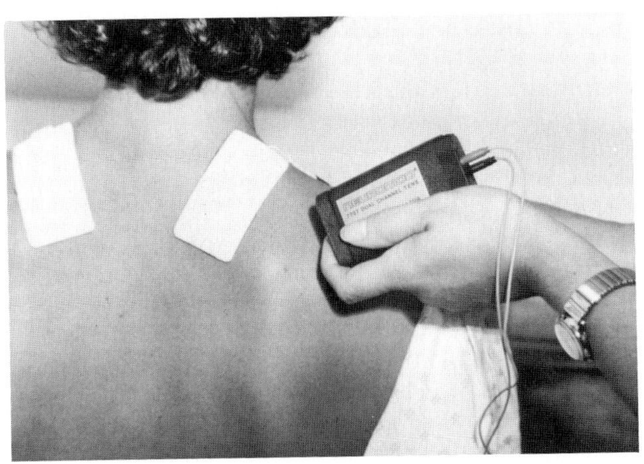

FIG. 43-11. A modern, battery-operated, solid state, single channel TENS unit being used for the relief of cervical pain using self-stick hypoallergenic skin electrodes. (Sister Kenny Institute, 1979).

major use of TENS continues to be pain relief (see Fig. 43-11). The recent development of better skin electrode systems has increased its value for this. As noted in Table 43-30 the use of TENS in cases of acute pain is significantly more effective than in cases of chronic pain, mainly because of overuse and overexpectation. TENS is of value over a period of time only when the pain is moderate, limited to a single area, and well-circumscribed. It is usually best to loan the patient a unit for a 2-week to 1-month clinical trial before purchase is suggested. Burton and Ray have found TENS to be of significant value in the treatment of pain due to peripheral bony metastases in cancer, if these are single.

Efficacy, precautions, and practical limitations of TENS have been reviewed by Burton.[75] Reasonable cautions include caution during use in patients with demand cardiac pacemakers (present pacemakers now have protective circuits) and avoiding the placement of electrodes over the carotid sinuses (to avoid vagovagal reflexes). The most common complication is skin reactions to electrodes (about 3–4%). This can be alleviated by changing the electrode placement site or using different types of electrodes. (Hyporeactive gel pad electrodes are now available.)

Important elements in the therapeutic success of TENS are experienced personnel working under a physician's supervision along with adequate patient education. TENS has had no adverse effects from long-term use. It is a safe, moderately expensive means of pain relief intended for problems of limited magnitude only.

DORSAL CORD NEUROSTIMULATION AND PERCUTANEOUS ELECTRICAL NEUROSTIMULATION

DCN was the first widely employed implanted neuroaugmentive device designed for pain relief (see Fig. 43-12). After improvements in operative technique and instrumentation, the major disadvantage was an inability to predict the degree of pain relief prior to surgical laminectomy and implantation in patients who had been previously medically and psychologically screened. Initial use of TENS to determine DCN value for pain relief has not been found reliable. This has been replaced by the use of twin percutaneous spiral-cord-stimulating electrodes placed in the epidural space through lumbar puncture needles under local anesthesia. Placement is performed in a special procedure suite under biplane fluoroscopic control. Trial stimulation is undertaken by moving the electrodes to different levels to determine various stimulation parameters. If good pain relief is found, the flexible neurostimulating electrodes are left in the epidural space, and fine wire extensions are carried through the skin.

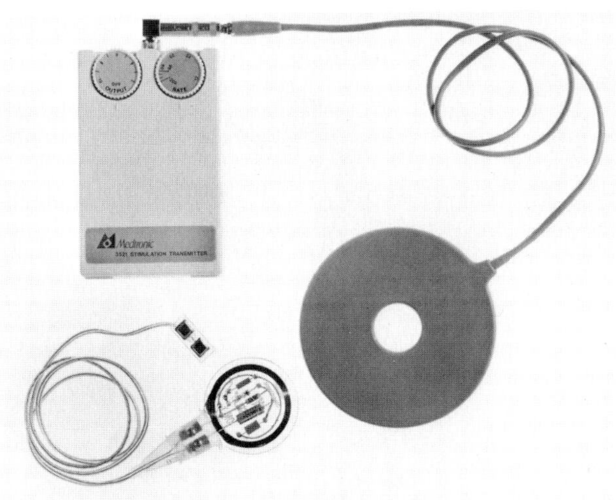

FIG. 43-12. The external and internal components of the DCN system consist of a power pack with attached RF antenna (attached to the skin) and a subcutaneously placed RF receiver connected to a two-plate platinum electrode. (Sister Kenny Institute, 1979)

These are then connected to a compact, battery-operated pulse generator so that the patient may test the system on an ambulatory basis over several days. Should the results remain positive, the system can be made permanent by surgical connection to a subcutaneous radio frequency receiver (see Fig. 43-13). This unit is powered by an external pulse generator. Systems using a totally implanted pulse generator are now under development. For a physically debilitated cancer patient, the percutaneous electrode extensions may be used alone for many months with negligible infection risk if topical antibiotics are applied daily to the wire emergence site.

Because of the success of PENS, the use of DCN has tended to be restricted to patients who have had good relief with PENS but in whom the system malfunctioned, usually owing to electrode movement.

PENS and DCN are best applied for the relief of unilateral somatic pain of a paleo–spinal–thalamic type. These systems are not capable of relieving *severe* pain and are of little value in relieving pain of visceral origin. However, experimental work in our department suggests that neurostimulation of the celiac plexus may be of value in controlling chronic visceral pain from cancer.

A 5-year follow-up survey by Burton on the long-term efficacy of spinal cord stimulation according to patient opinion, drug usage, and level of activity showed a good–to–excellent

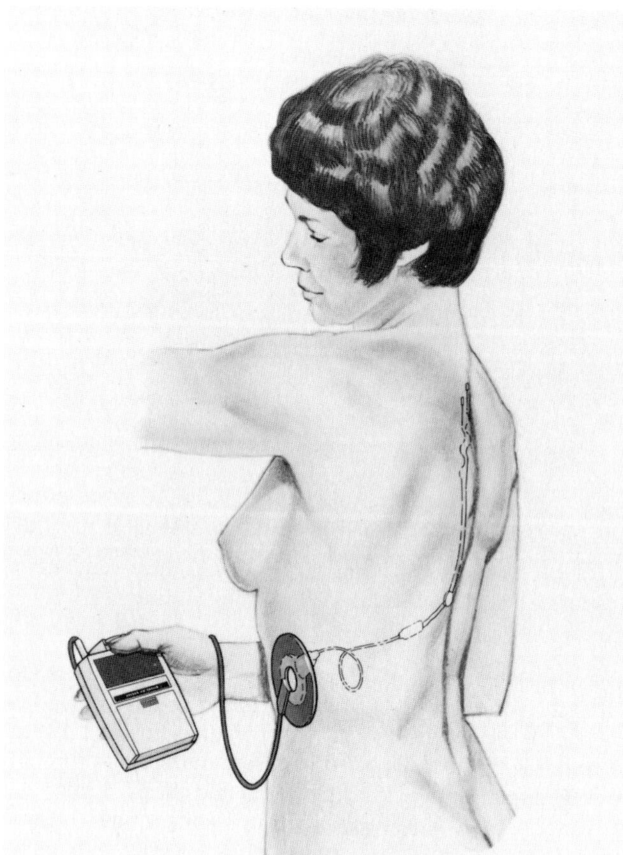

FIG. 43-13. A PENS system connected to a RF receiver. Electrode location in the thoracic area would be used for the relief of back and leg pain. (Sister Kenny Institute, 1979)

result in 43% of patients. No patient was made worse neurologically.[76] Pudenz has indicated "There seems to be no direct untoward effect from stimulation of the spinal cord, at appropriate stimulus threshold levels."[77]

Spinal stimulation is best employed in cancer patients with an intact nervous system. When previous destructive procedures like chordotomy have been employed, efficacy is markedly reduced. Care should also be exercised to rule out patients in whom distal metastases might produce additional pain sites beyond the area of influence of the implanted neurostimulator. Only DBS is presently capable of producing pain relief for these patients.

PERIPHERAL NERVE STIMULATION

PNS systems in which the neurostimulator electrode is wrapped around a peripheral mixed nerve have clinical value when cancer pain is limited to a single extremity. Recent improvements in electrodes have alleviated early problems of nerve constriction. Prior to the use of a PNS, a single or multichannel TENS should be attempted. Often, a good clinical result can be obtained by this simpler method. A significant disadvantage of PNS is the reportedly high incidence of muscle spasm. Pre-implant screening is also difficult, and for these reasons spinal cord stimulators tend to be the preferred device.

DEPTH BRAIN NEUROSTIMULATION

Cancer pain due to widespread metastases or having a midline or bilateral distribution represents one of the greatest therapeutic challenges to medical science. The chronic use of narcotic medications sacrifices personality and quality of life for relief of constant intractable pain.

Although DBS for pain relief is relatively new, centers in the United States, Sweden, France, and West Germany have now documented impressive results with periventricular and periaqueductal grey neurostimulation. Due to the basically low risk, the nondestructive nature of the procedure, and the magnitude of the problem, DBS may be the procedure of choice for the cancer patient with intractable pain and a reasonable life expectancy (more than a few months). There can be no greater personal reward in medicine than to see the re-emergence of a pain-free, cognizant human being following treatment with DBS, especially when the patient was previously obtruded and being treated with high doses of narcotic drugs.

From the papers presented on DBS at the Fourth Meeting of the European Society for Stereotaxic and Functional Neurosurgery* it is evident that this treatment modality

* Paris, July 12–14, 1979.

FIG. 43-14. A DBS system showing the subcortical electrode passing through a burr hole. It is connected to a subclavicular RF receiver. Often, these systems are not activated for more than two to three 30-minute periods a day to achieve total pain relief. (Sister Kenny Institute, 1979)

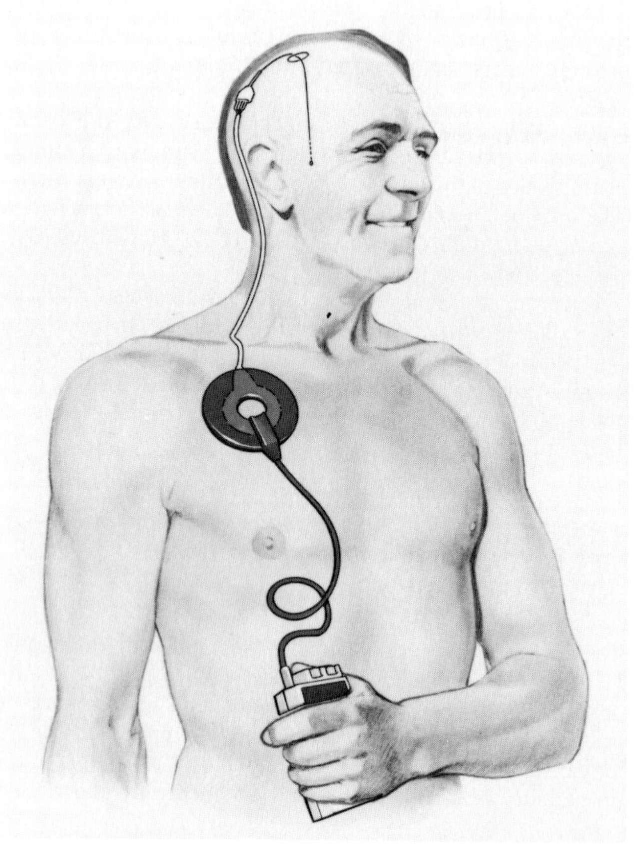

should be seriously considered whenever there is severe and functionally incapacitating pain, which is resistant to other forms of therapy. Success rates of 50 to 75% were reported at the meeting. Although the rate of complications was less than 5%, complications were severe and consisted of intracerebral and intraventricular hemorrhage, subgaleal infection, and meningitis.

DBS often does not produce complete pain relief in cancer patients, probably because of the mixing of neo- and paleospinal-thalamic somatic pain with elements of visceral discomfort.[78]

The present DBS system resembles most other neuroaugmentive devices (see Fig. 43-14). Through a burr hole, electrodes are placed at the target using a stereotaxic technique in which the ventricular system is visualized by injection of a radio-opaque material. (Techniques utilizing CT for this purpose are under development). A needle is passed to the target area and a fine, multicontact wire electrode is passed through the needle and left in place. Percutaneous extensions of the electrode are used for ambulatory testing. If the result is good, the system is internalized and an RF receiver is added.

A series of audiovisual presentations on these neuroaugmentive devices and methods of use has been prepared by Ray and is available through the Sister Kenny Institute for use by physicians, allied health personnel, and patients.[79]

SUMMARY

The field of neuroaugmentive surgery has now reached a point where both efficacy and safety of the systems employed can be determined.[80] This is reflected by the approval, by Medicare, of TENS, as well as peripheral nerve dorsal column and depth brain neurostimulator implantation coverage in the treatment of intractable pain according to guidelines recommended by the neurosurgical profession:[81]

> The implantation of the stimulator is used only as a late resort (if not a last resort) for patients with intractable pain.
>
> With respect to a), other modalities (pharmocological, surgical, physical, or psychological therapies) have been tried and did not prove satisfactory, or are judged to be unsuitable or contraindicated for the given patient.*
>
> Patients have undergone careful screening, evaluation and diagnosis by a multidisciplinary team prior to implantation. (Such screening must include psychological, as well as physical evaluation).
>
> All the facilities, equipment and professional and support personnel required for the proper diagnosis, treatment training and follow-up of the patient (including that required to satisfy condition c) must be available, and
>
> Demonstration of pain relief with a temporarily implanted electrode precedes permanent implantation.

The Medicare guidelines reflect the criteria required for successful application of these devices. When employed by skillful and experienced physicians in adequate medical environments, results tend to be significantly higher. A very important aspect of this success rate is complete and careful patient education by health professionals. Cancer disability is an unfortunate circumstance; superimposed intractable pain is a devastating complication which can now, in some cases, be reasonably alleviated by nondestructive, nonpharmacologic means.

* These modalities might be contraindicated in a cancer patient.

REFERENCES

1. Bonica JJ: Importance of the problem. International Symposium on Pain of Advanced Cancer. In Bonica JJ et al (eds): Advances in Pain Research and Therapy, Vol 2, pp 1–12. New York, Raven Press, 1979
2. Oster MW, Vizel M, Turgeon MS: Pain of terminal cancer patients. Arch Intern Med 138:1801–1802, 1978
3. Houde RW: The use and misuse of narcotics in the treatment of chronic pain. International Symposium on Pain. In Bonica JJ (ed): Advances in Neurology, Vol 4, pp 527–536. New York, Raven Press, 1974
4. Marks RM, Sachar EJ: Undertreatment of medical inpatients with narcotic analgesics. Ann Intern Med 78:173–181, 1973
5. Vandam CD: Analgesic drugs—the mild analgesics—the potent analgesics. N Engl J Med 286:20–23, 249–253, 1972
6. Bonica JJ: Introduction to management of pain of advanced cancer. International Symposium on Pain of Advanced Cancer. In Bonica JJ Albe-Fessard D (eds): Advances in Pain Research and Therapy, Vol 2, pp 115–130. New York, Raven Press, 1979
7. Lasanga L.: The clinical evaluation of morphine and its substitutes as analgesics. Pharmacol Rev 16:47–83, 1964
8. Houde RW: Medical treatment of oncological pain. In Bonica JJ et al (eds): Recent Advances on Pain, pp 168–188. Springfield, Illinois, Charles C Thomas, 1974
9. Moertel CG, Ahmann DL, Taylor WF et al: Relief of pain by oral medications: A controlled evaluation of analgesic combinations. JAMA 229:55–59, 1974
10. Catalano RB: The medical approach to management of pain caused by cancer. Semin Oncol 2:379–392, 1975
11. Houde RW: On assaying analgesics in man. In Knighton RS, Dumke PR (eds): Pain, pp 183–196. Boston, Little, Brown & Co, 1966
12. Twycross RG: The use of narcotic analgesics in terminal illness. J Med Ethics 1:10–17, 1975
13. Twycross RG: Diseases of the central nervous system. Relief of terminal pain. Med J 4:212–214, 1975
14. Beaver WT: Mild analgesics. A review of their clinical pharmacology. Am J Med Sci 250:577–604, 1965
15. Beaver WT: Mild analgesics. A review of their clinical pharmacology. (Part II). Am J Med Sci 251:576–599, 1966
16. Simon LS, Mills JA: Nonsteroidal antiinflammatory drugs. N Engl J Med 302:1179–1185, 1237–1243, 1980
17. Vane JR: Inhibition of prostaglandin synthesis as a mechanism of action for aspirin-like drugs. Nature (New Biol) 231:232–235, 1971
18. Martino G, Ventafridda V, Parini J et al: A controlled study on the analgesic activity of indoprofen in patients with cancer pain. In Bonica JJ, Albe-Fessard D (eds): Advances in Pain Research and Therapy, Vol 1, pp 573–578. New York, Raven Press, 1976
19. Moertel CG, Ahmann DL, Taylor WF et al: A comparative evaluation of marketed analgesic drugs. N Engl J Med 286:813–815, 1972
20. Hollister LE: Effective use of analgesic drugs. Annu Rev Med 27:431–446, 1976
21. Lewis JR: Misprescribing analgesics. JAMA 228:1115–1156, 1974
22. Edison GR: Letter: Hallucinations associated with pentazocine. N Engl J Med 281:447–448, 1969
23. Shimm DS, Logue GL, Maltbie AA et al: Medical management of chronic cancer pain. JAMA 241:2408–2412, 1979
24. Ettinger DS, Vitale PJ, Trump DL: Important clinical pharmacologic considerations in the use of methadone in cancer patients. Cancer Treat Rep 63:457–459, 1979
25. Twycross RG: Clinical experience with diamorphine in advanced malignant disease. Int J Clin Pharmacol 9:184–198, 1974
26. Anonymous: The Brompton Cocktail, Lancet 1:1220–1221, 1979
27. Glover DD, Lowry TF, Jacknowitz AI: Brompton's mixture in

alleviating pain of terminal neoplastic disease: Preliminary results. South Med J 73:278–282, 1980
28. Twycross RG: Choice of strong analgesic in terminal cancer: diamorphine or morphine? Pain 3:93–104, 1977
29. Melzack R, Mount BM, Gordon JM: The Brompton mixture versus morphine solution given orally: effects on pain. Can Med Assoc J 120:435–438, 1979
30. Beaver WT, Feise G: Comparison of the analgesic effects of morphine, hydroxyzine, and their combination in patients with postoperative pain. In Bonica JJ, Albe-Fessard D (eds): Advances in Pain Research and Therapy, Vol 1, pp 553–557. New York, Raven Press, 1976
31. Forrest WH Jr, Brown BW Jr, Brown CR et al: Dextroamphetamine with morphine for the treatment of postoperative pain. N Engl J Med 296:712–715, 1977
32. Montgomery BJ: Psychotropic drugs finding analgesic use. JAMA 240:1225, 1978
33. McGhee JL, Alexander MR: Phenothiazine analgesia—fact or fantasy? Am J Hosp Pharm 36:633–640, 1979
34. Bunney WE, Pert CB, Klee W et al: Basic and clinical studies of endorphins. Ann Intern Med 91:239–250, 1979
35. Chung SH, Dickenson A: Pain, enkephalin, and acupuncture. Nature 283:243–244, 1980
36. Hosobuchi Y, Li CH: The analgesic activity of human B-endorphin in man. Commun Psychopharmacol 2:33–37, 1978
37. Wang JK, Nauss LA, Thomas JE: Pain relief by intrathecally applied morphine in man. Anesthesiology 50:149–151, 1979
38. Oyama T, Jin T, Yamaya R et al: Profound analgesic effects of B-endorphin in man. Lancet 1:122–124, 1980
39. Carpenter MB: Human Neuroanatomy, p 245. Baltimore, Williams & Wilkins, 1976
40. Black P: Management of cancer pain: An overview. Neurosurgery 5:507, 1979
41. Mansuy L, Sindou M, Fischer G et al: Spino-Thalamic cordotomy in cancerous pain. Results of a series of 124 patients operated on by the direct posterior approach. Neurochirurgie 22:5, 437, 1976
42. Coggeshall RE: Afferent fibers in the ventral root. Neurosurgery 4:5, 443, 1979
43. Papo I, Luongo A: High cervical commissural myelotomy in the treatment of pain. J Neurol Neurosurg Psychiatry 39:7, 705, 1976
44. Cook AW, Kawakami Y: Commissural myelotomy. J Neurosurg 47:1, 1977
45. Frazier CH: Section of the antereolateral columns of the Spinal Cord for the relief of pain. A report of six cases, Arch Neurol Psychiatry 4:137, 1920
46. White JC, Sweet WH: Pain and the Neurosurgeon, p 695. Springfield, Charles C Thomas, 1969
47. White JC, Sweet WH: Pain and the Neurosurgeon, p 695. Springfield, Charles C Thomas, 1969
48. Rosomoff HL, Carroll F, Brown J et al: Percutaneous radiofrequency cervical cordotomy. Technique. J Neurosurgery 23:639, 1965
49. Mullan S, Harper PV, Hekmatpanak J et al: Percutaneous interruption of spinal pain tracts by means of a Strontium 90 needle. J Neurosurg 20:931, 1963
50. Mullan S: Percutaneous cordotomy for pain. Surg Clin North Am 46:3, 1966
51. Tasker RR: Percutaneous cervical cordotomy. Neurophysiology (Suppl) 39:2, 114, 1976–77
52. Steude U: Percutaneous chordotomy for the treatment of pain; technic, indications and results. Fortschr Med 94:11, 609, 1976
53. Grote W, Roosen K, Book WJ: High cervical percutaneous cordotomy in intractable pain. Neurochirurgia (Stuttg) 21:6, 209, 1978
54. Wilson CB, Fewer D: Role of neurosurgery in the management of patients with carcinoma of the breast. Cancer 28:1681, 1971
55. Levin AB, Benson RC Jr., Katz J et al: Chemical hypophysectomy for relief of bone pain in carcinoma of the prostate. J Urol 119:4, 517, 1978
56. Tindall GT, Payne NS, Nixon DW: Transspenoidal hypophysectomy for disseminated carcinoma of the prostate gland. Results in 53 patients. J Neurosurgery 50:3, 275, 1979
57. Tindall GT, Nixon DW, Christy JH et al: Pain relief in metastatic cancer other than breast and prostate gland following transsphenoidal hypophysectomy. A preliminary report. J Neurosurgery 47:5, 659, 1977
58. Larossa JT, Strong MS, Melby JC: Endocrinologically incomplete transethmoidal trans-sphenoidal hypophysectomy with relief of bone pain in breast cancer, N Engl J Med 298:24, 1332, 1978
59. Moricca G: Chemical hypophysectomy for cancer pain. Adv Neurol 4:707, 1974
60. Lipton S, Miles J, Williams N et al: Pituitary injection of alcohol for widespread cancer pain. Pain 5:1, 73, 1978
61. Mracek Z: Cervical tractotomy V, IX, X and VII and accompanying rhizotomy in incurable pain due to malignant tumors of the facial–cervical region. Zentralbl Neurochir 39:3, 311, 1978
62. Whisler WW, Voris HC: Mesencephalotomy for intractable pain due to malignant disease. Appl Neurophysiol 41:1–4, 52, 1978
63. Sweet WH: Controlled thermocoagulation of trigeminal ganglion and rootlets for differential destruction of pain fibers: Facial pain other than trigeminal neuralgia. Clin Neurosurg 23:96, 1976
64. White JC, Sweet WH: Pain and the Neurosurgeon, p 664. Springfield, Charles C Thomas, 1969
65. Zanes CP: Personal communication, July 30, 1979
66. Shealy CN, Mortimer JT, Reswick JB: Electrical inhibition of pain by stimulation of the dorsal columns: preliminary clinical report. Anesth Analg 46:489–491, 1967
67. Shealy CN, Mortimer JT, Hagfors NR: Dorsal column electroanalgesia. J Neurosurg 32:560–564, 1970
68. Ray CD (ed): Minneapolis pain seminar. Electrical stimulation of the human nervous system for the control of pain. Surg Neurol 4:61–204, 1973
69. Burton C: Dorsal column stimulation: Optimization of application. Surg Neurol 4:171–176, 1973
70. Hoppenstein R: Percutaneous implantation of chronic spinal cord electrodes for control of intractable pain. Preliminary report. Surg Neurol 4:195–198, 1973
71. Mazars GJ: Intermittent stimulation of nucleus ventralis posterolateralis for intractable pain. Surg Neurol 4:93–95, 1973
72. Ray CD: New electrical stimulation methods for therapy and rehabilitation. Ortho Rev 6:29–39, 1977
73. Melzak R, Wall PD: Pain mechanisms: A new theory science. 150:971–979, 1965
74. Wall PD, Sweet WH: Temporary abolition of pain in man. Science 155:108–109, 1967
75. Burton CV: Transcutaneous electrical nerve stimulation to relieve pain. Postgrad Med 59:105–108, 1976
76. Burton CV: Safety and clinical efficacy: Session on spinal cord stimulation. Neurosurgery 1:214–215, 1977
77. Pudenz RH: Adverse effects of electrical energy applied to the nervous system. J Appl Neurophysiol 1:190–191, 1977
78. Meyerson BA, Boethius J, Carlsson AM: Percutaneous central grau stimulation for cancer pain. Appl Neurophysiol 41:57–65, 1978
79. Ray CD (ed): Audio-visual series on neuroaugmentation. ES-2: Review of electrical stimulation. P-1: Pisces (PENS) implantation. DBS-1: Deep brain implantation. PP-1: Pisces for patient review. PDBS-1: Deep brain for patient review. Available from Education Dept, Sister Kenny Inst, 2727 Chicago Ave, Minneapolis, MN 55407
80. Burton CV, Ray CD, Nashold BS: Symposium on the safety and clinical efficacy of implanted neuroagumentive devices. Neurosurgery 1:185–232, 1977
81. Medicare, U.S. Department of Health, Education, and Welfare: Health Care Financing Administration, Part A. Intermediary Manual, Part 3. November 14, 1979

Philip A. Pizzo
Robert C. Young

CHAPTER 44

Management of Infections of the Cancer Patient

Infectious complications are a frequent cause of morbidity and the major cause of death in patients with cancer. The increased risk and severity of infectious sequelae result from the profound alteration of normal host defenses secondary to the patient's underlying malignancy and its treatment. A thorough understanding of the impaired host defenses which occur in the cancer patient, and the interaction of these defects with the patient's endogenous and exogenous microbial flora is essential for the successful recognition, effective management, and ultimate prevention of serious infectious complications.

IMPAIRED HOST DEFENSES OF THE CANCER PATIENT

INTEGUMENTARY AND MUCOSAL BARRIERS

The skin and mucosal surfaces comprise the primary host defense against invasion by endogenous and acquired microorganisms. The integrity of this physical barrier can be disrupted by the patient's tumor (*e.g.*, local invasion or obstruction) or by its treatment (*e.g.*, surgery, intravenous catheters, radiation, or chemotherapy). Lesions induced by these treatments provide a nidus for microbial colonization, a focus for local infection, and a potential portal for systemic invasion.

PHAGOCYTIC DEFENSES

The neutrophil and the monocyte–macrophage are the major cellular defenses against most bacteria and fungi.[1,2] Whether disease related or as a consequence of therapy, the degree of severe neutropenia is inversely related to the risk of serious infection (Table 44-1).[3] A significant drop in the lymphocyte count may also contribute to a heightened risk of infection, especially when both the lymphocyte and neutrophil counts are simultaneously depressed.[3]

In addition to quantitative defects, qualitative abnormalities of neutrophil function have been described in patients with hematologic malignancies. These include defects in chemotaxis, phagocytosis, bactericidal capacity, and the absence of the respiratory burst that usually accompanies phagocytosis.[4,5] While phagocytic capacity remains normal, decreased spontaneous migratory and chemotactic leukocyte functions have been described in untreated patients with lymphoma and carcinoma, suggesting the presence of a circulating inhibitor in the sera of these patients.[6] Cancer chemotherapy may also produce defects of neutrophil function. Corticosteroids, for example, can decrease phagocytosis and neutrophil migration.[8] The combination of prednisone with vincristine–asparaginase or 6-mercaptopurine–methotrexate has been shown to produce a significant decrease in the phagocytic and killing capability of leukocytes.[9] Although the mechanism is not clear, bactericidal activity may also be transiently impaired within the 3 months following cranio–spinal irradiation in patients with leukemia and may thus contribute to the infectious complications which occur during that period.[10]

The mature macrophage is more resistant to cytotoxic chemotherapy than the granulocyte and hence provides some residual phagocytic capacity during periods of severe neutropenia. In addition, the activated macrophage is also an important defense against mycobacteria, *Listeria*, *Brucella*, and several fungi, protozoans, and viruses.[2]

TABLE 44-1. Percentage of Cancer Patients Who Develop Serious Infections with Granulocytopenia and the Cumulative Risk of Infection with Prolonged Granulocytopenia

GRANULOCYTE LEVEL (PER MM³)		PERCENTAGE OF SERIOUS INFECTIONS (DURATION OF GRANULOCYTOPENIA IN WEEKS)							
Initial	*Change*								
1	2	3	*4*	6	*10*	*12*	*14*		
Any level	Any fall	12							
Any level	Fall to 2,000	2							
Any level	Fall to 1,500	5							
Any level	Fall to 1,000	10	30	45	50	65	70	85	100
Any level	Fall to 500	19							
Any level	Fall to <100	28	50	72	85	100			

(Adapted from Bodey *et al*, Ann Intern Med 61:328–340, 1966)

CELLULAR AND HUMORAL IMMUNITY

Patients with lymphoid malignancies (especially Hodgkin's disease) may also have abnormalities of cell-mediated immunity (*e.g.*, anergy, decreased PHA responsiveness) which may persist even after the underlying malignancy has been treated.[11,12] These defects are further aggravated by chemotherapy (*e.g.*, glucocorticosteroids), making such patients susceptible to certain viral (*e.g.*, *H. zoster*) or fungal (*e.g.*, *Cryptococcus*) infections.[8,13]

Cytotoxic chemotherapy has signficant adverse effects on both B- and T-cell functions, resulting in diminished opsonizing activity, inadequate agglutination and lysis of bacteria, and deficient neutralization of bacterial toxins.[14] Impaired antibody production has been described in untreated patients with chronic lymphocytic leukemia, multiple myeloma, and Hodgkin's disease.[15] Suppressor lymphocytes may also contribute to impaired antibody production in patients with multiple myeloma and Hodgkin's disease and may also relate to the fungal infections which occur in some of these patients.[16,17] In experimental animals, the glucocorticoid-induced defects in lymphocyte function and decreased neutralizing-antibody formation contribute to the increased lethality of fungal, protozoan, and viral infection. Similarly, high levels of IgG antibody to the O antigen of gram-negative bacilli exert an important protective role against infection by these organisms.[18,19] It may also be important that many drugs commonly used in cancer therapy have significant B-cell cytotoxicity and may thus contribute to impaired antibody formation.[20]

While various components of complement are important for host defense, including opsonization, chemotaxis, anaphylatoxin generation, and serum bactericidal activity, infectious sequelae specifically related to complement defects have not been described in cancer patients. However, the potential importance of serum complement is illustrated by its role in the successful treatment of experimental disseminated candidiasis.[21]

THE RETICULO–ENDOTHELIAL SYSTEM AND SPLENECTOMY

The spleen serves as both a mechanical filter and an early source of opsonizing activity. Splenectomized patients manifest diminished antibody production when challenged with particulate antigens, are deficient in tuftsin (the phagocytosis promoting peptide), and have decreased levels of IgM and properdin.[22–25] Consequently, splenectomized patients (*e.g.*, patients with Hodgkin's disease) are at increased risk for septicemia, usually with *S. pneumonia*, *N. meningitis*, or *H. influenza*. Septicemia in these patients is characteristically fulminant, with large numbers of organisms in the blood stream. While the incidence of postsplenectomy septicemia is especially significant in children and adolescents also receiving chemotherapy (range 1.4%–20%), bacteremia (with *S. pneumonia, H. influenza*) can occur even when patients are not granulocytopenic, suggesting that splenectomy is an important independent risk factor for cancer patients.[26–28] Splenectomy, however, does not appear to enhance the risk for most nonbacterial infections (*e.g.*, *H. zoster*).[29]

NUTRITION

Malnutrition is a frequent complication of cancer and its treatment, and it further contributes to the loss of integrity of the integumentary and mucosal barriers, impaired phagocytic capacity, decreased macrophage mobilization, and depressed lymphocyte function.[30] The anorexia and cachexia associated with cancer, therefore, merit aggressive nutritional support (*e.g.*, elemental diets, supplements, parenteral alimentation).[31]

THE EXOGENOUS AND ENDOGENOUS MICROBIAL FLORA

Unperturbed, the endogenous microbial flora exists as a carefully balanced synergistic microenvironment within the host. However, the majority (86%) of the infections which occur in cancer patients arise from this endogenous microbial flora, although 47% of the infecting organisms are acquired by the patient during hospitalization (the most frequent isolates being *Ps. aeruginosa, E. coli, K. pneumonia*, and *C. albicans*).[32] Certain acquired biotypes of Enterobacteriae are more likely to colonize the host, while acquisition of *Ps. aeruginosa* is especially important, since 40% to 68% of newly colonized patients may develop septicemia during subsequent periods of granulocytopenia.[33,34] Numerous sources may con-

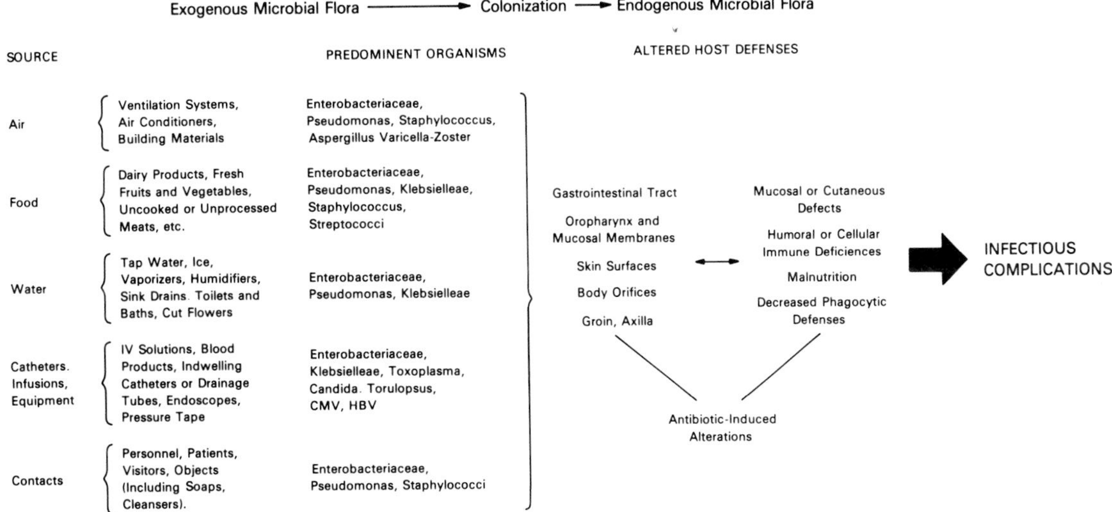

FIG. 44-1. Sources for nosocomial infection in high-risk patients.

tribute to the potential colonization of the hospitalized patient, including staff–patient and patient–patient transmission (most frequently due to the lack of careful handwashing techniques) and food, air, water, special equipment (*e.g.*, respirators or humidifiers), and medical or surgical procedures (Fig. 44-1).[35] Furthermore, interactions among different components of the host's endogenous microflora (*i.e.*, viruses with bacteria or protozoa) may also result in alterations of the microenvironment and consequent infectious complications (*e.g.*, synergistic gangrene of Meleney caused by combined infection with microaerophilic *Streptococcus* and *S. aureus* or the putative interaction of *T. gondii* and *P. carinii* with cytomegalovirus).[36] The host's endogenous microbial flora can also be perturbed by the antibiotic and chemotherapeutic agents frequently used to treat cancer patients, and when these microbial alterations occur in conjunction with the previously-described host defects, infectious sequelae may result.

INITIAL EVALUATION AND MANAGEMENT OF THE FEBRILE CANCER PATIENT

Fever is a common occurrence in cancer patients and can result from tumor necrosis, inflammation, transfusions, and drugs (including both chemotherapeutic and antimicrobial agents). While the patient's underlying malignancy can also occasionally cause fever (*e.g.*, Pel–Ebstein fever of Hodgkin's disease), the majority (55%–70%) of the fevers which occur in cancer patients appear to have an infectious etiology, especially when the patient is granulocytopenic (*i.e.*, PMN less than 500mm³).[37–42]

The initial evaluation and management of the febrile patient depend on the underlying malignancy and the degree of treatment-induced host compromise. For example, altered cellular immunity places the patient with Hodgkin's disease at increased risk for *H. zoster* infection or cryptococcal meningitis; patients who have undergone allogeneic bone marrow transplantation are at risk for severe interstitial pneumonia (especially with CMV and *Pneumocystis carinii*).[43–45] Patients with hematologic malignancies or lymphomas have generally been considered to be at greater risk for bacterial and fungal infections than are patients with solid tumors.[46–48] However, we have recently observed that as treatment schedules for patients with solid tumors have become more intensive and the duration of granulocytopenia more prolonged, the incidence, character, and outcome of the infections in these patients has become more similar to those observed in patients with leukemia.

While the evaluation of the non-immunosuppressed febrile cancer patient can proceed according to general medical principles, the detection of infection and the management of the febrile–granulocytopenic patient is complicated by two important factors: first, the presence of granulocytopenia markedly alters the host's inflammatory response, making it difficult to detect the presence of infection; second, an undetected and untreated infection can be rapidly fatal in the granulocytopenic cancer patient.[49–51]

Since the classic signs and symptoms of infection are likely to be absent in the granulocytopenic cancer patient (*e.g.*, pyuria may be detectable in only 11% of patients with a urinary tract infection or purulent sputum in only 8% of patients with pneumonia), the physician must take a careful history and perform a scrupulous physical examination, being especially attentive to subtle signs of inflammation.[49] Moreover, the physical exam may need to be repeated frequently, especially when an initial source of the infection is not discernible. Since the patient's endogenous microbial flora accounts for 86% of the infecting organisms, surveillance cultures (nose, throat, urine, and stool) should be considered along with at least two blood cultures (from different venipunctures).[32] Suspicious skin or other lesions should be aspirated or biopsied, and should be Gram-stained and cultured. If an intravenous needle or catheter is in place when the patient first becomes febrile, it must be considered a potential focus of infection and should be removed and cultured. A chest roentgenogram should also be performed as part of the initial patient evaluation.

Even with such a comprehensive evaluation, an infectious etiology is initially demonstrated in only 50% to 70% of febrile–granulocytopenic patients.[42] Moreover, definitive diagnosis may take days (presumably because of the low microbial inoculum) and some infections cannot be unequivocally diagnosed. While gallium scanning has been helpful in detecting occult infections in noncompromised patients, we have found them to be unreliable in granulocytopenic (less than 500 PMNs/mm^3) patients, presumably because lactoferrin from granulocytes is necessary to bind and localize the gallium to sites of infection. In the future, it may be possible to employ rapid diagnostic methods that are nonculture-dependent (*e.g.*, serum antigen detection or nuclear scintiscanning with labelled granulocytes).[52–55] At the present time, however, our technology does not always ensure early accurate diagnosis and, therefore, following the initial evaluation, it is imperative to initiate broad spectrum antibiotic therapy empirically.

Bacteria are responsible for most of the acute infections which occur in granulocytopenic patients. While virtually any organism (even presumed nonpathogens) can be the cause of an infection, the gram-negative bacilli (especially *E. coli, K. pneumonia*, and *Ps. aeruginosa*) predominate in most institutions. Gram-positive bacteria (especially *S. aureus* and *streptococci*) are also isolated frequently. Surprisingly, anaerobic organisms are an infrequent cause of infection in cancer patients. The relative distribution of these organisms varies from institution to institution. Of note is that several centers have recently observed a decrease in pseudomonas isolates, while other institutions have noted an increase in the isolation of gram-positive organisms (especially *S. aureus*).[56,57] This bacterial shift is reminiscent of the pattern of infection that was described in cancer patients during the 1950s and early 1960s.

Fungal infections (especially *Candida, Aspergillus,* and *Mucormycosis*) have been observed with increasing frequency, especially in patients with prolonged (*i.e.*, greater than 7 days) granulocytopenia. Unfortunately, these infections are both difficult to diagnose and to treat, and a high index of suspicion is essential to permit early intervention.[58,59]

In addition, antibiotic-sensitivity patterns may also vary among institutions, especially due to the selective pressure of excessive or indiscriminate antibiotic use. Hence, it is imperative for physicians to remain aware of possible changes in the microbial distribution and antibiotic sensitivity patterns at their institution.

The morbidity and mortality of infection are reduced from more than 50% to less than 20% when empiric broad-spectrum antibiotic therapy is initiated immediately after the expeditious diagnostic evaluation of the febrile–neutropenic cancer patient, whether or not a bacterial infection can be initially documented.[42,60] The particular antibiotic regimen selected for the initial empiric therapy of the febrile–granulocytopenic patient should satisfy the following criteria: the drug combination should "cover" the major pathogenic isolates observed at the particular hospital, the combination of antibiotics should be synergistic (or at least additive) and should contain at least one bactericidal agent (especially in neutropenic patients), the agents chosen should have the least possible organ toxicity, and the blood levels achieved should be carefully monitored (Table 44-2). Most institutions utilize either a two or three drug combination, generally consisting of a cephalosporin or a semisynthetic penicillin, and an aminoglycoside.[60,61] Recent studies have compared the therapeutic efficacy of two and three drug combinations, including newer antibiotic agents (*e.g.*, cephazolin, cephamandole, ticarcillin, tobramycin, amikacin) but to date, a clear superiority of one antibiotic combination has not been clearly established (Table 44-3).[62–66] New combinations (*e.g.*, trimethoprim-sulfamethioxazole plus ticarcillin) as well as the advent of the third generation cephalosporins (*e.g.*, cefotaxime, moxalactam, cefoperazone) may provide future therapeutic alternatives. At the NCI we presently use a three drug combination: cephalothin 170 mg/kg/day, I.V., q4h), gentamicin (6 mg/kg/day, I.V., q6h), and carbenicillin (500 mg/kg/day, I.V., q4h).

Following the initial evaluation and institution of empiric antibiotic therapy in the febrile–neutropenic cancer patient, the subsequent management depends on the identification (or the lack of identification) of the etiology for the fever and the duration of neutropenia. Between 1976 and 1979, we prospectively evaluated 754 episodes (in 261 patients) of fever (defined as three oral temperature elevations above 38°C during a 24-hour period, or a single oral temperature elevation of 38.5°C or higher) and neutropenia (less than 500 PMN/mm^3) at the NCI. A documented source of infection was definable within the first 7 days in 384 (51%) of these episodes. The remaining 370 episodes (49%) had no detectable infectious etiology and were, therefore, classified as FUO. The management of specific infections and patients with FUO is considered below.

TABLE 44-2. Nephrotoxic Drugs Used in Cancer Patients

CHEMOTHERAPEUTIC AGENTS	ANTIMICROBIAL AGENTS
Cis-dichlorodiammineplatinum	Cephalosporins
Methotrexate	Aminoglycosides
Streptozotocin	Antipseudomonal Penicillins
BCNU	Penicillinase-Resistant Penicillins
Methyl CCNU	Vancomycin
	Amphotericin-B
	Pentamidine isethionate

MANAGEMENT OF SPECIFIC INFECTIOUS COMPLICATIONS

SEPTICEMIA

Approximately one-fifth of the febrile episodes which occur in granulocytopenic cancer patients are due to septicemia. In most cancer centers, the gram-negative enteric bacilli (especially *Klebsiella, E. coli, Ps. aeruginosa*) represent the major pathogens. Infections due to gram-positive bacteria (especially *Staphylococci, Streptococci*) vary in their frequency, but in some institutions have surpassed gram-negative bacteria as the most frequent aerobic isolates.[56,57] The current mortality from septicemia ranges from 20% to 40%, but may approach 70% for patients with polymicrobial sepsis.[67,68] In addition, infections tend to be fulminant and deaths within the first 24 hours to 48 hours are common in untreated septic granulocytopenic cancer patients. Since septicemia, in the febrile–granulocytopenic cancer patient, cannot be reliably diagnosed by physical examination (*e.g.*, the fever pattern and the presence or absence of chills are not consistently predictive), rapid evaluation and the initiation of empiric antibiotic therapy is essential.[60] This approach has resulted in a significant decrease in the incidence, morbidity, and mortality from septicemia. While the degree of initial neutropenia is not of prognostic significance, the duration that the white blood count remains low may be related to outcome.

The subsequent antibiotic therapy of the patient with septicemia depends on the sensitivity of the microbial isolate. For patients with gram-negative septicemia, an aminoglycoside (*e.g.*, gentamicin, tobramicin, amikacin) is generally combined with a semisynthetic penicillin (*e.g.*, carbenicillin, ticarcillin). This combination is important, since an aminoglycoside alone is inadequate in the neutropenic patient, while the use of a semisynthetic penicillin alone may result in the development of microbial resistance (especially by *Ps. aeruginosa*). While the combination of an aminoglycoside and a semisynthetic penicillin (*e.g.*, carbenicillin, ticarcillin) is satisfactory for the majority of the gram-negative bacteria, many isolates of *Serratia* have multiple antibiotic resistance, although amikacin currently appears to be effective.[69] It is also imperative to serially monitor antibiotic levels (especially the aminoglycosides) initially and then at least weekly in order to minimize "breakthrough" bacteremia and decrease antibiotic-induced organ toxicity. The treatment of a gram-negative isolate which is resistant to the initial antibiotic regimen poses a major therapeutic dilemma but must be based upon *in vitro* sensitivity testing.

Treatment of gram-positive septicemia is successfully accomplished with a cephalosporin or with a penicillinase-resistant penicillin (*e.g.*, oxacillin, methicillin). Suprisingly, the morbidity and mortality of *S. aureus* septicemia is low in cancer patients (4% at the NCI), and nonhematogenous sequelae are infrequent, perhaps because of the early institution of antibiotics when cancer patients become febrile.[70,71] We have found that a 2 week to 3 week course of antibiotic therapy is adequate for the treatment of *S. aureus* septicemia if no clinical evidence of organ involvement is present and if the patient's granulocytopenia has resolved.[70] *S. epidermidis* has also been associated with serious infection in the cancer patient. The possibility of methicillin-resistant staphylococci should also be considered and, if necessary, the therapy appropriately modified (generally by instituting vancomycin 25 mg/kg/day to 40 mg/kg/day, I.V., q8h).

Serious Group A streptococcal infections are relatively infrequent in cancer patients, but deserve special consideration in the splenectomized patient.[26,27] Documented septicemia with *Streptococcus bovis*, while uncommon, is additionally important in view of its close association with carcinoma of the colon and should therefore heighten the clinician's suspicion of an underlying (and perhaps undetected) neoplasm.[72,73] Of concern, septicemia with *Corynebacterium diptheriae* and *Corynebacterium equi*, resistant to virtually all antimicrobials except vancomycin, has been recently described in cancer patients.[74,75]

We have recently observed that seven of 15 patients who remained granulocytopenic for more than 7 days and who were treated initially with a single (*i.e.*, narrow-spectrum) antibiotic for gram-positive septicemia developed a second (gram-negative) septicemic episode. In contrast, none of the 24 granulocytopenic patients who were treated for gram-positive septicemia with broad-spectrum antibiotics developed second bacterial infections, suggesting that the broad-spectrum antibiotic therapy used in these patients may have provided systemic prophylaxis during the period of prolonged granulocytopenia.[76]

Patients who become afebrile during therapy, and whose granulocytopenia resolves (PMN greater than 500/mm^3), appear to be adequately treated with 10 days to 14 days of antibiotics, irrespective of the particular organisms responsible for the septicemia. On the other hand, patients whose septicemia is associated with organ complications (*e.g.*, deep tissue cellulitis or osteomyelitis) may require 4 weeks to 6 weeks of antimicrobial therapy. The management of the patient with persistent granulocytopenia who remains febrile after a week of "appropriate" antibiotic therapy for the initial septic isolate is a perplexing problem. For these patients, the possibility of a second (occult) infection that is incompletely sensitive to the antibiotic regimen being used or the development of a supra-infection must be considered. However, the discontinuation of antibiotic therapy in these initially infected and still febrile–granulocytopenic patients is associated with a significant recurrence of septicemia (generally with the same organism or with an organism sensitive to the original antibiotic regimen), suggesting that continued antibiotic therapy is beneficial.[77] At the NCI we are currently exploring the risks and benefits of continued antibiotic therapy in patients with continuing granulocytopenia and fever, as well as the addition of empiric antifungal therapy for such high-risk patients.

In addition to antibiotic therapy, white blood cell transfusions may be of benefit to some patients with documented gram-negative septicemia.[78,79] However, granulocyte collection technology has been hindered by difficulty in collecting adequate numbers of functional granulocytes (approximately 10^{10} cells per day for an adult) since filtration leukapharesis methods (which yield the highest numbers of granulocytes) impair chemotactic and bactericidal functions, while sedimentation methods may result in suboptimal yields, thus raising questions regarding the utility of these transfusions. Since refinements in antibiotic management suggest that patients with gram-negative sepsis can recover without granulocyte transfusions if therapy is instituted promptly with antibiotics to which the organism is sensitive, and since controlled clinical trials have indicated that white blood cell transfusions are unnecessary for patients with short periods of granulocytopenia (less than 7 days), it is not possible to formulate general guidelines until more definitive data is available. We reserve granulocyte transfusion for patients with documented gram-negative septicemia, especially if the microbial isolate is unresponsive to antibiotics or if the duration of granulocytopenia (PMNs less than 500/mm^3) is

(Text continues on page 1684)

TABLE 44-3. Commonly Used Antimicrobial Agents in Cancer Patients

	TRADE NAME	MAJOR INDICATIONS	USUAL DAILY DOSAGE (IV)	DAILY DOSAGE SCHEDULE	USUAL MAXIMUM ADULT DOSE PER DAY
ANTIBIOTICS					
Penicillin G	Benzathin Permapen Bicillin	*S. pneumoniae, S. pyogenes, S. viridens, S. bovis, Nisseria,* most anaerobes (except *B. fragilis*)	25,500,000 units/kg	q 4 h	20 gm
PENICILLINASE RESISTANT					
Methicillin	Staphcillin, Celbenin	*S. aureus, Streptococci*	1–300 mg/kg	q 4 h	12 gm
Nafcillin	Unipen		1–300 mg/kg	q 4 h	12 gm
Oxacillin	Prostaphin, Bactocill		1–300 mg/kg	q 4 h	12 gm
AMINOPENICILLIN					
Ampicillin	Omipen Principen Polycillin Penbritin	*S. fecalis, L. monocytogenes, Hemophilus, E. coli, Salmonella, Proteus*	2–400 mg/kg	q 4 h	12 gm
ANTIPSEUDOMONAS					
Carbenicillin	Pyopen, Geopen	*Ps. aeruginosa, Enterobacter, Proteus, Serratia, Acinetobacter*	500 mg/kg	q 4 h	36 gm
Ticarcillin	Ticar	*Providentia,* most anaerobes	300 mg/kg	q 4 h	21 gm
CEPHALOSPORINS					
Cephalothin	Keflin	*E. coli, Klebsiella, Proteus, Hemophilus S. aureus, S. epidermidis, Streptococci*	170 mg/kg	q 4 h	12 gm
Cefazolin	Kefzol, Ancef	Similar to *Cephalothin,* more active against *Klebsiella, E. coli*	50 mg/kg	q 6 h	2–6 gm
Cephamandole	Mandol	More active against *Hemophilus, Klebsiella, E. coli, Proteus;* less active against Gram positive cocci	1–150 mg/kg	q 4 h	6-12 gm
AMINOGLYCOSIDES					
Gentamicin	Garamycin	*Ps. aeruginosa, Enterobacteriaceæ, Enterococcus* (with ampicillin)	3–6 mg/kg	q 6-8 h	
Tobramycin	Nebicin	Similar to Gentamicin	3–6 mg/kg	q 6-8 h	
Amikacin	Amikin	*Serratia, Proteus, Pseudomonas, Enterobacteriaceæ, Providentia*	15 mg/kg	q 8-12 h	
MISCELLANEOUS					
Chloramphenicol	Chloromycetin	*Hemophilus, B. fragilis, S. pneumonia, Nisseriae, Salmonella, Klebsiella,* most anaerobes, *Rickettsia*	50–100 mg/kg	q 6 h	3–6 gm

PEAK SERUM LEVEL (μg ml)	T ½ (HRS)		MODIFICATIONS FOR RENAL FAILURE (ADULTS)		ADDITIONAL COMMENTS
	Normal	*Renal Failure*	*Moderate* C_{CR} *10–50 ml/min*	*Severe* C_{CR} *<10 ml/min*	
2	0.5	2.5	NC	1,600,000 units q 6 h	
40	0.5	4	NC	2 gm q 8 h	Rare nephritis
	0.5	1.5	NC	NC	Rare SGOT elevation
6	0.5	1.0	NC	NC	Rare neutropenia, hepatotoxicity
3.5	1.0	8	NC	0.5–1 gm q 8 h	Diarrhea common Synergistic with aminoglycoside for Enterococcus
200	1.1	15	3 gm q 4 h	2 gm q 8 h	Synergistic with gentamicin for Pseudomonas. ↑ sodium load, hypokalemia
	1.2	15	2 gm q 4 h	2 gm q 8 h	Rare platelet dysfunction Should never be mixed in same bottle with aminoglycosides
80	0.5–0.8	2	1 gm q 4–6 h	1 gm q 8 h	Most Gram positive activity
135	1.5	20–40	0.5 gm q6–12 h	0.5 gm q 24–48 h	Longest half-life
36	0.3		1.2 gm q 6–8 h	0.5 gm q 8–12 h	
4–8	2.3	45–55	monitor serum levels		All aminoglycosides synergistic with penicillins or cephalosporins against Pseudomonas, Enterococcus, Staph, Strep, Enterobacteriaceæ All have renal and ototoxicity
4–8	2.3	45–55	monitor serum levels		
15–25	2.3	50–80	monitor serum levels		
12	4.1	4.2	NC	NC	Both idiosyncratic and dose related bone marrow toxicity Dosage must be reduced with hepatoxicity

(Table 44-3 continues on page 1684)

TABLE 44-3. Commonly Used Antimicrobial Agents in Cancer Patients (*Continued*)

	TRADE NAME	MAJOR INDICATIONS	USUAL DAILY DOSAGE (IV)	DAILY DOSAGE SCHEDULE	USUAL MAXI-MUM ADULT DOSE PER DAY
Erythromycin	Ilotycin Gluceptate	*Legionella, Mycoplasma*	30–50 mg/kg	q 6 h	6 gm
Clindamycin	Cleocin	*B. fragilis, Clostridia, S. pneumoniae, S. viridens, S. pyrogenes, S. aureus*	30 mg/kg	q 6 h	2400 mg
Vancomycin	Vancocin	*C. difficile, S. aureus, S. epidermidis, S. fecalis,* multiply resistant *Corynebacteria, S. bovis*	25–40 mg/kg	q 8-12	3 gm
Trimethoprim-Sulfamethoxazole (1–5 ratio)	Bactrim Septra	*P. carinii, S. aureus, S. pneumonia, S. pyogenes, Salmonella, Listeria, E. coli, Proteus, Serratia, Hemophilus, Nisseria*	10–20 mg/kg as trimethoprim	q 8-12	960 mg
ANTIPARASITICS					
Pentamidine Isethionate	Lomidine	*P. carinii*	4 mg/kg	Once/day	
Thiabendazole	Mintezol	*Strongloides, Visceral Larva Migrans*	50 mg/kg 2 days	q 12 h	3 gm
ANTIFUNGAL AGENTS					
Amphotericin B	Fungizone	*Candida, Aspergillus, Zygomycetes, Torulopsis, Cryptococcus, Histoplasma*	.05–1.0 mg/kg	Once/day	
5-Fluorocytosine	Flucytosine Ancobon	*Cryptococcus, Candida, Torulopsis, Chromomycosis*	50–150 mg/kg	q 6	
ANTIVIRAL AGENTS					
Adenine Arabinoside	Vidarabine	*H. simplex, Varicella, Zoster Virus, vaccinia*	10–20 mg/kg	12 hr infusion per day	

likely to exceed 7 days. Such patients receive continuous-flow centrifuge cells (most often from a family member), daily for at least 4 days, or until the patient becomes afebrile (see also Chapter 43, Section 2).

Fortunately, cardiovascular compromise secondary to endotoxemia has become less frequent with the early, aggressive antibiotic therapy of febrile–granulocytopenic patients. However, should signs of cardiovascular compromise develop, close monitoring is essential (including central venous and pulmonary wedge pressures), along with respiratory support and vigorous fluid and acid–base replacement, including adrenergic receptor blocking agents (dopamine), vasopressor (*e.g.*, norepinephrine), or vasodilating agents (*e.g.*, isoproterenol), to maintain an adequate cardiac output and avoid irreversible lactic acidosis.[80] High-dose corticosteroid analogs may be beneficial when instituted at the onset of bacteremic shock.[81]

Coagulation abnormalities are also frequently associated with septicemia, including a lowered platelet count, prolonged prothrombin and partial thromboplastin time, and a reduced level of fibrinogen. Patients who remain normotensive or who respond to initial antishock measures generally do not have significant bleeding sequelae associated with these abnormalities. However, disseminated intravascular coagulopathy (DIC) may occur in patients who remain hypotensive in spite of vigorous hydration with plasma expanders. Consumption

PEAK SERUM LEVEL (µg ml)	T ½ (HRS) Normal	T ½ (HRS) Renal Failure	MODIFICATIONS FOR RENAL FAILURE (ADULTS) Moderate C_{CR} 10–50 ml/min	Severe C_{CR} <10 ml/min	ADDITIONAL COMMENTS
0.4–1.8	1.4	5	NC	NC	Burning and phlebitis intravenously
10	2.4	6	NC	NC	Risk for pseudomembraneous enterocolitis (Treat with vancomycin)
25–50	6	9 days	1 gm q 36 h	1 gm q 10–14 days	Drug of choice for antibiotic (*C. difficile*) induced colitis
1.6–3.2	7½		10 mg/kg q 12 h	5 mg/kg q 12 h	May be useful for prophylaxis against *P. carinii* and bacteria
0.2	Very short				Very toxic hypotension, renal damage, sterile abscesses, hypo and hyperglycemia. Available only through CDC.
	1				Rare hepatoxicity. May cause nausea, vomiting, headache, dizziness
0.5–2.0	24	NC	NC	0.5 mg kg q 36 h	Dose modification necessary for patients with hepatic abnormalities. Major toxicities are fever, electrolyte disturbances. May be combined with 5 FC to treat Cryptococcal meningitis.
30	3.4	200	12–25 mg/kg once	Not given	Rapid resistance develops when used alone. Normal use is in conjunction with amphotericin Parenteral form investigational
3–4.1	3.3 hrs		No data	No data	Poorly soluble, necessitates large infusion volumes, mild bone marrow depression.

coagulopathy in these patients may respond to appropriate coagulation factor and platelet replacement, along with careful heparinization (*i.e.*, 50 units/kg to 100 units/kg. I.V. every 4 hours).[82]

Some episodes of septicemia in the cancer patient may be iatrogenic, associated with intravenous catheters (and hyperalimentation fluids), as well as secondary to hemodynamic monitoring, intra-arterial chemotherapy, or surgical procedures (*e.g.*, sigmoidoscopy, dental procedures, gastrointestinal or genitourinary endoscopy, or catheterization).[83-88] *S. viridens, S. aureus, Clostridia, Erwinia, S. marcesens*, anaerobes, or *C. albicans* are most often isolated in such patients. The patient may be nongranulocytopenic and therapy is generally successful if the nidus of infections is removed and appropriate therapy instituted.

RESPIRATORY TRACT INFECTIONS

SINUSES

Sinusitis in the cancer patient is primarily caused by bacteria or fungi. Patients with nasopharyngeal tumors who have obstruction of sinus drainage are at highest risk for acute or chronic episodes of sinusitis. Anaerobic infections deserve special consideration, and biopsy, culture, and initiation of appropriate antibiotic therapy (*e.g.*, clindamycin, 30 mg/kg/day to 40 mg/kg/day, q6h) are important.[89] Antral windows may be necessary to afford appropriate drainage. Neutropenic patients (especially when treated with prolonged broad-spectrum antibiotic therapy) are also at risk for fungal infections of the sinuses (especially *Aspergillus spp* or *mucor*) and suspicious cases require early biopsy and antifungal therapy.[90,91]

PULMONARY INFECTIONS

The lung is the most common site of serious infection in cancer patients. The diagnostic possibilities vary according to the patient's age, underlying malignancy, remission–relapse status, prior and current chemotherapy, radiation therapy, neutrophil count, microbial colonization, and presenting symptomatology. Although the ability to detect a pulmonary infiltrate radiographically may be difficult in the neutropenic patient, it is generally possible to place patients into one of four categories according to the type of infiltrate and the degree of neutropenia (Table 44-4):

Patchy or Localized Infiltrate in the Non-Neutropenic Patient

Infection in these patients is generally similar to that in the general population, and may be due to viruses (*e.g.*, RSV, parainfluenza, adenovirus), mycoplasma, or bacteria (*S. pneumonia, H. influenza*). Patients with pulmonary metastases are at risk for obstructive bronchopneumonias and may require bronchoscopy in addition to antibiotic therapy. It is important to recognize that the majority of these necrotizing pneumonias or lung abscesses are caused by anaerobic bacteria and should be treated with either penicillin or chloramphenicol.

Both tuberculous and atypical mycobacteria deserve consideration, especially in patients with carcinoma of the lung. Identification of the offending organism is important since the atypical mycobacteria are often resistant to available antituberculous agents. The infection frequently becomes apparent following immunosuppressive therapy (especially corticosteroids), suggesting a reactivation infection. The mortality of tuberculous infections ranges from 17% to 50% in cancer patients, and a high index of suspicion is important, since the pulmonary lesions may be confused with the underlying malignancy or other infectious etiologies.[92,93] Sputum should be cultured, and new infiltrates can often be successfully diagnosed by fiberoptic bronchoscopy and brush biopsy with minimal complications.[94] Tuberculin skin testing should be performed prior to chemotherapy in all patients. Reactive patients (who have not been previously adequately treated with isoniazid) should be treated prophylactically with isoniazid for approximately 1 year. Patients with radiographic and culture evidence (*e.g.*, positive sputum) for typical tuberculosis should be treated for at least 18 months to 24 months with at least two drugs (usually INH and ethambutal or rifampin). The possibility of chemotherapy-induced pneumonitis (*e.g.*, busulfan, cyclophosphamide, bleomycin) also deserves consideration in these patients.[95,96]

Interstitial Infiltrates in the Non-Neutropenic Patient

The protozoan *Pneumocystis carinii* is a frequent etiologic agent in this group of patients and has been responsible for a significant number of deaths in patients who are free of detectable cancer.[97] *P. carinii* has a global distribution and inactive cysts can be detected in asymptomatic patients. Furthermore, antibody to *P. carinii* is detectable in nearly

TABLE 44-4. Differential Diagnosis of Pneumonia in Cancer Patients

LOCALIZED INFILTRATE	DIFFUSE INFILTRATE
NON-NEUTROPENIC PATIENTS Bacteria: *S. pneumonia, Hemophilus, Mycobacteria* Mycoplasma Viruses: *RSV, adenovirus* Underlying tumor Drugs: *Busulfan, bleomycin, cyclophasphomide*	NON-NEUTROPENIC PATIENTS Parasites: *P. carinii, T. gondii, Strongloides* Bacteria: Mycobacteria, Nocardia, Legionella, Pittsburg Pneumonia Agent Mycoplasma Viruses: *H. simplex, V. Zoster, Cytomegalovirus*, measles, influenza, adenovirus Fungi: *Aspergillus, Candida, Zygomycetes, Cryptococcus* Radiation Pneumonitis Drugs
NEUTROPENIC PATIENTS Bacteria: Any Gram positive or Gram negative, Mycobacteria, Nocardia Fungi: *Aspergillus, Zygomycetes, Candida, Cryptococcus, Histoplasma* Virus: *H. simplex, V. Zoster* Drugs	NEUTROPENIC PATIENTS Bacteria: Any Gram positive or Gram negative, Mycobacteria, Nocardia, Legionella Mycoplasma Fungi: *Candida, Aspergillus, Zygomycetes, Cryptococcus, Histoplasma* Parasites: *P. carinii, T. gondii, Strongloides* Viruses: *H. simplex, V. Zoster, Cytomegalovirus*, measles, influenza, adenovirus. Radiation Pneumonitis Drugs

100% of normal children, suggesting that the pneumonias which occur in immunocompromised hosts are predominantly reactivation-infections.[98] While horizontal transmission of pneumocystis has not been conclusively demonstrated, several accounts of time–space clustering of infectious episodes suggest that patient–patient transmission may play a role in some cases of pneumocystic pneumonia.[99]

The most common clinical manifestations of pneumocystis include fever, cough, and tachypnea, generally with intercostal retractions and the absence of detectable rales. Chest radiograph shows a hazy, bilateral alveolar infiltrate which often begins at the hilus and spreads to the periphery. Arterial blood gases reflect a low P_aO_2, normal P_aCO_2, and alkaline pH. The clinical presentation can be indolent (1 month–2 months) or fulminant (4 days–5 days). Furthermore, the chest roentgenographic findings may occasionally be atypical (*e.g.*, lobar consolidation, effusion, and even nodular).

Untreated, pneumocystis carries a 100% mortality in cancer patients. While definitive diagnosis of pneumocystis requires histological or cytological demonstration of the thick-walled cysts (*e.g.*, with toluidine blue O or the methenamine–silver-nitrate method of Gomori), or of the thin-wall trophozoite cyst (by Gimesa, Wright, or Gram–Weigert staining), the recent demonstration that trimethoprim–sulfamethoxazole (TMP/SMX) is effective for pneumocystis pneumonia, has lessened the need for immediate biopsy of suspected cases.[100] Our current policy is to immediately initiate TMP/SMX (20 mg/kg as trimethoprim per day) in suspected cases. If stabilization or improvement does not occur within 48 hours to 72 hours, or if deterioration takes place, an open lung biopsy is performed to confirm the diagnosis. If pneumocysts are observed in the biopsy (suggesting possible resistance to TMP/SMX), the patient is switched to pentamidine iosthionate (4 mg/kg I.M. daily). In addition to appropriate antimicrobial therapy, the patient's respiratory function must be carefully monitored, and early intervention with respiratory support may be necessary.[100]

The newly described pneumonitis associated with *Legionella pneumophilia* or with the "Pittsburgh pneumonia agent" (PPA) also deserves consideration, since early therapy with erythromycin (and TMP/SMX for "PPA") may be lifesaving.[101–104]

CMV has also been associated with the severe interstitial pneumonia, especially in patients who have undergone allogeneic bone marrow transplantation, presumably due to reactivation of latent CMV secondary to intensive chemotherapy and the immunosuppressive effects of graft-*versus*-host disease. Approximately half of the patients undergoing allogeneic bone marrow transplantation have developed interstitial pneumonia, especially recipients who have a hematologic malignancy *versus* patients with aplastic anemia (62% *vs.* 35%). The pneumonia characteristically occurs within 3 months of transplantation (the median time of onset being 50 days post-transplantation), has been associated with CMV in approximately half of these cases, and is lethal in 65% of the patients.[45,105] In addition to the lung, extensive organ involvement may occur with CMV, including involvement of the liver, spleen, hematopoietic system (generally with atypical lymphocytosis), kidney, heart (myocarditis, pericarditis), CNS (peripheral neuropathy and Guillain–Barré syndrome), and ophthalmic system (optic nerve infiltration, retinitis). Such widespread disease, however, generally appears to be restricted to patients with end-stage malignancy. CMV has also been isolated in association with other infecting organisms, including *P. carinii,* bacteria, and even other herpes viruses.[106] Moreover, experimental studies in mice and clinical observation in humans suggest that CMV may predispose to supra-infections with bacteria or fungi.[107] This has suggested to some workers that a CMV vaccine may reduce the infection-related morbidity and mortality observed in some organ transplant recipients.[108] Diagnosis of CMV may be difficult. A fourfold rise of antibody titer (in association with suggestive symptoms) and the presence of IgM immunofluorescent antibody, has been suggested as diagnostic confirmation of CMV infection.[109] Since cultures may take up to 28 days to demonstrate cytopathic effects, aspiration or biopsy of definable lesions is generally required for seriously ill patients. Treatment with the purine nucleoside, 9-β-D-arabinofuranosyl adenine (Ara A) (both therapeutic and prophylactic) has been disappointing in patients with CMV pneumonitis; studies employing human interferon are currently in progress.[110,111]

The measles virus can also cause a severe pneumonia, which is either interstitial or nodular, in the compromised host. This pneumonia may occur either concomitant with the initial illness (fever, coryza, and rash) or may develop up to 6 months following the initial infection.[112] Diagnosis can be difficult and may necessitate lung biopsy (for specific immunofluorescent staining) and culture. Immunosuppressed patients who are seronegative for measles antibody and who have contact with measles should receive prophylactic gamma globulin (0.5 ml/kg, maximum dose 15 ml), as soon as possible after exposure. Treatment of measles in the cancer patient is supportive and prophylaxis should only include passive immunization, since live viral vaccines may result in severe complications in the immunosuppressed patient.[113]

While the incidence of influenza and other common upper respiratory viruses (RSV, adenoviruses, rhinovirus, enteroviruses) is not increased in frequency, they may be severe in cancer patients. The most frequent complication is secondary bacterial infection. Some centers routinely employ the killed influenza vaccine for cancer patients, although the antibody response to this vaccine may be significantly diminished in patients receiving chemotherapy.[114,115]

Patchy or Localized Infiltrate in the Neutropenic Patient

In addition to the organisms noted for non-neutropenic patients, opportunistic gram-negative bacteria (*e.g.*, *Klebsiella*, *Pseudomonas*) must be strongly considered in the patient who is neutropenic. Staphylococcal pneumonia can also be fulminant, although it is infrequent even in cancer patients with staph septicemia.[70]

Initial treatment in this setting should include broad-spectrum antibiotics, and if the patient fails to improve (or stabilize) within 48 hours to 72 hours after the initiation of therapy, further evaluation is mandatory to exclude other potentially treatable organisms. While diagnostic material can occasionally be obtained with transtracheal aspiration, bronchoscopy or percutaneous needle biopsy, the yield with these procedures rarely approaches 50%. Most centers, therefore, employ open lung biopsies as the most reliable method for visualizing the involved lung and directly obtaining tissue for culture and histology. In addition, this technique permits better control of bleeding at the biopsy site. Since patients who are candidates for open lung biopsy are often thrombocytopenic, appropriate hematologic preparation for surgery is vital. Elevation of the platelet count to a surgically safe level of 50,000/mm^3 can usually be accomplished by the infusion of 4 units to 8 units of platelet concentrates an hour prior to surgery. Maintenance of the platelet count at this level for the 24 hours following surgery with additional platelet concentrates minimizes any postoperative bleeding complications.

The higher bacteria, *Nocardia asteroides* and *N. brasiliensis*, can cause serious pneumonia in the cancer patient, most often presenting as either a lobar infiltrate or as miliary or cavitary lesions. Brain abscesses occur in approximately 30% of the patients. Thus, the constellation of fever, pneumonia, and CNS symptomatology should suggest the diagnosis of a *Nocardia* infection. Diagnosis depends upon culture of the organism from sputum, exudates, and abscesses. Microscopically, the organisms are branching partially acid-fast and filamentous. Skin lesions (usually subcutaneous abscesses) are also associated with *Nocardia*. Sulfonamides (*e.g.*, sulfadiazine, 4 gm/day to 6 gm/day for 4 months to 6 months) provide the most effective therapy for this infection, but mortality remains significant (30%) once the infection has become disseminated.[116] Favorable responses have also been observed with ampicillin plus erythromycin or with minocycline.

Fungal infections, however, constitute the greatest threat for the neutropenic patient who develops a new or progressive pulmonary infiltrate while receiving broad spectrum antibiotic therapy, often occurring as part of a disseminated infection (Table 44-5). *Candida* is the most common fungal infection. A characteristic radiographic appearance cannot be described, and the altered inflammatory response of the immunosuppressed patient may result in either a false negative chest roentgenogram or as perihilar densities and even a miliary pattern.[117] The presence of *Candida* in the sputum correlates poorly with overt infection. While a positive blood culture for *Candida* is highly correlated with invasive or disseminated infection in the immunocompromised patient, negative blood cultures are much more likely.[118]

TABLE 44-5. Fungal Organisms Encountered in Cancer Patients

CONDITION	ISOLATE
Hematopoietic malignancies or patients with neutropenia	*Candida, Aspergillus, Zygomycetes, Histoplasma, Torulopsis*
Hodgkin's disease and patients with cell-mediated immune defects	*Cryptococcus, Histoplasma, Coccidioides*
Patients receiving hyperalmentation	*Candida, Torulopsis*
Less common isolates in immunosuppressed patients	*Petriellidium boydii, Fusarium, Sporothrix*

Endophthalmitis, characterized by focal, white fluffy mound-like retinal lesions which can extend rapidly into the vitreous, has been associated with disseminated candidiasis.[119,120] While ophthalmologic examination is, therefore, an important part of the evaluation of high-risk patients, recent experimental data suggests that these retinal lesions are composed primarily of inflammatory cells and may not be as apparent in neutropenic patients.[121] Measurement of serum antibody or precipitins has proven unreliable; recently, encouraging results have been obtained with ELISA (enzyme-linked immunoadsorbent assay), ELISA-inhibition, or radioimmunoassay measurement of circulating fungal antigens.[122,123] In addition to *C. albicans, C. tropicalis* has also been recently recognized as a serious pathogen in immunosuppressed patients.[124]

In many centers, the incidence of aspergillosis has increased over the last decade, making it the second most frequent fungal infection in cancer patients.[59,125,126] The upper airway is the most frequent route of entry of these organisms, and clusters of nosocomial aspergillosis have occurred in hospitals where construction materials have been contaminated with aspergillus spores.[127] The pathologic hallmark of aspergillosis is blood vessel invasion, with consequent thrombosis and infarction. Aspergillus pneumonia in the immunocompromised host is commonly a rapidly invasive necrotizing bronchopneumonia, or a hemorrhagic infection with thrombosis of the pulmonary arteries and veins. Approximately half of these patients are also infected with other organisms (especially *Candida*) and a third of patients with aspergillus pneumonia have had a preceding bacterial pneumonia (especially *Pseudomonas*). A characteristic radiographic appearance for aspergillus pneumonia has not been described, but the development of a new pulmonary infiltrate in a neutropenic patient who is receiving broad-spectrum antibiotics should raise suspicion. Blood cultures are virtually never positive, even though disseminated infection occurs in 30% of patients. Although surveillance cultures of the nares may be helpful for early presumptive diagnosis, the definitive diagnosis of aspergillus pneumonia requires a lung biopsy and histologic examination.[128] Without prompt intervention, aspergillus pneumonia is virtually always fatal, especially if the underlying malignancy does not remit or bone marrow recovery occur. Recent reports of successful treatment of patients with aspergillus pneumonia when amphotericin is initiated early (even during profound neutropenia) are encouraging (see page 1689).[128,129]

The phycomycetes (especially *Mucor* and *Rhizopus*) are the third most frequent cause of invasive fungal infection in cancer patients.[130] Like aspergillus, the phycomycetes are acquired by way of the respiratory tract and cause a necrotizing bronchopneumonia or infarction secondary to vascular invasion or thrombosis. Dissemination to other organs (kidney, gastrointestinal tract, CNS, liver, pancreas, heart) may occur in as many as 50% of phycomycetes infections. Early biopsy of suspicious lesions and aggressive therapy (with amphotericin-B) are essential for infected patients.

Histoplasmosis can also cause serious pneumonia in the cancer patient, usually manifested as a miliary infiltrate.[131]

Infection is usually disseminated and the reticulo–endothelial system is generally so heavily infected that the resultant adenopathy, hepatosplenomegaly, and bone marrow involvement can sometimes be confused with the underlying malignancy.[132] Consequently, careful histological examination, of biopsies from the nodes, liver, or bone marrow, for the intracellular yeast forms using Giemsa or methanamine–silver staining is extremely important in the evaluation of suspected patients or those from endemic areas.[133]

Coccidioides imitis and *Cryptococcus neoformans* can also result in serious pneumonia and disseminated infections in cancer patients.[94,134,135] *Torulopsis glabrata,* a yeast that is closely related to *Cryptococcus* and *Candida,* has been increasingly isolated from cancer patients and associated with serious fungal infections. Infection with *T. glabrata* occurs predominantly in debilitated, neutropenic patients, but has also been associated with a foreign body (hyperalimentation catheter, urinary catheter).[136,137] The most common sites of infection are lung, kidney, and GI tract. Fungemia with this organism may occasionally produce an "endotoxin-like shock" syndrome. Because of its similarity to *Candida,* diagnosis of *T. glabrata* is difficult, and differentiation rests upon its smaller size and lack of pseudo-mycelia.

Treatment options for the patient with serious fungal disease are currently limited to a small number of drugs, the most reliable of which is amphotericin-B.[138] While amphotericin achieves a concentration in excess of the minimum inhibitory concentration (MIC) of virtually all the major fungal pathogens, it is associated with significant acute and delayed toxicity. Acutely, most patients experience fever, chills (sometimes with rigors), nausea, and vomiting. Less commonly, hypotension, bronchospasm, or seizures may occur in some patients. With continued administration, nephrotoxicity (including azotemia, elevated creatinine, mild renal tubular acidosis, and cylinduria) and electrolyte disturbances (especially hypokalemia) occurs. A decreased erythrocyte production often occurs after 22 days to 35 days of amphotericin therapy. Since most immunosuppressed patients who become candidates for amphotericin are already receiving nephrotoxic antibiotics, the decision to initiate therapy is often difficult. When therapy is instituted in the cancer patient, it is important to achieve an effective serum concentration of amphotericin as rapidly as possible. We initially administer a test dose of 1 mg of amphotericin to eligible patients; if tolerated, the remaining dose of 0.5 mg/kg/day is given within 8 hours to 12 hours. Patients receiving amphotericin are best kept warm and quiet. Premedication with acetomenophen, and the addition of hydrocortisone sodium succinate (25 mg to 50 mg) to the infusion bottle may reduce toxicity. The dose of 0.5 mg/kg (the therapeutic range is 0.4 mg/kg to 0.6 mg/kg) is administered over approximately 2 hours to 3 hours daily. The infusion should not be interrupted because of fever and chills since this is a self-limited reaction. We have found meperidine (Demerol) (0.5–1 mg/kg, I.V.) helpful in controlling the rigors, although the mechanism of action is unknown. Potassium supplementation is important and if toxicity is excessive, an every other day amphotericin schedule may be helpful. The total dose for disseminated infection remains unresolved but appears to be in the range of 1.5 g to 2 g. The combination of amphotericin with other agents (*e.g.*, rifampin, 5-fluorocytosine) is promising and may help to diminish toxicity.[139,140]

5-fluorocytosine (5FC) is an antimetabolite that has demonstrable *in vitro* efficacy against most fungi.[141] It can be administered orally (150 mg/kg/day, q6h), and is well absorbed. The data to support its efficacy as a single agent for the treatment of serious fungal infections in humans are meager. Of importance, is that *in vivo* resistance to 5FC develops rapidly. However, 5FC may be additive or synergistic with amphotericin-B.[140,141] Toxicity from 5FC includes nausea, vomiting, hepatotoxicity, and the risk of bone marrow depression.

Recently, the imidazole derivatives, miconazole and clotrimazole, have been successfully used for patients with chronic mucocutaneous candidiasis.[142,143] However, neither has yet demonstrated reliable efficacy in the neutropenic cancer patient with disseminated fungal disease. Newer derivatives (*e.g.*, econazole, ketoconazole) may hold promise for cancer patients.[138]

In view of the diagnostic difficulty and high mortality associated with invasive fungal infections in cancer patients, the role of early empiric therapy in high-risk patients is important. We have prospectively studied the utility of empiric amphotericin-B for patients who remain febrile and neutropenic in spite of a week of broad-spectrum antibiotics and for patients receiving antibiotics for a specific infection but who continue to remain febrile after 7 days of antibiotics and show evidence of colonization of their intestinal tracts with *Candida*. Our preliminary observations suggest that the empiric addition of amphotericin to the antibiotic regimen within the first two weeks of therapy significantly reduces fungal morbidity and mortality in patients with persistent fever and granulocytopenia, and that this strategy may be beneficial until more reliable early diagnostic methods are available.

The utility of granulocyte transfusions for disseminated fungal disease has not been demonstrated in humans, and we have recently observed increased frequency of acute respiratory deterioration when WBC transfusions are administered in conjunction with amphotericin-B.[144]

Interstitial Infiltrate in the Neutropenic Patient

In addition to *P. carinii* and CMV, gram-positive and gram-negative bacteria and several fungi can cause interstitial infiltrates in neutropenic patients. Hence, broad-spectrum antibiotics as well as TMP/SMX are empirically initiated in these patients. Again, failure of the patient to improve necessitates lung biopsy and consideration of antifungal therapy.

CARDIOVASCULAR INFECTIONS

Endocarditis is an infrequent complication of bacteremia in cancer patients, presumably because of the early initiation of empiric antibiotics in these patients.[70] On the other hand, endocarditis may suggest an underlying malignancy (*e.g.*, association of *S. bovis* with colon cancer).[72,73] Rarely, gram-negative organisms (*e.g.*, *Pseudomonas*) and fungi (*Candida*) are the cause of endocarditis in cancer patients.[145] Myocardial microabscesses occur more frequently (*e.g.*, *Candida*) and myocarditis may be associated with both viruses and protozoa (*i.e.*, toxoplasma). Since bacterial endocarditis is uncommon, protracted courses of antibiotics (*i.e.*, greater than 3 weeks) are generally unnecessary for the cancer patient with proven bacteremia who has responded to two weeks of antibiotic therapy.[70]

Peripheral vascular infections are also infrequent in cancer patients. However, vascular necrosis is characteristic of certain organisms (*e.g.*, *Pseudomonas, Aspergillus, Mucor*) and may result in a characteristic cutaneous necrosis.[146-148] *Aspergillus* can also produce an obstruction of the hepatic vein leading to a Budd–Chiari syndrome.[149]

GASTROINTESTINAL TRACT INFECTIONS

The GI tract is a major reservoir of microorganisms and is associated with several characteristic infectious complications and serves as a major portal for systemic infection during periods of host compromise.

ORAL MUCOSITIS

Ulceration of the oral mucosa frequently occurs with several commonly used chemotherapeutic agents (*e.g.*, methotrexate, 5-FU, actinomycin-D, doxorubicin). Colonization of drug-induced lesions by the indigenous aerobic or anaerobic oral flora may result in local infection, and in the neutropenic patient, may provide a portal for septicemia.[150] The vigorous use of mouth-cleansing salts and solutions (*e.g.*, equal parts of a non-irritating mouth wash, hydrogen peroxide, and water swished every 2 hours) may help to decrease or control the mucositis. Unfortunately the oral mucosa is a difficult site to decontaminate fully, and several organisms (*e.g.*, *C. albicans*) are especially problematic. While oral candidiasis (thrush) is predominantly a superficial infection, in severely neutropenic patients it may serve as a portal for systemic invasion. Oral nystatin is of only minimal benefit; patients with more extensive oral candidiasis, however, may respond to a short course of amphotericin-B (0.1 mg/kg/day to 0.5 mg/kg/day for 7 days). Recent experience with clotrimazole troches (50 mg, 5 times daily) is promising.[138] In addition to bacterial and fungal infections of the oropharynx, certain viruses (especially *H. simplex*) may be significant pathogens. Encouraging results with Ara-A have been observed in immunosuppressed patients with severe mucocutaneous lesions, although future studies are necessary to assure efficacy and safety.[131] The major hazards associated with intravenous Ara-A to date include fluid overload (primarily because of the low solubility of the compound) and the risk of bone marrow depression and immunosuppression. Preliminary observations with acycloguanine (Acyclovir), a new antiviral agent, are also promising.[152]

Esophagitis is characterized by dysphagia and burning retrosternal pain, usually associated with fever and neutropenia in a patient already receiving broad-spectrum antibiotic therapy. *C. albicans* is the most common etiologic agent, although *H. simplex*, bacterial organisms, or mixed infections can also produce these symptoms.[90,153] A characteristic cobblestone appearance of the distal esophageal mucosa is observed on a contrast esophagram, although this pattern does not discriminate among the various diagnostic possibilities. Since a short course of amphotericin-B (0.1 mg/kg/day to 0.5 mg/kg/day for 7 days) affords prompt relief for patients who have candida esophagitis, we empirically institute this therapy in symptomatic patients who have positive esophagrams. Patients who fail to improve, however, require esophagoscopy and biopsy to determine subsequent therapy.

INTRA-ABDOMINAL INFECTIONS

In addition to infection with the common intestinal flora, the cancer patient is also at risk for infection with GI pathogens (*e.g.*, *Salmonella*), as well as several unique intra-abdominal syndromes:[154]

Typhlitis is a necrotizing cellulitis of the cecum, usually presenting as an acute abdomen with severe right lower quadrant pain. Gram-negative bacilli (especially *Pseudomonas*) are most commonly responsible, and the mortality is high even with optimal antibiotic management. Surgical excision of the necrotic tissue (although risky in such patients) has been successful when combined with aggressive supportive management.[155,156]

Necrotizing enterocolitis, characterized by abdominal pain, distension, and intractable diarrhea, may occur with a variety of antibiotics, the most notable being clindamycin.[157] While the exact etiology is not defined, current evidence suggests that this is related to a toxin produced by *Clostridia difficile*, presumably as a consequence of antibiotic induced alterations of the microbial flora. Of note is that this toxin can be neutralized by the antitoxin from *Clostridia sardelli* and that the syndrome responds to oral vancomycin (500mg q6h for 7 days), to which *C. difficile* is sensitive.[158-160]

A *hyperinfection syndrome* manifested by nausea, diarrhea, abdominal pains, fever, and less commonly by dehydration and shock, can occur as a consequence of the invasion and ulceration of the intestinal tract by filariform larvae of *Strongyloides stercoralis* which undergo maturation (from the rhabditiform stage) as a consequence of chemotherapy. Treatment is with thiabendazole (25 mg/kg/day, in 2 divided doses, for 2 days).[161]

Finally, *clostridial peritonitis* in cancer patients can be fulminant, and is characterized by fever, tachycardia, and flank tenderness (which may extend to the axilla and thighs). The abdominal wall rapidly becomes ecchymotic and crepitant.[162] Aspiration of the cellulitis yields a cherry red fluid, the Gram stain of which shows the large gram-positive rods of clostridia. Aggressive therapy with high dose penicillin plus either clindamycin, chloramphenicol, or an aminoglycoside is essential.

Hepatitis can occur in the cancer patient as a primary infection (*e.g.*, hepatitis virus A,B, non–A,—non–B) or as a secondary infection (*e.g.*, CMV, EBV, *Herpes simplex*, toxoplasmosis). The hepatitis-B virus (HBV) and the non-A, non-B virus are the major causes of serum or transfusion related hepatitis. Diagnosis is aided by detection of specific viral antigens in the serum of infected patients, especially hepatitis-B surface antigen (HBsAg, which includes several subtypes), DNA-polymerase, and the hepatitis-Be antigen, all of which are present prior to and at the onset of clinical symptoms. HBsAg may be detected in the serum as early as 6 days after infection with HBV, although it is usually observed 29 days to 43 days after parenteral exposure, and 67 days to 82 days after oral exposure.[163] In patients with self-limited HBV infection, the DNA polymerase titer falls early and the HBsAg titer later in the clinical disease course, eventually being replaced by antibody to HBsAg and HBeAg.

HBV may result in: acute infection, chronic infection (including chronic "persistent" and chronic "active or aggressive" hepatitis), and an symptomatic carrier state (with or without mild hepatic disease). While the frequency of HBsAg is approximately 0.1% in the general population of the United States, it has been detected in 10% to 20% of children or adults with cancer.[164,165] This has largely been a consequence of multiple transfusions, although currently available sensitive screening tests have reduced this risk considerably. Nonparenteral transmission (*e.g.*, saliva, urine, feces, semen, effusions, CSF) also constitutes an important mechanism for infection. Immunosuppressive therapy may increase the risk of hepatitis as well as enhance the development of a chronic carrier state.[166]

Since many of the chemotherapeutic agents which are currently used in cancer treatment are either metabolized or excreted by the liver, altered hepatic function secondary to HBV hepatitis can seriously compromise the pharmacokinetics of administered chemotherapy. This is most pronounced for patients with chronic hepatitis, in whom even reduced dosages of chemotherapy may both permit the maintenance of the viral carrier state, and aggravate drug-induced hepatic injury.

Treatment of the patient with chronic active hepatitis remains controversial. The current recommendation is that immunosuppressive therapy be restricted to patients who are symptomatic and who have subacute hepatitis with multilobular necrosis and active cirrhosis.[167] Encouraging therapeutic results have more recently been observed using human leukocyte and fibroblast interferon for patients with chronic hepatitis.[168-171] Both short and long courses of interferon have been studied: a short course (10 days to 14 days) leads to a decreased serum level of DNA polymerase, HBcAg, anti-HBcAg and HBeAg; the hepatocyte HBcAg is also reduced. However, HBsAg remains unchanged and all virologic markers again become elevated following the termination of the interferon therapy. However, with 4 months to 5 months of continuous interferon therapy, HBsAg may be eliminated in some patients, without rebound after the discontinuation of therapy. Further study of the dose of interferon (or interferon inducers), and the schedule of administration, may enhance the utility of this therapy.

Because of the morbidity of HBV, trials using standard immune serum globulin have been compared with serum globulin containing either high titer or an intermediate titer of antibody to HBsAg for patients or medical staff who have been potentially inoculated with HBV. While earlier studies suggested that the high titer globulin was effective, recent observations suggest that it may merely delay the onset of hepatitis (up to 9 months), the incidence of hepatitis remaining unchanged at 7%.[172,173] High titer globulin (0.07 mg/kg) is currently recommended for patients or staff who have had a significant parenteral (or nonparenteral) inoculation or ingestion of HBV and who are also negative for anti-HBsAg.

A hepatitis-B vaccine has recently been prepared from formalin treated purified human HBsAg.[174,175] The need for this vaccine in cancer patients, however, may be lessening with the decreased incidence of HBV transmission in the population.

Evidence for a third hepatitis virus now exists from the reassessment of patients with chronic hepatitis and from the transmission of a plasma containing virus (not A or B) to chimpanzees.[176-180] Further study is underway to clarify the epidemiology and control of this newly discovered hepatitis virus.

PERIANAL INFECTIONS

Even minor tears or ulceration of the anorectal mucosa in the neutropenic patient can result in perirectal cellulitis, usually with gram-negative bacteria.[181] Fluctuance may be difficult to detect when the patient is neutropenic, but when present should be aspirated and cultured for both aerobic and anaerobic organisms. In addition to broad-spectrum systemic antibiotics, Sitz baths, warm peroxide compresses, low bulk diets, stool softeners and antidiarrheal agents may help to promote local healing and to prevent further inflammation. In the absence of "abscess" organization, surgical drainage is difficult and may aggravate local healing. Antibiotic therapy should be continued until complete local resolution has occurred, since these lesions can serve as a portal for infection during subsequent courses of chemotherapy and neutropenia. Patients who do not respond to therapy with a semisynthetic penicillin and an aminoglycoside may benefit from the addition of more specific anaerobic antibiotic therapy (*i.e.*, clindamycin or chloramphenicol). Continued lack of response after 48 hours to 72 hours of the addition of such specific anaerobic therapy in the neutropenic patient is an indication for granulocyte transfusions.

GENITOURINARY TRACT INFECTIONS

The risk of a urinary tract infection is increased by tumor obstruction, bladder atony due to cord compression by tumor, or catheterization. In addition to bacterial infection, the urinary tract may also become infected with *Candida albicans* or *Torulopsis* (especially in catheterized patients). Generally this is a superficial infection (*i.e.*, "bladder thrush"), and may be treated by instillation of amphotericin-B (50 mg in 1 liter of D5W per day) into the bladder, or with oral 5-fluorocytosine (100 mg/kg/day to 150 mg/kg/day, q6h). However, disseminated candidiasis may occur from a nidus in the bladder in neutropenic patients, necessitating a high index of suspicion (the presence of pseudohyphae in the urine is not diagnostic) and intervention with intravenous amphotericin-B.

While atypical genital infections have been rarely described in the compromised host, the patient with local tumor involvement (*e.g.*, ovarian, cervical) may encounter anaerobic infections necessitating specific antibiotic therapy (*i.e.*, clindamycin, chloramphenicol).

CUTANEOUS INFECTIONS

The integrity of this primary physical defense barrier is frequently disrupted in the cancer patient (*e.g.*, needle punctures, biopsies, surgery, radiation, chemotherapy). Consequently, local cutaneous infection with bacteria or fungi is not uncommon and may result in disseminated infection during periods of immunosuppression. Vigilant skin cleansing with iodophor solutions is essential prior to any procedure which may permit the introduction of potential pathogens. Careful attention to the physical examination of the skin in febrile cancer patients may yield a lesion from which a specific diagnosis can be made.

The skin can also become infected during bacteremia (*e.g., Ps. aeruginosa, A. hydrophilia, C. equi, S. marcesens*); fungemia (*e.g., Aspergillus, Candida, Mucor, C. neoformans,* H. *Capsulatum*); or viremia (*H. simplex* and *Varicella–Zoster Virus* (*VZV*)). Hence skin lesions may permit the early diagnosis of generalized infection, and fresh lesions should be aspirated (or biopsied) and the material cultured and examined with Gram stain, KOH, and modified acid-fast stain. If a viral process is suspected, the base of a fresh vesicle should be scraped, smeared on a microscope slide, stained with Wright or Giemsa and examined for multinucleated giant cells indicative of a herpes infection (Tzanck test). If indicated, vesicle fluid should be cultured and examined by electron microscopy. The diagnosis of vesicular lesions in the cancer patient is not only important for appropriate patient management, but also permits the physician to decide whether isolation is necessary for the protection of other patients and staff members.[182]

Primary varicella (chickenpox) is the most serious vesicular eruption in pediatric cancer patients, having a mortality of 7%.[183] The major complication is the visceral dissemination which occurs in 32% of patients. Pneumonia occurs in 79% of patients with visceral varicella, generally developing 3 days to 7 days after the onset of skin lesions, usually presenting as bilateral "fluffy" nodular infiltrates. Other target organs during disseminated V-Z infection include the liver, spleen, CNS, gastrointestinal tract, bone marrow, and lymph nodes. Secondary bacterial infection accounts for the additional severity of varicella dissemination. The risk for visceral dissemination is increased in patients receiving chemotherapy at the time of infection, especially when they are also lymphopenic (less than 500/mm^3).

Because of the severity of varicella infection in patients with cancer, attention has been directed at immunoprophylaxis, the most effective regimen being zoster immune globulin (ZIG), prepared from the sera of patients who have recently recovered from zoster and provided through the American Red Cross Blood Services. Administered within 72 hours of exposure, ZIG generally modifies the infection to a mild or subclinical form. Zoster immune plasma (ZIP) (10 ml/kg) is also effective, but is generally less available. Management of the sero-negative patient exposed to varicella (commonly from a household or playmate contact) should include the discontinuation of all chemotherapy, and the administration of ZIG (or ZIP) within 72 hours of exposure.[184,185] Chemotherapy should ideally be withheld in patients with documented exposure until the end of the incubation period (generally 21 days). In patients who develop overt varicella, immunosuppressive therapy should not be reinstituted until all the skin lesions have dried and scabbed.

Since Ara-A has shown encouraging results in the treatment of herpes zoster, it may be of potential benefit for primary viscerally-disseminated varicella, although careful clinical trials to confirm its efficacy are lacking. Early trials with the use of low-dose interferon are encouraging, and results from higher-dose interferon studies may provide an additional therapeutic option.[186] Supportive management and early treatment of secondary bacterial infection is critical for patients with established varicella.

Since varicella is very contagious, there is considerable risk of spread to other seronegative immunosuppressed patients. Therefore, extreme caution must be exercised in the management of potentially or overtly infected patients. An essential component of this resides in careful patient and parent education, and may necessitate absence from school when chickenpox has occurred in the classroom (generally for the 21-day incubation period). Parents should also be alerted not to bring their children to the clinic waiting room area if chickenpox is suspected, and if hospitalization is required, reverse isolation should be undertaken (ideally on a hospital floor where immunosuppressed patients are not located).[182] Furthermore, staff members should also be checked for a history of chicken pox (or tested serologically using the FAMA [fluorescent antibody against membrane antigen] or IAHA [Immune adherence hemagglutination] technique) to further minimize the possibility of nosocomial transmission.

Attempts have also been undertaken to develop a vaccine for VZV which might be protective for high risk patients. Although encouraging results have been obtained from studies in Japan, extreme caution must be exercised since a live vaccine may lead to severe acute side-effects in immunosuppressed patients, or in the case of a latent virus (like VZV), may result in serious zoster-like infections.[187]

The incidence of reactivation infection with VZV (*i.e.*, shingles) in cancer patients who are VZV seropositive ranges from 15% to 52% in contrast to an incidence of 5% in a general population (although this rate rises with increasing age to 16% by the ninth decade).[188,189] Radiation therapy contributes to the risk of developing zoster since the involved dermatome is often the site of prior irradiation. Unlike primary varicella, the mortality associated with zoster is low, even in the cancer patient (approximately 0.1%). However, the morbidity related to zoster is considerable, primarily because of dissemination or neurological complications. Dissemination of zoster outside the original dermatome occurs in 6.7% to 50% of infected patients. In addition to cutaneous lesions, viremia and visceral involvement (*e.g.*, gastrointestinal tract, myocardium, pulmonary) may occur.[190,191] The risk for dissemination appears to correlate with low levels of circulating antibody and a delay in the production of intravesicular interferon.[192]

Neurologic complications are a major cause of morbidity and include peripheral neuropathy, meningitis, and myelitis. Encephalitis may occur by way of direct viral spread (*i.e.*, along a cranial nerve) or may be "post-infectious." Generally, *H. zoster* encephalitis appears within 2 weeks of the time that the rash was noted (although it may occur one week before the rash and up to eight weeks after the cutaneous phase). A unique syndrome of ophthalmic zoster with contralateral hemiplegia has been described, particularly with crainial nerve involvement. Opthalmic zoster (without CNS complications) is associated with involvement of the nasociliary branch (which is suggested by zoster lesions at the tip of the nose). Post-herpetic neuralgia is a significant problem, particularly in older patients and occasionally lasts for months following the initial infection. Patients with post-herpetic neuralgia may derive symptomatic benefit from dilantin or tegretal.

Diagnosis of zoster is primarily based on the characteristic distribution of skin vesicles, a positive Tzanck prep or direct fluorescent-antibody stain to varicella–zoster antigen.

As with chickenpox, local skin care (*e.g.*, Domeboro's solution) and observation for secondary bacterial complications, are important considerations. Ara-A, administered at a dosage of 10 mg/kg for 12 hrs/day for 5 days, has been associated with accelerated cutaneous healing (evidenced by earlier viral clearance from vesicles, cessation of new vesicle formation, and more rapid healing of vesicles). A double-blind placebo controlled trial has recently shown that the early administration of human leukocyte interferon to immunosuppressed patients with VZV prevents both dermatomal spread of zoster as well as dissemination to distant cutaneous or visceral sites.[193] This effect was most apparent with higher doses of interferon (approximately 1.7×10^5 units to 5.1×10^5 units per kg per day). Therapy must be initiated prior to dissemination (*i.e.*, within 72 hours from onset of lesions) to be effective. The major side effects of interferon (especially at higher doses) include fever, malaise, and transient bone marrow depression (granulocytopenia and thrombocytopenia). A current limitation of interferon therapy is the lack of a readily available source of quantities sufficient for extensive clinical use, although this may be overcome with cloned interferon production.[168,194]

In addition to viral infections, serious iatrogenic cutaneous eruptions have occurred in cancer patients receiving immunotherapy with both BCG and MER. These are characterized by local abscesses, erythema nodosum, and occasionally by high fevers, hepatosplenomegaly, abnormal liver function, and pulmonary and bone marrow involvement.[195-197] The acute episode generally resolves within three weeks. Recent observations suggest that therapeutic intervention (*e.g.*, with isoniazid for BCGosis) may aggravate the hepatitis, and thus its use remains controversial.[196]

MUSCULOSKELETAL INFECTIONS

The musculoskeletal system is an uncommon primary site of infection in cancer patients. However, atypical infections such as deep pyomyositis (due to S. *aureus* or gram-negative organisms) have been described in both neutropenic and nonneutropenic leukemia patients.[198] Diagnosis may be difficult because of the minimal fluctuance (even in nonneutropenic patients) associated with these infections, thus necessitating a heightened index of suspicion. Treatment includes incision and drainage in addition to appropriate antibiotic therapy.

Crepitance and soft tissue tenderness should suggest an anaerobic infection, either with *Clostridia* or with the toxin producing *Bacillus cereus*.[199,200] Immediate intervention with debridement and antibiotics is essential, and hyperbaric oxygen may be used in some cases. In addition, other gas-forming organisms (*e.g., E. coli*) may cause a similar clinical syndrome.

Septic arthritis or osteomyelitis in the cancer patient may be due to gram-negative organisms (*e.g., Pseudomonas, Klebsiella, Salmonella, Eikinella*) or fungi (*Candida*) as well as the more common gram-positive bacterial pathogens. Early detection may be facilitated by bone scanning, but aspiration and culture are essential to define the microbiologic etiology and necessary therapy. Patients with local skeletal defects, or who have undergone extensive surgery (*e.g.*, amputation, soft tissue dissection), as well as patients with bacteremia or fungemia are considered at high risk, and should be carefully observed. Occasionally it may be difficult to differentiate osteomyelitis from tumor (*e.g.*, Ewing's sarcoma) or radionecrosis.

CENTRAL NERVOUS SYSTEM INFECTIONS

Central nervous system (CNS) infections are suprisingly infrequent in cancer patients, although the physician should be aware of several unique CNS infections which may occur as a consequence of the underlying disease or its treatment.[201]

MENINGITIS

While meningitis is surprisingly infrequent in neutropenic cancer patients, even minimal symptomatology (headache, meningismus, disorientation), should prompt a diagnostic lumbar puncture. Spinal fluid should be cultured for both bacteria (both aerobic and anaerobic) and fungi, and must be carefully examined with Gram stain and India ink preparation.[202] Patients with leukemia or lymphoma may have meningitis with *Listeria monocytogenes* or *Cryptococcal neoformans*. The presence of gram-positive rods in the spinal fluid of cancer patients should suggest the possibility of *Listeria* and appropriate therapy (intravenous ampicillin and carbenicillin) should be promptly initiated.[203] Splenectomized cancer patients appear to be at increased risk for meningitis.

Cryptococcal infections most often present as an insidious meningoencephalitis, headache being the most common symptom. Occasionally, patients have mental alterations, cranial nerve abnormalities, fever, nausea, or vomiting.[135] CSF examination reveals a mild mononuclear pleocytosis (generally 40 WBC/mm^3 to 400 WBC/mm^3) and decreased CSF glucose. Diagnosis includes the demonstration of organisms by India ink staining (positive in only 50%) and culture (the reliability of which may be enhanced by culturing 5 ml to 10 ml of spinal fluid). However, more than 85% of patients will have detectable polysaccharide cryptococcal antigen in their CSF and the presence of the antigen in CSF or serum permits a presumptive diagnosis of cryptococcal meningitis in 94% of patients.[204] A 67% rate of improvement or cure has recently been observed using the combination of intravenous amphotericin (0.3 mg/kg/day) with oral 5-FC (150 mg/kg/day, q6h).[140]

BRAIN ABSCESS

The presence of focal CNS findings in the febrile cancer patient should suggest a brain abscess. In addition to aerobic and anaerobic bacteria, nocardia and fungi are the most likely causes. The association of pulmonary lesions with focal neurological findings is suggestive of nocardia, aspergillus, mucor, candida.[90,116] Early diagnosis is essential (including EEG, CT scan, brain scan) since appropriate therapy (*e.g.*, surgery, sulfadiazine for nocardia, amphotericin for fungi) may be life-saving.

ENCEPHALITIS

Herpes simplex, varicella–zoster and measles are the most likely causes of viral encephalitis. Of importance, *H. simplex* (which may present with either focal or generalized symptomatology) has recently shown encouraging responsiveness to adenosine arabinoside (15 mg/kg/day over 12 hrs for 10 days).[205]

In addition to viruses, the obligate intracellular parasite, *Toxoplasma gondii,* also has a predilection for the CNS in the compromised host, most often presenting as a necrotizing encephalitis of the gray matter. The symptoms are protean and include mental confusion, headache, meningeal signs, cranial nerve palsey, and occasionally hemiparesis, convulsions, coma, and blindness.[206–208] Infection is rarely restricted to the CNS; also frequently seen are fever, lymphadenopathy, hepatosplenomegaly, hepatitis, pneumonitis, myocarditis, and pericarditis. Diagnosis depends on histological confirmation, serology, or culture. Lymph node biopsy may demonstrate the focal distention of the trabecular and subcapsular sinuses by monocyte-like cells. However, the demonstration of cysts does not confirm active infection, since cysts may also be found in asymptomatic patients. The Sabin–Feldman dye test may demonstrate a titer greater than 1:1000 early in the disease. However, an IgM indirect fluorescent antibody test may be more useful, since it rises within the first week after infection and does not depend on the presence of live cysts to be elevated. A low titer in the cancer patient must be interpreted carefully, since immunosuppression may alter the host's immunologic responsiveness.

The treatment of toxoplasmosis is generally successful if pyrimethamine and triple sulfonamide (usually in conjunction with folinic acid) are administered for at least 1 month.[207]

SHUNT INFECTIONS

Frequently, Ommaya reservoirs are being used to deliver chemotherapeutic drugs to patients with established CNS leukemia or malignancy. Some institutions are now using these shunts for the administration of prophylactic CNS therapy. Like any foreign body, these devices represent a potential source for infection. Fortunately, with scrupulous skin antisepsis, the incidence of shunt infections has been less than 10% in our experience.[209] Furthermore, although shunt infections do occur in a small number of patients (*e.g.*, those with corynebacteria or *Proprionobacteria acnes*), we have successfully used systemic and intrareservoir antibiotics as an alternative to reservoir removal (four of six patients), thus permitting uninterrupted shunt usage in these high-risk patients.

DEMENTIAS

One of the disconcerting sequelae of modern chemotherapy has been the occurrence of leukoencephalopathy. Many of these dementing processes can be related to intrathecal chemotherapy, especially the combination of radiation and methotrexate.[210] However, the recent awareness that slow virus infections can produce CNS deterioration in man has raised concern that some dementing processes may have a viral etiology. Adults with lymphoma and symptoms of progressive mental and emotional deterioration, (including decreased visual acuity, aphasia and both sensory and cerebellar signs) may have antibody to the human papilloma virus JC, suggesting the diagnosis of progressive multifocal leukoencephalopathy.[211]

UNEXPLAINED FEVER

The management of the neutropenic, febrile cancer patient whose initial evaluation has failed to demonstrate an infectious etiology remains a diagnostic and therapeutic dilemma. Continued empiric antibiotic therapy in these patients may obscure the diagnosis of a subclinical infection; may contribute to hypersensitivity reactions, hematologic toxicity, and renal and electrolyte abnormalities; and may increase the risk of developing a resistant microbial flora or suprainfection.[212] On the other hand, the premature discontinuation of antibiotics in the granulocytopenic patient may result in significant infectious morbidity and mortality. These patients with unexplained fever can be divided into low and high risk categories. The majority (61%) are at low risk, as defined by the resolution of neutropenia (PMN less than 500/mm^3) within 7 days following the initiation of empiric antibiotic therapy.[212] In our experience, none of these patients developed recurrence of fever or other infectious complications when the antibiotics were discontinued at the resolution of neutropenia; hence, a short course of empiric antibiotic therapy appears safe for these patients with fever of unknown origin (FUO).

In contrast, FUO patients with prolonged neutropenia (PMNs less than 500/mm^3 for greater than 7 days) should be considered in a "high risk" category. In the NCI series, 39% of the FUO patients were in this category, and these patients can be further subdivided into those who become afebrile (but who remain neutropenic) while receiving empiric antibiotic therapy, and patients who continue to remain febrile while receiving antibiotics. To test the advantages and disadvantages of continued antibiotic therapy in these patients, we randomly assigned high risk FUO patients to receive or not receive continued antibiotic therapy. None of the FUO patients who had become afebrile but who remained neutropenic and who were randomized on day 7 to continue antibiotics (until the neutropenia resolved) developed subsequent infectious sequelae. In contrast, 41% of the afebrile–neutropenic FUO patients randomized to discontinue empiric antibiotics developed fever and infection within a median of two days after stopping antibiotics. These observations suggest that it is beneficial to continue empiric antibiotics in FUO patients who have become afebrile but who have prolonged neutropenia. However, whether these antibiotics should be continued for the entire duration of the neutropenia, or for a limited (*e.g.*, 14 day) treatment course, is presently unknown and is currently under study.

The second high risk FUO group includes patients who continue to remain both febrile and neutropenic after 7 days of empiric antibiotics. For these patients, the possibility that the empiric antibiotic regimen is "controlling" an occult infection must be balanced against the possibility that the antibiotics are inadequate, or that a fungal infection is a primary or secondary complication. In addition to empiric antibiotic therapy, we are evaluating the additional utility of empiric antifungal therapy in these patients and our preliminary data suggest significant reduction of infectious complications when amphotericin is added after seven days of broad-spectrum antibiotics.[214]

PREVENTION OF INFECTION IN CANCER PATIENTS

The most effective method for the prevention of infection will be the development of cancer treatment programs which are tumor specific and which do not result in the compromise of host defenses. Until this goal is achieved, however, the physician is faced with less than perfect options. Nonetheless, considerable advances have been made in infection prevention through the application of common sense methods of hygiene, and modalities specifically directed at the compromised cancer patient.

GENERAL PRINCIPLES OF HYGIENE

Many of the organisms which ultimately cause infection in the cancer patient are acquired during hospitalization (Fig. 44-1). Since the medical staff may be one of the major vectors for microbial transmission between patients, the importance of careful handwashing techniques cannot be overemphasized. Attention to other simple procedures also helps to reduce the incidence of nosocomial infections, for example, careful skin cleansing with iodophor solutions prior to needle puncture, the limited use of indwelling or drainage catheters, careful cleansing of disrupted mucosal or cutaneous surfaces, and antisepsis of commonly used equipment (especially vaporizers and respiratory support devices). In addition, care must be exercised to prevent patients and staff from transmitting an infection to other immunocompromised patients by the appropriate isolation of contagious patients (*e.g.*, with chickenpox). Similar precautions with susceptible medical and nursing personnel must also be taken.

PREVENTION MODALITIES SPECIFIC FOR THE COMPROMISED HOST

During the past 15 years, attention has been primarily directed at suppressing or eliminating the patient's endogenous microbial flora and in preventing the acquisition of new pathogenic organisms. More recently, methods to bolster host defenses have been sought (Fig. 44-2). Each contributes to the control of infection in the cancer patient:

Suppression or Elimination of the Host's Microbial Flora

The most comprehensive method is the total protected environment approach which utilizes a laminar air flow room (LAFR) consisting of HEPA (high efficiency particulate air) filters, capable of removing particles from the air which are larger than 0.3μ with a greater than 99.97% efficacy (Fig. 44-3). The HEPA filters are placed behind an end wall of the room, through which air passes in a laminar fashion toward the opposite end of the unit, out and around a self-sanitizing plastic enclosure, and along the existing room walls toward a return plenum. When all surfaces of the room are completely disinfected, and if all objects which then enter the facility are steam or gas sterilized, a relatively sterile environment is achieved.[35] In order to avoid contamination, patients entering an LAFR must be fully decontaminated, usually with oral nonabsorbable antibiotics, cutaneous antiseptics, orificial antibiotics and a semisterile diet. This "total protected environment" (PE) results in a significant reduction of the patient's microbial burden. However, it takes 1 week to 3 weeks for the regimen to become fully effective, and in order to maintain a state of decontamination, patients must continue on the antibiotic and antisepsis regimen throughout the period of isolation. Furthermore, there are certain body sites (especially the oropharynx) which are very difficult to effectively decontaminate, and certain organisms (especially *Candida albicans*) which are very difficult to eliminate with currently available antimicrobial agents, irrespective of site. These limitations

FIG. 44-2. Methods currently employed to prevent infection in high-risk patients.

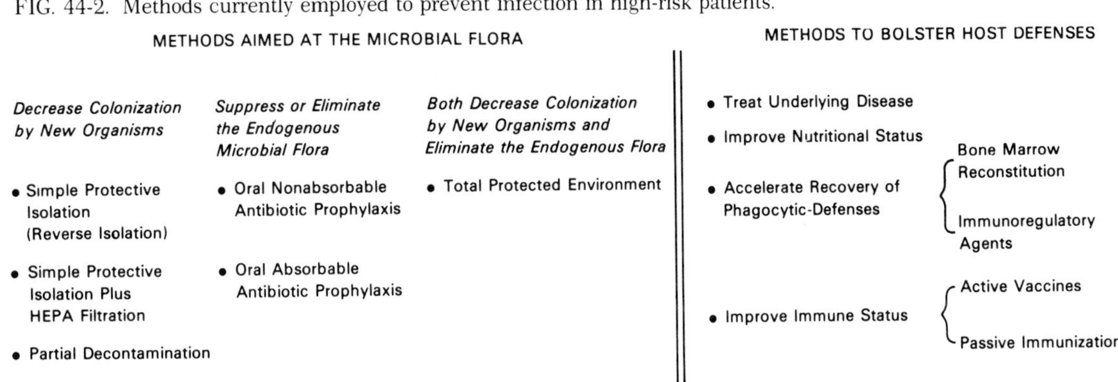

METHODS AIMED AT THE MICROBIAL FLORA
METHODS TO BOLSTER HOST DEFENSES
Decrease Colonization by New Organisms
Suppress or Eliminate the Endogenous Microbial Flora
Both Decrease Colonization by New Organisms and Eliminate the Endogenous Flora
• Simple Protective Isolation (Reverse Isolation)
• Simple Protective Isolation Plus HEPA Filtration
• Partial Decontamination
• Oral Nonabsorbable Antibiotic Prophylaxis
• Oral Absorbable Antibiotic Prophylaxis
• Total Protected Environment
• Treat Underlying Disease
• Improve Nutritional Status
• Accelerate Recovery of Phagocytic-Defenses
Bone Marrow Reconstitution
Immunoregulatory Agents
• Improve Immune Status
Active Vaccines
Passive Immunization

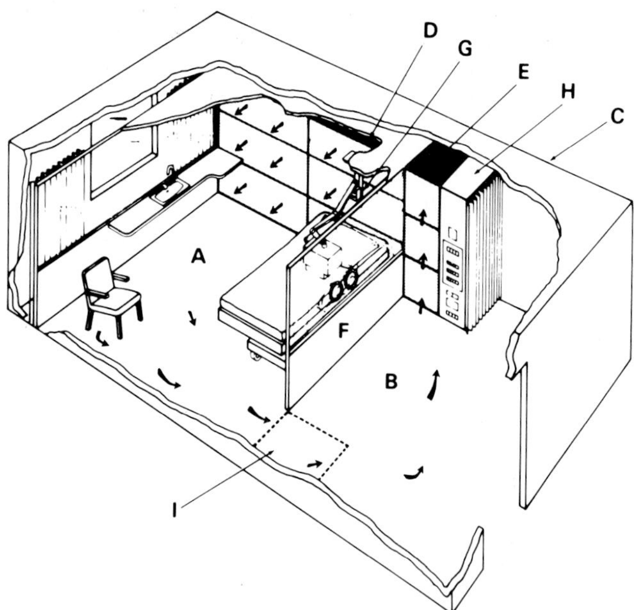

FIG. 44-3. Cross-section of a semi-portable laminar air flow room, housed within a standard hospital room: *A*, LAFR unit (sterile area); *B*, visitor area (not sterile); *C*, cross-section of entire hospital room housing the LAFR; *D*, HEPA filter wall. The *arrows* indicate the direction of air flow; *E*, air intake and blower unit which directs air through the HEPA filters; *F*, plastic or glass barrier separating the sterile LAFR from the outer anteroom (*B*); *G*, patient controls for nurse call, TV, etc.; *H*, control panel for the LAFR unit; *I*, air outflow area from the LAFR and entry into the LAFR.

reduce the overall efficacy of the PE. Nonetheless, the experience gained from clinical evaluations conducted during the last decade has consistently shown a significant reduction in the incidence of serious infections in profoundly granulocytopenic patients treated in a protected environment when compared with patients treated in a regular hospital setting. These obvious benefits of the protected environment must be evaluated in conjunction with the expense of the facility, which includes the need for a skilled nursing staff, sterile supply service, dieticians, housekeeping and maintenance services, and a microbiology laboratory. Furthermore, the social and psychological impact of isolation is considerable for severely ill patients, and occupational, psychological, and physical therapists must work conjointly with the medical and nursing staff in caring for these patients. These constraints and the expense of the prophylactic medications necessary for the total protected environment limit the general applicability of the PE such that the relative benefits of infection control accrued by the PE must be carefully balanced against its cost and utility. For the patient with cancer, the major utility of the protected environment resides in whether the reduced incidence of infection permits the administration of more intensive chemotherapy which might result in an increased remission rate and an improved duration of survival. A recent analysis of the utility of the protected environment for patients with acute leukemia failed to demonstrate a consistent improvement in remission rate or duration, even though infectious complications were deduced. Thus, the limiting factor appears to be the effectiveness of currently available chemotherapy rather than infection prevention. A number of solid tumors (*e.g.*, small cell carcinoma of the lung, non-Hodgkin's lymphoma, metastatic pediatric sarcomas) have been shown to respond favorably to initial combination chemotherapy, although patients who present with metastatic disease have a high recurrence rate, raising the possibility that early intensive chemotherapy might be effective in eliminating tumor cells resistant to lower dosages of chemotherapy. Since hematologic and extramedullary toxicity are the major limitations of intensive chemotherapy, the use of a protected environment permits the delivery of this therapy. Preliminary observations utilizing this strategy in adults with non-Hodgkin's lymphoma have shown an increased duration of remission in patients who received intensive chemotherapy and we have observed similar results in pediatric patients with metastatic Ewing's sarcoma and rhabdomyosarcoma.[215,216]

In a similar manner, the utility of the PE has been assessed for patients undergoing allogeneic bone marrow transplantation for aplastic anemia or acute leukemia. While isolated patients have a reduction in the bacterial and fungal infections which occur during the posttransplant period, the isolation regimen itself does not reduce the incidence of the severe interstitial pneumonitis which follows the transplantation, since this is presumably secondary to the reactivation of latent CMV as a sequel to immunosuppression and GvHD.[45]

As an alternative to the total protected environment, oral nonabsorbable antibiotics (*e.g.*, the combination of gentamicin, vancomycin, and nystatin) have been evaluated for the prevention of infection.[35,216] Although more than a dozen clinical trials have been conducted, a consistent benefit has not been observed. Even if these regimens prove useful, however, a disturbing increase in the incidence of aminoglycoside resistant isolates has been observed in centers where nonabsorbable antibiotics are frequently employed.

It has also been observed that the "partial decontamination" of the cancer patient (*i.e.*, the elimination of the aerobic flora but preservation of the anaerobic microbial flora) may protect the host from colonization with potentially pathogenic organisms, and hence diminish the incidence of infection during high risk periods.[217,218] This can be accomplished with a number of oral antibiotics, including naladixic acid, TMP/SMX, polymixin B, and amphotericin.

Finally, the utility of oral absorbable antibiotics has been suggested from the observation that patients receiving trimethoprim–sulfamethoxazole (TMP/SMZ) as prophylaxis against *P. carinii* pneumonia also had a decreased incidence of bacterial infection.[219] These observations have recently been extended to hospitalized adults who were randomly assigned to TMP/SMZ or a placebo. TMP/SMZ treated patients had a significantly reduced incidence of infection (especially bacteremias) during granulocytopenia when compared to a control group (19% *versus* 39%).[220] TMP/SMX has also been used in conjunction with nonabsorbable antibiotics and appears more effective in preventing infection than nonabsorbable antibiotics alone.[221] We are currently conducting a double-blind, prospectively randomized trial to investigate the role of TMP/SMX plus erythromycin in preventing fever or infection in patients with malignancy and preliminary observations suggest this regimen is useful in reducing fever and infection for patients receiving intensive chemotherapy, but further study is necessary.

Bolstering Host Defenses

Attempts to restore or supplement depleted host defenses have also been investigated. Recently, the value of cryopreserved autologous bone marrow in reconstituting hematopoiesis following intensive chemotherapy has been studied.[223] This technique appears capable of accelerating granulocyte recovery following marrow-ablative therapy. The value of this technology in decreasing the severity of infectious complications is under study.

Prophylactic granulocyte transfusions have also been employed in severely neutropenic patients to reduce the incidence of infection. While the initial results for patients receiving prophylactic granulocyte transfusions following bone marrow transplantation were encouraging, more recent studies suggest only equivocal benefit. Of concern, there appears to also be a serious risk for alloimmunization and CMV infection with prophylactic granulocyte transfusion programs.[216,224–225]

Recently, immune-adjuvants and other agents (*e.g.*, lithium carbonate) have been used to shorten the period of drug-induced neutropenia and thus potentially reduce the incidence and severity of infection.[227] Combined with prophylactic antibiotics, these agents may provide an important adjunct to infection prevention.

In addition to modulation of the granulocyte and macrophage–monocyte system, improved humoral, and cellular immunity has also been sought. Two bacterial vaccines have been evaluated in cancer patients: A lipopolysaccharide pseudomonas vaccine has been shown to result in a short-lived antibody response and some reduction in infection by pseudomonas. However, the adverse effects associated with the administration of this vaccine, and the declining incidence of pseudomonas infections in cancer patients, have limited the use of this preparation.[227] Recently, a pneumococcal polysaccharide vaccine has been tested in splenectomized patients who are at risk for fulminant septicemia. While the antibody response to this vaccine is disappointing in patients receiving combination chemotherapy, current studies are assessing the benefit of immunization prior to splenectomy and chemotherapy with more encouraging preliminary data.[20,228]

Passive immunization also deserves consideration since high levels of IgG antibody to the O antigen of gram-negative bacilli appear to have a protective effect against infection by these organisms.[18,19] We have also observed that cancer patients who succumb to gram-negative septicemia have a significantly lower level of antibody to the core glycoplipid of *Enterobacteriaciae*; the value of passive immunization with these antibodies is under investigation with promising preliminary results.[229–230]

The prevention or attenuation of several common viral illnesses can be accomplished if immune serum globulin or high-titer globulin is administered within 72 hours of exposure.[231] Patients exposed to hepatitis A, measles, rubella, or polio who are seronegative (and who have not been previously immunized) should be given standard immune globulin. Specific high-titer globulin should be administered to patients exposed to hepatitis B, chickenpox, vaccinia, or mumps.

Vaccination of the cancer patient against viruses has two problems: first, the antibody response of patients receiving chemotherapy is often inadequate, rendering active immunization of limited utility in cancer patients.[114,115] Secondly, the use of live vaccines may be associated with serious immediate or unanticipated delayed complications in the cancer patient and should, therefore, be avoided.[232]

In summary, the enormous experience gained in the management of infectious complications in cancer patients has resulted in a significant decrease in morbidity and mortality. Nonetheless, infection remains the most common cause of death and a significant impediment to cancer therapy. This necessitates a more accurate assessment of the factors which place the patient at risk for infection, as well as improved means for the early detection of occult infection in neutropenic patients. These diagnostic tests should be noninvasive, and specific (*e.g.*, based on the antigenic determinants of the infectious organism).

Improved treatment schedules will require development of less toxic antimicrobial agents in conjunction with improved methods for bolstering host defenses. Improved preventive methods are most important, including methods for altering the degree of host compromise, and methods for decreasing the endogenous microbial flora (*i.e.*, prophylactic antibiotics).

Clearly the most significant challenge is the development of effective cancer treatment methods which are tumor specific and which do not produce the significant compromise of host defenses which results in infectious complications.

REFERENCES

1. Stossel T: Phagocytosis. Clinical disorders of recognition and ingestion. Ann J Pathol 88:741–751, 1977
2. Poplack DG, Blaese MR: The mononuclear phagocytic system. In Stiehm E and Fulginetti V (eds): Immunologic Disorders of Infants and Children. Philadelphia, WB Saunders, pp 109–126, 1980
3. Bodey GP, Buckley M, Sathe YS et al: Quantitative relationships between circulating leukocytes and infection in patients with acute leukemia. Ann Intern Med 64:328–340, 1966
4. Strauss RR, Paul BB, Jacobs AA et al: The metabolic and phagocytic activities of leukocytes from children with acute leukemia. Cancer Res 30:480–488, 1970
5. Pickering LK, Anderson DC, Choi S et al: Leukocyte function in children with malignancy. Cancer 35:1365–1371, 1975
6. McCormack RT, Nelson RD, Bloomfield CD et al: Neutrophilic function in lymphoreticular malignancy. Cancer 44:920–926, 1979
7. Snyderman R, Seigler HF, Meadows L: Abnormalities of monocyte chemotaxis in patients with melanoma. Effects of immunotherapy and tumor removal. J Natl Cancer Inst 58:37–41, 1977
8. Cline MJ: Drugs and phagocytosis. N Engl J Med 291:1187–1188, 1974
9. Pickering LK, Ericsson CD, Kohl S: Effect of chemotherapeutic agents on metabolic and bactericidal activity of polymorphonuclear leukocytes. Cancer 42:1741–1746, 1978
10. Baehner RL, Neiburger RG, Johnson DG et al: Transient bactericidal defect of peripheral blood phagocytes from children with acute lymphoblastic leukemia receiving craniospinal irradiation. N Engl J Med 289:1209–1213, 1973
11. Young R, Corder M, Haynes H. Delayed hypersensitivity in Hodgkin's disease. A study of 103 untreated patients. Am J Med 52:63–72, 1972

12. Fisher RI, DeVita VT, Bostick F: Persistent immunologic abnormalities in long term survivors of advanced Hodgkin's disease. Ann Intern Med 92:595–599, 1980
13. Dale DC, Petersdorf RG: Corticosteroids and infectious disease. Med Clin North Am 57:1277–1287, 1973
14. Hersh EM, Gutterman JU, Mavligit GM: Effect of haematological malignancies and their treatment on host defense factors. Clin Haematol 5:425–448, 1976
15. Fahey JL, Scoggins R, Utz JP et al: Infection, antibody response and gamma globulin components in multiple myeloma and macroglobulinemia. Am J Med 35:698–707, 1973
16. Broder S, Waldmann TA: The suppressor-cell network in cancer. N Engl J Med 299:1281–1284, 1335–1342, 1978
17. Stobo JD, Paul S, Von Scoy RE et al: Suppressor thymus-derived lymphocytes in fungal infection. J Clin Invest 57:319–328, 1976
18. Zinner SH, McCabe WR: Effect of IgM and IgG antibody in patients with bacteremia due to gram-negative bacilli. J Infect Dis 133:37–45, 1976
19. McCabe WR, Kaijser B, Olling S et al: *Escherichiae coli* bacteremia: H and O antigens and serum sensitivity of strains from adults and neonates. J Infect Dis 138:33–41, 1978
20. Siber GR, Weitzman SA, Aisenberg AC et al: Impaired antibody response to pneumococcal vaccine after treatment for Hodgkin's disease. N Engl J Med 299:442–448, 1978
21. Gelfand JA, Hurley DL, Fauci AS et al: Role of complement in host defense against experimental disseminated candidiasis. J Infect Dis 138:9–16, 1978
22. Rowley DA: The formation of circulating antibody in the splenectomized human being following intravenous injection of heterologous erythocytes. J Immunol 65:515–521, 1950
23. Constantopoulos A, Najjar VA, Wish JB et al: Defective phagocytosis due to tuftsin deficiency in splenectomized subjects. Am J Dis Child 125:663–665, 1973
24. Schumacher MJ: Serum immunoglobulin and transferrin levels after childhood splenectomy. Arch Dis Child 45:114–117, 1970
25. Carlisle HN, Saslaw S: Properdin levels in splenectomized persons. Proc Soc Exp Biol Med 102:150–155, 1959
26. Donaldson SS, Glatstein E, Vosti KL: Bacterial infections in pediatric Hodgkin's disease. Relationship to radiation, chemotherapy, and splenectomy. Cancer 41:1949–1958, 1978
27. Chilcote RR, Baehner RL, Hammond D, the Investigators and Special Studies Committee of the Children's Cancer Study Group: Septicemia and meningitis in children splenectomized for Hodgkin's disease. N Engl J Med 295:798–800, 1976
28. Weitzman S, Aisenberg AC: Fulminant sepsis after the successful treatment of Hodgkin's disease. Am J Med 62:47–50, 1977
29. Schimpff SC, O'Connell MJ, Greene WH et al: Infections in 92 splenectomized patients with Hodgkin's disease. A clinical review. Am J Med 59:695–701, 1975
30. Donaldson SS, Lenon RA: Alterations of nutritional status. Impact of chemotherapy and radiation therapy. Cancer 43:2036–2052, 1979
31. Shib ME: Principles of nutritional therapy. Cancer 43:2093–2112, 1979
32. Schimpff SC, Young VM, Greene WH et al: Origin of infection in acute nonlymphocytic leukemia: significance of hospital acquisition of potential pathogens. Ann Intern Med 77:707–714, 1972
33. van der Waaij D, Tielemons-Speltie TM, de Houban-Roech AMJ: Infection by and distribution of biotypes of enterobacteriaceae species in leukaemic patients treated under ward conditions and in units for protective isolation in seven hospitals in Europe. Infection 5:188–194, 1977
34. Schimpff SC, Greene WH, Young VM et al: Significance of *Pseudomonas aeruginosa* in the patient with leukemia or lymphoma. J Infect Dis (Suppl) 130:S24–S31, 1974
35. Pizzo PA, Levine AS: The utility of protected environment regimens for the compromised host: A critical assessment. In Progress in Hematology, Vol X, pp 311–332. New York, Grune & Stratton, 1977
36. Mackowiak PA: Microbial synergism in human infections. N Engl J Med 298:21–26, 83–87, 1979
37. Sokal JE, Shimoaka K: Pyrogen in the urine of febrile patients with Hodgkin's disease. Nature 215:1183–1185, 1967
38. Browder AA, Hoff JA, Petersdorf RG: The significance of fever in neoplastic disease. Ann Intern Med 55:932–942, 1961
39. Klastersky J, Weerts D, Hensgens C et al: Fever of unexplained origin in patients with cancer. Eur J Cancer 9:649–656, 1973
40. Goodall PT, Vosti KL: Fever in acute myelogenous leukemia. Arch Intern Med 135:1197–1203, 1975
41. Rodriguez V, Burgess M, Bodey GP: Management of fever of unknown origin in patients with neoplasms and neutropenia. Cancer 32:1007–1012, 1973
42. The EORTC International Antimicrobial Therapy Project Group: Three antibiotic regimens in the treatment of infection in febrile granulocytopenic patients with cancer. J Infect Dis 137:14–29, 1978
43. Goodman R, Jaffe N, Filler R et al: Herpes zoster in children with stage I-III Hodgkin's disease. Radiology 118:429–431, 1976
44. Kaplan MS, Rosen PP, Armstrong D: Cryptococcosis in a cancer hospital. Clinical and pathological correlates in forty-six patients. Cancer 39:2265–2274, 1977
45. Winston DJ, Gale RP, Meyer DV: Infectious complications of human bone marrow transplantation. Medicine 58:1–31, 1979
46. Bodey GP, Rodriguez V, Chang HY et al: Fever and infection in leukemic patients. A study of 494 consecutive patients. Cancer 41:1610–1622, 1978
47. Feld R, Bodey GP: Infections in patients with malignant lymphoma treated with combination chemotherapy. Cancer 39:1018–1025, 1977
48. Bouza E, Burgaleta C, Golde DW: Infections in hairy cell leukemia. Blood 51:851–859, 1978
49. Sickles EA, Green WH, Wiernik PH: Clinical presentation of infection in granulocytopenic patients. Arch Intern Med 135:715–719, 1975
50. Schimpff S, Satterlee W, Young VM et al: Empiric therapy with carbenicillin and gentamicin for febrile patients with cancer and granulocytopenia. N Engl J Med 284:1061–1065, 1971
51. Umsaswasdi T, Middleman EA, Luna EA et al: Klebsiella bacteremia in cancer patients. Am J Med Sci 265:473–482, 1973
52. Brice JL, Tornabene TG, La Farce FM: Diagnosis of bacterial meningitis by gas-liquid chromatography. I. Chemotyping studies of *Streptococcus pneumoniae, Haemophilus influenzae, Neisseria meningitidis, Staphylococcus aureus,* and *E. coli.* J Infect Dis 140:443–452, 1979
53. Feigin RD, Wang M, Shackelford PG: Countercurrent immunoelectrophoresis of urine as well as of CSF and blood for diagnosis of bacterial meningitis. J Pediatr 89:773–775, 1976
54. Thakur ML, Lavender JP, Arnot RN et al: Indium-111-labeled autologous leukocytes in man. J Nucl Med 18:1014–1021, 1977
55. Wright DG, Pizzo PA, Jones AE: Studies on ^{67}Gallium uptake at sites of neutrophil exudation. Clin Res 27:360A, 1979
56. Pizzo PA, Ladisch SL, Gill F et al: Increasing incidence of gram-positive sepsis in cancer patients. Med Pediatr Oncol 5:241–244, 1978
57. Pizzo PA, Robichaud KF: Bacteremia in children with cancer. The impact of infection control studies. Infect Dis Rev (in press)
58. Edwards JE, Lehrer RI, Stiehm ER et al: Severe candidal infections. Clinical perspective, immune defense mechanisms and current concepts of therapy. Ann Intern Med 89:91–106, 1978
59. Young RC, Bennett JE, Vogel CL et al: Asperigillosis. The spectrum of the disease in 98 patients. Medicine 49:147–173, 1970
60. Schimpff SC, Aisner J: Empiric antibiotic therapy. Cancer Treat Rep 62:673–680, 1978
61. Klastersky J, Meunier-Carpentier F, Prevost JM: Significance of antimicrobial synergism for the outcome of gram-negative sepsis. Am J Med Sci 273:157–167, 1977
62. Lau WK, Young LS, Winston DJ et al: Comparative efficacy and toxicity of amikacin/carbenicillin versus gentamicin/carbenicillin in leukopenic patients. A randomized prospective trial. Am J Med 62:959–966, 1977

63. Vincent PC, Jennis F, Hilmer R et al: Tobramycin and cephalothin sodium in treatment of infected patients with acute leukemia. J Infect Dis 134:S170–S174, 1976
64. Feld R, Valdivieso M, Bodey GP et al: Comparison of amikacin and tobramycin in the treatment of infection in patients with cancer. J Infect Dis 135:61–66, 1977
65. Gurwith M, Brunton JL, Lank B et al: Granulocytopenia in hospitalized patients. II. A prospective comparison of two antibiotic regimens in the empiric therapy of febrile patients. Am J Med 64:127–132, 1978
66. Parry M, Neu HC: A comparative study of ticaricillin plus tobramycin versus carbenicillin plus gentamicin for the treatment of serious infections due to gram-negative bacilli. Am J Med 64:961–966, 1978
67. Singer C, Kaplan M, Armstrong D: Bacteremia and fungemia complicating neoplastic disease. A study of 364 cases. Am J Med 62:731–742, 1977
68. Mortensen BT, Mortensen N, Nissen NI: Clinical experience with bacteremia in patients with leukemia and allied neoplastic diseases. Chemotherapy 24:178–186, 1978
69. Yu VL: *Serratia marcescens*. Historical perspective and clinical review. N Engl J Med 300:887–893, 1979
70. Ladisch SL, Pizzo PA: *S. aureus* sepsis in children with cancer. Pediatr 61:231–234, 1978
71. Kilton LJ, Fossieck BE, Cohen MH: Bacteremia due to gram-positive cocci in patients with neoplastic disease. Am J Med 66:596–602, 1979
72. Klein RS, Recco RA, Catalono MT: Association of *Streptococcus bovis* with carcinoma of the colon. N Engl J Med 297:800–802, 1977
73. Klein RS, Catalano MT, Edberg SC et al: *Streptococcus bovis* septicemia and carcinoma of the colon. Ann Intern Med 91:560–562, 1979
74. Hande KR, Witebsky FG, Brown MS et al: Sepsis with a new species of *Corynebacterium*. Ann Intern Med 85:423–426, 1976
75. Berg R, Chmel H, Mayo J et al: *Corynebacterium equi* infection complicating neoplastic disease. Am J Clin Pathol 68:73–77, 1977
76. Pizzo PA, Ladsich SL, Robichaud K: Treatment of gram-positive septicemia in cancer patients. Cancer 45:206–207, 1980
77. Gill FA, Robinson R, MacLowry JD et al: The relationship of fever, granulocytopenia and antimicrobial therapy to bacteremia in cancer patients. Cancer 39:1704–1709, 1977
78. Herzig RH, Herzig GP, Graw RG Jr et al: Granulocyte transfusion therapy for gram-negative septicemia. N Engl J Med 296:701–705, 1977
79. Higby DJ, Burnett D: Granulocyte transfusions: current status. Blood 55:2–8, 1980
80. Winslow EJ, Loeb HS, Rahimtoola SH et al: Hemodynamic studies and results of therapy in 50 patients with bacteremic shock. Am J Med 54:421–432, 1973
81. Schumer W: Steroids in the treatment of clinical septic shock. Ann Surg 184:333–341, 1976
82. Corrigan JJ: Heparin therapy in bacterial septicemia. J Pediatr 91:695–700, 1977
83. Buxton AE, Highsmith AK, Garner JS et al: Contamination of intravenous infusion fluids: effects of changing administration sets. Ann Intern Med 90:764–768, 1979
84. Band JD, Maki DG: Infections caused by arterial catheters used for hemodynamic monitoring. Am J Med 67:735–741, 1979
85. Maki DG, McCormick RD, Uman SJ et al: Septic endarteritis due to intra-arterial catheters for cancer chemotherapy. I. Evaluation of an outbreak, II. Risk factors, clinical features and management, III. Guidelines for prevention. Cancer 44:1228–1240, 1979
86. Tully JL, Lew MA, Connor M, D'Orsi CJ: Clostridial sepsis following hepatic arterial infusion chemotherapy. Am J Med 67:707–710, 1979
87. LeFrock JL, Ellis CA, Turchik JB et al: Transient bacteremia associated with sigmoidoscopy. N Engl J Med 289:467–469, 1973
88. Pizzo PA, Ladish SL, Witebsky F: Alpha-hemolytic streptococci: Clinical significance in cancer patients. Med Pediatr Oncol 4:367–370, 1978
89. Frederich J, Baude AI: Anaerobic infection of the paranasal sinuses. N Engl J Med 290:135–137, 1974
90. Krick JA, Remington JS: Opportunistic invasive fungal infections in patients with leukemia and lymphoma. Clin Haematol 5:249–310, 1976
91. Eden OB, Santos J: Effective treatment for rhinopulmonary mucormycosis in a boy with leukemia. Arch Dis Child 54:557–559, 1979
92. Kaplan MH, Armstrong D, Rosen P: Tuberculosis complicating neoplastic disease. A review of 201 cases. Cancer 33:850–858, 1974
93. Feld R, Bodey GP, Groschel D: Mycobacteriosis in patients with malignant disease. Arch Intern Med 136:67–70, 1976
94. Lauver GL, Hasan FM, Morgan RB et al: The usefulness of fiberoptic bronchoscopy in evaluating new pulmonary lesions in the compromised host. Am J Med 66:580–585, 1979
95. Iacuone JJ, Wong KY, Bove KE et al: Acute respiratory illness in children with acute lymphoblastic leukemia. J Pediatr 90:915–919, 1977
96. Pascual RS, Mosher MB, Sikand RS: Effects of bleomycin on pulmonary function in man. Am Rev Resp Dis 108:211–217, 1973
97. Hughes WT. *Pneumocystis carinii* pneumonia. N Engl J Med 297:1381–1383, 1977
98. Meuwissen JH, Tauber I, Leewenberg ADEM et al: Parasitologic and serologic observations of infection with *Pneumocystis* in humans. J Infect Dis 136:4349, 1977
99. Ruebush TK, Weinstein RA, Baehner RL et al: An outbreak of Pneumocystis pneumonia in children with acute lymphocytic leukemia. Am J Dis Child 132:143–148, 1978
100. Hughes WT, Feldman S, Chudhary SC et al: Comparison of pentamidine-isethionate and trimethoprim-sulfamethoxazole in the treatment of *Pneumocystis carinii* pneumonia. J Pediatr 92:285–291, 1978
101. Singer C, Armstrong D, Rosen PP et al: Diffuse pulmonary infiltrates in immunosuppressed patients. Prospective study of 80 cases. Am J Med 66:100–119, 1979
102. Saravalatz LD, Burch KH, Fisher E et al: The compromised host and Legionnaire's disease. Ann Intern Med 90:533–537, 1979
103. Myerowitz RL, Pasculle AW, Dowling JN et al: Opportunistic lung infection due to "Pittsburg Pneumonia Agent." N Engl J Med 301:953–958, 1979
104. Rogers BH, Donowitz GR, Walker GK et al: Opportunistic pneumonia. A clinicopathological study of five cases caused by an unidentified acid-fast bacterium. N Engl J Med 301:959–961, 1979
105. Neiman PE, Reeves W, Ray G et al: A prospective analysis of interstitial pneumonia and opportunistic viral infection among recipients of allogeneic bone marrow grafts. J Infect Dis 136:754–767, 1977
106. Lemon SM, Hutt LM, Huang YT et al: Simultaneous infection with multiple herpes viruses. Am J Med 66:270–276, 1979
107. Rand KH, Pollard RB, Merigan TC: Increased pulmonary superinfections in cardiac transplant patients undergoing primary cytomegalovirus infection. N Engl J Med 298:951–953, 1978
108. Plotkin SA, Farquhar J, Hornberger E: Clinical trials of immunization with the Town 125 strain of human cytomegalovirus. J Infect Dis 134:470–475, 1976
109. Henson D, Siegel SE, Fuccillo DA et al: Cytomegalovirus infection during acute childhood leukemia. J Infect Dis 126:469–481, 1972
110. Kraemer KG, Neiman P, Reeves WC: Prophylactic adenine arabinoside following marrow transplantation. Transplant Proc 10:237–240, 1978
111. Pollard RB, Merigan TC: Perspectives for the control of cytomegalovirus infections in bone marrow transplant recipients. Transplant Proc 10:241–245, 1978
112. Siegel MM, Walter JK, Ablin AR: Measles pneumonia in childhood leukemia. Pediatr 60:38–40, 1977

113. Mitus A, Halloway A, Evans AE: Attenuated measles vaccine in children with acute leukemia. Am J Dis Child 103:413–418, 1962
114. Schafer AI, Churchill WH, Ames P et al: The influence of chemotherapy on response of patients with hematologic malignancies to influenza vaccine. Cancer 43:25–30, 1979
115. Schildt RA, Luedke DW, Kasai G et al: Antibody response to influenza immunization in adult patients with malignant disease. Cancer 44:1629–1635, 1975
116. Young LS, Armstrong D, Blevins A et al: *Nocardia asteroides* infection complicating neoplastic disease. Am J Med 50:356–367, 1971
117. Dubois PJ, Myerowitz RL, Allen CM. Patho-radiologic correlation of pulmonary candidiasis in immunosuppressed patients. Cancer 40:1026–1036, 1977
118. Young RC, Bennett JE, Geelhoed GW et al: Fungemia with compromised host resistance. A study of 70 cases. Ann Intern Med 80:605–612, 1974
119. Edwards JE Jr, Foos RY, Montgomerie JZ et al: Occular manifestations of candida septicemia: Review of seventy-six cases of hematogenous candida endophthalmitis. Medicine 53:47–75, 1974
120. Fishman LS, Griffin JR, Sapico FL et al: Hematogenous candida endophthalmitis—a complication of candidemia. N Engl J Med 286:675–681, 1972
121. Henderson DK, Vukalcic LJ, Hockey LJ: The effect of immunosuppression in experimental hematogenous candida endophthalmitis. 18th Interscience Conf on Antimicrob Agents Chemother 18:400, 1978
122. Glew RH, Buckley HR, Rosen HM et al: Serologic tests in the diagnosis of systemic candidiasis. Enhanced diagnostic accuracy with crossed immunoelectrophoresis. Am J Med 64:586–591, 1978
123. Segal E, Berg RA, Pizzo PA et al: Detection of candida antigen in the sera of patients with candidiasis by an ELISA inhibition technique. A preliminary report. J Clin Microbiol 10:116–118, 1979
124. Wingard JR, Merz WG, Saral R: *Candida tropicalis:* A major pathogen in immunocompromised patients. Ann Intern Med 91:539–543, 1979
125. Meyer RD, Young LS, Armstrong D, Yu B: Aspergillosis complicating neoplastic disease. Am J Med 54:6–15, 1973
126. Fraser DW, Ward JI, Ajello L et al: Aspergillosis and other systemic mycoses. The growing problem. JAMA 242:1631–1635, 1979
127. Aisner J, Schimpff SC, Bennett JE et al: *Aspergillus* infection in cancer patients. Association with fireproofing materials in new hospitals. JAMA 235:411–412, 1976
128. Aisner J, Schimpff SC, Wiernik PH: Treatment of invasive aspergillosis: relation of early diagnosis and treatment to response. Ann Intern Med 86:539–543, 1977
129. Pennington JE. Successful treatment of Aspergillus pneumonia in hematologic neoplasia. N Engl J Med 295:426–427, 1976
130. Meyer RD, Rosen P, Armstrong D: Phycomycosis complicating leukemia and lymphoma. Ann Intern Med 77:871–879, 1972
131. Kauffman CA, Israel KS, Smith JW et al: Histoplasmosis in immunosuppressed patients. Am J Med 64:923–931, 1978
132. Brodeur GM, Wilber RB, Melvin SL et al: Histoplasmosis mimicking childhood non-Hodgkin's lymphoma. Med Pediatr Oncol 7:77–81, 1979
133. Davies SF, McKenna RW, Sarosi GA: Trephine biopsy of the bone marrow in disseminated histoplasmosis. Am J Med 67:617–622, 1979
134. Deresinski SC, Stevens DA: Coccidioidomycosis in compromised hosts. Experience at Stanford University Hospital. Medicine 54:377–395, 1974
135. Kaplan MS, Rosen PP, Armstrong D: Cryptococcosis in a cancer hospital. Clinical and pathological correlates in forty-six patients. Cancer 39:2265–2274, 1977
136. Valdivieso M, Luna M, Bodey GP et al: Fungemia due to *Torulopsis glabrata* in the compromised host. Cancer 38:1750–1756, 1976
137. Aisner J, Schimpff SC, Sutherland JC et al: *Torulopsis glabrata* infection in patients with cancer. Increasing incidence and relationship to colonization. Am J Med 61:23–28, 1976
138. Medoff G, Kobayashi G: Strategies in the treatment of systemic fungal infections. N Engl J Med 302:140–156, 1980
139. Beggs WH, Sarosi GA, Andrews FA: Synergistic action of amphotericin B and rifampin on *Candida albicans*. Am Rev Respir Dis 110:671–673, 1974
140. Bennett JE, Dismukes WE, Duma RJ et al: Amphotericin B-flucytosine in cryptococcal meningitis. N Engl J Med 301:126–131, 1979
141. Bennett JF: Flucytosine. Ann Intern Med 86:319–322, 1977
142. Fischer TJ, Klein RB, Kershnar HE et al: Miconazole in the treatment of chronic mucocutaneous candidiasis. A preliminary report. J Pediatr 91:815–819, 1977
143. Kirkpatrick CH, Alling DW: Treatment of chronic oral candidiasis with clotrimazole trouches. A controlled clinical trial. N Engl J Med 299:1201–1203, 1978
144. Wright DG, Robichand K, Pizzo PA et al: Lethal pulmonary reactions associated with the combined use of amphotericin B and leukocyte transfusions. N Engl J Med, 304:1185–1189, 1981
145. Ihde DC, Roberts WC, Marr KC et al: Cardiac candidiasis in cancer patients. Cancer 41:2364–2371, 1978
146. Whitecar JP, Luna M, Bodey GP. *Pseudomonas* bacteremia in patients with malignant diseases. Am J Med Sci 260:216–223, 1970
147. Prystowsky SD, Vogelstein B, Ettinger DS et al: Invasive aspergillosis. N Engl J Med 295:655–658, 1976
148. Kramer BS, Hernandez AD, Reddick RL et al: Cutaneous infarction. Manifestations of disseminated mucormycosis. Arch Dermatol 113:1075–1076, 1977
149. Young RC: The Budd–Chiari syndrome caused by aspergillus. Arch Intern Med 124:754–757, 1969
150. Dreizen S, McCredie KB, Bodey G: Unusual mucocutaneous infections in immunosuppressed patients with leukemia. Postgrad Med 66:131–141, 1979
151. Ch'ien LT, Cannon NJ, Charamella LJ et al: Effect of adenine arabinoside on severe *Herpes hominis* infection in man. J Infect Dis 128:658–663, 1973
152. Selby PJ, Jameson B, Watson JG et al: Parenteral acyclovir therapy for herpes virus infections in man. Lancet ii:1267–1270, 1979
153. Buss DH, Scharyj M: Herpes virus infection of the esophagus and other visceral organs in adults. Incidence and clinical significance. Am J Med 66:457–462, 1979
154. Novak R, Feldman S: Salmonellosis in children with cancer. Am J Dis Child 133:298–300, 1979
155. Varki AP, Armitage JO, Feagler JR: Typhlitis in acute leukemia. Successful treatment by early surgical intervention. Cancer 43:695–697, 1979
156. Kies MS, Luedke DW, Boyd JF et al: Neutropenic enterocolitis. Two case reports of long term survival following surgery. Cancer 43:730–734, 1979
157. Dosik GM, Luna M, Valdivieso M et al: Necrotizing colitis in patients with cancer. Am J Med 67:646–656, 1979
158. Larson HE, Price AB, Honour P et al: *Clostridium difficile* and the aeiology of pseudomembraneous colitis. Lancet i:1063–1066, 1978
159. Bartlett JG, Chang TW, Gurwith M et al: Antibiotic-associated pseudomembraneous colitis due to toxin-producing clostridia. N Engl J Med 298:531–534, 1978
160. Tedesco F, Markham R, Gurwith M et al: Oral vancomycin for antibiotic-associated pseudomembraneous colitis. Lancet ii:226–228, 1978
161. Rassiga AA, Lowry JL, Forman WB: Diffuse pulmonary infection due to *Strongloides stercoralis*. JAMA 230:426–427, 1974
162. Wynne JW, Armstrong D: Clostridial septicemia. Cancer 29:215–221, 1972
163. Krugman S, Overby LR, Mushawar IK et al: Viral hepatitis, Type B. Studies on natural history and prevention re-examined. N Engl J Med 300:101–106, 1979
164. Wands JR, Walker JA, Davis TT et al: Hepatitis in an oncology unit. N Engl J Med 291:1371–1375, 1976

165. Tabor E, Gerety JR, Mott M et al: Prevalence of hepatitis B in a high-risk setting: A serologic study of patients and staff in a pediatric oncology unit. Pediatr 61:711–715, 1978
166. Berk PD, Jones A, Plotz PH et al: Corticosteroid therapy for chronic active hepatitis. Ann Intern Med 85:523–524, 1976
167. Editorial: Immunosuppressive therapy for chronic active hepatitis. Lancet ii:507–508, 1978
168. Dunnick J, Galasso GJ: Clinical trials with exogenous interferon. Summary of a meeting. J Infect Dis 139:109–123, 1979
169. Greenberg HB, Pollard RB, Lutwick LI et al: Effect of leukocyte interferon on hepatitis-B virus infection in patients with chronic active hepatitis. N Engl J Med 295:517–522, 1976
170. Desmyter J, Ray MB, DeGroote J et al: Administration of human fibroblast interferon in chronic hepatitis-B infection. Lancet ii:645–647, 1976
171. Dolen JG, Carter WA, Horozewicz JS et al: Fibroblast interferon treatment of a patient with chronic active hepatitis. Increased number of circulating T lymphocytes and elimination of rosette-inhibitory factor. Am J Med 67:127–130, 1979
172. Seeff LB, Wright EC, Zimmerman HJ et al: Type B hepatitis after needle-stick exposure: prevention with hepatitis B immune globulin. Ann Intern Med 88:285–293, 1978
173. Grady GF, Lee VA, Prince AM et al: Hepatitis B immune globulin for accidental exposures among medical personnel: final report of a multicenter controlled trial. J Infect Dis 138:625–638, 1978
174. Purcell RH, Gerin JC: Hepatitis B subunit vaccine. A preliminary report of safety and efficacy test in chimpanzees. Am J Med Sci 270:395–399, 1975
175. Gerety RJ, Tabor E, Purcell RH et al: Summary of an International Workshop on Hepatitis B vaccines. J Infect Dis 140:642–648, 1979
176. Meyers, JD, Dienstag JL, Purcell RH et al: Parenterally transmitted non-A, non-B hepatitis. An epidemic reassessed. Ann Intern Med 87:57–59, 1977
177. Hoofnagle HJ, Gerety RJ, Tabor E et al: Transmission of non-A, non-B hepatitis. Ann Intern Med 87:14–20, 1977
178. Berman M, Alter HJ, Isak KG et al: The chronic sequelae of non-A, non-B hepatitis. Ann Intern Med 91:1–6, 1979
179. Alter HJ, Purcell RH, Holland PV et al: Transmissible virus in non-A, non-B hepatitis. Lancet i:459–463, 1978
180. Tabor E, Gerety RJ, Drucker JA et al: Transmission of non-A, non-B hepatitis from man to chimpanzee. Lancet i:463–465, 1978
181. Schimpff SC, Wiernik PA, Block JB: Rectal abscesses in cancer patients. Lancet ii:844–847, 1972
182. Leclair JM, Zaia JA, Levin MJ et al: Airborne transmission of chickenpox in a hospital. N Engl J Med 302:450–453, 1980
183. Feldman S, Hughes WT, Daniel CB: Varicella in children with cancer: seventy-seven cases. Pediatr 56:388–397, 1975
184. Gershon AA, Steinberg S, Brunnell PA: Zoster immune globulin. A further assessment. N Engl J Med 290:243–245, 1975
185. Geiser CF, Bishop Y, Myers M et al: Prophylaxis of varicella in children with neoplastic disease: Comparative results with zoster immune plasma and gamma globulin. Cancer 35:1027–1030, 1975
186. Arvin AM, Feldman S, Merigan TC: Human leukocyte interferon in the treatment of varicella in children with cancer in preliminary controlled trial. Antimicrob Agents Chemother 13:605–607, 1978
187. Takahashi M, Otsuka T, Okuno Y et al: Live vaccine used to prevent the spread of varicella in children in hospital. Lancet ii:1288–1290, 1974
188. Feldman S, Hughes WT, Kim HY. Herpes zoster in children with cancer. Am J Dis Child 126:178–184, 1973
189. Reboul F, Donaldson SS, Kaplan HS: Herpes zoster and varicella infections in children with Hodgkin's disease. An analysis of contributing factors. Cancer 41:95–99, 1978
190. Feldman S, Chaudary S, Ossi M et al: A viremic phase for herpes zoster in children with cancer. J Pediatr 91:597–600, 1977
191. Myers MG: Viremia caused by varicella–zoster virus. Association with malignant progressive varicella. J Infect Dis 140:229–233, 1979
192. Stevens DA, Merigan TC: Interferon, antibody and other host factors in herpes zoster. J Clin Invest 51:1170–1178, 1972
193. Merigan TC, Rand KH, Pollard RB et al: Human leukocyte interferon for the treatment of herpes zoster in patients with cancer. N Engl J Med 298:981–987, 1978
194. Friedman PM: Antiviral activity of interferons. Bacteriol Rev 41:543–567, 1977
195. Ritch PS, McCredie KB, Gutterman JU et al: Disseminated BCG disease associated with immunotherapy by scarification in acute leukemia. Cancer 42:167–170, 1978
196. Rosenberg SA, Seipp C, Sears HF: Clinical and immunologic studies of disseminated BCG infection. Cancer 41:1771–1780, 1978
197. Voith MA, Lichtenfeld KM, Schimpff SC et al: Systemic complications of MER immunotherapy of cancer. Pulmonary granulomatosis and rash. Cancer 43:500–504, 1979
198. Blatt J, Reaman G, Pizzo PA. Pyomyositis in acute lymphocytic leukemia heralded by cutaneous vasculitis. Two case reports. Med Pediatr Oncol 7:237–239, 1979
199. Lehman TJA, Quinn JJ, Siegel S et al: *Clostridium septicum* infection in childhood leukemia. Report of a case and review of the literature. Cancer 40:950–953, 1977
200. Groschel D, Burges MA, Bodey GP. Gas gangrene-like infection with *Bacillus–cereus* in a lymphoma patient. Cancer 37:988–991, 1976
201. Chernik N, Armstrong D, Posner JB. Central nervous system infections in patients with cancer. Changing patterns. Cancer 40:268–274, 1977
202. Heerema MS, Ein ME, Musher DM et al: Anaerobic bacterial meningitis. Am J Med 67:219–227, 1979
203. Lavetter A, Leedom JM, Mathies AW et al: Meningitis due to *Listeria monocytogenes*. N Engl J Med 285:598–603, 1971
204. Diamond RD, Bennett JE. Prognostic factor in cryptococcal meningitis: A study in 111 cases. Ann Intern Med 80:176–181, 1974
205. Whitley RJ, Soong SJ, Dolin R et al: Adenine arabinoside therapy of biopsy-proven Herpes simplex encephalitis. N Engl J Med 297:289–294, 1977
206. Remington JS: Toxoplasmosis in the adult. Bull NY Acad Med 50:211–227, 1974
207. Ruskin J, Remington JS: Toxoplasmosis in the compromised host. Ann Intern Med 84:193–199, 1976
208. McLeod R, Berry PF, Marshall WH et al: Toxoplasmosis presenting as brain abscesses. Diagnosis by computerized tomography and cytology of aspirated purulent material. Am J Med 67:711–714, 1979
209. Bleyer WA, Pizzo PA, Spence AM et al: The Ommaya reservoir: Newly recognized complications and recommendations for insertion and use. Cancer 41:2431–2437, 1978
210. Pizzo PA, Poplack DG, Bleyer WA: The neurotoxicities of current leukemia therapy. Am J Pediatr Hematol Oncol 1:127–140, 1979
211. Narayan O, Penney JB, Johnson RJ et al: Etiology of progressive multifocal leukoencephalopathy. Identification of papovovirus. N Engl J Med 289:1278–1282, 1973
212. Pennington JE: Fever, neutropenia, and malignancy: a clinical syndrome in evolution. Cancer 39:1345–1349, 1977
213. Pizzo PA, Robichaud KJ, Gill FA et al: Duration of empiric antibiotic therapy in granulocytopenic cancer patients. Am J Med 67:194–200, 1979
214. Pizzo PA, Robichaud K, Simon R et al: Empiric antifungal therapy for cancer patients with prolonged fever and granulocytopenia. Proc Am Soc Clin Oncol 21:348, 1980
215. Bodey GP, Rodriguez V, Carbonillas F et al: Protected-environment prophylactic-antibiotic program for malignant lymphomas. Randomized trial during chemotherapy to induce remission. Am J Med 66:74–81, 1979
216. Storring RA, Jameson B, McElwain TJ et al: Oral non-absorbable antibiotics prevent infection in acute non-lymphoblastic leukaemia. Lancet ii:837–839, 1977
217. Guit HF, van Furth R: Partial antibiotic decontamination. Br Med J i:800–802, 1977
218. Sleijfer P Th, Mulder NH, de Vries-Hospers HG: Prevention of

infection in leukopenic patients by elimination of gram-negative bacteria and yeasts from the gastrointestinal tract. Congr Int Soc Hematol, Paris, 1978
219. Hughes WT, Kuhn S, Chaudhary S et al: Successful chemoprophylaxis for *Pneumocystis carinii* pneumonitis. N Engl J Med 297:1419–1426, 1977
220. Gurwith MJ, Brunton JL, Lank BA: A prospective controlled investigation of prophylactic trimethoprim/sulfamethoxazole in hospitalized granulocytopenic patients. Am J Med 66:248–256, 1979
221. Enno A, Catovsky D, Darrell J et al: Co-trimoxazole for the prevention of infection in leukemia. Lancet ii:395–397, 1978
222. Pizzo PA, Robichaud KJ, Edwards BK: A randomized clinical trial of Bactrim + Erythromycin vs. a placebo for preventing fever and infection in granulocytopenic cancer patients. 20th Interscience Conf Antimicrob Ag Chemother 334, 1980
223. Deisseroth A, Abrams RA: The role of autologous stem cell reconstitution in intensive therapy for resistant neoplasms. Cancer Treat Rep 63:461–471, 1979
224. Clift RA, Sanders JE, Thomas ED et al: Granulocyte transfusions for the prevention of infection in patients receiving bone marrow transplantation. N Engl J Med 298:1052–1057, 1978
225. Schiffer CA, Aisner J, Daly PA et al: Alloimmunization following prophylactic granulocyte transfusions. Blood 54:766–774, 1979
226. Lyman GH, Williams CC, Preston D: The use of lithium carbonate to reduce infection and leukopenia during systemic chemotherapy. N Engl J Med 302:257–260, 1980
227. Pennington JE, Reynolds HY, Wood RE et al: Use of a *Pseudomonas aeruginosa* vaccine in patients with acute leukemia and cystic fibrosis. Am J Med 58:629–635, 1975
228. Levine AM, Overturt G, Fields R et al: Response to pneumococcal vaccine in patients with Hodgkin's disease, lymphoma and myeloma. Am Assoc Cancer Res 686, 1979
229. Peter G, Pizzo PA, Robichaud K et al: Possible protective effect of circulating antibodies to the shared core glycolipid (CGL) of enterobacteriacae in children with malignancy. Soc Pediatr Res 13:466, 1979
230. Wolf JC, McCutchan JA, Ziegler EJ: Prophylactic antibody to core lipopolysaccharide in neutropenic patients. 19th Interscience Conf Antimicrob Ag Chemother 65, 1979
231. Stiehm ER: Standard and special human serum globulin as therapeutic agents. Pediatr 63:301–319, 1979
232. Davis LE, Bodian D, Price D et al: Chronic progressive poliomyelitis secondary to vaccination of an immunodeficient child. N Engl J Med 297:241–245, 1977

CHAPTER 45

Management of the Adverse Effects of Treatment

Hair Loss

CLAUDIA A. SEIPP

Alopecia can be a distressing side effect for patients receiving cancer therapy. The initial psychological impact of this loss can cause some patients to reject potentially curative therapy. It is important, therefore, for physicians and nurses to recognize the anxiety produced by this change and some methods that may be used to reduce stress.

Hair loss from radiation therapy to the head does not occur uniformly and seems to be dose dependent. Epilation can begin at doses of 500 rad, often progressing with spotty areas of baldness. Hair regrowth begins 8 to 9 weeks after therapy but is frequently different in character than the original hair.[1]

The amount of body hair lost by patients in any chemotherapeutic program is specific to the drug or combination of drugs administered, is time and dose related, and is reversible. Whether guidance for the provision of head covering is offered, or preventative measures are attempted through scalp hypothermia or occlusive scalp tourniquet, patients report that intervention by nurses and physicians is of great value in their adjustment to this alteration in body image.[2]

HEAD COVERING

Most patients will choose to cover their heads during the period of hair loss. Hair pieces and wigs are sometimes provided by hospitals or treatment centers. Hairpieces are tax-deductible medical expenses and are covered by some medical insurance policies.[3] Wigs should be chosen while the patient still has hair, both for the psychological effect and so that hair color and style can be matched.

In hot weather, patients may choose to wear hats, scarves, or turbans. Children often choose to wear caps or hats and some men prefer to shave their heads entirely rather than bother with a toupee. Patients will frequently help each other by suggesting alternatives. Cosmetologists may provide useful suggestions for other forms of makeup and for replacement of eyebrows and eyelashes.

Some investigators have attempted to prevent hair loss from chemotherapy through the use of a scalp tourniquet technique or by scalp hypothermia.

SCALP TOURNIQUET

The use of a scalp tourniquet was initially proposed for patients receiving vincristine. Since vinca alkaloids are rapidly cleared from the bloodstream, it was proposed that the superficial scalp veins could be temporarily occluded during administration of the drug, thus avoiding drug contact with hair follicles.[4] The pneumatic tourniquet procedure was extended for use to patients who received injections of cyclophosphamide, methotrexate, and 5-fluorouracil. Although "no alopecia" was reported in 20 consecutive patients receiving other drug regimens and scalp occlusion, this finding is not supported by a comparative research study.[5]

Concern for the condition of underlying tissues has led more recent investigators to use a narrow sphygmomonometer cuff wrapped about the head below the hairline. Uniform controlled pressures are able to be provided safely during administration of chemotherapy and for 15 minutes afterward at pressures 50 mmHg above systolic blood pressure. Good protection against the epilating effect of adriamycin at cumulative doses below 300 mg/m^2 when compared to an identical control group has been reported.[6]

The use of the scalp tourniquet is limited to drugs which are able to achieve plasma concentrations below epilation levels but within the maximum tolerance level of the tourniquet, usually 20 minutes.

The possibility that malignant cells are spared exposure to chemotherapy by the use of these techniques limits their usefulness.[7] For this reason, leukemia patients and patients with multiple myeloma are generally excluded from antiepilating procedures.

SCALP HYPOTHERMIA

Vasoconstriction can also be achieved through icing of the scalp. Refinements in technique have produced several commercially available ice turbans which can reduce scalp temperatures to 23°C to 24°C after 10 minutes. Some ice caps are designed to be disposable, to minimize the chance of infection and lessen the financial investment by the patient.

The ice turban is carefully applied to achieve uniform conformity to the scalp. It is put on 10 minutes prior to the infusion of doxorubicin (adriamycin) and is left in place for 30 minutes. Excellent protection against hair loss for patients receiving this drug at doses under 50 mg/m^2 per treatment has been reported.[8] This effect was maintained throughout a 6 month to 8 month treatment period with monthly drug cycles.

The use of methods which decrease scalp bloodflow during chemotherapy should be considered only in the treatment of cancers in which a risk for development of subsequent scalp metastasis does not exist.

Nausea and Vomiting

STEPHEN E. SALLAN
CAROL M. CRONIN

The present intensification of chemotherapy and radiation therapy programs has resulted in increased toxicity to cancer patients. Two of the most troublesome and commonly encountered toxicities are nausea and vomiting. Nausea, the feeling of the imminent need to vomit, and vomiting, the forceful expulsion of the gastric contents, are generally considered to be mild, self-limiting symptoms associated with numerous organic and psychiatric diseases. These symptoms, however, are often severe and prolonged in patients receiving cancer chemotherapy or radiation therapy and may result in either pronounced physiological debilitation, rendering the patient unfit for further treatment, or psychological distress such that the patient may refuse further treatment.

When vomiting can be anticipated, as with cancer chemotherapy, prophylatic therapy is much more effective than *post facto* treatment and oftentimes may completely inhibit the nausea–retching–vomiting cycle. An understanding of the physiology of vomiting, the principles of antiemetic therapy, and the pharmacology of antiemetic agents is important for the implementation therapy.

PHYSIOLOGY OF VOMITING

The act of vomiting is integrated by the vomiting center located in the medullary lateral reticular formation.[9] Efferent pathways include phrenic nerves to the diaphragm, spinal nerves to abdominal musculature, and visceral nerves to the stomach and esophagus (Fig. 45-1). The vomiting center receives afferent input from several sources: (1) the chemoreceptor trigger zone (CTZ), a distinct medullary center located in the floor of the fourth ventricle; (2) vagal and other sympathetic afferents from the viscera; (3) midbrain receptors of intracranial pressure; (4) the labyrinthine apparatus; and (5) higher CNS structures (*e.g.*, the limbic system). The nature of the interaction of toxic substances with the CTZ is unknown; once stimulated, the CTZ activates the vomiting

FIG. 45-1. Connections between the chemoreceptor trigger zone, vomiting center, and efferents of vomiting. (Newburger PE, Sallan SE: Symptom Control in Childhood Malignancy: Pain and Vomiting. From *Care of the Child with Cancer*. American Cancer Society, 1979)

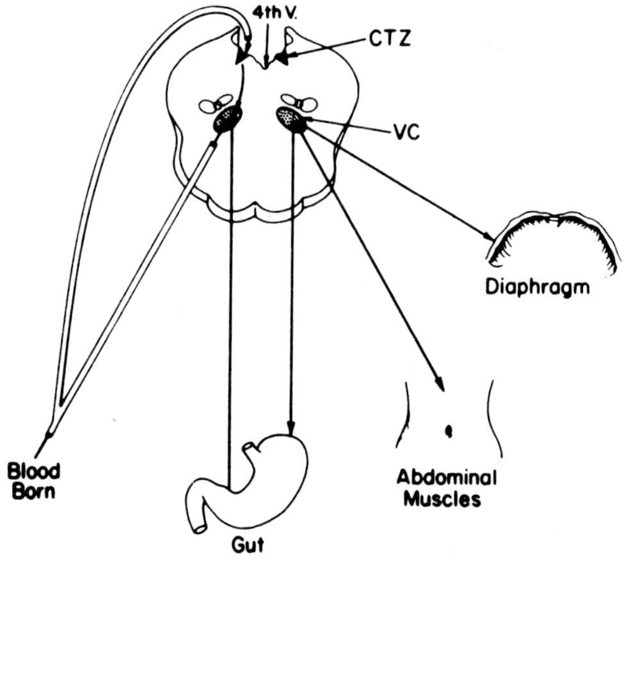

center to produce nausea and vomiting. The CTZ has no autonomous capability to produce vomiting.

Animal studies with CTZ ablation suggest that chemotherapeutic agents induce nausea and vomiting by CTZ stimulation.[10] Participation of the forebrain and peripheral mechanisms have also been demonstrated.[11] However, there are major species differences, so one can only infer the site of action in humans by extrapolation from animal studies and by clinical observation.[10] Radiation-induced nausea and vomiting appear to be mediated through both CTZ and peripheral mechanisms.[12]

The neurochemistry of vomiting remains obscure. The CTZ contains H_1 and H_2 histamine receptors, and its anatomic surroundings are rich in histamine. H_1 antagonists (*e.g.*, dimenhydrinate) have antiemetic activity limited to motion sickness and vestibular disorders.[10] H_2 antagonists are not effective antiemetics. Other neurotransmitters possibly involved in the control of vomiting are dopamine and acetylcholine. Apomorphine, the classic CTZ stimulant, has dopaminomimetic properties and its action is blocked by phenothiazines, which are potent dopamine blockers.[13] The phenothiazines also have anticholinergic and antihistaminic effects but their antiemetic efficacy correlates best with dopamine-blocking activity.[14] Nitrogen mustard, a potent emetic, has cholinergic activity, and centrally-acting anticholinergic drugs such as scopolamine are effective antiemetics.[15,16] A role for endogenous opiates is suggested by the mixed emetic–antiemetic effects of narcotic analgesics, which are blocked by naloxone, by the emetic properties of naloxone itself, and by the concentration of opiate receptors in the CTZ.[17,18]

PRINCIPLES OF ANTIEMETIC THERAPY

The basic principles of the treatment of nausea and vomiting are to identify and, if possible, treat the underlying cause and to initiate therapy before symptoms become established.

Patients with malignancy suffer from nausea and vomiting primarily as a result of therapy. However, there are uncommon but important non-iatrogenic emetic stimuli, including gastrointestinal inflammation or obstruction, increased intracranial pressure, infection, heart failure, and metabolic derangement.[10]

The psychological status of the patient also plays a major role in developing effective therapy. The efficacy of placebo and the disastrous effect of a vomiting roommate demonstrate the importance of suggestion.[19] Hypnosis may serve as an important adjunct, in combination with a good antiemetic regimen, in providing effective control of nausea and vomiting. Conditioned responses, such as vomiting upon arrival in the clinic, are difficult to control, but a setting that is free of the sight or smell of food removes at least one stimulus. Since anxiety abets nausea, reassurance, quiet, and privacy are also important adjuncts to therapy.

All of the antiemetic drugs are more effective when administered prophylactically, before the start of chemotherapy or radiation. This approach is particularly important in those patients who experience anticipatory (psychogenic) vomiting prior to receiving treatment. Once effective antiemetic therapy has been initiated, it is essential to continue the treatment on a scheduled regimen rather than on a "prn" basis in order to prevent the development of break-through vomiting. The duration of follow-up therapy should be individualized to each patient, based on previous patterns of nausea and vomiting.

Knowledge of the emetogenic potential and patterns of the various chemotherapeutic agents helps to predict the severity and duration of the anticipated symptoms.

All of these factors should be considered in the selection of a proper antiemetic agent (Table 45-1).

PHARMACOLOGIC THERAPY OF VOMITING

Antiemetic drugs can be classified into four general groups: phenothiazines, antihistamines, cannabinoids, and others (Table 45-2). At present, the phenothiazines are the most effective of the commercially available agents. At the usual therapeutic doses, many phenothiazines appear to depress CTZ activity and may also directly depress the vomiting center.[10] These drugs act on both the central and autonomic nervous systems and, in standard doses, usually do not produce marked cortical depression. They are widely distributed throughout the body and are 90% bound to plasma proteins. Metabolism is primarily by way of the liver, with metabolic products being excreted in the urine, bile, and feces.

Two distinct chemical classes of phenothiazines exist, each with their own therapeutic and toxic characteristics. The aliphatic class, of which chlorpromazine (Thorazine) is the prototype, has limited antiemetic activity and is associated with a high incidence of orthostatic hypotension, sedation, prolongation of the sedative effects of narcotics and barbiturates, and blood dyscrasias. The piperazine class, which includes prochlorperazine (Compazine), thiethylperazine (Torecan), and perphenazine (Trilafon) has pronounced antiemetic activity but is associated with an increased incidence of extrapyramidal effects. Although most clinicians prescribe prochlorperazine or chlorpromazine, thiethylperazine and

TABLE 45-1. Chemotherapeutic Agents with Emetogenic Potential*

AGENT	SEVERITY	TIME OF ONSET
cis-Platinum	↑	Late (2½ hours after chemo)†
Cytoxan		Late†
Actinomycin-D		Late (occasionally immediate)†
Nitrogen Mustard		Early, intermittent for approx. 6–10 hr
Adriamycin		Late (usually less severe in infants, toddlers)
Methotrexate		Late (occasionally immediate)
Azacytidine		Early (less common when given as continuous infusion)
Cytosine Abrabinoside		Rare
Procarbazine		Gastritis-like symptoms

*When used in combination, the emetogenic potential of each agent is additive.

†May be protracted.

TABLE 45-2. Suggested Antiemetics for Chemotherapy Induced Nausea and Vomiting

GENERIC NAME	TRADE NAME	CHEMICAL CLASS	AVAILABLE ROUTES	RECOMMENDED ADULT DOSES	REGIMEN
thiethylperazine	Torecan	piperazine phenothiazine	PO,PR,IM,IV*	10mg	every 6 hours initially, then every 8 hours
perphenazine	Trilafon	piperazine phenothiazine	PO,IM,IV	5mg parenterally 4mg orally	every 4 hours initially, then every 6 hours
prochlorperazine	Compazine	piperazine phenothiazine	IV,PR,IM,PO†	all 10 mg except 25 mg PR	every 6 hours
haloperidol	Haldol	butyrophenone	PO,IM	0.5–1.0mg	every 8 hours
dimenhydrinate	Dramamine	antihistamine	IM,IV,PR,PO†	50–100mg	every 4 hours administer IV over 15 minutes
benzquinamide	Emete-con	benzquinolizine	IM,IV	50mg IM 25mg IV‡	may repeat first dose in 1 hr, then every 3–4 hrs with IV, switch to IM as soon possible

*although widely used clinically, the intravenous administration of Torecan is not recommended by the manufacturer
‡syrups of both Dramamine (12.5mg/4cc) and Compazine (1mg/cc) are available
‡intravenous benzquinamide is contraindicated in patients with cardiovascular disease

perphenazine are much more effective agents, at least in experimental animals. Evidence in dogs indicates that perphenazine has a maximal efficacy at nontoxic doses 24-fold that of chlorpromazine and 8-fold that of prochlorperazine in preventing apomorphine-induced emesis.[20] Furthermore, perphenazine gains in its relative antiemetic activity as the emetic stimulus increases in intensity. It has been suggested that the increased antiemetic activity of perphenazine may be due to its greater affinity to and tighter binding with receptors in the CTZ. Thiethylperazine acts to decrease the incidence of nausea and vomiting as well as the severity of the symptoms, resulting in enhanced antiemetic activity. The major disadvantage of these agents is the development of extrapyramidal reactions or agitation, most commonly associated with intravenous administration. The incidence of these reactions can be decreased, however, by administering the I.V. solution slowly, over 45–60 minutes and by concomitant administration of an antihistamine such as diphenhydramine (Benadryl). Although promethazine (Phenergan) is an effective phenothiazine antiemetic for vestibular disorders, it does not exhibit the antiemetic activity necessary to control chemotherapy-induced vomiting.

Many antihistamines have antiemetic properites, but there is no correlation between antihistaminic potency and antiemetic activity.[21] Both dimenhydrinate (Dramamine) and diphenhydramine are effective antiemetics for motion sickness and may be used in combination with other antiemetic therapy to potentiate effectivness or to decrease toxicity.[22,23] The exact mechanism of action of these agents is unknown; however, they appear to act by blockade of labyrinthine impulses and they do not antagonize apomorphine-induced emesis.[24,25] Our clinical experience indicates that the antihistamines, particularly dimenhydrinate, may be effective in controlling the chronic nausea which often accompanies progressive disease, but we have not yet rigorously tested this hypothesis.

Trimethobenzamide (Tigan) is an ethanolamine antihistamine which exerts its primary action on the CTZ. Although it has been reported to be an effective antiemetic, some investigators have found it to be less effective than placebo.[26,27] Since its efficacy appears to be inversely proportional to the intensity of the emetic stimulus, we do not recommend its use for cancer chemotherapy-induced vomiting.[28]

The cannabinoids, the active ingredients of marijuana, have proven antiemetic properties. Delta-9-tetrahydrocannabinol (THC) has been shown to be more effective than both placebo and prochlorperazine for the prevention of vomiting in patients receiving antineoplastic drugs.[29,30] It is also effective in controlling radiation-induced nausea and vomiting.[31] Although the exact mechanism of action is unknown, THC is thought to exert its antiemetic effect through CNS depression. Interest in the cannabinoids has led to the development of synthetic analogues of THC. Nabilone, the first of the synthetics to be investigated, has proven to be more effective than prochlorperazine in patients receiving cancer chemotherapy.[32] Neurologic toxicity with chronic administration in dogs developed after completion of the human clinical trials, resulting in the withdrawal of this agent from further clinical use. However, such toxicity was found to be species specific, so the drug should be available for clinical use in the future. THC is now being distributed for use as an antiemetic by the National Cancer Institute and can be obtained by calling the Office of the Associate Director, Cancer Therapy Evaluation Division of Cancer Treatment, NCI. Two other agents, nabitan and levonantradol are presently being investigated and appear to exert significant antiemetic activity with limited toxicity.[33,34]

The agents that comprise the "other" class of antiemetics include haloperidol (Haldol), benzquinamide (Emete-con), and scopolamine.

Haloperidol, a non-phenothiazine tranquilizer, is an effective antiemetic in the treatment of post-operative nausea and vomiting and may be useful in patients receiving radiation therapy and cancer chemotherapy.[35,36] A butyrophenone derivative that is pharmacologically related to the piperazine class of phenothiazine, haloperidol is an effective antiemetic at relatively low doses, thus causing fewer side effects than phenothiazines.[37,38] Adult antiemetic doses range from 0.5 mg to 1.0 mg and are administered every 8 hours. The absence of hypotension and other side effects makes it a drug of choice for elderly or debilitated patients.[39] Its exact mechanism of antiemetic action is unknown, although it is thought to depress the CTZ. Animal studies have shown haloperidol to be 40 times more potent as an antiemetic and its duration of action four times longer than chlorpromazine.[40] Although numerous clinical trials have reported the antiemetic efficacy of haloperidol, primarily in postoperative patients, the Food and Drug Administration has not yet approved the use of haloperidol as an antiemetic.

Benzquinamide, a benzquinolizine derivative structurally unrelated to the phenothiazines or antihistamines, acts by depression of the CTZ. The antiemetic activity of this agent has been compared to prochlorperazine and was found to be equally effective in studies of postoperative patients and superior to the phenothiazines in general medical patients.[41,42] It appears to be relatively nontoxic with no hypotension or extrapyramidal reactions reported; the degree of somnolence associated with benzquinamide parallels that of the phenothiazines. We have administered this agent to a number of patients who were receiving antineoplastic drugs and had experienced adverse reactions to phenothiazines and have noted results varying from no antiemetic response to a complete control of nausea and vomiting.

Scopolamine is one of the oldest and most effective antiemetic agents currently available. It is a centrally-acting anticholinergic agent known to suppress motion sickness; however, its short duration of action and serious toxicity prevented its wide application.[43] The recently developed Transdermal Therapeutic System-Scopolamine® minimizes these unwanted pharmacological effects. This novel method for the systemic administration of scopolamine is comprised of small flexible membranes that adhere comfortably to the skin. Following placement behind the ear, the drug is absorbed through the skin into the bloodstream and is distributed throughout the body. The system provides controlled administration of drug at a predetermined rate for up to 3 days.[44] TTS-Scopolamine has been shown to provide effective antiemetic control for motion sickness and for high-dose methotrexate therapy, and has recently been approved for use in motion sickness by the Food and Drug Administration.[16,45,46]

All patients receiving chemotherapeutic agents should be started on a good antiemetic regimen prior to the administration of the chemotherapy. We suggest thiethylperazine or perphenazine as the initial agents of choice. They should be administered *parenterally* prior to chemotherapy and then continued on a scheduled regimen either parenterally or orally. Trilafon has been used successfully as a continuous infusion in the concentration of 5 mg/250 cc to be administered over 5 hours.For outpatient therapy, suppositories should be used for vomiting patients who cannot tolerate oral medication. If neither perphenazine nor thiethylperazine prove effective, haloperidol or benzquinomide should be tried. Addition of a barbiturate (pentobarbital, 50–150 mg I.V. or P.O.) to a phenothiazine regimen has been found to be clinically useful. Although the patient may continue to experience extensive vomiting, it appears to be less emotionally devastating. We have not encountered any aspiration of vomitus using barbiturates according to this regimen, but do not recommend it as standard practice. The addition of diphenhydramine to a phenothiazine regimen controls much of the agitation and restlessness associated with the phenothiazines; it may enhance the degree of somnolence experienced by the patient, but not as much as would a barbiturate.

For patients allergic to the phenothiazines, we recommend benzquinamide followed by dimenhydrinate or a barbiturate depending on the severity of vomiting.

Cardiac Toxicity

CHARLES E. MYERS

The management of cardiomyopathy has become a topic of considerable interest to the oncologist, predominantly as a result of the widespread use of the anthracycline antibiotics doxorubicin and daunorubicin. Clinical use of these agents is associated with both an acute and a chronic cardiomyopathy which is often debilitating and not infrequently fatal. For this reason, the major focus of this chapter will be on the cause, characteristics, and management of this anthracycline-induced myocardiopathy. It is important to note, however, that impaired cardiac function can be seen in cancer patients as a consequence of high-dose cyclophosphamide and mediastinal radiation therapy through an anterior port and secondary to iron overload from repeated transfusions.[47–49] The discussion in this chapter of how to evaluate a cardiomyopathy is certainly pertinent to these other syndromes.

RECOMMENDED APPROACH

Finally, it should be noted that the present chapter assumes the reader is acquainted with the material on the pharmacology of the anthracyclines presented in the chapter on clinical pharmacology (Chapter 6).

PATHOPHYSIOLOGY

In order to understand the assessment and treatment of anthracycline-induced cardiomyopathy, it is important to understand something of the mechanisms which regulate function in the normal heart and how anthracyclines alter this system.

In both skeletal and cardiac muscle, contraction results from a sequence of events that begins with depolarization of the cell membrane.[50] This electrical event results in the rapid release of free calcium within the muscle cell. The calcium released in turn binds to the actin–myosin complex, triggering contraction. Subsequent muscle relaxation is associated with removal of calcium from the actin–myosin complex secondary to binding to a variety of intracellular storage sites.

Skeletal muscle is organized into motor units, each with its own nerve supply and the force of contraction is regulated by the number of motor units activated. Cardiac muscle, on the other hand, is a functional syncitium in which every cardiac cell contracts with each heart beat. Instead, the force of contraction is modulated by the amount of calcium made available to the actin–myosin complex. This central role of calcium in regulating the force of myocardial contraction has interesting implications for the mechanism of anthracycline-induced cardiomyopathy.

Regulation of the myocardial calcium pool is governed by influx, efflux, and intracellular binding of that ion. Influx occurs predominantly during the slow wave of the action potential. Efflux is governed by a pump for which both sodium and calcium compete. As a consequence, events which increase intracellular sodium can lead to increased intracellular calcium through competition for this pump. Thus, inhibition of the cardiac membrane Na–K exchange pump by cardiac glycosides such as digoxin leads to increased sodium concentration which, through competition with calcium, leads to an increase in the latter. This increased calcium in turn leads to the expected increase in force of contraction. Inhibition of this same Na–K exchange pump by doxorubicin has been reported, but would be expected to result in increased, not decreased, contractility.[51] It is obvious that this effect is not directly related to the chronic cardiomyopathy which develops.

Intracellular binding of calcium appears to be the major factor regulating the availability of calcium to the contractile apparatus and thus the force of contraction on a beat-to-beat basis. The two most important sites of this binding are cardiac mitochondria and the sarcoplasmic reticulum. There is now considerable evidence that both of these sites are affected in the chronic cardiomyopathy. Dilation and distortion of the sarcoplasmic reticulum is one of the characteristic pathologic changes seen in the chronic cardiomyopathy.[52] Unfortunately, none of the modern biochemical techniques that have been used to study calcium binding to the sarcoplasmic reticulum have been applied to material from doxorubicin-treated hearts. In addition, significant changes in myocardial calcium metabolism have been demonstrated.[53] Finally, a number of laboratories have now shown alterations in the size and kinetics of the various myocardial calcium pools.[54,55] As a result of this body of evidence, there is a general concensus that alterations in myocardial calcium metabolism do occur after doxorubicin and that these alterations probably play a role in the impaired contractility of the chronic cardiomyopathy. At present, the major disagreements arise over what the mechanism is that creates these abnormalities in calcium physiology. While DNA intercalation appears to play a role in the antitumor effect of these agents, there is little evidence

TABLE 45-3. Biochemical Effects

1. Inhibition of Na–K ATPase
2. Direct membrane binding
3. Generation of semiquinone radical, superoxide, and hydrogen peroxide with peroxidation of membrane lipid
4. DNA intercalation
5. Alterations in myocardial calcium metabolism

of its involvement in the cardiomyopathy and, as a hypothesis, this fails to explain most of the unique properties of this toxicity. The two most likely hypotheses at present appear to be either direct alteration in membrane function by anthracyclines or drug-induced free radical damage.

Doxorubicin has been shown to bind to cell membranes and such binding has been shown to alter the morphology and fluidity of the membrane.[56,57] Furthermore, rapid changes in membrane function have also been reported.[58] Perhaps most interesting is a recent report that application of doxorubicin to the toad bladder results in the rapid onset of a transmembrane sodium current.[59] Of the components of the cell membrane, specific binding has been shown to the protein spectrin and to the phospholipid cardiolipin.[60] Cardiolipin is of interest because its concentration is high in the membranes of transformed cells and cardiac mitochondria. This association has led one group to propose it as the explanation for why these agents exhibit both cardiac toxicity and antitumor activity.[61] In spite of these observations, however, this hypothesis offers no concrete reason why binding of doxorubicin or other anthracyclines to a cell membrane should result in tumor cell death or in the kind of persistent chronic cardiomyopathy which is typical of these agents.

As originally articulated, the free radical hypothesis proposed that cardiac toxicity arises because cardiac sarcosomes and mitochondria activate anthracyclines to free radical intermediates which are themselves toxic and which also lead to production of superoxide and hydrogen peroxide.[62] In most tissues, superoxide and hydrogen peroxide are disposed of by way of the action of the enzymes superoxide dismutase, catalase, and glutathione peroxidase.[63] Cardiac tissue, however, contains very little catalase and, after doxorubicin administration, glutathione peroxidase activity declines. This leaves the heart with no known mechanism for detoxifying hydrogen peroxide.[64,65] Thus, doxorubicin would lead to oxygen radical generation at the same time as it abrogates one of the key remaining mechanisms for their removal.

One of the advantages of this hypothesis is that it leads to rather specific predictions as to the sequence of events in the development of the cardiomyopathy. Oxygen radicals readily damage cell membranes by way of lipid peroxidation. Thus, membrane function should be altered and specific products of lipid peroxidation should be found in the heart muscle. As we mentioned earlier, altered membrane function has been shown. In addition, evidence for peroxidation of cardiac lipids has been found in acute mouse experiments and in the hearts of patients treated with anthracyclines.[62,72]

A second aspect of this hypothesis is that it would predict that alterations in the quinone–hydroquinone functionalities in the B and C rings of the anthracyclines (see chapter on clinical pharmacology) should markedly affect cardiac toxicity. Recently, two derivatives have been prepared which test this hypothesis. Aclacinomycin lacks the 11-position hydroxyl and 5-imino-daunorubicin lacks the 5-position carbonyl. Both analogs have proved to be significantly less cardiotoxic than is doxorubicin.[67–69]

The third aspect of this hypothesis is the prediction that free radical scavengers, which dampen free radical reactions, should lessen the cardiac toxicity of doxorubicin in a variety of systems. Tocopherol, a known free radical scavenger, has been shown to have this effect.[62,40-72] Protection has been observed in a number of species, including chronic rabbit and pig models and acute mouse and rat models. *In vitro* tocopherol lessens the doxorubicin-induced rapid decay in isolated purkinje fiber function.[73] Other radical scavenging agents such as cystamine and *N*-acetyl-cysteine also have apparent protective activity.[75,76]

In spite of the apparent successes of the free radical hypothesis, it has a number of failings. It provides no explanation for the focal nature of the lesions seen on electron microscopy. It fails to explain, as currently formulated, the ability of chelating agents such as ICRF 159 and ICRF 187 to protect against cardiac damage.[77,78] Also none of the free radical scavengers tested thus far completely prevents cardiac damage in a chronic model and in certain models they appear inactive.[79] Finally, this hypothesis does not explain the diminished cardiac toxicity of certain anthracycline analogs such as AD32 or certain *N*-alkylated derivatives.

CLINICAL ASSESSMENT OF CARDIAC DAMAGE

The problem of how to assess the extent of doxorubicin-induced cardiac damage has been approached by two different paths. Perhaps the most direct has been that championed by Billingham and co-workers, who have depended on pathological grading of cardiac tissue obtained by endocardial biopsy. This contrasts with most of the other workers in the field who have attempted to assess the physiological function of the heart by a variety of techniques ranging from EKG to radionuclide cineangiography. In evaluating the results reported using the different approaches, it is important to recognize that pathology and function often have a complex, variable relationship in the heart. Hypoxia and electrolyte disturbances such as hyper- and hypocalcemia present examples of this dissociation between severity of pathologic change and altered performance. This is not just a theoretical consideration; we know that doxorubicin causes both structural change and major abnormalities in calcium metabolism. It is possible that pathologic grading and physiologic function may give discordant results. Caution should, therefore, be exercised when making comparisons between the two approaches.

PHYSIOLOGIC ASSESSMENT OF CARDIAC DYSFUNCTION

The clinical syndrome of anthracycline-induced cardiomyopathy is a direct consequence of reduced myocardial contractility. The goal of physiologic assessment is to provide an accurate means of measuring this change in contractility. Unfortunately, all the techniques currently available for the assessment of cardiac function suffer from an inability to separate changes in intrinsic contractility from extrinsic factors that affect cardiac performance. This occurs because the strength of myocardial contraction is conditioned by preload and afterload as well as intrinsic contractility. In cancer patients, load functions are by no means constant and can be affected by changes in hydration due to vomiting or fever or to blood volume changes from hemorrhage or transfusions. The clinician should keep all of these changes in mind when evaluating the results of cardiac function tests.

In addition to the above, physiologic tests can be divided according to whether they study the isovolemic phase of the cardiac cycle, which includes the period of time from the onset of electrical contraction to the opening of the aortic valve, or the ejection phase, which includes the period of time that the aortic valve is open. The isovolemic phase is one of rapidly changing pressure; therefore the most direct measure of this would be dP/dt obtained by cardiac catheterization. The ejection phase is one of rapidly changing volume and important direct measures here would be total volume ejected and peak dV/dt. Finally, because of a possible change in rate of relaxation induced by the anthracyclines, measurement of the rate of diastolic filling would be of value.

Table 45-4 lists the techniques that have been most commonly applied to the study of doxorubicin cardiomyopathy. Of these, measurement of systolic time interval has seen the widest use. As applied, the most common technique is to measure the ratio of the pre-ejection period to the duration of the ejection phase (PEP:LVET). It thus effectively compares the ratio of the two phases of contraction. This technique has a major disadvantage in that it is significantly affected by both preload and afterload. Thus, while patients treated with doxorubicin exhibit prolongation of the PEP:LVET, the measurements are associated with a large standard error.[80,81] As a result, a population of patients with known cardiomyopathy will have PEP:LVET measurements that overlap with a control population. These results may be improved if a patient may be used as his or her own control by comparing pre- and post-treatment PEP:LVET measurements. Even so, this technique leaves much to be desired, and better techniques are available.

Echocardiography has found wide use in cardiology for the measurement of valve motion, detection of pericardial effusions, and estimation of heart size. It offers accurate dimensional measurements with sampling rates which approach 1000/second. Unfortunately, this technique has its limitations as a means of following doxorubicin cardiomyopathy. Conventional M-mode echocardiography has a narrow angle of view and so can only yield the transverse cardiac diameter at a given level. Estimates of ventricular volume essential for calculation of ejection fraction or cardiac output require a series of assumptions about cardiac geometry which are always only approximately true and, under certain conditions, definitely in error. This technique is particularly sensitive to dyssynergy of ventricular wall motion. Two-dimensional echocardiography gives a view of a much larger part of the left ventricle and thus overcomes many of the above problems. The equipment currently available for two-dimensional echocardiography unfortunately gives measurements with much less accuracy than does the M-mode approach. Finally, accurate use of echocardiography demands well-trained, experienced technicians. However, with a well-trained technician, studies adequate for the quantitation of left ventricular dimensions will only be obtained in 60% to 70% of adults.[82] All of these problems mean that echocardiography is best limited to use in patients in whom a good study can be obtained, a pretreatment study is available for comparison, and ventricular dyssynergy has been ruled out.[78-85]

TABLE 45-4. Physiologic Tests of Cardiac Function

MODALITY USED	PERTINENT MEASUREMENT	PHASE OF CARDIAC CYCLE	VALUE CONSIDERED TO INDICATE CARDIOMYOPATHY	ADVANTAGES	DISADVANTAGES
Systolic time intervals	PEP/LVET	Both	a. Greater than .42–.45 b. Increase of over 0.07 from control	Simple to perform; inexpensive	Large standard error; affected severely by load factors
Echocardiography	Fractional shortening	Ejection	Less than 30%	Equipment widely available; personnel trained to perform tests widely available; inexpensive	30%–40% of adults cannot be studied; measurement of ventricular volumes subject to errors
EKG	QRS voltage	None	A drop in QRS voltage of 30% or greater	Simple to perform; inexpensive	Lacks adequate sensitivity; develops associated with the cardiomyopathy rather than predicts
Cardiac catheterization	Ejection fraction; cardiac output; pressure measurement	Both	Resting cardiac index of under 2.5 liters/min; exercise better under 5; pulmonary wedge pressure over 12 mm Hg; resting right ventricular end diastolic pressure under 12 mmHg	Allows comprehensive assessment of cardiac function	Invasive with the risks that this entails; expensive
Radionuclide cineangiocardiography	Ejection fraction; dV/dt during diastole and systole	Both	A drop of greater than 15% from pretreatment; ejection fraction of less than 45%; failure to increase EF by greater than 5% with exercise	Accurate measure of ventricular volumes; noninvasive; easy to obtain values at rest and with exercise	Expensive equipment

EKG changes are frequently noted after doxorubicin. Of these, a drop in QRS voltage is the only one to correlate with the development of the chronic cardiomyopathy.[86] This change presumably reflects diffuse damage and drop-out of contractile elements because it is usually a late change. The major disadvantage of this technique is that the drop in QRS voltage is often coincidental with the onset of cardiomyopathy. Changes in voltage are often associated with the appearance of an S3 gallop or other signs and symptoms of congestive heart failure. For this reason, the EKG changes serve only as another indication of the existence of a significant cardiomyopathy rather than as a sensitive index of early cardiac damage.

Cardiac catheterization obviously provides very complete information on cardiac function. It alone provides the opportunity to directly measure pressure and volume changes and provides a well-established technique for monitoring cardiac output as well. There are only a few disadvantages to this approach. First, estimation of ventricular volume does require assumptions of ventricular geometry, usually that of prolate ellipse. Second, it is an invasive technique with an established complication rate. Third, allergy to the contrast dyes used is a relatively common problem and would limit the technique to pressure measurements. In spite of these problems, this must be viewed as the most comprehensive of the techniques available.[80]

The final technique to be discussed is also the most recent to be developed. Radionuclide cineangiography depends upon labeling of the cardiac blood pool with radioactive technetium. Gamma-camera views are then taken at multiple times during a cardiac cycle. In the early radioisotope cardiac studies, long and short axes of the isotope ventricular image during end systole and end diastole were used to estimate volume and fraction of blood ejected.[87] The approach used in these calculations was similar to that used in cardiac catheterization with the same potentially faulty assumptions about cardiac geometry. More recently, the number of counts per minute over the ventricle has been assumed to be proportional to the ventricular blood volume.[88–90] This approach has the advantage of being more independent of ventricular geometry. By linking the gamma camera views to a simultaneously recorded electrocardiogram, it is possible to gain valuable information on ejection fraction, rates of ejection, diastolic filling, and dyssynergy of wall motion. Several workers have measured each of these parameters by both radionuclide cineangiography and cardiac catheterization. Typically, the correlation coefficient between the two techniques has been 0.9 or greater. Radionuclide cineangiography has the added advantage in that, through the use of a horizontal bicycle ergometer, it is possible to study the response of the heart to exercise load. Radionuclide cineangiography measurement of ejection fraction at rest and during exercise has proved to be of value in the study of coronary artery disease and idiopathic hypertrophic subaortic stenosis.[91,92] Recently, similar studies done in patients who received doxorubicin suggest that radionuclide cineangiography with exercise may be a very sensitive test for anthracycline cardiomyopathy.[93,94]

PATHOLOGIC ASSESSMENT OF CARDIAC DAMAGE

Pathologic assessment of doxorubicin cardiomyopathy is dependent upon the ability to obtain heart muscle biopsies in a reproducible and safe fashion. While cardiac biopsies have been done by both the transthoracic and transvenous route, the transvenous biopsy technique is currently the most accepted, primarily because of its lower rate of complication. Since the original report of the technique of transvenous endomyocardial biopsy by Sakakibara and Konno, this technique has evolved, in the hands of several groups, into a technique which allows the clinician to obtain multiple endocardial samples in an outpatient setting with minimal risk.[95] Mason and co-workers of Stanford have had the largest experience with this technique, with over 1300 biopsies having been performed, primarily for the purpose of diagnosis and management of cardiac transplant rejection. For that purpose, the technique has proved its value.[96] The value of the endocardial biopsy as a diagnostic tool in other diseases of the myocardium has been questioned by observers with considerable experience with the technique.[97] Specifically, it has not proven of value in the diagnosis or quantitation of idiopathic dilated cardiomyopathy or idiopathic hypertrophic cardiomyopathy. In each of the cases, the technique appears to be limited by the small amount of tissue obtained and the limited area of the myocardium biopsied, usually the septal surface of the right ventricle. More accurate information in these situations appears to be obtained by biopsies obtained at thoracotomy. In addition, there are problems with artifactual ultrastructural changes, especially at the edges of the biopsy. It is not clear at present whether similar problems will plague the use of this technique in the assessment of doxorubicin cardiomyopathy.

Evaluation of the transvenous endocardial biopsy as a diagnostic tool in the assessment of doxorubicin cardiomyopathy has been performed predominantly by Billingham, Mason, and Bristow at Stanford University.[98-100] This group has performed biopsies on over 50 patients after various total cumulative doses. These studies have been invaluable in that they provide the only human material free of autolytic change and this has aided clear definition of the pathologic picture. The reader is referred to the series of articles published by that group.[80,98-100] The major characteristics of the pathologic picture are the development of focal lesions in which both dilation of the sarcoplasmic reticulum and destruction of the myofibrils are prominant. The frequency of the focal lesions increases with total dose administered. There appears to be good correlation between biopsy severity and clinical congestive heart failure. In a smaller group of patients, these authors have compared pathologic grading of the endocardial biopsy score, systolic time intervals, echocardiography, and EKG with assessment of myocardial performance by cardiac catheterization.[80] Of these, only endocardial biopsy showed a good correlation with the results of cardiac catheterization. A recent abstract from this group does report a good agreement between the results of endomyocardial biopsy and radioisotope cineangiography.[101] It is difficult, at the present time, to put these results in perspective. The patients studied thus far are few in number. In addition, confirmation of these observations by other investigators would be of value. It should be noted that some workers have expressed skepticism about the ability to grade a focal pathologic process from a few biopsy specimens of only several cubic mm in volume.[97]

RISK FACTORS

Table 45-5 lists those factors which have been proposed as increasing the incidence of cardiomyopathy in patients receiving daunomycin or doxorubicin. Of these, the most clearly established is mediastinal radiation therapy. Billingham and co-workers have reported the results of endocardial biopsies in 12 patients who had mediastinal radiation 6 months to 14 years prior to receiving doxorubicin.[99] When these biopsies were compared to dose-matched controls, the irradiated patients had significantly higher pathologic scores. In addition to the typical doxorubicin-induced lesions, these biopsies exhibited endothelial damage in the capillaries and vessels characteristic of acute radiation damage. In parallel with these pathologic studies, a number of investigators have reported an increased incidence of cardiomyopathy in patients who have had mediastinal radiation therapy.[102,103]

Hypertension has been reported as a risk factor.[102] The data seen are most convincing for uncontrolled hypertension, and this may relate to increased afterload. Catecholamines may, however, also play a role. Pheochromocytoma has been associated in a case report with accelerated appearance of the cardiomyopathy, and Bristow and co-workers have proposed that doxorubicin-stimulated catecholamine release plays a critical role in the genesis of the cardiomyopathy.[104,105]

Both cyclophosphamide and mitomycin C have also been reported to lead to accelerated development of the cardiomyopathy, although here the data are less convincing than in the case of radiation and hypertension.[106,107] Cyclophosphamide, in high doses, is cardiotoxic and this toxicity may

TABLE 45-5. Risk Factors

1. Mediastinal radiation therapy
2. Uncontrolled hypertension
3. Administration of individual doses greater than 50 mg/m^2
4. Coadministration with either cyclophosphamide or mitomycin-C

be additive with that of the anthracyclines.[47] Mitomycin-C is of interest because it shares with the anthracyclines the ability to undergo redox cycling leading to the production of superoxide and hydrogen peroxide.[108]

Finally, the dose of doxorubicin given with each cycle of therapy appears also to be a risk factor. Most of the information on the cardiac toxicity of doxorubicin comes from patients treated with 50–75 mg/m² every 3 weeks to 4 weeks. Weiss and co-workers first reported lower cardiac toxicity when doxorubicin was given at the rate of 20 mg/m² per week.[109] These results led to the suggestion that cardiac toxicity developed only with the higher plasma levels associated with dosages equal to or greater than 50 mg/m². This hypothesis appears to have been confirmed in a randomized controlled trial in which endocardial biopsy was used as an endpoint.[110] At present, it is not clear whether the antitumor efficacy is preserved at the lower dose rates.

NATURAL HISTORY OF ANTHRACYCLINE CARDIAC TOXICITY

The clinician managing a patient receiving an anthracycline needs to be aware that these agents can cause acute cardiac toxicity as well as chronic cardiomyopathy and that this acute toxicity can have serious, even fatal, consequences. Arrythmias and conduction abnormalities are the most commonly noted manifestations of this acute toxicity.[111,112] They can range in severity from benign supraventricular tachycardias to complete heart block and ventricular tachycardia. The incidence of the more severe arrythmias is difficult to assess from the literature, but unexplained episodes of sudden death within a few days of having received a dose of doxorubicin has been noted in 1% of the patients so treated.[113] A comprehensive prospective Holten monitoring study would be of great value in defining this risk and perhaps identifying the characteristics of patients likely to develop life-threatening rhythm disturbances. A second aspect of this acute toxicity is the development of what has been called the myocarditis–pericarditis syndrome.[100] In its most severe manifestation, this syndrome is characterized by the onset of florid congestive heart failure associated with pericarditis developing within a short interval of a dose of doxorubicin. These patients can exhibit a variable course, which ranges from recovery of near normal function to rapid demise. Evidence suggests that this is merely a flagrant manifestation of a more subtle, clinically inapparent, acute drop in left ventricular function which can occur after doxorubicin. Thus, Singer and co-workers have reported that radionuclide cineangiography studies done at frequent intervals after doxorubicin may reveal a decrement in left ventricular function which reaches a nadir at 24 hours and is followed by a variable recovery.[114]

There has been considerable discussion as to whether these acute changes represent the antecedent of the chronic cardiomyopathy. It seems clear that the severity of transient arrythmias which develop after doxorubicin does not correlate with the subsequent development of the chronic cardiomyopathy.[111,112] The acute changes in the myocardial function ranging from the myocarditis–pericarditis syndrome to subclinical changes in ejection fraction are a different matter. It is already clear that patients who exhibit these changes can be left with a persistent deficit in myocardial function. In addition, endocardial biopsies and autopsy material have shown severe damage.[100] One must postulate either that doxorubicin can cause severe myocardial damage by two independent mechanisms or that the acute syndrome and the chronic cardiomyopathy are expressions of the same process. While the latter seems more likely, there is desperate need for good clinical studies which assess the relationship between these acute changes and chronic cardiomyopathy.

The chronic cardiomyopathy these agents cause has been the subject of intense investigative interest. However, the study of the natural history of this cardiomyopathy has been rendered difficult because most large patient populations treated with anthracyclines have had a short survival post-therapy. Thus, Von Hoff and colleagues were only able to provide significant numbers out to somewhat in excess of 250 days after the last drug treatment.[115,116] This picture is likely to change now that doxorubicin is being used in adjuvant chemotherapy of soft tissue sarcomas and breast cancer, where long survival after therapy may be expected.

From the information currently available, it is possible to construct a rather detailed picture of the natural history of this toxicity. Both endocardial biopsy and radionuclide angiocardiography show that the damage steadily accumulates with each dose of doxorubicin.[94,98] While there is considerable individual variation in the rate at which this damage develops, most patients will have moderate-to-severe pathologic damage and up to 50% will exhibit clear-cut functional impairment by the time they have received a total dose of 500 mg/m². Most of the patients destined to present with clinically apparent cardiomyopathy do so within a short time after the last adriamycin dose. Thus, Von Hoff et al noted 50% of the cases did so by 2 months and greater than 75% by 101 days.[115,116] One percent to 10% of the patients who received 550 mg/m² will develop clinically overt cardiomyopathy. Both endocardial biopsies and radionuclide cineangiocardiography seem to indicate that for most patients the degree of myocardial damage rapidly stabilizes. There appear to be exceptions; a few patients in the series reported by Alexander and co-workers clearly improved function as did those of Singer and associates.[94,114] In the opposite direction, we have observed a few patients whose congestive heart failure presented more than one year after the end of therapy.

The prognosis with clinically apparent doxorubicin cardiomyopathy is grave. Mortalities have ranged as high as 48%.[117] The likelihood of a fatal outcome is higher in patients who present in the first month off therapy than in those who present later.[103] While risk factors such as previous mediastinal radiation therapy, cyclophosphamide, or hypertension may increase the incidence of cardiomyopathy, there is no evidence that these make a fatal outcome more likely.

MANAGEMENT

Very little has been written on the management of the chronic cardiomyopathy and virtually no clinical trials exist on the subject. In the experience of the author, treatment of this cardiomyopathy differs little from the principles which govern the management of cardiomyopathies in general. Salt restriction and bed rest are the major tools at the clinician's disposal. Reduction of afterload, by agents that decrease peripheral vasculture resistance, has a sound physiologic basis and seems to be of clinical benefit in selected patients. As with most cardiomyopathies, the role of cardiac glycosides is unclear. At NCI, we have failed to see any improvement in ejection fraction in patients treated with digoxin, even though there appeared to be a clinical improvement in several patients so treated. These comments underline the difficulty in objectively assessing the value of therapy in this cardiomyopathy without benefit of a randomized clinical trial.

Gonadal Dysfunction

RICHARD L. SCHILSKY
RICHARD J. SHERINS

With the success of cytotoxic chemotherapy in the treatment of Hodgkin's disease, acute lymphocytic leukemia, germ cell testicular tumors, and other malignant and nonmalignant disorders have come new concerns for the long-term toxic effects of these therapies on normal host tissues. While many of the acute and chronic toxicities of antineoplastic drugs have been well defined, little attention has been paid to gonadal dysfunction resulting from anti-tumor therapy. In part, this lack of attention has stemmed from the absence of any immediate or life-threatening symptoms resulting from gonadal injury and, in part, it has reflected the absence, until recently, of a group of long-term cancer survivors who are concerned about their reproductive potential.

Many drugs used in the treatment of cancer have profound and often lasting effects on gonadal function. Both germ cell production and endocrine function may be affected. The magnitude of the effect can vary with the drug class or combination used in treatment; the total dose administered; and the age of the patient at the time of therapy.

CHEMOTHERAPY EFFECTS IN ADULT MEN

CLINICAL PATHOPHYSIOLOGY

Testicular function in adult men is particularly susceptible to injury by many chemotherapeutic agents. The primary histopathological lesion produced by the drugs studied to date is one of progressive dose-related depletion of the germinal epithelium lining the seminiferous tubule (Fig. 45-2).[118–126] Frequently, spermatocytes and spermatogonia disappear completely and only Sertoli cells remain lining the tubular lumen, a state described as germinal aplasia. The Leydig cells remain morphologically intact, although recent data suggest they may be functionally abnormal.[122,127]

The clinical accompaniments of germinal depletion (Table 45-6) are a marked reduction in testicular volume, severe oligospermia or azoospermia, and infertility.[123,124] Because the gonad regulates gonadotropin secretion, serum follicle stimulating hormone (FSH) and luteinizing hormone (LH) levels reflect the state of the seminiferous epithelium (Fig. 45-3). Germinal aplasia results in a fivefold increase in serum FSH levels (Fig. 45-4); and partial germinal depletion results in a lesser increase in FSH concentration, suggesting that the seminiferous tubule is the site of feedback inhibition of FSH secretion.[125] Thus, the serum FSH level serves as a marker for the presence of testicular germ cell loss. By contrast, serum LH and testosterone levels tend to remain within normal limits in the presence of germinal depletion. However, administration of LH-releasing hormone to patients with germinal aplasia results in an exaggerated LH response suggestive of subtle Leydig cell failure.[122,126,127]

FIG. 45-2. *A*, Testicular biopsy from a normal testis. *B*, Germinal aplasia. Note that the seminiferous tubules appear atrophic and only Sertoli cells line the seminiferous tubular lumens.

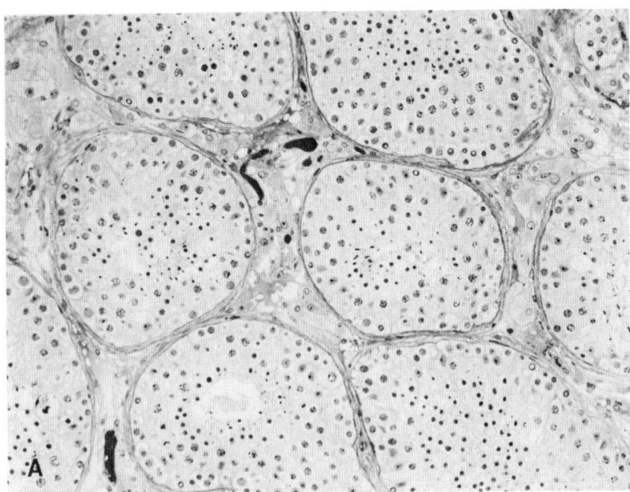

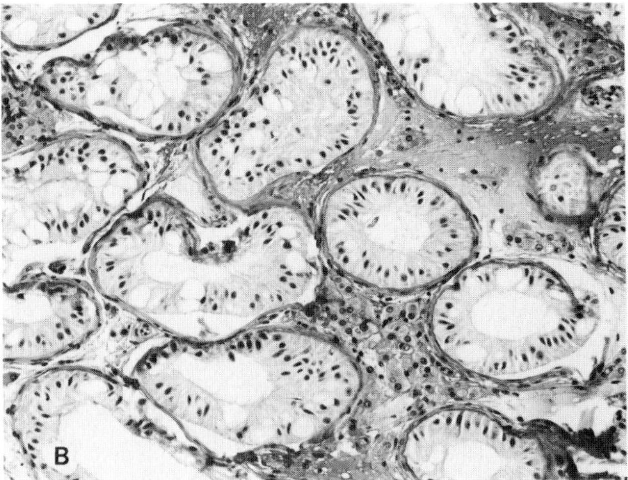

TABLE 45-6. Evaluation of Gonadal Function in Men Following Cancer Therapy

I. HISTORY

A. Sexual History

1. Pretreatment fertility history of both partners
2. Developmental: age of testicular descent, age of puberty, congenital anomalies of urinary tract or central nervous system
3. Surgical: orchiopexy, pelvic or retroperitoneal surgery, injury to genitals, spinal cord injury
4. Medical: venereal disease, mumps, renal disease, diabetes, epididymitis, tuberculosis, or other chronic illnesses
5. Drugs: many drugs interfere with spermatogenesis, erection, and ejaculation

II. CLINICAL AND LABORATORY FEATURES OF GERMINAL APLASIA

	TESTIS SIZE			HORMONE PROFILE		
	Length × width (cm)	*Volume* (cc)	SPERM COUNT (million/ml)	*FSH mIU/ml*	*LH mIU/ml*	*Testosterone ng/100 ml*
Normal Men	5.0 × 3.0	16–30	20–100	4–25	4–20	250–1200
Germinal Aplasia	3.7 × 2.3	8–15	0	25–90	8–25	200–700

SINGLE AGENTS

The anti-cancer agents most commonly associated with testicular germ cell depletion are listed in Table 45-7. Studies of men receiving single alkylating agents for lymphoma have been a major source of information about drug-related infertility. During alkylating agent therapy, the seminiferous epithelium is depleted in a dose-related fashion. Progressive but reversible oligospermia occurs in men receiving up to 400 mg of chlorambucil, while azoospermia and germinal aplasia occur in those patients treated with cumulative doses in excess of 400 mg.[121] Similarly, germinal aplasia is uncommon in patients receiving less than 6 g to 10 g of cyclophosphamide.[118] Vinblastine, doxorubicin, and procarbazine have all been implicated as being toxic to the germinal epithelium in both animals and man, although specific dose–toxicity relationships have not been established for these drugs.[128-130] Further prospective evaluation of the effects of these and

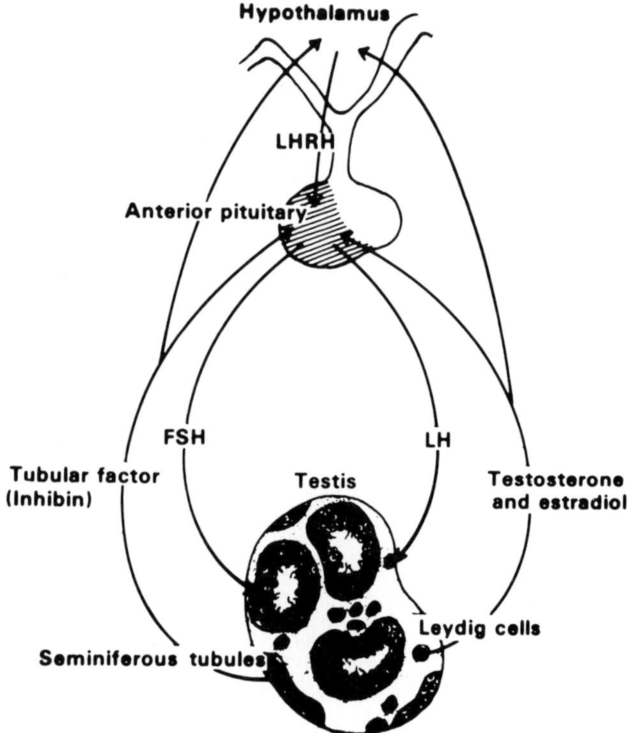

FIG. 45-3. Hypothalamic-pituitary-testicular interrelationships. Note that LH acts primarily on Leydig cells whereas FSH primarily affects the seminiferous tubules. (Sherins RJ, Winters SJ: Management of disorders of the testis. In Melmon K, Morelli HP (eds): Clinical Pharmacology: Basic Principles and Therapeutics, 2nd ed, p 582. New York, Macmillan, 1978)

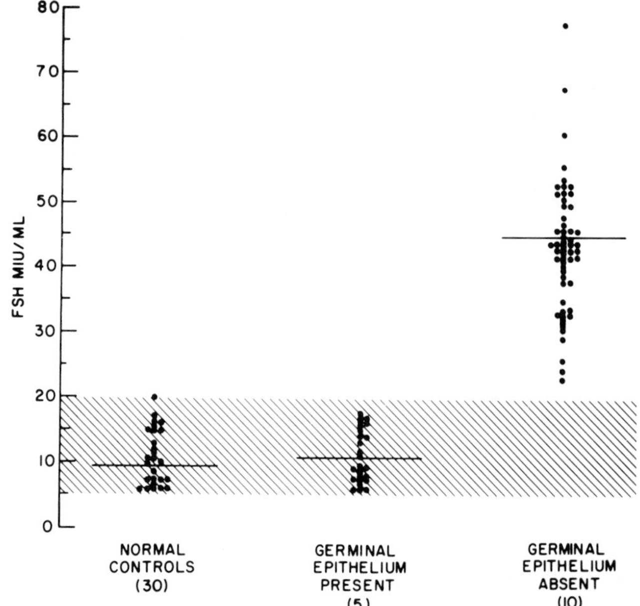

FIG. 45-4. Serum FSH levels in normal men and in men with germinal aplasia. (VanThiel DH, Sherins RJ, Myers GH et al: J Clin Invest 51:1009–1019, 1972)

TABLE 45-7. Antitumor Agents Associated with Testicular Germ Cell Depletion

DEGREE OF RISK	DRUG
Definite	Chlorambucil Cyclophosphamide Nitrogen mustard Busulfan Procarbazine
Probable	Doxorubicin Vinblastine Cytosine arabinoside
Unlikely	Methotrexate 5-Fluorouracil 6-Mercaptopurine Vincristine
Unknown	Bleomycin *cis*-Platinum Nitrosoureas

other single agents on testicular function is required to establish reliable data concerning the threshold drug dose above which seminiferous tubular damage becomes irreversible.

COMBINATION CHEMOTHERAPY

Combination drug regimens have a profound impact on spermatogenesis. The effects of nitrogen mustard, vincristine, procarbazine, and prednisone (MOPP) have been most carefully investigated and it is clear that more than 80% of men receiving this regimen develop azoospermia, germinal aplasia, testicular atrophy, and elevated serum FSH levels.[131-133] Recent evidence demonstrates that the use of procarbazine leads to particularly long-lasting testicular damage. Indeed, this drug alone induces germinal aplasia in adult male monkeys.[129,134]

Whereas the MOPP combination produces irreversible germinal aplasia in the majority of patients, this may not be true of other multimodal regimens currently in use. Cyclophosphamide and doxorubicin, when used as adjuvant chemotherapy for soft tissue sarcoma, appear to produce irreversible testicular damage only in men over 40 years of age or in men receiving concomitant irradiation proximal to the gonads. Similar drug doses, administered to younger patients, produce only transient, reversible elevations of serum FSH. These data suggest that, for some drug combinations, patient age is an important determinant of drug effects on the testis.[167]

CHEMOTHERAPY EFFECTS IN ADULT WOMEN

An assessment of the impact of cancer chemotherapy on ovarian function has been hampered by the relative inaccessibility of the ovary to biopsy and the resultant inability to obtain reliable estimates of the size of the germ cell population. One must rely primarily on menstrual and reproductive history and on determinations of serum hormone levels to assess the functional status of the ovary.

CLINICAL PATHOPHYSIOLOGY

Examination of the ovaries of women who have developed chemotherapy-related ovarian failure frequently reveals arrest of follicular maturation or frank destruction of ova and follicles.[135-137] Clinically, these patients become amenorrheic and may complain of menopausal symptoms of estrogen deficiency such as "hot flashes," vaginal dryness, and dyspareunia. Abnormally low circulating estrogen levels result in marked elevation of both serum FSH and LH, a manifestation of the loss of feedback inhibition of gonadotropin secretion consequent to drug-induced primary ovarian failure.

SINGLE AGENTS

Drugs most commonly associated with ovarian failure are shown in Table 45-8. Overall, at least 50% of women treated with single alkylating agents develop permanent ovarian failure and amenorrhea.[132,135,137,138-141]

Recent studies of the use of adjuvant chemotherapy in breast cancer patients have demonstrated that when amenorrhea occurs following such treatment, it is related to the age of the patient as well as to the total dose administered. Generally, patients older than 35–40 years of age at the time of treatment have a much greater likelihood of developing permanent amenorrhea following moderate doses of chemotherapy than do younger patients. Conversely, younger patients tolerate higher total drug doses prior to the onset of permanent amenorrhea. In one study, amenorrhea occurred following a mean cyclophosphamide dose of 5.2 g in all patients over 40 years whereas amenorrhea occurred in younger subjects only after a mean total dose of 9.3 g. Further, menses resumed within 6 months of discontinuing therapy in 50% of women under the age of 40 years.[142] Similar age-related phenomena have been noted following adjuvant chemotherapy with L-phenylalanine mustard.[143]

COMBINATION CHEMOTHERAPY

Most available information concerning the effects of combination chemotherapy regimens on ovarian function has come from the study of women receiving MOPP for Hodgkin's disease. Unlike the profound effects of this regimen on

TABLE 45-8. Antitumor Agents Associated with Ovarian Dysfunction

DEGREE OF RISK	DRUG
Definite	Cyclophosphamide L-phenylalanine mustard Busulfan Nitrogen mustard
Unlikely	Methotrexate 5-Fluorouracil 6-Mercaptopurine
Unknown	Doxorubicin Bleomycin Vinca alkaloids *cis*-Platinum Nitrosoureas Cytosine arabinoside

testicular function, MOPP produces ovarian dysfunction and amenorrhea in only 40% to 50% of treated women.[144–146] The frequency of ovarian injury is clearly related to the age of the patient at the time of treatment, with persistent amenorrhea occurring much more commonly in subjects older than 35–40 years of age. Ovarian dysfunction in younger patients appears to be related to the total chemotherapy dose administered, since permanent amenorrhea occurs in women receiving the highest cumulative drug doses. Continued long-term prospective follow-up of women who maintain normal menses following chemotherapy will be necessary to determine whether these patients are at risk for the development of premature ovarian failure and early menopause.

CHEMOTHERAPY EFFECTS IN CHILDREN

Evaluation of the effects of chemotherapy on gonadal function in children is particularly complex because of the variables introduced by the continuum of sexual development present in this patient population. Thus, knowledge of the pubertal status of the patient at the time of therapy and at the time of evaluation, along with recognition of the need to compare the results of hormonal evaluation to appropriate age-matched normal children, is required before definitive conclusions concerning drug effects can be drawn.

BOYS

Prior to the onset of puberty, the testicular germinal epithelium appears to be more resistant to moderate doses of alkylating agents than is the adult testis. Cyclophosphamide, in cumulative doses up to 20 g, produces only minor alterations in the testicular histology of prepubertal boys and no abnormalities in serum gonadotropins or testosterone levels.[147–149] However, at cumulative doses greater than 20 g, germinal aplasia has been documented.[150–152] Little information is available concerning the effects of other drugs on the immature testis, though recent data suggest that cytosine arabinoside in cumulative doses greater than 1 g/m^2 may be damaging to the germinal epithelium.[153]

Chemotherapy administered to male patients during puberty appears to have profound effects on both germ cell production and endocrine function. Following MOPP, gynecomastia, accompanied by elevation of serum FSH and LH levels and by low normal serum testosterone levels, has been noted in a majority of patients studied.[154] Testicular biopsy confirmed the occurrence of germinal aplasia in these patients as well. Thus, in contrast to prepubertal boys, chemotherapy administered during puberty may result in injury to both Leydig cells and the seminiferous epithelium, with gynecomastia being the clinical manifestation of this endocrine dysfunction. The reasons for the increased sensitivity to cytotoxic chemotherapy during puberty require further study.

GIRLS

Currently, there is a paucity of information available concerning the effects of cytotoxic drugs on the prepubertal and pubertal ovary. Post-mortem studies of ovarian histology of girls treated with chemotherapy have revealed a spectrum of results ranging from normal histology to arrest of follicular maturation and frank ovarian destruction.[147,155] From clinical studies, delay in menarche or interruption of menses in girls treated with single agent cyclophosphamide is very uncommon.[149,151,156,157] Studies of girls with acute lymphocytic leukemia treated with vincristine, methotrexate, and 6-mercaptopurine have revealed normal ovarian function in more than 80% of patients.[158] Thus, it would appear that the immature ovary is relatively insensitive to cytotoxic chemotherapy; however, follow-up of these patients will be required for many years to accurately determine the long-term effects of this therapy on reproductive potential.

RADIATION THERAPY

The complicated dosimetry of modern radiation therapy has made assessment of the impact of radiation therapy on gonadal function particularly difficult. If irradiated directly, both the testis and the ovary are highly radiosensitive organs. As little as 400 rad delivered in a single fraction to the testis or 1000 rad as a single dose to the ovary will cause irreversible gonadal destruction in most patients. Occasionally, however, late recovery of ovarian function may occur following irradiation, particularly in younger patients. Techniques to shield the gonads from the radiation beam have been employed during pelvic irradiation in an effort to ameliorate these toxic effects. During pelvic irradiation to an "inverted Y" field, lead shielding of the scrotum can decrease the dose delivered to the testis during treatment by at least 50%; however, it has been estimated that a cumulative dose of 100 rad to 200 rad will still reach the testis during a 4-week course of irradiation.[159] Since the dose is highly fractionated, it would be less likely to produce irreversible testicular damage. Thus, appropriate shielding is warranted in any circumstance where significant scrotal irradiation may occur. Similarly, oophoropexy (where the ovaries are surgically placed in the midline behind the uterus) and lead shielding are effective in preserving ovarian function in 50% to 60% of women receiving pelvic irradiation for Hodgkin's disease.[160]

Though gonadal shielding is commonly employed when the chance of testicular or ovarian irradiation may be high, there have been no studies performed to assess the dose received by the gonad when the treatment beam is directed to anatomically remote sites. The recent use of both chemotherapy and irradiation in combination for the therapy of soft tissue sarcoma suggests that radiation scatter, in the absence of gonadal shielding, can be an important contributor to gonadal toxicity. Thus, cyclophosphamide and doxorubicin, used as adjuvant chemotherapy, are associated with irreversible testicular injury only in those men under the age of 40 years who receive concomitant irradiation to the lower extremity proximal to the gonads.[167] Clearly, further studies of radiation dose received by the gonads during primary therapy of other sites are needed to determine the contribution of this therapy to gonadal dysfunction as well as to define the circumstances under which gonadal shielding is necessary.

COUNSELING

At the present time, infertility must be viewed as an unfortunate complication of cancer chemotherapy. Though much information has accumulated concerning the antifertility potential of alkylating agents, further study of other commonly used drugs such as doxorubicin, bleomycin, and *cis*-platinum is required to assess the impact of these agents on gonadal function. As new effective antitumor agents are introduced into clinical practice, additional screening for gonadal toxicity will become necessary. Further, long-term prospective studies of reproductive function in patients receiving cancer chemotherapy are needed to accurately assess the magnitude and duration of gonadal dysfunction to be expected from any therapeutic regimen.

Counseling of patients facing the high probability of chemotherapy-induced sterility is a difficult task. Several important points should be considered. Though the great majority of men will become infertile following cancer chemotherapy, it is currently impossible to predict if or when spermatogenesis might resume and standard contraceptive practices should therefore not be abandoned. Factors such as total drug dose administered and duration of time off therapy may be important determinants of reversibility as well as the type of drug or combination administered. Recent evidence suggests that the use of procarbazine in combination chemotherapy regimens may be associated with more long-lasting testicular damage than that seen with alkylating agents alone.[134] Return of spermatogenesis is uncommon before 1–2 years off chemotherapy has elapsed, but may be expected to occur within 4 years off therapy, if at all. Individual patients should be followed carefully with serial measurements of testicular volume, determinations of serum FSH, and semen analyses.

Pretreatment sperm banking may be valuable to some patients interested in having children following the completion of chemotherapy. Though the technology of freezing, preserving, and thawing human sperm has advanced considerably, ultimate conception rates using cryo-preserved semen remain only 50% to 60% due to loss of semen quality following thawing.[166,168,169] In addition, cancer patients may have decreased sperm counts or sperm motility prior to receiving any therapy which mitigates against successful semen preservation. For example, up to one-third of patients with Hodgkin's disease may be oligospermic prior to receiving any therapy.[161] Nevertheless, sperm banking can be offered to patients if they are properly informed of the cost:benefit ratio of the procedure.

While women older than 40 years of age frequently develop permanent chemotherapy-induced amenorrhea, many younger patients maintain normal menses throughout the treatment period or resume them shortly after therapy is discontinued. These patients, in particular, frequently have questions concerning the risks of spontaneous abortion and fetal abnormalities occurring in subsequent pregnancies. Though many anti-neoplastic agents are teratogenic, particularly if administered during the first trimester of pregnancy, most available information suggests that there is no increased incidence of spontaneous abortion or fetal abnormalities in the human previously treated with chemotherapy in comparison to the general population.[162–164] However, a recent study indicates that women previously treated with both chemotherapy and irradiation have a greater chance of pregnancy ending in abortion or with delivery of an abnormal child than do sibling controls.[165] At present, the available data are inadequate to assess the risk of genetic damage to germ cells posed by cancer chemotherapy. Careful studies over many years will be required before the true risks to subsequent generations are known.

Further information on gonadal dysfunction may be found in references 171–177.

Second Cancers

FREDERICK P. LI

It is ironic that some treatments for cancer also have the potential to induce new malignancies.[176,177] This section examines the role of chemotherapy, radiotherapy, and host susceptibility in the development of second cancers, and methodologic approaches to studies of these carcinogenic influences.

CHEMOTHERAPY

In 1971, the International Agency for Research on Cancer established a program to evaluate the available data on the carcinogenic risk of chemical agents.[178] To date, more than 400 chemicals have been examined for reported carcinogenic effects in animal experiments or epidemiologic studies. Among 54 chemicals investigated in relative detail in both experimental and human studies, 18 are considered to be carcinogenic for humans (Group 1), 18 are probably carcinogenic for humans (Group 2), and 18 could not be classified with regard to their carcinogenicity for humans (Group 3). Group 1 lists one cancer chemotherapeutic drug in current use (melphalan) and another (chlornaphazine) which is no longer employed clinically. The agents in Group 2 include chlorambucil and cyclophosphamide. These four drugs are alkylating agents, raising the possibility that other cancer chemotherapeutic agents in this class are also carcinogenic. However, data for most other alkylating agents have been anecdotal or inconclusive. In drug combinations associated with cancer development, the carcinogenic elements are often not known with certainty. None of the antimetabolites, vinca alkaloids, or antibiotics have been classified on the basis of available data as carcinogens for humans. Systematic follow-up studies of patients treated with newer agents and drug combinations should yield additional knowledge of their carcinogenic potential.

TABLE 45-9. Acute Nonlymphocytic Leukemia After Administration of Cytotoxic Drugs for Cancer and Non-Cancerous Diseases

	NUMBER DEVELOPING LEUKEMIA		
INITIAL DISEASE	*Drugs*	*Drugs and Radiotherapy*	*Total*
Multiple myeloma	33	21	54
Hodgkin's disease	7	26	33
Lymphoid disorders	14	7	21
Solid tumors	8	6	14
Non-cancerous diseases	12	–	12
All diagnoses	74	60	134

(Data reported before 1977, as summarized in Casciato DA, Scott, JL: Acute leukemia following prolonged cytotoxic agent therapy. Medicine 58:32–37,1979)

ACUTE LEUKEMIA

Melphalan, cyclophosphamide, and chlorambucil are associated with the development in humans of acute myelogenous leukemia and its variants. Casciato and Scott summarized 134 cases of acute nonlymphocytic leukemia associated with cancer chemotherapeutic drug treatments and reported before 1977 (Table 45-9).[179] All but 12 received the treatment for a malignancy. Sixty of them also had radiation therapy, and some received several drugs. The predominant drug was melphalan in 50 patients, chlorambucil in 30, and cyclophosphamide in 18. Between one and four leukemias were associated with other drugs: thio-TEPA, vinblastine, azothioprine, uracil mustard, urethrane, procarbazine, and methotrexate. The data were compiled mainly from case reports and small series. The total number of treated patients was not specified. The aggregate data suggest that melphalan, chlorambucil, and cyclophosphamide may be leukemogenic in humans, but provide no indications of risk of the complication.

In the last few years, studies have helped quantify the leukemogenic effects of several drug therapies for cancer. These reports have demonstrated excess risk of leukemia after treatment with alkylating agents for ovarian cancer, Hodgkin's disease, multiple myeloma, and polycythemia vera.

Ovarian Cancer Patients

Table 45-10 summarizes observed and expected numbers of acute nonlymphocytic leukemia found in three recent studies of patients treated for ovarian carcinomas. Reimer reported in 1977 on 5455 patients treated at 51 United States institutions for advanced ovarian carcinoma between 1970 and 1975.[180] Acute nonlymphocytic leukemia developed in 13 patients, whereas 0.6 cases were expected on the basis of number of patients, age, and follow-up duration. All 13 had received alkylating agents: melphalan alone in four patients, melphalan with another alkylating agent in two, chlorambucil in three, cyclophosphamide in two, thio-TEPA in one, and uracil mustard in one. Treatment duration ranged from 17 months to 90 months. None of the 13 also had radiotherapy for ovarian carcinoma. No excess of leukemias was found in a historical series treated between 1935 and 1972 primarily with surgery and radiotherapy. In another report in 1978, Einhorn evaluated 474 patients treated with melphalan for ovarian carcinoma.[181] Among 48 patients who received more than 300 mg of melphalan and survived more than three years, four developed acute nonlymphocytic leukemia. Only one of these patients had received radiotherapy. The expected number was not specified but was a fraction of one case of leukemia. In 1980, Pedersen-Bjergaard reported the development of acute nonlymphocytic leukemia in seven of 553 women treated for ovarian carcinoma with dihydroxybusulfan.[182] Treatment duration ranged between 12 months and 37 months. Concomitant radiotherapy had been administered to two of the seven women. The expected number was 0.04 cases of acute leukemia. In these and other studies, leukemia tended to develop in patients treated for long duration with high cumulative doses.

Acute leukemia has not been shown to be part of the natural history of ovarian carcinoma, and is likely a consequence of the alkylating agent therapy. Among ten other published case reports of acute leukemia after ovarian carcinoma, seven had received thio-TEPA. Additional therapies were chlorambucil in two of them and one each with cyclophosphamide and radiotherapy, methotrexate and fluorouracil, methotrexate, and methotrexate and cyclophosphamide.[182]. However, no excess cancers have been detected after adjuvant low-dose thio-TEPA therapy for breast cancer and colon cancer.[188,189]

Multiple Myeloma Patients

At least 15 patients with untreated multiple myeloma have developed acute leukemia.[185] It is uncertain whether these patients had plasma-cell leukemia or acute myelogenous leukemia.

Two recent studies have reported increased risk of acute leukemia after chemotherapy for multiple myeloma (Table 45-10). Gonzalez and coworkers reported in 1977 that acute leukemia developed in six of 476 multiple myeloma patients treated with melphalan and prednisone; some also received procarbazine, vincristine, carmustine, radiotherapy, or several agents. Therapy usually continued to relapse or death.[186] The observed incidence of acute leukemia was approximately 100-fold higher than expected. In 1979 Bergsagel and colleagues reported on a randomized study of 364 multiple myeloma patients treated with prednisone and three different schedules of melphalan, cyclophosphamide, and carmustine administered in combination or in sequence.[185] Acute leukemias developed in 14 patients, whereas 0.06 cases were expected. The actuarial risk of acute leukemia reached 17% at 50 months after treatment initiation, but the error of the estimate was not recorded.

Hodgkin's Disease Patients

A review in 1975 identified 93 patients with Hodgkin's disease and acute leukemia in the literature.[187] The two malignancies developed simultaneously in seven patients, suggesting that acute leukemia may be part of the natural history of Hodgkin's disease. However, magnitude of the intrinsic risk of acute leukemia and other second neoplasms in Hodgkin's disease patients is difficult to assess. Acute leukemia followed Hodg-

TABLE 45-10. Risk of Acute Leukemia in Patients Treated for Ovarian Cancer or Multiple Myeloma

SERIES	NUMBER TREATED	LEUKEMIAS OBSERVED: EXPECTED	MAJOR THERAPY*
OVARIAN CANCER			
Reimer, 1977	5455	13:0.6	Alkylating agents
Einhorn, 1978	474	4:<1	Melphalan
Pedersen-Bjergaard, 1980	553	7:.04	Dihydroxybusulfan
MULTIPLE MYELOMA			
Gonzalez, 1977	476	6:.06	Melphalan, prednisone
Bergsagel, 1979	364	14:.06	Melphalan, cyclophosphamide, carmustine

* Some patients in each series also received radiotherapy and other drugs.

kin's disease in the 86 remaining patients, most of whom had received radiotherapy and 37 of whom received some form of chemotherapy. The temporal relationship of the multiple primaries was reversed in other reported cases; that is, Hodgkin's disease developed during remission of acute leukemia.[188]

Recent studies of survivors of Hodgkin's disease show increased risk of second primary cancers, particularly acute nonlymphocytic leukemia and non-Hodgkin's lymphoma after combined modality treatments. Brody and co-workers reported that the risk of second neoplasms has increased in recent years in association with more intense therapy for Hodgkin's disease.[189] The cumulative risk of second malignancy after 5 years of follow-up was 1.2% among patients treated between 1950 and 1954 and 1960 and 1964, and was 4% among those treated between 1968 and 1972. The same trend was also observed at 10 years of follow-up. Among 23 second malignancies in that study, three were acute nonlymphocytic leukemia. Canellos and colleagues examined the relative risk of second cancer in relation to the form of therapy for Hodgkin's disease.[190] Sixteen of 452 treated patients developed second tumors. The relative risks were 1.6 for non-intensive therapy, approximately 4 for either intense radiotherapy or intense chemotherapy, 6 for intense chemotherapy followed by intense radiotherapy, and 18 for intense radiotherapy followed by intense chemotherapy for relapse. The intense chemotherapy was MOPP (mustine, vincristine, procarbazine, and prednisone) for at least six cycles. Two of six second cancers in the combined modality group were acute nonlymphocytic leukemia and at least two additional leukemias have developed among these patients.[191] Among 680 Hodgkin's disease patients treated at Stanford University, eight developed acute leukemia. These patients were among the subgroup of 330 patients who had received both radiotherapy and chemotherapy.[192] The actuarial risk of acute leukemia in this group at 10 years of follow-up was 3.9% (95% confidence limit, 0.2%–61%).[193] In addition, risk of non-Hodgkin's lymphoma was 4.4% among all Hodgkin's disease patients (confidence limit, 1%–15%) and 15.2% among the subgroup treated with combined modalities (4%–52%).[193] Excess risk of acute nonlymphocytic leukemia among Hodgkin's disease patients has also been reported by the Southwest Oncology Group (11 leukemias observed, 0.4 expected among 643 patients), Cancer and Acute Leukemia Group B (nine observed, 0.06 expected among 802 patients in complete remission of Hodgkin's disease), Manitoba University (two observed, 0.05 expected among 232 patients) and Odense University (three observed, 0.04 expected among 201 patients).[194–197] Most patients with leukemia had received combined modality treatment. Data of the Instituto Nazionale Tumori in Milan on 764 Hodgkin's disease patients showed 7.3% probability of second solid tumors and 2.4% probability of acute nonlymphocytic leukemia within ten years after initiation of therapy.[198] Seven of the nine patients who developed acute leukemia had received radiotherapy and MOPP (five cases) or MABOP (mustine, Adriamycin, bleomycin, vincristine, and prednisolone; two cases). The risk of acute leukemia after ten years was 5.4% among the 147 patients treated with MOPP and radiotherapy and 3.8% among 87 patients treated with MABOP and radiotherapy. No leukemia was observed in a third group of 55 patients treated with radiotherapy and ABVD (adriamycin, bleomycin, vinblastine, and dacarbazine). However, the expected number of cases, based on risk with the other treatments, is probably one for leukemia, and oncogenic potential of the three regimens may be comparable. Mustine and procarbazine are the suspected carcinogenic elements of MOPP therapy, but confirmatory single-agent data for humans are not available.

Acute leukemia has usually developed between 3 and 6 years after initiation of treatment for Hodgkin's disease.[179,190,192,198] A high proportion of patients were in complete remission of Hodgkin's disease at diagnosis of acute leukemia. Leukemia was often preceded by a preleukemic phase of peripheral blood cytopenia.[191–198] Cytogenetic studies have revealed a tendency to aneuploidy, particularly hypodiploidy involving B-group chromosomes.[199] Survival after onset of leukemia is a few months in nearly all instances.

Polycythemia Vera Patients

Acute nonlymphocytic leukemia tends to develop in patients with polycythemia rubra vera.[200] Therapy with ^{32}Ph has been implicated as a leukemogenic factor. In a randomized study of 431 evaluable polycythemia patients, acute leukemia developed in one of 134 treated with phlebotomy only, six of 156 treated with phosphorus-32 and phlebotomy, and 15 of 141 treated with chlorambucil and phlebotomy.[201] The findings suggest that chlorambucil was a potent leukemogenic factor, and the drug has been excluded from the therapeutic trial. Phosphorus-32 also appears to have a leukemogenic influence.[200,201]

BLADDER CANCER

Bladder cancer has been associated with the use of two antitumor drugs, chlornaphazine and cyclophosphamide.[178] Among 61 patients treated for polycythemia rubra vera with chlornaphazine in Denmark, ten developed bladder tumors and five had abnormal urine cytology.[202] The interval from treatment initiation to diagnosis of bladder cancer ranged between 3 years and 10 years. Three of the patients died from bladder cancer. Although nine of the ten patients had also received ^{32}Ph therapy, this agent alone was not associated with bladder cancer in a second series of polycythemia patients. Bladder cancer has also developed in a few Hodgkin's disease patients treated with chlornaphazine.[203] The carcinogenic effect of the chlornaphazine on the bladder may be the result of its chemical analogy to 2-naphthylamine, a known bladder carcinogen in humans.[178]

Hemorrhagic cystitis and bladder fibrosis are recognized complications of cyclophosphamide therapy. In addition, at least 18 patients have developed bladder cancer after cyclophosphamide treatments.[204, 205] Most were treated for a lymphoid malignancy and had a history of drug-associated hemorrhagic cystitis.[205,206] Duration of drug therapy was usually longer than 2 years, and interval to development of bladder cancer ranged from 3 years to 15 years.[207] Radiation and other forms of chemotherapy had also been given in some of them, and cigarette smoking was reported in others. In a study of 19,082 patients who had survived cancer for at least 5 years, 170 had received cyclophosphamide therapy and 18,912 had not.[204] Three among the 170 (1.8%) patients treated with cyclophosphamide developed bladder cancer, whereas 39 among the other 18,912 (0.2%) developed a second cancer in the bladder. These small numbers suggest a possible carcinogenic effect of cyclophosphamide on the human bladder.

OTHER ASSOCIATIONS

Among approximately 9000 renal transplant recipients, 32 developed non-Hodgkin's lymphoma whereas 1.3 cases were expected.[208] Most had histiocytic lymphomas and a high proportion were primary within the brain. The interval from transplantation to tumor development was less than 1 year in 13 of the patients. In addition, possible excess of hepatobiliary cancer, bladder cancer, leukemia, and skin cancers has also been noted, but the relative risks are small. Comparable findings of excess lymphomas and other cancers have also been reported after cardiac transplantation.[209] Nearly all renal transplant recipients received immunosuppressive therapy with azothioprine and corticosteroids. Additional treatments in some patients included actinomycin-D, antilymphocyte globulin, and radiotherapy. The role of the drugs in induction of lymphomas that start to appear within weeks after transplantation is unclear. Reports suggest that uremic patients in general may have a slightly increased risk of cancer.[210] In addition, the grafted kidney produces profound immunologic reactions, and lymphomas are a feature of diverse states of altered immunity. The immunologic disorders may be inborn, as in ataxia–telangiectasia, Wiskott–Aldrich syndrome and X-linked immunodeficiency, or acquired in transplant recipients or perhaps autoimmune diseases, such as systemic lupus erythematosus.[208] In these patients, the excess risk of lymphoma might be conferred by the underlying disease rather than drug treatment. Thus, some associations between cancer chemotherapy and subsequent neoplasia may not be causal, and isolated reports of second malignancies may be due to chance, host factors, or other influences.[211,212] Consistent excess of specific cancers after drug exposure is needed to establish an etiologic relationship. Induction of malignancies other than leukemia and bladder cancer by anticancer drugs remains unproven in humans. On the other hand, absence of carcinogenic risk for a treatment regimen is difficult to prove because of requirement of large sample size, and complete follow-up for decades. Furthermore, negative studies cannot exclude a carcinogenic effect with changes in dose, schedule, and treatment conditions, or administration in combination with other agents.

RADIOTHERAPY

Carcinogenic effects of ionizing radiation have been identified in studies of nuclear bomb survivors, occupationally irradiated workers, and patients treated for neoplasia and noncancerous diseases.[213,214] Investigators have examined the types of tumors induced by radiotherapy and time to tumor development. In addition, the effect of dose and the modifying influence of dose rate, fractionization, and quality of radiation have been evaluated. Analysis and interpretation of risk for humans have been hindered by incomplete radiation exposure data, few appropriate study populations, and confounding host factors. Experimental studies of radiation biology have yielded insights that may be applicable to humans.

Most data on radiation carcinogenesis are based on persons exposed to intermediate doses of hundreds of rad. A substantial proportion of these studies concerns the effects of partial-body radiotherapy for nonmalignant diseases.[215,216] The data show excess cancers after external-beam radiation to the scalp for tinea capitis, to the neck for thymic enlargement in infancy, to the spine for ankylosing spondylitis, to the pelvis for metropathia hemorrhagica, to the breasts for postpartum mastitis, and to the chest after pneumothorax therapy for pulmonary tuberculosis.[217–222] These patients and other persons exposed to comparable doses of radiation have developed excess cancers in diverse tissues within the radiation field. The data suggest that myeloid precursor cells and the thyroid may be more susceptible to neoplastic transformation. The female breast, lung, and salivary glands appear to have intermediate susceptibility. Other tissues have lower susceptibility, although cancer can be induced under appropriate conditions.[213,216] An apparent exception is chronic lymphocytic leukemia, which has not developed excessively among atomic bomb survivors and patients irradiated for ankylosing spondylitis.[219,223]

RADIOTHERAPY FOR CANCER

Data are scanty on radiation-induced malignancies among patients treated for cancer with thousands of rad. Evaluable studies have been carried out on patients with childhood cancers, Hodgkin's disease, and carcinoma of the cervix. Among 102 children with multiple cancers, the second malignancy was associated with radiotherapy in 69 instances.[224] Sarcomas of bone and soft tissues accounted for nearly one-half of the radiation-associated cancers. Several leukemias, lymphomas, and carcinomas of the skin and thyroid were also observed, whereas few had the common visceral carcinomas of adulthood. In 15 of the patients, hereditary retinoblastoma or other genetic predisposition to cancer was also present. A 20-fold excess risk of second cancer was found in a subgroup of these patients who had received orthovoltage radiotherapy.[225] Among Hodgkin's disease patients, radiation is associated with excess acute nonlymphocytic leukemia and non-Hodgkin's lymphoma, as indicated earlier in the discussion, but most had also received intense chemotherapy.[189–197] In addition, solid tumors have developed in Hodgkin's disease patients treated solely with radiotherapy, but no single tumor type predominated. Among patients irradiated for carcinomas of the cervix, no excess leukemia has been observed in several large studies.[226] In one series of 28,490 treated women, 13 leukemias were observed and 15.5 were expected.[226] A two-fold excess risk could be excluded by the data. Risk of any cancer after radiotherapy for cervical carcinoma has also been reported: 30 cancers were observed among 1563 patients, whereas 29 were expected.[227] No excess cancers in the irradiated pelvis were found.

Radiotherapy is used to treat virtually all forms of cancer. Large numbers of patients have received thousands of rad for the common cancers, such as carcinomas of the head and neck, lung, colon, breast, and endometrium. Small series of these patients have been reported to develop radiation-associated acute leukemia or sarcomas of bone and soft tissues.[228,229] However, high dose radiotherapy for cancer in adults has not been found to induce excess second primary carcinomas. Paucity of data in the literature may indicate low risk of radiation carcinogenesis after radiotherapy for cancer in doses of thousands of rad. Other explanations include high mortality from the initial cancer and co-morbid diseases, inadequate follow-up of treated patients, and failure to accurately diagnose second cancers.

TIME TO CANCER DIAGNOSIS

Cancers develop within irradiated tissues years to decades after exposure. Among atomic bomb survivors, the excess of acute leukemia was found within three years and peaked at 5 years to 8 years after irradiation.[223,230] Acute lymphocytic leukemia and chronic myelogenous leukemia have tended to develop earlier than acute myelogenous leukemia, which remains excessive three decades after the bombing.[223] The time to diagnosis of solid tumors among atom bomb survivors and other exposed groups has usually been longer than a decade.[213,231] The average time is longer than 15 years for radiation-induction of thyroid, breast, and urinary tract cancers.[218,231] In one study of survivors of childhood cancer, second cancer risk was higher at 15 years to 19 years of follow-up than during the preceding decade.[225] Among Hodgkin's disease patients, increased risk of second cancers has been detected during the first decade after radiotherapy, and data for longer follow-up periods are scanty. Palliative radiotherapy for other cancers rarely prolongs survival for many years, but improved prognosis with advances in therapy may result in rise in frequency of neoplastic complications in the future.

DOSE AND OTHER CONDITIONS OF EXPOSURE

The dose–hazard relationship for radiation cannot be stated with precision for humans.[213] Data for the effect of very high doses and low doses are particularly scanty. Thyroid cancer has been reported after 9 rad in children treated for tinea capitis, and after 3000 rad in Hodgkin's disease patients.[232,233]

Most studies for doses up to hundreds of rad are interpreted as showing a direct linear dose–hazard relationship, that is, doubling the dose doubles the cancer risk.[213] The slope of the line suggests one to ten excess cancers within irradiated tissues per million person-years of observation per rad. This linear absolute risk model assumes a fixed risk per rad that is applicable to a wide range of doses. The model has appeal for its simplicity and has been used extensively for purposes of radiation protection. An alternative relative risk model suggests that radiation increases cancer frequency by a fraction of the underlying cancer risk; for example, breast irradiation is more hazardous to females who have higher underlying breast cancer rates.[213] However, all dose–risk estimates for humans have wide confidence intervals and available data are also consistent with curvilinear dose–response models. Threshold dose for tumor induction is unresolved, and is not readily measured in human populations.[213] Possible requirement of multiple ionizing events for neoplastic transformation and modifying influence of endocrine, immunologic, and DNA-repair factors suggest that the relationship for gamma radiation may be curvilinear with a rising slope at lower doses.[234] At high doses, studies in laboratory animals suggest plateau or reduction in cancer risk, perhaps because transformed cells were also lethally damaged.[234] Studies in humans have shown no excess of cancers after intense radiotherapy for cervical carcinomas or no excess thyroid cancer after intense radioactive iodine treatments.[226,227,235] On the other hand, high-dose irradiation equivalent to thousands of rad is associated with development of second malignancies after Hodgkin's disease and childhood cancers.[189–198,224] Osteosarcoma risk also appears to increase with dose in the range of thousands of rad among retinoblastoma patients and persons who harbor internal emitters deposited in bone.[213,236] One explanation for the discrepancy is that human organs differ in susceptibility to carcinogenic effects of high-dose radiotherapy. Leukemia and thyroid cancer risk may be substantial at intermediate doses, but diminishes at high doses. On the other hand, bone cancer risk appears to be negligible at lower doses and rises with doses of thousands of rad. Other tissues could have different characteristics, but data are scanty.

Carcinogenic risk per rad is probably modified by dose rate, quality of radiation, and other conditions of exposure. Data on exposed humans are often incomplete, but dose–risk curves for leukemia differ for Hiroshima and Nagasaki. The higher slope for Hiroshima has been attributed to greater neutron contribution with high relative biologic effectiveness.[213,230] With external beam radiotherapy, the frequency of radiation-associated second cancers was higher at one center that employed orthovoltage equipment as compared with another that used megavoltage machines for treatment of childhood cancers.[225,237] Effects of protracted exposure in humans are difficult to measure but animal data suggest prolongation of gamma radiation may diminish the carcinogenic response.[234]

AGE AND SEX

Age at irradiation may influence the risk of radiogenic cancer and the type of tumor induced. Children who survived atomic bombing were more susceptible to leukemia, particularly acute lymphocytic leukemia.[213] Thyroid cancer risk may also be higher among irradiated children as compared with adults.[231] For breast cancer, the risk in women is high after chest irradiation between the ages of 15 years and 19 years and diminishes with increasing age.[226] Cancer rate in the opposite breast was not increased by scatter from radiotherapy for unilateral breast cancer in a study of 385 women, suggesting low risk for this exposure after childbearing ages.[238] Breast cancer is also uncommon among irradiated men of any age. Apparently, low risk of second neoplasms with irradiation for cancer may be due in part to the advanced age of many treated patients. Some of them have short survival because of age or disease, and the remainder who are adults may be less susceptible than children and adolescents to radiation carcinogenesis. In contrast, data on cancer induction by chemotherapeutic agents have come largely from studies of adults. Actinomycin-D has even been reported to reduce the risk of radiation carcinogenesis in children in a single report, but the combination was not protective in an animal model.[239,240]

DATA ANALYSIS AND BIAS

Observational bias may produce erroneous data on risk of chemotherapy- or radiotherapy-induced cancers. Second neoplasms can be difficult to diagnose, and must be distinguished from more common recurrences of the initial cancer. Reported cancer risk may be low because new lesions in cancer patients are usually assumed to be recurrences. The number of reports of treatment-associated leukemias may reflect, in part, ease of diagnosis in patients treated for solid tumors. Some second neoplasms are not readily classified as malignant or benign. For example, benign osteochondroma in irradiated bone may resemble osteosarcoma, and microscopic foci of carcinoma in irradiated thyroids have unknown biologic behavior.[241,242]

Bias in patient selection may markedly distort risk estimates. Patients with double primary cancers have two opportunities to be ascertained for study. Inclusion in a follow-up study of persons identified in connection with the second tumor will overestimate the cancer risk. In one series of 19 patients with second cancers, four were referred to the study institution only after development of the second cancer. The analysis excluded the four patients to avoid a 25% overestimate of the second cancer risk.[225] Several other patients were excluded from the analysis because recurrent disease or benign second tumor could not be excluded.[243]

In most published series, only a few patients developed treatment-associated cancers. For studies in Table 45-10, up to 100-fold excess risk of leukemia was reported on the basis of four to 14 affected patients who comprised 1% to 2% of the entire series. The observation of leukemia may have prompted the publications, whereas series without the complication were not reported. Point estimates of risk are particularly unstable at the longest follow-up interval because of small numbers, and confidence intervals should be presented. Risk is often measured in person-years of observation and compared with expected numbers calculated from appropriate age- and sex-specific cancer rates for the general population. The method assumes that the risk of cancer development is fairly stable during the follow-up interval. However, data suggest a latent period of longer than a decade for radiation induction of solid tumors in the general population. Follow-up data pertaining predominantly to the latent period will show a low cancer risk. A correction can be made through stratification of the risk estimate by follow-up interval, that is, risk at 0–4 years, 5–9 years, and 10–14 years after irradiation.[211,212,244]

HOST FACTORS

Second neoplasms may be due to factors other than chemotherapy and radiotherapy for cancer. Patients may develop second malignancies because of environmental carcinogens that can affect multiple organs.[245] For example, cigarette smokers develop excess cancers of the lung, larynx, and bladder, asbestos workers develop lung cancer and mesothelioma, and alcoholics develop liver cancer and oropharyngeal cancers. In addition, some cancer genes are associated with cancers at multiple sites.

More than 200 single-gene disorders have been associated with the development of benign or malignant tumors in humans.[246,247] A few of these genetic diseases, chiefly autosomal dominant diseases, predispose to more than one form of cancer (Table 45-11). Among the pharcomatoses, von Recklinghausen's neurofibromatosis, and tuberous sclerosis are usually associated with neural tumors. Recently, neurofibromatosis has also been described in association with childhood nonlymphocytic leukemia, Wilms' tumor, and rhabdomyosarcoma.[248] In the multiple endocrine neoplasia syndromes, the component neoplasms appear to share in common progenitor cells in the embryonic neural crest. Explanations for the constellation of neoplasms in Gardner's syndrome, Cowden's disease, and nevoid basal cell carcinoma syndrome are uncertain. Autosomal recessive chromosome breakage syndromes, genodermatoses, and immunodeficiency syndromes also predispose to cancer, but multiple primary cancers are rare in part because of shortened lifespan.[246,247] In xeroderma pigmentosum, sunlight accelerates the development of skin cancers, possibly because of defective excision repair of ultraviolet ray damage to DNA, but internal malignancies are not a characteristic feature.[249]

Knudson developed a two-mutation model for inheritance

TABLE 45-11. Autosomal Dominant Diseases Associated with Multiple Primary Neoplasms[246]

GENETIC DISEASE	PREDOMINANT TUMOR TYPES
MULTIPLE ENDOCRINE NEOPLASIA	
Type I	Parathyroid, pancreatic islet cells, pituitary
Type II	Medullary thyroid carcinoma, pheochromocytoma, parathyroid
Type III	Medullary thyroid carcinoma, pheochromocytoma, mucosal neuroma
PHACOMATOSES	
von Recklinghausen's neurofibromatosis	Brain tumors, peripheral nerve tumors, pheochromocytoma, childhood cancers
Tuberous sclerosis	Brain tumors, renal tumors
von Hippel-Lindau	Renal carcinoma, cerebellar hemangioblastoma
OTHER	
Hereditary retinoblastoma	Retinoblastoma, osteosarcoma
Nevoid basal cell carcinoma syndrome	Basal cell carcinomas, medulloblastoma, ovarian tumors
Gardner's syndrome	Colon cancer, sarcomas, carcinoma of ampulla of Vater
Cowden's disease	Carcinomas of breast, thyroid carcinoma, meningioma, hamartomas

of retinoblastoma, which subsequently was expanded to encompass Wilms' tumor, neuroblastoma, and several dominantly inherited cancers in adults.[250,251] According to the model, the first mutation in hereditary cancers has been transmitted from a parent. Cancers develop in the somatic cells that undergo a second mutation. Second mutations in several cells of one organ produce multifocal tumors or bilateral tumors in paired organs. The mutations in two organs produce double primary cancers. Hereditary cancers develop at earlier ages because the second mutation usually occurs in less time than the two mutations required to produce nonhereditary cancer in a single somatic cell. In hereditary retinoblastoma, bilateral eye tumors are common and may be followed by development of osteosarcoma in radiated or distal sites.

Some cancers tend to aggregate in families, and genetic influences have been postulated. For many cancers, risk of the same neoplasm among close relatives of affected patients is reported to be increased by two-fold to three-fold.[252] In addition, families have been reported with clusters in several generations of adenocarcinomas of the breast, ovary, colon, and endometrium. Up to 20% of cancer patients in some kindreds had multiple primary cancers.[252] A second family cancer syndrome involves sarcomas in childhood associated with breast cancer, leukemia, and brain tumors at early ages.[252] Other constellations have been reported in small series, but chance aggregation may be the explanation.[253] Fraumeni has suggested that cancers which tend to aggregate in families may also develop excessively as double primaries in one person.[252] Excluding patients with predisposing single gene diseases and family cancer syndromes, constitutional susceptibility to new neoplasms among cancer patients in general may not be increased.

Host factors can interact with environmental carcinogens. Age and sex have been shown to modify susceptibility to radiation carcinogenesis.[213] Genetic–environmental interactions have also been reported to alter susceptibility to certain multiple primary cancers. In patients irradiated for medulloblastoma associated with the nevoid basal cell carcinoma syndrome, skin cancers in the radiation field have developed within 6 months to 3 years after the treatment.[254] Earlier development of second cancer has also been reported for osteosarcoma associated with radiotherapy for the hereditary form of retinoblastoma.[354] *In vitro* studies have suggested that cultured fibroblasts from some retinoblastoma patients may be slightly more sensitive to the lethal effects of gamma radiation.[255] In ataxia–telangiectasia, the cells show marked *in vitro* sensitivity to radiation, and at least one patient developed radiation dermatitis and basal cell carcinoma after treatment for tinea capitis.[256]

COMMENT

Approximately 400,000 persons die of cancer annually in the United States. Only several dozen deaths due to the carcinogenic effects of cancer therapy have been reported each year. Cancer is a common and lethal disease, whereas neoplastic complications of therapy have been rare.

Many second cancers are diseases of medical progress resulting from treatment advances that prolong the lives of cancer patients. The carcinogenic effects of the treatments *per se* are difficult to determine and, to date, relatively few agents have been implicated. For most therapies with a carcinogenic potential, a few percent of patients develop cancer during each decade of survival and the benefits of treatment for lethal conditions clearly exceed the risks. Treatment-induced cancers include skin and thyroid cancer that are readily cured and have little clinical importance. Threat to life arises in patients who develop acute leukemia and solid tumors in vital organs. These lesions are usually resistant to further chemotherapy and radiotherapy and carry an ominous prognosis. To avoid these fatal complications, consideration has been given to alterative treatment regimens that eliminate potentially carcinogenic components. However, problems can arise from attempts to modify therapies that are curative or markedly prolong life of cancer patients. Carcinogenesis is only one of many adverse effects of cancer therapy, and overall risks and benefits need to be weighed to achieve the maximum likelihood of cure with reduced risk of complications. Risk of a second cancer may not be fully avoidable in patients with an underlying predisposition that is independent of therapy.

Periodic screening of treated cancer patients offers the hope of early detection of second cancers, but the benefits of earlier diagnosis of leukemia and some solid tumors have not been established. Reduction of risk of treatment-induced cancer by use of retinoids or other potential inhibitors of carcinogenesis merits evaluation.[257]

Individual case reports cannot establish carcinogenic effects of a treatment regimen. Nevertheless, these reports are useful in identifying therapies that require thorough follow-up evaluation of large series of treated patients. Case reports regarding newer agents, such as doxorubicin, nitrosoureas, bleomycin, procarbazine, and *cis*-platinum may be particularly informative.[176,258–260] In addition, follow-up studies should focus on adjuvant chemotherapy for breast cancer, combined modality treatment for testicular cancer and acute lymphocytic leukemia, and other therapies associated with highly favorable prognosis.[261-263]

REFERENCES

1. Moss WT, Brand WN, Battiford H: Radiation Oncology: Rationale, Techniques, Results, 5th ed, pp 57–58. St. Louis, CV Mosby, 1979
2. Wagner L, Bye MG: Body image and patients experiencing alopecia as a result of cancer chemotherapy. Cancer Nursing 2:5, 365–369
3. US-DHHS: "Chemotherapy and You." NIH Pub No 80–1136, Aug 1980
4. O'Brien R et al: Scalp tourniquet to lessen alopecia after Vincristine. N Engl J Med 283:1469, 1970
5. Lyons A: Letter: Prevention of hair loss by headband during cytotoxic therapy. Lancet 1:354, 1974
6. Lovejoy NC: Preventing hair loss during adriamycin therapy. Cancer Nursing 2:2, 117–121
7. Helson L: Letter: Vincristine and alopecia. N Engl J Med 284:6, 336
8. Dean JC, Salmon SE, Griffith KS: Prevention of doxorubicin-induced hair loss with scalp hypothermia. N Engl J Med 301:26, 1427–1429
9. Wang SC, Borison HL: A new concept of organization of the central emetic mechanism: Recent studies on the sites of action of apomorphine, copper sulfate, and cardiac glycosides. Gastroenterol 22:1–12, 1952
10. Wang SC: Emetic and antiemetic drugs. In Root WS, Hofmann FE (eds): Physiological Pharmacology, Vol. 2, pp 255–328. New York, Academic Press, 1965
11. Borison HL, Brand D, Orkand RK: Emetic action of nitrogen mustard in dogs and cats. Am J Physiol 192:410–416, 1958
12. Wang SC, Renzi AA, Chinn SI: Mechanism of emesis following X-irradiation. Am J Physiol 193:335–339, 1958
13. Jaffe JH, Martin WR: Narcotic analgesics and antagonists. In Goodman LS, Gilman A (eds): The Pharmacologic Basis of Therapeutics, 5th ed, pp 245–283. New York, Macmillan, 1975
14. Byck R: Drugs and the treatment of psychiatric disorders. In Goodman LS, Gilman A (eds): The Pharmacologic Basis of Therapeutics, 5th ed, pp 152–200. New York, Macmillan, 1975
15. Hunt CC, Philips FS: The acute pharmacology of methyl-bis(2-chloroethyl)amine. J Pharmacol Exp Ther 95:131–143, 1949
16. Sawicka J, Sallan SE: Transdermal Therapeutic System-Scopolamine®: Prevention of vomiting associated with cancer chemotherapy (abstr). Proc Am Soc Clin Oncol 18:302, 1977
17. Costello DJ, Borison HL: Naxolone blocks narcotic self-blockage of emesis in cats. J Pharmacol Exp Ther 203:222–230, 1977
18. Snyder SH: Opiate receptors in the brain. N Engl J Med 296:266–271, 1977
19. Parson JA, Webster JH, Dowd J: Evaluation of the placebo effect in the treatment of radiation sickness. Acta Radiol 56:129–140, 1961
20. Wang SC: Perphenazine, a potent and effective antiemetic. J Pharmacol Exp Ther 123:306–310, 1958
21. Chinn HI, Smith PK: Motion sickness. Pharmacol Rev 7:33–82, 1955
22. Gay LN, Carliner PE: The prevention and treatment of motion sickness. Bull Johns Hopkins Hosp 84:470–487, 1949
23. Nickerson M: Dramamine. Science 111:312–313, 1950
24. Jaju BP, Wang SC: Effects of diphenhydramine and dimenhydrinate on vestibular neuronal activity of act: A search for the locus of their antimotion sickness action. J Pharmacol Exp Ther 176:718–723, 1971
25. Wyant GM: A comparative study of eleven antiemetic drugs in dogs. Can Anesth Soc J 9:399–407, 1962
26. Bardfield P: A controlled double-blind study of trimethobenzamide, prochlorperazine and placebo. JAMA 196:796–798, 1966
27. Dobkin A, Evers W, Israel J: Double-blind evaluation of metoclopramide, trimethobenzamide and a placebo as postanesthetic antiemetics following methoxyglurane anaesthesia. Can Anaesth Soc J 15:80–91, 1968
28. Wolfson B, Torres-Kay M, Foldes F: Investigation of the usefulness of trimethobenzamide for the prevention of postoperative nausea and vomiting. Anesth Analg 41:172–177, 1962
29. Sallan SE, Zinberg NE, Frei E III: Antiemetic effect of delta-9-tetrahydrocannabinol in patients receiving cancer chemotherapy. N Engl J Med 293:795–797, 1975
30. Sallan SE, Cronin CM, Zelen M et al: Antiemetics in patients receiving chemotherapy for cancer. N Engl J Med 302:134–138, 1980
31. Davies GH, Weatherstone RM, et al: A pilot study of orally administered tetrahydrocannabinol in the management of patients undergoing radiotherapy for carcinoma of the bronchus. Br J Clin Pharmacol 1:301–306, 1974
32. Herman TS, Einhorn LH, Jones SE et al: Superiority of nabilone over prochlorperazine as an antiemetic in patients receiving cancer chemotherapy. N Engl J Med 300:1295–1297, 1979
33. Sallan SE, Cronin CM: Nabitan trials. (unpublished findings)
34. Sallan SE, Cronin CM: Levonantradol trials. (in press) J Clin Pharmacol 1981
35. Plotkin DA, Plotkin D, Okun R: Haloperidol in the treatment of nausea and vomiting due to cytotoxic drug administration. Curr Ther Res 15:599–602, 1973.
36. Cole DR, Duffy DF: Haloperidol for radiation sickness. NY State J Med 74:1558–1562, 1974
37. Barton M, Libonanti M, Cohen P: The use of haloperidol for treatment of postoperative nausea and vomiting—a double-blind placebo-controlled trial. Anesthesiology 42:508–512, 1975
38. Christman R, Weinstein R, Larose J: Low-dose haloperidol as antiemetic treatment in gastrointestinal disorders: A double-blind study. Curr Ther Res 16:1171–1176, 1974
39. Robbins E, Nagel J: Haloperidol parenterally for the treatment of vomiting and nausea from gastrointestinal disorders in a group of geriatric patients: Double-blind, placebo-controlled study. J Am Geriatr Soc 23:38–41, 1975
40. Tornetta F: Double-blind evaluation of haloperidol for antiemetic activity. Anesth Analg 51:964–967, 1972
41. Finn H, Urban B, Thomas J et al: Antiemetic efficacy of benzquinamide. NY State J Med 71:651–653, 1971
42. Medoff J: A double-blind evaluation of the antiemetic efficacy of benzquinamide. Curr Ther Res 12:706–710, 1970
43. Shaw JE, Bayne W, Schmitt LG: Clinical pharmacology of scopolamine. Clin Pharmacol Ther 19:115, 1976
44. Shaw JE, Chandrasekaran SK, Campbell PS et al: New procedures for evaluation cutaneous administration. In Drill VA, Lazar P (eds): Cutaneous Toxicity, pp 83–95. New York, Academic Press, 1977
45. Graybiel A, Knepton J, Shaw HE: Prevention of experimental motion sickness by scopolamine absorbed through the skin. Aviat Space Environ Med 47:1096–1100, 1976
46. Shaw JE, Schmitt LG, McCauley ME et al: Transdermally administered scopolamine for prevention of motion sickness in a vertical oscillator. Clin Pharmacol Ther 21:117, 1977

47. Buckner CD, Rudolph RH, Fefer A et al: High dose cyclophosphamide therapy for malignant disease. Cancer 29:357–365, 1972
48. Fajardo LF, Stewart RJ, Cohn KE: Morphology of radiation-induced heart disease. Arch Pathol 86:512–519, 1968
49. Buja LM, Roberts WC: Iron in the heart. Etiology and clinical significance. Am J Med 51:209–221, 1971
50. Braunwald E, Ross J: Control of cardiac performance. In Berne R, Sperelakis N, Geiger S (eds): Handbook of Physiology, Sec. 2, The Cardiovascular System, Vol 1, The Heart. Bethesda, Am Physiol Soc, 1979
51. Gozalvez M, Van Rossum GDV, Blanco MF: Inhibition of sodium–potassium-activated adenosine-5′-triphosphatase and ion transport by adriamycin. Cancer Res 39:257–261, 1979
52. Olson HM, Young DM, Prieur DJ et al: Electrolyte and morphologic alterations of myocardium in adriamycin-treated rabbits. Am J Pathol 77:439–454, 1974
53. Brockman E, Zbinden G: Effect of doxorubicin and rubidazone on respiratory function and Ca^{2+} transport in rat heart mitochondria. Toxicology Letters 3:29–34, 1979
54. Revis N, Marusic N: Sequestration of calcuium 45 by mitochondria from rabbit heart, liver and kidney after doxorubicin or digoxin, doxirubicin treatment. Exp Mol Pathol 31:440–451, 1979
55. Villani F, Piccinini F et al: Influence of adriamycin on calcium exchangeability in cardiac muscle and its modification by Ouabin. Biochem Pharmacol 27:985–987, 1978
56. Mikkelson RB, Lin PS, Wallach DF: Interaction of adriamycin with human red blood cells; a biochemical and morphological study. J Mol Med 2:33–40, 1977
57. Goldman R, Fashinetti T, Bach D et al: A differential interaction of daunomycin, adriamycin, and their derivatives with human erythrocytes and phospholipid bilayers. Biochim Biophys Acta 512:254–269, 1978
58. Murphree SA, Cunningham LS et al: Effects of adriamycin on surface properties of sarcoma 180 ascites cells. Biochem Pharmacol 25:1227–1235, 1976
59. Solie TN, Yunker C: Adriamycin-induced changes in translocation of sodium ions in transporting epithelial cells. Life Sci 22:1907–1910, 1978
60. Duarte-Karim M, Ruysschaert JM, Hildebrand J: Affinity of adriamycin to phospholipids—a possible explanation for cardiac mitochondrial lesions. Biochem Biophys Res Commun 71:658–663, 1978
61. Tritton TA, Murphree SA, Sartorelli AC: Adriamycin; a proposal on the specificity of drug action. Biochem Biophys Res Commun 84:802–808, 1978
62. Myers CE, Liss RH, Ifrim J et al: Adriamycin: The role of lipid peroxidation in cardiac toxicity and tumor response. Science 197:165–169, 1977
63. Chance B, Spies H, Boveris A: Hydroperoxide metabolism in mammalian tissue. Physiol Rev 59:527–605, 1979
64. Doroshow JA, Locker GY, Myers CE: The enzymatic defenses of the mouse heart against reactive oxygen metabolites: Alterations produced by doxorubicin. J Clin Invest 65:128–135, 1980
65. Revis NW, Marusic N: Glutathione peroxidase activity and selenium concentration in the hearts of doxorubicin-treated rabbits. J Mol Cell Cardiol 10:945–951, 1978
66. Lantz B, Adolfsson J, Langenlof B et al: Cardiomyopathy in leukemia with reference to rubidomycin cardiotoxicity. Cancer Chemother Pharmacol 2:95–99, 1979
67. Dantchev D, Slioussantchouk V, Paintrand M et al: Electron microscopic studies of the heart and light microscopic studies of golden hamsters with adriamycin, detorubicin, AD32 and aclacinomycin. Cancer Treat Rep 63:875–888, 1979
68. Pretronigro DP, McGinness JE, Koren MJ et al: Spontaneous generation of adriamycin semiguinone radicals at physiologic pH. Physiol Chem Phys 11:405–414, 1974
69. Tong GL, Henry DW, Acton EM: 5-Iminodaunorubicin. Reduced cardiotoxicity properties in an antitumor anthracycline. J Med Chem 22:34–39, 1979
70. Van Vleet JF, Greenwood L, Ferrans VJ et al: Effects of selenium-vitamin E on adriamycin-induced cardiomyopathy in rabbits. Am J Vet Res 39:997–1010, 1978
71. Herman EH, Ferrans VJ: Effect of vitamin E on the chronic doxorubicin toxicity in miniature swine. Fed Proc 39:3126, 1980
72. Sonneveld P: Effect of alpha-tocopherol on the cardiotoxicity of adriamycin in the rat. Cancer Treat Rep 62:1033–1035, 1978
73. Averbach S, Singer D: Adriamycin: Cellular electrophysiologic changes. Fed Proc 38:3998, 1979
74. Kishi T, Watanabe T, Folkers K: Prevention by forms of coenzyme Q of the inhibition by adriamycin of coenzyme Q10-dependent enzyme in mitochondria of the myocardium. Proc Natl Acad Sci 73:4653–4656, 1976
75. Olson RD, MacDonald JS, Harbison RD et al: Altered myocardial glutathione levels: A possible mechanism of adriamycin toxicity. Fed Proc 36:303, 1977
76. Doroshow JH, Locker GY, Myers CE: The prevention of doxorubicin cardiac toxicity by N-acetyl-L-cysteine. Proc AACR and ASCO 20:1035, 1979
77. Herman E, Botray R, Chadwick D: Modification of some of the toxic effects of daunomycin by pretreatment with the antineoplastic agent ICRF-159. Toxicol Appl Pharmacol 27:517–526, 1974
78. Herman E, Ardalan B, Bier C et al: Reduction of daunorubicin lethality and myocardial cellular alteration by pretreatment with ICRF 187 in Syrian golden hamsters. Cancer Treat Rep 63:89–92, 1979
79. Breed JGS, Zimmerman ANE, Dormans JAMA et al: Failure of the antioxidant vitamin E to protect against adriamycin-induced cardiotoxicity in the rabbit. Cancer Res 40:2033–2038, 1980
80. Mason JW, Bristow MR, Billingham ME et al: Invasive and noninvasive methods of assessing adriamycin cardiotoxic effects in man: Superiority of histopathologic assessment using endocardial biopsy. Cancer Treat Rep 62:857–864, 1978
81. Balcerzak SP, Christakis J, Lewis RD et al: Systolic time intervals in monitoring adriamycin-induced cardiotoxicity. Cancer Treat Rep 62:893–900, 1978
82. Gottdiener JS: Noninvasive assessment of cardiac dysfunction in the cancer patient. Cancer Treat Rep 62:949–954, 1978
83. Hutchinson RJ, Bailey C, Wood D et al: Systolic time intervals in monitoring for anthracycline cardiomyopathy in pediatric patients. Cancer Treat Rep 62:907–910, 1978
84. Ewy GA, Jones SE, Freedman MJ et al: Noninvasive cardiac evaluation of patients receiving adriamycin. Cancer Treat Rep 62:915–922, 1978
85. Henderson IC, Sloss LJ, Jaffe N et al: Serial studies of cardiac function in patients receiving adriamycin. Cancer Treat Rep 62:923–930, 1978
86. Minow RA, Benjamin RS, Lee ET et al: QRS voltage change with adriamycin administration. Cancer Treat Rep 62: 931–934, 1978
87. Zaret BL, Strauss HW, Hurley PJ et al: A scintiphotographic method for detecting regional ventricular dysfuncition in man. N Engl J Med 284:1165–1170, 1971
88. Federman J, Brown ML, Tancredi RG et al: Multiple-gated acquisition cardiac blood-pool isotope imaging. Mayo Clinic Proc 53:625–633, 1978
89. Green MV, Ostrow HG, Douglas MA et al: High temporal resolution EGG-gated scintigraphic angiocardiography. J Nucl Med 16:95–98, 1975
90. Burow RD, Strauss HW, Singleton R et al: Analysis of left ventricular function from multiple gated acquisition cardiac blood pool imaging: Comparison to contrast angiography. Circulation 56:1024–1028, 1977
91. Borer JS, Bacharach SL, Green MV et al: Real time radionuclide cineangiography in the noninvasive evaluation of global and regional left ventricular function at rest and during exercise in patients with coronary artery disease. N Engl J Med 296:839–844, 1977
92. Borer JS, Bacharach SL, Green MV et al: Obstructive versus nonobstructive asymmetric septal hypertrophy. Differences in left ventricular function with exercise. Am J Cardiol 41:379, 1978
93. Kennedy JW, Sorensen SG, Ritchie JL et al: Radionuclide angiography for the evaluation of anthracycline therapy. Cancer Treat Rep 62:941–944, 1978

94. Alexander J, Dainiak N, Berger HJ et al: Serial assessment of doxorubicin cardiotoxicity with quantitative radionuclide angiocardiography. N Engl J Med 300:278–283, 1979
95. Sakakibara S, Konno S: Endomyocardial biopsy. Jpn Heart J 3:537–543, 1962
96. Mason JW: Techniques for right and left ventricular endomyocardial biopsy. Am J Cardiol 41:887–892, 1978
97. Ferrans VJ, Roberts WC: Myocardial biopsy: A useful diagnostic procedure or only a research tool. Am J Cardiol 41:965–967, 1978
98. Bristow MR, Mason JW, Billingham ME et al: Adriamycin cardiomyopathy: Evaluation by phonography, endomyocardial biopsy and cardiac catheterization. Ann Intern Med 88:168–175, 1978
99. Billingham ME, Mason JW, Bristow MA et al: Anthracycline cardiomyopathy monitored by morphologic changes. Cancer Treat Rep 62:865–872, 1978
100. Bristow MR, Thompson PD, Martin RP et al: Early anthracycline cardiotoxicity. Am J Med 65:823–832, 1978
101. Bristow M: Rational system for cardiac monitoring in patients receiving anthracyclines. Proc Am Soc Clin Oncol 21:C-149, 1980
102. Billingham ME, Bristow MR, Glatstein E et al: Adriamycin cardiotoxicity: Endomyocardial biopsy evidence of enhancement by irradiation. Am J Surg Pathol 1:17–23, 1977
103. Minow RA, Benjamin RS, Lee ET et al: Adriamycin cardiomyopathy—risk factors. Cancer 39:1397–1402, 1977
104. Deasis DN, Ali KM, Soto A et al: Acute cardiac toxicity of antineoplastic agents as the first manifestation of pheochromocytoma. Cancer 42:2005–2008, 1978
105. Bristow MR, Billingham ME, Daniels JR: Histamine and catecholamine mediate adriamycin cardiotoxicity. Proc Am Assoc Cancer Res 20:477, 1979
106. Denine EP, Schmidt LM: Adriamycin-induced myopathies in the rhesus monkey with emphasis on cardiomyopathy. Toxicol Appl Pharmacol 33:162, 1975
107. Buzdar AO, Legha S, Tashima CK et al: Adriamycin and mitomycin C. Possible synergistic cardiotoxicity. Cancer Treat Rep 62:1005–1008, 1978
108. Tomasz M, Mercado CM, Olson J et al: The mode of interaction of mitomycin C with deoxyribonucleic acid and other polynucleotides *in vitro*. Biochemistry 13:4878–4881, 1974
109. Weiss AJ, Manthel RW: Experience with the use of adriamycin in combination with other anticancer agents using a weekly schedule, with particular reference to lack of cardiac toxicity. Cancer 40:2041–2052, 1977
110. Benjamin RS, Ewer MS, MacKay B et al: Endomyocardial biopsy study of anthracycline-induced cardiomyopathy—Detection, reversibility, and potential amelioration. Proc Am Soc Clin Oncol 20:C–335, 1979
111. Tan L, Etcubanas E, Wollner N et al: Adriamycin—an antitumor antibiotic in the treatment of neoplastic diseases. Cancer 32:9–17, 1973
112. Cortes EP, Lutman G, Wanka J et al: Adriamycin cardiotoxicity: A clinicopathologic correlation. Cancer Chemother Rep, Pt. 3, 6:215–225, 1975
113. O'Bryan R, Luce J, Talley R et al: Phase II evaluation of adriamycin in human neoplasia. Cancer 32:1–8, 1973
114. Singer JW, Narahara KA, Ritchie JL et al: Time- and dose-dependent changes in ejection fraction determined by radionuclide angiography after anthracycline therapy. Cancer Treat Rep 62:945–948, 1978
115. Von Hoff D, Layard DW et al: Risk factors for doxorubicin-induced congestive heart failure. Ann Intern Med 91:710–717, 1979
116. Von Hoff DD, Rozencweig M, Layard DW et al: Daunomycin-induced cardiotoxicity in children and adults. A review of 110 cases. Am J Med 62:200–210, 1977
117. Pratt CB, Ransom JL, Evans WE: Age-related adriamycin cardiotoxicity in children. Cancer Treat Rep 62:1381–1384, 1978
118. Fairley KF, Barrie JU, Johnson W: Sterility and testicular atrophy related to cyclophosphamide therapy. Lancet 1:568–569, 1972
119. Kumar R, Biggart JD, McEvoy J et al: Cyclophosphamide and reproductive function. Lancet 1:1212–1213, 1972
120. Miller DG: Alkylating agents and human spermatogenesis. JAMA 217:1662–1665, 1971
121. Richter P, Calamera JC, Morgenfeld MD et al: Effect of chlorambucil on spermatogenesis in the human with malignant lymphoma. Cancer 25:1026–1030, 1970
122. Jacobson RJ, Sagel J, Distiller LA et al: Leydig cell dysfunction in male patients with Hodgkin's disease receiving chemotherapy. Clin Res 26:437A, 1978
123. Cheviakoff J, Calamera JC, Morgenfeld M et al: Recovery of spermatogenesis in patients with lymphoma after treatment with chlorambucil. J Repro Fertil 33:155–157, 1973
124. Qureshi MJA, Goldsmith HJ, Pennington HJ et al: Cyclophosphamide therapy and sterility. Lancet 2:1290–1291, 1972
125. Van Thiel DH, Sherins RJ, Myers GH et al: Evidence for a specific seminiferous tubular factor affecting follicle-stimulating hormone secretion in man. J Clin Invest 51:1009–1019, 1972
126. Chapman RM, Sutcliffe SB, Rees LH et al: Cyclical combination chemotherapy and gonadal function. Lancet 1:285–289, 1979
127. Mecklenberg RS, Sherins RJ: Gonadotropin response to luteinizing hormone releasing hormone in men with germinal aplasia. J Clin Endocrinol Metabol 38:1005–1009, 1974
128. deCunha MF, Meistrich ML, Reid HL et al: Effect of chemotherapy on human sperm production. Proc Am Assoc Cancer Res 20:100, 1979
129. Sieber SM, Correa P, Dalgard DW et al: Carcinogenic and other adverse effects of procarbazine in nonhuman primates. Cancer Res 38:2125–2134, 1978
130. Vilar O: Effect of cytostatic drugs on human testicular function. In Mancini RE, Martini L (eds): Male Fertility and Sterility, pp 423–440. New York, Academic Press, 1974
131. Asbjornsen G, Molne K, Klepp O et al: Testicular function after combination chemotherapy for Hodgkin's disease. Scand J Hematol 16:66–69, 1976
132. Fosdick WM, Parsons JL, Hill DF: Long-term cyclophosphamide therapy in rheumatoid arthritis. Arthritis Rheum 11:151–161, 1968
133. Sherins RJ, DeVita VT: Effects of drug treatment of lymphoma on male reproductive capacity. Ann Intern Med 79:216–220, 1973
134. Roeser HP, Stochs AE, Smith AJ: Testicular damage due to cytotoxic drugs and recovery after cessation of therapy. Aust N Z J Med 8:250–254, 1978
135. Belohorsky B, Siracky J, Sandor L et al: Comments on the development of amenorrhea caused by myleran in cases of chronic myelosis. Neoplasma 4:397–402, 1960
136. Miller JJ, Williams GF, Leissring JC: Multiple late complications of therapy with cyclophosphamide including ovarian destruction. Am J Med 50:530–535, 1971
137. Sobrinho LG, Levine RA, DeConti RC: Amenorrhea in patients with Hodgkin's disease treated with antineoplastic agents. Am J Obstet Gynecol 109:135–139, 1971
138. Galton DAG, Till M, Wiltshaw E: Busulfan: Summary of clinical results. Ann NY Acad Sciences 68:967–973, 1958
139. Louis J, Limarzi LR, Best WR: Treatment of chronic granulocytic leukemia with myleran. Arch Intern Med 97:299–308, 1956
140. Uldall PR, Kerr DNS, Tacchi D: Sterility and cyclophosphamide. Lancet 1:693–694, 1972
141. Warne GL, Fairley KF, Hobbs JB et al: Cyclophosphamide-induced ovarian failure. N Engl J Med 289:1159–1162, 1973
142. Koyama H, Wada T, Nishizawa Y et al: Cyclophosphamide-induced ovarian failure and its therapeutic significance in patients with breast cancer. Cancer 39:1403–1409, 1977
143. Fisher B, Sherman B, Rockette H et al: L-phenylalanine mustard in the management of premenopausal patients with primary breast cancer. Cancer 44:847–857, 1979
144. Chapman RM, Sutcliffe SB, Malpas JS: Cytotoxic-induced ovarian failure in women with Hodgkin's disease I. Hormone function. JAMA 242:1877–1881, 1979
145. Morgenfeld MC, Goldberg V, Parisier H et al: Ovarian lesions due to cytostatic agents during the treatment of Hodgkin's disease. Surg Gynecol Obstet 134:826–828, 1972

146. Sherins R, Winokur S, DeVita VT et al: Surprisingly high risk of functional castration in women receiving chemotherapy for lymphoma. Clin Res 23:343, 1975
147. Arneil GC: Cyclophosphamide and the prepubertal testis. Lancet 2:1259–1260, 1972
148. Kirkland RT, Bongiovanni AM, Cornfeld D et al: Gonadotropin responses to luteinizing releasing factor in boys treated with cyclophosphamide for nephrotic syndrome. J Pediatr 89:941–944, 1976
149. Pennisi AJ, Grushkin CM, Lieberman E: Gonadal function in children with nephrosis treated with cyclophosphamide. Am J Dis Child 129:315–318, 1975
150. Etteldorf JN, West CD, Pitcock JA et al: Gonadal function, testicular histology, and meiosis following cyclophosphamide therapy in patients with nephrotic syndrome. J Pediatr 88:206–212, 1976
151. Lentz RD, Bergstein J, Steffes MW et al: Post-pubertal evaluation of gonadal function following cyclophosphamide therapy before and during puberty. J Pediatr 91:385–394, 1977
152. Rapola J, Koskimies O, Huttanen NP et al: Cyclophosphamide and the pubertal testis. Lancet 1:98–99, 1973
153. Lendon M, Hann IM, Palmer MK et al: Testicular histology after combination chemotherapy in childhood for acute lymphoblastic leukemia. Lancet 2:439–441, 1978
154. Sherins RJ, Olweny CLM, Ziegler JL: Gynecomastia and gonadal dysfunction in adolescent boys treated with combination chemotherapy for Hodgkin's disease. N Engl J Med 299:12–16, 1978
155. Himelstein-Braw R, Peters H, Faber M: Morphologic study of the ovaries of leukemic children. Br J Cancer 38:82–87, 1978
156. Chiu J, Drummond KN: Long-term followup of cyclophosphamide therapy in frequent relapsing minimal lesion nephrotic syndrome. J Pediatr 84:825–830, 1974
157. DeGroot GW, Faiman C, Winter JSD: Cyclophosphamide and the prepubertal gonad: A negative report. J Pediatr 84:123–125, 1974
158. Siris EJ, Leventhal BG, Vaitukaitis JL: Effects of childhood leukemia and chemotherapy on puberty and reproductive function in girls. N Engl J Med 294:1143–1146, 1976
159. Jackson HL, Hass AC, Sooby D et al: The gonadal exposure of boys and young men treated with inverted "Y" fields: It's reduction and genetic significance. Radiology 96:181–186, 1979
160. Ray GR, Trueblood HW, Enright LP et al: Oophoropexy: A means of preserving ovarian function following pelvic megavoltage radiotherapy for Hodgkin's disease. Radiology 96:175–180, 1970
161. Chapman RM, Sutcliffe SB et al: Male gonadal dysfunction in Hodgkin's disease. JAMA 245:1323–1328, 1981.
162. Johnson SA, Goldman JM, Hawkins DF: Pregnancy after chemotherapy for Hodgkin's disease. Lancet 2:93, 1979
163. Li FP, Fine W, Jaffe N et al: Offspring of patients treated for cancer in childhood. J Nat Cancer Inst 62:1193–1197, 1979
164. Van Thiel DH, Ross GT, Lipsett MB: Pregnancies after chemotherapy of trophoblastic neoplasms. Science 169:1326–1327, 1970
165. Holmes GE, Holmes FF: Pregnancy outcome of patients treated for Hodgkin's disease. Cancer 41:1317–1322, 1978
166. Ansbacher R: Artificial insemination with frozen spermatozoa. Fertil Steril 29:375–379, 1978
167. Shamberger RC, Sherins RJ, Rosenberg SA: The effects of postoperative adjuvant chemotherapy and radiotherapy on testicular function in men undergoing treatment for soft tissue sarcoma. Cancer 47:2368–2374, 1981
168. Curie-Cohen M, Luttrell L, Shapiro J: Current practice of artificial insemination by donor in the United States. N Engl J Med 300:585–590, 1979
169. Sherman JK: Synopsis of the use of frozen human semen since 1964: state of the art of human semen banking. Fertil Steril 24:397–412, 1973
170. Buchanan JD, Fairley KF, Barrie JU: Return of spermatogenesis after stopping cyclophosphamide therapy. Lancet 2:156–157, 1975
171. Blatt J, Mulvihill JJ, Ziegler JL et al: Pregnancy outcome following cancer chemotherapy. Am J Med 69:828–832, 1980
172. Blatt J, Poplack DG, Sherins RJ: Testicular function in boys after chemotherapy for acute lymphoplastic leukemia. N Engl J Med 304:1121–1124, 1981
173. Fox BW, Fox M: Biochemical aspects of the actions of drugs on spermatogenesis. Pharmacol Rev 19:21–57, 1967
174. Lu CC, Meistrich ML: Cytotoxic effects of chemotherapeutic drugs on mouse testis cells. Cancer Res 39:3575–3582, 1979
175. Schilsky RL, Lewis BJ, Sherins RJ et al: Gonadal dysfunction in patients receiving chemotherapy for cancer. Ann Intern Med 93:109–114, 1980
176. Sherins RJ, Howards SS: Male infertility. In Harrison JH (ed): Campbell's Urology, 4th ed, pp 715–776. Philadelphia, WB Saunders, 1978
177. Sieber SM, Adamson RH: Toxicity of antineoplastic agents in man: Chromosomal aberrations, antifertility effects, congenital malformations, and carcinogenic potential. Adv Cancer Res 22:57–155, 1975
176. Harris CC: A delayed complication of cancer therapy—Cancer. J Natl Cancer Inst 63:275–277, 1979
177. Sieber SM: The action of antitumor agents: A double-edged sword? Med Pediatr Oncol 3:123–131, 1977
178. IARC Working Group: An evaluation of chemicals and industrial processes associated with cancer in humans based on human and animal data: IARC monographs volumes 1 to 20. Cancer Res 40:1–12, 1980
179. Casciato DA, Scott JL: Acute leukemia following prolonged cytotoxic agent therapy. Medicine 58:32–47, 1979
180. Reimer RR, Hoover R, Fraumeni JF Jr et al: Acute leukemia after alkylating-agent therapy of ovarian cancer. N Engl J Med 297:177–181, 1977
181. Einhorn N: Acute leukemia after chemotherapy (melphalan). Cancer 41:444–447, 1978
182. Pedersen-Bjergaard J, Nissen NI, Sorensen HM et al: Acute non-lymphocytic leukemia in patients with ovarian carcinoma following long-term treatment with treosulfan (= dihydroxybusulfan). Cancer 45:19–29, 1980
183. Chan PYM, Sadoff L, Winkley JH: Second malignancies following first breast cancer in prolonged thiotepa adjuvant chemotherapy. In Salmon SE, Jones SE (eds): Adjuvant Therapy of Cancer, pp 597–607, Amsterdam, North-Holland Biomedical Press, 1977
184. Boice JD, Greene MH, Keehn RJ et al: Late effects of low-dose adjuvant chemotherapy in colorectal cancer. J Natl Cancer Inst 64:501–511, 1980
185. Bergsagel DE, Bailey AJ, Langley GR et al: The chemotherapy of plasma-cell myeloma and the incidence of acute leukemia. N Engl J Med 301:743–748, 1979
186. Gonzalez F, Trujillo JM, Alexanian R: Acute leukemia in multiple myeloma. Ann Intern Med 86:440–443, 1977
187. Rosner F, Grunwald H: Hodgkin's disease and acute leukemia. Am J Med 58:339–353, 1975
188. Woodruff RK, Brearley RL, Whitehouse JMA et al: Hodgkin's disease occurring during acute leukaemia in remission. Lancet 2:900–903, 1977
189. Brody RS, Schottenfeld D, Reid A: Multiple primary cancer risk after therapy for Hodgkin's disease. Cancer 40:1917–1926, 1977
190. Canellos GP, DeVita VT, Arseneau JC et al: Second malignancies complicating Hodgkin's disease in remission. Lancet 1:847–950, 1975
191. Canellos GP: Second malignancies complicating Hodgkin's disease in remission. Lancet 1:1294, 1975
192. Coleman CN, Williams CJ, Flint A et al: Hematologic neoplasia in patients treated for Hodgkin's disease. N Engl J Med 297:1249–1252, 1977
193. Krikorian JG, Burke JS, Rosenberg SA et al: Occurrence of non-Hodgkin's lymphoma after therapy for Hodgkin's disease. N Engl J Med 300:452–458, 1979
194. Toland DM, Coltman CA, Moon TE: Second malignancies complicating Hodgkin's disease: The Southwest Oncology Group experience. Cancer Clinical Trials 1:27–33, 1978
195. Pajak TF, Nissen NI, Stutzman L et al: Acute myeloid leukemia (AML) occurring during complete remission (CR) in Hodgkin's disease. Proc AACR and ASCO 20:394, 1979
196. Neufield H, Weinerman BH, Kemel S: Secondary malignant

neoplasms in patients with Hodgkin's disease. JAMA 239:2470–2471, 1978
197. Larsen J, Brincker H: The incidence and characteristics of acute myeloid leukaemia arising in Hodgkin's disease. Scand J Hematol 18:197–206, 1977
198. Valagussa P, Santoro A, Kenda R et al: Second malignancies in Hodgkin's disease: a complication of certain forms of treatment. Br Med J 280:216–219, 1980
199. Rowley JD, Golomb HM, Vardiman J: Nonrandom chromosomal abnormalities in acute nonlymphocytic leukemia in patients treated for Hodgkin disease and non-Hodgkin lymphomas. Blood 50:759–770, 1977
200. Bloomfield CD, Brunning RD: Acute leukemia as a terminal event in nonleukemic hematopoietic disorders. Semin Oncol 3:297–317, 1976
201. Silverstein MN, Goldberg JD, Balcerzak SP et al: The incidence of acute leukemia in a randomized clinical trial for polycythemia vera. Blood (Suppl) 54:209a, 1979
202. Theide T, Christensen BC: Bladder tumors induced by chlornaphazine. Acta Med Scand 185:133–137, 1969
203. Videbaek A: Chlornaphazin (Erysan) may induce cancer of the urinary bladder. Acta Med Scand 176:45–50, 1964
204. Fairchild WV, Spence CR, Solomon HD et al: The incidence of bladder cancer after cyclophosphamide therapy. J Urol 122:163–164, 1979
205. Plotz PH, Klippel JH, Decker JL et al: Bladder complications in patients receiving cyclophosphamide for systemic lypus erythematosus or rheumatoid arthritis. Ann Intern Med 91:221–223, 1979
206. Wall RL, Clausen KP: Carcinoma of the urinary bladder in patients receiving cyclophosphamide. N Engl J Med 293:271–273, 1975
207. Pearson RM, Soloway MS: Does cyclophosphamide induce bladder cancer? Urology 11:437–447, 1978
208. Fraumeni JF Jr, Hoover R: Immunosurveillance and cancer: epidemiologic observations. Natl Cancer Inst Monogr 47:121–126, 1977
209. Krikorian JG, Anderson JL, Bieber CP et al: Malignant neoplasms following cardiac transplantation. J Am Med Assoc 240:639–643, 1978
210. Matas AJ, Simmons RL, Kjellstrand CM et al: Increased incidence of malignancy in uremic patients and its significance to transplantation. Transplant Proc 9:1137–1140, 1977
211. Schoenberg BS, Myers MH: Statistical methods for studying multiple primary malignant neoplasms. Cancer 40:1892–1898, 1977
212. Brody RS, Schottenfeld D: Multiple primary cancers in Hodgkin's disease. Semin Oncol 7:187–201, 1080
213. National Academy of Sciences—National Research Council: The effects on populations of exposure to low levels of ionizing radiation. Washington, DC, National Academy of Sciences, 1972
214. International Commission on Radiological Protection: Annals of the ICRP. Oxford, Pergamon Press, 1977
215. Hutchison GB: Late neoplastic changes following medical irradiation. Radiology 105:645–652, 1977
216. Hutchison GB: Carcinogenic effects of medical irradiation. In Hiatt HH, Watson JD, Winsten JA (eds): Origins of Human Cancer, pp 501–507. Cold Spring Harbor Laboratory, 1977
217. Shore RE, Albert RE, Pasternak BS: Follow-up study of patients treated by X-ray epilation for tinea capitis. Arch Environ Health 31:21–28, 1976
218. Hempelmann LH, Hall WJ, Phillips M et al: Neoplasms in persons treated with x-rays in infancy: Fourth survey in 20 years. J Natl Cancer Inst 55:519–530, 1975
219. Court-Brown WM, Doll R: Mortality from cancer and other causes after radiotherapy for ankylosing spondylitis. Br Med J 2:1327–1332, 1965
220. Doll R, Smith PG: The long-term effects of X-irradiation in patients treated for metropathia haemorrhagica. Br J Radiol 41:362–368, 1968
221. Shore RE, Hempelmann LH, Kowaluk E et al: Breast neoplasms in women treated with X-rays for acute postpartum mastitis. J Natl Cancer Inst 59:813–822, 1977
222. Boice JD, Monson RR: Breast cancer in women after repeated fluoroscopic examinations of the chest. J Natl Cancer Inst 59:823–832, 1977
223. Bizzozero OJ, Johnson KG, Ciocco A et al: Radiation-related leukemia in Hiroshima and Nagasaki 1946–1964. II. Observations of type-specific leukemia, survivorship, and clinical behavior. Ann Intern Med 66:522–530, 1967
224. Meadows AT, D'Angio GJ, Mike V et al: Patterns of second malignant neoplasms in children. Cancer 40:1903–1911, 1977
225. Li FP, Cassady JR, Jaffe N: Risk of second tumors in survivors of childhood cancer. Cancer 35:1230–1235, 1975
226. Boice JD, Hutchison GB: Leukemia in women following radiotherapy for cervical cancer: ten year follow-up of an international study. J Natl Cancer Inst 65:115–129, 1980
227. Morton RF, Villasanta U: New cancers arising in 1,563 patients with carcinoma of the cervix treated by irradiation. Am J Obstet Gynecol 115:462–466, 1973
228. Rodriguez V, Bodey GP, Trujillo JM et al: Previous radiation exposure in patients with leukemia. Arch Intern Med 132:874–877, 1973
229. Kim JH, Chu FC, Woodard HQ et al: Radiation-induced soft-tissue and bone sarcoma. Radiology 129:501–508, 1978
230. Upton AC: Radiation effects. In Hiatt HH, Watson JD, Winsten JA (eds): Origins of Human Cancer, pp 474–500. Cold Spring Harbor Laboratory, 1977
231. Beebe GW, Kato H, Land CE: Studies of the mortality of A-bomb survivors. Radiat Res 75:138–201, 1978
232. Modan B, Ron E, Werner A: Thyroid cancer following scalp irradiation. Radiology 123:741–744, 1977
233. McDougall IR, Coleman CN, Burke JS et al: Thyroid carcinoma after high-dose external radiotherapy for Hodgkin's disease—Report of three cases. Cancer 45:2056–2060, 1980
234. Shellabarger CJ: Radiation carcinogenesis—laboratory studies. Cancer 37:1090–1096, 1976
235. Holm L, Dahlqvist I, Israelsson A et al: Malignant thyroid tumors after iodine-131 therapy—a retrospective cohort study. N Engl J Med 303:188–191, 1980
236. Sagerman RH, Cassady JR, Tretter P et al: Radiation induced neoplasia following external beam therapy for children with retinoblastoma. Am J Roentgenol Radium Ther Nucl Med 105:529–535, 1969
237. Haselow RE, Nesbit M, Dehner LP et al: Second neoplasms following megavoltage radiation in a pediatric population. Cancer 42:1185–1191, 1978
238. McCredie JA, Inch WR, Alderson M: Consecutive primary carcinomas of the breast. Cancer 35:1472–1477, 1975
239. D'Angio GJ, Meadows A, Mike V et al: Decreased risk of radiation-associated second malignant neoplasms in actinomycin-D-treated patients. Cancer 37:1177–1185, 1976
240. D'Angio GJ, Hahn EW, Feingold SM et al: Actinomycin D and radiation-associated mammary cancer (MCa) in rates. Proc AACR and ASCO 21:85, 1980
241. Tefft M, Vawter GF, Mitus A: Second primary neoplasms in children. Am J Roentgenol 103:800–822, 1968
242. Schneider AB, Favus MJ, Stachura ME et al: Incidence, prevalence and characteristics of radiation-induced thyroid tumors. Am J Med 64:243–252, 1978
243. Li FP: Second malignant tumors after cancer in childhood. Cancer 40:1899–1902, 1977
244. Makuch R, Simon R: Recommendations for the analysis of the effect of treatment on the development of second malignancies. Cancer 44:250–253, 1979
245. Wynder EL, Mushinski MH, Spivak JC: Tobacco and alcohol consumption in relation to the development of multiple primary cancers. Cancer 40:1872–1878, 1977
246. Mulvihill JJ: Genetic reperatory of human neoplasia. In Mulvihill JJ, Miller RW, Fraumeni JF Jr (eds): Genetics of Human Cancer. New York, Raven Press, 1977
247. Lynch HT, Frichot BC III: Skin, heredity, and cancer. Semin Oncol 5:67–84, 1978
248. McKeen EA, Bodurtha J, Meadows AT et al: Rhabdomyosarcoma complicating multiple neurofibromatosis. J Pediatr 94:173–174, 1979

249. Kraemer KH, Coon HG, Petinga RA et al: Genetic heterogeneity in xeroderma pigmentosum: complementation groups and their relationship to DNA repair rates. Proc Natl Acad Sci USA 72:59–63, 1975
250. Hethcote HW, Knudson AG Jr: Model for the incidence of embryonal cancers: application to retinoblastoma. Proc Natl Acad Sci USA 75:2453–2457, 1978
251. Knudson AG Jr, Strong LC, Anderson DE: Heredity and cancer in man. Prog Med Genet 9:113–158, 1973
252. Fraumeni JF Jr: Clinical patterns of familial cancer. In Mulvihill JJ, Miller RW, Fraumeni JF Jr (eds): Genetics of Human Cancer. New York, Raven Press, 1977
253. Moertel CG: Multiple primary malignant neoplasms. Cancer 40:1786–1792, 1977
254. Strong LC: Genetic and environmental interactions. Cancer 40:1861–1866, 1977
255. Weichselbaum RR, Nove J, Little JB: X-ray sensitivity of diploid fibroblasts from patients with hereditary or sporadic retinoblastoma. Proc Natl Acad Sci USA 75:3962–3964, 1978
256. Levin S, Perlov S: Ataxia-telangiectasia in Israel with observations on its relationship to malignant disease. Israel J Med Sci 7:1535–1541, 1971
257. Lotan R: Different susceptibilities of human melanoma and breast carcinoma cell lines to retinoic acid-induced growth inhibition. Cancer Res 39:1014–1019, 1979
258. Cohen RJ, Wiernik PH, Walker MD: Acute nonlymphocytic leukemia associated with nitrosourea chemotherapy: Report of two cases. Cancer Treat Rep 60:1257–1261, 1976
259. Harmon WE, Cohen HJ, Schneeberger EE et al: Chronic renal failure in children treated with methyl CCNU. N Engl J Med 300:1200–1203, 1979
260. Leopold WR, Miller EC, Miller JA: Carcinogenicity of antitumor cis-platinum(11) coordination complexes in the mouse and rat. Cancer Res 39:913–918, 1979
261. Walters TR: Childhood acute lymphocytic leukemia with a second primary neoplasm. Am J Pediatr Hematol Oncol 1:285–287, 1979
262. Lerner HJ: Acute myelogenous leukemia in patients receiving chlorambucil as long term adjuvant chemotherapy for stage II breast cancer. Cancer Treat Rep 62:1135–1138, 1978
263. Einhorn LH, Donohue J: Cis-diamminedichloroplatinum, vinblastine, and bleomycin combination chemotherapy in disseminated testicular cancer. Ann Intern Med 87:293–198, 1977

Joel A. DeLisa
Robert M. Miller
Rosalie Raps Melnick
Mary Ann Mikulic

CHAPTER 46

Rehabilitation of the Cancer Patient

Of the approximately 655,000 newly diagnosed cases of cancer in the U.S. each year, and the approximately 1.5 million Americans who are considered to be cured, a significant number will experience functional limitations due to their disease or its treatment.[1] In a random sample of 805 cancer patients, Lehmann demonstrated that a significant number of these patients had functional disabilities that could be treated by rehabilitation techniques.[2] The primary barrier to optimal rehabilitation in the cancer patient was failure to identify functional problems. Physicians in general were unfamiliar with the concepts of rehabilitation and its value for cancer patients, resulting in a lack of appropriate referrals. Table 46-1 identifies functional problems in cancer patients and the results of rehabilitation techniques.

Some of the rehabilitation concepts and techniques that can be used with cancer patients are described in this chapter. With a clear understanding of the principles and tools of rehabilitation, the primary care physician should be able to identify patients with functional problems and make appropriate rehabilitation referrals. Rehabilitation should start as soon as diagnosis is made and should be implemented throughout the entire spectrum of care, not only directly after the surgical or medical treatment.

Rehabilitation is best defined as the development of the disabled patient to the fullest physical, psychological, social, vocational, avocational, and educational potential. This should be consistent with physiologic and environmental limitations and realistic goals determined by the patient and the medical team. Rehabilitation enables the disabled to become independent in all aspects of life. Rehabilitation professionals and the patient share responsibility in achieving maximum independence, addressing illness management, along with the problems that might be encountered. Rehabilitation considers the affected anatomical site, histology, stage of cancer, treatments used, metastasis, patient age, and prognosis.

Emphasis is placed on the functional assessment of each patient, such as evaluating performance and activities of daily living (ADL). ADL include personal care (feeding, grooming, bathing, dressing), the mobility spectrum (bed mobility, transfers to and from bed, wheelchair, or commode, wheelchair propulsion, ambulation, stair climbing, and driving). Rehabilitation assessment includes evaluation of both psychological and social functioning to identify potential problems and resources.

Therapeutic interventions are directed toward maximizing functional capabilities and prevention of secondary complications. To attain the desired goals, the principles of energy conservation and work simplification are employed. For example, the housewife may be advised to change her work habits so that she uses a utility cart in table setting. Reorganization of the kitchen will improve work flow.

By following the specific physical treatment regimens, and the environment through work modification or adaptive equipment, improved function can be achieved. Patients may also be assisted in making behavioral changes to attain their psychological and social goals.

To remove some of the barriers in rehabilitation, Lehmann devised a successful model. This was to have the physiatrist provide the link between the clinical oncology team (radiation oncologist, general surgeon, medical oncologist, gynecologist, otolaryngologist, and other medical and surgical specialists) and the comprehensive rehabilitation team. All cancer patients were automatically screened by a trained cancer rehabilitation coordinator. Then, those with functional problems were seen by the physiatrist and appropriate specialists on the rehabilitation team.

Since rehabilitation is a holistic and comprehensive approach, the combined expertise of a multidisciplinary team is necessary. The multidisciplinary team uses an approach that accentuates the patient's remaining abilities. Team members evaluate patients according to their clinical specialty and then join in a team conference to develop a comprehensive functional problem list. It is usually led by the physician in charge. An individualized therapeutic rehabilitation plan is then defined and implemented so that the patient may function within the limitations of the disease.

The team must deal with death and dying, adjusting to radical fluctuations in patients' medical and psychological states. These can range from a sense of well-being to extreme pain and nausea sometimes brought on by the treatment. This can cause difficulties in determining clear and realistic performance expectations. Some cancer patients may remain dependent instead of striving for independence. Then the team must readjust its goals and expectations to avoid feelings of failure in the patient.

Patients are perceived as the co-managers of their rehabilitation. The successful team approach contains coordination, cooperation, and open communication.

TABLE 46-1. Percentage of People in Sample with One or More Rehabilitation Problems

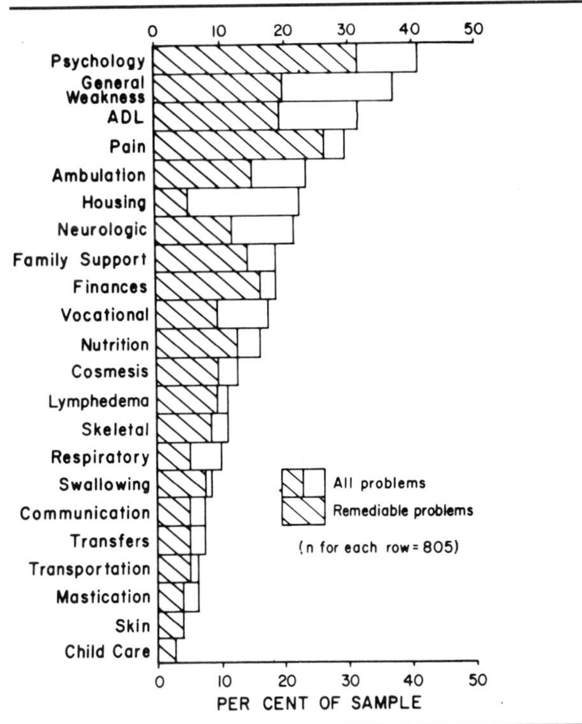

(Lehmann JF, DeLisa JA, Warren CG et al: Cancer rehabilitation: Assessment of need, development, and evaluation of a model of care. Arch Phys Med Rehabil 59:410–419, 1978)

THE OCCUPATIONAL THERAPIST

The occupational therapist can provide many services to cancer patients. These include the following:

1. Evaluation and training of self-care activities, such as dressing, eating, bathing, and personal hygiene to maximize independence, utilizing orthoses, or adaptive equipment, when necessary
2. Provide training in home management skills, providing simpler methods to minimize fatigue and conserve energy
3. Explore vocational skills and avocational interests; working with the vocational counselor when a change in employment is anticipated
4. Aid in maintaining and improving joint range of motion (ROM), muscle strength, endurance, and coordination.
5. Evaluate and train the patient in weak areas to compensate for those sensory and perceptual deficits
6. Evaluate the home and suggest modifications to provide a barrier-free environment
7. Assess driving habits and retrain when necessary, with the assistance of appropriate devices when necessary
8. Educate the family by demonstrating techniques designed to maintain maximum patient independence and to minimize overprotection
9. Train in the functional use of an upper extremity prosthesis.

THE PHYSICAL THERAPIST

The physical therapist assists the patient in functional restoration. Tasks may include the following:

1. Provide joint ROM measurements and exercises to maintain and increase ROM
2. Perform muscle strength evaluation and quantification
3. Evaluate sitting and standing balance, transfers, and ambulation, including wheelchair and bipedal. Progressive gait training may be offered and includes rough ground, ramps, and stairs
4. Offer exercises to increase strength, endurance, and coordination for either specific muscle groups or the entire body
5. Use of modalities, both superficial and deep heat and cold, as well as hydrotherapy techniques, electrical stimulation, traction, and massage
6. Aid in home evaluations to make the environment barrier-free and accessible

THE PROSTHETIST–ORTHOTIST

The prosthetist–orthotist is responsible for the design, fabrication, and fitting of the orthosis (brace) and prosthesis (artificial limb). The prosthetist–orthotist makes certain that the device functions and fits properly, and that the patient adjusts well to its presence. Patient and family instruction in the care of the prosthesis and follow-up maintenance and repair should also be stressed.

THE REHABILITATION NURSE

Rehabilitation nursing involves assessment of the health status of the individual and determines short- and long-range goals for the patient. The nurse provides information on the physical, social, and behavioral sciences and shows an awareness of attitudes toward the disabled.

Rehabilitation nursing therapy is similar to nursing in other settings. However, the functions of the rehabilitation nurse emphasize certain priorities related to promoting maximal function. The nurse must be constantly vigilant for any small skills and environmental modifications that can make the difference between dependence and independence. Nursing therapy is responsible for assessing the client and developing a nursing care plan which addresses, but is not limited to, the following.

1. Hygienic factors
2. Environmental factors (heat and noise, control of personal property, sanitation including infection control, and safety)
3. Assistance with adaptive equipment needed by patients to communicate, eat, move, eliminate, dress, and ambulate
4. Utilize specific preventive measures to minimize the effects of inactivity
5. Specify measures to promote optimal independence
6. Help the patient integrate the various therapies into their daily activities

THE SPEECH PATHOLOGIST

Patients with diagnosed carcinoma of the oral, nasal, pharyngeal, and laryngeal structures may have problems with speaking and swallowing. The speech pathologist can help in the following areas:

1. Evaluation and treatment of neurological communication problems
2. Vocal reeducation
3. Preoperative counseling prior to laryngectomy or glossectomy
4. Alaryngeal speech training (esophageal speech, or use of a prosthetic larynx)
5. Retraining speech in patients with intra-oral defects (*i.e.*, glossectomy, palatectomy)
6. Managing dysphagia

THE PSYCHOLOGIST

The psychologist helps the patient and significant others to psychologically prepare for full participation in rehabilitation. This can involve a number of activities, including:

1. Testing involving
   Personality, style (manipulative, dependent, dogmatic)
   Ways of dealing with stress
   Problem solving skills
   Psychological status (neurosis, psychosis)
2. Incorporation of the test results into the care plan
3. Counseling in
   Adjustment to body changes
   Development of problem solving skills
   Secondary problems caused by the disease and its treatment
   Adjustment to changes in sexual functioning and viable alternatives
   Death and dying
4. Testing of intelligence, memory, and perceptual functioning

THE SOCIAL WORKER

The social worker interacts with the patient, family, and rehabilitation team, and can assist in the following ways:

1. Evaluating the patient's total living situation, including life style, family, finances and community resources, and assess the impact of cancer on these areas
2. Maintaining a continuing relationship with the patient and family
3. Discussing arrangements and concerns about finances
4. Helping the family develop the skills needed to actively participate in treatment procedures in the home
5. Providing assistance in locating alternative living situations

THE VOCATIONAL COUNSELOR

Some major areas of responsibility for vocational counselors with respect to cancer patients include:

1. Evaluating vocational interests, aptitudes, and skills
2. Counseling patients who must shift to alternate occupations
3. Organizing activities, individual or group, to improve job related behaviors (*i.e.*, job interview skills, work skills, employer–employee relationship behaviors)
4. Acting as a liaison between agencies that provide training or job placement services and the patient
5. Providing counseling and education to potential employers of these patients

Other team members may include a psychiatrist, enterostomal therapist, maxillofacial prosthetist, dentist, dietitian, or chaplain.

PSYCHOLOGICAL, SOCIAL, VOCATIONAL, AND DISCHARGE PLANNING ISSUES

There are many possible psychological and social issues related to cancer rehabilitation. They can have a significant effect on rehabilitation, quality of life, and life styles, and are likely to begin with the first suspicion or diagnosis of cancer. These effects remain throughout the patient's lifetime. The type and magnitude of the concerns, fears, and problems will vary with the type and site of the cancer, and will fluctuate in intensity and focus throughout the course of the disease.

The effect of cancer and its treatment on the quality of life has been described by Devlin, Plant, and Griffith in an article on the aftermath of anorectal surgery.[3] They concluded that there is an "immense price paid in physical discomfort and in psychological and social trauma" and further that "society has determined life must be saved at all costs, and the skill of the surgeon is directed toward this end. We have shown that it is now time to look more closely at the costs and at those who bear them; more emphasis must now be placed on the quality of the life saved."[3] The rehabilitation team can offer assistance here by maximizing the patient's functional abilities.

Psychological and social concerns must be included in the treatment plan from the beginning by assessing psychological and social functioning at the onset. All team members must share responsibility for the psychosocial aspects of care.

Very few cancer patients receive vocational rehabilitation, though many would benefit from it. This may be due to the fact that in many states, the laws are written in such a way that cancer patients are ineligible for vocational rehabilitation benefits. Vocational assessment should then too be an integral part of the treatment from the beginning, with vocational needs identified early. Once these needs are known, appropriate recommendations and referrals can be made.

Early consideration of vocational aspects of rehabilitation may have a positive effect on the patient's adjustment to the disease and thus may increase the desire for rehabilitation. With this approach and careful data collection on the results of vocational rehabilitation there is the potential to change the laws that discriminate against cancer patients in vocational rehabilitation.

Medical intervention requires changes in the cancer patient's lifestyle. Even small skin lesions require changes like using skin creams, protective clothing, and staying out of the sun. Such changes range from minor inconveniences to radical changes in the patient's physical and intellectual functioning or appearance. These changes must be dealt with throughout the treatment and aggressively tackled as a part of rehabilitation. One of the main determinants in the success or failure of rehabilitation efforts will be the psychological condition of the patient and family. It can affect the patient's readiness to learn and the ability to work in therapy.

To wait until psychosocial problems arise is unfair to the patient and will unnecessarily impede recovery and rehabilitation. Ongoing preventive psychological intervention and social support helps to minimize problems and, in turn, improves the rehabilitation process.

Another area of psychological and social concern is physical body changes, their impact on the patient's self and body image, and social implications imposed by self or others. Loss of body parts or functions, intellectual changes, or treatment residuals are painful for the patient and often ignored by professionals, perhaps because of their own discomfort with these issues. This must be dealt with from the onset if the patient is to be truly ready for rehabilitation. It is incumbent upon the primary care physician to either provide counseling and education in these areas or refer the patient and the family to resource people who will.

Sexuality and sex-related issues are frequent concerns for patients with cancer. Some of these concerns are directly related to cancer or the effects of treatment (*e.g.*, impotence, paralysis, stomas, amputation). Others are related to how they feel about the cancer and its resulting physical or functional changes.

Regardless of the problem or its source, sexuality and sex-related issues deserve the full attention of appropriate health care providers. In some cases, the intervention is aimed at actual behavior considerations and changes, while in other cases the main requirement will be psychological intervention and adjustment See Chapter 12 for discussion of sexual dysfunction in cancer patients.

There are various psychological and social intervention procedures that should be under the guidance of trained professionals. A one–to–one interview with the psychologist and social worker is a good start. The format from then on will vary. Useful techniques may include ongoing individual counseling, psychiatric referral for medications, support groups with other cancer patients, family groups for spouse and children, couples counseling, and visits by previously rehabilitated patients. These should all be available and used appropriately throughout treatment, and as needed thereafter. If psychological and social intervention is needed and is not provided in a timely and appropriate manner, cancer treatment and rehabilitation can never be considered a success regardless of the medical results.

COMPLICATIONS OF INACTIVITY/DISUSE SYNDROME

Complications can add significantly to the patient's disability by decreasing functional abilities and necessitating more health care resources for maintenance. For example, prolonged bedrest can be harmful to the body because of its deconditioning effects. It may decompensate the patient who is marginally independent to the extent of requiring total care. Since it is easier to prevent than to treat these complications, prophylactic programs should be prescribed for all bed-ridden patients.[4]

Inactivity and immobilization can affect the following body systems: musculoskeletal, cardiovascular, respiratory, endocrine, urinary, digestive, and dermatological.[5] Inactivity and immobilization can also affect mental status, lead to psychological problems, and create situations that necessitate social work intervention. Since most of this data comes from studies on healthy volunteers, cancer patients whose immune response has been altered by the disease, or whose nerves and hematopoietic systems have been subjected to chemotherapy may be more susceptible.

Effect on the Musculoskeletal System

Musculoskeletal complications include contractures, decreased muscle strength, decreased endurance, and osteoporosis. A contracture is a limitation of active and passive joint ROM owing to a pathological condition, affecting the skin, subcutaneous tissue, muscle, ligament, joint capsule, or synovium. Contractures can impair mobility, self-care, and function. With motion impaired, more muscular energy is required to accomplish the musculoskeletal activity, causing rapid fatigue.[5]

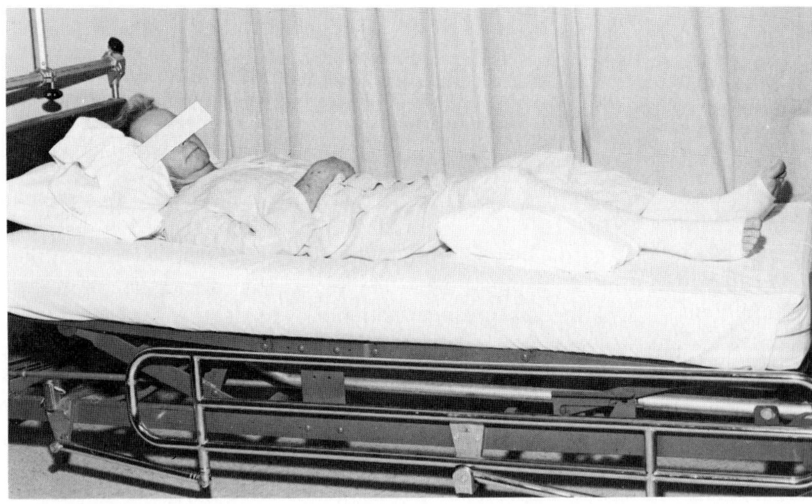

FIG. 46-1. Improper bed positioning (pillows under neck and knees) contributes to development of flexion contractures.

Connective tissue and its collagen fibers provide support for organs, binding their cells and tissues together. Collagen fibers will not maintain their optimal length unless they are frequently stretched, which normally occurs during body motion. If a muscle is immobilized in a shortened position, the collagen fibers will shorten and deformity may occur. The loose connective tissue may become dense, thus restricting ROM. Edema, stasis, and bleeding tend to increase the formation of this dense connective tissue. Dynamic muscle imbalance due to paralysis or spasticity that malpositions joints, and degenerative or ischemic muscle disease that causes structural changes can further increase the contracture development.

Improper bed positioning can also lead to problems. Soft mattresses or the use of pillows under the knees or behind the neck of a supine patient can exacerbate the development of flexion contractures (see Fig. 22-1). This can hamper bed mobility, transfers, ambulation, and cause backaches. Without bedrest precautions, it is common to see contractures with the hips flexed, abducted and externally rotated, knees flexed and feet plantar flexed. This inhibits standing and ambulation, which requires full ROM in hips, knees, and ankles.

These contractures can be prevented through good nursing care, using trochanteric roll, avoiding knee pillows, using a foot board and posterior leg splints, along with ROM exercises performed twice daily. ROM exercises can be performed by therapists, nurses, patients, or taught to family members. ROM exercises may be passive, as the therapist moves the extremity through the full ROM, or active-assistive, as the patient initiates and the therapist completes, taking the joint through its full ROM. Active ROM requires the patient to move the joint through its full ROM without assistance.

A hip flexion contracture is difficult to stretch, even when using ultrasound and static stretch. This is because it is hard to adequately stabilize the pelvis to obtain three-point pressure. Knee contractions greater than 15° can also be difficult to stretch manually, even with the use of heat. This is especially true in the elderly patient.

A patient confined to bed will lose muscle strength and endurance, and develop atrophy. In normal subjects, a muscle at complete rest (no muscle tension is exerted) will lose 10–15% of its physical strength weekly—approximately 3–5% daily.[5,6] A muscle immobilized for 3–5 weeks will lose half of its strength. Additional disease processes, pre-existing weakness, or age may further reduce strength. Conversely, it takes about 60 days to increase muscle strength 10%; hence, it is much easier to lose than to gain. Fortunately, muscle strength can be maintained if the normal muscle undergoes an isometric contraction at a tension that is 20–30% of maximum for several seconds daily.[6] If the tension generated by the contraction is less than 20% of maximum, strength continues to decrease. Motor strength is clinically measured by the manual muscle testing and grading scheme described in Table 46-2. Examples of exercises to maintain strength while bed-ridden are noted in Table 46-3 and in Figures 46-2, 46-3, and 46-4.

Endurance decreases from disuse. In fact, disuse affects endurance more than instantaneous strength, as it adversely affects blood supply and metabolic demand of the muscle.[5]

TABLE 46-2. Quantifying Manual Motor Strength

GRADE	TEST PERFORMANCE
5/5	Normal power. The muscle can move the joint through the full ROM, against gravity and against maximum resistance applied by the examiner.
4/5	The muscle can move the joint through the full ROM, against gravity and against some, but not full, examiner resistance.
3/5	The muscle can move the joint through the full ROM, against gravity, but with no examiner resistance.
2/5	The muscle can move the joint through full ROM, but only with gravity eliminated and no examiner resistance.
1/5	Contraction of the muscle can be seen or felt, but is of insufficient strength to produce movement even with gravity eliminated.
0/5	Complete paralysis. No visible or palpable contraction of the muscle even with gravity eliminated.

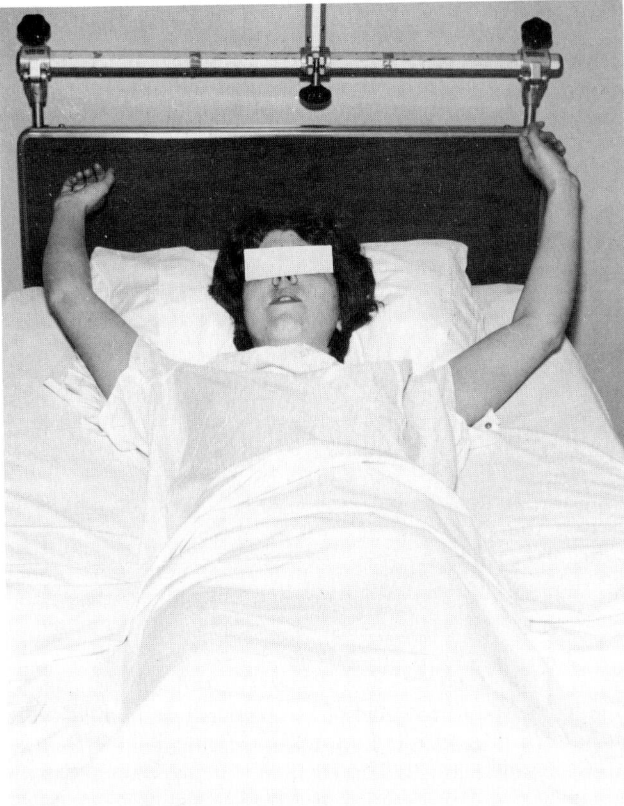

FIG. 46-2. To maintain active shoulder ROM in the supine position, the patient raises both arms out to the side, bends the elbow, and reaches behind the head. The sequence is completed by having the patient return the arms to the side

TABLE 46-3. Exercise for the Bed Rest Patient

1. Passive ROM to all extremities once or twice a day, depending on tightness and tone abnormalities, until patient is able to assist with exercises.
2. Have patient assist with all self care as soon as possible.
3. Active ROM may be accomplished unilaterally or bilaterally while in the supine position.

Shoulder:
a. Shrug shoulders in a circular motion
b. Raise arm above head, keeping elbow straight. Return arm to the side.
c. Raise arm out to the side; flex elbow and reach behind the head. Return arm to the side.
d. Grasp hands behind head, force elbows back and down.

Elbow:
a. With palms up, touch hand to shoulder, return with palm down.

Wrists:
a. Make circular motions with the wrist
b. Make an "O" with thumb and each finger

Fingers:
a. Squeeze a ball.
b. Make an "O" with thumb and each fingertip

Hip:
a. Raise one leg up at hip, keeping the knee straight, then relax. Repeat with the opposite leg.
b. Flex knee and hip up toward chest, relax. Repeat with opposite leg.
c. Flex knees up and place feet flat on the bed. Tighten buttock muscles, lifting buttocks up. Relax.
d. Perform isometric quadriceps sets
e. With the leg straight, move the leg out to side. Return. Repeat with opposite leg.
f. With the leg straight, roll the knee in and out.

Foot:
a. Dorsiflex and plantarflex the ankles
b. Make a circular motion with the feet.

Trunk:
a. With the hip and knees flexed and the feet flat on the bed, flex the chin and slowly curl up reaching for the knees. Hold 3–5 seconds, relax.

Hip and Trunk:
a. Flex knees and place feet flat on the bed. Tighten buttock muscles, lifting buttocks up. Hold for 3–5 seconds. Relax.
b. With the hips and knees flexed and feet flat on the bed, rotate both legs to the right, then to the left, keeping knees together.

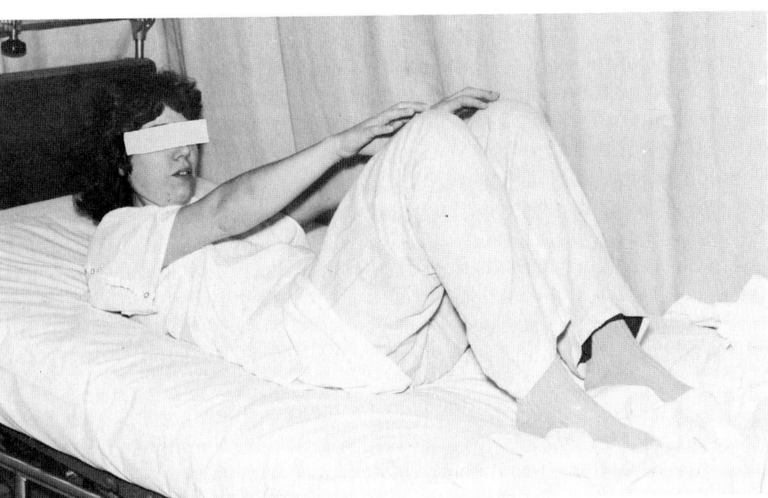

FIG. 46-3. Active ROM exercises for the trunk are performed while supine with the hips and knees flexed and the feet flat on the bed. The patient then flexes the chin and slowly curls up reaching for the knees. The patient holds for 3–5 seconds and then relaxes.

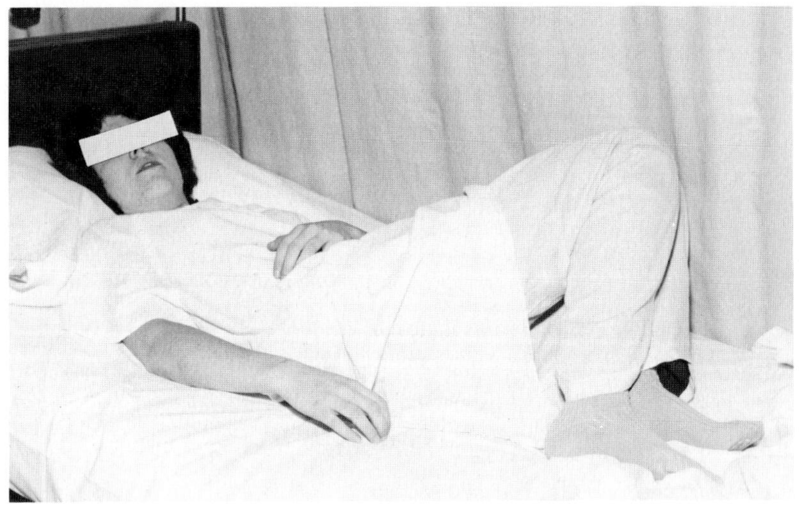

FIG. 46-4. Another hip and trunk active ROM exercise in the supine position is to have the hips and knees flexed with the feet flat on the bed, keeping the knees together. The legs are then rotated from the right to the left.

Reduced endurance may cause CNS fatigue, reduce patient motivation, and decrease the beneficial effects of rehabilitation.

Prescriptions for bedside exercises to maintain strength can prevent these complications. Such prescriptions should contain (1) type, (2) intensity, (3) duration, and (4) frequency of the exercise.

Effect on the Cardiovascular System

One of the most dramatic dangers of prolonged bedrest is the inability of the circulatory system to readjust to the upright position. When a normal person stands from the supine position, heart rate increases an average of 10–20 beats per minute.[7] Systolic blood pressure decreases an average of 14 mmHg and 500 cc of blood volume is redistributed from the thorax to the legs.[8]

The ability of normal subjects to adapt to the upright position may be lost or severely impaired after 3 weeks of forced bedrest, owing to impairment of the autonomic control of the heart and the peripheral circulation. It may occur faster in a patient receiving chemotherapy. In a study by Deitrick, after 3 weeks of forced bedrest, a significant increase of heart rate and decrease of pulse pressure of 40–70% was found from levels obtained in the horizontal resting position, and fainting episodes were frequent.[9] These normal subjects were unable to maintain stable pulse and blood pressure, despite a strong sympathetic response that was manifested by sweating, pallor, and restlessness. In reestablishing the normal orthostatic reflexes, it took 3–4 weeks after the subject became ambulatory for the pulse and blood pressure to return to prebedrest values. Older patients are more susceptible to these cardiovascular changes.

The specific therapies used to reestablish the orthostatic reflexes are (1) early mobilization of body parts not affected by the pathology, (2) active and passive ROM exercises, (3) utilization of the tilt table, and (4) use of an electric hospital bed.

With bedrest there are changes in blood volume and viscosity, which results in an increased risk of thrombophlebitis. Greenleaf found that the reduction in plasma volume can be limited by exercises, isotonic being more effective than isometric.[10]

Effect on the Respiratory System

Due to the splinting effect of the bed, breathing tends to be shallower and less frequent, with consequent reduced aeration of the posterior lungs. The clearance of secretions from the bronchial tree is decreased and there is atelectasis and an increased incidence of respiratory infection. Pulmonary embolus is another frequent complication. Early mobilization may help prevent some of these problems.

Effect on the Endocrine System

During bedrest, the anabolic process of tissue building is slowed, while the catabolic process that breaks down tissues is increased. An increase in catabolism of protein, which leads to a negative nitrogen balance, results in slow healing of wounds and decubitis.[9]

A negative calcium balance also exists after prolonged recumbency.[9] This is in part due to calcium being absorbed from bones that are not stressed by body weight or muscle contraction, and may result in osteoporosis. In osteoporetic bone, the strength and density are decreased, with resultant fractures. Exercise, activity, and diet can reduce this negative calcium balance.

Effect on the Urinary System

Inactivity can lead to the development of urinary retention, renal stones, and urinary tract infections. Difficulty in urinating is directly related to position. Incomplete emptying is a function of both the stasis in the entire urinary tract and decreased muscle functioning which interferes with bearing down to void.

Excessive calcium loss and its excretion in the urine, plus urinary stasis, predisposes a patient to stone formation. Other factors which contribute to stone formation are alkaline urine and decreased urine volume. Intervention should be directed toward maintaining adequate hydration, keeping urine pH acid and promoting complete bladder emptying in the upright position. These same interventions will decrease the likelihood of infection.

Effect on the Digestive System

Decrease in peristalsis is the primary deleterious effect of inactivity on the digestive system. This contributes to problems of anorexia and constipation. Reduction in one's energy requirements will affect one's appetite. Additionally, the bedfast patient is not likely to take in adequate fluid. Anorexia and dehydration also have an impact on the decrease in intestinal peristalsis and contribute to the development of constipation.

Intervention should include exercises to increase activity, surveillance of fluid and dietary intake and establishment of a bowel program. Bowel programs can be enhanced by taking advantage of the gastrocolic reflex (which is strongest after intake of a meal) abdominal massage, digital stimulation, and suppositories.[11]

Constipation, as a side effect of pain medication, may be a significant problem in cancer patients. It is not uncommon for these individuals to require laxatives in conjunction with their bowel program. Lactulose shows some promise in the treatment of chronic constipation and establishment of normal defecation patterns.[12]

Effect on the Skin

Reduced bed mobility due to general debilitation, painful movements, lethargy from pain medications, or a depressed psychological response frequently leads to skin breakdown over bony prominences. Comprehensive skin care programs should include both preventive techniques and specific treatments of decubitus or pressure ulcers.

Pressure ulcer is the preferred diagnostic term because it addresses the primary etiology. Obstruction of capillary flow and the accompanying ischemia are recognized as the mechanisms responsible for ulcer formation.[13] Capillary pressure is 32 mmHg and application of pressure exceeding this level produces capillary obstruction.[14] Pressures over bony prominences in the supine, sidelying, prone, and sitting positions far exceed 32 mmHg.[13,15] Tissue damage can be avoided if the pressure is intermittent and relieved at 5-minute intervals.[16]

Shear forces will also result in tissue necrosis. These exist when the bone and underlying tissues move and the skin is held in place. This commonly occurs when an individual is pulled up in bed, or when the head of the bed is elevated. Friction from mechanical forces to the epidermis also contributes to the formation of ulcers.[17]

Edema, or any other variable that alters normal cell metabolism, has the potential to alter the cellular response to ischemia and skin susceptibility to breakdown. Greater susceptibility also exists with a decrease in muscle mass and skin elasticity and with diminished food and fluid intake, all concomitants of immobility.

Although prevention is the best approach to the management of skin problems, even the most vigilant care may fail when the effects of the disease or its treatment render tissue incapable of withstanding even normal capillary pressure. Available body resting surfaces may be so limited that adequate turning and changes of position can not be affected.

Prevention requires recognition of the multiple risk factors, including paralysis, malnutrition, incontinence, lack of sensation, pain (especially if aggravated by movement), spasticity, edema, contractures, sedation, altered mental status, and psychological stress. Nutritional deficiencies reflected by hematocrit, hemoglobin, serum protein, iron, zinc, and vitamin C levels should be corrected.[18,19] Education of staff, patient, and family to the causes of skin breakdown, the identification of patients at risk, and knowledge of body sites most frequently involved are prerequisites of preventive care. Patients at risk should be protected by pressure-dispersing padding on operating tables during prolonged surgery, because their vulnerability is further increased under these conditions.

Observation is the key to prevention. Skin inspection techniques should be taught to patients or to significant others. Exposed areas should also be palpated for temperature increases and induration. The area exposed to excessive pressure will become erythematous following pressure release. If erythema and induration persist for more than 20 minutes, the exposure interval has been too long and the areas should be kept free of pressure until these conditions disappear. Graphs depicting duration of pressure and fade time permit analysis of individual response and the development of safe position-change schedules.

In addition to specific turning schedules, small shifts of weight or "pushups" will also contribute to the prevention of breakdown. This is especially significant when a patient can not be turned owing to the nature of the illness or injury, or for patients in chairs who are too weak to lift themselves off the chair frequently. Frequency of pushup varies from 5-minute to 15-minute intervals, depending on tissue tolerance. Electronic buzzers are available to assist in conditioning the patient to perform this necessary protective behavior. Massage to high pressure areas, exercise, and anti-embolic stockings may be used to improve circulation.

Numerous mechanical devices are employed in preventive skin management. Generally, these devices are intended to alter points of pressure at regular intervals or to provide a molding effect to disperse pressure over a wider area. None of these devices has proven totally effective in the prevention of pressure ulcers, and their use will not reduce the need for continuing intensive surveillance and observation.

Electric rotating beds are available but they are cumbersome and confining. Turning frames and circle electric beds may be considered for individuals who experience severe pain on movement. Alternating air mattresses are limited in that they only partially reduce pressure at intervals. For maximum effect the patient should be positioned directly over the air cells with only a sheet over the mattress, as pillows, sheepskin, and so forth will negate its effect. Other mattresses are designed to disperse pressure over larger surfaces. Water mattresses are more efficient in accomplishing this than any of the foam varieties, but caution must be exerted to establish and maintain adequate buoyancy.

Bed positioning techniques include elevation of heels and malleoli off the bed with pillows or foam. Pillows or split foam mattresses can provide a bridging effect to remove pressure

TABLE 46-4. Steps to Prevent the Development of Pressure Ulcers

1. Staff and patient/family education as to cause
2. Identification of patients at risk
   a. Decreased mobility—pain, paralysis, sedation
   b. Mental status—unconscious, anesthetized, confused
   c. Incontinence
   d. Malnutrition—nausea, hematocrit, serum protein, etc.
   e. Dehydration—vomiting, diarrhea, fever, poor intake
   f. Edema—circulatory impairments
3. Intensive surveillance for those at risk
   a. Monitoring of above risk factors
   b. Daily skin inspection (especially over bony prominences)
4. Institution of specific protective regimens
   a. Positioning and turning schedules
   b. Determine tissue tolerance to pressure (observe and record fade times)
   c. Pressure dispersion equipment (special mattresses and wheelchair pads)
   d. Reduce shear and friction (sheepskin, cornstarch)
   e. Pressure relief maneuvers: bridging over bony prominences, "pushups"
   f. Remove *all pressure* from reddened areas which do not fade in twenty minutes. *GET OFF THAT SPOT*

over the sacrum and trochanters. Pillows to support the patient in the desired position also add to general comfort. Sheepskin ads to comfort and reduces shear. Use of a lifting and turning sheet can reduce shear and friction. A light dusting of cornstarch can further reduce friction.

Wheelchair cushions reduce pressures exerted over the ischial tuberosities.[20] In a comparison of several types, Souther found that a 2-inch latex foam pad can significantly reduce ischial pressure; however, a water-filled cushion (Jobst Hydro-Float) was the most effective.[21] The height of the wheelchair footrest should be adjusted to permit pressure to be dispersed along the undersurface of the leg. The steps to prevent pressure ulcers are summarized in Table 46-4.

Treatment of pressure ulcers, when they do occur, should address the intrinsic factors discussed relative to prevention as well as local and surgical interventions. Forty-six agents have been identified in an analysis of local treatment, yet well-designed clinical and laboratory studies to evaluate proposed therapies are lacking.[22]

The basic tenets of treatment are (1) remove all pressure, (2) treat infection if present, (3) debride and keep the ulcer clean, and (4) protect from further injury. Topical antibiotics are not indicated because of the bacterial resistance factor. Debridement can be mechanical—by means of wet to dry dressings—surgical, or biochemical. A variety of debriding enzymes are useful. A combination of sutilains and collagenase appears to effect faster debridement. Recently, dextranomer beads (Debrisan) have shown some promise in cleaning wounds and promoting healing.[23] Pace reports clinical evidence of faster healing with local application of benzyl peroxide.[24] Surgical closure should be considered when lesions involve muscle, bone, or joints.

Psychological and Social Effects

Inactivity due to bedrest can lead to psychological and social problems which may require professional intervention, though awareness of potential problems may allow prevention. The patient on bedrest will need a degree of assistance with routine self-care and treatment-related duties. For brief periods of time, dependence may be satisfactory; however, if it is long term, psychological problems may develop.

For patients at home, bedrest can also cause problems for family members who take on added responsibilities. For patients without family assistance the recruitment of aides can be frustrating and expensive. The possible psychological and social impact of these frustrations and expenses on rehabilitation is evident and must be addressed early in treatment if preventive measures for the disuse syndrome are to be successful.

Another complication of total bedrest is social and intellectual isolation which may lead to depression, withdrawal, and anxiety. It also allows the patient to dwell on his or her situation, which may exacerbate existing psychological problems. Isolation must be minimized, and its effects treated to allow participation in rehabilitation.

BREAST CANCER

In the adult female, breast cancer accounts for more new cases and many more deaths than cancer of any other organ. This disease is rare in men, with about one case to every 100 to 120 in females.[1] Treatment usually involves removal of the breast with some or all of the axillary nodes. The pectoralis major and pectoralis minor muscles are removed during a standard radical mastectomy, which will affect shoulder strength. The pectoralis major is left intact in modified radical mastectomy and there is usually little functional shoulder deficit. Adjuvant therapy, including radiotherapy or chemotherapy, may lead to significant disability.

The disability may be minimized by rehabilitation beginning as soon as the diagnosis is made. The goals for rehabilitation of the post-mastectomy patient include:[25]

1. *Physical restoration*—obtain functional pain free use of the affected arm with full ROM
2. *Psychosocial rehabilitation*—to help the patient accept the loss of her breast and to help both the patient and significant others cope with their fears and anxieties concerning death and dying, physical attractiveness, and sexuality
3. *Cosmetic rehabilitation*—restoration of the external physical appearance by use of a temporary breast form, external breast prosthesis or breast reconstruction
4. *Occupational/vocational rehabilitation*—which includes patient education to prevent excessive edema and infection of the affected arm, as well as returning the patient to employment.

PHYSICAL RESTORATION

History and Physical

Physical rehabilitation of the patient with breast cancer focuses on preventive measures. It is important to know preoperatively whether the patient has had shoulder trauma, tendinitis, bursitis, arthritis, adhesive capsulitis, C5–C6 radiculopathy, or a rotator cuff tear on the same side as the proposed mastectomy. These conditions and any functional shoulder limitations will affect the rehabilitation outcome with respect to shoulder ROM and strength. It is essential to perform and record an exact musculoskeletal exam of the shoulder and upper extremity (UE), recording the shoulder ROM with respect to external rotation, internal rotation, abduction, extension, and forward flexion. Motor strength of the UE and scapulohumeral muscles must be recorded and any atrophy must be noted. UE baseline circumference measurements should be taken pre-operatively and at regular postoperative intervals to note the onset of lymphedema. The brachium is measured above the lateral epicondyle of the humerus and the antibrachium 3 inches below the lateral epicondyle. Measurements are also taken at the wrist and across the metacarpal phalangeal joints. Some centers will utilize volumetric measurement instead of circumference measurement.

UE deep tendon reflexes should be recorded and a careful sensory examination performed. Since both the long thoracic (serratus anterior) and thoracodorsal (latissimus dorsi) nerves may be injured with axillary node dissection, it is essential to check these muscles carefully both pre- and postoperatively.

The thoracodorsal nerve is often surrounded by metastatic nodes; consequently, it may be necessary to sacrifice the nerve.[26] However, the long thoracic nerve that innervates the serratus anterior usually does not have nodes running with it and should be spared, since its injury will result in medial winging of the scapula with weakness in forward flexion against resistance. Upward rotation of the scapula is almost completely abolished, thus limiting shoulder abduction and forward flexion.

Treatment

Patients first seen with far advanced disease may receive palliative radiation therapy followed by chemotherapy. Radiation fibrosis may cause marked limitation of shoulder ROM, arm lymphedema, and ulcerations of the skin, as well as brachial plexus injury with corresponding pain, and motor and sensory loss. These patients require an individualized, closely monitored rehabilitation plan to maximize function.[27]

The rehabilitation plan used for patients who have a normal shoulder (ROM and strength) and who will be receiving preoperative radiotherapy should include baseline goniometric shoulder ROM measurements, which should be reviewed periodically during the course of radiation. The patient should also be instructed in a home program to maintain ROM. These exercises are to be performed two to three times daily for 6 months, then at least daily for 1 or 2 years.[27] Patients who have restricted shoulder ROM and are receiving radiation should be placed on a daily supervised active assistive ROM program to obtain maximum function, and then shifted to a daily home program, possibly with heat and static stretch, that is closely supervised.[27]

For mastectomy patients, Degenshein suggests a postoperative position technique in which the arm is placed at right angles to the chest with the shoulder in external rotation, and a towel placed around the arm and pinned to the bedsheet. This keeps the elbow free.[28] Even if the arm is kept in this position for 24 to 48 hours, the patient will have a 90° painless abduction ROM at the shoulder and all internal and external rotation. In this posture, the arm is not pinned to the chest wall, thus reducing the risk of developing a frozen shoulder. Immediately after surgery, the arm should be compressed with an elastic wrap to minimize the development of edema.

In complicated cases, a suggested treatment plan would be referral to physical therapy on the third to fifth postoperative day, when wound healing has been well established. Before the physical therapy prescription is written, it is essential to consider the following:

1. Stage of wound healing
2. Adherence or lack of adherence of the skin grafts
3. Presence or absence of drainage tubes, and the amount of drainage
4. Local instability of the chest wall.

In the supine position, the amount of tension on the suture line is assessed as the patient is carefully progressed toward full passive ROM, especially in abduction, external rotation, and flexion. This will allow evaluation of shoulder mobility without applying undue tension to the surgical wound or mobilizing the skin flaps.

As mentioned earlier, one must consider the presurgical complications involving the musculoskeletal system of the affected extremity such as brachial plexus injury, long thoracic, or thoracodorsal nerve injury.[29] Electrodiagnostic studies may prove helpful in documenting the injury and predicting the prognosis for neurologic recovery.[30] These complications will obviously cause a modification in the postmastectomy rehabilitation prescription.

At the first therapy visit, the patient should be instructed in active ROM exercises for the elbow, wrist, and fingers of the involved extremity. One-handed ADLs, using the noninvolved arm, are also taught at this time.

By the fifth postoperative day, the suction catheters have usually been removed and the therapy program can be accelerated, as there is less risk of separation of the skin flaps and the formation of seromas. Active ROM exercises in the supine position to the affected shoulder should be initiated, avoiding stretch of the suture line. If needed, muscle relaxation exercises (*i.e.*, deep breathing exercises) can be taught to the patient to aid in decreasing muscle tension and improving pain tolerance. Isometric exercises to the biceps, triceps, forearm musculature, and the hand intrinsics should be initiated to improve the pumping efficiency of the affected extremity. These exercises should be performed with the affected arm wrapped and elevated. Isometric exercises to the rotated cuff musculature on the affected side should be taught in order to maintain the patient's strength. Positioning is utilized to gradually increase shoulder flexion, abduction, and external rotation. Simultaneously, maintenance active assistance ROM exercises should be performed on the unaffected extremity in order to avoid the complications of immobilization. Daily ROM and circumference measurement must be obtained and recorded to document the patient's progress and to look for evidence of postmastectomy lymphedema.

When the sutures have been removed, usually 9 to 12 days postoperatively, exercises can then be prescribed for the erect position. Progressive active and active assistive exercises are used to increase the ROM to 180° of forward flexion and abduction at the affected shoulder, and to obtain full range of external rotation. Wand exercises, use of the overhead pulley, and wall climbing exercises are designed to increase elevation (Fig. 46-5*A*, *B*, *C*). If the pectoralis group has been removed, progressive resistive exercises to the shoulder abductors and adductors are utilized to prevent possible shoulder dislocation. Wall weights or sandbags can be used to perform these exercises. If the patient has chest wall adhesions, skin mobilization, friction massage, and stretching of the subcutaneous fibrosis of the glenohumeral joint are prescribed.

To prevent swelling of the affected extremity, the arm should be elevated when sitting for an extended period of time. For elevation to be effective, it must be maintained for at least 30 minutes.

In individuals who have developed chronic capsulitis due to prolonged immobilization, diathermy modalities (short wave diathermy and ultrasound) can be very helpful when combined with active stretching at the shoulder. Diathermy is contraindicated in the presence of infection or carcinoma.[31]

Prior to discharge the patient must be able to demonstrate, the various exercises which have been prescribed to facilitate rehabilitation. With proper physical therapy, full ROM of the affected shoulder can be obtained; however, full muscular strength will not be obtained if the pectoralis major and minor have been removed and weakness will be noted in horizontal adduction.

PSYCHOLOGICAL ASPECTS OF MASTECTOMY

As with most amputations, the loss of a breast requires marked psychological and social adjustments. With the emphasis our culture places on the female breast, the resulting psychological and social problems may be extensive. Preventive intervention in these areas should begin before surgery and continue throughout treatment and rehabilitation. Intervention techniques should involve the patient and significant others, as the reaction of others to the patient and to the breast loss may affect the patient's attitude toward rehabilitation.

Pre-operatively, the patient should be encouraged to explore and express feelings, fears, and concerns, and begin to mourn the loss. During this time, potential psychological problems must be identified and treatment initiated. Some of the more common psychological and social problems are reactive depression, anger, frustration, resentment, feelings of being less of a "woman," and fear of death. These conditions may lead to withdrawal or flailing out at family, friends, and staff.

Intervention techniques can take a number of forms, ranging from educational classes to intensive individual psychotherapy. After initial professional assessment of the patient's psychological and social needs, treatment follow-up plans can be established. A group approach to psychological and social intervention can be very beneficial for patients and their families. Led by a professional, groups can allow for the exploration of feelings, sharing of problems and solutions, and personal growth. The sessions can also be educational, teaching breast self-examination, proper care of the affected extremity, and explanation of the surgical procedure. Successful mastectomy patients who have mastered their crisis and have made successful adjustments can be included. Also, different types of breast forms and suitable types of wearing apparel may be demonstrated. For some patients with acute psychiatric problems, group therapy may not be appropriate, and individual sessions must be utilized. Others may decline group participation.

COSMETIC REHABILITATION OF BREAST CANCER

Temporary breast forms are used by the patient until a permanent prosthesis is obtained. Permanent prostheses are usually not ordered until at least 8 weeks after surgery. Temporary breast forms can be made from such materials as fluff, cotton, lamb's wool, nylon stockings, or facial tissues. Permanent breast forms usually consist of foam rubber, liquid filled plastic, air filled plastic, synthetics, or cloth. These may be stock items or custom made.

The fitting of the permanent prosthesis must consider size, weight, symmetry, feel, comfort, and cost. Consultation with the American Cancer Society will be helpful in identifying local resources. It may be necessary to assist some patients in locating sources of modified clothing.

Breast reconstruction can technically be performed on any of these patients, even those who have received radiation therapy. Patient selection is based on the patient's general health and perception of the deformity.[32] The reconstruction may contribute to better and faster psychological adjustment for the patient. Some surgeons feel that breast reconstruction should be performed even in patients who have a poor prognosis. See Chapter 27 for further discussion of breast reconstruction.

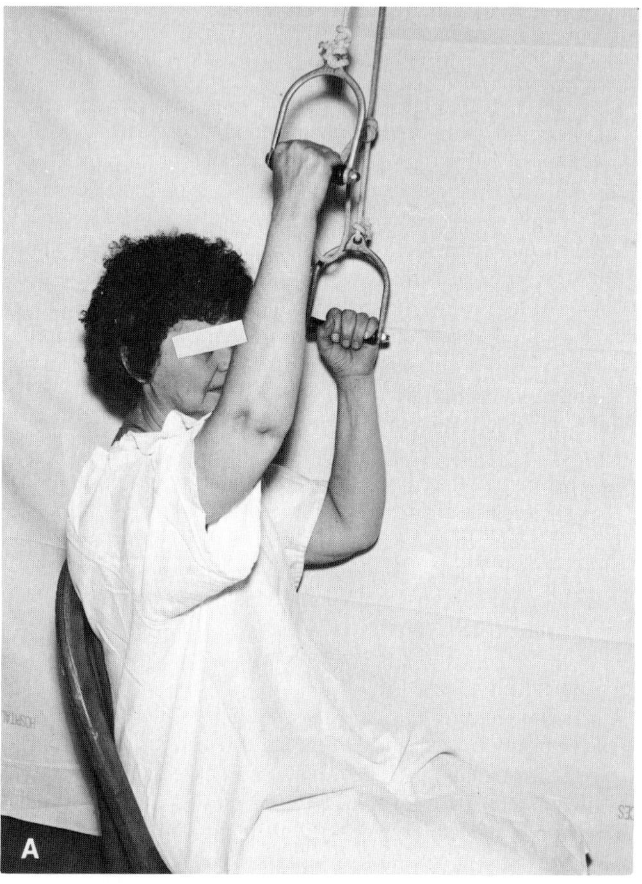

Reach to Recovery Program of the American Cancer Society

This is a voluntary program in which all of the volunteers have undergone mastectomy for breast cancer and have become successfully rehabilitated. This group aids the patient in physiological, psychological, and cosmetic rehabilitation. The volunteers will not see the patient unless it is requested by the physician, who may request all or a portion of the program.[33] When they visit the patient, they bring with them a kit containing a booklet of exercises for the affected shoulder, breast prostheses, and information about clothing. They also provide a temporary breast form and some exercise equipment. It is well to remember that not every patient is a candidate for this type of visit and some patients may even resent this approach.

POSTMASTECTOMY LYMPHEDEMA

Reports on the incidence of postmastectomy lymphedema vary from 6.7% to 62.5%.[34] Severe edema, which is defined as an increase of 35% in volume, occurs in approximately 10% of these patients.[35] The disability from lymphedema is proportional to its amount and disfigurement. It has never been explained why some mastectomy patients develop lymphedema and others do not. Some may go several years with no lymphedema, only to develop massive edema later for no known reason. Onset 6 months postmastectomy should arouse suspicion of occult infection or recurrent tumor.

Multiple factors such as radiation therapy, infection, delayed wound healing, surgical ablation of lymphatic nodes and vessels, fibrosis from radiation or chronic edema, thrombophlebitis, inadequate regeneration of lymphatic vessels or

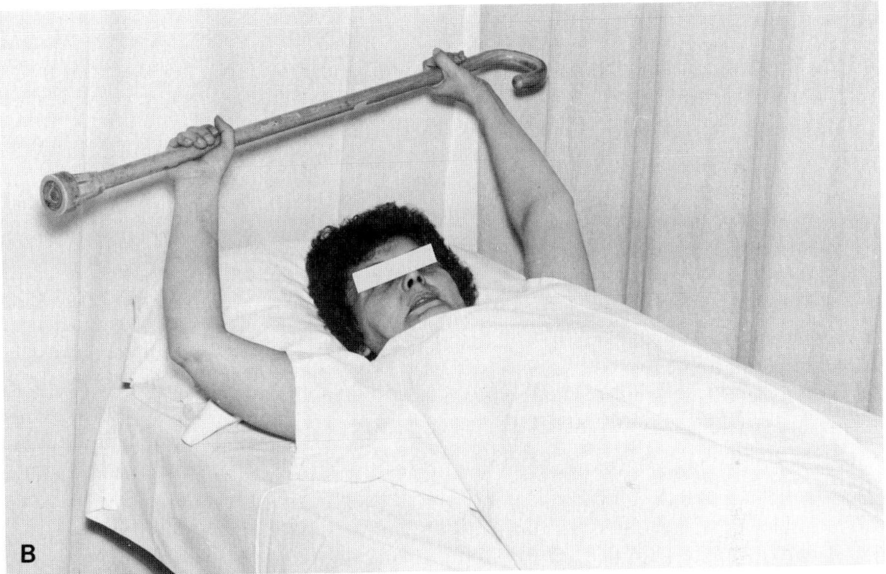

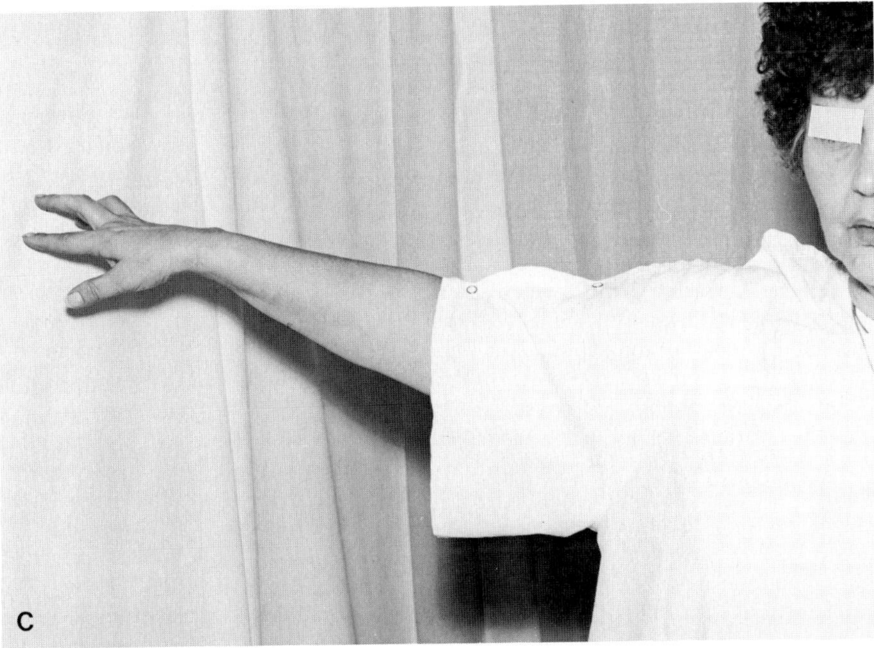

FIG. 46-5. Overhead pulley, wand exercises, and wall climbing exercises are used to obtain full shoulder ROM. *A*, Pulley; *B*, wand; *C*, wall climbing.

recurrent tumor have been suggested as possible etiological factors. However, it is generally believed that a combination of multiple factors is operating.[36,37] To help determine the pathology and aid with treatment it is important to know whether the cause of the lymphedema is disease of the lymphatics or venous system. Venograms and lymphangiography may aid in making this differential diagnosis.

Prevention is much better than any surgical or medical treatment designed to remedy the situation once it has occurred.[26] The axillary vein should not be damaged and prevention of infection is a necessity. Postoperatively, the arm should be elevated and a supervised exercise program to obtain full ROM should be initiated. Elastic compression bandage or sleeves are also helpful in preventing lymphedema.[38]

Multiple surgical procedures have been devised for treatment of lymphedema.[38,39] The aim of these surgical procedures has been to reestablish the lymphatic flow. The procedures are:

1. Lymphangioplasty, which creates new lymphatic pathways
2. Bridging procedures, which form a bypass of normal tissue with intact lymphatics over a disease or blocked area
3. Lymphaticovenous shunts, which develop an anastomosis between the lymph and venous systems[40]
4. Superficial to deep lymphatic anastomosis, which connects lymphatics by converting shaved pedical strips of deep fascia into bone or muscle[41]
5. Lysis of axillary vein adhesions[42]
6. Amputation, where the edema is severe and disabling, and the hand is nonfunctional

None of these procedures has proven to be universally successful or accepted. Goldsmith's intact omentum bridging transposition, in which the omentum with its rich lymphatic and vascular supply is pulled up through the subcutaneous tunnel in the chest wall and laid on the underlying muscle of the lymphedematous arm may possibly be most successful.[43]

Medical treatment of postmastectomy lymphedema includes elevation of the hand higher than the elbow, which in turn is higher than the shoulder.[44] To be effective, the elevation must persist for at least 30 minutes each session, and the frequency of elevation is determined by the clinical status. During all or part of the night the arm should be elevated while the patient is supine.

The patient should be instructed in isometric exercises of the affected arm and hand to increase the active muscle pump. To take advantage of gravity these should be done with the distal part of the extremity elevated higher than the proximal. The exercises are isometric, rather than isotonic, to reduce joint motion and cause less constriction.[38] The frequency of these isometric contractions needs to be determined by the patient's response during the therapy. An example would be isometric contractions for a second, then a 2-second to 3-second rest period, for a total of 20 contractions.[38] When established, this should be repeated frequently throughout the day. These isometric exercises need to be supplemented with isotonic exercises to obtain full shoulder ROM.

Pneumatic intermittent compression (pneumomassage) can be helpful in increasing the flow of fluid out of the limb. The most common one is produced by Jobst. It is composed of a number of cuffs which inflate, then deflate sequentially. This pumping results in milking the limb from the distal to the proximal points. The common adjustment settings for intervals of pressure are 45 seconds on and 15 seconds off.[45] The pressure setting is usually slightly lower than the diastolic blood pressure of the patient. In persistent cases, the circulation unit, when available, works better than the Jobst unit, as it inflates from distal to proximal, while the Jobst unit fills all at once. Both units empty simultaneously. The pressure phase forces the edema fluid up the lymphatic channels and the exhaust phase allows them to refill assisted by gravity in the slightly elevated limb. The treatment may vary from 2 hours twice daily, up to a maximum of 12 hours per day.[36] The duration of treatment depends upon the amount of lymphedema and its response to pneumomassage.[4] Rest periods may be necessary if problems such as nausea, pain, or finger tingling occur. Circumference measurements should be taken before and after each pneumatic compression session to document progress. Jewelry should be removed and a wrinkle-free, full-cuff, hand stockinette should be applied to absorb perspiration. It can be done on either an inpatient or an outpatient basis, but it is contraindicated if there is evidence of acute phlebitis, cellulitis, or recurrent carcinoma. Pitting edema seems to respond better than the brawny variety.

After each treatment, a figure-eight elastic wrap is used to provide compression and keep the fluid volume reduced. Instruction in proper figure-eight wrapping technique must be provided. The elastic wrap is applied upon rising.

When the volume of the affected arm and hand has been reduced and stabilized, a custom fitted, pressure gradiated, elastic sleeve should be provided. The patient should wear it throughout waking hours. To remain effective, it must be replaced every 2 to 3 months.[37] Prior to the replacement, it may become necessary once again to treat the patient with intermittent pneumatic compression before measuring for a new elastic sleeve. Some people find the elastic sleeve uncomfortable and others find it cosmetically unacceptable. For patients who, for social or occupational reasons, choose not to have an elastic sleeve, a Jobst home unit can be prescribed for daily use.

Diuretic therapy and salt restriction are used as an adjuvant therapy to the pneumatic compression, particularly for patients who live in hot humid areas, and in those with cardiovascular problems. A higher incidence of postmastectomy lymphedema has been noted with obese patients and weight loss should be encouraged.[46]

Lymphedema provides an excellent culture media, and low grade cellulitis (usually streptococcus) may occur. Erythromycin, 250 mg q.i.d. for 7 days, should be initiated at the first sign of infection.[29] Some physicians prescribe prophylactic erythromycin 48 hours before pneumomassage.

It is essential to remember that the programs discussed above are not rigid and will need to be modified for each patient. Upon discharge, the patient should have regular measurements, circumferential or volumetric, of the affected arm.

TABLE 46-5. Exercise Program for the Postmastectomy Patient

1. *3–5 days postoperative:* Patient is supine with operative side elevated and the arm wrapped
   a. Active ROM to the fingers, wrist and elbow on the operative side. Some examples of these exercises are:
      1. With palm up, touch hand to shoulder on operated side. Return with palm down.
      2. Make circular motions with wrist on operative side
      3. Make a fist, then straighten fingers on operated side (squeeze a ball).
   b. Active ROM of nonoperated UE.
2. *5 days postoperative:* Patient is supine with operated UE Ace wrapped.
   a. Isometric exercises to operated UE for strengthening, using opposite arm for assistance.
   b. Gentle, straight active shoulder ROM of operated side, *i.e.*, abduction—raise arm sideways and upward, keeping elbow straight.
   c. Continue with active elbow and hand exercises
   d. Relaxation breathing exercises
3. *9–12 days postoperative:* Or when sutures removed
   a. Active assistive shoulder ROM to the operated side, *i.e.*, sitting, overhead pulleys, clasp hands in front midline, raise arms forward and up as far as tolerated.
   b. Upper back isometrics in sitting position
   c. Active shoulder ROM of operated side in sitting position.

The patient must be educated to the performance and avoidance of specific behaviors to protect the arm. These are designed to avoid excessive use of the arm, constrictive clothing, local or generalized heating, and trauma.[29,47,48]

Some "DO's"

1. Wear canvas gloves when gardening, wear rubber gloves when cleaning utensils with steel wool.
2. Wear a loose rubber glove on this hand when washing dishes.
3. Wear a thimble when sewing.
4. Keep dress sleeves loose.
5. Wash the smallest break on the skin on the operative side with soap and water, cover it with a bandage.
6. Use an electric razor for shaving; avoid nicks and scrapes.
7. Keep the arm elevated when sitting
8. Apply a lanolin hand cream several times daily.
9. Contact the doctor if the arm on the operative side appears hot, reddened, or swollen.

Some "DON'T's"

1. Don't hold a cigarette in this hand.
2. Don't carry your purse or anything heavy with this arm.
3. Don't wear a wristwatch or other jewelry on this arm.
4. Don't cut or pick at cuticles or hangnails on this hand.
5. Don't work near thorny plants, or dig in the garden barehanded.
6. Don't reach into a hot oven with this arm.
7. Don't permit injections or vaccinations in this arm.
8. Don't permit blood to be drawn from this arm (an obvious exception would be if you were receiving chemotherapy and have no other veins remaining).
9. Don't allow your blood pressure to be taken in this arm.
10. Don't get sunburned, tan gradually.

Results of rehabilitation programs for postmastectomy lymphedema are widely reported in the literature. Zeissler has shown that 67% of 123 patients benefited from this type of treatment program.[37]

HEAD AND NECK CANCER

Areas of major functional concern in head and neck cancer patients include nutrition and deglutition problems, shoulder dysfunction, self-care consideration, altered speech communication, and disfigurement.

In planning for the rehabilitation needs of patients with head and neck cancer some pretreatment data must be gathered. This data base should include medical and social history, including lifestyle, nutritional habits, and intellectual learning ability. Head and neck cancer patients frequently have a long history of alcohol abuse and heavy smoking, the combination of which contributes to the development of squamous cell carcinoma in the head and neck.[49,50] These habits may also contribute to deterioration of intellectual functioning, noncompliant behavior and, possibly recurrent disease.[51] In order to improve the chances of cure and enhance compliance, the patient may need assistance in altering smoking and drinking habits.

NUTRITION AND DEGLUTITION

Because of the frequent impairment of the deglutitory mechanism, maintenance of optimal nutrition is a prime concern. Alterations in dentition, jaw musculature, tongue mobility, palatal function, taste appreciation, saliva, laryngeal and pharyngeal musculature, or esophageal function each contribute to potential deglutitory impairment.

An optimal nutritional state prior to and during treatment may enhance the patient's chances for recovery.[52] Generally, the patient's nutritional state is monitored by weight. High-protein dietary supplements may be encouraged in an attempt to affect weight gain. If weight declines in excess of 4.5 kg (10 pounds) a nasogastric tube is often inserted to provide primary nutritional needs or supplement what the patient can take by mouth.[53] (See Chapter 43 for discussion of nutritional management.)

Swallowing impairments are often anticipated in the course of treatment or in advancing disease, and gastrostomies or jejunostomies may be performed to provide nutritionally complete formulas and vitamin supplements.[54] Since canned formulas are very expensive, some patients are instructed in blenderized diets. The instructions should address nutritional education and procedural techniques relative to food preparation, cleaning, and storage to avoid spoilage.[55]

Radiation and chemotherapy in these patients present special problems in nutritional management and deglutition. Alteration in taste, noxious sensations, or loss of taste is common.[56] A decrease in salivary flow may lead to xerostomia. Saliva may be altered to a thick sticky consistency, interfering with swallowing and speech. Mucositis, loss of appetite, nausea, and esophagitis are common sequelae of these treatment modes.[57]

To counteract the above effects and reduce the likelihood of anorexia, careful dietary planning is necessary. Since red meat may taste rancid, fish, poultry, eggs, and dairy products can be substituted to provide the required protein.[56] Menus that emphasize gravy, sauces, and butter will help to compensate for the dry oral mucosa. An increase in total fluid intake will also aid the patient with decreased saliva, and dryness can be relieved by providing artificial saliva, sugarless gum, or sugarless lemon drops. Papain, a protylytic enzyme from papaya fruit, will dissolve thick secretions. Its effect can be obtained by dissolving a papase tablet in the mouth or coating a cotton swab with meat tenderizer and swabbing the mouth ten minutes prior to the meal.[58,59] Episodes of nausea can be minimized by providing the patient with frequent small meals, avoiding cooking fragrances, and by the use of anti-emetic drugs.[53] Pain from mucositis may contribute to an anorexic state. Viscous lidocaine (Xylocaine) ten minutes before a meal, or diphenhydramine (Benadryl) mixed with nondairy whipped cream and placed in the mouth acts as a soothing topical analgesic.[58]

The teeth are particularly susceptible to damage from radiation. Caries may result from the direct effect of irradiation on teeth or supporting structures. The alterations in salivary flow change bacterial flora and raise the oral pH, thus creating a medium for bacterial growth.[57] Dental consultation prior to radiation therapy with prophylaxis treatment can often prevent rampant caries. There is evidence to suggest that fluoride treatment can aid in the prevention of decay and also reduce postradiation hypersensitivity to the sensations of hot, cold, and sweet foods.[60]

Prior to radiation, all necessary tooth extractions in the field should be performed, and the gums allowed to heal. When extractions are required in an already radiated field, the risk of osteoradionecrosis is increased. Hence, all nonrestorable teeth and those in the direct path of radiation are usually removed.[57,61]

The risk of osteoradionecrosis is reduced when bone is covered by normal mucosa and contains healthy teeth. A program of oral hygiene should therefore be established prior to radiation therapy. Dentures should not be worn during therapy because of the risk of developing mucosal sores, and complete recovery of radiated mucosa should be allowed before dentures are refitted.[61]

Excision of structures important to swallowing during surgery has a greater influence on deglutition than impaired motility of residual structures.[62] Patients who have undergone either partial or total glossectomy will experience some disruption in the ability to move a bolus from the anterior to the posterior oral cavity, which is referred to as dysphagia mechanica.[59]

All partial and total glossectomy patients must be evaluated on an individual basis. It has been reported that patients with partial glossectomies have remarkable adaptation to swallowing, and in one series more than 50% of patients with total glossectomy were able to take adequate oral nutrition.[63,64]

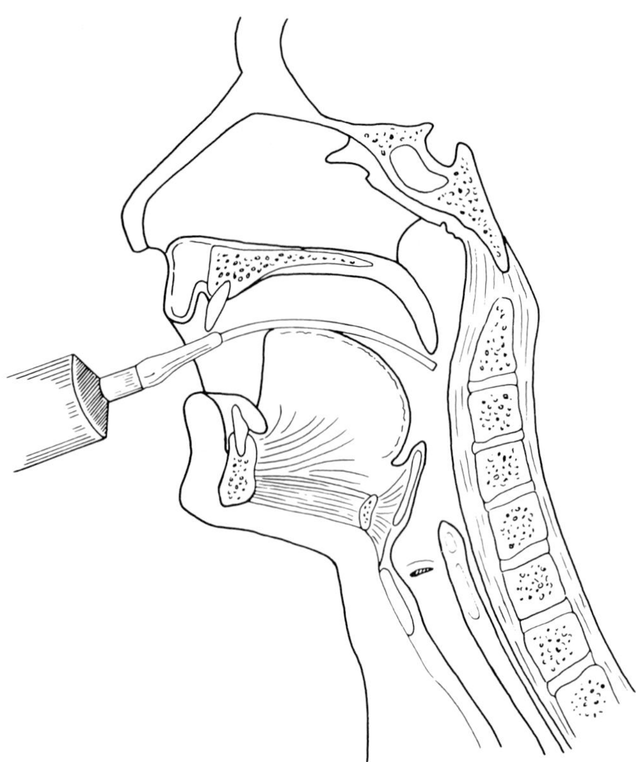

FIG. 46-6. Use of modified syringe to introduce fluids into oropharynx of patients with dysphagia mechanica.

Some may be able to take adequate liquid diets by adjusting body and head posture to allow for swallowing.[65] Others may need to adapt a large syringe, by attaching a length of tubing that reaches to the uvula, in order to place fluids in the oropharynx for swallowing (Fig. 46-6).[55] Soft foods that do not require mastication can be inserted into the mouth on a long-handled spoon or plunger and placed near the uvula to be swallowed.[59,65,66] Finger foods can be placed in the posterior mouth and manipulated by remaining muscles for swallowing. These patients should avoid food that falls apart in the mouth (corn, applesauce, dry ground meat) and include food that holds together (custards, pudding, ground meat combined with gravy).

Orogastric tube feedings can be used as either an intermediate mode of nutritional intake or a permanent solution for nutritional management. A lubricated feeding tube intermittently passed orally allows the patient to take canned or blenderized diets, all fluids, and medications. The patient's attempt to swallow the tube allows the deglutitory muscles to be exercised without risk of aspiration and free from the constant interference of a nasogastric tube.[58,65]

Other dysphagia mechanica patients have had resections of the soft or bony palate. The major problem in these cases is leakage of food and liquid through the defect into adjoining cavities. Prosthetic obturators designed to separate the cavities are often successful in solving these mechanical swallowing problems.[67] Again, these patients must be considered individually, since some patients with palatal defects are unable to manage nutritionally without tube feedings.

Patients who have undergone partial laryngectomies, especially those having had superglottic laryngectomies, are susceptible to aspiration because of interruption of the pharyngeal phase of swallowing. The incidence of persistent dysphagia in these patients has varied greatly among reports.[68–73] For those with superglottic laryngectomies who have the ability to learn and can intellectualize the swallowing act, a technique can be taught to protect the airway and minimize aspiration. The patient learns to (1) inhale before swallowing, (2) flex the neck, (3) consciously hold the breath while swallowing, and (4) gently cough or clear the throat immediately after the swallow is complete.[58]

SHOULDER DYSFUNCTION

The trapezius is the muscle most responsible for normal shoulder alignment, function and cosmesis. It can be divided functionally into upper, middle and lower fibers, and is innervated by the spinal accessory nerve and C_3, C_4, C_5 plexus (Table 46-6). This muscle is the primary upward rotator during shoulder abduction and forward flexion, and the main stabilizer of the scapula. With the loss of the trapezius during radical neck dissection due to excision of the nerve supply, the remaining scapular musculature is inadequate to maintain normal shoulder alignment and function. The deeper posterior scapular muscles lack the size and direction of pull to adequately oppose the action of the pectoral group (pectoralis major and minor), to stabilize the scapula during glenohumeral motion, or to support the weight of the affected arm when it hangs at the side. Muscles that are synergistic with the trapezius for one motion are unfortunately antagonistic during another. Hence, substitution for each function is not completely adequate, since the substituted muscles cannot perform shoulder abduction and forward flexion in a coordinated functional manner.[74]

Injury to the accessory nerve will affect shoulder function postoperatively. This is true whether the injury is partial, due to neuropraxia (physiologic bruise), or complete, with or without nerve continuity. Electrodiagnosis can be helpful in documenting and differentiating partial from complete nerve injury and in predicting prognosis.[30] Pre-operative shoulder pathology such as bursitis or adhesive capsulitis will affect postoperative shoulder function.

To test the trapezius, the patient must be examined with the clothes removed above the waist. One way to test the upper trapezius is to ask the patient to elevate the shoulder (shrug) against resistance. This test can give inaccurate results, however, since muscular patients may have a well-developed levator scapula that can provide this function, or the upper trapezius may be innervated anomalously by a branch from cervical roots 2–3.[27] To avoid misjudgement, it is better to view the patient from behind, with the arms relaxed at the side of the body and the shoulder at rest. With a weak or paralyzed trapezius, the scapula is displaced downward (drooped) and laterally (lateral winging), owing to the unopposed pull of the serratus anterior, and the superior angle is rotated further from the spine than the inferior angle.[27]

TABLE 46-6. The Function of the Various Positions of the Trapezius

PARTS OF THE TRAPEZIUS	FUNCTION
Upper fibers	Elevates scapula
Middle fibers	Retracts (adducts) scapula
Lower fibers	Depresses scapula
Upper and lower fibers	Upward rotator of scapula
All fibers	Hold the scapula tightly to the thoracic cage during movement of arm

Following sacrifice or injury of the accessory nerve, active ROM of the involved shoulder will have limited abduction in the horizontal position of only 60° to 70° with the scapula's upward rotation (Fig. 46-7).[75] A few very strong patients can abduct to 160° providing they move the arm forward 20° to 25° while abducting.[74] Patients who have anomalous innervation of the upper trapezius may have abduction to 160° but are unable to perform this horizontal abduction against resistance, owing to the weakness of the middle portion of the trapezius.[76]

The main antagonist of the trapezius is the pectoralis group. The resulting shoulder malalignment is mainly due to the pull of the unopposed pectoralis major when the trapezius is weakened or paralyzed, resulting in a contracture in the protracted (abducted) position. This pectoralis group shortening can be further complicated by deltopectoral flap healing, which aggravates the scapular protraction deformity. Hence, it is essential to prevent any contracture of the pectoralis muscle group in these patients. This will be discussed later.

A dropped shoulder is not only painful (because of stretch of the rhomboids, levator scapulae, and the denervated upper trapezius) and cosmetically unacceptable to many patients, but it has marked functional limitations, such as the inability to push, lift, or carry heavy objects. These patients are unable to actively reach shoulder level or above, and loading them at their maximum shoulder ROM produces and increases pain. These patients often find the shoulder problems to be the major long-term functional disability. For a laborer, it can mean the end of employment. This can be a devastating and painful problem to a patient who has had a bilateral radical neck dissection (Fig. 46-8). Whenever possible, the accessory nerve should be preserved, or a nerve graft used to replace the removed segment of nerve.

When patients have had the accessory nerve sacrificed or injured, the goals of the physical rehabilitation program are (1) to avoid contracture of the pectoralis group, (2) to unload the shoulder as early as possible after surgery to prevent or reduce shoulder and neck pain and to avoid stretch of the trapezius, and (3) to strengthen the levator scapulae, rhomboideus major and minor, and serratus anterior to improve scapular stability and facilitate shoulder elevation.[74]

Following surgery, shoulder external and internal ROM are usually preserved, but due to scapular instability, strength is decreased. Excessive shoulder internal rotation must be avoided, since this further protracts and depresses the shoulder, aggravating the disability, and may increase pain. Proper body mechanics and shoulder posture (shoulders back) are essential to maximize function and reduce pain.

The following general postoperative exercise scheme may need to be modified for each individual patient.[55]

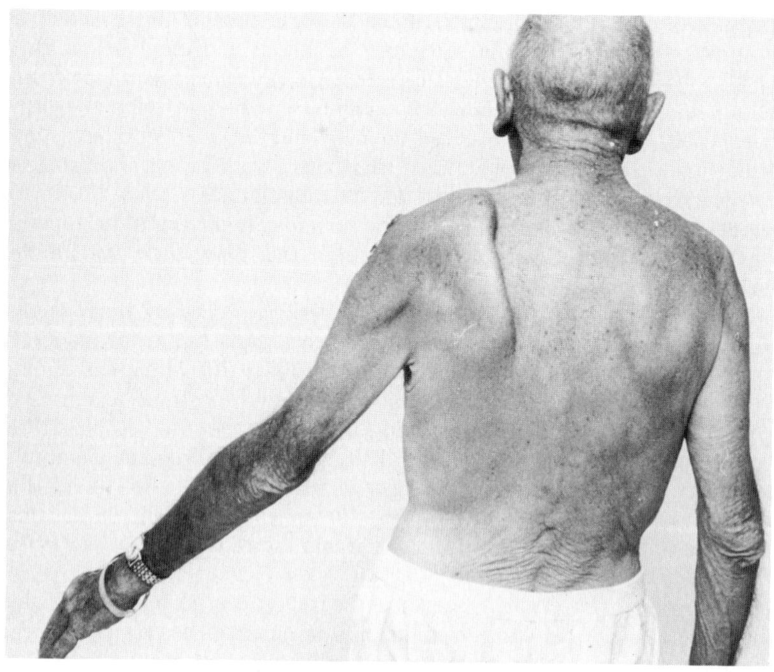

FIG. 46-7. Maximal active abduction in this patient following severance of accessory nerve.

WEEK 1 (4–8 DAYS AFTER SUTURE AND DRAIN REMOVAL). Emphasis is on proper bed positioning and maintaining full stretch of pectoralis muscle group. Treatment is at bedside.

- passive ROM in the supine position, to the limit of the graft, b.i.d.
- limit abduction to 90°

FIG. 46-8. Marked scapular protraction deformity which may be present following severance of both accessory nerves. *A*, Right view; *B*, front view.

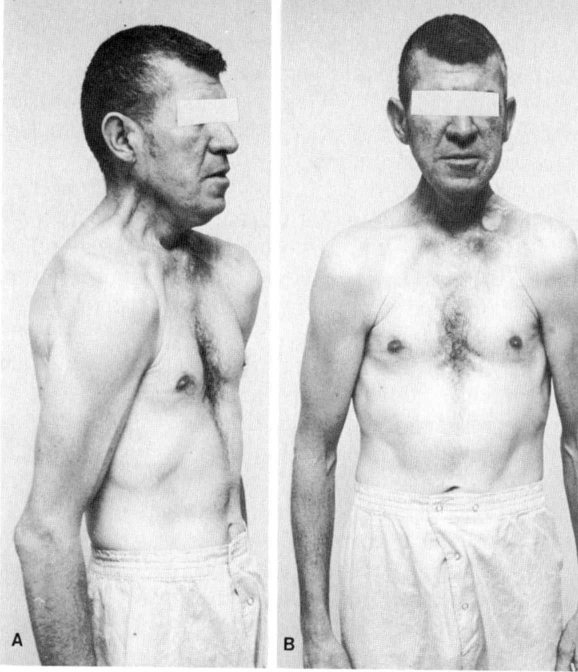

- do not depress or protract the scapula
- prescribe a sling for sitting and ambulation. This eliminates the gravitational pull on the shoulder muscles due to the weight of the arm and prevents stretching the trapezius
- train in performing ADLs with the unaffected arm

WEEKS 2–3 (21 DAYS). There may be a longer wait if the tissue has been irradiated since it heals slower. Treatment is in the therapy clinic.

- active assistive ROM exercises with gravity eliminated to limit of graft line, added to the passive exercise program. ROM is performed with patient in prone position to eliminate the pull of the clavicular head of the pectoralis major
- do not resist scapular depression and protraction, as this may strengthen these muscles and aggravate the deformity
- the sling is used when the patient is ambulating
- shoulder precautions are reviewed, avoiding rapid resistive movements and loading of the arm
- passive stretch of the pectoralis group is started about three weeks postoperatively
- active cervical flexion, extension, lateral bending, and rotation ROM are initiated. Skin flaps are watched carefully

WEEK 4 (1 MONTH PLUS). Active resistive (isometric) exercises are added to strengthen external rotation, horizontal abduction, scapular elevation, and retraction. The goal is to increase the strength and mechanical advantage of the serratus anterior, rhomboideus major and minor, levator scapulae, and middle trapezius muscles, and to obtain a balance between the strengthened muscles and the stretch of the pectoralis group to obtain a more satisfactory functional shoulder.

Manual stretch of skin graft (deltopectoral flap) may be necessary to prevent skin tightness in healing, which would further limit ROM and cause more scapular protraction. Body mechanics and instruction in the proper positioning of involved arm, as well as proper lift techniques should be stressed. Training with mirrors or videotape is often helpful.

Shoulder pain complaints are common after the patient is ambulatory. Pain is usually located along the medial border of the scapula and upper trapezius. The patient may develop other causes of shoulder pain such as bursitis, and these must be treated to prevent a frozen shoulder. Passive shoulder ROM must be maintained. As the patient's activity level increases, attention to shoulder deficits may also increase. Orthotic devices may be used, such as the Duncan shoulder harness. Villaneuva has developed an orthosis he feels is very helpful to patients whose vocation requires prolonged use of the affected arm in front of the body in an unsupported manner.[74] This orthosis is not cosmetically acceptable to all patients, however, and it may put pressure on the ulnar nerve in the axilla.

NECK DYSFUNCTION

During total radical neck dissection, the sternocleidomastoid, platysmus, omohyoid, and anterior digastric muscles will be removed, resulting in asymmetrical neck motion. This asymmetry may lead to pain and injury to the deep cervical musculature and fascia during rapid and resistive movements. Postoperatively, the patient may need to use the hand to stabilize the head when coming up to a sitting position. When the sutures are removed, a passive ROM program with stretch to the limits of the graft line should be prescribed. As healing progresses, active ROM can be initiated and progress to active resistive strengthening about the fourth week. Patients who have had bilateral radical neck dissection are unable to flex their heads against gravity. These patients cannot go from the supine to the sitting position without holding their heads or rolling to the side to stabilize their heads. Their cervical lateral musculature is much stronger than their forward flexors.

SELF-CARE CONSIDERATIONS

In addition to the modifications and considerations necessary to manage nutrition and swallowing, the head and neck cancer patient faces other life alterations through every phase of treatment. For example, patients undergoing chemotherapy often experience a loss of self-care independence owing to fatigue, general muscle weakness, and even loss of muscle mass.[77] Because of depressed bone marrow, they are at risk for infection. Daily activities should be modified in such a way as to conserve energy, stress safety, and encourage hygiene. Assistive devices like grab bars on toilets and tubs will aid in energy conservation and improve safety on transfers. ROM must be maintained through conservative exercise and the avoidance of complications from bedrest becomes a principal consideration.

ROM exercises should also be performed prophylactically to reduce restrictive movement brought on by irradiation of tissues.[77] Other self-care considerations for patients undergoing radiation therapy relate to the protection of irradiated tissues. For example, soap, ointments, salves, deodorants, perfumes, cologne, cosmetics, and other foreign substances should be avoided.[55] Though hair loss in radiated fields is common, shaving when necessary with an electric razor is safer than with a blade. When bathing, lukewarm water is recommended and the skin should be blotted dry. Clothing should be loose fitting around radiated areas.[55]

Head and neck surgery often involves either temporary or permanent creation of a tracheostome. Patient education regarding stoma care is vital. Swimming must be avoided and bathing must be done with care to avoid drowning. Showers should be taken while wearing a special protective bib. Since the air entering the tracheal stoma has not been humidified by the nose, mouth, and pharynx, most neck breathers require humidified air to prevent dryness and crusting that can block the airway. Patients must be gradually weaned from the continuous mist they received during the first days after surgery. Patients with permanent tracheostomes may eventually adjust to the dry air and may only need room humidifiers for sleeping.

With a tracheal stoma, patients are unable to occlude the glottis in order to perform the Valsalva maneuver. Since this maneuver is important in functional activities like defecation, lifting, and pushing, patients must learn to compensate. For example, during defecation, patients should occlude their stoma with a thumb to hold their breath and develop abdominal push.

Neck breathers should be instructed to wear medical alert bracelets and to carry medical data on their person. The American Cancer Society provides emergency cards for neck breathers that describe pulmonary resuscitation procedures, such as keeping the neck opening clear, giving mouth-to-neck breathing only, and giving oxygen to the neck when needed.

SPEECH COMMUNICATION

Speech is accomplished through the processes of cerebration, respiration, phonation, and articulation. The resonating cavities of the nose, mouth, and pharynx influence the acoustic product. Head and neck cancers and their treatment have the potential to interfere with one or more of these processes. For example, cancer of the larynx is frequently treated with total laryngectomy, thus diverting the respiratory system away from the oral articulators and eliminating the vocal apparatus.

For patients with laryngectomies, the conventional means of speech rehabilitation are esophageal speech or prosthetic devices. Esophageal voice is accomplished by training patients to force air into the esophagus by injection or suction methods, to trap the air in an esophageal reservoir, and to release the air in a controlled manner, allowing it to pass up through the remnants of the circopharyngeal sphincter. The esophagus, therefore, acts as a false lung, using trapped air under pressure to produce vibration of tissues at its uppermost end.[78] The resulting voice is then articulated in the usual manner of speech.

With good esophageal speech the product is remarkably similar to normal laryngeal speech.[79] A considerable number of patients, however, are unable to learn this method.[80] Failure may be due to problems of esophageal sphincter relaxation, scarring, or nerve damage. Pharyngectomy, along with laryngectomy, usually precludes esophageal speech.[79] Impaired intellectual ability and hearing loss interfere with the learning process. Abdominal distension, excessive flatulence and even

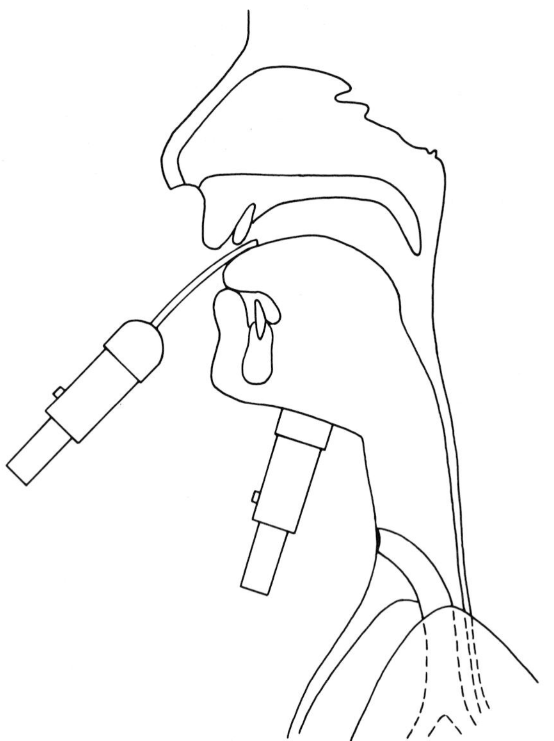

FIG. 46-9. Sound generated by an electrolarynx can be transmitted through the neck or introduced into the mouth directly by a short catheter.

peptic ulcers are sequelae related to aerophagia, a potential complication of esophageal speech.

Prosthetic devices, such as the electrolarynx or pneumatic external reed, are also available for speech rehabilitation. Some esophageal speakers use a prosthesis intermittently. The electrolarynx, either intra-oral or neck type, is the most commonly used speech aid (Fig. 46-9). A neck type electrolarynx is a battery powered tone generator that conveys sound through neck tissue to resonate within the oral cavity, where it can be articulated as speech.

When the neck is not suitable for transmitting the sounds because of edema or pain, an intra-oral electrolarynx can be used to transmit the generated tone directly into the mouth through a small catheter. In general, the speech produced by the neck type electrolarynx is more intelligible, but training with the intra-oral electrolarynx can begin almost immediately following surgery without stressing the neck wounds. Some speech pathologists advocate beginning speech rehabilitation with an intra-oral device, changing to the neck type when suture lines are well healed, and teaching esophageal speech, if indicated, when the patient starts to eat by mouth.[58]

The pneumatic external reed larynx diverts pulmonary air from the tracheostome past a vibrating membrane, reed, or rubber band (Fig. 46-10). The sound produced by the vibrator is directed into the mouth by way of a length of tubing and articulated as speech. Though some patients use this method of speech quite satisfactorily, many lack the respiratory support to drive the vibrator.[78]

A number of surgical procedures are being tried in an attempt to provide patients with a sound source following laryngectomy. One such method implants a transected trachea into the pharynx, forming a "neoglottis" at this junction.[81] Another procedure attempts to reconstruct a pseudolarynx from retained thyroid cartilage.[82] Some surgeons have reported success with the development of external appliances shunting air from the tracheostome through a surgically created pharyngocutaneous fistula.[83–85] Most recently, the placement of a one-way valved prosthesis through a controlled tracheal-esophageal fistula has been highly successful in achieving speech.

Rehabilitation of patients with laryngectomies should begin with pre-operative counseling. Some will benefit from a pre-operative visit by a person with a laryngectomy who has functional speech, while others will be discouraged by such a visit.[86] The American Cancer Society has booklets available that help explain anatomic and physiologic changes with a laryngectomy, and lists resources available to patients following treatment. Many communities have laryngectomy clubs or "lost chord clubs" that can serve as a useful resource for information and support as well as a social outlet for some patients with laryngectomies and their families.

Another group requiring speech rehabilitation is glossectomy patients. Skelly and her co-workers have shown that many patients with partial and total glossectomies can achieve intelligible speech with therapy.[64,87–90] Patients with partial glossectomies tend to use the remaining tongue stump for articulation and need to be taught modifications of normal articulatory patterns in order to improve speech intelligibility.[87] Total glossectomy patients must learn complex and varied substitutions to approximate phonemes that can be under-

FIG. 46-10. A pneumatic external voice prosthesis diverts air from the lungs to vibrate a membrane, reed, or rubber band and transmits the sound to the mouth.

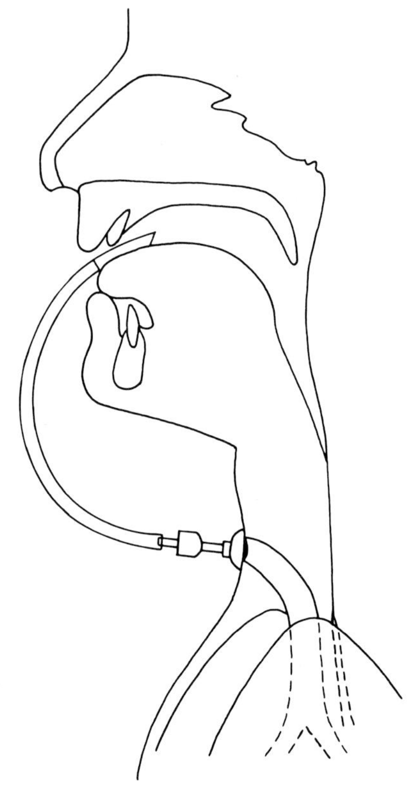

stood. Those with a total glossectomy must master the use of lips, cheeks, soft palate, mandible, and floor of the mouth to substitute for the missing tongue.[64,87]

Intelligible speech has been achieved in up to 50% of patients with total glossectomies, with 57% of these same patients able to swallow adequately.[64] In general, patients who learn to swallow without difficulty also develop intelligible speech.[64,87] Speech therapy may begin as soon as 10 days postoperatively, or as soon as wounds are healed. Early training consists of practice occluding the stoma and producing vocal tones.[64] The therapy is generally long and intense, with 6–8 months of elapsed time before usable gains in intelligibility occur.[89]

The total glossectomy patient learns to produce vowels by varying the degree of mandibular thrust.[90] Consonants are approximated by substituting sounds produced by the compensating articulators. For example, the phoneme /z/ can be approximated by creating bilabial tension and obstructing the airstream, and the phoneme /d/ can be produced by lower lip contact with the upper teeth or alveolar ridge.[87] Once these compensations are mastered, the therapist emphasizes consistency of substitution in order to improve intelligibility.[89] The most intelligible glossectomy speakers have the most consistent substitution while those with the least consistency have the poorest intelligibility scores.[90] Skelly reports that a group of eight patients with total glossectomies without dysphagia had intelligibility scores from 0% to 8% on single words at admission, and shifted to scores ranging from 18% to 42% following therapy.[87] For total glossectomy patients with dysphagia these clinicians advocate the teaching of an easily interpretable American Indian sign language called Amerind.[88]

DISFIGUREMENT

As more patients survive longer with head and neck cancers and as surgical procedures become necessarily more sophisticated and extensive, the need for restoring acceptable appearance and function presents an enormous challenge. In spite of tremendous advances in plastic surgery in the mouth and face, defects from orbital exenteration, removal of the external ear, and the loss of the entire nose can not be satisfactorily managed with plastic surgery alone.[27]

Presurgical consultation with a maxillofacial prosthodontist is necessary for the preparation or modification of the surgical site in order to facilitate retention of the prosthesis. This also allows the prosthodontist to obtain impressions and diagnostic casts of teeth and jaw arches and to collect necessary data regarding the mold, shade, and alignment of existing dentition.[67]

Surgical splints, stents, and obturators fabricated for use in the primary surgical procedure may be helpful in promoting healing and reducing the period of hospitalization.[27,67] In the case of maxillectomy, an obturator inserted at wound closure may permit early intelligible speech, limited chewing and swallowing.[67]

Interim prostheses are also devised to promote functional return following extensive surgery. For example, an interim obturator to fill palatal defects is fabricated once major healing has occurred. This interim palatal obturator generally extends into the defect to improve voice and stability of the prosthesis, and artificial teeth are included to aid in mastication.[27] Another example of interim prosthesis is one used to correct mandibular discontinuity after unilateral mandibular resection. The remaining mandible tends to drift toward the defect and rotate back, resulting in malocclusion. This can often be corrected by using simple hand pressure to guide the mandible to proper occlusion.[67] More severe malocclusions require a maxillomandibular guiding prosthesis to reinforce movement of the mandible away from the defect to functional occlusion.[27,67]

Some clinicians feel that because aged and debilitated patients often cannot tolerate staged extended surgical restoration, especially in the face, they are best treated by prosthetic rehabilitation.[91] The maxillofacial prosthodontist attempts to develop a facial prosthesis that is comfortable, natural in appearance, and durable. Acrylics, silicones, polyvinyl chlorides, and urethanes are most commonly used in the fabrication of these prostheses.[67,92] Regardless of the material used, the prosthesis has to be altered frequently, as the tissues change. Because the material wears out, the prosthesis should be replaced about once a year and a new facial moulage obtained as needed. Temporary removable facial prostheses are frequently used when delay of surgery is elected. These can also be used in cases of the uncontrolled primary, allowing the surgeon to remove the prosthesis and view the defect during follow-up.[91]

The most noticeable part of the facial prosthesis is the margin, and the maxillofacial prosthodontist tries to conceal this beneath hair, glasses, or natural facial lines.[67] These prostheses are usually held in place with skin adhesives, although glasses and intraoral prostheses can provide mechanical reinforcement for added stability. When a facial prosthesis approaches the oral cavity, retention problems are greater because of saliva leakage and movement of support structures.[67]

The psychological and social effects of head and neck cancer can be particularly severe owing to the visibility of the cancer and the effect of radiation and surgery. The psychological and social intervention must begin with diagnosis and supporting relationships should be developed. When more is known about the extent of the disease, the treatments for it, and the prognosis, individualized psychological and social intervention programs can be developed. Because of the poor prognosis for many of these patients, counseling services about death and dying should be available for the patients and significant others.

Staff members who work with these patients must be sensitive to the psychological needs of the patient and should convey attitudes of acceptance and support. Careful staff selection is appropriate and consideration should be given to providing staff members with psychological support.

BONE AND SOFT TISSUE MALIGNANCY: AMPUTATIONS, PATHOLOGIC FRACTURES

Soft tissue sarcomas are limited to the tissue around bone. They can sometimes be treated with surgical excision of the tumor and the muscular compartment in which it lies, leaving the bony skeleton intact. Disability relates to the specific functions of the muscle resected or to any residual instability of the extremity. Functional limitation can be decreased by proper muscle retraining, an orthosis for the lower extremity (LE) or a static or dynamic splint for the upper extremity (UE).[93]

Treatment of a highly malignant operable soft tissue cancer or a primary bone cancer sometimes involves amputation. The level of the amputation is dictated by the bone involved. Tumors of the foot are often treated with a below knee (BK) amputation, while those of the tibia or fibula usually require a midthigh amputation. Femur tumors require hip disarticulation or hemipelvectomy.[94] For far advanced disease, a hemicorporectomy may be performed.[95]

Patients with amputations due to cancer are usually younger (10–30 years of age) than those with amputations due to peripheral vascular disease.[96] The levels of amputation are higher, and most amputations involve the LE.

Pre-operatively, the patient should be counseled with respect to the disease process, the surgical procedure, and the level of amputation. Phantom sensation should be discussed. The rehabilitation plan should be presented, as well as the estimated time for prosthetic fitting and gait or UE training. If the amputation involves the LE, the pre-operative physical restoration program involves crutch walking prior to surgery, when the patient does not have a fear of falling, is not receiving analgesics, and has not developed deconditioning due to bedrest.[93] Most patients with amputations of the UE can be taught to perform one-handed self-care activities.

The time from operative decision to surgery is often very short, and most of the pre-operative rehabilitation is psychological preparation. The focus should be on reducing the patient's anxiety and fear, and on helping the patient begin to mourn the loss and to deal with the change in body image. The presurgical intervention might include introducing the patient to persons with amputations at similar levels, who have adjusted to the loss and the use of a prosthesis. These activities should continue after surgery.

SURGERY

Wound closure and surgical dressing techniques have advanced in the past few years and involve a rigid dressing with either immediate or early postoperative fitting of a temporary prosthesis. The rigid dressing consists of a thin wound dressing covered by a rigid plaster of Paris that conforms totally to the contours of the stump. Incorporated into the plaster of Paris is a coupling device with which the pylon and artificial foot may be attached.

Formation of edema in an amputated stump is the primary cause of stump pain and delayed healing. The rigid dressing properly applied prevents edema, even if the amputated limb is kept in the dependent position. These patients do not experience frequent phantom pain, although phantom sensations are still present.

For BK and above the knee (AK) amputations with immediate fit dressing, the pylon prosthesis is applied while the patient is on the operating table. In early fitting, the pylon is usually applied 10 days to 14 days after surgery, at the initial cast change when the drain is removed. For UE amputations, hip disarticulations, or hemipelvectomies, the rigid dressing can still be applied to promote more rapid wound healing.

Postoperatively, the patient with LE amputation should be instructed in progressive resistive exercises to the muscles of the opposite LE, as well as the crutch and shoulder depressor muscles of the UEs. Balancing exercises and gait training with the prosthesis should begin on the parallel bars. It is important to eventually train the patient to ambulate on rough terrain, ramps, stairs, and to get up from the floor.

The patient with an UE amputation should be taught one-handed techniques for self-care activities, ROM, and strengthening exercises of the remaining arm. If the dominant hand has been lost, training should be extended to include handwriting and dexterity. Driver retraining and evaluation for vocational rehabilitation should be considered.

It is imperative during the postoperative phase that the patient with LE amputation (BK, AK) not develop hip or knee flexion contractures on the operated side. These can result from muscle imbalance or poor bed positioning, that is, pillows placed under the AK stump or under the knee. A knee flexion contractor of greater than 15° or a hip flexion contracture of 30° to 40° may make it impossible to fit the patient with a satisfactory prosthesis.[97] If a stump is present, it should be moved through full ROM b.i.d. to help prevent contracture. The patient is also taught stump conditioning, skin care, and stump wrapping.

A prosthesis should be prescribed for any patient with a cancer-related amputation who desires one, provided the surgical wound has healed and ambulation is a reasonably safe goal. Residual malignant disease is not a contraindication to prosthetic prescription and the key consideration should be the patient's need, both functionally and psychologically. Each case has to be judged individually.

A prosthesis of functional value can be provided for any LE amputation. The type of prosthesis socket and its suspension may be of concern in patients with healing problems due to radiation or chemotherapy. Patients undergoing chemotherapy often experience weight fluctuations, resulting in rapid changes in stump size.[98] It is important to remember that prosthesis fitting must be determined individually with clinical circumstances, and with the experiences of the physician and prosthetist modifying the prescriptions.

The following generalizations in prosthetic prescription for common amputation levels can be made:

BK LEVEL. The prosthesis of choice for a patient with BK amputation is a patella tendon bearing (PTB) prosthesis with a solid ankle cushion heel (SACH) foot (Fig. 46-11). The socket may have a soft liner. This type of prosthesis is prescribed even for patients who are receiving chemotherapy, or who live a long way from any facility where prosthetic adjustments can be made.[98] It is desirable to delay the prosthetic fitting until the patient's weight has stabilized, otherwise the socket will need to be modified or replaced many times.[27] Prosthetic gait training for these patients is usually short and they usually ambulate without canes or crutches.

AK LEVEL. The patient with AK amputation is harder to fit prosthetically or to prescribe for a typical prosthesis. Radiated skin heals slower and maintenance of total contact without skin necrosis requires vigilance and meticulous skin

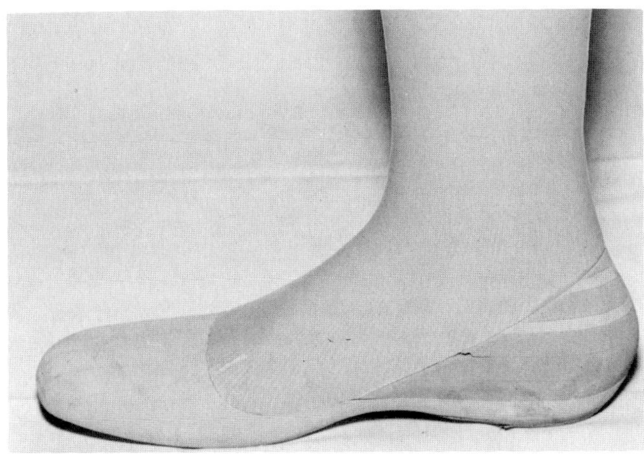

FIG. 46-11. SACH foot. Heel compresses at heel strike and acts as a shock absorber. In the BK prosthesis, a knee bending moment is generated and is controlled by the hamstrings, allowing the prosthesis to move forward at the knee to "foot flat" phase of gait.

care. The socket can be either a total contact quadrilateral suction socket, which is used for most peripheral vascular amputations, or a quadrilateral nonsuction socket suspended by a hip joint and pelvic belt or silesian bandage.[98]

The quadrilateral socket has an ischial and gluteal weight-bearing shelf which constitutes the proximal posterior socket wall. The lateral border is trimmed proximal to the trochanter. Anteriorly, it drops to the same level as the ischial gluteal seat, and on the medial border it runs posteriorly, also at the level of the ischial gluteal seat. The lateal wall is shaped to distribute forces generated by the hip abductors, necessary to prevent the pelvis from dropping on the contralateral side during stance on the prosthesis side.

The total contact provides support of the distal soft tissue, thus enhancing peripheral vascular return. The patient's ischial and gluteal area is maintained on the seat by a bulge in the anterior socket wall conforming to Scarpa's triangle. Relief is provided for the adductor longus tendon, and the area over the rectus femoris is fitted to avoid inhibition of active contraction of the muscle.

The term "suction socket" is used to identify an AK amputation socket that by intimate fit creates a vacuum within the socket. The negative pressure is maintained by a one-way valve that allows air to be expelled. The suction socket provides for self-suspension of the prosthesis, although axillary belts may be added. In the nonsuction socket, suspension is provided by a combination of the mechanical hip joint, the pelvic band, and a waist belt. A constant friction knee component, the more expensive hydraulic, hydracadence, or the Henschke-Mauch units can be prescribed.

After surgery, the patient with AK amputation may start with crutch walking and stump exercises. A temporary prosthesis is usually made about 2 weeks postoperatively, and the socket is replaced as often as variations in stump size require. After 6 weeks to 8 weeks, a nonsuction socket suspended by silesian bandage or pelvic belt can be prescribed. At 6 months to 8 months, when stump size has stabilized, a definite quadrilateral suction socket can be prescribed to replace the nonsuction one.[99] If a constant suction socket is provided, it is necessary to follow the patient very closely.

HIP DISARTICULATION LEVELS. Patients with hip disarticulation usually have a Canadian hip disarticulation prosthesis prescribed. In this prosthesis, the socket encircles the pelvis and provides for ischial weight-bearing on the amputated side. It has a free-swinging hip joint with an extension stop, and an articulated knee with an elastic strap that passes posterior to the hip and anterior to the mechanical knee, which provides for prosthetic hip and knee extension. These patients maintain their hip hiking and pelvic tilting musculature and their gait pattern is free of vaulting. They may need a cane when walking on uneven ground, grass, or thick carpets.[27]

HEMIPELVECTOMY LEVEL. With the hemipelvectomy procedure and the loss of pelvic bones, the patient's sitting surface is unstable. Special cushions need to be fabricated to allow the patient to have proper skeletal alignment while sitting to minimize the risk of scoliosis, back pain, and skin breakdowns. With removal of the ipsilateral pelvis and the loss of muscle insertions, hip hiking and pelvic tilting cannot be accomplished. Body weight is carried on soft tissue instead of bone, resulting in poor prosthetic stability.

The Canadian hemipelvectomy prosthesis can be prescribed for ambulation.[100] A cane or crutch is needed to assist in walking. The patient must vault in order for the leg to clear the floor during the swing phase of gait.[27] This prosthesis is heavy, unwieldy, and in patients whose weight fluctuates, there may be many fitting problems. Since ambulation with the prosthesis is slower than crutch walking without it, some patients prefer to ambulate on crutches and use the prosthesis only for special occasions.[101] With this level of amputation, neurogenic bladders are not common.[102]

HEMICORPORECTOMY LEVEL. Hemicorporectomy, or translumbar amputation, has been performed for advanced cancer in a final life-saving effort.[95,103] The amputation is usually between the L4 and L5 levels. The procedure requires the fecal stream to be diverted by a colostomy or an ileostomy. With the latter, continuous liquid drainage causes special prosthetic concerns. The urine is diverted by an ilioloop procedure, emptying into a collecting bag.

A sitting bucket prosthesis, mounted on a platform to allow the socket to rotate, allows the patient to sit and perform wheelchair ambulation. The following criteria must be fulfilled by the bucket prosthesis:[95,103]

1. Contact sufficient to support the soft tissue, but insufficient to cause increased intra-abdominal pressure with stomal herniation, nausea, or abdominal pain
2. No weight bearing or pressure on the tip of the vertebral column and sufficient distribution of weight bearing surfaces to prevent pressure necrosis
3. Independent transfer in and out of the socket.
4. No impedance of stomal drainage and easy access to the drainage bags
5. No restriction of respiratory capacity

A full prosthesis can also be made using a similar socket without the platform. It has free-swinging hip joints, locked knee joints, and SACH feet.[103] The prosthesis is suspended by a shoulder harness and the patient ambulates using bilateral forearm crutches and a swing-through gait pattern. These patients can drive an automobile using hand controls and a special harness to improve trunk stability.

INTERSCAPULOTHORACIC LEVEL. In patients undergoing interscapulothoracic amputation, a functional UE prosthesis is usually not feasible. It is too heavy, too noisy, and too difficult to stabilize on the remaining chest wall. There is a tendency for rotation and displacement when traction or pressure is applied. For patients who desire a nonfunctional cosmetic UE prosthesis, an appliance with a hand terminal device and cosmetic glove can be prescribed. For most patients, the easiest and most useful prosthesis is a cosmetic shoulder cap to support the clothing on the amputated side and provide symmetrical shoulder appearance.[93] Usually, a soft temporary cap is made and can be worn as soon as the sutures are removed, until a permanent prosthesis is provided.

SHOULDER DISARTICULATION LEVEL. A functional prosthesis can be prescribed for the individual with a shoulder disarticulation. It will have a double wall shoulder cap socket with the trim line 2.5 inches to 3 inches medial to the acromion, also medial to the deltopectoral groove. In addition, it will have a passive multiple action shoulder joint, a Hosmer forearm lift assist elbow unit, a flexion wrist unit, and a light aluminum terminal device. It uses a dual control system with a chest strap harness.

PSYCHOLOGICAL CONSIDERATIONS

Since patients with amputations due to cancer are usually young, the impact of the cancer and amputation on their education process and return to school may be significant and require professional intervention. The patient and family should be offered counseling about body image change, cancer related fears, full participation in rehabilitation, and how to deal with others around these issues. The teacher and classmates should also be provided with information on changes to expect and how to be supportive, while allowing the patient to be as independent as possible.

For cancer patients scheduled for any amputation, vocational considerations must be addressed from the beginning. If the amputation will necessitate adaptive changes in the work environment, they should be initiated. If a new job or retraining is needed postoperatively, this should also be addressed early to provide a tangible goal and to increase motivation for the overall rehabilitation process.

METASTATIC BONE CANCER

Bone pain from cancer is described as dull and aching in character. When more than half of the circumference of a weight-bearing bone has been destroyed, the patient will usually complain of pain when walking.

In managing metastatic bone tumors there is concern about pathological fractures, and their effect on function. Fractures are often spontaneous, or occur after minimal trauma. The fractures usually involve long bones (femur, humerus) as well as pelvis and ribs.[93] The sites of the metastases are often functionally significant.[104] Pathological fractures are caused by neoplastic lesions, usually metastatic, eroding large amounts of the bone and causing severe weakness of the remaining normal bony cortex. It is best to treat metastatic tumors before pathological fractures occur. Metallic stabilization of weakened bone should be considered whenever a third of the bone mass has been replaced by tumor.[104] Obviously, the decision to operate depends on the patient's health and desire to have the operation.

Intramedullary rods are used to augment the strength of the cancerous bone and, if used prophylactically, can stabilize a painful lesion, prevent fractures, and allow the patient functional use of the limb. These rods are usually combined with bone cement. Other procedures, such as total joint arthroplasty, resection arthroplasty, and allograft interposition techniques can also be used as methods of internal fixation, in order to increase the rate of rehabilitation.

For metastasis to spinal vertebrae, various surgical techniques and orthoses have been developed to provide stability, prevent neurologic damage, and relieve pain. For patients who have cervical vertebral involvement without neurological damage, a sternal occipital mandibular immobilization (SOMI) orthosis has been used for any level from the basilar occiput apophysis down to the T2 level (Fig. 46-12).[25] SOMI limits cervical flexion much more than extension.[105]

Bone metastasis of the thoracic spine can prove to be difficult to treat because mutliple bones are usually involved with the tumor, that is, the spine, ribs, sternum, clavicle, and scapula. It is often difficult to prescribe orthoses for patients with bone pain and fractures but no neurological deficits, as these involved bones are unreliable in providing support or counterpressure. For thoracic vertebral bony lesions without a neurological deficit, a Taylor orthosis with sternal instead of axillary pads is often prescribed.[27]

LUNG CANCER

Rehabilitation goals in patients with lung cancer are to prevent pulmonary disability following radiation or surgery by facilitating bronchial drainage, improving ventilation, and preventing postural deformity such as scoliosis.[106]

Surgery to remove cancerous lung tissue (thoracotomy, lobectomy, and pneumonectomy) may be associated with a postoperative limitation of pulmonary function and impairment of the mechanics of breathing. The decrease in respiratory reserve depends on the amount of lung tissue resected. Impairment of the mechanism of breathing is due to chest wall resection with transected muscles, pain, and bandaging all resulting in splinting.[107]

Pre-operative treatment is helpful, since many of these patients already have restricted pulmonary function which will only be aggravated by the thoracotomy and lung tissue resection. It is best prior to surgery to have the patient quit smoking, and try inhaled or oral bronchodilators. If the sputum is purulent, antibiotics should be prescribed.

The pre-operative rehabilitation program should emphasize breathing retraining to increase diaphragmatic excursion with a resultant reduction in the work of breathing, increased tidal

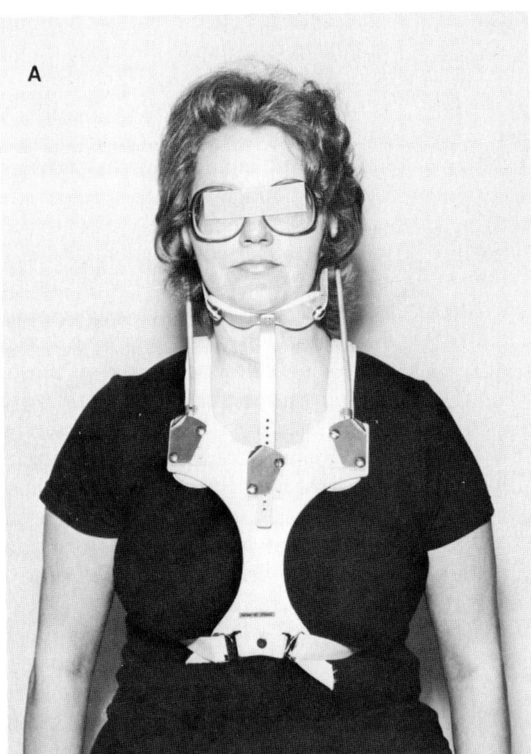

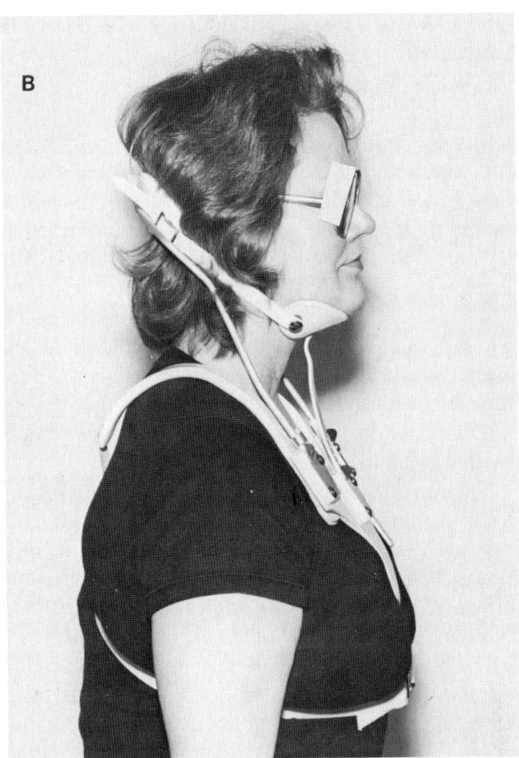

FIG. 46-12. The SOMI orthesis prevents cervical flexion and provides vertebral stability. *A*, Front view; *B*, side view.

volume, and improvement in the distribution of inspired gas.[108] Diaphragmatic abdominal breathing is usually combined with pursed lips breathing, which is an effective method of altering the respiratory pattern, slowing down the respiratory rate and decreasing airway collapse during expiration.[109] It is best to teach these exercises pre-operatively when there is no incision pain; however, some patients quickly revert to their old breathing patterns when not being supervised. Segmental breathing can be taught in order to allow certain areas to expand, and the lateral basal, posterior basal, and diaphragmatic areas should receive special attention.[110] These techniques are much harder for patients with pulmonary pathology than normal individuals.

Postural drainage is utilized to help clear bronchial secretions from a particular segment or lobe of the lung, and is most effective in patients who have bronchiectasis or an infiltrate. The frequency and duration of drainage is dependent on the patient's individual needs and tolerance.[111]

Pre-operatively, effective coughing is taught using correct respiratory control, rather than by simply increasing force or volume of expelled air.[96] It is best to have the patient fully inspire and cough two or three times in one breath.[111] This will allow evacuation throughout the tracheobronchial tree segments. Postoperatively, therapy begins as soon as the patient awakes. The intensity of the program will depend on the patient's overall medical condition, tolerance to exercise, and specific respiratory problem.[106]

Manual hand splinting of the chest by the patient or staff helps to reduce the patient's discomfort and apprehension, as incision pain plays a major role in cooperation with therapy. Initially, respiratory accessory muscle activity of the thorax and neck should be eliminated to further reduce discomfort. It is sensible to treat these patients 20 to 30 minutes after administration of analgesics, so they can comply with the therapeutic plan. The postoperative treatment program should include breathing exercises, positional drainage, and proper coughing. The intensity of the program depends on the patient's physical condition and response to exercise.

Chest percussion and vibration may be added to the program when they can be tolerated. These methods are used to loosen secretions that may adhere to the inner lumen of the small bronchi. Direct pressure to the wound site should be avoided and it should not be used in cases of suspected pneumothorax, chest trauma, rib fracture, or pathological fracture.[111] As the patient improves and the incisional pain decreases, a more active exercise program is initiated to restore ROM and muscle strength. The program will focus on correction and prevention of scoliosis and any ipsilateral shoulder restriction. Contracture of this shoulder could impede such ADLs as dressing, bathing, and grooming. In some patients, dyspnea may be so severe that it interferes with self-care and day-to-day activities, and they need to be instructed in energy conservation techniques.

Some of the extrapulmonary effects of lung cancer are peripheral neuropathies, myositis, cortical cerebellar degeneration, and the myasthenic syndrome. All of these will potentially affect the patient's ability to function with respect to ADLs and mobility. The problems stemming from the remote effects should be addressed in the comprehensive rehabilitation plan.

OSTOMIES FOR BOWEL AND BLADDER CANCER

Surgical treatment of bowel and bladder cancer may result in ostomies to divert feces and urine. For patients with ostomies, rehabilitation must address the individual's adjustment to a drastically altered self-concept, the ability to control elimination, and the need to learn ostomy management in a manner that facilitates optimum psychosocial function. Rehabilitation is a continuous and dynamic process designed to provide the patient the opportunity to learn necessary skills. When possible, this continuity should be provided by a nurse specialist or enterostomal therapist who is skillful in utilizing knowledge relative to body image, learning theories, and the effects of the disease and its treatment, and who is competent in all aspects of stoma management.

The concept of trained enterostomal therapists is credited to Dr. Rupert Turnbull of the Cleveland Clinic. Certification has been administered by their official organization, the International Association for Enterostomal Therapy, and presently includes individuals of diverse backgrounds, some with ostomies themselves.[112]

Acceptance of an altered body image, and learning self-care progresses faster if rehabilitation is initiated at the time of diagnosis. Clear explanations of the physical and functional outcome expectations of surgery should be given. While this is primarily the surgeon's role, the enterostomal therapist should help clarify and amplify the physiological and psychological consequences. Initially, the psychological impact of this information can interfere with the patient's ability to assimilate it, but it sets the stage for future interventions aimed at self-care independence. Persons who are ill-prepared pre-operatively will require more time, support, and assistance in their rehabilitation.[113] It has been demonstrated that patients provided with the continuous services of an enterostomal therapist have shorter hospital stays and require fewer home visits to attain successful management.[112]

To help the patient resolve conflicts and eventually accept an altered body image the following rehabilitation steps have been proposed:

1. Accepts the importance of viewing the operative site
2. Touches and explores the operative site
3. Accepts the necessity of learning to care for the stoma
4. Develops independence and competence in daily care
5. Re-integrates the new body image and adjusts to a possibly altered life style.[114]

This process may be modified by cultural attitudes and values and the patient's actual ability to perform the procedures.

Participation of an enterostomal therapist in the selection of the stoma site can also contribute to problem prevention. The stoma should be on a flat surface without creases and wrinkles, and away from scars, bony protuberances, the waistline, umbilicus, and other stomas. To best assess the site, the patient should be checked in the supine, sitting and forward-bending positions. The stoma should protrude about a half inch above the skin level to allow for more effective collection of liquid drainage.[115]

The procedural steps for teaching the behaviors to accomplish control of urine and feces should reflect the competence of the enterostomal therapist and the familiarity with the specific equipment and appliances to be utilized. The prescribed appliance system should be consistently available during hospitalization, at discharge, and in the community. The patient should be made aware of the various component parts and options and help select them. The care and use of each component should be explained to the patient.

About 50% of the patients with a descending or sigmoid colostomy are able to develop a natural evacuation at regular intervals, thus avoiding a collecting device. Other patients with colostomies may require irrigation to control elimination. This should be encouraged in those who had regular bowel movements prior to surgery, and who desire to try this method in order to avoid a collecting device. Patients whose bowel movements were irregular and unpredictable prior to surgery will most likely have to wear a collecting device, even if they use irrigation to stimulate bowel evacuation. Perforation due to colostomy irrigations may occur, although the risk can be reduced by using an irrigating cone, or inserting the catheter tip less than 5 cm.[115]

A typical colostomy irrigation program would involve training the bowel on a fixed daily, or every other day, schedule. The time chosen should be convenient and without distraction, taking usually an hour, to start. The gastrocolic reflex is stimulated by using food, or hot or cold liquids to increase peristalsis. The irrigation is used to stimulate the colon from below. A bag or can containing 500–1000 cc of lukewarm water is hung 60 cm above the stoma. The patient should sit on the toilet with the soiled appliance bag or dressing removed. An irrigation bag is attached with the long end in the toilet bowl and the water is then allowed to run through the tubing to remove all air. The lubricated cone or catheter is inserted into the stoma and the water is released to enter at a rate that is determined by the patient's comfort. Rapid distention of the bowel may produce cramps. It usually takes 5 minutes to 10 minutes for the water to run into the bowel. The return from the irrigation occurs in two stages. The first occurs with the removal of the cone or catheter, and drainage through the irrigation bag into the toilet bowl. Thirty minutes later the rest of the drainage occurs. Most persons will then remove the appliance, clean it, dry it, and cover the colostomy with a gauze pad.[115]

Bromley presented this rehabilitation process covering preoperative counseling to post-hospital follow-up, utilizing Orem's self-care theory.[116] Her interventions are designed to bring about a transition from dependence to independence, relative to ostomy management. Although limited to physical abilities immediately postoperatively, the patient is able to learn through the modeling of the enterostomal therapist. Explaining and giving information also prepare the patient for participation. Other learning concepts to be utilized in developing self-care include building in a measure of success for each session, positively reinforcing appropriate behaviors, and shaping these through stages of successive approximations from dependence to independence.[117]

A resource for patient information and psychological support is a member of the Ostomy Association, who will visit patients upon request. These volunteers all have ostomies, and can be located through the American Cancer Society. Another "normalizing" approach used in physical rehabilitation is to have patients wear their own clothing while still in the hospital. This practice can also resolve the patient's fears about visibility of appliances.

For the patient with an ostomy, skin care will always be important. During the operation, and immediately postoperatively, it is essential to avoid skin damage. Sutures must not be placed through the epidermis of the peristomal skin, and accumulation of blood and serum in the subcutaneous tissue adjacent to the stoma must be avoided. To avoid leakage, there must be an exact fit of the appliance to the skin around the stoma, leaving only an ⅛ inch to 1⁄16 inch margin between the stoma and the appliance edge, to allow for contraction and relaxation of the stoma. Any complaint of stomal itching or burning should be interpreted as leakage and the appliance must be changed immediately.[115]

The most common postoperative skin problems are maceration or candida infection. Skin maceration should be treated by covering the erosion with nonadherent bandage and topical steroid cream or spray. Candida infection will respond to nystatin powder.[115] Contact dermatitis may develop and should be treated by removing the irritant (adhesive tape or material comprising the appliance or the barrier), and by using local steroids. Folliculitis is best treated by trimming the hairs around the stoma, not by pulling them out or shaving them with a razor.[115]

Diet information for the colostomy and ileostomy patient should not consist of long lists of restrictive prohibitions but rather a more positive approach of experimenting to determine individual tolerance.[118] Foods that cause gas or diarrhea before surgery are likely to continue to be a problem. Patients with a colostomy should be advised to chew foods well to avoid constipation, especially nuts, seeds, popcorn, and celery. New foods should be tried one at a time to discover their effect on the ostomy. Patients on diabetic or antihypertensive diets should continue with them, following surgery.[115]

Gas is produced in an empty intestine and is a consequence of abdominal surgery. The gas, though harmless, is uncomfortable and embarrassing. Patients should avoid skipping meals to prevent an empty intestine. They should be informed that anxiety, gum chewing, candy sucking, and cigarette smoking will increase gas.[115]

Ileostomy patients may experience problems with fluids and electrolytes. When the terminal ileum is removed, vitamin B-12 supplements are required. Diarrhea, caused by infection (influenza), medications, or bowel irradiation, may lead to rapid dehydration in ileostomy patients. Urine output of less than 400 ml in 12 hours indicates impending dehydration and requires intravenous electrolytes.[115]

Discharge planning and follow-up are the real tests of hospital initiated rehabilitation programs. A smooth transition back to community living is dependent on early communication among the patient, family, hospital team, and community resource people. Written information for home reference should include instructions to reinforce teaching and sources of equipment, appropriate medication, and dietary information. Patients need printed material regarding the resumption of activities, including sexual intercourse, Ostomy Association information, follow-up appointments, and names of individuals to call for assistance. In some states, the American Cancer Society will contribute to the cost of equipment. Referrals to a home nursing service may enhance the transition. The community nurse, using technical knowledge and sensitivity, can further stimulate the resumption of normal activities. This nurse also brings a knowledge of community resources and how to coordinate them on behalf of the patient's optimal functioning in the community.

Unless there are complicating medical problems, most patients with ostomies should be able to return to their previous employment. This will not be true for many laborers, as heavy and prolonged lifting should be avoided.[115]

Although rapid changes in atmospheric pressure may produce more intestinal gas, there should be no travel restrictions with respect to the ostomy. The patient should take along any equipment required for routine ostomy care. Seat belts should be fastened below or well above the stoma.[115]

No special clothing is required, but too tight or too rigid clothing tends to put too much pressure on the stoma. The patient should be able to participate in all exercise and sports, and can even enjoy swimming, provided he uses a non-water-soluble appliance seal.[115]

SEXUAL FUNCTION

A major area of psychological concern for many patients with ostomies is sexual functioning. (For further discussion see Chapter 12.) Sexual problems which arise may be from the changes imposed by the cancer or the surgery, but more frequently arise from how the patient feels about and deals with the changes.[119]

People frequently confuse sex, sex acts, and sexuality. Trieschman describes the difference between these terms. She describes *sex* as referring to one of the primary drives, *sex act* as behavior involving the erogenous zones and genitalia, and *sexuality* combines these with aspects of personality, communication, and relationship patterns.[120]

For patients with ostomies, sexual problems most commonly will involve sexuality issues; however, for some males, impotence will result from the surgery itself. For both men and women, ostomy surgery will result in an altered body image. How they integrate this into their total being and self acceptance will determine the extent of the impact. If the person with the ostomy is not comfortable, it will be much more difficult for others to be; likewise, when others show overt negative reactions to the ostomy, it will make it much more difficult for the patient to be accepting of the ostomy and altered body image. Patients with ostomies and their significant others can be helped in these areas through counseling, and if appropriate, by meeting with other patients and their partners. Desensitization by a trained therapist to the ostomy and its disfigurement may also be beneficial.

Other ostomy-related concerns which can affect sexual functioning are the fears of odor, spillage, and of the appliances getting in the way. These problems can be minimized through education, careful self-care, experimentation, and experience. The quality of commercial products and appliances available for ostomy care is improving, as is our knowledge of care procedures. Education and counseling of these patients and their families can significantly increase their quality of life and add to the chance of success for their overall rehabilitation program.

CANCER OF THE BRAIN

Cancer of the central nervous system (CNS) represents only about 2% of all cancers, but up to 15% of patients with systemic cancer develop neurological symptoms.[121] The nervous system is susceptible to anatomic lesions and to toxic or destructive effects of surgery, chemotherapy, and radiation. Cancer of vital organs may also have a remote effect on the nervous system.[122]

Whether the patient has a primary brain tumor or metastatic lesions or the brain is affected by a treatment modality or remote cancer, the patient may have functional deficits that can be treated by a rehabilitation team. Among the problems that may be encountered in these patients are intellectual impairments, mobility deficits, ADL problems, and bowel and bladder incontinence. Rehabilitation should begin as soon as the diagnosis of cancer is made and initial steps taken to prevent further complications and minimize the impact of the deficit on the patient's quality of life. Rehabilitation goals and plans must consider the patient's prognosis. For some, gains in function may increase comfort and allow a degree of independence. The use of adaptive equipment, therapeutic exercise, self-care training, mobility training, or environmental modifications may significantly increase the quality of their remaining lives. In some, the prevention of complications may allow the patient time at home that would otherwise be missed.

The degree of deficit and ability to respond to rehabilitation measures may fluctuate during and following treatment. During radiation and chemotherapy there may be a decline in the patient's neurological or hematological condition, but completion of these therapies may result in cure or a marked improvement.

INTELLECTUAL IMPAIRMENTS

Changes in cognitive functions are common in patients with cancer of the brain. These deficits may be generalized and obvious, or local and difficult to detect. Since many rehabilitation techniques are dependent on learning and cooperation, all patients with brain cancer should be evaluated for cognitive changes. In many cases, the deficits themselves may not be subject to change, but the patient's rehabilitation plan should be developed by the team, patient, and significant others with full knowledge of their learning capabilities and weaknesses. For patients who cannot learn, the team should work with the care providers to develop a management plan.

When lesions are present in the left cerebral hemisphere, the communication and intellectual deficits of aphasia are common. Such patients should be evaluated by a speech pathologist to assess all language modalities, including speaking, writing and gesturing for expression, and listening and reading for comprehension. In addition to these language functions, other learning modalities should be assessed, including visual–spatial skills, memory, and problem solving. Since metastatic lesions are often focal, there may be residual language skills that can be used for communication. Patients should not be denied speech therapy if they can benefit from it, their prognosis warrants it, and they desire it. The greatest benefits, however, may be realized by organizing and educating the patient's family and care providers about the degree of impairment and prevention of patient frustration.

The patients with severe aphasia may be misleading, because they will frequently retain social or automatic speech, and use facial expressions and head nods in a seemingly appropriate manner. They "seem to understand everything." Careful examination will show that some of these patients are not able to follow even short, simple, spoken or written instructions, and cannot express themselves through any modality. In this case, their daily needs should be anticipated by the care providers, and the patient's daily schedule of activities organized into a routine. A consistent schedule helps to reduce the patient's requirements for speech and thus decreases frustration.

Talking to the patient with severe aphasia may be compared to the presentation of irritating static which interferes with the message being conveyed. For the most part, these patients do not have hearing impairments, and shouting only increases the irritation. When spoken directions are ineffective, one should use demonstration to communicate instructions. Some severely aphasic patients are able to learn self-care activities when the clinician demonstrates the performance in a stepwise fashion, and either eliminates or simplifies the verbal input. It is important not to isolate the patient by assuming more intellectual deficit than is present; therefore, each patient deserves careful assessment and an individualized plan.

The cognitive problems of cancer patients with right brain lesions are frequently missed because they often retain the ability to speak fluently. Their problems are generally related to visual–motor–perceptual and spatial difficulties that impair performance. They have problems judging form, distance, rate of movement, and the position of body parts. Up and down, left and right, and in and out are frequently confused. They may have problems performing simple actions like putting on a shirt, brushing teeth, or propelling a wheelchair through a doorway. The lack of initiation of action or performance becomes a major problem and they are often incorrectly described as obstinate, uncooperative, unmotivated, or depressed. Due to their good verbal skills, the rehabilitation potential of these patients can be overestimated, and with their impulsiveness and perceptual problems, they are unsafe. It is very important that their care providers are cognizant of the patient's limitations and understand the discrepancy between their language and performance.

Intellectual assessment of patients with right brain lesions usually demonstrates that they have retained the language modalities of speech and verbal comprehension. Hence, they follow spoken instructions better than demonstrated acts. Care providers should be instructed to talk the patient through activities that are otherwise performed incompletely, inaccurately, or with poor judgment. Patients may need specific spoken instructions to help them begin an activity such as eating, dressing, or wheelchair propulsion. Frequent verbal feedback is needed to help them complete the task safely.

Compared to the patient with aphasia, these patients are less likely to learn independent performance of self-care activities. Some eventually learn to talk themselves through a self-care task or use written cues to assist them in initiating and sequencing actions.[123]

Left side neglect is seen in some patients with right brain lesions. Unlike patients with visual field cuts, those with neglect do not turn to see stimuli in the left visual space. Neglect may involve all of the senses on the affected side, thus the patient ignores the speech of a visitor on the left, forgets about the left arm that may become caught in the spokes of a wheelchair, and misses food placed on the left half of a food tray. Some investigators have demonstrated that these patients do not generalize learning in order to compensate for this integrative impairment. They suggest that the patient should not be frustrated by expectations of learning, but managed by talking them through activities requiring attention to the left side very time the action is performed.[124]

It is possible for a patient to have good language and visual–perceptual skills, but to experience problems with recent memory, since the memory processes appear to need a totally functioning brain for maximum performance. These patients may recall details of past events, names of old acquaintances, and occasions long past, yet be unable to retain new information, which may drastically affect their rehabilitation program. Some patients with memory deficits can use written aids like a printed daily schedule and step-by-step instruction cards. As with other brain-damaged patients they need a fixed routine and predictable environment to reduce frustrations and ease management.

Early intellectual assessment is important for establishing a baseline of abilities that can be used to follow disease progression. For those patients who do not demonstrate significant cognitive impairments, the evaluation may identify preferred and stronger modalities of learning. This information assists the rehabilitation team in the development of techniques for teaching.

MOBILITY

Depending on the degree of paresis or plegia, the following therapy programs should be instituted to maximize function. These will have to be modified by the patient's desires, prognosis, and other medical diseases or complications. As mentioned earlier, proper bed positioning techniques and passive or active ROM are essential to avoid contractures that may further limit function. As strength returns to muscle groups, specific strengthening exercises, using resistive techniques, must be initiated.

Extremely weak patients need to work on bed mobility and practice coming to a sitting position. Sitting balance is essential for being able to transfer safely from the bed to the wheelchair, and from the wheelchair to the toilet, tub, or car. The most common transfers are the standing pivot and the sliding transfer described in detail by Stolov.[125] It is much easier to transfer to an equal height; hence, environmental modifications such as raised toilet seats and grab bars are essential. Some patients may require standby assistance with verbal cues to remind the patient to lock wheelchair brakes before transferring. Ambulation may be by wheelchair or bipedal, with or without aids, and the degree of independence may vary with the environment. The patient may be independent in a level home but need assistance for stairs, ramps, and uneven ground.

The best mode of ambulation for the patient may be the wheelchair. It is important to prescribe one that meets the patient's needs, taking into consideration cost, size, and special adaptive components such as removable armrests to facilitate side transfers, desk arms to permit the chair to fit under a table or desk, and detachable elevating leg rests for patients with LE edema. Thin, solid tires move easier on level, smooth surfaces, while balloon tires are better for thick carpeting, grass, or gravel. One can prescribe a manual one-arm drive or electric wheelchair, depending on the patient's needs and environment.[126] All wheelchairs must have brakes.

It is necessary to have free-standing balance before independent bipedal ambulation can be considered. Most patients want to walk, but some, such as those with severe cerebellar ataxia, are not safe. Most patients with hemiparesis, and many with hemiplegia, can be taught to walk using an ankle foot orthosis (AFO), provided they do not have significant hip or knee flexion contractures. The hemiplegic patient neurologically recovers in a proximal to distal distribution with an extensor synergy pattern present in the LE. To maximize this recovery, and minimize the effects of bed rest, the hip and knee extensors and hip abductor muscles should receive strengthening exercises. The dorsiflexors frequently do not return and the AFO compensates for this function. This orthosis works best with the ankle in the neutral position or with passive ROM to 5° dorsiflexion. It is important to actively range the ankle joint and prevent muscle imbalance, extensor synergy, and spasticity from developing static contractures.

The therapist works on free-standing balance with the patient within parallel bars and then, if safe, the patient progresses to walking within the bars using an AFO with the normal hand on the bar for support. Many assistive devices are available for walking, with the four-legged (quad) cane being the most common for the patient with hemiplegia or hemiparesis.[127] This allows a slow, wide-base gait in which much of the body weight is supported through the hand. Quad canes are difficult to use on stairs.Before discharge, the patient should be trained on stairs, ramps, and uneven ground, and getting up from the floor, for when a fall occurs. In this way, the patient and significant others will know the patient's safety limits and when assistance is needed.

ADL PROBLEMS

ADL retraining and management should be guided by the patient's prognosis, needs and desires, the degree of intellectual impairment, the presence of other diseases and complications, and the care provider's requirements and skills. In patients with poor prognosis, the aim should be to restore basic self-care functions to make their care easier. These small gains may take on major significance in terms of quality of life and allow the patient to die at home with dignity.

For patients who have lost the use of one UE, training in one-handed techniques may be indicated. Assistive aids are available in many forms that facilitate function and increase independence. Velcro strips instead of buttons may allow a patient to dress independently. Shoes can be modified for one-handed tying, and silverware, such as rocker knives or large-handled untensils, is available for self-feeding.[128] Some patients with rotator cuff paresis need slings to support the affected arm to prevent glenohumeral subluxation and shoulder pain.[93]

Bathing is a major problem for many hemiplegics because of the difficulty with bathtub transfers and in reaching all body parts. Tub benches with rubber suction cups for stability, and a grab bar on the wall, may allow tub transfers. Long-handled sponges and hand-held showers may allow the patient to wash all body parts and thereby minimize dependence.

When there is ataxia of the UEs a weighted wrist cuff may improve stability and coordination. Weighted utensils may assist independent eating.

Some patients with brain cancer will experience dysphagia. This may be due to a combination of spastic weakness of the deglutitory muscles and intellectual impairments (pseudobulbar dysphagia), or flaccid paralysis of the swallowing mechanism (paralytic dysphagia). The differential diagnosis of the dysphagia is important in developing the management plan.[59] Patients with pseudobulbar dysphagia need their intellectual deficits controlled by simplification of the environment and removal of distractions. If they have an adequate protective cough reflex, they can often be fed safely by being positioned upright with the neck flexed, and chin toward the chest. They are more apt to choke on liquids and foods that fall apart in the mouth, and will do better on textures that hold together as a single bolus. Liquids should be served either hot (avoid burning) or ice cold to help initiate swallowing. Many patients with paralytic dysphagia are unable to be fed safely and must receive nutrition by an alternative route, like a nasogastric or orogastric tube.

BOWEL AND BLADDER INCONTINENCE

Brain cancer that alters a patient's sensorium, mobility, communication, or performance can lead to bowel and bladder incontinence. Incontinence can prolong hospitalization, make nursing home placement difficult, or preclude home care. Further, it interferes with ambulation and ADL training.

In planning a program to control bowel incontinence, staff should take the patient's past bowel habits into consideration. The neurogenic bowel is trained by instituting a regular consistent program which utilizes the gastrocolic reflex, positioning on a stable commode, digital stimulation, bisacodyl (Ducolax) or glycerine rectal suppositories, consistent high fiber diet, and adequate fluids.[11] For patients who cannot be transferred easily from bed, disposable pads can be used. Medications to provide bulk or soften the stool, such as docusate sodium (Colace), may also be indicated. The goal of the program is to enable the individual to defecate at a predictable time and place, and to prevent accidents and social embarrassment.

A program to control urinary incontinence should establish a consistent daily schedule in which the patient is taken to the toilet or provided with a urinal or bedpan at regularly timed intervals. The male can often be managed by external condom drainage, although the confused patient does not permit it to remain in place.[129] The patient with a neurogenic bladder can be managed by establishing bladder training programs that address the findings of the complete bladder work-up, including urodynamic flow studies.[130] Intermittent in-and-out straight catheterization is preferred to an indwelling retention catheter, as this is more likely to keep the urine sterile. With fluid intake scheduled and restricted, voiding drills regularly performed, and appropriate medications used, voiding can be initiated and residuals decreased, provided there is no detrusor–external-sphincter dyssynergia.

For a hyperreflexic upper motor neuron bladder, propantheline bromide (Probanthine), an anticholenergic drug, can be prescribed to block the detrusor activity and enlarge bladder capacity. Bethencol (Urocholine), a cholenergic drug, can be used to stimulate the detrusor bladder musculature to contract in an areflexic lower motor neuron neurogenic bladder. When the bladder neck fails to relax during voiding, an alpha receptor blocker such as phenoxybenzamine chloride (Dibenzyline) will reduce the internal sphincter resistance. To reduce external-sphincter–detrusor dyssynergia, diazepam (Valium), baclofen (Lioresal), or dantrolene sodium (Dantrium) may be helpful.

SPINAL CORD TUMORS

Cancer of the spinal cord, whether primary or metastatic, can produce various forms of paralysis (paraparesis, paraplegia, quadriparesis, quadriplegia) with paraplegia or paraparesis the most common. Spinal metastasis is usually epidural and affects about 5% of patients with systemic cancer.[121]

The anatomical patterns of cord involvement result from either direct cord compression or ischemic compromise of the arterial blood supply to the spinal cord. The most common sites of spinal cord ischemia are T3 to T9 segments, where a marginal arterial blood supply is present.[131] Arterial compromise can give rise to sudden permanent paraplegia within hours, while direct cord compression is usually characterized by a slow, steady neurological progression over days to weeks. Early diagnosis, when there are soft neurologic signs (*i.e.*, radicular pain), is the key, as these patients may show reversibility of neurological deficits with irradiation and steroids.

The functional limitations of patients with spinal cord cancer vary greatly, depending on the level of the lesion and whether it is complete or incomplete with respect to motor and sensory functions. Rehabilitation treatment strategies and techniques are basically the same, whether the etiology is trauma or cancer. The patient's prognosis, endurance, mental outlook, and general medical condition may greatly modify the functional treatment plan.

With a complete spinal cord lesion, impairment of function to varying degrees is present in dressing, feeding, ambulation (wheelchair, bipedal, or automobile), transfers (off and on chairs, beds, toilets, and in and out of automobiles and bathtubs), and personal hygiene (bathing, grooming, and bowel and bladder functions). Higher level lesions and more complete lesions result in more extensive disabilities. Patients with high lesions are best treated in specialized centers that have expertise in treatment techniques and adaptive equipment to maximize function.

In assessing function, the adaptive patient's level of performance is described as follows:

1. *Independent*—the patient can perform the activity safely without any assistance
2. *Standby assistance*—the patient can perform the activity but is inconsistent and needs someone close by for safety
3. *Partial physical assistance*—the patient cannot complete the task without some actual physical assistance
4. *Unable to perform the activity*—the patient needs someone to perform the task

The following discussion will indicate specific root levels for complete spinal cord lesions and the optimal functional levels that can be obtained with training. Motivational problems, depression, contractures, decubitus, deconditioning, or other medical problems may prevent the patient from obtaining an optimal functional level.[132,133]

C2 THROUGH C4 LESIONS. These patients are completely dependent for all of their self-care activities and transfers. They can propel an electric wheelchair with a mouth wand, chin attachment, or by voice control. The C2 through C3 patients usually require tracheostomy and assisted ventilation. A battery power portable respirator can be fitted to the wheelchair. An environmental control system, which allows the patient to control a telephone, television, light switch, call button, and so forth, can be purchased. These patients require a full time attendant. Male patients usually have undergone an urethral sphincterotomy and wear an external collecting device consisting of a condom, a tube, and a collecting bag. Female patients use a continuous indwelling urinary catheter, since no satisfactory external collecting device exists for women.

C5 LESIONS. With training, these patients can propel their electric wheelchairs using a "joy stick." With their food cut and mobile arm supports, they can feed themselves, using a plate guard and universal cuff with a spoon, or by using an electric or carbon dioxide powered splint. They are totally dependent on an attendant for personal hygiene, dressing, transfers, and writing. They can be taught to type with a head wand. A few can be taught to drive with special adaptive vans. Male patients usually have a urethral sphincterotomy and use an external collecting device, while female patients have a continuous indwelling urinary catheter.

C6 THROUGH C7 LESIONS. The C6 root allows the patient to have wrist extension (dorsiflexion), and with the wrist-driven flexor hinge splint, patients can feed themselves, write, and drive, using hand controls and special vans. The wrist-driven flexor hinge orthosis uses dorsiflexion to create opposition of the thumb and the second and third fingers. Some patients may choose to eat using a universal cuff, which has a slot for a spoon or fork. The patient can also dress and bathe with partial assistance after training. The clothes usually have loops and Velcro closures to replace buttons and snaps. Transfers require standby assistance and a sliding board. Ambulation is independent using manual wheelchair with "quad" knobs, although some may require an electric wheelchair. These patients require an attendant. Males usually have a urethral sphincterotomy and wear an external collecting device, and females use an indwelling urinary catheter.

T1 THROUGH T2 LESIONS. This group, with proper training, can live alone, as they are independent in dressing, eating, personal hygiene, can drive an automobile with hand controls and trunk support. Ambulation is independent with a manual wheelchair. Transfers may require standby assistance and a sliding board. Female patients use continuous indwelling catheters and males usually require urethral sphincterotomies and an external collecting system.

T2 THROUGH T6 LESIONS. These patients have additional trunk stability. They can become independent in all self-care activities with training, and they ambulate independently in a manual wheelchair. Bipedal ambulation is not practical. They can drive with hand controls, but may require additional external trunk support. Female patients usually have a continuous indwelling urinary catheter and males a urethral sphincterotomy and external collecting system to control urinary leakage. An attendant is not usually required.

T7 THROUGH T12 LESIONS. These patients have greater trunk stability, and are independent in self-care activities. They ambulate independently, using a manual wheelchair, and drive with hand controls. Bilateral knee–ankle–foot orthosis (KAFO) can be prescribed for exercise and to allow the patient to obtain the upright posture. Excessive energy consumption makes bipedal ambulation impractical. Bowel and bladder function can become independent, although male patients usually wear external collection devices and may require sphincterotomy, and female patients may use absorbent pads. Attendance is not required.

L1 THROUGH L2 LESIONS. These patients, with training, are independent in all self-care activities, including bowel and bladder functions. Due to some dribbling, males may choose to wear an external collecting device and females may use absorbent pads. The patient can drive, using hand controls, and can ambulate, usually with a manual wheelchair. Bipedal ambulation with bilateral KAFOs and crutches or a walkerette, can be functional for short distances using a four point swing-through or swing-to-gait pattern. No attendant is necessary.

L4 THROUGH S1 LESIONS. These patients usually do not need wheelchairs, although they may desire them for long journeys. Independent bipedal ambulation is achieved using bilateral AFO's and two canes. After training, they will be independent in self-care activities, transfers, driving with hand controls, and bowel and bladder functions. They do not usually require urinary catheters. Male patient may use an external collecting system and female patients might wear an absorbent pad.

CRANIAL AND PERIPHERAL NERVES

These can also be injured by the cancer or its treatment. The functional deficit will depend on the function of the specific muscles innervated by that nerve, whether the lesion is complete or incomplete, any neural recovery, the training of other musculature, and the use of adaptive equipment which may substitute for the impaired function. Remote cancer effects on the nervous system such as encephalomyelitis, cerebellar dysfunction, subacute cerebellar degeneration, Eaton Lambert syndrome, and peripheral neuropathy may also result in significant disability.[119] The avoidance of the complications of inactivity and the use of therapeutic exercise, self-care training, adaptive equipment, and environmental modification can improve the patient's functional levels and quality of life.

PEDIATRIC CONSIDERATIONS

Many of the problems seen in the patient with cancer in the pediatric age group are similar to those seen in adults. For example, the weakness commonly seen in leukemia can be due to either the disease process or the peripheral neuropathy associated with the chemotherapy. Contractures could further impair mobility and self care skills, thus, they need to be prevented by ROM exercises and proper bed positioning. Fixed contractures that interfere with function should be treated with heat and static stretch. Adaptive equipment and environmental modification, as well as work simplification techniques are all utilized to conserve energy and improve function.

For children with cancer, many of their possible psychological and social problems related to the cancer, or the residual effects of surgery, chemotherapy or radiation, are similar to those previously discussed. Additional areas of psychological and social concern in pediatric patients include the reactions of parents and peers, and the school situation.

For parents, the fact that their child has cancer is very traumatic. Many issues may come to the surface, including feelings of guilt—"Could we have prevented this?"—fear for the child's survival, and anxiety over the treatment and its effects. It is remarkable that the child's attitude is usually extremely positive and that the parents are helped by this.[134]

The parents' plans for their healthy child's future, and the impact of the cancer and its treatment on that future, is also a factor in the patient's ability to cope. Cancer-related stress can put a strain on the parent's relationship and can alter the parent–child relationship, particularly in the direction of overprotectiveness. Health care providers must be cognizant of these issues, and keep track of how the parents are coping, as well as following the child's own progress.

Children can be very cruel to each other, as well as very understanding and accepting, depending on the circumstances. For children who are already experiencing anxiety and stress due to the cancer and the residuals of treatment, looking or acting differently can be very difficult, particularly if this fact is noted by peers. For children undergoing cancer treatment that will result in alterations in their physical appearance, it is important that health care providers help the young patient to be assimilated back into their peer group. Understanding and knowledgeable adults, such as the physician, parent, or other health care provider, should spend some time trying to explain the obvious changes to the patients and their friends. The intent is not to foster sympathy, but rather to develop understanding among the peer group about the body and functional changes observed, and enlisting their assistance to help rather than hinder the rehabilitation process. One way to do this is by working with schoolmates, perhaps the entire classroom, explaining briefly what has happened to the child, what changes to expect, areas where help may be needed, and areas where the child should be expected to function independently. The teacher may be recruited to help put the issue into perspective, but the parent or health care provider must explain the needed information to the teacher if this course of action is selected.

If the cancer or the effect of its treatment will interfere with the child's normal classroom performance, then adaptations must be made so that education can continue. This may include environmental changes or a tutor.

Children can be remarkably resilient after physical trauma, surgery, and illness. The adults in their environment frequently have a more difficult time in adjusting to and responding to the cancer-induced changes that can interfere with the child's rehabilitation. It is imperative that when cancer rehabilitation is in progress, professional counseling be available for the child as well as for the adults in the environment.

It would be extremely unfortunate if we were to find cases 10 or 20 years in the future where the cancer had been successfully treated, and physical rehabilitation provided, only to find that parents' attitudes and peer treatment had caused long-term psychological and social problems. A little treatment, and a little understanding at the right time, will go a long way toward helping the child with cancer develop along "normal" lines.

CONCLUSION

A limited number of forms of cancer and the rehabilitation aspects of treatment are covered in this chapter. For almost all forms of cancer, rehabilitation is a vital component of the treatment and care plan, and should be addressed in a multidisciplinary manner. The first step in selecting appropriate rehabilitation techniques is to identify what physical and functional limitations or deficits will result from the cancer or the treatment procedures. These areas then become the focal point for rehabilitation procedures. Keeping in mind special precautions necessary owing to the natures of radiation, surgery, chemotherapy, and cancer cells, rehabilitation procedures are similar to those used for other functional losses and deficits due to non-cancer reasons.

The rehabilitation process, whether for adults or children, should start as soon as the diagnosis is made. With an understanding of the rehabilitation techniques described in this chapter, physicians should be able to identify the patient in need of rehabilitation. They should be able to address the cancer patient's needs relative to prevention, specific therapy, and restoration. With a knowledge of rehabilitation concepts and expertise of team members, appropriate referrals can be made to ensure adequate rehabilitation of cancer patients. Rehabilitation programs should be individualized for each patient and designed to improve the quality of each life.

REFERENCES

1. Silverger E: Cancer statistics, 1979. Cancer 29:6–21, 1979
2. Lehmann JF, DeLisa JA, Warren CG et al: Cancer rehabilitation: assessment of need, development, and evaluation of a model of care. Arch Phys Med Rehabil 59:410–419, 1978
3. Devlin HB, Plant JA, Griffin M: Aftermath of surgery for anorectal cancer. Br Med J 3:413–418, 1971
4. Healey JE Jr, Villanueva R, Donovan ES: Principles of rehabilitation. In Holland JF, Frei E III (eds): Cancer Medicine, pp 1917–1929. Philadelphia, Lea and Febiger, 1973
5. Kottke FJ: The effects of limitation of activity upon the human body. JAMA 196:825–830, 1966
6. Muller EA: Influence of training and of inactivity on muscle strength. Arch Phys Med 51:449–462, 1970
7. Bevegard S, Holmgren A, Jonsson B: The effect of body position on the circulation at rest and during exercise, with special reference to the influence on the stroke volume. Acta Physiol Scand 49:279–298, 1960
8. Waterfield RL: The effect of posture on the volume of the leg. J Physiol 72:121–131, 1931
9. Deitrick JE, Whedon GD, Shorr E: Effects of immobilization upon various metabolic and physiologic functions of normal men. Am J Med 4:3–36, 1948
10. Greenleaf JE, Bernauer EM, Young HL et al: Fluid and electrolyte shifts during bed rest with isometric and isotonic exercise. J Appl Physiol 42:59–66, 1977
11. Taylor N, Berni R, Horning MR: Neurogenic bowel management. Am Fam Physician 7:126–128, 1973
12. The Medical Letter, Vol 22, No 1, Issue 548, p 2–3. Jan 11, 1980
13. Kosiak M: Etiology and pathology of decubitus ulcer. Arch Phys Med 40:62–69, 1959
14. Landis EM: Micro injection studies of capillary blood pressures in human skin. Heart 15:209–228, 1930
15. Lindan O, Greenway RM, Piazza JM: Pressure distribution on the surface of the human body. I. Evaluation in lying and sitting positions using a "Bed of springs and nails." Arch Phys Med 46:378–385, 1965
16. Kosiak M: A mechanical resting surface: its effect on the prevention of ischemic ulcers. Arch Phys Med Rehabil 56:547, 1975
17. Dinsdale SM: Decubitus ulcers: Role of pressure and friction in causation. Arch Phys Med Rehabil 55:147–152, 1974
18. Agate J: Pressure sores mechanical and medical factors. Nurs Mirror (Suppl) V 144, March 17, 1977
19. Kavchak-Keyes MA: Four proven steps for preventing debucitus ulcers. Nursing 7(9):58–61, 1977
20. deLateur BJ, Berni R, Hongladarom T et al: Wheelchair cushions designed to prevent pressure sores: an evaluation. Arch Phys Med Rehabil 57:129–135, 1976
21. Souther SG, Carr SD, Vistnes LM: Wheelchair cushions to reduce pressure under bony prominences. Arch Phys Med Rehabil 55:460–464, 1974
22. Mikulic MA: Decubitus: An analysis of current methods of prevention and treatment. Am J Nurs (in press)
23. McClemont EJ, Shand IG, Ramsay B: Pressure sores: a new method of treatment. Br J Clin Pract 33:21–25, 1979
24. Pace WE: Treatment of cutaneous ulcers with benzoyl peroxide. Can Med Assn J 115:1101–1106, 1976
25. Burdick D: Rehabilitation of the breast cancer patient. Cancer 36:645–648, 1975
26. Maier WP: The technique of modified radical mastectomy. Surg Gynecol Obstet 145:68–74, 1977
27. Villanueva R, Drane JB, Gunn AE et al: Rehabilitation of the cancer patient. In Clark RL, Howe CD (eds): Cancer Patient Care at M.D. Anderson Hospital and Tumor Institute, pp 671–691. Chicago, Year Book Medical Publishers, 1976
28. Degenshein GA: Mobility of the arm following radical mastectomy. Surg Gynecol Obstet 145:77, 1977
29. Nelson PA: Recent advances in treatment of lymphedema of the extremities. Geriatrics 21:162–173, 1966
30. DeLisa JA, Kraft GH, Ganes BM: Clinical electromyography and nerve conduction studies. Ortho Rev 7:75–84, 1978
31. Lehmann JH: Diathermy. In Krusen FH, Kottke, FJ, Elwood PM (eds): Handbook of Physical Medicine and Rehabilitation, 2nd ed, pp 273–345. Philadelphia, WB Saunders, 1971
32. Bostwick J III: Breast reconstruction: a comprehensive approach. Clin Plast Surg 6:143–162, 1979
33. Markel WM: Rehabilitation after mastectomy. Proc Natl Conf 7:851–852, 1973
34. Britton RC, Nelson PA: Causes and treatment of postmastectomy lymphedema of the arm: Report of 114 cases. JAMA 180:95–102, 1962
35. Farrow JH: Rehabilitation following radical breast surgery. Cancer 16:222–223, 1966
36. Leis HP Jr, Bowers WF, Dursi J: Postmastectomy edema of arm. N Y J Med 66:618–624, 1966
37. Zeissler RH, Rose GB, Nelson PA: Postmastectomy lymphedema: late results of treatment in 385 patients. Arch Phys Med Rehabil 53:159–166, 1972
38. Grabois M: Rehabilitation of the postmastectomy patient with lymphedema. Cancer 26:75, 1976
39. Stone EG, Hugo NE: Lymphedema. Surg Gynecol Obstet 135:625–631, 1972
40. Neilubowicz J, Olszewski W, Sokolowski J: Surgical lymphovenous shunts. J Cardiovasc Surg 9:262–267, 1968
41. Thompson N: The surgical treatment of chronic lymphoedema of the extremities. Surg Clin North Am 47:445–503, 1967
42. Larson NE, Crampton AR: A surgical procedure for postmastectomy edema. Arch Surg 106:475–481, 1973
43. Goldsmith HS, Santos R de Ros, Beatie EJ Jr: Omental transportation in the control of chronic lymphedema JAMA 203:1119–1121, 1968
44. Stillwell GK: Treatment of postmastectomy lymphedema. Mod Treat 6:396–412, 1969
45. Sanderson RG, Fletcher WS: Conservative management of primary lymphedema. Northwest Med 64:584–588, 1965
46. Treves N: An evaluation of the etiological factors of lymphedema following radical mastectomy: an analysis of 1007 cases. Cancer 10:444–459, 1957
47. Robbins GF, Markel WM: The postmastectomy lymphedematous arm. Med Ann DC 42:495–497, 1973
48. Robbins GF, Markel WM: The postmastectomy lymphedematous arm. J Med Assoc GA 62:319–321, 1973
49. Rothman KJ: The effect of alcohol consumption on risk of cancer of the head and neck. Laryngoscope (Suppl) 88:51–55, 1978
50. Lowry WS: Alcoholism in cancer of the head and neck. Laryngoscope 85:1275–1280, 1975
51. Dropkin MJ: Compliance in postoperative head and neck patients. Cancer Nurs 379–384, 1979
52. Van Pellon M: Feeding the cancer patient. Nursing 78:8(10):87–88, 1978
53. Bradford K: A practical application of nutrition for the patient with head and neck cancer. Cancer Bull 29(2):35–36, March/April, 1977
54. Aker S, Tilmont G, Harrison V: A guide to good nutrition during and after chemotherapy and radiation. Health Sci Learning Research Center, Fred Hutchinson Cancer Research Center, 1976
55. Dudgeon B, DeLisa J, Miller R: Head and neck cancer, a rehabilitation approach. Am J Occup Ther 34:243–251, 1980
56. DeWys WD, Walters K: Abnormalities of taste sensation in cancer patients. Cancer 36:1888–1896, 1975
57. Donaldson SS: Nutritional consequences of radiotherapy. Cancer Res 37:2407–2413, 1977
58. Larsen GL: Guidelines for head and neck rehabilitation. Fred Hutchinson Cancer Research Center, 1979
59. Larsen GL: Rehabilitating dysphagia: mechanica, paralytica, pseudobulbar. J Neurosurg Nurs 8(1):14–17, 1976
60. Keyes HM, McCasland JP: Techniques and results of a comprehensive dental care program in head and neck cancer patients. Int J Radiat Oncol Biol Phys 1:859–865, 1976

61. Mossman KL, Sheer AC: Complications of radiotherapy of head and neck cancer. Ear Nose Throat J 56:145–149, 1977
62. Doberneck RC, Antoine JE: Deglutition after resection of oral, laryngeal, and pharyngeal cancers. Surgery 75:87–90, 1974
63. Trible WM: The rehabilitation of deglutition following head and neck surgery. Laryngoscope 77:518–523, 1967
64. Donaldson RC, Skelly M, Paletta FX: Total glossectomy for cancer Am J Surg 116:585–590, 1968
65. Aguilar NV, Olson ML, Shedd DP: Rehabilitation of deglutition problems in patients with head and neck cancer. Am J Surg 138:501–507, 1979
66. Bobie RA: Rehabilitation of swallowing disorders. Am Fam Physician 17(5):84–95, 1978
67. Desjardins RP, Laney WR: Prosthetic rehabilitation after cancer resection in the head and neck. Surg Clin North Am 57:809–822, 1977
68. Staple TW, Ogura JH: Cineradiography of the swallowing mechanism following supraglottic subtotal laryngectomy. Radiology 87:226–230, 1966
69. Litton WB, Leonard JR: Aspiration after partial laryngectomy: cineradiographic studies. Laryngoscope 79:887–908, 1969
70. Weaver AW, Fleming SM: Partial laryngectomy: analysis of associated swallowing disorders. Am J Surg 136:486–489, 1978
71. Schoenrock LD, King AY, Everts EC et al: Hemilaryngectomy: deglutition evaluation and rehabilitation. Trans Am Acad Opthalmol Otolaryngol 76:752–757, 1972
72. Bocca E, Pignataro O, Mosciaro O: Supraglottic surgery of the larynx. Ann Otol 77:1005–1026, 1968
73. Som ML: Conservation surgery for carcinoma of the supraglottis. J Laryngol 84:655–678, 1970
74. Villanueva R: Orthosis to correct shoulder pain and deformity after trapezius palsy. Arch Phys Med Rehabil 58:30–34, 1977
75. Saunders WH, Johnson EW: Rehabilitation of the shoulder after radical neck dissection. Ann Otol Rhinol Laryngol 84:812–816, 1975
76. Imnan VT, Saunders JB de CM, Abbott LC: Observation of shoulder joint. J Bone Joint Surg 26:1–30, 1944
77. Villanueva R, Chandra A: The role of rehabilitation medicine in physical restoration of patients with head and neck cancer. Cancer Bull 29(2):46–54, 1977
78. Kelly D: Speech rehabilitation of the laryngectomized patient. Cancer Bull 29(2):39–41, 1977
79. Calcaterra TC, Zwitman DH: Vocal rehabilitation after partial or total laryngectomy. Calif Med 117:12–15, 1972
80. Shedd D: A brief survey of surgical speech rehabilitation research. Laryngoscope (Suppl) 88:88–93, 1978
81. Staffieri M, Serafini I: La Riabitazione Chiurgica della Voce e della Respirazione dopo Laringectomia Totale. ATTI del XXIX Congresso Nationale, Associazone Otologi Ospedalieri Italiani, Bologna, 28, 1976
82. Iwai H, Koike Y: Primary laryngoplasty. Arch Otorhinolaryngol (NY) 206:1–10, 1973
83. Taub S, Bergner LH: Air bypass voice prosthesis for vocal rehabilitation of laryngectomees. Am J Surg 125:748–756, 1973
84. Edwards N: Post-laryngectomy vocal rehabilitation using expired air and an external fistula method. Laryngoscope 85:690–699, 1975
85. Sisson GA, McConnel FM, Logemann JA et al: Voice rehabilitation after laryngectomy: results with the use of a hypopharyngeal prosthesis. Arch Otolaryngol 101:178–181, 1975
86. Gilchrist AG: Rehabilitation after laryngectomy. Acta Otolaryngol (Stockh) 75:511–518, 1973
87. Skelly M, Spector DJ, Donaldson RC et al: Compensatory physiologic phonetics for the glossectomee. J Speech Hear Disord 36:101–114, 1971
88. Skelly M, Donaldson RC, Fust RS et al: Changes in phonatory aspects of glossectomee intelligibility through vocal parameter manipulation. J Speech Heart Disord 37:379–389, 1972
89. Skelly M, Donaldson R, Schinsky L: Substitution consistency as a factor in glossectomee intelligibility. J Missouri Heart Assoc 5(3):21–23, 1972
90. Skelly M, Donaldson R: Rehabilitation of speech after total glossectomy. Presented to Twelfth World Congress of Rehabilitation International, Sydney, Australia, 1972
91. Drane J: Role of maxillofacial prosthetics. Cancer Bull 29(2):41–45, 1977
92. Gonzalez JB: Recently developed elastomers for facial prostheses. Mayo Clin Proc 53:423–431, 1978
93. Dietz JH Jr: The cancer patient after amputation of an extremity or neurologic disability: In Scottenfeld D (ed): Cancer Epidemiology and Prevention: Current Concepts, pp 511–521. Springfield Ill, Charles C Thomas, 1975
94. Campbell CJ: Indications and principles of amputation for bone sarcoma. Proc Natl Cancer Conf 6:757–767, 1970
95. deLateur BJ, Lehmann JF, Winterscheid LC et al: Rehabilitation of the patient after hemicorporectomy. Arch Phys Med Rehabil 50:11–16, 1969
96. Rusk MA (ed): Rehabilitation Medicine. 4th ed, pp 623–627. St Louis, CV Mosby, 1977
97. Murdock G: Levels of amputations and limiting factors. Ann R Coll Surg Engl 40(4):204–216, 1967
98. Muilenburg AL: Prosthetic considerations for the cancer amputee. In: Rehabilitation of the Cancer Patient, pp 65–73. Chicago, Year Book Medical Publishers, 1972
99. Jones RF: Amputee rehabilitation: basic principles in prosthetic assessment and fitting, Part 2. Med J Aust 2:331–335, 1977
100. Hampton F: Hemipelvectomy prosthesis. Artif Limbs 8:3–27, 1964
101. Sneppen O, Johansen T, Heerfordt J et al: Hemipelvectomy: postoperative rehabilitation assessed on the basis of 41 cases. Acta Orthop Scand 49:175–179, 1978
102. Nielsen M, Nielsen JB, Gerstenberg T et al: Bladder function after hemipelvectomy. Acta Orthop Scand 48:181–185, 1977
103. Simons BC, Lehmann JF, Taylor N et al: Prosthetic management of hemicorporectomy. Orthop Prosth 22:63–68, June 1968
104. Wirth CR: Metastatic bone cancer. Curr Probl Cancer 3(11):2–36, 1979
105. Fisher SV, Bowar JF, Awad EA et al: Cervical orthoses effect on cervical spine motion: roentgenographic and goniometric method of study. Arch Phys Med Rehabil 58:109–115, 1977
106. Hinterbuchner C: Rehabilitation of physical disability in cancer. NY State J Med 78:1066–1069, 1978
107. Dietz JH Jr: Rehabilitation of the cancer patient. Med Clin North Am 53:607–624, 1969
108. Lertzman MM, Cherniack RM: Rehabilitation of patients with chronic obstructive pulmonary disease. Am Rev Respir Dis 114:1145–1165, 1976
109. Petty TL: Pulmonary rehabilitation. Basis of respiratory disease. Am Thorac Soc 4(1):1–6, 1975
110. Zislis JM: Rehabilitation of the cancer patient. Geriatrics 25:150–158, 1970
111. Cassara EL: Chest physical therapy. Int Anesthesiol Clin 9(4):159–171, 1971
112. Frey GS: The effect of special preparation of the therapist on the rehabilitation of the ostomate. Int Assoc for Enterostomal Ther 6(3):26–28, 1979
113. Watson PG, Wood RY, Wechsler NL et al: Comprehensive care of the iliostomy patient. Nurs Clin North Am 11(3):427–444, 1976
114. Costello AM: Supporting the patient with problems relating to body image, pp 36–40. Proc Natl Conf Cancer Nursing, Chicago Am Cancer Soc, 1974
115. Guidelines for ostomy rehabilitation. In: Guidelines for Managing Cancer, developed by Fred Hutchinson Cancer Research Center, Section 5, 6, 1979
116. Bromley B: Applying Orem's self-care theory in enterostomal therapy. Am J Nurs 80–245:249, 1980
117. Fordyce WE: Psychological assessment and management. In Kursen FH, Kottke FJ, Ellwood PM (eds): Handbook of Physical Medicine and Rehabilitation, 2nd ed, pp 168–195. Philadelphia, WB Saunders, 1971
118. Gazzard BG, Saunders B, Dawson AM: Diets and stoma function. Br J Surg 65:642–644, 1978
119. Rosenbaum EG, Rosenbaum IR: A Comprehensive Guide for

Cancer Patients and Their Families. Palo Alto, Bull Publishing Co, 1980
120. Griffith ER, Trieschmann RB, Hohmann GW et al: Sexual dysfunction associated with physical disabilities. Arch Phys Med Rehabil 56:8–13, 1975
121. Posner JB: Neurological complications of systemic cancer. Med Clin North Am 63(4):783–800, 1979
122. Horstein S: Distal effects of neoplasm on the nervous system. Postgrad Med 50:85–90, 1971
123. Fowler RS Jr, Fordyce W: Adapting care for the brain damaged patient. Am J Nurs 72:1832–1835; 2056–2059, 1972
124. Stanton KM, Flowers CR, Kuhl PK et al: Language-oriented training program to teach compensation of left side neglect. Arch Phys Med Rehabil 60:540, 1979
125. Stolov WC: Progressive ambulation (mobility). Postgrad Med 47:229–235, 1970
126. Spiegler JH, Goldberg MJ: The wheelchair as a permanent mode of mobility. A detailed guide to prescription. I. Frame, armrest, and brakes. Am J Phys Med 47:315–316, 1968; II. Upholstery, leg supports, wheels and accessories. 48:25–37, 1969
127. Jebsen RH: Use and abuse of ambulation aids. JAMA 199:5–10, 1967
128. Hale G (ed): The Source Book for the Disabled. New York, Paddington Press, 1979
129. Kester NC, Block JM: Rehabilitation of patients after surgery for brain tumor. In Vinken PJ, Bryn GW (eds): Handbook of Clinical Neurology, vol 18, Part III: Tumors of the Brain and Skull, pp 523–529, Amsterdam, North Holland Publishing, 1975
130. Koff SA, Diokno AC, Lapides J: Neurogenic bladder dysfunction. Am Fam Phys 19:100–109, 1979
131. Gilbert H, Apuzzo M, Marshall L et al: Neoplastic epidural spinal cord compression: a current prospective. JAMA 240:2771–2773, 1978
132. Long C II, Lawton EB: Functional significance of spinal cord lesion level. Arch Phys Med 36:249–255, 1955
133. Symington DC, McKay DW: A study of functional independence in the quadriplegia patient. Arch Phys Med 47:378–392, 1966
134. Voute PA, Burgers JMV, Van Putten WJ et al: Amputations in children: Clinical indications and psychological implications. Arch Chir Neerlandicum 25:427–433, 1973

CHAPTER 47

Susan Molloy Hubbard
Claudia A. Seipp

Administration of Cancer Treatments: Practical Guide for Physicians and Oncology Nurses

THE EVOLUTION OF ROLES FOR ONCOLOGY NURSES

During the early 1970s, the need for skilled nurses who could share responsibility with physicians for the administration of chemotherapy limited clinical cancer research. At certain centers, investigators began to prepare nurses to participate in clinical trials, and a new and expanded role for nurses in research began to emerge.[1,2,3] Initially, guidance and supervision from experienced physicians were essential for the proper education of these nurses. These nurses learned directly about the natural history of cancer and the management of cancer patients from physicians at the bedside and in clinics.

Within 1 year, integration of a single cancer chemotherapy nurse into the primary care team in the Medicine Branch of the National Cancer Institute permitted a 25% increase in outpatient visits, although the number of physicians did not increase.[1] The chemotherapy nurse administered intravenous drugs to all outpatients and served as a resource person. Patient and staff acceptance of the nurse was excellent, and errors related to the administration of these drugs were reduced. Working as part of a research team, the nurse had opportunities to learn by participating in the collection, analysis, and publication of data. As her skills and knowledge increased, the chemotherapy nurse began to assume greater responsibility in educating patients about their disease and their treatment.[4]

At one large cancer center, a survey of growth over 6 years demonstrates that outpatient visits for intravenous chemotherapy by nurses have almost quadrupled, as have the number of clinical protocols and diseases under investigation.[5,6] Although the number of staff fellows and nurses has grown, their services have also expanded.[7–18] Nurses have developed and conducted structured educational programs for patients and hospital staff on chemotherapy, management of side-effects, and current progress in cancer treatment.

In cervical cancer detection studies, well-trained nurses screen women as accurately as physicians.[19,20] Nurse screening constituted a 46% decrease in overall cost.[21] Studies indicate that overall productivity in the private practice setting increased 26% to 31% when a nurse was a group practice member.[22]

Adult and pediatric nurse practioners with advanced preparation and skills can assume responsibility for selected cancer patients.[23,24,25] Under the general supervision of a senior oncologist, they provide and coordinate care within specific written guidelines, managing outpatients with chronic care needs, continuing or rehabilitative care needs, and those in the terminal stage of illness. They often manage patients receiving chemotherapy on established protocols. They order and administer drugs at major cancer centers.

The designations *clinical nurse specialist* and *nurse practitioner* indicate that these nurses have completed formalized educational programs at the master's level.[26-28] The increasing demand for cancer nurse specialists to provide expert care to patients utilizing advanced knowledge and clinical skills emphasizes the need to define this level of preparation.[29] Fourteen university programs currently exist for graduate education in cancer nursing.[30]

PRACTICAL ISSUES AFFECTING PATIENT CARE

INTRAVENOUS CHEMOTHERAPY

Oncology nurses now administer most chemotherapy, including phase I and phase II agents, in ambulatory care clinics. These nurses must know the diseases and drugs and must have a high level of clinical expertise and the ability to manage acute changes in the patient's condition as they evolve. Outpatient management permits the maintenance of a more normal lifestyle during cancer therapy, but it also requires that patients and their families be informed about the drugs, their side-effects, and any measures that can prevent or reduce unnecessary complications (Table 47-1 and Table 47-2).

The oncology nurse's role in IV therapy can be divided into five major areas: safe administration of chemotherapy, reduction of avoidable morbidity, patient education concerning care and maintenance of indwelling catheters, the procurement of blood components for therapeutic purposes, and the administration of intracavitary therapy.

The purpose of this section is to provide specific information about techniques that should be employed in the administration of chemotherapy, the types of cannulae and catheters that are available, and the requisite knowledge, judgment, and technical skills that a physician or nurse should have before administering cytotoxic drugs.[31]

Techniques

Patient preparation is an important step in intravenous technique. Position the patient comfortably for venipuncture and the infusion. School chairs with arm rests can be used although special chairs for use by phlebotomy teams are commercially available. The purpose and duration of the intravenous line should be reiterated even if a detailed explanation of the therapy has recently been provided. Orient the patient to the specific drugs as they are administered during the infusion and explain the need for any special safety precautions during or following the infusion. If the patient has had an axillary node dissection, venous circulation may be compromised, and the affected extremity should be avoided whenever possible. If the affected extremity must be used for IV therapy, maintenance of strict aseptic technique is especially important. Avoid veins in the lower extremities, especially in adults, where the risks of thrombophlebitis and embolism are great.

Base vein selection on the nature of the infusion and its duration. When prolonged infusions are planned, avoid veins located over areas of joint flexion, such as the antecubital fossa. Infiltration often occurs if the joint is moved. Large, easily accessible veins provide convenient venipuncture and decrease the risk of chemical phlebitis during the administration of irritating drugs. These veins are also ideal for direct injections (IV push); they are usually large, with rapid circulatory flow. The vein should follow a straight course for a distance that permits insertion of the needle or catheter. Base the needle gauge on the size of the vein. Palpate the vein for resilience; thrombosed veins feel hard and cordlike. When a prolonged need for IV therapy is anticipated, use distal sites initially. Inadvertent thrombosis in proximal sites may preclude further use of the vein until adequate collateral circulation has been established. Great care, therefore, must be exercised when administering irritating drugs through veins in the antecubital fossa. If venipuncture is difficult, or the needle's position is tenuous, infuse a sterile saline or D_5W solution to ensure that the needle is completely in the vein prior to the administration of chemotherapy. A tourniquet tied above the site of the venipuncture will slow down the infusion if the needle is in the vein. A venous return will be apparent if negative pressure is exerted in the tubing of the administration set.

The selection of a specific intravenous cannula depends on the purpose and length of the infusion, as well as on the size and condition of the patient's veins (Fig. 47-1). Scalp vein needles are employed for most short-term infusions. These steel needles are associated with a low incidence of septicemia and thrombophlebitis.[32] Scalp vein needles range from 25 to 16 gauge in diameter. They are manufactured with a short length of plastic tubing and a female Luer lock adaptor that connects to administration sets. They are also available with a self-sealing cap at the end of the tubing that permits use as heparin locks. The needle and bevel are short, reducing the risk of puncturing the posterior wall of the vein. Plastic wings provide stability and maximal control of the needle during insertion. A short strip of tape is placed over the plastic wings to anchor the needle. Then the tubing is looped and taped independently of the needle. This prevents a pull on the tubing from dislodging the needle. If a tissue vesicant is to be administered, the area above the venipuncture site should not be covered with tape until the agent has been infused. This allows the nurse close observation for evidence of extravasation. Armboards are useful for immobilizing an extremity when a long infusion is planned or sudden movements, such as sudden vomiting, are anticipated. Tape placed over the needle should not be secured to the armboard, nor should it tightly constrict any part of the hand or arm.

Short plastic or silicone catheters can facilitate prolonged therapy but they increase the risk of thrombophlebitis. To minimize the risk of infection, aseptic technique must be strict. Local anesthesia (ethyl alcohol spray or intradermally

(Text continues on page 1770)

TABLE 47-1. Cancer Chemotherapy Agents in Clinical Use

DRUG (SYNONYMS)	DOSE, ROUTE, AND SCHEDULE WHEN USED AS A SINGLE AGENT	ACUTE SIDE EFFECTS	COMMENTS AND PRECAUTIONS FOR SAFE ADMINISTRATION
ALKYLATING AGENTS			
Mechlorethamine (HN_2, nitrogen mustard mustargen)	0.4 mg/kg IV q 3–4 wks	Severe nausea & vomiting (N/V) occur in ½–2 hrs, lasting 2–12 hrs	Potent tissue vesicant; administer in established (IV) line, sodium thiosulfate may ↓ tissue damage. May cause chemical thrombophlebitis; use (IV) Solu-cortef 100 mg to ↓ reaction; may discolor vein. Allergic reactions may occur, but are rare.
	0.2–0.4 mg/kg intracavitary	Fever, chills, malaise	Pain common due to intense inflammatory reaction. Turn patient immediately to maximize drug distribution.
	10 mg in 60 ml water for topical use TIW then q wkly	–	Rubber or plastic gloves should be worn. May be given topically and intralesionally in mycosis fungoides. Hypersensitivity reactions can occur with topical use.
Cyclophosphamide (CYT), Cytoxan, Endoxan	500–1500 mg/m² (IV) q 3–4 wks 60–120 mg/m² (PO) qD continuous	N/V dose related in 6–12 hrs, may last 8–10 hrs Dizziness, rhinorrhea, sinus congestion may occur with rapid infusion of high doses	Fluid intake must be high to maintain adequate urine output in order to ↓ risk of hemorrhagic cystitis. D/C if dysuria or hematuria develop. Barbiturates, phenytoin may ↑ toxic effects by affecting activation by hepatic microsomal enyzmes. Inappropriate antidiuretic effect can occur at doses > 50 mg/kg. Alopecia in ≈ 50% with regrowth during continued Rx. Daily oral CYT may be taken in divided doses with meals.
L-phenylalanine mustard (L-PAM, Melphalan, Alkeran L-sarcolysin)	0.2 mg/kg (PO) qD × 5d q 4–6 wks or 0.05–0.1 mg/kg (PO) continuous	Chronic nausea/anorexia can occur	Well tolerated; little alopecia; take on empty stomach. (IV) preparation available. Delayed and cumulative myelotoxicity may occur.
Chlorambucil (Leukeran)	0.05–0.2 mg/kg (PO) qD continuous	Well tolerated	Occasional dermatitis; hepatotoxicity rare. Reliable absorption.
Busulfan (Myleran)	0.05–0.2 mg/kg (PO) qD continuous	Well tolerated	Reliable absorption; prolonged use associated with pulmonary fibrosis, gynecomastia, adrenal insufficiency; hyperpigmentation. Pregnancy has occurred during Rx. Effective contraceptives should be used.
Triethylene Thiophosphoramide (Thiotepa, TSPA TESPA)	0.2 mg/kg (IV) qD × 5 q 3–4 wks 1–10mg/m² intrathecal 10–60 mg q 3–4 wks intracavitary	Well tolerated	Can be given IM and SC or instilled into bladder. Poor oral absorption. Allergic reactions or dermatitis rare. Pain, N/V, headache can occur with intracavitary instillation.
NITROSOUREAS			
Carmustine (BCNU, BiCNU)	150–200 mg/m² (PO) q 4–6 wks	Severe N/V in 2–4 hrs lasting 4–6 hrs Burning and local pain Generalized flushing	Flushing and venous pain 2° to alcohol diluent, ↑ volume & ↓ rate to ↓ chemical thrombophlebitis. Phlebitis can be delayed by several days. Tissue vesicant; delayed and cumulative myelosuppression. Pulmonary and renal toxicity; hepatotoxicity in ≈ 20%. Refrigerate and protect from light. Enters CSF.
Lomustine (CCNU, CeeNU)	100–130 mg/m² (PO) q 4–6 wks	Moderate-severe N/V in 2–6 hrs	If taken at bedtime with antiemetics, N/V may be reduced; absorbed in ≈ 30 min. Alopecia, stomatitis. Renal toxicity with prolonged use.
Semustine (Methyl CCNU, MeCCNU, MCCNU)	150–200 mg/m² q 4–6 wks	Moderate-severe N/V 1–4 hrs	Taken on empty stomach at bedtime; Stomatitis, Renal failure has been seen with prolonged use.

TABLE 47-1. *(Continued)*

DRUG (SYNONYMS)	DOSE, ROUTE, AND SCHEDULE WHEN USED AS A SINGLE AGENT	ACUTE SIDE EFFECTS	COMMENTS AND PRECAUTIONS FOR SAFE ADMINISTRATION
NITROSOUREAS *(Continued)*			
Streptozoticin (STZ, Zanosar)	500 mg/m²k (IV) qD × 5 d q 3–4 wks or 1500 mg/m² (IV) q wk	Moderate-severe N/V 1–4 hrs Reactive hypoglycemia 2° to insulin release Burning and local pain	Administer with 1–2 liters hydration to nephrotoxicity. Check for glycosuria, proteinuria and hypophosphatemia prior to each dose. Slow infusion to ↓ local pain. Tissue vesicant; transient mild hepatotoxicity; mild anemia. Myelosuppression with prolonged use has occurred.
ANTIMETABOLITES			
Cytosine Arabinoside HCL (ARA-C, Cytosar HCL, Cytarabine HCL, Arabinosyl-cytosine)	100 mg/m² q 12 hrs (IV) or (SC) × 7–21 days 100 mg/m² continuous (IV) infusion × 10 days 20–30 mg/m² intrathecal	Dose and schedule dependent N/V	Less N/V with slow infusions; anorexia. Flu-like syndrome with fever and headache. Stomatitis; arthralgias; rashes. For intrathecal use reconstitute in Elliott's B solution; neurotoxicity with IT use common. Use with caution if hepatic dysfunction exists. Sensitivity to sunlight; use sunscreen. Alopecia.
5-Fluorouracil (5FU, Fluorouracil, Adrucil)	7.5–12 mg/kg (IV) × 5d then 12–15 mg/kg (IV) q wkly 20–30 mg/kg intra-arterial × 5–21 days (oral use investigational)	Dose and schedule dependent N/V	Promote oral hygiene; stomatitis in 5–8 days, preceded by sore mouth/tongue. Pharyngitis, diarrhea, proctitis may be severe. Interrupt Rx when GI toxicity appears. GI toxicity often immediately precedes myelotoxicity. Examine mouth prior to each dose. Diffuse hair thinning. Nail cracking and loss. Sensitivity to sunlight (use sunscreen) dermatitis; hyperpigmentation. Topical 5FU (Efudex) for malignant keratoses. ↑ toxicity post adrenalectomy. ↓ myelotoxicity with intraarterial use. Conjunctival irritation. Cerebellar ataxia; visual disturbances rare. Oral absorption erratic.
Methotrexate (MTX, amethopterin)	20–80 mg/m² (IV), (IM) (PO) 10–15 mg/m² intrathecally q wk	Mild-moderate nausea, Occasional vomiting Arachnoiditis, vomiting, fever, headache	Renal impairment delays excretion and ↑ systemic toxicity. Check renal function prior to use. Stomatitis with ulceration along any portion of GI tract. Interrupt Rx when stomatitis develops. Pulmonary and hepatotoxicity with prolonged use. Dilute preservative free MTX in Elliott's B solution for IT use. Omit systemic MTX when IT dose given. MTX levels in CSF should be monitored. MTX is protein bound; avoid sulfonamides, aspirin, tetracycline, phenytoin and chloral hydrate. They displace MTX from plasma proteins. MTX pneumonitis seen with prolonged administration. D/C MTX and initiate steroid Rx.
	High Dose MTX 2–10 gms/m² (IV) q 3–4 wks given as an infusion of 6–24 hrs duration followed by folinic acid rescue.	Mild-moderate N/V Allergic reactions and convulsions (rare) Fever, pneumothorax	Maintain urinary *p*H>6.5–7.0 and high urinary output to prevent precipitation of MTX in renal tubules. Adjust urinary *p*H with $NaHCO_3$; check urine *p*H q 3–6 hrs. Monitor BUN, creatinine, LFT prior to each dose. Use only preservative free MTX. Continue CF until plasma MTX <10^{-8} molar (0.45 micro grams/100 ml)
Folinic acid (Citrovorum factor, C.F., Leucovorin calcium)	15–25 mg q 3–6 hrs. (IV) or (PO) × 8–12 doses begun 2–6 hrs after end of MTX infusion.		

(Table continues on page 1768)

TABLE 47-1. (*Continued*)

DRUG (SYNONYMS)	DOSE, ROUTE, AND SCHEDULE WHEN USED AS A SINGLE AGENT	ACUTE SIDE EFFECTS	COMMENTS AND PRECAUTIONS FOR SAFE ADMINISTRATION
ANTIMETABOLITES (*Continued*)			
6–Mercaptopurine (6–MP, Purinethol)	1–2.5 mg/kg (PO) qD (IV) preparation investigational)	Nausea and anorexia Fever	6MP dose reduction to 25–33% if concurrent allopurinol is given; allopurinol inhibits 6MP degradation by xanthine oxidase. Hepatic or renal dysfunction requires dose reduction. Monitor for hepatotoxicity. Stomatitis and diarrhea at high dose.
6–Thioguanine (6TG, Thioguanine, Tabloid)	1–2 mg/kg (PO) qD	Well tolerated	Reduce dose if stomatitis/diarrhea develop. Full dose can be given with allopurinol. Monitor for hepatotoxicity.
5 Azacytadine (5–AC)	150–300 mg/m^2 (IV) 3–5d	Dose and schedule dependent N/V and diarrhea (Profound with rapid infusions) Fever Hypotension (with rapid infusion)	Continuous 24 hr infusions b N/V & diarrhea unstable after reconstitution; use in < 6 hrs; 24 hr infusions given as 4 six-hr infusions; can be given SC. Ringer's lactate provides optimal *p*H & stability. Stomatitis; hypophosphatemia; pruritic rash. Neurologic toxicity (weakness, lethargy) reported but rare. Hepatotoxicity rare but serious complication.
ANTITUMOR ANTIBIOTICS			
Dactinomycin (Actinomycin D, ACT-D, Cosmegen)	0.015 mg/kg (IV) × 5d q 3–4 wks	Moderate-severe N/V in 2–5 hrs lasting 12–24 hrs	Use preservative free diluent to prevent precipitation. Dosage calculated in micrograms. Tissue vesicant; administer in established (IV) line. N/V tends to ↓ with daily use; prolonged anorexia common. Severe radiation recall reactions with necrosis can occur. Acneiform rash, alopecia, hyperpigmentation, stomatitis, glossitis, diarrhea, proctitis.
Bleomycin (Bleo, Blenoxane)	5–15 units/m^2 (IV) (IM) SC q wkly or intralesional)	Mild N/V; anorexia Fever and chills (103–105° F) may → dehydration and hypotension Anaphylactic reactions (may be delayed)	Powder can be diluted in saline or sterile water (1–3 ml). Anaphylactoid reactions in 6% lymphoma patients; give test dose of 1–2 units and observe for 2–4 hrs. Pulmonary fibrosis; do not exceed 400 units total dose. Acetominophen and antihistamines may ↓ febrile reactions. Dose reduction if serum creat >1.5 mg/dl. Stomatitis; alopecia; hyperpigmentation; erythema of skin. Cutaneous toxicity may be severe and require cessation of Rx.
Doxorubicin hydrochloride (Adriamycin, ADM)	30–75/m^2 (IV) q 3–4 wks	Dose related N/V Local pain in small veins	Tissue vesicant; extravasation may require skin grafting. Dose reduction of 50–75% with hepatic dysfunction (bilirubin >1.5). Cardiotoxicity; limit total dose to 550 mg/m^2; reddish urine with ADM. Local erythema, with urticaria and pruritus can occur along vein. Recall reactions in irradiated sites, alopecia totalis in ≈3–4 wks. Stomatitis; proctitis. Bladder instillation well tolerated.
Daunomycin (Daunorubicin, Rubidomycin DNR, Cerubidine)	30–60 mg/m^2 (IV) × 3d q 3–4 wks	Moderate-severe N/V Local pain in small veins Allergic reactions	Tissue vesicant; cardiotoxicity; limit total dose to 550 mg/m^2. Dose reduction with hepatic dysfunction; reddish urine with DNR. Stomatitis and diarrhea unusual; alopecia common.
Mithramycin (Mithracin)	0.025–0.05 mg/kg (IV) qod to toxicity 0.025 mg/kg (IV) for tumor-related hypercalcemia	Moderate-severe N/V in 6 hrs lasting 12–24 hrs (N/V with 4–6 hr infusion) Fever No acute effects	Coagulation abnormalities and hemorrhage often preceded by flushing and epistaxis. CNS toxicity with neuromuscular excitability, headache; dermatitis. Azotemia and electrolyte abnormalities ↓ PO_2, K, Mg, Ca. Tissue vesicant; unstable in acidic solution dilute with sterile water D/C Rx if abnormal LFTs/RFTs develop.

TABLE 47-1. (*Continued*)

DRUG (SYNONYMS)	DOSE, ROUTE, AND SCHEDULE WHEN USED AS A SINGLE AGENT	ACUTE SIDE EFFECTS	COMMENTS AND PRECAUTIONS FOR SAFE ADMINISTRATION
PLANT ALKALOIDS			
Vincristine sulfate (Oncovin, VCR)	0.5–2 mg/m^2 (IV) q wk	N/V unusual	Tissue vesicant; biliary excretion; ↓ dose with hepatic dysfunction. Peripheral neuropathy, paresthesias; toxicity ↑ in elderly and immobile patients. Constipation, abdominal pain; ileus; use stool softeners. Vocal chord paresis; alopecia; hyponatremia and inappropriate ADH rare.
Vinblastine sulfate (Velban, VLB)	6 mg/m^2 (IV) q wk 0.1–0.4 mg/kg (IV) q wk	N/V unusual	Tissue vesicant; ↓ dose with hepatic dysfunction; stomatitis; myelotoxicity; neurotoxicity at high doses (>20 mg). Corneal ulceration if splashed into the eye.
VP-16 (Etoposide, VP-16-213 EPEG) [NSC 14150]	200–250 mg/m^2 (IV) q wk 50–60 mg/m^2 (IV) qd × 5 d q 2–4 wks 125–140 mg/m^2 (IV) (TIW) q 4 wks	Mild nausea Hypotension Fever, chills Anaphylactoid reactions Bronchospasm	Unstable in D_5W; may precipitate in saline solutions after 30 minutes. Use only clean solutions. Severe hypotension with rapid infusion; infuse over ½ hr.; check BP. Treat bronchospasm with antihistamines and d/c infusion. Oral formulation causes GI toxicity. N/V; diarrhea.
VM-26 (PTG, Thenylidene) [NCS 132819]	30 mg/m^2 (IV) qD × 5 100–130 mg/m^2 (IV) q wk	Hypotension Bronchospasm Fever, chills Anaphylaxis Mild N/V	Chemical thrombophlebitis common. Administer as 15–30 minute infusion. Use antihistamines if bronchospasm develops and D/C infusion. May be diluted in dextrose or saline solutions.
MISCELLANEOUS AGENTS			
L-Asparaginase (Elspar, Crasnitin, L-ASP, Asnase, Colaspase)	1000–20,000 U/m^2 q 10–14d	Moderate to severe N/V Fever, chills, urticaria Anaphylactic reactions	Anaphylaxis precautions; desensitization and skin testing may have value in preventing hypersensitivity reactions. Prophylactic antihistamines may control reactions; risk with repeated use. Malaise, anorexia, hepatotoxicity common within 2 wks. Hyperglycemia; coagulation abnormalities. CNS abnormalities with lethargy; pancreatitis, azotemia. Use only clear solutions.
Acridinyl-aniside (AMSA, M-AMSA) [NCS 156303]	90–120 mg/m^2 (IV) q 4 wks	Severe pain and burning in vein Moderate-severe N/V	Chemical thrombophlebitis; ↑ volume to 500 ml and ↓ rate to ↓ pain. Incompatible with D_5W. Urine turns orange. ↓ dose for hepatic dysfunction; renal toxicity. Stomatitis, diarrhea.
Cisplatin (Platinol, DDP)	60–120 mg/m^2 (IV) q 3–4 wks 15–20 mg/m^2 (IV) qD × 5d q 3–4 wks	Severe N/V in 1 hr lasting 6–24 hrs Anaphylactic reactions Convulsions	Anaphylactic reactions with tachycardia, hypotension, erythema, facial edema, wheezing—Rx with antihistamines with Solu–cortef then pretreat with same for future doses. Check creat clearance, BUN, lytes; renal toxicity; IV hydration and diuresis with furosemide and mannitol. Peripheral neuropathy, ophthalmic toxicity. ↓ Mg requiring oral or IM replacement to manage neuromuscular irritability.
Dacarbazine (DTIC, Imidazole-carboxamide)	150–250 mg/m^2 (IV) qD × 5d q 4 wks 1000–1200 mg/m^2 (IV) q 4 wks	Moderate to severe N/V in 1–3 hrs N/V with daily doses Local pain	Flu-like syndrome with fever myalgia and malaise lasting 7–10 days; facial flushing and paresthesias. Tissue vesicant; ↓ rate to ↓ pain. Protect from light. Metabolic activation by liver.
Hexamethyl-melamine (HMM, HXM) [NSC 13875]	6–12 mg/kg (PO) qD × 14–21d or continuous	Moderate-severe N/V	Gastrointestinal toxicity may be dose limiting at high doses. Neurotoxicity with peripheral neuropathies, agitation; confusion; hallucinations; petit mal seizures. May exacerbate vincristine related neuropathy.

(*Table continues on page 1770*)

TABLE 47-1. *(Continued)*

DRUG (SYNONYMS)	DOSE, ROUTE, AND SCHEDULE WHEN USED AS A SINGLE AGENT	ACUTE SIDE EFFECTS	COMMENTS AND PRECAUTIONS FOR SAFE ADMINISTRATION
MISCELLANEOUS AGENTS (*Continued*)			
Hydroxyurea (Hydrea)	25 mg/kg (PO) continuous 100 mg/kg (IV) qD × 3d	Minimal N/V	GI toxicity only at high doses >70 mg/kg. Pretreat patients with allopurinol as rapid fall in leukemic cells occurs in many patients.
Mitotane (O, p′ -DDD Lysodren)	2–10 g mo, (PO) qD continuous	Severe N/V	CNS toxicity with lethargy, vertigo, visual disturbance. Acute adrenal insufficiency. Allergic rash. Sensitivity to sunlight.
Procarbazine (Matulane, Natulan, Methylhydrazine)	100–200 mg/m^2 (PO) × 14d or continuous	Moderate-severe N/V which subsides with daily use	Sympathomimetics, tricyclic antidepressants, other MAO inhibitors and food rich in tyramine can cause acute hypertensive crisis. Advise patients to avoid alcohol—can cause antabuse-like reaction. Barbiturates, phenothiazines, antihistamines may cause ↑ CNS depression. Hypersensitivity reactions with fever, rash, urticaria, angioedema. CNS abnormalities, depression, nightmares, mania, psychosis (rare).
PALA (PALA disodium) [NSC Z24131]		Dose related N/V Diarrhea	Dermatitis with erythematous macular plaques >2000 mg/m^2 skin toxicity may be ↓ with prednisone 60 mg/qD.
HYPOXIC CELL SENSITIZERS			
Misonidozole [NSC 261037]	2.5–16 gms/m^2 (KO) or (IV) q wk (in divided doses)	Mild N/V	Peripheral neuropathy with paresthesias and ↓ DTRs, somnolence at higher doses. Adequate hydration appears to ↓ risk of toxicity. Occasional hypersensitivity reactions. (IV) preparation administered over 5 minutes. Phenytoin and other inducers of hepatic microsomal enzyme activity may alter misonidozole metabolism.

injected procaine) may be employed to prevent discomfort during insertion. Because inexperienced individuals may sever the tip of the catheter during insertion or removal, these catheters should be inserted only by experienced nurses. Use only radiopaque catheters; if a catheter tip is severed, it can be visualized radiographically.

The decision to utilize a heparin lock often is based on the condition of the patient's veins and the type of drugs that will be administered.[33] Agents that must be administered daily, but do not cause local tissue damage are suitable for administration through heparin locks. Following the insertion of the heparin lock, instill a dilute solution of sodium heparin (100 units/ml) into the self-sealing diaphragm of the device every 6 hours. This fills the tubing and the lumen of the needle with heparin to prevent coagulation of blood at the tip. Outpatients can learn to flush the heparin lock with heparin, using aseptic technique. Once taught how to take proper care of their heparin locks, patients who might otherwise remain hospitalized can be discharged to the outpatient clinic for their therapy.

Central Venous Catheters

A central venous catheter made of siliconized rubber (silastic) is used for the administration of parenteral nutrition solutions, which are hypertonic and highly irritating to peripheral veins. These catheters can also provide long-term access to the intravenous circulation of patients who need frequent blood withdrawal or frequent administration of drugs and blood products over prolonged periods.[34] However, catheters used for the administration of parenteral nutrition must not be utilized for blood withdrawal or drug administration. A separate line must be inserted. Small dacron cuffs are fused around the proximal surface of plain central venous catheters when frequent access to the venous circulation is anticipated. This is the major feature that distinguishes the Hickman (1.6 mm internal bore) and the Broviak (1.0 mm bore) catheters from other central venous catheters. These catheters are generally inserted into the cephalic or femoral vein in the operating room, under local anesthesia by physicians or specially trained nurses. The vessel is exposed through an

Over-the-needle catheter
(ONC)

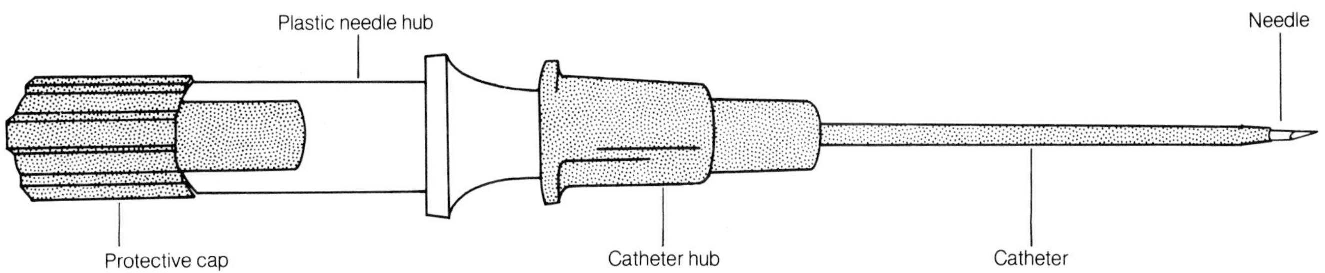

Inside-the-needle-catheter
(INC)

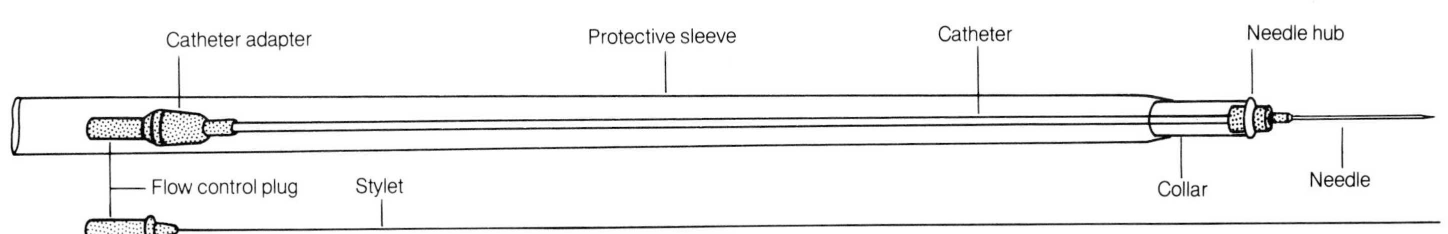

Winged-tip

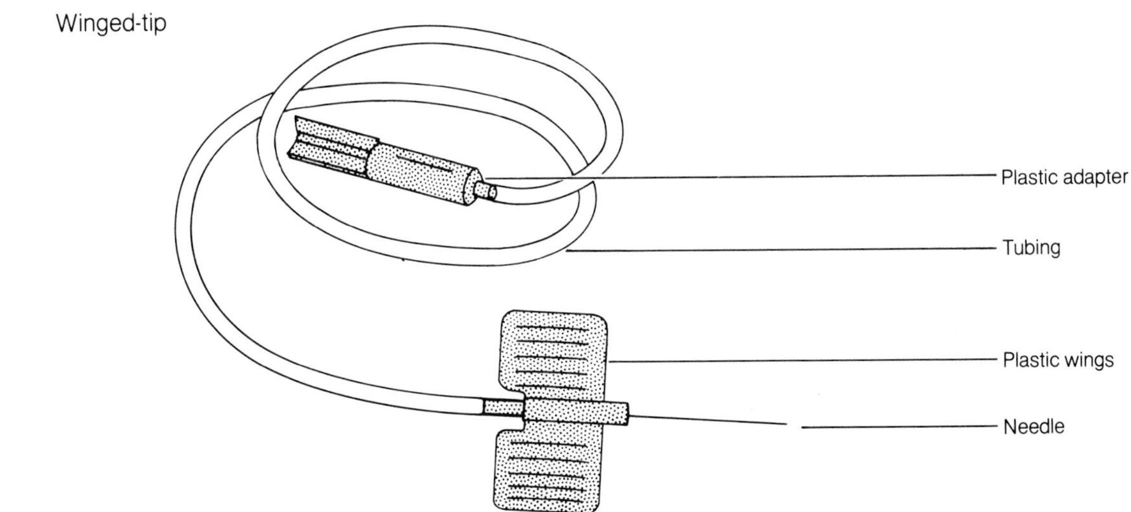

FIG. 47-1. A comparison of the major types of IV cannulae.

incision in the skin. A second, small incision is made distally so the cannula can be tunneled through the subcutaneous tissue to the site of the cut down and introduced into the vessel. The Dacron cuff elicits a fibroblastic reaction that anchors the catheter and provides a mechanical barrier against bacterial contamination.

The surgical team develops procedures for sterile dressing change and central line maintenance in cooperation with the infections control committee and pharmacy. Realistic procedures that can be taught to nursing personnel throughout the hospital must be initiated and rigorously enforced. To minimize serious complications, authority and accountability for these catheters must rest with a specialized team.[35] Team members see patients daily and initially perform all dressing changes and irrigations. Because patients and their families can be taught heparinization procedures and sterile catheter care by nurses, many can be followed as outpatients if their clinical condition permits discharge (Fig. 47-2).

Recent reports indicate that nurses may safely and effectively perform declotting of central venous catheters with fibrinolytic enzymes.[36] Urokinase has been shown to be safe and effective in dissolving clots that have formed in central lines. Failure to declot the line occurs only when the destruction is caused by precipitation of incompatible solutions. No adverse reactions to the declotting enzyme have been observed. Since inadvertent clotting of central catheters is the major complication that necessitates catheter removal, this technique may represent a major advance in catheter care.

Regional administration of chemotherapy may be performed when the majority of the arterial blood is supplied by a single artery that can be catheterized. Nurses ensure the maintenance of catheter sterility and often supervise the administration of drugs through the arterial line.[37]

Nurses play a major role in the procurement of white blood cells and platelets for transfusion to granulocytopenic and thrombocytopenic patients.[38] Leukapheresis and platelet-

FIG. 47-2. Sterile dressing changes for central venous lines[39,46]

Wash hands and don a mask.

If the patient's respiratory function will not be compromised, a second mask is sometimes placed loosely over the patient's mouth to prevent contamination from respiratory organisms.

Place the patient in a supine position, turning the patient's head away from the incision to make the site more accessible and to minimize the risk of contamination. Placing the patient flat decreases the risk of air embolism.

Open dressing set, don gloves.

Remove the old dressing taking care not to disturb the catheter. Carefully discard the soiled dressing into a plastic disposal bag taking care not to contaminate the area.

Examine the site for inflammation or discharge. Culture any drainage.

Change into new gloves or use "no touch technique" without gloves.

Clean the catheter site with acetone, using a circular motion which moves from the insertion site out to the periphery, discarding each sponge.

Clean the catheter site with povidone-iodine. Allow to dry.

Apply topical povidone-iodine ointment to the catheter insertion site and approximately 2cm along the catheter.

Cover the insertion site with a sterile 2″ × 2″ gauze sponge or vaseline gauze.

Paint the area with Skin Prep*™ protective dressing. Allow to dry.

Place partially occlusive dressing over the gauze, taking care not to contaminate the tape that will cover the sterile gauze sponge.

Take a piece of 1″ adhesive tape and cut a ½″ slit in the tape. Position the tape so that the catheter rests in the slit. This insures air occlusion and permits access to the hub of the catheter for tubing changes.

Secure and seal all tubing junctions. Label the dressing with the date and time.

Change dressing immediately if the dressing becomes wet or contaminated or the catheter develops a leak.

Dressings are routinely changed two to three times each week depending on institutional policies.

*Skin Prep™: Ingredients: Isopropyl alcohol 69%;
Poly-MVE/MA N-butyl nonoester, dimethyl phthalate
UNITED, Division of Howmedica, Inc.
P.O. Box 1970, Largo, Florida 33540

pheresis from normal donors are usually performed by nurses under the general supervision of an attending physician.

Infusion Pumps

When the timing of an infusion is an important variable, infusion pumps are valuable. They eliminate the need to count drops or adjust flow rates, and some models have alarm systems that are set off if the infusion infiltrates or the bottle of solution empties.[39] These pumps are especially useful when there is risk of harm if the solution infuses too quickly (*i.e.*, pediatric patients, parenteral nutrition solutions). Peristaltic pumps, such as the IVAC pump, control the rate of infusion. The pump stops automatically when a pre-set volume of fluid is infused and an alarm is sounded.

Continuous IV infusions may also be administered by nurses, using lightweight infusion pump systems, consisting of a cartridge mounted in a control unit.[40] Continuous infusion can be maintained at precise flow rates of 0.4 to 2.0 ml/hour with these devices. Closure-resistant tubing and a 0.2-micron filter ensure delivery of sterile fluid on a continuous basis. Since patients can be taught to change cartridges without risk of contamination, IV chemotherapy may be administered at home under the guidance and supervision of chemotherapy nurses. At one institution, 297 of 307 patients received full courses of continuous IV therapy as outpatients, using an indwelling silicone central venous catheter and a portable infusion pump.[41] The three percent who did not complete the course of therapy had treatment discontinued for reasons unrelated to infectious complications or technical problems. Success of the study was attributed to pump reliability and an extensive program of patient and family education, designed and taught by nurses.

OTHER ROUTES FOR PARENTERAL DRUG ADMINISTRATION

A unique method of drug administration has recently been developed for patients with tumors that remain localized to the intraperitoneal cavity, such as ovarian cancer.[42] Chemotherapy may be administered directly into the peritoneal cavity using a semipermanent, indwelling, silastic catheter. This catheter is also used for peritoneal dialysis in patients with renal failure. It is implanted under local anesthesia. Two liters of dialysate and chemotherapy are instilled (methotrexate, 5–fluorouracil or adriamycin) into the abdominal cavity. A 4-hour dwell time elapses before the dialysate is drained. Intraperitoneal therapy is generally administered continuously for 48 hours or once daily for 5 days. As in renal dialysis, instillation and drainage of the dialysate at the specified intervals can be easily managed by oncology nurses. Although the therapeutic value of intraperitoneal chemotherapy has not yet been firmly established, early clinical trials have demonstrated that the technique is tolerated. Repeated instillations are possible in almost all patients. Since the portal vein, the major route of drug egress, achieves high concentrations of drugs instilled into the peritoneal cavity, this technique is also under investigation in patients with colorectal cancer who are at great risk of developing hepatic metastases.

Drug administration by oncology nurses includes direct instillation of chemotherapy into the central venous system. Many pediatric oncology nurse practitioners perform lumbar punctures and intrathecal therapy. In addition to enhancing continuity of care, performance of such invasive procedures by consistent nurses can reduce the anxiety that children experience when primary physicians change frequently. Persistent central nervous system disease can be managed without frequent lumbar punctures when chemotherapy is directly instilled into a lateral ventricle utilizing an implantable reservoir, such as the Ommaya pump.[43] Nurses manage the care of these reservoirs and the administration of intraventricular chemotherapy. When administering drugs into the Ommaya reservoir, the following procedure is followed:*

place patient in a supine position; don mask and sterile gloves
shampoo hair with Phisohex and shave scalp over the reservoir
cleanse skin over reservoir with Phisohex three times
place sterile 4 × 4 gauze over reservoir and pump six times
prepare LP tray with Betadine, alcohol, syringes, scalp vein needle, and gauze sponges
change into new sterile gloves
prep skin over reservoir with Betadine (×3); allow Betadine to dry; prep area with alcohol; place sterile drape around reservoir
insert scalp vein needle into the reservoir; remove spinal fluid for laboratory studies
inject medication into reservoir using scalp vein needle and flush scalp vein tubing with Elliott's B solution
remove needle
pump reservoir six times
and dress puncture site with Betadine ointment and spot Band–aid

COMPLICATIONS OF PARENTERAL THERAPY

Infection is the most serious complication of parenteral therapy. Almost all infections are preventable if insertion and maintenance techniques preserve sterility. Most infections develop at the puncture site. Almost inevitably, the organisms involved are normal skin flora that have entered the body via the intravenous needle. In patients who are immunosuppressed or granulocytopenic, even organisms not usually considered pathogenic may cause fatal sepsis. Pay special attention to preserving the sterility of in-line filters, stopcocks, tubing, and solutions, especially those rich in glucose. Regular inspection of puncture sites for subtle evidence of infection is important in preventing nosocomial infections.

The most common complications associated with IV therapy in peripheral veins are thrombophlebitis and infiltration with extravasation of the infusate into surrounding tissues. In cancer patients receiving IV chemotherapy and/or broad-spectrum antibiotics that can irritate veins, these complications are often major problems. Whenever a patient complains of pain during an infusion, carefully inspect the site. If none of the signs of thrombophlebitis or infiltration reviewed are

* Nursing Department, Clinical Center, NIH, October, 1979

present, the nurse should slow the infusion and apply heat to the area, to determine if discomfort is caused by venous spasm. Heat will dilate the vessel, increase blood flow, and relieve pain related to venous spasm. Pain related to thrombophlebitis is not relieved by heat.

In addition to pain, thrombophlebitis causes erythema and tenderness along the length of the vessel. If inflammation is severe, the vessel will develop swelling, induration, and a tender palpable venous cord. Factors contributing to the development of thrombophlebitis include hypertonicity of the solution, irritating diluents such as alcohol, highly acidic or alkaline *p*H, particulate matter in the solution, traumatic cannula insertion, and infection.

Nitrogen mustard frequently produces a severe chemical thrombophlebitis and venous discoloration 1 to 3 days following administration, even when it is given through a running IV in a large vein. To ameliorate or prevent this reaction, add 100 mg hydrocortisone sodium succinate (Solu Cortef) to the intravenous solution that infuses as nitrogen mustard is given IV push. Compatibility studies have demonstrated that dextrose and saline solutions containing this steroid are compatible with both nitrogen mustard and vincristine sulfate, which are often given in combination.

Acridinylaniside (AMSA), Dacarbazine (DTIC), and carmustine (BCNU) also cause venous irritation and can produce severe pain and evidence of thrombophlebitis during and following infusion. Pain may be alleviated by increasing the volume of fluid in which the agent is diluted and slowing the rate of infusion. Application of cold packs to the arm during the infusion can also reduce discomfort.

If the needle is dislodged or a vein bursts during an infusion, infiltration and extravasation of the infusate into tissues may occur. Many chemotherapeutic agents, and solutions that are hypertonic, highly acidic, or alkaline, may cause serious tissue damage if extravasated. Although complaints of pain or burning are often early indicators of an infiltration, even potent tissue vesicants can extravasate without producing symptoms. Any evidence of infiltration, (blanching, edema, or loss of blood return) is sufficient to interrupt the infusion when a solution containing chemotherapy is administered. Even if the agent is not a vesicant, extravasation of the drug into tissues adversely affects drug absorption and can predispose the patient to infection.

The presence of a blood return or the absence of blanching or edema are not sufficient proof that all of the infusate is entering the vein. When the posterior wall of the vessel has been punctured during venipuncture, some infusate can extravasate. If enough of the needle's bevel remains in the vein, a good blood return may be apparent and obvious edema may be absent. To establish whether an infiltration has occurred, apply a tourniquet proximal to the site of the venipuncture to restrict blood flow through the vein. If fluid continues to infuse at the same rate despite the obstruction to venous return, there is extravasation.

When extravasation of an agent that causes tissue necrosis occurs, such as doxorubicin hydrochloride, the following procedures can ameliorate toxicity to local tissue:[44]

- immediately terminate the infusion and remove the intravenous needle
- apply an ice pack to induce local vasocontriction
- spray the affected area with ethyl chloride to anesthetize the skin
- inject 50 to 100 mg hydrocortisone sodium succinate directly into the infiltrated area using 25-gauge straight needles; multiple injections should be given to include the entire area
- cover the area with a film of 1% hydrocortisone cream and cover with gauze secured with paper tape
- apply ice packs to the affected area for 24 hours
- instruct patients to apply the steroid cream twice daily until all the erythema has resolved
- instruct patients to exercise the affected arm or hand

Patients are instructed to call the nurse or physician if pain is severe. This regimen has prevented tissue necrosis, ulceration, and loss of range of motion in our patients. Only mild tenderness and brawny skin discoloration have occurred. To permit immediate initiation of treatment, standard orders should be developed and be readily available.

Recent reports suggest that immediate IV administration of 8.5% sodium bicarbonate (5 ml) may also have a role in reducing toxicity to local tissue from doxorubicin hydrochloride extravasations.[45] The rationale for the administration of sodium bicarbonate is based on data on the binding of doxorubicin hydrochloride to cellular DNA and tissue.[46–47] Binding appears to be pH dependent, requiring an acidic environment. Following doxorubicin extravasations the use of sodium bicarbonate in patients has been reported beneficial.[47] When sodium bicarbonate was employed to ameliorate tissue necrosis in rats that received intradermal doxorubicin hydrochloride, toxicity was reduced.[48] Agents that cause tissue necrosis when extravasated are listed as vesicants in Table 47-1.

Alopecia is a common but distressing side-effect of cancer therapy. Although hair loss is not a life-threatening toxicity, it can be a devastating side-effect for patients. Concern about the psychological effect of alopecia has stimulated nurses to investigate the feasibility of preventing hair loss in patients.[49] Dean, Salmon, and Griffith have studied the effects of scalp hypothermia on doxorubicin-induced alopecia.[50] Scalp temperatures of 23° to 24°C can be achieved with the use of an ice turban after 10 minutes. The ice turban is applied for 35 to 40 minutes. Pharmacokinetic data indicate that plasma concentration falls rapidly over the first 30 minutes, but that there is a relatively long terminal half-life. Excellent protection at doses of 50 mg or less was reported. At doses greater than 60 mg, scalp hypothermia was less effective. The investigators reported that they would try to achieve lower scalp temperatures in future studies, hoping to improve protection from hair loss. The authors stated that scalp hypothermia was well tolerated when carried out repeatedly over a period of 6 to 8 months of treatment, but other investigators have indicated that scalp hypothermia is associated with psychological problems and loss of compliance after repeated icings. Studies to evaluate the psychological effect of scalp hypothermia should be performed before this intervention becomes widely advocated.

Knowledge and Skills

Knowledge about the anatomy and physiology of veins and arteries and the physiologic responses of veins to stimulation by the nervous system is essential for proficiency in intravenous therapy. Technical expertise must be demonstrated, and knowledge about safe administration and the management of complications must be evaluated, under the supervision of an experienced physician or nurse preceptor. Because chemotherapy nurses are expected to assume full responsibility for the administration of agents ordered by the oncologist, it is essential that they also have a sound understanding of pharmacology.

The creation of a satellite pharmacy, in our outpatient clinic, where drugs are mixed by a pharmacist in a laminar air flow cabinet, has eliminated the need for nurses to mix IV medications. This service enables the nurse to spend a greater amount of time teaching and counseling patients. Sterility of solutions is ensured, and delays in obtaining appropriate doses are minimal. The pharmacist's presence in the clinic permits the nurse to check drug doses and dilutions directly with the pharmacist and to resolve any questions.

LEGAL IMPLICATIONS OF EXPANDED NURSING ROLES IN CHEMOTHERAPY

The state laws that govern IV therapy and the administration of parenteral drugs by registered nurses vary because these functions were formerly considered areas of medical practice. To permit nurses to assume responsibilities in this area, a state usually adopts a consensus statement issued jointly by its medical society, nursing association, and hospital association.[51] Although the content varies from state to state, these policy statements acknowledge that medical and nursing practice overlap in IV therapy, and describe the shared legal accountabilities and liabilities. Each employer must establish standards of practice that ensure that a nurse is qualified by knowledge, skill, and experience to administer IV therapy.

The nurse must have a written order that is signed and dated by a physician specifying which patient is to be treated and the manner in which treatment is to be administered (*i.e.*, IV push, rapid infusion). The nurse can be held negligent if an incorrect drug or dosage is administered even if the physician's order is incorrect. Because many agents are prescribed on the basis of body surface area, a nomogram for the calculation of the individual patients' drug doses should be available to the nurse (see Appendix Fig. 1). Most institutions require a nurse to demonstrate a high level of knowledge and skill about drugs, their normal dose ranges, reconstitution, administration, physiologic effects, and toxicities, in a written and a practical examination prior to assuming responsibilities for drug administration.[51]

Negligence is defined as conduct that produces harm and falls below the standard of care for professional practice in a specific area. A chemotherapy nurse is expected to act with the care and skill that any responsible and prudent nurse would employ under similar circumstances. The oncology nurse has a legal responsibility to understand the purpose and effects of each chemotherapeutic agent that is prescribed for IV administration. If there is any doubt about the accuracy of the drug, the dosage, or the manner in which the drug is to be administered, the nurse must verify the order with the physician before carrying out the order. Otherwise the nurse assumes liability for negligence if harm to the patient results. The chemotherapy nurse cannot avoid legal liability even if the physician is sued and held liable.

Since many chemotherapeutic agents currently employed in cancer treatment are tissue vesicants if extravasated during IV administration, liability is a concern for the oncology nurse and physician. Should a malpractice suit be brought against a nurse following the extravasation of an agent that produced tissue necrosis, the following questions would be considered: (1) whether the policies or guidelines formulated by the employer for the IV administration of chemotherapy were followed; (2) whether the drug was administered in a prudent and proper manner, in accordance with the physician's orders; (3) whether the nurse terminated the IV infusion immediately if the patient complained of pain or burning; (4) whether the nurse exercised reasonable judgment before and during the infusion (*i.e.*, examining the site for evidence of infiltration); (5) whether the nurse took appropriate action to manage the extravasation or reaction; (6) whether the physician was informed promptly about the nature and severity of the reaction; and (7) whether the incident and therapeutic actions are described in the patient's medical record. In general, a chemotherapy nurse will not be held liable for harm that results to a patient if the policies and procedures developed as the standard of care have been followed. However, the nurse must also demonstrate that good clinical judgment was exercised throughout the infusion. If a nurse consults the physician promptly when a problem occurs, initiates appropriate measures to manage the adverse effects, documents objective findings and the therapeutic measures that were taken in the medical record, then the legal requirements for safe and prudent practice will be fulfilled. The physician is liable if it can be demonstrated that the nurse's knowledge and technical expertise were inadequate, or unevaluated; if adequate supervision was not provided, as recommended by the joint practice statement or institutional policies; or if the physician did not respond to the nurse's request for guidance or assistance.

The nurse may be held personally liable for any action that is deemed negligent or beyond the scope of the nurse's role, as defined by legal or institutional policies. Accordingly, each nurse should determine the advisability of obtaining individual malpractice insurance, based on a thorough understanding of the coverage provided by the employer. If full coverage for all legal fees and damages is provided by the employer, the need for a personal malpractice policy is minimal. If, however, the employer provides only enough coverage to protect itself in a malpractice suit, the nurse should obtain insurance through a commercial carrier or professional organization.

INFORMED CONSENT

Legal responsibility for obtaining consent, as discussed in Chapter 10, rests with the physician but is a legal and ethical responsibility shared by nurses. Although nurses do not assume primary responsibility for obtaining consent, they do have a responsibility to ensure that patients understand the nature of the treatment being offered. When serious questions or conflicts are identified, they must be related to the physician by the nurse, so that a valid consent can be obtained or reestablished. Nurses can be held liable for negligence in legal matters surrounding the adequacy of informed consent.

For cancer patients to give a valid consent for a procedure or treatment, they must understand their prognosis, and the alternatives that are open to them. Education must provide specific information about the way that therapy will be administered and the specific side effects that may be anticipated. The framework for this information is a basic understanding of the disease, the rationale for the staging evaluation and treatment modalities. Education about a specific therapy and its consequences should include information about immediate and long-term benefits as well as acute and chronic toxicities.

The exact information that is provided to a patient will vary in terms of extent and detail. Because patients receive information from multiple sources, it is axiomatic that consistency be maintained. When physicians rotate, the nurse's knowledge about patients, diseases, drugs, protocols, and the management of patients assumes great importance. Their experience and skills can ensure that the quality and continuity of care are maintained during periods of transition. This is especially important for patients who are managed as outpatients and must take steps to meet their potential needs for care at home.

FLOW SHEETS

If important data about a patient's clinical course are recorded concisely on a flow sheet, those caring for the patient can obtain a quick summary of significant events in the patient's course of treatment. In any clinical setting, the oncologist and the nurse benefit greatly from having previous observations available for review. Oncology nurses have played a major role in the development and maintenance of flow sheets (Fig. 47-3). Entries requiring explanation can be noted in the area designated for comments. A human figure to illustrate important clinical findings can be used to evaluate clinical change.

Flow sheets permit a brief summary of drugs administered, dose reductions, toxicity, response, and cumulative dosages. Fluctuations in hematologic, biochemical clinical parameters, specific tumor markers, and performance status can also be assessed. Rate of response, remission duration, and time to maximal response are readily calculated. Significant data can readily be taken from the flow sheet and computerized to permit rapid analysis of data, facilitating the early recognition of important trends during the clinical trials.

SURGERY

Changes in the philosophy of the surgical management of cancer patients have produced noticeable changes in traditional surgical nursing care. Although patients with cancer are initially admitted to a hospital for surgical procedures, many will receive several treatment modalities. Surgical nurses must therefore be prepared with the fundamentals of medical oncology, radiotherapy, and critical care nursing.[52]

PREOPERATIVE PREPARATION

Preparing patients for operations is a responsibility shared by the surgeon, anesthesiologist, and the surgical nursing staff. Patients and family members need information and clarification about the surgical procedure. The patient's primary nurse coordinates preoperative teaching, supplementing information from the physician and reinforcing the patient's knowledge base.

Preoperative assessment of the patient's likelihood to develop major wound complications should be made by nurses who will care for the patient in the postoperative period. This requires knowledge of the patient's diagnosis, staging evaluation, and proposed treatment plan. Knowledge of nutritional status and medications that the patient takes can provide important predictive information and should be obtained during the nursing history. Aspirin, anticoagulants, antihypertensives, hormones, antibiotics, chemotherapy, or steroids can contribute to surgical risk as can a history of alcohol, tobacco, or drug abuse.[53]

If devices or monitors are to be used in the postoperative period, teach the patient how they function preoperatively to avoid anxiety in the special care unit. Patients should be taught respiratory exercises and how to breathe with the ventilation devices preoperatively. Time spent teaching deep breathing and effective coughing can assist patient cooperation with respiratory exercises, despite incisional pain.[54] Temporary and permanent alterations in body functions should be reviewed preoperatively. Foley catheters, tracheotomy tubes, and colostomy or other drainage systems should be discussed.[55] Information on the availability of postoperative pain medication can relieve preoperative anxiety. Details about where the family can wait, when they can see the patient, and when they can talk to the surgeon should also be provided routinely.

POSTOPERATIVE CARE

Preoperative radiotherapy and chemotherapy increase the likelihood of problems to complicate wound healing, nutrition, physical rehabilitation, and sexual and psychological readjustments for patients in the post–operative period.

WOUND HEALING, INFECTION, AND HEMORRHAGE

In the immediate postoperative period, give priority to the prevention of complications at the site of the surgical wound. If skin flaps have been raised, tissue transferred, or free skin applied to the site, it is essential to maintain tissue viability by assuring that drainage tubes sutured into the wound are effective in removing blood, plasma, or air. Intact skin coverage is necessary to prevent infection, fistula formation, wound breakdown, and flap necrosis. Assessment of the viability of skin flaps requires skilled observations on the part of nurses.[56]

Normal hematologic defense mechanisms may be diminished or absent in the cancer surgical candidate.[57] The potential for hematoma or frank bleeding in the surgical wound must be recognized. The formation of a hematoma in the surgical wound or frank brisk bleeding in drainage tubing

NIH - 442-2 (REV. 10-77)

PROTOCOL NO.	TUMOR TYPE
CLIN. ASSOC.	STUDY CHAIRMAN

B.S. AREA		Date (Yr:
		Day on Study or Cycle/Day
THERAPY	DRUGS	
	OTHER	Radiotherapy
		Transfusions
		Antibiotics
HEMATOLOGY		WBC/mm^{3}x10^3
		Hgb g% or Hct %
		Platelets/mm^{3}x10^3
		Polys %/Lymphs %
		Bone marrow
CHEMISTRIES		Uric acid mg% Urinalysis
		Ca/PO$_4$mg%
		Alk.Phos.
		Bilirub, mg% tot.
		SGPT SGOT
		alb/Tot.prot g%
		LDH
		BUN/Creat. mg%
If any abnormal item can be designated tumor-related (T) or drug-related please include in appropriate box.	PHYSICAL	Wt. (kg) Ht. (cm)
		Performance (B)
		Liver, Spleen (cm)
		Neurologic
		Effusions, edema
	TUMOR (cm x cm)	Site 1 (C)
		Site 2 (C)
		Site 3 (C)
		New Lesions
	FOLLOWABLE DISEASE	Chest X-ray
		Bone Series
		Scan: Bone/Brain
		Scan: Liver
		EMI
		Ultrasound
		LAG IVP
	TOXICITY	GI (Specify) (A)
		Respiratory (Specify) (A)
		Neurologic (A)
		CV/GU (A)
		Other
PAT. STATUS		Overall Response (CR, PR, S, NR)
		% Regression

(C) Show Tumors 1,2,3,4,5, and code each with letters:

B = Bone S = Skin/SC H = Hepatic
C = CNS L = Lung M = Breast
N = Nodes P = Pleura O = Other(Specify)

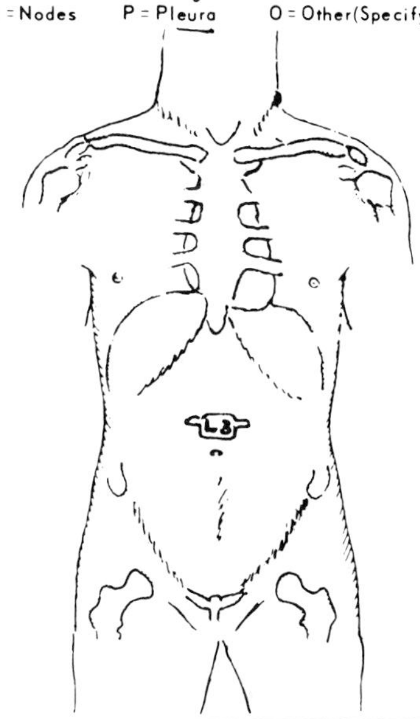

L3

REMARKS

PATIENT IDENTIFICATION

(A) TOXICITY
0 = None, normal
1 = Mild
2 = Moderate
3 = Pronounced
4 = Life threat
5 = Lethal

(B) PERFORMANCE
100 = Normal
90 = Minor signs or symptoms
80 = Normal activity with effort
70 = Unable to carry on normal activity but cares for self
60 = Requires occassional assistance with personal needs
50 = Requires considerable assistance and medical care
40 = Disabled
30 = Severely disabled and hospitalized
20 = Very sick; active supportive treatment necessary
10 = Moribund
0 = Death

DISTRIBUTION: Original to Chart; Canary - Study Chairman; Pink - Chemo-Nurse; Goldenrod - Clinical Associate

Page of pages

FIG. 47-3. Flow sheet.

demands surgical exploration and ligation of bleeding sites. Pressure dressings over amputation sites require frequent inspection for drainage and circulation. When the amputated stump is placed in an occlusive plaster dressing, the patient's signs and subjective symptoms must be carefully monitored.

Assess the potential for postoperative complications to develop in patients who have had radical head and neck explorations. Chyle leak, wound breakdown, and carotid artery rupture may necessitate emergency nursing interventions.[56] Emergency equipment near the patient's bedside should include a tracheotomy tray, pressure dressings, and bull-dog clamps for hemorrhage control.

Intake and output records must be designed to reflect the status of each separate drainage site. Visible chart flow sheets for a 24-hour period must be readily available to the surgeon. A typical example of this type of nursing work sheet is presented in Figure 47-4.

Compromise of host defense mechanisms in cancer patients increases the likelihood of a nosocomial infection to develop in the postoperative period. Length of hospitalization, stage of disease, and number of invasive procedures correlate directly with the frequency of infection.[58] Since the most frequent source of sepsis from nosocomial infection is the urinary tract, it is important to prevent postoperative bladder catheterization. Encourage male patients to stand at the bedside to void, women to use a toilet, and bladder credé.[59] If indwelling catheters are necessary, sterile, closed catheter drainage systems minimize infectious complications. Since poor respiratory ventilation accounts for a significant number of infectious complications, deep breathing exercises and early ambulatory activity should be encouraged.

WOUND DRAINAGE

Isolate the drainage from enterocutaneous fistulas from the skin so that the highly alkaline or acid fluids will not excoriate the surrounding tissues. Five basic guidelines have been proposed by enterostomal therapists for the management of these complicated surgical wounds, regardless of dimensions:[60]

- Cleaning and drying skin with a mild soap
- Use of a hypoallergic adhesive—an adhesive collodian spray or cement, stomahesive face plate, karaya ring
- Use of a skin barrier—Karayapaste, Stomahesive—silicone spray
- Use of a collecting pouch—many designs, most disposable
- Framing entire pouch with hypoallergic tape

Silicone rubber contoured face plates can be devised for more elaborate customizing by obtaining an impression with an alginate material that is often used for dental impressions. The impression is used to prepare a face plate for the drainage pouch with the same configuration as the wound and surrounding abdominal surface.[61] Respect for the fragile integrity of the skin must be provided through cleanliness, protection from irritants, and a well-fitted appliance.[62] Test all adhesive for skin sensitivity with each patient as well.

When a bowel enterostomy is made for primary control of a pelvic tumor, patients must adjust to permanent changes in bowel or bladder function. A positive attitude and an effective teaching program lead to confident self-care whether support is provided by a committed primary nurse or a specially trained enterostomal therapist. Detailed information and opportunities for practice sessions prior to discharge from the hospital reduce the frustration of dealing with this radical change in lifestyle.

A comprehensive care program includes emotional support in this period of crisis. Donovan and Pierce present a comprehensive illustrated section about ostomy care in their text.[63] In the preoperative period nurses must reassure patients and their families that they will receive all the help they need to cope with postoperative changes in bowel or bladder function. Sharing this information with a spouse or family member is often the most important contribution that a nurse can make to the patient's physical and emotional adjustments. When family members know what to expect, they can modify life in the home to facilitate long-term rehabilitation. Often visual teaching aids are the best approach.

Colostomy control varies with the level of surgical intervention, the practices of the surgeon, and individual patient needs. Diet, irrigation, and medication can often be synchronized to achieve control. However, not all colostomates can or should irrigate.[64]

The choice of an ostomy appliance is influenced by the nature of the drainage, anatomic considerations, and the patient's preferences and capacity for self-care. A variety of temporary and permanent appliances and supplies are available at an annual cost of approximately $150.[17] Before discharge, make patients aware of the ostomy association in their local area. Ostomates provide emotional support, education, and practical knowledge. They will visit patients in the hospital or at home to share experiences and to assist patients and families in the postoperative period. Most patients also benefit from community nursing services, to provide continuity of care after hospitalization.

RADIATION THERAPY

The nursing care of cancer patients undergoing radiotherapy involves education about the purpose, method of administration, prevention of complications, and management of unavoidable local or systemic toxicity. To perform these activities the nurse must have a working knowledge of the principles of radiotherapy, the relation between radiosensitivity and tissue tolerance, the onset and character of commonly encountered side-effects, and the measures that should be initiated to ameliorate toxicity. Facts about treatment techniques must often be reiterated and supplemented after discussions with the radiotherapist have been initiated. Knowledge about normal tissue tolerance in the radiation field enables the nurse to anticipate the onset and severity of side-effects.

Self-care measures taught by the radiotherapy nurse should be simple, easily carried out, and logical in relation to anticipated toxicities (Fig. 47-5).[65–67] Education of patients in self-care can decrease unnecessary morbidity and also provide concrete evidence to patients that they have an important and active role to play in their treatment. Care of normal tissues within radiation fields is generally outlined by the

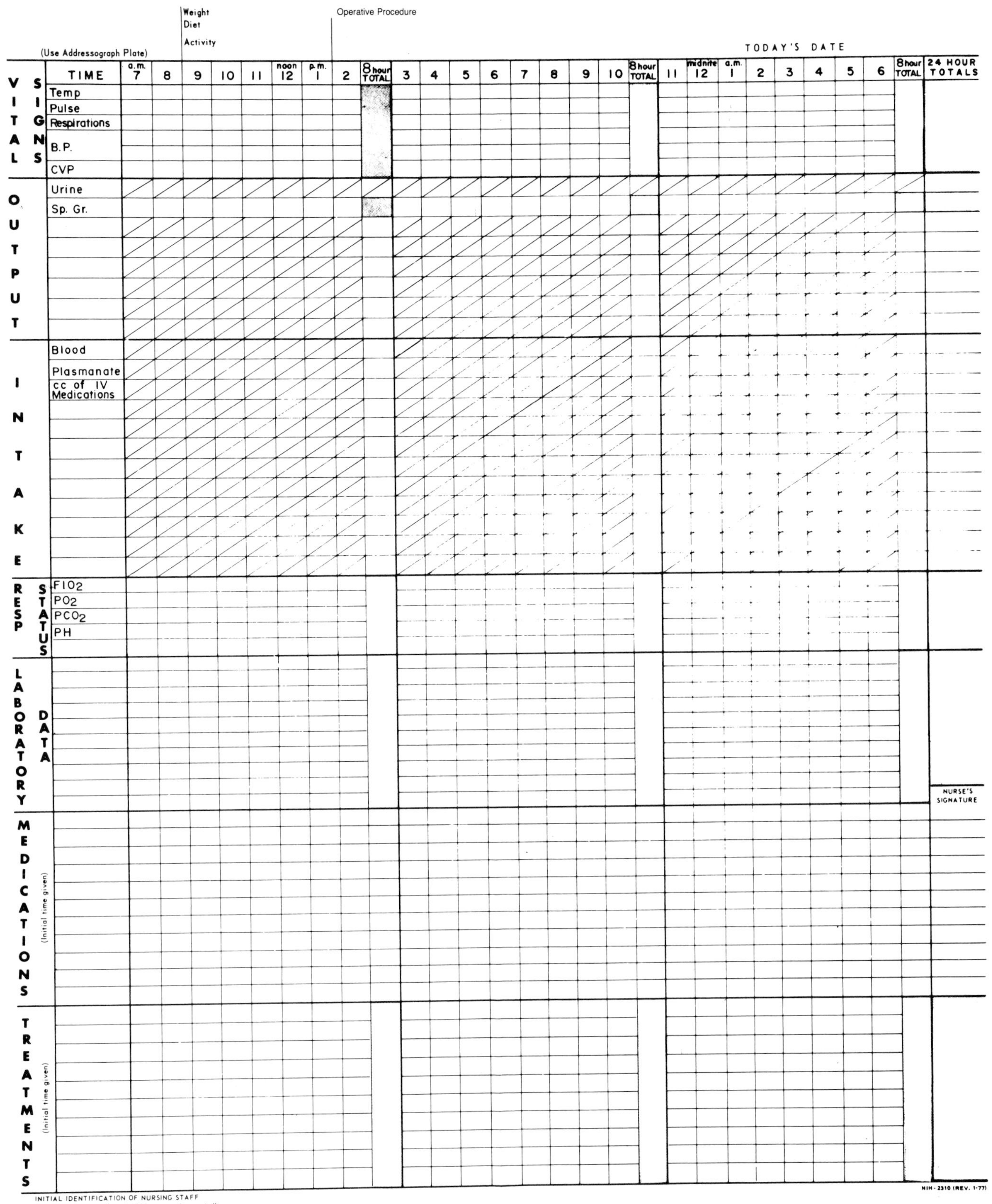

(Use Addressograph Plate)

Weight
Diet
Activity

Operative Procedure

TODAY'S DATE

	TIME	a.m. 7	8	9	10	11	noon 12	p.m. 1	2	8 hour TOTAL	3	4	5	6	7	8	9	10	8 hour TOTAL	11	midnite 12	a.m. 1	2	3	4	5	6	8 hour TOTAL	24 HOUR TOTALS
VITALS SIGNS	Temp																												
	Pulse																												
	Respirations																												
	B.P.																												
	CVP																												
OUTPUT	Urine																												
	Sp. Gr.																												
INTAKE	Blood																												
	Plasmanate																												
	cc of IV Medications																												
RESP STATUS	FIO2																												
	PO2																												
	PCO2																												
	PH																												
LABORATORY DATA																													NURSE'S SIGNATURE
MEDICATIONS (Initial time given)																													
TREATMENTS (Initial time given)																													

INITIAL IDENTIFICATION OF NURSING STAFF
(Sign signature once per sheet for 24 hour recording period)

NIH-2310 (REV. 1-77)

FIG. 47-4. Surgical flow sheet.

1. *Preventative Mouth Care*
   a. Assessment of the mouth daily
   b. Before and after meals and at bedtime:
      Brush with soft bristled toothbrush and toothpaste of choice
      Rinse with Cepacol mouthwash. Gentle flossing between teeth
   c. Use vaseline for lubricant on the lips to prevent dryness
2. *Mild Stomatitis*
   a. Culture the oral cavity
   b. Obtain CBC
   c. Order bland diet*
   d. Institute oral hygiene before and after meals and at bedtime
      Brush with soft brush
      Rinse with equal parts H_2O_2, Cepacol, H_2O
   e. Topical anesthetics when needed:
      Viscous xylocaine, Orabase, or a mix of equal parts Bendryl elixir/Maalox/1% Xylocaine viscous
   f. Use topical antibiotics, such as mycostatin
   g. Prescribe analgesics prn.
3. *Severe Stomatitis*
   a. Culture the oral cavity
   b. Bland liquid diet.* May need parenteral supplements.
   c. CBC
   d. Oral hygiene q 2–4 hours. Cleaning teeth and gums with Toothettes or H_2O/Cepacol/H_2O_2 mixture-soaked gauze.
   e. Use local anesthetics and systemic analgesics and antibiotics prn.

*Placing full diet in blender when only pureed foods are tolerated.
Ice cream, milkshakes, popsicles, gelatin, soft cheeses are well-tolerated.

FIG. 47-5. Protocol for oral care. (Beck S: Impact of a systematic oral care protocol on stomatitis after chemotherapy. Cancer Nurs 2:185–199, 1979)

radiation therapy nurse and may vary from one institution to another. Generally, these instructions are written so the materials can be taken home, reread, shared with family members, and reinforced.

A detailed discussion of the acute and chronic effects of radiotherapy on normal tissues can be found in Chapter 7 and throughout the book in discussions of radiotherapy for specific tumors. Guidelines for dietary support are provided in Chapter 43, and those for the amelioration of other adverse treatment effects are found in Chapter 45.

IMMUNOTHERAPY

It is important that nurses involved with patients in immunotherapeutic trials thoroughly understand principles of immunology in order to accurately assess patient responses.[69–70]

Evaluation of cell-mediated immune function can be performed with the application of several nonspecific intradermal skin test antigens. The responsibility for skin testing is frequently assumed by nurses who should be aware of the intention and expected results of their intervention. Nurses must be certain that authority for this practice has been specifically delegated to them through the institutions in which they are employed. Although the risks to the patient from skin testing are small, the possibility of anaphylaxis exists.[71]

Intradermal injections of five common agents are applied to the volar area of the forearms in adults and the paravertebral area in children. Ethyl chloride spray, a local anesthesic, can be applied immediately before the procedure. The skin tests are applied in a consistent predetermined order, 3 to 4 cm apart. Cleanse the skin surface with alcohol. Prepare each antigen in a separate tuberculin syringe with a small gauge (25–27 ga) needle. Common recall antigens include all or some of the following:

Trichophyton	1:30 dilution	use 0.1 ml
Purified Protein Derivatives (PPD)	5 TU (intermediate)	use 0.1 ml
Candida	1:100 dilution	use 0.1 ml
Streptokinase-Streptodornase (SKSD)	75 U	use 0.05 ml
Mumps		use 0.1 ml

Although some institutions measure the reactions more frequently, a reading at 48 hours is usually chosen for convenience. An accurate recording of the area of induration is made in two dimensions. Reactions to recall antigens can be considered positive when the diameter measures more

TABLE 47-2. Hormonal Agents

DRUG (SYNONYMS)	DOSE, ROUTE, AND SCHEDULE WHEN USED AS A SINGLE AGENT	COMMENTS AND PRECAUTIONS FOR SAFE ADMINISTRATION
ANDROGENS		
Fluoxymesterone (Halotestin)	10–30 mg/day (PO)	Patients may become sensitized to oil carriers; dosage reductions required for hepatic dysfunction; obstructive jaundice; ↑ appetite and weight gain; anorexia and N/V at high doses; hypercalcemia in immobilized patients, especially those with bone metastases; masculinization, hirsutism, acne, patchy alopecia, voice change, ↑ libido; sodium and fluid retention—monitor weight; low salt diet.
Calusterone (Methosarb)	40 mg (qid (PO) or 0.3 mg/kg/day (PO)	
Testolactone (Teslac)	250 mg (qid (PO) or 100 mg (IM) (TIW)	
Testosterone proprionate (Oreton propionate)	50–100 mg (IM) (TIW)	
Testosterone enanthate (Delatestryl)	600–1200 mg (IM) qW	
Dromostanolone propionate (Drolban)	100 mg (IM) (TIW)	
ESTROGENS		
Diethylstilbestrol (DES)	1–15 mg (PO) qD	N/V at high doses resembling morning sickness that often subsides with continued Rx; rapid rise in serum calcium in patients with bone metastases; sodium and fluid retention with hypertension → CHF and thromboembolic complications; monitor weight; low salt diet; feminization, gynecomastia, endometrial hypertrophy, uterine bleeding, areolar hyperpigmentation, urinary frequency; sensitization to oil carrier.
Fosfestrol (Stilbestrol diphosphate), Stilphostrol, Honvan	50–200 mg (PO) (tid) 500–1000 mg (IV) × 5d then 250–100 mg (IV) q wk	
Chlorotrianisene (TACE)	12–25 mg (PO) (tid)	
Conjugated equine estrogenic compound (Premarin)	1–10 mg (PO) (tid)	
Ethinyl Estradiol (Estinyl)	0.5–1 mg (PO) (tid)	
ANTI-ESTROGENIC COMPOUNDS		
Tamoxifen citrate (Nolvadex)	10–80 mg (PO) qD	Transient "flare" in skin, soft tissue and bone metastases, hypercalcemia; mild leukopenia and thrombocytopenia; vaginal discharge, bleeding and pruritus; corneal opacity and retinopathies with prolonged high doses >240 mg/day >1 year; induction of ovulation and lactation; hot flashes.
PROGESTINS		
Hydroxyprogesterone caproate (Delalutin)	1–2.5 qm (IM) (BIW)	Generally well tolerated; minimal fluid retention; some alopecia; occasional hypercalcemia patients with bone metastases; use with care in patients with hepatic dysfunction; thromboembolic phenomena.
Medroxyprogesterone acetate Provera (P.O.) Depoprovera (I.M.)	20–200 mg (PO) qD 200–800 mg (IM) (BIW)	
Megesterol acetate (Megase)	40–300 mg (PO) qD	

(*Table continues on page 1782*)

TABLE 47-2. *(Continued)*

DRUG (SYNONYMS)	DOSE, ROUTE, AND SCHEDULE WHEN USED AS A SINGLE AGENT	COMMENTS AND PRECAUTIONS FOR SAFE ADMINISTRATION
ADRENAL CORTICAL STEROIDS		Agents vary with respect to mineralocorticoid potency (sodium and fluid retention); intermittent administration can ↓ serious toxicity. Adrenalectomized patients must ↑ steroids in stress, infection; trauma; oral preparations irritate GI mucosa—administer with antacids. Side effects associated with prolonged use: Immunosuppression:— ↑ risk of infection GI ulceration and hemorrhage Hyperglycemia, diabetes, hyperlipidemia, weight gain Sodium and fluid retention, hypertension, edema, potassium wasting Emotional lability, euphoria, psychosis Muscle wasting, osteoporosis, aseptic necrosis of bones Glaucoma, cataracts Cushingoid appearance, acne Secondary amenorrhea, growth failure Suppression of adrenal function, necessitating slow withdrawal.
Prednisone (Deltasone)	40–60 mg/m^2 (PO) qD	
Prednisolone (Delta Cortef)	40–60 mg/m^2 (IM) qD	
Methylprednisolone (Medrol) Sodium succinate (Solumedrol) Acetate (Depomedrol)	10–25 mg (IV) or (IM)	
Hydrocortisone (Cortef-) Sodium succinate (Solu-cortef) Dexametrasone (Decadron)	0.5–16 mg (PO) (IV), (PO) or (IM) qD	
CHEMICAL ADRENALECTOMY		Skin rash within 5–7 days lasting 8 days Lethargy, somnolence Addisonian characteristics ↓ secretion of aldosterone with postural hypotension and ↓ Na Hypothyroidism, virilization Mild nausea, vertigo, nystagmus
Aminoglutethimide	750–2000 (PO) qD	

than 5 mm. When patients are provided with instructions and appropriate measuring tools, they can read and report their own skin test results.[72] The nurse then documents these results so the physician will have the readings for retrieval and interpretation.

Immunocompetence can also be measured by skin testing with a chemical antigen, dinitrochlorobenzene (DNCB), to which most individuals have never been exposed. Initial sensitization is performed with two solutions of different strengths; 0.1 ml of a 2000-mcg solution applied to one forearm and another dose of 50 mcg applied to the other. After an initial hypersensitivity response to the chemical at the sites, the immunocompetent host will produce a secondary flare 7 to 14 days later, or whenever challenged with DNCB at a later time.[73]

FIG. 47-6. Heaf gun. Multiple prong technique.

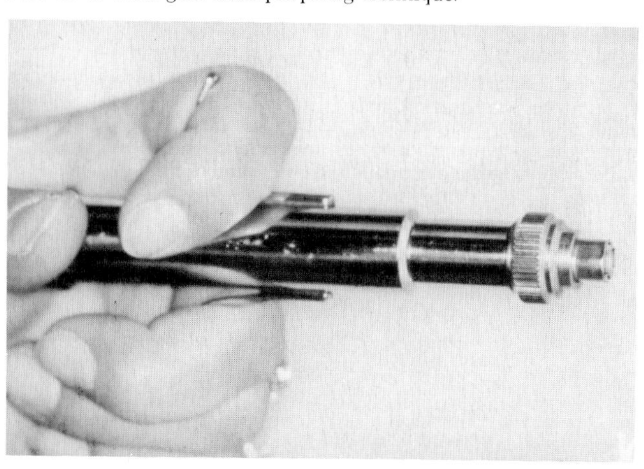

A variety of immunotherapeutic agents have been used in clinical trials. Three active nonspecific bacterial adjuvants have received more widespread use, however, and appear in Table 47-3.

Three methods of giving BCG intradermally have been employed. Although the intention and dose are similar, investigators prefer one procedure over another. The tine and heaf gun are familiar instruments for vaccination. Scarification grids are easily produced with a sharp needle as well (Figs. 47-6 to 47-8). In all cases, the skin preparation is identical and the BCG is dripped onto the wound.

Most immunotherapy patients are in adjuvant treatment programs. Many are in remission and receive immunotherapy in the outpatient area.[74] The nurse participating in a cancer immunotherapy program must assess patients for response and toxicity,[75] while assisting them to make adaptations in their lifestyle compatible with prolonged therapy. When there is no evidence of disease, compliance with an extended course of treatment can be difficult. If nurses recognize this conflict as a potential problem, they can assist patients to deal with their ambivalence.

TABLE 47-3. Active Non-Specific Immunotherapeutic Agents

AGENT	PREPARATION	ADMINISTRATION	SIDE EFFECTS	NURSING IMPLICATIONS
BCG (bacillus calmette—Guerin)	Pasteur, Tice, Glaxo, Trudeu, Phipps-strains, differ in ratio of live to dead organisms and storage. Freeze-dried preparations activated by specific diluent.	Intradermal: see photos near major lymph node drainage sites. Scarification / Heaf gun / 36 Tine Grid: $5 \times 5 cm^2$ area in 4 sites each application	Flaring, recall at old sites, itching, fever, malaise. Scarring is long lasting and permanent.	Astute observation of patient responses and accurate recording. Obligation to obtain specific information from investigators in order to support patient and family. Acetominophen 2 tabs q 4–6h for symptomatic relief fever, malaise.
		Skin prep with acetone. Injection into skin with applicator, inducing bleeding 1 ml. BCG solution dropped onto broken skin, mixed with blood. Dried with hair dryer. Occlusive, water proof dressing × 24h.		Cool compresses, talc for itching. Lidocaine topically if itching severe. Differentiate regional lymphadenitis from tumor mets with patient and family. Swimming and direct bathing after crust formed.
		Intracavitary Instillation abdominal-paracentesis pleural-thoracentesis	Fever chills	Turn patient side to side to distribute BCG in cavity. Patient usually quite ill. Supportive measures. Observation as above.
		bladder-instillation via urethral catheter 50 ml diluent, retained 3h before voiding		
		Intralesional—M.D. injects usually melanatic lesions	Local draining abscess at injection sites.	ASA, acetominophen prn. for fever, lymphadenitis.
		Oral—add to cranberry juice	Nausea	
		Aerosol—nebulizer	Fever, cough, persistent malaise	Careful nebulization technique. Treat as tbc. Nurse wears mask.
MER (methanol extraction residue of BCG) Non-viable	Total dose to 0.4 mg given in increments. Thoroughly mix solution before diluting with sterile water or NSS.	Rotating intradermal sites—causes severe local stinging with persistent reddening of surrounding tissues. Intralesional—by M.D.	Recall or flare of old sites. Lesions are painful, draining. Ulcers can be 0.5 cm deep.	Choose skin sites carefully. Deep and persistent scarring. Soothe local areas with cool wet soaks. Analgesia prescription prn.
C-Parvum (Corney-bacterium Parvum) Non-viable	2–4 mgm/injection	Subcutaneous-abdominal wall and/or IV solution over 30 minutes.	12 to 48 hour fever, chills, nausea, headache. Abdominal sites often painful. Can abscess if not kept in subcutaneous tissue.	Supportive measures as above.

Many new immunotherapeutic agents are under investigation in cancer research centers and frequently receive widespread recognition in the popular press. Nurses must familiarize themselves with new developments so that they can accurately answer patient queries and temper their enthusiasm with realistic expectations.

CONTINUING CARE

Thorough discharge planning can facilitate adjustment and continued recovery and is an important facet of patient rehabilitation. A skilled oncology nurse can provide assistance to patients and their families, then directing patients to appropriate resources.[76]

Ideally, discharge planning begins shortly after admission. Realistically, it begins as the patient recovers and shows signs that he no longer needs hospitalization. Often a nurse is the discharge-planning coordinator who identifies community resources for home care. With strong support from a community-based visiting health care team, many patients can be cared for in the home, even when their physical needs are great.[9,10,76–82] If home discharge is not feasible, the discharge coordinator must find appropriate extended-care facilities.

If the patient's condition deteriorates, a hospice may provide sensitive care for dying patients.[82–83] The types of resources

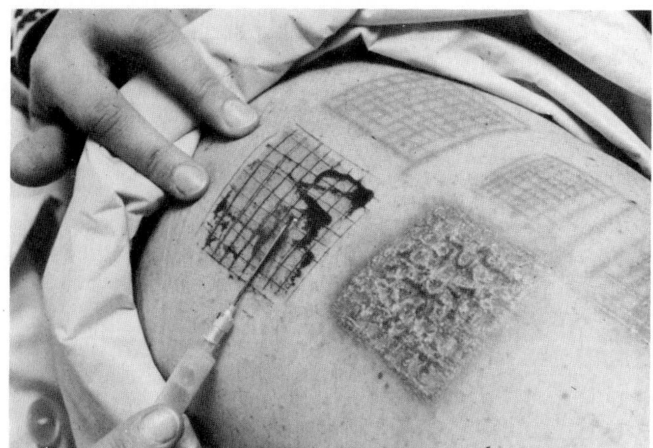

FIG. 47-7. Scarification. Skin scratching with old and recent sites (Courtesy of J. Baker)

available in any community and the roles played by nurses in these home-care programs vary widely. Communication is essential to avoid gaps in the provision of services and duplication of efforts.

The financial cost of cancer to a family is by no means limited to medical expense.[84-87] Nonmedical, out-of-pocket expenses are major sources of anxiety; unlike medical bills, these expenses are not reimbursable. Loss of income, transportation, food, babysitters, and miscellaneous expenses contribute to the financial cost associated with cancer treatment.

A major area of research interest to nurses is the development of programs that facilitate the delivery of good nursing care in the home. Such studies emphasize family members as primary care givers and the nurses as consultants who provide information and coordinate available community re-

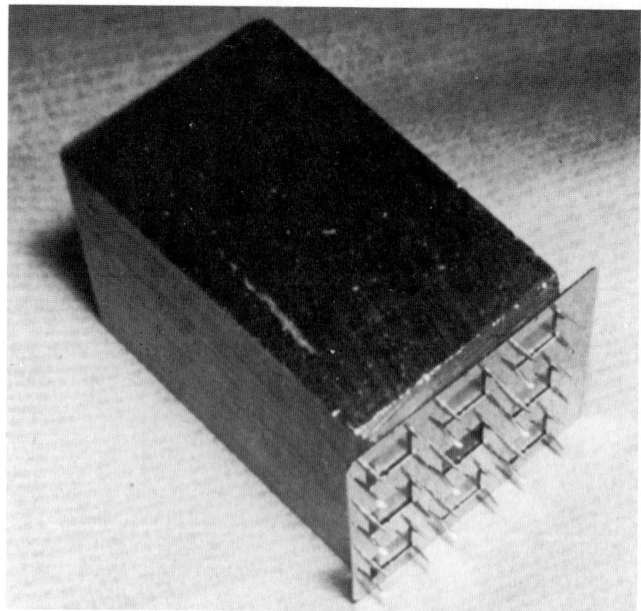

FIG. 47-8. Multiple tine injector. (Courtesy of W. Wood, M.D.)

sources. The need for nurses to conduct research to identify what learning needs are greatest, ways to improve patient education, to reduce disease and treatment-related morbidity, and to improve discharge planning is clear. Third-party coverage for care provided by nurses in outpatient clinics, in private offices, and in the home must be justified by data that prove such services decrease the cost of care or significantly improve the quality of care provided.[88] Contemporary oncology nurses should assume a responsibility in the design and performance of clinical trials to resolve the nursing care problems of cancer patients.

Nomogram for Determination of Body Surface Area from Height and Weight (Adults)[1]

Height

cm 200 — 79 in, 78, 195 — 77, 76, 190 — 75, 74, 185 — 73, 72, 180 — 71, 70, 175 — 69, 68, 170 — 67, 66, 165 — 65, 64, 160 — 63, 62, 155 — 61, 60, 150 — 59, 58, 145 — 57, 56, 140 — 55, 54, 135 — 53, 52, 130 — 51, 50, 125 — 49, 48, 120 — 47, 46, 115 — 45, 44, 110 — 43, 42, 105 — 41, 40, cm 100 — 39 in

Body surface area

2.80 m², 2.70, 2.60, 2.50, 2.40, 2.30, 2.20, 2.10, 2.00, 1.95, 1.90, 1.85, 1.80, 1.75, 1.70, 1.65, 1.60, 1.55, 1.50, 1.45, 1.40, 1.35, 1.30, 1.25, 1.20, 1.15, 1.10, 1.05, 1.00, 0.95, 0.90, 0.86 m²

Weight

kg 150 — 330 lb, 145 — 320, 140 — 310, 135 — 300, 290, 130, 280, 125, 270, 120, 260, 115, 250, 110, 240, 105, 230, 100 — 220, 95 — 210, 90 — 200, 190, 85, 180, 80, 170, 75, 160, 70, 150, 65, 140, 60, 130, 55, 120, 50 — 110, 105, 45 — 100, 95, 90, 40, 85, 80, 35, 75, 70, kg 30 — 66 lb

* Reproduction only by permission of the publishers of these *Scientific Tables*.

†) From the formula of DuBois and DuBois. *Arch. micrn. Med.* 17.863 (1916): $S = W^{0.696} \times H^{0.726} \times 71.84$, or $\log S = \log W \times 0.425 + \log H \times 0.725 + 1.8564$ (S = body surface in square centimeters. W = weight in kilograms. H = height in centimeters).

APPENDIX FIG. 1.

REFERENCES

1. Hubbard SM: The role of the chemotherapy nurse in medical oncology. Proceedings of the 11th annual meeting of ASCO 16:256, 1974
2. Hubbard SM: The practice of cancer nursing. In: American Cancer Society Proceedings of the Second National Conference on Cancer Nursing, pp 23–29. New York, American Cancer Society, 1977
3. Hubbard SM, Donehower M: The nurse in a cancer research setting. Semin Oncol 7:9-18, 1980
4. Moore P: Beyond the protocol. Oncol Nurs Forum 5:12–14, 1978
5. Miller SA: Institutional Growth. Oncol Nurs Forum 5:8-10, 1978
6. Hubbard SP, DeVita VT: Chemotherapy research nurse. Am J Nurs 76:560–565, 1976
7. Henke C: Emerging roles of the nurse in oncology. Semin Oncol 7:4–8, 1980
8. Supper V, Yarbro CH, Mayer-Scogna D: Nursing interventions in clinical research: A model program of nursing contributions to a cooperative study group. Oncol Nurs Forum 6:26–27, 1979
9. McKenzie S: The cancer care team in the community hospital. Supervisor Nurse 9:17–22, 1978
10. Coburn KM: Oncology nursing in the local community. Cancer Nurs 2:287–294, 1979
11. Thaney KM: The nurse in a community hospital setting. Semin Oncol 7:18–27, 1980
12. Belis L, Weiss, R, Trush D: The oncology clinic: A primary care facility. Cancer Nurs 3:47–52, 1980
13. Ryan L, Edwards RL, Rickles FR: A joint practice approach to cancer care, Oncol Nurs Forum 7:8, 1980
14. National Joint Practice Commission Statement on Joint Practice in Primary Care: Definitions and Guidelines. Chicago, 1977
15. Brown KC: Nature and scope of services: Joint practice. J Nurs Administration 7:13–15, 1977
16. "Joint Practice: A new dimension in nurse–physician collaboration." Am J Nurs 77(9):1466–1468, 1977
17. Jackson BS: The growing role of nurses in enterostomal therapy. Semin Oncol 7:48–55, 1980
18. Jackson BS: The clinical nurse specialist, the nursing department's case for the hospital administrator. Supervisor Nurse 4:29–36, 1973
19. Richards DB, Holcombe JK: The nurse's role in screening and cancer detection. Semin Oncol 7:56–62, 1980
20. White LN, Judkins AF, Cornelius JL et al: Screening of cancer by nurses. Cancer Nurs 2:15–20, 1978
21. Greenfield S, Komarff AL, Pass TM et al: Efficiency and cost of primary care by nurses and physician's assistants. N Engl J Med 298:305–309, 1978
22. Holmes G, Livingston G, Mills AL: Contributions of a nurse clinician to office practice productivity: Comparison of two solo practices. Health Serv Res 11:21–33, 1976
23. Maxwell MB: Nurse practitioner chemotherapy clinic. Cancer Nurs 2:211–218, 1979
24. Hershey N: Expanded roles for professional nurses. J Nurs Administration 3:30–33, 1973
25. Leitch C, Mitchell E: A State by State Report: The legal accommodations of nurses practicing in expanded roles. Nurse Practitioner 2:19–22, 1977
26. Georgeopoulos BS, Christman L: The clinical nurse specialists: A role model. Am J Nurs 70:1030–1039, 1970
27. Roy C, Oblog M: The practitioner movement—Towards the science of nursing. Am J Nurs 78:1698–1702, 1978
28. Mauksch IG: Nursing is coming of age . . . .Through the Practitioner movement. Am J Nurs 75:1834–1843, 1975
29. Craytor, J et al: The Master's Degree with a Speciality in Cancer Nursing Curriculum Guide and Role Definition. American Cancer Society, New York, 1979
30. Given B: Education of the oncology nurse: The key to excellent patient care. Semin Oncol 7:71–79, 1980
31. Plumer AL: Principles and practice of intravenous therapy. New York, Little, Brown and Co, 1975
32. Maki DG, Goldman DA, Rhame FS: Infection control in intravenous therapy. Ann of Intern Med 79:867–887, 1973
33. Hanson RL: Heparin lock or keep open IV? Am J Nurs 76:1102–1103, 1976
34. Bjeletich J, Hichman RO: The Hickman indwelling catheter. Am J Nurs 80:62–65, 1980
35. Maher MM et al: An improved needle adaptor for central venous catheters. J Parent Enter Nutr 3:2, 77–78, 1979
36. Lawson M, Bottino J, Hurtuvise M et al: Declotting central venous catheters by using fibrinolytic enzymes as a declotting agent. Proc Fifth Ann Cong Oncol Nurs Soc 5:64, 1980
37. Hobbs B, Ness S: Rationale for and long-term care of indwelling arterial infusion systems. Oncol Nurs Forum 4:6–8, 1977
38. Patterson P: Granulocyte transfusion: Nursing considerations. Cancer Nurs 3:101–104, 1980
39. Beaumont E: The new infusion pumps. Nursing 77:31–35, 1977
40. Buckles RG: New horizons in drug delivery. C-A 28:343–354, 1978
41. Schleper J, Lawson M, Bowen J et al: Outpatient intravenous chemotherapy delivered by portable infusion pumps. Proc Fifth Ann Cong Oncol Nurs Soc 5:64, 1980
42. Jones R, Myers C, Guarino A et al: High volume intraperitoneal chemotherapy ("belly bath") for ovarian cancer: Pharmacologic basis and early results. Cancer Chemother Pharmacol 1:161–166, 1978
43. Pochedly C: Treatment of meningeal leukemia. Hosp Pract 11:123–126, 1976
44. Barlock A, Howser D, Hubbard SM: Nursing management in adriamycin Extravasation. Am J Nurs 79:94–98, 1979
45. Swartz AJ: Chemotherapy extravasation. Cancer Nurs 2:405–408, 1979
46. Bowers DG, Lynch B: Adriamycin extravasation. Plast Reconstr Surg 61:86–92, 1978
47. Zweig J, Kasakow B: An apparently effective countermeasure for doxorubicin extravasation. JAMA 239:2116–2117, 1978
48. Dodds L: Use of sodium bicarbonate as a countermeasure for adriamycin extravasation. Clin Pharmacol Ther (in press)
49. Lovejoy NC: Preventing hair loss during adriamycin therapy. Cancer Nurs 2:117–122, 1979
50. Dean JC, Salmon SE, Griffith KS: Prevention of doxorubicin induced hair loss with scalp hypothermia. N Engl J Med 301:1427–1429, 1979
51. Creighton H: Law Every Nurse Should Know, 3rd ed. Philadelphia, WB Saunders, 1975
52. Hubbard SM: Neoplastic processes. In Medical–Surgical Nursing, New York, A conceptual approach. Jones DA, Girovec MM, Dunbard CF (eds): McGraw-Hill, 1978.
53. Schumann D: Preoperative measures to promote wound healing. Nurs Clin North Am 14:695, 1979
54. Byrne N: Critical care of the thoracic surgical patient. Cancer Nurs 1:2, 135–144, 1978
55. McConnell EA: How to truly help the patient with a radical neck dissection. Nursing '76 11:59–65, 1976
56. O'Dell AJ: Objectives and standards in the care of the patient with a radical neck dissection. Nurs Clin North Am 8(1):159–164, 1973
57. Guthrie TH, Long PP: Surgical nursing intervention in patients with hematological malignancies: An overview. Cancer Nurs 2(5):353–358, 1979
58. Gorrell CR: Frequency of infection in hospitalized patients with colon cancer. Presented at the 5th Annual Congress of the Oncology Nursing Society, San Diego, 1980
59. Aspinoll MJ: Scoring against nosocomial infections. Am J Nurs 78:1704–1707, 1978
60. Fowler E, Jeter KF, Schwartz AA: How to cope when your patient has an enterocutaneous fistula. Am J Nurs 80:426–429
61. Benifield JR et al: Custom-fitted appliances for intestinal fistulas. Am J Surg 136:279–281, 1978
62. Schumann D: How to help wound healing in your abdominal surgery patient. Nursing '80 10:4, 1980
63. Donovan MI, Perice SG: Cancer Care Nursing, pp. 156–195. New York, Appleton-Century-Crofts, 1976

64. Watt R: Colostomy irrigation: Yes or No? Am J Nurs 77:442–444, 1977
65. Smith DS, Chamorrow TP: Nursing care of patients undergoing combination chemotherapy and radiotherapy. Cancer Nurs 1(2):129–134, 1978
66. Thaney KM, Craytor JK, McNally JA: Radiation therapy, Ch 7. In Peterson BH, Kellogg CJ, (eds): Current Practice in Oncology Nursing, pp 80–87. St. Louis, CV Mosby, 1976
67. Dietz KA: Programmed Instruction: Cancer care radiation therapy; external radiation. Cancer Nurs 2(2):129–138, 2(3):233–244, 1979
68. Champagne EE, Kane NE: A teaching program for patients receiving interstitial radioactive iodine[125] for cancer of the prostate. Oncol Nurs Forum 7(1):12–15, 1980
69. Hersh EM, Gutterman JU, Mavligit G: Immunotherapy of Cancer in Man, pp. 90–94, Springfield, Il, Charles C Thomas, 1973
70. McCalla JL: Immunotherapy: concepts and nursing implications. In Kruse LC, Reese JL, Hart LK, (eds): Cancer, Pathophysiology, Etiology, and Management, Chapter 28. St. Louis, CV Mosby, 1979
71. Dean JC: Application and reading of skin tests. In Dorr DT, Fritz WL (eds): Cancer chemotherapy Handbook, Chapter 10. New York, Elsevier, 1980
72. Morris DL, Hersh EM, Gutterman JU et al: Recall antigen delayed-type hypersensitivity skin testing: Standardization of self reading by patients. Cancer Immunity and Immunotherapy 6:5–8, 1979
73. Coral FA: A perspective on cancer immunotherapy. In Kellog CJ, Sullivan BP (eds): Current Perspectives in Oncologic Nursing, vol II, 35–44. St. Louis, CV Mosby, 1978
74. Seipp CA: Immunotherapy for patients with osteogenic sarcoma: approaches to an Outreach Program. Oncol Nurs Forum 5:5–6, 1978
75. Cox KO, Ern M: Programmed instruction: Immunotherapy. Cancer Nurs 3:307–321, 1980
76. Whang MSY: Community resources for the cancer patient. In Burkhalter P, Donley DL, (eds): Dynamics of Oncology Nursing, pp 443–458. New York, McGraw-Hill, 1978
77. Hunter G, Johnson SH: Physical support systems for the homebound oncology patient. Oncol Nurs Forum 7:21–24, 1980
78. Martinson I: Home care for the dying child. Am J Nurs 77:1816–1817, 1977
79. Martinson I et al: Facilitating home care for dying children. Cancer Nurs 1:41–45, 1978
80. Michael S: Home IV therapy. Am J Nurs 78:1223–1226, 1978
81. Klopovich P, Suenram D, Cairns N: A common sense approach to caring for children with cancer: the community health nurse. Cancer Nurs 7:28–37, 1980
82. Benoliel J, McCorkle R: A holistic approach to terminal illness. Cancer Nurs 1:143–149, 1978
83. Paige RL, Looney JF: Hospice Care for the advanced cancer patient. Am J Nurs 77:1812–1815, 1977
84. McNaull F, Wheeler K: The cancer patient's financial concerns—An element in assessing nursing interventions. Oncol Nurs Forum 5:1–4, 1978
85. Cronk B, Mileo R: Cost of terminal care: Home, hospice vs hospital. Nursing Outlook 27(8):522–526, 1979
86. Lanky SB, Cairns N, Clark G et al: Childhood cancer and nonmedical costs of the illness. Cancer 43:403–408, 1979
87. Williams S, Weber H, Pooler J: IV. Cost containment: effect on clinical practice. Oncol Nurs Forum 7:32–33, 1980
88. Batey MV: V. Cost containment: Nursing research. Oncol Nurs Forum 7:33–34, 1980

CHAPTER 48

Newer Methods of Cancer Treatment

Section 1

Immunotherapy

WILLIAM D. TERRY
RICHARD J. HODES

Immunotherapy is the use of the immune system or its products to control, damage, or destroy malignant cells in patients with cancer. At the present time, immunotherapy is experimental and, despite a prolonged history, must be considered to be in the early stages of its development.

HISTORY

Human immunotherapy probably began in the late 1800s when Busch and Coley reported that streptococcal infections could cause necrosis of human tumors.[1,2] Coley injected streptococcal cultures into human tumors and reported a few remarkable regressions. In order to improve the safety of this treatment Coley switched to bacteria-free culture filtrates, first from streptococci, and then from mixtures of bacteria. These were known as Coley's Mixed Bacterial Toxins or Coley's Toxins.[3] Although Coley's treatments were based on the logical extension of a clinical observation, there was no theoretical framework within which to place these observations, and it was therefore impossible to generalize from these findings or to build upon them.

At the same time, however, information was accumulating about the specificity of antibodies, their ability to recognize subtle chemical differences and their apparent function in the control of infectious diseases. Based on this information Ehrlich, von Dungern, and others hypothesized that antibodies must also play a role in the control of cancer.[4,5] These workers made the assumption that cancer cells must, as a consequence of the malignant transformation, develop on their surface antigens (tumor antigens or tumor-associated antigens) that make them antigenically distinct from normal cells. Antibodies capable of specifically recognizing these antigens could thus control the growth of malignant cells. Such antibodies were viewed as having a surveillance function and assumed to eliminate almost all new malignant cells before they could proliferate and become clinically significant tumors. An expansion of this concept of the surveillance function of the humoral and cellular immune systems has been provided in more modern immunologic terms by Burnet.[6]

Surveillance hypotheses propose that the immune system is capable of controlling malignancy when only a small number of malignant cells are present. These hypotheses have been extended to include the proposal that the immune system can also influence malignant cell growth at a time when the tumor is clinically apparent and therefore consists of millions or billions of cells. Thus, the (as yet unproven) assumption that human tumors contain specific antigens, coupled with the hypothesis that the immune system can recognize these antigens, react against them and thereby destroy large numbers of tumor cells, became the theoretical underpinning for modern immunotherapy.

Sporadic attempts to stimulate immunity against tumor cells in patients with cancer continued through the early 20th century. A more systematic approach to the use of immunotherapy in skin cancer was established by Klein, who demonstrated that delayed hypersensitivity reactions elicited on or in skin cancers resulted in a high percentage of cases in permanent regression of these local lesions.[7–9] At about the same time, trials of immunotherapy in leukemia and melanoma were initiated and the era of modern immunotherapy was launched.[10,11]

As was already perceived at the time of Ehrlich, immune system functions are characterized by exquisite specificity. Much of modern immunology has been concerned with achieving insights into the mechanisms that underlie specific immune recognition. Of equal importance from the point of view of contemporary immunotherapy, however, is the fact that specific immune reactions, whether mediated by antibodies or cells, may have biologic consequences that are nonspecific. For example, the highly specific interaction of sensitized lymphoid cells with a soluble sensitizing agent produces a delayed hypersensitivity reaction.[12] The secondary consequences of this reaction are nonspecific; a variety of biologically active substances are released by the lymphoid cell and these substances activate a multiplicity of biologic systems.[13] Any delayed hypersensitivity reaction, regardless of the specific eliciting antigen, leads to the same set of biologic consequences.

Clinical immunotherapy has attempted to exploit both the specific and nonspecific attributes of the immune system to destroy malignant cells. As already noted, however, attempts to develop antitumor-specific immune reactions are based on the assumption that the malignant cell membrane contains antigens that distinguish malignant from normal cells. A thorough discussion of tumor antigens is beyond the scope of this chapter; for a review see reference 14. It can be stated, however, that there is no conclusive evidence indicating that human tumors, at the time they become clinically apparent, contain surface antigens that can be recognized by the immune system of the tumor-bearing patient, nor is there evidence that the immune system develops, or can be induced to develop, an effective immune response against such tumors. Much of clinical immunotherapy ignores this problem and proceeds on the assumptions that tumor antigens exist and that tumor-bearing patients can make an effective antitumor immune response.

Although neither human tumor antigens nor specific antitumor immune responses have been convincingly demonstrated, there are a number of immune response pathways and effector mechanisms that may be of relevance to immunotherapy. In principle, one of the most highly specific of these is the generation of antibodies directed against malignant cell antigens. Although such antibodies have been reported in humans, critical reevaluation has raised questions about previous conclusions.[15] If specific antitumor antibodies are produced, it is likely that they will be generated by T-cell dependent responses, requiring the participation of functional thymic-dependent (T) lymphocytes, as well as B-lymphocytes (from which antibody-forming cells differentiate) and most probably also requiring accessory cells capable of presenting tumor antigen to the immune system. Tumor-specific antibodies could produce antitumor effects by a number of mechanisms. Antibody-mediated complement-dependent lysis of malignant cells is perhaps the most direct of these mechanisms, but the effectiveness of this pathway is not well established *in vivo*. Antibody-dependent cell-mediated cytotoxicity (ADCC) is an alternative mechanism by which specific antibody might mediate antitumor effects.[16] The effector cells in ADCC are F_c receptor-bearing cells which have in varying circumstances been characterized as macrophages (or monocytes) or as null (non-T, non-B) lymphocytes. The specificity of ADCC killing is determined entirely by antibody, and does not reflect or require any antigen specificity of the effector cell involved. Thus, an antitumor antibody could coat tumor cells specifically and sensitize them to "nonspecific" destruction by ADCC effector cells.

Another highly specific immune mechanism for killing tumor cells involves thymus dependent (T) lymphocytes. Cytotoxic T-lymphocytes (CTL) active in vitro were initially characterized in systems specific for major transplantation antigens, and in that situation have been a useful in vitro model of allograft rejection.[17] Analogous T-cell mediated cytolysis has subsequently been described in a number of putative tumor-specific systems. It should be pointed out, however, that these experimental systems have in general not been optimal syngeneic tumor-specific systems, and have most frequently employed established tumor lines which have been passaged *in vitro* or *in vivo*. In a number of systems, CTL have been generated which were specific for lysis of a single tumor line; thus, cytotoxicity was not observed against "syngeneic" nonmalignant cells, nor against other tumor cell lines derived from the same inbred strain of experimental animal. In other instances, cross-reactivities among several tumor lines or with embryonic tissues have been observed.[18]

Recent experimental findings have led to an appreciation of a still more complex aspect of specific T-cell recognition by demonstrating that T cells, including CTL specific for syngeneic tumors, do not recognize antigens (such as tumor antigens) in isolation, but only in the context of "self" histocompatibility antigens on the cell surface.[18–21] The implications of this phenomenon for tumor immunotherapy are potentially significant. It is not clear, for example, whether the immunization of an individual with allogeneic tumor cells (on which tumor antigens would be presented in association with allogeneic histocompatibility determinants) would generate CTL capable of recognizing tumor antigen on tumor cells of the host type. Thus, even the most rigorous serologic definitions of tumor antigens and their cross-reactivities may not be adequate to predict the specificity of CTL for tumor-associated antigens. One seriously limiting factor in the study of tumor-specific CTL has been the difficulty of obtaining significant numbers of cytotoxic effector cells of adequate potency and specificity. In this respect, an interesting recent development has been the establishment in long-term tissue culture of continuous CTL lines capable of maintaining a high degree of specificity.[22,23] It may be anticipated that the establishment of tumor-specific CTL lines will be of considerable investigative value, and it is possible that such lines will be of therapeutic value as well in adoptive immunotherapy.

There are two categories of immune effector cells that seem to discriminate all malignant cells as a class from normal cells. Macrophages, after "activation" by a number of procedures, are active in cytostatic and cytolytic assays against malignant cells.[24-28] This activation can be accomplished by "nonspecific" pharmacologic or physical stimuli, or by the products of specifically activated immune T-lymphocytes. Macrophage-mediated activity therefore does not require antigen-specific priming. Effector activity is without apparent antigen specificity, in that tumor cells are affected independent of their etiology, histology, or strain of origin. Some specificity exists for macrophage effector activity, however, as many types of tumor cells are found to be susceptible *in vitro*, while most or all nonmalignant cells are not susceptible. Controversy exists about the nature of this specificity, since it is unclear whether macrophage effectors actually recognize determinants expressed only on malignantly transformed cells or whether, for example, all rapidly dividing cells are susceptible targets.[29] While the physiologic importance of these effects is not clear, they do represent a potential antitumor mechanism without the fine specificity of other immune pathways.

More recently, a phenomenon termed "natural killer" (NK) activity has been characterized in both animal and human systems.[30,31] The lineage of NK cells is distinct from that of macrophages, but is otherwise controversial, some investigators proposing that natural killers are of the T-cell lineage and others finding no such association. Although NK activity is not dependent upon prior immunization, it is modified by a number of pharmacologic agents. In particular, it has been noted that interferon and its inducers are potent enhancers of NK activity.[30] Susceptibility to NK effects varies widely among tumor lines, although this variability is without apparent correlation to detectable antigenicity. Certain normal lymphoid cell populations are also susceptible to NK effects. In experimental mice, differences have been reported among inbred strains in their relative abilities to mediate NK activity, and some evidence has been presented to suggest that this activity correlates with resistance to transplanted tumors.[31] This reported correlation represents the strongest circumstantial evidence for a physiologic role of NK cells *in vivo*. The mechanism that permits NK cells and macrophages to discriminate between normal and malignant cells is not known and it has not been well established that either cell plays a significant role in the control of malignant cell growth *in vivo*.

In recent years, it has been demonstrated that complex regulatory systems modulate many immune responses. Thus, even when adequate inducing stimuli are presented, and intact effector mechanisms exist, the ability to successfully activate these immune effector mechanisms is dependent on regulatory influences. While such regulatory influences can be mediated by a number of cell types, the most impressive examples of antigen-specific immune suppression have been T-cell mediated. Indeed, it has been demonstrated that suppressor T-cells can inhibit *in vivo* tumor rejection in a highly antigen specific manner.[32] Elegant experiments have further demonstrated that the concomitant induction of suppressor T-cells may be a contributing or permissive factor in tumor induction.[33,34] Moreover, treatment of tumor-bearing mice in a manner designed to eliminate suppressor T-cells has been reported to significantly retard tumor growth.[35] The potential presence of such immune suppression implies that in situations in which no antitumor immune response is demonstrable, it becomes critical to distinguish the absence of tumor antigens from other factors, such as immune suppression, interfering with the generation of such a response. The therapeutic implications of suppressor effects are two-fold, in that either selective elimination of existing suppressors or the induction of suppressor cells by immune intervention must be considered as potential consequences of immunotherapy. Other forms of suppression may be mediated by tumor-specific antibodies. Either alone or in antigen–antibody complexes, such antibodies appear to act by interfering with antitumor immune mechanisms and these blocking or enhancing effects may be reversible by the removal of antibodies or complexes.[36]

Just as effector mechanisms may be either highly antigen specific or may lack specificity, so immune suppressor cells may be either specific or nonspecific. In addition to antigen-specific suppressor T-cells, there are examples in experimental animals and in humans of nonspecific suppressor cells in tumor-bearing hosts. Such suppressor activity has been associated both with T-cells and with monocytes or macrophages, the identity of the suppressor cell depending in some instances upon the type of malignancy.[37] The immune suppression mediated by these suppressor cells has been broad and antigen-nonspecific, including the suppression of immunoglobulin synthesis, of mitogen-induced T-cell proliferation, and of proliferative and cytotoxic responses to alloantigens. Such broad immunosuppression might be expected to compromise overall host resistance, including both specific and nonspecific effector responses to tumor-associated determinants, and many of the non-tumor related agents used in immunotherapy have the effect of at least partially correcting this suppression.

The multiplicity of antigen specific and nonspecific antitumor effector mechanisms, as well as the complexity of regulatory events which modulate these effectors, has implications for tumor immunotherapy. Immunotherapy may be designed to activate any one of several effector mechanisms. For any mechanism, activation may be achieved in several ways. For example, an established tumor specific CTL response may be increased either by immunization with an immunogenic form of a given tumor antigen or with the administration of an immune adjuvant. An immunologic or pharmacologic therapy directed at the elimination of specific or nonspecific suppressor cells could, however, have an effect on the final response identical to that achieved by specific immunization or adjuvant stimulation.

The potential immune response of the host to malignancy is thus extremely complex. This complexity of both effector and regulatory mechanisms suggests a large number of potential immunotherapeutic interventions but also increases the difficulty in predicting the net effect of such interventions. It is clear that the current understanding of the immune response to malignant cells is only preliminary, and that a great deal must be learned by laboratory experimentation before this understanding can be optimally applied to clinical immunotherapy.

IMMUNOTHERAPEUTIC AGENTS

Many agents have been studied in humans in an attempt to develop effective immunotherapeutic materials (Table 48-1). These efforts have been plagued by the lack of firm information concerning which immunologic mechanisms (if any) may be of importance in controlling the growth of human cancer cells. A certain amount of information from animal experiments is helpful in identifying materials for testing in humans. Having selected an agent, however, it is impossible to design treatment schedules on other than empiric grounds. As opposed to chemotherapy or radiotherapy, where the maximum tolerable dose provides a starting point for the design of treatment, the maximum tolerable dose of an agent that acts on the immune system may suppress some immune functions while stimulating others, and, as has already been mentioned, the importance of the various functions in controlling human malignant cells is not known. As a consequence, empiric decisions have been made and wide variations in dose, frequency, and route of administration will be noted in the description of immunotherapeutic clinical trials.

The dilemma of the immunotherapist is further compounded by the fact that many of the agents used are biologicals, and are produced by techniques that result in batch-to-batch variation. There is no information concerning which characteristics of these products may be most important for immunotherapeutic effectiveness and there is, therefore, no way to monitor batch-to-batch consistency for relevant characteristics. In addition, a biological agent, such as the strain of *Mycobacterium bovis* known as Bacille Calmette Guérin (BCG), is available in many different substrains and these are each grown under different conditions and harvested and stored in different ways. Information does not exist which would permit a rational choice concerning the best methods for preparing and storing BCG preparations for any particular immunotherapeutic study.

TABLE 48-1. Agents Tested for Immunotherapeutic Effect in Humans

- I. Biologicals
  - A. Bacteria and Fungi
    1. Mycobacteria, primarily BCG
       - a. intact living
       - b. cell walls on oil droplets
       - c. cell wall skeletons on oil droplets
       - d. methanol extractable residue (MER)
       - e. Freund's adjuvant
    2. Nocardia rubra
       - a. cell wall skeletons
    3. Corynebacteria
       - a. formalin inactivated C. parvum
    4. Streptococci
       - a. OK-432
    5. Pseudomonas aeruginosa
    6. Streptomyces
       - a. Bestatin
    7. Lentinus edodes
       - a. Lentinan
    8. PSK
  - B. Mammalian Products
    1. Interferon
    2. Thymosin
    3. Immune RNA
    4. Malignant cell antigens
       - a. intact tumor cells
       - b. modified intact tumor cells Vibrio cholera neuraminidase (VCN)
       - c. tumor cell membranes or extracts
       - d. viral oncolysates
    5. Antibodies
       - a. antitumor (unblocking)
       - b. antiferritin
- II. Synthetic chemicals
    1. Levamisole
    2. Imexon
    3. Azimexon
    4. Tilorone
    5. Polyinosinic polycytidilic acid (Poly IC)
    6. Poly IC plus poly-L-lysine (Poly ICLC)
    7. Polyadenylic–polyuridylic acid (Poly AU)

BCG, BCG DERIVATIVES, AND NOCARDIA DERIVATIVES

An attenuated strain of *Mycobacterium bovis* was developed by Calmette and Guérin for use as a vaccine against human tuberculosis.[38] Bacille Calmette Guérin (or BCG) was shown to be a potent stimulant of the reticuloendotheial system and, since stimulation of this system was associated with prevention of tumor growth, BCG was assessed for antitumor activity in animals.[39–46]

When positive results with living BCG organisms were obtained, attempts were made to identify the portion of the organism responsible for antitumor activity. The methanol-extraction residue (MER) of phenolized BCG was shown to both stimulate the immune system and to inhibit tumor growth.[47–49] Further attempts to fractionate BCG led to preparations of disrupted organisms (BCG cell walls) which, when attached to oil droplets, retained the ability to inhibit tumor growth.[50,51] Further fractionation with removal of protein and lipid led to a preparation designated BCG cell wall skeleton, a complex of mycolic acid arabinogalactane—mucopeptide which retains the ability to stimulate the immune system and inhibit tumor growth.[52–56] Similar properties have been demonstrated for the cell wall skeleton of *Nocardia rubra*.[57–59] The toxic side effects of living BCG and the BCG derivatives depend upon dose, schedule, and route of administration. Disseminated BCG infections have been reported following the use of living BCG, a complication which could be avoided by using non-living alternative preparations.[60]

The mechanisms whereby BCG or BCG derivatives exert antitumor effects have not been established conclusively.[61–67] Lymphocytes sensitized against mycobacteria are stimulated to release cytotoxic lymphokines when exposed to mycobacterial antigens.[63–65] These lymphokines can also attract and activate macrophages.[66–68] As was already mentioned, activated macrophages appear to have cytostatic or cytotoxic effects on tumor cells but not on normal cells.[24–27,69,70]

CORYNEBACTERIUM PARVUM

Formalin-killed suspensions of the bacteria *Corynebacterium parvum (C. parvum)* or *C. granulosum* also stimulate the immune system and inhibit tumor growth in experimental animals.[71–77] The mechanisms responsible for these activities appear similar to those induced by BCG stimulation.[77,78]

OK-432

In animal experiments, it has been noted that β-hemolytic streptococci have anticancer effects and that the effects can be increased by treating the bacteria with penicillin and incubating them at 45°C.[79] OK-432 is the lyophilized form of this preparation and it has been studied extensively in animals where it appears to increase activation of macrophages and T-lymphocytes and induce interferon production.[86] Effects on the human immune system have also been reported following intradermal, intramuscular, intravenous, intraperitoneal, and intratumoral injections.[81] Preliminary studies of this material in the treatment of human cancer have been reported.[82]

PSEUDOMONAS AERUGINOSA

A heptavalent lipopolysaccharide *Pseudomonas aeruginosa* vaccine was tested for its ability to prevent intercurrent infections in patients with acute nonlymphoblastic leukemia. Unexpectedly, an unusually large number of long term remissions were noted in those patients receiving the vaccine.[83] A repeat study is in progress.

BESTATIN

Bestatin, a competitive inhibitor of aminopeptidase enzymes, is purified from culture filtrates of *Streptomyces olivoreticuli*.[84] This material increases cellular and humoral immune responses in animals and appears to retard tumor growth.[85] A phase I trial in which Bestatin was administered orally at 40 mg/m^2 per day three times a week for 2 weeks to patients with advanced solid tumors and depressed immune responses indicated that the drug increased NK cell activity and improved delayed hypersensitivity without causing any significant toxicity. No effect on tumor size was noted.[86]

LENTINAN

A polysaccharide isolated from Lentinus edodes has been shown to have antitumor activity.[87] Lentinan is a glucan of high molecular weight that does not appear to stimulate the reticuloendothelial system. Antitumor activity required the presence of T-cells in mice. Evaluable trials of lentinan in the treatment of human cancer have not been reported.

PSK

PSK is a polysaccharide extracted from the mycelia of the CM-101 strain of *Coriolus versicolor*. While it has been shown to stimulate certain immune responses in animals, evaluable trials of PSK in the treatment of cancer have not been reported.[88]

INTERFERON

Interferon refers to a family of glycoproteins, synthesized by many types of animal cells. Discovered in 1957, interferons are defined biologically by their ability to inhibit intracellular viral replication.[89] At least three interferons are secreted by human cells: leukocyte interferon, fibroblast interferon, and immune interferon. The last is synthesized primarily by T-lymphocytes and is less well-characterized than the others. Information about interferon properties and effects are contained in several reviews.[90-92]

Interferon is discussed as an immunotherapeutic agent because it augments lymphocyte cytotoxic activity *in vitro* and *in vivo*, and increases macrophage activity.[30,93-95] It also has antitumor effects and it is speculated that the antitumor effects are mediated at least in part through the immune system.[90] Considerable emphasis has been placed on the fact that interferon increases the cytotoxic activities of NK cells and that there may be a correlation between NK activity and tumor resistance.[30,96-99] A number of clinical trials of interferon have been performed. It must be noted that although the treatment material is referred to as "interferon" it is in fact a crude preparation that contains interferon and a variety of other biologically active substances.

In the first extensive study of the effectiveness of interferon in the treatment of human cancer, patients with osteogenic sarcoma and without evidence of metastases were treated with surgery or irradiation or both and then received intramuscular injections of preparations containing 3×10^6 I.U. of human leukocyte interferon activity daily for one month, then three times a week for an additional 17 months.[100] Twenty-eight patients received the interferon preparations; the results were compared with a nonrandomized concurrent control group representing all the other patients with osteosarcoma in Sweden who were entered in the cancer registry of the National Board of Health and Welfare of Sweden from 1972 to 1974. Actuarial curves showed a slight survival benefit for interferon-treated patients, but this is not of statistical significance. Since the trial was not prospectively randomized and since questions have been raised about the accuracy of the diagnoses in some of these patients, it should be considered that interferon preparations have not had an adequate trial in osteosarcoma.

Interferon preparations have also been studied in the treatment of patients with multiple myeloma.[101,102] Promising results were obtained in a pilot study in which eight patients, who had not received prior chemotherapy or radiotherapy, were injected with a partially purified preparation containing 3×10^6 I.U. of interferon intramuscularly daily for 16 weeks to 144 weeks. Five of the patients had a therapeutic response (either a decrease of the myeloma protein concentration by more than 50% of the pretreatment value or a decrease of urinary light chain excretion to less than 0.2 g per 24 hours, or more than a 50% decrease in the size of plasmacytomas). A prospective randomized trial was initiated and 66 patients who had never received cytostatic or radiation therapy were entered before the study was closed. Patients were randomly assigned to receive interferon alone or melphalan (0.25mg/km/day) and prednisolone every 6 weeks. At the end of a relatively short follow-up period, twenty-four of the patients treated with interferon had died or required a change in therapy while only ten of the chemotherapy patients had died or required a treatment alteration. These poor results led to discontinuation of the trial. In searching for a reason for the difference between the results of the pilot trial (five responses in eight evaluable patients) and the randomized trial (four responses in twenty-two evaluable patients) the investigators discovered that the method of interferon preparation had been modified to include a terminal lyophilization and that it was this modified interferon preparation that had been used in the randomized trial. Investigations of possible decreases in therapeutic efficacy owing to lyophilization are in progress. It must be concluded at this point, however, that the only randomized trial of interferon in multiple myeloma indicates that interferon is less effective than conventional chemotherapy.

Patients with multiple myeloma are also being treated with polyinosinic polycytidilic acid (poly IC) stabilized with poly-L-lysine (poly(ICLC)) as an inducer of interferon.[103] There are no reportable results at this time.

Poly(ICLC) is being studied in various leukemias, lymphomas and osteosarcoma, but only scattered results are available.[103] A randomized trial using the less stable interferon inducer, polyriboinosinic–polyribocytidilic acid (poly IC) has been carried out in acute myelogenous leukemia.[104] No significant differences in remission duration or survival were noted when comparing the 72 patients who received chemotherapy alone to the 40 patients who received chemotherapy plus poly IC.

In a pilot study of non-Hodgkin's lymphomas, one of seven evaluable patients with nodular lymphoma had a complete response (12 months duration) and two had partial responses (12 months and 6 months duration) when treated with a preparation containing 10×10^6 units of human leukocyte interferon intramuscularly daily for 30 days.[105,106] Additional studies in this disease are in progress.

Human leukocyte interferon has also been studied in patients with lung cancer. Sixteen patients received human leukocyte interferon, 3×10^6 units intramuscularly daily for 30 days. There were no objective responses.[107]

Juvenile laryngeal papillomatosis is a rare, nonmalignant disease which may be virus induced and can cause death due to airway obstruction.[108–111] Interferon is reported to control the growth of papillomas, presumably by way of its antiviral activity.[112,113] Poly(ICLC) has also been used successfully to control the growth of papillomas, presumably by inducing interferon production and limiting viral infection.[103]

There are, therefore, no convincing clinical trials indicating that preparations containing interferon activity are of therapeutic value for any form of human cancer. Further, since all studies are being performed with materials that contain many other biologically active substances, any clinical trials yielding positive results with these preparations will have to be repeated with pure interferon when it becomes available before it can be concluded that interferon is the effective agent.

THYMOSIN

Thymosin is the term given to extracts of calf thymus that contain certain biological properties. A partially purified fraction referred to as fraction 5 contains about a dozen heat stable polypeptides with molecular weights from 1,200 to 14,000.[114,115] Fraction 5 of thymosin causes increased reactivity in mixed lymphocyte and mitogen stimulation assays and increases the number of E-rosette forming lymphocytes in the peripheral blood of patients with depressed numbers of E-rosettes. The effects of thymosin fraction 5 have been studied in patients with various forms of immunodeficiency and cancer.[115,116]

ANTIBODIES TO TUMOR-ASSOCIATED ANTIGENS

If a particular antigen is expressed on tumor cells, and is expressed at a lower concentration or not at all on normal cells, it is possible to use antibodies against that antigen as a vehicle for delivering diagnostic reagents to the surface of cancer cells. The presence of high concentrations of carcinoembryonic antigen (CEA) on the surface of some tumor cells makes it possible to label anti-CEA antibody molecules with radioactive iodine and to use these radiolabeled antibodies, in combination with computer assisted photoscanning to visualize small tumor deposits.[117]

This technique can also be used to deliver treatment reagents. For example, anti-ferritin antibodies labeled with ^{131}I have been used to treat patients with primary liver malignancies.[118] Six of eight patients so treated have shown objective responses in a Phase I study but, since the radiolabeled ferritin was part of a complex treatment regimen including radiotherapy and chemotherapy and, since no patients received the radio-chemotherapy without the anti-ferritin, a treatment effect cannot be ascribed to the radiolabeled antibody.

IMMUNE RNA

It has been reported that RNA extracted from lymphoid tissues of immunized animals is able to increase the cell-mediated immunity of unimmunized animals against the immunizing antigen.[119] Experiments suggest that "immune RNA" from the lymphoid tissues of animals immunized against a cancer can, when incubated *in vitro* with lymphoid cells of animals from other species, transfer tumor specific immunity that is demonstrable when those lymphocytes are infused into unimmunized recipients.[120]

Immune RNA has been extracted from lymphoid tissues of non-human species that had been immunized with human tumors; the RNA was then injected into cancer patients[121,122] Neither toxicity nor objective regressions were reported. RNA has also been extracted from the lymphoid tissues of guinea pigs immunized against human renal cell carcinoma. The RNA was incubated *in vitro* with peripheral blood lymphocytes of patients with renal cell cancer.[123] Autologous lymphocytes were then infused into the patients and subsequent in vitro tests indicated increased cell-mediated cytotoxicity against renal carcinoma cells. Of six patients studied, one had a complete remission and two had partial remissions. It should be noted, however, that the clinical course of renal cell carcinoma is quite variable and a randomized trial with larger numbers of patients will be required before therapeutic efficacy can be established.

LEVAMISOLE

Tetramisole, a synthetic anti-helminthic with activity against nematodes, has been used extensively in animals and humans[124,125] Tetramisole was also reported to augment the protective effect of Brucella vaccine in mice.[126] The levorotatory analog of tetramisole, levamisole, was shown to have biologic properties similar to those of tetramisole, and most studies of clinical immunotherapy of cancer have been carried out with levamisole.

Levamisole increases phagocytosis, stimulates lymphoblast transformation, and increases delayed hypersensitivity reactions, primarily in circumstances where these functions are depressed. Levamisole does not, however, appear to directly affect tumor cell growth *in vitro*.[127]

IMEXON

Imexon is a synthetic chemical with effects on animal immune systems and animal cancers.[128,129] When administered intravenously to patients with advanced cancer, some evidence of effect on the immune system was obtained, but in about 20 percent of the patients there were significant toxic effects.[130] One patient with metastatic lung cancer and one with metastatic malignant melanoma entered sustained complete remissions following treatment with this drug.

AZIMEXON

Azimexon is chemically related to Imexon; both chemicals belong to a class of compounds called the 2-cynanaziridines. Azimexon has anti-cancer effects in animals, appears to stimulate components of the immune system and can be administered intravenously or orally to humans without toxicity.[131,132] Effects on human tumor growth have not been reported.

TILORONE

This compound is a basic ether of fluorenone that stimulates antibody production and also induces interferon.[133,134] Preliminary clinical studies have shown this drug to be moderately toxic and without apparent antitumor effect in humans.[135,136]

CLINICAL TRIALS

LEUKEMIAS AND LYMPHOMAS

Acute Lymphocytic Leukemia

Some of the earliest "modern" immunotherapy trials were carried out in patients with acute lymphocytic leukemia (ALL). In one of these trials (Table 48-2) patients brought into remission with chemotherapy were randomized to receive no further treatment, BCG, allogeneic irradiated leukemic blast cells, or BCG plus the blast cells.[10] While the ten control patients relapsed rapidly, the 20 patients receiving some form of immunotherapy survived much longer and seven of those 20 patients were in complete remission 10 years to 13 years after the beginning of treatment.[137] The number of patients studied was quite small and the treatment benefit seemed to be conferred about equally by any of the three types of immunotherapy.

Attempts have been made to confirm these findings by treating patients with BCG plus living allogeneic leukemic cells and comparing the results with those obtained from using chemotherapy alone, or by treating patients with BCG and comparing the results to those obtained with chemotherapy or with no further treatment (Table 48-2).[138-141] These four reports showed no evidence of a treatment effect caused by the immunotherapeutic agent. While none of these trials was an exact replica of the original Mathé study it is not clear which variables, if any, are responsible for the different results observed.

Levamisole has also been investigated in ALL.[142] Patients, 88% of whom were less than 16 years of age, were brought into remission and were subsequently randomized to receive chemotherapy (208 patients) or chemotherapy plus 100 mg/m² of levamisole daily (185 patients). Levamisole caused prolongation of remission duration and survival but only in that subgroup of patients considered to be "low risk" (less than 16 years of age and with a white blood count of less than 50,000 at the time of diagnosis). The effect is quite significant in this group; survival at 5 years was 60% for those receiving levamisole and only 35% in the control group. The data are

TABLE 48-2. Acute Lymphocytic Leukemia

AUTHOR (Reference Number)	RANDOMIZED	PATIENTS	STUDY DESIGN	NUMBER PATIENTS	RESULTS
Mathé(137)	Yes	All ages	No further treatment BCG (Pasteur) I.D. Cells* BCG + cells	10 8 5 7	10 controls relapsed rapidly. 7 of 20 immunotherapy patients in complete remission for 10–13 yrs.
Poplack(139)	Yes	Under 20 years	Chemotherapy Chemotherapy BCG (Pasteur) I.D. + cells†	24 11 21	No significant differences
Andrien(138)	Yes	Under 50 years	Chemotherapy BCG (Pasteur) I.D. + cells	34 30	No significant differences
Kay(141)	Yes	Children	No further treatment Chemotherapy BCG (Glaxo) I.D.	18 53 50	No significant differences
Heyn(140)	Yes	Children	No further treatment Chemotherapy BCG (Tice) I.D.	31 285 34	Remission duration significantly prolonged by chemotherapy
Pavlovsky(142)	Yes	Most under 15 years	Chemotherapy Chemotherapy + levamisole 100 mg/m²	208 185	1. Low risk; remission duration and survival prolonged 2. High risk; no significant difference

* Irradiated, allogeneic blast cells
† Viable, allogeneic blast cells

not presented for survival for all levamisole patients independent of risk category and, since a relationship between risk and treatment outcome was not predicted before the trial, additional studies will be required to substantiate the efficacy of levamisole in this disease.

Acute Myelogenous Leukemia

The effectiveness of various types of immunotherapy has been studied extensively in patients with acute myelogenous leukemia (AML). These studies can be grouped into those using an immunoadjuvant, those using an immunoadjuvant plus tumor cells and those using tumor cells alone (Table 48-3). Although it is tempting to make comparisons, it must be remembered that no one of the trials exactly replicates another. Variations exist in the chemotherapy used for remission induction, consolidation (if any) and maintenance, in the source, dose, schedule, and site of administration of the immunotherapeutic agents and in the statistical analyses applied.

In four studies, intradermal BCG has been administered in conjunction with chemotherapy during some portion of the first remission.[143–148] No consistent trend is noted in remission duration, but survival tends to be prolonged and in one study, is of borderline statistical significance. Intradermal BCG has also been given in the absence of maintenance chemotherapy and although median survival appears to be prolonged, the prolongation was not statistically significant.[149] BCG has also been given intravenously and a significant prolongation of survival reported.[150] MER has been given both during remission induction and during maintenance and no benefit was observed.[151]

BCG has been administered in combination with allogeneic blast cells in a number of trials.[152–160] In two of these trials, irradiated allogeneic blast cells were used; in a third trial, unirradiated viable allogeneic cells were administered.[152–157] A fourth trial used irradiated allogeneic blast, but did not administer chemotherapy during maintenance.[158–160] All four trials showed prolongation in median duration of remission and survival and three reported statistically significant prolongation of survival.[153,157,159] C. parvum has been given intravenously in combination with irradiated blast cells administered subcutaneously during remission without effect.[161]

The combination of irradiated blast cells and chemotherapy does not appear to produce better results than can be achieved by the same chemotherapy plus intravenous BCG.[162] It should be noted that the median survival obtained with intravenous BCG in this trial (73 weeks) is somewhat less than that reported in an earlier trial (96 weeks; see Table 48-3).[150]

Despite the many differences in these trials, some generalizations can be made. Of 11 trials in which BCG was given alone or in combination with allogeneic blast cells, eight report prolongation of median remission duration. The exceptions include the two trials using intravenous BCG and one using BCG intradermally.[148,150,162] In many instances the prolongations are quite short and in only one trial does it achieve statistical significance, but the trend seems to be consistent.[158–160] BCG, with or without cells, seems to prolong survival and does so to a statistically significant degree in five of the 11 trials. The prolongation of survival was at least partially attributable to increased survival after first relapse. In addition, increased survival has been associated with an increased rate of induction of second and subsequent remissions.[158] It should be noted that equally impressive effects have been obtained with BCG alone or BCG plus cells, suggesting that BCG may be responsible for whatever benefit is achieved. Nothing is known of the mechanisms whereby BCG prolongs survival or facilitates reinduction of remission after first relapse in AML. Studies designed to illuminate these mechanisms are needed.

A number of other approaches to the immunotherapy of AML are listed in Table 48-3. MER was administered intradermally along with chemotherapy during induction and maintenance without apparent effect.[151] The use of allogeneic blast cells digested with the enzyme neuraminidase (derived from *Vibrio cholera* organisms) has been assessed in combination with chemotherapy or chemotherapy plus MER.[163] No treatment benefit was noted. Neither intravenous *C. parvum* nor lysates of virus infected allogeneic blast cells have caused significant therapeutic effects.[161,164]

Despite the trends noted with BCG, none of the trials provides evidence that patients are being cured of AML by immunotherapeutic agents; rather, patients treated with BCG are living longer but ultimately die with disease.

AML is one of the few diseases in which an immunotherapeutic agent has produced a relatively consistent beneficial result. At the present time, it seems reasonable to conclude, therefore, that BCG exerts a small, positive treatment effect, primarily on survival, mediated through unknown, possibly non-immunologic mechanisms, when administered to adults in first remission from acute myelogenous leukemia.

Lymphomas

In one of the few evaluable studies of immunotherapy in patients with lymphoma, BCG has been assessed for activity in remission induction or maintenance of patients with Stage III or Stage IV non-Hodgkins lymphomas.[165,166] Patients were randomized to receive a four-drug combination, a five-drug combination or four of the five drugs plus intradermal Pasteur BCG during remission induction. Once in remission, all patients were rerandomized to no further treatment or BCG. The addition of BCG to chemotherapy during induction caused an increased complete response rate (from about 45% to 67%) and a marginally improved survival in patients with histiocytic lymphoma and an incresed survival in patients with nodular lymphoma.

Following chemotherapeutically induced disease reduction, patients with multiple myeloma have been randomized to receive maintenance chemotherapy (53 patients) or the same chemotherapy plus levamisole at 100 mg/m^2/day (58 patients).[167] Early results suggest significant prolongation of remission duration.

Solid Tumors

The immunotherapy of solid tumors may involve intratumoral injections of the primary tumor, regional application of the agent either pre- or postoperatively, or systemic administration.

TABLE 48-3. Acute Myelogenous Leukemia

AUTHOR (Reference Number)	RANDOMIZED	MAINTENANCE TREATMENT			STUDY DESIGN	NUMBER OF PATIENTS	MEDIAN REMISSION (Weeks)	MEDIAN SURVIVAL (Weeks)
		Chemo	*Adjuvant*	*AML Cells*				
Gutterman(143,144)	No, historical	+	BCG-Pasteur; I.D.*	–	C† C + I‡	24 14	52 (NS§) 85	96(S¶) >145
Hewlett(145)	Yes	+	BCG-Pasteur; I.D.	–	C C + I	25 20	55 (NS) 59	74 (NS) >55
Vogler(146,147)	Yes	+	BCG-Tice; I.D.	–	C C + I	33 25	32 (NS) 40	72 (NS) 93
Vogler(148)	Yes	+, –	BCG-Tice; I.D.	–	C I C + I	21 17 22	74 43 (NS) 39	78 83 (NS) NR**
Omura(149)	Yes	+, –	BCG-Tice; I.D.	–	No maintenance C I	32 35 30	26 30 (NS) 35	69 69 (NS) 96
Whittaker(150)	Yes	+	BCG-Glaxo; I.V.††	–	C C + I	24 21	35 (NS) 29	62 (S) 96
Cuttner(151)	Yes	+	MER; I.D.	–	C C + I	90 71	66 (NS) 67	97 (NS) 85
Powles(152,153)	No, alternate	+	BCG-Glaxo; I.D.	Irradiated, allogeneic blasts, S.C.‡‡	C C + I	22 28	27 (NS) 43	39 (S) 73
Peto(154,155)	Yes	+	BCG-Glaxo; I.D.	Irradiated, allogeneic blasts, S.C.	C C + I	24 47	21 (NS) 32	47 (NS) 70
Reizenstein (156,157)	Yes	+	BCG-Glaxo; I.D.	Viable, allogeneic blasts S.C.	C C + I	36 40	26 (NS) 43	58 (S) 99
Harris(158–160)	Yes	–	BCG-Glaxo; I.D.	Irradiated allogeneic blasts, S.C.	no maintenance	20 21	20 (S) 35	53 (S) 96
Gale(161)	Yes	+	C. parvum, I.V. (Burroughs-Wellcome)	Irradiated allogeneic blasts, S.C.	C C + I	31 15	69 (NS) 69	96 (NS) 91
Whittaker(162)	Yes	+	BCG-Glaxo; I.V.	Irradiated allogeneic blasts, S.C.	C + BCG C + cells	18 16	45 (NS) 29	73 (NS) 69
Sauter(164)	Yes	+	None	Viral oncolysate of allogeneic blasts, S.C.	C C + I	22 22	28 (NS) 28	52 (NS) 52

* I.D.—intradermal
† C.—chemotherapy
‡ I.—immunotherapy
§ NS—non-significant
¶ S—significant at least at $p = 0.05$
** NR—Not reached
†† I.V.—intravenous
‡‡ S.C.—subcutaneous

Melanoma Stage I

The effects of inducing delayed hypersensitivity reactions in or on skin cancers and the effects of direct intralesional injection of immune adjuvants, such as BCG, on melanoma and other tumors have been extensively studied.[8,168] The results, in general, suggested that this maneuver could lead to the eradication of local tumor deposits, but also indicated that there was no significant effect on disease course; patients continued to die with progressive systemic disease.

Results of experiments with intralesional BCG therapy of intradermal tumor transplants in guinea pigs led to the conclusion that this form of treatment might be beneficial in humans if the BCG were injected early in the course of the disease.[169] A clinical trial has been carried out to explore this possibility.[170]

Patients with primary malignant melanoma, clinical Stage I, were identified by punch or incisional biopsy. Patients with lesions which were Clark level IV or V, or level III and greater than 2.25 mm thick, were randomized to receive either immediate surgery or intralesional BCG followed by surgery. BCG (Trudeau Institute) was injected into the tumor remaining after biopsy; 3 weeks to 6 weeks later the tumor was removed with a wide excision and a regional lymph node dissection performed. Patients randomized to surgery also had wide excision of the tumor plus regional lymph node dissection.

Thirteen patients were randomized to each group. Of those receiving BCG, five recurred and three died, while the surgery alone group had ten recurrences and six deaths. This study was discontinued due to excessive morbidity resulting from BCG injections.[60] Although the number of patients studied was small, the results were encouraging and further study of this approach is indicated.

Melanoma Stage II

There have been conflicting reports concerning the effectiveness of BCG in the treatment of patients with Stage I (poor prognosis) or Stage II malignant melanoma. In an historically controlled study, patients with Stage II melanoma were given intradermal BCG and the results compared to those that had been obtained in prior years with patients in the same institution treated with surgery alone (Table 48-4).[171,172] The results were interpreted to show prolongation of disease-free interval and survival. A similar trial using a simultaneous but nonrandomized control also indicated that BCG lowered recurrence rate and increased survival.[173,174]

No consistent treatment effects have been found, however, in any of five randomized trials comparing BCG to no further treatment.[175-179] Morton reported that BCG caused a significant prolongation of survival after recurrence, a result similar to that observed with the use of BCG in acute myelogenous leukemia but the implication of the observation is not clear, especially since the effect appears to be eliminated in patients receiving tumor vaccine as well as BCG.[178] It would appear, therefore, that no significant benefit has been achieved with BCG used alone as a systemic agent in patients with Stage I (poor prognosis) or Stage II melanoma.

Levamisole has also been studied in Stage I/II melanoma. No differences were found in disease-free interval or survival between 90 patients randomized to recieve levamisole, 150 mg per day for 3 consecutive days every 2 weeks, and 90 patients receiving placebo.[180]

A number of randomized trials have yielded contradictory information concerning the usefulness of BCG in combination with a chemotherapeutic agent in the treatment of poor prognosis Stage I or Stage II melanoma. A large multi-institutional study, coordinated by the WHO Collaborating Center, randomized Stage I or II patients, after they had been rendered disease-free by surgery, to (1) no further treatment, (2) dacarbazine, (3) BCG intradermally or (4) dacarbazine plus intradermal BCG.[176] Preliminary analysis of results suggests that the chemotherapy alone increases remission duration significantly when compared to no further treatment, but that none of the other treatment arms have induced a significant treatment effect. In comparison, a smaller single institution study randomized the same types of patients to receive either (1) dacarbazine, (2) BCG intradermally or (3) the combination of dacarbazine plus BCG.[181,182] Analysis of these results suggested that chemotherapy alone was deleterious, and the investigators discontinued that arm of the study. Moreover, significant prolongation of survival was noted in the chemotherapy plus BCG group when compared to either form of treatment given alone.

This strikingly different chemotherapy result could be due to the smaller amount of chemotherapy given by Wood and associates. The WHO study gave dacarbazine intravenously, 200mg/m^2 per day for 5 days every 4 weeks for 2 years, while Wood and associates gave the same dose for only 3 days each month for 6 months, then every 2 months for 6 months and every 3 months during the second year. In addition, the distribution of 75% males and 25% females in the group of patients receiving dacarbazine alone in the Wood study might be expected to lead to a poorer result owing to the better prognosis of this disease in females.

Another randomized study of Stage I and Stage II melanoma patients has also failed to show significant advantage of BCG plus chemotherapy when compared to no further treatment.[183] The amount of dacarbazine given in this study was, however, much less than that used by Wood. The combination of dacarbazine (at doses similar to those used by WHO) and BCG has been compared to BCG alone, but only in patients with Stage II disease with a primary lesion on the trunk.[177] No differences in remission or survival were noted.

Thus the observation by Wood and associates that BCG plus dacarbazine produces a survival advantage in patients with Stage I or Stage II melanoma is not supported by the findings of Quirt, Cunningham, or the WHO. There are differences in the design of each of these studies which might account for the differences in results, but it seems reasonable to conclude that the combination of dacarbazine and BCG has not been established to have a treatment effect in patients with Stage I or Stage II melanoma.

Because melanoma is one of the human neoplasms suspected to contain tumor-associated antigens, tumor-related immunotherapy, using autologous or allogeneic tumor cells, has been attempted.[14] One study of this type was discontinued due to an apparent deleterious effect on patient survival.[184] Fifteen Stage II patients were randomized to receive no

TABLE 48-4. Melanoma

AUTHOR (Reference Number)	RAN-DOMIZED	STAGE	STUDY DESIGN	NUMBER OF PATIENTS	RESULTS
Gutterman(171,172)	No; historical	II	No further therapy BCG I.D. (Tice)	42	Remission duration and survival prolonged
Morton(174)	No; contem-pora-neous	II	No further therapy BCG I.D. (Tice)	42 84	Remission duration prolonged
Morton(178)	Yes	II	No further therapy BCG I.D. (Tice) BCG + tumor vaccine	46 45 49	No significant difference in remission duration. BCG alone, compared to other 2 groups, gives increased survival from recurrence; $p = 0.008$
Terry(179)	Yes	I, II	No further therapy Methyl CCNU BCG I.D. (Trudeau) BCG + tumor vaccine	43 46 47 45	No significant difference
Cunningham(177) (ECOG)	Yes	I, II	No further therapy BCG I.D. (Tice)	242 232	No significant difference
			BCG I.D. (Tice) Chemotherapy + BCG I.D.	86 89	No significant difference
Pinsky(175)	Yes	II	No further therapy BCG I.D. (Tice)	23 24	No significant difference
Beretta(176) (WHO)	Yes	I, II	No further therapy Chemotherapy BCG I.D. (Pasteur) Chemotherapy + BCG I.D.	157 188 173 178	Remission duration increased for chemotherapy compared to control; No other differences
Wood(181,182)	Yes	I, II	Chemotherapy BCG I.D. (Tice) Chemotherapy + BCG I.D.	20 65 (31) 56 (18)	Survival prolonged for chemotherapy + BCG compared to chemotherapy or BCG alone
Quirt(183)	Yes	I, II	No further therapy Chemotherapy + BCG I.D. (Connaught)	47 47	No significant difference
Spitler(180)	Yes	I, II	Placebo Levamisole 150 mg per day, 3 consecutive days, every other week	90 90	No significant difference

further therapy or immunization with 5×10^7 irradiated autologous tumor cells mixed with BCG and injected once intradermally. There appeared to be accelerated recurrences and an increased death rate in the patients injected with tumor cells. It is not clear whether the apparent poor result was related to therapy or represented a random fluctuation in clinical outcome.

In another study, autologous tumor cells were treated with the enzyme neuraminidase (derived from *Vibrio cholera* organisms) and irradiated with 10,000 rad. Neuraminidase removes sialic acid from polysaccharides and is reported to increase the immunogenicity of tumor cells.[185] These *Vibrio cholera* neuraminidase (VCN) treated cells (2×10^8 cells) were given along with BCG and the result compared to that obtained in patients randomized to receive no further treatment.[186] While no positive treatment effect was noted, no deleterious effect was noted either and it appears, therefore, that autologous tumor cells can be given without necessarily inducing rapid recurrence.

A major trial of specific immunotherapy has utilized allogeneic melanoma cells grown in tissue culture.[178] Three melanoma tumors were established in tissue culture and the cell lines were administered, with BCG, to patients with Stage II melanoma. Patients were randomized to receive no further therapy (46 patients), BCG intradermally (45 patients), or BCG intradermally plus a mixture of the three tumor cell lines (49 patients). No significant difference in remission duration or survival has been noted for patients receiving the vaccine.

A related trial has used the same three cell lines established by Morton.[179] Patients with poor prognosis Stage I or Stage II disease were randomized to receive no further treatment (43 patients), methyl-CCNU (46 patients), BCG (47 patients), or

BCG plus a tumor cell vaccine consisting of the three cell lines that had been treated with VCN (45 patients). Methyl-CCNU was given for 18 months; BCG or BCG plus cells were given for 2 years. No significant differences in remission duration or survival have been noted.

Thus, attempts at specific immunotherapy have not been shown to be effective in melanoma.

Very few attempts have been made to use antisera in the treatment of human cancer. *In vitro* studies have been interpreted to suggest that melanoma cells contain tumor antigens, that lymphocytes from melanoma patients are specifically cytotoxic for these melanoma cells, that serum from melanoma patients contains a factor, presumably antibody, that can block this cell-mediated cytotoxicity, and that serum from melanoma patients who have had spontaneous tumor regression, as well as serum from normal healthy North American blacks contains a factor (again presumably antibody) that can neutralize or unblock the blocking factor. A trial was carried out to study the effects of infusing plasma from blacks into patients with Stage II or Stage III melanoma.[187] No evidence of a treatment effect was noted.

Disseminated Melanoma

BCG, in conjunction with chemotherapy has also been studied extensively in patients with disseminated malignant melanoma. In only one of these trials have increases in response rate or survival been reported, and this trial was historically controlled.[188] Randomized trials using the same chemotherapy or different chemotherapy have not confirmed this result.[189,190] Other trials have been carried out using subcutaneous or intravenous *Corynebacterium parvum* and again no differences in objective response rate or survival have been noted.[189,191] Patients with metastatic melanoma have also been injected with irradiated allogeneic tumor cells mixed with BCG without apparent effect.[192]

The results of currently available immunotherapy in malignant melanoma are, therefore, quite disappointing. Intralesional injection of an immune adjuvant, such as BCG, into Stage I lesions may prove useful, but a definitive trial is required. No reproducible effects have been seen in patients with disseminated disease and benefits to patients with lymph node metastases are at best marginal.

Lung Cancer

Lung tumors are accessible for direct intratumoral injection and several investigators have explored this approach to immunotherapy.[193–197] In a prospective randomized study of patients with Stage I through Stage III non-small-cell lung cancer, the results of surgical removal alone have been compared with those obtained by first injecting the tumor mass with living BCG, waiting 2 to 3 weeks and then resecting the lesion (Table 48-5).[195] BCG was injected through a flexible fine needle passed through a fiberoptic bronchoscope. Isoniazid (INH) was administered to patients receiving BCG to assure that disseminated BCG infection did not develop, and was also administered to surgical controls to assure that INH was not causing a treatment effect. It is too early to evaluate the results of this trial but it is possible to state that the approach is feasible and the toxicity acceptable (one pneumothorax out of 32 patients injected, moderate fever and occasional peritumoral pneumonitis).

Feasibility has also been demonstrated in non-randomized trials using injections of living BCG (Glaxo) through a bronchoscope into endobronchial tumors and direct percutaneous injections into accessible lesions, as well as by using the cell wall skeleton of BCG or *Nocardia rubra* organisms and by using living BCG and BCG cell wall skeletons.[193,194,196,197] Although feasibility has been established, efficacy has not yet been evaluated.

Adjuvants have also been injected into the pleural space following resection of lung cancer. McKneally and co-workers entered 66 patients with Stage I non-small-cell lung cancer into a randomized study to determine whether BCG injected intrapleurally postoperatively affected time to recurrence or survival.[198] All patients received INH. Those patients receiving BCG and INH had statistically significant prolongation in time to recurrence ($p = 0.0003$) and time to death ($p = 0.02$) when compared with control patients who received only INH. No treatment effect was noted in patients with Stage II or III disease.

These encouraging results led the National Lung Cancer Study Group to conduct a larger trial in which control patients did not receive INH and the procedures used for staging patients were more likely to detect microscopic metastatic disease than those used by McKneally.[199] Patients categorized as Stage I in the cooperative trial are therefore more likely to have a better prognosis than those in the McKneally trial. Three-hundred-forty-six patients have been randomized to this trial and followed for a median of 313 days. No differences have been found in recurrence or survival. As expected, prognosis has been very good and if there are any treatment effects, they will only be detected with long-term follow-up of large numbers of patients.

Another randomized trial involving modifications of the McKneally protocol has reported no treatment effect following intrapleural BCG.[200] At this time, therefore, there has not been a confirmation of the original observation concerning the beneficial effect of intrapleural BCG.

Corynebacterium parvum has also been administered intrapleurally and intrapleural BCG has been studied in combination with oral levamisole.[199,201,202] No significant treatment benefits were detected in either trial.

Systemic administration of adjuvants or other putative immunotherapeutic agents has been studied in lung cancer. Levamisole has been reported to prolong survival in patients with resectable non-small-cell lung cancer.[203] All patients received 150 mg of levamisole, regardless of weight, for 3 consecutive days before thoracotomy and then for 3 consecutive days every other week after surgery. Life-table analysis showed little difference between the treated patients and those randomized to receive placebo. However, when only patients and controls whose body weights were low enough to make the administered dose equal to or greater than 2 mg/kg/day were compared, significant prolongation of remission duration and survival were noted. A similar trial was carried out by Anthony.[204] In this instance, however, some attempt was made to achieve a weight-related dose for all patients in the trial. Patients were randomized to receive placebo or

TABLE 48-5. Lung Cancer

AUTHOR (Reference Number)	RANDOMIZED	TYPE	STAGE	STUDY DESIGN	NUMBER OF PATIENTS	RESULTS
Matthay(195)	Yes	Non-small-cell	I, II, III	Surgery BCG I.T. + Surgery	23 32	Feasible; too early to interpret
McKneally(198)	Yes	Non-small-cell	I	Surgery + INH Surgery + INH + BCG I.P.	36 30	Remission duration and survival significantly prolonged
National Lung Cancer Study Group(199)	Yes	Non-oat-cell	I	Surgery + saline I.P. Surgery + INH + BCG I.P.	346	No difference between the two groups; code not broken
Baldwin(200)	Yes	All types	I	Surgery Surgery + INH + BCG I.P.	24 26	No difference
National Lung Cancer Study Group(199)	Yes	Adeno Ca. + large cell undifferentiated	II, III	Surgery + chemotherapy Surgery + INH + BCG I.P. + levamisole	41	One arm appears better; code not broken
Wright(202)	Yes	Non-small-cell	I, II, III	Surgery Surgery + BCG I.P. Surgery + BCG I.P. + levamisole	33 48 53	No differences for all stages analyzed together
National Lung Cancer Study Group(199)	Yes	Squamous	II, III	Surgery Surgery + Radiotherapy Surgery + Radiotherapy + levamisole	61	Too early; code not broken
Ludwig Cancer Research Center(201)	Yes	Non-small-cell	I, II	Surgery Surgery + C. parvum I.P.	196 204	No difference
Amery(203)	Yes	Non-small-cell	I, II, III	Surgery Surgery + levamisole 150 mg/day	115 96	Prolongation of remission and survival, but only for patients with lower body weight
Anthony(204)	Yes	All types	I, II, III	Surgery + placebo Surgery + levamisole approx. 2 mg/kg/day	118 99	No significant difference
Cohen(205)	Yes	Small cell	not specified	Chemotherapy Chemotherapy + thymosin 20 mg/M^2 Chemotherapy + thymosin 60 mg/M^2	26 14 27	Prolongation of survival of those patients receiving thymosin, 60 mg/m^2
Reid(206)	Yes	Non-small-cell	I, II	Surgery Surgery + BCG (Pasteur) I.D. Surgery + BCG + Irradiated allogeneic tumor cells	20 15 13	Too early to evaluate
Stewart(208)	Partially	All	I	Surgery + chemotherapy Surgery + tumor antigen + Freund's adjuvant Surgery + chemotherapy + tumor antigen + Freund's adjuvant	8 15 13	Prolongation of survival of patients receiving tumor antigen plus Freund's adjuvant
Takita(209)	Yes	Squamous cell	I, II	Surgery Surgery + tumor antigen + Freund's adjuvant Surgery + Freund's adjuvant	27 24 29	Prolongation of survival of patients receiving Freund's adjuvant

levamisole for 3 days before thoracotomy and 3 days every 2 weeks for 2 years with 100 mg/day if the patient's weight was less than 50 kg, 150 mg/day if the patient's weight was between 50 kg and 75 kg, and 200 mg/day if the patient's weight was greater than 75 kg. All these patients therefore received 2–3 mg/kg/treatment-day. The results showed no benefit from levamisole and actually showed an apparently higher postoperative mortality in levamisole-treated patients. The authors speculate that the pre-operative administration of levamisole may predispose to the development of autoimmune processes involving the heart or lungs.

The results obtained by Amery and Anthony appear to be contradictory and a large prospectively randomized trial using adequate, weight-related doses of levamisole may be required to resolve this issue.

Thymosin has been tested in patients with small cell anaplastic bronchogenic carcinoma.[205] Patients were randomized to receive 60 mg/m^2 or 20 mg/m^2 of thymosin fraction V given subcutaneously twice weekly, or to receive no thymosin. All patients received chemotherapy. Statistically significant prolongation of survival was reported for patients receiving the 60 mg/m^2 dose. The design of the trial, however, was not optimal and another randomized trial of the effects of thymosin plus chemotherapy compared to chemotherapy alone will be required before conclusions concerning efficacy can be made. It should be noted that thymosin fraction V is a crude preparation of a biological material and any future clinical trial will be confronted with the problems of how to be sure that the preparation used is comparable to the one used by Cohen and associates.

Tumor-related immunotherapy has been studied in lung cancer using both intact cells and tumor cell membrane extracts. In one study, patients with resected non-small-cell lung cancers were randomized to receive no further treatment, BCG, or BCG plus allogeneic tumor cells twice monthly for 2 years.[206] Single cell suspensions of allogeneic tumor cells were prepared from fresh surgical specimens, irradiated with 5000 rad and frozen in dimethyl-sulfoxide until used for intradermal and subcutaneous administration. Relatively few patients were studied and no significant survival advantage was demonstrated for either treatment group.

Attempts have also been made to extract lung tumor cell membrane fractions that might contain tumor antigens.[207] One study, using this type of preparation in combination with Freund's* complete adjuvant, reported significant prolongation of the survival of patients with resected stage I lung cancer of all histologic types.[208] Small numbers of patients were studied and the trial design was such that it will not be possible to determine whether treatment effects are due to the Freund's adjuvant or the "tumor antigen" preparation.

A related study, using a similar "tumor antigen" preparation, compared no further treatment to the effect caused by Freund's adjuvant alone or in combination with the "tumor antigen" in patients with resected Stage I or Stage II squamous cell lung cancer.[209] Significant prolongation of survival was reported for both treatment arms, suggesting that any treatment effect is due to the Freund's adjuvant and not to the "tumor antigen." The number of patients studied was small, however, and the duration of the trial so short that these results must be considered preliminary.

BCG, levamisole, thymosin, Freund's adjuvant, or Freund's adjuvant plus a "tumor antigen" preparation have all been reported to prolong either disease free interval or survival in lung cancer. None of these "positive" trials is definitive and additional trials will be required to test the validity of these preliminary observations.

Breast Cancer

Levamisole has been studied in patients with various stages of breast cancer.[210] Following surgery, patients with Stage II disease were randomized to receive radiotherapy alone or in combination with levamisole. Survival was somewhat longer in 40 patients receiving levamisole, but the difference is not statistically significant (Table 48-6). Similar results were seen in postoperative Stage III patients randomized to receive chemotherapy plus levamisole (19 patients), radiotherapy plus levamisole (20 patients), or chemotherapy plus radiotherapy plus levamisole (20 patients).[210] The two groups receiving chemotherapy plus levamisole appeared to have longer survival than the group receiving radiotherapy plus levamisole but the differences are not significant. These authors also report that patients with Stage IV disease achieve significant survival benefit from treatment with levamisole plus chemotherapy. In a randomized trial, 51 patients were treated with chemotherapy and 48 with the same chemotherapy plus levamisole. The latter group had considerably longer survival ($p = 0.001$).

Another trial of levamisole in combination with chemotherapy in Stage IV breast cancer also showed a prolongation in survival for those patients receiving levamisole.[211] The number of patients studied was small (29 in each group) and the authors point out that the results obtained with four of the levamisole-treated patients strongly influenced the outcome of the entire trial. Cautious interpretation of these data is therefore warranted.

Intradermal BCG has been studied in patients with Stage II or III breast cancer.[212] Patients were randomized to receive chemotherapy (102 patients) or chemotherapy plus BCG (98 patients). No significant differences were noted.

Preliminary results suggest that chemotherapy plus intradermal BCG prolongs survival in patients with Stage IV breast cancer.[213] A nonrandomized trial comparing chemotherapy (44 patients) to chemotherapy plus intradermal BCG (105 patients) in Stage IV disease also reported prolongation of patient survival.[214,215] Although large numbers of patients were studied, the absence of randomized controls makes interpretation difficult.

In some institutions, Stage III breast cancer is treated with radiotherapy alone. Prolongation of disease-free interval and survival was reported for 20 patients receiving levamisole after radiotherapy.[216,219] The numbers of patients studied were small and the study design called for alternating assignment of patients rather than random assignment. Confirmation of this trial is required.

Corynebacterium parvum in combination with chemotherapy appears to prolong survival in Stage IV patients, but

* Freund's adjuvant is a water-in-oil emulsion containing mycobacterial lipids in the oil phase.

TABLE 48-6. Breast Cancer

AUTHOR	RANDOMIZED	STAGE	TREATMENT	NUMBER OF PATIENTS	RESULTS
Klefstrom(210)	Yes	II	Placebo Levamisole	32 40	Survival improved; $p = 0.06$
La Cour(219)	Yes	T_2,T_3 $N_0N_1M_0$	Surgery + radiotherapy Surgery + radiotherapy + Poly A.U.	144 155	5-year survival increased from 74% to 86%; $p < 0.05$
Buzdar(212)	Yes	II	Chemotherapy Chemotherapy + BCG I.D.	62 58	No significant difference
Buzdar(212)	Yes	III	Chemotherapy Chemotherapy + BCG I.D.	37 38	No significant difference
Klefstrom(210)	Yes	III	Chemotherapy + levamisole Radiotherapy + levamisole Chemotherapy + radiotherapy + levamisole	19 20 20	No significant difference
Rojas(216)	No; alternate	III	Radiotherapy Radiotherapy + levamisole	23 20	Median survival increased from 22 to 41.5 months; $p < 0.05$
Klefstrom(210)	Yes	IV	Chemotherapy Chemotherapy + levamisole	51 48	Median survival improved from 19 mos to 36 mos; $p = 0.001$
Stephens(211)	Yes	IV	Chemotherapy Chemotherapy + levamisole	29 29	Median survival increased from 11.5 to 16.5 months; $p = 0.02$
Hortobagyi(215)	No; historical	IV	Chemotherapy Chemotherapy + BCG I.D.	44 105	Median survival increased from 15 to 21 months; $p = 0.02$
McCulloch(213)	Yes	IV	Chemotherapy Chemotherapy + BCG I.D.	25 24	Median survival increased from 10 to 16 months; $p < 0.05$
Pinsky(218)	Yes	IV	Chemotherapy Chemotherapy + C. parvum	23 24	Increased survival, but only for responders

only in those demonstrating a response (partial or complete tumor regression).[218] The number of patients studied was small.

Polyadenylic–polyuridylic acid (polyA·polyU) has been studied in 300 patients with operable breast cancer, with or without palpable lymph nodes, but without distant metastases.[219] Patients were treated with surgery (some also received radiotherapy) and were then randomized to receive intravenous polyA·polyU or intravenous saline (145 patients). Overall survival was significantly prolonged in the patients receiving polyA·polyU and survival rates compared favorably with those reported by Bonadonna for adjuvant chemotherapy. Further exploration of this approach seems warranted.

Colon Cancer

Verhaegan and associates have studied the use of oral levamisole in colon cancer.[220] A total of 60 patients was assigned (not randomized) to treatment or control groups following surgery that rendered them apparently disease free. The two groups were comparable for age, sex, primary tumor site (colon or rectum), and Duke's classification. The treatment group received levamisole 150 mg/daily for 3 consecutive days every 2 weeks for 2 years. The control group received no additional treatment following surgery.

Results indicated a beneficial effect of levamisole with 21 of 30 (70%) of levamisole patients alive after 5 years and only 13 of 30 (43%) control patients alive at that time. This is reported as a statistically significant result. The disease-free interval for the levamisole-treated patients was a year longer than that for controls (47 *versus* 35 months). This study must be interpreted with caution because it was not truly randomized and because the number of patients is relatively small.

On the assumption that lymph nodes draining a tumor site may be hyporeactive and that stimulation of these nodes might be beneficial, a trial of oral BCG in patients with colon or rectal cancer penetrating the bowel wall or involving regional lymph nodes or both has been initiated.[221] Following surgery, apparently disease-free patients were randomized to receive chemotherapy or the same chemotherapy plus 6×10^8 viable Connaught BCG organisms given by mouth every 2 weeks (Table 48-7). Treatment was for 1 year with patients followed to death. Those patients receiving chemoimmunotherapy appeared to have a longer disease-free interval, but the difference is not significant and patients are still being followed.

Patients with colorectal carcinoma and lymph node metastases (Dukes'C) treated with intradermal BCG alone or in combination with chemotherapy following surgery are reported to have significant prolongation of disease-free interval and survival.[222] This study utilized an historical surgical control group for comparison and until there is a comparable randomized trial, these results must be considered as a preliminary unconfirmed observation.

Levamisole is being studied in the treatment of patients with metastatic colon or rectal cancer.[223] Patients are random-

TABLE 48-7. Colon Cancer

AUTHOR (Reference Number)	RAN-DOMIZED	STAGES	STUDY DESIGN	NUMBER OF PATIENTS	RESULTS
Verhaegen(220)	No	A, B1, B2, C	Surgery Surgery and levamisole	30 30	Increased remission duration & survival; 70% *vs* 43% alive at 5 years
Panettiere(221)	Yes	C	Surgery Surgery + chemotherapy Surgery + chemotherapy + BCG (Connaught) P.O.	90 90 90	No significant differences
Mavligit(222)	No	C	Surgery Surgery + BCG I.D. Surgery + BCG + chemotherapy	48 64 73	Remission duration and survival of both treatment groups is better than that of controls
Borden(223)	Yes	Disseminated	Chemotherapy Chemotherapy + levamisole	45 40	Median survival increased from 44 to 81 weeks
Engstrom(225)	Yes	Disseminated	Chemotherapy Chemotherapy + BCG (Glaxo) I.D.	24 23	No significant difference in survival
Moertel(224)	Yes	Disseminated	Chemotherapy Chemotherapy + MER I.D.	92 89	No significant difference in survival

TABLE 48-8. Bladder Cancer

AUTHOR (Reference Number)	RAN-DOMIZED	TYPE	STAGES	STUDY DESIGN	NUMBER OF PATIENTS	RESULTS
Morales(226)	No; patient is own control	Transitional cell carcinoma of bladder	P1S to P1	BCG intravesical	26	Decreased frequency of recurrence after treatments; $p=0.00001$
Lamm(227)	Yes	Transitional cell carcinoma of bladder	All	Surgery Surgery + BCG intravesical + I.D.	24 23	Median remission duration increased from 12 to 19 months; $p=0.01$
Pinsky(228)	Yes	Multicentric bladder cancer	All	Fulguration Fulguration + BCG intravesical + I.D.	26 25	Remission duration increased; $p=0.01$ Decreased no. of tumors per month

ized to receive chemotherapy alone or in combination with levamisole. An interim analysis of this study showed a significantly increased median survival of 80.9 weeks for 40 patients receiving levamisole compared to a median survival of 43.7 weeks for 45 patients receiving chemotherapy alone.

Patients with advanced colorectal cancer have been treated with chemotherapy alone or in conjunction with MER. MER did not produce a treatment advantage and may have been associated with an increase of severe leukopenia.[224] Chemotherapy has also been compared to chemotherapy plus BCG in patients with advanced colon cancer and no treatment difference was noted.[225]

Bladder Cancer

Bladder cancer provides an opportunity to study the effects of immunotherapeutic agents on local recurrence. Patients with transitional cell carcinoma of the bladder and a history of multiple recurrences have been treated with intravesical instillations and intradermal injections of BCG given weekly for 6 weeks.[226] The number of recurrences following treatment was compared with that detected during a similar time interval prior to treatment. A significant reduction in tumor incidence was noted and 14 of 26 patients had no recurrences during the study interval (Table 48-8).

The same immunotherapeutic approach was assessed in a trial in which patients with resected transitional cell carcinoma were randomized to receive no further therapy or treatment with intravesical and intradermal BCG.[227] Time to recurrence was significantly prolonged by BCG. The number of patients with recurrent tumors was decreased from 46% to 22%; the number of episodes of recurrence was decreased from 19 to eight and the total number of individual recurrent tumors decreased from 67 to 17.

In a third study, patients have been randomized to treatment with fulguration or fulguration plus intravesical and intradermal BCG.[228] Again, a significant prolongation in time to recurrence and a significant decrease in the number of recurrent tumors per month were observed.

None of these studies has been in progress long enough to know whether the use of intravesical and intradermal BCG will lead to prolongation of survival. It is also not clear whether the observed treatment effects were due to the intravesical BCG, the intradermal BCG, or really required both. In all three studies, patients were treated for 6 weeks. Whether greater treatment benefit could be derived from a longer treatment course or from repeat courses remains to be determined. It can be reasonably concluded, however, that the combination of intravesical and intradermal BCG appears to decrease the frequency of recurrence and increase the time to recurrences of superficial bladder cancer. Additional studies to determine whether intravesical or intradermal BCG is the effective agent are required.

Miscellaneous Solid Tumors

BCG has been administered to patients with Stage III and Stage IV and recurrent ovarian carcinoma.[229] Patients were randomized to receive chemotherapy (65 patients) or the same chemotherapy plus Pasteur BCG (56 patients) intradermally for up to 2 years. The complete remission rate was better for patients receiving BCG and the median duration of survival was 22.3 months, significantly better than the 13.7 months achieved by patients on chemotherapy alone. Although survival appears to be prolonged, there is no evidence for long-term cures.

Patients with Stage IIB, Stage IIIB, and Stage IVA ovarian cancer confined to the pelvis or periaortic nodes or both have been randomized and treated with radiotherapy or radiotherapy plus intravenous *C. parvum.*[84,230] No significant differences in disease progression or survival have been noted.

By contrast, in a non-randomized pilot trial, intravenous *C. parvum* appeared to have a treatment effect on patients with Stage III ovarian cancer. Forty-five consecutive patients were treated with melphalan plus intravenous *C. parvum* (Wellcome) and the results compared to those obtained with groups of 63 and 58 patients with similar characteristics who were receiving melphalan alone.[231] The number of complete responses was increased by *C. parvum* and the median survival was increased from about 12 months in the two control groups to 25 months in patients receiving *C. parvum.*

Patients with squamous cell cancer of the head and neck have been treated with various forms of immunotherapy. Intralesional injections of BCG cell walls attached to mineral oil droplets have been used preoperatively.[232] Patients with $T_{1/2}$, $N_{0/1/2}$, M_0 were randomized to receive radical surgery alone or a single injection of the BCG cell wall preparation followed 24 days later by radical surgery. Twelve patients were randomized to each group and no significant difference in remission duration or survival had been noted at the time of this report.

In a randomized trial, 42 patients with head and neck cancer received conventional therapy while 37 were treated with conventional therapy plus levamisole.[233] The dosage of levamisole was not modified according to the weight of the patient. No treatment effect has been seen. The effects of intravenous, subcutaneous and intra-lymphnodal *C. parvum* plus radiotherapy have been compared to radiotherapy alone in head and neck cancer patients; no differences were noted.[234] In a study of tumor-related immunotherapy of sarcoma, patients with Stage I or Stage II skeletal or soft tissue sarcoma were randomized, following surgery, to treatment with chemotherapy alone or chemotherapy plus immunotherapy. Immunotherapy consisted of living BCG plus irradiated tissue culture cell lines derived from two soft tissue sarcomas and one osteogenic sarcoma.[235] At the time of the report, the trial was still in progress but no treatment effects had been noted.

CONCLUSIONS

Despite considerable effort, the contribution of immunotherapy to the treatment of cancer is, at this time, negligible. A few facts do seem to be established:

1. Delayed hypersensitivity reactions induced in a tumor lead to tumor necrosis. Whether this is a strictly local phenomenon or whether there is a systemic benefit derived from this immune destruction has not yet been established.
2. Intradermal or intravenous BCG appears to cause a small prolongation in remission duration and a somewhat longer prolongation of survival after relapse in acute myelogenous leukemia. The mechanism responsible for these effects is not known.
3. BCG decreases the frequency of recurrences in papillary carcinoma of the bladder. This is presumably due to immune-mediated tumor necrosis before the tumors become large enough to be clinically detected.

None of the other agents discussed in this chapter has had consistent therapeutic effects, although current preliminary reports of trials utilizing levamisole appear encouraging for several types of cancer.

It is not surprising that progress in clinical immunotherapy has been slow. Information critical to the development of a sound theoretical framework on which therapy could be based is lacking, and in the absence of this information, empiricism has been the rule. The number of potential variables in the host–tumor–therapy interaction is quite large and the probability of developing an effective treatment empirically is, therefore, correspondingly small. Additional information is required concerning the surface antigens of tumor cells, immune-system–tumor-cell interactions, and the regulation and control of immune system functions before rational judgements can be made on the probability that immunotherapy will be of value in the systemic treatment of cancer.

REFERENCES

1. Busch W: Verhandlungen arztlicher Gesellschaften. Berl Klin Wochenschr 5:137–138, 1868
2. Coley WB: Contributions to the knowledge of sarcoma. Ann Surg 14:199–220, 1891
3. Nauts HC, Fowler GA, Bagatko FH: A review of the influence of bacterial infection and of bacterial products (Coley's Toxins) on malignant tumors in man. Acta Med Scand (Suppl) 276:1–103, 1953

4. Ehrlich P: Uber den jetzigen Stand der Karzinomforschung. In Himmelweit F (ed): The Collected Papers of Paul Ehrlich, Vol II, pp 550–562. London, Pergamon Press, 1957
5. Ehrlich P: On immunity with special reference to cell life. Proc R Soc Lond 66:424–448, 1900
6. Burnet FM: The concept of immunological surveillance. Prog Exp Tumor Res 13:1–27, 1970
7. Klein E: Local cytostatic chemotherapy and immunotherapy. Geriatrics 23:154–175, 1968
8. Klein E: Hypersensitivity reactions at tumor sites. Cancer Res 29:2351, 1969
9. Klein EO, Holtermann H, Milgrom RW et al: Immunotherapy for accessible tumors utilizing delayed hypersensitivity reactions and separated components of the immune system. Med Clin North Am 60:389–418, 1976
10. Mathé G, Amiel JL, Schwarzenberg L et al: Active immunotherapy for acute lymphoblastic leukemia. Lancet i:697–699, 1969
11. Morton DL, Eilber FR, Malmgren RA et al: Immunological factors which influence response to immunotherapy in malignant melanoma. Surgery 68:158–164, 1970
12. Landsteiner K, Chase MW: Experiments on transfer of cutaneous sensitivity to simple compounds. Proc Soc Exp Med 49:688–690, 1942
13. David JR: Delayed hypersensitivity in vitro: Its mediation by cell-free substances formed by lymphoid cell-antigen interaction. Proc Natl Acad Sci 56:72–77, 1966
14. Rosenberg SA: Serologic Analysis of Human Cancer Antigens. New York, Academic Press, 1980
15. Rosenberg SA: Lysis of human normal and sarcoma cells in tissue culture by normal human sera. Implications for experiments in human immunology. J Natl Cancer Inst 58:1233–1238, 1977
16. Lovchik, JC, Hong R: Antibody-dependent cell-mediated cytolysis (ADCC): Analyses and projections. Prog Allergy 22:1–44, 1977
17. Hayry P, Andersson LC, Nordling S et al: Allograft response in vitro. Transplant Rev 12:91–140, 1972
18. Burton RC, Chism, SE, Warner NL: In vitro induction and expression of T-cell immunity to tumor-associated antigens. Contemp Top Immunobiol 8:69–106, 1978
19. Doherty PC, Blanden RV, Zinkernagel RM: Specificity of virus-immune effector T cells for H-2 K or H-2 D compatible interactions: Implications for H-antigen diversity. Transplant Rev 29:89–124, 1976
20. Shearer GM, Rehn TG, Schmitt-Verhulst A: Role of the major histocompatibility complex in the specificity of in vitro T-cell-mediated lympholysis against chemically-modified autologous lymphocytes. Transplant Rev 29:222–248, 1976
21. Chesebro B, Wehrly K: Studies on the role of the host immune response in recovery from Friend virus leukemia. II. Cell-mediated immunity. J Exp Med 143:85–99, 1976
22. Gillis S, Smith KA: Long term culture of tumor-specific cytotoxic T cells. Nature 268:154–156, 1977
23. von Boehmer H, Haas W, Pohlit H et al: T-cell clones: their use for the study of specificity, induction, and effector function of T-cells. Springer Semin Immunopathol 3:23–37, 1980
24. Holterman OA, Casale GP, Klein E: Tumor cell destruction by macrophages. J Med (Basel) 3:305–309, 1972
25. Alexander P: Activated macrophages and the anti-tumor action of BCG, Natl Cancer Inst Monogr 39:127–133, 1973
26. Hibbs JB Jr: Macrophage nonimmunologic recognition: target cell factors related to contact inhibition. Science 180:868–870, 1973
27. Keller R: Cytostatic elimination of syngeneic rat tumor cells in vitro by nonspecifically activated macrophages. J Exp Med 138:625–644, 1973
28. Fink MA: The Macrophage in Neoplasia. New York, Academic Press, 1976
29. Holterman OA, Lisafeld BA, Klein E et al: Cytocidal and cytostatic effects of activated peritoneal leukocytes. Nature 257:228–229, 1975
30. Herberman RB, Djeu JY, Kay HD et al: Natural killer cells: characteristics and regulation of activity. Immunol Rev 44:43–70, 1979
31. Kiessling R, Wigzell H: An analysis of the murine NK cell as to structure, function, and biological relevance. Immunol Rev 44:165–208, 1979
32. Fujimoto S, Greene MI, Sehon AH: Regulation of the immune response to tumor antigens. I. Immunosuppressor cells in tumor-bearing hosts. J Immunol 116:791–799, 1976
33. Fisher MS, Kripke ML: Systemic alteration induced in mice by ultraviolet light irradiation and its relationship to ultraviolet carcinogenesis. Proc Natl Acad Sci 74:1688–1692, 1977
34. Spellman CW, Daynes RA: Modification of immunological potential by ultraviolet radiation. II. Generation of suppressor cells in short-term UV-irradiated mice. Transplantation 24:120–126, 1977
35. Greene MI, Dorf ME, Pierres M et al: Reduction of syngeneic tumor growth by an anti-I-J alloantiserum. Proc Natl Acad Sci 74:5118–5121, 1977
36. Sjogren HO, Hellstrom I, Bansal SC et al: Elution of "blocking factors" from human tumors, capable of abrogating tumor-cell destruction by specifically immune lymphocytes. Int J Cancer 9:274–283, 1972
37. Waldmann TA, Broder S: Suppressor cells in the regulation of the immune response. In Schwartz RS (ed): Progress in Clinical Immunology, pp 155–199. Grune & Stratton, 1977
38. Guěrin C: The history of BCG. In Rosenthal RG (ed): Vaccination against Tuberculosis, pp 48–53. Boston, Little, Brown & Co, 1957
39. Biozzi G, Benacerraf B, Grumbach F et al: Etude de l'activité granulopexique du systeme reticulo-endothelial au cours de l'infection tuberculeuse experimentale de la souris. Ann Inst Pasteur (Paris) 87:291–300, 1954
40. Bradner WT, Clarke DA, Stock CC: Stimulation of host mice defense against experimental cancer. I. Zymosan and sarcoma 180 in mice. Cancer Res 18:347–351, 1958
41. Halpern BN, Biozzi G, Stiffel C et al: Effet de la stimulation du systéme réticulo-endotheleal par l'inoculation du bacille de Calmette-Guérin sur le développement de l'epithélioma atypique T-8 de Guérin chez le rat. C R Soc Biol (Paris) 153:919–923, 1959
42. Biozzi G, Stiffel C, Halpern BN et al: Effet de l'inoculation du bacille de Calmette-Guérin sur le développement de la tumeur ascitique d'Ehrlich chez la souris. C R Soc Biol (Paris) 153:987–989, 1959
43. Old LJ, Clarke DA, Benacerraf B: Effect of Bacillus Calmette-Guérin infection on transplanted tumours in the mouse. Nature (London) 184:291–292, 1959
44. Old LJ, Clarke DA, Benacerraf B et al: The reticuloendothelial system and the neoplastic process. Ann NY Acad Sci 88:264–280, 1960
45. Old LJ, Benacerraf B, Clarke DA et al: The role of the reticuloendothelial system in the host reaction to neoplasia. Cancer Res 21:1281–1300, 1961
46. Old LJ, Clarke DA, Benacerraf B et al: Effect of prior splenectomy on the growth of sarcoma 180 in normal and Bacillus Calmette-Guérin infected mice. Experientia 18:335–336, 1962
47. Weiss DW, Bonhag RS, Leslie P: Studies on the heterologous immunogenicity of a methanol-insoluble fraction of attenuated tubercle bacille (BCG). II. Protection against tumor isografts. J Exp Med 124:1039–1065, 1966
48. Weiss DW: MER and other mycobacterial fractions in the immunotherapy of cancer. Med Clin North Am 60:473–497, 1976
49. Weiss DW: Host mechanisms for control of tumor growth that can be modulated by nonspecific immunotherapy. In: Immunotherapy of Human Cancer, p 41–61. The University of Texas System Cancer Center, M.D. Anderson Hospital and Tumor Institute, 22nd annual Clinical Conference on Cancer, New York, Raven Press, 1978
50. Ribi E, Meyer TJ, Azuma I et al: Mycobacterial cell wall components in tumor suppression and regression. Natl Cancer Inst Monogr 39:115–119, 1973
51. Zbar B, Ribi E, Meyer T et al: Immunotherapy of cancer:

Regression of established intradermal tumor after intralesional injection of mycobacterial cell walls attached to oil droplets. J Natl Cancer Inst 52:1571–1577, 1974

52. Azuma I, Ribi EE, Meyer TJ et al: Biologically active components from mycobacterial cell walls. I. Isolation and composition of cell wall skeleton and component P3. J Natl Cancer Inst 52:95–101, 1974
53. Azuma I, Taniyama T, Hirao F et al: Antitumor activity of cell-wall skeletons and peptidoglycolipids on mycobacteria and related microorganisms in mice and rabbits. Gan 65:493–505, 1974
54. Yamamura Y, Yoshizaki K, Azuma I et al: Immunotherapy of human malignant melanoma with oil-attached BCG cell-wall skeleton. Gan 66:355–363, 1975
55. Tokuzen R, Okabe M, Nakahare W et al: Effect of Nocardia and Mycobacterium cell-wall skeleton on autochthonous tumor graft. Gan 66:433–435, 1975
56. Yoshimoto T, Azuma I, Sakatani M et al: Effect of oil-attached BCG cell-wall skeleton on the induction of pleural fibrosarcomas in mice. Gan 67:441–445, 1975
57. Azuma I, Taniyama T, Hirao F et al: Antitumor activity of cell-wall skeletons and peptidoglycolipids of mycobacteria and related microorganisms in mice and rabbits. Gan 65:493–505, 1974
58. Azuma I, Taniyama T, Yamawaki M et al: Adjuvant and antitumor activities of *Nocardia* cell-wall skeletons. Gan 67:733–736, 1976
59. Azuma I, Yamawaki M, Yasumoto K et al: Antitumor activity of *Nocardia* cell wall skeleton preparations in transplantable tumors in syngeneic mice and patients with malignant pleurisy. Cancer Immunol Immunother 4:95–100, 1978
60. Rosenberg SA, Seipp C, Sears HF: Clinical and immunologic studies of disseminated BCG infection. Cancer 41:1771–1780, 1978
61. Baldwin RW, Pimm MV: BCG in tumor immunotherapy. In Klein G, Weinhouse S (eds): Advances in Cancer Research, Vol 28, pp 91–147. New York, Academic Press, 1978
62. Tokunaga T, Kataoka T, Nakamura RM et al: Mode of antitumor action of BCG. Gan 21:59–72, 1978
63. Heise ER, Weiser RS: Factors in delayed sensitivity: Lymphocyte and macrophage cytotoxins in the tuberculin reaction. J Immunol 103:570–576, 1969
64. Meltzer MS, Bartlett GL: Cytotoxicity in vitro by products of specifically stimulated spleen cells: Susceptibility of tumor cells and normal cells. J Natl Cancer Inst 49:1439–1443, 1972
65. Holm G, Stejskal V, Perlmann P: Cytotoxic effects of activated lymphocytes and their supernatants. Clin Exp Immunol 14:169–179, 1973
66. Snyderman R, Altman LC, Hausman MS et al: Human mononuclear leukocyte chemotaxis: A quantitative assay for humoral and cellular chemotactic factors. J Immunol 108:857–860, 1972
67. David JR: Lymphocyte mediators and cellular hypersensitivity. N Engl J Med 288:143–149, 1973
68. David JR, Lawrence HS, Thomas L: Delayed hypersensitivity in vitro. II. Effect of sensitive cells on normal cells in the presence of antigen. J Immunol 93:274–278, 1964
69. Keller R: Susceptibility of normal and transformed cell lines to cytostatic and cytocidal effects exerted by macrophages. J Natl Cancer Inst 56:369–374, 1976
70. Nathan CF: The role of oxidative metabolism in the cytotoxicity of activated macrophages after pharmacologic triggering. In Terry WD, Yamamura Y (eds): Immunobiology and Immunotherapy of Cancer. New York, Elsevier, pp 345–355
71. Woodruff MFA, Boak JL: Inhibitory effect of injection of *Corynebacterium parvum* on the growth of tumor transplants in isogenic hosts. Br J Cancer 20:345–355, 1966
72. Currie GA, Bagshawe KD: Active immunotherapy with *Corynebacterium parvum* and chemotherapy in murine fibrosarcomas. Brit Med J 1:541–544, 1970
73. Olivotto M, Bomford R: In vitro inhibitions of tumor cell growth and DNA synthesis by peritoneal and lung macrophages from mice injected with *Corynebacterium Parvum*. Int J Cancer 13:478–488, 1974
74. Scott MT: Corynebacterium parvum as a therapeutic antitumor agent in mice. II. Local injection. J Natl Cancer Inst 53:861–865, 1974
75. Halpern B: Corynebacterium Parvum: Applications in Experimental and Clinical Oncology. New York, Plenum Press, 1975
76. Likhite V, Halpern B: Lasting rejection of mammary adenocarcinoma cell tumors in DBA/2 mice with intratumor injection of killed *Corynebacterium Parvum*. Cancer Res 34:341–344, 1975
77. Milas L, Scott MT: Antitumor activity of *Corynebacterium Parvum*. In Advances in Cancer Research, Vol 26, pp 257–306. Klein G, Weinhouse S (eds): Academic Press, New York, 1978
78. Tuttle RL, North RJ: Mechanisms of antitumor action of *Corynebacterium parvum*: Nonspecific tumor cell destruction at site of an immunologically mediated sensitivity reaction to *C. parvum*. J Natl Cancer Inst 55:1403–1411, 1975
79. Okamoto H, Shoin S, Koshimura S et al: Studies on the anticancer and streptolysin S-forming abilities of hemolytic streptococci. A review. Jpn J Microbiol 11:323–334, 1967
80. Matsubara S, Suzuki F, Ishida N: Inductions of immune interferon in mice treated with a bacterial immunopotentiator OK 432. Cancer Immunol Immunother 6:41–45, 1979
81. Uchida A, Hoshino T: Reduction of suppressor cells in cancer patients treated with OK 432 immunotherapy. Int J Cancer (in press)
82. Micksche M, Kokoschka EM, Jakesz R et al: Phase I study with streptococcus pyogenes preparation (OK 432). In Terry WD, Rosenberg SA (eds): Immunotherapy of Human Cancer. New York, Elsevier, 1981
83. Gee TS, Dowling MD, Cunningham I et al: Evaluation of *Pseudomonas aeruginosa* vaccine for prolongation of remissions in adults with acute nonlymphoblastic leukemia treated with the L-12 protocol: A preliminary report. In Terry WD, Windorst D (eds): Immunotherapy of Cancer: Present Status of Trials in Man, pp 415–422. New York, Raven Press, 1978
84. Umezawa H, Ishizuka M, Aoyagi T et al: Enhancement of delayed-type hypersensitivity by Bestatin, an inhibitor of aminopeptidase B and Leucine aminopeptidase. J Antibiot 29:857–859, 1976
85. Bruley-Rosset M, Florentin I, Kiger N et al: Restoration of impaired immune functions of aged animals by chronic bestatin treatment. Immunology 38:75–83, 1979
86. Serrou B, Cupissol D, Flad H et al: Phase I evaluation of Bestatin in patients bearing advanced solid tumors. In Terry WD, Rosenberg SA (eds): Immunotherapy of Human Cancer. New York, Elsevier, 1981
87. Maeda YY, Hamuro J, Yamada Y et al: The nature of immunopotentiation by the anti-tumor polysaccharide lentinan and the significance of biogenic amines in its action. In: Immunopotentiation, Ciba Foundation Symposium 18, pp 259–286. New York, North Holland-Elsevier
88. Ikikawa T, Udhara N, Maeda YY et al: Antitumor activity of aqueous extracts of edible mushrooms. Cancer Res 29:734–735, 1969
89. Isaacs A, Lindenmann J: Virus interference: I. The interferon. Proc R Soc Biol 147:258–267, 1957
90. Gresser I, Tovey MG: Antitumor effects of interferon. Biochim Biophys Acta 516:231–247, 1978
91. Borden EC: Interferons: Rational for clinical trials in neoplastic disease. Ann Intern Med 91:472–479, 1979
92. Krim M: Towards tumor therapy with interferons, Part I. Interferons: Production and properties. Blood 55, 5:711–721, 1980
93. Lindahl P, Leary P, Gresser I: Enhancement by interferon of the specific cytotoxicty of sensitized lymphocytes. Proc Natl Acad Sci USA 69:721–725, 1972
94. Zarling JM, Sosman J, Eskra L et al: Enhancement of T cell cytotoxic responses by purified human fibroblast interferon. J Immunol 121:2002–2004, 1980
95. Gresser I: Antitumor effects of interferon. In Becker F (ed): Cancer—A Comprehensive Treatise, Vol 5, pp 521–571. New York, Plenum Press, 1977
96. Einhorn S, Blomgren H, Strander H: Interferon and spontaneous cytotoxicity in man: II. Studies in patients receiving exogenous leukocyte interferon. Acta Med Scand 204:477–484

97. Gidlund M, Orn A, Wigzell H: Enhanced NK cell activity in mice injected with interferon and interferon inducers. Nature 273:759–761, 1978
98. Karre K, Klein GO, Kiessling R: Low natural *in vitro* resistance to syngeneic leukemias in natural killer-deficient mice. Nature 284:624–626, 1980
99. Talmadge JE, Meyers KM, Prieur DJ et al: Role of NK cells in tumor growth and metastasis in *beige* mice. Nature 284:622–624, 1980
100. Strander H, Cantell K, Ingimarsson S et al: 1977. Interferon treatment of osteogenic sarcoma: A clinical trial. In Chirigos MA (ed): Modulation of Host Immune Resistance in the Prevention or Treatment of Induced Neoplasias. Fogarty International Center Proceedings #28:377–381, 1977. DHEW Publication No. (NIH) 77-893
101. Mellstedt H, Bjorkholm M, Johansson B et al: Interferon therapy in myelomatosis. Lancet i:245–248, 1979
102. Mellstedt H, Aahre A, Bjorkholm M et al: Interferon therapy of patients with myeloma. In Terry, WD, Rosenberg SA (eds): Immunotherapy of Human Cancer. New York, Elsevier, 1981
103. Levine AS, Durie B, Lampkin B et al: Interferon induction, toxicity, and clinical efficacy of poly (ICLC) in hematologic malignancies and other tumors. In Terry WD, Rosenberg SA (eds): Immunotherapy of Human Cancer. New York, Elsevier, 1981
104. McIntyre OR, Rai K, Glidewell E et al: Polyriboinosinic: Polyribocytidylic acid as an adjunct to remission maintenance therapy in acute myelogenous leukemia. In Terry WD, Windhorst D (eds): Immunotherapy of Cancer: Present Status of Trials in Man, pp 423–431. New York, Raven Press, 1978
105. Merigan TC, Sikora K, Breeden JH et al: Preliminary observations on the effect of human leukocyte interferon in non-Hodgkin's lymphoma. N Engl J Med 299:1449–1453, 1978
106. Gallagher JG, Louie AC, Sikora K et al: The evaluation of human leukocyte interferon in patients with non-Hodgkin's lymphoma and Hodgkin's disease: A phase II study. In Terry WD, Rosenberg SA (eds): Immunotherapy of Human Cancer. New York, Elsevier, 1981
107. Krown SE, Stoopler MB, Gralla RJ et al: Phase II trial of human leukocyte interferon in non-small cell lung cancer—Preliminary results. In Terry WD, Rosenberg SA (eds): Immunotherapy of Human Cancer. New York, Elsevier, 1981
108. Majoros M, Parkhill EM, Devine KD: Papillomas of the larynx in children. A clinicopathologic study. Am J Surg 108:470–479, 1964
109. zur Hausen H: Oncogenic herpes viruses. Biochim Biophys Acta 47:25–53, 1975
110. zur Hausen H: Papilloma viruses and squamous cell carcinomas in man. Perspect Virol 10:93–102, 1978
111. zur Hausen H: Human papilloma viruses and their possible role in squamous cell carcinomas. Curr Top Microbiol Immunol 78:1–30, 1978
112. Einhorn S, Strander H: Interferon therapy for neoplastic diseases in man in vitro and in vivo studies. In Stinebring W, Chapple P (eds): Human Interferon Production and Clinical Use, pp 159–174. New York, Plenum Press, 1977
113. Haglund S, Lundquist PG, Ingimarsson S et al: Interferon therapy in juvenile laryngeal papillomatosis. In Terry WD, Rosenberg SA (eds): Immunotherapy of Human Cancer. New York, Elsevier, 1981
114. Hooper JA, McDaniel MC, Thurman GB et al: The purification and properties of bovine thymosin. Ann NY Acad Sci 249:125–144, 1975
115. Goldstein AL, Cohen GH, Rossio JL et al: Use of thymosin in the treatment of primary immunodeficiency diseases and cancer. Med Clin North Am 60:591–606, 1976
116. Goldstein AL, Marshall GD, Rossio JL: Thymosin therapy: Approach to immunoreconstitution in immunodeficiency diseases and cancer. In Terry WD, Rosenberg SA (eds): Immunotherapy of Human Cancer, pp 173–179. New York, Raven Press, 1978
117. Goldenberg DM, Deland F, Kim E et al: Use of radiolabelled antibodies to carcinoembryonic antigen for the detection and localization of diverse cancers by external photoscanning. N Eng J Med 298:1384–1388, 1978
118. Order SE, Klein JL Ettinger D et al: Radiolabelled antibody to tumor associated proteins. In Terry WD, Rosenberg SA (eds): Immunotherapy of Human Cancer. New York, Elsevier, 1981
119. Mannick JA, Egdahl RH: Transfer of heightened immunity to skin homografts by lymphoid RNA. J Clin Invest 43:2166–2177, 1964
120. Deckers PJ, Pilch YJ: Transfer of immunity to tumor isografts by the systemic administration of xenogeneic "immune" RNA. Nature 231:181–183, 1971
121. Pilch YH, Ramming KP, deKernion J: Clinical trials of immune RNA in the immunotherapy of cancer. In Terry WD, Windhorst D (eds): Immunotherapy of Cancer: Present Status of Trials in Man, pp 539–555. New York, Raven Press, 1978
122. Ramming KP, deKernion JB: Immune RNA therapy for renal cell carcinoma: survival and immunologic monitoring. Ann Surg 186:459–467, 1977
123. Richie JP, Wang BS, Steele GD et al: Xenogeneic immune RNA therapy in advanced renal cell carcinoma: Phase I trial. In press in Terry WD, Rosenberg SA (eds): Immunotherapy of Human Cancer. New York, Elsevier, 1981
124. Thienpont D, Vanparijs OFJ, Raeymaekers AHM et al: Tetramisole (R8299), a new, potent broad-spectrum antihelminthic. Nature 209:1084–1086, 1966
125. Chirigos MA (ed): Modulation of host immune resistance in the prevention or treatment of induced neoplasias. In: Fogarty International Center Proceeding No 28, DHEW Publication No (NIH) 77–893, 1974
126. Renoux G, Renoux M: Effet immunostimulant d'un imidothiazole dans l'immunisation des souris contre l'infection par Brucella abortus. Comptes Rendus. Acad Sci Paris 272:349–350, 1971
127. Brugmans J, Symoens J: The effects of levamisole on host defense mechanisms: A review. In Chirigos MA (ed): Modulation of Host Immune Resistance in the Prevention or Treatment of Induced Neoplasias, pp 3–16. DHEW Publication No (NIH) 77-893, 1974
128. Ziegler AE, Bicker U, Hebold G: Experimental investigations on increased resistance to infections with *Candida albicans* and *Staphylococcus aureus Smith* by 4-imino-1, 4-diazobicyclo-(3.1.0)-hesane-2-on BM 06.002 (Prop. INN Imexon) in mice. Exp Pathol 14S:321–327, 1977
129. Bicker U, Fuhse P: Carcinostatic action of 2-cyanaziridines against a sarcoma in rats. Exp Pathol 10:279–284, 1975
130. Micksche M, Kokoschka EM, Sagaster P et al: Phase I study for a new immunostimulating drug, BM 06002, in man. In: Immune Modulation and Control of Neoplasia by Adjuvant Therapy. Prog Cancer Res Ther 7:403–413, 1978
131. Bicker U: Immunomodulating effects of BM 12531 in animals and tolerance in man. Cancer Treat Rep 62:1987–1996, 1978
132. Goutner A, Schwarzenberg L, Mathe G: Phase I study of azimexon in immunodepressed cancer patients. In Terry WD, Rosenberg SA (eds): Immunotherapy of Human Cancer. New York, Elsevier, 1981
133. Albrecht WL: Tilorone and analogs: Physiochemical and antiviral properties. In Chirigos MA (ed): Modulation of Host Immune Resistance in the Prevention or Treatment of Induced Neoplasias, pp 83–87. DHEW Publication No (NIH) 77–893, 1974
134. Munson AE, Munson JA, Regelson W et al: Effect of tilorone hydrochloride and congeners on reticuloendothelial system, tumors, and the immune response. Cancer Res 32:1397–1403, 1972
135. Israel L, Miller P, Edelstein R. Antitumor activity of tilorone in man: A preliminary report. In Chirigos MA (ed): Modulation of Host Immune Resistance in the Prevention or Treatment of Induced Neoplasias, pp 145–152. DHEW Publication No (NIH) 77–893, 1974
136. Richter P, Wampler GL, Kuperminc M et al: Tilorone: Phase II study. In Chirigos MA (ed): Modulation of Host Immune Resistance in the Prevention or Treatment of Induced Neoplasias pp 141–143. DHEW Publication No (NIH) 77–893, 1974

137. Mathé G, Schwarzenberg L, De Vassal F et al: Chemotherapy followed by active immunotherapy in the treatment of acute lymphoid leukemias for patients of all ages: Results of ICIG acute lymphoid leukemia protocols 1, 9, and 10; prognostic factors, and therapeutic implications. In: Terry WD, Windhorst D (eds): Immunotherapy of Cancer: Present Status of Trials in Man. New York, Raven Press, 1978
138. Andrien JM, Beumer-Jockmans MP, Bury J et al: Immunotherapy versus chemotherapy as maintenance treatment of acute lymphoblastic leukemia. In Terry WD, Windhorst W (eds): Immunotherapy of Cancer: Present Status of Trials in Man, pp 471–480. New York, Raven Press, 1978
139. Poplack DG, Leventhal BG, Simon R et al: Treatment of acute lymphatic leukemia with chemotherapy alone or chemotherapy plus immunotherapy. In Terry WD, Windhorst W (eds): Immunotherapy of Cancer: Present Status of Trials in Man, pp 497–501. New York, Raven Press, 1978
140. Heyn RM, Joo P, Karon M et al: BCG in the treatment of acute lymphocytic leukemia. In Terry WD, Windhorst W, (eds): Immunotherapy of Cancer: Present Status of Trials in Man, pp 503–512. New York, Raven Press, 1978
141. Kay HEM: Acute lymphoblastic leukemia: 5-year follow-up of the Concord trial. In Terry WD, Windhorst W (eds): Immunotherapy of Cancer: Present Status of Trials in Man, pp 493–496. New York, Raven Press, 1978
142. Pavlovsky S, Garay G, Muriel FS et al: Levamisole therapy during maintenance of remission in patients with acute lymphoblastic leukemia. In Terry WD, Rosenberg SA (eds): Immunotherapy of Human Cancer. New York, Elsevier, 1981
143. Gutterman JU, Rodriguez V, McCredie KB et al: Chemoimmunotherapy of acute myeloblastic leukemia: Four-year follow-up with BCG. In Terry, WD, Windhorst D (eds): Immunotherapy of Cancer: Present Status of Trials in Man, pp 375–381. New York, Raven Press, 1978
144. Gutterman JU, Hersh EM, Rodriguez V et al: Chemoimmunotherapy of adult acute leukemia. Prolongation of remission in myeloblastic leukemia with BCG. Lancet 2:1405–1409, 1974
145. Hewlett JS, Balcerzak S, Gutterman JU et al: Remission maintenance in adult acute leukemia with and without BCG. A southwest oncology group study. In Terry WD, Windhorst D, (eds): Immunotherapy of Cancer: Present Status of Trials in Man, pp 383–390. New York, Raven Press, 1978
146. Vogler WR, Bartolucci AA, Omura GA, et al: Randomized clinical trial of remission induction, consolidation and chemoimmunotherapy maintenance in adult acute myeloblastic leukemia. Cancer Immunol Immunother 3:163–170, 1978
147. Vogler WR, Bartolucci AA, Omura GA et al: A randomized clinical trial of BCG in myeloblastic leukemia. In Terry WD, Windhorst D, (eds): Immunotherapy of Cancer: Present Status of Trials in Man, pp 365–374. New York, Raven Press, 1978
148. Vogler WR, Winton EF, Gordon DA et al: A phase III trial comparing Bacillus Calmette-Guerin (BCG), Cytosine Arabinoside and Daunorubicin with a combination of BCG, Cytosine Arabinoside and Daunorubicin for maintenance therapy in acute myeloblastic leukemia. In Terry WD, Rosenberg SA, (eds): Immunotherapy of Human Cancer. New York, Elsevier, 1981
149. Omura GA, Vogler WR, LeFante J: BCG Immunotherapy of acute myelogenous leukemia. In Terry WD, Rosenberg SA (eds). Immunotherapy of Human Cancer. New York, Elsevier, 1981
150. Whittaker JA, Slater AJ: The immunotherapy of acute myelogenous leukemia using intravenous BCG. Br J Haematol 35:263–273, 1977
151. Cuttner J, Glidewell O, Holland JF: A controlled trial of chemoimmunotherapy of acute myelocytic leukemia with MER. In Terry WD, Rosenberg SA (eds): Immunotherapy of Human Cancer. New York, Elsevier, 1981
152. Powles RL, Russell J, Lister TA, et al: Immunotherapy for acute myelogenous leukemia: A controlled clinical study 2½ years after entry of the last patient. Br J Cancer 35:265–272, 1977
153. Powles RL, Russell J, Lister TA et al: Immunotherapy for acute myelogenous leukemia: Analysis of a controlled clinical study 2½ years after entry of the last patient. In Terry WD, Windhorst W (eds): Immunotherapy of Cancer: Present Status of Trials in Man, pp 315–326. New York, Raven Press, 1978
154. Peto R: Immunotherapy of acute myeloid leukemia. In Terry WD, Windhorst D, (eds): Immunotherapy of Cancer: Present Status of Trials in Man, pp 341–346. New York, Raven Press, 1978
155. Medical Research Council. Immunotherapy of acute myeloid leukemia. Br J Cancer 37:1–14, 1978
156. Reizenstein P, Brenning G, Engstedt L et al: Effect of immunotherapy on survival and remission duration in acute nonlymphatic leukemia. In Terry WD, Windhorst W (eds): Immunotherapy of Cancer: Present Status of Trials in Man, pp 329–339, New York, Raven Press, 1978
157. Reizenstein P, Andersson B, Bjorkholm M et al: BCG plus leukemic cell therapy of patients with acute myelogenous leukemia. Effect in groups with high and low remission rates. In Terry WD, Rosenberg SA (eds): Immunotherapy of Human Cancer. New York, Elsevier, 1981
158. Harris R, Zuhrie SR, Freeman CB et al: Active immunotherapy in acute myelogenous leukemia and the induction of second and subsequent remissions. Br J Cancer 37:282–287, 1978
159. Harris R, Zuhrie SR, Freeman CB et al: A successful randomized trial of immunotherapy alone versus no maintenance treatment in acute myelogenous leukemia. In Terry WD, Rosenberg SA (eds): Immunotherapy of Human Cancer. New York, Elsevier, 1981
160. Zuhrie SR, Harris R, Freeman CB et al: Immunotherapy alone versus no maintenance treatment in acute myelogenous leukaemia. Br J Cancer 41:272–288, 1980
161. Gale RP, Foon KA, Yale C et al: Immunotherapy of acute myelogenous leukemia. In Terry WD, Rosenberg SA (eds): Immunotherapy of Human Cancer. New York, Elsevier, 1981
162. Whittaker JA, Bailey-Wood R, Hutchins S: Active immunotherapy for the treatment of acute myelogenous leukemia. In Terry WD, Rosenberg SA (eds): Immunotherapy of Human Cancer. New York, Elsevier, 1981
163. Holland JF, Beski JG: Comparison of chemotherapy with chemotherapy plus VCN-treated cells in acute myelocytic leukemia. In Terry WD, Windhorst D (eds): Immunotherapy of Cancer: Present Status of Trials in Man, pp 347–352. New York, Raven Press, 1978
164. Sauter C, Caballi F, Lindenmann J et al: Viral Oncolysis: Its application in maintenance treatment of acute myelogenous leukemia. In Terry WD, Windhorst D (eds): Immunotherapy of Cancer: Present Status of Trials in Man, pp 355–362. New York, Raven Press, 1978
165. Jones SE, Salmon SE, Fisher R: 1979. Adjuvant immunotherapy with BCG in non-Hodgkin's lymphoma: A Southwest Oncology Group controlled clinical trial. In Jones SE, Salmon SE (eds): Adjuvant Therapy of Cancer II, pp 163–172. New York, Grune & Stratton, 1979
166. Jones SE: Chemoimmunotherapy of malignant lymphoma. In Terry WD, Rosenberg SA (eds): Immunotherapy of Human Cancer. New York, Elsevier, 1981
167. Salmon SE, Alexanian R, Dixon D: Chemoimmunotherapy for multiple myeloma: Effect of levamisole during maintenance. In Terry WD, Rosenberg SA (eds): Immunotherapy of Human Cancer. New York, Elsevier, 1981
168. Rosenberg SA, Rapp HJ: Intralesional immunotherapy of melanoma with BCG. Med Clin North Am 60:419–430, 1976
169. Zbar B, Bernstein ID, Bartlett GL et al: Immunotherapy of cancer: Regression of intradermal tumors and prevention of growth of lymph node metastases after intralesional injection of living Mycobacterium bovis. J Natl Cancer Inst 49:119–130, 1972
170. Rosenberg SA, Rapp H, Terry WD et al: Intralesional BCG therapy of patients with primary stage I melanoma. In Terry WD, Rosenberg SA (eds): Immunotherapy of Human Cancer. New York, Elsevier, 1981
171. Gutterman JU, Mavligit GM, Reed RC et al: Immunology and immunotherapy of human malignant melanoma: Historic review and perspectives for the future. Semin Oncol 2:155–174, 1975

172. Gutterman JU, Mavligit GM, McBride CM et al: Postoperative immunotherapy for recurrent malignant melanoma: An updated report. In Terry WD, Windhorst D (eds): Immunotherapy of Cancer: Present Status of Trials in Man, pp 35–55. New York, Raven Press, 1978
173. Eilber FR, Morton DL, Holmes EC et al: Adjuvant immunotherapy with BCG in treatment of regional lymph node metastases from malignant melanoma. N Engl J Med 294:237–240, 1976
174. Morton DL, Holmes EC, Eilber FR et al: Adjuvant immunotherapy of malignant melanoma: Preliminary results of a randomized trial in patients with lymph node metastases. In Terry WD, Windhorst D (eds): Immunotherapy of Cancer: Present Status of Trials in Man, pp 57–63. New York, Raven Press, 1978
175. Pinsky CM, Hirshaut Y, Wanebo HJ et al: Surgical adjuvant immunotherapy with BCG in patients with malignant melanoma: Results of a prospective randomized trial. In Terry WD, Windhorst D (eds): Immunotherapy of Cancer: Present Status of Trials in Man, pp 27–32. New York, Raven Press, 1978
176. Beretta G: 1981. Controlled study for prolonged chemotherapy, immunotherapy and chemotherapy plus immunotherapy as an adjuvant to surgery in malignant melanoma. Reporting for the WHO Collaborating Centres for Evaluation of Methods of Diagnosis and Treatment of Melanoma. In Terry WD, Rosenberg SA (eds): Immunotherapy of Human Cancer. New York, Elsevier, 1981
177. Cunningham TJ, Schoenfeld D, Nathanson L et al: A controlled ECOG study of adjuvant therapy (BCG, BCG-DTIC) in patients with stage I and II malignant melanoma—1980. In Terry WD, Rosenberg SA (eds): Immunotherapy of Human Cancer. New York, Elsevier, 1981
178. Morton DL, Holmes EC, Eilber FR et al: Adjuvant immunotherapy of malignant melanoma: Results of a randomized trial in patients with lymph node metastases. In Terry WD, Rosenberg SA (eds): Immunotherapy of Human Cancer. New York, Elsevier, 1981
179. Terry WD, Hodes RJ, Rosenberg SA et al: Treatment of stage I and II malignant melanoma with adjuvant immunotherapy of chemotherapy: Preliminary analysis of a prospective randomized trial. In Terry WD, Rosenberg SA (eds): Immunotherapy of Human Cancer. New York, Elsevier, 1981
180. Spitler LE, Sagebiel R, Allen R et al: Levamisole in melanoma. In Terry WD, Rosenberg SA (eds): Immunotherapy of Human Cancer. New York, Elsevier, 1981
181. Wood WC, Cosimi AB, Carey RW et al: Randomized trial of adjuvant therapy for "high risk" primary malignant melanoma. Surgery 83:677–681, 1978
182. Wood WC, Cosimi AB, Carey RW et al: Adjuvant chemoimmunotherapy in stage I and II melanoma. In Terry WD, Rosenberg SA (eds): Immunotherapy of Human Cancer. New York, Elsevier, 1981
183. Quirt IC, Kersey PA, Baker MA et al: Adjuvant chemoimmunotherapy with DTIC and BCG in patients with poor prognosis primary malignant melanoma and completely resected recurrent melanoma. In Terry WD, Rosenberg SA (eds): Immunotherapy of Human Cancer. New York, Elsevier, 1981
184. McIllmurray MB, Embleton MJ, Reeves WG et al: Controlled trial of active immunotherapy in management of stage IIB malignant melanoma. Br Med J 1:540–542, 1977
185. Sanford BH, Codington JF: Further studies on the effect of neuraminidase on tumor cell transplantability. Tissue Antigens 1:153–161, 1971
186. Simmons RL, Aranha GV, Gunnarsson A et al: Active specific immunotherapy for advanced melanoma utilizing neuraminidase-treated autochthonous tumor cells. In Terry WD, Rosenberg SA (eds): Immunotherapy of Cancer: Present Status of Trials in Man, pp 123–133. New York, Raven Press, 1978
187. Wright PW, Hellstrom KE, Hellstrom I et al: Serotherapy of malignant melanoma. In Terry WD, Rosenberg SA (eds): Immunotherapy of Cancer: Present Status of Trials in Man, pp 135–143. New York, Raven Press, 1978
188. Gutterman JU, Hersh EM, Mavligit et al: Chemoimmunotherapy of disseminated malignant melanoma with BCG: Follow-up report. In Terry WD, Windhorst D (eds): Immunotherapy of Cancer: Present Status of Trials in Man, pp 103–112. New York, Raven Press, 1978
189. Beretta G: Controlled study with imidazole-carboxamide (DTIC), DTIC + Bacillus Calmette-Guerin (BCG), and DTIC + Corynebacterium parvum (CP) in advanced malignant melanoma. Reporting for the WHO Collaborating Centres for Evaluation of Methods of Diagnosis and Treatment of Melanoma. In Terry WD, Rosenberg SA (eds): Immunotherapy of Human Cancer. New York, Elsevier, 1981
190. Costanzi JJ: Chemotherapy and BCG in the treatment of disseminated malignant melanoma. In Terry WD, Windhorst D (eds): Immunotherapy of Cancer: Present Status of Trials in Man, pp 87–94. New York, Raven Press, 1978
191. Presant CA, Bartolucci AA, Smalley RV et al: Malignant Melanoma: Intravenous Corynebacterium parvum with DTIC and cyclophosphamide. In Terry WD, Rosenberg SA (eds): Immunotherapy of Human Cancer. New York, Elsevier, 1981
192. Mastrangelo MJ, Bellet RE, Berd D et al: A randomized prospective trial comparing Methyl-CCNU + Vincristine to Methyl- CCNU + Vincristine + BCG + Allogeneic Tumor Cells in patients with metastatic malignant melanoma. In Terry WD, Windhorst D (eds): Immunotherapy of Cancer.: Present Status of Trials in Man, pp 95–102. New York, Raven Press, 1978
193. Hayata Y, Ohbo K, Ogawa I et al: Immunotherapy for lung cancer cases using BCG or BCG cell-wall skeleton: Intratumoral injections. Gan Monogr 21:151–160, 1978
194. Holmes EC, Ramming KP, Golub SH et al: Intralesional BCG in pulmonary tumors. In Terry WD, Rosenberg SA (eds): Immunotherapy of Human Cancer. New York, Elsevier, 1981
195. Matthay RA, Mahler DA, Mitchell MS et al: 1981. Intratumoral BCG immunotherapy prior to surgery for carcinoma of the lung: Preliminary results. In Terry WD, Rosenberg SA (eds): Immunotherapy of Human Cancer. New York, Elsevier, 1981
196. Yamamura Y: Adjuvant immunotherapy of lung cancer with BCG cell wall skeleton. In Terry WD, Rosenberg SA (eds): Immunotherapy of Human Cancer. New York, Elsevier, 1981
197. Yamamura Y: Phase I study with nocardia rubra cell wall skeleton. In Terry WD, Rosenberg SA (eds): Immunotherapy of Human Cancer. New York, Elsevier, 1981
198. McKneally MF, Maver C, Kausel HW et al: Four year follow-up on the Albany experience with intrapleural BCG in lung cancer. In Terry WD, Rosenberg SA (eds): Immunotherapy of Human Cancer. New York, Elsevier, 1981
199. The National Lung Cancer Study Group. Surgical adjuvant immunotherapy in non-oat cell carcinoma. In Terry WD, Rosenberg SA (eds): Immunotherapy of Human Cancer. New York, Elsevier, 1981
200. Baldwin RW, Iles PB, Langman MJS et al: 1981. Intrapleural BCG in lung cancer treatment. In Terry WD, Rosenberg SA (eds): Immunotherapy of Human Cancer. New York, Elsevier, 1981
201. The Ludwig Lung Cancer Study Group. Intrapleural corynebacterium parvum as adjuvant therapy in operable bronchogenic non-small cell carcinoma: A preliminary report. In Terry WD, Rosenberg SA (eds): Immunotherapy of Human Cancer. New York, Elsevier, 1981
202. Wright PW, Hill LD, Peterson AV et al: Adjuvant immunotherapy with intrapleural BCG and levamisole in patients with resected, non-small cell lung cancer. In Terry WD, Rosenberg SA (eds): Immunotherapy of Human Cancer. New York, Elsevier, 1981
203. Amery WK, Cosemans J, Gooszen HC et al: Four-year results from double-blind study of adjuvant levamisole treatment in resectable lung cancer. In Terry WD, Rosenberg SA (eds): Immunotherapy of Human Cancer. New York, Elsevier, 1981
204. Anthony HM: The Yorkshire trial of adjuvant therapy with levamisole in surgical lung cancer. In Terry WD, Rosenberg SA (eds): Immunotherapy of Human Cancer. New York, Elsevier, 1981
205. Cohen MH, Chretien PB, Johnston-Early A et al: Thymosin

fraction V prolongs survival of intensively treated small cell lung cancer patients. In Terry WD, Rosenberg SA (eds): Immunotherapy of Human Cancer. New York, Elsevier, 1981
206. Reid JW, Perlin E, Oldham RK et al: Immunotherapy of carcinoma of the lung with intradermal BCG and allogeneic tumor cells: A clinical trial. In Terry WD, Rosenberg SA (eds): Immunotherapy of Human Cancer. New York, Elsevier, 1981
207. Hollinshead AC, Stewart THM, Herberman RB: Delayed hypersensitivity reactions to soluble membrane antigens of human malignant lung cells. J Natl Cancer Inst 52:327–338, 1974
208. Stewart THM, Hollinshead AC, Harris JE et al: Specific active immunotherapy of stage I lung cancer patients. In Terry WD, Rosenberg SA (eds): Immunotherapy of Human Cancer. New York, Elsevier, 1981
209. Takita H, Hollinshead AC, Bhayana JN et al: Adjuvant specific active immunotherapy of squamous cell lung carcinoma. In Terry WD, Rosenberg SA (eds): Immunotherapy of Human Cancer. New York, Elsevier, 1981
210. Klefstrom P, Holsti P, Grohn P et al: Combination of levamisole immunotherapy with conventional treatments in breast cancer. In Terry WD, Rosenberg SA (eds): Immunotherapy of Human Cancer. New York, Elsevier, 1981
211. Stephens EJW, Wood HF, Mason B: The influence of levamisole on the survival of patients with end-stage mammary carcinoma treated with chemotherapy. In Terry WD, Rosenberg SA (eds): Immunotherapy of Human Cancer. New York, Elsevier, 1981
212. Buzdar AU, Blumenschein GR, Hortobagyi GN et al: Adjuvant chemotherapy with 5-fluorouracil, Adriamycin, and Cyclophosphamide, with or without BCG immunotherapy in stage II or III breast cancer. In Terry WD, Rosenberg SA (eds): Immunotherapy of Human Cancer. New York, Elsevier, 1981
213. McCulloch PB, Poon M, Dent PB et al: A stratified randomized trial of 5 F. U., Adriamycin, and Cyclophosphamide alone or with BCG in stage IV breast cancer. In Terry WD, Rosenberg SA (eds): Immunotherapy of Human Cancer. New York, Elsevier, 1981
214. Gutterman JU, Cardenas JO, Blumenschein GR et al: Chemoimmunotherapy of advanced breast cancer: Prolongation of remission and survival with BCG. Br Med J 2:1222–1225, 1976
215. Hortobagyi GN, Gutterman JU, Blumenschein GR et al: Chemoimmunotherapy of advanced breast cancer with BCG. In Terry WD, Windhorst D (eds): Immunotherapy of Cancer: Present Status of Trials in Man, pp 655–668. New York, Raven Press, 1978
216. Rojas AF, Mickiewicz E, Feierstein JN et al: Levamisole in advanced human breast cancer. Lancet 1:211–215, 1976
217. Rojas AF, Feierstein JN, Glait HM et al: Levamisole action in breast cancer stage III. In Terry WD, Windhorst D (eds): Immunotherapy of Cancer: Present Status of Trials in Man, pp 635–645. New York, Raven Press, 1978
218. Pinsky CM, DeJager RL, Wittes RE et al: Corynebacterium parvum as adjuvant to combination chemotherapy in patients with advanced breast cancer: Preliminary results of a prospective randomized trial. In Terry WD, Windhorst D (eds): Immunotherapy of Cancer: Present Status of Trials in Man, pp 647–654. New York, Raven Press, 1978
219. Lacour J, Lacour F, Spira A et al: Adjuvant immunotherapy with Polyadenylic–Polyuridylic acid (Poly A Poly U) in operable breast cancer. In Terry WD, Rosenberg SA (eds): Immunotherapy of Human Cancer. New York, Elsevier, 1981
220. Verhaegen H, De Cree J, De Cock W et al: Levamisole therapy in patients with colorectal cancer. In Terry WD, Rosenberg SA (eds): Immunotherapy of Human Cancer. New York, Elsevier, 1981
221. Panettiere FJ, Chen TT: The SWOG colon adjuvant study of chemotherapy with and without oral BCG: An update. In Terry WD, Rosenberg SA (eds): Immunotherapy of Human Cancer. New York, Elsevier, 1981
222. Mavligit GM, Gutterman JU, Burgess MA et al: Prolongation of postoperative disease-free interval and survival in human colorectal cancer by BCG or BCG plus 5-fluorouracil. Lancet 1:871–876, 1976
223. Borden EC, Davis TE, Crowley JJ et al: Interim analysis of a trial of levamisole and 5-Fluorouracil in metastatic colorectal carcinoma. In Terry WD, Rosenberg SA (eds): Immunotherapy of Human Cancer. New York, Elsevier, 1981
224. Moertel CG, O'Connell MJ, Ritts RE et al: A controlled evaluation of combined immunotherapy (MER–BCG) and chemotherapy for advanced colorectal cancer. In Terry WD, Windhorst D (eds): Immunotherapy of Cancer: Present Status of Trials in Man, pp 573–586. New York, Raven Press, 1978
225. Engstrom PF, Paul AR, Catalano RB et al: Fluorouracil versus Fluorouracil + BCG in colorectal adenocarcinoma. In Terry WD, Windhorst D (eds): Immunotherapy of Cancer: Present Status of Trials in Man, pp 587–596. New York, Raven Press, 1978
226. Morales A, Ersil A: Adjuvant BCG immunotherapy in the prophylaxis and treatment of non-invasive bladder cancer. In Terry WD, Rosenberg SA (eds): Immunotherapy of Human Cancer. New York, Elsevier, 1981
227. Lamm DL, Thor DE, Harris SC et al: Intravesical and percutaneous BCG immunotherapy of recurrent superficial bladder cancer. In Terry WD, Rosenberg SA (eds): Immunotherapy of Human Cancer. New York, Elsevier, 1981
228. Pinsky CM, Camacho FJ, Kerr D et al: Treatment of superficial bladder cancer with intravesical Bacillus Calmette–Guerin (BCG). In Terry WD, Rosenberg SA (eds): Immunotherapy of Human Cancer. New York, Elsevier, 1981
229. Alberts DS, Mason NL, O'Toole R et al: A randomized trial of adriamycin-cyclophosphamide plus BCG versus adriamycin–cyclophosphamide therapy of advanced ovarian cancer. In Terry WD, Rosenberg SA (eds): Immunotherapy of Human Cancer. New York, Elsevier, 1981
230. DiSaia PJ, Gall S, Levy D et al: A preliminary report on the treatment of women with cervical cancer, stages IIB, IIIB, and IVA confined to the pelvis and/or periaortic nodes with radiotherapy alone versus radiotherapy plus immunotherapy (intravenous C-Parvum), phase III. In Terry WD, Rosenberg SA (eds): Immunotherapy of Human Cancer. New York, Elsevier, 1981
231. Gall SA, Creasman WT, Blessing JA et al: Chemoimmunotherapy in primary stage III ovarian epithelial cancer: A gynecological oncology group study. In Terry WD, Rosenberg SA (eds): Immunotherapy of Human Cancer. New York, Elsevier, 1981
232. Bier J, Bitter K, Pickartz H et al: Intratumoral therapy with BCG-cell-wall preparation in patients with head and neck cancer. In Terry WD, Rosenberg SA (eds): Immunotherapy of Human Cancer. New York, Elsevier, 1981
233. Pinsky CM, Hilal EY, Wanebo HJ et al: Randomized trial of levamisole in patients with squamous cell carcinoma of head and neck: Preliminary results. In Terry WD, Rosenberg SA (eds): Immunotherapy of Human Cancer. New York, Elsevier, 1981
234. Cheng V S-T, Suit HD, Wang CC et al: Clinical trial of C parvum (i. ln. and i.v.) and radiation therapy in the treatment of head and neck carcinoma. In Terry WD, Rosenberg SA (eds): Immunotherapy of Human Cancer. New York, Elsevier, 1981
235. Eilber FR, Morton DL: Specific and nonspecific immunotherapy as an adjunct to chemotherapy and surgery in skeletal and soft tissue carcinoma. In Terry WD, Rosenberg SA (eds): Immunotherapy of Human Cancer. New York, Elsevier, 1981

Section 2

Hyperthermia

GEORGE M. HAHN

Historically, attempts to treat malignancies by elevating body temperatures go back many years.[1,2] In part, the rationale for this approach is based on the well-documented occurrences of spontaneous remissions in patients who had episodes of high fevers. This subject was reviewed extensively by Selawry and co-workers, who found that out of 450 reported spontaneous remissions of histologically proven malignancies, 150 were associated with development of acute fevers resulting from concurrent diseases such as malaria or typhus.[3] Similarly, Huth observed that one-third of spontaneous remissions of lymphomas in children was also associated with fevers.[4] Lymphoma remissions were never of long duration, but several "cures" of carcinomas and sarcomas have been described. Not surprisingly, such results have led to attempts to utilize intentional infections or other pyrogens for the induction of high fevers in patients with malignancies. Probably the most prominent of these studies was carried out by Coley.[5-7] Quite impressive results were obtained by him through the use of bacterial toxins, particularly against osteosarcomas.[8] Whether or not these successes resulted exclusively or even primarily from the induction of fevers or perhaps involved a nonspecific host immune response is a matter of some controversy. Whatever the reasons for the observed antitumor effects, these results have been the motivational basis for a variety of experiments on animal tumors to determine the effects of heat on transplanted and spontaneous cancers. Prominent among the older studies are those of Westermark, Jares and Warren, Overgaard and Okkels, and Crile.[9-14] Particularly, Crile's rather remarkable studies showed that some transplanted tumors could be destroyed without accompanying destruction of normal tissue, provided the appropriate temperature–time profile was employed.

BIOLOGICAL BASIS

While the phenomenological studies just described, without doubt, maintained and accentuated interest in hyperthermia as a tool against neoplasia, the current interest in this modality of treatment is based on more fundamental biological studies. These have demonstrated that exposure of cells to elevated temperatures generates survival curves not too different from those seen for irradiated cells. There is some evidence, though controversial, that the process of malignant transformation may be invariably accompanied by some level of heat sensitization.[15] There exists clear evidence that the milieu in the interior of some tumors, characterized as it is by low pH and low oxygen and nutrient availability, causes cells to become much more rapidly inactivated by temperatures in excess of about 42°C than are cells in normal tissue. Furthermore, equally good evidence has shown that heat accentuates the effects of irradiation and many chemotherapeutic agents by a variety of mechanisms. Some of the key experimental results will be reviewed here.

Initial survival curves from heat-treated mammalian cells were obtained by Westra and Westra and Dewey, who showed that survival curves of Chinese hamster cells, when exposed to elevated temperatures for various lengths of time, had a shoulder followed by a portion of the survival curve that was linear when plotted against the logarithm of surviving fraction.[16,17] Above 43°C, the time required to inactivate cells to a given survival level was reduced by a factor of two for every degree of increased temperature. A biologically fascinating modification of temperature response, which may also have considerable clinical implications, was shown by Henle and Leeper, and Gerner and Schneider.[18,19] Chinese hamster cells and HeLa cells, when exposed to a nonlethal dose of heat, subsequently develop a transient thermal tolerance. During this tolerant state, which may last up to several days, the cells are appreciably more heat resistant than cells which have never been exposed to elevated temperatures. Recently, it has also been demonstrated that thermotolerance can be induced *in vivo,* both in tumors and in normal tissue.[20,21] Several studies have shown that pH values lower than about 7.0 cause cells to become very heat sensitive.[22-25] Survival curves obtained by Gerweck are shown in Fig. 48-1. In addition to sensitizing cells, low pH appears to delay or eliminate the development of thermal tolerance. Metabolic deprivation sensitizes cells to heat, as does chronic hypoxia.[26,27] However, cells made acutely hypoxic respond in the same way as do

FIG. 48-1. Survival of CHO cells heated at 42° C. These survival curves demonstrate the development of thermal tolerance at pH 7.0 as evidenced by the reduced efficiency of cell killing after about 120 minutes of exposure. At pH 6.7, all killing is increased even at short exposure times and the development of tolerance is either inhibited or delayed. Many studies have indicated that the interstitial fluid in tumors is at a lower point, perhaps as low as 6.7, than that of normal tissue which is at pH 7.4.[24]

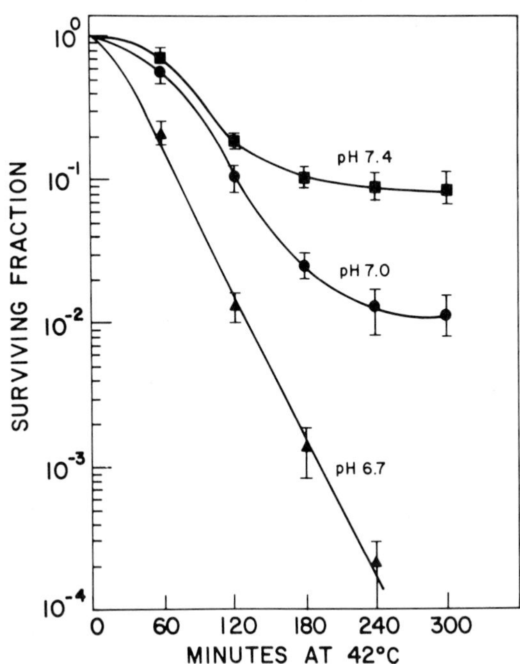

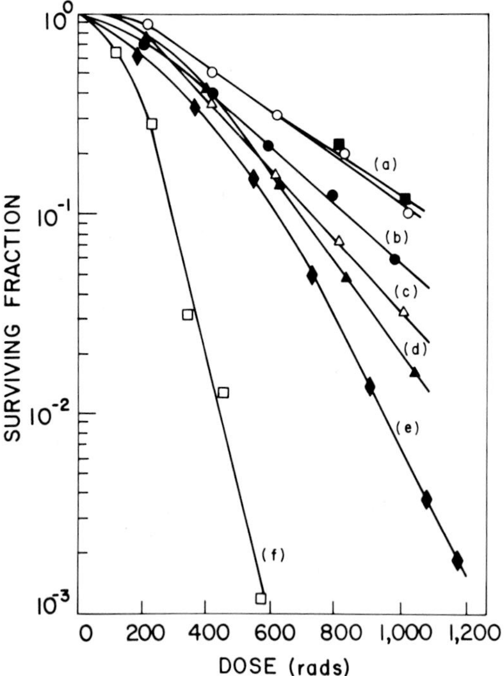

FIG. 48-2. Survival curves of Chinese hamster cells (V-79) irradiated at a dose rate of 3.3 rads/min (a-d, f) at various temperatures or at 360 rads/min at 0°(e). a: 34 and 37°; b: 39°; c: 40°; d: 41°; f:42°. The increasing cytotoxicity with increasing temperature between 37 and 41° is interpreted as progressive inhibition of recovery from sub-lethal damage. Such recovery is completely blocked at 0° (curve e). At 42° there is toxicity from an x-ray and heat interaction which presumably is in addition to inhibition of recovery.[29]

FIG. 48-3. EMT-6 cells exposed *in vitro* to x-irradiation alone or in conjunction with 43° C (60 min). a: x-ray only, b: x-ray immediately followed by heat, c: heat immediately followed by x-ray. The effect of heat alone is shown by the intercepts of (a) and (b) with the 0 dose axis. In some other cell lines the relative sensitizing effects of heating before or after x-ray are reversed.[31]

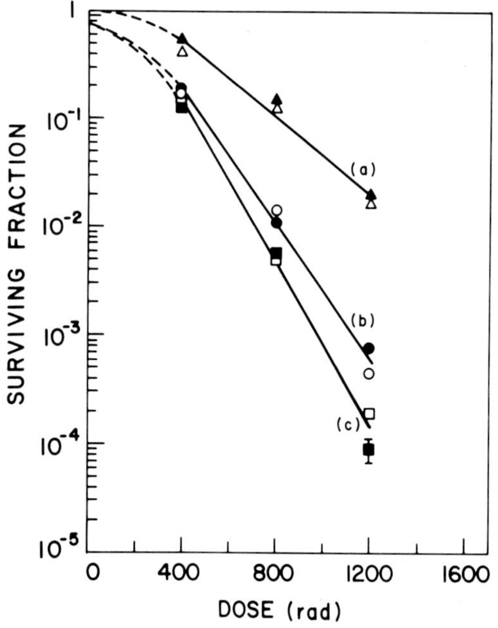

well-oxygenated cells.[28] Under no circumstances does hypoxia seem to confer heat resistance on cells, in marked contrast to the protection that lack of oxygen provides against ionizing radiations.

The radiation response of mammalian cells is modified by heat in a variety of ways. At low dose rates, temperatures in the region of 39° to 41°, which by themselves kill few if any cells, sharply increase the effectiveness of irradiation (Fig. 48-2).[29]

This has been interpreted as demonstrating that heat interferes with recovery from sublethal damage.[30] Indeed, direct test by a two fraction experiment with cells held at the elevated temperature between roentgenographic exposures verified this hypothesis. At higher temperatures, the radiation response is modified, even though irradiation may be at high dose rates.[16,17] Sensitization is maximum if the irradiation is carried out during the heating period. However, heating immediately before or after radiation still produces considerable potentiation (Fig. 48-3). An increasing time interval between the two insults decreases the magnitude of this interaction.[31] Elevated temperatures can also modify or abolish recovery from potentially lethal damage, that is, the increase in survival of cells kept in a noncycling environment after the exposure to radiation.[32] Finally, hyperthermia can accentuate the cytotoxic efficacy of many drugs, sometimes dramatically so.[33] This increased effectiveness may manifest itself as a continuous change of the rate at which cells are inactivated (most alkylating agents, nitrosoureas, or *cis*-platinum) or there may be a threshold temperature, 43°C for Chinese hamster cells, which must be exceeded before marked synergism can be demonstrated (bleomycin, doxorubicin, amphotericin-B). However, depending upon timing of the treatments, heat exposure may also render cells more drug resistant (actinomycin-D, doxorubicin). There are also many compounds which, at low doses, are nontoxic at 37°C but at similar concentration become potent cell killers at elevated temperatures. Among such "thermal sensitizers" are drugs rich in sulfhydryl groups, cysteamine for example, and several agents whose only known common effect on cells is that of "fluidizing" membranes, such as aliphatic alcohols and various anesthetics.[31,34-36] Examples of several temperature-drug interactions are shown in Fig. 48-4.

ANIMAL EXPERIMENTS

The cellular experiments, particularly those involving pH and nutrients, have indicated that many cells in solid tumors should be more at risk to heat than cells of normal tissue; and, in fact, studies with a variety of mouse tumor systems have shown that heating periods of 10 minutes to 1 hour at temperatures ranging from 42°C to 45°C can cause tumor regression or tumor cures.[11,37-39] Furthermore, these studies have demonstrated that it is the temperature–time profile *per se* that is important and not the way temperature is generated. Results for four tumor systems treated identically are shown in Fig. 48-5. The spectrum of heat sensitivities of various tumors is obvious. While a 30-minute exposure at 45°C of EMT 6 tumors cures 100% of animals, a similar exposure of mice bearing a transplanted radiation-induced fibrosarcoma

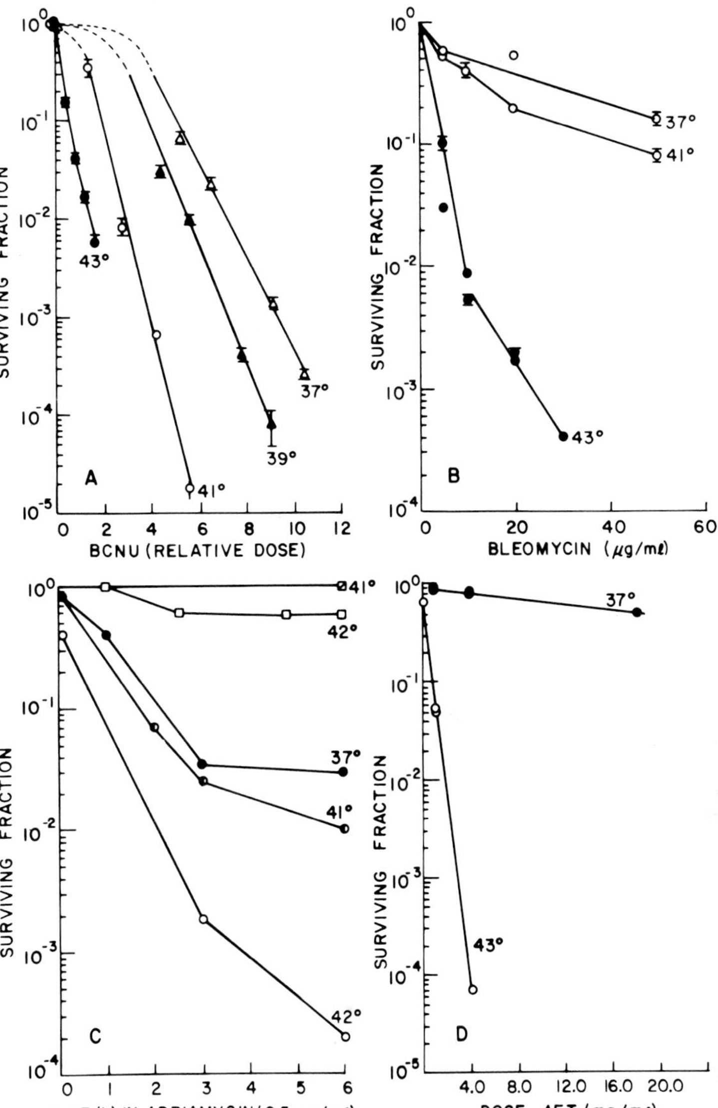

FIG. 48-4. Thermochemotherapy: Survival curves of cells exposed *in vitro* to drugs at various temperatures. Panels A, B, and D show dose response curves of Chinese hamster cells (HA1) exposed to graded doses of drugs for 60 min at the indicated temperature. Panel C is a time response of EMT-6 cells exposed to a fixed dose (0.5 μg/ml) of adriamycin. In panel C, the top two curves marked 41° and 42° are survival curves obtained in the absence of drug. In panel A the dose is presented in terms of relative units of BCNU; these units are approximately 1 μg/ml, but are corrected for drug inactivation by hydrolysis at the temperature of interest. 1-(2-chloroethyl)-3-cyclohexyl-1-nitrosourea (BCNU) is an example of a drug whose rate of cell inactivation follows simple Arrhenius kinetics. Bleomycin and adriamycin both exhibit thresholds at 42–43° C. S-(2-aminoethyl)isothiouronium bromide HCL (AET) is an example of a thermic sensitizer, showing little or no cell killing at 37°, but major cytotoxic activity at elevated temperatures.[33]

(RIF) rarely if ever cures any of the mice. However, a large number of temporary regressions are seen even for the heat-resistant tumors.

Studies from Robinson's group have shown clearly that the influence of a relatively mild heat exposure on radiation sensitivity of tumors can be appreciable.[40] In Fig 48-6 the change of a single roentgen dose required to cure 50% of animals bearing a mammary carcinoma (TCD_{50}) is shown. While a dose of over 5000 rad is required to cure 50% of unheated tumors, a 1 hour exposure to 43°C reduces that dose by a factor of about three. Since all mouse tumors examined to date contain hypoxic cells, Robinson's data implies clearly that the combined heat–radiation treatment was extremely effective in dealing with these. This conclusion is strengthened by results showing that for fractioned therapy, the advantage of heating is reduced. However, even there Faria and Hahn have shown that two treatments of 44.5°C (45 min), which cause very little normal tissue damage, can reduce the TCD_{50} of a fractionated course of radiotherapy by about 2000 rad.[41] In that study the timing of the heat treatments was such as to utilize hyperthermia and irradiation as independent modalities; the possibility that heat sensitized tumor or normal cells was minimized. This study indicated that hyperthermia and ionizing radiations are most effective against different components of the tumor cell population. In other words, with respect to tumor eradication the two modalities are quite complementary in function. Furthermore, consistent with an earlier finding of Field and associates, the kinetics of heat-induced normal tissue damage were very different from those seen after irradiation.[42] This may very well mean that the two modalities induce different types of tissue toxicities.

There are relatively few studies that analyze the quantitative response of murine tumors after thermochemotherapy. Typical results obtained by Marmor and co-workers with the heat-resistant RIF tumors are shown in Fig. 48-7.[43,80] In general, drugs that show more than additive cell killing *in vitro* also show more than additive antitumor effects, providing drug and heat treatments are given simultaneously. Drugs which offer the greatest potential in combination with localized

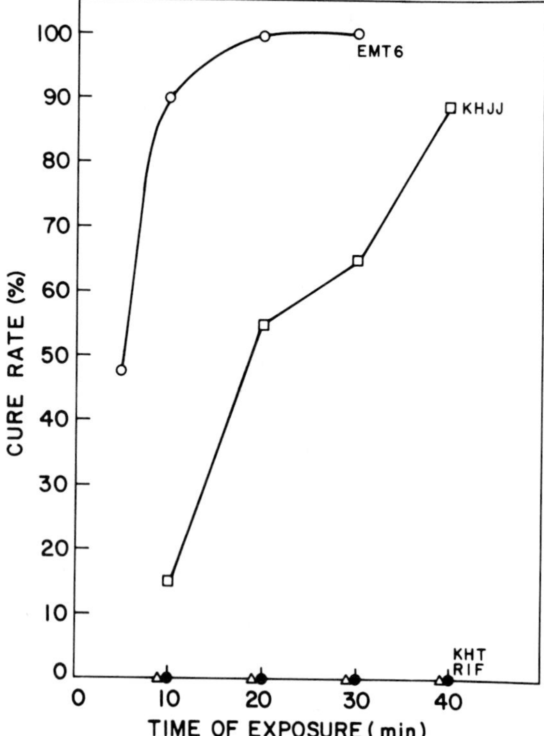

FIG. 48-5. Cure rates of several murine tumors treated with localized hyperthermia (44°) under standardized conditions. Tumors were implanted into the flanks of either Balb/c mice (EMT-6 and KHJJ) or C_3H mice (KHT, RIF). Neoplasms weighing between 100–150 mg were uniformly heated by currents induced by a capacitively coupled radiofrequency system at 13.56 MHz. Although KHT and RIF tumors exposed for 40 min regressed routinely, these always regrew within a few days after treatment. EMT-6 and KHJJ data[47] (1978). KHT and RIF data unpublished.

FIG. 48-6. Reduction by heat of a single x-ray dose required to cure 50% of tumor-bearing mice. C_3H mice carrying a transplantable mammary carcinoma were heated for one hour at the indicated temperatures. Irradiation was carried out during heating in such a way that the heating periods before and after irradiation were equalized. The TCD_{50} is the x-ray dose required to permanently sterilize the tumors of 50% of the experimental animals.[40]

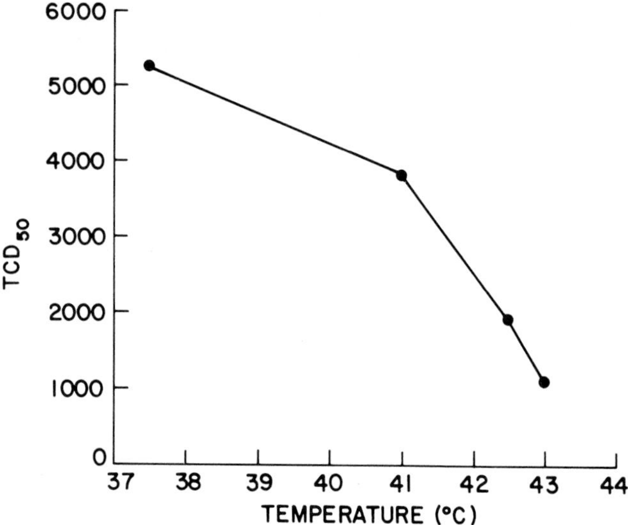

heating are: BCNU, bleomycin, *cis*-platinum, and Methyl-CCNU.

The problem of normal tissue damage, either by heat itself or by heat plus radiation, has been the subject of several studies, although none exists examining drug–heat interactions.[44] The design of studies was such as to yield almost surely conservative answers. The reason for this is that the mouse tissues chosen, skin and ear, and also cartilage in the tail of the rat, may very likely be unusually heat sensitive. For example, mouse ear is normally at a temperature of about 29°C. Cells adapted to such a low temperature tend to become quite heat sensitive, as was demonstrated in tissue culture experiments.[45] Additionally, the skin can be cooled during treatment to prevent it from reaching temperatures which would lead to thermal damage.

In any case, what has been demonstrated by the normal tissue studies is that temperature–time profiles that have the potential of being tumoricidal may also leave some normal tissue damage. These results have been analyzed by Field and associates.[42,81] Obviously, if hyperthermia is to be an effective tool for the treatment of cancers, the question of normal tissue damage becomes extremely important. Perhaps for these studies the mouse (or rat) is an unfortunate experimental model. Heating of tumors in these animals is relatively simple, and uniform heating of such tumors requires only unsophisticated equipment. The tumor can be placed in a position where it can be heated easily, and the site of the tumor can be chosen to coincide with the capability of the heating equipment. The mouse itself appears to be unusually heat sensitive. Whole body studies have shown that exposures to 41°C or 42°C temperature of mice for periods exceeding 1 hour turn are almost invariably fatal. By this criterion at least, large animals, including humans, are considerably more heat resistant.

For these reasons and others, studies with large animals appear to be highly desirable. Unfortunately, there are only a few of these in the literature. Dickson and co-workers showed that radio frequency heating of the VX 2 carcinoma in rabbits can lead to a high percentage of cures.[46] (The technique of radio frequency heating will be described in a later section.) Two studies have examined the effects of localized heating on spontaneous tumors on dogs and cats.[47,48] The findings of Marmor and associates are illustrated in Table 48-9. Both complete and partial remissions were induced by the heat treatments. These were 43°C for one hour, repeated six times over a 3 week period. Most of the animals had been treated previously, unsuccessfully, by one or two other modalities and were then referred to Stanford by veterinarians on the San Francisco peninsula. Interestingly, the histologies of the tumors and the type of "patients" closely mirror those seen in Phase I human studies. Tumors were heated by ultrasound and examples of temperature distributions obtained are shown in Fig. 48-8. Perhaps the most important finding of the study was that a treatment protocol which can induce complete remissions in the sizable number of dog and cat tumors, even in advanced "patients," appear to cause no serious normal tissue damage. Precaution is in order, however, because follow-up was short in most of these animals, usually only a few months. Any long-term normal tissue damage would not have been detected.

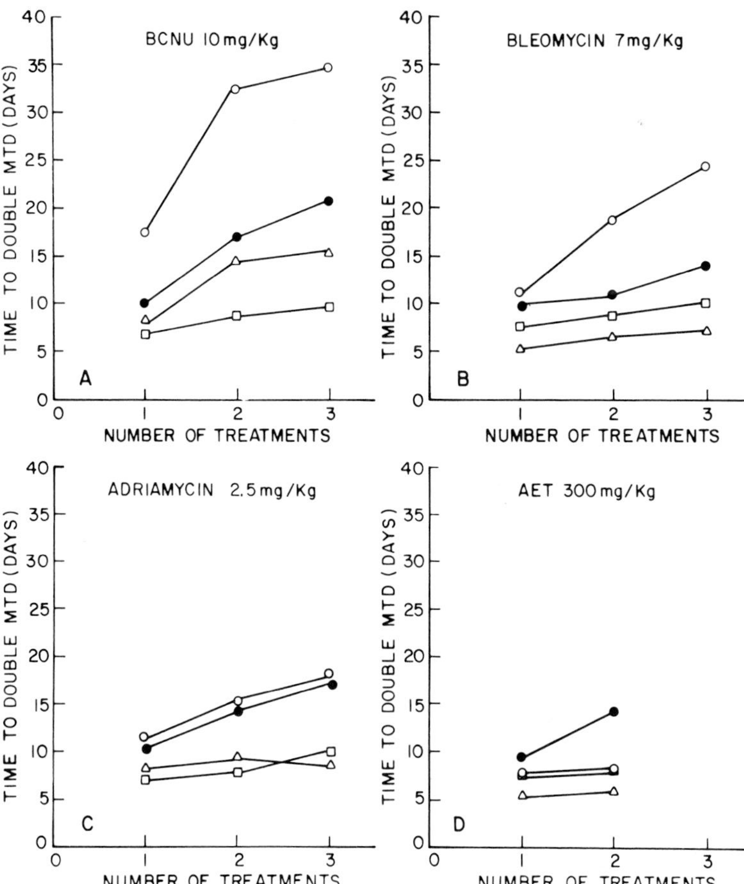

FIG. 48-7. Thermochemotherapy: Response of RIF tumors to combinations of hyperthermia and drugs. C_3H mice bearing RIF tumors, weighing between 100 and 150 mg were heated to indicated temperatures as described in Fig. 5. Once equilibrium temperature was reached, some animals were injected with drug, others with diluent only. A final group was heated but injected with drug 24 hr after heating. Tumor dimensions were measured daily and mean tumor diameter (MTD) calculated. The time required for MTDs to double is plotted on the ordinate. □——□ heat (43°, 30 min) and diluent only. △——△ drug and diluent; ●——● heat and drug separated by 24 hr; ○——○ heat and drug given simultaneously. The combined treatment shows clear potentiation for BCNU and bleomycin; none for adriamycin or AET at the dosages employed.[53]

What about other adverse effects of hyperthermia? There are two studies which indicate that localized heating may accelerate the rate of dissemination of cancer.[49,50] Neither of these is very convincing. In the experiments of Dickson and Ellis, 90% of rats bearing Yoshida sarcoma died of their hyperthermic treatment. In the few survivors, the duration of survival was much reduced from unheated controls (16± 2.5 days *versus* 26± 3.1 days). However, the treatment, which killed 90% of the animals, must have severely traumatized the survivors. The animals may, therefore, have had a reduced capacity of mounting a host response against the disseminated Yoshida sarcoma cells. Very likely, that impairment, rather than the effect of hyperthermia *per se*, was responsible for the result. The second study employed retrospective controls, which were not handled in the same way as the hyperthermic group. It is well known that manual

TABLE 48-9. Treatment of spontaneous tumors in dogs and cats with ultrasound

PATHOLOGY	COURSES	ANIMALS	COMPLETE REGRESSION	PARTIAL REGRESSION	NO EFFECT
Squamous cell carcinoma	8	7	3	4	1
Fibrosarcoma	5	5	0	1	4
Perianal adenocarcinoma	3	3	0	1	2
Mastocytoma	2	1	0	2	0
Osteogenic sarcoma	1	1	0	0	1
Mammary carcinoma	1	1	0	0	1
Liposarcoma	1	1	0	0	1
Hemangiosarcoma	1	1	0	1	0
TOTAL	22	20	3	9	10
PERCENT (all courses)			14	41	45

(Marmor J, Pounds D, Hahn N et al: Treating spontaneous tumors in dogs and cats by ultrasound-induced hyperthermia. Int J Radiat Oncol Biol Phys 4:967–973, 1978)

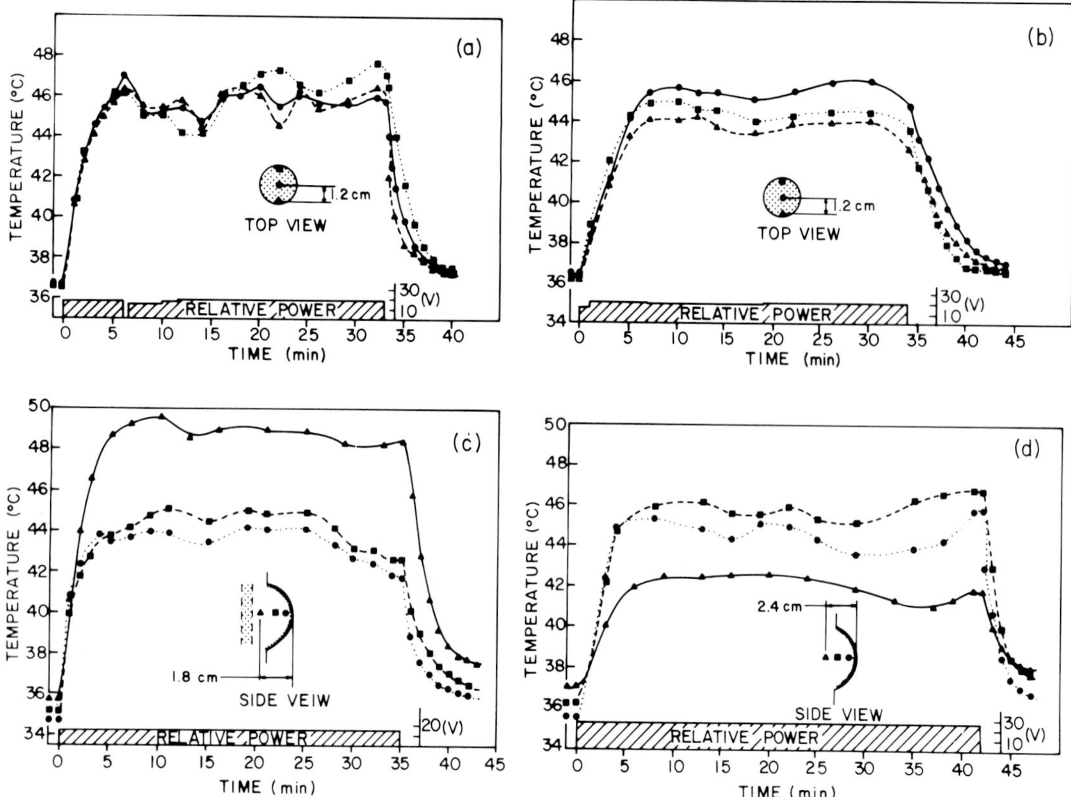

FIG. 48-8. Temperature distributions in human tumors. Lesions were heated with ultrasound (2 MHz, app 1.5 W/cm^2) and temperature measured by thermocouples. Panels a and b show horizontal, panels b and c vertical distributions; a and c, squamous cell carcinoma metastatic to scalp, b and d squamous cell carcinoma of the neck. In panel a, note how the temperature distribution is modified by the presence of bone.[43]

manipulation of tumor-bearing sites can increase the rate of metastasis. There are three studies which show either no such effect or a *reduced* rate of metastasis resulting from localized heating, though Yerushalmi found an increased incidence of metastases after *whole body* hyperthermia.[51-53] This important area deserves more attention than it has seen in the past.

HUMAN STUDIES

This section is divided into two parts: whole body and regional or localized hyperthermia.

WHOLE BODY HYPERTHERMIA

Recent attempts to use whole body heating for the treatment of widely disseminated cancers are due to Pettigrew and his associates.[54-56] In the United States, most of the early work was that of Larkin and Bull and their groups.[57-59] In general, all investigators report a fair number of objective responses (Table 48-10, showing published results from Larkin's group), though most of these appear to be of short durations.

Perhaps because of these short-term remissions, attempts have been made to combine whole body hyperthermia with either localized radiation therapy or with chemotherapy. Typical treatment regimens consisted of at least two hours at a temperature of 41.5°C to 42°C. Higher temperatures are said to involve an unacceptable degree of risk to the patients due to brain damage. For those also receiving radiation therapy, at least four such hyperthermia exposures were carried out. Again citing data from Larkin's results, chemotherapy with 5-FU, DTIC, and cyclophosphamide seemed to increase the rate of objective responses (59% *versus* 52%), though a larger number of patients will be needed to establish statistical significance. Analysis of biochemical and hematological data indicated that for the three drugs employed in the study, no increase in toxicity was observed for the combined modalities over that seen with heat alone. Problems encountered at the maximum temperature tolerated (42°C) centered primarily on liver damage, particularly in patients with histories of alcoholism. At least two fatalities were attributable to extensive liver necrosis.

REGIONAL OR LOCALIZED HYPERTHERMIA

Localized hyperthermia is not limited to 42°C. In fact, some data indicate that considerably higher temperatures (perhaps 45°C or even higher) may be desirable.[60] Reports on studies involving hyperthermia alone as a mode of treating cancer patients are rare. Additionally, some of the published data are difficult to evaluate, either because of insufficient detail about

TABLE 48-10. (*A*) Typical results achieved with whole body hyperthermia

PRIMARY SITE	NUMBER OF PATIENTS	RESPONSE		
		Objective	*Subjective*	*None*
Lung	22	6	4	8
Melanoma	13	8		5
Kidney	7	1		6
Colon	8	3	1	3
Prostate	5	2	1	2
Stomach	4	1	2	1
Soft-tissue sarcoma	4	2		2
Hematological	4	4		
Breast	2	1	1	
Pancreas	2		1	1
Osteosarcoma	2		1	1
Ovary	1			
Small intestine	1			
Thyroid	1	1		
Head and Neck	1	1		
Multiple myeloma	1	1		
TOTAL	78	31	11	29

(*B*) Response rates of treatment with total body hyperthermia alone or in combination

	NUMBER OF PATIENTS	NUMBER RESPONDING	PERCENT RESPONSE
TBH* alone	42	22	52
TBH and drugs	29	17	59
TBH and radiation	4	2	50
TBH and immunotherapy	6	4	67

* TBH, total-body hyperthermia
(Larkin J: A clinical investigation of total-body hyperthermia as cancer therapy. Cancer Res 39:2252–2254, 1979)

methods of heating or thermometry, or because of the rather large claims made on the basis of very little data. (One such paper is modestly entitled "The cure of cancer: a preliminary hypothesis.")[61] Marmor and associates have examined the effects of ultrasound induced hyperthermia on localized, surface accessible malignancies.[53] Equipment limitations severely restricted the study. Tumors that could be heated adequately were limited to 4 cm in diameter and 3 cm in depth. Temperature measurement was by means of thermocouples embedded in 29-gauge needles. These were inserted into the tumors and the temperature was monitored continuously. A partial response was defined as a 50% (or greater) reduction in tumor mass lasting at least 2 weeks, while a complete response was recorded if there was clinical disappearance of the lesion for a similar minimum time. Treatment was 30 minutes at temperatures between 43°C and 45°C; a course consisted of six treatments. Tumor sites were primarily head and neck, with squamous cell carcinoma the most frequently encountered histology. All patients had had extensive therapy before being given hyperthermia; frequently, tumors were local recurrences in areas that had been heavily irradiated.

Overall response rate was 54%, with a complete response rate of 12%; these results are summarized in Table 48-11. Adverse effects, except for minor, local burns at the site of thermocouple insertions, were essentially nil. This was true even in patients whose tumor was located in areas that had received up to 11,000 rad of radiation.[47] The response rate of tumors in irradiated areas tended to be higher than that of lesions in previously unirradiated areas. Multiple courses of six heat treatments each were well tolerated; no additional normal tissue damage was observed in patients receiving retreatment. However, the same caution is appropriate here as was in the outbred animal study; follow-up was short, usually a few months (maximum about 2 years), so that long-term effects again may not have been observed. Very similar overall results were observed by Kim and Hahn, who utilized radio frequency induced currents for heating.[62] These investigators also compared effects of heat plus radiation with that of radiation alone. The response rate to the combined treatments was appreciably higher than that for radiotherapy alone (Table 48-12). Furthermore, these authors state that "patients who were treated with conventional fractionation, 200 to 300 rad/treatment, showed no disproportionate skin reaction from the radiation therapy alone."[62]

Chemotherapy in combination with hyperthermia has seen primary use for the perfusion of extremities, particularly in melanoma patients. Two groups having done such work extensively are those of Cavalieri and of Stehlin.[63–67] A typical technique is that described by Tonak and co-workers.[68] For the perfusion of lower extremities, the iliac artery and vein are first exposed. These vessels are then cannulated and connected with an oxygenator. The isolated extremity can now be perfused utilizing a pump oxygenator in series with

TABLE 48-11. Objective Tumor Responses Following Localized Ultrasound Hyperthermia of Superficial Human Neoplasms

HISTOLOGY	PRIMARY SITE	NUMBER OF PATIENTS	NUMBER OF COURSES OF TREAT-MENT	RESPONSES CR(%)	PR(%)	NE(%)
Squamous cell carcinoma	Head and neck	9	12	1(8)	7(58)	4(33)
	Lung	1	1	0	1	0
Adenocarcinoma	Ovary	2	2	0	1	1
	Breast	1	2	0	0	2
	Uterus	1	1	0	1	0
	Nose	1	1	0	0	1
Lymphomas	DHL	2	2	0	0	2
	Mycosis fungoides	1	2	2	0	0
Melanoma		1	1	0	0	1
Medullary carcinoma	Thyroid	1	1	0	1	0
Neurofibrosarcoma		1	1	0	0	1
TOTAL		21	26	3(12)	11(42)	12(46)

CR—Complete Response: clinical disappearance of tumor within the heated area: PR—Partial Response: >50% decrease in tumor volume within the heated area: NE—No Effect: <50% decrease in tumor volume, stasis or growth of tumor within the heated area. DHL—Diffuse Histiocytic Lymphoma.

(Marmor J, Kozak D, Hahn G: Effects of systemically administered bleomycin or Adriamycin with local hyperthermia on primary tumor and lung metastases. Cancer Treat Rep 63:1279–1290, 1979)

TABLE 48-12 Combination hyperthermia and radiation therapy

HISTOLOGY	NUMBER OF PATIENTS	COMPLETE RESPONSE RT	RFH + RT	MEDIAN FOLLOW-UP (Months)
Mycosis fungoides*	14	2/12	10/12	18
Lymphoma cutis*	5	1/5	4/5	12
Kaposi sarcoma*	7	3/7	4/7	18
Malignant melanoma†	22	5/19	19/22	9
Chondrosarcoma†	1	0/1	1/1	7
Others†	5	1/3	3/5	6
TOTAL	54	12/49 (26%)	42/54 (78%)	

RT—radiation therapy
RFH—radio frequency heating

* In these radiation sensitive tumors, regressions were routinely seen in both groups. In the column headed RT, the fraction of lesions which did not recur during follow-up period is indicated. Under RFH + RT are listed the number of similarly non-recurring responses, plus the number of cases where recurrences were observed, but at later times than in matched lesions receiving RT only.

† For these relatively radiation resistant tumors, complete regressions are tabulated without regard to time of possible recurrence.

(Kim J, Hahn E: Clinical and biological studies of localized hyperthermia. Cancer Res 39:2258–2261, 1979)

a heat exchanger. Stehlin advocates continuous monitoring of both blood and muscle temperature, with the latter held to a maximum of 40°C, while blood is raised to 43.3°C.[65] Drugs used include melphalan, and melphalan plus actinomycin-D.[67,68] Impressive long-term survival data of melanoma patients have been provided by Stehlin's group. Their experience in treatment of this disease with hyperthermic perfusion goes back to 1967 (Table 48–13). Thermochemotherapy perfusion of extremities appears to be a safe, useful procedure for melanomas, osteogenic sarcomas, and soft tissue sarcomas. Very surprisingly, the literature contains no reports on combinations of local heating (as opposed to regional) with chemotherapy, either with curative or palliative intent.

TECHNICAL ASPECTS OF HYPERTHERMIA

INDUCTION OF HYPERTHERMIA

Whole body heating techniques described in the literature range from the coating of patients with paraffin, coupled with breathing of hot air, to the utilization of water blankets, to insulation of patients' metabolic heat and the addition of external heat to skin tolerance by a high-flow, low-pressure water suit controlled by a microprocessor, to whole body perfusion by extracorporeally heated blood.[54,55,57,59,69] While some of the systems have become quite sophisticated, employing feedback loops actuated by one or several sensors, conceptually and technically, whole body heating presents relatively few difficulties. Similarly, regional hyperthermic perfusion, as described in the last section, is carried out routinely by the groups mentioned, as well as others. It also presents no overwhelming obstacles.

The major technical problems existing today are associated with localized heating. At the same time, localized heating either by itself or as an adjunct to conventional modalities, offers the greatest possibilities for improving the treatment of cancer. One of the major reasons why this appears to be the case relates to the low net blood exchange rate between many tumors and their adjacent normal tissues. Blood flow values in many tumors, particularly large tumors, appear to be reduced by factors of two or three from that of normal tissue.[70,71] If heating is accomplished by deposition of energy, then even in the absence of preferential absorption, the tumor should rise to a higher temperature than its environment, because blood flow accounts for about 80% of heat transfer in normal tissue.

Heating of arbitrary volumes of tissue involves not only energy deposition in the tumor, but equally important, sparing of normal tissue to the point where the danger of creating unwanted hot spots is negligible. There are two physical approaches for appropriately heating deep-seated tumors: electromagnetic and ultrasound. Each of these has its advantages and disadvantages. For a more detailed discussion see reference 72. In general, ultrasound appears to be optimal for the precise heating of volumes up to 5 × 5 × 5 cm³ and at depths up to 15 cm. (However, lung and perhaps brain lesions cannot be heated with equipment currently being constructed.) Two systems to do this have recently been developed: one jointly by Stanford and the Hewlett-Packard Corporation; the other at MIT.[73] The former involves six transducers, operating at about 300 KHz optically focused and aligned by way of an ultrasound reflection system. The other is a sophisticated, computer-controlled scanning unit which, in principle, can be used to heat volumes of almost arbitrary shape (though not arbitrary volume). Both units are currently undergoing clinical evaluations.

Electromagnetic apparati vary from microwave units operating anywhere between 100 and 2200 MHz, to capacitively or inductively coupled radio frequency current generators. These can operate at frequencies down to about 400 KHz. In some situations, the implanting of electrodes for direct-current heating is quite feasible.[74] This is particularly attractive for combined hyperthermia–brachytherapy.[48] Here the radioactive implants can also serve as electrodes. There are now several commercial units available, both microwave and radio frequency, though with one or two possible exceptions, these have not undergone extensive clinical tests. The availability of electromagnetic heating equipment is changing so rapidly that any details presented here would very likely be outdated by publication time.

THERMOMETRY

Currently all temperature-measuring equipment utilizes invasive techniques.[75,76] Thermistors and thermocouples implanted in small (29-gauge) needles are commercially available. These are inserted directly into the tissue of interest and perform quite satisfactorily when used in conjunction with ultrasound. However, metallic probes pose special problems for electromagnetic heating devices. Eddy currents generated on the surface of embedded needles can induce enough noise into the electronics of the thermometer to introduce errors of several degrees' magnitude. This problem can be minimized by placing the needles at right angles to anticipated current flow, by appropriate filtering of the thermistors' or thermocouples' output signal and by carefully shielding all open leads, and particularly by the use of high-resistance leads. Another difficulty, frequently not appreciated, is the distortion and concentration of current flow in the immediate neighborhood of any metallic sensor. The latter might read the "correct" temperature, that is, the temperature in its vicinity but, because of field distortion, the temperature might not be representative of the value even at a small distance away from the probe. For these reasons, several nonmetallic, nondisturbing probes have been developed. Some of these either are, or soon will become, commercially available.[76,82] All of these employ fiber optics to introduce a test beam of light onto either liquid or solid crystals, and from the magnitude of the reflected light beam, also obtained by fiber optic techniques, the temperature at the sensor can be deduced. The biggest problem today is size; probes of less than about 1 mm in diameter have yet to be constructed.

The ideal temperature sensing unit would be noninvasive. In principle, the estimation of temperature changes is possible from ultrasound velocity measurements. Several investigators are currently performing studies to determine the feasibility of combining velocity measurements with computerized reconstruction tomography in order to produce two- (or three-) dimensional maps of temperature distributions.[77–79] Obviously, such data, if produced on-line during treatment, could aid immensely in the hyperthermic treatment of tumors. Unfortunately, it is likely that it will be several years before an instrument of this type could be available for clinical evaluation.

TABLE 48-13. 5-Year Survivals of Melanoma Patients Treated with Perfusions of Melphalan at Elevated Temperatures

STAGE OF DISEASE	NUMBER OF PATIENTS	SURVIVAL RATE (%)
I	70	86.3 from perfusion
II, IIIA, IIIB and IIIAB	73	52.5 from perfusion
IIIA	30	74.0 from initial treatment for IIIA disease*

* Average follow-up for these 30 patients is 79.5 months.
(Stehlin J, Giovanella B, de Ipolyi P: Results of eleven years' experience with heated perfusion for melanoma of the extremities. Cancer Res 39:2225–2257, 1979)

FUTURE PROSPECT OF HYPERTHERMIA

WHOLE BODY HYPERTHERMIA

Since this is the only form of heat treatment potentially able to deal with widely disseminated disease, there is no doubt that attempts to utilize it will continue and involve additional groups. As the technology of inducing body temperatures is rapidly becoming simpler and easier to use, whole body hyperthermia in conjunction with radiotherapy will become feasible and very likely will be used against traditionally radioresistant tumors. A major need for advancing these and various other aspects of whole body hyperthermia is the development of an adequate animal model. As has been pointed out earlier, mice and rats are simply too heat sensitive to serve as useful models.

Regional hyperthermic perfusion may already be on its way to being an accepted treatment modality; here the advances should come in the direction of the utilization of different drugs (*e.g.*, BCNU and *cis*-platinum) and perhaps in the development of techniques for the treatment of specific organs such as the liver. One could conceive of multiple regional treatments involving a stepwise approach to whole body treatment. This might have an advantage in reducing the temperature limitation associated with current whole body treatment.

LOCALIZED HYPERTHERMIA

For localized hyperthermia several attractive avenues appear. First of all, for those patients having localized recurrences in field irradiated to normal tissue tolerance, hyperthermia offers an additional and effective treatment. There is no reason, save the lack of available adequate equipment, why such patients should not routinely be treated by hyperthermia now. Localized hyperthermia has a very definite role in palliative chemotherapy; it can aid in the rapid shrinking of specific life-endangering or painful lesions. Perhaps as heat–drug interactions become more widely appreciated, more rapid clinical usage will develop in this area.

However, the major use of hyperthermia should develop in conjunction with radiotherapy. There are several reasons for this. The two modalities act in a complementary way on the cellular level and this complementarity is accentuated by the physiology of many solid tumors. Radiation therapy is frequently the treatment of choice against localized disease, and it is against isolated, solid lesions that heat has maximum effect. Assuming that equipment development and availability advances at its current rate, within the next 3 years to 5 years many radiotherapy centers will offer hyperthermia as a routine adjunct for the treatment of at least the relatively radioresistant tumors and possibly in conjunction with the treatment of other lesions.

REFERENCES

1. Busch W: Uber den Einfluss, Welchen Heftigere Erysipeln auf Organisierte Neubildungen Ausuben. Verhandl Naturh Preuss Rhein Wesphal 23:28–30, 1866
2. Fehleisen: Die Atiologie des Erysipels. T Fischer-Verlag, Berlin, 1883
3. Selawry O, Goldstein M, McCormick T: Hyperthermia in tissue-cultured cells of malignant origin. Cancer Res 17:785–791, 1957
4. Huth E: Die Rolle der bakteriellen Infection bei Spontanremission maligner Tumoren und Leukosen. In Korpereigene Abwehr und bosartige Geschwultste (Lampert, H, Selawry, O., eds) ULM: Hsug. 23–37, 1957
5. Coley W: The treatment of malignant tumors by repeated inoculations of erysipelas—With a report of ten original cases. Am J Med Sci 105:487–511, 1893
6. Coley W: Treatment of inoperable malignant tumors with the toxines of erysipelas and the bacillus prodigiosus. Am J Med Sci 108:50–66, 1894
7. Coley W: A report of recent cases of inoperable sarcoma successfully treated with mixed toxins of erysipelas and bacillus prodigiosus. Surg Gynecol Obstet 13:174–190, 1911
8. Coley-Nauts H, Swife W, Coley B: The treatment of malignant tumors by bacterial toxins as developed by the late William B. Coley, MD reviewed in light of modern research. Cancer Res 6:205–216, 1946
9. Westermark F: Uber die Behandlung des ulcerierenden Cervixcarcinoms mittels Konstanter Warme. Zbl Gynak 22:1335–1339, 1898
10. Jares J, Warren S: Physiological effects of radiation; I. A study of the in vitro effect of high fever temperatures upon certain experimental animal tumors. Am J Roentgenol 41:685, 1939
11. Overgaard K, Overgaard J: Investigations on the possibility for a thermic tumor therapy I. Eur J. Cancer 8:67–78, 1972
12. Crile G: Heat as an adjunct to the treatment of cancer. Experimental Studies. Cleveland Clin Q 28:75–89, 1961
13. Crile G: Selective destruction of cancers after exposure to heat. Ann Surg 156:404–407, 414–416, 1962
14. Crile G: The effects of heat and radiation on cancer implanted in the feet of mice. Cancer Res 23:372–380, 1963
15. Giovanella B, Stehlin J, Morgan A: Selective lethal effect of supranormal temperatures on human neoplastic cells. Cancer Res 36:3944–3950, 1976
16. Westra A: The influence of radiation on the capacity of in vitro cultured mammalian cells to proliferate. Published in Academic Doctoral Theses, University of Amsterdam, Holland, June 2, 1971
17. Westra A, Dewey W: Variation in sensitivity to heat shock during the cell cycle of Chinese hamster cells in vitro. Int J Radiat Biol 19:467–477, 1971
18. Henle K, Leeper D: Interaction of hyperthermia and radiation in CHO Cells: Recovery kinets. Radiat Res 66:505–518, 1976
19. Gerner E, Schneider M: Induced thermal resistance in Hela cells. Nature 256:500–502, 1976
20. Hahn G, VanKersen I: unpublished data, 1980
21. Law M, Coultas P, Field S: Induced thermal resistance in the mouse ear. Br J Radiol 52:308–314, 1979
22. Ardenne M von, Chaplain R: Selektionsteigerung der Strahlentherapeutischen Wirkung durch manipulierte Tumorubersauerung und Warme. Naturwiss 55:448, 1968
23. Gerweck L, Rottinger E: Enhancement of mammalian cell sensitivity to hyperthermia by pH alteration. Radiat Res 67:508–511, 1976
24. Gerweck L: Modifications of cell lethality at elevated temperatures—the pH effect. Radiat Res 70:224–235, 1977
25. Overgaard J: Influence of extracellular pH on the viability and morphology of tumor cells exposed to hyperthermia. J Nat Cancer Inst 56:1243–1250, 1976
26. Hahn G: Metabolic aspects of the role of hyperthermia in mammalian cell inactivation and their possible relevance to cancer treatments. Cancer Res 34:3117–3123, 1974
27. Dewey W, Thrall D, Gillette E: Hyperthermia and radiation—A selective thermal effect on chronically hypoxic tumor cells in vivo. Int J Radiat Oncology Biol Phys 2:99–103, 1977
28. Power J, Harris J: Response of extremely hypoxic cells to hyperthermia: Survival and oxygen enhancement ratios for exponential and plateau-phase cultures. Radiology 123:767–770, 1977
29. Ben-Hur E: Thermally enhanced radiosensitivity of cultured Chinese hamster cells. Nature (New Biol) 238:209–211, 1972
30. Ben-Hur E, Elkind M: Thermally enhanced radioresponse of cultured Chinese hamster cells: damage and repair of single-stranded DNA and a DNA complex. Radiat Res 59:484–495, 1974

31. Li G, Hahn G, Shiu E: Cytotoxicity of commonly used solvents at elevated temperatures. J Cell Physiol 93:331–334, 1977
32. Li G, Evans R, Hahn G: Modifications and inhibition of repair of potentially lethal X-ray damage by hyperthermia. Radiat Res 67:491–501, 1976
33. Hahn G: Potential for therapy of drugs and hyperthermia. Cancer Res 39:2264–2268, 1979
34. Kapp D, Hahn G: Thermosensitization by sulfhydryl compounds of exponentially growing chinese hamster cells. Cancer Res 39:4630–4635, 1979
35. Yatvin M: Influence of membrane lipid composition on hyperthermia and radiation killing of cells. Radiat Res 70:610, 1977
36. Yau T, Kim S, Crissman H: Selection and characterization of a variant of murine L5178Y lymphoma resistant to local anesthetics. J Cell Physiol 99:239–246, 1979
37. Mendecki J, Friedenthal E, Botstein C: Effects of microwave-induced local hyperthermia on mammary adenocarcinoma in C3H mice. Cancer Res 36:2113–2114, 1976
38. Marmor J, Hahn N, Hahn G: Tumor cure and cell survival after localized radiofrequency heating. Cancer Res 37:879–883, 1977
39. Marmor J, Hilerio F, Hahn G: Tumor eradication and cell survival after localized hyperthermia induced by ultrasound. Cancer Res 39:2166–2171, 1979
40. Robinson J, Wizenberg M, Edsack E et al: Thermally enhanced radiocurability of mammary tumors in C3H mice. Presented at the International Biophysics Congress, Moscow, August 1972
41. Faria and Hahn: unpublished data, 1980
42. Field S, Hume S, Low M et al: Some effects of combined hyperthermia and ionizing radiation on normal tissues. Int Symp on Radiobiol Research Needed for the Improvement of Radiother, 1976
43. Marmor J, Pounds D, Postic T et al: Treatment of superficial human neoplasms by local hyperthermia induced by ultrasound. Cancer 43:196–205, 1979
44. Field S: The response of normal tissue to hyperthermia alone or in combination with X-rays, pp 37–48. Cancer Ther by Hyperthermia and Radiation, 1978
45. Li G, Hahn G: Adaptation to different growth temperatures modifies some mammalian cell survivor responses. Exp Cell Res 128:475–480, 1980
46 Dickson J, Shah S, Waggott D et al: Tumor eradications in the rabbit by radiofrequency heating. Cancer Res 37:2162–2169, 1977
47. Marmor J, Hahn G: Ultrasound heating in previously irradiated sites. Int J Radiat Oncol Biol Phys 4:1029–1030, 1978
48. Miller R, Connor W, Heusinkveld R et al: Prospects for hyperthermia in human cancer therapy. Radiology 123:489–495, 1977
49. Dickson J, Ellis H: Stimulation of tumor cell dissemination by raised temperature (42°C) in rats with transplanted yoshida tumours. Nature 248:354–358, 1974
50. Walker A, McCallum H, Wheldon T et al: Promotion of metastasis of C3H mouse mammary carcinoma by local hyperthermia. Br J Cancer 38:561–564, 1978
51. Schechter M, Stowe S, Moroson H: Effects of hyperthermia on primary and metastatic tumor growth and host immune response in rats. Cancer Res 38:498–502, 1978
52. Yerushalmi A: Influence on metastatic spread of whole-body or local tumor hyperthermia. Eur J Cancer 12:455–463, 1974
53. Marmor J, Kozak D, Hahn G: Effects of systemically administered bleomycin or adriamycin with local hyperthermia on primary tumor and lung metastases. Cancer Treat Rep 63:1279–1290, 1979
54. Pettigrew R, Gatt J, Ludgate C et al: Circulatory and biochemical effects of whole body hyperthermia. Br Med J 4:679–682, 1974
55. Pettigrew R, Galt J, Ludgate C et al: Clinical effects of whole-body hyperthermia in advanced malignancy. Br Med J 4:679–682, 1974
56. Pettigrew R: Cancer therapy by whole body heating, pp 282–288. Int Symp on Cancer Ther by Hyperthermia and Radiation, 1975
57. Larkin J, Edwards W, Smith D et al: Systemic thermotherapy: description of a method and physiologic tolerance in clinical subjects. Cancer 40:3155–3159, 1977
58. Larkin J: A clinical investigation of total-body hyperthermia as cancer therapy. Cancer Res 39:2252–2254, 1979
59. Bull J: Summary of the informal discussion of animal models and clinical studies. Cancer Res 39:2262–2263, 1979
60. Storm F, Harrison W, Élliott R et al: Normal tissue and solid tumor effects of hyperthermia in animal models and clinical trials. Cancer Res 39:2245–2251, 1979
61. Holt J: The cure of cancer a preliminary hypothesis. Aust Radiol 18:15–17, 1974
62. Kim J, Hahn E: Clinical and biological studies of localized Hyperthermia. Cancer Res 39:2258–2261, 1979
63. Cavaliere R, Ciocatto E, Giovanella B et al: Selective heat sensitivity of cancer cells (biochemical and clinical studies). Cancer 20:1351–1381, 1967
64. Cavaliere R, Moricca G, Caputo A: Regional hyperthermia by perfusion. International symposium on cancer therapy by hyperthermia and radiation 251–265, 1975
65. Stehlin J: Hyperthermic perfusion with chemotherapy for cancer of the extremities. Surg Gynecol Obstet 129:305–308, 1969
66. Stehlin J, Giovanella B, de Ipolyi P et al: Results of hyperthermic perfusion for melanoma of the extremities. Surg Gynecol Obstet 140:339–348, 1975
67. Stehlin J, Giovanella B, de Ipolyi P et al: Results of eleven years' experience with heated perfusion for melanoma of the extremities. Cancer Res 39:2255–2257, 1979
68. Tonak J, Muhe E, Groitl H et al: Chemotherapy by regional perfusion, pp 340–341. Cancer Ther by Hyperthermia and Radiation, 1978
69. Parks L, Minaberry D, Smith D et al: Treatment of far-advanced bronchogenic carcinoma by extracorporeally-induced systemic hyperthermia. J Thorac Cardiovasc Surg 78:883–892, 1979
70. Hahn G: The use of microwaves for the hyperthermic treatment of cancer: Advantages and disadvantages. Photochem Photobiol Rev 3:277–301, 1978
71. Mantyla M: Regional blood flow in human tumors. Cancer Res 39:2304–2306, 1979
72. Hahn G, Kernahan P, Martinez A et al: Some heat transfer problems associated with heating by ultrasound, microwaves or radiofrequency. N Y Acad Sci 1980
73. Lele P: A strategy for localized chemotherapy of tumors using ultrasonic hyperthermia. Ultrasound Med Biol 5:95–97, 1979
74. Doss J: Use of RF fields to produce hyperthermia in animal tumors, pp 226–227. Int Symp Cancer Ther by Hyperthermia and Radiation, 1975
75. Cetas T, Connor W, Boone M: Thermal dosimetry: Some biophysical considerations, pp 3–12. In Streffer G et al (eds): Cancer Therapy by Hyperthermia and Radiation. Baltimore: Urban & Schwarzenberg, 1978
76. Christensen D: Thermal dosimetry and temperature measurements. Cancer Res 39:2325–2327, 1979
77. Johnson S, Greenleaf J, Samayoa W et al: Reconstruction of three dimensional velocity fields and other parameters by acoustic raytracins. Ultrasonics Symposium Proceedings, IEEE Cat No 75, CHO 994–995, 1975
78. Bowen T, Connor W, Nasoui R et al: Measurement of the temperature dependence of the velocity of ultrasound in soft tissue. Ultrasonics Symposium Proceedings, IEEE Cat No 75:CHO 994–995, 1975
79. Sachs T, Tanney C: A two-beam acoustic system for tissue analysis. Phys Med Biol 22:327–340, 1977
80. Marmor J, Pounds D, Hahn N et al: Treating spontaneous tumors in dogs and cats by ultrasound-induced hyperthermia. Int J Radiat Oncol Biol Phys 4:967–973, 1978
81. Field S, Hume S, Law M et al: The response of tissues to combined hyperthermia and X-rays. Br J Radiol 50:129–134, 1977
82. Cetas T, Connor W: Thermometry considerations in localized hyperthermia. Med Phys 5:79–91, 1978

Section 3

Radiation Sensitizers and Protectors

THEODORE L. PHILLIPS

Over the past two decades most of the major advances made in radiotherapeutic techniques and subsequent results have been because of improvements in equipment and physical dose distribution; it is likely that such benefits are approaching a plateau. Further advances in the efficacy of radiotherapy in controlling regional and local disease and advances in reducing the morbidity of radiotherapy will depend in the future on biologic, rather than physical, improvements. Among the most exciting of the newer methods to be applied in cancer therapy is the use of combined radiation and chemical modifiers.

The knowledge that has been gained in radiation chemistry and cellular radiobiology over the past 20 years has led to an understanding of the initial radiochemical lesions which occur in the cells. This understanding has led to the realization that these lesions could be modified by chemical compounds that interact with reactive species at the time of irradiation. Two major classes of such compounds have been identified, the hypoxic cell sensitizers and the sulfhydryl-containing radioprotectors.

The recognition that hypoxic cells were abundant in tumors and were up to three times more resistant to radiation led to early attempts at circumventing this potential problem. Although hyperbaric chambers have proven successful in certain tumor sites, they are cumbersome and expensive and apparently do not cause full oxygenation in all tumors. The discovery of chemicals to replace oxygen in this function of sensitizing hypoxic cells constitutes a major advance. This chapter will deal at length with the effect of hypoxia on cells and their possible modification of this effect through hypoxic cell sensitizers.

The recognition that sulfhydryl compounds present at the time of irradiation could aid in the repair of initial radiochemical lesions led to the design of compounds which eventually showed activity *in vivo* in protecting aerated, rather than hypoxic, cells. The further discovery of protective compounds which were selectively concentrated in certain normal tissues has stimulated the advances in this field and led to early clinical applications.

It will be seen that the hypoxic cell sensitizers and the radioprotectors offer the potential for great improvement in the efficacy of radiotherapy and a decrease in its morbidity. In addition, recent discoveries suggest that these compounds may also modify the effects of cytotoxic chemotherapy.

SENSITIZERS

RADIATION EFFECTS AT THE CELLULAR AND SUBCELLULAR LEVEL

Radiation kills cells primarily through the deposition of energy in the DNA and associated protein molecules which make up the chromatin material of mammalian cells. Photons, the primary radiation source used in clinical radiotherapy, interact with tissue to produce accelerated electrons which deposit their energy as ion pairs. These short-lived ion pairs may be created in a biologic molecule, such as DNA, or in the abundant cellular water.

These two types of initial events are known as the direct and indirect effect. Indirect effects mediated through water account for more than half of the energy deposition and result in the formation of hydroxyl and hydrogen free radicals and hydrated electrons. These species then interact, returning the situation to normal, or may interact with biologically important molecules, such as DNA, to cause secondary breaks in that substance, leading to the indirect effect. Such radicals may be formed on the DNA itself, leading to breakage (direct effect). Lesions caused in DNA which lead to cell death result from single and double-stranded DNA breaks. It is likely that the lethal lesion is an unrepaired double-stranded DNA break, which leads to chromosome misrepair or non-union. This lesion then leads to loss of vital genetic information after

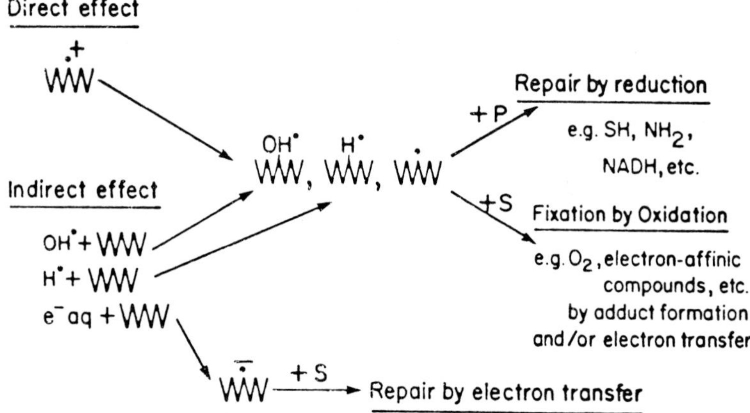

FIG. 48-9. Redox processes in cellular radiobiology. (Chapman JD, Gillespie CJ): Radiation-induced events and their timescale in mammalian cells. Adv Radiat Biol

several cell divisions and the subsequent loss of reproductive integrity of the cells.

After the initial radiochemical events the cellular target molecule contains free radical species, either hydroxyl or hydrogen radicals or an unpaired outer electron. This is a highly excited state with a short lifetime. It may be repaired by reduction, through the presence of a radical reducing species, such as sulfhydryls, amino, and other groups, or fixed by oxidation, through reaction with oxygen, or by electron affinic compounds by adduct formation or electron transfer. These reactions are shown schematically in Fig. 48-9. Through the presence of oxygen or other electron affinic compounds, cellular radiosensitivity is greatly increased.

Experiments with bacteria and more recently mammalian cells have shown that the survival curves for cells are changed to a great degree by the presence of oxygen. The slope of such curves changes by a factor of up to 3, and it is clear that oxygen is primarily dose modifying. Chronic severe hypoxia may also interfere with repair of sublethal damage. The presence of hypoxic cells in tumors can alter their response to increasing doses of radiation. In Fig. 48-10 can be seen examples for the experimental EMT6/S.F. tumor grown as a large tumor in the mouse flank or as small nodules in the lung. Also shown is the response when the cells are removed from the flank tumor and irradiated *in vitro*. Even small pulmonary metastatic tumors contain a portion of cells which yield a shallower slope in the terminal portion of the survival curve. The slope and position of this portion of the curve is related to the percentage of hypoxic cells and to the severity of their hypoxia. From such curves it can be deduced that the larger tumor contains approximately 30% hypoxic cells and the smaller tumor approximately 3%.

Soon after the recognition that hypoxia caused increased radioresistance, it was postulated that hypoxia could account for the difficulty in control of larger tumors by radiotherapy. Studies by Gray and others revealed that hypoxic cells were more resistant to radiation and suggested from histologic evaluation that human tumors contained large zones of hypoxia.[1] The zone of hypoxia appears related to the distance between a viable patent capillary and the center of a tumor cord. Oxygen is able to diffuse approximately 150–200 μ from the capillary, at which point it is completely utilized by the intervening cells. This leads to a typical pattern of tumor growth in which central necrotic zones are seen in tumor cords with peripheral vessels and tumor cords are seen with central vessels in which peripheral necrosis is observed. In addition, tumor vasculature is abnormal, causing fluctuations in flow patterns and leading to frequent closing down of flow in many areas and resultant transient hypoxia.

Based on these observations, clinicians in the United Kingdom and elsewhere in the world began trials of hyperbaric oxygen administration. These trials involved pressurizing patients at 3 to 4 atmospheres of oxygen for 30 minutes to 40 minutes prior to irradiation in the chamber. In many instances it could be shown that the oxygen content in hypoxic zones of tumors was increased and that in some animal tumors this led to a marked reduction in the radiation dose required for control. On the other hand, many animal tumors were not sensitized by hyperbaric oxygen, probably due to physiologic responses of the animal to the high pressure exposure. In spite of this problem, clinical trials in head and neck cancer and in carcinoma of the cervix have been positive with increased local control and survival in patients treated under hyperbaric oxygen.[2,3] Because of the great difficulty and expense and the physiologic response negating the hyperbaric effect in many patients, attempts were made early on to devise another method of increasing cell sensitivity in hypoxic cells.

DEVELOPMENT OF HYPOXIC CELL SENSITIZERS

In the early 1960s Adams and others proposed that not only oxygen but other electron affinic compounds would be capable of sensitizing cells to radiation through fixation of the free radicals in DNA by oxidation. Using the recently improved tools of radiochemistry, they determined the electron affinity of a number of compounds and were able to classify compounds according to electron affinity. They found that highly electron-affinic compounds could sensitize hypoxic bacteria *in vitro* and discovered that there was a clear-cut relationship between electron affinity and potency as a hypoxic cell sensitizer.[4] In the late 1960s compounds were found which sensitized mammalian cells *in vitro*, but which were initially

FIG. 48-10. Dose response curves for EMT6/S.F. tumor cells irradiated as lung nodules *in situ* (■), as a flank tumor *in situ* (●), and as a single cell suspension prepared from flank tumors (▲). (Fu KK, Phillips TL, Wharam MD: Radiation response of artificial pulmonary metastases of the EMT6 tumor. Int J Radiat Oncol Biol Phys 1:257–260, 1976)

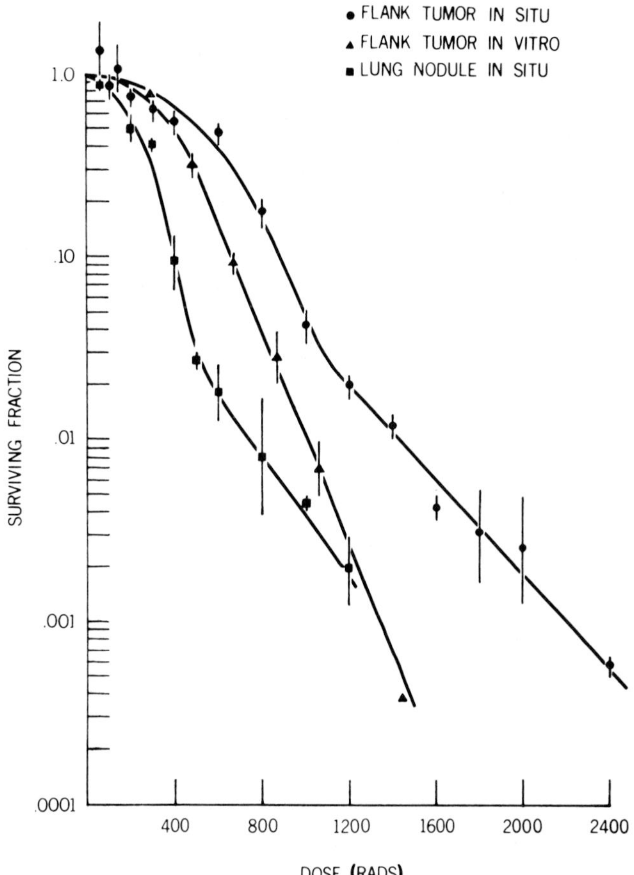

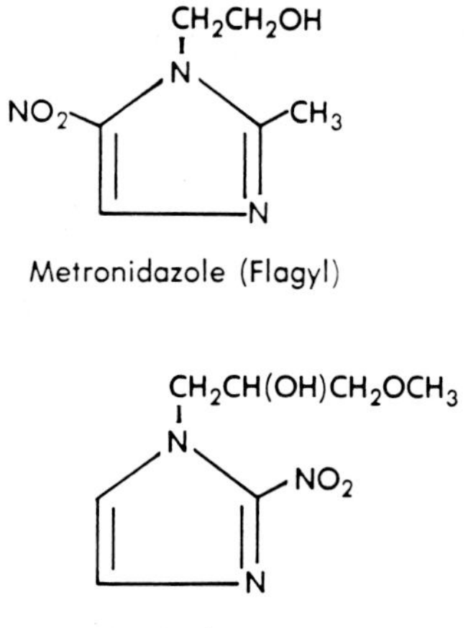

Metronidazole (Flagyl)

Misonidazole (Ro-07-0582)

FIG. 48-11. Chemical structures of metronidazole and misonidazole.

ineffective *in vivo*. The nitrofurans were found to be outstanding sensitizers of hypoxic cells with almost the same increase in sensitivity as could be yielded by oxygen.[5] Again, these proved ineffective *in vivo*.

Through the work of Adams and his colleagues, it became evident that successful hypoxic cell sensitizers would have to meet a number of criteria: (1) high electron affinity; (2) absence of toxicity to aerated cells at concentrations showing high hypoxic cell radiation sensitization; (3) ability to sensitize mammalian cells under conditions of hypoxia *in vitro;* (4) ability to reach pharmacologic concentrations throughout the body with a sufficiently long half-life to allow tumor penetration; (5) sufficient lipophilicity to allow full tumor penetration; (6) absence of whole animal toxicity at concentrations sufficient to cause significant tumor sensitization; (7) absence of cell cycle variation in effectiveness; and (8) sensitization with small daily fractions.[6,7,49]

Finally in the early 1970s two classes of compounds were found which met all of these criteria.[8] The 5-nitroimidazoles and the 2-nitroimidazoles were found in cells *in vitro* to be excellent sensitizers of hypoxic cells. The 5-nitro compounds appeared to be significantly less potent, with approximately ten-fold higher concentrations required for the same degree of sensitization as that for 2-nitro compounds in most instances. Both metronidazole, a commonly used antitrichomonad, and misonidazole (formerly Ro-07-0582) were potent sensitizers *in vitro* and *in vivo*. Their structure is shown in Fig. 48-11. Misonidazole had been developed as a competitive product to metronidazole as an antitrichomonad, but proved to show significant toxicity in large animal testing and had been dropped. The effect of misonidazole on the survival of cells irradiated *in vitro* is shown in Fig. 48-12.

Shortly ater the demonstrations of activity of these compounds *in vitro,* they were extensively tested against a wide range of rodent tumors *in vitro*.[7,9-13] Table 48-14 summarizes data available on tumor sensitizer enhancement ratios. The sensitizer enhancement ratio is the ratio by which sensitivity of cells in nitrogen is increased. Oxygen increases sensitivity by a factor of 2.8 to 3. It can be seen from this tabulation that these hypoxic cell sensitizers are unique in that they sensitize essentially all animal tumors known to contain hypoxic cells. There is no evidence of a differential effect due to the tumor histologic type or site. There is no effect of cell cycle, with cells in or out of cycle or in any stage of the cell cycle equally sensitized, if hypoxic. The degree of enhancement observed is evident when tumor regrowth and tumor control experiments are reviewed (Figs. 48-13, 48-14).

The sensitization of all tumors known to contain hypoxic cells led to the rapid introduction of these compounds into clinical trials in Canada and the United Kingdom. Urtasun began the study of metronidazole, first for maximum tolerance and pharmacology and then in a randomized clinical trial in the treatment of malignant gliomas.[14-16] Dische and his colleagues at the Mount Vernon Hospital explored the toxicity of misonidazole, first in human volunteers and then in volunteer patients looking for the pharmacology, toxicology, and the ability of the compound to sensitize artificially hypoxic skin, as well as to enhance the response of multiple subcutaneous metastases.[17-20]

The design of clinical trials with hypoxic cell sensitizers is somewhat different than that for conventional chemotherapy. When a compound is first introduced, it goes through Phase I testing in which its maximum tolerated dose is established and in which the dose limiting toxicities are identified. Hypoxic cell sensitizer testing generally involves the use of patients who are otherwise receiving radiotherapy for palliative purposes, thus justifying the administration of a potentially

FIG. 48-12. Survival curves for oxygenated and hypoxic V79-379A cells irradiated in the presence of 1 and 10 mM misonidazole. Note that at 10 mmoles the sensitivity of hypoxic cells approaches that of cells irradiated in air. (Adams GE, Flockhart IR, Smithen CE et al): Electron-Affinic Sensitization. VII. A correlation between structures, one-electron reduction potentials, and efficiencies of nitroimidazoles as hypoxic cell radiosensitizers. Radiat Res 67:9–20, 1976

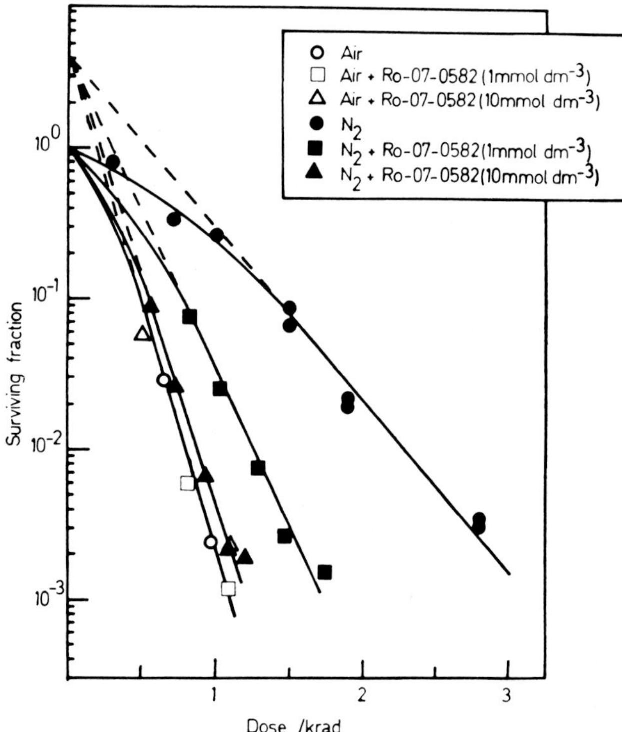

TABLE 48-14. Animal Tumor Enhancement *IN VIVO*

EXPERIMENTER	TUMOR	ASSAY	ENHANCEMENT WITH RO-07-0582 0.2–0.3 mg/g	ENHANCEMENT WITH RO-07-0582 1 mg/g	ENHANCEMENT WITH METRONIDAZOLE 1 mg/g
Begg	CBA fast sarcoma F; ld* >10% + hypoxia	Regrowth, loss of 125-IUdR	1.0	1.6	1.3
Denekamp and Harris	CBA carcinoma NT; 3d −6%	Regrowth delay	>1.4	1.9	1.6
Hewett	WHT squamous carcinoma D ld 18%	Cell dilution *in vivo,*	1.0		
McNally	CBA fast sarcoma F ld >10%	Cell dilution *in vitro*	1.3	2.2	–
Peters	WHT intraderm. squamous ca G ld 0.3%	Cure	1.9	1.8	–
Rauth (Toronto)	C_3H sarcoma KHT; 2d 6%	Cell dilution Lung colonies	1.2–1.3	1.8	1.5
Sheldon, Foster, and Fowler	C_3H 1st generation transplant of spontaneous mammary carcinoma; 6d 10%	Cure	1.3	1.8	1.3
Sheldon	WHT anaplastic carcinoma MT line transplant 1.5d 50%	Cure	1.8	2.0	1.5
Denekamp and Stewart	WHT bone sarcoma 2 2.5 d –	Regrowth delay	–	1.8	–
Stone and Withers	MDAH-MCa-4 mammary carcinoma 2.5 d 20–25%	Cure	–	2.3	1.5
Brown	MDAH-MCa-4 mammary carcinoma 4d 20–25%	Cure	1.8–2.0	2.3	1.3
Brown	EMT6 tumor 3.5d 30%	Cell dilution *in vitro*	2.4–2.7	2.9	2.1

* Doubling time, days
+ Percent hypoxic cells

toxic compound. The Phase I studies are also designed to elucidate the pharmacology of the compound and establish that adequate tumor drug levels are achieved for sensitization.

The second phase of testing involves the establishment of the efficacy of specific combinations of hypoxic cell sensitizer and radiotherapy. The nature of radiotherapy requires multiple treatments and thus the drug must be administrable over a number of weeks with several dosages per week. The maximum tolerated dose must not only be worked out for single doses but for multiple doses and then must be applied in conjunction with a specific radiotherapy regimen in a specific disease site. From the Phase II trials currently completed with misonidazole, it is evident that each disease site imposes limitations on patient tolerance of the drug and on specific radiation fractionation patterns and that Phase II studies are needed to establish the tolerance of both drug and radiation regimen. If the study includes 30 to 40 patients, it can also be established with statistical validity that the response rate is at least as good as prior historical controls, thus allowing a subsequent randomized comparison with conventional radiotherapy.

Phase III studies are then built upon successful Phase II studies with the derived radiation–sensitizer combination contrasted at the same tumor site and stage with conventional radiotherapy. In some trials, an altered fractionation scheme with sensitizer may be compared to conventional treatment or altered schemes may be compared with and without the sensitizer, while in others conventional radiotherapy may be compared with and without the drug.

SENSITIZER DOSE-RESPONSE RELATIONSHIPS

As with oxygen, the sensitizer enhancement ratio is concentration dependent. With misonidazole in most cultured cell systems and tumors *in vivo,* maximal enhancement occurs at approximately 500–1000 μg/ml of medium or per gram of tumor. This compares to 2–5 millimolar in concentration. The concentration *versus* sensitizer enhancement curve is not linear, however, and there is a rather steep rise at low concentrations with enhancement of 1.5 evident at less than 50 μg/ml and 2.0 at approximately 300 μg/ml (Fig. 48-15). Significant enhancement of response has been shown in rodent tumors with concentrations in the tumor of approximately 25 μg/ml.[11,21] From this it would appear that concentrations between 50 and 100 μg/ml would be optimum in the serum, considering that tumor concentrations range from 50% and 80% of serum concentrations in most studies of human tumors.

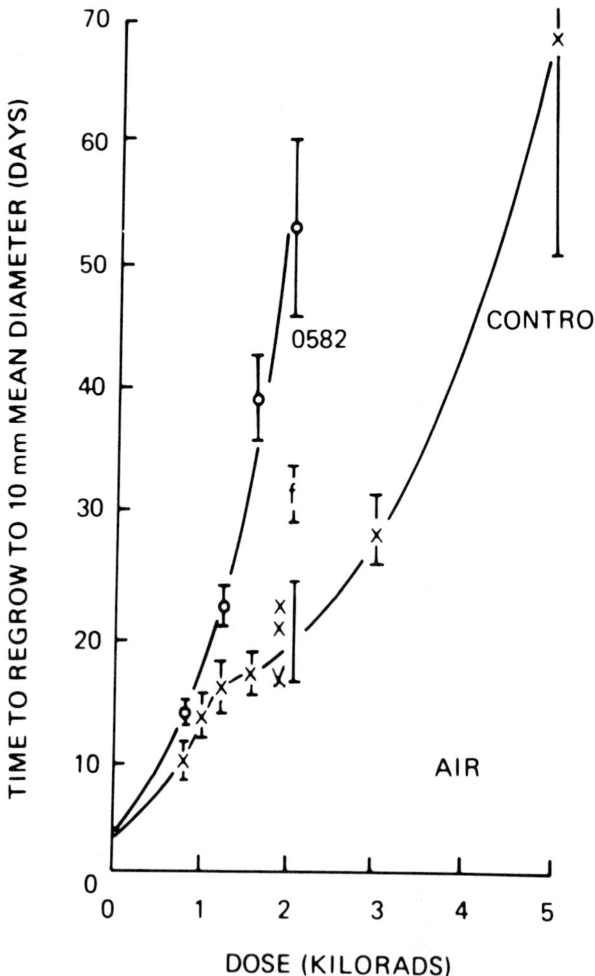

FIG. 48-13. Time required for experimental tumors to regrow to a 10 mm mean diameter as a function of roentgen ray dose for tumors in air-breathing mice. The curve to the right is a control and the one to the left is for animals irradiated 15 minutes after IP injection of 1 mg/gm of misonidazole. (Denekamp J, Harris SR: Tests of two electron-affinic radiosensitizers *in vivo* using regrowth of an experimental carcinoma. Radiat Res 61:191–205, 1975)

INITIAL CLINICAL TRIALS WITH MISONIDAZOLE

The rodent testing with misonidazole revealed that the 50% lethal dose was approximately 1.5 to 1.8 mg/gm with an acute syndrome leading to death within a few hours or days, in some cases associated with convulsions. Testing in dogs at large doses over protracted times had revealed degeneration of the brainstem and cerebellum, and thus it was suspected that neurotoxicity might ensue after prolonged misonidazole administration.

In the British studies, volunteers were initially given single doses of misonidazole, up to quite high levels without any significant toxicity other than acute nausea and in some cases vomiting.[19] Administration was then started with doses several times weekly over 3 weeks to 6 weeks in both Britain and in Canada.[18,22] In Canada, Urtasun had previously started trials with metronidazole at rather large doses and had established the dose limiting toxicity to be primarily nausea and vomiting, had established the pharmacologic distribution and active penetration of the drug into tumor, cerebrospinal fluid, and brain, and had begun a trial of metronidazole in malignant gliomas.[14–16]

Dische, in England, continued his studies with the introduction of misonidazole into a number of radiation trials following the establishment of the pharmacologic distribution and tumor levels.[23] Parallel with these efforts, Urtasun began administration of misonidazole in Canada and Kogelnik began it in Austria.[24–26] These authors noted that there was significant peripheral neuropathy with multiple administrations of misonidazole in addition to acute nausea and vomiting following larger individual drug doses.

In initial reports the neurotoxicity was peripheral sensory neuropathy with no reports of motor lesions. One episode of convulsions was observed in the early British trials.

U.S. trials of misonidazole as an hypoxic cell sensitizer began in July, 1977, under the sponsorship of the Radiation Therapy Oncology Group.[27,28] These studies were designed to establish the maximum tolerated dose of misonidazole with a number of administration schemes. Emphasis was placed on the establishment of the maximum tolerated drug dose over 3-week and 6-week courses for use in palliative and curative regimens. Patients were initially given one drug dose weekly for 3 weeks or 6 weeks and then subsequent patients were given two and three drug administrations per week for the 3-week or 6-week course. Later extensions of the Phase I U.S. study involved daily administration over 1 week to 2 weeks and, finally, 6 weeks.[29]

The U.S. Phase I study involved pharmacology, toxicology, and limited efficacy testing. Patients were selected with normal hematologic and blood chemistry values and who had reasonably good functional status. All were receiving palliative radiotherapy for metastatic or advanced local disease.

Pharmacologic evaluation revealed that misonidazole was well absorbed orally in the form utilized (originally, enteric-coated tablets and, later, capsules). There was a plateau of serum concentration between 2 hours and 4 hours and then excretion with a half-life of 13–14 hours. A typical misonidazole absorption and excretion curve is shown in Fig. 48-16. The majority of the patients studied in the U.S. Phase I trial were evaluated by high performance liquid chromatography, which identified a primary metabolite of misonidazole, desmethylmisonidazole, also known as Ro-05-9963. Cultured cells and animal testing have revealed that this is an equally effective hypoxic cell sensitizer with misonidazole; thus the two concentrations may be combined in estimating enhancement ratios.

Urinary excretion studies (Fig. 48-17) revealed that two-thirds of the drug identifiable in the urine was excreted as the metabolite, rather than the parent compound. This more polar substance was more readily excreted with a shorter half-life than that of the parent compound. Only one-third of the administered compound could be detected in the urine in any of the patients evaluated. Rarely was any compound found in the stool. The majority of the compound is broken down into further products, which were not identified and which may involve opening of the ring structure. These studies indicated that misonidazole would reach excellent blood levels, would be present for prolonged periods, and would have areas under the curve rather long for ideal radiosensitization in that

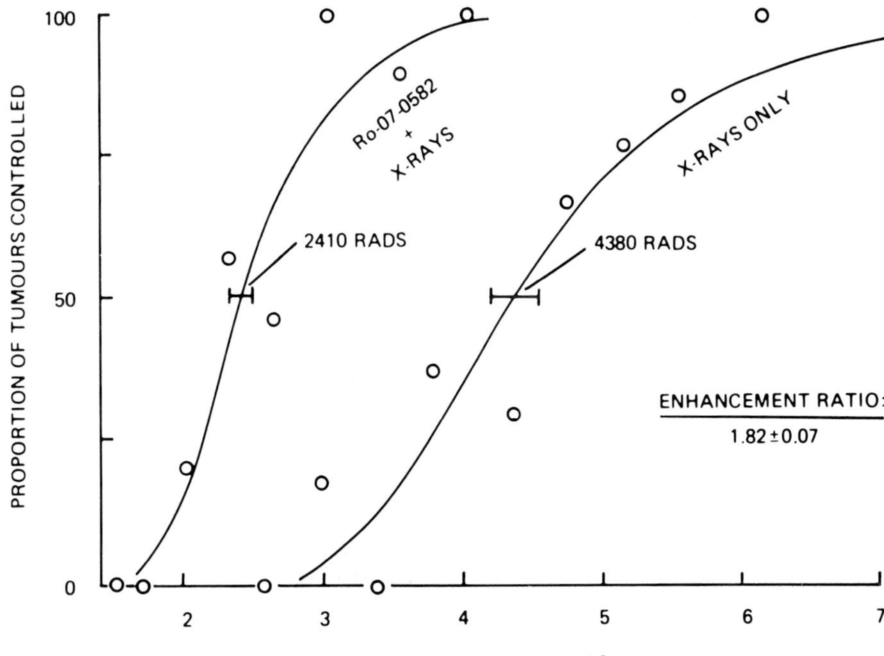

FIG. 48-14. Proportion of tumors controlled at 150 days following irradiation as a function of radiation dose. The curve to the right represents animals treated with x-rays alone and the curve to the left represents animals treated 30 minutes after IP injection of misonidazole 1 mg/gm. (Sheldon PW, Foster JL, Fowler JF: Radiosensitization of C3H mouse mammary tumours by a 2-nitroimidazole drug. Br J Cancer 30:560–565, 1974)

significant exposures of the patient to drug levels would occur after radiation was delivered at peak concentration. The majority of patients showed tumor drug levels approximately 80% of the serum level four hours after oral administration.

Serum levels were generally reproducible from one patient to the other and from one dose to another. Table 48-15 summarizes the misonidazole serum levels *versus* dose administered observed in the Phase I trial in the U.S. These concentrations could be expected to lead to good sensitizer enhancement ratios. If one assumes that tumor concentration is similar to that in the serum, enhancement ratios might be predicted as shown in Fig. 48-18. In this figure previously published data by Dische has been superimposed on the plasma concentrations and patient doses administered in the Phase I trial.[18] It can be seen that at 1 g/m² enhancement on the order of 1.4 and at 2.5 g/m² 1.7 can be expected.

FIG. 48-15. The sensitizer enhancement ratio as a function of drug concentration in medium (for the *in vitro* data indicated by dotted lines) or for four different tumors (indicated by the data points). The tumor values fall close to those for V79 cells *in vitro* and indicates significant enhancement at concentrations less than 50 μg/ml. (Denekamp J: Testing of hypoxic cell radiosensitizers *in vivo*. Can Clin Tr 3:139–148, 1980)

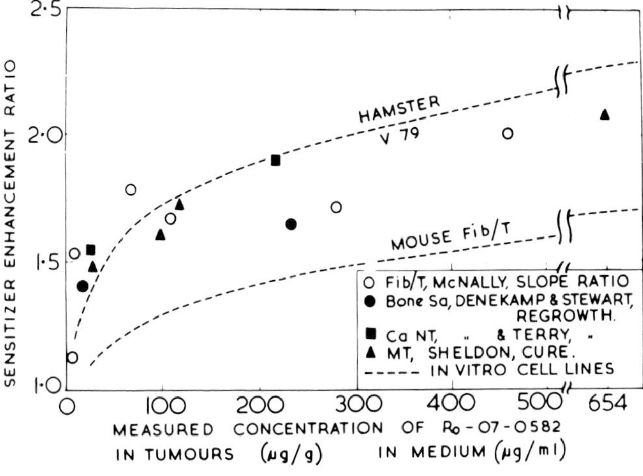

FIG. 48-16. Serum levels of misonidazole (Ro-07-0582) and desmethylmisonidazole (Ro-05-9963) following an oral dose of 2 g/m². Closed circles with numbers in parentheses indicate additional points at the time of other administrations. (Wasserman TH, Phillips TL, Johnson RJ et al.: Initial United States clinical and pharmacologic evaluation of misonidazole (Ro-07-0582), an hypoxic cell radiosensitizer. Int J Radiat Oncol Biol Phys 5:775–786, 1979)

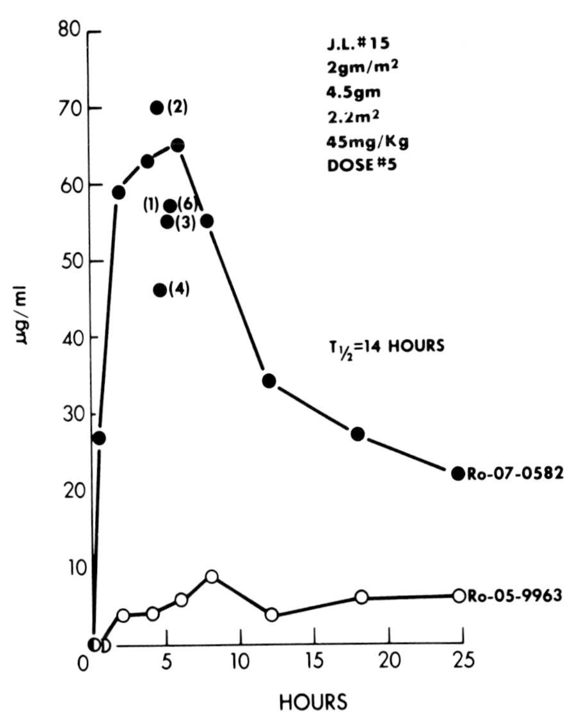

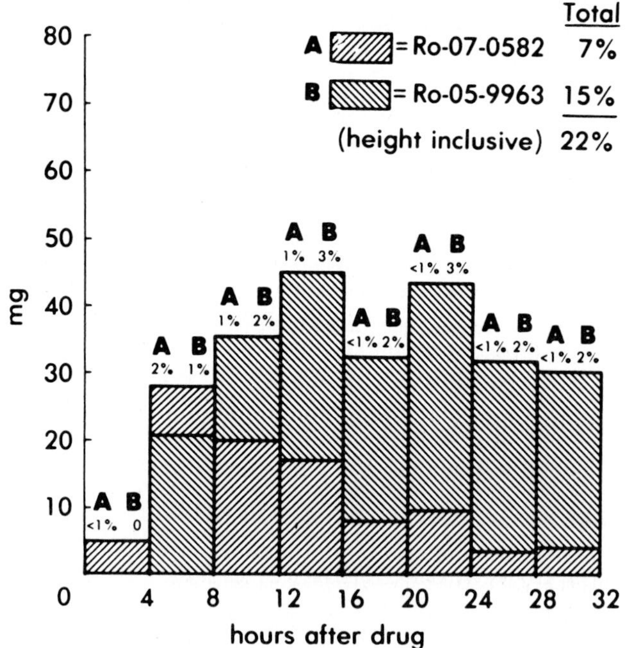

FIG. 48-17. Urinary excretion of misonidazole and desmethylmisonidazole as measured by high performance liquid chromatography with 4-hour urine collections after a dose of 1 g/m². (Phillips TL, Wasserman TH, Johnson RJ et al.: The hypoxic cell sensitizer programme in the United States. Br J Cancer 37:276–280 (suppl III) 1978)

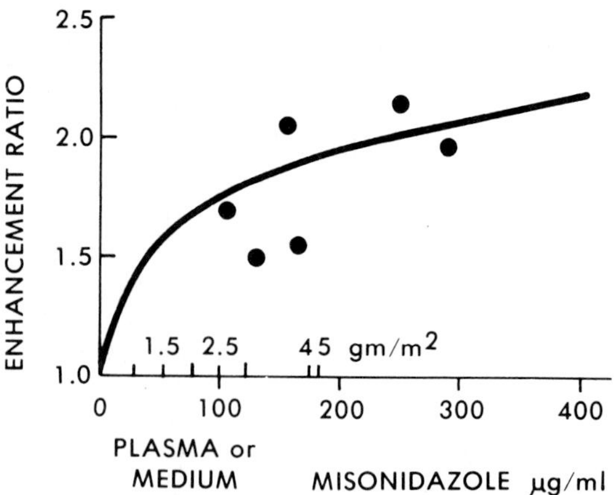

FIG. 48-18. Concentration of misonidazole related to orally administered dose and expected sensitizer enhancement ratio. Closed circles represent experimental points obtained with artificially hypoxic human skin and the line the results of cell culture studies. (Dische S: Hypoxic cell sensitizers in radiotherapy. Int J Radiat Oncol Biol Phys 4:157–160, 1978)

As in the British studies, neurotoxicity proved to be the major side-effect associated with misonidazole administration. Nausea and vomiting was experienced by 48 of 102 patients in the Phase I study. It was associated to some extent with concurrent radiotherapy, but was significantly increased in incidence at doses above 2 g/m².

Peripheral neuropathy was observed and was found to be not only sensory but, at higher doses, motor as well. The incidence at total doses below 9 g/m² was 9 of 34 patients and at doses above 9 g/m² 40 of 65 patients. The overall incidence was 49%. Severe grades with motor, as well as prolonged sensory changes and paresthesias occurred at doses of 12 g/m² and greater.

Central nervous system effect, including somnolence and confusion with transient coma, was noted in nine instances. All severe central nervous system effects occurred at doses above 9 g/m². In addition to the CNS effects, ototoxicity was noted in the form of decreased hearing and transient deafness in nine patients. Both encephalopathy and ototoxicity were rarely seen in the absence of preceding peripheral neuropathy, which can act as a warning sign for cessation of drug administration.

Patients taking dexamethasone and phenytoin sodium had a significantly lower incidence of neuropathy than did patients taking similar total doses in administration schemes without the administration of these two additional compounds. Phenytoin sodium appears to shorten the half-life of misonidazole.[50,51]

When proper adjustments are made for the reduction in toxicity caused by phenytoin sodium and dexamethasone, the maximum tolerated doses appeared to be approximately 10.5 g/m² in 3 weeks and 12 g/m² in 6 weeks. Patients taking dexamethasone and phenytoin sodium because of brain tumors or brain metastases may receive somewhat higher doses of misonidazole.

Although Phase I tests are not designed for efficacy, a

TABLE 48-15. R.T.O.G. Phase I Study—Relationship of Dose to Mean 4–6 Hour Serum Level

DOSE (g/m²)	NUMBER OF DOSES (Determinations)	MEAN 4–6 HR SERUM LEVEL (µg/ml) (0582 + 9963)	STANDARD DEVIATION	OBSERVED RANGE
1.0	17	30	+/− 9	21–57
1.25	116	46	+/− 6	31–61
1.5	78	60	+/− 18	16–95
1.75	18	70	+/− 18	39–107
2.0	99	76	+/− 14	51–120
2.5	43	98	+/− 23	35–148
3.0	25	116	+/− 26	39–155
4.0	8	175	+/− 56	83–238
5.0	7	183	+/− 60	91–245

number of observations were made in the British, Canadian, and American studies. Thomlinson and Dische compared the response of several patients with multiple subcutaneous metastases, irradiating with and without misonidazole and observing regression and regrowth.[20] In several patients, there was a significant increase in the regrowth delay in lesions treated in conjunction with misonidazole. Urtasun found in his randomized Phase II study of malignant gliomas that patients treated in nine fractions with radiation alone *versus* radiation plus metronidazole experienced significantly prolonged median survival when treated with metronidazole.[15] Both groups, however, received somewhat low radiation doses and exhibited median survival times poorer than in some other trials with higher total radiation doses. In the Phase I U.S. study, five patients received radiation alone as contrasted to radiation plus misonidazole for multiple metastatic lesions.[29] In all cases, the response of the lesions treated with misonidazole using the same radiation scheme was greater than for radiation alone. Rather large radiation fractions and misonidazole doses of 2 g/m^2 or greater were employed.

CURRENT CLINICAL TRIALS

Clinical evaluations of misonidazole in the Phase II and Phase III mode are now going on in a number of countries. Those conducting Phase III randomized trials include the United States, the United Kingdom, Europe (through the EORTC), and South Africa. Randomized trials in Britain are evaluating carcinoma of the lung, cervix, head, and neck and malignant gliomas.

In the United States a large series of Phase II and Phase III trials is underway through the Radiation Therapy Oncology Group and trials are beginning in a number of other cooperative groups. A large Phase III trial in malignant gliomas is underway in the Brain Tumor Study Group.

Phase II studies, which were designed to establish the efficacy and tolerance of a given radiation–misonidazole combination have been completed in a number of sites by the RTOG. All five studies involving gliomas, head and neck cancer, brain metastases, liver metastases, and lung cancer employed rather large misonidazole doses with large radiation fractions, used either throughout the course for metastatic disease or once per week in more limited disease. The head and neck trial was unique in using two radiation fractions on one day to take advantage of the long misonidazole half-life.

The malignant glioma study was noteworthy in that the median survival time was 52 weeks, which is long contrasted to a number of other prior trials of radiation only and equal to survival seen with radiation plus chemotherapy, which was not utilized in this trial. Excellent response rates were seen in the head and neck, brain metastasis and liver metastasis studies, and the complete response rates and control seen in the lung study were at least equal to prior irradiation results in the RTOG. All of these studies were felt to warrant further investigation as experimental arms in randomized trials.

Additional Phase II studies are underway in order to determine in which other sites randomized trials may be indicated and to finalize a successful radiation–misonidazole combination. Although the treatment of hemibody metastases has yielded a number of responses and significant palliation, it has not shown many objective partial or complete responses. This will likely be replaced by a fractionated hemibody study. Treatment of advanced or recurrent melanomas and sarcomas with large radiation fractions has yielded modest responses after conversion of the study from once weekly to twice weekly irradiation, but it is not clear that these large fractions are advantageous in this particular type of disease. Although carcinoma of the bladder has responded well to the large fractions employed in the Phase II study, there have been significant bowel complications and this study has now been closed for derivation of a new fractionation scheme. Retreatment of central nervous system tumors has been very rewarding, with a high number of complete responses, suggesting this as an arm in a future study of initial disease, as well as for the treatment of recurrences. Problems have been encountered in the treatment of locally advanced carcinoma of the esophagus with oral misonidazole because of difficulty in drug administration. Use of a similar radiation fractionation scheme at the National Cancer Institute with I.V. misonidazole has shown excellent tumor response. Altered fractionation schemes in head and neck cancer are being explored in a randomized Phase II study to establish the potential next arm for head and neck trials. In carcinoma of the cervix, altered fractionation of 400 rad twice weekly was found unpopular within the group and is now to be opened as a study of conventional fractionation in carcinoma of the cervix with daily misonidazole. One thousand rad monthly for advanced pelvic cancer is being explored as a palliative measure.

A number of Phase II studies have yielded Phase III studies including gliomas, head and neck cancer, lung cancer, and brain metastases. These are based on the closed Phase II studies previously mentioned. One trial is a study designed for more limited lung carcinoma (non-oat-cell) with conventional fractionation with and without daily misonidazole. Additional Phase III studies compare 300 rad × 7 with and without misonidazole for hepatic metastases and investigate conventional radiotherapy with and without daily misonidazole in advanced carcinoma of the cervix.

An overview of the current Phase II clinical trials with misonidazole reveals that there is apparent increased effectiveness of radiation with sensitizer at a number of sites. It is likely that the benefit is modest at the total doses now deliverable, that is, 12 g/m^2. Clearly the ideal radiosensitizer has not been developed. One would like to deliver up to ten times as much sensitizer as is possible with misonidazole to achieve enhancement ratios of 2 to 3 with every radiation fraction over an entire 6-week course. Thus the development of new analogs is a major concern.

NEW DRUG DEVELOPMENT

The Division of Cancer Treatment of the National Cancer Institute has established a Radiation Sensitizer/Protector Working Group, which acts as a subcommittee of its Drug Development Decision Network. This committee has been working for a number of years to elucidate principles by which more ideal radiosensitizers would be developed, tested and evaluated in the clinic. At this point it is clear that the limiting toxicity is neurotoxicity, both central and peripheral. A number of animal models have been evolved which allow prediction of neurotoxicity through the evaluation of performance of rodents on devices such as the rotorod, the performance of dogs after protracted administration, and a unique test of the effects on peripheral nerves through quantitative cytochemical evaluation of lysosomal enzyme activity. These studies and concomitant pharmacologic studies by Brown and colleagues have led to the prediction that compounds with a lower lipophilicity than misonidazole will yield significantly reduced neurotoxicity.[30,31] These compounds exhibit lower brain-to-tumor ratios than misonidazole and lower concentrations in peripheral nerve, as well as brain. Initial testing in dogs carried out by the DCT's Toxicology Branch reveals that the first compound with a lower lipophilicity, desmethylmisonidazole (mentioned above), can be delivered in doses 2.5 to 3 times higher in dogs than misonidazole.

Brown and Lee have carried out an extensive evaluation of the effect of drug lipophilicity and pharmacologic alterations on tumor enhancement and toxicity, which has led to the development of a number of new, promising compounds.[6] A number of these analogs are shown in Table 48-16. Variation in the side chain at the one position on the 2-nitroimidazole ring yields marked variations in the partition coefficient. All of the compounds, except for the last one, SR-2530, have proven to be good hypoxic cell sensitizers, while SR-2530 shows poor tumor access and poor sensitization *in vivo*. These changes in partition coefficient have yielded marked decreases in penetration of the brain and CSF, as studied in dogs, and marked increases in the acute LD_{50} in mice.

From this and other work, it was predicted that Ro-05-9963, the metabolite observed in humans, would have a shorter half-life and lower access to the brain with lower toxicity. It is about to enter Phase I clinical testing. From the other compounds listed, SR-2508 and SR-2555 have been identified as having potential and are soon to enter large animal testing for toxicity. Eventually it is hoped that the goal of a compound with a therapeutic ratio ten times higher than misonidazole will be achieved.

In addition to the potential for deriving an effective, nontoxic sensitizer through manipulations of the pharmacologic distribution are attempts to modify the chemical structure. It is possible that electron affinity may be dissociated from neurotoxicity and attempts are underway to synthesize compounds which might achieve those ends.

CYTOTOXICITY

In addition to their properties as hypoxic cell sensitizers at concentrations non-toxic to normal aerated cells, the hypoxic cell sensitizers have been discovered to show significant cytotoxicity after chronic exposure to hypoxic cells.[22,32] *In vitro,* an exposure to 5 mmol concentration of misonidazole for 2 hours will begin a significant cell kill. Longer exposures then yield exponential cell kill. It has been shown in a number of systems *in vivo* as well that high concentrations for long periods cause the kill of tumor cells in the hypoxic compartment. In general, the concentrations and exposures required are larger than those currently achievable with clinically administrable doses in humans.

In addition to cytotoxicity, prolonged exposure to high concentrations of misonidazole appears to cause cellular lesions which lead to elimination of the shoulder on the radiation dose–response curve and thus increased radiosensitivity of cells so treated to small radiation fractions. It has been theorized that a toxic metabolite is produced in hypoxic cells during their exposure to misonidazole. This metabolite is not produced during exposure of aerated cells to misonidazole, and it appears diffusable to adjacent aerated cells.

Chronic exposures to misonidazole not only sensitize cells to radiation, but also sensitize cells to hyperthermia exposure. Hyperthermia also leads to enhanced cell kill by misonidazole in the hypoxic fraction. In addition to these observations, there has been the recent exciting observation that misonidazole exposure of cells apparently increases their sensitivity to cytotoxic chemotherapy.

INTERACTION WITH ALKYLATING AGENTS AND OTHER CYTOTOXIC CHEMOTHERAPY

Recently Rose and associates and Stratford and associates have demonstrated increased cytotoxicity of alkylating agent

TABLE 48-16. Various 2-Nitroimidazoles and Their Attributes

COMPOUND DESIGNATION NUMBER)	STRUCTURE*	MOLECULAR WEIGHT	PARTITION COEFFICIENT (P)	E^1 (mV)	ACUTE LD_{50} (mg/g)
Ro-07-0269	—$CH_2CHOHCH_2C1$	205	1.5	−384	~0.18
Ro-07-0913	—$CH_2CHOHCH_2OEt$	215	1.27	−391	>1.1
SR-2514	—CH_2CH_2NO | HC1	263	0.82	−390	−0.9
Ro-07-0741	—$CH_2CHOHCH_2F$	189	0.44	−383	−0.9
Misonidazole	—$CH_2CHOHCH_2OMe$	201	0.43	−389	1.8(1.3–2.6)
Desmethylmisonidazole	—$CH_2CHOHCH_2OH$	187	0.13	−389	3.1(2.2–4.4)
SR-2512	—$CH_2CH_2SOCH_3$	203	0.060	–	~2.0
SR-2508	—$CH_2CONHCH_2CH_2OH$	214	0.046	−388	4.9(4.3–5.6)
SR-2555	—$CH_2CON(CH_2CH_2OH)_2$	258	0.026	−398	>7.7
SR-2530	—$CH_2CONHCH_2CHOHCH_2OH$	244	0.014	−392	>6.1

* Structure of the side chain at the 1- position of the 2-nitroimidazole ring.

chemotherapy *in vitro* and, later, in tumors *in vivo* following exposure to misonidazole.[33,34] In more recent abstracts Clement, Johnson, and Wodinsky also were able to demonstrate enhanced cell kill with a number of cytotoxic chemotherapeutic agents, including cyclophosphamide and melphalan.[35] Preliminary results from these and other laboratories suggest that not only cyclophosphamide and melphalan but also nitrosoureas, 5-fluorouracil, and other compounds may give enhanced tumor kill when administered in conjunction with high doses of misonidazole. On the other hand, in almost every case, increased toxicity of cytotoxic compounds can be shown when they are administered with misonidazole, and with the exceptions of cyclophosphamide and melphalan it would appear that enhancement of bone marrow and general toxicities may be similar to that of tumor response.

The mechanisms by which misonidazole may enhance response to alkylating agents is as yet unclear. There is no question that pre-exposure to high concentrations of misonidazole sensitize cells *in vitro* to subsequent alkylating agent chemotherapy, much as it does to subsequent radiation. It has not been demonstrated unequivocally, however, that this occurs *in vivo*. It is also clear from limited pharmacologic studies that administration of misonidazole significantly alters alkylating agent pharmacology. If the enhanced response is due to production of a toxic product in tumor hypoxic zones, then a differential enhanced effect could be expected. On the other hand, pharmacologic prolongation of alkylating agent half-life may yield equal increases in effect in tumor and vulnerable normal tissue.

Combined misonidazole and cytotoxic chemotherapy remains an exciting but unproven possibility warranting the onset of careful Phase I clinical testing.

PROTECTORS

INITIAL RADIOBIOLOGIC EVENTS

As for hypoxic cell sensitizers, it is in the initial radiochemical events that the potential application of radioprotectors is found. As shown in Fig. 48-9, the radicals formed in the target molecule, in all probability DNA and associated protein, may be repaired by reduction, rather than fixed by oxidation. Almost all cells contain significant sulfhydryl compounds in the nonprotein fractions and these participate in such protective activities. Depletion of such sulfhydryls can be shown to cause significant cellular sensitization. The addition of exogenous sulfhydryl compounds will significantly protect aerated cells, but has only a small effect in hypoxic cells. From these observations it is likely that repair by reduction competes with fixation by oxidation. The addition of sulfhydryl containing compounds to the intracellular milieu might protect oxic cells to a much greater degree than hypoxic cells, much as electron affinic compounds sensitize hypoxic cells but not aerated cells.

Protection against ionizing radiation by sulfhydryl containing compounds was first described by Patt and colleagues in the late 1940s.[36] Soon thereafter, this mechanism was recognized by the military as a potential method for protecting troops against radiation exposure in atomic warfare. A number of large synthesis programs were undertaken in an attempt to find highly effective, orally administered compounds. One such effort was mounted by the United States Army Medical Research and Development Command which catalogued several hundred thousand compounds and studied several thousand in much greater detail.

From this program came a number of promising compounds, many of which were in the thiophosphate class.[37] They generally contained the active sulfhydryl in conjunction with an aminopropyl group and in that sense resembled cysteine and cysteamine, some of the early compounds. A number of these agents are summarized in Table 48-17. WR-2721 appears to be the most efficacious in terms of its therapeutic ratio in that it shows significant protection at doses far below its maximum tolerated level. In addition, the relationship between dose and the dose reduction factor is not linear, with much steeper increases in protection occurring at low concentrations.

DIFFERENTIAL NORMAL TISSUE PROTECTION

The use of a protective compound in clinical oncology can only be predicated upon the presence of a differential effect on normal tissue *vis-a-vis* tumor. If normal tissue could be protected against radiation, then total radiation doses could be increased yielding enhanced tumor cell kill with no increased price in normal tissue damage. As mentioned previously, it was to be expected on a radiochemical basis that protection would be less in hypoxic cells than aerated

TABLE 48-17. Chemical Structure of Cysteamine-Related Thiophosphate Radioprotective Compounds

DESIGNATION	CHEMICAL NAME	STRUCTURE
MEA	β-mercaptoethylamine (cysteamine)	$H_2NCH_2CH_2SH$
WR-2529	3-(2-mercaptoethylamino) propionamide ρ-toluenesulfonate	O ‖ $HSCH_2CH_2NH$ $CH_2CH_2CNH_2 \mid CH_3C_6H_4SO_3H$
WR-2721	S-2-(3-aminopropylamino) ethyl phosphorothioic acid hydrate	$H_2NCH_2CH_2CH_2$ $NHCH_2CH_2S$ $PO_3H_2 \mid XH_20$
WR-2823	S-2-(5-aminopentylamino) ethyl phosphorothioic acid monohydrate	$H_2N(CH_2)_5$ $NHCH_2CH_2S$ $PO_3H_2 \mid H_20$
WR-638	Sodium hydrogen S-(2-aminoethyl) phosphorothioate	O ‖ $H_2NCH_2CH_2S$ P—(OH) (ONa)

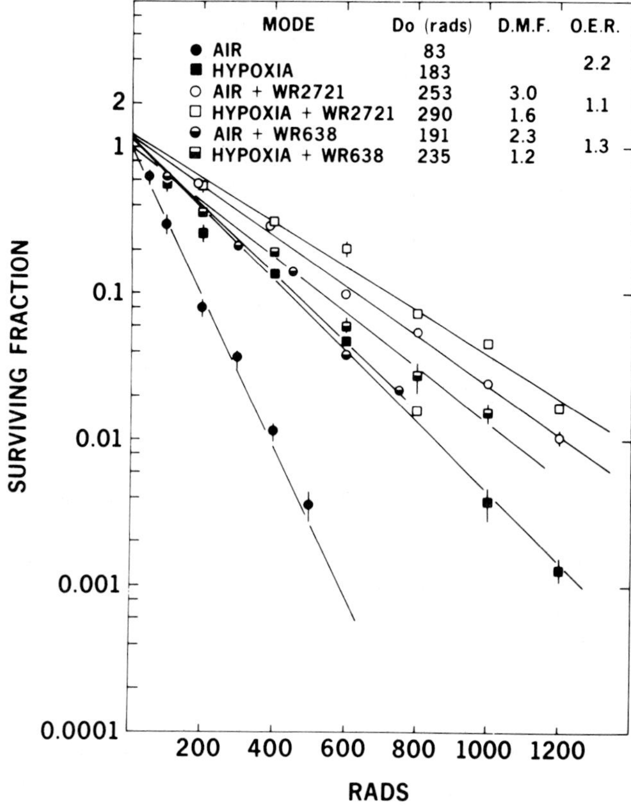

FIG. 48-19. Survival of mouse CFUs bone marrow cells as a function of radiation dose and chemical radioprotector administration. Treatment was delivered in the donor mouse, breathing air or made hypoxic through the breathing of 5.5% nitrogen. Note the very low OER for CFUs irradiated in the presence of WR-2721 and the markedly low dose modifying factor for both protectors shown in hypoxic cells. (Harris JW, Phillips TL: Radiobiological and biochemical studies of thiophosphate radioprotective compounds related to cysteamine. Radiat Res 46:362–379, 1971)

cells. This is indeed the case as shown in Fig. 48-19 from experiments by Harris and Phillips.[38] It can be seen that artificially hypoxic bone marrow CFUs are protected to a significantly lesser degree than aerated CFUs, leading to a reduction in the oxygen enhancement ratio. This alone might be adequate basis for potential clinical trials of such protectors, but of course one would need to fear protection of the aerated portion of a tumor, which may represent 70% to 90% of the tumor cells.

Yuhas and Storer observed that WR-2721, in contrast to cysteamine, appeared to cause differential protection of normal tissue in terms of skin reaction, as compared to tumor response.[39] In later work, Yuhas discovered that WR-2721 appears actively concentrated by a process that may be facilitated diffusion in normal tissues, whereas it reaches slowly increasing concentrations over several hours in tumor.[40] Thus for time periods of 30 minutes to 60 minutes after intravenous or intraperitoneal injection, concentrations will be far higher in most normal tissues than in tumor. This pharmacologic effect can then be added to that of the decreased protection in hypoxic cells, leading to the conclusion that very significant differential radioprotection should occur.

TABLE 48-18. Tissue Blood Ratios for WR-2721 in Mouse* and Dog† (Thirty Minutes Postinjection)

TISSUE	MOUSE	DOG
Liver	5.3	3.1
Spleen	2.5	2.2
Kidney	3.9	19
Lung	3.3	1.4
Muscle	1	0.7
Bone marrow	3.5‡	1.5
Brain	0.1	0.03
Small intestine	3.3	1.3
Thymus	1.6	1.3
Adrenal	3.1[c]	2
Heart	2.4	0.9

* 100 mg/kg. Blood level = 49 μg/ml.
† 21 mg/kg. Blood level = 21 μg/ml.
‡ Rat 70 mg/kg. Blood level = 46 μg/ml.
(Washburn LC, Rafter JJ, Hayes RL: Prediction of the effective radioprotective dose of WR-2721 in humans through an interspecies tissue distribution study. Radiats Re 566:100–105, 1976)

It has been shown that WR-2721 must be dephosphorylated to be activated as a protector. In the serum it is rapidly absorbed by normal tissues or bound to serum proteins. Compound entering cells is dephosphorylated and activated. There is no systematic evidence that activation occurs to a lesser extent in tumor than normal tissue, and it is thought that a membrane activity may exclude the drug from tumor early after injection while allowing it into normal tissues for binding.

OBSERVED PROTECTIVE CAPACITY IN NORMAL TISSUES

The degree of protection which can be achieved by WR-2721 is by no means uniform. Although a significant variation in the concentration of WR-2721 can be found in a range of normal tissues, as shown in Table 48-18, these concentrations are not reflected in the same dose modifying or dose reduction factors, as shown in Table 48-19 and in Fig. 48-20.[41–43] The central nervous system is not protected because the drug does not reach significant concentrations in this organ because of its low lipophilicity. On the other hand, good concentrations are seen in lung and kidney, while rather low dose reduction factors have been observed. This may be related to the location

TABLE 48-19. WR-2721 Dose Modifying Factors for Critical Type 1 Normal Tissues

TISSUE	ACUTE DMF	CHRONIC DMF
Brain	1.0	–
Spinal cord	–	–
Lung	–	1.2
Heart	–	–
Stomach	–	–
Small intestine	1.8 – 2.1	–
Large bowel	–	–
Liver (chromosomes)	–	2.7
Kidney	–	1.5
Bone marrow LD_{50}	2.2 – 2.7	–
Bone marrow CFU	3.0	–

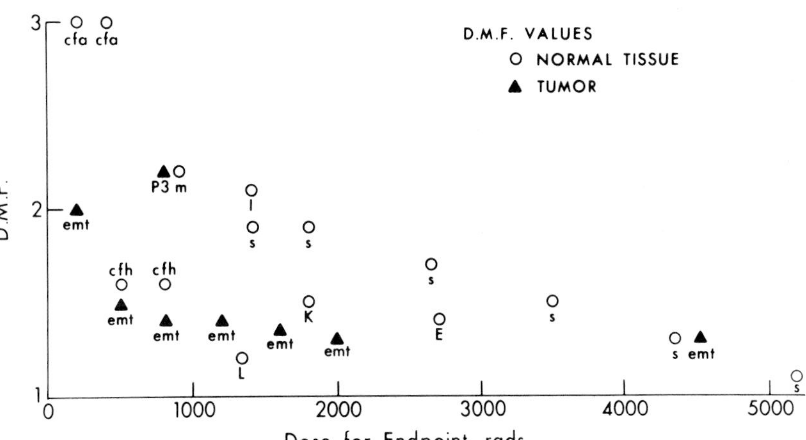

FIG. 48-20. Dose modifying factor values for normal tissue and tumor as a function of the dose size required for a given endpoint in control animals. (*cfa* = aerated CFUs; *cfh* = hypoxic CFUs; *emt* = EMT6/S.F. carcinoma; *P3* = P388 leukemia; *I* = intestinal crypts; *L* = lung $LD_{50/160}$; *K* = kidney $LD_{50/365}$; *s* = skin reaction grade, days 16–40; *E* = esophageal $LD_{50/28}$; *m* = $LD_{50/30}$ in DBA/2 mice). (Phillips TL, Kane L, Utley JF: Radioprotection of tumor and normal tissues by thiophosphate compunds. Cancer 32:528–535, 1973)

of drug within cells or specific cells within the tissue in these organs, leading to a high overall uptake with low uptake in the cells determining tissue damage.

From animal studies it can be concluded that WR-2721 will show significant protection in bone marrow, skin, mucous membranes, and salivary glands and in the lining of the small intestine. Protection of the liver and, to a lesser extent, the kidney is also evident. This compound would appear of potential usefulness in the treatment of head and neck cancer and the treatment of abdominal malignancies, as well as with hemibody and whole body radiation where its significant bone marrow protection will be important.

EARLY CLINICAL TESTING

Although the U.S. Army Drug Development Program brought WR-2721 to early Phase I human testing in volunteers, it was conducted with an oral compound that achieved only limited results. More recently exploration of administration to humans has been carried out in Japan with an intravenous compound. From small and large animal studies, it is to be expected that the side-effects will include potential nausea and vomiting, as well as hypotension secondary to the ganglionic blocking activity of WR-2721. In the Japanese studies, the major toxicity that was observed with doses up to 100 mg/m² was some nausea and vomiting. The Japanese reported anecdotal observations of decreased reactions in the oral mucosa.[44]

U.S. Phase I studies with intravenous compound were begun at the University of New Mexico with a local IND and locally derived compound. This study has currently escalated single doses to 450 m/m².[45] The only associated side-effect has been transient nausea and vomiting which is eliminated by somewhat slower drug infusion. At this concentration protection equal to 150 mg/kg in rodents may be expected.

FIG. 48-21. *A*, Response of CFUs treated *in situ* prior to transplantation by cyclophosphamide alone IV or cyclophosphamide IV preceded 30 minutes by WR-2721 IP at a dose two-thirds of the LD_{50}. *B*, Tumor growth curves for the EMT6/S.F. tumor treated with saline alone or saline plus WR-2721 as compared to growth after treatment by cyclophosphamide alone intravenously at a dose of 250 mg/kg or the same dose preceded 30 minutes by a dose of 500 mg/kg WR-2721.

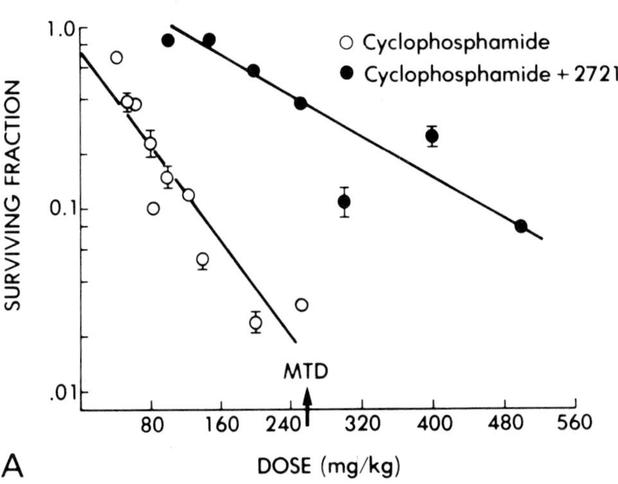

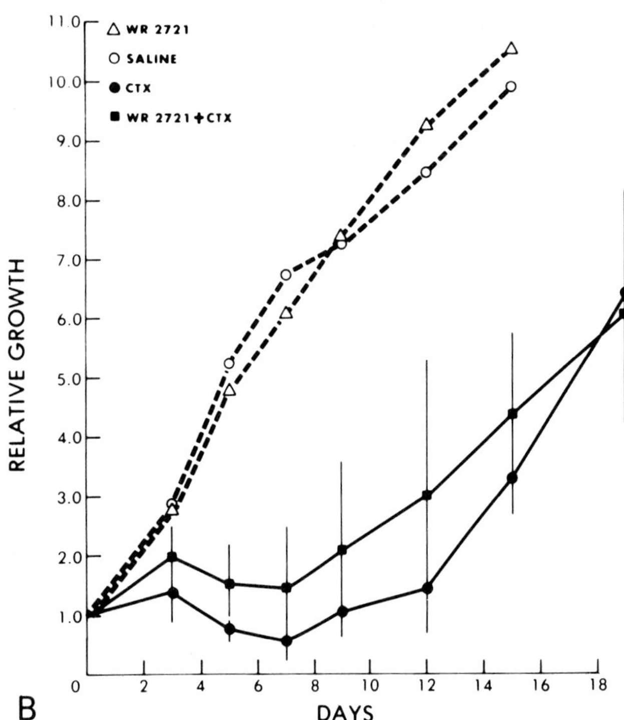

FUTURE CLINICAL TRIALS

The Radiation Therapy Oncology Group has designed an extensive Phase I evaluation of WR-2721 to build upon the experience of the University of New Mexico trial. It will escalate doses with a schedule ranging from five times to one time per week over 3 weeks and then over 7 weeks to find the maximum tolerated dose with each administration schedule that might be associated with clinical radiotherapy. Although some observations may be made in a Phase I study as to reduced radiation reactions, it is essential to employ conventional radiation doses and first establish the drug's dose-limiting toxicity. It is not yet clear whether this toxicity will be a cumulative one or the daily limitations of associated nausea, vomiting, hypotension, or inanition.

Phase II studies with radioprotectors are far different than those for cytotoxic drugs or sensitizers. In these studies, the maximum tolerated drug dose for a given radiation regimen has been established and it is then necessary to establish the maximum tolerated radiation dose. Tissues must be selected which are known to concentrate WR-2721 and which have been protected in animal studies. Thus Phase II studies may well be directed toward head and neck cancers and abdominal malignancies, such as liver metastases, ovarian cancer, and GI cancers. Phase II studies will employ a fixed WR-2721 dose with radiation doses escalating from the conventional by 5% to 10% increments to doses that yield similar degrees of acute and late radiation reactions as experienced by historical controls.

Such information derived from Phase II studies can then be used to design Phase III trials in which the efficacy of conventional radiation therapy will be compared to the efficacy and toxicity of radiation therapy using augmented doses in conjunction with the protector, WR-2721.

NEW DRUG DEVELOPMENT

Although the exact dose-limiting toxicity for multiple WR-2721 administrations has not yet been elucidated, it is to be expected that there will be a dose-limiting toxicity. Thus it may be necessary to derive less toxic compounds that can be administered at higher concentrations, yielding higher dose reduction factors. In addition it is clear that WR-2721 does not protect brain or spinal cord and that protection of the lung is poorer than average. Thus a drug development program must concentrate on analogs which yield protection in these structures. Obviously any drug development program must keep in mind the need for differential protection and any structure function alterations must leave residual differential uptake in normal tissue.

At this point it is not clear to what extent potential development might be to alter the lipophilicity and thus the pharmacology of the compound. Some alteration may be permissible, allowing increased uptake in the brain without loss of differential radioprotection. Other possible routes include alterations of the molecule leading to differential metabolism to an active form in normal tissue as compared to tumor.

INTERACTION WITH ALKYLATING AGENT CHEMOTHERAPY

Many years ago it was observed that certain sulfhydryl containing compounds could protect against the effect of mustard gas. This potential application of sulfhydryl compounds was ignored for many years until the recent rediscovery of the phenomenon by Yuhas.[46] He postulated that the differential uptake seen for WR-2721 in normal tissues as compared to tumors could yield differential protection of normal tissues against alkylating agent toxicity. In experiments, he demonstrated that chemotherapeutic agent distribution was uniform between tumor and normal tissue, while WR-2721 concentrations were far higher in normal tissue. These findings predicted differential protection and, indeed, this was the case.

Yuhas has demonstrated for mechlorethamine, nitrogen mustard, cyclophosphamide, and *cis*-platinum that essentially no protection occurs in a range of tumor systems as measured by regrowth assay. He has shown protection of bone marrow as determined by the $LD_{50/30}$, protection against skin reactions in conjunction with combined chemotherapy and radiation, and protection against renal injury secondary to multiple doses of *cis*-platinum.[47]

In our laboratory we have shown that WR-2721 protects bone marrow CFUs against *cis*-platinum, cyclophosphamide, nitrogen mustard, and BCNU, whereas it causes no significant protection of the EMT6 tumor to these agents as measured by regrowth.[48] In recent experiments, we have also shown significant protection of intestinal crypt cells against toxicity by doxorubicin, *cis*-platinum, and BCNU. Thus far, no protection against doxorubicin cardiotoxicity has been observed. Yet to be tested are the potential for WR-2721 to protect against alkylating agent and nitrosourea pulmonary damage and cyclophosphamide damage to the bladder among others. There is no evidence as yet that WR-2721 protects against anything but alkylation.

From the data so far available, it appears that clinical trials are warranted with combinations of WR-2721 and cyclophosphamide, melphalan, nitrogen mustard, and *cis*-platinum. This development is obviously in its early formative stages because of the need to complete Phase I testing of WR-2721 alone and to establish in Phase I testing that there is, indeed, protection against significant alkylating agent toxicities in humans. If successful, this approach may allow for significant increases in cytotoxic chemotherapy doses and, it is hoped, concomitant increases in tumor response rates.

SUMMARY

The identification of the basic mechanisms involved in radiation killing of cells through the understanding of radiation chemistry and radiation biology has allowed for the elucidation of a number of modifying mechanisms. In particular, the repair of target molecule free radicals by reduction and their fixation by oxidation provide the potential for augmentation of the results of clinical radiotherapy.

A wide range of compounds have now been discovered which

exhibit electron affinity and which can mimic oxygen in their ability to sensitize the hypoxic cells of tumor to radiation. More recently, these compounds have shown suggestive evidence that they may differentially sensitize tumors to alkylating agent chemotherapy as well.

The use of sulfhydryl-containing compounds to repair free radical lesions in the DNA of aerated normal tissues has proven possible. There appears to be a differential effect on normal tissue *versus* tumor through increased drug uptake of certain compounds in normal tissues *vis-a-vis* tumor and through the decreased protective efficacy of these compounds in hypoxic cells. More recently, it has been demonstrated that sulfhydryl-containing radioprotective compounds are also active in protecting cells against toxic effects of alkylating agent chemotherapy.

It would appear that in the near future extensive combinations of radiation, cytotoxic chemotherapy, hypoxic cell sensitizers, and radioprotectors may yield significant improvements in the therapeutic ratio and in the control of tumors.

REFERENCES

1. Gray LH, Conger AD, Ebert M et al: The concentration of oxygen dissolved in tissues at the time of irradiation as a factor in radiotherapy. Br J Radiol 26:638–648, 1953
2. Henk JM, Smith CW: Radiotherapy and hyperbaric oxygen in head and neck cancer. Lancet ii:104–105, 1977
3. Watson ER, Halnan KE, Dische S: Hyperbaric oxygen and radiotherapy: A Medical Research Council trial in carcinoma of the cervix. Br J Radiol 51:879–887, 1978
4. Adams GE, Cooke MS: Electron-affinic sensitization. I. A structural basis for chemical radiosensitizers in bacteria. Int J Radiat Oncol Biol Phys 15:457–471, 1969
5. Chapman JD, Reuvers AP, Borsa J et al: Nitroheterocyclic drugs as selective radiosensitizers of hypoxic mammalian cells. Cancer Chemother Rep 58:559–570, 1974
6. Brown JM, Lee WW: Pharmacokinetic considerations in radiosensitizer development. Cancer Clin Trials (in press)
7. Committee for Radiation Oncology Studies: Research plan for radiation oncology: radiation sensitizers. Cancer (suppl) 37:2062–2070, 1976
8. Asquith JC, Watts ME, Patel K et al: Electron-affinic sensitization. V. Radiosensitization of hypoxic bacteria and mammalian cells in vitro by some nitroimidazoles and nitropyrazoles. Radiat Res 60:108–118, 1974
9. Denekamp J, Harris SR: Tests of two electron-affinic radiosensitizers in vivo using regrowth of an experimental carcinoma. Radiat Res 61:191–205, 1975
10. Denekamp J, Stewart FA: Sensitization of mouse tumors using fractionated X-irradiation. Br J Cancer (suppl) 37:259–263, 1978
11. Denekamp J: Testing of hypoxic cell radiosensitizers in vivo. Cancer Clin Trials 3:139–148, 1980
12. Sheldon PW, Foster JL, Fowler JF: Radiosensitization of C_3H mouse mammary tumours by a 2-nitroimidazole drug. Br J Cancer 30:560–565, 1974
13. Sheldon PW, Hill SA, Foster JL et al: Radiosensitization of C_3H mouse mammary tumours using fractionated doses of X-rays with the drug Ro-07-0582. Br J Radiol 49:76–80, 1976
14. Urtasun RC, Sturmwind J, Rabin H et al: "High-dose" metronidazole: A preliminary pharmacological study prior to its investigational use in clinical radiotherapy trials. Br J Radiol 47:297–300, 1974
15. Urtasun R, Band P, Chapman JD et al: Radiation and high-dose metronidazole in supratentorial glioblastomas. N Engl J Med 294:1364–1367, 1976
16. Urtasun RC, Band PR, Chapman JD et al: Metronidazole as a radiosensitizer. N Engl J Med 295:901–902, 1976
17. Dische S, Gray AJ, Zanelli GD: Clinical testing of the radiosensitiser Ro-07-0582. II. Radiosensitization of normal and hypoxic skin. Clin Radiol 27:159–166, 1976
18. Dische S, Saunders MI, Lee ME et al: Clinical testing of the radiosensitizer Ro-07-0582: Experience with multiple doses. Br J Cancer 35:567–579, 1977
19. Gray AJ, Dische S, Adams GE et al: Clinical testing of the radiosensitizer Ro-07-0582. I. Dose tolerance, serum and tumour concentrations. Clin Radiol 27:151–157, 1976
20. Thomlinson RH, Dische S, Gray AJ et al: Clinical testing of the radiosensitizer Ro-07-0582. III. Response of tumours. Clin Radiol 27:167–174, 1976
21. McNally NJ, Denekamp J, Sheldon P et al: Radiosensitization by misonidazole (Ro-07-0582). The importance of timing and tumor concentration of sensitizer. Radiat Res 73:568–580, 1978
22. Hall EJ, Miller R, Astor M et al: The nitroimidazoles as radiosensitizers and cytotoxic agents. Br J Cancer (suppl) 37:120–123, 1978
22. Whitmore GF, Gulyas S, Varghese AJ: Sensitizing and toxicity properties of misonidazole and its derivatives. Br J Cancer (suppl) 37:115–119, 1978
23. Dische S: Hypoxic cell sensitizers in radiotherapy. Int J Radiat Oncol Biol Phys 4:157–160, 1978
24. Urtasun RC, Band P, Chapman JD et al: Clinical phase I study of the hypoxic cell radiosensitizer Ro-07-0582, a 2-nitroimidazole derivative. Radiology 122:801–804, 1977
25. Urtasun RC, Partington J, Koziol D et al: A comparison of metronidazole and misonidazole: blood and tumor tissue distribution, toxicity and efficacy. Cancer Clin Treat (in press)
26. Kogelnik HD: Clinical experience with misonidazole. High dose fractions versus low doses. Cancer Clin Treat 3:179–186, 1980
27. Phillips TL, Wasserman TH, Johnson RJ et al: The hypoxic cell sensitizer programme in the United States. Br J Cancer (suppl) 37:276–280, 1978
28. Wasserman TH, Phillips TL, Johnson RJ et al: Initial United States clinical and pharmacologic evaluation of misonidazole (Ro-07-0582), an hypoxic cell radiosensitizer. Int J Radiat Oncol Biol Phys 5:775–786, 1979
29. Phillips TL, Wasserman TH, Johnson RJ et al: Final report on the United States phase I clinical trial of the hypoxic cell radiosensitizer, misonidazole. Cancer (in press)
30. Brown JM, Yu NY, Cory MJ et al: In vivo evaluation of the radiosensitizing and cytotoxic properties of newly synthesized electron-affinic drugs. Br J Cancer (suppl.) 37:206–211, 1978
31. Brown JM, Workman P: Partition coefficient as a guide to the development of radiosensitizers which are less toxic than misonidazole. Radiat Res 82:171–190, 1980
33. Rose CM, Millar JL, Peacock JH et al: The effect of misonidazole on in vivo tumor cell kill in Lewis lung carcinoma treated with melphalan or cyclophosphamide. Cancer Clin Treat (in press)
34. Stratford IJ, Adams GE, Horsman MR et al: The interaction of misonidazole with radiation, chemotherapeutic agents or heat: A preliminary report. Cancer Clin Treat 3:231–236, 1980
35. Clement JJ, Johnson RK, Wodinsky I: Enhancement of antitumor activity of some alkylating agents by the radiation sensitizer misonidazole (abstr #1165), AACR Proceedings 21:291, 1980
36. Patt HM, Tyree EB, Straube RL et al: Cysteine protection against X-irradiation. Science 110:213–214, 1949
37. Yuhas JM, Storer JB: Chemoprotection against three modes of radiation death in the mouse. Int J Radiat Biol 15:233–237, 1969
38. Harris JW, Phillips TL: Radiobiological and biochemical studies of thiophosphate radioprotective compounds related to cysteamine. Radiat Res 46:362–379, 1971
39. Yuhas JM, Storer JB: Differential chemoprotection of normal and malignant tissues. J Natl Cancer Inst 42:331–335, 1969
40. Yuhas JM: Active vs passive absorbtion kinetics as the basis for selective protectors of normal tissues against alkylating agents by WR-2721. Cancer Res (in press)
41. Washburn LC, Rafter JJ, Hayes RL: Prediction of the effective radioprotective dose of WR-2721 in humans through an interspecies tissue distribution study. Radiat Res 66:100–105, 1976
42. Phillips TL, Kane LJ, Utley JF: Radioprotection of tumor and

normal tissues by thiophosphate compounds. Cancer 32:528–535, 1973
43. Phillips TL: Rationale for initial clinical trials and future development of radioprotectors. Cancer Clin Treat 3:165–173, 1980
44. Sugahara T, Tanaka Y: Clinical experiences of chemical radiation protection in tumor radiotherapy in Japan. Cancer Clin Treat (in press)
45. Kligerman M, Yuhas JM: (personal communication)
46. Yuhas JM: Differential protection of normal and malignant tissues against the cytotoxic effects of mechlorethamine. Cancer Treat Rep 63:971–976, 1979
47. Yuhas JM, Spellman JM, Culo F: The role of WR-2721 in radiotherapy and/or chemotherapy. Cancer Clin Treat 3:211–216, 1980
48. Wasserman TH, Phillips TL, Ross G et al: Differential protection against cytotoxic chemotherapeutic effects on bone marrow CFU/s and EMT-6 carcinoma by WR-2721. Cancer Treat Rep (submitted)
49. Adams GE, Flockhart IR, Smithen CE et al: Electron-affinic sensitization. VII. A correlation between structures, one-electron reduction potentials, and efficiencies of nitroimidazoles as hypoxic cell radiosensitizers. Radiat Res 67:9–20, 1976
50. Wasserman TH, Urtasun R, Schwade JG et al: The neurotoxicity of misonidazole: Potential modifying role of phenytoin sodium and dexamethasone Br J Radiol 53:172–173, 1980
51. Workman P: Effects of pretreatment with phenobarbitone and phenytoin on the pharmacokinetics and toxicity of misonidazole in mice. Br J Cancer 40:335–353, 1979

Section 4

Photosensitizers

THOMAS J. DOUGHERTY
KENNETH R. WEISHAUPT
DONN G. BOYLE

The term "photoradiation therapy" (PRT), in the context of this review, describes the use of photosensitizing drugs to treat malignant tumors. A photosensitizer may be considered to be a material capable of causing light-induced reactions in molecules which do not absorb the light. Phototherapy, photochemotherapy, and photodynamic therapy have all been used to describe the same procedure, but some of these terms have been used in a broader context to describe any therapy utilizing light, sometimes in conjunction with a drug and sometimes not, such as with phototherapy in the treatment of hyperbilirubinemia. Without attempting to judge the merits of any of these terms to refer to photosensitization as a treatment of malignant disease, in this article, the term "photoradiation therapy" (PRT) will be used exclusively for this purpose, since its meaning is unequivocal.

An ideal photosensitizer for treatment of malignant disease would be one which (1) has no systemic toxicity; (2) is taken up and retained only by malignant tissue; (3) absorbs at, and is efficient in destroying, malignant tissue at wavelengths not absorbed by tissue. Currently, there is no such ideal photosensitizer known. Until one is found, work progresses with certain photosensitizing drugs which may approach the ideal closely enough to have therapeutic benefit at least in certain situations. While there is no photosensitizer presently known to be taken up or retained only by malignant tissue, there are several potentially useful photosensitizers for which such a tumor-specific characteristic has been claimed, such as berberine sulfate, fluoroscein, eosin, tetracycline, acridine orange and several porphyrins.[1–10] Among this group, the porphyrins have been most extensively investigated.

Policard first noted in 1924 that some human and animal tumors fluoresced upon illumination with a Wood's lamp.[6] The red fluorescence was attributed to endogenous porphyrins arising from secondary infection by hemolytic bacteria. In 1942, Auler and Banzer noted characteristic red porphyrin fluorescence in rat tumors, but not in normal tissues, following systemic injections of hematoporphyrin, a non-metallic porphyrin derived from hemoglobin.[7] Figge and co-workers demonstrated the generality of this apparent tumor localization characteristic of hematoporphyrin by examining various types of induced and transplanted tumors in mice.[8] They found porphyrin fluorescence in several types of sarcomas and carcinomas, as well as in lymph nodes, traumatized tissues and embryonic tissues. In 1960, Lipson introduced hematoporphyrin derivative (Hpd), a material prepared by an acetic-acid–sulfuric-acid treatment of hematoporphyrin, according to Schwartz, and which was shown to have a superior tumor localizing property to that of hematoporphyrin.[9–11] Fluorescence in human tumors due to systemically injected Hpd, was demonstrated first in 1961 by Lipson in nine cases of bronchial and esophageal tumors.[12] In a subsequent study by Lipson of 50 patients with suspected bronchogenic tumors, an 80% correlation of tumor fluorescence with biopsy-proven malignancy was found.[13] Lipson also demonstrated Hpd fluorescence in cervical lesions.[14] In a large study of Hpd localization reported in 1968, Gregorie and his group studied 226 patients with suspected squamous cell or adenocarcinoma.[15] They found a 77% correlation of fluorescence with biopsy-proven malignancy for squamous lesions and an 84% correlation for adenocarcinoma. There were 23% and 16% false negatives, respectively, for squamous cell and adenocarcinoma tumors. Except for fluorescence in traumatized tissues, embryonic tissue and lymph nodes, all workers indicated that normal tissues did not demonstrate fluorescence due to hematoporphyrin or Hpd. However, in 1979, Gomer and Dougherty showed that following intraperitoneal injection of ^{14}C-Hpd or ^{3}H-Hpd in mice, distribution at 3 hours was as follows: liver ~ kidney > spleen > lung > transplanted mammary tumor > skin > muscle.[16] At 24 hours, a similar distribution was found except that Hpd in the lung was lower than that in the tumor.

Currently, Hpd is being studied for localization of early bronchogenic tumors by Sanderson and Cortese at the Mayo Clinic and by Profio and Doiron at the University of California at Santa Barbara, in conjunction with Balchum from the University of South California and King from the University of Alberta.[17–20] These groups are using modified bronchoscopes with special fiber optics and filter systems for detection of Hpd fluorescence in very small tumors in the lung. Early results by these groups are very promising and indicate that lesions of the order of 1 mm to 2 mm may be localized.

While several other porphyrins are able to accumulate in cells *in vitro,* aside from hematoporphyrin or Hpd, only tetraphenylporphine sulfonate (TPPS) has shown to have this capability *in vivo.*[21–24] TPPS shows tumor localization properties in animal tumors similar to those of Hpd, and in fact has been shown to accumulate to an even higher degree in malignant tissue. For example, ^{14}C or ^{3}H-Hpd has a maximum level of 5 μ to 8 μ porphyrin per gram tumor tissue (transplanted mouse mammary carcinoma) occurring 24 hours following 10 mg/kg injected intraperitoneally, whereas maximum TPPS levels of 20 μg/g were found by Musser in S-180 tumors following 10 mg/kg injected intraperitoneally.[24] In addition, experimental tumors in mice respond to light treatment following systemic TPPS in a way similar to that when Hpd is injected.[25] However, the prolonged serum half-life of TPPS demonstrated in mice (>30 hours for 10 mg/kg *versus* 3 hours for 10 mg/kg Hpd) has precluded its use clinically since photosensitivity likely would be very prolonged (see below).[16]

Finally, it is interesting to note that there are reports indicating that injected Hpd may cause fluorescence of premalignant lesions, such as CIS lesions in cervix and bladder, as well as in frank malignancy.[26,27]

Having obtained a therapeutically useful level of a photosensitizer in a tumor, it is desirable to be able to activate it using wavelengths not absorbed by tissue, but only by the photosensitizing drug itself. However, since some tissue components absorb throughout the entire visible spectrum, such as melanin, hemoglobin and oxyhemoglobin, this requirement is not completely attainable although it is approachable at least in some tissues.[28] Visible wavelengths greater than 600 nm are least absorbed by skin and other tissue components and would, therefore, be least attenuated if light were applied through the skin or other tissues to treat lesions. In this regard, again, the porphyrins discussed above are most useful since nonmetallic porphyrins demonstrate weak absorption in the red (600 nm–700 nm). Dougherty and co-workers measured the percent transmission of light from a HeNe laser (632.8 nm) through an excised rat tumor.[29] They found that approximately 10% of directly transmitted light reached 1 cm and approximately 30% of transmitted plus reflected light reached this distance. It should be noted that there was no skin involved in these measurements nor any circulating blood. Measurements of this type are complicated by the large scattering component of the tissues and, aside from this rather crude measurement, no data relating to light dosimetry in tissue other than skin are available.[30]

TREATMENT OF TUMORS WITH PHOTOSENSITIZERS

The first attempt to use photosensitization to treat cancer was reported in 1903 when Tappenier and Jesionek used topical eosin and sunlight to treat skin tumors.[31] While they noted some regression of the lesions, there were no further reports from this group. It was not until the early 1970s that interest in such therapy was revived. In 1972 and 1975, Diamond and associates reported that hematoporphyrin, injected systemically into rats bearing subcutaneously transplanted glioma tumors, caused extensive tumor necrosis when the lesion was exposed to white light.[32,33] Neither the light nor porphyrin had any effect alone. In 1973 and 1974, Dougherty and associates reported that fluorescein and green light (488 nm) retarded the growth of subcutaneously implanted mammary tumors in mice.[34,35] In 1974, Tomson and colleagues reported that acridine orange, given orally to mice with epithelial tumors, sensitized such tumors to light from an argon laser.[5]

The first reported instances of complete tumor eradication of experimental tumors were in 1975 when it was reported that Hpd in conjunction with locally applied red light, delivered one day after the drug, prevented recurrences for at least 90 days in about half of the mice with subcutaneous mammary tumors.[36] Also, in 1975 Kelly and co-workers demonstrated that Hpd activated by white light caused necrosis of human bladder carcinoma transplanted into immunosuppressed mice. They further demonstrated that the normal bladder epithelium, also transplanted into the mice, was not destroyed by the light applied following systemic Hpd.[27] In 1976, Kelly and Snell reported treatment of a human bladder carcinoma following intravenous Hpd by transmitting white light transurethrally through a quartz rod.[37] The patient had multicentric nodules and only a small area (approximately 3 cm in diameter) was illuminated. It was noted that after 2 days there was histological evidence of tumor destruction in the treated area and unchanged tumor in untreated areas.

The group at Roswell Park Memorial Institute has been studying response of a wide variety of malignant tumors in humans, generally metastatic, to photoradiation therapy (PRT) utilizing Hpd as the photosensitizing drug. First reports appeared in 1978 and 1979.[29,38] The initial study was designed primarily to assess toxicity and tumor response. Most patients had extensive, distant disease not treated by PRT. Most had progressing disease following one or several conventional modalities such as surgery, radiotherapy, and chemotherapy. Recently, Forbes, at the University of Adelaide, Australia, Treurniet-Donker, at the Rotterdamsch Radio-Therapeutisch Instituut, and Kennedy, at the Ontario Research Foundation, Kingston, have initiated similar studies. Table 48-20 summarizes all results known to date regarding responses of various types of tumors.

Follow-up ranged from 2 days to 3 years. The majority of lesions responded to treatment. Unlike ionizing radiation, response to PRT frequently is seen a short time after treatment (1 day to 2 days) with lesions appearing grossly necrotic and hemorrhagic. The longest follow-up to date is approximately 3 years for a woman who had metastatic breast carcinoma lesions recurrent after surgery, radiotherapy, and several courses of chemotherapy. Before treatment by PRT, she had several superficial lesions localized mainly on the left lateral chest wall and left supraclavicular area. The entire left chest wall was treated by PRT in two sessions, 2 weeks apart. To date she has not had recurrence in the photoradiation field. However, approximately 9 months after PRT treatment, she was treated with an antiestrogen drug for a metastatic supraclavicular node.

TABLE 48-20. Types of Tumors Treated by PRT*

TUMOR TYPE	NUMBER OF PATIENTS	NUMBER OF RESPONSES†
Angiosarcoma	1	1
Basal cell carcinoma‡	5	5
Breast carcinoma	35	34
Chondrosarcoma	1	1
Colon carcinoma	3	2
Endometrial carcinoma	1	1
Glioma‡	3	1
Kaposi's sarcoma‡	2	2
Liposarcoma	1	0
Malignant melanoma		
pigmented	6	1
non-pigmented	6	6
Mycosis fungoides‡	4	3
Ovarian carcinoma	1	1
Parotid carcinoma	2	2
Prostatic carcinoma	1	1
Renal cell carcinoma	1	0
Retinoblastoma	1	1
Squamous cell carcinoma‡	3	3

* Unless otherwise indicated, tumors were metastatic. Data compiled by Dougherty (Roswell Park Memorial Institute), Forbes (University of Adelaide, Australia), Kennedy (Ontario Cancer Foundation, Kingston Clinic, Canada), and Treurniet-Donker (Rotterdam Radio-Therapeutisch Instituut, Netherlands).

† Response indicates biopsy-proven necrosis or reduction in size by at least 50%.

‡ Primary lesions or recurrent in primary site.

Normal tissue (skin) response was also assessed in this group of patients in order to judge therapeutic effect. In most cases, this was done on areas of normal skin within the light field during treatment of tumor lesions. In some cases, remote areas of skin were treated as well. Several combinations of Hpd dose, time between drug administration and light treatment and light dose were found which caused tumor response with acceptable damage to normal skin. If light treatment was given too soon after Hpd administration or if the light dose was too high, skin necrosis occurred. An updated assessment of these variables is shown in Table 48-21.

The light source for the early group of patients treated at Roswell Park was a 5 KW xenon arc lamp with filtration to remove ultraviolet, infrared, and visible wavelengths below 600 nm. This is based on the premise that while the porphyrin absorbs more strongly in the blue–green portion of the spectrum, these wavelengths are unable to penetrate skin sufficiently, in most instances, to be effective.[30] When absorbed in cells, Hpd absorbs between 620 nm and 640 nm.[39] This filtered xenon lamp produces 85% of the emitted energy between 600 nm and 700 nm and 15% in the infrared. Recent results in the laboratory and on patients indicate that this small fraction of infrared radiation does not contribute significantly to the response of either tumor or normal skin, although this point needs further investigation. When treating lesions in or under the skin, the normal tissue effects are the major factor limiting the light dose. The maximum tolerable light dose, found not to result in unacceptable skin damage, was 2000 mw-min/cm^2 (120 J/cm^2) delivered no sooner than the third day following 2.5 mg/kg and no sooner than 4 days following 3.5 mg/kg. This dose could be delivered in either 20 minutes or 10 minutes without noticeable differences in response. From biopsy samples taken following treatment, it was estimated that this light dose caused coagulation necrosis to a depth of about 1.5 cm to 2.0 cm in tumor lesions treated through the skin. It is clear, however, that sufficient variability exists from patient to patient that adjustments in light dose are frequently necessary.

Aside from skin toxicity due to overtreatment with the therapeutic light, all patients were ultra-sensitive to bright light, especially sunlight both outside and inside. They were cautioned to remain out of bright sunlight for at least 30 days and to then start exposure cautiously. Those who did not do so experienced mild to severe edema to exposed areas. One patient also had slight sloughing of skin on the face. In this context, a difference among patients in drug retention in skin is evident. Some patients experienced no difficulty in the sun 30 days after receiving the drug, while a few continued to experience difficulty for several months. Hepatic function appeared normal in all cases. Besides this phototoxicity, patients with very extensive disease, treated by PRT, may experience mild to severe pain, usually controllable and of short duration, although in some cases, discomfort may last several weeks. In addition, such patients may experience toxicity due to necrotizing tissue, such as spiking fever and infection.

We are currently evaluating other light sources for PRT. One is a bank of special fluorescent lamps emitting approximately 35% of their energy between 600 nm and 650 nm, the remainder being in the infrared. These lamps were assembled and provided to us by GTE Sylvania Corporation. In order to remove wavelengths below 600 nm, we have added a plastic ruby filter sheet of the type used in graphic arts. This system provides 14 mw/cm^2 of energy over an area of 2000 cm^2 and allows treatment of an entire chest wall in a single field, although treatment times range up to 2 hours for a single treatment.

A third light source offering certain unique advantages is a dye-laser, operating near 633 nm. This system consists of an argon laser "pumping" a dye laser with Rhodamine-B dye. The dye-laser is operated without the tuning wedge necessary to obtain bandwidths of less than 1.0 nm. Since the absorption of Hpd in this range is broad (620 nm–640 nm), advantage can be taken of the increased power obtained by removing the wedge and utilizing a larger portion of the Rhodamine-B emission. Using an 18-watt argon laser, approximately 3 watts of red light can be obtained from the dye-laser. While the total effective power available from the laser is not much different from the other light sources, it provides all the power in a 0.5 mm beam easily coupled into a single quartz fiber optic light guide. Our present system uses a low-loss 200 μM quartz core fiber which can be coupled to the laser with an efficiency of as much as 85%. Because of the low-loss characteristics of the fiber, its length has little effect on emitted power. This light delivery fiber provides great flexibility in providing light to areas reached only with difficulty with the static light source. However, its major advantage is that the fiber is small enough to be inserted into the biopsy channel of endoscopes or through small needles, thus for the first time allowing for light delivery directly to a tumor site without intervening tissue.

TABLE 48-21. Effect of PRT Variables on Skin and Tumor Response*

HPD DOSE (mg/kg)	TIME INTERVAL† (DAYS)	INCIDENT LIGHT DOSE (mw-min/cm²)‡	TUMOR RESPONSE''	SKIN RESPONSE
2.5	1	2000–4000	Necrosis	Necrosis
	2	2000–4000	Necrosis	Severe edema to necrosis
	3	1000	Partial to complete necrosis	Moderate edema
	3	2000	Necrosis	Moderate to severe edema
	4–7	2000	Partial to complete necrosis	None to moderate edema
3.5	1 → 3	2000	Necrosis	Necrosis
	4 → 6	1000	Necrosis	Moderate to severe edema
	6 → 10	1000–1500	None to partial necrosis	Moderate edema

* Tumors were metastatic cutaneous or subcutaneous chest wall nodules, ranging in size from 0.5 cm to 2.0 cm. More highly pigmented lesions responded less strongly. These responses are general and may vary from patient to patient.

† Interval between Hpd injection and light treatment.

‡ Light source was a filtered Xe arc lamp emitting 1100 mw/cm² between 600 nm and 700 nm. The light dose from the laser, emitting near 635 nm at 60 mw/cm² leading to an essentially equivalent result, would be one-half of these values.

'' The skin was outside the tumor area. In some cases skin in the tumor area responded more strongly. Also heavily irradiated (ionizing) skin may show enhanced response although only if chronic radiation-changes are evident. Varying degrees of erythema accompanied all responses.

The only other photosensitizer evaluated for treatment of malignant disease is methoxsalen (8-methoxypsoralen) for patients suffering from mycosis fungoides, a malignancy of the lymphoreticular system manifested by various stages of skin lesions. The general procedure had been originally developed by Parrish and associates to treat psoriasis and combined oral methoxsalen with ultraviolet light between 320 nm and 390 nm (UVA).[40] Studies by Gilchrest and co-workers, Roenigk and Lowe and co-workers included patients in various stages of disease, most of whom had recurred after various other therapies such as topical nitrogen mustard, electron beam therapy, or chemotherapy.[41–43] Patients ingested approximately 0.6 mg/kg methoxsalen 2 hours prior to light therapy. Light dose was determined by that amount which produced minimal erythema in a test area of normal skin determined 48 to 72 hours after exposure. One to four treatments per week were used until clearing of lesions became evident, at which point the frequency was reduced. Light exposures were between 1 joule/cm² and 16 joule/cm² (17–267 mw-min/cm²), generally starting low and gradually increasing to maintain the minimum erythemic dose as skin pigmentation increased. The number of treatments ranged from ten to 76. Significant improvement was seen clinically and histologically, in most cases, although relapse was a frequent occurrence and may be due to the presence of malignant cells deep in the dermis not reached by the U.V. light. Thus, Lowe and associates recommend maintenance therapy to control recurrence.[43] While not necessarily a preferred primary treatment for advanced mycosis fungoides, as compared to electron beam therapy for instance, it compares favorably with topical chemotherapy and apparently can be used after other therapies have failed.

CURRENT STUDIES OF PRT

Since the 1978 and 1979 reports, additional patients with metastatic breast carcinoma involving the chest wall have been treated by PRT at Roswell Park, by Forbes at the University of Adelaide, Australia, and by Treurniet-Donker at the Rotterdamsch Radio-Therapeutisch Instituut in the Netherlands.

As previously, all patients had failed to respond or experienced recurrence on prior conventional therapy. The latter patients have been treated with a variety of light sources of the types described above, depending on the particular situation. The total number of patients in this group, for whom benefit can be assessed, beyond whatever psychological benefit there may be from controlling isolated lesions in patients with extensive disease, is 16 out of a total of 35. As indicated above, the selection of most patients early in the study precluded long-term assessment or even short-term benefit. Follow-up times range to 3 years (one case) with the average being about 6 months. Of the 16 patients, eight showed recurrence in treated areas (and frequently outside of treated areas, as well), 2 months to 9 months after treatment, five have shown no recurrence in treated areas up to 9 months (the one patient treated 3 years ago received an anti-estrogen drug 9 months later due to a recurrent supraclavicular node), one showed no response and the other two remain under treatment. In one case, no attempt has been made at complete eradication, since the disease had recurred in an area which had previously received a very high dose of ionizing radiation and showed some skin necrosis and telangiectasis before PRT. There were 40 to 50 palpable lesions in an area of approximately 200 cm². In this patient, a low light dose (1000 mw-min/cm²) has been applied to this area and has resulted in tumor control without extensive skin damage. Over a 1-year period, a few lesions have reappeared and have responded well to repeated PRT. After three courses of PRT, in this period of time, no skin changes beyond those present prior to PRT, have been observed. This palliative treatment appears to be quite appropriate in this patient who had exhausted most other options.

Recurrence of lesions in treated areas is a frequent finding. Although we note that patients who have received two treatments approximately 2 weeks apart are less likely to recur, the number of patients is much too small to draw conclusions. However, it is clear that patients receiving steroids demonstrate skin responses below the average for a given set of treatment conditions. While the mechanism of this modification of response is not known, it may be that tumor response is also reduced (*e.g.*, by more rapid drug clearance). This point needs further clarification.

Although follow-up is short, we conclude that PRT can benefit patients who have disease localized to one side of the chest wall and of moderate size and extension, particularly if other therapies are not feasible. Prior conventional therapy appears not to preclude a good response, although in several patients who received very high doses of ionizing radiation and had obvious resultant skin changes, there was an enhanced acute effect of PRT on the skin. However, even in these patients, once the acute effect subsided, there have been no apparent long-term effects (maximum follow-up is 3 years). Hyperpigmentation in the treatment field is a common side effect whether or not there was prior radiotherapy.

Patients with extensive disease may or may not benefit from treatment. Although the bank of fluorescent lamps makes treatment feasible, there are several problems encountered with such patients. Frequently, the chest wall is so covered by ulcerating lesions that there is no normal skin remaining. Destruction of the lesion risks perforation through the chest wall. Second, the patients frequently experience severe pain from rapid destruction of a large mass of tumor over a large area. They are likely to show spiking fever and prolonged lethargy (1 month or more). Also, such patients are likely to have involved supraclavicular and axillary nodes not reachable by PRT, at least as currently applied. The possible benefit to this group of patients remains to be assessed. It is possible that palliation in such patients may be achieved using fractionation procedures, although effective fractionation procedures for PRT remain to be established.[38]

Application of PRT to various malignancies is being studied by several investigators. Our group at Roswell Park has shown recently that the activating light from the laser can be delivered directly to the tumor site by inserting the light delivery fiber through a needle placed into the tumor. Using this technique on primary tumors in cats and dogs, promising results have been obtained (Table 48-22). The ability to completely eradicate certain osteogenic sarcoma lesions without side-effects is promising.

From this work it is evident that there is a limit of approximately 5 cc to 10 cc of tumor tissue which can be effectively treated by a single fiber insertion. Thus, larger tumors require multiple insertions of the fiber or perhaps better, multiple fibers inserted simultaneously in order to achieve an adequate light dose over the entire mass. Also, it is clear that although the light from a single fiber is scattered throughout a relatively large volume of tissue (in fact, the reflected light observable on the surface is frequently over an area exceeding 10 cm²), there is "overkill" in the immediate vicinity of the fiber and "underkill" at the extremity. Also, there may be thermal effects within the immediate vicinity of the fiber tip owing to the extremely high light intensity at this point. To some extent, this problem may be solvable using fibers that diffuse the light at the tip, although even in this case, multiple fibers would be desirable. In addition, proper placement of the fibers requires a knowledge of the physics of light distribution in tissues (*i.e.*, dosimetry).

In addition to duplicating the Roswell Park experience in applying PRT to metastatic breast carcinoma, Forbes has used the fiber implants to advantage in several other types of tumors in humans. While these results are very preliminary, they demonstrate the potentially wide applicability of PRT. For example, he has succeeded in treating lesions in the brain and in the bronchus. Brain tumors were treated by placing the light delivery fiber from the laser directly into the lesion exposed at operation, 5 days after the patient received 2.5 mg/kg or 5.0 mg/kg Hpd. One patient had two such procedures and, in one case, as much visible tumor was removed surgically as possible prior to light treatment. Patients tolerated the treatment without noticeable side effects. In one case, histological examination at autopsy revealed extensive necrosis in the tumor lesion, with a sharp margin between necrotic and viable tumor tissue. The other patients are surviving and evaluation is continuing. Although results of interstitial PRT on brain tumors remain to be assessed, this treatment apparently can be carried out safely in such cases. In the bronchus, one patient was treated by Forbes 5 days post 5.0 mg/kg Hpd by inserting the light-delivery fiber directly into the lesion through a needle that had been inserted through the chest wall guided by 2-dimensional radiological techniques. The patient suffered no side-effects and roentgenographic examination indicated a short-lived reduction in the tumor mass. Forbes has also treated such lesions by delivering the fiber directly to the lesion through a bronchoscope. Apparent complete eradication of a recurrent 5 cm ovarian lesion in the pelvis and involving the vaginal vault has been achieved by Forbes using a similar technique. This required 11 fiber insertions in order to adequately expose the entire mass. The first few treatments were delivered on day 3 and day 4 following 5.0 mg/kg Hpd and the remainder on day 15. In these treatments, Forbes has used 200 mw to 300 mw of red light delivered through the fiber from the laser (approximately 633 nm), generally for 20 minutes to 30 minutes at each insertion. While the time interval is clearly too short to reasonably assess the ultimate results of such therapy, Forbes has demonstrated that it is both feasible and safe to treat a variety of life-threatening lesions by this technique, with the expectation that improved methodology may lead to their eradication or control.

Equally promising results are being obtained by Kennedy at the Kingston Clinic of the Ontario Cancer Foundation. Kennedy, using externally applied red light, has succeeded in eradicating large squamous cell carcinoma lesions in the

TABLE 48-22. Response of Primary Dog/Cat Tumors to PRT*

TUMOR TYPE/LOCATION/SIZE	ANIMAL	NUMBER OF TREATMENTS†	RESULTS	FOLLOW-UP
Osteogenic Sarcoma/Mandible 2.5 × 2.5 cm	Cat	1	Complete clearance. No side effects	2½ yr
Osteogenic Sarcoma/Sinus Cavity, Hard Palate 3.0 × 3.5 cm	Dog	2	Complete clearance. No side effects.	8 mo
Osteogenic Sarcoma/Tibia 7.5 × 6.5 cm	Dog	2	No response.	–
Osteogenic Sarcoma/Tibia 5 × 2 cm	Dog	1	Approximately ¼–½ cleared.	1 mo
Squamous Cell/Sinus Cavity 2.0 × 1.0 cm	Cat	4	Apparent complete response; followed by rapid regrowth.	3 mo
Squamous Cell/Hard Palate 2 × 3 cm	Dog	7	Apparent complete response; followed by rapid regrowth.	2 mo
Sebacious Gland/Face 3 × 3 cm	Dog	2	90% cleared after first treatment — retreated.	1 mo
Mast Cell Sarcoma/Chest Wall 2.5 × 2.5 cm	Dog	1	Complete clearance. No side effects.	6 mo
Fibrosarcoma/Leg Several Lesions 0.5 to 3.5 cm	Dog	1	Clearance followed by regrowth at periphery.	1 mo
Prostatic Carcinoma Metastatic to Pelvis 4 × 4 cm	Dog	1	50% clearance.	2 wk Followed by euthanasia due to deteriorated condition.
Melanoma/Mouth 4 × 2 cm 3 × 2 cm	Cat	5	Amelanotic lesion cleared after second treatment; melanotic lesion required 5 treatments; died of metastatic disease; no local disease at autopsy.	1 yr

* Animals received 5.0 mg/kg Hpd two days prior to treatment.
† Multiple insertions of the light delivery fiber from the laser were used for lesions larger than 1 cm diameter. Conditions were 200–600 mw at 625–640 nm for 20–60 minutes. In some cases external light was applied also from the laser.

sinus cavity of patients who had failed surgery, radiotherapy, and chemotherapy. This was accomplished by using multiple PRT treatments (six or more) to slowly shrink the large masses. Sufficient time between treatments (2–3 weeks) was allowed for tumor sloughing or, in some instances, the necrotic tissue was removed prior to the subsequent treatment. A similar approach has been successful in treating a recurrent retinoblastoma tumor involving the eye socket in a child. Kennedy has also found, as reported by Dougherty, that basal cell carcinoma lesions can be effectively treated by PRT.

MODE OF ACTION

Since Hpd is currently the only photosensitizer known to be effective against malignant tumors (aside from methoxsalen), consideration of mechanism is limited to this particular porphyrin. At this early stage in the use of Hpd, it is fair to say that specific molecular mechanisms are largely unknown. However, there is information on certain aspects of its mode of action. The overall aspects are fairly complicated and relate to the pharmacokinetics of the drug itself, the various chemical events elicited when the drug is photoactivated in tissue, and the biologic response of various tissues to these events.

Since numerous investigators have reported specific tumor fluorescence following Hpd administration, it is clearly important to attempt to understand the extent and mechanism of this action. Gomer and Dougherty, using radioactively tagged Hpd, demonstrated that the distribution in mice was quite different from that indicated by fluorescence and that liver, kidney, and spleen accumulated higher levels of the drug than did the transplanted mammary carcinoma tumors (Table 18-23).[16] The ^{14}C-Hpd gave essentially the same values as found for ^{3}H-Hpd, thus ruling out exchange. Recent results from this group have demonstrated that the Sarcoma-180 tumor accumulates levels of ^{3}H-Hpd similar to that of the carcinomas. Further, we have found that hematoporphyrin (from which Hpd is prepared) accumulates to levels very similar to those of Hpd in mouse tissues and tumors, as judged by tritium assay, yet hematoporphyrin does not sensitize the mouse tumors to photo-destruction. Further, both porphyrins have a high quantum efficiency for singlet oxygen formation in solution ($\Phi_{1O_2} > 0.75$), the apparent cytotoxic agent.[44] In order to understand this apparent anomaly, we have used autoradiographic methods to study the inter- and intra-distribution of ^{3}H-Hpd in mouse tissue as a function of time after injection.[45] Animals with either the SMT-F or S-180 tumors were injected with 5 mg/kg to 50 mg/kg of ^{3}H-

Hpd and tissues were examined at various times thereafter. The half-life for serum clearance was approximately 3 hours. At 3 hours postinjection, all tissues examined (liver, kidney, spleen, skin, stomach, lung, tumor) demonstrated widely distributed (stroma and parenchyma) levels of tritium, although a preference for the vascular stroma and connective tissue of the tumors of approximately 5:1 was evident. Liver, at this time, showed a higher level in certain areas, apparently Kupffer cells. None of the tissues excluded the porphyrin. However, a clear difference between normal and malignant tissues was evident at longer times following injection of Hpd. Beginning at 12 hours and clearly evident at 24 hours after injection, normal tissues had largely cleared the porphyrin from the parenchymal cells while retaining it in cells of the reticuloendothelial system, that is, in Kupffer cells in the liver and in red pulp macrophages in spleen and connective tissue. It was noted that the liver, kidney, and spleen appeared to sequester essentially all of the material in the phagocytic cells since the level between 3 hours and 24 hours was essentially unchanged (Table 48-23). In contrast to the normal tissues, the tumors did not demonstrate any change in drug distribution between 3 hours and 7 days (the longest time of examination). Tumor cells appeared to retain Hpd for an inordinately long time after injection, as did liver and spleen. The only other cells which appeared to have this property were reticuloendothelial cells, particularly macrophages of the connective tissue, although it is possible that fibroblasts may also retain the drug for extended times. This latter point is not well established.

Comparison of the Hpd data with that for ^{3}H-hematoporphyrin revealed that this latter porphyrin readily entered the vascular stroma of normal and malignant tissues of the mouse but did not enter parenchymal cells whether in normal or malignant tissue. In fact, the distribution pattern of hematoporphyrin in tissues is similar to that of albumin examined by ^{131}I tagging. This protein, to which both porphyrins bind strongly, in general, is not found to enter parenchymal cells but is largely retained in vascular stroma as is ^{3}H-hematoporphyrin.[46] The uniqueness of Hpd, therefore, appears to be its ability to enter cells of all kinds and be retained in reticuloendothelial cells and tumor cells long after it has cleared from the serum. While the retention of Hpd in reticuloendothelial cells is presumably related to normal phagocytic processes, the reason for retention in tumor cells is not known. We have found that these tumor cells do not phagocytize ^{131}I-albumin. Conceivably, other proteins that strongly bind Hpd may be phagocytized. While it is possible that tumor cells have a specific, strong binding site for Hpd, this is unlikely in view of our studies of cells in culture. For example, CHO (from normal hamster ovary fibroblasts), L929 (from normal mouse fibroblasts), HeLa (from human malignant cervical carcinoma) and PC-1 (from human malignant lung carcinoma) cells demonstrate no differences in rate of Hpd accumulation, equilibrium levels, or efflux rate when examined under similar conditions in suspension culture.[46] Also, V-79 cells (normal hamster fibroblasts), CHO and HeLa cells in monolayer cultures, all exhibit similar behavior toward Hpd, as do primary cultures of embryonic mouse fibroblasts and macrophages.[47] It should be noted that Mossman and associates have reported that mixed cultures of HeLa cells and normal cervical epithelium cells exhibit preferential fluorescence of the HeLa cells following Hpd exposure. However, we have noted a considerable variation in fluorescence of cultured cells containing similar levels of Hpd.

When mouse tumors containing Hpd are exposed to light (600 nm–700 nm), a series of changes can be seen starting immediately after exposure. The earliest changes seen histologically are around the tumor vessels, where the porphyrin level is highest. These are coagulation of red cells within the vessels and death of cells nearest the vessels. Tumor cells remote from the vessels, while not grossly damaged at this time, appear to be less well packed. Electron micrographs demonstrate that some tumor cells, closest to the vessels, have become devoid of cytoplasmic contents which can be seen leaking into the interstitial fluid.[45] However, at this time, the endothelial cells appear intact. By 3 hours after treatment, the entire tumor shows gross hemorrhage and massive destruction of tumor cells.

TABLE 48-23. ^{3}H-Hpd Levels in DBA/$_2$ Mice (μg/g or μg/ml)*

TIME AFTER INJECTION	SERUM	SMT-F MAMMARY TUMOR†	LIVER	KIDNEY	SPLEEN	LUNG	SKIN	MUSCLE
1	6.17(1)	2.63	13.97 ± 1.03 (2)	12.08 ± 1.04 (2)	10.66 ± 0.40 (2)	4.99 ± 1.62 (4)	2.53 ± 0.46 (2)	1.63 ± 0.35 (2)
4	9.49 ± 0.7 (3)	5.35	22.17 ± 3.26 (3)	17.55 ± 0.21 (3)	9.26 ± 1.23 (3)	5.84 ± 1.02 (3)	3.20 ± 1.22 (2)	1.56 ± 0.19 (3)
17	2.15 ± 0.68 (5)	6.8	22.48 ± 1.98 (5)	19.13 ± 2.23 (5)	8.79 ± 1.07 (5)	–	–	0.38 ± 0.57 (5)
24	1.48 ± 0.19 (7)	7.3	22.14 ± 2.68 (7)	13.53 ± 2.25 (7)	8.53 ± 0.98 (7)	2.74 ± 0.77 (7)	2.06 ± 0.03 (2)	0.60 ± 0.45 (7)
48	0.64 ± 0.1 (3)	6.7	26.17 ± 2.38 (3)	12.06 ± 0.88 (3)	9.90 ± 0.10 (3)	2.52 ± 0.27 (3)	1.96 ± 0.46 (3)	0.87 ± 0.20 (3)
72	0.38 ± 0.07 (2)	8.3	18.56 ± 2.60 (2)	9.25 ± 3.56 (2)	8.36 ± 1.59 (2)	2.17 ± 0.21 (2)	1.42 ± 0.66 (2)	0.93 ± 0.31 (2)

* ± S.D.; Numbers in parenthesis are number of samples; 10 mg/kg ^{3}Hpd, i.p.

† Corrected for increase in tumor volume.

The apparent cytotoxic agent responsible for cellular destruction is singlet oxygen formed by energy transfer from the excited porphyrin;

$$P + h\nu \rightarrow P^*(S)$$
$$P^*(S) \rightarrow P^*(T)$$
$$O_2 + P^*(T) \rightarrow P + {}^1O_2^*$$
$${}^1O_2^* \rightarrow O_2$$
$${}^1O_2^* + T \rightarrow T(O_2)$$

where P represents porphyrin, $P^*(S)$ and $P^*(T)$ represent excited prophyrin singlet and triplet states, respectively, ${}^1O_2^*$ represents singlet oxygen, T represents cellular target, and $T(O_2)$ indicates oxidized target. Evidence for this mechanism is the protection from light of cells in culture containing both Hpd and isobenzofuran, an effective singlet oxygen trap.[44] However, this material may be capable also of trapping free radicals. Also, Moan and co-workers have demonstrated an enhanced cytotoxic effect of photo-activated hematoporphyrin where D_2O is substituted for H_2O in the media of cultured cells, an effect frequently considered to be proof of singlet oxygen involvement.[49] A similar experiment has not yet been reported for Hpd. Further, removal of oxygen from the atmopshere over cell cultures prevents destruction due to Hpd plus light and clamping off blood flow in the legs of mice with leg tumors before and during illumination prevents tumor response due to Hpd plus light. It seems likely that formation of singlet oxygen is just the start of a long chain of events, probably including many oxygen radicals, leading to cell destruction.

While the cellular target (or targets) leading to destruction of the cells is not known, it is likely that the cell membrane plays an important role. Kessel has shown that several porphyrins in cell culture can cause photoactivated inhibition of membrane transport properties.[50] Also, we find that cultured cells demonstrate a high degree of ${}^{51}Cr$ leakage following Hpd plus light. For example, there is an order of magnitude more ${}^{51}Cr$ leakage from V-79 cells following Hpd plus light than occurs from these cells following a dose of ionizing radiation sufficient to lead to a similar cellular survival level.[51] However, preliminary experiments, carried out in our laboratory, indicate DNA strand breaks also occur due to photoactivated Hpd. Conversely to the ${}^{51}Cr$ effects, the degree of DNA strand breaks is an order of magnitude less than that due to an ionizing radiation dose sufficient to lead to the same survival level. It has been reported by Kessel and by Dubbleman that cross linking of membrane proteins occurs in cells exposed to light following accumulation of certain porphyrins.[50,51] Kessel has also shown that cellular binding is a prerequisite to photoactivated effects on cells, even though in principle, externally generated singlet oxygen has a long enough lifetime in solution (1μ second) to collide many times with the cell membrane and indeed diffuse to any potential cellular target.[21] Also, it should be noted that while the cell membrane may be an important target for singlet oxygen, Hpd is distributed throughout the cell as follows: soluble fraction of cytoplasm, 60% to 70%, mitochondrial fraction, 13% to 15%, microsomes, 7% to 13%, and nuclei, 4% to 9%.[53]

We have demonstrated that both normal tissue and the SMT-F tumor in mice are capable of repairing photoradiation damage. With a given dose of light, delivered either as a single dose or in two equal fractions with a 3-hour interval, reduced damage is apparent in the normal mouse foot and in the SMT-F tumor.[54,55] The kinetics of this repair remain to be evaluated, particularly as they relate to normal and malignant tissues.

FUTURE APPLICABILITY OF PRT TO CANCER THERAPY

PRT has yet to be proven to be a curative treatment for malignant disease. Clearly, several types of solid tumors respond to treatment and complete necrosis with eradication of lesions has been demonstrated by several groups. Equally clearly, the results are short-term and methods primitive. The fact that PRT can be applied safely, in areas previously receiving maximum tolerable doses of ionizing radiation, may offer considerable incentive for further development. Also, the preliminary data indicate that certain radio-resistant tumors such as osteogenic sarcoma, may be responsive to PRT.

In many ways PRT is in a stage similar to the early days of radiotherapy; it is known that the method can eradicate tumors, but how to do this for the maximum benefit of the patient remains to be determined. Major questions remain. Do all types of tumors take up Hpd and to what extent? What is the appropriate drug dose? How long after injection should the light be delivered? What is the light dose required to eradicate a given lesion? How can this light be effectively delivered and measured? Are multiple treatments preferrable to a single treatment? Can the light dose be effectively fractionated? What are the repair capabilities of normal and malignant tissue?

It is interesting to note that while Hpd has been used clinically since 1961, its structure remains unknown.[12] Considering the rather unique capabilities of this material, this is surprising. A search for better photosensitizers should be made in order to obtain drugs with better tissue distribution and, in particular, photosensitizers that would clear tissue faster to prevent or reduce photosensitivity reactions due to sunlight. This is especially important in using such materials for tumor localization, since such patients are frequently active and treated on an outpatient basis.

Current technology with lasers and fiber optics make it feasible to deliver high intensity light to almost any site in the body through needles, endoscopes, or at surgery. This will allow PRT to be used to treat life-threatening malignant disease which may not be responsive to current modalities. For example, could PRT be used to treat resectable or non-resectable portions of lesions in the brain or pancreas?

Since PRT is a local treatment, it likely will be desirable to use it in combination with systemic treatment or in combination with ionizing radiation or hyperthermia. Many of these studies are currently underway.

REFERENCES

1. Mellors RC, Glassman A, Papanicolaou GN: A microfluorimetric scanning method for the detection of cancer cells in smears of exfoliated cells. Cancer 5:458–468, 1952

2. Moore GE: Diagnosis and localization of brain tumors; a clinical and experimental study employing fluorescent and radioactive tracer methods. Springfield, Illinois, Charles C Thomas, 1953
3. Santamaria L, Prino G: The photodynamic substances and their mechanism of action. In Gallo U, Santamaria L (eds): Research Progress in Organic Biological and Medicinal Chemistry, Vol I, pp 260–336. Milan, Societa Editoriale Farmacentia, 1964
4. Rall DD, Loo TL, Lane M et al: Appearance and persistence of fluorescent material in tumor tissue after tetracycline administration. J Natl Cancer Inst, 19:79–86, 1957
5. Tomson SH, Emmett EA, Fox SH: Photodestruction of mouse epithelial tumors after acridine orange and argon laser. Cancer Res 34:3124–3127, 1974
6. Policard A: Etudes sur les aspects offerts par des tumeur experimentales examinee a la lumiere de woods. CR Soc Biol 91:1423–1424, 1924
7. Auler H, Banzer G: Untersuchungen uber die rolle der prophine bei geschwulstkranken menschen und tieren. Z Krebsforsch 53:65–68, 1942
8. Figge FHJ, Weiland GS, Manganiello LOJ: Cancer detection and therapy. Affinity of neoplastic embryonic and traumatized regenerating tissues for porphyrins and metalloporphyrins. Proc Soc Exptl Biol Med 68:640–641, 1948
9. Schwartz S: (Private communication and as quoted in Ref 10, p 1)
10. Lipson RL: The photodynamic and fluorescent properties of a particular hematoporphyrin derivative and its use in tumor detection. Master's Thesis, University of Minnesota, 1960
11. Lipson RL, Baldes EJ, Olsen AM: The use of a derivative of hematoporphyrin in tumor detection. J Natl Cancer Inst 26:1–8, 1961
12. Lipson RL, Baldes EJ, Olsen AM: Hematoporphyrin derivative: A new aid of endoscopic detection of malignant disease. J Thorac Cardiovasc Surg 42:623–629, 1961
13. Lipson RL, Baldes EJ, Olsen AM: A further evaluation of the use of hematoporphyrin derivative as a new aid for the endoscopic detection of malignant disease. Dis Chest 46:676–679, 1964
14. Lipson RL, Pratt JH, Baldes EJ et al: Hematoporphyrin derivative for the detection of cervical cancer. Obstet Gynecol 24:78–84, 1964
15. Gregorie HB Jr, Horger EO, Ward JL et al: Hematoporphyrin derivative fluorescence in malignant neoplasms. Ann Surg 167:829–828, 1968
16. Gomer CJ, Dougherty TJ: Determination of ^{3}H- and ^{14}C hematoporphyrin derivative distribution in malignant and normal tissue. Cancer Res 39:146–151, 1979
17. Kinsey JH, Cortese DA, Sanderson DR: Detection of hematoporphyrin fluorescence during fiver-optic bronchoscopy to localize early bronchogenic carcinoma. Mayo Clinic Proc 53:594–600, 1978
18. Cortese DA, Kinsey JH, Woolnen LB et al: Clinical application of a new endoscopic technique for detection of in-situ bronchial carcinoma. Mayo Clin Proc 54:635–642, 1979
19. Dioron DR, Profio AE, Vincent RG et al: Fluorescence bronchoscopy for detection of lung cancer. Chest 76:27–32, 1979
20. Profio AE, Doiron DR, King EG: Laser fluorescence bronchoscope for localization of occult lung tumors. Med Phys 6:523–525, 1979
21. Kessel D: Effects of photoactivated prophyrins on cell surface of leukemia L1210 cells. Biochem 16:3443–3449, 1977
22. Winkelman J: The distribution of tetraphenylporphine sulfonate in the tumor-bearing rat. Cancer Res 22:589–596, 1962
23. Winkelman J, Slater G, Grossman J: The concentration in tumor and other tissue of parentally administered tritium and ^{14}C-labelled tetraphenylporphine sulfonate. Cancer Res 27:2060–2064, 1967
24. Musser DA, Wagner JM, Datta-Gupta N: The distribution of tetraphenylporphine sulfonate ($TPPS_4$) and tetracarboxyphenylporphine (TCPP) in tumor-bearing mice. J Natl Cancer Inst 61:1397–1403, 1978
25. Dougherty TJ: (Unpublished results) 1974
26. Kyriazis GA, Balin H, Lipson RL: Hematoporphyrin derivative fluorescence test colposcopy and colpophotography in the diagnosis of atypical metaplasia, dysplasia and carcinoma in-situ of the cervix uteri. Am J Obstet Gynecol 117:375–380, 1973
27. Kelly JF, Snell ME, Berenbaum MC: Photodynamic destruction of human bladder carcinoma. Br J Cancer 31:237–244, 1975
28. Edwards E, Duntley SQ: Spectrophotometry of living human skin. J Invest Dermatol 16:311, 1951
29. Dougherty TJ, Kaufman JE, Goldfarb A et al: Photoradiation therapy for the treatment of malignant tumors. Cancer Res 38:2628–2635, 1978
30. Everett MA, Yeargers E, Sayre RM et al: Penetration of epidermis by ultraviolet rays. Photochem Photobiol I, 533–542, 1962
31. Tappenier H, Jesionek A: Therapeutische versuche mit fluoreszierenden stoffe. Muench Med Wochschr 1:2042–2044, 1903
32. Diamond I, Granelli S, McDonagh AF et al: Photodynamic therapy of malignant tumors. Lancet 2:1175–1177, 1973
33. Granelli SG, Diamond I, McDonagh AF et al: Photochemotherapy of glioma cells by visible light and hematoporphyrin. Cancer Res 35:2567–2570, 1975
34. Dougherty TJ: Photoradiation therapy, Abstracts of the American Chemical Society Meeting, No 014, Chicago, Illinois, Sept 1973
35. Dougherty TJ: Activated dyes as anti-tumor agents. J Natl Cancer Inst 51:1333–1336, 1974
36. Dougherty TJ, Grindey GB, Fiel R et al: Photoradiation therapy II. Cure of animal tumors with hematoporphyrin and light. J Natl Cancer Inst 55:115–119, 1975
37. Kelly JF, Snell ME: Hematoporphyrin derivative: A possible aid in the diagnosis and therapy of carcinoma of the bladder. J Urol 115:150–151, 1976
38. Dougherty TJ, Lawrence G, Kaufman JE et al: Photoradiation in the treatment of recurrent breast carcinoma. J Natl Cancer Inst 62:231–237, 1979
39. Dougherty TJ: (unpublished results) 1975
40. Parrish JA, Fitzpatrick TB, Tanenbaum L et al: Photochemotherapy of psoriasis with oral methoxsalen and long-wave ultraviolet light. N Engl J Med 291:1207–1222, 1974
41. Gilchrest BA, Parrish JA, Tanenbaum L et al: Oral methoxalen photochemotherapy of mycosis fungoides. Cancer 38:683–689, 1976
42. Roenigk, H: Photochemotherapy for mycosis fungoides. Arch Dermatol 113:1047–1051, 1977
43. Lowe NJ, Cripps DJ, Dufton PA et al: Photochemotherapy for mycosis fungoides. Arch Dermatol 115:50–53, 1979
44. Weishaupt KR, Gomer CJ, Dougherty TJ: Identification of singlet oxygen as the cytotoxic agent in photo-inactivation of a murine tumor. Cancer Res 36:2326–2329, 1976
45. Bugelski PJ: Morphologic aspects of the photosensitizing effects and distribution of hematoporphyrin derivative in experimental tumors and cultured cells. PhD Thesis submitted to the Graduate School, State University of New York at Buffalo, 1980
46. Chang CT, Dougherty TJ: Photoradiation therapy: Kinetics and thermodynamics of porphyrin uptake and loss in normal and malignant cells in culture. Radiat Res 74:498–499, 1978
47. Henderson BW, Dougherty TJ: (Unpublished results) 1980
48. Mossman BT, Gray MJ, Silberman L et al: Identification of neoplastic versus normal cells in human cervical cell culture. J Obstet Gynecol 43:635–639, 1974
49. Moan J, Pettersen EO, Christensen T: The mechanism of photodynamic inactivation of human cells in-vitro in the presence of hematoprophyrin. Br J Cancer 39:398–401, 1979
50. Kessel D: Effects of photo-activated porphyrins in cell surface properties. Biochem Soc Trans 5:139–140, 1977
51. Gomer CJ, Bellnier DA, Dougherty TJ: (unpublished results) 1979
52. Dubbelman TMAR, DeGoeij AFOM, van Steveninck J: Protoporphyrin-sensitized photodynamic modification of proteins in isolated human red blood cell membranes. Photochem Photobiol 28:197–204, 1978
53. Gomer CJ: Evaluation of in-vivo tissue localization and in-vitro photosensitization reactions of hematoporphyrin derivative. PhD Thesis submitted to the Graduate School, State University of New York at Buffalo, 1978
54. Dougherty TJ, Borcicky D, Weiskaupt KR et al: Repair of damage in experimental and clinical photoradiation. Proc Am Assoc Cancer Res 18:44, 1977
55. Michalakes C, Weiskaupt KR, Dougherty TJ: (unpublished results) 1980

Section 5

Densely Ionizing Particle Radiation Therapy

DAVID A. PISTENMAA

Motivation for the investigation of particle beam radiation therapy is based upon the potential of this method of treatment to increase the rates of local and regional control of malignant neoplasms. The expected advantages of particle beam radiotherapy are based upon the improved physical dose distributions achievable with protons, helium ions, negative π-mesons (pions), and heavy ions and the demonstrated increased biological effectiveness of neutrons, helium ions, pions, and heavy ions. The improved physical dose distributions available with charged particle irradiation provide an opportunity to circumvent one of the most common reasons for the failure of photon irradiation to eradicate cancer locally or regionally. This is the inability to deliver an adequate radiation dose with photons to the target (tumor containing) volume because of the limited tolerance to radiation of the normal tissues surrounding the tumor.

The increased biological effectiveness of irradiation with beams of neutrons, helium ions, pions, or heavy ions provides an opportunity to overcome another common reason for the failure of photon irradiation to eradicate cancer. This is the inability to eradicate tumors in a substantial fraction of patients despite delivery of a radiation dose with photons which is, however, adequate to eradicate some tumors in that group of patients. It is hypothesized that the most common reason for the latter observation is the presence of foci of hypoxic or anoxic tumor cells which are much more resistant to photon or electron irradiation than are oxygenated cells.

Because of these physical or biological properties, treatment with particle beams is expected to have a major impact on the management of patients by improving the local and regional control of cancers. The types of patients who are expected to benefit from radiation therapy with any one particle beam will vary depending upon the physical or biological property, or combination thereof, of the specific particle. The improved physical dose distributions theoretically achievable with protons, helium ions, pions, and heavy ions may be of benefit to: (a) patients whose treatment is compromised by unacceptable acute morbidity (nausea, vomiting, and diarrhea) of photon irradiation; (b) patients who would experience a high frequency of severe late complications if doses sufficient to eradicate a high percentage of tumors were given; (c) patients who are scheduled to undergo chemotherapy in conjunction with radiotherapy and in whom particle beam radiotherapy would improve their tolerance to chemotherapy by preserving more bone marrow; (d) patients whose immunological systems might contribute to the success of treatment and in whom particle beam irradiation would give a lower dose to lymphoid organs; and (e) patients in whom a surgical procedure in the irradiated region is planned or later becomes necessary and in whom the lower dose to normal tissues surrounding the tumor volume with particle beam irradiation would be expected to decrease postoperative complications.

Treatment with neutrons or with charged particles having an increased biological effect (pions and heavy ions) may be of benefit to patients with: (a) tumors in which hypoxic or anoxic cells are, in fact, a cause of failure of conventional photon radiation therapy and (b) patients whose tumors are moderately resistant to treatment with photons and electrons but which might be more sensitive to particle beam radiation doses, for the same amount of or less normal tissue injury, because of differences in the repair of sublethal and potentially lethal damage and in cell cycle sensitivity.

If particle beam radiation therapy does improve local and regional control rates, this modality will assume even greater significance in the future when it is expected that improved detection methods will result in the recognition of more tumors prior to the development of distant metastases and also as advances in chemotherapy increase the likelihood of eradicating disseminated microscopic foci of cancer. In addition, for selected disease sites, particle beam radiation may become an alternative to treatment with surgery alone or with surgery in combination with photon irradiation thereby preserving normal anatomy and physiological function.

The following section will examine in more detail the physical or biological properties of beams of neutrons, protons, helium ions, pions, or heavy ions that offer significant promise for improved local and regional control of tumors. That section will also address several other clinically relevant considerations, including tumor and organ delineation, patient positioning and immobilization during treatment, and the incorporation of corrections for tissue density inhomogeneities into treatment calculations. The succeeding section will review the scope and preliminary observations of the particle beam clinical research program in the United States. The final section will discuss the interrelationships among the investigation of particle beam radiation therapy and other research efforts to improve the local and regional control of malignancies.

PHYSICAL AND BIOLOGICAL PROPERTIES OF PARTICLE BEAMS

Although dose distributions achievable with electron beams offer significant advantages compared to photon beams for the treatment of many patients with superficial tumors, the dose distributions achievable with beams of protons, helium ionos, pions, or heavy ions are superior for both superficial and deeply seated tumors. Therapeutic electron beams are a readily available feature of many modern linear accelerators and therefore will not be discussed in this chapter. In contrast to equipment for the production of therapeutic electron or photon beams, the equipment required to produce beams of neutrons and charged heavy particles for cancer treatment is much more complex and expensive.[1]

Beams of neutrons for radiotherapy can be generated either by bombarding a target containing tritium (T) with accelerated deuterium (D) ions in a D–T generator or by bombarding a suitable target such as beryllium (Be) with protons (p) or deuterons (d) accelerated in a cyclotron or linear accelerator. The D–T generator produces a monoenergetic 14 MeV neutron beam whereas the proton on beryllium (p → Be) and deuteron on beryllium (d → Be) reactions produce neutron beams with a spectrum of energies which can be modified somewhat by filtering. The neutron beam produced by bombarding a beryllium target with 42 MeV protons penetrates tissues slightly better than does the 14 MeV beam from a D–T generator.

The production of beams of protons, helium ions, and heavy ions such as ^{12}C, ^{20}Ne, ^{38}Si, and ^{40}Ar with sufficient energy to treat deeply seated tumors in patients requires increasingly sophisticated equipment with increasing mass of the particle.[1] A linear accelerator or cyclotron could be used to produce a therapeutic proton beam, whereas only a cyclotron would be practical for the final acceleration of helium and heavier ions.

A pion beam for radiotherapy can be produced in a suitable target by either a 500 MeV (or greater) energy electron beam or a proton beam of similar energy.[2] A linear accelerator or cyclotron facility for pion radiotherapy would be comparable in cost to a heavy ion radiotherapy facility.[1]

PHYSICAL PROPERTIES OF PARTICLE BEAMS

The physical characteristics of particle beams which are of clinical interest relate to the properties of beam attenuation and the pattern of energy deposition on a microscopic scale. The latter property is termed linear energy transfer (LET) and is expressed as keV per micron (keV/μ). Beams of neutrons, uncharged particles with a mass approximately 2000 times that of the electron, are attenuated exponentially in matter and therefore give dose distributions similar to those achieved with cobolt-60 (^{60}Co) or 6 mV roentgen radiation machines, depending upon the energy of the neutrons. Because neutrons scatter significantly and are also more difficult to collimate than photons, the physical dose distributions attainable with neutron beams are less satisfactory than those with megavoltage roentgen beams. However, the higher linear energy transfer by neutrons compared to photons produces significantly greater biological effects for the same physical dose. The LET spectrum is slightly different for neutron beams of different energies and it generally changes, but only slightly, for each beam with depth of penetration in tissues.[3] These factors must be taken into consideration when planning clinical studies or comparing results at institutions with beams of different energies.

The charged particles that are of interest for clinical application are protons, helium ions, pions, and a number of heavy ions. Protons are singly charged particles with a mass approximately 2000 times that of the electron. Helium ions are doubly charged particles with a mass approximately 4 times that of the proton. Negative π-mesons (pions) are singly charged particles with a mass 273 times that of the electon. Heavy ions of interest include carbon-12 (^{12}C), neon-20 (^{20}Ne), silicon-28 (^{28}Si), and argon-40 (^{40}Ar). They can be highly charged, depending upon the number of electrons stripped from the atom. In comparison to the exponential attenuation in matter of photon and neutron beams, charged particle beams have a definite range determined by their initial momentum and modified slightly by range straggling. The range, expressed in g/cm^2, varies for different materials and for different tissues in the body. When the charged particles reach the end of their range, there is an intense burst of ionization (Bragg peak), which is considerably more dense than the ionization in the plateau (entrance) region which would correspond in a patient to the distance from the surface of the body to the beginning of the target (tumor) volume. Pion and proton beams have a particularly attractive physical property in that the ionization produced by them in the plateau region is comparable to that produced by photons. However, when a pion reaches the end of its trajectory it is captured by an atom which subsequently disintegrates producing a number of densely ionizing (high LET) charged particles, high energy neutrons, and photons (star formation). The high LET radiations enhance the biological effectiveness of a pion beam in the peak region which would coincide with the target volume. Proton beams exhibit a Bragg peak with slightly increased biological effectiveness but no star formation.

The stopping region of charged particle beams can be made to conform to a designated treatment volume either by selecting particles with the proper initial incident energy or by interposing absorber materials between the source of the particles and the patient to modulate the energy (range) of the particle beam as it strikes the surface of the body. Thus, normal tissues at penetration depths greater than that of the target volume will receive no radiation from the primary particle beam but may experience a small radiation dose from secondary (fragmentation) particles or, in the case of pions, from beam contaminants (electrons and muons) and from neutrons produced in the star region. Charged particle beams therefore have the potential of delivering an increased radiation dose to the target volume relative to that in the adjacent normal tissues. This is illustrated in Fig. 48-22 which shows the relative ability to treat a designated target (tumor) volume from one direction with photons, neutrons, and several charged particles.

Fig. 48-22 also illustrates another principle related to treatment with pions, helium ions, and heavy ions. The greater the mass of the charged particle, the narrower the Bragg peak and the greater the intensity of high LET events therein. This differential energy absorption between the peak and the plateau is partially lost, however, if the stopping region must be broadened in order to encompass a large treatment volume. When this is necessary, the high LET peak events are diluted by the generally lower LET events common to the plateau region. This reduces the differential biological effect between the peak and plateau regions (peak-to-plateau ratio). This is an extremely important consideration for particle beam radiation because the biological effects of the beams are strongly correlated with the proportion of high LET events.[4]

BIOLOGICAL PROPERTIES OF PARTICLE BEAMS

As mentioned earlier, protons do not have a significantly greater biological effect than photons, whereas neutrons, helium ions, pions, and heavy charged particles do because of their higher rate of energy loss. There are many phenomena which explain the increased biological effectiveness of high

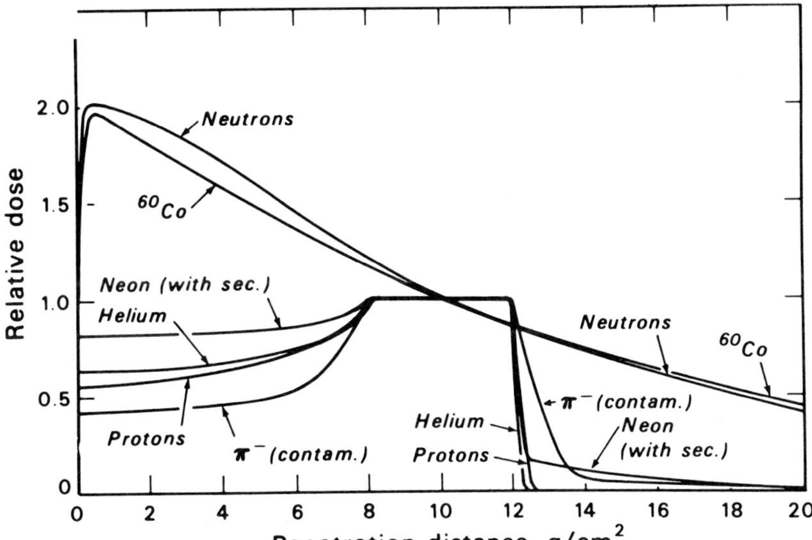

FIG. 48-22. Depth-dose curves calculated or measured for ^{60}Co gamma rays, neutrons, and various charged particles calculated or measured to deliver a unit dose to a 4 g/cm^2 wide region (8–12 g/cm^2) centered at a depth of 10.0 g/cm^2. Both gamma rays and neutrons give a high dose in the entrance region (0–8 g/cm^2) as well as a substantial dose in the 12–20 g/cm^2 region beyond the target volume. On the other hand, all of the charged particles give a lower dose in the entrance region than in the target volume and a negligible or very low dose beyond it. (Tobias CA, Lyman JT, Lawrence JA: Progress in Atomic Medicine: Recent Advances in Nuclear Medicine, Vol 3, pp 167–218. New York, Grune and Stratton, 1971)

LET radiations as observed *in vitro* and in animal tumor systems.[5,6]

One of the most important biological characteristics of high LET radiations compared to photons is the decrease in sensitivity of tumor cell killing to the oxygen concentration at the time of irradiation.[1,5] This is illustrated in Fig, 48-23. This effect of oxygen is termed the oxygen enhancement ratio (OER) which is the ratio of the dose required to achieve a specific response in anoxic cells to that required to achieve the same response with aerobic cells. For low LET radiations the OER is 2.5–3.0, whereas for high LET radiations the OER decreases with increasing LET rates and approaches 1 as the LET rate exceeds approximately 100 keV/μ as shown in Fig. 48-24.[6] Therefore, if, as hypothesized, hypoxic or anoxic cells contribute to the failure to eradicate certain tumors by low LET radiations, then the high LET radiations offer significant potential for the treatment of such malignancies.

Since the OER is the ratio of the killing of anoxic cells to the killing of aerobic cells by one type of radiation under specific conditions, it is important to compare the OER for a particle beam with the OER for photon irradiation under identical conditions. The ratio of the OER for roentgen rays to the OER for particle irradiation is termed the oxygen gain factor (OGF) and is an indication of the potential benefit of particle beam radiotherapy.[1] Since hypoxic or anoxic cells are generally not present in normal tissues, the OGF is an indication of expected differential response of tumor cells compared to normal tissues within or near the high-dose treatment volume. Although the oxygen effect has been well documented *in vitro* and has been demonstrated in experimental animal tumors, it is at this point strongly suspected, but not yet proven, to be a factor in the treatment of human tumors.

In addition to the oxygen effect, other factors which may contribute to the greater effectiveness of high LET compared to low LET radiation therapy include the following: (1) there

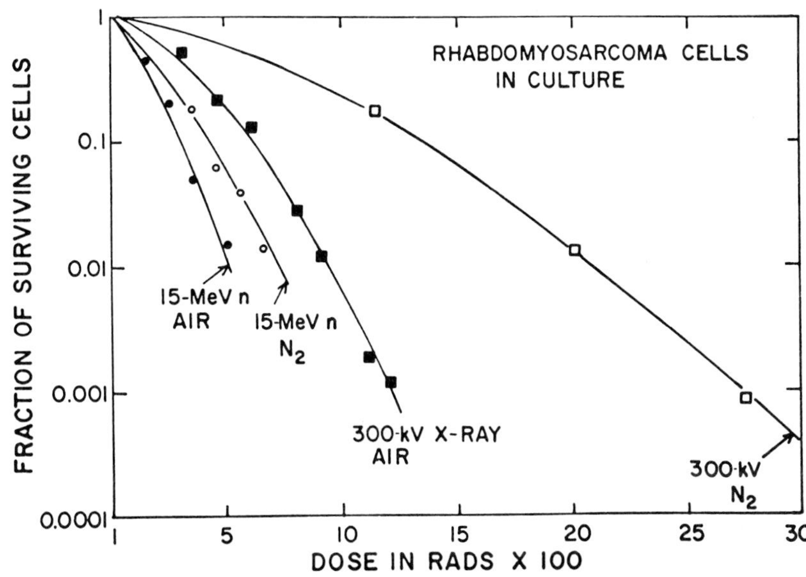

FIG. 48-23. Survival curves for cells irradiated by 300 kV x-rays 15-MeV neutrons under aerated and hypoxic conditions. (Barendsen GW: Response of cultured cells, tumors and normal tissues to radiations of different linear energy transfer. Curr Top Radiat Res 4:295, 1968)

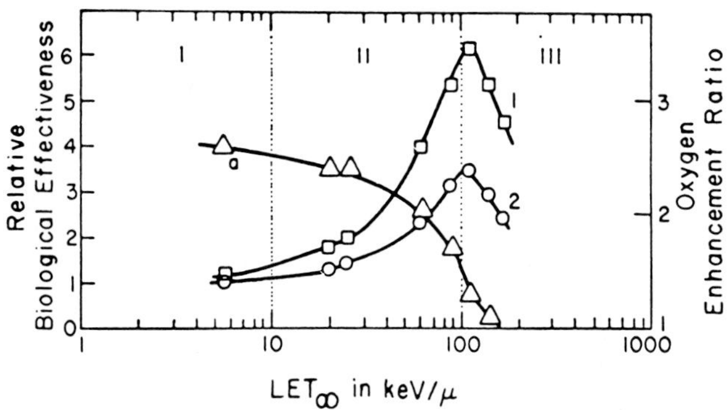

FIG. 48-24. Variations of RBE and OER as a function of LET derived from survival curves of cultured human kidney cells irradiated with alpha particles and deuterons. RBE curves I and II correspond to survival fractions of 0.5 and 0.01, respectively. Curve *a* represents the variation of OER with LET. (Barendsen GW: Radiobiological dose-effect relations for radiation characterized by a wide spectrum of LET; Implications for their application in radiotherapy. Los Alamos Scientific Laboratory Report LA-5180-C:120, 1972)

is greater cell killing than with the same dose of low LET radiation, (2) there is less repair of both sublethal and potentially lethal radiation damage in cells after high LET irradiation than after low LET irradiation, (3) there is less variation in cell killing as a function of position in the cell replication cycle with high compared to low LET irradiation, and (4) there is relatively greater sensitivity of cells of high ploidy than of euploid cells to high LET radiations.[1] This differential biological effect of various types of radiations is termed the relative biological effectiveness (RBE). RBE is defined as the ratio of the dose of reference radiation (generally 250 kV roentgen rays) to produce a given response divided by the dose of high LET radiation required to produce the same response. This comparison must be carried out under identical experimental or clinical conditions and radiation schedules. The RBE increases gradually with increasing LET up to approximately 100 keV/μ after which it decreases slightly with higher LET rates as shown in Fig. 48-23.

Because of the relationships between LET and OER as well as with RBE, it is highly desirable to achieve a homogeneous distribution of the high LET ionization events throughout the target volume when treating with helium ions, pions, and heavy ions. This will insure that the biologically effective dose distributions for these particles will be more predictable and be more likely to produce the favorable results expected of particle beam radiation therapy.[4]

CLINICAL CONSIDERATIONS

In order to exploit the potential advantages of particle beam radiation therapy, one must pay careful attention to all of the details inherent in sophisticated megavoltage roentgen radiation treatment. In fact, the increased biological effect of high LET radiations on normal as well as malignant tissues and the influence of tissue density inhomogeneities on charged particle dose distributions warrant even more complex planning of treatments than is necessary to achieve the best megavoltage radiation therapy results.

The objective of comparing particle beam radiation therapy with the best conventional megavoltage radiation therapy is to ascertain whether a higher rate of local–regional tumor control can be achieved for the same level of normal tissue complications. The improved physical dose distributions possible with charged particles may make it feasible to spare parts of organs, including even part of the circumference of a hollow organ. In order to realize this advantage of particle beam radiation therapy, it is essential to use the latest diagnostic imaging technology, especially computerized tomography, for delineating tumors and normal organs.[7-10] It is important to determine the location of tumors and normal organs in all treatment positions because both external and internal anatomical relationships change with changes in body position, such as supine *versus* prone or both *versus* lateral decubitus positions. In order to carry out many treatments planned with great precision, it will be necessary to use sophisticated patient immobilization devices to insure the accuracy of each treatment and the reproducibility of treatments during the course of therapy.

In terms of delivering the radiation dose, the tumorcidal dose range for most kinds of tumors is often quite close to the range of radiation doses for which there is a significant probability of producing injury in one or more adjacent normal tissues.[2] The dose–response curve for tumor eradication as well as that for normal tissue injury is usually a rather steep sigmoidal function of radiation dose. The steepness of this dose–response curve is such that an increase in dose of 10% to 15% might give an increase of 40% to 60% in the local control rate. Thus, the goal for charged particle beam radiation therapy is to achieve a slightly higher biologically effective dose in the target volume while maintaining a low risk of injury to nearby normal tissues.

Neutron beam therapy offers only the advantage of an increased biologically effective dose. One must hope that the potential additional effects of neutrons on tumor cells, as discussed above, will give greater tumor-cell killing for the same acceptable low level of normal tissue injury experienced with aggressive photon radiation therapy.

A consideration of great importance to charged particle beam radiation therapy and, to a lesser extent, neutron therapy is the correction of dose calculations for tissue density inhomogeneities.[7] Because charged particles have a finite range which is determined by the stopping power of the medium through which they pass, the stopping power of all of the tissues in the particle beam path must be known or accurately estimated for precise treatment calculations. Tissue density information obtained from modern computerized tomographic (CT) scanners provides an excellent first approximation to the information necessary for particle beam treatment calculations.[7] Thus, in addition to providing excellent information for the delineation of tumors and normal organs, CT scan cross-sections provide the necessary information for accurate corrections for tissue inhomogeneities.[7,8] Density information from CT scan cross-sections can also be used to correct neutron beam dose calculations for the increased beam transition through lung tissue and eventually may be useful for refining calculations in patients who have an abundance of adipose tissue. Because there is preferential absorption of energy from neutron beams in hydrogenated materials, there is an increased risk of injury to tissues with high lipid concentrations such as the brain and spinal cord as well as in adipose tissues.[11]

CLINICAL RESEARCH

The ultimate goal of the particle beam radiation therapy clinical research program is to ascertain whether that modality is superior to conventional photon radiation therapy for the treatment of tumors in different parts of the body. Because of the preliminary status of nearly all prospective randomized clinical trials with all particle beams, the experience at Hammersmith Hospital, London, in the treatment of head and neck cancers stands out as the most encouraging endorsement of high LET radiation therapy.[12] Between July, 1971, and September, 1976, 133 patients with advanced cancers of the head and neck were randomized to receive treatment with either photons or neutrons. Sixty-three patients received photon radiation therapy either at Hammersmith Hospital or at referring institutions, while 70 patients received neutron therapy at Hammersmith Hospital. With a minimum follow-up of 2 years, 53 of the 70 patients (75%) receiving neutron therapy had permanent local control whereas only 12 of the 63 patients (19%) treated with photons had local control.[12] Complications were observed in ten of the 70 patients (15%) treated with neutrons but in only one of the 63 patients (2%) treated with photons.[12] Both of these differences were statistically significant at the $p < 0.05$ level. Although the survival rates at 2 years for the groups treated with neutrons and photons were 28% and 15%, respectively, the differences were not significant.[12] The much higher local control rate achieved with neutrons compared to photons provided motivation for the initiation of a number of prospective randomized clinical trials with neutrons in this country. This section will review the facilities and equipment available in the United States for clinical research with particle beams and will review the scope and preliminary results of ongoing particle beam clinical research.

RESOURCES FOR CLINICAL RESEARCH

In order to understand the handicaps under which particle beam radiation therapy has been conducted in the United States through 1980, it is essential to consider the limitations in patient treatment at the various facilities. The important parameters to consider in comparing particle beam and photon treatment techniques are beam delivery, beam characteristics, beam availability, and accessibility of the facility to patients and physicians.

Table 48-24 lists the present and planned particle beam radiation therapy facilities. As shown in Table 48-24, all operational facilities have limitations in beam delivery compared to isocentric rotational megavoltage linear accelerators. Except for the Lewis Research Center cyclotron, which has both horizontally and vertically oriented beams, the neutron therapy facilities all have horizontally oriented beams. The proton, helium ion, and heavy ion facilities all have only horizontally oriented beams, whereas the pion facility has only a vertically oriented beam. If the patient can sit in a chair or stand during his treatment sessions, the horizontal fixed beam is adequate for most clinical situations. However, if the patient cannot tolerate sitting or standing in a rigid, precisely reproducible fashion, treatment with multiple radiation fields becomes extremely difficult and the potential advantages of particle beam therapy can be lost. There are difficulties in executing multiple-field treatment with a vertically oriented particle beam, because the patient must be changed from the supine to prone position for anterior–posterior opposed fields or to lateral decubitus positions if lateral fields are to be employed.

As noted earlier, planning of treatments and calculations must be performed for each position in most patients, because changes may occur in both internal and external anatomical relationships. Other characteristics of particle beams which have posed problems for clinical research to date are the depth of penetration and dose rate. Because of the poor depth–dose characteristics of the neutron beam at the University of Washington, it has been difficult at that facility to treat deeply seated tumors, especially in obese patients. The proton beam at the Harvard cyclotron has a maximum depth of penetration of 15.9 cm in water, thereby restricting the selection of patients to those with tumors at depths less than that or compromising the use of multiple fields as would be done with megavoltage roentgen rays. The pion dose rate of 5 rad to 10 rad per minute, depending upon the treatment volume, at Los Alamos dictates treatment times on the order of 15 minutes to 30 minutes for a single field when delivering a dose equivalent to a conventional 200 rad photon fraction. Even longer treatment times would be necessary if a pion treatment schedule were designed to have fewer treatments with higher daily doses.

In most facilities, use of the cyclotron or proton linear accelerator is shared with physics research programs. Even though the clinical research programs have enjoyed a high priority in terms of beam time and scheduling, there have often been limitations on the number of days per week on which treatment can be delivered. This compromises the ability to study multiple daily fractionation schedules with particle beams. A different problem with beam availability limits the total number of patients that can be treated with pions at Los Alamos and with heavy ions at Lawrence Berkeley Laboratory. At both facilities the total beam time is limited to 7 months or less each year primarily because of inadequate funds to meet increased energy costs but also to perform maintenance and to prepare for physics experiments. Another problem often encountered at facilities with relatively antiquated physics machines is unexpected shutdowns, often requiring weeks or months to repair.

A major logistical problem results from the remoteness of most particle beam therapy facilities from clinical centers as shown in Table 48-24. This causes great inconvenience to patient and physician and is often a limiting factor in patient selection.

In recognition of all of the above limitations in conducting particle beam radiation therapy research at facilities initially designed and constructed for physics research, the National Cancer Institute has funded development of cyclotron neutron therapy facilities at the M. D. Anderson Hospital and Tumor Institute, the University of California at Los Angeles, and the

TABLE 48-24. Characteristics of Particle Beam Therapy Facilities in the United States

LOCATION	STATUS	CHARACTERISTICS OF EQUIPMENT AND FACILITY
A. Neutron Therapy Facilities		
Cleveland Clinic Foundation Lewis Research Center (NASA) Cleveland, Ohio	Operational	Physics cyclotron; horizontal and vertical treatment beams; 42 MeVp-Be or 25 MeVp-Be; 45 minutes from Cleveland Clinic
Fermi National Accelerator Laboratory (Fermilab) Batavia, Illinois	Operational	Physics machine; (injector for synchrotron); horizontal treatment beam; 66 MeVp-Be; 30 miles from downtown Chicago
Fox Chase Cancer Center and University of Pennsylvania Philadelphia, Pennsylvania	Under Construction Operational in Early 1981	D–T generator designed for clinical use; isocentric treatment capability; 14 MeV neutrons from D–T reaction; in Fox Chase Cancer Center
M. D. Anderson Hospital and Tumor Institute University of Texas Houston, Texas	Under Construction Operational in Early 1981	Cyclotron therapy system designed for clinical use; one isocentric treatment beam and one horizontal beam; 42 MeVp-Be; in M. D. Anderson Hospital
University of California Wadsworth VA Medical Center Los Angeles, California	Under Construction Operational in 1982 or Early 1983	Cyclotron therapy system designed for clinical use; dedicated cyclotron for clinical use; one isocentric treatment beam and one horizontal beam; 42 MeVp-Be; to be in Wadsworth VA Medical Center
University of Washington Seattle, Washington	Operational Will Close in 1982	Physics cyclotron adapted for clinical use; horizontal treatment beam; 22 MeVd-Be; on campus—10 minutes from University Hospital
	Under Construction Operational in 1982 or Early 1983	Cyclotron therapy system designed for clinical use; one isocentric treatment beam and one horizontal beam; 48 MeVp-Be (variable energy 32–48 MeV); to be in University Hospital
B. Proton Therapy Facility		
Massachusetts General Hospital (MGH) Harvard University Cyclotron Cambridge, Massachusetts	Operational	Physcis cyclotron; 160 MeV protons; two horizontal treatment beams; 20 minutes from MGH
C. Negative π-Meson (Pion) Therapy Facility		
Los Alamos Meson Physics Facility Los Alamos, New Mexico	Cancer patient treatment in 1982	Physics proton linear accelerator; vertical pion beam; pion range up to 28 cm in water; 75 miles from Albuquerque
D. Helium and Heavy Ion Therapy Facilities	Helium and Heavy Ion Therapy Facilities	
University of California Lawrence Berkeley Laboratory Berkeley, California	Helium Ions Operational	Physics synchrocyclotron; 930 MeV helium ions; horizontal treatment beam; 12 miles from UC Hospital (San Francisco)
	Heavy Ions Operational	Physics machine (combination of a heavy ion linear accelerator and a synchrotron); high energy beams of ^{12}C, ^{20}Ne, or other ions; two horizontal treatment beams; 12 miles from UC Hospital

University of Washington in Seattle as shown in Table 48-24. In addition, NCI will support clinical research with D–T generator at the Fox Chase Cancer Center and at the University of Pennsylvania, Philadelphia. All three cyclotrons and the D–T generator will be dedicated solely to clinical use, will provide state of the art flexibility in neutron beam delivery, and will have depth dose and dose rate charcteristics suitable for treatment of tumors in most anatomical sites. In addition, all four facilities will be adjacent to major medical centers to facilitate the conduct of clinical research.

CLINICAL STUDIES AND RESULTS

Clinical studies with neutrons have been conducted in the United States since 1972 when they were initiated at M. D. Anderson Hospital. This research, as well as pretherapeutic and clinical research at each of the particle facilities, has been funded primarily by the National Cancer Institute. Extensive financial assistance has also been provided by the Department of Energy in the way of facilities, support services, utilities, and beam time at the Los Alamos Meson Physics Facility, Fermilab, and Lawrence Berkeley Laboratory. Since January, 1977, the Radiation Therapy Oncology Group, a clinical cooperative group supported by NCI, has provided support for the particle beam clinical trials to include: (1) coordination of scientific activities, including the design and implementation of protocols; (2) administrative support for entry of patients into studies, collection, and tabulation of data, distribution of protocols, assistance to study chairman, compilation and distribution of reports, and arranging meetings of study participants; (3) quality control activities; and (4) administrative support for the pathology committee and other scientific committees as needed.

The total number of patients treated in part or totally by particle beams in the United States is shown in Table 48-25.

TABLE 48-25. Approximate Number of Patients Treated Totally Or In Part By Particle Beams In The USA (September 1980)

PARTICLE BEAM	PILOT AND PHASE I/II STUDIES	PHASE III*	TOTAL
Neutrons	1846	465	2311
Protons	198	11	209
Helium and Heavy Ions	236	19	255
Pions	161	7	168

* A comparable number of patients have been treated on control arms.

As of this writing, 2311 patients have been treated with neutrons and 632 patients have been treated with charged particles. Of the 2311 patients treated with neutrons, 465 (20.1%) have been treated in Phase III prospective randomized protocols. Of the 565 patients treated with neutrons in RTOG Phase I, II, or III studies, 363 (64.2%) have received mixed beam therapy (usually two neutron and three photon treatments per week), 119 patients (21.1%) have received neutron boosts after photon irradiation, and 83 patients (14.7%) have been treated only with neutrons. The protocols by which patients have been treated are shown in Table 48-26. As shown in Table 48-26, 932 patients have been treated with photons or neutrons on RTOG protocols, 832 (89.3%) on prospective randomized Phase III studies, and 100 (10.7%) on Phase I and Phase II studies. Only three RTOG protocols have accessioned 100 or more patients each, and only one protocol (76-11) has been closed. Because patients are still being accessioned to all protocols except 76-11 and the follow-up is limited on all protocols, the results of all studies are preliminary. Interim evaluations of the studies on malignant gliomas, head and neck cancers, and cancers of the cervix are summarized below.

RTOG protocol 76-11, activated on July 1, 1976, was designed to compare boost therapy with neutrons to that with photons for patients with malignant gliomas. All patients

TABLE 48-26. Status of Entry of Patients into Particle Beam Therapy Studies in the United States (September, 1980)

PROTOCOL TITLE	PROTOCOL NUMBER	DATE ACTIVATED	STATUS	NUMBER OF PATIENTS ASSIGNED TO STUDY
A. Neutrons				
Phase III Study of Malignant Gliomas	RTOG 76-11	8/01/76	Closed 9/80	165
Phase III Study of Squamous Cell Carcinoma of the Uterine Cervix	RTOG 76-08	10/01/76	Active	101
Phase III Study of Potentially Operable Squamous Cell Carcinomas of the Oral Cavity, Pharynx, and Larynx	RTOG 76-09	10/01/76	Active	79
Phase III Study of Squamous Cell Carcinoma of the Oral Cavity, Pharynx, and Larynx	RTOG 76-10	10/01/76	Active	277
Phase II Study of Neutrons Alone or with Photons (i.e., Mixed Beam) or of Either in Combination with Surgery for Stage B1 (Grade III or IV) or Stage B2, C and D1 (Any Grade) Urinary Bladder Carcinima	RTOG 77-05	7/01/77	Active	34
Phase III Study of Neutrons Alone or in Combination with Photons for Clinical Stage C Adenocarcinoma of the Prostate	RTOG 77-04	7/07/77	Active	65
Phase II Study of Carcinoma of the Esophagus	RTOG 77-09	8/09/77	Active	47
Phase I/II Study of Localized, Non-resectable, Non-oat Cell Cancer of the Lung	RTOG 78-07	6/15/78	Active	16
Phase III Study of Supplemental Neutron Therapy for Squamous Cell Carcinoma of the Oral Cavity, Pharynx, and Larynx Treated with Radiation Only	RTOG 78-08	6/15/78	Active	78
Phase III Study of Fast Neutron and Mixed Beam (Neutron/Photon) Radiation Therapy in the Treatment of Localized, Inoperable Non-oat Cell Cancer of the Lung (Squamous Cell, Adenocarcinoma and Large Cell Undifferentiated Types)	RTOG 79-07	7/09/79	Active	39
Phase I/II Study of Misonidazole Combined with Neutrons for Treatment of Malignant Gliomas	RTOG 79-03	7/16/79	Active	15
Phase III Study of Adenocarcinoma of the Pancreas	RTOG 79-21	2/01/80	Active	16
TOTAL				932

(Table 48-26 continues on page 1852)

TABLE 48-26. Status of Entry of Patients into Particle Beam Therapy Studies in the United States (September, 1980) (*Continued*)

	PROTOCOL TITLE	PROTOCOL NUMBER	DATE ACTIVATED	STATUS	NUMBER OF PATIENTS ASSIGNED TO STUDY
B.	Protons				
	Pilot and Local Phase I/II and III		1973		209
C.	Helium and Heavier Ions				
	Seven LBL-BAHIA[a] Pilot Studies		1976 or later	Closed	119
	Phase I/II Study of Ocular Melanoma	NCOG 7081 RTOG 79-08	3/19/79 7/09/79	Active Active	26 0
	Phase I/II Study of Esophageal Cancer (Stages I & II)	NCOG 3E81 RTOG 79-09	12/20/78 7/09/79	Active Active	19 0
	Phase I/II Study of Advanced or Recurrent Malignant Neoplasms Using Heavy Charged Particle Radiation	NCOG 0R81 RTOG 79-11	3/19/79 7/09/79	Active Active	68 2
	Phase III Study of Pancreatic Adenocarcinoma Using Conventional Radiotherapy + 5FU or Heavy Charged Particle Therapy + 5FU	NCOG 3P81 RTOG 79-10	8/31/78 7/09/79	Active Active	34 0
	Phase I/II Study of Pancreatic Carcinoma with Heavy Ions	VASOG 79-01	1/01/80	Active	2
	TOTAL				270†
D.	Pions				
	Pilot Studies	–	1973	Closed	9
	Phase I/II Study of Solid Tumors	RTOG 79-23	10/01/74	Active	133
	Phase I/II Study of Metastatic Tumors	RTOG 79-24	11/01/76	Active	19
	Phase III Study of T3 and T4 Transitional Cell Carcinoma of the Bladder	RTOG 78-26	6/01/77	Active	1
	Phase III Study of Adenocarcinoma of the Rectum or Rectosigmoid (Inoperable or Recurrent)	RTOG 78-25	6/01/79	Active	3
	Phase III Study of Carcinoma of the Oral Cavity (Excluding Lip) and Pharynx	RTOG 78-28	6/01/79	Active	8
	TOTAL				173

[a] Bay Area Heavy Ion Association

† 15 photons only in NCOG 3P81; 155 helium only; 50 helium boost; 4 carbon; 9 neon; 1 argon; 6 carbon boost; 3 neon boost; 27 more than one ion.

received 5000 photon rad to the whole brain in 5 weeks to 5½ weeks and then were randomized to receive either 1500 photon rad in 1½ weeks to 2 weeks or a neutron dose equivalent to 1500 photon rad to the whole brain in 1½ weeks to 2 weeks. The objectives of the study were to compare the two arms in terms of survival, the time to recurrence, and the tolerance of normal tissues. The study had accrued 165 patients before closure in September 1980. Although a preliminary analysis unadjusted for prognostic factors of 131 evaluable patients showed no significant difference in survival between the two arms, conclusions must await the final analysis.[13]

RTOG protocol 76-08, activated on October 1, 1976, has accessioned 104 patients in a study of mixed beam neutron therapy in patients with squamous carcinomas of the cervix; FIGO Stages IIB, III, or IVA with negative lymph nodes on lymphangiography; or selective lymphadenectomy. The patients are randomized initially to photon irradiation or to mixed neutron and photon irradiation to a photon dose of 5000 rad (or the equivalent thereof with photons and neutrons) in 5 weeks to 5½ weeks. The mixed beam arm consists of two neutron and three photon treatments per week. When clinically appropriate, the pelvic irradiation if followed by 4000 mg-hours to 5000 mg-hours of radium. If treatment with radium is not possible, an external beam boost of 1000 rad to 1600 rad in 1 week to 1½ weeks with photons or the equivalent mixed beam dose is given to a reduced volume. The objectives of the study are to compare the two arms in terms of (a) survival, (b) local tumor control, and (c) severity of complications. A preliminary analysis of 75 patients treated between February, 1977, and August, 1979, at M. D. Anderson Hospital in accordance with the protocol showed no significant differences by all three criteria with an average follow-up of 24 months (range 9–39 months).[14] Patient accrual will continue.

RTOG protocol 76-10, activated October 1, 1976, has accessioned 282 patients into a prospective randomized study of the role of neutron therapy in the treatment of patients with Stage T2-4, NO-3 squamous cell carcinoma of the oral cavity, oropharynx, supraglottic larynx, and hypopharynx for patients to be treated by radiotherapy alone. The protocol initially had three arms as follows: (A) 26 to 32 neutron fractions over 7 weeks to 8 weeks delivering total doses of 1950 rad at Seattle and 2400 rad at Fermilab; (B) three photon treatments per week for a total dose of 4500 rad in association with two neutron fractions per week to a total of 730 neutron rad at Seattle and 900 neutron rad at Fermilab over 6½ weeks to 8 weeks; and (C) 33 to 40 photon fractions delivering 6600 rad to 7400 rad over 6½ weeks to 8 weeks. Before Arm A was dropped in December, 1979, because of poor patient accrual (only 23 patients), an institution could choose to treat patients on either two or three arms, one of which had to be the all photon arm. The objectives of this study are to assess survival, local tumor control, and the frequency and severity of complications. An interim analysis has been made of 73 patients treated in accordance with the protocol at M. D. Anderson Hospital between January 1977 and February 1979 (average follow-up of 22 months with a range of 10 months to 36 months). Of the 41 patients treated on the mixed beam arm, 25 patients (61%) had local control and 20 patients (49%) were alive compared to 47% local control (15/32) and 25% survival (8 of 32 patients) in the photon arm.[15] Although both local control and survival are better in the mixed beam group, only the latter is statistically significant at this time.[15] The complication rates in both arms were low and showed no difference. The RTOG study will remain open until approximately December, 1981, with a projected total accrual of 360 patients.

Although only the preliminary results of the head and neck study show improved local control and survival with mixed beam therapy, they complement the promising results of the randomized trial at Hammersmith Hospital comparing neutrons and photons in the treatment of patients with advanced cancers of the head and neck which have already been mentioned.[12] In addition, there is increasing evidence from other studies that also suggests the potential for improving local and regional tumor control with neutron therapy. The efficacy of neutron beams when used alone to eradicate cancer locally is reflected in excellent rates of local control in the treatment of tumors in several sites, including inoperable soft tissue sarcomas, carcinoma of the stomach, and malignant gliomas.[16–21] The apparent complete eradication of tumor cells in patients with malignant astrocytomas is extremely encouraging and also challenging because of the need to reduce the associated normal tissue injury.[11,22] Several studies combining neutron and photon treatments, generally two neutron and three photon treatments each week, have produced rewarding regressions and local control rates for cancers of the oropharynx, metastatic cervical adenopathy from squamous cell carcinomas of the head and neck region, advanced carcinomas of the major salivary glands, and carcinomas of the pancreas.[18,23–25]

The major problem experienced to date in the neutron therapy investigations has been an increasing incidence of normal tissue injury with increasing neutron doses.[26] This was anticipated in these studies as well as in other studies which are designed to establish the tolerance of normal tissues to a new treatment modality. Although these adverse normal tissue reactions with high neutron doses have led to the treatment of most patients by the mixed beam or neutron boost techniques, it is expected that treatment with neutrons alone will resume after the tolerance of normal tissues has been established for the neutron beams at the new clinically dedicated neutron therapy facilities.

The small number of patients treated entirely with neutrons in the randomized studies reflects the previously described difficulties encountered in executing neutron therapy with physics machines. In addition, the differences in biological effectiveness among the neutron beams at the present clinical facilities has impeded the establishment of tolerance doses for many normal tissues.[27] With the establishment of the three cyclotron neutron generators of comparable energy and the change of the energy at the Lewis Research Center cyclotron to MeV(p-Be), there will be an opportunity to conduct studies at four institutions using the same neutron energy to compare the efficacy of treatment with neutrons alone to that with photons.

Although the proton and helium ion beams at the Harvard cyclotron and Lawrence Berkeley Laboratory, respectively, have been used extensively for two or more decades in the treatment of pituitary tumors, investigations into the use of those charged particle beams for the treatment of cancer did not begin in earnest until the mid-1970s.[28–30] As shown in Table 48-25, only 632 cancer patients have been treated in part or totally in the USA with charged particle beams. Phase III studies with the charged particle beams are just getting underway as shown in Table 48-26. The ongoing proton beam studies are emphasizing the treatment of ocular melanomas, prostatic carcinoma, soft tissue sarcomas, and other selected tumors for which the dose-localizing properties of the proton beam may provide a significant advantage.[31,32] The ongoing studies with the helium ion beam are also exploring the dose-localizing potential of that beam in the treatment of carcinomas of the esophagus, pancreas, and stomach; ocular melanomas; malignant gliomas; and tumors in other selected sites.[28] Randomized studies to evaluate the dose-localizing advantages of these particles and especially the associated increased biological advantages of helium ions and eventually heavy ions are planned.

Randomized studies with pions are just getting underway for carcinoma of the bladder, carcinomas of the oral cavity and pharynx, and adenocarcinomas of the rectum—sites in which encouraging responses to pions were seen in the Phase I and Phase II studies.[33] Because favorable responses were also seen in patients with malignant gliomas and prostatic carcinomas, randomized studies are being considered for these sites as well.

SUMMARY

In the preceding sections, the rationale for particle beam radiotherapy, the scope of the clinical research program, and preliminary results therefrom were presented. Although the preliminary results of neutron therapy are not so encouraging

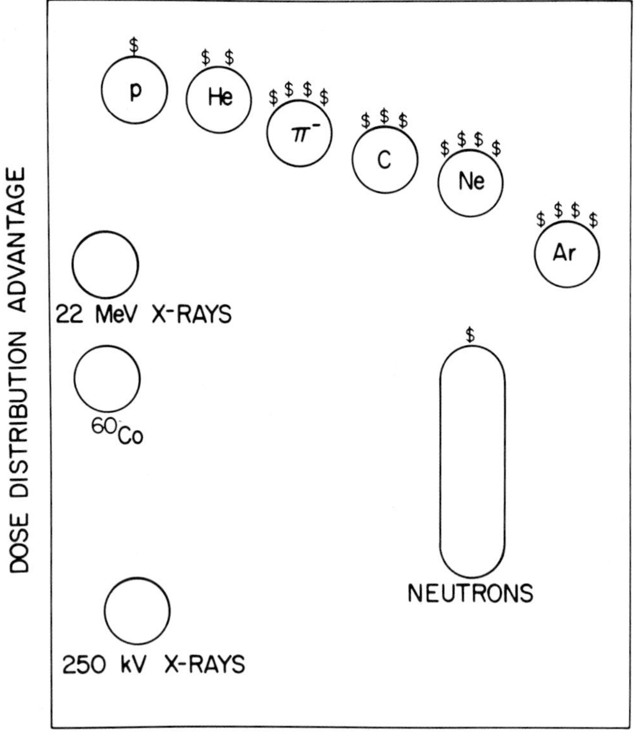

FIG. 48-25. Schematic presentation of the relative merits of low and high energy photons, ^{60}Co gamma rays, neutrons, and various charged particles. The relative positions of the particles will vary in different clinical situations depending upon many factors such as the size of the target volume, the size of the patient, and the anatomic location of the tumor. (Raju MR: Heavy Particle Radiotherapy, p 463. New York, Academic Press)

as would have been anticipated from the results of pretherapeutic studies, it is too soon to expect conclusive results because of the small number of patients treated in prospective randomized studies and because of the physical limitation of facilities. As noted earlier, neutron therapy systems designed specifically for the treatment of patients will be available at two facilities in early 1981 and at two more institutions in 1982. Even with these new facilities, only a relatively small number of patients will be treated yearly. Thus, the research program to evaluate the role of neutrons in cancer therapy will require many years.

In the United States, the opportunity to evaluate charged particle beam radiation therapy, despite its promise, is severely handicapped because of the physical limitations of the equipment and, in turn, the small number of patients that can be treated annually with each charged particle beam. It should be noted that the technology for sophisticated planning of treatments with charged particles has just recently become available.[16,17,26] This will insure that the maximum yield of information about the efficacy of charged particle beams for the treatment of cancer will be obtained from the limited resources. Despite these limitations, the United States has a unique opportunity to evaluate the contributions of all particle beams being considered for improved local and regional control of cancers because of the range of equipment available. It is possible to study the potential advantages of an increased biological effect by itself (neutrons), the advantages of improved clinical dose distributions alone (protons), and the advantages of having both an increased biological effect and an improved physical dose distribution (helium ions, pions, and heavy ions). The relative merits of the various particles compared to each other and to photons are shown in Fig. 48-25. It will be important to evaluate these potential advantages of the various particle beams in the actual treatment of patients with cancers.[34] This comparison will assist in the development of recommendations with regard to the types and numbers of additional clinically dedicated facilities which should be made available for continued clinical investigations and eventually for the routine treatment of patients.

As discussed earlier, the number of patients who stand to benefit from improved local and regional control of cancer is expected to increase with time because of continued population growth, more frequent detection of tumors at an early stage, and the development of chemotherapeutic agents for the treatment of microscopic metastases. For these reasons, it is essential to continue basic and pretherapeutic as well as clinical research with neutrons and charged particles and to expand these studies to include an evaluation of the use of radiation modifiers in conjunction with particle beam radiation therapy. There are also numerous questions to answer with regard to continued research with particle beams by themselves. Clinical observations have shown that late effects of neutron beam therapy are more severe than would have been expected from the observed acute effects.[26,35] Thus, although improved tumor control is expected with particle beam radiation therapy, the possibility of adverse effects on normal tissue, especially those occurring long after treatment, must be defined carefully. In addition to continued observations in conjunction with clinical studies, these investigations, should be performed definitively in animals for a wide range of time, dose, fractionation, and volume factors. These considerations are extremely important in particle beam radiation therapy, both with regard to effects on tumors and normal tissues. Because of the large number of alternative schedules for using particle beams alone or in conjunction with photons (particles and photons on alternating days, particles and photons on each treatment day, and photons supplemented by a particle beam boost sometime during the course of treatment), it will be necessary to investigate these possible alternatives in the laboratory and then to evaluate the most promising schedules in Phase I and Phase II clinical studies. It will also be important to understand the correlation of biological effects and the LET spectrum of particle beams as the ability to incorporate tissue density inhomogeneity corrections into treatment calculations is refined. Such refinements will be necessary to fully exploit the potential advantages of particle beam radiation therapy and to fairly compare this new modality to sophisticated photon radiation therapy.

The National Cancer Institute is sponsoring a program to develop radiation modifiers to include chemical sensitizers, hypoxic cell radiosensitizers, radioprotectors, and hyperthermia. All of these modifiers, when used in conjunction with photon irradiation, have the potential of improving the local and regional control of cancers. There is also considerable potential for the use of radiation modifiers with particle beam

TABLE 48-27. Particle Beam Therapy Patient Referral Information

INSTITUTIONS ACCEPTING PATIENTS FOR RESEARCH STUDIES	TYPE OF PARTICLE BEAM	TELEPHONE NUMBER
At Present		
Cleveland Clinic Lewis Research Center (NASA) Cleveland, Ohio	Neutrons	(216) 444-5570
Fermi National Accelerator Laboratory (Fermilab) Batavia, Illinois	Neutrons	(312) 840-3865
University of Washington Seattle, Washington	Neutrons	(206) 543-3390
Massachusetts General Hospital (MGH) Harvard University Cambridge, Massachusetts	Protons	(617) 726-8150
University of California Lawrence Berkeley Laboratory Berkeley, California	Helium and Heavy Ions	(415) 486-6325
Fox Chase Cancer Center & University of Pennsylvania Philadelphia, Pennsylvania	Neutrons	(215) 728-2582
Starting in Late 1982		
M. D. Anderson Hospital and Tumor Institute University of Texas Houston, Texas	Neutrons	(713) 792-3410
Starting in Late 1983		
University of California Wadsworth VA Medical Center Los Angeles, California	Neutrons	(213) 825-9304

radiation therapy. Radioprotectors should be especially efficacious in treatment with neutrons where relatively poor dose distributions carry a higher risk of normal tissue injury. Radiosensitizers might further enhance the increased biological effectiveness of neutrons on hypoxic or anoxic cells. Although proton beams have no increased biological effect, the improved physical dose distributions achievable with these particles might be enhanced by the use of radiosensitizers or radioprotectors or both. Radiosensitizers and radioprotectors may also complement the clinical use of helium ions, pions, and heavy ions. The use of these radiation modifiers as well as chemical sensitizers and hyperthermia should be explored in the laboratory and eventually in the clinic. Emphasis in the clinical research program initially, however, should be on a comparison of particle beam radiation therapy with the best conventional photon radiation therapy to establish the effectiveness of the various particle beams. It would then be appropriate to evaluate the role of radiation modifiers in conjunction with particle beam therapy as well as with photon radiation therapy in prospective randomized trials.

Because of the high cost of clinically dedicated particle beam facilities, the cost effectiveness of their contributions to the overall treatment of cancer eventually will have to be considered. First, however, it is essential to establish the real contributions, if any, of particle beam radiation therapy. If this cannot be established, there is no need to pursue the question of cost effectiveness. It is hoped that the particle beam radiation therapy research program will define an important role for particle beams in the treatment of cancer and that the problem posed for health care administration will show how to provide this treatment modality for the patients needing such treatment.

Information for physicians who would like to refer patients for particle beam radiation therapy studies is presented in Table 48-27.

REFERENCES

1. A Report from The Committee for Radiation Oncology Studies (CROS) and its Particle Subcommittee: Proposal for a program in particle-beam radiation therapy in the United States. Cancer Clin Trials 1(3):153, 1978
2. Kaplan HS, Schwettman HA, Fairbank WM et al: A hospital-based superconducting accelerator facility for negative pi-meson beam radiotherapy. Radiology 108(1):159, 1973
3. Oliver GD, Grant WH, Smathers JB: Radiation quality of fields produced by 16-, 30-, and 50-MeV deuterons on beryllium. Radiat Res 61:366, 1975
4. Pistenma DA, Li GC, Bagshaw MA: The desirability of treatment with multiple fields of charged heavy particle therapy. Phys Med Biol 23(4):610, 1978

5. Barendsen GW: Response of cultured cells, tumors and normal tissues to radiations of different linear energy transfer. Curr Top Radiat Res 4:295, 1968
6. Barendsen GW: Radiobiological dose-effect relations for radiation characterized by a wide spectrum of LET: Implication for their application in radiotherapy. Los Alamos Scientific Laboratory Report LA-5180-C:120, 1972
7. Chen GTY, Singh RP, Castro JR et al: Treatment planning for heavy ion radiotherapy. Int J Radiat Oncol Biol Phys 5(10):1809, 1979
8. Hogstrom KR, Smith AR, Simon SL et al: Static pion beam treatment planning of deep seated tumors using computerized tomographic scans. Int J Radiat Oncol Biol Phys 5(6):875, 1979
9. Stewart JR, Hicks JA, Boone MLM et al: Computed tomography in radiation therapy: Report of the Committee for Radiation Oncology Studies, subcommittee on CT scanning and radiation therapy. Int J Radiat Oncol Biol Phys 4:313, 1978
10. Tsujii H, Bagshaw MA, Smith AR et al: Localization of structures for pion radiotherapy by computerized tomography and orthodiagraphic projection. Int J Radiat Oncol Biol Phys 6(3):319, 1980
11. Laramore GE, Griffin TW, Gerdes AJ et al: Fast neutron and mixed (neutron/photon) beam teletherapy for grades III and IV astrocytomas. Cancer 42(1):96, 1978
12. Catterall M, Bewley DK, Sutherland I: Second report on results of a randomised clinical trial of fast neutrons compared with x or gamma rays in treatment of advanced tumours of head and neck. Br Med J 1:1642, 1977
13. Griffin TW (personal communication)
14. Morales PH, Hussey DH, Maor MH et al: Preliminary report of the M.D. Anderson Hospital randomized trial of neutron and photon irradiation for locally advanced carcinoma of the uterine cervix. Int J Radiat Oncol Biol Phys (to be submitted)
15. Maor MH, Hussey DH, Fletcher GH et al: Fast neutron therapy for locally advanced head and neck tumors. Int J Radiat Oncol Biol Phys (in press)
16. Catterall M, Bloom HJG, Ash DV et al: Fast neutrons compared with megavoltage x-rays in the treatment of patients with supratentorial glioblastoma: A controlled pilot study. Int J Radiat Oncol Biol Phys 6(3):261, 1980
17. Catterall M, Kingsley D, Lawrence G et al: The effects of fast neutrons on inoperable carcinoma of the stomach. Gut 16:150, 1975
18. Laramore GE, Blasko JC, Griffin TW et al: Fast neutron teletherapy for advanced carcinomas of the oropharynx. Int J Radiat Oncol Biol Phys 5(10):1821, 1979
19. Ornitz R, Herskovic A, Schell M et al: Treatment experience: locally advanced sarcomas with 15 MeV fast neutrons. Cancer 45(11):2712, 1980
20. Parker RG, Berry HC, Gerdes AJ et al: Fast neutron beam radiotherapy of glioblastoma multiforme. Am J Roentgenol 127:331, 1976
21. Salinas R, Hussey DH, Fletcher GH et al: Experience with fast neutron therapy for locally advanced sarcomas. Int J Radiat Oncol Biol Phys 6(3):267, 1980
22. Shaw CM, Sumi SM, Alvord EC et al: Fast-neutron irradiation of glioblastoma multiforme. J Neurosurg 49:1, 1978
23. Al-Abdulla ASM, Hussey DH, Olson MH et al: Preliminary report of combined x-ray and fast neutron therapy for carcinoma of the pancreas. Int J Radiat Oncol Biol Phys (in press)
24. Griffin TW, Laramore GE, Parker RG et al: An evaluation of fast neutron beam teletherapy of metastatic cervical adenopathy from squamous cell carcinomas of the head and neck region. Cancer 42(6):2517, 1978
25. Henry LW, Blasko JC, Griffin TW et al: Evaluation of fast neutron teletherapy for advanced carcinomas of the major salivary glands. Cancer 44(3):814, 1979
26. Ornitz RD, Bradley EW, Mossman KL et al: Clinical observations of early and late normal tissue injury in patients receiving fast neutron irradiation. Int J Radiat Oncol Biol Phys 6:273, 1980
27. Hall EJ, Withers HR, Geraci JP et al: Radiobiological intercomparisons of fast neutron beams used for therapy in Japan and the United States. Int J Radiat Oncol Biol Phys 5(2):227, 1979
28. Castro JR, Quivey JM, Lyman JT et al: Current status of clinical particle radiotherapy at Lawrence Berkeley Laboratory. Cancer 46(4):633, 1980
29. Kjellberg RN, Shintani A, Frantz AG et al: Proton beam therapy in acromegaly. N Engl J Med 278:689, 1968
30. Lawrence, JH, Chong CY, Born JL et al: Endocrine and Non-Endocrine Hormone Producing Tumors, p 39. Chicago, Yearbook Medical Publishers, 1973
31. Suit HD, Goitein M, Tepper JE et al: Clinical experience and expectation with protons and heavy ions. Int J Radiat Oncol Biol Phys 3:115, 1977
32. Suit HD, Goitein M, Tepper J et al: Exploratory study of proton radiation therapy using large field techniques and fractionated dose schedules. Cancer 35(6):1646, 1975
33. Kligerman MM, von Essen CF, Khan MK et al: Experience with pion radiotherapy. Cancer 43(3):1043, 1979
34. Raju MR: Heavy Particle Radiotherapy, p 463. New York, Academic Press, 1980
35. Withers HR, Flow BL, Huchton JI et al: Effect of dose fractionation on early and late skin responses to y-rays and neutrons. Int J Radiat Oncol Biol Phys 3:227, 1977
36. Tobias CA, Lyman JT, Lawrence JA: Progress in Atomic Medicine: Recent Advances in Nuclear Medicine, Vol 3, p 167–218. New York, Grune & Stratton, 1971

Section 6

Intraoperative Radiation Therapy

ALFRED L. GOLDSON

Intraoperative radiotherapy (IOR) is the radiation treatment of a surgically exposed tumor with an roentgen ray or particle beam during an operation.

IOR originated more than 40 years ago in the United States and Germany, but the current interest in IOR must be credited to the work of Abe at Kyoto University in Japan and to our work at Howard University in Washington, D.C.[1-4]

Although detailed assessment of the value of IOR for specific tumors and stages is not possible at this time, we believe that an outline of the future place of IOR in cancer management can be presented.

RATIONALE

The basic rationale for IOR is the well-established observation, that higher doses,* provided they are tolerated, result in better tumor control and that IOR permits the safe delivery of higher doses than other radiotherapeutic techniques.

The delivery of a higher dose with IOR is possible for two reasons: The first reason is, that in IOR, many highly

* In comparing the doses used in IOR with those used in fractionated external radiotherapy, one must make allowances for the lesser biological effect of fractionated doses. For many reactions 2000 rad single dose is approximately equivalent to 6000 rad given in 30 fractions over 6 weeks. It is with this assumption, that we talk about "higher" doses with IOR.

radiosensitive organs such as the skin, the intestines and the lungs can be mechanically pulled out of the radiation beam. The second reason for the delivery of a higher dose is the possibility to limit the radiation beam more precisely to the tumor area than with a small beam or rotational external therapy or with interstitial implants. With these two techniques, which also aim at higher tumor doses, considerable radiation outside of the target area is unavoidable.

The strict limitation of the radiation effect to the tumor area might prove of special benefit for pediatric tumors such as Wilm's tumor, neuroblastoma, and embryonal rhabdomyosarcoma. Almost complete sparing is possible of the bones, which should prevent stunting of bone growth and bone marrow depression.

Besides the higher dose, which can be delivered by the better sparing of adjacent radiosensitive organs, intra-operative radiotherapy has a number of other advantages over the competing radiotherapeutic techniques: compared with external therapy with small multiple fields or with rotational techniques, IOR has the important advantage of direct visualization of the tumor and the ease of beam direction. Even with transverse axial tomograms and sophisticated computer techniques, the radiation cannot be limited with the same simplicity, efficiency and certainty to the tumor area as with IOR. In other words, the probability of a "geographical miss" is much higher in external beam therapy than in intraoperative radiotherapy.

Another advantage of intra-operative radiotherapy over external beam therapy is that the decision on the volume to be irradiated can be made on the basis of a direct examination by both the surgeon and radiotherapist. Such surgical–radiotherapeutic teamwork is rarely achieved in external radiation therapy.

Compared with interstitial implants, there are two advantages of IOR: the first is the better possibility to treat lymph node areas. This is difficult to do with implants because the areas are large, there is not enough tissue to implant, and normal organs such as the intestines may receive excessive radiation, because they come to lay directly on the implanted site. The second advantage of IOR is the absence of radiation protection problems after the treatment with IOR. With interstitial implants, cumbersome radiation safety precautions have to be taken, even if the implanted activity is low.

Further advantages of IOR over the competing radiotherapeutic techniques lie in the possibility to apply radioprotective or radiosensitizing maneuvers, which will be briefly discussed later.

The principal disadvantage of IOR is the lack of fractionation. While there are distinct biological and practical advantages from fractionation of radiotherapy, it appears quite possible, that the better spatial distribution of IOR could compensate for it. Furthermore, it is of course possible to combine IOR with fractionated external beam therapy and in this way to obtain the benefits of fractionation. In this combination, IOR would be essentially a "boost therapy."

EQUIPMENT

Most of the present day IOR is given in radiation therapy rooms equipped with electron beam accelerators. The patient is usually brought from the operating room to the radiotherapy room while under anesthesia. Obviously, this is a makeshift arrangement, which exposes the patient to an additional risk; and the transport through unsterile areas jeopardizes the sterility.

The only fully integrated facility for intra-operative radiotherapy at present is the one at Howard University Hospital. Part of it is shown in Fig. 48-26. This facility is a surgically modified super-voltage treatment suite, 25 × 25 feet in dimension. It houses a Varian Clinac 18 MeV Linear Accelerator, with a 500 rad per minute output at 100 cm distance. It has electron beam capabilities of 6, 9, 12, 15 and 18 MeV as well as a 10 MeV photon beam. Modifications of the accelerator room for surgery included special circuits for all electrical equipment including accelerator and treatment couch, conductive flooring, separate air circulation, and a special nitrous oxide, oxygen and suction column.

TECHNIQUE

In our IOR facility, surgery and intraoperative radiotherapy are performed in the same room. General anesthesia is used on all patients. They are placed on a standard operating room table. Operating room tables are a little harder to position for IOR than special radiotherapy couches but they are more flexible. They also adapt to the Trendelenburg position, which is essential for anesthesia emergencies. The surgical technique for IOR is essentially the same as for other operations. If indicated, the radiosensitive organs should be sufficiently mobilized to pull them out of the radiation beam. After histological confirmation of the malignancy by frozen section as much of the tumor as possible is excised. The size and shape of the treatment collimators or applicators are selected to give 1 cm to 2 cm margin of apparently normal tissue. The optimal energy of electrons is determined by the depth of invasion of the tumor. Single doses of 1000 rad to 3000 rad are usually given, calculated for the 90% isodose.

During irradiation, which takes 2 minutes to 6 minutes, all personnel leave the treatment room. Vital signs, including EKG, pulse, and respiration are monitored remotely by television and by a multichannel oscilloscope in the control room. During IOR the surgical team can scrub again and is ready to begin the closure as soon as IOR is completed. Following irradiation, silver clips are placed, which aid in the postoperative monitoring of the tumor shrinkage. They are also useful for beam direction for postoperative irradiation. The surgical proceedings are then completed and the patient is taken to the recovery room where standard postoperative care is initiated. No radiation precautions are required after IOR.

CLINICAL EXPERIENCE

Table 48-28 shows the number of patients with various tumors, which have been treated by IOR according to our information. The data on the Japanese experience have been gained from a summary paper of Abe, Takahashi, Adachi, and Yoshii as well as from personal visits of the major Japanese IOR centers.[5] (Kyoto University Hospital, Dr. Abe; Komagome Cancer Hospital, Tokyo, Dr. T. Matsuda; and Chiba Cancer Center, Dr. M. Nakano and Dr. T. Todoroki).

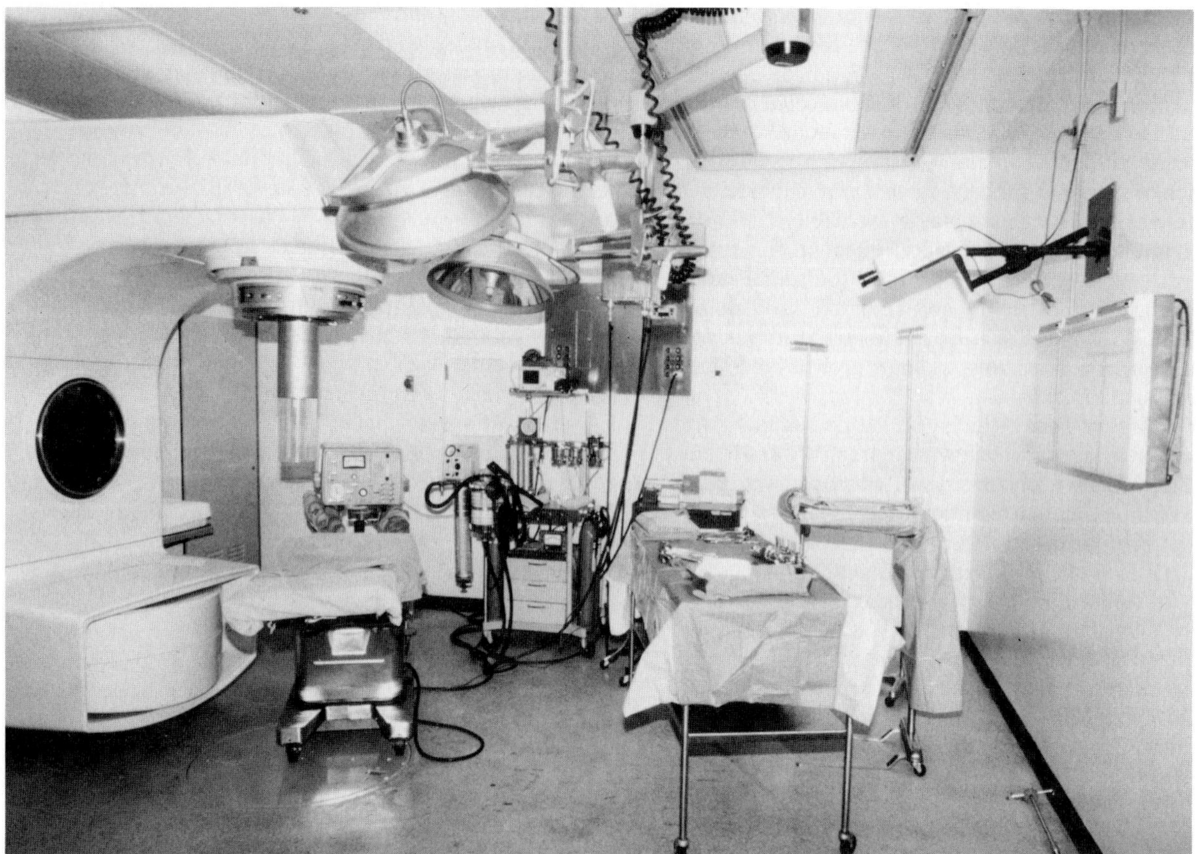

FIG. 48-26. Howard University Intraoperative Radiotherapy (IOR) facility. One of the four supervoltage therapy rooms of the Department of Radiotherapy is completely equipped as an operating room. The operation is started and completed in this room. The electron beams of a Varian 18 MeV linear accelerator are used.

TABLE 48-28. Patients Treated with Intra-operative Radiotherapy in Japanese Hospitals to April, 1979, and at Howard University from November, 1976, to March, 1980

TYPE OF CANCER	JAPANESE EXPERIENCE *Number of Patients*	*Number of Hospitals*	*HOWARD UNIVERSITY, NUMBER OF PATIENTS*
Stomach	183	10	3
Bladder	171	10	3
Pancreas	108	14	16
Biliary tract	59	12	1
Lung	51	3	4
Brain	36	3	0
Soft tissues	28	7	0
Uterus	21	2	12
Prostate	26	6	0
Colon	13	2	1
Rectum	10	2	0
Mediastinum	9	?	0
Ovary	8	2	0
Esophagus	3	3	1
Breast	0	0	2
Others	6	?	2
TOTAL	728	26	44

Our own data cover the 3½-year period from November, 1976, through March, 1980. At the time of this writing, IOR has also been initiated at two other USA hospitals, namely the Massachusetts General Hospital in Boston and the Hospital of the National Cancer Institute in Bethesda, Maryland.

The results are difficult to evaluate, because the number of patients in most tumor categories is still small, not enough time has elapsed, many different hospitals are involved and no controlled clinical trials have been conducted. In the language of chemotherapy, these are only "Phase I Toxicity Trials."

Cancer of the stomach (186 patients) is the cancer most frequently treated with IOR. Abe and associates in a recent review of their 78 patients treated with IOR, reported that he had three 5-year survivors in his subgroup of 14 patients, who had incomplete resection.[3] His largest subgroup were 50 patients, in which IOR was given to the lymph nodes around the celiac axis after subtotal gastrectomy. Compared with historical controls in his own hospital, Abe et al noted marked improvement of survival in all stages except Stage I. He reported no serious sequelae in the 2600 rad to 3500 rad dose range.

Cancer of the urinary bladder (173 patients) accounts for the second largest number of patients treated with IOR. Of the 171 patients treated in Japan, 117 (68%) received IOR at the Tokyo Cancer Center after resection of the primary bladder cancer. In other Japanese hospitals IOR was used as primary treatment for 40 patients with bladder cancer. This is recommended only if the tumor can be encompassed by a treatment cone of 4 cm diameter. Doses of 3000 rad to 3500 rad are advised for treatment of primary bladder cancer.

Cancer of the pancreas (121 patients) is the third most frequently treated cancer. IOR of pancreas cancer has excited special interest in the United States since treatment with other methods is disappointing. Thirty-six percent of our patients treated with IOR had pancreatic cancer.

We have recently reviewed in detail the experience with our first 15 patients with unresectable pancreas cancer treated by intraoperative radiotherapy.[6,10] Ten of our 15 patients had liver metastases at the time of the IOR, and the others had lesions larger than 6 cm in greatest dimensions. The median survival of our group was 6 months and only one of these patients is still alive at 12 months. No complications were encountered, if the dose was kept under 3000 rad. The most encouraging finding in our group was that local recurrences in the treated area were not observed.

Abe and associates have recently reported a median survival of 3 months for their six patients with pancreas cancer. Matsuda[3,7] had seven deaths within 4 months among his 12 patients with pancreas cancer. However, one of his patients is alive after 3 years and 2 months. He reported pain relief in 71% of his patients.

Cancer of the biliary tract (60 patients) is the fourth most frequently treated cancer. As in cancer of the pancreas, all patients had unresectable tumors and no one survived 5 years. Complications have not been observed. Worthwhile palliation has been reported for the Japanese series.

Cancer of the lung (55 patients) is the fifth most frequent cancer treated with IOR. The many different types of lung cancer and the various clinical settings, in which they received IOR, precludes conclusions as to the value of IOR in lung cancer. The four patients whom we treated received their IOR after resection of the primary, to the hilar and mediastinal nodes. This appears as an attractive combined surgical–radiotherapeutic procedure, because these nodes are frequently involved and because their resection is difficult. However, the radiosensitivity of the esophagus, which in our experience is about 2500 rad for IOR, limits the dose that can be delivered. One of our patients, who had cancerous mediastinal lymph nodes proven by mediastinoscopy, was found at autopsy 6 months later to be free of disease in the mediastinum, although he expired from widespread metastases.

Cancer of the brain (36 patients) is the sixth most frequent cancer treated with IOR. All of these patients were treated in Japan, most by Matsuda at the Komagome Cancer Hospital in Tokyo.[7] His usual technique was to give pre-operatively 3600 rad to 4000 rad by external radiotherapy. At the operation, the tumor was removed as far as possible followed by 1000 rad to 2000 rad of IOR. There were no complications at these dose levels. Matsuda's longest survivor with glioblastoma multiforme was alive 3 years and 3 months after this procedure.

Soft tissue sarcoma (28 patients) was the seventh most frequent cancer treated by IOR. In all patients, IOR was given after resection of the primary or of the recurrence. Abe and associates reported with this combination a local control in 73% of their patients.[5] They recommended a dose range of 3500 rad to 4000 rad.

Cancer of the uterus (33 patients) was the eighth most frequent cancer treated with IOR. Twenty-one of these were treated in Japan, but we lack details on this group. Our own group consists of 12 patients, eight with cancer of the cervix, and four with cancer of the endometrium. All our patients received IOR to the para-aortic nodes prior to conventional radiotherapy or surgery to the primary. We have already reported this study, which was carried out in cooperation with Dr. Delgado of Georgetown University.[8] All small intestines could be displaced in these studies from the intraoperative radiotherapy beam and doses from 1000 rad to 2500 rad were tolerated without complications. In contrast, external radiotherapy to the para-aortic nodes in biologically comparable doses carries a serious risk of radiation damage to the intestines. Our studies in dogs showed no damage of the aorta or the vena cava for doses of up to 4000 rad. It might, therefore, be possible to use high doses in the para-aortic node area, and to treat effectively lymph node metastases of testicular and other cancers, which spread to the para-aortic nodes.

Cancer of the prostate (26 patients) is the ninth most frequent cancer treated with IOR. All this experience has been collected in Japan; we are using interstitial implants in prostatic cancer. A small diameter applicator is used for intraoperative radiotherapy, which is inserted either by the transpubic or by the perineal route. The limit to the dose is determined by the radiation tolerance of the rectum.

Cancer of the colon (14 patients) is the tenth most frequent cancer treated with IOR. Abe and associates have recently reported the details of their eight colon cancer patients.[3] Two in whom the primary was not resected and another two patients, in whom the resection was incomplete, had a median survival of only 10 months and all were dead in 18 months. Of the three patients in whom the tumor was resected and only the infiltrated tumor bed was irradiated, one is alive 9 years and the other 10 years after intraoperative radiotherapy.

Other cancers (41 patients) which have been treated by IOR in Japan include cancers of the colon, rectum, mediastinum, ovary, esophagus, small intestine, orbit, oral cavity, and testis.

Among the other cancers, which we have treated by IOR at Howard University, were two patients with small cancers of the breast, who refused more radical procedures. These two patients received IOR immediately following the resection of the primary. They have done well and have developed no complications. We feel that for minimal breast cancer excision supplemented by IOR is as promising as supplemental interstitial implantation or postoperative radiotherapy, and that it has practical advantages as well as cosmetic advantages.

In evaluating the clinical experience, it is noteworthy that about ⅔ of all IOR has been given to the tumor bed or to the lymph node areas or to both after conventional treatment of the primary by surgery or radiotherapy. The use of IOR as an adjunct to cancer surgery emerges, therefore, as the most important indication of IOR. It is conceivable that IOR immediately following surgery could become a routine in major hospitals, after the benefits are more clearly documented and more suitable machines for IOR become available. One may even speculate that the use of IOR could lead in time to less radical cancer operations.

For the treatment of unresectable cancers, especially of pancreas cancer, not too much can be expected with present techniques, since the dose, which can be delivered, is limited by the radiosensitivity of the duodenum, which cannot be avoided. It is hoped that the use of radioprotective maneuvers, to be described in the following section, might permit higher doses and result in improved rates for cure and palliation.

FUTURE

While the clinical experience is not sufficient to determine the value of IOR for cancer management, it seems to be assured that IOR will occupy an important niche in the cancer armamentarium. However, much work remains to be done before IOR can be put to wider use.

The first requirement is the more accurate *determination of the tolerances of the normal tissues to the single doses used in IOR*. The large body of data on tolerance of organs and tissues to radiation has been mainly collected with fractionated radiation. It is urgent to conduct animal studies with single, well-localized radiation doses for all organs, which may be in the IOR beam.

The second requirement for the wider use of IOR is the *exploration of the special possibilities for radioprotection and radiosensitization*.

Radioprotection of the radiosensitive intestines against IOR doses of 2000 rad was achieved in our studies in rats by clamping the afferent artery shortly before and during the IOR.[9] Cooling of radiosensitive organs during the IOR may yield a similar protective effect. Chemical radioprotectors such as WR2721 may also be useful especially for intra-arterial injection, even if they are too toxic for systemic use; their systemic effect could be neutralized by counteracting drugs.

Radioprotection appears most promising for treatment of carcinoma of the pancreas (protection of the duodenum), for treatment of the hilar and mediastinal nodes in lung cancer (protection of the esophagus) and for the prostate (protection of the rectum).

Radiosensitization is another possibility to improve the effectiveness of IOR. Chemical radiosensitizer such as metronidazole and misonidazole, discussed in detail in one of the preceding chapters, could be used. They would be probably more effective and less toxic if injected intra-arterially shortly before the IOR. They might show a better effect with the larger doses used in IOR.

Another unusual opportunity exists in IOR for the use of *hyperthermia*, because it is relatively easy to maintain the desired temperature selectively in the surgically exposed tumor area during the short period of IOR and at the one occasion. A circumscribed hyperthermia cannot be obtained to the same degree for external radiotherapy. Fractionated external radiation also requires many hyperthermia applications.

The third requirement for the wider use of IOR is the *development of machines for IOR, which can be used in existing operating rooms*. We have explored the use of roentgen ray machines for this purpose. Fig. 48-27 shows the depth–dose curves of roentgen ray machines, which could be used in existing operating rooms. The machine with the lowest energy would be a 50 kV Contact Therapy Machine produced by the Philips Company. This machine has been used in the early trials with IOR, and might be useful even today for small tumor nests and small lymph node areas.[1,2] Its great advantage is that it can be rolled into any operating room and can be plugged into any existing outlet, that the room does not require additional radiation protection and that the cost is low.

Another machine to consider would be a roentgen ray machine in the 100 kV range. Operating rooms, which have the required ³⁄₁₆ inch of lead protection for diagnostic roentgen ray machines, could use a 100 kV therapy machine without modifications. In fact, the existing diagnostic machines in such operating rooms could be easily modified for therapy. In our hospital, for instance, four of the 12 operating rooms are equipped with ceiling-suspended 100 kV roentgen ray machines.

One might also consider the so called "Orthovoltage Machines" which have energies of 200 kV to 300 kV. This energy range would ordinarily give too much dose in the depth, but by using such machines at short distances one can, as indicated in Fig. 48-27, get similar curves as with a 100 kV roentgen ray machine at about 20 cm distance. The great disadvantage of these machines is the much greater lead thickness of the walls, which is required for protection, and which usually requires structural alterations of the building. The advantages over the 100 kV roentgen ray machines are the higher dose rates and the lower dose in bone. However, these advantages do not seem important enough to go to the problems and expenses of a 200 kV to 300 kV instillation.

In comparing the depth dose curves for roentgen beams in

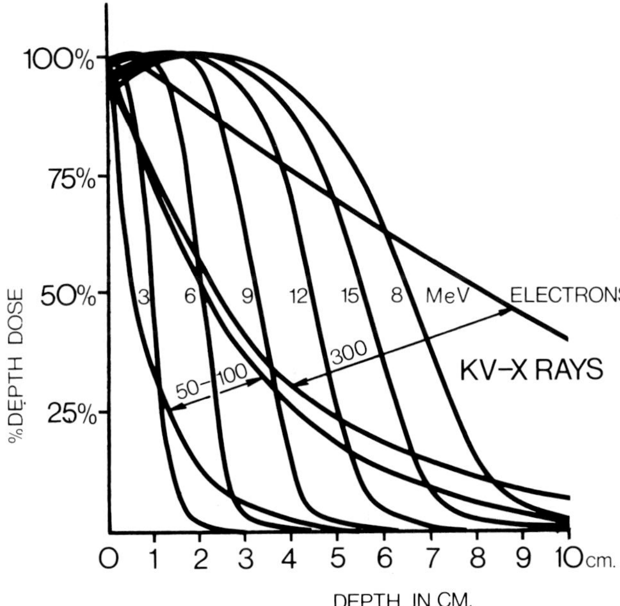

FIG. 48-27. Depth dose curves for electron beams and roentgen rays for intraoperative radiotherapy (IOR). The electron beams are clearly superior for IOR, but 50–100 KV x-ray machines may provide a suitable compromise between expense of the IOR facility and desirable beam characteristic, especially for the treatment of micrometastases. (The curves for 50–100 KV and the curves for 300 KV indicate the range of depth doses for different distances).

Fig. 48-27 with the depth dose curves of the electron beams of our linear accelerator, it is apparent, that roentgen rays no matter what energy are a poor second choice to electrons for intra-operative radiotherapy. The key advantage of IOR, namely the exact limitation of the radiation effect to the tumor volume is lost with roentgen rays. This appears especially important for the treatment of unresectable cancers. For the treatment of micrometastases and small tumor nests, a roentgen ray machine in the 50 kV to 100 kV region may however be an acceptable compromise.

In view of the great advantages of electron beams for IOR we have urged for the last years the manufacturers of linear accelerators to produce a "electron beam therapy only" version for IOR. According to our measurements, such a version would require not much more lead protection of the room than for 100 kV roentgen ray machines. This would make it feasible to install the electron beam accelerator in existing operating rooms. In our opinion, a stationary, downward directed beam would be adequate, since the usual operating table permits sufficient movement to angle the beam relative to the patient. A stationary electron beam machine would also take up much less space in the operating room than the rotating accelerator. The photon beams available in the presently produced accelerators are of no value for IOR. In our experience, a maximum electron energy of 15 MeV or even of 12 MeV would be sufficient. It is hoped that with the rapid progress in electronics such an electron beam machine for operating rooms will be produced soon, since without it the full potential of IOR cannot be realized.

SUMMARY

Intraoperative Radiotherapy (IOR) is a recently revived surgical–radiotherapeutic team approach. It permits to deliver higher doses to the primary and to the lymph node areas than other radiotherapeutic techniques.

Preliminary clinical studies with IOR in 28 hospitals with 772 patients indicate that IOR is a safe and effective procedure for local tumor control, if the tolerance of the normal tissues is not exceeded.

For the future, the most important tasks are studies to determine the tolerance doses of various organs to IOR more precisely, to test radioprotective and radiosensitizing maneuvers and to develop machines for IOR, which can be used in existing operating rooms.

REFERENCES

1. Pack G, Livingston E: Palliative irradiation of gastric cancer. In Pack G, Livingston E (eds): Treatment of Cancer and Allied Diseases, vol II pp 1100–1102. New York, 1940
2. Henschke U, Henschke G: Zur Technik der Operationsbestrahlung. Strahlenther 74:223–239, 1944
3. Abe M, Takahashi M, Yabumoto E et al: Clinical experience with intraoperative radiotherapy of locally advanced cancers. Cancer 45:40–48, 1980
4. Goldson A: Preliminary clinical experience with intraoperative radiotherapy. J Natl Med Assoc 70:493–495, 1978
5. Abe M, Takahashi M, Adachi H et al: Intraoperative radiotherapy of malignant diseases in Japan. Paper presented at the third "High LET and Allied Areas in Radiotherapy" Seminar under the US–JAPAN COOPERATIVE RESEARCH PROGRAM, May 22–23, Kyoto University Club House, Kyoto, Japan, 1979
6. Goldson A: Techniques and indications for intraoperative radiotherapy of pancreatic carcinoma. In Cohn I (ed): Pancreatic Cancer: New Directions in Therapeutic Management, pp 23–29. New York, Masson Publishing, 1981
7. Matsuda T: (personal communication)
8. Goldson A, Delgado G, Hill L: Intraoperative radiation of the paraaortic nodes in cancer of the uterine cervix. Obstet Gynecol 52:713–717, 1978
9. Henschke U, Chang F, Choppala J, Kovi J: Increase in radiation tolerance of the small intestine by Arterial Clamping. J Natl Med Assoc 68:67–70, 1076
10. Goldson A, Ashayer E, Roux V: Single high-dose intraoperative electrons for advanced-stage pancreatic cancer: Phase I Pilot Study. Int J Radiat Oncol Biol Physiol (in press)

Section 7

Transcatheter Management of the Cancer Patient

SIDNEY WALLACE
VINCENT P. CHUANG

The treatment of patients with neoplastic diseases by intra-arterial infusion and devascularization has been employed for two to three decades with less than dramatic results.[1–8] The renewed interest has been stimulated by the diagnostic radiologist as the interventional radiologist utilizing percutaneous transcatheter intra-arterial infusion and occlusion. These percutaneous techniques allow ready access to the vascular supply of the neoplasm with an associated decrease in morbidity and mortality when compared with the surgical approach.[9] The availability of new chemotherapeutic and embolic agents has encouraged further exploration of the therapeutic potential of these procedures.

TECHNIQUE

The standard angiographic techniques for catheterization are employed. Selective catheterization of the specific vessel supplying the neoplasm is preferable for optimal infusion and essential for embolization and occlusion. Most frequently, 5-French or 6.5-French polyethylene catheters are introduced through the femoral artery. The brachial artery is the alternate avenue for prolonged infusions of 5 days or more and for those vessels difficult to cannulate from the femoral route. Bilateral femoral artery puncture with internal iliac artery catheterization is frequently necessary for pelvic infusions. Aqueous heparin (15,000 to 25,000 units) is given each day during the infusion to maintain a $1\frac{1}{2}$-fold prolongation of the clotting parameters to minimize thrombotic complications. Acetylsalicylic acid, 650 mg twice a day, is given in an attempt to decrease platelet aggregation; it is to be hoped that this minimizes the thrombogenic complications of prolonged catheter placement.

INFUSION

The rationale for intra-arterial infusion is the exposure of the neoplasm to a high local concentration of the chemotherapeutic agent, as compared with the intravenous administration, without an increase in toxicity.[10,11] Most cytotoxic agents have a steep dose–response curve, that is, the higher the concentration of drug, the higher the antitumor effect.[11] The systemic concentration and, therefore, the systemic toxicity will usually be the same whether the agent is delivered intra-arterially or intravenously.[12] Neoplasms refractory to systemic chemotherapy may respond to arterial infusion of the same agent at the same dose rate.

The cytotoxic agents delivered by the intra-arterial route include 5-fluorouracil (5FU), floxuridine (FUDR), doxorubicin, methotrexate, *cis*-diamminedichloroplatinum (CDDP), cytoxan, imidazole carboxamide (DTIC), vincristine, vinblastine, mitomycin-C, VP-16, phenylalanine mustard, actinomycin-D, vindesine, and AMSA. Prior to the use of a new agent intra-arterially, laboratory experimentation is necessary to determine the tolerable dose to the patient, the organ, and the artery infused.

Catheter placement should be monitored to insure the desired distribution of chemotherapeutic agents. The injection of isotopes, ^{99m}Tc-macroaggregated albumin, at the same rate as the infusion provides a more accurate evaluation of distribution.[13]

EMBOLIZATION

The materials available for embolization include: autologous clot and tissue; clot modified by thrombin, epsilon aminocaproic acid (Amicar), heat, and so on; absorbable gelatin sponge (Gelfoam, Oxycel); (Ivalon); cyanoacrylates; silastic and metallic spheres; silicone and silicone rubber; (Ethibloc); microfibrillaa collagen hemostat (Avitene); sodium tetradecyl sulphate (Sotradecol); lyophylized porcine dura mater; balloon catheters and detachable balloons; and metallic devices such as brushes and stainless steel coils.[14–22,81] The combination of particulate emboli for the peripheral vascular bed of the neoplasm and central occlusion of the major supplying vessel is superior to either component alone. In general, at M. D. Anderson Hospital (MDAH), peripheral embolization is accomplished with absorbable gelatin sponge particles or polyvinyl alcohol foam (Ivalon) granules and central occlusion with absorbable gelatin sponge segments and steel coils (Figs. 48-28, 48-29, 48-30).[13,16,23–27]

The indications for transcatheter embolization of neoplasms are: (1) to control hemorrhage, (2) pre-operative, to facilitate resection by decreasing blood loss and operating time, (3) to inhibit tumor growth, (4) to relieve pain by decreasing tumor bulk, and (5) perhaps to stimulate an immune response to the ischemic neoplasm.

CONTROL OF HEMORRHAGE

The control of hemorrhage in patients with neoplastic diseases is often life-saving and may allow the opportunity for more specific antitumor therapy by surgery, radiation, or chemotherapy.[28–31]

Gastrointestinal

The intravenous infusion of vasopressin, the preferred treatment for bleeding from esophageal varices, is at times effective in the management of diffuse gastrointestinal hemorrhage as seen in patients with leukemia.[14,32] Intra-arterial vasopressin is usually ineffective in the control of gastrointestinal bleeding from the malignant neoplasms but is used in the treatment of hemorrhage of benign etiology in the cancer patient. Gastrointestinal bleeding from neoplasms of the liver, stomach, duodenum, and rectosigmoid, as well as radiation changes, especially in the rectum, is more readily controlled

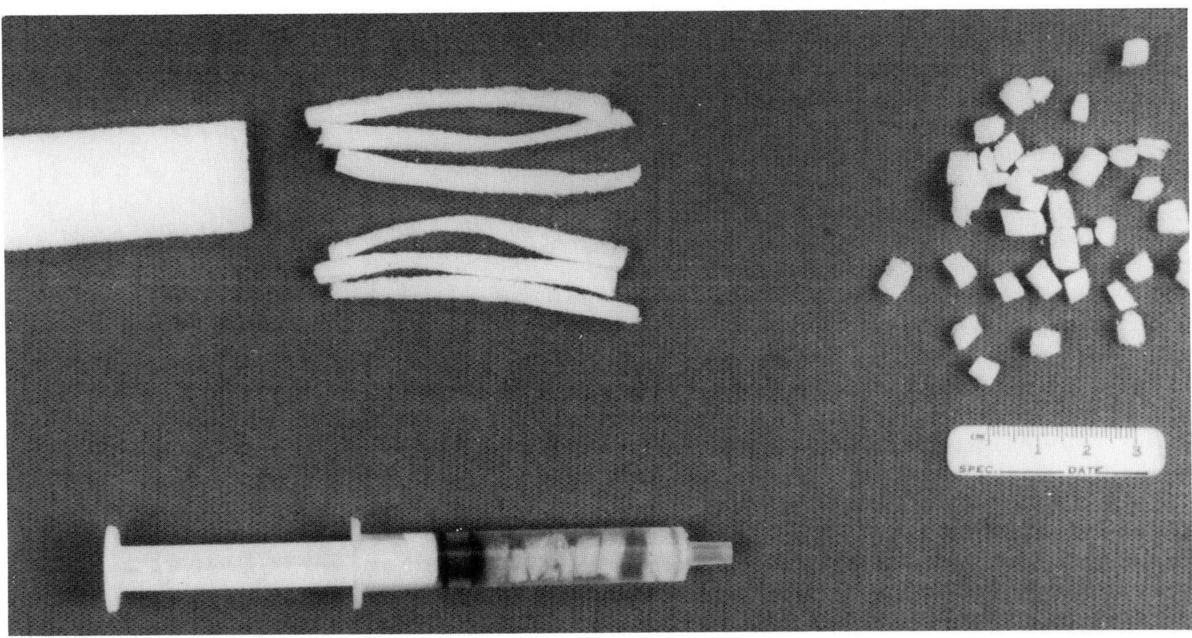

FIG. 48-28. Gelfoam is sliced into cubes and strips for arterial embolization. Five to ten pieces of Gelfoam cubes are loaded at a time into either a 1 ml or 3 ml syringe with saline or contrast material and injected into the artery for peripheral occlusion. When the arterial flow slows, Gelfoam strips are used.

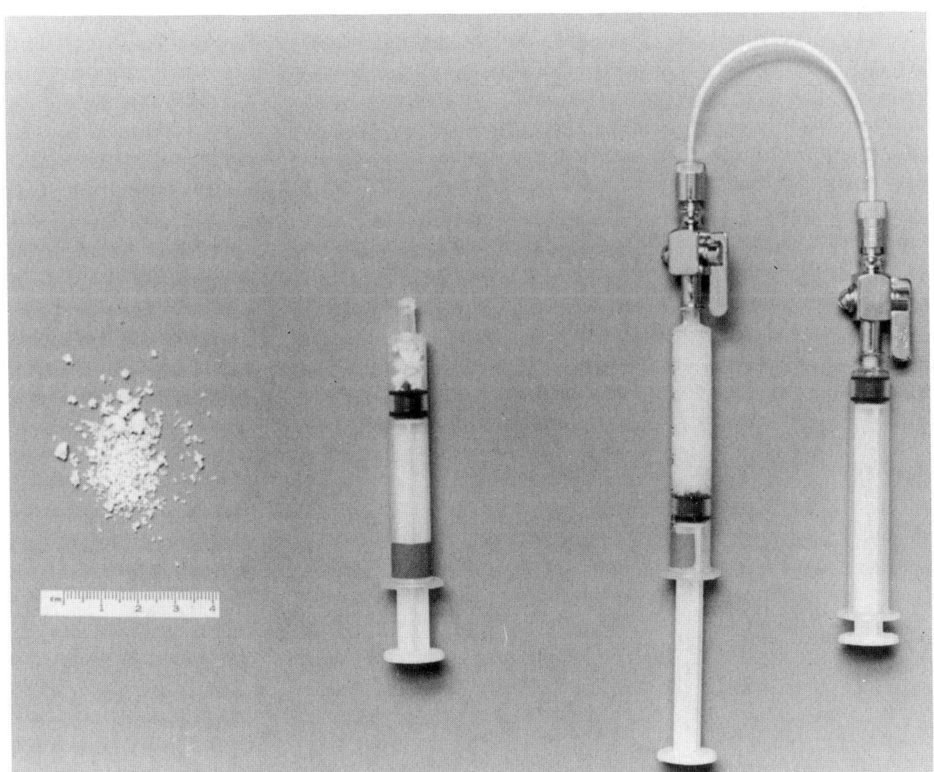

FIG. 48-29. To the *right*, Ivalon (polyvinyl alcohol foam) particles in dry form. In the *center*, mg of Ivalon are loaded in a 3 ml syringe. To the *left*, several ml of saline are added to the syringe and the Ivalon particles are injected back and forth through a connecting tube to obtain a uniform suspension.

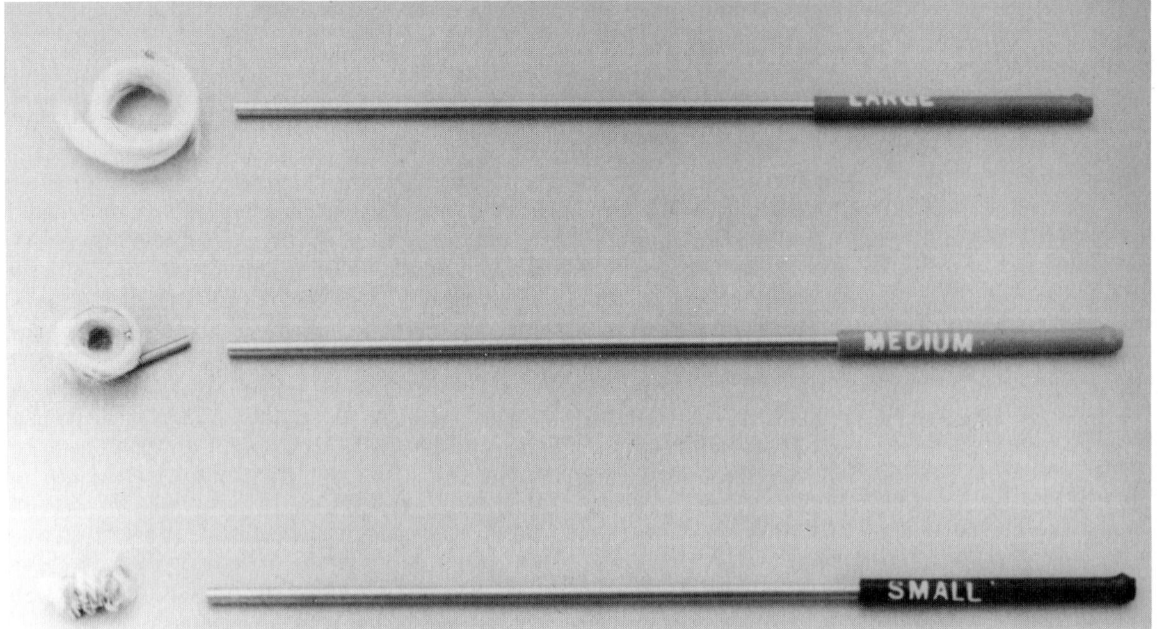

FIG. 48-30. New coils. The coils are housed inside metal cartridges. When pushed out of the cartridges with a guide wire, the coils resume a spring-like configuration. Three sizes are available: 3mm, 5mm, and 8mm in helical diameter.

by embolization of the left gastric, gastroduodenal, hepatic, superior and inferior pancreaticoduodenal, inferior mesenteric, and internal iliac arteries.[15,28,30,33]

Genitourinary

Hemorrhage from neoplasms of the genitourinary tract has been successfully treated by intra-arterial embolization. This has been accomplished in patients with neoplasms of the bladder, uterine cervix, and corpus. Bleeding caused by radiation cystitis may be controlled by bilateral internal iliac artery embolization.[24,34,35]

RENAL CARCINOMA

Approximately 15,000 Americans were stricken by renal carcinoma and 7,500 succumbed to this disease in 1978. Renal carcinoma accounts for about 3% of all cases of malignant disease. There are about 3.5 new cases per 100,000 people per year in this country and they involve males nearly twice as frequently as females. Eighty-six percent to 89% of all renal malignant tumors are adenocarcinomas, the remainder being tumors of the renal pelvis and capsule.

Therapeutic management of renal carcinoma depends upon the extent and, therefore, the stage of the patient's disease. Approximately 33% of the patients will present with the neoplasm confined by the renal capsule, Stage I. Of those neoplasms over 6.5 cm in diameter, one series noted lymph node metastases in over 50%. The 5-year survival rate of patients with Stage I disease is about 60%. Stage II neoplasms include those extending through the capsule into the perinephric fat. The presence of regional lymph node metastases or a tumor thrombus in the renal vein or inferior vena cava signifies Stage III disease. The 5-year survival rate for patients with Stage II or III renal carcinoma ranges from 30% to 35%. At the time of diagnosis, 25% to 57% of patients with renal cell carcinoma will have metastatic disease, Stage IV, with a 5-year survival rate of 8% to 11%. In 642 patients with renal cell carcinoma seen at MDAH, sites of clinically determined metastases were distributed as follows: lungs, 69%; bone, 43%; liver, 14%; brain, 7%; lymph nodes, 5%; skin, 4%; and thyroid, spermatic cord, vagina, breast, and nasopharynx in less than 1%. The median survival rates according to these sites of metastases are: lungs, 6 months; liver, 3 months; brain, 2.5 months; and bone, 15 months. More than 80% of patients with renal carcinoma and metastases are dead at one year.[36-39]

SPONTANEOUS REGRESSION

Renal carcinoma has been considered one of the more common types of malignant disease that undergoes spontaneous regression, but this is rare. It has been reported in 40 to 60 cases, usually in males with pulmonary metastases who have been treated by nephrectomy. The rarity of this phenomenon has been emphasized by Montie and associates, who found that only four cases occurred after nephrectomy of 474 patients with metastatic disease, an incidence of 0.8%.[38] In view of the fact that the operative mortality rate following nephrectomy performed in patients with metastatic diseases ranges from 2.3% to 10%, there appears to be no justification for performing the procedure merely in the hope of affecting a spontaneous regression.[36,37,39,40]

RENAL ARTERY EMBOLIZATION

Transcathether intra-arterial embolization of renal neoplasms was initially suggested by Lalli, Peterson, and Bookstein in 1969.[41] Lang, employing radioactive gold grains as emboli, noted a decrease in the size of renal carcinoma in 20 patients.[42] Almgard and associates reported encouraging results after autologous muscle tissue embolization of renal neoplasms.[43] As part of the therapeutic management at MDAH, 100 patients with renal carcinoma have undergone transcatheter intra-arterial tumor embolization utilizing absorbable gelatin sponge and stainless steel coils (Fig. 48-31).[44,45]

Results and Discussion

The 100 patients were divided into three groups based upon the extent of disease and the therapeutic management. Group I consisted of 25 patients with regionally advanced tumors without metastases, Stage I through Stage III, who were treated by embolization 1 day to 6 days prior to surgery to facilitate the operative procedure. Twenty-four hours to, preferably, 72 hours yielded optimal conditions for the operative procedure. With tumors greater than 7 cm, especially if hypervascular (65%–80% of renal carcinomas are hypervascular), dilated tortuous veins usually cover the surface of the neoplasm and the renal hilum. Regional lymph node metastases and a tumor thrombus in the renal vein or inferior vena cava may impede access to the renal artery. Pre-operative renal artery occlusion with resultant collapse of the renal veins facilitated nephrectomy. The major hilar veins are ligated first. With intravenous tumor thrombus, the hazards of tumor embolization were reduced and the thrombectomy was facilitated. The infarcted neoplasm and kidney were edematous, creating a more definable plane with the renal bed. These factors reduced blood loss and decreased operating time. For neoplasms less than 7 cm in diameter, it is not as yet considered advisable to subject the patient to the morbidity associated with embolization. Of the 25 patients with local disease treated by embolization and nephrectomy, 15 patients are alive with a median survival of 24 months and a range of 4.5 months to 47 months.

In Group II were 49 patients with limited metastases treated according to a planned protocol and medroxyprogesterone acetate (Depo-Provera) (400 mg I.M. twice a week). The embolization was usually done 4 days to 7 days prior to nephrectomy. Because a response to this combined approach is usually observed within 4.5 months, the patients are not considered for evaluation until that length of time has elapsed. All 49 patients satisfy the criteria for evaluation. In this group, 35 patients had pulmonary metastases; 22 of these patients had metastases that were confined to the lungs. The renal carcinomas were hypervascular in 82%, and the mean size was 12.0 cm in greatest diameter as defined by angiography. Renal vein invasion was found in three and inferior vena caval extension in two patients. Of this group of 49 patients with metastases, primarily pulmonary, the median survival is 14 months, in contrast to 6 months for a control group treated by nephrectomy alone. A response was noted in 18 of the 49 patients (36%) (Fig. 48-32). Seven responses were complete, with the disappearance of all metastases for 9 months to 15 months. Three remain in complete remission. Of the seven patients, four are alive after 7 months to 44 months, and three died 14 months to 19 months after nephrectomy. Five patients had partial responses (PR, 50% or greater reduction in all lesions). One of these five patients is still alive after 41 months while four have died after 12 months to 24 months. Six patients experienced measurable regression of less than 50%, or stabilization (S), for longer than 12 months. Five of these six patients are alive after 15 months to 44 months and one died 17 months after nephrectomy. In view of the survival statistics, the stabilization of the disease was considered a response. Of the 18 responders, nine are still alive with a median follow-up of 25 months.

Twenty-six patients treated by embolization without nephrectomy comprised Group III. These patients were not candidates for surgery because of their general medical condition or extensive tumor involvement. Metastases frequently were present in the liver or brain. Also included in this group were patients with contralateral renal or diffuse abdominal metastases. Palliative infarction was done either to control gross hematuria or persistent flank pain or both. The median survival of this group was 4 months. Because of the ominous prognosis of patients with liver metastases (3 months), a new therapeutic protocol has been instituted. Hepatic artery embolization is performed first, followed in 4 weeks to 6 weeks by renal tumor infarction, nephrectomy, and medroxyprogesterone acetate (Provera). One patient treated in this manner had 90% necrosis of the hepatic metastases documented by surgery and histopathology. Further study is necessary to evaluate this approach.

Complications

Although the complications discussed here are those seen with renal artery embolization, they do occur to varying degrees with embolization in general. Virtually all patients undergoing renal artery occlusion experience flank pain of 24 hours to 48 hours duration, requiring narcotics for relief. The narcotics are given intravenously in aliquots of 25 mg of meperidine (Demerol) during embolization. *Fever* up to 40°C almost always accompanies the pain, lasting as long as 5 days, but antibiotics are seldom needed. *Anorexia, nausea,* and *vomiting* may occur for 3 to 5 days, requiring symptomatic management. In a few patients, *paralytic ileus* requires nasogastric suction and intravenous fluids. *Hypertension* occurs in many patients during embolization and lasts 2 hours to 4 hours. No patient has experienced persistent hypertension.

Major complications have been relatively few. *Renal failure* occurred in two patients, in one of whom it was irreversible. This was believed to be related to the large volume of contrast material (300 cc) and to the infarction that was performed at the same time. These two events have been separated by at least 24 hours without another episode of failure. *Renal abscess* complicated occlusion in one patient, and another patient had gas in the retroperitoneal space presumably due to tumor necrosis. In the presence of a urinary tract infection or calculi, antibiotics are given before and after embolization.

Unintentional embolization of the gelatin sponge and steel coils is always a potential complication.[80] Loss of a coil into

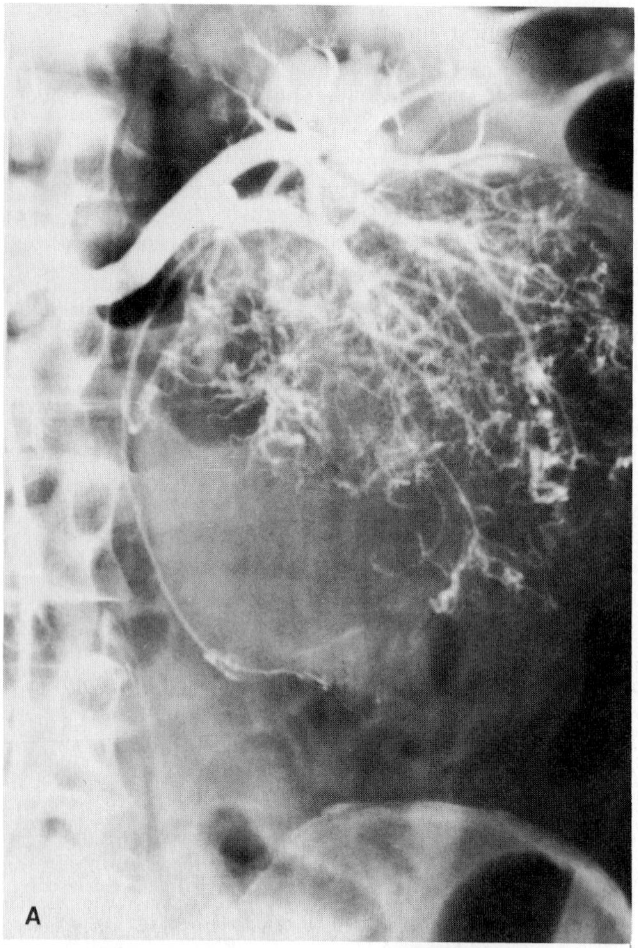

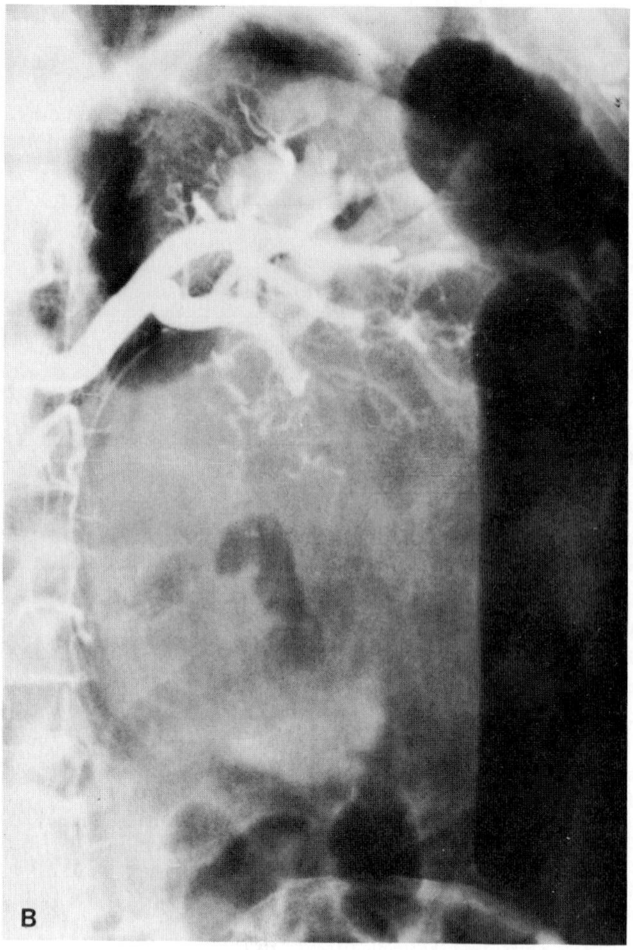

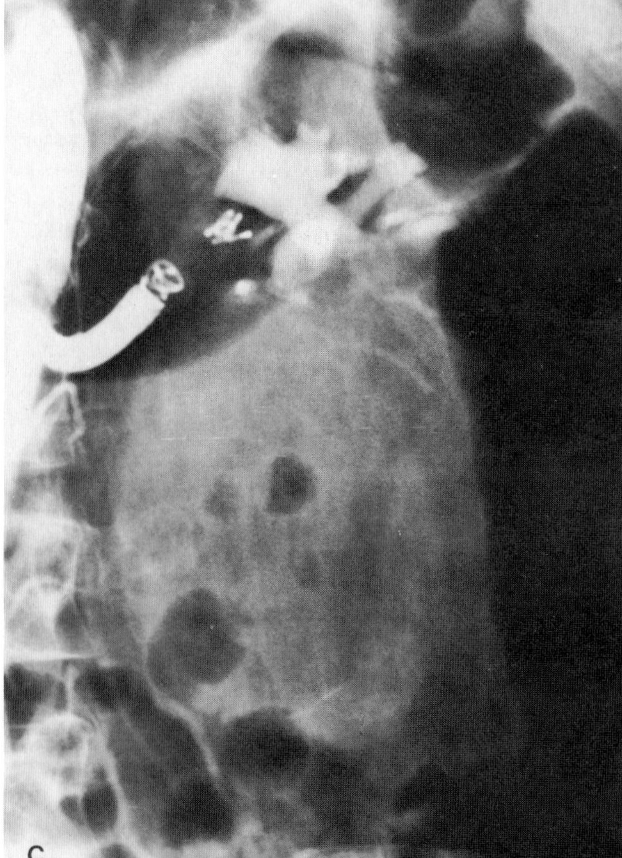

FIG. 48-31. Renal carcinoma infarction. *A,* Left renal arteriogram reveals a hypervascular neoplasm in the lower aspect of left kidney, typical of a renal cell carcinoma. *B,* Following Gelfoam embolization, the tumor vessels as well as the segmental and interlobar arteries are occluded. *C,* Coils are used for central occlusion of the left kidney.

the aorta occurred in two patients. Chuang has extracted an errant steel coil with a Dormier basket, while Habighorst used a Fogarty catheter. Surgery was reported necessary for the removal of a coil that migrated to the opposite renal artery after occlusion of a renal carcinoma.[47-49]

LIVER

Primary and secondary neoplasms localized to an anatomical segment or lobe of the liver are best treated by resection if the patient is a surgical candidate and the remainder of the liver is normal.[3] Unfortunately, these circumstances are relatively uncommon and the morbidity and mortality of resection are high. The duration of life after discovery of primary hepatic cancer without treatment is usually only 3 months to 6 months.

The liver is the major organ most frequently involved by metastatic disease. The patient's hepatic metastases rather than the primary neoplasm usually govern the course of the disease as well as the survival. One-half to two-thirds of the patients who die of cancer of the gastrointestinal tract, pancreas, breast, and ovary, and one-third of the patients who die of lung and kidney cancers have liver metastases. The median survival for patients with untreated liver metastases from carcinoma of the colon is 150 days; from the stomach, 60 days; and from the pancreas, 50 days. In view of this ominous prognosis, an aggressive therapeutic approach by the interventional radiologist is justified. The transcatheter management of hepatic neoplasms, whether primary or secondary, by infusion and occlusion offers viable therapeutic alternatives.

HEPATIC ARTERY INFUSION (HAI)

Intra-arterial infusion of chemotherapeutic agents has been utilized to treat hepatic neoplasms for approximately two decades.[1,6,50] Several modifications have been made to improve its effectiveness, including: (1) meticulous and persistent efforts in selective hepatic artery catheter placement, which is accomplished in 95%; (2) higher concentration of chemotherapeutic agents delivered over shorter infusion periods of 2 hours to 5 days, depending upon the regimen; (3) repeated cycles of HAI every 4 weeks to 6 weeks; and (4) in the event of multiple hepatic arteries, hepatic flow redistribution.

REDISTRIBUTION OF HEPATIC FLOW

The classical distribution of the hepatic artery originating from the celiac artery occurs in approximately 55% of the population. Michels has described ten major anatomical variations.[51] The incidence of aberrant right hepatic artery is 26% and that of the left hepatic artery is 28%. These aberrant arteries can originate from the left gastric artery, the superior mesenteric, or branches from both.

Redistribution of hepatic arterial flow, in the presence of multiple hepatic arteries, is accomplished by selective occlusion of certain of the hepatic arteries so that the entire supply originates from one artery (Fig. 48-33).[30,52] This facilitates the technical aspects of hepatic arterial infusion and allows for

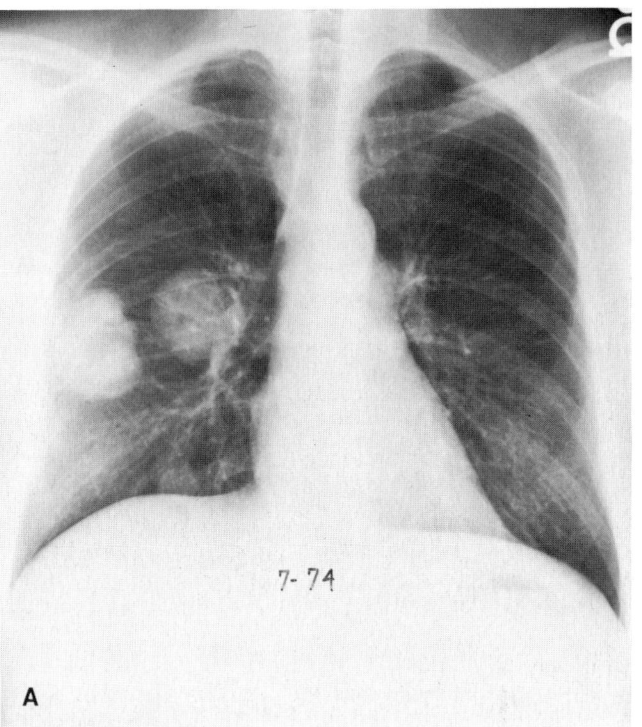

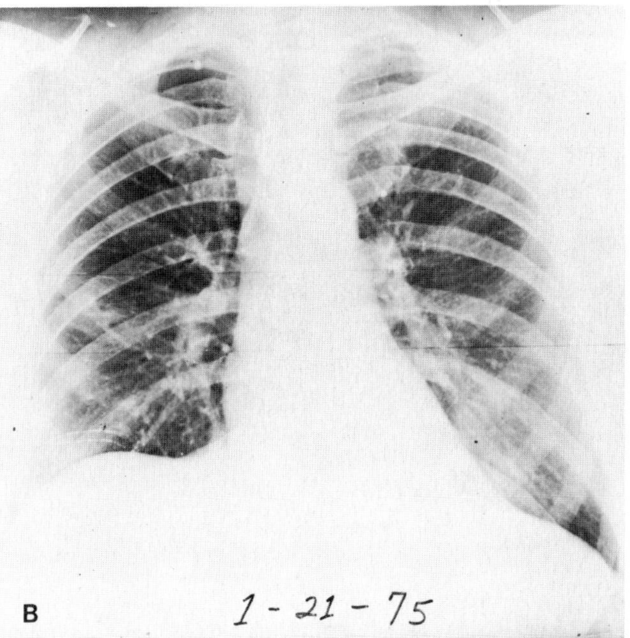

FIG. 48-32. Response of pulmonary metastasis to infarction, nephrectomy, and hormonal therapy. *A*, Metastatic nodules in right lung in a patient with carcinoma of kidney. The kidney was embolized, a nephrectomy was performed 5 days later, and depo-Provera was given. *B*, Six months later, the pulmonary metastases completely resolved.

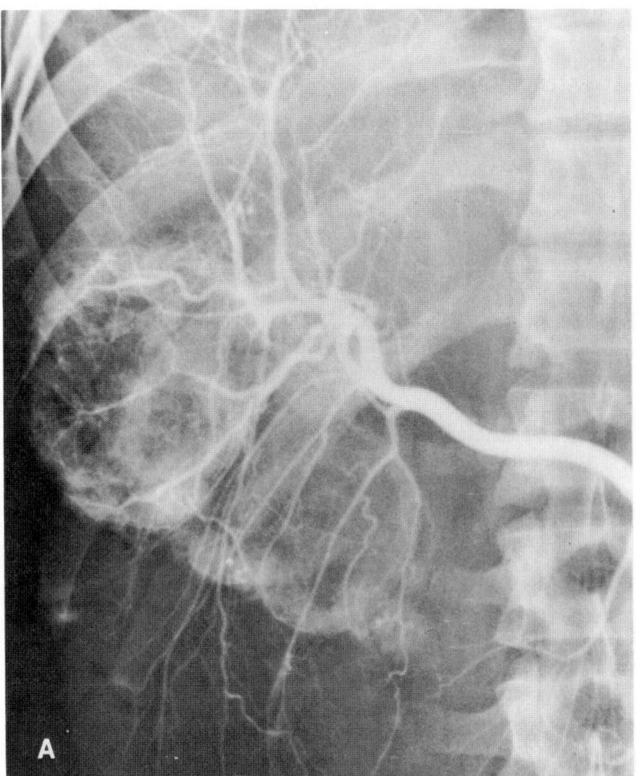

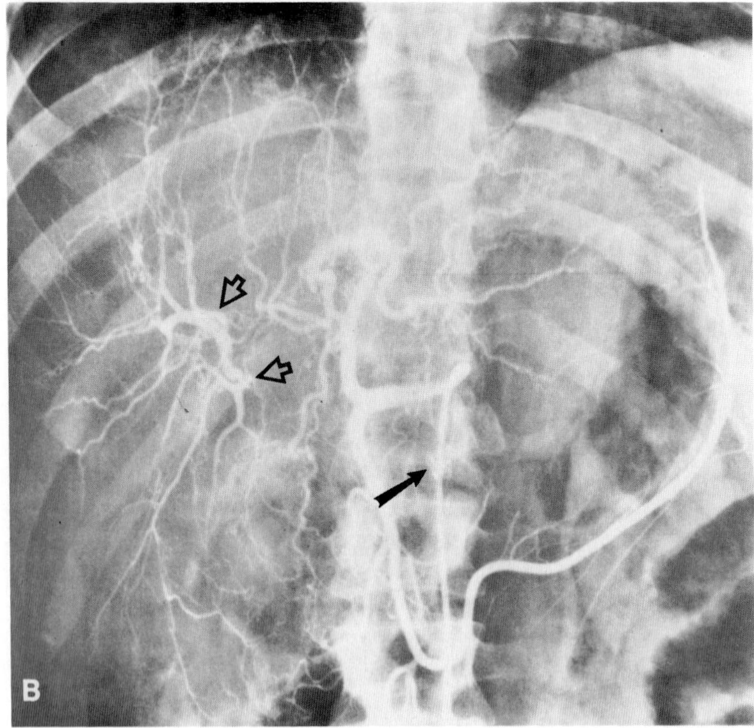

FIG. 48-33. Hepatic flow redistribution. *A*, Right hepatic arteriogram reveals metastatic melanoma in the right lobe of the liver. The replaced right hepatic artery originates from the superior mesenteric artery. *B*, The replaced right hepatic artery was embolized with a coil (*closed arrow*). The left hepatic arteriogram (through celiac artery) reveals redistribution of flow from the left hepatic artery through intrahepatic colaterals to the right hepatic artery (*open arrows*)

delivery of the chemotherapeutic agent to the entire liver. This is done by using stainless steel coils with attached (Dacron) strands. The development of intrahepatic collaterals is instantaneous in most cases.[53,54] Following hepatic arterial redistribution, the catheter is repositioned into the patent artery and the infusion is begun. The efficacy of the intrahepatic collateral arterial infusion has been demonstrated by the regression of neoplasm in both the lobe receiving native and that receiving collateral circulation. The mechanism related to the response in the lobe receiving collaterals might be due to either the effect of the chemotherapy or the reduced flow through the collaterals.

SELECTION OF DRUGS

Administration of mitomycin-C (MTC), 15 mg/m^2 over a 2 hour to 24 hour period, and of floxuridine (FUDR), 100 mg/m^2 per day for a 5-day continuous infusion, is the present protocol for hepatic metastases from colorectal carcinoma.[7] Doxorubicin 60 mg/m^2 to 75 mg/m^2 given over the course of 5 days in three pulses of 20 mg/m^2 to 25 mg/m^2 each, is added to the above for a primary hepatocellular neoplasm or metastases from a variety of primary carcinomas. For metastases from breast carcinoma, soft tissue sarcomas, and melanomas, *cis*-diamminedichloroplatinum (CDDP), 120 mg/m^2, is infused over 2 hours.[55] Doxorubicin and heparin are incompatible and should not be infused at the same time through the same catheter.

Results

HAI of metastatic colon carcinoma comprises our most extensive experience. These patients are treated with mitomycin-C and floxuridine (FUDR) for at least three cycles. The response rate, as defined by the angiographic measurement of tumor size, was 55% PR and 12% CR. The median survival rate from the time of the initiation of HAI as a first line therapy in comparison with the intravenous route did not significantly improve. However, with HAI as a second line of therapy following failure of intravenous FUDR and mitomycin-C, there was significant prolongation of life from 7 months to 14 months.[7] In patients treated with CDDP for metastases confined to the liver from carcinoma of the breast, the response rate was 30% (CR 10%; PR 20%).

The results of HAI are not optimal. The limitations of HAI are largely due to the lack of effective antitumor agents. In the event of failure to respond after three cycles, or in the absence of effective agents, hepatic artery embolization is undertaken.

Complications

Hepatic artery trauma is associated with superselective catheterization, a higher concentration of chemotherapeutic agents over a shorter infusion time, or a combination of these factors.[1,6,56,57] Vascular trauma resulted in a 17% incidence of occlusion and 6% aneurysm.[58]

The arterial blood supply to the stomach, duodenum, gallbladder, and pancreas also originates from the hepatic artery. Unavoidable infusion of the gastroduodenal and the right gastric arteries has resulted in gastrointestinal symptoms of dyspepsia in 11.6% of the patients; some of them had documented gastritis, gastric and duodenal ulcers, cholecystitis, and pancreatitis.[58]

HEPATIC ARTERY OCCLUSION (HAE)

The nutritive blood supply to the liver originates from the hepatic artery (30%) and the portal vein (70%). Primary and secondary hepatic neoplasms receive their blood supply almost exclusively from the hepatic artery (90%). Markowitz suggested the use of hepatic artery ligation for the management of patients with hepatic neoplasms.[4] Following hepatic artery ligation, there is a 90% decrease of tumor blood flow and a 30% to 40% decrease of flow to normal parenchyma, which allows selective destruction of the tumor without apparent damage to the normal liver.[2,3,5,59] The response to surgical ligation is usually temporary due to the rapid development of collateral circulation.[53,54]

Devascularization of a hepatic neoplasm can be achieved percutaneously by combined peripheral embolization of particulate material (Gelfoam, Ivalon, *etc.*) and central occlusion with steel coils (Fig. 48-34). This method can be used: (1) in patients with unresectable primary hepatic neoplasms; (2) pre-operatively, to facilitate surgery of a resectable neoplasm; (3) in metastatic neoplasms that fail to respond to chemotherapy; (4) as the initial management of certain metastases usually refractory to chemotherapy and (5) to control pain and hemorrhage of an hepatic neoplasm.

Since 1972, 88 HAEs have been performed in our institution. This has been accomplished utilizing gelatin sponge or steel coils or both in 72 instances. More recently, polyvinyl alcohol foam (Ivalon) particles have been added in 16 for more permanent peripheral embolization.[16] Proximal hepatic artery occlusion, usually with coils, was similar to hepatic artery ligation, and collateral circulation invariably occurred. Peripheral HAE with absorbable gelatin sponge frequently recanalized within days to months and repeated embolizations were required. Combined peripheral and proximal HAE had more persistent effects; however, collateral supply eventually formed. Our initial experience with polyvinyl alcohol foam (Ivalon) particles suggests a significant improvement in the attempt to more permanently and more effectively occlude the vascular supply to the hepatic neoplasm.[16]

Results and Discussion

The effectiveness of the 72 HAEs in 49 patients is difficult to evaluate because embolization was frequently performed as the last resort after all other therapy failed. The reference point for comparison is difficult but essential to establish, that is, from the initial diagnosis, from the initiation of chemotherapy, or from the time of hepatic artery embolization. In our series, the survival time of these patients was calculated from the time of HAE after failure of chemotherapy in the majority of cases. Twenty-six patients expired with a median survival time of 7 months and a range of 5 days to 24 months. Sixteen patients are still alive and have a median survival of 11 months with a range of 6 months to 54 months. Seven patients are lost to follow-up. These results suggest that this modality has something to offer in the management of hepatic neoplasms.

Complications

The post-embolization syndrome consists of nausea, vomiting, paralytic ileus, pain, and fever. This was experienced by the majority of patients and was similar to that observed after renal infarction. Transient elevation of liver function tests was seen in most patients. Lactic dehydrogenase (LDH) and serum glutamic oxaloacetic transaminase (SGOT) were elevated for 1 day to 5 days and frequently returned to near pre-embolization levels in 1 week to 2 weeks. The alkaline

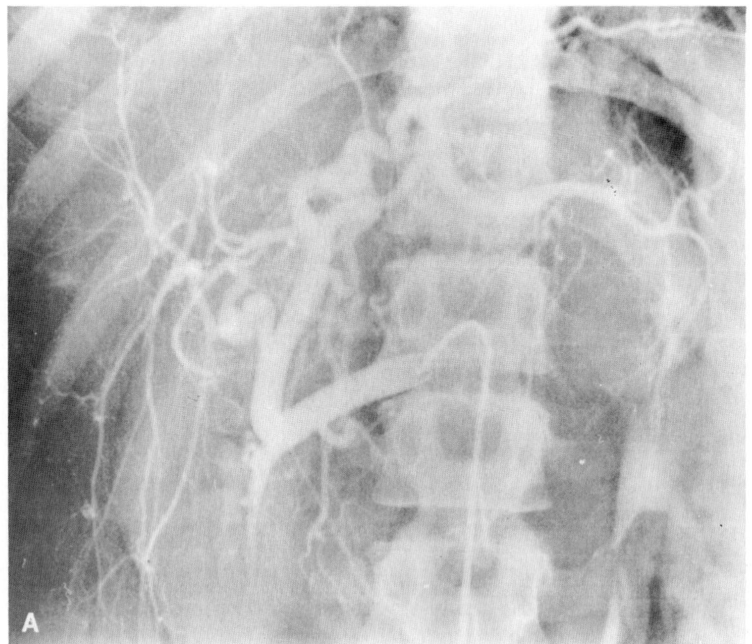

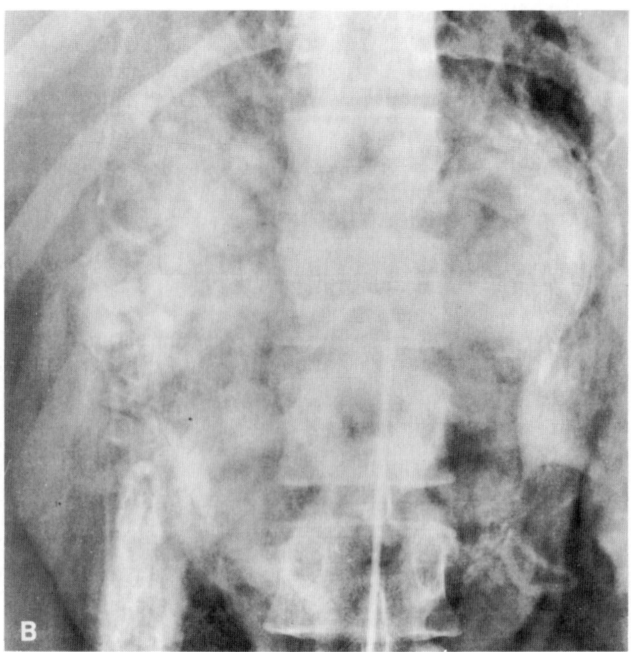

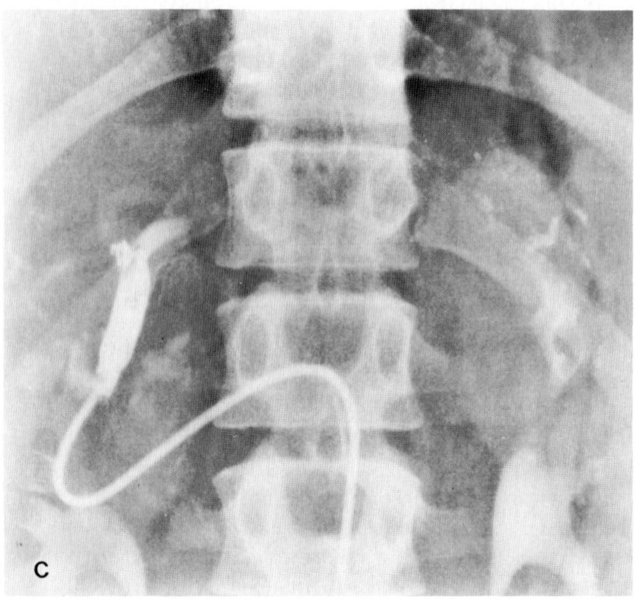

FIG. 48-34. Hepatic neoplasm embolization. *A*, Common hepatic arteriogram reveals markedly enlarged left and midhepatic arteries with multiple tumor vessels in the left lobe. *B*, The hepatogram phase shows hypervascular mass occupying the entire left lobe, consistent with a hepatoma. *C*, Selective embolization of mid and left hepatic artery was done using Ivalon particles, Gelfoam, and coils.

phosphatase was also elevated but returned more slowly. No patient in this series developed liver abscess or died as the result of liver necrosis.

BONE

In the management of primary and secondary neoplasms of bone, the interventional radiologist can make a significant contribution. Intraarterial infusion of chemotherapy has been employed in malignant bone tumors for local management of pain and in selected cases preoperatively for limb salvage procedures.[72,78,79] Transcatheter arterial occlusion has also been effective in the relief of pain from metastases, especially from renal carcinoma; pre-operatively, to decrease vascularity prior to resection; as well as definitive therapy for giant cell tumors (GCT) and aneurysmal bone cyst (ABC).[60,61]

INTRA-ARTERIAL INFUSION

The 3-year disease-free survival rate of patients with osteosarcoma treated by surgery alone or in combination with radiation therapy is usually 20% and never more than 40%.[62–65] Chemotherapy utilizing high dose methotrexate with citrovorum factor rescue, *cis*-diamminedichloroplatinum-II (CDDP), or doxorubicin administered as a single agent or in a multi-agent regimen usually in combination with amputation, has resulted in the eradication of established metastases, destruction of primary tumors, and increase in disease-free survival to 55% in 3 years.[64–71]

Advances achieved with chemotherapy have been instrumental in investigating, when applicable, more conservative methods for treatment of the primary neoplasm, short of amputation. Although systemic chemotherapy has been effective in the management of pulmonary metastases, the need for better control of the primary tumor was undertaken by the intra-arterial infusion, usually of CDDP, in an attempt to control the primary sarcoma.[72]

Fourteen patients, ten males and four females 12 years to 73 years of age, were treated by the intra-arterial infusion of CDDP. Of the 14 patients, 12 had primary osteosarcomas, one had recurrence, and one had metastases. The neoplasms were located in the innominate bone in six patients, in the femur in four, in the sarcum in two, and one each in the tibia and radius. Four of the 14 patients had pulmonary metastases prior to intra-arterial infusion of CDDP.

CHEMOTHERAPY

CDDP was infused at a dosage of 80 mg/m^2 to 150 mg/m^2 (usually 120 mg/m^2) over a 2-hour period with vigorous hydration and mannitol diuresis.[66,67,69] Infusion was repeated every 3 to 4 weeks for 3 to 4 cycles.

Results and Discussion

Standard criteria cannot be employed to define the response in bone tumors. Consequently, the response must be subdivided into that assessed by clinical means, including radiographic techniques, and that by histopathologic criteria in those cases in which tissue is available. Eight of 14 patients (57%) had angiographic improvement as defined by a decrease or disappearance of the tumor vascularity. An improved angiogram reflected partial or complete remission, which was indicated by the good correlation with histologic material and the prolonged responses in those who did not undergo surgical resections. The latter findings also substantiated the value of multiple needle biopsies in estimating response.

The response of 57% to intra-arterial infusion of CDDP compared favorably with the systemically administered CDDP response of 21% from combined series previously reported.[72,67,69] Despite the increased local concentration of intra-arterial CDDP, systemic levels are no different from those achieved with intravenous therapy.[12] No responding patients developed pulmonary metastases while receiving intra-arterial CDDP.

The eight responders are all alive with a follow-up period of 14 months to 21 months (median 17.5 months); six of them have no evaluable disease at present. Of the six nonresponders, all died of disease from 3 months to 14 months (median 6.5 months).

In those four patients treated by intra-arterial CDDP prior to local resection for limb preservation, either complete or partial response occurred with at least 50% destruction of the tumor. Since a customized endoprosthesis required 8 weeks to 12 weeks to prepare, it was necessary to maintain local tumor control pre-operatively for this period of time. Intra-arterial CDDP was successful in accomplishing this goal. All four with limb salvage procedures are alive with no evidence of disease, although the follow-up is still short (Fig. 48-35).

Other malignant bone tumors, including chondrosarcoma, malignant fibrous histiocytoma, and malignant giant cell tumors, have been treated in a similar fashion.

Complications

The complication in this group of patients included nausea and vomiting in all patients; skin reaction with edema, pain, and discoloration in 2 patients; and transient diastolic hypertension in 4 pediatric patients. Although CDDP is known to have auditory and neurologic toxicity, none developed in this series.

ARTERIAL EMBOLIZATION

Arterial embolization of tumors of bone for the alleviation of pain was suggested by Feldman and co-workers in the management of a patient with metastases to the ilium from an unknown primary neoplasm.[73] Relief of discomfort and some degree of calcification were also noted in a patient at M. D. Anderson Hospital with an aneurysmal bone cyst of the sacrum, after bilateral internal iliac artery ligation.

METASTATIC RENAL CARCINOMA

Nine patients with renal carcinoma metastases to bone were managed by embolization after failing to respond to radiation therapy.[60,61] The osteolytic metastases were in the ilium in four patients, the proximal femur in three, the lumbar spine in one, and the base of the skull in one. Six of these patients failed previous treatment. The three other patients were managed pre-operatively by embolization to reduce vascularity and decrease blood loss during curettage, methacrylate instillation, and internal hip fixation.

Of the six patients who underwent embolization for control of pain, one had complete relief, three had marked relief, one had moderate relief, and one had mild relief of pain. The alleviation of pain began within 12 hours to several days after embolization. The duration of relief ranged from 1 month to 6 months.

In the three patients who had embolization pre-operatively, there was a minimal blood loss at surgery in comparison to that usually noted with renal metastases. This greatly facilitated the operative procedure and pain was alleviated in all three patients, who ambulated soon after the operation.

BENIGN BONE TUMORS

Ten patients, nine females and one male with ages ranging from 13 years to 46 years, were treated definitively by embolization.[61] Seven of the neoplasms were in the sacrum or ilium, or both, two were in the lumbar spine, and one was in the proximal humerus. Eight of the neoplasms were histologically giant cell tumors (GCT), one was an aneurysmal bone cyst (ABC), and one had elements of both. All have had a previous attempt at management by surgery, radiation, or a combination of both.

Pain relief was experienced by seven of the ten patients; increased calcification as a manifestation of healing of the neoplasm was observed in five. One patient had an initial

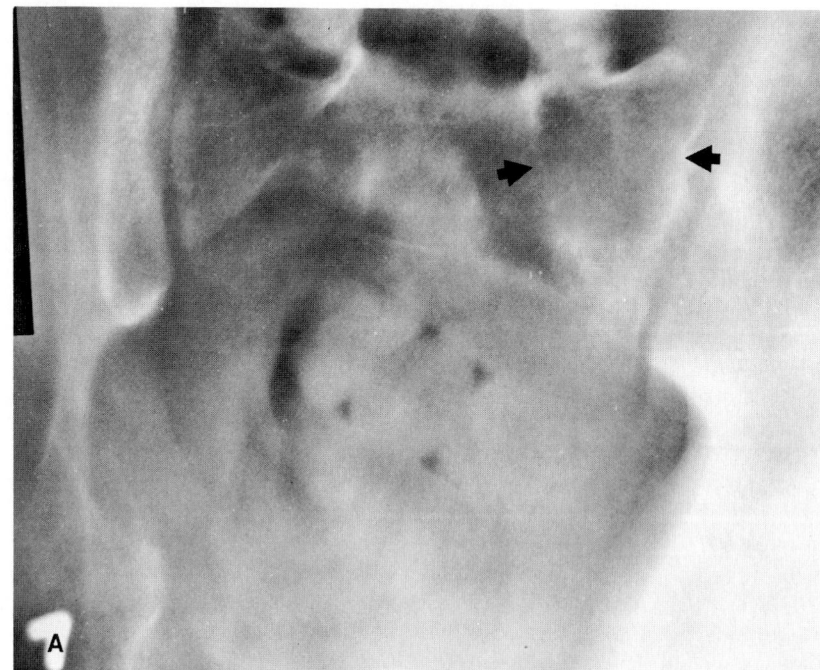

FIG. 48-35. Osteosarcoma infusion. *A,* A lytic lesion (*arrows*) in the left wing of sacrum. The patient previously had right lower extremity amputation for an osteosarcoma of right femur. Percutaneous biopsy of the sacral lesion confirmed the diagnosis of recurrent osteosarcoma. *B,* On the initial pelvic arteriogram, the catheter is placed in the left lateral sacral artery which originates from the posterior trunk of left internal iliac artery and supplies the entire tumor. Multiple tumor vessels and stain are noted (*arrows*). *C,* Following three courses of intra-arterial infusion of *cis*-platinum, the tumor vessels and stain completely disappeared and the lateral sacral artery became thrombosed at its origin (*arrow*). Complete pain relief was observed 48 hours after the first course of infusion. *D,* Follow-up tomography of the sacrum. Increased calcification of the lesion (*arrows*) is noted, indicative of healing. The patient is still alive without evaluable disease for 20 months. ▶

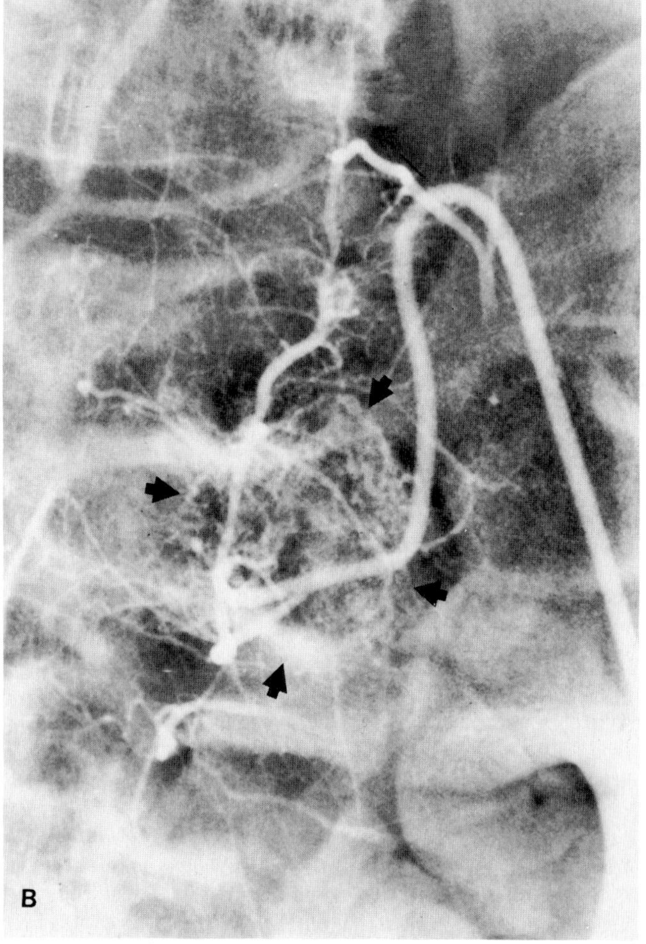

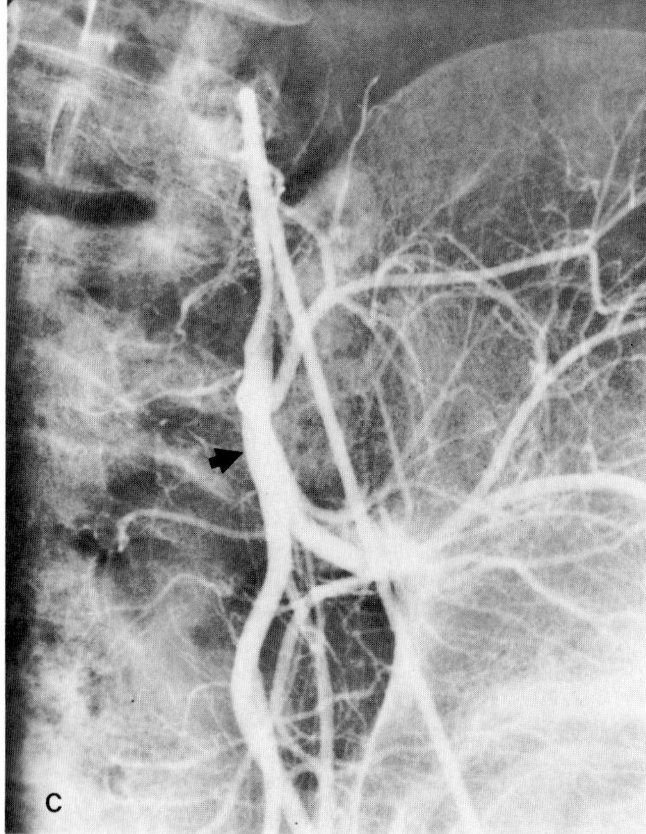

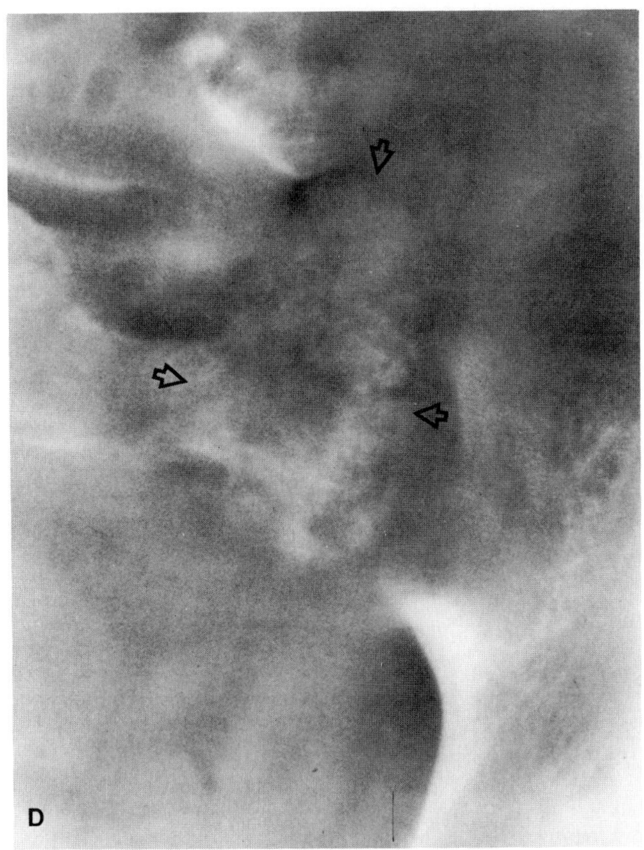

response but was lost to follow-up after four months. Six of the ten patients responded to arterial embolization and occlusion, a 60% success rate, and have been asymptomatic during a follow-up of 4 months to 55 months. In one patient, the embolization performed 1 year prior to resection reduced the size of the tumor and resulted in calcification of the margin, thus facilitating surgery (Fig. 48-36).

Complications

Two of the ten patients had complications related to the embolization: one had foot drop; one experienced transient numbness in the lateral aspect of the foot.

NEOPLASMS OF EXTREMITIES

Intra-arterial infusion of neoplasms of the extremities is readily accomplished by the transfemoral approach. For the lower extremity, the contralateral femoral artery is punctured and the ipsilateral femoral is catheterized in an antegrade fashion over the aortic bifurcation. This approach has been utilized in the management of recurrent melanoma, soft tissue tumors and, as has already been described, bone tumors. The dramatic response of four of nine patients with recurrent malignant melanoma to the infusion of CDDP has stimulated further exploration of this approach.[8,55]

PELVIC NEOPLASMS

Bilateral internal iliac artery infusion of chemotherapeutic agents has been utilized to treat advanced carcinoma of the bladder, cervix, prostate, ovary, and recurrent colorectal carcinoma, which at times has been associated with pelvic lymph node metastases. Internal iliac artery infusion has also been used in the management of soft tissue tumors and malignant neoplasms of bone, as previously described.

BLADDER CARCINOMA

Carcinoma of the urinary bladder comprises 2% of malignant disease and strikes 28,000 Americans each year. Its mortality rate is greater than that of carcinoma of the cervix. Ninety-seven percent of all bladder tumors are epithelial in origin, with 90% transitional cell carcinoma, 6% to 7% squamous cell carcinoma, and 1% to 2% adenocarcinoma.

Eighteen patients with advanced bladder carcinoma, Stage D_2 (extensive carcinoma with lymph node invasion beyond the origin of the common iliac arteries), were treated with intra-arterial *cis*-platinum alone or in combination with systemic chemotherapy (CISCA).[74] Of the 18 patients, there were 12 males and six females whose ages ranged from 32 years to 78 years. Thirteen of the 18 patients had transitional cell carcinoma, two had anaplastic carcinoma, two had squamous cell carcinoma, and one had signet ring adenocarcinoma. Nine patients had previous radiation therapy with recurrence in 3 months to 24 months following therapy. Cystectomy with loop diversion had been part of the definitive management in five patients. Prior or concomitant chemotherapy had been administered to ten patients.

Cis-diamminedichloroplatinum (CDDP) was infused at a dosage of 80 mg/m^2 to 120mg/m^2 over a 24-hour period with the patient on vigorous hydration and mannitol diuresis. If tolerated, the infusion technique was repeated every 4 weeks for a total of three courses, at which time the status of the patient was re-evaluated. Additional courses were given on occasion. In patients who failed to respond to CDDP infusion or developed drug toxicity, another therapeutic regime was instituted. FAM (5-fluorouracil, adriamycin, and mitomycin-C) was the alternative approach and was given to two patients. This included the intra-arterial administration of 5FU 1000 mg/m^2 per day for 5 days, and the intravenous delivery through a subclavian venous line of doxorubicin, 20 mg/m^2 per day for 3 days, and mitomycin-C, 5 mg/m^2 per day for 2 days.

The responses of these 18 patients can be divided into four groups. Three patients treated after surgery or radiation therapy had removed all measurable traces of the disease were considered as adjuvant treatment. Of the remaining 15 patients, there were six CRs, three PRs, and six failures, for a response rate of 60%. The survival lengths ranged from 26 weeks to 104 weeks with a median survival length, thus far, of 52 weeks. This compares well with a median survival of 13 weeks without chemotherapy and 19 weeks with chemotherapy prior to the combination of CDDP, adriamycin, and Cytoxan (CISCA).[75-77] CISCA has succeeded in achieving an overall response rate of 50%, usually of pulmonary metastases, and a median survival of approximately 40 weeks. The

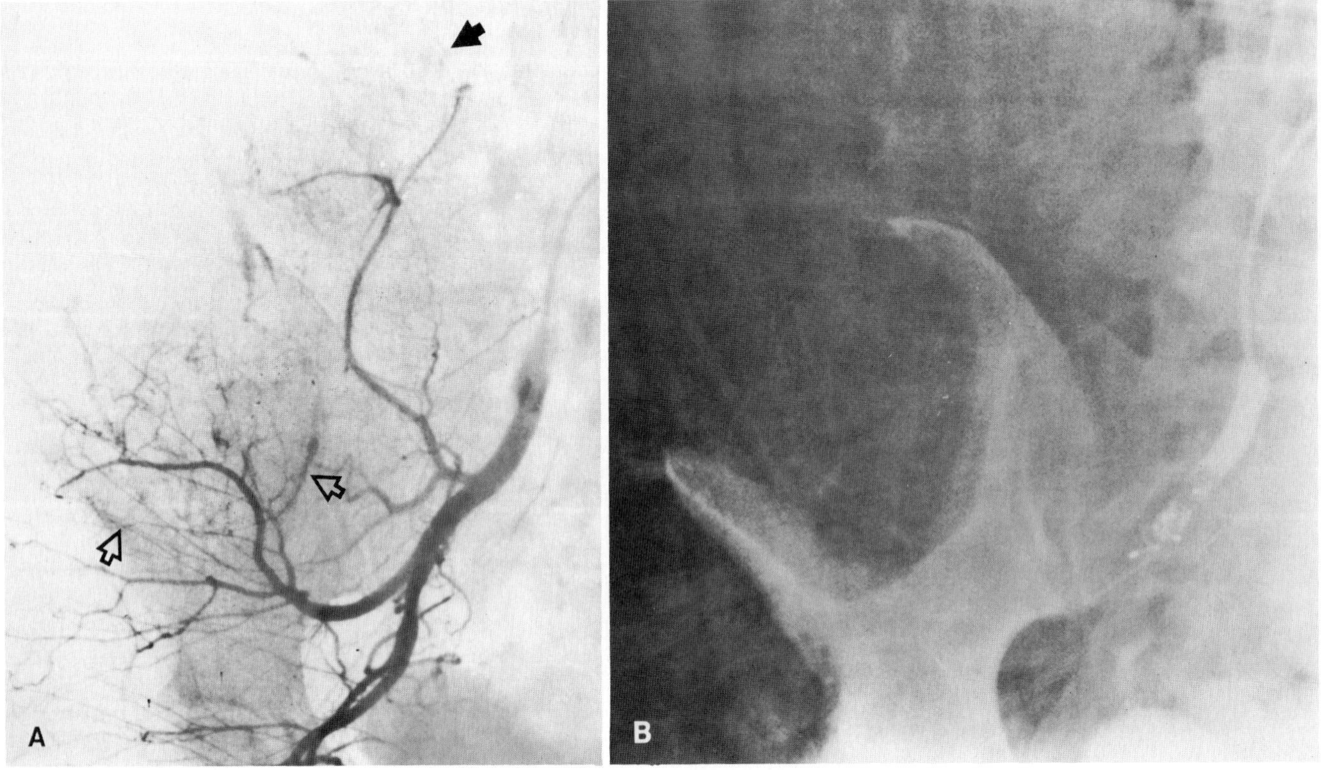

FIG. 48-36. Infusion of aneurysmal bone cyst with giant cell tumor components. *A*, Subtraction film of right internal iliac arteriogram demonstrates a hypervascular tumor of the right ilium (*open arrows*) and its adjacent soft tissue mass (*closed arrows*). *B*, Following embolization with Gelfoam and coils, the right internal iliac artery is occluded at its origin. *C*, Thirteen months following arterial embolization, calcification along the margin of the tumor is seen. The patient had complete relief of pain clinically. The lesion was resected and the patient has been asymptomatic for 38 months.

FIG. 48-37. Transitional cell carcinoma of the bladder. *A*, The bladder lesion was primarily on the right and posterior and difficult to distend. *B*, Following intra-arterial CDDP there is good distensibility and no obvious residual neoplasm.

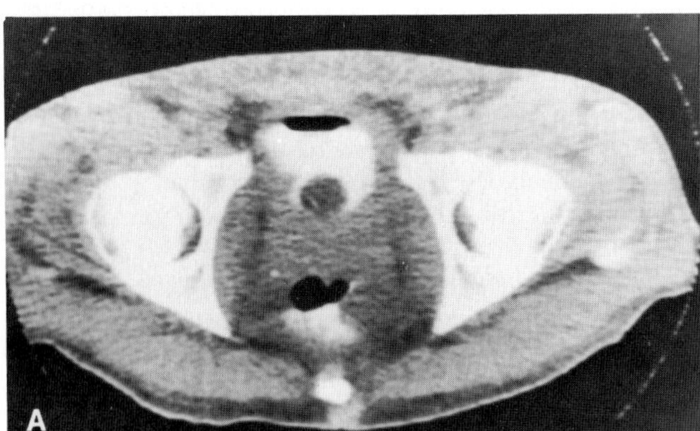

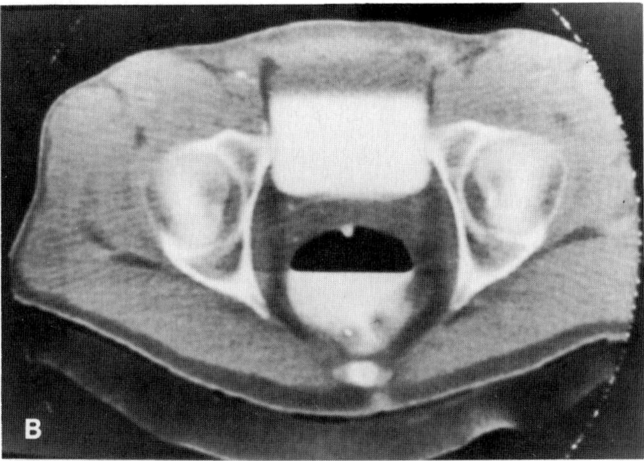

primary lesion is rarely controlled and pelvic and retroperitoneal lymph nodes are seldom sterilized by CISCA (Fig. 48-37).[75]

Complications

Two patients experienced acute tubular necrosis, which responded to medical management. An embolus to the lower extremity occurred in one patient shortly after catheterization but resolved spontaneously. Seven patients experienced transient peripheral neuritis, sensory in six and mixed motor and sensory in one. Both patients receiving intra-arterial 5-fluorouracil had erythematous skin reactions which accompanied each infusion and persisted for 2 weeks.

CARCINOMA OF THE CERVIX

Nine patients with squamous cell carcinoma of the uterine cervix were treated by bilateral internal iliac artery infusion of CDDP.[76] Six of these patients had unresectable pelvic recurrences following radiation therapy and three had previously untreated, large volume primary tumors. Only three patients (33%) experienced partial responses, including two patients with pelvic recurrences and one with a previously untreated tumor. The durations of response were 6 months, 4 months, and 3 months. One of these three patients developed progressive disease after 6 months and died 13 months after the initiation of chemotherapy. The 4-month responder is currently alive with progressive disease after 20 months. The previously untreated patient demonstrated a marked reduction in tumor volume and, after three infusions of CDDP, began radiation therapy. She remains free of disease at 7 months following the initiation of therapy.

Although a 33% response rate is not dramatic, the percutaneous intra-arterial route of administration will be pursued, employing other combinations of chemotherapeutic agents.

CONCLUSION

The application of interventional radiology in the cancer patient is in its infancy. Further exploration depends in part upon the availability of more effective chemotherapeutic agents. Even more important are the interest and ingenuity of the interventional radiologist. In addition, the interventional radiologist must assume a new role of more active participation in patient management. This is associated with greater commitment and responsibility for the patient's welfare. The patients and medical community must appreciate this new role and must become aware of the increased risks as well as the rewards.

REFERENCES

1. Ansfield FJ, Ramariz G, Skibba JL et al: Intrahepatic arterial infusion with 5-Fluorouracil. Cancer 28:1147–1151, 1971
2. Fortner JG, Mulcar RJ, Solis A et al: Treatment of primary and secondary liver cancer by hepatic artery ligation and infusion chemotherapy. Am Surg 178:162–172, 1973
3. Lee YTN: Nonsystemic treatment of metastatic tumors of the liver—a review. Med Pediatr Oncol 4:185–203, 1978
4. Markowitz J: The hepatic artery. Surg Gynecol Obstet 95:644, 1952
5. Nilsson LA: Therapeutic hepatic artery ligation in patients with secondary liver tumors. Rev Surg 23:374–376, 1966
6. Oberfield RA, McCaffrey JA, Pilio T et al: Prolonged and continuous percutaneous intra-arterial hepatic infusion chemotherapy in advanced metastatic liver adenocarcinoma from colorectal primary. Cancer 44:414–423, 1979
7. Patt YZ, Mavligit GM, Chuang VP et al: Percutaneous hepatic arterial infusion (HAI) of Mitomycin C and Floxuridine (FUDR)—An effective treatment for metastatic colorectal carcinoma in the liver. Cancer 46:261–265, 1980
8. Pritchard JD, Mavligit GM, Wallace S et al: Regression of regionally advanced malignant melanoma after arterial infusion with cis-platinum and actinomycin-D. Clin Oncol 5:179–182, 1979
9. Wallace S: Interventional radiology. Cancer 37:517–531, 1976
10. Ensminger WD, Rosovsky A, Raso V et al: A clinical– pharmacological evaluation of hepatic arterial infusions of 5-Fluoro-2'-Deoxyuridine and 5-Fluorouracil. Cancer Res 38:3784–3792, 1978
11. Frei E III: Effect of dose and schedule on response. In Holland JF, Frei E III (eds): Cancer Medicine, pp 717–730. Philadelphia, Lea & Febiger, 1973
12. Stewart DJ, Benjamin RS, Siefert W et al: Clinical pharmacology of intra-arterial cis-diamminedichloroplatinum (II) (abstr C-76). Proc Am Assoc Cancer Res Am Soc Clin Oncol 1980;21
13. Kaplan WD, D'Orsi CJ, Ensminger WD et al: Intra-arterial radionuclide infusion: A new technique to assess chemotherapy perfusion patterns. Cancer Treatment Rep 62:699–703, 1978
14. Athanasoulis CA, Baum S, Waltman AC et al: Control of acute gastric mucosal hemorrhage. Intra-arterial infusion of posterior pituitary extract. N Engl J Med 290:597–603, 1974
15. Bookstein JJ, Chlosta EM, Foley D et al: Transcatheter hemostasis of gastrointestinal bleeding using modified autogenous clot. Radiology 113:277–285, 1974
16. Chaung VP, Soo CS, Wallace S: Ivalon embolization in abdominal neoplasms. Am J Roentgenol 136:723–733, 1981
17. Doppman LJ, Zapol W, Pierce JL: Transcatheter embolization with a silicone rubber preparation—Experimental observations. Invest Radiol 6:304–309, 1971
18. Dotter CT: Selective instant arterial thrombosis with isobutyl cyanoacrylate. Work in progress at the 59th Scientific Assembly and Annual Meeting of the Radiological Society of North America, Chicago, Illinois, 1973
19. Kerber CW, Bank WO, Horton JA: Polyvinyl alcohol foam: prepackaged emboli for therapeutic embolization. Am J Roentgenol 130:1193–1194, 1978
20. Tadavarthy SM, Moller JH, Amplatz M: Polyvinyl alcohol (Ivalon)—a new embolic material. Am J Roentgenol 125:609–616, 1975
21. White RI Jr, Giargiana FA Jr, Bell W: Bleeding duodenal ulcer control selective arterial embolization with autologous blood clot. JAMA 229:546–548, 1974
22. White RI Jr, Kaufman SL, Barth KH et al: Therapeutic embolization with detachable silicone balloons. JAMA 241:1257–1260, 1979
23. Anderson JH, Wallace S, Gianturco C et al: "Mini" Gianturco stainless steel coils for transcatheter vascular occlusion. Radiology 132:301–303, 1979
24. Bree RL, Goldstein HM, Wallace S: Transcatheter embolization of the internal iliac artery in the management of neoplasms of the pelvis. Surg Gynecol Obstet 143:597–601, 1976
25. Chuang VP, Wallace S, Gianturco C: A new improved coil for tapered tip catheter for arterial occlusion. Radiology 135:507–509, 1980
26. Gianturco C, Anderson JH, Wallace S: Mechanical devices for arterial occlusion. Am J Roentgenol 124:428–435, 1975
27. Wallace S, Gianturco C, Anderson JH et al: Therapeutic vascular occlusion utilizing steel coil technique: Clinical applications. Am J Roentgenol 127:381–387, 1976

28. Goldstein HM, Medellin H, Ben-Menachem Y et al: Transcatheter arterial embolization in the management of bleeding in the cancer patient. Radiology 115:603–608, 1975
29. Goldstein HM, Wallace S, Anderson JH et al: Transcatheter occlusion of abdominal tumors. Radiology 120:539–545, 1976
30. Granmayeh M, Wallace S, Schwarten D: Transcatheter occlusion of the gastroduodenal artery. Radiology 131:59–64, 1979
31. Rosch J, Dotter CT, Brown MJ: Selective arterial embolization—A new method for control of acute gastrointestinal bleeding. Radiology 120:303–306, 1972
32. Baum S, Nusbaum M: The control of gastrointestinal hemorrhage by selective mesenteric arterial infusion of vasopressin. Radiology 98:497–505, 1971
33. Chuang VP, Wallace S, Zornoza J et al: Transcatheter arterial occlusion in the management of rectosigmoidal bleeding. Radiology 133:605–609, 1979
34. Kobayashi I, Kusano S, Matsubayashi T et al: Selective embolization of the vesical artery in the management of massive bladder hemorrhage. Radiology 136:345–348, 1980
35. Schwartz PE, Goldstein HM, Wallace S et al: Control of arterial hemorrhage using percutaneous arterial catheter technique in patients with gynecologic malignancy. Gynecol Oncol 3:2760–2788, 1975
36. Johnson DE, Kaesler KE, Samuels ML: Is nephrectomy justified in patients with metastatic renal carcinoma? J Urol 114:27–29, 1975
37. Lokich JJ, Harrison JH: Renal cell carcinoma: Natural history and chemotherapeutic experience. J Urol 114:371–374, 1975
38. Montie JE, Stewart BH, Straffon RA et al: The role of adjunctive nephrectomy in patients with metastatic renal cell carcinoma. J Urol 117:272–275, 1977
39. Skinner DG, Colvin RB, Vermillion CD et al: Diagnosis and management of renal cell carcinoma: A clinical and pathologic study of 309 cases. Cancer 28:1165–1177, 1971
40. Johnson DE, Samuels ML: Chemotherapy for metastatic renal carcinoma. In *Cancer Chemotherapy—Fundamental Concepts and Recent Advances,* pp 493–503. (Proc Univ Texas System Cancer Center, M. D. Anderson Hosp & Tumor Inst 19th Annual Clin Conf on Cancer, 1975). Chicago, Year Book Medical Publishers, 1975
41. Lalli AF, Peterson N, Bookstein JJ: Roentgen guided infarction of kidney and lung—A potential therapeutic technique. Radiology 93:434–435, 1969
42. Lang EK: Superselective arterial catheterization as vehicle for delivering radioactive infarct particles to tumors. Radiology 98:391–399, 1971
43. Almgard LE, Fernstron I, Haverling M et al: Treatment of renal adenocarcinoma by embolic occlusion of the renal circulation. Br J Urol 45:474–479, 1973
44. Goldstein HM, Medellin H, Beydoun MT et al: Transcatheter embolization of renal cell carcinoma. Am J Roentgenol 123:557–562, 1975
45. Wallace S, Chuang VP, Swanson DA et al: Embolization of renal carcinoma—Experience with 100 patients. Radiology 138: 563–570, 1981
47. Chuang VP: Nonoperative retrieval of Gianturco coils from abdominal aorta. Am J Roentgenol 132:996–997, 1979
48. Habighorst VLV, Krentz W, Klug B et al: Spiralembolication der Niermarterie nach Gianturco. Fortschr Roentgenstr 128:47–51, 1978
49. Wirthlin LS, Gross WS, James TP et al: Renal artery occlusion from migration of stainless steel coils. JAMA 243:2064–2065, 1980
50. Sullivan RD, Norcross JW, Watkins E Jr: Chemotherapy of metastatic liver cancer by prolonged hepatic artery infusion. N Engl J Med 270:321, 1964
51. Michels NA: Blood Supply and Anatomy of the Upper Abdominal Organs, p 581. Philadelphia, JB Lippincott, 1955
52. Chaung VP, Wallace S: Hepatic arterial redistribution for intra-arterial infusion of hepatic neoplasms. Radiology 135:295–299, 1980
53. Koehler RE, Karobkin M, Lewis F: Arteriographic demonstration of collateral arterial supply to the liver after hepatic artery ligation. Radiology 117:49–54, 1975
54. Reuter RS, Redman RH: Gastrointestinal Angiography, pp 308. Philadelphia, WB Saunders, 1977
55. Calvo DB, Patt YZ, Wallace S et al: Phase I-II trial of percutaneous intra-arterial cis-diamminedichloroplatinum (II) for regionally confined malignancy. Cancer 45:1278–1283, 1980
56. Clouse ME, Ahmed R, Ryan RB et al: Complications of long term transbrachial hepatic arterial infusion chemotherapy. Am J Roentgenol 129:799–803, 1977
57. Goldman ML, Bilbao MK, Rosch G et al: Complications of indwelling chemotherapy catheters. Cancer 37:1983–1990, 1975
58. Chuang VP, Wallace S: Current status of transcatheter management of neoplasms. Cardiovasc Intervent Radiol 3:256–267, 1980
59. Mori W, Masuda M, Miyanaga T: Hepatic artery ligation and tumor necrosis in the liver. Surgery 59:359–363, 1966
60. Chuang VP, Wallace S, Swanson D et al: Arterial occlusion in the management of pain from metastatic renal carcinoma. Radiology 133:611–614, 1979
61. Wallace S, Granmayeh M, deSantos LA et al: Arterial occlusion of pelvic bone tumors. Cancer 43:322–328, 1979
62. Gehan EA, Sutow WW, Uribe-Botero G et al: The M. D. Anderson Experience, pp 271–282. In Terry W, Windhorst D (eds): Immunotherapy of Cancer: Present Status of Treatment in Man, New York, Raven Press, 1978
63. Marcove RC, Mike V, Hajek JV et al: Osteogenic sarcoma under the age of twenty-one. A review of 145 operative cases. J Bone Joint Surg 52:411–423, 1970
64. Sutow WW: Primary adjuvant chemotherapy in osteosarcoma. The Cancer Bulletin 30:178–181, 1978
65. Taylor WF, Ivins JC, Dahlin DC: Osteogenic sarcoma experience at the Mayo Clinic, pp 257–269. In Terry W, Windhorst D (eds): Immunotherapy of Cancer: Present Status of Treatment in Man. New York, Raven Press, 1978
66. Baum E, Greenberg L, Gaynon P et al: Use of cis-platinum diammine dichloride (CDDP) in osteogenic sarcoma (OS) in children, (Abstr C315) Proc Am Assoc Cancer Res Am Soc Clin Oncol 1978;19:385
67. Hayes DM, Cvitkovic E, Golbey RB et al: High dose Cis-platinum diammine dichloride. Amelioration of renal toxicity by Mannitol diuresis. Cancer 39:1372–1381, 1977
68. Jaffe N: High-dose methotrexate therapy in osteogenic sarcoma. Chemioterapia Oncologica 3:234–242, 1978
69. Ochs J, Freeman AJ, Douglass HO et al: Cis-dichlorodiammine-platinum (II) in advanced osteogenic sarcoma. Cancer Treat Rep 62:239–245, 1978
70. Rosen G, Niremberg A, Juergens H et al: Phase-II trial of cis-platinum in osteogenic sarcoma, (abstr C299). Proc Am Assoc Cancer Res Am Soc Clin Oncol 1979;20–363
71. Sutow WW, Gehan EA, Dyment PG et al: Multidrug adjuvant chemotherapy for osteosarcoma: Interim report of the Southwest Oncology Group Studies. Cancer Treat Rep 62:265–269, 1978
72. Chuang VP, Wallace S, Benjamin RS et al: Multimodal approach to osteosarcoma: Emphasis on intra-arterial cis-diamminedichloro-platinum II and limb preservation. Cardiovasc Intervent Radiol (in press)
73. Feldman F, Casarella WJ, Dick HM et al: Selective intra-arterial embolization of bone tumors. A useful adjunct in the management of selected lesions. Am J Roentgenol 123:130–139, 1975
74. Wallace S, Chuang VP, Samuels ML et al: Transcatheter intra-arterial infusion of chemotherapy in advanced bladder cancer. Cancer (in press)
75. Samuels ML, Moran ME, Johnson DE et al: CISCA combination chemotherapy for metastatic carcinoma of the bladder, pp 101–106. In Johnson DE, Samuels ML (eds): Cancer of the Genitourinary Tract. New York, Raven Press, 1979
76. Carlson JA Jr, Freedman RS, Wallace S et al: Intra-arterial cis-platinum in the management of squamous cell carcinoma of the uterine cervix (submitted for publication)
76. Sternberg JR, Bracken RB, Handel PB et al: Combination chemotherapy (CISCA) for advanced urinary tract carcinoma. JAMA 238:2282–2287,

77. Yagoda A: Phase II trials in bladder cancer at Memorial Sloan-Kettering Cancer Center, 1975–1978. In Johnson DE, Samuels ML (eds): Cancer of the Genitourinary Tract, pp 107–119. New York, Raven Press, 1979
78. Jaffe N, Watts H, Fellows KE et al: Local en bloc resection for limb preservation. Cancer Treat Rep 62:217–223, 1978
79. Rosen G, Murphy ML, Hovos AG et al: Chemotherapy, en bloc resection, and prosthetic bone replacement in the treatment of osteogenic sarcoma. Cancer 37:1–11, 1976
80. Woodside J, Schwartz H, Bergreen P: Peripheral embolization complicating bilateral renal infarction with Gelfoam. Am J Roentgenol 126:1033–1034, 1976
81. Anderson JH, Chica G, Wallace S et al: Experimental studies with transcatheter vascular occlusion, pp 57–65. In Johnson DE, Samuels ML (eds): Cancer of the Genitourinary Tract. New York, Raven Press, 1979

CHAPTER 49 **Jane E. Henney**

Unproven Methods of Cancer Treatment

"In all matters relating to disease, credulity remains a permanent fact uninfluenced by civilization or education."
William Osler

Each year approximately one million Americans are diagnosed as having cancer.[1] Many of these individuals, along with scores of others who think or fear that they have cancer, will invest countless hours and billions of dollars exploring alternatives to scientifically proven methods of cancer diagnosis and management.[2] This search for alternative forms of therapy is not only costly in time and money, but in terms of human life. In at least 41% of cases, medically sound therapies offer the patient the best possibility of increased survival and cure and always offer the best chance of palliation.[3] Many laymen are unaware, however, that such results are possible and turn to alternative unproven therapies assuming that their condition is hopeless. A more disturbing situation has also recently occurred, for some alternatives to conventional cancer therapy are also being touted as cancer preventatives.[4] Initially, these commodities are being purchased by individuals interested in promoting their own health. They fear the possible development of cancer and are often medically naive and, therefore, unaware that the products they consume have carcinogenic properties such as mutagenicity, as demonstrated by a positive Ames test as well as other potentials for inducing ill health.[5-]

Several questions naturally arise regarding this age-old, but currently rapidly expanding, problem of therapies that are widely promoted treatments but scientifically unproven. For example, what motivates a well-meaning group of men and women to seek substitute forms of therapy? Who offers these alternatives and how are they promoted? What is the scope of options? Finally, what can reputable health professionals do to counter this trend and ensure an informed consumer?

WHAT MOTIVATES THE PATIENT TO SEEK ALTERNATIVES

The basic psychological climate that makes the pursuit of scientifically unproven methods appealing to cancer victims is a complex one. Probably the prime motivator to seek alternatives to conventional therapy is fear.[8] A Gallup poll conducted in 1976 revealed that cancer is one of the chief concerns to the American public. One thousand, five-hundred-forty-eight men and women were surveyed; 58% of the persons interviewed stated that cancer was the disease they feared most. This was followed by blindness, feared most by 21%, and heart disease, feared most by 10%.[9] This fear arises because cancer is often equated with a rapid, painful course eventuating in death. Thus, to both the healthy individual or the diagnosed cancer patient, fear of suffering and dying are foremost.

The patient faces another series of fears arising from the

sometimes difficult cancer treatments presently offered by the medical establishment. Surgery may, by necessity, be radical and result in cure with permanent disfigurement; radiotherapy is psychologically threatening to many patients, for it can neither be seen or felt. Chemotherapy, like radiotherapy, is often attended by a variety of side-effects, including malaise, alopecia, stomatitis, severe nausea, vomiting, and diarrhea.

Nearly all cancer patients fear that even if a remission is induced, failure may occur. Those patients who seek care from reputable health professionals cannot be guaranteed a cure by the physician. This conservative approach, which is well-grounded in reality and not in false hopes or promises, nevertheless accomplishes little in alleviating the fears and anxieties of the patient.

The group of people who seek therapy outside the conventional arena tends to be suspicious of reputable methods and the medical profession. Many people are deeply disillusioned with science and technology. The physician, who to many represents an authority figure and uses a language that often is perceived as mysterious, has the potential to rebuff a population of patients who are understandably apprehensive. Promoters of alternatives, on the other hand, are often viewed by these same patients and their families as courageous leaders willing to go against the grain of the system and possessed of a self-defined "truth." The language they speak and the techniques used to illustrate the advisability of the products they suggest are geared to the lay person.[10]

Unproven therapies and the context in which they are administered also offer the individual patient an opportunity to become involved. This participation offers the patient the opportunity to at least in part control his or her own care. The patient does not passively turn decision making over to the authoritarian figure of the doctor, but rather actively exerts the partial but necessary control for himself and his destiny and thus, feelings of self-sufficiency and independence are maintained. These feelings may, in some ways, account for the subjective improvement that is often noted by patients who have received such therapy.

PROMOTERS AND THE METHODS THEY USE

Sponsors of these scientifically unfounded treatments vary greatly. Their educational background ranges from individuals trained in the scientific or legal disciplines at prestigious institutions to lay people with little formal educational training. Some may be genuinely motivated to help a sick person, or they may be unscrupulous in seeking adventure and profits by exploiting patients who genuinely are seeking help.

No matter what the educational background, common personality traits and methods for promoting the product in question appear to be shared by the advocates of these alternatives. Frequently, these promoters claim that a conspiracy exists at some level of the state or federal government or organized American medicine to keep these "cures" from the American people. This phenomenon was particularly evidenced in those who promoted Krebiozen in the 1960s (see section on DRUGS). Another tactic frequently used by the promoter is to claim that these bastions of the "establishment" do not want to lose the business generated by cancer patients.[11]

The promoter is usually quite skilled in the use of pamphlets, books, and sophisticated audiovisual techniques, rather than scientific meetings or refereed journals, to advertise his methods. Individual patient testimonials, rather than substantive data developed in a well-controlled and designed clinical trial, are frequently used to support the claims that are made. Promoters such as those who promoted the Hoxsey method (see section on Drugs), have been known to use spurious data based on claims of a "cured" cancer patient who, in fact, never had cancer or patients who may have obtained a remission from conventional therapy and concurrently or subsequently self-administered an alternative mode of therapy but chose to believe the latter has been responsible for the cure.

Another way of advertising alternative therapies, in recent years, has been for individuals promoting such therapies to enter the clinics and wards of reputable institutions and distribute literature and solicit recently diagnosed cancer patients to abandon the scientifically well-grounded management plan proposed for them in favor of an alternative method often promoted as being natural and nontoxic. This same type of information is supplied to the friends and relatives of the patient. These well-meaning family members, in turn, often exert subtle but very real pressure on the patient to seek the alternative. The patient is made to feel that he or she would be "letting friends or relatives down" not to participate in alternative therapy and this decision would result in abandonment. For the already psychologically traumatized patient, this fear of isolation is intolerable.

The distribution of the message by those who promote such methods not only reaches the patient directly but by a variety of indirect routes. Promoters are now taking advantage of sophisticated computerized technology and have developed the capability to generate mass mailings. This mailing network can be used to influence the political and legislative arena, for it can generate funding for political candidates and lawmakers who support such efforts or exert pressure on elected officials or the practicing oncologist who does not accept such treatment methods.[12,13]

When promoting an unproven method, the specific "cure" or method for detecting whether cancer is present in any part of body is advertised as unique. The theories rendered by the promoter to explain the efficacy of these methods are often quite complex, as is the case with laetrile (see section on Drugs) but are not supportable with scientific evidence. Promoters also commonly exhibit an unwillingness to disclose methods of preparation of the product, but claim a unique way to prepare and formulate the product in question.

Unfortunately, when patients who have sought alternative therapy fail to respond, they are disregarded by the promoter who claims the patients have either had insufficient faith or have failed to follow directions or have sought the cure too late, or have constitutional resistance.[10] Thus, the promoter attributes all failures to the patient rather than to the product.

WHAT ARE THE ALTERNATIVES OFFERED?

The most commonly promoted alternatives are devices, diets, and drugs. Recently, combinations of the two, specifically diets and drugs, have been at the forefront of scientifically unproven methods. There has also been a growing interest in creating a highly structured framework for the cancer patient who seeks alternative therapy. It is this phantom framework that provides a milieu in which the patient can actively participate and retain a sense of self-control and actualization. The following sections list specific examples of some of the most prominent methods promoted in this country over the past 50 years. Table 49-1 lists many of the other devices, diets, drugs, and techniques that have captured some degree of attention by the United States populace during the 20th century.

TABLE 49-1. Scientifically Unproven Methods Promoted for the Diagnosis or Treatment of Cancer

Alkylizing punch
Almonds
Aloe vera plant
Anticancergen Z50-zuccalalytic test
Antineol
Asparagus oil
Bacteria enema
Bamfolin (S.N.K.)
Bio medical detoxification therapy
Bonifacio anticancer goat serum
Cancer lipid concentrate and the malignancy index
Carcalon
Carcin
Carrot/celery juice
Carzodelan
Cedar cones
CH-23
Chamonils
Chaparrel tea
Chase dietary method
Coffee enemas
Coley's mixed toxins
Collodanrum and bichloracetic acid—Kahlenberg
Compound X
Contreras method
Crofton immunization
Diamond carbon compound
DMSO (haematoxylin dissolved in dimethyl sulfoxide)
Esterlit
Ferguson plant products
Fresh cell therapy
Fresh defatted bile capsules
Frost method
Gerson method
Glover serum
Goat's milk
Grape diet
H-11
Hadley vaccine and blood and skin tests
Hemacytology index (HCL)
Hendricks natural immunity therapy
Hoxley method
Hubbard E meter and Hubbard electrometer
Iscador-mistletoe
Issels combination therapy
Kanfer neuromuscular handwriting test
KC555
Kelly malignancy index (ecology therapy)
Kallzyne
Koch treatment
Krebiozen
Lewis methods
Livingston vaccine
Makar: intradermal cancer tests (ICT)
M-P virus
Marijuana
Millet bread
Milluve
Mucorhicin
Multiple enzyme therapy
Naessens
Olive oil
Oncon juice
Orgone energy devices
Polonine
Rand vaccine
Revici cancer control
Samuels casual therapy/ endogenous endocrinotherapy/Daussets method
Sanders treatment
Snake meat
Snake oil capsules
Staphylococcus phage lysate
Sunflower seeds
Ultraviolet blood irradiation—intravenous treatment
Unpolished brown rice
unsulfured raisins
Vitamin B-15 pangamic acid
Zen macrobiotic diet

DEVICES

Mechanical devices that have not been scientifically proven to be useful in either the diagnosis or treatment of cancer have ranged from simple boxes containing a jumble of electric wiring to quite complex technology. This type of scientifically unproven methodology was more prevalent in the earlier part of this century when the country was transfixed by the possibilities of high technology.

OSCILLOCLAST

Dr. Albert Abrams of San Francisco was one of the leading proponents of devices that were alleged to be useful in the diagnosis and treatment of cancer. His testing, known as "Radionics," proposed that electrons are basic biological units and disease is a disharmony of electronic oscillation. Abrams proposed that the devices he developed could adjust these oscillations and thus detect and treat disease. Physicians from throughout the country submitted blood samples dried on a piece of blotting paper to Abrams' "College of Electronic Medicine." This blood sample was then placed by Abrams in a simple device composed of a box with a slot cut in the side and a series of lights and dials. Metal plates were connected to the box and were held by a technician who was termed a "reagent" and who purportedly served as a detector for any radiation emanating from the dried blood sample. The operator held a wand and if the wand focused on a particular location this was said to be an "electronic reaction." From this reaction the operator allegedly could determine the type of disease and recommend treatment with one of the many treatment machines that were available for sale. These simplistic machines were purported to cure not only cancer, but syphilis and tuberculosis as well.

This machinery was still being distributed as recently as 1958, by Fred Hart who operated Abrams' Electronic Medical Foundation after Dr. Abrams' death. An injunction was brought against Hart and the Electronic Medical Foundation in that year in the District Court in San Francisco. A complete investigation by the Food and Drug Administration provided evidence that the machines could not distinguish between colored water and blood, or the blood of a living man from that of a dead man. Although it is now illegal to use such a machine, a few of them remain in active use.[14]

THE HUBBARD E-METER

During the 1950s, following the publication of his book, *Dianetics: The Modern Science of Mental Healing*, L. Ronald Hubbard founded the Hubbard Dianetic Research Foundation in Elizabeth, New Jersey. In Dianetics, the conscious and the unconscious mind are referred to as the analytical and the reactive mind, respectively. The analytical mind is seen by Hubbard and his followers to be a perfect computing apparatus except for occasional mistakes known as "engrams." These engrams are purportedly recorded by the unconscious or reactive mind when the analytical mind "isn't looking." Such engrams can be erased if a person's mind is audited and the patient returns to the track of time in which the engram or mistakes occurred.

Hubbard E-Meters are the devices used by followers of Hubbard to "audit" people who have any mental, emotional, or physical problems. The device is a battery-operated skin galvanometer-type device and have been labeled by those who advocate such treatment to state that these machines are effective for the diagnosis, prevention, treatment, detection, and elimination of all mental, nervous, psychosomatic and physical ailments, including cancer.[14,15]

THE DROWN RADIO THERAPEUTIC INSTRUMENT

The developer of this device was Dr. Ruth Drown. She contended that the device she had invented was based on the Abrams Electronic Reaction theory and would be used for both diagnosing and treating a wide variety of diseases ranging from cancer to loss of memory.

The complex device consisted of a collection of dials, terminal posts, and an ammeter or voltmeter. By placing one drop of patient's blood on a blotter, Drown claimed crystals were formed. These crystals were then to be used in a similar fashion to the crystals in the early radio receiving sets. By activating the device to the proper wave length, Drown claimed a diagnosis could be made. Once the accurate diagnosis was made, she could then use the device to send "healing waves" to the patient, no matter the location, and effect a cure.[14]

DIETS

Interest in diet and nutrition has long held both medical and popular attention. This interest has provided an avenue for those who would promote scientifically unproven methods of treatment for cancer victims. A change in dietary habits appeals to many, for the habits of eating and what one chooses to eat give a patient back some degree of independence and the opportunity to exert control. Even though many of these diet regimens may be harmless, some have the potential for increasing the toxic effects of other scientifically unproven methods (See section on Combination Therapy) and can, if used exclusively to treat the cancer, will almost certainly result in no benefit at all to the cancer victim. Although many dietary methods have been purported to be useful in the treatment of cancer, the following have dominated the attention and interest of cancer victims.

GRAPE DIET

In the late 1920s, Johanna Brandt, who had received a Doctor of Naturopathy and an Honorary Degree of Philosophy of Naturopathy, published a book, *The Grape Cure*. This publication stated that the Grape Diet was a treatment for cancer and practically all other human diseases.[16]

This treatment involved the consumption of a diet made up almost exclusively of grapes. A typical day on the grape diet would consist of the intake of 2 ounces to 8 ounces of grapes, beginning at 8:00 A.M. and repeating every 2 hours; until seven meals of grapes had been consumed. Only water was permitted in addition to the grapes. The entire program consisted of "(1) the exclusive Grape Diet for 1 to 2 weeks; (2) the gradual introduction of other fresh fruits and sour milk; (3) the raw diet, including raw vegetables, salads, and fruits, with dried fruits, nuts, milk products, honey, and olive oil; and (4) under favorable circumstance, one cooked meal at midday; during which no liquid, salad, or fruits should be eated."[17] In addition to taking in grapes in huge quantities, grape poultices, gargles, enemas, or douches were also recommended. Although not popular today, as late as 1969 this diet was being promoted as a successful treatment for cancer.

GERSON DIET

Dr. Max Gerson was a German physician who specialized in internal medicine and nerve diseases. Three events were to change his conventional medical practice to one which supported a method not well-grounded in the scientific method. Dr. Gerson had suffered migraine headaches for many years. He devised a special diet which he believed cured this condition. In the late 1920s, he developed yet another dietary treatment that he claimed to be efficacious in the treatment of tuberculosis.[18] Finally, he gave this latter dietary recommendation, with minor modification, to a patient who allegedly was suffering from cancer of the biliary tract and who subsequently claimed to be cured; following the dietary treatment recommended.[19]

Gerson translated this alleged success into a treatment for all cancer patients.[20] The dietary recommendations were based on "(1) detoxification of the whole body; (2) providing the essential contents of potassium; (3) adding oxidizing enzymes continuously as long as they are not reactivated and built in the body (in the form of green leaf juice and fresh calf's liver juice)."[21,22]

The diet and its preparation were outlined in minute detail. For instance, no foodstuffs could be eaten other than fresh fruits and vegetables (which had been chopped by a machine sold by Dr. Gerson) and oatmeal. No aluminum utensils or pressure cookers were to be used in the preparation of food and it was further recommended that no steam be allowed to escape during the preparation of any of these dishes. Specifically taboo were the use of tobacco and alcohol and any products containing sodium, including salt and sodium bicarbonate and all spices.

Only after 6 weeks of this spartan-like diet were patients allowed any protein. This was permitted only in the form of milk products. In addition to the diet, Gerson recommended medication including niacin, brewer's yeast, fresh defatted bile in capsules, liver and iron capsules, dicalcium phosphate and viosterol, injections or crude liver extract intramuscularly, Lugol's solution and thyroid extract, and coffee enemas.[21,22]

Despite many patients' rigorous attention to following this detailed regimen that was based on an elaborate but unsupportable theory and the persistent promotion by many of Gerson's followers, reviews of small series of cases failed to support that the method had any antitumor properties.[22]

DIETARY SUPPLEMENTS

Total diet control as illustrated in the previous examples is only one side of the nutritional coin that is exploited by those who would promote scientifically unproven methods. Additive components such as vitamins, both genuine and fraudulent, are increasingly advocated as beneficial in the treatment or prevention of cancer. Vitamins seem to have particular appeal to the public, for who has not heard from the mass media, or as a child more directly from parents, that to "take your vitamins" will be rewarded not only with immediate approval but by a healthy body and long life.

Two vitamins currently proported to have antitumor properties are megadoses of vitamin C and vitamin A. Another substance, pangamic acid, marketed as a vitamin with antitumor properties but meeting neither any of the criteria of a vitamin nor demonstrating antitumor effect is currently enjoying a vogue among those who promote scientifically unproven treatments.

Vitamin C

Vitamin C as a treatment for cancer has been widely advocated by Ewan Cameron, a Scottish physician, and the prestigious two-time winner of the Nobel Prize, Linus Pauling. According to Cameron, cancer cells release an enzyme, hyaluronidase, which is capable of destroying the substances that give integrity to the normal cell. Cameron, therefore, theorizes that if one could reduce the hyaluronidase production or in some way strengthen the cellular cement of cells, collagen, then growth of malignancies could be greatly inhibited.[23] Linus Pauling's contribution relates to the latter part of the theory, for he suggests that vitamin C is capable of providing reinforcement and strength to the collagen. Cameron and Pauling put this hypothesis to a clinical test in Cameron's native Scotland. One hundred patients were given 10 g of ascorbic acid per day and were matched with 100 historical controls who had not received the drug. The results of this study were reported by these two investigators to be positive; the treated patients had a mean survival time approximately 300 days greater than that of the control group. Moreover, some patients who had received vitamin C remained alive several years after they were considered untreatable.[24]

When approached by Linus Pauling to duplicate these results in a double-blind clinical evaluation of vitamin C, the National Cancer Institute declined to sponsor such a trial for the following reason: many patients in the original Cameron and Pauling study had tumors in which standard treatment was available but were denied this therapy in favor of the testing of an experimental agent based on theory alone. The National Cancer Institute recommended that vitamin C be tested, but in a fashion similar to that used for other anticancer agents. This testing was conducted at the Mayo Clinic. After completing the study, the Mayo investigators concluded that the use of high-dose vitamin C in patients with advanced cancer who have previously received irradiation or chemotherapy could not be recommended, for no benefit either subjectively or objectively had been observed in the treated group.[25] Following this first study, these same investigators are currently conducting a study in patients who have advanced cancer, but in whom no known treatment is considered standard.

Vitamin A

The use of vitamin A either alone or in combination for the treatment of cancer has been popularized in the past decade.[26] Theories as to the mechanism of action vary greatly, from enzyme destruction to enhancement of the immune mechanism. The dosages that are commonly advocated, that is, 300,000 to 3,000 I.U. of vitamin A palmitate are not without hazard, for they are 10 times to 100 times above those levels associated with vitamin A toxicity.

Pangamic Acid—"Vitamin B-15"

Although vitamin B-15 was patented in 1949 and sold under the name of Pangamet, pangamic acid, also referred to as vitamin B-15, has enjoyed a resurgence of popularity and is being widely promoted as helpful against a variety of diseases, including cancer. There is, however, no evidence to date that this substance is either a vitamin, for it meets none of the standard criteria, or that it is effective in the treatment of any disease state. An analysis of the original material indicated that its composition was that of lactose. Samples of the material now sold have been analyzed and contain varying amounts of dimethylglycine hydrochloride, DMG. Studies further indicate that when DMG is mixed with sodium nitrate, a substance similar to saliva, and incubated, the material is positive in the Ames test.[27]

DRUGS

Although scientifically unproven methods have been a part of our history for centuries, by far the most common alternative is that which takes the form of a drug or "medicine." Four such drugs have dominated in each of the past four decades in the United States. These drugs illustrate not only a wide range of alternatives that have been offered, but also many of the methods and techniques used by those who promote such compounds.

1940s: KOCH TREATMENT

Dr. William F. Koch, of Detroit, was the major promoter of a cancer cure in the 1940s. He worked through an organization which went by the name of "Christian Medical Research League." Although repeated analyses of Koch's Treatment indicated that the solution was distilled water, Koch continued to insist that there was an "active" ingredient, glyoxylide, in the water. It was claimed that this ingredient was so potent that it had to be diluted, 1 part glyoxylide to 1 trillion parts of water. Although no firm evidence existed that the treatment had any anticancer effect, many lay persons and an estimated 3000 health team members actively promoted the solution's merits. In fact, when Koch was prosecuted on two occasions in 1943 and 1946, over 100 persons testified in defense of Koch and his "cure," claiming that the product was effective in treatment of over 69 different diseases, cancer in particular. Both of these attempts at prosecution ended in mistrials. In 1948, Koch retired and moved to South America, but the

Koch treatment continued to be promoted by the Christian Medical Research League until the early 1950s.[28]

1950s: HOXSEY TREATMENT

Harvey Hoxsey, of Dallas, during the 1950s promoted two medicines for the treatment of cancer. These were commonly referred to as "pink medicine" and "black medicine." The former was composed of lactated pepsin and potassium iodine, while the latter was cascara in an extract of prickly ash bark, buckthorn bark, red clover blossoms, burberry root, burdock root, licorice root, pokeweed, and alfalfa. Not only could patients obtain these "medicines" from the Hoxey Clinic in Dallas, but a package deal of a physical examination and blood and urine tests were offered by the clinic. These tests routinely revealed that potential clients indeed had cancer and a lifetime supply of the two "medicines" was offered for purchase.

Some 400 patients who claimed to have had cancer that was cured by the Hoxsey method were reviewed by the inspectors of the Food and Drug Administration in the late 1950s. After close scrutiny of this group it became clear that one group had either been self-diagnosed or never had a biopsy indicating cancer and a second group had received conventional forms of therapy, had been cured, and had later sought the Hoxsey treatment for fear the tumor had returned. The third group comprised those who received the therapy but continued to demonstrate clinically apparent tumor or those who had died. In 1960, a Federal Court injunction finally halted the sale of this product which had grossed over $50 million for the promoters.[28]

1960s: KREBIOZEN

Krebiozen, unlike the Koch treatment and Hoxsey remedy, was much more sinister, for it had the sponsorship of prestigious Andrew C. Ivy, M.D., Ph.D., Vice President, and Professor Emeritus of the University of Illinois. Ivy had been introduced to Dr. Steven Durovic in the late 1940s. Durovic was a Yugoslavian physician who had established the Institute Biologica Duga in Buenos Aires with his brother. The Institute was the site of production for a substance named kositerin, which was supposedly efficacious for the treatment of hypertension. This material was said to have come from the blood of horses that had been inoculated with *Actinomycosis bovis*, which causes a disease commonly known as "lumpy jaw." Durovic informed Ivy that the substance also had antitumor properties. In animal experiments using 12 dogs and cats, Dr. Durovic had reportedly observed the "clearing" of disease from seven, and the remaining five animals had improved.[29] Instead of putting Durovic's observation to the test of the scientific method, which requires results that can be duplicated, Ivy proceeded to inject not only himself with the substance but also a colleague, Louis Krasno, M.D., Ph.D., and the first patients in August, 1949.

Within 18 months, Ivy announced the results of his clinical experiments at a press conference. The results were recorded in a pamphlet published by the Krebiozen Foundation, rather than in a refereed scientific publication. The pamphlet stated that of the 22 patients treated, eight of the patients had died, but these deaths were not attributed to cancer. It was learned later that two additional patients had died after the publication of the pamphlet, but prior to the meeting: Ivy failed to mention this at the time of the conference. Attempts were made at a number of institutions to confirm the positive results that had been reported, but to no avail.[30] When confronted with this data, Krebiozen supporters claimed that a conspiracy by organized American medicine was keeping this cure from the American public.

Claims continued by the Foundation that the majority of patients achieved objective improvement due to the administration of this drug and they began to seek a "fair test" for Krebiozen. In 1961, the Foundation gave the National Cancer Institute records of clinical data on 4200 cancer patients and 10 mg of Krebiozen. After careful study, officials at the National Cancer Institute concluded that more substantial data would be required before a decision would be made regarding the further clinical testing of Krebiozen.[31]

Analysis of separate samples that had been obtained by the Food and Drug Administration and the National Cancer Institute revealed that the substance was creatine monohydrate in mineral oil. Other lots of the "drug" subsequently evaluated by the FDA proved to be only mineral oil.[32] The FDA initiated litigation and a federal grand jury investigation resulted in an indictment of Ivy, the Durovic brothers, and the Krebiozen Research Foundation on 49 counts of fraud and conspiracy. Despite voluminous evidence to the contrary, all were acquitted.[33]

The acquittal did not alter the Food and Drug Administration ruling that the interstate distribution of Krebiozen was illegal. To demonstrate their objection to the position the FDA had taken, Krebiozen supporters demonstrated at several federal agencies. Members of Congress were also in support of the reversal of the FDA policy. A public hearing was held and the decision by the FDA was upheld.

In the midst of this turmoil, the Krebiozen Research Foundation gave the NCI the records of 504 patients who were considered to be the "best cases" in the Foundation's file. After a thorough review of data submitted, and additional data provided by the Food and Drug Administration officials who ferreted out the hospital and physician's records, pathology reports, and death certificates on the 504 patients, a panel of 24 experts was assembled in August, 1963. These experts were to evaluate the complete data set, using the standard criteria for evaluating a response. Of the 504 patients records submitted, 216 were found to be inadequate for evaluation. Only two patients of the remaining 288 were considered to have had tumor regression which might have been attributed to Krebiozen. These results were within the probability of spontaneous regression, an occurrence not unknown in the field of cancer. The committee, therefore, recommended that no further clinical trials be initiated.[31]

An additional investigation of the Krebiozen Foundation was undertaken by the FDA following this first review. This second analysis involved the records of 4307 patients. Unfortunately, 2781 of these records were inevaluable because of overlapping treatments, lack of proof of diagnosis, inadequate documentation, and lack of similar standard prerequisites needed for acceptable evaluation. Of the remaining 1526 evaluable cases, three patients were noted to have obtained a partial remission of the tumor. However, one remission was of two weeks "duration," one remission was a reduction in size of a primary breast cancer from which large biopsies were taken during treatment, and a third was a 50% decrease in size of a lymph node approximately ¾ inch in diameter, although a coexistent cancer seen in the chest roentgenogram was not restudied by film. Thus, each of these attempts failed to confirm the positive reports of the Krebiozen advocates.[31]

1970s: LAETRILE

Until recently laetrile was one of the most widely known and publicized scientifically unproven method of cancer treatment.[34] The term "laetrile" is a general one, denoting a variety of cyanogenic glucosides. Although this spectrum of cyanogenic glucosides provides a fertile ground for debate and an obvious rationalization for why a particular product does not produce the promised favorable results, the majority of laetrile samples analyzed are composed of amygdalin, a D-mandelonitrile-B-D-glucoside-6-B-D-glucoside, and some degree of impurities. This chemical substance is present in a variety of food products, including apricot pits, almonds, macademia nuts, apples, cherries, peaches, and pears.[35,36]

Amygdalin was first isolated by Robiquet and Boutron in 1830 and the chemical properties were later described by Liebig and Wohler in 1837.[37,38] The synthesis was reported in 1924 followed by a description of amygdalin's biochemical properties by Vierhover and Mack in 1935.[36] They reported that during *in vitro* hydrolysis with emulsion and dilute acid, one molecule of HCN and benzaldehyde and two molecules of glucose were released. Further, in toxicity studies in dogs and rabbits, the rate of release of HCN was dependent on the concentration of an enzyme group, collectively termed emulsion. This rate had a direct correlation with the onset of cyanide symptoms and death in the test animals.[36,39]

It was not until the late 1940s that Dr. E. T. Krebs, Sr., first proposed a medical use for amygdalin to treat cancer patients and coined the word "laetrile" to describe the form of the mandelonitrile compound. Interestingly, Krebs' original intention with the chemical was to find a substance capable of altering the taste of smuggled whiskey during the Prohibition.[40] His son, E. R. Krebs, Jr., later obtained a patent on laetrile and claimed that laetrile exhibited antitumor properties on the basis of the unproven hypothesis known as the "trophoblastic theory of malignancy" or the "unitarian theory of the origin of neoplasms."[41,42] In brief, this theory is that cancer arises out of misguided trophoblastic cells that migrate to different parts of the body during the early embyronic development of the human. Although these cells have the potential to transform into malignant cells, the intrinsic release of normal pancreatic enzymes prevents this from occurring. Another control that is necessary in helping keep this transformation from occurring is an extrinsic control, amygdalin (laetrile). The direct antitumor activity that the promoters claim for laetrile is allegedly due to release of hydrogen cyanide within the cancer cell by the action of β-gludosidase on amygdalin. Further, the antitumor activity of hydrogen cyanide is claimed to be augmented by benzaldehyde, which is also released from amygdalin by the action of β-glucosidase. The mechanism of action described by those who advocate laetrile states that this dramatic cell-killing action of hydrogen cyanide affects *only* malignant cells, for these cells lack the necessary enzymes, rhodaneses, to fight the highly potent poison, but do have high concentration of the releasing enzyme, glucoronidase, which acts to potentiate the hydrogen cyanide. Normal cells, on the other hand, are claimed to have high levels of rhodaneses, which convert the cyanide released to thiocyanate and low quantities of glucoronidase, which are needed to release the hydrogen cyanide. These cells are therefore protected. Unfortunately, this theory lacks scientific validation, for careful measurements of both glucuronidase and rhodanese in a variety of normal and malignant mammalian tissues has failed to reveal these differences.[43,44]

For the medical community, much more disconcerting than the lack of validation for an elaborate and imaginative scientific theory has been the repeated lack of objective evidence for any significant antitumor activity in animal model systems. Results have been negative not only in the transplantable animal tumor systems but also in the "spontaneous" or naturally developing animal tumors and the xenograft system, in which human tumors are grown in athymic nude mice.[45-50] Recent results in cell culture systems have indicated that even though laetrile is capable of producing a 50% inhibition of colony formation by both normal and leukemic cells, it only achieves this at doses that are well in excess of those known to produce fatality in humans.[51]

Likewise, clinical data relative to laetrile have been insufficient to warrant a high priority for further evaluation of the compound.[52-55] Two retrospective studies that sought data as to laetrile's antitumor efficacy have been conducted. The first occurred in 1953, when the California Cancer Commission initiated an uncontrolled retrospective study of laetrile in 44 outpatients. Laetrile proponents declined to be involved in the study unless they were allowed to direct it. Patients with a variety of tumor types were included, but only one patient was alive and free of disease at the time of the study. Interestingly, the initial diagnosis on this patient was unconfirmed by biopsy.[56] The Commission concluded from the results of the study that laetrile, at best, could be viewed as a poor anticancer agent.

From the time of this first retrospective analysis until the second in 1977, many events relative to laetrile occurred. Among the more noteworthy was the legal action taken by the Food and Drug Administration against many of the proponents of laetrile. In 1962, Krebs, Jr., pled guilty to five counts of violating the new drug provisions of the federal Food, Drug, and Cosmetic Act. In 1965, Krebs, Sr., agreed to a permanent court injunction against further distribution of the drug and informed the court he was going out of business. In spite of this pledge, in 2 months time he was back in court to plead "no contest" to criminal contempt charges stating he had disobeyed a restraining order which prohibited shipment of laetrile in interstate commerce. Again, in January, 1966, Krebs Sr., pleaded guilty to a contempt charge of shipping laetrile in violation of an injunction. In

February of the same year, he was given a suspended sentence of one year by a California U.S. District Court for failing to register as a producer of the drug, laetrile.

During this decade marked with legal proceedings for the laetrile proponents, a liaison was established between the Krebs and Andrew McNaughton. McNaughton's Foundation had been the distributor of laetrile in Canada. In the spring of 1970, an Investigational New Drug Application (IND) was filed with the Food and Drug Aministration by the McNaughton Foundation. On April 20, the Food and Drug Administration assigned IND 6734 to the McNaughton Foundation of California. However, after an expedited review of the application by the FDA, during April, 1978 a 10-day pretermination notice that outlined specific deficiencies in the application was issued to the McNaughton Foundation as well as a notice to stop all ongoing clinical studies until the deficiencies in the application were addressed. When the sponsor failed to respond, the IND terminated in May, 1970.[57] Following this denial to proceed with the clinical study of laetrile under the auspices of IND 6734, the FDA had an *ad hoc* Committee of Oncology consultants review the IND submission from the McNaughton Foundation. It was the stated opinion of these experts that there is "no acceptable evidence of therapeutic effect to justify clinical trials. . . ."[57] Despite these seemingly overwhelming conclusions of the scientific community, interest in obtaining laetrile by members of the lay public from sources outside the United States continued to increase. Promoters of laetrile employed many of the same techniques used by previous advocates of scientifically unproven methods, including public meetings, press conferences, patient testimonials, and the like, but also began the heretofore uncommon practice of distributing pamphlets and other materials to patients early in their diagnosis when they were institutionalized.

In July, 1978, the courts once again became involved with laetrile. This time, their goal was not only to try one of the promoters, but also to consider whether the federal rules and regulations that apply to all investigational drugs should apply to compounds like laetrile. That is to say, should it be required that drugs used for cancer victims be capable of meeting the usual FDA standards of safety and efficacy. The United States District Court in Oklahoma presided over by Judge Luther Bohanon ruled in the case of Rutherford vs. the United States of America that such terms have no meaning in the context of a "terminally ill" patient.[58] The Court failed to address itself to the fact that the plaintiff, Rutherford, rather than suffering from "terminal cancer" had suffered from a polypoid adenocarcinoma of the colon and had likely been cured by the original cautery that he had received.[59] Judge Bohanon left the designation of terminally ill to any licensed medical practitioner and thereby, authorized the intravenous administration of this compound. This injunction, although upheld by the United States Court of Appeals for the 10th Circuit was later overturned by higher courts, but led to a cascade of legislation in 23 states by representatives who sought to "legalize" laetrile and make it available for their constituents.[60-62]

With this escalated level of public interest and concern, and the knowledge that as many as 50,000 to 75,000 U.S. cancer patients were seeking laetrile therapy, and further that many of these patients were leaving therapies that were known to be effective, the National Cancer Institute initiated the second retrospective study to determine possible laetrile anticancer activity.[63,64]

Over 440,000 letters were sent to health professionals soliciting case histories of laetrile users. In addition, letters were sent to many laetrile promoters, prescribers, and users requesting similar case histories. Of the 93 cases received from these sources, only 68 were considered complete. These cases were then reviewed by a panel of non-NCI expert oncologists. The panel was "blinded" from the treatment used in each case considered. Of the 68 patients who had received laetrile, two were judged by the panel to have obtained a complete remission and four a partial remission. Although these results could be explained by a variety of non-laetrile factors, anticancer activity attributable to laetrile was also felt to be possible.[65]

Thus, during the summer of 1978, the National Cancer Institute once again considered laetrile as a possible candidate for clinical evaluation. As the major developer of anticancer drugs in this country, the National Cancer Institute considers thousands of compounds each year for potential development. To warrant clinical evaluation a compound must demonstrate one or more of the following characteristics:

1. Evidence of antitumor activity in the cell culture and animal tumor screening systems (The level of activity observed when laetrile had been tested in both the *in vitro* and *in vivo* systems had been insufficient on prior occasions to suggest further testing.);
2. Unique mechanism of action (Although the elaborate theory espoused by the laetrile proponents had never been scientifically validated, there was reason to suspect that laetrile could act as a radiosensitizer, for radiation energy could break the cyanide bond and thus produce *in situ* radiosensitization);
3. Evidence of clinical activity (Drugs developed outside the United States are often tested in humans earlier than in the U.S. When these tests indicate positive results, further development of the drug in this country is warranted. Laetrile had evidenced only a minimal level of such activity as demonstrated by the data from the NCI retrospective study).

With the modest evidences of possible antitumor activity but the compelling need to provide reliable prospective clinical information on this controversial compound to the patients afflicted with cancer and to the physicians, allied health professionals, and friends whose advice is sought by cancer patients, the National Cancer Institute submitted an investigational new drug application to the Food and Drug Administration in December 1978. After a lengthy review of this submission, the Food and Drug Administration gave approval in January 1980, and the first prospective clinical trial of laetrile began in the spring of 1980. The data generated from this clinical trial subjected laetrile to the same scientific scrutiny used for testing all other anticancer agents and was conducted by investigators expert in the area of anticancer drug development.

The investigators first conducted a limited pharmacology/toxicity study that involved six cancer patients. Five of the six patients experienced few toxic effects that could be ascribed to laetrile or to the special diet. A sixth patient, however, did show clinical evidence of cyanide toxicity after consuming large quantities of almonds. The conclusion of this study was not that laetrile is safe, but that in the doses and manner given in this trial it was safe to proceed with the Phase II study.[66]

One hundred seventy-eight patients were then entered in the Phase II study. One hundred fifty-six received laetrile according to the original protocol and were evaluated for anti-tumor response. An additional 14 patients received higher doses of both laetrile and supplemental vitamins. In neither group was their substantive benefit in terms of anti-tumor response, improvement in symptoms related to cancer, or extension of lifespan.[67] This evaluation has shed light on an issue kept clouded by controversy over the past decade.

Combination Therapy

Another facet that adds to the complexity of the laetrile question is that the promoters have begun to administer the drug in combination with an array of enzymes and vitamins known as the "laetrile diet" or "total metabolic therapy." Indeed, recently laetrile promoters have also tried unsuccessfully to establish laetrile as a vitamin, B-17, and cancer as a state of vitamin deficiency, rather than the original claims that gave strong emphasis to laetrile's role as a drug with antitumor properties. This approach, plus the use of a multiple-factored single therapy, has served to deemphasize laetrile as a central issue and instead to diffuse the controversy, for it now becomes plausible that not using or misusing any one of the components could upset the balance of providing the promised cure. The laetrile diet commonly consists of nutritional guidelines that encourage the use of enzymes, megadoses of vitamins, particularly A and C (as previously described), minerals, enhancements of the immune system, adequate rest and exercise, and consideration of the mind-body relationship of each patient through the use of meditation techniques.[68,69] Unfortunately for cancer patients, those who promote such attractive therapies have never put any of these therapies, either alone or in combination, to a rigorous scientific test for validation.

ROLE OF THE HEALTH PROFESSIONAL

Each of the examples cited serves to remind the health professional who cares for the cancer patient that fears of the diagnosis, disease process, treatment, and death are very real and provide a prime opportunity for those at the margins of science who would fraudulently promote diagnostic methods or treatments that have not been subjected to careful testing. Nostrums that have enjoyed a vogue have generally attempted to borrow on the validity of other similar methods that were concurrently under scientific testing.

Health professionals, primarily physicians and nurses, are often asked to discuss not only methods under scientific testing but also diets, devices, or drugs that have not undergone such testing with an inquiring cancer patient or family member. One can best deal with these queries if they are approached with an open and direct, yet nonjudgmental attitude. It is of prime importance to delineate for those who seek such information the scientific rationale from the promotional efforts that are used to support any drug, device, or diet. Patients should be aware that all treatments currently used by the medical community were at one stage of development "unproven methods." Each, however, has been subjected to the careful approach required by the scientific method. It is also important to provide the inquirer with information relative to the criteria used for selecting the drugs, devices, or diets that will be subjected to a clinical study. Most patients and family members can understand that not all methods proposed by either the scientific or the lay community can be subjected to scientific scrutiny at the same time or the same rate, but that those with the greatest possibility of success, as defined by the preclinical screening tests used, receive the highest priority for further development and clinical testing. In all such encounters the physician or nurse should not lose patience but should view them as yet another opportunity to extend acceptance, hope, and comfort to those under his or her care.

Should scientifically unproven methods come to the attention of the physician or nurse and further information is needed or scientific investigation is felt by the health professional to be warranted, the American Society of Clinical Oncology or the American Cancer Society should be contacted. Both organizations have standing committees on new or unproven methods of treatment that keep current information regarding such practices. If the health professional feels that further scientific investigation of the method is warranted, the National Cancer Institute should be contacted.

If a physician or nurse encounters unproven methods or promotional techniques that he or she feels warrants further legal investigation, the local health department, consumer protection office, and medical society should be notified. Federal agencies and national organizations that are also involved in the investigation, regulation, or reporting of such practices are the Food and Drug Administration, Federal Trade Commission, United States Postal Service, Consumer Product Safety Commission, and the American Medical Association.

REFERENCES

1. Cancer Facts and Figures. American Cancer Society, 1977
2. Young JH: Health quackery a depressing boom industry. American Council on Science and Health News and Views, 1980
3. Axtel LM, Asire AJ, Myers MH (eds): Cancer Patient Survival, Report No. 5, DHEW publication (NIH), 7-992, 1976
4. McNaughton Foundation: Physician's Handbook of Vitamin B-17 Therapy. Science Press International, Sausalito, 1973
5. Lewis JP: Laetrile. West J Med 127:55, 1977
6. Selby LA, Mengers RW, Houser EC et al: Outbreak of swine malformations associated with wild black cherries, Prunus serotina. Arch Environ Health 22:496, 1971
7. Fenselau C, Pallante S, Batziner RP et al: Mandelonitrile beta-glucuronide: Synthesis and characterization, Science 198:625, 1977
8. Ingelfinger FJ: Cancer! Alarm! Cancer! N Engl J Med 293:1319, 1975
9. Most feared diseases. Parade Magazine. February 6, 1977

10. American Cancer Society: Unproven Methods of Cancer Management. New York, The American Cancer Society, 1971
11. Markle GE, Peterson JC, Wagenfield MD: Notes from the cancer underground: participation in the laetrile movement. Social Science Medicine 12:31, 1978
12. Barrett S, Knight G: The Health Robbers. Philadelphia, George Stickler, 1976
13. Herbert V: Laetrile: The cult of cyanide-promoting poison for profit. Am J Clin Nutri 32:1121–1158, 1979
14. Milstead JL, Davis JB, Dobelle M: Quackery in the Medical Device Field. Proceedings Second National Congress on Medical Quackery, pp 30–35, 1963
15. Anonymous, Hubbard E-Meter, Hubbard: Electrometer. CA 16:214–215, 1966
16. Brandt J: The Grape Cure. New York, Harmony Centre, 1928
17. Anonymous, Unproven Methods of Cancer Mangement—Grape Diet. CA 24:144–146, 1974
18. Gerson's cancer treatment. JAMA 132:645–646, 1946
19. Gerson M: The cure of advanced cancer by diet therapy: A summary of 30 years of clinical experimentations. Physiol Chem & Physico 10: pp 449–464, 1978
20. Gerson M: Muencl Med Woclenscler 72:967, 1930
21. Cancer News Journal, March/April 1972
22. Anonymous. Unproven methods of cancer management—Gerson method of treatment for cancer. CA 23:314–317, 1973
23. Cameron E: Hyaluronidase and Cancer. New York, Pergamon Press, 1966
24. Cameron E, Pauling L: Supplemental ascorbate in the supportive treatment of cancer prolongation of survival time in terminal human cancer. Proc Natl Acad Sci USA 73:3685–3689, 1976
25. Creagan ET, Moertel CG, O'Fallon JR et al: Vitamin C (Ascorbic acid) therapy to benefit patients with advanced cancer; a controlled trial. N Engl J Med 301:687–690, pp 687–690, 1979
26. Hoefer JH: The importance of vitamin A and protolytic enzymes in cancer therapy. In Heinsohn DL (ed): Cancer Metabolic Therapy and Laetrile. Sevierville, Tennessee, Crescent Publishing, 1977
27. Check WA: Vitamin B-15—whatever it is, it won't help. JAMA 243:2473–2480, 1980
28. Janssen WF: Cancer quackery—The past in the present. Semin Oncol 6:526–536, 1979
29. Durovic S: Cancer and Krebiozen: A new concept in cancer. Today's Japan, Orient/West 6:51–55, 1961
30. A status report on Krebiozen, Council on Pharmacy and Chemistry. JAMA 147:864–873, 1951
31. Holland JF: The Krebiozen story—Is cancer quackery dead? JAMA 200:213–218, 1967
32. Unproven methods of cancer management: Krebiozen and Carcolon. CA 23:111–115, 1973
33. Complaint 67-3255. Criminal Contempt. North District of Illinois, 1-16-69
34. Holden C: Laetrile: "quack" cancer remedy still brings hope to suffering. Science 193:982–985, 1976
35. Greenberg DM: The vitamin fraud in cancer quackery. West J Med 122:345–348, 1975
36. Vierhover A, Mack H: Biochemistry of amygdalin. Am J Pharm 107:397–450, 1935
37. Robiquet, B: Les amandes ameres et l'huile volatile qu'elles fournissent. Ann Clin Phys 44:352–382, 1830
38. Liebiz J, Wohler F: Uber die Bildung des Bittermandelols. Annalen der Chemie und Pharmacie 22:1–24, 1837
39. Dorr RT, Paxinos J: The current status of Laetrile. Ann Intern Med 89:389–397, 1978
40. Culbert ML: Freedom from Cancer. The Amazing Story of Vitamin B-17, or Laetrile New York, Pocket Books, 1977
41. Beard J: Embryological aspects and etiology of carcinoma. Lancet 1:1758–1761, 1902
42. Beard HH: A New Approach to the Conquest of Cancer, Rheumatic and Heart Diseases. New York, Pageant Press, 1958
43. Conchie J, Findley J, Levvy GA: Mammalian glycosidases: Distribution in the body. Biochem 71:318–325, 1959
44. Gal EM, Fung FH, Greenberg DM: Studies on the biological action of malononitriles II. Distribution of rhodanese (transulfurase) in the tissues of normal and tumor-bearing animals and the effect of malononitriles thereon, Cancer Res 12:574–579, 1952
45. Hill JJ II, Shine TE, Hill HZ et al: Failure of amygdalin to arrest B16 melanoma and BW5141 AKR leukemia. Cancer Res 36:2102–2107, 1976
46. Laster WR Jr, Schabel FM Jr: Experimental studies of the antitumor activity of amygdalin M.F. (NSC–15780) alone and in combination with B glucosidase (NSC–128056), Cancer Chemotherapy Rep 59:951–965, 1975
47. Wodinsky I, Swiniarski J: Antitumor activity of amygdalin set on a spectrum of transplantable rodent tumors. Cancer Chemother Rep 59:939–950, 1975
48. Stock CC, Tarnowski GS, Schmid FA et al: Antitumor tests of amygdalin in transplantable animal tumor systems. J Surg Oncol 10:81–88, 1978
49. Stock CC, Martin DS, Suguira K et al: Antitumor tests of amygdalin in spontaneous animal tumor systems, J Surg Oncol 10:89–123, 1978
50. Ovejira AA, Houchens DP, Barker AD et al: Inactivity of DL-amygdalin against human breast and colon tumor xenografts in athymic (nude) mice, Cancer Treat Rep 62:576–578, 1978
51. Koeffler PH, Lowe L, Golde D: Amygdalin (Laetrile): Effect of clonogenic cells from human myeloid leukemia cell lines and normal human marrow. Cancer Treat Rep 64:105–110, 1980
52. Navarrow MD: The mechanism of action and therapeutic effects of laetile in cancer. J Philipp Med Assoc 33:620–627, 1957
53. Navarro MP: Laetrile therapy in cancer. Phillip J Cancer 4:204–209, 1962
54. Tasca M: Clinical observations on the therapeutic effects of a cyanogenetic glucuronoside (sic) in cases of human malignant neoplasms. Gaz Med Ital 118:153–159, 1959
55. Morrone JA: Chemotherapy of inoperable cancer. Exp Med Surg 20:299–308, 1962
56. California Medical Association, Cancer Commission: The treatment of cancer with "Laetriles." Calif Med 78:320–326, 1953
57. Edwards CC: Statement before the Subcommittee on Intergovernmental Operations, pp 21–22, June 9, 1970
58. Rutherford vs. United States, 399 F Suppl 1208 (WD Oklahoma, 1975)
59. Anonymous: "Cured" cancer patient proselytizes for laetrile. Med World News 14:18, 1976
60. Rutherford vs. United States, 542 F. 2d 1137 (10th Cir 1976)
61. United States vs. Rutherford, No 78–605, June 18, 1979
62. The twenty-three states are: Alaska, Arizona, Colorado, Delaware, Florida, Idaho, Illinois, Indiana, Kansas, Louisiana, Maryland, Montana, Nevada, New Hampshire, New Jersey, North Dakota, Oklahoma, Oregon, South Dakota, Texas, Washington, Kentucky, and West Virginia.
63. Diamond GEB. Cancer research: Who profits? Harvard Political Review 5:17–21, 1977
64. Speech delivered by Mr. Robert Bradford. Workshop on Metabolic Therapy, Amygdalin and Cancer. Newark, New Jersey, February 4–5, 1978
65. Ellison NM, Byar DP, Newell GR: Special report on laetrile: the NCI laetrile review. N Engl J Med 299:549–552, 1978
66. Moertel CG, Ames MM, Jovach JS et al: A pharmacologic and toxicological study of amygdalin. JAMA 255:591–594, 1978
67. Moertel C, Rubin J, Sarna G et al: A phase II trial of amygdalin (laetrile) in the treatment of human cancer. Proc Am Soc Clin Oncol 22:383, 1981
68. Physicians Handbook of Vitamin B-17, 2nd ed, pp 6–32. Therapy Science Press International, 1975
69. Richardson JA, Griffin P: Laetrile Case Histories, p 112. New York, Bantam Books, 1977

Index

Numerals in italics *indicate a figure;* "t" *following a page number indicates a table.*